drug
facts and comparisons®

1998 edition

drug facts and comparisons®

1998 edition

Facts and Comparisons®
St. Louis
A **Wolters Kluwer** Company

Drug Facts and Comparisons,® 1998 Edition

ISBN 0-57439-034-1
ISSN 0277-9714

Printed in the United States of America

Published by
Facts and Comparisons®
111 West Port Plaza, Suite 300
St. Louis, Missouri 63146-3098
314/878-2515
Toll free Customer Service 1-800-223-0554

Contributing Review Panel

Jonathan Abrams, MD
Professor of Medicine
Cardiology Division
University of New Mexico
Albuquerque, New Mexico

Ezra A. Amsterdam, MD, FACC
Professor, Internal Medicine
Director
Cardiac Care Unit
University of California at Davis and Sacramento
School of Medicine and Medical Center

Danial E. Baker, PharmD
Associate Professor of Pharmacy Practice
Director, Drug Information Center
Washington State University College of Pharmacy
Spokane, Washington

Julie K. Baltz, PharmD
Clinical Research Pharmacist
National Cancer Institute
Bethesda, Maryland

Jimmy D. Bartlett, OD, DOS
Professor of Optometry and Pharmacology
Schools of Optometry and Medicine
University of Alabama at Birmingham

Dale Berg, MD
Instructor of Medicine
Medical College of Wisconsin
Milwaukee, Wisconsin

Lawrence R. Borgsdorf, PharmD
Pharmacist Specialist – Ambulatory Care
Kaiser Permanente
Bakersfield, California

Daniel L. Brown, PharmD
Director of Pharmacy Services
Merced Community Medical Center
Merced, California

R. Keith Campbell, RPh, FAPP
Associate Dean/Professor of Pharmacy
Washington State University
College of Pharmacy
Pullman, Washington

Daniel T. Casto, PharmD
Clinical Pharmacy Program
University of Texas Health Science Center
San Antonio, Texas

Sonja Chandler, PharmD, MS
MD Anderson Cancer Center
Texas Medical Center
Division of Pharmacy
Houston, Texas

Melvin D. Cheitlin, MD
Professor of Medicine
University of California, San Francisco, Cardiology Division
Associate Chief, Cardiology Division
San Francisco General Hospital
San Francisco, California

Stephen L. Dahl, PharmD
University of Missouri – Kansas City
School of Medicine
Kansas City, Missouri

Richard J. Duma, MD, PhD
Infectious Disease Division
Halifax Medical Center
Daytona Beach, Florida

Kathryn M. Edwards, MD
Department of Pediatrics
Vanderbilt University Medical School
Nashville, Tennessee

LTC Michael S. Edwards, PharmD
US Army Medical Department
Washington, DC

Mary J. Ferrill, PharmD
Assistant Professor
Drug Information Specialist
University of the Pacific
School of Pharmacy
Stockton, California

N. Rex Ghormley, OD, FAAO
Contact Lens and Vision Care Consultants, President
St. Louis, Missouri

Thomas A. Golper, MD
Professor of Medicine
Medical Director & Director of Clinical Research
Division of Nephrology
University of Arkansas for Medical Sciences
Little Rock, Arkansas

John D. Grabenstein, EdM, MS, FASHP
Pharmaceutical Policy Division
School of Pharmacy, CB#7340
University of North Carolina
Chapel Hill, North Carolina

Ellen L. Hamburg, PharmD
Associate Professor of Clinical Pharmacy
Arnold and Marie Schwartz College of Pharmacy and Health Sciences of Long Island University
State University of New York
Health Sciences Center at Brooklyn
Brooklyn, New York

Edward A. Hartshorn, PhD
Clinical Professor
University of Texas at Austin, College of Pharmacy
University of Texas Medical Branch at Galveston
Galveston, Texas

Gary A. Holt, MEd, PhD, RPh
Assistant Professor of Pharmacy
School of Pharmacy
Northeast Louisiana University
Monroe, Louisiana

Siret D. Jaanus, PhD
Acting Chairman
Department of Biomedical Sciences
State University of New York
State College of Optometry
New York, New York

Robert E. Kates, PharmD, PhD
President
Analytical Solutions, Inc.
Sunnyvale, California

Julio R. Lopez, PharmD
Assistant Professor, School of Pharmacy, University of the Pacific
Assistant Clinical Professor, School of Pharmacy, University of California, San Francisco
Director, Drug Information Center, VA Medical Center
Martinez, California

Susan O'Donoghue, MD
Associate Director, Cardiac Arrhythmia Center
Washington Hospital Center
Washington, DC

Richard M. Oksas, PharmD, MPh
Pharmaceutical Consultant
Medication Information Service
Torrance, California

Edward V. Platia, MD
Director, Cardiac Arrhythmia Center
Washington Hospital Center
Professor of Medicine
George Washington University School of Medicine

Michael T. Reed, PharmD
Associate Professor of Clinical Pharmacy
Arnold and Marie Schwartz College of Pharmacy and Health Sciences of Long Island University
Brooklyn, New York
The Mount Sinai Medical Center
New York, New York

J. James Rowsey, MD
Professor and Chairman
Department of Ophthalmology
University of South Florida College of Medicine
Tampa, Florida

Frederick L. Ruben, MD
Infectious Disease Division
Montefiore University Hospital
University of Pittsburgh
Pittsburgh, Pennsylvania

Mary Beth Shirk, PharmD
Clinical Pharmacy Specialist, Pain Management
The Ohio State University Medical Center
Columbus, Ohio

Burgunda V. Sweet, PharmD
Clinical Pharmacist, Home Medication Infusion Service
The University of Michigan Hospitals
Ann Arbor, Michigan

Udho Thadani, MBBS, FRCP(C), FACC
Professor of Medicine
Vice Chief of Cardiology and Director of Clinical Research
University of Oklahoma Health Sciences Center
Oklahoma City, Oklahoma

Robert A. Wild, MD
Chief, Section of Research & Education in Women's Health
Department of Obstetrics and Gynecology
University of Oklahoma Health Sciences Center
Oklahoma City, Oklahoma

Thom J. Zimmerman, MD, PhD
Chairman of Department of Ophthalmology and Visual Sciences
Professor of Pharmacology & Toxicology
University of Louisville

Preface

Drug Facts and Comparisons® provides a broad range of drug information to fulfill the everyday needs of practicing healthcare professionals. Developed in 1945 by pharmacist Erwin K. Kastrup, *Facts and Comparisons®* was designed to provide objective information in a format to facilitate comparisons of drug products. Although the basic concepts remain the same, the content of *Drug Facts* continues to evolve to reflect the changing information needs of health-care professionals.

Drug Facts and Comparisons®, a loose-leaf text, is kept up-to-date through the issue of monthly updates. The Annual Bound Edition of *Facts and Comparisons* was first published in 1978. In 1982, the title became *Drug Facts and Comparisons®*, which better describes the nature of the reference.

This edition incorporates 50 new drugs: Adapalene *(Differin),* Albendazole *(Albenza),* Amlexanox *(Aphthasol),* Anagrelide HCl *(Agrylin),* Atorvastatin *(Lipitor),* Azelastine *(Astelin),* Betaine Anhydrous *(Cystadane),* Bismuth Subsalicylate, Metronidazole, Tetracycline HCl Combination *(Helidac),* Brimonidine Tartrate *(Alphagan),* Butenafine *(Mentax),* Cabergoline *(Dostinex),* Cidofovir *(Vistide),* Clonidine HCl *(Duraclon),* Danaparoid *(Orgaran),* Donepezil *(Aricept),* Factor IX Concentrate *(Benefix),* Fexofenadine HCl *(Allegra),* Fosfomycin Tromethamine *(Monurol),* Fosphenytoin *(Cerebyx),* Glatiramer Acetate *(Copaxone),* Hydrocortisone Buteprate *(Pandel),* Imiquimod *(Aldara),* Irinotecan *(Camptosar),* Invermectin *(Stromectol),* Levofloxacin *(Levaquin),* Meropenem *(Merrem IV),* Midodrine HCl *(ProAmatine),* Miglitol *(Glyset),* Mirtazapine *(Remeron),* Nelfinavir Mesylate *(Viracept),* Nevirapine *(Viramune),* Nilutamide *(Nilandron),* Olanzapine *(Zyprexa),* Olopatadine *(Patanol),* Penciclovir *(Denavir),* Pentosan Polysulfate Sodium *(Elmiron),* Ranitidine Bismuth Citrate *(Tritec),* Remifentanil HCl *(Ultiva),* Reteplase *(Retevase),* Ropivacaine *(Naropin),* Samarium Sm 153 *(Quadramet),* Sparfloxacin *(Zagam),* Tiludronate *(Skelid),* Topiramate *(Topamax),* Trandolapril *(Mavik),* Troglitazone *(Rezulin),* Valproic Acid *(Depacon),* Valsartan *(Diovan),* Zafirlukast *(Accolate),* Zileuton *(Zyflo).*

Significant new indications added include: Alendronate *(Fosamax)* for osteolytic bone metastases, Alfentanil *(Alfenta)* for monitored anesthesia care, Alteplase *(Activase)* for acute ischemic stroke, Bleomycin Sulfate *(Blenoxane)* for the treatment of malignant pleural effusion, Bupropion *(Zyban)* for smoking cessation treatment, Clarithromycin for increased urinary flow and improvement of symptoms of BPH, Epoetin Alfa *(Epogen)* for reduction of allogeneic blood transfusion in surgery patients, Lansoprazole *(Prevacid)* for maintenance of healed duodenal ulcers, Piperacillin Sodium/Tazobactam Sodium *(Zosyn)* for nosocomial pneumonia, Podofilox *(Condylox)* for treatment of anogenital warts, Sumatriptan Succinate *(Imitrex)* for cluster headaches.

Sections that have undergone major revisions include: Alkylating Agents, Anthelmintics, Anticoagulants, Antihyperlipidemics, Cephalosporins, 5HT3 Receptor Antagonists, Growth Hormones, HMG-CoA Reductase Inhibitors, *H. Pylori* Agents, Low Molecular Weight Heparins, MAOIs, Orphan Drugs, SSRIs, Tetracyclic Compounds, Thrombolytic Enzymes, Topical Anti-Infectives/Antibiotics, Tricyclic Compounds.

As this edition goes to press, we begin the process of revision for the 1999 edition. As always, *Drug Facts and Comparisons®* remains dedicated to fulfilling the drug information needs of healthcare professionals. Comments, criticisms and suggestions are always welcome.

S.K.H.

Table of Contents

Introduction

Drug Facts and Comparisons® *(DFC)* is a comprehensive drug information compendium. Organized by therapeutic drug classes, the format is designed to provide a wide scope of drug information in a manner that facilitates comparisons among drugs. A comprehensive index, a detailed table of contents for each chapter and extensive cross referencing enable the reader to quickly locate needed information. All readers are urged to review the following information to assure efficient and effective use of *DFC*.

Editorial Policy

The principal editorial guidelines are: Accurate, unbiased information; concise, standardized presentation; comparative, objective format; timely delivery. Review of FDA-approved product labeling, thousands of biomedical journal articles and textbooks, and policies and recommendations from many authoritative and official groups (eg, Centers for Disease Control; National Academy of Sciences; Joint National Committee on Detection, Evaluation, and Treatment of High Blood Pressure; National Heart, Lung and Blood Institute; American Thoracic Society; National Cancer Institute; Food and Drug Administration) form the base of evaluation of information for *DFC*.

Editorial policy is guided by the distinguished Facts and Comparisons® Editorial Advisory Panel. This is an authoritative group of nationally and internationally recognized clinicians, scientists, physicians, pharmacists and pharmacologists. Pages for *DFC* are reviewed by these eight panel members, and many other prominent health-care professionals provide review in their specific areas of expertise. Indications and dosage recommendations are FDA-approved unless otherwise specified. Legitimate "unlabeled" uses and dosages are included when appropriate and given special emphasis. Input from a special panel of drug interaction experts is also a feature.

This collection of wisdom is then molded and refined into the *DFC* monographs and product listings. Many sources of drug information are constantly monitored so that *DFC* contains the most comprehensive, current drug information data base available. There is not a more complete text available presenting such clinical prescribing and drug product information.

Most of the products listed are protected by letters of patent, and their names are trademarked and registered by the firm whose name appears with the product. The product distributor is given in parentheses next to the brand name who may or may not be the actual manufacturer or fabricator of the final dosage form. When more than one company distributes a generic product, the generic product name is listed, followed by "Various, eg," in parentheses with a selected list of distributors. Listing of specific products is an indication only of market availability, and is not an endorsement or recommendation.

Products that contain the same active ingredients are listed together for comparison and as an aid in product selection. However, drug product interchange is regulated by state laws; listing of products together does not imply that products are therapeutically equivalent or legally interchangeable. Caution is particularly advised when attempting to compare extended-release or delayed-release dosage forms.

Organization:

Information in *DFC* is organized by therapeutic use. Each of the 12 chapters is divided into groups and subgroups to facilitate comparisons of drugs and drug products with similar uses. The first page of each chapter provides a detailed outline, including page references of the information presented in that chapter.

Products most similar in content or use are listed together. This format of presenting the FACTS makes it easy to make COMPARISONS of identical, similar or related products. Because drugs are listed by use, some drugs with multiple uses may be listed in more than one section of the book.

Index:

The alphabetical index includes page references for all drugs by their generic name, brand name, synonyms, common abbreviations and therapeutic group names. Generic names are listed in bold type face for easy identification. A separate index is included with the COLOR LOCATOR.

Drug Monographs:

Prescribing information is presented in comprehensive drug monographs. General information on a group of closely related drugs (eg, ACE inhibitors) may be presented in a group monograph. Specific information relating to a particular drug is presented in an individual monograph under the generic name of the drug. All monographs are divided into sections identified with bold titles for ease in locating the desired information.

Actions: This section gives a brief summary of the known pharmacologic and pharmacokinetic properties.

Indications: All indications or uses listed are FDA-approved unless specifically designated as "Unlabeled uses."

Contraindications: This section specifies those conditions in which the drug should NOT be used.

Warnings and Precautions: These sections list conditions in which use of the drug may be hazardous, precautions to observe and parameters to monitor during therapy.

Drug Interactions: A brief summary of documented, clinically significant drug-drug, drug-lab test and drug-food interactions is provided.

Adverse Reactions: Reported adverse reactions are presented. Incidence data on adverse effects are included when available.

Overdosage: The clinical manifestations of toxicity and treatment of overdosage are given for most agents.

Patient Information: Essential information required by the patient for safe and effective self-administration of the medication is included.

Administration and Dosage: Dosage ranges and methods of administration are presented.

Product Listings:

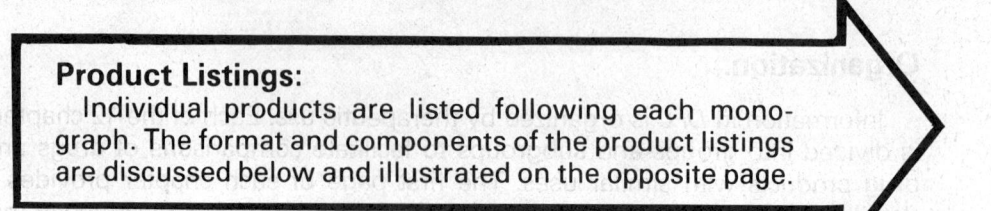

Individual products are listed following each monograph. The format and components of the product listings are discussed below and illustrated on the opposite page.

1. Cross references to the appropriate drug monograph(s) for complete prescribing information appear at the beginning of the monograph.
2. Products are grouped by dosage form or strength.
3. Identical brand name products are listed in alphabetical order.
4. The name of the distributor is given in parentheses next to the product name.
5. Products available by their generic name from multiple sources are indicated as available from (Various) distributors and in selected cases, specific generic manufacturers are listed.
6. Package sizes are given for all dosage forms and strengths of each product.
7. Product identification imprint codes are listed in parentheses.
8. Distribution status of products is indicated as *Rx* or *otc*.
9. Controlled substances are designated by their schedule (*c-II*, *c-III*, *c-IV*, or *c-V*).
10. Sugar free liquid preparations are designated by *sf*.
11. Combination products are listed in tables to facilitate comparisons. Products most similar in formulation are listed next to each other.
12. Products with identical formulations are listed together.

HYDROCHLOROTHIAZIDE

(1) For complete prescribing information, refer to the Thiazides and Related Diuretics group monograph.

Administration and Dosage:

Edema: Initial – 25 to 200 mg daily for several days, or until dry weight is attained.

Maintenance – 25 to 100 mg daily or intermittently. Refractory patients may require up to 200 mg daily.

Hypertension: Initial – 25 mg daily as a single dose. The dose may be increased to 50 mg daily as a single or two divided doses. Doses > 50 mg are often associated with marked reductions in serum potassium. Patients usually do not require doses > 50 mg daily when combined with other antihypertensives.

Infants and children: Usual dosage is 2.2 mg/kg (1 mg/lb) daily in two doses. Pediatric patients with hypertension only rarely will benefit from doses > 50 mg daily.

Infants (< 6 months) – Up to 3.3 mg/kg (1.5 mg/lb) daily in two doses.

Infants (6 months to 2 years of age) – 12.5 to 37.5 mg daily in two doses. Base dosage on body weight.

Children (2 to 12 years of age) – 37.5 to 100 mg daily in two doses. Base dosage on body weight.

Rx	**Hydrochlorothiazide** (Various, eg, Geneva, Major, Schein, Zenith) (5)	**Tablets:** 25 mg (2)	In 30s, 100s, 500s, 1000s, 5000s, UD 32s and UD 100s.
(8) *Rx*	**Esidrix** (Ciba)		Lactose, sucrose. (Ciba 22). Pink, scored. In 100s.
Rx	**HydroDIURIL** (Merck)		(6) Lactose. (MSD 42). Peach, scored. In 100s and 1000s.
Rx	**Hydro-Par** (Parmed)		Peach, scored. In 1000s.
Rx	**Oretic** (Abbott) (4)		Lactose. White. In 100s, 1000s and UD 100s.
Rx	**Hydrochlorothiazide** (Various, eg, Danbury, Geneva, Major, Schein, Zenith)	**Tablets:** 50 mg	In 30s, 100s, 500s, 1000s, 5000s and UD 100s. (7)
Rx	**Esidrix** (Ciba)		Lactose, sucrose. (Ciba 46). Yellow, scored. In 100s and consumer pack

COUGH PREPARATIONS

Antitussive Combinations, Liqui

		Product & Distributor	Decongestant	Antihistamine	Antitussive
(11)	(9) c-v	**Prometh w/ Codeine Syrup** (Various, eg, Barre-National, Goldline, Moore, URL)		6.25 mg promethazine HCl	10 mg codeine phosphate
	(3) c-v	**Pentazine VC w/Codeine Liquid** (Century)			
	c-v	**Phenergan with Codeine Syrup** (Wyeth-Ayerst)			
	c-v	**Pherazine w/ Codeine Syrup** (Halsey)			
	c-v	**Tricodene Cough & Cold Liquid** (Pfeiffer)		12.5 mg pyrilamine maleate	8.2 mg codeine phosphate
	c-III sf	**S-T Forte 2 Liquid** (Scot-Tussin)		2 mg chlorphenir-amine maleate	2.5 mg hydrocodone bitartrate
	(12) otc	**Effective Strength Cough Formula Liquid** (Barre-National)		2 mg chlorphenir-maleate	15 mg dextromethorphan HBr
	otc	**Primatuss Cough Mixture 4 Liquid** (Rugby)			
	otc sf	**Scot-Tussin DM Liquid** (Scot-Tussin)			
	(10) otc sf	**Tricodene Sugar Free Liquid** (Pfeiffer)		2 mg chlorphenir-amine maleate	10 mg dextromethorphan HBr

Color Locator

The Color Locator is an aid in identifying tablets and capsules by their appearance. The products pictured include commonly used prescription drug products. Because of the similarity in size, shape and color of products with significantly different ingredients, product identification should be confirmed by checking the identifying imprints.

Organization

Products are arranged by dosage form, color, size and shape. Every effort has been made to accurately reproduce the color of each product. However, variations will occur and exact reproductions are sometimes not possible. See the Table of Contents below for dosage form arrangement. The index begins on page CL-41.

Contents

Each product pictured is identified with the product trade name, strength and manufacturer. For products with a product identification code imprint, the imprint is included following the manufacturer's name. Products are also indicated as prescription (℞) or controlled substance (C-II, C-III, C-IV or C-V).

Slight variations of color and ID code may occur. Drug manufacturers are expanding the use of product imprints to identify products by name or ID code. During this transition, various lots of the same product may have differing imprints. The ID code following the manufacturer name may not appear on all products pictured.

Table of Contents

CL-2 Light Yellow to Yellow-Gold Tablets

℞
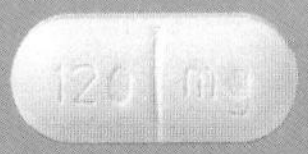

Cardizem 120 mg
Hoechst Marion Roussel 120

℞
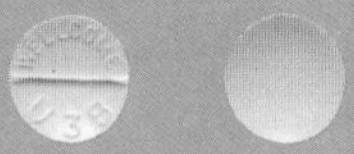
Thioguanine 40 mg
Glaxo Wellcome U3B

℞
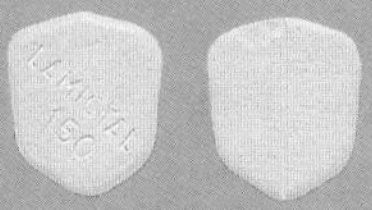
Lamictal 150 mg
Glaxo Wellcome 150

℞
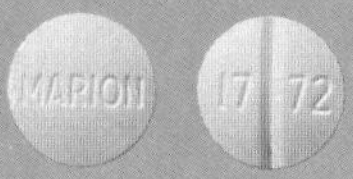

Cardizem 60 mg
Hoechst Marion Roussel 1772

℞
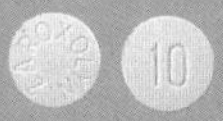

Zaroxolyn 10 mg
Medeva 10

℞
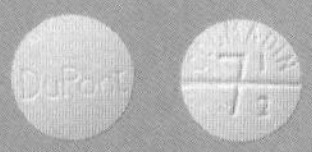
Coumadin 7.5 mg
DuPont 7 1/2

℞
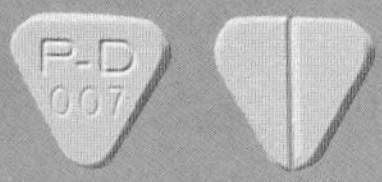

Dilantin Infatab 50 mg
Parke-Davis P-D 007

℞
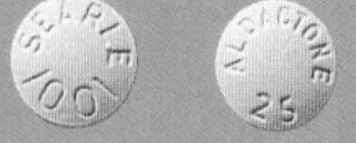
Aldactone 25 mg
Searle 1001 25

℞
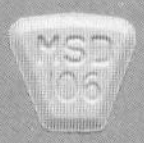

Prinivil 10 mg
Merck MSD 106

℞
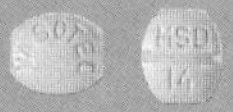
Vasotec 2.5 mg
Merck MSD 14

℞
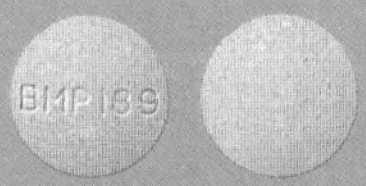

Augmentin '125' Chewable
SmithKline Beecham BMP 189

℞
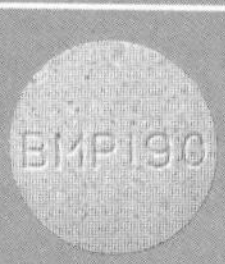

Augmentin '250' Chewable
SmithKline Beecham BMP 190

C-II
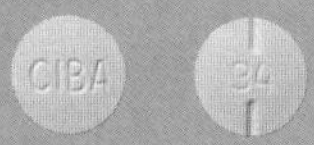

Ritalin 20 mg
Ciba 34

C-II
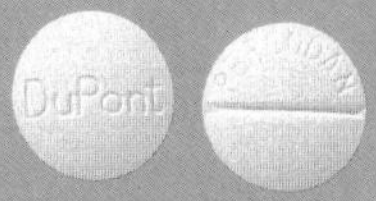

Percodan
DuPont

℞
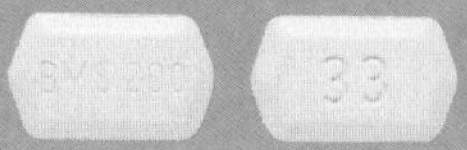

Serzone 200 mg
B-M Squibb BMS 200 33

℞
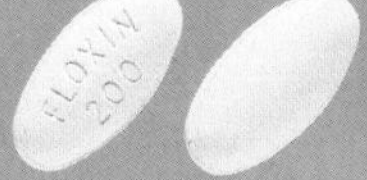
Floxin 200 mg
McNeil 200

℞
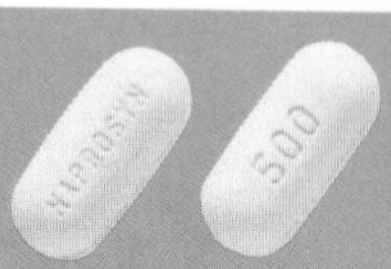

Naprosyn 500 mg
Roche 500

℞
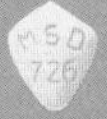
Zocor 5 mg
Merck MSD 726

℞
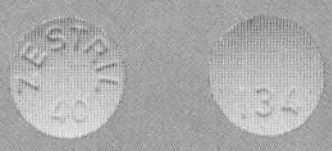
Zestril 40 mg
Zeneca 40 134

℞
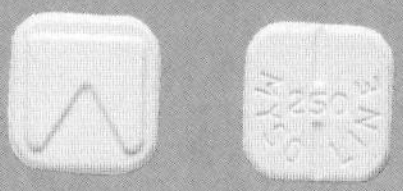
Mysoline 250 mg
Wyeth-Ayerst 250

℞
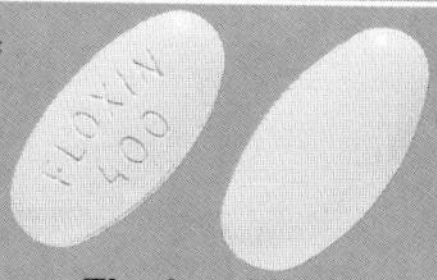

Floxin 400 mg
McNeil 400

℞
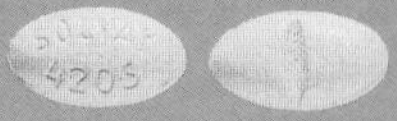
Luvox 50 mg
Solvay 4205

C-II
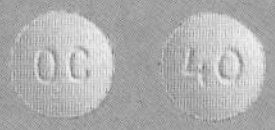

OxyContin 40 mg
Purdue Pharma OC 40

℞
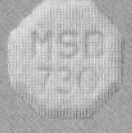

Mevacor 10 mg
Merck MSD 730

Yellow-Gold to Yellow Tablets

℞
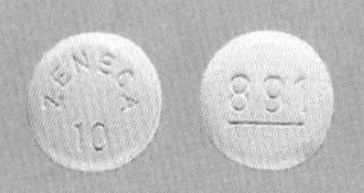
Sular 10 mg
Zeneca 10 891

℞
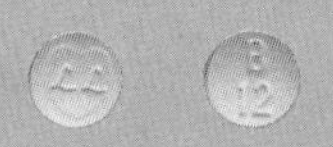
Ziac 2.5/6.25
Lederle LL B12

℞
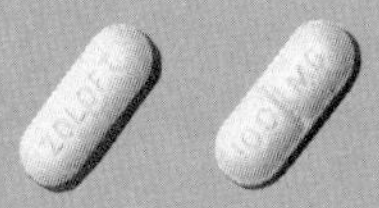
Zoloft 100 mg
Roerig 100

℞
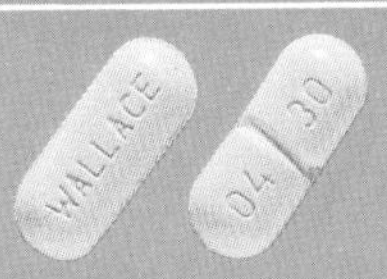
Felbatol 400 mg
Wallace 04 30

℞
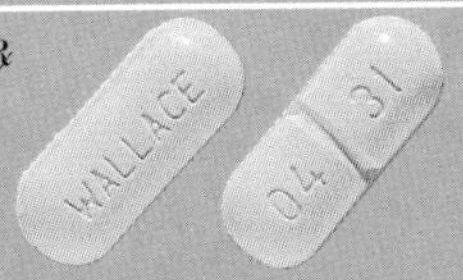
Felbatol 600 mg
Wallace 04 31

℞
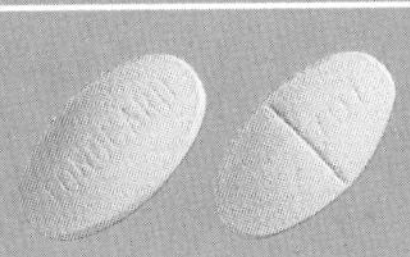
Tonocard 400 mg
Astra Merck 707

℞
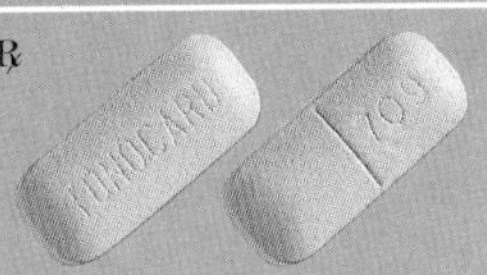
Tonocard 600 mg
Astra Merck 709

℞
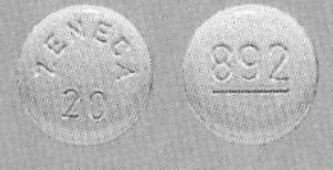
Sular 20 mg
Zeneca 20 892

℞
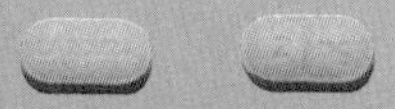
Cardura 2 mg
Roerig 2

℞
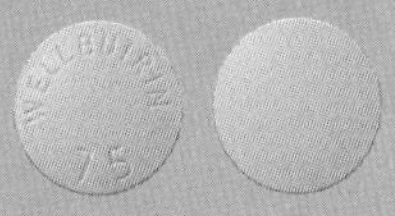
Wellbutrin 75 mg
Glaxo Wellcome 75

℞
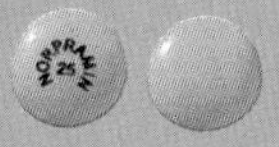
Norpramin 25 mg
Hoechst Marion Roussel 25

℞
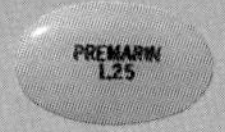
Premarin 1.25 mg
Wyeth-Ayerst 1.25

℞
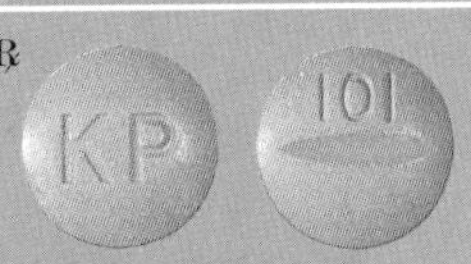
Azulfidine 500 mg
Pharmacia & Upjohn KP 101

℞
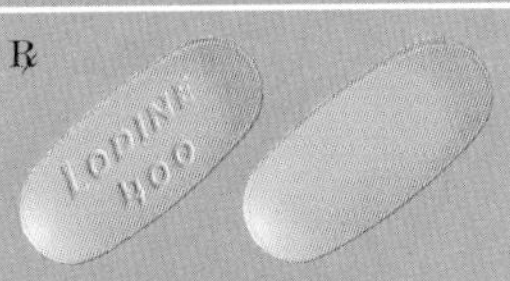
Lodine 400 mg
Wyeth-Ayerst 400

℞
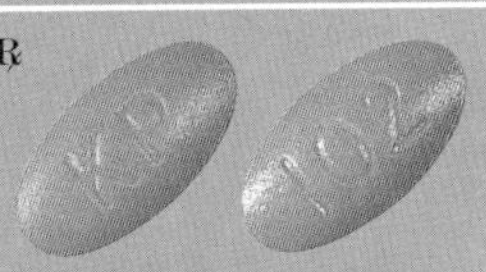
Azulfidine EN-tabs 500 mg
Pharmacia & Upjohn KP 102

℞
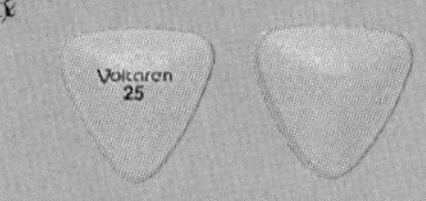
Voltaren 25 mg
Ciba 25

℞
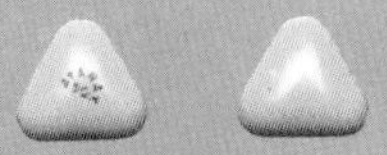
Atarax 50 mg
Roerig 50

℞
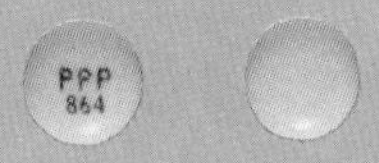
Prolixin 2.5 mg
Apothecon PPP 864

℞
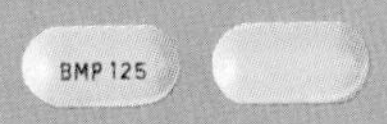
Menest 0.3 mg
SmithKline Beecham BMP 125

℞
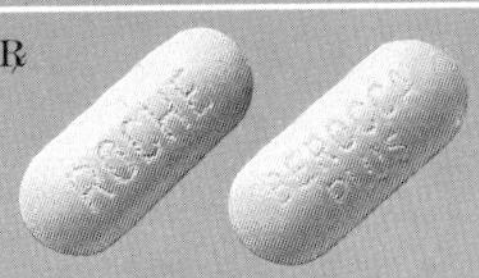
Berocca Plus
Roche

℞
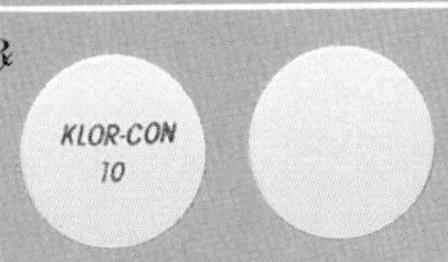
Klor-Con 10 10 mEq
Upsher-Smith 10

℞
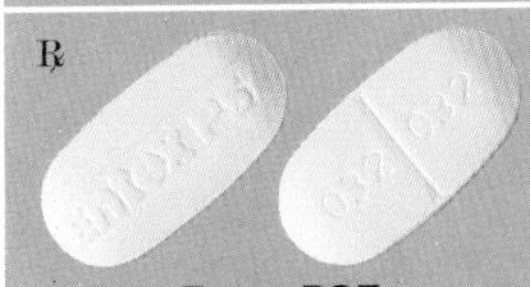
Entex PSE
Dura 032

℞
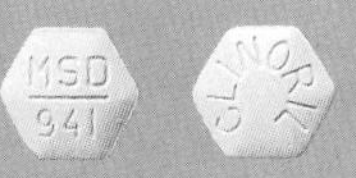
Clinoril 150 mg
Merck MSD 941

℞
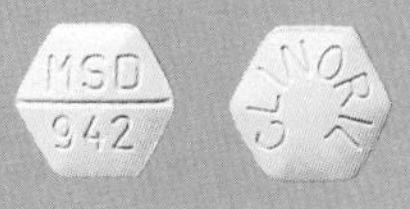
Clinoril 200 mg
Merck MSD 942

Yellow Tablets

℞
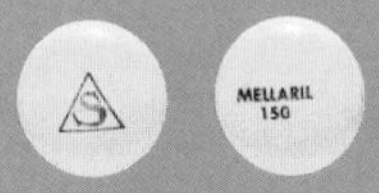

Mellaril 150 mg
Sandoz 150

℞
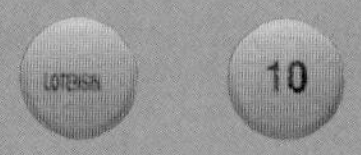

Lotensin 10 mg
Ciba 10

℞
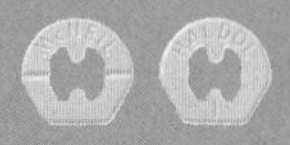

Haldol 1 mg
McNeil 1

℞
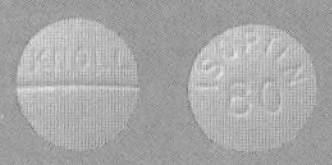

Isoptin 80 mg
Knoll 80

℞
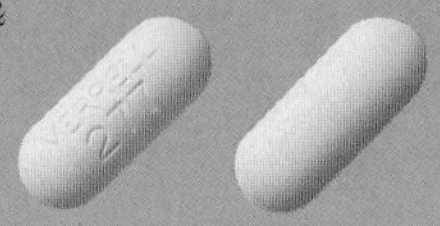

Hiprex 1 g
Hoechst Marion Roussel 277

℞
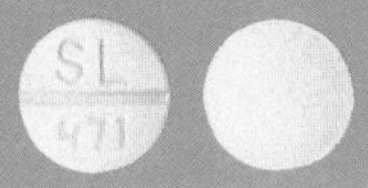

Propranolol 80 mg
Sidmak SL 471

℞
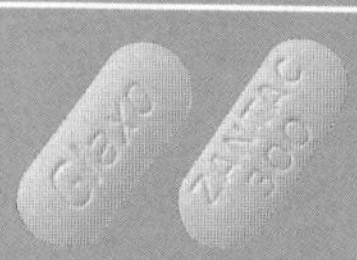

Zantac 300 mg
Glaxo Wellcome 300

℞
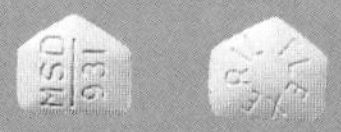

Flexeril 10 mg
Merck MSD 931

℞
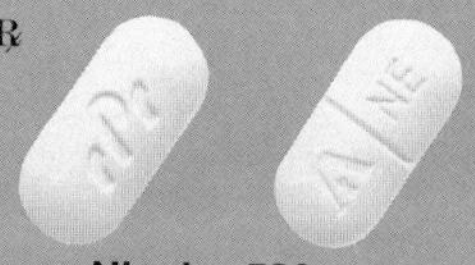

Nicolar 500 mg
Rhone-Poulenc Rorer NE

℞
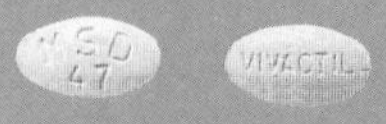

Vivactil 10 mg
Merck MSD 47

℞
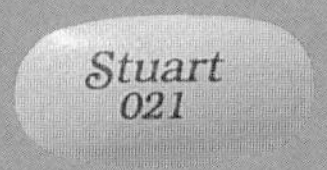

Stuartnatal Plus
Wyeth-Ayerst 021

℞
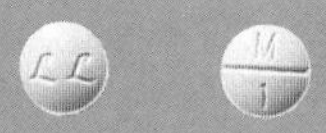

Rheumatrex 2.5 mg
Lederle LL M1

℞
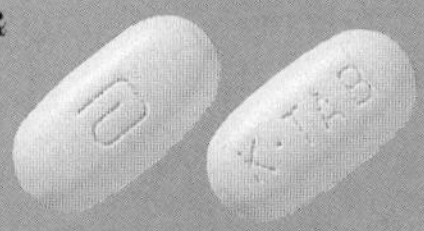

K-Tab 10 mEq
Abbott

℞
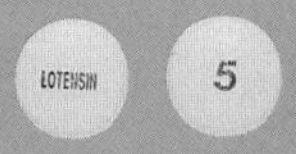

Lotensin 5 mg
Ciba 5

℞
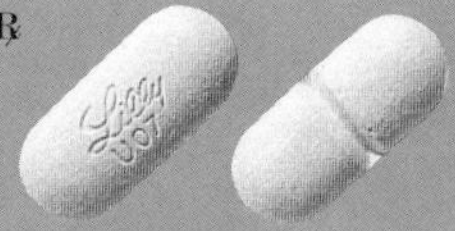

Dymelor 500 mg
Lilly U07

℞
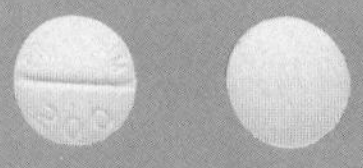

Proloprim 200 mg
Glaxo Wellcome 200

℞
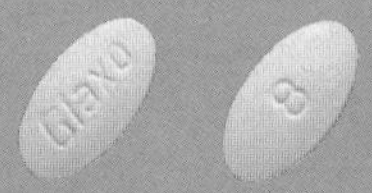

Zofran 8 mg
Glaxo Wellcome 8

℞
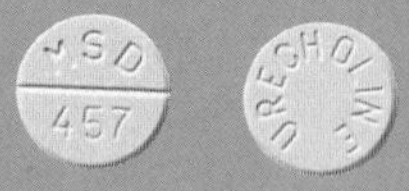

Urecholine 25 mg
Merck MSD 457

℞
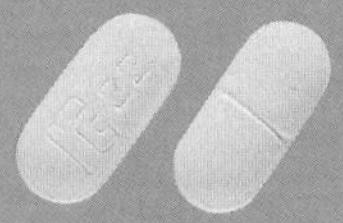

Levatol 20 mg
Schwarz Pharma RC 22

℞
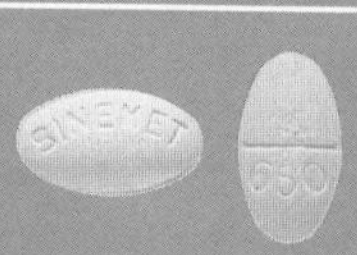

Sinemet-25/100
DuPont 650

℞
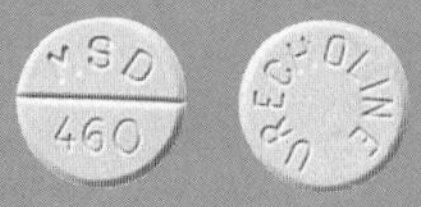

Urecholine 50 mg
Merck MSD 460

℞
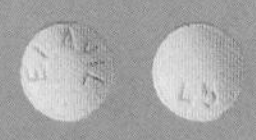

Elavil 25 mg
Zeneca 45

℞

Cantil 25 mg
Hoechst Marion Roussel 37

C-IV
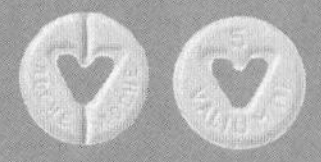

Valium 5 mg
Roche 5

℞

Levothroid 100 mcg
Forest Pharm 100

℞
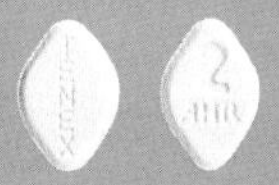
Tenex 2 mg
Robins AHR 2

℞

Decadron 0.5 mg
Merck MSD 41

℞

Clozaril 100 mg
Sandoz 100

℞
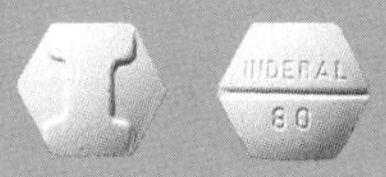

Inderal 80 mg
Wyeth-Ayerst I 80

℞
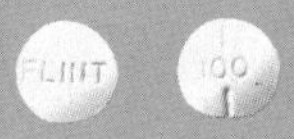

Synthroid 0.1 mg
Knoll Flint 100

℞
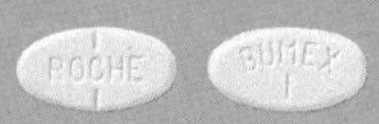

Bumex 1 mg
Roche 1

℞
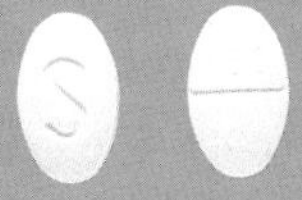
Sorbitrate 10 mg
Zeneca S 780

℞
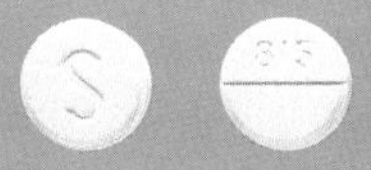

Sorbitrate 10 mg Chewable
Zeneca S 815

℞

Imuran 50 mg
Glaxo Wellcome 50

℞

Risperdal 3 mg
Janssen R 3

C-II
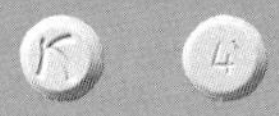

Dilaudid 4 mg
Knoll K 4

C-IV
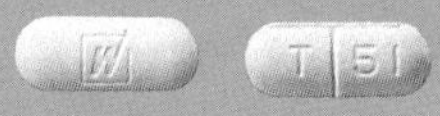

Talwin NX
Sanofi Winthrop W T51

C-II

Ritalin 5 mg
Ciba 7

℞
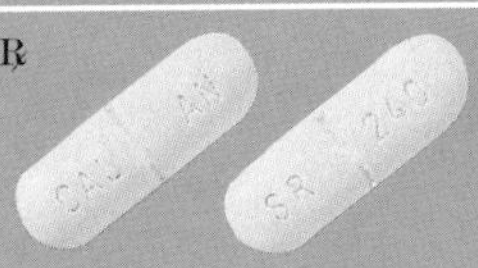
Calan SR 240 mg
Searle SR 240

℞
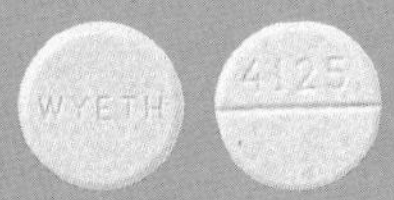

Isordil Tembids 40 mg
Wyeth-Ayerst 4125

℞
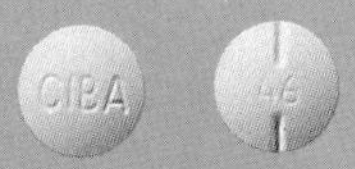

Esidrix 50 mg
Ciba 46

℞

Lanoxin 0.125 mg
Glaxo Wellcome Y3B

℞
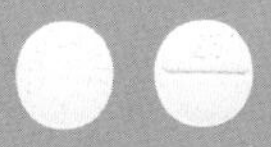
Clozaril 25 mg
Sandoz 25

℞
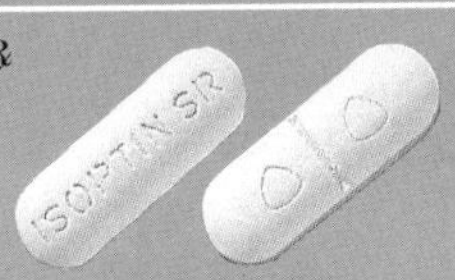

Isoptin SR 240 mg
Knoll SR

℞
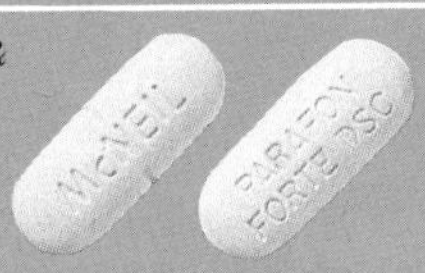

Parafon Forte DSC 500 mg
McNeil DSC

℞

Sorbitrate 5 mg Chewable
Zeneca S 810

℞
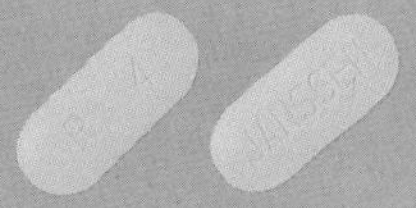
Risperdal 4 mg
Janssen R 4

℞

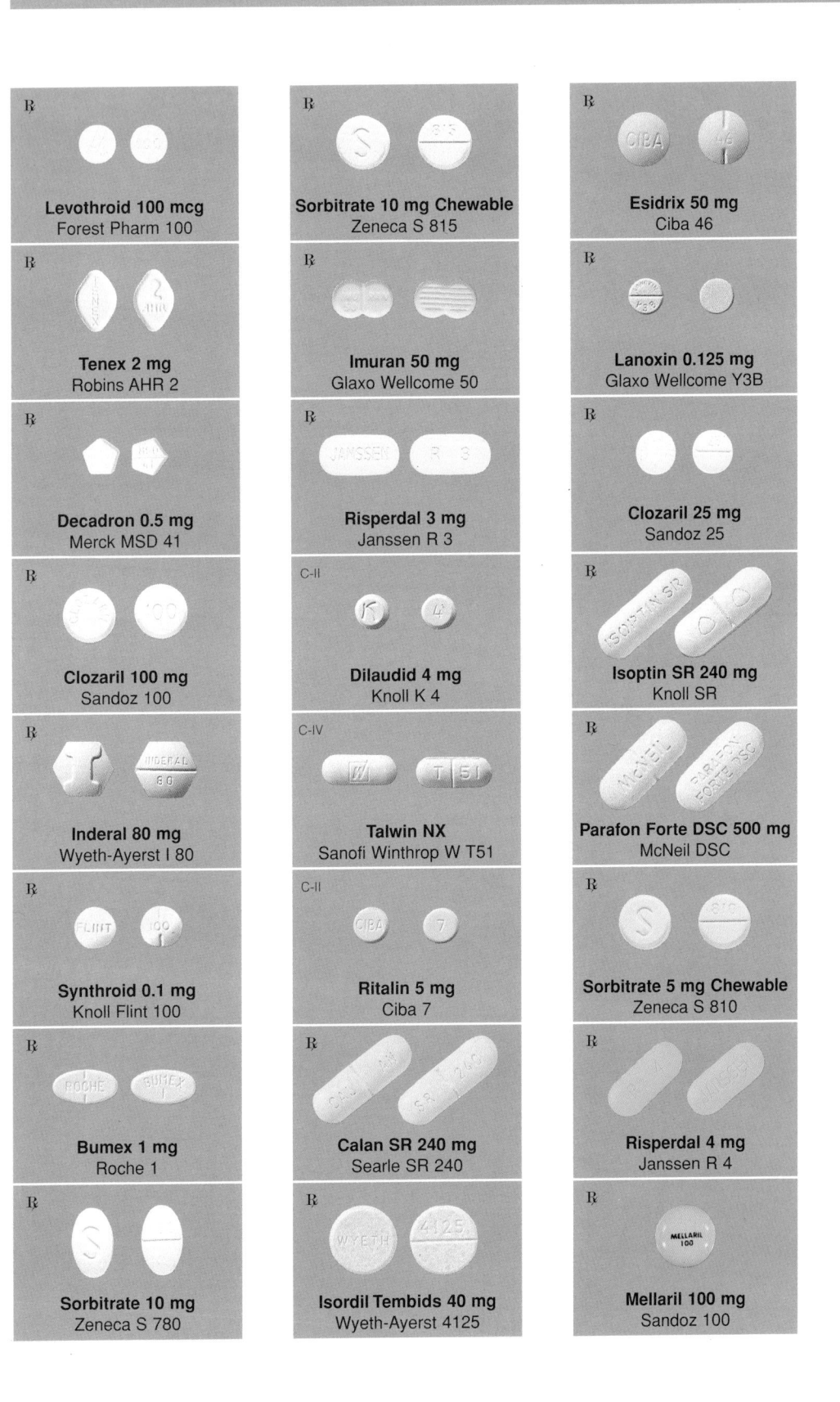

Mellaril 100 mg
Sandoz 100

CL-6 Yellow-Green to Green Tablets

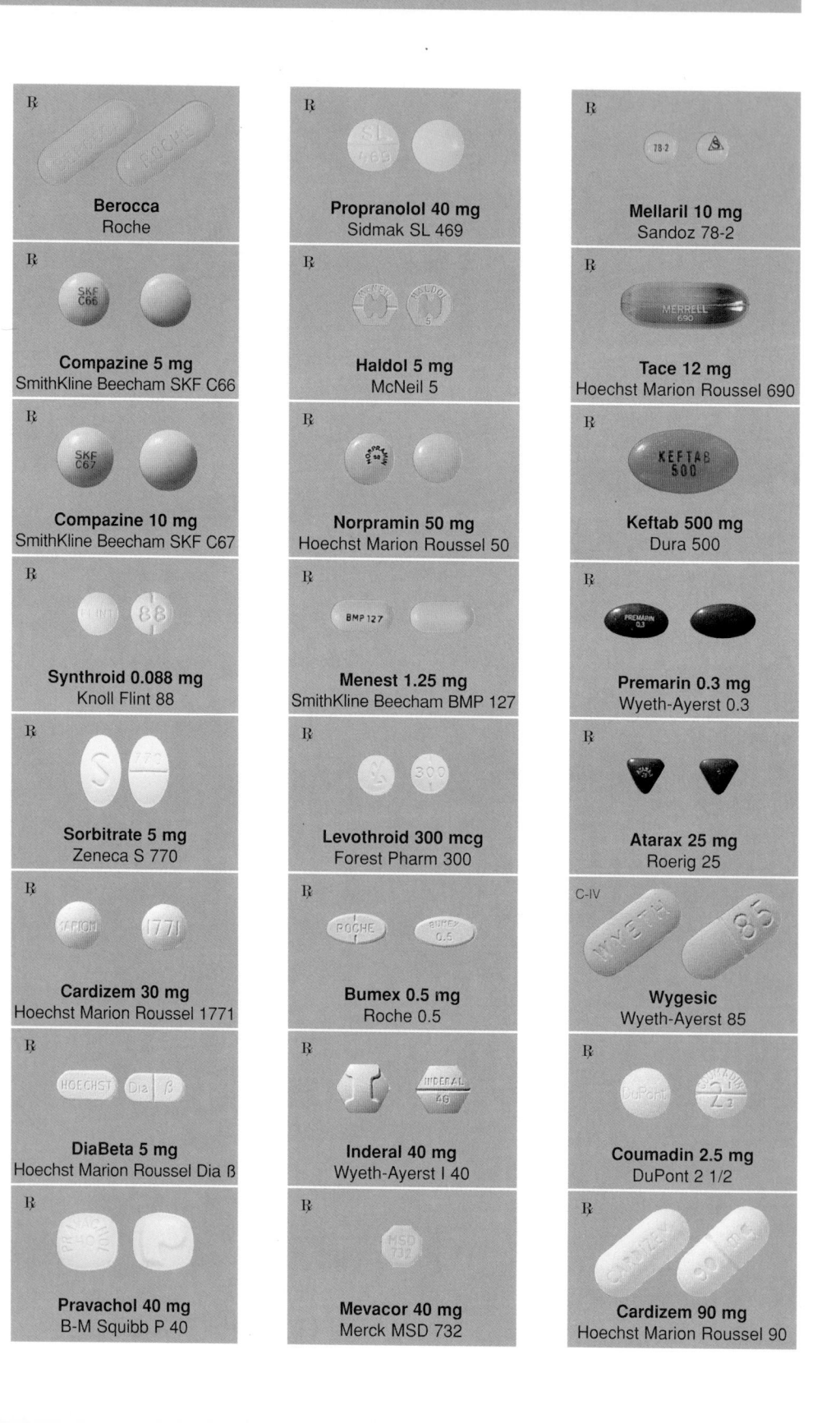

℞

Berocca
Roche

℞

Propranolol 40 mg
Sidmak SL 469

℞

Mellaril 10 mg
Sandoz 78-2

℞

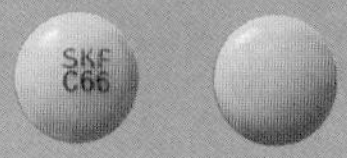

Compazine 5 mg
SmithKline Beecham SKF C66

℞

Haldol 5 mg
McNeil 5

℞

Tace 12 mg
Hoechst Marion Roussel 690

℞

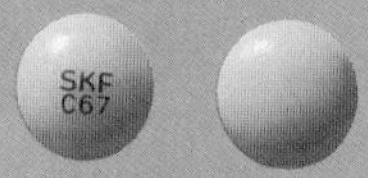

Compazine 10 mg
SmithKline Beecham SKF C67

℞

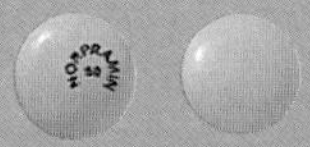

Norpramin 50 mg
Hoechst Marion Roussel 50

℞

Keftab 500 mg
Dura 500

℞

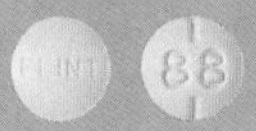

Synthroid 0.088 mg
Knoll Flint 88

℞

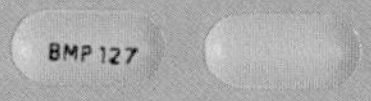

Menest 1.25 mg
SmithKline Beecham BMP 127

℞

Premarin 0.3 mg
Wyeth-Ayerst 0.3

℞

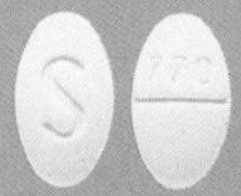

Sorbitrate 5 mg
Zeneca S 770

℞

Levothroid 300 mcg
Forest Pharm 300

℞

Atarax 25 mg
Roerig 25

℞

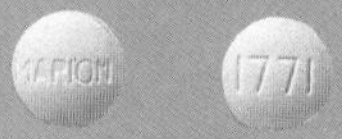

Cardizem 30 mg
Hoechst Marion Roussel 1771

℞

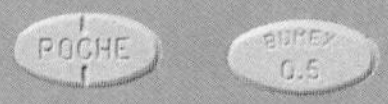

Bumex 0.5 mg
Roche 0.5

C-IV

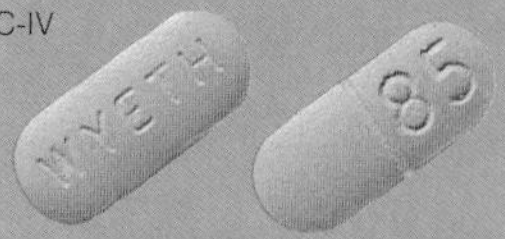

Wygesic
Wyeth-Ayerst 85

℞

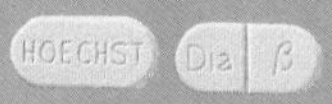

DiaBeta 5 mg
Hoechst Marion Roussel Dia ß

℞

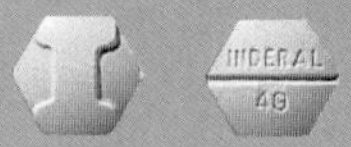

Inderal 40 mg
Wyeth-Ayerst I 40

℞

Coumadin 2.5 mg
DuPont 2 1/2

℞

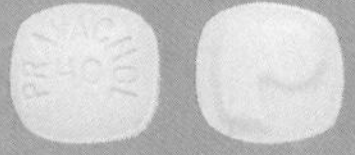

Pravachol 40 mg
B-M Squibb P 40

℞

Mevacor 40 mg
Merck MSD 732

℞

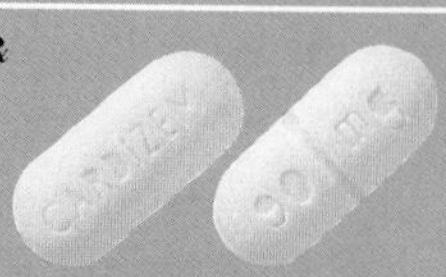

Cardizem 90 mg
Hoechst Marion Roussel 90

℞
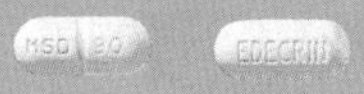
Edecrin 50 mg
Merck MSD 90

℞
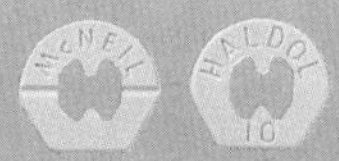
Haldol 10 mg
McNeil 10

℞
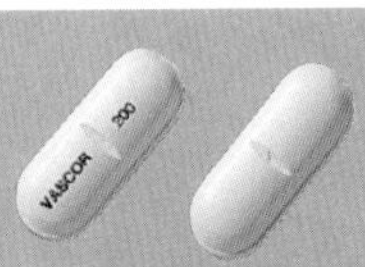
Vascor 200 mg
McNeil 200

℞
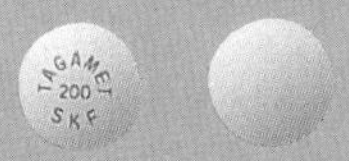
Tagamet 200 mg
SmithKline Beecham SKF 200

℞
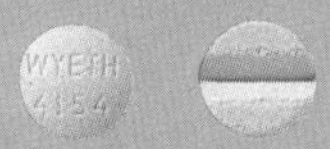
Isordil Titradose 20 mg
Wyeth-Ayerst 4154

℞
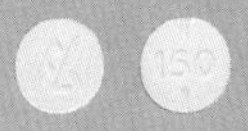
Levothroid 150 mcg
Forest Pharm 150

℞
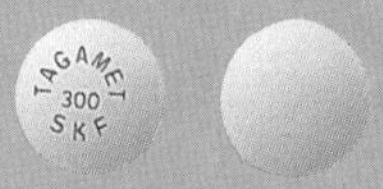
Tagamet 300 mg
SmithKline Beecham SKF 300

℞
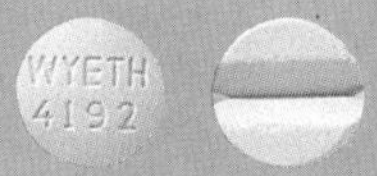
Isordil Titradose 40 mg
Wyeth-Ayerst 4192

℞
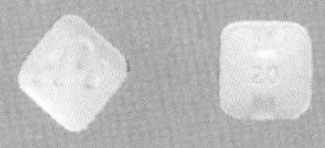
Hygroton 50 mg
Rhone-Poulenc Rorer H 20

℞
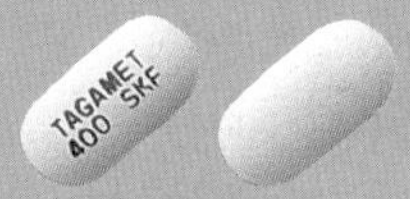
Tagamet 400 mg
SmithKline Beecham 400 SKF

℞
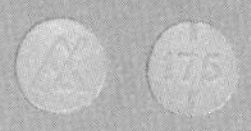
Levothroid 175 mcg
Forest Pharm 175

C-II
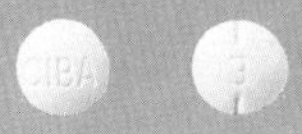
Ritalin 10 mg
Ciba 3

℞
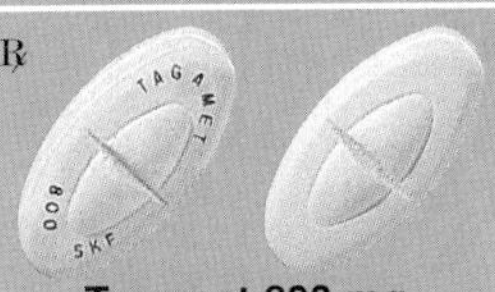
Tagamet 800 mg
SmithKline Beecham 800 SKF

℞
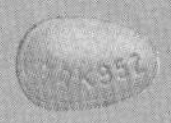
Cozaar 50 mg
Merck MRK 952

℞
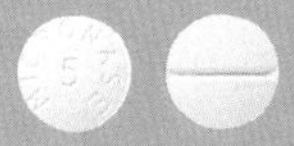
Micronase 5 mg
Pharmacia & Upjohn 5

℞
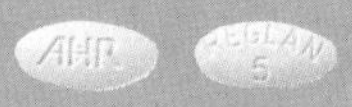
Reglan 5 mg
Robins AHR 5

C-II
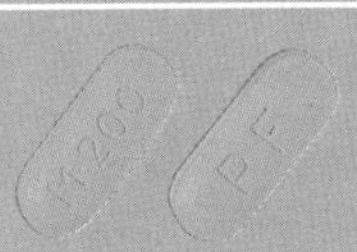
MS Contin 200 mg
Purdue Frederick PF M200

℞
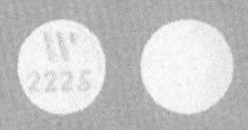
Cystospaz 0.15 mg
PolyMedica W 2225

℞
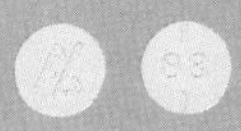
Levothroid 88 mcg
Forest Pharm 88

℞
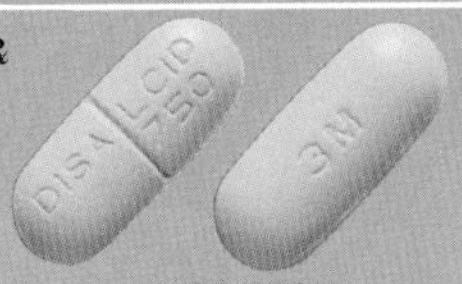
Disalcid 750 mg
3M Pharm 750

℞
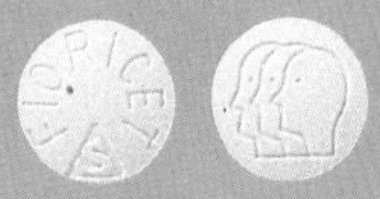
Fioricet
Sandoz S

℞
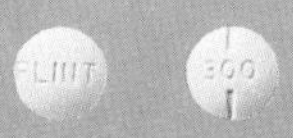
Synthroid 0.3 mg
Knoll Flint 300

℞
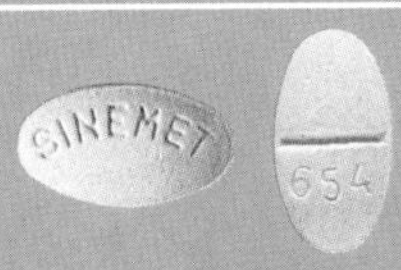
Sinemet-25/250
DuPont 654

C-IV
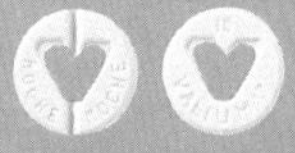
Valium 10 mg
Roche 10

Blue Tablets

℞

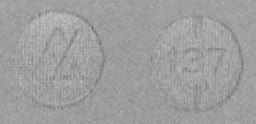

Levothroid 137 mcg
Forest Pharm 137

℞

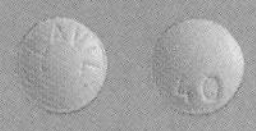

Elavil 10 mg
Zeneca 40

℞

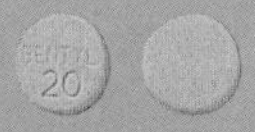

Bentyl 20 mg
Hoechst Marion Roussel 20

℞

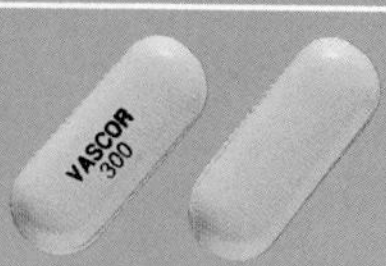

Vascor 300 mg
McNeil 300

℞

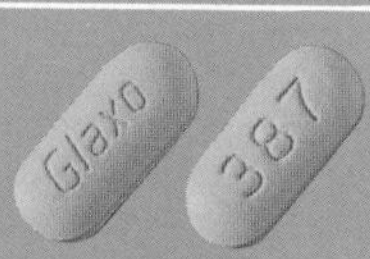

Ceftin 250 mg
Glaxo Wellcome 387

℞

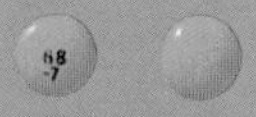

Norpramin 10 mg
Hoechst Marion Roussel 68-7

℞

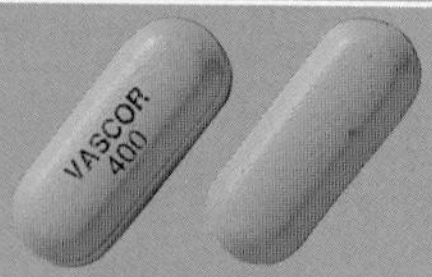

Vascor 400 mg
McNeil 400

℞

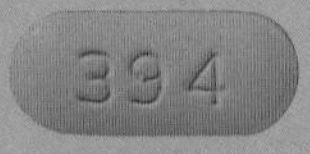

Ceftin 500 mg
Glaxo Wellcome 394

℞

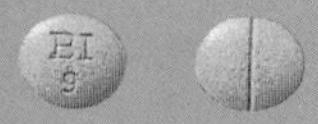

Combipres 0.2 mg
Boehringer Ingelheim BI 9

℞

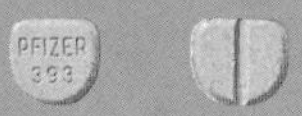

Diabinese 100 mg
Pfizer 393

℞

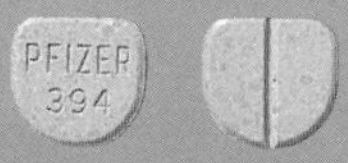

Diabinese 250 mg
Pfizer 394

℞

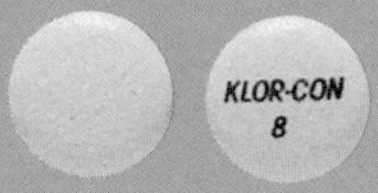

Klor-Con 8 8 mEq
Upsher-Smith 8

℞

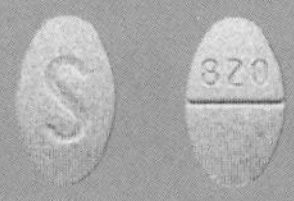

Sorbitrate 20 mg
Zeneca S 820

℞

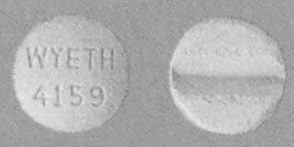

Isordil Titradose 30 mg
Wyeth-Ayerst 4159

℞

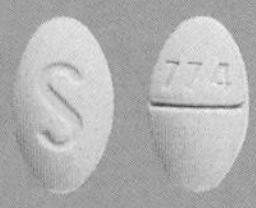

Sorbitrate 40 mg
Zeneca S 774

℞

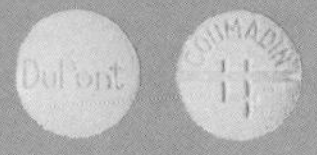

Coumadin 4 mg
DuPont 4

℞

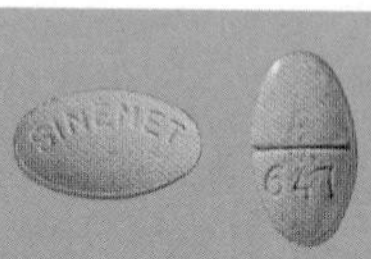

Sinemet-10/100
DuPont 647

℞

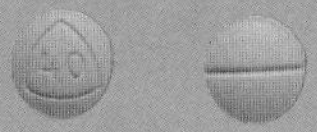

Isoptin 40 mg
Knoll 40

℞

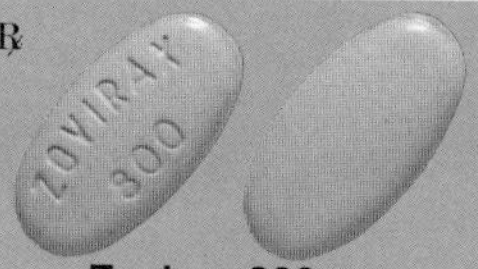

Zovirax 800 mg
Glaxo Wellcome 800

℞

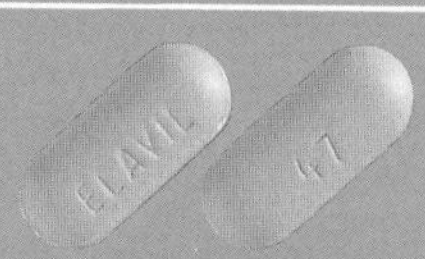

Elavil 150 mg
Zeneca 47

℞

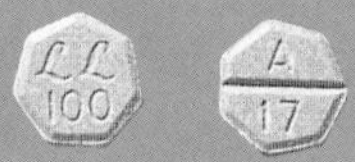

Asendin 100 mg
Lederle LL 100 A17

C-IV

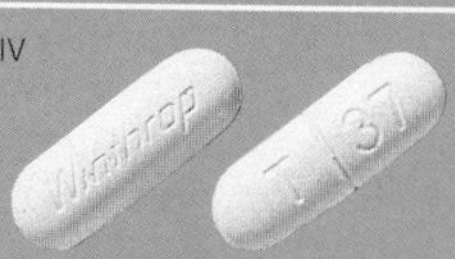

Talacen
Sanofi Winthrop T37

℞

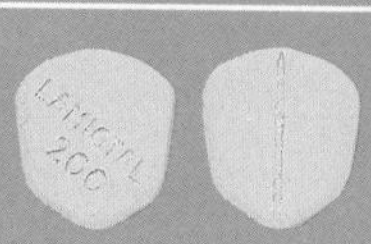

Lamictal 200 mg
Glaxo Wellcome 200

C-III

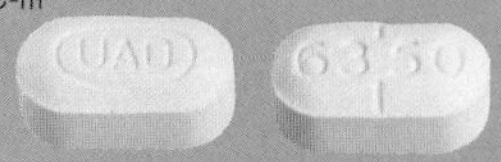

Lorcet 10/650
UAD 6350

℞
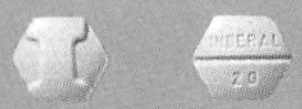
Inderal 20 mg
Wyeth-Ayerst I 20

℞
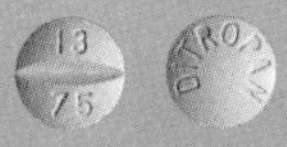
Ditropan 5 mg
Hoechst Marion Roussel 1375

℞
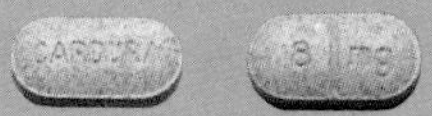
Cardura 8 mg
Roerig 8

C-IV
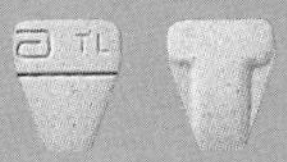
Tranxene 3.75 mg
Abbott TL

℞
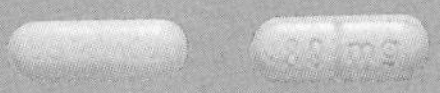
Betapace 80 mg
Berlex 80

℞
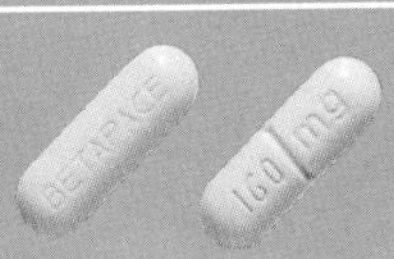
Betapace 160 mg
Berlex 160

℞
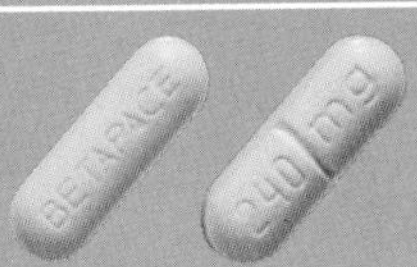
Betapace 240 mg
Berlex 240

℞
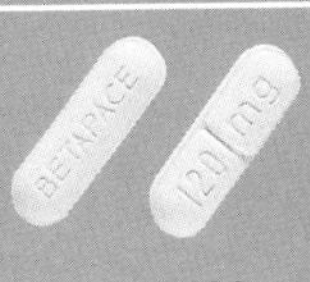
Betapace 120 mg
Berlex 120

℞
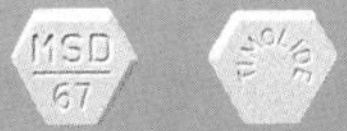

Timolide 10/25
Merck MSD 67

℞
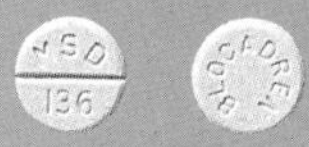
Blocadren 10 mg
Merck MSD 136

℞
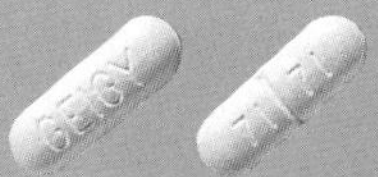
Lopressor 100 mg
Ciba Geigy 71 71

℞
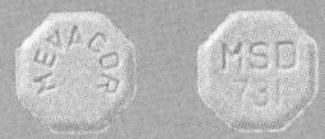
Mevacor 20 mg
Merck MSD 731

℞
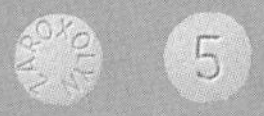

Zaroxolyn 5 mg
Medeva 5

C-IV
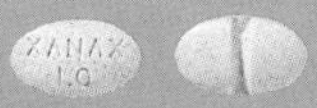
Xanax 1 mg
Pharmacia & Upjohn 1.0

℞
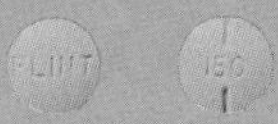
Synthroid 0.15 mg
Knoll Flint 150

℞
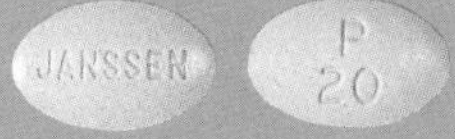

Propulsid 20 mg
Janssen P 20

℞
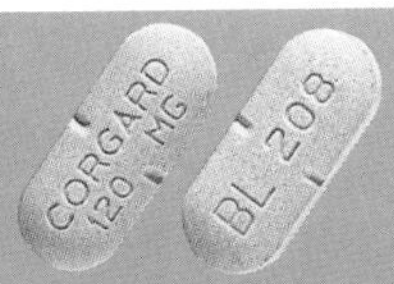

Corgard 120 mg
B-M Squibb 120 BL 208

℞
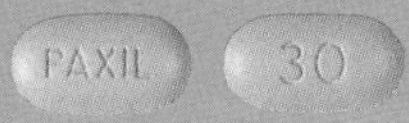

Paxil 30 mg
SmithKline Beecham 30

℞
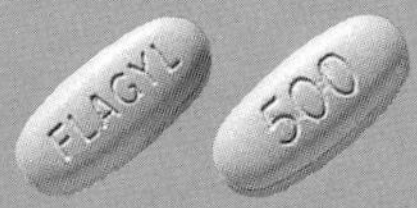

Flagyl 500 mg
Searle 500

℞
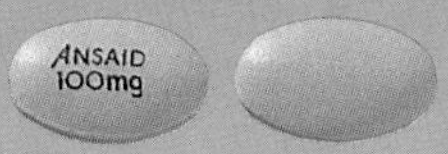

Ansaid 100 mg
Pharmacia & Upjohn 100

℞
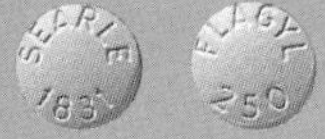
Flagyl 250 mg
Searle 1831 250

℞
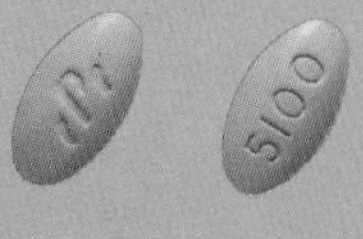

Penetrex 200 mg
Rhone-Poulenc Rorer 5100

℞
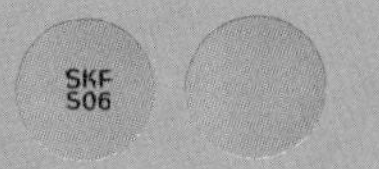

Stelazine 5 mg
SmithKline Beecham SKF S06

℞
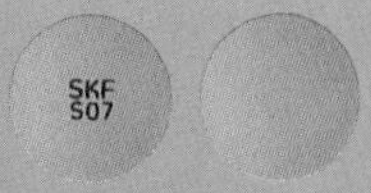

Stelazine 10 mg
SmithKline Beecham SKF S07

Blue to Pink Tablets

℞
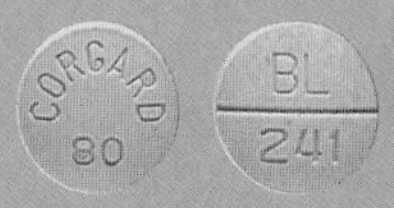
Corgard 80 mg
B-M Squibb 80 BL 241

℞
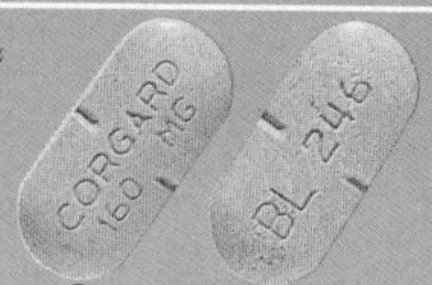
Corgard 160 mg
B-M Squibb 160 BL 246

℞
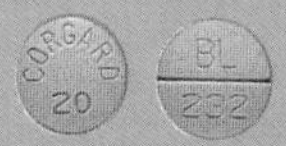
Corgard 20 mg
B-M Squibb 20 BL 232

℞
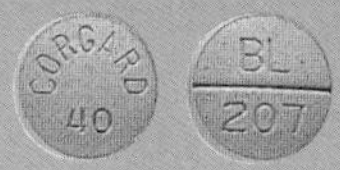
Corgard 40 mg
B-M Squibb 40 BL 207

C-II
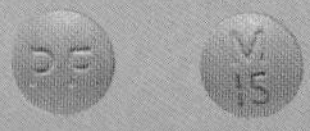
MS Contin 15 mg
Purdue Frederick PF M 15

℞
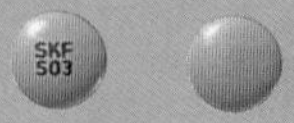
Stelazine 1 mg
SmithKline Beecham SKF S03

℞
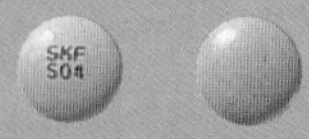
Stelazine 2 mg
SmithKline Beecham SKF S04

℞
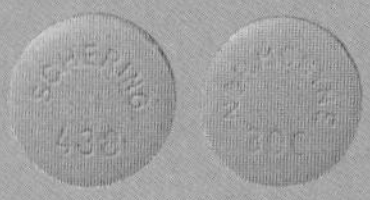
Normodyne 300 mg
Schering 438 300

℞
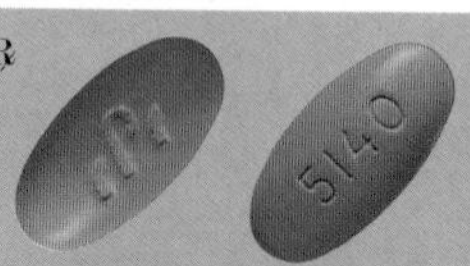
Penetrex 400 mg
Rhone-Poulenc Rorer 5140

℞
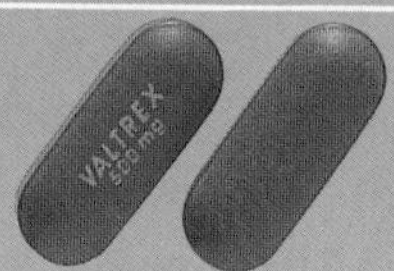
Valtrex 500 mg
Glaxo Wellcome 500

C-IV
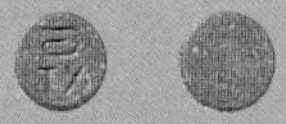
Tranxene-SD 11.25 mg
Abbott TX

℞
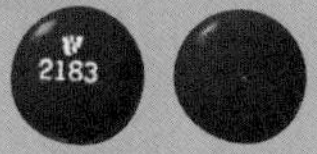
Urised
PolyMedica W 2183

℞
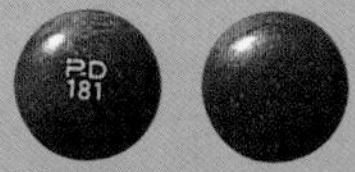
Pyridium 200 mg
Parke-Davis P-D 181

℞
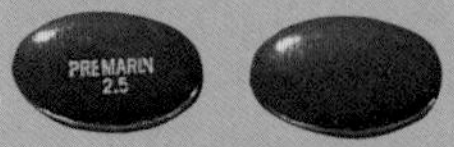
Premarin 2.5 mg
Wyeth-Ayerst 2.5

C-II
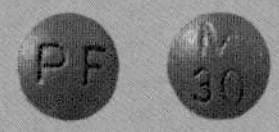
MS Contin 30 mg
Purdue Frederick PF M 30

℞
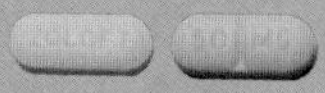
Zoloft 50 mg
Roerig 50

℞
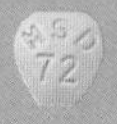
Proscar 5 mg
Merck MSD 72

℞
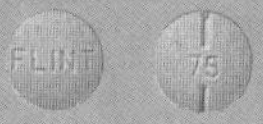
Synthroid 0.075 mg
Knoll Flint 75

℞
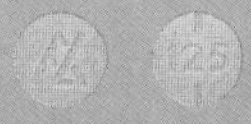
Levothroid 125 mcg
Forest Pharm 125

℞
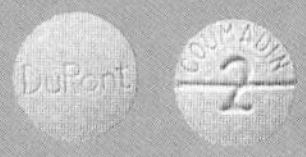
Coumadin 2 mg
DuPont 2

℞
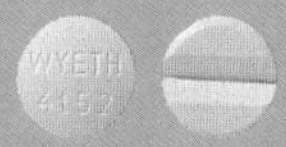
Isordil Titradose 5 mg
Wyeth-Ayerst 4152

℞
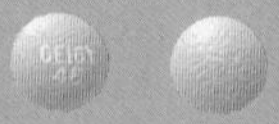
PBZ-SR 100 mg
Ciba Geigy 48

℞
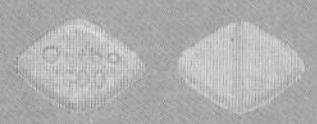
Ortho-Est 1.25 mg
Ortho 1800

C-III
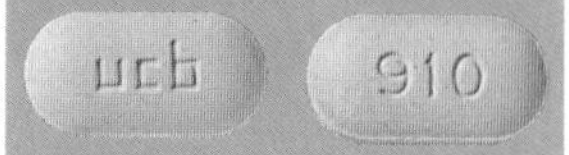
Lortab 10/500
UCB Pharma 910

℞
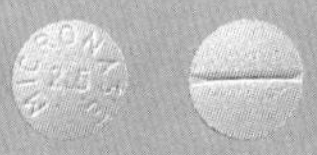
Micronase 2.5 mg
Pharmacia & Upjohn 2.5

℞
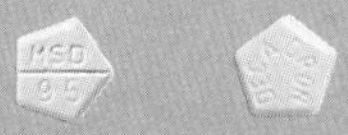
Decadron 1.5 mg
Merck MSD 95

℞
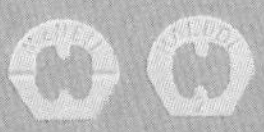
Haldol 2 mg
McNeil 2

℞
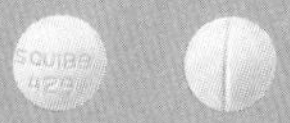
Florinef Acetate 0.1 mg
Apothecon Squibb 429

℞
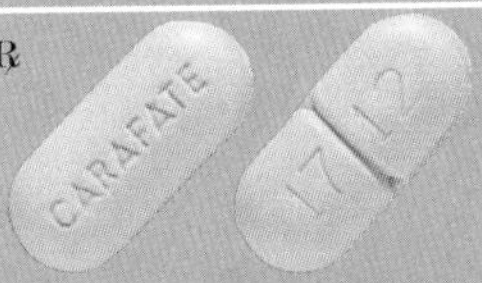

Carafate 1 g
Hoechst Marion Roussel 1712

℞
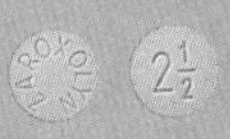
Zaroxolyn 2.5 mg
Medeva 2 1/2

℞
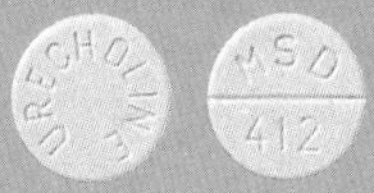

Urecholine 10 mg
Merck MSD 412

C-IV
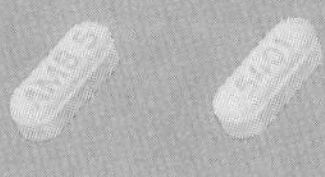
Ambien 5 mg
Searle AMB 5 5401

℞
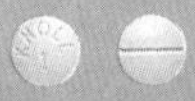
Mavik 1 mg
Knoll 1

℞
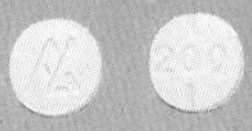
Levothroid 200 mcg
Forest Pharm 200

℞
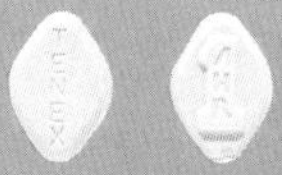
Tenex 1 mg
Robins AHR 1

℞
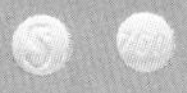
Sorbitrate 5 mg Sublingual
Zeneca S 760

℞
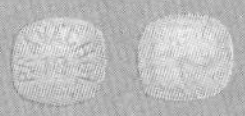
Pravachol 10 mg
B-M Squibb P 10

℞
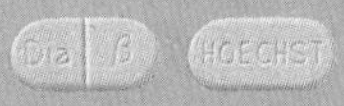

DiaBeta 2.5 mg
Hoechst Marion Roussel Dia ß

℞
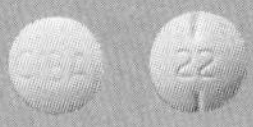
Esidrix 25 mg
Ciba 22

C-II
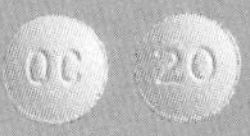

OxyContin 20 mg
Purdue Pharma OC 20

℞
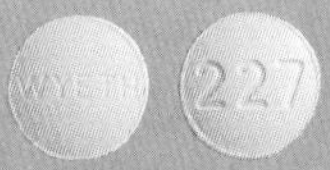

Phenergan 50 mg
Wyeth-Ayerst 227

℞
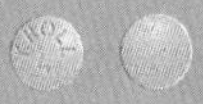
Mavik 4 mg
Knoll 4

℞
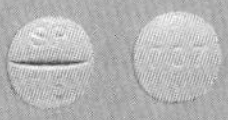
Univasc 7.5 mg
Schwarz Pharma SP 7.5 707

℞
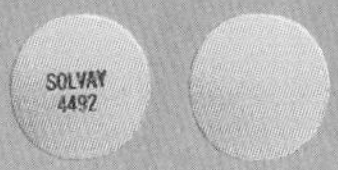

Lithobid Slow-Release 300 mg
Solvay 4492

℞
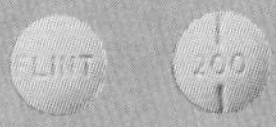
Synthroid 0.2 mg
Knoll Flint 200

℞
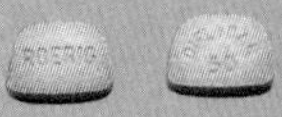
Diflucan 50 mg
Roerig 50

℞
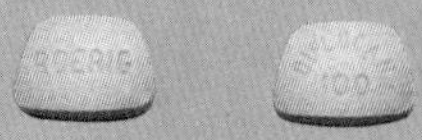
Diflucan 100 mg
Roerig 100

℞
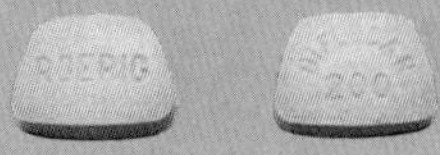
Diflucan 200 mg
Roerig 200

Pink Tablets

℞

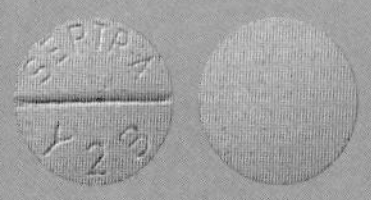

Septra 80/400
Glaxo Wellcome Y2B

℞

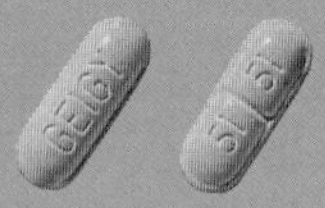

Lopressor 50 mg
Ciba Geigy 51 51

℞

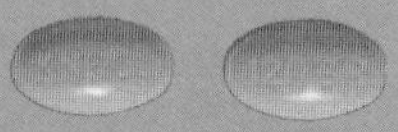

Isoptin SR 120 mg
Knoll 120 SR

℞

Septra DS 160/800
Glaxo Wellcome O2C

℞

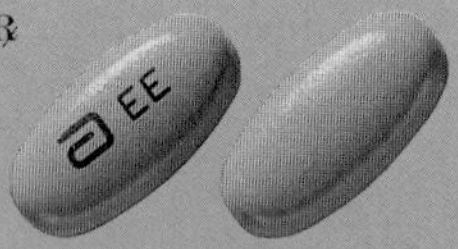

E.E.S. 400 400 mg
Abbott EE

℞

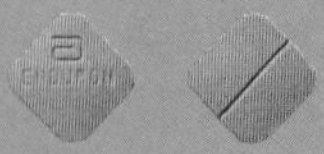

Enduron 5 mg
Abbott

℞

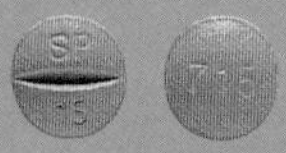

Univasc 15 mg
Schwarz Pharma SP 15 715

℞

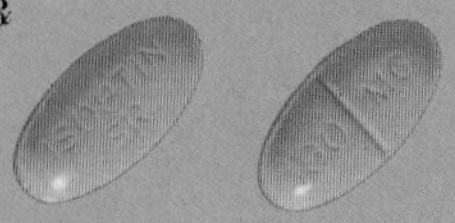

Isoptin SR 180 mg
Knoll SR 180

℞

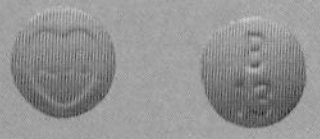

Ziac 5/6.25
Lederle LL B13

℞

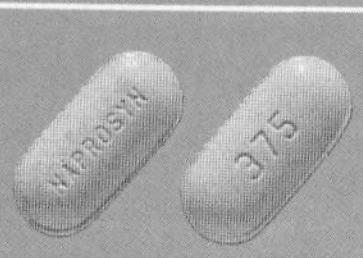

Naprosyn 375 mg
Roche 375

℞

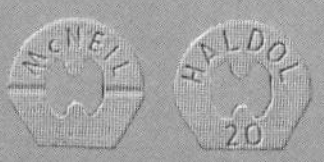

Haldol 20 mg
McNeil 20

℞

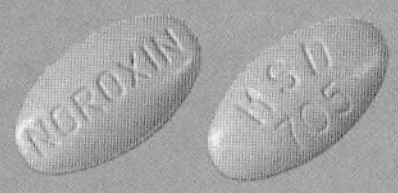

Noroxin 400 mg
Merck MSD 705

℞

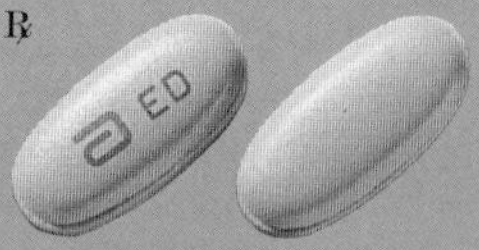

Ery-Tab 500 mg
Abbott ED

℞

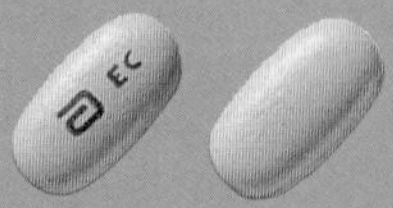

Ery-Tab 250 mg
Abbott EC

℞

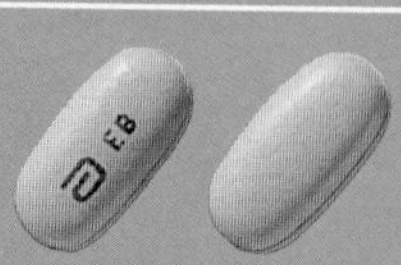

Erythromycin 250 mg
Abbott EB

℞

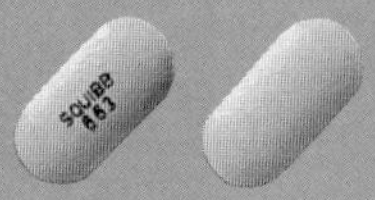

Sumycin 250 mg
Apothecon Squibb 663

℞

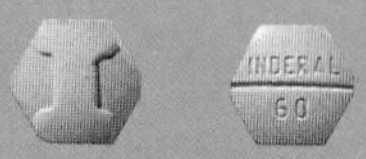

Inderal 60 mg
Wyeth-Ayerst I 60

℞

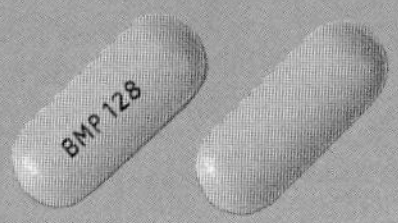

Menest 2.5 mg
SmithKline Beecham BMP 128

℞

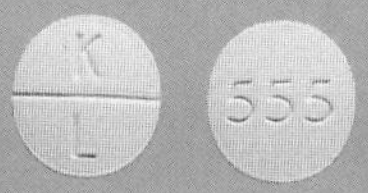

Yohimex 5.4 mg
Kramer KL 555

℞

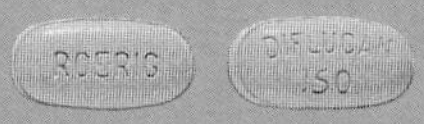

Diflucan 150 mg
Roerig 150

℞

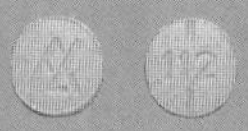

Levothroid 112 mcg
Forest Pharm 112

℞

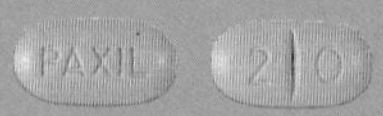

Paxil 20 mg
SmithKline Beecham 20

℞

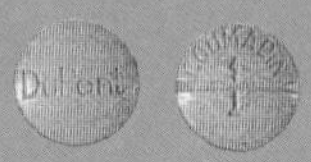

Coumadin 1 mg
DuPont 1

℞

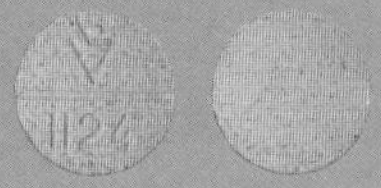

Dilor G
Savage 1124

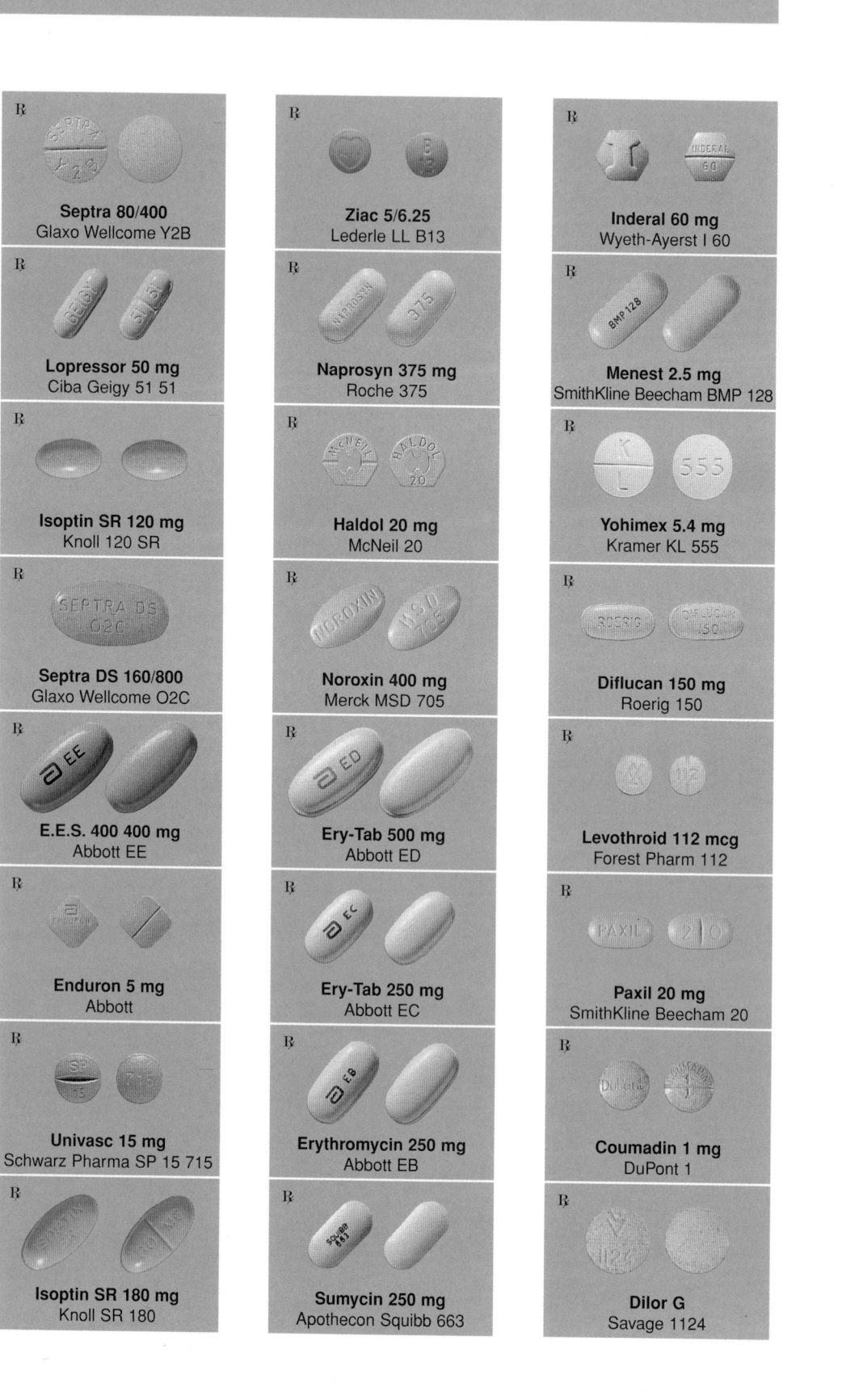

Pink to Red Tablets

℞

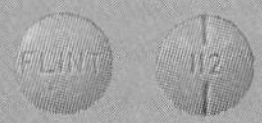

Synthroid 0.112 mg
Knoll Flint 112

℞

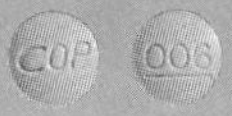

Luride Lozi-Tabs 1 mg
Colgate COP 006

℞

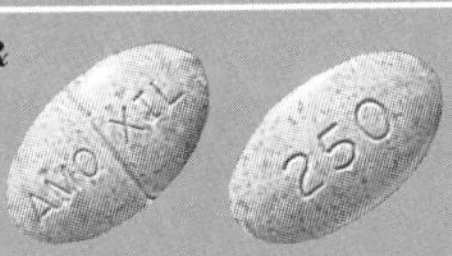

Amoxil 250 mg Chewable
SmithKline Beecham 250

℞

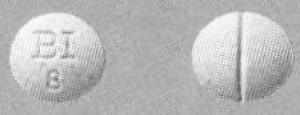

Combipres 0.1 mg
Boehringer Ingelheim BI 8

C-IV

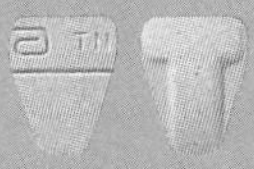

Tranxene 15 mg
Abbott TN

℞

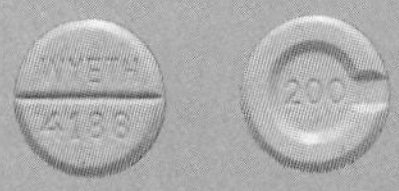

Cordarone 200 mg
Wyeth-Ayerst C 200 4188

℞

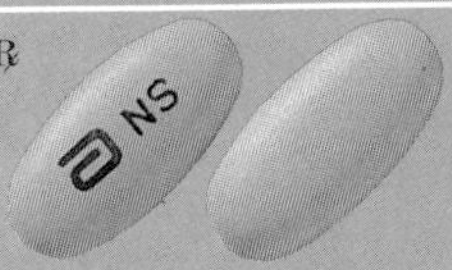

Depakote 500 mg
Abbott NS

℞

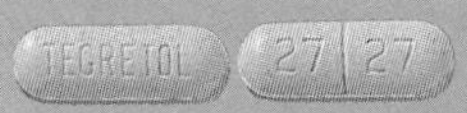

Tegretol 200 mg
Ciba 27 27

℞

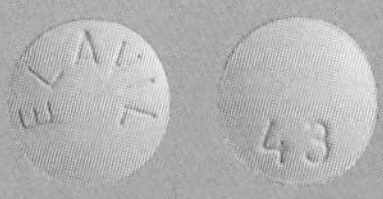

Elavil 100 mg
Zeneca 43

℞

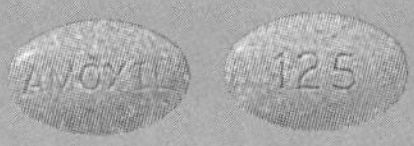

Amoxil 125 mg Chewable
SmithKline Beecham 125

℞

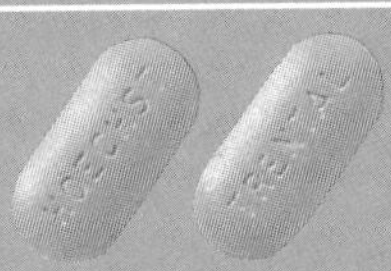

Trental 400 mg
Hoechst Marion Roussel

℞

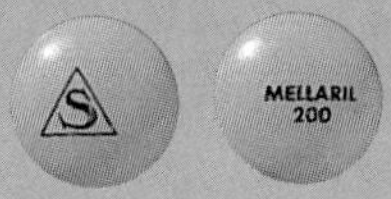

Mellaril 200 mg
Sandoz 200

℞

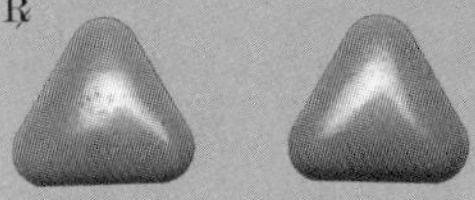

Atarax 100 100 mg
Roerig 100

℞

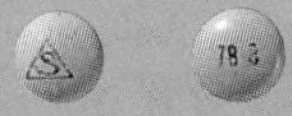

Mellaril 15 mg
Sandoz 78-8

℞

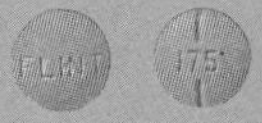

Synthroid 0.175 mg
Knoll Flint 175

℞

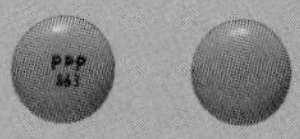

Prolixin 1 mg
Apothecon PPP 863

℞

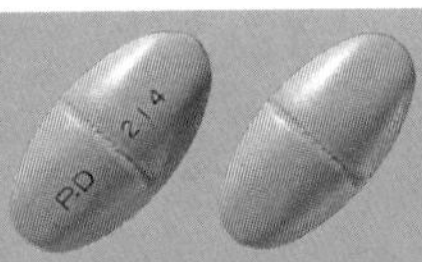

Choledyl SA 400 mg
Parke-Davis P-D 214

℞

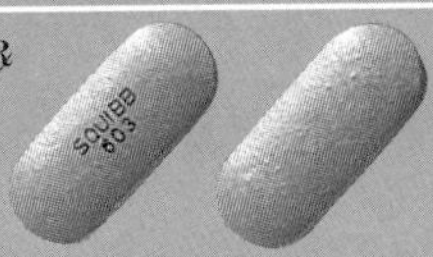

Sumycin 500 mg
Apothecon Squibb 603

℞

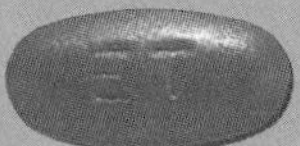

Erythrocin 500 mg
Abbott ET

℞

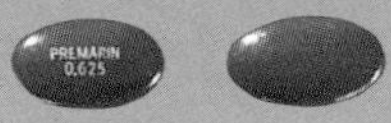

Premarin 0.625 mg
Wyeth-Ayerst 0.625

℞

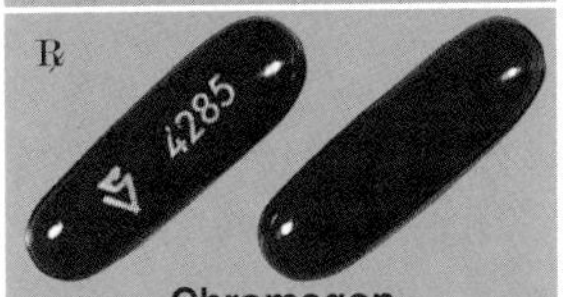

Chromagen
Savage 4285

℞

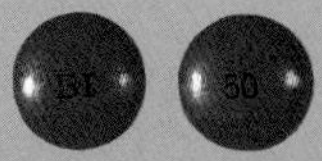

Serentil 50 mg
Boehringer Ingelheim BI 50

℞

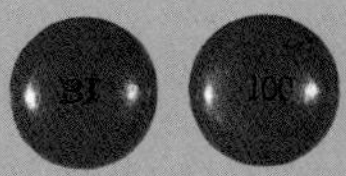

Serentil 100 mg
Boehringer Ingelheim BI 100

℞

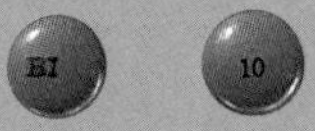

Serentil 10 mg
Boehringer Ingelheim BI 10

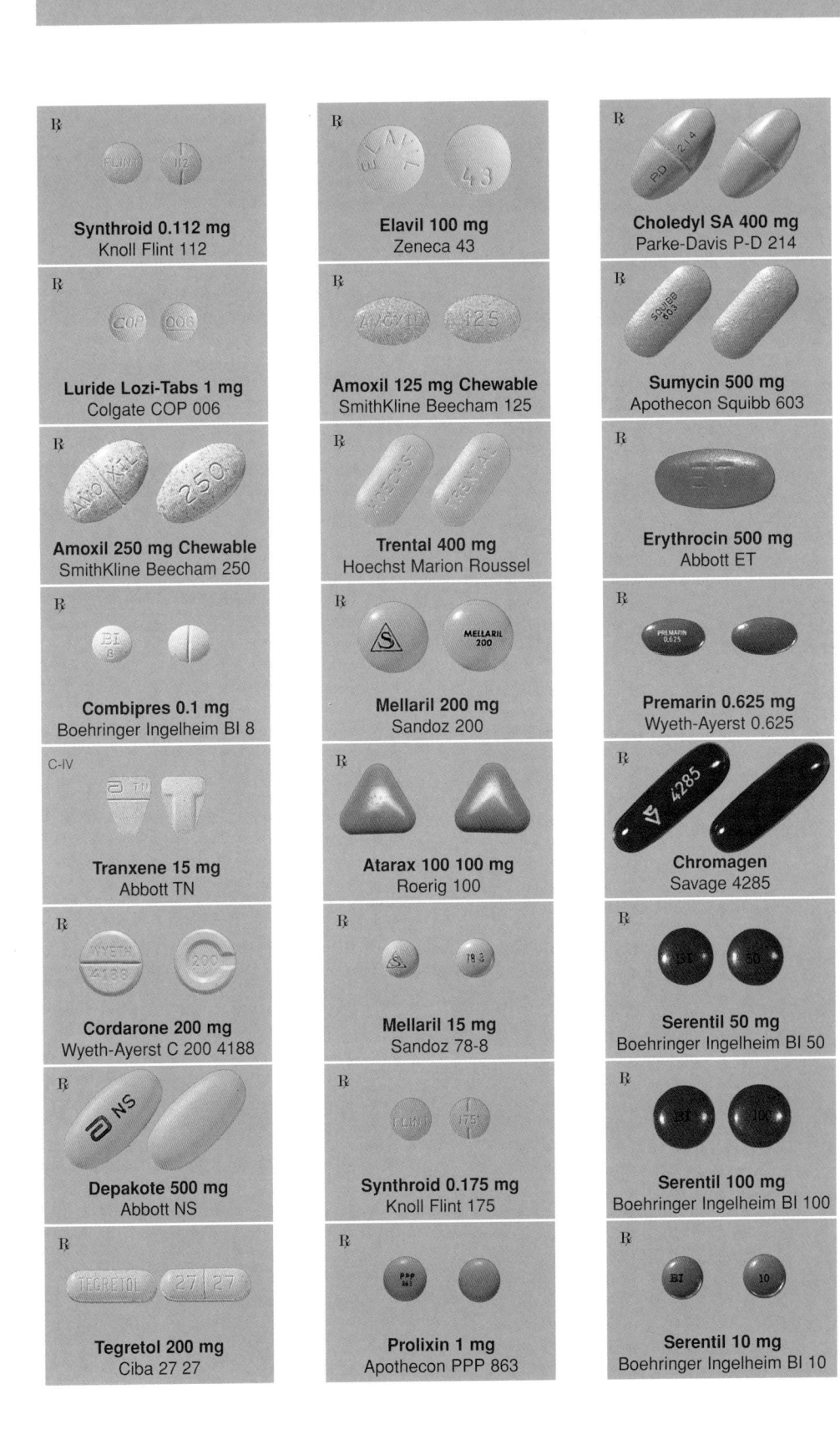

Red to Peach Tablets

℞
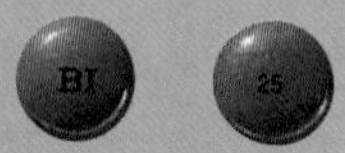
Serentil 25 mg
Boehringer Ingelheim BI 25

℞
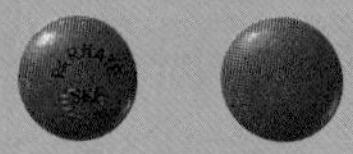
Parnate 10 mg
SmithKline Beecham SKF

℞
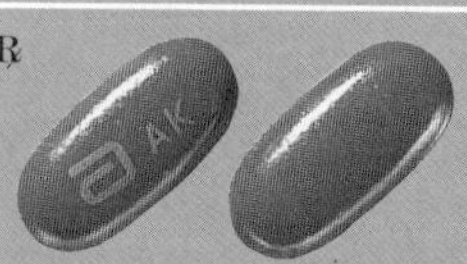
Iberet-Folic-500
Abbott AK

℞
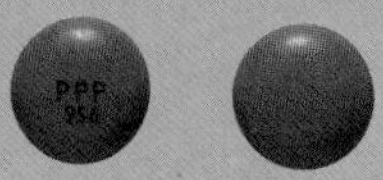
Prolixin 10 mg
Apothecon PPP 956

℞
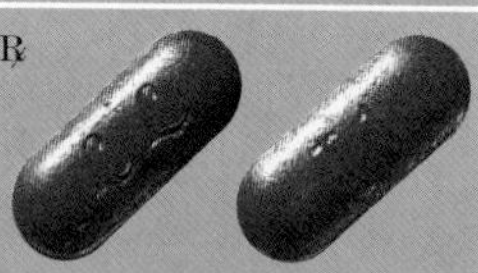
TriHEMIC 600
Lederle LL T1

℞
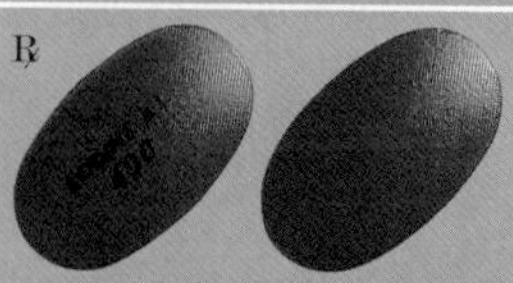
Lodine XL 400 mg
Wyeth-Ayerst 400

℞
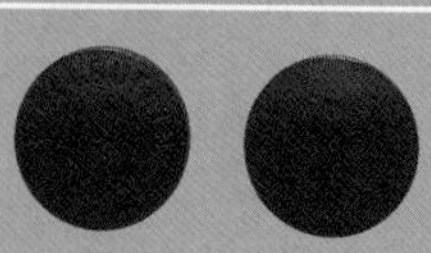
Wellbutrin 100 mg
Glaxo Wellcome 100

C-III
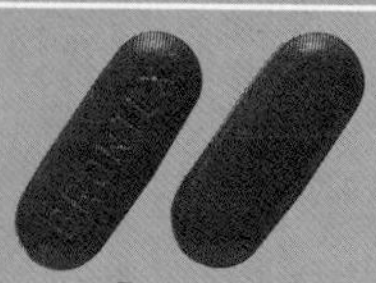
Brontex
Procter & Gamble

℞
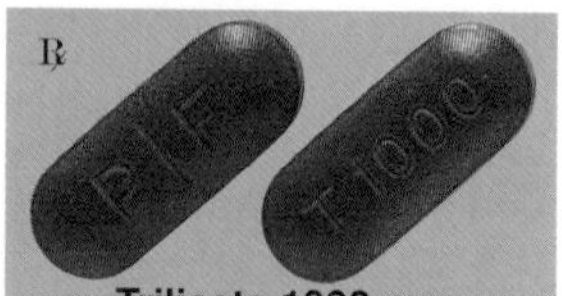
Trilisate 1000 mg
Purdue Frederick PF T1000

C-IV
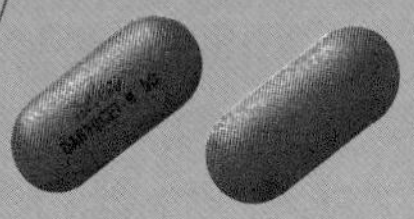
Darvocet-N 50
Lilly 50

℞
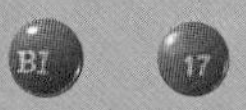
Persantine 25 mg
Boehringer Ingelheim BI 17

℞
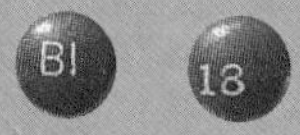
Persantine 50 mg
Boehringer Ingelheim BI 18

℞
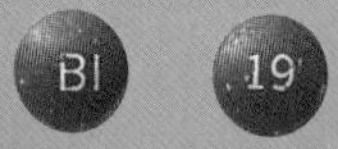
Persantine 75 mg
Boehringer Ingelheim BI 19

℞
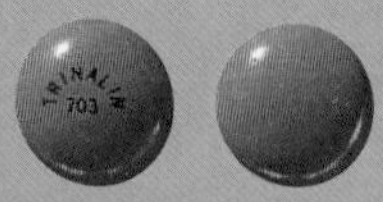
Trinalin Repetabs
Key 703

℞

Fero-Folic-500
Abbott AJ

℞
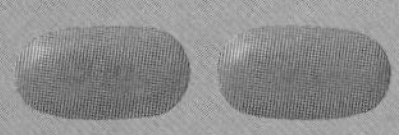
Depakote 125 mg
Abbott NT

℞
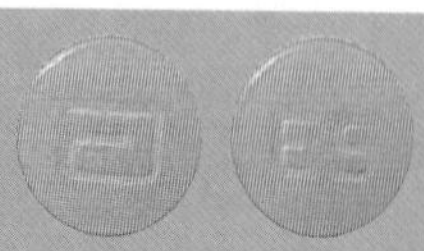
Erythrocin 250 mg
Abbott ES

℞
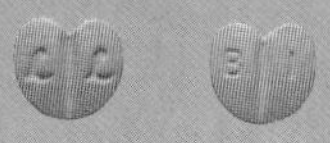
Zebeta 5 mg
Lederle LL B1

℞
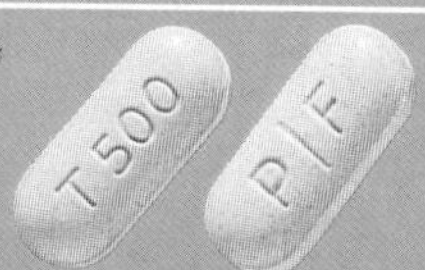
Trilisate 500 mg
Purdue Frederick T500 PF

C-IV
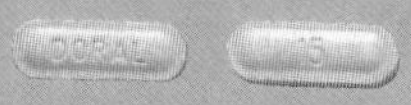
Doral 15 mg
Wallace 15

C-IV
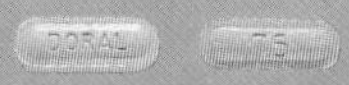
Doral 7.5 mg
Wallace 7.5

℞
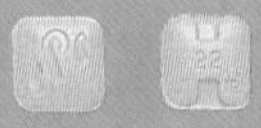
Hygroton 25 mg
Rhone-Poulenc Rorer H 22

℞
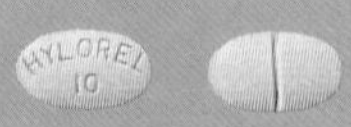
Hylorel 10 mg
Medeva 10

℞
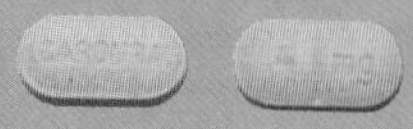
Cardura 4 mg
Roerig 4

℞

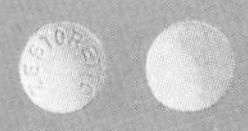

Zestoretic 10 mg/12.5 mg
Zeneca

℞

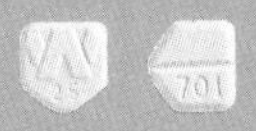

Effexor 25 mg
Wyeth-Ayerst 25 701

℞

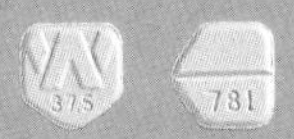

Effexor 37.5 mg
Wyeth-Ayerst 37.5 781

℞

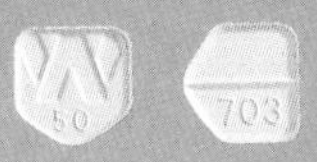

Effexor 50 mg
Wyeth-Ayerst 50 703

℞

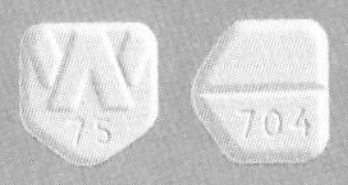

Effexor 75 mg
Wyeth-Ayerst 75 704

℞

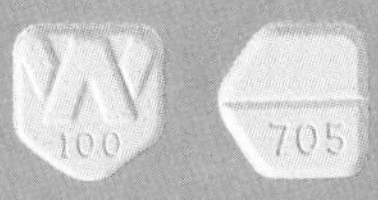

Effexor 100 mg
Wyeth-Ayerst 100 705

℞

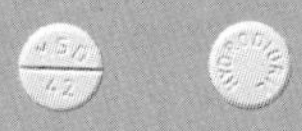

HydroDIURIL 25 mg
Merck MSD 42

℞

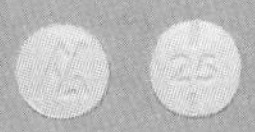

Levothroid 25 mcg
Forest Pharm 25

℞

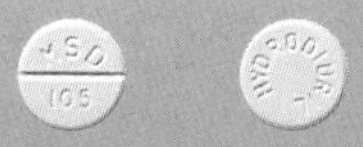

HydroDIURIL 50 mg
Merck MSD 105

℞

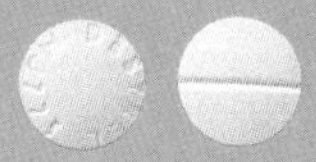

Desyrel 50 mg
Mead Johnson MJ 775

℞

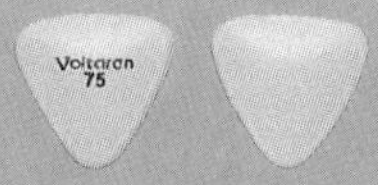

Voltaren 75 mg
Ciba 75

℞

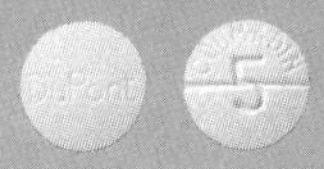

Coumadin 5 mg
DuPont 5

℞

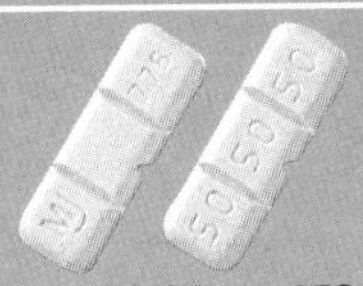

Desyrel Dividose 150 mg
Mead Johnson MJ 778 50

℞

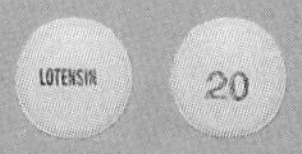

Lotensin 20 mg
Ciba 20

℞

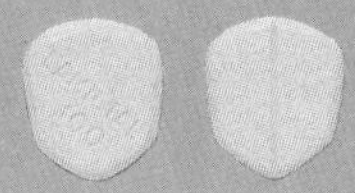

Lamictal 100 mg
Glaxo Wellcome 100

℞

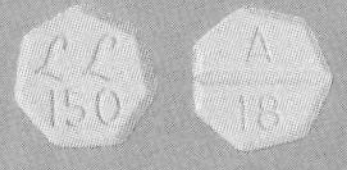

Asendin 150 mg
Lederle LL 150 A18

C-IV

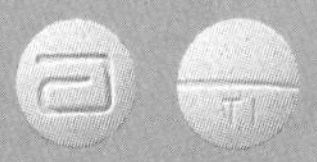

Cylert 37.5 mg
Abbott TI

℞

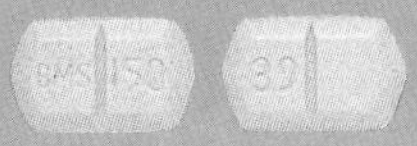

Serzone 150 mg
B-M Squibb BMS 150 39

℞

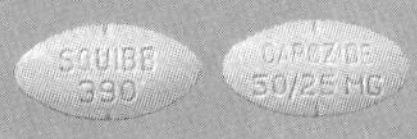

Capozide 50/25
B-M Squibb 390 50/25

℞

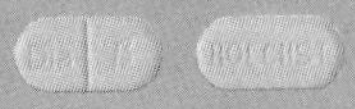

DiaBeta 1.25 mg
Hoechst Marion Roussel Dia ß

℞

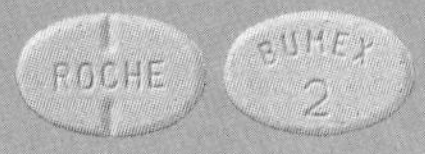

Bumex 2 mg
Roche 2

℞

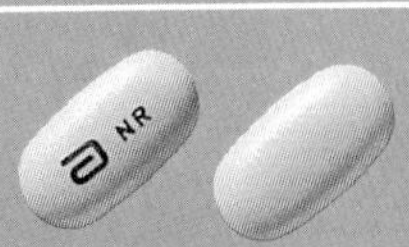

Depakote 250 mg
Abbott NR

℞

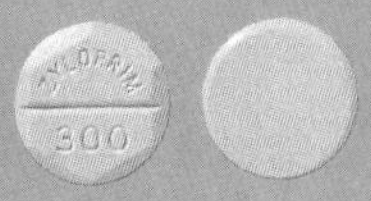

Zyloprim 300 mg
Glaxo Wellcome 300

℞

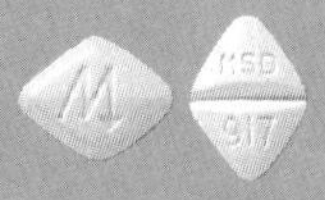

Moduretic
Merck MSD 917

Peach to Orange Tablets

℞

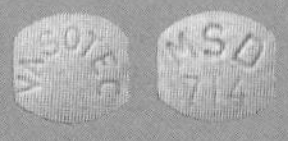

Vasotec 20 mg
Merck MSD 714

℞

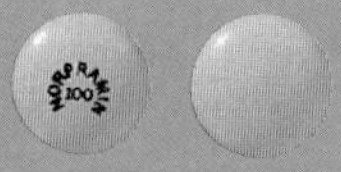

Norpramin 100 mg
Hoechst Marion Roussel 100

℞

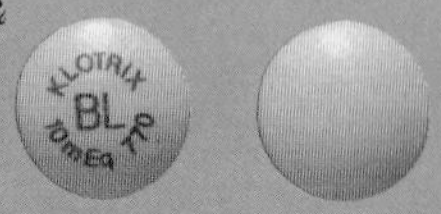

Klotrix 10 mEq
Bristol BL 770

℞

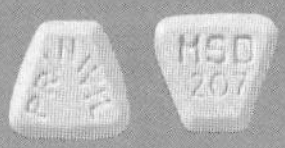

Prinivil 20 mg
Merck MSD 207

℞

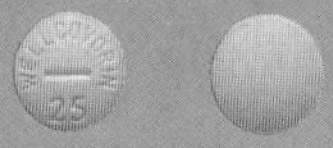

Wellcovorin 25 mg
Glaxo Wellcome 25

C-II

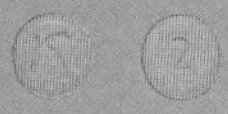

Dilaudid 2 mg
Knoll 2

℞

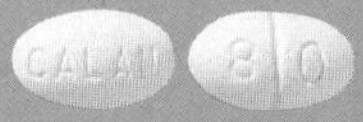

Calan 80 mg
Searle 80

℞

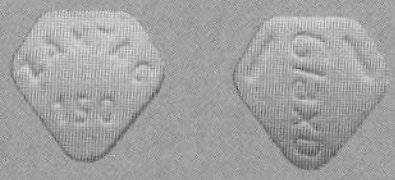

Zantac 150 mg
Glaxo Wellcome 150

℞

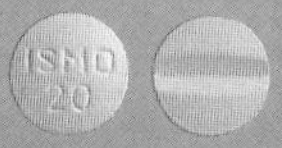

ISMO 20 mg
Wyeth-Ayerst 20

C-II

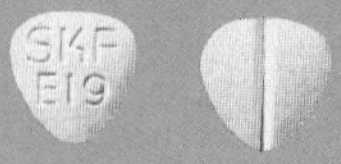

Dexedrine 5 mg
SmithKline Beecham SKF E19

℞

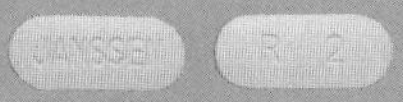

Risperdal 2 mg
Janssen R 2

℞

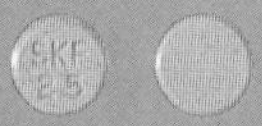

Vontrol 25 mg
SmithKline Beecham SKF 25

℞

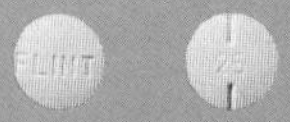

Synthroid 0.025 mg
Knoll Flint 25

℞

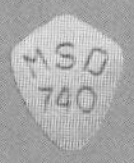

Zocor 20 mg
Merck MSD 740

℞

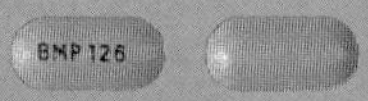

Menest 0.625 mg
SmithKline Beecham BMP 126

℞

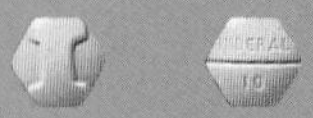

Inderal 10 mg
Wyeth-Ayerst I 10

℞

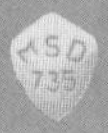

Zocor 10 mg
Merck MSD 735

℞

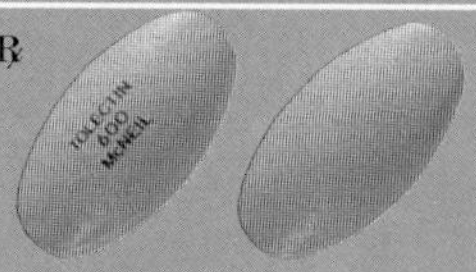

Tolectin 600 600 mg
McNeil 600

℞

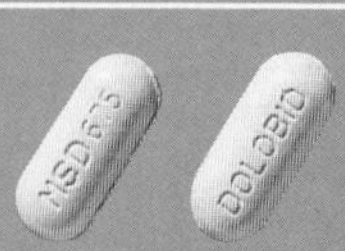

Dolobid 250 mg
Merck MSD 675

℞

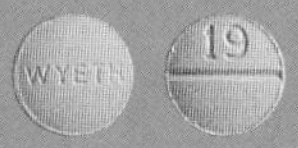

Phenergan 12.5 mg
Wyeth-Ayerst 19

℞

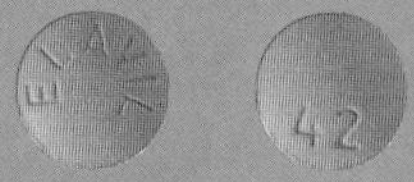

Elavil 75 mg
Zeneca 42

℞

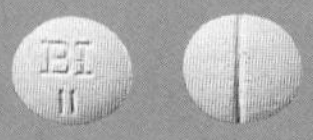

Catapres 0.3 mg
Boehringer Ingelheim BI 11

℞

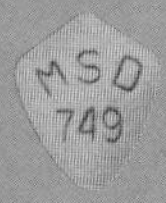

Zocor 40 mg
Merck MSD 749

℞

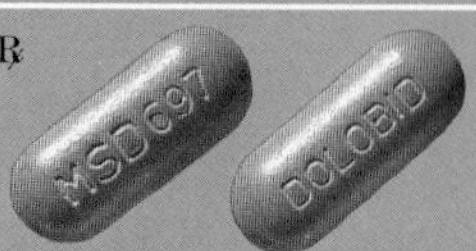

Dolobid 500 mg
Merck MSD 697

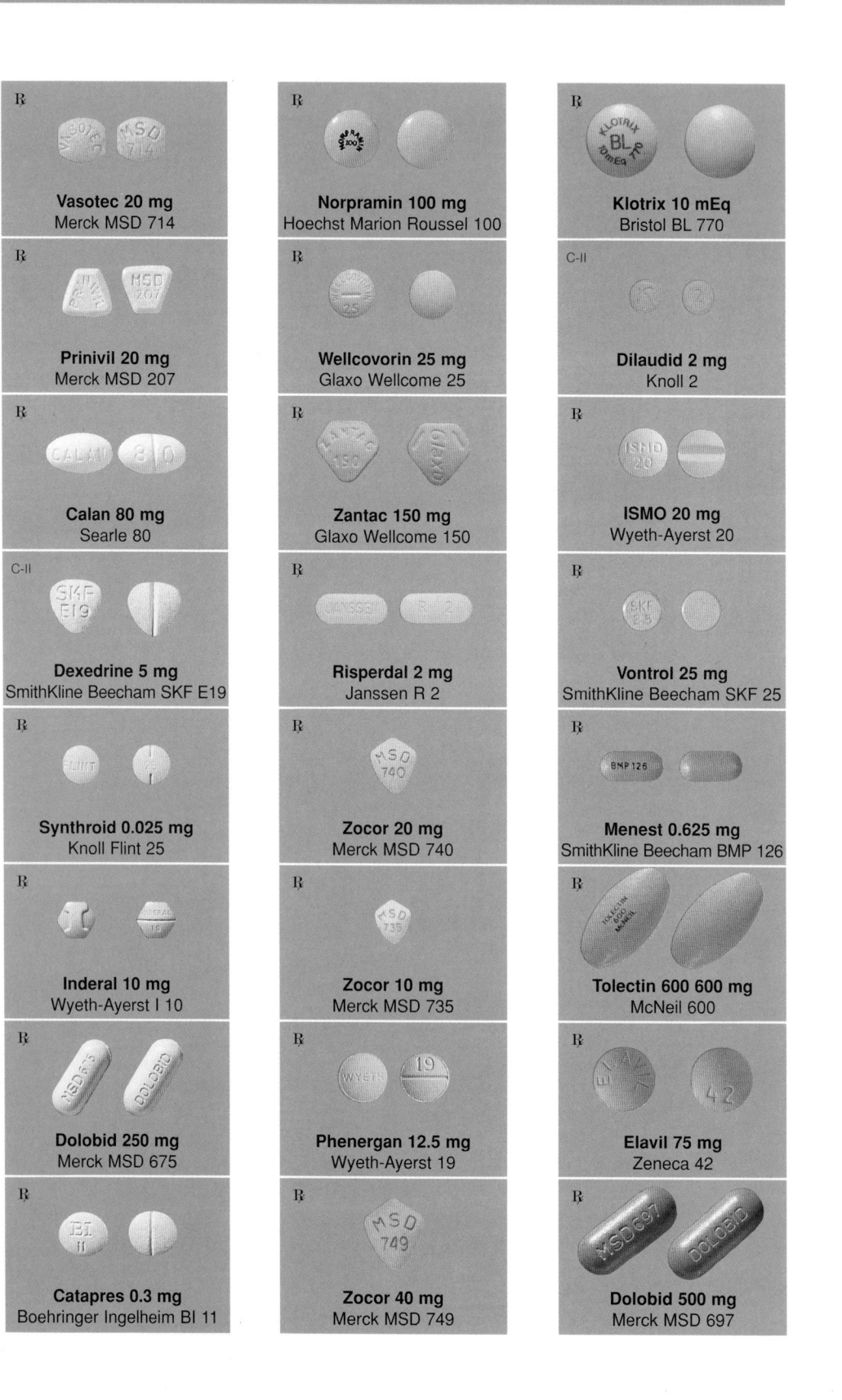

℞

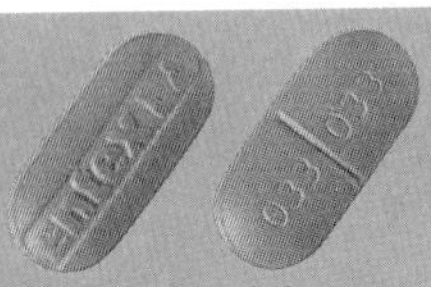

Entex LA
Dura 033 033

℞

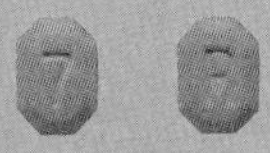

Lozol 1.25 mg
Rhone-Poulenc Rorer 7 R

℞

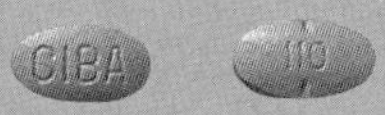

Ludiomil 25 mg
Ciba 110

℞

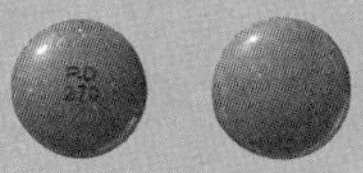

Nardil 15 mg
Parke-Davis P-D 270

℞

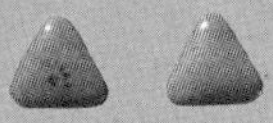

Atarax 10 mg
Roerig 10

℞

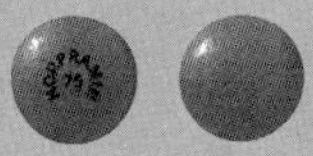

Norpramin 75 mg
Hoechst Marion Roussel 75

C-IV

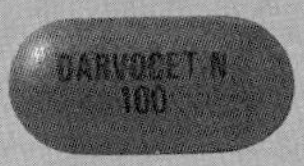

Darvocet-N 100
Lilly 100

℞

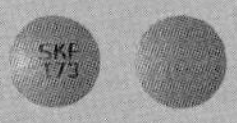

Thorazine 10 mg
SmithKline Beecham SKF T73

℞

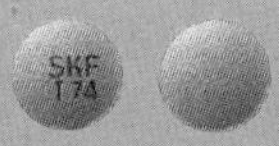

Thorazine 25 mg
SmithKline Beecham SKF T74

℞

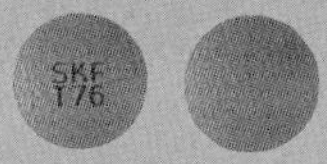

Thorazine 50 mg
SmithKline Beecham SKF T76

℞

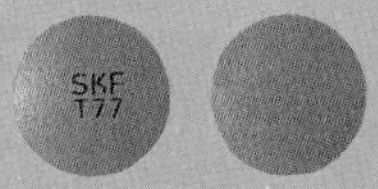

Thorazine 100 mg
SmithKline Beecham SKF T77

℞

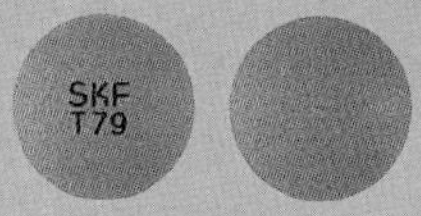

Thorazine 200 mg
SmithKline Beecham SKF T79

C-II

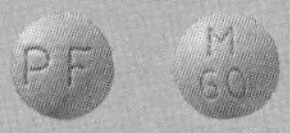

MS Contin 60 mg
Purdue Frederick PF M 60

℞

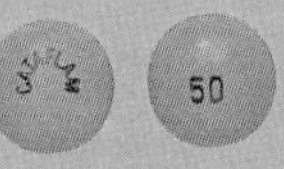

Cataflam 50 mg
Ciba 50

℞

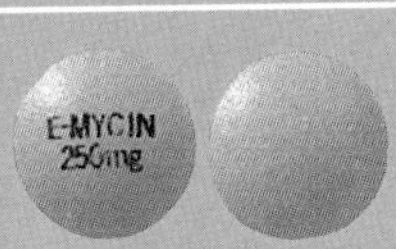

E-Mycin 250 mg
Knoll 250

℞

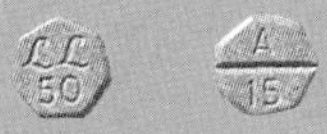

Asendin 50 mg
Lederle LL 50 A15

℞

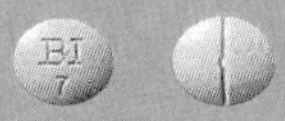

Catapres 0.2 mg
Boehringer Ingelheim BI 7

℞

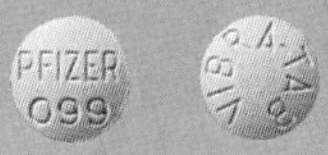

Vibra-Tabs 100 mg
Pfizer 099

℞

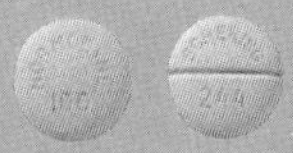

Normodyne 100 mg
Schering 100 244

℞

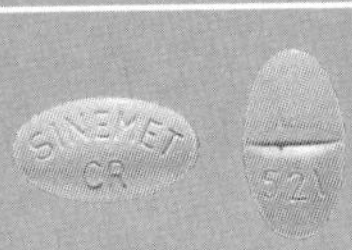

Sinemet CR-50/200
DuPont 521

℞

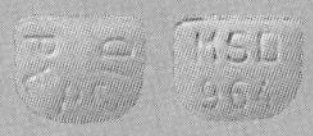

Pepcid 40 mg
Merck MSD 964

℞

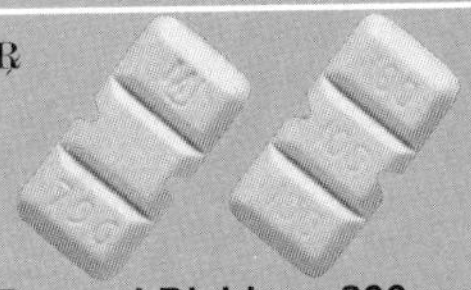

Desyrel Dividose 300 mg
Mead Johnson MJ 796 100

C-IV

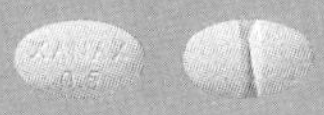

Xanax 0.5 mg
Pharmacia & Upjohn 0.5

℞

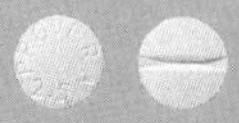

Provera 2.5 mg
Pharmacia & Upjohn 2.5

Brown Tablets

℞

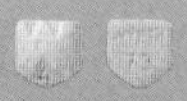

Wytensin 4 mg
Wyeth-Ayerst W4 73

℞

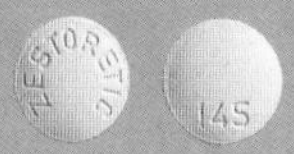

Zestoretic 20 mg/25 mg
Zeneca 145

C-IV

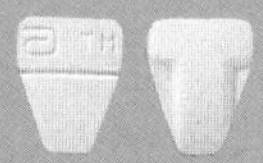

Tranxene 7.5 mg
Abbott TM

℞

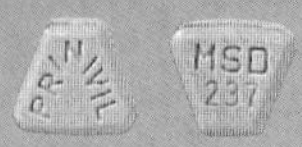

Prinivil 40 mg
Merck MSD 237

℞

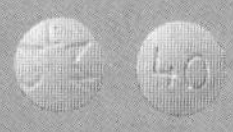

Calan 40 mg
Searle 40

℞

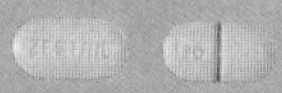

Zestril 5 mg
Zeneca 130

℞

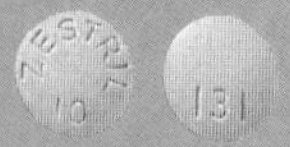

Zestril 10 mg
Zeneca 10 131

℞

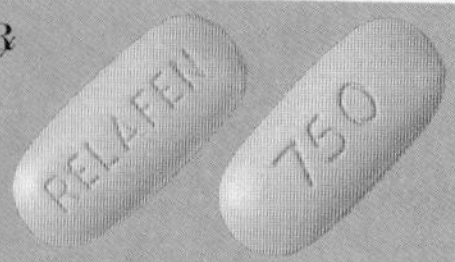

Relafen 750 mg
SmithKline Beecham 750

℞

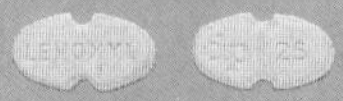

Levoxyl 25 mcg
Jones Medical dp 25

℞

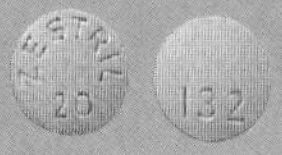

Zestril 20 mg
Zeneca 20 132

℞

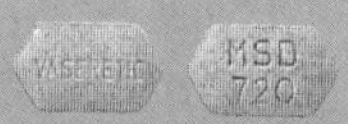

Vaseretic 10-25
Merck MSD 720

℞

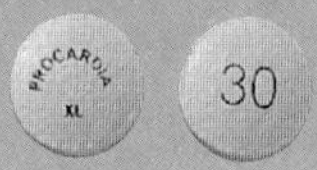

Procardia XL 30 mg
Pratt Pfizer 30

℞

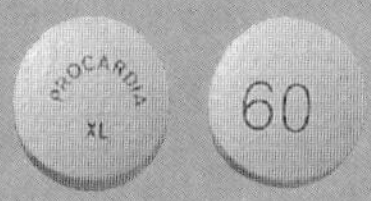

Procardia XL 60 mg
Pratt Pfizer 60

℞

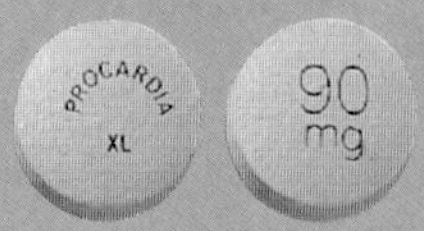

Procardia XL 90 mg
Pratt Pfizer 90

℞

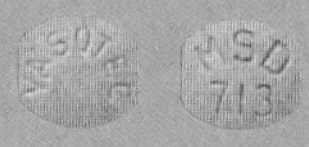

Vasotec 10 mg
Merck MSD 713

℞

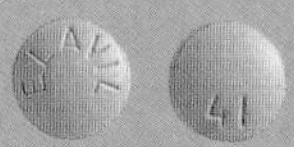

Elavil 50 mg
Zeneca 41

℞

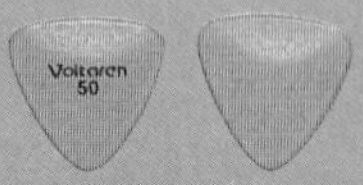

Voltaren 50 mg
Ciba 50

℞

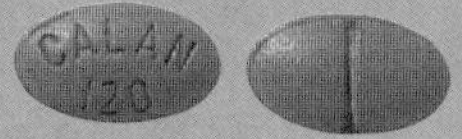

Calan 120 mg
Searle 120

℞

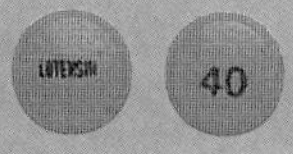

Lotensin 40 mg
Ciba 40

℞

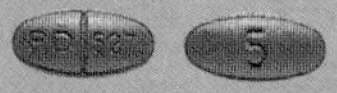

Accupril 5 mg
Parke-Davis PD 527 5

℞

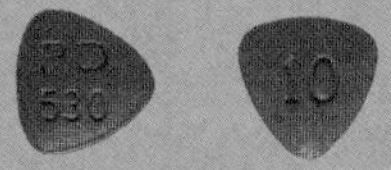

Accupril 10 mg
Parke-Davis P-D 530 10

℞

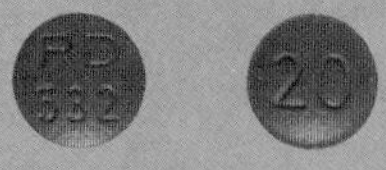

Accupril 20 mg
Parke-Davis P-D 532 20

℞

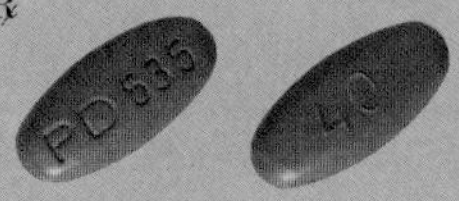

Accupril 40 mg
Parke-Davis P-D 535 40

℞

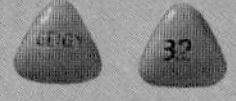

Tofranil 10 mg
Ciba Geigy 32

℞

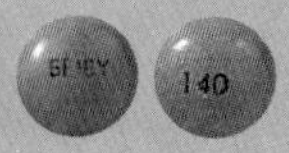

Tofranil 25 mg
Ciba Geigy 140

℞

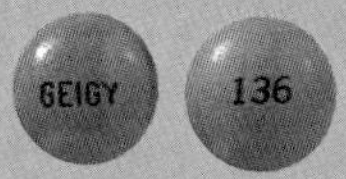

Tofranil 50 mg
Ciba Geigy 136

℞

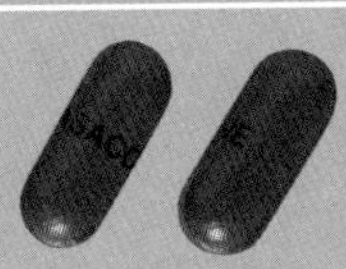

Asacol 400 mg
Procter & Gamble NE

℞

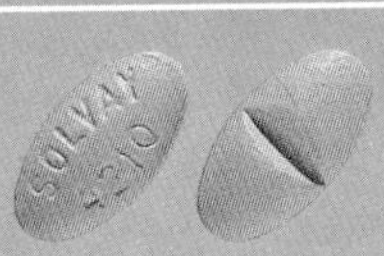

Luvox 100 mg
Solvay 4210

℞

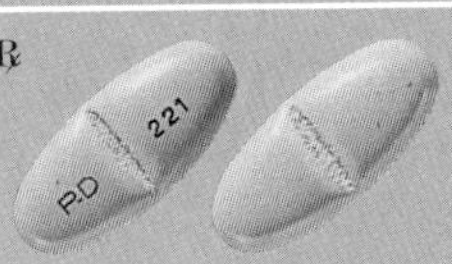

Choledyl SA 600 mg
Parke-Davis P-D 221

℞

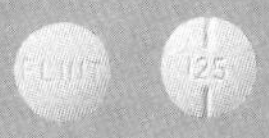

Synthroid 0.125 mg
Knoll Flint 125

℞

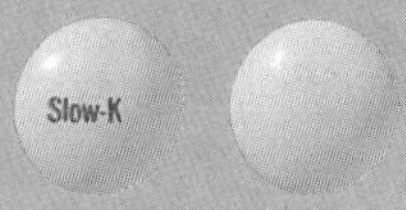

Slow-K 8 mEq
Ciba

℞

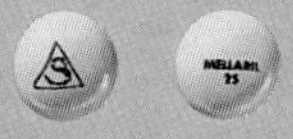

Mellaril 25 mg
Sandoz 25

℞

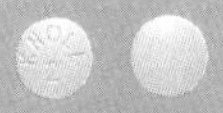

Mavik 2 mg
Knoll 2

℞

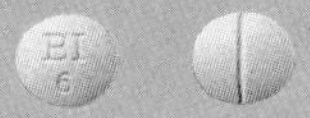

Catapres 0.1 mg
Boehringer Ingelheim BI 6

℞

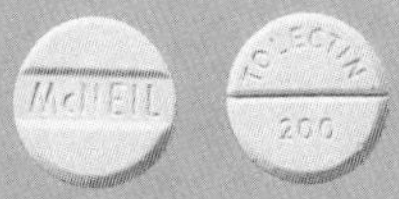

Tolectin 200 200 mg
McNeil 200

℞

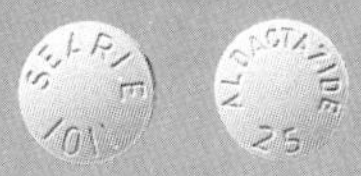

Aldactazide 25/25
Searle 1011 25

℞

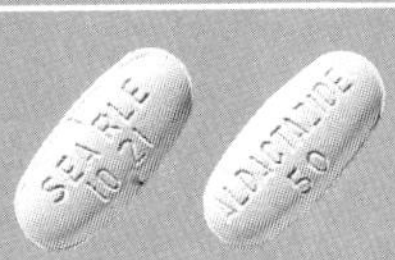

Aldactazide 50/50
Searle 1021 50

℞

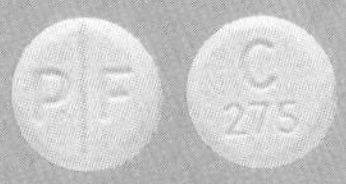

Cardioquin 275 mg
Purdue Frederick PF C275

℞

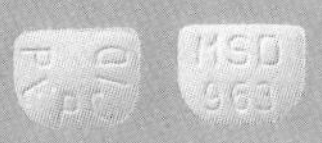

Pepcid 20 mg
Merck MSD 963

℞

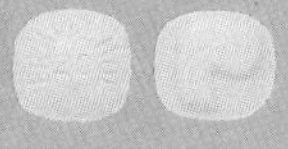

Pravachol 20 mg
B-M Squibb P 20

℞

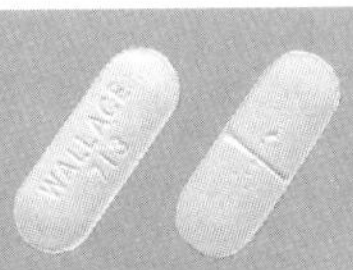

Rynatan
Wallace 713

℞

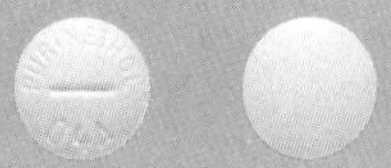

Purinethol 50 mg
Glaxo Wellcome 04A

C-IV

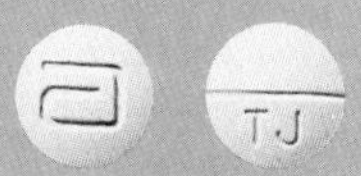

Cylert 75 mg
Abbott TJ

C-II

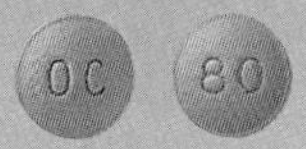

OxyContin 80 mg
Purdue Pharma OC 80

℞

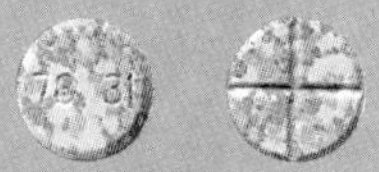

Bellergal-S
Sandoz 78-31

℞

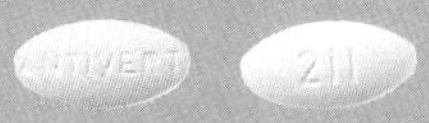

Antivert/25 25 mg
Roerig 211

C-III

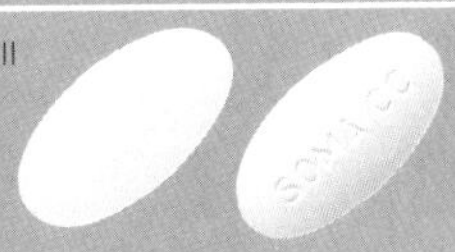

Soma Compound w/ Codeine
Wallace 2403 CC

℞

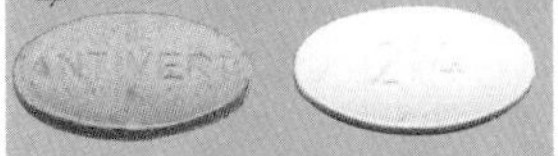

Antivert/50 50 mg
Roerig 214

CL-20 Multi-Colored to White Round Tablets

℞
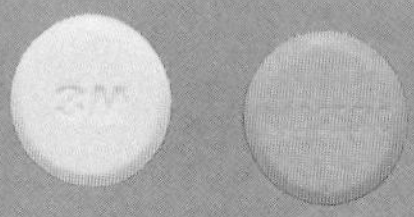
Norgesic
3M Pharm

℞
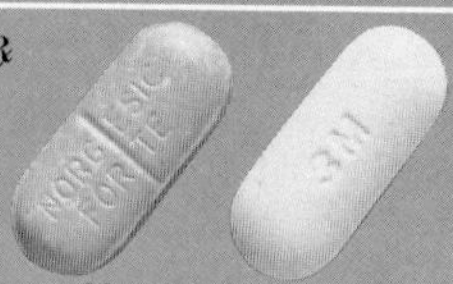
Norgesic Forte
3M Pharm

C-III
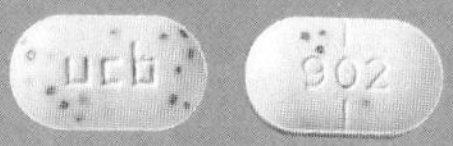
Lortab 5/500
UCB Pharma 902

C-III
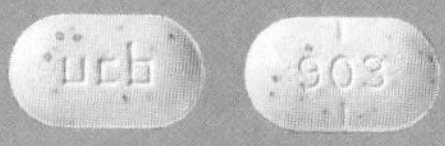
Lortab 7.5/500
UCB Pharma 903

C-IV
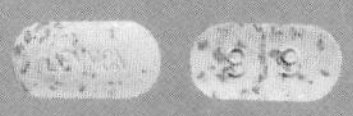
Adipex-P 37.5 mg
Gate Lemmon 99

℞
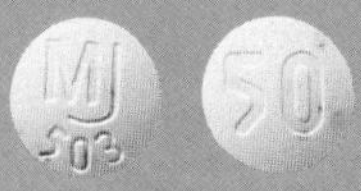
Cytoxan 50 mg
BMSOI MJ 503 50

℞
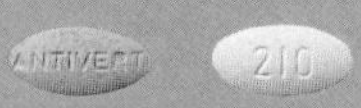
Antivert 12.5 mg
Roerig 210

℞
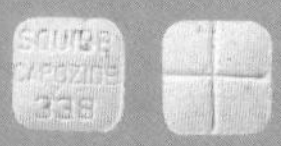
Capozide 25/15
B-M Squibb 338

℞
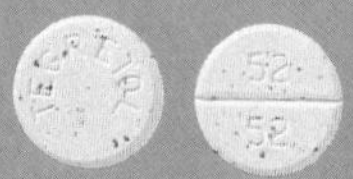
Tegretol 100 mg Chewable
Ciba 52 52

℞
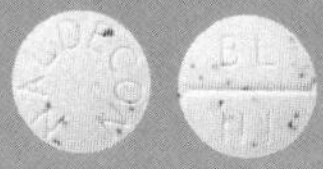
Naldecon
Apothecon BL N1

C-III
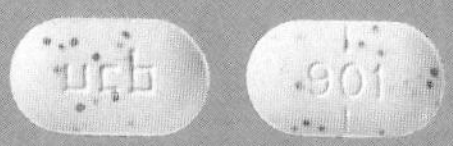
Lortab 2.5/500
UCB Pharma 901

℞
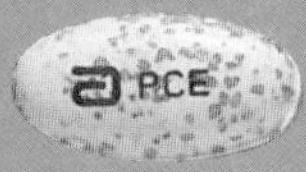
PCE 333 mg
Abbott

℞
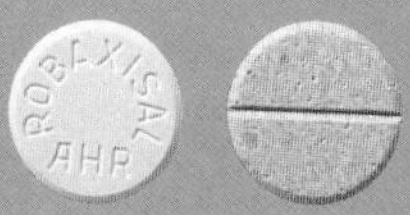
Robaxisal
Robins AHR

℞
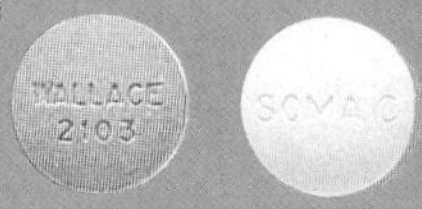
Soma Compound
Wallace 2103

C-II
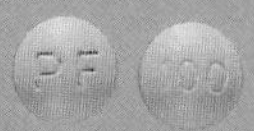
MS Contin 100 mg
Purdue Frederick PF 100

℞
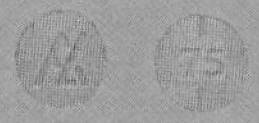
Levothroid 75 mcg
Forest Pharm 75

℞
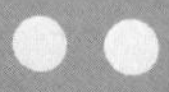
Nitrostat 0.3 mg
Parke-Davis

℞
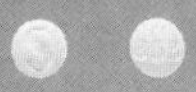
Sorbitrate 2.5 mg Sublingual
Zeneca S 853

℞

Prinivil 2.5 mg
Merck 15

℞
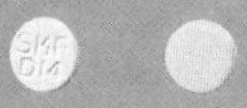
Cytomel 5 mcg
SmithKline Beecham SKF D14

C-V
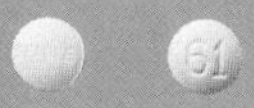
Lomotil
Searle 61

℞
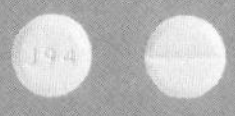
Tapazole 5 mg
Jones Medical J94

℞
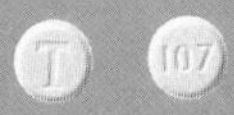
Tenormin 25 mg
Zeneca T 107

C-II
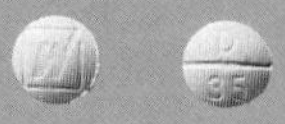
Demerol 50 mg
Sanofi Winthrop WD 35

℞

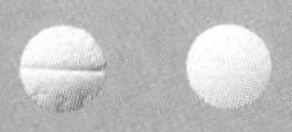

Myleran 2 mg
Glaxo Wellcome K2A

℞

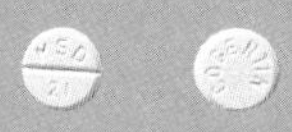

Cogentin 0.5 mg
Merck MSD 21

℞

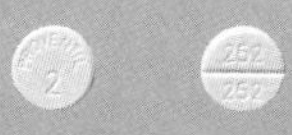

Proventil 2 mg
Schering 2 252

℞

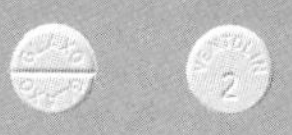

Ventolin 2 mg
Glaxo Wellcome 2

℞

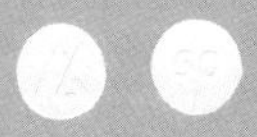

Levothroid 50 mcg
Forest Pharm 50

℞

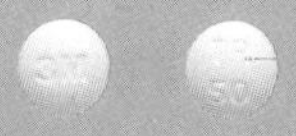

Tambocor 50 mg
3M Pharm TR 50

℞

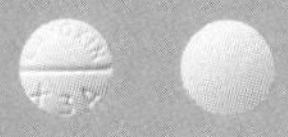

Lanoxin 0.25 mg
Glaxo Wellcome X3A

℞

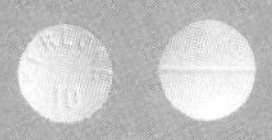

Kerlone 10 mg
Searle 10

℞

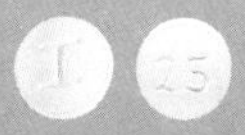

Imitrex 25 mg
Glaxo Wellcome I 25

℞

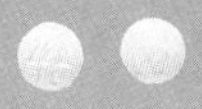

Armour Thyroid 1/4 gr
Forest Pharm A TC

℞

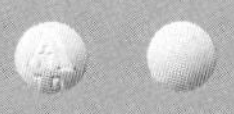

Armour Thyroid 1/2 gr
Forest Pharm A TD

℞

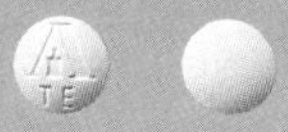

Armour Thyroid 1 gr
Forest Pharm A TE

℞

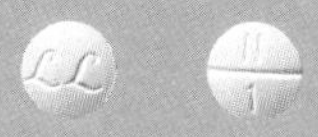

Neptazane 50 mg
Lederle LL N1

C-IV

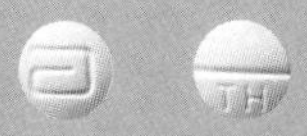

Cylert 18.75 mg
Abbott TH

℞

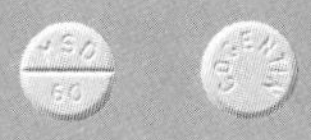

Cogentin 2 mg
Merck MSD 60

℞

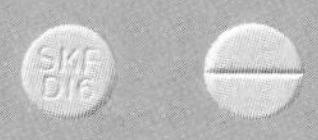

Cytomel 25 mcg
SmithKline Beecham SKF D16

℞

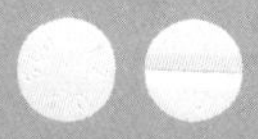

Monoket 10 mg
Schwarz Pharma 610 10

℞

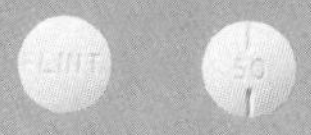

Synthroid 0.05 mg
Knoll Flint 50

℞

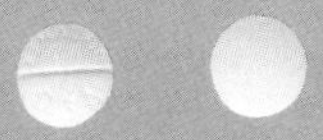

Kemadrin 5 mg
Glaxo Wellcome S3A

℞

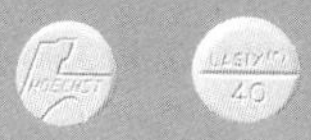

Lasix 40 mg
Hoechst Marion Roussel 40

℞

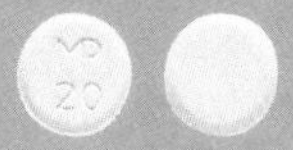

Ergoloid Mesylate 1 mg
Mutual MP 20

℞

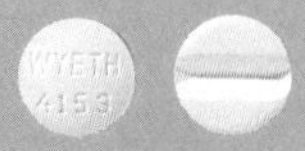

Isordil Titradose 10 mg
Wyeth-Ayerst 4153

℞

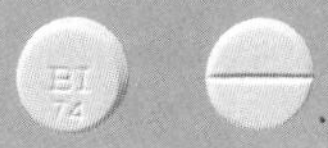

Alupent 10 mg
Boehringer Ingelheim BI 74

℞

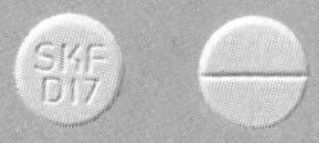

Cytomel 50 mcg
SmithKline Beecham SKF D17

White Round Tablets

C-IV

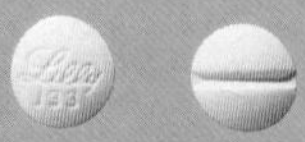

Phenobarbital 100 mg
Lilly J33

℞

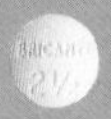

Bricanyl 2.5 mg
Hoechst Marion Roussel 2 1/2

℞

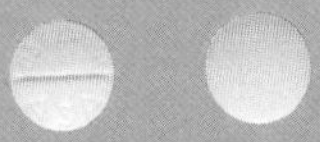

Daraprim 25 mg
Glaxo Wellcome A3A

℞

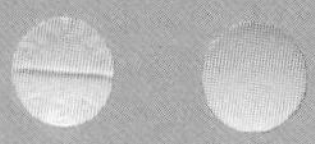

Alkeran 2 mg
Glaxo Wellcome A2A

℞

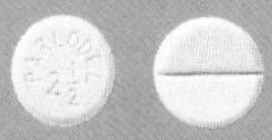

Parlodel 2.5 mg
Sandoz 2 1/2

℞

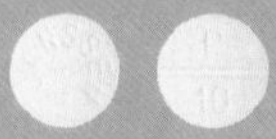

Propulsid 10 mg
Janssen P 10

℞

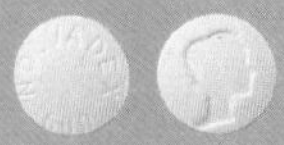

Nolvadex 10 mg
Zeneca 600

℞

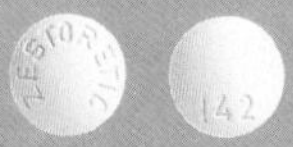

Zestoretic 20 mg/12.5 mg
Zeneca 142

℞

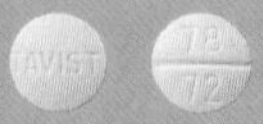

Tavist 2.68 mg
Sandoz 78 72

℞

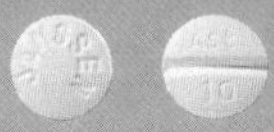

Hismanal 10 mg
Janssen AST 10

℞

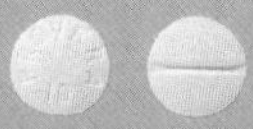

Provera 10 mg
Pharmacia & Upjohn 10

℞

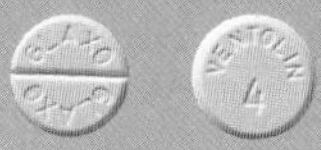

Ventolin 4 mg
Glaxo Wellcome 4

℞

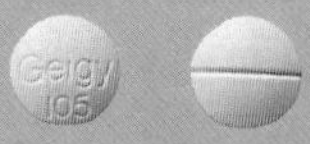

Brethine 5 mg
Ciba Geigy 105

C-II

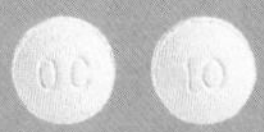

OxyContin 10 mg
Purdue Pharma OC 10

℞

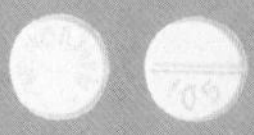

Tenormin 50 mg
Zeneca 105

℞

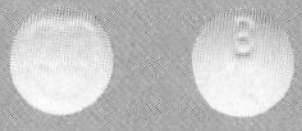

Ziac 10/6.25
Lederle LL B14

℞

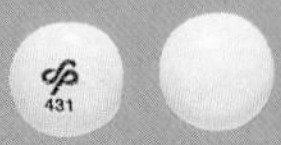

Proventil Repetabs
Schering 431

C-II

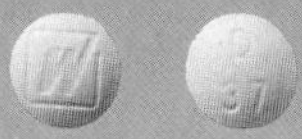

Demerol 100 mg
Sanofi Winthrop WD 37

℞

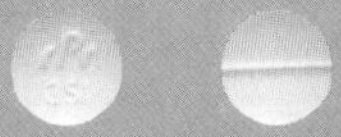

Slo-Phyllin 100 mg
Rhone-Poulenc Rorer 351

℞

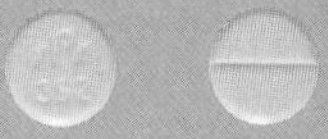

Slo-Phyllin 200 mg
Rhone-Poulenc Rorer 352

℞

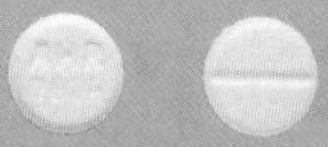

Robinul 1 mg
Robins AHR 7824

℞

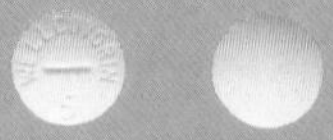

Wellcovorin 5 mg
Glaxo Wellcome 5

℞

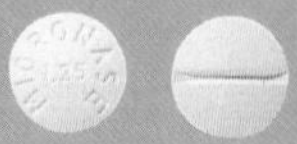

Micronase 1.25 mg
Pharmacia & Upjohn 1.25

℞

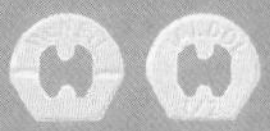

Haldol 0.5 mg
McNeil 1/2

White Round Tablets

℞

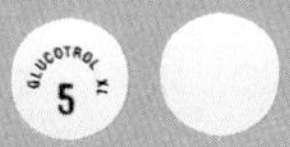

Glucotrol XL 5 mg
Pratt Pfizer 5

℞

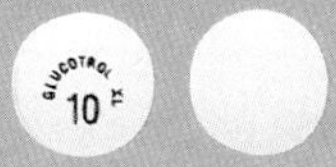

Glucotrol XL 10 mg
Pratt Pfizer 10

℞

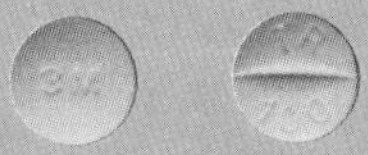

Tambocor 100 mg
3M Pharm TR 100

℞

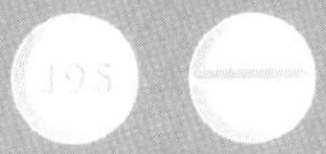

Tapazole 10 mg
Jones Medical J95

℞

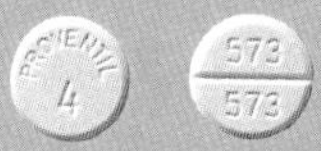

Proventil 4 mg
Schering 4 573

℞

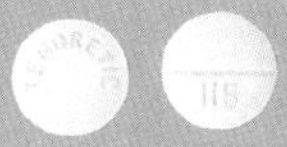

Tenoretic 50
Zeneca 115

℞

Norflex 100 mg
3M Pharm 221

C-IV

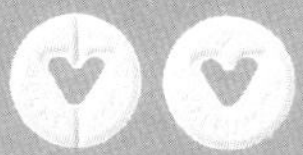

Valium 2 mg
Roche 2

℞

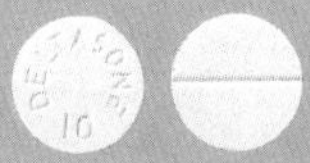

Deltasone 10 mg
Pharmacia & Upjohn 10

℞

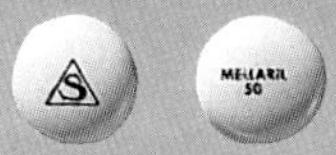

Mellaril 50 mg
Sandoz 50

℞

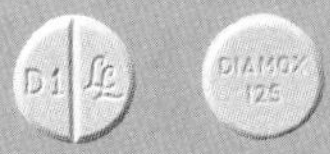

Diamox 125 mg
Lederle D1 LL 125

℞

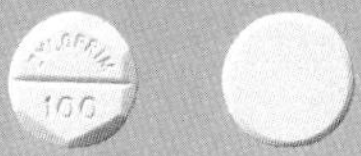

Zyloprim 100 mg
Glaxo Wellcome 100

℞

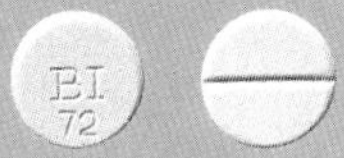

Alupent 20 mg
Boehringer Ingelheim BI 72

℞

Monoket 20 mg
Schwarz Pharma 620 20

℞

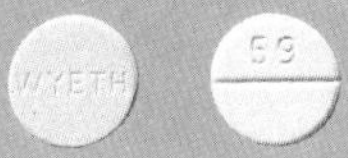

Pen•Vee K 250 mg
Wyeth-Ayerst 59

℞

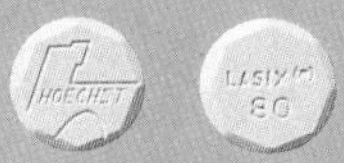

Lasix 80 mg
Hoechst Marion Roussel 80

℞

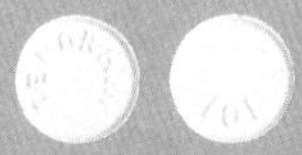

Tenormin 100 mg
Zeneca 101

℞

Fosamax 10 mg
Merck MRK 936

℞

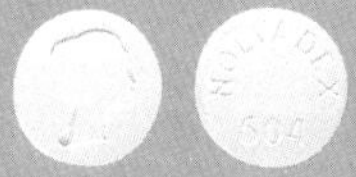

Nolvadex 20 mg
Zeneca 604

℞

Accolate
Zeneca 20

℞

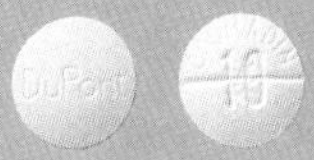

Coumadin 10 mg
DuPont 10

℞

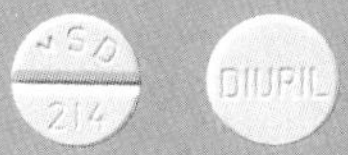

Diuril 250 mg
Merck MSD 214

℞

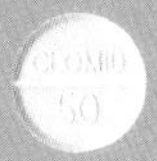

Clomid 50 mg
Hoechst Marion Roussel 50

℞

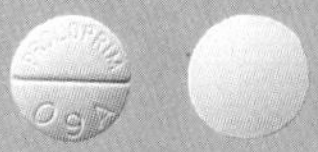

Proloprim 100 mg
Glaxo Wellcome O9A

CL-24 White Round Tablets

℞

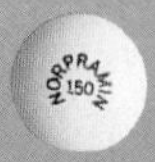

Norpramin 150 mg
Hoechst Marion Roussel 150

℞

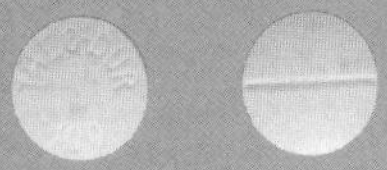

Theo-Dur 100 mg
Key 100

℞

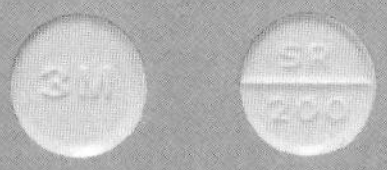

Theolair-SR 200 mg
3M Pharm SR 200

℞

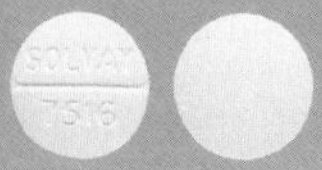

Lithotabs 300 mg
Solvay 7516

℞

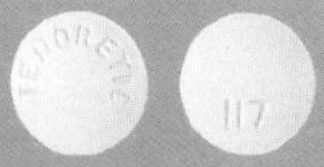

Tenoretic 100
Zeneca 117

℞

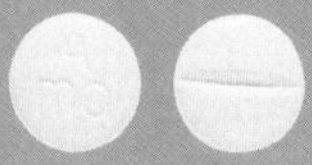

Toprol-XL 50 mg
Astra A MO

℞

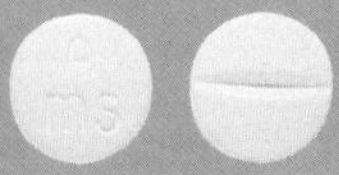

Toprol-XL 100 mg
Astra A MS

℞

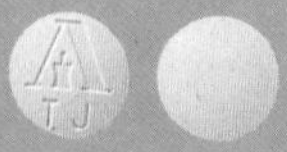

Armour Thyroid 1-1/2 gr
Forest Pharm A TJ

℞

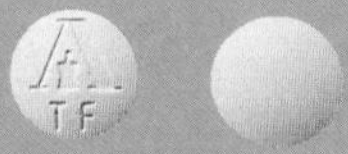

Armour Thyroid 2 gr
Forest Pharm A TF

℞

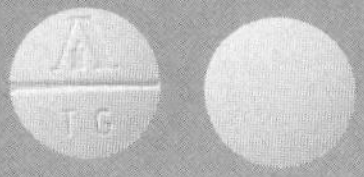

Armour Thyroid 3 gr
Forest Pharm A TG

℞

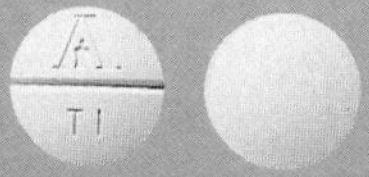

Armour Thyroid 5 gr
Forest Pharm A TI

℞

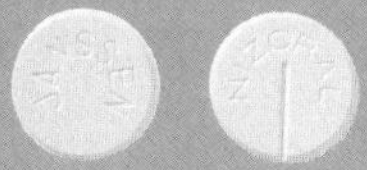

Nizoral 200 mg
Janssen

℞

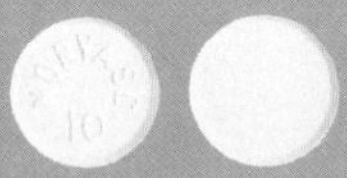

Norvasc 10 mg
Pfizer 10

℞

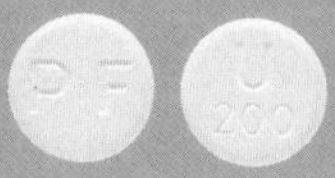

T-Phyl 200 mg
Purdue Frederick PF U200

℞

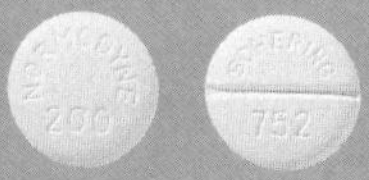

Normodyne 200 mg
Schering 200 752

℞

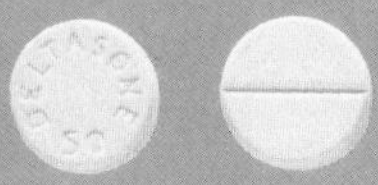

Deltasone 50 mg
Pharmacia & Upjohn 50

C-III

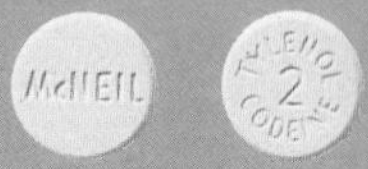

Tylenol w/Codeine No. 2
McNeil 2

C-III

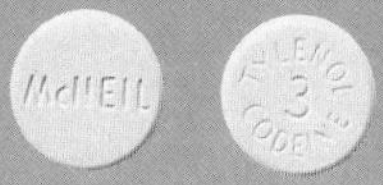

Tylenol w/Codeine No. 3
McNeil 3

C-III

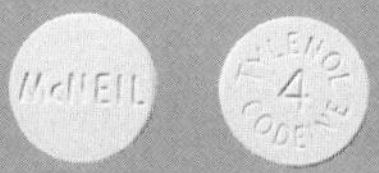

Tylenol w/Codeine No. 4
McNeil 4

℞

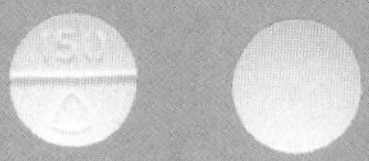

Rythmol 150 mg
Knoll 150

℞

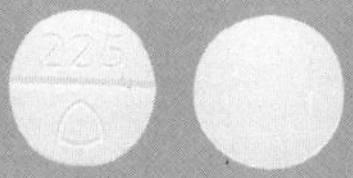

Rythmol 225 mg
Knoll 225

℞

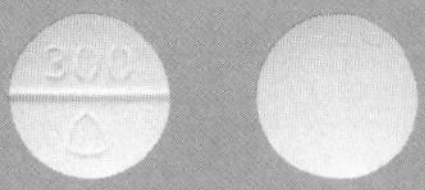

Rythmol 300 mg
Knoll 300

℞

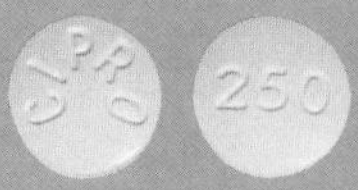

Cipro 250 mg
Bayer Corp 250

℞

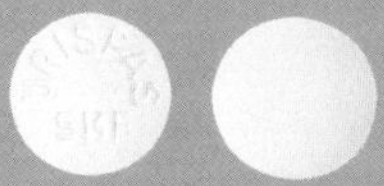

Urispas 100 mg
SmithKline Beecham SKF

℞
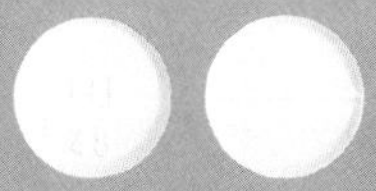

Respbid 250 mg
Boehringer Ingelheim BI 48

℞
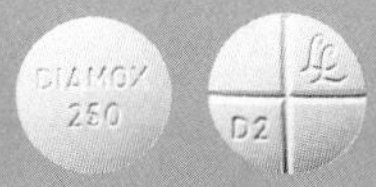

Diamox 250 mg
Lederle 250 D2 LL

℞
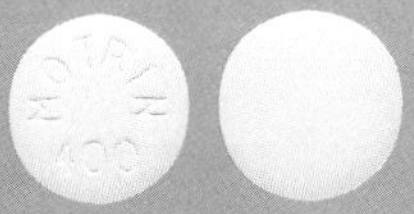

Motrin 400 mg
Pharmacia & Upjohn 400

℞
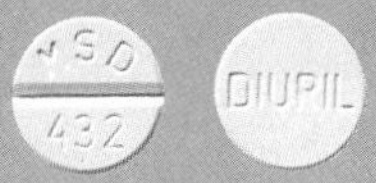

Diuril 500 mg
Merck MSD 432

℞
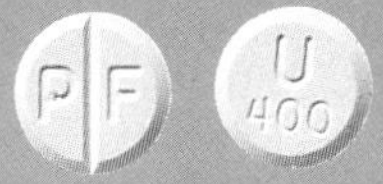

Uniphyl 400 mg
Purdue Frederick PF U400

℞
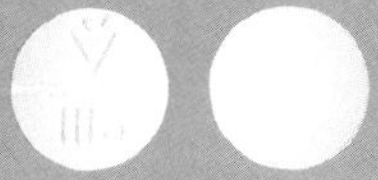

Dilor-400 400 mg
Savage 1116

℞
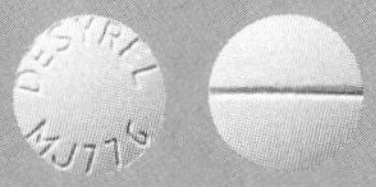

Desyrel 100 mg
Mead Johnson MJ 776

℞
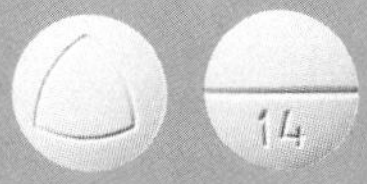

Quadrinal
Knoll 14

℞
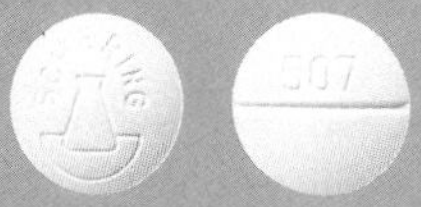

Fulvicin P/G 250 mg
Schering 507

C-III
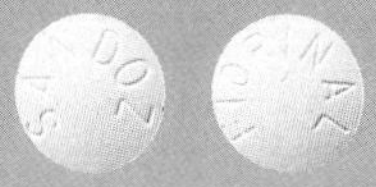

Fiorinal
Sandoz

℞
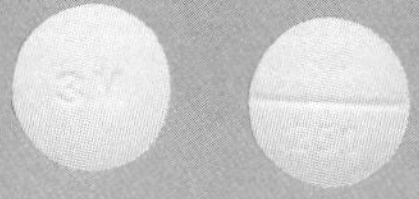

Theolair-SR 250 mg
3M Pharm SR 250

℞
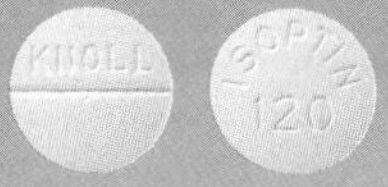

Isoptin 120 mg
Knoll 120

℞
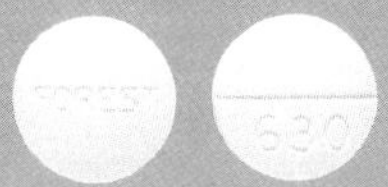

Esgic
Forest Pharm 630

℞
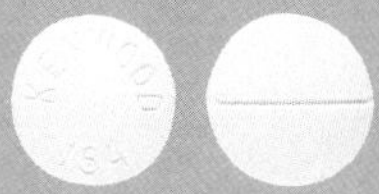

Deconamine
Kenwood/Bradley 184

℞
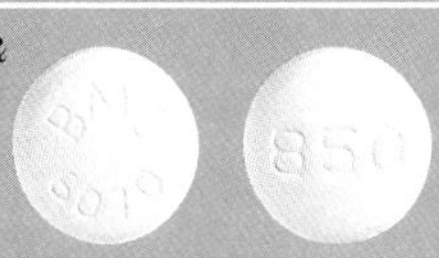

Glucophage 850 mg
B-M Squibb BMS 6070 850

℞
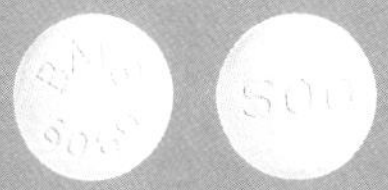

Glucophage 500 mg
B-M Squibb BMS 6060 500

℞
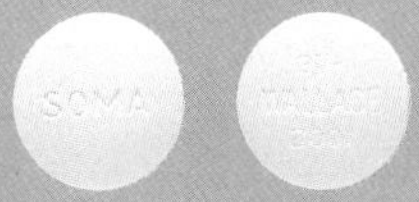

Soma 350 mg
Wallace 37-2001

℞
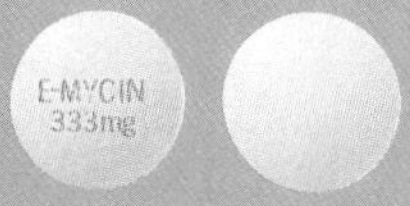

E-Mycin 333 mg
Knoll 333

℞
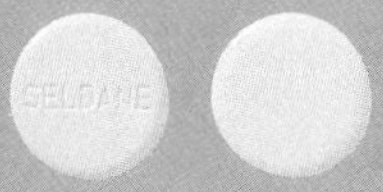

Seldane 60 mg
Hoechst Marion Roussel

℞
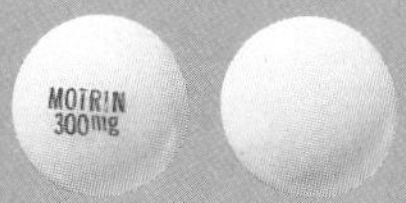

Motrin 300 mg
Pharmacia & Upjohn 300

C-II
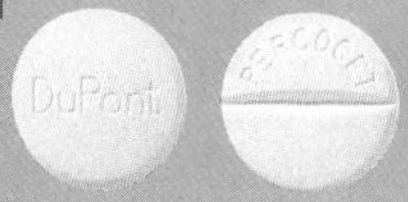

Percocet
DuPont

℞
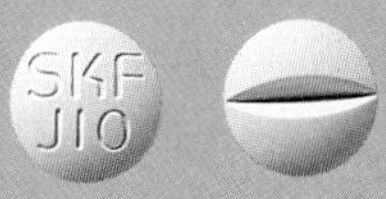

Eskalith CR 450 mg
SmithKline Beecham SKF J10

℞
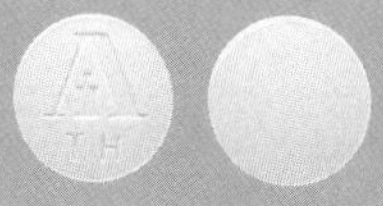

Armour Thyroid 4 gr
Forest Pharm A TH

℞
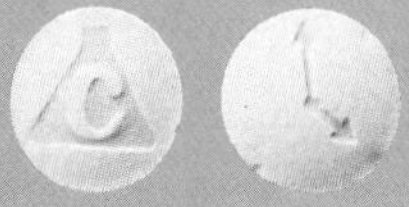

Quinaglute 324 mg SR
Berlex C

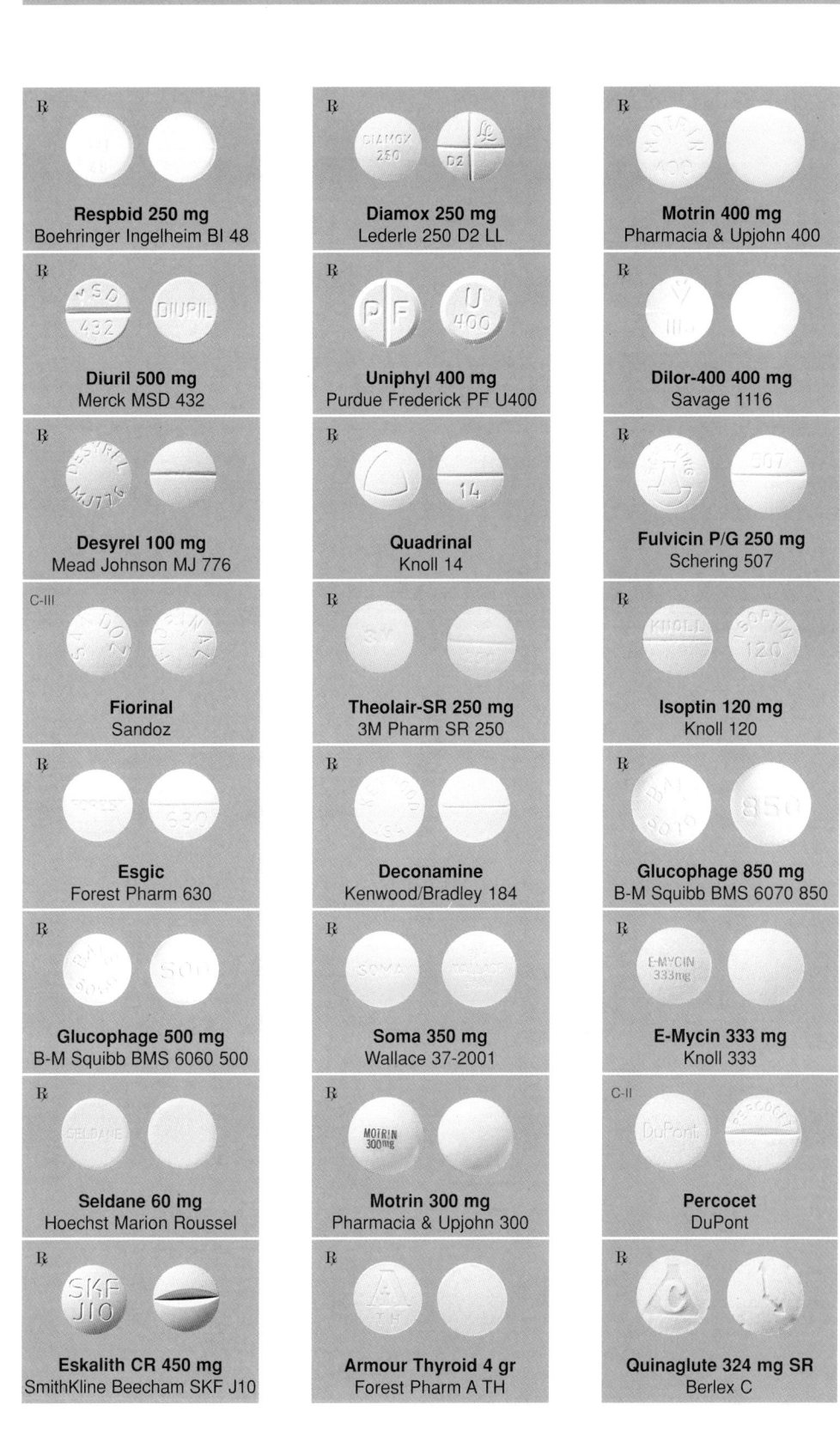

CL-26 White Round to Odd-Shaped Tablets

℞

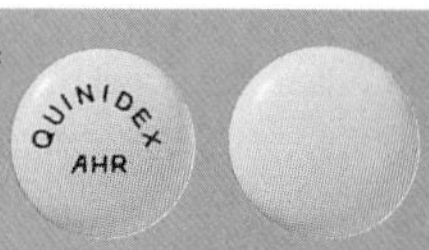

Quinidex Extentabs 300 mg
Robins AHR

℞

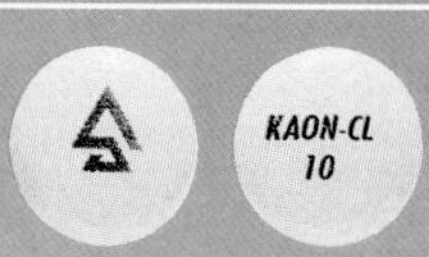

Kaon-CL 10 10 mEq
Savage 10

℞

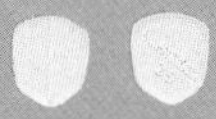

Lamictal 25 mg
Glaxo Wellcome 25

C-IV

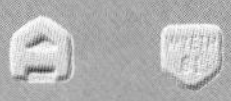

Ativan 0.5 mg
Wyeth-Ayerst A 81

C-IV

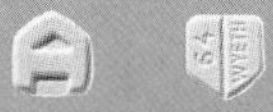

Ativan 1 mg
Wyeth-Ayerst A 64

C-IV

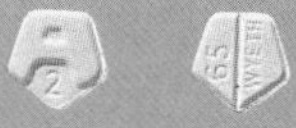

Ativan 2 mg
Wyeth-Ayerst A2 65

℞

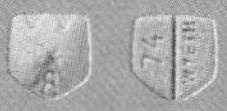

Wytensin 8 mg
Wyeth-Ayerst W8 74

℞

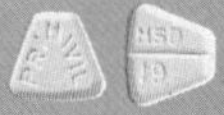

Prinivil 5 mg
Merck MSD 19

℞

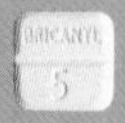

Bricanyl 5 mg
Hoechst Marion Roussel 5

℞

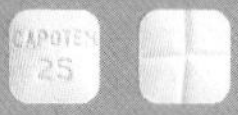

Capoten 25 mg
B-M Squibb 25

℞

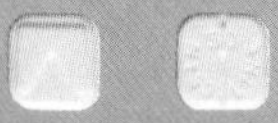

Mysoline 50 mg
Wyeth-Ayerst 50

℞

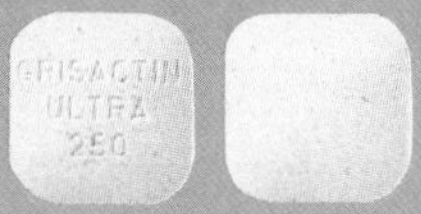

Grisactin Ultra 250 mg
Wyeth-Ayerst 250

℞

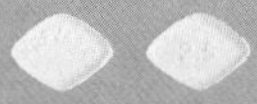

Norvasc 2.5 mg
Pfizer 2.5

℞

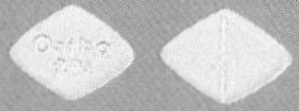

Ortho-Est 0.625 mg
Ortho 1801

℞

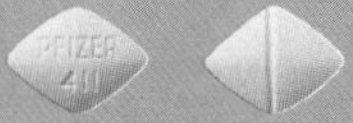

Glucotrol 5 mg
Pratt Pfizer 411

℞

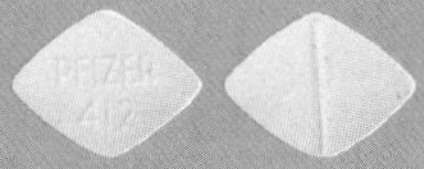

Glucotrol 10 mg
Pratt Pfizer 412

℞

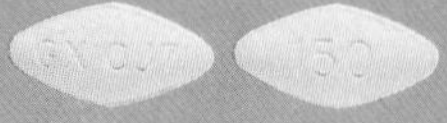

Epivir 150 mg
Glaxo Wellcome GX CJ7 150

℞

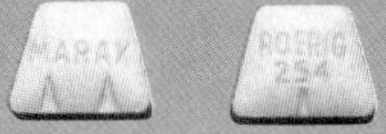

Marax
Roerig 254

℞

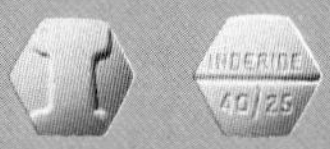

Inderide 40/25
Wyeth-Ayerst I 40/25

℞

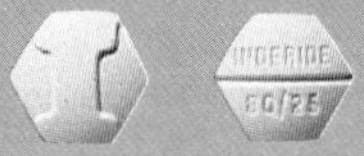

Inderide 80/25
Wyeth-Ayerst I 80/25

℞

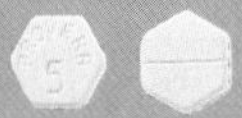

Provera 5 mg
Pharmacia & Upjohn 5

℞

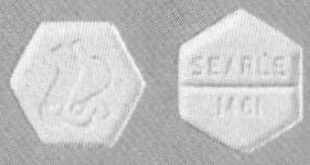

Cytotec 200 mcg
Searle 1461

℞

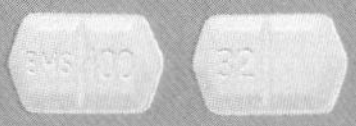

Serzone 100 mg
B-M Squibb BMS 100 32

℞

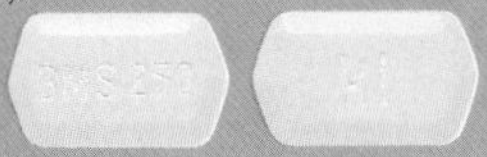

Serzone 250 mg
B-M Squibb BMS 250 41

℞
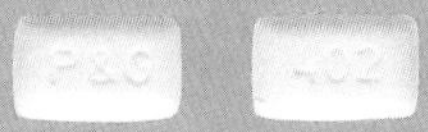
Didronel 200 mg
Procter & Gamble 402

℞
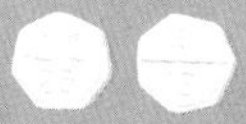
Asendin 25 mg
Lederle LL 25 A13

℞
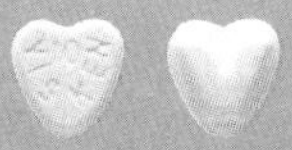
Visken 10 mg
Sandoz 10 V

℞
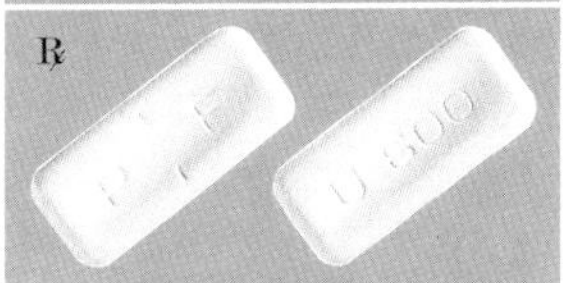
Uniphyl 600 mg
Purdue Frederick PF U 600

℞
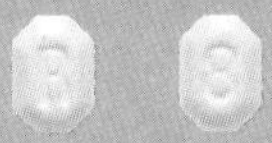
Lozol 2.5 mg
Rhone-Poulenc Rorer R 8

℞
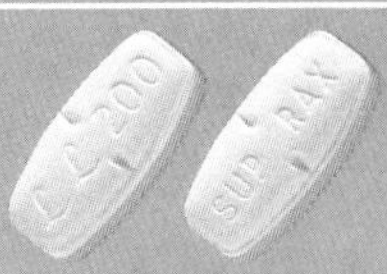
Suprax 200 mg
Lederle LL 200

℞
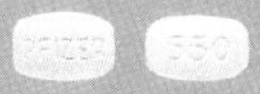
Zyrtec 5 mg
Pfizer 550

℞
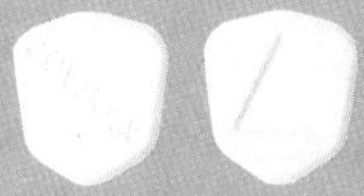
Zovirax 400 mg
Glaxo Wellcome

℞
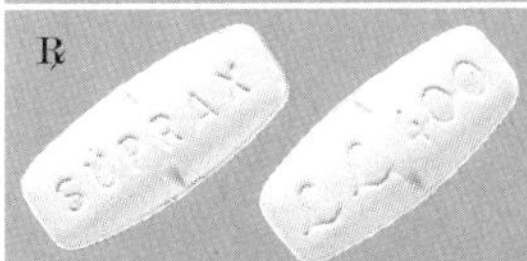
Suprax 400 mg
Lederle LL 400

℞
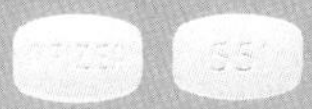
Zyrtec 10 mg
Pfizer 551

℞

Demi-Regroton
Rhone-Poulenc Rorer R32

℞

Lasix 20 mg
Hoechst Marion Roussel

℞
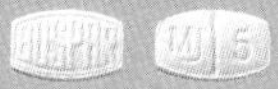
BuSpar 5 mg
B-M Squibb MJ 5

℞
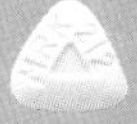
Fosamax 40 mg
Merck MRK 212

℞
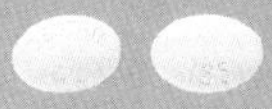
Zestril 2.5 mg
Zeneca 2 1/2 135

℞
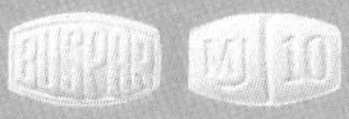
BuSpar 10 mg
B-M Squibb MJ 10

C-II

Dilaudid 8 mg
Knoll 8

℞
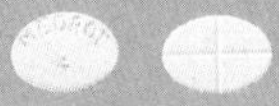
Medrol 4 mg
Pharmacia & Upjohn 4

℞
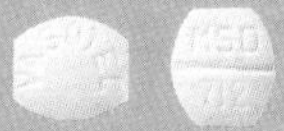
Vasotec 5 mg
Merck MSD 712

℞
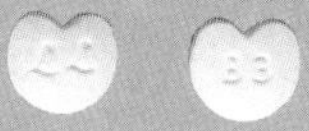
Zebeta 10 mg
Lederle LL B3

℞
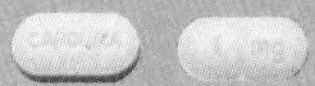
Cardura 1 mg
Roerig 1

℞
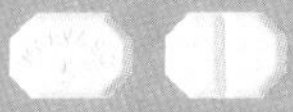
Norvasc 5 mg
Pfizer 5

℞
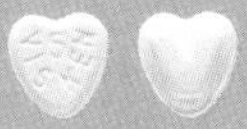
Visken 5 mg
Sandoz 5 V

℞
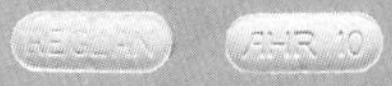
Reglan 10 mg
Robins AHR 10

White Oval Tablets

C-IV

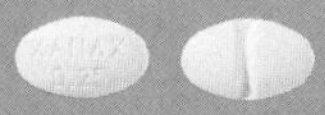

Xanax 0.25 mg
Pharmacia & Upjohn 0.25

℞

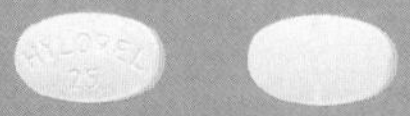

Hylorel 25 mg
Medeva 25

℞

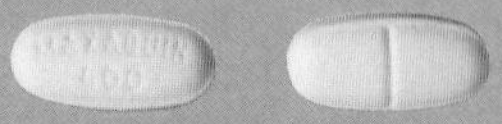

Maxaquin 400 mg
Searle 400

℞

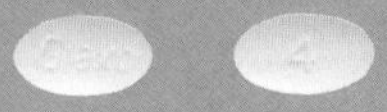

Zofran 4 mg
Glaxo Wellcome 4

℞

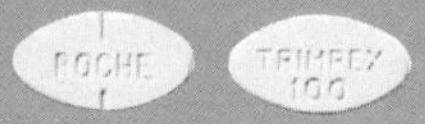

Trimpex 100 mg
Roche 100

℞

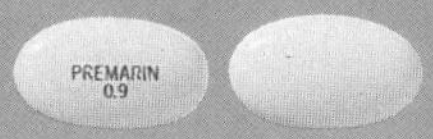

Premarin 0.9 mg
Wyeth-Ayerst 0.9

℞

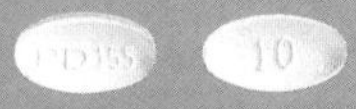

Lipitor 10 mg
Parke-Davis PD155 10

℞

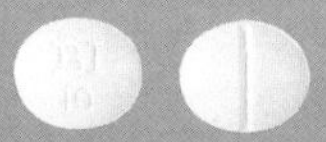

Combipres 0.3 mg
Boehringer Ingelheim BI 10

℞

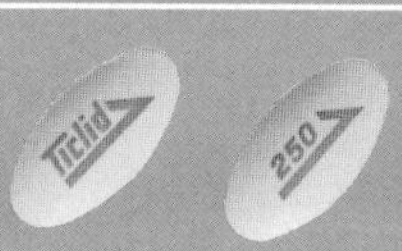

Ticlid 250 mg
Roche 250

℞

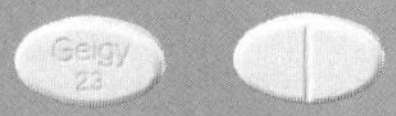

Lioresal 10 mg
Ciba Geigy 23

℞

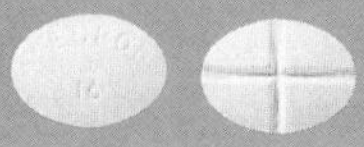

Medrol 16 mg
Pharmacia & Upjohn 16

℞

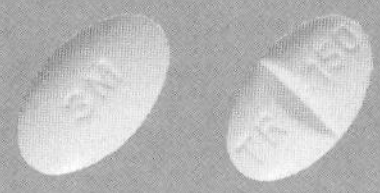

Tambocor 150 mg
3M Pharm TR 150

℞

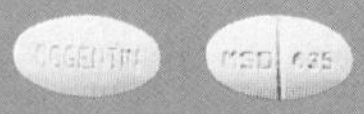

Cogentin 1 mg
Merck MSD 635

℞

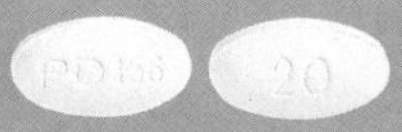

Lipitor 20 mg
Parke-Davis PD156 20

℞

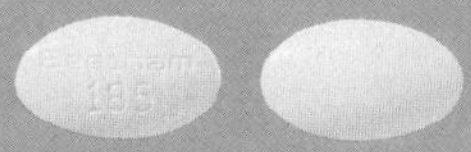

Beepen-VK 250 mg
SmithKline Beecham 185

℞

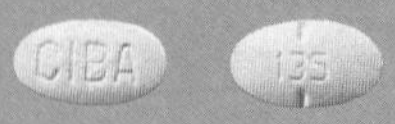

Ludiomil 75 mg
Ciba 135

℞

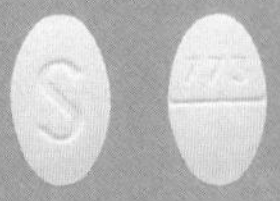

Sorbitrate 30 mg
Zeneca S 773

℞

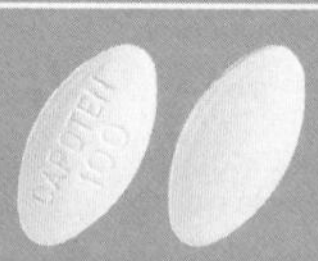

Capoten 100 mg
B-M Squibb 100

℞

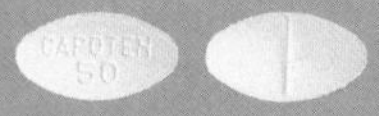

Capoten 50 mg
B-M Squibb 50

℞

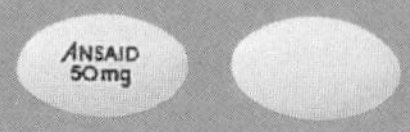

Ansaid 50 mg
Pharmacia & Upjohn 50

℞

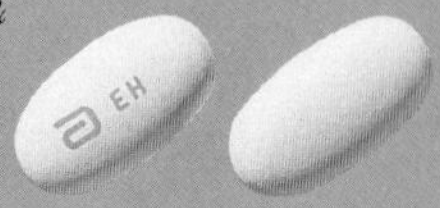

Ery-Tab 333 mg
Abbott EH

℞

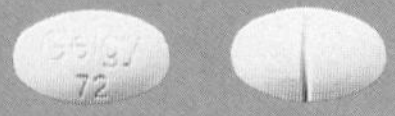

Brethine 2.5 mg
Ciba Geigy 72

℞

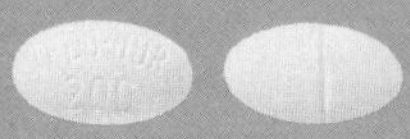

Theo-Dur 200 mg
Key 200

℞

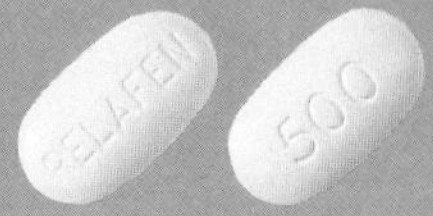

Relafen 500 mg
SmithKline Beecham 500

C-III
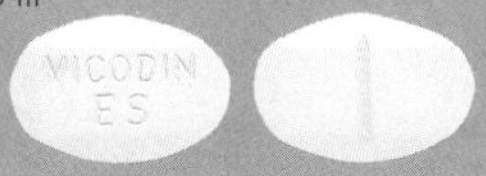
Vicodin ES
Knoll

℞
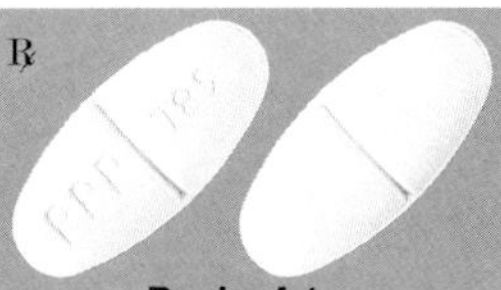
Duricef 1 g
B-M Squibb PPP 785

℞
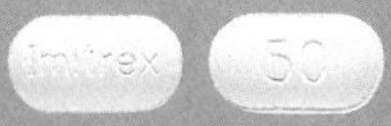
Imitrex 50 mg
Glaxo Wellcome 50

℞
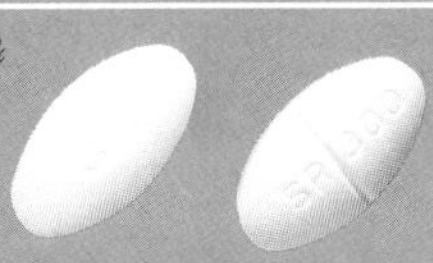
Theolair-SR 300 mg
3M Pharm SR 300

℞
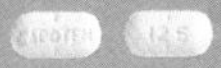
Capoten 12.5 mg
B-M Squibb 12.5

℞
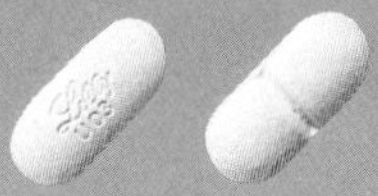
Dymelor 250 mg
Lilly U03

℞
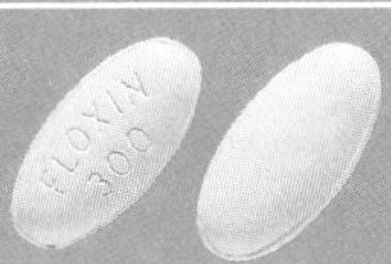
Floxin 300 mg
McNeil 300

C-II
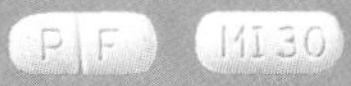
MSIR 30 mg
Purdue Frederick PF MI 30

℞
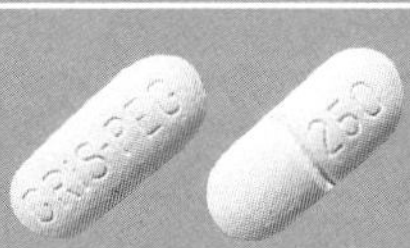
Gris-PEG 250 mg
Allergan Herbert 250

℞
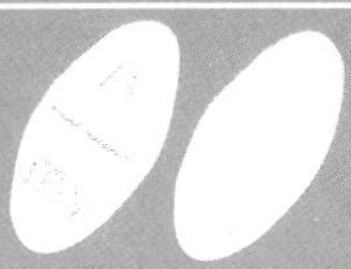
Toprol-XL 200 mg
Astra A MY

C-IV
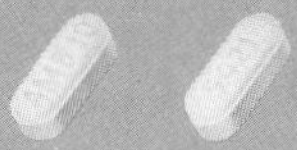
Ambien 10 mg
Searle AMB 10 5421

℞
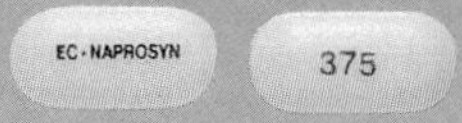
EC-Naprosyn 375 mg
Roche 375

℞
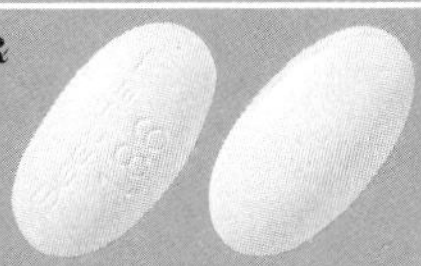
Beepen-VK 500 mg
SmithKline Beecham 186

℞
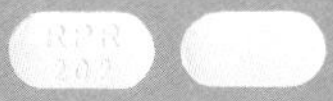
Rilutek 50 mg
Rhone-Poulenc Rorer RPR 202

℞
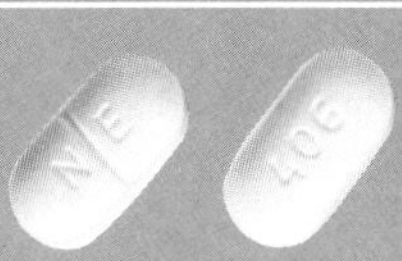
Didronel 400 mg
Procter & Gamble NE 406

℞
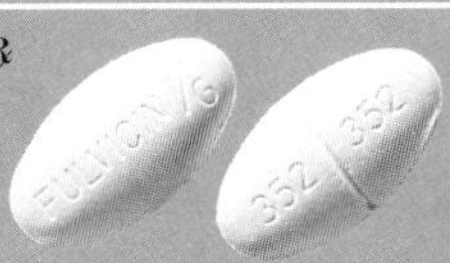
Fulvicin P/G 330 mg
Schering 352

℞
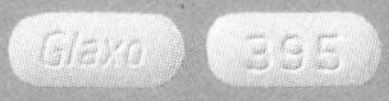
Ceftin 125 mg
Glaxo Wellcome 395

℞
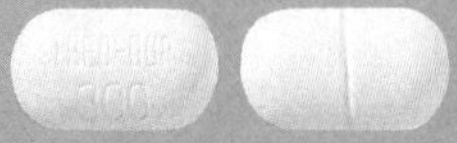
Theo-Dur 300 mg
Key 300

℞
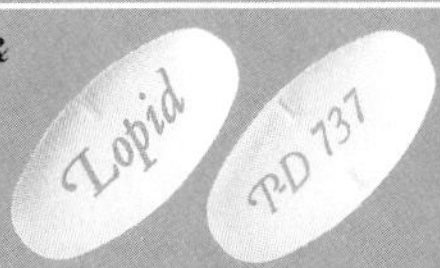
Lopid 600 mg
Parke-Davis P-D 737

℞
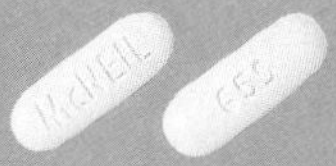
Ultram 50 mg
McNeil 659

℞
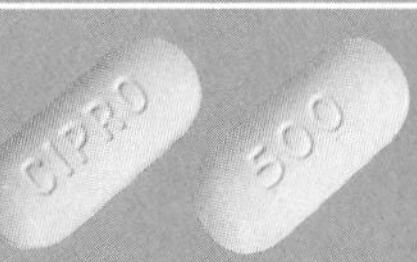
Cipro 500 mg
Bayer Corp 500

℞
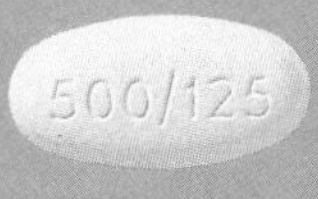
Augmentin '500'
SmithKline Beecham 500/125

℞

Risperdal 1 mg
Janssen R 1

℞
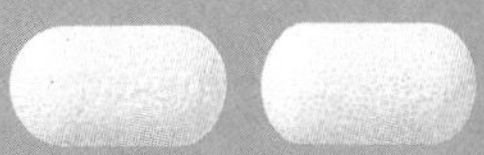
K-Dur 10 10 mEq
Key 10

C-III

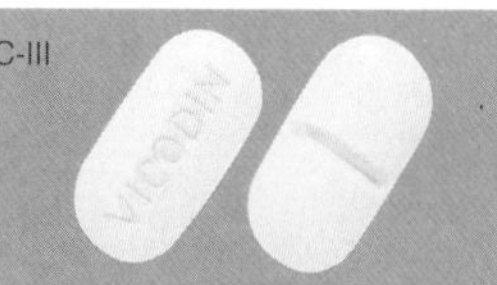

Vicodin
Knoll

℞

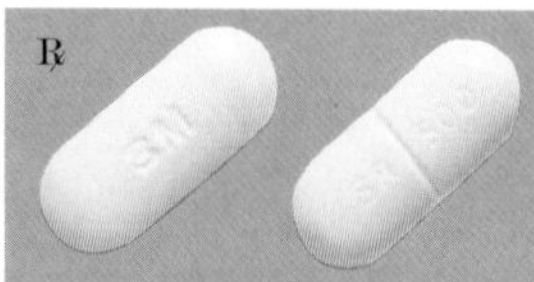

Theolair-SR 500 mg
3M Pharm SR 500

℞

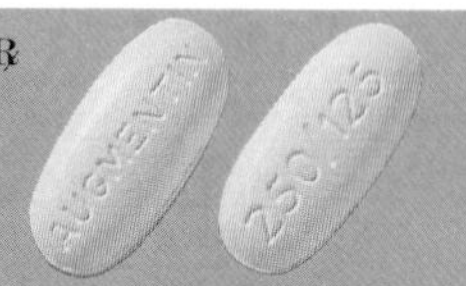

Augmentin '250'
SmithKline Beecham 250/125

℞

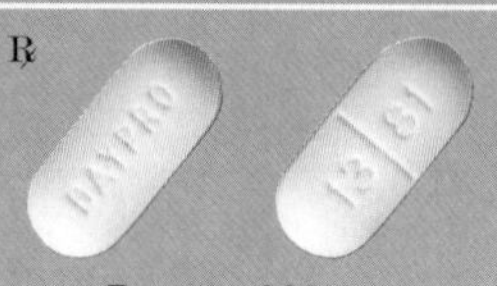

Daypro 600 mg
Searle 1381

℞

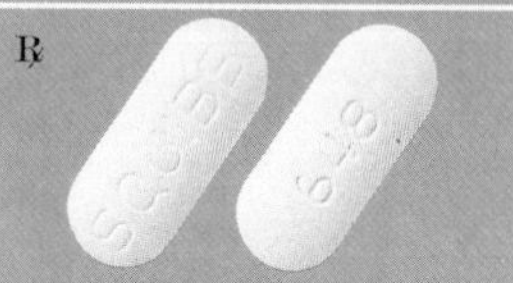

Veetids 500 mg
Apothecon Squibb 648

℞

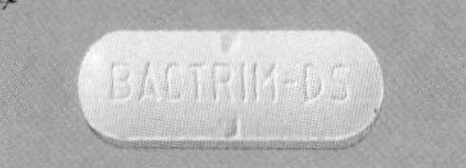

Bactrim DS
Roche 01

C-III

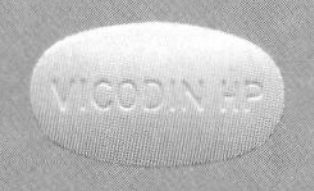

Vicodin HP
Knoll

℞

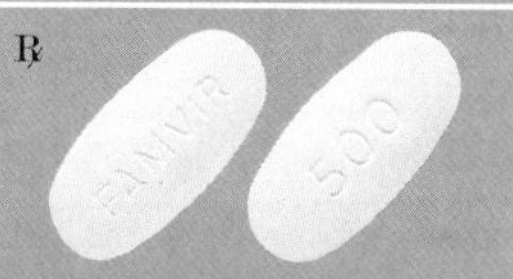

Famvir 500 mg
SmithKline Beecham 500

℞

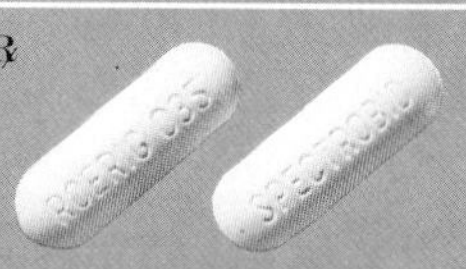

Spectrobid 400 mg
Roerig 035

℞

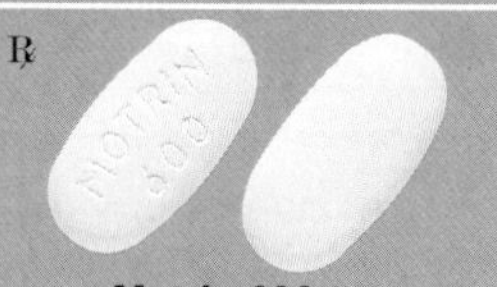

Motrin 600 mg
Pharmacia & Upjohn 600

℞

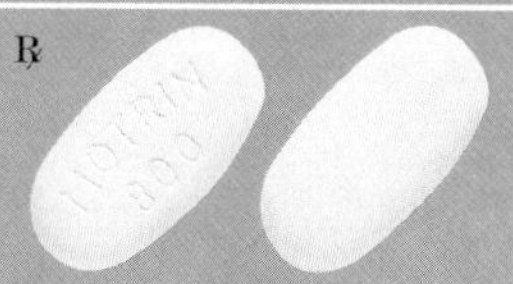

Motrin 800 mg
Pharmacia & Upjohn 800

℞

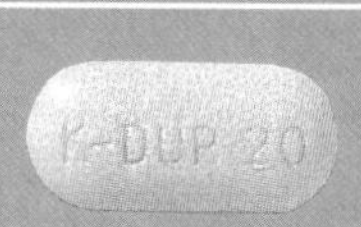

K-Dur 20 20 mEq
Key 20

℞

Seldane-D
Hoechst Marion Roussel

C-III

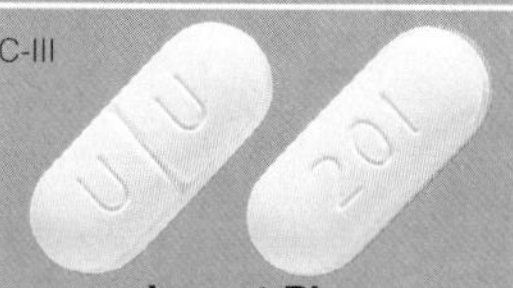

Lorcet Plus
UAD UU 201

℞

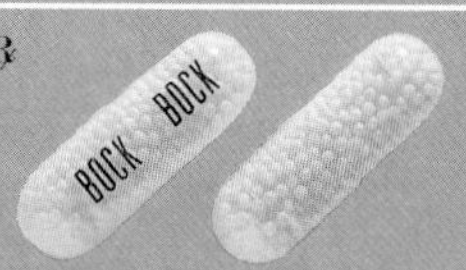

Poly-Histine-D Ped Caps
Sanofi Winthrop Bock

℞

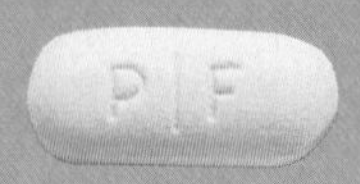

Trilisate 750 mg
Purdue Frederick PF T750

℞

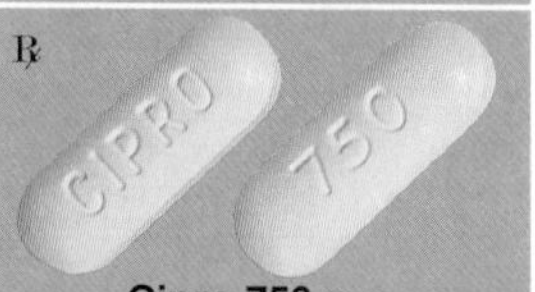

Cipro 750 mg
Bayer Corp 750

C-IV

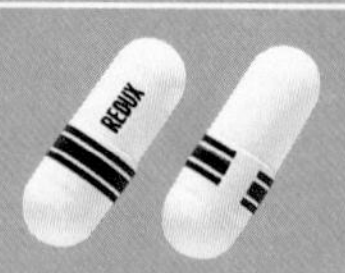

Redux 15 mg
Wyeth-Ayerst

℞

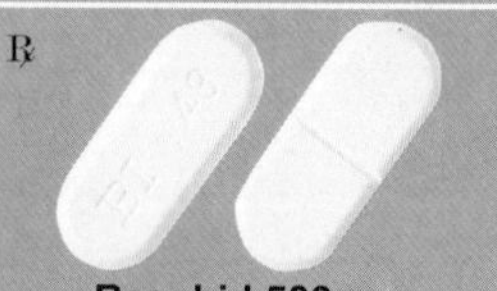

Respbid 500 mg
Boehringer Ingelheim BI 49

℞

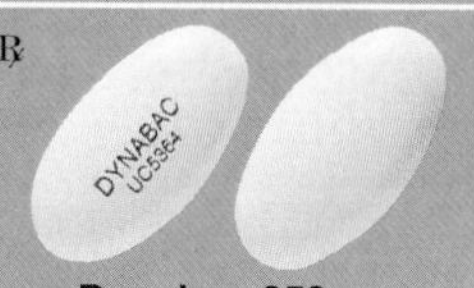

Dynabac 250 mg
Sanofi Winthrop UC5364

℞

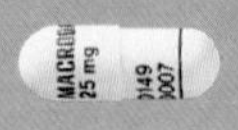

Macrodantin 25 mg
Procter & Gamble 0149 0007

℞

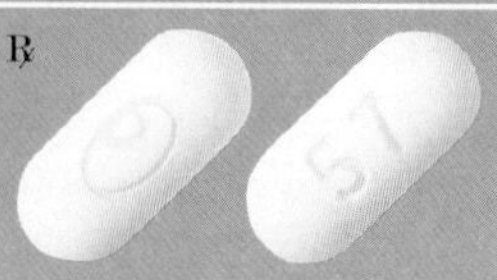

ZORprin 800 mg
Knoll 57

℞

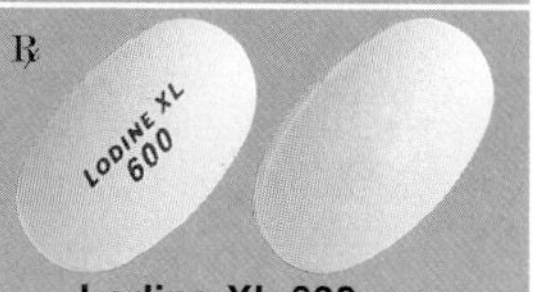

Lodine XL 600 mg
Wyeth-Ayerst 600

℞

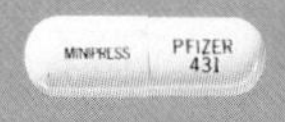

Minipress 1 mg
Pfizer 431

℞
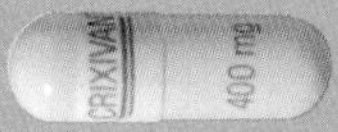

Crixivan 400 mg
Merck

℞
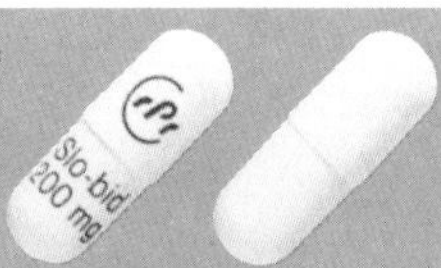

Slo-Bid 200 mg
Rhone-Poulenc Rorer 200

℞
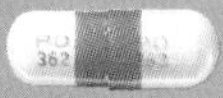
Dilantin Kapseals 100 mg
Parke-Davis P-D 362

℞
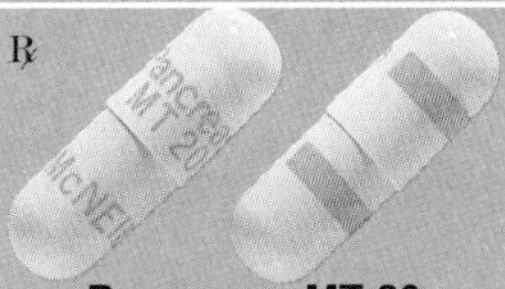
Pancrease MT 20
McNeil MT 20

℞
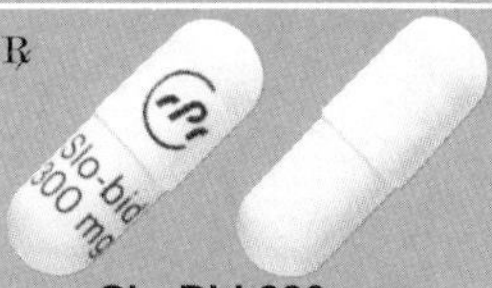
Slo-Bid 300 mg
Rhone-Poulenc Rorer 300

℞
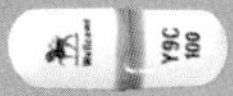

Retrovir 100 mg
Glaxo Wellcome Y9C 100

℞
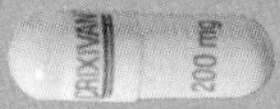

Crixivan 200 mg
Merck

℞
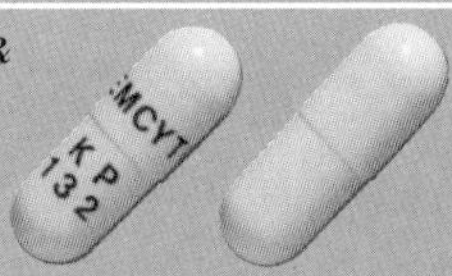
Emcyt
Pharmacia & Upjohn KP 132

℞

Dilantin Kapseals 30 mg
Parke-Davis P-D 365

℞
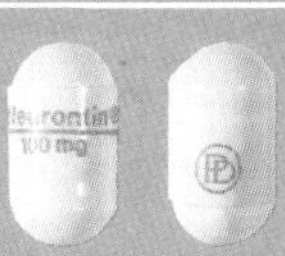
Neurontin 100 mg
Parke-Davis 100

℞
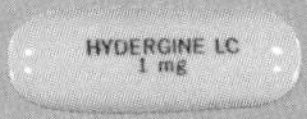

Hydergine LC 1 mg
Sandoz LC 1

℞
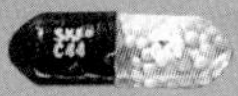
Compazine Spansule 10 mg
SmithKline Beecham SKF C44

℞
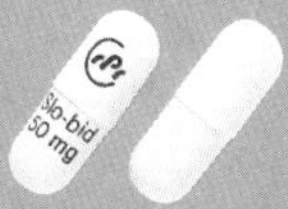

Slo-Bid 50 mg
Rhone-Poulenc Rorer 50

℞
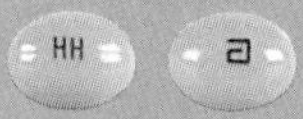

Hytrin 1 mg
Abbott HH

℞
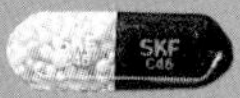

Compazine Spansule 15 mg
SmithKline Beecham SKF C46

℞
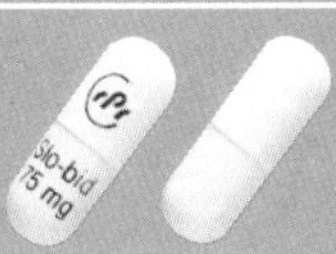

Slo-Bid 75 mg
Rhone-Poulenc Rorer 75

℞
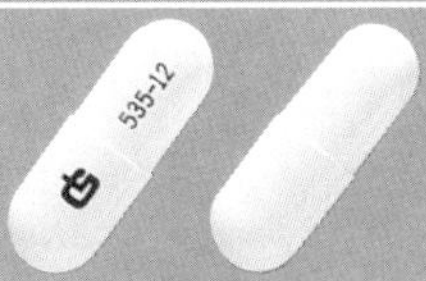

Esgic
Forest Pharm 535-12

℞
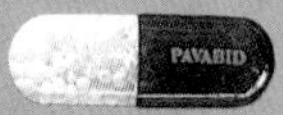

Pavabid 150 mg
Hoechst Marion Roussel 1555

℞
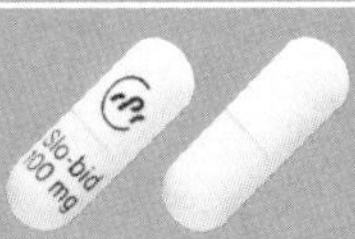

Slo-Bid 100 mg
Rhone-Poulenc Rorer 100

℞
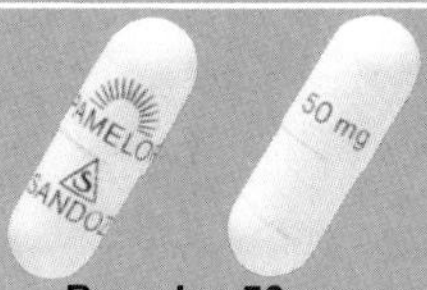

Pamelor 50 mg
Sandoz 50

C-II
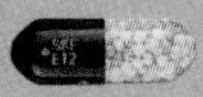
Dexedrine 5 mg
SmithKline Beecham SKF E12

℞
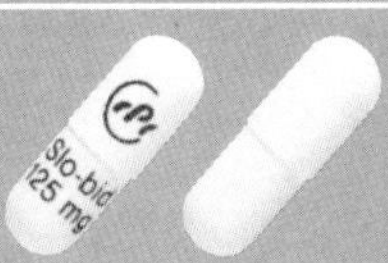

Slo-Bid 125 mg
Rhone-Poulenc Rorer 125

℞
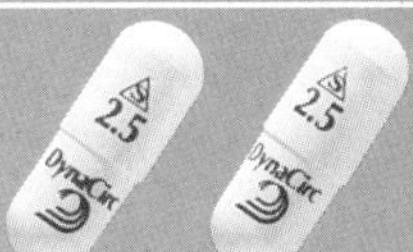

DynaCirc 2.5 mg
Sandoz 2.5

C-II
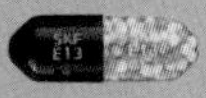
Dexedrine 10 mg
SmithKline Beecham SKF E13

Brown to Yellow Capsules

C-II

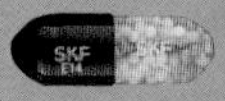

Dexedrine 15 mg
SmithKline Beecham SKF E14

℞

Axid 300 mg
Lilly 3145 300

℞

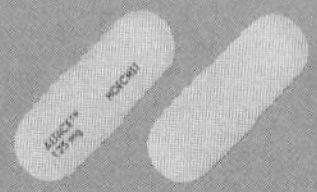

Altace 1.25 mg
Hoechst Marion Roussel 1.25

℞

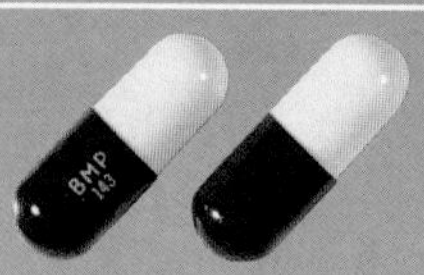

Bactocill 250 mg
SmithKline Beecham BMP 143

℞

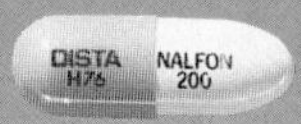

Nalfon 200 mg
Dista H76 200

℞

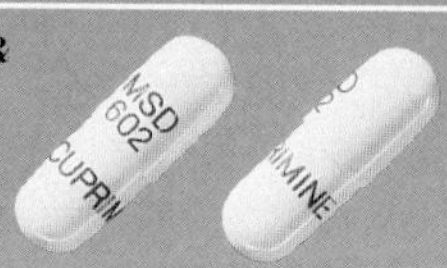

Cuprimine 250 mg
Merck MSD 602

℞

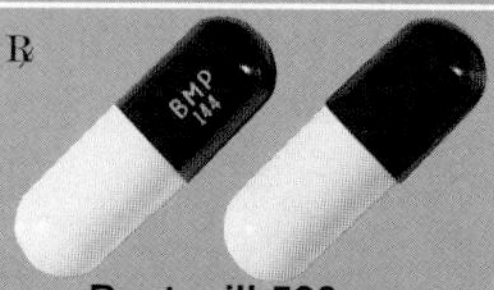

Bactocill 500 mg
SmithKline Beecham BMP 144

℞

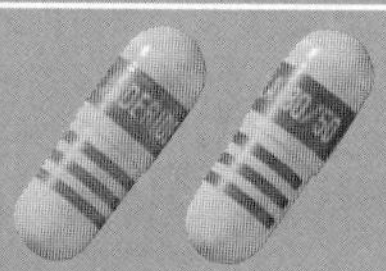

Inderide LA 80/50
Wyeth-Ayerst 80/50

℞

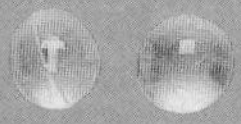

Tessalon Perles 100 mg
Forest Pharm T

℞

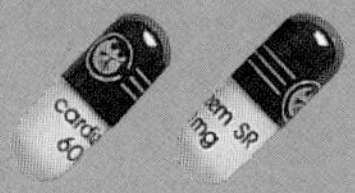

Cardizem SR 60 mg
Hoechst Marion Roussel 60

℞

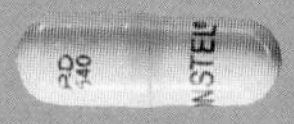

Ponstel 250 mg
Parke-Davis P-D 540

℞

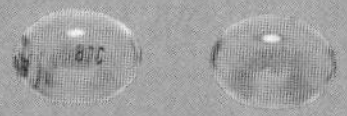

Lanoxicaps 0.1 mg
Glaxo Wellcome B2C

℞

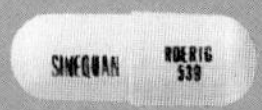

Sinequan 75 mg
Roerig 539

℞

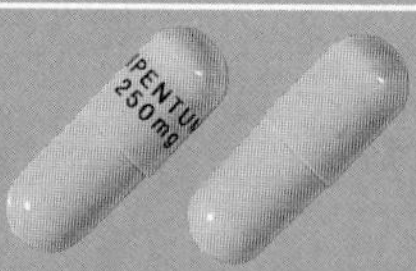

Dipentum 250 mg
Pharmacia & Upjohn 250

℞

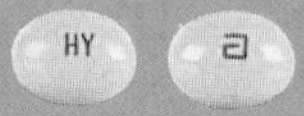

Hytrin 2 mg
Abbott HY

℞

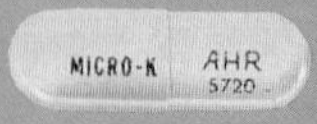

Micro-K Extencaps 8 mEq
Robins AHR 5720

℞

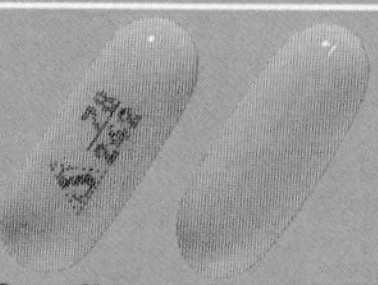

Sandimmune 50 mg
Sandoz 78 242

℞

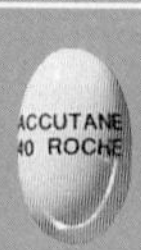

Accutane 40 mg
Roche 40

℞

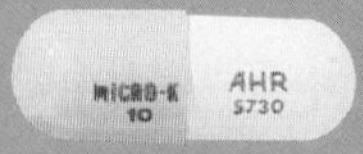

Micro-K 10 Extencaps 10 mEq
Robins 10 AHR 5730

℞

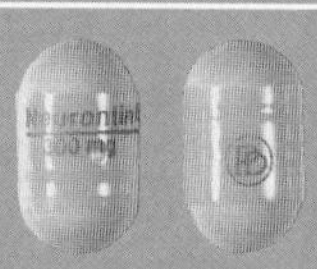

Neurontin 300 mg
Parke-Davis 300

C-II

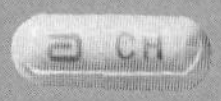

Nembutal Sodium 100 mg
Abbott CH

℞

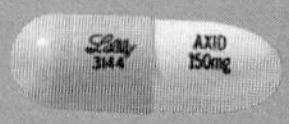

Axid 150 mg
Lilly 3144 150

℞

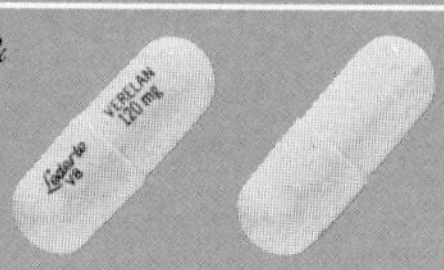

Verelan 120 mg
Lederle V8 120

℞

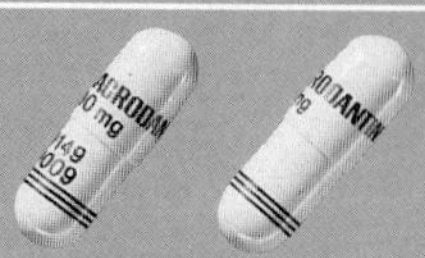

Macrodantin 100 mg
Procter & Gamble 0149 0009

℞

Terramycin 250 mg
Pfizer 073

℞

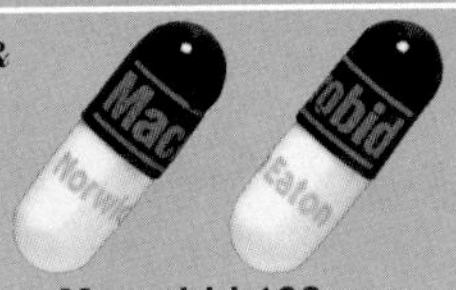

Macrobid 100 mg
Procter & Gamble

℞

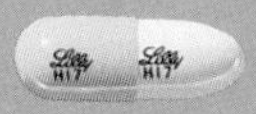

Aventyl HCl 10 mg
Lilly H17

℞

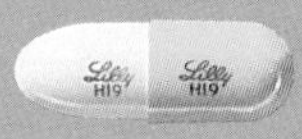

Aventyl HCl 25 mg
Lilly H19

℞

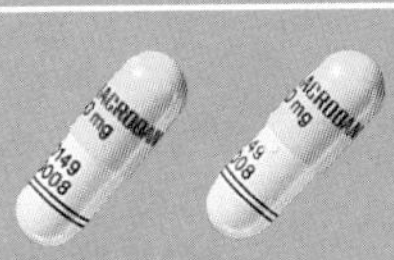

Macrodantin 50 mg
Procter & Gamble 0149 0008

℞

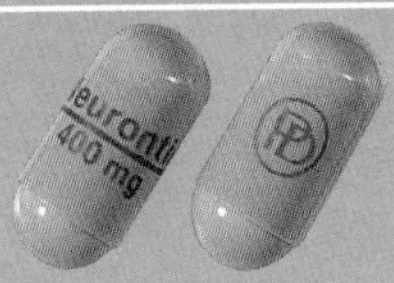

Neurontin 400 mg
Parke-Davis 400

℞

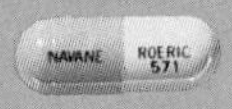

Navane 1 mg
Roerig 571

℞

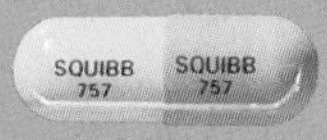

Pronestyl 500 mg
Princeton Squibb 757

C-IV

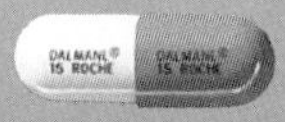

Dalmane 15 mg
Roche 15

℞

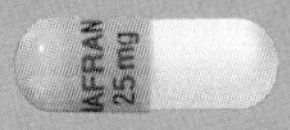

Anafranil 25 mg
Ciba 25

℞

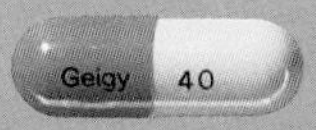

Tofranil-PM 100 mg
Ciba Geigy 40

℞

Nalfon 300 mg
Dista H77

℞

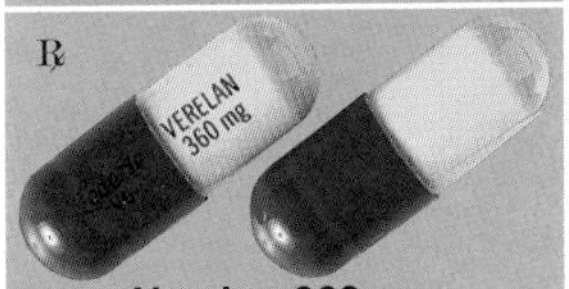

Verelan 360 mg
Lederle V6

℞

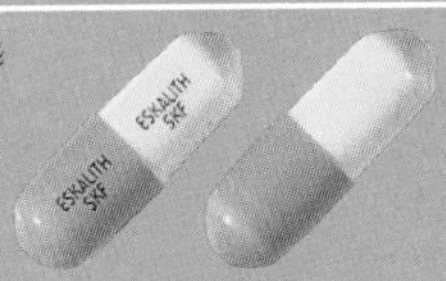

Eskalith 300 mg
SmithKline Beecham SKF

℞

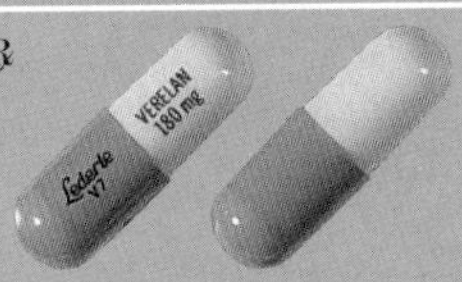

Verelan 180 mg
Lederle V7 180

℞

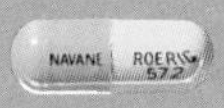

Navane 2 mg
Roerig 572

℞

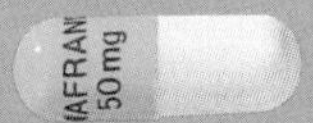

Anafranil 50 mg
Ciba 50

℞

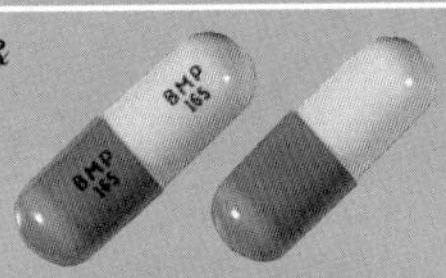

Dycill 250 mg
SmithKline Beecham BMP 165

℞

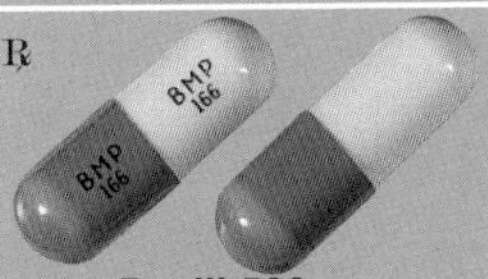

Dycill 500 mg
SmithKline Beecham BMP 166

℞

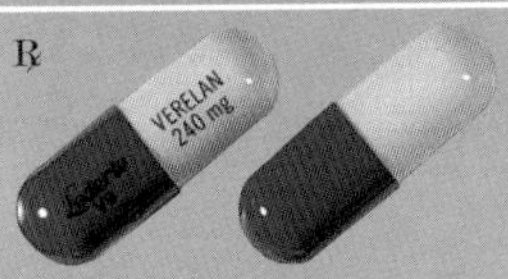

Verelan 240 mg
Lederle V9 240

C-III

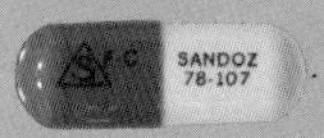

Fiorinal w/Codeine
Sandoz F-C 78-107

℞

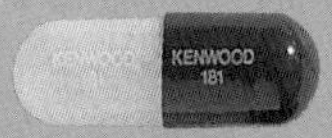

Deconamine SR
Kenwood/Bradley 181

℞

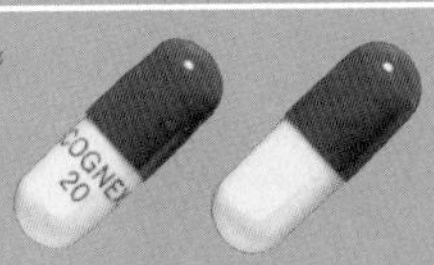

Cognex 20 mg
Parke-Davis 20

℞

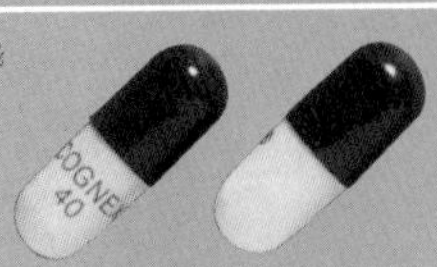

Cognex 40 mg
Parke-Davis 40

Yellow to Green Capsules

℞

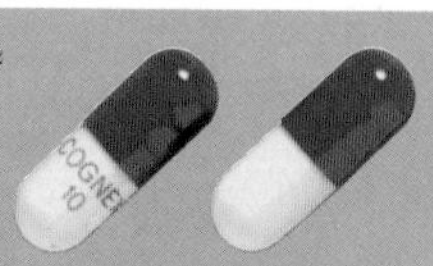

Cognex 10 mg
Parke-Davis 10

℞

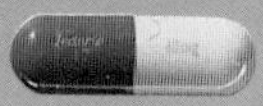

Loxitane 10 mg
Lederle L2 10

℞

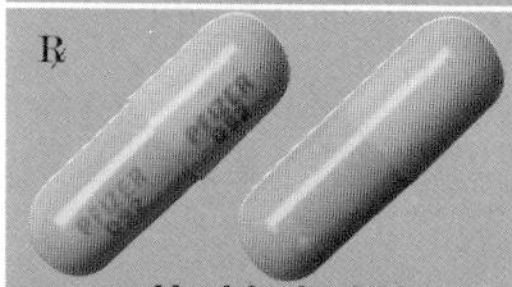

Urobiotic-250
Roerig 092

℞

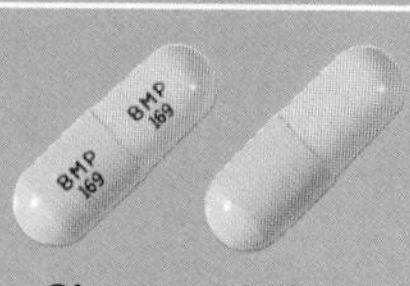

Cloxapen 250 mg
SmithKline Beecham BMP 169

℞

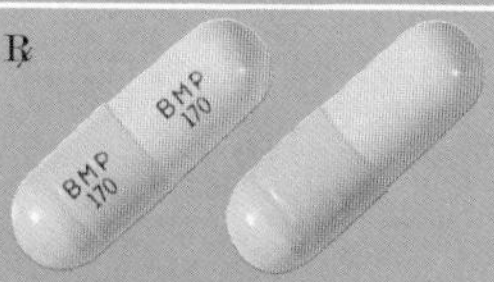

Cloxapen 500 mg
SmithKline Beecham BMP 170

℞

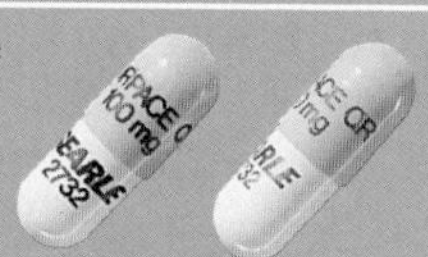

Norpace CR 100 mg
Searle 2732 100

℞

Prozac 10 mg
Dista 3104 10

℞

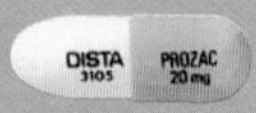

Prozac 20 mg
Dista 3105 20

C-IV

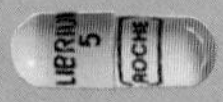

Librium 5 mg
Roche 5

C-IV

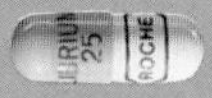

Librium 25 mg
Roche 25

℞

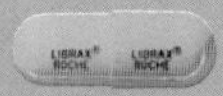

Librax
Roche

℞

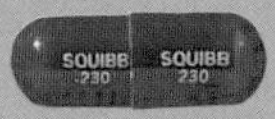

Trimox 250 mg
Apothecon Squibb 230

℞

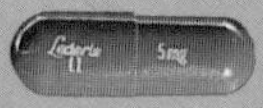

Loxitane 5 mg
Lederle L1 5

℞

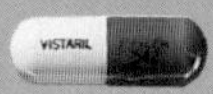

Vistaril 50 mg
Pfizer 542

℞

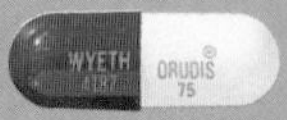

Orudis 75 mg
Wyeth-Ayerst 4187 75

℞

Keflex 250 mg
Dista H69 250

℞

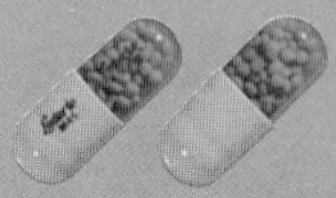

Minocin 50 mg
Lederle M45

℞

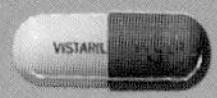

Vistaril 25 mg
Pfizer 541

℞

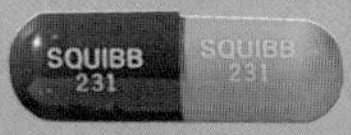

Trimox 500 mg
Apothecon Squibb 231

C-III

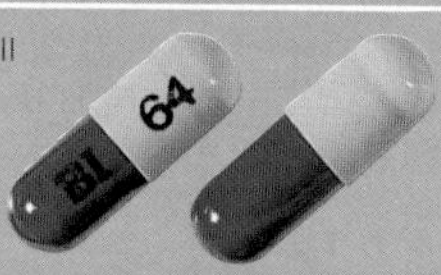

Prelu-2 105 mg
Boehringer Ingelheim BI 64

℞

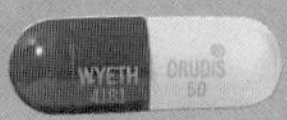

Orudis 50 mg
Wyeth-Ayerst 4181 50

℞

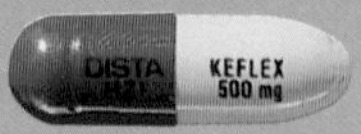

Keflex 500 mg
Dista H71 500

C-III

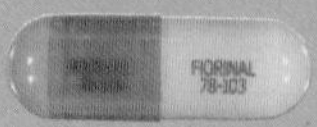

Fiorinal
Sandoz 78-103

℞

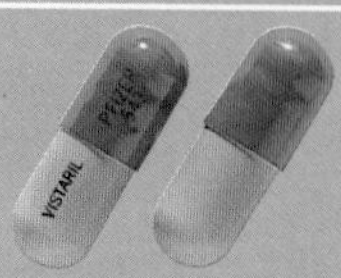

Vistaril 100 mg
Pfizer 543

℞
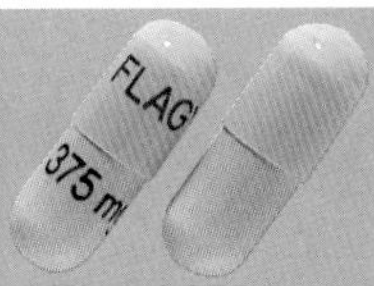
Flagyl 375 mg
Searle 375

℞
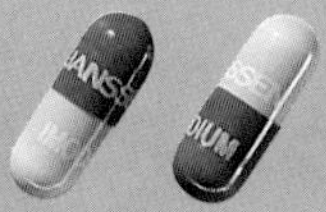
Imodium 2 mg
Janssen

℞
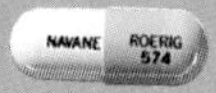

Navane 10 mg
Roerig 574

℞
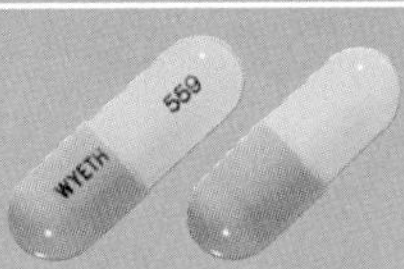

Wymox 250 mg
Wyeth-Ayerst 559

℞
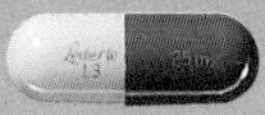
Loxitane 25 mg
Lederle L3 25

℞
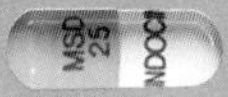
Indocin 25 mg
Merck MSD 25

℞
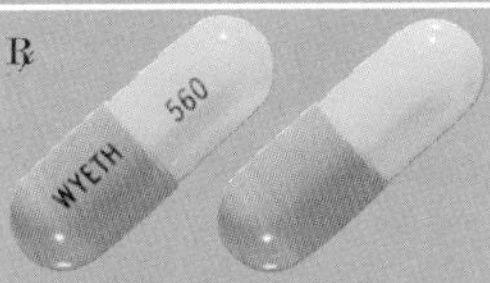

Wymox 500 mg
Wyeth-Ayerst 560

℞
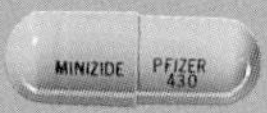

Minizide 1
Pfizer 430

℞
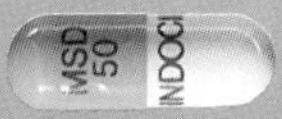

Indocin 50 mg
Merck MSD 50

℞
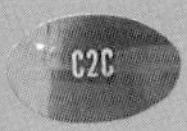

Lanoxicaps 0.2 mg
Glaxo Wellcome C2C

℞
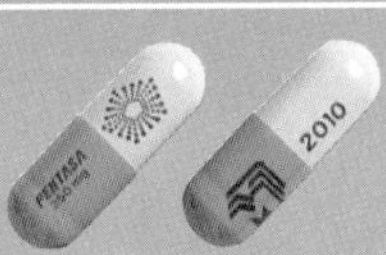

Pentasa 250 mg
Hoechst Marion Roussel 2010

℞
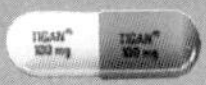
Tigan 100 mg
SmithKline Beecham 100

C-IV
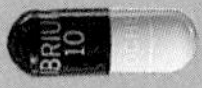
Librium 10 mg
Roche 10

℞
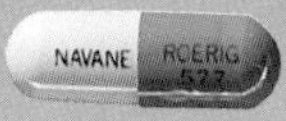

Navane 20 mg
Roerig 577

℞

Dynapen 250 mg
Apothecon Bristol 7893

℞
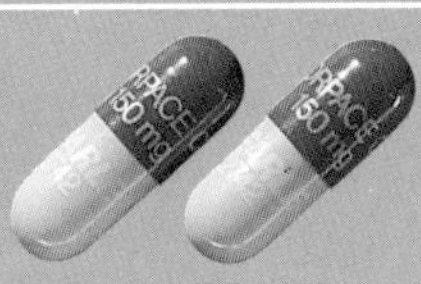
Norpace CR 150 mg
Searle 2742 150

℞
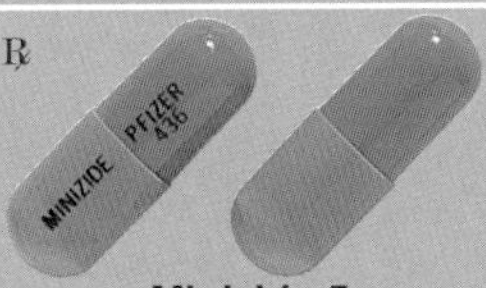

Minizide 5
Pfizer 436

℞

Dynapen 500 mg
Apothecon Bristol 7658

℞
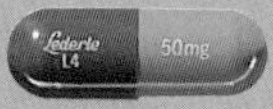

Loxitane 50 mg
Lederle L4 50

℞
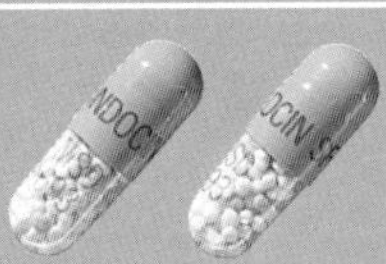
Indocin SR 75 mg
Merck MSD 693

℞

Minipress 5 mg
Pfizer 438

℞
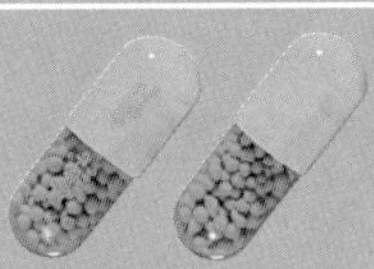
Minocin 100 mg
Lederle M46

C-IV
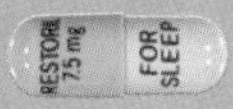

Restoril 7.5 mg
Sandoz 7.5

℞
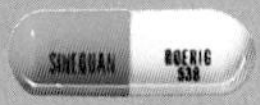

Sinequan 100 mg
Roerig 538

Blue Capsules

C-II
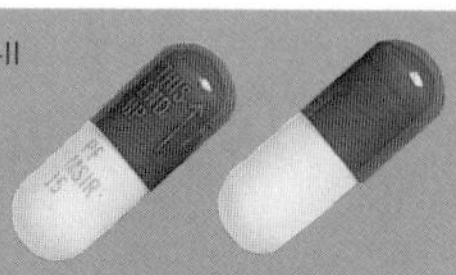
MSIR 15 mg
Purdue Frederick PF 15

℞
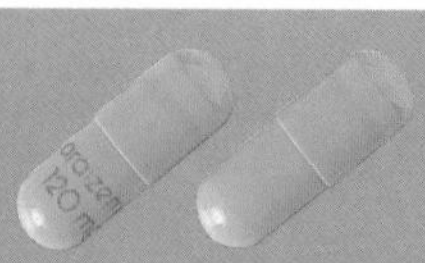
Cardizem CD 120 mg
Hoechst Marion Roussel

C-III
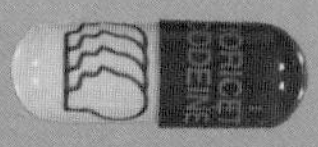
Fioricet w/Codeine
Sandoz

℞
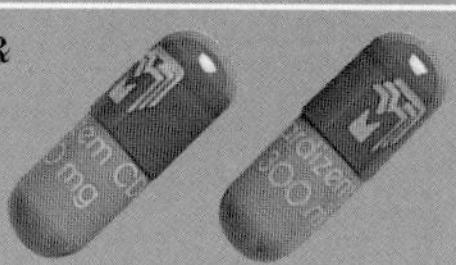
Cardizem CD 300 mg
Hoechst Marion Roussel 300

℞
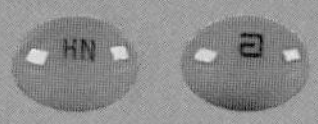

Hytrin 10 mg
Abbott HN

℞
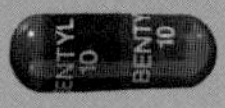
Bentyl 10 mg
Hoechst Marion Roussel 10

C-III
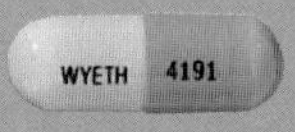

Synalgos-DC
Wyeth-Ayerst 4191

℞
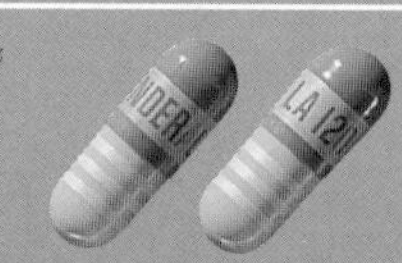
Inderal LA 120 mg
Wyeth-Ayerst 120

℞
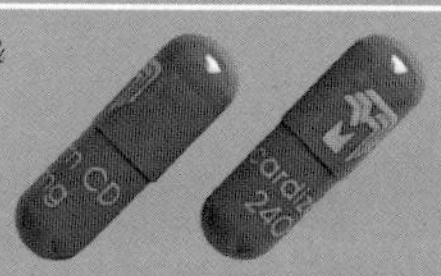
Cardizem CD 240 mg
Hoechst Marion Roussel 240

℞
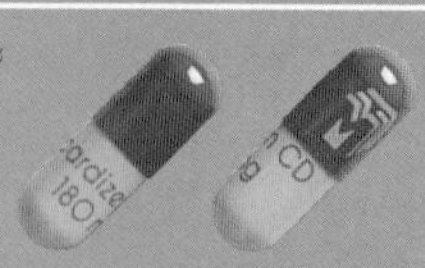
Cardizem CD 180 mg
Hoechst Marion Roussel 180

℞
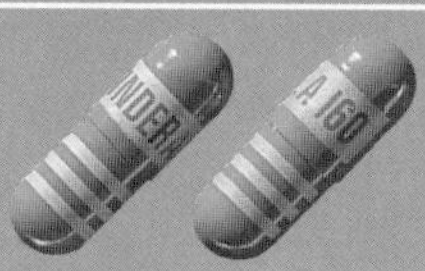
Inderal LA 160 mg
Wyeth-Ayerst 160

℞
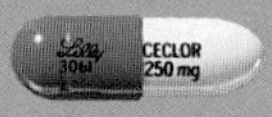

Ceclor 250 mg
Lilly 3061 250

℞
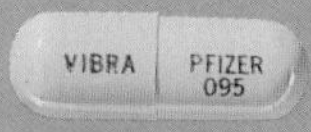

Vibramycin 100 mg
Pfizer 095

℞
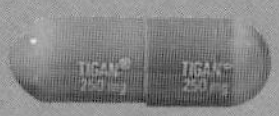
Tigan 250 mg
SmithKline Beecham 250

℞

Ceclor 500 mg
Lilly 3062 500

℞

Zovirax 200 mg
Glaxo Wellcome 200

℞
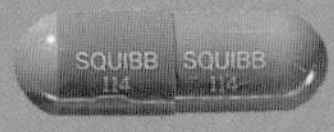

Velosef 500 mg
Apothecon Squibb 114

℞
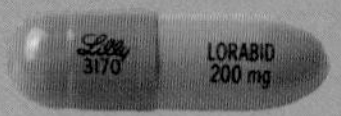

Lorabid 200 mg
Lilly 3170 200

℞
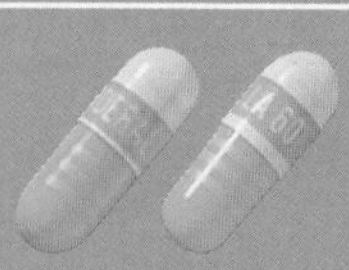
Inderal LA 60 mg
Wyeth-Ayerst 60

℞
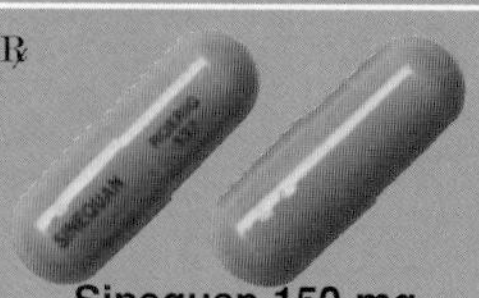
Sinequan 150 mg
Roerig 537

℞
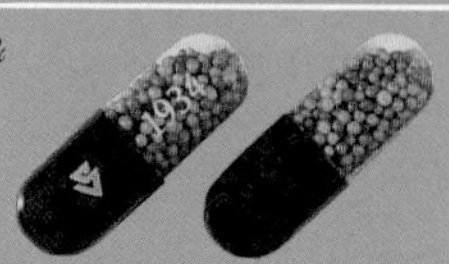
Brexin LA
Savage 1934

℞
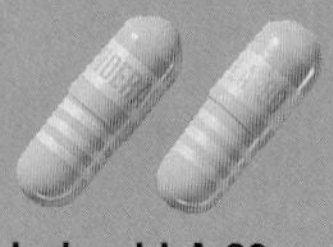
Inderal LA 80 mg
Wyeth-Ayerst 80

℞
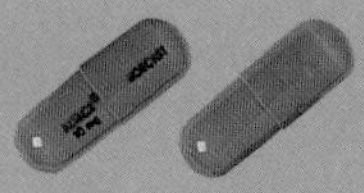
Altace 10 mg
Hoechst Marion Roussel 10

C-II
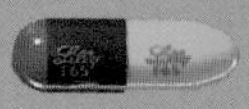
Tuinal 100 mg
Lilly F65

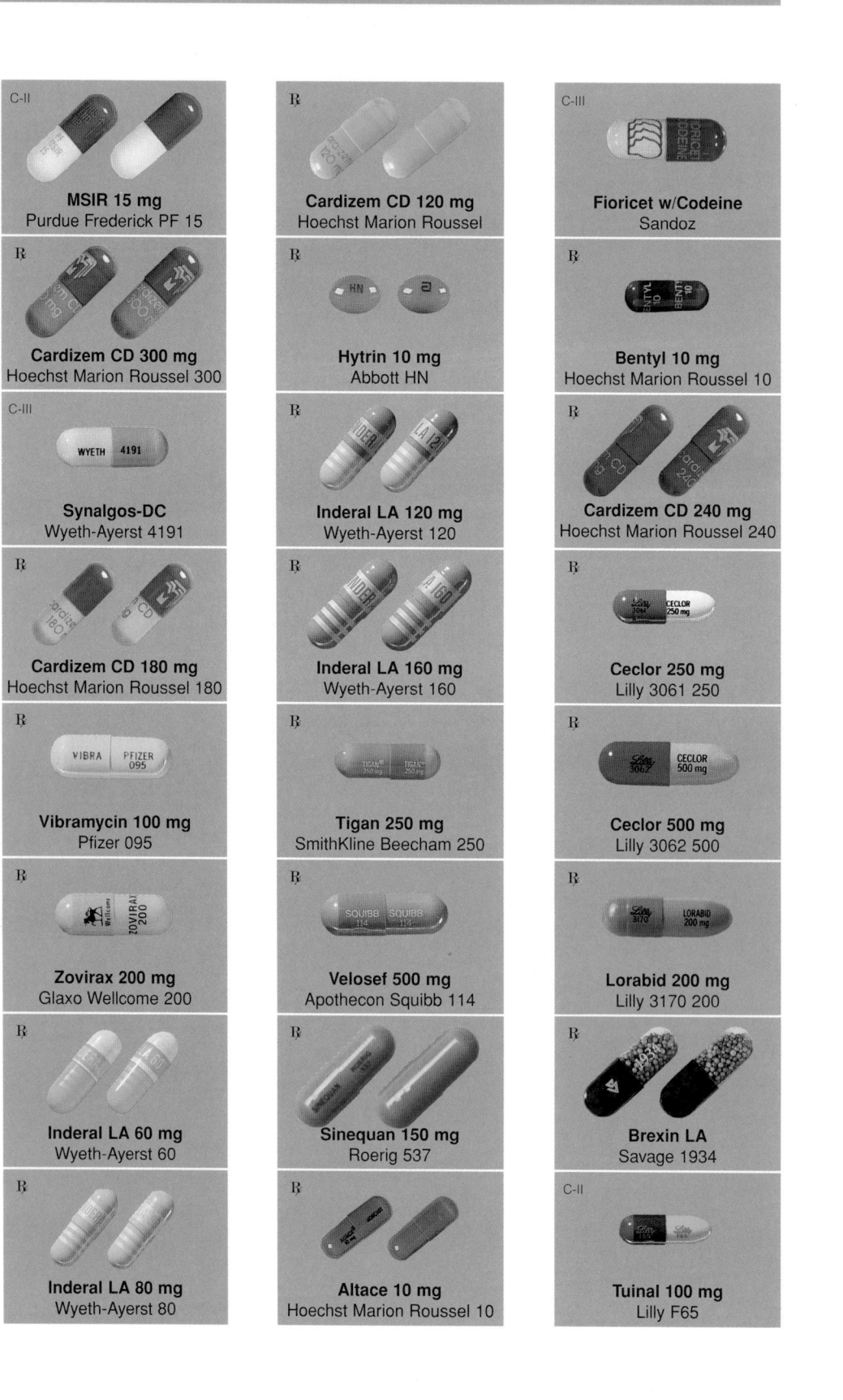

℞

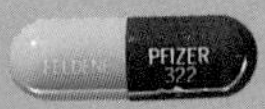

Feldene 10 mg
Pfizer 322

C-IV

Restoril 30 mg
Sandoz 30

℞

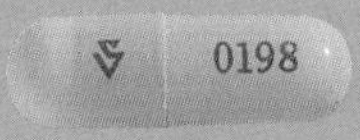

Axocet
Savage 0198

C-II

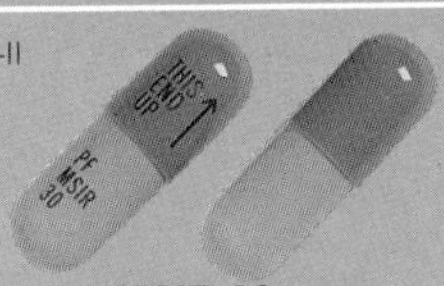

MSIR 30 mg
Purdue Frederick PF 30

℞

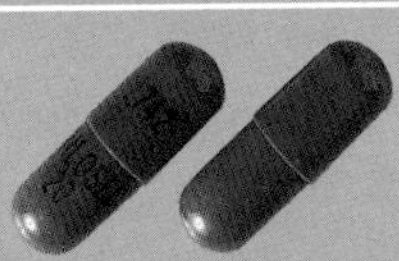

Prilosec 20 mg
Astra Merck 742 20

℞

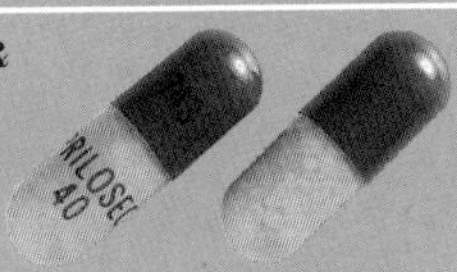

Prilosec 40 mg
Astra Merck 743 40

℞

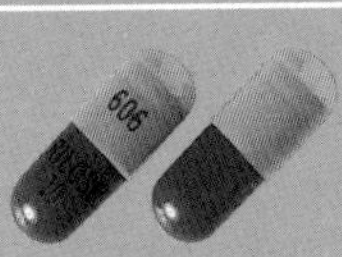

Prilosec 10 mg
Astra Merck 606 10

℞

Sinequan 50 mg
Roerig 536

℞

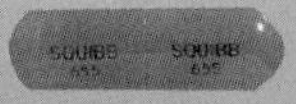

Sumycin 250 mg
Apothecon Squibb 655

℞

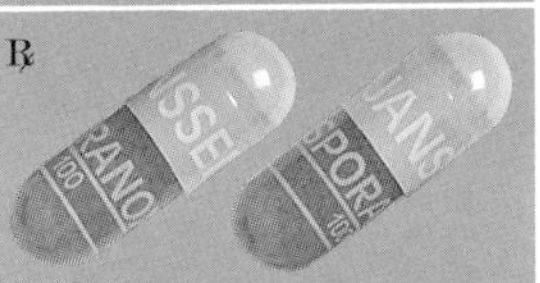

Sporanox 100 mg
Janssen 100

℞

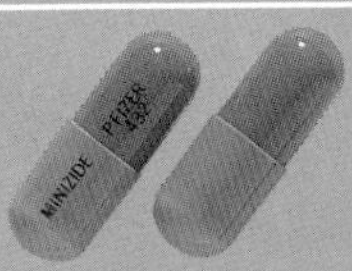

Minizide 2
Pfizer 432

℞

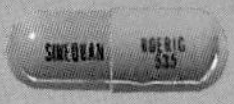

Sinequan 25 mg
Roerig 535

℞

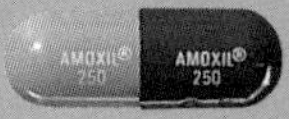

Amoxil 250 mg
SmithKline Beecham 250

℞

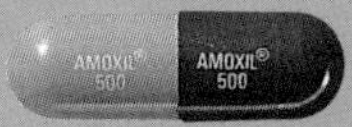

Amoxil 500 mg
SmithKline Beecham 500

℞

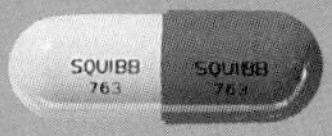

Sumycin 500 mg
Apothecon Squibb 763

℞

Minipress 2 mg
Pfizer 437

C-IV

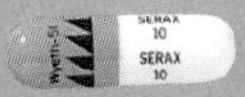

Serax 10 mg
Wyeth-Ayerst 51

℞

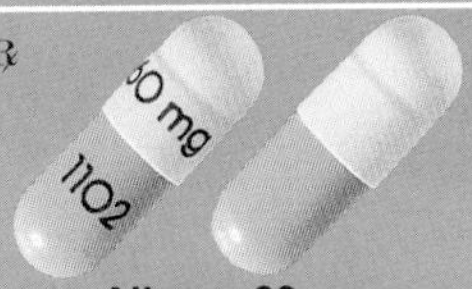

Allegra 60 mg
Hoechst Marion Roussel 1102

℞

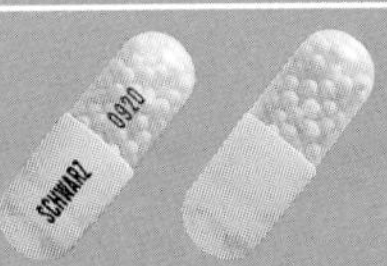

Dilatrate SR 40 mg
Schwarz Pharma 0920

℞

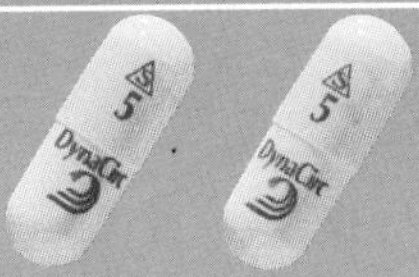

DynaCirc 5 mg
Sandoz 5

C-IV

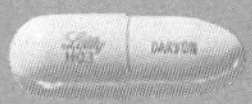

Darvon 65 mg
Lilly H03

℞

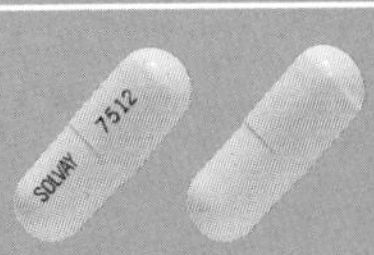

Lithonate 300 mg
Solvay 7512

℞

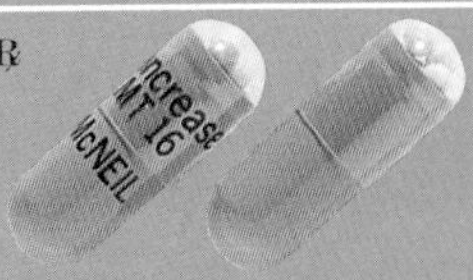

Pancrease MT 16
McNeil MT 16

℞

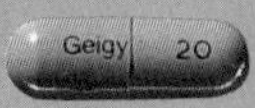

Tofranil-PM 75 mg
Ciba Geigy 20

Pink to Red Capsules

℞
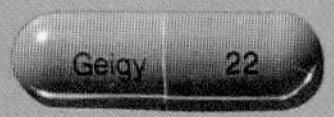

Tofranil-PM 150 mg
Ciba Geigy 22

℞

VePesid 50 mg
BMSOI 3091

℞
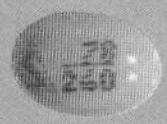
Sandimmune 25 mg
Sandoz 78-240

℞
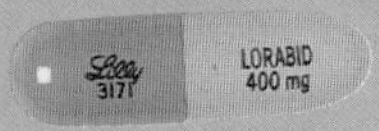

Lorabid 400 mg
Lilly 3171 400

℞
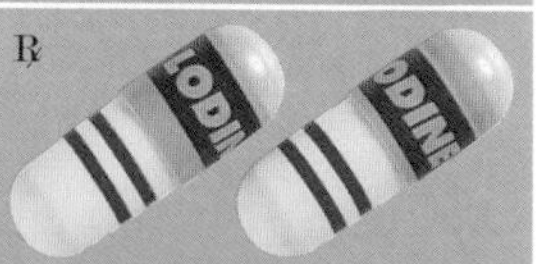
Lodine 200 mg
Wyeth-Ayerst

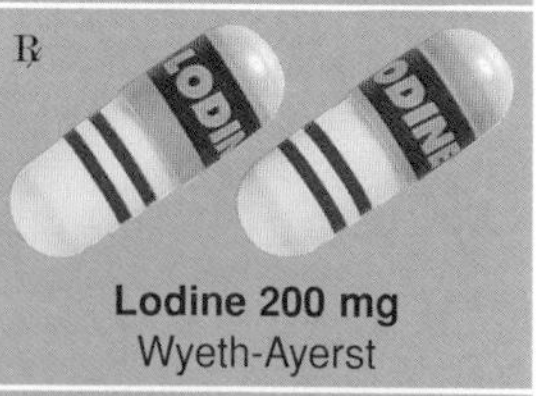

℞
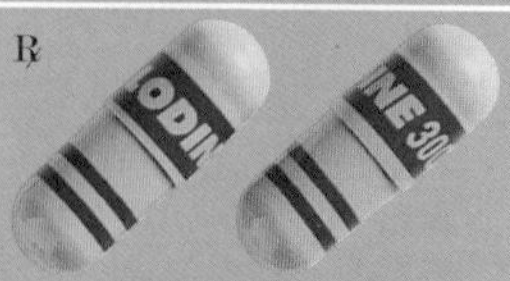
Lodine 300 mg
Wyeth-Ayerst 300

℞
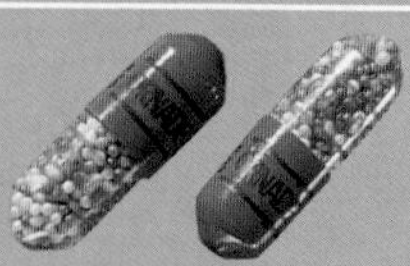
Ornade Spansules
SmithKline Beecham SKF

℞
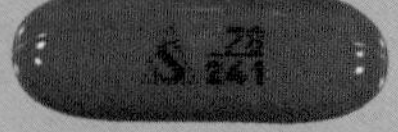
Sandimmune 100 mg
Sandoz 78 241

℞
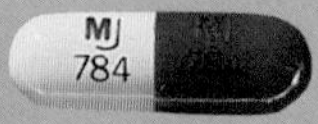

Duricef 500 mg
B-M Squibb MJ 784

C-IV
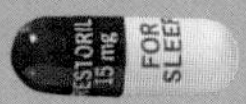

Restoril 15 mg
Sandoz 15

℞
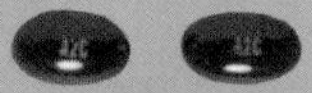
Lanoxicaps 0.05 mg
Glaxo Wellcome A2C

℞
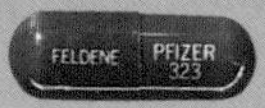

Feldene 20 mg
Pfizer 323

℞
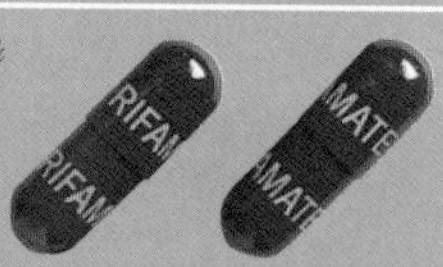
Rifamate
Hoechst Marion Roussel

℞
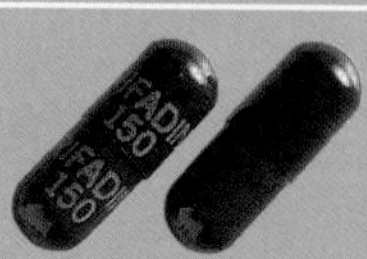
Rifadin 150 mg
Hoechst Marion Roussel 150

℞
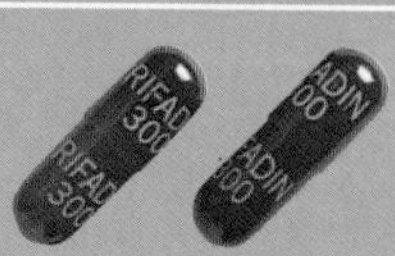
Rifadin 300 mg
Hoechst Marion Roussel 300

℞
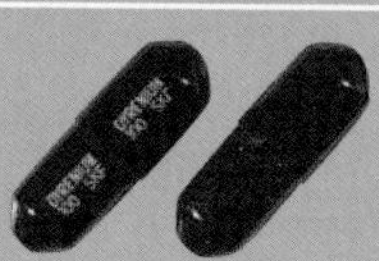
Dyrenium 100 mg
SmithKline Beecham 100 SKF

℞
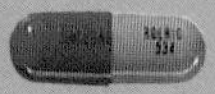
Sinequan 10 mg
Roerig 534

℞
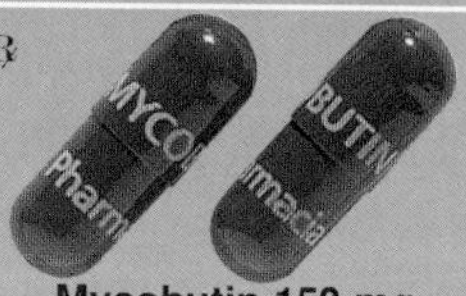
Mycobutin 150 mg
Pharmacia & Upjohn

℞
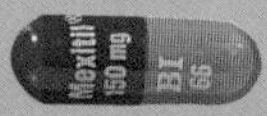
Mexitil 150 mg
Boehringer Ingelheim BI 66

℞
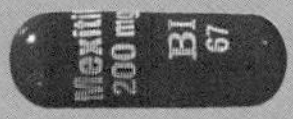
Mexitil 200 mg
Boehringer Ingelheim BI 67

℞
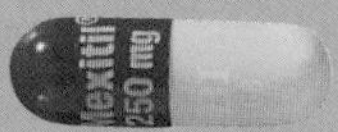
Mexitil 250 mg
Boehringer Ingelheim BI 68

℞
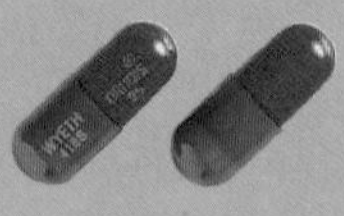
Orudis 25 mg
Wyeth-Ayerst 4186 25

℞
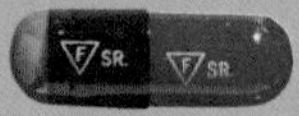
Extendryl SR.
Fleming F SR

℞
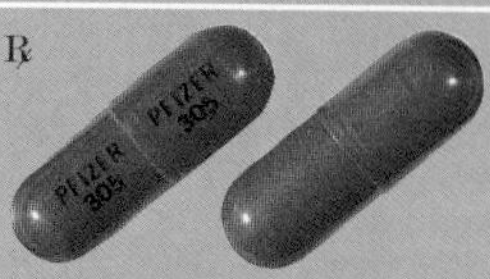
Zithromax 250 mg
Pfizer 305

℞
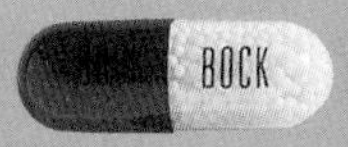

Poly-Histine-D Caps
Sanofi Winthrop Bock

℞

Dyazide
SmithKline Beecham

℞
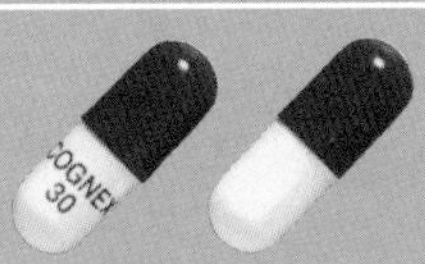

Cognex 30 mg
Parke-Davis 30

℞
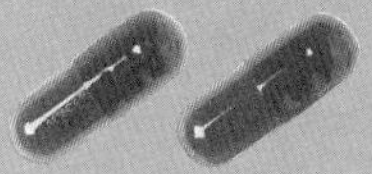
Altace 5 mg
Hoechst Marion Roussel 5

℞
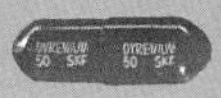

Dyrenium 50 mg
SmithKline Beecham 50 SKF

℞
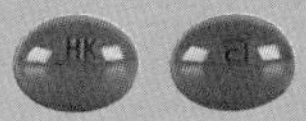

Hytrin 5 mg
Abbott HK

℞
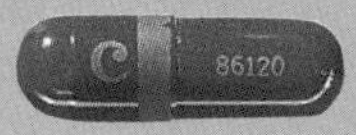

Midrin
Carnrick C 86120

℞

Ilosone 250 mg
Dista H09 250

C-IV
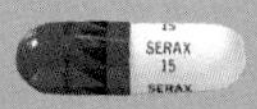

Serax 15 mg
Wyeth-Ayerst 6

℞

Procardia 10 mg
Pratt Pfizer 260

℞
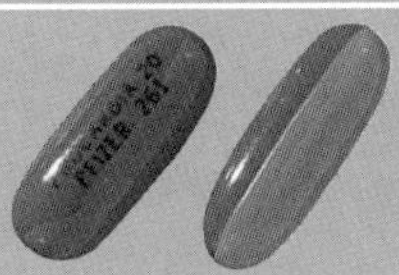
Procardia 20 mg
Pratt Pfizer 20 261

℞
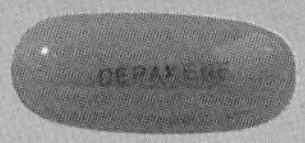

Depakene 250 mg
Abbott

℞
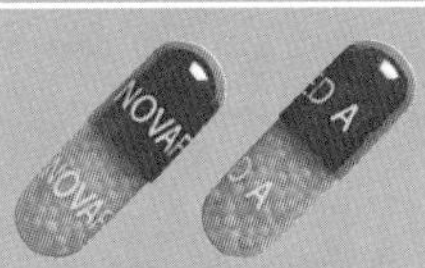
Novafed A
Hoechst Marion Roussel

℞
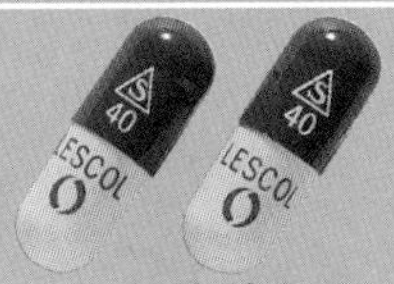

Lescol 40 mg
Sandoz 40

℞
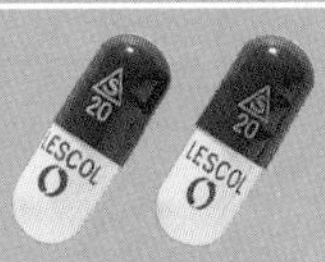

Lescol 20 mg
Sandoz 20

C-IV
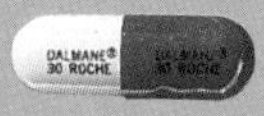

Dalmane 30 mg
Roche 30

℞
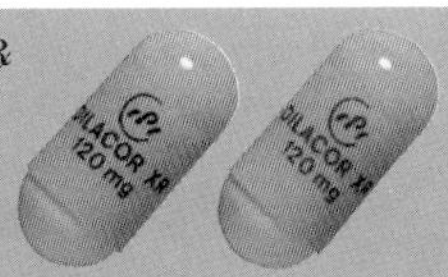

Dilacor XR 120 mg
Rhone-Poulenc Rorer 120

℞

Diamox Sequels 500 mg
Lederle D3

℞
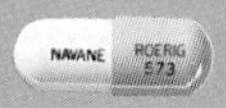

Navane 5 mg
Roerig 573

℞
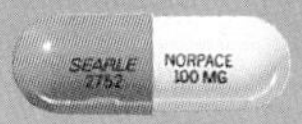

Norpace 100 mg
Searle 2752 100

℞
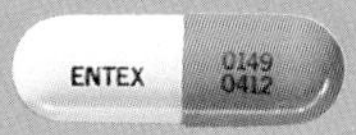

Entex
Dura 0149 0412

℞
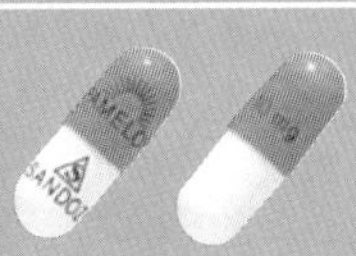
Pamelor 10 mg
Sandoz 10

℞
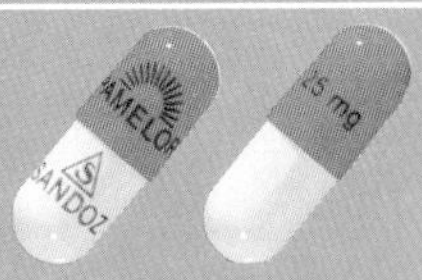

Pamelor 25 mg
Sandoz 25

℞
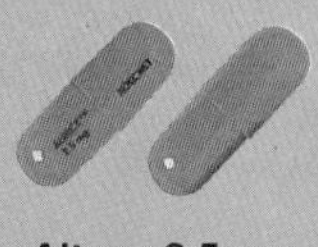
Altace 2.5 mg
Hoechst Marion Roussel 2.5

℞
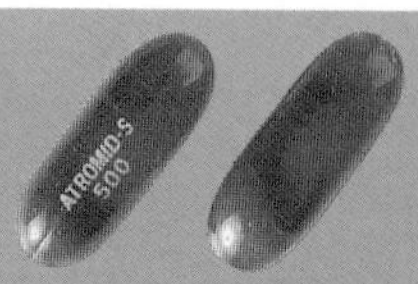

Atromid-S 500 mg
Wyeth-Ayerst 500

℞
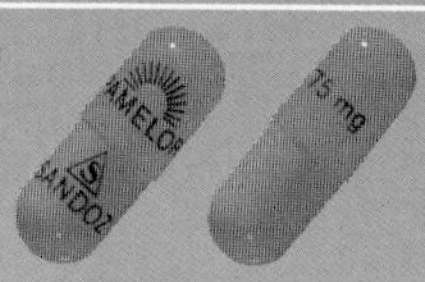

Pamelor 75 mg
Sandoz 75

℞
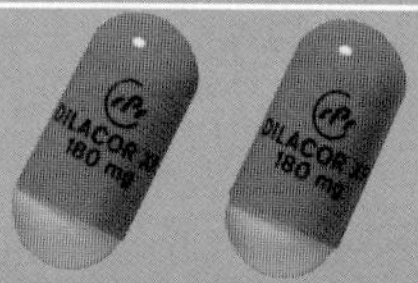

Dilacor XR 180 mg
Rhone-Poulenc Rorer 180

℞
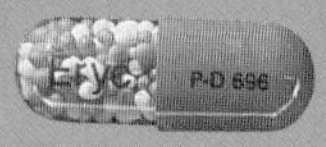

ERYC 250 mg
Parke-Davis P-D 696

℞
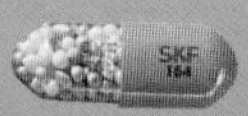

Thorazine Spansule 75 mg
SmithKline Beecham SKF T64

℞
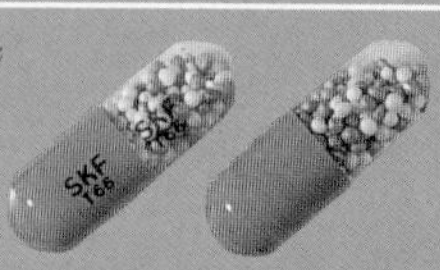

Thorazine Spansule 150 mg
SmithKline Beecham SKF T66

℞
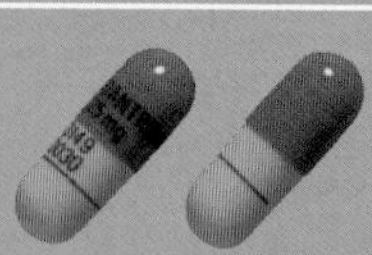
Dantrium 25 mg
Procter & Gamble 0149 0030

℞
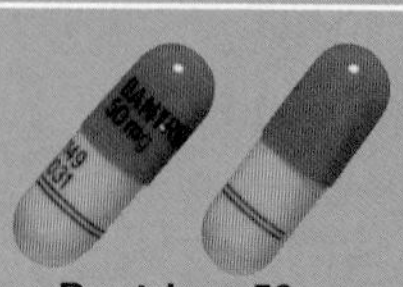
Dantrium 50 mg
Procter & Gamble 0149 0031

℞
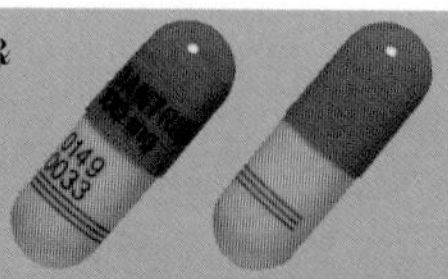

Dantrium 100 mg
Procter & Gamble 0149 0033

℞
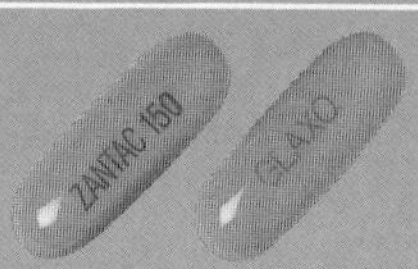

Zantac 150 GELdose 150 mg
Glaxo Wellcome 150

℞
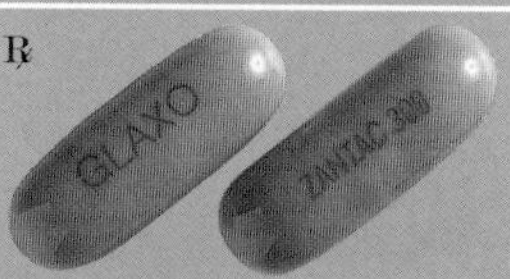

Zantac 300 GELdose 300 mg
Glaxo Wellcome 300

℞
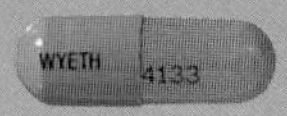

Surmontil 50 mg
Wyeth-Ayerst 4133

℞
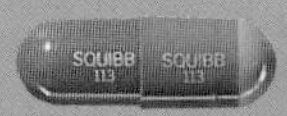

Velosef 250 mg
Apothecon Squibb 113

℞

Sectral 200 mg
Wyeth-Ayerst 4177 200

℞
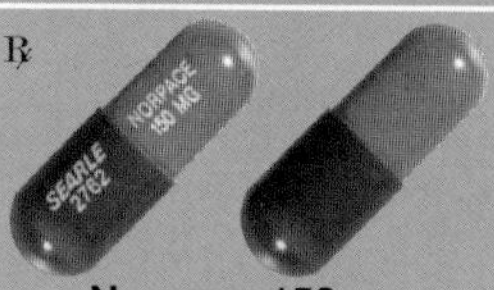

Norpace 150 mg
Searle 2762 150

℞

Sectral 400 mg
Wyeth-Ayerst 4179 400

℞
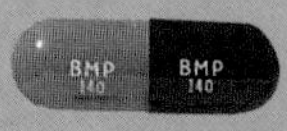

Totacillin 250 mg
SmithKline Beecham BMP 140

℞
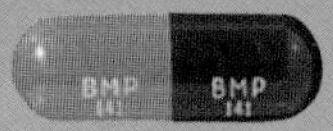

Totacillin 500 mg
SmithKline Beecham BMP 141

℞
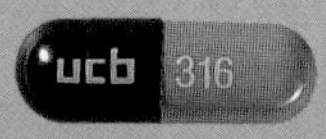

Vicon Forte
UCB Pharma 316

℞
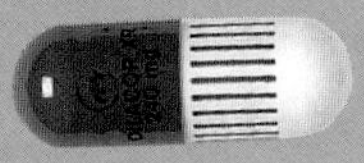
Dilacor XR 240 mg
Rhone-Poulenc Rorer 240

℞
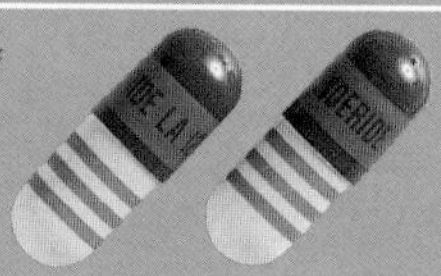
Inderide 120/150
Wyeth-Ayerst

℞
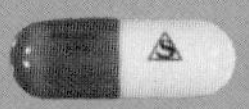
Parlodel 5 mg
Sandoz 5

℞
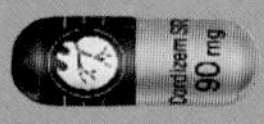

Cardizem SR 90 mg
Hoechst Marion Roussel 90

℞
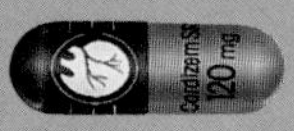

Cardizem SR 120 mg
Hoechst Marion Roussel 120

chapter 1

nutritional products

RECOMMENDED DIETARY ALLOWANCES OF VITAMINS AND MINERALS

Recommended Dietary Allowances (RDA) are published by the Food and Nutrition Board, National Research Council-National Academy of Sciences, as a guide for nutritional problems and to provide standards of good nutrition for different age groups. They are revised periodically.

The RDA values are *not requirements;* they are *recommended* daily intakes of certain essential nutrients. Based on available scientific knowledge, they are believed to be adequate for known nutritional needs for most *healthy* persons under usual environmental stresses. The recommended allowances vary for age and sex, with extra allowances for women during pregnancy and lactation. The most commonly used RDA values (the "reference male" and "reference female") are those of adults 23 to 50 years of age. With the exception of energy (kilocalories), the RDA provide for individual requirement variations and prevent symptoms of clinical deficiency of 97% of the population.

RDA have been established for many essential nutrients; however, present knowledge of human nutritional needs of pantothenic acid and biotin is incomplete. Therefore, to ensure adequate nutrient intake, obtain the recommended allowances from as varied a selection of foods as possible. Nutritionists suggest that dietary planning include regular intake of each of the four basic food groups:

1.) Milk, cheese, dairy products – Minimum 2 servings/day.
2.) Meat, poultry, fish, beans – Minimum 2 servings/day.
3.) Vegetables, fruit – Minimum 4 servings/day.
4.) Bread, cereal (whole-grain and enriched or fortified) – Minimum 4 servings/day.

Such a balance, in sufficient quantities will provide about 1200 kcal, enough protein, and most of the vitamins and minerals required daily. A person may increase nutrient and energy intake by consuming larger quantities (or more servings/day) of the four basic food groups. Nutrient and energy intake may also be increased by selecting food from the fifth group, fats-sweets-alcohol, which provides mainly energy.

RDA quantities apply only to healthy persons and are not intended to cover therapeutic nutritional requirements in disease or other abnormal states (ie, metabolic disorders, weight reduction, chronic disease, drug therapy). Although certain single nutrients in larger quantities may have pharmacologic actions, these are unrelated to nutritional functions. There is no convincing evidence that consuming excessive quantities of single nutrients will cure or prevent nonnutritional diseases.

The "official" listings of United States Recommended Daily Allowances (US-RDAs) should not be confused with the RDA values. US-RDA are derived from the 1968 RDA and serve as legal standards for nutritional labeling of food and dietary food and dietary supplement products controlled by the Food and Drug Administration. Generally, they represent the higher value of the male or female RDA and are grouped into only three age brackets plus one category for pregnant or lactating women. Prior to 1972, these allowances were erroneously listed as minimum daily requirements (MDR). A second fallacy perpetuated by US-RDA labeling of foods is the implication that a food is defective if it does not contain all the officially established nutrients in their full US-RDA quantities. No individual food is nutritionally complete, but several foods together should complement each other to provide maximal nutrient balance and to minimize naturally occurring toxic principles consumed from any individual foodstuff.

The Recommended Dietary Allowances (RDA) for adult males and adult females are included in each individual vitamin monograph. The following table presents the listing of vitamin and mineral RDA values for all age groups as published in Recommended Dietary Allowances, 10th Edition, National Academy of Sciences, Washington, D.C., 1989.

RECOMMENDED DIETARY ALLOWANCES[1]

Patient Parameters						Fat-Soluble Vitamins				Water-Soluble Vitamins							Minerals						
Age (years) or Condition	Weight[2] (kg)	Weight[2] (lb)	Height[2] (cm)	Height[2] (in)	Protein g	Vitamin A μg RE[3]	Vitamin D IU[4]	Vitamin E IU[5]	Vitamin K μg	Ascorbic Acid (C) mg	Thiamine (B_1) mg	Riboflavin (B_2) mg	Niacin (B_3) mg	Pyridoxine (B_6) mg	Folate μg	Cyanocobalamin (B_{12}) μg	Calcium mg	Phosphorus mg	Magnesium mg	Iron mg	Zinc mg	Iodine μg	Selenium μg
Infants																							
0.0-0.5	6	13	60	24	13	375	300	4	5	30	0.3	0.4	5	0.3	25	0.3	400	300	40	6	5	40	10
0.5-1	9	20	71	28	14	375	400	6	10	35	0.4	0.5	6	0.6	35	0.5	600	500	60	10	5	50	15
Children																							
1-3	13	29	90	35	16	400	400	9	15	40	0.7	0.8	9	1	50	0.7	800	800	80	10	10	70	20
4-6	20	44	112	44	24	500	400	10	20	45	0.9	1.1	12	1.1	75	1	800	800	120	10	10	90	20
7-10	28	62	132	52	28	700	400	10	30	45	1	1.2	13	1.4	100	1.4	800	800	170	10	10	120	30
Males																							
11-14	45	99	157	62	45	1000	400	15	45	50	1.3	1.5	17	1.7	150	2	1200	1200	270	12	15	150	40
15-18	66	145	176	69	59	1000	400	15	65	60	1.5	1.8	20	2	200	2	1200	1200	400	12	15	150	50
19-24	72	160	177	70	58	1000	400	15	70	60	1.5	1.7	19	2	200	2	1200	1200	350	10	15	150	70
25-50	79	174	176	70	63	1000	200	15	80	60	1.5	1.7	19	2	200	2	800	800	350	10	15	150	70
51 +	77	170	173	68	63	1000	200	15	80	60	1.2	1.4	15	2	200	2	800	800	350	10	15	150	70
Females																							
11-14	46	101	157	62	46	800	400	12	45	50	1.1	1.3	15	1.4	150	2	1200	1200	280	15	12	150	45
15-18	55	120	163	64	44	800	400	12	55	60	1.1	1.3	15	1.5	180	2	1200	1200	300	15	12	150	50
19-24	58	128	164	65	46	800	400	12	60	60	1.1	1.3	15	1.6	180	2	1200	1200	280	15	12	150	55
25-50	63	138	163	64	50	800	200	12	65	60	1.1	1.3	15	1.6	180	2	800	800	280	15	12	150	55
51 +	65	143	160	63	50	800	200	12	65	60	1	1.2	13	1.6	180	2	800	800	280	10	12	150	55
Pregnant					60	800	400	15	65	70	1.5	1.6	17	2.2	400	2.2	1200	1200	320	30	15	175	65
Lactating – 1st 6 mo.					65	1300	400	18	65	95	1.6	1.8	20	2.1	280	2.6	1200	1200	355	15	19	200	75
2nd 6 mo.					62	1200	400	16	65	90	1.6	1.7	20	2.1	260	2.6	1200	1200	340	15	16	200	75

Reproduced from: *Recommended Dietary Allowances,* 10th edition, 1989, National Academy of Sciences, National Academy Press, Washington, DC.

[1] The allowances, expressed as average daily intakes over time, are intended to provide for individual variations among most normal persons as they live in the US under usual environmental stresses. Diets should be based on a variety of common foods in order to provide other nutrients for which human requirements have been less well defined.

[2] Weights and heights of Reference Adults are actual medians for the US population of the designated age, as reported by NHANES II. The median weights and heights of those under 19 years of age were taken from Hamill PV et al. *Am J Clin Nutr* 1979;32:607-29. The use of these figures does not imply that the height-to-weight ratios are ideal.

[3] Retinol equivalents. 1 retinol equivalent = 1 μg retinol or 6 μg β-carotene.

[4] As cholecalciferol. 10 μg cholecalciferol = 400 IU of vitamin D.

[5] α-Tocopherol equivalents. 1 mg d-α-tocopherol = α-TE = 1.49 IU.

Fat-Soluble Vitamins

VITAMIN A

Actions:

Pharmacology: Vitamin A is found only in animal sources; it occurs in high concentrations in the liver of the cod, halibut, tuna and shark. It is also prepared synthetically. Absorption from an aqueous vehicle is greater than from an oily solution.

One IU vitamin A is equal to 0.3 mcg all-trans-retinol. Vitamin A activity is expressed as retinol equivalents (RE). One RE has the activity of 1 mcg all-*trans*-retinol (3.33 IU), 6 mcg (10 IU) β-carotene or 12 mcg carotenoid provitamins. Beta-carotene (provitamin A) is converted to retinol primarily in the intestinal mucosa.

Retinol combines with opsin, the rod pigment in the retina, to form rhodopsin, which is necessary for visual adaptation to darkness. Vitamin A prevents growth retardation and preserves the integrity of epithelial cells. Deficiency is characterized by nyctalopia (night blindness), keratomalacia (corneal necrosis), keratinization and drying of skin, lowered resistance to infection, retardation of growth, thickening of bone, diminished production of cortical steroids, and fetal malformations.

Pharmacokinetics: Vitamin A is fat soluble; absorption requires bile salts, pancreatic lipase and dietary fat. It is transported in blood to the liver by chylomicrons of the lymph. Normal serum vitamin A is 80 to 300 IU/ml. It is stored (primarily as palmitate) both in parenchymal liver cells and in non-parenchymal fat-storing cells in the liver. The normal adult liver contains ≈ 100 to 300 mcg/g, providing 2 years' requirements of vitamin A. Vitamin A is mobilized from liver stores and transported in plasma as retinol, bound to retinol-binding protein (RBP).

The excretion pathways are uncertain; a major portion appears to be excreted in the bile bound to a glucuronide and a small amount is excreted in the urine.

Indications:

Treatment of vitamin A deficiency: Deficiencies occur rarely in well nourished individuals; conditions which may cause vitamin A deficiency include: Biliary tract or pancreatic disease, sprue, colitis, hepatic cirrhosis, celiac disease, regional enteritis, extreme dietary inadequacy and partial gastrectomy and cystic fibrosis.

Parenteral administration is indicated when oral administration is not feasible as in anorexia, nausea, vomiting, preoperative and postoperative conditions, or in the "malabsorption syndrome" with accompanying steatorrhea.

Contraindications:

Hypervitaminosis A; oral use in malabsorption syndrome; hypersensitivity; IV use.

Warnings:

Renal function impairment: Vitamin A toxicity and elevated plasma calcium and alkaline phosphatase concentrations have been reported in chronic renal failure patients undergoing hemodialysis.

Pregnancy: Category C. Safety of amounts exceeding 5000 IU oral or 6000 IU parenteral daily during pregnancy has not been established. Avoid use of vitamin A in excess of the RDA during normal pregnancy. Animal reproduction studies have shown fetal abnormalities associated with overdosage in several species. One case of an infant with congenital renal anomalies has been reported.

Lactation: The US-RDA of vitamin A is 6000 units for nursing mothers. Human milk supplies sufficient vitamin A for infants unless maternal diet is grossly inadequate.

Precautions:

Closely supervise prolonged daily administration over 25,000 IU. Evaluate vitamin A intake from fortified foods, dietary supplements, self-administered drugs and prescription drug sources.

Blood level assays are not a direct measure of liver storage. Liver storage should be adequate before discontinuing therapy.

Single vitamin A deficiency is rare. Multiple vitamin deficiency is expected in any dietary deficiency.

Acne: Efficacy of large systemic doses of vitamin A in the treatment of acne has not been established; in view of the potential for toxicity, avoid this use. However, see topical vitamin A (tretinoin) and isotretinoin individual monographs.

Drug Interactions:

Cholestyramine may reduce absorption of vitamin A due to the reduced availability of fat-solubilizing bile salts.

Mineral oil use may interfere with the intestinal absorption of vitamin A.

Oral contraceptives significantly increase plasma vitamin A levels.

Adverse Reactions:

See Overdosage. Anaphylactic shock and death have been reported after IV use.

Fat-Soluble Vitamins

VITAMIN A

Overdosage:

Toxicity manifestations depend on patient's age, dosage, duration of administration, RBP levels and the liver's ability to store or secrete vitamin A.

Acute toxicity: Signs of increased intracranial pressure develop in 8 to 12 hours; cutaneous desquamation follows in a few days. A 25,000 IU/kg dose has caused acute toxicity.

Infants – Doses of > 350,000 IU.

Adults – Doses of > 2 million IU.

Chronic toxicity: 4000 IU/kg administered for 6 to 15 months.

Infants (3 to 6 months old) – 18,500 IU (water dispersed) daily for 1 to 3 months.

Adults – 1 million IU daily for 3 days, 50,000 IU daily for longer than 18 months or 500,000 IU daily for 2 months.

Hypervitaminosis A syndrome generally manifests as a cirrhotic-like liver syndrome. The following have been reported as manifestations of chronic overuse:

Body as a whole – Malaise; lethargy; night sweats; abdominal discomfort; jaundice; anorexia; vomiting.

Musculoskeletal – Slow growth; hard tender cortical thickening over radius and tibia; migratory arthralgia; premature closure of epiphysis; bone pain.

CNS – Irritability; headache; vertigo; increased intracranial pressure as manifested by bulging fontanelles, papilledema and exophthalmos.

Dermatologic – Lip fissures; drying and cracking skin; alopecia; scaling; massive desquamation; increased pigmentation; generalized pruritus; erythema; inflammation of the tongue, lips and gums.

Miscellaneous – Hypomenorrhea; hepatosplenomegaly; edema; leukopenia; vit. A plasma levels > 1200 IU/dl; polydipsia; polyuria; hypercalcemia.

Treatment: Discontinue vitamin A. If hypercalcemia persists, give IV saline, prednisone and calcitonin. Perform liver function tests; liver damage may be permanent.

Patient Information:

Avoid prolonged use of mineral oil and cholestyramine while taking this drug.

Do not exceed recommended dosage, especially during pregnancy. Notify physician if signs of overdosage (eg, nausea, vomiting, anorexia, malaise, dry/cracking skin/lips, irritability, hair loss) or bulging fontanelle in infants occur.

Administration and Dosage:

Recommended dietary allowances (RDA): Adult males, 1000 mcg RE; adult females, 800 mcg RE (RE = retinol equivalents: 1 RE = 1 mcg retinol or 6 mcg β-carotene).

For a complete listing of RDA by age, sex or condition, refer to the RDA table.

Treatment of deficiency states:

Adults and children (> 8 years old) –

Severe deficiency with xerophthalmia: 500,000 IU/day for 3 days, followed by 50,000 IU/day for 2 weeks.

Severe deficiency: 100,000 IU/day for 3 days, then 50,000 IU/day for 2 weeks.

Follow-up therapy: Adults - 10,000 to 20,000 IU/day for 2 months.

Children (1 to 8 years old) – 5000 to 10,000 IU/day for 2 months.

Parenteral (IM): Adults - 100,000 IU/day for 3 days, 50,000 IU/day for 2 weeks.

Children (1 to 8 years old) – 17,500 to 35,000 IU/day for 10 days.

Infants – 7500 to 15,000 IU/day for 10 days.

otc	**Aquasol A** (Astra USA)	**Drops:** 5000 IU/0.1 ml	In 30 ml w/dropper.
otc	**Palmitate-A 5000** (Akorn)	**Tablets:** 5000 IU vitamin A	In 100s.
otc	**Vitamin A** (Various, eg, Lilly, Schein)	**Capsules:** 10,000 IU	In 100s, 250s and 1000s.
Rx[1]	**Vitamin A** (Various, eg, Lilly, Rugby, Schein)	**Capsules:** 25,000 IU	In 100s, 250s, 500s and 1000s.
Rx	**Aquasol A** (Astra USA)		Red. In 100s.
Rx[1]	**Vitamin A** (Various, eg, Major, Rugby, Schein)	**Capsules:** 50,000 IU	In 100s, 250s, 500s and 1000s.
Rx	**Del-Vi-A** (Del-Ray)		Amber. In 100s.
Rx	**Aquasol A** (Astra USA)		Red. In 100s and 500s.
Rx	**Aquasol A** (Astra USA)	**Injection:** 50,000 IU/ml	In 2 ml vials.[2]

[1] Some products may be available *otc* according to distributor discretion.

[2] With 0.5% chlorobutanol, polysorbate 80, butylated hydroxyanisole and butylated hydroxytoluene.

Fat-Soluble Vitamins

VITAMIN D

Actions:

Pharmacology: Vitamin D is a fat-soluble vitamin derived from natural sources such as fish liver oils or from conversion of provitamins (ergosterol and 7-dehydrocholesterol) derived from foodstuffs. One USP unit or one IU vitamin D activity is equal to 0.025 mcg vitamin D_3 (1 mg = 40,000 units). "Vitamin D" refers to both ergocalciferol (D_2) and cholecalciferol (D_3). Vitamin D_2, essentially a plant vitamin, is used in fortified milk and cereals. Natural supplies of vitamin D depend on ultraviolet light for conversion of 7-dehydrocholesterol to vitamin D_3 or ergosterol to vitamin D_2.

Vitamin D is hydroxylated by the hepatic microsomal enzymes to 25-hydroxyvitamin D (25-[OH]-D_3 or calcifediol). Calcifediol is hydroxylated primarily in kidney to 1, 25-dihydroxy-vitamin D (1, 25-$[OH]_2$-D_3 or calcitriol). Calcitriol is believed to be the most active form of vitamin D_3 in stimulating intestinal calcium and phosphate transport.

Dihydrotachysterol is a synthetic reduction product of tachysterol, a close isomer of vitamin D. Dihydrotachysterol is hydroxylated in liver to 25-hydroxydihydrotachysterol, the major circulating active form of the drug. It does not undergo further hydroxylation by kidney, and therefore is the analog of 1,25-dihydroxy-vitamin D.

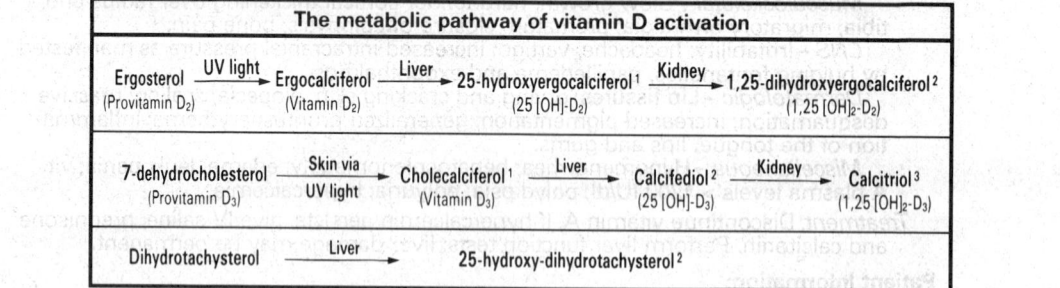

The metabolic pathway of vitamin D activation						
Ergosterol (Provitamin D_2)	—UV light→	Ergocalciferol (Vitamin D_2)	—Liver→	25-hydroxyergocalciferol[1] (25 [OH]-D_2)	—Kidney→	1,25-dihydroxyergocalciferol[2] (1,25 $[OH]_2$-D_2)
7-dehydrocholesterol (Provitamin D_3)	—Skin via UV light→	Cholecalciferol[1] (Vitamin D_3)	—Liver→	Calcifediol[2] (25 [OH]-D_3)	—Kidney→	Calcitriol[3] (1,25 $[OH]_2$-D_3)
Dihydrotachysterol	—Liver→	25-hydroxy-dihydrotachysterol[2]				

[1] The kidney, in the absence of PTH, converts vitamin D_3 to 24,25$(OH)_2$-D_3, which is much less active than 1,25$(OH)_2$-D_3.
[2] Major transport form of vitamin D; minor intrinsic activity. [3] Physiologically active forms.

Physiological function – Vitamin D is considered a hormone. Although not a natural human hormone, vitamin D_2 apparently can substitute for D_3 in every metabolic step. Vitamin D, in conjunction with PTH and calcitonin, regulates calcium homeostasis. Vitamin D metabolites promote active absorption of calcium and phosphorus by the small intestine, increase rate of accretion and resorption of minerals in bone and promote resorption of phosphate by renal tubules. Vitamin D is also involved in magnesium metabolism.

Vitamin D deficiency leads to progressive hearing loss, rickets in children and osteomalacia in adults. Vitamin D reverses symptoms of nutritional rickets or osteomalacia unless permanent deformities have occurred. Response to vitamin D varies, as seen in idiopathic hypercalcemia at one extreme and vitamin D-resistant rickets at the other.

Pharmacokinetics:

Absorption – Vitamin D is readily absorbed from the small intestine. Vitamin D_3 may be absorbed more rapidly and more completely than vitamin D_2. Bile is essential for adequate absorption. Absorption is reduced in liver or biliary disease and steatorrhea.

Distribution – Stored chiefly in the liver, vitamin D is also found in fat, muscle, skin and bones. In plasma, it is bound to alpha globulins and albumin.

Metabolism – There is a 10 to 24 hour lag between administration of ergocalciferol and onset of its action. Maximal hypercalcemic effects occur about 4 weeks after using a daily fixed dose; duration of action can be ≥ 2 months. Serum half-life of calcifediol is ≈ 16 days. Elimination half-life of calcitriol is 3 to 6 hours; pharmacologic activity persists 3 to 5 days. Dihydrotachysterol has a rapid onset of effect and is less persistent after treatment cessation.

Excretion – The primary route of excretion of vitamin D is in the bile; only a small percentage is found in the urine.

Fat-Soluble Vitamins

VITAMIN D

Indications:

Refer to individual product listings.

Contraindications:

Hypercalcemia; evidence of vitamin D toxicity; malabsorption syndrome; hypervitaminosis D; abnormal sensitivity to the effects of vitamin D; decreased renal function.

Warnings:

Hypersensitivity to vitamin D may be one etiological factor in infants with idiopathic hypercalcemia. In these cases, severely restrict vitamin D intake.

Concomitant calcium administration: Adequate dietary calcium is necessary for clinical response to vitamin D therapy.

Monitoring: Dosage adjustment is required as soon as there is clinical improvement. Individualize dosage. Start therapy at the lowest possible dose and do not increase without careful monitoring of the serum calcium. Estimate daily dietary calcium intake and adjust the intake when indicated. Patients with normal renal function taking calcitriol should avoid dehydration. Maintain adequate fluid intake. In vitamin D-resistant rickets, the range between therapeutic and toxic doses is narrow. When high therapeutic doses are used, follow progress with frequent serum and urinary calcium, phosphate and urea nitrogen determinations.

Periodically determine serum calcium, phosphate, magnesium and alkaline phosphatase; monitor 24 hour urinary calcium and phosphate, especially in hypoparathyroid and dialysis patients. During the initial phase, determine serum calcium twice weekly. Maintain serum calcium levels between 9 and 10 mg/dl.

Hypercalcemia: The product of serum calcium multiplied by phosphate (Ca x P) should not exceed 70; exceeding the solubility product may result in precipitation of calcium phosphate. Progressive hypercalcemia due to overdosage may require emergency attention. Chronic hypercalcemia can lead to generalized vascular calcification, nephrocalcinosis and other soft tissue calcification. Radiographic or slit lamp evaluation of suspect anatomical regions may be useful for early detection.

In patients with normal renal function, chronic hypercalcemia may be associated with an increase in serum creatinine. While this is usually reversible, it is important to pay careful attention to factors which may lead to hypercalcemia.

A fall in serum alkaline phosphatase levels usually precedes hypercalcemia and may indicate impending hypercalcemia. Should hypercalcemia develop, discontinue the drug immediately. After achieving normocalcemia, readminister at a lower dosage.

Renal function impairment: The kidneys of uremic patients cannot adequately synthesize calcitriol, the active hormone formed from precursor vitamin D. Resultant hypocalcemia and secondary hyperparathyroidism are a major cause of the metabolic bone disease of renal failure. However, other bone-toxic substances which accumulate in uremia (eg, aluminum) may also contribute.

The beneficial effect of calcitriol in renal osteodystrophy appears to result from correction of hypocalcemia and secondary hyperparathyroidism. It is uncertain whether calcitriol produces other independent beneficial effects. In patients with renal osteodystrophy accompanied by hyperphosphatemia, maintain a normal serum phosphorus level by dietary phosphate restriction or administration of aluminum gels to prevent metastatic calcification.

Because of the effect on serum calcium, administer to patients with renal stones only when potential benefits outweigh possible hazards.

Pregnancy: Category C. Safety of amounts in excess of 400 IU/day is not established. Avoid doses greater than the RDA during a normal pregnancy. Animal studies have shown fetal abnormalities associated with hypervitaminosis D. Calcifediol and calcitriol are teratogenic in animals when given in doses several times the human dose. The offspring of a woman administered 17 to 36 mcg/day of calcitriol (17 to 144 times the recommended dose) during pregnancy manifested mild hypercalcemia in the first two days of life which returned to normal at day 3. There are no adequate and well controlled studies in pregnant women; use during pregnancy only if the potential benefits outweigh the potential hazards to the fetus.

Lactation: Vitamin D is excreted in breast milk in limited amounts. In a mother given large doses of vitamin D, 25-hydroxycholecalciferol appeared in the milk and caused hypercalcemia in the child. Monitoring of the infant's serum calcium concentration is required in that case. Exercise caution when giving to a nursing mother.

Children: Safety and efficacy in children of doses exceeding the RDA and in children undergoing dialysis have not been established. Pediatric doses must be individualized and monitored under close medical supervision.

Fat-Soluble Vitamins

VITAMIN D

Precautions:

Use caution in patients with coronary disease, renal function impairment and arteriosclerosis, especially in the elderly.

Concomitant vitamin D intake: Evaluate vitamin D ingested in fortified foods, dietary supplements and other concomitantly administered drugs. It may be necessary to limit dietary vitamin D and its derivatives during treatment.

Hypoparathyroidism: May need calcium, parathyroid hormone, dihydrotachysterol.

Tartrazine sensitivity: Some of these products contain tartrazine, which may cause allergic-type reactions (including bronchial asthma) in susceptible individuals. Although incidence of sensitivity is low, it is frequently seen in patients with aspirin hypersensitivity. Products containing tartrazine are identified in product listings.

Drug Interactions:

Vitamin D Drug Interactions

Precipitant drug	Object drug*		Description
Vitamin D	Antacids, magnesium-containing	↑	Hypermagnesemia may develop in patients on chronic renal dialysis.
Vitamin D	Digitalis glycosides	↑	Hypercalcemia in patients on digitalis may precipitate cardiac arrhythmias.
Vitamin D	Verapamil	↑	Atrial fibrillation has recurred when supplemental calcium and calciferol have induced hypercalcemia.
Cholestyramine	Vitamin D	↓	Intestinal absorption of vitamin D may be reduced.
Mineral oil	Vitamin D	↓	Absorption of vitamin D is reduced with prolonged use of mineral oil.
Phenytoin, Barbiturates	Vitamin D	↓	Half-life of vitamin D may be decreased.
Thiazide diuretics	Vitamin D	↑	Hypoparathyroid patients on vitamin D may develop hypercalcemia due to thiazide diuretics.

* ↑ = Object drug increased. ↓ = Object drug decreased.

Adverse Reactions:

Early: Weakness; headache; somnolence; nausea; vomiting; dry mouth; constipation; muscle pain; bone pain; metallic taste.

Late: Polyuria; polydipsia; anorexia; irritability; weight loss; nocturia; mild acidosis; reversible azotemia, generalized vascular calcification, nephrocalcinosis; conjunctivitis (calcific); pancreatitis; photophobia; rhinorrhea; pruritus; hyperthermia; decreased libido; elevated BUN; albuminuria; hypercholesterolemia; elevated AST and ALT; ectopic calcification; hypertension; cardiac arrhythmias; overt psychosis (rare).

In clinical studies on hypoparathyroidism and pseudohypoparathyroidism, hypercalcemia was noted on at least one occasion in about 1 in 3 patients and hypercalciuria in about 1 in 7. Elevated serum creatinine levels were observed in about 1 in 6 patients (approximately one half of whom had normal levels at baseline).

Overdosage:

Symptoms: Administration to patients in excess of their daily requirements can cause hypercalcemia, hypercalciuria and hyperphosphatemia. Concomitant high intake of calcium and phosphate may lead to similar abnormalities. Doses of 60,000 IU/day can cause hypercalcemia.

Hypercalcemia leads to anorexia, nausea, weakness, weight loss, vague aches and stiffness, constipation, diarrhea, mental retardation, tinnitus, ataxia, hypotonia, depression, amnesia, disorientation, hallucinations, syncope, coma, anemia and mild acidosis. Impairment of renal function may cause polyuria, nocturia, hypercalciuria, polydipsia, reversible azotemia, hypertension, nephrocalcinosis, generalized vascular calcification, irreversible renal insufficiency or proteinuria. Widespread calcification of soft tissues, including heart, blood vessels, renal tubules and lungs can occur. Bone demineralization (osteoporosis) may occur in adults; decline in average linear growth rate and increased bone mineralization may occur in infants and children (dwarfism). Effects can persist ≥ 2 months after ergocalciferol treatment, 1 month after cessation of dihydrotachysterol therapy, 2 to 4 weeks for calcifediol and 2 to 7 days for calcitriol. Death can result from cardiovascular or renal failure.

Fat-Soluble Vitamins

VITAMIN D

Treatment of hypervitaminosis D with hypercalcemia consists of immediate withdrawal of the vitamin, a low calcium diet, generous fluid intake and urine acidification along with symptomatic and supportive treatment.

Hypercalcemic crisis with dehydration, stupor, coma and azotemia requires more vigorous treatment. The first step is hydration; saline IV may quickly and significantly increase urinary calcium excretion. A loop diuretic (eg, furosemide) may be given with the saline infusion to further increase calcium excretion. Other measures include administration of citrates, sulfates, phosphates, corticosteroids, EDTA and plicamycin. Persistent or markedly elevated serum calcium levels may be corrected by dialysis against a calcium-free dialysate. With appropriate therapy, and when no permanent damage has occurred, recovery is probable.

Treatment: of accidental overdosage consists of general supportive measures. Refer to General Management of Acute Overdosage. If ingestion is discovered within a short time, emesis or gastric lavage may be of benefit. Mineral oil may promote fecal elimination. Treat hypercalcemia as outlined above.

Patient Information:

Compliance with dosage instructions, diet and calcium supplementation are essential.

Swallow whole; do not crush or chew.

Eating a balanced diet and periodic exposure to sunlight usually satisfies normal vitamin D requirements. Never use vitamin supplements as a substitute for a balanced diet.

Notify physician if any of the following occurs: Weakness, lethargy, headache, anorexia, weight loss, nausea, vomiting, abdominal cramps, diarrhea, constipation, vertigo, excessive thirst, excessive urine output, dry mouth or muscle or bone pain.

Avoid concurrent prolonged use of mineral oil. If on chronic renal dialysis, avoid magnesium-containing antacids while taking this drug. See Drug Interactions.

Administration and Dosage:

Individualize dosage. The effectiveness of therapy is predicated on adequate daily intake of calcium either by calcium supplementation or proper dietary measures. Refer to the Recommended Dietary Allowances table for a complete listing of RDAs.

DIHYDROTACHYSTEROL (DHT)

Complete prescribing information for these products begins in the Vitamin D group monograph.

Dihydrotachysterol is a synthetic reduction product of tachysterol, a close isomer of vitamin D; 1 mg is approximately equivalent to 3 mg (120,000 IU) vitamin D_2.

Indications:

Treatment of acute, chronic and latent forms of postoperative tetany, idiopathic tetany and hypoparathyroidism.

Administration and Dosage:

Initial dose: 0.8 to 2.4 mg daily for several days.

Maintenance dose: 0.2 to 1 mg daily, as required, for normal serum calcium levels. Average dose is 0.6 mg daily. May be supplemented with oral calcium.

Rx	**DHT** (Roxane)	**Tablets:** 0.125 mg	Lactose, sucrose. (54 280). White. In 50s and UD 100s.
		0.2 mg	Lactose, sucrose. (54 903). Pink. In 100s and UD 100s.
		0.4 mg	Lactose, sucrose. (54 772). White. In 50s.
		Intensol Solution: 0.2 mg/ml	20% alcohol. In 30 ml w/dropper.
Rx	**Hytakerol** (Winthrop Pharm.)	**Capsules:** 0.125 mg	In 50s.
		Oral Solution: 0.25 mg/ml in oil	In 15 ml.

Fat-Soluble Vitamins

CALCITRIOL (1,25 dihydroxycholecalciferol; 1,25 $[OH]_2$–D_3)

Complete prescribing information for these products begins in the Vitamin D group monograph.

Indications:

Management of hypocalcemia in patients on chronic renal dialysis.

May reduce elevated parathyroid hormone levels in some patients.

Unlabeled uses: Calcitriol, orally (0.5 mcg/day for 6 months) and topically (0.5 mcg/g petrolatum once daily for 8 weeks), decreased the severity of psoriatic lesions in patients with psoriasis vulgaris.

Administration and Dosage:

Dialysis patients: 0.25 mcg/day. If a satisfactory response is not observed, increase dosage by 0.25 mcg/day at 4 to 8 week intervals. During this titration period, obtain serum calcium levels at least twice weekly; if hypercalcemia is noted, discontinue use until normocalcemia is attained.

Patients with normal or only slightly reduced serum calcium levels may respond to doses of 0.25 mcg every other day. Most patients undergoing hemodialysis respond to doses between 0.5 and 1 mcg/day.

Oral calcitriol may normalize plasma ionized calcium in some uremic patients, yet fail to suppress parathyroid hyperfunction. In these individuals with autonomous parathyroid hyperfunction, oral calcitriol may be useful to maintain normocalcemia, but has not been shown to be adequate treatment for hyperparathyroidism.

Hypoparathyroidism: Initial dose is 0.25 mcg/day given in the morning. If a satisfactory response in the biochemical parameters and clinical manifestations of the disease is not observed, increase dose at 2 to 4 week intervals. During the dosage titration period, obtain serum calcium levels at least twice weekly and, if hypercalcemia is noted, immediately discontinue use until normocalcemia ensues. Carefully consider lowering dietary calcium intake.

Adults and children (≥ 6 years) – 0.5 to 2 mcg daily.

(1 to 5 years) – 0.25 to 0.75 mcg daily. The number of treated patients with pseudohypoparathyroidism < 6 years of age is too small to make dosage recommendations.

Rx	**Rocaltrol** (Roche)	**Capsules:** 0.25 mcg	Sorbitol. (Rocaltrol 0.25 Roche). Light orange. In 30s and 100s.
		0.5 mcg	Sorbitol. (Rocaltrol 0.5 Roche). Dark orange. In 100s.
Rx	**Calcijex** (Abbott)	**Injection:** 1 mcg/ml	In 1 ml amps.
		2 mcg/ml	In 1 ml amps.

CALCIFEDIOL (25–hydroxycholecalciferol; 25 [OH]–D_3)

Complete prescribing information for these products begins in the Vitamin D group monograph.

Indications:

Management of metabolic bone disease or hypocalcemia in patients on chronic renal dialysis.

Increases serum calcium levels and decreases alkaline phosphatase, parathyroid hormone levels, subperiosteal bone resorption, histological signs of hyperparathyroid bone disease and mineralization defects in some patients.

Administration and Dosage:

Initial dose: 300 to 350 mcg/week, administered daily or on alternate days. If a satisfactory response is not obtained, dosage may be increased at 4 week intervals. During this period, obtain serum calcium levels at least weekly; if hypercalcemia is noted, discontinue use until normocalcemia is attained.

Some patients with normal serum calcium levels may respond to doses of 20 mcg every other day. Most patients respond to doses between 50 and 100 mcg/day or between 100 and 200 mcg on alternate days.

Rx	**Calderol** (Organon)	**Capsules:** 20 mcg	White. In 60s.
		50 mcg	Orange. In 60s.

Fat-Soluble Vitamins

ERGOCALCIFEROL (D_2)

Complete prescribing information for these products begins in the Vitamin D group monograph.

Ergocalciferol 1.25 mg provides 50,000 IU of vitamin D activity.

Indications:

Treatment of refractory rickets (also known as vitamin D-resistant rickets), familial hypophosphatemia and hypoparathyroidism.

Administration and Dosage:

Recommended dietary allowances (RDAs): Adults (< 25 years) 400 IU; (> 25 years) 200 IU. For a complete listing of RDAs by age, sex and condition, refer to the RDA table. Daily dosage of 400 IU satisfies requirements for all age groups, unless there has been exposure to ultraviolet irradiation.

Individualize dosage. The range between therapeutic and toxic doses is narrow.

Blood calcium, phosphorus and BUN determinations must be made every 2 weeks or more frequently if necessary. X-ray bones monthly until the condition is corrected and stabilized. Ensure adequate calcium intake. Maintain serum calcium concentration between 9 and 10 mg/dl.

Vitamin D resistant rickets: 12,000 to 500,000 IU daily.

Hypoparathyroidism: 50,000 to 200,000 IU/day plus 500 mg elemental calcium 6 times daily.

Familial hypophosphatemia: 10,000 to 80,000 IU daily plus 1 to 2 g/day elemental phosphorus.

IM therapy: Required in patients with GI, liver or biliary disease associated with malabsorption of vitamin D.

otc	**Calciferol Drops** (Schwarz Pharma Kremers Urban)	**Liquid:** 8000 IU per ml	In 60 ml[1].
otc	**Drisdol Drops** (Winthrop Pharm.)		In 60 ml[1].
Rx	**Vitamin D** (Various, eg, Dixon-Shane, Major, Moore, Rugby, Schein, URL)	**Capsules:** 50,000 IU	In 100s and 1000s.
Rx	**Drisdol** (Winthrop Pharm.)		Tartrazine. In 50s.
Rx	**Calciferol** (Schwarz Pharma Kremers Urban)	**Tablets:** 50,000 IU	Sugar. (KU 1). Yellow. Oval. In 100s.
Rx	**Calciferol** (Schwarz Pharma Kremers Urban)	**Injection:** 500,000 IU per ml	In 1 ml amps.[2]

[1] In propylene glycol.
[2] In sesame oil.

CHOLECALCIFEROL (D_3)

Complete prescribing information for these products begins in the Vitamin D group monograph.

Cholecalciferol 1 mg provides 40,000 IU vitamin D activity.

Indications:

Dietary supplement, treatment of vitamin D deficiency or prophylaxis of deficiency.

Unlabeled uses: Hypocalcemic tetany and hypoparathyroidism.

Administration and Dosage:

400 to 1000 IU daily.

otc *sf*	**Delta-D** (Freeda)	**Tablets:** 400 IU D_3	In 250s and 500s.
otc *sf*	**Vitamin D_3** (Freeda)	**Tablets:** 1000 IU D_3	In 100s.

Fat-Soluble Vitamins

VITAMIN E

Actions:

Pharmacology: Although the exact biochemical mechanisms of vitamin E in the body are unclear, it is an essential element of human nutrition. Many of its actions are related to its antioxidant properties. Vitamin E may protect cellular constituents from oxidation and prevent the formation of toxic oxidation products; it preserves red blood cell (RBC) wall integrity and protects them against hemolysis; it may act as a cofactor in enzyme systems. Enhancement of vitamin A utilization and suppression of platelet aggregation have also been attributed to vitamin E.

Clinical deficiency of vitamin E is rare, since adequate amounts are supplied in the normal diet. Sources of vitamin E include vegetable oils, vegetable shortening and margarine. Other food sources include leafy vegetables, milk, eggs and meats. Absorption depends on the ability to digest and absorb fat; bile is essential. There is no single storage organ, but adipose tissue, liver and muscle account for most of the body's tocopherol.

Low tocopherol levels have been noted in: Premature infants; severe protein-calorie malnourished infants with macrocytic megaloblastic anemia; prolonged fat malabsorption (ie, cystic fibrosis, hepatic cirrhosis, sprue); malabsorption syndromes (ie, celiac disease, GI resections); acanthocytosis; patients with abetalipoproteinemia. Low levels of vitamin E make the erythrocyte more susceptible to destruction by oxidants. Vitamin E deficiency may result in hemolysis; also consider the possibility of deficiency in spino-cerebellar syndromes.

Vitamin E requirements – The daily vitamin E requirement is related to the dietary intake of polyunsaturated fatty acids (PUFA), primarily linoleic acid. Vitamin E requirements may be increased in patients taking large doses of iron; diets containing selenium, sulfur-amino acids or antioxidants may decrease the daily requirement. Vitamin E supplementation has been effective in preventing the hemolytic anemia and relieving the edema and skin lesions which develop in low birthweight premature infants fed artificial formulas containing iron and high concentrations of PUFA. Commercial infant formulas currently available provide an adequate ratio of vitamin E to PUFA; formulas for premature infants have a lower level of iron to preclude interference with vitamin E use. Thus, there is no longer a need to routinely administer vitamin E supplementation to prevent anemia.

Indications:

Treatment of vitamin E deficiency.

Unlabeled uses: Vitamin E has been used in certain premature infants to reduce the toxic effects of oxygen therapy on the lung parenchyma (bronchopulmonary dysplasia) and the retina (retrolental fibroplasia). It has also been used to prevent hemolytic anemia in infants, and has been investigated for the prevention of periventricular hemorrhage in premature infants.

It has also been used in cancer, skin conditions, nocturnal leg cramps, sexual dysfunction, heart disease, aging, premenstrual syndrome and to increase athletic performance. However, data does not support use of vitamin E in these conditions.

Contraindications:

Vitamin E should not be administered IV, since the role of IV vitamin E in the deaths of 38 infants receiving the drug remains unclear.

Drug Interactions:

Oral anticoagulants: The hypoprothrombinemic effects may be increased, possibly with bleeding.

Adverse Reactions:

Hypervitaminosis E symptoms include fatigue, weakness, nausea, headache, blurred vision, flatulence and diarrhea.

Patient Information:

Swallow capsules whole; do not crush or chew.

Fat-Soluble Vitamins

VITAMIN E

Administration and Dosage:

Recommended dietary allowances (RDAs): Adult males, 15 IU; adult females, 12 IU. For a complete listing of RDAs by age, sex and condition, refer to the RDA table.

The potencies of the several forms of vitamin E vary; therefore, dosage is usually standardized in International Units (IU), based on activity. The following table indicates the relative potency of 1 mg of the various forms of vitamin E available:

Relative Potencies of Vitamin E	
1 mg dl-alpha tocopheryl acetate = 1 IU	1 mg d-alpha tocopherol = 1.49 IU
1 mg dl-alpha tocopherol = 1.1 IU	1 mg d-alpha tocopheryl acid succinate = 1.21 IU
1 mg d-alpha tocopheryl acetate = 1.36 IU	1 mg dl-alpha tocopheryl acid succinate = 0.89 IU

Free tocopherols can be oxidized and destroyed under adverse conditions; the esters available, acetate and succinate, are very stable in light. Keep in a dry, airtight container.

otc	**Vitamin E** (Various, eg, Schein)	**Tablets:** 200 IU[1]	In 100s.
		400 IU[1]	In 50s and 100s.
otc	**Vitamin E** (Various, eg, Dixon-Shane, Geneva Marsam, Schein)	**Capsules:** 100 IU[1]	In 100s, 250s, 500s and 1000s.
		200 IU[1]	In 100s, 250s, 500s and 1000s.
		400 IU[1]	In 50s, 60s, 90s, 100s, 250s, 500s, 1000s.
		500 IU[1]	In 100s and 1000s.
		600 IU[1]	In 60s, 100s, 250s and 1000s.
		1000 IU[1]	In 30s, 50s, 60s, 100s, 250s, 500s & 1000s.
otc	**Aquasol E** (Astra)	**Capsules:** 73.5 mg[2]	In 100s.
otc sf	**E-200 I.U. Softgels** (Nature's Bounty)	**Capsules:** 147 mg[2]	In 100s.
otc sf	**Amino-Opti-E** (Tyson)	**Capsules:** 165 mg[3]	In 100s.
otc	**Aquasol E** (Astra)	**Capsules:** 400 IU[1]	In 30s.
otc	**E-400 I.U. in a Water Soluble Base** (Nature's Bounty)		In 100s.
otc sf	**Vita-Plus E Softgels** (Scot-Tussin)	**Capsules:** 400 IU[1]	In 100s.
otc sf	**E-Complex-600** (Nature's Bounty)	**Capsules:** 600 IU[1]	In 50s.
otc sf	**E-1000 I.U. Softgels** (Nature's Bounty)	**Capsules:** 1000 IU[1]	In 50s.
otc	**One A Day Extras Vitamin E** (Bayer)	**Capsules, soft gel:** 400 IU vitamin E	(One A Day). In 60s.
otc	**Aquasol E** (Astra)	**Drops:** 50 mg[4] per ml	In 12 and 30 ml.

[1] Form of vitamin E unknown; content given in IU.
[2] As d-alpha tocopheryl acetate.
[3] As d-alpha tocopheryl acid succinate.
[4] As dl-alpha tocopheryl acetate.

Water-Soluble Vitamins

THIAMINE HCl (B_1)

Actions:

Pharmacology: Thiamine combines with adenosine triphosphate (ATP) to form thiamine pyrophosphate, a coenzyme. Its role in carbohydrate metabolism is the decarboxylation of pyruvic and alpha keto acids. An increase in serum pyruvic acid is one sign of the deficiency state. The need for thiamine is greater when the carbohydrate content of the diet is high. Significant B_1 depletion can occur in 3 weeks of total thiamine dietary absence.

Pharmacokinetics: Maximum oral absorption is 8 to 15 mg daily. Oral absorption may be increased by administering in divided doses with food. Tissue stores are saturated when intake exceeds minimal requirement ($\approx$ 1 mg/day); excess thiamine is excreted in urine. With normal renal function, 80% to 96% of an IV dose is excreted in urine.

Clinical trials: Beriberi, a deficiency state, is characterized by GI manifestations, peripheral neurologic changes and cerebral deficits. *Wet beriberi* includes cardiovascular symptoms characterized by dyspnea on exertion, palpitations, ECG abnormalities and high-output cardiac failure.

Wernicke's encephalopathy is characterized by horizontal nystagmus, bilateral sixth nerve palsy, ataxia and confusion. Conditions associated with development are excessive alcohol consumption, prolonged IV feeding, hyperemesis gravidarum, anorexia nervosa, prolonged fasting, refeeding after starvation and gastric plication.

Indications:

Treatment or prophylaxis of thiamine deficiency.

Parenteral: When the oral route is not feasible (eg, anorexia, nausea, vomiting, severe alcoholism, preoperative and postoperative conditions); impaired GI absorption in malabsorption syndromes; beriberi.

Unlabeled uses: Oral thiamine has been studied as a mosquito repellant; further verification is needed.

Contraindications:

Hypersensitivity to thiamine.

Warnings:

Sensitivity reactions can occur. Deaths have resulted from IV use. An intradermal test dose is recommended in patients with suspected sensitivity.

Wernicke's encephalopathy: Thiamine deficient patients may experience a sudden onset or worsening of Wernicke's encephalopathy following glucose administration; in suspected thiamine deficiency, administer thiamine before or along with dextrose-containing fluids.

Single vitamin B_1 deficiency is rare. Suspect multiple vitamin deficiencies.

Pregnancy: Category A (parenteral). Studies have not shown an increased risk of fetal abnormalities if administered during pregnancy. The possibility of fetal harm appears remote; however, use during pregnancy only if clearly needed.

Lactation: It is not known whether this drug is excreted in breast milk. Use with caution in nursing women.

Adverse Reactions:

Feeling of warmth; pruritus; urticaria; weakness; sweating; nausea; restlessness; tightness of the throat; angioneurotic edema; cyanosis; pulmonary edema; hemorrhage into the GI tract; cardiovascular collapse; death.

Parenteral: Some tenderness and induration may follow IM use.

Water-Soluble Vitamins

THIAMINE HCl (B_1)

Administration and Dosage:

Recommended dietary allowances (RDAs): Adult males, 1.2 to 1.5 mg; adult females, 1.1 mg. Thiamine is recommended at 0.5 mg/1000 Kcal intake. For a complete listing of RDAs by age, sex and condition, refer to the RDA table.

Wet beriberi with myocardial failure: Treat as an emergency cardiac condition. Administer 10 to 30 mg IV 3 times daily.

Beriberi: 10 to 20 mg IM 3 times/day for 2 weeks. Give an oral therapeutic multivitamin containing 5 to 10 mg thiamine daily for 1 month to achieve body tissue saturation.

Incompatibility: B_1 is unstable in neutral or alkaline solutions; do not use in combination with alkaline solutions (eg, **carbonates, citrates, barbiturates, erythromycin lactobionate IV**). Solutions containing sulfites are incompatible with thiamine.

otc	**Thiamine HCl** (Various, eg, Dixon-Shane, Freeda, Geneva Marsam, Genetco, Lilly, Major, Nature's Bounty, Purepac, Rugby, Schein)	**Tablets:** 50 mg	In 100s, 200s, 1000s and UD 100s.
		100 mg	In 100s, 250s, 500s, 1000s and UD 100s.
		250 mg	In 100s, 250s, 1000s and UD 100s & 1000s.
		500 mg	In 100s and 1000s.
otc	**Thiamilate** (Tyson)	**Tablets, enteric coated:** 20 mg	In 100s.
Rx	**Thiamine HCl** (Various, eg, Dixon-Shane, Elkins-Sinn, Goldline, Lilly, Major)	**Injection:** 100 mg per ml	In 1 ml amps and syringes and 1, 2, 10 and 30 ml vials.

[1] With 0.5% chlorobutanol.

RIBOFLAVIN (B_2)

Actions:

Pharmacology: Riboflavin functions in the body as a coenzyme in the forms of flavin adenine dinucleotide (FAD) and flavin mononucleotide (FMN), which play a vital metabolic role in numerous tissue respiration systems. Symptoms of riboflavin deficiency include corneal vascularization, cheilosis, glossitis and seborrheic dermatitis, especially in skin folds. Corneal vascularization is usually accompanied by itching and burning, blepharospasm and photophobia.

Indications:

Treatment and prevention of riboflavin deficiency.

Precautions:

Riboflavin deficiency seldom occurs alone and is often associated with deficiency of other B vitamins and protein.

Patient Information:

Riboflavin may cause a yellow/orange discoloration of the urine.

Administration and Dosage:

Recommended Dietary Allowances (RDAs): Adult males, 1.4 to 1.8 mg; adult females, 1.2 to 1.3 mg. For a complete listing of RDAs by age, sex or condition, refer to the RDA table.

Treatment of deficiency states: 5 to 25 mg daily.

otc	**Riboflavin** (Various, eg, Freeda, IDE, Nature's Bounty, Rugby)	**Tablets:** 25 mg	In 100s and 250s.
		50 mg	In 100s, 500s and 2500s.
		100 mg	In 100s, 250s and 500s.

Water-Soluble Vitamins

CALCIUM PANTOTHENATE (B_5; Pantothenic Acid)

Actions:

Pharmacology: Pantothenic acid is a precursor of coenzyme A, which is a cofactor for a variety of enzyme-catalyzed reactions involving transfer of acetyl groups. It is associated with oxidative metabolism of carbohydrates; gluconeogenesis; synthesis of fatty acids, sterols, steroid hormones and porphyrins.

Pantothenic acid deficiency has not been recognized in humans with a normal diet, due to the ubiquitous occurrence of this vitamin in ordinary foods. However, a deficiency syndrome was experimentally induced in volunteers. Symptoms included fatigue, headache, sleep disturbances, abdominal cramps, nausea and flatulence. Paresthesias in the extremities, muscle cramps and impaired coordination also occurred.

Indications:

Pantothenic acid deficiency.

Administration and Dosage:

The magnitude of need is not definitely known. From 4 to 7 mg/day has been recommended for adults.

otc	**Calcium Pantothenate** (Various, eg, Freeda, Rugby, Schein)	**Tablets:** 100 mg	In 100s.
		250 mg	In 100s.
		500 mg	In 100s.
otc *sf*	**Calcium Pantothenate** (Freeda)	**Tablets:** 25 mg	In 250s and 500s.
otc *sf*	**Calcium Pantothenate** (Freeda)	**Tablets:** 218 mg	In 100s, 250s and 500s.
		545 mg	In 100s, 250s and 500s.

Water-Soluble Vitamins

NIACIN (B_3; Nicotinic Acid)

Actions:

Pharmacology: Niacin, vitamin B_3, is the common name for nicotinic acid. Nicotinic acid functions in the body as a component of two coenzymes: NAD (nicotinamide adenine dinucleotide, coenzyme I) and NADP (nicotinamide adenine dinucleotide phosphate, coenzyme II), which serve a role in oxidation-reduction reactions essential for tissue respiration. Nicotinic acid is present in NAD and NADP in its active form, nicotinamide (niacinamide). The niacin deficiency state *pellagra* is characterized by mucous membrane, GI and CNS manifestations, a triad often referred to as dermatitis, diarrhea and dementia.

Although nicotinic acid and nicotinamide function identically as vitamins, their pharmacologic effects differ. In large doses (up to 6 g/day), nicotinic acid is effective in reduction of serum lipids (both LDL cholesterol and triglycerides; see Antihyperlipidemic Agents introduction). The mechanism of this action may involve: Decreased production of VLDL by the liver; inhibition of lipolysis in adipose tissue; decreased esterification of triglycerides by the liver; increased action of lipoprotein lipase. In large doses, peripheral vasodilation is produced, predominantly in the cutaneous vessels of the face, neck and chest. Nicotinic acid causes a release of histamine, which acts directly on peripheral vessels, producing vasodilation and increased blood flow. Nicotinamide does not affect blood lipid levels or cardiovascular system.

Pharmacokinetics: Niacin is rapidly absorbed from the GI tract; peak serum concentrations usually occur within 45 minutes. The plasma elimination half-life is about 45 minutes. The major metabolites include nicotinuric acid, N-methyl-nicotinamide and 2–pyridone. Approximately ⅓ of an oral dose is excreted unchanged in the urine.

The following prescribing information pertains primarily to therapeutic uses of niacin in doses exceeding basic nutritional intake (RDA levels).

Indications:

Correction of niacin acid deficiency; prevention and treatment of pellagra.

Nicotinic acid: Adjunctive therapy in patients with significant hyperlipidemia who do not respond adequately to diet and weight loss (see Antihyperlipidemic Agents).

Contraindications:

Hepatic dysfunction; active peptic ulcer.

Warnings:

Schizophrenia: There is no convincing evidence to support the use of megadoses of nicotinic acid in the treatment of schizophrenia as part of what is referred to as "orthomolecular psychiatry." Furthermore, high doses are associated with considerable toxicity, including liver damage, hypotension, peptic ulceration, hyperglycemia, hyperuricemia, dermatoses, cardiac arrhythmias, tachycardia, heartburn, nausea, vomiting, diarrhea and other effects commonly seen with lower doses such as flushing and pruritus.

Pregnancy: (Category C if used in doses above the RDA). Use doses in excess of nutritional requirements during pregnancy or lactation only when clearly needed and when potential benefits outweigh potential hazards to the fetus or nursing infant.

Children: Safety and efficacy in children have not been established in doses which exceed nutritional requirements.

Precautions:

Monitoring: Monitor liver function tests and blood glucose frequently.

Closely observe patients with coronary disease, gallbladder disease, a history of jaundice, liver disease, peptic ulcer or arterial bleeding.

Diabetes: Observe diabetic or potential diabetic patients closely for decreased glucose tolerance. Adjustment of diet or hypoglycemic therapy may be necessary.

Gout: Elevated uric acid levels have occurred; use caution in patients predisposed to gout.

Flushing appears frequently with oral therapy and may occur within the first 2 hours of administration. This is transient and will usually subside with continued therapy. The flush response can be attenuated with a dose of a prostaglandin inhibitor, such as aspirin, administered at a dose of approximately 325 mg 30 minutes to 1 hour before the niacin administration.

Tartrazine sensitivity: Some of these products contain tartrazine, which may cause allergic-type reactions (including bronchial asthma) in susceptible individuals. Although the incidence of tartrazine sensitivity in the general population is low, it is frequently seen in patients who also have aspirin hypersensitivity. Specific products containing tartrazine are identified in the product listings.

Water-Soluble Vitamins

NIACIN (B_3; Nicotinic Acid)

Drug Interactions:

Lovastatin: Coadministration of niacin may have resulted in rhabdomyolysis in one patient.

Sulfinpyrazone's uricosuric effect may be inhibited by nicotinic acid.

Adverse Reactions:

Flushing (see Precautions), pruritus and GI distress appear frequently with nicotinic acid oral therapy.

GI: Activation of peptic ulcer; nausea; vomiting; abdominal pain; diarrhea.

The hepatotoxicity of nicotinic acid (including cholestatic jaundice) has occurred with as little as 750 mg/day for < 3 months. Hepatitis occurred with sustained release nicotinic acid with as little as 500 mg/day for 2 months. Crystalline (non-sustained release) niacin may be less hepatotoxic.

Dermatologic: Severe generalized flushing; sensation of warmth; keratosis nigricans; pruritus; skin rash; dry skin; itching; tingling.

Body as a whole: Toxic amblyopia; hypotension; transient headache; atrial fibrillation and other cardiac arrhythmias; decreased glucose tolerance.

Lab test abnormalities: Decreased glucose tolerance; abnormalities of hepatic function tests; hyperuricemia.

Patient Information:

Cutaneous flushing and a sensation of warmth, especially in the area of the face, neck and ears, may occur within the first 2 hours. Itching or tingling and headache may also occur. These effects are transient and will usually subside with continued therapy.

May cause GI upset; take with meals.

If dizziness (postural hypotension) occurs, avoid sudden changes in posture.

Extended release products: Swallow whole; do not break, crush or chew.

Administration and Dosage:

Recommended Dietary Allowances (RDAs): Adult males, 15 to 20 mg; adult females, 13 to 15 mg. Niacin is recommended at 6.6 mg/1000 Kcal intake. For a complete listing of RDAs by age, sex and condition, refer to the RDA table.

Oral: Begin therapy with small doses and increase dose in gradual increments, observing for adverse effects and efficacy.

Niacin deficiency – up to 100 mg/day.
Pellagra – Up to 500 mg/day.
Hyperlipidemia – 1 to 2 g 3 times daily. Do not exceed 6 g/day.

Parenteral: Use only for vitamin deficiencies (not for treatment of hyperlipidemia) and when oral therapy is impossible. The length of parenteral treatment depends upon the patient's response and upon how soon oral medication and a complete and well balanced diet may be taken. Administer by slow IV injection, SC or IM. The IV route is recommended whenever possible.

otc	**Nicotinic Acid (Niacin)** (Various)	**Tablets:** 25 mg	In 100s, 1000s and UD 100s.
otc[1]	**Nicotinic Acid (Niacin)** (Various, eg, Freeda, Nature's Bounty)	**Tablets:** 50 mg	In 100s, 200s, 250s, 300s, 500s, 1000s and UD 100s, 250s and 1000s.
otc[1]	**Nicotinic Acid (Niacin)** (Various, eg, Dixon-Shane, Freeda, Nature's Bounty, Schein)	**Tablets:** 100 mg	In 100s, 250s, 300s, 500s, 1000s and UD 100s, 250s and 1000s.
otc[1]	**Nicotinic Acid (Niacin)** (Various, eg, Nature's Bounty)	**Tablets:** 250 mg	In 100s and 1000s.
otc[1]	**Nicotinic Acid (Niacin)** (Various, eg, Major)	**Tablets:** 500 mg	In 100s, 250s, 500s and 1000s.
Rx	**Niacor** (Upsher-Smith)		(Niacor). White, scored. In 100s.
Rx	**Nicolar** (Rhone-Poulenc Rorer)		Tartrazine. (NE). Yellow, scored. In 100s.

Water-Soluble Vitamins

NIACIN (B_3; Nicotinic Acid)

otc *sf*	**Slo-Niacin** (Upsher-Smith)	**Tablets, timed release:** 250 mg	Pink. In 100s and 1000s.
otc *sf*	**Slo-Niacin** (Upsher-Smith)	**Tablets, timed release:** 500 mg	Pink. In 100s and UD 100s.
otc *sf*	**Slo-Niacin** (Upsher-Smith)	**Tablets, timed release:** 750 mg	Pink. In 100s.
otc[1]	**Nicotinic Acid** (Niacin) (Various, eg, Dixon-Shane, Geneva Marsam, Goldline, Major, Moore, Schein, Vitarine)	**Capsules, timed release:** 125 mg	In 100s and 1000s.
otc	**Nicobid Tempules** (Rhone-Poulenc Rorer)		(2835/USV). Black/ clear. In 100s.
otc[1]	**Nicotinic Acid** (Niacin) (Various, eg, Dixon-Shane, Geneva Marsam, Major, Nature's Bounty, Parmed, Rugby, Schein, Vitarine)	**Capsules, timed release:** 250 mg	In 100s and 1000s.
otc	**Nicobid Tempules** (Rhone-Poulenc Rorer)		(2840/USV). Green/ clear. In 100s.
otc[1]	**Nicotinic Acid** (Niacin) (Various, eg, Dixon-Shane, Major, Moore, Parmed, Rugby, Vitarine)	**Capsules, timed release:** 400 mg	In 100s and 1000s.
otc	**Nia-Bid** (Roberts/Hauck)		In 100s.
otc	**Niacels** (Hauck)		In 100s.
otc	**Nico-400** (Jones Medical)		In 100s.
Rx	**Nicotinic Acid** (Niacin) (Various, eg, Goldline, Major, Nature's Bounty, Rugby, Schein)	**Capsules, timed release:** 500 mg	In 100s and 250s.
otc	**Nicobid Tempules** (Rhone-Poulenc Rorer)		(2841/USV). Blue/ white. In 100s.
otc	**Nicotinex** (Fleming)	**Elixir:** 50 mg/5 ml	14% alcohol. Sherry wine base. In pt and gal.
Rx	**Nicotinic Acid** (Niacin) (Various)	**Injection:** 100 mg/ml	In 30 ml vials.

[1] Some products may be available *Rx*, according to distributor discretion.

NICOTINAMIDE (Niacinamide)

Actions:

Pharmacology: Nicotinamide is used by the body as a source of niacin. Lipid metabolism, tissue respiration and glycogenolysis require nicotinamide. Nicotinamide does not have hypolipidemic or vasodilating effects.

Indications:

Prophylaxis and treatment of pellagra.

Administration and Dosage:

Therapeutic dose is 50 mg 3 to 10 times daily.

otc[1]	**Nicotinamide (Niacinamide)** (Various, eg, Freeda, Nature's Bounty, Rugby, Schein, Sidmak, UDL, Vangard, Vitarine)	**Tablets:** 50 mg	In 100s, 1000s and UD 100s.
		100 mg	In 100s, 1000s and UD 100s.
		125 mg	In 100s, 500s and 1000s.
		250 mg	In 100s, 500s and 1000s.
		500 mg	In 100s and 1000s.

[1] Some products may be available *Rx*, according to distributor discretion.

Water-Soluble Vitamins

PYRIDOXINE HCl (B_6)

Actions:

Pharmacology: Vitamin B_6 activity in natural substances , pyridoxine in plants, and pyridoxal or pyridoxamine in animals, are converted to physiologically active forms of vitamin B_6, pyridoxal phosphate (codecarboxylase) and pyridoxamine phosphate.

Vitamin B_6 acts as a coenzyme in the metabolism of protein, carbohydrates and fat. In protein metabolism, it participates in the decarboxylation of amino acids; conversion of tryptophan to niacin or serotonin (5-hydroxytryptamine); and deamination, transamination and transulfuration of amino acids. In carbohydrate metabolism, it is responsible for the breakdown of glycogen to glucose-1-phosphate.

The total adult body pool consists of 16 to 25 mg pyridoxine. The need for pyridoxine increases with the amount of protein in the diet.

Pharmacokinetics: Pyridoxine is readily absorbed from the GI tract. Its biologic half-life appears to be 15 to 20 days. Vitamin B_6 is degraded to 4–pyridoxic acid in the liver. This metabolite is excreted in the urine.

Indications:

Pyridoxine deficiency, including: Inadequate diet; drug-induced deficiency (eg, isoniazid, hydralazine, oral contraceptives); inborn errors of metabolism (eg, B_6-dependent seizures or B_6-responsive anemia).

The parenteral route is indicated when oral use is not feasible (eg, anorexia, nausea, vomiting, preoperative and postoperative conditions, impaired GI absorption).

Unlabeled uses:

Hydrazine poisoning. Although experience is limited, reversal of neurologic symptoms and CNS depression have been reported.

Premenstrual syndrome (PMS) has been treated with pyridoxine 40 to 500 mg/day, but with conflicting results.

Hyperoxaluria type I (and oxalate kidney stones) has been treated with pyridoxine in low doses (25 to 300 mg/day).

Nausea and vomiting in pregnancy is sometimes treated with pyridoxine.

Contraindications:

Sensitivity to pyridoxine.

Warnings:

Pregnancy: Category A. Pyridoxine requirements are increased during pregnancy and lactation. Pyridoxine varies in concentration in breast milk in response to changes in maternal intake of the vitamin. Use doses in excess of the RDA for lactating females with caution. Pyridoxine may inhibit lactation by prolactin suppression.

Children: Safety and efficacy have not been established for use in children.

Precautions:

Pyridoxine deficiency alone is rare; multiple vitamin deficiencies can be expected in any inadequate diet. Some drugs may result in increased pyridoxine requirements, including: Cycloserine, hydralazine, isoniazid, oral contraceptives and penicillamine.

Drug abuse and dependence: Noted in adults withdrawn from 200 mg/day.

Drug Interactions:

Pyridoxine Drug Interactions

Precipitant drug	Object drug*		Description
Pyridoxine	Levodopa	⬇	Pyridoxine reduces levodopa's effectiveness by increasing its peripheral metabolism; therefore, lower levels are available for CNS penetration. Avoid supplemental vitamins that contain > 5 mg pyridoxine per daily dose.
Pyridoxine	Phenobarbital	⬇	Phenobarbital serum levels may be decreased.
Pyridoxine	Phenytoin	⬇	Phenytoin serum levels may be decreased.

* ⬇ = Object drug decreased.

Adverse Reactions:

Sensory neuropathic syndromes; unstable gait; numb feet; awkwardness of hands; perioral numbness; decreased sensation to touch, temperature and vibration; paresthesia; somnolence; low serum folic acid levels.

Water-Soluble Vitamins

PYRIDOXINE HCl (B_6)

Overdosage:

Ataxia and severe sensory neuropathy have occurred in patients who had consumed pyridoxine (50 mg to 2 g) over a long period of time. When pyridoxine is discontinued, symptoms will lessen. It may take 6 months for sensation to normalize.

Administration and Dosage:

Recommended Dietary Allowances (RDAs): Adult males, 1.7 to 2 mg; adult females, 1.4 to 1.6 mg. Requirements are greater in persons having certain genetic defects or those receiving INH or oral contraceptives. For a complete listing of RDAs by age, sex and condition, see the RDA table.

Dietary deficiency: 10 to 20 mg daily for 3 weeks. Follow-up treatment is recommended daily for several weeks with an oral therapeutic multivitamin containing 2 to 5 mg pyridoxine. Correct poor dietary habits and encourage an adequate, well balanced diet.

Vitamin B_6 dependency syndrome: May require a therapeutic dosage of as much as 600 mg/day and 30 mg/day for life.

Deficiencies due to isoniazid: Some advocate pyridoxine prophylaxis for all isoniazid patients; others advocate prophylaxis only for those predisposed to neuropathy. Recommended prophylactic doses range from 6 to 100 mg daily, but the lower doses appear more common. Treatment of established neuropathy requires 50 to 200 mg daily.

INH poisoning (> 10 g), give an equal amount of pyridoxine: 4 g IV followed by 1 g IM every 30 minutes. Pyridoxine can be toxic, but doses of 70 to 357 mg/kg have been administered without incident.

otc	**Pyridoxine HCl** (Various, eg, Geneva Marsam)	**Tablets:** 25 mg	In 100s and 1000s.
otc	**Nestrex** (Fielding)		Dextrose. In 100s.
otc	**Pyridoxine HCl** (Various, eg, Geneva Marsam, Moore)	**Tablets:** 50 mg	In 100s and 1000s.
otc	**Pyridoxine HCl** (Various, eg, Moore, Schein)	**Tablets:** 100 mg	In 100s and 1000s.
otc	**Vitamin B_6** (Mission)	**Tablets, timed release:** 100 mg	In 100s.
Rx	**Pyridoxine HCl** (Various, eg, Major, Moore, Schein)	**Injection:** 100 mg/ml	In 10 and 30 ml vials.

[1] With 1.5% benzyl alcohol.

CYANOCOBALAMIN (B_{12})

Vitamin B_{12} is essential to growth, cell reproduction, hematopoiesis and nucleic acid and myelin synthesis. For use of vitamin B_{12} in treatment of pernicious anemia, see monograph in Blood Modifiers section.

Indications:

Nutritional vitamin B_{12} deficiency.

These products are NOT indicated for treatment of pernicious anemia.

Contraindications:

Hypersensitivity to cyanocobalamin.

Administration and Dosage:

Recommended Dietary Allowances (RDAs): Adults, 2 mcg. For a complete listing of RDAs by age, sex and condition, refer to the RDA table.

Nutritional deficiency: 25 to 250 mcg/day.

otc	**Vitamin B_{12}** (Various, eg, Dixon-Shane, Geneva, Rugby, Schein)	**Tablets:** 25 mcg	In 100s.
		50 mcg	In 100s and 1000s.
		100 mcg	In 100s and 1000s.
		250 mcg	In 100s.
otc	**Ener-B** (Nature's Bounty)	**Nasal gel:** 400 mcg/unit	In 0.1 ml units (12s)

Water-Soluble Vitamins

PARA-AMINOBENZOIC ACID (PABA)

Actions:

Pharmacology: This accessory food factor is found naturally associated with B complex vitamins. Small amounts are present in cereal, eggs, milk and meats. Detectable amounts are normally found in human blood, spinal fluid, urine and sweat.

PABA is a component of several biological systems and participates in a number of biologic processes. It is believed that PABA has an antifibrosis action due to mediation of increased oxygen uptake at the tissue level. Pathological fibrosis is believed to occur from either too much serotonin or too little monoamine oxidase (MAO) activity over a period of time. MAO requires an adequate supply of oxygen to function properly. By increasing oxygen supply at the tissue level, PABA enhances MAO activity and prevents, or causes, regression of fibrosis. These effects are speculative.

Indications:

Aminobenzoate potassium: "Possibly effective" in the treatment of scleroderma, dermatomyositis, morphea, linear scleroderma, pemphigus and Peyronie's disease.

Topical PABA is useful as a sunscreen (see Sunscreens section).

Contraindications:

Concurrent sulfonamide use (PABA inhibits the bacteriostatic activity of sulfonamides).

Warnings:

Renal function impairment: Use cautiously.

Pregnancy: Category C. Safety for use has not been established. Use only when clearly needed and when potential benefits outweigh potential hazards to the fetus.

Lactation: Use only when clearly needed.

Precautions:

Anorexia or nausea: Should anorexia or nausea occur, interrupt therapy until the patient is eating normally again. This avoids the possibility of hypoglycemia.

Hypersensitivity: If a hypersensitivity reaction occurs, discontinue the drug. Refer to Management of Acute Hypersensitivity Reactions.

Drug Interactions:

PABA Drug Interactions

Precipitant drug	Object drug*		Description
PABA	Dapsone	⬇	Dapsone's antimalarial effect may be antagonized by PABA due to interference with its primary mechanism of action.
PABA	Procainamide	⟷	PABA inhibits procainamide conversion to N-acetylprocainamide and it inhibits renal excretion of N-acetylprocainamide.

* ⬇ = Object drug decreased. ⟷ = Undetermined effect.

Water-Soluble Vitamins

PARA-AMINOBENZOIC ACID (PABA)

Adverse Reactions:

Anorexia, nausea, fever and rash (see Precautions).

Overdosage:

Nausea and vomiting are the most common events associated with overdose. Depression of the leukocyte count and an alleged fatal case of toxic hepatitis have occurred.

Administration and Dosage:

Take with food. Take tablets with an adequate amount of liquid to prevent GI upset.

Adults: 12 g daily in 4 to 6 divided doses. As a dietary supplement, take one tablet daily.

Children: 1 g/10 lb (4.55 kg) daily in divided doses.

Storage/Stability: Store powder in a tight, light-resistant container.

otc	**Para-Aminobenzoic Acid** (Various, eg, Freeda, Paddock, Rugby)	**Tablets:** 100 mg	In 100s and 250s.
		500 mg	In 100s.
		Powder	In 120 g.
Rx	**Potaba** (Glenwood)	**Tablets:** 500 mg[1]	In 100s and 1000s.
		Capsules: 500 mg[1]	In 250s and 1000s.
		Envules (Powder): 2 g[1]	In 50s.
		Powder[1]	In 100 g and 1 lb.

[1] As aminobenzoate potassium.

Water-Soluble Vitamins

VITAMIN C (Ascorbic Acid)

Actions:

Pharmacology: Vitamin C is an essential vitamin in man; however, its exact biological functions are not fully understood. It is essential for the formation and the maintenance of intercellular ground substance and collagen, for catecholamine biosynthesis, for synthesis of carnitine and steroids, for conversion of folic acid to folinic acid and for tyrosine metabolism.

The deficiency state *scurvy* is characterized by degenerative changes in the capillaries, bone and connective tissues. Mild vitamin C deficiency symptoms may include faulty bone and tooth development, gingivitis, bleeding gums and loosened teeth. Febrile states, chronic illness and infection increase the need for ascorbic acid. Premature and immature infants require relatively large amounts of the vitamin. Hemovascular disorders, burns and delayed fracture and wound healing are indications for an increase in daily intake.

Absorption of dietary ascorbate from the intestines is nearly complete. Vitamin C is readily available in citrus fruit, tomatoes, potatoes and leafy vegetables.

Indications:

Prevention and treatment of scurvy. Parenteral administration is desirable in an acute deficiency or when absorption of oral ascorbic acid is uncertain.

Unlabeled uses: Vitamin C in high doses has been advocated for prevention of the common cold, for treatment of asthma, atherosclerosis, wounds, schizophrenia and for treatment of cancer; however, clinical data do not justify these uses.

Vitamin C (≥ 2 g/day) may be used as a urinary acidifier with methenamine therapy. Data regarding the efficacy of ascorbic acid for this purpose are conflicting. Failure to significantly lower urine pH may be attributed to inadequate dosage (< 2 g/day).

Vitamin C in doses of at least 150 mg has been used to control idiopathic methemoglobinemia (less effective than methylene blue).

Warnings:

Excessive vitamin C doses: Diabetics, patients prone to recurrent renal calculi, those undergoing stool occult blood tests and those on sodium restricted diets or anticoagulant therapy should not take excessive doses of vitamin C over an extended period of time.

Pregnancy: Category C. It is not known whether ascorbic acid can cause fetal harm or can affect reproduction capacity. Give to pregnant women only if clearly needed.

Do not administer ascorbic acid to pregnant women in excess of the amount needed for treatment. The possibility of the fetus adapting to high levels of the vitamin could result in a scorbutic condition after birth when the intake drops to normal levels. This action is controversial.

Lactation: Administer with caution to a nursing mother. Ascorbic acid is excreted in breast milk, but does not necessarily increase in response to increasing doses.

Precautions:

Tartrazine sensitivity: Some of these products contain tartrazine, which may cause allergic type reactions (including bronchial asthma) in susceptible individuals. Although the incidence of sensitivity is low, it is frequently seen in patients who also have aspirin hypersensitivity. Specific products containing tartrazine are identified in the product listings.

Sulfite sensitivity: Some of these products contain sulfites which may cause allergic-type reactions in certain susceptible people. The overall prevalence of sulfite sensitivity in the general population is unknown and probably low. Sulfite sensitivity is seen more frequently in asthmatic than in nonasthmatic people.

Drug Interactions:

Contraceptives, oral and estrogens: Ascorbic acid increases serum levels of estrogen and estrogen contained in oral contraceptives, possibly resulting in adverse reactions.

Warfarin: The anticoagulant action of warfarin may be reduced.

Drug/Lab test interactions: Large doses (> 500 mg) of vitamin C may cause false-negative urine **glucose determinations.**

No exogenous vitamin C should be ingested for 48 to 72 hours before conducting amine-dependent stool **occult blood** tests, as false-negative results may occur.

Water-Soluble Vitamins

VITAMIN C (Ascorbic Acid)

Adverse Reactions:

Large doses may cause diarrhea and precipitation of cystine, oxalate or urate renal stones if the urine becomes acidic during therapy.

Transient mild soreness may occur at the site of IM or SC injection. Too rapid IV administration may cause temporary faintness or dizziness.

Administration and Dosage:

Recommended Dietary Allowances (RDAs): Adults, 60 mg. For a complete listing of RDAs by age, sex and condition, refer to the RDA table.

Administer IV, IM or SC. Avoid too rapid IV injection. Absorption and utilization are somewhat more efficient with the IM route, which is usually preferred.

Infants: Average daily protective requirement is 30 mg. The usual curative dose is 100 to 300 mg daily, continued as long as clinical symptoms persist or until saturation, as indicated by excretion tests, has been attained.

Premature infants: May require 75 to 100 mg/day.

Adults: The average protective dose is 70 to 150 mg daily. For scurvy, 300 mg to 1 g daily is recommended. However, up to 6 g/day has been administered parenterally to normal adults without evidence of toxicity.

Enhanced wound healing – Doses of 300 to 500 mg daily for 7 to 10 days both preoperatively and postoperatively are adequate, although considerably larger amounts have been recommended.

Burns – Individualize dosage. For severe burns, daily doses of 1 to 2 g are recommended.

In other conditions in which the need for vitamin C is increased, 3 to 5 times the daily optimum allowances appears adequate.

ASCORBIC ACID

Complete prescribing information for these products begins in the Vitamin C group monograph.

otc	**Ascorbic Acid** (Various, eg, Lannett)	**Tablets**: 25 mg	In 1000s.
otc	**Ascorbic Acid** (Various, eg, Goldline, Lannett)	**Tablets**: 50 mg	In 1000s and UD 100s.
otc	**Ascorbic Acid** (Various, eg, Century, Dixon-Shane, Lannett, UDL, West-Ward)	**Tablets**: 100 mg	In 100s, 500s, 1000s and UD 100s.
otc	**Ascorbic Acid** (Various, eg, Approved Pharm[1], Dixon-Shane, Geneva Marsam, Lannett, Moore, UDL, West-Ward)	**Tablets**: 250 mg	In 30s, 100s, 500s, 1000s and UD 100s.
otc	**Ascorbic Acid** (Various, eg, Approved Pharm[1], Century, Dixon-Shane, Geneva Marsam, Lannett, Lederle, Roxane, Rugby, UDL, West-Ward)	**Tablets**: 500 mg	In 100s, 250s, 500s, 1000s and UD 100s.
otc	**One A Day Extras Vitamin C** (Bayer)	**Tablets**: 500 mg	(One A Day). Lactose. In 100s.
otc	**Ascorbic Acid** (Various, eg, Approved Pharm.[1])	**Tablets**: 1000 mg	In 50s and 100s.
otc	**SunKist Vitamin C** (Ciba)	**Tablets, chewable**: 60 mg	Sorbitol, sucrose, lactose. Orange flavor. In 11s.
otc	**Ascorbic Acid** (Various, eg, Rugby)	**Tablets, chewable**: 100 mg	In 100s, 250s and 1000s.
otc	**Flavorcee** (Hudson)		Orange flavor. In 100s.

Water-Soluble Vitamins

ASCORBIC ACID

otc	**Ascorbic Acid** (Various, eg, Dixon-Shane, Geneva Marsam)	**Tablets, chewable:** 250 mg	In 100s and 1000s.
otc	**Flavorcee** (Hudson)		Orange flavor. In 250s.
otc	**Ascorbic Acid** (Various, eg, Dixon-Shane, Scientific Nutrition)	**Tablets, chewable:** 500 mg	In 90s, 100s and 1000s.
otc	**Flavorcee** (Hudson)		With rose hips. Sodium free. In 90s.
otc	**Ascorbic Acid** (Various, eg, Approved Pharm.[1])	**Tablets, timed release:** 500 mg	In 100s.
otc sf	**Ascorbic Acid Caplets**[1] (Approved Pharm.)	**Tablets, timed release:** 1000 mg	Sodium free. In 50s, 100s and 250s.
otc sf	**Ascorbic Acid Caplets** (Approved Pharm.)	**Tablets, timed release:** 1500 mg	Rose hips. Sodium free. In 50s.
otc	**SunKist Vitamin C** (Ciba)	**Caplets:** 500 mg	In 60s.
otc	**Ascorbic Acid** (Various, eg, Geneva Marsam)	**Capsules, timed release:** 500 mg	In 100s
otc	**Ascorbicap** (ICN)		Tartrazine. In 50s and 250s.
otc	**Cebid Timecelles** (Hauck)		In 100s.
otc	**Cevi-Bid** (Geriatric)		In 30s, 100s and 500s.
otc sf	**N'ice Vitamin C Drops** (SmithKline Beecham Consumer)	**Lozenges:** 60 mg	Menthol, sorbitol and tartrazine. Orange, lemon and grape flavors. In 16s.
otc sf	**C-Crystals** (Nature's Bounty)	**Crystals:** 5 g per teaspoon	In 180 g.
otc sf	**Vita-C** (Freeda)	**Crystals:** 4 g per teaspoonful	Sodium free. In 100 and 500 g.
otc sf	**Dull-C** (Freeda)	**Powder:** 4 g per teaspoonful	Sodium free. In 100 and 500 g.
otc	**Ce-Vi-Sol** (Mead Johnson Nutritional)	**Liquid:** 35 mg per 0.6 ml	5% alcohol. In 50 ml w/dropper.
otc	**Cecon** (Abbott)	**Solution:** 100 mg per ml	In 50 ml w/dropper.
otc	**Ascorbic Acid** (Various, eg, Rugby)	**Syrup:** 500 mg per 5 ml	In 120 and 480 ml.
Rx	**Ascorbic Acid** (Various, eg, Loch, Lyphomed, Pasadena)	**Injection:** 250 mg per ml	In 2 ml amps and 2 and 30 ml vials.
Rx	**Ascorbic Acid** (Various, eg, American Regent, Major, Pasadena, Schein)		In 2 ml amps and 50 ml vials.

[1] With or without rose hips.
[2] With 0.5% sodium hydrosulfite.

Water-Soluble Vitamins

SODIUM ASCORBATE

Complete prescribing information for these products begins in the Vitamin C group monograph.

otc sf	**Sodium Ascorbate** (Freeda)	**Tablets**: 585 mg (equiv. to 500 mg ascorbic acid)	Buffered. In 100s, 250s and 500s.
otc sf	**Sodium Ascorbate** (Freeda)	**Crystals**: 1020 mg (equiv. to 900 mg ascorbic acid) per ¼ teaspoonful	Buffered. In 120 and 480 g.
Rx	**Sodium Ascorbate** (Various, eg, Interstate)	**Injection**: 250 mg/ml (equiv. to 222 mg/ml ascorbic acid)	In 30 ml vials.
Rx	**Cenolate** (Abbott)	**Injection**: 562.5 mg per ml (equiv. to 500 mg/ml ascorbic acid)	In 1 and 2 ml amps.[1]

[1] With 0.5% sodium hydrosulfite.

CALCIUM ASCORBATE

Complete prescribing information for these products begins in the Vitamin C group monograph.

otc sf	**Calcium Ascorbate** (Freeda)	**Tablets**: 610 mg (equiv. to 500 mg ascorbic acid)	Buffered. Sodium free. In 100s, 250s and 500s.
otc sf	**Calcium Ascorbate** (Freeda)	**Powder**: 1 g (equiv. to 826 mg ascorbic acid) per ¼ teaspoonful	Buffered. In 120, 480 g.

Water-Soluble Vitamins

ASCORBIC ACID COMBINATIONS

Complete prescribing information for these products begins in the Vitamin C group monograph.

otc	**Chewable C** (Approved Pharm.)	**Tablets, chewable:** 100 mg vitamin C as sodium ascorbate and ascorbic acid	Sugar, fructose. Orange flavor. In 100s.
otc	**Chewable C** (Approved Pharm.)	**Tablets, chewable:** 250 mg vitamin C as sodium ascorbate and ascorbic acid	Orange flavor. In 100s.
otc	**Chewable C** (Approved Pharm.)	**Tablets, chewable:** 300 mg vitamin C as ascorbic acid and sodium ascorbate with rose hips	Lemon flavor. In 100s.
otc	**Chewable C** (Approved Pharm.)	**Tablets, chewable:** 500 mg vitamin C as sodium ascorbate and ascorbic acid	Orange flavor. In 100s.
otc	**SunKist Vitamin C** (Ciba)	**Tablets, chewable:** 250 mg vitamin C as sodium ascorbate and ascorbic acid	Fructose, sorbitol, sucrose, lactose. Orange flavor. In 60s.
otc	**SunKist Vitamin C** (Ciba)	**Tablets, chewable:** 500 mg vitamin C as sodium ascorbate and ascorbic acid	Fructose, sorbitol, sucrose, lactose. Orange flavor. In 60s.
otc	**C-Max** (Bio-Tech)	**Tablets, gradual release:** 1000 mg vitamin C, 40 mg magnesium, 5 mg zinc, 10 mg potassium, 1 mg manganese and 10 mg pectin in a rose hips base	In 100s.
otc	**Vicks Vitamin C Drops** (Richardson-Vicks)	**Lozenges:** 60 mg vitamin C as sodium ascorbate and ascorbic acid	Orange or lemon flavor. In 14s and 30s.

Water-Soluble Vitamins

BIOFLAVONOIDS (Vitamin P)

Citrus bioflavonoids, formerly referred to as Vitamin P, are derived from the rind of green citrus fruits, and are also found in rose hips and black currants.

These products were previously used to decrease capillary permeability and fragility and were classified as hemostatic agents. Their mechanism of action is unknown.

Unlabeled uses: This group of compounds has been widely used for many diseases including: Rheumatic fever; decidual bleeding in pregnancy; habitual abortion; poliomyelitis; prevention of hemorrhage in anticoagulated patients; rheumatoid arthritis; periodontal disease; diabetic retinitis; various thrombocytopenic and nonthrombocytopenic hemorrhagic disorders; herpes labialis. Unfortunately, many of these uses have not been tested in controlled clinical trials; hence, *there is little evidence that they are effective for any indication. There is no established need in human nutrition.*

otc	**Citro-Flav 200** (Goldline)	**Capsules**: 200 mg citrus bioflavonoids complex	In 100s.
otc sf	**Pan C-500** (Freeda)	**Tablets**: 100 mg hesperidin, 100 mg citrus bioflavonoids, and 500 mg vitamin C	Sodium free. In 100s, 250s and 500s.
otc	**Amino-Opti-C** (Tyson)	**Tablets, sustained release**: 250 mg lemon bioflavonoids, rutin, hesperidin, 1000 mg vitamin C and rose hips powder	In 100s.
otc sf	**C Factors "1000" Plus** (Solgar)	**Tablets**: 1000 mg vitamin C with rose hips, 250 mg citrus bioflavonoids, 50 mg rutin, 25 mg hesperidin complex	Sodium free. Capsule shape. In 50s, 100s and 250s.
otc	**Peridin-C** (Beutlich)	**Tablets**: 150 mg hesperidin complex, 50 mg hesperidin methyl chalcone (bioflavonoids) and 200 mg ascorbic acid	In 100s and 500s.
otc sf	**Span C** (Freeda)	**Tablets**: 300 mg citrus bioflavonoids and 200 mg vitamin C (ascorbic acid; from rose hips)	Sodium free. In 100s, 250s and 500s.
otc sf	**Flavons-500** (Freeda)	**Tablets**: 500 mg citrus bioflavonoids complex and hesperidin complex	Sodium free. In 100s and 250s.
otc sf	**C Speridin** (Marlyn)	**Tablets, sustained release**: 100 mg hesperidin, 100 mg lemon bioflavonoids and 500 mg ascorbic acid	In 100s.
otc sf	**Super Complex C–500 Caplets** (Approved Pharm.)	**Tablets**: 25 mg citrus hesperidin complex; 100 mg citrus bioflavonoid complex; 50 mg rutin; 500 mg ascorbic acid; 100 mg rose hips, acerola, green pepper and black currant concentrate	Sodium free. In 100s.
otc sf	**Citrus-flav C 500** (Fibertone)	**Tablets**: 200 mg citrus bioflavonoids complex, 200 mg vitamin C, 40 mg hesperidin complex, 50 mg acerola, 10 mg rutin in a citrus base of orange and lemon powder, grapefruit concentrate powder and citrus pectin	Sodium free. In 100s and 250s.

Water-Soluble Vitamins

BIOFLAVONOIDS (Vitamin P)

otc	**Bio-Acerola C Complex** (Solgar)	**Wafers**: 500 mg vitamin C, 10 mg citrus bioflavonoids, 5 mg rutin in a natural base of acerola, rose hips, buckwheat, black currant and green pepper concentrate powders	Cane sugar. Cherry flavoring. In 50s and 100s.
otc	**Super Citro Cee** (Marlyn)	**Tablets, sustained release**: 500 mg lemon bioflavonoids, 50 mg rutin, 500 mg ascorbic acid and 500 mg rose hips powder	In 50s, 100s and 200s.
otc sf	**Ester-C Plus** (Solgar)	**Capsules**: 500 mg vitamin C, 25 mg citrus bioflavonoid complex, 10 mg acerola, 10 mg rose hips, 5 mg rutin, 62 mg calcium	Sodium free. In 50s.
otc sf	**Extra Potency Ester-C Plus** (Solgar)	**Tablets**: 1000 mg vitamin C, 200 mg citrus bioflavonoid complex, 25 mg acerola, 25 mg rutin, 25 mg rose hips, 125 mg calcium	Sodium free. In 30s.
otc sf	**Ester-C Plus Multi-Mineral** (Solgar)	**Capsules**: 425 mg vitamin C, 50 mg citrus bioflavonoid complex, 12.5 mg acerola, 12.5 mg rose hips, 5 mg rutin, 25 mg calcium, 13 mg magnesium, 12.5 mg potassium, 2.5 mg zinc	Sodium free. In 60s.
otc sf	**Quercetin** (Freeda)	**Tablets**: 50 mg bioflavonoid (from eucalyptus)	Sodium free. In 100s and 250s.
		250 mg bioflavonoid (from eucalyptus)	Sodium free. In 100s and 250s.

CALCIUM

For information on parenteral calcium products, refer to Intravenous Nutritional Therapy, Electrolytes section.

Actions:

Pharmacology: Calcium is the fifth most abundant element in the body; the major fraction is in bone. It is essential for the functional integrity of the nervous and muscular systems, for normal cardiac function, for cell permeability and for blood coagulation. It also functions as an enzyme cofactor and affects the secretory activity of endocrine and exocrine glands.

Adequate calcium intake is particularly important during periods of bone growth in childhood and adolescence, and during pregnancy and lactation. An adeauate supply of calcium is necessary in adults, especially those over 40 years of age, to prevent a negative calcium balance which may contribute to the development of osteoporosis.

Patients with advanced renal insufficiency exhibit phosphate retention and some degree of hyperphosphatemia. The retention of phosphate plays a pivotal role in causing secondary hyperparathyroidism associated with osteodystrophy and soft tissue calcification. Calcium acetate, when taken with meals, combines with dietary phosphate to form insoluble calcium phosphate which is excreted in the feces.

Elemental Calcium Content of Calcium Salts

Calcium salt	% Calcium	mEq Ca^{++}/g
Calcium glubionate	6.5	3.3
Calcium gluconate	9.3	4.6
Calcium lactate	13	9.2
Calcium citrate	21	12
Calcium acetate	25	12.6
Tricalcium phosphate	39	19.3
Calcium carbonate	40	20

Calcium must be in a soluble, ionized form to be absorbed. Solubility (except calcium lactate) is increased by acidic pH. Give with meals to maximize acidity and solubility. Differences in absorption and bioavailability between various calcium salts appear to exist, as well as between different preparations of the same salt.

Indications:

As a dietary supplement when calcium intake may be inadequate (eg, childhood and adolescence, chronic renal failure, pregnancy, lactation, postmenopausal females, the aged).

In the treatment of calcium deficiency states which may occur in diseases such as: Tetany of newborn; end stage renal disease, mild to moderate renal insufficiency; renal osteodystrophy; acute and chronic hypoparathyroidism; pseudohypoparathyroidism; postmenopausal and senile osteoporosis; rickets and osteomalacia. Some studies have suggested that the use of calcium citrate is more effective than calcium carbonate in the treatment of postmenopausal osteoporosis.

Calcium acetate (PhosLo): Control of hyperphosphatemia in end stage renal failure; does not promote aluminum absorption.

Unlabeled uses: Calcium supplementation may lower blood pressure in some hypertensive patients with indices suggesting calcium "deficiency." However, other hypertensives may experience a pressor response.

In one study, calcium administration significantly reduced premenstrual symptoms of fluid retention, pain and negative affect.

Contraindications:

Renal calculi; hypophosphatemia; hypercalcemia.

Warnings:

PhosLo: End stage renal failure patients may develop hypercalcemia when given calcium with meals. Do not give other calcium supplements concurrently with *PhosLo*. Chronic hypercalcemia may lead to vascular and other soft tissue calcification. Monitor serum calcium levels twice weekly during the early dose adjustment period. Do not allow serum calcium times phosphate product to exceed 66.

Pregnancy: Category C (PhosLo). It is not known whether *PhosLo* can cause fetal harm when administered to a pregnant woman or can affect reproduction capacity. Give to a pregnant woman only if clearly needed.

Precautions:

Hypercalcemia/hypercalciuria may result when therapeutic amounts are given for prolonged periods; it is most likely to occur in hypoparathyroid patients receiving high doses of vitamin D. Avoid by frequent monitoring of plasma and urine calcium levels. For symptoms and treatment refer to the vitamin D monograph.

CALCIUM

Calcium citrate:

Renal function impairment – Avoid concurrent aluminum-containing antacids.

Drug Interactions:

Calcium Drug Interactions			
Precipitant	Object drug*		Description
Thiazide diuretics	Calcium salts	⬆	Hypercalcemia resulting from renal tubular reabsorption, or bone release of calcium by thiazides may be amplified by exogenous calcium.
Calcium salts	Atenolol	⬇	Mean peak plasma levels and bioavailability of atenolol may be decreased, possibly resulting in decreased beta blockade.
Calcium salts	Iron salts	⬇	GI absorption of iron may be reduced.
Calcium carbonate	Quinolones	⬇	The bioavailability of norfloxacin may be reduced; ciprofloxacin and ofloxacin do not appear to be affected.
Calcium salts	Sodium polystyrene sulfonate	⬇	Coadministration in patients with renal impairment may result in an unanticipated metabolic alkalosis and a reduction of the resin's binding of potassium.
Calcium salts	Tetracyclines	⬇	The absorption and serum levels of tetracyclines are decreased; a decreased anti-infective response may occur.
Calcium salts	Verapamil	⬇	Clinical effects and toxicities of verapamil may be reversed.

* ⬆ = Object drug increased. ⬇ = Object drug decreased.

Drug/Food interactions: Diets high in dietary fiber have been shown to decrease absorption of calcium due to decreased transit time in the GI tract and complexing of fiber with the calcium.

Adverse Reactions:

GI disturbances are rare. Mild hypercalcemia ($Ca^{++} > 10.5$ mg/dl) may be asymptomatic or manifest itself as: Anorexia; nausea; vomiting; constipation; abdominal pain; dry mouth; thirst; polyuria. More sever hypercalcemia ($Ca^{++} > 12$ mg/dl) is associated with confusion, delirium, stupor and coma.

The risk of hypercalcemia with calcium acetate may be less than that of calcium carbonate and calcium citrate.

Overdosage:

Administration of *PhosLo* in excess of the appropriate daily dosage can cause severe hypercalcemia (see Adverse Reactions). Severe hypercalcemia can be treated by acute hemodialysis and discontinuing therapy.

Patient Information:

Notify physician if any of the following occurs: Anorexia, nausea, vomiting, constipation, abdominal pain, dry mouth, thirst or polyuria.

Take with or following meals to enhance absorption.

Take with a large glass of water.

Administration and Dosage:

Recommended Dietary Allowances (RDAs): Adults (25 to > 51 years of age), 800 mg. For a complete listing of RDAs by age, sex and condition, refer to the RDA table.

Dietary supplement: The usual daily dose is 500 mg to 2 g, 2 to 4 times daily.

An NIH Consensus Development conference recommends a calcium intake for adults of 1000 to 1500 mg/day to reduce bone loss associated with aging.

PhosLo: 2 tablets with each meal. The dosage may be increased to bring the serum phosphate value < 6 mg/dl, as long as hypercalcemia does not develop. Most patients require 3 to 4 tablets with each meal.

CALCIUM GLUBIONATE, 6.5% calcium.

Complete prescribing information for these products begins in the Calcium group monograph.

otc	**Neo-Calglucon** (Sandoz)	**Syrup**: 1.8 g calcium glubionate (115 mg calcium) per 5 ml	Saccharin, sorbitol, sucrose. In 480 ml.

CALCIUM GLUCONATE, 9% calcium.

Complete prescribing information for these products begins in the Calcium group monograph.

otc	**Calcium Gluconate** (Various, eg, Dixon-Shane, Genetco, Lannett, Lilly, Major, Roxane, Rugby, Schein, URL, West-Ward)	**Tablets**: 500 mg (45 mg calcium)	In 100s, 1000s and UD 100s.
		650 mg (58.5 mg calcium)	In 100s, 1000s and UD 100s.
		975 mg (87.75 mg calcium)	In 100s, 500s, 1000s and UD 100s.
		1 g (90 mg calcium)	In 1000s.

CALCIUM LACTATE, 13% calcium.

Complete prescribing information for these products begins in the Calcium group monograph.

otc	**Calcium Lactate** (Various, eg, Dixon-Shane, Geneva Marsam, Rugby)	**Tablets**: 325 mg (42.25 mg calcium)	In 1000s.
		650 mg (84.5 mg calcium)	In 100s and 1000s.

CALCIUM CITRATE, 21% calcium.

Complete prescribing information for these products begins in the Calcium group monograph.

otc	**Citracal** (Mission)	**Tablets**: 950 mg (200 mg calcium)	In 100s.
otc	**Citracal Liquitab** (Mission)	**Tablets, effervescent**: 2376 mg (500 mg calcium)	Aspartame (12 mg phenylalanine). Citrus flavor. In 30s.

CALCIUM ACETATE, 25% calcium.

Complete prescribing information for these products begins in the Calcium group monograph.

otc	**Calphron** (Nephro-Tech)	**Tablets**: 667 mg (169 mg calcium)	In 200s.
Rx	**PhosLo** (Braintree)		In 200s.

TRICALCIUM PHOSPHATE (Calcium Phosphate, Tribasic), 39% calcium.

Complete prescribing information for these products begins in the Calcium group monograph.

otc *sf*	**Posture** (Whitehall)	**Tablets**: 1565.2 mg (600 mg calcium)	In 60s.

CALCIUM CARBONATE, 40% calcium.

Complete prescribing information for these products begins in the Calcium group monograph.

For calcium carbonate antacids, see the Antacids monograph.

otc sf	**FemCal** (Freeda)	**Tablets:** 250 mg (100 mg calcium)	100 IU vitamin D_3, B, 100 mg Mg, Mn, Si. Kosher. In 100s and 250s.
otc	**Calcium Carbonate** (Various, eg, Rugby)	**Tablets:** 650 mg (260 mg calcium)	In 1000s.
otc sf	**Calciday-667** (Nature's Bounty)	**Tablets:** 667 mg (266.8 mg calcium)	In 60s.
otc	**Calcium Carbonate** (Roxane)	**Tablets:** 1.25 g (500 mg calcium)	Film coated. In 100s and UD 100s.
otc	**Os-Cal 500** (SK-Beecham)		Corn syrup. (OsCal). In 60s and 120s.
otc sf	**Oyst-Cal 500** (Goldline)		Tartrazine. Lime green. Film coated. Oblong. In 60s, 120s and 1000s.
otc sf	**Oystercal 500** (Nature's Bounty)		In 60s.
otc	**Oyster Shell Calcium-500** (Vangard)		In 100s, UD 100s and 640s.
otc	**Calcium 600** (Various, eg, Dixon-Shane, Major, Rugby, Schein)	**Tablets:** 1.5 g (600 mg calcium)	In 60s, 120s and 1000s.
otc	**Cal-Plus** (Geriatric Pharm.)		In 100s.
otc sf	**Caltrate 600** (Lederle)		(LL C 600). Film coated. In 60s.
otc	**Gencalc 600** (Goldline)		White. Film coated. Oblong. In 60s.
otc	**Nephro-Calci** (R & D)		In 100s and 500s.
otc	**Caltrate, Jr.** (Lederle)	**Tablets, chewable:** 750 mg (300 mg calcium)	(LL). Orange flavor. In 60s.
otc	**Calci-Chew** (R & D)	**Tablets, chewable:** 1.25 g (500 mg calcium)	Sugar. Assorted flavors. In 100s.
otc	**Os-Cal 500** (SK-Beecham)		Dextrose. (OsCal). Bavarian cream/coconut flavor. In 60s.
otc	**Oysco 500** (Rugby)		In 60s.
otc	**Tums 500** (SK-Beecham)		Sucrose, < 4 mg sodium. Cherry flavor. In 60s.
otc	**Cal-Guard Softgels** (Rugby)	**Capsules:** 125 mg calcium (50 mg calcium)	In 60s.
otc	**Calci-Mix** (R & D)	**Capsules:** 1250 mg powdered calcium carbonate (500 mg calcium)	To be mixed with food. In 100s.
otc	**Calcium Carbonate** (Roxane)	**Oral Suspension:** 1.25 g (500 mg calcium) per 5 ml	Sorbitol. In 500 ml and UD 5 ml.
otc	**Cal Carb-HD** (Konsyl Pharm)	**Powder:** 6.5 g (2400 mg calcium) per packet	Simethicone. In 210 g bottles and 7 g packets.
otc	**Florical** (Mericon)	**Capsules and tablets:** 364 mg calcium carbonate (145.6 mg calcium) and 8.3 mg sodium fluoride *Dose:* 1 capsule or tablet daily.	In 100s and 500s.

PHOSPHORUS REPLACEMENT PRODUCTS

For information on parenteral phosphate, refer to the monograph in the IV Nutritional Therapy section.

Actions:

Pharmacology: Phosphorus is an important component of all cells in the body; 80% to 85% of body phosphorus is present in the skeletal system. The remainder functions intracellularly for 1) Energy transport and production in the form of ATP and ADP; 2) phospholipids in cell membranes responsible for nutrient transport; 3) part of nucleic acids (RNA, DNA); 4) buffering systems and calcium transport.

Phosphate administration lowers urinary calcium levels and increases urinary phosphate levels and urinary pyrophosphate inhibitor. Orthophosphates appear to decrease the aggregation and number of oxalate crystals in the urine of calculous patients.

Indications:

Dietary supplements of phosphorus, particularly if the diet is restricted or if needs are increased.

Contraindications:

Addison's disease; hyperkalemia; acidification of urine in urinary stone disease; patients with infected urolithiasis or struvite stone formation; severely impaired renal function (< 30% of normal); presence of hyperphosphatemia.

Warnings:

Pregnancy: Category C. It is not known whether this product can cause fetal harm or can affect reproduction capacity when administered to a pregnant woman. Use only when clearly needed.

Lactation: It is not known whether this drug is excreted in breast milk. Exercise caution when administering to a nursing woman.

Precautions:

Monitoring: The following determinations are important in patient monitoring (other tests may be warranted in some patients): Renal function; serum calcium; serum phosphorus; serum potassium; serum sodium. Monitor at periodic intervals during therapy.

Sodium/Potassium restriction: Use with caution if patient is on sodium or potassium restricted diet. These products provide significant amounts of sodium or potassium.

Special risk patients: Use with caution when the following medical problems exist: Cardiac disease (particularly in digitalized patients); acute dehydration; renal function impairment or chronic renal disease; extensive tissue breakdown; myotonia congenita; cardiac failure; cirrhosis of the liver or severe hepatic disease; peripheral and pulmonary edema; hypernatremia; hypertension; preeclampsia; hypoparathyroidism; osteomalacia; acute pancreatitis; rickets (rickets may benefit from phosphate therapy; however, use caution).

Kidney stones: Warn patients with kidney stones of the possibility of passing old stones when phosphate therapy is started.

Drug Interactions:

Phosphate Drug Interactions

Precipitant drug	Object drug*		Description
Antacids	Phosphates	⬇	Antacids containing magnesium, aluminum or calcium may bind the phosphate and prevent its absorption.
Calcium Vitamin D	Phosphates	⬇	The effects of phosphates may be antagonized in the treatment of hypercalcemia.
Potassium-containing agents Potassium-sparing diuretics	Phosphates	⬆	Hyperkalemia may occur with concurrent use. Periodically monitor patient's serum potassium level.

* ⬆ = Object drug increased. ⬇ = Object drug decreased.

PHOSPHORUS REPLACEMENT PRODUCTS

Adverse Reactions:

Individuals may experience a mild laxative effect for the first few days. If this persists, reduce the daily intake until this effect subsides, or, if necessary, discontinue use.

GI upset (eg, diarrhea, nausea, stomach pain, vomiting) may occur with phosphate therapy. The following side effects have been reported less frequently: Headaches; dizziness; mental confusion; seizures; weakness or heaviness of legs; unusual tiredness or weakness; muscle cramps; numbness, tingling, pain or weakness of hands or feet; numbness or tingling around lips; fast or irregular heartbeat; shortness of breath or troubled breathing; swelling of feet or lower legs; unusual weight gain; low urine output; unusual thirst; bone and joint pain (possible phosphate-induced osteomalacia). High serum phosphate levels may increase the incidence of extraskeletal calcification.

Administration and Dosage:

Recommended dietary allowances (RDAs): Adults, 800 to 1200 mg. For a complete listing of RDAs by age, sex and condition, refer to the RDA table.

In the product table, contents given per capsule, tablet or 75 ml reconstituted liquid.

Capsules must be reconstituted. Do *not* swallow capsules. Refer to manufacturers' labeling for reconstitution of capsules and powder.

	Product and distributor	Phosphorus		Potassium		Sodium		Recommended adult dose	How supplied
		mg	mM	mg	mEq	mg	mEq		
Rx	**Uro-KP-Neutral[1] Tablets** (Star)	250	8	49.4	1.27	250.5	10.9	1 or 2 tablets 4 times daily with full glass of water	Peach. Film coated. Capsule shape. In 100s.
Rx	**K-Phos Neutral[2] Tablets** (Beach)	250	8	45	1.1	298	13		(Beach 1125). White, scored. Film coated. Capsule shape. In 100s and 500s.
otc sf	**Neutra-Phos[3] Powder** (Willen)	250	8	278	7	164	7	1 capsule or 1 powder packet reconstituted in 75 ml water 4 times daily. Provides 250 mg phosphorus per dose (1 g daily)	Fruit flavor. In 64 g bottle and 1.25 g packets.
otc sf	**Neutra-Phos-K[4] Powder** (Willen)	250	8	556	14.25	0	0		In 71 g bottle and 1.45 g packets (100s).

[1] From disodium and dipotassium phosphate anhydrous and monobasic sodium anhydrous.

[2] From dibasic sodium phosphate anhydrous, monobasic sodium phosphate and monobasic potassium phosphate monohydrate.

[3] From monobasic and dibasic sodium and potassium phosphates.

[4] From dibasic and monobasic potassium phosphates.

FLUORIDE

Actions:

Pharmacology: Sodium fluoride acts systemically before tooth eruption, and topically posteruption, by increasing tooth resistance to acid dissolution, by promoting remineralization and by inhibiting the cariogenic microbial process. Acidulation provides greater topical fluoride uptake by dental enamel than neutral solutions. Phosphate protects enamel from demineralization by the acidulated formulation. Topical application of fluoride works superficially on enamel and plaque, and can reduce dental caries by 30% to 40%. Fluoride supplements may reduce the incidence of caries by up to 60%.

Pharmacokinetics: Fluoride is absorbed in the GI tract, lungs and skin. About 90% of oral fluoride is absorbed in the stomach. Absorption is related to solubility; sodium fluoride is almost completely absorbed. Calcium, iron or magnesium ions may delay absorption. Following ingestion, 50% of fluoride is deposited in bone and teeth. The major route of excretion is the kidneys; it is also excreted by sweat glands, the GI tract and in breast milk.

Indications:

Prevention of dental caries: Both neutral and acidulated phosphate fluoride effectively control dental decay. Use where water supplies are low in fluoride (< 0.7 ppm). Fluoride also controls rampant dental decay which frequently follows xerostomia-producing radiotherapy of head and neck tumors.

In communities without fluoridated water, the American Dental Association's Council on Dental Therapeutics recommends continuing fluoride supplements until the age of 13; the American Academy of Pediatrics recommends supplementation until 16 years of age.

Unlabeled uses: Sodium fluoride may be effective in treating osteoporosis. Doses (as fluoride) up to 60 mg daily or more are used in conjunction with calcium supplements, vitamin D or estrogen. However, large doses may result in a higher frequency of side effects. Some data suggest that doses < 50 mg/day are efficacious with fewer adverse reactions. No commercially available products contain high sodium fluoride doses for this use; therefore a large number of tablets would be required to obtain this dosage. Fluoride supplementation is not recommended for the prophylaxis of osteoporosis due to the potential for increased incidence of fractures (see Precautions).

Contraindications:

When the fluoride content of drinking water exceeds 0.7 ppm; low sodium or sodium free diets; hypersensitivity to fluoride.

Do not use 1 mg tablets in children < 3 years old or when the drinking water fluoride content is ≥ 0.3 ppm. Do not use 1 mg/5 ml rinse (as a supplement) in children < 6 years old.

Warnings:

Pregnancy: Consult physician before using.

Lactation: Consult physician before using.

Children: See Contraindications.

Precautions:

Fractures: Some epidemiological studies suggest that the incidence of certain types of bone fractures (crippling skeletal fluorosis) may be higher in some communities with naturally high or adjusted fluoride levels. However, other studies have not detected increased incidence of bone fractures. Crippling skeletal fluorosis is more common in parts of the world with high natural fluoride (> 10 ppm), but is extremely rare in the US.

Mucositis: Gingival tissues may be hypersensitive to some flavors or alcohol.

Tartrazine sensitivity: Some of these products contain tartrazine, which may cause allergic-type reactions (including bronchial asthma) in susceptible individuals. Although the incidence of tartrazine sensitivity in the general population is low, it is frequently seen in patients who also have aspirin hypersensitivity. Specific products containing tartrazine are identified in the product listings.

Drug Interactions:

Drug/Food interactions: Incompatibility of dairy foods with systemic fluoride has occurred due to formation of calcium fluoride, which is poorly absorbed.

FLUORIDE

Adverse Reactions:

Dermatologic: Eczema; atopic dermatitis; urticaria; allergic rash and other idiosyncrasies (rare).

Body as a whole: Gastric distress; headache; weakness. Rinses and gels containing stannous fluoride may produce surface staining of the teeth; this does not occur with nonstannous fluoride topical preparations. Acidulated fluoride may dull porcelain and composite restorations.

Overdosage:

Chronic overdosage of fluorides may result in dental fluorosis (a mottling of tooth enamel) and osseous changes.

Acute overdosage:

Symptoms – In children, acute ingestion of 10 to 20 mg sodium fluoride may cause excessive salivation and GI disturbances; 500 mg may be fatal. The oral lethal dose is 70 to 140 mg/kg (5 to 10 g in adults).

GI – Salivation, nausea, abdominal pain, vomiting and diarrhea are frequent due to conversion of sodium fluoride to corrosive hydrofluoric acid in the stomach.

CNS – Because of the calcium-binding effect of fluoride, CNS irritability, paresthesias, tetany, convulsions and respiratory and cardiac failure may occur. Fluoride has a direct toxic action on muscle and nerve tissue, and it interferes with many enzyme systems.

Hypocalcemia, hypoglycemia and delayed hyperkalemia are frequent laboratory findings.

Treatment: Usual supportive measures. Refer to General Management of Acute Overdosage. Precipitate the fluoride by using gastric lavage with 0.15% calcium hydroxide. Administer IV glucose in saline for a forced diuresis; IV calcium may be indicated for tetany. Administer calcium IM (10 ml of 10% calcium gluconate, 5 ml in children) every 4 to 6 hours until recovery is complete. Maintain electrolytes, normal blood pH and adequate urine output. Removing fluoride with dialysis and hemoperfusion may also be beneficial.

Patient Information:

Tablets and drops: Milk and other dairy products may decrease absorption of sodium fluoride; avoid simultaneous ingestion.

Tablets: Dissolve in the mouth, chew, swallow whole, add to drinking water or fruit juice or add to water for use in infant formulas or other food.

Drops: Take orally, undiluted, or mix with fluids or food.

Rinses and gels are most effective immediately after brushing or flossing and just prior to sleep. Expectorate any excess. Do not swallow. Do not eat, drink or rinse mouth for 30 minutes after application.

Notify dentist if teeth become mottled.

Administration and Dosage:

Use according to directions accompanying the product.

Fluoride Dosage

Route/Age	Daily dose
Oral:	
Fluoride content of drinking water (< 0.3 ppm):	
<2 years	0.25
2 to 3 years	0.5 mg
3 to 12 years	1 mg
Fluoride content of drinking water (0.3 - 0.7 ppm):	
< 2 years	0.125 mg
2 to 3 years	0.25 mg
3 to 14 years	0.25 - 0.75 mg
Topical (rinse):	
Children (6 to 12 years)	5 to 10 ml[1]
Adults and children (> 12 years)	10 ml[1]

[1] Use once daily (*Point-Two,* once weekly) after thoroughly brushing teeth and rinsing mouth. Rinse around and between teeth for 1 minute, then spit out.

FLUORIDE, ORAL

Complete prescribing information begins in the Fluoride group monograph.

Rx *sf*	**Luride Lozi-Tabs** (Colgate-Hoyt)	**Tablets, chewable:** 0.25 mg	Vanilla flavor. In 120s.
Rx	**Sodium Fluoride**[1] (Various, eg, Major, Rugby)	**Tablets, chewable:** 0.5 mg (from 1.1 mg sodium fluoride)	In 1000s.
Rx	**Fluoritab** (Fluoritab)		Dye free. Pineapple flavor. In 1000s and 5000s.
Rx *sf*	**Luride Lozi-Tabs** (Colgate-Hoyt)		Grape and assorted fruit flavors. In 120s. Grape also in 1200s.
Rx *sf*	**Pharmaflur 1.1** (Pharmics)		Grape flavor. In 120s.
Rx	**Sodium Fluoride**[1] (Various, eg, Geneva, Major, Rugby, Schein)	**Tablets, chewable:** 1 mg (from 2.2 mg sodium fluoride)	In 100s, 1000s and UD 1000s.
Rx	**Fluoritab** (Fluoritab)		Dye free. Pineapple and cherry flavors in 100s and 5000s. 1000s (cherry only).
Rx	**Karidium** (Lorvic)		White. In 180s and 1000s.
Rx *sf*	**Luride Lozi-Tabs** (Colgate-Hoyt)		Cherry and assorted fruit flavors. In 120s and 1000s. Cherry also in 5000s.
Rx *sf*	**Luride-SF Lozi-Tabs** (Colgate-Hoyt)		In 120s.
Rx *sf*	**Pharmaflur** (Pharmics)		Cherry flavor. In 1000s.
Rx *sf*	**Pharmaflur df** (Pharmics)		Dye free. Cherry flavor. In 120s.
Rx	**Fluoride** (Kirkman)	**Tablets:** 1 mg (from 2.2 mg sodium fluoride)	In 1000s.
Rx *sf*	**Flura** (Kirkman)		In 100s and 1000s.
Rx	**Karidium** (Lorvic)		White. In 180s and 1000s.
Rx	**Sodium Fluoride** (Rugby)	**Drops:** 0.125 mg per drop (from ≈ 0.275 mg sodium fluoride)	In 30 ml.
Rx	**Karidium** (Lorvic)		In 30 and 60 ml w/dropper.
Rx *sf*	**Fluoritab** (Fluoritab)	**Drops:** 0.25 mg per drop (from 0.55 mg sodium fluoride)	In 22.8 ml.
Rx	**Flura-Drops** (Kirkman)		In 30 ml.
Rx *sf*	**Pediaflor** (Ross)	**Drops:** 0.5 mg per ml (from 1.1 mg sodium fluoride)	< 0.5% alcohol, sorbitol. Cherry flavor. In 50 ml w/dropper.
Rx *sf*	**Luride** (Colgate)		Peach flavor. In 50 ml.
Rx *sf*	**Fluoride Loz** (Kirkman)	**Lozenges:** 1 mg (from 2.2 mg sodium fluoride)	In 1000s.
Rx	**Flura-Loz** (Kirkman)		Raspberry flavor. In 100s and 1000s.
Rx *sf*	**Phos-Flur** (Colgate-Hoyt)	**Solution:**[2] 0.2 mg per ml (from 0.44 mg sodium fluoride)	Cherry flavor. In 250, 500 ml & gal. Cinnamon (w/saccharin), grape, wintergreen flavors. In 500 ml.

[1] May be regular or chewable.
[2] May be used as a rinse or supplement.

FLUORIDE, TOPICAL

Complete prescribing information for these products begins in the Fluoride group monograph.

otc	**ACT** (Johnson & Johnson)	**Rinse**: 0.02% (from 0.05% sodium fluoride)	7% alcohol. In 90, 360 and 480 ml.
otc	**Fluorigard** (Colgate-Palmolive)		6% alcohol. Tartrazine. In 180, 300 & 480 ml.
otc *sf*	**MouthKote F/R** (Parnell)	**Rinse**: 0.04% sodium fluoride	Benzyl alcohol, sorbitol, menthol, EDTA. In 237 ml.
Rx	**Fluorinse** (Oral-B)	**Rinse**: 0.09% (from 0.2% sodium fluoride)	Alcohol free. Mint and cinnamon flavors. In 480 ml.
Rx	**Point-Two** (Colgate-Hoyt)		6% alcohol. Mint flavor. In 240 ml and gal.
Rx	**PreviDent Rinse** (Colgate Oral)	**Rinse**: 0.2% neutral sodium fluoride	6% alcohol. Mint flavor. In 250 ml and gal (with pump dispenser).
Rx	**Gel Kam** (Scherer)	**Gel**: 0.1% (from 0.4% stannous fluoride)	Cinnamon flavor. In 65 and 122 g and 105 g (Dental Therapy-Pak [2]).
otc	**Gel-Tin** (Young Dental)		Lime, grape, cinnamon, raspberry, mint and orange flavors. In 60 g.
otc	**Stop** (Oral-B)		Grape, cinnamon, bubblegum, piña colada and mint flavors. In 120 g.
Rx	**Karigel** (Lorvic)	**Gel**: 0.5% (from 1.1% sodium fluoride)	pH 5.6. Orange flavor. In 30, 130 and 250 g.
Rx	**Karigel-N** (Lorvic)		Neutral pH. In 24 and 120 g.
Rx	**Prevident** (Colgate-Hoyt)		Mint, berry, cherry and fruit sherbet flavors. In 24 and 60 g. Lime flavor in 60 g.
Rx	**Thera-Flur** (Colgate-Hoyt)	**Gel-Drops**: 0.5% (from 1.1% sodium fluoride)	pH 4.5. Lime flavor. In 24 ml.
Rx	**Thera-Flur-N** (Colgate-Hoyt)		Neutral pH. In 24 ml.
Rx	**Luride** (Colgate Oral)	**Gel**: 1.2% (from sodium fluoride and hydrogen fluoride)	Mint flavor. In 7 g.
Rx	**Minute-Gel** (Oral-B)	**Gel**: 1.23% (as acidulated phosphate fluoride)	Spearmint, strawberry, grape, apple-cinnamon, cherry cola and bubblegum flavors. In 480 ml.

ZINC SUPPLEMENTS

For information on parenteral zinc, refer to the monograph in the IV Nutritional Therapy section.

Actions:

Pharmacology: Normal growth and tissue repair depend upon adequate zinc. Zinc acts as an integral part of several enzymes important to protein and carbohydrate metabolism.

Zinc deficiency manifestations include: Anorexia; growth retardation; impaired taste and olfactory sensation; hypogonadism; alopecia; hepatosplenomegaly; dwarfism; rashes; cutaneous lesions; glossitis; stomatitis; blepharitis; paronychia; impaired healing.

Pharmacokinetics: Zinc salts are poorly absorbed from the GI tract; 20% to 30% of dietary zinc is absorbed. The major stores of zinc are in skeletal muscle and bone; zinc is also found in hair, nails, prostate, spermatazoa and the choroid of the eye. The main excretion route is through the intestine. Only minor amounts are lost in the urine (≈ 2%).

Indications:

As a dietary supplement; use to treat or prevent zinc deficiencies.

Unlabeled uses: For acrodermatitis enteropathica and delayed wound healing associated with zinc deficiency, doses of 220 mg zinc sulfate 3 times daily are used. Zinc sulfate has also been used to treat acne, rheumatoid arthritis and Wilson's disease. However, data conflict and are insufficient to recommend these uses.

In one study, zinc gluconate appeared to significantly shorten the duration of the common cold. Patients (n = 65) dissolved one tablet containing 23 mg zinc (one-half tablet for children) in the mouth every 2 hours until all symptoms were absent for 6 hours; 11% were asymptomatic within 12 hours, 22% within 24 hours. Zinc sulfate should not be used. Further study is needed.

Contraindications:

Pregnancy (see Warnings); lactation.

Warnings:

Excessive intake in healthy persons may be deleterious. Eleven healthy men who ingested 150 mg zinc twice daily for 6 weeks showed significant impairment of lymphocyte and polymorphonuclear leukocyte functions and a significant decrease in high-density lipoproteins (HDL). No clinical side effects were seen during the study.

Pregnancy: Although zinc deficiency during pregnancy has been associated with adverse perinatal outcomes, other studies report no such occurrences. Therefore, since zinc deficiency is very rare, the routine use of zinc supplementation during pregnancy is not recommended. However, a dietary zinc intake of 15 mg/day is recommended.

Lactation: Breast milk concentrations of zinc decrease over time following delivery; extra dietary intake of zinc of 7 mg/day for the first 6 months of lactation and 4 mg/day during the second 6 months are recommended.

Precautions:

Do not exceed prescribed dosage; will cause emesis if administered in single 2 g doses.

Drug Interactions:

Zinc Drug Interactions			
Precipitant drug	Object drug *		Description
Zinc salts	Fluoroquinolones	⬇	The GI absorption and serum levels of some fluoroquinolones may be decreased, possibly resulting in a decreased anti-infective response.
Zinc salts	Tetracyclines	⬇	The GI absorption and serum levels of tetracyclines may be decreased, possibly resulting in a decreased anti-infective response. Doxycycline does not appear to be affected.

* ⬇ = Object drug decreased.

Drug/Food interactions: Bran products (including brown bread) and some foods (eg, protein, phytates, some minerals) may decrease zinc absorption.

Adverse Reactions:

Nausea; vomiting.

ZINC SUPPLEMENTS

Overdosage:

Symptoms: Nausea; severe vomiting; dehydration; restlessness; sideroblastic anemia (secondary to zinc-induced copper deficiency).

Treatment: Reduce dosage or discontinue to control symptoms.

Patient Information:

If GI upset occurs, take with food, but avoid foods high in calcium, phosphorus or phytate.

Administration and Dosage:

Recommended dietary allowances (RDAs): Adults, 12 to 15 mg. For a complete listing of RDAs by age, sex and condition, refer to the RDA table.

Dietary supplement: Average adult dose is 25 to 50 mg zinc daily. Take zinc with food to avoid gastric distress; however, some studies indicate that ingestion with some foods (eg, those that contain bran, phytates, protein, some minerals) may inhibit zinc absorption.

ZINC SULFATE (23% zinc)

Complete prescribing information for these products begins in the Zinc Supplements group monograph.

otc	**Zinc 15** (Mericon)	**Tablets:** 66 mg (15 mg zinc)	In 100s.
otc	**Orazinc** (Mericon)	**Tablets:** 110 mg (25 mg zinc)	In 100s.
otc	**Zinc Sulfate** (Various, eg, Rugby)	**Tablets:** 200 mg (45 mg zinc)	In 1000s.
Rx	**Zinc Sulfate** (Various)	**Capsules:** 220 mg (50 mg zinc)	In 100s, 1000s and UD 100s.
otc	**Orazinc** (Mericon)		In 100s and 1000s.
otc	**Verazinc** (Forest)		In 100s.
otc	**Zinc-220** (Alto)		Pink and blue. In 100s, 1000s and UD 100s.
Rx	**Zincate** (Paddock)		In 100s and 1000s.

ZINC GLUCONATE (14.3% zinc)

Complete prescribing information for these products begins in the Zinc Supplements group monograph.

otc	**Zinc Gluconate** (Various, eg, IDE)	**Tablets:** 10 mg (1.4 mg zinc)	In 250s.
otc	**Zinc Gluconate** (Various, eg, IDE)	**Tablets:** 15 mg (2 mg zinc)	In 250s.
otc	**Zinc Gluconate** (Various, eg, IDE, Major, Mission, Moore)	**Tablets:** 50 mg (7 mg zinc)	In 100s and 250s.
otc	**Zinc Gluconate** (Major)	**Tablets:** 78 mg (11 mg zinc)	In 100s and 300s.

COMPLEX ZINC CARBONATES

Complete prescribing information for these products begins in the Zinc Supplements group monograph.

otc	**Zinc** (Sublingual Products)	**Liquid:** 15 mg/ml	Fructose, corn syrup solids, sorbitol, parabens. Fruit flavor. In 30 ml with dropper.

ZINC COMBINATIONS

otc	**Zinc Lozenges** (Zenith-Goldline)	**Lozenges:** 23 mg	Fructose. In 30s.

MAGNESIUM

For information on parenteral magnesium, refer to the monographs in the IV Nutritional Therapy and Anticonvulsant sections.

Actions:

Pharmacology: Magnesium is an electrolyte which is necessary in a number of enzyme systems, phosphate transfer, muscular contraction and nerve conduction. Magnesium deficiency may occur in: Malabsorption syndromes; prolonged diarrhea or steatorrhea; vomiting; pancreatitis; aldosteronism; renal tubular damage; chronic alcoholism; vomiting; pancreatitis; aldosteronism; renal tubular damage; prolonged IV therapy with magnesium-free solutions; diuretic therapy; during hemodialysis; renal tubular damage; disorders associated with hypokalemia and hypocalcemia; in patients on digitalis therapy. While there are large stores of magnesium present intracellularly and in bone in adults, these stores often are not mobilized sufficiently to maintain plasma levels; therefore serum levels may not reflect total magnesium stores.

Indications:

As a dietary supplement.

Unlabeled uses: A pyridoxine/magnesium oxide combination has been used to prevent recurrence of calcium oxalate kidney stones.

Oral magnesium gluconate may be a cost-effective and clinically effective alternative to oral ritodrine as a tocolytic for continued inhibition of contractions following parenteral magnesium sulfate. Further study is needed.

Warnings:

Pregnancy: There is weak evidence that magnesium supplementation reduces the risk of poor perinatal outcome. However, since magnesium deficiency is rare, there appears to be no need for routine supplementation during pregnancy.

Precautions:

Renal disease: Do not use without physician supervision due to potential accumulation.

Excessive dosage may cause diarrhea and GI irritation.

Drug Interactions:

Magnesium Drug Interactions

Precipitant drug	Object drug*		Description
Magnesium salts	Aminoquinolones	⬇	The absorption and therapeutic effect of the aminoquinolines may be decreased.
Magnesium salts	Digoxin	⬇	Magnesium salts may absorb digoxin in the GI tract, decreasing its bioavailability; however, this has only been reported for magnesium-containing antacids.
Magnesium salts	Nitrofurantoin	⬇	Adsorption of nitrofurantoin onto magnesium salts may occur, decreasing the bioavailability and possibly the anti-infective effect of nitrofurantoin.
Magnesium salts	Penicillamine	⬇	The GI absorption of penicillamine may be decreased, possibly decreasing its pharmacologic effects; however this has only been reported for magnesium-containing antacids.
Magnesium salts	Tetracyclines	⬇	The GI absorption and serum levels of tetracyclines may be decreased; a decreased antimicrobial response may occur.

* ⬇ = Object drug decreased.

MAGNESIUM

Overdosage:

Symptoms: Hypermagnesemia following oral ingestion in the absence of renal disease is unlikely; however, it may occur with overdosage. Symptoms may include: Hypotension, nausea, vomiting, urinary retention, bradycardia, cutaneous vasodilation (3 to 9 mEq/L); ECG changes, hyporeflexia, secondary CNS depression (5 to 10 mEq/L); respiratory changes, coma (> 9 to 10 mEq/L); asystolic arrest (> 14 to 15 mEq/L).

Treatment: Reversal of toxicity with calcium is immediate but transient. Dialysis is the treatment of choice (both peritoneal and hemodialysis).

Administration and Dosage:

1 g Mg = 83.3 mEq (41.1 mmol).

Dietary supplement: 54 to 483 mg/day in divided doses. Refer to product labeling.

Recommended dietary allowances (RDAs):

Adult – Males, 350 to 400 mg; females, 280 to 300 mg. For a complete listing of RDAs by age, sex and condition, refer to the RDA table.

Magnesium-containing antacids may also be used; refer to the Antacids monograph.

otc	**Mag-200** (Optimox)	**Tablets:** 400 mg magnesium (oxide)	In 120s.
otc	**Mag-Ox 400** (Blaine)	**Tablets:** 400 mg magnesium oxide (241.3 mg magnesium)	Scored. In 100s and 1000s.
otc	**Almora** (Forest)	**Tablets:** 500 mg magnesium gluconate (27 mg magnesium)	In 100s.
otc	**Magonate** (Fleming)		In 100s and 1000s.
otc	**Magtrate** (Mission)	**Tablets:** 500 mg magnesium gluconate (29 mg magnesium	In 100s.
otc sf	**Chelated Magnesium** (Freeda)	**Tablets:** 500 mg magnesium amino acids chelate (100 mg magnesium)	In 100s, 250s and 500s.
otc	**Slow-Mag** (Searle)	**Tablets, sustained release:** 535 mg magnesium chloride hexahydrate (64 mg magnesium)	In 60s.
otc	**Mag-Tab SR** (Niche)	**Caplets, sustained release:** 84 mg magnesium (as lactate)	In 60s and 100s.
otc	**Uro-Mag** (Blaine)	**Capsules:** 140 mg magnesium oxide (84.5 mg magnesium)	In 100s and 1000s.
otc	**Magonate** (Fleming)	**Liquid:** 54 mg/5 ml magnesium (as gluconate)	Melon flavor. In pt and gal.

MANGANESE

For information on parenteral manganese, refer to the monograph in the IV Nutritional Therapy section.

Actions:

Pharmacology: Manganese is a cofactor in many enzyme systems; it stimulates synthesis of cholesterol and fatty acids in the liver and influences mucopolysaccharide synthesis. It is concentrated in mitochondria, primarily of the pituitary gland, pancreas, liver, kidney and bone.

Indications:

As a dietary supplement.

Administration and Dosage:

20 to 50 mg daily.

The need for manganese in human nutrition has been established, but no RDA has been determined. Manganese deficiency is unlikely because dietary intake usually satisfies the need; therefore, 2 to 5 mg/day via the diet is recommended.

otc sf	**Chelated Manganese** (Freeda)	**Tablets:** 20 mg	In 100s, 250s and 500s.
		50 mg	In 100s, 250s and 500s.

POTASSIUM REPLACEMENT PRODUCTS

For information on parenteral potassium, refer to the IV Nutritional Therapy section.

Actions:

Pharmacology: Potassium, the principal intracellular cation of most body tissues, participates in a number of essential physiological processes, such as maintenance of intracellular tonicity and a proper relationship with sodium across cell membranes, cellular metabolism, transmission of nerve impulses, contraction of cardiac, skeletal and smooth muscle, acid-base balance and maintenance of normal renal function. Normal potassium serum levels range from 3.5 to 5 mEq/L. The active ion transport system maintains this gradient across the plasma membrane.

mEq/g of Various Potassium Salts	
Potassium salt	mEq/g
Potassium gluconate	4.3
Potassium citrate	9.8
Potassium bicarbonate	10
Potassium acetate	10.2
Potassium chloride	13.4

Potassium homeostasis – The potassium concentration in extracellular fluid is normally 4 to 5 mEq/L; the concentration in intracellular fluid is approximately 150 to 160 mEq/L. Plasma concentration provides a useful clinical guide to disturbances in potassium balance. By producing large differences in the ratio of intracellular to extracellular potassium, relatively small absolute changes in extracellular concentration may have important effects on neuromuscular activity.

Despite wide variations in dietary intake of potassium (eg, 40 to 120 mEq/day), plasma potassium concentration is normally stabilized within the narrow range of 4 to 5 mEq/L by virtue of close renal regulation of potassium balance. Renal potassium excretion is accomplished largely by potassium secretion in the distal portion of the nephron; essentially all filtered potassium is reabsorbed in the proximal tubule. The potassium that appears in the urine is added to the filtrate by a distal process of sodium-cation exchange. Fecal excretion of potassium is normally only a few mEq per day and does not play a significant role in potassium homeostasis.

Natural potassium sources – Foods rich in potassium include: Beef; veal; ham; chicken; turkey; fish; milk; bananas; dates; prunes; raisins; avocado; watermelon; canteloupes; apricots; molasses; beans; yams; broccoli; brussels sprouts; lentils; potatoes; spinach.

Hypokalemia – Gradual potassium depletion may occur whenever the rate of potassium loss through renal excretion or GI loss exceeds the rate of potassium intake. Potassium depletion is usually a consequence of prolonged therapy with oral diuretics, primary or secondary hyperaldosteronism, diabetic ketoacidosis, severe diarrhea (especially if associated with vomiting) or inadequate replacement during prolonged parenteral nutrition. Potassium depletion due to these causes is usually accompanied by a concomitant deficiency of chloride and is manifested by hypokalemia and metabolic alkalosis.

The use of potassium salts in patients receiving diuretics for uncomplicated essential hypertension is often unnecessary when such patients have a normal diet. However, if hypokalemia occurs, dietary supplementation with potassium-containing foods may be adequate. In more severe cases, potassium salt supplementation may be indicated.

Potassium depletion sufficient to cause 1 mEq/L drop in serum potassium requires a loss of about 100 to 200 mEq potassium from the total body store.

Symptoms: Weakness; fatigue; ileus; tetany; polydipsia; flaccid paralysis or impaired ability to concentrate urine (in advanced cases). ECG may reveal atrial and ventricular ectopy, prolongation of QT interval, ST segment depression, conduction defects, broad or flat T waves or appearance of U waves.

Indications:

Treatment of hypokalemia in the following conditions: With or without metabolic alkalosis; digitalis intoxication; familial periodic paralysis; diabetic acidosis; diarrhea and vomiting; surgical conditions accompanied by nitrogen loss, vomiting, suction drainage, diarrhea and increased urinary excretion of potassium; certain cases of uremia; hyperadrenalism; starvation and debilitation; corticosteroid or diuretic therapy.

Prevention of potassium depletion when dietary intake is inadequate in the following conditions: Patients receiving digitalis and diuretics for congestive heart failure; significant cardiac arrhythmias; hepatic cirrhosis with ascites; states of aldosterone excess with normal renal function; potassium-losing nephropathy; certain diarrheal states.

When hypokalemia is associated with alkalosis, use potassium chloride. When acidosis is present, use the bicarbonate, citrate, acetate or gluconate potassium salts.

POTASSIUM REPLACEMENT PRODUCTS

Unlabeled uses: In patients with mild hypertension, the use of potassium supplements (24 to 60 mmol/day) appears to result in a long-term reduction of blood pressure.

Contraindications:

Severe renal impairment with oliguria or azotemia; untreated Addison's disease; hyperkalemia from any cause (eg, systemic acidosis, acute dehydration, extensive tissue breakdown); adynamia episodica hereditaria; acute dehydration; heat cramps; patients receiving potassium-sparing diuretics (spironolactone, triamterene or amiloride) or aldosterone-inhibiting agents.

Solid dosage forms of potassium supplements are contraindicated in any patient in whom there is cause for arrest or delay in tablet passage through the GI tract. Wax matrix potassium chloride preparations have produced esophageal ulceration in cardiac patients with esophageal compression due to an enlarged left atrium; give potassium supplementation as a liquid preparation to these patients.

Warnings:

Hyperkalemia: In patients with impaired potassium excretion, potassium salts can produce hyperkalemia or cardiac arrest. This occurs most commonly in patients given IV potassium, but may also occur in patients given oral potassium. Potentially fatal hyperkalemia can develop rapidly and may be asymptomatic.

Hyperkalemia may be manifested only by an increased serum potassium concentration and characteristic ECG changes (eg, peaking of T waves, loss of P wave, depression of ST segment, prolongation of the QT interval, lengthened P-R interval, widened QRS complex). However, the following may also occur: Parasthesias; heaviness; muscle weakness and flaccid paralysis of the extremities; listlessness; mental confusion; decreased blood pressure; shock; cardiac arrhythmias; heart block.

In response to a rise in the concentration of body potassium, renal excretion of the ion is increased. With normal kidney function, it is difficult to produce potassium intoxication by oral administration. However, administer potassium supplements with caution, since the amount of deficiency and corresponding daily dose is unknown. Frequently monitor the clinical status, periodic ECG and serum potassium levels. This is particularly important in patients receiving digitalis and in patients with cardiac disease. There is a hazard in prescribing potassium in digitalis intoxication manifested by atrioventricular (AV) conduction disturbance.

GI lesions: Potassium chloride tablets have produced stenotic or ulcerative lesions of the small bowel and death. These lesions are caused by a concentration of potassium ion in the region of a rapidly dissolving tablet, which injures the bowel wall and produces obstruction, hemorrhage or perforation. The reported frequency of small bowel lesions is much less with wax matrix tablets (< 1 per 100,000 patient-years) and microencapsulated tablets than with enteric coated tablets (40 to 50 per 100,000 patient-years). Upper GI bleeding, esophageal ulceration and stricture, gastric ulceration and lower GI ulceration have occurred with wax matrix preparations. The total number of GI lesions is < 1 per 47,000 patient-years. Discontinue either type of tablet immediately and consider the possibility of bowel obstruction or perforation if severe vomiting, abdominal pain or distention or GI bleeding occurs.

Patients at greatest risk for developing potassium chloride-induced GI lesions include: The elderly, the immobile and those with scleroderma, diabetes mellitus, mitral valve replacement, cardiomegaly or esophageal stricture/compression.

Reserve slow release potassium chloride preparations for patients who cannot tolerate liquids or effervescent potassium preparations, or for patients in whom there is a problem of compliance with these preparations.

Some studies suggest the "microencapsulated" preparations are less likely to cause GI damage; however, evidence conflicts and a specific recommendation of one solid oral product over another (wax matrix or microencapsulated) cannot be made. Avoid enteric coated products.

Metabolic acidosis and hyperchloremia: In some patients (eg, those with renal tubular acidosis), potassium depletion is rarely associated with metabolic acidosis and hyperchloremia. Replace with potassium bicarbonate, citrate, acetate or gluconate.

Renal function impairment requires careful monitoring of the serum potassium concentration and appropriate dosage adjustment.

Pregnancy: Category C. It is not known whether potassium salts can cause fetal harm when administered to a pregnant woman or can affect reproduction capacity. Give to a pregnant woman only if clearly needed.

Lactation: It is not known whether this drug is excreted in breast milk. Exercise caution when administering to a nursing woman. The normal potassium content of breast milk is ≈ 13 mEq/L. As long as body potassium is not excessive, the contribution of potassium salts should have little or no effect on the level of breast milk.

Children: Safety and efficacy for use in children have not been established.

POTASSIUM REPLACEMENT PRODUCTS

Precautions:

Monitoring: When blood is drawn for analysis of plasma potassium, it is important to recognize that artificial elevations can occur after improper venipuncture technique or as a result of in vitro hemolysis of the sample.

Hypokalemia is ordinarily diagnosed by demonstrating potassium depletion in a patient and by a careful clinical history. In interpreting the serum potassium level, consider that acute alkalosis can produce hypokalemia in the absence of a deficit in total body potassium, while acute acidosis can increase the serum potassium concentration to the normal range, even in the presence of a reduced total body potassium. Treatment, particularly in the presence of cardiac disease, renal disease or acidosis, requires careful attention to acid-base balance and monitoring of serum electrolytes, ECG and clinical status of the patient.

The administration of concentrated dextrose or sodium bicarbonate may cause an intracellular potassium shift. This may cause hypokalemia which, in turn, may lead to serious cardiac arrhythmias.

Giving potassium to hypokalemic hypertensives may lower blood pressure.

Tartrazine sensitivity: Some of these products contain tartrazine, which may cause allergic-type reactions (including bronchial asthma) in susceptible individuals. Although the incidence of tartrazine sensitivity in the general population is low, it is frequently seen in patients who also have aspirin hypersensitivity. Specific products containing tartrazine are identified in the product listings.

Drug Interactions:

Potassium Preparation Drug Interactions			
Precipitant drug	Object drug*		Description
ACE inhibitors	Potassium preparations	↑	Concurrent use may result in elevated serum potassium concentrations in certain patients.
Potassium-sparing diuretics	Potassium preparations	↑	Potassium-sparing diuretics will increase potassium retention and can produce severe hyperkalemia.
Potassium preparations	Digitalis	↑	In patients receiving digoxin, hypokalemia may result in digoxin toxicity. Therefore, use caution if discontinuing a potassium preparation in patients maintained on digoxin.

* ↑ = Object drug increased.

In addition, potassium citrate, a urinary alkalinizer, may affect the renal excretion and pharmacologic effects of various agents (refer to the Citrate and Citric Acid Solutions monograph).

Adverse Reactions:

Most common: Nausea, vomiting, diarrhea, flatulence and abdominal discomfort due to GI irritation are best managed by diluting the preparation further, by taking with meals or by dose reduction.

Rare: Skin rash.

Most severe: Hyperkalemia; GI obstruction, bleeding, ulceration or perforation.

Overdosage:

For symptoms and treatment of potassium overdosage and hyperkalemia, refer to the monograph in the IV Nutritional Therapy section.

Patient Information:

May cause GI upset; take after meals or with food and with a full glass of water.

Do not chew or crush tablets; swallow whole.

Oral liquids, soluble powders and effervescent tablets: Mix or dissolve completely in 3 to 8 ounces of cold water, juice or other suitable beverage and drink slowly.

Following release of potassium chloride, the expended wax matrix, which is not absorbable, can be found in the stool. This is no cause for concern.

Do not use salt substitutes concurrently, except on the advice of a physician.

Notify physician if tingling of the hands and feet, unusual tiredness or weakness, a feeling of heaviness in the legs, severe nausea, vomiting, abdominal pain or black stools (GI bleeding) occurs.

Administration and Dosage:

The usual dietary intake of potassium ranges between 40 to 150 mEq/day.

Individualize dosage. Usual range is 16 to 24 mEq/day for the prevention of hypokalemia to 40 to 100 mEq/day or more for the treatment of potassium depletion.

Potassium intoxication may result from any therapeutic dosage.

POTASSIUM REPLACEMENT PRODUCTS

Rx	**Kaon-Cl** (Adria)	**Tablets, controlled release:** 6.7 mEq (500 mg) potassium chloride in a wax matrix	Tartrazine, sucrose. (Adria/307). Yellow. Sugar coated. In 100s, 250s & 1000s.
Rx	**Potassium Chloride** (Various, eg, Abbott, Geneva, Goldline, Major, Rugby, Warner Chilcott)	**Tablets, controlled release:** 8 mEq (600 mg) potassium chloride in a wax matrix	In 100s and 1000s.
Rx	**Klor-Con 8** (Upsher-Smith)		Blue. Film coated. In 100s, 500s and UD 100s.
Rx	**Slow-K** (Summit)		(Slow-K). Sucrose. Buff. Sugar coated. In 100s, 1000s and UD 100s.
Rx	**K⁺8** (Alra)	**Tablets, extended release:** 8 mEq potassium chloride	In 100s and 500s.
Rx	**K + 10** (Alra)	**Tablets, controlled release:** 10 mEq (750 mg) potassium chloride in a wax matrix	Film coated. In 100s, 500s, 1000s and UD 100s.
Rx	**Kaon Cl-10** (Adria)		Sucrose. (Adria/304). Green. Sugar coated. Capsule shape. In 100s, 500s, 1000s and Stat-Pak 100s.
Rx	**Klor-Con 10** (Upsher-Smith)		Yellow. Film coated. In 100s, 500s and UD 100s.
Rx	**Klotrix** (Bristol)		Orange. Film coated. In 100s, 1000s and UD 100s.
Rx	**K-Tab** (Abbott)		Yellow. Film coated. Oval. In 100s, 1000s, 5000s and Abbo-Pac 100s.
Rx	**Potassium Chloride** (Various, eg, Major, Rugby)	**Tablets, extended release:** 750 mg potassium chloride equivalent to 10 mEq potassium in a wax matrix	In 100s and 1000s.
Rx	**K-Dur 10** (Key)	**Tablets, controlled release:** 750 mg microencapsulated potassium chloride equivalent to 10 mEq potassium	(K-Dur 10). White. Oblong. In 100s and UD 100s.
Rx	**Ten-K** (Summit)		White, scored. Capsule shaped. Polymeric coated crystals. In 100s, 500s and UD 100s.
Rx	**K-Dur 20** (Key)	**Tablets, controlled release:** 1500 mg microencapsulated potassium chloride equivalent to 20 mEq potassium	(K-Dur 20). White, scored. Oblong. In 100s, 500s, 1000s and UD 100s.
otc	**Potassium Gluconate** (Various, eg, Rugby)	**Tablets:** 500 mg potassium gluconate (83.45 mg potassium)	In 100s and 1000s.
otc	**Potassium Gluconate** (Mission)	**Tablets:** 595 mg potassium gluconate (99 mg potassium)	In 100s.
Rx	**K + Care ET** (Alra)	**Tablets, effervescent:** 20 mEq potassium (from potassium bicarbonate)	Saccharin. In 30s and 100s.
Rx *sf*	**Klorvess** (Sandoz)	**Tablets, effervescent:** 20 mEq potassium (from potassium chloride and bicarbonate and lysine hydrochloride)	Sodium free. Saccharin. White. In 60s and 1000s.

POTASSIUM REPLACEMENT PRODUCTS

Rx	**K&bullet2;Lyte/Cl** (Bristol)	**Tablets, effervescent**: 25 mEq potassium (from potassium Cl and bicarbonate, l-lysine monohydrochloride and citric acid)	Saccharin, docusate sodium. Fruit punch or citrus flavor. In 30s, 100s and 250s.
Rx	**K&bullet2;Lyte/Cl 50** (Bristol)	**Tablets, effervescent**: 50 mEq potassium (from potassium Cl and bicarbonate, l-lysine monohydrochloride and citric acid)	Saccharin, docusate sodium. Fruit punch or citrus flavor. In 30s & 100s.
Rx	**K + Care ET** (Alra)	**Tablets, effervescent**: 25 mEq potassium (from potassium bicarbonate)	Saccharin. Orange or lime flavor. In 30s and 100s.
Rx	**Effer-K** (Nomax)	**Tablets, effervescent**: 25 mEq potassium (as bicarbonate and citrate)	Saccharin. Orange or lime flavor. In 30s, 100s & 250s.
Rx	**Effervescent Potassium** (Rugby)		Saccharin. Lime, orange or fruit punch flavors. In 30s.
Rx *sf*	**Klor-Con/EF** (Upsher-Smith)		Saccharin. Orange flavor. In 30s and 100s.
Rx	**K&bullet2;Lyte** (Bristol)		Saccharin, docusate sodium, dextrose. Orange or lime flavor. In 30s, 100s and 250s.
Rx	**K&bullet2;Lyte DS** (Bristol)	**Tablets, effervescent**: 50 mEq potassium (from potassium bicarbonate and citrate and citric acid)	Saccharin, docusate sodium, lactose. Orange or lime flavor. In 30s and 100s.
Rx	**Micro-K Extencaps** (Robins)	**Capsules, controlled release**: 600 mg potassium chloride equivalent to 8 mEq potassium. Microencapsulated particles	(Micro-K AHR/5720). Orange. In 100s, 500s and UD 100s.
Rx	**Potassium Chloride** (Various, eg, EtheX, Goldline, Major, Moore, Parmed, Rugby, Schein, Warner-Chilcott)	**Capsules, controlled release**: 10 mEq (750 mg) potassium chloride. Microencapsulated particles	In 100s and 500s.
Rx	**K-Lease** (Adria)		(13/308). Green. In 100s, 500s, 1000s and 2500s.
Rx	**K-Norm** (Fisons)		Sugar. (K-Norm 10). Clear. In 100s and 500s.
Rx	**Micro-K 10 Extencaps** (Robins)		(Micro-K 10 AHR/ 5730). Orange/white. In 100s, 500s and UD 100s.

POTASSIUM REPLACEMENT PRODUCTS

Rx	**Potassium Chloride** (Various, eg, Barre-National, Geneva, Major, Parmed, PBI, Rugby, Schein)	**Liquid**: 20 mEq/15 ml potassium and chloride (10%KCl)	In pt and gal.
Rx *sf*	**Cena-K** (Century)		In pt and gal.
Rx	**Kaochlor 10%** (Adria)		5% alcohol, tartrazine, saccharin, sorbitol, sucrose. Citrus flavor. In 480 ml.
Rx *sf*	**Kaochlor S-F** (Adria)		5% alcohol, saccharin. Fruit flavor. In 480 ml.
Rx *sf*	**Kay Ciel** (Forest)		4% alcohol. In 118 ml, pt and gal.
Rx	**Klorvess** (Sandoz)		0.75% alcohol. Saccharin, sucrose. Cherry flavor. In 480 ml.
Rx *sf*	**Potasalan** (Lannett)		4% alcohol. Orange flavor. In pt and gal.
Rx	**Rum-K** (Fleming)	**Liquid**: 30 mEq/15 ml potassium and chloride (15% KCl)	Butter-rum flavor. In pt and gal.
Rx	**Potassium Chloride** (Various, eg, Barre-National, Geneva, Major, PBI, Rugby, Schein)	**Liquid**: 40 mEq/15 ml potassium and chloride (20% KCl)	In pt and gal.
Rx *sf*	**Cena-K** (Century)		In pt and gal.
Rx *sf*	**Kaon-Cl 20%** (Adria)		5% alcohol, saccharin. Cherry flavor. In 480 ml.
Rx	**Potassium Gluconate** (Various, eg, Major, PBI)	**Liquid**: 20 mEq/15 ml potassium (as potassium gluconate)	In 118 ml, pt, gal and UD 5 and 15 ml (100s).
Rx *sf*	**Kaon** (Adria)		5% alcohol. Saccharin. Grape flavor. In 480 ml.
Rx	**Kaylixir** (Lannett)		5% alcohol. Saccharin. In pt and gal.
Rx	**K-G Elixir** (Geneva)		5% alcohol. In 480 ml.
Rx	**Tri-K** (Century)	**Liquid**: 45 mEq/15 ml potas- sium (from potassium acetate, potassium bicarbonate and potassium citrate)	In pt and gal.
Rx	**Twin-K** (Boots)	**Liquid**: 20 mEq/15 ml potas- sium (as potassium gluconate & potassium citrate)	Sorbitol, saccharin. In 480 ml.
Rx *sf*	**Kolyum** (Fisons)	**Liquid**: 20 mEq potassium and 3.4 mEq chloride/ 15 ml (from potas-sium gluconate and potassium chloride)	Sorbitol, saccharin. Cherry flavor. In pt and gal.
Rx	**K + Care** (Alra)	**Powder**: 15 mEq potassium chloride per packet	Saccharin. Fruit or orange flavor. In 30s and 100s.

POTASSIUM REPLACEMENT PRODUCTS

Rx	**Potassium Chloride** (Various, eg, Geneva, Schein)	**Powder**: 20 mEq potassium chloride per packet	In 30s and 100s.
Rx *sf*	**Gen-K** (Goldline)		Orange/fruit flavor. In 30s.
Rx *sf*	**Kay Ciel** (Forest)		Saccharin. In 30s and 100s.
Rx	**K + Care** (Alta)		Saccharin. Fruit or orange flavor. In 30s and 100s.
Rx	**K-Lor** (Abbott)		Saccharin. Fruit flavor. In 30s and 100s.
Rx *sf*	**Klor-Con** (Upsher-Smith)		Saccharin. Fruit flavor. In 30s and 100s.
Rx	**Micro-K LS** (Robins)		Extended-release. Sucrose. In 30s and 100s.
Rx	**K + Care** (Alra)	**Powder**: 25 mEq potassium chloride per packet	Saccharin. Orange flavor. In 30s and 100s.
Rx *sf*	**Klor-Con/25** (Upsher-Smith)		Saccharin. Fruit flavor. In 30s, 100s and 250s.
Rx	**K &bullet2; Lyte/Cl** (Mead-J)	**Powder**: 25 mEq potassium chloride per dose	Fruit punch flavor. In 225 g (30 doses).
Rx *sf*	**Klorvess Effervescent Granules** (Sandoz)	**Powder**: 20 mEq each potassium & chloride (potassium chloride, bicarbonate and citrate & lysine hydrochloride)/packet	Sodium free. Saccharin. In 30s.

Salt Replacement Products

SODIUM CHLORIDE

For information on parenteral sodium products, refer to the monograph in the IV Nutritional Therapy section.

Indications:

Prevention or treatment of extracellular volume depletion, dehydration or sodium depletion (eg, due to excessive salt restriction); aid in the prevention of heat prostration.

Warnings:

Acclimatization: Inappropriate salt administration in an effort to acclimatize to a hot environment can be dangerous. Balanced electrolytes and adequate hydration are essential.

Salt tablets may pass through the GI tract undigested. Avoid their use in treating heat cramps since they may cause vomiting, pooling of oral fluids and potassium depletion. Use oral salt solutions instead.

Pregnancy: Seek professional advice before using these products.

Lactation: Seek professional advice before using these products.

Precautions:

Supplementation: Individuals with adequate dietary sodium intake and normal renal function should not require sodium chloride supplementation. Balanced electrolyte supplements may be preferred to prevent hypokalemia.

Use with caution in the presence of congestive heart failure, kidney dysfunction, peripheral or pulmonary edema or preeclampsia.

Overdosage:

Symptoms: Overdosage may cause serious electrolyte disturbances. Ingestion of large amounts of sodium chloride irritates the GI mucosa and may result in nausea, vomiting, diarrhea and abdominal cramps. Edema is a sign of excess total body sodium.

Manifestations of hypernatremia may include:

Neurologic – Irritability; restlessness; weakness; obtundation progressing to convulsions and coma.

Cardiovascular – Hypertension; tachycardia; fluid accumulation.

Respiratory – Pulmonary edema; respiratory arrest.

Treatment includes usual supportive measures. Refer to General Management of Acute Overdosage. Use appropriate measures to empty the stomach. Magnesium sulfate may be given as a cathartic. Provide an adequate airway and ventilation. Maintain vascular volume and tissue perfusion.

Administration and Dosage:

Refer to specific product labeling for dosage guidelines.

otc	**Sodium Chloride** (Purepac)	**Tablets:** 650 mg	In 100s.
otc	**Sodium Chloride** (Various)	**Tablets:** 1 g	In 100s and 1000s.
otc	**Sodium Chloride** (Lilly)	**Tablets:** 2.25 g	In 100s and 500s.
otc	**Slo-Salt-K** (Mission)	**Tablets, slow release:** 410 mg sodium chloride and 150 mg potassium chloride in wax matrix	In 1000s.

ORAL ELECTROLYTE MIXTURES

Actions:

Pharmacology: Used properly, mixtures with electrolytes, water and glucose prevent dehydration or achieve rehydration, and maintain strength and feeling of well being. They contain sodium, chloride, potassium and bicarbonate to replace depleted electrolytes and restore acid-base balance. Glucose facilitates sodium transport, which aids in sodium and water absorption.

Indications:

For maintenance of water and electrolytes following corrective parenteral therapy for severe diarrhea; for maintenance to replace mild to moderate fluid losses when food and liquid intake are discontinued; to restore fluid and minerals lost in diarrhea and vomiting in infants and children.

Contraindications:

Severe, continuing diarrhea or other critical fluid losses; intractable vomiting; prolonged shock, renal dysfunction (anuria, oliguria). These require parenteral therapy.

Administration and Dosage:

Individualize dosage. Follow the guidelines listed on the product labeling.

Ricelyte: Children < 2 years of age: Consult physician.

Children ≥ 2 years of age – Administer every 3 to 4 hours, up to 2 quarts per day.

Resol: Individualize dosage based on extent of weight loss and dehydration as assessed by the physician.

Pedialyte/Rehydralyte: Offer frequently in amounts tolerated. Adjust total daily intake to meet individual needs, based on thirst and response to therapy. In the following table, suggested intakes for replacement are based on fluid losses of 5% or 10% of body weight, including maintenance requirement.

Pedialyte/Rehydralyte Dosage for Infants/Young Children

	Weight (approx.)			*Rehydralyte*	
Age	kg	lb	*Pedialyte oz/day*	Replacement for 5% dehydration (oz/day)	Replacement for 10% dehydration (oz/day)
2 wks	3.2	7	13-16	18-21	23-26
3 mos	6	13	28-32	38-42	48-52
6 mos	7.8	17	34-40	47-53	60-66
9 mos	9.2	20	38-44	53-59	68-74
1 yr	10.2	23	41-46	58-63	75-80
1.5 yr	11.4	25	45-50	64-69	83-88
2 yr	12.6	28	48-53	69-74	90-95
2.5 yr	13.6	30	51-56	74-79	97-102
3 yr	14.6	32	54-58	78-82	102-106
3.5 yr	16	35	56-60	83-87	110-114
4 yr	17	38	57-62	85-90	113-118

Extemporaneous oral rehydration solution (developed by the World Health Organization) To be added to 1 L water. Follow physician's administration instructions.

	Na+/Cl–	K+	Citrate	Glucose
Source	NaCl or table salt	KCl or potassium salt[1]	sodium bicarbonate (baking soda)	Glucose or sucrose (cane sugar)
Weight (g)	3.5	1.5	2.5	20[2]
Household measure	0.5 tsp	0.25 tsp	0.5 tsp	2 tbsp[3]
mmol/L	90/80	20	30	111

[1] See potassium salt substitutes.
[2] If sucrose is used, 40 g.
[3] If sucrose is used, 4 tbsp.

ORAL ELECTROLYTE MIXTURES

		Electrolyte content (mEq/L)									
	Product	Na^+	K^+	Cl^-	Citrate	Ca^{++}	Mg^{++}	Phosphate	Other Content	Calories per fl. oz.	How Supplied
otc	**Rehydralyte Solution** (Ross)	75	20	65	30				25 g/L dextrose	3	In 240 ml ready-to-use.
otc	**Infalyte Oral Solution** (Mead Johnson)	50	25	45	34				30 g/L rice syrup solids	4.2	Fruit flavor. In ≈ 1 L ready-to-use.
otc	**Resol Solution** (Wyeth-Ayerst)	50	20	50	34	4	4	5	20 g/L glucose	2.5	In 240 ml ready-to-use.
otc	**Naturalyte** (UBI)	45	20	35	48				25 g/L dextrose		Unflavored, fruit or bubble gum flavors. In 240 ml and 1 L.
otc	**Pedialyte Solution** (Ross)	45	20	35	30				25 g/L dextrose	3	Regular or fruit flavor. In 240 & 960 ml ready-to-use.
otc	**Pedialyte Freezer Pops** (Ross)	45	20	35	30				25 g/L dextrose, phenylalanine, aspartame	3	Grape, cherry, orange and blue raspberry flavors. In 2.1 fl oz ready-to-freeze pops (16s).
otc	**Pediatric Electrolyte** (Goldline)	45	20	35	48				25 g/L dextrose	3	Fruit and bubble gum flavors. In 1 L.

Systemic Alkalinizers

CITRATE AND CITRIC ACID SOLUTIONS

Actions:

Pharmacology: Citrate and citric acid solutions are systemic and urinary alkalinizers. Preparations containing potassium citrate are preferred in patients requiring potassium or those who require sodium restriction. Conversely, sodium citrate may be administered when potassium is undesirable or contraindicated. Potassium citrate and sodium citrate are capable of buffering gastric acidity (pH > 2.5). The effects are essentially those of chlorides before absorption, and subsequently, those of bicarbonates.

Pharmacokinetics: Potassium citrate and sodium citrate are absorbed and metabolized to potassium bicarbonate and sodium bicarbonate, thus acting as systemic alkalinizers. The citric acid is metabolized to carbon dioxide and water; therefore, it has only a transient effect on systemic acid-base status. It functions as a temporary buffer component.

Oxidation is virtually complete; < 5% of the citrates are excreted in the urine unchanged.

Indications:

Treatment of chronic metabolic acidosis, particularly when caused by renal tubular acidosis.

Conditions where long-term maintenance of an alkaline urine is desirable, in treatment of patients with uric acid and cystine calculi of the urinary tract and in conjunction with uricosurics in gout therapy to prevent uric acid nephropathy.

Nonparticulate neutralizing buffers.

Contraindications:

Severe renal impairment with oliguria, azotemia or anuria; untreated Addison's disease; adynamia episodica hereditaria; acute dehydration; heat cramps; severe myocardial damage; hyperkalemia.

Sodium citrate: Sodium restricted patients.

Warnings:

Pregnancy: Polycitra-K is not expected to cause fetal harm when administered in dosages that will not result in hyperkalemia.

Lactation: Exercise caution when administered to a nursing woman.

Precautions:

Urolithiasis: Citrate mobilizes calcium from bones and increases its renal excretion; this, along with the elevated urine pH, may predispose to urolithiasis.

Hyperkalemia/Alkalosis: Patients with low urinary output and abnormal renal mechanisms may develop hyperkalemia or alkalosis, especially in the presence of hypocalcemia.

Sodium salts: Use cautiously in patients with cardiac failure, hypertension, impaired renal function, peripheral and pulmonary edema and preeclampsia. Monitor serum electrolytes, particularly the serum bicarbonate level, in patients with renal disease.

GI effects: Dilute with water to minimize GI injury associated with the oral ingestion of concentrated potassium salts. Take after meals to avoid saline laxative effect.

Drug Interactions:

Urinary Alkalinizer Drug Interactions

Precipitant drug	Object drug *		Description
Urinary alkalinizers (eg, potassium citrate, sodium citrate)	Chlorpropamide Lithium Methenamine Methotrexate Salicylates Tetracyclines	⬇	Urinary alkalinizers may increase the excretion and decrease the serum levels of these agents, possibly decreasing their pharmacologic effects.
Urinary alkalinizers (eg, potassium citrate, sodium citrate)	Anorexiants Flecainide Mecamylamine Quinidine Sympathomimetics	⬆	Urinary alkalinizers may decrease the excretion and increase the serum levels of these agents, possibly increasing their pharmacologic effects.

* ⬆ = Object drug increased. ⬇ = Object drug decreased.

Systemic Alkalinizers

CITRATE AND CITRIC ACID SOLUTIONS

Adverse Reactions:

Hyperkalemia: Listlessness, weakness, mental confusion, tingling of extremities and other symptoms associated with high serum potassium. Hyperkalemia may exhibit the following ECG abnormalities: Disappearance of the P wave; widening or slurring of the QRS complex; changes of the ST segment; tall peaked T waves.

Overdosage:

Symptoms: Overdosage with sodium salts may cause diarrhea, nausea, vomiting, hypernoia (excessive mental activity) and convulsions. Overdosage with potassium salts may cause hyperkalemia and alkalosis, especially in the presence of renal disease. Treat hyperkalemia immediately, because lethal levels can be reached in a few hours.

Treatment: For treatment of hyperkalemia, refer to the Potassium monograph in the IV Nutritional Therapy section; for treatment of sodium overdosage, refer to the Sodium Chloride monograph in the Salt Replacement Products section.

Patient Information:

Dilute with water; follow with additional water, if desired.

Take after meals.

Notify physician if diarrhea, nausea, stomach pain, vomiting or convulsions occur.

Administration and Dosage:

Dilute in water before taking; follow with additional water, if desired. Monitor urinary pH with Hydrion paper (pH 6 to 8) or *Nitrazine* paper (pH 4.5 to 7.5).

Dosage:

Adults – 15 to 30 ml diluted with water, after meals and before bedtime.

Children – 5 to 10 ml diluted with water, after meals and before bedtime. The solution, not the crystals, is recommended for pediatric administration since dosage can be more easily regulated.

Neutralizing buffer: A single dose of 15 ml diluted with 15 ml water.

Rx sf	**Polycitra-K** (Willen)	**Crystals**: 1100 mg potassium citrate monohydrate and 334 mg citric acid monohydrate per 5 ml when reconstituted. (2 mEq potassium per ml and is equivalent to 2 mEq bicarbonate)	In UD packets (100) to make 15 ml when reconstituted.
Rx	**Cytra-3** (Cypress)	**Syrup**: 550 mg potassium citrate monohydrate, 500 mg sodium citrate dihydrate, 334 mg citric acid monohydrate per 5 ml (1 mEq potassium and 1 mEq sodium per ml and is equivalent to 2 mEq bicarbonate).	Sugar free. In 16 oz. bottles.
Rx	**Polycitra** (Willen)		Sugar. Alcohol free. In 473 ml.
Rx	**Cytra-LC** (Cypress)	**Solution**: 550 mg potassium citrate monohydrate, 500 mg sodium citrate dihydrate, 334 mg citric acid monohydrate per 5 ml (1 mEq potassium and 1 mEq sodium per ml and is equivalent to 2 mEq bicarbonate).	In 16 oz. bottles.
Rx sf	**Polycitra-LC** (Willen)		Alcohol free. In 473 ml.
Rx	**Cytra-K** (Cypress)	**Solution**: 1100 mg potassium citrate monohydrate and 334 mg citric acid monohydrate per 5 ml. (2 mEq potassium per ml and is equivalent to 2 mEq bicarbonate)	Alcohol free. In 473 ml.
Rx sf	**Polycitra-K** (Willen)		Alcohol free. In 473 ml.
Rx	**Oracit** (Carolina Medical Products)	**Solution**: 490 mg sodium citrate and 640 mg citric acid per 5 ml. (1 mEq sodium per ml and is equivalent to 1 mEq bicarbonate)	Parabens. In 500 ml and UD 15 and 30 ml.
Rx sf	**Bicitra** (Willen)	**Solution**: 500 mg sodium citrate dihydrate and 334 mg citric acid monohydrate per 5 ml. (1 mEq sodium per ml and is equivalent to 1 mEq bicarbonate)	Alcohol free. In 120 and 473 ml, gal and UD 15 and 30 ml.
Rx	**Cytra-2** (Cypress)		Grape flavored. In 16 oz. bottles.

Systemic Alkalinizers

SODIUM BICARBONATE

For information on parenteral sodium bicarbonate products, refer to the monograph in the IV Nutritional Therapy section.

One g of sodium bicarbonate provides 11.9 mmol sodium and 11.9 mmol bicarbonate.

Indications:

A gastric, systemic and urinary alkalinizer.

Precautions:

Use cautiously in patients with edematous sodium-retaining states, congestive heart failure or renal impairment. Prolonged therapy may lead to systemic alkalosis.

Administration and Dosage:

Usual dose is 325 mg to 2 g, 1 to 4 times daily. Maximum daily intake is 16 g (200 mEq) in patients < 60 years old and 8 g (100 mEq) in those older than 60 years of age.

otc	**Sodium Bicarbonate** (Various, eg, Rugby)	**Tablets:** 325 mg	In 1000s.
		650 mg	In 1000s.
		Powder	In 120 and 300 g and 1 lb.

VITAMIN A & D COMBINATIONS

	Product & Distributor	A IU	D IU	C mg	Content Given Per	Other Content and How Supplied
otc	**White Cod Liver Oil Concentrate Capsules** (Schering-Plough)	10,000	400		capsule	Vitamin E. In 40s and 100s.
otc	**Super D Perles** (Roberts)					In 100s.
otc	**Vitamin A & D Tablets** (Nature's Bounty)	10,000	400		tablet	In 100s.
otc	**White Cod Liver Oil Concentrate w/ Vitamin C Tablets** (Schering-Plough)	4,000	200	50	chewable tablet	Tartrazine, sugar. In 100s.
otc	**White Cod Liver Oil Concentrate Tablets** (Schering-Plough)	4,000	200		chewable tablet	Tartrazine, sugar. In 100s.
otc sf	**Tri-Vi-Sol Drops** (Mead J Nutritional)	1,500	400	35	1 ml	In 30 and 50 ml w/dropper.
otc	**Tri-Vitamin Infants' Drops** (Schein)					Pineapple flavor. In 50 ml w/dropper.
otc sf	**Vi-Daylin ADC Drops** (Ross)					< 0.5% alcohol, parabens. Pineapple flavor. In 50 ml.
otc	**Cod Liver Oil Capsules** (Various, eg, Apothecon, Goldline, IDE, Moore, Nature's Bounty, Rugby, Bristol-Myers Squibb)	1,250	≈ 135		capsule	In 100s, 250s and 1000s.
otc	**Scott's Emulsion** (SK-Beecham)	1,250	100		5 ml	Benzyl alcohol, parabens. In 187.5 and 375 ml.
otc	**Cod Liver Oil USP** (Humco)	1,000	100		g	In 120 ml, pt and gal.
otc	**Cod Liver Oil Liquid USP** (Various, eg, Apothecon, Humco, Purepac, Bristol-Myers Squibb)	850	85		g	In 120 and 360 ml and pt.

CALCIUM AND VITAMIN D

CALCIUM AND VITAMIN D

Content given per tablet or softgel.

	Product and Distributor	Ca[1] mg	D IU	P mg	Other Content and How Supplied
otc	**Calcium Carbonate 600 mg + Vitamin D Tablets** (Major)	600	125		In 72s.
otc	**Calcium with Vitamin D Tablets** (Schein)				Green. Oval. In 60s.
otc sf	**Calcium 600 + D Tablets** (Nature's Bounty)				In 60s.
otc sf	**Caltrate 600 + Iron/Vitamin D Tablets** (Lederle)				18 mg Fe.[2] (LL). Film coated. Capsule shape. In 60s.
otc sf	**Posture-D Tablets** (Whitehall)				Scored. Film coated. In 60s.
otc sf	**Caltrate 600 + D Tablets** (Lederle)	600	200		(Caltrate). In 60s.
otc sf	**Caltrate Plus Tablets** (Lederle)				7.5 mg Zn, Mg, Cu, Mn, B. (Caltrate). In 60s.
otc sf	**Super Calcium '1200' Softgels** (Schiff)				In 60s and 120s.
otc	**Calcium 600 with Vitamin D Tablets** (Mission)	600	100		In 60s.
otc sf	**Calel D Tablets** (Rhone-Poulenc Rorer)	500	200		In 75s.
otc sf	**Desert Pure Calcium** (Cal•White Mineral Co.)	500	125		Film coated. Oval. In 200s.
otc	**Os-Cal 500 + D Tablets** (SK-Beecham)	500	125		Parabens, EDTA. In 60s and 120s.
otc sf	**Oyster Calcium 500 mg + D Tablets** (Nion)				In 120s.
otc sf	**Oyster Calcium Tablets** (Nature's Bounty)	375	200		800 IU vitamin A. In 100s.
otc	**Citracal Caplets + D** (Mission)	315	200		In 60s.
otc	**Caltro Tablets** (Geneva)	250	125		Green. In 100s and 1000s.
otc	**Os-Cal 250 + D Tablets** (SK-Beecham)				Parabens, EDTA. In 100s and 240s.
otc	**Oysco D Tablets** (Rugby)				In 100s, 250s and 1000s.
otc	**Oyst-Cal-D Tablets** (Goldline)				Tartrazine. Green. Film coated. In 100s, 240s and 1000s.
otc sf	**Oyster Calcium with Vitamin D Tablets** (Nion)				In 100s.
otc sf	**Oystercal-D 250 Tablets** (Nature's Bounty)				In 100s and 250s.
otc	**Oyster Shell Calcium with Vitamin D Tablets** (Major)				In 100s, 1000s and UD 100s.
otc	**Amino-Min-D Capsules** (Tyson)	250	100		7.5 mg Fe, 5.6 mg Zn, Mg, I, Mn, Cu, K, Cr, Se, betaine HCl, glutamic acid HCl. In 100s.
otc sf	**FemCal Tablets** (Freeda)				100 mg Mg, Mn, Si, B. Kosher. In 100s and 250s.
otc	**Calcet Tablets** (Mission)	152.8	100		In 100s.
otc sf	**Bone Meal Tablets** (Nion)	236		118	In 250s.
otc sf	**Super CalciCaps Tablets** (Nion)	400	133	42	In 90s and 180s.

CALCIUM AND VITAMIN D

CALCIUM AND VITAMIN D

	Product and Distributor	Ca[1] mg	D IU	P mg	Other Content and How Supplied
otc	**Dical-D Wafers** (Abbott)	232	200	180	Chewable. Sucrose, dextrose. Vanilla flavor. In 51s.
otc	**CalciCaps Tablets** (Nion)	125[3]	67	60	In 100s and 500s.
otc	**CalciCaps with Iron Tablets** (Nion)				7 mg Fe.[4] Tartrazine. In 100s and 500s.
otc	**Dical-D Tablets** (Abbott)	117[5]	133	90	In 100s.
otc	**Dical CapTabs** (Rugby)				Sucrose. In 1000s.
otc	**Diostate D Tablets** (Roberts)	114	133	88	Tartrazine, sucrose. In 100s.

[1] Expressed in mg elemental calcium.
[2] As ferrous fumarate.
[3] Dibasic calcium phosphate, calcium gluconate and calcium carbonate.
[4] As ferrous gluconate.
[5] Dibasic calcium phosphate hydrous as anhydrous.

VITAMIN COMBINATIONS, MISCELLANEOUS, WITH C

VITAMIN COMBINATIONS, MISCELLANEOUS, WITH C

Content given per capsule, tablet or ml.

	Product and Distributor	A IU	E mg	B_3 mg	C mg	Other Content	How Supplied
otc	**Antiox** (Mayrand)	42,000[1]	100[5]		120		In 60s.
otc	**A.C.N. Tablets** (Person & Covey)	25,000		25	250		In 100s.
otc	**Ocuvite Extra** (Storz)	6000	50[5]		200	40 mg Zn, 40 mg B_3, 3 mg B_2, Cu, Se, Mn, L-glutathione	In 50s.
otc	**Pro Skin Capsules** (Marlyn)	6250[6]	100[3]		100	10 mg B_5, 10 mg Zn, Se	In 60s.
otc	**Protegra Softgels** (Lederle)	5000[1]	200[5]		250	7.5 mg Zn, Cu, Se, Mn	In 50s.
otc	**Theragran AntiOxidant** (BM-Squibb)	5000[1]	200[5]		250	Mn, Cu, Zn, Se	In 50s.
otc	**OcuCaps Caplets** (Akorn)	5000[1]	182[2]		400	40 mg Zn, 5 mg L-glutathione, sodium pyruvate, Cu, Se	In 60s.
otc	**Ocuvite Tablets** (Lederle)	5000[1]	30[3]		60	40 mg Zn, Cu, 40 mcg Se, lactose	In 60s.
otc *sf*	**C & E Softgels** (Nature's Bounty)		400[2]		500		In 50s.
otc *sf*	**Vitamin C + E Caplets** (Triage)		400[3]		500		Protein coated. In 50s.
otc	**Ecee Plus Tablets** (Edwards)		165[4]		100	70 mg Mg sulfate, 80 mg Zn sulfate	In 100s.
otc	**Sublingual C & Niacin Liquid** (Pharmaceutical Lab)			20	180	Fructose, sorbitol	In 30 ml.

[1] As beta carotene.
[2] In IU; as mixed tocopherols complex.
[3] As dl-alpha tocopheryl acetate.
[4] As d-alpha tocopheryl acid succinate.
[5] Form of vitamin E unknown; content given in mg.
[6] As beta, alpha and gamma carotene and lycopenes.

VITAMIN COMBINATIONS, MISCELLANEOUS

VITAMIN COMBINATIONS, MISCELLANEOUS

Content given per capsule, tablet or ml.

	Product and Distributor	Ca[1] mg	E mg	B_6 mg	C mg	Other Content	How Supplied
otc sf	**Ze Caps Capsules** (Everett)		200[2]			9.6 mg Zn (as gluconate), sorbitol	In 60s.
otc sf	**Dolomite Tablets** (Nature's Bounty)	130				78 mg Mg	In 100s and 250s.
otc	**Beelith Tablets** (Beach)			20		362 mg Mg	In 100s.
otc sf	**Chelated Calcium Magnesium Tablets** (Nature's Bounty)	500				250 mg Mg	Protein coated. In 50s and 100s.
otc sf	**Calcium Magnesium Zinc Tablets** (Nature's Bounty)	333				133 mg Mg, 8.3 mg Zn	In 100s.
otc sf	**KLB6 Softgels** (Nature's Bounty)			3.5		100 mg soya lecithin, 25 mg kelp, 40 mg cider vinegar	In 100s.
otc	**Ultra KLB6 Tablets** (Nature's Bounty)			16.7		400 mg lecithin, 33.3 mg kelp, 80 mg cider vinegar	In 100s.
otc sf	**Mag-Cal Tablets** (Fibertone)	416.7[3] 166.7[1]				66.7 IU D_3, 83.3 mg Mg, Cu, Mn, K, Zn	In 180s.
otc sf	**Bo-Cal Tablets** (Fibertone)	250				125 mg Mg, 100 IU D_3, B	In 120s.
otc sf	**Oesto-Mins Powder**[4] (Tyson)	250			500	250 mg Mg, 45 mg K, 100 IU vitamin D	In 200 g.
otc sf	**Multi-Mineral Tablets** (Nature's Bounty)	166.7				75.7 mg P, 25 mcg I, 3 mg Fe, 66.7 mg Mg, 0.33 mg Cu, 2.5 mg Zn, 12.5 mg K, 8.3 mg Mn	In 100s.
otc sf	**Mag-Cal Mega Tablets** (Freeda)	400				800 mg Mg	Kosher. In 100s and 250s.
otc sf	**Super CalciCaps M-Z Tablets** (Nion)	400				133 mg Mg, 5 mg Zn, 1667 mg vitamin A, 133 IU vitamin D, Se	In 90s.

[1] Calcium content expressed in mg elemental calcium.
[2] As dl-alpha tocopheryl acetate.
[3] Carbonate.
[4] Content given per 4.5 g.

B VITAMIN COMBINATIONS, ORAL

Content given per capsule, tablet or 5 ml.

	Product & Distributor	B_1 mg	B_2 mg	B_3 mg	B_5 mg	B_6 mg	B_{12} mcg	FA mg	Other Content	How Supplied
otc sf	**B Complex-150 Tablets** (Nion)	150	150	150	150	150	150	0.4	150 mcg biotin, 100 mg PABA, 150 mg choline bitartrate, 150 mg inositol	Sustained-release. In 30s.
otc	**B 100 Tablets** (Fibertone)	100	100	100	100	100	100	0.4	50 mcg biotin, 100 mg PABA, 100 mg choline bitartrate, 100 mg inositol	Sustained-release. In 100s.
otc sf	**B-100 Tablets** (NBTY)	100	100	100	100	100	100	0.1	100 mcg d-biotin, 100 mg base of PABA, choline, inositol and lecithin	In 50s and 100s.
otc	**Mega-B Tablets** (Arco)								100 mg PABA, 100 mg inositol, 100 mcg d-biotin, 100 mg choline bitartrate and lecithin	In 100s.
otc sf	**Super Quints-50 Tablets** (Freeda)	50	50	50	50	50	50	0.4	30 mg PABA, 50 mcg d–biotin, 50 mg inositol	Kosher. In 100s, 250s and 500s.
otc sf	**B Complex-50 Tablets** (Nion)								50 mcg biotin, 50 mg PABA, 50 mg choline bitartrate, 50 mg inositol	Sustained-release. In 100s.
otc sf	**B-50 Tablets** (NBTY)	50	50	50	50	50	50	0.1	50 mcg d-biotin, PABA, choline bitartrate, inositol	In 50s and 100s.
otc sf	**Vital B-50 Tablets** (Goldline)									Timed release. In 60s.
otc	**Iso-B Capsules** (Tyson)	25	25	75	125	50	100	0.2	2.5 mg pyridoxal 5 phosphate, 50 mg PABA, 50 mg inositol, 125 mg choline bitartrate, 100 mcg biotin	In 120s.

B VITAMIN COMBINATIONS, ORAL

	Product & Distributor	B_1 mg	B_2 mg	B_3 mg	B_5 mg	B_6 mg	B_{12} mcg	FA mg	Other Content	How Supplied
otc	**Neurodep-Caps Capsules** (Medical Products)	125				125	1000			In 50s.
otc	**Apatate Liquid** (Kenwood/Bradley)	15				0.5	25			Cherry flavor. In 120 and 240 ml.
otc	**Apatate Tablets** (Kenwood/Bradley)	15				0.5	25			Chewable. Cherry flavor. In 50s.
otc	**Secran Liquid** (Scherer)	10		10			25		17% alcohol	In 480 ml.
otc	**Orexin Tablets** (Roberts)	8.1				4.1	25		Saccharin	Chewable. In 100s.
otc *sf*	**B-Complex and B-12 Tablets** (NBTY)	7	14	4.5			25		10 mg protease	In 90s.
otc	**Surbex Filmtabs** (Abbott)	6	6	30	10	2.5	5			Film coated. In 100s.
otc	**Apetil Liquid** (Kenwood/Bradley)	1.7	0.3	6.7		2.5	5		14.6 mg Zn, Mg, Mn, l-lysine, sucrose, parabens, sorbitol	Alcohol free. In 237 ml.
otc	**B-Complex with B-12 Tablets** (Major)	3	2	20	0.1	1	5			In 100s.
otc *sf*	**B-Complex with B-12 Tablets** (Goldline)	1.5	1.7	20	10	2	6	0.4		In 100s.
otc	**Almebex Plus B_{12} Liquid** (Dayton)	1	2	5		0.4	5		33 mg choline, parabens, sucrose	In 473 ml with vitamin B_{12} in separate glass container.
otc *sf*	**B-Complex Elixir** (Nion)	2.3	1	6.7		0.3			10% alcohol, sorbitol	Orange flavor. In 240 and 480 ml.

B VITAMIN COMBINATIONS, ORAL

	Product & Distributor	B_1 mg	B_2 mg	B_3 mg	B_5 mg	B_6 mg	B_{12} mcg	FA mg	Other Content	How Supplied
otc	**Geravim Elixir** (Major)	0.83	0.42	8.3	1.67	0.17	0.17		I, 2.5 mg Fe, Mg, 0.3 mg Zn, choline, Mn, 18% alcohol, corn syrup, methylparaben, sorbitol	In pt and gal.
otc	**Gevrabon Liquid** (Lederle)								2.5 mg Fe, choline, I, Mg, Mn, 0.3 mg Zn, 18% alcohol, sucrose	In 480 ml.
otc	**Vitamin-Mineral-Supplement Liquid** (Pennex)								I, 2.5 mg Fe, Mg, 0.3 mg Zn, Mn, choline, 18% alcohol, sorbitol, methylparaben, corn syrup	Sherry wine flavor. In 473 ml.
Rx	**Senilezol Liquid** (Edwards)	0.42	0.42	1.67	0.83	0.17	0.83		3.3 mg ferric pyrophosphate, 15% alcohol, sucrose, methylparaben	In 473 ml.
otc	**Eldertonic Liquid** (Mayrand)	0.17	0.19	2.22	1.11	0.22	0.67		1.7mg Zn, Mg, Mn, 13.5% alcohol	In 240ml, pt and gal.
otc	**Geroton Forte Liquid** (Kenwood/Bradley)	1.5	1.7	20	10	2	6		15 mg Zn, 2 mg Mg, 2 mg Mn, 13.5% alcohol, methylparaben, sucrose	In 473 ml.
otc sf	**Brewers Yeast Tablets** (NBTY)	0.06	0.02	0.2						In 250s.
Rx	**Megaton Elixir** (Hyrex)			4.4	1.1	0.44	1.33	0.1	4 mg Fe, Mn, 1.7 mg Zn, 13% alcohol, parabens, sucrose	Sherry wine flavor. In 473 ml.
Rx	**May-Vita Elixir** (Mayrand)								4 mg Fe, Mn, 1.7 mg Zn, 13% alcohol	In 473 ml.

B VITAMINS, PARENTERAL

Content given per ml.

	Product & Distributor	B_1 mg	B_2 mg	B_3 mg	B_5 mg	B_6 mg	Other Content	How Supplied
Rx	**B-Ject-100 Injection**(Hyrex)	100	2	100	2	2		In 30 ml vials.[1]
Rx	**Vitamin B Complex 100 Injection**(McGuff)							In 10 and 30 ml vials.[1]

[1] May contain benzyl alcohol.

B VITAMINS WITH VITAMIN C, PARENTERAL

Content given per ml.

	Product & Distributor	B_1 mg	B_2 mg	B_3 mg	B_5 mg	B_6 mg	B_{12} mcg	C mg	Other Content	Content Given Per	How Supplied
Rx	**Key-Plex Injection** (Hyrex)	50	5	125	6	5	1000	50	Benzyl alcohol	1 ml	In 10 ml multiple dose vials.
Rx	**Lypholized Vitamin B Complex & Vitamin C with B_{12} Injection** (McGuff)										In 10 ml vials.
Rx	**Neurodep Injection** (Medical Products)										In 10 ml vials.
Rx	**Vicam Injection** (Keene)										In 10 ml vials.

B VITAMIN COMBINATIONS

B VITAMINS WITH VITAMIN C, ORAL

B VITAMINS WITH VITAMIN C, ORAL
Content given per capsule, tablet or 5 ml.

	Product & Distributor	B_1 mg	B_2 mg	B_3 mg	B_5 mg	B_6 mg	B_{12} mcg	C mg	Other Content	How Supplied
otc sf	**Enviro-Stress Tablets** (Vitaline)	50	50	100	50	50	25	600	0.4 mg FA, 30 mg Zn, 30 IU vitamin E, Mg, Se, PABA	Slow release. In 90s and 1000s.
otc sf	**T-Vites Tablets** (Freeda)	25	25	150	25	25		100	30 mcg biotin, PABA, K, Mg carbonate, 2 mg Mn and 20 mg Zn gluconate	Kosher. In 100s.
otc sf	**Beminal 500 Tablets** (Whitehall)	25	12.5	100	20	10	5	500	Lactose	In 100s.
otc	**ThexForte Caplets** (Lee)	25	15	100	10	5		500		In 75s.
otc	**Vicon-C Capsules** (Whitby)	20	10	100	20	5		300	Mg, 80 mg Zn sulfate	Yellow/orange. Banded. In 60s and UD 100s.
otc sf	**Viogen-C Capsules** (Goldline)								Mg, 50 mg dried Zn sulfate, tartrazine	In 100s.
otc	**Allbee-T Tablets** (Robins)	15.5	10	100	23	8.2	5	500	Lactose, desiccated liver	In 100s.
Rx	**B-C With Folic Acid Tablets** (Geneva)	15	15	100	18	4	5	500	0.5 mg folic acid	Orange. Oblong. In 100s.
Rx	**Berocca Tablets** (Roche)								0.5 mg folic acid, sugar	(Berocca Roche). Light green. Capsule shaped. In 100s and 500s.
Rx	**B-Plex Tablets** (Goldline)								0.5 mg folic acid	In 100s.
Rx	**Formula B Tablets** (Major)									In 250s.
Rx	**Strovite Tablets** (Everett)								0.5 mg folic acid, lactose	In 100s.

B VITAMINS WITH VITAMIN C, ORAL

B VITAMINS WITH VITAMIN C, ORAL

	Product & Distributor	B_1 mg	B_2 mg	B_3 mg	B_5 mg	B_6 mg	B_{12} mcg	C mg	Other Content	How Supplied
otc	**Allbee with C Caplets** (Robins)	15	10.2	50	10	5		300	Saccharin, lactose	In 130s.
otc	**Nion B Plus C Caplets** (Nion)									In 100s.
otc	**Therapeutic B Complex with C Capsules** (Upsher-Smith)									Yellow/green. In UD 100s.
otc	**B-Complex/Vitamin C Caplets** (Geneva)									Yellow. In 100s.
otc	**Econo B & C Caplets** (Vangard)									In 100s and UD 100s.
otc	**Arcobee with C Caplets** (NBTY)								Tartrazine	In 100s.
otc *sf*	**B-C-Bid Caplets** (Roberts)									In 100s.
otc *sf*	**Farbee with Vitamin C Caplets** (Major)									In 100s, 130s and 1000s.
otc *sf*	**Gen-bee with C Caplets** (Goldline)									In 130s and 1000s.
otc	**Vita-Bee with C Captabs** (Rugby)									In 100s and 1000s.

B VITAMIN COMBINATIONS

B VITAMINS WITH VITAMIN C, ORAL

B VITAMINS WITH VITAMIN C, ORAL

	Product & Distributor	B_1 mg	B_2 mg	B_3 mg	B_5 mg	B_6 mg	B_{12} mcg	C mg	Other Content	How Supplied
otc *sf*	**Superplex T Tablets** (Major)	15	10	100	20	5	10	500		In 100s.
otc	**Surbex-T Filmtabs** (Abbott)									Orange. In 100s.
otc	**High Potency N-Vites Tablets** (Nion)									In 100s.
otc	**Surbu-Gen-T Tablets** (Goldline)									In 100s.
otc	**Probec-T Tablets** (Roberts)	12.2	10	100	18.4	4.1	5	600	Sucrose	In 60s.
otc	**3 mg Biotin Forte Tablets** (Vitaline)	10	10	40	10	25	10	200	3 mg biotin, 800 mcg FA, 30 mg Zn	In 60s and 1000s.
otc	**Extra Strength 5 mg Biotin Forte Tablets** (Vitaline)	10	10	40	10	25	10	100	5 mg biotin, 800 mcg FA	In 60s and 1000s.
otc	**B Complex + C Tablets** (Various, eg, Nion)	15	10	100	20	5	10	500		Timed release. In 100s.
otc	**Surbex with C Filmtabs** (Abbott)	6	6	30	10	2.5	5	250	Lactose	Film coated. In 100s.
otc	**Sublingual B Total Liquid** (Pharmaceutical Lab)		1.7	20	30	2	1000	60	Sorbitol	Alcohol free. In 30 ml with dropper.
Rx	**Nephplex Rx Tablets** (Nephro-Tech)	1.5	1.7	20	10	10	6	60	1 mg FA, 300 mcg d–biotin	In 100s.
Rx	**Nephro-Vite Rx Tablets** (R & D)									(RD 12). Yellow. Film coated. In 100s.
otc	**Nephro-Vite Vitamin B Complex and C Supplement Tablets** (R & D)								800 mcg FA, 300 mcg d-biotin	(RD 02). Yellow. Film coated. In 100s.
Rx	**Nephrocaps Capsules** (Fleming)	1.5	1.7	20	5	10	6	100	1 mg FA, 150 mcg biotin	Black. Oval. In 100s.
otc	**Stress B Complex with Vitamin C Tablets** (Mission)	13.8	10	50		4.1		300	15 mg Zn	Timed- release. In 60s.

MULTIVITAMINS, PARENTERAL

	Product & Distributor	Content[1] given per	A IU	D IU	E IU	B_1 mg	B_2 mg	B_3 mg	B_5 mg	B_6 mg	B_{12} mcg	C mg	biotin mcg	FA mg	Other Content and How Supplied
Rx	**Berocca Parenteral Nutrition** (Roche)	1 ml	3,300	200	10[2]	3	3.6	40	15	4	5	100	60	0.4	In 2 vial or ampule sets: Soln 1[3] (1 or 2 ml) and soln 2[3] (1 or 2 ml).
Rx	**M.V.I.-12 Injection** (Astra)	5 ml													In 2 vial sets: Vial 1[4] (5 ml single dose or 50 ml multiple dose) and vial 2[5] (5 ml single dose or 50 ml multiple dose).
Rx	**M.V.I.-12 Unit Vial** (Astra)	10 ml													In 10 ml two chambered vials.[4]
Rx	**M.V.I. Pediatric** (Astra)	5 ml	2,300	400	7[2]	1.2	1.4	17	5	1	1	80	20	0.14	200 mcg vitamin K_1 and 375 mg mannitol. In single and multiple dose vials.[6]
Rx	**Multi Vitamin Concentrate Injection** (Lyphomed)	5 ml	10,000	1,000	5[2]	50	10	100	25	15		500			In 5 ml vials.[5]
Rx	**B Complex with C and B-12 Injection** (Goldline)	1 ml				50	5	125	6	5	1,000	50			1% benzyl alcohol. In 10 ml multiple dose vials.

[1] After combining vials, if necessary.
[2] As dl-alpha tocopheryl acetate.
[3] With propylene glycol, EDTA and 1% benzyl alcohol.
[4] With propylene glycol, polysorbate 80 and polysorbate 20.
[5] With propylene glycol.
[6] With polysorbate 20 and polysorbate 80.

MULTIVITAMINS, CAPSULES AND TABLETS

Content given per capsule or tablet.

For a comparison of the potencies of the various forms of vitamin E, see the vitamin E monograph.

	Product & Distributor	A IU	D IU	E IU	B_1 mg	B_2 mg	B_3 mg	B_5 mg	B_6 mg	B_{12} mcg	C mg	FA mg	Other Content and How Supplied
otc sf	**Multi 75 Tablets** (Fibertone)	25,000	500	150[1]	75	75	75	75	75	75	250	0.4	50 mg Ca, 10 mg Fe, biotin, I, Mg, 15 mg Zn, Cu, PABA, K, Mn, Cr, Se, Mo, B, Si, choline bitartrate, inositol, rutin, lemon bioflavonoid complex, hesperidin complex, betaine HCl. Timed-release. In 60s and 90s.
otc	**Oncovite** (Mission)	10,000	400	200	0.37	0.5	5	2.5	25	1.5	500	0.4	Sugar. 7.5 mg Zn. In 100s.
otc sf	**Quintabs Tablets** (Freeda)	10,000	400	29[2]	25	25	100	25	25	25	300	0.1	Inositol, PABA. Kosher. In 100s and 250s.
otc	**Ru-lets M 500 Tablets** (Rugby)	10,000	400	30[3]	15	10	100	20	5	12	500		Mg, 20 mg Fe, Cu, 1.5 mg Zn, Mn, I. Film-coated. In 100s.
otc	**Nutrox Capsules** (Tyson)	10,000		150[4]	25	25	50	22			80		L-cysteine, taurine, glutathione, 15 mg zinc oxide, Se. In 90s.
otc	**Optilets-500 Filmtabs** (Abbott)	50,000	400	30[3]	15	10	100	20	5	12	500[5]		Film-coated. In 120s.
otc	**Adavite Tablets** (Hudson)	5,000	400	30[2]	3	3.4	30	10	3	9	90	0.4	35 mcg biotin, 1250 IU beta carotene. In 130s.
otc	**Theravee Tablets** (Vangard)	5,500	400	30[2]	3	3.4	30	10	3	9	120	0.4	15 mcg biotin. In 100s and UD 100s.
otc	**One-A-Day Men's Vitamin Tablets** (Bayer)	5,000	400	45[2]	2.25	2.55	20	10	3	9	200	0.4	(One-A-Day). In 60s and 100s.

MULTIVITAMINS, CAPSULES AND TABLETS

	Product & Distributor	A IU	D IU	E IU	B_1 mg	B_2 mg	B_3 mg	B_5 mg	B_6 mg	B_{12} mcg	C mg	FA mg	Other Content and How Supplied
otc sf	**Therapeutic Tablets** (Goldline)	5,000	400	30[3]	3	3.4	20	10	3	9	90	0.4	30 mcg d-biotin. In 100s and 130s.
otc	**Theragran Caplets** (Mead-Johnson)												30 mcg biotin, lactose, sucrose. In 100s.
otc	**Therems Tablets** (Rugby)	5,000	400	30[3]	3	3.4	30	10	3	9	120	0.4	15 mcg biotin, 1250 IU beta carotene. In 130s and 1000s.
otc	**Theravim Tablets** (NBTY)	5,000	400	30[2]	3	3.4	30	10	3	9	90	0.4	1250 IU beta carotene, 35 mcg biotin. In 130s.
otc sf	**One-A-Day Essential Tablets** (Bayer)	5,000	400	30[2]	1.5	1.7	20	10	2	6	60	0.4	In 75s and 130s.
otc	**One-Tablet-Daily Tablets** (Various, eg, Goldline)												In 365s and 1000s.
otc	**Tab-A-Vite Tablets** (Major)			30[3]									In 30s, 100s, 250s, 1000s and UD 100s.
otc	**Dayalets Filmtabs** (Abbott)	5,000	400	30[3]	1.5	1.7	20		2	6	60	0.4	Film-coated. In 100s.
otc sf	**Vita-Bob Softgel Capsules** (Scot-Tussin)												In 100s.
otc	**Sigtab Tablets** (Roberts)	5,000	400	15[2]	10.3	10	100	20	6	18	333	0.4	Sucrose. In 90s and 500s.
otc	**Zymacap Capsules** (Roberts)	5,000	400	15[2]	2.25	2.6	30	15	3	9	90	0.4	In 90s.
otc	**Unicap Capsules** (Upjohn)	5,000	400	30[2]	1.5	1.7	20		2	6	60	0.4	Tartrazine. In 120s.
otc	**Multi-Day Tablets** (NBTY)	5,000	400	30[2]	1.5	1.7	20	10	2	6	60	0.4	In 100s.
otc sf	**Unicap Tablets** (Upjohn)	5,000	400	15[2]	1.5	1.7	20		2	6	60	0.4	Tartrazine. In 120s.
otc	**Unicap Jr. Chewable Tablets** (Upjohn)												Sucrose. In 120s.

MULTIVITAMINS, CAPSULES AND TABLETS

	Product & Distributor	A IU	D IU	E IU	B_1 mg	B_2 mg	B_3 mg	B_5 mg	B_6 mg	B_{12} mcg	C mg	FA mg	Other Content and How Supplied
otc	**Multivitamins Capsules** (Solvay)	5,000	400	10[3]	2.5	2.5	20	5	0.5	2	50		(0032–1204). Oval. Brown. In 100s and UD 100s.
otc	**Vita-Kid Chewable Wafers** (Solgar)	10,000	400	10[5]	2	2	10		2	5	100	0.3	In 50s and 100s.
otc	**Hexavitamin Tablets** (Various, eg, Upsher-Smith)	5,000	400		2	3	20				75		In 100s, 1000s and UD 100s.
otc	**Therabid Tablets** (Mission)	5,000	200	30[2]	15	10	100	20	10	5	500		In 60s.
otc sf	**Oxi-Freeda Tablets** (Freeda)			150[2]	20	20	40	20	20	10	100		5000 IU beta carotene, glutathione, L-cysteine, Se, 15 mg Zn. Kosher. In 100s and 250s.
otc	**Sesame Street Plus Extra C Tablets** (McNeil)	2,750	200	10[2]	0.75	0.85	10	5	0.7	3	80	0.2	Sucrose, lactose. Chewable. Character shapes. In 50s.
otc sf	**Bugs Bunny with Extra C Children's Tablets** (Bayer)	2,500	400	15[2]	1.05	1.2	13.5		1.05	4.5	250	0.3	Chewable. Fruit flavors. In 60s.
otc	**Flintstones Plus Extra C Children's Tablets** (Bayer)												Chewable. Character shapes. In 60s and 100s.
otc	**Garfield Plus Extra C Chewable Tablets** (Menley & James)												Sucrose, lactose. Character shapes. In 60s.
otc sf	**Sunkist Multi-Vitamins + Extra C Tablets** (Ciba)												5 mcg vitamin K, sorbitol, aspartame, phenylalanine. Citrus flavor. In 60s.

MULTIVITAMINS, CAPSULES AND TABLETS

	Product & Distributor	A IU	D IU	E IU	B_1 mg	B_2 mg	B_3 mg	B_5 mg	B_6 mg	B_{12} mcg	C mg	FA mg	Other Content and How Supplied
otc	**Animal Shapes Tablets** (Major)	2,500	400	15[2]	1.05	1.2	13.5		1.05	4.5	60	0.3	In 100s and 250s.
otc	**Flintstones Children's Tablets** (Bayer)												Sucrose. Chewable. Character shapes. In 60s and 100s.
otc	**Garfield Chewable Tablets** (Menley & James)												Sucrose, lactose. Character shapes. In 60s.
otc	**Fruity Chews Tablets** (Goldline)												Sucrose. Chewable. In 100s.
otc	**Bounty Bears Tablets** (NBTY)												In 100s.
otc	**Poly-Vi-Sol Tablets** (Mead-Johnson)												Sugar. Chewable. Peter Rabbit shapes. In 60s.
otc	**Vi-Daylin Tablets** (Ross)			15[3]									Sucrose. Chewable. Cherry flavor. In 100s.
otc	**Allbee C-800 Tablets** (Robins)			45[2]	15	17	100	25	25	12	800		Lactose. (AHR). Elliptical. In 60s.
otc	**Stress Formula Vitamins Capsules and Tablets** (Various, eg, Goldline, NBTY)			30[2]	10	10	100	20	5	12	500	0.4	**Capsules**: 45 mcg biotin. In 100s. **Tablets**: 45 mcg biotin. In 60s.
otc	**Stress Formula w/Zinc Tablets** (Various, eg, Goldline, NBTY)												45 mcg biotin, 23.9 mg Zn, Cu. In 60s.

MULTIVITAMINS, CAPSULES AND TABLETS

	Product & Distributor	A IU	D IU	E IU	B_1 mg	B_2 mg	B_3 mg	B_5 mg	B_6 mg	B_{12} mcg	C mg	FA mg	Other Content and How Supplied
otc	**Stress Formula 600 Tablets** (Vangard)			30[3]	15	10	100	20	5	12	500	0.4	45 mcg biotin. In UD 100s.
otc	**Stresstabs Tablets** (Lederle)			30[3]	10	10	100	20	5	12	500	0.4	45 mcg biotin. In 60s.
Rx	**Cefol Filmtab Tablets** (Abbott)			30[3]	15	10	100	20	5	6	750	0.5	Green. Film coated. In 100s.

[1] As d-alpha tocopherol.
[2] Form of vitamin E unknown.
[3] As dl-alpha tocopheryl acetate.
[4] As d-alpha tocopheryl acid succinate.
[5] As d-alpha tocopheryl succinate.

MULTIVITAMINS, DROPS AND LIQUIDS

For a comparison of the potencies of various forms of vitamin E, see the Vitamin E monograph.

	Product & Distributor	Content Given Per	A IU	D IU	E IU	B_1 mg	B_2 mg	B_3 mg	B_5 mg	B_6 mg	B_{12} mcg	C mg	Other Content	How Supplied
otc	**Certagen Liquid** (Goldline)	15 ml	2,500	400	30[1]	1.5	1.7	20	10	2	6	60	6.6% alcohol. 300 mcg biotin, 9 mg Fe, 3 mg Zn, Cr, I, Mn, Mo	In 237 ml.
otc	**Syrvite Liquid**[1] (Various, eg, Major)	5 ml	2,500	400	15[3]	1.05	1.2	13.5		1.05	4.5	60		In 480 ml.
otc	**Daily Vitamins Liquid** (Rugby)												Sugar, parabens, corn syrup, < 0.5% alcohol	In 237 and 473 ml.
otc	**Vi-Daylin Multivitamin Liquid** (Ross)				15[4]								≤ 0.5% alcohol, glucose, sucrose, methylparaben	Lemon/orange flavor. In 240 and 480 ml.
otc sf	**LKV Infant Drops** (Freeda)	0.6 ml	2,500	400	5[3]	1	1	10	3	1	4	50	75 mcg biotin	In 60 ml after mixing powder and liquid.
otc	**ADEKs Pediatric Drops** (Scandipharm)	1 ml	1500	400	40[6]	0.5	0.6	6	3	0.6	4	45	0.1 mg vitamin K, 15 mcg biotin, 5 mg zinc, 1 mg beta carotene	In 60 ml.
otc	**Poly-Vi-Sol Drops** (Mead Johnson)	1 ml	1,500	400	5[3]	0.5	0.6	8		0.4	2	35		In 30 and 50 ml.
otc sf	**Baby Vitamin Drops** (Goldline)													Alcohol free. In 50 ml.
otc sf	**Poly-Vitamin Drops** (Schein)				5[4]									Alcohol free. In 50 ml.

MULTIVITAMINS, DROPS AND LIQUIDS

	Product & Distributor	Content Given Per	A IU	D IU	E IU	B_1 mg	B_2 mg	B_3 mg	B_5 mg	B_6 mg	B_{12} mcg	C mg	Other Content	How Supplied
otc sf	**Vi-Daylin Multivitamin Drops** (Ross)	1 ml	1,500	400	5[5]	0.5	0.6	8		0.4	1.5	35	< 0.5% alcohol, methylparaben, EDTA	Fruit flavor. In 50 ml.
otc	**Theragran Liquid** (Mead-Johnson)	5 ml	5,000	400		10	10	100	21.4	4.1	5	200	Sucrose, methylparaben	In 120 ml.
otc	**Thera Multi-Vitamin Liquid** (Major)	5 ml	10,000	400		10	10	100	21.4	4.1	5	200	Sucrose, methylparaben	In 118 ml.
otc	**Theravite Liquid** (Barre-National)												Sugar, methylparaben	In 118 ml.

[1] May contain alcohol.
[2] As dl-alpha tocopheryl acetate.
[3] Form of vitamin E unknown.
[4] As d-alpha tocopheryl acetate.
[5] As d-alpha tocopheryl acid succinate.
[6] As d-alpha tocopheryl polyethylene glycol-1000 succinate.

MULTIVITAMINS WITH IRON

These products contain supplemental iron; products containing therapeutic amounts of iron (> 25 mg) with vitamins are listed in the blood modifiers section.

For a comparison of the potencies of various forms of vitamin E, see the Vitamin E monograph.

Content given per capsule, tablet or liquid dose.

	Product & Distributor	Fe[1] mg	A IU	D IU	E IU	B_1 mg	B_2 mg	B_3 mg	B_5 mg	B_6 mg	B_{12} mcg	C mg	FA mg	Other Content and How Supplied
otc sf	**Unicap Plus Iron Tablets** (Upjohn)	22.5	5000	400	30[2]	1.5	1.7	20	10	2	6	60	0.4	Ca. In 120s.
otc	**Femiron Multi-Vitamins and Iron Tablets** (Menley & James)	20	5000	400	15[2]	1.5	1.7	20	10	2	6	60	0.4	In 35s, 60s and 90s.
otc	**Dayalets + Iron Filmtabs** (Abbott)	18	5000	400	30[3]	1.5	1.7	20		2	6	60	0.4	Film coated. In 100s.
otc sf	**One-Tablet-Daily with Iron** (Goldline)	18	5000	400	30[3]	1.5	1.7	20	10	2	6	60	0.4	In 100s.
otc	**Tab-A-Vite + Iron Tablets** (Major)													Tartrazine. In 100s.
otc sf	**Multi-Day Plus Iron Tablets** (NBTY)	18	5000	400	15[2]	1.5	1.7	20		2	6	60	0.4	In 100s.
otc	**Vi-Daylin Multivitamin + Iron Tablets** (Ross)	12	2500	400	15[3]	1.05	1.2	13.5		1.05	4.5	60	0.3	Chewable. Orange flavor. In 100s.
otc	**Sesame Street Plus Iron Tablets** (McNeil-CPC)	10	2750	200	10[2]	0.75	0.85	10	5	0.7	3	40	0.2	Chewable. Character shapes. In 50s.

MULTIVITAMINS WITH IRON

	Product & Distributor	Fe[1] mg	A IU	D IU	E IU	B_1 mg	B_2 mg	B_3 mg	B_5 mg	B_6 mg	B_{12} mcg	C mg	FA mg	Other Content and How Supplied
otc	**Animal Shapes + Iron Tablets** (Major)	15	2500	400	15[3]	1.05	1.2	13.5		1.05	4.5	60	0.3	In 100s and 250s.
otc	**Bounty Bears Plus Iron Tablets** (NBTY)				15[2]									Chewable. In 100s.
otc *sf*	**Bugs Bunny Plus Iron Tablets** (Bayer)													Chewable. In 60s.
otc	**Children's SunKist Multivitamins + Iron Tablets** (Ciba)													5 mcg vitamin K_1, sorbitol, aspartame, phenylalanine, tartrazine. Citrus flavor. In 60s.
otc	**Flintstones Plus Iron Tablets** (Bayer)													Chewable. Character shapes. In 60s and 100s.
otc	**Garfield Plus Iron Tablets** (Menley & James)													Sucrose, lactose. Chewable. Character shapes. In 60s.
otc	**Fruity Chews with Iron Tablets** (Goldline)													Sucrose. In 100s.
otc	**Vi-Daylin Multivitamin + Iron Liquid** (Ross)	10	2500	400	15[4]	1.05	1.2	13.5		1.05	4.5	60		Per 5 ml. ≤ 0.5% alcohol, glucose, sucrose, parabens. Lemon/lime flavor. In 237 and 473 ml.
otc *sf*	**Baby Vitamin Drops with Iron** (Goldline)	10	1500	400	5[2]	0.5	0.6	8		0.4		35		Per 1 ml. In 50 ml.
otc	**Poly-Vi-Sol with Iron Drops** (Mead-Johnson)													Per 1 ml. In 50 ml.
otc	**Polyvitamin Drops with Iron** (Various, eg, Rugby)													Per 1 ml. In 50 ml.
otc *sf*	**Multi-Vit Drops w/Iron** (Barre-National)													Per 1 ml. Methylparaben. In 50 ml.
otc *sf*	**Vi-Daylin Multivitamin + Iron Drops** (Ross)													Per 1 ml. Methylparaben, < 0.5% alcohol. Fruit flavor. In 50 ml.

MULTIVITAMINS WITH IRON

<table>
<tr><th></th><th>Product & Distributor</th><th>Fe[1] mg</th><th>A IU</th><th>D IU</th><th>E IU</th><th>B_1 mg</th><th>B_2 mg</th><th>B_3 mg</th><th>B_5 mg</th><th>B_6 mg</th><th>B_{12} mcg</th><th>C mg</th><th>FA mg</th><th>Other Content and How Supplied</th></tr>
<tr><td>otc
sf</td><td>Vi-Daylin ADC Vitamins + Iron Drops (Ross)</td><td rowspan="2">10</td><td rowspan="2">1500</td><td rowspan="2">400</td><td rowspan="2"></td><td rowspan="2"></td><td rowspan="2"></td><td rowspan="2"></td><td rowspan="2"></td><td rowspan="2"></td><td rowspan="2"></td><td rowspan="2">35</td><td rowspan="2"></td><td>Per 1 ml. Methylparaben. Fruit flavor. In 50 ml.</td></tr>
<tr><td>otc</td><td>Tri-Vi-Sol with Iron Drops (Mead-Johnson)</td><td>Per 1 ml. Fruit-like flavor. In 50 ml.</td></tr>
<tr><td>otc</td><td>Simron Plus Capsules (SmithKline Beecham)</td><td>10</td><td></td><td></td><td></td><td></td><td></td><td></td><td></td><td>1</td><td>3.3</td><td>50</td><td>0.1</td><td>Parabens. In 100s.</td></tr>
</table>

[1] Iron content expressed in mg elemental iron.
[2] Form of vitamin E unknown.
[3] As dl-alpha tocopheryl acetate.
[4] As d-alpha tocopheryl acid succinate.

MULTIVITAMINS WITH IRON AND OTHER MINERALS

For a comparison of the potencies of various forms of vitamin E, see the Vitamin E monograph.

Content given per capsule, tablet or 5 ml.

	Product & Distributor	Fe[1] mg	A IU	D IU	E IU	B_1 mg	B_2 mg	B_3 mg	B_5 mg	B_6 mg	B_{12} mcg	C mg	FA mg	Other Content	How Supplied
otc	**One-Tablet-Daily with Minerals** (Goldline)	18	5,000	400	30[2]	1.5	1.7	20	10	2	6	60	0.4	Ca, Cl, Cr, Cu, I, K, Mg, Mn, Mo, P, Se, 30 mcg biotin, 15 mg Zn	In 100s and 1000s.
otc	**Theravee-M Tablets** (Vangard)	27	5,000	400	30[2]	3	3.4	30	10	3	9	120	0.4	Ca, Cl, Cr, Cu, K, I, Mg, Mn, Mo, Se, 15 mg Zn, P, 15 mcg biotin, 2,500 IU beta carotene	In 100s, 1000s and UD 100s.
otc	**Therems-M Tablets** (Rugby)	27	5,000[3]	400	30[2]	3	3.4	20	10	3	9	90	0.4	Ca, Cl, Cr, Cu, I, K, Mg, Mn, Mo, P, Se, 15 mg Zn, 30 mcg biotin	In 130s and 1000s.
otc	**Adavite-M Tablets** (Hudson)				30[4]									Ca, Cl, Cr, Cu, I, K, Mg, Mn, Mo, P, Se, 15 mg Zn, 30 mcg biotin	In 130s.
otc *sf*	**Therapeutic-M Tablets** (Goldline)				30[2]									Ca, Cl, Cr, Cu, I, K, Mg, Mn, Mo, P, Se, 15 mg Zn, 30 mcg biotin	In 1000s.
otc	**Theravim-M Tablets** (NBTY)				30[4]									Ca, Cl, Cr, Cu, I, K, Mg, Mn, Mo, P, Se, 15 mg Zn, 30 mcg biotin	In 130s.
Rx	**Bacmin Tablets** (Marnel)	27	5,000		30[2]	20	20	100	25	25	50	500	0.8	Cr, Cu, Mg, Mn, 22.5 mg Zn, 0.15 mg biotin	(EV201). Dark red. In 100s.
otc	**Multi-Day with Calcium and Extra Iron Tablets** (NBTY)	27	5,000	400	30[4]	1.5	1.7	20	10	2	6	60	0.4	Ca, 15 mg Zn, tartrazine	In 100s.

MULTIVITAMINS WITH IRON AND OTHER MINERALS

	Product & Distributor	Fe[1] mg	A IU	D IU	E IU	B_1 mg	B_2 mg	B_3 mg	B_5 mg	B_6 mg	B_{12} mcg	C mg	FA mg	Other Content	How Supplied
otc *sf*	**Total Formula Tablets** (Vitaline)	20	10,000	400	30[4]	15	15	25	25	25	25	100	0.4	Ca, Cr, Cu, I, K, Mg, Mn, Mo, P, Se, Si, V, vitamin K, 300 mcg biotin, 30 mg Zn, choline, bioflavonoids, hesperidin, inositol, PABA, rutin	In 90s and 100s.
otc *sf*	**Total Formula-2 Tablets** (Vitaline)														With boron. In 60s.
otc	**Optilets-M-500 Filmtabs** (Abbott)	20	5,000	400	30[2]	15	10	100	20	5	12	500		Cu, I, Mg, Mn, 1.5 mg Zn	Film coated. In 120s.
otc *sf*	**Unicap T Tablets** (Upjohn)	18	5,000	400	30[4]	10	10	100	25	6	18	500	0.4	Cu, I, K, Mn, Se, 15 mg Zn, tartrazine	In 60s.
otc *sf*	**Avail Tablets** (Menley & James)	18	5,000	400	30[4]	2.25	2.55	20		3	9	90	0.4	Ca, Cr, I, Mg, Se, 22.5 mg Zn	In 60s.
otc *sf*	**Decagen Tablets** (Goldline)	18	5,000	400	30[2]	1.7	2	20	10	3	6	60	0.4	Ca, Cl, Cr, Cu, B, I, K, Mg, Mn, Mo, Ni, P, Se, Si, Sn, V, 15 mg Zn, vitamin K, 30 mcg biotin	In 130s.
otc	**Myadec Tablets** (Parke-Davis)													30 mcg biotin, vitamin K, Ca, P, I, Mg, Cu, 15 mg Zn, Mn, K, Cl, Cr, Mo, Se, Ni, Si, V, B, Sn	In 130s.
otc	**Nova-Dec Tablets** (Rugby)													Ca, Cr, Cu, I, Mg, Mo, Mn, P, Se, K, 15 mg Zn, vitamin K, Cl, Ni, Sn, Si, V, B, 30 mcg biotin	In 130s.

MULTIVITAMINS WITH IRON AND OTHER MINERALS

	Product & Distributor	Fe[1] mg	A IU	D IU	E IU	B_1 mg	B_2 mg	B_3 mg	B_5 mg	B_6 mg	B_{12} mcg	C mg	FA mg	Other Content	How Supplied
otc	**Centrum Jr. with Iron Tablets** (Lederle)	18	5,000	400	30[4]	1.5	1.7	20	10	2	6	60	0.4	Ca, Cr, Cu, I, Mg, Mn, Mo, P, 15 mg Zn, 45 mcg biotin, vitamin K	Chewable. In 60s.
otc	**Cerovite Tablets** (Rugby)													Ca, Cl, Cr, Cu, I, K, Mg, Mn, Mo, Ni, P, Se, Si, Sn, V, 30 mcg biotin, vitamin K, 15 mg Zn	In 130s.
otc *sf*	**Children's SunKist Multivitamins Complete Tablets** (Ciba)													Ca, 10 mg Zn, 40 mcg biotin, vitamin K_1, Cu, I, K, Mg, Mn, P, sorbitol, aspartame, phenylalanine, tartrazine.	Chewable. Citrus flavor. In 60s.
otc *sf*	**Daily-Vite w/Iron & Minerals Tablets** (Rugby)													Ca, Cl, Cr, Cu, I, K, Mg, Mn, Mo, P, Se, 15 mg Zn, biotin, vitamin K	In 100s.
otc	**Flintstones Complete Tablets** (Bayer)													Ca, Cu, I, Mg, P, 15 mg Zn, 40 mcg biotin	Chewable. In 60s and 120s.
otc *sf*	**Unicap M Tablets** (Upjohn)													Ca, Cu, I, K, Mn, P, 15 mg Zn, tartrazine	In 120s.
otc	**One-A-Day Maximum Formula Tablets** (Bayer)													Ca, Cl, Cr, Cu, I, K, Mg, Mn, Mo, P, Se, 15 mg Zn, 30 mcg biotin	(One-A-Day). In 60s and 100s.
otc	**Garfield Complete with Minerals Tablets** (Menley & James)													Ca, Cu, I, Mg, P, 15 mg Zn, 40 mcg biotin, sorbitol, aspartame, phenylalanine	Chewable. In 60s.

MULTIVITAMINS WITH IRON AND OTHER MINERALS

	Product & Distributor	Fe[1] mg	A IU	D IU	E IU	B_1 mg	B_2 mg	B_3 mg	B_5 mg	B_6 mg	B_{12} mcg	C mg	FA mg	Other Content	How Supplied
otc	**Stuart Formula Tablets** (J & J-Merck)	5	5,000	400	10[2]	1.5	1.7	20		1	3	50	0.1	Ca, Cu, I	In 100s.
otc	**Unicomplex-T & M Tablets** (Rugby)	18	5,000	400	30[4]	10	10	100	25	6	18	500	0.4	Ca, Cu, I, K, Mn, P, 15 mg Zn	In 90s and 1000s.
otc	**Gevral Tablets** (Lederle)	18	5,000		30[2]	1.5	1.7	20		2	6	60	0.4	Ca, I, Mg, P, lactose, parabens, sucrose	In 100s.
otc	**Cerovite Jr. Tablets** (Rugby)	18	5,000	400	15[4]	1.5	1.7	20	10	2	6	60	0.4	Cu, I, Mg, Zn, Mn, Mo, 45 mcg biotin, Cr, sugar	In 60s.
otc	**Multi-Day Plus Minerals Tablets** (NBTY)	18	6,500	400	30[2]	1.5	1.7	20	10	2	6	60	0.4	Ca, Cl, Cr, Cu, I, K, Mg, Mn, Mo, P, Se, 15 mg Zn, 30 mcg biotin	In 100s.
otc *sf*	**Hair Booster Vitamin Tablets** (NBTY)	18						35	100		6		0.4	Cu, I, Mn, 15 mg Zn, inositol, PABA, protein, choline bitartrate	In 60s.
otc *sf*	**Quintabs-M Tablets** (Freeda)	15	10,000	400	50[4]	30	30	150	30	30	30	300	0.4	Ca, Cu, Mg, Mn, Se, 30 mg Zn, PABA, K	Kosher. In 100s, 250s and 500s.
otc	**Generix-T Tablets** (Goldline)	15	10,000	400	5.5[4]	15	10	100	10	2	7.5	150		Cu, I, Mg, Mn, 1.5 mg Zn	In 100s.
otc	**Multilex T & M Tablets** (Rugby)														Sugar. In 100s and 1000s.
otc *sf*	**Multilex Tabs** (Rugby)	15	10,000	400	5.5[2]	10	5	30	10	1.7	3	100		Cu, I, Mg, Mn, 1.5 mg Zn	In 100s.
otc	**Vitarex Tablets** (Pasadena)	15	10,000	200	15[4]	15	10	100	20	5	5	250		Ca, Cu, I, K, Mg, Mn, P, 10 mg Zn	In 100s.
otc	**Fosfree Tablets** (Mission)	29	3,000	300		9	4	21	2	5	4	100		351 mg Ca	Sugar. In 120s.

MULTIVITAMINS WITH IRON AND OTHER MINERALS

	Product & Distributor	Fe^1 mg	A IU	D IU	E IU	B_1 mg	B_2 mg	B_3 mg	B_5 mg	B_6 mg	B_{12} mcg	C mg	FA mg	Other Content	How Supplied
otc sf	**Monocaps Tablets** (Freeda)	14	10,000	400	15^5	15	15	41	15	15	15	125	0.1	Ca, Cu, I, K, Mg, Mn, Se, 12 mg Zn, 15 mcg biotin, L-lysine, PABA, lecithin	Kosher. In 100s, 250s and 500s.
otc	**Vita-Plus H Softgels (Capsules)** (Scot-Tussin)	13.4	5,000	400	3^2	3	2.5	20	5	1.5	2.5	50		Ca, K, Mg, Mn, P, 1.4 mg Zn	In 100s.
otc	**Circavite-T Tablets** (Circle)	12	10,000	400	15^2	10.3	10	100	18.4	4.1	5	200		Cu, I, Mg, Mn, 1.5 mg Zn	Maroon. In 100s.
otc	**Vigomar Forte Tablets** (Marlop Pharm)	12	10,000	400	15^4	10	10	100	20	5	5	200		I, Mg, Cu, Mn, 1.5 mg Zn	In 100s.
otc	**Poly-Vi-Sol w/Iron Tablets** (Mead-Johnson)	12	2,500	400	15^4	1.05	1.2	13.5		1.05	4.5	60	0.3	Cu, 8 mg Zn, sugar	Chewable. Peter Rabbit shapes. Fruit flavors. In 100s.
otc sf	**Vitalets Tablets** (Freeda)	10	5,000	400	5^4	2.5	0.9	20	3	2	5	60		25 mcg biotin, Mn, Ca	Chewable. Fruit flavors and unflavored. Kosher. In 100s and 250s.
otc sf	**Unicap Sr. Tablets** (Upjohn)	10	5,000	200	15^4	1.2	1.4	16	10	2.2	3	60	0.4	Ca, Cu, I, K, Mg, Mn, P, 15 mg Zn	In 120s.
otc sf	**Geritol Extend Caplets** (SmithKline-Beecham)	10	3,333	200	15^4	1.2	1.4	15		2	2	60	0.2	Vitamin K, Ca, I, Mg, Se, 15 mg Zn	In 40s and 100s.
otc	**Advanced Formula Centrum Liquid** (Lederle)	9	2,500	400	30^2	1.5	1.7	20	10	2	6	60		300 mcg biotin, Cr, I, Mn, Mo, 3 mg Zn, 6.7% alcohol, sucrose	In 236 ml.

MULTIVITAMINS WITH IRON AND OTHER MINERALS

	Product & Distributor	Fe[1] mg	A IU	D IU	E IU	B_1 mg	B_2 mg	B_3 mg	B_5 mg	B_6 mg	B_{12} mcg	C mg	FA mg	Other Content	How Supplied
otc *sf*	**Hi-Po-Vites Tablets** (Hudson)	6	10,000	400	13[5]	25	25	50	12.5	15	50	150	0.4	B, Ca, Cr, Cu, I, K, Mg, Mn, Mo, P, Se, 5 mg Zn, 1 mg biotin, bioflavonoids, bone meal, PABA, choline bitartrate, betaine, inositol, lecithin, desiccated liver, rutin	In 100s.
otc *sf*	**Ultra Vita Time Tablets** (NBTY)														In 100s.
otc *sf*	**Formula VM-2000 Tablets** (Solgar)	5	12,500	200	100[4]	50	50	50	50	50	50	150	0.2	B, Ca, Cr, Cu, I, K, Mg, Mn, Mo, Se, 7.5 mg Zn, betaine, 50 mcg biotin, choline, bioflavonoids, amino acids, hesperidin, inositol, l-glutathione, PABA, rutin	In 30s, 60s, 90s and 180s.
otc	**M.V.M. Capsules** (Tyson and Associates)	3.6	400		60[2]	20	10	10	100	31	160	50	0.08	Ca, Cr, Cu, I, K, Mg, Mo, 6 mg Zn, 160 mcg biotin, PABA, Mn, Se, tryptophan	In 150s.
otc *sf*	**Maximum Red Label Tablets** (Vitaline)	3.3	2,500	67	66.7[4]	16.7	8.3	31.7	66.7	16.7	16.7	200	0.13	Ca, Cr, Cu, I, K, Mg, Mn, Mo, Se, Si, V, 5 mg Zn, 50 mcg biotin, choline, inositol, bioflavonoids, l-lysine, PABA	In 180s.

MULTIVITAMINS WITH IRON AND OTHER MINERALS

	Product & Distributor	Fe[1] mg	A IU	D IU	E IU	B_1 mg	B_2 mg	B_3 mg	B_5 mg	B_6 mg	B_{12} mcg	C mg	FA mg	Other Content	How Supplied
otc	**Androvite Tablets** (Optimox)	3	4,167	67	67[5]	8.3	8.3	8.3	16.7	16.7	20.8	167	0.06	PABA, inositol, biotin, betaine, B, Cr, Cu, I, Mg, Mn, Se, 8.3 mg Zn, pancreatin, hesperidin, rutin	In 180s.
otc sf	**ProCycle Gold Tablets** (Cyclin Pharm)	3	833.3	67	67	1.7	1.7	3.3	1.7	3.3	21	30	0.07	167 mg Ca, 2.5 mg Zn, B, Cu, Cr, I, Mg, Mn, Se, PABA, inositol, rutin, biotin, hesperidin, pancreatin, betaine	In 100s.
otc	**Opticare PMS Tablets** (Standard Drug)	2.5	2,083	17[6]	14[5]	4.2	4.2	4.2	4.2	50	10.4	250	0.03	Cr, Cu, I, K, Mg, Mn, Se, 4.2 mg Zn, 10.4 mcg biotin, choline bitartrate, bioflavonoids, inositol, PABA, rutin, Ca, amylase activity, protease activity, lipase activity, betaine, tartrazine	In 150s.
otc	**4 Hair Softgel Capsules** (Marlyn)	2.5	1,250		10[4]			5	25	1.5	44	25	33.3	250 mcg biotin, I, Mg, Cu, 7.5 mg Zn, choline bitartrate, inositol, Mn, methionine, PABA, B, L-cysteine, tyrosine, Si	In 60s.

[1] Iron content expressed in mg elemental iron.
[2] As dl-alpha tocopheryl acetate.
[3] From acetate and beta carotene.
[4] Form of vitamin E unknown.
[5] As d-alpha tocopheryl acid succinate.
[6] As cholecalciferol.

MULTIVITAMINS WITH FLUORIDE, CAPSULES AND TABLETS

Used for prophylaxis of vitamin deficiencies and as an aid in the prevention of dental caries in infants and children where the fluoride content of the drinking water does not exceed 0.7 ppm. For complete prescribing information on fluoride-containing products, refer to the Fluoride group mongraph.

Content given per capsule or tablet.

For a comparison of the potencies of various forms of vitamin E, see the Vitamin E monograph.

	Product & Distributor	F[1] mg	A IU	D IU	E IU	B_1 mg	B_2 mg	B_3 mg	B_5 mg	B_6 mg	B_{12} mcg	C mg	FA mg	Other Content and How Supplied
Rx	**Adeflor M Tablets** (Kenwood/Bradley)	1	6,000	400		1.5	2.5	20	10	10	2	100		250 mg Ca, 30 mg Fe, sorbitol, sucrose. Pink. Elliptical. In 100s.
Rx	**Mulvidren-F Softab Tablets** (Wyeth-Ayerst)	1	4,000	400		1.6	2	10	2.8	1	3	75		Saccharin. (Stuart 710). Chewable. Orange, scored. In 100s.
Rx	**Poly Vitamins Fluoride Tablets**[2] (Various, eg, Goldline, Rugby, Schein)	1	2,500	400	15[3]	1.05	1.2	13.5		1.05	4.5	60	0.3	In 100s.
Rx	**Chewable Multivitamins w/Fluoride Tablets** (Moore)				15[4]									Sucrose. Fruit flavor. In 100s.
Rx	**Florvite Tablets** (Everett)													Sucrose. Chewable. Fruit flavors. In 100s.
Rx	**Florvite + Iron Chewable Tablets** (Everett)													12 mg Fe, Cu, 10 mg Zn, sucrose. Cherry flavor. In 100s.
Rx	**Poly-Vi-Flor Tablets 1.0 mg** (Mead-Johnson)													Sucrose. Chewable. In 100s and 1000s.
Rx	**Poly-Vi-Flor with Iron 1.0 mg Tablets** (Mead-Johnson)													Cu, 12 mg Fe, 10 mg Zn, sucrose. Chewable. In 100s and 1000s.
Rx	**Polyvitamin Fluoride Tablets w/Iron** (Various, eg, Rugby, Schein)													Cu, 12 mg Fe, 10 mg Zn. Chewable. In 100s.
Rx	**Soluvite C.T. Tablets** (Pharmics)													Chewable. In 100s.
Rx	**Polytabs-F Tablets** (Major)													Chewable. In 100s and 1000s.
Rx	**Vi-Daylin/F Chewable Multivitamin Tablets** (Ross)													Chewable. In 100s.
Rx	**Vi-Daylin/F Multivitamins + Iron Chewable Tablets** (Ross)													12 mg Fe, sucrose. Cherry flavor. In 100s.

MULTIVITAMINS WITH FLUORIDE, CAPSULES AND TABLETS

	Product & Distributor	F[1] mg	A IU	D IU	E IU	B_1 mg	B_2 mg	B_3 mg	B_5 mg	B_6 mg	B_{12} mcg	C mg	FA mg	Other Content and How Supplied
Rx	**Tri-Vi-Flor 1.0 mg Tablets** (Mead-Johnson)	1	2,500	400								60		Sucrose. Chewable. Fruit flavor. In 100s.
Rx	**Chewable Triple Vitamins with Fluoride Tablets** (Major)													Dextrose, sucrose. Fruit flavor. In 100s.
Rx	**Trivitamin Fluoride Tablets** (Schein)													Sucrose. Chewable. Fruit flavor. In 100s.
Rx	**Half Strength Florvite with Iron Tablets** (Everett)	0.5	2,500	400	15[4]	1.05	1.2	13.5		1.05	4.5	60	0.3	Cu, 12 mg Fe, 10 mg Zn, sucrose. Chewable. Cherry flavor. In 100s.
Rx	**Poly Vitamins w/Fluoride 0.5 Tablets**[2] (Various, eg, Goldline, Rugby, Schein)													In 100s and 1000s.
Rx	**Florvite Tablets Half Strength** (Everett)													Sucrose. Chewable. In 100s.
Rx	**Poly-Vi-Flor 0.5 mg Tablets** (Mead-Johnson)													Lactose, sucrose. Chewable. Fruit flavor. In 100s.
Rx	**Poly-Vi-Flor 0.5 mg w/Iron Tablets** (Mead-Johnson)													Cu, 12 mg Fe, 10 mg Zn, lactose, sucrose. Chewable. Fruit flavor. In 100s.
Rx	**Polyvitamins w/Fluoride 0.5 mg and Iron Tablets** (Rugby)													Cu, 12 mg Fe, 10 mg Zn, sucrose. Chewable. Cherry flavor. In 100s.
Rx	**Poly-Vi-Flor Tablets 0.25 mg** (Mead-Johnson)	0.25	2,500	400	15[4]	1.05	1.2	13.5		1.05	4.5	60	0.3	Lactose, sucrose. Chewable. Fruit flavor. In 100s.
Rx	**Poly-Vi-Flor 0.25 mg Tablets w/Iron** (Mead-Johnson)													Cu, 12 mg Fe, 10 mg Zn, lactose, sucrose. Chewable. Fruit flavor. In 100s.

[1] Fluoride content expressed in mg elemental fluoride.
[2] May be chewable.
[3] Form of vitamin E unknown.
[4] As dl–alpha tocopheryl acetate.

MULTIVITAMINS WITH FLUORIDE DROPS

For complete prescribing information on fluoride-containing products, refer to the Fluoride group monograph.

For a comparison of the potencies of the various forms of vitamin E, see the vitamin E monograph.

	Product & Distributor	Content Given Per	F[1] mg	A IU	D IU	E IU	B_1 mg	B_2 mg	B_3 mg	B_5 mg	B_6 mg	B_{12} mcg	C mg	Other Content and How Supplied
Rx	**Polyvitamin w/Fluoride Drops** (Various, eg, Rugby, Schein)	1 ml	0.5	1,500	400	5[2]	0.5	0.6	8		0.4	2	35	In 50 ml.
Rx	**Florvite Drops** (Everett)					5[3]								Fruit flavor. In 50 ml.
Rx	**Poly-Vi-Flor 0.5 mg Drops** (Mead-Johnson)					5[4]								Fruit flavor. In 50 ml.
Rx	**Poly-Vi-Flor with Iron 0.5 mg Drops** (Mead-Johnson)	1 ml	0.5	1,500	400	5[4]	0.5	0.6	8		0.4		35	10 mg Fe[5]. Fruit flavor. In 50 ml.
Rx	**Florvite + Iron Drops** (Everett)													10 mg Fe[5]. In 50 ml.
Rx	**Multivitamin with Fluoride Drops** (Major)	1 ml	0.5	1,500	400	4.1[4]	0.5	0.6	8		0.4	2	35	In 50 ml.
Rx	**ADC with Fluoride Drops** (Various, eg, Hi-Tech, Major)	1 ml	0.5	1,500	400								35	Methylparaben. In 50 ml.
Rx	**Tri-A-Vite F Drops** (Major)													In 50 ml.
Rx	**Triple Vitamin ADC w/Fluoride Drops** (Nilor Pharm)													In 50 ml.
Rx	**Tri-Vi-Flor 0.5 mg Drops** (Mead-Johnson)													Fruit flavor. In 50 ml.
Rx	**Tri-Vitamin w/Fluoride Drops** (Rugby)													In 50 ml.
Rx	**Tri Vit w/Fluoride 0.5 mg Drops** (Barre-National)													In 50 ml.
Rx *sf*	**Trivitamin Fluoride 0.5 mg Drops** (Various, eg, Schein)													Alcohol free. In 50 ml.

MULTIVITAMINS WITH FLUORIDE DROPS

	Product & Distributor	Content Given Per	F[1] mg	A IU	D IU	E IU	B_1 mg	B_2 mg	B_3 mg	B_5 mg	B_6 mg	B_{12} mcg	C mg	Other Content and How Supplied
Rx *sf*	**Polyvitamin Fluoride Drops** (Various, eg, Goldline, Hi-Tech, Major, Rugby, Schein)	1 ml	0.25	1,500	400	5[3]	0.5	0.6	8		0.4	2	35	Alcohol free. In 50 ml.
Rx	**Poly-Vi-Flor 0.25 mg Drops** (Mead-Johnson)					5[4]								Fruit flavor. In 50 ml.
Rx	**Florvite Drops** (Everett)					5[2]								Fruit flavor. In 50 ml.
Rx	**Multivitamin and Fluoride Drops** (Major)													In 50 ml.
Rx	**Polyvitamin Drops w/Iron and Fluoride** (Various, eg, Goldline, Hi-Tech, Rugby, Schein)	1 ml	0.25	1,500	400	5[4]	0.5	0.6	8		0.4		35	10 mg Fe[5]. In 50 ml.
Rx	**Florvite + Iron Drops** (Everett)													10 mg Fe[5]. Fruit flavor. In 50 ml.
Rx	**Poly-Vi-Flor with Iron 0.25 mg Drops** (Mead-Johnson)													10 mg Fe[5]. In 50 ml.
Rx *sf*	**Vi-Daylin/F Multivitamin Drops** (Ross)													Methylparaben, < 0.1% alcohol. Fruit flavor. In 50 ml.
Rx *sf*	**Vi-Daylin/F Multivitamin + Iron Drops** (Ross)													10 mg Fe[5], < 0.1% alcohol, methylparaben. Fruit flavor. In 50 ml.

MULTIVITAMINS WITH FLUORIDE DROPS

	Product & Distributor	Content Given Per	F[1] mg	A IU	D IU	E IU	B_1 mg	B_2 mg	B_3 mg	B_5 mg	B_6 mg	B_{12} mcg	C mg	Other Content and How Supplied
Rx	**Tri-Flor-Vite with Fluoride Drops** (Everett)	1 ml	0.25	1,500	400								35	In 50 ml.
Rx	**Tri-Vi-Flor 0.25 mg Drops** (Mead-Johnson)													Fruit flavor. In 50 ml.
Rx *sf*	**Trivitamin Fluoride Drops** (Various, eg, Schein)													Alcohol free. In 50 ml.
Rx *sf*	**Vi-Daylin/F ADC Vitamins Drops** (Ross)													≈ 0.3% alcohol, parabens. Fruit flavor. In 50 ml.
Rx	**Soluvite-f Drops** (Pharmics)	0.6 ml												In 57 ml.
Rx	**Tri-Vi-Flor 0.25 mg with Iron Drops** (Mead-Johnson)	1 ml												10 mg Fe[5]. In 50 ml.
Rx *sf*	**Vi-Daylin/F ADC + Iron Drops** (Ross)													10 mg Fe[5], methylparaben. Fruit flavor. In 50 ml.
Rx	**Tri Vit w/Fluoride 0.25 mg Drops** (Barre-National)													In 50 ml.
Rx	**Apatate w/Fluoride Liquid** (Kenwood/Bradley)	5 ml	0.5				15				0.5	25		Cherry flavor. In 120 ml.

[1] Fluoride content expressed in mg elemental fluoride.
[2] As dl–alpha tocopheryl acetate.
[3] Form of vitamin E unknown.
[4] As d-alpha tocopheryl acid succinate.
[5] Iron content expressed in mg elemental iron.

MULTIVITAMINS WITH CALCIUM AND IRON

Content given per tablet or capsule.

For a comparison of the potencies of the various forms of vitamin E, see the vitamin E monograph.

	Product & Distributor	Ca[1] mg	Fe[1] mg	A IU	D IU	E mg	B_1 mg	B_2 mg	B_3 mg	B_5 mg	B_6 mg	B_{12} mcg	C mg	FA mg	Other Content	How Supplied
otc *sf*	**One-A-Day Women's Formula Tablets** (Bayer)	450	27	5,000	400	30[2]	1.5	1.7	20	10	2	6	60	0.4	15 mg Zn, tartrazine	In 60s and 100s.
otc *sf*	**Women's Daily Formula Capsules** (Kavon Co)	450	25	5,000	400	30[2]	1.7	1.7	20	10	4	6	60	0.4	25 mg Zn, parabens	In 60s and 130s.
otc *sf*	**K.P.N. Tablets** (Freeda)	333[3]	11	2,667	133	10[2]	2	2	10	3.3	0.83	2	33	0.27	Cu, I, K, Mg, Mn, 6.7 mg Zn, bioflavonoids	Kosher. In 100s and 250s.
Rx	**Mynatal Capsules** (ME Pharm)	300	65	5,000	400	30[4]	3	3.4	20	10	10	12	120	1	30 mcg biotin, Cr, Cu, I, Mg, Mn, Mo, 25 mg Zn	In 100s and 500s.
Rx	**Prenatal Z Tablets** (Ethex)	300	65	5,000	400	30[4]	3	3	20		12.2	12	80	1	I, Mg, 20 mg Zn	Delayed-release. (Ethex 218). Blue. Oval. Film-coated. In 100s.
Rx	**Prenate 90 Tablets** (Bock)	250	90	4,000	400	30[2]	3	3.4	20		20	12	120	1	DSS, Cu, I, 25 mg Zn	Dye free. Delayed-release. (Bock PN90). Film-coated. In 100s.
Rx	**Mynate 90 Plus Caplets** (ME Pharm)															Delayed-release. In 100s.
Rx	**Prenatal MR 90 Tablets** (Ethex)															Delayed-release. (Ethex 212). Oval. Film coated. In 100s.

MULTIVITAMINS WITH CALCIUM AND IRON

	Product & Distributor	Ca[1] mg	Fe[1] mg	A IU	D IU	E mg	B_1 mg	B_2 mg	B_3 mg	B_5 mg	B_6 mg	B_{12} mcg	C mg	FA mg	Other Content	How Supplied
Rx	**Par-F Tablets** (Pharmics)	250	60	5,000	400	30[2]	3	3.4	20	10	12	12	120	1	Cu, I, Mg, 15 mg Zn	In 100s.
Rx	**Materna Tablets** (Lederle)	250	60	5,000	400	30[4]	3	3.4	20	10	10	12	100	1	Cr, Cu, I, Mg, Mn, Mo, 25 mg Zn, 30 mcg biotin, lactose, parabens, sucrose	In 100s.
Rx	**Mynatal FC Caplets** (ME Pharm)					30[2]									30 mcg biotin, 25 mg Zn, I, Mg, Cr, Cu, Mo, Mn	In 100s.
Rx	**Mynatal P.N. Forte Caplets** (ME Pharm)	250	60	5,000	400	30[2]	3	3.4	20		4	12	80	1	25 mg Zn, I, Mg, Cu	In 100s.
Rx	**Niferex-PN Forte Tablets** (Central)					30[4]									Cu, I, Mg, 25 mg Zn	(Central 10). Dye free. White. Capsule shape. Film-coated. In 100s.
Rx	**Prenatal Maternal Tablets** (Ethex)	250	60	5,000	400	30[2]	2.9	3.4	20	10	12.2	12	100	1	Cr, Cu, I, Mg, Mn, Mo, 25 mg Zn, 30 mcg biotin	In 100s.
Rx	**Marnatal-F Tablets** (Marnel)	250	60	4,000	400	30[4]	3	3.4	20		5	12	100	1	Mg, 25 mg Zn, Cu, I	(Marnatal-F). Lt. pink. Film-coated. In 30s and 100s.
Rx	**Pramilet FA Tablets** (Ross)	250	40	4,000	400		3	2	10	1	3	3	60	1	Cu, I, Mg, Zn	Film coated. In 100s.
otc	**Os-Cal Fortified Tablets** (SmithKline-Beecham)	250	5	1,668	125	0.8[4]	1.7	1.7	15		2		50		Mg, Mn, 0.5 mg Zn, parabens, EDTA	In 100s.
Rx sf	**O-Cal f.a. Tablets** (Pharmics)	200	66	5,000	400	30[2]	3	3	20		4	12	90	1	1.1 mg F, Mg, I, Cu, 15 mg Zn	In 100s.

MULTIVITAMINS WITH CALCIUM AND IRON

	Product & Distributor	Ca[1] mg	Fe[1] mg	A IU	D IU	E mg	B_1 mg	B_2 mg	B_3 mg	B_5 mg	B_6 mg	B_{12} mcg	C mg	FA mg	Other Content	How Supplied
Rx	**Stuartnatal Plus Tablets** (Wyeth-Ayerst)	200	65	4,000	400	22[2]	1.84	3	20		10	12	120	1	2 mg Cu, 25 mg Zn	(Wyeth 792). Kosher. Lt. yellow. Capsule shape. In 100s.
Rx	**Prenatal Plus** (Goldline)															In 100s.
Rx	**Prenatal Plus w/ Betacarotene Tablets** (Rugby)	200	65	4,000	400	11	1.84	3	20		10	12	120	1	25 mg Zn, Cu	In 100s and 500s.
Rx	**Prenatal Plus-Improved Tablets** (Rugby)	200	65	4,000	400	11[2]	1.5	3	20		10	12	120	1	Cu, 25 mg Zn	In 100s.
Rx	**Prenatal-1 + Iron Tablets** (Various, eg, ESI, Goldline, Qualitest, Schein)															In 100s and 500s.
Rx	**Par-Natal Plus 1 Improved Tablets** (Parmed)															In 500s.
Rx	**Lactocal-F Tablets** (Laser)	200	65	4,000	400	30[4]	3	3.4	20		5	12	100	1	Cu, I, Mg, 15 mg Zn	(Laser 173). White. Oval. Film-coated. In 100s and 1000s.
Rx	**Prenatal Z Advanced Formula** (Ethex)	200	65	3,000	400	10	1.5	1.6	17		2.2	2.2	70	1	175 mcg potassium iodide, 100 mg magnesium oxide, 15 mg zinc oxide	In 100s.

MULTIVITAMINS WITH CALCIUM AND IRON

	Product & Distributor	Ca[1] mg	Fe[1] mg	A IU	D IU	E mg	B_1 mg	B_2 mg	B_3 mg	B_5 mg	B_6 mg	B_{12} mcg	C mg	FA mg	Other Content	How Supplied
Rx	**Natalins Rx Tablets** (Mead-Johnson)	200	60	4,000	400	15[2]	1.5	1.6	17	7	4	2.5	80	1	30 mcg biotin, 25 mg Zn, Cu, Mg	(MJ 702). White. Oval. In 100s and 1000s.
Rx	**Mynatal Rx Caplets** (ME Pharm)															In 100s.
Rx	**Prenatal Rx w/ Beta-Carotene Tablets** (Rugby)														30 mcg biotin, 3 mg Cu, 100 mg Mg, 25 mg Zn	In 100s and 500s.
Rx	**Prenatal Rx Tablets** (Various, eg, Ethex, Goldline, Moore, Qualitest, Schein)														30 mcg biotin, Cu, Mg, 25 mg Zn	In 100s and 500s.
Rx	**Natarex Prenatal Tablets** (Major)	200	60	4,000	400	15[4]	1.5	1.6	17	7	4	2.5	80	1	Cu, Mg, 25 mg Zn, 30 mcg biotin	In 100s.
otc	**Prenatal w/Folic Acid Tablets** (Geneva)	200	60	4,000	400	11[2]	1.5	1.7	18		2.6	4	100	0.8	25 mg Zn	Salmon. Oval. In 100s.
otc	**Prenatal-S Tablets** (Goldline)					11[4]										In UD 100s.
otc	**Prenavite Tablets** (Rugby)															In 100s and 500s.
otc	**Stuart Prenatal Tablets** (Wyeth-Ayerst)	200	60	4,000	400	11[4]	1.8	1.7	18		2.6	4	100	0.8	25 mg Zn	Kosher. In 100s.
Rx	**Nestabs FA Tablets** (Fielding)	200	36	5,000	400	30[2]	3	3	20		3	8	120	1	I, 15 mg Zn	In 100s.
otc	**Nestabs Tabs** (Fielding)	200	36	5,000	400	30[2]	3	3	20		3	8	120	0.8	I, 15 mg Zn	In 100s.
otc	**Natalins Tablets** (Mead Johnson)	200	30	4,000	400	15[4]	1.5	1.6	17		2.6	2.5	70	0.5	Mg, Cu, 15 mg Zn	In 100s.
otc	**Nutricon Tablets** (Pasadena)	200	20	2,500	200	15[5]	1.5	1.5	10	5	2	5	50	0.4	Cu, I, Mg, 3.75 mg Zn, 150 mcg biotin	In 120s.

MULTIVITAMINS WITH CALCIUM AND IRON

	Product & Distributor	Ca[1] mg	Fe[1] mg	A IU	D IU	E mg	B_1 mg	B_2 mg	B_3 mg	B_5 mg	B_6 mg	B_{12} mcg	C mg	FA mg	Other Content	How Supplied
otc	**Sigtab-M Tablets** (Roberts)	200	18	6,000	400	45[2]	5	5	25	.015	3		100	0.4	Vitamin K, P, Mg, 45 mcg biotin, Cu, 15 mg Zn, I, Mn, K, Cl, Mo, Se, Cr, Ni, Sn, V, Si, B	In 100s.
Rx	**Mission Prenatal Rx Tablets** (Mission)	175	60	8,000	400		4	2	20	10	20	8	240	1	Cu, I, 15 mg Zn	In 100s.
otc	**Centrum, Jr. + Extra Calcium Tablets** (Lederle)	160	18	5,000	400	30[2]	1.5	1.7	20	10	2	6	60	0.4	Cr, Cu, I, Mg, Mn, Mo, P, 15 mg Zn, vitamin K, 45 mcg biotin, sugar	Chewable. Fruit flavor. In 60s.
otc	**Calcet Plus Tablets** (Mission)	152.8	18	5,000	400	30[2]	2.25	2.55	30	15	3	9	500	0.8	15 mg Zn, sugar	In 60s.
otc	**My-Vitalife Capsules** (ME Pharm)	130	27	6,500	400	30[2]	1.5	1.7	20	10	2	6	60	0.4	Cr, Cu, K, I, Mg, Mn, Mo, P, Se, 15 mg Zn, 30 mcg biotin	In 60s.
otc	**Centrum, Jr. + Extra C Tablets** (Lederle)	108	18	5,000	400	30[2]	1.5	1.7	20	10	2	6	300	0.4	Cr, Cu, I, Mg, Mn, Mo, P, 15 mg Zn, vitamin K, 45 mcg biotin, sugar, lactose	Chewable. Fruit flavor. In 60s.
otc sf	**Bugs Bunny Complete Tablets** (Bayer)	100	18	5,000	400	30[4]	1.5	1.7	20	10	2	6	60	0.4	40 mcg biotin, Cu, I, Mg, P, aspartame, phenylalanine, 15 mg Zn	Chewable. Fruit flavor. In 60s.

MULTIVITAMINS WITH CALCIUM AND IRON

	Product & Distributor	Ca[1] mg	Fe[1] mg	A IU	D IU	E mg	B_1 mg	B_2 mg	B_3 mg	B_5 mg	B_6 mg	B_{12} mcg	C mg	FA mg	Other Content	How Supplied
otc	**4 Nails Softgel Capsules** (Marlyn)	167	3	833	67	10[2]	3.3	1.7	8.3	8.3	8.3	8.3	10	33.3	8.3 mcg biotin, P, I, Mg, Cu, 3.3 mg Zn, Cr, Mn, methionine, inositol, choline bitartrate, Se, PABA, protein isolate, gelatin, lecithin, unsaturated fatty acid, predigested protein, L-cysteine, B mucopolysaccharides, silicon amino acid chelate, S	In 60s.
otc	**Optimox Prenatal Tablets** (Optimox)	100	5	833	67	2[6]	0.5	0.6	6.7	3.3	0.73	0.87	30	0.13	Cr, Cu, I, Mg, Mn, Se, 3.17 mg Zn	In 360s.
otc	**Gynovite Plus Tablets** (Optimox)	83	3	833	67	67[6]	1.7	1.7	3.3	1.7	3.3	21	30	0.07	B, betaine, biotin, Cr, Cu, hesperidin, I, inositol, Mg, Mn, PABA, pancreatin, rutin, Se, 2.5 mg Zn	In 100s.
otc	**Sesame Street Complete Tablets** (McNeil-CPC)	80	10	2,750	200	10[4]	0.75	0.85	10	5	0.7	3	40	0.2	15 mg biotin, Cu, I, Mg, 8 mg Zn, lactose	Sucrose. Chewable. Fruit flavor. In 50s.

MULTIVITAMINS WITH CALCIUM AND IRON

	Product & Distributor	Ca[1] mg	Fe[1] mg	A IU	D IU	E mg	B_1 mg	B_2 mg	B_3 mg	B_5 mg	B_6 mg	B_{12} mcg	C mg	FA mg	Other Content	How Supplied
otc sf	**Hipotest Tablets** (Marlop Pharm)	53.5	50	10,000	400	12.5[6]	25	25	50	13	15	50	150		Choline, betaine, PABA, rutin, bioflavonoids, 1 mg biotin, desiccated liver, bone meal, Cu, Mg, Mn, 2.2 mg Zn, I, P, lecithin	In 100s
otc sf	**Maxi-Vite Tablets** (Goldline)	53.5	1.5	10,000	400	15[2]	10	10	100	20	5	5	200	0.4	1 mcg biotin, I, P, Cu, Mg, Mn, 1.5 mg Zn, PABA, rutin, glutamic acid, inositol, choline bitartrate, bioflavanoids, L-lysine, betaine, lecithin	In 60s.
otc	**Theragran-M Caplets** (Mead Johnson)	40	27	5,000	400	30[4]	3	3.4	20	10	3	9	90	0.4	Cl, Cr, Cu, I, K, Mg, Mn, Mo, P, Se, 15 mg Zn, 30 mcg biotin, lactose, sucrose	In 90s, 130s, 180s and 200s.

MULTIVITAMINS WITH CALCIUM AND IRON

	Product & Distributor	Ca[1] mg	Fe[1] mg	A IU	D IU	E mg	B_1 mg	B_2 mg	B_3 mg	B_5 mg	B_6 mg	B_{12} mcg	C mg	FA mg	Other Content	How Supplied
otc	**Ondrox Tablets** (Unimed)	25	3	2,000	100	17[2]	0.25	0.28	3.33	1.67	0.33	1	41.7	0.67	5 mcg biotin, I, Mg, Cu, P, vitamin K, K, Cr, Mn, Mo, Se, V, B, Si, 2.5 mg Zn, bioflavanoids, K, inositol, N-acetylcysteine, L-glutathione, L-methionine, L-glutamine, taurine	Sustained-release. In 60s and 180s.
Rx	**Mynatal PN Captabs** (ME Pharm)	125	60	4,000	400		3	3	10		2	3	50	1	18 mg Zn	Blue. Film-coated. In 100s.

[1] Calcium and iron content expressed in mg elemental calcium and iron.
[2] Form of vitamin E unknown.
[3] As calcium carbonate and gluconate.
[4] As dl-alpha tocopheryl acetate.
[5] As d-alpha tocopheryl acetate.
[6] As d-alpha tocopheryl acid succinate.

MULTIVITAMINS WITH MINERALS

Content given per capsule, tablet or 5 ml.

For a comparison of the potencies of various forms of vitamin E, see the Vitamin E monograph.

	Product & Distributor	A IU	D IU	E IU	B_1 mg	B_2 mg	B_3 mg	B_5 mg	B_6 mg	B_{12} mcg	C mg	FA mg	Zn[1] mg	Other Content	How Supplied
otc	**Vademin-Z Capsules** (Roberts/Hauck)	12,500	50	50[2]	10	5	25	10	2		150		2.6	Mg, Mn	In 60s.
otc sf	**Super Hi Potency Tablets** (Nion)	10,000	400	150[3]	75	75	75	75	75	75	250	0.4	15	Betaine, 75 mcg biotin, Ca, Fe, hesperidin, I, K, Mg, Mn, Se[4]	In 100s.
otc sf	**Total Formula-3 without Iron Tablets** (Vitaline)	10,000	400	30[5]	15	15	25	25	25	25	100	0.4	30	Ca, Cr, Cu, I, K, Mg, Mn, Mo, V, B, Se, Si, vitamin K, 300 mcg biotin, hesperidin[4]	In 60s and 1000s.
Rx	**Vicon Forte Capsules** (Whitby)	8000		50[6]	10	5	25	10	2	10	150	1	18	Mg, Mn, lactose	(Whitby 316). Orange/black. In 60s, 500s and UD 100s.
otc sf	**ICAPS Time Release Tablets** (Ciba Vision)	7000		100[6]		20					200		14.25	Cu, Se	In 60s and 120s.
otc sf	**ICAPS Plus Tablets** (Ciba Vision)	6000		60[6]		20					200		14.25	Cu, Se, Mn	In 60s, 120s and 180s.
otc	**Garfield Complete with Minerals Tablets** (Menley & James)	5000	400	30[6]	1.5	1.7	20	10	2	6	60	0.4	15	Fe, Ca, Cu, P, I, Mg, 40 mcg biotin, aspartame, phenylalanine	Chewable. Character shapes. In 60s.
otc	**PowerMate Tablets** (Green Turtle Bay)[7]	5000		100[6]			12.5				250		2.5	Se, n-acetyl-L-cysteine	In 50s.
otc	**One-A-Day Extras Antioxidant Softgel Capsules** (Bayer)	5000		200[6]							250		7.5	Cu, Se, Mn, tartrazine	(One-A-Day). In 50s.
otc	**Vi-Zac Capsules** (Whitby)	5000		50[6]							500		18	Lactose	Orange/banded. In 60s.
otc sf	**Glutofac Caplets** (Kenwood/Bradley)	5000		30[6]	15	10	50	20	50		300		5	Ca, Cr, Cu, Fe, K, Mg, Mn, P, Se	In 90s.
otc	**OCuSoft VMS Tablets** (OCuSoft)	5000		30[6]							60			Cu, Se, 40 mg Zn	Film coated. In 60s.

MULTIVITAMINS WITH MINERALS

	Product & Distributor	A IU	D IU	E IU	B_1 mg	B_2 mg	B_3 mg	B_5 mg	B_6 mg	B_{12} mcg	C mg	FA mg	Zn[1] mg	Other Content	How Supplied
Rx	**Zincvit Capsules** (Kenwood/Bradley)	5000	50	50[6]	10	5	25		2		300	1	9.2	Mg, Mn	(Ram/Ram). Aqua green. In 60s.
otc	**ADEKs Tablets** (Scandipharm)	4000	400	150[6]	1.2	1.3	10	10	1.5	12	60	0.2	1.1	Vitamin K, 50 mcg biotin, 3 mg beta carotene, fructose	Chewable. Tan. Capsule shape. In 60s.
Rx	**Eldercaps Capsules** (Mayrand)	4000	400	25[6]	10	5	25	10	2		200	1	15.8	Mg, Mn	In 100s.
otc	**Vicon Plus Capsules** (Whitby)	4000		50[6]	10	5	25	10	2		150		18	Mg, Mn, lactose	In 60s.
otc sf	**Kenwood Therapeutic Liquid** (Kenwood/Bradley)	3333	133	1.5[8]	2	1	20	2	0.33		50			Ca, K, Mg, Mn, P	Alcohol free. In 240 ml.
otc	**Flintstones Plus Calcium Tablets** (Bayer)	2500	400	15[6]	1.05	1.2	13.5		1.05	4.5	60	0.3		200 mg Ca, sorbitol	Chewable. Character shapes. In 60s.
otc sf	**Maximum Green Label Tablets** (Vitaline)	2500	16.7	66.7[5]	16.7	8.3	31.7	66.7	16.7	16.7	200	0.13	5	Ca, Cr, I, K, Mg, Mn, Mo, Se, Si, V, 50 mcg biotin, SOD, L–lysine[4]	In 180s.
otc sf	**Maximum Blue Label Tablets** (Vitaline)													Ca, Cr, Cu, I, K, Mg, Mn, Mo, Se, Si, V, 50 mcg biotin, SOD, L–lysine[4]	In 180s.
otc sf	**PowerVites Tablets** (Green Turtle Bay)[7]	2500	150	12.5[3]	6.3	6.3	25	25	12.5	6.3	125	0.15	2.5	B, Ca, Mg, Cu, Cr, Mn, K, Se, betaine, hesperidin, biotin[4]	In 40s, 100s and 200s.
otc sf	**Vita-PMS Tablets** (Bajamar)	2083	16.7	16.7[3]	4.2	4.2	4.2	4.2	50	10.4	250	0.33	4.2	Mg, Ca, Cu, Mn, K, Se, Cr, I, Fe, biotin, betaine[4]	In 100s.
otc	**Po-Pon-S Tablets** (Shionogi)	2000	100	5[6]	5	3	35	15	4	6	100			Ca, P	Sugar coated. In 60s and 240s.
otc	**Maxovite Tablets** (Tyson)	2083	16.7	16.7[3]	5	4.2	4.2	4.2	54.2	10.8	250	0.33	5	Ca, Cr, Cu, Fe, I, K, Mg, Mn, Se, 11.7 mcg biotin[4]	Sustained release. In 120s and 240s.

MULTIVITAMINS WITH MINERALS

	Product & Distributor	A IU	D IU	E IU	B_1 mg	B_2 mg	B_3 mg	B_5 mg	B_6 mg	B_{12} mcg	C mg	FA mg	Zn[1] mg	Other Content	How Supplied
otc sf	**Vita-PMS Plus Tablets** (Bajamar)	667	16.7	16.7[3]	4.2	4.2	4.2	4.2	16.7	10.4	250	0.33	4.2	Mg, Ca, Cu, Mn, K, Se, Cr, I, Fe, biotin, betaine[4]	In 100s.
otc sf	**Stress 600 w/Zinc Tablets** (Nion)			45[8]	20	10	100	25	10	25	600	0.4	5.5	Cu, 45 mcg biotin	In 60s.
otc	**Mediplex Tabules (Tablets)** (US Pharm)			60[8]	25	10	100	25	10	25	300		4	Cu, Mg, Mn	In 100s.
otc	**Bee-Zee Tablets** (Rugby)			45[8]	15	10.2	100	25	10	6	600		5.2		In 60s.
otc sf	**Z-gen Tablets** (Goldline)														In 60s.
otc	**Z-Bec Tablets** (Robins)			45[6]									22.5	Parabens	In 60s, 500s and Dis–Co pack 100s.
otc	**Surbex 750 with Zinc Tablets** (Abbott)			30[8]	15	15	100	20	20	12	750	0.4	22.5		Film coated. In 50s.
otc sf	**Stress B-Complex Tablets** (Moore)			30[8]	15	10	100	20	5	12	500	0.4	23.9	Cu, 45 mcg biotin	In 60s.
otc	**Stresstabs + Zinc Tablets** (Lederle)			30[6]	10	10	100	20	5	12	500	0.4	23.9	Cu, 45 mcg biotin	In 60s.

[1] Zinc content expressed in mg elemental zinc.
[2] As dl-alpha tocopheryl succinate.
[3] As d-alpha tocopherol.
[4] Also contains bioflavonoids, choline, inositol, PABA and rutin.
[5] As d-alpha tocopheryl succinate.
[6] Form of vitamin E unknown.
[7] The Green Turtle Bay Vitamin Co., P.O. Box 642, Summit, NJ 07902; (908) 277–2240.
[8] As dl-alpha tocopheryl acetate.

GERIATRIC SUPPLEMENTS WITH MULTIVITAMINS AND MINERALS

Content given per capsule, tablet or 5 ml.

For a comparison of the potencies of various forms of vitamin E, see the Vitamin E monograph.

	Product & Distributor	A IU	D IU	E IU	B_1 mg	B_2 mg	B_3 mg	B_5 mg	B_6 mg	B_{12} mcg	C mg	Fe[1] mg	FA mg	Ca[1] mg	Zn mg	Other Content	How Supplied
otc sf	**Mega VM-80 Tablets** (NBTY)	10,000	1000	100[2]	80	80	80	80	80	80	250	1.2	0.4	4.5	3.58	Choline, inositol, 80 mcg biotin, PABA, bioflavonoids, betaine, hesperidin, Cu, I, K, Mg, Mn, Se	In 60s and 100s.
otc	**Vita-Plus G Softgel Capsules** (Scot-Tussin)	5000	400	10[3]	5	5	15	5	1	1	50	3.3		145	0.5	K, Mg, Mn, P, I, Cu, choline, l-lysine, inositol	In 100s.
Rx	**Cezin-S Capsules** (UAD)	10,000	50	50[4]	10	5	50	10	2		200		0.5		18	Mg, Mn	In 100s.
otc	**One-A-Day 55 Plus Tablets** (Bayer)	6000	400	60[2]	4.5	3.4	20	20	6	25	120		0.4	220	15	30 mcg biotin, vitamin K, I, Mg, Cu, Cr, Se, Mo, Mn, K, Cl	(One-A-Day). In 50s and 80s.
otc	**Cerovite Senior Tablets** (Rugby)	6000	400	45[3]	1.5	1.7	20	10	3	25	60	9	0.2	200	15	30 mcg biotin, Cu, I, Mg, P, Cl, Cr, Mn, Mo, Ni, Se, Si, V, K, vitamin K	In 60s.
otc	**Centrum Silver Tablets** (Lederle)	5000	400	45[2]	1.5	1.7	20	10	3	25	60	4	0.4	200	15	30 mcg biotin, Cu, I, Mg, P, B, Cl, Cr, Mn, Mo, Ni, Se, Si, V, K, vitamin K	In 60s, 100s and 180s.
otc	**Certagen Senior Tablets** (Goldline)	6000	400	45[3]	1.5	1.7	20	10	3	25	60	3	0.2	80	15	30 mcg biotin, Cl, Cr, Cu, I, Mg, Mn, Mo, Ni, P, K, Se, Si, V, vitamin K	In 60s.
otc sf	**Certa-Vite Golden Tablets** (Major)	6000	400	45[3]	1.5	1.7	20	10	3	25	60			200	15	30 mcg biotin, Cl, Cr, Cu, I, K, Mg, Mn, Mo, Ni, P, Se, Si, V, vitamin K, tartrazine	In 60s.
otc	**Gerimed Tablets** (Fielding)	5000	400	30[2]	3	3	25		2	6	120			370	15	P	In 60s.
Rx	**Strovite Plus Caplets** (Everett)	5000		30[3]	20	20	100	25	25	50	500	9	0.8		22.5	150 mcg biotin, Cr, Cu, Mg, Mn	(EV201). Dark red. In 100s.

GERIATRIC SUPPLEMENTS WITH MULTIVITAMINS AND MINERALS

	Product & Distributor	A IU	D IU	E IU	B_1 mg	B_2 mg	B_3 mg	B_5 mg	B_6 mg	B_{12} mcg	C mg	Fe[1] mg	FA mg	Ca[1] mg	Zn mg	Other Content	How Supplied
otc sf	**Ultra-Freeda Tablets** (Freeda)	4166	133	66.7[2]	16.7	16.7	33	33	16.7	33	333	2	0.27	27	1.1	Choline, inositol, bioflavonoids, PABA, 100 mcg biotin, Cr, I, K, Mg, Mn, Mo, Se	In 90s, 180s and 270s.
otc sf	**Iron Free Ultra-Freeda Tablets** (Freeda)	4166	133	66.7[2]	16.7	16.7	33	33	16.7	33	333		0.27	27	1.1		In 90s, 180s and 270s.
otc	**Optivite P.M.T. Tablets** (Optimox)	2083	†	16.6[4]	4.2	4.2	4.2	4.2	50	10.4	250	2.5	0.03	†	4.2	Choline, Cr, Cu, I, K, Mg, Mn, Se, bioflavonoids, betaine, PABA, pancreatin, rutin, inositol, biotin	In 180s.
otc	**Hep-Forte Capsules** (Marlyn)	1200		10[2]	1	1	10	2	0.5	1	10		0.06		0.5	Choline, inositol, biotin, dl–methionine, desiccated liver, liver concentrate, liver fraction number 2	In 100s, 300s and 500s.
otc	**Vigortol Liquid** (Rugby)				0.8	0.4	8.3	1.7	0.2	0.2		0.3			0.3	Choline, I, Mg, Mn, 18% alcohol, sugar, methylparaben	Sherry wine flavor. In 473 ml.
otc	**Gerivite Liquid** (Goldline)															Choline, I, Mg, Mn, 18% alcohol, methylparaben, sorbitol	Rum and sherry wine flavors. In 473 ml.
otc	**Viminate Liquid** (Various, eg, Moore)				2.5	1.25	25	5	0.5	0.5		7.5			1	Choline, I, Mg, Mn	In 480 ml.
otc	**Geroton Forte Liquid** (Kenwood/Bradley)				0.2	0.2	2.2	1.1	0.2	0.7					0.4	Mg, Mn, 13.5% alcohol, sucrose, methylparaben	In 473 ml.
otc	**Geravite Elixir** (Roberts-Hauck)				0.3	0.4	33.3			3.3						L–lysine, 15% alcohol, parabens, sorbitol, sucrose	Wine flavor. In 480 ml.

† Amount not supplied by manufacturer.
[1] Calcium and iron content expressed in mg elemental calcium and iron.
[2] Form of vitamin E unknown.
[3] As dl-alpha tocopheryl acetate.
[4] As d-alpha tocopheryl acid succinate.

LIPOTROPICS WITH VITAMINS

Content given per capsule or tablet.

	Product & Distributor	Choline (mg)	Inositol (mg)	Methionine (mg)	B_1 mg	B_2 mg	B_3 mg	B_5 mg	B_6 mg	B_{12} mcg	C mg	Other Content	How Supplied
otc	**Lipogen Capsules** (Various, eg, Rugby)	111[1]	†		0.33	0.33	3.33	1.7	0.33	1.7	100	Bioflavonoids, sorbitol, lecithin	In 60s.
otc	**Lipogen Caplets** (Goldline)	111	111		0.33	0.33	3.33	1.7	0.33	1.7	20	1667 IU vitamin A (as beta carotene), 10 IU vitamin E,[2] 10 mg Zn, Cu, Se	In 100s.
otc	**Lipotriad Caplets** (Numark)	†	†		1.5	1.7	20	10	2	6	60	5000 IU vitamin A (as beta carotene), 30 IU E,[2] 30 mg Zn, Cu, Se	In 60s.
otc	**Lipoflavonoid Caplets** (Numark)	111	111		0.33	0.33	3.33	1.66	0.33	1.66	100	100 mg lemon bioflavonoid complex	In 100s and 500s.
otc *sf*	**Cholinoid Capsules** (Goldline)	111[1]	111		0.33	0.33	3.33	1.7	0.33	1.7	100	100 mg lemon bioflavonoid complex	In 100s.
otc	**Liponol Capsules** (Rugby)	240[1]	83	110	3	3	10	2	2	2		56 mg desiccated liver, 30 mg liver concentrate, sorbitol, lecithin	In 60s.
otc *sf*	**Methatropic Capsules** (Goldline)											86 mg desiccated liver	In 100s.
otc *sf*	**Cholidase Tablets** (Freeda)	450[1]	150						2.5	5		7.5 mg vitamin E[3]	In 100s.

† Amount not supplied by manufacturer.
[1] From choline bitartrate.
[2] Form of vitamin E unknown.
[3] As d-alpha tocopherol.

INTRAVENOUS NUTRITIONAL THERAPY

Intravenous nutritional therapy is required when normal enteral feeding is not possible or is inadequate for nutritional requirements. Specific nutritional requirements and administration mode depend on the nutritional status of the patient and the duration of parenteral therapy. To meet IV nutritional requirements, one or more of the following nutrients may be required:

Protein Substrates
- Amino Acids - General Formulations
- Amino Acids - Renal Failure Formulations
- Amino Acids - Hepatic Failure/Encephalopathy Formulations
- Amino Acids - Metabolic Stress Formulations

Energy Substrates
- Dextrose
- IV Fat Emulsion

Electrolytes
Vitamins
Trace Metals

The following general discussion reviews peripheral and central administration routes, and provides basic guidelines for use of various components of IV nutritional therapy.

PERIPHERAL PARENTERAL NUTRITION:

Peripheral protein sparing: Amino acids with maintenance electrolytes (with or without dextrose) prevent protein catabolism, for short periods of time, in patients with adequate body fat and no clinically significant protein malnutrition. Lipolysis provides energy from oxidation of free fatty acids and ketone bodies; minimal nitrogen is lost since proteolysis does not occur. For peripheral IV infusion, 1 to 1.5 g/kg/day of amino acids achieves optimal fat mobilization and spares protein catabolism.

ProcalAmine is a unique product that provides a physiological ratio of biologically useable essential and nonessential amino acids, glycerin (glycerol) and maintenance electrolytes. Glycerin preserves body protein and participates as an active energy substrate through its phosphorylation to α-glycerophosphate.

Peripheral total parenteral nutrition (TPN) is for patients requiring parenteral nutrition when the central venous route is not indicated. Amino acids with electrolytes, combined with 5% or 10% dextrose and used with IV fat emulsions (and usually vitamins and trace metals), reduce protein catabolism in patients moderately catabolic or depleted and minimize liver glycogen depletion. Peripheral infusions may provide inadequate maintenance requirements for those with greatly increased metabolic demands or severe nutritional deficiencies requiring repletion. May add oral calories as tolerated.

CENTRAL TOTAL PARENTERAL NUTRITION: Amino acids combined with hypertonic dextrose and IV fat emulsions infused via a central venous catheter promote protein synthesis in hypercatabolic or severely depleted patients or those requiring long-term parenteral nutrition. Appropriate electrolytes, vitamins and trace minerals are added to provide total parenteral nutrition.

Actions:

Pharmacology:

Amino acids promote the production of proteins (anabolism) needed for synthesis of structural components, reduce the rate of protein breakdown (catabolism), promote wound healing and act as buffers in the extracellular and intracellular fluids.

Dextrose is a source of calories; nonprotein calories are required for efficient use of amino acids. It decreases protein and nitrogen losses, promotes glycogen deposition and prevents ketosis (see individual monograph).

IV fat emulsions provide a mixture of fatty acids to be used as a source of energy and to prevent essential fatty acid deficiency (EFAD) (see individual monograph).

Fluid/Electrolytes/Trace metals are provided to compensate for normal sensible and insensible losses, as well as the additional losses often present in patients requiring parenteral nutrition (see individual section).

Indications:

Parenteral nutrition is indicated to prevent nitrogen and weight loss or to treat negative nitrogen balance when: (1) The alimentary tract, by the oral, gastrostomy or jejunostomy route, cannot or should not be used; (2) GI absorption of protein is impaired by obstruction, inflammatory disease or its complications or antineoplastic therapy; (3) bowel rest is needed because of GI surgery or its complications such as ileus, fistulae or anastomotic leaks; (4) metabolic requirements for protein are substantially increased, as with extensive burns, infections, trauma or other hypermetabolic states; (5) morbidity and mortality may be reduced by replacing amino acids lost from tissue breakdown, thereby preserving tissue reserves, as in acute renal failure; (6) tube feeding methods alone cannot provide adequate nutrition.

INTRAVENOUS NUTRITIONAL THERAPY

After the patient's nutritional deficits, reserves and current status are assessed, set rational and precise nutritional goals. Dosage, route of administration and concomitant infusion of nonprotein calories depend on nutritional and metabolic status, anticipated duration of parenteral nutritional support and vein tolerance.

Peripheral parenteral nutrition: Administration of nutritional solutions through peripheral veins is appropriate if caloric needs are minimal, if they can be partially met by enteral alimentation, if nutritional therapy will only be required for 5 to 14 days, or if central venous access is not feasible.

Central parenteral nutrition: Amino acids, with hypertonic dextrose and IV fat emulsions infused via central venous catheter, promote protein synthesis in the hypercatabolic or severely depleted or in those requiring long-term parenteral nutrition.

Specific disease states in which TPN requires special considerations are:

Renal failure
Acute metabolic stress
Hepatic failure/Hepatic encephalopathy
See individual sections for specific discussions.

Total nutrient admixtures (TNA): A combination of amino acids, dextrose and lipids in one container has been used. Also known as multicomponent admixtures, all-in-one, 3-in-1 or triple mix, TNA offers the advantage of substituting some dextrose calories with lipids, reducing carbohydrate-related complications (eg, impaired glucose control). It also appears to be used better by the liver due to continuous lipid administration, and is less likely to interfere with immune functions. See also admixture incompatibilities/compatibilities under Administration and Dosage.

Contraindications:

Protein substrates: Hypersensitivity to any component; decreased (subcritical) circulating blood volume; inborn errors of amino acid metabolism (eg, maple syrup urine disease, isovaleric acidemia); anuria.

General amino acid formulations: Severe renal failure or liver disease; hepatic coma or encephalopathy; metabolic disorders involving impaired nitrogen utilization.

Renal failure formulations: Severe electrolyte and acid-base imbalance; hyperammonemia.

Hepatic failure/Hepatic encephalopathy formulations: Anuria.

High metabolic stress formulations: Anuria; hyperammonemia; hepatic coma; severe electrolyte or acid-base imbalance.

Warnings:

Prevention of complications: IV nutritional therapy may be associated with complications that can be prevented or minimized by careful attention to solution preparation, administration and patient monitoring. It is essential to follow a carefully prepared protocol based on current medical practices, preferably administered by an experienced team.

Amino acid metabolism: Hyperchloremic metabolic acidosis may result from amino acids provided as hydrochloride salts that release hydrochloride when utilized. To prevent or control this, supply a portion of the cations as acetate or lactate salts. Sodium and potassium phosphates are also available.

Hepatic function impairment may result in serum amino acid imbalances, metabolic alkalosis, prerenal azotemia, hyperammonemia, stupor and coma. Instances of asymptomatic hyperammonemia have occurred in patients without overt liver dysfunction. Amino acid products specifically formulated for patients with hepatic failure are discussed separately in this section. Give conservative doses of amino acids to patients with known or suspected hepatic dysfunction.

Hyperammonemia occurs most often in children and adults with renal or hepatic disease and results from a diminished ability to handle a protein load. It is of special significance in infants as it can result in mental retardation. This reaction is dose-related and more likely to develop during prolonged therapy; treatment involves adjusting the dosage or decreasing amino acids.

Ketosis – Administration of amino acids without carbohydrates may result in the accumulation of ketones; correct ketonemia by administering carbohydrates.

Infection control: Parenteral nutrition is associated with a constant risk of sepsis. Careful, aseptic technique in the preparation of solutions and insertion and maintenance of central venous catheters is imperative. A 0.22 micron filter is often recommended to block particulate matter and bacteria. Presence of *Staphylococcus* or *Candida* suggests catheter sepsis. Early symptoms of infection include fever, chills, glucose intolerance and a change in the level of consciousness.

If other sources are not apparent and if fever persists, change solution, delivery system and catheter site. Culture catheter tip and draw blood cultures.

INTRAVENOUS NUTRITIONAL THERAPY

Pregnancy: Category C. It is not known whether IV nutritional therapy can cause fetal harm when given to a pregnant woman or can affect reproduction capacity. Use only when clearly needed and potential benefits outweigh hazards to the fetus.

Lactation: Exercise caution when administering to a nursing woman.

Children: The effect of amino acid infusions without dextrose on carbohydrate metabolism of children is not known. Use special caution in pediatric patients with acute renal failure, especially low birth weight infants. Laboratory and clinical monitoring must be extensive and frequent.

Precautions:

Monitoring: Laboratory monitoring and clinical evaluation are necessary before and during use. Do not withdraw venous blood for blood chemistries through the same peripheral infusion site; interference with estimations of nitrogen-containing substances may occur. The following general protocol is suggested:

General Patient Monitoring During IV Nutritional Therapy
Baseline studies: CBC, platelet count, prothrombin time, weight, body length and head circumference (in infants), electrolytes, CO_2, BUN, glucose, creatinine, total protein, cholesterol, triglycerides (if on fat emulsion), uric acid, bilirubin, alkaline phosphatase, LDH, AST, albumin and other appropriate parameters.
Daily studies during stabilization (average 3 to 5 days): Urine glucose, acetone and ketones each shift, intake/output, weight, plasma and urine osmolarity, electrolytes, trace elements, CO_2, BUN, creatinine.
Routine studies after stabilization: *Daily* - Intake/output, weight, urine glucose and osmolarity and ketones.
Two to three times weekly - Electrolytes, BUN, blood glucose, plasma transaminases, bilirubin, blood acid-base status, ammonia, creatinine.
Weekly: CBC, prothrombin time, plasma total protein and fractions, hemoglobin, body length and head circumference (in infants), cholesterol, triglycerides, uric acid, albumin, LDH, AST, alkaline phosphatase.
Periodic: Nitrogen balance, trace elements, total lymphocyte count, iron status.

BUN: IV amino acid infusion may induce a rise in BUN, especially in GI bleeding or impaired hepatic or renal function. Perform appropriate laboratory tests periodically; discontinue if BUN exceeds normal postprandial limits and continues to rise. A modest rise in BUN normally results from increased protein intake. Azotemic patients should not receive amino acids without regard to total nitrogen intake.

Protein sparing – If daily increases in BUN (range, 10 to 15 mg/dl) for > 3 days occur, discontinue protein sparing therapy and institute a regimen with full nonprotein caloric substrates.

Cardiac effects: Avoid circulatory overload, particularly in patients with cardiac insufficiency. In patients with myocardial infarction, infusion of amino acids should always be accompanied by dextrose; in anoxia, free fatty acids cannot be used by the myocardium, and energy must be produced anaerobically from glycogen or glucose.

Hypertonic solutions containing dextrose should not be administered by peripheral vein infusions. Do not use hypertonic solutions in the presence of intracranial or intraspinal hemorrhage or if the patient is already dehydrated.

Glucose imbalances:

Hyperglycemia – Glucose intolerance is the most common metabolic complication; metabolic adaptation to large glucose loads requires up to 72 hours, although severely septic or hypermetabolic patients may not be able to handle the glucose load. A too rapid infusion of amino acid-carbohydrate mixtures may result in hyperglycemia, glycosuria and a hyperosmolar syndrome, characterized by mental confusion and loss of consciousness. Reducing the administration rate, decreasing the dextrose concentration or administering insulin will minimize these reactions.

Hyperglycemia may not be reflected by glycosuria in renal failure. Therefore, determine blood glucose frequently, often every 6 hours, to guide dosage of dextrose and insulin if required. Infusion of hypertonic dextrose carries a greater risk of hyperglycemia in low birth weight or septic infants.

Excess carbohydrate calories may result in fatty infiltration of the liver. Excess carbon dioxide from too much glucose can compromise weaning hypermetabolic patients from mechanical ventilation or can precipitate acute respiratory failure.

Rebound hypoglycemia may result from sudden cessation of a concentrated dextrose solution due to continued endogenous insulin production. Withdraw parenteral nutrition mixtures slowly. Administer a solution containing 5% or 10% dextrose when hypertonic dextrose infusions are abruptly discontinued.

Essential fatty acid deficiency (EFAD) results from long-term fat-free IV feeding; symptoms include dry, scaly skin, eczematous rash, hair loss, poor wound healing and fatty degeneration of the liver. In adults, administer at least 500 ml fat emulsion per week to prevent EFAD (see individual monograph).

Electrolyte abnormalities: Intracellular ion deficits may arise due to two mechanisms. As protein is used for increased energy demands in a catabolic patient, intracellular ions are lost. In addition, as anabolism occurs, ions are employed in building new cells. Focus attention on supplying adequate potassium, phosphate, magnesium and calcium. Observe patients for clinical signs of paresthesias, neuromuscular weakness and changes in level of consciousness; monitor laboratory results.

The presence of impaired renal function, pulmonary disease, or cardiac insufficiency presents danger of retention of fluids.

Sodium – Use solutions containing sodium ions cautiously in patients with CHF, severe renal insufficiency, and edema with sodium retention.

Potassium – Use solutions containing potassium ions cautiously in patients with hyperkalemia or severe renal failure, and in conditions in which potassium retention is present.

Acetate – Use solutions containing acetate ions cautiously in patients with metabolic or respiratory alkalosis and in those conditions in which there is an increased level or impaired utilization of this ion, such as severe hepatic insufficiency.

Cancer chemotherapy patients: The American College of Physicians discourages the routine use of parenteral nutrition in patients undergoing cancer chemotherapy since no benefit has been determined (ie, there was no improvement in overall or short-term survival and no greater improvement in chemotherapy response).

Sulfite sensitivity: Some of these products contain sulfites which may cause allergic-type reactions including anaphylactic symptoms and life-threatening or less severe asthmatic episodes in certain susceptible persons. The overall prevalence of sulfite sensitivity in the general population is unknown and probably low. Sulfite sensitivity is seen more frequently in asthmatic or atopic persons.

Drug Interactions:

Tetracycline, because of its antianabolic activity, may reduce the protein sparing effects of infused amino acids.

Adverse Reactions:

Catheter complications: Phlebitis and venous thrombosis may occur at the site of venipuncture or along the vein. If this occurs, discontinue use or choose another administration site. Use of large peripheral veins, inline filters and slower infusion rates may reduce the incidence of local venous irritation. Infection at the injection site and extravasation may occur.

Nausea, fever and flushing of the skin have occurred.

Metabolic complications include: Metabolic acidosis and alkalosis; hypophosphatemia; hypocalcemia; osteoporosis; glycosuria; hyperglycemia; hypo- or hypermagnesemia; osmotic diuresis; dehydration; hypervolemia; rebound hypoglycemia; hypo- or hypervitaminosis; electrolyte imbalances; hyperammonemia; elevated hepatic enzymes.

Phosphorus deficiency may lead to impaired tissue oxygenation and acute hemolytic anemia. Relative to calcium, excessive phosphorus intake can precipitate hypocalcemia with cramps, tetany and muscular hyperexcitability.

Complications known to occur from the placement of central venous catheters are pneumothorax, hemothorax, hydrothorax, artery puncture and transection, injury to the brachial plexus, malposition of the catheter, formation of arteriovenous fistula, phlebitis, thrombosis and air and catheter embolus.

Reactions reported in clinical studies as a result of infusion of the parenteral fluid were water weight gain, edema, increase in BUN and mild acidosis.

Administration and Dosage:

Total daily dose depends on daily protein requirements and on the patient's metabolic and clinical responses. The determination of nitrogen balance and accurate daily body weights, corrected for fluid balance, are probably the best means of assessing protein requirements. In addition, guide dosage by the patient's fluid intake limits, glucose and nitrogen tolerances and metabolic and clinical response.

INTRAVENOUS NUTRITIONAL THERAPY

Protein: Recommended dietary allowances of protein are approximately 0.9 g/kg for a healthy adult and 1.4 to 2.2 g/kg for healthy growing infants and children. Protein and caloric requirements in traumatized or malnourished patients may be substantially increased. Daily doses of approximately 1 to 1.5 g/kg for adults and 2 to 3 g/kg for infants are generally sufficient to promote positive nitrogen balance, although higher doses may be required in severely catabolic states. Such higher doses require frequent laboratory evaluation.

Energy requirements: To ensure proper caloric intake, estimate required calorie and energy needs using basal metabolic rate; also consider energy expenditure and disease states. The energy required for proper amino acid utilization is derived from glycogenolysis, lipolysis or infusion of dextrose or fat emulsions. After glycogen is depleted, in the absence of exogenous calories, fat becomes the major energy source. Parenteral amino acids will not be retained and utilized for anabolic purposes unless adequate nonprotein calories are provided simultaneously.

IV fat emulsion should comprise no more than 60% of the total caloric intake, with carbohydrates and amino acids comprising the remaining 40% or more.

Electrolyte requirements: In adults, ≈ 60 to 180 mEq of potassium, 10 to 30 mEq of magnesium and 10 to 40 mM of phosphate per day appear necessary to achieve optimum metabolic response; individualize each requirement. Give sufficient quantities of the major extracellular electrolytes, sodium, calcium and chloride. (Calcium prevents hypocalcemia that may accompany phosphate administration.) Consider content of amino acid infusion when calculating daily electrolyte intake.

HepatAmine contains < 3 mEq chloride/L and ≤ 10 mM/L of phosphate. Some patients, especially hypophosphatemics, may require additional phosphate.

Fluid balance: Provide sufficient water to compensate for insensible, urinary and other (eg, nasogastric suction, fistula drainage, diarrhea) fluid losses. Average daily adult fluid requirements are between 2500 and 3000 ml, but may be much higher with losses such as fistula drainage or in burn patients.

Vitamin therapy: If a patient's nutritional intake is primarily parenteral, provide vitamins (especially the water soluble vitamins). Iron is added to the solution or given IM in depot form as indicated. Folic acid and vitamin K are required additives.

Pediatric requirements are constrained by the greater relative fluid and caloric requirements per kg of the infant. Amino acids are best administered in a 2.5% concentration. For most pediatric patients, 2.5 g amino acids/kg/day with dextrose alone or with IV fat calories of 100 to 130 kcal/kg/day are recommended for maintenance. Start with nutritional solution of half strength at a rate of about 60 to 70 ml/kg/day. Within 24 to 48 hours, the volume and concentration of the solution can be increased until full strength pediatric solution is given at a rate of 125 to 150 ml/kg/day.

A basic central line solution for pediatric use should contain 25 g of amino acids and 200 to 250 g of glucose per 1000 ml. Such a solution given at a rate of 145ml/kg/day provides 100 to 130 kcal/kg/day.

Give supplemental electrolytes and vitamins (including agents such as carnitine) as needed. Iron is more critical in infants because of increasing red cell mass needed for growth. Monitor serum lipids for EFAD in patients maintained on fat-free TPN.

To ensure the precise delivery of the small volumes of fluid necessary, use accurately calibrated and reliable infusion systems.

Preparation/stability of solutions: Aseptically prepare solutions under a laminar flow hood. Use promptly after mixing. Store under refrigeration for a brief period of time only (< 24 hours). Do not exceed 24 hours for administration time of a single bottle.

Admixture incompatibilities/compatibilities: Because of the potential for incompatibility in the complex formulations, keep additives to a minimum. Do not administer simultaneously with *blood* through the same infusion site because of possible pseudoagglutination. *Antibiotics, steroids* and *pressor agents* should not be added to these solutions. *Bleomycin* is incompatible with amino acids.

Vitamins, electrolytes, trace minerals, heparin and *insulin* are compatible with these solutions.

Total nutrient admixture (TNA; all-in-one; 3-in-1; triple mix): The combination of amino acids, dextrose and lipids (also known as total nutrient admixture) in one container is generally compatible. When utilizing this type of admixture, consider the following: (1) The order of mixing is important – add amino acids to the fat emulsion or the dextrose; (2) do not add the electrolytes directly to the fat emulsion – add them to the dextrose or amino acids first; (3) TNAs with electrolytes will eventually aggregate; (4) if not used immediately, refrigerate.

Administration sets: Replace all IV sets every 24 hours. Follow appropriate guidelines for care and maintenance of long-term indwelling catheters (eg, Broviac or Hickman).

Protein Substrates

AMINO ACID INJECTION (General formulations)

For a complete discussion of the use of protein substrates as a compound of intravenous nutritional therapy, refer to the IV Nutritional Therapy general monograph.

Actions:

Pharmacology: Crystalline amino acid injections are hypertonic solutions of balanced essential and nonessential l–amino acids; d–amino acids are not readily utilized by the body. Depending on the amount of caloric supplementation, these amino acids provide a substrate for protein synthesis (anabolism) or enhance conservation of existing body protein (protein sparing effect).

Administration and Dosage:

Peripheral protein sparing: Administer amino acids in a dose of 1 to 1.7 g/kg/day via a peripheral vein. If daily increases in BUN in the range of 10 to 15 mg/dl for > 3 days occur, discontinue and implement a regimen with full nonprotein calorie substrates.

ProcalAmine – Approximately 3 L/day will provide 90 g of amino acids, 390 nonprotein calories and recommended daily intake of principal intra- and extracellular electrolytes for the stable patient. In adults, begin with 3 L on the first day with close monitoring of the patient.

Peripheral vein administration: Mix amino acid injections with low concentrations of dextrose solutions (5% or 10%) and administer by peripheral vein with fat emulsions.

Central vein administration: Typically, 500 ml amino acid injection mixed with 500 ml concentrated dextrose injection, electrolytes and vitamins is administered over an 8 hour period.

Strongly hypertonic mixtures of amino acids and dextrose may be safely administered by continuous infusion only through a central venous catheter with the tip located in the superior vena cava. The initial rate of IV infusion should be 2 ml/min and may be increased gradually to the maximum required dose, as indicated by frequent determinations of urine and blood sugar levels. May be started with infusates containing lower concentrations of dextrose and gradually increased to estimated caloric needs as the patient's glucose tolerance increases. If the administration rate falls behind schedule, do not attempt to "catch up" to planned intake. Do not exceed 24 hours administration time for a single bottle. In addition to meeting protein needs, the administration rate is also governed by the patient's glucose tolerance, especially during the first few days of therapy.

Protein Substrates

CRYSTALLINE AMINO ACID INFUSIONS

	Aminosyn 3.5% (Abbott)	Aminosyn II 3.5% (Abbott)	Aminosyn 5% (Abbott)	Aminosyn II 5% (Abbott)	Travasol 5.5% (Clintec)	TrophAmine 6% (McGaw)
Amino Acid Concentration	3.5%	3.5%	5%	5%	5.5%	6%
Nitrogen (g/100 ml)	0.55	0.54	0.79	0.77	0.925	0.93
Amino Acids (Essential) (mg/100 ml)						
Isoleucine	252	231	360	330	263	490
Leucine	329	350	470	500	340	840
Lysine	252	368	360	525	318	490
Methionine	140	60	200	86	318	200
Phenylalanine	154	104	220	149	340	290
Threonine	182	140	260	200	230	250
Tryptophan	56	70	80	100	99	120
Valine	280	175	400	250	252	470
Amino Acids (Nonessential) (mg/100 ml)						
Alanine	448	348	640	497	1140	320
Arginine	343	356	490	509	570	730
Histidine[1]	105	105	150	150	241	290
Proline	300	253	430	361	230	410
Serine	147	186	210	265		230
Taurine						15
Tyrosine	31	95	44	135	22	140
Aminoacetic Acid (Glycine)	448	175	640	250	1140	220
Glutamic Acid		258		369		300
Aspartic Acid		245		350		190
Cysteine						< 14
Electrolytes (mEq/L)						
Sodium	7	16.3		19.3		5
Potassium			5.4			
Chloride					22	< 3
Acetate	46	25.2	86	35.9	48	56
Phosphate (mM/L)						
Osmolarity (mOsm/L)	357	308	500	438	575	525
Supplied in (ml)	1000[2]	1000[3]	500[4] 1000[4]	500[3] 1000[3]	500[5] 1000[5] 2000[5]	500[6]
Labeled Indications						
Peripheral Parenteral Nutrition	Yes	Yes	Yes	Yes	Yes	Yes
Central TPN	No	No	Yes	Yes	Yes	Yes
Protein Sparing	Yes	Yes	Yes	Yes	Yes	No

Protein Substrates

CRYSTALLINE AMINO ACID INFUSIONS

	Aminosyn 7% (Abbott)	**Aminosyn-PF 7%** (Abbott)	**Aminosyn II 7%** (Abbott)	**Aminosyn 8.5%** (Abbott)
Amino Acid Concentration	7%	7%	7%	8.5%
Nitrogen (g/100 ml)	1.1	1.07	1.07	1.34
Amino Acids (Essential) (mg/100 ml)				
Isoleucine	510	534	462	620
Leucine	660	831	700	810
Lysine	510	475	735	624
Methionine	280	125	120	340
Phenylalanine	310	300	209	380
Threonine	370	360	280	460
Tryptophan	120	125	140	150
Valine	560	452	350	680
Amino Acids (Nonessential) (mg/100 ml)				
Alanine	900	490	695	1100
Arginine	690	861	713	850
Histidine[1]	210	220	210	260
Proline	610	570	505	750
Serine	300	347	371	370
Taurine		50		
Tyrosine	44	44	189	44
Aminoacetic Acid (Glycine)	900	270	350	1100
Glutamic Acid		576	517	
Aspartic Acid		370	490	
Cysteine				
Electrolytes (mEq/L)				
Sodium		3.4	31.3	
Potassium	5.4			5.4
Chloride				35
Acetate	105	32.5	50.3	90
Phosphate (mM/L)				
Osmolarity (mOsm/L)	700	586	612	850
Supplied in (ml)	500[4]	250[7] 500[7]	500[3]	500[4] 1000[4]
Labeled Indications				
Peripheral Parenteral Nutrition	Yes	Yes	Yes	Yes
Central TPN	Yes	Yes	Yes	Yes
Protein Sparing	Yes	No	Yes	Yes

Protein Substrates

CRYSTALLINE AMINO ACID INFUSIONS

	Aminosyn II 8.5% (Abbott)	**Travasol 8.5 without electrolytes** (Clintec)	**FreAmine III 8.5%** (McGaw)
Amino Acid Concentration	8.5%	8.5%	8.5%
Nitrogen (g/100 ml)	1.3	1.43	
Amino Acids (Essential) (mg/100 ml)			
Isoleucine	561	406	590
Leucine	850	526	770
Lysine	893	492	620
Methionine	146	492	450
Phenylalanine	253	526	480
Threonine	340	356	340
Tryptophan	170	152	130
Valine	425	390	560
Amino Acids (Nonessential) (mg/100 ml)			
Alanine	844	1760	600
Arginine	865	880	810
Histidine[1]	255	372	240
Proline	614	356	950
Serine	450		500
Taurine			
Tyrosine	230	34	
Aminoacetic Acid (Glycine)	425	1760	1190
Glutamic Acid	627		
Aspartic Acid	595		
Cysteine			< 20
Electrolytes (mEq/L)			
Sodium	33.3		10
Potassium			
Chloride		34	< 3
Acetate	61.1	73	72
Phosphate (mM/L)			10
Osmolarity (mOsm/L)	742	890	810
Supplied in (ml)	500[3] 1000[3]	500[8] 1000[8] 2000[8]	500[9] 1000[9]
Labeled Indications			
Peripheral Parenteral Nutrition	Yes	Yes	Yes
Central TPN	Yes	Yes	Yes
Protein Sparing	Yes	Yes	Yes

Protein Substrates

CRYSTALLINE AMINO ACID INFUSIONS

	TrophAmine 10% (McGaw)	Aminosyn 10% (Abbott)	Aminosyn-PF 10% (Abbott)	Aminosyn II 10% (Abbott)	Aminosyn (pH6) 10% (Abbott)
Amino Acid Concentration	10%	10%	10%	10%	10%
Nitrogen (g/100 ml)	1.55	1.57	1.52	1.53	1.57
Amino Acids (Essential) (mg/100 ml)					
Isoleucine	820	720	760	660	720
Leucine	1400	940	1200	1000	940
Lysine	820	720	677	1050	720
Methionine	340	400	180	172	400
Phenylalanine	480	440	427	298	440
Threonine	420	520	512	400	520
Tryptophan	200	160	180	200	160
Valine	780	800	673	500	800
Amino Acids (Nonessential) (mg/100 ml)					
Alanine	540	1280	698	993	1280
Arginine	1200	980	1227	1018	980
Histidine[1]	480	300	312	300	300
Proline	680	860	812	722	860
Serine	380	420	495	530	420
Taurine	25		70		
Tyrosine	240	44	40	270	44
Aminoacetic Acid (Glycine)	360	1280	385	500	1280
Glutamic Acid	500		620	738	
Aspartic Acid	320		527	700	
Cysteine	< 16				
Electrolytes (mEq/L)					
Sodium	5		3.4	45.3	
Potassium		5.4			2.7
Chloride	< 3				
Acetate	97	148	46.3	71.8	111
Phosphate (mM/L)10					
Osmolarity (mOsm/L)	875	1000	829	873	993
Supplied in (ml)	500[6]	500[4] 1000[4]	1000[10]	500[3] 1000[3]	500[11] 1000[11]
Labeled Indications					
Peripheral Parenteral Nutrition	Yes	Yes	Yes	Yes	Yes
Central TPN	Yes	Yes	Yes	Yes	Yes
Protein Sparing	No	Yes	No	Yes	Yes

Protein Substrates

CRYSTALLINE AMINO ACID INFUSIONS

	Travasol 10% (Clintec)	FreAmine III 10% (McGaw)	Novamine (Clintec)	Novamine 15% (Clintec)	Aminosyn II 15% (Abbott)
Amino Acid Concentration	10%	10%	11.4%	15%	15%
Nitrogen (g/100 ml)	1.65	1.53	1.8	2.37	2.3
Amino Acids (Essential) (mg/100 ml)					
Isoleucine	600	690	570	749	990
Leucine	730	910	790	1040	1500
Lysine	580	730	900	1180	1575
Methionine	400	530	570	749	258
Phenylalanine	560	560	790	1040	447
Threonine	420	400	570	749	600
Tryptophan	180	150	190	250	300
Valine	580	660	730	960	750
Amino Acids (Nonessential) (mg/100 ml)					
Alanine	2070	710	1650	2170	1490
Arginine	1150	950	1120	1470	1527
Histidine[1]	480	280	680	894	450
Proline	680	1120	680	894	1083
Serine	500	590	450	592	795
Taurine					
Tyrosine	40		30	39	405
Aminoacetic Acid (Glycine)	1030	1400	790	1040	750
Glutamic Acid			570	749	1107
Aspartic Acid			330	434	1050
Cysteine		< 24			
Electrolytes (mEq/L)					
Sodium		10			62.7
Potassium					
Chloride	40	< 3			
Acetate	87	≈89	114	151	107.6
Phosphate (mM/L)		10			
Osmolarity (mOsm/L)	1000	≈ 950	1057	1388	1300
Supplied in (ml)	250[12,13] 500[12,13] 1000[12,13] 2000[12]	500[9] 1000[9]	500[14] 1000[14]	500[14] 1000[14]	2000[15]
Labeled Indications					
Peripheral Parenteral Nutrition	Yes	Yes	Yes	Yes	Yes
Central TPN	Yes	Yes	Yes	Yes	Yes
Protein Sparing	Yes	Yes	Yes	No	No

[1] Histidine is considered an essential amino acid in infants and in renal failure.
[2] With 7 mEq/L sodium from the antioxidant sodium hydrosulfite.
[3] Includes 20 mg/dl sodium hydrosulfite.
[4] Includes 5.4 mEq/L potassium from the antioxidant potassium metabisulfite.
[5] With ≈ 3 mEq/L sodium bisulfite.
[6] With < 50 mg sodium metabisulfite per 100 ml.
[7] From the antioxidant sodium hydrosulfite.
[8] With 3 mEq/L sodium bisulfite.
[9] With < 0.1 g sodium bisulfite per 100 ml.
[10] With 230 mg sodium hydrosulfite per 100 ml.
[11] Potassium derived from the antioxidant potassium metabisulfite.
[12] Acetate in Viaflex container = 60 mEq/L; osmolarity is 970 mOsm/L.
[13] Sizes also come in Viaflex containers.
[14] With 30 mg sodium metabisulfite.
[15] With 60 mg sodium hydrosulfite per 100 ml.

Protein Substrates

CRYSTALLINE AMINO ACID INFUSIONS WITH ELECTROLYTES

	ProcalAmine (McGaw)	**FreAmine III 3% w/Electrolytes** (McGaw)	**Aminosyn 3.5% M** (Abbott)	**Aminosyn II 3.5% M** (Abbott)	**3.5% Travasol w/Electrolytes** (Clintec)	**5.5% Travasol w/Electrolytes** (Clintec)
Amino Acid Concentration	3%	3%	3.5%	3.5%	3.5%	5.5%
Nitrogen (g/100 ml)	0.46	0.46	0.55	0.54	0.591	0.925
Amino Acids (Essential) (mg/100 ml)						
Isoleucine	210	210	252	231	168	263
Leucine	270	270	329	350	217	340
Lysine	220	220	252	368	203	318
Methionine	160	160	140	60	203	318
Phenylalanine	170	170	154	104	217	340
Threonine	120	120	182	140	147	230
Tryptophan	46	46	56	70	63	99
Valine	200	200	280	175	161	252
Amino Acids (Nonessential) (mg/100 ml)						
Alanine	210	210	448	348	728	1140
Arginine	290	290	343	356	364	570
Histidine[1]	85	85	105	105	154	241
Proline	340	340	300	253	147	230
Serine	180	180	147	186		
Tyrosine			31	95	14	22
Glycine	420	420	448	175	728	1140
Glutamic Acid				258		
Aspartic Acid				245		
Cysteine	< 20	< 20				
Electrolytes (mEq/L)						
Sodium	35	35	47	36	25	70
Potassium	24	24.5	13	13	15	60
Magnesium	5	5	3	3	5	10
Chloride	41	41	40	37	25	70
Acetate	47	44	58	25	52	102
Phosphate (mM/L)	3.5	3.5	3.5	3.5	7.5	30
Osmolarity (mOsm/L)	735	≈ 405	477	425	450	850
Nonprotein Calories (g/100 ml) (glycerin)	3					
Supplied in (ml)	1000[2]	1000[3]	1000[4]	1000[5]	500[6] 1000[6]	500[6] 1000[6] 2000[6]
Labeled Indications						
Peripheral Parenteral Nutrition	Yes	Yes	Yes	Yes	Yes	Yes
Central TPN	No	No	No	No	No	Yes
Protein Sparing	Yes	Yes	Yes	Yes	Yes	Yes

Protein Substrates

CRYSTALLINE AMINO ACID INFUSIONS WITH ELECTROLYTES

	Aminosyn 7% w/Electrolytes (Abbott)	Aminosyn II 7% with Electrolytes (Abbott)	Aminosyn 8.5% w/Electrolytes (Abbott)	Aminosyn II 8.5% with Electrolytes (Abbott)	FreAmine III 8.5% w/Electrolytes (McGaw)	Travasol 8.5% w/Electrolytes (Clintec)	Aminosyn II 10% with Electrolytes (Abbott)
Amino Acid Concentration	7%	7%	8.5%	8.5%	8.5%	8.5%	10%
Nitrogen g/100 ml	1.1	1.07	1.34	1.3	1.3	1.43	1.53
Amino Acids (Essential) (mg/100 ml)							
Isoleucine	510	462	620	561	590	406	660
Leucine	660	700	810	850	770	526	1000
Lysine	510	735	624	893	620	492	1050
Methionine	280	120	340	146	450	492	172
Phenylalanine	310	209	380	253	480	526	298
Threonine	370	280	460	340	340	356	400
Tryptophan	120	140	150	170	130	152	200
Valine	560	350	680	425	560	390	500
Amino Acids (Nonessential) (mg/100 ml)							
Alanine	900	695	1100	844	600	1760	993
Arginine	690	713	850	865	810	880	1018
Histidine[1]	210	210	260	255	240	372	300
Proline	610	505	750	614	950	356	722
Serine	300	371	370	450	500		530
Tyrosine	44	189	44	230		34	270
Glycine	900	350	1100	425	1190	1760	500
Glutamic Acid		517		627			738
Aspartic Acid		490		595			700
Cysteine					< 20		
Electrolytes (mEq/L)							
Sodium	70	76	70	80	60	70	87
Potassium	66	66	66	66	60	60	66
Magnesium	10	10	10	10	10	10	10
Chloride	96	86	98	86	60	70	86
Acetate	124	50	142	61	125	141	72
Phosphate (mM/L)	30	30	30	30	20	30	30
Osmolarity (mOsm/L)	1013	869	1160	999	1045	1160	1130
Supplied in (ml)	500[7]	500[8]	500[7]	500[8]	500[9] 1000[9]	500[6] 1000[6] 2000[6]	1000[8]
Labeled Indications							
Peripheral Parenteral Nutrition	Yes	Yes	Yes	Yes	Yes	Yes	Yes
Central TPN	Yes	Yes	Yes	Yes	Yes	Yes	Yes
Protein Sparing	Yes	Yes	Yes	Yes	Yes	Yes	Yes

[1] Histidine is considered an essential amino acid in infants and in renal failure.
[2] With < 50 mg K+ metabisulfite and 3 mEq Ca/L.
[3] With < 0.05 g of the antioxidant potassium metabisulfite.
[4] Includes 7 mEq/L sodium from the antioxidant sodium hydrosulfite.
[5] With 20 mg sodium hydrosulfite per 100 ml.
[6] With 3 mEq/L sodium bisulfite.
[7] Includes 5.4 mEq/L potassium from the antioxidant potassium metabisulfite.
[8] Includes sodium from the antioxidant sodium hydrosulfite.
[9] With < 0.1 g sodium bisulfite per 100 ml.

Protein Substrates

CRYSTALLINE AMINO ACID INFUSIONS WITH DEXTROSE

	Travasol 2.75% in 5% Dextrose[1] (Clintec)	Travasol 2.75% in 10% Dextrose[1] (Clintec)	Travasol 2.75% in 25%Dextrose[1] (Clintec)	Aminosyn II 3.5% in 5% Dextrose[1] (Abbott)	Aminosyn II 3.5% in 25% Dextrose[1] (Abbott)
Amino Acid Concentration	2.75%	2.75%	2.75%	3.5%	3.5%
Dextrose Concentration	5%	10%	25%	5%	25%
Nitrogen (g/100 ml)	0.46	0.46	0.46	0.54	0.54
Amino Acids (Essential) (mg/100 ml)					
Isoleucine	132	132	132	231	231
Leucine	170	170	170	350	350
Lysine	159	159	159	368	368
Methionine	159	159	159	60	60
Phenylalanine	170	170	170	104	104
Threonine	115	115	115	140	140
Tryptophan	50	50	50	70	70
Valine	126	126	126	175	175
Amino Acids (Nonessential) (mg/100 ml)					
Alanine	570	570	570	348	348
Arginine	285	285	285	356	356
Histidine[2]	120	120	120	105	105
Proline	115	115	115	252	252
Serine				186	186
Tyrosine	11	11	11	94	94
Aminoacetic Acid (Glycine)	570	570	570	175	175
Glutamic Acid				258	258
Aspartic Acid				245	245
Cysteine					
Electrolytes (mEq/L)					
Sodium				18	18
Potassium					
Magnesium					
Chloride	11	11	11		
Acetate	16	16	16	25.2	25.2
Phosphate (mM/L)					
Osmolarity (mOsm/L)	530	785	1540	585	1515
Supplied in (ml)	500 ml with 500 ml dextrose	500 ml with 500 ml dextrose	500 ml with 500 ml dextrose	1000 ml with 1000 ml dextrose[3]	500 ml with 500 ml dextrose[3]
Labeled Indications					
Peripheral Parenteral Nutrition	Yes	Yes	Yes	Yes	No
Central TPN	Yes	Yes	Yes	No	Yes

Protein Substrates

CRYSTALLINE AMINO ACID INFUSIONS WITH DEXTROSE

	Travasol 4.25% in 5% Dextrose[1] (Clintec)	Aminosyn II 4.25% in 10% Dextrose[1] (Abbott)	Travasol 4.25% in 10% Dextrose[1] (Clintec)	Aminosyn II 4.25% in 20% Dextrose[1] (Abbott)
Amino Acid Concentration	4.25%	4.25%	4.25%	4.25%
Dextrose Concentration	5%	10%	10%	20%
Nitrogen (g/100 ml)	0.7	0.65	0.7	0.65
Amino Acids (Essential) (mg/100 ml)				
Isoleucine	203	280	203	280
Leucine	263	425	263	425
Lysine	246	446	246	446
Methionine	246	73	246	73
Phenylalanine	263	126	263	126
Threonine	178	170	178	170
Tryptophan	76	85	76	85
Valine	195	212	195	212
Amino Acids (Nonessential) (mg/100 ml)				
Alanine	880	422	880	422
Arginine	440	432	440	432
Histidine[2]	186	128	186	128
Proline	178	307	178	307
Serine		225		225
Tyrosine	17	115	17	115
Aminoacetic Acid (Glycine)	880	212	880	212
Glutamic Acid		314		314
Aspartic Acid		298		298
Cysteine				
Electrolytes (mEq/L)				
Sodium		19		19
Potassium				
Magnesium				
Chloride	17		17	
Acetate	22	30.6	22	30.6
Phosphate (mM/L)				
Osmolarity (mOsm/L)	680	894	935	1295
Supplied in (ml)	500 ml with 500 ml dextrose	1000 ml w/1000 ml dextrose[3]	500 ml with 500 ml dextrose	1000 ml with 1000 ml dextrose[3]
Labeled Indications				
Peripheral Parenteral Nutrition	Yes	Yes	Yes	No
Central TPN	Yes	No	Yes	Yes

Protein Substrates

CRYSTALLINE AMINO ACID INFUSIONS WITH DEXTROSE

	Aminosyn II 4.25% in 25% Dextrose[1] (Abbott)	Travasol 4.25% in 25% Dextrose[1] (Clintec)	Aminosyn II 5% in 25% Dextrose[1] (Abbott)
Amino Acid Concentration	4.25%	4.25%	5%
Dextrose Concentration	25%	25%	25%
Nitrogen (g/100 ml)	0.65	0.65	0.77
Amino Acids (Essential) (mg/100 ml)			
Isoleucine	280	203	330
Leucine	425	263	500
Lysine	446	246	525
Methionine	73	246	86
Phenylalanine	126	263	149
Threonine	170	178	200
Tryptophan	85	76	100
Valine	212	195	250
Amino Acids (Nonessential) (mg/100 ml)			
Alanine	422	880	496
Arginine	432	440	509
Histidine[2]	128	186	150
Proline	307	178	361
Serine	225		265
Tyrosine	115	17	135
Aminoacetic Acid (Glycine)	212	880	250
Glutamic Acid	314		369
Aspartic Acid	298		350
Cysteine			
Electrolytes (mEq/L)			
Sodium	19		22.2
Potassium			
Magnesium			
Chloride		17	
Acetate	30.6	22	35.9
Phosphate (mM/L)			
Osmolarity (mOsm/L)	1536	1690	1539
Supplied in (ml)	750 and 1000 ml and 750 and 1000 ml dextrose[3]	500 ml with 500 ml dextrose[3]	500, 750 and 1000 ml and 500, 750 and 1000 ml dextrose[3]
Labeled Indications			
Peripheral Parenteral Nutrition	No	Yes	No
Central TPN	Yes	Yes	Yes

[1] Solution composition represents admixture of dual-chamber *Quick Mix* or *Nutrimix* container.
[2] Histidine is considered an essential amino acid in infants and in renal failure.
[3] With 30 mg sodium hydrosulfite per 100 ml.

Protein Substrates

CRYSTALLINE AMINO ACID INFUSIONS WITH ELECTROLYTES IN DEXTROSE

	Aminosyn II 3.5% M[1] **in 5% Dextrose**[2] (Abbott)	**Aminosyn II 4.25% M**[1] **in 10% Dextrose**[2] (Abbott)
Amino Acid Concentration	3.5%	4.25%
Dextrose Concentration	5%	10%
Nitrogen (g/100 ml)	0.535	0.65
Amino Acids (Essential) (mg/100 ml)		
Isoleucine	231	280
Leucine	350	425
Lysine	368	446
Methionine	60	73
Phenylalanine	104	126
Threonine	140	170
Tryptophan	70	85
Valine	175	212
Amino Acids (Nonessential) (mg/100 ml)		
Alanine	348	422
Arginine	356	432
Histidine[3]	105	128
Proline	252	307
Serine	186	225
Tyrosine	94	115
Aminoacetic Acid (Glycine)	175	212
Glutamic Acid	258	314
Aspartic Acid	245	298
Cysteine		
Electrolytes (mEq/L)		
Sodium	41	43.7
Potassium	13	13
Magnesium	3	3
Chloride	36.5	36.5
Acetate	25.1	30.5
Phosphorus (mM/L)	3.5	3.5
Osmolarity (mOsm/L)	616	919
Supplied in (ml)	500 and 1000 ml and 500 and 1000 ml dextrose[4]	500 ml and 500 ml dextrose[4]
Labeled Indications		
Peripheral Parenteral Nutrition	Yes	Yes
Central TPN	No	Yes
Protein Sparing	No	No

[1] With maintenance electrolytes.
[2] Solution composition represents admixture of *Nutrimix* dual-chamber container.
[3] Histidine is considered an essential amino acid in infants and in renal failure.
[4] With 30 mg sodium hydrosulfite per 100 ml.

AMINO ACID FORMULATIONS FOR RENAL FAILURE

For a complete discussion of the use of protein substrates for intravenous nutritional therapy, refer to the general monograph.

Actions:

Pharmacology: Patients with renal decompensation have different amino acid requirements than those with normal renal function. Use in uremic patients is based on the minimal requirements for each of the 8 essential amino acids. These products contain histidine, an amino acid considered essential for infant growth and for uremic patients.

In renal failure, nonspecific nitrogen-containing compounds are broken down in the intestine. The ammonia formed is absorbed and incorporated by the liver into nonessential amino acids, provided essential amino acid requirements are being met. Exogenously supplying only essential amino acids allows urea nitrogen to be recycled which can serve as a precursor for nonessential amino acid synthesis. Therefore, administration to uremic patients, particularly those who are protein deficient, results in the utilization of retained urea, and may be followed by a drop in BUN and resolution of many azotemic symptoms.

Infusion of essential amino acids and hypertonic dextrose promotes protein synthesis, improves cellular metabolic balance, decreases the rate of rise of BUN and minimizes deterioration of serum potassium, magnesium and phosphorus balance in patients with impaired renal function. This therapy may decrease morbidity associated with acute renal failure and promote earlier return of renal function. Although controversial, these formulations may have no clinically significant advantage over the general formulations containing both essential and nonessential amino acids in most uremic patients.

Indications:

For nutritional support of uremic patients, particularly when oral nutrition is impractical, not feasible or insufficient.

Essential amino acid injection does not replace dialysis and conventional supportive therapy in patients with renal failure. To promote urea reutilization, provide adequate calories with minimal amounts of essential amino acids and restrict the intake of nonessential nitrogen.

Children: Use with caution in pediatric patients, especially low birth weight infants, due to limited clinical experience. Laboratory and clinical monitoring must be extensive and frequent. Use a low initial dose and increase slowly.

The absence of arginine in *NephrAmine* and *Aminess* may accentuate the risk of hyperammonemia in infants. *Aminosyn-RF* and *RenAmin* contain arginine.

Administration and Dosage:

Provide adequate calories simultaneously. Administer essential amino acid/dextrose mixtures by continuous infusion through a central venous catheter. Use slow initial infusion rates, generally 20 to 30 ml/hour for the first 6 to 8 hours. Increase by 10 ml/hour each 24 hours, up to a maximum of 60 to 100 ml/hour.

Administration rate is governed by the patient's nitrogen, fluid and glucose tolerance. Uremic patients are frequently glucose intolerant, especially in association with peritoneal dialysis, and may require exogenous insulin to prevent hyperglycemia. To prevent rebound hypoglycemia when hypertonic dextrose infusions are abruptly discontinued, administer a 5% dextrose solution.

Adults:

Aminosyn-RF – 300 to 600 ml. Mix 300 ml with 500 ml of 70% dextrose to provide a solution of 1.96% essential amino acids in 44% dextrose (calorie:nitrogen ratio = 504:1).

Aminess – 400 ml. Mix 400 ml with 500 ml of 70% dextrose to yield a solution of 2.3% essential amino acids in 39% dextrose (calorie:nitrogen ratio = 450:1).

NephrAmine – 250 to 500 ml. Mix 250 ml w/500 ml of 70% dextrose to yield solution of 1.8% essential amino acids in 47% dextrose (calorie:nitrogen ratio = 744:1).

RenAmin – 250 to 500 ml.

Children: Individualize dosage. A dosage of 0.5 to 1 g/kg/day will meet the requirements of the majority of pediatric patients. Use a low initial daily dosageand increase slowly; > 1 g/kg/day is not recommended.

Protein Substrates

AMINO ACID FORMULATIONS FOR RENAL FAILURE

	Aminosyn-RF 5.2% (Abbott)	Aminess 5.2% (Clintec)	5.4% NephrAmine (McGaw)	RenAmin (Clintec)
Amino Acid Concentration	5.2%	5.2%	5.4%	6.5%
Nitrogen (g/100 ml)	0.79	0.66	0.65	1
Amino Acids (Essential) (mg/100 ml)				
Isoleucine	462	525	560	500
Leucine	726	825	880	600
Lysine	535	600	640	450
Methionine	726	825	880	500
Phenylalanine	726	825	880	490
Threonine	330	375	400	380
Tryptophan	165	188	200	160
Valine	528	600	640	820
Histidine	429	412	250	420
Amino Acids (Nonessential) (mg/100 ml)				
Cysteine			< 20	
Arginine	600			630
Alanine				560
Proline				350
Glycine				300
Serine				300
Tyrosine				40
Electrolytes (mEq/L)				
Sodium			5	
Acetate	≈ 105	50	≈ 44	60
Potassium	5.4			
Chloride			< 3	31
Osmolarity (mOsm/L)	475	416	435	600
Supplied in (ml)	300[1]	400[2]	250[3]	250[4] 500[4]

[1] With 60 mg potassium metabisulfite per 100 ml.
[2] In 500 ml bottle.
[3] With < 0.05 g sodium bisulfite per 100 ml.
[4] With ≈ 3 mEq sodium bisulfite.

Protein Substrates

AMINO ACID FORMULATIONS FOR HIGH METABOLIC STRESS

For a complete discussion of the use of protein substrates as a compound of intravenous nutritional therapy, refer to the IV Nutritionals monograph.

Actions:

Pharmacology: These are mixtures of essential and nonessential amino acids with high concentrations of branched chain amino acids (BCAA): isoleucine, leucine, valine.

Acute metabolic stress is characterized by increased urinary nitrogen excretion and hyperglycemia; glucose utilization and fat store mobilization are impaired. The primary substrates used to meet energy requirements of muscle are BCAAs.

Indications:

To prevent nitrogen loss or treat negative nitrogen balance in adults if: (1) The alimentary tract, by oral, gastrostomy or jejunostomy route, cannot or should not be used, or adequate protein intake is not feasible by these routes; (2) GI protein absorption is impaired; or (3) nitrogen homeostasis is substantially impaired as with severe trauma or sepsis.

Administration and Dosage:

Daily amino acid doses of ≈ 1.5 g/kg for adults with adequate calories generally satisfy protein needs and promote positive nitrogen balance. May need higher doses in severely catabolic states. Fat emulsion may help meet energy requirements.

For severely catabolic, depleted patients or those requiring long-term TPN, consider central venous nutrition. Start with infusates containing lower dextrose concentrations; gradually increase dextrose to estimated caloric needs as glucose tolerance increases. *FreAmine HBC* 750 ml and 250 ml 70% dextrose or 500 ml *Aminosyn-HBC* 7% and 500 ml concentrated dextrose, with added electrolytes, trace metals and vitamins, may be given over 8 hours. *BranchAmin* 4% must be admixed with a complete amino acid injection, with or without a concentrated caloric source.

For moderately catabolic, depleted patients in whom central venous route is not indicated, may infuse diluted *FreAmine HBC* or *Aminosyn-HBC* 7% with minimal caloric supplementation by peripheral vein; supplement, if desired, with fat emulsion.

Usual administration of 4% BCAA Injection is used as a supplement to parenteral nutrition solutions to achieve an amino acid solution that is ≈ 50% w/w BCAA. One method for achieving this ratio is the admixture of two volumes of 4% BCAA Injection at 4 g/dl concentration with one volume of an amino acid solution of 8 to 10 g/dl concentration. The supplemental amino acid mixture is given with energy substrates to provide at least 35 kcal/kg ideal body weight as nonprotein calories.

AMINO ACID FORMULATION IN HEPATIC FAILURE/HEPATIC ENCEPHALOPATHY

Actions:

Pharmacology: This formulation is a mixture of essential and nonessential amino acids with high concentrations of the BCAAs, isoleucine, leucine and valine.

Hepatic failure/Hepatic encephalopathy – Etiopathology of hepatic encephalopathy is unknown and multifactorial. Rationale for BCAA therapy is based on studies in which BCAA infusions reversed abnormal plasma amino acid pattern characterized by lower BCAA levels and elevated aromatic amino acids and methionine. Normalization of these amino acids improved mental status and EEG patterns. Nitrogen balance was significantly improved and mortality reduced in these typically protein-intolerant patients who received substantial amounts of protein equivalents.

Indications:

For the treatment of hepatic encephalopathy in patients with cirrhosis or hepatitis. Provides nutritional support for patients with these diseases of the liver who require parenteral nutrition and are intolerant of general purpose amino acid injections, which are contraindicated in patients with hepatic coma.

Administration and Dosage:

Give 80 to 120 g amino acids (12 to 18 g nitrogen)/day. Typically, 500 ml *HepatAmine* with ≈ 500 ml 50% dextrose and electrolytes and vitamins is given over 8 to 12 hours. This results in total daily fluid intake of ≈ 2 to 3 L. Patients with fluid restrictions may only tolerate 1 to 2 L. Although nitrogen requirements may be higher in severely hypercatabolic or depleted patients, provision of additional nitrogen may not be possible due to fluid intake limits, nitrogen or glucose intolerance.

Use slow initial infusion rates; gradually increase to 60 to 125 ml/hr.

Peripheral vein administration is indicated with or without parenteral carbohydrate calories for patients in whom the central venous route is not indicated and who can consume adequate calories enterally. Prepare infusates by dilution of *HepatAmine* with Sterile Water for Injection or 5% to 10% Dextrose to prepare isotonic or slightly hypertonic solutions; accompany with adequate caloric supplementation.

Protein Substrates

AMINO ACID FORMULATION FOR HIGH METABOLIC STRESS AND IN HEPATIC FAILURE/ HEPATIC ENCEPHALOPATHY

	STRESS FORMULATION			HEPATIC FORMULATION
	4% BranchAmin (Clintec)	**FreAmine HBC 6.9%** (McGaw)	**Aminosyn-HBC 7%** (Abbott)	**HepatAmine** (McGaw)
Amino Acid Concentration	4%	6.9%	7%	8%
Nitrogen (g/100 ml)	0.443	0.97	1.12	1.2
Amino Acids (Essential) (mg/100 ml)				
Isoleucine	1380	760	789	900
Leucine	1380	1370	1576	1100
Lysine		410	265	610
Methionine		250	206	100
Phenylalanine		320	228	100
Threonine		200	272	450
Tryptophan		90	88	66
Valine	1240	880	789	840
Amino Acids (Nonessential) (mg/100 ml)				
Alanine		400	660	770
Arginine		580	507	600
Histidine[1]		160	154	240
Proline		630	448	800
Serine		330	221	500
Tyrosine			33	
Glycine		330	660	900
Cysteine		< 20		< 20
Electrolytes (mEq/L)				
Sodium		10	7[4]	10
Chloride		< 3		< 3
Acetate		≈ 57	72	≈ 62
Phosphate (mM/L)				10
Osmolarity (mOsm/L)	316	620	665	785
Supplied in (ml)	500	750[2,3]	500[4] 1000[4]	500[2]
Labeled Indications				
Peripheral Parenteral Nutrition	Yes[5]	Yes	Yes	Yes
Central TPN	Yes[5]	Yes	Yes	Yes

[1] Histidine is considered an essential amino acid in infants and in renal failure.
[2] With < 100 mg sodium bisulfite/100 ml.
[3] In 1000 ml bottles.
[4] With 60 mg sodium hydrosulfite.
[5] Must be admixed with a complete amino acid injection.

Protein Substrates

CYSTEINE HCl

For a complete discussion of the use of protein substrates as a component of intravenous nutritional therapy, refer to the IV Nutritionals monograph.

Actions:

Pharmacology: Cysteine is a sulfur-containing amino acid. It is synthesized from methionine via the trans-sulfuration pathway in the adult, but newborn infants lack the enzyme necessary to effect this conversion. Therefore, cysteine is generally considered an essential amino acid in infants.

Metabolism of cysteine produces pyruvate and inorganic sulfate as end products. Cysteine is introduced directly into the pathway of carbohydrate metabolism at the pyruvate stage with all three carbons convertible to glucose. The sulfur is primarily transformed to inorganic sulfate, which is introduced into complex polysaccharides among other structural components.

In premixed solutions of crystalline amino acids, cysteine is relatively unstable over time, eventually converting to insoluble cystine. To avoid such precipitation, cysteine is provided as an additive for use with crystalline amino acid solutions immediately prior to administration.

Indications:

Use only after dilution as an additive to Aminosyn to meet the IV amino acid nutritional requirements of infants receiving total parenteral nutrition.

Administration and Dosage:

Use only after dilution in *Aminosyn.* Combine each 0.5 g of cysteine with 12.5 g of amino acids, such as that present in 250 ml of *Aminosyn* 5%, then dilute with 250 ml of 50% Dextrose or lesser volume as indicated. Equal volumes of *Aminosyn* 5% and 50% Dextrose produce a final solution containing *Aminosyn* 2.5% and 25% Dextrose, which is suitable for administration by central venous infusion.

Storage: Avoid excessive heat. Do not freeze. Begin administration of the final admixture within 1 hour of mixing; otherwise, immediately refrigerate the mixture and use within 24 hours.

Rx	**Cysteine HCl** (Various, eg, Abbott, Gensia)	**Injection:** 50 mg per ml	In 10 ml additive syringe and single dose vials.

Carbohydrates

DEXTROSE (d-GLUCOSE)

Actions:

Pharmacology: A source of calories and fluids in patients unable to obtain adequate oral intake. Parenterally injected dextrose undergoes oxidation to carbon dioxide and water, and provides 3.4 calories per gram of d–glucose monohydrate (molecular weight 198.17). A 5% solution is isotonic and is administered by IV infusion into peripheral veins. Concentrated dextrose infusions are used to provide increased caloric intake with less fluid volume; they may be irritating if given by peripheral infusions. Therefore, administer highly concentrated solutions only by central venous catheters.

Dextrose injections may induce diuresis. Dextrose is readily metabolized, may decrease body protein and nitrogen losses, promotes glycogen deposition, and decreases or prevents ketosis if sufficient doses are provided.

Caloric Content and Osmolarity of the Various Concentrations of Dextrose

Dextrose concentration		Caloric content	Osmolarity
%	g/L	(Cal/L)	(mOsm/L)
2.5	25	85	126
5	50	170	253
10	100	340	505
20	200	680	1010
25	250	850	1330
30	300	1020	1515
40	400	1360	2020
50	500	1700	2525
60	600	2040	3030
70	700	2380	3535

Indications:

2.5%, 5% and 10%: Used for peripheral infusion to provide calories whenever fluid and caloric replacement are required.

25% (hypertonic): Acute symptomatic episodes of hypoglycemia in the neonate or older infant to restore depressed blood glucose levels and control symptoms.

50%: Used in the treatment of insulin hypoglycemia (hyperinsulinemia or insulin shock) to restore blood glucose levels.

10%, 20%, 30%, 40%, 50%, 60% and 70% (hypertonic): For infusion after admixture with other solutions such as amino acids.

Unlabeled uses: Hypertonic solutions of 25% to 50% have been used as a sclerosing agent for the treatment of varicose veins, as an irritant to produce adhesive pleuritis and to reduce cerebrospinal pressure and cerebral edema caused by delirium tremens or acute alcohol intoxication.

Contraindications:

In diabetic coma while blood sugar is excessively high.

Concentrated solutions: When intracranial or intraspinal hemorrhage is present; in the presence of delirium tremens in dehydrated patients; in patients with severe hydration, anuria, hepatic coma or glucose-galactose malabsorption syndrome.

Warnings:

Fluid/Solute overload: Dextrose solutions IV can cause fluid or solute overload resulting in dilution of serum electrolyte concentrations, overhydration, congested states or pulmonary edema.

Hypertonic dextrose solutions may cause thrombosis if infused via peripheral veins; therefore, administer via a central venous catheter.

Diabetes mellitus: Use dextrose-containing solutions with caution in patients with subclinical or overt diabetes mellitus or carbohydrate intolerance.

Rapid administration of hypertonic solutions may produce significant hyperglycemia or hyperosmolar syndrome, especially in patients with chronic uremia or carbohydrate intolerance.

Pregnancy: Category C. It is not known whether dextrose can cause fetal harm when administered to a pregnant woman or can affect reproduction capacity. Use only when clearly needed. Dextrose crosses the placenta; however, insulin does not cross the placenta and the fetus is responsible for its own insulin production in response to the dextrose. Therefore, administer dextrose to a pregnant woman with caution. One report recommends an infusion rate of 3.5 to 7 g/hour since doses > 10 g/hr cause increases in fetal insulin.

Carbohydrates

DEXTROSE (d-GLUCOSE)

Lactation: Exercise caution when administering dextrose to a nursing woman.

Children: Use with caution in infants of diabetic mothers, except as may be indicated in hypoglycemic neonates.

Precautions:

Monitoring: Perform clinical evaluations and laboratory determinations to monitor fluid balance, electrolyte concentrations and acid-base balance.

Hyperglycemia and glycosuria may be functions of rate of administration or metabolic insufficiency. To minimize these conditions, slow the infusion rate, monitor blood and urine glucose; if necessary, administer insulin. When concentrated dextrose infusion is abruptly withdrawn, administer 5% or 10% dextrose to avoid rebound hypoglycemia.

Extravasation: Administer so that extravasation does not occur. If thrombosis occurs during administration, stop injection and correct.

Hypokalemia: Excessive administration of potassium free solutions may result in significant hypokalemia. Add potassium to dextrose solutions and administer to fasting patients with good renal function, especially those on digitalis therapy.

Vitamin B complex deficiency may occur with dextrose administration.

Drug Interactions:

Corticosteroids: Cautiously administer parenteral fluids, especially those containing sodium ions, to patients receiving corticosteroids or corticotropin.

Adverse Reactions:

Febrile response; infection at the injection site; tissue necrosis; venous thrombosis or phlebitis extending from the site of injection; extravasation; hypovolemia; hypervolemia; dehydration; mental confusion or unconsciousness. These may occur because of the solution or administration technique. Use the largest available peripheral vein and a well placed small bore needle.

Hypertonic solutions are more likely to cause irritation; administer into larger central veins. Significant hyperglycemia, hyperosmolar syndrome and glycosuria may occur with too rapid administration of hypertonic solutions.

Overdosage:

In the event of a fluid or solute overload during parenteral therapy, reevaluate the patient's condition and institute appropriate corrective treatment.

Administration and Dosage:

Do not administer concentrated solutions SC or IM.

The concentration and dose depend on the patient's age, weight and clinical condition. Add electrolytes based on fluid and electrolyte status.

The maximum rate at which dextrose can be infused without producing glycosuria is 0.5 g/kg/hour. About 95% is retained when infused at 0.8 g/kg/hour.

Insulin-induced hypoglycemia: Determine blood glucose before injecting dextrose. In emergencies, promptly administer without waiting for pretreatment test results.

Adults – 10 to 25g. Repeated doses may be required in severe cases.

Neonates – 250 to 500 mg/kg/dose (5 to 10 ml of 25% dextrose in a 5 kg infant) to control acute symptomatic hypoglycemia.

Severe cases or older infants – Larger or repeated single doses up to 10 or 12 ml of 25% dextrose may be required. Subsequent continuous IV infusion of 10% dextrose may be needed to stabilize blood glucose levels.

Admixture incompatibilities: Additives may be incompatible. When introducing additives, use aseptic technique, mix thoroughly and do not store.

Do not administer dextrose simultaneously with blood through the same infusion set because pseudoagglutination of red cells may occur.

Storage/Stability: Do not use unless solution is clear. Discard unused portion. Protect from freezing and extreme heat.

Carbohydrates

DEXTROSE (d-GLUCOSE)			
Rx	**D-2.5-W** (Various, eg, Abbott, Clintec)	2.5%	In 1000 ml.
Rx	**D-5-W** (Various, eg, Abbott, Clintec, IMS, McGaw)	5%	In 25, 50, 100, 150, 250, 500 and 1000 ml vials and 10 ml syringes, 25 ml fill in 150 ml, 50 ml fill in 250 ml and 100 ml fill in 250 ml vials.
Rx	**D-10-W** (Various, eg, Abbott, Clintec, Elkins-Sinn, McGaw, Solopak, Winthrop)	10%	In 3 ml amps, 250, 500 and 1000 ml vials, 17 ml fill in 20 ml, 500 ml fill in 1000 ml, and 1000 ml fill in 2000 ml vials.
Rx	**D-20-W** (Various, eg, Abbott, Clintec, McGaw)	20%	In 500 ml vials, 500 ml fill in 1000 ml and 1000 ml fill in 2000 ml.
Rx	**D-25-W** (Various, eg, Abbott, IMS)	25%	In 10 ml syringes.
Rx	**D-30-W** (Various, eg, Abbott, Clintec, McGaw)	30%	In 500 and 1000 ml, 500 ml fill in 1000 ml and 1000 ml fill in 2000 ml.
Rx	**D-40-W** (Various, eg, Abbott, Clintec, McGaw)	40%	In 500 and 1000 ml, 500 ml fill in 1000 ml and 1000 ml fill in 2000 ml.
Rx	**D-50-W** (Various, eg, Abbott, Astra, Clintec, IMS, McGaw, Lyphomed, Pasadena, Schein)	50%	In 500, 1000 and 2000 ml and 50 ml amps, vials and syringes and 500 ml fill in 1000 ml and 1000 ml fill in 2000 ml.
Rx	**D-60-W** (Various, eg, Abbott, Clintec, McGaw)	60%	In 500 and 1000 ml, 500 ml fill in 1000 ml and 1000 ml fill in 2000 ml.
Rx	**D-70-W** (Various, eg, Abbott, Clintec, McGaw)	70%	In 70, 1000 and 2000 ml, 500 ml fill in 1000 ml and 1000 ml fill in 2000 ml.

Carbohydrates

ALCOHOL (ETHANOL) IN DEXTROSE INFUSIONS

For specific information on dextrose, refer to the individual monograph.

Actions:

Pharmacology: Alcohol in dextrose solutions are an intravenous source of carbohydrate calories that restore blood glucose levels. Each ml of alcohol provides 5.6 calories; each gram of d–glucose monohydrate provides 3.4 calories. Dextrose may aid in minimizing liver glycogen depletion and exerts a protein-sparing action.

Pharmacokinetics: Ethyl alcohol is metabolized at a rate of ≈ 10 to 20 ml/hour. Sedative effects of alcohol occur if infusion rate exceeds metabolism rate. Dextrose (d-glucose) can be infused at a maximum of ≈ 0.5 to 0.85 g/kg/hour without producing significant glycosuria. Thus, the maximum rate that alcohol can be infused without producing sedative effects is well below maximum rate of dextrose utilization. Alcohol is metabolized (mostly in liver) to acetaldehyde or acetate; oxidation rate is linear with time. Starvation lowers metabolism rate and insulin increases it.

Indications:

Increasing caloric intake and replenishing fluids.

Unlabeled uses:

Premature labor – Infusion of a 10% solution of ethyl alcohol IV causes a decrease in uterine activity during labor, presumably by inhibiting the release of oxytocin from the posterior pituitary, and has been used to prevent premature delivery. However, this use has largely been replaced by other therapies (eg, β-adrenergic therapy).

Contraindications:

Epilepsy; urinary tract infection; alcoholism; diabetic coma.

Warnings:

Special risk patients: Use alcohol cautiously in shock, following cranial surgery and in actual or anticipated postpartum hemorrhage.

Diabetic patients: Alcohol decreases blood sugar in these patients. In the untreated diabetic, the rate of alcohol metabolism is slowed.

Vitamin deficiencies: As a nutrient, alcohol supplies only calories; given alone it may cause or potentiate vitamin deficiencies and liver function disturbances.

IV administration can cause fluid or solute overload resulting in dilution of serum electrolyte concentrations, overhydration, congested states or pulmonary edema.

Extravasation: Avoid extravasation during IV administration; do not give SC.

Pseudoagglutination/Hemolysis: Do not administer simultaneously with blood because of possibility of pseudoagglutination or hemolysis.

Renal/Hepatic function impairment: Use alcohol cautiously.

Pregnancy: Category C. It is not known whether alcohol can cause fetal harm when administered to a pregnant woman or can affect reproduction capacity. Use only when clearly needed. It crosses the placenta rapidly and enters fetal circulation.

Fetal Alcohol Syndrome (FAS) a pattern of fetal anomalies, is associated with chronic maternal alcohol consumption of 60 to 75 ml absolute alcohol (4 to 5 drinks) per day; mild FAS is associated with ingestion of as little as 30 ml per day. Features of FAS involve craniofacial, limb, growth, and CNS anomalies. Other reported problems involve cardiac and urogenital defects, liver abnormalities and hemangiomas. Behavioral problems may be long-term. Moderate drinking (> 1 ounce absolute alcohol twice/week) is associated with second trimester spontaneous abortions.

Administration of alcohol prior to delivery may cause intoxication and depression of the newborn.

Lactation: Alcohol passes freely into breast milk approximately equivalent to maternal serum levels; however, effects on the infant are generally insignificant until maternal blood levels reach 300 mg/dl. The American Academy of Pediatrics considers alcohol use in the mother compatible with breastfeeding, although adverse effects may occur.

Alcohol may cause potentiation of severe hypoprothrombic bleeding, a pseudo-Cushing syndrome and a reduction in the milk-ejecting response.

Children: Safety and efficacy are not established. See Administration and Dosage.

Precautions:

Monitoring: Clinical evaluation and periodic laboratory determinations are necessary to monitor changes in electrolyte concentrations and fluid and acid-base balance.

Administer slowly and observe patient for restlessness or narcosis.

Gout: Alcohol increases serum uric acid and can precipitate acute gout.

Carbohydrates

ALCOHOL (ETHANOL) IN DEXTROSE INFUSIONS

Drug Interactions:

The following interactions may occur with alcohol administration. Those interactions that may only occur with long-term oral alcohol ingestion have not been included.

Alcohol Drug Interactions			
Precipitant drug	Object drug*		Description
Barbiturates Benzodiazepines Chloral hydrate Glutethimide Meprobamate Metoclopramide Phenothiazines	Alcohol	⬆	Increased CNS depressant effects may occur.
Cephalosporins[1] Chlorpropamide Disulfiram Furazolidone Metronidazole Procarbazine	Alcohol	⬆	A disulfiram-like reaction consisting of facial flushing, lightheadedness, weakness, sweating, tachycardia, nausea or vomiting may occur.
Alcohol	Antidiabetic agents (insulin, phenformin, sulfonylureas)	⬆	Because of altered glucose metabolism, the pharmacologic effects of these agents may be increased by alcohol resulting in hypoglycemia. In addition, alcohol may contribute to the lactic acidosis that is sometimes observed following phenformin administration. Both hypo- and hyperglycemia have occurred with sulfonylureas and alcohol.
Alcohol	Bromocriptine	⬆	Intolerance of bromocriptine due to the severity of side effects has occurred with concurrent alcohol.
Alcohol	Salicylates	⬆	Alcohol may potentiate aspirin-induced GI blood loss and bleeding time prolongation.

* ⬆ = Object drug increased.

[1] Those agents with a methyltetrazolethiol moiety.

Adverse Reactions:

Fever; injection site infection; venous thrombosis or phlebitis; extravasation; hypervolemia. These may occur because of the solution or administration technique.

Alcoholic intoxication may occur with too rapid infusion. Vertigo, flushing, disorientation (especially in elderly patients), or sedation may also occur. An alcoholic odor may be noted on the breath. Generally, these effects can be avoided by slowing the rate of infusion. Too rapid infusion of hypertonic solutions may cause local pain and, rarely, excessive vein irritation. Use the largest available peripheral vein and a well placed small bore needle.

Overdosage:

In the event of alcoholic intoxication or sedation, slow the infusion or discontinue temporarily. If overhydration or solute overload occurs, reevaluate the patient and institute appropriate corrective measures.

Administration and Dosage:

Administer by slow IV infusion only; do not give SC. Individualize dosage. The average adult can metabolize approximately 10 ml/hour (200 ml of 5% solution or 100 ml of 10% solution). The usual adult dosage is 1 to 2 L and rarely exceeds 3 L of a 5% solution in a 24 hour period. Children may be given 40 ml/kg/24 hours or from 350 to 1000 ml, depending on size and clinical response.

Storage/Stability: Do not use unless solution is clear and seal is intact. Discard unused portion. Protect from freezing and extreme heat.

	Product/Distributor	Cal/L	mOsm/L	How Supplied
Rx	**5% Alcohol and 5% Dextrose in Water** (Abbott, Clintec)	450	1114	In 1000 ml.
Rx	**5% Alcohol and 5% Dextrose in Water** (McGaw)		1125	In 1000 ml.
Rx	**10% Alcohol and 5% Dextrose in Water** (McGaw)	720	1995	In 1000 ml.

Lipids

INTRAVENOUS FAT EMULSION

Refer to the general discussion beginning in the IV Nutritional Therapy monograph.

Warning:

Deaths in preterm infants after infusion of IV fat emulsions have occurred. Autopsy findings included intravascular fat accumulation in the lungs. Treatment of premature and low birth weight infants with IV fat emulsion must be based on careful benefit-risk assessment. Strict adherence to the recommended total daily dose is mandatory; hourly infusion rate should be as slow as possible and should not exceed 1 g/kg in 4 hours. Premature and small for gestational age infants have poor clearance of IV fat emulsion and increased free fatty acid plasma levels following fat emulsion infusion; therefore, administer less than the maximum recommended doses in these patients to decrease the likelihood of IV fat overload. Monitor the infant's ability to eliminate the infused fat from the circulation (such as triglycerides or plasma free fatty acid levels). The lipemia must clear between daily infusions.

Actions:

Pharmacology: Intravenous fat emulsions are prepared from either soybean or safflower oil and provide a mixture of neutral triglycerides, predominantly unsaturated fatty acids. The major component of fatty acids are linoleic, oleic, palmitic, stearic and linolenic acids; see product listings for content. In addition, these products contain 1.2% egg yolk phospholipids as an emulsifier and glycerol to adjust tonicity. The emulsified fat particles are approximately 0.4 to 0.5 microns in diameter, similar to naturally occurring chylomicrons. IV fat emulsions are isotonic and may be given by central or peripheral venous routes.

These products are metabolized and utilized as a source of energy, causing an increase in heat production, decrease in respiratory quotient and an increase in oxygen consumption following use. The infused fat particles are cleared from the blood stream in a manner thought to be comparable to the clearing of chylomicrons.

Essential Fatty Acid Deficiency (EFAD) – Linoleic, linolenic and arachidonic acids are essential in humans. Linoleic acid, the metabolic precursor to both linolenic and arachidonic acid, cannot be synthesized in vivo. When there is a deficiency of linoleic acid, the enzyme system that converts linoleic acid to arachidonic acid (a tetraene) acts on oleic acid to synthesize eicosatrienoic acid (a triene) which lacks the physiologic functions of arachidonic acid. Biochemically, EFAD is defined as a triene to tetraene ratio > 0.4. Clinical manifestations of EFAD include scaly dermatitis, alopecia, growth retardation, poor wound healing, thrombocytopenia and fatty liver. IV fat emulsion prevents or reverses biochemical and clinical manifestations of EFAD.

Indications:

Source of calories and essential fatty acids for patients requiring parenteral nutrition for extended periods of time (usually for > 5 days).

Source of essential fatty acids when a deficiency occurs.

Contraindications:

Disturbance of normal fat metabolism such as pathologic hyperlipemia, lipoid nephrosis or acute pancreatitis, if accompanied by hyperlipemia. Egg yolk phospholipids are present; do not give to patients with severe egg allergies.

Warnings:

Special risk patients: Exercise caution in severe liver damage, pulmonary disease, anemia, blood coagulation disorders, or when there is danger of fat embolism.

Pregnancy: Category C. It is not known whether IV fat emulsions can cause fetal harm when administered to a pregnant woman or can affect reproduction capacity. Use only when clearly needed.

Precautions:

Monitoring: When IV fat emulsion is administered, monitor the patient's capacity to eliminate the infused fat from the circulation. The lipemia must clear between daily infusions. Closely monitor the hemogram, blood coagulation, liver function tests, plasma lipid profile and platelet count (especially in neonates). Discontinue use if a significant abnormality in any of these parameters is attributed to therapy.

Jaundiced or premature infants: Use with caution because free fatty acids displace bilirubin bound to albumin.

Too rapid administration can cause fluid or fat overloading. This can result in dilution of serum electrolyte concentrations, overhydration, pulmonary edema, impaired pulmonary diffusion capacity or metabolic acidosis.

Lipids

INTRAVENOUS FAT EMULSION

Adverse Reactions:

Most frequent: Sepsis due to administration equipment and thrombophlebitis due to vein irritation from concurrently administered hypertonic solutions. These adverse reactions are inseparable from the TPN procedure with or without IV fat emulsion.

Less frequent (more directly related to IV fat emulsion):

Immediate (acute) (< 1%) – Dyspnea; cyanosis; hyperlipemia; hypercoagulability; nausea; vomiting; headache; flushing; increase in temperature; sweating; sleepiness; chest and back pain; slight pressure over the eyes; dizziness; irritation at the infusion site; thrombocytopenia in neonates (rare).

Long-term (chronic) – Hepatomegaly; jaundice due to central lobular cholestasis; splenomegaly; thrombocytopenia; leukopenia; transient increases in liver function tests; overloading syndrome (focal seizures, fever, leukocytosis, splenomegaly and shock).

The deposition of brown pigmentation in the reticuloendothelial system (the so-called "IV fat pigment") has occurred. Cause and significance of this phenomenon are unknown.

Overdosage:

Stop the infusion until visual inspection of the plasma, determination of triglyceride concentrations or measurement of plasma light-scattering activity by nephelometry indicates the lipid has cleared. Reevaluate the patient and institute appropriate corrective measures.

Administration and Dosage:

Total parenteral nutrition: As part of TPN, administer IV via a peripheral vein or by central venous catheter. Fat emulsion should comprise no more than 60% of the patient's total caloric intake, with carbohydrates and amino acids comprising the remaining 40% or more of caloric intake.

Adults –

10%: Initial infusion rate is 1ml/min for the first 15 to 30 minutes. If no adverse reactions occur, the infusion rate can be increased to 2 ml/min. Infuse only 500 ml the first day and increase dose the following day. Do not exceed a daily dosage of 2.5 g/kg.

20%: Initial infusion rate is 0.5 ml/min for the first 15 to 30 minutes. Infuse only 250 ml (Liposyn II;) or 500 ml *(Intralipid)* the first day and increase dose the following day. Do not exceed a daily dosage of 3 g/kg.

Children:

10% – Initial infusion rate is 0.1 ml/min for the first 10 to 15 minutes.

20% – Initial infusion rate is 0.05 ml/min for the first 10 to 15 minutes.

If no untoward reactions occur, increase rate to 1 g/kg in 4 hours. Do not exceed daily dosage of 3 g/kg.

The dosage for premature infants starts at 0.5 g fat/kg/24 hours (5 ml *Intralipid* 10%; 2.5 ml *Intralipid* 20%) and may be increased in relation to the infant's ability to eliminate fat. The maximum dosage recommended by the American Academy of Pediatrics is 3 g fat/kg/24 hours.

Fatty acid deficiency: To correct EFAD, supply 8% to 10% of the caloric intake by IV fat emulsion to provide an adequate amount of linoleic acid (4% of caloric intake as linoleate).

Fat emulsion is supplied in single dose containers; do not store partially used bottles or resterilize for later use. Do not use filters. Do not use any bottle in which there appears to be separation of the emulsion.

Fat emulsions may be simultaneously infused with amino acid-dextrose mixtures by means of a Y–connector located near the infusion site using separate flow rate controls for each solution. Keep the lipid infusion line higher than the amino acid-dextrose line. Since the lipid emulsion has a lower specific gravity, it may be taken up into the amino acid-dextrose line.

Fat emulsions may also be infused through a separate peripheral site.

Lipids

INTRAVENOUS FAT EMULSION

Total nutrient admixture (TNA): IV fat emulsions are compatible with dextrose and amino acids, when properly mixed, for use in TPN therapy. This is also referred to as all-in-one, 3-in-1 and triple-mix. The following proper mixing sequence must be followed to minimize pH-related problems by ensuring that typically acidic dextrose injections are not mixed with lipid emulsions alone: (1) Transfer dextrose injection to the TPN admixture container; (2) transfer amino acid injection; (3) transfer the IV fat emulsion.

Amino acid injection, dextrose injection and the IV fat emulsion may be simultaneously transferred to the admixture container. Use gentle agitation to avoid localized concentration effects. Additives must not be added directly to the fat emulsion and in no case should the fat emulsion be added to the TPN container first. Shake bags gently after each addition to minimize localized concentration. If evacuated glass containers are used, add the dextrose and amino acid injections first, followed by the fat emulsion and then additives. Shake bottles gently after each addition.

Use these admixtures promptly; store under refrigeration (2° to 8°C; 36° to 46°F) for ≤ 24 hours and use completely within 24 hours after removal from refrigeration.

The prime destabilizers of emulsions are excessive acidity (low pH) and inappropriate electrolyte content. Give careful consideration to additions of divalent cations (calcium and magnesium) which cause emulsion instability. Amino acid solutions exert a buffering effect protecting the emulsion.

Inspect the admixture carefully for "breaking or oiling out" of the emulsion, which is described as the separation of the emulsion and can be visibly identified by a yellowish streaking or the accumulation of yellowish droplets in the admixed emulsion. Also examine the admixture for particulates. The admixture must be discarded if any of the above is observed.

Heparin may be added to activate lipoprotein lipase at a concentration of 1 or 2 units/ml prior to administration.

Lipid-containing fluids have a propensity to extract phthalates from phthalate-plasticized polyvinyl chloride (PVC). Although the amount is very small and no adverse clinical effects have been reported from administration of such amounts of phthalate, consider administration through a nonphthalate infusion set. Commercially available products may be accompanied by nonphthalate infusion sets.

Product & Distributor	Oil (%) Safflower	Soybean	Fatty acid content (%) Linoleic	Oleic	Palmitic	Linolenic	Stearic	Egg yolk phospholipids (%)	Glycerin (%)	Calories/ml	Osmolarity (mOsm/L)	How Supplied
Intralipid[1] 10% (Clintec)		10	50	26	10	9	3.5	1.2	2.25	1.1	260	In 50, 100, 250 and 500 ml.
Intralipid[1] 20% (Clintec)		20	50	26	10	9	3.5	1.2	2.25	2	260	In 50, 100, 250 and 500 ml.
Liposyn II[2] 10% (Abbott)	5	5	65.8	17.7	8.8	4.2	3.4	1.2	2.5	1.1	276	In 100, 200 and 500 ml.
Liposyn II[2] 20% (Abbott)	10	10	65.8	17.7	8.8	4.2	3.4	1.2	2.5	2	258	In 200 and 500 ml.
Liposyn III[2] 10% (Abbott)		10	54.5	22.4	10.5	8.3	4.2	1.2	2.5	1.1	284	In 100, 200 and 500 ml.
Liposyn III[2] 20% (Abbott)		20	54.5	22.4	10.5	8.3	4.2	1.2	2.5	2	292	In 200 and 500 ml.

[1] Store at 25°C (77°F) or below; do not freeze.

[2] Store at 30°C (86°F) or below; do not freeze.

Electrolytes

SODIUM CHLORIDE

For information on oral sodium chloride, refer to Minerals and Electrolytes, Oral section.

Actions:

Pharmacology: Normal osmolarity of the extracellular fluid ranges between 280 to 300 mOsm/L; it is primarily a function of sodium and its accompanying ions, chloride and bicarbonate. Sodium chloride is the principal salt involved in maintenance of plasma tonicity. One g of sodium chloride provides 17.1 mEq sodium and 17.1 mEq chloride.

Hyponatremia (< 135 mEq/L): Symptoms may include weakness, nausea, disorientation, lethargy and headache; severe cases may progress to seizures and coma.

Indications:

For parenteral restoration of sodium ion in patients with restricted oral intake. Sodium replacement is specifically indicated in patients with hyponatremia or low salt syndrome. Sodium Chloride may also be added to compatible carbohydrate solutions such as Dextrose in Water to provide electrolytes.

Sodium Chloride Injections are also indicated as pharmaceutic aids and diluents for the infusion of compatible drug additives.

0.9% Sodium Chloride (Normal Saline), which is isotonic, restores both water and sodium chloride losses. Other indications for parenteral 0.9% saline include: Diluting or dissolving drugs for IV, IM or SC injection; flushing of IV catheters; extracellular fluid replacement; treatment of metabolic alkalosis in the presence of fluid loss and mild sodium depletion; as a priming solution in hemodialysis procedures and to initiate and terminate blood transfusions without hemolyzing red blood cells.

0.45% Sodium Chloride (Hypotonic) is primarily a hydrating solution and may be used to assess the status of the kidneys, since more water is provided than is required for salt excretion. It may also be used in the treatment of hyperosmolar diabetes where the use of dextrose is inadvisable and there is a need for large amounts of fluid without an excess of sodium ions.

3% or 5% Sodium Chloride (Hypertonic) is used in hyponatremia and hypochloremia due to electrolyte and fluid loss replaced with sodium-free fluids; drastic dilution of body water following excessive water intake; emergency treatment of severe salt depletion.

Bacteriostatic Sodium Chloride: Only for diluting or dissolving drugs for IV, IM or SC injection. See Contraindications and Warnings.

Concentrated Sodium Chloride: As an additive in parenteral fluid therapy for use in patients who have special problems of sodium electrolyte intake or excretion. It is intended to meet the specific requirements of the patient with unusual fluid and electrolyte needs. After available clinical and laboratory information is considered and correlated, determine the appropriate number of milliequivalents of Concentrated Sodium Chloride Injection, USP and dilute for use.

Contraindications:

Hypernatremia; fluid retention; when the administration of sodium or chloride could be clinically detrimental.

3% and 5% sodium chloride solutions: Elevated, normal or only slightly decreased plasma sodium and chloride concentrations.

Bacteriostatic sodium chloride: Newborns (see Warnings); for fluid or sodium chloride replacement.

Warnings:

Fluid/solute overload: Excessive amounts of sodium chloride by any route may cause hypokalemia and acidosis. Administration of IV solutions can cause fluid or solute overload resulting in dilution of serum electrolyte concentrations, congestive heart failure (CHF), overhydration, congested states or acute pulmonary edema, especially in patients with cardiovascular disease and in patients receiving corticosteroids or corticotropin or drugs that may give rise to sodium retention. The risk of dilutional states is inversely proportional to the electrolyte concentration. The risk of solute overload causing congested states with peripheral and pulmonary edema is directly proportional to the electrolyte concentration.

Infusion of > 1 L of isotonic (0.9%) sodium chloride may supply more sodium and chloride than normally found in serum, resulting in hypernatremia; this may cause a loss of bicarbonate ions, resulting in an acidifying effect. Infusion during or immediately after surgery may result in excessive sodium retention.

Hypertonic solutions: When administered peripherally, slowly infuse through a small bore needle placed well within the lumen of a large vein to minimize venous irritation. Carefully avoid infiltration.

SODIUM CHLORIDE

Bacteriostatic Sodium Chloride: Do not use in newborns. Benzyl alcohol as a preservative in Bacteriostatic Sodium Chloride Injection has been associated with toxicity in newborns. This toxicity may result from both high cumulative amounts (mg/kg) of benzyl alcohol and the limited detoxification capacity of the neonate liver. These solutions have not been reported to cause problems in older infants, children and adults. It is estimated that a 30 ml IV dose may be given to adults without toxic effects. Data are unavailable on the toxicity of other preservatives in newborns. Use preservative-free Sodium Chloride Injection for flushing intravascular catheters. Where a sodium chloride solution is required for preparing or diluting medications for use in newborns, use only preservative-free 0.9% Sodium Chloride.

Concentrated Sodium Chloride Injection is hypertonic and must be diluted before use. Inadvertent direct injection or absorption of concentrated Sodium Chloride Injection may give rise to sudden hypernatremia and such complications as cardiovascular shock, CNS disorders, extensive hemolysis, cortical necrosis of the kidneys and severe local tissue necrosis (if administered extravascularly). Do not use unless solution is clear.

Surgical patients should seldom receive salt-containing solutions immediately following surgery unless factors producing salt depletion are present. Because of renal retention of salt during surgery, additional electrolyte given IV may result in fluid retention, edema and overloading of the circulation.

Renal function impairment: Infusions of sodium ions may result in excessive sodium retention; administer with care.

Pregnancy: Category C. It is not known whether sodium chloride can cause fetal harm when given to a pregnant woman or can affect reproduction capacity. Use only if clearly needed.

Lactation: It is not known whether sodium chloride is excreted in breast milk. Exercise caution when administering sodium chloride to a nursing woman.

Children: Safety and efficacy have not been established.

Precautions:

Monitoring: Clinical evaluation and periodic laboratory determinations are necessary to monitor changes in fluid balance, electrolyte concentrations and acid-base balance during prolonged parenteral therapy or whenever the condition of the patient warrants such evaluation. Significant deviations from normal concentrations may require tailoring of the electrolyte pattern.

Extraordinary electrolyte losses (eg, during protracted nasogastric suction, vomiting, diarrhea, GI fistula drainage) may necessitate additional electrolyte supplementation. Supply additional essential electrolytes, minerals and vitamins as needed.

Hypokalemia may result from excessive administration of potassium-free solutions.

Special risk patients: Administer cautiously to patients with decompensated cardiovascular, cirrhotic and nephrotic disease, circulatory insufficiency, hypoproteinemia, hypervolemia, urinary tract obstruction, CHF and to patients with concurrent edema and sodium retention, those receiving corticosteroids or corticotropin and those retaining salt.

Elderly or postoperative patients: Exercise care in administering sodium-containing solutions in renal or cardiovascular insufficiency, with or without CHF.

3% and 5% sodium chloride solutions: Infuse very slowly and use with caution to avoid pulmonary edema; observe patients constantly.

Adverse Reactions:

Reactions due to solution or technique of administration: Febrile response; local tenderness; abscess; tissue necrosis or infection at injection site; venous thrombosis or phlebitis extending from injection site; extravasation; hypervolemia.

Hypernatremia may be associated with edema and exacerbation of CHF due to retention of water, resulting in expanded extracellular fluid volume.

Ion excess/deficit: Symptoms may result from an excess or deficit of one or more of the ions present in the solution; therefore, frequent monitoring of electrolyte levels is essential. If infused in large amounts, chloride ions may cause a loss of bicarbonate ions, resulting in an acidifying effect.

Postoperative salt intolerance: Symptoms include cellular dehydration, weakness, disorientation, anorexia, nausea, distention, deep respiration, oliguria, increased BUN.

Too rapid infusion of hypertonic solutions may cause local pain and venous irritation. Adjust rate of administration according to tolerance. Use of the largest peripheral vein and a well-placed small bore needle is recommended. (See Warnings.)

Electrolytes

SODIUM CHLORIDE

If an adverse reaction occurs, discontinue the infusion, evaluate the patient, institute appropriate countermeasures and save remainder of the fluid for examination.

Overdosage:

Parenteral preparations are unlikely to pose a threat of sodium chloride or fluid overload except possibly in newborn or very small infants. If these occur, reevaluate the patient and institute appropriate corrective measures.

Administration of too much sodium chloride may result in serious electrolyte disturbances with resulting retention of water, edema, loss of potassium and aggravation of an existing acidosis.

When intake of sodium chloride is excessive, excretion of crystalloids is increased in an attempt to maintain normal osmotic pressure. Thus there is increased excretion of potassium and of bicarbonate and, consequently, a tendency toward acidosis. There is also a rapid elimination of any foreign salt, such as iodide and bromide, being used for therapy.

Administration and Dosage:

Individualize dosage. Frequent laboratory determinations and clinical evaluation are essential to monitor changes in fluid balance, blood glucose and electrolytes.

In the average adult, daily requirements of sodium and chloride are met by the infusion of 1 L of 0.9% sodium chloride (154 mEq each of sodium and chloride). Base fluid administration on calculated maintenance or replacement fluid requirements.

Do not use plastic container in series connection.

If administration is controlled by a pumping device, take care to discontinue pumping action before the container runs dry or air embolism may result.

IV catheters: Prior to and after administration of the medication, entirely flush the catheter with 0.9% Sodium Chloride for Injection. Use in accord with any warnings or precautions appropriate to the medication being administered.

Calculation of sodium deficit: To calculate the amount of sodium that must be administered to raise serum sodium to the desired level, use the following equation (TBW = total body water): Na deficit (mEq) = TBW (desired – observed plasma Na).

Base the repletion rate on the degree of urgency in the patient. Use of hypertonic saline (eg, 3% or 5%) will correct the deficit more rapidly.

Concentrated Sodium Chloride: The dosage as an additive in parenteral fluid therapy is predicated on specific requirements of the patient. The appropriate volume is then withdrawn for proper dilution. Having determined the mEq of sodium chloride to be added, divide by four to calculate the number of ml to be used. Withdraw this volume and transfer into appropriate IV solutions such as 5% Dextrose Injection. The properly diluted solution may be given IV.

Admixture incompatibilities: Some additives may be incompatible. Consult a pharmacist. When Sodium Chloride Injections are used as diluents for infusion of compatible drug additives, refer to dosage and administration information accompanying additive drugs. Check specific references for any possible incompatibility with sodium chloride.

To minimize the risk of possible incompatibilities arising from mixing this solution with other additives that may be prescribed, inspect the final infusate for cloudiness or precipitation immediately after mixing, prior to administration and periodically during administration. Do not store.

Stability and storage: Replace IV apparatus at least once every 24 hours. Use only if solution is clear. Protect from freezing; avoid excessive heat. Store at 15° to 30°C (59° to 86°F). Brief exposure up to 40°C (104°F) does not adversely affect product.

Electrolytes

SODIUM CHLORIDE INTRAVENOUS INFUSIONS FOR ADMIXTURES

		Sodium (mEq/L)	Chloride (mEq/L)	Osmolarity (mOsm/L)	How Supplied
Rx	**0.45% Sodium Chloride** (**½ Normal Saline**) (Various, eg, Abbott, Astra, Clintec, McGaw)	77	77	≈ 155	In 25, 50, 150, 250, 500 and 1000 ml.
Rx	**0.9% Sodium Chloride** (**Normal Saline**) (Various, eg, Abbott, Astra, Clintec, Elkins -Sinn, Gensia, McGaw, Lyphomed, Rugby, Smith & Nephew SoloPak)	154	154	≈ 310	In 2, 3, 5, 10, 20, 25, 30, 50, 100, 150, 250, 500, 1000ml and 2 ml fill in 3 ml.
Rx	**3% Sodium Chloride** (Various, eg, Clintec, McGaw)	513	513	1030	In 500 ml.
Rx	**5% Sodium Chloride** (Various, eg, Abbott, Clintec, McGaw)	855	855	1710	In 500 ml.

SODIUM CHLORIDE DILUENTS

Rx	**Bacteriostatic Sodium Chloride Injection**[1] (Various, eg, American Regent, Elkins-Sinn, Lyphomed, Major, Rugby)	0.9% sodium chloride	In 2, 10, and 30 ml.

[1] With benzyl alcohol or parabens.

CONCENTRATED SODIUM CHLORIDE INJECTION

Not for direct infusion. *Must* be diluted before use.

Rx	**Sodium Chloride Injection** (Various, eg, Abbott, IMS, Lyphomed)	14.6% sodium chloride	In 20, 40 and 200 ml.
Rx	**Sodium Chloride Injection** (Various, eg, American Regent, Gensia, IMS, Lyphomed, Pasadena)	23.4% sodium chloride	In 30, 50, 100 and 200 ml.

Electrolytes

POTASSIUM SALTS

For information on oral potassium, refer to Mineral and Electrolytes, Oral section. For information on potassium phosphate, refer to specific monograph in this section.

Actions:

Pharmacology: The principal intracellular cation, potassium is essential for maintenance of intracellular tonicity; transmission of nerve impulses; contraction of cardiac, skeletal and smooth muscle; and maintenance of normal renal function. Potassium participates in carbohydrate utilization and protein synthesis and is critical in regulating nerve conduction and muscle contraction, particularly in the heart.

Hypokalemia – Gradual potassium depletion occurs via renal excretion, through GI loss or because of inadequate intake (excretion > intake). Depletion usually results from diuretic therapy, primary or secondary hyperaldosteronism, diabetic ketoacidosis, severe diarrhea (especially if associated with vomiting) or inadequate replacement during prolonged parenteral nutrition.

Potassium depletion sufficient to cause 1 mEq/L drop in serum potassium requires a loss of about 100 to 200 mEq of potassium from the total body store.

Symptoms: Weakness; fatigue; ileus; polydipsia; flaccid paralysis or impaired ability to concentrate urine (in advanced cases).

ECG may reveal premature atrial and ventricular contractions, prolongation of QT interval, ST segment depression, broad and flat T waves or appearance of U waves. Severe cases may lead to muscular weakness, paralysis, respiratory failure.

Pharmacokinetics: Normally about 80% to 90% of potassium intake is excreted in urine with the remainder voided in stool and, to a small extent, in perspiration. Kidneys do not conserve potassium well; during fasting or in patients on a potassium-free diet, potassium loss from the body continues, resulting in potassium depletion. A deficiency of either potassium or chloride will lead to a deficit of the other.

Indications:

Prevention and treatment of moderate or severe potassium deficit when oral replacement therapy is not feasible.

Potassium acetate is useful as an additive for preparing specific IV fluid formulas when patient needs cannot be met by standard electrolyte or nutrient solutions.

Also indicated for marked loss of GI secretions by vomiting, diarrhea, GI intubation or fistulas; prolonged diuresis; prolonged parenteral use of potassium-free fluids (eg, normal saline, dextrose solutions); diabetic acidosis, especially during vigorous insulin and dextrose treatment; metabolic alkalosis; attacks of hereditary or familial periodic paralysis; hyperadrenocorticism; primary aldosteronism; overmedication with adrenocortical steroids, testosterone or corticotropin; healing phase of scalds or burns; cardiac arrhythmias, especially due to digitalis glycosides.

Contraindications:

Diseases where high potassium levels may be encountered; hyperkalemia; renal failure and conditions in which potassium retention is present; oliguria or azotemia; anuria; crush syndrome; severe hemolytic reactions; adrenocortical insufficiency (untreated Addison's disease); adynamica episodica hereditaria; acute dehydration; heat cramps; hyperkalemia from any cause; early postoperative oliguria except during GI drainage.

Warnings:

Potassium intoxication: Do not infuse rapidly. High plasma concentrations of potassium may cause death through cardiac depression, arrhythmias or arrest. Monitor potassium replacement therapy whenever possible by continuous or serial ECG. In addition to ECG effects, local pain and phlebitis may result when a > 40 mEq/L concentration is infused.

Renal impairment or adrenal insufficiency may cause potassium intoxication. Potassium salts can produce hyperkalemia and cardiac arrest. Potentially fatal hyperkalemia can develop rapidly and be asymptomatic. Use with great caution, if at all.

Concentrated potassium solutions are for IV admixtures only; do not use undiluted. Direct injection may be instantaneously fatal.

Metabolic alkalosis: Potassium depletion is usually accompanied by an obligatory loss of chloride resulting in hypochloremic metabolic alkalosis. Treat the underlying cause of potassium depletion and administer IV potassium chloride.

Use solutions containing acetate ion carefully in metabolic or respiratory alkalosis, and when there is an increased level or impairment of utilization of this ion.

Metabolic acidosis: Treat associated hypokalemia with an alkalinizing potassium salt (eg, bicarbonate, citrate, gluconate, acetate).

Electrolytes

POTASSIUM SALTS

Musculoskeletal/Cardiac effects: When serum sodium or calcium concentration is reduced, moderate elevation of serum potassium may cause toxic effects on the heart and skeletal muscle. Weakness and later paralysis of voluntary muscles, with consequent respiratory distress and dysphagia, are generally late signs, sometimes significantly preceding dangerous or fatal cardiac toxicity.

Renal function impairment: Normal kidney function permits safe potassium therapy. Although temporary elevation of serum potassium level due to renal insufficiency secondary to dehydration or shock may mask an intracellular potassium deficit, do not replenish potassium until renal function is reestablished by overcoming dehydration and shock. Discontinue potassium-containing solutions if signs of renal insufficiency develop during infusions.

Pregnancy: Category C. It is not known whether potassium salts can cause fetal harm when administered to a pregnant woman or can affect reproduction capacity. Give to a pregnant woman only if clearly needed.

Lactation: Exercise caution when administering to a nursing woman.

Precautions:

Monitoring: Close medical supervision with frequent ECGs and serum potassium determinations. Plasma levels are not necessarily indicative of tissue levels.

Special risk patients: Use with caution in the presence of cardiac disease, particularly in digitalized patients or in the presence of renal disease, metabolic acidosis, Addison's disease, acute dehydration, prolonged or severe diarrhea, familial periodic paralysis, hypoadrenalism, hyperkalemia, hyponatremia and myotonia congenita.

Fluid/Solute overload: IV administration can cause fluid or solute overloading resulting in dilution of serum electrolyte concentrations, overhydration, congested states or pulmonary edema.

The risk of dilutional states is inversely proportional to the electrolyte concentration of administered parenteral solutions. The risk of solute overload causing congested states with peripheral and pulmonary edema is directly proportional to the electrolyte concentrations of such solutions.

Drug Interactions:

Potassium Preparation Drug Interactions			
Precipitant drug	Object drug*		Description
ACE inhibitors	Potassium preparations	⬆	Concurrent use may result in elevated serum potassium concentrations in certain patients.
Potassium-sparing diuretics/ potassium-containing salt substitutes	Potassium preparations	⬆	Potassium-sparing diuretics and potassium-containing salt substitutes will increase potassium retention and can produce severe hyperkalemia.
Potassium preparations	Digitalis	⬆	In patients on digoxin, hypokalemia may result in digoxin toxicity. Use caution if discontinuing a potassium preparation in patients maintained on digoxin.

* ⬆ = Object drug increased.

Adverse Reactions:

Hyperkalemia: Adverse reactions involve the possibility of potassium intoxication. Signs and symptoms include: Paresthesias of extremities; flaccid paralysis; muscle or respiratory paralysis; areflexia; weakness; listlessness; mental confusion; weakness and heaviness of legs; hypotension; cardiac arrhythmias; heart block; ECG abnormalities such as disappearance of P waves, spreading and slurring of the QRS complex with development of a biphasic curve and cardiac arrest. See Overdosage.

GI: Nausea; vomiting; abdominal pain; diarrhea.

Reactions due to solution or technique of administration: Febrile response; infection at injection site; venous thrombosis; phlebitis extending from injection site; extravasation; hypervolemia; hyperkalemia; venospasm.

Overdosage:

If excretory mechanisms are impaired or if potassium is administered too rapidly IV, potentially fatal hyperkalemia can result (see Contraindications and Warnings). It is important to consider the entire clinical picture and not rely solely on potassium levels since only extracellular potassium can be measured, yet intracellular potassium accounts for 98% of the total body amount.

Electrolytes

POTASSIUM SALTS

Symptoms: Mild (> 5.5 to 6.5 mEq/L) to moderate (> 6.5 to 8 mEq/L) hyperkalemia may be asymptomatic and manifested only by increased serum potassium concentration and characteristic ECG changes. Other symptoms include muscular weakness, progressing to flaccid quadriplegia and respiratory paralysis; however, these generally do not develop unless potassium concentrations exceed 8 mEq/L. Dangerous cardiac arrhythmias often occur before onset of complete paralysis. Note that hyperkalemia produces symptoms paradoxically similar to those of hypokalemia.

ECG – Progressive increase in height and peaking of T waves; lowering of the R wave; decreased amplitude and ultimate disappearance of P waves; prolongation of PR interval and QRS complex; shortening of the QT interval; and finally, ventricular fibrillation and death.

Treatment: Terminate potassium administration. Monitor ECG. Infusion of combined dextrose and insulin in a ratio of 3 g dextrose to 1 unit regular insulin may be administered to shift potassium into cells. Administer sodium bicarbonate 50 to 100 mEq IV to reverse acidosis and also produce an intracellular shift. Give 10 to 100 ml calcium gluconate or calcium chloride 10% to reverse ECG changes. To remove potassium from the body use sodium polystyrene sulfonate resin or hemodialysis or peritoneal dialysis.

In digitalized patients, too rapid lowering of serum potassium can cause digitalis toxicity (see Drug Interactions).

Administration and Dosage:

mEq/g of Various Potassium Salts

Potassium salt	mEq/g
Potassium acetate	10.2
Potassium chloride	13.4
Dibasic potassium phosphate[1]	11.5
Monobasic potassium phosphate[1]	7.3

[1] Commercial preparations of potassium phosphate injection contain a mixture of both mono- and dibasic salts (see Potassium Phosphate monograph).

Do not administer undiluted potassium. Potassium preparations must be diluted with suitable large volume parenteral solutions, mixed well and given by slow IV infusion.

Too rapid infusion of hypertonic solutions may cause local pain and, rarely, vein irritation. Adjust rate of administration according to tolerance. Use of the largest peripheral vein and a small bore needle is recommended.

The usual additive dilution of potassium chloride is 40 mEq/L of IV fluid. The maximum desirable concentration is 80 mEq/L, although extreme emergencies may dictate greater concentrations.

In critical states, potassium chloride may be administered in saline (unless saline is contraindicated) since dextrose may lower serum potassium levels by producing an intracellular shift.

Avoid "layering" of potassium by proper agitation of the prepared IV solution. Do not add potassium to an IV bottle in the hanging position.

Individualize dosage. Guide dosage and rate of infusion by ECG and serum electrolyte determinations. The following may be used as a guide:

Potassium Dosage/Rate of Infusion Guidelines

Serum K+	Maximum infusion rate	Maximum concentration	Maximum 24 hour dose
> 2.5 mEq/L	10 mEq/hr	40 mEq/L	200 mEq
< 2 mEq/L	40 mEq/hr	80 mEq/L	400 mEq

Add electrolytes to the mixed solutions only after considering electrolytes already present and potential incompatibilities such as calcium and phosphate or sulfate.

Children: IV infusion up to 3 mEq/kg or 40 mEq/m^2/day. Adjust volume of administered fluids to body size.

Electrolytes

POTASSIUM ACETATE

Must be diluted before use.

Rx	**Potassium Acetate** (Various, eg, Abbott, American Regent, IMS, Lyphomed)	**Injection**: 2 mEq/ml	In 20, 50 and 100 ml vials.
Rx	**Potassium Acetate** (Various, eg, Lyphomed, McGuff)	**Injection**: 4 mEq/ml	In 50 ml vials.

POTASSIUM CHLORIDE FOR INJECTION CONCENTRATE

Concentrate *must* be diluted before use.

Rx	**Potassium Chloride** (McGaw)	**Injection**: 2 mEq/ml	In 250 and 500 ml.
Rx	**Potassium Chloride** (Various, eg, Abbott, Baxter, Lyphomed)	**Injection**: 10 mEq	In 5, 10, 50 and 100 ml vials and 5 ml additive syringes.
Rx	**Potassium Chloride** (Various, eg, Abbott, American Regent, Baxter, Lyphomed)	**Injection**: 20 mEq	In 10 and 20 ml vials, 10 ml additive syringes, 10 ml amps.
Rx	**Potassium Chloride** (Various, eg, Abbott, Baxter, Lyphomed)	**Injection**: 30 mEq	In 15, 20, 30 and 100 ml vials and 20 ml additive syringes.
Rx	**Potassium Chloride** (Various, eg, Abbott, American Regent, Baxter, Lyphomed, McGuff)	**Injection**: 40 mEq	In 20, 30, 50 and 100 ml vials, 20 ml amps, 20 ml additive syringes.
Rx	**Potassium Chloride** (Various, eg, American Regent, McGuff)	**Injection**: 60 mEq	In 30 ml vials.
Rx	**Potassium Chloride** (Various, eg, Lyphomed)	**Injection**: 90 mEq	In 30 ml vials.

Electrolytes

CALCIUM

For information on oral calcium, refer to the Minerals and Electrolytes, Oral section.

Actions:

Pharmacology: Calcium is the fifth most abundant element in the body with > 99.5% of total body stores in skeletal bone. It is essential for the functional integrity of the nervous and muscular systems, for normal cardiac contractility and the coagulation of blood. It also functions as an enzyme cofactor and affects the secretory activity of endocrine and exocrine glands. Normal levels are 8.5 to 10.5 mg/dl.

Hypocalcemia –

Symptoms: Tetany; paresthesias; laryngospasm; muscle spasms; seizures (usually grand mal); irritability; depression; psychosis; prolonged QT interval; intestinal cramps and malabsorption; respiratory arrest. Prolonged hypocalcemia may be associated with ectodermal defects including the nails, skin and teeth.

Pharmacokinetics: Approximately 80% of body calcium is excreted in the feces as insoluble salts; urinary excretion accounts for the remaining 20%.

Indications:

Hypocalcemia: For a prompt increase in plasma calcium levels (eg, neonatal tetany and tetany due to parathyroid deficiency, vitamin D deficiency, alkalosis); prevention of hypocalcemia during exchange transfusions; conditions associated with intestinal malabsorption.

Calcium chloride and gluconate: Adjunctive therapy in the treatment of insect bites or stings, such as Black Widow spider bites to relieve muscle cramping; sensitivity reactions, particularly when characterized by urticaria; depression due to overdosage of magnesium sulfate; acute symptoms of lead colic; rickets; osteomalacia.

Calcium chloride: To combat the deleterious effects of severe hyperkalemia as measured by ECG, pending correction of increased potassium in the extracellular fluid.

Cardiac resuscitation – Particularly after open heart surgery, when epinephrine fails to improve weak or ineffective myocardial contractions.

Calcium gluconate: To decrease capillary permeability in allergic conditions, nonthrombocytopenic purpura and exudative dermatoses such as dermatitis herpetiformis; for pruritus of eruptions caused by certain drugs; in hyperkalemia, calcium gluconate may aid in antagonizing the cardiac toxicity, provided the patient is not receiving digitalis therapy.

Unlabeled uses: Calcium salts have been used to treat verapamil overdose, treat acute hypotension from verapamil and prevent initial hypotension in patients requiring verapamil for whom decreases in blood pressure could be detrimental.

Contraindications:

Hypercalcemia; ventricular fibrillation; digitalized patients.

Warnings:

Extravasation: **Calcium chloride** and **gluconate** can cause severe necrosis, sloughing and abscess formation with IM or SC admininstration. Take great care to avoid extravasation or accidental injection into perivascular tissues.

Hypocalcemia of renal insufficiency: **Calcium chloride** is an acidifying salt and is therefore usually undesirable for treating this condition.

Pregnancy: Category C. It is not known whether this drug can cause fetal harm when given to a pregnant woman or can affect reproduction capacity. Use only when clearly needed.

Lactation: It is not known whether **calcium gluconate** is excreted in breast milk. Exercise caution when administering to a pregnant woman.

Precautions:

Cardiovascular effects: It is particularly important to prevent a high concentration of calcium from reaching the heart because of the danger of cardiac syncope.

Electrolytes

CALCIUM

Drug Interactions:

Calcium Drug Interactions			
Precipitant	Object drug*		Description
Thiazide diuretics	Calcium salts	↑	Hypercalcemia resulting from renal tubular reabsorption, or bone release of calcium by thiazides may be amplified by exogenous calcium.
Calcium salts	Atenolol	↓	Mean peak plasma levels and bioavailability of atenolol may be decreased, possibly resulting in decreased beta blockade.
Calcium salts	Digitalis glycosides	↑	Inotropic and toxic effects are synergistic; arrhythmias may occur, especially if calcium is given IV. Avoid IV calcium in patients on digitalis glycosides; if necessary, give slowly in small amounts.
Calcium salts	Sodium polystyrene sulfonate	↓	Coadministration in patients with renal impairment may result in an unanticipated metabolic alkalosis and a reduction of the resin's binding of potassium.
Calcium salts	Verapamil	↓	Clinical effects and toxicities of verapamil may be reversed.

* ↑ = Object drug increased. ↓ = Object drug decreased.

Drug/Lab test interactions: Transient elevations of plasma 11-hydroxy-corticosteroid levels (Glenn-Nelson technique) may occur when IV calcium is administered, but levels return to control values after 1 hour. In addition, IV calcium gluconate can produce false-negative values for serum and urinary magnesium.

Adverse Reactions:

IM administration: Mild local reactions may occur (**calcium gluceptate**). Local necrosis and abscess formation may occur with **calcium gluconate,** and severe necrosis and sloughing may occur with IM or SC administration of **calcium chloride.**

IV administration: Rapid IV administration may cause bradycardia, sense of oppression, tingling, metallic, calcium or chalky taste or "heat waves". Rapid IV **calcium gluconate** may cause vasodilation, decreased blood pressure, cardiac arrhythmias, syncope and cardiac arrest. **Calcium chloride** injections cause peripheral vasodilation and a local burning sensation; blood pressure may fall moderately.

Overdosage:

Symptoms: Inadvertent systemic overloading with calcium ions can produce an acute hypercalcemic syndrome characterized by a markedly elevated plasma calcium level, weakness, lethargy, intractable nausea and vomiting, coma and sudden death.

Treatment: It may be life-saving to rapidly lower blood calcium to safe levels. It is now agreed the most effective therapy is IV sodium chloride infusion plus potent natriuretic agents, (eg, furosemide). Sodium competes with calcium for reabsorption in the distal renal tubule and furosemide potentiates this effect. Together they markedly increase renal calcium clearance and reduce hypercalcemia.

Administration and Dosage:

Elemental Calcium Content of Calcium Salts		
Salt	% Calcium	mEq/g
Calcium chloride	27.3	13.6
Calcium gluconate	9.3	4.65
Calcium gluceptate	8.2	4.1

Calcium gluconate is generally preferred over calcium chloride as it is less irritating.

IV: Warm solutions to body temperature and give slowly (0.5 to 2 ml/min); stop if patient complains of discomfort. Resume when symptoms disappear. Following injection, patient should remain recumbent for a short time. Repeated injections may be needed because of the rapid calcium excretion. Inject **calcium chloride** and **gluconate** through a small needle into a large vein to minimize venous irritation.

IM administration of **calcium gluceptate** and **gluconate** may be tolerated; however, *reserve this route for emergencies when technical difficulty makes IV injection impossible.* Administer **calcium gluconate** only by the IV route and **calcium chloride** by the IV or intraventricular route.

Electrolytes

CALCIUM

Admixture incompatibilities: Calcium salts should not generally be mixed with **carbonates, phosphates, sulfates** or **tartrates** in parenteral admixtures; they are conditionally compatible with potassium phosphates, depending on concentration. Calcium ions will chelate **tetracycline.**

CALCIUM GLUCONATE

1 g (10 ml) contains 93 mg (4.65 mEq) calcium.

Administration and Dosage:

For IV use only, either directly or by infusion; SC or IM injection may cause severe necrosis and sloughing. Do not exceed a rate of 0.5 to 2 ml/minute. Calcium gluconate may also be administered by intermittent infusion at a rate not exceeding 200 mg/min, or by continuous infusion. Discontinue injection if the patient complains of discomfort. Do not use IM, as abscess formation and local necrosis may occur.

Adults: 2.3 to 9.3 mEq (5 to 20 ml) as required. Dosage range is 4.65 to 70 mEq/day.

Children: 2.3 mEq/kg/day or 56 mEq/m^2/day, well diluted; give slowly in divided doses.

Infants: Not more than 0.93 mEq (2 ml).

Emergency elevation of serum calcium:

Adults – 7 to 14 mEq (15 to 30.1 ml) IV.

Children – 1 to 7 mEq (2.2 to 15 ml).

Infants – < 1 mEq (2.2 ml). Depending on patient response, these doses can be repeated every 1 to 3 days.

Hypocalcemic tetany:

Adults – 4.5 to 16 mEq of calcium (9.7 to 34.4 ml) may be given IM until therapeutic response occurs.

Children – 0.5 to 0.7 ,mEq/kg (1.1 to 1.5 ml/kg) IV 3 or 4 times daily or until tetany is controlled.

Neonates – 2.4 mEq/kg/day (5.2 ml/kg/day) in divided doses.

Hyperkalemia with secondary cardiac toxicity: Administer IV to provide 2.25 to 14 mEq (4.8 to 30.1 ml) while monitoring ECG. If necessary, repeat doses after 1 to 2 min.

Magnesium intoxication:

Adults – Initial dose is 4.5 to 9 mEq (9.7 to 19.4 ml) IV. Adjust subsequent doses to patient response. If IV use is not possible, give 2 to 5 mEq (4.3 to 10.8 ml) IM.

Exchange transfusion:

Adults – Approximately 1.35 mEq (2.9 ml) IV concurrent with each 100 ml of citrated blood.

Neonates – Administer IV at a dosage of 0.45 mEq (1 ml)/100 ml of exchanged citrated blood.

Stability: If precipitation has occurred in syringes, do not use. If precipitation is present in vials or amps dissolve by heating to 80°C (146°F) in a dry heat oven for a minimum of 1 hour. Shake vigorously; allow to cool to room temperature. Do not use if precipitate remains.

Rx	**Calcium Gluconate** (Various, eg, American Regent, Astra, Elkins-Sinn, IDE, IMS, Lyphomed, McGuff, Rugby)	**Injection:** 10%	In 10 ml amps and syringes, 10 and 50 ml single dose vials and 100 and 200 ml pharmacy bulk vials.[1]

[1] Not for direct infusion; dilute prior to use.

CALCIUM GLUCEPTATE

1.1 g (5 ml) contains 90 mg (4.5 mEq) calcium.

Administration and Dosage:

IM: 2 to 5 ml (0.44 to 1.1 g). Inject 5 ml (1.1 g) doses in the gluteal region or, in infants, in the lateral thigh.

IV: 5 to 20 ml (1.1 to 4.4 g). Warm solution to body temperature and administer slowly (≤ 2 ml/min).

Exchange transfusions in newborns: 0.5 ml (0.11 g) after every 100 ml of blood exchanged.

Storage/stability: Do not administer unless solution is clear; do not use if crystals are present. Discard unused portion.

Rx	**Calcium Gluceptate** (Abbott)	**Injection:** 1.1 g per 5 ml	In 5 ml amps and 5 ml fill in 10 ml vial.[2]

[2] With 5 mg/ml monothioglycerol.

Electrolytes

CALCIUM CHLORIDE

1 g (10 ml) contains 273 mg (13.6 mEq) calcium.

Administration and Dosage:

For IV use only. Injection is irritating to veins and must not be injected into tissues, since severe necrosis and sloughing may occur. Avoid extravasation. Administer slowly (not to exceed 0.5 to 1 ml/minute).

Intraventricular administration – In cardiac resuscitation, injection may be made into the ventricular cavity; do not inject into the myocardium. Intraventricular injection may be administered by personnel who are well trained in the technique and familiar with possible complications. Break off the IV needle supplied with the syringe and replace with a suitable intracardiac needle by affixing it firmly to the Luer taper provided on the syringe. After the injection has been completed, remove the needle/syringe assembly from the injection site by grasping the needle at the Luer fitting.

The intraventricular dose usually ranges from 200 to 800 mg (2 to 8 ml).

Hypocalcemic disorders:

Adults – 500 mg to 1 g at intervals of 1 to 3 days, depending on response of patient or serum calcium determinations. Repeated injections may be required.

Children – 0.2 ml/kg up to 1 to 10 ml/day.

Magnesium intoxication: Give 500 mg promptly; observe patient for signs of recovery before further doses are given.

Hyperkalemic ECG disturbances of cardiac function: Adjust dosage by constant monitoring of ECG changes during administration.

Cardiac resuscitation:

Adults – Dose ranges from 500 mg to 1 g IV or 200 to 800 mg injected into the ventricular cavity.

Children – 0.2 ml/kg.

Rx	**Calcium Chloride** (Various, eg, Abbott, American Regent, Astra, IMS, Lyphomed, Moore, VHA)	**Injection:** 10%	In 10 ml amps, vials and syringes.

CALCIUM PRODUCTS COMBINED, PARENTERAL

Rx	**Calphosan** (Glenwood)	**Injection:** 50 mg calcium glycerophosphate and 50 mg calcium lactate per 10 ml in sodium chloride solution (0.08 mEq Ca/ml)	In 60 ml vials.[1]

[1] With 0.25% phenol.

Electrolytes

MAGNESIUM

For information on oral magnesium, refer to the Minerals and Electrolytes, Oral section. For information on the use of magnesium sulfate as an anticonvulsant, refer to the monograph in the Anticonvulsants section.

Actions:

Pharmacology: Magnesium is a cofactor in a number of enzyme systems, and is involved in neurochemical transmission and muscular excitability. As a nutritional adjunct in hyperalimentation, the precise mechanism of action is uncertain.

Magnesium deficiency is rare in well nourished individuals, except in malabsorption syndromes. Magnesium deficiency may occur in malabsorption syndromes, chronic alcoholism, malnutrition, intestinal bypass surgery, diuretic therapy, severe diarrhea, prolonged nasogastric suction, steatorrhea, during hemodialysis, diabetes mellitus, pancreatitis, primary aldosteronism and renal tubular damage. Early symptoms of hypomagnesemia (< 1.5 mEq/L) may develop as early as 3 to 4 days or within weeks. Predominant deficiency effects are neurological (eg, muscle irritability, clonic twitching, tremors). Hypocalcemia and hypokalemia often follow low serum levels of magnesium. While large stores of magnesium are found intracellularly and in bone in adults, they often are not mobilized sufficiently to maintain plasma levels. Parenteral magnesium therapy repairs the plasma deficit and causes deficiency signs and symptoms to cease. The normal adult body contains 20 to 30 g (2000 mEq) magnesium.

Magnesium prevents or controls convulsions by blocking neuromuscular transmission and decreasing the amount of acetylcholine liberated at the end plate by the motor nerve impulse. Magnesium is said to have a depressant effect on the CNS, but it does not adversely affect the mother, fetus or neonate when used as directed in eclampsia or preeclampsia. Normal plasma magnesium levels range from 1.5 to 2.5 mEq.

Magnesium acts peripherally to produce vasodilation. With low doses, only flushing and sweating occur; larger doses cause a lowering of blood pressure and CNS depression. The central and peripheral effects of magnesium poisoning are antagonized by IV administration of calcium.

One g of magnesium sulfate provides 8.12 mEq of magnesium.

Hypermagnesemia – As plasma magnesium rises above 4 mEq/L, the deep tendon reflexes are first decreased and then disappear as the plasma level approaches 10 mEq/L. At this level respiratory paralysis may occur. Heart block also may occur at this or lower plasma levels of magnesium. Serum magnesium concentrations in excess of 12 mEq may be fatal.

Pharmacokinetics: IM injection results in therapeutic plasma levels within 60 minutes and persists for 3 to 4 hours. IV doses provide immediate effects that last for 30 minutes. Effective anticonvulsant serum levels range from 2.5 to 7.5 mEq/L. Magnesium is excreted by the kidneys at a rate proportional to the plasma concentration and glomerular filtration.

Indications:

Hypomagnesemia: Magnesium sulfate is used as replacement therapy in magnesium deficiency especially in acute hypomagnesemia accompanied by signs of tetany similar to those observed in hypocalcemia. In such cases, the serum magnesium (Mg^{++}) level is usually below the lower limit of normal (1.5 to 2.5 or 3 mEq/L) and the serum calcium (Ca^{++}) level is normal (4.3 to 5.3 mEq/L) or elevated.

Total parenteral nutrition patients may develop hypomagnesemia (< 1.5 mEq/L) without supplementation. Magnesium is added to correct or prevent hypomagnesemia.

Preeclampsia/eclampsia/nephritis (magnesium sulfate): Prevention and control of convulsions of severe preeclampsia and eclampsia and for control of hypertension, encephalopathy and convulsions associated with acute nephritis in children (see monograph in Anticonvulsants, Miscellaneous section).

Unlabeled uses: Inhibition of premature labor (tocolytic); however, it is not a first-line agent.

In suspected acute myocardial infarction patients immediately after admission to counteract post-infarctional hypomagnesemia and subsequent arrhythmias.

Magnesium IV is effective as a bronchodilator and, therefore, may be useful in some asthmatic patients.

Since magnesium deficiency may play a role in chronic fatigue syndrome, it has been suggested that magnesium administration may be beneficial in this condition; however, there are conflicting reports and further study is needed.

Electrolytes

MAGNESIUM

Contraindications:

Magnesium sulfate: Heart block or myocardial damage; IV magnesium to patients with preeclampsia during the 2 hours preceding delivery.

Magnesium chloride: Renal impairment; marked myocardial disease; coma.

Warnings:

Renal function impairment: Because magnesium is excreted by the kidneys, use with caution. Parenteral use in the presence of renal insufficiency may lead to magnesium intoxication.

Elderly: Geriatric patients often require reduced dosage because of impaired renal function. In patients with severe impairment, dosage should not exceed 20 g in 48 hours. Monitor serum magnesium in such patients.

Pregnancy: Category A. Studies in pregnant women have not shown that magnesium sulfate injection increases the risk of fetal abnormalities if administered during all trimesters of pregnancy. If this drug is used during pregnancy, the possibility of fetal harm appears remote. However, because studies cannot rule out the possibility of harm, use during pregnancy only if clearly needed.

When administered by continuous IV infusion (especially for > 24 hours preceding delivery) to control convulsions in toxemic mothers, the newborn may show signs of magnesium toxicity, including neuromuscular or respiratory depression (see Overdosage).

Lactation: Since magnesium is distributed into milk during parenteral magnesium sulfate administration, use with caution in nursing women.

Children: Safety and efficacy in children have not been established.

Precautions:

Monitoring: Maintain urine output at a level of ≥ 100 ml every 4 hours. Monitor serum magnesium levels and clinical status to avoid overdosage in preeclampsia. See Overdosage for serum level/toxicity relationships.

Clinical indications of safe dosage regimen include presence of the patellar reflex (knee jerk) and absence of respiratory depression (≈ 16 breaths or more/min). Serum magnesium levels usually sufficient to control convulsions range from 3 to 6 mg/dl (2.5 to 5 mEq/L). Strength of deep tendon reflexes begins to diminish when magnesium levels exceed 4 mEq/L. Reflexes may be absent at 10 mEq/L, where respiratory paralysis is possible. Keep an injectable calcium salt immediately available to counteract potential hazards of magnesium intoxication in eclampsia.

Flushing/Sweating: Administer with caution if flushing or sweating occurs.

Hypomagnesemia: Do not administer magnesium sulfate injection unless hypomagnesemia is confirmed.

Drug Interactions:

Neuromuscular blocking agents, nondepolarizing: Neuromuscular blocking effects may be increased by concurrent magnesium sulfate. Prolonged respiratory depression with extended periods of apnea may occur.

Adverse Reactions:

Adverse effects are usually the result of magnesium intoxication and include: Flushing; sweating; hypotension; stupor; depressed reflexes; flaccid paralysis; hypothermia; circulatory collapse; cardiac and CNS depression proceeding to respiratory paralysis (the most life-threatening effect).

Hypocalcemia with signs of tetany secondary to magnesium sulfate therapy for eclampsia has occurred.

Overdosage:

Symptoms: Sharp drop in blood pressure and respiratory paralysis. ECG changes may include increased PR interval, increased QRS complex and prolonged QT interval. Disappearance of the patellar reflex is a useful clinical sign to detect the onset of magnesium intoxication.

Although patients usually tolerate high concentrations of magnesium in plasma, there are occasional instances when cardiac consequences may be seen in the form of complete heart block at concentrations well below 10 mEq/L.

Other signs include muscle weakness, hypotension, sedation and confusion. As plasma concentrations of magnesium begin to exceed 4 mEq/L, deep-tendon reflexes are decreased and may be absent at levels approaching 10 mEq/L.

When magnesium sulfate injection is administered parenterally in doses that are sufficient to induce hypermagnesemia, the drug has a depressant effect on the CNS and, via the peripheral neuromuscular junction, on muscle.

Electrolytes

MAGNESIUM

Approximate Correlation of Magnesium Toxicity vs Serum Level	
Serum level (mEq/L)	Effect
1.5 to 2.5	Normal serum concentration
4 to 7	"Therapeutic" level for preeclampsia/ eclampsia/convulsions
7 to 10	Loss of deep tendon reflexes, hypotension, narcosis
12 to 15	Respiratory paralysis
> 15	Cardiac conduction affected. PR interval lengthening, QRS widening, dysrhythmias
> 25	Cardiac arrest

Treatment: Provide artificial ventilation until a calcium salt (10 to 20 ml of a 5% solution, diluted with isotonic Sodium Chloride for Injection if desired) can be injected IV to antagonize the effects of magnesium. A dose of 5 to 10 mEq calcium will usually reverse the respiratory depression and heart block. Physostigmine 0.5 to 1 mg SC may be helpful. Peritoneal dialysis or hemodialysis are also effective.

Hypermagnesemia in the newborn may require resuscitation and assisted ventilation via endotracheal intubation or intermittent positive pressure ventilation as well as IV calcium.

Administration and Dosage:

IV administration: Do not exceed 1.5 ml/min of a 10% concentration (or its equivalent), except in cases of severe eclampsia with seizures. Dilute IV infusion solutions to a concentration of ≤ 20% prior to IV administration. The most commonly used diluents are 5% Dextrose Injection and 0.9% Sodium Chloride Injection.

IM administration: Deep IM injection of the undiluted (50%) solution is appropriate for adults, but dilute to ≤ 20% concentration prior to IM injection in children.

Admixture incompatibilities: Magnesium sulfate in solution may result in a precipitate formation when mixed with solutions containing: Alcohol (in high concentrations); alkali carbonates and bicarbonates; alkali hydroxides; arsenates; barium; calcium; clindamycin phosphate; heavy metals; hydrocortisone sodium succinate; phosphates; polymyxin B sulfate; procaine HCl; salicylates; strontium; tartrates.

Hyperalimentation: Maintenance requirements are not precisely known. Maintenance dose range:

Adults – 8 to 24 mEq/day.
Infants – 2 to 10 mEq/day.

Mild magnesium deficiency:

Adults – 1 g (8.12 mEq; 2 ml of 50% solution) IM every 6 hours for 4 doses (total of 32.5 mEq/24 hours).

Severe hypomagnesemia:

IM – As much as 2 mEq/kg (0.5 ml of 50% solution) within 4 hours if necessary.

IV – 5 g (≈ 40 mEq)/L of 5% Dextrose Injection or 0.9% Sodium Chloride solution, infused over 3 hours. In treatment of deficiency states, observe caution to prevent exceeding renal excretory capacity.

Seizures associated with preeclampsia/eclampsia/nephritis: Refer to Anticonvulsants, Miscellaneous for complete dosing information.

Rx	**Magnesium Chloride** (Various, eg, American Regent, McGuff)	**Injection**: 20% (1.97 mEq/ml)	In 50 ml multiple dose vials.
Rx	**Magnesium Sulfate** (Various, eg, Astra, Lyphomed, Pasadena)	**Injection**: 10% (0.8 mEq/ml)	In 20 and 50 ml vials and 20 ml amps.
Rx	**Magnesium Sulfate** (Various, eg, Abbott)	**Injection**: 12.5% (1 mEq/ml)	In 20 ml vials.
Rx	**Magnesium Sulfate** (Various, eg, Abbott, American Regent, Astra, IMS, Lyphomed, McGuff, Pasadena, Smith & Nephew Solopak)	**Injection**: 50% (4 mEq/ml)	In 2, 5, 10, 20 and 50 ml vials, 5 and 10 ml syringes, 2 and 10 ml amps.

SODIUM BICARBONATE

For information on oral sodium bicarbonate, refer to Minerals and Electrolytes, Oral.

Actions:

Pharmacology: Increases plasma bicarbonate; buffers excess hydrogen ion concentration; raises blood pH; reverses the clinical manifestations of acidosis.

One g sodium bicarbonate provides 11.9 mEq each of sodium and bicarbonate.

Pharmacokinetics: Sodium bicarbonate in water dissociates to provide sodium (Na^+) and bicarbonate (HCO_3^-) ions. Sodium is the principal cation of extracellular fluid. Bicarbonate is a normal constituent of body fluids and normal plasma level ranges from 24 to 31 mEq/L. Plasma concentration is regulated by the kidney. Bicarbonate anion is considered "labile" since, at a proper concentration of hydrogen ion (H^+), it may be converted to carbonic acid (H_2CO_3), then to its volatile form, carbon dioxide (CO_2), excreted by lungs. Normally, a ratio of 1:20 (carbonic acid: bicarbonate) is present in extracellular fluid. In a healthy adult with normal kidney function, almost all the glomerular filtered bicarbonate ion is reabsorbed; < 1% is excreted in urine.

Indications:

Metabolic acidosis: In severe renal disease, uncontrolled diabetes, circulatory insufficiency due to shock, anoxia or severe dehydration, extracorporeal circulation of blood, cardiac arrest and severe primary lactic acidosis where a rapid increase in plasma total CO_2 content is crucial. Treat metabolic acidosis in addition to measures designed to control the cause of the acidosis (eg, insulin in uncomplicated diabetes, blood volume restoration in shock). Since an appreciable time interval may elapse before all ancillary effects occur, bicarbonate therapy is indicated to minimize risks inherent to acidosis itself.

At one time it was suggested to administer bicarbonate during cardiopulmonary resuscitation following cardiac arrest; however, recent evidence suggests that little benefit is provided and its use may be detrimental. For treatment of acidosis in this clinical situation, concentrate efforts on restoring ventilation and blood flow. According to the American Heart Association guidelines, use as a last resort after other standard measures have been utilized.

Urinary alkalinization: In the treatment of certain drug intoxications (eg, salicylates, lithium) and in hemolytic reactions requiring alkalinization of the urine to diminish nephrotoxicity of blood pigments.

Severe diarrhea which is often accompanied by a significant loss of bicarbonate.

Neutralizing additive solution: To reduce the incidence of chemical phlebitis and patient discomfort due to vein irritation at or near the infusion site by raising the pH of IV acid solutions.

Contraindications:

Losing chloride by vomiting or from continuous GI suction; receiving diuretics known to produce a hypochloremic alkalosis; metabolic and respiratory alkalosis; hypocalcemia in which alkalosis may produce tetany, hypertension, convulsions or congestive heart failure (CHF); when sodium use could be clinically detrimental.

Neutralizing additive solution: Do not use as a systemic alkalinizer.

Warnings:

Cardiac effects:

Cardiac arrest – The risk of rapid infusion must be weighed against the potential for fatality due to acidosis.

CHF – Since sodium accompanies bicarbonate, use cautiously in patients with CHF or other edematous or sodium-retaining states.

Fluid/Solute overload: IV administration can cause fluid or solute overloading resulting in dilution of serum electrolyte concentrations, overhydration, congested states or pulmonary edema. The risk of dilutional states is inversely proportional to the electrolyte concentrations of administered parenteral solutions. The risk of solute overload causing congested states with peripheral and acute pulmonary edema is directly proportional to the electrolyte concentrations of such solutions. Rapid or excessive administration of Sodium Bicarbonate Injection may produce tetany due to a decrease in ionized calcium and hypokalemia as potassium reenters the cells. Hypertonic solutions may cause vein damage. Avoid extravasation.

Neonates and children (< 2 years old): Rapid injection (10 ml/min) of hypertonic sodium bicarbonate solutions may produce hypernatremia, a decrease in cerebrospinal fluid pressure and possible intracranial hemorrhage. Do not administer > 8mEq/kg/day. A 4.2% solution is preferred for such slow administration.

Electrolytes

SODIUM BICARBONATE

Renal function impairment: Administration of solutions containing sodium ions may result in sodium retention. Use with caution. Also use cautiously in oliguria or anuria.

Elderly: Exercise particular care when administering sodium-containing solutions to elderly or postoperative patients with renal or cardiovascular insuffiency, with or without CHF.

Pregnancy: Category C. It is not known whether sodium bicarbonate can cause fetal harm when administered to a pregnant woman. Use only if clearly needed.

Lactation: It is not known whether this drug is excreted in breast milk. Exercise caution when administering to a nursing woman.

Precautions:

Monitoring: Adverse reactions may result from an excess or deficit of one or more of the ions in the solution; frequent monitoring of electrolyte levels is essential.

Avoid overdosage and alkalosis by giving repeated small doses and periodic monitoring by appropriate laboratory tests.

Potassium depletion may predispose to metabolic alkalosis, and coexistent hypocalcemia may be associated with carpopedal spasm as the plasma pH rises. Minimize by treating electrolyte imbalances prior to or concomitantly with bicarbonate.

Chloride loss: Patients losing chloride by vomiting or GI intubation are more susceptible to developing severe alkalosis if given alkalinizing agents.

Neutralizing additive solution: Administer this solution promptly. When introducing additives, mix thoroughly and do not store. Raising pH of IV fluids with neutralizing additive solution will only reduce incidence of chemical irritation caused by infusate; it will not diminish any foreign body effects caused by needle or catheter.

Extraordinary electrolyte losses such as may occur during protracted nasogastric suction, vomiting, diarrhea or GI fistula drainage may necessitate additional electrolyte supplementation.

Drug Interactions:

Sodium Bicarbonate Drug Interactions

Precipitant drug	Object drug*		Description
Sodium bicarbonate	Chlorpropamide Lithium Methotrexate Salicylates Tetracyclines	⬇	The renal clearance of these agents may be increased due to alkalinization of the urine, possibly resulting in a decreased pharmacologic effect.
Sodium bicarbonate	Anorexiants Flecainide Mecamylamine Quinidine Sympathomimetics	⬆	The renal clearance of these agents may be decreased due to alkalinizaton of the urine, possibly resulting in increased pharmacologic or toxic effects.

* ⬆ = Object drug increased. ⬇ = Object drug decreased.

Adverse Reactions:

Symptoms: Extravasation of IV hypertonic solutions of sodium bicarbonate may cause chemical cellulitis (because of their alkalinity), with tissue necrosis, ulceration or sloughing at the site of infiltration. Prompt elevation of the part, warmth and local injection of lidocaine or hyaluronidase are recommended to prevent sloughing.

Too rapid infusion of hypertonic solutions may cause local pain and venous irritation. Adjust the rate of administration according to tolerance. Use of the largest peripheral vein and a well placed small bore needle is recommended.

Too rapid or excessive administration may result in hypernatremia and alkalosis accompanied by hyperirritability or tetany. Hypernatremia may be associated with edema and exacerbation of CHF due to the retention of water, resulting in an expanded extracellular fluid volume.

Reactions that may occur because of the solution or the technique of administration include febrile response, infection at the site of injection, venous thrombosis or phlebitis extending from the injection site, extravasation and hypervolemia.

SODIUM BICARBONATE

Treatment: If an adverse reaction does occur, discontinue the infusion, evaluate the patient, institute appropriate therapeutic countermeasures and save the remainder of the fluid for examination if deemed necessary.

Overdosage:

Symptoms: Excessive or too rapid administration may produce alkalosis. Severe alkalosis may be accompanied by hyperirritability or tetany.

Treatment: Discontinue sodium bicarbonate. Control symptoms of alkalosis by rebreathing expired air from a paper bag or rebreathing mask or, if more severe, by parenteral injections of calcium gluconate (to control tetany and hyperexcitability). Correct severe alkalosis by IV infusion of 2.14% ammonium chloride solution, except in patients with hepatic disease, in whom ammonia use is contraindicated. Sodium chloride (0.9%) IV or potassium chloride may be indicated if there is hypokalemia.

Administration and Dosage:

Administer IV or SC following dilution to isotonicity (1.5%). For IV administration, suitable concentrations range from 1.5% (isotonic) to 8.4% (undiluted), depending on the clinical condition and requirements of the patient. Suitable dilution can be calculated from the following formula:

$$\text{conc}_1 \times \text{volume}_1 = \text{conc}_2 \times \text{volume}_2$$

Thus, $8.4\% \times 50\text{ ml} = 1.5\% \times 280\text{ ml}$; or $7.5\% \times 50\text{ ml} = 1.5\% \times 250\text{ ml}$; or $4.2\% \times 10\text{ ml} = 1.5\% \times 28\text{ ml}$.

The diluent may be Sterile Water for Injection, Sodium Chloride Injection, 5% Dextrose or other standard electrolyte solutions. For SC administration, an isotonic solution (1.5%) of sodium bicarbonate can be prepared by diluting 1 ml (84 mg) of 8.4% solution with 4.6 ml Sterile Water for Injection. For 7.5% solution, dilute 1 ml (75 mg) with 4 ml Sterile Water for Injection. For 4.2% solution, dilute 1ml (42 mg) with 1.8 ml Sterile Water for Injection.

Cardiac arrest: Bicarbonate administration in this situation may be detrimental. See Indications. Administer according to results of arterial blood pH and $PaCO_2$ and calculation of base deficit. Flush IV lines before and after use.

Adults – A rapid IV dose of 200 to 300 mEq of bicarbonate, given as a 7.5% or 8.4% solution. Observe caution where rapid infusion of large quantities of bicarbonate is indicated. Bicarbonate solutions are hypertonic and may produce an undesirable rise in plasma sodium concentration. In cardiac arrest, however, the risks from acidosis exceed those of hypernatremia.

In emergencies, administer 300 to 500 ml of 5% sodium bicarbonate injection as rapidly as possible without overalkalinizing the patient. To avoid overalkalinizing a patient whose own body mechanisms for correcting metabolic acidosis may be maximally stimulated, only one-third to one-half of the calculated dose is administered as rapidly as indicated by the patient's cardiovascular and fluid balance status. Then, redetermine serum pH and bicarbonate concentration.

Infants (≤ 2 years of age) – 4.2% solution for IV administration at a rate not to exceed 8 mEq/kg/day to guard against the possibility of producing hypernatremia, decreasing CSF pressure and inducing intracranial hemorrhage.

Initial dose – 1 to 2 mEq/kg/min given over 1 to 2 minutes followed by 1 mEq/kg every 10 minutes of arrest. If base deficit is known, give calculated dose of 0.3 × kg × base deficit. If only 7.5% or 8.4% sodium bicarbonate is available, dilute 1:1 with 5% Dextrose in Water before administration.

Severe metabolic acidosis: Administer 90 to 180 mEq/L (≈ 7.5 to 15 g) at a rate of 1 to 1.5 L during the first hour. Adjust to patient's needs for further management.

Electrolytes

SODIUM BICARBONATE

Less urgent forms of metabolic acidosis: Sodium Bicarbonate Injection may be added to other IV fluids. The amount of bicarbonate to be given to older children and adults over a 4 to 8 hour period is approximately 2 to 5 mEq/kg, depending on the severity of the acidosis as judged by the lowering of total CO_2 content, blood pH and clinical condition. Initially, an infusion of 2 to 5 mEq/kg over 4 to 8 hours will produce improvement in the acid-base status of the blood.

Alternatively, estimates of the initial dose of sodium bicarbonate may be based on the following equation:

$$0.5\ (L/kg) \times \text{body weight (kg)} \times \text{desired increase in serum } HCO_3^-\ (mEq/L) = \text{bicarbonate dose (mEq)}$$

or

$$0.5\ (L/kg) \times \text{body weight (kg)} \times \text{base deficit (mEq/L)} = \text{bicarbonate dose (mEq)}.$$

The next step of therapy is dependent on the clinical response of the patient. If severe symptoms have abated, reduce frequency of administration and dose.

If the CO_2 plasma content is unknown, a safe average dose of sodium bicarbonate is 5 mEq (420 mg)/kg.

It is unwise to attempt full correction of a low total CO_2 content during the first 24 hours, since this may accompany an unrecognized alkalosis due to delayed readjustment of ventilation to normal. Thus, achieving total CO_2 content of about 20 mEq/L at the end of the first day will usually be associated with a normal blood pH. Further modification of the acidosis to completely normal values usually occurs in the presence of normal kidney function when and if the cause of the acidosis can be controlled. Total CO_2 brought to normal or above normal within the first day may be associated with grossly alkaline blood pH.

If administration is controlled by a pumping device, discontinue pumping action before the container runs dry or air embolism may result.

Neutralizing additive solution: One vial of neutralizing additive solution added to 1 L of any of the commonly used parenteral solutions including Dextrose, Sodium Chloride, Ringer's, etc, will increase the pH to a more physiologic range (specific pH may vary slightly).

Note – Some products such as amino acid solutions and multiple electrolyte solutions containing dextrose will not be brought to near physiologic pH by the addition of sodium bicarbonate neutralizing additive solution. This is due to the relatively high buffer capacity of these fluids.

Admixture incompatibilities: Avoid adding sodium bicarbonate to parenteral solutions containing **calcium**, except where compatibility is established; precipitation or haze may result. **Norepinephrine** and **dobutamine** are incompatible.

Storage/Stability: Store at 15° to 30°C (59° to 86°F). Avoid excessive heat. Protect from freezing. Brief exposure up to 40°C does not adversely affect the product. Replace administration apparatus at least once every 24 hours.

Electrolytes

SODIUM BICARBONATE

Rx	**Sodium Bicarbonate** (Abbott)	**Injection**: 4.2% (0.5 mEq/ml)	In 10 ml (5 mEq) syringes.
Rx	**Sodium Bicarbonate** (Astra)		In 2.5 and 5 ml fill in 5 and 10 ml syringes.
Rx	**Sodium Bicarbonate** (Lyphomed)		In 10 ml (5 mEq) *Bristoject* syringes.
Rx	**Sodium Bicarbonate** (Abbott)	**Injection**: 5% (0.6 mEq/ml)	In 500 ml[1] (297.5 mEq).
Rx	**Sodium Bicarbonate** (Baxter)		In 500 ml (297.5 mEq).
Rx	**Sodium Bicarbonate** (McGaw)		In 500 ml[1](297.5 mEq).
Rx	**Sodium Bicarbonate** (Abbott)	**Injection**: 7.5% (0.9 mEq/ml)	In 50 ml (44.6 mEq) amps and 50 ml (44.6 mEq) syringes.
Rx	**Sodium Bicarbonate** (American Regent)		In 50 ml (44.6 mEq) vials.
Rx	**Sodium Bicarbonate** (Astra)		In 44.6 ml fill in 50 ml syringes.
Rx	**Sodium Bicarbonate** (Lyphomed)		In 50 ml (44.6 mEq) single-dose vials, 50 ml (44.6 mEq) *Bristoject* syringes and 200 ml (179 mEq) *MaxiVials.*
Rx	**Sodium Bicarbonate** (Abbott)	**Injection**: 8.4% (1 mEq/ml)	In 50 ml (50 mEq) fliptop vials and 10 ml (10 mEq) and 50 ml (50 mEq) syringes.
Rx	**Sodium Bicarbonate** (American Regent)		In 50ml (50 mEq) vials.
Rx	**Sodium Bicarbonate** (Astra)		In 10 and 50 ml syringes.
Rx	**Sodium Bicarbonate** (Lyphomed)		In 50 ml (50 mEq) vials and 10 and 50 mEq Bristoject syringes.
Rx	**Neut** (Abbott)	**Neutralizing Additive Solution**[2]: 4% (0.48 mEq/ml)	In 5 ml (2.4 mEq) fliptop and pintop vials.[1]
Rx	**Sodium Bicarbonate** (Lyphomed)	**Neutralizing Additive Solution**[2]: 4.2% (0.5 mEq/ml)	In 5 ml fill in 6 ml vials (2.5 mEq).

[1] With EDTA.

[2] For use as a neutralizing additive solution to acidic large volume parenterals.

Electrolytes

SODIUM LACTATE

Complete prescribing information for these products begins in the Sodium Bicarbonate monograph.

Actions:

Pharmacology: One liter of Molar sodium lactate (isotonic) administered IV is potentially equivalent in alkalinizing effect to approximately 280 ml of 5% sodium bicarbonate. One g of sodium lactate provides 8.9 mEq of sodium and of lactate.

Pharmacokinetics: Sodium lactate is metabolized to bicarbonate in the liver. The alkalinizing effects of sodium lactate result from simultaneous removal of lactate and hydrogen ions. Lactate is metabolized to glycogen and ultimately converted to carbon dioxide and water in the liver. The conversion of sodium lactate to bicarbonate requires 1 to 2 hours.

Indications:

As an alkalinizing agent for the treatment of metabolic acidosis resulting from starvation, acute infections, diabetic acidosis, diarrhea and vomiting, or renal failure.

Warnings:

Hepatic function impairment/severe illness: Conversion of lactate to bicarbonate may be impaired in the severely ill and in persons with hepatic disease.

Severe acidosis: Not intended nor effective for correcting severe acidotic states that require immediate restoration of plasma bicarbonate levels. Sodium lactate has no advantage over sodium bicarbonate and may be detrimental in the management of lactic acidosis.

Rx	**1/6 Molar Sodium Lactate** (Various, eg, Abbott, Baxter, McGaw)	**Injection** 167 mEq/L each of sodium and lactate ions	In 500 and 1000 ml.

SODIUM ACETATE

Complete prescribing information for these products begins in the Sodium Bicarbonate monograph.

Actions:

Pharmacology: The acetate ion is metabolized to bicarbonate almost on an equimolar basis. Metabolism occurs outside the liver. One g of sodium acetate provides 7.3 mEq of sodium and of acetate.

Indications:

Useful in acidotic states. Used as a source of sodium in large volume IV fluids to prevent or correct hyponatremia in patients with restricted intake. Useful for preparing IV fluid formulas when patient needs cannot be met by standard electrolyte or nutrient solutions.

Rx	**Sodium Acetate** (Various, eg, Abbott, American Regent, Lyphomed)	**Injection**: 2 mEq each of sodium and acetate per ml (16.4%)	In 20, 50 and 100 ml vials.
Rx	**Sodium Acetate** (Various, eg, American Regent, LyphoMed)	**Injection**: 4 mEq each of sodium and acetate per ml (32.8%)	In 50 and 100 ml vials.

Electrolytes

TROMETHAMINE

Actions:

Pharmacology: Tromethamine, a highly alkaline, sodium-free organic amine, acts as a proton acceptor to prevent or correct acidosis. When administered IV as a 0.3 M solution, it combines with hydrogen ions from carbonic acid to form bicarbonate and a cationic buffer. It also acts as an osmotic diuretic, increasing urine flow, urinary pH and excretion of fixed acids, carbon dioxide and electrolytes.

Pharmacokinetics: At pH 7.4, 30% of tromethamine is not ionized and therefore is capable of reaching equilibrium in total body water. This portion may penetrate cells and may neutralize acidic ions of the intracellular fluid. The drug is rapidly eliminated by the kidneys; ≥ 75% appears in urine after 8 hours and the remainder within 3 days.

Indications:

Prevention and correction of systemic acidosis in the following conditions: Metabolic acidosis associated with cardiac bypass surgery; correction of acidity of Acid Citrate Dextrose (ACD) blood in cardiac bypass surgery; cardiac arrest.

Contraindications:

Anuria; uremia.

Warnings:

Administer slowly: Correct only the existing acidosis; avoid overdosage and alkalosis.

Duration of therapy: Because clinical experience has been limited generally to short-term use, do not administer for > 1 day except in a life-threatening situation.

Respiratory depression, although infrequent, may be more likely in patients with chronic hypoventilation or those treated with drugs which depress respiration. Large doses may depress ventilation due to increased blood pH and reduced CO_2 concentration. Adjust dosage so that blood pH does not increase above normal. If respiratory acidosis is present concomitantly with metabolic acidosis, the drug may be used with mechanical assistance to ventilation.

Perivascular infiltration of this highly alkaline solution may cause inflammation, vascular spasms and tissue damage (eg, necrosis, sloughing, chemical phlebitis, thrombosis). Place the needle within the largest available vein and infuse slowly (see Adverse Reactions).

Hemorrhagic hepatic necrosis has occurred in newborns when a hypertonic solution of tromethamine was administered via the umbilical vein.

Renal function impairment demands extreme care because of potential hyperkalemia and possible decreased excretion of tromethamine. Monitor ECG and serum potassium.

Pregnancy: Category C. It is not known whether tromethamine can cause fetal harm when administered to a pregnant woman or can affect reproduction capacity. Give to a pregnant woman only if clearly needed.

Children: Severe hemorrhagic liver necrosis has occurred in neonates.

Hypoglycemia may occur when administered to premature or even full term neonates.

Precautions:

Monitoring: Measure blood pH, pCO_2, bicarbonate, glucose and electrolytes before, during and after administration.

Electrolytes

TROMETHAMINE

Adverse Reactions:

Generally, side effects are infrequent. Transient depression of blood glucose; respiratory depression, hemorrhagic hepatic necrosis (see Warnings).

Local: Local reactions that may occur because of the solution or the technique of administration include: Febrile response; infection at injection site; venous thrombosis or phlebitis extending from the site of extravasation; hypervolemia.

Overdosage:

Symptoms: Overdosage, in terms of total drug or too rapid administration, may cause alkalosis, overhydration, solute overload and severe prolonged hypoglycemia (several hours).

Treatment: Discontinue infusion and institute appropriate countermeasures.

Administration and Dosage:

Administer by slow IV infusion, by addition to pump oxygenator ACD blood or other priming fluid, or by injection into the ventricular cavity during cardiac arrest.

For peripheral vein infusion, use a large needle in the largest antecubital vein or place an indwelling catheter in a large vein of an elevated limb to minimize chemical irritation by the alkaline solution.

Avoid overtreatment (alkalosis). Measure pretreatment and subsequent blood values (eg, pH, pCO_2, pO_2, glucose, electrolytes) and urinary output to monitor dosage and progress of treatment. Limit dosage to increase blood pH to normal limits (7.35 to 7.45) and to correct acid-base derangements. Drug retention may occur, especially in patients with impaired renal function.

Dosage may be estimated from the buffer base deficit of the extracellular fluid (mEq/L) using the Siggaard-Andersen nomogram. The following formula is a general guide:

Tromethamine solution (ml of 0.3M) = body weight (kg) × base deficit (mEq/L) × 1.1*

Determine need for additional solution by serial measurements of existing base deficit.

Acidosis during cardiac bypass surgery: Average dose of approximately 9 ml/kg (2.7 mEq/kg or 0.32 g/kg). A total single dose of 500 ml (150 mEq or 18 g) is adequate for most adults. Larger single doses (up to 1000 ml) may be required in severe cases. Do not exceed individual doses of 500 mg/kg over a period of not less than 1 hour.

Acidity of ACD priming blood: Stored blood has a pH range from 6.22 to 6.8. Use from 0.5 to 2.5 g (15 to 77 ml) added to each 500 ml of ACD blood to correct acidity. Usually, 2 g (62 ml) added to 500 ml of ACD blood is adequate.

Acidosis associated with cardiac arrest: Administer at the same time that other standard resuscitative measures are being applied.

If the chest is open, inject 2 to 6 g (62 to 185 ml) directly into the ventricular cavity. Do not inject into the cardiac muscle. If the chest is not open, inject from 3.6 to 10.8 g (111 to 333 ml) into a large peripheral vein. Additional amounts may be required to control systemic acidosis persisting after cardiac arrest is reversed.

Stability/Storage: Highly alkaline solutions may erode glass; discard solutions of tromethamine 24 hours after reconstitution. Protect from freezing and extreme heat.

Rx	**Tham** (Abbott)	**Injection:** 18 g (150 mEq) per 500 ml (0.3M)	In 500 ml single dose container.[1]

[1] With acetic acid.

* Factor of 1.1 accounts for an approximate reduction of 10% in buffering capacity due to sufficient acetic acid to lower pH of the 0.3M solution without electrolytes to ≈ 8.6.

PHOSPHATE

Actions:

Pharmacology: A prominent component of all body tissues, phosphorus participates in bone deposition, regulation of calcium metabolism, buffering effects on acid-base equilibrium and various enzyme systems. In the extracellular fluid, phosphate exists as both a monovalent and a divalent form, the ratio of which is pH-dependent.

Normal serum inorganic phosphate levels are as follows:

Adults: 3 to 4.5 mg/dl.

Children: 4 to 7 mg/dl.

Hypophosphatemia –

Moderate (serum level ≤ 2.5 mg/dl): Symptoms include muscle weakness, malaise, paresthesias, CNS irritability, confusion, obtundation.

Severe (serum level < 1 mg/dl): Seizures, coma, respiratory failure, hemolytic anemia, rhabdomyolysis, tremors, platelet and leukocyte dysfunction.

Pharmacokinetics: Phosphate infused IV is excreted in the urine. Plasma phosphate is filtered by the renal glomeruli, and > 80% is actively reabsorbed by the tubules.

Indications:

A source of phosphate to add to large volume IV fluids, to prevent or correct hypophosphatemia in patients with restricted oral intake.

Additive for preparing specific IV fluid formulas when needs of patient cannot be met by standard electrolyte or nutrient solutions.

Contraindications:

High phosphate or low calcium levels.

Potassium phosphate: Hyperkalemia.

Sodium phosphate: Hypernatremia.

Warnings:

Electrolyte intoxication: To avoid phosphate, sodium or potassium intoxication, infuse solutions slowly.

Hypocalcemic tetany: Infusions of high concentrations of phosphate reduce serum calcium and produce symptoms of hypocalcemic tetany. Monitor calcium levels.

Cardiac effects: Use sodium phosphate with caution in patients with cardiac failure or who are on other edematous or sodium-retaining medications. Use potassium phosphate with caution in the presence of cardiac disease, particularly in digitalized patients. High plasma concentrations of potassium may cause death through cardiac depression or arrhythmias.

Adrenal insufficiency: Administration of phosphate products in patients with adrenal insufficiency may cause sodium or potassium phosphate intoxication.

Renal function impairment: Administration may cause sodium or potassium phosphate intoxication.

Hepatic function impairment: Use sodium phosphate with caution in patients with cirrhosis.

Pregnancy: Category C. It is not known whether sodium phosphate can cause fetal harm when administered to a pregnant woman or can affect reproduction capacity. Give phosphate to a pregnant woman only if clearly needed.

Lactation: It is not known whether this drug is excreted in breast milk. Exercise caution when administering to a nursing woman.

Precautions:

Monitoring: Guide replacement therapy by the serum inorganic phosphate level and the limits imposed by the accompanying sodium or potassium ion.

Drug Interactions:

For information on drug interactions involving potassium, refer to the Potassium Salts monograph in this section.

Electrolytes

PHOSPHATE

Adverse Reactions:

Phosphate intoxication results in reciprocal hypocalcemic tetany.

Overdosage:

Potassium phosphate may cause combined potassium and phosphate intoxication.

Symptoms: Paresthesias of the extremities; flaccid paralysis; listlessness; confusion; weakness and heaviness of the legs; hypotension; cardiac arrhythmias; heart block; ECG abnormalities (eg, disappearance of P waves, spreading and slurring of the QRS complex with development of a biphasic curve, cardiac arrest).

Treatment: Immediately discontinue infusions. Restore depressed serum calcium levels; reduce elevated potassium levels.

Administration and Dosage:

Commercial injections are mixtures of the monobasic and dibasic salt forms. To avoid confusion, prescribe and dispense in terms of millimoles (mM) of phosphorus.

For IV use only. Dilute and thoroughly mix in a larger volume of fluid. Individualize dosage. Monitor serum sodium (or potassium), inorganic phosphorus and calcium levels.

Total parenteral nutrition (TPN): Approximately 10 to 15 mM of phosphorus (equivalent to 310 to 465 mg elemental phosphorus) per liter of TPN solution is usually adequate to maintain normal serum phosphate; larger amounts may be required in hypermetabolic states. Consider the amount of sodium (or potassium) which accompanies the addition of phosphate; monitor serum electrolytes and ECG.

Infants receiving TPN – 1.5 to 2 mM/kg/day.

Rx	**Potassium Phosphate** (Various, eg, Abbott, American Regent, Lyphomed)	**Injection:** Provides 3 mM phosphate and 4.4 mEq potassium per ml	In 5, 10, 15, 30, and 50 ml vials.
Rx	**Sodium Phosphate** (Various, eg, Abbott, American Regent, Lyphomed)	**Injection:** Provides 3 mM phosphate and 4 mEq sodium per ml	In 10, 15, 30 and 50 ml vials.

Electrolytes

AMMONIUM CHLORIDE

Actions:

Pharmacology: When loss of hydrogen and chloride ions occurs, serum bicarbonate and pH rise and serum potassium falls. The ammonium ion is converted into urea in the liver. The liberated hydrogen and chloride ions in blood and extracellular fluid result in decreased pH and corrected alkalosis. Ammonium chloride also lowers urinary pH which increases the excretion rate of basic drugs (eg, amphetamines, quinidine).

One g ammonium chloride provides 18.7 mEq of chloride.

Indications:

Treatment of hypochloremic states and metabolic alkalosis.

Contraindications:

Renal function impairment; hepatic function impairment (see Warnings); metabolic alkalosis due to vomiting of hydrochloric acid when it is accompanied by loss of sodium (excretion of sodium bicarbonate in the urine).

Warnings:

Hepatic function impairment, severe (as occurs in uremia, cirrhosis or hepatitis): The liver may fail to convert the ammonia to urea. This may result in marked ammonia retention with intoxication and hepatic coma.

Pregnancy: Category C. It is not known whether this drug can cause fetal harm when administered to a pregnant woman or affect reproductive capacity. Use only if clearly needed.

Precautions:

Ammonium toxicity: Observe patients receiving ammonium chloride for symptoms of ammonia toxicity (eg, pallor, sweating, irregular breathing, retching, bradycardia, cardiac arrhythmias, local and general twitching, tonic convulsions, coma).

Use with caution in primary respiratory acidosis, and high total CO_2 and buffer base.

Administer slowly IV to avoid pain, toxic effects and local irritation at the venipuncture site and along the course of the vein.

Adverse Reactions:

Serious metabolic acidosis (see Overdosage).

Rapid IV administration may cause pain or irritation at the injection site or along the vein.

Reactions which may occur because of solution or administration technique include: Febrile response; injection site infection; venous thrombosis or phlebitis extending from injection site; extravasation; hypervolemia (from large volume diluent).

Overdosage:

Symptoms: Serious degree of metabolic acidosis; confusion; disorientation; coma.

Treatment:

Acidosis – Administer sodium bicarbonate or sodium lactate.

Administration and Dosage:

Administer by slow IV infusion.

Dosage depends on the patient's condition and tolerance. Add the contents of one to two vials (100 to 200 mEq) to 500 or 1000 ml isotonic (0.9%) Sodium Chloride Injection. Do not exceed a concentration of 1% to 2% ammonium chloride or an administration rate of 5 ml/min in adults (≈ 3 hours for infusion of 1000 ml). Monitor dosage by repeated serum bicarbonate determinations.

Storage/Stability: Avoid excessive heat; protect from freezing. When exposed to low temperatures, concentrated solutions may crystallize. If crystals form, warm the solution to room temperature in a water bath prior to use.

Rx	**Ammonium Chloride** (Abbott)	**Injection:** 26.75% (5 mEq/ml) To be diluted before infusion	In 20 ml (100 mEq) vials.[1]

[1] With 2 mg EDTA.

TRACE METALS

Actions:

Pharmacology:

Chromium – Trivalent chromium is part of glucose tolerance factor, an essential activator of insulin-mediated reactions. Chromium helps maintain normal glucose metabolism and peripheral nerve function.

Serum chromium is bound to transferrin (siderophilin). Administration of chromium supplements to chromium deficient patients can result in normalization of the glucose tolerance curve from the diabetic-like curve typical of chromium deficiency. This response is viewed as a more meaningful indicator than serum chromium levels.

Copper serves as a cofactor for serum ceruloplasmin, an oxidase necessary for proper formation of the iron carrier protein, transferrin. Copper also helps maintain normal rates of red and white blood cell formation. The daily turnover of copper through ceruloplasmin is approximately 0.5 mg.

Iodine – Absorption from the GI tract is rapid and complete. Skin and lungs can also absorb iodine. On administration, iodide equilibrates in extracellular fluids and although all body cells contain iodide, it is specifically concentrated by the thyroid gland, which is estimated to contain 7 to 8 mg total iodine.

Other important organs to take up iodide are salivary glands, gastric mucosa, choroid plexus, skin, hair, mammary glands and placenta. Iodine in saliva and gastric mucosal secretions is reabsorbed and recycled. The circulating iodine is hormonal thyroxine of which 30 to 70 mcg is protein bound and 0.5 mcg is free thyroxine.

Manganese serves as an activator for several enzymes. During minimal intake, 20 mcg/day is retained. Manganese is bound to a specific transport protein, transmanganin, and is widely distributed, but it concentrates in mitochondria-rich tissues such as brain, kidney, pancreas and liver.

Molybdenum is a constituent of the enzymes xanthine oxidase, sulfite oxidase and aldehyde oxidase. Tissue storage of molybdenum varies with the intake levels and is affected by the amount of copper and sulfate in the diet. Consistent levels are observed in liver, kidney and adrenal cortex.

Selenium is part of glutathione peroxidase which protects cell components from oxidative damage due to peroxides produced in cellular metabolism.

Pediatric conditions, Keshan disease and Kwashiorkor have been associated with low dietary intake of selenium. The conditions are endemic to geographic areas with low selenium soil content. Dietary supplementation with selenium salts reduces the incidence of the conditions among affected children.

Zinc serves as a cofactor for > 70 different enzymes. Zinc facilitates wound healing, helps maintain normal growth rates, normal skin hydration and the senses of taste and smell. Zinc resides in muscle, bone, skin, kidney, liver, pancreas, retina, prostate and particularly in the red and white blood cells. Zinc binds to plasma albumin, α_2–macroglobulin and some plasma amino acids including histidine, cysteine, threonine, glycine and asparagine.

At plasma levels < 20 mcg/dl, dermatitis followed by alopecia has been reported for TPN patients.

TRACE METALS

The following table summarizes deficiency symptoms, excretion routes and normal plasma levels for various trace metals. The serum level at which deficiency symptoms appear for many of these elements is not well defined.

Trace Metals: Deficiency/Excretion/Plasma Levels

Trace metal	Symptoms of deficiency	Excretion	Normal plasma levels
Copper	Leukopenia, neutropenia, anemia, decreased ceruloplasmin levels, impaired transferrin formation of secondary iron deficiency, skeletal abnormalities, defective tissue formation.	Bile (80%), intestinal wall (16%), urine (4%)	80-163 mcg/dl
Chromium	Impaired glucose tolerance, peripheral neuropathy, ataxia, confusion.	Kidneys (3-50 mcg/day), bile	1-5 mcg/L[1]
Iodine	Impaired thyroid function, goiter, cretinism.	Kidneys, bile	0.5-1.5 mcg/dl
Manganese	Nausea, vomiting, weight loss, dermatitis, changes in growth and hair color.	Bile; if obstruction present, then pancreatic juice or return to intestinal lumen. Urine (negligible)	6-12 mcg/L (whole blood)
Molybdenum	Tachycardia, tachypnea, headache, night blindness, nausea, vomiting, central scotomas, edema, lethargy, disorientation, coma, hypermethioninemia, hypouricemia, hypouricuria, low urinary excretion of inorganic sulfate and elevated urinary excretion of thiosulfate.	Primarily renal, some biliary	nd
Selenium	Muscle pain & tenderness, cardiomyopathy, Kwashiorkor, Keshan disease.	Urine, feces, lungs, skin	nd
Zinc	Diarrhea, apathy, depression, parakeratosis, hypogeusia, anorexia, dysosmia, geophagia, hypogonadism, growth retardation, anemia, hepatosplenomegaly, impaired wound healing.	90% in stools; urine, perspiration	100 ± 12 mcg/dl

[1] Not considered a meaningful index of tissue stores.
nd = No data

Indications:
Supplement to IV solutions given for TPN.

Contraindications:
Do not give undiluted by direct injection into a peripheral vein because of the potential for infusion phlebitis, tissue irritation and potential to increase renal loss of minerals from a bolus injection.

Molybdenum without copper supplement: Copper-deficient patients. See Warnings.

Warnings:
Renal failure or biliary tract obstruction: Metals may accumulate. Serial determinations of serum trace metal concentrations may be a valuable guideline.

Consider the possibility of **copper** and **manganese** retention in patients with biliary tract obstruction. Ancillary routes of manganese excretion include pancreatic secretions or reabsorption into the lumen of the duodenum, jejunum or ileum.

Adjust, reduce or omit use in renal dysfunction or GI malfunction. Consider contributions from blood transfusions. Frequently determine plasma levels.

Wilson's disease: Avoid administering **copper** supplements to patients with this genetic disorder of copper metabolism.

Decreased serum levels: Administration of **copper** in the absence of **zinc** and of zinc in the absence of copper may cause decreases in plasma levels. Perform periodic determinations of plasma zinc and copper for subsequent administrations.

TRACE METALS

Copper deficiency: **Molybdenum** promotes tissue **copper** mobilization and increases urinary copper excretion; excessive amounts produce a copper deficiency. Frequently check the metabolism of copper in patients receiving molybdenum.

Multiple trace element solutions present a risk of overdosage when the need for one trace element is appreciably higher than that for the other trace elements in the formulation. Administration of trace metals as separate entities may be required.

Hypersensitivity: Sensitization to **iodides** and deaths due to anaphylactic shock after use have occurred (see Adverse Reactions). Evaluate patient for hypersensitivity before initiating TPN. If patient develops a reaction, withdraw TPN immediately and institute appropriate measures. Refer to Management of Acute Hypersensitivity.

Pregnancy: Category C. It is not known whether trace metals can cause fetal harm or can affect reproductive capacity. Give to a pregnant woman only if clearly needed.

Molybdenum crosses the placenta. Presence of **selenium** in placenta and umbilical cord blood has been reported.

Precautions:

Replacement trace metal therapy beyond maintenance requirements may be necessary in protracted vomiting or diarrhea, in patients with fistula drainage or nasogastric suction or in acute catabolic states.

Diabetes mellitus: In assessing the contribution of chromium supplements to maintenance of glucose homeostasis, consider that the patient may be diabetic.

Iodine is readily absorbed through skin, lungs and mucous membranes. Give consideration to the environment, topical skin disinfection and wound treatment practices with surgical swabs and solutions containing iodine and povidone iodine. Air in the coastal areas is known to contain more iodine than inland areas.

Benzyl alcohol: Some of these products contain benzyl alcohol, which has been associated with a fatal "gasping" syndrome in premature infants.

Adverse Reactions:

Symptoms of toxicity are unlikely to occur at recommended doses.

Hypersensitivity to **iodides** may result in angioneurotic edema, cutaneous and mucosal hemorrhages, fever, arthralgia, lymph node enlargement and eosinophilia. See Warnings.

Overdosage:

Chromium: Nausea, vomiting, GI ulcers, renal/hepatic damage, convulsions, coma.

Copper: Prostration, behavior change, diarrhea, progressive marasmus, hypotonia, photophobia, hepatic damage and peripheral edema have occurred with a serum copper level of 286 mcg/dl. Penicillamine is an effective antidote.

Iodine: Symptoms of chronic poisoning include metallic taste, sore mouth, increased salivation, coryza, sneezing, swelling of the eyelids, severe headache, pulmonary edema, tenderness of salivary glands, acneiform skin lesions and skin eruptions. Abundant fluid and salt intake helps in elimination of iodides.

Manganese: "Manganese madness", irritability, speech disturbances, abnormal gait, headache, anorexia, apathy and impotence.

Molybdenum: Gout-like syndrome with increased blood levels of molybdenum, uric acid and xanthine oxidase.

No data on treatment of molybdenosis in humans is available. Among animals, treatment with copper, sulfate ions and tungsten enhances excretion of molybdenum. The sulfur-containing amino acids, methionine and cysteine, may afford limited protection.

Selenium: Toxicity symptoms include hair loss, weak nails, dermatitis, dental defects, GI disorders, nervousness, mental depression, metallic taste, vomiting and garlic odor of breath and sweat. Acute poisoning due to ingestion has resulted in death with histopathological changes including fulminating peripheral vascular collapse, internal vascular congestion, diffusely hemorrhagic, congested and edematous lungs and brick-red color gastric mucosa. Death was preceded by coma. No effective antidote is known.

Zinc: Single IV doses of 1 to 2 mg/kg have been given to adult leukemic patients without toxic manifestations. However, acute toxicity was reported in an adult when 10 mg zinc was infused over 1 hour on each of 4 consecutive days. Profuse sweating, decreased consciousness, blurred vision, tachycardia (140/min) and marked hypothermia (94.2°F) on the fourth day were accompanied by a serum zinc concentration of 207 mcg/dl. Symptoms abated within 3 hours.

TRACE METALS

Patients receiving an inadvertent overdose (50 to 70 mg zinc/day) developed hyperamylasemia (557 to 1850 Klein units; normal, 130 to 310).

Death resulted from 1683 mg zinc IV over 60 hours to a 72-year-old patient. Symptoms included hypotension (80/40 mm Hg), pulmonary edema, diarrhea, vomiting, jaundice and oliguria with a serum zinc level of 4184 mcg/dl.

Calcium supplements may confer a protective effect against zinc toxicity.

Administration and Dosage:

Administer IV after dilution. Frequently monitor plasma levels and clinical status.

Preparation: Trace metals are usually physically compatible together, and with the electrolytes usually present in amino acid/dextrose solution used for TPN.

ZINC

Complete prescribing information begins in the Trace Metals group monograph.

Administration and Dosage:

Metabolically stable adults: 2.5 to 4 mg/day. Add 2 mg/day for acute catabolic states.

Stable adults with fluid loss from the small bowel: Give an additional 12.2 mg zinc per L of TPN solution, or an additional 17.1 mg per kg of stool or ileostomy output.

Full-term infants and children (≤ 5 years of age): 100 mcg/kg/day.

Premature infants (birth weight < 1500 g and up to 3 kg): 300 mcg/kg/day.

Rx	**Zinc Sulfate** (Various, eg, American Regent, Loch, Lyphomed, McGuff, Raway)	**Injection:** 1 mg/ml (as sulfate [as 4.39 mg heptahydrate or 2.46 mg anhydrous])	In 10 and 30 ml vials.
Rx	**Zinca-Pak** (Smith & Nephew SoloPak)		In 10 and 30[1] ml vials.
Rx	**Zinc Sulfate** (Various, eg, Loch, Raway)	**Injection:** 5 mg/ml (as 21.95 mg sulfate)	In 5 and 10 ml vials.
Rx	**Zinca-Pak** (Smith & Nephew SoloPak)		In 5 ml vials.
Rx	**Zinc** (Various, eg, Abbott)	**Injection:** 1 mg/ml (as 2.09 mg chloride)	In 10 ml vials.

[1] With 0.9% benzyl alcohol.

COPPER

Complete prescribing information begins in the Trace Metals group monograph.

Administration and Dosage:

Adults: 0.5 to 1.5 mg/day.

Children: 20 mcg/kg/day.

Rx	**Copper** (Abbott)	**Injection:** 0.4 mg/ml (as 1.07 mg cupric Cl)	In 10 ml vials.
Rx	**Cupric Sulfate** (Various, eg, American Regent, Loch, Lyphomed)	**Injection:** 0.4 mg/ml (as 1.57 mg sulfate)	In 10 and 30 ml vials.
Rx	**Cupric Sulfate** (Various, eg, Loch, LyphoMed)	**Injection:** 2 mg/ml (as 7.85 mg sulfate)	In 10 ml vials.

MANGANESE

Complete prescribing information begins in the Trace Metals group monograph.

Administration and Dosage:

Adults: 0.15 to 0.8 mg/day.

Children: 2 to 10 mcg/kg/day.

Rx	**Manganese Chloride** (Various, eg, Abbott)	**Injection:** 0.1 mg/ml (as 0.36 mg manganese chloride)	In 10 ml vials.
Rx	**Manganese Sulfate** (Various, eg, American Regent, Lyphomed)	**Injection:** 0.1 mg/ml (as 0.31 mg sulfate)	In 10 and 30 ml vials.

Trace Metals

MOLYBDENUM

Complete prescribing information for these products begins in the Trace Metals group monograph.

Administration and Dosage:

Metabolically stable adults: 20 to 120 mcg/day. For pediatric patients, calculate the additive dosage level by extrapolation.

Deficiency state resulting from prolonged TPN support: 163 mcg/day for 21 days reverses deficiency symptoms without toxicity.

Rx	**Ammonium Molybdate** (Various, eg, American Regent)	**Injection:** 25 mcg/ml (as 46 mcg/ml ammonium molybdate tetrahydrate)	In 10 ml vials.
Rx	**Molypen** (Lyphomed)		In 10 ml vials.

CHROMIUM

Complete prescribing information for these products begins in the Trace Metals group monograph.

Administration and Dosage:

Adults: 10 to 15 mcg/day.

Metabolically stable adults with intestinal fluid loss: 20 mcg/day.

Children: 0.14 to 0.2 mcg/kg/day.

Rx	**Chromium** (Various, eg, Abbott, McGuff)	**Injection:** 4 mcg/ml (as 20.5 mcg chromic chloride hexahydrate)	In 10 and 30 ml vials.
Rx	**Chromic Chloride** (Various, eg, Lyphomed)		In 10 and 30[1] ml vials.
Rx	**Chromium Chloride** (Various, eg, American Regent, Raway)		In 10 and 30 ml vials.
Rx	**Chroma-Pak** (Smith & Nephew SoloPak)		In 10 and 30[1]ml vials.
Rx	**Chromic Chloride** (Various)	**Injection:** 20 mcg/ml (as 102.5 mcg chromic chloride hexahydrate)	In 10 ml vials.
Rx	**Chroma-Pak** (Smith & Nephew SoloPak)		In 5 ml vials.

[1] With 0.9% benzyl alcohol.

SELENIUM

Complete prescribing information for these products begins in the Trace Metals group monograph.

Administration and Dosage:

Metabolically stable adults: 20 to 40 mcg/day.

Deficiency state resulting from prolonged TPN support: 100 mcg/day for 24 and 31 days, respectively, reverses deficiency symptoms without toxicity.

Children: 3 mcg/kg/day.

Rx	**Selenium** (Various, eg, American Regent, McGuff)	**Injection:** 40 mcg/ml (as 65.4 mcg selenious acid)	In 10 ml vials.
Rx	**Sele-Pak** (Smith & Nephew SoloPak)		In 10 and 30[1] ml vials.
Rx	**Selepen** (Lyphomed)		In 10 and 30[1] ml vials.

[1] With 0.9% benzyl alcohol.

IODINE

Complete prescribing information for these products begins in the Trace Metals group monograph.

Administration and Dosage:

Metabolically stable adults: 1 to 2 mcg/kg/day (normal adults, 75 to 150 mcg/day).

Pregnant and lactating women; growing children: 2 to 3 mcg/kg/day.

Rx	**Iodopen** (Lyphomed)	**Injection:** 100 mcg/ml (as 118 mcg sodium iodide)	In 10 ml vials.

Trace Metals

TRACE METAL COMBINATIONS

Complete prescribing information begins in the Trace Metals group monograph.

Administration and Dosage:

See manufacturers' product labeling for individual dosing information.

Therapeutic supplements to provide replacement for extraordinary losses of individual trace metals may be added.

Content given per ml solution.

	Product and Distributor	Chromium (as chloride) mcg	Copper (as sulfate) mcg	Iodine (as sodium iodine) mcg	Manganese (as sulfate) mg	Selenium (as selenious acid) mcg	Zinc (as sulfate) mg	How Supplied
Rx	**Pedtrace-4** (Fujisawa)	0.85	0.1		0.025		0.5	In 3 and 10 ml vials.
Rx	**Multiple Trace Element Neonatal** (American Regent)	0.85	0.1		0.025		1.5	In 2 ml vials.
Rx	**Neotrace-4** (Fujisawa)							In 2 ml vials.
Rx	**PedTE-PAK-4** (SoloPak)	1	0.1		0.025		1	In 3 ml vials.
Rx	**P.T.E.-4** (Fujisawa)							In 3 ml vials.
Rx	**Multiple Trace Element Pediatric** (American Regent)	1	0.1		0.03		0.5	In 10 ml vials.
Rx	**Trace Metals Additive in 0.9% NaCl** (Abbott)	2	0.2[1]		0.16[1]		0.8[1]	In 5, 10, 50 ml vials, 5 ml syringes.
Rx	**M.T.E.-4** (Fujisawa)	4	0.4		0.1		1	In 3, 10 and 30[2] ml vials.
Rx	**MulTE-PAK-4** (SoloPak)							In 3, 10 and 30 ml vials.
Rx	**Multiple Trace Element** (American Regent)							In 3 and 10 ml vials.
Rx	**Multiple Trace Element Concentrated** (American Regent)	10	1		0.5		5	In 1 and 10 ml vials.
Rx	**ConTE-PAK-4** (SoloPak)							In 1, 10[2] and 30[2] ml vials.
Rx	**M.T.E.-4 Concentrated** (Fujisawa)							In 1 and 10[2] ml vials.
Rx	**PTE-5** (Fujisawa)	1	0.1		0.025	15	1	In 3 and 10 ml vials.
	M.T.E.-5 (Fujisawa)	4	0.4		0.1	20	1	In 10 ml vials.
Rx								
Rx	**MulTE-PAK-5** (SoloPak)							In 3 and 10 ml vials.
Rx	**Multiple Trace Element with Selenium** (American Regent)							In 3, 10 and 30[2] ml vials.

Trace Metals

TRACE METAL COMBINATIONS

	Product and Distributor	Chromium (as chloride) mcg	Copper (as sulfate) mcg	Iodine (as sodium iodine) mcg	Manganese (as sulfate) mg	Selenium (as selenious acid) mcg	Zinc (as sulfate) mg	How Supplied
Rx	**M.T.E.-5 Concentrated** (Fujisawa)	10	1		0.5	60	5	In 1 and 10^2ml vials.
Rx	**Multiple Trace Element with Selenium Concentrated** (American Regent)							In 1 ml fill in 2 ml vials and 10^2 ml vials.
Rx	**Multitrace-5 Concentrate** (American Regent)							In 1 ml single-dose and 10 ml multiple-dose vials[2].
Rx	**M.T.E.-6** (Fujisawa)	4	0.4	25	0.1	20	1	In 10 ml vials.
Rx	**M.T.E.-7**[3] (Fujisawa)							In 10 ml vials.
Rx	**M.T.E.-6 Concentrated** (Fujisawa)	10	1	75	0.5	60	5	In 1 and 10^2 ml vials.

[1] As chloride.
[2] With 0.9% benzyl alcohol.
[3] With 25 mcg molybdenum.

TRACE METALS AND ELECTROLYTE COMBINATIONS

Administration and Dosage:

Not for direct infusion. These concentrated solutions are for IV admixtures only. Dilute to appropriate strength with suitable IV fluid prior to administration.

Adults: Add 20 ml/L (40 ml of double electrolyte products per 2 L) amino acid/dextrose solution (TPN) or other suitable IV solution.

Trace Elements (mg/ml)	**Tracelyte** (Lyphomed)	**Tracelyte w/ Double Electrolytes** (Lyphomed)	**Tracelyte-II** (Lyphomed)	**Tracelyte-II w/ Double Electrolytes** (Lyphomed)
Chromium (as chloride) (mcg/ml)	0.6	0.3	0.6	0.3
Copper (as sulfate)	0.06	0.03	0.06	0.03
Manganese (as sulfate)	0.015	0.0075	0.015	0.0075
Zinc (as sulfate)	0.15	0.075	0.15	0.075
Electrolytes (mEq/ml)				
Acetate	2.03	2.03	1.475	1.475
Calcium	0.25	0.25	0.225	0.225
Chloride	1.675	1.675	1.75	1.75
Gluconate	0.25	0.25		
Magnesium	0.4	0.4	0.25	0.25
Potassium	2.025	2.025	1	1
Sodium	1.25	1.25	1.75	1.75
Osmolarity (mOsm/L)	7570	7570	6200	6200
How Supplied	20 ml vials[1]	40 ml vials[2]	20 ml vials[1]	40 ml vials[2]

[1] To prepare 1 liter solution.
[2] To prepare 2 liter solution.

Intravenous Replenishment Solutions

COMBINED ELECTROLYTE SOLUTIONS

Electrolyte content given in mEq/L.

	Product & Distributor	Na^+	K^+	Ca^{++}	Mg^{++}	Cl^-	Lactate	Acetate	Gluconate	Citrate	Osmolarity (mOsm/L)	How Supplied
Rx	**Plasma-Lyte 56**[1] (Baxter)	40	13		3	40		16			111	In 1000 ml.
Rx	**Ringer's Injection** (Various, eg, Abbott, Baxter, McGaw)	≈ 147	4	≈ 4		≈ 156					≈ 310	In 250, 500 and 1000 ml.
Rx	**Lactated Ringer's Injection** (Various, eg, Abbott, Baxter, McGaw)	130	4	3		≈ 109	28				≈ 273	In 150, 250, 500 and 1000 ml.
Rx	**Plasma-Lyte R**[1] (Baxter)	140	10	5	3	103	8	47			312	In 1000 ml.
Rx	**Isolyte S pH 7.4**[3,4] (McGaw)	141	5		3	98		27	23		295	In 500 and 1000 ml.
Rx	**Normosol-R**[5] (Abbott)	140	5		3	98		27	23		295	In 500 and 1000 ml.
Rx	**Normosol-R pH 7.4**[6] (Abbott)										295	In 500 and 1000 ml.
Rx	**Plasma-Lyte 148**[1] (Baxter)										294	In 500 and 1000 ml.
Rx	**Plasma-Lyte A pH 7.4**[4] (Baxter)										294	In 500 and 1000 ml.
Rx	**0.15% Potassium Chloride in 0.9% Sodium Chloride Injection** (Various, eg, Baxter, McGaw)	154	20			174					≈ 350	In 1000 ml.

Intravenous Replenishment Solutions

COMBINED ELECTROLYTE SOLUTIONS

	Product & Distributor	Na^+	K^+	Ca^{++}	Mg^{++}	Cl^-	Lactate	Acetate	Gluconate	Citrate	Osmolarity (mOsm/L)	How Supplied
Rx	**0.22% Potassium Chloride in 0.9% Sodium Chloride Injection** (McGaw)	154	30			184					365	In 1000 ml.
Rx	**0.3% Potassium Chloride in 0.9% Sodium Chloride Injection** (Various, eg, Baxter, McGaw)	154	40			194					≈ 390	In 1000 ml.

[1] pH ≈ 5.5.
[2] pH ≈ 6.7.
[3] With 1 mEq/L phosphate.
[4] pH ≈ 7.4.
[5] pH ≈ 5.5-7.
[6] pH ≈ 7.2-7.8.
[7] pH ≈ 6.

Intravenous Replenishment Solutions

COMBINED ELECTROLYTE CONCENTRATES

These concentrated solutions are not for direct infusion. They are for prescription compounding of IV admixtures only. Dilute to appropriate strength with suitable IV fluid prior to administration. Electrolyte concentrations listed are based on amount when diluted in one liter. Osmolarity is based on the concentrate.

Electrolyte content given in mEq/L after dilution.

	Product & Distributor	Na^+	K^+	Ca^{++}	Mg^{++}	Cl^-	Acetate	Gluconate	Osmolarity (mOsm/L)	How Supplied
Rx	**Hyperlyte** (McGaw)	25	≈ 40	5	8	≈ 33	≈ 41	5	6015	In 25 ml fill in 30 ml vials.
Rx	**Lypholyte** (Lyphomed)								7562	In 20, 40, 100 and 200 ml flip-top vials.
Rx	**Multilyte-40** (Lyphomed)								6015	In 25 ml flip-top vials.
Rx	**Nutrilyte** (American Regent)								7562	In 20 and 100 ml.
Rx	**Lypholyte-II** (Lyphomed)	35	20	4.5	5	35	29.5		6200	In 20 & 40 ml single dose flip-top vials & 100 and 200 ml flip-top vials.
Rx	**TPN Electrolytes** (Abbott)	35	20	4.5	5	35	29.5		6200	In 20 ml flip-top vials.
Rx	**Nutrilyte II** (American Regent)	35	20	4.5	5	35	29.5		6212	In 20 and 100 ml vials.
Rx	**TPN Electrolytes II** (Abbott)	18	18	4.5	5	35	10.5		4320	In 20 ml flip-top and pintop vials and 20 ml syringes.
Rx	**TPN Electrolytes III** (Abbott)	25	40.6	5	8	33.5	40.6	5	7520	In 20 ml flip-top and pintop vials and 20 ml syringes.
Rx	**Hyperlyte CR** (McGaw)	25	20	5	5	30	30		5500	In 250 ml Super-Vials.
Rx	**Hyperlyte R** (McGaw)	25	20	5	5	30	25		4205	In 25 ml fill in 30 ml vials.
Rx	**Multilyte-20** (Lyphomed)								4205	In 25 ml flip-top vials.

Intravenous Replenishment Solutions

DEXTROSE-ELECTROLYTE SOLUTIONS
Electrolyte content given in mEq/L.

	Product & Distributor	Dextrose (g/L)	Calories (Cal/L)	Na^+	K^+	Ca^{++}	Mg^{++}	Cl^-	Phosphate	Lactate	Acetate	Gluconate	Osmolarity (mOsm/L)	Other Content & How Supplied
Rx	**Dextrose 2.5% with 0.45% Sodium Chloride** (Various, eg, Abbott, Baxter, McGaw)	25	85	77				77					280	In 250, 500 and 1000 ml.
Rx	**Dextrose 5% with 0.11% Sodium Chloride** (McGaw)	50	170	19				19					290	In 500 ml.
Rx	**Dextrose 5% with 0.2% Sodium Chloride** (Various, eg, Abbott, Baxter, McGaw)	50	170	34-38.5				34-38.5					320-330	In 250, 500 and 1000 ml.
Rx	**Dextrose 5% with 0.33% Sodium Chloride** (Various, eg, Abbott, Baxter, McGaw)	50	170	51-56				51-56					355-365	In 250, 500 and 1000 ml.
Rx	**Dextrose 5% with 0.45% Sodium Chloride** (Various, eg, Abbott, Baxter, McGaw)	50	170	77				77					≈ 405	In 250, 500 and 1000 ml.
Rx	**Dextrose 5% with 0.9% Sodium Chloride** (Various, eg, Baxter, McGaw)	50	170	154				154					≈ 560	In 250, 500 and 1000 ml.
Rx	**Dextrose 10% with 0.2% Sodium Chloride** (Various, eg, Abbott, McGaw)	100	340	34-38.5				34-38.5					575-582	In 250 and 500 ml.
Rx	**Dextrose 10% with 0.3% Sodium Chloride** (Abbott)	100	340	51				51					607	In 250 ml.
Rx	**Dextrose 10% with 0.45% Sodium Chloride** (McGaw)	100	340	77				77					660	In 1000 ml.
Rx	**Dextrose 10% with 0.9% Sodium Chloride** (Various, eg, Abbott, Baxter, McGaw)	100	340	154				154					813	In 500 and 1000 ml.

Intravenous Replenishment Solutions

DEXTROSE-ELECTROLYTE SOLUTIONS

	Product & Distributor	Dextrose (g/L)	Calories (Cal/L)	Na^+	K^+	Ca^{++}	Mg^{++}	Cl^-	Phosphate	Lactate	Acetate	Gluconate	Osmolarity (mOsm/L)	Other Content & How Supplied
Rx	**0.179% Potassium Chloride in 5% Dextrose and Lactated Ringer's** (Baxter)	50	170	130	24	3		129		28			565	In 1000 ml.
Rx	**0.328% Potassium Chloride in 5% Dextrose and Lactated Ringer's** (Baxter)	50	170	130	44	3		149		28			605	In 1000 ml.
Rx	**Potassium Chloride 0.075% in D-5-W** (Various, eg, Baxter, McGaw)	50	170		10			10					≈ 272	In 1000 ml.
Rx	**Potassium Chloride 0.15% in D-5-W** (Various, eg, Baxter, McGaw)	50	170		20			20					≈ 293	In 1000 ml.
Rx	**Potassium Chloride 0.224% in D-5-W** (Baxter)	50	170		30			30					312	In 1000 ml.
Rx	**Potassium Chloride 0.3% in D-5-W** (Baxter)	50	170		40			40					333	In 500 and 1000 ml.
Rx	**0.075% Potassium Chloride in 5% Dextrose and 0.2% NaCl** (Various, eg, Abbott, Baxter)	50	170	34-38.5	10			44-48.5					340-349	In 1000 ml.
Rx	**0.15% Potassium Chloride in 5% Dextrose and 0.2% Sodium Chloride** (Various, eg, Abbott, Baxter, McGaw)	50	170	34-38.5	20			54-58.5					360-370	In 250, 500 and 1000 ml.
Rx	**0.22% Potassium Chloride in 5% Dextrose and 0.2% NaCl** (Various, eg, Abbott, Baxter, McGaw)	50	170	34-38.5	30			64-68.5					380-389	In 1000 ml.
Rx	**0.3% Potassium Chloride in 5% Dextrose and 0.2% Sodium Chloride** (Various, eg, Abbott, Baxter, McGaw)	50	170	34-38.5	40			74-78.5					400-409	In 1000 ml.

Intravenous Replenishment Solutions

DEXTROSE-ELECTROLYTE SOLUTIONS

	Product & Distributor	Dextrose (g/L)	Calories (Cal/L)	Na^+	K^+	Ca^{++}	Mg^{++}	Cl^-	Phosphate	Lactate	Acetate	Gluconate	Osmolarity (mOsm/L)	Other Content & How Supplied
Rx	**0.15% Potassium Chloride in 5% Dextrose and 0.33% Sodium Chloride** (Various, eg, Abbott, Baxter, McGaw)	50	170	51-56	20			71-76					395-405	In 500 and 1000 ml.
Rx	**0.224% Potassium Chloride in 5% Dextrose & 0.33% NaCl** (Various, eg, Abbott, Baxter)	50	170	51-56	30			81-86					415-425	In 1000 ml.
Rx	**0.3% Potassium Chloride in 5% Dextrose and 0.33% Sodium Chloride** (Various, eg, Abbott, Baxter)	50	170	51-56	40			91-96					434-446	In 1000 ml.
Rx	**0.075% Potassium Chloride in 5% Dextrose and 0.45% Sodium Chloride** (Various, eg, Baxter, McGaw)	50	170	77	10			87					≈ 425	In 1000 ml.
Rx	**0.15% Potassium Chloride in 5% Dextrose and 0.45% Sodium Chloride** (Various, eg, Baxter, McGaw)	50	170	77	20			97					≈ 445	In 500 and 1000 ml.
Rx	**0.22% Potassium Chloride in 5% Dextrose and 0.45% Sodium Chloride** (Various, eg, Baxter, McGaw)	50	170	77	30			107					≈ 465	In 1000 ml.
Rx	**0.3% Potassium Chloride in 5% Dextrose and 0.45% Sodium Chloride** (Various, eg, Baxter, McGaw)	50	170	77	40			117					≈ 490	In 1000 ml.
Rx	**0.15% Potassium Chloride in 5% Dextrose and 0.9% Sodium Chloride** (Various, eg, Baxter, McGaw)	50	170	154	20			174					≈ 600	In 1000 ml.
Rx	**0.22% Potassium Chloride in 5% Dextrose and 0.9% Sodium Chloride** (McGaw)	50	170	154	30			184					620	In 1000 ml.

Intravenous Replenishment Solutions

DEXTROSE-ELECTROLYTE SOLUTIONS

	Product & Distributor	Dextrose (g/L)	Calories (Cal/L)	Na^+	K^+	Ca^{++}	Mg^{++}	Cl^-	Phosphate	Lactate	Acetate	Gluconate	Osmolarity (mOsm/L)	Other Content & How Supplied
Rx	**0.15% Potassium Chloride in 10% Dextrose and 0.2% Sodium Chloride** (McGaw)	100	340	34	20			54					615	In 250 ml.
Rx	**0.3% Potassium Chloride in 5% Dextrose and 0.9% Sodium Chloride** (Various, eg, Baxter, McGaw)	50	170	154	40			194					≈ 640	In 1000 ml.
Rx	**Isolyte G with 5% Dextrose** (McGaw)	50	170	65	17			149					555	70 mEq NH_4^+ In 1000 ml.[1]
Rx	**5% Dextrose and Electrolyte #75** (Baxter)	50	180	40	35			48	15	20			402	In 250, 500 and 1000 ml.
Rx	**Isolyte M with 5% Dextrose** (McGaw)	50	170	38	35			44	15		20		400	In 500 ml.[1]
Rx	**Dextrose 5% in Ringer's** (Various, eg, Abbott, Baxter, McGaw)	50	170	≈147	4	≈4.5		≈156					≈560	In 150, 250, 500 and 1000 ml.
Rx	**Dextrose 2.5% in Half-Strength Lactated Ringer's** (Various, eg, Abbott, Baxter, McGaw)	25	≈89	≈65.5	2	≈1.5		≈55		14			≈264	In 250, 500 and 1000 ml.
Rx	**Dextrose 5% in Lactated Ringer's** (Various, eg, Abbott, Baxter, McGaw)	50	170-180	130	4	3		109-112		28			525-530	In 250, 500 and 1000 ml.
Rx	**5% Dextrose and Electrolyte No. 48** (Baxter)	50	180	25	20		3	24	3	23			348	In 250, 500 and 1000 ml.
Rx	**Isolyte H with 5% Dextrose** (McGaw)	50	170	42	13		3	39			17		370	In 500 and 1000 ml.[1]
Rx	**Normosol-M and 5% Dextrose** (Abbott)	50	170	40	13		3	40			16		363	In 500 and 1000 ml.
Rx	**Plasma-Lyte 56 and 5% Dextrose** (Baxter)													In 500 and 1000 ml.
Rx	**Isolyte P with 5% Dextrose** (McGaw)	50	170	25	20		3	23	3		23		350	In 250 amd 500 ml.[1]

Intravenous Replenishment Solutions

DEXTROSE-ELECTROLYTE SOLUTIONS

	Product & Distributor	Dextrose (g/L)	Calories (Cal/L)	Na^+	K^+	Ca^{++}	Mg^{++}	Cl^-	Phosphate	Lactate	Acetate	Gluconate	Osmolarity (mOsm/L)	Other Content & How Supplied
Rx	**Isolyte S with 5% Dextrose** (McGaw)	50	170	142	5		3	98			30	23	555	In 1000 ml.[1]
Rx	**Normosol-R and 5% Dextrose** (Abbott)	50	185	140	5		3	98			27	23	552	In 500 & 1000 ml.[2]
Rx	**Plasma-Lyte 148 and 5% Dextrose** (Baxter)	50	190	140	5		3	98			27	23	547	In 500 and 1000 ml.
Rx	**10% Dextrose with Electrolytes** (Abbott)	100	340	80	20		6	80	7 (mM)			21	730	In 500 ml in 1000 ml partial fill container.[2]
Rx	**10% Dextrose and Electrolyte No. 48** (Baxter)	100	*	25	20		3	24	3	23			600	In 250 ml.[1]
Rx	**Isolyte R with 5% Dextrose** (McGaw)	50	170	41	16	5	3	40			24		380	In 1000 ml.[1]
Rx	**Plasma-Lyte M and 5% Dextrose** (Baxter)	50	180	40	16	5	3	40		12	12		377	In 500 and 1000 ml.
Rx	**Plasma-Lyte R and 5% Dextrose** (Baxter)	50	181	140	10	5	3	103		8	47		564	In 1000 ml.[1]
Rx	**Isolyte E with 5% Dextrose** (McGaw)	50	170	141	10	5	3	103			49		565	8 mEq citrate. In 1000 ml.[1]

[1] With sodium bisulfite.
[2] With sodium metabisulfite.
* Not indicated by manufacturer.

INTRAVENOUS NUTRITIONAL THERAPY

Intravenous Replenishment Solutions

HYPERTONIC DEXTROSE SOLUTIONS WITH ELECTROLYTES

Electrolyte content given in mEq/L.

	Product & Distributor	Dextrose (g/L)	Calories (Cal/L)	Na+	K+	Ca++	Mg++	Cl–	Phosphate	Lactate	Acetate	Gluconate	Osmolarity (mOsm/L)	Other Content & How Supplied
Rx	**50% Dextrose with Electrolyte Pattern N** (McGaw)	500	1700	90	80		16	150	28				2875	16 mEq sulfate. In 500 ml in 1000 ml partial fill containers.[1]
Rx	**50% Dextrose with Electrolyte Pattern A** (McGaw)	500	1700	84	40	10	16	115				13	2800	16 mEq sulfate. In 500 ml in 1000 ml partial fill containers.[2]

[1] With sodium metabisulfite.
[2] With sodium bisulfite.

INVERT SUGAR-ELECTROLYTE SOLUTIONS

Invert sugar is composed of equal parts of dextrose (glucose) and fructose (levulose). It has the same caloric value as dextrose but is more rapidly utilized. Fructose augments utilization of dextrose. Used for nonelectrolyte fluid and caloric replacement.

Refer to dextrose monograph for further information.

Electrolyte content given in mEq/L.

	Product & Distributor	Invert Sugar (g/L)	Calories (Cal/L)	Na+	K+	Ca++	Mg++	Cl-	Phosphate	Lactate	Osmolarity (mOsm/L)	How Supplied
Rx	**5% Travert and Electrolyte No. 2** (Baxter)	50	196	56	25		6	56	12.5	25	449	In 1000 ml.[1]
Rx	**10% Travert and Electrolyte No. 2** (Baxter)	100	384	56	25		6	56	12.5	25	726	In 1000 ml.[1]

[1] With sodium bisulfite.

LACTOBACILLUS

Actions:

Pharmacology: A viable culture of the naturally occurring metabolic products produced by *Lactobacillus acidophilus* and *L bulgaricus.*

Indications:

Dietary supplement.

Unlabeled uses: Treatment of uncomplicated diarrhea, including that due to antibiotic therapy. The FDA has determined that these ingredients are not generally recognized as safe and effective as antidiarrheal drug products.

Treatment of acute fever blisters (cold sores).

Contraindications:

Allergy to milk or sensitivity to lactose.

Warnings:

Children: Unless directed by a physician, do not use in children < 3 years old.

Precautions:

Fever: Unless directed by physician, do not use for > 2 days or in the presence of high fever.

Administration and Dosage:

Bacid: 2 capsules 2 to 4 times daily. Must be refrigerated.

Lactinex:

Granules – 1 packet added to or taken with cereal, food, milk, fruit juice or water 3 or 4 times daily. Must be refrigerated.

Tablets, chewable – 4 tablets 3 or 4 times daily. May follow each dose with a small amount of milk, fruit juice or water.

Moredophilus: 1 tsp daily with liquid. Store at room temperature.

Pro-Bionate:

Capsules – 1 capsule 1 to 3 times daily.

Powder – ¼ to 1 tsp 1 to 3 times daily.

Superdophilus: ¼ to 1 tsp 1 to 3 times daily.

otc	**Bacid** (Ciba)	**Capsules**: Cultured strain ≥ 500 million viable *L acidophilus*	Mineral oil. In 50s and 100s.
otc *sf*	**Kala** (Freeda)	**Tablets**: 200 million units soy-based *L acidophilus*	In 100s, 250s and 500s.
otc	**Lactinex** (Becton Dickinson)	**Granules**: Mixed culture of *L acidophilus and L bulgaricus*	In 1 g packets (12s).
		Tablets, chewable: Mixed culture of *L acidophilus and L bulgaricus*	Lactose, sucrose and mineral oil. In 50s.
otc *sf*	**MoreDophilus** (Freeda)	**Powder**: 4 billion units of acidophilus-carrot derivative per g.	In 120 g.
otc	**Pro-Bionate** (Natren)	**Powder**: 2 billion *Lactobacillus acidophilus* strain NAS per g.	In 52.5 and 90 g.
		Capsules: 2 billion *Lactobacillus acidophilus* strain NAS per g.	In 30s and 60s.
otc	**Superdophilus** (Natren)	**Powder**: 2 billion *Lactobacillus acidophilus* strain DDS-1 per g.	In 37.5, 75 and 135 g.

Amino Acids

GLUTAMIC ACID

Indications:

Dietary supplement.

Administration and Dosage:

500 to 1000 mg daily or as directed. Take with liquids.

otc	**Glutamic Acid** (Various, eg, Freeda)	**Tablets:** 500 mg	In 100s and 500s.
otc	**Glutamic Acid** (J.R. Carlson)	**Powder**	In 100 g bottles.

L-LYSINE

Actions:

Pharmacology: An essential amino acid which improves utilization of vegetable proteins.

Indications:

Dietary supplement.

Unlabeled uses: Oral L-lysine has been promoted as treatment and as a prophylactic agent in herpes simplex infections; however, controlled studies do not support these claims.

Administration and Dosage:

312 to 1500 mg daily.

otc	**L-Lysine** (Various, eg, Rugby)	**Tablets:** 312 mg	In 100s.
otc	**Enisyl** (Person & Covey)	**Tablets:** 334 mg	In 100s.
otc	**L-Lysine** (Various, eg, Goldline, Moore, Mission, Pasadena, Rugby, Schein, URL)	**Tablets:** 500 mg	In 100s.
otc	**Enisyl** (Person & Covey)		In 100s and 250s.
otc	**L-Lysine** (Approved Pharm.)	**Tablets:** 1000 mg	In 60s.
otc	**L-Lysine** (Various, eg, Miller, Tyson & Assoc.)	**Capsules:** 500 mg	In 100s and 250s.

METHIONINE

Indications:

Dietary supplement.

Administration and Dosage:

500 mg daily. The recommended daily allowance has not been established.

Rx	**Methionine** (Various, eg, Schein)	**Tablets:** 500 mg	In 100s, 500s and 1000s.
Rx	**Methionine** (Tyson and Assoc.)	**Capsules:** 500 mg	In 30s.

THREONINE

Indications:

Dietary supplement.

Administration and Dosage:

500 mg daily, preferably on an empty stomach, or as directed.

otc	**Threonine** (Freeda)	**Tablets:** 500 mg	In 100s and 250s.
otc	**Threonine** (Various, eg, Solgar, Tyson & Assoc.)	**Capsules:** 500 mg	In 60s.

Amino Acids Combinations

AMINO ACIDS WITH VITAMINS AND MINERALS

otc	**Dequasine** (Miller)	**Tablets**: 20 mg L-lysine, 100 mg L–cysteine, 50 mg dl–methionine, 200 mg vitamin C, 5 mg iron. Cu, I, Mg, Mn, Zn. *Dose: 1 tablet daily.*	In 100s.
otc sf	**NeuRecover-LT** (NeuroGenesis)	**Capsules**: 375 mg vitamin D, L–phenylalanine, 50 mg L–glutamine, 277.7 IU vitamin A, 0.375 mg B_1, 0.85 mg B_2, 1.25 mg B_5, 1 mg B_6, 1 mcg B_{12}, 0.03 mg FA, 30 mg C, 0.05 mg biotin, 10 mg B_3, 50 mg Ca, 25 mg Mg, 0.01 mg Cr. *Dose: 2 capsules 3 times daily.*	Yeast and preservative free. In 42s and 180s.
otc sf	**NeuroSlim** (NeuroGenesis/ Matrix)	**Capsules**: 500 mg vitamin D, L–phenylalanine, 15 mg L–glutamine, 25 mg L–tyrosine, 10 mg L–carnitine, 10 mg L–arginine pyroglutamate, 10 mg L–ornithine/L-aspartate, 0.033 mg Cr, 0.012 mg Se, 0.33 mg vitamin B_1, 5 mg B_2, 3.3 mg B_3, 0.33 mg B_5, 0.33 mg B_6, 1 mcg B_{12}, 5 IU E, 0.05 mg biotin, 0.066 mg FA, 1 mg Fe, 2.5 mg Zn, 35 mg Ca, 0.25 mg I, 0.33 mg Cu, 25 mg Mg. *Dose: 6 capsules daily.*	Yeast and preservative free. In 42s and 180s.
otc sf	**NeuRecover-DA** (NeuroGenesis/ Matrix)	**Capsules**: 460 mg vitamin D, L-phenylalanine, 25 mg L–glutamine, 333.3 IU vitamin A, 2.417 mg B_1, 0.85 mg B_2, 33 mg B_3, 15 mg B_5, 3 mg B_6, 5 mcg B_{12}, 0.067 mg FA, 100 mg C, 5 IU E, 0.05 mg biotin, 25 mg Ca, 0.01 mg Cr, 1.5 mg Fe, 25 mg Mg, 2.5 mg Zn. *Dose: 2 capsules 3 times daily.*	Yeast and preservative free. In 42s and 180s.
otc sf	**NeuRecover-SA** (NeuroGenesis/ Matrix)	**Capsules**: 250 mg vitamin D, L–phenylalanine, 150 mg L–tyrosine, 50 mg L-glutamine, 1.67 mg vitamin B_1, 2.5 mg B_2, 16.7 mg B_3, 15 mg B_5, 3.3 mg B_6, 5 mcg B_{12}, 0.067 mg FA, 100 mg C, 25 mg Ca, 0.01 mg Cr, 1.5 mg Fe, 25 mg Mg, 5 mg Zn. *Dose: ≤ 6 capsules daily.*	Yeast and preservative free. In 42s and 180s.

Amino Acids Combinations

AMINO ACIDS WITH VITAMINS AND MINERALS

otc	**Herpetrol** (Alva)	**Tablets**: L-lysine, vitamin A, E, B_2, C and Zn. *Dose: 4 tablets daily until symptoms subside.*	In 42s and 84s.
otc	**A/G-Pro** (Miller)	**Tablets**: 542 mg protein hydrolysate (45% amino acids), 50 mg L–lysine, 12.5 mg dl–methionine, 16.7 mg vitamin C, 0.33 mg B_6, 1.66 mg iron. Cu, I, K, Mg, Mn, Zn. *Dose: 2 tablets 3 times daily before meals.*	In 180s.
otc	**Jets** (Freeda)	**Tablets, chewable**: 300 mg lysine, 25 mg vitamin C, 25 mcg B_{12}, 5 mg B_6, 10 mg B_1.	In 30s, 250s and 500s.
otc	**Ondrox** (Unimed)	**Tablets, sustained release**: 100 IU D, L-glutathione, L-methionine, L-glutamine, taurine, N-acetylcysteine, 333 IU vitamin A, 1667 IU beta carotene, 16.7 IU E, 41.7 mg C, 66.7 mg folic acid, 0.25 mg B^1, 0.28 mg B^2, 3.3 mg B^3, 0.33 mg B^6, 1 mcg B^{12}, 5 mcg biotin, 1.7 mg B^5, I, Fe, Ca, Mg, Cu, 2.5 mg Zn, P, vitamin K, K, Cr, Mn, Mo, Se, Omega 3 oils, V, B, Si, citrus bioflavonoids, sodium benzoate, potassium sorbate, BHT, inositol, propyl gallate	In 60s and 180s.
otc	**PDP Liquid Protein** (Wesley Pharm.)	**Liquid**: 15 g protein (from hydrolyzed animal collagen), L-tryptophan and 72 calories per 30 ml. *Dose: 30 ml daily.*	Sorbitol, saccharin. Cherry flavor. In qt.

Amino Acid Derivatives

LEVOCARNITINE (L-Carnitine)

Actions:

Pharmacology: L-carnitine is a naturally occurring amino acid derivative, synthesized from methionine and lysine, required in energy metabolism. It facilitates long-chain fatty acid entry into cellular mitochondria, delivering substrate and subsequent energy production and can promote the excretion of excess organic or fatty acids in patients with defects in fatty acid metabolism or specific organic acidopathies that bioaccumulate acyl CoA esters. Commercial synthesis of carnitine produces a D and L racemic mixture. In the biologic system, only the L isomer is present. The D isomer has pharmacologic effects but does not participate in lipid metabolism.

Primary carnitine deficiency is a rare inborn error of metabolism in which biosynthesis or use of L-carnitine is impaired and normal dietary sources (eg, meat, milk) are inadequate or ineffectual in compensating for the deficiency. Primary systemic carnitine deficiency results in impairment in fatty acid metabolism, and manifests itself as elevated triglycerides and free fatty acids, diminished ketogenesis, lipid infiltration of liver and muscle and low plasma, RBC or tissue levels of L-carnitine. Severe chronic deficiency may be associated with hypoglycemia, progressive myasthenia, hypotonia, lethargy, hepatomegaly, encephalopathy, hepatic coma, cardiomegaly, congestive heart failure, cardiac arrest, neurologic disturbances and, in infants, impaired growth and development.

Secondary carnitine deficiency can be a consequence of inborn errors of metabolism. L-carnitine may alleviate the metabolic abnormalities of patients with inborn errors that result in accumulation of toxic organic acids. Conditions for which this effect was demonstrated are: Glutaric aciduria II, methyl malonic aciduria, propionic acidemia and medium chain fatty acyl CoA dehydrogenase deficiency. Autointoxication occurs in these patients due to the accumulations of acyl CoA compounds that disrupt intermediary metabolism. The subsequent hydrolysis of the acyl CoA compound to its free acid results in acidosis that can be life-threatening. L-carnitine clears the acyl CoA compound by formation of acyl carnitine which is quickly excreted. L-carnitine deficiency is defined biochemically as abnormally low plasma levels of free carnitine < 20 mcmol/L at age > 1 week post-term and may be associated with low tissue or urine levels. Further, this condition may be associated with a ratio of plasma ester/free L-carnitine levels > 0.4 or abnormally elevated levels of esterified L-carnitine in the urine. In premature infants and newborns, secondary deficiency is defined as plasma free L–carnitine levels below age-related normal levels.

Pharmacokinetics:

Absorption/Distribution – L-carnitine tablets are bioequivalent to the oral solution. Following the administration of 1980 mg twice daily, the maximum plasma concentration (Cmax) was 80 nmol/ml and the time to maximum concentration (Tmax) occurred at 3.3 hours. There were no significant differences for AUC and urinary excretion observed between these two formulations. Approximately 76% of free L–carnitine is eliminated in the urine. Using plasma levels uncorrected for endogenous L-carnitine, the mean distribution half-life was 0.585 hours and the mean apparent terminal elimination half-life was 17.4 hours following a single IV dose.

The absolute bioavailability from tablets and oral solution was determined compared to the bioavailability from the injection. After correction for circulating endogenous levels in the plasma, absolute bioavailability was 15.1% from the tablets and 15.9% from the oral solution.

Total body clearance (dose/AUC including endogenous baseline levels) was a mean of 4 L/hr. Endogenous baseline levels were not subtracted since total body clearance does not distinguish between exogenous sources and endogenously synthesized L–carnitine. Volume of distribution of the IV administered dose above baseline endogenous levels was calculated to be a mean of 29 L (approximately 0.39 L/kg) which is an underestimate of the true volume of distribution since plasma L-carnitine is known to equilibrate slowly with, for instance, muscle L-carnitine. L-carnitine is not bound to plasma protein or albumin.

LEVOCARNITINE (L-Carnitine)

Metabolism/Excretion – Adult male volunteers administered a dose of L-carnitine following 15 days of a high carnitine diet and additional carnitine supplement, excreted 58% to 65% of the administered dose in 5 to 11 days in the urine and feces. Maximum concentration in serum occurred from 2 to 4.5 hours after drug administration. Major metabolites found were trimethylamine N-oxide, primarily in urine (8% to 49% of the administered dose) and [^{3}H]-γ-butyrobetaine, primarily in feces (0.44% to 45% of the administered dose). Urinary excretion of carnitine was 4% to 8% of the dose. Fecal excretion of total carnitine was < 1% of total carnitine excretion.

After attainment of steady state following 4 days of L-carnitine tablets (1980 mg every 12 hours) or oral solution (2000 mg every 12 hours), urinary excretion was a mean of 2107 and 2339 mcmol, respectively, equivalent to 8.6% and 9.4%, respectively, of the orally administered doses (uncorrected for endogenous urinary excretion). After a single IV dose (20 mg/kg) prior to multiple oral doses, urinary excretion was 6974 mcmol, equivalent to 75.6% of the intravenously administered dose (uncorrected for endogenous urinary excretion).

Indications:

Primary systemic carnitine deficiency.

Secondary carnitine deficiency: Acute and chronic treatment of patients with an inborn error of metabolism that results in secondary carnitine deficiency.

Unlabeled uses:

L-carnitine appears effective in modifying abnormal plasma lipoprotein patterns. Most studies have dealt with hemodialysis patients. Carnitine apparently normalizes the abnormal lipid profile produced by loss of plasma L-carnitine (53% to 78%) in the hemodialysis procedure.

It has also been used to improve athletic performance, and may be of use in valproate toxicity.

Warnings:

Carnitine deficiency: D, L-carnitine, sold in health food stores as vitamin BT, competitively inhibits L-carnitine and can cause a deficiency.

Pregnancy: Category B. There are no adequate and well controlled studies in pregnant women. Use during pregnancy only if clearly needed.

Lactation: It is not known whether L-carnitine is excreted in breast milk. However, carnitine is a normal component of breast milk. Decide whether to discontinue nursing or to discontinue the drug, taking into account the importance of the drug to the mother.

Precautions:

Monitoring should include periodic blood chemistries, vital signs, plasma carnitine concentrations and overall clinical condition.

Adverse Reactions:

Most common: Transient GI complaints (41%) including: Nausea, vomiting, abdominal cramps, diarrhea; avoid by slow consumption or greater dilution of liquid. Decreasing dosage may diminish or eliminate drug-related body odor (11%) or GI symptoms.

Mild myasthenia has occurred in uremic patients on D, L-carnitine but not L-carnitine.

Overdosage:

Treatment includes usual supportive measures. Refer to General Management of Acute Overdosage.

Amino Acid Derivatives

LEVOCARNITINE (L-Carnitine)

Administration and Dosage:

Solution:

Adults – Give 1 to 3 g/day for a 50 kg subject. Use higher doses with caution. Start dosage at 1 g/day, and increase slowly while assessing tolerance and response.

Children: 50 to 100 mg/kg/day. Give higher doses with caution. Start dosage at 50 mg/kg/day, and increase slowly to a maximum of 3 g/day while assessing tolerance and therapeutic response.

Give alone or dissolve in drinks or liquid food. Space doses evenly (every 3 or 4 hours), preferably with or after meals; consume slowly to maximize tolerance.

Tablets:

Adults – 990 mg 2 or 3 times a day, depending on clinical response.

Infants and children – Between 50 and 100 mg/kg/day, in divided doses, with a maximum of 3 g/day. Dosage depends on clinical response.

Injection: Administer IV. Give 50 mg/kg as a slow 2 to 3 minute bolus injection or by infusion. Often a loading dose is given in patients with severe metabolic crisis followed by an equivalent dose over the following 24 hours. Administer every 3 or 4 hours, and never < 6 hours either by infusion or by IV injection. Use a range of 50 mg/kg for all subsequent daily doses or as therapy may require. The highest dose administered has been 300 mg/kg.

Obtain a plasma carnitine level prior to beginning therapy. Monitor weekly and monthly as well, including blood chemistries, vital signs, plasma carnitine concentrations (plasma free carnitine levels should be between 35 and 60 mcmol/L) and overall clinical condition.

Storage: Store amps at room temperature (25°C; 77°F) in original carton until use to protect from light. Discard unused portion since it contains no preservatives.

Rx	**Carnitor** (Sigma-Tau)	**Tablets**: 330 mg	In 90s.
otc	**L-Carnitine** (Various, eg, R & D Labs, Tyson)	**Capsules**: 250 mg	In 30s and 60s.
Rx	**Carnitor** (Sigma-Tau)	**Solution**: 100 mg per ml	Sucrose. Cherry flavor. In 118 ml.
Rx	**VitaCarn** (Kendall McGaw)		Sucrose. Cherry flavor. In 118 ml.
Rx	**Carnitor** (Sigma-Tau)	**Injection**: 1 g/5 ml	In 5 ml single-dose amps.[1]

[1] Preservative free.

LIPOTROPIC PRODUCTS

The need for lipotropics in human nutrition is not established. The lipotropic factors choline, inositol and betaine, not proven therapeutically valuable, have been used for treatment of liver disorders and disturbed fat metabolism.

Choline (trimethylethanolamine), a component of the major phospholipid, lecithin, demonstrates lipotropic action, functions as a methyl group donor and is a precursor of the neurochemical transmitter, acetylcholine. Choline and lecithin (because of its choline content) have been advocated for tardive dyskinesia, Huntington's chorea, Tourette's syndrome, Friedreich's ataxia, presenile dementia, fatty liver and cirrhosis. Intestinal bacteria metabolize choline to trimethylamine, which imparts an unpleasant odor to the breath and body. Lecithin does not produce this odor. Choline also causes clinical depression in some patients.

Inositol, an isomer of glucose, is present in cell membrane phospholipids and plasma lipoproteins. No specific role in human nutrition has been established.

Linoleic and linolenic acid are polyunsaturated fatty acids that serve as precursors of important biochemical compounds, such as arachidonic acid, which gives rise to a wide variety of prostaglandins. Linoleic acid is regarded as an essential fatty acid because it cannot be synthesized in vivo and because it has a defined metabolic significance; it helps support normal growth and development and prevent essential fatty acid deficiency (EFAD). The metabolic significance of linolenic acid is unclear. Use of these precursors to alter disease states requires more research.

CHOLINE

Administration and Dosage:

650 mg to 2 g daily or as directed.

otc	**Choline** (Various, eg, Approved, Rugby)	**Tablets**: 250 mg, 300 and 500 mg	In 100s.
		650 mg	In 90s and 100s.
otc	**Choline Bitartrate** (Various, eg, City Chem, Fibertone, Spectrum)	**Tablets**: 250 mg	In 100s, 250s, 500s, 1000s.
		Powder	In 120 g and 1 lb.
Rx	**Choline Chloride** (Various, eg, Baker, Biochemical, City Chem, Spectrum)	**Powder**	In 120 and 500 g and 1 and 5 lb.
otc	**Choline Dihydrogen** Citrate (Freeda)	**Tablets**: 650 mg	In 250s.
		Powder:	In 120 g and 1 lb.

INOSITOL

Administration and Dosage:

1 to 3 g daily in divided doses.

otc	**Inositol** (Various, eg, Biochemical, Freeda, Nature's Bounty, Rugby)	**Tablets**: 250 mg	In 100s.
		500 mg	In 100s.
		650 mg	In 90s and 100s.
		Powder	In 25, 60, 100, 120, 500 g & lb.

LIPOTROPIC COMBINATIONS

otc	**Lecithin** (Various, eg, Approved, Dixon-Shane, Goldline, Moore, Nature's Bounty, Rugby, Schein, West-Ward)	A source of choline, inositol, phosphorus, linoleic & linolenic acids. *Dose:* 1-2 caps/day.	
		Capsules: 420 mg	In 60s.
		1.2 g	In 100s, 250s, 1000s.
		Tablets: 1.2 g	In 50s.
		Granules	In 210, 240, 420 g & lb.
		Liquid	In 480 ml.
otc	**PhosChol** (American Lecithin)	Phosphatidylcholine (highly purified lecithin)	
		Softgels: 565 mg	In 100s and 300s
		900 mg	In 100s and 300s.
		Liq conc.: 3000 mg/5 ml	In 240 and 480 ml.
otc	**Pertropin** (Lannett)	**Capsules**: 7 mins. linolenic acid, other essential unsaturated free fatty acids, 5 IU vitamin E. *Dose:* 1 or 2 capsules 3 or 4 times daily.	In 100s.

OMEGA-3 (N-3) POLYUNSATURATED FATTY ACIDS

Cold water fish oils contain large amounts of omega-3 (N-3) polyunsaturated fatty acids, eicosapentaenoic acid (EPA) and docosahexaenoic acid (DHA). Diets high in omega-3 fatty acids may lower very low-density lipoproteins (VLDL), triglyceride and total cholesterol concentrations; increase concentrations of high-density lipoproteins (HDL); prolong bleeding times; decrease platelet aggregation; reduce plasma fibrinogen (data conflict); inhibit leukocyte function.

Studies on the effects of omega-3 fatty acids on the lipoproteins closely associated with atherosclerosis (LDL and HDL) show variable results and require further investigation.

Some studies have actually shown an increase in LDL-cholesterol levels in patients and healthy subjects receiving omega-3 fatty acids at doses currently recommended by the manufacturers (4.6 to 13.3 g/day). Although the optimal dose has not been established, significant effects of the omega-3 fatty acids may only be observed with 20 g or more per day. Some of the available products also contain cholesterol and saturated fat, which may play a role in the increased LDL-cholesterol levels.

Patients on diets with high levels of fish oils have increased EPA levels and decreased arachidonic acid levels in plasma lipids and platelet membranes. Also, increased synthesis of prostaglandin I_3 and decreased platelet synthesis of thromboxane A_2 have been noted. Prostaglandin I_3, an antiaggregation substance, and thromboxane A_2, a potent stimulator of platelet aggregation and secretion, are usually in balance. It is believed EPA is utilized by vessel walls to synthesize prostaglandin I_3, and arachidonic acid is utilized by platelets to synthesize thromboxane A_2. Therefore, the higher EPA levels and lower arachidonic acid levels produced by a diet high in fish oils could cause decreased platelet aggregation. Vitamin E in the product could also contribute to decreased platelet aggregation.

Indications:

Omega-3 fatty acids may be used as nondrug dietary supplements for patients at early risk of coronary artery disease primarily because of effects on platelets and lipids.

The American Heart Association recommends consumption of fish; however, it does not find justification for fish oil capsule supplementation.

Unlabeled uses: Omega-3 fatty acids have been studied as adjunctive treatment of rheumatoid arthritis (20 g/day have been used). These agents may also be of benefit in the treatment of psoriasis (10 to 15 g/day); however, data is conflicting. Omega-3 fatty acids (18 g/day) may be beneficial in preventing early restenosis after coronary angioplasty in combination with dipyridamole and aspirin in high risk male patients.

Warnings:

Diarrhea has occurred in patients taking 4 to 6 capsules per day.

Increased bleeding time and inhibition of platelet aggregation have occurred. Use caution in patients receiving **anticoagulants** or **aspirin**.

Diabetes mellitus: In one study the fasting and mean glucose levels increased and insulin secretion was impaired in six patients with non-insulin dependent diabetes mellitus (NIDDM) following 1 month of omega-3 fatty acid administration (5.4 g/day). However, increased insulin sensitivity in NIDDM patients has occurred. Use with caution in NIDDM patients.

Pregnancy: Until further information is available, do not use omega-3 fatty acids in these patients.

Children: Until further information is available, do not use omega-3 fatty acids in these patients.

Administration and Dosage:

Nutritional supplement: 1 to 2 capsules 3 times daily with meals.

OMEGA-3 (N-3) POLYUNSATURATED FATTY ACIDS

	Product/ Distributor	mg/ capsule	N-3 fat content (mg) EPA	DHA	Other Content	How Supplied
otc *sf*	**Promega Pearls Softgels** (Parke-Davis)	600	168	72	<2 mg cholesterol, 1 IU vitamin E[1] < 2% RDA of vitamins A, B_1, B_2, B_3, Fe and Ca	In 60s and 90s.
otc	**Cardi-Omega 3 Capsules** (Thompson Medical)	1000	180	120	< 2% RDA of vitamins A, B_1, B_2, B_3, C, D, Fe and Ca	Sodium free. Peppermint flavor. In 60s.
otc *sf*	**EPA Capsules** (Nature's Bounty)				1 IU vitamin E[1]	In 50s and 100s.
otc	**Max EPA Capsules** (Various, eg, Jones Medical, Moore, Rexall, Schein)				5 mg cholesterol, < 2% RDA of vitamins A, B_1, B_2, B_3, C, Ca, Fe	In 60s, 90s & 100s.
otc *sf*	**Promega Softgels** (Parke-Davis)	1000	280	120	< 1 mg cholesterol, 1 IU vitamin E[1] (6% RDA), vitamins A, B_1, B_2, B_3, Ca & Fe (< 2% RDA)	Sodium free. In 30s and 60s.
otc *sf*	**Sea-Omega 50 Softgels** (Rugby)	1000	300	200	1 IU vitamin E[1]	Sodium free. In 50s.
otc	**Sea-Omega 30 Softgels** (Rugby)	1200	180	140	2 IU vitamin E[1]	In 100s.
otc	**Marine Lipid Concentrate Softgels** (Vitaline)	1200	360	240	5 IU vitamin E[1]	Sodium free. In 90s.
otc	**SuperEPA 1200 Softgels** (Advanced Nutritional)	1200	360	240	5 IU vitamin E[1]	In 60s, 90s and 180s.
otc	**SuperEPA 2000 Capsules** (Advanced Nutritional)	1000	563	312	20 IU vitamin E[1].	In 30s, 60s and 90s.

[1] As d-alpha tocopherol.

ENTERAL NUTRITIONAL THERAPY

Enteral nutrition products may be administered orally, via nasogastric tube, via feeding gastrostomy or via needle-catheter jejunostomy. The defined formula diets may be monomeric or oligomeric (amino acids or short peptides and simple carbohydrates) or polymeric (more complex protein and carbohydrate sources) in composition. Modular supplements are used for individual supplementation of protein, carbohydrate or fat when formulas do not offer sufficient flexibility.

There are different criteria for evaluating and categorizing these products; no single system of classification is ideal. Caloric density, generally in the range of 1, 1.5 or 2 Cal/ml, influences the density of other nutrients. Protein content is also a major determinant. Osmolality may be important in patients who experience diarrhea and cramping with high osmolality formulas. Consider products with low fat content in patients with significant malabsorption, hyperlipidemia or severe exocrine pancreatic insufficiency. Medium chain triglycerides are a useful energy source in patients with malabsorption, but do not provide essential fatty acids. Lactose, poorly tolerated by patients lacking lactase activity, has been eliminated from many of the nutritionally complete enteral formulas. In general, with the exception of lactose or specific allergies (eg, corn, gluten), the source of the protein or carbohydrate is not critical. Various amounts of vitamins, electrolytes and minerals are included in the formulations. Consider sodium and potassium content in patients with renal or hepatic disease. Also, consider vitamin K content in patients receiving warfarin, since the hypoprothrombinemic effect may be decreased. Although many of the products have been formulated to contain lesser amounts of vitamin K, caution is still warranted.

Some enteral preparations list the osmolality or osmolarity of the formula at standard dilution. However, when the term osmolarity is used, it cannot be determined whether the osmolarity was calculated from osmolality or if the term osmolarity is being used erroneously. Also, when samples of a specific product from the same lot or different lots were reconstituted, or if the powder was reconstituted by using the provided scoop vs reconstitution by weight, there was a wide variation in osmolality. Be aware of these potential discrepancies when utilizing osmolality information.

Cost of products is influenced by composition (oligomeric or polymeric) and form (ready-to-use or powder). In general, polymeric products cost less than oligomeric products. The form of the product indirectly affects its cost due to the amount of labor involved in preparation.

Specialized formulas are indicated for specific disease states and may be nutritionally incomplete.

Hepatic failure/encephalopathy formulas contain high concentrations of branched chain amino acids (BCAA) and low concentrations of aromatic amino acids (AAA) in an attempt to correct the abnormal plasma amino acid profiles.

Renal failure formulas contain only essential amino acids as the source of protein.

Trauma or high stress formulas contain high concentrations of BCAA, but unlike the hepatic products, are not restricted in the amounts of AAA.

Monitoring of patients receiving enteral nutritional therapy includes the following: Weight, fluid balance, serum electrolytes, glucose tolerance, liver and renal function, albumin and general condition. Watch for GI overload or obstruction and abdominal distention; check tube placement for proper position. Initiate therapy with a slow but gradual advancement in administration rate.

Several case reports and single-dose studies suggest that phenytoin administration during enteral nutritional therapy may result in decreased phenytoin concentrations; however, this has not been substantiated. Monitor phenytoin concentrations in these patients. Consider giving phenytoin 2 hours before and after the enteral feeding, or stopping the enteral therapy for 2 hours before and after phenytoin administration.

Enteral Nutritional Product Categories	
Modular Supplements	*Defined Formulas*
Protein	Milk-based formulas
Carbohydrate	Specialized formulas
Fat	Hepatic failure/encephalopathy
	Renal failure
	Trauma/stress
	Pulmonary
	Nutritionally complete, lactose free formulas

Content listed is based on standard dilutions. Refer to manufacturer's literature for mixing directions, other dilutions and storage conditions.

Modular Supplements

PROTEIN PRODUCTS

otc	**Gevral Protein** (Lederle)	**Powder:** Ca caseinate and sucrose. Each cup (≈26 g) contains: 15.6 g protein, 7.05 g carbohydrate, 0.52 g fat, < 50 mg Na, ≥ 13 mg K and 95.3 Calories *Dose:* 26 g in 8 oz liquid.	< 1% alcohol. In 8 oz and 5 lb.
otc	**ProMod** (Ross)	**Powder:** D-whey protein concentrate and soy lecithin. Each 26.4 g provides 20 g protein, 2.4 g fat, 2.68 g carbohydrate, 176 mg Ca, 60 mg Na, 260 mg K, 132 mg P and 112 Calories *Dose:* Add 1 scoop (6.6 g) to liquid, food or enteral formula.	In 275 g cans.
otc	**Propac** (Sherwood)	**Powder:** Each tablespoon (4 g) contains 3 g protein (from whey protein), 0.24 g carbohydrate from lactose, 0.32 g fat, 2 mg Cl, 20 mg K, 9 mg Na, 14 mg Ca, 12 mg P, 2 mg Mg and 16 Calories *Dose:* Add 1 tablespoon to liquid.	In 20 g packets and 350 g cans.

GLUCOSE POLYMERS

These glucose polymers are derived from cornstarch by hydrolysis.

Indications:

Supplies calories in persons with increased caloric needs or persons unable to meet their caloric needs with usual food intake. Supplies carbohydrate calories in protein, electrolyte and fat restricted diets. Also used to increase the caloric density of traditional foods, liquid and tube feedings.

Administration and Dosage:

Add to foods or beverages or mix in water. Small, frequent feedings are more desirable than large amounts given infrequently. May be used for extended periods with diets containing all other essential nutrients, or as an oral adjunct to IV administration of nutrients. Not a balanced diet; do not use as a sole source of nutrition.

Content given per 100 ml liquid or 100 g powder.

	Product & Distributor	CHO (g)	Calories	Sodium (mg)	Chloride (mg)	Potassium (mg)	Calcium (mg)	Phosphorus (mg)	How Supplied
otc	**Polycose Liquid** (Ross)	50	200	70	140	6	20	3	In 126 ml.
otc	**Polycose Powder** (Ross)	94	380	110	223	10	30	5	In 350 g.
otc	**Modocal Powder** (Mead Johnson Nutritional)	95[1]	380	70	150	< 10		—	In 368 g.[2]
otc	**Sumacal Powder** (Sherwood)	95[1]	380	100	210	< 39	< 20	< 31	In 400 g.[2]

[1] Maltodextrin.

[2] Contains 0.4 g/100 g minerals (ash).

Modular Supplements

CORN OIL

Indications:

Increasing caloric intake.

Precautions:

Use in the presence of gallbladder disease or diabetes only on the advice of a physician.

Administration and Dosage:

Adults: 45 ml 2 to 4 times daily, after or between meals.

Children: 30 ml 1 to 4 times daily, after or between meals.

otc	**Lipomul** (Roberts)	**Liquid**: 10 g corn oil per 15 ml in a vehicle containing polysorbate 80, glyceride phosphates and 6.3 mg saccharin (from sodium saccharin) with 0.05% sodium benzoate, 0.05% benzoic acid, 0.07% sorbic acid, BHA and vitamin E. Each serving (45 ml) contains 270 Calories and 30 g fat.	Citrus-vanilla flavor. In 473 ml.

SAFFLOWER OIL

Indications:

Dietary management of patients requiring caloric supplementation (ie, fatty acid deficiencies). Supplies essential fatty acids.

Precautions:

Use in the presence of gallbladder disease or diabetes only on the advice of a physician.

Do not administer to patients with a severe malabsorption syndrome.

Administration and Dosage:

Oral: May give by tablespoon. Flavor additives may improve patient acceptance.

Tube feeding: Can be added to a patient's formula depending upon the degree of caloric supplementation needed.

Shake well before using.

otc	**Microlipid** (Sherwood)	**Emulsion**: 50% fat emulsion. Safflower oil, polyglycerol esters of fatty acids, soy lecithin, xanthan gum and ascorbic acid. Contains 4500 Calories and 500 g fat per L. *Osmolality* - 60 mOsm/kg water	In 120 ml.

MEDIUM CHAIN TRIGLYCERIDES (MCT)

Osmolality: Medium chain triglycerides are more rapidly hydrolyzed than conventional food fat, require less bile acid for digestion, are carried by the portal circulation and are not dependent on chylomicron formation or lymphatic transport. Does not provide essential fatty acids.

Indications:

A special dietary supplement for use in the nutritional management of patients who cannot efficiently digest and absorb conventional long chain food fats.

Precautions:

Hepatic cirrhosis: In persons with advanced cirrhosis, large amounts of MCT may elevate blood and spinal fluid levels of medium chain fatty acids (MCFA) due to impaired hepatic clearance of MCFA which are rapidly absorbed via the portal vein. These elevated levels have caused reversible coma and precoma in subjects with advanced cirrhosis, particularly with portacaval shunts. Use with caution in persons with hepatic cirrhosis and complications such as portacaval shunts or tendency to encephalopathy.

Administration and Dosage:

15 ml, 3 to 4 times per day. Mix with fruit juices, use on salads and vegetables, incorporate into sauces or use in cooking or baking. Do not use plastic containers or utensils.

otc	**MCT** (Mead Johnson Nutritionals)	**Oil:** Lipid fraction of coconut oil consisting primarily of the triglycerides of C_8 ($\approx$ 67%) and C_{10} ($\approx$ 23%) saturated fatty acids. Contains 115 Calories/15 ml	In qt.

Defined Formula Diets

MILK-BASED FORMULAS

See individual product listings for specific labeled indications.

	Product & Distributor	Content per Liter: Protein g	Protein Source	Carbohydrate g	Carbohydrate Source	Fat g	Fat Source	Na (mg)	K (mg)	mOsm/ kg H_2O	Cal/ ml	Other Content	How Supplied
otc	**Sustacal Powder**[1] (Mead Johnson Nutritionals)	87.5	nonfat milk, whole milk (vanilla flavor)	200	sugar, corn syrup solids, lactose (vanilla flavor)	2.9	butter (vanilla flavor)	133 (60 mEq)	4042 (104 mEq)	unknown	1.2	Vit A, B_1, B_2, B_3, B_5, B_6, B_{12}, C, D, E, Ca, Cl, Cu, Fe, I, Mg, Mn, P, Zn[2]	Vanilla flavor. In 57 g packets (4s) and 1 lb cans. Chocolate flavor. In 57 g packets (4s).
otc	**Lonalac Powder** (Mead Johnson Nutritionals)	53.1	casein	74	lactose	55.2	coconut oil	40 (1.7 mEq)	1958 (50 mEq)	360	1	Vit A, B_1, B_2, B_3, Ca, Cl, Mg, P	In 1 lb cans.
otc	**Meritene Powder**[3] (Sandoz Nutrition)	69.2	nonfat milk, whole milk, Ca caseinate, amino acids	119	sugar, hydrolyzed corn starch, fructose	34	soy lecithin	1077 (47 mEq)	2808 (72 mEq)	690	1.06	Vit A, B_1, B_2, B_3, B_5, B_6, B_{12}, C, D, E, K, Ca, Cl, Cu, Fe, I, Mg, Mn, P, Zn[4]	Plain (sugar free), chocolate, eggnog, vanilla and milk chocolate flavors. In 1 and 4.5 lb.
otc	**Compleat Regular Formula Liquid** (Sandoz Nutrition)	43	beef, nonfat milk, amino acids	130	fruits and vegetables, maltodextrin	43	beef, corn oil, mono- and diglycerides	1300 (56.5 mEq)	1400 (36 mEq)	450	1.07	Vit A, B_1, B_2, B_3, B_5, B_6, B_{12}, C, D, E, K, Ca, Cl, Cr, Cu, Fe, I, Mg, Mn, Mo, P, Se, Zn[4]	In 250 ml ready-to-use cans.
otc	**Forta Shake Powder**[5] (Ross)	9	nonfat milk	26	sucrose	< 1	unknown	115 (5 mEq)	440 (11.3 mEq)	NA	140	Vit A, B_1, B_2, B_3, B_5, B_6, B_{12}, C, D, E, Ca, Cu, Fe, I, Mg, Mn, P, Zn[2]	Vanilla, strawberry and eggnog flavors. In 470 g cans. Dutch chocolate flavor. In 530 g cans.

Defined Formula Diets

MILK-BASED FORMULAS

	Product & Distributor	Content per Liter: Protein g	Protein Source	Carbohydrate g	Carbohydrate Source	Fat g	Fat Source	Na (mg)	K (mg)	mOsm/ kg H_2O	Cal/ ml	Other Content	How Supplied
otc	**Ensure Pudding**[6] (Ross)	6.8	nonfat milk	34	sucrose, modified food starch	9.7	partially hydrogenated soybean oil	240	330	unknown	250	850 IU vitamin A, 68 IU D, 7.7 IU E, 12 mcg K, 15.4 mg C, 68 mcg folic acid, 0.25 mg B_1, 0.29 mg B_2, 0.34 mg B_6, 1.1 mcg B_{12}, 3.4 mg B_3, choline, biotin, 1.7 mg B_5, 220 mg Cl, 200 mg Ca, 3.83 mg Zn, 3.06 mg Fe, P, Mg, I, Mn, Cu, tartrazine	Vanilla, chocolate, tapioca and butterscotch flavors. In 150 g cans.
otc	**Sustacal Pudding**[6] (Mead Johnson Nutritionals)	6.8	nonfat milk, amino acids	32	sugar, lactose, modified food starch	9.5	partially hydrogenated soy oil	120 (5.2 mEq)	320 (8.2 mEq)	NA	240	Vit A, B_1, B_2, B_3, B_5, B_6, B_{12}, C, D, E, Ca, Cl, Cu, Fe, I, Mg, Mn, P, Zn^2, tartrazine (vanilla flavor)	Vanilla, chocolate and butterscotch flavors. In 150 g.

Defined Formula Diets

MILK-BASED FORMULAS

	Product & Distributor	Content per Liter								mOsm/ kg H_2O	Cal/ ml	Other Content	How Supplied
		Protein		Carbohydrate		Fat		Na	K				
		g	Source	g	Source	g	Source	(mg)	(mg)				
otc	**Nepro Liquid** (Ross)	6.6	Ca, Mg and Na caseinates	51.1	sucrose, hydrolyzed cornstarch	22.7	high-oleic safflower oil, soy oil	197	251	NA	2	Vit A, D, E, C, B_1, B_3, B_5, B_6, B_{12}, I, biotin, FA, Na, K, Cl, Ca, P, Mg, Mn, Cu, Zn, Fe, Se[8]	Lactose free. Vanilla flavor. In 240 ml ready-to-use cans.
otc	**Sustagen Powder**[7] (Mead Johnson Nutritionals)	24	nonfat milk, whole milk, Ca caseinate, amino acids	66	dextrose, lactose, corn syrup solids, sugar (chocolate)	3.5	milk fat	220 (9.6 mEq)	710 (18.2 mEq)	1130	1.9	Vit A, B_1, B_2, B_3, B_5, B_6, B_{12}, C, D, E, K, Ca, Cl, Cu, Fe, I, Mg, Mn, P, Zn[4]	Vanilla and chocolate flavors. In 1 lb.
otc	**Nutraloric Powder**[3] (Nutraloric)	91.5	Na and Ca caseinates	175	corn syrup solids, fructose	125	soybean oil, soy lecithin, mono- and diglycerides	874 (38 mEq)	3166.2 (81 mEq)	unknown	2.2	Vit A, B_1, B_2, B_3, B_5, B_6, B_{12}, C, D, E, K, Ca, Cl, Cu, Fe, I, Mg, Mn, P, Zn[4]	Chocolate, strawberry, banana nut and vanilla flavors. In 1 lb.

[1] Content given for powder mixed with skim milk.
[2] Also contains folic acid and biotin.
[3] Content given for powder mixed with whole milk.
[4] Also contains folic acid, biotin and choline.
[5] Content given per serving (42 g mix).
[6] Content given per serving (150 g).
[7] Content given per serving (100 g).
[8] Content given per serving (240 ml).

Defined Formula Diets

SPECIALIZED FORMULAS

See individual product listings for specific labeled indications.

		Content per Liter											
		Protein		Carbohydrate		Fat							
	Product & Distributor	g	Source	g	Source	g	Source	Na (mg)	K (mg)	mOsm/kg H_2O	Cal/ml	Other Content	How Supplied
otc	**Amin-Aid Instant Drink Powder**[1] (McGaw)	6.6	amino acids (including phenylalanine)	124.3	maltodextrins, sucrose	15.7	partially hydrogenated soybean oil, lecithin, mono- and diglycerides	< 115 (5 mEq)	NA	700	2	Tartrazine (lemon-lime flavor)	*For acute or chronic renal failure.* Lemon-lime, orange, berry and strawberry flavors. In 156 g packets (12s).
otc	**Boost** [11] (Mead Johnson)	10	unknown	35	unknown	7	unknown	130	400	unknown	240	Vit A, C, D, E, B_1, B_2, B_3, B_5, B_6, B_9, B_{12}, biotin, Ca, P, I, Mg, Zn, Cu, sugar, corn syrup	Vanilla, chocolate, strawberry and mocha flavors. In 237 ml.
otc	**Suplena Liquid** (Ross)	29.6	Ca and Na caseinates, carnitine, taurine	252.5	hydrolyzed corn starch, sucrose	95	high-oleic safflower oil, soy oil, soy lecithin	775 (34 mEq)	1104 (28.3 mEq)	unknown	2	Vit A, B_1, B_2, B_3, B_5, B_6, B_{12}, C, D, E, K, Ca, Cl, Cu, Fe, I, Mg, Mn, P, Se, Zn^2	*For renal conditions.* Vanilla flavor. In 240 ml ready-to-use cans.
otc	**Hepatic-Aid II Instant Drink Powder**[3] (McGaw)	15	amino acids (high BCAA, low AAA)	57.3	maltodextrins, sucrose	12.3	partially hydrogenated soybean oil, lecithin, mono- and diglycerides	< 115 (5 mEq)	unknown	560	1.2	May contain tartrazine	*For chronic liver disease.* Chocolate, eggnog and custard flavors. In 93 g packets (12s).

Defined Formula Diets

SPECIALIZED FORMULAS

	Product & Distributor	Protein g	Protein Source	Carbohydrate g	Carbohydrate Source	Fat g	Fat Source	Na (mg)	K (mg)	mOsm/kg H_2O	Cal/ml	Other Content	How Supplied
otc	**Accupep HPF Powder** (Sherwood)	40	hydrolyzed lactalbumin	188	maltodextrin	10	MCT oil (fractionated coconut oil), corn oil, mono- and diglycerides	680 (29.6 mEq)	1150 (29.5 mEq)	490	1	Vit A, B_1, B_2, B_3, B_5, B_6, B_{12}, C, D, E, K, Ca, Cl, Cu, Fe, I, Mg, Mn, P, Zn[2,4]	*For GI conditions.* In 128 g packets.
otc	**Cyclinex-2 Powder**[5] (Ross)	15	amino acids (including carnitine, phenylalanine, tryptophan)	40	hydrolyzed cornstarch	20.7	palm oil, hydrogenated coconut oil, soy oil, mono- and diglycerides	1175 (51.1 mEq)	1830 (47 mEq)	NA	480	Vit A, B_1, B_2, B_3, B_5, B_6, B_{12}, C, D, E, K, inositol, Cl, Cu, I, Mg, Mn, P, Se, Zn, Ca, Fe[2]	*For urea cycle disorder or gyrate atrophy.* Nonessential amino acid free. In 325 g.
otc	**Glutarex-2 Powder**[5] (Ross)	30	amino acids (including carnitine and phenylalanine)	30	hydrolyzed cornstarch	15.5	palm oil, hydrogenated coconut oil, soy oil, mono- and diglycerides	880 (38.3 mEq)	1370 (35 mEq)	NA	410	Vit A, B_1, B_2, B_3, B_5, B_6, B_{12}, C, D, E, inositol, K, Cl, Cu, I, Mg, Mn, P, Se, Zn, Ca, Fe[2]	*For glutaric aciduria type* I. Lysine- and tryptophan-free. In 325 g.
otc	**Hominex-2 Powder**[5] (Ross)	30	amino acids (including carnitine, phenylalanine, tryptophan)	30	hydrolyzed cornstarch	15.5	palm oil, hydrogenated coconut oil, soy oil, mono- and diglycerides	880 (38.3 mEq)	1370 (35.1 mEq)	NA	410	Vit A, B_1, B_2, B_3, B_5, B_6, B_{12}, C, D, E, K, inositol, Cl, Cu, I, Mg, Mn, P, Se, Zn [2]	*For vitamin B_6-nonresponsive homocystinuria or hypermethioninemia.* Methionine free. In 325 g.

Defined Formula Diets

SPECIALIZED FORMULAS

	Product & Distributor	Content per Liter: Protein g	Protein Source	Carbohydrate g	Carbohydrate Source	Fat g	Fat Source	Na (mg)	K (mg)	mOsm/ kg H_2O	Cal/ ml	Other Content	How Supplied
otc	**l-Valex-2 Powder**[5] (Ross)	30	carnitine, phenylalanine, tryptophan, amino acids	30	hydrolyzed cornstarch	15.5	palm oil, hydrogenated coconut oil, soy oil, mono- and diglycerides	880 (38.3 mEq)	1370 (35.1 mEq)	NA	410	Vit A, B_1, B_2, B_3, B_5, B_6, B_{12}, C, D, E, K, inositol, Ca, Cl, Cu, I, Mg, Mn, P, Se, Zn^2	*For disorder of leucine catabolism.* Leucine free. In 325 g.
otc	**Ketonex-2 Powder**[5] (Ross)	30	carnitine, phenylalanine, tryptophan, amino acids	30	hydrolyzed cornstarch	15.5	palm oil, hydrogenated coconut oil, soy oil, mono- and diglycerides	880 (38.3 mEq)	1370 (35.1 mEq)	NA	410	Vit A, B_1, B_2, B_3, B_5, B_6, B_{12}, C, D, E, K, inositol, Ca, Cl, Cu, I, Mg, Mn, P, Se, Zn^2	*For maple syrup urine disease (MSUD).* Isoleucine, leucine and valine free. In 325 g.
otc	**Phenex-2 Powder**[5] (Ross)	30	amino acids (including carnitine, tryptophan)	30	hydrolyzed cornstarch	15.5	palm oil, hydrogenated coconut oil, soy oil, mono- and diglycerides	880 (38.3 mEq)	1370 (35.1 mEq)	NA	410	Vit A, B_1, B_2, B_3, B_5, B_6, B_{12}, C, D, E, K, inositol, Ca, Cl, Cu, I, Mg, Mn, P, Se, Zn^2	*For phenylketonuria (PKU).* Phenylalanine free. In 325 g.
otc	**Propimex-2 Powder**[5] (Ross)	30	amino acids (including carnitine, phenylalanine, tryptophan)	30	hydrolyzed cornstarch	15.5	palm oil hydrogenated coconut oil, soy oil, mono- and diglycerides	880 (38.3 mEq)	1370 (35.1 mEq)	NA	410	Vit A, B_1, B_2, B_3, B_5, B_6, B_{12}, C, D, E, K, inositol, Ca, Cl, Cu, I, Mg, Mn, P, Se, Zn^2	*For propionic or methylmalonic acidemia.* Methionine and valine free. In 325 g.

Defined Formula Diets

SPECIALIZED FORMULAS

	Product & Distributor	Content per Liter: Protein g	Protein Source	Carbohydrate g	Carbohydrate Source	Fat g	Fat Source	Na (mg)	K (mg)	mOsm/ kg H_2O	Cal/ ml	Other Content	How Supplied
otc	**Tyrex-2 Powder**[5] (Ross)	30	amino acids (including carnitine, tryptophan)	30	hydrolyzed cornstarch	15.5	palm oil, hydrogenated coconut oil, soy oil	880 (38.3 mEq)	1370 (35.1 mEq)	NA	410	Vit A, B_1, B_2, B_3, B_5, B_6, B_{12}, C, D, E, K, inositol, Ca, Cl, Cu, I, Mg, Mn, P, Se, Zn[2]	*For tyrosinemia type* II. Phenylalanine and tyrosine free. In 325 g.
otc	**Travasorb Renal Diet Powder** (Clintec)	23	crystalline amino acids	270.5	glucose oligosaccharides, sucrose	17.7	MCT (fractionated cocount oil), sunflower oil, soy lecithin	unknown	unknown	590	1.35	Vit B_1, B_2, B_3, B_5, B_6, C[2]	*For acute renal failure.* Apricot and strawberry flavors. In 120 g packets (6s).
otc	**Immun-Aid Powder**[6] (McGaw)	18.5	lactalbumin, amino acids (including carnitine, phenylalanine, taurine)	60	maltodextrins	11	medium chain triglycerides, canola oil	290 (12.6 mEq)	530 (13.6 mEq)	460	500	VitA, B_1, B_2, B_3, B_5, B_6, B_{12}, C, D, E, K, Ca, Fe, Cl, Cu, Cr, I, Mg, Mn, Mo, P, Se, Zn[2]	*For immunocompromised patients.* Custard flavor. In 123 g packets (24s).
otc	**Glucerna Liquid** (Ross)	41	amino acids (including carnitine, taurine), Ca and Na caseinate	93	hydrolyzed cornstarch, fructose, soy fiber	55	high-oleic safflower oil, soy oil, soy lecithin	917 (40 mEq)	1542 (40 mEq)	375	1	Vit A, B_1, B_2, B_3, B_5, B_6, B_{12}, C, D, E, K, Cl, Ca, P, Mg, I, Mn, Cu, Zn, Fe, Se, Cr, Mo[2]	*For abnormal glucose tolerance.* Vanilla flavor. In 240 ml ready-to-use cans and 1 liter ready-to-hang feeding containers.

Defined Formula Diets

SPECIALIZED FORMULAS

		Content per Liter											
		Protein		Carbohydrate		Fat							
	Product & Distributor	g	Source	g	Source	g	Source	Na (mg)	K (mg)	mOsm/ kg H_2O	Cal/ ml	Other Content	How Supplied
otc	**Stresstein Powder** (Sandoz Nutrition)	70	amino acids (including 44% BCAA, phenylalanine, tryptophan)	170	maltodextrins	28	MCT, soybean oil, polyglycerol esters of fatty acids	1300 (56.5 mEq)	2200 (56.4 mEq)	910	1.2	Vit A, B_1, B_2, B_3, B_5, B_6, B_{12}, C, D, E, K, Ca, P, I, Fe, Mg, Cu, Zn, Cl, Mn, Se, Cr, Mo[2]	*For moderately and severely stressed patients.* In 102 g packets (36s).
otc	**TraumaCal Liquid** (Mead Johnson Nutritionals)	83	Ca and Na caseinate, amino acids (including phenylalanine, tryptophan)	195	corn syrup, sugar	69	soybean oil, MCT (fractionated coconut oil), lecithin	1200 (52 mEq)	1400 (36 mEq)	490	1.5	Vit A, B_1, B_2, B_3, B_5, B_6, B_{12}, C, D, E, K, Ca, P, I, Fe, Mg, Mn, Cu, Zn, Cl[2]	*For moderately and severely stressed patients.* Lactose free. Vanilla flavor. In 237 ml ready-to-use cans.
otc	**Pulmocare Liquid**[7] (Ross)	62	Ca and Na caseinate, amino acids (including carnitine, taurine)	104	hydrolyzed cornstarch, sucrose	92	corn oil, soy lecithin, canola oil, MCT (fractionated coconut oil), high-oleic safflower oil	1292 (56 mEq)	1708 (44 mEq)	475	1.5	Vit A, B_1, B_2, B_3, B_5, B_6, B_{12}, C, D, E, K, Cl, Ca, P, Mg, I, Mn, Cu, Zn, Fe, Se, Cr, Mo[2]	*For pulmonary patients.* Lactose free. Vanilla and strawberry flavors. In 240 ml ready-to-use cans and 1 liter ready-to-hang containers.
otc	**Respalor Liquid** (Mead Johnson Nutritionals)	75	Ca and Na caseinate	146	corn syrup, sugar	70	MCT (fractionated coconut oil), soy lecithin, canola oil	1250 (54 mEq)	1458 (37 mEq)	580	1.5	Vit A, B_1, B_2, B_3, B_5, B_6, B_{12}, C, D, E, K, Cl, Ca, P, Mg, I, Mn, Cu, Zn, Fe, Se, Cr, Mo[2]	*For pulmonary patients.* Lactose free. Vanilla flavor. In ready-to-use 240 ml.

Defined Formula Diets

SPECIALIZED FORMULAS

		Content per Liter											
		Protein		Carbohydrate		Fat							
	Product & Distributor	g	Source	g	Source	g	Source	Na (mg)	K (mg)	mOsm/ kg H_2O	Cal/ ml	Other Content	How Supplied
otc	**Regain Medical Nutrition Bar**[8] (NCI Medical Foods)	15	whey protein isolate, Ca caseinate, amino acids (including phenylalanine, tryptophan)	53	fructose, maltodextrin, cellulose, rice	7	cottonseed, soybean and canola oils, glycerin, soy lecithin	95 (4.13 mEq)	65 (1.6 mEq)	NA	330	Vit A, B_1, B_2, B_3, B_5, B_6, B_{12}, C, D, E, K, Ca, P, Mg, I, Cu, Zn, Fe [9,10]	*For impaired renal function.* Lactose free. Vanilla, strawberry and malt flavors with cocoa coating. In 85 g.
otc	**Peptamen Liquid** (Carnation)	40	enzymatically hydrolyzed whey proteins, amino acids (including carnitine, taurine)	127.2	maltodextrin, starch	39.2	MCT (fractionated coconut oil), sunflower oil, soy lecithin	500 (22 mEq)	1252 (32 mEq)	270	1	Vit A, B_1, B_2, B_3, B_5, B_6, B_{12}, C, D, E, K, Cl, Ca, P, Mg, I, Mn, Cu, Zn, Fe, Se, Cr, Mo[2]	*For GI impairment.* Unflavored. In ready-to-use 250 ml cans and 500 ml, 1 L and 1.5 L UltraPak bags.

[1] Content given per 156 g package.
[2] Also contains folic acid, biotin and choline.
[3] Content given per ≈ 93 g packets.
[4] Also contains ash.
[5] Content given per 100 g.
[6] Content given per 123 g.
[7] Content given for vanilla flavor.
[8] Content given per 85 g bar.
[9] Also contains folic acid and biotin.
[10] Also contains cocoa.
[11] Content given per 237 ml.
[12] Content given per 240 ml.

Defined Formula Diets

LACTOSE FREE PRODUCTS

See individual product listings for specific labeled indications.

		Content per Liter											
		Protein		Carbohydrate		Fat		Na	K				
	Product & Distributor	g	Source	g	Source	g	Source	(mg)	(mg)	mOsm/ kg H_2O	Cal/ ml	Other Content	How Supplied
otc	**Nepro Liquid** (Clintec)	69.7	Ca, Mg and Na caseinates	214.6	sucrose, hydrolyzed cornstarch	95.3	90% high-oleic safflower oil, 10% soy oil	215	1054	NA	2	Vit A, B_1, B_3, B_5, B_6, B_{12}, biotin, FA, Na, K, Cl, Ca, P, Mg, Mn, I, Cu, Zn, Fe, Se	Vanilla flavor. In 240 ml ready-to-use-cans.
otc	**Reabilan Liquid** (Elan)	31.5	whey peptides, caseinates	131.5	maltodextrins, tapioca starch	39	MCT (fractionated coconut oil), oenothera biennis oil, soya oil, soya lecithin	702 (31 mEq)	1252 (32 mEq)	350	1	Vit A, B_1, B_2, B_3, B_5, B_6, B_{12}, C, D, E, Ca, P, I, Fe, Mg, Cu, Zn, Cl, Mn, Se, Cr[1]	Gluten free. In ready-to-use 375 ml cans.
otc	**Choice dm** (Mead Johnson Nutritionals)	10.6	unknown	25	unknown	12	unknown			unknown	1	Vit A, D, E, K, C, FA, B_1, B_2, B_3, B_5, B_6, B_{12}, biotin, Ca, P, I, Fe, Mg, Cu, Zn, Mn, Cl, K, Na, Se, Cr, Mo, sucrose	Vanilla flavor. In 240 ml ready-to-use cans.
otc	**Travasorb MCT Powder** (Clintec Nutrition)	49.6	lactalbumin, Na and K caseinate	122.8	corn syrup solids	33	sunflower oil, MCT (fractionated coconut oil)	350 (15.2 mEq)	1000 (26 mEq)	250	1	Vit A, B_1, B_2, B_3, B_5, B_6, B_{12}, C, D, E, K, Ca, Cl, Cu, Fe, I, Mg, Mn, P, Zn[1]	Gluten free. Unflavored. In 94.2 g packets.

Defined Formula Diets

LACTOSE FREE PRODUCTS

	Product & Distributor	Protein g	Protein Source	Carbohydrate g	Carbohydrate Source	Fat g	Fat Source	Na (mg)	K (mg)	mOsm/ kg H_2O	Cal/ ml	Other Content	How Supplied
otc	**Vitaneed Liquid** (Sherwood)	40	pureed beef, Ca and Na caseinate, dietary fiber from soy	128	maltodextrin, pureed fruits and vegetables	40	corn oil, soy lecithin	630 (27.4 mEq)	1250 (32 mEq)	300	1	Vit A, B_1, B_2, B_3, B_5, B_6, B_{12}, C, D, E, K, Ca, Cl, Cu, Fe, I, Mg, Mn, P, Zn[1]	In 250 ml cans and 1 L pre-filled closed system containers.
otc	**Travasorb HN Powder** (Clintec Nutrition)	45	enzymatically hydrolyzed lactalbumin	175	glucose oligosaccharides	13	MCT (fractionated coconut oil), sunflower oil	921 (40 mEq)	1170 (30 mEq)	560	1	Vit A, B_1, B_2, B_3, B_5, B_6, B_{12}, C, D, E, K, Ca, Cl, Cu, Fe, I, Mg, Mn, P, Zn[1]	Gluten free. Unflavored. In 88.2 g packets.
otc	**Travasorb STD Powder** (Clintec Nutrition)	30	enzymatically hydrolyzed lactalbumin	190	glucose oligosaccharides	14	MCT (fractionated coconut oil), sunflower oil	921 (40 mEq)	1170 (30 mEq)	560	1	Vit A, B_1, B_2, B_3, B_5, B_6, B_{12}, C, D, E, K, Ca, Cl, Cu, Fe, I, Mg, Mn, P, Zn[1]	Gluten free. Unflavored. In 88.2 g packets.
otc	**Lipisorb Powder** (Mead Johnson Nutritionals)	35	Na caseinate, carnitine	117	corn syrup solids, sucrose	48	MCT, corn oil, soy lecithin	733 (32 mEq)	1250 (32 mEq)	320	1	Vit A, B_1, B_2, B_3, B_5, B_6, B_{12}, C, D, E, K, Ca, Cl, Cu, Fe, I, Mg, Mn, P, Zn[1]	Vanilla flavor. In 1 lb.
otc	**Introlan Half-Strength Liquid** (Elan Pharma)	22.5	Na and Ca caseinate	70	maltodextrin	18	corn oil, MCT, soy lecithin	345 (15 mEq)	585 (15 mEq)	150	0.5	Vit A, B_1, B_2, B_3, B_5, B_6, B_{12}, C, D, E, K, Ca, Cl, Cu, Cr, Fe, I, Mg, Mn, Mo, P, Se, Zn[1]	Gluten free. Unflavored. In 1 L closed system containers. Also available with color check.

(Columns Protein through Fat: Content per Liter.)

Defined Formula Diets

LACTOSE FREE PRODUCTS

	Product & Distributor	Content per Liter								mOsm/ kg H_2O	Cal/ ml	Other Content	How Supplied
		Protein		Carbohydrate		Fat		Na (mg)	K (mg)				
		g	Source	g	Source	g	Source						
otc	**Replete-Oral Liquid** (Clintec Nutrition)	62.5	K and Ca caseinate	113.2	maltodextrin, sucrose	34	corn oil, soy lecithin	500 (22 mEq)	1560 (40 mEq)	350	1	Vit A, B_1, B_2, B_3, B_5, B_6, B_{12}, C, D, E, K, Ca, Cl, Cu, Fe, I, Mg, Mn, P, Zn[1]	Gluten free. Vanilla flavor. In 250 ml ready-to-use cans.
otc	**Attain Liquid** (Sherwood)	40	Na and Ca caseinate	135	maltodextrin	35	MCT, corn oil, soy lecithin	805 (35 mEq)	1600 (41 mEq)	300	1	Vit A, B_1, B_2, B_3, B_5, B_6, B_{12}, C, D, E, K, Ca, Cl, Cu, Fe, I, Mg, Mn, P, Zn, Cr, Se, Mo[1]	In 250 ml cans and 1 L closed system containers.
otc	**Profiber Liquid** (Sherwood)	40	Na and Ca caseinate, dietary fiber from soy	132	hydrolyzed cornstarch	40	corn oil, soy lecithin	730 (32 mEq)	1250 (32 mEq)	300	1	Vit A, B_1, B_2, B_3, B_5, B_6, B_{12}, C, D, E, K, Ca, Cl, Cr, Cu, Fe, I, Mg, Mn, Mo, P, Se, Zn[1]	In 250 ml cans and 1 L pre-filled closed system containers.
otc	**Impact Liquid** (Sandoz Nutrition)	56	Na and Ca caseinate, L–arginine	130	hydrolyzed cornstarch	28	structured lipids from palm kernel oil and sunflower oil, refined menhaden oil, hydroxylated soy lecithin	1100 (48 mEq)	1300 (33 mEq)	375	1	Vit A, B_1, B_2, B_3, B_5, B_6, B_{12}, C, E, D, K, Ca, Fe, P, I, Mg, Zn, Cu, Cl, Mn, Se, Cr, Mo[1]	In 250 ml ready-to-use cans.

Defined Formula Diets

LACTOSE FREE PRODUCTS

	Product & Distributor	Content per Liter								mOsm/ kg H_2O	Cal/ ml	Other Content	How Supplied
		Protein		Carbohydrate		Fat		Na (mg)	K (mg)				
		g	Source	g	Source	g	Source						
otc	**Nutren 1.0 Liquid** (Clintec Nutrition)	40	K and Ca caseinates, taurine, carnitine	127	maltodextrin, corn syrup solids	38	MCT (fractionated coconut oil), corn oil, soy lecithin, canola oil	500 (21.7 mEq)	1252 (32 mEq)	300-390	1	Vit A, B_1, B_2, B_3, B_5, B_6, B_{12}, C, D, E, K, Ca, Cl, Cr, Cu, Fe, I, Mg, Mn, Mo, P, Se, Zn[1]	Gluten free. Unflavored and vanilla, chocolate and strawberry flavors. In 250 ml and UltraPak prefilled bags in 1 and 1.5 L.
otc	**Sustacal Liquid** (Mead Johnson Nutritionals)	60.4	Ca and Na caseinate, soy protein isolate	138	sugar, corn syrup	23	partially hydrogenated soy oil, soy lecithin	1000 (40 mEq)	2042 (52.4 mEq)	NA	1	Vit A, B_1, B_2, B_3, B_5, B_6, B_{12}, C, D, E, K, Ca, P, I, Fe, Mg, Cu, Zn, Mn, Cl[1]	Vanilla, chocolate, strawberry and eggnog flavors. In 240, 360 ml and qt ready-to-use cans.
otc	**Tolerex Powder** (Sandoz Nutrition)	20.6	free amino acids (phenylalanine, tryptophan)	226.3	predigested carbohydrates	1.45	safflower oil	468 (20.4 mEq)	1172 (30.1 mEq)	550	1	Vit A, B_1, B_2, B_3, B_5, B_6, B_{12}, C, D, E, K, Ca, P, I, Fe, Mg, Cu, Zn, Mn, Se, Mo, Cr, Cl.[1]Citric Acid[3]	vanilla, raspberry, orange-pineapple, lemon-lime, Cherry-Vanilla flavor. In 80 g packets (6s).
otc	**Vivonex T.E.N. Powder** (Sandoz Nutrition)	38.2	free amino acids (phenylalanine and tryptophan)	205	unknown	2.77	linoleic acid	460 (20 mEq)	782 (20 mEq)	630	1	Vit A, B_1, B_2, B_3, B_5, B_6, B_{12}, C, D, E, K, Ca, P, I, Fe, Mg, Cu, Zn, Mn, Se, Mo, Cr, Cl[1]	In 80.4 g packets.

Defined Formula Diets

LACTOSE FREE PRODUCTS

	Product & Distributor	Content per Liter								mOsm/kg H_2O	Cal/ml	Other Content	How Supplied
		Protein		Carbohydrate		Fat		Na	K				
		g	Source	g	Source	g	Source	(mg)	(mg)				
otc	**Portagen Powder** (Mead Johnson Nutritionals)	23.3	Na caseinate, amino acids (including taurine, carnitine)	77	corn syrup solids, sucrose	32	MCT (fractionated coconut oil), corn oil, soy lecithin	367 (16 mEq)	833 (21 mEq)	NA	unknown	Vit A, B_1, B_2, B_3, B_5, B_6, B_{12}, C, D, E, K, inositol, Ca, P, I, Fe, Mg, Cu, Zn, Mn, Cl[1]	In 1 lb cans.
otc	**Vital High Nitrogen Powder** (Ross)	41.7	essential amino acids (including phenylalanine, tryptophan), partially hydrolyzed whey, meat and soy	184.7	hydrolyzed cornstarch, sucrose	10.8	safflower oil, MCT (fractionated coconut oil), mono- and diglycerides, soy lecithin	566.7 (24.6 mEq)	1400 (36 mEq)	500	1	Vit A, B_1, B_2, B_3, B_5, B_6, B_{12}, C, D, E, K_1, Ca, P, Mg, Fe, Cu, Zn, Mn, I, Cl, folic acid, biotin, choline[1]	Vanilla flavor. In 79 g packets.
otc	**TwoCal HN Liquid** (Ross)	83	Na and Ca caseinates	214.2	hydrolyzed cornstarch, sucrose	90	MCT (fractionated coconut oil), corn oil, soy lecithin	1292 (56 mEq)	2417 (62 mEq)	unknown	2	Vit A, B_1, B_2, B_3, B_5, B_6, B_{12}, C, D, E, K, Ca, P, Mg, Fe, Cr, Cu, Se, Zn, Mn, Mo, I, Cl[1]	Vanilla flavor. In ready-to-use 240 ml cans.
otc	**Entrition HN EntriPak Liquid** (Clintec)	44	Na and Ca caseinates, soy protein isolate	114	maltodextrin	41	corn oil, soy lecithin, mono- and diglycerides	645 (28 mEq)	1579 (40 mEq)	300	1	Vit A, B_1, B_2, B_3, B_5, B_6, B_{12}, C, D, E, K, Ca, Cl, Cu, Fe, I, Mg, Mn, P, Zn[1]	Unflavored. In 1 liter closed feeding pouch systems.

Defined Formula Diets

LACTOSE FREE PRODUCTS

	Product & Distributor	Content per Liter: Protein g	Protein Source	Carbohydrate g	Carbohydrate Source	Fat g	Fat Source	Na (mg)	K (mg)	mOsm/ kg H_2O	Cal/ ml	Other Content	How Supplied
otc	**Precision High Nitrogen Diet Powder**[4] (Sandoz Nutrition)	12.5	egg white solids	62	maltodextrin, sucrose	0.36	MCT, partially hydrogenated soybean oil, mono-and diglycerides	280 (12.2 mEq)	260 (6.7 mEq)	525	1.05	Vit A, B_1, B_2, B_3, B_5, B_6, B_{12}, C, D, E, K, Ca, P, I, Fe, Mg, Cu, Zn, Cl, Mn, Se, Cr, Mo[1], tartrazine	Citrus flavor. In 87.9 g packets (10s).
otc	**Criticare HN Liquid** (Mead Johnson Nutritionals)	38	enzymatically hydrolyzed casein, amino acids (including phenylalanine, tryptophan)	220	maltodextrin, modified cornstarch	5.3	safflower oil, mono- and diglycerides	630 (27 mEq)	1320 (34 mEq)	650	1.06	Vit A, B_1, B_2, B_3, B_5, B_6, B_{12}, C, D, E, K, Ca, P, I, Fe, Mg, Cu, Zn, Mn, Cl[1]	Unflavored. In 240 ml ready-to-use bottles.
otc	**Isocal Liquid** (Mead Johnson Nutritionals)	34	Ca and Na caseinates, soy protein isolate	135	maltodextrin	44	soy oil, MCT (fractionated coconut oil), soy lecithin	530 (23 mEq)	1320 (34 mEq)	270	1.06	Vit A, B_1, B_2, B_3, B_5, B_6, B_{12}, C, D, E, K, Ca, P, I, Fe, Mg, Cu, Zn, Mn, Cl, Se, Cr, Mo[1]	In 240, 360 ml and qt ready-to-use cans, 1 L ready-to-hang containers and 240 ml bottles.
otc	**Isocal HN Liquid** (Mead Johnson Nutritionals)	44	Ca and Na caseinate, soy protein isolate, amino acids (including taurine, carnitine)	123	maltodextrin	45	soy oil, MCT (fractionated coconut oil)	930 (40 mEq)	1610 (41 mEq)	270	1.06	Vit A, B_1, B_2, B_3, B_5, B_6, B_{12}, C, D, E, K, Ca, P, I, Fe, Mg, Cu, Zn, Mn, Cl, Se, Cr, Mo[1]	Vanilla flavor. In 240 ml and qt ready-to-use cans. Unflavored. In 1 L ready-to-hang bottles.

Defined Formula Diets

LACTOSE FREE PRODUCTS

	Product & Distributor	Content per Liter: Protein g	Protein Source	Carbohydrate g	Carbohydrate Source	Fat g	Fat Source	Na (mg)	K (mg)	mOsm/ kg H_2O	Cal/ ml	Other Content	How Supplied
otc	**Reabilan HN Liquid** (Elan)	58.2	whey peptides, casein peptides, taurine	158	maltodextrins, tapioca starch	52	MCT (fractionated coconut oil), oenothera biennis oil, soya oil, soya lecithin	1000 (43.5 mEq)	1661 (42.4 mEq)	490	1.3	Vit A, B_1, B_2, B_3, B_5, B_6, B_{12}, C, D, E, K, Ca, P, I, Fe, Mg, Cu, Zn, Mn, Cl, Se, Cr, Mo[1]	Gluten free. In ready-to-use 375 ml cans.
otc	**Isolan Liquid** (Elan)	40	caseinates	144	maltodextrin	36	MCT, corn oil	690 (30 mEq)	1170 (30 mEq)	300	1.06	Vit A, B_1, B_2, B_3, B_5, B_6, B_{12}, C, D, E, K, Ca, P, I, Fe, Mg, Cu, Zn, Mn, Cl, Se, Cr, Mo[1]	Gluten free. Unflavored. In 237 ml ready-to-use open system containers and 1 L closed system containers.
otc	**Isotein HN Powder**[5] (Sandoz Nutrition)	20	Na and Ca caseinate, lactalbumin, amino acids (including tryptophan, phenylalanine)	46.7	maltodextrin, fructose	10	MCT, hydrogenated soybean oil, mono- and diglycerides	183 (8 mEq)	317 (8.1 mEq)	300	1.19	Vit A, B_1, B_2, B_3, B_5, B_6, B_{12}, C, D, E, K, Ca, P, I, Fe, Mg, Cu, Zn, Mn, Cl, Se, Cr, Mo[1]	Gluten free. Vanilla flavor. In 87 g packets (36s).
otc	**Jevity Liquid** (Ross)	44	Ca and Na caseinate, soy fiber, carnitine, taurine	150.8	hydrolyzed cornstarch	35	MCT (fractionated coconut oil) canola oil, high-oleic safflower oil, soy lecithin	917 (40 mEq)	1542 (40 mEq)	300	1.06	Vit A, B_1, B_2, B_3, B_5, B_6, B_{12}, C, D, E, K, Ca, P, Mg, Fe, Mn, Cu, Zn, I, Cl, Se, Cr, Mo[1]	In 240 ml and qt ready-to-use cans and 1 L ready-to-hang bottles.

Defined Formula Diets

LACTOSE FREE PRODUCTS

	Product & Distributor	Content per Liter: Protein g	Protein Source	Carbohydrate g	Carbohydrate Source	Fat g	Fat Source	Na (mg)	K (mg)	mOsm/ kg H_2O	Cal/ ml	Other Content	How Supplied
otc	**Resource Liquid** (Sandoz Nutrition)	37	Ca and Na caseinate, soy protein isolate, amino acids (including phenylalanine and tryptophan)	145	sugar, hydrolyzed cornstarch	37	corn oil, soy lecithin	886 (39 mEq)	1603 (41 mEq)	430	1.06	Vit A, B_1, B_2, B_3, B_5, B_6, B_{12}, C, D, E, K, Ca, P, I, Fe, Mg, Cu, Zn, Mn, Cl[1]	*Gluten free.* Vanilla, chocolate and strawberry flavors. In 240 ml ready-to-use Tetra-Brik paks.
otc	**Osmolite Liquid** (Ross)	37	Ca and Na caseinate, soy protein isolate, carnitine, taurine	143	hydrolyzed cornstarch	37	MCT (fractionated coconut oil), canola oil, high-oleic safflower oil, soy lecithin	625 (27 mEq)	1000 (26 mEq)	300	1.06	Vit A, B_1, B_2, B_3, B_5, B_6, B_{12}, C, D, E, K, Cl, Ca, Cr, P, Se, Mg, I, Mn, Mo, Cu, Zn, Fe[1]	Unflavored. In 240 ml and qt ready-to-use cans and 1 L ready-to-hang containers.
otc	**Introlite Liquid** (Ross)	22.2	Na and Ca caseinates	70.5	hydrolyzed cornstarch	18.4	MCT (fractionated coconut oil), corn oil, soy oil, soy lecithin	930 (40 mEq)	1570 (40 mEq)	200	0.53	Vit A, B_1, B_2, B_3, B_5, B_6, B_{12}, C, D, E, K, Cl, Ca, P, Mg, I, Mn, Cu, Zn, Fe, Se, Cr, Mo[1]	In 1 L ready-to-use ready-to-hang containers.
otc	**Osmolite HN Liquid** (Ross)	44	Ca and Na caseinate, soy protein isolate, carnitine, taurine	140	hydrolyzed cornstarch	35	MCT (fractionated coconut oil), high-oleic safflower oil, soy lecithin, canola oil	917 (40 mEq)	1541 (40 mEq)	300	1.06	Vit A, B_1, B_2, B_3, B_5, B_6, B_{12}, C, D, E, K, Cl, Ca, Cr, P, Se, Mg, I, Mn, Mo, Cu, Zn, Fe[1]	In 240 ml and qt ready-to-use cans and 1 L ready-to-hang containers.

Defined Formula Diets

LACTOSE FREE PRODUCTS

	Product & Distributor	Content per Liter								mOsm/ kg H_2O	Cal/ ml	Other Content	How Supplied
		Protein		Carbohydrate		Fat							
		g	Source	g	Source	g	Source	Na (mg)	K (mg)				
otc	**Sustacal Basic Liquid** (Mead Johnson Nutritionals)	37	unknown	147	unknown	35	unknown	833 (36.2 mEq)	1583 (41 mEq)	unknown	1	Vit A, B_1, B_2, B_3, B_5, B_6, B_{12}, C, D, E, K, Cl, Ca, P, Mg, I, Mn, Cu, Zn, Fe[1]	Chocolate, vanilla and strawberry flavors. In 240 ml.
otc	**Nutrilan Liquid** (Elan)	38	caseinates	143	maltodextrin	37	MCT, corn oil	632.5 (27.5 mEq)	1057 (27.1 mEq)	320	1.06	Vit A, B_1, B_2, B_3, B_5, B_6, B_{12}, C, D, E, K, Cl, Ca, P, Mg, I, Mn, Cu, Zn, Fe, Se, Cr, Mo[1]	Chocolate, vanilla and strawberry flavors. In ready-to-use 240 ml TetraPak open system containers.
otc	**Ensure Liquid and Powder**[6] (Ross)	37	Ca and Na caseinate, soy protein isolate	143	corn syrup, sucrose	37	corn oil, soy lecithin	833 (36.2 mEq)	1542 (40 mEq)	470	1.06	Vit A, B_1, B_2, B_3, B_5, B_6, B_{12}, C, D, E, K, Cl, Ca, Cr, P, Se, Mn, Mo, I, Mg, Cu, Zn, Fe[1]	Vanilla, chocolate, coffee, blackwalnut, strawberry and eggnog flavors. In 240 ml and qt ready-to-use cans and 400 g powder.
otc	**Ensure HN Liquid** (Ross)	44	Ca and Na caseinate, soy protein isolate	140	corn syrup, sucrose	35	corn oil, soy lecithin	792 (34 mEq)	1042 (40 mEq)	470	1.06	Vit A, B_1, B_2, B_3, B_5, B_6, B_{12}, C, D, E, K, Cl, Ca, P, Mg, Fe, Mn, Cu, Zn, I[1]	Vanilla flavor. In 240 ml and qt ready-to-use cans. Chocolate flavor. In 240 ml ready-to-use cans.

Defined Formula Diets

LACTOSE FREE PRODUCTS

	Product & Distributor	Content per Liter								mOsm/ kg H_2O	Cal/ ml	Other Content	How Supplied
		Protein		Carbohydrate		Fat		Na	K				
		g	Source	g	Source	g	Source	(mg)	(mg)				
otc	**Ensure High Protein Liquid** (Ross)	50.4	Ca and Na caseinates, soy protein isolate	129.4	sucrose, maltodextrin	25.2	safflower oil, canola oil, soy oil	1218	2100	unknown	1	Vit A, B_1, B_2, B_3, B_5, B_6, B_{12}, C, D, E, K_1, Ca, Cl, Cr, Cu, Fe, I, Mg Mn, Mo, P, Se, Zn, folic acid	Banana, chocolate, wild berry and vanilla flavors. In 237 ml.
otc	**Ultracal Liquid** (Mead Johnson Nutritional)	44	Ca and Na caseinate, soy fiber, oat fiber, taurine, carnitine	123	maltodextrin	45	MCT (fractionated coconut oil), canola oil, mono- and diglycerides, soy lecithin	930 (40 mEq)	1610 (41 mEq)	310	1.06	Vit A, B_1, B_2, B_3, B_5, B_6, B_{12}, C, D, E, K, Ca, P, I, Fe, Mg, Cu, Zn, Mn, Cl, Se, Cr, Mo[1]	Vanilla flavor. In 240 ml and qt ready-to-use cans and 1 L ready- to-hang containers.
otc	**Compleat Modified Formula Liquid** (Sandoz Nutrition)	43	beef, Ca caseinate, amino acids (including phenylalanine, tryptophan)	140	maltodextrin, pureed fruits & vegetables	37	canola oil, mono- and diglycerides	1000 (43.5 mEq)	1400 (36 mEq)	300	1.07	Vit A, B_1, B_2, B_3, B_5, B_6, B_{12}, C, D, E, K, Ca, P, I, Fe, Mg, Cu, Zn, Cl, Mn, Se, Cr, Mo[1]	In ready-to-use 250 ml cans and 1000 and 1500 ml closed system containers.
otc	**Ensure with Fiber Liquid** (Ross)	39	Ca and Na caseinate, soy protein isolate, soy fiber	160	hydrolyzed cornstarch, sucrose	37	corn oil, soy lecithin	833 (36 mEq)	1667 (43 mEq)	480	1.1	Vit A, B_1, B_2, B_3, B_5, B_6, B_{12}, C, D, E, K, Cl, Ca, P, Mg, Fe, Mn, Cu, Zn, I, Se, Cr, Mo[1]	Vanilla and chocolate flavors. In 240 ml and qt (vanilla only) ready-to-use cans.

Defined Formula Diets

LACTOSE FREE PRODUCTS

	Product & Distributor	Content per Liter: Protein g	Protein Source	Carbohydrate g	Carbohydrate Source	Fat g	Fat Source	Na (mg)	K (mg)	mOsm/ kg H_2O	Cal/ ml	Other Content	How Supplied
otc	**Fiberlan Liquid** (Elan)	50	Na and Ca caseinates	160	maltodextrin	40	MCT, corn oil, soy lecithin	920 (40 mEq)	1560 (40 mEq)	310	1.2	Vit A, B_1, B_2, B_3, B_5, B_6, B_{12}, C, D, E, K, Cl, Ca, P, Mg, Fe, Mn, Cu, Zn, I, Se, Cr, Mo[1]	Gluten free. Unflavored. In ready-to-use 237 ml open system containers and 1 L unflavored closed system containers.
otc	**Precision LR Diet Powder**[7] (Sandoz Nutrition)	7.5	egg white solids, amino acids (including phenylalanine, tryptophan)	71	maltodextrin, sucrose	0.45	MCT, partially hydrogenated soybean oil, mono- and diglycerides	200 (8.7 mEq)	250 (6.4 mEq)	510	1.1	Vit A, B_1, B_2, B_3, B_5, B_6, B_{12}, C, D, E, K, Ca, P, I, Fe, Mg, Cu, Zn, Mn, Se, Cr, Mo, Cl[1], tartrazine	Cholesterol and gluten free. Orange, cherry and vanilla flavors. In 90 g packets.
otc	**Isosource Liquid** (Sandoz Nutrition)	43	Ca and Na caseinate, soy protein isolate	170	hydrolyzed cornstarch	41	MCT, canola oil, soy lecithin	1200 (52.2 mEq)	1700 (44 mEq)	360	1.2	Vit A, B_1, B_2, B_3, B_5, B_6, B_{12}, C, D, E, K, Ca, Cl, Cu, Fe, I, Mg, Mn, P, Zn, Se, Cr, Mo[1]	Fiber and gluten free. Vanilla flavor. In ready-to-use 250 ml cans, 240 ml TetraBrik packs and 1 and 1.5 L closed system containers.

Defined Formula Diets

LACTOSE FREE PRODUCTS

	Product & Distributor	Content per Liter								mOsm/ kg H_2O	Cal/ ml	Other Content	How Supplied
		Protein		Carbohydrate		Fat		Na (mg)	K (mg)				
		g	Source	g	Source	g	Source						
otc	**Nitrolan Liquid** (Elan)	60	caseinates	160	maltodextrin	40	MCT, corn oil, soy lecithin	690 (30 mEq)	1170 (30 mEq)	310	1.24	Vit A, B_1, B_2, B_3, B_5, B_6, B_{12}, C, D, E, K, Ca, P, I, Fe, Mg, Cu, Zn, Cl, Mn, Se, Cr, Mo[1]	Gluten free. Unflavored. In ready-to-use 240 ml open system containers and 1 L closed system containers with or without color check.
otc	**Isosource HN Liquid** (Sandoz Nutrition)	53	Ca and Na caseinate, soy protein isolate, amino acids (including phenylalanine, tryptophan)	160	hydrolyzed cornstarch	41	MCT, canola oil, soy lecithin	1100 (48 mEq)	1700 (44 mEq)	330	1.2	Vit A, B_1, B_2, B_3, B_5, B_6, B_{12}, C, D, E, K, Ca, P, I, Fe, Mg, Cu, Zn, Cl, Mn, Se, Cr, Mo[1]	Vanilla flavor. In ready-to-use 250 ml cans, 240 ml TetraBrik packs and 1 and 1.5 ml closed system containers.
otc	**Comply Liquid** (Sherwood)	60	Ca and Na caseinate	180	maltodextrin, sucrose[8]	60	corn oil, soy lecithin	1100 (48 mEq)	1850 (47 mEq)	410	1.5	Vit A, B_1, B_2, B_3, B_5, B_6, B_{12}, C, D, E, K, Ca, Cl, Cu, Fe, I, Mg, Mn, P, Zn[1]	Unflavored. In 250 ml cans. Vanilla, orange and banana flavors. In 250 ml cans and 1000 ml prefilled systems.

Defined Formula Diets

LACTOSE FREE PRODUCTS

	Product & Distributor	Content per Liter: Protein g	Protein Source	Carbohydrate g	Carbohydrate Source	Fat g	Fat Source	Na (mg)	K (mg)	mOsm/ kg H_2O	Cal/ ml	Other Content	How Supplied
otc	**Nutren 1.5 Liquid** (Clintec Nutrition)	60	Ca K and Na caseinate	169.2	maltodextrin	67.6	MCT (fractionated coconut oil), corn oil, canola oil, soy lecithin	752 (33 mEq)	1872 (48 mEq)	410-590	1.5	Vit A, B_1, B_2, B_3, B_5, B_6, B_{12}, C, D, E, K, Ca, Cl, Cu, Fe, I, Mg, Mn, P, Zn, Cr, Mo, Se[1]	Gluten free. Unflavored and vanilla and chocolate flavors. In 250 ml ready- to- use cans. Unflavored. In 1 L prefilled closed system containers.
otc	**Ensure Plus Liquid**[9] (Ross)	54.2	Ca and Na caseinate, soy protein isolate	197.1	corn syrup, sucrose	53	corn oil, soy lecithin	1042 (45.3 mEq)	1917 (49 mEq)	690	1.5	Vit A, B_1, B_2, B_3, B_5, B_6, B_{12}, C, D, E, K, Cl, Ca, P, Mg, Mn, I, Fe, Cu, Zn, Cr, Se, Mo[1]	Chocolate, vanilla, eggnog, strawberry and coffee flavors. In ready-to-use 240 ml and qt cans and 1 L ready-to-hang containers.
otc	**Resource Plus Liquid**[9] (Sandoz Nutrition)	55	Ca and Na caseinate, soy protein isolate	200	hydrolyzed cornstarch, sugar	53	corn oil, soy lecithin	1266 (55 mEq)	2068 (53 mEq)	600	1.5	Vit A, B_1, B_2, B_3, B_5, B_6, B_{12}, C, D, E, K, Ca, P, I, Fe, Mg, Cu, Zn, Cl, Mn[1]	Gluten free. Vanilla, chocolate and strawberry flavors. In 240 ml ready-to-use Brik-Paks.

Defined Formula Diets

LACTOSE FREE PRODUCTS

	Product & Distributor	Content per Liter											
		Protein		Carbohydrate		Fat		Na	K	mOsm/	Cal/	Other	How Supplied
		g	Source	g	Source	g	Source	(mg)	(mg)	kg H_2O	ml	Content	
otc	**Sustacal Plus Liquid** (Mead Johnson Nutritionals)	61	Ca and Na caseinate, amino acid (including phenylalanine, tryptophan)	190	corn syrup solids, sugar	58	corn oil, soy lecithin	850 (37 mEq)	1480 (38 mEq)	480	1.52	Vit A, B_1, B_2, B_3, B_5, B_6, B_{12}, C, D, E, K, Ca, P, I, Fe, Mg, Cu, Zn, Mn, Cl, Cr, Se, Mo[1]	Eggnog, chocolate and vanilla flavors. In 240 ml ready-to-use cans.
otc	**Ensure Plus HN Liquid** (Ross)	62	Ca and Na caseinate, soy protein isolate, amino acid (including carnitine, taurine)	197	hydrolyzed cornstarch, sucrose	49	corn oil, soy lecithin	1167 (51 mEq)	1792 (46 mEq)	unknown	1.5	Vit A, B_1, B_2, B_3, B_5, B_6, B_{12}, C, D, E, K, choline, Cl, Ca, P, Mg, I, Mn, Cu, Zn, Fe, Se, Cr, Mo[1]	Vanilla and chocolate flavors. In 240 ml ready-to-use cans and 1 L ready-to-hang containers.
otc	**Ultralan Liquid** (Elan)	60	caseinates	202	maltodextrin	50	MCT, corn oil	1035 (45 mEq)	1755 (45 mEq)	610	1.5	Vit A, B_1, B_2, B_3, B_5, B_6, B_{12}, C, D, E, K, Cl, Ca, P, Mg, I, Mn, Cu, Zn, Fe, Se, Cr, Mo[1]	Gluten free. Unflavored. In ready-to-use 1000 ml NewPak closed system containers with and without color check.

Defined Formula Diets

LACTOSE FREE PRODUCTS

	Product & Distributor	Protein g	Protein Source	Carbohydrate g	Carbohydrate Source	Fat g	Fat Source	Na (mg)	K (mg)	mOsm/ kg H_2O	Cal/ ml	Other Content	How Supplied
otc	**Advera** (Ross)	60	soy protein hydrolysate, sodium caseinate, 127 mg/L carnitine, 212 mg/L taurine	215.8	hydrolized cornstarch, sucrose	22.8	canola oil, medium-chain triglycerides (fractionated coconut oil), refined deodorized sardine oil	1046	2827	unknown	1.3	8.9 g dietary fiber (from soy fiber), vit A, D, E, K, C, folic acid, B_1, B_2, B_3, biotin, B_5, B_6, B_{12}, Cl, Ca, Zn, Fe, P, Mg, I, Mn, Cu, Se, Cr, Mo, choline	*For dietary management in HIV infection or AIDS.* Gluten free. Chocolate and orange cream flavors. In 240 ml cans.
otc	**Magnacal Liquid** (Sherwood)	70	Ca and Na caseinate	250	maltodextrin, sucrose	80	partially hydrogenated soy oil, soy lecithin, mono- and diglycerides	1000 (43.5 mEq))	1250 (32 mEq)	590	2	Vit A, B_1, B_2, B_3, B_5, B_6, B_{12}, C, D, E, K, choline, Ca, Cl, Cu, Fe, I, Mg, Mn, P, Zn[10]	Vanilla flavor. In ready-to-use 120 and 240 ml bottles and 250 ml cans.
otc	**Isocal HCN Liquid** (Mead Johnson Nutritionals)	75	Ca and Na caseinate, amino acids (including phenylalanine, tryptophan)	200	corn syrup	102	soy oil, MCT (fractionated coconut oil), soy lecithin	800 (35 mEq)	1700 (43 mEq)	640	2	Vit A, B_1, B_2, B_3, B_5, B_6, B_{12}, C, D, E, K, Ca, P, I, Fe, Mg, Cu, Zn, Mn, Cl, Se, Cr, Mo[1]	Vanilla flavor. In 240 ml ready-to-use cans.

Defined Formula Diets

LACTOSE FREE PRODUCTS

	Product & Distributor	Content per Liter								mOsm/kg H_2O	Cal/ml	Other Content	How Supplied
		Protein		Carbohydrate		Fat		Na (mg)	K (mg)				
		g	Source	g	Source	g	Source						
otc	**Nutren 2.0 Liquid** (Clintec Nutrition)	80	Ca and K caseinate, amino acids	196	maltodextrin, corn syrup solids, sucrose	106	MCT (fractionated coconut oil), corn oil, soy lecithin, canola oil	1000 (44 mEq)	2500 (64 mEq)	710	2	Vit A, B_1, B_2, B_3, B_5, B_6, B_{12}, C, D, E, K, Ca, Cl, Cu, Fe, I, Mg, Mn, P, Zn, Cr, Se, Mo[1]	Gluten free. Vanilla flavor. In 250 ml ready-to-use cans.
otc	**Forta Drink Powder**[10] (Ross)	5	whey protein concentrate	15	sucrose, pineapple juice solids	< 1	unknown	50 (2.2 mEq)	70 (1.8 mEq)	NA	85	Vit A, B_1, B_2, B_3, B_5, B_6, B_{12}, C, D, E, Ca, Cu, Fe, I, Mg, Mn, P, Zn[1]	Orange and fruit punch flavors. In 482 g cans.
otc	**Neocate One + Liquid**[11] (SHS)	≈ 2.5	amino acids	14.6	sucrose, maltodextrin	3.5	fractionated coconut oil, canola oil, high oleic sunflower oil	20 (0.9 mEq)	93 (2.4 mEq)	835	100	Vit A, B_1, B_2, B_3, B_5, B_6, B_{12}, C, D, E, K, Ca, Cl, Cr, Cu, Fe, I, Mg, Mn, Mo, Se, Zn, FA, biotin, choline, inositol	Gluten free. Orange and pineapple flavors. In 237 ml with straw.

[1] Also contains folic acid, biotin and choline.
[2] Content given per orange flavor.
[3] Vanilla flavor does not contain citric acid.
[4] Content given per 87.9 g packet.
[5] Content given per 87 g packet.
[6] Content given per ready-to-use liquid.
[7] Content given per 90 g packet.
[8] Unflavored does not contain sucrose.
[9] Content given per vanilla flavor.
[10] Content given per serving (24 ml).Content given per 100 ml.

INFANT FOODS

Uses: Formula for bottle-fed infants; as a supplement to breast-feeding.
See individual product listings for specific labeled indications.

Precautions:

In conditions where the infant is losing abnormal quantities of one or more electrolytes, it may be necessary to supply electrolytes from sources other than the formula. With premature infants weighing < 1500 g at birth, it may be necessary to supply an additional source of sodium, calcium and phosphorus during the period of very rapid growth.

	Product & Distributor	Dilution	Content per Dilution: Protein g	Protein Source	Carbohydrate g	Carbohydrate Source	Fat g	Fat Source	Na (mg)	K (mg)	Cal	Other Content	How Supplied
otc	**Enfamil Human Milk Fortifier Powder** (Mead Johnson Nutritionals)	4 packets (3.8 g) added to breast milk	0.7	whey protein, Na caseinate	2.7	corn syrup solids, lactose	< 0.1	unknown	7 (0.3 mEq)	15.6 (0.4 mEq)	14	Vit A, B_1, B_2, B_3, B_5, B_6, B_{12}, C, D, E, K, Ca, P, Zn, Mg, Mn, Cu, Cl[1]	In 0.96 g packets (100s).
otc	**Enfamil Premature Formula Liquid** (Mead Johnson Nutritionals)	150 ml	3	nonfat milk, whey protein concentrate, amino acids	11.1	corn syrup solids, lactose	5.1	soy oil, MCT (fractionated coconut oil), mono- and diglycerides, linoleic acid	39 (1.7 mEq)	103 (2.6 mEq)	80	Vit A, B_1, B_2, B_3, B_5, B_6, B_{12}, C, D, E, K, inositol, Ca, P, Mg, Zn, Fe, Mn, Cu, I, Cl[1]	In 90 ml nursettes.
otc	**Enfamil Liquid and Powder** (Mead Johnson Nutritionals)	1 liter	15	nonfat milk, reduced minerals whey	69	lactose	37.3	soy and coconut oils, soy lecithin, mono- and diglycerides, high-oleic sunflower oil, palm olein, linoleic acid	180 (7.8 mEq)	720 (18.4 mEq)	667	Vit A, B_1, B_2, B_3, B_5, B_6, B_{12}, C, D, E, K, inositol, Ca, P, Mg, Zn, Fe, Mn, Cu, I, Cl[1]	In 390 ml concentrate, 240 ml and 1 qt ready-to-use cans 90 , 180 and 240 ml nursettes and 1 and 2 lb powder.
otc	**Carnation Good-Start Liquid and Powder** (Carnation)	1 liter	16	reduced minerals whey, taurine	74.4	lactose, maltodextrin	34.5	palm olein, soy oil, coconut oil, high-oleic safflower oil	162 (7 mEq)	663 (17 mEq)	0.68	Vit A, B_1, B_2, B_3, B_5, B_6, B_{12}, C, D, E, K, inositol, Ca, Mg, P, Zn, Fe, Mn, Cu, I, Cl[1]	In 390 ml concentrated liquid, 1 qt ready-to-feed containers and 360 g powder.

INFANT FOODS

	Product & Distributor	Dilution	Content per Dilution									Other Content	How Supplied
			Protein		Carbohydrate		Fat		Na	K			
			g	Source	g	Source	g	Source	(mg)	(mg)	Cal		
otc	**PediaSure Liquid** (Ross)	1 liter	30	Na caseinate, whey protein concentrate, taurine, carnitine	108	hydrolyzed cornstarch, sucrose	49	high-oleic safflower oil, soy oil, MCT (fractionated coconut oil, mono- and diglycerides, soy lecithin	375 (16.3 mEq)	1292 (33 mEq)	1000	Vit A, B_1, B_2, B_3, B_5, B_6, B_{12}, C, D, E, K, inositol, Ca, Mg, P, Zn, Fe, Mn, Cu, I, Cl, Cr, Mo, Se[1]	Gluten free. Vanilla flavor. In ready-to-use 240 ml cans.
otc	**Enfamil Next Step Liquid and Powder** (Mead Johnson Nutritionals)	1 liter	17.3	nonfat milk	74	corn syrup solids, lactose	33.3	palm olein, soy oil, coconut oil, high- oleic sunflower oil, linoleic acid	273 (11.9 mEq)	867 (22.2 mEq)	100	Vit A, B_1, B_2, B_3, B_5, B_6, B_{12}, C, D, E, K, inositol, Ca, Mg, P, Zn, Fe, Mn, Cu, I, Cl, Se[1]	In 390 ml concentrate, 1 qt ready-to-use liquid and 360 and 720 g powder.
otc	**Carnation Follow-Up Formula Liquid and Powder** (Carnation)	1 liter	17.3	nonfat milk	88	corn syrup	27.3	palm olein, coconut oil, high oleic safflower oil, soy lecithin, soy oil	260 (11.5 mEq)	900 (23 mEq)	676	Vit A, B_1, B_2, B_3, B_5, B_6, B_{12}, C, D, E, K, inositol, Ca, Mg, P, Zn, Fe, Mn, Cu, I, Cl[1]	In 390 ml concentrate, 1 qt ready-to-feed containers and 360 g powder.

[1] Also contains folic acid, biotin and choline.

INFANT FOODS WITH IRON

See individual product listings for specific labeled indications.

	Product & Distributor	Dilution	Content per Dilution										Other Content	How Supplied
			Protein		Carbohydrate		Fat		Iron (mg)	Na (mg)	K (mg)	Cal		
			g	Source	g	Source	g	Source						
otc	**Lofenalac Powder** (Mead Johnson Nutritionals)	1 liter	22	casein hydrolysate, amino acids (including tryptophan, taurine, carnitine	54.2	corn syrup solids, modified tapioca starch	16.3	corn oil	12.5	313 (14 mEq)	680 (17.4 mEq)	667	Vit A, B_1, B_2, B_3, B_5, B_6, B_{12}, C, D, E, K, inositol, Ca, P, Mg, Zn, Mn, Cu, I, Cl[1]	Low phenylalanine. In 1 lb powder.
otc	**Similac w/Iron Liquid and Powder** (Ross)	1 liter	15	nonfat milk, taurine	72.3	lactose	37	Coconut oil, corn oil, soy oil, mono- and diglycerides, soy lecithin, linoleic acid	12	180 (8 mEq)	700 (18 mEq)	676	Vit A, B_1, B_2, B_3, B_5, B_6, B_{12}, C, D, E, K, inositol, Ca, P, Mg, Zn, Mn, Cu, I, Cl[1]	In 390 ml concentrate, 240 ml and 1 qt ready-to-use cans, 120 and 240 ml nursettes and 1 lb powder.
otc	**SMA Iron Fortified Liquid and Powder** (Wyeth-Ayerst)	1 liter	15	nonfat milk, reduced minerals whey, taurine	71	lactose	35.3	oleo, coconut, safflower, sunflower and soybean oils, soy lecithin, linoleic acid	12	147 (6.4 mEq)	553 (14.2 mEq)	667	Vit A, B_1, B_2, B_3, B_5, B_6, B_{12}, C, D, E, K, Ca, P, Mg, Cl, Cu, Zn, Mn, I[1]	In 384 ml concentrate, ready-to-use 240 ml and 1 qt and 1 and 2 lb powder.
otc	**Enfamil w/Iron Liquid and Powder** (Mead Johnson Nutritionals)	1 liter	15	nonfat milk, reduced minerals whey	69	lactose	37	soy and coconut oils, soy lecithin, mono- and diglycerides, palm olein, high-oleic sunflower oil, linoleic acid	12.5	180 (8 mEq)	720 (18.4 mEq)	666	Vit A, B_1, B_2, B_3, B_5, B_6, B_{12}, C, D, E, K, inositol, Ca, P, Mg, Zn, Mn, Cu, I, Cl[1]	In 390 ml concentrate, ready-to-use 240 ml and 1qt , 180 ml nursettes and 1 and 2 lb powder.

INFANT FOODS WITH IRON

	Product & Distributor	Dilution	Content per Dilution										Other Content	How Supplied
			Protein		Carbohydrate		Fat		Iron	Na	K	Cal		
			g	Source	g	Source	g	Source	(mg)	(mg)	(mg)			
otc	**Gerber Baby Formula with Iron Liquid and Powder** (Gerber)	1 liter	15	nonfat milk	71	lactose	36	palm olein, soy oil, coconut oil, high oleic sunflower oil, soy lecithin, mono- and diglycerides, linoleic acid	12	220 (10 mEq)	720 (19 mEq)	667	Vit A, B_1, B_2, B_3, B_5, B_6, B_{12}, C, D, E, K, inositol, Ca, P, Mg, Zn, Mn, Cu, I, Cl[1]	In 390 ml concentrate, 1 qt ready-to-use and 1 lb powder.
otc	**Bonamil Infant Formula w/Iron Powder or Liquid** (Wyeth-Ayerst)	150 ml	2.3	nonfat milk, taurine	10.7	lactose	5.4	soybean oil, coconut oil, soy lecithin, linoleic acid	1.8	27	93	100	Vit A, B_1, B_2, B_3, B_5, B_6, B_{12}, C, D, E, K, biotin, choline, Ca, P, Mg, Zn, Mn, Cu, I, Cl, folic acid	In 453 g powder or 946 ml ready-to-feed liquid

[1] Also contains folic acid, biotin and choline

SPECIALIZED INFANT FOODS

See individual product listings for specific labeled indications.

	Product & Distributor	Dilution	Content per Dilution										Other Content	How Supplied
			Protein		Carbohydrate		Fat		Iron	Na	K	Cal		
			g	Source	g	Source	g	Source	(mg)	(mg)	(mg)			
otc	**Soyalac Liquid and Powder** (Nutricia-Loma Linda)	per 100 calories	3.1	soybean extract	10	corn syrup, sucrose	5.5	soy oil, linoleic acid	1.5	‡	‡	667	unknown	Lactose free. In 390 ml concentrate, 1 qt ready-to-use and 420 g powder.

SPECIALIZED INFANT FOODS

	Product & Distributor	Dilution	Content per Dilution										Other Content	How Supplied
			Protein		Carbohydrate		Fat		Iron (mg)	Na (mg)	K (mg)	Cal		
			g	Source	g	Source	g	Source						
otc	**I-Soyalac Liquid and Powder** (Nutricia-Loma Linda)	per 100 calories	3.1	soy protein isolate, amino acids	10	sucrose, tapioca dextrin, potato maltodextrin	5.5	soy oil, linoleic acid	1.9	‡	‡	100	unknown	Corn syrup solids and lactose free. In 390 ml concentrate and 1 qt ready-to-use and 420 g powder.
otc	**Alimentum Liquid** (Ross)	1 liter	19	casein hydrolysate, amino acids (including tryptophan, taurine, carnitine)	69	sucrose, modified tapioca starch	36	MCT (fractionated coconut oil), safflower oil, soy oil	12	297 (13 mEq)	798 (21 mEq)	676	Vit A, B_1, B_2, B_3, B_5, B_6, B_{12}, C, D, E, K, inositol, Ca, Cl, Cu, I, Mg, Mn, P, Zn[1]	*For infants and children with severe food allergies, sensitivity to intact protein, protein maldigestion or fat malabsorption.* Corn and lactose free. In ready-to-use 240 and 360 ml.

SPECIALIZED INFANT FOODS

	Product & Distributor	Dilution	Content per Dilution										Other Content	How Supplied
			Protein		Carbohydrate		Fat		Iron (mg)	Na (mg)	K (mg)	Cal		
			g	Source	g	Source	g	Source						
otc	**Isomil Liquid and Powder** (Ross)	1 liter	17	soy protein isolate, amino acids (including carnitine)	70	corn syrup, sucrose, cornstarch[2]	37	corn, soy and coconut oils, mono- and diglycerides, soy lecithin	12	297 (13 mEq)	730 (18.4 mEq)	676	Vit A, B_1, B_2, B_3, B_5, B_6, B_{12}, C, D, E, K, inositol, Ca, P, Mg, Zn, Mn, Cu, I, Cl[1]	*For infants and children who are allergic or sensitive to cow's milk, lactose intolerant or deficient or are galactosemic.* Lactose free. In 390 ml concentrate, 120 ml nursing bottles, 240 ml and 1 qt ready-to-use and 420 g powder.
otc	**Isomil SF Liquid** (Ross)	1 liter	18	soy protein isolate, amino acids (including carnitine)	68.3	hydrolyzed cornstarch	37	soy oil, coconut oil, mono- and diglycerides, soy lecithin, linoleic acid	12	297 (13 mEq)	730 (19 mEq)	676	Vit A, B_1, B_2, B_3, B_5, B_6, B_{12}, C, D, E, K, inositol, Ca, P, Cu, Mg, Zn, Mn, I, Cl[1]	*For infants and children with an allergy sensitivity to cow's milk protein or intolerance to sucrose.* Sucrose and lactose free. In 390 ml concentrate.
otc	**Nursoy Liquid and Powder** (Wyeth-Ayerst)	1 liter	21	soy protein isolate, methionine	69	sucrose	36	oleo, coconut, safflower and soybean oils, soy lecithin	11.5	200 (9 mEq)	700 (18 mEq)	667	Vit A, B_1, B_2, B_3, B_5, B_6, B_{12}, C, D, E, K, inositol, Ca, P, Cl, Mg, Mn, Cu, Zn, I[1]	In 390 ml concentrate, 1 qt ready-to-use and 1 lb powder.

SPECIALIZED INFANT FOODS

	Product & Distributor	Dilution	Content per Dilution											Other Content	How Supplied
			Protein		Carbohydrate		Fat		Iron (mg)	Na (mg)	K (mg)	Cal			
			g	Source	g	Source	g	Source							
otc	**Pregestimil Powder** (Mead Johnson Nutritionals)	1 liter	18.7	enzymatically hydrolyzed casein, amino acids (including tryptophan, taurine, carnitine)	69	corn syrup solids, modified corn starch, dextrose	37.3	corn oil, MCT (fractionated coconut oil), high-oleic safflower oil, linoleic acid	12.5	260 (11.3 mEq)	726 (19 mEq)	667		Vit A, B_1, B_2, B_3, B_5, B_6, B_{12}, C, D, E, K, inositol, Ca, P, Cu, Mg, Zn, Mn, I, Cl[1]	*For infants with severe malabsorption disorders.* In 1 lb powder.
otc	**Nutramigen Liquid and Powder** (Mead Johnson Nutritionals)	1 liter	19	enzymatically hydrolyzed casein, amino acids (including tryptophan, taurine, carnitine)	89.3	corn syrup solids, modified cornstarch	26	corn oil, soy oil, linoleic acid	12.5	313 (14 mEq)	727 (19 mEq)	667		Vit A, B_1, B_2, B_3, B_5, B_6, B_{12}, C, D, E, K, inositol, Ca, P, Cu, Mg, Zn, Mn, I, Cl[1]	*For infants and children sensitive to intact proteins of milk and other foods.* Lactose and sucrose free. In 1 lb powder, 390 ml concentrate and 1 qt ready-to-use.
otc	**ProSobee Liquid and Powder**- (Mead Johnson Nutritionals)	1 liter	20	soy protein isolate, amino acids (including taurine, carnitine)	67	corn syrup solids	35.3	linoleic acid, coconut, corn and soy oil, palm olein, high oleic sunflower oils[3]	12.5	240 (10.5 mEq)	813 (21 mEq)	667		Vit A, B_1, B_2, B_3, B_5, B_6, B_{12}, C, D, E, K, inositol, Ca, P, Cu, Mg, Zn, Mn, I, Cl[1]	*For infants with a family history of allergies.* Sucrose, milk and lactose free. In 390 ml concentrate, 240 ml and 1 qt ready-to-use and 420 g powder.

SPECIALIZED INFANT FOODS

	Product & Distributor	Dilution	Content per Dilution										Other Content	How Supplied
			Protein		Carbohydrate		Fat		Iron (mg)	Na (mg)	K (mg)	Cal		
			g	Source	g	Source	g	Source						
otc	**Similac PM 60/40 Low-Iron Liquid** (Ross)	1 liter	15.6	whey protein concentrate, Na caseinate, carnitine, taurine	68	lactose	37	coconut oil, mono- and diglycerides, soy oil, linoleic acid	1.5	160 (7 mEq)	573 (15 mEq)	100	Vit A, B_1, B_2, B_3, B_5, B_6, B_{12}, C, D, E, K, inositol, Ca, P, Cu, Mg, Zn, Mn, I, Cl	*For infants who are predisposed to hypocalcemia or those who would benefit from lowered mineral levels.* In 120 ml bottles.
otc	**Similac Low-Iron Liquid and Powder** (Ross)	1 liter	14.3	nonfat milk, taurine	72	lactose	36	Corn, coconut and soy oils, mono- and diglycerides, soy lecithin, linoleic acid	1.5	180 (7.8 mEq)	700 (17.9 mEq)	676	Vit A, B_1, B_2, B_3, B_5, B_6, B_{12}, C, D, E, K, inositol, Ca, P, Cu, Mg, Zn, Mn, I, Cl[1]	In 390 ml concentrate, 240 ml and 1 qt ready-to-use, 120 and 240 ml nursettes and 1 lb powder.
otc	**RCF Liquid** (Ross)	1 liter	39.3	soy protein isolate, amino acids (including carnitine and taurine)	0.08	unknown	71	soy oil, coconut oil, mono- and diglycerides, soy lecithin	3	579 (25.2 mEq)	1429 (37 mEq)	818	Vit A, B_1, B_2, B_3, B_5, B_6, B_{12}, C, D, E, K, inositol, Ca, P, Cu, Mg, Zn, Mn, I, Cl[1]	Carbohydrate free. In 390 ml concentrate.
otc	**Lactofree Liquid and Powder** (Mead Johnson Nutritionals)	1 liter	14.7	milk protein isolate, taurine, carnitine	69.3	corn syrup solids	37	palm olein, soy, coconut and high -oleic sunflower oils, linoleic acid	12	200 (9 mEq)	733 (19 mEq)	676	Vit A, B_1, B_2, B_3, B_5, B_6, B_{12}, C, D, E, K, inositol, Ca, P, Cu, Mg, Zn, Mn, I, Cl, Se[1]	Lactose free. In 1 qt ready-to-use liquid, 390 ml concentrate and 400 g powder.

SPECIALIZED INFANT FOODS

	Product & Distributor	Dilution	Content per Dilution										Other Content	How Supplied
			Protein		Carbohydrate		Fat		Iron (mg)	Na (mg)	K (mg)	Cal		
			g	Source	g	Source	g	Source						
otc	**Gerber Baby Low Iron Formula Liquid and Powder** (Gerber)	1 liter	15	nonfat milk, taurine	71.3	lactose	36	palm olein, soy, coconut and high-oleic sunflower oil, soy lecithin, mono- and diglycerides, linoleic acid	3.3	220 (9.6 mEq)	720 (18.5 mEq)	667	Vit A, B_1, B_2, B_3, B_5, B_6, B_{12}, C, D, E, K, inositol, Ca, P, Cu, Mg, Zn, Mn, I, Cl[1]	In ready-to-use qt, 150 ml concentrate and 1 and 2 lb powder.
otc	**SMA Lo-Iron Infant Formula** (Wyeth Ayerst)	1 liter	15	nonfat milk, reduced minerals whey, taurine	71	lactose	353	oleo oil, coconut oil, high oleic safflower or sunflower oil, soybean oil, soy lecithin, linoleic acid	1.3	147 (6.4 mEq)	553 (14.2 mEq)	667	Vit A, B_1, B_2, B_3, B_5, B_6, B_{12}, C, D, E, K, inositol, Ca, P, Cu, Mg, Zn, Mn, I, Cl[1]	In 390 ml concentrate, 1 qt ready-to-use liquid and 1 lb powder.
otc	**Gerber Soy formula Liquid and Powder** (Gerber)	1 liter	20	soy protein isolate, amino acids (including taurine, carnitine)	67	corn syrup solids, sugar	35.3	palm olein, soy, coconut and high oleic sunflower oils, soy lecithin, mono- and diglycerides, linoleic acid	12	313 (14 mEq)	767 (20 mEq)	667	Vit A, B_1, B_2, B_3, B_5, B_6, B_{12}, C, D, E, K, inositol, Ca, P, Cu, Mg, Zn, Mn, I, Cl[1]	In 1 qt ready-to-use, and 420 g powder.

SPECIALIZED INFANT FOODS

	Product & Distributor	Dilution	Protein g	Protein Source	Carbohydrate g	Carbohydrate Source	Fat g	Fat Source	Iron (mg)	Na (mg)	K (mg)	Cal	Other Content	How Supplied
otc	**Pro-Phree Powder** (Ross)	100 g powder[4]	NA	NA	60	hydrolyzed cornstarch	31	palm oil, hydrogenated coconut oil, soy oil, mono- and diglycerides, linoleic acid	11.9	250 (11 mEq)	875 (22.4 mEq)	520	Vit A, B_1, B_2, B_3, B_5, B_6, B_{12}, C, D, E, K, inositol, Ca, P, Cu, Mg, Zn, Mn, I, Cl, Se[1,5]	*For nutritional support of infants and toddlers who require extra calories, minerals, vitamins and/or protein restriction.* Protein free. In 350 g powder.
otc	**Propimex-1 Powder** (Ross)	100 g powder[4]	15	amino acids (including carnitine, phenylalanine, tryptophan, taurine)	46.3	hydrolyzed cornstarch	24	palm oil, hydrogenated coconut oil, soy oil, mono- and diglycerides, linoleic acid	9	190 (8.3 mEq)	675 (18 mEq)	480	Vit A, B_1, B_2, B_3, B_5, B_6, B_{12}, C, D, E, K, inositol, Ca, P, Cu, Mg, Zn, Mn, I, Cl, Se[1]	*For nutritional support of infants and toddlers with propionic or methylmalonic acidemia.* Methionine- and valine -free. In 350 g powder.
otc	**Tyromex-1 Powder** (Ross)	100 g powder[4]	15	amino acids (including tryptophan, taurine, carnitine)	46.3	hydrolyzed cornstarch	29	palm oil, hydrogenated coconut oil, soy oil, mono- and diglycerides, linoleic acid	9	190 (8.3 mEq)	675 (17.3 mEq)	480	Vit A, B_1, B_2, B_3, B_5, B_6, B_{12}, C, D, E, K, inositol, Ca, P, Cu, Mg, Zn, Mn, I, Cl, Se[1]	*For nutritional support of infants and toddlers with tyrosinemia type* I. Phenylalanine, tyrosine and methionine free. In 350 g powder.

SPECIALIZED INFANT FOODS

	Product & Distributor	Dilution	Content per Dilution: Protein g	Protein Source	Carbohydrate g	Carbohydrate Source	Fat g	Fat Source	Iron (mg)	Na (mg)	K (mg)	Cal	Other Content	How Supplied
otc	**Ketonex-1 Powder** (Ross)	100 g powder[4]	15	amino acids (including phenylalanine, tryptophan, carnitine, taurine)	46.3	hydrolyzed cornstarch	24	palm oil, hydrogenated coconut oil, soy oil, mono-and diglycerides, linoleic acid	9	190 (8.3 mEq)	675 (17.3 mEq)	480	Vit A, B_1, B_2, B_3, B_5, B_6, B_{12}, C, D, E, K, inositol, Ca, P, Cu, Mg, Zn, Mn, I, Cl, Se[1]	*For nutritional support of infants and toddlers with maple syrup urine disease (MSUD).* Isoleucine, leucine and valine free. In 350 g powder.
otc	**Glutarex-1 Powder** (*Ross*)	100 g powder[4]	15	amino acids (including carnitine, phenylalanine, taurine)	47	hydrolyzed cornstarch	24	palm oil, hydrogenated coconut oil, soy oil, mono- and diglycerides, linoleic acid	9	190 (8.3 mEq)	675 (17.3 mEq)	480	Vit A, B_1, B_2, B_3, B_5, B_6, B_{12}, C, D, E, K, inositol, Ca, P, Cu, Mg, Zn, Mn, I, Cl, Se[1]	*Nutritional support of infants and toddlers with glutaric aciduria type* I. Lysine and tryptophan free. In 350 g powder.
otc	**Hominex-1 Powder** (Ross)	100 g powder[4]	15	amino acids (including phenylalanine, tryptophan, taurine, carnitine)	46.3	hydrolyzed cornstarch	24	palm oil, hydrogenated coconut oil, soy oil, mono- and diglycerides, linoleic acid	9	190 (8.3 mEq)	675 (17.3 mEq)	480	Vit A, B_1, B_2, B_3, B_5, B_6, B_{12}, C, D, E, K, inositol, Ca, P, Cu, Mg, Zn, Mn, I, Cl, Se[1]	*Nutritional support of infants and toddlers with vitamin B_6-nonresponsive homocystinuria or hypermethioninemia.* Methionine free. In 350 g powder.

SPECIALIZED INFANT FOODS

	Product & Distributor	Dilution	Content per Dilution										Other Content	How Supplied
			Protein		Carbohydrate		Fat							
			g	Source	g	Source	g	Source	Iron (mg)	Na (mg)	K (mg)	Cal		
otc	**I-Valex-1 Powder** (Ross)	100 g powder[4]	15	amino acids (including carnitine, phenylalanine, tryptophan, taurine)	46.3	hydrolyzed cornstarch	24	palm oil, hydrogenated coconut oil, soy oil, mono- and diglycerides, linoleic acid	9	190 (8.3 mEq)	675 (17.3 mEq)	480	Vit A, B_1, B_2, B_3, B_5, B_6, B_{12}, C, D, E, K, inositol, Ca, P, Cu, Mg, Zn, Mn, I, Cl, Se[1]	*Nutritional support of infants and toddlers with a disorder of leucine catabolism.* Leucine free. In 350 g.
otc	**Cyclinex-1 Powder** (Ross)	100 g powder[4]	7.5	amino acids (including phenylalanine, tryptophan, carnitine, taurine)	52	hydrolyzed cornstarch	27	palm oil, hydrogenated coconut oil, soy oil, mono- and diglycerides, linoleic acid	10	215 (9.3 mEq)	760 (19.4 mEq)	515	Vit A, B_1, B_2, B_3, B_5, B_6, B_{12}, C, D, E, K, inositol, Ca, P, Cu, Mg, Zn, Mn, I, Cl, Se[1]	*For nutritional support of infants and toddlers with a urea cycle disorder or gyrate atrophy.* Nonessential amino acid free. In 350 g.
otc	**Phenex-1 Powder** (Ross)	100 g powder[4]	15	amino acids (including tryptophan, taurine, carnitine)	46.3	hydrolyzed cornstarch	24	palm oil, hydrogenated coconut oil, soy oil, mono- and diglycerides	9	190 (8.3 mEq)	675 (17.2 mEq)	480	Vit A, B_1, B_2, B_3, B_5, B_6, B_{12}, C, D, E, K, inositol, Ca, P, Cu, Mg, Zn, Mn, I, Cl, Se[1]	*Nutritional support of infants and toddlers with phenylketonuria (PKU).* Phenylalanine free. In 350 g.

SPECIALIZED INFANT FOODS

	Product & Distributor	Dilution	Content per Dilution										Other Content	How Supplied
			Protein		Carbohydrate		Fat		Iron (mg)	Na (mg)	K (mg)	Cal		
			g	Source	g	Source	g	Source						
otc	**Isomil DF** (Ross)	per 100 calories	2.7	soybean solids, amino acids	10.1	corn syrup, sucrose	5.5	soy oil, coconut oil	1.8	44 (1.9 mEq)	108 (2.8 mEq)	676	Vit A, B_1, B_2, B_3, B_5, B_6, B_{12}, C, D, E, K, inositol, Ca, P, Cu, Mg, Zn, Mn, I, Cl, Se[1]	*For management of diarrhea in infants and toddlers.* Lactose free. In 960 ml, pre-diluted, ready-to-use cans.

* ‡ Amount Unknown.
[1] Also contains folic acid, biotin and choline
[2] Concentrate contains cornstarch.
[3] Ready-to-use contains soy lecithin and mono- and diglycerides.
[4] Content given from unreconstituted powder.
[5] Contains trace amounts of taurine and carnitine.

Food Modifiers

LACTOSE

These products are used as modifiers for infant formulas or as dietary supplements.

otc	**Lactose** (Various, eg, Humco, Paddock)	**Powder**	In 1 lb.

CALCIUM CASEINATE

otc	**Casec** (Mead Johnson Nutritionals)	**Powder:** Contains 88 g protein, 1.6 g calcium, 120 mg sodium, 2 g fat and 370 calories per 100 g	In 75 g.

LACTASE ENZYME

Indications:

To digest lactose contained in milk for patients with lactose intolerance.

Administration and Dosage:

Liquid: 5 to 15 drops per qt of milk, based on lactose conversion level desired.

Tablets: 1 to 3 tablets with the first bite of dairy food. *Lactaid* may be chewed or swallowed; do not take more than 6 tablets at a time.

Capsules: 1 or 2 capsules taken with milk or dairy products. If the patient is severely intolerant to lactose, increase dosage until a satisfactory dose is achieved.

otc	**LactAid** (McNeil)	**Liquid:** Beta-D-galactosidase derived from *Kluyveromyces lactis yeast* (≥ 1250 neutral lactase units per 5 drop dosage)	Glycerol, water, inert yeast. In units of 12, 30 and 75 one quart dosages at 5 drops/ dose.
		Tablets: ≥ 3000 FCC lactase units of beta-D-galactosidase from *Aspergillis oryzae*	Capsule shape. In 12s, 100s and UD 50s.
otc	**Lactrase** (Schwarz Pharma Kremers Urban)	**Capsules:** 250 mg standardized enzyme lactase	(Kremers Urban 505). Orange/white. In 100s and blister-pack 10s and 30s.
otc	**SureLac** (Caraco)	**Tablets, chewable:** 3000 FCC lactase units	May contain Sorbitol or mannitol. In 60s.
otc	**Dairy Ease** (Sterling Health)	**Tablets, chewable:** 3300 FCC lactase units	Mannitol. In 26, 40, 60 and 100s.

ALPHA-D-GALACTOSIDASE ENZYME

Actions:

Pharmacology: Alpha-D-galactosidase enzyme hydrolyzes raffinose, verbascose and stachyose into the digestible sugars sucrose, fructose, glucose and galactose.

Indications:

Treatment of gassiness or bloating as a result of eating a variety of grains, cereals, nuts, seeds or vegetables containing the sugars raffinose, stachyose or verbascose. This includes all or most legumes and all or most cruciferous vegetables (eg, oats, wheat, beans, peas, lentils, peanuts, soy-content foods, pistachios, broccoli, brussels sprouts, cabbage, carrots, corn, onions, squash, cauliflower).

Precautions:

Galactosemics should not use without physician advice since one of the breakdown sugars is galactose.

Administration and Dosage:

Use 3 to 8 drops per average serving. Approximately 5 drops on the first portion of food consumed will deal with the entire subsequent portion. Use a higher or lower number of drops depending on the quantity of food eaten, levels of alpha-linked sugars in the food and the gas-producing propensity and tolerance of the person.

otc	**Beano** (AK Pharma)	**Liquid:** Alpha-D-galactosidase-derived from *Aspergillus niger* (≥ 175 galactose units per 5 drop dosage)	Glycerol. In 75 serving size at 5 drops per dose.
		Tablets: Alpha-galactosidase enzyme derived from *Aspergillus niger*	Cornstarch, sucrose, hydrogenated cottonseed oil, sorbitol. In 12s, 30s and 100s.

chapter 2

blood modifiers

IRON-CONTAINING PRODUCTS, ORAL

Actions:

Pharmacology: Iron, an essential mineral, is a component of hemoglobin, myoglobin and a number of enzymes. The total body content of iron is approximately 50 mg/kg in men (3.5 g in the average 70 kg man) and 35 mg/kg in women. Iron is primarily stored as hemosiderin or ferritin, found in the reticuloendothelial cells of the liver, spleen and bone marrow. Approximately two-thirds of total body iron is in the circulating red blood cell mass in hemoglobin, the major factor in oxygen transport.

Pharmacokinetics:

Absorption/Distribution – The average dietary intake of iron is 18 to 20 mg/day; however, only about 10% of this iron is absorbed (1 to 2 mg/day) in individuals with adequate iron stores. Absorption is enhanced (20% to 30%) when storage iron is depleted or when erythropoiesis occurs at an increased rate. Iron is primarily absorbed from the duodenum and upper jejunum by an active transport mechanism. The ferrous salt form is absorbed three times more readily than the ferric form. The common ferrous salts (sulfate, gluconate, fumarate) are absorbed almost on a milligram-for-milligram basis, but differ in the content of elemental iron. Sustained release or enteric coated preparations reduce the amount of available iron; absorption from these doseforms is reduced because iron is transported beyond the duodenum. Dose also influences the amount of iron absorbed. The amount of iron absorbed increases progressively with larger doses; however, the percentage absorbed decreases. Food can decrease the absorption of iron by 40% to 66%; however, gastric intolerance may often necessitate administering the drug with food.

Excretion – Iron is transported via the blood and bound to transferrin. The daily loss of iron from urine, sweat and sloughing of intestinal mucosal cells amounts to approximately 0.5 to 1 mg in healthy men. In menstruating women, ≈ 1 to 2 mg is the normal daily loss.

Elemental Iron Content of Iron Salts

Iron salt	% Iron
Ferrous sulfate	20
Ferrous sulfate, exsiccated	≈ 30
Ferrous gluconate	≈12
Ferrous fumarate	33

Indications:

For the prevention and treatment of iron deficiency anemias.

Unlabeled uses: Iron supplementation may be required by most patients receiving epoetin therapy. Failure to administer iron supplements (oral or IV) during epoetin therapy can impair the hematologic response to epoetin.

Contraindications:

Hemochromatosis; hemosiderosis; hemolytic anemias.

Warnings:

Chronic iron intake: Individuals with normal iron balance should not take iron chronically.

Precautions:

Intolerance: Discontinue use if symptoms of intolerance appear.

GI effects: Occasional GI discomfort, such as nausea, may be minimized by taking with meals and by slowly increasing to the recommended dosage.

Tartrazine sensitivity: Some of these products contain tartrazine, which may cause allergic-type reactions (including bronchial asthma) in susceptible individuals. Although the incidence of tartrazine sensitivity in the general population is low, it is frequently seen in patients who also have aspirin hypersensitivity. Specific products containing tartrazine are identified in the product listings.

Sulfite sensitivity: Some of the products contain sulfites, which may cause allergic-type reactions (eg, hives, itching, wheezing, anaphylaxis) in certain susceptible persons. Although the overall prevalence of sulfite sensitivity in the general population is probably low, it is seen more frequently in asthmatics or in atopic nonasthmatic persons. Specific products containing sulfites are identified in the product listings.

IRON-CONTAINING PRODUCTS, ORAL

Drug Interactions:

Iron Salts Drug Interactions

Precipitant drug	Object drug *		Description
Antacids	Iron salts	⬇	GI absorption of iron may be reduced.
Ascorbic acid	Iron salts	⬆	Ascorbic acid may enhance the absorption of iron from the GI tract; however, this increase may not be significant.
Chloramphenicol	Iron salts	⬆	Serum iron levels may be increased.
Cimetidine	Iron salts	⬇	GI absorption of iron may be reduced.
Iron salts	Levodopa	⬇	Levodopa appears to form chelates with iron salts, decreasing levodopa absorption and serum levels.
Iron salts	Methyldopa	⬇	Extent of methyldopa absorption may be decreased, possibly resulting in decreased efficacy.
Iron salts	Penicillamine	⬇	Marked reduction in GI absorption of penicillamine may occur, possibly due to chelation.
Iron salts	Quinolones	⬇	GI absorption of quinolones may be decreased due to formation of a ferric ion-quinolone complex.
Iron salts	Tetracyclines	⬇	Coadministration may decrease absorption and serum levels of tetracyclines. Absorption of iron salts may also be decreased.
Tetracyclines	Iron salts	⬇	

* ⬆ = Object drug increased ⬇ = Object drug decreased

Drug/Food interactions: Eggs and milk inhibit iron absorption. Coffee and tea consumed with a meal or 1 hour after a meal may significantly inhibit the absorption of dietary iron; clinical significance has not been determined. Administration of calcium and iron supplements with food can reduce ferrous sulfate absorption by one-third. If combined iron and calcium supplementation is required, iron absorption is not decreased if calcium carbonate is used and the supplements are taken between meals.

Adverse Reactions:

GI irritation; anorexia; nausea; vomiting; constipation; diarrhea. Stools may appear darker in color.

Iron-containing liquids may cause temporary staining of the teeth. Dilute the liquid to reduce this possibility. When iron-containing drops are given to infants, some darkening of the membrane covering the teeth may occur.

Overdosage:

Symptoms: The oral *lethal* dose of elemental iron is about 200 to 250 mg/kg; however, considerably less has been fatal. Symptoms may present when 30 to 60 mg/kg is ingested. Acute poisoning will produce symptoms in four stages:

1) Within 1 to 6 hours: Lethargy; nausea; vomiting; abdominal pain; tarry stools; weak-rapid pulse; hypotension; dehydration; acidosis; coma.

2) If not immediately fatal, symptoms may subside for about 24 hours.

3) Symptoms return 12 to 48 hours after ingestion and may include: Diffuse vascular congestion; pulmonary edema; shock; acidosis; convulsions; anuria; hyperthermia; death.

4) If patient survives, in 2 to 6 weeks after ingestion, pyloric or antral stenosis, hepatic cirrhosis and CNS damage may be seen.

Treatment: Maintain proper airway, respiration and circulation. If the patient is a candidate for emesis, induce with syrup of ipecac; follow with gastric lavage using tepid water or 1% to 5% sodium bicarbonate to convert the ferrous sulfate to ferrous carbonate, which is poorly absorbed and less irritating. Systemic chelation therapy with deferoxamine is generally recommended for patients with serum iron levels > 300 mg/dl; IM therapy may suffice, but severe poisoning (ie, shock, coma) may require IV administration (see deferoxamine mesylate in the Antidotes section). Oral use of deferoxamine is controversial and generally discouraged. Saline cathartics may be used. Specific treatment for shock, convulsions, acidosis and renal failure may be necessary. Treatment includes usual supportive measures. Refer to General Management of Acute Overdosage.

Patient Information:

Take on an empty stomach; if GI upset occurs, take after meals or with food.

Avoid coadministration with antacids, tetracyclines or fluoroquinolones.

IRON-CONTAINING PRODUCTS, ORAL

Drink liquid iron preparations in water or juice and through a straw to prevent tooth stains.

Medication may cause black stools, constipation or diarrhea.

Do not chew or crush sustained release preparations.

Administration and Dosage:

Recommended Dietary Allowances (RDAs): Adult males (≥ 19 years old) – 10 mg; adult females (11 to 50 years old) – 15 mg, (≥ 51 years old) – 10 mg; pregnancy – 30 mg; lactation – 15 mg. For a complete listing of RDAs by age, sex or condition, refer to the RDAs section in the Nutrionals Chapter.

Iron replacement therapy in deficiency states:

Adults – 100 to 200 mg (2 to 3 mg/kg) elemental iron daily in three divided doses is the usual therapeutic dose.

Children (2 to 12 years) – 3 mg/kg/day in 3 to 4 divided doses; (6 months to 2 years) – up to 6 mg/kg/day in 3 to 4 divided doses.

Infants – 10 to 25 mg daily in 3 to 4 divided doses.

The length of iron therapy depends upon the cause and severity of the iron deficiency. In general, approximately 4 to 6 months of oral iron therapy is required to reverse uncomplicated iron deficiency anemias.

Iron supplementation: Consider only in individuals with documented risk factors for iron deficiency.

Pregnancy – 30 mg elemental iron daily (not taken with meals) should be adequate to meet the daily requirement of the last 2 trimesters.

FERROUS SULFATE

For complete prescribing information, refer to the Iron-Containing Products, Oral group monograph.

20% elemental iron.

otc	**Mol-Iron** (Schering-Plough)	**Tablets:** 195 mg (39 mg iron)	Sugar. In 100s.
otc	**Feratab** (Upsher-Smith)	**Tablets:** 300 mg (60 mg iron)	In 100s.
otc	**Ferrous Sulfate** (Various, eg,Geneva, Major, Parmed, Rugby, Schein)	**Tablets:** 324 mg (65 mg iron)	Plain or enteric coated. In 100s, 1000s, 5000s and UD 100s.
otc	**Fe^{50}** (Northampton Medical)	**Caplets:** 160 mg (50 mg iron)	PEG. In 100s.
otc	**Ferrous Sulfate** (Various, eg, Geneva, Parmed, Rugby)	**Capsules:** 250 mg (50 mg iron)	In 100s and 1000s.
otc	**Ferospace** (Hudson)		In 60s.
otc	**Fero-Gradumet Filmtab** (Abbott)	**Tablets, timed release:** 525 mg (105 mg iron)	Castor oil. Red. Film coated. In 100s.
otc	**Fer-In-Sol** (Mead Johnson Nutritionals)	**Syrup:** 90 mg (18 mg iron) per 5 ml	Sugar, sorbitol, sodium bisulfite. 5% alcohol. In pt.
otc	**Ferrous Sulfate** (Various, eg, Barre, Goldline, Major, Rugby, Schein)	**Elixir:** 220 mg (44 mg iron) per 5 ml	In pt and gal.
otc	**Feosol** (SmithKline-Beecham)		Saccharin, sucrose, glucose. 5% alcohol. In pt.
otc	**Ferrous Sulfate** (Various, eg, Barre, Major, Schein)	**Drops:** 75 mg (15 mg iron) per 0.6 ml	In 50 ml.
otc	**Fer-gen-sol** (Goldline)		Sucrose, sorbitol, 0.2% alcohol. In 50 ml.
otc	**Fer-In-Sol** (Mead Johnson Nutritionals)		Sugar, sorbitol, sodium bisulfite, 0.2% alcohol. In 50 ml w/dropper.
otc	**Fer-Iron** (Rugby)		Sugar, sorbitol, sodium bisulfite, 0.2% alcohol. In 50 ml.

FERROUS SULFATE EXSICCATED

For complete prescribing information, refer to the Iron-Containing Products, Oral group monograph.

Dried ferrous sulfate is prepared by exposing well crushed crystals of ferrous sulfate to 70° to 80°F (21° to 27°C) stirring frequently, and then powdering. This salt is more stable in air than the fully hydrated ferrous sulfate. Contains ≈ 30% elemental iron.

otc	**Fer-In-Sol** (Mead Johnson Nutritionals)	**Capsules:** 190 mg (60 mg iron)	Lecithin. In 100s.
otc	**Feosol** (SmithKline-Beecham)	**Tablets:** 200 mg (65 mg iron)	Glucose. Triangular. In 100s, 1000s and UD 100s.
otc	**Feosol** (SmithKline-Beecham)	**Capsules, timed release:** 159 mg (50 mg iron)	Sucrose. (Feosol). In 30s, 60s, 500s and UD 100s.
otc	**Ferrous Sulfate** (Various, eg, Parmed)	**Capsules, timed release:** 250 mg dried ferrous sulfate equivalent (50 mg iron)	In 100s and 1000s.
otc	**Ferralyn Lanacaps** (Lannett)		Red and clear. In 100s, 500s and 1000s.
otc	**Ferra-TD** (Goldline)		Red and clear. In 100s and 1000s.
otc	**Slow FE** (Ciba Consumer)	**Tablets, slow release:** 160 mg (50 mg iron)	Lactose. (Ciba). In 30s, 60s and 100s.

FERROUS GLUCONATE

For complete prescribing information, refer to the Iron-Containing Products, Oral group monograph.

11.6% elemental iron.

otc	**Ferrous Gluconate** (Various, eg, Major, Parmed, Rugby)	**Tablets:** 300 mg (34 mg iron)	In 100s and 1000s.
otc	**Fergon** (Winthrop Consumer)	**Tablets:** 320 mg (37 mg iron)	Sucrose. In 100s and 1000s.
otc	**Ferralet (Mission)**		In 100s.
otc	**Ferrous Gluconate** (Various, eg, Dixon-Shane, Geneva, Goldline, Schein, URL)	**Tablets:** 325 mg (38 mg iron)	In 100s and 1000s.
otc	**Ferralet Slow Release** (Mission)	**Tablets, sustained release:** 320 mg (37 mg iron)	In 30s.
otc	**Simron** (SmithKline Beecham)	**Capsules, soft gelatin:** 86 mg (10 mg iron)	Maroon. In 100s.
otc	**Fergon** (Winthrop Consumer)	**Elixir:** 300 mg (34 mg iron) per 5 ml	7% alcohol, glucose, saccharin. In pt.

FERROUS FUMARATE

For complete prescribing information, refer to the Iron-Containing Products, Oral group monograph.

33% elemental iron.

otc	**Femiron** (Menley & James)	**Tablets:** 63 mg (20 mg iron)	In 40s and 120s.
otc	**Fumerin** (Laser)	**Tablets:** 195 mg (64 mg iron)	Sugar coated. In 100s and 1000s.
otc	**Ferrous Fumarate** (Mission)	**Tablets:** 200 mg (66 mg iron)	Sugar. In 100s.
otc	**Fumasorb** (MiLance)		In 30s and 60s.
otc	**Ircon** (Kenwood)		In 100s.
otc	**Hemocyte** (U.S. Pharm.)	**Tablets:** 324 mg (106 mg iron)	In 100s.
otc	**Ferrous Fumarate** (Various, eg, Major, Rugby, Schein)	**Tablets:** 325 mg (106 mg iron)	In 1000s.
otc	**Ferretts** (Pharmics)		Sugar. In 100s.
otc	**Nephro-Fer** (R & D Labs)	**Tablets:** 350 mg (115 mg iron)	In 100s.
otc sf	**Ferro-Sequels** (Lederle)	**Tablets, timed release:** 150 mg (50 mg iron)	Lactose. In 30s, 100s, 1000s and UD 100s.
otc	**Feostat** (Forest)	**Tablets, chewable:** 100 mg (33 mg iron)	Chocolate flavor. In 100s and 1000s.
otc	**Span-FF** (Lexis)	**Capsules, controlled release:** 325 mg (106 mg iron)	Sucrose. In 60s, 100s and 500s.
otc	**Feostat** (Forest)	**Suspension:** 100 mg (33 mg iron) per 5 ml	In 240 ml.
otc	**Feostat** (Forest)	**Drops:** 45 mg (15 mg iron) per 0.6 ml	In 60 ml.

POLYSACCHARIDE-IRON COMPLEX

For complete prescribing information, refer to the Iron-Containing Products, Oral group monograph.

otc	**Niferex** (Central)	**Tablets:** 50 mg iron	Brown. Film coated. In 100s.
otc	**Hytinic** (Hyrex)	**Capsules:** 150 mg iron	In 50s and 500s.
otc	**Niferex-150** (Central)		(Central). Orange and brown. In 100s and 1000s.
otc	**Nu-Iron 150** (Mayrand)		In 100s.
otc	**Polysaccharide Iron Complex** (Various, eg, URL)		In 100s.
otc sf	**Niferex** (Central)	**Elixir:** 100 mg iron per 5 ml	10% alcohol. Dye free. In 240 ml.
otc sf	**Nu-Iron** (Mayrand)		10% alcohol. In 237 ml.

MODIFIED IRON PRODUCTS

For complete prescribing information, refer to the Iron-Containing Products, Oral group monograph.

otc	**Ferocyl** (Hudson)	**Tablets, sustained release:** 150 mg ferrous fumarate (50 mg iron) and 100 mg docusate sodium	In 100s.
otc	**Ferro-Docusate T.R.** (Parmed)	**Capsules, timed release:** 150 mg ferrous fumarate (50 mg iron) and 100 mg docusate sodium	Sucrose. In 100s.
otc	**Ferro Dok TR** (Major)		In 100s.
otc	**Ferro-DSS S.R.** (Geneva Marsam)		Green. In 100s.

IRON WITH VITAMIN C

For complete prescribing information, refer to the Iron-Containing Products, Oral group monograph.

ASCORBIC ACID (VITAMIN C) may enhance the absorption of iron.

Content given per capsule or tablet.

	Product and Distributor	Dose Form	Fe (mg)	Vitamin C: Ascorbic Acid (mg)	Vitamin C: Sodium Ascorbate (mg)	Other Content & How Supplied
otc	**Mol-Iron With Vitamin C** (Schering-Plough)	**Tablets**	39[1]	75		Sugar. In 100s.
otc	**Ferancee-HP** (J&J-Merck)		110[2]	600[3]		Red. Film coated. Oval. In 60s.
otc	**Vitron-C-Plus** (Ciba Consumer)		132[2]	250		Lactose. In 100s.
otc	**Nifrex with Vitamin C** (Central)	**Tablets, Chewable**	50[4]	100	169	In 50s.
otc	**Vitron-C** (Ciba Consumer)		66[2]	125		Saccharin. Fruit flavor. In 100s and 1000s.
otc	**Ferancee** (J&J-Merck)		67[2]	150[3]		Sugar, saccharin, tartrazine. In 100s.
Rx	**Cevi-Fer** (Geriatric Pharm.)	**Tablets and Capsules, Timed Release**	20[2]	300		1 mg folic acid. In 30s and 100s.
otc	**Irospan** (Fielding)		60[1]	150		In 100s (Tablets) and 60 (Capsules).
otc	**Ferromar** (Marnel)		65[2]	200[3]		In 100s
otc	**Fe-O.D.** (Trimen)		100[2]	500		In 100s.
otc	**Fero-Grad-500** (Abbott)		105[1]		500	Red. Film coated. In 100s, 500s and UD 100s.
otc	**Hemaspan** (Bock)		110[2]	200[3]		20 mg DSS. (Bock 330). Tan. In 30s and 100s.

[1] From ferrous sulfate.
[2] From ferrous fumarate.
[3] Form of vitamin C unknown.
[4] From polysaccharide-iron complex.

IRON DEXTRAN

Warning:

The parenteral use of complexes of iron and carbohydrates has resulted in fatal anaphylactic-type reactions. Deaths associated with such administration have been reported; therefore, use iron dextran injection only in those patients in whom the indications have been clearly established and laboratory investigations confirm an iron deficient state not amenable to oral iron therapy.

Actions:

Pharmacology: Iron dextran, a hematinic agent, is a complex of ferric hydroxide and dextran for IM or IV use. The iron dextran complex is dissociated by the reticuloendothelial system, and the ferric iron is transported by transferrin and incorporated into hemoglobin and storage sites.

Indications:

For treatment of patients with documented iron deficiency in whom oral administration is unsatisfactory or impossible.

Unlabeled uses: Iron supplementation may be required by most patients receiving epoetin therapy. Failure to administer iron supplements (oral or IV) during epoetin therapy can impair the hematologic response to epoetin.

Contraindications:

Hypersensitivity to the product; all anemias not associated with iron deficiency.

Warnings:

Maximum dose: 2 ml of undiluted iron dextran is the maximum recommended daily dose.

Delayed adverse reactions: The following pattern of signs/symptoms has been reported as a delayed (1 to 2 days) reaction at recommended doses: Modest-high fever; chills; backache; headache; myalgia; malaise; nausea; vomiting; dizziness. These reactions have been reported in an unexpectedly high incidence with certain batches. Therefore, in estimating the benefit/risk of treatment for an individual patient, assume that such a delayed reaction may occur.

Hypersensitivity: Have epinephrine immediately available in the event of acute hypersensitivity reactions. (Usual adult dose: 0.5 ml of a 1:1000 solution by SC or IM injection.) Refer to Management of Acute Hypersensitivity Reactions.

Hepatic function impairment: Use this preparation with extreme caution in the presence of serious impairment of liver function.

Carcinogenesis: A risk of carcinogenesis may exist for the IM injection of iron-carbohydrate complexes. Such complexes produce sarcoma when large doses are injected in rats, mice, and rabbits and possibly in hamsters.

The long latent period between the injection of a potential carcinogen and the appearance of a tumor makes it impossible to accurately measure the risk in humans. There have been, however, several reports describing tumors at the injection site in humans who previously received iron-carbohydrate complexes IM.

Pregnancy: In animal studies, iron dextran during pregnancy caused an increase in the number of stillbirths and fetal anomalies, fetal edema and a decrease in neonatal survival. In addition, the fetus can obtain from 80% to 90% of the iron administered to the pregnant dam during the third trimester. Whether this represents a danger to the fetus and whether the drug is effective in treating maternal iron deficiency under these circumstances is not known. Therefore, do not use in pregnancy or in women of child-bearing potential unless potential benefits outweigh possible hazards.

Precautions:

Iron overload: Unwarranted therapy with parenteral iron will cause excess storage of iron with the consequent possibility of exogenous hemosiderosis. Such iron overload is particularly apt to occur in patients with hemoglobinopathies and other refractory anemias which might be erroneously diagnosed as iron deficiency anemia.

Allergies/Asthma: Use with caution in patients with history of significant allergies/asthma.

Arthritis: Patients with iron deficiency anemia and rheumatoid arthritis may have an acute exacerbation of joint pain and swelling following IV administration.

Adverse Reactions:

Anaphylactic reactions including fatal anaphylaxis; other hypersensitivity reactions (dyspnea, urticaria, other rashes, itching, arthralgia, myalgia and febrile episodes); variable degree of soreness and inflammation at or near injection site, including sterile abscesses (IM); brown skin discoloration at injection site (IM); lymphadenopathy; local phlebitis at injection site (IV); peripheral vascular flushing with overly rapid

IRON DEXTRAN

IV administration; hypotensive reaction; possible arthritic reactivation in patients with quiescent rheumatoid arthritis; leukocytosis, frequently with fever, headache, backache, dizziness, malaise, transitory paresthesias, nausea and shivering.

Administration and Dosage:

Iron deficiency anemia:

Dosage – Use periodic hematologic determinations as a guide. Iron storage may lag behind the appearance of normal blood morphology. Although there are significant variations in body build and weight distribution among males and females, the following table and formula represent a convenient means for estimating the total iron required. This requirement reflects the amount of iron needed to restore hemoglobin to normal or near normal levels plus an additional 50% allowance to provide replenishment of iron stores in most individuals with moderately or severely reduced levels of hemoglobin.

The formula should not be used for patients weighing ≤ 30 pounds (adjustments have been made in the table values to account for the lower normal hemoglobins for those patients weighing ≤ 30 pounds).

Note: The table and accompanying formula are applicable for dosage determinations only in patients with iron deficiency anemia; they are not to be used for dosage determinations in patients requiring iron replacement for blood loss.

Iron Dextran Dosage Determination for Iron Deficiency Anemia

$$\frac{\text{mg blood iron}}{\text{lb body weight}} = \frac{\text{ml blood}}{\text{lb body weight}} \times \frac{\text{g hemoglobin}}{\text{ml blood}} \times \frac{\text{mg iron}}{\text{g hemoglobin}}$$

a) Blood volume .... 8.5% body weight

b) Normal hemoglobin (males and females)
 > 30 pounds .... 14.8 g/dl
 ≤ 30 pounds .... 12 g/dl

c) Iron content of hemoglobin 0.34%

d) Hemoglobin deficit

e) Weight

Based on the above factors, individuals with normal hemoglobin levels will have approximately 20 mg of blood iron per pound of body weight.

Total Amount of Iron Dextran Required (to the nearest ml) for Restoration of Hemoglobin and Replacement of Depleted Iron Stores, Based on Observed Hemoglobin and Body Weight

Patient weight		Amount required (ml) based on observed hemoglobin			
lb	kg	4 g/dl	6 g/dl	8 g/dl	10 g/dl
10	4.5	3	3	2	2
20	9.1	7	6	4	3
30	13.6	10	8	7	5
40	18.1	18	14	11	8
50	22.7	22	18	14	10
60	27.2	26	21	17	12
70	31.8	31	25	19	14
80	36.3	35	28	22	16
90	40.8	39	32	25	18
100	45.4	44	35	28	20
110	49.9	48	39	30	21
120	54.4	53	42	33	23
130	59	57	46	36	25
140	63.5	61	50	39	27
150	68.1	66	53	41	29
160	72.6	70	57	44	31
170	77.1	74	60	47	33
180	81.7	79	64	50	35

IRON DEXTRAN

The total amount of iron (in mg) required to restore hemoglobin to normal levels and to replenish iron stores may be approximated from the following formula:

$$0.3 \times \text{body weight in lb} \times \left(100 - \frac{\text{hemoglobin [g/dl]} \times 100}{14.8}\right)$$

To calculate dose in ml, divide this result by 50.

Administration:

IV injection – The total amount of iron dextran required for the treatment of iron deficiency anemia is determined from the preceding formula or table (see Dosage section).

Test dose: Prior to administering the first therapeutic dose, give all patients an IV test dose of 0.5 ml. Although anaphylactic reactions known to occur following administration are usually evident within a few minutes or sooner, it is recommended that a period of ≥ 1 hour elapse before the remainder of the initial therapeutic dose is given.

Individual doses of ≤ 2 ml may be given on a daily basis until the calculated total amount required has been reached.

Give undiluted and slowly (≤ 1 ml/min).

IM injection – The total amount required for the treatment of iron deficiency anemia is determined from the preceding formula or table (see Dosage section).

Test dose: Prior to administering the first therapeutic dose, give all patients an IM test dose of 0.5 ml administered in the same recommended test site and by the same technique as described for IV injection. Although anaphylactic reactions known to occur following administration are usually evident within a few minutes or sooner, it is recommended that a period of ≥ 1 hour elapse before the remainder of the initial therapeutic dose is given.

If no adverse reactions are observed, the injection can be given according to the following schedule until the calculated total amount required has been reached. Each day's dose should ordinarily not exceed 0.5 ml (25 mg iron) for infants < 10 lb, 1 ml (50 mg iron) for children < 20 lb and 2 ml (100 mg iron) for other patients.

Inject only into the muscle mass of the upper outer quadrant of the buttock (never into the arm or other exposed areas) and inject deeply with a 2 or 3 inch 19 or 20 gauge needle. If the patient is standing, have them bear their weight on the leg opposite the injection site, or if in bed, have them in a lateral position with injection site uppermost. To avoid injection or leakage into the subcutaneous tissue, a Z-track technique (displacement of the skin laterally prior to injection) is recommended.

Iron replacement for blood loss: Some individuals sustain blood losses on an intermittent or repetitive basis. Such blood losses may occur periodically in patients with hemorrhagic diatheses (eg, familial telangiectasia, hemophilia, GI bleeding) and on a repetitive basis from procedures such as renal hemodialysis. Direct iron therapy in these patients toward replacement of the equivalent amount of iron represented in the blood loss. The table and formula described under *Iron deficiency anemia* are not applicable for simple iron replacement values.

Quantitative estimates of the individual's periodic blood loss and hematocrit during the bleeding episode provide a convenient method for the calculation of the required iron dose.

The following formula is based on the approximation that 1 ml of normocytic, normochromic red cells contains 1 mg elemental iron:

Replacement iron (in mg) = Blood loss (in ml) x hematocrit

Example: Blood loss of 500 ml with 20% hematocrit

Replacement iron = 500 x 0.2 = 100 mg

$$\text{Iron dextran dose} = \frac{100 \text{ mg}}{50} = 2 \text{ ml}$$

Rx	**InFeD** (Schein)	**Injection**: 50 mg iron per ml (as dextran)[1]	In 2 ml amps and 10 ml vials.
Rx	**DexFerrum** (American Regent)		In 2 ml single dose vials.

[1] With ≈ 0.9% sodium chloride.

IRON WITH VITAMINS

For complete prescribing information, refer to the Iron—Containing Products, Oral group monograph.

In these products:

IRON in combination with *FOLIC ACID* is used to treat iron deficiency anemia in conjunction with certain nutritional deficiencies.

B COMPLEX vitamins function as coenzymes in carbohydrate, protein or amino acid metabolism, synthesis of DNA and other molecules, maturation of red blood cells, nerve cell function or oxidation-reduction reactions.

ASCORBIC ACID (Vitamin C) may enhance the absorption of iron.

For specific indications, refer to individual product labeling.

Warnings:

Pernicious anemia: Folic acid alone is improper therapy in the treatment of pernicious anemia and other megaloblastic anemias where vitamin B_{12} is deficient. Where anemia exists, establish its nature and determine underlying causes.

Folic acid, especially in doses > 0.1 mg daily, may obscure pernicious anemia, in that hematologic remission may occur while neurological manifestations remain progressive. Concomitant parenteral therapy with vitamin B_{12} may be necessary in patients with deficiency of vitamin B_{12}.

Precautions:

Sulfite sensitivity: Some products contain sulfites that may cause allergic-type reactions including anaphylactic symptoms and life-threatening or less severe asthmatic episodes in susceptible persons. The overall prevalence in the general population is unknown and probably low. It is seen more frequently in asthmatic or atopic nonasthmatic persons.

IRON WITH VITAMINS

For complete prescribing information, refer to the Iron With Vitamins Introduction.

Content given per capsule or tablet.

	Product & Distributor	Fe mg	A IU	D IU	E IU	B_1 mg	B_2 mg	B_3 mg	B_5 mg	B_6 mg	B_{12} mcg	C mg	FA mg	Other Content and How Supplied
Rx	**Hemocyte-F Tablets** (US Pharm.)	106[1]											1	Maroon. In 100s.
Rx	**Nephro-Fer Rx Tablets** (R & D)	106.9[1]											1	(RD33). Brown. Oval. Film coated. In 120s.
otc	**Ircon-FA Tablets** (Kenwood)	82[1]											0.8	In 100s.

IRON WITH VITAMINS

	Product & Distributor	Fe mg	A IU	D IU	E IU	B_1 mg	B_2 mg	B_3 mg	B_5 mg	B_6 mg	B_{12} mcg	C mg	FA mg	Other Content and How Supplied
otc	**Slow FE Slow Release Iron with Folic Acid Tablets** (Ciba)	50[3]											0.4	Lactose. In 20s.
otc	**Tolfrinic Tablets** (B.F. Ascher)	200[1]									25	100		Lactose. Dark brown. Film coated. In 100s.
Rx	**Niferex-150 Forte Capsules** (Central)	150[4]									25		1	(44). Red, brown and white. In 100s and 1000s.
otc	**Fero-Folic-500 Filmtabs** (Abbott)	105[3]										500	0.8	Controlled release. Red. Film coated. In 100s and 500s.
Rx	**Fumatinic Capsules** (Laser)	90[1]									15	100	1	Sustained release. Red and orange. In 100s.
otc	**Ferralet Plus Tablets** (Mission)	46[5]									25	400	0.8	Sugar. In 60s.
otc	**Generet-500 Tablets** (Goldline)	105[3]				6	6	30	10	5	25	500[6]		Timed release. In 60s.
otc	**Iberet-500 Filmtabs** (Abbott)													Controlled release. Red. Film coated. In 60s, 100s and Abbo-Pac 100s.
otc	**Iberet Filmtabs** (Abbott)	105[3]				6	6	30	10	5	25	150[6]		Controlled release. Film coated. In 60s.
otc	**Iron-Folic 500 Tablets** (Major)	105[3]				6	6	30	10	5	25	500[6]	0.8	Timed release. In 100s and 500s.
otc	**Vita-Feron** (Vitaline)	150									6		0.8	In 90s.
Rx	**Nephro-Vite Rx + Fe Tablets** (R & D)	100[1]				1.5	1.7	20	10	10	6	60[2]	1	300 mcg d-biotin. Lactose. (RD 23). Brown. Oval. Film coated. In 120s.
Rx	**Nephplex Rx Tablets** (Nephro-Tech)	66[1]				1.5	1.7	20	10	10	6	60	1	300 mcg d-biotin. In 100s.

IRON WITH VITAMINS

	Product & Distributor	Fe mg	A IU	D IU	E IU	B_1 mg	B_2 mg	B_3 mg	B_5 mg	B_6 mg	B_{12} mcg	C mg	FA mg	Other Content and How Supplied
Rx	**Prenatal Plus w/ Betacarotene** (Rugby)	65	4000	400	11	1.8	3	20		10	12	120	1	Ca, Zn, Cu. In 100s and 500s.
Rx	**Advanced Formula Zenate** (Solvay)	65[1]	4000	400	10[9]	1.5	1.6	17		2.2	2.2	70	1	Ca, I, Mg, Se, 15 mg Zn. In 100s.
otc	**Gerivites Tablets** (Rugby)	50[7]	5000	400	30[8]	1.5	1.7	20	10	2	300	60	0.4	Ca, Cl, Cr, Cu, I, K, Mg, Mn, Mo, Ni, Se, Si, P, 15 mg Zn. In 40s.
Rx	**Hemocyte Plus Tablets** (US Pharm.)	106[1]				10	6	30	10	5	15	200[6]	1	Cu, Mg, Mn, 18.2 mg Zn. In 100s.
Rx	**Iberet-Folic-500 Filmtabs** (Abbott)	105[3]				6	6	30	10	5	25	500[6]	0.8	Controlled release. Red. Film coated. In 60s.
otc sf	**Parvlex Tablets** (Freeda)	100[1]				20	20	20	1	10	50	50[2]	0.1	Cu, Mn. In 100s and 250s.
Rx	**Tabron Tablets** (Parke-Davis)	100[1]			30[9]	6	6	30	10	5	25	500	1	50 mg DSS, parabens. Film sealed. In 100s.
otc	**Prenatal H.P.** (Mission)	30	4,000	400		4	2	10	1	20	2	100	0.8	50 mg Ca. Sugar. In 100s.
Rx	**Prenatal Rx** (Mission)	29.5[1]	3,000	400		4	2	20	10	20	8	240[2]	1	175 mg Ca, 2 mg Cu, 0.3 mg I, 15 mg Zn. In 100s.
otc	**Allbee C-800 Plus Iron Tablets** (Robins)	27[1]			45[8]	15	17	100	25	25	12	800	0.4	Lactose. Red. Film coated. Elliptical. In 60s.
otc	**Surbex 750 with Iron Filmtabs** (Abbott)	27[10]			30[9]	15	15	100	20	25	12	750[6]	0.4	Film coated. In 50s.
otc	**Theragran Stress Formula Tablets** (Mead Johnson)	27[1]			30[9]	15	15	100	20	25	12	600	0.4	45 mcg biotin. In 75s.

IRON WITH VITAMINS

	Product & Distributor	Fe mg	A IU	D IU	E IU	B_1 mg	B_2 mg	B_3 mg	B_5 mg	B_6 mg	B_{12} mcg	C mg	FA mg	Other Content and How Supplied
otc sf	**StressForm "605" with Iron Tablets** (NTBY)	27[7]			30[8]	15	15	100	20	5	12	605	0.4	45 mcg biotin. In 60s.
otc	**Stress Formula w/Iron Tablets** (Goldline)	27[1]			30[9]	10	10	100	20	5	12	500[2]	0.4	45 mcg biotin. In 60s.
otc	**Stress Formula with Iron Tablets** (NTBY)	27[7]			30[8]	10	10	100	20	5	12	500	0.4	45 mcg biotin. In 60s.
otc	**Stresstabs + Iron Tablets** (Lederle)	18[1]			30[9]	10	10	100	20	5	12	500	0.4	45 mcg biotin. (LL S2). Orange-red. Capsule shape. Film coated. In 60s.
Rx	**Niferex-PN Tablets** (Central)	60[4]	4,000	400		3	3	10		2	3	50[6]	1	Ca, 18 mg Zn. Blue. Film coated. Oval. In 30s, 100s and 1000s.
Rx	**Nu-Iron V Tablets** (Mayrand)													Ca. Maroon. Film coated. In 100s.
Rx	**B C w/Folic Acid Plus Tablets** (Geneva)	27[1]	5,000		30[9]	20	20	100	25	25	50	500	0.8	0.15 mg biotin, Cr, Cu, Mg, Mn, 22.5 mg Zn. In 100s.
Rx	**Berocca Plus Tablets** (Roche)													0.15 mg biotin, Cr, Cu, Mg, Mn, 22.5 mg Zn. (Berocca Plus/Roche). Yellow. Capsule shape. In 100s.
Rx	**Berplex Plus Tablets** (Schein)													0.15 mg biotin, Cr, Cu, Mg, Mn, Zn. In 100s.
Rx	**Formula B Plus Tablets** (Major)													0.15 mg biotin, Cr, Cu, Mg, Mn, Zn. In 100s and 500s.
otc	**Mission Prenatal H.P. Tablets** (Mission)	30[5]	4,000	400		5	2	10	1	25	2	100	0.8	Ca, sugar. In 100s.
otc	**Mission Prenatal F.A. Tablets** (Mission)	30[5]	4,000	400		5	2	10	1	10	2	100	0.8	Ca, 15 mg Zn, sugar. In 100s.

IRON WITH VITAMINS

	Product & Distributor	Fe mg	A IU	D IU	E IU	B_1 mg	B_2 mg	B_3 mg	B_5 mg	B_6 mg	B_{12} mcg	C mg	FA mg	Other Content and How Supplied
otc	**Mission Prenatal Tablets** (Mission)	30[5]	4,000	400		5	2	10	1	3	2	100	0.4	Ca, sugar. In 100s.
otc	**Iromin-G Tablets** (Mission)	30[5]	4,000	400		5	2	10	1	20.6	2	100	0.8	Ca, sugar. In 100s.
Rx	**Nestabs FA Tablets** (Fielding)	36[1]	5,000	400	30[8]	3	3	20		3	8	120	1	Ca, I, 15 mg Zn. In 100s.
Rx *sf*	**Vitafol Caplets** (Everett)	65[1]	6,000	400	30[11]	1.1	1.8	15		2.5	5	60	1	Ca. (EV0072). Film coated. In 100s and 1000s.
otc	**Compete Tablets** (Mission)	27[5]	5,000	400	45[9]	2	2.6	30		20.6	9	90	0.4	22.5 mg Zn, sugar. In 100s.
otc *sf*	**Freedavite Tablets** (Freeda)	10[1]	5000	400	3[9]	5	3	25	5	2	2	60		Choline, inositol, potassium iodide, Ca, Cu, K, Mg, Mn, Se, 0.2 mg Zn. In 100s and 250s .
otc	**Mission Surgical Supplement Tablets** (Mission)	27[5]	5000	400	45[9]	2.5	2.6	30	16.3	3.6	9	500		22.5 mg Zn, sugar. In 100s.
otc	**Therapeutic-H Tablets** (Goldline)	66.7[1]	8333	133	5[9]	3.3	3.3	33.3	11.7	3.3	50	100[6]	0.33	Cu, Mg. In 100s.
otc	**Thera Hematinic Tablets** (Major)													Cu, Mg. In 250s and 1000s.
otc	**Theravee Hematinic Tablets** (Vangard)	66.7[7]	8333	133	5[9]	3.3	3.3	33.3	11.7	3.3	50	100	0.33	Cu, Mg. In UD 100s.

IRON WITH VITAMINS

	Product & Distributor	Fe mg	A IU	D IU	E IU	B_1 mg	B_2 mg	B_3 mg	B_5 mg	B_6 mg	B_{12} mcg	C mg	FA mg	Other Content and How Supplied
Rx	**Theragran Hematinic Tablets** (Apothecon)	66.7[1]	1400	140	5[9]	3.3	3.3	33.3	11.7	3.3	50	100[6]	0.33	Ca, Cu, Mg, lactose, sucrose, sodium bisulfite. In 90s.
otc sf	**Yelets Tablets** (Freeda)	20[1]	10,000	400	10[8]	10	10	25	10	10	10	100	0.1	PABA, lysine, glutamic acid, Ca, I, Mg, Mn, Se, 4 mg Zn. In 100s and 250s.
Rx	**Zodeac-100 Tablets** (Econo Med)	60[1]	8000	400	30[8]	1.7	2	20	11	4	8	120	1	300 mcg biotin, Ca, Cu, I, Mg, 15 mg Zn. Orange. Film coated. In 100s.
otc sf	**Geritol Complete Tablets** (SK-Beecham)	18[7]	6000	400	30[9]	1.5	1.7	20	10	2	6	60	0.4	45 mcg biotin, Ca, Cl, Cr, Cu, I, K, Mg, Mn, Mo, Ni, P, Se, Si, Sn, V, Zn, vitamin K. In 14s, 40s, 100s and 180s.
otc sf	**Geriot Tablets** (Goldline)	50[12]	6000	400	30[9]	1.5	1.7	20	10	2	6	60	0.4	45 mcg biotin, Ca, Cl, Cr, Cu, I, K, Mg, Mn, Mo, Ni, P, Se, Si, Sn, V, Zn, vitamin K. In 100s.
otc	**Thera-M Tablets** (Various, eg, Major)	27[7]	5000	400	30[8]	3	3.4	20	10	3	9	90	0.4	30 mcg biotin, 15 mg Zn, P, Ca, Cu, Cr, Se, Mo, K, Cl, I, Mg, Mn. In 130s and 1000s.
otc	**Multi-Vitamin Mineral w/Beta-Carotene Tablets** (Mission)	27[1]	5000	400	30[8]	2.25	2.6	20	10	3	9	90	0.4	0.45 mg biotin, Ca, Cl, Cr, Cu, I, K, Mg, Mn, Mo, P, Se, 15 mg Zn, vitamin K_1. In 130s.

IRON WITH VITAMINS

	Product & Distributor	Fe mg	A IU	D IU	E IU	B_1 mg	B_2 mg	B_3 mg	B_5 mg	B_6 mg	B_{12} mcg	C mg	FA mg	Other Content and How Supplied
otc	**CertaVite Tablets** (Major)	18[1]	5000	400	30[9]	1.5	1.7	20	10	2	6	60	0.4	30 mcg biotin, Ca, P, I, Mg, Cu, Mn, K, Cl, Cr, Mo, Se, Ni, Si, Sn, V, B, vitamin K_1, 15 mg Zn. In 130s and 300s.
otc sf	**ABC to Z Tablets** (NTBY)													30 mcg biotin, Ca, Cl, Cr, Cu, I, K, Mg, Mn, Mo, Ni, P, Se, Si, Sn, V, Zn, vitamin K_1. In 100s.
otc	**Advanced Formula Centrum Tablets** (Lederle)													30 mcg biotin, B, Ca, Cl, Cr, Cu, I, K, Mg, Mn, Mo, Ni, P, Se, Si, Sn, V, 15 mg Zn, vitamin K_1. In 60s, 130s and 200s.
otc sf	**Certagen Tablets** (Goldline)													30 mcg biotin, B, Ca, Cl, Cr, Cu, I, K, Mg, Mn, Mo, Ni, P, Se, Si, Sn, V, 15 mg Zn, vitamin K_1. In 100s and 1000s.
otc	**Cerovite Advanced Formula Tablets** (Rugby)													30 mcg biotin, Ca, Cl, Cr, Cu, I, K, Mg, Mn, Mo, Ni, P, Se, Si, Sn, V, 15 mg Zn, vitamin K_1. In 130s.
Rx	**Nephron FA** (Nephro-Tech)	200[1]				1.5	1.7	20	10	10	6	40	1	300 mcg biotin, 75 mg docusate sodium. In 100s.

[1] From ferrous fumarate.
[2] From ascorbic acid.
[3] From ferrous sulfate.
[4] From polysaccharide-iron complex.
[5] From ferrous gluconate.
[6] As sodium ascorbate.
[7] Form of iron content unknown.
[8] Form of vitamin E content unknown.
[9] As dl-alpha tocopheryl acetate.
[10] From ferrous sulfate, exsiccated.
[11] As d-alpha tocopherol succinate.
[12] From carbonyl iron.

IRON WITH VITAMINS, LIQUIDS

For complete prescribing information, refer to the Iron With Vitamins Introduction.

Content given per 15 ml.

	Product & Distributor	Fe mg	B_1 mg	B_2 mg	B_3 mg	B_5 mg	B_6 mg	B_{12} mcg	C mg	FA mg	Other Content	How Supplied
Rx sf	**Niferex Forte Elixir** (Central)	300[1]						75		3	10% alcohol, sorbitol	In 120 ml.
Rx sf	**Nu-Iron Plus Elixir** (Mayrand)										10% alcohol	Dye free. In 237 ml.
Rx	**Hemocyte Plus Elixir** (US Pharm)	12[1]			13.3	3.3	1.3	4		0.33	5 mg zinc, 1.3 mg Mn, 4.3% alcohol, sucrose, parabens	Sherry wine flavor. In 473 ml.
otc	**Trophite + Iron Liquid** (Menley & James)	60[2]	30					75			Saccharin, glucose, parabens	In 120 ml.
Rx	**Vitafol Syrup** (Everett)	90[2]			39.9		6	25.02		0.75		Raspberry-mint flavor. In 473 ml.
otc sf	**Vitalize SF Liquid** (Scot-Tussin)	66[2]	30				15	75			300 mg L-lysine, sorbitol	Alcohol and dye free. In 120 ml.
otc sf	**Kovitonic Liquid** (Freeda)	42[2]	5				10	30		0.1	10 mg L-lysine, sorbitol	In 120 and 240 ml.
otc	**Geritol Tonic Liquid** (SmithKline Beecham)	18[2]	2.5	2.5	50	2	0.5				25 mg methionine, 50 mg choline bitartrate, 12% alcohol	In 120 and 360 ml.
otc	**Iberet-Liquid** (Abbott)	78.75[3]	4.5	4.5	22.5	7.5	3.75	18.75	112.5		1% alcohol, sorbitol, parabens	Raspberry-mint flavor. In 240 ml.
otc	**Iberet-500 Liquid** (Abbott)	78.75[3]	4.5	4.5	22.5	7.5	3.75	18.75	375		Sorbitol, sucrose, parabens	Citrus flavor. In 240 ml.

[1] From polysaccharide-iron complex.
[2] From ferric pyrophosphate.
[3] From ferrous sulfate.

IRON AND LIVER COMBINATIONS

For complete prescribing information refer to the Iron—Containing Products, Oral group monograph.

IRON and LIVER combinations are recommended for iron deficiency anemia in conjunction with certain nutritional deficiencies.

Precautions:

The ingredients in these products are not sufficient, nor are they intended, for the treatment of pernicious anemia. The use of folic acid without adequate vitamin B_{12} therapy in patients with pernicious anemia may result in hematologic remission, but neurological progression.

Benzyl alcohol: Some parenteral products contain benzyl alcohol, which has been associated with a fatal "gasping syndrome" in premature infants.

LIVER (concentrate, fraction or desiccated) is used as a source of vitamin B complex.

B COMPLEX VITAMINS function as coenzymes in nutrient metabolism and maturation of red blood cells.

ASCORBIC ACID (Vitamin C) may enhance the absorption of iron.

IRON AND LIVER COMBINATIONS, CAPSULES AND TABLETS

For complete prescribing information, refer to the Iron and Liver Combinations introduction.

Content given per capsule or tablet.

	Product & Distributor	Fe mg	Liver	B_1 mg	B_2 mg	B_3 mg	B_5 mg	B_6 mg	B_{12} mcg	C mg	Other Content	How Supplied
Rx	**Feocyte Tablets** (Dunhall)	110[1]	15 mg (desiccated)					2	50	100	0.8 mg folic acid, Cu	Prolonged action. In 100s and 1000s.
otc sf	**I-L-X B_{12} Caplets** (Kenwood)	37.5[2]	130 mg (desiccated)	2	2	20			12	120		In 100s.

[1] From ferrous fumarate, ferrous gluconate and ferrous sulfate, dried.

[2] From *Ferronyl* carbonyl iron.

IRON AND LIVER COMBINATIONS, LIQUIDS

Refer to the general discussion of these products in the Iron and Liver Combinations introduction.

Content given per 15 ml.

	Product & Distributor	Fe mg	Liver	B_1 mg	B_2 mg	B_3 mg	B_5 mg	B_6 mg	B_{12} mcg	Other Content	How Supplied
otc	**Liquid Geritonic** (Geriatric Pharm)	105[1]	375 mg liver fraction 1	3	3	30		0.3	9	60 mg inositol, 180 mg glycine, 375 mg yeast concentrate, Ca, I, K, Mg, Mn, P, 20% alcohol	In 240 ml and gal.
otc	**I-L-X B_{12} Elixir** (Kenwood/Bradley)	102[1]	98 mg liver fraction 1	5	2	10			10	8% alcohol	In 240 ml.
otc	**I-L-X Elixir** (Kenwood/Bradley)	70[2]	98 mg liver concentrate 1:20	5	2	10				8% alcohol	In 240 ml.

[1] From iron ammonium citrate, brown.
[2] From ferrous gluconate.

IRON AND LIVER COMBINATIONS, PARENTERAL

Refer to the general discussion of this product in the Iron and Liver Combinations introduction.

Administration and Dosage:

1 to 2 ml IM 1 to 3 times weekly.

	Product & Distributor	Fe mg	Liver[1] mcg	B_1 mg	B_2 mg	B_3 mg	B_5 mg	B_6 mg	B_{12} mcg	Other Content	How Supplied
Rx	**Hytinic** (Hyrex)	3[2]	1		0.75	50	1.25		15	2% procaine HCl, 2% benzyl alcohol	In 30 ml vials.

[1] B_{12} equivalent.
[2] From ferrous gluconate.

IRON WITH VITAMIN B_{12} AND INTRINSIC FACTOR

These products contain Intrinsic Factor derived from stomach extract to promote the absorption of vitamin B_{12}. For treatment of anemias that respond to hematinics, including pernicious anemia and other megaloblastic anemias and also iron deficiency anemia.

Content given per capsule.

	Product & Distributor	Fe mg	B_{12}[1] mcg	IFC[2]	B_1 mg	B_2 mg	B_3 mg	C mg	FA mg	Other Content	How Supplied
Rx	**Pronemia Hematinic Capsules** (Lederle)	115[3]	15	75 mg				150	1	Parabens	(LL P9). Maroon. In 30s.
Rx	**Contrin Capsules** (Geneva)	110[3]	15	240 mg				75	0.5		In 100s.
Rx	**Ferotrinsic Capsules** (Rugby)										In 100s, 500s and 1000s.
Rx	**Foltrin Capsules** (Vitarine)										(PP-5380). Maroon/red. In 100s and 1000s.
Rx	**Livitrinsic-f Capsules** (Goldline)										In 100s and 1000s.
Rx	**Trinsicon Capsules** (Whitby)										(Whitby/Trinsicon). Pink and red. In 60s, 500s and UD 100s.
Rx	**TriHemic 600 Tablets** (Lederle)	115[3]	25 mcg B_{12}	75 mg IFC				600	1	50 mg DSS, 30 IU vitamin E[6].	(LL T1). Red. Film coated. Capsule shape. In 30s and 500s.
Rx	**Chromagen Capsules** (Savage)	66[3]	10 mcg B_{12}	100 mg desiccated stomach substance				250			Maroon. In 100s and 500s.

[1] B_{12} activity derived from cobalamin or liver.
[2] Intrinsic factor as concentrate or from stomach preparations.
[3] From ferrous fumarate.
[4] From ferrous gluconate.
[5] One NF unit of *vitamin B_{12} with Intrinsic Factor Concentrate* (IFC) contains ≤ 15 mcg B_{12} and 300 mg IFC.
[6] From dl-alpha-tocopheryl acetate.

FOLIC ACID (Folacin; Pteroylglutamic Acid; Folate)

Actions:

Pharmacology: Exogenous folate is required for nucleoprotein synthesis and maintenance of normal erythropoiesis. Folic acid stimulates production of red and white blood cells and platelets in certain megaloblastic anemias. Folic acid is the precursor of tetrahydrofolic acid, which is involved as a cofactor for transformylation reactions in the biosynthesis of purines and thymidylates of nucleic acids. Impairment of thymidylate synthesis in patients with folic acid deficiency is thought to account for the defective deoxyribonucleic acid (DNA) synthesis that leads to megaloblast formation and megaloblastic and macrocytic anemias.

Pharmacokinetics: Dietary folic acid is present in foods (eg, liver, dried beans, peas, lentils, oranges, whole-wheat products, vegetables such as asparagus, beets, broccoli, brussels sprouts and spinach), primarily as reduced folate polyglutamate. It must undergo hydrolysis, reduction and methylation in the GI tract before it is absorbed. Conversion to tetrahydrofolate, the active form, is B_{12}-dependent; supplies are maintained by food and enterohepatic recirculation. Oral synthetic folic acid is a monoglutamate and is completely absorbed following administration, even in the presence of malabsorption syndromes.

Folic acid appears in the plasma ≈ 15 to 30 minutes after an oral dose; peak levels are generally reached within 1 hour. After IV administration, the drug is rapidly cleared from the plasma. Cerebrospinal fluid levels are several times greater than serum levels of the drug. Folic acid is metabolized in the liver to 7,8–dihydrofolic acid and eventually to 5,6,7,8–tetrahydrofolic acid. Tetrahydrofolic acid derivatives are distributed to all body tissues but are stored primarily in the liver. Normal serum levels of total folate have been reported to be 5 to 15 ng/ml; normal CSF levels are ≈ 16 to 21 ng/ml. Normal erythrocyte folate levels have been reported to range from 175 to 316 ng/ml. In general, folate serum levels < 5 ng/ml indicate folate deficiency, and levels < 2 ng/ml usually result in megaloblastic anemia.

After a single oral dose of 100 mcg of folic acid in a limited number of healthy adults, only a trace amount of the drug appeared in the urine. An oral dose of 5 mg in one study and a dose of 40 mcg/kg in another study resulted in ≈ 50% of the dose appearing in the urine. After a single oral dose of 15 mg, up to 90% of the dose was recovered in the urine. A majority of the metabolic products appeared in the urine after 6 hours; excretion was generally complete within 24 hours. Small amounts of orally administered folic acid have also been recovered in the feces.

Indications:

Megaloblastic anemia: Treatment of megaloblastic anemias due to a deficiency of folic acid as seen in tropical or nontropical sprue, anemias of nutritional origin, pregnancy, infancy or childhood.

Contraindications:

Treatment of pernicious anemia and other megaloblastic anemias where vitamin B_{12} is deficient (not effective).

Warnings:

Pernicious anemia: Folic acid in doses > 0.1 mg daily may obscure pernicious anemia in that hematologic remission can occur while neurologic manifestations remain progressive.

Except during pregnancy and lactation, folic acid should not be given in therapeutic doses > 0.4 mg daily until pernicious anemia has been ruled out. Patients with pernicious anemia receiving > 0.4 mg folic acid daily who are inadequately treated with vitamin B_{12} may show reversion of the hematologic parameters to normal, but neurologic manifestations due to vitamin B_{12} deficiency have been ruled out or are being adequately treated with cobalamin. Daily doses exceeding the Recommended Dietary Allowance should not be included in multivitamin preparations; if therapeutic amounts are necessary, folic acid should be given separately.

There is a potential danger in administering folic acid to patients with undiagnosed anemia, since folic acid may obscure the diagnosis of pernicious anemia by alleviating the hematologic manifestations of the disease while allowing the neurologic complications to progress. This may result in severe nervous system damage before the correct diagnosis is made. Adequate doses of vitamin B_{12} may prevent, halt or improve the neurologic changes caused by pernicious anemia.

Benzyl alcohol, contained in some of these products as a preservative, has been associated with a fatal "gasping syndrome" in premature infants.

Elderly: A recent study observed that homocysteine concentrations increase with age and low levels of folate and vitamins B_6 and B_{12}. Data suggest that high homocysteine levels may correlate with the development of occlusive vascular disease which may increase the risk of MI. Therefore, it may be prudent to consider the status of folate in persons > 65 years of age.

FOLIC ACID (Folacin; Pteroylglutamic Acid; Folate)

Pregnancy: Category A. Pregnant women are more prone to develop folate deficiency as reflected in larger dosage recommendations. Folate-deficient mothers may be more prone to complications of pregnancy and fetal abnormalities, including fetal anomalies, placental abruption, toxemia, abortions, placenta previa, low-birth-weight and premature delivery. Folic acid is usually indicated in the treatment of megaloblastic anemias of pregnancy. Folic acid requirements are markedly increased during pregnancy. The Recommended Dietary Allowance of folate during pregnancy is 0.4 mg/day.

Studies in pregnant women have not shown that folic acid increases the risk of abnormalities if administered during pregnancy. If the drug is used during pregnancy, the possibility of fetal harm appears remote. Because studies cannot rule out the possibility of harm, use folic acid during pregnancy only if clearly needed.

However, the US Public Health Service has recently recommended the use of folic acid in women of childbearing age to reduce the incidence of neural tube defects (NTDs). This is based on several studies that reported a > 50% reduced risk of NTDs in women who received 0.4 mg folic acid prior to conception and during early pregnancy. According to the US Public Health Service, all women of childbearing age in the US who are capable of becoming pregnant should consume 0.4 mg of folic acid per day for the purpose of reducing their risk of having a pregnancy affected with spina bifida or other NTDs. Because the effects of high intakes are not well known but include complicating the diagnosis of vitamin B_{12} deficiency, care should be taken to keep total folate consumption at < 1 mg/day, except under physician supervision. Women who have had a prior NTD-affected pregnancy are at high risk of having a subsequent affected pregnancy. When these women are planning to become pregnant, they should consult their physicians for advice.

Lactation: Folic acid is excreted in breast milk; milk:plasma ratio equals ≈ 0.02.

During lactation, folic acid requirements are markedly increased; however, amounts present in human milk are adequate to fulfill infant requirements, although supplementation may be needed in low-birth-weight infants, in those who are breastfed by mothers with folic acid deficiency (50 mcg daily), or in those with infections or prolonged diarrhea.The Recommended Dietary Allowance of folate during lactation is 0.26 to 0.28 mg/day.

Drug Interactions:

Folic Acid Drug Interactions			
Precipitant drug	Object drug*		Description
Aminosalicylic acid	Folic acid	⬇	Decreased serum folate levels may occur during concurrent use.
Contraceptives, oral	Folic acid	⬇	Oral contraceptives may impair folate metabolism and produce folate depletion, but the effect is mild and unlikely to cause anemia or megaloblastic changes.
Dihydrofolate reductase inhibitors (eg, methotrexate, trimethoprim)	Folic acid	⬇	A dihydrofolate reductase deficiency caused by administration of folic acid antagonists may interfere with folic acid utilization.
Sulfasalazine	Folic acid	⬇	Signs of folate deficiency have occurred.
Folic acid	Hydantoins	⬇	An increase in seizure frequency and a decrease in serum concentration to subtherapeutic levels have been reported in patients receiving folic acid (particularly 5 to 30 mg/day) with phenytoin. **Phenytoin** may cause a decrease in serum folate levels, and may produce symptoms of folic acid deficiency in 27% to 91% (but clinically important megaloblastic anemia in < 1%) of patients on long-term therapy. If folic acid is required, a higher dose of phenytoin may be needed.

* ⬇ = Object drug decreased.

Adverse Reactions:

Folic acid is relatively nontoxic in man. Rare instances of allergic responses to folic acid preparations have occurred and have included erythema, skin rash, itching, general malaise and respiratory difficulty due to bronchospasm. One patient experienced symptoms suggesting anaphylaxis following injection of the drug.

GI: Anorexia, nausea, abdominal distention, flatulence and a bitter or bad taste have been reported in patients receiving 15 mg folic acid daily for 1 month.

FOLIC ACID (Folacin; Pteroylglutamic Acid; Folate)

CNS: Altered sleep patterns, difficulty in concentrating, irritability, overactivity, excitement, mental depression, confusion and impaired judgement were reported in patients receiving 15 mg daily.

Miscellaneous: Allergic sensitization has been reported.

Decreased vitamin B_{12} serum levels may occur in patients receiving prolonged folic acid therapy.

Patient Information:

Take only under medical supervision.

Administration and Dosage:

Give orally, except in severe intestinal malabsorption. Although most patients with malabsorption cannot absorb food folates, they are able to absorb folic acid given orally.

Parenteral administration is not advocated but may be necessary in some individuals (eg, patients receiving parenteral or enteral alimentation). Give IM, IV or SC if disease is very severe or GI absorption is very severely impaired. Doses > 0.1 mg should not be used unless anemia due to vitamin B_{12} deficiency has been ruled out or is being adequately treated with cobalamin. Daily doses > 1 mg do not enhance the hematologic effect, and most of the excess is excreted unchanged in the urine.

Usual therapeutic dosage: Up to 1 mg daily. Resistant cases may require larger doses.

Maintenance: When clinical symptoms have subsided and the blood picture has normalized, use the dosage below. Never give < 0.1 mg/day. Keep patients under close supervision and adjust maintenance dose if relapse appears imminent. In the presence of alcoholism, hemolytic anemia, anticonvulsant therapy or chronic infection, the maintenance level may need to be increased.

Infants – 0.1 mg/day.
Children (< 4 years of age) – Up to 0.3 mg/day.
Adults and children (> 4 years of age) – 0.4 mg/day.
Pregnant and lactating women – 0.8 mg/day.

Recommended Dietary Allowances (RDAs): Adult males, 0.15 to 0.2 mg/day; females, 0.15 to 0.18 mg/day.

For a complete listing of RDAs by age and sex, refer to the RDA table in the Nutritionals chapter.

Stability: At concentrations usually used for parenteral nutrition, folate will remain stable in solution providing the pH of the solution remains above 5.

otc[1]	**Folic Acid** (Various, eg, Fibertone, Major, Rugby)	**Tablets:** 0.4 mg	In 100s.
otc[1]	**Folic Acid** (Various, eg, Fibertone, Rugby)	**Tablets:** 0.8 mg	In 100s.
Rx	**Folic Acid** (Various, eg, Genetco, Geneva, Goldline, Halsey, Major, Moore, Paddock, Parmed, Qualitest, Rugby)	**Tablets:** 1 mg	In 30s, 100s, 1000s and UD 100s.
Rx	**Folic Acid** (LyphoMed)	**Injection:** 5 mg/ml	In 10 ml vials.[2]
Rx	**Folvite** (Lederle)		In 10 ml vials.[3]

[1] Although most folic acid products carry the *Rx* legend, products which provide 0.4 mg or less (or 0.8 mg for pregnant or lactating women) may be *otc* items.
[2] With 1.5% benzyl alcohol and EDTA.
[3] With 1.5% benzyl alcohol.

LEUCOVORIN CALCIUM (Folinic Acid; Citrovorum Factor)

Actions:

Pharmacology: Leucovorin is one of several active, chemically reduced derivatives of folic acid. It is useful as an antidote to drugs which act as folic acid antagonists. Leucovorin is a mixture of the diasteroisomers of the 5-formyl derivative of tetrahydrofolic acid (THF). The biologically active compound of the mixture is the l-isomer, known as citrovorum factor or folinic acid. Leucovorin does not require reduction by the enzyme dihydrofolate reductase in order to participate in reactions utilizing folates as a source of "one-carbon" moieties. l-Leucovorin is rapidly metabolized to 1,5-methyltetrahydrofolate, which can, in turn, be metabolized via other pathways back to 5,10-methyl-ene-tetrahydrofolate, which is converted to 5-methyltetrahydrofolate by an irreversible, enzyme-catalyzed reduction using the cofactors $FADH_2$ and NADPH.

Administration of leucovorin can counteract the therapeutic and toxic effects of folic acid antagonists such as methotrexate (MTX), which act by inhibiting dihydrofolate reductase.

In contrast, leucovorin can enhance the therapeutic and toxic effects of fluoropyrimidines used in cancer therapy, such as 5-fluorouracil (5-FU). Concurrent administration of leucovorin does not appear to alter the plasma pharmacokinetics of 5-FU. 5–FU is metabolized to fluorodeoxyuridylic acid, which binds to and inhibits the enzyme thymidylate synthase (an enzyme important in DNA repair and replication). The reduced folate, 5,10-methylenetetetrahydrofolate, acts to stabilize the binding of fluorodeoxyuridylic acid to thymidylate synthase and thereby enhances the inhibition of this enzyme.

Pharmacokinetics:

Leucovorin Pharmacokinetics[1]

Parameter	IV	IM	Oral
Total reduced folates:			
Mean peak conc. (ng/ml)	1259 (range, 897-1625)	436 (range, 240 to 725)	393 (range, 160 to 550)
Mean time to peak	10 min	52 min	2.3 hrs
Terminal half-life	6.2 hrs	6.2 hrs	5.7 hrs
5-Methyl-THF[2]			
Mean peak conc. (ng/ml)	258	226	367
Mean time to peak	1.3 hrs	2.8 hrs	2.4 hrs
5-Formyl-THF[3]			
Mean peak conc. (ng/ml)	1206	360	51
Mean time to peak	10 min	28 min	1.2 hrs

[1] Following administration of a 25 mg dose.
[2] The major metabolite to which leucovorin is primarily converted in the intestinal mucosa and which becomes the predominant circulating form of the drug.
[3] The parent compound.

The initial rise in total reduced folates is primarily due to the parent compound (5–formyl-THF). A sharp drop in parent compound follows and coincides with the appearance of the active metabolite (5-methyl-THF).

Following IV administration, the area under the plasma concentration vs time curves (AUC) for l-leucovorin, d-leucovorin and 5-methyl-THF were 28.4 ± 3.5, 956 ± 97 and 129 ± 12 mg • min/L. When a higher dose of d,l-leucovorin was used, similar results were obtained. The d-isomer persisted in plasma at concentrations greatly exceeding those of the l-isomer. There was no difference between IM and IV administration in the AUC for total reduced folates, 5-formyl-THF or 5-methyl-THF. The AUC of total reduced folates after oral administration was 92% of the AUC after IV administration.

Following oral administration leucovorin is rapidly absorbed and expands the serum pool of reduced folates. At a dose of 25 mg, almost 100% of the l-isomer but only 20% of the d-isomer is absorbed. Oral absorption of leucovorin is saturable at doses > 25 mg. The apparent bioavailability of leucovorin was 97% for 25 mg, 75% for 50 mg and 37% for 100 mg.

LEUCOVORIN CALCIUM (Folinic Acid; Citrovorum Factor)

Clinical trials: In a randomized clinical study in patients with advanced metastatic colorectal cancer, three treatment regimens were compared. Leucovorin 200 mg/m^2 and 5-FU 370 mg/m^2 vs leucovorin 20 mg/m^2 and 5-FU 425 mg/m^2 vs 5-FU 500 mg/m^2. All drugs were given by slow IV infusion daily for 5 days repeated every 28 to 35 days. Response rates were 26%, 43% and 10% for the high-dose leucovorin, low-dose leucovorin and 5-FU alone groups, respectively. Respective median survival times were 12.2 months, 12 months and 7.7 months. The low-dose leucovorin regimen gave a significant improvement in weight gain of > 5%, relief of symptoms and improvement in performance status. The high-dose regimen gave a significant improvement in performance status and trended toward improvement in weight gain and in relief of symptoms.

In a second randomized clinical study, the 5-FU monotherapy was replaced by a regimen of sequentially administered MTX, 5-FU and leucovorin. Response rates with leucovorin 200 mg/m^2 and 5-FU 370 mg/m^2 vs leucovorin 20 mg/m^2 and 5-FU 425 mg/m^2 vs sequential MTX and 5-FU and leucovorin were, respectively, 33%, 31% and 4%. Respective median survival times were 402 days, 418 days and 223 days. No significant difference in weight gain of > 5% or in improvement in performance status was seen between the treatment arms.

Indications:

Oral and parenteral: Leucovorin "rescue" after high-dose methotrexate therapy in osteosarcoma.

To diminish the toxicity and counteract the effects of impaired methotrexate elimination and of inadvertent overdosages of folic acid antagonists (eg, pyrimethamine, trimethoprim).

Parenteral: Treatment of megaloblastic anemias due to folic acid deficiency when oral therapy is not feasible.

In combination with 5-fluorouracil to prolong survival in the palliative treatment of patients with advanced colorectal cancer.

Contraindications:

Pernicious anemia and other megaloblastic anemias secondary to the lack of vitamin B_{12} (see Warnings).

Warnings:

Anemias: Leucovorin is improper therapy for pernicious anemia and other megaloblastic anemias secondary to the lack of vitamin B_{12}. A hematologic remission may occur while neurologic manifestations continue to progress.

5-Fluorouracil dosage/toxicity: Leucovorin enhances the toxicity of 5-FU. When these drugs are administered concurrently in the palliative therapy of advanced colorectal cancer, the dosage of 5-FU must be lower than usually administered. Although the toxicities observed in patients treated with the combination of leucovorin plus 5-FU are qualitatively similar to those observed in patients treated with 5-FU alone, GI toxicities (particularly stomatitis and diarrhea) are observed more commonly and may be more severe and of prolonged duration in patients treated with the combination.

In a controlled trial, toxicity, primarily GI, resulted in 7% of patients requiring hospitalization when treated with 5-FU alone or 5-FU in combination with 200 mg/m^2 leucovorin and 20% when treated with 5-FU in combination with 20 mg/m^2 leucovorin. In another trial, hospitalizations related to treatment toxicity also appeared to occur more often in patients treated with low-dose leucovorin/5-FU combination than in patients treated with the high-dose combination (11% vs 3%). Therapy with leucovorin/5-FU must not be initiated or continued in patients who have symptoms of GI toxicity of any severity, until those symptoms have completely resolved. Patients with diarrhea must be monitored with particular care until the diarrhea has resolved, as rapid clinical deterioration leading to death can occur. In an additional study utilizing higher weekly doses of 5-FU and leucovorin, elderly or debilitated patients were found to be at greater risk for severe GI toxicity.

Since leucovorin enhances the toxicity of 5-FU, administer the combination for advanced colorectal cancer under the supervision of a physician experienced in the use of antimetabolite cancer chemotherapy. Take particular care in the treatment of elderly or debilitated colorectal cancer patients, as these patients may be at increased risk of severe toxicity.

Methotrexate concentrations: Monitoring of the serum MTX concentration is essential in determining the optimal dose and duration of treatment with leucovorin. Delayed MTX excretion may be caused by a third space fluid accumulation (ie, ascites, pleural effusion), renal insufficiency or inadequate hydration. Under such circumstances, higher doses of leucovorin or prolonged administration may be indicated. Doses higher than those recommended for oral use must be given IV.

LEUCOVORIN CALCIUM (Folinic Acid; Citrovorum Factor)

Calcium content: Because of the calcium content of the leucovorin solution, inject no more than 160 mg/min IV (16 ml of a 10 mg/ml, or 8 ml of a 20 mg/ml solution per minute).

Folic acid antagonist overdosage: In the treatment of accidental overdosages of folic acid antagonists (eg, pyrimethamine, trimethoprim), administer leucovorin as promptly as possible. As the time interval between antifolate administration (eg, MTX) and leucovorin rescue increases, leucovorin's effectiveness in counteracting toxicity decreases.

Benzyl alcohol: Because of the benzyl alcohol contained in the 1 ml amp and in certain diluents used for leucovorin injection, when doses > 10 mg/m^2 are administered, reconstitute leucovorin injection with Sterile Water for Injection, USP, and use immediately (see Administration and Dosage). Benzyl alcohol has been associated with a fatal "Gasping Syndrome" in premature infants.

Pregnancy: Category C. It is not known whether leucovorin can cause fetal harm when administered to a pregnant woman or can affect reproduction capacity. Give to a pregnant woman only if clearly needed.

Lactation: It is not known whether this drug is excreted in breast milk. Exercise caution when administering to a nursing woman.

Precautions:

Parenteral administration is preferable to oral dosing if there is a possibility that the patient may vomit or not absorb the leucovorin. Leucovorin has no effect on nonhematologic toxicities of MTX such as the nephrotoxicity resulting from drug or metabolite precipitation in the kidney.

Monitoring: Obtain a CBC with differential and platelets prior to each treatment with the leucovorin/5-FU combination. During the first two courses a CBC with differential and platelets must be repeated weekly and thereafter once each cycle at the time of anticipated WBC nadir. Perform electrolyte and liver function tests prior to each treatment for the first three cycles, then prior to every other cycle. Institute dosage modifications of 5-FU as follows, based on the most severe toxicities:

5-Fluorouracil Dosage Modifications Based on Toxicities			
Diarrhea or stomatitis	WBC/mm^3 nadir	Platelets/mm^3 nadir	5-FU dose
Moderate	1000-1900	25,000-75,000	decrease 20%
Severe	< 1000	< 25,000	decrease 30%

If no toxicity occurs, the 5-FU dose may increase 10%.

Defer treatment until WBCs are 4000/mm^3 and platelets are 130,000/mm^3. If blood counts do not reach these levels within 2 weeks, discontinue treatment. Follow up patients with physical examination prior to each treatment course and with appropriate radiological examination as needed. Discontinue treatment when there is clear evidence of tumor progression.

Drug Interactions:

Leucovorin Drug Interactions			
Precipitant drug	Object drug*		Description
Leucovorin	Anticonvulsants	⬇	Folic acid in large amounts may counteract the antiepileptic effect of phenobarbital, phenytoin and primidone, and increase the frequency of seizures in susceptible children. Although this interaction has not been reported with leucovorin, consider the possibility when using these drugs concomitantly.
Leucovorin	5-Fluorouracil	⬆	Leucovorin may enhance the toxicity of 5-FU (see Warnings).
Leucovorin	Methotrexate	⬇	Small quantities of systemically administered leucovorin enter the CSF primarily as 5-methyltetrahydrofolate and remain 1 to 3 orders of magnitude lower than the usual MTX concentrations following intrathecal administration. However, high doses of leucovorin may reduce the efficacy of intrathecally administered MTX.

* ⬆ = Object drug increased. ⬇ = Object drug decreased.

LEUCOVORIN CALCIUM (Folinic Acid; Citrovorum Factor)

Adverse Reactions:

Allergic sensitization, including anaphylactoid reactions and urticaria, has been reported following administration of both oral and parenteral leucovorin. No other adverse reactions have been attributed to the use of leucovorin alone.

The following table summarizes significant adverse events occurring in 316 patients treated with the leucovorin/5-FU combinations compared with 70 patients treated with 5-FU alone for advanced colorectal carcinoma.

Adverse Reactions with the Leucovorin/5-Fluorouracil Combination						
	High leucovorin[1]/5-FU (n=155)		Low leucovorin[2]/5-FU (n=161)		5-FU alone (n=70)	
Adverse reaction	Any[3] (%)	Grade 3+[4] (%)	Any[3] (%)	Grade 3+[4] (%)	Any[3] (%)	Grade 3+[4] (%)
Leukopenia	69	14	83	23	93	48
Thrombocytopenia	8	2	8	1	18	3
Infection	8	1	3	1	7	2
Nausea	74	10	80	9	60	6
Vomiting	46	8	44	9	40	7
Diarrhea	66	18	67	14	43	11
Stomatitis	75	27	84	29	59	16
Constipation	3		4	–	1	–
Lethargy/Malaise/ Fatigue	13	3	12	2	6	3
Alopecia	42	5	43	6	37	7
Dermatitis	21	2	25	1	13	–
Anorexia	14	1	22	4	14	–
Hospitalization for toxicity		5%		15%		7%

[1] High leucovorin = 200 mg/m^2.
[2] Low leucovorin = 20 mg/m^2.
[3] Any = Percentage of patients reporting toxicity of any severity.
[4] Grade 3+ = Percentage of patients reporting toxicity of Grade 3 or higher.

Overdosage:

Excessive amounts of leucovorin may nullify the chemotherapeutic effect of folic acid antagonists (eg, pyrimethamine, trimethoprim).

Administration and Dosage:

Oral administration of doses > 25 mg is not recommended.

Advanced colorectal cancer: Either of the following two regimens is recommended:

1) Leucovorin 200 mg/m^2 by slow IV injection over a minimum of 3 minutes, followed by 5-FU 370 mg/m^2 by IV injection.

2) Leucovorin 20 mg/m^2 by IV injection followed by 5-FU 425 mg/m^2 by IV injection.

Treatment is repeated daily for 5 days. This 5 day treatment course may be repeated at 4 week (28 day) intervals for 2 courses and then repeated at 4 to 5 week (28 to 35 day) intervals provided that the patient has completely recovered from the toxic effects of the prior treatment course.

In subsequent treatment courses, adjust the dosage of 5-FU based on patient tolerance of the prior treatment course. Reduce the daily dosage of 5-FU by 20% for patients who experienced moderate hematologic or GI toxicity in the prior treatment course, and by 30% for patients who experienced severe toxicity (see Precautions). For patients who experienced no toxicity in the prior treatment course, 5-FU dosage may be increased by 10%. Leucovorin dosages are not adjusted for toxicity.

Several other doses and schedules of leucovorin/5-FU therapy have also been evaluated in patients with advanced colorectal cancer; some of these alternative regimens may also have efficacy in the treatment of this disease. However, further clinical research will be required to confirm the safety and efficacy of these alternative treatment regimens.

Leucovorin rescue after high-dose MTX therapy: The recommendations for leucovorin rescue are based on an MTX dose of 12 to 15 g/m^2 administered by IV infusion over 4 hours (see Methotrexate monograph). Leucovorin rescue at a dose of 15 mg (≈ 10 mg/m^2) every 6 hours for 10 doses starts 24 hours after the beginning of the MTX infusion. In the presence of GI toxicity, nausea or vomiting, administer leucovorin parenterally.

Determine serum creatinine and MTX levels at least once daily. Continue leucovorin administration, hydration and urinary alkalinization (pH of ≥ 7) until the MTX

LEUCOVORIN CALCIUM (Folinic Acid; Citrovorum Factor)

level is < 5 x 10^{-8}M (0.05 micromolar). Adjust the leucovorin dose or extend leucovorin rescue based on the following guidelines:

Guidelines for Leucovorin Rescue Dosage and Administration

Clinical situation	Laboratory findings	Leucovorin dosage/duration
Normal MTX elimination	Serum MTX level ≈ 10 micromolar at 24 hrs after administration, 1 micromolar at 48 hrs, and < 0.2 micromolar at 72 hours	15 mg orally, IM or IV every 6 hrs for 60 hrs (10 doses starting at 24 hrs after start of MTX infusion)
Delayed late MTX elimination	Serum MTX level remaining > 0.2 micromolar at 72 hrs and > 0.05 micromolar at 96 hrs after administration	Continue 15 mg orally, IM or IV every 6 hrs, until MTX level is < 0.05 micromolar
Delayed early MTX elimination or evidence of acute renal injury	Serum MTX level of ≥ 50 micromolar at 24 hrs, or ≥ 5 micromolar at 48 hrs after administration or a ≥ 100% increase in serum creatinine level at 24 hrs after MTX administration (eg, an increase from 0.5 mg/dl to ≥ 1 mg/dl)	150 mg IV every 3 hrs, until MTX level is < 1 micromolar; then 15 mg IV every 3 hrs until MTX level is < 0.05 micromolar

Patients who experience delayed early MTX elimination are likely to develop reversible renal failure. In addition to appropriate leucovorin therapy, these patients require continuing hydration and urinary alkalinization, and close monitoring of fluid and electrolyte status, until the serum MTX level has fallen to < 0.05 micromolar and the renal failure has resolved.

Some patients will have abnormalities in MTX elimination or renal function following administration, which are significant but less severe than the abnormalities described in the table above. These abnormalities may or may not be associated with significant clinical toxicity. If significant clinical toxicity is observed, extend leucovorin rescue for an additional 24 hours (total of 14 doses over 84 hours) in subsequent courses of therapy. Always consider the possibility that the patient is taking other medications which interact with MTX (eg, medications which may interfere with MTX elimination or binding to serum albumin) when laboratory abnormalities or clinical toxicities are observed.

Impaired MTX elimination or inadvertent overdosage: Begin leucovorin rescue as soon as possible after an inadvertent overdosage and within 24 hours of MTX administration when there is delayed excretion (see Warnings). Administer leucovorin 10 mg/m^2 IV, IM or orally every 6 hours until the serum MTX level is < 10^{-8}M. In the presence of GI toxicity, nausea or vomiting, administer leucovorin parenterally.

Determine serum creatinine and MTX levels at 24 hour intervals. If the 24 hour serum creatinine has increased 50% over baseline or if the 24 or 48 hour MTX level is > 5 x 10^{-6}M or > 9 x 10^{-7}M, respectively, increase the dose of leucovorin to 100 mg/m^2 IV every 3 hours until the MTX level is < 10^{-8}M.

Use hydration (3 L/day) and urinary alkalinization with sodium bicarbonate solution concomitantly. Adjust the bicarbonate dose to maintain the urine pH at ≥ 7.

Folic acid antagonist overdosage: Recommended dose to counteract hematologic toxicity from folic acid antagonists with less affinity for mammalian dihydrofolate reductase than MTX (eg, pyrimethamine, trimethoprim) is 5 to 15 mg/day.

Megaloblastic anemia due to folic acid deficiency: ≤ 1 mg leucovorin/day. There is no evidence that doses > 1 mg/day have greater efficacy than 1 mg doses; also, loss of folate in urine becomes roughly logarithmic as the amount given exceeds 1 mg.

Storage/Stability: Leucovorin powder for injection contains no preservative. Reconstitute with Bacteriostatic Water for Injection, USP, which contains benzyl alcohol, or with Sterile Water for Injection, USP. When reconstituted with Bacteriostatic Water for Injection, USP, the resulting solution must be used within 7 days. If the product is reconstituted with Sterile Water for Injection, USP, it must be used immediately.

Because of the benzyl alcohol contained in the 1 ml amp and in Bacteriostatic Water for Injection, USP, when doses > 10 mg/m^2 are administered, reconstitute the leucovorin amps with Sterile Water for Injection, USP, and use immediately. Because of the calcium content of the leucovorin solution, inject no more than 160 mg/min IV (16 ml of a 10 mg/ml, or 8 ml of a 20 mg/ml solution per minute). Protect from light.

LEUCOVORIN CALCIUM (Folinic Acid; Citrovorum Factor)

Rx	**Leucovorin Calcium** (Various, eg, Barr, Lederle)	**Tablets**: 5 mg (as calcium)	In 30s, 100s and UD 50s.
Rx	**Wellcovorin** (Glaxo Wellcome)		Lactose. (Wellcovorin 5). Off-white, scored. In 20s, 100s and UD 50s.
Rx	**Leucovorin Calcium** (Lederle)	**Tablets**: 15 mg (as calcium)	Lactose. (LL 15 C 35). Yellowish-white, scored. Oval, convex. In 12s, 24s and UD 50s.
Rx	**Leucovorin Calcium** (Barr)	**Tablets**: 25 mg (as calcium)	(485). Light green. In 25s.
Rx	**Wellcovorin** (Glaxo Wellcome)		Lactose. (Wellcovorin 25). Peach, scored. In 25s and UD 10s.
Rx	**Leucovorin Calcium** (Lederle)	**Injection**: 3 mg/ml (as calcium)	In 1 ml amps.[1]
Rx	**Leucovorin Calcium** (Lederle)	**Powder for Injection**: 50 mg/vial (as calcium)[2]	In vials.
Rx	**Leucovorin Calcium** (Lederle)	**Powder for Injection**: 100 mg/vial (as calcium)[2]	In vials.
Rx	**Wellcovorin** (Glaxo Wellcome)		In vials.
Rx	**Leucovorin Calcium** (Lederle)	**Powder for Injection**: 350 mg/vial (as calcium)[2]	In vials.

[1] With 0.9% benzyl alcohol.
[2] Preservative free.

VITAMIN B_{12}

Actions:

Pharmacology: Vitamin B_{12} (cyanocobalamin and hydroxocobalamin) is essential to growth, cell reproduction, hematopoiesis and nucleoprotein and myelin synthesis. Its physiologic role is associated with methylation, participating in nucleic acid and protein synthesis. Cyanocobalamin participates in red blood cell formation through activation of folic acid coenzymes. Cyanocobalamin has hematopoietic activity apparently identical to that of the anti-anemia factor in purified liver extract. Hydroxocobalamin (vitamin B_{12a}), an analog of cyanocobalamin in which a hydroxyl radical replaces the cyano radical, functions the same as cyanocobalamin.

The normal range of plasma B_{12} is 200 to 750 pg/ml, which represents about 0.1% of the total body content. The total daily loss ranges from 2 to 5 mcg. Because of its slow rate of utilization and considerable body stores, vitamin B_{12} deficiency may take many months to appear.

The average diet supplies about 5 to 15 mcg/day of vitamin B_{12}. Vitamin B_{12} is bound to intrinsic factor during transit through the stomach; separation occurs in the terminal ileum in the presence of calcium, and vitamin B_{12} enters the mucosal cell for absorption. It is then transported by specific B_{12} binding proteins, transcobalamin I and II. Transcobalamin II is the delivery protein for vitamin B_{12}. In addition, approximately 1% of the total amount ingested is absorbed by simple diffusion, but this mechanism is significant only with large doses.

For use of oral vitamin B_{12} in the treatment of nutritional deficiency, see the monograph in the Nutritionals chapter.

Pharmacokinetics: Absorption of vitamin B_{12} depends on the presence of sufficient intrinsic factor and calcium. In general, absorption of oral B_{12} is inadequate in malabsorptive states and in pernicious anemia (unless intrinsic factor is simultaneously administered).

Cyanocobalamin is rapidly absorbed from IM and SC injection sites; the plasma level peaks within 1 hour. Once absorbed, it is bound to plasma proteins, stored mainly in the liver and is slowly released when needed to carry out normal cellular metabolic functions. Within 48 hours after injection of 100 to 1000 mcg of vitamin B_{12}, 50% to 98% of the dose appears in the urine. The major portion is excreted within the first 8 hours. More rapid excretion occurs with IV administration; there is little opportunity for liver storage.

Hydroxocobalamin (vitamin B_{12a}) is more highly protein bound and is retained in the body longer than cyanocobalamin. However, it has no advantage over cyanocobalamin. Administration of hydroxocobalamin has resulted in antibody formation to the hydroxocobalamin-transcobalamin II complex and thus cyanocobalamin may be preferred.

Indications:

Vitamin B_{12} deficiency due to malabsorption syndrome as seen in pernicious anemia; GI pathology, dysfunction or surgery; fish tapeworm infestation; malignancy of pancreas or bowel; gluten enteropathy; sprue; small bowel bacterial overgrowth; total or partial gastrectomy; accompanying folic acid deficiency.

Increased vitamin B_{12} requirements associated with pregnancy, thyrotoxicosis, hemolytic anemia, hemorrhage, malignancy and hepatic and renal disease.

Vitamin B_{12} absorption test (Schilling test).

Cyanocobalamin (oral) is used for nutritional vitamin B_{12} deficiency (see monograph in Vitamins section).

Unlabeled uses: Hydroxocobalamin has been used to prevent and to treat cyanide toxicity associated with sodium nitroprusside. It lowers red blood cell and plasma cyanide concentrations by combining with cyanide to form cyanocobalamin, which is nontoxic and excreted in the urine.

Contraindications:

Hypersensitivity to cobalt, vitamin B_{12} or any component of these products.

Warnings:

Inadequate response: Parenteral administration is preferred for pernicious anemia. Avoid the IV route.

A blunted or impeded therapeutic response may be due to infection, uremia, bone marrow suppressant drugs (ie, chloramphenicol), concurrent iron or folic acid deficiency or misdiagnosis.

Vitamin B_{12} deficiency allowed to progress for > 3 months may produce permanent degenerative lesions of the spinal cord.

Optic nerve atrophy: Patients with early Leber's disease (hereditary optic nerve atrophy) treated with cyanocobalamin suffer severe and swift optic atrophy.

VITAMIN B_{12}

Hypokalemia and sudden death may occur in severe megaloblastic anemia which is treated intensely.

Benzyl alcohol: Some of these products contain benzyl alcohol, which has been associated with a fatal "gasping syndrome" in premature infants.

Pregnancy: Category C (parenteral). Adequate and well controlled studies have not been performed in pregnant women. However, B_{12} is an essential vitamin and needs are increased during pregnancy. The National Academy of Sciences has recommended that 2.2 mcg/day should be consumed during pregnancy.

Lactation: Vitamin B_{12} is excreted in breast milk in concentrations that approximate the mother's vitamin B_{12} blood level. Amounts of B_{12} recommended by the Food and Nutrition Board, National Academy of Sciences-National Research Council (2.6 mcg daily) should be consumed during lactation.

Children: The Food and Nutrition Board, National Academy of Sciences-National Research Council recommends a daily intake of 0.3 to 0.5 mcg/day for infants < 1 year of age and 0.7 to 1.4 mcg/day for children 1 to 10 years of age.

Precautions:

Monitoring: During treatment of severe megaloblastic anemia, monitor serum potassium levels closely for the first 48 hours and replace potassium if necessary. Obtain reticulocyte counts, hematocrit and vitamin B_{12}, iron and folic acid plasma levels prior to treatment and between the fifth and seventh days of therapy, and then frequently until the hematocrit is normal. If folate levels are low, also administer folic acid. Continue periodic hematologic evaluations throughout the patient's lifetime.

Test dose: Anaphylactic shock and death have occurred after parenteral vitamin B_{12} administration. Give an intradermal test dose in patients sensitive to the cobalamins.

Folate: Doses > 10 mcg daily may produce hematologic response in patients with folate deficiency. Indiscriminate use may mask the true diagnosis of pernicious anemia.

Doses of folic acid > 0.1 mg/day may result in hematologic remission in patients with vitamin B_{12} deficiency. Neurologic manifestations will not be prevented with folic acid, and if not treated with vitamin B_{12}, irreversible damage will result.

Single deficiency (vitamin B_{12} alone) is rare. Expect multiple vitamin deficiency in any dietary deficiency.

Polycythemia vera: Vitamin B_{12} deficiency may suppress the signs of polycythemia vera. Treatment with vitamin B_{12} may unmask this condition.

Vegetarian diets containing no animal products (including milk products or eggs) do not supply any vitamin B_{12}. Vegetarians should take oral vitamin B_{12} regularly.

Stomach carcinoma: Pernicious anemia patients have about 3 times the incidence of stomach carcinoma as the general population; perform appropriate tests for this condition when indicated.

Immunodeficient patients: Vitamin B_{12} malabsorption may occur in patients with AIDS or HIV infection. Consider monitoring vitamin B_{12} levels in these patients.

Drug Interactions:

Vitamin B_{12} Drug Interactions

Precipitant drug	Object drug*		Description
Aminosalicylic acid	Vitamin B_{12}	⬇	Biologic and therapeutic action of vitamin B_{12} may be reduced. An abnormal Schilling test and symptoms of vitamin B_{12} deficiency may also occur.
Chloramphenicol	Vitamin B_{12}	⬇	The hematologic effects of vitamin B_{12} may be decreased in patients with pernicious anemia.
Colchicine Alcohol	Vitamin B_{12}	⬇	Colchicine or excessive alcohol intake (longer than 2 weeks) may cause malabsorption of vitamin B_{12}.

* ⬇ = Object drug decreased.

Drug/Lab test interactions: Methotrexate, pyrimethamine and most antibiotics invalidate folic acid and vitamin B_{12} diagnostic microbiological blood assays.

Adverse Reactions:

The following reactions are associated with parenteral vitamin B_{12}:

Hypersensitivity: Anaphylactic shock and death.

Cardiovascular: Pulmonary edema; congestive heart failure early in treatment; peripheral vascular thrombosis.

Dermatologic: Itching; transitory exanthema.

VITAMIN B_{12}

Miscellaneous: Feeling of swelling of the entire body; mild transient diarrhea; polycythemia vera; pain at injection site; severe and swift optic nerve atrophy (see Warnings).

Patient Information:

Patients with pernicious anemia will require monthly injections of vitamin B_{12} for the rest of their lives. Failure to do so will result in return of the anemia and in development of incapacitating and irreversible damage to the nerves of the spinal cord.

A well balanced dietary intake is necessary; correct poor dietary habits.

Do not take folic acid instead of vitamin B_{12} because folic acid may prevent anemia, but allow progression of subacute combined degeneration.

HYDROXOCOBALAMIN, CRYSTALLINE (Vitamin B_{12})

For complete prescribing information, refer to the Vitamin B_{12} monograph.

Administration and Dosage:

Administer IM only. The recommended dosage is 30 mcg/day for 5 to 10 days, followed by 100 to 200 mcg monthly. Children may be given a total of 1 to 5 mg over 2 or more weeks in doses of 100 mcg, then 30 to 50 mcg every 4 weeks for maintenance. Institute concurrent folic acid therapy at the beginning of treatment if needed.

Rx	**Hydroxocobalamin** (Various, eg, Major)	**Injection:** 1000 mcg/ml	In 30 ml.
Rx	**Hydro Cobex** (Pasadena)		In 30 ml vials.
Rx	**Hydro-Crysti-12** (Roberts Hauck)		In 30 ml.
Rx	**LA-12** (Hyrex)		In 30 ml.

CYANOCOBALAMIN CRYSTALLINE

For complete prescribing information, refer to the Vitamin B_{12} monograph.

Administration and Dosage:

Addisonian pernicious anemia: Parenteral therapy is required for life; oral therapy is not dependable. Administer 100 mcg daily for 6 or 7 days by IM or deep SC injection. If there is clinical improvement and a reticulocyte response, give the same amount on alternate days for 7 doses, then every 3 to 4 days for another 2 to 3 weeks. By this time, hematologic values should have become normal. Follow this regimen with 100 mcg monthly for life. Administer folic acid concomitantly if needed.

Other patients with vitamin B_{12} deficiency: In seriously ill patients, administer both vitamin B_{12} and folic acid. It is not necessary to withhold therapy until the precise cause of B_{12} deficiency is established. For hematologic signs, children may be given 10 to 50 mcg/day for 5 to 10 days followed by 100 to 250 mcg/dose every 2 to 4 weeks; for neurologic signs, 100 mcg/day for 10 to 15 days, then once or twice weekly for several months, possibly tapering to 250 to 1000 mcg monthly by 1 year.

Oral – Up to 1000 mcg/day. Oral vitamin B_{12} therapy is not usually recommended for vitamin B_{12} deficiency. The maximum amount of vitamin B_{12} that can be absorbed from a single oral dose is 1 to 5 mcg. The percent absorbed decreases with increasing doses.

IM or SC – 30 mcg daily for 5 to 10 days followed by 100 to 200 mcg monthly. Larger doses (eg, 1000 mcg) have been recommended, even though a larger amount is lost through excretion. However, it is possible that a greater amount is retained, allowing for fewer injections.

Schilling test: The flushing dose is 1000 mcg IM.

Storage: Protect parenterals from light. Avoid freezing.

CYANOCOBALAMIN CRYSTALLINE

otc	**Vitamin B_{12}** (Goldline)	**Tablets**: 500 mcg	Pink. In 100s.
		1000 mcg	Pink. In 100s.
Rx	**Vitamin B_{12}** (Various, eg, Goldline, Rugby)	**Injection**: 100 mcg per ml	In 30 ml vials.
Rx	**Vitamin B_{12}** (Various, eg, American Regent, Geneva, Goldline, Major, Pasadena, Rugby, Schein, Warner Chilcott)	**Injection**: 1000 mcg per ml	In 10 and 30 ml multi-dose vials.
Rx	**Crystamine** (Dunhall)		In 10 and 30 ml multi-dose vials[1]
Rx	**Crysti 1000** (Roberts Hauck)		In 10 ml vials.
Rx	**Cyanoject** (Mayrand)		In 10 and 30 ml[1].
Rx	**Cyomin** (Forest)		In 30 ml multi-dose vials[1].
Rx	**Rubesol-1000** (Central)		In 10 and 30 ml vials[1].

[1] With benzyl alcohol.

LIVER PREPARATIONS

For complete prescribing information, refer to the Vitamin B_{12} monograph.

Actions:

Pharmacology: Crude liver extracts are a source of vitamin B_{12} (extrinsic factor). However, since liver extracts may cause serious sensitization, purified crystalline cyanocobalamin is the preferred source of vitamin B_{12} in deficiency states.

PARENTERAL LIVER PREPARATIONS

For complete prescribing information, refer to the Vitamin B_{12} monograph.

Administration and Dosage:

Inject IM only.

Rx	**Liver, Crude** (Various, eg Merit)	**Injection**: 2 mcg B_{12} per ml	In 30 ml vials.

PARENTERAL LIVER COMBINATIONS

For complete prescribing information, refer to the Vitamin B_{12} monograph.
Content given per ml.

	Product & Distributor	Liver Inj. B12 Equiv. (mcg)	Cryst. B12 (mcg)	FA (mg)	How Supplied
Rx	**Liver Combo No. 5** (Rugby)	10	100	0.4	In 10 ml vials.[1]

[1] With phenol.

PHYTONADIONE (K_1, Phylloquinone, Methylphytyl Napthoquinone)

Warning:

IV use: Severe reactions, including fatalities, have occurred during and immediately after IV injection, even with precautions to dilute the injection and to avoid rapid infusion. These severe reactions resemble hypersensitivity or anaphylaxis, including shock and cardiac or respiratory arrest. Some patients exhibit these severe reactions on receiving vitamin K for the first time. Therefore, restrict the IV route to those situations where other routes are not feasible and the serious risk involved is justified.

Actions:

Pharmacology: Vitamin K promotes the hepatic synthesis of active prothrombin (factor II), proconvertin (factor VII), plasma thromboplastin component (factor IX) and Stuart factor (factor X). The mechanism by which vitamin K promotes formation of these clotting factors involves the hepatic post-translational carboxylation of specific glutamate residues to gamma-carboxylglutamate residues in proteins involved in coagulation, thus leading to their activation.

Phytonadione (vitamin K_1) is a lipid-soluble synthetic analog of vitamin K. Phytonadione possesses essentially the same type and degree of activity as the naturally occurring vitamin K.

Pharmacokinetics: Phytonadione is only absorbed from the GI tract via intestinal lymphatics in the presence of bile salts. Although initially concentrated in the liver, vitamin K is rapidly metabolized and very little tissue accumulation occurs. Little is known about the metabolic fate of vitamin K. Almost no free unmetabolized vitamin K appears in bile or urine.

Parenteral phytonadione is generally detectable within 1 to 2 hours. Phytonadione usually controls hemorrhage within 3 to 6 hours. A normal prothrombin level may be obtained in 12 to 14 hours. Oral phytonadione exerts its effect in 6 to 10 hours.

The US daily allowances for vitamin K have not been officially established, but have been estimated to be 10 to 20 mcg for infants, 15 to 100 mcg for children and adolescents and 70 to 140 mcg for adults. Usually, dietary vitamin K will satisfy these requirements, except during the first 5 to 8 days of the neonatal period. Naturally occurring vitamin K is found in various foods, including cabbage, cauliflower, kale, spinach, fish, liver, eggs, meats, cereal grain products, fruits and milk and dairy products.

Recommended Dietary Allowances as published by the National Academy of Sciences are as follows: Adult males, 45 to 80 mcg/day; adult females, 45 to 65 mcg/day. For a complete listing of RDA by age, sex or condition, refer to the RDA table in the Nutritionals chapter.

Indications:

Coagulation disorders due to faulty formation of factors II, VII, IX and X when caused by vitamin K deficiency or interference with vitamin K activity.

Oral: Anticoagulant-induced prothrombin deficiency (see Warnings); hypoprothrombinemia secondary to salicylates or antibacterial therapy; hypoprothrombinemia secondary to obstructive jaundice and biliary fistulas, but only if bile salts are administered concomitantly with phytonadione.

Parenteral: Anticoagulant-induced prothrombin deficiency; hypoprothrombinemia secondary to conditions limiting absorption or synthesis of vitamin K (eg, obstructive jaundice, biliary fistula, sprue, ulcerative colitis, celiac disease, intestinal resection, cystic fibrosis of the pancreas, regional enteritis); drug-induced hypoprothrombinemias due to interference with vitamin K metabolism (eg, antibiotics, salicylates); prophylaxis and therapy of hemorrhagic disease of the newborn.

Contraindications:

Hypersensitivity to any component of the product.

Warnings:

Oral anticoagulant-induced hypoprothrombinemia: Vitamin K will not counteract the anticoagulant action of heparin.

Phytonadione promotes synthesis of prothrombin by the liver. Immediate coagulant effect should not be expected. It takes a minimum of 1 to 2 hours for a measurable improvement in the prothrombin time (PT).The prothrombin test is sensitive to the levels of factors II, VII and X. Fresh plasma or blood transfusions may be required for severe blood loss or lack of response to vitamin K.

PHYTONADIONE (K_1, Phylloquinone, Methylphytyl Napthoquinone)

With phytonadione use and anticoagulant therapy indicated, the patient is faced with the same clotting hazards prior to starting anticoagulant therapy. Phytonadione is not a clotting agent, but overzealous therapy may restore original thromboembolic phenomena conditions. Keep dosage as low as possible and check PT regularly.

Hepatic function impairment: Hypoprothrombinemia due to hepatocellular damage is not corrected by administration of vitamin K. Repeated large doses of vitamin K are not warranted in liver disease if the initial response is unsatisfactory (Koller test). Failure to respond to vitamin K may indicate a coagulation defect or a condition unresponsive to vitamin K. In hepatic disease, large doses may further depress liver function.

Paradoxically, giving excessive doses of vitamin K or its analogs in an attempt to correct hypoprothrombinemia associated with severe hepatitis or cirrhosis may actually result in further depression of the prothrombin concentration.

Pregnancy: Category C. Vitamin K crosses the placenta. It is not known whether vitamin K can cause fetal harm when administered to a pregnant woman or can affect reproduction capacity. Use only if clearly needed.

Lactation: Vitamin K is excreted in breast milk. Consider this if the drug must be used in a nursing mother.

Children: Safety and efficacy in children have not been established. Hemolysis, jaundice and hyperbilirubinemia in newborns, particularly in premature infants, have been reported with vitamin K. These effects may be dose-related. Therefore, do not exceed recommended dose.

Precautions:

Benzyl alcohol contained in some products has been associated with toxicity in newborns. Specific products containing benzyl alcohol are identified in the product listings.

Drug Interactions:

Vitamin K Drug Interactions			
Precipitant drug	Object drug*		Description
Vitamin K	Anticoagulants	⬇	Anticoagulant effects are antagonized by vitamin K. Temporary resistance to oral anticoagulants may result. It may be necessary to increase the anticoagulant dose.
Mineral oil	Vitamin K	⬇	Mineral oil may decrease GI absorption of vitamin K with concurrent oral administration.

* ⬇=Object drug decreased.

Adverse Reactions:

Allergic reactions: Anaphylactoid reactions may occur.

Parenteral administration: Rarely, pain, swelling and tenderness at the injection site; after repeated injections, erythematous, indurated pruritic plaques have occurred. These have rarely progressed to scleroderma-like lesions that have persisted for long periods. In other cases, these lesions have resembled erythema perstans.

Transient "flushing sensations" and "peculiar" sensations of taste; rarely, dizziness, rapid and weak pulse, profuse sweating, brief hypotension, dyspnea and cyanosis.

Hyperbilirubinemia has been observed in the newborn following administration of phytonadione. This has occurred rarely and primarily with doses above those recommended (see Warnings).

Deaths have occurred after IV administration (see boxed warning).

Administration and Dosage:

If possible, discontinue or reduce the dosage of drugs interfering with coagulation mechanisms (eg, salicylates, antibiotics) as an alternative to phytonadione. The severity of the coagulation disorder should determine whether the immediate administration of phytonadione is required in addition to discontinuation or reduction of interfering drugs.

Inject SC or IM when possible. In older children and adults, inject IM in the upper outer quadrant of the buttocks. In infants and young children, the anterolateral aspect of the thigh or the deltoid region is preferred. When IV administration is unavoidable, inject very slowly, not exceeding 1 mg/min.

PHYTONADIONE (K_1, Phylloquinone, Methylphytyl Napthoquinone)

Anticoagulant-induced prothrombin deficiency in adults: 2.5 to 10 mg or up to 25 mg (rarely, 50 mg) initially. Determine subsequent doses by PT response or clinical condition. If in 6 to 8 hours after parenteral administration (or 12 to 48 hours after oral administration) the PT has not been shortened satisfactorily, repeat dose. If shock or excessive blood loss occurs, transfusion of blood or fresh frozen plasma may be required.

Hemorrhagic disease of the newborn:

Prophylaxis – Single IM dose of 0.5 to 1 mg within 1 hour after birth. This may be repeated after 2 to 3 weeks if the mother has received anticoagulant, anticonvulsant, antituberculous or recent antibiotic therapy during her pregnancy. Twelve to 24 hours before delivery, 1 to 5 mg may be given to the mother.

Oral doses of 2 mg are adequate for prophylaxis.

Treatment – 1 mg SC or IM. Higher doses may be necessary if the mother has been receiving oral anticoagulants. Empiric administration of vitamin K_1 should not replace proper laboratory evaluation. A prompt response (shortening of the PT in 2 to 4 hours) is usually diagnostic of hemorrhagic disease of the newborn; failure to respond indicates another diagnosis or coagulation disorder. Give blood or blood products such as fresh frozen plasma if bleeding is excessive. This therapy does not correct the underlying disorder; give phytonadione concurrently.

Hypoprothrombinemia due to other causes in adults: 2.5 to 25 mg (rarely, up to 50 mg); amount and route of administration depends on severity of condition and response obtained. Avoid oral route when clinical disorder would prevent proper absorption. Give bile salts with tablets when endogenous supply of bile to GI tract is deficient.

Storage: Protect from light at all times.

Rx	**Mephyton** (Merck)	**Tablets**: 5 mg	Lactose. (MSD 43 Mephyton). Yellow, scored. In 100s.
Rx	**AquaMEPHYTON** (Merck)	**Injection (aqueous colloidal solution):** 2 mg per ml	In 0.5 ml amps.[1]
Rx	**Phytonadione** (IMS)		In 0.5 ml *Min-I-ject* prefilled syringes.
Rx	**AquaMEPHYTON** (Merck)	**Injection (aqueous dispersion)**: 10 mg per ml	In 1 ml amps[1] and 2.5 and 5 ml vials.[1]

[1] With polyoxyethylated fatty acid derivative, dextrose and benzyl alcohol.

EPOETIN ALFA (Erythropoietin; EPO)

Actions:

Pharmacology: Erythropoietin is a glycoprotein that stimulates red blood cell production. It is produced in the kidney and stimulates the division and differentiation of erythroid progenitors in bone marrow. Epoetin alfa, a 165 amino acid glycoprotein manufactured by recombinant DNA technology, has the same biological effects as endogenous erythropoietin. It has a molecular weight of 30,400 daltons and is produced by mammalian cells into which the human erythropoietin gene is introduced. The product contains the identical amino acid sequence of natural erythropoietin.

Endogenous production of erythropoietin is regulated by the level of tissue oxygenation. Hypoxia and anemia generally increase the production of erythropoietin, which in turn stimulates erythropoiesis. In healthy subjects, plasma erythropoietin levels range from 0.01 to 0.03 U/ml and increase up to 100- to 1000-fold during hypoxia or anemia. In patients with chronic renal failure (CRF), erythropoietin production is impaired; this deficiency is the primary cause of their anemia.

Epoetin alfa stimulates erythropoiesis in anemic patients on dialysis and those who do not require regular dialysis. The first evidence of a response to epoetin alfa administration is an increase in the reticulocyte count within 10 days, followed by increases in the red cell count, hemoglobin and hematocrit, usually within 2 to 6 weeks. Once the hematocrit reaches the suggested target range (30% to 36%), that level can be sustained by epoetin alfa therapy in the absence of iron deficiency and concurrent illnesses.

The rate of hematocrit increase varies between patients and is dependent upon the dose of epoetin alfa within a therapeutic range of ≈ 50 to 300 U/kg 3 times weekly; a greater biologic response is not observed at doses > 300 U/kg 3 times weekly. Other factors affecting rate and extent of response include availability of iron stores, baseline hematocrit and concurrent medical problems. Responsiveness in HIV-infected patients is dependent on the endogenous serum erythropoietin level prior to treatment. Patients with levels ≤ 500 mU/ml receiving zidovudine (AZT) ≤ 4200 mg/week may respond; patients with levels > 500 mU/ml do not appear to respond. In four trials, 60% to 80% of patients had levels ≤ 500 mU/ml. Response is manifested by reduced transfusion requirements and increased hematocrit.

Pharmacokinetics: Epoetin alfa IV is eliminated via first-order kinetics with a circulating half-life of 4 to 13 hours in patients with CRF. Within the therapeutic dosage range, detectable levels of plasma erythropoietin are maintained for ≥ 24 hours. After SC administration of epoetin alfa to patients with CRF, peak serum levels are achieved within 5 to 24 hours after administration and decline slowly thereafter. There is no apparent difference in half-life between patients not on dialysis (serum creatinine > 3) and patients maintained on dialysis. The half-life in healthy volunteers is ≈ 20% shorter than in CRF patients.

Clinical trials: The rate of increase in hematocrit is dependent upon the dose of epoetin alfa administered and individual patient variation.

Hematocrit Increase Based on Epoetin Alfa Dose in Chronic Renal Failure Patients

Starting dose (3 times weekly, IV)	Hematocrit increase	
	Hematocrit points/ day	Hematocrit points/ 2 weeks
50 U/kg	0.11	1.5
100 U/kg	0.18	2.5
150 U/kg	0.25	3.5

Over this dosage range, ≈ 95% of all patients responded with a clinically significant increase in hematocrit, and by the end of ≈ 2 months of therapy, virtually all patients were transfusion-independent. Once the target hematocrit was achieved, the maintenance dose was individualized.

Dialysis patients – Thirteen clinical studies were conducted involving IV administration to a total of 1010 anemic patients on dialysis for 986 patient-years of epoetin alfa therapy. In the three largest trials, the median maintenance dose necessary to maintain the hematocrit between 30% to 36% was ≈ 75 U/kg 3 times weekly. In the US multicenter Phase III study, ≈ 65% of the patients required doses of ≤ 100 U/kg 3 times weekly to maintain their hematocrit at ≈ 35%. Almost 10% of patients required ≤ 25 U/kg 3 times weekly, and ≈ 10% required a dose of > 200 U/kg 3 times weekly to maintain their hematocrit at this level.

EPOETIN ALFA (Erythropoietin; EPO)

Patients with CRF not requiring dialysis – Four clinical trials were conducted in 181 epoetin alfa-treated patients for ≈ 67 patient-years of experience. These patients responded to therapy in a manner similar to that of patients on dialysis. These patients demonstrated a dose-dependent and sustained increase in hematocrit when epoetin alfa was administered either IV or SC. Doses of 75 to 150 U/kg/week maintain hematocrits of 36% to 38% for up to 6 months. Correcting the anemia of progressive renal failure will allow patients to remain active even though their renal function continues to decrease.

Zidovudine-treated HIV-infected patients – In four placebo controlled trials enrolling 297 anemic (hematocrit < 30%) HIV-infected (AIDS) patients receiving concomitant therapy with zidovudine, epoetin alfa reduced the mean cumulative number of units of blood transfused per patient by ≈ 40% in patients with endogenous erythropoietin levels ≤ 500 mU/ml (n = 89) vs placebo. Among those patients who required transfusions at baseline, 43% epoetin alfa vs 18% placebo were transfusion-independent during the second and third months of therapy. Epoetin alfa therapy also resulted in significant increases in hematocrit compared with placebo. There was a statistically significant reduction in transfusion requirements in epoetin alfa-treated patients whose mean weekly zidovudine dose was ≤ 4200 mg/week. In patients whose prestudy endogenous serum erythropoietin levels were > 500 mU/ml, epoetin alfa therapy did not reduce transfusion requirements or increase hematocrit.

Cancer patients on chemotherapy – In double-blind trials involving 131 anemic cancer patients, 72 were treated with concomitant non-cisplatin-containing chemotherapy regimens and 59 received cisplatin-containing regimens. Patients received either epoetin alfa 150 units/kg or placebo SC 3 times weekly for 12 weeks. Epoetin therapy was associated with a significantly greater hematocrit response than placebo. Mean number of units of blood transfused per patient after the first month of therapy was significantly lower with epoetin alfa, and the proportion of patients transfused during months 2 and 3 of therapy combined was significantly lower with epoetin alfa vs placebo (22% vs 43%). Patients with lymphoid and solid cancers and those without tumor infiltration of the bone marrow respond to epoetin alfa.

Surgery – Epoetin alfa has been studied in a placebo controlled, double-blind trial enrolling 316 patients scheduled for major, elective orthopedic hip or knee surgery who were expected to require ≥ 2 units of blood and who were not able or willing to participate in an autologous blood donation program. They received 300 U/kg epoetin alfa, 100 U/kg epoetin alfa or placebo by SC injection for 10 days before surgery, on the day of surgery and for four days after surgery. All patients received oral iron and a low dose postoperative warfarin regimen.

Treatment with epoetin alfa 300 U/kg significantly reduced the risk of allogeneic transfusion in patients with a pretreatment hemoglobin of > 10 to ≤ 13 g/dl; 5/31 (16%) of epoetin alfa 300 U/kg, 6/26 (23%) of epoetin alfa 100 U/kg and 13/29 (45%) of placebo-treated patients were transfused.

Indications:

Treatment of anemia associated with CRF, including patients on dialysis (end-stage renal disease) and patients not on dialysis, to elevate or maintain the red blood cell level (as manifested by the hematocrit or hemoglobin determinations) and to decrease the need for transfusions.

Not intended for patients who require immediate correction of severe anemia. Epoetin alfa may obviate the need for maintenance transfusions but is not a substitute for emergency transfusion.

Treatment of anemia related to zidovudine therapy in HIV-infected patients: To elevate or maintain the red blood cell level (as manifested by the hematocrit or hemoglobin determinations) and to decrease the need for transfusions in these patients when the endogenous erythropoietin level is ≤ 500 mU/ml and the dose of zidovudine is ≤ 4200 mg/week.

Not indicated for the treatment of anemia in HIV-infected patients caused by other factors such as iron or folate deficiencies, hemolysis or GI bleeding that should be managed appropriately.

Treatment of anemia in cancer patients on chemotherapy: Treatment of anemia in patients with non-myeloid malignancies where anemia is caused by the effect of concomitantly administered chemotherapy. It is intended to decrease the need for transfusions in patients who will be receiving chemotherapy for a minimum of 2 months.

Reduction of allogeneic blood transfusion in surgery patients: For the treatment of anemic patients (hemoglobin > 10 to ≤ 13 g/dl) scheduled to undergo elective, noncardiac, nonvascular surgery to reduce the need for allogeneic blood transfusions. Epoetin alfa is indicated for patients at high risk for perioperative transfusions with significant, anticipated blood loss.

EPOETIN ALFA (Erythropoietin; EPO)

Unlabeled uses: Pruritus associated with renal failure.

Contraindications:

Uncontrolled hypertension; hypersensitivity to mammalian cell-derived products or to human albumin.

Warnings:

Anemia: Not intended for CRF patients who require correction of severe anemia; epoetin alfa may obviate the need for maintenance transfusions but is not a substitute for emergency transfusion. Not indicated for treatment of anemia in HIV-infected patients or cancer patients caused by other factors such as iron or folate deficiencies, hemolysis or GI bleeding that should be managed appropriately.

Epoetin alfa is not indicated for anemic patients who are willing to donate autologous blood.

Hypertension: Up to 80% of patients with CRF have a history of hypertension. Do not treat patients with uncontrolled hypertension; monitor blood pressure adequately before initiation of therapy. Although there does not appear to be any direct pressor effects of epoetin, blood pressure may rise during therapy. During the early phase of treatment when the hematocrit is increasing, ≈ 25% of patients on dialysis may require initiation of, or increases in, antihypertensive therapy. Hypertensive encephalopathy and seizures have occurred in CRF patients treated with epoetin.

Take special care to closely monitor and aggressively control blood pressure in epoetin-treated patients. Advise patients of the importance of compliance with antihypertensive therapy and dietary restrictions. If blood pressure is difficult to control by initiation of appropriate measures, the hematocrit may be reduced by decreasing or withholding the epoetin dose. A clinically significant decrease in hematocrit may not be observed for several weeks. It is recommended that the epoetin dose be decreased if the hematocrit increase exceeds 4 points in any 2–week period because of the possible association of excessive rate of rise of hematocrit with an exacerbation of hypertension.

In chronic renal failure patients on hemodialysis with clinically evident ischemic heart disease or CHF, manage the hematocrit carefully, not to exceed 36%.

In contrast to CRF patients, epoetin alfa has not been linked to exacerbation of hypertension, seizures and thrombotic events in HIV-infected patients. However, withhold epoetin alfa in these patients if pre-existing hypertension is uncontrolled, and do not start until blood pressure is controlled.

Hypertension associated with a significant increase in hematocrit, has been noted rarely in cancer patients receiving epoetin alfa. Nevertheless, monitor blood pressure carefully, particularly in patients with an underlying history of hypertension or cardiovascular disease.

Seizures: The relationship to seizures is uncertain. The baseline incidence of seizures in the untreated dialysis population appears to be 5% to 10% per patient-year. There have been 47 seizures in 1010 patients on dialysis treated with epoetin alfa with an exposure of 986 patient-years for a rate of ≈ 0.048 events per patient-year. In patients on dialysis, there appeared to be a higher incidence of seizures during the first 90 days of therapy (occurring in ≈ 2.5% of patients) when compared with subsequent 90–day periods. Monitor the presence of premonitory neurologic symptoms closely. Patients should avoid potentially hazardous activities such as driving or operating heavy machinery during this period.

Because the relationship between seizures and the rate of rise of hematocrit is uncertain, decrease the dose of epoetin alfa if the hematocrit increase exceeds 4 points in any 2–week period.

Growth factor potential: The possibility that epoetin alfa can act as a growth factor for any tumor type, particularly myeloid malignancies, cannot be excluded.

EPOETIN ALFA (Erythropoietin; EPO)

Thrombotic events: During hemodialysis, patients treated with epoetin alfa may require increased anticoagulation with heparin to prevent clotting of the artificial kidney. Clotting of the vascular access (A-V shunt) has occurred at an annualized rate of ≈ 0.25 events per patient-year on epoetin alfa therapy, a rate which appears to be no higher than that seen in untreated patients.

Overall, for patients with CRF (whether on dialysis or not) in whom the target hematocrit was 32% to 40%, other thrombotic events (eg, myocardial infarction, cerebrovascular accident, transient ischemic attack) have occurred at an annualized rate of < 0.04 events per patient-year of epoetin alfa. The risk of thrombotic events, including vascular access thromboses, was significantly increased in patients with ischemic heart disease or CHF receiving epoetin alfa therapy with the goal of reaching a normal hematocrit (42%) as compared with a target hematocrit of 30%. Monitor patients with pre-existing vascular disease closely.

In one study, 4 out of 7 deaths were associated with thrombotic events. Weigh the anticipated benefits of epoetin alfa treatment against the potential for increased risks associated with therapy.

There have been rare reports of serious or unusual thromboembolic events including migratory thrombophlebitis, microvascular thrombosis, pulmonary embolus, and thrombosis of the retinal artery and temporal and retinal veins. A causal relationship has not been established.

Heart disease/congestive heart failure (CHF): In chronic renal failure patients on hemodialysis with clinically evident ischemic heart disease or CHF, manage the hematocrit carefully, not to exceed 36%.

Hypersensitivity: Skin rashes and urticaria are rare, mild and transient. There is no evidence of antibody development to erythropoietin, including those receiving epoetin alfa for > 4 years. Nevertheless, if an anaphylactoid reaction occurs, immediately discontinue the drug and initiate appropriate therapy. Refer to Management of Acute Hypersensitivity Reactions.

In > 125,000 patients treated with epoetin alfa, there have been rare reports of potentially serious allergic reactions including urticaria with associated respiratory symptoms or circumoral edema, or urticaria alone. Most reactions occurred in situations where a causal relationship could not be established. Many of these patients resumed therapy without recurrence of symptoms, some in conjunction with antihistamine pretreatment. However, symptoms recurred with rechallenge in a few instances, suggesting that allergic reactivity, although rare, may occasionally be associated with epoetin alfa therapy.

Two zidovudine-treated, HIV-infected patients had urticarial reactions within 48 hours of their first exposure to medication. One was treated with epoetin alfa and one was treated with placebo. Both patients had positive immediate skin tests against their medication with a negative saline control. The basis for this apparent pre-existing hypersensitivity to components of the formulation is unknown but may be related to HIV-induced immunosuppression or prior exposure to blood products.

Pregnancy: Category C. Adverse effects occurred in rats when given epoetin in doses 5 times the human dose. There are no adequate and well controlled studies in pregnant women. Use in pregnancy only if the potential benefit justifies the potential risk to the fetus. In some female patients, menses have resumed following epoetin alfa therapy; discuss the possibility of pregnancy and evaluate need for contraception.

Lactation: It is not known whether epoetin alfa is excreted in breast milk. Exercise caution when administering to a nursing woman.

Children: Safety and efficacy have not been established.

EPOETIN ALFA (Erythropoietin; EPO)

Precautions:

Monitoring:

Patients with CRF not requiring dialysis – Monitor blood pressure and hematocrit no less frequently than for patients maintained on dialysis. Closely monitor renal function and fluid and electrolyte balance, as an improved sense of well-being may obscure the need to initiate dialysis in some patients.

Determine the hematocrit twice a week until it has stabilized in the target range and the maintenance dose has been established. After any dose adjustment, determine the hematocrit twice weekly for at least 2 to 6 weeks until the hematocrit has stabilized; then monitor at regular intervals.

Perform complete blood count with differential and platelet counts regularly. Modest increases have occurred in platelets and white blood cell counts, but values remained within normal ranges.

Monitor serum chemistry values (including blood urea nitrogen [BUN], uric acid, creatinine, phosphorus and potassium) regularly. In patients on dialysis, modest increases occurred in BUN, creatinine, phosphorus and potassium. In some patients, modest increases in serum uric acid and phosphorus were observed. The values remained within the ranges normally seen in patients with CRF. Also monitor renal function and fluid and electrolyte balance as an improved sense of well-being may obscure the need to initiate dialysis in some patients.

Zidovudine-treated, HIV-infected patients – Measure hematocrit once a week until it is stabilized; measure periodically thereafter.

Iron evaluation – During therapy, absolute or functional iron deficiency may develop. Functional iron deficiency, with normal ferritin levels but low transferrin saturation, is presumably caused by the inability to mobilize iron stores rapidly enough to support increased erythropoiesis. Transferrin saturation should be at least 20%, and ferritin should be at least 100 ng/ml. Prior to and during therapy, evaluate the patient's iron status, including transferrin saturation (serum iron divided by iron binding capacity) and serum ferritin. Virtually all patients will eventually require supplemental iron to increase or maintain transferrin saturation to levels that will adequately support epoetin alfa-stimulated erythropoiesis.

Hematology: The elevated bleeding time characteristic of CRF decreases toward normal after correction of anemia in epoetin alfa-treated patients. Reduction of bleeding time also occurs after correction of anemia by transfusion.

Allow sufficient time to determine a patient's responsiveness before adjusting the dose. Because of the time required for erythropoiesis and the red cell half-life, an interval of 2 to 6 weeks may occur between the time of a dose adjustment (initiation, increase, decrease or discontinuation) and a significant change in hematocrit.

Porphyria exacerbation has been observed rarely in epoetin alfa-treated patients with CRF. However, epoetin alfa has not caused increased urinary excretion of porphyrin metabolites in healthy volunteers, even in the presence of a rapid erythropoietic response. Nevertheless, use with caution in patients with known porphyria.

Bone marrow fibrosis is a complication of CRF and may be related to secondary hyperparathyroidism or unknown factors. The incidence of bone marrow fibrosis was not increased in a study of patients on dialysis who were treated with epoetin alfa for 12 to 19 months, compared with controls.

Delayed or diminished response: If the patient fails to respond or to maintain a response to doses within the recommended range, consider and evaluate the following etiologies:

1.) Functional iron deficiency may develop with normal ferritin levels but low transferrin saturation (< 20%), presumably caused by the inability to mobilize iron stores rapidly enough to support increased erythropoiesis. Virtually all patients will eventually require supplemental iron therapy.
2.) Underlying infectious, inflammatory or malignant processes.
3.) Occult blood loss.
4.) Underlying hematologic diseases (eg, thalassemia, refractory anemia or other myelodysplastic disorders).
5.) Vitamin deficiencies: Folic acid or vitamin B_{12}.
6.) Hemolysis.
7.) Aluminum intoxication.
8.) Osteitis fibrosa cystica.
9.) Increase in zidovudine dosage.

Lipid profile: In one study, total cholesterol, apoprotein B and serum triglycerides fell significantly after initiation of epoetin therapy.

EPOETIN ALFA (Erythropoietin; EPO)

Diet: As the hematocrit increases and patients experience an improved sense of well-being, reinforce the importance of compliance with dietary guidelines and frequency of dialysis.

Hyperkalemia is not uncommon in patients with CRF. In patients on dialysis, hyperkalemia has occurred at an annualized rate of ≈ 0.11 episodes per patient-year of epoetin alfa therapy, often in association with poor compliance to medication, dietary guidelines and frequency of dialysis.

Dialysis management: Therapy with epoetin alfa results in an increase in hematocrit and a decrease in plasma volume that could affect dialysis efficiency. This has not adversely affected dialyzer function or the efficiency of high-flux hemodialysis.

Renal function: In short-term trials (< 1 year) in patients with CRF not on dialysis, changes in creatinine and creatinine clearance were not significantly different in epoetin alfa-treated patients, compared with placebo-treated patients.

Benzyl alcohol: Benzyl alcohol is contained in some of these products as a preservative, has been associated with a fatal "gasping syndrome" in premature infants.

Adverse Reactions:

CRF patients: Epoetin alfa is generally well tolerated. The following adverse reactions are frequent sequelae of CRF and are not necessarily caused by epoetin alfa therapy:

Epoetin Alfa Adverse Reactions in CRF Patients

Adverse reaction	Epoetin alfa (n = 200)	Placebo (n = 135)	Adverse reaction	Epoetin alfa (n = 200)	Placebo (n = 135)
Hypertension	24%	19%	Skin reaction (administration site)	7%	12%
Headache	16%	12%	Asthenia	7%	12%
Arthralgia	11%	6%	Dizziness	7%	13%
Nausea	11%	9%	Clotted access	7%	2%
Edema	9%	10%	Seizure	1.1%	1.1%
Fatigue	9%	14%	CVA/TIA	0.4%	0.6%
Diarrhea	9%	6%	Myocardial infarction	0.4%	1.1%
Vomiting	8%	5%			
Chest pain	7%	9%			

Most common – Incidence (number of events per patient-year) in patients on dialysis (> 567 patients): Hypertension (0.75); headache (0.4); tachycardia (0.31); nausea/vomiting (0.26); clotted vascular access (0.25); shortness of breath (0.14); hyperkalemia, diarrhea (0.11). Events that occurred within hours of administration of epoetin alfa were rare, mild and transient, and included injection site stinging in dialysis patients and flu-like symptoms (eg, arthralgias, myalgias).

Hypersensitivity – Skin rashes, urticaria (rare, mild and transient). See Warnings.

Miscellaneous – Seizures. See Warnings.

Zidovudine-treated HIV-infected patients: Adverse experiences were consistent with the progression of HIV infection.

Epoetin Alfa Adverse Reactions in Zidovudine-Treated Patients

Adverse reaction	Epoetin alfa (n = 144)	Placebo (n = 153)	Adverse reaction	Epoetin alfa (n = 144)	Placebo (n = 153)
Pyrexia	38%	29%	Shortness of breath	14%	13%
Fatigue	25%	31%	Asthenia	11%	14%
Headache	19%	14%	Skin reaction (injection site)	10%	7%
Cough	18%	14%	Dizziness	9%	10%
Diarrhea	16%	18%	Seizures[1]	2.5%[2]	*
Rash	16%	8%	Hypersensitivity[1]	rare	*
Nausea	15%	12%			
Congestion, respiratory	15%	10%			

* Incidence unknown.
[1] See Warnings.
[2] Within the first 10 days of therapy.

EPOETIN ALFA (Erythropoietin; EPO)

Surgery patients:

Adverse Reactions in Surgery Patients Treated with Epoetin Alfa

Event	300 U/kg (n = 112)[1]	100 U/kg (n = 101)[1]	Placebo (n = 103)[1]	600 U/kg (n = 73)[2]	300 U/kg (n = 72)[2]
Pyrexia	51%	50%	60%	47%	42%
Nausea	48%	43%	45%	45%	58%
Constipation	43%	42%	43%	51%	53%
Skin reaction (injection site)	25%	19%	22%	26%	29%
Vomiting	22%	12%	14%	21%	29%
Skin pain	18%	18%	17%	5%	4%
Pruritus	16%	16%	14%	14%	22%
Insomnia	13%	16%	13%	21%	18%
Headache	13%	11%	9%	10%	19%
Dizziness	12%	9%	12%	11%	21%
Urinary tract infection	12%	3%	11%	11%	8%
Hypertension	10%	11%	10%	5%	10%
Diarrhea	10%	7%	12%	10%	6%
Deep venous thrombosis[3]	10%	3%	5%	0%[4]	0%[4]
Dyspepsia	9%	11%	6%	7%	8%
Anxiety	7%	2%	11%	11%	4%
Edema	6%	11%	8%	11%	7%

[1] Study included patients undergoing orthopedic surgery treated with epoetin alfa or placebo for 15 days.
[2] Study including patients undergoing orthopedic surgery treated with epoetin alfa 600 U/kg weekly × 4 or 300 U/kg daily × 15.
[3] See Warnings.
[4] Determined by clinical symptoms.

Cancer patients on chemotherapy: Adverse reactions were consistent with the underlying disease state.

Epoetin Alfa Adverse Reactions in Cancer Patients

Adverse reaction	Epoetin alfa (n = 63)	Placebo (n = 68)	Adverse reaction	Epoetin alfa (n = 63)	Placebo (n = 68)
Pyrexia	29%	19%	Shortness of breath	13%	9%
Diarrhea	21%	7%	Paresthesia	11%	6%
Nausea	17%	32%	Upper respiratory infection	11%	4%
Vomiting	17%	15%	Dizziness	5%	12%
Edema	17%	1%	Trunk pain	3%	16%
Asthenia	13%	16%			
Fatigue	13%	15%			

Overdosage:

The maximum amount that can be safely administered in single or multiple doses has not been determined. Doses of ≤ 1500 U/kg 3 times weekly for 3 to 4 weeks have been given without any direct toxic effects.

Epoetin alfa can cause polycythemia if the hematocrit is not carefully monitored and the dose appropriately adjusted. If the suggested target range is exceeded, epoetin alfa may be temporarily withheld until the hematocrit returns to the target range; therapy may then be resumed using a lower dose (see Administration and Dosage). If polycythemia is of concern, phlebotomy may be indicated to decrease the hematocrit.

Patient Information:

Home dialysis patients: In those situations in which the physician determines that a home dialysis patient can safely and effectively self-administer epoetin alfa, instruct the patient as to the proper dosage and administration. Refer patients to the full "Information for Home Dialysis Patients" section supplied with the product.

Inform patients of the signs and symptoms of allergic drug reaction and advise them of appropriate actions.

EPOETIN ALFA (Erythropoietin; EPO)

Thoroughly instruct the patient in the importance of proper disposal and caution against reuse of needles, syringes or drug product. Make available a puncture-resistant container for disposal of used syringes and needles. Dispose of the full container according to directions provided by the physician.

Administration and Dosage:

CRF patients:

General Therapeutic Guidelines in CRF Patients for Epoetin Alfa	
Starting dose	50 to 100 U/kg 3 times weekly IV or SC
Reduce dose when:	1) Hematocrit approaches 36% or 2) Hematocrit increases > 4 points in any 2 week period.
Increase dose if:	Hematocrit does not increase by 5 to 6 points after 8 weeks of therapy and hematocrit is below suggested target range.
Maintenance dose	Individualize.
Suggested target hematocrit range	30% to 36%

Epoetin alfa may be given either as an IV or SC injection. In patients on hemodialysis, epoetin usually has been administered as an IV bolus 3 times/week. While the administration is independent of the dialysis procedure, epoetin may be administered into the venous line at the end of the dialysis procedure to obviate the need for additional venous access. In patients with CRF not on dialysis, epoetin may be given either as an IV or SC injection.

Home hemodialysis patients who have been judged competent by their physicians to self-administer epoetin without medical or other supervision may give themselves either an IV or SC injection. Home peritoneal dialysis patients may give themselves an SC injection.

Pre-therapy iron evaluation – Prior to and during therapy, evaluate the patient's iron stores, including transferrin saturation and serum ferritin. Virtually all patients will eventually require supplemental iron. See Precautions.

Dose adjustment – Following therapy, a period of time is required for erythroid progenitors to mature and be released into circulation resulting in an eventual increase in hematocrit. Additionally, red blood cell survival time affects hematocrit and may vary because of uremia. As a result, the time required to elicit a clinically significant change in hematocrit (increase or decrease) following any dose adjustment may be 2 to 6 weeks.

Dose adjustment should not be made more frequently than once a month, unless clinically indicated. After any dose adjustment, determine the hematocrit twice weekly for at least 2 to 6 weeks.

- If the hematocrit is increasing and approaching 36%, reduce the dose to maintain the suggested target hematocrit range. If the reduced dose does not stop the rise in hematocrit and it exceeds 36%, temporarily withhold doses until the hematocrit begins to decrease, then reinitiate at a lower dose.
- At any time, if the hematocrit increases by > 4 points in a 2–week period, immediately decrease the dose. After the dose reduction, monitor the hematocrit twice weekly for 2 to 6 weeks and make further dose adjustments as outlined in the maintenance dose section.
- If a hematocrit increase of 5 to 6 points is not achieved after an 8–week period and iron stores are adequate (see Delayed or diminished response), the dose may be incrementally increased. Further increases may be made at 4– to 6–week intervals until the desired response is attained.

Maintenance – Individualize dosage for each patient on dialysis.

Dialysis patients: Median dose is 75 U/kg 3 times weekly (range, 12.5 to 525 U/kg 3 times weekly).

Nondialysis CRF patients: Dose of 75 to 150 U/kg/week has maintained hematocrits of 36% to 38% for up to 6 months.

Delayed or diminished response – Over 95% of patients with CRF responded with clinically significant increases in hematocrit, and virtually all patients were transfusion-independent within ≈ 2 months of initiation of therapy.

If a patient fails to respond or maintain a response, consider other etiologies and evaluate as clinically indicated. See Precautions for discussion of delayed or diminished response.

EPOETIN ALFA (Erythropoietin; EPO)

Zidovudine-treated, HIV-infected patients: Determine endogenous serum erythropoietin level prior to transfusion. Patients taking zidovudine with erythropoietin levels > 500 mU/ml are unlikely to respond.

Initial dose – For patients with serum erythropoietin levels ≤ 500 mU/ml who are receiving a dose of zidovudine ≤ 4200 mg/week, the recommended starting dose is 100 U/kg as an IV or SC injection 3 times weekly for 8 weeks.

If the response is not satisfactory in terms of reducing transfusion requirements or increasing hematocrit after 8 weeks of therapy, the dose can be increased by 50 to 100 U/kg 3 times weekly. Evaluate response every 4 to 8 weeks thereafter and adjust the dose accordingly by 50 to 100 U/kg increments 3 times weekly. If patients have not responded satisfactorily to a 300 U/kg dose 3 times weekly, it is unlikely that they will respond to higher doses.

Monitor hematocrit weekly during the dose adjustment phase of therapy.

Maintenance dose – When the desired response is attained, titrate the dose to maintain the response based on factors such as variations in zidovudine dose and the presence of intercurrent infectious or inflammatory episodes. If hematocrit exceeds 40%, stop the dose until hematocrit drops to 36%. When resuming treatment, reduce the dose by 25%, then titrate to maintain desired hematocrit.

Cancer patients on chemotherapy:

Starting dose – 150 units/kg SC 3 times weekly. In general, patients with lower baseline serum erythropoietin levels responded more vigorously to epoetin. Treatment of patients with grossly elevated erythropoietin levels (eg, > 200 mU/ml) is not recommended. Monitor hematocrit on a weekly basis until it is stable.

Dose adjustment – If response is not satisfactory in terms of reducing transfusion requirement or increasing hematocrit after 8 weeks of therapy, the dose may be increased up to 300 units/kg 3 times weekly. If patients do not respond, it is unlikely that they will respond to higher doses. If hematocrit exceeds 40%, hold the dose until it falls to 36%. Reduce dose by 25% when treatment is resumed and titrate to maintain desired hematocrit. If initial dose includes a very rapid hematocrit response (eg, increase of > 4 percentage points in any 2–week period), reduce the dose.

Surgery: Prior to initiating treatment with epoetin alfa, obtain a hemoglobin to establish that it is > 10 to ≤ 13 g/dl. The recommended dose is 300 U/kg/day SC for 10 days before surgery, on the day of surgery and for 4 days after surgery.

An alternate dose schedule is 600 U/kg SC in once-weekly doses (21, 14 and 7 days before surgery) plus a fourth dose on the day of surgery.

All patients should receive adequate iron supplementation. Initiate iron supplementation no later than the beginning of treatment with epoetin alfa and continue throughout the course of therapy.

Preparation: Do not shake. Prolonged vigorous shaking may denature the glycoprotein, rendering it biologically inactive.

Admixture incompatibility – Do not give in conjunction with other drug solutions. However, at time of SC administration, epoetin alfa may be admixed in a syringe with Bacteriostatic 0.9% Sodium Chloride Injection with Benzyl Alcohol 0.9% (Bacteriostatic Saline) at a 1:1 ratio. The Benzyl Alcohol acts as a local anesthetic that may ameliorate SC injection site discomfort.

Single-dose 1 ml vial – Contains no preservative. Use only one dose per vial; do not re-enter the vial. Discard unused portions.

Multi-dose 2 ml vial – Contains preservative. Store at 2° to 8°C (36° to 46°F) after initial entry and between doses. Discard 21 days after initial entry.

Storage/Stability: Store at 2° to 8°C (36° to 46°F). Do not freeze or shake.

Rx	**Epogen** (Amgen)	**Injection:** 2000 units/ml	In 1 ml vials.[1]
Rx	**Procrit** (Ortho Biotech)		In 1 ml vials.[1]
Rx	**Epogen** (Amgen)	**Injection:** 3000 units/ml	In 1 ml vials.[1]
Rx	**Procrit** (Ortho Biotech)		In 1 ml vials.[1]
Rx	**Epogen** (Amgen)	**Injection:** 4000 units/ml	In 1 ml vials.[1]
Rx	**Procrit** (Ortho Biotech)		In 1 ml vials.[1]
Rx	**Epogen** (Amgen)	**Injection:** 10,000 units/ml	In 1 ml vials[1] and 2 ml multidose vials.[2]
Rx	**Procrit** (Ortho Biotech)		In 1 ml vials[1] and 2 ml multidose vials.[2]
Rx	**Epogen** (Amgen)	**Injection:** 20,000 units/ml	In 1 ml multidose vials.[2]
Rx	**Procrit** (Ortho Biotech)		In 1 ml multidose vials.[2]

[1] Single-dose vials. Preservative free with 2.5 mg albumin (human) per ml.
[2] Preserved with 1% benzyl alcohol. With 2.5 mg albumin (human) per ml.

FILGRASTIM (Granulocyte Colony Stimulating Factor; G-CSF)

Actions:

Pharmacology: Filgrastim is a human granulocyte colony stimulating factor (G-CSF), produced by recombinant DNA technology. Filgrastim is produced by *Escherichia coli* bacteria inserted with the human G-CSF gene. G-CSF regulates the production of neutrophils within the bone marrow; endogenous G-CSF is a glycoprotein produced by monocytes, fibroblasts and endothelial cells. It has minimal direct in vivo or in vitro effects on the production of other hematopoietic cell types.

Colony stimulating factors are glycoproteins that act on hematopoietic cells by binding to specific cell surface receptors and stimulating proliferation, differentiation commitment and some end-cell functional activation. Endogenous G-CSF is a lineage-specific CSF with selectivity for neutrophil lineage. It is not species-specific and primarily affects neutrophil progenitor proliferation, differentiation and selected end-cell functional activation (including enhanced phagocytic ability, priming of the cellular metabolism associated with respiratory burst, antibody-dependent killing, and increased expression of functions associated with cell surface antigens).

Pharmacokinetics: Absorption and clearance follow first-order pharmacokinetics without apparent concentration dependence. A positive linear correlation occurs between the parenteral dose and both the serum concentration and area under the concentration-time curve (AUC). Continuous IV infusion of 20 mcg/kg filgrastim over 24 hours resulted in mean and median serum concentrations of ≈ 48 and 56 ng/ml, respectively. Subcutaneous (SC) administration of 3.45 and 11.5 mcg/kg resulted in maximum serum concentrations of 4 and 49 ng/ml, respectively, within 2 to 8 hours. The volume of distribution averaged 150 ml/kg in both healthy subjects and cancer patients. The elimination half-life in both healthy subjects and cancer patients was ≈ 3.5 hours. Clearance rates were ≈ 0.5 to 0.7 ml/min/kg. Single parenteral doses or daily IV doses, over a 14 day period, resulted in comparable half-lives. The half-lives were similar for IV administration (231 minutes following doses of 34.5 mcg/kg) and for SC administration (210 minutes following doses of 3.45 mcg/kg). Continuous 24 hour IV infusions at 20 mcg/kg over an 11 to 20 day period produced steady-state serum concentrations of filgrastim with no evidence of drug accumulation over the time period investigated.

Clinical trials:

Myelosuppressive chemotherapy – Filgrastim is safe and effective in accelerating the recovery of neutrophil counts following a variety of chemotherapy regimens. In a randomized, double-blind, placebo controlled trial, patients with small cell lung cancer received filgrastim or placebo. Filgrastim prevented infection as manifested by febrile neutropenia, decreased hospitalization and decreased IV antibiotic usage.

Bone marrow transplant (BMT) – In two separate randomized, controlled trials, patients with Hodgkin's and non-Hodgkin's lymphoma were treated with myeloablative chemotherapy and autologous bone marrow transplantation (ABMT). A statistically significant reduction in the median number of days of severe neutropenia (absolute neutrophil count [ANC] < 500/mm^3) occurred in the filgrastim group vs controls. In one study, the number of days of febrile neutropenia was also reduced, as well as reductions in the number of hospitalization days and antibiotic use. Similar results were noted in myeloid and non-myeloid malignancies, breast cancer, malignant melanoma, acute lymphoblastic leukemia and germ cell tumor with ABMT.

Mobilization of peripheral blood progenitor cells (PBPC) was studied in 50 heavily pre-treated patients with non-Hodgkin's lymphoma, Hodgkin's disease or acute lymphoblastic leukemia. Colony-forming-unit/granulocyte macrophage (CFU-GM) was used as the marker for engraftable PBPC. Both the CFU–GM and CD34+ cells reached a maximum on day 5 at > 10-fold over baseline and then remained elevated with leukapheresis.

Engraftment – In a randomized unblinded study of patients with Hodgkin's disease or non-Hodgkin's lymphoma undergoing myeloablative chemotherapy, 27 patients received filgrastim-mobilized PBPC followed by filgrastim and 31 patients received ABMT followed by filgrastim. Patients in the filgrastim-mobilized PBPC group had significantly fewer days of platelet transfusions, shorter time to a sustained platelet count, shorter time to recovery, fewer days of red blood cell transfusions and a shorter duration of post-transplant hospitalization.

FILGRASTIM (Granulocyte Colony Stimulating Factor; G-CSF)

Indications:

Cancer patients:

Myelosuppressive chemotherapy – To decrease the incidence of infection, as manifested by febrile neutropenia, in patients with non-myeloid malignancies receiving myelosuppressive anti-cancer drugs associated with a significant incidence of severe neutropenia with fever.

Bone marrow transplant (BMT) – To reduce the duration of neutropenia and neutropenia-related clinical sequelae (eg, febrile neutropenia) in patients with non-myeloid malignancies undergoing myeloablative chemotherapy followed by BMT.

Peripheral Blood Progenitor Cell (PBPC) Collection – For the mobilization of hematopoietic progenitor cells into the peripheral blood for leukapheresis collection. Mobilization allows for collection of increased progenitor cell numbers capable of engraftment compared with collection by leukapheresis without mobilization or bone marrow harvest. After myeloablative chemotherapy, the transplantation of an increased number of progenitor cells can lead to more rapid engraftment, decreasing the need for supportive care.

Severe chronic neutropenia (SCN): Chronic administration to reduce the incidence and duration of sequelae of neutropenia (eg, fever, infections, oropharyngeal ulcers) in symptomatic patients with congenital, cyclic or idiopathic neutropenia.

Unlabeled uses: Filgrastim may be beneficial in AIDS (0.3 to 3.6 mcg/kg/day), aplastic anemia (800 to 1200 mcg/m^2/day), hairy cell leukemia, myelodysplasia (15 to 500 mcg/m^2/day), drug-induced and congenital agranulocytosis, alloimmune neonatal neutropenia.

Contraindications:

Hypersensitivity to *E. coli*-derived proteins, filgrastim or any product components.

Warnings:

Hypothyroidism: In one study, two patients with pre-existing antibodies to thyroid microsomes and to thyroglobulin and with normal thyroid function and size developed transient hypothyroidism and goiter that required thyroxine therapy.

Hypersensitivity: Allergic-type reactions have occurred on initial or subsequent treatment in < 1 in 4000 patients treated with filgrastim. These have generally been characterized by systemic symptoms involving at least two body systems, most often skin (rash, urticaria, facial edema), respiratory (wheezing, dyspnea) and cardiovascular (hypotension, tachycardia). Some reactions occurred on initial exposure. Reactions tended to occur within the first 30 minutes after administration and appeared to occur more frequently in patients receiving IV filgrastim. Rapid resolution of symptoms occurred in most cases after administration of antihistamines, steroids, bronchodilators or epinephrine. Symptoms recurred in > 50% of patients who were rechallenged. Refer also to Management of Acute Hypersensitivity Reactions.

Pregnancy: Category C. There are no adequate and well controlled studies in pregnant women. Use during pregnancy only if the potential benefit justifies the potential risk to the fetus.

Lactation: It is not known whether filgrastim is excreted in breast milk. Exercise caution if administering to a nursing woman.

Children: Serious long-term risks associated with daily filgrastim have not been identified in pediatric patients ages 4 months to 17 years with SCN.

The safety and efficacy in neonates and patients with autoimmune neutropenia of infancy have not been established.

In the cancer setting, 12 pediatric patients with neuroblastoma have received up to six cycles of cyclophosphamide, cisplatin, doxorubicin and etoposide chemotherapy concurrently with filgrastim. In this population, filgrastim was well tolerated. There was one report of palpable splenomegaly associated with filgrastim therapy, however, the only consistently reported adverse event was musculoskeletal pain, which was no different from the experience in the adult population.

FILGRASTIM (Granulocyte Colony Stimulating Factor; G-CSF)

Precautions:

Monitoring:

Myelosuppressive chemotherapy – Obtain complete blood count (CBC) and platelet counts prior to chemotherapy, and at regular intervals (twice per week) during therapy to avoid leukocytosis and to monitor the neutrophil count. Following cytotoxic chemotherapy, the neutrophil nadir occurred earlier during cycles when filgrastim was administered and WBC differentials demonstrated a left shift, including the appearance of promyelocytes and myeloblasts. In addition, the duration of severe neutropenia was reduced and was followed by an accelerated recovery in the neutrophil counts. Therefore, regular monitoring of WBC counts, particularly at the time of the recovery from the post-chemotherapy nadir, is recommended in order to avoid excessive leukocytosis. In clinical studies, therapy was discontinued when the ANC $\geq$ 10,000/mm^3 after the expected chemotherapy-induced nadir.

BMT – Obtain CBC and platelet counts at a minimum of 3 times per week following marrow infusion to monitor the recovery of marrow reconstitution.

SCN – It is essential that serial complete blood cell counts with differential and platelet counts, and an evaluation of bone marrow morphology and karyotype be performed prior to initiation of therapy. The use of filgrastim prior to confirmation of SCN may impair diagnostic efforts and may thus impair or delay evaluation and treatment of an underlying condition, other than SCN, causing the neutropenia. During the initial 4 weeks of filgrastim therapy and during the 2 weeks following any dose adjustment, perform a CBC with differential and platelet count twice weekly. Once a patient is clinically stable, perform a CBC with differential and platelet count monthly.

Simultaneous use with chemotherapy and radiation: The safety and efficacy of filgrastim given simultaneously with cytotoxic chemotherapy or radiotherapy have not been established. Because of the potential sensitivity of rapidly dividing myeloid cells to cytotoxic chemotherapy, do not use filgrastim 24 hours before to 24 hours after the administration of cytotoxic chemotherapy (see Administration and Dosage).

Growth factor potential: Filgrastim is a growth factor that primarily stimulates neutrophils. However, the possibility that filgrastim can act as a growth factor for any tumor type, particularly myeloid malignancies, cannot be excluded. Therefore, exercise caution in using this drug in any malignancy with myeloid characteristics.

Leukocytosis: White blood cell counts of $\geq$ 100,000/mm^3 were observed in $\approx$ 2% of patients receiving doses > 5 mcg/kg/day. There were no reports of adverse events associated with this degree of leukocytosis. In order to avoid potential complications of excessive leukocytosis, CBC is recommended twice per week during therapy (see Monitoring).

Premature discontinuation of therapy: A transient increase in neutrophil count is typically seen 1 to 2 days after therapy initiation. However, for a sustained therapeutic response, continue therapy until the post-setnadir ANC = 10,000/mm^3. Therefore, premature discontinuation of therapy prior to recovery from the expected neutrophil nadir is generally not recommended (see Administration and Dosage).

Hematologic effects: Because of the potential of receiving higher doses of chemotherapy, the patient may be at greater risk of thrombocytopenia, anemia and nonhematologic consequences of increased chemotherapy doses. Fewer than 6% of patients had thrombocytopenia (< 50,000/mm^3) during therapy, most of whom had a pre-existing history of thrombocytopenia. In most cases, thrombocytopenia was managed by dose reduction or interruption. An additional 5% of patients had platelet counts between 50,000 to 100,000/mm^3. There were no associated serious hemorrhagic sequelae in these patients. Regular monitoring of the hematocrit and platelet count is recommended. Furthermore, exercise care in the use of filgrastim in conjunction with other drugs known to lower the platelet count. In septic patients, be alert to the possibility of adult respiratory distress syndrome, due to the possible influx of neutrophils at the inflammation site.

FILGRASTIM (Granulocyte Colony Stimulating Factor; G-CSF)

Cardiac events (eg, myocardial infarctions, arrhythmias) have occurred in 11 of 375 cancer patients receiving filgrastim; the relationship to filgrastim therapy is unknown. However, closely monitor patients with pre-existing cardiac conditions.

Medullary bone pain occurred in 24% of patients. This bone pain was generally of mild to moderate severity, and could be controlled in most patients with nonnarcotic analgesics; infrequently, bone pain was severe enough to require narcotic analgesics. Bone pain occurred more frequently in patients treated with higher doses (20 to 100 mcg/kg/day) administered IV, and less frequently in patients treated with lower SC doses (3 to 10 mcg/kg/day).

Cutaneous vasculitis: There have been rare reports of cutaneous vasculitis in patients receiving filgrastim. In most cases the severity was moderate or severe. Most reports involved patients with severe chronic neutropenia receiving long-term therapy. Symptoms of vasculitis generally developed simultaneously with an increase in the ANC and abated when the ANC decreased. Many patients were able to continue therapy at a reduced dose.

Drug Interactions:

Drug interactions have not been fully evaluated. Drugs which may potentiate the release of neutrophils, such as lithium, should be used with caution.

Adverse Reactions:

Myelosuppressive chemotherapy: In clinical trials, the most adverse experiences were the sequelae of the underlying malignancy or cytotoxic chemotherapy. Medullary bone pain, reported in 24% of patients, was the only consistently observed adverse reaction attributed to therapy (see Precautions).

Spontaneously reversible elevations in uric acid, lactate dehydrogenase and alkaline phosphatase occurred in 27% to 58% of patients receiving filgrastim therapy following cytotoxic chemotherapy; increases were generally mild to moderate. Transient decreases in blood pressure (< 90/60 mmHg), which did not require clinical treatment, were reported in 7 of 176 patients.

Filgrastim Adverse Reactions in Patients Receiving Myelosuppressive Chemotherapy (%)

Adverse reactions	Filgrastim (n = 384)	Placebo (n = 257)
Nausea/Vomiting	57	64
Skeletal pain	22	11
Alopecia	18	27
Diarrhea	14	23
Neutropenic fever	13	35
Mucositis	12	20
Fever	12	11
Fatigue	11	16
Anorexia	9	11
Dyspnea	9	11
Headache	7	9
Cough	6	8
Skin rash	6	9
Chest pain	5	6
Generalized weakness	4	7
Sore throat	4	9
Stomatitis	5	10
Constipation	5	10
Pain (unspecified)	2	7

BMT: In clinical trials, the adverse reactions reported were those typically seen in patients receiving intensive chemotherapy followed by bone marrow transplantation. The most common events included stomatitis, nausea and vomiting, generally of mild-to-moderate severity and considered unrelated to filgrastim. In the randomized studies of BMT, the following occurred more frequently in patients treated with filgrastim than controls: Nausea (10%); vomiting (7%); hypertension (4%); rash (12%); peritonitis (2%); renal insufficiency, capillary leak syndrome (rare); erythema nodosum of moderate severity (1 patient).

FILGRASTIM (Granulocyte Colony Stimulating Factor; G-CSF)

PBPC Collection: Decreased platelet counts (97%); anemia (65%); mild to moderate musculoskeletal symptoms (44%); medullary bone pain (33%); headache (7%); increases in alkaline phosphatase (21%); increases in neutrophil counts; white blood cell > 100,000/mm^3 (rare).

SCN: Mild to moderate bone pain, readily controlled with non-narcotic analgesics (≈ 33%); palpable splenomegaly (≈ 30%); epistaxis (15%; associated with thrombocytopenia in 2%); anemia (≈ 10%, but in most cases appeared to be related to frequent diagnostic phlebotomy, chronic illness or concomitant medications); monosomy, splenomegaly (< 3%); myelodysplasia or myeloid leukemia (≈ 3%); injection site reaction, rash, hepatomegaly, arthralgia, osteoporosis, increase in LDH, cutaneous vasculitis, hematuria/proteinuria, exacerbation of some pre-existing skin disorders (eg, psoriasis), alopecia (infrequent); abdominal/flank pain (infrequent); thrombocytopenia (see Precautions).

Lab test abnormalities:

Lab test abnormalities – In clinical trials, the following laboratory results were observed. Cyclic fluctuations in the neutrophil counts were frequently observed in congenital or idiopathic neutropenia after initiation of filgrastim therapy. Platelet counts were generally at the upper limits of normal prior to therapy. With filgrastim therapy, platelet counts decreased but usually remained within normal limits. Early myeloid forms were noted in peripheral blood in most patients, including the appearance of metamyelocytes and myelocytes. Promyelocytes and myeloblasts were noted in some patients. Relative increases were occasionally noted in the number of circulating eosinophils and basophils. No consistent increases were observed with filgrastim therapy. Increases were observed in serum uric acid, lactic dehydrogenase and serum alkaline phosphatase.

Overdosage:

To avoid the potential risks of excessive leukocytosis, discontinue therapy if the ANC surpasses 10,000/mm^3 after the ANC nadir has occurred. Doses that increase the ANC > 10,000/mm^3 may not result in any additional clinical benefit.

The maximum tolerated dose of filgrastim has not been determined. Efficacy was demonstrated at 4 to 8 mcg/kg/day in a study of non-myeloablative chemotherapy. Patients in the BMT study received up to 138 mcg/kg/day without toxic effects, although there was a flattening of the dose response curve above daily doses of > 10 mcg/kg/day. Discontinuation of therapy in patients receiving myelosuppressive chemotherapy usually results in a 50% decrease in circulating neutrophils within 1 to 2 days, with a return to pretreatment levels in 1 to 7 days.

Patient Information:

If the patient can safely and effectively self-administer filgrastim, instruct the patient as to the proper dosage and administration. Refer patients to the full "Information for Patients" section included with the product information; it is not a disclosure of all or possible intended effects.

Administration and Dosage:

Approved by the FDA in February 1991.

Myelosuppressive chemotherapy: Recommended starting dose is 5 mcg/kg/day, given as a single daily injection by SC bolus injection, by short IV infusion (15 to 30 minutes) or by continuous SC or IV infusion. Obtain CBC and platelet count before instituting therapy; monitor twice weekly during therapy. Doses may be increased in increments of 5 mcg/kg for each chemotherapy cycle according to duration and severity of the ANC nadir.

Administer no earlier than 24 hours after cytotoxic chemotherapy and not in the 24 hours before administration of chemotherapy. Give daily for up to 2 weeks until ANC has reached 10,000/mm^3 following the expected chemotherapy-induced neutrophil nadir. Duration of therapy needed to attenuate chemotherapy-induced neutropenia may depend on the myelosuppressive potential of the chemotherapy regimen employed. Discontinue therapy if the ANC surpasses 10,000/mm^3 after the expected chemotherapy-induced neutrophil nadir (see Precautions). In clinical trials, efficacy was observed at doses of 4 to 8 mcg/kg/day.

FILGRASTIM (Granulocyte Colony Stimulating Factor; G-CSF)

BMT: Recommended dose following BMT is 10 mcg/kg/day given as an IV infusion of 4 or 24 hours or as a continuous 24 hour SC infusion. For patients receiving BMT, administer the first dose of filgrastim at least 24 hours after cytotoxic chemotherapy and at least 24 hours after bone marrow infusion.

During the period of neutrophil recovery, titrate the daily dose against the neutrophil response as follows:

Filgrastim Dose Based on Neutrophil Response

Absolute neutrophil count	Filgrastim dose adjustment
When ANC > 1000/mm³ for 3 consecutive days	Reduce to 5 mcg/kg/day[1]
If ANC remains > 1000/mm³ for 3 more consecutive days	Discontinue filgrastim
If ANC decreases to < 1000/mm³	Resume at 5 mcg/kg/day

[1] If ANC decreases to < 1000/mm³ at any time during the 5 mcg/kg/day administration, increase filgrastim to 10 mcg/kg/day and follow the steps in the table.

PBPC collection: 10 mcg/kg/day SC, either as a bolus or a continuous infusion. It is recommended that filgrastim be given for at least 4 days before the first leukapheresis procedure and continued until the last leukapheresis. Administration of filgrastim for 6 to 7 days with leukaphereses on days 5, 6 and 7 was found to be safe and effective.

SCN:

Starting dose –

Congenital neutropenia: 6 mcg/kg twice daily SC every day.

Idiopathic or cyclic neutropenia: 5 mcg/kg as a single injection SC every day.

Dose adjustments – Chronic daily administration is required to maintain clinical benefit. ANC should not be used as the sole indication of efficacy. Individually adjust the dose based on the patient's clinical course as well as ANC. Reduce the dose if the ANC is persistently > 10,000/mm³.

Dilution of solution: If required, filgrastim may be diluted in 5% Dextrose Solution. Filgrastim diluted to concentrations between 5 and 15 mcg/ml should be protected from adsorption to plastic materials by addition of albumin (human) to a final concentration of 2 mg/ml. When diluted in 5% Dextrose or 5% Dextrose plus albumin, filgrastim is compatible with glass bottles, PVC and polyolefin IV bags and polypropylene syringes. Dilution to a final concentration of < 5 mcg/ml is not recommended at any time. Do not dilute with saline at any time; product may precipitate.

Admixture incompatibilities: Amphotericin B; cefonicid; cefoperazone; cefotaxime; cefoxitin; ceftizoxime; ceftriaxone; cefuroxime; clindamycin; dactinomycin; etoposide; fluorouracil; furosemide; heparin; mannitol; metronidazole; methylprednisolone; mezlocillin; mitomycin; prochlorperazine; piperacillin; thiotepa.

Storage/Stability: Refrigerate at 2° to 8°C (36° to 46°F). Do not freeze. Avoid shaking. Prior to injection, filgrastim may be allowed to reach room temperature for a maximum of 24 hours. Discard any vial left at room temperature for > 24 hours. Use only one dose per vial; do not re-enter the vial.

Filgrastim injection repackaged in 1 ml plastic tuberculin syringes stored at 2° to 8°C (36° to 46°F) remain sterile for 7 days.

Rx	**Neupogen** (Amgen)	**Injection:** 300 mcg/ml[1]	Preservative free. In 1 and 1.6 ml single-dose vials.

[1] With 0.59 mg acetate, 50 mg mannitol, 0.004% *Tween* 80 and 0.035 mg Na/ml in Water for Injection.

SARGRAMOSTIM (Granulocyte Macrophage Colony Stimulating Factor; GM-CSF)

Actions:

Pharmacology: Sargramostim is a recombinant human granulocyte-macrophage colony stimulating factor (rhu GM-CSF) produced by recombinant DNA technology in a yeast (*S. cerevisiae*) expression system. GM-CSF is a hematopoietic growth factor that stimulates proliferation and differentiation of hematopoietic progenitor cells. Sargramostim is a glycoprotein of 127 amino acids. The amino acid sequence differs from the natural human GM-CSF by substituting leucine at position 23; the carbohydrate moiety may be different from the native protein.

GM-CSF belongs to a group of growth factors termed colony stimulating factors that support survival, clonal expansion and differentiation of hematopoietic progenitor cells. GM-CSF induces partially committed progenitor cells to divide and differentiate in the granulocyte-macrophage pathways.

GM-CSF can activate mature granulocytes and macrophages. GM-CSF is a multilineage factor and, in addition to dose-dependent effects on the myelomonocytic lineage, can promote the proliferation of megakaryocytic and erythroid progenitors. Other factors are also required to induce complete maturation in these two lineages. The various cellular responses (division, maturation, activation) are induced through GM-CSF binding to specific receptors expressed on the cell surface of target cells.

The biological activity of GM-CSF is species-specific. Chemotactic, antifungal and antiparasitic activities of granulocytes and monocytes are increased by exposure to sargramostim. Sargramostim increases the cytotoxicity of monocytes toward certain neoplastic cell lines and activates polymorphonuclear neutrophils to inhibit the growth of tumor cells.

Pharmacokinetics: In eight patients receiving 250 mcg/m^2 of sargramostim by 2 hour IV infusion, serum concentration ranged from 120 to 1500 pg/ml at the termination of the infusion. Then the serum levels decreased with a mean initial half-life and terminal half-life of ≈ 11 minutes and 1.6 hours, respectively, while the mean area under the plasma concentration-time curve (AUC) was 5.35 mcg/ml/hr. When the same patients were treated with 250 mcg/m^2 sargramostim SC, serum levels peaked at 3 hours and ranged between 100 and 1500 pg/ml. The serum levels decreased with a mean terminal half-life and terminal half-life of ≈ 2.6 hours, while the mean AUC was 4.65 mcg/ml/hr. The mean serum levels remained > 100 pg/ml for 12 hours after the SC injection and 6 hours after the 2 hour infusion.

Clinical trials:

Acute myelogenous leukemia (AML) – The safety and efficacy in the treatment of AML were evaluated in a multi-center, randomized, double-blind placebo controlled trial of 99 newly diagnosed adult patients (55 to 70 years of age) receiving induction with or without consolidation. A combination of standard doses of daunorubicin (days 1 to 3) and ara-C (days 1 to 7) was administered during induction and high dose ara-C was administered days 1 to 6 as a single course of consolidation. Sargramostim significantly shortened the median duration of ANC < 500/mm^3 by 4 days and < 1000/mm^3 by 7 days. Following induction, 75% of patients receiving sargramostim achieved ANC > 500/mm^3 by day 16 compared with day 25 for patients receiving placebo. The incidence of severe infections and deaths associated with infections was significantly reduced in patients who received sargramostim.

Mobilization of peripheral blood progenitor cells (PBPC) and engraftment – Mobilization of PBPC and myeloid reconstitution post-transplant were compared between four groups of patients (n = 196) receiving sargramostim for mobilization and a historical control group who did not receive any mobilization treatment. Sequential cohorts received sargramostim. The cohorts differed by dose (125 or 250 mcg/m^2/day), route (IV over 24 hours or SC) and use of post-transplant sargramostim. Leukaphereses were initiated for all mobilization groups after the WBC reached 10,000/mm^3. PBPCs from patients treated at the 250 mcg/m^2/day dose had a significantly higher number of granulocyte-macrophage colony-forming units (CFU-GM) than those collected without mobilization. After transplantation, mobilized subjects had shorter times to myeloid engraftment, and fewer days between transplantation and the last platelet transfusion compared to non-mobilized subjects.

Bone marrow transplant (BMT) failure or engraftment delay – In one study, 140 patients experiencing graft failure following allogeneic or autologous BMT were evaluated in comparison with 103 historical controls; 163 had lymphoid or myeloid leukemia, 24 had non-Hodgkin's lymphoma (NHL), 19 had Hodgkin's disease and 37 had other diseases (eg, aplastic anemia, myelodysplasia, nonhematologic malignancy). Three categories of patients were eligible: 1) Patients displaying a delay in engraftment; 2) patients displaying a delay in engraftment who had evidence of an active infection; and 3) patients who lost their marrow graft after a transient engraftment.

SARGRAMOSTIM (Granulocyte Macrophage Colony Stimulating Factor; GM-CSF)

One hundred day survival was improved in patients treated with sargramostim after graft failure following either autologous or allogeneic BMT. In addition, the median survival was improved by > 2-fold. Median survival of patients treated with sargramostim after autologous failure was 474 days vs 161 days for the historical patients. After allogeneic failure, median survival was 97 days vs 35 days, respectively. Improvement in survival was better in patients with fewer impaired organs.

Indications:

Acceleration of myeloid recovery in patients with non-Hodgkin's lymphoma (NHL), acute lymphoblastic leukemia (ALL) and Hodgkin's disease undergoing autologous bone marrow transplantation (BMT).

BMT failure or engraftment delay: For patients who have undergone allogeneic or autologous BMT in whom engraftment is delayed or has failed.

Survival benefit may be relatively greater in those patients who demonstrate one or more of the following characteristics: Autologous BMT failure or engraftment delay; no previous total body irradiation; malignancy other than leukemia; or a multiple organ failure score ≤ 2.

Induction chemotherapy in acute myelogenous leukemia (AML): For use following induction chemotherapy in older patients with AML to shorten neutrophil recovery time and reduce severe and life-threatening infections resulting in death. Safety and efficacy have not been established in AML patients < 55 years of age.

Mobilization and following transplantation of autologous PBPC: For mobilization of hematopoietic progenitor cells into peripheral blood collection by leukapheresis. Mobilization allows collection of increased progenitor cells capable of engraftment compared with collection without mobilization. After myeloablative chemotherapy, the transplantation of an increased number of progenitor cells can lead to rapid engraftment which may decrease the need for supportive care. Myeloid reconstitution is further accelerated by administration following PBPC transplantation.

Myeloid reconstitution after allogeneic BMT: For acceleration of myeloid recovery in patients undergoing allogeneic BMT from human lymphocyte antigen (HLA)-matched related donors. Safety and efficacy have been established in accelerating myeloid engraftment, reducing the incidence of bacteremia and other culture positive infections and shortening the median duration of hospitalization.

Unlabeled uses: GM-CSF has been used in the following conditions:

To increase WBC counts in patients with myelodysplastic syndromes and in AIDS patients receiving zidovudine.

To decrease nadir of leukopenia secondary to myelosuppressive chemotherapy and decrease myelosuppression in preleukemic patients.

To correct neutropenia in aplastic anemia patients.

To decrease transplantation-associated organ system damage, particularly in the liver and kidney (consistent with the observation that the duration of neutropenia correlates with organ system injury).

Contraindications:

Excessive leukemic myeloid blasts in the bone marrow or peripheral blood (≥ 10%); known hypersensitivity to GM-CSF, yeast-derived products or any component of the product; simultaneous administration with cytotoxic chemotherapy or radiotherapy, or administration 24 hours preceding or following chemotherapy or radiotherapy.

Warnings:

Cardiovascular symptoms: Occasional transient supraventricular arrhythmia has occurred during administration, particularly in patients with a previous history of cardiac arrhythmia. However, these arrhythmias have been reversible after discontinuation of sargramostim. Use with caution in patients with preexisting cardiac disease.

Respiratory symptoms: Sequestration of granulocytes in the pulmonary circulation has occurred following sargramostim infusion, occasionally with dyspnea. Give special attention to respiratory symptoms during or immediately following infusion, especially in patients with pre-existing lung disease. In patients displaying dyspnea during administration, reduce the rate of infusion by half. Subsequent IV infusions may be administered following the standard dose schedule with careful monitoring. If respiratory symptoms worsen despite infusion rate reduction, discontinue infusion. Administer with caution in patients with hypoxia.

Fluid retention: In patients with pre-existing pleural and pericardial effusions, administration of sargramostim may aggravate fluid retention; however, fluid retention associated with or worsened by sargramostim has been reversible after interruption or dose reduction with or without diuretic therapy. Use with caution in pre-existing fluid retention, pulmonary infiltrates or congestive heart failure.

SARGRAMOSTIM (Granulocyte Macrophage Colony Stimulating Factor; GM-CSF)

Hypersensitivity: Use appropriate precautions during parenteral administration of recombinant proteins in case an allergic or untoward reaction occurs. Transient rashes and local injection site reactions have occasionally been observed. Serious allergic or anaphylactic reactions have been reported rarely. If any anaphylactoid reaction occurs, immediately discontinue and initiate appropriate therapy. Refer to Management of Acute Hypersensitivity Reactions.

Renal/Hepatic function impairment: In some patients with preexisting renal or hepatic dysfunction, sargramostim has induced elevation of serum creatinine or bilirubin and hepatic enzymes. Dose reduction or interruption has resulted in a decrease to pretreatment values. Biweekly monitoring of renal and hepatic function in patients with renal or hepatic dysfunction prior to treatment is recommended.

Pregnancy: Category C. It is not known whether sargramostim can cause fetal harm or affect reproduction capacity when administered to a pregnant woman. Give to a pregnant woman only if clearly needed.

Lactation: It is not known whether sargramostim is excreted in breast milk. Exercise caution when administering to a nursing woman.

Children: Safety and efficacy have not been established; however, available data indicate that sargramostim does not exhibit any greater toxicity in children than in adults. A total of 124 pediatric subjects between the ages of 4 months and 18 years have been treated with 60 to 1000 mcg/m^2/day IV and 4 to 1500 mcg/m^2/day SC.

Precautions:

Benzyl alcohol: Benzyl alcohol as a preservative has been associated with a fatal "gasping syndrome" in premature infants.

Growth factor potential: Sargramostim is a growth factor that primarily stimulates normal myeloid precursors. However, the possibility that sargramostim can act as a growth factor for any tumor type, particularly myeloid malignancies, cannot be excluded. Exercise caution when using this drug in any malignancy with myeloid characteristics. Should disease progression be detected, discontinue therapy.

First dose effects: A syndrome with respiratory distress, hypoxia, flushing, hypotension, syncope or tachycardia has occurred rarely following the first use. These signs have resolved with symptomatic treatment and usually do not recur with subsequent doses in the same cycle of treatment.

Increase in peripheral blood counts: Stimulation of marrow precursors with sargramostim may result in a rapid rise in WBC count. If the ANC > 20,000 cells/mm^3 or if the platelet count > 500,000/mm^3, interrupt administration or reduce the dose by half. Base the decision to reduce the dose or interrupt treatment on the clinical condition of the patient. Excessive blood counts have returned to normal or baseline levels within 3 to 7 days following cessation of therapy. Perform biweekly monitoring of CBC with differential (including examination for the presence of blast cells) to preclude development of excessive counts.

Purged bone marrow: Sargramostim is effective in accelerating myeloid recovery in patients receiving bone marrow purged by anti-B lymphocyte monoclonal antibodies. Data obtained from uncontrolled studies suggest that if in vitro marrow purging with chemical agents causes a significant decrease in the number of responsive hematopoietic progenitors, the patient may not respond to sargramostim. When the bone marrow purging process preserves a sufficient number of progenitors, a beneficial effect of sargramostim on myeloid engraftment has occurred.

Previous exposure to chemotherapy/radiotherapy: In patients who have received extensive radiotherapy to hematopoietic sites for the treatment of primary disease in the abdomen or chest before autologous BMT, or have been exposed to multiple myelotoxic agents (eg, alkylating agents, anthracycline antibiotics, antimetabolites), the effect of sargramostim on myeloid reconstitution may be limited.

Concomitant use with chemotherapy and radiotherapy: Because of potential sensitivity of rapidly dividing hematopoietic progenitor cells to cytotoxic chemotherapeutic or radiologic therapies, do not administer within 24 hours preceding or following chemotherapy or radiotherapy (see Contraindications).

Monitoring: Sargramostim can induce variable increases in WBC or platelet counts. To avoid potential complications of excessive leukocytosis (WBC > 50,000 cells/mm^3; ANC > 20,000 cells/mm^3), perform a CBC twice weekly during therapy. Biweekly monitoring of renal and hepatic function in patients with renal or hepatic dysfunction prior to initiation of treatment is recommended. Carefully monitor body weight and hydration status during administration (see Warnings).

Drug Interactions:

Drugs which may potentiate the myeloproliferative effects of sargramostim, such as lithium and corticosteroids, should be used with caution.

SARGRAMOSTIM (Granulocyte Macrophage Colony Stimulating Factor; GM-CSF)

Adverse Reactions:

Sargramostim Adverse Reactions (%)[1]					
Adverse reaction	Sargramostim (n = 184)	Placebo (n = 180)	Adverse reaction	Sargramostim (n = 184)	Placebo (n = 180)
Cardiovascular			*Hemic/Lymphatic*		
Hypertension	25-34	32	Hyperglycemia	25	23
Hemorrhage	23-29	30-43	Thrombocytopenia	19	34
Cardiac event	23	32	Leukopenia	17	29
Edema	13-34	11-35	Hypomagnesemia	15	9
Hypotension	13	26	Petechia	6	11
Peripheral edema	11-15	7-21	Agranulocytosis	6	11
Tachycardia	11	9	*Musculoskeletal*		
Pericardial effusion	4	1	Bone pain	21	5
Pleural effusion	1	0	Arthralgia	11	4
Capillary leak syndrome	< 1	-	*Respiratory*		
			Pulmonary event	48	64
CNS			Pharyngitis	23	13
Neuro-clinical	42	53	Lung disorder	20	23
Neuro-motor	25	26	Epistaxis	17	16
Neuro-psych	15	26	Dyspnea	15-28	14-31
CNS disorder	11	16	Rhinitis	11	14
Paresthesia	11	13	*Miscellaneous*		
Insomnia	11	9	Fever	77-95	74-96
Anxiety	11	2	Liver event	77	83
Neuro-sensory	6	11	Mucous membrane disorder	75	78
Dermatologic			Infection	65	68
Skin events	77	45	Metabolic disorder	58	49
Rash	44-70	38-73	Malaise	57	51
Alopecia	37-73	45-74	Weight loss	37	28
Pruritus	23	13	Headache	36	36
GI			Chills	19-25	20-26
Nausea	58-90	55-96	Coagulation event	19	21
Diarrhea	52-89	53-82	Asthenia	17-66	20-51
Vomiting	46-85	34-90	Pain	17	36
Abdominal pain	38	23	Chest pain	15	9
GI disorder	37	47	Liver damage	13	14
Stomatitis	24-62	29-63	Allergy	12	15
Dyspepsia	17	20	Sepsis	11	14
Anorexia	13-54	11-58	Eye hemorrhage	11	0
Hematemesis	13	7	Back pain	9	18
Dysphagia	11	7	Weight gain	8	21
GI hemorrhage	11-27	5-33	Sweats	6	13
Constipation	8	11	*Lab test abnormalities*		
Abdominal distention	4	13	High glucose	41	49
GU			Low albumin	27	36
GU event	50	57	High BUN	23	17
Bilirubinemia	30	27	High cholesterol	17	8
Urinary tract disorder	14	13	Increased creatinine	15	14
Hematuria	9	21	Increased ALT	13	16
Kidney function, abnormal	8	10	Increased alkaline phosphatase	8	14
Hemic/Lymphatic					
Blood dyscrasia	25	27	Low calcium	2	7

[1] Data pooled from separate studies, including allogeneic BMT patients, AML patients and following BMT or peripheral stem cell transplantation.

In some patients with preexisting renal or hepatic dysfunction enrolled in uncontrolled clinical trials, administration of sargramostim has induced elevation of serum creatinine or bilirubin and hepatic enzymes (see Warnings); headache (26%); pericardial effusion (25%); arthralgia (21%); myalgia (18%).

SARGRAMOSTIM (Granulocyte Macrophage Colony Stimulating Factor; GM-CSF)

The most frequent adverse events were fever, asthenia, headache, bone pain, chills and myalgia. These systemic events were generally mild or moderate and were usually prevented or reversed by the administration of analgesics and antipyretics such as acetaminophen. In these uncontrolled trials, other infrequent events reported were dyspnea, peripheral edema and rash. Reports of events occurring with marketed sargramostim include arrhythmia, eosinophilia, hypotension, injection site reactions, pain (including abdominal, back, chest and joint pain) tachycardia, thrombosis and transient liver function abnormalities.

Overdosage:

The maximum amount that can be safely administered in single or multiple doses has not been determined. Doses ≤ 100 mcg/kg/day (4000 mcg/m²/day or 16 times the recommended dose) were administered to 4 patients for 7 to 18 days.

Symptoms: Increases in WBC ≤ 200,000 cells/mm³ were observed. Adverse events reported were dyspnea, malaise, nausea, fever, rash, sinus tachycardia, headache and chills. All these events were reversible after discontinuation of sargramostim.

Treatment: Discontinue therapy and carefully monitor the patient for WBC increase and respiratory symptoms.

Administration and Dosage:

Approved by the FDA in March 1991.

Myeloid reconstitution after autologous or allogeneic BMT: 250 mcg/m²/day for 21 days as a 2 hour IV infusion beginning 2 to 4 hours after the autologous bone marrow infusion, and ≥ 24 hours after the last dose of chemotherapy and 12 hours after the last dose of radiotherapy. If a severe adverse reaction occurs, reduce or temporarily discontinue the dose until the reaction abates. If blast cells appear or progression of the underlying disease occurs, discontinue the treatment. Interrupt or reduce dose by half if the ANC > 20,000 cells/mm³. Patients should not receive sargramostim until the post-marrow infusion ANC is < 500 cells/mm³.

To avoid potential complications of excessive leukocytosis (WBC > 50,000 cells/mm³; ANC > 20,000 cells/mm³), a CBC with differential is recommended twice weekly during therapy. Interrupt or reduce the dose by half if the ANC > 20,000 cells/mm³.

Neutrophil recovery following chemotherapy in AML: 250 mcg/m²/day IV over a 4 hour period starting ≈ day 11 or 4 days following the completion of induction chemotherapy, if the day 10 bone marrow is hypoplastic with < 5% blasts. If a second cycle of induction chemotherapy is necessary, administer ≈ 4 days after the completion of chemotherapy if the bone marrow is hypoplastic with < 5% blasts. Continue sargramostim until an ANC > 1500/mm³ for 3 consecutive days or a maximum of 42 days. Discontinue immediately if leukemic regrowth occurs. If a severe adverse reaction occurs, reduce the dose by 50% or temporarily discontinue the dose until the reaction abates.

Mobilization of PBPC: 250 mcg/m²/day IV over 24 hours or SC once daily. Continue at the same dose through the period of PBPC collection. The optimal schedule for PBPC collection has not been established. In clinical studies, collection of PBPC was usually begun by day 5 and performed daily until protocol specified targets were achieved (see Clinical trials, Mobilization of PBPC and Engraftment). If WBC > 50,000 cells/mm³, reduce the dose by 50%. If adequate numbers of progenitor cells are not collected, other mobilization therapy should be considered.

Post peripheral blood progenitor cell transplantation: 250 mcg/m²/day IV over 24 hours or SC once daily beginning immediately following infusion of progenitor cells and continuing until an ANC > 1500 for 3 consecutive days is attained.

BMT failure or engraftment delay: 250 mcg/m²/day for 14 days as a 2 hour IV infusion. The dose can be repeated after 7 days off therapy if engraftment has not occurred. If engraftment still has not occurred, a third course of 500 mcg/m²/day for 14 days may be tried after another 7 days off therapy. If there is still no improvement, it is unlikely that further dose escalation will be beneficial. If a severe adverse reaction occurs, the dose can be reduced or temporarily discontinued until the reaction abates. If blast cells appear or disease progression occurs, discontinue the treatment.

SARGRAMOSTIM (Granulocyte Macrophage Colony Stimulating Factor; GM-CSF)

Preparation:

1.) Reconstitute with 1 ml Sterile Water for Injection, with or without preservatives.
2.) During reconstitution, direct the Sterile Water for Injection at the side of the vial and gently swirl the contents to avoid foaming during dissolution. Avoid excessive or vigorous agitation; do not shake.
3.) Perform dilution for IV infusion in 0.9% Sodium Chloride Injection. If the final concentration is < 10 mcg/ml, add albumin (human) at a final concentration of 0.1% to the saline prior to addition of sargramostim to prevent adsorption to the components of the drug delivery system. For a final concentration of 0.1% albumin (human), add 1 mg albumin (human) per 1 ml 0.9% Sodium Chloride Injection.
4.) Do not use an in-line membrane filter for IV infusion.
5.) In the absence of compatibility and stability information, do not add other medication to infusion solutions containing sargramostim. Use only 0.9% Sodium Chloride Injection to prepare IV infusion solutions.

Storage/Stability: Refrigerate the sterile powder, the reconstituted solution and the diluted solution for injection at 2° to 8°C (36° to 46°F). Do not freeze or shake.

Solutions reconstituted without preservatives must be administered within 6 hours following mixing. Discard reconstituted solutions with preservatives after 20 days.

Rx	**Leukine** (Immunex)	**Powder for injection, lyophilized:** 250 mcg	Preservative free. In single-use vials.[1]
		500 mcg	Preservative free. In single-use vials.[1]

[1] With 40 mg mannitol, 10 mg sucrose, 1.2 mg tromethamine and 0.9% benzyl alcohol.

ANTIPLATELET AGENTS

Venous thrombi consist mainly of fibrin and red blood cells. Arterial thrombi are composed mainly of platelet aggregates. Theoretically, anticoagulant drugs should be effective for reducing risks involved with venous thrombi formation and antiplatelet drugs should be more effective for reducing risks of arterial thrombi formation.

The drugs most commonly used for their antiplatelet effects are aspirin, sulfinpyrazone, dipyridamole and ticlopidine.

DIPYRIDAMOLE

Actions:

Pharmacology: It is believed that platelet reactivity and interaction with prosthetic cardiac valve surfaces, resulting in abnormally shortened platelet survival time, is a significant factor in thromboembolic complications occurring in connection with prosthetic heart valve replacement. Dipyridamole lengthens abnormally shortened platelet survival time in a dose-dependent manner.

Dipyridamole is a platelet adhesion inhibitor, although the mechanism of action has not been fully elucidated. The mechanism may relate to: 1) Inhibition of red blood cell uptake of adenosine, itself an inhibitor of platelet reactivity, 2) phosphodiesterase inhibition leading to increased cyclic-3′, 5′-adenosine monophosphate within platelets and 3) inhibition of thromboxane A_2 formation which is a potent stimulator of platelet activation.

Hemodynamics – In animals, intraduodenal doses of 0.5 to 4 mg/kg dipyridamole produced dose-related decreases in systemic and coronary vascular resistance leading to decreases in systemic blood pressure and increases in coronary blood flow. Onset of action in animals was about 24 minutes and effects persisted for about 3 hours.

In humans, the same qualitative hemodynamic effects have been observed. However, acute IV administration of dipyridamole may worsen regional myocardial perfusion distal to partial occlusion of coronary arteries.

Pharmacokinetics:

Metabolism – Following an oral dose of dipyridamole, the average time to peak concentration is about 75 minutes. The decline in plasma concentration fits a two-compartment model. The α half-life (the initial decline following peak concentration) is $\approx$ 40 minutes. The β half-life (the terminal decline in plasma concentration) is $\approx$ 10 hours. Dipyridamole is highly bound to plasma proteins. It is metabolized in the liver where it is conjugated as a glucuronide and excreted with the bile.

Clinical trials: In three randomized controlled clinical trials involving 854 patients who had undergone surgical placement of a prosthetic heart valve, dipyridamole with warfarin decreased the incidence of postoperative thromboembolic events by 62% to 91% compared to warfarin alone. In three additional studies involving 392 patients taking dipyridamole and coumarin-like anticoagulants, the incidence of thromboembolic events ranged from 2.3% to 6.9%. Dipyridamole does not influence prothrombin time or activity measurements when administered with warfarin.

Indications:

Thromboembolic complications: Adjunct to coumarin anticoagulants in the prevention of postoperative thromboembolic complications of cardiac valve replacement.

Unlabeled uses: At one time, dipyridamole was indicated as a "possibly effective" long-term therapy for chronic angina pectoris. The FDA, however, has withdrawn approval for this indication.

Dipyridamole in combination with aspirin has been commonly used in the prevention of myocardial reinfarction and reduction of mortality post MI. However, combination therapy appears to be no more beneficial than the use of aspirin alone.

Warnings:

Fertility impairment: A significant reduction in number of corpora lutea with consequent reduction in implantations and live fetuses was observed at 155 times the maximum recommended human dose.

Pregnancy: Category B. There are no adequate and well-controlled studies in pregnant women. Use during pregnancy only if clearly needed.

Lactation: Dipyridamole is excreted in breast milk. Exercise caution when administering to a nursing woman.

Children: Safety and efficacy in children < 12 years of age have not been established.

Precautions:

Hypotension: Use with caution in patients with hypotension since it can produce peripheral vasodilation.

DIPYRIDAMOLE

Adverse Reactions:

Adverse reactions at therapeutic doses are usually minimal and transient. With long-term use, initial side effects usually disappear. The following reactions were reported in two heart valve replacement trials comparing dipyridamole and warfarin therapy to either warfarin alone or warfarin and placebo: Dizziness (13.6%); abdominal distress (6.1%); headache, rash (2.3%); diarrhea; vomiting; flushing; pruritus; angina pectoris, liver dysfunction (rare).

On those uncommon occasions when adverse reactions have been persistent or intolerable, they have ceased on withdrawal of the medication.

Overdosage:

Symptoms: Hypotension, if it occurs, is likely to be of short duration, but a vasopressor may be used if necessary. In animals, symptoms of acute toxicity included ataxia, decreased locomotion, diarrhea, emesis and depression.

Treatment: Since dipyridamole is highly protein bound, dialysis is not likely to be of benefit.

Administration and Dosage:

Adjunctive use in prophylaxis of thromboembolism after cardiac valve replacement: The recommended dose is 75 to 100 mg, 4 times daily as an adjunct to the usual warfarin therapy. Please note that aspirin is not to be administered concomitantly with coumarin anticoagulants, which are indicated for use with dipyridamole in the prevention of thromboembolic complications (see Indications).

Rx	**Dipyridamole** (Various, eg, Barr, Geneva, Genetco, Goldline, Moore, Schein)	**Tablets:** 25 mg	In 90s, 100s, 500s, 1000s, 5000s and UD 100s,
Rx	**Persantine** (Boehringer Ingelheim)		(Bl/17). Orange, sugar coated. In 100s, 1000s and UD 100s.
Rx	**Dipyridamole** (Various, eg, Barr, Geneva, Genetco, Goldline, Moore, Schein)	**Tablets:** 50 mg	In 100s, 500s, 1000s and UD 100s,
Rx	**Persantine** (Boehringer Ingelheim)		(Bl/18). Orange, sugar coated. In 100s, 1000s and UD 100s.
Rx	**Dipyridamole** (Various, eg, Barr, Geneva, Genetco, Goldline, Moore, Schein)	**Tablets:** 75 mg	In 100s, 500s, 1000s and UD 100s.
Rx	**Persantine** (Boehringer Ingelheim)		(Bl/19). Orange, sugar coated. In 100s, 500s and UD 100s.

TICLOPIDINE HCl

Ticlopidine was approved by the FDA in October 1991.

Warning:

Neutropenia defined as an absolute neutrophil count (ANC) < 1200 neutrophils/mm³ occurred in 50 of 2048 (2.4%) stroke patients who received ticlopidine in clinical trials. Neutropenia is calculated as follows: ANC = WBC x % neutrophils.

Severe neutropenia (< 450 neutrophils/mm³) or agranulocytosis occurred in 17 patients (0.8%) who received ticlopidine. When the drug was discontinued, the neutrophil counts returned to normal (> 1200 neutrophils/mm³) within 1 to 3 weeks.

Mild to moderate neutropenia (451 to 1200 neutrophils/mm³) occurred in 33 patients (1.6%) who received ticlopidine. Eleven of the patients discontinued treatment and recovered within a few days. In the remaining 22 patients, the neutropenia was transient and did not require discontinuation of therapy.

The onset of severe neutropenia occurred 3 weeks to 3 months after the start of therapy with no documented cases of severe neutropenia beyond that time. The bone marrow typically showed a reduction in myeloid precursors. It is therefore essential that CBCs and white cell differentials be performed every 2 weeks starting from the second week to the end of the third month of therapy, but more frequent monitoring is necessary for patients whose absolute neutrophil counts have been consistently declining or are 30% less than the baseline count.

If clinical evaluation and repeat laboratory testing confirm the presence of neutropenia, discontinue the drug. In clinical trials, when therapy was discontinued immediately upon detection of neutropenia, the neutrophil counts returned to normal within 1 to 3 weeks.

After the first 3 months of therapy, CBCs need to be obtained only for patients with signs or symptoms suggestive of infection.

Actions:

Pharmacology: Ticlopidine is a platelet aggregation inhibitor. When taken orally, ticlopidine causes a time and dose-dependent inhibition of both platelet aggregation and release of platelet granule constituents, as well as a prolongation of bleeding time. Ticlopidine interferes with platelet membrane function by inhibiting ADP-induced platelet-fibrinogen binding and subsequent platelet-platelet interactions. The effect on platelet function is irreversible for the life of the platelet.

In healthy volunteers, substantial inhibition (> 50%) of ADP-induced platelet aggregation is detected within 4 days after administration of ticlopidine 250 mg twice daily, and maximum platelet aggregation inhibition (60% to 70%) is achieved after 8 to 11 days. Lower doses cause less and more delayed platelet aggregation inhibition, while doses > 250 mg twice daily give little additional effect on platelet aggregation, but an increased rate of adverse effects. After discontinuation of ticlopidine, bleeding time and other platelet function tests return to normal within 2 weeks in the majority of patients. At the recommended therapeutic dose (250 mg twice daily), ticlopidine has no known significant pharmacological actions in man other than inhibition of platelet function and prolongation of the bleeding time.

Pharmacokinetics: Ticlopidine is rapidly absorbed (> 80%), with peak plasma levels occurring at approximately 2 hours after dosing, and is extensively metabolized. Administration after meals results in a 20% increase in the area under the plasma concentration-time curve (AUC).

Ticlopidine displays non-linear pharmacokinetics and clearance decreases markedly on repeated dosing. In older volunteers, the apparent half-life after a single 250 mg dose is about 12.6 hours; with repeat dosing at 250 mg twice daily, the terminal elimination half-life rises to 4 to 5 days and steady-state levels of ticlopidine in plasma are obtained after ≈ 14 to 21 days.

Ticlopidine binds reversibly (98%) to plasma proteins, mainly to serum albumin and lipoproteins. The binding to albumin and lipoproteins is nonsaturable over a wide concentration range. Ticlopidine also binds to alpha-1 acid glycoprotein; at concentrations attained with the recommended dose, ≤ 15% in plasma is bound to this protein.

Ticlopidine is metabolized extensively by the liver; only trace amounts of intact drug are detected in the urine. Following an oral dose, 60% is recovered in the urine and 23% in the feces. Approximately, one-third of the dose excreted in the feces is intact ticlopidine, possibly excreted in the bile. Ticlopidine is a minor component in plasma (5%) after a single dose, but at steady state is the major component (15%). Approximately 40% to 50% of the metabolites circulating in plasma are covalently bound to plasma proteins, probably by acylation. Although analysis of urine and plasma indicates at least twenty metabolites, no metabolite which accounts for the activity of ticlopidine has been isolated.

TICLOPIDINE HCl

Clearance decreases with age. Steady-state trough values in elderly patients (mean age 70 years) are about twice those in young populations.

Hepatically impaired patients – The average plasma concentration in patients with advanced cirrhosis was slightly higher than that seen in older subjects.

Renally impaired patients – Patients with mildly (creatinine clearance [Ccr] 50 to 80 ml/min) or moderately (Ccr 20 to 50 ml/min) impaired renal function were compared to healthy subjects (Ccr 80 to 150 ml/min). AUC values of ticlopidine increased by 28% and 60% in mild and moderately impaired patients, respectively, and plasma clearance decreased by 37% and 52%, respectively, but there were no statistically significant differences in ADP-induced platelet aggregation. Bleeding times showed significant prolongation only in the moderately impaired patients.

Clinical trials:

Patients experiencing stroke precursors – In a trial comparing ticlopidine and aspirin (The Ticlopidine Aspirin Stroke Study; TASS), 3069 patients (1987 men, 1082 women) who had experienced such stroke precursors as transient ischemic attack (TIA), transient monocular blindness (amaurosis fugax), reversible ischemic neurological deficit or minor stroke were randomized to ticlopidine 250 mg twice daily or aspirin 650 mg twice daily. The study was designed to follow patients for at least 2 and up to 5 years. Over the duration of the study, ticlopidine significantly reduced the risk of fatal and nonfatal stroke by 24% from 18.1 to 13.8 per 100 patients followed for 5 years, compared to aspirin. During the first year, when the risk of stroke is greatest, the reduction in risk of stroke (fatal and nonfatal) compared to aspirin was 48%; the reduction was similar in men and women.

Patients who had a completed atherothrombotic stroke – In a trial comparing ticlopidine with placebo (The Canadian American Ticlopidine Study; CATS) 1073 patients who had experienced a previous atherothrombotic stroke were treated with ticlopidine 250 mg twice daily or placebo for up to 3 years. Ticlopidine significantly reduced the overall risk of stroke by 24% from 24.6 to 18.6 per 100 patients followed for 3 years, compared to placebo. During the first year, the reduction in risk of fatal and nonfatal stroke over placebo was 33%.

Indications:

To reduce the risk of thrombotic stroke (fatal or nonfatal) in patients who have experienced stroke precursors, and in patients who have had a completed thrombotic stroke.

Because ticlopidine is associated with a risk of neutropenia/agranulocytosis, which may be life-threatening (see Warnings), reserve for patients who are intolerant to aspirin therapy where indicated to prevent stroke.

Unlabeled uses: Ticlopidine has also been utilized in various other conditions; further study is needed:

Ticlopidine Unlabeled Uses

Condition	Result
Intermittent claudication	Improved maximum walking and pain-free distance
Chronic arterial occlusion	Improved lower extremity ulcer healing, vascular improvement
Subarachnoid hemorrhage	Reduced incidence of neurological deficit
Uremic patients with AV shunts or fistulas	Reduced incidence of vascular occlusion
Open heart surgery	Preoperative use reduces degree of platelet count drop during extracorporeal circulation
Coronary artery bypass grafts	Decreased graft occlusion
Primary glomerulonephritis	Reduced degree of proteinuria and hematuria, improved creatinine clearance
Sickle cell disease	Reduced incidence, duration, severity of infarctive crises

Contraindications:

Hypersensitivity to the drug; presence of hematopoietic disorders such as neutropenia and thrombocytopenia; presence of a hemostatic disorder or active pathological bleeding (such as bleeding peptic ulcer or intracranial bleeding); severe liver impairment.

Warnings:

Thrombocytopenia: Rarely, thrombocytopenia may occur in isolation or together with neutropenia. If clinical evaluation and repeat laboratory testing confirm the presence of thrombocytopenia (< 80,000 cells/mm^3), discontinue the drug.

TICLOPIDINE HCl

Cholesterol elevation: Ticlopidine therapy causes increased serum cholesterol and triglycerides. Serum total cholesterol levels are increased 8% to 10% within 1 month of therapy and persist at that level. The ratios of lipoprotein subfractions are unchanged.

Hematological effects: Rare cases of pancytopenia and thrombotic thrombocytopenia purpura, some of which have been fatal, have occurred.

Anticoagulant drugs: If a patient is switched from an anticoagulant or fibrinolytic drug to ticlopidine, discontinue the former drug prior to ticlopidine administration.

Renal function impairment: There is limited experience in patients with renal impairment. In controlled clinical trials, no unexpected problems have been encountered in patients having mild renal impairment and there is no experience with dosage adjustment in patients with greater degrees of renal impairment. Nevertheless, for renally impaired patients it may be necessary to reduce ticlopidine dosage or discontinue it altogether if hemorrhagic or hematopoietic problems are encountered (see Pharmacokinetics).

Hepatic function impairment: Because of limited experience in patients with severe hepatic disease, who may have bleeding diatheses, the use of ticlopidine is not recommended.

Elderly: Clearance of ticlopidine is somewhat lower in elderly patients and trough levels are increased. No overall differences in safety or efficacy were observed between elderly patients and younger patients, but greater sensitivity of some older individuals cannot be ruled out.

Pregnancy: Category B. Doses of 400 mg/kg in rats, 200 mg/kg/day in mice and 100 mg/kg in rabbits produced maternal toxicity as well as fetal toxicity, but there was no evidence of a teratogenic potential of ticlopidine. There are no adequate and well controlled studies in pregnant women. Use during pregnancy only if clearly needed.

Lactation: Ticlopidine is excreted in the milk of rats. It is not known whether this drug is excreted in human breast milk. Because of the potential for serious adverse reactions in nursing infants from ticlopidine, decide whether to discontinue nursing or to discontinue the drug, taking into account the importance of the drug to the mother.

Children: Safety and efficacy in patients < 18 years of age have not been established.

Precautions:

Increased bleeding risk: Use with caution in patients who may be at risk of increased bleeding from trauma, surgery or pathological conditions. If it is desired to eliminate the antiplatelet effects of ticlopidine prior to elective surgery, discontinue the drug 10 to 14 days prior to surgery. Increased surgical blood loss has occurred in patients undergoing surgery during treatment with ticlopidine. In TASS and CATS it was recommended that patients have ticlopidine discontinued prior to elective surgery. Several hundred patients underwent surgery during the trials, and no excessive surgical bleeding was reported.

Prolonged bleeding time is normalized within 2 hours after administration of 20 mg methylprednisolone IV. Platelet transfusions may also be used to reverse the effect of ticlopidine on bleeding.

GI bleeding: Ticlopidine prolongs template bleeding time. Use with caution in patients who have lesions with a propensity to bleed (such as ulcers). Use drugs that might induce such lesions with caution in patients on ticlopidine.

Drug Interactions:

The dose of drugs metabolized by hepatic microsomal enzymes with low therapeutic ratios, or being given to patients with hepatic impairment, may require adjustment to maintain optimal therapeutic blood levels when starting or stopping concomitant therapy with ticlopidine.

Ticlopidine Drug Interactions			
Precipitant drug	Object drug*		Description
Antacids	Ticlopidine	⬇	Administration of ticlopidine after antacids has resulted in an 18% decrease in ticlopidine plasma levels.
Cimetidine	Ticlopidine	⬆	Chronic cimetidine administration has reduced the clearance of a single ticlopidine dose by 50%.
Ticlopidine	Aspirin	⬆	Ticlopidine potentiated the effect of aspirin on collagen-induced platelet aggregation. Ticlopidine-mediated inhibition of ADP-induced platelet aggregation is not affected. Coadministration is not recommended.
Ticlopidine	Digoxin	⬇	Digoxin plasma levels may be slightly decreased (≈ 15%).
Ticlopidine	Theophylline	⬆	Theophylline elimination half-life was significantly increased (from 8.6 to 12.2 hr) with a comparable reduction in total plasma clearance in healthy volunteers.

* ⬆ = Object drug increased ⬇ = Object drug decreased

Drug/Food interaction: The oral bioavailability of ticlopidine is increased by 20% when taken after a meal. Administer with food to maximize GI tolerance.

Adverse Reactions:

Adverse reactions were relatively frequent, with > 50% of patients reporting at least one. Most (30% to 40%) involved the GI tract. Most adverse effects are mild, but 21% of patients discontinued therapy because of an adverse event, principally diarrhea, rash, nausea, vomiting, GI pain and neutropenia. Most adverse effects occur early in the course of treatment, but a new onset of adverse effects can occur after several months.

Ticlopidine Adverse Reactions vs Aspirin and Placebo (%)			
Adverse reaction	Ticlopidine (n = 2048)	Aspirin (n = 1527)	Placebo (n = 536)
Any reaction	60	53.2	34.3
Diarrhea	12.5	5.2	4.5
Nausea	7	6.2	1.7
Dyspepsia	7	9	0.9
Rash	5.1	1.5	0.6
GI pain	3.7	5.6	1.3
Neutropenia	2.4	0.8	1.1
Purpura	2.2	1.6	0
Vomiting	1.9	1.4	0.9
Flatulence	1.5	1.4	0
Pruritus	1.3	0.3	0
Dizziness	1.1	0.5	0
Anorexia	1	0.5	0
Abnormal liver function test	1	0.3	0

GI: Ticlopidine therapy has been associated with a variety of GI complaints including diarrhea and nausea. The majority of cases are mild, but about 13% of patients discontinued therapy. They usually occur within 3 months of initiation of therapy and typically are resolved within 1 to 2 weeks without discontinuation of therapy. If the effect is severe or persistent, discontinue therapy.

Hemorrhagic: Ticlopidine has been associated with a number of bleeding complications such as ecchymosis, epistaxis, hematuria, conjunctival hemorrhage, GI bleeding and perioperative bleeding. Intracerebral bleeding was rare with an incidence no greater than that seen with comparable agents (ticlopidine 0.5%, aspirin 0.6%, placebo 0.75%).

TICLOPIDINE HCl

Rash: Ticlopidine has been associated with a maculopapular or urticarial rash (often with pruritus). Rash usually occurs within 3 months of initiation of therapy, with a mean onset time of 11 days. If drug is discontinued, recovery occurs within several days. Many rashes do not recur on drug rechallenge. There have been rare reports of severe rashes.

Miscellaneous: Adverse reactions occurring in 0.5% to 1% of patients: GI fullness; urticaria; headache; asthenia; pain; epistaxis; tinnitus.

In addition, rarer, relatively serious events have also been reported: Pancytopenia; hemolytic anemia with reticulocytosis; allergic pneumonitis; systemic lupus (positive ANA); peripheral neuropathy; vasculitis; serum sickness; arthropathy; hepatitis; cholestatic jaundice; nephrotic syndrome; myositis; hyponatremia; immune thrombocytopenia; thrombocytopenic thrombotic purpura.

Lab test abnormalities: Elevations of alkaline phosphatase and transaminases generally occurred within 1 to 4 months of therapy initiation. The incidence of elevated alkaline phosphatase (> 2 times upper limit of normal) was 7.6% in ticlopidine patients, 6% in placebo patients, and 2.5% in aspirin patients. The incidence of elevated AST (> 2 times upper limit of normal) was 3.1% in ticlopidine patients, 4% with placebo and 2.1% with aspirin. Occasionally patients developed minor elevations in bilirubin. Perform liver function testing whenever liver dysfunction is suspected, particularly during the first 4 months of treatment.

Overdosage:

One case of deliberate overdosage has been reported. A 38-year-old male took a single 6000 mg dose (equivalent to 24 standard 250 mg tablets). The only abnormalities reported were increased bleeding time and increased ALT. No special therapy was instituted and the patient recovered without sequelae.

Single oral doses of 1600 and 500 mg/kg were lethal to rats and mice, respectively. Symptoms of acute toxicity were GI hemorrhage, convulsions, hypothermia, dyspnea, loss of equilibrium and abnormal gait.

Patient Information:

A decrease in the number of white blood cells (neutropenia) can occur, especially during the first 3 months of treatment. If neutropenia is severe, it could result in an increased risk of infection. It is critically important to obtain the scheduled blood tests to detect neutropenia. Patients should contact their physician if they experience any indication of infection such as fever, chills or sore throat, all of which may be consequences of neutropenia.

It may take longer than usual to stop bleeding when taking ticlopidine. Patients should report any unusual bleeding to their physician. Patients should tell physicians and dentists that they are taking ticlopidine before any surgery is scheduled and before any new drug is prescribed.

Promptly report side effects such as severe or persistent diarrhea, skin rashes or subcutaneous bleeding, or any signs of cholestasis, such as yellow skin or sclera, dark urine or light colored stools.

Take ticlopidine with food or just after eating in order to minimize GI discomfort.

Administration and Dosage:

Recomended dose: 250 mg twice daily taken with food.

Rx	**Ticlid** (Syntex)	**Tablets:** 250 mg	(Ticlid 250). White. Oval. Film coated. In 30s and UD 100s.

ABCIXIMAB

Actions:

Pharmacology: Abciximab is the Fab fragment of the chimeric human-murine monoclonal antibody 7E3. Abciximab binds to the intact glycoprotein IIb/IIIa (GPIIb/IIIa) receptor of human platelets, which is a member of the integrin family of adhesion receptors and the major platelet surface receptor involved in platelet aggregation. The drug inhibits platelet aggregation by preventing the binding of fibrinogen, von Willebrand factor and other adhesive molecules to GPIIb/IIIa receptor sites on activated platelets. The mechanism is thought to involve steric hindrance or conformational effects to block access of large molecules to the receptor rather than interacting directly with the RGD (arginine 10 glycine-aspartic acid) binding site.

IV administration of single bolus doses from 0.15 to 0.3 mg/kg produced rapid, dose-dependent inhibition of platelet function as measured by ex vivo platelet aggregation in response to adenosine diphosphate (ADP) or by prolongation of bleeding time. At the two highest doses (0.25 and 0.3 mg/kg) at 2 hours post injection, > 80% of the GPIIb/IIIa receptors were blocked and platelet aggregation in response to 20 mcM ADP was almost abolished. The median bleeding time increased to over 30 minutes at both doses compared with a baseline value of ≈ 5 minutes.

IV administration of a single bolus dose of 0.25 mg/kg followed by a continuous 10 mcg/min infusion for periods of 12 to 96 hours produced sustained high grade GPIIb/IIIa receptor blockade (≥ 80%) and inhibition of platelet function for the duration of the infusion in most patients. Results in patients who received the 0.25 mg/kg bolus followed by a 5 mcg/min infusion for 24 hours showed a similar initial receptor blockade and inhibition of platelet aggregation, but the response was not maintained throughout the infusion period.

Low levels of GPIIb/IIIa receptor blockade are present for up to 10 days following cessation of the infusion. Bleeding time returned to ≤ 12 minutes within 12 hours following the end of infusion in 75% of patients and within 24 hours in 90%. Ex vivo platelet aggregation in response to 5 mcM ADP returned to > 50% of baseline within 24 hours following the end of infusion in 34% of patients and within 48 hours in 72%. In response to 20 mcM ADP, ex vivo platelet aggregation returned to ≥ 50% of baseline within 24 hours in 62% of patients and within 48 hours in 88%.

Pharmacokinetics: Following IV bolus administration, free plasma concentrations of abciximab decrease rapidly with an initial half-life of < 10 minutes and a second phase half-life of about 30 minutes, probably related to rapid binding to the platelet receptors. Platelet function generally recovers over the course of 48 hours, although abciximab remains in the circulation for up to 10 days in a platelet-bound state. IV administration of a 0.25 mg/kg bolus dose of abciximab followed by continuous infusion of 10 mcg/min produces almost constant free plasma concentrations throughout the infusion. At the termination of the infusion period, free plasma concentrations fall rapidly for about 6 hours and then decline at a slower rate.

Clinical trials: Patients (n = 2099) undergoing percutaneous transluminal coronary angioplasty or atherectomy (PTCA) who were at high risk for abrupt closure of the treated coronary vessel were randomly allocated to one of three treatments: 1) Abciximab bolus (0.25 mg/kg) followed by an infusion (10 mcg/min) for 12 hours (bolus plus infusion group); 2) abciximab bolus (0.25 mg/kg) followed by a placebo infusion (bolus group) or; 3) a placebo bolus followed by a placebo infusion (placebo group). Patients at high risk during or following PTCA were defined as those with unstable angina or a non-Q-wave myocardial infarction (n = 489), those with an acute Q-wave MI within 12 hours of symptom onset (n = 66) and those who were at high risk because of coronary morphology or clinical characteristics as defined in ACC/AHA criteria (n = 1544). Treatment was initiated 10 to 60 minutes before the onset of PTCA. All patients initially received an IV heparin bolus (10,000 to 12,000 units) and boluses of up to 3000 units thereafter to a maximum of 20,000 units during PTCA. Heparin infusion was continued for 12 hours to maintain a therapeutic elevation of activated partial thromboplastin time (APTT, 1.5 to 2.5 times normal). Unless contraindicated, aspirin (325 mg) was administered orally 2 hours prior to the planned procedure and then once daily.

The primary endpoint was the occurrence of any of the following events within 30 days of PTCA: Death, MI or the need for urgent intervention for recurrent ischemia (ie, urgent PTCA, urgent coronary artery bypass graft [CABG] surgery, a coronary stent or an intra-aortic balloon pump). The 4.5% lower incidence of the primary endpoint in the bolus plus infusion treatment group, compared with the placebo group, was statistically significant, whereas the 1.3% lower incidence in the bolus treatment group was not. A lower incidence of the primary endpoint was observed in the bolus plus infusion treatment arm for all three high-risk subgroups: Patients with unstable angina, patients presenting within 12 hours of the onset of symptoms of an acute MI and patients with other high-risk clinical or morphologic characteristics. The treatment effect was largest in the first two subgroups and smallest in the third subgroup.

Mortality was uncommon and similar rates were observed in all arms. The rate of acute MI was significantly lower in the groups treated with abciximab. While 80% of MIs in the study were non-Q-wave infarctions, patients in the bolus plus infusion arm experienced a lower incidence of both Q-wave and non-Q-wave infarctions. The primary endpoint events in the bolus plus infusion treatment group were reduced mostly in the first 48 hours and this benefit was sustained through 30 days and 6 months. At the 6 month follow-up visit, this event rate remained lower in the bolus plus infusion arm (12.3%) than in the placebo arm (17.6%).

Indications:

Platelet aggregation inhibition: Adjunct to percutaneous transluminal coronary angioplasty or atherectomy (PTCA) for the prevention of acute cardiac ischemic complications in patients at high risk for abrupt closure of the treated coronary vessel.

Abciximab is intended for use with aspirin and heparin.

Contraindications:

Because abciximab increases the risks of bleeding (see Warnings), it is contraindicated in the following clinical situations: Active internal bleeding; recent (within 6 weeks) GI or GU bleeding of clinical significance; history of cerebrovascular accident (CVA) within 2 years or CVA with a significant residual neurological deficit; bleeding diathesis; administration of oral anticoagulants within 7 days unless prothrombin time is < 1.2 times control; thrombocytopenia (<100,000 cells/mcl); recent (within 6 weeks) major surgery or trauma; intracranial neoplasm, arteriovenous malformation or aneurysm; severe uncontrolled hypertension; presumed or documented history of vasculitis; use of IV dextran before PTCA or intent to use it during PTCA; hypersensitivity to any component of this product or to murine proteins.

Warnings:

Bleeding: Abciximab is associated with an increased frequency of major bleeding complications (see Contraindications) including retroperitoneal bleeding, spontaneous GI and GU bleeding and bleeding at the arterial access site. In the following conditions, clinical data suggest that the risks of major bleeds due to therapy may be increased and should be weighed against the anticipated benefits: Patients who weigh < 75 kg; patients > 65 years old; history of prior GI disease; patients receiving thrombolytics; heparin anticoagulation.

The following conditions are also associated with an increased risk of bleeding in the angioplasty setting which may be additive to that of abciximab: PTCA within 12 hours of the onset of symptoms for acute MI; prolonged PTCA (lasting > 70 minutes); failed PTCA.

Should serious bleeding occur that is not controllable with pressure, stop the infusion of abciximab and any concomitant heparin.

Bleeding sites – Therapy with abciximab requires careful attention to all potential bleeding sites (including catheter insertion, arterial and venous puncture, cutdown, needle puncture, GI, GU and retroperitoneal sites).

Femoral artery access site: Abciximab is associated with an increase in bleeding rate particularly at the site of arterial access for femoral sheath placement. Use care when attempting vascular access so that only the anterior wall of the femoral artery is punctured, avoiding a Seldinger technique for obtaining sheath access. Avoid femoral vein sheath placement unless needed. While the vascular sheath is in place, maintain patients on complete bed rest with the head of the bed ≤ 30° and restrain the affected limb in a straight position.

Discontinue heparin at least 4 hours prior to arterial sheath removal. Following sheath removal, apply pressure to the femoral artery for at least 30 minutes using either manual compression or a mechanical device for hemostasis. Apply a pressure dressing following hemostasis. Maintain the patient on bed rest for 6 to 8 hours following sheath removal or discontinuation of abciximab, whichever is later.

Frequently check the sheath insertion site and distal pulses of affected leg(s) while the femoral artery sheath is in place, and for 6 hours after femoral artery sheath removal. Measure any hematoma and monitor for enlargement.

General nursing care: Arterial and venous punctures, IM injections and use of urinary catheters, nasotracheal intubation, nasogastric tubes and automatic blood pressure cuffs should be minimized. When obtaining IV access, avoid non-compressible sites (eg, subclavian or jugular veins). Consider saline or heparin locks for blood drawing. Document and monitor vascular puncture sites. Provide gentle care when removing dressings.

ABCIXIMAB

High-risk patients: Patients at high risk for abrupt closure include those undergoing PTCA with at least one of the following conditions: Unstable angina or a non-Q-wave MI; an acute Q-wave MI within 12 hours of the onset of symptoms.

Other high-risk clinical or morphologic characteristics include: Two type B lesions in the artery to be dilated; one type B lesion in the artery to be dilated in a woman of at least 65 years of age; one type B lesion in the artery to be dilated in a patient with diabetes mellitus; one type C lesion in the artery to be dilated; angioplasty of an infarct-related lesion within 7 days of MI.

Hypersensitivity: Administration of abciximab may result in human anti-chimeric antibody (HACA) formation that can cause allergic or hypersensitivity reactions (including anaphylaxis), thrombocytopenia or diminished benefit upon readministration of abciximab. Patients with HACA titers may have allergic or hypersensitivity reactions when treated with other diagnostic or therapeutic monoclonal antibodies. Anaphylaxis may occur at any time during administration. If it does, immediately stop administration of abciximab and initiate standard appropriate resuscitative measures (refer to Management of Acute Hypersensitivity Reactions).

Pregnancy: Category C. It is not known whether abciximab can cause fetal harm when administered to a pregnant woman or can affect reproduction capacity. Give to a pregnant woman only if clearly needed.

Lactation: It is not known whether this drug is excreted in breast milk or absorbed systemically after ingestion. Exercise caution when abciximab is administered to a nursing woman.

Children: Safety and efficacy in children have not been established.

Precautions:

Monitoring: Before infusion of abciximab, measure platelet count, prothrombin time and APTT to identify pre-existing hemostatic abnormalities. During and after treatment, closely monitor platelet counts and extent of heparin anticoagulation, as assessed by activated clotting time or APTT (see Thrombocytopenia).

Concomitant therapy: In a clinical trial, abciximab was used concomitantly with heparin and aspirin. Because abciximab inhibits platelet aggregation, use caution when it is used with other drugs that affect hemostasis, including thrombolytics, oral anticoagulants, nonsteroidal anti-inflammatory drugs, dipyridamole and ticlopidine.

Low molecular weight dextran and oral anticoagulants were usually given for the deployment of a coronary stent. In the 11 patients who received low molecular weight dextran with abciximab, 5 had major bleeding events and 4 had minor bleeding events.

Thrombocytopenia: Monitor platelet counts prior to treatment, 2 to 4 hours following the bolus dose of abciximab and at 24 hours or before discharge, whichever is first. If a patient experiences an acute platelet decrease (eg, decrease to < 100,000 cells/mcl or a decrease of at least 25% from pretreatment value), determine additional platelet counts. These platelet counts should be drawn in separate tubes containing EDTA, citrate or heparin to exclude pseudothrombocytopenia due to in vitro anticoagulant interaction. If true thrombocytopenia is verified, immediately discontinue abciximab and appropriately monitor and treat the condition. For patients with thrombocytopenia in the clinical trial, a daily platelet count was obtained until it returned to normal. If a patient's platelet count dropped to 60,000 cells/mcl, heparin and aspirin were discontinued. If a patient's platelet count dropped below 50,000 cells/mcl, platelets were transfused.

Restoration of platelet function: In the event of serious uncontrolled bleeding or the need for surgery (especially major procedures within 48 to 72 hours of treatment with abciximab), determine a bleeding time. Preliminary evidence suggests that platelet function may be restored, at least in part, with platelet transfusions.

ABCIXIMAB

Adverse Reactions:

Abciximab Adverse Reactions (%)		
Adverse reaction	Placebo (n = 681)	Bolus + infusion (n = 678)
Cardiovascular		
Hypotension	12	21.1
Bradycardia	2.9	5.2
GI		
Nausea	16	18.4
Vomiting	9	11.4
Hemic/Lymphatic		
Anemia	0.4	1.2
Leukocytosis	0.1	1
CNS		
Hypesthesia	0.3	1
Confusion	0	0.6
Respiratory		
Pleural effusion/Pleurisy	0.2	1.3
Pneumonia	0.4	1
Miscellaneous		
Pain	2.6	3.4
Peripheral edema	0.4	1.6
Abnormal vision	0.1	0.7

Bleeding: The most common complication of abciximab therapy is bleeding (see Warnings). Treatment was associated with statistically significant increases in both major and minor bleeding events and in bleeding requiring transfusions. Major bleeding events were defined as either an intracranial hemorrhage or a decrease in hemoglobin > 5 g/dl. Minor bleeding events included spontaneous gross hematuria, spontaneous hematemesis, observed blood loss with a hemoglobin decrease of > 3 g/dl or a decrease in hemoglobin of at least 4 g/dl without an identified bleeding site.

Major bleeding events occurred most commonly in patients treated with the bolus plus infusion regimen (14% vs 11.1% with bolus only, 6.6% with placebo). Ten patients who had major bleeding events died (two patients had deaths attributable to bleeding; both had a hemorrhagic stroke). Approximately 70% of abciximab-treated patients with major bleeding had bleeding at the arterial access site in the groin. Abciximab-treated patients also had a higher incidence of major bleeding events from GI, GU, retroperitoneal and other sites. Excess spontaneous major organ bleeding occurred primarily in patients weighing ≤ 75 kg who received abciximab.

Abciximab treatment was not associated with excess major bleeding in patients who underwent CABG surgery. The incidence of CABG surgery-related major blood loss was similar in all 3 groups (3% to 5%). Some patients with prolonged bleeding times received platelet transfusions to correct the bleeding time prior to surgery.

Minor bleeding occurred in 16.9%, 15.4% and 9.8% of patients receiving bolus plus infusion, bolus only or placebo, respectively.

Thrombocytopenia: Patients treated with abciximab were more likely to experience decreases in platelet counts and to require platelet transfusions than patients treated with placebo . Patients with decrease of platelets to < 50,000 cells/mcl, 1.6% with abciximab vs 0.7% with placebo; patients with decrease of platelets to < 100,000 cells/mcl, 5.2% with abciximab vs 3.4% with placebo; patients who received platelet transfusions, 5.5% with abciximab vs 2.6% with placebo (see Precautions).

Human anti-chimeric antibody development (HACA): HACA may appear in response to the administration of abciximab. Positive responses occurred in 6.5% of the patients in the bolus plus infusion group vs 0% with placebo. There was no excess of hypersensitivity or allergic reactions related to abciximab treatment compared with placebo treatment (see Warnings).

Cardiovascular: Atrial fibrillation/flutter (3.5%); vascular disorder (1.8%); pulmonary edema (1.5%); complete AV block (1.3%); supraventricular tachycardia, weak pulse (1%); palpitation (0.7%); intermittent claudication, pericardial effusion (0.4%); limb embolism, pulmonary embolism, ventricular arrhythmia (0.3%).

GI: Diarrhea (0.9%); constipation, ileus (0.3%).

Hematologic/Lymphatic: Hemolytic anemia, petechiae (0.3%).

CNS: Abnormal thinking (2.1%); dizziness (1.8%); coma (0.4%); brain ischemia, insomnia (0.3%).

ABCIXIMAB

Musculoskeletal: Myopathy (0.4%); cellulitis, myalgia (0.3%).

GU: Urinary tract infection (1.9%); urinary retention (0.4%); abnormal renal function (0.3%).

Miscellaneous: Dysphonia (0.3%); pruritus (0.3%).

Overdosage:

There has been no experience of overdosage. It is recommended that infusion be discontinued after 12 hours to avoid effects of prolonged platelet receptor blockade.

Administration and Dosage:

Approved by the FDA on December 22, 1994.

Abciximab is intended for use in patients undergoing PTCA. The safety and efficacy of abciximab have only been investigated with concomitant administration of heparin and aspirin.

Failed PTCAs: In patients with failed PTCAs, stop the continuous infusion of abciximab because there is no evidence for abciximab efficacy in that setting.

Serious bleeding: In the event of serious bleeding that cannot be controlled by compression, discontinue abciximab and heparin (see Warnings).

The recommended dosage is an IV bolus of 0.25 mg/kg administered 10 to 60 minutes before the start of PTCA, followed by a continuous IV infusion of 10 mcg/min for 12 hours.

Administration instructions:

1.) Do NOT use preparations of abciximab containing visibly opaque particles.
2.) Anticipate hypersensitivity reactions whenever protein solutions such as abciximab are administered. Epinephrine, dopamine, theophylline, antihistamines and corticosteroids should be available for immediate use. If symptoms of an allergic reaction or anaphylaxis appear, stop the infusion and give appropriate treatment (see Warnings).
3.) Withdraw the necessary amount of abciximab (2 mg/ml) for bolus injection through a sterile, non-pyrogenic, low protein-binding 0.2 or 0.22 micron filter into a syringe. Administer the bolus 10 to 60 minutes before the procedure.
4.) Withdraw 4.5 ml of abciximab for the continuous infusion through a sterile, non-pyrogenic, low protein-binding 0.2 or 0.22 micron filter into a syringe. Inject into 250 ml of sterile 0.9% saline or 5% dextrose and infuse at a rate of 17 ml/hr (10 mcg/min) for 12 hours via a continuous infusion pump equipped with an in-line sterile, non-pyrogenic, low protein-binding 0.2 or 0.22 micron filter. Discard the unused portion at the end of the 12-hour infusion.

Admixture incompatibilities: Administer in a separate IV line; no other medication should be added to the infusion solutions. No incompatibilities have been observed with glass bottles or polyvinyl chloride bags and administration sets.

Storage/Stability: Store vials at 2° to 8°C (36° to 46°F). Do not freeze, shake or use beyond the expiration date. Discard any unused portion left in the vial.

Rx	**ReoPro** (Lilly)	**Injection:** 2 mg/ml abciximab	In buffered solution of 0.01 M sodium phosphate, 0.15 M NaCl and 0.001% polysorbate 80. In 5 ml vials.

ANAGRELIDE HCl

Actions:

Pharmacology: The mechanism by which anagrelide reduces blood platelet count is under investigation. Studies support a hypothesis of dose-related reduction in platelet production resulting from a decrease in megakaryocyte hypermaturation. In blood withdrawn from healthy volunteers treated with anagrelide, a disruption was found in the postmitotic phase of megakaryocyte development and a reduction in megakaryocyte size and ploidy. At therapeutic doses, anagrelide does not produce significant changes in white cell counts or coagulation parameters and may have a small but clinically insignificant effect on red cell parameters. Platelet aggregation is inhibited in people at doses higher than those required to reduce platelet count. Anagrelide inhibits cyclic AMP phosphodiesterase and ADP- and collagen-induced platelet aggregation.

Pharmacokinetics:

Absorption/Distribution – Anagrelide plasma levels peaked at 5 ng/ml at ≈ 1 hour, decreased rapidly during the first 6 to 8 hours and then declined more slowly. At fasting and at a dose of 0.5 mg, the plasma half-life is 1.3 hours, terminal elimination half-life is ≈ 3 days and the volume of distribution is 12 L/kg. Anagrelide does not accumulate in plasma after repeated administration. Bioavailability is reduced by food.

Metabolism/Excretion – Anagrelide is extensively metabolized before elimination in urine. The drug is extensively metabolized; < 1% is recovered unchanged in the urine. Following oral administration, > 70% of the dose was recovered in urine and 10% in the feces. Based on limited data, there appears to be a trend towards dose linearity between doses of 0.5 mg and 2 mg.

Clinical trials: A total of 551 patients with essential thrombocythemia (ET) were treated with anagrelide in three clinical trials. The mean duration of anagrelide therapy for study patients was 65 weeks; 23% of patients received treatment for 2 years. In one study, 274 ET patients were treated with anagrelide starting at doses of 0.5 to 2.0 mg every 6 hours. The dose was increased if the platelet count was still high but did not exceed 12 mg/day. Efficacy was defined as reduction of platelet count to or near physiologic levels (150,000 to 400,000/mcl). The criteria for defining subjects as "responders" were reduction in platelets for ≥ 4 weeks to ≤ 600,000/mcl or by ≥ 50% from baseline value.

Decrease in Mean Platelet Count Over Time with Anagrelide

		Weeks				Years		
	Baseline	4	12	24	48	2	3	4
Mean*	1045	627	537	506	508	501	474	464
N	274	265	245	206	179	139	76	11

* x 10^3/mcl.

In another study, 139 patients who had baseline symptoms thought to be secondary to thrombocythemia (eg, headache, dizziness, neurological or visual symptoms) and who were treated for ≤ 1 year with anagrelide, showed a significant reduction in frequency of symptoms at 1 year compared with the first month of treatment.

Indications:

Essential thrombocythemia (ET): For the treatment of patients with ET to reduce the elevated platelet count and the risk of thrombosis and to ameliorate associated symptoms.

Warnings:

Cardiovascular: Use with caution in patients with known or suspected heart disease only if the potential benefits outweigh the potential risks. Because of the positive inotropic effects and side effects of anagrelide, a pretreatment cardiovascular examination is recommended along with careful monitoring during treatment. Therapeutic doses of anagrelide may cause cardiovascular effects, including vasodilation, tachycardia, palpitations and congestive heart failure.

Thrombocytopenia: Platelet counts < 100,000/mcl occurred in 35 patients, and reduction < 50,000/mcl occurred in 7 of the 551 ET patients while on anagrelide therapy. Thrombocytopenia promptly recovered upon discontinuation of anagrelide.

ANAGRELIDE HCl

Renal toxicity: Of the 551 ET patients studied, 10 were found to have renal abnormalities. Six of the 10 experienced renal failure (≈ 1%) while on anagrelide treatment; in two, the renal failure was possibly related to anagrelide treatment. The remaining four were found to have preexisiting renal impairment and were successfully treated with anagrelide. Doses ranged from 1.5 to 6 mg/day with exposure periods of 2 to 12 months. Serum creatinines remained within normal limits, and no dose adjustment was required because of renal insufficiency.

Renal function impairment: It is recommended that patients with renal insufficiency (creatinine ≥ 2 mg/dl) receive anagrelide when the potential benefits of therapy outweigh the potential risks. Monitor patients closely for signs of renal toxicity while receiving anagrelide.

Hepatic function impairment: It is recommended that patients with evidence of hepatic dysfunction (bilirubin, AST or measures of liver function > 1.5 times the upper limit of normal) receive anagrelide when the potential benefits of therapy outweigh the potential risks. Monitor patients closely for signs of hepatic toxicity while receiving anagrelide.

Pregnancy: Category C. A fertility and reproductive performance study performed in female rats revealed that anagrelide at oral doses of ≥ 60 mg/kg/day (49 times the recommended maximum human dose) disrupted implantation and exerted adverse effect on embryo/fetal survival.

Five women became pregnant while on anagrelide treatment at doses of 1 to 4 mg/day. Treatment was stopped as soon as it was realized that they were pregnant. All delivered healthy babies. There are no adequate and well-controlled studies in pregnant women. Use anagrelide during pregnancy only if the potential benefit justifies the potential risk to the fetus.

Lactation: It is not known whether this drug is excreted in breast milk. Decide whether to discontinue nursing or to discontinue the drug, taking into account the importance of the drug to the mother.

Children: The safety and efficacy of anagrelide in patients < 16 years old have not been established. Anagrelide has been used successfully in eight pediatric patients (age range 8 to 17 years), including three patients with essential thrombocythemia, who were treated at a dose of 1 to 4 mg/day.

Precautions:

Monitoring: Anagrelide therapy requires close clinical supervision of the patient. While the platelet count is being lowered (usually during the first 2 weeks of treatment), monitor blood counts (hemoglobin, white blood cells), liver function (AST, ALT) and renal function (serum creatinine, BUN).

Blood pressure – In nine subjects receiving a single 5 mg dose of anagrelide, standard blood pressure fell an average of 22/15 mmHg, usually accompanied by dizziness. Only minimal changes in blood pressure were observed following a 2 mg dose.

Interruption of therapy – In general, interruption of anagrelide treatment is followed by an increase in platelet count. After sudden stoppage of therapy, the increase in platelet count can be observed within 4 days.

Drug Interactions:

Sucralfate: A single case report suggests sucralfate may interfere with anagrelide absorption.

Drug/Food interactions: When a 0.5 mg dose was taken after food, bioavailability was modestly reduced by an average of 13.8%, and plasma half-life slightly increased (to 1.8 hours), when compared to the same subjects in the fasting state. The peak plasma level was lowered by ≈ 45% and delayed by 2 hours.

Adverse Reactions:

While most reported adverse reactions during anagrelide therapy have been mild in intensity and have decreased in frequency with continued therapy, serious adverse events reported in patients with ET and in patients with thrombocythemias of other etiologies include: Congestive heart failure; myocardial infarction; cardiomyopathy; cardiomegaly; complete heart block; atrial fibrillation; cerebrovascular accident; pericarditis; pulmonary infiltrates; pulmonary fibrosis; pulmonary hypertension; pancreatitis; gastric/duodenal ulceration; seizure. The most common adverse events for treatment discontinuation were headache, diarrhea, edema, palpitations and abdominal pain.

ANAGRELIDE HCl

Anagrelide Adverse Reactions (≥ 5%)			
Adverse reaction	% (n = 551)	Adverse reaction	% (n = 551)
Cardiovascular		*Miscellaneous*	
Palpitations	27.2	Headache	44.5
Chest Pain	7.8	Asthenia	22.1
Tachycardia	7.3	Edema	19.8
GI		Pain	14.7
Diarrhea	24.3	Dizziness	14.5
Abdominal pain	17.4	Dyspnea	10.5
Nausea	15.1	Rash, including urticaria	7.8
Flatulence	10.5	Paresthesia	7.3
Vomiting	7.4	Peripheral Edema	7.1
Dyspepsia	6.4	Back pain	6.4
Anorexia	5.8	Malaise	5.8

Other adverse reactions (< 5%):

Body as a whole: Fever; flu symptoms; chills; neck pain; photosensitivity.

Cardiovascular: Arrhythmia; hemorrhage; cardiovascular disease; cerebrovascular accident; angina pectoris; heart failure; postural hypotension; vasodilation; migraine; syncope.

CNS: Depression; somnolence; confusion; insomnia; hypertension; nervousness; amnesia.

Dermatologic: Pruritus; skin disease; alopecia.

GI: Constipation; GI distress; GI hemorrhage; gastritis; melena; aphthous stomatitis; eructations; nausea; vomiting.

GU: Dysuria; hematuria.

Hematologic: Anemia; thrombocytopenia (see Warnings); ecchymosis; lymphadenoma.

Musculoskeletal: Arthralgia; myalgia; leg cramps.

Respiratory: Rhinitis; epistaxis; respiratory disease; sinusitis; pneumonia; bronchitis; asthma.

Special senses: Amblyopia, abnormal vision, tinnitus, visual field abnormality, diplopia.

Miscellaneous: Elevated liver enzymes (see Warnings); dehydration.

Overdosage:

Symptoms: Single oral doses of anagrelide at 2500, 1500 and 200 mg/kg in mice, rats and monkeys, respectively, were not lethal. Symptoms of acute toxicity were: Decreased motor activity in mice and rats and softened stools and decreased appetite in monkeys.

There are no reports of overdosage with anagrelide. Platelet reduction from anagrelide therapy is dose-related; therefore, thrombocytopenia, which can potentially cause bleeding, is expected from overdosage. Should overdosage occur, cardiac and central nervous system toxicity can also be expected.

Treatment: In case of overdosage, close clinical supervision of the patient is required; this especially includes monitoring of the platelet count for thrombocytopenia. Decrease dosage or stop, as appropriate, until the platelet count returns to within the normal range.

Patient Information:

Anagrelide is not recommended in women who are or may become pregnant. It may cause fetal harm when administered to a pregnant woman. If this drug is used during pregnancy or if the patient becomes pregnant while taking this drug, apprise the patient of the potential harm to the fetus. Instruct women of childbearing potential that they must not be pregnant and that they should use contraception while taking anagrelide.

ANAGRELIDE HCl

Administration and Dosage:

Approved by the FDA on March 17, 1997.

Initiate treatment with anagrelide under close medical supervision. The recommended starting dose is 0.5 mg 4 times/day or 1 mg twice/day; maintain for ≥ 1 week, then adjust to the lowest effective dosage required to reduce and maintain platelet count < 600,000/mcl ideally to the normal range. Increase the dosage by ≤ 0.5 mg/day in any 1 week. Dosage should not exceed 10 mg/day or 2.5 mg in a single dose. Individualize the decision to treat asymptomatic young adults with essential thrombocythemia.

To monitor the effect of anagrelide and prevent the occurrence of thrombocytopenia, perform platelet counts every 2 days during the first week of treatment and at least weekly thereafter until the maintenance dosage is reached.

Typically, platelet count begins to respond within 7 to 14 days at the proper dosage. Most patients will experience an adequate response at a dose of 1.5 to 3 mg/day. Closely monitor patients with known or suspected heart disease, renal insufficiency or hepatic dysfunction.

Rx	**Agrylin** (Roberts)	**Capsules:** 0.5 mg	Lactose. Opaque, white. (ROBERTS 063). In 100s.
		1 mg	Lactose. Opaque, gray. (ROBERTS 064). In 100s.

ANTICOAGULANTS

Blood coagulation resulting in the formation of a stable fibrin clot involves a cascade of proteolytic reactions involving the interaction of clotting factors, platelets and tissue materials. Clotting factors (see table) exist in the blood in inactive form and must be converted to an enzymatic or activated (a) form before the next step in the clotting mechanism can be stimulated. Each factor is stimulated in turn until an insoluble fibrin clot is formed.

Two separate pathways, intrinsic and extrinsic, lead to the formation of a fibrin clot. Both pathways must function for hemostasis.

Intrinsic pathway: All the protein factors necessary for coagulation are present in circulating blood. Clot formation may take several minutes and is initiated by activation of factor XII.

Extrinsic pathway: Coagulation is activated by release of tissue thromboplastin, a factor not found in circulating blood. Clotting occurs in seconds because factor III bypasses the early reactions.

Refer to the complete coagulation pathway.

Anticoagulants used therapeutically include fractionated and unfractionated heparin, warfarin (a coumarin derivative) and anisindione (an indandione derivative).

Blood Clotting Factors

Factor	Synonym	Vitamin K-dependent
I	Fibrinogen	no
II	Prothrombin	yes
III	Tissue thromboplastin, tissue factor	no
IV	Calcium	no
V	Labile factor, proaccelerin	no
VII	Proconvertin	yes
VIII	Antihemophilic factor, AHF	no
IX	Christmas factor, plasma thromboplastin component, PTC	yes
X	Stuart factor, Stuart-Prower factor	yes
XI	Plasma thromboplastin antecedent, PTA	no
XII	Hageman factor	no
XIII	Fibrin stabilizing factor, FSF	no
HMW-K	High molecular weight Kininogen, Fitzgerald factor	no
PL	Platelets or phospholipids	no
PK	Prekallikrein, Fletcher factor	no
Protein C[1]		yes
Protein S[2]		yes

[1] Partially responsible for inhibition of the extrinsic pathway. Inactivates factors V and VIII and promotes fibrinolysis. Activity declines following warfarin administration.

[2] A cofactor to accelerate the anticoagulant activity of protein C. Decreased levels occur following warfarin administration.

ANTICOAGULANTS

COAGULATION PATHWAY

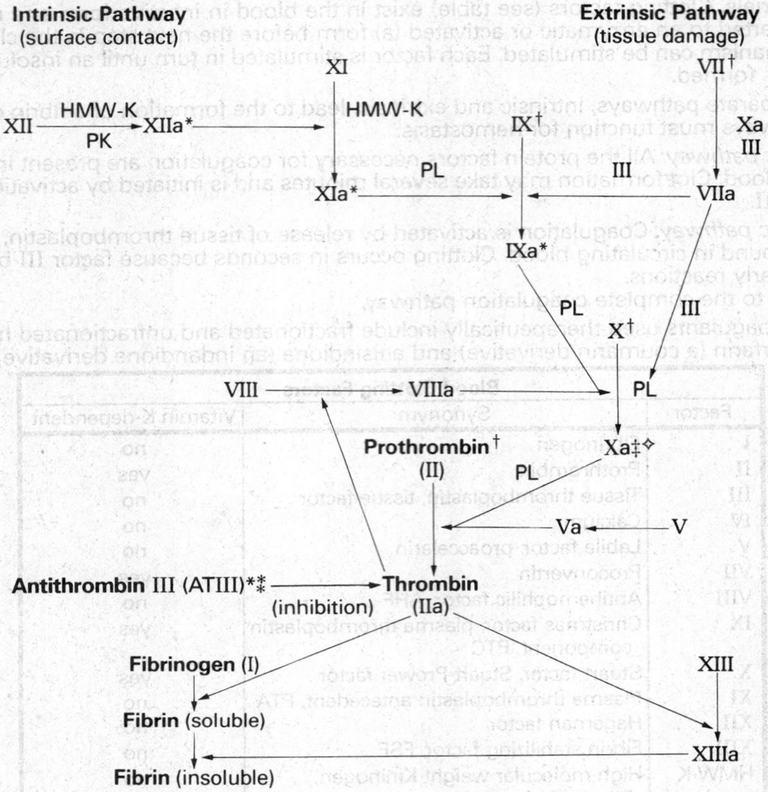

* Major site of activity for unfractionated heparin
† Site of activity for warfarin and anisindione
‡ Major site of activity for fractionated heparin
⁑ Minor site of activity for fractionated heparin
✧ Minor site of activity for fractionated heparin

LOW MOLECULAR WEIGHT HEPARINS

Actions:

Pharmacology: Enoxaparin (fragments of 2000 to 8000 daltons) and dalteparin (fragments of 2000 to 9000 daltons) are low molecular weight heparins (LMWHs) obtained by depolymerization of unfractioned porcine heparin. They have antithrombotic properties. They enhance the inhibition of Factor Xa and thrombin by antithrombin III and potentiate preferentially the inhibition of coagulation factor Xa, while only slightly affecting thrombin and clotting time (eg, activated partial thromboplastin time [APTT] or prothrombin time [PT]).

Pharmacokinetics:

Low Molecular Weight Heparins Pharmacokinetics					
Drug	Mean Bioavailability (%)	Mean T_{max}[1] (hrs)	Mean Vd (L)	Mean Cl (ml/min)	Mean t½ (hrs)
Dalteparin	87	4	7	20	4
Enoxaparin	92	4	6	25	4.5

[1] Time to peak anti-Xa activity.

Indications:

Prevention of deep vein thrombosis (DVT) which may lead to pulmonary embolism following hip/knee surgery (enoxaparin) or for patients undergoing abdominal surgery who are at risk for thromboembolic complications (dalteparin).

Unlabeled uses: For systemic anticoagulation in venous and arterial thromboembolic complications.

Contraindications:

Hypersensitivity to LMWHs, heparin or pork products; active major bleeding; thrombocytopenia associated with positive in vitro tests for antiplatelet antibody in the presence of an LMWH.

Warnings:

Route of administration: For SC administration only: do not administer IM.

Interchangeability with heparin: LMWHs cannot be used interchangeably (unit for unit) with unfractionated heparin or other LMWHs.

Spinal/Epidural anesthesia: As with other anticoagulants, there have been rare cases of neuraxial hematomas reported with the concurrent use of **enoxaparin** and spinal/epidural anesthesia resulting in long-term or permanent paralysis. The risk of these rare events may be higher with the use of post-operative indwelling epidural catheters.

Hemorrhage: Use LMWHs, like other anticoagulants, with extreme caution in patients who have an increased risk of hemorrhage, such as those with severe uncontrolled hypertension, bacterial endocarditis, congenital or acquired bleeding disorders, active ulceration and angiodysplastic GI disease, hemorrhagic stroke or shortly after brain, spinal or ophthalmological surgery. As with other anticoagulants, bleeding can occur at any site during therapy with an LMWH. Search for a bleeding site if an unexpected drop in hematocrit or blood pressure occurs.

Thrombocytopenia: Thrombocytopenia occurred in < 1% of patients using **dalteparin** (platelet counts of < 50,000/mm^3 or < 100,000/mm^3) and in ≈ 2% of **enoxaparin**-treated patients (platelet counts < 100,000/mm^3 and > 50,000/mm^3).

Use extreme caution in patients with a history of heparin-induced thrombocytopenia. Closely monitor thrombocytopenia of any degree.

Renal/Hepatic function impairment: Use **dalteparin** with caution in patients with severe liver or kidney insufficiency.

Delayed elimination of **enoxaparin** may occur with renal function impairment. Use with caution.

Elderly: Delayed elimination of **enoxaparin** may occur. Use with caution.

Pregnancy: Category B. There are no adequate and well controlled studies in pregnant women. Use during pregnancy only if clearly needed.

Lactation: It is not known whether these drugs are excreted in breast milk. Exercise caution when administering to a nursing woman.

Children: Safety and efficacy in children have not been established.

Precautions:

Monitoring: Periodic routine complete blood counts, including platelet count and stool occult blood tests, are recommended during the course of treatment. No special monitoring of blood clotting times (eg, APTT) is needed.

LOW MOLECULAR WEIGHT HEPARINS

Retinopathy: Use **dalteparin** with caution in patients with hypertensive or diabetic retinopathy.

Thromboembolic event: If a thromboembolic event should occur despite LMWH prophylaxis, discontinue the drug and initiate appropriate therapy.

Special risk patients: Use with care in patients with bleeding diatheses, uncontrolled arterial hypertension or a history of recent GI ulceration and hemorrhage.

Drug Interactions:

Anticoagulants/Platelet inhibitors: Use LMWHs with care in patients receiving oral anticoagulants or platelet inhibitors (eg, aspirin, salicylates, NSAIDs, dipyridamole, sulfinpyrazone, ticlopidine) because of increased risk of bleeding.

Drug/Lab test interactions: Asymptomatic increases in transaminase levels (AST and ALT) greater than three times the upper limit of normal of the laboratory reference range have been reported (1.7% and 4.3% of patients, respectively, during treatment with **dalteparin** and 2 of 10 healthy subjects and in up to 4% of patients during treatment with **enoxaparin**). Similar significant increases in transaminase levels have been observed in patients treated with heparin and other LMWHs. Such elevations are fully reversible and are rarely associated with increases in bilirubin. Because transaminase determinations are important in the differential diagnosis of myocardial infarction, liver disease and pulmonary emboli, interpret elevations that might be caused by LMWHs with caution.

Adverse Reactions:

Hemorrhage: The incidence of hemorrhagic complications during prophylactic use has been low.

Enoxaparin: The following rates of major bleeding events have been reported during clinical trials with enoxaparin, heparin and placebo in patients undergoing knee/hip replacement surgery.

Major Bleeding Episode[1]: Enoxaparin vs Heparin vs Placebo			
Parameter	Enoxaparin (n = 786)	Heparin (n = 541)	Placebo (n = 50)
Dose	30 mg q 12 hr	15,000 units q 24 hr	
Incidence	4%	6%	4%

[1] Bleeding complication considered major if accompanied by a significant clinical event or if hemoglobin decreased by ≥ 2 g/dl or transfusion of ≥ 2 units of blood products was required.

Dalteparin – The most commonly reported side effect is hematoma at the injection site. The incidence of bleeding may increase with higher dosages.

The following table summarizes adverse bleeding events that occurred in clinical trials that studied dalteparin 2500 and 5000 IU administered once daily to abdominal surgery patients.

Adverse Bleeding Events with Dalteparin (%)				
Bleeding event	Dalteparin 2500 IU/24 hr	Dalteparin 5000 IU/24 hr	Heparin 10,000 IU/24 hr	Placebo
Post-op transfusion	5.7 to 8.9	12.1 to 15.9	7.9 to 12.7	7.1
Wound hematoma	0.1 to 3.4	0.4 to 2.4	1.2 to 3.9	2.6
Reoperation due to bleeding	0.2 to 1.3	0.8 to 1.2	0.4 to 0.8	1.3
Injection site hematoma	0.2 to 4.7	5.4 to 7.1	1.1 to 9.5	1.1

Thrombocytopenia:

Enoxaparin – Thrombocytopenia occurred in ≈ 2% of enoxaparin-treated patients (platelet counts 50,000 to 100,000/mm^3). Platelet counts < 50,000/mm^3 occurred at a rate of 0.1% in patients given enoxaparin.

Dalteparin – Thrombocytopenia (platelet counts of < 50,000 to 100,000/mm^3) occurred in < 1% of patients.

Miscellaneous:

Dalteparin – Pain at injection site for dalteparin 2500 IU qd and 5000 IU qd is 0 to 1.1% and 1.8 to 4.5%, respectively. Allergic reactions (eg, pruritus, rash, fever, injection site reaction, bullous eruption), skin necrosis (rare); anaphylactoid reactions (few cases).

Enoxaparin – Mild local irritation, pain, hematoma and erythema may follow SC injection; fever (5%); nausea (3%).

LOW MOLECULAR WEIGHT HEPARINS

Overdosage:

Symptoms: An excessive amount may lead to dose-related hemorrhagic complications.

Treatment: Effects of LMWHs may generally be stopped by the slow IV injection of protamine sulfate (1% solution) at a dose of 1 mg for every 100 anti-Xa IU of dalteparin or 1 mg for every mg of enoxaparin. A second infusion of 0.5 mg protamine per 100 anti-Xa IU of dalteparin or per 1 mg of enoxaparin may be administered if the APTT measured 2 to 4 hours after the first infusion remains prolonged. Even with these additional doses of protamine, the APTT may remain more prolonged than would usually be found following administration of conventional heparin. In all cases, the anti-Factor Xa activity is never completely neutralized (maximum, 60% to 75%). Take particular care to avoid overdosage with protamine.

Administration of protamine sulfate can cause severe hypotensive and anaphylactoid reactions. Because fatal reactions, often resembling anaphylaxis, have been reported, give protamine only when resuscitation techniques and treatment of anaphylactic shock are readily available.

Patient Information:

Contact the physician if you experience bleeding, bruising, dizziness, lightheadedness, itching, rash, fever, swelling or difficulty breathing.

Injections are given around the navel, upper thigh or buttocks. The injection site must be changed daily.

Use proper technique; inject deep under the skin, not into muscle.

If excessive bruising occurs at the injection site, it may be lessened by an ice cube massage of the site prior to injection.

ENOXAPARIN SODIUM

For complete prescribing information, refer to the Low Molecular Weight Heparins group monograph.

Indications:

Prevention of deep vein thrombosis (DVT): For prevention of DVT, which may lead to pulmonary embolism, following hip or knee replacement surgery.

Unlabeled uses: For systemic anticoagulation in venous and arterial thromboembolic complications.

Administration and Dosage:

Approved by the FDA on March 29, 1993.

Administration: Administer by SC injection only.

Adults: In patients undergoing hip replacement, the recommended dose is 30 mg twice daily administered by SC injection, with the initial dose given within 12 to 24 hours post-operatively provided hemostasis has been established. Continue treatment throughout the period of postoperative care until the risk of deep vein thrombosis has diminished. Up to 14 days administration has been well tolerated in controlled clinical trials. The average duration of administration is 7 to 10 days.

Screen all patients prior to prophylactic administration of enoxaparin to rule out a bleeding disorder. There is usually no need for daily monitoring of the effect of enoxaparin in patients with normal presurgical coagulation parameters.

Systemic anticoagulation: 1 mg/kg SC twice daily.

SC injection technique: Administer while patients are lying down; administer by deep SC injection. To avoid the loss of drug, do not expel the air bubble from the syringe before the injection. Alternate administration between the left and right anterolateral and left and right posterolateral abdominal wall. Introduce the whole length of the needle into a skin fold held between the thumb and forefinger; hold the skin fold throughout the injection. To minimize bruising, do not rub the injection site after completion of the injection.

Admixture incompatibility: Do not mix with other injections or infusions.

Storage/Stability: Store at ≤ 25°C (77°F). Do not freeze.

Rx	**Lovenox** (Rhone-Poulenc Rorer)	**Injection**: 30 mg/0.3 ml[1]	In packs of 10 prefilled syringes with a 26 gauge x ½ inch needle.

[1] Preservative free. Anti-Factor Xa activity of ≈ 3000 IU (with reference to the WHO First International Low Molecular Weight Heparin Reference Standard).

DALTEPARIN SODIUM

For complete prescribing information, refer to the Low Molecular Weight Heparins group monograph.

Indications:

Prophylaxis of deep vein thrombosis (DVT): For prophylaxis of DVT, which may lead to pulmonary embolism, in patients undergoing abdominal surgery who are at risk for thromboembolic complications.

Unlabeled uses: For systemic anticoagulation in venous and arterial thromboembolic complications.

Administration and Dosage:

Approved by the FDA on December 22, 1994 (1S classification).

Administration: Dalteparin is administered by SC injection. Do not administer by IM injection.

Adults: In patients undergoing abdominal surgery with a risk of thromboembolic complications, administer 2500 IU each day, SC only, starting 1 to 2 hours prior to surgery and repeated once daily for 5 to 10 days postoperatively. Dosage adjustment and routine monitoring of coagulation parameters are not required if these dosage and administration recommendations are followed.

High risk patients: In patients at high risk for thromboembolic complications (eg, malignancy), administer 5000 IU, SC only, the evening before surgery and repeat once daily for 5 to 10 days postoperatively. Alternatively, in patients with malignancy, the first 5000 IU dose can be administered as 2500 IU SC 1 to 2 hours prior to surgery with an additional 2500 IU SC dose 12 hours later and then 5000 IU once daily for 5 to 10 days.

Systemic anticoagulation: 200 IU/kg SC daily or 100 IU/kg SC twice daily.

SC injection technique: Administer while patient is sitting or lying down. Administer by deep SC injection. Dalteparin may be injected in a U-shaped area around the navel, the upper outer side of the thigh or the upper outer quadrangle of the buttock. Vary the injection site daily. When the area around the navel or the thigh is used, use the thumb and forefinger to lift up a fold of skin while giving the injection. Insert the entire length of the needle at a 45° to 90° angle.

Admixture incompatibility: Do not mix with other injections or infusions unless specific compatibility data are available that support such mixing.

Storage/Stability: Store at controlled room temperature, 20° to 25°C (68° to 77°F).

Rx	**Fragmin** (Pharmacia)	**Solution:** 2500 anti-Factor Xa IU/0.2 ml	Preservative free.
		5000 anti-Factor Xa IU/0.2 ml	Preservative free. In single dose prefilled syringes.

Glycosaminoglycans

DANAPAROID SODIUM

Actions:

Pharmacology: Danaparoid sodium injection is an antithrombotic agent. The average molecular weight is ≈ 5500 daltons. Danaparoid is a low molecular weight sulfated glycosaminoglycans (low molecular weight heparinoid) extracted from porcine mucosa. Danaparoid prevents fibrin formation in the coagulation pathway via thrombin generation inhibition by anti-Xa and anti-IIa (thrombin) effects. The anti-Xa and anti-IIa activity ratio is > 22; inactivation of factor Xa is mediated by antithrombin-III (AT-III) while factor IIa inactivation is mediated by both AT-III and heparin cofactor II (HC II). Danaparoid has only minor effects on platelet function and platelet aggregability.

Because of its predominant anti-Xa activity, danaparoid has little effect on clotting assays (eg, prothrombin time [PT], partial thromboplastin time [PTT]). Danaparoid has minimal effect on fibrinolytic activity and bleeding time.

Cross-sensitivity studies involving patients with Type II heparin-induced thrombocytopenia indicate that danaparoid has a much lower in vitro cross-reactivity in platelet aggregation tests than the low molecular weight heparins and dalteparin sodium.

Pharmacokinetics:

Absorption – By SC route of administration, danaparoid is ≈ 100% bioavailable, compared with the same dose administered IV. The maximum anti-Xa activity (T_{max}) occurred at ≈ 2 to 5 hours.

For single SC doses of 750, 1500, 2250 and 3250 anti-Xa units of danaparoid, the mean peak plasma anti-Xa activities were 102.4, 206.1, 283.9 and 403.4 mU/ml, respectively.

Excretion – The mean value for the terminal half-life was ≈ 24 hours and the clearance was 0.36 L/hr. Clearance was affected by body surface area in that the higher the body surface, the faster the clearance. Danaparoid is mainly eliminated via the kidneys. In patients with severely impaired renal function, the half-life of elimination of plasma anti-Xa activity may be prolonged. Monitor such patients carefully.

Clinical trials: In a European multicenter double-blind trial, danaparoid was compared with placebo in 196 patients undergoing elective hip replacement surgery. The administration of danaparoid for 7 to 14 days post-operatively significantly reduced the overall incidence of DVT to 15% (15/98 patients), compared with the incidence of 57% (56/98 patients) observed with placebo.

In a US multicenter trial, danaparoid was compared with warfarin in 396 patients undergoing elective hip replacement. A significant reduction in the overall incidence of DVT was observed with danaparoid (14.6%; 29/199 patients) compared with warfarin (26.9%; 53/197 patients).

Indications:

Prophylaxis of post-operative deep venous thrombosis (DVT): For the prophylaxis of post-operative DVT, which may lead to pulmonary embolism (PE), in patients undergoing elective hip replacement surgery.

Unlabeled uses: Danaparoid has been used clinically in the treatment of thromboembolism and to produce anticoagulation during hemodialysis, hemofiltration during cardiovascular operation and in pregnant patients at increased risk of thrombosis. It may represent a useful replacement for heparin in patients with heparin-induced thrombocytopenia, but further investigation will be necessary if the difficulties in monitoring and neutralizing its anticoagulant effects are to be overcome.

Contraindications:

Severe hemorrhagic diathesis (eg, hemophilia and idiopathic thrombocytopenic purpura); active major bleeding state, including hemorrhagic stroke in the acute phase; hypersensitivity to danaparoid; Type II thrombocytopenia associated with a positive in vitro test for antiplatelet antibody in the presence of danaparoid; patients with known hypersensitivity to pork products.

Warnings:

IM injection: Danaparoid is not intended for IM administration.

Interchangeability: Because a specific standard for the anti-Xa activity of danaparoid is used, the anti-Xa unit activity of danaparoid is not equivalent to that described for heparin or low-molecular weight heparin. Therefore, danaparoid cannot be dosed interchangeably (unit for unit) with either heparin or low-molecular weight heparins.

Hemorrhage: Hemorrhage can occur at virtually any site in patients receiving danaparoid. An unexplained fall in hematocrit or fall in blood pressure should lead to serious consideration of a hemorrhagic event. Use danaparoid, like anticoagulants, with extreme caution in disease states in which there is increased risk of hemor-

Glycosaminoglycans

DANAPAROID SODIUM

rhage, such as severe uncontrolled hypertension, acute bacterial endocarditis, congenital or acquired bleeding disorders, active ulcerative and angiodysplastic gastrointestinal disease, non-hemorrhagic stroke, shortly after brain, spinal or ophthalmological surgery and post-operative indwelling epidural catheter use.

Renal/Hepatic function impairment: Consider the risks and benefits of danaparoid carefully before use in patients with severely impaired renal function or hemorrhagic disorders (see Administration and Dosage).

Pregnancy: Category B. There are no adequate and well controlled studies in pregnant women. Use danaparoid during pregnancy only if clearly needed.

Lactation: It is not known whether danaparoid is excreted in breast milk. Exercise caution when danaparoid is administered to a nursing woman.

Children: Safety and efficacy in pediatric patients have not been established.

Precautions:

Monitoring: Danaparoid has only a small effect on factor IIa (thrombin) activity, therefore routine coagulation tests (eg, prothrombin time [PT], activated partial thromboplastin time [APTT], kaolin cephalin clotting time [KCCT], whole blood clotting time [WBCT] and thrombin time [TT]) are unsuitable for monitoring danaparoid activity at recommended doses.

Periodic complete blood counts (CBC), including platelet count, and stool occult blood tests are recommended during the course of treatment.

Hypersensitivity: Danaparoid contains sodium sulfite which may cause allergic-type reactions, including anaphylactic symptoms and life-threatening or less severe asthmatic episodes in certain susceptible people. The overall prevalence of sulfite sensitivity in the general population is unknown and probably low. Sulfite sensitivity is seen more frequently in asthmatic than in non-asthmatic patients.

Thrombocytopenia: Danaparoid shows a low cross-reactivity with antiplatelet antibodies in individuals with Type II heparin-induced thrombocytopenia. No cases of white-clot syndrome or cases of Type II thrombocytopenia have been reported in clinical studies for the prophylaxis of DVT in patients receiving multiple doses of danaparoid ≥ 14 days.

Drug Interactions:

Anticoagulants: Use with caution in patients receiving oral anticoagulants or platelet inhibitors. Monitoring of anticoagulant activity of oral anticoagulants by prothrombin time and thrombotest is unreliable ≤ 5 hours after danaparoid administration.

Adverse Reactions:

The following table summarizes adverse bleeding events that occurred in clinical trials which studied danaparoid injection compared with placebo, warfarin and other agents (heparin, heparin/DHE, acetylsalicylic acid, dextran and low-molecular weight heparins).

Glycosaminoglycans

DANAPAROID SODIUM

Blood Loss and Transfusions DVT and PE Prophylaxis for Orthopedic Hip Surgery All Patients Treated

Blood loss and transfusions	Total	Danaparoid	Placebo	Warfarin	Other[1]
Intraoperative blood loss (ml)					
Males	596	330	27	141	98
Females	1259	686	66	219	288
Postoperative blood loss (ml)					
Males	580	318	45	88	129
Females	1256	639	122	80	415
Transfusions (units PRBCs)					
Males	462	258	35	87	82
Females	1152	604	92	177	279

[1] "Other" includes the following active reference agents: Heparin; heparin/DHE; acetylsalicylic acid; dextran; low-molecular weight heparins.

Danaparoid Adverse Reactions

Adverse experience	Danaparoid n = 645	Placebo n = 135	Warfarin n = 243	Other[1] n = 168
CNS				
Insomnia	20	0	32	0
Headache	17	1	13	0
Dizziness	15	0	14	0
GI				
Nausea	92	3	78	8
Constipation	73	0	70	2
Vomiting	19	3	20	3
Dermatologic				
Rash	31	0	18	2
Pruritus	25	1	14	0
Miscellaneous				
Fever	143	1	138	3
Injection site pain	49	4	0	34
Peripheral edema	21	0	19	4
Joint disorder	17	0	15	0
Urinary tract infection	17	1	5	5
Edema	17	0	14	2
Asthenia	15	0	10	1
Anemia	14	3	5	5
Urinary retention	13	0	14	1

[1] "Other" includes the following active reference agents: Heparin; heparin/DHE; acetylsalicylic acid; dextran; low-molecular weight heparins.

Incidence of Adverse Experiences (≥ 2%) DVT and PE Prophylaxis Indication

Adverse experience	Danaparoid n = 2383 (%)	Placebo n = 276 (%)	Warfarin n = 421 (%)	Other[1] n = 1163 (%)
Injection site pain	327 (13.7)	53 (19.2)	0 (0)	153 (13.2)
Pain	207 (8.7)	0 (0)	202 (48)	20 (1.7)
Fever	173 (7.3)	1 (0.4)	150 (35.6)	21 (1.8)

Glycosaminoglycans

DANAPAROID SODIUM

Incidence of Adverse Experiences (≥ 2%) DVT and PE Prophylaxis Indication				
Adverse experience	Danaparoid n = 2383 (%)	Placebo n = 276 (%)	Warfarin n = 421 (%)	Other[1] n = 1163 (%)
Nausea	98 (4.1)	3 (1.1)	79 (18.8)	13 (1.1)
Urinary tract infection	96 (4)	3 (1.1)	27 (6.4)	65 (5.6)
Constipation	83 (3.5)	0 (0)	73 (17.3)	3 (0.3)
Rash	51 (2.1)	0 (0)	25 (5.9)	5 (0.4)
Infection	51 (2.1)	3 (1.1)	0 (0)	47 (4)

[1] "Other" includes the following active reference agents: Heparin; heparin/DHE; acetylsalicylic acid; dextran; low-molecular weight heparins.

Overdosage:

Single SC doses of danaparoid at 3800 anti-Xa units/kg (20.5 times the recommended human dose) and 15200 anti-Xa units/kg (82 times the recommended human dose) were lethal to female and male rats, respectively. Symptoms of acute toxicity after IV dosing were respiratory depression, prostration and twitching.

Symptoms: Accidental overdosage following administration of danaparoid may lead to bleeding complications.

Treatment: The effects of danaparoid on anti-Xa activity cannot be antagonized with any known agent at this time. Although protamine sulfate partially neutralizes the anti-Xa activity of danaparoid and can be safely coadministered, there is no evidence that protamine sulfate is capable of reducing severe non-surgical bleeding during treatment with danaparoid. In the event of serious bleeding, discontinue danaparoid and administer blood or blood product transfusions as needed. Withdrawal of danaparoid may be expected to restore the coagulation balance without rebound phenomenon.

Administration and Dosage:

Approved by the FDA on December 24, 1996.

Usual adult dosage: In patients undergoing hip replacement surgery, the recommended dose of danaparoid is 750 anti-Xa units twice daily administered by SC injection beginning 1 to 4 hours pre-operatively, and then not sooner than 2 hours after surgery. Continue treatment throughout the period of post-operative care until the risk of deep vein thrombosis has diminished. The average duration of administration in clinical trials was 7 to 10 days, up to 14 days.

Renal function impairment: Carefully monitor patients with serum creatinine ≥ 2 mg/dl.

Administration: Administer SC and not by IM injection. SC injection technique: Have the patient lie down and administer by deep SC injection using a fine needle (25 to 26 gauge) to minimize tissue trauma. Alternate administration between the left and right anterolateral and left and right posterolateral abdominal wall. Introduce the whole length of the needle into a skin fold held gently between the thumb and forefinger; hold the skin fold throughout the injection and neither pinch nor rub afterwards.

Storage/Stability: Store ampules at a temperature of 2° to 30°C (36° to 86°F). Store syringes at a refrigerated temperature of 2° to 8°C (36° to 46°F). Protect from light.

Rx	**Organan** (Organon)	**Injection:** 750 anti-Xa units/0.6 ml	Sodium sulfite. In single-dose ampules and prefilled syringes. In 10s.

Glycosaminoglycans

HEPARIN

Actions:

Pharmacology: Commercial preparations of heparin are derived from bovine lung or porcine intestinal mucosa; although chemical and biological differences exist, there are no clinical differences in the antithrombotic effects. The anticoagulant potency of heparin is standardized by bioassay and is expressed in "units" of activity. Because the number of units per milligram vary, express dosage only in "units." (Heparin sodium should contain not less than 140 heparin units/mg.)

The major rate-limiting step in the coagulation cascade is the activation of factor X, which is involved in both intrinsic and extrinsic pathways (refer to the Anticoagulant introduction). Small amounts of heparin in combination with antithrombin III (ATIII) inhibit thrombosis by inactivating factor Xa and inhibiting the conversion of prothrombin to thrombin. Once active thrombosis has developed, larger amounts of heparin in combination with heparin cofactor (HC-II) can inhibit further coagulation by inactivating thrombin and preventing the conversion of fibrinogen to fibrin. In combination with ATIII, heparin inactivates activated coagulation factors IX, X, XI, XII, plasmin, kallikrein and thrombin, inhibiting conversion of fibrinogen to fibrin. The heparin-antithrombin III complex is 100 to 1000 times more potent as an anticoagulant than antithrombin III alone. Heparin also prevents the formation of a stable fibrin clot by inhibiting the activation of factor XIII (the fibrin stabilizing factor). Other effects include the inhibition of thrombin-induced activation of factors V and VIII and variable inhibitions of platelet aggregates.

Commercial products contain both low and high molecular weight heparin fractions. Low molecular weight heparin has a greater inhibitory effect on factor Xa and less antithrombin activity than the high molecular weight fraction.

Heparin inhibits reactions that lead to clotting, but does not significantly alter the concentration of the normal clotting factors of blood. Although clotting time is prolonged by full therapeutic doses, in most cases it is not measurably affected by low doses of heparin. Bleeding time is usually unaffected. The drug has no fibrinolytic activity; it will not lyse existing clots, but it can prevent extension of existing clots.

Heparin also enhances lipoprotein lipase release, (which clears plasma of circulating lipids), increases circulating free fatty acids and reduces lipoprotein levels.

Pharmacokinetics:

Absorption/Distribution – Heparin is not adsorbed from the GI tract and must be given IV or SC. An IV bolus results in immediate anticoagulant effects, the anticoagulant response to heparin at therapeutic doses is not linear but increases disproportionately both in its intensity and duration with increasing dose. Peak plasma levels of heparin are achieved 2 to 4 hours following SC use, although there are considerable individual variations. Once absorbed, heparin is distributed in plasma and is extensively and nonspecifically protein bound.

Metabolism/Excretion – Heparin is rapidly cleared from plasma with an average half-life of 30 to 180 minutes. Half-life is dose-dependent and non-linear and may be disproportionately prolonged at higher doses (30 min at 25 u/kg versus150 minutes at 400 u/kg). Heparin is partially metabolized by liver heparinase and the reticuloendothelial system. There may be a secondary site of metabolism in the kidneys. Apparent volume of distribution is 40 to 60 ml/kg. In patients with deep venous thrombosis, plasma clearance is more rapid and half-life is shorter than in patients with pulmonary embolism. Heparin half-life may be prolonged in liver disease. Heparin is excreted in urine as unchanged drug (up to 50%) particularly after large doses. Some urinary degradation products have anticoagulant activity.

Indications:

Thrombosis/Embolism: Prophylaxis and treatment of venous thrombosis and its extension; pulmonary embolism; peripheral arterial embolism; atrial fibrillation with embolization.

Coagulopathies: Diagnosis and treatment of acute and chronic consumption coagulopathies (disseminated intravascular coagulation [DIC]).

Prophylaxis: Low dose regimen for prevention of postoperative deep venous thrombosis (DVT) and pulmonary embolism in patients undergoing major abdominothoracic surgery or patients who are at risk of developing thromboembolic disease.

According to National Institutes of Health Consensus Development Conference, low-dose heparin is treatment of choice as prophylaxis for DVT and pulmonary embolism in urology patients > 40 years old; pregnant patients with prior thromboembolism; stroke patients; those with heart failure, acute MI or pulmonary infection; also recommended as suggested prophylaxis in high-risk surgery patients, moderate and high-risk gynecologic patients without malignancy, neurology patients with extracranial problems and patients with severe musculoskeletal trauma.

Glycosaminoglycans

HEPARIN

Clotting prevention: Prevention of clotting in arterial and heart surgery, blood transfusions, extracorporeal circulation, dialysis procedures and blood samples.

Unlabeled uses: Prophylaxis of left ventricular thrombi and cerebrovascular accidents post-MI.

Continuous infusion for treatment of myocardial ischemia in unstable angina refractory to conventional treatment. Heparin decreases the number of anginal attacks and silent ischemic episodes and reduces the daily duration of ischemia. Intermittent heparin is not as effective.

Prevention of cerebral thrombosis in the evolving stroke.

As an adjunct in treatment of coronary occlusion with acute myocardial infarction (MI). Although there is some controversy regarding the efficacy of heparin therapy with concurrent antiplatelet therapy (eg, aspirin) in the prevention of rethrombosis/reocclusion after primary thrombolysis with thrombolytics (eg, alteplase, anistreplase, streptokinase) during acute MI, it is recommended by the American College of Cardiology and the American Heart Association. Generally, administer heparin IV immediately after thrombolytic therapy, usually within 2 to 8 hours (depending on the thrombolytic used), and maintain the infusion for at least 24 hours. Begin aspirin therapy immediately as soon as the patient is admitted, and continue its administration.

Contraindications:

Hypersensitivity to heparin; severe thrombocytopenia; uncontrolled bleeding (except when it is due to DIC); any patient for whom suitable blood coagulation tests cannot be performed at the appropriate intervals (there is usually no need to monitor coagulation parameters in patients receiving low-dose heparin).

Warnings:

IM administration should be avoided because of the danger of hematoma formation.

Hemorrhage can occur at virtually any site in patients receiving heparin. An unexplained fall in hematocrit, fall in blood pressure or any other unexplained symptom should lead to serious consideration of a hemorrhagic event. An overly prolonged coagulation test or bleeding can usually be controlled by withdrawing the drug. Signs and symptoms will vary according to the location and extent of bleeding and may be present as paralysis, headache, chest, abdomen, joint or other pain, shortness of breath, difficulty breathing or swallowing, unexplained swelling or unexplained shock. GI or urinary tract bleeding may indicate an underlying occult lesion. Certain hemorrhagic complications may be difficult to detect.

Adrenal hemorrhage resulting in acute adrenal insufficiency has occurred. Discontinue therapy in patients who develop signs and symptoms of acute adrenal hemorrhage or insufficiency. Initiation of therapy should not depend on laboratory confirmation of diagnosis, since any delay in an acute situation may result in death.

Ovarian (corpus luteum) hemorrhage has developed in a number of reproductive age women receiving anticoagulants. If unrecognized, this may be fatal.

Retroperitoneal hemorrhage may occur.

Germinal matrix-intraventricular hemorrhage occurs fourfold higher in low-birth-weight infants receiving heparin therapy.

Use heparin with extreme caution in disease states in which there is increased danger of hemorrhage. These include:

Cardiovascular – Subacute bacterial endocarditis; severe hypertension.

CNS – During and immediately following spinal tap, spinal anesthesia or major surgery, especially of the brain, spinal cord or eye.

Hematologic – Hemophilia; some vascular purpuras; thrombocytopenia.

GI – Ulcerative lesions, diverticulitis or ulcerative colitis; continuous tube drainage of the stomach or small intestine.

Obstetric – Menstruation.

Other – Liver disease with impaired hemostasis; severe renal disease.

Hyperlipidemia: Heparin may increase free fatty acid serum levels by induction of lipoprotein lipase. The catabolism of serum lipoproteins by this enzyme produces lipid fragments rapidly processed by the liver. Patients with dysbetalipoproteinemia (type III) cannot catabolize the lipid fragments, resulting in hyperlipidemia.

Benzyl alcohol, contained in some of these products as a preservative, has been associated with a fatal "gasping syndrome" in premature infants.

Resistance: Increased resistance to the drug is frequently encountered in fever, thrombosis, thrombophlebitis, infections with thrombosing tendencies, MI, cancer and postoperative states.

Glycosaminoglycans

HEPARIN

Thrombocytopenia has occurred in patients receiving heparin with a reported incidence of up to 30%. The development of thrombocytopenia does not necessarily imply a causal relationship. Often patients have other potential causes for thrombocytopenia; they can be ill, receiving several medications or in a postoperative phase. Exclude these potential causes for thrombocytopenia before implicating heparin. The incidence of heparin-associated thrombocytopenia is higher with bovine than with porcine heparin (15.6% vs 5.8%). The severity also appears to be related to heparin dosage, with low-dose therapy resulting in fewer complications.

Early thrombocytopenia (Type I) develops 2 to 3 days after starting heparin, tends to be mild and is due to a direct action of heparin on platelets.

Delayed thrombocytopenia (Type II) develops 7 to 12 days after either low-dose or full-dose heparin, can have serious consequences and may reflect the presence of an immunoglobulin that induces platelet aggregation.

Mild thrombocytopenia (platelet count > 100,000/mm^3) may remain stable or reverse even if heparin is continued. However, closely monitor thrombocytopenia of any degree. If a count falls < 100,000/mm^3 or if recurrent thrombosis develops, discontinue heparin. If continued heparin therapy is essential, administration of heparin from a different organ source can be reinstituted with caution.

White clot syndrome – Patients may develop new thrombus formation in association with thrombocytopenia resulting from irreversible aggregation of platelets induced by heparin, the so-called "white clot syndrome." The process may lead to severe thromboembolic complications (eg, skin necrosis, gangrene of the extremities possibly leading to amputation, MI, pulmonary embolism, stroke, possibly death). Monitor platelet counts before and during therapy. If significant thrombocytopenia occurs, immediately terminate heparin and institute other therapeutic measures.

Hypersensitivity: Give heparin to patients with documented hypersensitivity only in life-threatening situations. Before a therapeutic dose is given, a trial dose may be advisable. Have epinephrine 1:1000 immediately available. Refer to Management of Acute Hypersensitivity Reactions.

Vasospastic reactions may develop 6 to 10 days after starting therapy and last 4 to 6 hours. The affected limb is painful, ischemic and cyanotic. An artery to this limb may have been recently catheterized. After repeated injections, the reaction may gradually increase to generalized vasospasm with cyanosis, tachypnea, feeling of oppression and headache. Protamine sulfate has no marked effect. Itching and burning, especially on the plantar side of the feet, is possibly based on a similar allergic vasospastic reaction. Chest pain, elevated blood pressure, arthralgias or headache have also been reported in the absence of definite peripheral vasospasm.

Elderly: A higher incidence of bleeding has occurred in women > 60 years of age.

Pregnancy: Category C. Safety for use during pregnancy has not been established. Heparin does not cross the placenta. However, its use during pregnancy has been associated with 13% to 22% unfavorable outcomes, including stillbirths and prematurity. This contrasts with a 31% incidence with coumarin derivatives. Heparin is probably the preferred anticoagulant during pregnancy, but it is not risk free. Heparin-induced osteoporosis has occurred, including collapse of vertebrae. Use with caution during pregnancy, especially during the last trimester and during the immediate postpartum period, because of the risk of maternal hemorrhage.

Lactation: Heparin is not excreted in breast milk.

Children: See Administration and Dosage. Safety and efficacy have not been determined in newborns; germinal matrix intraventricular hemorrhage occurs more often in low-birth-weight infants receiving heparin.

Use heparin lock flush solution with caution in infants with disease states in which there is an increased danger of hemorrhage. The use of the 100 unit/ml concentration is not advised because of bleeding risk, especially in low-birth-weight infants.

Precautions:

Monitoring: The most common test used to monitor heparin's effect is Activated Partial Thromboplastin Time (APTT). The APTT is widely used, quick, easily done and reproducible. Other tests used include Activated Coagulation Time (ACT) and Lee White-Whole Blood Clotting Time (WBCT). The ACT is also rapid and readily available. The WBCT is time consuming and unreliable; it is used as a standard with which to compare newer tests. If the coagulation test is unduly prolonged or if hemorrhage occurs, discontinue the drug promptly (see Overdosage). Perform periodic platelet counts, hematocrit and tests for occult blood in stool during the entire course of therapy, regardless of route of administration.

HEPARIN

Hyperkalemia may develop, probably due to induced hypoaldosteronism. Use with caution in patients with diabetes or renal insufficiency. Monitor patient closely.

Drug Interactions:

Heparin Drug Interactions			
Precipitant drug	Object drug*		Description
Cephalosporins	Heparin	↑	Several parenteral cephalosporins have caused coagulopathies; this might be additive with heparin, possibly increasing the risk of bleeding.
Nitroglycerin	Heparin	↓	The pharmacologic effects of heparin may be decreased, although information on the interaction is conflicting.
Penicillins	Heparin	↑	Parenteral penicillins can produce alterations in platelet aggregation and coagulation tests. These effects might be additive with heparin, possibly increasing the risk of bleeding.
Platelet inhibitors (eg, ibuprofen, indomethacin, dipyridamole, hydroxychloroquine, NSAIDs, ticlopidine phenylbutazone, aspirin, dextran)	Heparin	↑	An increased risk of bleeding is possible during concurrent administration due to interference with platelet aggregation.
Digitalis tetracyclines nicotine antihistamines	Heparin	↓	May partially counteract the anticoagulant action of heparin sodium.
Streptokinase	Heparin	↓	Relative resistance to heparin anticoagulation following administration of streptokinase as a systemic thrombolytic agent may occur.

* ↑ = Object drug increased. ↓ = Object drug decreased.

Drug/Lab test interactions: Significant elevations of **aminotransferase** (AST and ALT) levels have occurred in a high percentage of patients. Cautiously interpret aminotransferase increases that might be caused by heparin.

Adverse Reactions:

Hemorrhage is the chief complication (≤ 10%). See Warnings.

Local: Avoid IM use. Local irritation, erythema, mild pain, hematoma or ulceration may follow deep SC use, but are more common after IM use. Histamine-like reactions and subcutaneous and cutaneous necrosis have been observed.

Hypersensitivity:

Most common – Chills; fever; urticaria.

Rare – Asthma; rhinitis; lacrimation; headache; nausea; vomiting; shock; anaphylactoid reactions. Allergic vasospastic reactions with painful, ischemic, cyanotic limbs may develop 6 to 10 days after starting therapy and last 4 to 6 hours. Whether these are identical to thrombocytopenia-associated complications is undetermined. See Warnings.

Miscellaneous: Thrombocytopenia (see Warnings); osteoporosis (after long-term, high doses); cutaneous necrosis, suppressed aldosterone synthesis, delayed transient alopecia, priapism, rebound hyperlipidemia (after discontinuation).

Overdosage:

Symptoms: Bleeding is the chief sign of heparin overdosage. Nosebleeds, hematuria or tarry stools may be the first sign of bleeding. Easy bruising or petechial formations may precede frank bleeding.

Treatment: Protamine sulfate (1% solution) will neutralize heparin (see individual monograph). Each mg of protamine neutralizes ≈ 100 USP heparin units.

Administration and Dosage:

Give by intermittent IV injection, continuous IV infusion or deep SC (ie, above the iliac crest of abdominal fat layer) injection. Avoid IM injection.

Glycosaminoglycans

HEPARIN

Continuous IV infusion is generally preferable due to the higher incidence of bleeding complications with other routes.

Adjust dosage according to coagulation test results prior to each injection. Dosage is adequate when WBCT is ≈ 2.5 to 3 times control value, or when APTT is 1.5 to 2 times normal.

When given by continuous IV infusion, perform coagulation tests every 4 hours in the early stages. When administered by intermittent IV infusion, perform coagulation tests before each dose during early stages and at appropriate intervals thereafter. After deep SC injection, perform tests 4 to 6 hours after the injections.

General heparin dosage guidelines: Although dosage must be individualized, the following guidelines may be used:

Heparin Dosage Guidelines

Method of administration	Frequency	Recommended dose[1]
Subcutaneous[2]	Initial dose	10,000 – 20,000 units[3]
	Every 8 hours	8,000 – 10,000 units
	Every 12 hours	15,000 – 20,000 units
Intermittent IV	Initial dose	10,000 units[4]
	Every 4 to 6 hours	5,000 – 10,000 units[4]
IV Infusion	Initial dose	In 1000 ml 0.9% sodium chloride.
	Continuous	20,000 – 40,000 units/day[3]

[1] Based on a 68 kg (150 lb) patient.
[2] Use a concentrated solution.
[3] Immediately preceded by IV loading dose of 5,000 units.
[4] Administer undiluted or in 50 to 100 ml 0.9% NaCl.

Heparin Dosage for DVT Treatment

PTT (secs)	Action	Rate change
< 45	5,000 units bolus	increase by 250 units/hr
45 to 54	—	increase by 150 units/hr
55 to 85	—	no change
86 to 110	stop infusion × 1 hr	decrease by 150 units/hr
> 110	stop infusion × 1 hr	decrease by 250 units/hr

Children: In general, the following dosage schedule may be used as a guideline:

Initial dose – 50 units/kg IV bolus.

Maintenance dose – 100 units/kg/dose IV drip every 4 hours, or 20,000 units/m^2/24 hours continuous IV infusion.

Low-dose prophylaxis of postoperative thromboembolism: Low-dose heparin prophylaxis, prior to and after surgery, will reduce the incidence of postoperative DVT in the legs and clinical pulmonary embolism. Give 5000 units SC 2 hours before surgery and 5000 units every 8 to 12 hours thereafter for 7 days or until the patient is fully ambulatory, whichever is longer. Administer by deep SC injection above the iliac crest or abdominal fat layer, arm or thigh using a concentrated solution. Use a fine guage needle (25 to 26 guage) to minimize tissue trauma. Reserve such prophylaxis for patients > 40 years of age undergoing major surgery. Exclude patients on oral anticoagulants or drugs that affect platelet function (see Drug Interactions) or in patients with bleeding disorders, brain or spinal cord injuries, spinal anesthesia, eye surgery or potentially sanguineous operations.

If bleeding occurs during or after surgery, discontinue heparin and neutralize with protamine sulfate. If clinical evidence of thromboembolism develops despite low-dose prophylaxis, give full therapeutic doses of anticoagulants until contraindicated. Prior to heparinization, rule out bleeding disorders; perform appropriate coagulation tests just prior to surgery. Coagulation test values should be normal or only slightly elevated at these times.

Surgery of the heart and blood vessels: Give an initial dose of not less than 150 units/kg to patients undergoing total body perfusion for open heart surgery. Often, 300 units/kg is used for procedures < 60 minutes and 400 units/kg is used for procedures > 60 minutes.

Extracorporeal dialysis: Follow equipment manufacturers' operating directions.

Glycosaminoglycans

HEPARIN

Blood transfusion: Add 400 to 600 units per 100 ml whole blood to prevent coagulation. Add 7500 units to 100 ml 0.9% Sodium Chloride Injection (or 75,000 units/L of 0.9% Sodium Chloride Injection); from this sterile solution, add 6 to 8 ml per 100 ml whole blood. Perform leukocyte counts on heparinized blood within 2 hours of addition of heparin. Do not use heparinized blood for isoagglutinin, complement, erythrocyte fragility tests or platelet counts.

Laboratory samples: Add 70 to 150 units per 10 to 20 ml sample of whole blood to prevent coagulation of sample. (See *Blood transfusion*.)

Clearing intermittent infusion (heparin lock) sets: To prevent clot formation in a heparin lock set, inject dilute heparin solution (Heparin Lock Flush Solution, USP; or a 10 to 100 units/ml heparin solution) via the injection hub to fill the entire set to the needle tip. Replace this solution each time the heparin lock is used. Aspirate before administering any solution via the lock to confirm patency and location of needle or catheter tip. If the administered drug is incompatible with heparin, flush the entire heparin lock set with sterile water or normal saline before and after the medication is administered; following the second flush, the dilute heparin solution may be reinstilled into the set. Consult the set manufacturer's instructions.

Because repeated injections of small doses of heparin can alter APTT, obtain a baseline APTT prior to insertion of a heparin lock set.

Preparation of solution: Slight discoloration does not alter potency.

When heparin is added to infusion solution for continuous IV administration, invert container ≥ 6 times to ensure adequate mixing and to prevent pooling of heparin.

Converting to oral anticoagulant therapy: Perform baseline coagulation tests to determine prothrombin activity when heparin activity is too low to affect prothrombin time (PT) or the International Normalized Ratio (INR). For immediate anticoagulant effect, give heparin in usual therapeutic doses. When results of initial prothrombin determinations are known, initiate the oral anticoagulant in the usual amount. Perform coagulation tests and prothrombin activity at appropriate intervals. To ensure continuous anticoagulation, continue full heparin therapy for several days after PT or INR has reached therapeutic range. Heparin therapy may then be discontinued. Measure PT or INR ≥ 6 hours after last IV bolus dose and 24 hours after last SC dose of heparin. If continuous IV heparin infusion is used, PT or INR can usually be measured at any time. When prothrombin activity reaches the desired therapeutic range, discontinue heparin and continue oral anticoagulants.

HEPARIN SODIUM INJECTION, USP

For complete prescribing information, refer to the Heparin Group Monograph.
A sterile solution of heparin sodium in water for injection.

		Multiple Dose Vials-	
Rx	**Heparin Sodium** (Various, eg, Elkins-Sinn, Fujisawa, Pasadena, Solopak, Pharmacia & Upjohn)	**Injection:** 1000 units per ml	In 1, 10 and 30 ml vials.
Rx	**Heparin Sodium** (Abbott)	**Injection:** 2000 units per ml	In 5 and 10 ml vials.
Rx	**Heparin Sodium** (Abbott)	**Injection:** 2500 units per ml	In 5 and 10 ml vials.
Rx	**Heparin Sodium** (Various, eg, Elkins-Sinn, Fujisawa, Pasadena, Schein, Pharmacia & Upjohn, URL)	**Injection:** 5000 units per ml	In 1 and 10 ml vials.
Rx	**Heparin Sodium** (Various, eg, Elkins-Sinn, Lilly, Fujisawa, Pasadena, Schein, Phamacia & Upjohn)	**Injection:** 10,000 units per ml	In 0.5, 1, 4, 5 and 10 ml vials.

Glycosaminoglycans

HEPARIN SODIUM INJECTION, USP

Rx	**Heparin Sodium** (Various, eg, Pasadena, Schein)	**Injection:** 20,000 units per ml	In 1, 2 and 5 ml vials.
Rx	**Heparin Sodium** (Various, eg, Pasadena, Schein)	**Injection:** 40,000 units per ml	In 1, 2 and 5 ml vials.
		Single Dose Ampules and Vials	
Rx	**Heparin Sodium** (Various, eg, Fujisawa)	**Injection:**1000 units per ml.	In 1 ml vials.
Rx	**Heparin Sodium** (Various, eg, Fujisawa, Sanofi Winthrop)	**Injection:** 5000 units per ml	In 1 ml vials.
Rx	**Heparin Sodium** (Various, eg, Fujisawa, Pasadena, Pharmacia & Upjohn, Sanofi Winthrop)	**Injection:** 10,000 units per ml	In 1 ml vials.
Rx	**Heparin Sodium** (Various, eg, Fujisawa, Pasadena, Schein)	**Injection:** 20,000 units per ml	In 1 ml vials.
Rx	**Heparin Sodium** (Various, eg, Pasadena)	**Injection:** 40,000 units per ml	In 1 ml vials.
		Unit-Dose	
Rx	**Heparin Sodium**[1] (Elkins-Sinn)	**Injection:** 1000 units per dose	In 1, 10 and 30 ml Dosette vials.[2]
Rx	**Heparin Sodium**[1] (Wyeth-Ayerst)		In 1 ml Tubex.[2]
Rx	**Heparin Sodium**[1] (Wyeth-Ayerst)	**Injection:** 2500 units per dose	In 1 ml Tubex.[2]
Rx	**Heparin Sodium**[1] (Elkins-Sinn)	**Injection:** 5000 units per dose	In 1 and 10 ml vial.[2]
Rx	**Heparin Sodium**[1] (Wyeth-Ayerst)		In 0.5 and 1 ml Tubex.[2]
Rx	**Heparin Sodium**[1] (Sanofi Winthrop)		In 1 ml fill in 2 ml Carpuject.[2]
Rx	**Heparin Sodium**[1] (Wyeth-Ayerst)	**Injection:** 7500 units per dose	In 1 ml Tubex.[2]
Rx	**Heparin Sodium**[1] (Elkins-Sinn)	**Injection:** 10,000 units per dose	In 0.5, 1 and 4 ml vials.[2]
Rx	**Heparin Sodium**[1] (Wyeth-Ayerst)		In 1 ml Tubex.[2]
Rx	**Heparin Sodium**[1] (Wyeth-Ayerst)	**Injection:** 20,000 units per dose	In 1 ml Tubex.[2]

[1] From porcine intestinal mucosa.
[2] With benzyl alcohol.

HEPARIN SODIUM AND SODIUM CHLORIDE

For complete prescribing information, refer to the Heparin Group Monograph.

Rx	**Heparin Sodium**[1] **and 0.9% Sodium Chloride** (Baxter Healthcare)	**Injection:** 1000 units	In 500 ml Viaflex.
		2000 units	In 1000 ml Viaflex.
Rx	**Heparin Sodium**[1] **and 0.45% Sodium Chloride** (Abbott)	**Injection:** 12,500 units	In 250 ml.[2]
		25,000 units	In 250 and 500 ml.[2]

[1] From porcine intestinal mucosa.
[2] With EDTA.

HEPARIN SODIUM LOCK FLUSH SOLUTION

For complete prescribing information, refer to the Heparin Group Monograph.

Used as an IV flush to maintain patency of indwelling IV catheters in intermittent IV therapy or blood sampling; not intended for therapeutic use.

Rx	**Heparin Lock Flush** (Various, eg, Abbott, Fujisawa, Solopak, Sanofi Winthrop, Wyeth-Ayerst)	**Injection:** 10 units per ml	In 1, 2, 5, 10, 30 and 50 ml vials; 1, 2, 2.5, 3, 5 ml disp. syringe.
Rx	**Hep-Lock**[1] (Elkins-Sinn)		In 1, 2 ml Dosette vials; 1, 2.5 ml Dosette cartridge needle units; 10, 30 ml vials.[2]
Rx	**Hep-Lock U/P**[1] (Elkins-Sinn)		Preservative free. In 1 ml Dosette vials.
Rx	**Heparin Lock Flush** (Various, eg, Abbott, Fujisawa, Solopak, Sanofi Winthrop, Wyeth-Ayerst)	**Injection:** 100 units per ml	In 1, 2, 5, 10, 30 and 50 ml vials; 1 ml amps; 1, 2, 2.5, 3, 5 ml disp. syringe.
Rx	**Hep-Lock**[1] (Elkins-Sinn)		In 1, 2 ml Dosette vials; 1, 2.5 ml Dosette cartridge needle units; 10, 30 ml vials.[2]
Rx	**Hep-Lock U/P**[1] (Elkins-Sinn)		Preservative free. In 1 ml Dosette vials.

[1] From porcine intestinal mucosa.
[2] With benzyl alcohol.

COUMARIN AND INDANDIONE DERIVATIVES

Actions:

Pharmacology: Coumarins (dicumarol and warfarin) and indandiones (anisindione) interfere with the hepatic synthesis of vitamin K-dependent clotting factors (refer to the Anticoagulant introduction) which results in an in vivo depletion of clotting factors VII, IX, X and II (prothrombin). Anticoagulant effects are dependent on the half-lives of these clotting factors, which are 6, 24, 48 to 72 and 60 hours, respectively. Hence, the reduction in the rate of synthesis of the clotting factors determines the clinical response. Although factor VII is quickly depleted and an initial prolongation of the prothrombin time (PT) is seen in 8 to 12 hours, maximum anticoagulation (thus, antithrombotic effects) is not approached for 3 to 4 days as the other factors are depleted and the drug achieves steady state.

Oral anticoagulants have no direct effect on an established thrombus, nor do they reverse ischemic tissue damage. However, once thrombosis has occurred, anticoagulant treatment may prevent further extension of the formed clot and prevent secondary thromboembolic complications which may result in serious and possibly fatal sequelae.

Warfarin is available as a racemic mixture containing the R(+) and S(–) enantiomers in equal proportions; however, the S-isomer is 2 to 5 times more potent as an anticoagulant than the R-isomer.

Pharmacokinetics:

Absorption – The oral anticoagulants are generally rapidly and completely absorbed. Although serum levels are easily attained, therapeutic effect is more dependent on depletion of clotting factors; duration of effect may vary more in relation to their half-lives.

Distribution – Oral anticoagulants are highly bound to plasma proteins (97% to > 99%), primarily albumin. Therefore, potential exists for interaction with other drugs capable of displacing these agents from binding sites. (See Drug Interactions.)

Metabolism/Excretion – These agents are metabolized by hepatic microsomal enzymes and are excreted primarily in the urine as inactive metabolites.

Various Pharmacokinetic Parameters of Oral Anticoagulants

Oral anticoagulant	Half-life (days)	Peak activity (days)	Duration[1] (days)
Coumarin derivatives			
Warfarin	1-2.5[2]	3-4	2-5
Dicumarol	1-2	1.5-2	5-6
Indandione derivative			
Anisindione	3-5	2-3	1-3

[1] Following drug discontinuation
[2] S-isomer ≈ 2 days; R-isomer ≈ 1.33 days

Indications:

Warfarin/Anisindione/Dicumarol: Prophylaxis and treatment of venous thrombosis and its extension; prophylaxis and treatment of atrial fibrillation with embolization; prophylaxis and treatment of pulmonary embolism.

Warfarin: Prophylaxis or treatment of the thromboembolic complications associated with atrial fibrillation.

Anisindione/Dicumarol: As an adjunct in the treatment of coronary occlusion.

Unlabeled uses: Oral anticoagulants have been used to prevent recurrent transient ischemic attacks and to reduce the risk of recurrent MI, but data conflict. Warfarin has shown potential benefit as an adjunct in the treatment of small-cell carcinoma of the lung, given concomitantly with chemotherapy and radiation.

Contraindications:

Pregnancy (see Warnings); hemorrhagic tendencies; hemophilia; thrombocytopenic purpura; leukemia; recent or contemplated surgery of the eye or CNS, major regional lumbar block anesthesia or surgery resulting in large, open surfaces; patients bleeding from the GI, respiratory or GU tract; threatened abortion; aneurysm (cerebral, dissecting aortic); ascorbic acid deficiency; history of bleeding diathesis; prostatectomy; continuous tube drainage of small intestine; polyarthritis; diverticulitis; emaciation; malnutrition; cerebrovascular hemorrhage; eclampsia/preeclampsia; blood dyscrasias; severe uncontrolled or malignant hypertension; severe renal or hepatic disease; pericarditis and pericardial effusion; subacute bacterial

COUMARIN AND INDANDIONE DERIVATIVES

endocarditis; visceral carcinoma; following spinal puncture and other diagnostic or therapeutic procedures (eg, IUD insertion) with potential for uncontrollable bleeding; history of warfarin-induced necrosis.

Warnings:

Intolerance to coumarins: Reserve **anisindione** for patients who cannot tolerate coumarins.

Monitoring:

Prothrombin time (PT) – Treatment is highly individualized. Control dosage by periodic determination of PT or other suitable coagulation tests (eg, INR, APTT) Whole blood clotting and bleeding times are not effective measures. Monitor PT daily during the initiation of therapy and whenever any other drug is added to or discontinued from therapy which may alter the patient's response (see Drug Interactions). Once stabilized, monitor PT every 4 to 6 weeks.

International Normalized Ratio (INR) – Thromboplastins vary greatly in their responsiveness to the anticoagulant effects, differing not only between manufacturers but from lot to lot as well.

A system of standardizing the PT was introduced by the World Health Organization in 1983. It is based on the determination of an International Normalized Ratio which provides a common basis for PT results and interpretations of therapeutic ranges. The INR is derived from calibrations of commercial thromboplastin reagents against a sensitive human brain thromboplastin, the International Reference Preparation (IRP). For a discussion of the relationship between PT and INR in clinical practice, refer to Administration and Dosage.

In long-term therapy with anticoagulants, perform periodic laboratory evaluation of organ systems, including hematopoietic, renal and hepatic studies.

Hemorrhage/necrosis: The most serious risks associated with anticoagulant therapy are hemorrhages in any tissue or organ and, less frequently, necrosis or gangrene of skin and other tissues; this has resulted in death or permanent disability. The risk of hemorrhage is related to the intensity and duration of therapy. Necrosis appears to be associated with local thrombosis and usually appears within a few days of the start of therapy. In severe cases, debridement or amputation of the affected tissue, limb, breast or penis has been reported. Diagnose carefully to determine whether necrosis is caused by an underlying disease. Discontinue therapy when anticoagulants are the suspected cause; consider heparin therapy.

Hemorrhagic tendency may be manifested by hematuria, skin petechiae, hemorrhage into or from a wound or ulcerating lesion or petechial and purpuric hemorrhages throughout the body. Caution patients to report any signs of bleeding, bruising, red or dark brown urine or black or red stools. Examine patients daily and test urine to detect hematuria. Bleeding complications in the GU tract may range in severity from microscopic to gross hematuria to extensive uterine hemorrhage. When an ulcerative lesion of the GI tract is suspected or when therapy is administered postoperatively to patients who have had an operative procedure on the GI tract, examine stools frequently for evidence of hemorrhage into the bowel. GI hemorrhage may be secondary to peptic ulceration or silent neoplasm and is responsible for 25% of all deaths caused by oral anticoagulant therapy.

Bleeding during anticoagulant therapy does not always correlate with prothrombin activity. Bleeding that occurs when PT or INR is in the therapeutic range warrants investigation; it may unmask a previously unsuspected lesion (eg, tumor, ulcer).

Independent risk factors that may provide a basis for predicting major bleeding with anticoagulants include: ≥ 65 years of age; history of stroke; history of GI bleeding; serious comorbid condition (eg, recent MI, renal insufficiency, severe anemia); atrial fibrillation.

Ovarian hemorrhage – Reports indicate that a woman receiving short- or long-term therapy with heparin or warfarin may be at risk of developing ovarian hemorrhage at the time of ovulation. Observe caution when dicumarol is administered because of similar actions.

"Purple toe syndrome" – Anticoagulant therapy may enhance the release of atheromatous plaque emboli, thereby increasing the risk of complications from systemic cholesterol microembolization including the "purple toe syndrome." Discontinuation of therapy is recommended when such phenomena are observed. While the "purple toe syndrome" is reported to be reversible, other complications of microembolization may not be.

Excessive uterine bleeding may occur, but menstrual flow is usually normal. Women may be at risk of developing ovarian hemorrhage at the time of ovulation.

Adrenal hemorrhage with resultant acute adrenal insufficiency has occurred. Discontinue therapy if signs and symptoms of acute adrenal hemorrhage or

COUMARIN AND INDANDIONE DERIVATIVES

insufficiency develop. Measure plasma cortisol levels and promptly institute aggressive IV corticosteroid therapy. Do not depend on laboratory confirmation of diagnosis before initiating therapy; any delay in an acute situation may result in death.

Special risk patients: There is an increased risk with use of anticoagulants in the following conditions: Trauma; infection (concomitant antibiotic therapy may alter intestinal flora); renal insufficiency; prolonged dietary insufficiencies (eg, sprue, vitamin K deficiency); severe to moderate hypertension; polycythemia vera; vasculitis; Major regional lumbar block anesthesia; subacute bacterial endocarditis; open wound, visceral carcinoma; active tuberculosis; history of ulcerative disease of the GI tract and during the postpartum period; severe allergic disorders; anaphylactic disorders; indwelling catheters; severe diabetes; surgery or trauma resulting in large exposed raw surfaces. Thoroughly evaluate the benefits vs the enhanced risk of hemorrhage, thrombosis or embolization.

Use with caution in patients with active tuberculosis, severe diabetes, history of ulcerative disease of the GI tract and during menstruation and the postpartum period.

Protein C deficiency: Known or suspected hereditary, familial or clinical deficiency in protein C has been associated with necrosis following warfarin therapy. Tissue/skin necrosis may occur in the absence of protein C deficiency. Concurrent anticoagulation therapy with heparin for 4 to 7 days before initiation of warfarin therapy may minimize the incidence of this reaction. Discontinue therapy when warfarin or dicumarol is the suspected cause of developing necrosis. Suspect this condition if there is a history of recurrent episodes of thromboembolic disorders in the patient or in the family. Consider heparin therapy for anticoagulation.

Congestive heart failure (CHF): Patients with CHF may become more sensitive to dicumarol, thereby requiring more frequent laboratory monitoring and reduced doses of dicumarol.

Agranulocytosis and hepatitis have been associated with **anisindione** use. Perform liver function and blood studies periodically. Instruct patients to report to the physician symptoms such as marked fatigue, chills, fever or sore throat; discontinue the drug promptly since these symptoms may signal the onset of severe toxicity. If leukopenia or evidence of hypersensitivity occurs, discontinue the drug. Test the urine periodically for albumin whenever anisindione is used because of the possibility of renal damage.

Rebound hypercoagulability was thought to occur upon sudden anticoagulant withdrawal, but has not been reproducible. Also there is no evidence that thrombosis will recur following abrupt withdrawal. Therefore, tapering the dose to discontinuation appears unnecessary, although tapering the dose gradually over 3 to 4 weeks is recommended if possible.

Hypersensitivity: Delayed reactions are rare and occur within 1 to 3 months following the start of anisindione. Discontinue the medication at the first sign of hypersensitivity reactions. Symptoms include:

Dermatologic – Erythema to macular or eczematous rash; fatal exfoliative dermatitis; exudative erythema multiforme; alopecia.

Hematologic – Eosinophilia; leukopenia; thrombocytopenia; agranulocytosis; pancytopenia; neutropenia.

Renal – Nephropathy; nephritis; acute tubular necrosis; nephrotic azotemia; oliguria; anuria; albuminuria.

GI – Enanthema with diarrhea; severe stomatitis; ulcerative colitis; paralytic ileus.

Hepatic – Mixed hepatocellular damage; cholestasis; hepatitis; jaundice.

Other – Microadenopathy; fever.

Renal/Hepatic function impairment: Use with caution.

Elderly: May be more sensitive to these agents.

Pregnancy: Category X. Oral anticoagulants pass the placental barrier. Fetal hemorrhage (possibly fatal), embryopathy (fetal warfarin syndrome), optic atrophy, brain abnormalities including dorsal midline dysplasia characterized by agenesis of the corpus callosum, Dandy-Walker malformation and midline cerebellar atrophy, eye abnormalities, mental retardation, blindness, diaphragmatic hernia, hydrocephaly, microcephaly, spontaneous abortion (10%), stillbirth (8%), nasal hypoplasia, CNS defects (10%) and prematurity may occur.

Although rare, teratogenic reports following in utero exposure to warfarin include urinary tract anomalies such as single kidney, asplenia, anenchephaly, spina bifida, cranial nerve palsey, cardiac defects and congenital heart disease, polydactyly, deformities of toes, corneal leukoma, cleft palate, cleft lip and schizencephaly. Low birth weight and growth retardation have also been reported. Approximately 30% of exposed fetuses may experience a problem related to anticoagulants.

If a patient becomes pregnant during therapy, apprise her of the potential risks to the fetus and discuss the possibility of terminating the pregnancy. If oral anticoagulants are used in pregnant women, do not administer during the first trimester and discontinue prior to labor and delivery.

Some clinicians suggest the replacement of oral anticoagulants with heparin therapy before term. Heparin is withheld during early labor and reinstituted 6 hours postpartum. After 5 to 7 days, therapy with oral anticoagulants may be resumed if indicated.

Lactation: **Warfarin and dicumarol** appear in breast milk in an inactive form. Infants nursed by warfarin-treated mothers had no change in PT. Dicumarol causes a prothrombinopenic state in the nursing infant. Effects in premature infants have not been evaluated.

Children: Safety and efficacy in children < 18 years old have not been established. Oral anticoagulants may be beneficial in children with rare thromboembolic disorder secondary to other disease states such as the nephrotic syndrome or congenital heart lesions. Heparin is the initial anticoagulant of choice because of its immediate onset of action.

Precautions:

Patient selection: Use care in the selection of patients to ensure cooperation, especially from alcoholic, senile or psychotic patients.

Enhanced anticoagulant effects: Endogenous factors that may result in an increased response to the oral anticoagulants or an increased PT or INR include: Carcinoma; hepatic disorders including hepatitis or obstructive jaundice; biliary fistula; febrile states; preparatory bowel sterilization; elevated temperature; recent surgery; X-ray therapy; vitamin K deficiency; steatorrhea; CHF; diarrhea; poor nutritional state or collagen disease; hyperthyroidism; initial hypoprothrombinemia; increased age; malabsorption; vascular damage. Female and elderly patients are more sensitive to these agents.

Decreased anticoagulant effects: Endogenous factors that may reduce the response to the oral anticoagulants or decrease the PT or INR include: Edema; hyperlipidemia; diabetes mellitus; hypothyroidism; hereditary resistance to oral anticoagulants; pregnancy; hypercholesterolemia.

Drug Interactions:

The oral anticoagulants have a great potential for clinically significant drug interactions. Warn all patients about potential hazards and instruct against taking **any** drug, including nonprescription products, without the advice of a physician or pharmacist. In addition, advise against sudden change in life habits (eg, drastic change in diet or alcohol consumption).

Careful monitoring and appropriate dosage adjustments usually will permit combination therapy. Critical times during therapy occur when an interacting drug is added to or discontinued from a patient stabilized on anticoagulants.

COUMARIN AND INDANDIONE DERIVATIVES

Oral Anticoagulant Drug Interactions

Precipitant drug		Object drug*		Description
Acetaminophen Androgens Beta blockers Chlorpropamide Clofibrate Corticosteroids Cyclophosphamide Dextrothyroxine Disulfiram Erythromycin Fluconazole Gemfibrozil Glucagon Hydantoins[1]	Influenza virus vaccine Isoniazid Ketoconazole Miconazole Moricizine Propoxyphene Quinolones Streptokinase Sulfonamides Tamoxifen Thioamines Thyroid hormones Urokinase	Anticoagulants	↑	These agents may increase the anticoagulant effect. The risk of bleeding may be increased. The mechanism of the interaction is unknown or complicated.
Amiodarone Chloramphenicol Cimetidine Ifosfamide[2] Lovastatin Metronidazole Omeprazole	Phenylbutazones[2] Propafenone Quinidine Quinine SMZ-TMP Sulfinpyrazone	Anticoagulants	↑	These agents may increase the anticoagulant effect of warfarin or anisindione caused by inhibition of the anticoagulant's hepatic metabolism. The risk of bleeding may be increased.
Chloral hydrate Loop diuretics Nalidixic acid		Anticoagulants	↑	These agents may increase the anticoagulant effect of warfarin or anisindione caused by displacement from binding sites. The risk of bleeding may be increased.
Aminoglycosides Mineral oil Tetracyclines Vitamin E		Anticoagulants	↑	These agents may increase the anticoagulant effect of warfarin or anisindione caused by interference with vitamin K. The risk of bleeding may be increased.
Cephalosporins[3] Diflunisal NSAIDs Penicillins Salicylates		Anticoagulants	↑	These agents may increase the anticoagulant effect of warfarin and increase the risk of bleeding caused by effects on platelet function, and, in the case of NSAIDs, GI irritant effects.
Ascorbic acid Dicloxacillin Ethanol[4] Ethchlorvynol	Griseofulvin Nafcillin Sucralfate Trazodone	Anticoagulants	↓	These agents may decrease the anticoagulant effect of warfarin or anisindione. The mechanism of the interaction is unknown.
Aminoglutethimide Barbiturates Carbamazepine	Etretinate Glutethimide Rifampin	Anticoagulants	↓	These agents may decrease the anticoagulant effect of warfarin or anisindione caused by induction of the anticoagulant's hepatic microsomal enzymes.

COUMARIN AND INDANDIONE DERIVATIVES

Oral Anticoagulant Drug Interactions				
Precipitant drug		Object drug*		Description
Cholestyramine[5] Contraceptives, oral[6] Estrogens[6]	Thiopurines[7] Spironolactone[8] Thiazide diuretics[8] Vitamin K[9]	Anticoagulants	↓	These agents may decrease the anticoagulant effect of warfarin or anisindione by various mechanisms.

* ↑ = Object drug increased. ↓ = Object drug decreased.
1 Hydantoin serum levels may also be increased.
2 May also displace the anticoagulant from protein binding sites.
3 Those agents with a methyltetrazolethiol side chain.
4 Chronic consumption may increase the clearance of the anticoagulant; moderate to small doses do not alter the anticoagulant effect.
5 Reduced anticoagulant absorption and possibly increased elimination.
6 Rarely, increased risk of thromboembolism; this is in contrast to intended effect.
7 Thiopurine-induced increase in synthesis or activation of prothrombin.
8 Diuretic-induced hemoconcentration of clotting factors.
9 Vitamin K overcomes interference of vitamin K-dependent clotting factors by anticoagulants.

Drug/Lab test interactions: Dicumarol and indandione anticoagulants, including anisindione, or their metabolites may cause red-orange discoloration of alkaline urine; this may interfere with spectrophotometrically determined urinary laboratory tests.

Adverse Reactions:

Hemorrhage is the principal adverse effect of oral anticoagulants; skin necrosis has occurred rarely (see Warnings). Hemorrhage from any tissue or organ is a consequence of the anticoagulant effect. The signs and symptoms will vary according to the location and degree or extent of the bleeding. Hemorrhagic complications may present as: Paralysis; headache; chest, abdomen, joint or other pain; shortness of breath; difficult breathing or swallowing; unexplained swelling; unexplained shock. Therefore, consider the possibility of hemorrhage in evaluating the condition of any anticoagulated patient with complaints that do not indicate an obvious diagnosis.

Other adverse reactions include: Nausea; diarrhea; pyrexia; dermatitis; exfoliative dermatitis; urticaria; alopecia; sore mouth; mouth ulcers; priapism (causal relationship not established); paralytic ileus and intestinal obstruction from submucosal or intramural hemorrhage.

Anisindione: Dermatitis has been the only reported reaction consistently associated with anisindione. The following reactions have been reported with other indandione anticoagulants and therefore might also occur with anisindione: Headache; sore throat; blurred vision; paralysis of accommodation; steatorrhea; hepatitis; liver damage; renal tubular necrosis; albuminuria; anuria; myeloid immaturity; leukocyte agglutinins; red cell aplasia; atypical mononuclear cells; leukopenia; leukocytosis; red-orange urine; anemia; thrombocytopenia; eosinophilia; agranulocytosis; jaundice.

Warfarin: Other side effects are infrequent and include:

Dermatologic – Necrosis or gangrene of the skin and other tissues (see Warnings).

GI – Vomiting; anorexia; abdominal cramping; diarrhea; hepatotoxicity; cholestatic jaundice.

Dicumarol: Adrenal hemorrhage (see Warnings); excessive uterine bleeding has occured but menstrual flow is usually normal; abdominal cramping; "purple toes" syndrome; hypersensitivity; leukopenia; vomiting.

Miscellaneous – Fever; systemic cholesterol microembolization ("purple toes" syndrome, see Warnings); ovarian hemorrhage (see Warnings); hypersensitivity reactions (see Warnings).

Overdosage:

Symptoms:

Early – Microscopic hematuria; excessive menstrual bleeding; melena; petechiae; oozing from superficial injuries (eg, nicks made by shaving, bleeding from gums after brushing teeth, excessive bruising).

Treatment: Excessive anticoagulation, with or without bleeding, is readily controlled by discontinuing therapy and, if necessary, by administration of oral or parenteral phytonadione (Vitamin K_1; see individual monograph).

COUMARIN AND INDANDIONE DERIVATIVES

In excessive prothrombinopenia with mild or no bleeding, omission for 24 to 48 hours may suffice; if necessary, give small doses of oral or SC phytonadione (2 to 10 mg). If minor bleeding persists or progresses to frank bleeding, give 5 to 25 mg IV phytonadione. A dose of > 25 mg will make the patient refractory to further anticoagulation for a few days. Such use of phytonadione reduces response to subsequent anticoagulant therapy; therefore, use caution in determining the need for this vitamin. A hypercoagulable state may occur following the rapid reversal of a prolonged PT, APTT or INR. Smaller doses (5 to 15 mg) of phytonadione may be sufficient, except in cases of severe hemorrhage.

In emergency situations, clotting factors can be returned to normal by administering 200 to 500 ml of fresh frozen plasma or by giving commercial Factor IX complex. Consider fresh whole blood transfusions in cases of severe bleeding or prothrombinopenic states unresponsive to Vitamin K_1. Purified Factor IX preparations should not be used because they cannot increase the levels of prothrombin. Factor VII and Factor X are also depressed along with the levels of Factor IX as a result of warfarin treatment. Packed red blood cells may also be given if significant blood loss has occurred. Carefully monitor infusions of blood or plasma to avoid precipitating pulmonary edema in elderly patients or patients with heart disease.

Resumption of anticoagulant administration reverses the effect of phytonadione and a therapeutic PT or INR can again be obtained by careful dosage adjustment.

The following is a suggested approach for treatment of overanticoagulated patients:

Overanticoagulation Treatment Approach

INR	Is patient bleeding?	Is rapid reversal indicated?	Intervention
< 6	No	No	Hold the next few doses of anticoagulant, resume when INR is in therapeutic range.
6-10	Yes/No	Yes	0.5-1 mg K_1 SC; decrease in INR within 8 hours, INR in therapeutic range in 24 hours; give 0.5 mg dose K_1 SC if needed at 24 hour INR. Resume warfarin at a lower dose.
10-20	Yes/No	Yes	3-5 mg K_1 SC; decrease in INR within 6 hours[1]; repeat dose if needed.
> 20 ± urgent	Yes/No	Yes	10 mg K_1 slow IV over 20-30 minutes; check INR in 6 hours; may repeat dose every 12 hours if needed per INR[1]; supplement with plasma or Prothrombin Replacement Complex Core (PCC) if required.
> 20 and life-threatening	Yes/No	Yes	PCC with 10 mg K_1 slow IV over 20-30 minutes, repeated[1] prn per INR.

[1] If continued warfarin therapy is indicated, administer heparin until effects of K_1 have been reversed and patient becomes responsive to warfarin.

Patient Information:

Dosing is highly individual and may have to be adjusted several times based on lab test results. Strict adherence to prescribed dosage schedule is necessary.

Do not take or discontinue any other medication, except on advice of physician or pharmacist. Avoid alcohol, salicylates and drastic changes in dietary habits.

Anisindione may cause a red-orange discoloration of alkaline urine.

Notify physician if unusual bleeding or bruising, red or dark brown urine (blood), red or tar black stools or diarrhea occurs. Also report bleeding from the gums or nose, patches of discoloration or bruises on the arms, legs or toes, or excessive bleeding following minor cuts (eg, while shaving).

Do not change brands without consulting a physician or pharmacist.

Discuss with physician any plan to become pregnant or report any pregnancy promptly.

Consult physician before undergoing dental work or elective surgery.

COUMARIN AND INDANDIONE DERIVATIVES

Administration and Dosage:

Dosage: Individualize dosage. Adjust the dosage based on the results of the one stage PT. Different thromboplastin reagents vary substantially in their responsiveness to warfarin-induced effects on PT. To define the appropriate therapeutic regimen it is important to be familiar with the sensitivity of the thromboplastin reagent used in the laboratory and its relationship to the International Reference Preparation (IRP), a sensitive thromboplastin reagent prepared from human brain.

Early clinical studies of oral anticoagulants, which formed the basis for recommended therapeutic ranges of 1.5 to 2.5 times control PT, used sensitive human brain thromboplastin. When using the less sensitive rabbit brain thromboplastins commonly employed in PT assays today, adjustments must be made to the targeted PT range that reflect this decrease in sensitivity. Available clinical evidence indicates that prolongation of the PT to 1.2 to 1.5 times control, when measuring with the less sensitive thromboplastin reagents, is sufficient for prophylaxis and treatment of venous thromboembolism and minimizes the risk of hemorrhage associated with more prolonged PT values. In cases where the risk of thromboembolism is great, such as in patients with recurrent systemic embolism, maintain a PT of 1.5 to 2 times control. A ratio of > 2 appears to provide no additional therapeutic benefit in most patients and is associated with a higher risk of bleeding.

For the three commercial rabbit brain thromboplastins currently used in North America, a PT ratio of 1.3 to 2 is equivalent to an INR of 2 to 4. For other thromboplastins, the INR can be calculated as:

$$\text{INR} = (\text{observed PT ratio})^{\text{ISI}}$$

where the ISI (International Sensitivity Index) is the calibration factor and is available from the manufacturers of the thromboplastin reagent and observed PT ratio is:

$$\frac{\text{PT observed}}{\text{mean normal PT}}$$

Following are the recommended therapeutic ranges for oral anticoagulant therapy from the American College of Chest Physicians (ACCP) and the National Heart, Lung and Blood Institute (NHLBI):

ACCP/NHLBI Recommended Therapeutic Range for Oral Anticogulant Therapy

Condition	PT Ratio[1]	INR
Acute MI[2]	1.3 to 1.5	2 to 3
Atrial fibrillation[2]	1.3 to 1.5	2 to 3
Mechanical prosthetic valves	1.5 to 2	3 to 4.5
Pulmonary embolism, treatment	1.3 to 1.5	2 to 3
Systemic embolism		
Prevention	1.3 to 1.5	2 to 3
Recurrent	1.5 to 2	3 to 4.5
Tissue heart valves[2]	1.3 to 1.5	2 to 3
Valvular heart disease[2]	1.3 to 1.5	2 to 3
Venous thrombosis		
Prophylaxis (high-risk surgery)	1.3 to 1.5	2 to 3
Treatment	1.3 to 1.5	2 to 3

[1] ISI of 2.4
[2] To prevent systemic embolism

Loading dose: Heparin is preferred if rapid anticoagulation is necessary. Administer oral anticoagulants at anticipated maintenance dosage levels or a slightly higher loading dose (eg, 5-10 mg/day of warfarin for 2 to 4 days); then adjust the daily dosage based on the results of PT or INR determinations. Use of a large loading dose (eg, 30 mg warfarin) may increase incidence of bleeding complications; it does not offer more rapid protection vs thrombi formation, and is not recommended.

Transfer from heparin therapy: Because there is a delayed onset of oral anticoagulant effects, give heparin and warfarin simultaneously from the first day, or alternatively, start warfarin on the third to sixth day of heparin therapy. Use concurrent therapy until a therapeutic PT or INR is achieved.

Elderly: Lower dosages are recommended.

COUMARIN AND INDANDIONE DERIVATIVES

Duration of therapy: In the determination of the duration of long-term anticoagulant therapy, consider history of recurrent thromboembolism, underlying diseases, reason for anticoagulant therapy (eg, atrial fibrillation) and risks of adverse effects.

Treatment during dentistry and surgery (warfarin/dicumarol): The management of patients who undergo dental and surgical procedures requires close liaison between attending physicians, surgeons and dentists. In patients who must be anticoagulated prior to, during or immediately following dental or surgical procedures, adjusting the dosage to maintain the PT at the low end of the therapeutic range (or maintain the corresponding INR value) may safely allow for continued anticoagulation. Limit the operative site to permit effective use of local measures for hemostasis. Under these conditions, dental and surgical procedures may be performed without undue risk of hemorrhage.

Minidose warfarin may be beneficial as prophylaxis against venous thrombosis after major surgery. In one study, 1 mg daily given before surgery (mean 20 days) significantly lowered the incidence of DVT compared to controls; there was no difference between the 1 mg/day and the full-dose anticoagulation group. APTT and PT were not prolonged beyond normal on the day of surgery using the minidose therapy.

Coumarin and Indandione Derivatives

WARFARIN SODIUM

For complete prescribing information, refer to the Coumarin and Indandione Derivatives group monograph.

Administration and Dosage:

Approved by the FDA June 8, 1954.

Oral:

Induction – Initiate with 5-10 mg/day for 2 to 4 days; adjust daily dosage according to PT or INR determinations. Use of a large loading dose (eg, 30 mg) may increase the incidence of hemorrhagic and other complications, does not offer more rapid protection against thrombi formation and is not recommended.

Elderly/Debilitated patients or patients with increased sensitivity: Use lower dose.

Maintenance – 2 to 10 mg daily, based on PT or INR.

Bioequivalency problems have been documented for warfarin sodium products marketed by different manufacturers. Brand interchange is not recommended.

Storage/Stability – Protect from light. Store in carton until contents have been used. Store at controlled room temperature (59°-86°F; 15°-30°C). Dispense in a tight, light-resistant container.

Injectable: Warfarin injection provides an alternative administration route for patients who cannot receive oral drugs. The IV dosages would be the same as those that would be used orally if the patient could take the drug by the oral route. Administer as a slow bolus injection over 1 to 2 minutes into a peripheral vein. It is not recommended for IM administration. Reconstitute the vial with 2.7 ml sterile Water for Injection and inspect for particulate matter and discoloration immediately prior to use. Do not use if either particulate matter or discoloration is noted. After reconstitution, warfarin for injection is chemically and physically stable for 4 hours at room temperature. It does not contain any antimicrobial preservative and care must be taken to assure the sterility of the prepared solution. The vial is not recommended for multiple use; discard unused solution.

Rx	**Coumadin** (DuPont)	**Tablets:** 1 mg	Lactose. (Coumadin 1 DuPont). Pink, scored. In 100s, 1000s and UD 100s.
		2 mg	Lactose. (Coumadin 2 DuPont). Lavender, scored. In 30s, 100s, 1000s and UD 100s.
		2.5 mg	Lactose. (Coumadin 2½ DuPont). Green, scored. In 30s, 100s, 1000s and UD 100s.
		3 mg	Lactose. (Coumadin 3 DuPont). Tan, scored. In 100s, 1000s and UD 100s.
		4 mg	Lactose. (Coumadin 4 DuPont). Blue, scored. In 100s, 1000s and UD 100s.
		5 mg	Lactose. (Coumadin 5 DuPont). Peach, scored. In 30s, 100s, 1000s and UD 100s.
		6 mg	Lactose. (Coumadin 6 DuPont). Teal, scored. In 100s, 1000s and UD 100s.
		7.5 mg	Lactose. (Coumadin 7½ DuPont). Yellow, scored. In 100s and UD 100s.
		10 mg	Dye free. Lactose. (Coumadin 10 DuPont). White, scored. In 100s and UD 100s.
		Powder for Injection, lyophilized: 2 mg	Mannitol. In 5 mg vials.

Coumarin and Indandione Derivatives

ANISINDIONE

For complete prescribing information, refer to the Coumarin and Indandione Derivatives group monograph.

Administration and Dosage:

300 mg the first day, 200 mg the second day, 100 mg the third day and 25 to 250 mg daily for maintenance.

Storage/Stability: Store between 15° and 25°C (59° and 77°F).

Rx	**Miradon** (Schering)	**Tablets:** 50 mg	Lactose. (ANK or 795). Pink, scored. In 100s.

DICUMAROL

For complete prescribing information, refer to the Coumarin and Indandione Derivatives group monograph.

Administration and Dosage:

Induction: The dosage range for the average adult with normal prothrombin activity ranges from 200 to 300 mg the first day.

Maintenance: On subsequent days the dosage ranges from 25 to 200 mg.

Storage/Stability: Store at < 70°F (25°C).

Rx	**Dicumarol** (Abbott)	**Tablets:** 25 mg	Lactose. In 100s.

PROTAMINE SULFATE

Actions:

Pharmacology: Protamines are strongly basic simple proteins of low molecular weight, rich in arginine. They occur in sperm of salmon and certain other fish species. Given alone, protamine sulfate has a weak anticoagulant effect. However, when given with heparin (strongly acidic), a stable salt forms resulting in loss of anticoagulant activity of both drugs.

Pharmacokinetics: Protamine sulfate has a rapid onset of action. The half-life of protamine is shorter than that of heparin, therefore repeated doses are sometimes required. Heparin is neutralized within 5 minutes after IV injection. The metabolic fate of the heparin-protamine complex is not known, but one theory is that protamine sulfate in the heparin-protamine complex may be partially metabolized or may be cleaved by fibrinolysin, thus freeing heparin.

Indications:

Treatment of heparin overdosage.

Contraindications:

Hypersensitivity to the drug.

Warnings:

Recurrent bleeding: Hyperheparinemia or bleeding has occurred in some patients 30 minutes to 18 hours after cardiac surgery (under cardiopulmonary bypass) in spite of complete neutralization of heparin by adequate doses of protamine at the end of the operation. Therefore, observe patients closely after cardiac surgery. Administer additional doses of protamine sulfate if indicated by coagulation studies, such as the heparin titration test with protamine activated clotting time (ACT) or activated partial thromboplastin time (APTT) and the plasma thrombin time.

Excessively rapid administration can cause severe hypotensive and anaphylactoid reactions. Have facilities available to treat shock.

Pulmonary edema: High-protein, noncardiogenic pulmonary edema associated with the use of protamine has occurred in patients on cardiopulmonary bypass who are undergoing cardiovascular surgery. The etiologic role of protamine in the pathogenesis of this condition is uncertain, and multiple factors have been present in most cases. The condition has been reported in association with administration of certain blood products, other drugs, cardiopulmonary bypass alone and other etiologic factors. It is difficult to treat, and it can be life-threatening.

Circulatory collapse, severe and potentially irreversible, associated with myocardial failure and reduced cardiac output, can also occur. The mechanism(s) of this reaction and the role played by concurrent factors are unclear.

Hypersensitivity: Patients with a history of allergy to fish may develop hypersensitivity reactions; although, to date, no relationship has been established between allergic reactions to protamine and fish allergy.

Previous exposure to protamine through use of protamine-containing insulins or during heparin neutralization may predispose susceptible individuals to the development of untoward reactions from the subsequent use of this drug. Reports of the presence of antiprotamine antibodies in the serums of infertile or vasectomized men suggest that some of these individuals may react to the use of protamine sulfate.

Complement activation by the heparin-protamine complexes, release of lysosomal enzymes from neutrophils, and prostaglandin and thromboxane generation have been associated with the development of anaphylactoid reactions. Fatal anaphylaxis has been reported in one patient with no prior history of allergies. Give protamine only when resuscitation techniques and treatment of anaphylactic and anaphylactoid shock are readily available. Have epinephrine 1:1000 immediately available. Refer to Management of Acute Hypersensitivity Reactions.

Pregnancy: Category C. It is not known whether the drug can cause fetal harm when administered to a pregnant woman or can affect reproduction capacity. Administer to a pregnant woman only if clearly needed.

Lactation: It is not known whether this drug is excreted in breast milk. Administer cautiously to a nursing mother.

Children: Safety and efficacy in children have not been established.

Precautions:

Anticoagulant effects: Because of the anticoagulant effect, do not give > 50 mg over a short period unless a larger requirement is necessary.

Adverse Reactions:

Sudden fall in blood pressure; bradycardia; transitory flushing and feeling of warmth; dyspnea; nausea; vomiting; lassitude; back pain in conscious patients undergoing such procedures as cardiac catheterization; anaphylaxis that may result in severe res-

PROTAMINE SULFATE

piratory distress, capillary leak and noncardiogenic pulmonary edema (see Warnings); acute pulmonary hypertension; circulatory collapse; hypersensitivity (see Warnings).

Overdosage:

Symptoms: Overdose of protamine sulfate may cause bleeding. Protamine has a weak anticoagulant effect caused by an interaction with platelets and with many proteins including fibrinogen. Distinguish this effect from the rebound anticoagulation that may occur 30 minutes to 18 hours following the reversal of heparin with protamine.

Rapid administration of protamine is more likely to result in bradycardia, dyspnea, a sensation of warmth, flushing and severe hypotension. Hypertension has also occurred.

The median lethal dose of protamine sulfate in mice is 50 mg/kg. Serum concentrations of protamine sulfate are not clinically useful. Information is not available on the amount of drug in a single dose that is associated with overdosage or is likely to be life-threatening.

Treatment: In managing overdosage, consider the possibility of multiple drug overdoses, interaction among drugs and unusual drug kinetics.

Replace blood loss with blood transfusions or fresh frozen plasma. If the patient is hypotensive, consider fluids, epinephrine, dobutamine or dopamine. Refer to Management of Acute Overdosage.

Administration and Dosage:

Protamine sulfate 1 mg neutralizes ≈ 90 units of heparin activity derived from lung tissue or ≈ 115 units derived from intestinal mucosa.

Because heparin disappears rapidly from circulation, the protamine dose required also decreases rapidly with time elapsed since IV heparin injection. For example, if protamine is given 30 minutes after heparin, half the usual dose may be sufficient.

Give very slowly IV over 10 minutes in doses not to exceed 50 mg. Guide dosage by blood coagulation studies.

Incompatibilities: Certain antibiotics, including several cephalosporins and penicillins.

Prepared solution: Protamine sulfate injection is for use without further dilution; if further dilution is desired, use Dextrose 5% in Water or normal saline.

Storage/Stability: Refrigerate at 2° to 8°C (36° to 46°F); do not store diluted solutions; they contain no preservative.

Rx	**Protamine Sulfate** (Various, eg, Elkins-Sinn, Lilly, Fujisawa)	**Injection:** 10 mg/ml	Preservative-free. In 5 and 25 ml amps and 5 and 25 ml vials.

ALTEPLASE, RECOMBINANT

Actions:

Pharmacology: Alteplase, a tissue plasminogen activator (tPA) produced by recombinant DNA, is used in the management of acute myocardial infarction (AMI), acute ischemic stroke and pulmonary embolism (PE). It is a sterile, purified glycoprotein of 527 amino acids. It is synthesized using the complementary DNA for natural human tissue-type plasminogen activator obtained from a human melanoma cell line.

Biological potency, determined by an in vitro clot lysis assay, is expressed in International Units. The specific activity is 580,000 IU/mg.

Mechanism – Alteplase is an enzyme (serine protease) that has the property of fibrin-enhanced conversion of plasminogen to plasmin. It produces limited conversion of plasminogen in the absence of fibrin. When introduced into the systemic circulation at pharmacologic concentration, alteplase binds to fibrin in a thrombus and converts the entrapped plasminogen to plasmin. This initiates local fibrinolysis with limited systemic proteolysis. Following administration of 100 mg, there is a decrease (16% to 36%) in circulating fibrinogen. In a controlled trial, 8 of 73 patients (11%) receiving alteplase (1.25 mg/kg over 3 hours) experienced a decrease in fibrinogen to < 100 mg/dl.

Pharmacokinetics:

Absorption/Distribution – Because of its large molecular size, alteplase cannot easily diffuse across biological membranes and must be given parenterally, usually IV. Maximal plasma concentrations of 3 to 4 mg/L are achieved after standard administration of 90 to 100 mg doses. Steady-state concentrations for the initial infusion period were 45% higher when administered in an accelerated regimen.

Metabolism/Excretion – Alteplase is cleared rapidly from plasma at a rate of 380 to 570 ml/min, primarily by the liver. More than 50% of the drug present in plasma is cleared within 5 minutes after the infusion has been terminated, and ≈ 80% is cleared within 10 minutes. Initial volume of distribution is 2.8 to 4.6 L, and it approximately doubles at steady-state. Total body clearance is 34.3 to 38.4 L/hr.

Clinical trials:

3–hour infusion in AMI patients – Coronary occlusion because of thrombus is present in the infarct-related coronary artery in ≈ 80% of patients experiencing a transmural myocardial infarction (MI) evaluated ≤ 4 hours of onset of symptoms.

In patients studied in a controlled trial with coronary angiography at 90 and 120 minutes following infusion, infarct artery patency was observed in 71% and 85% of patients (n = 85), respectively. In a second study, patients received coronary angiography prior to and following infusion within 6 hours of symptoms; after the commencement of therapy in 71% of 83 patients, reperfusion of the obstructed vessel occurred ≤ 90 minutes.

Accelerated infusion in AMI patients – Accelerated infusion of alteplase was studied in an international, multi-center trial (GUSTO) that randomized 41,021 patients with AMI to four thrombolytic regimens. Entry criteria included onset of chest pain within 6 hours of treatment and ST segment elevation of ECG. The regimens included accelerated infusion of alteplase (≤ 100 mg over 90 minutes) plus IV heparin (n = 10,396); streptokinase (SK) (1.5 million units over 60 minutes) plus IV heparin (n = 10,410); or streptokinase (as above) plus subcutaneous (SC) heparin (n = 9841). A fourth regimen combined alteplase and streptokinase. Aspirin and heparin use was directed by the GUSTO study protocol as follows: All patients were to receive 160 mg chewable aspirin administered as soon as possible, followed by 160 to 325 mg daily. Intavenous heparin was directed to be a 5000 U IV bolus initiated as soon as possible, followed by a 1000 IU/hour continous IV infusion for at least 48 hours; subsequent heparin therapy was at the discretion of the attending physician. Subcutaneous heparin was directed to be 12,500 IU administered 4 hours after initiation of SK therapy, followed by 12,500 IU twice daily for 7 days or until discharge, whichever came first.

Subgroup analysis of patients by age, infarct location, time from symptom onset to thrombolytic treatment showed consistently lower 30–day mortality for the alteplase accelerated infusion group. For patients > 75 years of age, a predefined subgroup of 12% of patients enrolled, the incidence of stroke was 4% for the alteplase-accelerated infusion group, 2.8% for SK (IV) and 3.2% for SK (SC); the incidence of combined 30–day mortality or nonfatal stroke was 20.6% for accelerated infusion of alteplase 21.5% for SK (IV) and 22% for SK (SC).

Pulmonary emboli – In a comparative randomized trial (n = 45), 59% of 22 patients treated with alteplase (100 mg over 2 hours) experienced moderate or marked lysis of pulmonary emboli when assessed by pulmonary angiography 2 hours after treatment initiation. Alteplase patients also experienced a significant reduction in pulmonary embolism-induced pulmonary hypertension within 2 hours of treatment. Pulmonary perfusion at 24 hours was significantly improved.

Acute ischemic stroke – Depending upon the stroke assessment scale, recovery with minimal or no disability occurred in 11% to 12.6% more alteplase-treated patients than in those receiving placebo. Secondary analyses demonstrated consistent functional and neurological improvement within all stroke scales.

Indications:

AMI: Management of AMI in adults for the improvement of ventricular function following AMI, the reduction of the incidence of congestive heart failure and the reduction of mortality associated with AMI. Initiate treatment as soon as possible after the onset of AMI symptoms.

Acute ischemic stroke: Management of acute ischemic stroke in adults for improving neurological recovery and reducing the incidence of disability. Initiate treatment only within 3 hours after the onset of stroke symptoms and after exclusion of intracranial hemorrhage by a cranial computerized tomography (CT) scan or other diagnostic imaging method sensitive for the presence of hemorrhage (see Contraindications).

Pulmonary embolism (PE): Management of acute massive PE in adults, for the lysis of acute PE, defined as obstruction of blood flow to a lobe or multiple segments of the lungs, and for the lysis of PE accompanied by unstable hemodynamics (eg, failure to maintain blood pressure without supportive measures).

Confirm the diagnosis by objective means, such as pulmonary angiography or noninvasive procedures such as lung scanning.

Unlabeled uses: In patients with unstable angina pectoris, alteplase may result in coronary thrombolysis and reduction of ischemic events. Alteplase has been used successfully to clear thrombi in central venous catheters (2 mg injected as a bolus into the blocked catheter); in occlusion of small blood vessels by microthrombi; and in the management of peripheral arterial thrombo-embolism (0.5 to 1 mg/hour intra-arterially). Although, more studies are needed, alteplase has been shown to be effective in restoring blood flow to frostbitten limbs (0.075 mg/kg/hour for 6 hours).

Contraindications:

AMI or PE: Active internal bleeding; history of cerebrovascular accident; (≤ 2 months) intracranial or intraspinal surgery or trauma; intracranial neoplasm, arteriovenous malformation or aneurysm; bleeding diathesis; severe uncontrolled hypertension.

Acute ischemic stroke: Evidence of intracranial hemorrhage on pretreatment evaluation; suspicion of subarachnoid hemorrhage; recent intracranial surgery or serious head trauma or recent previous stroke; history of intracranial hemorrhage; uncontrolled hypertension at time of treatment (eg, > 185 mmHg systolic or >110 mmHg diastolic); seizure at the onset of stroke; active internal bleeding; intracranial neoplasm, arteriovenous malformation or aneurysm; bleeding diathesis (see Warnings).

Warnings:

Bleeding is the most common complication. The bleeding associated with thrombolytic therapy can be divided into two broad categories:

1.) Internal bleeding involving the GI tract, GU tract, retroperitoneal, intracranial sites or respiratory tract.

2.) Superficial or surface bleeding, observed mainly at invaded or disturbed sites (eg, venous cutdowns, arterial punctures, sites of recent surgical intervention).

The concomitant use of heparin anticoagulation may contribute to the bleeding. Some of the hemorrhagic episodes occurred ≥ 1 day after alteplase effects had dissipated but while heparin therapy was continuing.

As fibrin is lysed during therapy, bleeding from recent puncture sites may occur. Therefore, thrombolytic therapy requires careful attention to all potential bleeding sites (including catheter insertion sites, arterial and venous puncture sites, cutdown sites and needle puncture sites). Avoid IM injections and nonessential handling of the patient during treatment with alteplase. Perform venipunctures carefully and only as required. Minimize arterial and venous punctures.

Should an arterial puncture be necessary during an infusion, it is preferable to use an upper extremity vessel accessible to manual compression. Apply pressure for ≥ 30 minutes, apply a pressure dressing and check the puncture site frequently for bleeding evidence. Avoid noncompressible arterial puncture (ie, avoid internal jugular and subclavian punctures to minimize noncompressible site bleeding).

If serious bleeding (not controllable by local pressure) occurs, terminate the infusion and any concomitant heparin. Protamine can be given to reverse heparin effects.

In the following conditions, the risks of therapy may be increased and weighed against the anticipated benefits:

- Recent (≤ 10 days) major surgery (eg, coronary artery bypass graft, obstetrical delivery, organ biopsy, previous puncture of noncompressible vessels
- Cerebrovascular disease
- Recent (≤ 10 days) GI or GU bleeding
- Recent (≤ 10 days) trauma
- Hypertension: ≥ 180 mmHg systolic or ≥ 110 mmHg diastolic

ALTEPLASE, RECOMBINANT

- Likelihood of left heart thrombus (eg, mitral stenosis with atrial fibrillation)
- Acute pericarditis
- Subacute bacterial endocarditis
- Hemostatic defects including secondary to severe hepatic or renal disease
- Significant liver dysfunction
- Pregnancy
- Diabetic hemorrhagic retinopathy or other ophthalmic hemorrhaging
- Septic thrombophlebitis or occluded AV cannula at seriously infected site
- Advanced age (eg, > 75 years old)
- Patients currently receiving oral anticoagulants, eg, warfarin sodium
- Any other condition in which bleeding constitutes a significant hazard or would be particularly difficult to manage because of its location

Bleeding diathesis: Bleeding diathesis includes, but is not limited to: Current use of oral anticoagulants (eg, warfarin sodium) with prothrombin time (PT) > 15 seconds; administration of heparin ≤ 48 hrs preceding stroke onset with an elevated activated partial thromboplastin time (aPTT) at presentation; platelet count < 100,000/mm^3.

If serious bleeding in a critical location (intracranial, GI, retroperitoneal, pericardial) occurs, immediately discontinue alteplase andheparin therapy.

Cholesterol embolism has been reported rarely in patients treated with all thrombolytic agents; the incidence is unknown. This serious condition, which can be lethal, is associated with invasive vascular procedures (eg, cardiac catheterization, angiography, vascular surgery) or anticoagulant therapy. Clinical features of cholesterol embolism may include livedo reticularis, "purple toe" syndrome, acute renal failure, gangrenous digits, hypertension, pancreatitis, MI, cerebral infarction, spinal cord infarction, retinal artery occlusion, bowel infarction and rhabdomyolysis.

Arrhythmias may result from coronary thrombolysis associated with reperfusion. These arrhythmias (such as sinus bradycardia, accelerated idioventricular rhythm, ventricular premature depolarizations, ventricular tachycardia) are not different from those often seen in the ordinary course of AMI and may be managed with standard antiarrhythmic measures. Have antiarrhythmic therapy for bradycardia or ventricular irritability available when infusions of alteplase are administered.

Pulmonary embolism (PE): The treatment of PE with alteplase has not been shown to constitute treatment of underlying deep vein thrombosis. Consider the possible risk of reembolization caused by lysis of underlying deep venous thrombi.

Acute ischemic stroke: The risks of alteplase therapy to treat acute ischemic stroke may be increased in the following conditions and weighed against the anticipated benefits: Severe neurological deficit (eg, NIHSS > 22) at presentation (increases risk of intracranial hemorrhage) and major early infarct signs on a computerized cranial tomography (CT) scan (eg, substantial edema, mass effect of midline shift).

In patients without recent use of oral anticoagulants or heparin, initiate alteplase treatment prior to the availability of coagulation study results. However, discontinue infusion if either a pretreatment PT > 15 seconds or an elevated aPTT is identified.

In acute ischemic stroke, neither the incidence of intracranial hemorrhage nor the benefits of therapy are known in patients treated with alteplase > 3 hours after the onset of symptoms. Therefore, do not treat patients with acute ischemic stroke > 3 hours after symptom onset.

Cerebral edema: Administering alteplase 3 to 4 hours after a major ischemic stroke may cause cerebral edema with fatal brain herniation.

Neurological deficit: The safety and efficacy of treatment with alteplase in patients with minor neurological deficit or with rapidly improving symptoms prior to the start of alteplase administration has not been evaluated.

Elderly: In AMI patients, the proportional benefit of thrombolytic therapy decreases with increasing age. However, mortality rates remain considerably lower in elderly alteplase-treated patients, than elderly patients (> 76 years) excluded from thrombolytic therapy.

Alteplase-treated elderly patients (> 77 years) with acute ischemic stroke have an increased risk for symptomatic intracranial hemorrhage (ICH) within the first 36 hours, total ICH and all-cause 90–day mortality. Nevertheless, efficacy analyses suggest a reduced but favorable clinical outcome for elderly alteplase-treated patients.

Pregnancy: Category C. It is not known whether alteplase can cause fetal harm when administered to a pregnant woman or affect reproduction capacity. Give to a pregnant woman only if clearly needed.

Lactation: It is not known whether alteplase is excreted in breast milk. Exercise caution when administering to nursing women.

Children: Safety and efficacy for use in children have not been established.

ALTEPLASE, RECOMBINANT

Precautions:

Monitoring: With coadministration of heparin or aspirin, monitor for bleeding especially at arterial puncture sites. Control and monitor blood pressure frequently during and following alteplase administration to manage acute ischemic stroke.

Implement standard management of MI or PE concomitantly with treatment.

Hypersensitivity: There is no experience with readministration of alteplase. If an anaphylactoid reaction occurs, discontinue the infusion immediately and initiate appropriate therapy. Refer to Management of Acute Hypersensitivity Reactions.

Sustained antibody formation in patients receiving one dose of alteplase has not been documented, but readminister with caution. Detectable antibody levels (single point measurement) were reported in one patient but subsequent antibody test results were negative.

Laboratory tests: During therapy, if coagulation tests or measures of fibrinolytic activity are performed, the results may be unreliable unless specific precautions are taken to prevent in vitro artifacts. Alteplase present in blood in pharmacologic concentrations remains active in vitro. This can lead to degradation of fibrinogen in blood samples removed for analysis. Collection of blood samples in the presence of aprotinin (150 to 200 units/ml) can, to some extent, mitigate this phenomenon.

Drug Interactions:

In addition to bleeding associated with heparin and vitamin K antagonists, drugs that alter platelet function, such as aspirin, dipyridamole and abciximab, may increase risk of bleeding if given prior to, during or after alteplase therapy (see Administration and Dosage).

Heparin has been given with and after alteplase infusions to reduce risk of rethrombosis. Either heparin or alteplase may cause bleeding complications; carefully monitor for bleeding, especially at arterial puncture sites (see Administration and Dosage).

Adverse Reactions:

Bleeding (most frequent):

Incidence of Significant Bleeding with Alteplase	
	Total Dose
Site of Bleeding	≤100 mg/3 hr
GI	5%
GU	4%
Ecchymosis	1%
Retroperitoneal	< 1%
Epistaxis	< 1%
Gingival	< 1%

The incidence of intracranial hemorrhage (ICH) in AMI patients treated with alteplase is as follows:

Incidence of Intracranial Bleeding with Alteplase		
Dose	Patients	%
100 mg, 3 hours	3272	0.4
≤ 100 mg, accelerated	10,396	0.7
150 mg	1779	1.3
1 to 1.4 mg/kg	237	0.4

Accelerated infusion: All strokes (1.6%); nonfatal stroke (0.9%); hemorrhagic stroke (0.7%). The incidence of all strokes, as well as that for hemorrhagic stroke, increased with increasing age.

Miscellaneous: Occasional mild hypersensitivity reactions (eg, anaphylactoid reaction, laryngeal edema, rash), urticaria (rare); cholesterol embolization (rare, see Warnings); cerebral edema (see Warnings); bradycardia; cardiogenic shock; arrhythmias; pulmonary edema; heart failure; cardiac arrest; recurrent ischemia; reinfarction; myocardial rupture; mitral regurgitation; pericardial effusion; pericarditis; cardiac tamponade; venous thrombosis and embolism; electromechanical dissociation.Nausea, vomiting, hypotension and fever are frequent sequelae of MI and may or may not be attributable to therapy.

Administration and Dosage:

For IV administration only.

Acute myocardial infarction (AMI): Administer as soon as possible after the onset of symptoms. Do not use a dose of 150 mg because it has been associated with an increase in intracranial bleeding.

ALTEPLASE, RECOMBINANT

Accelerated infusion – The recommended total dose is based upon patient weight, ≤ 100 mg. For patients weighing > 67 kg, the recommended dose administered is 100 mg as a 15 mg IV bolus, followed by 50 mg infused over the next 30 minutes and then 35 mg infused over the next 60 minutes.

For patients weighing ≤ 67 kg, the recommended dose is administered as a 15 mg IV bolus, followed by 0.75 mg/kg infused over the next 30 minutes not to exceed 50 mg and then 0.50 mg/kg over the next 60 minutes not to exceed 35 mg.

The safety and efficacy of this accelerated infusion of alteplase regimen has only been investigated with concomitant administration of heparin and aspirin.

3–hour infusion – 100 mg given as 60 mg (34.8 million IU) in the first hour (with 6 to 10 mg given as a bolus over the first 1 to 2 minutes), 20 mg (11.6 million IU) over the second hour and 20 mg (11.6 million IU) over the third hour. For smaller patients (< 65 kg), use a dose of 1.25 mg/kg given over 3 hours as described above.

Concomitant administration – Although the use of anticoagulants during and following alteplase has been shown to be of equivocal benefit, heparin has been given concomitantly for ≥ 24 hours in > 90% of patients. Aspirin or dipyridamole has been given either during or following heparin treatment (see Drug Interactions).

Acute ischemic stroke: The recommended dose is 0.9 mg/kg (maximum of 90 mg) infused over 60 minutes with 10% of the total dose administered as an initial IV bolus over 1 minute. The safety and efficacy of this regimen with concomitant administration of heparin and aspirin during the first 24 hours after symptom onset has not been investigated. Doses > 0.9 mg/kg may be associated with an increased incidence of ICH. Do not use doses > 0.9 mg/kg (maximum 90 mg) in the management of acute ischemic stroke.

Pulmonary embolism: 100 mg administered by IV infusion over 2 hours. Institute or reinstitute heparin therapy near the end of or immediately following the alteplase infusion when the partial thromboplastin time or TT returns to twice normal or less.

Reconstitution: Reconstitute only with Sterile Water for Injection without preservatives. Do not use Bacteriostatic Water for Injection. The reconstituted preparation results in a colorless to pale yellow transparent solution. Slight foaming upon reconstitution is usual; standing undisturbed for several minutes is usually sufficient to allow dissipation of any large bubbles.

50 mg vial – Do not use if vacuum is not present. Reconstitute with a large bore needle (eg, 18–gauge), directing the stream of Sterile Water for Injection into the lyophilized cake.

100 mg vial – Use transfer device provided for reconstitution. 100 mg vials do not contain vacuum.

Admixture compatability: May be administered as reconstituted at 1 mg/ml. As an alternative, the reconstituted solution may be further diluted immediately before administration with an equal volume of 0.9% Sodium Chloride Injection or 5% Dextrose Injection to yield a concentration of 0.5 mg/ml.

Admixture incompatibilities: Do not add other medications to infusion solution.

Storage/Stability: Store lyophilized alteplase at controlled room temperature not to exceed 30°C (86°F) or under refrigeration (2° to 8°C; 36° to 46°F). During extended storage, protect from excessive exposure to light.

The solution may be used for direct IV administration within 8 hours following reconstitution when stored between 2° and 30°C (36° and 86°F). Avoid excessive agitation during dilution; mix by gentle swirling or slow inversion. Do not use other infusion solutions.

Rx	**Activase** (Genentech)	**Lyophilized powder for injection:** 50 mg (29 million IU)/vial[1]	In vials with diluent (50 ml Sterile Water for Injection) and vacuum.
		100 mg (58 million IU)/vial[1]	In vials with diluent (100 ml Sterile Water for Injection) and one transfer device.
	Activase (Genentech)	**Lyophilized powder for injection:** 50 mg (29 million IU)/vial[1]	In vials with diluent (50 ml Sterile Water for Injection) and vacuum.
		100 mg (58 million IU)/vial[1]	In vials with diluent (100 ml Sterile Water for Injection) and one transfer device.

[1] With L-arginine, phosphoric acid and polysorbate 80.

RETEPLASE, RECOMBINANT

Actions:

Pharmacology: Reteplase is a non-glycosylated deletion mutein of tissue plasminogen activator (tPA) containing 355 of the 527 amino acids of native tPA. It is produced by recombinant DNA technology in *Escherichia coli.* It catalyzes the cleavage of endogenous plasminogen to generate plasmin. Plasmin in turn degrades the fibrin matrix of the thrombus, thereby exerting its thrombolytic action.

Pharmacokinetics: Based on the measurement of thrombolytic activity, reteplase is cleared from plasma at a rate of 250 to 450 ml/min, with an effective half-life of 13 to 16 minutes. Reteplase is cleared primarily by the liver and kidney.

Clinical trials: In three studies, patients were treated with aspirin (initial doses of 160 to 350 mg and subsequent doses of 75 to 350 mg) and heparin (a 5000 IU IV bolus prior to administration of reteplase, followed by a 1000 IU/hr continuous IV infusion for ≤ 24 hours).

Reteplase vs streptokinase – Reteplase (10 + 10 U) was compared with streptokinase (1.5 million units over 60 minutes) in a double-blind, randomized, European study. Effects upon mortality rates at 35 days were studied in 6010 patients treated within 12 hours of the symptom onset of acute myocardial infarction (AMI). Incidence of selected outcomes including 35–day mortality, 6–month mortality, combined outcome of 35–day mortality or nonfatal stroke within 35 days, heart failure and cardiogenic shock was less with reteplase patients. The total incidence of stroke was similar between the groups; however, more reteplase-treated patients experienced hemorrhagic strokes than streptokinase-treated patients.

Reteplase vs alteplase – Two arteriographic studies were performed using open-label administration of the study agents and a blinded review of the arteriograms. Patients were treated within either 6 or 12 hours of the onset of symptoms. In the first study, reteplase (in doses of 10 + 10 U, 15 U or 10 + 5 U) was compared with a 3–hour regimen of alteplase (100 mg administered over 3 hours). In the second study, reteplase (10 + 10 U) was compared with an accelerated regimen of alteplase (100 mg administered over 1.5 hours). The follow-up arteriogram was performed at a median of 8 (study 1) and 5 (study 2) days following the administration of the thrombolytics. In study 1, the best patency results were obtained with the 10 + 10 U reteplase dose. In study 2, the percentage of patients with partial or complete flow and the percentage of patients with complete flow was significantly higher with reteplase than with alteplase at 90 minutes after the initiation of therapy. In both clinical trials, the reocclusion rates were similar for reteplase and alteplase.

Indications:

Acute myocardial infarction (AMI): The management of AMI in adults for the improvement of ventricular function following AMI, the reduction of the incidence of congestive heart failure and the reduction of mortality associated with AMI. Initiate treatment as soon as possible after the onset of AMI symptoms.

Contraindications:

Active internal bleeding; history of cerebrovascular accident; recent intracranial or intraspinal surgery or trauma (see Warnings); intracranial neoplasm, arteriovenous malformation or aneurysm; bleeding diathesis or severe uncontrolled hypertension because thrombolytic therapy increases the risk of bleeding.

Warnings:

Bleeding: The most common complication encountered during therapy is bleeding. Bleeding sites include both internal sites (intracranial, retroperitoneal, GI, GU or respiratory) and superficial sites (venous cutdowns, arterial punctures, sites of recent surgical intervention). The concomitant use of heparin anticoagulation may contribute to bleeding. In clinical trials, some of the hemorrhage episodes occurred ≥ 1 day after the effects of reteplase had dissipated but while heparin therapy was continuing. Should serious bleeding (not controllable by local pressure) occur, terminate concomitant anticoagulant therapy. In addition, do not give the second bolus of reteplase if serious bleeding occurs before it is administered.

The overall incidence of any bleeding event in patients treated with reteplase in clinical studies (n = 3805) was 21%. The severity and incidence of bleeding events were comparable for reteplase and the thrombolytic agents.

RETEPLASE, RECOMBINANT

Injection sites – As fibrin is lysed during reteplase therapy, bleeding from recent injection sites may occur. Therefore, thrombolytic therapy requires careful attention to all potential bleeding sites (including catheter insertion sites, arterial and venous puncture sites, cutdown sites and needle puncture sites). Avoid noncompressible arterial puncture and internal jugular and subclavian venous punctures to minimize bleeding from noncompressible sites. Should an arterial puncture be necessary during the administration of reteplase, it is preferable to use an upper extremity vessel that is accessible to manual compression. Apply pressure for ≥ 30 minutes, apply a pressure dressing and check the puncture site frequently for evidence of bleeding.

Avoid IM injections and nonessential handling of the patient during treatment. Perform venipunctures carefully and only as required.

High risk conditions – Carefully evaluate each patient being considered for reteplase therapy and weigh the benefits against the potential risks. In the following conditions, the risks of reteplase therapy may be increased and should be weighed against the anticipated benefits.

- Recent major surgery (eg, coronary artery bypass graft, obstetrical delivery, organ biopsy)
- Previous puncture of noncompressible vessels
- Cerebrovascular disease
- Recent GI or GU bleeding
- Recent trauma
- Hypertension: Systolic BP ≥ 180 mmHg or diastolic BP ≥ 110 mmHg
- Likelihood of left heart thrombus (eg, mitral stenosis with atrial fibrillation)
- Acute pericarditis
- Subacute bacterial endocarditis
- Hemostatic defects including secondary to severe hepatic or renal disease
- Severe hepatic or renal dysfunction
- Pregnancy
- Diabetic hemorrhagic retinopathy or other ophthalmic hemorrhaging
- Septic thrombophlebitis or occluded AV cannula at a seriously infected site
- Advanced age
- Patients currently receiving oral anticoagulants (eg, warfarin sodium)
- Any other condition in which bleeding constitutes a significant hazard or would be particularly difficult to manage because of its location

Cholesterol embolization: Cholesterol embolism has been reported rarely in patients treated with thrombolytic agents; the true incidence is unknown. This serious condition, which can be lethal, is also associated with invasive vascular procedures (eg, cardiac catheterization, angiography, vascular surgery) or anticoagulant therapy. Clinical features of cholesterol embolism may include livedo reticularis, "purple toe" syndrome, acute renal failure, gangrenous digits, hypertension, pancreatitis, myocardial infarction, cerebral infarction, spinal cord infarction, retinal artery occlusion, bowel infarction and rhabdomyolysis.

Arrhythmias: Coronary thrombolysis may result in arrhythmias associated with reperfusion. These arrhythmias (eg, sinus bradycardia, accelerated idioventricular rhythm, ventricular premature depolarizations, ventricular tachycardia) are not different from those often seen in the ordinary course of AMI and should be managed with standard antiarrhythmic measures. Have antiarrhythmic therapy for bradycardia or ventricular irritability available when reteplase is administered.

Pregnancy: Category C. There are no adequate and well controlled studies in pregnant women. The most common complication of thrombolytic therapy is bleeding and certain conditions, including pregnancy, can increase this risk. Use reteplase during pregnancy only if the potential benefit justifies the potential risk to the fetus.

Lactation: It is not known whether reteplase is excreted in breast milk. Exercise caution when reteplase is administered to a nursing woman.

Children: Safety and efficacy have not been established.

Precautions:

Readministration: There is no experience with patients receiving repeat courses of therapy with reteplase. Reteplase did not induce the formation of reteplase specific antibodies in any of the ≈ 2400 patients who were tested for antibody formation. If an anaphylactoid reaction occurs, initiate appropriate therapy and do not give the second bolus of reteplase.

Drug Interactions:

In addition to bleeding associated with heparin and vitamin K antagonists, drugs that alter platelet function (eg, aspirin, dipyridamole and abciximab) may increase the risk of bleeding if administered prior to or after reteplase therapy.

RETEPLASE, RECOMBINANT

Antithrombotics: Heparin and aspirin have been administered concomitantly with and following the administration of reteplase in the management of AMI. Because heparin, aspirin or reteplase may cause bleeding complications, careful monitoring for bleeding is advised, especially at arterial puncture sites.

Drug/Lab test interactions: Administration of reteplase may cause decreases in plasminogen and fibrinogen. During reteplase therapy, if coagulation tests or measurements of fibrinolytic activity are performed, the results may be unreliable unless specific precautions are taken to prevent in vitro artifacts. Reteplase is an enzyme that when present in blood in pharmacologic concentrations remains active under in vitro conditions. This can lead to degradation of fibrinogen in blood samples removed for analysis. Collection of blood samples in the presence of PPACK (chloromethylketone) at 2 micromolar concentrations was used in clinical trials to prevent in vitro fibrinolytic artifacts.

Adverse Reactions:

Bleeding:

Reteplase Hemorrhage Rates (%)[1]

Bleeding site	Occurence rate
Injection site	4.6 to 48.6
GI	1.8 to 9
GU	0.9 to 9.5
Anemia, site unknown	0.9 to 2.6
Intracranial hemorrhage	0.8 to 2.4

[1] See Warnings.

The following adverse events are frequent sequelae of myocardial infarction and may not be attributable to therapy.

Cardiovascular: Cardiogenic shock; arrhythmias (eg, sinus bradycardia, accelerated idioventricular rhythm, ventricular premature depolarizations, supraventricular tachycardia, ventricular tachycardia, ventricular fibrillation); AV block; heart failure; cardiac arrest; recurrent ischemia; reinfarction; myocardial rupture; mitral regurgitation; pericardial effusion; pericarditis; cardiac tamponade; hypotension; electromechanical dissociation.

Miscellaneous: Pulmonary edema; venous thrombosis and embolism; nausea; vomiting; fever; serious allergic or anaphylactoid reactions (rare).

Administration and Dosage:

Reteplase is for IV administration only. Reteplase is administered as a 10 + 10 U double-bolus injection. Each bolus is administered as an IV injection over 2 minutes. The second bolus is given 30 minutes after initiation of the first bolus injection. Give each bolus injection via an IV line in which no other medication is being simultaneously injected or infused. Do not add any other medications to the injection solution.

Admixture incompatibility: Do not administer heparin and reteplase simultaneously in the same IV line. If reteplase is to be injected through an IV line containing heparin, flush Normal Saline or 5% Dextrose Solution through the line prior to and following the reteplase injection. Do not add other medications to the solution.

Reconstitution: Reconstitute only with Sterile Water for Injection (without preservatives) immediately before use. The reconstituted preparation results in a colorless solution containing 1 U/ml. Slight foaming is not unusual; allowing the vial to stand undisturbed for several minutes will usually allow dissipation of any large bubbles.

Storage/Stability: Use the solution within 4 hours after reconstitution. Store at 2° to 30°C (36° to 86°F). Keep kit sealed prior to use to protect lyophilisate from light. Store the kit at 2° to 25°C (36° to 77°F).

Rx	**Retavase** (Boehringer Mannheim)	**Powder for injection, lyophilized:** 10.8 IU (18.8 mg) reteplase[1]	Preservative-free. In kits.[2]

[1] With 940.7 mg L-arginine

[2] Each kit includes a package insert, 2 single-use reteplase vials of 10.8 U (18.8 mg), 2 single-use diluent vials for reconstitution (10 ml Sterile Water for Injection), 2 sterile 10 ml syringes with 20–gauge needle attached, 2 sterile dispensing pins, 2 sterile 20–gauge needles for dose administration and 2 alcohol swabs.

THROMBOLYTIC ENZYMES

Warning:

Consider thrombolytic therapy in situations where the potential benefits outweigh the risk of potentially serious hemorrhage. With internal bleeding, it may be more difficult to manage than that which occurs with conventional anticoagulant therapy.

Institute treatment as soon as possible after onset of pulmonary embolism, preferably within 7 days. Any delay in instituting lytic therapy to evaluate the effect of heparin decreases the potential for optimal efficacy.

Institute **urokinase** therapy within 6 hours of onset of symptoms of coronary artery thrombosis associated with evolving transmural myocardial infarction (MI).

Actions:

Pharmacology:

Urokinase, a protein of human origin, acts on the endogenous fibrinolytic system. It converts plasminogen to the enzyme plasmin. Plasmin degrades fibrin clots, fibrinogen and other plasma proteins. Intravenous infusion for lysis of pulmonary embolism is followed by increased fibrinolytic activity. This effect disappears within a few hours after discontinuation, but a decrease in plasma levels of fibrinogen and plasminogen and an increased amount of circulating fibrin(ogen) degradation products (FDP) may persist for 12 to 24 hours. There is a lack of correlation between embolus resolution and changes in coagulation and fibrinolytic assay results. Because FDP has an anticoagulant effect, bleeding may be difficult to control.

Streptokinase acts with plasminogen to produce an "activator complex" that converts plasminogen to plasmin. Plasmin degrades fibrin clots as well as fibrinogen and other plasma proteins. Intravenous infusion of streptokinase is followed by increased fibrinolytic activity, which decreases plasma fibrinogen levels for 24 to 36 hours. The hyperfibrinolytic effect disappears within a few hours after discontinuation, but a prolonged thrombin time may persist for up to 24 hours because of the decrease in plasma levels of fibrinogen and an increase in the amount of circulating FDP. Depending upon the dosage and duration of infusion of streptokinase, the thrombin time will decrease to less than two times the normal control value within 4 hours and return to normal by 24 hours.

Intravenous administration reduces blood pressure and total peripheral resistance with a corresponding reduction in cardiac afterload. Streptokinase administered by the intracoronary route results in thrombolysis, usually within 1 hour, and ensuing reperfusion results in limitation of infarct size, improvement of cardiac function and reduction of mortality. Spontaneous reperfusion is known to occur. Data from one study show that 73% of the streptokinase-treated patients and 47% of the placebo-allocated patients reperfused during hospitalization.

Variable amounts of circulating antistreptokinase antibody are present in individuals as a result of recent streptococcal infections. The recommended dosage schedule usually obviates the need for antibody titration.

Anistreplase, the p-anisoylated derivative of the lys-plasminogen-streptokinase activator complex, is an inactive derivative of a fibrinolytic enzyme with the catalytic center of the activator complex temporarily blocked by an anisoyl group. The anisoyl group does not decrease the high fibrin-binding ability of the complex. Anistreplase is made in vitro from lys-plasminogen and streptokinase. Anistreplase differs from the complex initially formed in vivo upon administration of streptokinase; the latter complex contains predominantly glu-plasminogen. In solution, deacylation of anistreplase starts immediately and the enzymatically active lys-plasminogen-streptokinase activator complex is progressively formed. The production of plasmin from plasminogen by deacylated anistreplase can take place in the bloodstream or within the thrombus; the latter process is catalytically more efficient, but both may contribute to thrombolysis.

Pharmacokinetics: Streptokinase and urokinase are administered by IV or intracoronary infusion. Anistreplase is given IV only. IV infusion of urokinase is cleared rapidly by the liver; serum half-life is ≤ 20 minutes. Expect patients with impaired liver function (eg, cirrhosis) to show a prolongation in half-life. Small fractions of urokinase are excreted in bile and urine. The half-life of the streptokinase activator complex is ≈ 23 minutes; the complex is inactivated, in part, by antistreptococcal antibodies. The mechanism of elimination is clearance by sites in the liver; no metabolites of streptokinase have been identified.The half-life of fibrinolytic activity of the circulating anistreplase is 70 to 120 minutes (mean, 94 minutes).

Clinical trials:

Streptokinase – In the GISSI study, the reduction in mortality was time dependent; there was a 47% reduction in mortality among patients treated within 1 hour of the onset of chest pain, a 23% reduction among patients treated within 3 hours and a 17% reduction among patients treated between 3 and 6 hours.

The rate of reocclusion of the infarct-related vessel has been reported to be ≈ 15% to 20%. When the reinfarctions were evaluated in studies involving 8800 streptokinase-treated patients, the overall rate was 3.8% (range, 2% to 15%). In over 8500 control patients, the rate of reinfarction was 2.4%.

Studies with thrombolytic therapy for pulmonary embolism show no significant difference in lung perfusion scan between the thrombolysis group and the heparin group at 1-year follow-up.

For deep vein thrombosis (DVT), the combined results of five randomized studies show no residual thrombotic material in 60% to 75% of streptokinase-treated patients vs 10% treated with heparin. Thrombolytic therapy also generally preserves venous valve function, avoiding the pathology that produces the clinical post-phlebitic syndrome that occurs in 90% of the DVT patients treated with heparin.

Anistreplase – Randomized, controlled studies have demonstrated that anistreplase reduces mortality when administered within 6 hours of the onset of the symptoms of acute myocardial infarction (AMI). The benefit of mortality reduction occurs acutely and is maintained for at least 1 year.

In a double-blind, randomized trial of anistreplase vs heparin bolus, left ventricular function was improved and infarction size reduced. About 3 weeks after, mean infarct size was 24% lower in anistreplase patients than in heparin patients.

Anistreplase vs streptokinase – In two studies, anistreplase and intracoronary streptokinase were compared in patients with angiographically proven coronary artery occlusion. Reperfusion occurred ≈ 45 minutes after the start of therapy for both treatment groups. When therapy was initiated within 4 hours of onset of AMI symptoms, reperfusion rates of 59% (n = 87) and 68% (n = 41) were observed for anistreplase compared with 59% (n = 85) and 70% (n = 43) for streptokinase. Of those patients who had coronary artery reperfusion, angiographically demonstrated reocclusion occurred within 24 hours in 3% to 4% of those treated with anistreplase and in 7% to 12% of those treated with streptokinase.

Indications:

Urokinase:

Pulmonary embolism – For the lysis of acute massive pulmonary emboli defined as obstruction of blood flow to a lobe or multiple segments of the lung and for the lysis of pulmonary emboli accompanied by unstable hemodynamics (ie, failure to maintain blood pressure without supportive measures).

Coronary artery thrombosis – Urokinase has been reported to lyse acute thrombi obstructing coronary arteries associated with evolving transmural MI. The majority of patients who received urokinase by intracoronary infusion within 6 hours following onset of symptoms showed recanalization of the involved vessel.

It has not been established that intracoronary administration of urokinase during evolving transmural MI results in salvage of myocardial tissue, nor that it reduces mortality. The patients who might benefit from this therapy cannot be defined.

IV catheter clearance – To restore patency to IV catheters, including central venous catheters, obstructed by clotted blood or fibrin.

Streptokinase:

Acute evolving transmural MI – For use in the management of acute myocardial infarction (AMI) in adults, the lysis of intracoronary thrombi, the improvement of ventricular function and the reduction of mortality with AMI when administered by IV or intracoronary route, as well as for reduction of infarct size and congestive heart failure. Earlier administration is correlated with greater clinical benefit.

Pulmonary embolism – For the lysis of objectively diagnosed (angiography or lung scan) pulmonary emboli involving obstruction of blood flow to a lobe or multiple segments, with or without unstable hemodynamics.

Deep vein thrombosis (DVT) – For the lysis of objectively diagnosed (preferably ascending venography), acute, extensive thrombi of the deep veins such as those involving the popliteal and more proximal vessels.

Arterial thrombosis and embolism – Streptokinase is not indicated for arterial emboli originating from the left side of the heart because of the risk of new embolic phenomena such as cerebral embolism.

Occluded AV cannulae – An alternative to surgical revision for clearing totally or partially occluded arteriovenous cannulae.

Anistreplase:

Management of acute myocardial infarction (AMI) in adults, for the lysis of thrombi obstructing coronary arteries, the reduction of infarct size, the improvement of ventricular function following AMI and the reduction of mortality associated with AMI. Initiate treatment as soon as possible after the onset of AMI symptoms.

THROMBOLYTIC ENZYMES

Contraindications:

Active internal bleeding; history of cerebrovascular accident, intracranial or intraspinal surgery or trauma (within 2 months); recent trauma including cardiopulmonary resuscitation; intracranial neoplasm, arteriovenous malformation or aneurysm; known bleeding diathesis; severe uncontrolled arterial hypertension; severe allergic reaction to this product.

Anistreplase: Severe allergic reactions to either anistreplase or streptokinase.

Warnings:

Bleeding can be placed into two broad categories: Superficial or surface bleeding observed mainly at invaded or disturbed sites (eg, venous cutdowns, arterial punctures, sites of recent surgical intervention); and internal bleeding involving the GI tract, GU tract or vagina, or occurring IM, or at retroperitoneal or intracranial sites.

Minor bleeding occurs often, mainly at invaded or disturbed sites. Do not reduce dose when lytic therapy is continued; use local measures to control minor bleeding (apply pressure for at least 30 minutes, then apply a pressure dressing).

Several fatalities due to intracranial or retroperitoneal hemorrhage have occurred. Should uncontrollable bleeding occur, immediately discontinue infusion. Slowing the rate of administration will not help correct the bleeding. If necessary, manage blood loss and reverse the bleeding tendency with whole blood (fresh blood preferably), packed red blood cells and cryoprecipitate or fresh frozen plasma. Do not use dextran. Although the use of aminocaproic acid as an antidote in humans has not been documented, consider it in an emergency.

Following high-dose, brief-duration IV **streptokinase** therapy in AMI, severe bleeding complications requiring transfusion are extremely rare (0.3% to 0.5%), and combined therapy with low dose aspirin dose not appear to increase the risk of major bleeding. The addition of aspirin to streptokinase may cause a slight increase in the risk of minor bleeding (3.1% without aspirin vs 3.9% with aspirin).

Thrombolytic enzymes will cause lysis of hemostatic fibrin deposits such as those occurring at needle puncture sites; bleeding may occur. To minimize the risk of bleeding during treatment, venipunctures and physical handling of the patient should be performed carefully and as infrequently as possible; avoid IM injections.

Avoid invasive arterial procedures before and during treatment. Should an arterial puncture be necessary (except for intracoronary administration), upper extremity vessels are preferable.

High risk patients: Carefully evaluate each patient being considered for therapy and weigh anticipated benefits against potential risks associated with therapy.

In the following conditions, the risks of thrombolytic enzyme therapy may be increased and should be weighed against the anticipated benefits:

- Recent (within 10 days) major surgery (eg, coronary artery bypass graft, obstetrical delivery, organ biopsy, previous puncture of noncompressible vessels)
- Cerebrovascular disease
- Recent GI or GU bleeding (within 10 days)
- Recent trauma (within 10 days) including cardiopulmonary resuscitation
- Hypertension: Systolic BP ≥ 180 mmHg or diastolic BP ≥ 110 mmHg
- Likelihood of left heart thrombus (eg, mitral stenosis with atrial fibrillation)
- Subacute bacterial endocarditis
- Acute pericarditis
- Hemostatic defects including secondary to severe hepatic or renal disease
- Pregnancy
- Age > 75 years
- Diabetic hemorrhagic retinopathy or other ophthalmic hemorrhaging
- Septic thrombophlebitis or occluded AV cannula at seriously infected site
- Patients currently receiving oral anticoagulants (eg, warfarin sodium)
- Any other condition in which bleeding constitutes a significant hazard or would be particularly difficult to manage because of its location

Confirm the diagnosis of pulmonary embolism by objective means, such as pulmonary angiography via an upper extremity vein, or non-invasive procedures such as lung scanning.

Fever: Symptomatic treatment is usually sufficient. Use acetaminophen rather than aspirin.

Guillain-Barré syndrome: Although a cause-and-effect relationship has not been established, several case reports suggest that **streptokinase** induces immunological responses that may initiate this syndrome.

Respiratory: There have been reports of respiratory depression in patients receiving **streptokinase**. In some cases, it was not possible to determine whether the respiratory depression was associated with streptokinase or was a symptom of the underlying process. If respiratory depression is associated with streptokinase, the occurence is believed to be rare.

IV catheter clearance: If catheters are occluded by substances other than blood fibrin clots, such as drug precipitates, **urokinase** is not effective. Avoid excessive pressure when urokinase is injected into the catheter. Force could rupture the catheter or expel the clot into the circulation.

Arrhythmias may result from coronary thrombolysis associated with reperfusion. Reperfusion of the right coronary artery may carry a higher risk. These arrhythmias (such as sinus bradycardia, accelerated idioventricular rhythm, ventricular premature depolarizations, ventricular tachycardia) are not different from those often seen in the ordinary course of AMI and may be managed with standard antiarrhythmic measures. It is recommended that antiarrhythmic therapy be available when injections of thrombolytic enzymes are administered. Carefully monitor for arrhythmias during and immediately following administration of **streptokinase** for AMI.

Hypotension, sometimes severe, not secondary to bleeding or anaphylaxis may occur during or soon after IV **streptokinase** (1% to 10%) and **anistreplase**. Monitor patients and, should symptomatic or alarming hypotension occur, administer appropriate treatment. This may include a decrease in the IV streptokinase infusion rate. Smaller hypotensive effects are common and have not required treatment.

Non-cardiogenic pulmonary edema has been reported rarely in patients treated with **streptokinase.** The risk of this appears greatest in patients who have large MIs and are undergoing thrombolytic therapy by the intracoronary route.

Polyneuropathy has been rarely temporally related to the use of **streptokinase** with some cases described as Guillain-Barré syndrome.

Anticoagulant and antiplatelets after treatment for MI: In the treatment of AMI, aspirin has been shown to reduce the incidence of reinfarction and stroke. The addition of aspirin to **streptokinase** causes a minimal increase in the risk of minor bleeding (3.9% vs 3.1%) but does not appear to increase the incidence of major bleeding. The use of anticoagulants following streptokinase administration increases the risk of bleeding but has not been shown to be of unequivocal clinical benefit. Therefore, whereas the use of aspirin is recommended unless otherwise contraindicated, the use of anticoagulants should be decided by the treating physician.

Anticoagulation after IV treatment for other indications: Continuous IV infusion of heparin, without a loading dose, has been recommended following termination of **streptokinase,** infusion for treatment of pulmonary embolism or DVT to prevent rethrombosis. The effect of streptokinase on thrombin time (TT) and activated partial thromboplastin time (APTT) will usually diminish within 3 to 4 hours after streptokinase therapy, and heparin therapy without a loading dose can be initiated when the TT or the APTT is less than twice the normal control value.

Cholesterol embolism has occurred rarely in patients treated with all types of thrombolytic agents; the true incidence is unknown. This serious condition, which can be lethal, is also associated with invasive vascular procedures (eg, cardiac catheterization, angiography, vascular surgery) or anticoagulant therapy. Clinical features of cholesterol embolism include livedo reticularis, "purple toe" syndrome, acute renal failure, gangrenous digits, hypertension, pancreatitis, MI, cerebral infarction, spinal cord infarction, retinal artery occlusion, bowel infarction and rhabdomyolysis.

Pulmonary embolism: Should pulmonary embolism or recurrent pulmonary embolism occur during **streptokinase** therapy, complete the planned course of treatment in an attempt to lyse the embolus. While pulmonary embolism may occasionally occur during streptokinase treatment, the incidence is no greater than when patients are treated with heparin alone.

Hypersensitivity: Anaphylactic and anaphylactoid reactions have been observed rarely in patients treated with IV **streptokinase** (≤ 0.1%) and **anistreplase.** Fever and shivering, occurring in 1% to 4% of patients, are the most commonly reported allergic reactions with IV **streptokinase** in AMI.

Mild or moderate allergic reactions may be managed with concomitant antihistamine or corticosteroid therapy. Severe allergic reactions require immediate discontinuation of **streptokinase** with adrenergic, antihistamine or corticosteroid agents administered IV as required. Refer to the Acute Management of Hypersensitivity.

Skin testing may identify patients at risk for immediate-type allergic reactions to **streptokinase.** Manage mild or moderate reactions with concomitant antihistamine or corticosteroid therapy.

Elderly: **Anistreplase** was found to have a favorable risk/benefit profile in elderly patients (> 65 years, n = 940) who participated in clinical trials.

THROMBOLYTIC ENZYMES

Pregnancy: (*Category B – Urokinase).* Safety for use during pregnancy has not been established. Use only when clearly needed and when the potential benefits outweigh the potential hazards to the fetus.

(*Category C – Streptokinase/Anistreplase).* It is not known whether streptokinase or anistreplase can cause fetal harm when administered to a pregnant woman or can affect reproduction capacity. Use in pregnancy only if clearly needed.

Lactation:

Urokinase/Anistreplase – It is not known whether these drugs are excreted in breast milk. Exercise caution when administering to a nursing woman.

Children: Safety and efficacy for use in children have not been established.

Precautions:

Monitoring: Before therapy, determine hematocrit, platelet count, TT, aPTT, prothrombin time (PT) or fibrinogen levels. Discontinue heparin unless it is to be used with **urokinase** for intracoronary administration. The TT or aPTT should be less than twice the normal control value before therapy. Following the infusion, before (re)instituting heparin, the TT or aPTT should be less than twice the normal control value.

Resistance: Because of the increased likelihood of resistance due to antistreptokinase antibody, **streptokinase** and **anistreplase** may not be effective if administered ≥ 5 days (streptokinase between 5 days and 12 months and anistreplase between 5 days and 6 months) of prior streptokinase or anistreplase administration or streptococcal infections (ie, streptococcal pharyngitis, acute rheumatic fever or acute glomerulonephritis secondary to a streptococcal infection).

The incidence of hematomas/bruising was somewhat greater with repeat doses, but the adverse event profile was similar to that of patients who received one dose.

IV infusion: During infusion, decreases in the plasminogen and fibrinogen levels and an increase in the FDP level (the latter two prolong the clotting times of coagulation tests) will generally confirm the existence of lysis. Results do not, however, reliably predict either efficacy or risk of bleeding. Frequently observe the clinical response and check the vital signs (ie, pulse, temperature, respiratory rate and blood pressure) at least every 4 hours. Do not take the blood pressure in the lower extremities to avoid dislodging possible deep vein thrombi. Monitor therapy by performing the TT, PT, aPTT or fibrinogen ≈ 4 hours after initiation of therapy.

Intracoronary artery infusion: During studies, laboratory monitoring of hemostatic parameters during intracoronary artery infusion of **streptokinase** or **urokinase** showed minimal changes, if any. Heparin was continued or instituted following therapy and monitored accordingly.

Drug Interactions:

Anticoagulants and antiplatelet agents: Thrombolytic enzymes, alone or in combination with these agents, may cause bleeding complications; carefully monitor. Antiplatelet agents increased the incidence of bleeding events similarly in patients treated with anistreplase or non-thrombolytic therapy. There was no evidence of a synergistic effect of combined **anistreplase** and antiplatelet agents on bleeding events. In addition, there was no difference in the incidence of hemorrhagic cerebrovascular accidents in anistreplase-treated patients who did or did not receive aspirin.

Drug/Lab test interactions: IV administration of **streptokinase** and **anistreplase** will cause marked decreases in plasminogen and fibrinogen and increases in TT, aPTT and PT which normalize within 12 to 24 hours. These changes may also occur in some patients with intracoronary administration of streptokinase. Results of coagulation tests or measures of fibrinolytic activity performed during anistreplase therapy may be unreliable unless specific precautions are taken to prevent in vitro artifacts. Anistreplase, when present in blood in pharmacologic concentrations, remains active under in vitro conditions. This can lead to degradation of fibrinogen in blood samples removed for analysis. Collection of blood samples in the presence of aprotinin (2000 to 3000 KIU/ml) can, to some extent, mitigate this phenomenon.

Adverse Reactions:

Bleeding: There are two types: *Minor* (superficial or surface bleeding) and *major* (internal, severe bleeding). See Warnings.

Allergic reactions:

Urokinase – No evidence of induced antibody formation exists. Mild allergic reactions (eg, bronchospasm, skin rash) have been reported. Anaphylaxis is rare. Fever, chills, rigors, nausea or vomiting, transient hypotension or hypertension, dyspnea, tachycardia, cyanosis, back pain, hypoxemia and acidosis have been reported together and separately. Rare cases of MI with unknown causal relationship have also been reported.

THROMBOLYTIC ENZYMES

Anistreplase – Anaphylactic and anaphylactoid reactions (0.2%); urticaria, itching, flushing, rashes and eosinophilia have been occasionally observed. A delayed purpuric rash occurred in 0.3% of patients and may be associated with arthralgia, ankle edema, GI symptoms, mild hematuria, mild proteinuria and vasculitis. The syndrome was self-limiting and without long-term sequelae. See Warnings.

An unknown causal relationship (may also be associated with AMI or other therapy) reported in clinical trials: Chills, fever, headache, shock, cardiac rupture, chest pain, emboli, purpura, sweating, nausea or vomiting, thrombocytopenia, elevated transaminase levels, arthralgia, agitation, dizziness, paresthesia, tremor, vertigo, dyspnea, lung edema (< 10%); Guillain Barré syndrome, adult respiratory distress syndrome, low back pain (rare).

Cardiovascular: Arrhythmia/conduction disorders (38%); hypotension (10.4%). See Warnings.

Streptokinase – Anaphylactic and anaphylactoid reactions (0.1%); minor breathing difficulty; bronchospasm; periorbital swelling; urticaria; itching; flushing; nausea; headache; musculoskeletal pain; pulmonary edema; delayed hypersensitivity reactions (eg, vasculitis and interstitial nephritis) (see Warnings); angioneurotic edema, facial hematoma, low back pain (rare).

UROKINASE

For complete prescribing information, refer to the Thrombolytic Enzymes group monograph.

Administration and Dosage:

Pulmonary embolism: Administer via a constant infusion pump capable of delivering a total volume of 195 ml.

Give a priming dose of 4400 IU/kg (2000 IU/lb) as an admixture of urokinase with either 0.9% Sodium Chloride Injection or 5% Dextrose Injection at a rate of 90 ml/hour over 10 minutes. Follow by continuous infusion of 4400 IU/kg/hr (2000 IU/lb/hr) at a rate of 15 ml/hour for 12 hours. Some admixture will remain in the tubing at the end of an infusion pump delivery cycle; therefore, perform the following flush procedure to ensure administration of the total dose: Administer a solution of 0.9% Sodium Chloride Injection or 5% Dextrose Injection, approximately equal in amount to the volume of the tubing in the infusion set, via the pump to flush the admixture from the entire length of the infusion set. Pump the flush solution at the continuous infusion rate of 15 ml/hr.

At the end of therapy, treat with continuous heparin IV infusion to prevent recurrent thrombosis. Do not begin heparin until TT has decreased to less than twice the normal control value (≈ 3 to 4 hours after completing infusion).

Lysis of coronary artery thrombi: Prior to the infusion of urokinase, administer a bolus dose of heparin ranging from 2500 to 10,000 units IV. Consider prior heparin administration when calculating the heparin dose for this procedure. Following the bolus dose of heparin, infuse the prepared solution into the occluded artery at a rate of 4 ml/min (6000 IU/min) for ≤ 2 hours. In a clinical study, the average total dose of urokinase used for lysis of coronary artery thrombi was 500,000 IU.

To determine therapy response, periodic angiography during the infusion is recommended. It is suggested that the angiography be repeated at ≈ 15 minute intervals.

Continue therapy until the artery is maximally opened, usually 15 to 30 minutes after the initial opening. Following the infusion, determine coagulation parameters. It is advisable to continue heparin therapy after the artery is opened.

IV catheter clearance: When the following procedure is used to clear a central venous catheter, instruct the patient to exhale and hold his breath when the catheter is not connected to IV tubing or a syringe to prevent air from entering the catheter.

Disconnect the IV tubing from the catheter hub and attach an empty 10 ml syringe. Determine occlusion of the catheter by gently attempting to aspirate blood from the catheter with the 10 ml syringe. If aspiration is not possible, remove the syringe and attach a 1 ml tuberculin syringe filled with prepared urokinase to the catheter. Slowly and gently inject an amount of solution equal to the volume of the catheter. Remove the tuberculin syringe and connect an empty 5 ml syringe to the catheter. Wait ≥ 5 minutes before attempting to aspirate the drug and residual clot with the 5 ml syringe. Repeat aspiration attempts every 5 minutes. If the catheter is not open within 30 minutes, cap the catheter; allow urokinase to remain in the catheter 30 to 60 minutes before attempting to aspirate again. A second injection of urokinase may be necessary in resistant cases.

When patency is restored, aspirate 4 to 5 ml of blood to ensure removal of all drug and residual clot. Remove the blood-filled syringe, and replace it with a 10 ml syringe filled with 0.9% Sodium Chloride Injection. Gently irrigate the catheter with this solution to ensure patency of the catheter. Remove the 10 ml syringe, and reconnect sterile IV tubing to the catheter hub.

UROKINASE

Preparation of solution: Reconstitute three 250,000 IU vials with 5 ml Sterile Water for Injection. It is important to reconstitute only with Sterile Water for Injection without preservatives. Do not use Bacteriostatic Water for Injection. The solution should be slightly straw-colored. For further dilution procedures, consult the manufacturer's literature. To minimize formation of filaments, avoid shaking the vial during reconstitution. Roll and tilt the vial to enhance reconstitution. The solution may be terminally filtered (eg, through a ≤ 0.45 micron cellulose membrane filter). Do not add other medications to this solution. Because urokinase contains no preservatives, do not reconstitute until immediately before use. Discard any unused portion of the reconstituted material.

Storage/Stability:

Injection – Store powder at 2° to 8°C (35° to 47°F).

Catheter clearance – Store powder below 25°C (77°F). Avoid freezing.

Rx	**Abbokinase** (Abbott)	**Powder for Injection, lyophilized:** 250,000 IU/vial[1]	In vials.
Rx	**Abbokinase Open-Cath** (Abbott)	**Powder for catheter clearance**[2]	In single-dose 1 and 1.8 ml *Univials.*
🍁	**Abbokinase** (Abbott)	**Powder for Injection, lyophilized:** 250,000 IU/vial[1]	In 5 ml vials.
🍁	**Abbokinase Open-Cath** (Abbott)	**Powder for catheter clearance:** 5000 IU/ml	In 1 ml vials.

[1] With 25 mg mannitol, 250 mg albumin (human) and 50 mg sodium chloride.

[2] With 5 mg gelatin and 15 mg mannitol, 1.7 mg sodium chloride and 4.6 mg monobasic sodium phosphate anhydrous/ml when reconstituted.

STREPTOKINASE

For complete prescribing information, refer to the Thrombolytic Enzymes group monograph.

Administration and Dosage:

Acute evolving transmural MI: Administer as soon as possible after symptom onset. The greatest benefit in mortality reduction was observed when streptokinase was administered within 4 hours, but statistically significant benefit has been reported up to 24 hours.

IV infusion – Administer a total dose of 1,500,000 IU within 60 minutes.

Intracoronary infusion – Administer 20,000 IU by bolus followed by 2000 IU/min for 60 minutes for a total dose of 140,000 IU.

Pulmonary embolism, DVT, arterial thrombosis or embolism: Institute treatment as soon as possible after thrombotic event onset, preferably no later than 7 days after onset. Any delay in instituting lytic therapy to evaluate the effect of heparin therapy decreases the potential for optimal efficacy. Because human exposure to streptococci is common, antibodies to streptokinase (streptokinase resistance) are found normally. Thus, a loading dose of streptokinase sufficient to neutralize the resistance is required. A dose of 250,000 IU streptokinase infused into a peripheral vein over 30 minutes was appropriate in > 90% of patients. If the TT, aPTT or PT after 4 hours of therapy is < 1½ times the baseline, discontinue streptokinase.

Streptokinase Dosages

Indication	Loading dose	IV Infusion Dosage/Duration
Pulmonary embolism	250,000 IU over 30 min	100,000 IU/hr for 24 hrs (72 hrs if concurrent DVT is suspected).
Deep vein thrombosis	250,000 IU over 30 min	100,000 IU/hr for 72 hrs
Arterial thrombosis or embolism	250,000 IU over 30 min	100,000 IU/hr for 24 to 72 hrs

Arteriovenous cannula occlusion: Before using, try to clear the cannula by syringe technique, using heparinized saline solution. Slowly instill 250,000 IU in 2 ml solution into each occluded limb of the cannula. Clamp off cannula limb(s) for 2 hrs. Observe closely for adverse effects. After treatment, aspirate contents of infused cannula limb(s), flush with saline, reconnect cannula.

Reconstitution: Reconstitute with 5 ml Sodium Chloride Injection. Although Normal Saline is the usual diluent, 5% Dextrose Injection may also be used. For dissolution, gently swirl the vial. Avoid shaking to prevent foaming. Adjust the concentrate by addition of the same diluent.

STREPTOKINASE

Slight flocculation (thin translucent fibers) of reconstituted streptokinase occurs occasionally. Slowly add 5 ml Sodium Chloride Injection or 5% Dextrose Injection to the vial or bottle, directing the diluent at the side of the bottle or vial rather than into the drug powder. Roll and tilt gently to reconstitute. Avoid shaking.

Vial – If necessary, total volume may be increased to a maximum of 500 ml in glass or 50 ml in plastic containers.

Bottle – Administer by infusion pump. The reconstituted solution can be filtered through a 0.8 mcg or larger pore size filter.

Arteriovenous cannula – Slowly reconstitute contents of the 250,000 IU, vacuum-packed vial with 2 ml Sodium Chloride Injection or 5% Dextrose Injection.

Storage/Stability: Store unopened vials at room temperature (15° to 30°C or 59° to 86°F). The solution may be used for direct IV administration within 8 hours following reconstitution if stored at 2° to 8°C (36° to 46°F). Discard unused reconstituted drug. Do not add other medication to streptokinase.

Rx	**Kabikinase** (Pharmacia)	**Powder for Injection, lyophilized:** 250,000 IU and 750,000 IU/vial	No preservatives. In 8 ml vials.[1]
		1,500,000 IU/vial	No preservatives. In 10 ml vials.
Rx	**Streptase** (Astra)	**Powder for Injection, lyophilized**[2]: 250,000 IU and 750,000 IU/vial	No preservatives. In 6.5 ml vials.
		1,500,000 IU/vial	No preservatives. In 6.5 ml vials and 50 ml infusion bottle.
	Kabikinase (Pharmacia)	**Powder for Injection, lyophilized**[3]: 250,000 IU/vial and 750,000 IU/vial	In 8 ml vials.
		1,500,000 IU/vial	In 10 ml vials.
	Streptase (Hoechst-Roussel)	**Powder for Injection, lyophilized**[2]: 250,000 IU and 750,000 IU/vial	In 6.5 ml vials.
		1,500,000 IU/vial	In 6.5 ml vials and 68 ml infusion bottles.

[1] With 11 mg sodium l-glutamate and 14.5 mg albumin (human)/100,000 IU streptokinase.

[2] With 25 mg cross-linked gelatin polypeptides, 25 mg sodium l-glutamate and 100 mg normal serum albumin (human).

[3] With albumin (human), disodium phosphate anhydrous, sodium dihydrogen phosphate anhydrous and sodium-l-glutamate anhydrous.

ANISTREPLASE (Anisoylated Plasminogen Streptokinase Activator Complex; APSAC)

For complete prescribing information, refer to the Thrombolytic Enzymes group monograph.

Administration and Dosage:

Administer as soon as possible after the onset of symptoms. The recommended dose is 30 units of anistreplase administered only by IV injection over 2 to 5 minutes into an IV line or vein.

Reconstitution: Slowly add 5 ml of Sterile Water for Injection, by directing the stream of fluid against the side of the vial. Gently roll the vial, mixing the dry powder and fluid. Do not shake. Try to minimize foaming. The reconstituted preparation is a colorless to pale yellow transparent solution. Withdraw the entire contents of the vial.

Admixture incompatibility: Do not further dilute the reconstituted solution before administration or adding to any infusion fluids. Do not add other medications to the vial or syringe containing anistreplase.

Storage/Stability: Store lyophilized anistreplase between 2° to 8°C (36° to 46°F). If not administered within 30 minutes of reconstitution, discard.

Rx	**Eminase** (Roberts)	**Powder for injection, lyophilized**: 30 units[1]	Preservative free. In vials.[2]

[1] Potency is expressed in anistreplase units using an anitreplase-specific reference standard not comparable with other fibrinolytic units.

[2] With 100 mg mannitol, 46 mg L-lysine and 30 mg albumin (human).

PENTOXIFYLLINE

Actions:

Pharmacology: Pentoxifylline, a tri-substituted xanthine derivative, produces dose-related hemorheologic effects, and its metabolites improve blood flow by decreasing blood viscosity and improving erythrocyte flexiblity. Leukocyte properties of hemorheologic importance have been modified in animal and in vitro human studies. Pentoxifylline has been shown to increase leukocyte deformability and to inhibit neutrophil adhesion and activation. Tissue oxygen levels have been shown to be significantly increased by therapeutic doses of pentoxifylline in patients with peripheral arterial disease.

Pharmacokinetics:

Absorption/Distribution – After administration of the 400 mg controlled release tablet, plasma levels of the parent compound and its metabolites reach their maximum within 2 to 4 hours. Food intake shortly before dosing delays absorption of an immediate-release dosage form but does not affect total absorption. After oral administration in an aqueous solution, pentoxifylline is almost completely absorbed. Plasma levels of the parent compound and its metabolites peak within 1 hour.

Metabolism/Excretion – Pentoxifylline undergoes a first-pass effect. The major metabolites are Metabolite I and Metabolite V with plasma levels 5 and 8 times greater, respectively, than pentoxifylline. Following oral administration of aqueous solutions, the pharmacokinetics of the parent compound and Metabolite I are dose-related and not proportional (non-linear), with half-life and area under the blood level time curve (AUC) increasing with dose. The elimination kinetics of Metabolite V are not dose-dependent. Plasma half-lives of pentoxifylline and its metabolites are 0.4 to 0.8 hours and 1 to 1.6 hours, respectively. There is no evidence of accumulation or enzyme induction. The main biotransformation product is Metabolite V and excretion is primarily urinary. Essentially no parent drug is found in the urine. Less than 4% of the dose is recovered in feces.

Elderly: AUC was increased and elimination rate decreased in an older population (60 to 68 years) compared with younger individuals (22 to 30 years).

Indications:

Intermittent claudication on the basis of chronic occlusive arterial disease of the limbs. It improves function and symptoms but does not replace definitive therapy.

Unlabeled uses: Pentoxifylline was found superior to placebo in improving psychopathological symptoms in patients with cerebrovascular insufficiency. The drug has also been studied in diabetic angiopathies and neuropathies, transient ischemic attacks, leg ulcers, sickle cell thalassemias, strokes, high-altitude sickness, asthenozoospermia, acute and chronic hearing disorders, severe idiopathic recurrent aphthous stomatitis (400 mg three times a day for 1 month), eye circulation disorders and Raynaud's phenomenon.

Contraindications:

Patients with recent cerebral or retinal hemorrhage; intolerance to pentoxifylline or methylxanthines (eg, caffeine, theophylline, theobromine).

Warnings:

Hemorrhage: Patients with risk factors complicated by hemorrhage (eg, recent surgery, peptic ulceration) should have periodic exams for bleeding including hematocrit or hemoglobin.

Renal function impairment: The clearance of pentoxifylline is reduced in patients with renal impairment, possibly resulting in toxicity. A lower dosage may be necessary in these patients.

Pregnancy: Category C. Animal studies showed no fetal malformation. Increased resorption was seen in rats of the 576 mg/kg group. No adequate studies exist in pregnant women. Use only if clearly needed.

Lactation: Pentoxifylline and its metabolites are excreted in breast milk. Because of the potential for tumorigenicity seen in rats, decide whether to discontinue nursing or discontinue the drug, taking into account the importance of the drug to the mother.

Children: Safety and efficacy for use in children are not established.

Precautions:

Arterial disease of the limbs: Patients with chronic occlusive arterial disease of the limbs frequently show other manifestations of arteriosclerotic disease. There have been occasional reports of angina, hypotension and arrhythmia. Periodic systemic blood pressure monitoring is recommended, especially in patients receiving concomitant antihypertensive therapy.

PENTOXIFYLLINE

Drug Interactions:

Pentoxifylline Drug Interactions			
Precipitant drug	Object drug*		Description
Pentoxifylline	Warfarin	⬆	Although a causal relationship has not been established, there have been reports of bleeding and prolonged prothrombin time (PT) in patients receiving pentoxifylline with or without anticoagulants or platelet aggregation inhibitors. Frequently monitor PT in patients on warfarin.
Pentoxifylline	Theophylline	⬆	Concomitant administration of pentoxifylline-containing drugs leads to increased theophylline levels and theophylline toxicity in some individuals. Monitor patients closely for signs of toxicity and adjust theophylline dosage as necessary.
Pentoxifylline	Antihypertensives	⬆	Small decreases in blood pressure have been observed in some patients treated with pentoxifylline, periodically monitor systemic blood pressure for patients receiving concomitant antihypertensive therapy. If indicated, reduce dosage of the antihypertensive agents.

Adverse Reactions:

Rare (causal relationship unknown): Arrhythmia, tachycardia, anaphylactoid reactions, hepatitis, increased liver enzymes, jaundice, decreased serum fibrinogen, pancytopenia, aplastic anemia, leukemia, purpura, thrombocytopenia.

Cardiovascular: Angina/chest pain (0.3%); edema, hypotension, dyspnea (< 1%).

GI: Dyspepsia (2.8%); nausea (2.2%); vomiting (1.2%); belching/flatus/bloating (0.6%); anorexia, cholecystitis, constipation, dry mouth/thirst (< 1%).

CNS: Dizziness (1.9%); headache (1.2%); tremor (0.3%); anxiety, confusion, depression, seizures (< 1%).

Respiratory: Epistaxis, flu-like symptoms, laryngitis, nasal congestion (< 1%).

Dermatologic: Brittle fingernails, pruritus, rash, urticaria, angioedema (< 1%).

Ophthalmic: Blurred vision, conjunctivitis, scotomata (< 1%).

Miscellaneous: Earache, bad taste, excessive salivation, leukopenia, malaise, sore throat/swollen neck glands, weight change (< 1%).

Overdosage:

Symptoms: Apparently dose-related, usually occur 4 to 5 hours after ingestion and last ≈ 12 hours. Flushing, hypotension, nervousness, tremors, convulsions, somnolence, loss of consciousness, fever and agitation have occurred. Bradycardia (30 to 40 beats/min) with first and second degree AV block occurring after 2 hours in a patient who ingested 4 to 6 g; first degree AV block persisted until 16 hours after admission.

Treatment: Treat with gastric lavage and administer activated charcoal. Monitor ECG and blood pressure. In addition to symptomatic treatment, support respiration, maintain blood pressure, treat cardiac arrhythmias and control convulsions as required.

Administration and Dosage:

Take 400 mg 3 times daily with meals. If GI and CNS side effects occur, decrease to 400 mg twice daily. If side effects persist, discontinue. While therapeutic effects may be seen within 2 to 4 weeks, continue treatment for ≥ 8 weeks.

Rx	**Trental** (Hoechst Marion Roussel)	**Tablets, controlled release:** 400 mg	(Trental.) Pink. Film coated. Oblong. In 100s, bulk pack 5000s and UD 100s.

ANTITHROMBIN III (HUMAN)

Actions:

Pharmacology: Antithrombin III (human), produced from pooled human plasma of healthy donors, is a glycoprotein of molecular weight 58,000 and consists of 425 amino acids in a single polypeptide chain crosslinked by three disulfide bridges. Antithrombin III is identical with heparin cofactor I, a factor in plasma necessary for heparin to exert its anticoagulant effect. The quantity of antithrombin III in 1 ml of normal pooled human plasma is conventionally taken as one unit. The potency assignment has been determined with a standard calibrated against a World Health Organization (WHO) Antithrombin III Reference Preparation.

Each unit of plasma used to produce this product has been tested and found nonreactive for hepatitis B surface antigen (HBsAg) and negative for antibody to human immunodeficiency virus (HIV) by FDA-approved tests. In addition, antithrombin III has been heat-treated in solution at 60°C (140°F) for ≥ 10 hours.

Antithrombin III is a major coagulation inhibitor in blood. It inactivates thrombin and the activated forms of Factors IX, X, XI and XII (ie, all coagulation enzymes except Factor VIIa and Factor XIIIa). The concentration of antithrombin III in normal plasma has been estimated from 0.1 to 0.2 g/L. Antithrombin III levels are usually expressed as a percentage of a reference plasma.

In subjects with hereditary antithrombin III deficiency, the levels of antithrombin III are ≈ 50% of the level in normal human plasma. These subjects have a high risk of thromboembolic disease even at an early age. Surgery and pregnancy are significant factors precipitating venous thrombosis in antithrombin III deficient patients. Give antithrombin III (human) as replacement treatment in patients with hereditary antithrombin III deficiency in connection with surgical or obstetrical procedures or when they suffer from thromboembolism.

Pharmacokinetics: The mean biological half-life in three patients with hereditary antithrombin III deficiency and one healthy subject was 3 days. The half-life of antithrombin III is decreased by concurrent heparin treatment (see Drug Interactions).

Clinical trials: In clinical studies, 39 patients with hereditary antithrombin III deficiency were treated with antithrombin III on 60 separate occasions. In each case, antithrombin III was given prophylactically or therapeutically. In 68% of the treatments, the doses were between 30 and 50 IU/kg/day, and the duration of therapy was 2 to 8 days (range, 1 day to 20 weeks). Twenty women were given 47 prophylactic treatments during delivery and postpartum; 12 had previous thromboembolic complications. Further, seven women were treated during abortion; all patients had at least two previous incidences of thromboembolism. In cases treated with antithrombin III, there was no incidence of thrombosis. The same results were obtained when nine surgical patients were treated (13 operations). There was no thrombosis in connection with treatment, although seven patients had previous thrombosis. Additionally, 11 patients were treated for acute thrombosis. Five patients were treated with heparin alone without disappearance of soreness, swelling and pain. Addition of antithrombin III to the regimen reduced the thrombotic signs. The remaining six patients were treated with antithrombin III in combination with oral anticoagulants or heparin. In all cases but one, the clinical signs of acute thrombosis were reduced or eliminated after the combined treatment.

Indications:

Antithrombin III deficiency: Treatment of patients with hereditary antithrombin III deficiency in connection with surgical or obstetrical procedures or when they suffer from thromboembolism. Determine dosage so that the antithrombin III level in plasma is maintained at > 80%. (See Precautions and Administration and Dosage sections.)

Warnings:

HBsAg and HIV: This product is prepared from pooled units of human plasma. The risk of viral infection from this product cannot be totally eliminated. Each unit of plasma used to make this product has been tested and found nonreactive for HBsAg and negative for antibody to HIV by FDA-approved tests. These testing procedures are used to eliminate high-risk plasma donors, and a heat treatment step (60°C [140°F] for ≥ 10 hours in solution) in the manufacturing process is designed to reduce the risk of transmitting viral infections. However, test methods are not sensitive enough to detect all units of potentially infectious plasma, and treatment methods have not been shown to be totally effective in eliminating viral infectivity from this product.

Individuals who receive multiple infusions of blood or plasma products may develop signs or symptoms of some viral infections, particularly non-A, non-B hepatitis.

ANTITHROMBIN III (HUMAN)

Neonatal thromboembolism: Immediately after birth, measure the antithrombin III level in neonates of parents with hereditary antithrombin III deficiency . Fatal neonatal thromboembolism, such as aortic thrombi in children of women with hereditary antithrombin III deficiency has occurred. It is recommended that testing and treatment with antithrombin III of such neonates be discussed with an expert on coagulation.

Pregnancy: Category C. It is not known whether antithrombin III can cause fetal harm when administered to a pregnant woman or can affect reproductive capacity. Give to a pregnant woman only if clearly needed. Studies in pregnant women have not shown that antithrombin III increases the risk of fetal abnormalities if administered during the third trimester of pregnancy. Antithrombin III concentrates have been used in 23 full-term pregnancies; all resulted in deliveries with no neonatal complications and with healthy children.

Children: Only a few neonates and children have been treated with antithrombin III. Safety and efficacy in children have not been established.

Precautions:

Thrombosis: Inform subjects with antithrombin III deficiency about the risk of thrombosis in connection with pregnancy and surgery and about the inheritance of the disease.

Recommended rate of infusion is 50 IU/min (1 ml/min); do not exceed 100 IU/min (2 ml/min). One healthy subject became dyspneic after a rapid IV injection (1500 IU in 5 minutes), and his blood pressure increased.

Antithrombin III *deficiency diagnosis:* Base the diagnosis of hereditary antithrombin III deficiency on a clear family history of venous thrombosis as well as decreased plasma antithrombin III levels and the exclusion of acquired deficiency. Monitor antithrombin III plasma levels during the treatment period.

Antithrombin III in plasma may be measured with amidolytic assays by using synthetic chromogenic substrates or with clotting assays or with immunoassays. The latter does not detect all congenital antithrombin III deficiencies.

Drug Interactions:

Heparin: The anticoagulant effect of heparin is enhanced by concurrent antithrombin III in patients with hereditary antithrombin III deficiency. Thus, in order to avoid bleeding, reduce heparin dosage during antithrombin III treatment.

Adverse Reactions:

No adverse reactions occurred in clinical trials in hereditary antithrombin III deficient patients. However, 2 of 65 patients, with acquired antithrombin III deficiency with severe disseminated intravascular coagulation, exhibited diuretic and vasodilatory effects. In one case, the recorded decrease in arterial systolic blood pressure was 25 mmHg. The other decrease was not recorded.

Overdosage:

Antithrombin III levels of 150% to 210% have been found in a few patients, and no signs or symptoms of complications have been identified.

Administration and Dosage:

Each bottle of antithrombin III (human) is labeled with antithrombin III (AT-III) content expressed in International Units (IU). The quantity of antithrombin III in 1 ml of normal pooled human plasma is conventionally taken as one unit. The potency assignment has been determined with a standard calibrated against a World Health Organization (WHO) Antithrombin III Reference Preparation.

The amount of antithrombin III required to restore the recipient to a normal level varies with the circumstances and patient. Individualize dosage according to the needs of the patient. Consider the weight of the patient, the degree of the deficiency and the desired level of antithrombin III to be achieved. Base the dose on the medical judgment of the physician and on laboratory control values.

After the first dose, the antithrombin III level should increase to ≈ 120% of normal. Thereafter, maintain at levels > 80%. This may be achieved by administration of maintenance doses once every 24 hours. Initially and until the patient is stabilized, measure the antithrombin III level at least twice a day, thereafter once a day and always immediately before the next infusion.

ANTITHROMBIN III (HUMAN)

The administration of 1 IU/kg raises the level of AT-III by 1% to 2.1% depending on the condition of the patient. Thus, an initial loading dose may be calculated from the following formula (assuming a plasma volume of 40 ml/kg).

$$\text{Dosage Units} = \frac{[\text{desired AT-III level (\%)} - \text{baseline AT-III level (\%)}] \times \text{body weight (kg)}}{1\%/(\text{IU/kg})}$$

Thus, if a 70 kg individual has a baseline AT-III level of 57%, the initial dose would be (120% – 57%) × 70/1 = 4410 IU.

Measure plasma AT-III levels preceding and 30 minutes after the dose, and calculate the in vivo recovery. If the recovery differs from an anticipated rise of 1% for each IU/kg administered, modify the formula accordingly. For example, if in the above example, the plasma level measured 30 minutes after the infusion is 147%, then the increases in AT-III measured per each 1 IU/kg administered is (147% – 57%) × 70 kg/4410 units = 1.43% rise for each IU/kg.

The above recommendations for dosing are provided only as a general guideline for therapy. Individualize the exact loading and maintenance dosages and dosing intervals for each subject based on the individual clinical conditions, response to therapy and actual plasma AT-III levels achieved. Perform laboratory tests to assure that the desired levels are achieved.

When an infusion of antithrombin III is indicated for a patient with hereditary deficiency to control an acute thrombotic episode or to prevent thrombosis following surgical or obstetrical procedures, raise the antithrombin III level to normal and maintain this level for 2 to 8 days depending on the indication for treatment, type and extensiveness of surgery, the patient's medical condition and history and the physician's judgment. Base concomitant administration of heparin in each of these situations on the medical judgment of the physician.

Reconstitution: Dissolve the powder in 10 ml Sterile Water for Injection. Gently swirl the vial to dissolve the powder. Do not shake. Bring the solution to room temperature, and administer within 3 hours following reconstitution. Antithrombin III may be infused over 5 to 10 minutes. Administer IV.

Alternately, reconstitute with 0.9% Sodium Chloride Injection or 5% Dextrose Injection. After reconstitution, antithrombin III may be further diluted with the same diluent.

Rx	**ATnativ** (Hyland)	**Powder for injection, lyophilized:** 500 IU of antithrombin III (human)	In 50 ml infusion bottle with 10 ml Sterile Water for Injection.

ANTIHEMOPHILIC FACTOR (Factor VIII; AHF)

Actions:

Pharmacology: Antihemophilic factor (AHF) is a protein found in normal plasma necessary for clot formation. Administration of AHF can temporarily correct the coagulation defect of patients with classical hemophilia (hemophilia A). It is needed for transformation of prothrombin (Factor II) to thrombin by the intrinsic pathway.

Indications:

Classical hemophilia (hemophilia A), in which there is a deficiency of the plasma clotting factor, Factor VIII. Provides a means of temporarily replacing the missing clotting factor to correct or prevent bleeding episodes or perform surgery.

Contraindications:

Hypersensitivity to mouse, hamster or bovine protein (see Precautions).

Warnings:

von Willebrand's disease: Not effective in controlling the bleeding of patients with von Willebrand's disease.

Hepatitis and AIDS: AHF is prepared from human plasma; the risk of transmitting hepatitis or AIDS is present. The individual units of plasma are nonreactive when tested for hepatitis B surface antigen. In addition, these products are heated during manufacturing to reduce the risk of hepatitis transmission (including some non-A, non-B hepatitis).

Patients who have not received multiple infusions of blood or plasma products are very likely to develop signs or symptoms of some viral infections, especially non-A or non-B hepatitis, after introduction of clotting factor concentrates. For such patients, especially those with mild hemophilia, use single donor products. For patients with moderate or severe hemophilia who have received numerous infusions of blood or blood products, the risk of hepatitis is small.

Human T-lymphocyte virus type III/lymphadenopathy-associated virus (HIV) is the virus believed to cause AIDS. Donor screening tests for antibodies to HIV are available and are used to screen donated blood. Positive tests are further screened. Antibodies develop in infected individuals within 2 to 3 months of infection.

Pregnancy: Category C. Safety for use during pregnancy has not been established. Use only if clearly needed.

Children: AHF is safe and effective for use in children of all ages, including neonates.

Precautions:

Factor VIII inhibitor: Approximately 10% of patients with hemophilia develop inhibitors to Factor VIII. In patients with inhibitors, the response to AHF may be greatly reduced, and patients with high inhibitor levels may not respond to AHF. Anti-inhibitor complex is available.

Hemolysis: AHF contains naturally occurring blood group specific antibodies (Anti-A and Anti-B isoagglutinins). When large or frequently repeated doses are needed in patients of blood group A, B or AB, intravascular hemolysis may occur; monitor the hematocrit and Direct Coombs' test. Correct hemolytic anemia with compatible group O red blood cells.

Monoclonal antibody-derived Factor VIII:

Formation of antibodies to mouse protein – Although no hypersensitivity reactions have been observed, they may possibly occur due to trace amounts of mouse protein (less than 50 ng per 100 AHF activity units).

Laboratory tests: Assure that adequate AHF levels have been reached and are maintained. If the AHF level fails to reach expected levels or if bleeding is not controlled after apparently adequate dosage, inhibitors may be present. The presence of inhibitors can be demonstrated and quantitated in terms of AHF units neutralized by each ml of plasma or by the total estimated plasma volume. After sufficient dosage to neutralize inhibitor, additional dosage produces predicted clinical response.

Adverse Reactions:

Headache; somnolence; lethargy; acute hemolytic anemia; increased bleeding tendency; hyperfibrinogenemia (rare); flushing, diarrhea, fatigue, epistaxis (occurred in only one patient); dizziness; sore throat; cold feet; taste perversion; slight hypotension; nonspecific rash.

Allergic reactions: Hives, fever, urticaria, mild chills, nausea, stinging at the infusion site, tightness of the chest, hypotension and anaphylaxis may occur.

ANTIHEMOPHILIC FACTOR (Factor VIII; AHF)

Administration and Dosage:

Administer IV only. Use a plastic syringe; solutions may stick to the surface of glass.

Individualize dosage. The dose depends on patient weight, severity of the deficiency, severity of hemorrhage, presence of inhibitors and the Factor VIII level desired. Clinical effect on the patient is the most important factor of therapy. When inhibitors are present, dosage requirements are extremely variable; determine by clinical response. It may be necessary to administer more AHF to obtain the desired result.

There is a linear dose-response relation with an approximate yield of 2% rise in Factor VIII activity for each unit of Factor VIII/kg transfused. The following formulas provide a guide for dosage calculations:

$$\text{Expected Factor VIII increase (in \% of normal)} = \frac{\text{AHF/IU administered} \times 2}{\text{body weight (in kg)}}$$

$$\text{AHF/IU required} = \text{body weight (kg)} \times \text{desired Factor VIII increase (\% normal)} \times 0.5$$

Follow therapy with Factor VIII level assays. It may be dangerous to assume any certain level has been reached without direct evidence.

Prophylaxis of spontaneous hemorrhage: The level of Factor VIII required to prevent spontaneous hemorrhage is approximately 5% of normal; 30% of normal is the minimum required for hemostasis following trauma and surgery. Mild superficial or early hemorrhages may respond to a single dose of 10 AHF/IU/kg, leading to a rise of approximately 20% Factor VIII level. In patients with early hemarthrosis (mild pain, minimal or no swelling, erythema, warmth and minimal or no joint limitation), if treated promptly, even smaller doses may be adequate.

Mild hemorrhage: Do not repeat therapy unless further bleeding occurs. Minor episodes generally subside with a single infusion if level ≥ 20% of normal is attained.

Moderate hemorrhage and minor surgery require plasma Factor VIII level to be raised to 30% to 50% of normal for optimum hemostasis. This usually requires an initial dose of 15 to 25 AHF/IU/kg; if further therapy is required, administer a maintenance dose of 10 to 15 AHF/IU/kg every 12 to 24 hours.

Severe hemorrhage: For life-threatening bleeding, or hemorrhage involving vital structures (CNS, retropharyngeal and retroperitoneal spaces, iliopsoas sheath), raise the Factor VIII level to 80% to 100% of normal. Administer an initial AHF dose of 40 to 50 AHF/IU/kg and a maintenance dose of 20 to 25 AHF/IU/kg every 8 to 12 hours.

Major surgery procedures require a dose of AHF sufficient to achieve a level of 80% to 100% of normal; give 1 hour before the procedure. Check the Factor VIII level prior to surgery to assure the level is achieved. Maintain the Factor VIII level at a daily minimum of at least 30% of normal for a healing period of 10 to 14 days.

Dental extraction: The Factor VIII level should be raised to 50% immediately prior to the procedure.

Rate of administration: Administer preparations IV at a rate of ≈ 2 ml/minute. Can be given at up to 10 ml/min. As a precaution, determine the pulse rate before and during administration of the AHF concentrate. Should a significant increase of pulse rate occur, reduce the rate of administration or discontinue.

Storage: Refrigerate between 2° to 8°C (35° to 46°F). Do not freeze. After reconstitution, do not refrigerate; give within 3 hours.

Rx	**Alphanate** (Alpha Therapeutics)	**Injection:** A solvent detergent treated lyophilized concentrate of Factor VIII. When reconstituted, contains ≥ 10 IU FVIII:C/mg total protein, 0.5 to 1 g/100 ml albumin (human), ≤ 10 mmol Ca/L, ≤ 750 mcg glycine/IU FVIII:C, ≤ 2 U heparin/ml, ≤ 55 mmol histidine/L, ≤ 0.6 mg imidazole/ml, ≤ 300 mmol arginine/L.	≤ 0.25 mcg TNBP/IU FVIII:C. In single dose vials with diluent.
		When reconstituted, contains ≥ 1 IU FVIII:C/mg total protein, 0.5 to 1 g/100 ml albumin (human), ≤ 10 mmol Ca/L, ≤ 750 mcg glycine/IU FVIII:C, ≤ 2 U heparin/ml, ≤ 55 mmol histidine/L, ≤ 0.6 mg imidizole/ml, ≤ 300 mmol arginine/L, ≤ 0.25 mcg TNBP/IU.	≤ 10 mEq Na/vial. In single dose vials with diluent.

ANTIHEMOPHILIC FACTOR (Factor VIII; AHF)

Rx	**Antihemophilic Factor (Porcine) Hyate:C** (Speywood)	**Injection**: A freeze-dried concentrate of Antihemophilic Factor VIII:C. Each vial contains 400 to 700 porcine units.	In vials.
Rx	**Bioclate** (Centeon[4])	**Injection**: Concentrated recombinant Antihemophilic Factor. When reconstituted, contains 12.5 mg/ml albumin (human), 1.5 mg/ml PEG 3350, 55 mM histidine, 0.2 mg/ml Ca^{++}.	180 mEq Na/L. In 250, 500 and 1000 IU per single-dose bottle w/diluent, double-ended needle and 18 gauge needle.
Rx	**Helixate** (Centeon[4])	**Injection**: A stable dried concentrate of Antihemophilic Factor (recombinant). When reconstituted, contains 10 to 30 mg/ml glycine, ≤ 500 mcg/1000 IU imidazole, 2 to 5 mM $CaCl$, 100 to 130 mEq/L chloride, 4 to 10 mg/ml albumin (human).	100 to 130 mEq Na/L. In 250, 500 and 1000 IU with diluent[1], double-ended needle, filter needle and administration set.
Rx	**Hemofil M** (Baxter Healthcare)	**Injection**: A stable dried preparation of Antihemophilic Factor in concentrated form. When reconstituted, contains ≈ 12.5 mg/ml albumin (human).	In 10, 20 and 30 ml with diluent.[1,2]
Rx	**Humate-P** (Centeon)	**Injection**: A pasteurized, purified lyophilized concentrate of antihemophilic factor (human).	In single dose vials with diluent.[1,3]
Rx	**Koate-HP** (Bayer)	**Injection**: A stable dried concentrate of Antihemophilic Factor. When reconstituted, contains ≤ 5 U/ml heparin, ≤ 0.05 M glycine, ≤ 5 ppm TNBP, ≤ 5 ppm TNBP, ≤ 3 mM $CaCl$, ≤1 ppm aluminum, ≤ 0.06 M histidine, ≤ 10 mg/ml albumin (human).	With Sterile Water for Injection, double-ended transfer needle, filter needle and administration set. In 250, 500, 1000 and 1500 IU bottles.[1]
Rx	**Kogenate** (Bayer)	**Injection**: A stable dried concentration of Antihemophilic Factor (recombinant). When reconstituted, contains 10 to 30 mg/ml glycine, ≤ 500 mcg/1000 IU imidazole, 2 to 5 mM $CaCl$, 100 to 130 mEq/L chloride, 4 to 10 mg/ml albumin (human).	100 to 130 mEq Na/L. In single-dose bottles[1]w/diluent, double-ended transfer needle, filter needle and administration set.
Rx	**Monoclate-P** (Centeon)	**Injection**: A stable concentrate of Factor VIII: C. When reconstituted, contains ≈ 300 to 450 mmol sodium ions and ≈ 2 to 5 mmol calcium (as chloride) per L, ≈ 1% to 2% albumin (human), 0.8% mannitol, 1.2 mmol histidine and < 50 ng/100 AHF activity units mouse protein.	With diluent, double-ended needle, vented filter spike, winged infusion set and alcohol swabs.
Rx	**Profilate HP** (Alpha Therapeutic)	A stable freeze-dried concentrate of Antihemophilic Factor VIII:C (human) that has been suspended in heptane.	In single dose vials with diluent and needles.
Rx	**Recombinate** (Baxter)	Concentrated recombinant Antihemophilic Factor. When reconstituted, contains 12.5 mg/ml albumin (human), 1.5 mg PEG, 180 mEq/L sodium, 55 mM histidine, 0.2 mg/ml calcium.	In single dose 250, 500 and 1000 IU bottles[1] with diluent and needles.

[1] Actual number of AHF units are indicated on the vials.
[2] When reconstituted, contains 1.5 mg/ml PEG 3350, 0.055 M histidine, 0.03 M glycine and less than 10 ng/100 AHF activity units of mouse protein.
[3] Each 100 IU contains 60 to 100 mg glycine, 14 to 28 mg sodium citrate, 8 to 16 mg NaCl, 16 to 24 mg albumin (human), 4 to 20 mg of other proteins and 20 to 44 mg total proteins.
[4] Centeon, 1020 First Avenue, King of Prussia, PA 19406–1310, 800–683–1288.

ANTI-INHIBITOR COAGULANT COMPLEX

Actions:

Pharmacology: Anti-Inhibitor coagulant complex is prepared from pooled human plasma and contains variable amounts of activated and precursor clotting factors. Kinin generating system factors are also present; it is standardized by its ability to correct the clotting time of Factor VIII deficient plasma or Factor VIII deficient plasma containing inhibitors to Factor VIII.

Approximately 10% of individuals with hemophilia (ie, hemophilia A; Factor VIII deficiency) have laboratory-measurable inhibitors to Factor VIII. The treatment depends upon the existing level of inhibitor, whether or not the patient responds to infusions of Antihemophilic Factor (AHF) with increased inhibitor levels (anamnestic rise in Factor VIII antibody) and the severity of the bleeding episode.

Indications:

Factor VIII inhibitors: Patients with Factor VIII inhibitors who are bleeding or who are to undergo surgery.

Treat patients with anti-inhibitor coagulant complex whose present Factor VIII inhibitor levels are > 10 Bethesda Units (BU), and whose inhibitor levels are known to rise to > 10 BU following treatment with AHF.

Patients whose present Factor VIII inhibitor levels are between 2 and 10 BU and whose inhibitor levels remain in this range following treatment with AHF may be treated with either AHF or anti-inhibitor coagulant complex, depending on the patient's clinical history and severity of the bleeding episode.

Patients with Factor VIII inhibitor levels of < 2 BU whose inhibitor levels are known to remain at ≤ 2 BU following treatment with AHF may be treated with appropriate doses of AHF.

For patients who have low levels of Factor VIII inhibitor and whose history does not include adequate laboratory indications of an anamnestic response to AHF, base the treatment of choice on clinical judgment. In patients having noncritical or minor bleeding episodes, the use of anti-inhibitor coagulant complex will maintain the inhibitor at a low level and allow the use of other coagulant therapeutic agents in subsequent major emergencies.

Contraindications:

Signs of fibrinolysis; disseminated intravascular coagulation (DIC); patients with a normal coagulation mechanism.

Warnings:

Infectious disease transmission: Products are prepared from large pools of human plasma. Such plasma may contain the causative agents of viral hepatitis, AIDS or other viral diseases. Each unit of source plasma used in preparation is nonreactive for hepatitis B surface antigen (HBsAg) and human immunodeficiency virus (HIV) antibody by FDA-approved tests. In addition, *Feiba VH Immuno* has been subjected to a vapor heat treatment during the manufacturing process to reduce the risk of transmitting viral infections. However, no procedure is totally effective in eliminating viral infectivity.

Viral infections: Individuals who have not received multiple infusions of blood or plasma products are very likely to develop signs or symptoms of certain viral infections, especially non-A, non-B hepatitis.

Anamnestic responses with rise in Factor VIII inhibitor titer occurred in 20% of cases.

Lab tests: Tests used to control efficacy such as APTT, WBCT and TEG do not correlate with clinical improvement. Appearance of hemostatic improvement may occur without reduction of partial thromboplastin time. However, expect prothrombin time to be shortened.Attempts at normalizing these values by increasing the dose of anti-inhibitor coagulant complex may not be successful and are strongly discouraged because of the potential hazard of producing disseminated intravascular coagulation (DIC) by overdosage.

Hypersensitivity reaction: Refer to Management of Acute Hypersensitivity Reactions.

Hepatic function impairment: Give special caution and consideration to the use of *Autoplex T* in individuals with preexisting liver disease.

Pregnancy: Category C. It is not known whether the drug can cause fetal harm when administered to a pregnant woman or can affect reproduction capacity. Use only if clearly needed.

Children: No data are available for *Feiba VH Immuno* regarding use in newborns. For *Autoplex T,* give special caution and consideration to use in newborns. A higher morbidity and mortality may be associated with hepatitis.

ANTI-INHIBITOR COAGULANT COMPLEX

Precautions:

Disseminated intravascular coagulation (DIC): If signs of DIC occur, including changes in blood pressure and pulse rate, respiratory distress, chest pain and cough, stop the infusion and monitor the patient. Laboratory indications include prolonged thrombin time, prothrombin time and partial thromboplastin time tests, decreased fibrinogen concentration, decreased platelet count or the presence of fibrin split products.

Identification of clotting deficiency caused by the presence of Factor VIII inhibitors is essential before initiating administration of anti-inhibitor coagulant complex.

Reconstitution/Infusion time: If the infusion of the concentrate occurs > 1 hr following reconstitution, there may be increased prekallikrein activator (PKA) and consequent hypotension.

Drug Interactions:

Epsilon-aminocaproic acid (EACA) or tranexamic acid: The concomitant use of anti-inhibitor coagulant complex with such agents is not recommended because only limited data are available on the administration of these highly activated prothrombin complex products together with antifibrinolytic agents.

Adverse Reactions:

A rapid rate of infusion may cause headache, flushing and changes in pulse rate and blood pressure.

Laboratory and clinical signs of DIC have occasionally been observed following high doses (single infusion of > 100 U/kg and daily doses of 200 U/kg). Monitor patients on these doses carefully (see Precautions).

Hypersensitivity: Fever, chills, indications of protein sensitivity, signs and symptoms of high prekallikrein activity (changes in blood pressure or pulse rate); allergic reactions from mild, short-term urticarial rashes to severe anaphylactoid reactions.

Administration and Dosage:

One unit of Factor VIII Correctional Activity is the quantity of activated prothrombin complex that, upon addition to an equal volume of Factor VIII deficient or inhibitor plasma, will correct the clotting time (ellagic acid-activated partial thromboplastin time) to 35 seconds (normal).

Administer by IV injection or drip only.

Dosage range: 25 to 100 Factor VIII correctional units/kg, depending upon the severity of hemorrhage. If no hemostatic improvement is observed at ≈ 6 hours following the initial administration, repeat the dosage. Adjust subsequent dosages and administration intervals according to the patient's clinical response.

Joint hemorrhage: 50 to 100 U/kg at 12-hour intervals. Continue until clear signs of clinical improvement appear (eg, pain relief, swelling reduction, joint mobilization).

Mucous membrane bleeding: 50 U/kg at 6-hour intervals under careful monitoring of visible bleeding site with repeated measurements of hematocrit. If hemorrhage does not stop, increase to 100 U/kg at 6-hour intervals; do not exceed 200 U/kg/day.

Soft tissue hemorrhage: For serious soft tissue bleeding, such as retroperitoneal bleeding, 100 U/kg at 12-hour intervals. Do not exceed 200 U/kg/day.

Other severe hemorrhages, such as CNS bleeding, have been effectively treated with doses of 100 U/kg at 12-hour intervals. Anti-inhibitor coagulant complex may be indicated at 6-hour intervals until clear clinical improvement is achieved.

Rate of administration: Initially infuse at 2 ml/min. The rate may be gradually increased to 10 ml/min.

Children: Check fibrinogen levels prior to initial infusion; monitor during treatment.

Storage/Stability: Refrigerate the unreconstituted complex between 2° to 8°C (35° to 46°F). Avoid freezing. Do not refrigerate after reconstitution. Complete administration within 1 hour (*Autoplex T*) to 3 hours (*Feiba VH Immuno*) after reconstitution.

Rx	**Autoplex T** (Baxter Healthcare)	Dried anti-inhibitor coagulant complex. Maximum of 2 units heparin & 2 mg polyethylene glycol/ml reconstituted material. Heat treated.	In vials w/diluent, needles. Each bottle is labeled with the units of Factor VIII correctional activity it contains.
Rx	**Feiba VH Immuno** (Immuno-US)	Freeze-dried anti-inhibitor coagulant complex. Heparin free. Vapor heated.	In vials w/diluent, needles. Each bottle is labeled with the units of Factor VIII inhibitor bypassing activity it contains.

FACTOR IX CONCENTRATES

Actions:

Pharmacology: Factor IX is activated by factor VII in the extrinsic coagulation pathway as well as by factor XIa in the intrinsic coagulation pathway. Activated factor IX, in combination with activated factor VIII, activates factor X. This results in the conversion of prothrombin to thrombin. Thrombin then converts fibrinogen to fibrin, and a clot can be formed.

Factor IX is the specific clotting factor deficient in patients with hemophilia B and in patients with acquired factor IX deficiencies.

Naturally low levels of vitamin K-dependent clotting factors may also be found in vitamin K deficiency and in severe liver disease.

Factor IX concentrate preparations may be in the form of complexes or purified proteins. Factor IX Complex, also known as prothrombin complex concentrate (PCC), is a combination of the vitamin K-dependent clotting factors II (prothrombin), VII, IX and X and is derived from human plasma. Purified protein preparations contain either undetectable, non-therapeutic levels of plasma clotting factors (II, VII and X) or are inherently devoid of these factors (recombinant preparation).

The administration of Factor IX Concentrate raises Factor IX plasma levels, thus minimizing the hazards of hemorrhage in patients with Factor IX deficiency. Plasma levels of factors II, VII and X may be increased following administration of the Complex preparation.

Pharmacokinetics: The mean half-life of Factor IX administered to Factor IX deficient patients is ≈ 22 hours (range from 11 to 36 hours). Normal hemostasis is achieved when plasma levels are 10% to 25%. The mean increase in circulating factor IX activity after IV infusion is 0.67 to 1.15 IU/dL rise per IU/kg body weight.

Indications:

Factor IX deficiency (hemophilia B [Christmas disease]): To prevent or control bleeding episodes. Do not use in mild Factor IX deficiency if fresh frozen plasma is effective. (See individual monograph for product specifications).

Contraindications:

Known hypersensitivity to mouse protein (mononine).

Warnings:

Hepatitis and AIDS: Human-derived Factor IX products are prepared from pooled units of human plasma that may contain the causative agents of hepatitis and other viral and infectious diseases. Prescribed manufacturing procedures utilized at the plasma collection centers, plasma testing facilities and the fractionation facility are designed to reduce the risk of transmitting viral infection. However, the risk of viral infectivity from these products cannot be totally eliminated.

Individuals receiving human-derived plasma product infusions are likely to develop signs or symptoms of a viral infection, especially non-A, non-B hepatitis. Single donor fresh plasma may be appropriate. Scientific opinion encourages hepatitis B and hepatitis A vaccination at birth or diagnosis for patients with hemophilia.

Thrombosis: The administration of human factor IX concentrates containing factors II, VII, IX and X has been associated with the development of thromboembolic complications; signs include change in pulse rate, blood pressure, respiratory distress, chest pain and cough. Even though factor IX contains no coagulation factor other than factor IX, the potential risk of thrombosis and DIC observed with other products containing factor IX should be recognized. Because of the potential risk of thromboembolic complications, exercise caution when administering these products to patients with liver disease, post-operative patients, neonates or patients at risk of thromboembolic phenomena or DIC. In each of these situations, weigh the benefit of treatment against the risk of these complications.

Disseminated intravascular coagulation (DIC): If signs of DIC occur, stop the infusion promptly. To reduce the risk of enhancing intravascular coagulation, do not attempt to raise Factor IX or Factor VII levels to > 50% of normal. If it is necessary to raise the patient's Factor IX or Factor VII level higher than 50% of normal, monitor infusion to detect signs and symptoms of DIC. Do not use in known liver disease when there is any suspicion of DIC or fibrinolysis.

Hypersensitivity: Although no hypersensitivity reactions have been observed, because *Mononine* contains trace amounts of mouse protein, the possibility exists that patients treated with *Moninine* may develop hypersensitivity to the mouse protein. Refer to Management of Acute Hypersensitivity Reactions.

Pregnancy: Category C. It is not known whether Factor IX can cause fetal harm when administered to a pregnant woman. Give to a pregnant woman only if clearly needed.

Children: Safe and effective in children with hemophilia B (see Administration and Dosage).

FACTOR IX CONCENTRATES

Precautions:

Monitoring: In normal clinical practice there is variability among patients and their clinical conditions. Therefore, monitor the Factor IX level of each patient frequently during replacement therapy. For surgical interventions in particular, precise monitoring of the Factor IX replacement therapy using the Factor IX activity assay is advised.

Adverse Reactions:

The use of high doses of Factor IX Concentrates may be associated with myocardial infarction, DIC, venous thrombosis and pulmonary embolism (see Warnings).

Rapid infusion rate: Headache, flushing, changes in blood pressure or pulse rate, transient fever, chills, tingling, urticaria, nausea and vomiting may occur. Symptoms disappear promptly upon discontinuation. Except in the most reactive individuals, the infusion may be resumed at a slower rate.

Pyrogenic reactions: Chills and fever (particularly when large doses are used).

Patient Information:

Advise patients of the early signs of hypersensitivity reactions including hives, generalized urticaria, tightness of the chest, wheezing, hypotension and anaphylaxis. Advise patients to discontinue use of the product and contact their physician if these symptoms occur.

Administration and Dosage:

Factor IX Deficiency (Hemophilia B [Christmas disease]): For IV use only. One International Unit (IU) is defined as the activity present in 1 ml of average normal fresh plasma. The potency is standardized in terms of Factor IX content.

When reconstitution of Factor IX Concentrate is complete, its infusion should commence within 3 hours. However, begin the infusion as promptly as is practical.

The amount of Factor IX Concentrate required to restore normal hemostasis varies with circumstances and patient. Administer sufficient drug to achieve and maintain a plasma level of ≥ 20% until hemostasis is achieved. Dosage depends on the degree of deficiency and desired hemostatic level of the deficient factor. Use the following formula as a guide to calculate dosage or estimate the expected percentage increase obtained from a given dose:

Units required to raise blood level percentages:

Recombinant Factor IX –

1.2 IU/kg × body weight (kg) × desired increase (% of normal)

Human-derived Factor IX –

1 IU/kg × body weight (kg) × desired increase (% of normal).

If a 70 kg (154 lb) patient needs a 25% increase in Factor IX,
give 1 unit/kg × 70 kg × 25 = 1750 units.

As a general rule, one unit of human-derived Factor IX activity per kg will increase the circulating level of Factor IX by 1% of normal, and one IU of recombinant Factor IX per kg of body weight will increase the circulatory activity of Factor IX by 0.8 IU/dL. Determine exact dosage based on the physician's judgment of circumstances, patient condition, degree of deficiency and the desired level of Factor IX to be achieved. If inhibitors to Factor IX appear, use sufficient additional dosage to overcome the inhibitors.

In preparation for and following surgery, maintain levels > 25% for at least a week. Use laboratory control to assure such levels. To maintain levels > 25% for a reasonable time, calculate each dose to raise levels to 40% to 60% of normal.

To maintain an elevated level of the deficient factor, repeat dosage as needed. Clinical studies suggest relatively high levels may be maintained by daily or twice daily doses, while the lower effective levels may require injections only once every 2 or 3 days. A single dose may stop a minor bleeding episode.

Factor VII Deficiency (Proplex T only): Units required to raise blood level percentages:

0.5 unit/kg × body weight (in kg) × desired increase (% of normal).

Repeat dose every 4 to 6 hours as needed.

If a 70 kg (154 lb) patient with a Factor VII level of 0% needs to be elevated to 25%, give 0.5 unit/kg × 70 kg × 25 = 875 units.

FACTOR IX CONCENTRATES

Dosage guidelines may be derived from the following table:

Pharmacology of Vitamin K-Dependent Coagulation Factors						
	Hemostatic level[1] > % normal		Dosage/kg			
Factor	Minor spontaneous hemorrhage	Major trauma or surgery	Initial (loading)	Maintenance (daily)	Half-life (hrs)	% Increase in plasma level/dose of 1 U/kg
IX	10-15	20-25	40-60 IU	10-20 IU	20-30	≈ 1
II	10-15	20-40	40 U	15-20 U	50-80	-
VII	5-10	10-20	5-10 U	5 U qid	5	1.2-2.7
X	5-10	15-20	10-15 U	10 U	25-60	1.9

[1] In general, 25% is the minimal hemostatic level for patients during surgery or severe accidental trauma. The range of values in normal clinical practice is likely to be much wider than those shown above. This is because of differences between patients, clinical condition and type of assay employed.

Factor VIII Deficiency (Hemophilia A; Proplex T, Konyne 80 only): Employ dosage levels approximating 75 IU/kg.

Anti-Inhibitor Coagulant Complex is recommended when hemarthroses occurring in hemophiliacs with inhibitors to Factor VII cannot be resolved by administration of Factor IX Complex and in other types of bleeding episodes in Factor VII-inhibitor patients.

Inhibitor patients: For bleeding in hemophilia A patients with inhibitors to Factor VIII, administer 75 IU/kg.

Rate of administration varies with the individual product; adapt to response of the patient. Infuse slowly. Rates of ≈ 100 to 200 IU/min or 2 to 3 ml/min are suggested. If headache, flushing or changes in pulse rate or blood pressure appear, stop the infusion until symptoms subside, then resume at a slower rate.

Storage/Stability: Refrigerate between 2° to 8°C (35° to 46°F). Do not freeze.

Rx	**AlphaNine SD** (Alpha Therapeutic)	Dried plasma fraction of Factors II, VII, IX and X.[1] Solvent detergent treated. Virus filtered.	In single dose vials with diluent, needle and filter.[2]
Rx	**Benefix** (Genetics Inst.)	Nonpyrogenic lyophilized powder preparation. Purified protein produced by recombinant DNA for use in therapy of Factor IX deficiency.	In 250, 500 or 1000 IU/single dose vial with diluent, needle, filter, infusion set and alcohol swabs.
Rx	**Konyne 80** (Bayer)	Dried plasma fraction of coagulation Factors II, VII, IX and X.[1] Heparin free. Heat treated.	In 20 & 40 ml vials with diluent and needles.
Rx	**Hemonyne** (Lennod)	Dried plasma fraction of coagulation Factors II, VII, IX and X.[1] Heparin free. Heat treated.	In 20 & 40 ml vials with diluent and needles.
Rx	**Mononine** (Centeon)[3]	When reconstituted, each ml contains 100 IU Factor IX with nondetectable levels of Factors II, VII and X with ≈ 10mM histidine, ≈ 3% mannitol, ≤ 50 ng mouse protein per 100 IU Factor IX activity units.	In single dose vials with diluent, double-ended needle, vented filter spike, winged infusion set and alcohol swabs.[3]
Rx	**Profilnine SD** (Alpha Therapeutic)	Dried plasma fraction of coagulation Factors II, VII, IX and X.[1] Heparin free. Solvent detergent treated.	In single dose vials with diluent.
Rx	**Proplex T** (Baxter Healthcare)	Dried plasma fraction of coagulation Factors II, VII, IX and X.[1] Heat treated.	In 30 ml vials with diluent and needles.[4]

[1] Actual number of units shown on each bottle.
[2] Contains heparin and dextrose.
[3] Contains heparin.
[4] Centeon, 1020 First Avenue, King of Prussia, PA 19406-1310, 800-683-1288.

AMINOCAPROIC ACID

Actions:

Pharmacology: Inhibits fibrinolysis via inhibition of plasminogen activator substances and, to a lesser degree, through antiplasmin activity.

Pharmacokinetics: The drug is absorbed rapidly following oral administration. Peak plasma levels occur 0.75 to 1.65 hours after an oral dose. A single IV dose has a duration of action less than 3 hours. After prolonged administration, it distributes throughout both the extravascular and intravascular compartments and readily penetrates red blood and other tissue cells.

A major portion of the compound is recovered unmetabolized in the urine. Renal clearance is high (about 75% of the creatinine clearance).

Indications:

Excessive bleeding: Treatment of excessive bleeding resulting from systemic hyperfibrinolysis and urinary fibrinolysis. In life-threatening situations, fresh whole blood transfusions, fibrinogen infusions and other emergency measures may be required.

Unlabeled uses: Oral or IV aminocaproic acid, 36 g/day in six divided doses, has been used to prevent recurrence of subarachnoid hemorrhage (SAH).

In the management of amegakaryocytic thrombocytopenia, the need for platelet transfusion may be decreased by use of aminocaproic acid 8 to 24 g/day for 3 days to 13 months.

To abort and prevent attacks of hereditary angioneurotic edema.

In patients with acute promyelocytic leukemia who develop coagulopathy associated with low levels of alpha-2-plasmin inhibitor.

To reduce post-surgical bleeding complications in patients undergoing cardiopulmonary bypass procedures (eg, 5 g IV followed by 1 g/hr infusions for 6 to 8 hours).

As a bladder irrigant to control bleeding following transurethral resection of the prostate and intractable bladder hemorrhage due to radiation- or cyclophosphamide-induced cystitis.

Contraindications:

Evidence of an active intravascular clotting process.

Disseminated intravascular coagulation (DIC): It is important to differentiate between hyperfibrinolysis and DIC because aminocaproic acid administered to a patient with DIC may produce potentially fatal thrombus formation. Criteria which may characterize hyperfibrinolysis include platelet count (normal), protamine paracoagulation (negative) and euglobulin clot lysis (abnormal). Do not use aminocaproic acid in the presence of DIC without concomitant heparin.

Warnings:

Upper urinary tract bleeding: Administration may cause intrarenal obstruction in the form of glomerular capillary thrombosis, or clots in the renal pelvis and ureters. Do not use in hematuria of upper urinary tract origin, unless possible benefits outweigh risks.

Benzyl alcohol, a preservative used in these products, has been associated with toxicity in newborns and is not recommended for use in newborns.

Pregnancy: Category C. Safety for use during pregnancy has not been established. Use in women of childbearing potential and particularly during early pregnancy only when clearly needed and when the potential benefits outweigh the potential hazards to the fetus.

Precautions:

Hyperfibrinolysis: Aminocaproic acid inhibits both plasminogen activator substances and, to a lesser degree, plasmin activity. Do not administer without a definite diagnosis or laboratory findings indicative of hyperfibrinolysis (hyperplasminemia).

Cardiac, hepatic or renal disease: Administer with caution to these patients. Animal pathology has shown endocardial hemorrhages, myocardial fat degeneration and kidney concretions. Skeletal muscle weakness with necrosis of muscle fibers has been reported rarely. Consider the possibility of cardiac muscle damage when skeletal myopathy occurs. Monitor CPK levels in patients on long-term therapy; discontinue use if a rise in CPK is noted. Restrict use to patients in whom the potential benefits outweigh the potential hazards.

One case of cardiac and hepatic lesions occurred following 2 g of aminocaproic acid every 6 hours for a total dose of 26 g. Death was due to continued cerebral vascular hemorrhage. Necrotic changes in the heart and liver were noted at autopsy.

Clotting: Fibrinolysis is a normal process, presumably active at all times to ensure the fluidity of blood. Inhibition of fibrinolysis by aminocaproic acid may theoretically result in clotting or thrombosis. In the few reported cases, it appears that such intravascular clotting was more likely due to the patient's preexisting condition (eg, the presence of DIC), rather than to aminocaproic acid.

AMINOCAPROIC ACID

Extravascular clots formed in vivo may not undergo spontaneous lysis as do normal clots.

Fertility impairment: Impairment of fertility consistent with the antifibrinolytic activity of aminocaproic acid has been suggested in some rodent studies.

Drug Interactions:

Oral contraceptives or estrogens: An increase in clotting factors leading to a hypercoagulable state may be produced by coadministration.

Drug/Lab test interactions: Serum **potassium** may be elevated by aminocaproic acid, especially in impaired renal function.

Adverse Reactions:

GI: Nausea; cramps; diarrhea.

Musculoskeletal: Malaise. Myopathy characterized by weakness, fatigue, elevated serum enzymes such as creatine phosphokinase (CPK), rhabdomyolysis associated with myoglobinuria and renal failure have been reported.

CNS: Dizziness; tinnitus; headache; delirium; hallucinations; weakness. Two cases of convulsions following IV administration have been reported.

Miscellaneous: Conjunctival suffusion; nasal stuffiness; skin rash; renal failure; thrombophlebitis; hypotension.

There have been some reports of dry ejaculation during the period of treatment. This occurred only in hemophilia patients who received the drug after undergoing dental surgical procedures. Symptoms resolved in all patients within 24 to 48 hours of completion of therapy.

There have been reports of an increased incidence of certain neurological deficits (eg, hydrocephalus, cerebral ischemia, cerebral vasospasm) associated with use of fibrinolytic agents in the treatment of SAH. All of these events have also been described as part of the natural course of SAH, or as a consequence of diagnostic procedures such as angiography. Drug relatedness remains unclear.

Administration and Dosage:

Plasma levels: An initial dose of 5 g orally or IV, followed by 1 to 1.25 g hourly, should achieve and sustain drug plasma levels at 0.13 mg/ml. This is the concentration apparently necessary for inhibition of fibrinolysis. Administration of more than 30 g/24 hours is not recommended.

IV: Administer by infusion, using compatible IV vehicles (eg, Sterile Water for Injection, normal saline, 5% Dextrose or Ringer's Solution). Rapid IV injection undiluted into a vein is not recommended; hypotension, bradycardia or arrhythmias may result. For treatment of acute bleeding syndromes, give 4 to 5 g in 250 ml of diluent by infusion during the first hour, followed by continuous infusion at the rate of 1 to 1.25 g/hour in 50 ml of diluent. Continue for 8 hours or until bleeding is controlled.

Oral: If the patient can take oral medications, follow an identical dosage regimen.

For the treatment of acute bleeding syndromes due to elevated fibrinolytic activity, administer 5 g orally during the first hour of treatment, followed by a continuing rate of 1 to 1.25 g per hour. Continue this method of treatment for about 8 hours or until bleeding has been controlled.

Rx	**Aminocaproic Acid** (Various, eg, Abbott, American Regent)	**Injection**: 250 mg/ml	In 20 ml vials.
Rx	**Amicar** (Immunex)		In 20 and 96 ml vials.[1]
Rx	**Amicar** (Immunex)	**Tablets**: 500 mg	(LL A10). White, scored. In 100s.
		Syrup: 250 mg/ml	Saccharin and sorbitol. Raspberry flavor. In pint.

[1] With 0.9% benzyl alcohol.

TRANEXAMIC ACID

Actions:

Pharmacology: Tranexamic acid is a competitive inhibitor of plasminogen activation, and at much higher concentrations, a noncompetitive inhibitor of plasmin. It has actions similar to aminocaproic acid. Tranexamic acid is ≈ 10 times more potent in vitro than aminocaproic acid.

Tranexamic acid in a concentration of 1 mg/ml blood does not aggregate platelets in vitro; concentrations ≤ 10 mg/ml have no influence on platelet count, coagulation time or various coagulation factors in whole blood or citrated blood. On the other hand, tranexamic acid in concentrations of 1 and 10 mg/ml blood prolongs thrombin time.

Pharmacokinetics:

Absorption/Distribution – Absorption of tranexamic acid after oral use is ≈ 30% to 50%; bioavailability is not affected by food. The peak plasma level 3 hours after 1 g orally is 8 mg/L and after 2 g, 15 mg/L. An antifibrinolytic concentration of drug remains in different tissues for ≈ 17 hours and in serum up to 7 or 8 hours.

Tranexamic acid diffuses rapidly into joint fluid and the synovial membrane. In the joint fluid, the same concentration is obtained as in the serum. The biological half-life in the joint fluid is ≈ 3 hours.

The concentration of tranexamic acid in a number of other tissues is lower than in blood. Tranexamic acid concentration in cerebrospinal fluid is ≈ 10% that of plasma. The drug passes into the aqueous humor where the concentration is ≈ 10% of the plasma concentration.

Tranexamic acid has been detected in semen where it inhibits fibrinolytic activity but does not influence sperm migration.

The protein binding of tranexamic acid to plasminogen is ≈ 3% at therapeutic plasma levels. It does not bind to serum albumin.

Metabolism/Excretion – After an IV dose of 1 g, the plasma concentration time curve shows a triexponential decay with a half-life of ≈ 2 hours for the terminal elimination phase. The initial volume of distribution is ≈ 9 to 12 L. Urinary excretion is the main route of elimination via glomerular filtration. Overall renal clearance is equal to overall plasma clearance (110 to 116 ml/min), and > 95% of the dose is excreted unchanged in the urine. Excretion of tranexamic acid is ≈ 90% at 24 hours after IV administration of 10 mg/kg. After oral administration of 10 to 15 mg/kg, the cumulative urinary excretion at 24 and 48 hours is 39% and 41% of the ingested dose, respectively, or 78% and 82% of the absorbed material, respectively. Only a small fraction is metabolized. After oral administration, 1% of the dicarboxylic acid and 0.5% of the acetylated compound are excreted.

Indications:

Hemorrhage: For short-term use (2 to 8 days) in hemophilia patients to reduce or prevent hemorrhage, and to reduce the need for replacement therapy during and following tooth extraction.

Unlabeled uses: Tranexamic acid has been used for many hemostatic purposes including prevention of bleeding after surgery or trauma (eg, tonsillectomy and adenoidectomy, prostatic surgery and cervical conization), and to prevent rebleeding of subarachnoid hemorrhage. It has also been used to treat primary or IUD-induced menorrhagia, gastric and intestinal hemorrhage, recurrent epistaxis and hereditary angioneurotic edema. Tranexamic acid has been used with systemic therapy topically as a mouthwash to reduce bleeding after oral surgery in patients on anticoagulant therapy. The drug also inhibits induced hyperfibrinolysis during thrombolytic treatment with plasminogen activators.

Contraindications:

Acquired defective color vision: Prohibits measuring one endpoint of toxicity (see Warnings).

Subarachnoid hemorrhage: Cerebral edema and cerebral infarction may be caused by tranexamic acid in patients with subarachnoid hemorrhage.

Warnings:

Retinal changes: No retinal changes have been reported in patients treated with tranexamic acid for weeks to months in clinical trials. However, focal areas of retinal degeneration have developed in cats, dogs, rabbits and rats following oral or IV tranexamic acid at doses between 126 and 1600 mg/kg/day (3 to 40 times the recommended human dose) from 6 days to 1 year. The incidence of such lesions has varied from 25% to 100% and was dose-related. At lower doses, some lesions are reversible.

TRANEXAMIC ACID

Visual abnormalities, often poorly characterized, are the most frequently reported post-marketing adverse reaction in Sweden. For patients who are to be treated for longer than several days, perform an ophthalmological examination (including visual acuity, color vision, eyeground and visual fields) before and at regular intervals during treatment. Discontinue tranexamic acid if changes are found.

Renal function impairment: Reduce the dose in patients who have renal insufficiency because of accumulation.

Carcinogenesis: Leukemia in male mice receiving tranexamic acid up to 5 g/kg/day may have been related to treatment.

Hyperplasia of the biliary tract and cholangioma and adenocarcinoma of the intrahepatic biliary system have been reported in one strain of rats after dietary administration exceeding the maximum tolerated dose for 22 months. Subsequent similar studies in a different strain of rat have failed to show hyperplastic/neoplastic changes in the liver.

Pregnancy: Category B. There are no adequate and well controlled studies in pregnant women. However, tranexamic acid passes the placenta and appears in cord blood at concentrations approximately equal to maternal concentrations. Use only if clearly needed.

Lactation: Tranexamic acid is present in breast milk at 1% of the corresponding serum levels. Exercise caution when administering to nursing women.

Children: The drug has had limited use in children, principally in connection with tooth extraction. Limited data suggest that dosing instructions for adults can be used for children needing tranexamic acid therapy.

Adverse Reactions:

Giddiness has been reported occasionally.

Hypotension has been observed when IV injection is too rapid. Do not inject more rapidly than 1 ml/minute; this reaction has not been reported with oral use.

GI: Nausea, vomiting and diarrhea occur, but disappear when dosage is reduced.

Overdosage:

There is no known case of overdosage. Symptoms may be nausea, vomiting, hypotension or orthostatic hypotension. Treatment includes the usual supportive measures. Refer to General Management of Acute Overdosage.

Administration and Dosage:

For dental extraction in patients with hemophilia: Immediately before surgery, substitution therapy is given with tranexamic acid, 10 mg/kg IV. After surgery, give 25 mg/kg orally 3 to 4 times daily for 2 to 8 days.

Alternative: Give 25 mg/kg orally, 3 to 4 times/day beginning 1 day prior to surgery.

Parenteral: 10 mg/kg 3 to 4 times daily for patients unable to take oral medication.

Impaired renal function (moderate to severe): The following dosages are recommended:

Tranexamic Acid Dosage		
Serum creatinine (μmol/L)	IV Dose	Tablets
120-250 (1.36-2.83 mg/dl)	10 mg/kg bid	15 mg/kg bid
250-500 (2.83-5.66 mg/dl)	10 mg/kg/day	15 mg/kg/day
> 500 (> 5.66 mg/dl)	10 mg/kg every 48 hours or 5 mg/kg every 24 hours	15 mg/kg every 48 hours or 7.5 mg/kg every 24 hours

Preparation of solution: For IV infusion, tranexamic acid may be mixed with most solutions for infusion such as electrolyte, carbohydrate, amino acid and dextran solutions. Prepare mixture the same day solution is to be used. Heparin may be added to solution for injection. Do NOT mix with blood. This drug is a synthetic amino acid; do NOT mix with solutions containing penicillin.

Rx	**Cyklokapron** (Kabi Pharmacia)	**Tablets:** 500 mg	(CY). White. In 100s.
		Injection: 100 mg per ml	In 10 ml amps.

APROTININ

Actions:

Pharmacology: Aprotinin is a natural protease inhibitor obtained from bovine lung with a variety of effects on the coagulation system. It inhibits plasmin and kallikrein, thus directly affecting fibrinolysis. It also inhibits the contact phase activation of coagulation which both initiates coagulation and promotes fibrinolysis. In addition to these effects on the clotting and lysis cascades in blood, aprotinin preserves the adhesive glycoproteins in the platelet membrane, making them resistant to damage from the increased plasmin levels and mechanical injury that occur during cardiopulmonary bypass (CPB). The net effect is to inhibit both fibrinolysis and turnover of coagulation factors and to decrease bleeding, although the precise mechanism of this effect is unclear.

Patients undergoing cardiac surgery with extracorporeal circulation by a heart-lung machine develop adverse changes of their blood components, blood cells and specific coagulation proteins. These changes cause a transient hemostatic defect during the intraoperative and immediate postoperative period which may result in diffuse bleeding despite correct surgical technique. At times, this blood loss is severe enough to require multiple blood transfusions and even surgical re-exploration.

Pharmacokinetics:

Distribution – After IV injection, rapid distribution of aprotinin occurs into the total extracellular space, leading to a rapid initial decrease in plasma concentration. Following this distribution phase, a plasma half-life of about 150 minutes is observed. At later time points (ie, > 5 hours after dosing) there is a terminal elimination phase with a half-life of about 10 hours.

Average steady-state intraoperative plasma concentrations were 250 KIU/ml in patients (n = 20) treated during cardiac surgery by administration of the following dosage regimen: 2 million KIU IV loading dose, 2 million KIU into the pump prime volume and 500,000 KIU/hour of operation as continuous IV infusion (Regimen A). Average steady-state intraoperative plasma concentrations were 137 KIU/ml (n = 10) after administration of exactly half of Regimen A.

Metabolism/Excretion – Following a single IV dose, ≈ 25% to 40% is excreted in the urine over 48 hours. After a 30 minute infusion of 1 million KIU, ≈ 2% is excreted as unchanged drug. After a larger dose of 2 million KIU infused over 30 minutes, urinary excretion of unchanged aprotinin accounts for ≈ 9% of the dose. In animals, aprotinin is accumulated primarily in the kidney. After being filtered by the glomeruli, it is actively reabsorbed by the proximal tubules in which it is stored in phagolysosomes. Aprotinin is slowly degraded by lysosomal enzymes. The physiological renal handling is similar to that of other small proteins (eg, insulin).

Clinical trials: Two placebo controlled, double-blind studies were conducted involving 236 patients undergoing repeat coronary artery bypass graft (CABG) surgery, of whom 209 were valid for efficacy analysis. The following treatments were used in the studies: Regimen A (aprotinin: 2 million KIU IV loading dose, 2 million KIU into the pump prime volume, 500,000 KIU/hour of surgery as a continuous IV infusion); Regimen B (aprotinin: 1 million KIU IV loading dose, 1 million KIU into the pump prime volume, 250,000 KIU/hour of surgery as a continuous IV infusion [exactly one-half of Regimen A]); and placebo (normal saline). Fewer patients receiving either regimen of aprotinin required any donor blood compared to placebo (pooled data): Regimen A, 30% to 42%; Regimen B, 47%; placebo, 72% to 77%. The number of units of donor blood required by patients was also reduced by both regimens (data listed by study 1 and study 2, respectively): Regimen A, 1.8 units (range, 0 to 24) and 0.4 units (range, 0 to 5); Regimen B, 2 units (range, 0 to 18); placebo, 3.5 units (range, 0 to 34) and 3.3 units (range, 0 to 20).

Study 2 also included 151 patients undergoing primary CABG surgery; 74 of the patients receiving aprotinin and 67 receiving placebo were valid for efficacy analysis. Fewer patients receiving aprotinin required any donor blood, and number of units of donor blood required was also reduced: Regimen A, 38% and 1.1 units (range, 0 to 10), respectively; placebo, 52% and 2.1 units (range, 0 to 15), respectively.

In these studies there was no diminution of benefit with age. Male and female patients received benefits from aprotinin in terms of a reduction in the average number of units of donor blood transfused. Male patients did better than females in terms of the percentage of patients who required any donor blood transfusions. However, the number of female patients studied was small.

A double-blind, randomized study compared aprotinin (n = 28) and placebo (n = 23) in primary cardiac surgery patients (mainly CABG) requiring cardiopulmonary bypass who were treated with aspirin within 48 hours of surgery. The mean total blood loss (1209.7 ml vs 2532.3 ml) and the mean number of units of packed red blood cells transfused (1.6 units vs 4.3 units) were significantly less in the aprotinin group compared to the placebo group.

APROTININ

In a randomized, placebo controlled study of aprotinin Regimen A vs placebo in 212 patients undergoing primary aortic or mitral valve replacement or repair, no benefit was found for aprotinin in terms of the need for transfusion or the number of units of blood required.

Indications:

CABG patients (reduction of blood loss/need for transfusion): For prophylactic use to reduce perioperative blood loss and the need for blood transfusion in patients undergoing cardiopulmonary bypass in the course of repeat coronary artery bypass graft (CABG) surgery.

In selected cases of primary CABG surgery where the risk of bleeding is especially high (impaired hemostasis, eg, presence of aspirin or other coagulopathy) or where transfusion is unavailable or unacceptable.

The selected use of aprotinin in primary CABG patients is based on the risk of renal dysfunction and on the risk of anaphylaxis (should a second procedure be needed).

Contraindications:

Hypersensitivity to aprotinin.

Warnings:

Hypersensitivity: Patients who experience any allergic reaction to the test dose of aprotinin (see Precautions) should not receive further administration of the drug. Even after the uneventful administration of the 1 ml test dose, or without previous exposure to aprotinin, the full therapeutic dose may cause anaphylaxis. The symptoms of hypersensitivity-type reactions can range from skin eruptions, itching, dyspnea, nausea and tachycardia to fatal anaphylactic shock with circulatory failure. If hypersensitivity reactions occur during injection or infusion, stop administration immediately and initiate emergency treatment. Refer to Management of Acute Hypersensitivity Reactions. Patients with a history of allergic reactions to drugs or other agents may be at greater risk of developing an allergic reaction.

Pregnancy: Category B. There are no adequate and well controlled studies in pregnant women. Use during pregnancy only if clearly needed.

Children: Safety and efficacy have not been established.

Precautions:

Test dose: All patients treated with aprotinin should first receive a test dose to assess the potential for allergic reactions. Administer the 1 ml test dose of aprotinin IV at least 10 minutes prior to the loading dose. Particular caution is necessary when administering aprotinin (even test doses) to patients who have received aprotinin in the past because of the risk of anaphylaxis (see Warnings). In re-exposure cases, IV administration of an antihistamine is recommended shortly before the loading dose of aprotinin.

Loading dose: Give the loading dose of aprotinin IV to patients in the supine position over a 20 to 30 minute period. Rapid IV administration of aprotinin can cause a transient fall in blood pressure (see Administration and Dosage).

Renal failure/mortality: An increase in both renal failure and mortality compared to age-matched historical controls has been reported in patients receiving aprotinin while undergoing deep hypothermic circulatory arrest in connection with surgery of the aortic arch. The strength of this association is uncertain because there are no data from randomized studies to confirm or refute these findings.

Hepatic disease: No pharmacokinetic data from patients with pre-existing hepatic disease treated with aprotinin are available.

Whole blood clotting time: Aprotinin prolongs whole blood clotting time of heparinized blood as determined by the *Hemochron* method or similar surface activation methods. In the event of prolonged extracorporeal circulation, patients may require additional heparin, even in the presence of activated clotting time (ACT) levels that appear to represent adequate anticoagulation. Therefore, in patients on cardiopulmonary bypass (CPB) who are receiving aprotinin, the standard system of monitoring heparinization during CPB, by keeping the ACT > 400 to 450 seconds, may lead to inadequate anticoagulation. In patients undergoing cardiopulmonary bypass with aprotinin therapy, employ standard loading doses of heparin. However, administer additional heparin either in a fixed-dose regimen based on patient weight and duration of CPB, or on the basis of heparin levels measured by a method, such as protamine titration, that is not affected by aprotinin.

APROTININ

Drug Interactions:

Aprotinin Drug Interactions			
Precipitant drug	Object drug*		Description
Aprotinin	Captopril	⬇	In a study of nine patients with untreated hypertension, aprotinin IV infused in a dose of 2 million KIU over 2 hours blocked the acute hypotensive effect of 100 mg captopril.
Aprotinin	Fibrinolytic agents	⬇	Aprotinin is known to have antifibrinolytic activity and, therefore, may inhibit the effects of fibrinolytic agents.
Aprotinin	Heparin	⬆	Aprotinin, in the presence of heparin, has been found to prolong the activated clotting time. However, aprotinin should not be viewed as a heparin-sparing agent (see Precautions).

* ⬆ = Object drug increased. ⬇ = Object drug decreased.

Adverse Reactions:

Aprotinin is generally well tolerated. The adverse events reported are frequent sequelae of open-heart surgery and are not necessarily attributable to aprotinin therapy.

Aprotinin Adverse Reactions (%)		
Adverse reaction	Aprotinin (n = 364)	Placebo (n = 235)
Any event	70	70
Atrial fibrillation	25	22
Myocardial infarction	10	7
Heart failure	8	6
Atrial flutter	7	4
Ventricular tachycardia	5	4
Fever	5	3
Hypotension	4	4
Pneumonia	4	3
Respiratory disorder	4	3
Heart arrest	3	1
Congestive heart failure	3	1
Supraventricular tachycardia	3	3
Kidney failure	3	1
Sepsis	3	2
Apnea	3	2
Confusion	3	2
Heart block	2	1
Shock	2	1
Asthma	2	0
Dyspnea	2	0

Other adverse reactions included: Phlebitis, kidney tubular necrosis (1.4%); convulsion, cerebral embolism (0.8%); liver damage, acute kidney failure, cerebrovascular accident, lung edema, hemolysis, allergic reaction (0.5%); pericarditis; ventricular fibrillation; pleural effusion; pneumothorax. In a pooled analysis of three placebo controlled studies, in patients undergoing cardiopulmonary bypass, there was a trend toward an increased incidence of myocardial infarction in patients given aprotinin. Further, in the study of patients undergoing primary or repeat CABG (Study 2), a trend was seen toward an increased incidence of saphenous vein graft closure in patients who received aprotinin Regimen A vs placebo. No increase in mortality in the aprotinin group was observed.

Lab test abnormalities: Pooled data from three placebo controlled studies showed a statistically significant increase in the incidence of postoperative renal dysfunction in the aprotinin treated group. The incidence of serum creatinine elevations ≥ 0.5 mg/dl above baseline was 23% in aprotinin (Regimen A) patients vs 12% with placebo. In patients undergoing CABG procedures only, the rates were 20% in the aprotinin group and 13% in the placebo group. Postoperative renal dysfunction was observed somewhat more frequently in association with primary cardiac valve procedures (30% for aprotinin Regimen A and 14% for Regimen B vs 8% for placebo). In the majority of instances, the renal dysfunction was not severe and was reversible.

APROTININ

A total of 4% of aprotinin-treated (Regimen A) patients and 1% of the placebo group had a serum creatinine increase of ≥ 2 mg/dl above the preoperative value.

Patients with baseline elevations in serum creatinine were not at increased risk of developing postoperative renal dysfunction following aprotinin treatment. In aprotinin-treated patients, there was a mean increase in creatinine of 0.16 mg/dl after the high-dose regimen (A) and a mean increase of 0.05 mg/dl after the low-dose regimen (B).

Serum glucose – In the hours after cardiopulmonary bypass surgery, the serum glucose was increased; however, the average serum glucose increase in patients treated with the high-dose regimen (61 mg/dl) was less than in the placebo-treated group (78 mg/dl).

Serum transaminases – There was a significantly greater incidence of treatment emergent abnormal liver function tests in all aprotinin-treated (Regimen A and Regimen B) patients (6%) compared to placebo-treated patients (2%). The percent of primary CABG patients developing an elevation of ALT > 1.8 times the upper limit of normal was not higher in the aprotinin-treated group compared to placebo. Among the repeat CABG patients, the percent of subjects developing an elevation of ALT of this magnitude was significantly higher in the aprotinin-treated group. This suggests an indirect effect possibly related to the risk of repeated surgery and attendant myocardial dysfunction rather than a primary drug effect. There were no differences between drug and placebo groups in the incidence of elevated ALT > 3 times the upper limit of normal.

Serum creatine kinase (CK) – There was a trend toward an increased incidence of elevated serum CK with increased MB fractions in aprotinin-treated patients.

Partial thromboplastin time (PTT) and activated clotting time (ACT) – Significant elevations in the PTT and ACT in aprotinin-treated patients are expected in the hours after surgery due to circulating concentrations of aprotinin, which are known to inhibit activation of the intrinsic clotting system by contact with a foreign surface, a method used in these tests (see Precautions).

Hypersensitivity: Anaphylactic reactions in patients receiving aprotinin have been reported in < 0.5% of cases. Such reactions are more likely to occur with repeated administration (see Warnings).

Reported Incidence of Anaphylaxis with Aprotinin Treatment				
	No prior aprotinin exposure		Prior aprotinin exposure	
Studies	Total	Fatal	Total	Fatal
US controlled studies	0/398	0/398	0/0	0/0
Foreign controlled studies	7/1996	1/1996	0/0	0/0
US open studies	0/299	0/299	1/6	1/6
Foreign open studies	3/1873	1/1873	1[1]	0/0
Foreign marketing	5/140,000	1/140,000	13/7000	4/7000

[1] Patient was treated a second time in violation of study protocol.

Overdosage:

The maximum amount of aprotinin that can be safely administered in single or multiple doses has not been determined. Doses up to 17.5 million KIU have been administered within a 24 hour period without any apparent toxicity. There is one poorly documented case, however, of a patient who received a large, but not well determined, amount of aprotinin (in excess of 15 million KIU) in 24 hours. The patient, who had preexisting liver dysfunction, developed hepatic and renal failure postoperatively and died. The autopsy showed hepatic necrosis and extensive renal tubular and glomerular necrosis. The relationship of these findings to aprotinin therapy is unclear.

Administration and Dosage:

Approved by the FDA on December 29, 1993 (1P classification).

Dosage regimens:

Regimen A – 2 million KIU IV loading dose, 2 million KIU into the pump prime volume, 500,000 KIU/hr of operation as continuous IV infusion.

Regimen B – 1 million KIU IV loading dose, 1 million KIU into the pump prime volume, 250,000 KIU/hr of operation as continuous IV infusion.

Aprotinin given prophylactically in both dose regimens A and B to high-risk patients undergoing repeat CABG surgery significantly reduced the donor blood transfusion requirement relative to placebo treatment. The experience with the lower dose of aprotinin Regimen B is, however, limited. Regimen A appeared more effective than Regimen B in patients given aspirin preoperatively.

APROTININ

Aprotinin is supplied as a solution containing 10,000 KIU/ml, which is equal to 1.4 mg/ml. Administer all IV doses of aprotinin through a central line. Do not administer any other drug using the same line. Both regimens include a 1 ml test dose, a loading dose, a dose to be added to the priming fluid of the cardiopulmonary bypass circuit ("pump prime" dose) and a constant infusion dose. Regimen A is described in the table below:

Aprotinin Dosage: Regimen A[1]			
Test dose	Loading dose	"Pump prime" dose	Constant infusion dose
1 ml (1.4 mg or 10,000 KIU)	200 ml (280 mg or 2 million KIU)	200 ml (280 mg or 2 million KIU)	50 ml/hr (70 mg/hr or 500,000 KIU/hr)

[1] Regimen B is exactly half of Regimen A; however, both regimens include a 1 ml test dose.

Administer the 1 ml test dose IV at least 10 minutes before the loading dose. With the patient in a supine position, the loading dose is given slowly over 20 to 30 minutes, after induction of anesthesia but prior to sternotomy. When the loading dose is complete, it is followed by the constant infusion dose, which is continued until surgery is complete and the patient leaves the operating room. The "pump prime" dose is added to the priming fluid of the cardiopulmonary bypass circuit, by replacement of an aliquot of the priming fluid, prior to the institution of cardiopulmonary bypass. Total doses of > 7 million KIU have not been studied in controlled trials.

Renal function impairment: In clinical trials, patients with mildly elevated pretreatment serum creatinine levels did not have a notably higher incidence of clinically significant post-treatment elevations in serum creatinine following aprotinin Regimen A compared to placebo. Changes in aprotinin pharmacokinetics with age or impaired renal function are not great enough to require any dose adjustment.

Admixture incompatibility: Aprotinin is incompatible in vitro with corticosteroids, heparin, tetracyclines and nutrient solutions containing amino acids or fat emulsion. If aprotinin is to be given concomitantly with another drug, administer each drug separately through different venous lines or catheters.

Storage/Stability: Protect from freezing. Store between 2° and 25°C (36° and 77°F).

Rx	**Trasylol** (Bayer)	**Injection:** 10,000 KIU[1]/ml	In 100 and 200 ml vials.[2]

[1] KIU = Kallikrein Inhibitor Units.

[2] With 9 mg sodium chloride per ml.

THROMBIN, TOPICAL

Actions:

Pharmacology: Thrombin directly converts fibrinogen to fibrin, requiring no intermediate physiological agent for its action. Commercially available thrombin is derived from bovine sources. Blood fails to clot in the rare cases where the primary clotting defect is absence of fibrinogen itself. The speed with which thrombin clots blood depends on its concentration. For example, the contents of a 5000 unit vial dissolved in 5 ml of saline diluent is capable of clotting an equal volume of blood in less than a second or 1000 ml in less than a minute.

Indications:

Hemostasis: As an aid in hemostasis wherever oozing blood and minor bleeding from capillaries and small venules is accessible.

In conjunction with absorbable gelatin sponges for hemostasis in various types of surgery.

Contraindications:

Sensitivity to any product components or to material of bovine origin.

Warnings:

Do not inject: Thrombin must not be injected or otherwise allowed to enter large blood vessels. Extensive intravascular clotting and even death may result.

Hypersensitivity: Thrombin is an antigenic substance and has caused sensitivity and allergic reactions when injected into animals. Refer to Management of Acute Hypersensitivity Reactions.

Pregnancy: Category C. It is not known whether the drug can cause fetal harm when administered to a pregnant woman or can affect reproduction capacity. Safety for use during pregnancy has not been established. Use only when clearly needed and when the potential benefits outweigh the potential hazards to the fetus.

Children: Safety and efficacy for use in children have not been established.

Adverse Reactions:

Allergic reactions may be encountered in persons known to be sensitive to bovine materials.

Administration and Dosage:

Preparation of solution: Prepare in Sterile Distilled Water or Isotonic Saline. The intended use determines the strength of the solution. For general use in plastic surgery, dental extractions, skin grafting, neurosurgery, etc, solutions containing ≈ 100 units/ml are frequently used. Where bleeding is profuse, as from cut surfaces of liver and spleen, concentrations as high as 1000 to 2000 units/ml may be required. It may often be advantageous to use thrombin in dry form on oozing surfaces.

Topical use: The recipient surface should be sponged (not wiped) free of blood before thrombin is applied. A spray may be used or the surface may be flooded using a sterile syringe and small gauge needle. The most effective hemostasis results when the thrombin mixes freely with the blood as soon as it reaches the surface. In instances where thrombin in dry form is needed, the vial is opened and the dried thrombin is then broken up into a powder. Avoid sponging of treated surfaces to ensure that the clot remains securely in place.

Use in conjunction with adsorbable gelatin sponge: Immerse sponge strips in the thrombin solution. Knead the sponge strips vigorously to remove trapped air, thereby facilitating saturation of the sponge. Apply saturated sponge to bleeding area. Hold in place for 10 to 15 seconds with a pledget of cotton or a small gauze sponge.

Storage/Stability:

Thrombostat – Store at room temperature 15° to 30°C (59° to 86°F).

Thrombinar and Thrombin JMI – Refrigerate at 2° to 8°C (36° to 46°F).

Thrombogen – Use solution immediately upon reconstitution. If necessary, refrigerate at 2° to 8°C (36° to 46°F) for up to 3 hours.

THROMBIN, TOPICAL

Rx	**Thrombinar** (Jones Medical)	**Powder**	Preservative free. In 1000[1], 5000[2], or 50,000[1] unit vials.
Rx	**Thrombin-JMI** (Jones Medical)	**Powder**	In 10,000, 20,000 and 50,000 unit vials.
Rx	**Thrombogen** (Johnson & Johnson)	**Powder**	In 1000, 5000[3], 10,000[4] or 20,000[4] unit vials.
Rx	**Thrombostat** (Parke-Davis)	**Powder**	In 5000[5], 10,000[6] or 20,000[6] unit vials.

[1] With 50% mannitol and 45% sodium chloride.
[2] With 50% mannitol, 45% sodium chloride and Sterile Water for Injection diluent.
[3] With Isotonic Saline diluent and transfer needle.
[4] With Isotonic Saline diluent. benzethonium chloride and transfer needle. Also in spray kit.
[5] With Isotonic Saline diluent containing 0.02 mg benzethonium chloride per ml.
[6] With Isotonic Saline diluent containing 0.02 mg benzethonium chloride per ml. Also in spray kit.

MICROFIBRILLAR COLLAGEN HEMOSTAT

Actions:

Pharmacology: Microfibrillar collagen hemostat (MCH) is an absorbable topical hemostatic agent prepared as a dry, sterile, fibrous, water insoluble, partial hydrochloric acid salt of purified bovine corium collagen.

In contact with a bleeding surface, MCH attracts platelets which adhere to the fibrils and undergo the release phenomenon to trigger aggregation of platelets into thrombi in the interstices of the fibrous mass. The effect on platelet adhesion and aggregation is not inhibited by heparin in vitro. Platelets of patients with clinical thrombasthenia do not adhere to the hemostat in vitro. However, in clinical trials, it was effective in 50 of 68 patients receiving aspirin. It cannot control bleeding due to systemic coagulation disorders. Institute appropriate therapy to correct the underlying coagulopathy prior to use of the drug. It is tenaciously adherent to surfaces wet with blood, but excess material not involved in the hemostatic clot may be removed by teasing or irrigation, usually without restarting bleeding.

MCH stimulates a mild, chronic cellular inflammatory response. When implanted in animal tissues, it is absorbed in less than 84 days and does not predispose to stenosis at vascular anastomotic sites. These findings have not been confirmed in humans. In human studies of hemostasis in osteotomy cuts, it does not interfere with bone regeneration or healing.

Indications:

Hemostasis: Used in surgical procedures as an adjunct to hemostasis when control of bleeding by ligature or conventional procedures is ineffective or impractical.

Contraindications:

Closure of skin incisions; it may interfere with the healing of the skin edges due to simple mechanical interposition of dry collagen.

Bone surfaces to which prosthetic materials are to be attached with methylmethacrylate adhesives. By filling porosities of cancellous bone, MCH may significantly reduce the bond strength of methylmethacrylate adhesives.

Warnings:

Sterilization: MCH is inactivated by autoclaving. Ethylene oxide reacts with bound hydrochloric acid to form ethylene chlorohydrin.

Infection: The presence of the hemostat does not enhance or initiate experimental staphylococcus wound infections to a greater or lesser extent than control agents. The effects on experimental wounds contaminated with a gram-negative aerobic rod and an anaerobic non-spore-forming bacteria are currently under investigation. Use in contaminated wounds may enhance infection.

Pregnancy: There are no well controlled studies in pregnant women. Safety for use during pregnancy has not been established. Use only when clearly needed and when the potential benefits outweigh the potential hazards to the fetus.

Precautions:

Excess material: After several minutes, remove excess material; this is usually possible without the reinitiation of active bleeding. Failure to remove excess material may result in bowel adhesion or mechanical pressure sufficient to compromise the ureter. In otolaryngological surgery, precautions against aspiration should include removal of all excess dry material and thorough irrigation of the pharynx.

MICROFIBRILLAR COLLAGEN HEMOSTAT

Antibodies: Contains a low level of intercalated bovine serum protein which reacts immunologically as does beef serum albumin (BSA). Increases in anti-BSA titer have been observed following treatment. About two-thirds of individuals exhibit antibody titers because of ingestion of food products of bovine origin. Intradermal skin tests have occasionally shown weak positive reactions to BSA or MCH, but these have not been correlated with IgG titers to BSA. Tests have failed to demonstrate clinically significant elicitation of antibodies of the IgE class against BSA following therapy.

Blood from operative sites: Fragments of MCH may pass through filters of blood scavenging systems. Therefore, avoid reintroduction of blood from operative sites treated with MCH.

Autologous blood salvage circuits: MCH should not be used in conjunction with autologous blood salvage circuits.

Handling: Avoid spillage on nonbleeding surfaces, particularly in abdominal or thoracic viscera.

Adverse Reactions:

Most serious: Potentiation of infection (including abscess formation, hematoma, wound dehiscence and mediastinitis).

Body as a whole: Adhesion formation; allergic reaction; foreign body reaction; subgaleal seroma (single case).

The use of MCH in dental extraction sockets increases the incidence of alveolalgia. Transient laryngospasm due to aspiration of dry materials has been reported following use in tonsillectomy.

Administration and Dosage:

This product should not be resterilized. It is not for injection or intraocular use. Moistening or wetting with saline or thrombin impairs its hemostatic efficacy. It should be used dry. Discard any unused portion.

Fibrous form: Must be applied directly to the source of bleeding. Because of its adhesiveness, it may seal over the exit site of deeper hemorrhage and conceal an underlying hematoma as in penetrating liver wounds.

Surface preparation – Compress with dry sponges immediately prior to application of the dry product, then apply pressure over the hemostat with a dry sponge; the length of time varies with the force and severity of bleeding. A minute may suffice for capillary bleeding (eg, skin graft donor sites, dermatologic curettage), but 3 to 5 or more minutes may be required for brisk bleeding (eg, splenic tears) or high pressure leaks in major artery suture holes.

Control of oozing from cancellous bone – Pack firmly into the spongy bone surface. After 5 to 10 minutes, tease excess away; this can usually be accomplished with blunt forceps and is facilitated by wetting with sterile 0.9% saline solution and irrigation. If breakthrough bleeding occurs in areas of thin application, apply additional hemostat. The amount required depends on the severity of bleeding.

Capillary bleeding – 1 g is usually sufficient for a 50 cm^2 area. Thicker coverage is required for more brisk bleeding.

Application – Adheres to wet gloves, instruments or tissue surfaces. To facilitate handling, use dry smooth forceps. Do not use gloved fingers to apply pressure.

Non-woven web form: In neurosurgical and other procedures, apply small squares to bleeding areas; then cover the sites with moist cottonoid "patties". To prevent wetting of the MCH, and to apply needed pressure, hold a suction tip against the cottonoid for one to several minutes, depending on the briskness of bleeding. After 5 to 10 minutes, remove excess MCH by teasing and irrigation.

Rx	**Avitene Hemostat** (Davol)	**Non-woven web form:** 70 mm x 70 mm x 1 mm, 70 mm x 35 mm x 1 mm and 35 mm x 35 mm x 1 mm.	In sterile blister packs of 6s and 12s.
Rx	**Hemopad** (Astra)	**Fibrous absorbable collagen hemostat:** 2.5 cm x 5 cm, 5 cm x 8 cm and 8 cm x 10 cm.	In 10s.
Rx	**Hemotene** (Astra)	**Fibrous absorbable collagen hemostat:** 1 g	In dispenser pack of 5s.

ABSORBABLE GELATIN SPONGE

Actions:

Pharmacology: A sterile, pliable surgical sponge prepared from purified gelatin solution and capable of absorbing and holding many times its weight of whole blood.

When implanted into tissues, it is absorbed completely within 4 to 6 weeks without inducing excessive scar tissue formation. When applied to bleeding areas of nasal, rectal or vaginal mucosa, it completely liquefies within 2 to 5 days.

Indications:

Hemostasis: Surgical procedures as an adjunct to hemostasis when control of bleeding by ligature or conventional procedures is ineffective or impractical.

Also used in oral and dental surgery as an aid in providing hemostasis.

In open prostatic surgery, insertion into the prostatic cavity provides hemostasis.

Contraindications:

Closure of skin incisions (may interfere with the healing of skin edges); control of postpartum bleeding or menorrhagia.

Warnings:

Sterilization: Do not resterilize by heat, since heating may change absorption time. Ethylene oxide is not recommended for resterilization; it may be trapped in the interstices of the foam and trace amounts may cause burns or irritation to tissue.

Precautions:

Infection: Not recommended in the presence of infection. If signs of infection or abscess develop in the area where the sponge has been placed, reoperation may be necessary to remove the infected material and allow drainage.

Compression: Sponge may expand and impinge on nearby structures. When placing into cavities or closed tissue spaces, use minimal preliminary compression; avoid overpacking.

Adverse Reactions:

Sponge may form infection and abscess (see Precautions). Giant cell granuloma in the brain has occurred at implantation site, as well as brain and spinal cord compression due to sterile fluid accumulation. Excessive fibrosis and prolonged fixation of the tendon were seen when the sponge was used about a tendon juncture.

Administration and Dosage:

Hemostasis: Apply dry or saturated with NaCl injection. When bleeding is controlled, leave pieces in place. Since sponge causes little more cellular infiltration than the blood clot, the wound may be closed over it. When applied, the sponge will stay in place until it liquefies. When applied dry, compress pieces before application to bleeding surface, then hold in place with moderate pressure for 10 to 15 seconds. When used with saline solutions, immerse in solution, withdraw, squeeze to remove the air bubbles present and replace in solution where it will swell to original size. If it does not, remove and knead vigorously until all air is expelled. Leave piece wet, or blot to dampness on gauze, and apply to bleeding point. Hold in place with moderate pressure with a cotton pledget or small gauze sponge until hemostasis results.

Dentistry: When used dry, roll between fingers and lightly compress to diameter of cavity or socket. After insertion, apply light finger pressure for 1 or 2 min. When used moist, immerse in NaCl solution, then remove, squeeze thoroughly to remove air bubbles and replace in solution where it will swell to original size. Take from solution, blot on sterile gauze to remove excess fluid and place in cavity or wound.

Prostatectomy cones are designed for use with the Foley bag catheter.

Storage/Stability: Once package is opened, contents are subject to contamination.

Rx	**Gelfoam** (Upjohn)	**Sponges**: Size 12: 2 x 6 cm x 3 or 7 mm	In 4s and 12s (7 mm only).
		Size 50: 8 x 6.25 cm	In 4s.
		Size 100: 8 x 12.5 cm	In regular and compressed. In 6s.
		Size 200: 8 x 25 cm	In 6s.
		Packs: Size 2: 40 x 2 cm	In single jars.
		Size 6: 40 x 6 cm	In 6s.
		Dental pk: Size 4: 2 x 2 cm	In 15s.
		Prostatectomy cones: Size 13: 5″ diameter	In 6s.
		Size 18: 7″ diameter	In 6s.

ABSORBABLE GELATIN FILM, STERILE

Actions:

Pharmacology: A sterile, absorbable gelatin film for use in neurosurgery, thoracic and ocular surgery.

In the dry state, it has the appearance and texture of cellophane of equivalent thickness; when moistened, it assumes a rubbery consistency and can then be cut to the desired size and fitted to rounded or irregular surfaces. The rate of absorption after implantation ranges from 1 to 6 months, depending on the size of the implant and the site of implantation. Pleural and muscle implants are completely absorbed in 8 to 14 days; dural and ocular implants usually require at least 2 to 5 months for complete absorption. The absence of undue tissue reactions, with the consequent decreased likelihood of developing adhesions, has been of particular value in the case of dural and ocular implants.

Indications:

Neurosurgery: As a dural substitute; absorbable gelatin film is nonconducive to undue inflammatory reaction and absorbable at a rate slow enough to permit dural regeneration and healing of the arachnoid layer. Its use in patients undergoing craniotomies reportedly prevented the development of meningocerebral adhesions, thereby reducing the risk of postoperative sequelae.

Thoracic surgery: In the repair of pleural defects in connection with thoracotomies, thoracoplasties and extrapleural procedures, implantation has been followed by minimal tissue reaction and subsequent closure of the defect by ingrowth of regenerating pleural and fibrous tissue across the gradually resorbed implant.

Ocular surgery: In glaucoma filtration operations (ie, iridencleisis and trephination), extraocular muscle surgery and diathermy or scleral "buckling" operations for retinal detachment. There is a remarkable lack of cellular reaction to the film implanted subconjunctivally or used as a seton into the anterior chamber. Evidence shows that implants help prevent formation of adhesions between contiguous ocular structures.

Contraindications:

Since the rate of absorption is likely to be increased in the presence of purulent exudation, do not implant in grossly contaminated or infected surgical wounds.

Administration and Dosage:

Preparation: Immerse in sterile saline solution; soak until quite pliable; cut to the desired size and shape; apply as follows:

Covering dural defects: Place over the surface of the brain. Tuck the edges of the implant beneath the dura and the wound; close the wound in the usual manner. If desired, the film can be sutured loosely to the dura. The moist film tears easily.

Covering pleural defects: Place over the defect and anchor in place by means of small interrupted sutures.

As a seton in iridencleisis: Place a small piece (≈ 4 mm x 10 mm) over the prolapsed iris pillar parallel to the limbus; Tenon's capsule and the conjunctiva are then closed with continuous absorbable sutures closely spaced to assure tight wound closure.

Diathermy or scleral "buckling" operations: Place film over the sclera, then suture the muscle and the conjunctiva over the underlying film.

Extraocular muscle surgery: Place film over and beneath the muscle before Tenon's capsule and the conjunctiva are closed in layers.

Storage/Stability: Once the envelopes have been opened, contents are subject to contamination. To ensure sterility, use immediately after withdrawal from the envelope. Store at room temperature 15° to 30°C (59° to 86°F).

Rx	**Gelfilm** (Upjohn)	100 mm x 125 mm	In 1s.
Rx	**Gelfilm Ophthalmic** (Upjohn)	25 mm x 50 mm	In 6s.

ABSORBABLE GELATIN POWDER, STERILE

Actions:

Pharmacology: Possesses hemostatic properties. When implanted in tissues, it is absorbed completely in 4 to 6 weeks without excessive scar tissue formation. When applied to bleeding areas of skin or nasal, rectal or vaginal mucosa, it completely liquefies within 2 to 5 days and is nonirritating.

Indications:

Hemostasis: Gelatin powder, made into a paste by the addition of sterile saline solution, is indicated in the control of bleeding from capillary, venous and arteriolar bleeding by pressure when ligatures or other conventional procedures are ineffective or impractical.

Unlabeled uses: Gelatin powder has been used to stimulate granulation in the treatment of small ulcers, chronic leg ulcers, decubitus ulcers or other oozing lesions.

Contraindications:

Closure of skin incisions (it may interfere with the healing of skin edges); intravascular compartment use because of risk of embolization; control of postpartum bleeding or menorrhagia.

Warnings:

Sterilization: Do not resterilize by heat; heating may change its absorption time.

Ethylene oxide is not recommended for resterilization, as it may be trapped in the interstices of the foam.

Precautions:

Infection: Use is not recommended in the presence of infection. If signs of infection or abscess develop in an area where gelatin powder has been placed, reoperation may be necessary to remove the infected material and allow drainage.

Blood dyscrasias: Not recommended as the sole hemostatic agent in patients with blood dyscrasias characterized by abnormal bleeding. Employ concurrent therapeutic measures.

Compression: Avoid use in bony cavities because swelling may interfere with normal function and may result in compression necrosis of surrounding tissues.

Adverse Reactions:

The powder may act as a nidus for infection and abscess formation. Giant cell granuloma in the brain has been reported at the site of implantation, as well as compression of the brain and spinal cord as a result of accumulation of sterile fluid.

Excessive fibrosis and prolonged fixation of the tendon were seen when gelatin powder was used about the tendon juncture in the repair of severed tendons.

Fever without infection; hematoma, encapsulation of fluid, toxic shock syndrome in nasal surgery and failure of absorption and hearing loss during tympanoplasty have been reported. Also, during laminectomy operation, multiple neurologic events (eg, cauda equina syndrome, spinal stenosis, meningitis, arachnoiditis, headaches, paresthesias, pain, bladder and bowel dysfunction, impotence) have been reported.

Administration and Dosage:

Hemostasis: Open jar and pour contents (1 g) carefully into a sterile beaker. A putty-like paste is prepared by adding a total of approximately 3 to 4 ml of sterile saline to the powder. Avoid dispersion of the powder by compressing with gloved fingers into the bottom of the beaker, and then kneading to the desired consistency. The paste may then be smeared or pressed against the cut surface. Use the minimum amount possible to produce hemostasis. When bleeding stops, remove excess. It may be left in place and the wound closed over it. It should be removed, whenever possible, after use in laminectomy procedures and from foramina in bone, once hemostasis is achieved.

Storage/Stability: Store at room temperature. Use as soon as the package is opened and discard the unused contents.

Rx	**Gelfoam** (Upjohn)	**Powder**	In 1 g jars.

OXIDIZED CELLULOSE

Actions:

Pharmacology: An absorbable hemostatic agent prepared from cellulose by a special process that converts it into polyanhydroglucuronic acid (cellulosic acid). Oxidation of cellulose yields an absorbable product of known acidity, soluble in alkali.

Provides hemostatic action when applied to sites of bleeding. The mechanism of action is not completely understood, but it appears to be a physical effect rather than any alteration of the normal physiologic clotting mechanism. On contact with blood, oxidized cellulose becomes a dark reddish-brown or almost black, tenacious, adhesive mass. It conforms and adheres readily to the bleeding surface. After 24 to 48 hours, it becomes gelatinous and can be removed, usually without causing additional bleeding. If left in situ, absorption depends on several factors, including the amount used, degree of saturation with blood and the tissue bed.

Oxidized cellulose swells upon contact with blood; the resultant pressure adds to its hemostatic action. It does not enter the normal clotting mechanism; however, within a few minutes of contact with blood, it forms an artificially produced clot in the bleeding area.

Bactericidal effects – The hemostat is bactericidal in vitro against many gram-positive and gram-negative organisms including aerobes and anaerobes: *Staphylococcus aureus, S epidermidis, Micrococcus luteus, Streptococcus pyogenes* Group A and B, *S salivarius, Bacillus subtilis, Proteus vulgaris, Corynebacterium xerosis, Mycobacterium phlei, Clostridium tetani, Branhamella catarrhalis, Escherichia coli, Klebsiella aerogenes, Lactobacillus* sp, *Salmonella enteritidis, Shigella dysenteriae, Serratia marcescens, C perfringens, Bacteroides fragilis, Enterococcus, Enterobacter cloacae, Pseudomonas aeruginosa, P stutzeri* and *Proteus mirabilis.* In contrast to other hemostatic agents, it does not tend to enhance experimental infection.

Indications:

Hemorrhage: Used adjunctively in surgical procedures to assist in the control of capillary, venous and small arterial hemorrhage when ligation or other conventional methods of control are impractical or ineffective. Also indicated for use in oral surgery and exodontia.

Contraindications:

Packing or wadding as a hemostatic agent; packing or implantation in fractures or laminectomies (it interferes with bone regeneration and can cause cyst formation); control of hemorrhage from large arteries or on nonhemorrhagic serous oozing surfaces since body fluids other than whole blood (eg, serum) do not react with oxidized cellulose to produce satisfactory hemostatic effects; do not use around the optic nerve and chiasm; as a wrap in vascular surgery because it has a stenotic effect.

Warnings:

Sterilization: Do not autoclave; autoclaving causes physical breakdown.

Surgery: Not intended as a substitute for careful surgery and proper use of sutures and ligatures.

Contaminated wound: Closing oxidized cellulose in a contaminated wound without drainage may lead to complications and should be avoided.

Application/Removal: The hemostatic effect is greater when applied dry; therefore, do not moisten with water or saline. Do not impregnate with materials such as buffering or hemostatic substances. Its hemostatic effect is not enhanced by the addition of thrombin; the activity of thrombin is destroyed by the low pH of the product. If used temporarily to line the cavity of large open wounds, place so as not to overlap the skin edges.

May be left in situ when necessary, but remove it once hemostasis is achieved. It must always be removed if used in, around or in proximity to foramina in bone, areas of bony confine, the spinal cord or the optic nerve and chiasm; by swelling, it may cause nerve damage by pressure in a bony confine. Paralysis has been reported when used around the spinal cord, particularly in surgery for herniated intervertebral disc. Remove from open wounds by forceps or by irrigation with sterile water or saline solution after bleeding has stopped.

Infections: Although it is bactericidal against a wide range of pathogenic microorganisms, it is not a substitute for systemic antimicrobial agents to control or prevent postoperative infections. Do not impregnate with anti-infective agents.

OXIDIZED CELLULOSE

Precautions:

Packing: Apply by loosely packing against the bleeding surface. Avoid wadding or packing tightly, especially within the bony enclosure of the CNS and within other relatively rigid cavities where swelling may interfere with normal function or possibly cause necrosis.

Use sparingly to control bleeding in open reduction of fractures and in cancellous bone. To minimize the possibility of interference with callus formation and the theoretical chance of cyst formation, remove any excess after bleeding is controlled.

Urological procedures: Use minimal amounts and exercise care to prevent plugging of the urethra, ureter or catheter.

Since absorption is prevented in chemically cauterized areas, its use should not be preceded by application of silver nitrate or any other escharotic chemicals.

Otorhinolaryngologic surgery: Exercise care so that none of the material is aspirated by the patient (eg, controlling hemorrhage after tonsillectomy; controlling epistaxis).

Adverse Reactions:

Encapsulation of fluid and foreign body reactions, with or without infection, have been reported.

Possible prolongation of drainage in cholecystectomies and difficulty passing urine per urethra after prostatectomy have been reported. There has been one report of a blocked ureter after kidney resection.

Burning has been reported when applied after nasal polyp removal and after hemorrhoidectomy. Headache, burning, stinging and sneezing in epistaxis and other rhinological procedures and stinging when applied on surface wounds (varicose ulcerations, dermabrasions and donor sites) have also been reported. These are believed to be due to the low pH of the product.

Intestinal obstruction has occurred, due to transmigration of a bolus of oxidized cellulose from gallbladder bed to terminal ileum or to adhesions in a loop of denuded intestine to which oxidized cellulose had been applied.

Miscellaneous: Necrosis of nasal mucous membrane or perforation of nasal septum due to tight packing; urethral obstruction following retropubic prostatectomy and introduction of oxidized cellulose within enucleated prostatic capsule.

Administration and Dosage:

Withdraw hemostat from the container with dry sterile forceps. Minimal amounts of an appropriate size are laid on the bleeding site or held firmly against the tissues until hemostasis is obtained.

Storage/Stability: Discard opened, unused oxidized cellulose. It cannot be resterilized.

Rx	**Oxycel** (Becton-Dickinson)	**Pads:** 3″ x 3″, 8 ply	In 10s.
		Pledgets: 2″ x 1″ x 1″	
		Strips: 18″ x 2″, 4 ply	
		5″ x ½″, 4 ply	
		36″ x ½″, 4 ply	
Rx	**Surgicel** (Johnson & Johnson)	**Strips:** 2″ x 14″	In 1s.
		4″ x 8″	
		2″ x 3″	
		½″ x 2″	
		Surgical Nu-knit: 1″ x 1″	In 1s.
		3″ x 4″	
		6″ x 9″	

PLASMA PROTEIN FRACTIONS

Actions:

Pharmacology: The plasma protein fractions include plasma protein fraction 5% (83% albumin with alpha and beta globulins), normal serum albumin 5% and normal serum albumin 25%.

The albumin fraction of human blood has two known functions: Maintenance of plasma colloid osmotic pressure and carrier of intermediate metabolites in the transport and exchange of tissue products. It comprises about 50% to 60% of the plasma proteins and provides approximately 70% to 80% of their colloid osmotic pressure. Thus, it is important in regulating the volume of circulating blood; its loss is critical, particularly in shock with hemorrhage or reduced plasma volume. When plasma volume is reduced, an adequate amount of albumin quickly restores the volume in most instances. Twenty-five grams of albumin is the osmotic equivalent of approximately 2 units (500 ml) of fresh frozen plasma; or 100 ml of normal serum albumin 25% provides about as much plasma protein as does 500 ml plasma or 2 pints whole blood. Normal serum albumin 5% is osmotically equivalent to an approximately equal volume of citrated plasma. The 25% albumin solution is osmotically equivalent to 5 times the volume of citrated plasma.

Plasma protein fraction is effective in the maintenance of a normal blood volume, but it has not been proven effective to maintain oncotic pressure. When the circulating blood volume has been depleted, the hemodilution following albumin administration persists for many hours. In individuals with normal blood volume, it usually lasts only a few hours. The half-life of albumin is 15 to 20 days with a turnover of $\approx$ 15 g per day.

Albumin 5% increases the circulating plasma volume by approximately equal to the amount infused. Albumin 25% draws about 3.5 times its volume of additional fluid into the circulation within 15 minutes except when the patient is dehydrated. Both 5% and 25% decrease blood viscosity.

There is no evidence that normal serum albumin (human) interferes with normal coagulation mechanisms. Antibodies, especially isoagglutinins, have been removed, enabling the product to be used without regard to the patient's blood group or blood factors.

Unlike whole blood or plasma, plasma protein fractions are free of the danger of homologous serum hepatitis, because these solutions are heat treated at 60°C (140°F) for 10 hours; thus, the possibility of transmitting serum hepatitis is reduced to a minimum. No crossmatching is required and the absence of cellular elements removes the risk of sensitization with repeated infusions.

Indications:

Unless the condition responsible for the hypoproteinemia can be corrected, albumin in any form can provide only symptomatic relief or supportive treatment.

Shock due to burns, trauma, surgery and infections; in the treatment of injuries of such severity that shock, although not immediately present, is likely to ensue; in other similar conditions where the restoration of blood volume is urgent.

In cases in which there has been a considerable loss of red blood cells, transfusion with whole blood or red blood cells is indicated.

For the earliest emergency treatment of shock, it may be more convenient to have 25% normal serum albumin available because it is so highly concentrated. However, the concentrated solution depends (for its maximum osmotic effect) on holding additional fluids in the circulation, which are drawn from the tissues or administered separately; if patient is dehydrated, maximum effect cannot be obtained without additional fluids. Therefore, for routine hospital use, normal serum albumin 5% may be preferred, as maximum osmotic effect is obtained with no additional fluids.

Albumin 25% with appropriate crystalloids may offer therapeutic advantages in oncotic deficits or in long-standing shock where treatment has been delayed. Removal of ascitic fluid from the patient with cirrhosis may cause changes in cardiovascular function and even result in hypovolemic shock.

Burns: Albumin 5% or plasma protein 5% may be used in conjunction with adequate infusions of crystalloid to prevent hemoconcentration and to combat the water, protein and electrolyte losses which usually follow serious burns. After 24 hours, albumin 25% can be used to maintain plasma colloid osmotic pressure.

Hypoproteinemia: In clinical situations usually associated with a low concentration of plasma protein and, consequently, a reduced volume of circulating blood.

Normal serum albumin 5% or plasma protein fraction 5% may be used in hypoproteinemic patients, providing sodium restriction is not a problem. If sodium restriction is imperative, use 25% normal serum albumin.

For acute complications of chronic hypoproteinemia, use albumin 25% possibly in conjunction with a diuretic.

PLASMA PROTEIN FRACTIONS

Adult respiratory distress syndrome (ARDS): Characterized by deficient oxygenation caused by pulmonary interstitial edema complicating shock and postsurgical conditions. When clinical signs are those of hypoproteinemia with a fluid volume overload, albumin 25%, together with a diuretic, may play a role in therapy.

Cardiopulmonary bypass: Preoperative dilution of the blood using albumin and crystalloid is safe and well tolerated. Although the limit to which the hematocrit and plasma protein concentration can be safely lowered has not been defined, it is common to achieve a hematocrit of 20% and a plasma albumin concentration of 2.5 g/100 ml.

Acute liver failure with or without coma: Administration of albumin may serve the double purpose of supporting the colloid osmotic pressure of the plasma as well as binding excess plasma bilirubin. Albumin 25% may be considered.

Sequestration of protein rich fluids: This occurs in such conditions as acute peritonitis, pancreatitis, mediastinitis and extensive cellulitis. The magnitude of loss into the third space may require treatment of reduced volume or oncotic activity with albumin.

Erythrocyte resuspension: Albumin may be required to avoid excessive hypoproteinemia during certain types of exchange transfusion or with the use of very large volumes of previously frozen or washed red cells.

Acute nephrosis: Certain patients may not respond to cyclophosphamide or steroid therapy. A loop diuretic and albumin 25% may help control the edema and the patient may then respond to steroid treatment.

Renal dialysis: Albumin 25% may be of value in treating shock or hypotension.

Hyperbilirubinemia and erythroblastosis fetalis: Albumin can be a useful adjunct in exchange transfusions; it reduces the necessity for reexchange and increases the amount of bilirubin removed with each transfusion, lessening risk of kernicterus.

Contraindications:

A history of allergic reactions to albumin; severe anemia; cardiac failure; the presence of normal or increased intravascular volume; patients on cardiopulmonary bypass.

In chronic nephrosis, infused albumin is promptly excreted by the kidneys with no relief of the chronic edema or effect on the underlying renal lesion. It is of occasional use in the rapid "priming" diuresis of nephrosis. Similarly, in hypoproteinemic states associated with chronic cirrhosis, malabsorption, protein losing enteropathies, pancreatic insufficiency and undernutrition, the infusion of albumin as a source of protein nutrition is not justified.

Warnings:

Pregnancy: Category C. Safety for use has not been established. Use only when clearly needed and when the potential benefits outweigh the hazards to the fetus.

Precautions:

Concomitant blood administration: When large quantities of albumin are given, supplement with or replace by whole blood to combat relative anemia.

Not a substitute for whole blood in situations where the oxygen carrying capacity of whole blood is required in addition to plasma volume expansion. Contains no recognized blood coagulating factors and should not be used for control of hemorrhage due to deficiencies or defects in the clotting mechanism.

Hypotension: Rapid infusion (> 10 ml/min) may produce hypotension. Monitor blood pressure during use and slow or discontinue infusion if hypotension occurs. Vasopressors may also help correct the hypotension.

Hemorrhage: Supplement albumin with hemodilution. When circulating blood volume has been reduced, hemodilution following the administration of albumin persists for many hours. In patients with a normal blood volume, hemodilution lasts for a much shorter period.

Shock: Monitor blood pressure frequently. Widening of the pulse pressure is correlated with an increase in stroke volume or cardiac output.

Dehydration: Patients with marked dehydration require additional fluids.

Special risk patients: Use with caution in patients with hepatic or renal failure because of the added protein load.

Certain patients (eg, those with congestive cardiac failure, renal insufficiency or with stabilized chronic anemia) are at risk of developing circulatory overload. Rapid infusion may cause vascular overload with resultant pulmonary edema. Monitor for signs of increased venous pressure.

Use caution in patients with low cardiac reserve or with no albumin deficiency. A rapid increase in plasma volume may cause circulatory embarrassment or pulmonary edema.

PLASMA PROTEIN FRACTIONS

The quick rise in blood pressure that may follow administration of albumin after injuries or surgery necessitates observation to detect bleeding points that may have failed to bleed at the lower blood pressure; otherwise, new hemorrhage and shock may occur.

Adverse Reactions:

Allergic or pyrogenic reactions characterized primarily by fever and chills. Flushing, urticaria, back pain, headache, rash, nausea, vomiting, increased salivation and febrile reactions, tachycardia, hypotension, and changes in respiration, pulse and blood pressure have also been reported. If such reactions occur, discontinue the infusion and institute appropriate therapy.

Cardiovascular: Hypotension (see Precautions). In addition, rapid administration may result in vascular overload, dyspnea and pulmonary edema.

PLASMA PROTEIN FRACTION

For complete prescribing information, refer to the Plasma Protein Fractions group monograph.

Administration and Dosage:

Contains 130 to 160 mEq/L sodium.

Administer by IV infusion, preferably through an area of skin at some distance from any site of infection or trauma.

Hypovolemic shock: The initial dose may be 250 or 500 ml. The rate of infusion and volume of total dose depend on the patient's condition and response. Infusion at rates exceeding 10 ml/min may result in hypotension. Monitor blood pressure during administration; slow or stop infusion if sudden hypotension occurs.

In infants and young children, it may be used in the initial therapy of shock due to dehydration or infection. Infuse a dose of 10 to 15 ml/lb (20 to 30 ml/kg), at a rate ≤ 10 ml per minute. Repeat, depending upon the patient's condition and response.

Hypoproteinemia: Daily doses of 1000 to 1500 ml (50 to 75 g of protein) are appropriate; larger doses may be necessary in severe hypoproteinemia with continuing loss of plasma proteins. In these and other normovolemic patients, the rate of administration should not exceed 5 to 8 ml per minute; monitor such patients for signs of hypervolemia, which include dyspnea, pulmonary edema, abnormal rise in blood and central-venous pressure.

Adjust the rate of infusion in accordance with the clinical response.

If edema is present or if large amounts of protein are continuously lost, it may be preferable to use concentrated (25%) Normal Serum Albumin because of the greater amount of protein in a given volume. However, unless the pathology responsible for the hypoproteinemia can be corrected (as by proper diet in malnutrition), plasma derivatives can provide only symptomatic relief or supportive treatment.

Preparation: Ready for use without further preparation; may be administered without regard to the recipient's blood group or type.

Admixture compatibility: The solution is compatible with the usual IV solutions of carbohydrates or electrolytes, as well as whole blood and packed red cells. However, certain solutions containing protein hydrosylates amino acid solutions or alcohol must not be infused through the same administration set, as these combinations may cause the proteins to precipitate.

Storage/Stability: Store at room temperature, not exceeding 30°C (86°F). Do not use if the solution is turbid or has been frozen, if there is a sediment in the bottle or if more than 4 hours have elapsed after the container has been entered. Contains no preservative, so the contents of each bottle should be used on one occasion only. Destroy unused portions to prevent the possibility of use of contaminated solutions.

Rx	**Plasmanate** (Bayer)	**Injection:** 5%	In 50, 250 and 500 ml vials.
Rx	**Plasma-Plex** (Centeon)[1]		In 50, 250 and 500 ml vials with injection set.
Rx	**Plasmatein** (Alpha Therapeutic)		In 250 and 500 ml vials with injection set.
Rx	**Protenate** (Baxter Healthcare)		In 250 and 500 ml vials.

[1] Centeon, 1020 First Avenue, King of Prussia, PA 19406–1310, 800–683–1288.

ALBUMIN HUMAN (Normal Serum Albumin), 5%

For complete prescribing information, refer to the Plasma Protein Fractions group monograph.

Administration and Dosage:

Contains 130 to 160 mEq/L sodium.

Administer by IV infusion and without further dilution.

Infusion rate: Since albumin in this concentration provides additional fluid for plasma volume expansion when used in patients with normal blood volume, infusion rate should be slow enough to prevent too rapid expansion of plasma volume.

Shock: In the treatment of a patient in shock with greatly reduced blood volume, albumin 5% may be given as rapidly as necessary to improve clinical condition and restore normal blood volume. In adults, an initial dose of 500 ml of the 5% albumin solution is given as rapidly as tolerated. If response within 30 minutes is inadequate, an additional 500 ml of 5% albumin solution may be given. For pediatric use, 50 ml would be appropriate. In neonates and infants, albumin 5% may be given in large amounts. The recommended dose is 10 to 20 ml/kg. Guide therapy by the clinical response, blood pressure and assessment of relative anemia. If more than 1000 ml are given, or if hemorrhage has occurred, the administration of whole blood or red blood cells may be desirable.

In patients with slightly low or normal blood volume, give at a rate of 1 to 2 ml/min. Usual administration rate for children is one-quarter to one-half the adult rate.

Burns: After a burn injury (usually beyond 24 hours), there is a correlation between the amount of albumin infused and the resultant increase in plasma colloid osmotic pressure. In severe burns, immediate therapy usually includes large volumes of crystalloid, with lesser amounts of 5% albumin solution to maintain an adequate plasma volume. After the first 24 hours, the ratio of albumin to crystalloid may be increased to establish and maintain a plasma albumin level of about 2.5 g ± 0.5 g/100 ml or a total serum protein level of about 5.2 g/100 ml. However, an optimal regimen for severe burns is not established. Duration of therapy is decided by loss of protein from burned areas and in urine. Do not consider albumin as a source of nutrition.

Hypoproteinemia: The infusion of albumin as a nutrient in the treatment of chronic hypoproteinemia is not recommended. In acute hypoproteinemia, 5% albumin may be used in replacing the protein lost in hypoproteinemic conditions. However, if edema is present or if large amounts of albumin are lost, albumin 25% is preferred because of the greater amount of protein in the concentrated solution.

Preparation for administration: Swab stopper top immediately after removing seal with suitable antiseptic prior to entering vial. Inspect visually for particulate matter and discoloration.

Storage/Stability: Store at room temperature not exceeding 30°C (86°F). Do not freeze.

Rx	**Albuminar-5** (Centeon)[1]	**Injection:** 5%	In 50, 250, 500 and 1000 ml vials.
Rx	**Albutein 5%** (Alpha Therapeutic)		In 250 and 500 ml vials.
Rx	**Buminate 5%** (Baxter Healthcare)		In 250 and 500 ml vials.
Rx	**Normal Serum Albumin (Human) 5% Solution** (Immuno-US)		In 50, 250 and 500 ml vials with IV set.
Rx	**Plasbumin-5** (Bayer)		In 50, 250 and 500 ml vials.
Rx	**Albunex** (Mallinckrodt)		In 5, 10 and 20 ml single dose vials.

[1] Centeon, 1020 First Avenue, King of Prussia, PA 19406-1310, 800-683-1288.

ALBUMIN HUMAN (Normal Serum Albumin), 25%

For complete prescribing information, refer to the Plasma Protein Fractions group monograph.

Administration and Dosage:

Contains 130 to 160 mEq/L sodium. Administer by IV infusion.

Preparation: May be given undiluted or diluted in normal saline. If sodium restriction is required, administer either undiluted or diluted in a sodium free carbohydrate solution such as 5% Dextrose in Water.

Hypoproteinemia with or without edema: Unless the underlying pathology responsible for the hypoproteinemia can be corrected, IV use of albumin 25% is purely symptomatic or supportive. The usual daily dose of albumin for adults is 50 to 75 g and for children 25 g. Patients with severe hypoproteinemia who continue to lose albumin may require larger quantities. Since hypoproteinemic patients usually have approximately normal blood volumes, administration rate should not exceed 2 ml/minute, as more rapid injection may precipitate circulatory embarrassment and pulmonary edema. If slower administration is desired, 200 ml of 25% albumin may be mixed with 300 ml of 10% glucose solution and administered by continuous drip at a rate of 100 ml/hour. Although diuresis may occur soon after administration, best results are obtained if albumin is continued until the normal serum protein level is regained.

Burns: After a burn injury (usually beyond 24 hours) there is a correlation between the amount of albumin infused and the resultant increase in plasma colloid osmotic pressure. The aim should be to maintain the plasma albumin concentration in the region of 2.5 ± 0.5 g/100 ml, with a plasma oncotic pressure of 20 mm Hg (equivalent to a total plasma protein concentration of 5.2 g/100 ml). This can be achieved by the IV administration of albumin 25%. The duration of therapy is decided by the loss of protein from the burned areas and in the urine. In addition, oral or parenteral feeding with amino acids should be initiated, as albumin should not be considered a source of nutrition.

Duration of treatment varies, depending upon the extent of protein loss through renal excretion, denuded areas of skin and decreased albumin synthesis. Attempts to raise albumin levels > 4 g/100 ml may result in increased rates of catabolism.

Shock: Determine initial dose by the patient's condition and response to treatment. Guide therapy by degree of venous and pulmonary congestion or hematocrit measurements.

Greatly reduced blood volume – Administer as rapidly as desired. If the initial response is inadequate, (ie, if pulse rate remains above 100/min, the blood pressure below 10 cm water, or if acrocyanosis or cold sweat is present) additional albumin may be given 15 to 30 minutes following the first dose.

Slightly low or normal blood volume – The rate of administration should be 1 ml/minute. If there is continued loss of protein, it may be desirable to give whole blood or other blood fractions.

Erythrocyte resuspension: About 25 g of albumin per liter of erythrocytes is commonly used, although the requirements in preexistent hypoproteinemia or hepatic impairment can be greater. Albumin 25% is added to the isotonic suspension of washed red cells immediately prior to transfusion.

Acute nephrosis: A loop diuretic and 100 ml albumin 25% repeated daily for 7 to 10 days may control edema and the patient may then respond to steroid treatment.

Renal dialysis: The usual volume administered is about 100 ml; avoid fluid overload. These patients cannot tolerate substantial volumes of salt solution.

Hyperbilirubinemia and erythroblastosis fetalis: The use of albumin in exchange transfusions reduces the necessity for reexchange and increases the amount of bilirubin removed with each transfusion. Administer 1 g/kg 1 to 2 hours before transfusion.

Storage/Stability: Store at room temperature not exceeding 30°C (86°F). Do not freeze.

Rx	**Albuminar-25** (Centeon)[1]	**Injection:** 25%	In 20, 50 and 100 ml vials.
Rx	**Albutein 25%** (Alpha Therapeutic)		In 20, 50 and 100 ml vials.
Rx	**Buminate 25%** (Baxter Healthcare)		In 20, 50 and 100 ml vials.
Rx	**Normal Serum Albumin (Human) 25% Solution** (Immuno-US)		In 20, 50 and 100 ml vials with IV set.
Rx	**Plasbumin-25** (Bayer)		In 20, 50 and 100 ml vials.

[1] Centeon, 1020 First Avenue, King of Prussia, PA 19406-1310, 800-683-1288.

DEXTRAN 1

Actions:

Pharmacology: Clinical dextran is not antigenic, but its structure is similar to other antigenic polysaccharides. Some polysaccharide-reacting antibodies may cross-react with clinical dextran, forming antibody-antigen complexes that can trigger an anaphylactic reaction. This may occur in patients who have never received clinical dextran, but have enough dextran-reacting antibodies (DRA) to form large immune complexes. Dextran 1, a monovalent hapten, reacts with dextran-reactive immunoglobulin (IgG) without bridge formation and with no tendency for the formation of large immune complexes. A molar excess of monovalent hapten, given just before a clinical IV dextran solution, competitively prevents the formation of immune complexes with polyvalent clinical dextrans and impedes anaphylaxis. During the initial phase of a clinical dextran infusion, protection is effected by hapten inhibition. During the later phase and the following day, protection is exerted by dextran molecules in clinical dextran solutions because an antigen excess develops in the circulation and only small nonanaphylactogenic immune complexes can be formed. An additional injection of dextran 1 is recommended if ≥ 48 hours have elapsed since the previous infusion of clinical dextran.

Dextran-induced anaphylactic reactions have an incidence range of 0.002% to 0.025% per unit used (0.002% to 0.013% for dextran 40 and 0.017% to 0.025% for dextran 60/75). By means of hapten inhibition, the incidence is 15 to 20 times lower.

Pharmacokinetics: Because of its low molecular weight (MW = 1000), dextran 1 is rapidly and completely excreted by glomerular filtration. After IV injection of a single 20 ml dose, ≈ 50% is cleared from the blood within 30 minutes. Mean urinary elimination half-life was 41 ± 11 minutes in 12 healthy individuals.

Indications:

Serious anaphylactic reactions to dextran: Prophylaxis of serious anaphylactic reactions to IV infusion of clinical dextran. Mild dextran-induced anaphylactic (allergic) reactions are not prevented by dextran 1.

Contraindications:

Do not give dextran 1 if IV use of clinical dextran solutions is contraindicated. This includes marked hemostatic defects of all types or hemorrhagic tendencies, marked cardiac decompensation and renal disease with severe oliguria or anuria.

Warnings:

Cardiac effects: Severe hypotension and bradycardia have been reported.

Pregnancy: Category B. In rabbits, doses 35 to 70 times the human dose increased the incidence of fetal resorption, post-implantation fetal loss, retardation of fetal long-bone ossification and marginal fetal growth retardation. There are no adequate and well controlled studies in pregnant women. Use only if clearly needed.

Lactation: It is not known whether dextran 1 is excreted in breast milk. Exercise caution when administering to nursing women.

Precautions:

Reactions: If any reaction occurs, do not administer clinical dextran solutions.

Adverse Reactions:

Cutaneous (0.016%); moderate hypotension (systolic BP > 60 mm Hg; 0.014%); bradycardia (< 60 bpm) with moderate hypotension (0.013%); nausea, pallor, shivering (0.011%); bradycardia (0.004%); bradycardia with severe hypotension (systolic BP < 60 mm Hg; 0.001%). Do not give subsequent infusion if adverse reactions occur.

Overdosage:

The drug is rapidly cleared by renal excretion. Any overdosage, therefore, should be of short duration and of minimal consequence.

Administration and Dosage:

For IV use only. Do NOT dilute or admix with clinical dextran.

Adults: 20 ml (150 mg/ml) IV rapidly, 1 to 2 min before IV infusion of clinical dextran.

Children: 0.3 ml/kg in a corresponding manner.

The time interval between administration of dextran 1 and clinical dextran solutions should not exceed 15 min; if a longer period elapses, repeat dextran 1 dose. Repeat dextran 1 injection if 48 hours have elapsed since the last infusion of clinical dextran. Administer 1 to 2 min before every IV clinical dextran infusion.

May give IV through Y injection site if minimally diluted with primary solution. Do not give through an IV set used to infuse clinical dextran. May give through heparin lock.

Storage/Stability: Do not exceed 25°C (77°F). Protect from freezing.

Rx	**Promit** (Medisan)	**Injection:** 150 mg per ml	In 20 ml vials.

HETASTARCH (Hydroxyethyl Starch; HES)

Actions:

Pharmacology: Hetastarch (HES) is a complex mixture of ethoxylated amylopectin molecules of various sizes; average molecular weight (MW) is 450,000 (range, 10,000 to > 1 million). Colloidal properties of 6% HES approximate those of human albumin. After IV infusion, plasma volume expands slightly in excess of volume infused and decreases over 24 to 36 hours. Hemodynamic status will decrease after 24 hours. Adding HES to whole blood increases the erythrocyte sedimentation rate and improves the efficiency of granulocyte collection by centrifugal means.

Pharmacokinetics: Molecules < 50,000 MW are rapidly eliminated renally; ≈ 33% appear in urine in 24 hours. Larger molecules are broken down; ≈ 90% of the dose is eliminated (avg. half-life, 17 days; the remainder has a half-life of 48 days). The hydroxyethyl group remains intact and attached to glucose units when excreted.

Indications:

Shock: Adjunct for plasma volume expansion in shock due to hemorrhage, burns, surgery, sepsis or other trauma.

Leukapheresis: Adjunct to improve harvesting and increase yield of granulocytes.

Contraindications:

Severe bleeding disorders; severe cardiac failure; renal failure with oliguria or anuria.

Warnings:

Blood/Plasma substitute: Not a substitute for blood or plasma, as it does not have oxygen-carrying capacity or contain plasma proteins (eg, coagulation factors).

Coagulation effects: Large volumes may alter coagulation and result in transient prolongation of prothrombin time (PT), partial thromboplastin time (PTT), bleeding and clotting times, decreased hematocrit and excessive dilution of plasma proteins.

Leukapheresis: Slight declines in platelet count and hemoglobin levels have been observed in donors undergoing repeated leukapheresis procedures due to the volume expanding effects of hetastarch. Hemoglobin levels usually return to normal within 24 hours. Hemodilution by hetastarch and saline may also result in 24 hour declines of total protein, albumin, calcium and fibrinogen values.

Hypersensitivity: Anaphylactoid reactions (periorbital edema, urticaria, wheezing) have been reported. If these occur, discontinue the drug. If necessary, give antihistamines. See Management of Acute Hypersensitivity Reactions. Also, use caution when administering HES to a person allergic to corn.

Pregnancy: Category C. Safety for use has not been established. Use only when clearly needed and when potential benefits outweigh potential hazards to the fetus.

Lactation: It is not known whether hetastarch is excreted in breast milk. Exercise caution when administering to a nursing woman.

Children: Safety and efficacy have not been established.

Precautions:

Monitoring: During leukapheresis, monitor CBC, total leukocyte and platelet counts, leukocyte differential count, hemoglobin, hematocrit, PT and PTT.

Special risk patients: The possibility of circulatory overload exists. Take special care in patients with impaired renal clearance and when the risk of pulmonary edema or congestive heart failure is increased. Indirect bilirubin levels increased in two subjects receiving multiple infusions; levels returned to normal by 96 hours after infusion. Total bilirubin remained normal. Observe caution in liver disease.

Adverse Reactions:

Vomiting; mild temperature elevation; chills; itching; submaxillary and parotid glandular enlargement; mild influenza-like symptoms; headache; muscle pain; peripheral edema of the lower extremities; allergic reactions (see Warnings).

Administration and Dosage:

Administer by IV infusion only. Total dosage and rate of infusion depend upon the amount of blood lost and the resultant hemoconcentration.

Plasma volume expansion: The usual amount is 500 to 1000 ml. Total dosage does not usually exceed 1500 ml/day (20 ml/kg). In acute hemorrhagic shock, rates approaching 20 ml/kg/hour may be used.

Leukapheresis: In continuous flow centrifugation (CFC) procedures, 250 to 700 ml is typically infused at a constant fixed ratio of 1:8 to 1:13 to venous whole blood.

Storage/Stability: Store at room temperature not exceeding 40°C (104°F). Do not freeze. Do not use if solution is turbid deep brown or if crystalline precipitate forms.

Rx	**Hespan** (DuPont Pharma)	**Injection:** 6 g per 100 ml in 0.9% sodium chloride	In 500 ml IV infusion bottle.

DEXTRAN, LOW MOLECULAR WEIGHT (Dextran 40)

Actions:

Pharmacology: Dextran 40 is a branched polysaccharide plasma-volume expander with an average molecular weight of 40,000 (range 10,000 to 90,000). A 2.5% solution of dextran 40 is equivalent in colloid osmotic pressure to normal plasma. Generally, plasma volume is increased onefold to twofold over the volume of dextran 40 infused. The extent and duration of volume expansion produced will depend on the preexisting blood volume, rate of infusion and rate of dextran clearance by the kidneys.

Pharmacokinetics: Dextran 40 is evenly distributed in the vascular system. Its distribution according to molecular weight shifts toward higher molecular weights as the smaller molecules are excreted by the kidney. Approximately 50% administered to a normovolemic subject is excreted in the urine within 3 hours, 60% within 6 hours and 75% within 24 hours. The remaining 25% is partly hydrolyzed and excreted in the urine, partly excreted in the feces and partly oxidized. Unexcreted dextran molecules diffuse into the extravascular compartment and are temporarily taken up by the reticuloendothelial system. Some of these molecules are returned to the intravascular compartment via the lymphatics. Dextran is slowly degraded to glucose by the enzyme dextranase.

Adjunctive therapy in shock – Enhances blood flow, particularly in the microcirculation, by a combination of the following mechanisms: Increases blood volume, venous return and cardiac output; decreases blood viscosity and peripheral vascular resistance; reduces aggregation of erythrocytes and other cellular elements of blood by coating them and maintaining their electronegative charges.

Administration to a patient in shock usually increases blood volume, central venous pressure, cardiac output, stroke volume, arterial blood pressure, pulse pressure, capillary perfusion, venous return and urinary output; it also decreases blood viscosity, heart rate, peripheral resistance and mean transit time and prevents or reverses cellular aggregation. Hematocrit is lowered in proportion to the infusion volume.

The intense but relatively short-lived plasma expansion volume produced by dextran 40 is advantageous in the treatment of early shock because it acts rapidly to correct hypovolemia while allowing control of the plasma volume. If overexpansion occurs, the discontinuation of the infusion will result in a decline in plasma volume due to loss of dextran from the intravascular space.

Priming solution for extracorporeal circulation – Dextran 40's advantages over homologous blood and other priming fluids include: Decreased destruction of erythrocytes and platelets; reduced intravascular hemagglutination; maintenance of electronegativity of erythrocytes and platelets.

Prophylaxis against venous thrombosis and thromboembolism – The infusion of dextran 40 during and after surgical trauma reduces the incidence of deep venous thrombosis (DVT) and pulmonary embolism (PE) in surgical patients subject to procedures with a high incidence of thromboembolic complications. Dextran 40 simultaneously inhibits mechanisms essential to thrombus formation such as vascular stasis and platelet adhesiveness, and alters the structure and lysability of fibrin clots.

Dextran 40 increases cardiac output, arterial, venous and microcirculatory flow and reduces mean transit time, chiefly by expanding plasma volume, by reducing blood viscosity through hemodilution and by reducing red cell aggregation.

Indications:

Shock: Adjunctive treatment of shock or impending shock due to hemorrhage, burns, surgery or other trauma. The solution is for emergency treatment when whole blood products are not available; it is not a substitute for whole blood or plasma proteins.

Priming fluid: As a priming fluid, either as the sole primer or as an additive, in pump oxygenators during extracorporeal circulation.

DVT/PE prophylaxis: Prophylaxis against DVT and PE in patients undergoing procedures associated with a high incidence of thromboembolic complications, such as hip surgery.

Contraindications:

Hypersensitivity to dextran; marked hemostatic defects of all types (eg, thrombocytopenia, hypofibrinogenemia), including those caused by drugs (eg, heparin, warfarin); marked cardiac decompensation; renal disease with severe oliguria or anuria.

Decreased urinary output, secondary to shock, is not a contraindication unless there is no improvement in urine output after the initial dose.

If administration of sodium or chloride could be clinically detrimental, 10% Dextran in 0.9% Sodium Chloride Injection is contraindicated.

DEXTRAN, LOW MOLECULAR WEIGHT (Dextran 40)

Warnings:

Anaphylaxis: Antigenicity of dextrans is directly related to their degree of branching. Because dextran 40 has a low degree of branching, it is relatively free of antigenic effect. Hypersensitivity reactions have, however, been reported (see Adverse Reactions). Infrequently, severe and fatal anaphylactoid reactions (eg, marked hypotension, cardiac and respiratory arrest) have been reported. Most of these reactions occurred early in the infusion period in patients not previously exposed to IV dextran and have appeared after administration of as little as 10 ml. Stop infusion immediately if an anaphylactoid reaction is imminent. Refer to Management of Acute Hypersensitivity Reactions. In circulatory collapse due to anaphylaxis, institute rapid volume substitution with an agent other than dextran. Dextran 1 is indicated for prophylaxis of serious anaphylactic reactions to dextran infusions.

Fluid imbalance: These products are colloid hypertonic solutions and will attract water from the extravascular space. Poorly hydrated patients will need additional fluid therapy. If given in excess, vascular overload could occur. This can be avoided by monitoring central venous pressure.

Administration of dextran IV can cause fluid or solute overloading, resulting in dilution of serum electrolyte concentrations, overhydration, congested states or pulmonary edema. The risk of dilutional states is inversely proportional to electrolyte concentrations of administered parenteral solutions.

Hemorrhage: Use with caution in patients with active hemorrhage; the increase in perfusion pressure and improved microcirculatory flow may result in additional blood loss.

Avoid administering infusions that exceed the recommended dose, as a dose-related increase in the incidence of wound hematoma, wound seroma, wound bleeding, distant bleeding (hematuria and melena) and pulmonary edema has been observed.

Hematologic effects: Use with caution in patients with thrombocytopenia. Hematocrit should not be depressed below 30% by volume. When large volumes of dextran are administered, plasma protein levels will be decreased. Do not give dextran 40 to patients with marked thrombocytopenia or hypofibrinogenemia.

In individuals with normal hemostasis, dosages of up to 15 ml/kg or > 1000 ml may prolong bleeding time and decrease coagulation due to depressed platelet function. Dosages in this range also markedly decrease factor VIII; they also decrease factors V and IX to a slightly greater degree than would be expected from hemodilution alone. Because these changes tend to be more pronounced following trauma or major surgery, observe all patients for early signs of bleeding complications.

Special risk patients: Use solutions containing sodium ions with great care, if at all, in patients with congestive heart failure, severe renal insufficiency, in clinical states in which edema exists with sodium retention (particularly in postoperative or elderly patients) and in patients receiving corticosteroids.

Use dextrose-containing solutions with caution in overt or known subclinical diabetes mellitus.

Renal function impairment: Renal excretion causes elevation of the specific gravity of the urine. In the presence of adequate urine flow, only minor elevations occur, but in patients with diminished urine flow, urine viscosity and specific gravity can be increased markedly. As osmolarity is only slightly affected by the presence of dextran molecules, assess a patient's state of hydration by determination of urine or serum osmolarity. If signs of dehydration are noted, administer additional fluids. An osmotic diuretic such as mannitol is useful in maintaining adequate urine flow.

Renal failure, sometimes irreversible, has been reported. While the preexisting clinical condition of these patients could account for the oliguria or anuria, it is possible that dextran use may have contributed to its development. Evidence of tubular vacuolization (osmotic nephrosis) has been found following administration. The exact clinical significance is unknown.

In patients with diminished renal function, use of solutions containing sodium ions may result in sodium retention. Excessive doses may precipitate renal failure.

Pregnancy: Category C. Safety for use during pregnancy has not been established. Use only when clearly needed and when the potential benefits outweigh the potential hazards to the fetus.

Lactation: It is not known whether this drug is excreted in breast milk. Exercise caution when dextran 40 is administered to a nursing woman.

DEXTRAN, LOW MOLECULAR WEIGHT (Dextran 40)

Precautions:

Monitoring: Urine output should be carefully monitored. Usually, an increase in urine output occurs in oliguric patients after administration. If no increase is observed after the infusion of 500 ml, discontinue the drug until adequate diuresis develops spontaneously or can be induced by other means.

Exercise care to prevent a depression of the hematocrit below 30%.

Infusion of dextran may lead to excessive dilution of red blood cells and plasma proteins, dilution of other blood constituents (platelets, fibrinogen) or dilutional acidosis caused by dilution of the bicarbonate ion.

Bleeding complications: Observe patients for early signs of bleeding complications, particularly following surgery, major trauma or if anticoagulant drugs are being administered.

Drug Interactions:

Drug/Lab test interactions: Blood sugar determinations that employ high concentrations of acid (acetic or sulfuric) may cause hydrolysis of dextran; falsely elevated glucose assays may be reported in patients receiving dextran. In other laboratory tests, the presence of dextran may result in the development of turbidity, which can interfere with bilirubin assays in which alcohol has been employed, in total protein assays employing biuret reagent and in blood sugar determinations with the ortho-toluidine method. Consider withdrawal of blood for chemical laboratory tests prior to initiating therapy.

Blood typing and crossmatching procedures employing enzyme techniques may give unreliable readings if the samples are taken after infusion. Other blood typing and crossmatching procedures are not affected. Draw blood samples for the above determinations prior to initiating infusion or, alternatively, inform the laboratory that the patient has received dextran so that suitable assay methods can be applied.

Occasional abnormal renal and hepatic function values have been reported following IV use. The specific effect on renal and hepatic function could not be determined, as most of these patients had also undergone surgery or cardiac catheterization.

Adverse Reactions:

Hypersensitivity: Mild cutaneous eruptions, generalized urticaria, hypotension, nausea, vomiting, headache, dyspnea, fever, tightness of the chest, bronchospasm, wheezing and, rarely, anaphylactoid (allergic) shock (see Warnings).

Miscellaneous: Reactions which may occur because of the solution or the technique of administration include febrile response, infection at the injection site, venous thrombosis or phlebitis extending from the injection site, extravasation and hypervolemia.

Hypernatremia may be associated with edema and exacerbation of congestive heart failure due to the retention of water, resulting in expanded extracellular fluid volume.

If solutions containing sodium chloride are infused in large volumes, chloride ions may cause a loss of bicarbonate ions, resulting in an acidifying effect.

Administration and Dosage:

For IV use only.

Adjunctive therapy in shock: Total dosage during the first 24 hours should not exceed 20 ml/kg. The first 10 ml/kg should be infused rapidly, with the remaining dose being administered more slowly. Monitor the central venous pressure frequently during the initial infusion. Should therapy continue beyond 24 hours, total daily dosage should not exceed 10 ml/kg, and therapy should not continue beyond 5 days.

Hemodiluent in extracorporeal circulation: The dosage employed in the priming fluid will vary with the volume of pump oxygenator employed. It may be added as sole primer or as an additive. Generally, 10 to 20 ml/kg are added to the perfusion circuit. Do not exceed total dosage of 20 ml/kg; this can be limited and controlled by adding other priming fluids.

Prophylactic therapy of venous thrombosis and thromboembolism: Select dosage according to the risk of thromboembolic complications (eg, type of surgery and duration of immobilization). In general, initiate treatment during surgery. Administer 500 to 1000 ml (approximately 10 ml/kg) on the day of the operation. Continue treatment at a dose of 500 ml/day for an additional 2 to 3 days. Thereafter, and according to the risk of complications, 500 ml may be administered every second or third day during the period of risk for up to 2 weeks.

Children: The best guide is the body weight or surface area, and the total dosage should not exceed 20 ml/kg.

Storage/Stability: Store at a constant temperature between 15° to 30°C (59° to 86°F). Protect from freezing.

DEXTRAN, LOW MOLECULAR WEIGHT (Dextran 40)

Rx	**Dextran 40** (McGaw)	**Injection**: 10% dextran 40 in 0.9% sodium chloride	In 500 ml.
Rx	**Gentran 40** (Baxter)		In 500 ml.
Rx	**10% LMD** (Abbott)		In 500 ml.
Rx	**Rheomacrodex** (Medisan)		In 500 ml.
Rx	**Dextran 40** (McGaw)	**Injection**: 10% dextran 40 in 5% dextrose	In 500 ml.
Rx	**Gentran 40** (Baxter)		In 500 ml.
Rx	**10% LMD** (Abbott)		In 500 ml.
Rx	**Rheomacrodex** (Medisan)		In 500 ml.

DEXTRAN, HIGH MOLECULAR WEIGHT (Dextran 70 and 75)

Actions:

Pharmacology: Dextrans are synthetic polysaccharides used to approximate the colloidal properties of albumin. Dextran 70 has an average molecular weight (MW) of 70,000 (range 20,000 to 200,000), and dextran 75 has an average MW of 75,000. Dextran 70 improves blood pressure, pulse rate, respiratory exchange and renal function in patients with hypovolemia or hypotensive shock. IV infusion results in an expansion of plasma volume slightly in excess of volume infused and decreases from this maximum over the next 24 hours. This plasma volume expansion improves hemodynamic status for ≥ 24 hours.

Pharmacokinetics: Dextran molecules below 50,000 molecular weight are eliminated by renal excretion, with approximately 50% appearing in the urine in 24 hours in the normovolemic patient. The remaining dextran is enzymatically degraded to glucose at a rate of about 70 to 90 mg/kg/day. This is a variable process.

Indications:

Shock: Treatment of shock or impending shock due to surgery or other trauma, hemorrhage or burns. Intended for emergency treatment only when whole blood or blood products are not available; do not regard as a substitute for whole blood or plasma proteins. It should not replace other forms of therapy known to be of value in the treatment of shock.

Contraindications:

Hypersensitivity to dextran; marked hemostatic defects of all types (thrombocytopenia, hypofibrinogenemia, etc), including those induced by drugs; marked cardiac decompensation; renal disease with severe oliguria or anuria; severe congestive heart failure, pulmonary edema and severe bleeding disorders; where use of sodium or chloride could be clinically detrimental.

Warnings:

Anaphylaxis: Severe and fatal anaphylactoid reactions (eg, marked hypotension, cardiac and respiratory arrest) have occurred early in the infusion period in patients not previously exposed to IV dextran. Stop infusion immediately if an anaphylactoid reaction is imminent, provided that other means of sustaining the circulation are available. Refer to Management of Acute Hypersensitivity Reactions. In circulatory collapse due to anaphylaxis, institute rapid volume substitution with an agent other than dextran. Antihistamines may be effective in relieving some symptoms. Dextran 1 is indicated for prophylaxis of serious anaphylactic reactions associated with dextran infusions.

Hematologic effects: In individuals with normal hemostasis, dosages approximating 15 ml/kg or > 1000 ml prolong bleeding time and decrease coagulation due to depressed platelet function; use with caution in patients with thrombocytopenia. Such dosages also markedly decrease factor VIII and decrease factor V and factor IX more than would be expected from hemodilution alone. These changes tend to be more pronounced following trauma or major surgery; observe patients for early signs of bleeding complications. Transient prolongation of bleeding time may occur following doses > 1000 ml, particularly if the patient is on concomitant anticoagulation therapy. Take care to prevent depression of hematocrit below 30% by volume. When large volumes of dextran are given, plasma protein level will be decreased.

Special risk patients: Use solutions containing sodium ions with great care, if at all, in patients with congestive heart failure, pulmonary edema, severe renal insufficiency, patients receiving corticosteroids or corticotropin and in clinical states in which edema exists with sodium retention. Circulatory overload may occur. Exercise special care in patients with impaired renal clearance.

Exercise care in patients with pathological abdominal conditions and in those undergoing bowel surgery.

Fluid imbalance: Fluid or solute overloading may occur, resulting in dilution of serum electrolyte concentrations, overhydration, congested states (CHF) and peripheral or pulmonary edema. The risk of dilutional states is inversely proportional to the electrolyte concentration of administered parenteral solutions.

The risk of solute overload causing congested states with peripheral and pulmonary edema is directly proportional to electrolyte concentrations of such solutions.

Monitoring central venous blood pressure is recommended to detect overexpansion of blood volume. When signs of overexpansion appear, discontinuing IV infusion allows blood volume to readjust and decline, primarily by loss of fluid to urine.

Pregnancy: Category C. Safety for use during pregnancy has not been established. There are no adequate and well controlled studies in pregnant women. Use only when clearly needed and when potential benefits outweigh potential hazards.

Lactation: It is not known whether this drug is excreted in breast milk. Exercise caution when administering to a nursing woman.

DEXTRAN, HIGH MOLECULAR WEIGHT (Dextran 70 and 75)

Precautions:

Monitoring: Urine output should be carefully observed. An increase in urine output usually occurs in oliguric patients after the administration of dextran. If no increase is observed after the infusion of 500 ml of dextran, discontinue the drug until adequate diuresis develops spontaneously or can be provoked by other means.

Bleeding complications: Observe patients for early signs of bleeding complications, particularly following surgery or major trauma, or if anticoagulant drugs are being administered.

Drug Interactions:

Drug/Lab test interactions: Blood sugar determinations that employ high concentrations of acid (acetic or sulfuric) may cause hydrolysis of dextran; falsely elevated glucose assays may be reported in patients receiving dextran. In other laboratory tests, the presence of dextran may result in the development of turbidity, which can interfere with bilirubin assays in which alcohol has been employed, in total protein assays employing biuret reagent and in blood sugar determinations with the ortho-toluidine method.

Blood typing and crossmatching procedures employing enzyme techniques may give unreliable readings if the samples are taken after infusion. If blood is drawn after the infusion, the saline-agglutination and indirect antiglobulin methods may be used for typing and crossmatching. Draw blood samples for the above determinations prior to initiating infusion or, alternatively, inform the laboratory that the patient has received dextran so that suitable assay methods can be applied.

Adverse Reactions:

Infusion technique: Reactions which may occur because of the solution or the technique of administration include febrile response, infection at the injection site, venous thrombosis or phlebitis extending from the injection site, extravasation and hypervolemia. If a reaction develops, discontinue use and treat accordingly.

Hypersensitivity: Allergic reactions include urticaria, nasal congestion, wheezing, tightness of the chest, dyspnea, mild hypotension and, rarely, anaphylactoid (allergic) shock (see Warnings).

Miscellaneous: Sudden marked hypotension; nausea; vomiting; fever; joint pains.

Hypernatremia may be associated with edema and exacerbation of congestive heart failure due to water retention, resulting in expanded extracellular fluid volume.

If solutions containing sodium chloride are infused in large volumes, chloride ions may cause a loss of bicarbonate ions, resulting in an acidifying effect.

Administration and Dosage:

Administer by IV infusion only. Total dose and rate of infusion depend upon the magnitude of fluid loss and the resultant hemoconcentration. It is suggested that the total dosage not exceed 20 ml/kg during the first 24 hours.

Adults: The amount usually administered is 500 to 1000 ml, which may be given at a rate of from 20 to 40 ml/minute in an emergency.

Children: The best guide to dosage is the body weight or surface area of the patient; total dosage should not exceed 20 ml/kg.

No additives should be delivered via plasma volume expanders.

Storage/Stability: The solution has no bacteriostat; discard partially used containers. The solution must be clear. Store at a constant temperature not > 25°C (77°F).

Rx	**Dextran 75** (Abbott)	**Injection:** 6% dextran 75 in 0.9% sodium chloride	In 500 ml.
Rx	**Dextran 70** (McGaw)	**Injection:** 6% dextran 70 in 0.9% sodium chloride	In 500 ml.
Rx	**Gentran 70** (Baxter)		In 500 ml.
Rx	**Macrodex** (Medisan)		In 500 ml.
Rx	**Dextran 75** (Abbott)	**Injection:** 6% dextran 75 in 5% dextrose	In 500 ml.
Rx	**Gendex 75** (Lennod)		In 500 ml.
Rx	**Macrodex** (Medisan)	**Injection:** 6% dextran 70 in 5% dextrose	In 500 ml.

HEMIN

> **Warning:**
> Hemin for injection should only be used by physicians experienced in the management of porphyrias in hospitals where the recommended clinical and laboratory diagnostic and monitoring techniques are available.
> Consider hemin therapy after an appropriate period of alternate therapy (ie, 400 g glucose/day for 1 to 2 days).

Actions:

Pharmacology: Hemin for injection is an enzyme inhibitor derived from processed red blood cells. It was known previously as hematin. The term hematin has been used to describe the chemical reaction product of hemin and sodium carbonate solution. Hemin is an iron-containing metalloporphyrin.

Porphyrias are rare metabolic disorders that, as a group, represent disturbances of heme synthesis and are differentiated on the basis of specific enzymatic defects. Porphyrias are characterized clinically by neurologic (psychoses, seizures, paresis) or cutaneous (photosensitivity) manifestations, and chemically by overproduction of porphyrins or their precursors. Porphyrins are byproducts of heme synthesis; heme is the iron-containing constituent of hemoglobin and respiratory pigments and is produced and required by nearly every body tissue. Heme limits the hepatic or marrow synthesis of porphyrin, which is likely due to inhibition of delta-aminolevulinic acid synthetase, the enzyme that limits the rate of porphyrin/heme biosynthetic pathway. However, the exact mechanism by which hematin produces symptomatic improvement in patients with acute episodes of the hepatic porphyrias is not known.

Pharmacokinetics: Following IV administration of hematin in non-jaundiced patients, an increase in fecal urobilinogen can be observed, which is roughly proportional to the amount of hematin administered. This suggests an enterohepatic pathway as at least one route of elimination. Bilirubin metabolites are also excreted in the urine following hematin injections.

Clinical trials: Hemin therapy for the acute porphyrias is not curative. After discontinuation of treatment, symptoms generally return, although remission may be prolonged. Some neurological symptoms have improved weeks to months after therapy, although little or no response was noted at the time of treatment.

Indications:

Porphyria: For the amelioration of recurrent attacks of acute intermittent porphyria temporally related to the menstrual cycle in susceptible women. Manifestations such as pain, hypertension, tachycardia, abnormal mental status and mild to progressive neurologic signs may be controlled in selected patients.

Similar findings have been reported in other patients with acute intermittent porphyria, porphyria variegata and hereditary coproporphyria.

Contraindications:

Hypersensitivity to hemin; porphyria cutanea tarda.

Warnings:

Pregnancy: Category C. Safety for use during pregnancy has not been established. Use only when clearly needed and when the potential benefits outweigh the potential hazards to the fetus.

Lactation: It is not known whether hemin for injection is excreted in breast milk. Safety for use in the nursing mother has not been established.

Children: Safety and efficacy for use in children have not been established.

Precautions:

Monitoring: Drug effect will be demonstrated by a decrease in urinary concentration of one or more of the following compounds: ALA (delta-aminolevulinic acid); UPG (uroporphyrinogen); PBG (porphobilinogen coproporphyrin).

Neuronal damage: Clinical benefit depends on prompt administration. Attacks of porphyria may progress to irreversible neuronal damage. Hemin therapy is intended to prevent an attack from reaching the critical stage of neuronal degeneration. This agent is not effective in repairing neuronal damage.

Renal effects: Reversible renal shutdown has been observed where an excessive hematin dose (12.2 mg/kg) was administered in a single infusion. Oliguria and increased nitrogen retention occurred, although the patient remained asymptomatic. No worsening of renal function has been seen with use of recommended dosages.

Diagnostic tests: Before beginning therapy, diagnose the presence of acute porphyria using the following criteria: Presence of clinical symptoms and positive Watson-Schwartz or Hoesch test.

HEMIN

Drug Interactions:

Hemin Drug Interactions			
Precipitant drug	Object drug*		Description
Hemin	Anticoagulants	↑	Hemin has exhibited transient, mild anticoagulant effects during clinical studies; therefore, avoid concurrent anticoagulant therapy. The extent and duration of the hypocoagulable state has not been established.
Barbiturates Estrogens Steroid metabolites	Hemin	↔	These agents increase the activity of delta-aminolevulinic acid synthetase. Because hemin therapy limits the rate of porphyria/heme biosynthesis, possibly by inhibiting the enzyme delta-aminolevulinic acid synthetase, avoid use of these agents.

* ↑ = Object drug increased. ↔ = Undetermined effect.

Adverse Reactions:

Phlebitis with or without leukocytosis and with or without mild pyrexia has occurred after administration of hematin through small arm veins.

There has been one report of coagulopathy. This patient exhibited prolonged prothrombin time, partial thromboplastin time, thrombocytopenia, mild hypofibrinogenemia, mild elevation of fibrin split products and a 10% fall in hematocrit.

Overdosage:

Reversible renal shutdown has been observed in a case where an excessive hematin dose (12.2 mg/kg) was administered in a single infusion (see Precautions). Treatment of this case consisted of ethacrynic acid and mannitol.

Administration and Dosage:

For IV use only. Use a large arm vein or a central venous catheter to avoid phlebitis.

Before administering hemin for injection, consider alternate therapy (ie, 400 g glucose/day for 1 to 2 days). If improvement is unsatisfactory for the treatment of acute attacks of porphyria, administer an IV infusion containing a dose of 1 to 4 mg/kg/day of hematin over a period of 10 to 15 minutes for 3 to 14 days, based on clinical signs. In more severe cases, this dose may be repeated no earlier than every 12 hours. Give no more than 6 mg/kg in any 24 hour period.

Preparation of solution: Reconstitute by adding 43 ml of Sterile Water for Injection to the dispensing vial. Shake well for a period of 2 to 3 minutes to aid dissolution.

After reconstitution, each ml contains the equivalent of approximately 7 mg hematin (301 mg hemin/43 ml), 5 mg sodium carbonate (215 mg/43 ml) and 7 mg sorbitol (301 mg/43 ml). The drug may be administered directly from the vial.

Hemin Solution Preparation
Dosage Calculation Table
1 mg hematin equivalent = 0.14 ml
2 mg hematin equivalent = 0.28 ml
3 mg hematin equivalent = 0.42 ml
4 mg hematin equivalent = 0.56 ml

Because reconstituted hemin is not transparent, any undissolved particulate matter is difficult to see; therefore, terminal filtration through a sterile 0.45 micron or smaller filter is recommended.

Admixture incompatibility: Do not add any drug or chemical agent fluid admixture unless its effect on the chemical and physical stability has first been determined.

Storage/Stability: Because this product contains no preservative and undergoes rapid chemical decomposition in solution, do not reconstitute until immediately before use. Store lyophilized powder frozen until time of use. Discard any unused portion.

Rx	**Panhematin** (Abbott)	**Powder for Injection:** 301 mg hemin per vial (equivalent to 7 mg hematin per ml) after reconstitution with 43 ml Sterile Water for Injection.	Preservative free. With 300 mg sorbitol. In 2 ml vials.

SODIUM PHENYLBUTYRATE

Actions:

Pharmacology: Sodium phenylbutyrate is a pro-drug and is rapidly metabolized to phenylacetate. Phenylacetate is a metabolically-active compound that conjugates with glutamine via acetylation to form phenylacetylglutamine. Phenylacetylglutamine is excreted then by the kidneys. On a molar basis, it is comparable to urea (each containing two moles of nitrogen). Therefore, phenylacetylglutamine provides an alternate vehicle for waste nitrogen excretion.

Pharmacokinetics:

Absorption – Peak plasma levels of phenylbutyrate occur within 1 hour after a single dose of 5 g sodium phenylbutyrate powder with a C_{max} of 195 mcg/ml and for the tablets, a C_{max} of 218 mcg/ml under fasting conditions. The effect of food on phenylbutyrate's absorption is unknown.

Excretion – A majority of the administered compound (≈ 80% to 100%) is excreted by the kidneys within 24 hours as the conjugation product, phenylacetylglutamine. For each gram of sodium phenylbutyrate administered, it is estimated that between 0.12 to 0.15 g of phenylacetylglutamine nitrogen is produced.

Hepatic function impairment: In patients who did not have urea cycle disorders, but had impaired hepatic function, the metabolism and excretion of sodium phenylbutyrate were not affected.

Pharmacokinetic studies have not been conducted in the primary patient population (neonates, infants and children), but pharmacokinetic data were obtained from normal adult subjects.

Following oral administration of 5 g, measurable plasma levels of phenylbutyrate and phenylacetate were detected 15 and 30 min after dosing, respectively, and phenylacetylglutamine was detected shortly thereafter. The pharmacokinetic parameters for phenylbutyrate for C_{max} (mcg/ml), T_{max} (hours) and elimination half-life were 195, 1 and 0.76 hours, respectively, and for phenylacetate 45.3, 3.55 and 1.29 hours, respectively. The major sites for metabolism are the liver and kidney.

In patients with urea cycle disorders, sodium phenylbutyrate decreases elevated plasma ammonia and glutamine levels. It increases waste nitrogen excretion in the form of phenylacetylglutamine.

The pharmacokinetic parameters, AUC and C_{max} for both plasma phenylbutyrate and phenylacetate were about 30% to 50% greater in females than in males.

Indications:

Cycle disorders: Sodium phenylbutyrate is indicated as adjunctive therapy in the chronic management of patients with urea cycle disorders involving deficiencies of carbamoyl phosphate synthetase (CPS), ornithine transcarbamoylase (OTC) or argininosuccinic acid synthetase (AAS). It is indicated in all patients with neonatal-onset deficiency (complete enzymatic deficiency, presenting within the first 28 days of life). It is also indicated in patients with late-onset disease (partial enzymatic deficiency, presenting after the first month of life) who have a history of hyperammonemic encephalopathy. It is important that the diagnosis be made early and treatment initiated immediately to improve survival. Any episode of acute hyperammonemia should be treated as a life-threatening emergency.

Contraindications:

Management of acute hyperammonemia, which is a medical emergency.

Warnings:

Fluid retention: Use with great care, if at all, in patients with CHF or severe renal insufficiency, and in clinical states in which there is sodium retention with edema.

Pre-existing neurologic impairment: Reversal of pre-existing neurologic impairment is not likely to occur with treatment, and neurologic deterioration may continue.

Acute hyperammonemic encephalopathy recurred in the majority of patients.

Long-term: Sodium phenylbutyrate may be required life-long unless orthotopic liver transplantation is elected.

Renal/Hepatic function impairment: Sodium phenylbutyrate is metabolized in the liver and kidney, and phenylacetylglutamine is primarily excreted by the kidney. Use caution when administering the drug to patients with hepatic or renal insufficiency.

Pregnancy: Category C. It is not known whether sodium phenylbutyrate can cause fetal harm when administered to a pregnant woman or can affect reproduction capacity. Give sodium phenylbutyrate to a pregnant woman only if clearly needed.

Lactation: It is not known whether this drug is excreted in breast milk. Because many drugs are excreted in breast milk, exercise caution when administering sodium phenylbutyrate to a nursing woman.

Children: The use of tablets for neonates, infants and children ≤ 20 kg is not recommended (see Administration and Dosage).

SODIUM PHENYLBUTYRATE

Precautions:

Monitoring: Maintain plasma levels of ammonia, arginine, branched-chain amino acids and serum proteins within normal limits, and maintain plasma glutamine at levels < 1000 mcmol/L. Periodically monitor serum drug levels of phenylbutyrate and its metabolites, phenylacetate and phenylacetylglutamine.

Drug Interactions:

Probenecid is known to inhibit the renal transport of many organic compounds, including hippuric acid, and may affect renal excretion of the conjugation product of sodium phenylbutyrate, as well as its metabolite.

Corticosteroids may cause the breakdown of body protein and increase plasma ammonia levels.

Haloperidol/Valproate may cause hyperammonemia.

Adverse Reactions:

Amenorrhea/menstrual dysfunction (23%); decreased appetite (4%); body odor (probably caused by the metabolite phenylacetate), bad taste or taste aversion (3%).

Other adverse events reported in ≤ 2% of patients:

GI: Abdominal pain; gastritis; nausea; vomiting; constipation; rectal bleeding; peptic ulcer disease; pancreatitis (one patient).

Hematologic: Aplastic anemia; ecchymosis (one patient).

Cardiovascular: Arrhythmia; edema (one patient).

CNS: Depression; neurotoxicity (somnolence, fatigue and lightheadedness; less frequently, headache, dysgeusia, hypoacusis, disorientation, impaired memory and exacerbation of a pre-existing neuropathy). These adverse events were mainly mild in severity. The acute onset and reversibility when the phenylacetate infusion was discontinued suggest a drug effect.

Miscellaneous: Headache; syncope; weight gain; renal tubular acidosis; rash.

Lab test abnormalities:

Metabolic – Acidosis (14%); alkalosis, hyperchloremia (7%); hypophosphatemia (6%); hyperuricemia, hyperphosphatemia (2%); hypernatremia, hypokalemia (1%).

Nutritional – Hypoalbuminemia (11%); decreased total protein (3%).

Hepatic – Increased alkaline phosphatase (6%); increased liver transaminases (4%); hyperbilirubinemia (1%).

Hematologic – Anemia (9%); leukopenia, leukocytosis (4%); thrombocytopenia (3%); thrombocytosis (1%).

Overdosage:

No adverse experiences have been reported involving overdoses of sodium phenylbutyrate in patients with urea cycle disorders.

Treatment: In the event of an overdose, discontinue the drug and institute supportive measures. Hemodialysis or peritoneal dialysis may be beneficial.

Administration and Dosage:

Tablets: For oral use only. It is indicated for children weighing > 20 kg or adults.

Usual dose – 450 to 600 mg/kg/day in patients weighing < 20 kg, or 9.9 to 13 g/m^2/day in larger patients. Take in equally divided amounts with each meal (eg, three times daily). The safety and efficacy of doses > 20 g/day (40 tablets) has not been established.

Powder: For oral use via mouth, gastrostomy or nasogastric tube only. Mix with food (solid or liquid). Avoid acidic beverages. Each level teaspoon dispenses 3.2 g of powder and 3 g of sodium phenylbutyrate. Each level tablespoon dispenses 9.1 g of powder and 8.6 g of sodium phenylbutyrate. Shake lightly before use.

Usual dose – 450 to 600 mg/kg/day in patients weighing < 20 kg, or 9.9 to 13 g/m^2/day in larger patients. Take in equally divided amounts with each meal or feeding, four to six times daily. The safety and efficacy of doses > 20 g/day has not been established.

Storage/Stability: Store at room temperature, 15° to 30°C (59° to 86°F). After opening, keep bottle tightly closed.

Rx	**Buphenyl** (Ucyclyd Pharma)	**Tablets:** 500 mg	(UCY 500). Off-white, oval. In 250s and 500s.
		Powder: 3.2 g (3 g sodium phenylbutyrate) per tsp	In 500 and 950 ml bottles. Measurers provided.
		9.1 g (8.6 g sodium phenylbutyrate) per tbsp	In 500 and 950 ml bottles. Measurers provided.

chapter 3

hormones

ESTROGENS

For estrogens recommended for their antineoplastic action in prostatic carcinoma, refer to the estrogen section in the Antineoplastics chapter.

This general discussion applies to all estrogens; consider when using any estrogen.

Warning:

Estrogens have been reported to increase the risk of endometrial carcinoma.

Three independent studies have shown an increased risk of endometrial cancer in postmenopausal women exposed to exogenous estrogens for prolonged periods. This risk was independent of the other known risk factors. Incidence rates of endometrial cancer have increased sharply since 1969, which may relate to the rapidly expanding use of estrogens during the last decade. The prognosis for survival of endometrial cancer, however, is better in an estrogen user. This may be an issue of detection.

The risk of endometrial cancer in estrogen users was 4.5 to 13.9 times greater than in nonusers and appears to depend on duration of treatment and dose. Therefore, when estrogens are used for the treatment of menopausal symptoms, use the lowest dose and discontinue medication as soon as possible. When prolonged treatment is indicated, reassess the patient at least annually by endometrial sampling to determine the need for continued therapy. Cyclic administration of low doses of estrogen may carry less risk than continuous administration.

Close clinical surveillance of all women taking estrogens is important. In undiagnosed persistent or recurring abnormal vaginal bleeding, exclude malignancy.

There is no evidence that "natural" estrogens are more or less hazardous than "synthetic" estrogens at equiestrogenic doses.

Do not use estrogens during pregnancy.

The use of female sex hormones (both estrogens and progestins) during early pregnancy may seriously damage the offspring. Females exposed in utero to diethylstilbestrol (DES) have an increased risk of developing vaginal or cervical cancer, estimated at $\leq$ 4 per 1000 exposures. Furthermore, a high percentage of such exposed women (30% to 90%) have vaginal adenosis (epithelial changes of vagina and cervix). Although histologically benign, it is not known if they are precursors of malignancy. Similar data are not available for other estrogens or progestins, but it cannot be presumed that they would not induce similar changes.

There have also been congenital anomalies reported in male offspring whose mothers ingested the drug. The primary abnormalities have been related to structural problems of the GU tract and to abnormal semen quality. The effect of these lesions on carcinoma development and fertility is yet to be determined.

Several reports suggest an association between intrauterine exposure to female sex hormones and congenital anomalies, including congenital heart defects and limb reduction defects. One study estimated a 4.7-fold increased risk of limb reduction defects in infants exposed in utero to sex hormones (oral contraceptives, hormone withdrawal tests for pregnancy or attempted treatment for threatened abortion). Some of these exposures involved only a few days of treatment. The risk of limb reduction defects in exposed fetuses is somewhat less than 1 per 1000. No studies are definitive.

Female sex hormones have been used during pregnancy to treat threatened or habitual abortion. There is considerable evidence that estrogens are ineffective for these indications.

If estrogens are used during pregnancy, or if the patient becomes pregnant while taking estrogens, inform her of the potential risks to the fetus.

Actions:

Pharmacology: Although six different natural estrogens have been isolated from the human female, only three are present in significant quantities: Estradiol, estrone and estriol. The most potent and major secretory product of the ovary, estradiol, is rapidly oxidized to estrone. Hydration of estrone produces the much weaker estriol. The estrogenic potency of estradiol is 12 times estrone's and 80 times estriol's.

ESTROGENS

Estrogens, important in developing and maintaining female reproductive system and secondary sex characteristics, promote growth and development of vagina, uterus, fallopian tubes and breasts. They affect release of pituitary gonadotropins; cause capillary dilatation, fluid retention, protein anabolism and thin cervical mucus; inhibit or facilitate ovulation; prevent postpartum breast discomfort. Indirectly, they contribute to: Shaping the skeleton (conserving calcium and phosphorus and encouraging bone formation); maintenance of tone and elasticity of urogenital structures; changes in epiphyses of long bones that allow for pubertal growth spurt and its termination; growth of axillary and pubic hair; pigmentation of nipples and genitals.

Estrogens induce proliferation in the epithelium of the fallopian tubes, endometrium, cervix, vagina and mucosa of the GI tract and increase vascularity. Estrogens are responsible for vaginal acidity caused by deposition of glycogen in vaginal epithelium. They encourage cornification of superficial vaginal cells to give a characteristic vaginal smear.

In the preovulatory phase, estrogens produce changes in the tubular mucosa and stimulate the contraction and motility of the fallopian tubes to promote the ovum transport. Estrogens restore the endometrium, including its coiled arteries, after menstruation, but do not induce the glands to secrete. An endometrium suddenly deprived of estrogen breaks down and bleeds. The growth and secretory activity of cervical epithelium are determined in part by estrogens which also modify the physical and chemical properties of cervical mucus.

Menstruation – Decline of estrogenic activity at the end of the menstrual cycle can induce menstruation, although cessation of progesterone secretion does the same to an estrogen-primed endometrium. However, in the preovulatory or nonovulatory cycle, estrogen withdrawal is the primary determinant of the onset of menstruation.

Menopause – The cessation of cyclic function is the basic ovarian event in the menopause. Functional changes can be attributed to depletion of follicles, although a few follicles persist after the last menses.

The beginning of menopause is marked by hot flushes, decreasing frequency and quality of ovulation, associated with skips and delays of menses or variable periods of amenorrhea and later by decreasing estrogen secretion. The declining estrogen secretion is accompanied by signs and symptoms of hormone deficits in the estrogen-dependent organs, including pituitary, uterus, cervix, vagina and breasts. Pituitary gonadotropin secretion rises, reflected by increased quantities of gonadotropin in blood and urine. The endometrium becomes atrophic, myometrial mass decreases and the vaginal epithelium becomes thin as, deficient in glycogen, it fails to become keratinized. The ovarian stroma producing androgens persist at variable amounts of time.

Coronary heart disease – Observational studies consistently support the hypothesis that postmenopausal estrogen use reduces the risk of severe coronary heart disease. An estrogen-induced change in HDL levels may play a role and direct effects on the vessel wall. Randomized clinical trials are awaiting outcome.

Pharmacokinetics:

Absorption/Distribution – Absorption of most natural estrogens and their derivatives from the GI tract is complete. The limited oral effectiveness of natural estrogens and their esters is due to their metabolism. In estrogen-responsive tissues (female genital organs, breasts, hypothalamus, pituitary), estrogen classically binds to tissue-specific receptor proteins in the cytoplasm. The resulting estrogen-protein complex penetrates the nuclear membrane and ultimately binds to materials in the cell nucleus. This activates RNA synthesis and various proteins and enzymes that in turn affect characteristic changes in responsive tissues. Many other effects of estrogen cannot be explained by this classic mechanism. About 80% of estradiol is bound to sex hormone binding globulin; most of the rest is loosely bound to albumin and about 2% is unbound. Estrone is highly bound to protein as it circulates in the blood, primarily as a conjugate with sulfate.

Transdermal system: In contrast to oral estradiol, the skin metabolizes estradiol via the transdermal system only to a small extent. Therefore, transdermal use produces therapeutic serum levels of estradiol with lower circulating levels of estrone and estrone conjugates, and requires smaller total doses. Transdermal use produces mean serum estradiol concentrations comparable to those produced by daily oral administration at about 20 times the daily transdermal dose.

Metabolism/Excretion – Metabolism and inactivation occur primarily in the liver. During cyclic passage through the liver, estrogens are degraded to less active estrogenic compounds conjugated with sulfuric and glucuronic acids. Some estrogens are excreted into bile, reabsorbed from intestines and returned to the liver via the portal venous system. Water soluble estrogen conjugates, strongly acidic, are ionized in body fluids, which favor excretion in urine; tubular reabsorption is minimal.

ESTROGENS

Indications:

Moderate to severe vasomotor symptoms associated with menopause: The primary indication is to treat hot flushes. Sleep deprivation associated with this can aggravate depression. Estrogens are not the drug of choice for treating depression.

Atrophic vaginitis; kraurosis vulvae.

Female hypogonadism; female castration; primary ovarian failure.

Breast cancer: Palliation only in selected women and men or those with metastatic disease.

Prostatic carcinoma: Palliative therapy of advanced disease.

Osteoporosis: Conjugated estrogens are indicated in postmenopausal women, with evidence of loss or deficiency of bone mass, to retard further bone loss and estrogen-deficiency-induced osteoporosis. Use with other important measures such as diet, calcium and physiotherapy. A more favorable benefit/risk ratio exists if women have had a hysterectomy; there is no risk of endometrial carcinoma.

Bone loss is increased in many women following menopause, but there is no clear way to identify those women who will develop osteoporotic fractures. Estrogens can reduce rate of bone loss in postmenopausal women and reduce bone fractures. Women who have had an early surgical menopause (oophorectomy) appear to be at increased risk for osteoporosis development.

The FDA has also approved the use of the other oral short-acting estrogens (DES, esterified estrogens, estradiol, ethinyl estradiol and estropipate) in the treatment of osteoporosis.

Abnormal uterine bleeding due to hormonal imbalance in the absence of organic pathology (conjugated estrogens, parenteral).

Unlabeled uses: Oral DES is an effective postcoital contraceptive when given in doses of 25 mg twice daily for 5 days if therapy is started no later than 72 hours after intercourse. Although the FDA has indicated that use of DES as an emergency treatment (not as a routine method of birth control) is approvable, no manufacturer currently holds an approved NDA for this use. Ethinyl estradiol, conjugated estrogens and other estrogens have also been evaluated for postcoital contraception.

Ethinyl estradiol – A 5 mcg tablet is being investigated for use in the treatment of Turner's syndrome. Gynex (now Bio-Technology) received orphan status for this product in July 1988.

Contraindications:

Breast cancer, except in appropriately selected patients being treated for metastatic disease; estrogen-dependent neoplasia; undiagnosed abnormal genital bleeding; active thrombophlebitis or thromboembolic disorders; history of thrombophlebitis, thrombosis or thromboembolic disorders associated with previous estrogen use (except when used in treatment of breast or prostatic malignancy); known or suspected pregnancy (see Warning Box).

Warnings:

Induction of malignant neoplasms: Estrogens may increase the risk of endometrial carcinoma (see Warning Box). Long-term continuous administration of estrogens in some animals increased the frequency of carcinomas of the breast, cervix, vagina and liver. There is now evidence that estrogens increase the risk of carcinoma of the endometrium in humans. Closely monitor patients with an intact uterus for signs of endometrial cancer, and take appropriate diagnostic measures to rule out malignancy in the event of persistent or recurring abnormal vaginal bleeding.

There is no evidence that estrogens given to postmenopausal women increase the risk of breast cancer, although a recent report has raised this possibility. A prospective study of 23,244 women ≥ 35 years of age reported the relative risk of breast cancer increased 10% in women receiving estrogens for menopausal symptoms. The study concluded that ≥ 9 years of estrogen replacement treatment, use of estradiol, or estrogen-progestin combinations were associated with an increased risk. Other studies conflict.

Gallbladder disease: There is a 2–fold to 3–fold increase in risk of gallbladder disease in women receiving postmenopausal estrogens. This may be related to large doses.

Effects similar to those caused by estrogen-progestin oral contraceptives (OCs): Most of the serious adverse effects of OCs have NOT been documented as consequences of postmenopausal estrogen therapy. This may reflect the comparatively low doses of estrogen used in postmenopausal women. There is an increased risk of thrombosis in men receiving estrogens for prostatic cancer and in women receiving estrogens for postpartum breast engorgement, presumably because large doses are used in therapy.

Elevated blood pressure is common but is less frequent with estrogen replacement therapy than with OC use.

ESTROGENS

Thromboembolic disease – OC users have an increased risk of thromboembolic and thrombotic vascular diseases, including thrombophlebitis, pulmonary embolism, stroke and myocardial infarction. Cases of retinal thrombosis, mesenteric thrombosis and optic neuritis have been reported. The risk of several of these adverse reactions is dose-related. An increased risk of postsurgical thromboembolic complications has also been reported. If feasible, discontinue high dose estrogens at least 4 weeks before surgery associated with an increased risk of thromboembolism or during prolonged immobilization.

An increased rate of thromboembolic and thrombotic disease in postmenopausal users of estrogens has not been found, but such an increase may be present in some subgroups of women or in those receiving relatively large doses. Therefore, do not use in persons with active thrombophlebitis or thromboembolic disorders or in persons with a history of such disorders associated with estrogen use (except in treatment of malignancy).

Large doses (conjugated estrogens 5 mg/day), comparable to those used to treat prostate and breast cancer, have increased risk of nonfatal MI, pulmonary embolism and thrombophlebitis in men. When such estrogen doses are used, the thromboembolic and thrombotic adverse effects associated with OC use are a clear risk.

Hypercalcemia: Estrogens may lead to severe hypercalcemia in patients with breast cancer and bone metastases. If this occurs, discontinue the drug and take appropriate measures to reduce the serum calcium level.

Glucose tolerance: Usual replacement doses of estrogen improve insulin sensitivity.

Hepatic function impairment: Patients with a history of jaundice during pregnancy have an increased risk of recurrence while on estrogen-containing OCs. If jaundice develops in any patient on estrogen, discontinue medication and investigate the cause. Estrogens may be poorly metabolized in impaired liver function; use with caution.

Pregnancy: Category X. See Warning Box.

Lactation: Estrogens have been shown to decrease the quantity and quality of breast milk and may be excreted in breast milk. Administer only when clearly needed.

Children: Safety and efficacy are not established. Because of effects on epiphyseal closure, use judiciously in young patients in whom bone growth is incomplete.

Precautions:

History/physical exam: Before initiating estrogens, take complete medical and family history. Pretreatment and periodic history and physical exams every 12 months should include blood pressure, breasts, abdomen, pelvic organs and a Papanicolaou smear. Generally, do not prescribe for > 1 year between physical examinations.

Estropipate vaginal cream: Rule out gonorrhea or neoplasia before prescribing estropipate vaginal cream. Treat trichomonal, monilial or bacterial infection with appropriate anti-microbial therapy.

Excessive estrogenic stimulation: Certain patients may develop undesirable manifestations of excessive estrogenic stimulation (eg, abnormal or excessive uterine bleeding, mastodynia). Advise the pathologist of estrogen therapy when relevant specimens are submitted.

Fluid retention: Estrogens may cause some degree of fluid retention; conditions which might be influenced by this factor (eg, epilepsy, migraine and cardiac or renal dysfunction) require careful observation.

Calcium and phosphorus metabolism is influenced by estrogens; use caution in patients with metabolic bone diseases associated with hypercalcemia or in renal insufficiency.

Endometrial hyperplasia: Prolonged unopposed estrogen therapy may increase risk of endometrial hyperplasia.

Acute intermittent porphyria may be precipitated by estrogens.

Benzyl alcohol, contained in some of these products as a preservative, has been associated with a fatal "gasping syndrome" in premature infants.

Photosensitivity: Photosensitization (photoallergy or phototoxicity) may occur; therefore, caution patients to take protective measures against exposure to ultraviolet or sunlight (eg, sunscreens, protective clothing) until tolerance is determined.

Tartrazine sensitivity: Some of these products contain tartrazine which may cause allergic-type reactions (including bronchial asthma) in susceptible individuals. Although the incidence of sensitivity is low, it is frequently seen in patients who also have aspirin hypersensitivity. Specific products containing tartrazine are identified in the product listings.

ESTROGENS

Drug Interactions:

Estrogen Drug Interactions			
Precipitant drug	Object drug*		Description
Estrogens	Anticoagulants, oral	⬇	Estrogens may theoretically reduce the hypoprothrombinemic effect of anticoagulants.
Estrogens	Antidepressants, tricyclic	⬌	Pharmacologic effects of these agents may be altered by estrogens; the effects of this interaction may depend on the dose of the estrogen. An increased incidence of toxic reactions may also occur.
Barbiturates rifampin	Estrogens	⬇	Barbiturates, rifampin and other agents that induce hepatic microsomal enzymes with concomitant estrogens may produce lower estrogen levels than expected.
Estrogens	Corticosteroids	⬆	Estrogen coadministration may reduce the clearance and increase the elimination half-life of corticosteroids.
Estrogens	Dantrolene	⬌	While a definite drug interaction with dantrolene has not yet been established, observe caution with concomitant use. Hepatotoxicity has occurred more often in women > 35 years of age receiving dantrolene and estrogen.
Hydantoins	Estrogens	⬇	Breakthrough bleeding, spotting and pregnancy have resulted when these medications were used concurrently. A loss of seizure control has also been suggested and may be due to fluid retention.
Estrogens	Hydantoins		

* ⬆ = Object drug increased. ⬇ = Object drug decreased. ⬌ = Undetermined effect.

Drug/Lab test interactions: Certain endocrine and liver function tests may be affected by estrogen-containing OCs. Expect these similar changes with larger doses:

Increased sulfobromophthalein retention.

Increased prothrombin and factors VII, VIII, IX and X; decreased antithrombin III; increased norepinephrine-induced platelet aggregability.

Increased thyroid binding globulin (TBG) leading to increased circulating total thyroid hormone, as measured by PBI, T_4 by column or T_4 by radioimmunoassay. Free T_3 resin uptake is decreased, reflecting the elevated TBG; free T_4 concentration is unaltered.

Impaired glucose tolerance; decreased pregnanediol excretion; reduced response to metyrapone test; reduced serum folate concentration; increased serum triglyceride and phospholipid concentration.

Adverse Reactions:

See Warnings regarding induction of neoplasia, adverse effects on the fetus, increased incidence of gallbladder disease and adverse effects similar to those of OCs.

CNS: Headache; migraine; dizziness; mental depression; chorea; convulsions.

Dermatologic: Chloasma or melasma (may persist when drug is discontinued); erythema nodosum/multiforme; hemorrhagic eruption; urticaria; dermatitis; photosensitivity.

GI: Nausea; vomiting; abdominal cramps; bloating; cholestatic jaundice; colitis; acute pancreatitis.

GU: Breakthrough bleeding; spotting; change in menstrual flow; dysmenorrhea; premenstrual-like syndrome; amenorrhea during and after treatment; vaginal candidiasis; change in cervical eversion and degree of cervical secretion; cystitis-like syndrome; hemolytic uremic syndrome; endometrial cystic hyperplasia.

Local: Pain at injection site; sterile abscess; postinjection flare; redness and irritation at application site with the estradiol transdermal system (17%); rash (rare).

Ophthalmic: Steepening of corneal curvature; intolerance to contact lenses.

Miscellaneous: Aggravation of porphyria; edema; changes in libido; breast tenderness, enlargement or secretion.

Overdosage:

Serious ill effects have not been reported following ingestion of large doses of estrogen-containing OCs by young children. Overdosage of estrogen may cause nausea; withdrawal bleeding may occur in females.

ESTROGENS

Patient Information:

Patient package insert is available with products.

Diabetic patients: Notify physician if any of the following occur: Pain in the groin or calves of the legs; sharp chest pain or sudden shortness of breath; abnormal vaginal bleeding; missed menstrual period or suspected pregnancy; lumps in the breast; sudden severe headache, dizziness or fainting; vision or speech disturbance; weakness or numbness in an arm or leg; severe abdominal pain; yellowing of the skin or eyes; severe depression.

May cause photosensitivity (sensitivity to sunlight). Avoid prolonged exposure to the sun and other ultraviolet light. Use sunscreens and wear protective clothing until tolerance is determined.

Administration and Dosage:

Given cyclically for short-term use only: For treatment of moderate to severe vasomotor symptoms, atrophic vaginitis or kraurosis vulvae associated with the menopause, administer the lowest effective dose; discontinue medication as promptly as possible. Administration should be cyclic (eg, 3 weeks on and 1 week off). Attempt to discontinue or taper medication at 3 to 6 month intervals.

Cyclical: Female hypogonadism or castration; primary ovarian failure; osteoporosis.

Chronic: Inoperable progressing prostatic cancer, inoperable progressing breast cancer in appropriately selected men and postmenopausal women (see Indications).

Continued therapy with estrogen alone may induce functional uterine bleeding.

Concomitant progestin therapy: Addition of a progestin for 10 to 13 or more days of a cycle of estrogen has lowered the incidence of endometrial hyperplasia. Morphological and biochemical studies of endometrium suggest that 10 to 13 days of progestin are needed to provide maximal maturation of the endometrium and to eliminate any hyperplastic changes. It is not established whether this will provide protection from endometrial carcinoma. There may be additional risks with the inclusion of progestin in estrogen replacement regimens, including adverse effects on cardiovascular endothelium and carbohydrate and lipid metabolism. Choice of progestin, cyclic or continuous mode, and dosage may be important in minimizing risks.

Refer to product listings for dosages of individual agents.

ESTRONE

For complete prescribing information, refer to the Estrogens group monograph.

Administration and Dosage:

Administer IM only. Shake vial and syringe well prior to withdrawal and injection (using a 21 to 23 gauge needle) to properly suspend medication.

Cyclically:

Replacement therapy of estrogen deficiency associated conditions (eg, hypogonadism, female castration, primary ovarian failure) – Initial relief of symptoms may be achieved through the administration of 0.1 to 1 mg of estrone weekly in single or divided doses. Some patients may require 0.5 to 2 mg weekly.

Senile vaginitis and kraurosis vulvae – Generally, 0.1 to 0.5 mg 2 or 3 times/week.

Abnormal uterine bleeding due to hormone imbalance – May respond to brief courses of intensive therapy. Usual dose range is 2 to 5 mg daily for several days.

Chronically:

Inoperable progressing prostatic cancer – For palliation in prostatic cancer, use estrone at 2 to 4 mg, 2 or 3 times per week. If a response to therapy is going to occur, it should be apparent within 3 months of beginning therapy. If a response does occur, continue the hormone until the disease is again progressive.

Inoperable progressing breast cancer in appropriately selected men and postmenopausal women – 5 mg ≥ 3 times per week according to severity of pain.

Rx	**Estrone Aqueous** (Various, eg, Keene)	**Injection:** 2 mg per ml	In 10 and 30 ml vials.
Rx	**Aquest** (Dunhall)		In 10 ml vials.[1]
Rx	**Estrone Aqueous** (Various, eg, Moore, Rugby, URL)	**Injection:** 5 mg per ml	In 10 ml vials.
Rx	**Estrone 5** (Keene)		In 10 ml vials.[1]
Rx	**Kestrone 5** (Hyrex)		In 10 ml vials.[1]
Rx	**Estrogenic Substance Aqueous** (Various, eg, Veratex)	**Injection:** 2 mg per ml estrogenic substance or estrogens (mainly estrone)	In 10 and 30 ml vials.

[1] With sodium carboxymethylcellulose, povidone, benzyl alcohol and methyl- and propylparabens.

ESTRADIOL TRANSDERMAL SYSTEM

For complete prescribing information, refer to the Estrogens group monograph.

Indications:

Moderate to severe vasomotor symptoms associated with menopause; female hypogonadism; female castration; primary ovarian failure; atrophic conditions caused by deficient endogenous estrogen production, such as atrophic vaginitis and kraurosis vulvae; prevention of osteoporosis (loss of bone mass).

Administration and Dosage:

Initiation of therapy:

Treatment of menopausal symptoms – Start with the 0.05 mg system applied to the skin twice weekly. Adjust dose as necessary to control symptoms. Use the lowest dosage necessary to control symptoms, especially in women with an intact uterus. Make attempts to taper or discontinue the drug at 3 to 6 month intervals.

Prophylaxis to prevent postmenopausal bone loss – Initiate with 0.05 mg/day as soon as possible after menopause. Adjust dosage if necessary to control concurrent menopausal symptoms. Discontinuation may reestablish natural rate of bone loss.

In women who are not taking oral estrogens, start treatment immediately. In women who are currently taking oral estrogens, start treatment 1 week after withdrawal of oral therapy or sooner if symptoms reappear in < 1 week.

Therapeutic regimen: Therapy may be given continuously in patients who do not have an intact uterus. In patients with an intact uterus, therapy may be given on a cyclic schedule (eg, 3 weeks therapy followed by 1 week off).

Estraderm and *Vivelle* are applied twice a week; *Climara* patch lasts for 7 days.

Studies of the addition of a progestin for ≥ 7 days of a cycle of estrogen use show a lowered incidence of endometrial hyperplasia. Studies of endometrium suggest that 10 to 14 days of progestin are needed to provide maximal maturation of the endometrium and to eliminate any hyperplastic changes. Whether this will provide protection from endometrial carcinoma has not been clearly established. Additional risks, including adverse effects on carbohydrate and lipid metabolism, impairment of glucose tolerance, and possible enhancement of mitotic activity in breast epithelial tissue may be associated with the inclusion of progestin in estrogen replacement regimens. The choice of progestin and dosage may be important in minimizing these adverse effects.

Application of system: Place adhesive side of the system on a clean, dry area on the trunk of the body (including the buttocks and abdomen). Do not apply to breasts. Rotate application site with an interval of at least 1 week between applications to a particular site. The area should not be oily, damaged or irritated. Avoid the waistline, since tight clothing may rub the system off. Apply the system immediately after opening the pouch and removing the protective liner. Press firmly in place with the palm for ≈10 seconds. Make sure there is good contact, especially around the edges. In the unlikely event that a system should fall off, the same system may be reapplied. If necessary, apply a new system. In either case, continue the original treatment schedule.

ESTRADIOL TRANSDERMAL SYSTEM

	Product/ Distributor	Release rate (mg/24 hr)	Surface area (cm^2)	Total estradiol content (mg)	How Supplied
Rx	**FemPatch** (Parke-Davis)	0.025	30	10.3	In 4s.
Rx	**Vivelle** (Ciba)	0.0375	11	3.28	Calendar Packs (8 and 24 systems).
Rx	**Alora** (Procter & Gamble)	0.05	18	1.5	Calendar Packs (8 and 24 systems).
Rx	**Climara** (Berlex)		12.5	3.9	In 4s.
Rx	**Estraderm** (Ciba)		10	4	Calendar Packs (8 and 24 systems).
Rx	**Vivelle** (Ciba)		14.5	4.33	Calendar Packs (8 and 24 systems).
Rx	**Alora** (Procter & Gamble)	0.075	27	2.3	Calendar Packs (8 and 24 systems).
Rx	**Vivelle** (Ciba)		22	6.57	Calendar Packs (8 and 24 systems).
Rx	**Alora** (Procter & Gamble)	0.1	36	3	Calendar Packs (8 and 24 systems).
Rx	**Climara** (Berlex)		25	7.8	In 4s.
Rx	**Estraderm** (Ciba)		20	8	Calendar Packs (8 and 24 systems).
Rx	**Vivelle** (Ciba)		29	8.66	Calendar Packs (8 and 24 systems).

ESTRADIOL ORAL

For complete prescribing information, refer to the Estrogens group monograph.

Administration and Dosage:

Moderate to severe vasomotor symptoms, vulva/vaginal atrophy associated with menopause, female hypogonadism, female castration, primary ovarian failure: Initiate treatment with 1 or 2 mg/day; adjust to control presenting symptoms. Titrate to determine the minimal effective dose for maintenance therapy.

Prostatic cancer (androgen-dependent, inoperable, progressing): Administer 1 to 2 mg 3 times daily. Judge the effectiveness of therapy by phosphatase determinations and by symptomatic improvement of the patient.

Breast cancer (inoperable, progressing): Given in appropriately selected men and women, the usual dose is 10 mg 3 times daily for at least 3 months.

Osteoporosis prevention: Administer cyclically (eg, 23 days on and 5 days off) 0.5 mg/day as soon as possible after menopause. Adjust dosage if necessary to control concurrent menopausal symptoms. Discontinuation may re-establish natural rate of bone loss.

Rx	**Estrace** (Bristol Myers-Squibb)	**Tablets**: 0.5 mg micronized estradiol	Lactose. White, scored. In 100s.
		1 mg micronized estradiol	Lactose. Lavender, scored. In 100s and 500s.
		2 mg micronized estradiol	Tartrazine, lactose. Turquoise, scored. In 100s and 500s.

ESTRADIOL VALERATE IN OIL

For complete prescribing information, refer to the Estrogens group monograph.

Provides 2 to 3 weeks of estrogenic effect from a single IM injection.

Administration and Dosage:

For IM injection only.

Moderate to severe vasomotor symptoms, atrophic vaginitis or kraurosis vulvae associated with menopause, female hypogonadism, female castration or primary ovarian failure: 10 to 20 mg every 4 weeks.

Prostatic carcinoma: 30 mg or more every 1 or 2 weeks.

Rx	**Estradiol Valerate** (Various, eg, Goldline)	**Injection**: 10 mg/ml	In 10 ml vials.
Rx	**Delestrogen** (Mead Johnson)		In 5 ml vials.[1]
Rx	**Estradiol Valerate** (Various, eg, Goldline, Schein, Steris)	**Injection**: 20 mg/ml	In 10 ml vials.
Rx	**Delestrogen** (Mead Johnson)		In 5 ml vials and 1 ml Unimatic Single Dose syringe.[2]
Rx	**Dioval XX** (Keene)		In 10 ml vials.[2]
Rx	**Estra-L 20** (Pasadena)		In 10 ml vials.[2]
Rx	**Gynogen L.A. "20"** (Forest)		In 10 ml vials.[2]
Rx	**Valergen 20** (Hyrex)		In 10 ml vials.[2]
Rx	**Estradiol Valerate** (Various, eg, IDE, Goldline, Schein, Steris)	**Injection**: 40 mg/ml	In 10 ml vials.
Rx	**Delestrogen** (Mead Johnson)		In 5 ml vials.[2]
Rx	**Dioval 40** (Keene)		In 10 ml vials.[2]
Rx	**Estra-L 40** (Pasadena)		In 10 ml vials.[2]
Rx	**Valergen 40** (Hyrex)		In 10 ml vials.[2]

[1] In sesame oil with chlorobutanol.

[2] In castor oil with benzyl benzoate and benzyl alcohol.

CONJUGATED ESTROGENS, ORAL

For complete prescribing information, refer to the Estrogens group monograph.

Administration and Dosage:

Administer cyclically (3 weeks of daily estrogen and 1 week off) for all indications except selected cases of carcinoma.

Moderate to severe vasomotor symptoms associated with menopause: 1.25 mg/day. If the patient has not menstruated in 2 months or more, administration is started arbitrarily. If the patient is menstruating, begin administration on day 5 of bleeding.

Atrophic vaginitis and atrophic urethritis associated with menopause: 0.3 to 1.25 mg or more daily, depending on tissue response of the patient.

Female hypogonadism: 2.5 to 7.5 mg daily, in divided doses for 20 days, followed by a rest period of 10 days. If bleeding does not occur by the end of this period, repeat dosage schedule. The number of courses of estrogen therapy necessary to produce bleeding may vary, depending on the responsiveness of the endometrium.

If bleeding occurs before the end of the 10 day period, begin a 20 day estrogen-progestin cyclic regimen with estrogen, 2.5 to 7.5 mg daily in divided doses. During the last 5 days of estrogen therapy, give an oral progestin. If bleeding occurs before this regimen is concluded, discontinue therapy and resume on the fifth day of bleeding.

Female castration and primary ovarian failure: 1.25 mg/day. Adjust according to severity of symptoms and patient response. For maintenance, adjust to lowest effective level.

Osteoporosis: 0.625 mg/day, cyclically.

Mammary carcinoma (for palliation): 10 mg 3 times daily for at least 3 months.

Prostatic carcinoma (for palliation): 1.25 to 2.5 mg 3 times daily. Effectiveness can be judged by phosphatase determinations as well as by symptomatic improvement.

Rx	**Premarin** (Wyeth-Ayerst)	**Tablets:** 0.3 mg	Sucrose. Green. Oval. In 100s and 1000s.
		0.625 mg	Sucrose. Maroon. Oval. In 100s, 1000s and UD 100s.
		0.9 mg	Sucrose. White. Oval. In 100s.
		1.25 mg	Sucrose. Yellow. Oval. In 100s, 1000s and UD 100s.
		2.5 mg	Sucrose. Purple. Oval. In 100s and 1000s.

CONJUGATED ESTROGENS, PARENTERAL

For complete prescribing information, refer to the Estrogens group monograph.

Administration and Dosage:

Treatment of abnormal uterine bleeding due to hormonal imbalance in the absence of organic pathology. Administration IV produces a more rapid response and is preferred. Usual dose is one 25 mg injection IV or IM. Repeat in 6 to 12 hours if necessary. Inject slowly to obviate the occurrence of flushes.

Compatibility: Infusion of conjugated estrogens with other agents is not recommended. In emergencies, however, when an infusion has already been started, make the injection into the tubing just distal to the infusion needle. Solution is compatible with normal saline, dextrose and invert sugar solutions. It is not compatible with protein hydrolysate, ascorbic acid or any solution with an acid pH.

Storage/Stability: Before reconstitution, refrigerate at 2° to 8°C (36° to 46°F). Use the reconstituted solution within a few hours. Refrigerated reconstituted solution is stable for 60 days. Do not use if darkening or precipitation occurs.

Rx	**Premarin Intravenous** (Wyeth-Ayerst)	**Injection:** 25 mg conjugated estrogens	In *Secules*[1] (vials), each with 5 ml sterile diluent.[2]

[1] With 200 mg lactose, 0.2 mg simethicone and 12.2 mg sodium citrate.
[2] With 2% benzyl alcohol.

ESTERIFIED ESTROGENS

For complete prescribing information, refer to the Estrogens group monograph.

These products contain 75% to 85% sodium estrone sulfate and 6% to 15% sodium equilin sulfate, in such proportion that the total of these two components is not less than 90% of the total esterified estrogens content.

Administration and Dosage:

Moderate to severe vasomotor symptoms, atrophic vaginitis or kraurosis vulvae associated with menopause: Cyclic therapy for short-term use. Average dose is 0.3 to 1.25 mg daily. Adjust dosage to the lowest effective level and discontinue as soon as possible.

Female hypogonadism: Administer 2.5 to 7.5 mg daily in divided doses for 20 days followed by a 10 day rest period. If bleeding does not occur by the end of this period, repeat the same dosage schedule. The number of courses of estrogen therapy necessary to produce bleeding varies, depending on endometrial responsiveness.

If bleeding occurs before the end of the 10 day period, begin a 20 day estrogen-progestin cyclic regimen of 2.5 to 7.5 mg daily in divided doses for 20 days. During the last 5 days of estrogen therapy, give an oral progestin. If bleeding occurs before this regimen is concluded, discontinue therapy; resume on the fifth day of bleeding.

Female castration and primary ovarian failure: Give 1.25 mg daily, cyclically.

Prostatic carcinoma (inoperable, progressing): 1.25 to 2.5 mg 3 times a day. Judge the effectiveness of therapy by symptomatic response and phosphatase determinations.

Breast cancer (inoperable, progressing): In appropriately selected men and postmenopausal women, give 10 mg 3 times a day for at least 3 months.

Rx	**Estratab** (Solvay Pharm.)	**Tablets:** 0.3 mg	(Solvay 1014). Blue. Sugar coated. In 100s.
Rx	**Menest** (SmithKline Beecham)		(BMP 125). Yellow. Film coated. In 100s.
Rx	**Estratab** (Solvay Pharm.)	**Tablets:** 0.625 mg	(Solvay 1022). Yellow. Sugar coated. In 100s and 1000s.
Rx	**Menest** (SmithKline Beecham)		(BMP 126). Orange. Film coated. In 100s.
Rx	**Estratab** (Solvay Pharm.)	**Tablets:** 1.25 mg	(Solvay 1024). Orange-red. Sugar coated. In 100s and 1000s.
Rx	**Menest** (SmithKline Beecham)		(BMP 127). Green. Film coated. In 100s.
Rx	**Estratab** (Solvay Pharm.)	**Tablets:** 2.5 mg	(Solvay 1025). Lt. purple. Sugar coated. In 100s.
Rx	**Menest** (SmithKline Beecham)		(BMP 128). Pink. Film coated. In 50s.

ESTROPIPATE (Piperazine Estrone Sulfate)

For complete prescribing information, refer to the Estrogens group monograph.

Estropipate is crystalline estrone solubilized as the sulfate and stabilized with piperazine.

Administration and Dosage:

Moderate to severe vasomotor symptoms, vulval and vaginal atrophy associated with menopause: Give cyclically for short-term use. The lowest dose and regimen that will control symptoms should be chosen. Usual dosage range is 0.625 to 5 mg/day.

Female hypogonadism, female castration or primary ovarian failure: Administer cyclically, 1.25 to 7.5 mg/day for the first 3 weeks, followed by a rest period of 8 to 10 days. Repeat if bleeding does not occur by the end of the rest period. The duration of therapy necessary to produce withdrawal bleeding will vary according to the responsiveness of the endometrium. If satisfactory withdrawal bleeding does not occur, give an oral progestin in addition to estrogen during the third week of the cycle.

Osteoporosis prevention: 0.625 mg daily for 25 days of a 31 day cycle per month.

Rx	**Estropipate** (Various, eg, Rugby, Schein, Watson)	**Tablets**: 0.625 mg (equiv. to 0.75 mg estropipate)	In 100s.
Rx	**Ortho-Est** (Ortho)		Lactose. White. Diamond shape. In 100s.
Rx	**Ogen** (Upjohn)		Lactose. Yellow, scored. In 100s.
Rx	**Estropipate** (Various, eg, Rugby, Schein, Watson)	**Tablets**: 1.25 mg (equiv. to 1.5 mg estropipate)	In 100s and 500s.
Rx	**Ortho-Est** (Ortho)		Lactose. Lavender. Diamond shape. In 100s.
Rx	**Ogen** (Upjohn)		Lactose. Peach, scored. In 100s.
Rx	**Estropipate** (Various, eg, Rugby, Watson)	**Tablets**: 2.5 mg (equiv. to 3 mg estropipate)	In 100s.
Rx	**Ogen** (Upjohn)		Lactose. Blue, scored. In 100s.

QUINESTROL

For complete prescribing information, refer to the Estrogens group monograph.

Administration and Dosage:

Quinestrol is stored in body fat, slowly released over several days and metabolized to ethinyl estradiol.

Moderate to severe vasomotor symptoms associated with menopause, atrophic vaginitis, kraurosis vulvae, female hypogonadism, female castration and primary ovarian failure: Initially, 100 mcg daily for 7 days; follow with 100 mcg once weekly for maintenance starting 2 weeks after treatment begins. Increase dosage to 200 mcg/week if the therapeutic response is not desirable or optimal.

Rx	**Estrovis** (Parke Davis)	**Tablets**: 100 mcg	Lactose. In 100s.

ETHINYL ESTRADIOL

For complete prescribing information, refer to the Estrogens group monograph.

Administration and Dosage:

Moderate to severe vasomotor symptoms associated with menopause: Usual dosage range is 0.02 to 0.05 mg/day. The effective dose may be as low as 0.02 mg every other day. Dosage schedule for early menopause, while spontaneous menstruation continues, is 0.05 mg once/day for 21 days followed by a 7 day rest period. May add a progestational agent during the latter part of the cycle.

For initial treatment of late menopause, the same regimen is indicated with 0.02 mg for the first few cycles, after which the 0.05 mg dosage may be substituted. In more severe cases, such as those due to surgical and roentgenologic castration, give 0.05 mg 3 times daily at the start of treatment. With adequate clinical improvement, usually obtainable in a few weeks, dosage may be reduced to 0.05 mg/day. A progestational agent may be added during the latter part of a planned cycle.

Female hypogonadism: 0.05 mg 1 to 3 times daily during the first 2 weeks of a theoretical menstrual cycle. Follow with a progestin during the last half of the arbitrary cycle. Continue for 3 to 6 months. The patient is then untreated for 2 months. Prescribe additional therapy if the cycle cannot be maintained without hormonal therapy.

Cancer of the female breast (inoperable, progressing): In appropriately selected postmenopausal women, 1 mg 3 times daily given chronically for palliation.

Prostatic carcinoma (inoperable, progressing): 0.15 to 2 mg/day given chronically for palliation.

Rx	**Estinyl** (Schering)	**Tablets:** 0.02 mg	(Schering ER or 298). Beige. Sugar coated. In 100s and 250s.
		0.05 mg	(Schering EM or 070). Pink. Sugar coated. In 100s and 250s.
		0.5 mg	(Schering EP or 150). Peach, scored. In 100s.

DIETHYLSTILBESTROL (DES)

For complete prescribing information, refer to the Estrogens group monograph.

Administration and Dosage:

Prostatic carcinoma (inoperable, progressing): Given chronically, the usual dosage is 1 to 3 mg/day initially, increased in advanced cases; dosage may later be reduced to an average of 1 mg/day.

Breast cancer (inoperable, progressing): Given chronically in appropriately selected men and postmenopausal women, the usual dosage is 15 mg/day.

Rx	**Diethylstilbestrol** (Lilly)	**Tablets:** 1 mg	In 100s.
		5 mg	In 100s.

CHLOROTRIANISENE

For complete prescribing information, refer to the Estrogens group monograph.

Administration and Dosage:

Moderate to severe vasomotor symptoms associated with menopause: 12 to 25 mg/day given cyclically for 30 days; one or more courses may be prescribed.

Atrophic vaginitis and kraurosis vulvae: 12 to 25 mg/day cyclically for 30 to 60 days.

Female hypogonadism: 12 to 25 mg/day given cyclically for 21 days. May be followed immediately by 100 mg progesterone IM or by an oral progestin during the last 5 days of therapy. Next course may begin on the fifth day of induced uterine bleeding.

Prostatic carcinoma (inoperable, progressing): Given chronically, the usual dose is 12 to 25 mg/day.

Rx	**Tace** (Hoechst Marion Roussel)	**Capsules:** 12 mg	Tartrazine. (Merrell 690). Green. In 100s.
		25 mg	Tartrazine. (Merrell 691). Two-tone green. In 60s.

ESTRADIOL CYPIONATE IN OIL

For complete prescribing information, refer to the Estrogens group monograph.

Administration and Dosage:

Moderate to severe vasomotor symptoms associated with menopause: Usual dosage range is 1 to 5 mg IM, every 3 to 4 weeks.

Female hypogonadism: 1.5 to 2 mg IM at monthly intervals.

Rx	**Estradiol Cypionate** (Various, eg, Goldine, Moore, Rugby, Schein, Steris)	**Injection:** 5 mg per ml	In 10 ml vials.
Rx	**depGynogen** (Forest)		In 10 ml vials.[1]
Rx	**Depo-Estradiol Cypionate** (Upjohn)		In 5 ml vials.[1]
Rx	**DepoGen** (Hyrex)		In 10 ml vials.[1]
Rx	**Estro-Cyp** (Keene)		In 10 ml vials.[1]

[1] In cottonseed oil with chlorobutanol.

ESTROGEN COMBINATIONS, ORAL

Estrogens are used to alleviate symptoms associated with the menopausal syndrome. For complete prescribing information, see group monograph.

Meprobamate and **chlordiazepoxide** are antianxiety agents used to treat concomitant symptoms of anxiety (see individual monographs).

Administration and Dosage:

One tablet 3 times a day in 21 day courses followed by a 1 week rest period.

Rx	**PMB 200** (Wyeth-Ayerst)	**Tablets:** 0.45 mg conjugated estrogens and 200 mg meprobamate	Lactose, sucrose. Green. Oblong. In 60s.
Rx	**PMB 400** (Wyeth-Ayerst)	**Tablets:** 0.45 mg conjugated estrogens and 400 mg meprobamate	Lactose, sucrose. Pink. Oblong. In 60s.
Rx	**Menrium 5-2** (Roche)	**Tablets:** 0.2 mg esterified estrogens and 5 mg chlordiazepoxide	Lactose, sucrose. Light green. In 100s.
Rx	**Menrium 5-4** (Roche)	**Tablets:** 0.4 mg esterified estrogens and 5 mg chlordiazepoxide	Lactose, sucrose. Dark green. In 100s.
Rx	**Menrium 10-4** (Roche)	**Tablets:** 0.4 mg esterified estrogens and 10 mg chlordiazepoxide	Lactose, sucrose. Purple. In 100s.

MISCELLANEOUS ESTROGENS, VAGINAL

For complete prescribing information, refer to the Estrogens group monograph.

Actions:

Pharmacology: Depletion of endogenous estrogens occurs postmenopausally from a decline in ovarian function and may cause symptomatic vulvovaginal epithelial atrophy (atrophic vaginitis). The signs and symptoms of these atrophic changes may be alleviated by the topical application of an estrogenic hormone.

Indications:

Treatment of atrophic vaginitis and kraurosis vulvae associated with the menopause.

Warnings:

Vaginal bleeding: Because absorption through the vaginal mucosa may exist, uterine bleeding might be provoked by excessive administration in menopausal women. Cytologic study, endometrial assessment/sampling or D and C may be required to differentiate this uterine bleeding from carcinoma. Breast tenderness and vaginal discharge due to mucus hypersecretion may result from excessive estrogenic stimulation; endometrial bleeding may occur if use is suddenly discontinued.

Patient Information:

Patient package insert is available with product.

Insert high into vagina (≈ length of applicator) with applicator provided.

Administration and Dosage:

Treatment of atrophic vaginitis, kraurosis vulvae associated with the menopause. Choose the lower dose that will control symptoms and discontinue medication as promptly as possible. Make attempts to discontinue or taper medication at 3 to 6 month intervals.

Estropipate and conjugated estrogens – Administer cyclically; 3 weeks on and 1 week off. Give ½ to 2 g daily of conjugated estrogens and 2 to 4 g daily of estropipate intravaginally depending on severity of condition.

Estradiol – 2 to 4 g daily for 2 weeks. Gradually reduce to one-half initial dosage for a similar period. A maintenance dose of 1 g 1 to 3 times a week may be used after restoration of the vaginal mucosa has been achieved.

Dienestrol – Usual dosage is 1 applicator once or twice daily for 1 or 2 weeks, then reduce to initial dosage for a similar period. A maintenance dosage of 1 applicator 1 to 3 times a week may be used after restoration of vaginal mucosa has been achieved.

Rx	**Ogen** (Abbott)	**Cream:** 1.5 mg estropipate per g	In 42.5 g with applicator.
Rx	**Estrace** (Mead Johnson)	**Cream:** 0.1 mg estradiol per g in a nonliquefying base	In 42.5 g with applicator.
Rx	**Premarin** (Wyeth-Ayerst)	**Cream:** 0.625 mg conjugated estrogens per g in a nonliquefying base	In 42.5 g with or w/o calibrated applicator.
Rx	**Ortho Dienestrol** (Ortho Pharm.)	**Cream:** 0.01% dienestrol	In 78 g with or w/o applicator.
Rx	**Estring** (Pharmacia & Upjohn)	**Vaginal ring:** 2 mg estradiol	In single packs.

PROGESTINS

For progestins recommended only for antineoplastic action in endometrial carcinoma, see megestrol acetate and medroxyprogesterone acetate in the Antineoplastics chapter.

Warning:

Progestins have been used beginning with the first trimester of pregnancy to prevent habitual abortion or treat threatened abortion; however, there is no adequate evidence that such use is effective. There is evidence of potential harm to the fetus when given during the first 4 months of pregnancy. Therefore, the use of such drugs during the first 4 months of pregnancy is not recommended.

The cause of abortion is generally a defective ovum, which progestational agents could not be expected to influence. In addition, progestational agents have uterine relaxant properties that may cause a delay in spontaneous abortion when given to patients with fertilized defective ova.

Several reports suggest an association between intrauterine exposure to progestational drugs in the first trimester of pregnancy and genital abnormalities in male and female fetuses, and congenital anomalies, including congenital heart defects and limb-reduction defects. One study estimated that there is a 4.7–fold increased risk of limb-reduction defects in infants exposed in utero to sex hormones. The risk of hypospadias, 5 to 8 per 1,000 male births in the general population, may be approximately doubled with exposure to these drugs. There are insufficient data to quantify the risk to exposed female fetuses, but because some of the more androgenic variety of these drugs induce mild virilization of the external genitalia of the female fetus, and because of the increased association of hypospadias in the male fetus, it is prudent to avoid use of these drugs during the first trimester.

If the patient is exposed to progestational drugs during the first 4 months of pregnancy or if she becomes pregnant while taking this drug she should be apprised of the potential risks to the fetus.

Actions:

Pharmacology: Progesterone, a principle of corpus luteum, is the primary endogenous progestational substance. Progestins (progesterone and derivatives) transform proliferative endometrium into secretory endometrium. They inhibit (at the usual dose range) or facilitate through positive feedback the secretion of pituitary gonadotropins, which in turn prevents follicular maturation and ovulation or alternatively promotes it for the "primed" follicle. They also inhibit spontaneous uterine contractions as well as other smooth muscles throughout the body. Progestins may demonstrate some anabolic or androgenic activity.

Pharmacokinetics: Absorption of oral tablets and parenteral oily solutions of progestins is rapid; however, the hormone undergoes prompt hepatic transformation.

Indications:

Amenorrhea; abnormal uterine bleeding; endometriosis; contraception; AIDS wasting syndrome (megestrol acetate). Refer to the product listings for specific indications of individual agents.

Unlabeled uses: Medroxyprogesterone acetate (10 mg/day) has been used in the treatment of menopausal symptoms and to stimulate respiration in obstructive sleep apnea (60 to 120 mg/day) and other forms of chronic hypoventilation.

Adding progestin for ≥ 7 days of a cycle of estrogen replacement for menopause has lowered incidence of endometrial hyperplasia. Morphological and biochemical endometrium studies suggest 10 to 13 days of progestin provide maximal maturation of endometrium, and eliminate any hyperplastic changes. It is not clear whether this provides protection from endometrial carcinoma. There may be additional risks with progestin in estrogen replacement regimens, including adverse effects on carbohydrate and lipid metabolism. Choice of progestin and dosage may be important in minimizing these adverse effects.

Progesterone suppositories (rectal or vaginal, 200 to 400 mg twice daily) have been used in premenstrual syndrome (PMS). Some studies report no improvements in PMS symptoms with progesterone suppositories vs placebo; however, these studies may have had methodologic flaws. One controlled trial suggested oral progesterone (100 mg in the morning, 200 mg at night for 10 days during the luteal phase) improved PMS symptoms. Further controlled studies are needed.

Progesterone has been used successfully in premature labor in late stages of pregnancy. Progesterone suppositories have been used during the luteal phase to the end of the first trimester to decrease spontaneous abortions in previous aborters and in anovulatory women receiving clomiphene citrate or human menopausal gonadotropins, and in luteal phase defects to improve fertility (see Warning Box).

PROGESTINS

Norethindrone (5 mg/day) appears to be effective in the treatment of hyperparathyroidism associated with mild hypercalcemia in postmenopausal women.

Contraindications:

Hypersensitivity to progestins; thrombophlebitis, thromboembolic disorders, cerebral hemorrhage or patients with a history of these conditions; impaired liver function or disease; carcinoma of the breast or genital organs; undiagnosed vaginal bleeding; missed abortion; as a diagnostic test for pregnancy.

Warnings:

Ophthalmologic effects: Discontinue medication pending examination if there is a sudden partial or complete loss of vision, or if there is sudden onset of proptosis, diplopia or migraine. If papilledema or retinal vascular lesions are present, discontinue use.

Thrombotic disorders (thrombophlebitis, cerebrovascular disorders, retinal thrombosis, pulmonary embolism) occasionally occur in patients taking progestins; be alert to the earliest manifestations of the disease. If these occur or are suspected, discontinue the drug immediately. However, this has not been shown to occur more often than that seen in a control group.

Pregnancy: Category D (progesterone injection); Category X (norethindrone acetate). Use is not recommended (see Warning Box).

Lactation: Detectable amounts of progestins enter the milk of mothers receiving these agents. The effect on the nursing infant has not been determined.

Medroxyprogesterone does not adversely affect lactation and may increase milk production and duration of lactation if given in the puerperium.

Precautions:

Pretreatment physical examination should include breasts and pelvic organs, as well as Papanicolaou smear. Advise the pathologist of progestin therapy when relevant specimens are submitted. In cases of irregular vaginal bleeding, consider nonfunctional causes. Adequately diagnose all cases of vaginal bleeding.

Fluid retention may occur; therefore, conditions influenced by this factor (epilepsy, migraine, asthma, cardiac or renal dysfunction) require careful observation.

Depression: Observe patients who have a history of psychic depression and discontinue the drug if depression recurs to a serious degree.

Menopause: The age of the patient constitutes no absolute limiting factor, although treatment with progestins may mask the onset of the climacteric.

Benzyl alcohol, contained in some of these products as a preservative, has been associated with a fatal "gasping syndrome" in premature infants.

Photosensitivity: Photosensitization (photoallergy or phototoxicity) may occur; therefore, caution patients to take protective measures (ie, sunscreens, protective clothing) against exposure to ultraviolet light or sunlight until tolerance is determined.

Drug Interactions:

Drug Interactions			
Precipitant drug	Object drug*		Description
Aminoglutethimide	Medroxyprogesterone	⬇	Aminoglutethimide may increase the hepatic metabolism of medroxyprogesterone, possibly decreasing its therapeutic effects.
Rifampin	Norethindrone	⬇	Rifampin may reduce the plasma levels of norethindrone via hepatic microsomal enzyme induction, possibly decreasing its pharmacologic effects.

* ⬇ = Object drug decreased.

Drug/Lab test interactions: Laboratory test results of hepatic function, coagulation tests (increase in prothrombin, Factors VII, VIII, IX and X), thyroid, metyrapone test and endocrine functions, may be affected by progestins.

A decrease in glucose tolerance has been observed in a small percentage of patients on estrogen-progestin combination drugs. The mechanism is obscure but appears to be related to the more androgenic progestins; observe diabetic patients who are receiving progestin therapy.

Pregnanediol determination may be altered by the use of progestins.

PROGESTINS

Adverse Reactions:

CNS: Insomnia; somnolence; mental depression.

Dermatologic: Rash (allergic) with and without pruritus; acne; melasma or chloasma; photosensitivity. A small percentage of patients have local reactions at the site of injection. Progesterone is irritating at the injection site whether the oil or aqueous vehicle is used; however, the aqueous preparation is particularly painful.

GI: Changes in weight (increase or decrease); nausea.

GU: Breakthrough bleeding; spotting; change in menstrual flow; amenorrhea; changes in cervical eversion, cervical secretions.

Miscellaneous: Breast changes (tenderness); masculinization of the female fetus; edema; cholestatic jaundice; pyrexia.

Medroxyprogesterone acetate: Sensitivity reactions ranging from pruritus and urticaria to generalized rash; alopecia; hirsutism.

For information concerning adverse reactions associated with combined estrogen-progestin therapy, refer to the Oral Contraceptives group monograph.

Patient Information:

Patient package insert is available with product.

If GI upset occurs, take with food.

Diabetic patients: Glucose tolerance may be decreased; monitor urine sugar closely and report any abnormalities to physician.

Notify physician if pregnancy is suspected or if any of the following occurs: Sudden severe headache; visual disturbance; numbness in an arm or leg.

May cause photosensitivity (sensitivity to sunlight). Avoid prolonged exposure to the sun and other ultraviolet light. Use sunscreens and wear protective clothing until tolerance is determined.

PROGESTERONE

For complete prescribing information, refer to the Progestins group monograph.

Administration and Dosage:

For IM use. The drug is irritating at the injection site.

Amenorrhea: Administer 5 to 10 mg daily for 6 to 8 consecutive days. If ovarian activity has produced a proliferative endometrium, expect withdrawal bleeding 48 to 72 hours after the last injection. Spontaneous normal cycles may follow.

Functional uterine bleeding: Administer 5 to 10 mg daily for 6 doses. Bleeding should cease within 6 days. When estrogen is also given, begin progesterone after 2 weeks of estrogen therapy. Discontinue injections when menstrual flow begins.

Progesterone is available as a micronized powder for prescription compounding and, therefore, given orally.

Rx	**Progesterone In Oil** (Various, eg, Goldline, Lilly, Rugby, Schein, URL)	**Injection:** 50 mg per ml	In sesame or peanut oil with benzyl alcohol. In 10 ml vials.	1+
Rx	**Progesterone** (Various, eg, Cyclin, Gallipot)	**Powder**	In 1, 10, 25 and 100 g.	1+

MEDROXYPROGESTERONE ACETATE

For complete prescribing information, refer to the Progestins group monograph.

For information on parenteral medroxyprogesterone acetate, refer to the monograph in the Antineoplastics section.

The duration of action of medroxyprogesterone is prolonged and variable.

Administration and Dosage:

Secondary amenorrhea: 5 to 10 mg daily for 5 to 10 days. A dose for inducing an optimum secretory transformation of an endometrium that has been adequately primed with either endogenous or exogenous estrogen is 10 mg daily for 10 days. Start therapy any time. Withdrawal bleeding usually occurs 3 to 7 days after therapy ends.

Abnormal uterine bleeding due to hormonal imbalance in the absence of organic pathology: 5 to 10 mg daily for 5 to 10 days, beginning on the 16th or 21st day of the menstrual cycle. To produce an optimum secretory transformation of an endometrium that has been adequately primed with either endogenous or exogenous estrogen, give 10 mg daily for 10 days, beginning on the 16th day of the cycle. Withdrawal bleeding usually occurs 3 to 7 days after discontinuing therapy. Patients with recurrent episodes of abnormal uterine bleeding may benefit from planned menstrual cycling with medroxyprogesterone acetate.

MEDROXYPROGESTERONE ACETATE

Rx	**Cycrin** (ESI Pharma)	**Tablets:** 2.5 mg	In 100s
Rx	**Provera** (Upjohn)		(Provera 2.5). Orange, scored. In 25s, 30s and 100s.
Rx	**Cycrin** (ESI Pharma)	**Tablets:** 5 mg	In 100s
Rx	**Provera** (Upjohn)		(Provera 5.0). White, scored. Hexagonal. In 25s, 30s and 100s.
Rx	**Medroxyprogesterone Acetate** (Various, eg, Balan)	**Tablets:** 10 mg	In 30s, 40s, 50s, 60s, 100s, 250s, 500s and UD 100s.
Rx	**Amen** (Carnrick)		(C/AMEN). Peach/white, layered, scored. In 50s, 100s & 1000s.
Rx	**Curretab** (Solvay Pharm.)		(RR 1007). White, scored. In 50s.
Rx	**Provera** (Upjohn)		(Upjohn 50). White, scored. In 25s, 30s, 100s, 500s & Dosepak 10s.

HYDROXYPROGESTERONE CAPROATE IN OIL

For complete prescribing information, refer to the Progestins group monograph.

Hydroxyprogesterone, a long-acting progestin, has a 9 to 17 day duration of action.

Administration and Dosage:

For IM use.

Amenorrhea (primary and secondary); dysfunctional uterine bleeding; metrorrhagia: Usual adult dose is 375 mg.

Production of secretory endometrium and desquamation: Test for continuous endogenous estrogen production (medical D and C). Usual adult dose is 125 to 250 mg given on tenth day of cycle; repeat every 7 days until suppression is no longer desired.

Rx	**Hydroxyprogesterone Caproate** (Various, eg, Steris)	**Injection:** 125 mg per ml	In 10 ml vials.
Rx	**Hydroxyprogesterone Caproate** (Various, eg, Rugby, Schein)	**Injection:** 250 mg per ml	In 5 ml vials.
Rx	**Hylutin** (Hyrex)		In 5 ml vials.[1]
Rx	**Hyprogest 250** (Keene)		In 5 ml vials.[1]

[1] In castor oil with benzyl benzoate and benzyl alcohol.

NORETHINDRONE ACETATE

For complete prescribing information, refer to the Progestins group monograph.

Administration and Dosage:

Amenorrhea; abnormal uterine bleeding due to hormonal imbalance in the absence of organic pathology: Give 2.5 to 10 mg daily for 5 to 10 days during the second half of the menstrual cycle.

Endometriosis:

Initial dose – 5 mg/day for 2 weeks; increase in increments of 2.5 mg/day every 2 weeks until 15 mg/day is reached. Therapy may be held at this level for 6 to 9 months or until breakthrough bleeding demands temporary termination.

Rx	**Aygestin** (Wyeth-Ayerst)	**Tablets:** 5 mg	Scored. In 50s and cycle pack 10s.

MEGESTROL ACETATE

For complete prescribing information, refer to the Progestins group monograph. Megestrol is also used for advanced carcinoma of the breast or endometrium; refer to the monograph in the Antineoplastics chapter.

Actions:

Pharmacology: Several investigators have reported on the appetite enhancing property of megestrol acetate and its possible use in cachexia. The precise mechanism by which megestrol produces effects in anorexia and cachexia is unknown.

Clinical trials: Two clinical trials compared megestrol at doses of 100, 400 and 800 mg/day vs placebo in AIDS patients (n = 195) with anorexia/cachexia and significant weight loss. The percent of patients gaining ≥ 5 lbs at maximum weight gain in 12 study weeks was statistically significantly greater for the 800 mg (64%) and 400 mg (57%) groups than for the placebo group (24%). In 12 study weeks (from baseline to last evaluation), mean weight increased in the 800 mg group by 7.8 lbs, the 400 mg group by 4.2 lbs, the 100 mg group by 1.9 lbs and decreased in the placebo group by 1.6 lbs. Changes in body composition during the 12 study weeks showed increases in non-water body weight in the megestrol-treated groups. Greater percentages of megestrol-treated patients showed an improvement in appetite in the 800 mg group (89%), the 400 mg group (68%) and the 100 mg group (72%) than in the placebo group (50%).

The second trial compared megestrol 800 mg/day vs placebo in AIDS patients (n = 65) with anorexia/cachexia and significant weight loss. Patients in the 800 mg group had a statistically significantly larger increase in mean maximum weight change than patients in the placebo group. From baseline to study week 12, mean weight increased by 11.2 lbs in the megestrol-treated group and decreased 2.1 lbs in the placebo group. Changes in body composition showed increases in non-water weight in the megestrol group. A greater percentage of megestrol patients (67%) than placebo patients (38%) showed an improvement in appetite at last evaluation during the 12 study weeks.

Indications:

Appetite enhancement in AIDS patients: Treatment of anorexia, cachexia or an unexplained significant weight loss in patients with a diagnosis of acquired immunodeficiency syndrome (AIDS).

Tumors: Palliative treatment of advanced carcinoma of the breast or endometrium (refer to the monograph in the Antineoplastics chapter).

Contraindications:

As a diagnostic test for pregnancy; known or suspected pregnancy; prophylactic use to avoid weight loss.

Warnings:

HIV-infected women: Although megestrol has been used extensively in women for endometrial and breast cancers, its use in HIV-infected women has been limited. All the women in the clinical trials reported breakthrough bleeding.

Children: Safety and efficacy have not been established.

Precautions:

Causes of weight loss: Institute therapy with megestrol for weight loss only after treatable causes of weight loss are sought and addressed. These treatable causes include possible malignancies, systemic infections, GI disorders affecting absorption and endocrine, renal or psychiatric diseases.

Thromboembolic disease: Use with caution in patients with a history of thromboembolic disease.

Long-term use: Long-term treatment may increase the risk of respiratory infections and may cause secondary adrenal suppression.

MEGESTROL ACETATE

Adverse Reactions:

Megestrol Adverse Reactions (%)[1]		
Adverse reaction	Megestrol	Placebo
Diarrhea	8-15	8-15
Impotence	4-14	≤ 3
Rash	4-12	3-9
Flatulence	≤ 9	3-9
Hypertension	≤ 8	0
Asthenia	2-6	3-8
Insomnia	1-6	0
Nausea	≤ 5	3-9
Anemia	≤ 5	≤ 6
Fever	1-6	3
Libido decreased	≤ 5	≤ 3
Dyspepsia	≤ 3	≤ 5
Hyperglycemia	≤ 6	≤ 3
Headache	1-10	3-6
Pain	≤ 4	5-6
Vomiting	≤ 4	3-9
Pneumonia	≤ 2	3-6
Urinary frequency	≤ 2	≤ 5

[1] Data pooled from several studies. Percentages listed for megestrol without regard to specific dosage.

Body as a whole: Abdominal pain, chest pain, infection, moniliasis, sarcoma (1% to 3%).

Cardiovascular: Cardiomyopathy, palpitation (1% to 3%).

CNS: Paresthesia, confusion, convulsion, depression, neuropathy, hypesthesia, abnormal thinking (1% to 3%).

Dermatologic: Alopecia, herpes, pruritus, vesiculobullous rash, sweating, skin disorder (1% to 3%).

GI: Constipation, dry mouth, hepatomegaly, increased salivation, oral moniliasis (1% to 3%).

GU: Albuminuria, urinary incontinence, urinary tract infection, gynecomastia (1% to 3%).

Respiratory: Dyspnea, cough, pharyngitis, lung disorder (1% to 3%).

Miscellaneous: Leukopenia, amblyopia, LDH increased, edema, peripheral edema (1% to 3%).

Patient Information:

Use as directed by the physician.

Report any adverse reaction experiences while taking this medication.

Use contraception while taking this medication if capable of becoming pregnant; notify physician if you become pregnant while taking this medication.

Administration and Dosage:

Initial dose is 800 mg/day (20 ml/day). Shake container well before using. In clinical trials evaluating different dose schedules, daily doses of 400 and 800 mg/day were found to be clinically effective. A plastic dosage cup with 10 and 20 ml markings is provided for convenience.

Storage/Stability: Store at or below 25°C (77°F) and dispense in a tight container. Protect from heat.

Rx	**Megestrol Acetate** (Roxane)	**Tablets**: 20 mg	In 100s and UD 100s.
		40 mg	In 100s and UD 100s.
Rx	**Megace** (Mead Johnson Oncology)	**Suspension**: 40 mg/ml	≤0.06% alcohol, sucrose. Lemon-lime flavor. In 236.6 ml.

ESTROGENS AND PROGESTINS COMBINED

For complete prescribing information, refer to the Estrogens and Progestins group monographs.

Consider the information given for Oral Contraceptives (see group monograph) when using these products.

Actions:

Pharmacology: This dual hormone therapy is indicated for the treatment of endometriosis and hypermenorrhea and for the production of cyclic withdrawal bleeding.

Administration and Dosage:

Endometriosis: 5 to 10 mg daily for 2 weeks, beginning on day 5 of menstrual cycle. Administer this daily dose continuously (without cyclic interruption); increase by 5 or 10 mg increments at 2 week intervals, up to 20 mg/day. Continue this dose for 6 to 9 months. Increase further (up to 40 mg/day) if breakthrough bleeding occurs.

Hypermenorrhea: For emergency control of severe cases: 20 to 30 mg/day until bleeding is controlled, then reduce to 10 mg and continue through day 24 of cycle. Withdrawal flow usually will begin 2 or 3 days later. Cyclic withdrawal flow may be produced after treatment by giving 5 to 10 mg/day from day 5 through day 24 of the next 2 or 3 cycles.

Rx	**Enovid 10 mg** (Searle)	**Tablets:** 150 mcg mestranol and 9.85 mg norethynodrel	(Searle 10 101). Coral. In 50s.
Rx	**Enovid 5 mg** (Searle)	**Tablets:** 75 mcg mestranol and 5 mg norethynodrel	(Searle 5 51). Pink. In 6 Calendar-pak 20s and bottles of 100.
Rx	**Premphase** (Wyeth-Ayerst)	**Tablets:** 0.625 mg conjugated estrogens and 5 mg medroxyprogesterone acetate	Lactose, sucrose. Maroon, oval (estrogen tablets). Lactose. (Cycrin). Lt purple, oval, scored (medroxyprogesterone acetate tablets). In blister-card 28s (14 of each).
Rx	**Prempro** (Wyeth-Ayerst)	**Tablets:** 0.625 mg conjugated estrogens and 2.5 mg medroxyprogesterone acetate	Lactose, sucrose. Peach, oval. In blister-card 14s.

ORAL CONTRACEPTIVES

Actions:

Pharmacology: Oral contraceptives (OCs) include estrogen-progestin combos and progestin-only products.

Progestin-only – The mechanism by which progestin-only contraceptives prevent conception is not completely known, but they alter the cervical mucus, exert a progestational effect on the endometrium, apparently producing cellular changes that renders the endometrium hostile to implantation by a fertilized ovum (egg) and, in some patients, suppress ovulation.

Combination OCs inhibit ovulation by suppressing the gonadotropins, follicle-stimulating hormone (FSH) and luteinizing hormone (LH). Additionally, alterations in the genital tract, including cervical mucus (which inhibits sperm penetration) and the endometrium (which reduces the likelihood of implantation), may contribute to contraceptive effectiveness.

These products differ in the type and relative potency of the components and in the relative predominance of estrogenic or progestational activity. Their ultimate effects are related to combined estrogenic, progestational, androgenic and anti-estrogenic effects.

Progestins may modify the effects of estrogens; these effects depend on the type or amount of progestin present and the ratio of progestin to estrogen. Dosage, potency, length of administration and concomitant estrogen administration contribute to total progestational potency, making it difficult to establish equivalent doses of progestins. The total estrogenic potency of an OC is based on the combined effects of the estrogen and the estrogenic/antiestrogenic/androgenic effect of the progestin. The table in the Administration and Dosage section summarizes the effects of the various progestins.

Contraceptive efficacy – The following table gives pregnancy rates reported for various means of contraception. Efficacy in most cases depends greatly upon degree of compliance and user reliability. No other contraceptive drug or device except levonorgestrel implant and medroxyprogesterone injection approaches the efficacy of the combined oral contraceptives.

Pregnancy Rates for Various Means of Contraception (%)[1]

Method of contraception	Lowest expected[2]	Typical[3]
Oral Contraceptives		3
Combined	0.1	nd
Progestin-only	0.5	nd
Mechanical/Chemical		
Levonorgestrel implant	0.2	0.2
Medroxyprogesterone injection	0.3	0.3
IUD		
Progesterone	2	nd
Copper T 380A	0.8	nd
Condom		
Without spermicide	2	12
With spermicide[4]	1.8	4-6
Spermicide alone	3	21
Diaphragm (with spermicidal cream or gel)	6	18
Vaginal sponge		
Nulliparous	6	18
Multiparous	9	28
Female condom	2-4	12-25
Periodic abstinence (ie, rhythm; all methods)	1-9	20
Sterility		
Vasectomy	0.1	0.15
Tubal ligation	0.2	0.4
No contraception	85	85

nd = No data.

[1] During first year of continuous use.

[2] Best guess of percentage expected to experience an accidental pregnancy among couples who initiate a method and use it consistently and correctly.

[3] A "typical" couple who initiate a method and experience an accidental pregnancy.

[4] Used as a separate product (not in condom package).

ORAL CONTRACEPTIVES

There are three types of combination OCs: Monophasic, biphasic and triphasic. The biphasic and triphasic OCs are intended to deliver hormones in a fashion similar to physiologic processes.

Monophasic – Fixed dosage of estrogen to progestin throughout the cycle.

Biphasic – Amount of estrogen remains the same for the first 21 days of the cycle. Decreased progestin:estrogen ratio in first half of cycle allows endometrial proliferation. Increased ratio in second half provides adequate secretory development.

Triphasic – Estrogen amount remains the same or varies throughout cycle. Progestin amount varies.

Noncontraceptive health benefits – The following health benefits related to the use of combination OCs are supported by epidemiological studies that largely utilized OC formulations containing estrogen doses ≥ 35 mcg or 50 mcg mestranol.

Effects on menses: Increased menstrual cycle regularity; decreased blood loss and decreased incidence of iron deficiency anemia; decreased incidence of dysmenorrhea.

Effects related to inhibition of ovulation: Decreased incidence of functional ovarian cysts and ectopic pregnancies.

Other effects: Decreased incidence of fibroadenomas and fibrocystic disease of the breast; acute pelvic inflammatory disease; endometrial cancer; ovarian cancer (OC use is the only known method of prevention for ovarian cancer).

Pharmacokinetics:

Estrogens – Ethinyl estradiol is rapidly absorbed with peak concentrations attained in 1 to 2 hours. It undergoes considerable first-pass elimination. Mestranol is demethylated to ethinyl estradiol. Ethinyl estradiol is approximately 98% bound to plasma albumin. Half-life varies from 6 to 20 hours. It is excreted in bile and urine as conjugates, and undergoes some enterohepatic recirculation.

Progestins – Peak concentrations of norethindrone occur 0.5 to 4 hours after oral administration; it undergoes first-pass metabolism with an overall bioavailability around 65%. Levonorgestrel reaches peak concentrations between 0.5 to 2 hours, does not undergo a first-pass effect and is completely bioavailable. Norethindrone and levonorgestrel are chiefly metabolized by reduction followed by conjugation. Desogestrel is rapidly and completely absorbed and converted into 3–keto-desogestrel, the biologically active metabolite. Relative bioavailability is ≈ 84%. Maximum concentrations of the metabolite are reached at 1.4 ± 0.8 hours. Norgestimate is well absorbed; peak serum concentrations are observed within 2 hours followed by a rapid decline to levels generally below assay within 5 hours. However, a major metabolite, 17–deacetyl norgestimate, appears rapidly in serum with concentrations greatly exceeding that of the parent. Both norethynodrel and ethynodiol diacetate are converted to norethindrone. Progestins are bound both to albumin (79% to 95%) and to sex hormone binding globulin. Terminal half-life of the progestins are as follows: Norethindrone, 5 to 14 hours; levonorgestrel, 11 to 45 hours; desogestrel (metabolite), 38 ± 20 hours; norgestimate (metabolite), 12 to 30 hours.

Indications:

Contraceptive: For the prevention of pregnancy.

Because of the positive association between amount of estrogen and progestin in OCs and the risk of vascular disease and thromboembolism, minimizing exposure to these agents is in keeping with good principles of therapeutics. For any particular combination, prescribe the dosage regimen which contains the least amount of estrogen and progestin compatible with a low failure rate and needs of the individual patient. Start new patients on preparations containing ≤ 35 mcg estrogen.

Unlabeled uses: Ovral (50 mcg ethinyl estradiol and 0.5 mg norgestrel) in high doses has been used successfully as a postcoital contraceptive or "morning after" pill. Patients are given 2 tablets within 72 hours of unprotected intercourse at the initial visit and 2 tablets 12 hours later.

Contraindications:

Thrombophlebitis; thromboembolic disorders; history of deep-vein thrombophlebitis; cerebral vascular disease; myocardial infarction; coronary artery disease; known or suspected breast carcinoma or estrogen-dependent neoplasia; carcinoma of endometrium or other; hepatic adenomas/carcinomas (see Warnings); past or present angina pectoris; undiagnosed abnormal genital bleeding; known or suspected pregnancy (see Warnings); cholestatic jaundice of pregnancy/jaundice with prior pill use.

ORAL CONTRACEPTIVES

Warnings:

Cigarette smoking increases the risk of cardiovascular side effects from OCs. This risk increases with age and with heavy smoking (≥ 15 cigarettes per day) and is quite marked in women > 35 years of age. Women who use OCs should not smoke.

Risks of OC use: The use of OCs is associated with increased risk of thromboembolism, stroke, MI, hepatic neoplasia and gallbladder disease, although risk of serious morbidity or mortality is very small in healthy women without underlying risk factors. Risk of morbidity/mortality increases significantly in the presence of other underlying risk factors such as hypertension, hyperlipidemias, obesity and diabetes.

Mortality associated with all methods of birth control is low and below that associated with childbirth, with the exception of OC use in women ≥ 35 who smoke and ≥ 40 who do not smoke. In 1989 the Fertility and Maternal Health Drugs Advisory Committee recommended that although cardiovascular disease risk may be increased with OC use after age 40 in healthy non-smoking women (even with the newer low-dose formulations), there are also greater potential health risks associated with pregnancy in older women and with the alternative surgical and medical procedures that may be necessary if such women do not have access to effective and acceptable means of contraception. Therefore, the committee recommended that the benefits of low-dose OC use by healthy non-smoking women > 40 years of age may outweigh the possible risks.

In a recent Nurse's Health Study spanning 12 years and 1.3 million person-years of follow-up (166,755 women aged 30 to 55 years), it was concluded that use of OCs is safe, and there is no evidence to indicate that use for long durations adversely affect long-term risk for mortality. Results were adjusted for age, body mass index and smoking.

The following table lists the annual number of birth-related or method-related deaths associated with control of fertility according to age.

Estimated Annual Number of Deaths[1] due to Various Contraceptive Methods or to Pregnancy if Method Fails

Method	Age					
	15-19	20-24	25-29	30-34	35-39	40-44
No fertility control[2]	7	7.4	9.1	14.8	25.7	28.2
OCs, non-smoker[3]	0.3	0.5	0.9	1.9	13.8	31.6
OCs, smoker[3]	2.2	3.4	6.6	13.5	51.1	117.2
IUD[3]	0.8	0.8	1	1	1.4	1.4
Condom[2]	1.1	1.6	0.7	0.2	0.3	0.4
Diaphragm/ Spermicide[2]	1.9	1.2	1.2	1.3	2.2	2.8
Periodic abstinence[2]	2.5	1.6	1.6	1.7	2.9	3.6

[1] Among 100,000 non-sterile women, within 1 year of use.
[2] Deaths are birth-related.
[3] Deaths are method-related.

Thromboembolic and cardiovascular problems: Be alert to the earliest symptoms of thromboembolic and thrombotic disorders. Should any of these occur or be suspected, discontinue the drug immediately. Relative risk of users compared to nonusers is 3 for the first episode of superficial venous thrombosis, 4 to 11 for deep vein thrombosis or pulmonary embolism and 1.5 to 6 for women with predisposing conditions for venous thromboembolic disease. The incidence of deep vein thrombosis appears lower in white patients with type O blood (there is no causal relationship established). The estimated risk of hemorrhagic stroke is 2 times greater in OC users; the risk of thrombotic stroke is 10 times greater.

Risk of thromboembolism, including coronary thrombosis, appears to be directly related to estrogen dose used; however, estrogen quantity may not be the sole factor involved.

Myocardial infarction (MI) risk associated with OC use is increased. The greater the number of underlying risk factors for coronary artery disease (cigarette smoking, hypertension, hypercholesterolemia, obesity, diabetes) the higher the risk of developing MI; OC use is an additional risk factor. The risk is very low in women < 30 years of age. It is estimated that the relative risk of heart attack for current OC users is 2 to 6.

ORAL CONTRACEPTIVES

Long-term use – Data suggest that the increased risk of MI persists after discontinuation of long-term OC use; the highest risk group includes women 40 to 49 years old who used OCs for ≥ 5 years.

Smoking – OC users who also smoke have about a fivefold increased risk of fatal infarction compared to nonsmoking users, but a 10- to 12-fold increased risk compared to nonusers who do not smoke. Mortality rates associated with circulatory disease increase substantially in smokers, especially in those ≥ 35 years of age who use OCs.

Cerebrovascular diseases – OCs increase the risks of cerebrovascular events (thrombotic and hemorrhagic strokes), although, in general, the risk is greatest in hypertensive women > 35 years of age who also smoke. Relative risk of thrombotic strokes ranges from 3 (normotensive users) to 14 (severe hypertensive users). Relative risk of hemorrhagic stroke for OC users is 1.2 for nonsmokers, 7.6 for smokers, 1.8 for normotensives and 25.7 for severe hypertensives; for nonuser smokers, risk is 2.6.

Vascular disease – A positive association is observed between the amount of estrogen and progestin in OCs and the risk of vascular disease. A decline in serum high density lipoproteins (HDL) has occurred with progestins. Because estrogens increase HDL cholesterol, the net effect depends on a balance achieved between doses of estrogen and progestin and the androgenic activity of the progestin.

Age – The risk of cerebrovascular and circulatory disease in OC users is substantially increased in women ≥ 35 years of age with other risk factors (eg, smoking, uncontrolled hypertension, hypercholesterolemia [LDL 190], obesity, diabetes). Current clinical practice involves use of lower-estrogen dose formulations combined with careful restriction of OC use to women who do not have the various risk factors listed.

Postsurgical thromboembolism risk is increased 2– to 4-fold. If possible, discontinue OCs at least 2 to 4 weeks before and 2 weeks after surgery as OCs are associated with an increased risk of thromboembolism.

Subarachnoid hemorrhage has been increased by OC use. Smoking alone increases the incidence of these accidents; smoking and OC use appear to work together to produce a combined risk greater than either alone.

Persistence of risk – An increased risk may persist for at least 6 years after discontinuation of OC use for cerebrovascular disease and at least 9 years for MI in users 40 to 49 years of age who had used OCs ≥ 5 years; this risk was not demonstrated in other age groups. This information is based on studies that used OC formulations containing ≥ 50 mcg estrogen.

NOTE – The associations between OCs and cardiovascular disease are based on epidemiological studies whose conclusions have been criticized for several reasons: National trends of cardiovascular mortality are incompatible with these risk estimates; excess deaths may not be attributable entirely to smoking; the clinical diagnosis of thromboembolism is often unreliable.

Ocular lesions such as optic neuritis or retinal thrombosis have been associated with the use of OCs. Discontinue medication if there is unexplained loss of vision, onset of proptosis or diplopia, papilledema or retinal vascular lesions.

Carcinoma: Numerous epidemiological studies have been performed on the incidence of breast, endometrial, ovarian and cervical cancer in women using OCs. While there are conflicting reports, the overall evidence in the literature suggests that use of OCs is not associated with an increase in the risk of developing any cancer, regardless of age and parity of first use. The Cancer and Steroid Hormone study also showed no latent effect on the risk of breast cancer for at least a decade following long-term use. Some studies have shown a slightly increased relative risk of developing breast cancer, although most studies have not shown such a risk, and methodologies of earlier studies have been questioned. According to the CDC, there is a small subset of premenopausal-associated breast cancers, but there is no proof of cause and effect; there is no association with the postmenopausal variety.

Some studies suggest that OC use has been associated with an increase in the risk of cervical intraepithelial neoplasia in some populations of women. Other epidemiologic studies have suggested an increased risk of cervical dysplasia and carcinoma in long-term pill users; the incidence quadrupled when OCs were taken for > 10 years. However, there continues to be controversy about the extent to which such findings may be due to differences in sexual behavior and other factors.

In spite of many studies of the relationship between OC use and breast and cervical cancers, a cause and effect relationship has not been established.

Studies have reported an increased risk of endometrial carcinoma associated with the prolonged use of estrogen in postmenopausal women. However, the risk appears to be decreased in OC users due to the progestin component. In fact, there is a protective effect; users appear about half as likely to develop ovarian and endometrial cancer as women who have never used OCs.

ORAL CONTRACEPTIVES

There appears to be no increased risk of breast cancer in OC users or any subgroup of users, although the CDC states that there may be an association with a subset of young, premenopausal users. There is no increased risk of breast cancer in OC users with prior benign breast disease. Another study suggests that use prior to the first full-term pregnancy was associated with a significant relative risk of breast cancer especially when OC use began before age 25.

Close clinical surveillance of all women taking OCs is essential; they should be reexamined at least once a year. In all cases of undiagnosed persistent or recurrent abnormal vaginal bleeding, rule out malignancy. Monitor women with a strong family history of breast cancer or who have breast nodules, fibrocystic disease of the breast, cervical dysplasia or abnormal mammograms.

Hepatic lesions (adenomas, focal nodular hyperplasia, hepatocellular carcinoma, etc): Benign and malignant hepatic adenomas have been associated with the use of OCs. Severe abdominal pain, shock or death may be due to rupture and hemorrhage of a liver tumor. Fortunately this is quite rare, and there may be some association with higher dose mestranol preparations or duration (greater after 4 years or more) of OC use. While hepatic adenoma is uncommon, consider it in women presenting with abdominal pain and tenderness, abdominal mass or shock. A few cases of hepatocellular carcinoma have been reported in women taking OCs long-term; however, an association has not been established.

Pregnancy test: Do not administer progestin-only products or progestin-estrogen combinations to induce withdrawal bleeding as a test for pregnancy.

Gallbladder disease: Earlier studies have reported an increased risk of gallbladder surgery in users of OCs. More recent studies, however, have shown that the relative risk of developing gallbladder disease among OC users may be minimal. These recent findings may be related to the use of OC formulations containing lower estrogen and progestin doses.

Carbohydrate metabolism: Glucose tolerance may decrease, which is directly related to estrogen dose. Progestins increase insulin secretion, create insulin resistance and cause glucose intolerance, these effects varying with different agents. High-dose estrogens may create a state of hyperinsulinism. However, OCs appear to have no effect on fasting blood glucose in nondiabetic women. Observe prediabetic and diabetic patients receiving OCs. In a recent study, OC users were less likely to develop diabetes than nonusers.

Lipid profile: Triglycerides may increase. Some progestins decrease HDL, while some estrogens increase HDL. Because the net effect of an OC depends on a balance achieved between doses of the agents, consider this when choosing a product.

Elevated blood pressure and hypertension may occur within a few months of beginning use. The prevalence increases with the duration of use and age. Incidence of hypertension may directly correlate with increasing dosages of progestin.

Women with a history of hypertension, preexisting renal disease or hypertension-related diseases during pregnancy, familial tendency to hypertension or its consequences, or a history of excessive weight gain or fluid retention during the menstrual cycle may be more likely to develop elevated blood pressure; closely monitor these patients. Discontinue the OC if elevated blood pressure occurs. High blood pressure returns to normal in most women after OC discontinuation.

Headaches: Onset or exacerbation of migraine or development of headache of a new pattern which is recurrent, persistent or severe, requires OC discontinuation and evaluation.

Bleeding irregularities: Breakthrough bleeding (BTB), spotting and amenorrhea are frequent reasons for discontinuing OCs. In BTB, consider nonhormonal causes. In undiagnosed persistent or recurrent abnormal vaginal bleeding, rule out pregnancy or malignancy. If pathology has been excluded, time or formulation change may resolve the problem. Changing to an OC with a higher estrogen content may minimize menstrual irregularity, but consider the increased risk of thromboembolic disease. Consider short-term estrogen supplements.

It was thought that women with a history of oligomenorrhea or secondary amenorrhea or young women without regular cycles may tend to remain anovulatory or become amenorrheic after discontinuation of OCs; however, this is not certain. Other factors may play a role in the development of amenorrhea after OC withdrawal, including stress, previous menstrual irregularity, psychiatric conditions and marked weight loss. Also, the incidence may have been much higher when higher-dose products were used more regularly. Advise patients of this possibility.

Progestin-only products are more likely to cause an alteration in menstrual patterns. Amount and duration of flow, cycle length, BTB, spotting and amenorrhea varies. Bleeding irregularities occur more frequently with progestin-only products than with combination OCs.

ORAL CONTRACEPTIVES

Risks of use immediately preceding pregnancy: Some extensive epidemiological studies have revealed no increased risk of birth defects in OC users prior to pregnancy.

Menopause: Treatment with OCs may mask the onset of the climacteric.

Fertility impairment may occur in women discontinuing OCs; however, impairment diminishes with time. In nulliparous women aged 25 to 29 years, the effect is negligible after 48 months. Among nulliparous women 30 to 34, impairment persists up to 72 months and appears more severe. For parous women the effect is negligible and short-lived after cessation of contraception.

Pregnancy: Category X. Rule out pregnancy before initiating or continuing the OCs, and always consider it if withdrawal bleeding does not occur. Rule out pregnancy before continuing OCs for any patient who has missed 2 consecutive periods. If the patient has not adhered to the prescribed schedule, consider the possibility of pregnancy at the time of the first missed period, and withhold further use until pregnancy has been ruled out. If pregnancy is confirmed, apprise the patient of the potential risks to the fetus. The majority of recent studies do not indicate a teratogenic effect, particularly cardiac anomalies and limb reduction defects, when OCs are taken inadvertently during early pregnancy.

The use of female sex hormones (such as estrogens) during early pregnancy may seriously damage the offspring (see the Warning box in the Estrogens monograph). However, there is no conclusive evidence that OC use is associated with an increase in birth defects when taken inadvertently during early pregnancy. Previously, a few studies reported that OCs might be associated with birth defects, but these findings have not been seen in more recent studies. Nevertheless, do not use during pregnancy unless clearly necessary.

Ectopic pregnancy as well as intrauterine pregnancy may occur in contraceptive failures. In progestin-only OC failures, the ratio of ectopic to intrauterine pregnancies is higher than in women who are not receiving OCs, since the drugs are more effective in preventing intrauterine than ectopic pregnancies.

Lactation: Oral contraceptives may interfere with lactation, decreasing both the quantity and the quality of breast milk. Furthermore, a small fraction of the hormones in OCs are excreted in breast milk. A few adverse effects on the nursing infant have been reported, including jaundice and breast enlargement. If possible, defer use until the infant has been weaned; however, in some situations breastfeeding is the only real alternative.

Precautions:

Monitoring: Take a complete medical and family history prior to initiation of therapy. Physical examination before initiation of OCs may be deferred if requested by the patient and judged appropriate by the physician. Pretreatment and periodic exams should include blood pressure, breasts, abdomen and pelvic organs, including Pap smear. Perform preventative measures (ie, ensure up-to-date vaccinations) and screening, which should include total and HDL cholesterol within 5 year intervals. Advise the pathologist of OC therapy when relevant specimens are submitted. Do not prescribe for > 1 year without another physical exam.

Lipid disorders: Closely follow women taking OCs who are being treated for lipidemias. Some progestins may elevate LDL levels and decrease HDL levels (see Warnings), making hyperlipidemia control more difficult. Consider witholding the OC if the dyslipidemia does not respond (ie, LDL of 190).

Uterine fibroids: Preexisting uterine leiomyomata (uterine fibroids) may increase in size. However, there is no evidence of this with low-dose OCs. In addition, data from Great Britain indicates that the risk of developing uterine fibroids is actually reduced with OC use.

Depression: The incidence of depression in OC users ranges from < 5% to 30%. Pyridoxine deficiency may be a factor in the depression. Pyridoxine 25 to 50 mg per day has been recommended. In patients with history of depression, discontinue if depression recurs to a serious degree. Patients becoming significantly depressed should discontinue medication to determine if symptom is drug-related.

Pyridoxine deficiency: OC users may have relative pyridoxine deficiency; clinical significance is unknown.

Fluid retention: OCs may cause fluid retention; prescribe with caution and monitor patients with conditions which might be aggravated by fluid retention (eg, convulsive disorders; migraine syndrome; asthma; cardiac, hepatic or renal dysfunction).

Hepatic function: Patients with a history of jaundice during pregnancy have an increased risk of recurrence of jaundice; if jaundice develops, discontinue use. Steroid hormones may be poorly metabolized in patients with liver dysfunction; administer with caution.

ORAL CONTRACEPTIVES

Contact lens wearers who develop changes in vision or lens tolerance should be assessed by an ophthalmologist; consider temporary or permanent cessation of wear.

Serum folate levels may be depressed by therapy. Although OCs may impair folate metabolism, the effect is mild and unlikely to cause anemia or megaloblastic changes in women who have a good dietary folate intake. Since the pregnant woman is predisposed to folate deficiency, a woman who becomes pregnant shortly after stopping therapy may have a greater chance of developing folate deficiency and its attendant complications. Folic acid supplements are recommended.

Acute intermittent porphyria: Estrogens have been reported to precipitate attacks of acute intermittent porphyria; use with caution in susceptible patients.

Vomiting/Diarrhea: Several cases of OC failure have been reported in association with vomiting or diarrhea. If significant GI disturbance occurs, a back-up method of contraception for the remainder of the cycle is recommended.

Sexually transmitted diseases (STDs): Advise patients that OCs do not protect against HIV infection and other STDs.

Photosensitivity: Photosensitization (photoallergy or phototoxicity) may occur; therefore, caution patients to take protective measures against exposure to ultraviolet or sunlight (ie, sunscreens, protective clothing) until tolerance is determined.

Tartrazine sensitivity: Some of these products contain tartrazine, which may cause allergic-type reactions (including bronchial asthma) in susceptible individuals. Although the incidence of tartrazine sensitivity in the general population is low, it is frequently seen in patients who also have aspirin hypersensitivity. Specific products containing tartrazine are identified in the product listings.

Drug Interactions:

Oral Contraceptive Drug Interactions

Precipitant drug	Object drug*		Description
Contraceptives, oral	Acetaminophen	⬇	Onset of acetaminophen's effect may be delayed or decreased slightly, but the ultimate effect does not appear to be significantly affected.
Contraceptives, oral	Anticoagulants	⟷	Since OCs can increase levels of certain circulating clotting factors and reduce antithrombin III levels, therapeutic efficacy of the anticoagulants may be decreased by OCs. However, both an increased and decreased effect has occurred.
Contraceptives, oral	Antidepressants, tricyclic Benzodiazepines[1] Beta blockers Caffeine Corticosteroids Theophyllines	⬆	The hepatic metabolism of these agents may be decreased by OCs, resulting in increased therapeutic effects or toxicity.
Contraceptives, oral	Benzodiazepines	⬇	OCs may increase the clearance of the benzodiazepines that undergo glucuronidation (lorazepam, oxazepam, temazepam) due to increased metabolism.
Contraceptives, oral	Clofibrate	⬇	OCs may increase the elimination of clofibric acid, the active form of clofibrate.
Contraceptives, oral	Salicylates	⬇	OCs may increase the metabolic clearance of salicylates, possibly decreasing their therapeutic effect.
Antibiotics	Contraceptives, oral	⬇	Coadministration of griseofulvin, penicillins or tetracyclines with OCs may decrease the pharmacologic effects of the OCs, possibly due to altered steroid gut metabolism secondary to changes in the intestinal flora. Menstrual irregularities (spotting, breakthrough bleeding) and pregnancy may occur. An alternate or additional form of birth control may be advisable during concomitant use. OCs and troleandomycin may be associated with an increased frequency of intrahepatic cholestasis.

ORAL CONTRACEPTIVES

Oral Contraceptive Drug Interactions			
Precipitant drug	Object drug*		Description
Barbiturates Hydantoins[2] Rifampin	Contraceptives, oral	⬇	These agents may increase the hepatic metabolism of the OCs via hepatic microsomal enzyme induction, possibly resulting in decreased effectiveness of the OC; menstrual irregularities (spotting, breakthrough bleeding) and pregnancy may occur. An alternate or additional form of birth control may be advisable during concomitant use.

* ⬆ = Object drug increased. ⬇ = Object drug decreased. ⬌ = Undetermined effect.

[1] Those agents metabolized by oxidation.

[2] Pharmacologic effects of the hydantoins may also be altered.

Drug/Lab test interactions: Estrogen-containing OCs may cause the following alterations in serum, plasma or blood, unless specified otherwise.

Increased – Sulfobromophthalein retention; factors I (prothrombin), VII, VIII, IX, X; decreased tissue plasminogen, fibrinogen; norepinephrine-induced platelet aggregation; thyroid binding globulin (TBG), leading to increased total thyroid hormone (as measured by protein bound iodine or T_4 by column or radioimmunoassay); transcortin; corticosteroid levels; triglycerides and phospholipids; ceruloplasmin; aldosterone; amylase; gamma-glutamyltranspeptidase; iron binding capacity; transferrin; prolactin; renin activity; vitamin A.

Decreased – Antithrombin III; free T_3 resin uptake; response to metyrapone test; folate; glucose tolerance; albumin; cholinesterase; haptoglobin; zinc; vitamin B_{12}.

Adverse Reactions:

Breast changes: Tenderness; enlargement; secretion; diminution in lactation when given immediately postpartum.

CNS: Migraine; mental depression.

Dermatologic: Melasma; rash (allergic).

GI: Nausea and vomiting (occurring in approximately 10% to 30% of patients during the first cycle, less common with low doses, and majority resolve in 3 months); abdominal cramps; bloating; cholestatic jaundice.

GU: Breakthrough bleeding (majority, > 80%, resolve in 3 months); spotting; change in menstrual flow; amenorrhea during and after treatment; change in cervical erosion and cervical secretions; invasive cervical cancer; vaginal candidiasis.

Ophthalmic: Changes in corneal curvature (steepening); contact lens intolerance; neuro-ocular lesions (eg, retinal thrombosis, optic neuritis).

Serious: See Warnings. Thrombophlebitis and venous thrombosis with or without embolism; pulmonary embolism; coronary thrombosis; MI; cerebral thrombosis; arterial thromboembolism; cerebral hemorrhage; hypertension; gallbladder disease; congenital anomalies; hepatic adenomas or benign liver tumors; hepatocellular carcinoma; mesenteric thrombosis; Budd-Chiari syndrome.

Miscellaneous: Edema; weight change (increase or decrease); reduced carbohydrate tolerance; prevalence of cervical chlamydia trachomatis may be increased.

The following associations have been neither confirmed nor refuted: Premenstrual syndrome; cataracts; changes in libido; chorea; changes in appetite; cystitis-like syndrome; headache; nervousness; dizziness; hirsutism; loss of scalp hair; erythema multiforme; erythema nodosum; hemorrhagic eruption; vaginitis; renal function impairment; (hemolytic uremic syndrome); porphyria; rhinitis; fatigue; itching; anemia; pancreatitis; hepatitis; colitis; gingivitis; lupus erythematosus or lupus-like syndromes; sickle cell disease; cerbrovascular disease with mitral valve prolapse; rheumatoid arthritis; malignant melanoma; endometrial, cervical and breast carcinoma (conflicting data; see Warnings); herpes gestationis; malignant hypertension; pulmonary embolism; colonic Crohn's disease; pituitary tumors; ECG abnormalities; acne.

Overdosage:

Serious ill effects have not been reported following acute overdosage of OCs in young children. Overdosage may cause nausea. Withdrawal bleeding may occur in females.

Patient Information:

Patient package insert available with product.

To achieve maximum contraceptive effectiveness, take OCs exactly as directed at intervals not exceeding 24 hours, preferably at the same time each day. Take tablets regularly with a meal or at bedtime. Efficacy depends on strict adherence to the dosage schedule. For missed doses, see Administration and Dosage.

ORAL CONTRACEPTIVES

May cause spotting or breakthrough bleeding during the first few months of therapy; if bleeding occurs in > 1 cycle or lasts more than a few days, notify physician.

Use an additional method of birth control until after the first week of administration in the initial cycle, or for the entire cycle if vomiting or diarrhea occurs.

Inform patients that OCs do not protect against HIV infection and other STDs.

Administration and Dosage:

Product choice: Only low-dose pills should be routinely used now; there is rarely a need for 50 mcg estrogen component tablets.

Sunday-Start packaging: If the instructions recommend starting the regimen on Sunday, take the first tablet on the first Sunday after menstruation begins. If menstruation begins on Sunday, take the first tablet on that day.

21-Day regimen: Day 1 of the cycle is the first day of menstrual bleeding. Take 1 tablet daily for 21 days, beginning on day 5 of cycle. No tablets are taken for 7 days; whether bleeding has stopped or not, start a new course of 21 days. Withdrawal flow will normally occur about 3 days after the last tablet is taken. Follow the schedule whether flow occurs as expected, or whether spotting or BTB occurs during the cycle.

28-Day regimen: To eliminate the need to count the days between cycles, some products contain 7 inert or iron-containing tablets to permit continuous daily dosage during the entire 28-day cycle. Take the 7 tablets on the last 7 days of the cycle.

Biphasic and triphasic OCs: Follow instructions on the dispensers or packs; these are clearly marked, usually indicating where to start on the regimen and in what order to take the pills (usually marked with arrows), along with the appropriate week numbers. If there is any question, detailed instructions are provided in the specific package insert. As with the monophasic OCs, 1 tablet is taken each day; however, as the color of the tablet changes, the strength of the tablet also changes (ie, the estrogen/progestin ratio varies).

Missed dose: While there is little likelihood of ovulation occurring if only 1 tablet is missed, the possibility of spotting or bleeding is increased. The possibility of ovulation occurring increases with each successive day that scheduled tablets are missed. This is particularly likely to occur if ≥ 2 consecutive tablets are missed. Any time ≥ 1 active tablets have been missed, use another method of contraception for the balance of the cycle until tablets have been taken for 7 consecutive days. If a patient forgets to take 1 or more tablets, the following is suggested:

One tablet – Take it as soon as remembered, or take 2 tablets the next day; alternatively take 1 tablet, discard the other missed tablet, continue as scheduled and use another form of contraception until menses.

Two consecutive tablets – Take 2 tablets as soon as remembered with the next pill at the usual time, or take 2 tablets daily for the next 2 days, then resume the regular schedule. Use an additional form of contraception for the 7 days after pills are missed, preferably for the remainder of the cycle.

Three consecutive tablets – Begin a new compact of tablets, starting on day one of the cycle after the last pill was taken or starting 7 days after the last tablet was taken. Use an additional form of birth control until pills have been taken for 7 consecutive days, preferably for the remainder of the cycle.

Switching brands: If the patient switches brands of OCs, wait 7 days to start the new pack (21–day regimen) or start the next pack on the day after the last "reminder" pill (28–day regimen).

Bleeding that resembles menstruation occurs rarely. Persistent bleeding not controlled by this method indicates the need for re-examination of the patient; consider nonhormonal causes. If pathology has been excluded, time or a change to another formulation may solve the problem.

Missed menstrual period: 1. If the patient has not adhered to the prescribed dosage regimen, consider possible pregnancy after the first missed period; withhold OCs until ruling out pregnancy.

2. If the patient has adhered to the prescribed regimen and misses 2 consecutive periods, rule out pregnancy before continuing the contraceptive regimen.

After several months of treatment, menstrual flow may reduce to a point of virtual absence. This reduced flow may occur as a result of medication, and is not indicative of pregnancy.

Postpartum administration in non-nursing mothers may begin at the first postpartum examination (4 to 6 weeks), regardless of whether spontaneous menstruation has occurred. Also, start no earlier than 4 to 6 weeks after a midtrimester pregnancy termination. Immediate postpartum use is associated with increased risk of thromboembolism. If possible, nursing mothers should defer taking OCs until the infant is weaned (see Warnings). Note that early resumption of ovulation may occur if bromocriptine has been used for prevention of lactation.

ORAL CONTRACEPTIVES

Dosage adjustments: Side effects noted during the initial cycles may be transient; if they continue, dosage adjustments may be indicated. Many side effects are related to the potency of the estrogen or progestin in the products. Some effects may be related to the relative dominance of either the estrogenic or progestational component. The following table summarizes these dose-related side effects.

Achieving Proper Hormonal Balance In An Oral Contraceptive			
Estrogen		Progestin	
Excess	Deficiency	Excess	Deficiency
Nausea, bloating Cervical mucorrhea, polyposis Melasma Hypertension Migraine headache Breast fullness or tenderness Edema	Early or midcycle breakthrough bleeding Increased spotting Hypomenorrhea	Increased appetite Weight gain Tiredness, fatigue Hypomenorrhea Acne, oily scalp[1] Hair loss, hirsutism[1] Depression Monilial vaginitis Breast regression	Late breakthrough bleeding Amenorrhea Hypermenorrhea

[1] Result of androgenic activity of progestins.

Pharmacological Effects of Progestins Used in Oral Contraceptives[1]				
	Progestin	Estrogen	Antiestrogen	Androgen
Norgestrel/levonorgestrel	+++	0	++	+++
Desogestrel	+++	0/+	+++	0/+
Norgestimate	+++	0	+++	0
Ethynodiol diacetate	++	+[2]	+[2]	++
Norethindrone acetate	+	+	+++	++
Norethindrone	+	+[2]	+[2]	++
Norethynodrel	+	+++	0	0

[1] *Symbol Key: +++ pronounced effect ++ moderate effect + slight effect 0 no effect*

[2] Has estrogenic effect at low doses; may have antiestrogenic effect at higher doses.

Minimize the above effects by adjusting the estrogen/progestin balance or dosage. The following table categorizes products by both their estrogenic and progestational activity. Because overall activity is influenced by the interaction of components, including androgenic and antiestrogenic activity, it is difficult to precisely classify products; placement in the table is only approximate. Differences between products within a group are probably not clinically significant.

ORAL CONTRACEPTIVES

Estimated Relative Oral Contraceptive Estrogen/Progestin Activity

←PROGESTINS→	←ESTROGENS→ Low		←ESTROGENS→ Intermediate
High			Ovral
Intermediate	Demulen 1/35 Desogen Levlen	Lo/Ovral Nordette Ortho-Cyclen	Demulen 1/50
Low	*Monophasic* Brevicon Genora 0.5/35 Genora 1/35 Genora 1/50 Loestrin 21 1/20 Loestrin Fe 1/20 Loestrin 21 1.5/30 Loestrin Fe 1.5/30 Modicon	Nelova 0.5/35 E Nelova 1/35 E Nelova 1/50 M Norethin 1/35 E Norethin 1/50 M Norinyl 1 = 35 Norinyl 1 = 50 Ortho-Novum 1/35 Ortho-Novum 1/50	*Monophasic* Ovcon-35 Ovcon-50
Low	*Biphasic* Nelova 10/11	Ortho-Novum 10/11	
Low	*Triphasic* Ortho-Novum 7/7/7 Tri-Levlen	Tri-Norinyl Triphasil	

MONOPHASIC ORAL CONTRACEPTIVES

For complete prescribing information, refer to the Oral Contraceptives group monograph.

The combination therapy products are listed in order of decreasing estrogen content.

	Product & Distributor	Estrogen (mcg)	Progestin (mg)	How Supplied
Rx	**Genora 1/50** (Rugby)	50 mestranol	1 norethindrone	Lactose. White. In 21s (3s) and 28s (6s). With 7 peach inert tablets in the 28s.
Rx	**Nelova 1/50M** (Warner Chilcott)	50 mestranol	1 norethindrone	Lactose (active tablets). (WC 942). Light blue. In 6 packs of 21s & 28s. With 7 white inert tablets (WC 937) in the 28s.
Rx	**Norethin 1/50M** (Roberts)	50 mestranol	1 norethindrone	Sucrose (inert tablets). In 6 tablet dispensers of 21s and 28s. White with 7 blue inert tablets in the 28s.
Rx	**Norinyl 1 + 50** (Syntex)	50 mestranol	1 norethindrone	Lactose. White. In Wallette 21s and 28s. With 7 orange inert tablets in the 28s.
Rx	**Ortho-Novum 1/50** (Ortho Pharm.)	50 mestranol	1 norethindrone	Lactose. (Ortho 150). Yellow. In Dialpak and Veridate 21s and 28s. With 7 green inert tablets in the 28s.
Rx	**Ovcon-50** (Mead Johnson Labs)	50 ethinyl estradiol	1 norethindrone	Lactose. Yellow. In 6 compact cartons of 21s and 28s. With 7 green inert tablets in the 28s.
Rx	**Demulen 1/50** (Searle)	50 ethinyl estradiol	1 ethynodiol diacetate	Sucrose (inert tablets). (Searle 71). White. In 6 and 24 Compack 21s and 28s. With 7 pink inert tablets (Searle P) in the 28s.
Rx	**Zovia 1/50E** (Watson)	50 ethinyl estradiol	1 ethynodiol diacetate	Pink. In 21s and 28s. With 7 white inert tablets in the 28s.
Rx	**Ovral** (Wyeth-Ayerst)	50 ethinyl estradiol	0.5 norgestrel	Lactose. (Wyeth 56). White. In 6 Pilpak 21s and 28s. With 7 pink inert tablets (Wyeth 445) in the 28s.

MONOPHASIC ORAL CONTRACEPTIVES

	Product & Distributor	Estrogen (mcg)	Progestin (mg)	How Supplied
Rx	**Genora 1/35** (Rugby)	35 ethinyl estradiol	1 norethin-drone	Lactose. Pale blue. In blister packs of 21s (3s) or 28s (6s). With 7 peach inert tablets in the 28s.
Rx	**Nelova 1/35E** (Warner Chilcott)			Lactose (active tablets). (WC 930). Dark yellow. In 6 packs of 21s and 28s. With 7 white inert tablets (WC 937) in the 28s.
Rx	**Norethin 1/35E** (Roberts)			Sucrose (inert tablets). White. In 6 packs of 21s and 28s. With 7 blue inert tablets in the 28s.
Rx	**Norinyl 1 + 35** (Syntex)			Lactose. Yellow-green. In Wallette 21s and 28s. With 7 orange inert tablets in the 28s.
Rx	**Ortho-Novum 1/35** (Ortho Pharm.)			Lactose. (Ortho 135). Peach. In Dialpak and Veridate 21s and 28s. With 7 green inert tablets in the 28s.
Rx	**Brevicon** (Syntex)		0.5 norethin-drone	Lactose. Blue. In Wallette 21s and 28s. With 7 orange inert tablets in the 28s.
Rx	**Genora 0.5/35** (Rugby)			Lactose. White. In 21s and 28s. With 7 peach inert tablets in the 28s.
Rx	**Modicon** (Ortho Pharm.)			Lactose. (Ortho 535). White. In Dialpak 21s and 28s and Veridate 28s. With 7 green inert tablets in the 28s.
Rx	**Nelova 0.5/35E** (Warner Chilcott)			Lactose (active tablets). (WC 929). Light yellow. In 6 packs of 21s and 28s. With 7 white inert tablets (WC 937) in the 28s.
Rx	**Ovcon-35** (Mead Johnson Labs)	35 ethinyl estradiol	0.4 norethin drone	Lactose. Peach. In 6 compact cartons of 21s and 28s. With 7 green inert tablets in the 28s.
Rx	**Ortho-Cyclen** (Ortho Pharm.)		0.25 norgesti-mate	Lactose. (Ortho 250). Blue. In Dialpak and Veridate 21s and 28s. With 7 green inert tablets in the 28s.
Rx	**Demulen 1/35** (Searle)		1 ethynodiol diacetate	Sucrose (inert tablets). (Searle 151). White. In 6 and 24 Compack 21s and 28s. With 7 blue inert tablets (Searle P) in the 28s.
Rx	**Zovia 1/35E** (Watson)			Lt. pink. In 21s and 28s. With 7 white inert tablets in the 28s.

MONOPHASIC ORAL CONTRACEPTIVES

	Product & Distributor	Estrogen (mcg)	Progestin (mg)	How Supplied
Rx	**Loestrin 21 1.5/30** (Parke-Davis)	30 ethinyl estradiol	1.5 norethindrone acetate	Lactose, sugar (active tablets). Green. In 5 packs of 21s.
Rx	**Loestrin Fe 1.5/30** (Parke-Davis)			Lactose, sugar (active tablets), sucrose (inert tablets). Green with 7 brown tablets (75 mg ferrous fumarate/tab). In 5 packs of 28s.
Rx	**Lo/Ovral** (Wyeth-Ayerst)		0.3 norgestrel	Lactose. (Wyeth 78). White. In 6 Pilpak 21s and 28s. With 7 pink inert tablets (Wyeth 486) in the 28s.
Rx	**Desogen** (Organon)		0.15 desogestrel	Lactose. (T R 5 Organon). White with 7 green inert tablets (K H 2 Organon). In recyclable plastic dispenser 28s.
Rx	**Ortho-Cept** (Ortho)			Lactose. (Ortho D 150). Orange with 7 green inert tablets in the 28s. In Dialpak and Veridate 21s and 28s.
Rx	**Levlen** (Berlex)		0.15 levonorgestrel	Lactose. (B 21). Light orange. In 3 slidecase dispenser 21s and 28s. With 7 pink inert tablets (B 28) in the 28s.
Rx	**Levora 15/30-21** (SCS)			Lactose. (15/30 SCS). White tablets. In 21s.
Rx	**Levora 0.15/30-28** (SCS)			Lactose. (15/30 SCS). White tablets. In 21s. With 7 peach inerts.
Rx	**Nordette** (Wyeth-Ayerst)			Lactose. (Wyeth 75). Light orange. In 6 Pilpak 21s and 28s. With 7 pink inert tablets (Wyeth 486) in the 28s.
Rx	**Alesse-21** (Wyeth-Ayerst)	20 ethinyl estradiol	0.1 levonorgestrel	Lactose. (W 912). Pink. In 21s.
Rx	**Alesse-28** (Wyeth-Ayerst)			Lactose. (W 912). Pink. In 21s. (Inactive) Lactose. (W 650). Lt. green. In 7s.
Rx	**Loestrin 21 1/20** (Parke-Davis)	20 ethinyl estradiol	1 norethindrone acetate	Lactose, sugar. White. In 5 packs of 21s.
Rx	**Loestrin Fe 1/20** (Parke-Davis)			Lactose, sugar (active tablets), sucrose (inert tablets). White with 7 brown tablets (75 mg ferrous fumarate/tab). In 5 packs of 28s.

BIPHASIC ORAL CONTRACEPTIVES

For complete prescribing information, refer to the Oral Contraceptives group monograph.

The combination therapy products are listed in order of decreasing estrogen content.

	Product	*Phase 1:*	*Phase 2:*	How Supplied
Rx	**Jenest-28** (Organon)	0.5 mg norethindrone, 35 mcg ethinyl estradiol (7 white tablets)	1 mg norethindrone, 35 mcg ethinyl estradiol (14 peach tablets)	Lactose. White = (ORG 07). Peach = (ORG 14). Green = (ORG). In 6 Cyclic Tablet Dispensers of 28 tablets.
Rx	**Nelova 10/11** (Warner Chilcott)	0.5 mg norethindrone, 35 mcg ethinyl estradiol (10 light yellow tablets)	1 mg norethindrone, 35 mcg ethinyl estradiol (11 dark yellow tablets)	Lactose (active tablets). Light yellow = (WC 929). Dark yellow = (WC 930). In 6 packs of 21s and 28s. With 7 white inert tablets (WC 937) in the 28s.
Rx	**Ortho-Novum 10/11** (Ortho Pharm.)	0.5 mg norethindrone, 35 mcg ethinyl estradiol (10 white tablets)	1 mg norethindrone, 35 mcg ethinyl estradiol (11 peach tablets)	Lactose. White = (Ortho 535). Peach = (Ortho 135). In Dialpak 21s and 28s and Veridate 29s. With 7 green inert tablets in the 28s.

TRIPHASIC ORAL CONTRACEPTIVES

For complete prescribing information, refer to the Oral Contraceptives group monograph.

The combination therapy products are listed in order of decreasing estrogen content.

	Product	*Phase 1*	*Phase 2*	*Phase 3*	How Supplied
Rx	**Tri-Norinyl** (Syntex)	0.5 mg norethindrone, 35 mcg ethinyl estradiol (7 blue tablets)	1 mg norethindrone, 35 mcg ethinyl estradiol (9 yellow-green tablets)	0.5 mg norethindrone, 35 mcg ethinyl estradiol (5 blue tablets)	Lactose. 28-day has 7 orange inert tabs. In Wallette 21s and 28s.
Rx	**Ortho- Novum 7/7/7** (Ortho Pharm.)	0.5 mg norethindrone, 35 mcg ethinyl estradiol (7 white tablets)	0.75 mg norethindrone, 35 mcg ethinyl estradiol, (7 light peach tablets)	1 mg norethindrone, 35 mcg ethinyl estradiol, (7 peach tablets)	Lactose. White = (Ortho 535). Light peach = (Ortho 75). Peach = (Ortho 135). 28-day has 7 green inert tabs. In Dialpak and Veridate 21s and 28s.
Rx	**Tri-Levlen** (Berlex)	0.05 mg levonorgestrel, 30 mcg ethinyl estradiol, (6 brown tablets)	0.075 mg levonorgestrel, 40 mcg ethinyl estradiol (5 white tablets)	0.125 mg levonorgestrel, 30 mcg ethinyl estradiol (10 light yellow tablets)	Lactose. Brown = (B 95). White = (B 96). Light yellow = (B 97). 28-day has 7 light green placebo tablets (B 11). In 3 and 6 Slidecase dispenser 21s and 28s.
Rx	**Triphasil** (Wyeth-Ayerst)				Lactose. Brown = (W 641). White = (W 642). Light yellow = (W 643). 28-day has 7 light green inert tabs (W 650). In 3 dial dispensers (21s) and 3 compacts and 6 pack refills (28s).
Rx	**Ortho Tri-Cyclen** (Ortho Pharm.)	0.18 mg norgestimate, 35 mcg ethinyl estradiol (7 white tablets)	0.215 mg norgestimate, 35 mcg ethinyl estradiol (7 light blue tablets)	0.25 mg norgestimate, 35 mcg ethinyl estradiol (7 blue tablets)	Lactose. White = (Ortho 180). Light blue = (Ortho 215). Blue = (Ortho 250). 28-day has 7 green inert tablets. In Dialpak and Veridate 21s and 28s.
Rx	**Estrosep 21** (Parke-Davis)	1 mg norethindrone acetate, 20 mcg ethinyl estradiol (5 triangle tablets)	1 mg norethindrone acetate, 30 mcg ethinyl estradiol (7 square tablets)	1 mg norethindrone acetate, 35 mcg ethinyl estradiol (9 round tablets)	White. In 21s.

TRIPHASIC ORAL CONTRACEPTIVES

	Product	*Phase 1*	*Phase 2*	*Phase 3*	How Supplied
Rx	**Estrosep Fe** (Parke-Davis)	1 mg norethindrone acetate, 20 mcg ethinyl estradiol (5 triangle tablets)	1 mg norethindrone acetate, 30 mcg ethinyl estradiol (7 square tablets)	1 mg norethindrone acetate, 35 mcg ethinyl estradiol (9 round tablets)	White. Also has 7 brown 75 mg ferrous fumarate tablets. In 28s.

PROGESTIN-ONLY PRODUCTS

For complete prescribing information, refer to the Oral Contraceptives group monograph.

Administration and Dosage:

Administer daily, starting on the first day of menstruation. Take one tablet at the same time each day, every day of the year.

Postpartum administration: May be initiated no earlier than 4 weeks postpartum; however, consider the increased risk of thromboembolic disease associated with the postpartum period.

Missed dose:

One tablet – Take as soon as remembered, then take next tablet at regular time.

Two consecutive tablets – Do not take the missed tablets; discard and take the next tablet at the regular time (*Micronor* and *Nor-Q.D.*), or take 1 of the missed tablets, discard the other and take daily tablet at usual time (*Ovrette*).

Three consecutive tablets – Discontinue immediately.

Use an additional method of contraception if 2 or more tablets are missed until menses appears or pregnancy is ruled out. If menses does not occur within 45 days, regardless of circumstances, discontinue drug, use a nonhormonal method of contraception and rule out pregnancy. Because of the slightly higher failure rate of the progestin-only products, a more conservative approach is to discontinue the regimen if only 1 tablet is missed and use other nonhormonal contraceptive methods until menses occurs or pregnancy is ruled out.

Rx	**Micronor** (Ortho Pharm.)	**Tablets:** 0.35 mg norethindrone	Lactose. (Ortho 0.35). Lime. In Dialpak and Veridate 28s.
Rx	**Nor-Q.D.** (Syntex)		Lactose. Yellow. In dispenser 42s (6s).
Rx	**Ovrette** (Wyeth-Ayerst)	**Tablets:** 0.075 mg norgestrel	Lactose. (Wyeth 62). Yellow. In 6 Pilpak 28s.

LEVONORGESTREL IMPLANTS

Actions:

Pharmacology: Levonorgestrel implants are a set of six flexible closed capsules made of *Silastic* (dimethylsiloxane/methylvinylsiloxane copolymer), each containing 36 mg of the progestin levonorgestrel in an insertion kit to facilitate implantation. The capsules are sealed with *Silastic* adhesive (polydimethylsiloxane) and sterilized.

The initial dose is about 85 mcg/day, followed by a decline to about 50 mcg/day by 9 months, and to about 35 mcg/day by 18 months, with a further decline thereafter to about 30 mcg/day. The implant is a progestin-only product and does not contain estrogen. It is a totally synthetic and biologically active progestin which exhibits no significant estrogenic activity and is highly progestational. For further information, refer to the Progestins group monograph.

Diffusion of levonorgestrel through the wall of each capsule provides a continuous low dose of the progestin. Resulting blood levels are substantially below those generally observed among users of combination oral contraceptives containing the progestins norgestrel or levonorgestrel. Because of the range of variability in blood levels and variation in individual response, blood levels alone are not predictive of the risk of pregnancy in an individual woman.

Pharmacokinetics: Levonorgestrel concentrations among women show considerable variation. They reach a maximum, or near maximum, within 24 hours after placement with mean values of 1600 ± 1100 pg/ml. Levels decline rapidly over the first month partially due to a circulating protein, SHBG, that binds levonorgestrel and is depressed by the presence of levonorgestrel. Mean levels decline to values of around 400 pg/ml at 3 months to 258 ± 95 pg/ml at 60 months.

Concentrations decreased with increasing body weight by a mean of 3.3 pg/ml/kg. After capsule removal, mean concentrations drop to < 100 pg/ml by 96 hours and to below assay sensitivity (50 pg/ml) by 5 to 14 days. Fertility rates return to levels comparable to those seen in the general population of women using no method of contraception. Circulating concentrations can be used to forecast the risk of pregnancy only in a general statistical sense. Mean concentrations associated with pregnancy have been 210 ± 60 pg/ml. However, in clinical studies, 20% of women had one or more values below 200 pg/ml but an average annual gross pregnancy rate of < 1 per 100 women through 5 years.

Annual and 5 Year Cumulative Pregnancy Rates Per 100 Levonorgestrel Implant Users by Weight

	Year					
Weight	1	2	3	4	5	Cumulative
< 50 kg (< 110 lbs)	0.2	0	0	0	0	0.2
50-59 kg (110-130 lbs)	0.2	0.5	0.4	2	0.4	3.4
60-69 kg (131-153 lbs)	0.4	0.5	1.6	1.7	0.8	5
≥ 70 kg (≥ 154 lbs)	0	1.1	5.1	2.5	0	8.5
All	0.2	0.5	1.2	1.6	0.4	3.9

The lowest expected failure rate for levonorgestrel implants during the first year of use is < 1. The efficacy of the implant does not depend on patient compliance. For pregnancy rates for various other means of contraception, see the Oral Contraceptives Group Monograph.

Indications:

Prevention of pregnancy. The implant system is a long-term (up to 5 years) reversible contraceptive system. Remove the capsules by the end of the 5th year; new capsules may be inserted at that time if continuing contraceptive protection is desired.

Contraindications:

Active thrombophlebitis or thromboembolic disorders; undiagnosed abnormal genital bleeding; known or suspected pregnancy; acute liver disease; benign or malignant liver tumors; known or suspected carcinoma of the breast.

Warnings:

The following warnings are based on experience with levonorgestrel implants. For other warnings, refer to the Oral Contraceptives group monograph.

Bleeding irregularities: Most women can expect some variation in menstrual bleeding patterns. Irregular menstrual bleeding, intermenstrual spotting, prolonged episodes of bleeding and spotting, and amenorrhea occur in some women. Irregular bleeding patterns could mask symptoms of cervical or endometrial cancer. Overall, these irregularities diminish with continuing use. Since some users experience periods of amenorrhea, missed menstrual periods cannot serve as the only means of identifying early pregnancy. Perform pregnancy tests whenever a pregnancy is suspected. After a pattern of regular menses, ≥ 6 weeks of amenorrhea may signal pregnancy. If pregnancy occurs, the capsules must be removed.

LEVONORGESTREL IMPLANTS

Although bleeding irregularities have occurred in clinical trials, proportionately more women had increases rather than decreases in hemoglobin concentrations, a difference that was highly statistically significant. This finding generally indicates that reduced menstrual blood loss is associated with the use of levonorgestrel implants. In rare instances, blood loss did result in hemoglobin values consistent with anemia.

Delayed follicular atresia: If follicular development occurs, atresia of the follicle is sometimes delayed and the follicle may continue to grow beyond the size it would attain in a normal cycle. These enlarged follicles cannot be distinguished clinically from ovarian cysts. In the majority of women, enlarged follicles will spontaneously disappear and should not require surgery. Rarely, they may twist or rupture, sometimes causing abdominal pain; surgical intervention may be required.

Ectopic pregnancies have occurred among levonorgestrel implant users, although clinical studies have shown no increase in the rate of ectopic pregnancies per year among users as compared with users of no method or of IUDs. The incidence among users was 1.3 per 1000 woman-years, a rate significantly below the rate that has been estimated for non-contraceptive users in the US (2.7 to 3 per 1000 woman-years). The risk of ectopic pregnancy may increase with the duration of use and, possibly, with increased weight of the user. Any patient who presents with lower abdominal pain must be evaluated to rule out ectopic pregnancy.

Ocular lesions: There have been clinical case reports of retinal thrombosis associated with the use of oral contraceptives. Although it is believed that this adverse reaction is related to the estrogen component of oral contraceptives, remove the capsules if there is unexplained partial or complete loss of vision, onset of proptosis or diplopia, papilledema or retinal vascular lesions. Undertake appropriate diagnostic and therapeutic measures immediately.

Foreign body carcinogenesis: Rarely, cancers have occurred at the site of foreign body intrusions or old scars. None has been reported in levonorgestrel implant clinical trials. In rodents highly susceptible to such cancers, the incidence decreases with decreasing size of the foreign body. Because of the resistance of human beings to these cancers and because of the small size of the capsules, the risk to users is judged to be minimal.

Thromboembolic disorders: Patients who develop active thrombophlebitis or thromboembolic disease should have the levonorgestrel capsules removed. Also consider removal in women who will be immobilized for a prolonged period due to surgery or other illnesses.

Lactation: Steroids are not the contraceptives of first choice for lactating women. Levonorgestrel has been identified in breast milk. No significant effects were observed on the growth or health of infants whose mothers used the implants beginning 6 weeks after parturition in comparative studies with mothers using IUDs or barrier methods.

Precautions:

Physical examination and follow-up: Take a complete medical history and physical examination prior to the implantation or re-implantation of levonorestrel implants and at least annually during its use. These physical examinations should include special reference to the implant site, blood pressure, breasts, abdomen and pelvic organs, including cervical cytology and relevant laboratory tests. In case of undiagnosed, persistent or recurrent abnormal vaginal bleeding, conduct appropriate diagnostic measures to rule out malignancy. Carefully monitor women with a strong family history of breast cancer or who have breast nodules.

Carbohydrate and lipid metabolism: An altered glucose tolerance characterized by decreased insulin sensitivity following glucose loading has been found in some users of combination and progestin-only oral contraceptives. The effects of the levonorgestrel implants on carbohydrate metabolism appear to be minimal. In a study in which pretreatment serum glucose levels were compared with levels after 1 and 2 years of use, no statistically significant differences in mean serum glucose levels were evident 2 hours after glucose loading. The clinical significance of these findings is unknown but carefully observe diabetic and prediabetic patients.

Closely follow women who are being treated for hyperlipidemias. Some progestins may elevate LDL levels and render the control of hyperlipidemias more difficult. Although lipoprotein levels were altered in several clinical studies with the levonorgestrel implants, the long-term clinical effects of these changes have not been determined. A decrease in total cholesterol levels has occurred in all lipoprotein studies and reached statistical significance in several. Both increases and decreases in HDL levels have been reported in clinical trials. LDL and triglyceride levels also decreased from pretreatment values.

LEVONORGESTREL IMPLANTS

Liver function: If jaundice develops consider removing the capsules. Steroid hormones may be poorly metabolized in patients with impaired liver function.

Fluid retention: Steroid contraceptives may cause some degree of fluid retention. Prescribe with caution, and only with careful monitoring, in patients with conditions which might be aggravated by fluid retention.

Emotional disorders: Consider removing the capsules in women who become significantly depressed since the symptom may be drug-related. Carefully observe women with a history of depression and consider removal if depression recurs to a serious degree.

Contact lens wearers who develop changes in vision or in lens tolerance should be assessed by an ophthalmologist.

Insertion and removal: To be sure that the woman is not pregnant at the time of capsule placement and to assure contraceptive efficacy during the first cycle of use, insert the capsules during the first 7 days of the cycle or immediately following an abortion. Insertion is not recommended before 6 weeks postpartum in breastfeeding women.

Insertion and removal are not difficult procedures but instructions must be followed closely. It is strongly advised that all health care professionals who insert and remove the capsules be instructed in the procedures before they attempt them. A proper insertion just under the skin will facilitate removals. Proper insertion and removal should result in minimal scarring. If the capsules are placed too deeply, they can be harder to remove. If all capsules cannot be removed at the first attempt, try removal later when the site has healed. Bruising may occur at the implant site during insertion or removal. In some women, hyperpigmentation occurs over the implantation site but is usually reversible following removal.

Infection at the implant site has been uncommon (0.7%). Attention to aseptic technique and proper insertion and removal of the capsules reduces the possibility of infection. If infection occurs, institute suitable treatment. If infection persists, remove the capsules.

Expulsion of capsules is uncommon. It occurs more frequently when placement of the capsules is extremely shallow, too close to the incision, or when infection is present. Replacement of an expelled capsule must be accomplished using a new sterile capsule. If infection is present, treat and cure before replacement. Contraceptive efficacy may be inadequate with < 6 capsules.

Provisions for removal: Advise women that the capsules will be removed at any time for any reason. The removal should be done on such request or at the end of 5 years of usage by personnel instructed in the removal technique.

Drug Interactions:

Carbamazepine and phenytoin: Reduced efficacy (pregnancy) has occurred. Warn users of the possibility of decreased efficacy with use of any related drugs.

Drug/Lab test interactions: Certain endocrine tests may be affected by levonorgestrel implants: Sex hormone binding globulin concentrations are decreased; thyroxine concentrations may be slightly decreased and triiodothyronine uptake increased.

Adverse Reactions:

Gross annual discontinuation and continuation rates of levonorgestrel implant users are summarized in the following table:

Annual and 5 Year Cumulative Discontinuation/Continuation Rates Per 100 Levonorgestrel Implant Users

Parameter	Year 1	Year 2	Year 3	Year 4	Year 5	Cumulative
Pregnancy	0.2	0.5	1.2	1.6	0.4	3.9
Bleeding irregularities	9.1	7.9	4.9	3.3	2.9	25.1
Medical (excluding bleeding irregularities)	6	5.6	4.1	4	5.1	22.4
Personal	4.6	7.7	11.7	10.7	11.7	38.7
Continuation	81	77.4	79.2	76.7	77.6	29.5

LEVONORGESTREL IMPLANTS

Levonorgestrel Implant Adverse Reactions During First Year of Use	
Adverse Reaction	Incidence (%)
Many bleeding days or prolonged bleeding	27.6
Spotting	17.1
Amenorrhea	9.4
Irregular (onsets of) bleeding	7.6
Frequent bleeding onsets	7
Removal difficulties affecting subjects (based on 849 removals)	6.2
Scanty bleeding	5.2
Breast discharge	≥5
Cervicitis	≥ 5
Musculoskeletal pain	≥ 5
Abdominal discomfort	≥ 5
Leukorrhea	≥ 5
Vaginitis	≥ 5
Pain or itching near implant site (usually transient)	3.7
Infection at implant site	0.7

Miscellaneous: Headache; nervousness; nausea; dizziness; adnexal enlargement; dermatitis; acne; change of appetite; mastalgia; weight gain; hirsutism; hypertrichosis; scalp hair loss.

Overdosage:

Overdosage can result if > 6 capsules are in situ. Remove all implanted capsules before inserting a new set. Overdosage may cause fluid retention with its associated effects and uterine bleeding irregularities.

Patient Information:

Provide the patient with a copy of the patient labeling to help describe the characteristics of the system. Advise the patient that the prescribing information is available to them at their request. It is recommended that prospective users be fully informed about the risks and benefits associated with the use of the system, with other forms of contraception, and with no contraception at all. It is also recommended that prospective users be fully informed about the insertion and removal procedures. Health care providers may wish to obtain informed consent from all patients in light of the techniques involved with insertion and removal.

Administration and Dosage:

Levonorgestrel implants consist of six Silastic capsules; each capsule is 2.4 mm in diameter and 34 mm in length and each contains 36 mg levonorgestrel. The total administered (implanted) dose is 216 mg. Perform implantation of all six capsules during the first 7 days of the onset of menses. Insertion is subdermal in the midportion of the upper arm about 8 to 10 cm above the elbow crease. Distribute capsules in a fan-like pattern, about 15° apart, for a total of 75°. Proper insertion will facilitate later removal. (See section on Insertion/Removal under Precautions and in the package literature included with the product.)

Rx	**Norplant System** (Wyeth-Ayerst)	**Kit:** Set of 6 capsules each containing 36 mg levonorgestrel	Also includes trocar, scalpel, forceps, syringe, 2 syringe needles, pkg of skin closures, 3 pkgs of gauze sponges, stretch bandages and surgical drapes.

INTRAUTERINE PROGESTERONE CONTRACEPTIVE SYSTEM

Actions:

Pharmacology: The *Progestasert* system, a T–shaped unit that contains a reservoir of 38 mg progesterone, is indicated for intrauterine contraception. The mechanism of action has not been demonstrated. Hypotheses include progesterone-induced inhibition of sperm capacitation or survival and alteration of the uterine milieu to prevent nidation. During use of the system, the endometrium shows progestational influence. Progesterone from the system suppresses proliferation of the endometrial tissue (an antiestrogenic effect). Following removal of the system, the endometrium rapidly returns to its normal cyclic pattern and can support pregnancy.

Pharmacokinetics: Contraceptive effectiveness is enhanced by continuous release of progesterone into the uterine cavity at an average rate of 65 mcg/day for 1 year. The mechanism is local, not systemic. The concentrations of luteinizing hormone, estradiol and progesterone in systemic venous plasma follow regular cyclic patterns, indicative of ovulation during use of the system. For pregnancy rates for various means of contraception, refer to the Oral Contraceptives group monograph.

Indications:

Intrauterine contraception in women who have had at least one child, are in a stable, mutually monogamous relationship, and have no history of pelvic inflammatory disease (PID).

Unlabeled uses: This system has been used in the treatment of menorrhagia.

Contraindications:

Pregnancy or suspected pregnancy; previous ectopic pregnancy; presence or history of PID; patient or partner has multiple sexual partners; sexually transmitted disease; postpartum endometritis or infected abortion; pelvic surgery; abnormalities which result in uterine distortion or uteri that measure < 6 cm or > 10 cm by sounding; uterine or cervical malignancy, including an unresolved abnormal Pap smear; genital bleeding of unknown etiology; vaginitis or cervicitis unless infection has been completely controlled and is nongonococcal and non-chlamydial; incomplete involution of the uterus following abortion or childbirth; previously inserted intrauterine device (IUD) still in place; genital actinomycosis; conditions or treatments associated with increased susceptibility to infections with microorganisms (eg, leukemia, diabetes, AIDS); IV drug abuse.

Warnings:

Pelvic infection: An increased risk of PID associated with IUD use has been reported; the highest rate occurs shortly after insertion and up to 4 months thereafter. Teach patients to recognize the symptoms of PID and ectopic pregnancy. Pelvic infection may occur with an IUD in situ, and may result in tubo-ovarian abscesses or general peritonitis. If this occurs, remove the IUD and institute appropriate antibiotic treatment. PID can result in tubal damage and occlusion, threatening future fertility or predisposing to ectopic pregnancy. PID may be asymptomatic but still result in tubal damage and its sequelae.

Following diagnosis of PID, initiate antibiotic therapy promptly and remove the progesterone IUD. Guidelines for treatment are available from the CDC.

Genital actinomycosis has been associated primarily with long-term IUD use.

Embedment: Partial penetration or lodging of an IUD in the endometrium can result in difficult removal. In some cases, this can result in IUD fragmentation, necessitating surgical removal.

Perforation, partial or total, of the uterine wall or cervix may occur. If perforation occurs, remove the device. Adhesions, foreign body reactions, peritonitis, cystic masses in the pelvis, intestinal penetrations, local inflammatory reaction with abscess formation and erosion of adjacent viscera and intestinal obstruction may result if the IUD is left in the peritoneal cavity.

Mortality risks: Refer to the Oral Contraceptives group monograph for risk of death associated with various methods of contraception.

Pregnancy: Long-term effects on the fetus are unknown.

Septic abortion may be increased, associated in some instances with septicemia, septic shock and death in patients becoming pregnant with an IUD in place, usually in the second trimester. If pregnancy occurs with a system in situ, remove it if the thread is visible or, if removal is difficult, consider termination of the pregnancy.

Continuation of pregnancy – If pregnancy is maintained and the system remains in situ, warn the patient of the increased risk of spontaneous abortion and sepsis, including death, and premature labor and delivery. Advise her to report immediately all abnormal symptoms, such as flu-like syndrome, fever, chills, abdominal cramping and pain, bleeding or vaginal discharge; generalized symptoms of septicemia may be insidious.

INTRAUTERINE PROGESTERONE CONTRACEPTIVE SYSTEM

Congenital anomalies – Systemically administered sex steroids, including progestational agents, have been associated with an increased risk of congenital anomalies. It is not known whether there is an increased risk of such anomalies when pregnancy is continued with this system in place.

Ectopic pregnancy – The *Progestasert* system acts in the uterus to prevent uterine pregnancy, but it does not prevent either ovulation or ectopic pregnancy. Therefore, a pregnancy that occurs while a patient is using an IUD is much more likely to be ectopic. Determine whether ectopic pregnancy has occurred in patients with delayed menses or unilateral pelvic pain.

In clinical trials of the progesterone system, 1 of 3.6 pregnancies in parous women and 1 of 6.2 pregnancies in nulliparous women were ectopic. The per-year risk of ectopic pregnancy in progesterone system users is ≈ 1 ectopic pregnancy in 200 users per year. This risk is approximately the same as in noncontracepting, sexually active women.

In two clinical studies, for the first year the risk of ectopic pregnancy was approximately 6 times higher among women using progesterone systems than among women using copper systems. Over 2 years, the risk of an ectopic pregnancy with the progesterone-releasing IUD was about 10 times higher than that with copper-releasing IUDs.

Women who have previously had acute PID subsequently have an eightfold to tenfold greater than normal risk of ectopic pregnancy (see Pelvic Infection). Multiple sexual partners or a partner with multiple sexual partners, previous pelvic surgery, endometritis, endometriosis and retrograde menstruation have also been recognized as risk factors for ectopic pregnancy.

Precautions:

Prior to insertion, complete a medical and social history, and determine risk of ectopic pregnancy because of previous PID. Perform pelvic examination, Pap smear, gonorrhea and chlamydia culture and, if indicated, tests for other sexually transmitted diseases. Carefully sound the uterus prior to insertion to determine the degree of patency of the endocervical canal and the internal os, and the direction and depth of the uterine cavity. Occasionally, severe cervical stenosis may be encountered. The uterus should sound to a depth of 6 to 10 cm. Inserting the system into a uterine cavity measuring < 6.5 cm may increase the incidence of expulsion, bleeding and pain.

To reduce the possibility of insertion in the presence of an undetermined pregnancy, insert during or shortly following menstruation.

Cervicitis or vaginitis: Postpone use in these patients until infection has cleared and until the cervicitis has been shown not to be due to gonorrhea or chlamydia.

Involution of uterus: Do not insert postpartum or postabortion until involution of the uterus is completed. Incidence of perforation (see Warnings) and expulsion is greater if involution is not completed. Involution may be delayed in nursing mothers.

Anemia: Use cautiously in those who have anemia or history of menorrhagia or hypermenorrhea. Patients experiencing menorrhagia or metrorrhagia following IUD insertion may be at risk of developing hypochromic microcytic anemia.

Syncope, bradycardia or other neurovascular episodes may occur during insertion or removal, especially in patients previously disposed to these conditions or cervical stenosis.

Valvular or congenital heart disease patients are more prone to develop subacute bacterial endocarditis. The use of the IUD may represent a potential source of septic emboli.

Reexamine patient shortly after the first postinsertion menses, since an IUD may be expelled or displaced, but definitely within 3 months after insertion. Thereafter, perform an annual examination.

Replace the device every 12 months, since the level of contraceptive efficacy after this time decreases.

Remove the device for the following reasons: Menorrhagia/metrorrhagia-producing anemia; pelvic infection; endometritis; genital actinomycosis; intractable pelvic pain; dyspareunia; pregnancy; endometrial or cervical malignancy; uterine or cervical perforation; increase of length of the threads extending from the cervix or any other indication of partial expulsion. If retrieval threads are not visible, they may have retracted into the uterus or have been broken; therefore, consider the system displaced and remove. After menstrual period, determine that the threads still protrude from the cervix. Caution patients not to pull on the threads. If partial expulsion occurs, removal is indicated and a new system may be inserted.

Bleeding and cramps may occur during the first few weeks after insertion; if symptoms continue or are severe, consult physician.

INTRAUTERINE PROGESTERONE CONTRACEPTIVE SYSTEM

Prophylactic antibiotics may be considered prior to IUD insertion to decrease the risk of PID; however, the utility of this treatment is still under evaluation. Regimens include doxycycline 200 mg orally 1 hour before insertion or erythromycin 500 mg orally 1 hour before and 6 hours after insertion.

Drug Interactions:

Anticoagulants: Use IUDs with caution in patients receiving anticoagulants or having a coagulopathy.

Adverse Reactions:

Endometritis; spontaneous abortion; septic abortion; septicemia; perforation of uterus and cervix; pelvic infection; cervical erosion; vaginitis; leukorrhea; pregnancy; ectopic pregnancy; uterine embedment; difficult removal; complete or partial expulsion; intermenstrual spotting; prolongation of menstrual flow; anemia; amenorrhea or delayed menses; pain and cramping; dysmenorrhea; backaches; dyspareunia; neurovascular episodes including bradycardia and syncope secondary to insertion; fragmentation of IUD; tubo-ovarian abscess; tubal damage; fetal damage and congenital anomalies. Perforation into the abdomen followed by peritonitis, abdominal adhesions, intestinal penetration, intestinal obstruction, local inflammatory reaction, abscess formation and erosion of adjacent viscera, and cystic masses in the pelvis have occurred. Some of these adverse reactions can lead to loss of fertility, partial or total removal of reproductive organs, hormonal imbalance or death.

Patient Information:

Patient package insert and patient instructions available with product. The patient must read and initial each section of the Patient Information Leaflet, and the Informed Choice Statement must be signed by the patient and by the physician.

Notify physician if any of the following occurs: Abnormal or excessive bleeding; severe cramping; abnormal or odorous vaginal discharge; fever or flu-like syndrome; pain; genital lesions or sores; missed period.

Administration and Dosage:

Insert a single system into the uterine cavity. Contraceptive effectiveness is retained for 1 year, and the system must be replaced 1 year after insertion. See manufacturer's literature for insertion and removal instructions.

Rx	**Progestasert** (Alza)	**Intrauterine System:** T-shaped unit containing a reservoir of 38 mg progesterone with barium sulfate dispersed in medical grade silicone fluid.	In 6s w/inserters.

MEDROXYPROGESTERONE ACETATE

Medroxyprogesterone is also used for secondary amenorrhea and abnormal uterine bleeding (see the Progestins monograph) and as an antineoplastic (see monograph in Antineoplastics chapter).

Actions:

Pharmacology: Medroxyprogesterone, when administered IM at the recommended dose to women every 3 months, inhibits the secretion of gonadotropins which, in turn, prevents follicular maturation and ovulation and results in endometrial thinning. These actions produce its contraceptive effect.

Pharmacokinetics: Following a single 150 mg IM dose, medroxyprogesterone concentrations increase for approximately 3 weeks to reach peak plasma concentrations of 1 to 7 ng/ml. The levels then decrease exponentially until they become undetectable (< 100 pg/ml) between 120 to 200 days following injection. The apparent half-life following IM administration is approximately 50 days.

Women with lower body weights conceive sooner than women with higher body weights after discontinuing medroxyprogesterone.

The effect of hepatic or renal disease on the pharmacokinetics of medroxyprogesterone is unknown.

Clinical trials: In five clinical studies the 12 month failure rate for the group of women treated with medroxyprogesterone was 0 (no pregnancies reported) to 0.7 by Life-Table method. Pregnancy rates with contraceptive measures are typically reported for only the first year of use. The effectiveness of medroxyprogesterone is dependent on the patient returning every 3 months for re-injection.

Indications:

Prevention of pregnancy. It is a long-term injectable contraceptive in women when administered at 3 month intervals.

Contraindications:

Known or suspected pregnancy or as a diagnostic test for pregnancy; undiagnosed vaginal bleeding; known or suspected malignancy of breast; active thrombophlebitis, or current or past history of thromboembolic disorders, or cerebral vascular disease; liver dysfunction or disease; hypersensitivity to medroxyprogesterone or any of its other ingredients.

Warnings:

Bleeding irregularities: Most women using medroxyprogesterone experience disruption of menstrual bleeding patterns. Altered menstrual bleeding patterns include irregular or unpredictable bleeding or spotting, or rarely, heavy or continuous bleeding. If abnormal bleeding persists or is severe, institute appropriate investigation to rule out the possibility of organic pathology, and institute appropriate treatment when necessary.

As women continue using medroxyprogesterone, fewer experience intermenstrual bleeding and more experience amenorrhea. By month 12 amenorrhea was reported by 57% of women, and by month 24 amenorrhea was reported by 68% of women.

Bone mineral density changes: Use of medroxyprogesterone may be considered among the risk factors for development of osteoporosis. The rate of bone loss is greatest in the early years of use and then subsequently approaches the normal rate of age-related fall.

Thromboembolic disorders: Be alert to the earliest manifestations of thrombotic disorders (thrombophlebitis, pulmonary embolism, cerebrovascular disorders and retinal thrombosis). If any of these occur or are suspected, do not readminister the drug.

Ocular disorders: Do not readminister pending examination if there is a sudden partial or complete loss of vision or if there is a sudden onset of proptosis, diplopia or migraine. If examination reveals papilledema or retinal vascular lesions, do not readminister.

Carcinogenesis: Long-term case-controlled surveillance of users found slight or no increased overall risk of breast cancer and no overall increased risk of ovarian, liver or cervical cancer and a prolonged, protective effect of reducing the risk of endometrial cancer in the population of users.

An increased relative risk of 2.19 of breast cancer has been associated with the use of medroxyprogesterone in women whose first exposure to the drug was within the previous 4 years and who were < 35 years of age. However, the overall relative risk for ever-users was only 1.2.

A statistically insignificant increase in relative risk estimates of invasive squamous cell cervical cancer has been associated with the use of medroxyprogesterone in women who were first exposed before the age of 35 years.

MEDROXYPROGESTERONE ACETATE

Pregnancy: Category X. Infants from accidental pregnancies that occur 1 to 2 months after injection of medroxyprogesterone may be at an increased risk of low birth weight, which in turn is associated with an increased risk of neonatal death. The attributable risk is low because such pregnancies are uncommon.

A significant increase in incidence of polysyndactyly and chromosomal anomalies was observed among infants of medroxyprogesterone users, the former being most pronounced in women < 30 years of age. The unrelated nature of these defects, the lack of confirmation from other studies, the distant preconceptual exposure to medroxyprogesterone, and the chance effects due to multiple statistical comparisons, make a causal association unlikely.

Children exposed to medroxyprogesterone in utero and followed to adolescence showed no evidence of any adverse effects on their health including their physical, intellectual, sexual or social development.

Several reports suggest an association between intrauterine exposure to progestational drugs in the first trimester of pregnancy and genital abnormalities in male and female fetuses. The risk of hypospadias (5 to 8 per 1000 male births in the general population) may be approximately doubled with exposure to these drugs. There are insufficient data to quantify the risk to exposed female fetuses, but because some of these drugs induce mild virilization of the external genitalia of the female fetus and because of the increased association of hypospadias in the male fetus, it is prudent to avoid the use of these drugs during the first trimester of pregnancy.

To ensure that medroxyprogesterone is not administered inadvertently to a pregnant woman, it is important that the first injection be given only during the first 5 days after the onset of a normal menstrual period, within 5 days postpartum if not breastfeeding and at the sixth week postpartum if breastfeeding (see Administration and Dosage).

Ectopic pregnancy – Be alert to the possibility of an ectopic pregnancy among women using medroxyprogesterone who become pregnant or complain of severe abdominal pain.

Lactation: Detectable amounts of the drug have been identified in the milk of mothers receiving medroxyprogesterone. In nursing mothers treated with medroxyprogesterone, milk composition, quality and amount are not adversely affected. Infants exposed to medroxyprogesterone via breast milk have been studied for developmental and behavioral effects through puberty; no adverse effects have been noted.

Precautions:

Physical examination: The pretreatment and annual history and physical examination should include special reference to breast and pelvic organs, as well as a Papanicolaou smear.

Fluid retention: Because progestational drugs may cause some degree of fluid retention, conditions that might be influenced by this condition (eg, epilepsy, migraine, asthma, cardiac or renal dysfunction) require careful observation.

Weight changes: There is a tendency for women to gain weight while on medroxyprogesterone therapy. From an initial average body weight of 136 lbs, women who completed 1 year of therapy gained an average of 5.4 lbs, women who completed 2 years of therapy gained an average of 8.1 lbs, women who completed 4 years gained an average of 13.8 lbs and women who completed 6 years gained an average of 16.5 lbs. Two percent of women withdrew from a large-scale clinical trial because of excessive weight gain.

Return of fertility: Medroxyprogesterone has a prolonged contraceptive effect. It is expected that 68% of women who do become pregnant may conceive within 12 months, 83% may conceive within 15 months and 93% may conceive within 18 months from the last injection. The median time to conception for those who do conceive is 10 months following the last injection with a range of 4 to 31 months, and is unrelated to the duration of use.

CNS disorders and convulsions: Carefully observe patients who have a history of psychic depression; do not readminister if the depression recurs.

There have been a few reported cases of convulsions. Association with drug use or preexisting conditions is not clear.

Carbohydrate metabolism: A decrease in glucose tolerance has been observed in some patients. The mechanism of this decrease is obscure. For this reason, carefully observe diabetic patients during therapy.

Liver function: If jaundice develops, consider not readministering the drug.

Drug Interactions:

Aminoglutethimide may significantly depress the serum concentrations of medroxyprogesterone. Warn users of the possibility of decreased efficacy with the use of this or any related drugs.

MEDROXYPROGESTERONE ACETATE

Drug/Lab test interactions: The following laboratory tests may be affected by medroxyprogesterone: Plasma and urinary steroid levels are decreased (eg, progesterone, estradiol, pregnanediol, testosterone, cortisol); gonadotropin levels are decreased; sex-hormone binding globulin concentrations are decreased; protein bound iodine and butanol extractable protein bound iodine may increase; T_3 uptake values may decrease; coagulation test values for prothrombin (Factor II), and Factors VII, VIII, IX, and X may increase. Sulfobromophthalein and other liver function test values may be increased; the effects of medroxyprogesterone acetate on lipid metabolism are inconsistent. Both increases and decreases in total cholesterol, triglycerides, low-density lipoprotein (LDL) cholesterol, and high-density lipoprotein (HDL) cholesterol have been observed.

Adverse Reactions:

Menstrual irregularities (bleeding or amenorrhea), weight changes, headache, nervousness, abdominal pain or discomfort, asthenia (weakness or fatigue), dizziness (> 5%); decreased libido or anorgasmia, backache, leg cramps, depression, nausea, insomnia, leukorrhea, acne, vaginitis, pelvic pain, breast pain, no hair growth or alopecia, bloating, rash, edema, hot flashes, arthralgia (1% to 5%); galactorrhea, melasma, chloasma, convulsions, changes in appetite, GI disturbances, jaundice, GU infections, vaginal cysts, dyspareunia, paresthesia, chest pain, pulmonary embolus, allergic reactions, anemia, drowsiness, syncope, dyspnea, asthma, tachycardia, fever, excessive sweating and body odor, dry skin, chills, increased libido, excessive thirst, hoarseness, pain at injection site, blood dyscrasia, rectal bleeding, changes in breast size, breast lumps or nipple bleeding, axillary swelling, breast cancer, prevention of lactation, sensation of pregnancy, lack of return to fertility, paralysis, facial palsy, scleroderma, osteoporosis, uterine hyperplasia, cervical cancer, varicose veins, dysmenorrhea, hirsutism, accidental pregnancy, thrombophlebitis, deep vein thrombosis (< 1%).

Patient Information:

Patient labeling is included with each single dose vial. Give prospective users this labeling and inform them about the risks and benefits associated with the use of medroxyprogesterone, as compared with other forms of contraception or with no contraception at all.

Advise patients at the beginning of treatment that their menstrual cycle may be disrupted and that irregular and unpredictable bleeding or spotting results, and that this usually decreases to the point of amenorrhea as treatment continues, without other therapy being required.

Administration and Dosage:

Shake the vial vigorously just before use to ensure that the dose being administered represents a uniform suspension.

The recommended dose is 150 mg every 3 months administered by deep IM injection in the gluteal or deltoid muscle. To increase assurance that the patient is not pregnant at the time of the first administration, give this injection only during the first 5 days after the onset of a normal menstrual period; within 5 days postpartum if not breastfeeding; or, if breastfeeding, at 6 weeks postpartum. If the period between injections is > 14 weeks, determine that the patient is not pregnant before administering the drug.

Rx	**Depo-Provera** (Upjohn)	**Injection:** 150 mg/ml	In 1 ml vials.[1]

[1] With 28.9 mg PEG 3350, 2.41 mg polysorbate 80, 8.68 mg sodium chloride, 1.37 mg methylparaben and 0.15 mg propylparaben.

ANDROGENS

An androgenic agent used in the therapy of carcinoma of the breast is listed under Antineoplastic Agents: Testolactone. (See individual monograph.) Effective February 27, 1991, this agent was switched to a *c-iii* status by the DEA because of its abuse potential.

Actions:

Pharmacology: Testosterone, produced by the Leydig cells of the testis, is the primary natural androgen. In women, small amounts are synthesized by the ovary and adrenal cortex. Fluoxymesterone and methyltestosterone are synthetic derivatives of testosterone which have predominant anabolic and minor androgenic activity. Esterification (enanthate and propionate) prolongs the duration of action as the esters are hydrolyzed in vivo to free testosterone. Alkylation (methyltestosterone and fluoxymesterone) and halogenation at position 9 (fluoxymesterone) increase the pharmacologic activity per unit weight compared to oral testosterone.

In many tissues, the activity of testosterone appears to depend on reduction to dihydrotestosterone, which binds to cytosol receptor proteins. The steroid-receptor complex is transported to the nucleus where it initiates transcription events and cellular changes related to androgen action.

Endogenous androgens are responsible for the normal growth and development of the male sex organs and for maintenance of secondary sex characteristics. These effects include the growth and maturation of the prostate, seminal vesicles, penis and scrotum; the development of male hair distribution, such as beard, pubic, chest and axillary hair; laryngeal enlargement; vocal cord thickening; alterations in body musculature and fat distribution. These drugs also cause retention of nitrogen, sodium, potassium, phosphorus and decreased urinary excretion of calcium. The anabolic effects of androgens increase protein anabolism and decrease protein catabolism. Nitrogen balance is improved only when there is sufficient intake of calories and protein.

Androgens are responsible for the growth spurt of adolescence and for the termination of linear growth by fusion of the epiphyseal growth centers. In children, exogenous androgens accelerate linear growth rates, but may cause a disproportionate advancement in bone maturation. Use over long periods may result in fusion of the epiphyseal growth centers and termination of growth process. Androgens have been reported to stimulate production of red blood cells by enhancing production of erythropoietic stimulating factor.

During administration of exogenous androgens, endogenous testosterone release is inhibited through feedback inhibition of pituitary luteinizing hormone (LH). Large doses of exogenous androgens may suppress spermatogenesis through feedback inhibition of pituitary follicle stimulating hormone (FSH).

Pharmacokinetics:

Absorption –

Oral: Testosterone is metabolized by the gut and 44% is cleared by the liver in the first pass. Doses as high as 400 mg/day are needed to achieve clinically effective blood levels for full replacement therapy. The synthetic androgens (methyltestosterone and fluoxymesterone) are less extensively metabolized by the liver and have longer half-lives. They are more suitable than testosterone for oral administration. Buccal administration permits methyltestosterone to be absorbed directly into the systemic venous return so that the unmetabolized hormone is carried directly into the tissues. The buccal tablets have approximately twice the potency of oral methyltestosterone; peak serum concentrations are attained about 1 hour after buccal and 2 hours after oral administration.

IM: Testosterone esters are less polar than free testosterone. Testosterone esters in oil injected IM are absorbed slowly from the lipid phase; thus, testosterone cypionate and enanthate can be given at intervals of 2 to 4 weeks. Suspensions of testosterone or its esters in aqueous media may cause local irritation and the rate of absorption is not always uniform.

Distribution – Testosterone in plasma is about 98% bound to a specific testosterone-estradiol binding globulin. Generally, the amount of binding globulin will determine the percentage of free and bound testosterone; the free testosterone concentration will determine its half-life. There are considerable variations in the reported half-life of testosterone, ranging from 10 to 100 minutes. The half-life of testosterone cypionate IM is approximately 8 days; for oral fluoxymesterone, it is ≈ 9.2 hours; and for methyltestosterone it is 2.5 to 3 hours.

Metabolism/Excretion – Inactivation of testosterone occurs primarily in the liver. About 90% of a testosterone dose is excreted in the urine as conjugates of testosterone and its metabolites; about 6% of a dose is excreted in the feces.

ANDROGENS

Indications:

Males: For replacement therapy in hypogonadism associated with a deficiency or absence of endogenous testosterone. Prior to puberty, androgen replacement therapy is needed for development of secondary sexual characteristics. Prolonged treatment is required to maintain sexual characteristics in these and other males who develop testosterone deficiency after puberty. Appropriate adrenal cortical and thyroid hormone replacement therapy are still necessary, however, and are of primary importance.

Primary hypogonadism (congenital or acquired) – Testicular failure due to cryptorchidism, bilateral torsion, orchitis, vanishing testis syndrome or orchidectomy.

Hypogonadotropic hypogonadism (congenital or acquired) – Idiopathic gonadotropin or luteinizing hormone releasing hormone (LHRH) deficiency or pituitary-hypothalamic injury from tumors, trauma or radiation.

Delayed puberty – To stimulate puberty in carefully selected males with clearly delayed puberty. These patients usually have a familial pattern of delayed puberty that is not secondary to a pathological disorder; puberty is expected to occur spontaneously at a relatively late date. Brief treatment with conservative doses may be justified if these patients do not respond to psychological support. Discuss the potential adverse effect on bone maturation with the patient and parents prior to androgen administration. To assess the effect of treatment on the epiphyseal centers, obtain an x-ray of the hand and wrist to determine bone age every 6 months.

Impotence and male climacteric symptoms (methyltestosterone) – For treatment when conditions are secondary to androgen deficiency.

Females:

Metastatic cancer – May be used secondarily in women with advancing inoperable metastatic (skeletal) breast cancer who are 1 to 5 years postmenopausal. Primary goals of therapy include ablation of the ovaries. This treatment has been used in premenopausal women with breast cancer who have benefited from oophorectomy and have a hormone-responsive tumor.

Postpartum breast pain/engorgement – Androgens (methyltestosterone, fluoxymesterone and testosterone propionate) have been used for the management of postpartum breast pain and engorgement, but there is no satisfactory evidence that they prevent or suppress lactation.

Androgens are not effective (lack of substantial evidence) in treating fractures or managing surgery, convalescence or functional uterine bleeding or enhancement of athletic performance (see Warnings).

Unlabeled uses: In one study, weekly injections of testosterone enanthate 200 mg maintained safe, stable, effective and reversible contraception for at least 12 months in healthy fertile men rendered azoospermic.

A transdermal formulation of testosterone has been studied and may be an effective alternative to injections as a means of treating primary hypogonadism.

Contraindications:

Patients with serious cardiac, hepatic or renal diseases; hypersensitivity to the drug; in men with carcinomas of the breast or prostate; pregnancy (see Warnings); sensitivity/allergy to mercury compounds (*Histerone*).

Warnings:

Athletic performance: Although the anabolic steroids are generally the agents that are abused for enhancement of athletic performance, these agents have also been used for such purposes. However, these drugs are not safe and effective for this use and have a potential risk of serious side effects.

Product interchange: Do not use testosterone cypionate interchangeably with testosterone propionate because of differences in duration of action.

Breast cancer and immobilized patients: Androgen therapy may cause hypercalcemia by stimulating osteolysis. In cancer patients, hypercalcemia may indicate progression of bony metastasis. If hypercalcemia occurs, discontinue the drug.

Hepatic effects: Prolonged use of high doses of androgens has been associated with the development of potentially life-threatening peliosis hepatis, hepatic neoplasms and hepatocellular carcinoma.

Cholestatic hepatitis and jaundice occur with fluoxymesterone and methyltestosterone at relatively low doses. If cholestatic hepatitis with jaundice appears with use of any androgen, or if liver function tests become abnormal, discontinue the androgen and determine the etiology. Drug-induced jaundice is reversible when the medication is discontinued.

Oligospermia and reduced ejaculatory volume may occur after prolonged administration or excessive dosage.

ANDROGENS

Edema, with or without congestive heart failure, may be a serious complication in patients with preexisting cardiac, renal or hepatic disease. Use with caution in epilepsy, migraine or other conditions that may be aggravated by fluid retention. In addition to discontinuation of the drug, diuretic therapy may be required. If the administration of testosterone enanthate is restarted, use a lower dose.

Gynecomastia frequently develops and occasionally persists in patients being treated for hypogonadism. Use with caution in patients with preexisting gynecomastia.

Bone maturation: Use cautiously in healthy males with delayed puberty. Monitor bone maturation by assessing bone age of the wrist and hand every 6 months.

Carcinogenesis: Testosterone has induced cervical-uterine tumors in mice; these tumors metastasized in some cases. Injection of testosterone into some strains of female mice may increase their susceptibility to hepatoma. There are rare reports of hepatocellular carcinoma in patients receiving long-term therapy with androgens in high doses. Drug withdrawal did not lead to tumor regression in all cases.

Elderly: Elderly males treated with androgens may be at an increased risk of developing prostatic hypertrophy and prostatic carcinoma. Marked increase in libido may occur.

Pregnancy: Category X. Androgens are contraindicated in women who are or who may become pregnant. They cause virilization of the external genitalia of the female fetus (eg, clitoromegaly, abnormal vaginal development and fusion of genital folds to form a scrotal-like structure). The degree of masculinization is related to the amount of drug given and the age of the fetus. Masculinization is most likely to occur in the female fetus when androgens are given in the first trimester. If the patient becomes pregnant while taking these drugs, apprise her of the potential hazards to the fetus.

Lactation: It is not known whether androgens are excreted in breast milk. Decide whether to discontinue nursing or to discontinue the drug, taking into account the importance of the drug to the mother.

Children: Use androgens very cautiously in children; the drugs should only be given by specialists who are aware of the adverse effects on bone maturation.

Androgens may accelerate bone maturation without producing compensatory gain in linear growth. This adverse effect may result in compromised adult stature. The younger the child, the greater the risk of compromising final mature height.

Benzyl alcohol-containing products have been associated with a fatal "gasping syndrome" in premature infants. Refer to product listings.

Precautions:

Monitoring: Frequently determine urine and serum calcium levels during the course of therapy in women with disseminated breast carcinoma.

Because of the hepatotoxicity associated with the use of methyltestosterone and fluoxymesterone, periodically perform liver function tests.

Make periodic (every 6 months) x-ray examinations of bone age during treatment of prepubertal males to determine the rate of bone maturation and the effects of the androgen therapy on the epiphyseal centers.

Check hemoglobin and hematocrit periodically for polycythemia in patients who are receiving high doses of androgens.

Virilization: Observe women for signs of virilization (deepening voice, hirsutism, acne, clitoromegaly and menstrual irregularities). Discontinue therapy at the time of evidence of mild virilism to prevent irreversible virilization. Virilization is usual following high-dose androgens and is not prevented by concomitant use of estrogens. Some virilization should be tolerated during treatment for breast carcinoma.

Patients with benign prostatic hypertrophy may develop acute urethral obstruction. Priapism or excessive sexual stimulation may develop. Oligospermia may occur after prolonged administration or excessive dosage. If any of these effects appear, stop administration. If restarted, use a lower dosage. Avoid stimulation to the point of increasing nervous, mental and physical activities beyond the patient's cardiovascular capacity.

Acute intermittent porphyria: Androgens have precipitated attacks of acute intermittent porphyria; use cautiously in patients known to have this condition.

Hypercholesterolemia: Serum cholesterol may be altered during therapy; use caution in patients with a history of myocardial infarction or coronary artery disease. Perform serial determinations of serum cholesterol and adjust therapy accordingly.

Tartrazine sensitivity: Some of these products contain tartrazine, which may cause allergic-type reactions (including bronchial asthma) in susceptible individuals. Although the incidence of tartrazine sensitivity in the general population is low, it is frequently seen in patients who also have aspirin hypersensitivity. Specific products containing tartrazine are identified in the product listings.

ANDROGENS

Drug Interactions:

Anticoagulants: The anticoagulant effect may be potentiated by 17-alkyl testosterone derivatives (eg, fluoxymesterone, methyltestosterone). Although the non-17-alkylated agent (testosterone) appears safer, at least one case report described a similar interaction. Avoid the combination with 17-alkyl derivatives if possible.

Imipramine: Coadministration with methyltestosterone resulted in a dramatic paranoid response in four of five patients.

Drug/Lab test interactions:

Thyroid function tests – Decreased levels of thyroxine-binding globulin, resulting in decreased total T_4 serum levels and increased resin uptake of T_3 and T_4. Free thyroid hormone levels remain unchanged, and there is no clinical evidence of thyroid dysfunction.

Adverse Reactions:

Female:

Most common – Amenorrhea and other menstrual irregularities; inhibition of gonadotropin secretion and virilization, including deepening voice and clitoral enlargement. The latter usually is not reversible after androgens are discontinued. When administered to a pregnant woman, androgens cause virilization of external genitalia of the female fetus.

Male: Gynecomastia; excessive frequency and duration of penile erections; decreased ejaculatory volume. Oligospermia may occur at high dosages.

Body as a whole: Inflammation and pain at the site of IM injection; stomatitis with buccal preparations; increased serum cholesterol.

CNS: Increased or decreased libido; headache; anxiety; depression; generalized paresthesia; sleep apnea syndrome.

Electrolyte Disturbance: Retention of sodium, chloride, water, potassium, calcium and inorganic phosphates. Hypercalcemia may occur, particularly in immobile patients and in those patients with metastatic breast carcinoma.

GI: Nausea; cholestatic jaundice; alterations in liver function tests; rarely, hepatocellular neoplasms, peliosis hepatis.

Hematologic: Suppression of clotting factors II, V, VII and X; polycythemia.

Hypersensitivity: Skin manifestations; rarely, anaphylactoid reactions; rash.

Skin and appendages: Hirsutism; male pattern baldness; acne; seborrhea.

Patient Information:

Oral tablets: May cause GI upset.

Buccal tablets: Do not swallow; allow to dissolve between the gum and cheek; avoid eating, drinking or smoking while tablet is in place.

Notify physician if nausea, vomiting, swelling of the extremities (edema), priapism or jaundice occurs.

Females: Notify physician if hoarseness, deepening of the voice, male-pattern baldness, hirsutism, acne or menstrual irregularities occur.

TESTOSTERONE, SHORT-ACTING

For complete prescribing information, refer to the Androgens group monograph.

Administration and Dosage:

For IM use only. Administer deep in the gluteal muscle. Do not inject IV. Shake well.

Suggested dosage for androgens varies depending on age, sex and diagnosis of the patient. Adjust dosage according to response and appearance of adverse reactions.

Androgen replacement therapy: The guideline dose is 25 to 50 mg 2 to 3 times weekly.

Delayed puberty: Dosages are generally in the lower ranges and for a limited duration (eg, 4 to 6 months). Various regimens have been used to induce pubertal changes in hypogonadal males. Some experts advocate lower initial doses, gradually increasing the dose as puberty progresses, with or without a decrease to maintenance levels. Other experts emphasize that higher dosages are needed to induce pubertal changes and lower dosages can be used for maintenance after puberty. Consider the chronological and skeletal ages when determining initial dose and adjusting dose.

Other suggested doses are as follows (injection in oil):

Growth stimulation in Turner syndrome or constitutional delay of puberty – 40 to 50 mg/m^2/dose monthly for 6 months.

Male hypogonadism – Initiation of pubertal growth, 40 to 50 mg/m^2/dose monthly until the growth rate falls to prepubertal levels (approximately 5 cm/year); during terminal growth phase, 100 mg/m^2/dose monthly until growth ceases; maintenance virilizing dose, 100 mg/m^2/dose twice monthly or 50 to 400 mg/dose every 2 to 4 weeks.

Palliation of mammary cancer – Usual dose is 50 to 100 mg 3 times a week. Follow women with metastatic breast carcinoma closely because androgen therapy occasionally appears to accelerate the disease. Thus, many experts prefer to use the shorter-acting androgen preparations rather than those with prolonged activity for treating breast carcinoma, particularly during the early stages of androgen therapy.

Postpartum breast engorgement (testosterone propionate): 25 to 50 mg for 3 to 4 days, starting at the time of delivery.

TESTOSTERONE (IN AQUEOUS SUSPENSION)

For complete prescribing information, refer to the Testosterone, Short-Acting monograph.

c-iii	**Testosterone Aqueous** (Various)	**Injection**: 25 mg per ml	In 10 ml vials.
c-iii	**Testosterone Aqueous** (Various)	**Injection**: 50 mg per ml	In 10 and 30 ml vials.
c-iii	**Testosterone Aqueous** (Various, eg, Goldline)	**Injection**: 100 mg per ml	In 10 ml vials.
c-iii	**Testandro** (Redur Co.)		In 10 ml vials.[1]
c-iii	**Histerone 100** (Roberts Hauck)		In 10 ml vials.[1]
c-iii	**Tesamone** (Dunhall)		In 10 ml vials.[1]

[1] With sodium carboxymethylcellulose, methylcellulose, povidone, DSS and thimerosal.

TESTOSTERONE PROPIONATE (IN OIL)

For complete prescribing information, refer to the Testosterone, Short-Acting monograph.

c-iii	**Testosterone Propionate** (Various, eg, Geneva, Goldline, Schein, Steris)	**Injection**: 100 mg per ml	In 10 ml vials.

TESTOSTERONE, LONG-ACTING

For complete prescribing information, refer to the Androgens group monograph.

The enanthate and cypionate esters provide therapeutic effects for about 4 weeks.

Administration and Dosage:

For IM use only. Individualize dosage. In general, more than 400 mg/month is not required because of the prolonged action of the preparation.

Male hypogonadism:

Replacement therapy (eunuchism) – 50 to 400 mg every 2 to 4 weeks.

Males with delayed puberty: 50 to 200 mg every 2 to 4 weeks for a limited duration.

Palliation of inoperable breast cancer in women: 200 to 400 mg every 2 to 4 weeks. Androgen therapy occasionally appears to accelerate metastatic breast carcinoma.

NOTE: Use of a wet needle or wet syringe may cause the solution to become cloudy; however, this does not affect the potency of the material.

Storage: Warming and shaking vial redissolves crystals that may have formed.

TESTOSTERONE ENANTHATE (IN OIL)

For complete prescribing information, refer to the Testostrone, Long-Acting monograph.

c-III	**Testosterone Enanthate** (Various, eg, Schein, Steris)	**Injection:** 100 mg per ml	In 10 ml vials.
c-III	**Testosterone Enanthate** (Various, eg, Geneva, Schein, Steris)	**Injection:** 200 mg per ml	In 10 ml vials.
c-III	**Andro L.A. 200** (Forest)		In 10 ml vials.[1]
c-III	**Andropository-200** (Rugby)		In 10 ml vials.
c-III	**Delatestryl** (BioTechnology General)		In 5 ml vials and 1 ml single dose syringes.[1]
c-III	**Durathate-200** (Roberts Hauck)		In 10 ml vials.[1]
c-III	**Everone 200** (Hyrex)		In 10 ml vials.[1]

[1] In sesame oil with chlorobutanol.

TESTOSTERONE CYPIONATE (IN OIL)

For complete prescribing information, refer to the Testosterone, Long-Acting monograph.

c-III	**Testosterone Cypionate** (Various, eg, Geneva, Goldline, Keene, Schein, Steris)	**Injection:** 100 mg per ml	In 10 ml vials.
c-III	**depAndro 100** (Forest)		In 10 ml vials.[1]
c-III	**Depotest 100** (Hyrex)		In 10 ml vials.[1]
c-III	**Depo-Testosterone** (Upjohn)		In 10 ml vials.[2]
c-III	**Duratest-100** (Roberts Hauck)		In 10 ml vials.[1]
c-III	**Testosterone Cypionate** (Various, eg, Geneva, Goldline, Keene, Schein, Steris)	**Injection:** 200 mg per ml	In 10 ml vials.
c-III	**depAndro 200** (Forest)		In 10 ml vials.[2]
c-III	**Depotest 200** (Hyrex)		In 10 ml vials.[2]
c-III	**Depo-Testosterone** (Upjohn)		In 1 and 10 ml vials.[2]
c-III	**Duratest-200** (Roberts Hauck)		In 10 ml vials.[2]

[2] In cottonseed oil with benzyl alcohol.

[3] In cottonseed oil with benzyl benzoate and benzyl alcohol.

TESTOSTERONE TRANSDERMAL SYSTEM

For complete prescribing information, refer to the Androgens group monograph.

Actions:

Pharmacology:

Testoderm – Following placement of *Testoderm* on scrotal skin, the serum testosterone concentration rises to a maximum at 2 to 4 hours and returns toward baseline within approximately 2 hours after system removal. Serum levels reach a plateau at 3 to 4 weeks. The testosterone levels achieved with *Testoderm* generally are within the range for normal men.

Scrotal skin is at least five times more permeable to testosterone than other skin sites. *Testoderm* will not produce adequate serum testosterone concentration if it is applied to nongenital skin.

Androderm – Following application to non-scrotal skin, testosterone is continuously absorbed during the 24 hour dosing period. Daily application of 2 systems at approximately 10:00 p.m. results in a serum testosterone concentration profile that mimics the normal circadian variation observed in healthy young men. Maximum concentrations occur in the early morning hours with minimum concentrations in the evening.

Indications:

Replacement therapy in males for conditions associated with a deficiency or absence of endogenous testosterone.

Primary hypogonadism (congenital or acquired) – Testicular failure due to cryptorchidism, bilateral torsion, orchitis, vanishing testis syndrome, orchidectomy, Klinefelter's syndrome, chemotherapy or toxic damage from alcohol or heavy metals. These men usually have low serum testosterone levels and gonadotropins (FSH, LH) above the normal range.

Secondary hypogonadotropic hypogonadism (congenital or acquired) – Idiopathic gonadotropin or LHRH deficiency or pituitary-hypothalamic injury from tumors, trauma or radiation. These men have low testosterone serum levels but have gonadotropins in the normal or low range.

Appropriate adrenal cortical and thyroid hormone replacement therapy may be necessary in patients with multiple pituitary or hypothalamic abnormalities.

Administration and Dosage:

Testoderm: Patients should start therapy with a 6 mg/day system applied daily; if scrotal area is inadequate, use a 4 mg/day system. Place the patch on clean, dry, scrotal skin. Dry-shave scrotal hair for optimal skin contact. Do not use chemical depilatories. The system should be worn 22 to 24 hours.

After 3 to 4 weeks of daily system use, blood should be drawn 2 to 4 hours after system application for determination of serum total testosterone. Because of variability in analytical values among diagnostic laboratories, this laboratory work and later analyses for assessing the effect of the transdermal testosterone therapy should be performed at the same laboratory.

If patients have not achieved desired results by the end of 6 to 8 weeks of use, consider another form of testosterone replacement therapy.

Androderm: The usual starting dose is 2 systems applied nightly for 24 hours, providing a total dose of 5 mg/day.

Apply the adhesive side of the system to a clean, dry area of the skin on the back, abdomen, upper arms or thighs. Avoid bony prominences, such as the shoulder and hip areas. Do NOT apply to the scrotum. Rotate the sites of application, with an interval of 7 days between applications to the same site. The area selected should not be oily, damaged or irritated.

Apply the system immediately after opening the pouch and removing the protective release liner. Press the system firmly in place, making sure there is good contact with the skin, especially around the edges.

To ensure proper dosing, the morning serum testosterone concentration may be measured following system application the previous evening. If the serum concentration is outside the normal range, repeat sampling with assurance of proper system adhesion as well as appropriate application time. Confirmed serum concentrations outside the normal range may require increasing the dosage regimen to 3 systems, or decreasing the regimen to 1 system, maintaining nightly application. Because of variability in analytical values among diagnostic laboratories, this laboratory work and any later analysis for assessing the effect of therapy should be performed at the same laboratory so results can be more easily compared.

Non-virilized patient – Dosing may be initiated with 1 system nightly.

Storage – Do not store outside the pouch provided. Damaged systems should not be used. The drug reservoir may be burst by excessive pressure or heat. Discard systems in household trash in a manner that prevents accidental application or ingestion by children, pets or others.

TESTOSTERONE TRANSDERMAL SYSTEM

	Product/Distributor	Release rate (mg/24 hr)	Surface area (cm^2)	Total testosterone content (mg)	How Supplied
c-III	**Testoderm** (Alza)	4	40	10	In 30s.
		6	60	15	In 30s.
c-III	**Androderm** (SmithKline Beecham)	2.5	37	12.2	In 60s.

METHYLTESTOSTERONE

For complete prescribing information, refer to the Androgens group monograph.

Absorption through buccal mucosa into systemic circulation provides twice the androgenic activity of oral tablets.

Administration and Dosage:

Males:

Hypogonadism, male climacteric and impotence – 10 to 40 mg/day orally.

Androgen deficiency – 10 to 50 mg/day orally (5 to 25 mg buccal).

Postpubertal cryptorchidism – 30 mg/day orally.

Females:

Postpartum breast pain and engorgement – 80 mg/day orally for 3 to 5 days.

Breast cancer – 50 to 200 mg/day orally (25 to 100 mg buccal).

c-III	**Methyltestosterone** (Various, eg, Goldline, Major)	**Tablets**: 10 mg	In 100s and 1000s.
c-III	**Android-10** (ICN Pharm)		(BP 958). Green. In 100s.
c-III	**Oreton Methyl** (Schering)		Lactose. (Schering 311). White. In 100s.
c-III	**Methyltestosterone** (Various, eg, Goldline, Major, Rugby)	**Tablets**: 25 mg	In 100s and 1000s.
c-III	**Android-25** (ICN Pharm)		(BP 996). Yellow. In 100s.
c-III	**Methyltestosterone** (Various, eg, Goldline)	**Tablets (Buccal)**: 10 mg	In 100s.
c-III	**Oreton Methyl** (Schering)		(Schering 970). Lavender. Oval. In 100s.
c-III	**Testred** (ICN Pharm)	**Capsules**: 10 mg	(ICN 0901). Red. In 100s.
c-III	**Virilon** (Star)		(Virilon 10 mg). Black and clear. In 100s and 1000s.

FLUOXYMESTERONE

For complete prescribing information, refer to the Androgens group monograph.

Administration and Dosage:

Males:

Hypogonadism – 5 to 20 mg daily.

Females:

Inoperable breast carcinoma – 10 to 40 mg daily in divided doses. Continue for 1 month for a subjective response and 2 to 3 months for an objective response.

Prevention of postpartum breast pain and engorgement – 2.5 mg shortly after delivery. Then administer 5 to 10 mg daily in divided doses for 4 to 5 days.

c-III	**Halotestin** (Upjohn)	**Tablets**: 2 mg	Tartrazine, lactose, sucrose. (Halotestin 2). Peach, scored. In 100s.
c-III	**Halotestin** (Upjohn)	**Tablets**: 5 mg	Tartrazine, lactose, sucrose. (Upjohn 19). Lt. green, scored. In 100s.
c-III	**Fluoxymesterone** (Various, eg, Major, Parmed, Rugby)	**Tablets**: 10 mg	In 100s.
c-III	**Halotestin** (Upjohn)		Tartrazine, lactose, sucrose. (Halotestin 10). Green, scored. In 30s and 100s.

FINASTERIDE

Actions:

Pharmacology: Finasteride, a synthetic 4-azasteroid compound, is a competitive and specific inhibitor of steroid 5α-reductase, an intracellular enzyme that converts testosterone into the potent androgen 5α-dihydrotestosterone (DHT). It has no affinity for the androgen receptor. The 5α-reduced steroid metabolites in blood and urine are decreased after administration of finasteride.

Progressive enlargement of the prostate gland is often associated with urinary symptoms and a decrease in urine flow, although a precise correlation between increased gland size and symptoms has not been demonstrated. Benign prostatic hyperplasia (BPH) produces symptoms in the majority of men > 50 years of age and its prevalence increases with age.

The development of the prostate gland is dependent on the potent androgen DHT. The enzyme 5α-reductase metabolizes testosterone to DHT in the prostate gland, liver and skin. DHT induces androgenic effects by binding to androgen receptors in the cell nuclei of these organs.

A single 5 mg oral dose produces a rapid reduction in serum DHT concentration, with maximum effect observed 8 hours after the first dose. The suppression of DHT is maintained throughout the 24 hour dosing interval and with continued treatment. Daily dosing at 5 mg/day for up to 24 months reduces the serum DHT concentration by ≈ 70%. The median circulating level of testosterone increases by 10% but remains within the physiologic range.

Adult males with genetically inherited 5α-reductase deficiency also have decreased levels of DHT. Except for the associated urogenital defects present at birth, no other clinical abnormalities related to 5α-reductase deficiency have been observed in these individuals. These individuals have a small prostate gland throughout life and do not develop BPH.

In patients with BPH treated with finasteride (1 to 100 mg/day) for 7 to 10 days prior to prostatectomy, an ≈ 80% lower DHT content was measured in prostatic tissue removed at surgery compared to placebo; testosterone tissue concentration was increased up to 10 times over pretreatment levels. Intraprostatic content of prostate-specific antigen (PSA) was also decreased. In healthy male volunteers treated with finasteride for 14 days, discontinuation of therapy resulted in a return of DHT levels to pretreatment levels in ≈ 2 weeks.

In patients with BPH, finasteride had no effect on circulating levels of cortisol, estradiol, prolactin, thyroid-stimulating hormone or thyroxine, nor did it affect the plasma lipid profile. Increases of ≈ 10% were observed in luteinizing hormone (LH), follicle-stimulating hormone (FSH) and testosterone levels in patients receiving finasteride, but levels remained within the normal range. In healthy volunteers the hypothalamic-pituitary-testicular axis was not affected.

Pharmacokinetics: Finasteride is well absorbed after oral administration, with absolute bioavailability in humans of 63% (range, 34% to 108%). Following an oral dose, a mean of 39% was excreted in the urine in the form of metabolites; 57% was excreted in the feces. The major compound isolated from urine was the monocarboxylic acid metabolite; virtually no unchanged drug was recovered. The t-butyl side chain monohydroxylated metabolite has been isolated from plasma. These metabolites possess no more than 20% of the 5α-reductase inhibitory activity of finasteride. The half-life of finasteride is 4.7 to 7.1 hours.

Finasteride undergoes extensive hepatic metabolism through oxidative pathways to inactive compounds that are eliminated primarily through the bile; the mean urinary recovery of the parent drug within 24 hours of a dose was only 0.04%. In a study in 15 healthy male subjects, the mean bioavailability of a 5 mg tablet was 63%. Maximum finasteride plasma concentration averaged 37 ng/ml and was reached 1 to 2 hours postdose. The mean plasma elimination half-life was 6 hours (range, 3 to 16 hours). Following an IV infusion, mean plasma clearance was 165 ml/min and mean steady-state volume of distribution was 76 L. The bioavailability of finasteride was not affected by food. Approximately 90% is bound to plasma proteins. Finasteride crosses the blood-brain barrier.

There is a slow accumulation phase after multiple dosing. After dosing with 5 mg/day for 17 days, plasma concentrations were 47% and 54% higher than after the first dose in men 45 to 60 years old (n = 12) and ≥ 70 years old (n = 12), respectively; mean trough concentrations were 6.2 and 8.1 ng/ml, respectively. Although steady state was not reached in this study, mean trough plasma concentration in another study in patients with BPH (mean age, 65 years) receiving 5 mg/day was 9.4 ng/ml after > 1 year of dosing.

The elimination rate of finasteride is decreased in the elderly, but no dosage adjustment is necessary. The mean terminal half-life in subjects ≥ 70 years of age was ≈ 8 hours (range, 6 to 15 hours) compared to 6 hours (range, 4 to 12 hours) in subjects 45 to 60 years of age. As a result, mean AUC (0 to 24 hr) after 17 days of dosing was 15% higher in subjects ≥ 70 years of age.

FINASTERIDE

No dosage adjustment is necessary in patients with renal insufficiency. Urinary excretion of metabolites was decreased in patients with renal impairment. This decrease was associated with an increase in fecal excretion of metabolites. Plasma concentrations of metabolites were significantly higher in patients with renal impairment. However, finasteride has been well tolerated in BPH patients with normal renal function receiving up to 80 mg/day for 12 weeks where exposure of these patients to metabolites would presumably be much greater.

In 16 subjects receiving 5 mg/day, concentrations in semen ranged from undetectable (< 1 ng/ml) to 21 ng/ml. Based on a 5 ml ejaculate volume, the amount of finasteride in ejaculate was estimated to be < 1/50 of the dose of finasteride (5 mcg) that had no effect on circulating DHT levels in adults.

Clinical trials: In two double-blind, placebo controlled, 12 month studies in patients with BPH treated with 5 mg/day, statistically significant regression of the enlarged prostate gland was noted at the first evaluation at 3 months and was maintained during the studies. In both studies, the maximum urinary flow rates showed statistically significant increases from baseline in patients treated from week 2 throughout the 12 month studies.

Symptomatic improvement was also evaluated in these multicenter studies. The obstructive symptoms evaluated were hesitancy, feeling of incomplete bladder emptying, interruption of urinary stream, impairment of size and force of urinary stream and terminal urinary dribbling. The total symptom score also included straining to start urinary flow, dysuria, frequency of clothes wetting and urgency to urinate. On a scale of 0 (absence of all symptoms) to 36 (worst response for all symptoms), the mean baseline total symptom scores for the two studies were 10.1 and 10.6. From week 2 the scores of the patients treated with finasteride were numerically lower than those of placebo and remained so throughout the 12 month study.

In both of these 12 month studies, patients treated with finasteride 5 mg had progressively decreasing prostate volumes, increasing maximum urinary flow rates and improvement of BPH symptoms, suggesting an arrest in the disease process.

Indications:

Benign prostatic hyperplasia (BPH): Treatment of symptomatic BPH. There is a rapid regression of the enlarged prostate gland in most treated patients; ≈ 60% experience an increase in urinary flow and > 30% experience improvement in symptoms of BPH.

Unlabeled uses: Finasteride is being investigated as adjuvant monotherapy following radical prostatectomy. Other potential uses include prevention of the progression of first-stage prostate cancer, treatment of male pattern baldness, acne and hirsutism; however, studies are needed to assess these uses.

Contraindications:

Hypersensitivity to finasteride or any component of this product; pregnancy, lactation, children (see Warnings).

Warnings:

Duration of therapy: A minimum of 6 months of treatment may be necessary to determine whether an individual will respond to finasteride. It is not possible to identify prospectively those patients who will respond.

Patient evaluation: Prior to initiating therapy, perform appropriate evaluation to identify other conditions that might mimic BPH, such as infection, prostate cancer, stricture disease, hypotonic bladder or other neurogenic disorders.

Hepatic function impairment: Use caution in those patients with liver function abnormalities since finasteride is metabolized extensively in the liver.

Pregnancy: Category X. In female rats, low doses of finasteride administered during pregnancy have produced abnormalities of the external genitalia in male offspring. Finasteride is contraindicated in women who are or may become pregnant. Because of the ability of 5α-reductase inhibitors to inhibit the conversion of testosterone to DHT, finasteride may cause abnormalities of the external genitalia of a male fetus of a pregnant woman who receives finasteride. If this drug is used during pregnancy, or if pregnancy occurs while taking this drug, apprise the woman of the potential hazard to the male fetus.

It is not known whether the amount of finasteride that could potentially be absorbed by a pregnant woman through either direct contact with crushed finasteride tablets or from the semen of a patient taking finasteride can adversely affect a developing male fetus. Therefore, because of the potential risk to a male fetus, a woman who is pregnant or who may become pregnant should not handle crushed finasteride tablets. In addition, when the male patient's sexual partner is or may become pregnant, the patient should either avoid exposure of his partner to semen or he should discontinue finasteride.

FINASTERIDE

Lactation: It is not known whether finasteride is excreted in breast milk.

Children: Safety and efficacy have not been established.

Precautions:

Prostate cancer evaluation: Perform digital rectal examinations, as well as other evaluations for prostate cancer, on patients with BPH prior to initiating therapy and periodically thereafter. Although currently not indicated for this purpose, serum PSA is being increasingly used as one of the components of the screening process to detect prostate cancer. Generally, a baseline PSA > 10 ng/ml (*Hybritech*) prompts further evaluation and consideration of biopsy; for PSA levels between 4 and 10 ng/ml, further evaluation is generally considered advisable. A baseline PSA < 4 ng/ml does not exclude the diagnosis of prostate cancer.

Finasteride causes a decrease in serum PSA levels in patients with BPH even in the presence of prostate cancer. Consider this reduction of PSA levels when evaluating PSA laboratory data; it does not suggest a beneficial effect of finasteride on prostate cancer. In controlled clinical trials, finasteride did not appear to alter the rate of prostate cancer detection.

Carefully evaluate any sustained increases in PSA levels while on finasteride, including consideration of non-compliance to therapy.

Obstructive uropathy: As not all patients demonstrate a response to finasteride, carefully monitor patients with a large residual urinary volume or severely diminished urinary flow for obstructive uropathy. They may not be candidates for this therapy.

Drug Interactions:

Theophylline: In 12 healthy volunteers, finasteride 5 mg/day for 8 days significantly increased theophylline clearance by 7% and decreased its half-life by 10% after IV aminophylline administration. These changes were not clinically significant.

Drug/Lab test interactions: When PSA laboratory determinations are evaluated, consider the fact that PSA levels are decreased in patients treated with finasteride.

Adverse Reactions:

Finasteride is generally well tolerated; adverse reactions usually have been mild and transient. The following reactions have occurred: Impotence (3.7%); decreased libido (3.3%); decreased volume of ejaculate (2.8%); breast tenderness and enlargement; hypersensitivity reactions, including lip swelling and skin rash.

In North American and international clinical trials, 1.3% of patients were discontinued due to adverse experiences; only 1 of these patients (0.2%) discontinued therapy because of a sexual adverse experience.

Overdosage:

Patients have received single doses up to 400 mg and multiple doses up to 80 mg/day for 3 months without adverse effects.

Significant lethality was observed in male and female mice at single oral doses of 1500 mg/m^2 (500 mg/kg) and in female and male rats at single oral doses of 2360 mg/m^2 (400 mg/kg) and 5900 mg/m^2 (1000 mg/kg), respectively.

Patient Information:

Crushed finasteride tablets should not be handled by a woman who is pregnant or who may become pregnant because of the potential for absorption of finasteride and the subsequent potential risk to the male fetus. Similarly, when the male patient's sexual partner is or may become pregnant, the patient should either avoid exposure of his partner to semen or he should discontinue finasteride.

Inform patients that the volume of ejaculate may be decreased in some patients during treatment. This decrease does not appear to interfere with normal sexual function. However, impotence and decreased libido may occur.

Administration and Dosage:

Approved by the FDA on June 19, 1992.

The recommended dose is 5 mg once a day, with or without meals.

Although early improvement may be seen, at least 6 to 12 months of therapy may be necessary to assess whether a beneficial response has been achieved. Perform periodic follow-up evaluations to determine whether a clinical response has occurred.

Renal function impairment/elderly: No dosage adjustment is necessary.

Storage/Stability: Store at room temperature < 30°C (86°F). Protect from light and keep container tightly closed.

Rx	**Proscar** (Merck)	**Tablets:** 5 mg	Lactose. (MSD 72 Proscar). Blue. Film coated. Apple shape. In unit-of-use 30s and 100s and UD 100s.

ANABOLIC STEROIDS

These agents are derived from, or are closely related to, the androgen testosterone (see Androgens group monograph); they have androgenic as well as anabolic activity. Although these products possess a high-anabolic, low-androgenic activity ratio, the dissociation of anabolic from androgenic effects is incomplete and variable. Effective February 27, 1991, these agents were switched to a ***c-iii*** status by the DEA because of their abuse potential.

Warning:

Peliosis hepatis, a condition in which liver and sometimes splenic tissue is replaced with blood-filled cysts, has occurred in patients receiving androgenic anabolic steroids. These cysts, are sometimes present with minimal hepatic dysfunction, have been associated with liver failure. They are often not recognized until life-threatening liver failure or intra-abdominal hemorrhage develops. Withdrawal of drug usually results in complete disappearance of lesions.

Liver cell tumors: Most often these tumors are benign and androgen-dependent, but fatal malignant tumors have occurred. Withdrawal of drug often results in regression or cessation of tumor progression. However, hepatic tumors associated with androgens or anabolic steroids are much more vascular than other hepatic tumors and may be silent until life-threatening intra-abdominal hemorrhage develops.

Blood lipid changes associated with increased risk of atherosclerosis are seen in patients treated with androgens and anabolic steroids. These changes include decreased high-density lipoprotein and sometimes increased low-density lipoprotein. The changes may be very marked and could have a serious impact on the risk of atherosclerosis and coronary artery disease.

Actions:

Pharmacology: Anabolic steroids promote body tissue-building processes and reverse catabolic or tissue depleting processes. Administer adequate calories and protein to achieve positive nitrogen balance. Whether this balance is of primary benefit in the utilization of protein-building dietary substances is not established.

During exogenous administration of anabolic androgens, endogenous testosterone release is inhibited through inhibition of pituitary luteinizing hormone (LH). At large doses, spermatogenesis may be suppressed through feedback inhibition of pituitary follicle-stimulating hormone (FSH).

The androgenic properties of anabolic agents may cause serious disturbances of growth and sexual development when given to young children. They suppress the gonadotropic functions of the pituitary and may exert a direct effect on testes.

Indications:

Refer to individual product monographs for approved indications of specific products.

Anemia: Androgens stimulate erythropoiesis and may be of value in the treatment of certain types of anemia.

Hereditary angioedema: Prophylactic use may decrease frequency and severity of attacks.

Metastatic breast cancer: For control of metastatic breast cancer in women.

Contraindications:

Hypersensitivity to anabolic steroids; male patients with prostate or breast carcinoma; carcinoma of the breast in females with hypercalcemia; nephrosis; the nephrotic phase of nephritis; pregnancy (see Warnings); to enhance physical appearance or athletic performance (see Warnings).

Warnings:

Athletic performance is questionably modified by these agents and studies yield equivocal results. The athlete's motivation to use these steroids includes 1) increased muscle mass and strength; 2) decreased muscle recovery time allowing more frequent weight training; 3) decreased healing time after muscle injury; 4) increased aggressiveness. The increase in muscle size and weight gain is partially attributed to the increased sodium and water retention. Evidence suggests that if anabolic steroids increase lean muscle mass, the muscle tissue may be deficient in phosphate and structurally flawed. Although some athletes, previously trained in weight lifting, who continue intensive weight training and maintain a high-protein, high-calorie diet during steroid use may derive some benefit such as increased strength (due to reaching a chronic catabolic state), the serious health hazards associated with anabolic steroids minimize any real or perceived gain in performance. Effects of these agents may persist for up to 6 months after the last dose. Adverse effects may be serious and irreversible.

ANABOLIC STEROIDS

Steroid regimens used are often referred to as "stacking", "pyramiding" or "cycling". "Stacking", or "stacking the pyramid", describes the concurrent use of two or more agents at the same time, either using high doses or varying the dosage, possibly including both oral and injectable forms. This regimen is tapered upward, then downward, generally over 4 to 18 weeks, followed by a drug-free period over several months. "Pyramiding" follows the same concept but generally involves the use of a single agent. "Cycling" refers to the drug-free period which is used to aid in the preparation of an upcoming event in the hopes that the athlete will peak at the time of the contest. These regimens are used to achieve an optimal anabolic effect while minimizing side effects and detection during competition. Dosages used may be as high as 40 times the therapeutic amounts.

An abuse or addiction syndrome is now being recognized with the chronic use of these drugs. Long-term use can lead to a preoccupation with drug use, difficulty stopping despite side effects and drug craving. A type of withdrawal syndrome may be noted as well when drug levels fluctuate, with symptoms that are similar to those seen with alcohol, cocaine and narcotic withdrawal. To detect steroid use or abuse, be aware of physical, psychological and behavioral changes. Aggressive behavior is common in abusers.

In addition, athletes may ingest other drugs in an attempt to counteract short-term side effects of the steroids (eg, diuretics to minimize sodium and fluid retention).

Elderly: Geriatric patients treated with anabolic steroids may be at increased risk for the development of prostatic hypertrophy and prostatic carcinoma.

Pregnancy: Category X. Contraindicated because of possible fetal masculinization.

Lactation: It is not known whether anabolic steroids are excreted in breast milk. Because of the potential for serious adverse reactions in nursing infants, decide whether to discontinue nursing or to discontinue the drug.

Children: The adverse consequences of giving androgens to young children are not fully understood, but the possibility of causing serious disturbances does exist; weigh the possible benefits before instituting therapy in young children.

Anabolic agents may accelerate epiphyseal maturation more rapidly than linear growth in children, and the effect may continue for 6 months after the drug has been stopped. Therefore, monitor therapy by x-ray studies at 6 month intervals to avoid the risk of compromising adult height.

Safety and efficacy in children with hereditary angioedema or metastatic breast cancer (rarely found) have not been established.

Benzyl alcohol-containing products have been associated with a fatal "gasping syndrome" in premature infants. Refer to product listings.

Precautions:

Virilization in the female may occur. If amenorrhea or menstrual irregularities develop during treatment, discontinue the drug until etiology is determined.

Leukemia has been observed in patients with aplastic anemia treated with **oxymetholone**, but the role of oxymetholone is unclear.

Edema, with or without congestive heart failure, may occur. Concomitant administration of an adrenal steroid or ACTH may increase the edema. Use caution in patients with cardiac, renal or hepatic disease, epilepsy, migraine or other conditions that may be aggravated by fluid retention.

Hypercalcemia may develop both spontaneously and as a result of hormonal therapy in women with disseminated breast carcinoma. Perform frequent urine and serum calcium level examinations. If hypercalcemia occurs, discontinue the drug.

Diabetics: Monitor carefully. Tolerance to glucose may be altered. Monitor urine or blood sugar closely.

Seizure disorders: Patients may note an increase in seizure frequency.

Drug Interactions:

Anticoagulants: The anticoagulant effect may be potentiated by 17-alkyl testosterone derivatives (eg, anabolic steroids). Avoid this combination if possible.

Sulfonylureas: The hypoglycemic action may be enhanced by methandrostenolone. Monitor blood glucose and observe patients for signs of hypoglycemia.

Drug/Lab test interactions:

Glucose tests – Anabolic steroids have altered glucose tolerance tests. Monitor diabetics closely and adjust the insulin or oral hypoglycemic dosage accordingly.

Thyroid function tests – Decrease in protein-bound iodine (PBI), thyroxine-binding capacity, radioactive iodine uptake and an increase in T_3 uptake by resin; free thyroxine levels remain normal.

Miscellaneous – Altered metyrapone test.

ANABOLIC STEROIDS

Adverse Reactions:

CNS: Excitation; insomnia; habituation; depression.

Electrolyte Disturbance: Retention of sodium, chloride, water, potassium, phosphates and calcium; ankle swelling; decreased glucose tolerance.

Endocrine: Virilization is the most common undesirable effect. Acne occurs especially in women and prepubertal males. Anabolic steroids inhibit gonadotropin secretion.

Prepubertal males – The first signs of virilization are phallic enlargement and an increase in frequency of erections.

Postpubertal males – Acne; inhibition of testicular function with oligospermia; gynecomastia; testicular atrophy; chronic priapism; epididymitis; bladder irritability; change in libido; impotence.

Females – Hirsutism; acne; hoarseness or deepening of the voice; clitoral enlargement; change in libido; menstrual irregularities; male-pattern baldness. Voice changes, hirsutism and clitoral enlargement are usually not reversible even after prompt discontinuation. The use of estrogens with androgens will not prevent virilization in females. Masculinization of the fetus has occurred.

GI: Nausea; vomiting; diarrhea; cholestatic jaundice; hepatic necrosis; death; hepatocellular neoplasms and peliosis hepatis (long-term therapy; see Warning Box).

Lab test abnormalities:

Liver function tests – BSP retention; increased AST, serum bilirubin and alkaline phosphatase.

Blood coagulation tests – May suppress clotting factors II, V, VII and X and increase prothrombin time.

Miscellaneous – Increased creatinine and creatine excretion; increased serum cholesterol.

Miscellaneous: Premature closure of epiphyses in children; choreiform movement; increased serum cholesterol; increased serum levels of low-density lipoproteins and decreased levels of high-density lipoproteins.

Patient Information:

Diabetic patients: Glucose tolerance may be altered; monitor urine sugar closely and report abnormalities to physician.

Female patients: Notify physician if hoarseness, deepening of the voice, male-pattern baldness, hirsutism, menstrual irregularities or acne occurs.

May cause nausea or GI upset.

Notify physician if nausea, vomiting, changes in skin color or ankle swelling occurs.

OXYMETHOLONE

For complete prescribing information, refer to the Anabolic Steroids group monograph.

Indications:

Anemias caused by deficient red cell production, acquired or congenital aplastic anemia, myelofibrosis and hypoplastic anemias due to the administration of myelotoxic drugs.

Administration and Dosage:

Anemias: 1 to 5 mg/kg/day. The usual effective dose is 1 to 2 mg/kg/day. Individualize dosage. Response is not often immediate; give for a minimum trial of 3 to 6 months. Following remission, some patients may be maintained without the drug, while others may be maintained on an established lower daily dosage. Continuous maintenance is usually necessary in patients with congenital aplastic anemia.

c-III	**Anadrol-50** (Syntex)	**Tablets:** 50 mg	Lactose. (Syntex 2902). White, scored. In 100s.

STANOZOLOL

For complete prescribing information, refer to the Anabolic Steroids group monograph.

Indications:

Hereditary angioedema: Prophylactic use to decrease frequency and severity of attacks.

Administration and Dosage:

Individualize dosage. Initial dosage is 2 mg 3 times a day. After a favorable response is obtained in terms of prevention of edematous attacks, decrease dosage at intervals of 1 to 3 months to a maintenance dosage of 2 mg/day. Some patients may be successfully managed on a 2 mg alternate day schedule. During the dose adjusting phase, closely monitor patient response, particularly if there is a history of airway involvement.

The prophylactic dose to be used prior to dental extraction, or other traumatic or stressful situations, has not been established and may be substantially larger.

Attacks of hereditary angioedema are generally infrequent in childhood, and the risks from stanozolol administration are substantially increased. Therefore, long-term prophylactic therapy is generally not recommended in children; consider the benefits and risks involved.

c-III	**Winstrol** (Winthrop Pharm.)	**Tablets:** 2 mg	Lactose. (W 53). Pink, scored. In 100s.

OXANDROLONE

For complete prescribing information, refer to the Anabolic Steroids group monograph.

Indications:

Adjunctive therapy to promote weight gain after weight loss following extensive surgery, chronic infections, or severe trauma, and in some patients who, without definite pathophysiologic reasons, fail to gain or to maintain normal weight; to offset the protein catabolism associated with prolonged administration of corticosteroids; for relief of the bone pain frequently accompanying osteoporosis.

Unlabeled uses: Alcoholic hepatitis.

Orphan drug designation – Short stature associated with Turner syndrome; HIV wasting syndrome and HIV-associated muscle weakness.

Treatment IND – Constitutional delay of growth and puberty, which commonly is diagnosed when the height, pubertal development and bone age of an otherwise healthy adolescent are significantly below average for their chronological age.

Administration and Dosage:

Individualize dosage. Use intermittent therapy.

Adults: 2.5 mg 2 to 4 times daily. However, since the response of individuals to anabolic steroids varies, a daily dosage of as little as 2.5 mg or as much as 20 mg may be required to achieve the desired response. A course of therapy of 2 to 4 weeks is usually adequate. This may be repeated intermittently as indicated.

Children: Total daily dosage is ≤ 0.1 mg/kg or ≤ 0.045 mg/lb. this may be repeated intermittently as indicated.

c-III	**Oxandrin** (Gynex)	**Tablets:** 2.5 mg	Lactose. (Gynex 1111). White, oval, scored. In 100s.

NANDROLONE PHENPROPIONATE

For complete prescribing information, refer to the Anabolic Steroids group monograph.

Indications:

Control of metastatic breast cancer in women.

Administration and Dosage:

Inject deeply IM, preferably into the gluteal muscle.

If possible, therapy should be intermittent. Duration of therapy depends on patient response and adverse reactions.

Adults: 50 to 100 mg weekly, based on therapeutic response.

c-III	**Nandrolone Phenpropionate** (Various, eg, Lyphomed, Major)	**Injection (In Oil):** 25 mg per ml	In 5 ml vials.
c-III	**Durabolin** (Organon)		In 5 ml vials.[1]
c-III	**Nandrolone Phenpropionate** (Various, eg, Keene, Major, Rugby)	**Injection (In Oil):** 50 mg per ml	In 2 ml vials.
c-III	**Durabolin** (Organon)		In 2 ml vials.[1]
c-III	**Hybolin Improved** (Hyrex)		In 2 ml vials.[1]

[1] In sesame oil with benzyl alcohol.

NANDROLONE DECANOATE

For complete prescribing information, refer to the Anabolic Steroids group monograph.

Indications:

Management of the anemia of renal insufficiency. This drug increases hemoglobin and red cell mass. Surgically induced anephric patients may be less responsive.

Administration and Dosage:

If possible, therapy should be intermittent. Duration of therapy depends on response of the condition and appearance of adverse reactions.

Inject deeply IM, preferably into the gluteal muscle.

Anemia of renal disease:

Women – 50 to 100 mg per week.

Men – 100 to 200 mg per week.

Children (2 to 13 years) – Average dose is 25 to 50 mg every 3 to 4 weeks.

c-III	**Nandrolone Decanoate** (Various, eg, Goldline, Rugby, Schein)	**Injection (In Oil):** 50 mg per ml	In 2 ml vials.
c-III	**Deca-Durabolin** (Organon)		In 2 ml vials[1] and 1 ml syringes.[1]
c-III	**Hybolin Decanoate-50** (Hyrex)		In 2 ml vials.[1]
c-III	**Neo-Durabolic** (Hauck)		In 2 ml vials.[1]
c-III	**Nandrolone Decanoate** (Various, eg, Goldline, Lyphomed, Major, Rugby, Schein, URL)	**Injection (In Oil):** 100 mg per ml	In 2 ml vials.
c-III	**Deca-Durabolin** (Organon)		In 2 ml vials[1] and 1 ml syringes.[1]
c-III	**Hybolin Decanoate-100** (Hyrex)		In 2 ml vials.[1]
c-III	**Nandrolone Decanoate** (Various, eg, Lyphomed, Major, Schein)	**Injection (In Oil):** 200 mg per ml	In 1 ml vials.
c-III	**Androlone-D 200** (Keene)		In 1 ml vials.[1]
c-III	**Deca-Durabolin** (Organon)		In 1 ml vials[1] and 1 ml syringes.[1]
c-III	**Neo-Durabolic** (Hauck)		In 1 ml vials.[1]

[1] In sesame oil with benzyl alcohol.

POSTERIOR PITUITARY HORMONES

Actions:

Pharmacology: Posterior pituitary secretions include oxytocin and vasopressin, polypeptides containing eight amino acids. Oxytocin is formed primarily in the paraventricular nuclei and vasopressin in the supraoptic nuclei of the hypothalamus. They are then transported in combination with a carrier protein, neurophysin, to accumulate in nerve endings in the posterior pituitary gland. Under appropriate stimuli, they are released from nerve endings and absorbed into adjacent capillaries.

Vasopressin exhibits its most marked activity on the renal tubular epithelium, where it promotes water resorption of (antidiuretic hormone effect) and smooth muscle contraction throughout the vascular bed (vasopressor effects). Vasoconstriction is marked in portal and splanchnic vessels, somewhat less in peripheral, coronary, cerebral, and pulmonary vessels and slight in intrahepatic vessels. Vasopressin, and to a lesser extent, oxytocin, enhances GI motility and tone.

Neurogenic or central diabetes insipidus is a disorder of water metabolism that results from a partial or complete deficiency in the production and secretion of vasopressin from the neurohypophysis. Nephrogenic or peripheral diabetes insipidus results from an insensitivity of the renal tubules to the action of antidiuretic hormone. Vasopressin and its synthetic analogs are the principal treatment of neurogenic diabetes insipidus, but are ineffective in treating the nephrogenic variant.

Vasopressin is a purified form of the posterior pituitary, having only pressor and antidiuretic hormone (ADH) activity. Vasopressin may be obtained from natural sources or by chemical synthesis. The synthetic derivatives, lypressin and desmopressin, act principally as ADH, possessing little pressor activity, and are relatively free of oxytocic activity. Desmopressin has a longer duration of action.

Posterior Pituitary Hormone Products

Agent	Indications	Route	Concentration
Vasopressin Derivatives			
Vasopressin	Diabetes insipidus Post-op abdominal distention	Parenteral	20 u/ml
Lypressin	Diabetes insipidus	Nasal spray	0.185 mg/ml
Desmopressin	Diabetes insipidus	Nasal Parenteral	0.1 mg/ml 4 mcg/ml
	Nocturnal enuresis Renal capacity testing	Nasal	0.1 mg/ml
	Hemophilia A von Willebrand's disease (Type I)	Nasal Parenteral	1.5 mg/ml 4 mcg/ml
Oxytocics[1]			
Oxytocin	Initiate/augment labor 2nd trimester abortion Postpartum hemorrhage	Parenteral	10 u/ml
	Initial milk let-down	Nasal	40 u/ml
Ergonovine	Postpartum/postabortal hemorrhage Migraine headache	Oral Parenteral	0.2 mg 0.2 mg/ml
Methylergonovine	Postpartum/postabortal hemorrhage	Oral Parenteral	0.2 mg 0.2 mg/ml

[1] Other agents with oxytocic effects on the uterus used to induce abortion are discussed under Abortifacients.

Pharmacokinetics:

Oxytocin exerts its most marked activity in inducing uterine muscle contraction and inducing contraction of the lacteal glands, which results in milk ejection in lactating women. Uterine motility is controlled by a variety of biochemical and regulatory processes including cAMP, calcium, prostaglandins and oxytocin. The mechanism of oxytocin-facilitated smooth muscle contraction is poorly understood. The sensitivity of the uterus to oxytocin increases gradually during gestation, then increases sharply before parturition.

Naturally derived oxytocin, no longer commercially available, has been replaced by synthetic oxytocin. Oxytocin is most frequently used to induce or improve uterine contractions in labor. Ergot derivatives (ergonovine and methylergonovine) are also used for oxytocic effects on uterine muscle. These agents are most appropriately used to prevent postpartum uterine atony and hemorrhage.

POSTERIOR PITUITARY HORMONES

VASOPRESSIN (8-Arginine-Vasopressin)

Refer to the general discussion of these products in the Posterior Pituitary Hormones introduction.

Actions:

Pharmacology: Possesses vasopressor and antidiuretic hormone (ADH) activity.

Pharmacokinetics: Following IM or SC injection, the duration of antidiuretic activity for vasopressin aqueous solution is 2 to 8 hours. Most is metabolized and rapidly destroyed in liver and kidneys. Vasopressin aqueous solution has a plasma half-life of about 10 to 20 minutes. After 4 hours, about 5% of an SC dose is excreted unchanged in urine.

Indications:

Diabetes insipidus: Neurogenic diabetes insipidus.

Abdominal distention/roentgenography: Prevention and treatment of postoperative abdominal distention and in abdominal roentgenography to dispel interfering gas shadows.

Unlabeled uses: Vasopressin infusions (IV or selective intra-arterial) are used to manage bleeding esophageal varices at a dosage of 0.2 units/min initially, increased to 0.4 units/min if bleeding continues. Maximum recommended dose is 0.9 units/min.

Contraindications:

Anaphylaxis or hypersensitivity to vasopressin or its components.

Warnings:

Vascular disease: Use with extreme caution in patients with vascular disease (especially coronary artery disease) since even small doses may precipitate anginal pain; with larger doses, consider the possibility of MI.

Water intoxication: Vasopressin may produce water intoxication. Early signs of drowsiness, listlessness and headaches precede terminal coma and convulsions.

Vasoconstriction/Necrosis: Severe vasoconstriction and local tissue necrosis may result if vasopressin extravasates during IV infusion. Gangrene of the extremities, tongue necrosis and ischemic colitis may occur during treatment of esophageal varices.

Chronic nephritis with nitrogen retention contraindicates use until reasonable nitrogen blood levels have been attained.

Hypersensitivity: Local or systemic allergic reactions may occur in hypersensitive individuals (see Adverse Reactions). Anaphylaxis (cardiac arrest or shock) has been observed shortly after injection. Refer to Management of Acute Hypersensitivity Reactions.

Pregnancy: Category C. It is not known whether vasopressin causes fetal harm when administered to a pregnant woman or affects reproductive capacity. Administer to a pregnant woman only if clearly needed. Doses sufficient for an antidiuretic effect are not likely to produce tonic uterine contractions that could be harmful to the fetus or threaten the continuation of the pregnancy.

Lactation: Exercise caution when giving to a nursing woman.

Precautions:

Monitoring: Electrocardiograms and fluid and electrolyte status determinations are recommended at intervals during therapy.

Special risk patients: Use vasopressin cautiously in the presence of epilepsy, migraine, asthma, heart failure or any state in which a rapid increase in extracellular water may result in further compromise.

Drug Interactions:

Vasopressin Drug Interactions			
Precipitant drug	Object drug*		Description
Carbamazepine	Vasopressin	↑	Carbamazepine, which potentiates ADH, may potentiate the effects of vasopressin.
Chlorpropamide	Vasopressin	↑	Chlorpropamide, which potentiates ADH, may potentiate the effects of vasopressin.

* ↑ = Object drug increased.

Adverse Reactions:

Hypersensitivity: Tremor; sweating; vertigo; cardiac arrest; circumoral pallor; "pounding" in head; abdominal cramps; passage of gas; nausea; vomiting; urticaria and bronchial constriction (see Warnings).

POSTERIOR PITUITARY HORMONES

VASOPRESSIN (8-Arginine-Vasopressin)

Overdosage:

Treat water intoxication with water restriction and temporary withdrawal of vasopressin until polyuria occurs. Severe water intoxication may require osmotic diuresis with mannitol, hypertonic dextrose, or urea alone or with furosemide.

Patient Information:

Side effects such as skin blanching, abdominal cramps and nausea may be reduced by taking 1 or 2 glasses of water with the dose. These side effects usually are not serious and will probably disappear within a few minutes.

Administration and Dosage:

May be given IM or SC.

Adults: 5 to 10 units usually elicit full physiologic response. Give IM at 3 or 4 hour intervals as needed. Reduce dosage proportionately for children.

Diabetes insipidus:

Intranasal – The injection solution may be administered intranasally on cotton pledgets, by nasal spray or dropper. Individualize dosage.

Parenteral – 5 to 10 units 2 or 3 times daily as needed.

Abdominal distention: To prevent or relieve postoperative distention, give 5 units initially; increase to 10 units at subsequent injections, if necessary. Give IM at 3 or 4 hour intervals. Reduce dosage proportionately for children. These recommendations also apply to distention complicating pneumonia or other acute toxemias.

Abdominal roentgenography: Administer 2 injections of 10 units each. Give 2 hours and ½ hour, respectively, before films are exposed. An enema may be given prior to first dose.

Rx	**Vasopressin** (American Regent)	**Injection:** 20 pressor units/ml	With 0.5% chlorobutanol. In 0.5, 1 and 10 ml vials.
Rx	**Pitressin Synthetic** (Parke-Davis)		With 0.5% chlorobutanol. In 0.5 and 1 ml amps and vials.

LYPRESSIN (8–Lysine Vasopressin)

Refer to the general discussion of these products in the Posterior Pituitary Hormones introduction.

Actions:

Pharmacology: Lypressin is a synthetic lysine vasopressin analog that possesses antidiuretic activity with little vasopressor or oxytocic effect. The onset of antidiuretic effect is prompt, peaks in 30 to 120 minutes and has a duration of 3 to 8 hours.

Indications:

Diabetes insipidus: For the control or prevention of the symptoms and complications of neurogenic diabetes insipidus (including polydipsia, polyuria and dehydration). Useful in patients who have become unresponsive to other therapy or who experience local or systemic reactions, allergic reactions or other undesirable effects (eg, excessive fluid retention) from preparations of animal origin.

Warnings:

Hypersensitivity: Test patients with known sensitivity to antidiuretic hormones.

Pregnancy: Safety for use during pregnancy is not established. Use only when clearly needed and when potential benefits outweigh potential hazards to the fetus.

Precautions:

Cardiovascular effects: Cardiovascular pressor effects are minimal or absent when administered as a nasal spray in therapeutic doses. Nevertheless, use cautiously when such effects would be undesirable; mild blood pressure elevation has been noted in unanesthetized subjects who received IV lypressin. Large doses intranasally may cause coronary artery constriction; use caution in treating patients with coronary artery disease.

Upper respiratory conditions: Effectiveness may decrease in the presence of nasal congestion, allergic rhinitis and upper respiratory infections because of decreased absorption by the nasal mucosa; larger doses or adjunctive therapy may be required.

POSTERIOR PITUITARY HORMONES

LYPRESSIN (8–Lysine Vasopressin)

Drug Interactions:

Lypressin Drug Interactions

Precipitant drug	Object drug*		Description
Carbamazepine	Lypressin	↑	Carbamazepine, which potentiates ADH, may potentiate the effects of lypressin.
Chlorpropamide	Lypressin	↑	Chlorpropamide, which potentiates ADH, may potentiate the effects of lypressin.

* ↑ = Object drug increased.

Adverse Reactions:

Reactions have been infrequent and mild.

Local: Rhinorrhea; nasal congestion; irritation and pruritus of the nasal passages; nasal ulceration; periorbital edema with itching.

Systemic: Headache; conjunctivitis; heartburn secondary to excessive intranasal use; abdominal cramps and increased bowel movements. Inadvertent inhalation has resulted in substernal tightness, coughing and transient dyspnea. Hypersensitivity manifested by a positive skin test has occurred.

Overdosage:

Overdosage has caused marked, but transient fluid retention.

Patient Information:

Review administration technique with patient. Spray into nostril(s) as directed.

To ensure that a uniform, well-diffused spray is delivered, have the patient hold the bottle upright while in a vertical position with head upright.

Notify physician if drowsiness, listlessness, headache, shortness of breath, heartburn, nausea, abdominal cramps or severe nasal congestion or irritation occurs.

Administration and Dosage:

Administer 1 or 2 sprays to one or both nostrils whenever frequency of urination increases or significant thirst develops. One spray provides approximately 2 Posterior Pituitary (Pressor) Units. The usual dosage for adults and children is 1 or 2 sprays into each nostril 4 times daily. An additional bedtime dose helps eliminate nocturia not controlled with regular daily dosage. For patients requiring more than 2 sprays per nostril every 4 to 6 hours, reduce the time between doses rather than increase the number of sprays at each dose. More than 2 or 3 sprays in each nostril is usually wasted; the unabsorbed excess will drain posteriorly (by way of the nasopharynx) into the digestive tract where it will be inactivated.

The spray permits individualization of dosage necessary to control the symptoms of diabetes insipidus. Patients quickly learn to regulate dosage in accordance with their degree of polyuria and thirst; once determined, daily requirements remain fairly stable for months or years. Dosage has ranged from 1 spray per day at bedtime to 10 sprays into each nostril every 3 to 4 hours. Larger doses may represent greater severity of disease or other phenomena, such as poor nasal absorption. Large doses may also be due to the presence of mixed hypothalamic-hypophyseal and nephrogenic diabetes insipidus, the latter being unresponsive to antidiuretic hormone.

Rx	**Diapid** (Sandoz)	**Nasal Spray:** 0.185 mg lypressin (equivalent to 50 USP Posterior Pituitary [Pressor] Units)/ml	In 8 ml bottles.[1]

[1] With methyl and propyl parabens, sorbitol solution, glycerin and chlorobutanol.

POSTERIOR PITUITARY HORMONES

DESMOPRESSIN ACETATE (1-Deamino-8-D-Arginine Vasopressin)

Refer to the general discussion of these products in the Posterior Pituitary Hormones introduction.

Actions:

Pharmacology: A synthetic analog of arginine vasopressin, the naturally occurring human antidiuretic hormone (ADH) provides a prompt onset of action with a long duration. The antidiuretic action is more specific and more prolonged than that of the natural hormone or lypressin. The plasma half-life of lypressin is 17 to 35 minutes. Urine volume is reduced, and urine osmolality is increased.

The change in structure of arginine vasopressin to desmopressin acetate results in less vasopressor activity and decreased action on visceral smooth muscle relative to enhanced antidiuretic activity. Consequently, clinically effective antidiuretic doses are usually below the threshold for effects on vascular or visceral smooth muscle.

Desmopressin produces a dose-related increase in Factor VIII levels. The increase is rapid, becoming evident in ≤ 30 minutes and peaking in 90 to 120 minutes. The Factor VIII-related antigen and ristocetin cofactor activity are also increased to a smaller degree.

Pharmacokinetics:

Injection – Biphasic half-lives of desmopressin acetate are 7.8 and 75.5 minutes for the fast and slow phases, respectively, compared with 2.5 and 14.5 minutes for lysine vasopressin. When administered by injection, desmopressin has an antidiuretic effect ≈ 10 times that of an equivalent dose administered intranasally.

Intranasal – The half-life of the nasal spray is between 3.3 and 3.5 hours, over the range of intranasal doses, 150 to 450 mcg. Plasma concentrations of the nasal spray are maximal at ≈ 40 to 45 minutes after dosing. The bioavailability of the nasal spray when administered by the intranasal route as a 1.5 mg/ml solution is between 3.3% and 4.1%. Plasminogen activator activity increases rapidly after IV infusion, but clinically significant fibrinolysis has not occurred.

Oral – The bioavailability of the tablets is ≈ 5% and 0.15% compared with intranasal and IV desmopressin, respectively. The time to reach maximum plasma levels ranges from 0.9 to 1.5 hours following oral or intranasal administration, respectively. Following administration of tablets, the onset of antidiuretic effect occurs at around 1 hour, and it reaches a maximum at ≈ 4 to 7 hours based on the measurement of increased urine osmolality. The plasma half-life of desmopressin follows a monoexponential time course with $t_{1/2}$ values of 1.5 to 2.5 hours which is independent of dose. Increasing oral doses produces dose-dependent increases in the plasma levels of desmopressin tablets.

Clinical trials: In one study, the tablets and intranasal formulation were compared during an 8–hour dosing interval at steady-state. The doses administered to 36 hydrated (water loaded) healthy male adult volunteers every 8 hours were 0.1, 0.2 and 0.4 mg orally and 0.01 mg intranasally by rhinal tube.

With respect to the mean values of total urine volume decrease and maximum urine osmolality increase from baseline, the 0.4 and 0.2 mg oral dose produced between 95% to 110% and 84% to 99% of pharmacodynamic activity, respectively, when compared with the 0.01 mg intranasal dose.

While both the 0.2 mg and 0.4 mg oral doses are considered pharmacodynamically similar to the 0.01 mg intranasal dose, the pharmacodynamic data on an intersubject basis was highly variable and, therefore, individual dosing is recommended.

In another study in diabetes insipidus patients, the tablet and intranasal formulations were compared over a 12–hour period. Ten fluid-controlled patients < 18 years of age were administered tablet doses of 0.2 and 0.4 mg and intranasal doses of 10 and 20 mcg.

All four dose formulations have a similar, pronounced pharmacodynamic effect on urine volume and urine osmolality. At 2 hours after study drug administration, mean urine volume was 4 ml/min and urine osmolality was > 500 mOsm/kg. Mean plasma osmolality remained relatively constant over the time course recorded (0 to 12 hours).

Indications:

DDAVP:

Primary nocturnal enuresis (intranasal only) – May be used alone or adjunctive to behavioral conditioning or other nonpharmacological intervention. It is effective in some cases that are refractory to conventional therapies.

Central cranial diabetes insipidus (intranasal, oral and parenteral) – ADH replacement therapy in the management of central cranial (neurogenic) diabetes insipidus and for temporary polyuria and polydipsia following head trauma or surgery in the pituitary region. Ineffective for the treatment of nephrogenic diabetes insipidus.

POSTERIOR PITUITARY HORMONES

DESMOPRESSIN ACETATE (1-Deamino-8-D-Arginine Vasopressin)

Hemophilia A (intranasal and parenteral) with Factor VIII levels > 5%. Desmopressin will often maintain hemostasis in patients with hemophilia A during surgery and postoperatively when administered 30 minutes prior to procedure. The drug will also stop bleeding in hemophilia A patients with episodes of spontaneous or trauma-induced injuries such as hemarthroses, IM hematomas or mucosal bleeding.

von Willebrand's disease (Type I) (intranasal and parenteral) – Mild to moderate classic von Willebrand's disease (Type I) with Factor VIII levels > 5%. Hemostasis in these patients can often be maintained during surgery and postoperatively when the drug is administered 30 minutes prior to the procedure. Episodes of spontaneous or trauma-induced injuries such as hemarthroses, IM hematomas or mucosal bleeding can usually be stopped.

Stimate:

Hemophilia A with Factor VIII coagulant activity levels > 5%. Desmopressin will also stop bleeding in patients with hemophilia A with episodes of spontaneous or trauma-induced injuries such as hemarthroses, intramuscular hematomas or mucosal bleeding.

von Willebrand's disease (Type I) – Mild to moderate classic von Willebrand's disease (Type I) with Factor VIII levels > 5%. Desmopressin will also stop bleeding in mild to moderate von Willebrand's disease patients with episodes of spontaneous or trauma-induced injuries such as hemarthroses, intramuscular hematomas, mucosal bleeding or menorrhagia.

Unlabeled uses:

Intranasal – Treatment of chronic autonomic failure (eg, nocturnal polyuria, overnight weight loss, morning postural hypotension).

Contraindications:

Hypersensitivity to desmopressin acetate or its components.

Intranasal delivery may be inappropriate where there is an impaired level of consciousness.

Warnings:

Hemophilia A: Not indicated for treatment of hemophilia A with Factor VIII levels ≤ 5%, for the treatment of hemophilia B or in patients who have Factor VIII antibodies. Some patients with Factor VIII levels between 2% to 5% may be treatable.

von Willebrand's disease: Patients who are least likely to respond are those with severe homozygous von Willebrand's disease with Factor VIII coagulant activity, Factor VIII antigen and von Willebrand's factor (ristocetin cofactor) activities < 1%. Other patients may respond in a variable fashion, depending on the type of molecular defect.

Not indicated for the treatment of severe classic von Willebrand's disease (Type I) and when an abnormal molecular form of Factor VIII antigen is evident.

Do not use for Type IIB von Willebrand's disease; may induce platelet aggregation.

Test dose: Before the initial therapeutic administration of the nasal spray, the physician should establish that the patient shows an appropriate change in the coagulation profile following a test dose of intranasal administration.

Water intoxication: Caution very young and elderly patients to ingest only enough fluid to satisfy thirst to decrease the potential occurrence of water intoxication and hyponatremia. Pay particular attention to the possibility of the rare occurrence of an extreme decrease in plasma osmolality that may result in seizures, that could lead to coma.

Hypersensitivity reactions: Rare severe allergic reactions have been reported with desmopressin. Anaphylaxis has been reported with IV administration but not with intranasal or oral (tablets).

Pregnancy: Category B. Several publications of desmopressin acetate's use in the management of diabetes insipidus during pregnancy are available. However, there are no adequate and well controlled studies in pregnant women. Safety and efficacy for use during pregnancy has not been established. Use only when clearly needed and when the potential benefits outweigh potential hazards to the fetus. Published reports stress that, as opposed to preparations containing the natural hormones, desmopressin in antidiuretic doses has no uterotonic action, but the physician will have to weigh possible therapeutic advantages against possible danger in each case.

Lactation: Safety for use in nursing women has not been established. Patients receiving desmopressin for diabetes insipidus have been reported to breast feed without apparent problems in the infant. A single study in postpartum women showed

POSTERIOR PITUITARY HORMONES

DESMOPRESSIN ACETATE (1-Deamino-8-D-Arginine Vasopressin)

little, if any, change in breast milk following a 10 mcg intranasal dose. However, there have been no controlled studies in nursing mothers. Exercise caution when administering desmopressin to a nursing woman.

Children: Infants and children require careful fluid intake restriction to prevent possible hyponatremia and water intoxication.

Intranasal desmopressin has been used in children with diabetes insipidus, and the tablets have been used safely in children (≥ 4 years of age) with diabetes insipidus for periods ≤ 44 months. If desmopressin is used in the very young, adjust the dose individually, with attention to the danger of an extreme decrease in plasma osmolality leading to hyponatremia with possible convulsions. Initiate doses at 0.05 ml (intranasal) or 0.05 mg (oral).

Pediatric Use of Desmopressin Acetate	
Indication/Doseform	Safety and effectiveness not proven in children less than age:
Central cranial diabetes insipidus	
Intranasal	Adjust dosage (*DDAVP*)
Oral	4 years
Parenteral	12 years
Hemophilia A	
Intranasal	11 months (*Stimate*)
Oral	Not indicated.
Parenteral	3 months
Primary nocturnal enuresis	
Intranasal	6 years (*DDAVP*)
Oral	Not indicated.
Parenteral	Not indicated.
von Willebrand's disease	
Intranasal	11 months (*Stimate*)
Oral	Not indicated.
Parenteral	3 months

Precautions:

Monitoring:

Diabetes insipidus – Monitor urine volume/osmolality and plasma osmolality.

Hemophilia A – Determine Factor VIII coagulant activity before injecting desmopressin for hemostasis; if the activity is < 5% of normal, do not rely on desmopressin. Other tests to assess patient status include levels of Factor VIII coagulant, Factor VIII antigen and ristocetin cofactor and activated partial thromboplastin time (APTT).

von Willebrand's disease – Assess levels of Factor VIII coagulant, Factor VIII antigen and ristocetin cofactor. Skin bleeding time may also be helpful.

Cardiovascular effects: High intranasal dosage has infrequently produced a slight elevation of blood pressure that disappeared with dosage reduction. This effect has not been observed with single oral doses ≤ 0.6 mg. Use with caution in coronary artery insufficiency or hypertensive cardiovascular disease. Desmopressin injection has infrequently produced changes in blood pressure causing either a slight elevation in blood pressure or a transient fall in blood pressure and a compensatory increase in heart rate. Use the drug with caution in patients with coronary artery insufficiency or hypertensive cardiovascular disease.

Nasal mucosa changes (eg, scarring, edema, discharge, blockage, congestion, severe atrophic rhinitis), cranial surgery (eg, transphenoidal hypophysectomy) and nasal packing compromise intranasal delivery; consider administering IV.

Thrombotic events: There have been rare reports of thrombotic events (thrombosis, acute cerebrovascular thrombosis, acute myocardial infarction) following desmopressin injection in patients predisposed to thrombus formation. No causality has been determined; however, use the drug with caution in these patients.

Decreased response: There are reports of an occasional change in response to intranasal desmopressin with time, usually > 6 months. Some patients may show a decreased responsiveness, others a shortened duration of effect. There is no evidence this effect is because of the development of binding antibodies but it may be because of a local inactivation of the peptide. No lessening of effect has been seen in the 46 patients who were treated with desmopressin tablets for 12 to 44 months and no serum antibodies to desmopressin were detected.

POSTERIOR PITUITARY HORMONES

DESMOPRESSIN ACETATE (1-Deamino-8-D-Arginine Vasopressin)

Fluid/Electrolyte imbalance: Use with caution in patients with conditions associated with fluid and electrolyte imbalance, such as cystic fibrosis, because these patients are prone to hyponatremia.

Drug Interactions:

Desmopressin Drug Interactions			
Precipitant drug	Object drug*		Description
Desmopressin	Pressor agents	↑	Although desmopressin pressor activity is very low, use large intranasal doses or parenteral doses as large as 0.3 mcg/kg cautiously with other pressor agents.
Carbamazepine	Desmopressin	↑	Carbamazepine, which potentiates ADH, may potentiate the effects of desmopressin.
Chlorpropamide	Desmopressin	↑	Chlorpropamide, which potentiates ADH, may potentiate the effects of desmopressin.

* ↑ = Object drug increased.

Adverse Reactions:

Intranasal (DDAVP): Adverse reactions that disappear with dosage reduction include: abdominal pain (mild); facial flushing; headache (transient); nasal congestion; nausea; rhinitis. Other adverse reactions include: Asthenia; chills; conjunctivitis; cough; dizziness; epistaxis; eye edema; GI disorder; lacrimation disorder; nosebleed; nostril pain; sore throat; upper respiratory infections.

Intranasal (Stimate): Adverse reactions include: Agitation; balanitis; chest pain; chills; dizziness; dyspepsia; edema; insomnia; itchy or light sensitive eyes; pain; palpitations; somnolence; tachycardia; vomiting; warm feeling.

Parenteral: Adverse reactions that disappear with dosage reduction include: Abdominal pain (mild); facial flushing; headache (transient); nausea; vulval pain. Other adverse reactions include: Anaphylaxis (rare); blood pressure changes; burning pain; edema; erythema (local).

Oral: In long-term clinical studies in which patients with diabetes insipidus were followed for periods ≤ 12 to 44 months of tablet therapy, transient increases in AST ≤ 1.5 times the upper limit of normal occurred. Elevated AST returned to the normal range despite continued use of tablets.

Overdosage:

Symptoms: Abdominal pain, dyspnea, facial flushing, fluid retention, headache and mucous membrane irritation may occur.

Treatment: Reduce the dosage, decrease the frequency of use or withdraw the drug according to the severity of the condition. There is no known specific antidote.

Patient Information:

Patient instructions provided with intranasal product; review administration with patient.

If bleeding is not controlled, contact the physician.

Notify physician if headache, shortness of breath, heartburn, nausea, abdominal cramps or vulval pain occurs.

Intranasal: Inform patients that the bottle accurately delivers 25 or 50 doses. Discard any solution remaining after 25 or 50 doses because the amount delivered thereafter may be substantially less than prescribed. Do not attempt to transfer remaining solution to another bottle.

Administration and Dosage:

Primary nocturnal enuresis: Individualize dosage.

Initial dose (≥ 6 years of age) – 20 mcg (0.2 ml) intranasally at bedtime. Adjustment ≤ 40 mcg is suggested if the patient does not respond. Some patients may respond to 10 mcg and adjustment to that lower dose may be done if the patient has shown a response to 20 mcg. It is recommended that one-half of the dose be administered per nostril. Adequately controlled studies have not been conducted beyond 4 to 8 weeks.

POSTERIOR PITUITARY HORMONES

DESMOPRESSIN ACETATE (1-Deamino-8-D-Arginine Vasopressin)

Central cranial diabetes insipidus:

Intranasal – The nasal tube delivery system is supplied with a flexible calibrated plastic tube (rhinyle). Draw solution into the rhinyle. Insert one end of tube into nostril; blow on the other end to deposit solution deep into nasal cavity. The nasal spray pump may also be used.

Adults: 0.1 to 0.4 ml daily, either as a single dose or divided into 2 or 3 doses. Most adults require 0.2 ml daily in 2 divided doses. Adjust morning and evening doses separately for an adequate diurnal rhythm of water turnover.

Children (3 months to 12 years): 0.05 to 0.3 ml daily, either as a single dose or in 2 divided doses.

Parenteral – Administer SC or by direct IV injection.

Adults: 0.5 to 1 ml daily in 2 divided doses, adjusted separately for an adequate diurnal rhythm of water turnover. For patients switching from intranasal to IV, the comparable IV antidiuretic dose is approximately one-tenth the intranasal dose. Estimate response by adequate sleep duration and adequate but not excessive water turnover.

Oral – The dosage must be determined for each individual patient and adjusted according to the diurnal pattern of response. Estimate response by adequate duration of sleep and adequate, not excessive, water turnover. Begin therapy 12 hours after the last intranasal dose for patients previously on intranasal therapy. Observe patients closely during the initial dose titration period and measure appropriate safety parameters to assure adequate response. Monitor patient at regular intervals during therapy to assure adequate antidiuretic response. Implement modifications in dosage regimen as necessary to assure adequate water turnover.

Adults: Begin with 0.05 mg 2 times a day and adjust individually to their optimum therapeutic dose. Separately adjust each dose for an adequate diurnal rhythm of water turnover. Increase or decrease total daily dosage (range, 0.1 to 1.2 mg divided 2 or 3 times a day) as needed to obtain adequate antidiuresis.

Children: Begin dosing with 0.05 mg. Careful fluid intake restrictions in children is required to prevent hyponatremia and water intoxication.

Hemophilia A and von Willebrand's disease (Type I):

Parenteral – Administer 0.3 mcg/kg diluted in sterile physiologic saline; infuse IV slowly over 15 to 30 minutes. In adults and children weighing > 10 kg, use 50 ml diluent; in children weighing ≤ 10 kg, use 10 ml. Monitor blood pressure and pulse during infusion. If used preoperatively, administer 30 minutes prior to the procedure.

Determine the necessity for repeat dose or use of any blood products for hemostasis by laboratory response and patient's clinical condition. Consider the tendency toward tachyphylaxis with repeating dose more than every 48 hours.

Intranasal – Administer by nasal insufflation, 1 spray per nostril, to provide a total dose of 300 mcg. In patients weighing < 50 kg, 150 mcg administered as a single spray provided the expected effect on Factor VIII coagulant activity, Factor VIII ristocetin cofactor activity and skin bleeding time. If used preoperatively, administer 2 hours prior to the scheduled procedure.

The necessity for repeat administration or use of any blood products for hemostasis should be determined by laboratory response as well as the clinical condition of the patient. Consider the tendency toward tachyphylaxis (lessening of response) with repeated administration given more frequently than every 48 hours.

The nasal spray pump only delivers doses of 10 mcg (*DDAVP*) or 150 mcg (*Stimate*). If doses other than these are required, consider nasal tube delivery or injection.

The *Stimate* spray pump must be primed prior to the first use. To prime pump, press down 4 times. Discard the bottle after 25 doses since the amount delivered thereafter per spray may be substantially < 150 mcg of drug.

POSTERIOR PITUITARY HORMONES

DESMOPRESSIN ACETATE (1-Deamino-8-D-Arginine Vasopressin)

Storage/Stability:

Intranasal – Refrigerate nasal solution at 2° to 8°C (36° to 46°F). Nasal solution will maintain stability for ≤ 3 weeks when stored at room temperature (22°C; 72°F).

Injection – Store at room temperature between 15° to 30°C (59° to 86°F). Avoid exposure to excessive heat or light.

Rx	**DDAVP** (Rhone-Poulenc Rorer)	**Tablets**: 0.1 mg	Lactose. (DDAVP 01). White. In 100s.
		0.2 mg	Lactose. (DDAVP 02). White. In 100s.
Rx	**DDAVP** (Rhone-Poulenc Rorer)	**Nasal Solution**: 0.1 mg/ml (0.1 mg equals 400 IU arginine vasopressin)	**Nasal spray pump**: 9 mg NaCl/ml. In 2.5 or 5 ml bottle[1] with spray pump (25 or 50 doses of 10 mcg each, respectively).
			Rhinal tube delivery system: 9 mg NaCl/ml. In 2.5 ml vials[1] with applicator tubes.
Rx	**Stimate** (Armour)	**Nasal solution**: 1.5 mg/ml	9 mg NaCl/ml. In 2.5 ml bottle[1] (25 doses of 150 mcg each).
Rx	**DDAVP** (Rhone-Poulenc Rorer)	**Injection**: 4 mcg/ml	9 mg NaCl/ml. In 1 ml amps and 10 ml multiple dose vials.[1]

[1] With 5 mg chlorobutanol per ml.

ESTROGEN AND ANDROGEN COMBINATIONS

ESTROGEN AND ANDROGEN COMBINATIONS

Refer to group monographs on Androgens and Estrogens for complete prescribing information.

Indications:

Moderate to severe vasomotor symptoms associated with menopause in patients not improved with estrogens alone.

There is no evidence that estrogens are effective for nervousness or depression which may occur during menopause; do not use to treat these conditions.

Postpartum breast engorgement: Although estrogens have been widely used to prevent postpartum breast engorgement, controlled studies indicate the incidence of significant painful engorgement is low and usually responsive to analgesic or other supportive therapy. Because of the potential increased risk of puerperal thromboembolism associated with large doses of estrogens, carefully weigh the benefits to be derived from their use.

In June 1989, the FDA's Fertility and Maternal Health Drugs Advisory Committee unanimously recommended that these agents should not be used for prevention of postpartum breast engorgement.

ESTROGEN AND ANDROGEN COMBINATIONS, PARENTERAL

For complete prescribing information, refer to the Estrogen and Androgen Combinations group monograph.

Rx	**Testosterone Cypionate and Estradiol Cypionate** (Schein)	**Injection (In Oil):** 2 mg estradiol cypionate and 50 mg testosterone cypionate per ml	In 10 ml multi-dose vials.[1]
Rx	**depAndrogyn** (Forest)		In 10 ml multi-dose vials.[1]
Rx	**Depo-Testadiol** (Roberts)		In 10 ml vials.[1]
Rx	**Depotestogen** (Hyrex)		In 10 ml multi-dose vials.[1]
Rx	**Duo-Cyp** (Keene)		In 10 ml multi-dose vials.[1]
Rx	**Duratestrin** (Hauck)		In 10 ml vials.[1]
Rx	**Test-Estro Cypionates** (Rugby)		In 10 ml multi-dose vials.[1]
Rx	**Valertest No. 1** (Hyrex)	**Injection (In Oil):** 4 mg estradiol valerate and 90 mg testosterone enanthate per ml	In 10 ml vials.[2]

[1] With chlorobutanol in cottonseed oil.
[2] With chlorobutanol in sesame oil.

ESTROGEN AND ANDROGEN COMBINATIONS, ORAL

For complete prescribing information, refer to the Estrogen and Androgen Combinations group monograph.

Rx	**Premarin with Methyltestosterone** (Wyeth-Ayerst)	**Tablets:** 1.25 mg conjugated estrogens and 10 mg methyltestosterone	(879). Yellow. In 100s.
Rx	**Premarin with Methyltestosterone** (Wyeth-Ayerst)	**Tablets:** 0.625 mg conjugated estrogens and 5 mg methyltestosterone	(878). White. In 100s.
Rx	**Estratest** (Solvay)	**Tablets:** 1.25 mg esterified estrogens and 2.5 mg methyltestosterone	Lactose, sucrose, parabens. (Solvay 1026). Dark green. Sugar coated. Capsule shape. In 100s and 1000s.
Rx	**Menogen** (Breckenridge)		(NE 570). Dark green, capsule shape. In 100s.
Rx	**Estratest H.S.** (Solvay)	**Tablets:** 0.625 mg esterified estrogens and 1.25 mg methyltestosterone	Lactose, sucrose, parabens. (Solvay 1023). Light green. Sugar coated. Capsule shape. In 100s.
Rx	**Menogen H.S.** (Breckenridge)		(NE 560). Light green, capsule shape. In 100s.

CLOMIPHENE CITRATE

Actions:

Pharmacology: Clomiphene, an orally administered nonsteroidal agent, may induce ovulation in selected anovulatory women. Therapy appears to mediate ovulation through increased output of pituitary gonadotropins, which stimulates the maturation and endocrine activity of the ovarian follicle and the subsequent development and function of the corpus luteum. Clomiphene binds to estrogenic receptors in the cytoplasm and decreases the number of available estrogenic receptors (antiestrogen). The hypothalamus and pituitary interpret the false signal that estrogen levels are low and respond by increasing the secretion of luteinizing hormone (LH), follicle stimulating hormone (FSH) and gonadotropins. This results in ovarian stimulation.

Criteria for ovulation include an ovulation peak of estrogen excretion followed by a biphasic basal body temperature curve; urinary excretion of pregnanediol at post-ovulatory levels and endometrial histologic findings characteristic of the luteal phase.

Pharmacokinetics: Clomiphene is readily absorbed orally and is excreted principally in the feces. Excretion averaged 51% of the dose after 5 days. Drug appears in the feces 6 weeks after administration, suggesting that the remaining drug/metabolites are slowly excreted from a sequestered enterohepatic recirculation pool.

Clinical trials: In 11 studies appearing between 1964 and 1978, pregnancy occurred in 30.6% of 5413 patients with ovulatory dysfunction who received clomiphene citrate.

Indications:

Treatment of ovulatory failure in patients desiring pregnancy whose partners are fertile and potent.

Unlabeled uses: Clomiphene has been used to treat male infertility (50 to 400 mg/day for 2 to 12 months); however, this use is controversial, and further study is needed.

Contraindications:

Liver disease, history of liver dysfunction or abnormal bleeding of undetermined origin; pregnancy (see Warnings); uncontrolled thyroid or adrenal dysfunction; organic intracranial lesion (eg, pituitary tumor); ovarian cysts or enlargement not due to polycystic ovarian syndrome; abnormal uterine bleeding must be evaluated prior to therapy. It is important to detect neoplastic lesions.

Warnings:

Criteria for therapy: To start clomiphene therapy, the following criteria must be met: Normal liver function; normal levels of endogenous estrogen (as estimated from vaginal smears, endometrial biopsy, assay of urinary estrogen or from bleeding in response to progesterone) provide a favorable prognosis for treatment. A reduced estrogen level, although less favorable, does not preclude successful therapy.

Primary pituitary/ovarian failure: Therapy is ineffective in patients with primary pituitary or ovarian failure. Clomiphene cannot be substituted for appropriate therapy of other disturbances leading to ovulatory dysfunction (eg, thyroid or adrenal disease).

Multiple pregnancy: The incidence of multiple pregnancies was increased during those cycles in which clomiphene citrate was given. Among 2369 pregnancies, 92.1% were single and 6.9% were twins. Less than 1% of the reported deliveries resulted in triplets or more. Of these multiple pregnancies, 96% to 99% resulted in the births of live infants. Advise the patient of the frequency and potential hazards of multiple pregnancy before starting treatment.

Ophthalmologic effects: Blurring or other visual symptoms may occasionally occur; patients should use caution when driving or operating machinery, particularly in variable lighting. If visual symptoms occur, discontinue treatment and refer the patient for a complete ophthalmologic evaluation.

Pregnancy: Although no direct effect of clomiphene on the human fetus has been reported, do not administer in cases of suspected pregnancy; fetal effects have been reported in animals.

Birth defects – From 2369 delivered and reported pregnancies associated with clomiphene administration, 58 infants had birth defects. Eight of the 58 infants were born to 7 of 158 mothers who received clomiphene during the first 6 weeks after conception. Also, there were birth defects in 4 conceptions in the abortion/stillbirth category, in 14 of 357 infants from multiple pregnancies, and in 39 of 1697 infants from single pregnancies. Eight liveborn infants failed to survive.

CLOMIPHENE CITRATE

Defects included congenital heart lesions (8 infants), Down's syndrome (5 infants), club foot (4 infants), congenital gut lesions (4 infants), hypospadias (3 infants). Each of the following defects reportedly affected 2 infants each: Microcephaly, harelip and cleft palate, congenital hip defect, hemangioma and undescended testes. The following also occurred: Polydactyly (both of twins), conjoined twins with teratomatous malformation, patent ductus arteriosus, amaurosis (blindness), arteriovenous fistula, inguinal hernia, umbilical hernia, syndactyly, pectus excavatum, myopathy, dermoid cyst of scalp, omphalocele, spina bifida occulta, ichthyosis, persistent lingual frenulum and 7 infants with multiple somatic defects.

In addition to investigational studies, during the first 42 months of commercial availability of clomiphene, information was received on 7 infants with birth defects from 7 pregnancies. These reported defects were: Down's syndrome, adactyly of one hand, achondroplasia, anterior pituitary agenesis and multiple somatic lesions (3 infants).

Precautions:

Diagnosis prior to therapy: A complete pelvic examination is mandatory prior to treatment; repeat before each course. Do not administer in the presence of an ovarian cyst; further enlargement may occur. The incidence of endometrial carcinoma and ovulatory disorders increases with age. Perform an endometrial biopsy before starting therapy. If abnormal bleeding is present, full diagnostic measures are mandatory.

Ovarian overstimulation/enlargement: To minimize the hazard associated with occasional abnormal ovarian enlargement, use the lowest effective dose. Some patients with polycystic ovary syndrome may have an exaggerated response to usual doses. Mid-cycle ovarian pain may be accentuated. With higher or prolonged dosage, ovarian enlargement and cyst formation may occur more frequently and the luteal phase of the cycle may be prolonged. Maximal enlargement of the ovary, whether physiologic or abnormal, does not occur until several days after discontinuation of the drug. Examine patients who complain of pelvic pain after receiving clomiphene. If ovaries are enlarged, do not give additional therapy until they return to pretreatment size; reduce the dosage or duration of the next course. Ovarian enlargement and cyst formation regress spontaneously a few days or weeks after discontinuing therapy. Unless surgical indication for laparotomy exists, manage such cystic enlargement conservatively. Rarely, massive ovarian enlargement has occurred, including a patient with polycystic ovary syndrome taking 100 mg/day for 14 days.

Ophthalmic effects: Symptoms are usually described as "blurring" spots or flashes (scintillating scotomata). They correlate with increasing total dose and disappear within a few days or weeks after discontinuation. These symptoms appear to be due to intensification and prolongation of after-images. They often first appear or are accentuated with exposure to a more brightly lit environment. While measured visual acuity is not generally affected, one patient taking 200 mg/day developed visual blurring on day 7 of treatment, progressing to severe diminution of visual acuity by day 10. Vision returned to normal on the third day after treatment was stopped. Ophthalmologically definable scotomata and electroretinographic retinal function changes have also occurred.

The following conditions have also been reported in association with clomiphene therapy; cause and effect relationship has neither been proven nor disproven: Posterior capsular cataract (all in investigational studies) (4), detachment of the posterior vitreous (1), spasm of retinal arteriole (1) and thrombosis of temporal arteries of retina (1).

Hydatiform mole has been reported in 8 patients receiving clomiphene (includes 4 reported in original 2369 investigational pregnancies). A causal relationship has not been established.

Drug Interactions:

Drug/Lab test interactions:

BSP laboratory studies – Greater than 5% retention of bromsulphalein (BSP) has been reported in approximately 10% to 20% of patients. Retention was usually minimal, but was elevated during prolonged clomiphene administration or with apparently unrelated liver disease. In some patients, preexisting BSP retention decreased even though clomiphene was continued. Other liver function tests were usually normal.

CLOMIPHENE CITRATE

Adverse Reactions:

At recommended dosage, side effects are not prominent, infrequently interfere with treatment and are dose-related.

Vasomotor flushes (10.4%) resembling menopausal "hot flushes" are usually not severe and disappear promptly after treatment is discontinued.

Abdominal symptoms: Abdominal discomfort, distention, bloating (5.5%); abnormal uterine bleeding (1.25%). May resemble ovulatory (mittelschmerz) or premenstrual phenomena or discomfort due to ovarian enlargement.

Abnormal ovarian enlargement (14%) is infrequent at recommended dosage (see Precautions).

Miscellaneous: Nausea, vomiting (2.2%); breast tenderness (2.1%); visual symptoms (1.5%); headache (1.3%); dizziness, lightheadedness (1%); nervousness, insomnia (0.77%); increased urination (0.7%); depression, fatigue (0.7%); urticaria, allergic dermatitis (0.6%); weight gain (0.4%); reversible hair loss (0.3%); ophthalmic effects (see Precautions).

Patient Information:

Notify physician if bloating, stomach or pelvic pain, blurred vision, jaundice, hot flushes, breast discomfort, headache, nausea and vomiting occur.

May cause dizziness, lightheadedness and visual disturbances; observe caution while driving or performing other tasks requiring alertness, coordination or physical dexterity.

Administration and Dosage:

Choose patients only after careful diagnostic evaluation. Ovulation and pregnancy are more attainable on 100 mg/day for 5 days. As dosage increases, however, ovarian overstimulation and other side effects may increase. A correlation may exist between dosage and multiple births.

Initial therapy: First course is 50 mg/day for 5 days. Start at any time in patients who have had no recent uterine bleeding. If progestin-induced bleeding is planned, or if spontaneous uterine bleeding occurs prior to therapy, start the regimen on or about the fifth day of the cycle. If ovulation occurs with this dosage, there is no advantage to increasing the dose in subsequent cycles of treatment. Special treatment with lower doses over a shorter duration is recommended if unusual sensitivity to pituitary gonadotropin is suspected, including patients with polycystic ovary syndrome.

Second course of therapy: Increase the dose in patients not responding to the first course. If ovulation has not occurred after the first course, administer a second course of 100 mg/day for 5 days; do not increase this dosage or duration of therapy. Start this course as early as 30 days after the previous one.

Third course of therapy: The majority of patients who are going to respond will respond to the first course of therapy; 3 courses are an adequate therapeutic trial. If ovulatory menses has not yet occurred, reevaluate diagnosis. Further treatment is not recommended in patients who do not exhibit evidence of ovulation.

Pregnancy: Before starting therapy, advise patients that multiple pregnancy is possible and poses potential hazards. Properly timed coitus is important for good results. The likelihood of conception diminishes with each succeeding course of therapy. If pregnancy has not been achieved after 3 ovulatory responses, further treatment is not recommended. Long–term cyclic therapy is not recommended.

Rx	**Clomiphene Citrate** (Various, eg, Lemmon)	**Tablets:** 50 mg	In 10s and 30s.
Rx	**Clomid** (Hoechst Marion Roussel)		(Clomid 50). White, scored. In 30s.
Rx	**Milophene** (Milex)		(M50). White, scored. In 30s.
Rx	**Serophene** (Serono)		White, scored. In 10s and 30s.

UROFOLLITROPIN

Actions:

Pharmacology: Urofollitropin is a preparation of gonadotropin extracted from the urine of postmenopausal women. Urofollitropin stimulates ovarian follicular growth in women who do not have primary ovarian failure. Treatment in most instances results only in follicular growth and maturation. In order to effect ovulation in the absence of endogenous LH surge, human chorionic gonadotropin (HCG) must be given following the administration of urofollitropin when clinical and laboratory assessment of the patient indicate that sufficient follicular maturation has occurred.

Indications:

Ovulation induction: Urofollitropin and HCG are given sequentially for the induction of ovulation in patients with polycystic ovarian disease who have an elevated LH/FSH ratio and who have failed to respond to adequate clomiphene citrate therapy.

Urofollitropin and HCG may also be used to stimulate the development of multiple follicles in ovulatory patients undergoing Assisted Reproductive Technologies (ART) such as in vitro fertilization.

Follicle stimulation: Urofollitropin and HCG may also be used to stimulate the development of multiple follicles in ovulatory patients undergoing Assisted Reproductive Technologies (ART) such as in vitro fertilization.

Contraindications:

High levels of both LH and FSH indicating primary ovarian failure; overt thyroid or adrenal dysfunction; an organic intracranial lesion such as a pituitary tumor; the presence of any cause of infertility other than anovulation; abnormal bleeding of undetermined origin; ovarian cysts or enlargement not due to polycystic ovary syndrome; hypersensitivity to urofollitropin; pregnancy (see Warnings).

Warnings:

Administration: Urofollitropin should only be used by physicians who are thoroughly familiar with infertility problems. It is a potent gonadotropic substance capable of causing mild to severe adverse reactions. Use with great care.

Overstimulation of the ovary:

Ovarian enlargement – To minimize the hazard associated with the occasional abnormal ovarian enlargement associated with urofollitropin-HCG therapy, use the lowest dose consistent with expectation of good results. Careful monitoring of ovarian response can further minimize the risk of overstimulation.

Mild to moderate uncomplicated ovarian enlargement, which may be accompanied by abdominal distention or abdominal pain, occurs in approximately 20% of those treated with urofollitropin and HCG, and generally regresses without treatment within 2 or 3 weeks.

Ovarian Hyperstimulation Syndrome (OHSS) – The hyperstimulation syndrome is characterized by severe ovarian enlargement, abdominal pain/distention, nausea, vomiting, diarrhea, dyspnea and oliguria, and may be accompanied by ascites, pleural effusion, hypovolemia, electrolyte imbalance, hemoperitoneum and thromboembolic events. OHSS occurred in 6% of patients in trials.

If hyperstimulation occurs, stop treatment and hospitalize the patient. This syndrome develops rapidly within 24 hours to several days and generally occurs during the 7 to 10 days immediately following treatment. Hemoconcentration associated with fluid loss into the abdominal cavity has occurred and should be assessed in the following manner: 1) Fluid intake and output, 2) weight, 3) hematocrit, 4) serum and urinary electrolytes, 5) urine specific gravity, 6) BUN and creatinine and 7) abdominal girth. Perform these determinations daily or more often if the need arises. Treatment is primarily symptomatic and consists of bed rest, fluid and electrolyte replacement and analgesics. The ascitic, pleural and pericardial fluids should never be removed because of the potential danger of injury.

Hemoperitoneum from ruptured ovarian cysts is usually the result of pelvic examination. If this does occur, and if bleeding becomes such that surgery is required, design the surgical treatment to control bleeding and retain as much ovarian tissue as possible.

Intercourse should be prohibited in patients in whom significant ovarian enlargement occurs after ovulation because of the danger of hemoperitoneum resulting from ruptured ovarian cysts.

Pulmonary conditions: Serious pulmonary conditions (eg, atelectasis, acute respiratory distress syndrome) have been reported.

UROFOLLITROPIN

Arterial thromboembolism: Thromboembolic events both in association with, and separate from the OHSS, have been reported. Intravascular thrombosis and embolism, which may originate in venous or arterial vessels, can result in reduced blood flow to critical organs or the extremities. Sequelae of such events have included venous thrombophlebitis, pulmonary embolism, pulmonary infarction, cerebral vascular occlusion (stroke) and arterial occlusion resulting in loss of limb. In rare cases, thromboembolic events have resulted in death.

Multiple births: Reports of multiple pregnancies have been associated with urofollitropin-HCG treatment, including triplet and quintuplet gestations. In clinical studies, 83% of the pregnancies following therapy resulted in single births and 17% in multiple births. Advise the patient of the potential risk of multiple births before starting treatment.

Pregnancy: Category X. Contraindicated in pregnancy. In clinical trials, three incidents of chromosomal abnormalities and four birth defects were reported following urofollitropin-HCG therapy for stimulation prior to in vitro fertilization.

Lactation: It is not known if this drug is excreted in breast milk. Exercise caution if administering to a nursing mother.

Precautions:

Selection of patients: Give careful attention to diagnosis in candidates for therapy. Before treatment is instituted, perform a thorough gynecologic and endocrinologic evaluation including a hysterosalpingogram (to rule out uterine and tubal pathology) and documentation of anovulation by means of basal body temperature, serial vaginal smears, examination of cervical mucus, determination of serum or urinary progesterone, determination of urinary pregnanediol and endometrial biopsy. Patients with tubal pathology should receive the drug only if enrolled in an in vitro fertilization program. Exclude primary ovarian failure by the determination of gonadotropin levels. Make careful examination to rule out early pregnancy. Patients in late reproductive life have a greater predilection to endometrial carcinoma and a higher incidence of anovulatory disorders. Perform cervical dilation and curettage for diagnosis before starting therapy. Evaluate partner's fertility potential.

Ovulation confirmation: Treatment results in follicular growth and maturation to effect ovulation in the absence of an endogenous LH surge. HCG is given following the administration of urofollitropin when clinical assessment indicates sufficient follicular maturation has occurred. This is indirectly estimated by the estrogenic effect upon the target organs. With serum or urinary estrogen determinations and ultrasonography, the estrogenic effect is an acceptable means for monitoring the growth and development of follicles, timing HCG administration and minimizing the risk of hyperstimulation. Clinically confirm ovulation, with the exception of pregnancy, by indirect indices of progesterone production. The indices most generally used are a rise in basal body temperature, increase in serum progesterone and menstruation following the shift in basal body temperature.

Other clinical parameters that may have potential use for monitoring urofollitropin therapy include changes in the vaginal cytology, appearance and volume of the cervical mucus, sinnbarkeit and ferning of the cervical mucus.

Adverse Reactions:

The following adverse reactions are listed in decreasing order of potential severity: Pulmonary and vascular complications (see Warnings); Ovarian Hyperstimulation Syndrome (see Warnings); adnexal torsion (as a complication of ovarian enlargement; mild to moderate ovarian enlargement; abdominal pain; sensitivity to urofollitropin (febrile reactions which may be accompanied by chills, musculoskeletal aches, joint pains, malaise, headache and fatigue have occurred. It is not clear whether or not these were pyrogenic responses or possible allergic reactions); ovarian cysts; GI symptoms (nausea, vomiting, diarrhea, abdominal cramps, bloating); pain, rash, swelling or irritation at the site of injection; breast tenderness; headache; dermatological symptoms (dry skin, body rash, hair loss, hives); hemoperitoneum has been reported during menotropins therapy and, therefore, may also occur during urofollitropin therapy.

Overdosage:

Aside from possible hyperstimulation and multiple gestations (see Warnings), little is known concerning the consequences of acute overdosage.

Patient Information:

Prior to therapy, inform patients of the following: Duration of treatment and monitoring required; possible adverse reactions; risk of multiple births.

UROFOLLITROPIN

Administration and Dosage:

Individualize dosage.

Initial dose: 75 IU/day IM urofollitropin for 7 to 12 days, followed by 5,000 to 10,000 U of HCG one day after the last urofollitropin dose. Administration of urofollitropin may exceed 12 days if inadequate follicle development is indicated by estrogen or ultrasound measurement. Treat the patient until estrogenic activity is equivalent to or greater than that of a normal individual. If the ovaries are abnormally enlarged on the last day of therapy, do not give HCG in this course of therapy; this reduces the chances of developing hyperstimulation syndrome. If there is evidence of ovulation but no pregnancy, repeat this dosage regimen for at least two more courses before increasing the dose to 150 IU of FSH per day for 7 to 12 days. Follow this dose with 5,000 to 10,000 U of HCG one day after the last urofollitropin dose. If evidence of ovulation is present, but pregnancy does not ensue, repeat the same dose for two more courses. Larger doses are not recommended.

During treatment with urofollitropin and HCG and during a 2 week post-treatment period, examine patients at least every other day for signs of excessive ovarian stimulation. Stop administration if the ovaries become abnormally enlarged or if abdominal pain occurs. Most ovarian hyperstimulation occurs after treatment discontinuation and reaches its maximum at 7 to 10 days postovulation.

Encourage the couple to have intercourse daily, beginning on the day prior to HCG administration until ovulation is apparent from determining progestational activity.

For Assisted Reproductive Technologies, therapy with urofollitropin should be initiated in the early follicular phase (cycle day 2 or 3) at a dose of 150 IU per day, until sufficient follicular development is attained. In most cases, therapy should not exceed ten days.

Preparation of solution: Dissolve contents of 1 ampule in 1 to 2 ml sterile saline; administer IM immediately. Discard unused reconstituted material.

Storage: Store at 3° to 25°C (37° to 77°F). Protect from light.

Rx	**Metrodin** (Serono)	**Powder for Injection:** 0.83 mg (75 IU FSH activity) per amp[1]	With 2 ml amp sodium chloride injection. In 1, 10 and 100 ampuls.
		1.66 mg (150 IU FSH activity) per amp[1]	With 2 ml amp sodium chloride injection. In 1 ampule.
Rx	**Fertinex** (Serono)	**Powder for Injection, lyophilized:** 75 IU	In 1, 10 and 100 ampules with diluent.
		Powder for Injection, lyophilized: 150 IU	In 1 ampule with diluent.

[1] With 10 mg lactose, in a lyophilized form.

MENOTROPINS

Actions:

Pharmacology: Menotropins is a purified preparation of gonadotropins extracted from the urine of postmenopausal women. It is biologically standardized for follicle stimulating hormone (FSH) and luteinizing hormone (LH) activities.

Women – Produces ovarian follicular growth in women who do not have primary ovarian failure. Treatment results only in follicular growth and maturation. To effect ovulation, human chorionic gonadotropin (HCG) is given following menotropins when clinical assessment indicates sufficient follicular maturation.

Men – Menotropins administered concomitantly with HCG for at least 3 months induces spermatogenesis in men with primary or secondary pituitary hypofunction who have achieved adequate masculinization with prior HCG therapy.

Indications:

Women: Menotropins and HCG are given sequentially for induction of ovulation and pregnancy in the anovulatory infertile patient, in whom the cause of anovulation is functional and not due to primary ovarian failure.

Menotropins and HCG may be used to stimulate development of multiple follicles in ovulatory patients participating in an in vitro fertilization program.

Men: Menotropins and concomitant HCG are given for stimulation of spermatogenesis in men with primary or secondary hypogonadotropic hypogonadism due to a congenital factor or prepubertal hypophysectomy and in men with secondary hypogonadotropic hypogonadism due to hypophysectomy, craniopharyngioma, cerebral aneurysm or chromophobe adenoma.

Contraindications:

Women: High gonadotropin level indicating primary ovarian failure; overt thyroid and adrenal dysfunction; any cause of infertility other than anovulation; abnormal bleeding of undetermined origin; ovarian cysts or enlargement not due to polycystic ovary syndrome; organic intracranial lesion such as pituitary tumor; pregnancy.

Men: Normal gonadotropin levels indicating normal pituitary function; elevated gonadotropin levels indicating primary testicular failure; infertility disorders other than hypogonadotropic hypogonadism.

Warnings:

Physician use: This drug should be used only by physicians thoroughly familiar with infertility problems. Menotropins can cause mild to severe adverse reactions in women.

Hypersensitivity reactions: Hypersensitivity/anaphylactic reactions associated with menotropin administration have been reported in some patients. These reactions presented as generalized urticaria, facial edema, angioneurotic edema or dyspnea suggestive of laryngeal edema.

Pregnancy: Category X. Menotropins may cause fetal harm. Birth defects occurred in 5 of 287 pregnancies. Do not use during pregnancy.

Precautions:

Diagnosis prior to therapy:

Women – Perform a thorough gynecologic and endocrinologic evaluation, including a hysterosalpingogram. Document anovulation. Rule out primary ovarian failure and early pregnancy. Patients in late reproductive life have a greater predilection to endometrial carcinoma and a higher incidence of anovulatory disorders. Perform a cervical dilation and curettage before starting therapy in such patients. Evaluate the partner's fertility potential.

Men – Document lack of pituitary function. Prior to therapy, patients have low testosterone levels and low or absent gonadotropin levels. Patients with primary hypogonadotropic hypogonadism will have subnormal development of masculinization; those with secondary hypogonadotropic hypogonadism will have decreased masculinization.

Overstimulation of the ovary: To minimize the hazard of abnormal ovarian enlargement, use the lowest effective dose. Mild to moderate uncomplicated ovarian enlargement, with or without abdominal distention or abdominal pain, occurs in ≈ 20% of those treated with HCG and menotropins and generally regresses without treatment in 2 to 3 weeks. The hyperstimulation syndrome characterized by sudden ovarian enlargement and ascites, with or without pain or pleural effusion, occurs in ≈ 0.4% of patients at recommended doses. The overall incidence of this syndrome is about 1.3%.

MENOTROPINS

Hyperstimulation syndrome develops rapidly and generally occurs within 2 weeks following treatment; if it occurs, discontinue treatment and hospitalize patient. Hemoconcentration associated with fluid loss in the abdominal cavity has occurred; thoroughly assess by daily determination of fluid intake and output, weight, hematocrit, serum and urinary electrolytes, urine specific gravity, BUN, creatinine and abdominal girth. Treatment is primarily symptomatic and consists of bedrest, fluid and electrolyte replacement and analgesics. Never remove ascitic fluid because of the potential for injury to the ovary. Hemoperitoneum may occur from ruptured ovarian cysts, usually as a result of pelvic examination. If bleeding requires surgery, design the surgery to control bleeding and to retain as much ovarian tissue as possible. Prohibit intercourse when significant ovarian enlargement occurs after ovulation.

Multiple births: Pregnancies following therapy with HCG and menotropins resulted in 80% single births; 15% resulted in twins and 5% of pregnancies produced 3 or more conceptuses. Advise patient of the frequency and potential hazards of multiple pregnancy.

Pulmonary/Vascular complications: Serious pulmonary conditions (eg, atelectasis, acute respiratory distress syndrome) have been reported. In addition, thromboembolic events both in association with, and separate from, the Ovarian Hyperstimulation Syndrome have been reported following menotropin therapy. Intravascular thrombosis and embolism, which may originate in venous or arterial vessels, can result in reduced blood flow to critical organs or the extremities. Sequelae of such events have included venous thrombophlebitis, pulmonary embolism, pulmonary infarction, cerebral vascular occlusion (stroke) and arterial occlusion resulting in loss of limb. In rare cases, pulmonary complications or thromboembolic events have resulted in death.

Adverse Reactions:

Women: Ovarian enlargement, ovarian cysts, adnexal torsion (as a complication of ovarian enlargement); hyperstimulation syndrome; hemoperitoneum; hypersensitivity (see Warnings); febrile reactions; fever; chills; musculoskeletal aches; joint pains; nausea; headaches; malaise; pulmonary and vascular complications (see Precautions); abdominal pain; vomiting; diarrhea; abdominal cramps; bloating; pain, rash, swelling or irritation at injection site; body rashes; dizziness; tachycardia; dyspnea; tachypnea; ectopic pregnancy.

Men: Occasional gynecomastia, breast pain, mastitis, nausea, abnormal lipoprotein fraction, abnormal AST and ALT (occasional), erythrocytosis (Hct 50%, Hgb 17.8 g%, in one patient).

Administration and Dosage:

Women: Treatment results only in follicular growth and maturation. To effect ovulation, HCG must be given following menotropins when clinical assessment indicates sufficient follicular maturation. This is indirectly estimated by the estrogenic effect on target organs (ie, changes in the vaginal smear, appearance and volume of cervical mucus, spinnbarkeit, ferning of cervical mucus). Urinary excretion of estrogens is a more reliable index of follicular maturation.

The clinical confirmation of ovulation, with the exception of pregnancy, is by indirect indices of progesterone production. These include rise in basal temperature; increase in serum progesterone; menstruation following a shift in basal temperature.

Initial dosage – Individualize dosage. Initial IM dose is 75 IU FSH/75 IU LH (1 amp) per day, for 7 to 12 days; follow by 10,000 IU HCG 1 day after the last dose of menotropins. Do not exceed 12 days of menotropins administration. Treat the patient until indices of estrogenic activity are equal to or greater than those of the normal individual. Urinary estrogen determinations are useful as a guide to therapy. If the total estrogen excretion is < 100 mcg/24 hours or if the estriol excretion is < 50 mcg/24 hours prior to HCG administration, hyperstimulation syndrome is less likely to occur. If the estrogen values are greater than 150 mcg/24 hours, it is not advisable to administer HCG because the hyperstimulation syndrome is more likely to occur. If the ovaries are abnormally enlarged on the last day of menotropins therapy, do not administer HCG in this course.

The couple should have intercourse daily, beginning on the day prior to HCG administration, until ovulation occurs. Take care to ensure insemination.

Repeat dosage – If there is evidence of ovulation, but no pregnancy, repeat the regimen for at least 2 more courses before increasing the dose to 150 IU FSH/150 IU LH (2 amps) per day for 7 to 12 days. Follow by 10,000 IU HCG 1 day after the last dose of menotropins. Two amps of menotropins per day is the most effective dose. If evidence of ovulation is present, but pregnancy does not ensue, repeat the same dose for 2 more courses but larger doses are not recommended.

MENOTROPINS

During treatment with menotropins and HCG and for 2 weeks post-treatment, examine patients at least every other day for signs of excessive ovarian stimulation. Stop treatment if the ovaries become abnormally enlarged or if abdominal pain occurs. Hyperstimulation usually occurs after treatment has been discontinued and reaches its maximum 7 to 10 days postovulation.

Men: Prior to therapy with menotropins and HCG, pretreat with HCG alone (5,000 IU 3 times a week). Continue HCG for a sufficient period to achieve serum testosterone levels within the normal range and masculinization (ie, appearance of secondary sex characteristics). Pretreatment may require 4 to 6 months. The recommended dose is 1 amp menotropins IM 3 times a week and HCG 2,000 IU twice a week. Continue therapy for a minimum of 4 months to ensure detecting spermatozoa in ejaculate.

If the patient has not responded with increased spermatogenesis at the end of 4 months, continue treatment with 1 amp 3 times a week or increase dose to 2 amps (150 IU FSH/150 IU LH) 3 times a week, with the HCG dose unchanged.

Preparation of solution: Dissolve contents of 1 amp in 1 to 2 ml sterile saline. Administer IM immediately. Discard any unused portion.

Storage/Stability: Lyophilized powder may be refrigerated or stored at room temperature, 3° to 25°C (37° to 77°F).

Rx	**Pergonal** (Serono)	**Powder for Injection, lyophilized**: 75 IU FSH activity, 75 IU LH activity	In 2 ml amps.[1]
Rx	**Humegon** (Organon)		In vials with 2 ml NaCl injection.[2]
Rx	**Pergonal** (Serono)	**Powder for Injection, lyophilized**: 150 IU FSH activity, 150 IU LH activity	In 2 ml amps.[1]
Rx	**Humegon** (Organon)		In vials with 2 ml NaCl injection.[2]

[1] With 10 mg lactose in a lyophilized form.

[2] With 10.5 mg lactose, 0.25 mg monosodium phosphate, 0.25 mg disodium phosphate.

CHORIONIC GONADOTROPIN (HCG)

> **Warning:**
> HCG has no known effect on fat mobilization, appetite, sense of hunger or body fat distribution. HCG has NOT been demonstrated to be effective adjunctive therapy in the treatment of obesity. There is no substantial evidence that it increases weight loss beyond that resulting from caloric restriction, that it causes a more attractive or "normal" distribution of fat or that it decreases the hunger and discomfort associated with calorie restricted diets.

Actions:

Pharmacology: Human chorionic gonadotropin (HCG), a polypeptide hormone produced by the human placenta, is composed of an α and β subunit. The α subunit is essentially identical to the α subunits of the human pituitary gonadotropins, luteinizing hormone (LH) and follicle stimulating hormone (FSH), as well as to the α subunit of human thyroid stimulating hormone (TSH). The β subunits of these hormones differ in amino acid sequence.

HCG's action is virtually identical to pituitary LH's, although HCG appears to have a small degree of FSH activity as well. It stimulates production of gonadal steroid hormones by stimulating interstitial cells (Leydig cells) of testis to produce androgens, and the corpus luteum of the ovary to produce progesterone. Androgen stimulation in males leads to development of secondary sex characteristics and may stimulate testicular descent when no anatomical impediment is present. The descent is usually reversible when HCG is discontinued. During the normal menstrual cycle, LH participates with FSH in development and maturation of the normal ovarian follicle, and the mid-cycle LH surge triggers ovulation; HCG can substitute for LH in this function. During a normal pregnancy, HCG secreted by the placenta maintains the corpus luteum after LH secretion decreases, supporting continued estrogen and progesterone secretion and preventing menstruation.

Indications:

Prepubertal cryptorchidism not due to anatomical obstruction. HCG is thought to induce testicular descent in situations when descent would have occurred at puberty. HCG may help predict whether orchiopexy will be needed in the future. In some cases, descent following HCG administration is permanent, but in most cases the response is temporary. Therapy is usually instituted between the ages of 4 and 9.

Hypogonadism: Selected cases of hypogonadotropic hypogonadism (hypogonadism secondary to a pituitary deficiency) in males.

Ovulation induction: Induction of ovulation in the anovulatory, infertile woman in whom the cause of anovulation is secondary and not due to primary ovarian failure, and who has been appropriately pretreated with human menotropins.

Contraindications:

Precocious puberty; prostatic carcinoma or other androgen-dependent neoplasm; prior allergic reaction to chorionic gonadotropin; pregnancy (see Warnings).

Warnings:

Use for infertility: HCG should be used in conjunction with human menopausal gonadotropins only by physicians experienced with infertility problems.

Pregnancy: Category X. HCG may cause fetal harm when administered to a pregnant woman. Combined HCG/PMS (pregnant mare's serum) therapy has been noted to induce high incidences of external congenital anomalies in the offspring of mice, in a dose-dependent manner. The potential extrapolation to humans has not been determined.

Lactation: It is not known whether this drug is excreted in breast milk. Exercise caution when HCG is administered to a nursing woman.

Children: Safety and efficacy in children < 4 years of age have not been established.

Precautions:

Precocious puberty: Induction of androgen secretion by HCG may induce phallic enlargement; testicular enlargement and redness; development of pubic hair; agressive behavior. These changes are reversible within 4 weeks of the last injection.

Fluid retention: Since androgens may cause fluid retention, use HCG with caution in patients with epilepsy, migraine, asthma, cardiac or renal disease.

Adverse Reactions:

Headache; irritability; restlessness; depression; fatigue; edema; precocious puberty; gynecomastia; pain at injection site; agressive behavior; ovarian hyperstimulation syndrome; ovarian malignancy (rare); enlargement of pre-existing ovarian cysts and possible rupture; arterial thromboembolism.

CHORIONIC GONADOTROPIN (HCG)

Ovulation induction: The principal serious adverse reactions with this indication are: Ovarian hyperstimulation (sudden ovarian enlargement); ascites with or without pain and pleural effusion; rupture of ovarian cysts with resultant hemoperitoneum; multiple births; arterial thromboembolism.

Administration and Dosage:

For IM use only. There is a marked variance of opinion concerning dosage regimens. The regimen employed will depend on the indication, age and weight of the patient and the physician's preference. The following regimens have been advocated.

Prepubertal cryptorchidism not due to anatomical obstruction:

1.) 4000 USP units, 3 times weekly for 3 weeks.
2.) 5000 USP units every second day for 4 injections.
3.) 15 injections of 500 to 1000 USP units over a period of 6 weeks.
4.) 500 USP units, 3 times weekly for 4 to 6 weeks. If this course is not successful, start another course 1 month later, giving 1000 USP units per injection.

Selected cases of hypogonadotropic hypogonadism in males:

1.) 500 to 1000 USP units 3 times a week for 3 weeks, followed by the same dose twice a week for 3 weeks.
2.) 1000 to 2000 USP units, 3 times weekly.
3.) 4000 USP units 3 times weekly for 6 to 9 months; reduce dosage to 2000 USP units 3 times weekly for an additional 3 months.

Induction of ovulation and pregnancy: In the anovulatory, infertile woman in whom the cause of anovulation is secondary and not due to primary ovarian failure, and who has been appropriately pretreated with human menotropins (see Menotropins monograph) - 5,000 to 10,000 USP units 1 day following the last dose of menotropins.

The following products consist of lyophilized powder, with or without diluent, to prepare solutions for injection providing the indicated number of units of HCG. Refer to manufacturers' labeling for preparation and storage.

Rx	**Chorionic Gonadotropin** (Various, eg, Goldline, Lyphomed, Rugby, Steris)	**Powder for Injection:** 5,000 units per vial with 10 ml diluent (to make 500 units per ml)	In 10 ml vials.
Rx	**A.P.L.** (Wyeth-Ayerst)		In 10 ml vials.[1]
Rx	**Chorex-5** (Hyrex)		In 10 ml vials.[2]
Rx	**Profasi** (Serono)		In 10 ml vials.[2]
Rx	**Chorionic Gonadotropin** (Various, eg, Goldline, Lyphomed, Rugby, Steris)	**Powder for Injection:** 10,000 units per vial with 10 ml diluent (to make 1,000 units per ml)	In 10 ml vials.
Rx	**A.P.L.** (Wyeth-Ayerst)		In 10 ml vials.[1]
Rx	**Chorex-10** (Hyrex)		In 10 ml vials.[2]
Rx	**Choron 10** (Forest)		In 10 ml vials.[2]
Rx	**Gonic** (Hauck)		In 10 ml vials.[2]
Rx	**Pregnyl** (Organon)		In 10 ml vials.[3]
Rx	**Profasi** (Serono)		In 10 ml vials.[2]
Rx	**Chorionic Gonadotropin** (Various, eg, Goldline, Lyphomed, Steris)	**Powder for Injection:** 20,000 units per vial with 10 ml diluent (to make 2,000 units per ml)	In 10 ml vials.
Rx	**A.P.L.** (Wyeth-Ayerst)		In 10 ml vials.[1]

[1] With benzyl alcohol, < 0.2% phenol and lactose.
[2] With mannitol and 0.9% benzyl alcohol.
[3] With 0.9% benzyl alcohol.

GONADORELIN ACETATE

Actions:

Pharmacology: Gonadorelin acetate is used for the induction of ovulation in women with primary hypothalamic amenorrhea. Gonadorelin acetate is a synthetic decapeptide that is identical in amino acid sequence to endogenous gonadotropin-releasing hormone (GnRH) synthesized in the human hypothalamus and in various neurons terminating in the hypothalamus.

Under physiologic conditions, GnRH is released by the hypothalamus in a pulsatile fashion. The primary effect of GnRH is the synthesis and release of luteinizing hormone (LH) in the anterior pituitary gland. GnHR also stimulates the synthesis and release of follicle stimulating hormone (FSH), but this effect is less pronounced. LH and FSH subsequently stimulate the gonads to produce steroids which are instrumental in regulating reproductive hormonal status. Unlike human menopausal gonadotropin (hMG) which supplies pituitary hormones, pulsatile administration of gonadorelin replaces defective hypothalamic secretion of GnRH. The pulsatile administration of gonadorelin approximates the natural hormonal secretory pattern, causing pulsatile release of pituitary gonadotropins. Accordingly, gonadorelin is useful in treating conditions of infertility caused by defective GnRH stimulation from the hypothalamus.

Pharmacokinetics: Following IV injection of GnRH into healthy subjects or hypogonadotropic patients, plasma GnRH concentrations rapidly decline with initial and terminal half-lives of 2 to 10 min and 10 to 40 min, respectively. High clearance values (500 to 1500 L/day) and low volumes of distribution (10 to 15 L) were calculated. The pharmacokinetics of GnRH in healthy subjects and in hypogonadotropic patients were similar. GnRH was rapidly metabolized to various biologically inactive peptide fragments which are readily excreted in urine. Renal failure, but not hepatic disease, prolonged the half-life and reduced the clearance of GnRH.

Clinical trials: The following information summarizes clinical efficacy of gonadorelin acetate administered by pulsatile IV injection to 44 patients with primary hypothalamic amenorrhea: 93% (41/44) were ovulatory with gonadorelin acetate therapy, 62% (24/39) became pregnant (five did not desire pregnancy), and 100% (7/7) of those failing past attempts at ovulation induction by other methods were ovulatory on gonadorelin.

Indications:

Primary hypothalamic amenorrhea treatment.

Gonadorelin HCl (*Factrel*), a related polypeptide hormone, is indicated for evaluating the functional capacity and response of the gonadotropes of the anterior pituitary and for evaluating residual gonadotropic function of the pituitary following removal of a pituitary tumor by surgery or irradiation. See individual monograph in In Vivo Diagnostic Aids section.

Contraindications:

Women with any condition that could be exacerbated by pregnancy (eg, pituitary prolactinoma); sensitivity to gonadorelin acetate, gonadorelin HCl or any component of the product; patients who have ovarian cysts or causes of anovulation other than those of hypothalamic origin; any condition that may be worsened by reproductive hormones, such as a hormonally dependent tumor, since gonadorelin is intended to initiate events including the production of reproductive hormones (eg, estrogens and progestins).

Warnings:

Ovarian hyperstimulation, a syndrome of sudden ovarian enlargement, ascites with or without pain, or pleural effusion, has occurred (< 1%). This may be related to pulse dosage or concomitant use of other ovulation stimulators. Hyperstimulation may be a greater risk in patients where spontaneous variations in endogenous GnRH secretion occur.

Therapy with gonadorelin acetate should be conducted by physicians familiar with pulsatile GnRH delivery and the clinical ramifications of ovulation induction. If hyperstimulation should occur, discontinue therapy; spontaneous resolution can be expected. The preservation of the endogenous feedback mechanisms (pulsatile therapy) makes severe hyperstimulation (with ascites and pleural effusion) rare. However, be aware of the possibility and be alert for any evidence of ascites, pleural effusion, hemoconcentration, rupture of a cyst, fluid or electrolyte imbalance or sepsis.

Among 268 patients participating in clinical trials, one case of moderate hyperstimulation has been reported, but this cycle included the concomitant use of clomiphene citrate. In contrast, menotropins (hMG) with hCG have been variously reported to cause some degree of hyperstimulation in up to 50% of conception cycles, and severe hyperstimulation may occur in up to 1.3% of all cycles.

GONADORELIN ACETATE

Multiple pregnancy is a possibility (12%); minimize by careful attention to the recommended doses and ultrasonographic monitoring of the ovarian response to therapy, including follicle formulation. Multiple follicle development and spontaneous termination of pregnancy have occurred. Following a baseline pelvic ultrasound, conduct follow-up studies at a minimum on day 7 and day 14 of the therapy.

Asepsis: As with any IV medication, scrupulous attention to asepsis is important. The infusion area must be monitored as with all indwelling parenteral approaches. Change the cannula and IV site at 48-hour intervals.

Pregnancy: Category B. Studies in pregnant women have shown that gonadorelin acetate does not increase the risk of abnormalities when administered during the first trimester of pregnancy. The possibility of fetal harm appears remote if the drug is used during pregnancy. In clinical studies, 47 pregnant patients have used gonadorelin acetate during the first trimester of pregnancy (51 pregnancies) and the drug had no apparent adverse effect on the course of pregnancy. Reports on infants born to these women reveal no adverse effects or complications attributable to gonadorelin acetate. Nevertheless, use during pregnancy only for maintenance of the corpus luteum in ovulation induction cycles.

Lactation: It is not known whether the drug is excreted in breast milk. There is no indication for use of gonadorelin acetate in a nursing woman.

Children: Safety and efficacy in children < 18 years of age have not been established.

Precautions:

Monitoring: Following a diagnosis of primary hypothalamic amenorrhea, initiation of gonadorelin acetate therapy may be monitored by: Ovarian ultrasound – baseline, therapy day 7, therapy day 14; mid-luteal phase serum progesterone; clinical observation of infusion site at each visit as needed; physical examination including pelvic at regularly scheduled visits.

Differential diagnosis: Proper diagnosis is critical for successful treatment with gonadorelin. It must be established that hypothalamic amenorrhea or hypogonadism is due to a deficiency in quantity or pulsing of endogenous GnRH. The diagnosis of hypothalamic amenorrhea or hypogonadism is based on the exclusion of other causes of the dysfunction, since there is no practical technique to directly assess hypothalamic function. Prior to initiation of therapy, rule out disorders of general health, reproductive organs, anterior pituitary and central nervous system, other than abnormalities of GnRH secretion.

Lutrepulse pump is required. Provide the patient with detailed oral and written instructions regarding infusion pump usage and potential sepsis in order to minimize the frequency of infusion pump malfunction and inflammation, infection, mild phlebitis or hematoma at the catheter site.

Drug Interactions:

Ovulation stimulators should not be used concomitantly with gonadorelin acetate.

Adverse Reactions:

Adverse reactions have been reported in approximately 10% of treatment regimens. Ten of 268 patients interrupted therapy because of an adverse reaction but subsequently resumed treatment. One other subject did not resume treatment.

Ovarian hyperstimulation: In clinical studies involving 268 women, one case of moderate ovarian hyperstimulation occurred (see Warnings).

Multiple pregnancy: In clinical studies, 11 of 89 pregnancies (12%) were multiple (10 sets of twins, 1 set of triplets). See Warnings.

Local (Use of the infusion pump): Inflammation; infection; mild phlebitis; hematoma at the catheter site.

Anaphylaxis (bronchospasm, tachycardia, flushing, urticaria, induration of injection site) has been reported with the related polypeptide hormone gonadorelin HCl (*Factrel*). (See individual monograph in In Vivo Diagnostic Aids Section.)

Overdosage:

Continuous, non-pulsatile exposure to gonadorelin acetate could temporarily reduce pituitary responsiveness. If the pump should malfunction and deliver the entire contents of the 3.2 mg system, no harmful effects would be expected. Bolus doses as high as 3000 mcg of gonadorelin HCl have not been harmful. Pituitary hyperstimulation and multiple follicle development can be minimized by adhering to recommended doses and appropriate monitoring of follicle formation (see Warnings).

Patient Information:

Patient instructions included with kit; also includes physician package insert and pump manual.

GONADORELIN ACETATE

Administration and Dosage:

Primary hypothalamic amenorrhea: 5 mcg every 90 minutes (range, 1 to 20 mcg). This is delivered by *Lutrepulse* pump using the 0.8 mg solution at 50 mcl per pulse (see physician pump manual); 68% of the 5 mcg every 90 minute regimens induced ovulation in patients with primary hypothalamic amenorrhea.

The *Lutrepulse* pump can deliver 2.5, 5, 10 or 20 mcg of gonadorelin acetate every 90 minutes. The recommended treatment interval is 21 days. Some may be refractory to this dose. It may be necessary to raise the dose cautiously, and in stepwise fashion if there is no response after three treatment intervals. Carefully monitor all dose changes for inappropriate response. Some women may require a reduction in the recommended dose of 5 mcg.

The following table can be used to individualize the dose per pulse:

Gonadorelin Acetate Dose per Pulse			
Vial	Diluent	Volume/pulse	Dose/pulse
0.8 mg	8 ml	25 mcl	2.5 mcg
0.8 mg	8 ml	50 mcl	5 mcg
3.2 mg	8 ml	25 mcl	10 mcg
3.2 mg	8 ml	50 mcl	20 mcg

The response to gonadorelin acetate usually occurs within 2 to 3 weeks after therapy initiation. When ovulation occurs with the *Lutrepulse* pump in place, continue therapy for another 2 weeks to maintain the corpus luteum. A comparison of gonadorelin acetate to hCG or hCG plus gonadorelin acetate for corpus luteum maintenance revealed the following information:

Corpus Luteum Maintenance with Gonadorelin Acetate			
	hCG (n = 63)	Gonadorelin (n = 26)	hCG plus gonadorelin (n = 25)
Delivered	68%	73%	76%
Aborted	32%	27%	24%

Gonadorelin alone was able to maintain the corpus luteum during pregnancy.

Gonadorelin is to be reconstituted aseptically with 8 ml of diluent for gonadorelin acetate immediately prior to use and transfered to the plastic reservoir. First withdraw 8 ml of the saline diluent and then inject it onto the lyophile (drug product) cake. Shake for a few seconds to produce a solution which should be clear, colorless, and free of particulate matter. If particulate matter or discoloration are present, the solution should not be used. A pre-sterilized reservoir (bag) with the infusion catheter set supplied with the kit is filled with the reconstituted solution and administered IV using the *Lutrepulse* pump. Set the pump to deliver 25 or 50 mcl of solution, based upon the dose selected, over a pulse period of 1 minute and at a pulse frequency of 90 minutes. The 8 ml of solution will supply 90 minute pulsatile doses for approximately 7 consecutive days.

Storage: Store at controlled room temperature (15° to 30°C; 59° to 86°F).

Rx	**Lutrepulse** (Ferring)	**Powder for Injection (lyophilized)**: 0.8 and 3.2 mg	In 10 ml vials. In kits containing 10 ml diluent, catheter and tubing, four IV cannula units, syringe and needle, four alcohol swabs, elastic belt and 9V battery; also includes *Lutrepulse Pump* kit with pump, two 9V batteries, 3V lithium battery, physician pump manual and package insert.

NAFARELIN ACETATE

Actions:

Pharmacology: Nafarelin acetate is a potent agonistic analog of gonadotropin-releasing hormone (GnRH). At the onset of administration, nafarelin stimulates the release of the pituitary gonadotropins, LH and FSH, resulting in a temporary increase of ovarian steroidogenesis. Repeated dosing abolishes the stimulatory effect on the pituitary gland. Twice daily administration leads to decreased secretion of gonadal steroids by about 4 weeks; consequently, tissues and functions that depend on gonadal steroids for their maintenance become quiescent.

When used regularly in girls and boys with central precocious puberty (CPP), nafarelin suppresses LH and sex steroid hormone levels to prepubertal levels, affects a corresponding arrest of secondary sexual development, and slows linear growth and skeletal maturation. In some cases, initial estrogen withdrawal bleeding may occur, generally within 6 weeks after initiation of therapy. Thereafter, menstruation should cease. In clinical studies the peak response of LH to GnRH stimulation was reduced from a pubertal to a prepubertal response (< 15 mIU/ml) within 1 month.

Linear growth velocity, commonly pubertal in children with CPP, is reduced in most children within the first year of treatment to values of ≤ 5 to 6 cm/year. Children with CPP are frequently taller than their chronological age peers; height for chronological age approaches normal in most children during the second or third year of treatment. Skeletal maturation rate is usually abnormal in children with CPP; in most children, bone age velocity approaches normal during the first year of treatment. This results in a narrowing of the gap between bone age and chronological age, usually by the second or third year. Mean predicted adult height increases.

Pharmacokinetics:

Absorption/Distribution – Nafarelin is rapidly absorbed into systemic circulation after intranasal administration. Maximum serum concentrations are achieved between 10 and 45 minutes. In adults, following a single dose of 200 mcg base, the observed average peak concentration is 0.6 ng/ml, whereas following a single dose of 400 mcg base, the observed average peak concentration is 1.8 ng/ml. In children, following a single dose of 400 mcg base, the observed peak concentration 2.2 ng/ml, whereas following a single 600 mcg dose the observed peak concentration is 6.6 ng/ml. Bioavailability from a 400 mcg dose averaged 2.8%. The average serum half-life following intranasal administration is approximately 3 hours in adults and 2.5 hours in children. About 80% is bound to plasma proteins.

Metabolism/Excretion – After SC use, 44% to 55% of dose was recovered in urine and 18.5% to 44.2% in feces. About 3% of dose appears unchanged in urine. Serum half-life of metabolites is about 85.5 hours. Activity of the six identified metabolites, nafarelin metabolism by nasal mucosa, and pharmacokinetics in hepatic and renal impairment have not been determined.

Clinical trials:

Endometriosis – In controlled clinical studies, nafarelin doses of 400 and 800 mcg/day for 6 months were comparable to danazol 800 mg/day in relieving the clinical symptoms of endometriosis (pelvic pain, dysmenorrhea and dyspareunia) and in reducing the size of endometrial implants as determined by laparoscopy.

Nafarelin 400 mcg/day induced amenorrhea in ≈ 65%, 80% and 90% of the patients after 60, 90 and 120 days, respectively. Most of the rest reported only light bleeding or spotting. In post-treatment months 1, 2 and 3, normal cycles resumed in 4%, 82% and 100%, respectively, of those who did not become pregnant.

At the end of treatment, 60% of patients who received 400 mcg/day were symptom free, 32% had mild symptoms, 7% had moderate symptoms and 1% had severe symptoms. Of the 60% of patients who had complete symptom relief, 17% had moderate symptoms 6 months after treatment was discontinued, 33% had mild symptoms, 50% remained symptom free and no patient had severe symptoms.

There is no evidence that nafarelin enhances or decreases pregnancy rates.

CPP – In clinical trials, breast development was arrested or regressed in 82% of girls, and genital development was arrested or regressed in 100% of boys. Because pubic hair growth is largely controlled by adrenal androgens (unaffected by nafarelin), its development was arrested or regressed only in 54% of girls and boys.

Reversal of nafarelin's suppressive effects occurs in all children with CPP, and consists of appearance or return of menses, return of pubertal gonadotropin and gonadal sex steroid levels, or advancement of secondary sexual development. Semen analysis was normal in the two ejaculated specimens obtained thus far from boys who have been taken off therapy to resume puberty. Fertility has not been documented by pregnancies and the effect of long-term use on fertility is not known.

Indications:

Endometriosis, including pain relief and reduction of endometriotic lesions. Experience has been limited to women ≥ 18 years of age treated for 6 months.

Central precocious puberty (gonadotropin-dependent) in children of both sexes.

NAFARELIN ACETATE

Contraindications:

Hypersensitivity to GnRH, GnRH-agonist analogs or any excipients in the product; undiagnosed abnormal vaginal bleeding; pregnancy and lactation (see Warnings).

Warnings:

Establish diagnosis of CPP before treatment is initiated. Suspect CPP if premature development of secondary sexual characteristics occurs at or before age 8 in girls and 9 in boys, and is accompanied by significant advancement of bone age or poor adult height prediction. Confirm by pubertal gonadal sex steroid levels and pubertal LH response to stimulation by native GnRH. In females, pelvic ultrasound usually reveals enlarged uterus and ovaries, the latter often with multiple cystic formations. Brain magnetic resonance imaging or CT-scanning can detect hypothalamic or pituitary tumors, or anatomical changes associated with increased intracranial pressure. Exclude other causes of sexual precocity, such as congenital adrenal hyperplasia, testotoxicosis, testicular tumors or other autonomous feminizing or masculinizing disorders by proper clinical hormonal and diagnostic imaging examinations.

Regular monitoring is needed to assess both patient response as well as compliance. This is particularly important during the first 6 to 8 weeks of treatment to assure that suppression of pituitary-gonadal function is rapid. Begin assessment of growth velocity and bone age velocity within 3 to 6 months of treatment initiation.

Some patients may not show suppression of pituitary-gonadal axis by clinical or biochemical parameters. This may be due to lack of compliance with recommended treatment regimen and may be rectified by recommending that dosing be done by caregivers. If compliance problems are excluded, reconsider possible gonadotropin independent sexual precocity and conduct appropriate examinations. If compliance problems are excluded and gonadotropin-independent sexual precocity is not present, may increase dose to 1800 mcg/day as 600 mcg 3 times a day.

Hypersensitivity: Reactions have occurred in 0.2% of subjects or patients. Refer to Management of Acute Hypersensitivity Reactions.

Carcinogenesis/Fertility impairment: Carcinogenicity studies of nafarelin were conducted in rats (24 months) at doses up to 100 mcg/kg/day and mice (18 months) at doses up to 500 mcg/kg/day using IM doses (up to 110 times and 560 times the maximum recommended human intranasal dose, respectively). As seen with other GnRH agonists, nafarelin induced proliferative responses (hyperplasia or neoplasia) of endocrine organs. At 24 months, there was an increase in the incidence of pituitary tumors (adenoma/carcinoma) in high-dose female rats and a dose-related increase in male rats. Pancreatic islet cell adenomas increased in both sexes, as did benign testicular and ovarian tumors in treated groups. There were dose-related increases in benign adrenal medullary tumors in treated female rats and Harderian gland tumors in male mice. Pituitary adenomas increased in high-dose female mice. No metastases of these tumors were observed. Tumorigenicity in rodents is particularly sensitive to hormonal stimulation.

In reproduction studies in male and female rats, fertility suppression fully reversed when treatment was discontinued after continuous use for up to 6 months.

Pregnancy: Category X. IM nafarelin was administered to rats throughout gestation at 0.4, 1.6 and 6.4 mcg/kg/day (about 0.5, 2 and 7 times the maximum recommended human intranasal dose). An increase in major fetal abnormalities was observed in 4/80 fetuses at the highest dose. A similar, repeat study at the same doses in rats, and studies in mice and rabbits at doses up to 600 mcg/kg/day and 0.18 mcg/kg/day, respectively, failed to demonstrate an increase in fetal abnormalities. In rats and rabbits, there was a dose-related increase in fetal mortality and a decrease in fetal weight with the highest dose. The effects on rat fetal mortality are expected consequences of the alterations in hormonal levels brought about by the drug.

Safe use in pregnancy is not clinically established. Before starting treatment, exclude pregnancy. When used regularly at the recommended dose, nafarelin usually inhibits ovulation and stops menstruation. Contraception is not assured, however, particularly if patients miss successive doses. Patients should use nonhormonal methods of contraception. Advise patients that if they miss successive doses, breakthrough bleeding or ovulation may occur with the potential for conception. They should see their physician if they believe they may be pregnant. If used during pregnancy or if a patient becomes pregnant during treatment, discontinue the drug and apprise patient of potential risk to the fetus.

Lactation: It is not known whether nafarelin is excreted in breast milk. The effects on lactation or the nursing infant are not determined, do not give to nursing mothers.

Children: Nafarelin is used in children for CPP.

NAFARELIN ACETATE

Precautions:

Menstruation: Since menstruation should stop with effective doses of nafarelin, the patient should notify her physician if regular menstruation persists. Patients missing successive doses of nafarelin may experience breakthrough bleeding.

Bone density loss: The induced hypoestrogenic state results in a small loss in bone density over the course of treatment, some of which may not be reversible. During one 6 month treatment period, this bone loss should not be important. In patients with major risk factors for decreased bone mineral content such as chronic alcohol or tobacco use, strong family history of osteoporosis, or chronic use of drugs that can reduce bone mass such as anticonvulsants or corticosteroids, nafarelin may pose an additional risk. Weigh risks and benefits carefully before nafarelin is instituted. Repeated courses of GnRH analogs are not advisable in patients with major risk factors for loss of bone mineral content (see Adverse Reactions).

Intercurrent rhinitis patients should consult their physician for the use of a topical nasal decongestant. If the use of a topical nasal decongestant is required during treatment with nafarelin, the decongestant must be used at least 2 hours after nafarelin dosing to decrease the possibility of reducing drug absorption.

Retreatment for endometriosis is not recommended since safety data beyond 6 months are not available.

Ovarian cysts: As with other drugs that stimulate the release of gonadotropins or that induce ovulation in adult women with endometriosis, ovarian cysts have occurred in the first 2 months of therapy. Many, but not all, of these events occurred in women with polycystic ovarian disease. These cystic enlargements may resolve spontaneously, generally by about 4 to 6 weeks of therapy, but in some cases may require discontinuation of drug or surgical intervention. Relevance in children is unknown.

Drug Interactions:

Drug/Lab test interactions: Administration of nafarelin in therapeutic doses results in suppression of the pituitary-gonadal system. Normal function is usually restored within 4 to 8 weeks after treatment is discontinued. Therefore, diagnostic tests of pituitary gonadotropic and gonadal functions conducted during treatment and up to 4 to 8 weeks after discontinuation of nafarelin therapy may be misleading.

Adverse Reactions:

CPP: In clinical trials, 2.6% reported symptoms suggestive of drug sensitivity, such as shortness of breath, chest pain, urticaria, rash and pruritus. In these patients treated for an average of 41 months and as long as 80 months (6.7 years), adverse events most frequently reported consisted largely of episodes occurring during the first 6 weeks of treatment as a result of the transient stimulatory action of nafarelin upon the pituitary-gonadal axis: Acne (10%); transient breast enlargement, vaginal bleeding (8%); emotional lability (6%); transient increase in pubic hair (5%); body odor (4%); seborrhea (3%). Hot flashes, common in adult women treated for endometriosis, occurred in only 3% of treated children and were transient. Other adverse events included: Rhinitis (5%); white or brownish vaginal discharge (3%).

In one male patient with concomitant congenital adrenal hyperplasia, and who had discontinued treatment 8 months previously to resume puberty, adrenal rest tumors were found in the left testis. Relationship to nafarelin is unlikely.

Regular examination of the pituitary gland of children during long-term nafarelin therapy as well as during the post-treatment period has occasionally revealed changes in the shape and size of the pituitary gland. These changes include asymmetry and enlargement of the pituitary gland, and a pituitary microadenoma has been suspected in a few children.

Endometriosis: As would be expected with a drug that lowers serum estradiol levels, the most frequent adverse reactions were related to hypoestrogenism. In controlled studies comparing nafarelin (400 mcg/day) and danazol (600 or 800 mg/day), adverse reactions most frequently reported and thought to be drug-related are listed in the following table.

Adverse Reactions of Nafarelin Acetate vs Danazol During Treatment for Endometriosis (≈ %)		
Adverse reaction	Nafarelin (n = 203)	Danazol (n = 147)
Hypoestrogenic:		
Hot flashes	90	69
Libido decrease	22	7
Vaginal dryness	19	7
Headaches	19	21
Emotional lability	15	18
Insomnia	8	4
Androgenic:		
Acne	13	20
Myalgia	10	23
Breast size reduced	10	16
Edema	8	23
Seborrhea	8	17
Weight gain	8	28
Hirsutism	2	6
Libido increased	1	6
Miscellaneous:		
Nasal irritation	10	3
Depression	2	5
Weight loss	1	3

Other adverse reactions (< 1%) – Paresthesia; palpitations; chloasma; eye pain; maculopapular rash; urticaria; asthenia; lactation; breast engorgement; arthralgia. In formal clinical trials, immediate hypersensitivity possibly or probably related to nafarelin occurred in 3 (0.2%) of 1509 patients or healthy subjects (see Warnings).

Bone density changes – After 6 months of nafarelin, vertebral trabecular bone density and total vertebral bone mass decreased by an average 8.7% and 4.3%, respectively, compared to pretreatment. There was partial post-treatment recovery of bone density; average trabecular bone density and total bone mass were 4.9% and 3.3% less than pretreatment, respectively. Total vertebral bone mass decreased by a mean of 5.9% at the end of treatment. Mean total vertebral mass 6 months after post-treatment was 1.4% below pretreatment levels. There was little, if any, decrease in mineral content in compact bone of the distal radius and second metacarpal. Use for > 6 months or in the presence of other known risk factors for decreased bone mineral content may cause additional bone loss. (See Precautions.)

Lab test abnormalities –

Plasma enzymes: AST and ALT levels were more than twice the upper limit of normal in only one patient each. There was no other clinical or laboratory evidence of abnormal liver function, and levels returned to normal in both patients after treatment was stopped.

Lipids: At enrollment, 9% of the patients in the nafarelin 400 mcg/day group and 2% of the patients in the danazol group had total cholesterol values > 250 mg/dl. These patients also had cholesterol values > 250 mg/dl at the end of treatment.

Of patients whose pretreatment cholesterol values were < 250 mg/dl, 6% on nafarelin and 18% on danazol had post-treatment values > 250 mg/dl.

Mean pretreatment values for total cholesterol from all patients were 191.8 mg/dl with nafarelin and 193.1 mg/dl with danazol. After treatment, mean total cholesterol values were 204.5 mg/dl with nafarelin and 207.7 mg/dl with danazol.

Triglycerides were increased above the upper limit of 150 mg/dl in 12% of the patients who received nafarelin and in 7% of the patients who received danazol.

At the end of treatment, no nafarelin patients had abnormally low HDL cholesterol fractions (< 30 mg/dl) vs 43% of danazol patients. No nafarelin patients had abnormally high LDL cholesterol fractions (> 190 mg/dl) vs 15% of those on danazol. There was no increase in the LDL/HDL ratio in nafarelin patients, but there was an approximate twofold increase in the LDL/HDL ratio in danazol patients.

Other changes (10% to 15%): Nafarelin was associated with elevated plasma phosphorous and eosinophil counts, and decreased serum calcium and WBC counts. Danazol was associated with an increase in hematocrit and WBC.

NAFARELIN ACETATE

Overdosage:

There is no clinical evidence of adverse effects following overdose of GnRH analogs. Based on animal studies, nafarelin is not absorbed after oral administration.

Patient Information:

An information pamphlet for patients is included with the product.

Patients with intercurrent rhinitis should consult their physician about use of a topical nasal decongestant. Do not use until at least 2 hours after nafarelin.

Avoid sneezing during or immediately after dosing; this may impair drug absorption.

Endometriosis: Notify physician if regular menstruation persists. Breakthrough bleeding or ovulation may occur if successive doses are missed. Use a nonhormonal method of contraception during treatment.

Do not use if pregnant or breastfeeding, or if undiagnosed abnormal vaginal bleeding or allergies to any of the ingredients exist.

CPP: Reversibility of nafarelin's suppressive effects has been demonstrated by appearance or return of menses, by return of pubertal gonadotropin and gonadal sex steroid levels, or by advancement of secondary sexual development. Semen analysis was normal in two ejaculated specimens obtained thus far from boys taken off therapy to resume puberty. Fertility has not been documented by pregnancies; the effect of long-term use on fertility is not known.

Adequately counsel patients and their caregivers to ensure full compliance; irregular or incomplete daily doses may result in stimulation of the pituitary-gonadal axis.

During the first month of treatment, some signs of puberty (eg, vaginal bleeding, breast enlargement) may occur. This is the expected initial effect. Such changes should resolve soon after the first month. If it does not resolve within the first 2 months, this may be due to lack of compliance or the presence of gonadotropin-independent sexual precocity. If both possibilities are definitively excluded, the dose may be increased to 1800 mcg/day as 600 mcg 3 times/day.

Administration and Dosage:

Approved by the FDA in 1990.

Endometriosis: 400 mcg/day. One spray (200 mcg) into one nostril in the morning and one spray into the other nostril in the evening. Start treatment between days 2 and 4 of the menstrual cycle.

For patients with persistent regular menstruation after months of treatment, the dose may be increased to 800 mcg daily. The 800 mcg dose is given as 1 spray into each nostril in the morning (a total of 2 sprays) and again in the evening.

The recommended duration of administration is 6 months. Retreatment is not recommended since safety data are not available. If symptoms recur after a course of therapy, and further treatment nafarelin is contemplated, assess bone density before retreatment begins to ensure that values are within normal limits.

If the use of a topical decongestant is necessary during treatment with nafarelin, the decongestant should not be used until at least 2 hours after nafarelin dosing.

At 400 mcg/day, a bottle of nafarelin provides a 30 day (about 60 sprays) supply. If the daily dose is increased, increase the supply to the patient to ensure uninterrupted treatment for the recommended duration of therapy.

Central precocious puberty: 1600 mcg/day. The dose can be increased to 1800 mcg daily if adequate suppression cannot be achieved at 1600 mcg/day.

The 1600 mcg dose is achieved by 2 sprays (400 mcg) into each nostril in the morning (4 sprays) and 2 sprays into each nostril in the evening (4 sprays), a total of 8 sprays per day. The 1800 mcg dose is achieved by 3 sprays (600 mcg) into alternating nostrils 3 times a day, a total of 9 sprays per day. The patient's head should be tilted back slightly, and 30 seconds should elapse between sprays.

If the prescribed therapy has been well tolerated by the patient, continue treatment of CPP until resumption of puberty is desired.

There appeared to be no significant effect of rhinitis on the systemic bioavailability of nafarelin; however, if the use of a nasal decongestant for rhinitis is necessary, do not use the decongestant until at least 2 hours following nafarelin.

Avoid sneezing during or immediately after dosing with nafarelin, if possible, since this may impair drug absorption.

At 1600 mcg/day, a bottle of nafarelin provides about a 7 day supply (about 56 sprays). If the daily dose is increased, increase the supply to the patient to ensure uninterrupted treatment for the duration of therapy.

Storage: Store upright at room temperature. Protect from light.

Rx	**Synarel** (Syntex)	**Nasal Sol:** 2 mg/ml (as base)	In 10 ml bottle with metered spray pump (delivers ≈ 200 mcg/spray).[1]

[1] With benzalkonium chloride, glacial acetic acid and sorbitol.

HISTRELIN ACETATE

Actions:

Pharmacology: Histrelin, a gonadotropin releasing hormone (GnRH or LHRH) agonist, is a potent inhibitor of gonadotropin secretion when administered daily in therapeutic doses. Histrelin contains a synthetic nonapeptide agonist of the naturally occurring gonadotropin releasing hormone. The analog possesses a greater potency than the natural sequence hormone. Following an initial stimulatory phase, chronic SC administration desensitizes responsiveness of the pituitary gonadotropin which, in turn, causes a reduction in ovarian and testicular steroidogenesis.

Although animal studies have shown that *acute* administration of histrelin results in stimulation of the reproductive system, *chronic* administration in the rat delays sexual development, inhibits estrous cyclicity and pregnancy, reduces reproductive organ weight and inhibits ovarian and testicular steroidogenesis in a reversible fashion. In the rabbit, chronic administration resulted in decreased reproductive organ weights.

In human studies, chronic administration controls the secretion of pituitary gonadotropins resulting in decreased sex steroid levels and in the regression of secondary sexual characteristics in children with precocious puberty. In girls, menses cease, serum estradiol levels are decreased to prepubertal levels, linear growth velocities decrease, skeletal maturation is slowed and adult height predictions increase. In boys, testicular steroidogenesis is inhibited and testicular volume is reduced.

Continuous administration to patients with central precocious puberty can be monitored by standard GnRH testing and by serial determinations of sex steroid levels. The decreases in LH, FSH and sex steroid levels are evident within 3 months of therapy initiation.

Indications:

For control of the biochemical and clinical manifestations of central precocious puberty. Only patients with centrally mediated precocious puberty (either idiopathic or neurogenic, and occurring before age 8 in girls or 9.5 years in boys) should receive treatment. Patients must be able to maintain compliance with a *daily* regimen of injections.

Contraindications:

Hypersensitivity to any components of the product; pregnancy, lactation (see Warnings).

Warnings:

Inadequate control: Non-compliance with drug regimen or inadequate dosing may result in inadequate control of the pubertal process. The consequences of poor control include the return of pubertal signs such as menses, breast development and testicular growth. The long-term consequences of inadequate control of gonadal steroid secretion are unknown, but may include a further compromise of adult stature.

Hypersensitivity: Serious hypersensitivity reactions (angioedema, urticaria) have been reported following histrelin administration. Clinical manifestations may include: Cardiovascular collapse; hypotension; tachycardia; loss of consciousness; angioedema; bronchospasm; dyspnea; urticaria; flushing; pruritus. If any allergic reaction occurs, discontinue therapy. Serious acute hypersensitivity reactions may require emergency medical treatment. Refer to Management of Acute Hypersensitivity Reactions.

Carcinogenesis/Fertility impairment: Carcinogenicity studies were conducted in rats for 2 years at doses of 5, 25, or 150 mcg/kg/day (up to 15 times the human dose) and in mice for 18 months at doses of 20, 200, or 2000 mcg/kg/day (up to 200 times the human dose). As seen with other GnRH agonists, histrelin was associated with an increase in tumors of hormonally responsive tissues. There was a significant increase in pituitary adenomas in rats. There was an increase in pancreatic islet cell adenomas in treated female rats and a non-dose-related increase in testicular Leydig cell tumors (highest incidence in the low-dose group). In mice, there was a significant increase in mammary gland adenocarcinomas in all treated females. In addition, there were increases in stomach papillomas in male rats given high doses, and an increase in histiocytic sarcomas in female mice at the highest dose.

Fertility studies have been conducted in rats and monkeys given SC daily doses of histrelin up to 180 mcg/kg for 6 months and full reversibility of fertility suppression was demonstrated.

HISTRELIN ACETATE

Pregnancy: Category X. Histrelin is contraindicated in women who are or may become pregnant while receiving the drug. There was increased fetal size and mortality in rats and increased fetal mortality in rabbits after histrelin administration. Other responses included dystocia, a greater incidence of unilateral hydroureter and incomplete ossification in rat fetuses. When administered to rabbits on days 6 to 18 of pregnancy at doses of 20 to 80 mcg/kg/day (2 to 8 times the human dose), histrelin produced early termination of pregnancy and increased fetal death. In rats given histrelin on days 7 to 20 of pregnancy at doses of 1 to 15 mcg/kg/day (0.1 to 1.5 times the human dose) there was an increase in fetal resorptions. The effects on fetal mortality are expected consequences of the alterations in hormonal levels brought about by the drug. If this drug is inadvertently used during pregnancy or in the rare event that a patient becomes pregnant while taking this drug, apprise the patient of the potential hazard to the fetus.

Lactation: It is not known if this drug is excreted in breast milk. Because of the potential for serious adverse reactions in nursing infants, do not give to nursing women.

Children: Safety and efficacy in children < 2 years of age have not been established.

Precautions:

Monitoring: Perform an initial pelvic ultrasound to exclude other conditions before treating with histrelin. Monitor the patient carefully after 3 months and every 6 to 12 months thereafter by serial clinical evaluations, repeated height measurements, bone age determinations (yearly), and serial GnRH testing to document that gonadotropin responsiveness of the pituitary remains prepubertal while on therapy. During the initial agonistic phase of treatment, the patient may demonstrate transient increases in breast tissue, moodiness, vaginal secretions or testicular volume. After this initial agonistic phase (usually 1 to 3 weeks), control of the biochemical and physical manifestations of puberty should remain as long as chronic therapy is in effect. Discontinue treatment when the onset of puberty is desired. Following the discontinuation of treatment, document the onset of normal puberty. In addition, monitor patients to assess menstrual cyclicity, reproductive function and ultimate adult height.

Physical and endocrinologic evaluation: Before treatment is instituted, perform a thorough physical and endocrinologic evaluation which includes:

1.) Height and weight as baseline for serial monitoring.
2.) Hand and wrist x-ray for bone age determination, to document advanced skeletal age, and as baseline for serially monitoring predicted height.
3.) Total sex steroid level (estradiol or testosterone).
4.) Adrenal steroid level, to exclude congenital adrenal hyperplasia.
5.) Beta-human chorionic gonadotropin level, to rule out a chorionic gonadotropin-secreting tumor.
6.) GnRH stimulation test, to demonstrate activation of the hypothalamic-pituitary-gonadal (HPG) axis.
7.) Pelvic/adrenal/testicular ultrasound, to rule out a steroid-secreting tumor and to document gonadal size for serial monitoring.
8.) Computerized tomography of the head, to rule out previously undiagnosed intracranial tumor.

HPG axis reactivation: Studies in rats and monkeys have indicated that all of the known biochemical and antifertility effects of histrelin are reversible. Because children who have received histrelin have not been followed long enough to ensure reactivation of the HPG axis following long-term therapy, use histrelin only when the benefits to the patient outweigh the potential risks. In addition, advise the patient or guardian that hypogonadism may result if the HPG axis fails to reactivate after the drug is discontinued.

HISTRELIN ACETATE

Adverse Reactions:

At least one adverse experience was reported for 139 of the 183 (76%) children in clinical studies of central precocious puberty. Three of the 183 children (2%) stopped therapy due to a hypersensitivity reaction. The following reactions have occurred in patients treated for precocious puberty (n = 183) as well as various other indications (n = 196).

Cardiovascular: Vasodilation (35%); edema (2% to 3%); palpitations, tachycardia, epistaxis, hypertension, migraine headache, pallor (1% to 3%).

CNS: Headache (22%); mood changes, nervousness, dizziness, depression, libido changes, insomnia, anxiety (1% to 10%); paresthesia, cognitive changes, syncope, somnolence, lethargy, impaired consciousness, tremor, hyperkinesia, anxiety (1% to 3%); convulsions (increased frequency), hot flashes/flushes (2%); conduct disorder (1%).

Dermatologic: Reactions at medication site such as redness, swelling and itching (12% to 45%); acne, rash (3% to 10%); sweating (1% to 10%); urticaria (4%); keratoderma, pruritus, pain, dyschromia, alopecia (1% to 3%); erythema (1%).

Endocrine: Vaginal dryness (12%); leukorrhea (2% to 6%); metrorrhagia, breast pain/edema (1% to 10%); breast discharge, decreased breast size, tenderness of female genitalia (2% to 3%); goiter, hyperlipidemia, anemia, glycosuria (1%).

GI: GI/abdominal pain, nausea, vomiting, diarrhea, flatulence, decreased appetite, dyspepsia (2% to 12%); GI cramps/distress, constipation, decreased appetite, thirst, gastritis (1% to 3%).

GU: Vaginal bleeding (usually only one episode within 1 to 3 weeks of starting therapy lasting several days) (22%); irritation/odor/pruritus/infections/pain/hypertrophy of the female genitalia, vaginitis, dysmenorrhea (1% to 10%); dyspareunia, polyuria, dysuria, urinary frequency, incontinence, hematuria, nocturia (1% to 3%).

Hypersensitivity: Acute generalized hypersensitivity reactions (angioedema, urticaria) have occurred (see Warnings).

Musculoskeletal: Arthralgia, joint stiffness, muscle cramp (3% to 10%); muscle stiffness, myalgia (2% to 3%); pain, hypotonia (1%).

Respiratory: Upper respiratory infection, pharyngitis, respiratory congestion, cough (1% to 10%); asthma, breathing disorder, rhinorrhea, bronchitis, sinusitis (2% to 3%); hyperventilation (1% to 3%).

Special senses: Visual disturbances (2% to 6%); ear congestion (2% to 3%); abnormal pupillary function, otalgia, hearing loss, polyopia, photophobia (1% to 3%).

Miscellaneous: Pyrexia (3% to 14%); various body pains, weight gain, fatigue, viral infection (1% to 10%); chills, malaise, purpura (1% to 3%).

Overdosage:

Histrelin up to 200 mcg/kg (rats, rabbits) or 2000 mcg/kg (mice) resulted in no systemic toxicity. This represents 20 to 200 times the maximal recommended human dose of 10 mcg/kg/day.

Patient Information:

Patient information is provided in each 7 day kit.

Prior to therapy, inform patients and their families of the importance of complying with the schedule of single, *daily* injections, given at approximately the same time each day. If injections are not given daily, the pubertal process may be reactivated. Histrelin contains no preservative. Inform patients that vials are to be used once and any unused solution is to be discarded. Allow medication to reach room temperature before injecting. Rotate daily injections through different body sites (upper arms, thighs, abdomen).

Make patients aware of the required monitoring of their condition and of the potential risks of therapy. Within the first month of therapy, girls being treated with histrelin may experience a light menstrual flow. This menstrual flow is common and likely is related to the lower estrogen levels brought about by treatment, and the withdrawal of estrogen support from the endometrium.

Irritation, redness or swelling at the injection sites may occur. If these reactions are severe or do not go away, notify the physician.

Advise the patients and their families to discontinue the drug and seek medical attention at the first sign of skin rash, urticaria, rapid heartbeat, difficulty in swallowing and breathing, or any swelling which may suggest angioedema (see Warnings).

HISTRELIN ACETATE

Administration and Dosage:

Approved by the FDA in December 1991.

Central precocious puberty: 10 mcg/kg given as a single, daily SC injection. If prepubertal levels of sex steroids or a prepubertal gonadotropin response to GnRH testing are not achieved within the first 3 months of treatment, reevaluate the patient. Doses > 10 mcg/kg/day have not been evaluated in clinical trials. Vary injection site daily.

Storage/Stability: Histrelin contains no preservative. Vials are to be used once. Any unused solution is to be discarded. Store refrigerated at 2° to 8°C (36° to 46°F) and protect from light. Remove vial from packaging only at time of use. Allow vial to reach room temperature before injecting contents.

Rx	**Supprelin** (Roberts)	**Injection**: 120 mcg/0.6 ml (200 mcg/ml peptide base)	In 30 day kit of single use 0.6 ml vials.[1]
		300 mcg/0.6 ml (500 mcg/ml peptide base)	In 30 day kit of single use 0.6 ml vials.[1]
		600 mcg/0.6 ml (1000 mcg/ml peptide base)	In 30 day kit of single use 0.6 ml vials.[1]

[1] With 0.9% sodium chloride and 10% mannitol. Preservative free. With 7 syringes and needles.

DANAZOL

Actions:

Pharmacology: A synthetic androgen derived from ethisterone, danazol suppresses the pituitary-ovarian axis by inhibiting the output of pituitary gonadotropins. It also has weak, dose-related androgenic activity and is not estrogenic or progestational. Danazol depresses the output of both follicle-stimulating hormone (FSH) and luteinizing hormone (LH). Danazol acts by direct enzymatic inhibition of sex steroid synthesis and competitively inhibits binding of steroids to their cytoplasmic receptors in target tissues. Generally, the pituitary suppressive action is reversible. Ovulation and cyclic bleeding usually return within 60 to 90 days after therapy is discontinued.

In endometriosis, danazol alters the normal and ectopic endometrial tissue so that it becomes inactive and atrophic. Complete resolution of endometrial lesions occurs in the majority of cases. Changes in vaginal cytology and cervical mucus reflect the suppressive effect of danazol on the pituitary-ovarian axis.

Hereditary angioedema – Danazol prevents attacks of the disease characterized by episodic edema of the abdominal viscera, extremities, face and airway. In addition, danazol partially or completely corrects the primary biochemical abnormality of hereditary angioedema. It increases the levels of the deficient C1 esterase inhibitor (C1EI), thereby increasing the serum levels of the C4 component of the complement system.

Pharmacokinetics: Blood levels of danazol do not increase proportionately with increases in dose. When the dose is doubled, plasma levels increase only about 35% to 40%.

Indications:

Endometriosis: For the treatment of endometriosis amenable to hormonal management.

Fibrocystic breast disease: Most cases of symptomatic fibrocystic breast disease may be treated by simple measures (eg, padded bras and analgesics). Pain and tenderness may be severe enough to warrant suppression of ovarian function. Danazol is usually effective in decreasing nodularity, pain and tenderness, but it alters hormone levels; recurrence of symptoms is very common after cessation of therapy.

Hereditary angioedema: For the prevention of attacks of angioedema (cutaneous, abdominal, laryngeal) in males and females.

Unlabeled uses: Danazol has been used to treat precocious puberty, gynecomastia and menorrhagia. It has also been studied in the treatment of iodiopathic immune thrombocytopenia, lupus-associated thrombocytopenia and autoimmune hemolytic anemia.

Contraindications:

Undiagnosed abnormal genital bleeding; markedly impaired hepatic, renal or cardiac function.

Pregnancy and lactation.

Warnings:

Carcinoma of the breast should be excluded before initiating therapy for fibrocystic breast disease. Nodularity, pain and tenderness due to fibrocystic disease may prevent recognition of underlying carcinoma; therefore, if any nodule persists or enlarges during treatment, rule out carcinoma.

Long-term experience with danazol is limited. Long-term therapy with other steroids alkylated at the 17 position has been associated with serious toxicity (cholestatic jaundice, peliosis hepatis). Similar toxicity may develop after long-term danazol. Determine the lowest dose that will provide adequate protection. If the drug was begun for exacerbation of angioneurotic edema due to trauma, stress or another cause, consider decreasing or withdrawing therapy periodically.

Androgenic effects may not be reversible even when the drug is discontinued. Watch patients closely for signs of virilization.

Pregnancy: Use a nonhormonal method of contraception. If a patient becomes pregnant during treatment, discontinue use. Continuing treatment may result in androgenic effects in the fetus, which has been limited to clitoral hypertrophy and labial fusion of the external genitalia in the female fetus. If a patient becomes pregnant while taking danazol, apprise her of the potential risks to the fetus.

Precautions:

Fluid retention: Conditions influenced by edema (eg, epilepsy, migraine, cardiac or renal dysfunction) require careful observation.

Hepatic dysfunction has been reported; perform periodic liver function tests.

Semen should be checked for volume, viscosity, sperm count and motility every 3 to 4 months, especially in adolescents.

DANAZOL

Drug Interactions:

Insulin requirements may increase in diabetics. Abnormal glucose tolerance tests may be seen.

Warfarin: Prolongation of prothrombin time has been reported with concomitant use.

Adverse Reactions:

Androgenic: Acne; edema; mild hirsutism; decrease in breast size; deepening of the voice; oily skin or hair; weight gain; rarely, clitoral hypertrophy or testicular atrophy.

Hepatic: Dysfunction (elevated serum enzymes or jaundice) has been reported in patients receiving 400 mg/day or more.

Hypoestrogenic: Flushing; sweating; vaginitis (itching, dryness, burning and vaginal bleeding); nervousness; emotional lability.

The following have been reported, but the causal relationship is not confirmed:

Allergic – Skin rashes; rare nasal congestion.

CNS – Dizziness; headache; sleep disorders; fatigue; tremor; rarely, paresthesia of extremities, visual disturbances, anxiety, depression and changes in appetite.

GI – Gastroenteritis; rarely, nausea, vomiting and constipation.

GU – Rarely, hematuria.

Musculoskeletal – Muscle cramps or spasms; joint lock-up; joint swelling; pain in back, neck or legs.

Other: Hair loss; change in libido; elevated blood pressure; chills; pelvic pain; carpal tunnel syndrome.

Patient Information:

Notify physician if masculinizing effects occur (eg, abnormal growth of facial or other fine body hair, deepening of the voice).

Use nonhormonal contraceptive measures during therapy. Discontinue use if pregnancy is suspected.

Administration and Dosage:

Endometriosis: Begin therapy during menstruation or make sure the patient is not pregnant. Administer 800 mg/day in 2 divided doses to best achieve amenorrhea and rapid response to painful symptoms. Downward titration to a dose sufficient to maintain amenorrhea may be considered depending upon response. Initially, for mild cases, give 200 to 400 mg in 2 divided doses. Individualize dosage. Continue therapy uninterrupted for 3 to 6 months; may extend to 9 months. If symptoms recur after termination, treatment can be reinstituted.

Fibrocystic breast disease: Begin therapy during menstruation or make sure patient is not pregnant. Dosage ranges from 100 to 400 mg/day in 2 divided doses.

Breast pain and tenderness are usually relieved by the first month and eliminated in 2 to 3 months; elimination of nodularity requires 4 to 6 months of uninterrupted therapy. Regular or irregular menstrual patterns, and amenorrhea each occur in approximately ⅓ of patients treated with 100 mg and higher doses. Approximately 50% of patients may have recurring symptoms within 1 year; treatment may be reinstituted.

Hereditary angioedema: Individualize dosage. Recommended starting dose is 200 mg 2 or 3 times a day. After a favorable initial response, determine continuing dosage by decreasing the dosage by 50% or less at intervals of 1 to 3 months or longer if frequency of attacks prior to treatment dictates. If an attack occurs, increase dosage by up to 200 mg/day. During the dose adjusting phase, monitor response closely, particularly if patient has a history of airway involvement.

Rx	**Danazol** (Various, eg, Geneva, Goldline, Moore, Parmed, Rugby)	**Capsules:** 200 mg	In 50s, 100s and 500s.
Rx	**Danocrine** (Sanofi Winthrop)	**Capsules:** 50 mg	(Winthrop D03 50 mg). Orange/white. In 100s.
		Capsules: 100 mg	(Winthrop D04 100 mg). Yellow. In 100s.
		Capsules: 200 mg	(Danocrine Winthrop DO5 200 mg). Orange. In 100s.

GROWTH HORMONE

Actions:

Pharmacology: Somatrem and somatropin are purified polypeptide hormones of recombinant DNA origin. Somatrem contains the identical sequence of 191 amino acids constituting pituitary-derived human growth hormone plus an additional amino acid, methionine. Somatropin's amino acid sequence is identical to that of a human growth hormone of pituitary origin.

Linear growth – The primary action is the stimulation of linear growth. This effect is demonstrated in patients lacking adequate endogenous growth hormone production. Somatrem and somatropin are therapeutically equivalent to endogenous growth hormone. Short-term clinical studies in normal adults show equivalent pharmacokinetics. Treatment of growth hormone deficient children results in an increase in growth rate and insulin-like growth factor/somatomedin-C (IGF-I) levels similar to that seen with human growth hormone (pituitary origin).

Skeletal growth – These agents stimulate skeletal growth in pediatric patients with growth hormone deficiency. The measurable increase in body length after administration of somatropin or human growth hormone results from its effect on the epiphyseal growth plates of long bones. Concentrations of IGF-I, which may play a role in skeletal growth, are low in the serum of growth hormone deficient children but increase during treatment. Elevations in mean serum alkaline phosphatase concentrations are seen.

Cell growth – The number of skeletal muscle cells is markedly decreased in short-stature children lacking endogenous growth hormone compared with healthy children. Treatment with growth hormone increases the number and size of muscle cells.

Organ growth – Growth hormone influences internal organ size and increases red cell mass.

Protein metabolism – Linear growth is facilitated in part by increased cellular protein synthesis. Nitrogen retention, as demonstrated by a decline in urinary nitrogen excretion and blood urea nitrogen (BUN), follows the initiation of growth hormone therapy. Treatment with somatrem or somatropin results in a similar decline in BUN.

Carbohydrate metabolism – Children with hypopituitarism sometimes experience fasting hypoglycemia that is improved by somatropin therapy. Large doses of growth hormone may impair glucose tolerance. Administration of growth hormone to normal adults results in increased serum insulin levels. Although the precise mechanism by which these drugs induce insulin resistance is not known, it is attributed to a decrease in insulin sensitivity. An increase in serum glucose levels is observed during somatropin treatment.

Lipid metabolism – Administration of growth hormone results in reduction in body fat stores, lipid mobilization and increased plasma fatty acids. Mean cholesterol levels decreased in patients treated with somatropin.

Mineral metabolism – Retention of sodium, potassium and phosphorus induced by growth hormone administration is thought to be caused by cell growth. Serum levels of inorganic phosphate increase in patients with growth hormone deficiency after somatropin or somatrem therapy because of metabolic activity associated with bone growth as well as increased tubular reabsorption of phosphate by the kidney. Serum calcium is not significantly altered. Although calcium excretion in the urine is increased, there is a simultaneous increase in calcium absorption from the intestine.

Connective tissue metabolism – Growth hormone stimulates the synthesis of chondroitin sulfate and collagen as well as the urinary excretion of hydroxyproline.

Pharmacokinetics: Absorption – Following SC administration of 0.1 mg/kg somatropin in healthy men, a mean peak concentration (C_{max}) of 56.1 ng/ml occurred at a mean time of 7.5 hrs. The extent of absorption was 626 ng•hr/ml and closely compares with that of somatrem (590 ng•hr/ml). The absolute bioavailability of somatropin is 75% and 63% after SC and IM administration, respectively.

Distribution – The volume of distribution of somatropin after IV injection is about 0.07 L/kg. The mean terminal half-life after IV administration of rhGH is 19.5 minutes.The AUC of somatropin is similar regardless of injection site. In healthy and growth hormone-deficient adults and children, the IM and SC pharmacokinetic profiles of somatropin are similar regardless of type of growth hormone or dosing regimen used.

Metabolism – Growth hormone localizes to highly perfused organs, most notably liver and kidney. In the kidney, growth hormone is filtered by the glomerulus, reabsorbed in the proximal tubule and is broken down within renal cells into amino acids that return to the circulation. A small number of dose-ranging studies suggest that clearance and AUC of somatropin is proportional to dose in the therapeutic dose range. The mean half-life of IV somatropin is 0.36 hours, whereas SC and IM administered somatropin have mean half-lives of 3.8 and 4.9 hours, respectively.

GROWTH HORMONE

Excretion – In healthy volunteers, mean clearance is 0.14 L/hr/kg. Clearance of rhGH after IV administration in healthy adults and children is reported to be in the range of 116 to 1/4 ml/hr/kg. Consistent with the role of the liver and kidney as major elimination organs for exogenously administered human growth hormone, there is a reduction in growth hormone clearance in patients with severe liver or kidney dysfunction.

Indications:

Growth failure associated with chronic renal insufficiency: Treatment of children who have growth failure associated with chronic renal insufficiency up to the time of renal transplantation. Use in conjunction with optimal management of chronic renal insufficiency.

Growth failure (except Serostim): Long-term treatment of children who have growth failure caused by a lack of adequate endogenous growth hormone secretion.

Turner Syndrome (Nutropin and Nutropin AQ only): Long-term treatment of short stature associated with Turner Syndrome.

Cachexia (Serostim only): Treatment of AIDS wasting or cachexia.

Somatropin deficiency syndrome (Humatrope only): Replacement of endogenous somatropin in adults with somatropin deficiency syndrome who meet the following criteria: 1) Biochemical diagnosis of somatropin deficiency syndrome, by means of a negative response to a standard growth hormone stimulation test [maximum peak < 5 ng/ml when measured by RIA (polyclonal antibody) or < 2.5 ng/ml when measured by IRMA (monoclonal antibody)]; and 2) *Adult onset:* Patients who have somatropin deficiency syndrome, either alone or with multiple hormone deficiencies (hypopituitarism), as a result of pituitary disease, hypothalamic disease, surgery, radiation therapy; or *childhood onset:* Patients who were growth hormone-deficient during childhood who have somatropin deficiency syndrome confirmed as an adult before replacement therapy with somatropin is started.

Unlabeled: Short children due to Intrauterine Growth Retardation (IUGR), 0.5 to 5.1 U/m^2 for ≤ 18 months.

Contraindications:

Subjects with closed epiphyses; sensitivity to benzyl alcohol (diluent supplied with some products is Bacteriostatic Water for Injection, benzyl alcohol preserved); evidence of tumor activity or active neoplasia (intracranial lesions must be inactive and antitumor therapy completed prior to instituting therapy; discontinue if there is evidence of tumor activity, recurrent tumor growth or neoplasia); sensitivity to m-cresol or glycerin (diluent supplied with *Humatrope;* see Administration and Dosage).

Warnings:

Weight loss: Reevaluate treatment for AIDS wasting or cachexia in patients who continue to lose weight in the first 2 weeks of treatment.

HIV: Recombinant human growth hormone (rhGH) has been shown to potentiate HIV replication in vitro at concentrations ranging from 50 to 250 ng/ml. There was no increase in virus production when the antiretroviral agents, zidovudine, didanosine or lamivudine were added to the culture medium. Additional in vitro studies have shown that rhGH does not interfere with the antiviral activity of zalcitabine or stavudine. In controlled clinical trials, no significant growth hormone-associated increase in viral burden was observed. However, the protocol required all participants to be on concomitant nucleoside analogue therapy for the duration of the study. In view of the potential for acceleration of virus replication, it is recommended that HIV+ patients be maintained on nucleoside analogue therapy for the duration of serostim therapy.

Increased tissue turgor: Swelling (particularly in the hands and feet) and musculoskeletal discomfort (pain, swelling or stiffness) may occur during treatment with serostim but may resolve spontaneously with analgesic therapy or after reducing the frequency of dosing.

Carpal tunnel syndrome may occur during treatment with serostim. If the symptoms of carpal tunnel syndrome do not resolve by decreasing the weekly number of doses of serostim, it is recommended that treatment be discontinued.

Benzyl alcohol: The diluents supplied with some products contain benzyl alcohol as a preservative. Benzyl alcohol has been associated with a fatal "gasping syndrome" in premature intants.

Pregnancy: Category B (serostim only). Category C. Give to a pregnant woman only if clearly needed.

Lactation: It is not known whether somatropin is excreted in breast milk. Exercise caution when administering to a nursing mother.

GROWTH HORMONE

Children: Available literature data suggest that rhGH clearances are similar in adults and children.

Precautions:

Monitoring: Thyroid – Serum levels of inorganic phosphorus, alkaline phosphatase and parathyroid hormone (PTH) may increase with somatropin therapy. Changes in thyroid hormone laboratory measurements may develop during treatment in children who lack adequate endogenous growth hormone secretion. Untreated hypothyroidism prevents optimal response to therapy. Therefore, periodically test thyroid function and treat with thyroid hormone when indicated.

Diabetes: Insulin resistance may be induced by growth hormone. Closely monitor patients with diabetes or glucose intolerance during somatropin therapy.

Intracranial lesion: Frequently monitor patients with growth hormone deficiency secondary to an intracranial lesion for progression or recurrence of the underlying disease process. In pediatric patients, clinical literature has demonstrated no relationship between somatropin replacement therapy and CNS tumor recurrence. In adults, it is unknown whether there is any relationship between somatropin replacement therapy and CNS tumor recurrence.

Skin lesion: Carefully monitor patients for any malignant transformation of skin lesions.

Slipped capital epiphysis: Periodically examine patients with growth failure secondary to chronic renal insufficiency for evidence of renal osteodystrophy progression. Slipped capital femoral epiphysis or avascular necrosis of the femoral head may be seen in children with advanced renal osteodystrophy, and it is uncertain whether these problems are affected by growth hormone therapy. Obtain x-rays of the hip prior to initiating therapy. Physicians and parents should be alert to the development of a limp or complaints of hip or knee pain in patients treated with growth hormone. Slipped capital femoral epiphysis may occur more frequently in patients with endocrine disorders or in patients undergoing rapid growth.

Gynecomastia occurs in about 70% of boys during puberty, but prepubertal gynecomastia is rare. When gynecomastia does occur before puberty, there is usually evidence of endogenous or exogenous estrogenic stimulation.

Intracranial hypertension (IH) with papilledema, visual changes, headache, nausea or vomiting has been reported in a small number of patients treated with growth hormone products. Symptoms usually occurred within the first 8 weeks of the initiation of therapy. In all cases, IH-associated signs and symptoms resolved after termination of therapy or a reduction of the growth hormone dose. Funduscopic examination of patients is recommended at the initiation and periodically during the course of growth hormone therapy.

Renal transplant: No studies have been performed of somatropin (*Nutropin*) therapy in children who have received renal transplants. Treatment of patients with functioning renal allografts is not indicated.

Antibody production: As with all protein pharmaceuticals, a small percentage of patients may develop antibodies to the protein. Growth hormone antibody binding capacities < 2 mg/L have not been associated with growth attenuation. In some cases when binding capacity exceeds 2 mg/L, growth attenuation has been observed. In general, growth hormone antibodies are not neutralizing and do not interfere with the growth response. In addition to an evaluation of compliance with the prescribed treatment program and thyroid status, test for antibodies to human growth hormone in any patient who fails to respond to therapy.

Drug Interactions:

Glucocorticoid therapy may inhibit growth-promoting effect. Carefully adjust the glucocorticoid replacement dose in patients with coexisting ACTH deficiency to avoid an inhibitory effect on growth.

Drug/Lab test interactions: Changes in thyroid hormone laboratory measurements may develop during somatropin treatment in children who lack adequate endogenous growth hormone secretion (see Precautions).

GROWTH HORMONE

Adverse Reactions:

Leukemia has occurred in a small number of children receiving somatropin or somatrem; however, the relationship is uncertain.

Immunologic:

Somatrem – Approximately 30% to 40% of patients developed persistent antibodies. One of 84 subjects treated for 6 to 36 months developed antibodies associated with high binding capacities and failed to respond. In patients who had been previously treated with pituitary-derived growth hormone, 1 of 22 subjects developed persistent antibodies (see Precautions).

Somatropin – Approximately 2% of patients developed antibodies. Of the 232 patients receiving somatropin for ≥ 6 months, 4.7% had serum binding of radiolabeled growth hormone in excess of twice the binding observed in control sera. In comparison, 74.5% of 106 patients treated for ≥ 6 months with somatrem in a similar trial had serum binding of radiolabeled growth hormone of at least twice that of the binding observed in control sera. (see Precautions).

Miscellaneous:

Nutropin AQ – Mild and transient peripheral edema (infrequent); carpal tunnel syndrome, increased growth of pre-existing nevi, gynecomastia, pancreatitis (rare).

Somatropin –

Adults: Headache; localized muscle pain; weakness; mild hyperglycemia; glucosuria; mild, transient edema early during treatment (2.5%).

Pediatrics: Injection site pain (infrequent).

Overdosage:

Acute overdosage could lead initially to hypoglycemia and subsequently to hyperglycemia. Long-term overdosage could result in signs and symptoms of gigantism or acromegaly consistent with the known effects of excess human growth hormone.

Patient Information:

Inform patients being treated with growth hormone or their parents of the potential benefits and risks associated with treatment.

If home use is desired, give instructions on appropriate use, including a review of the contents of the patient information insert. Thoroughly instruct patients or parents in the importance of proper disposal and caution against any reuse of needles and syringes.

SOMATREM

For complete prescribing information, refer to the Growth Hormone group monograph.

Administration and Dosage:

Individualize dosage. Up to 0.1 mg/kg (0.26 IU/kg) SC or IM 3 times/week is recommended. Do not exceed a weekly dosage of 0.30 mg/kg (≈ 0.90 IU/kg) because of the potential risk of known effects of excess human growth hormone.

Preparation of solution: Reconstitute each 5 mg or 10 mg vial with 1 to 5 ml or 1 to 10 ml, respectively, of Bacteriostatic Water for Injection (benzyl alcohol preserved) only; aim the stream of diluent against the glass wall of the vial. Do not shake. Do not inject if solution is cloudy. Use a small enough syringe so that the prescribed dose can be drawn from the vial with reasonable accuracy. Use a needle of sufficient length (≥ 1 inch) to ensure that the injection reaches the muscle layer.

Newborns – Benzyl alcohol as a preservative has been associated with toxicity (see Warnings). When administering to newborns, reconstitute with Water for Injection. Use only one dose per vial; discard the unused portion. The pH after reconstitution is ≈ 7.8.

Store at 2° to 8°C (36° to 46°F). Use reconstituted vials in 14 days. Avoid freezing.

Rx	**Protropin** (Genentech)	**Powder for injection, lyophilized:** 5 mg (≈ 13 IU) per vial[1]	In cartons of 2 vials and 10 ml multi-dose vial of diluent.[2]
		10 mg (≈ 26 IU) per vial[3]	In cartons of 2 vials and two 10 ml multi-dose vials of diluent.[2]
(Canada)	**Protropin** (Genentech)	10 mg (≈ 26 IU) per vial[3]	In cartons of 2 vials and two 10 ml multi-dose vials of diluent.[2]

[1] With 40 mg mannitol.
[2] Bacteriostatic Water for Injection with benzyl alcohol.
[3] With 80 mg mannitol.

SOMATROPIN

For complete prescribing information, refer to the Growth Hormone group monograph.

Administration and Dosage:

Individualize dosage. Do not continue therapy if final height is achieved or epiphyseal fusion occurs. Evaluate patients who fail to respond adequately while on somatropin therapy to determine the cause of unresponsiveness.

Reconstitution technique (except Genotropin): To reconstitute somatropin, inject the diluent into the vial, aiming the liquid against the glass vial wall. Swirl the vial with a gentle rotary motion until contents are dissolved completely. The solution should be clear immediately after reconstitution. Do not administer if the reconstituted product is cloudy immediately after reconstitution or refrigeration.

Occasionally, after refrigeration, you may notice that small colorless particles of protein are present in the solution. This is not unusual for solutions containing proteins. Allow the vial to come to room temperature and gently swirl. Do not use if the solution is cloudy.

Genotropin: A dose of 0.16 to 0.24 mg/kg/week is recommended. The weekly dose should be divided into six to seven SC injections. Administer in the thigh, buttocks or abdomen; rotate the site of SC injections daily to help prevent lipoatrophy.

Reconstitution – Supplied as a powder, filled in a two-chamber cartridge with the active substance in the front chamber and the diluent in the rear chamber. A reconstitution device is used to co-mix the diluent and the lyophilized powder. Follow the directions for reconstitution provided with each device. Gently tip the cartridge upside down a few times until the contents are completley dissolved. Do not shake.

Storage/Stability: Before reconstitution, refrigerate at 2° to 8°C (36° to 46°F). Do not freeze. Protect from light. The 1.5 mg cartridge reconstituted with diluent may be refrigerated for only ≤ 24 hours because it contains no preservative. Use once and discard any remaining solution.

The 5.8 mg and 13.8 mg cartridges are reconstituted with a diluent containing a preservative. After reconstitution, they may be stored under refrigeration for up to 14 days.

Humatrope:

Pediatric patients – The recommended weekly dosage is 0.18 mg/kg (0.54 IU/kg). Divide into equal doses given either on 3 alternate days or 6 times per week. The maximal replacement weekly dosage is 0.3 mg/kg (0.9 IU/kg) divided into equal doses given on 3 alternate days. Administer by SC or IM injection. Individualize dosage and administration schedule.

Adult patients – The recommended dosage at the start of therapy is ≤ 0.006 mg/kg/day (0.018 IU/kg/day) given as a daily SC injection. The dose may be increased according to individual patient requirements to a maximum of 0.0125 mg/kg/day (0.0375 IU/kg/day).

Reconstitute each 5 mg vial with 1.5 to 5 ml of diluent supplied.

Storage/Stability: Before reconstitution, powder and diluent are stable when refrigerated at 2° to 8°C (36° to 46°F). Somatropin is stable for ≤ 14 days after reconstitution when stored in a refrigerator at 2° to 8° C (36° to 46°F). Avoid freezing.

Nutropin/Nutropin AQ:

Growth hormone deficiency (GHD) – A weekly dosage of 0.3 mg/kg (≈ 0.90 IU/kg) SC is recommended.

Chronic renal insufficiency (CRI) – A weekly dosage of 0.35 mg/kg (≈ 1.05 IU/kg) SC is recommended. Therapy may be continued up to the time of renal transplantation.

In order to optimize therapy for patients who require dialysis, the following guidelines for an injection schedule are recommended: 1) Hemodialysis patients should receive their injection at night just prior to going to sleep or at least 3 to 4 hours after their hemodialysis to prevent hematoma formation caused by the heparin; 2) Chronic Cycling Peritoneal Dialysis (CCPD) patients should receive their injection in the morning after they have completed dialysis; 3) Chronic Ambulatory Peritoneal Dialysis (CAPD) patients should receive their injection in the evening at the time of the overnight exchange.

Turner Syndrome – A weekly dosage of ≤ 0.375 mg/kg (≈ 1.125 IU/kg) divided into equal doses 3 to 7 times/week by SC injection is recommended.

Reconstitute each 5 mg vial with 1 to 5 ml or each 10 mg vial with 1 to 10 ml of Bacteriostatic Water for Injection (benzyl alcohol preserved) only.

SOMATROPIN

Newborns: Benzyl alcohol has been associated with toxicity (see Warnings). When administering to newborns, reconstitute with Water for Injection. Use only one dose per vial; discard the unused portion. The pH after reconstitution is ≈ 7.4.

Storage/Stability: Before reconstitution, vials and diluent are stable when refrigerated at 2° to 8°C (36° to 46°F). Avoid freezing the diluent.

Reconstituted vials are stable for up to 14 days stored in a refrigerator at 2° to 8°C (36° to 46°F). Avoid freezing.

Nutropin AQ – Vial contents are stable for 28 days after initial use when stored at 2° to 8°C (36° to 46°F). Avoid freezing the vial.

Serostim: Administered SC daily at bedtime according to the following dosage recommendations:

Serostim Dosage Recommendations	
Weight Range	Dose[1]
> 55 kg	6 mg SC daily
45 - 55 kg	5 mg SC daily
35 - 45 kg	4 mg SC daily

[1] Based on an ≈ daily dosage of 0.1 mg/kg.

In patients who weigh < 35 kg, administer at a dose of 0.1 mg/kg SC daily at bedtime.

Dose reductions for side effects related to treatment, which are unresponsive to symptomatic treatment, may be effected by reducing the total daily dose or the number of doses given per week.

Reconstitute each vial with 1 ml Sterile Water for Injection.

Storage/Stability: Before reconstitution, store powder and diluent at room temperature, 15° to 30°C (59° to 86°F). Use within 24 hours after reconstitution with diluent. Refrigerate the reconstituted solution at 2° to 8°C (36° to 46°F).

Norditropin: The recommended dosage is 0.024 to 0.034 mg/kg SC 6 to 7 times/week. Give the injections in the thighs and vary the injection site on the thigh on a rotating basis.

Reconstitute each 4 mg or 8 mg vial with the 2 ml diluent.

Storage/Stability: Before and after reconstitution, refrigerate at 2° to 8°C (36° to 46°F). Do not freeze. Avoid direct light. Use reconstituted vials within 14 days after dissolution.

Rx	**Genotropin** (Pharmacia)	**Powder for injection, lyophilized:** 1.5 mg (≈ 4 IU)/ml	Preservative free. In 1.5 mg Intra-Mix two-chamber cartridge with pressure-release needle. In 5s.
	Norditropin (Novo Nordisk)	**Powder for injection, lyophilized:** 4 mg (≈ 12 IU)/vial	In vials[1] with diluent.[2]
	Nutropin (Genentech)	**Powder for injection, lyophilized:** 5 mg (≈ 13 IU)/vial	In cartons of 2 vials[3] with a 10 ml multiple-dose vial of diluent.[4]
	Humatrope (Lilly)	**Powder for injection, lyophilized:** 5 mg (≈ 15 IU)/vial	In vials[5] w/ 5 ml diluent.[2]
🍁	**Humatrope** (Lilly)	**Powder for injection, lyophilized:** 5 mg (≈ 15 IU)/vial	In vials[5] w/ 5 ml diluent.[2]

SOMATROPIN

Rx	**Genotropin** (Pharmacia)	**Powder for injection, lyophilized:** 5.8 mg (≈ 15 IU)/ml	In 5.8 mg Intra-Mix two-chamber cartridge and pressure release needle. In 1s, 5s.
	Serostim (Serono)	**Powder for injection, lyophilized:** 6 mg (≈ 15 IU)/ml	Sucrose. In single-use vials with diluent.
	Norditropin (Novo Nordisk)	**Powder for injection, lyophilized:** 8 mg (≈ 24 IU)/vial	In vials[6] with diluent.[1]
	Nutropin (Genentech)	**Powder for injection, lyophilized:** 10 mg (≈ 26 IU)/vial	In cartons of 2 vials[7] with two 10 ml multiple-dose vials of diluent.[4]
	Nutropin AQ (Genentech)	**Injection:** 10 mg (≈ 30 IU)/vial	In cartons of 6 vials with one 2 ml vial[4,8] (5 mg/ml).

[1] Water for injection with 1.5% benzyl alcohol.
[2] Water for Injection with 0.3% m-cresol and 1.7% glycerin.
[3] With 45 mg mannitol and 1.7 mg glycine.
[4] Bacteriostatic Water for Injection with benzyl alcohol.
[5] With 25 mg mannitol and 5 mg glycine.
[6] With 44 mg mannitol and 8.8 mg glycine.
[7] With 90 mg mannitol and 3.4 mg glycine.
[8] With 17.4 mg sodium chloride, 5 mg phenol, 4 mg polysorbate 20 and 10 mM sodium citrate.

OCTREOTIDE ACETATE

Actions:

Pharmacology: Octreotide acetate is a long-acting octapeptide with pharmacologic actions similar to those of the natural hormone somatostatin. It is an even more potent inhibitor of growth hormone, glucagon and insulin than somatostatin. Like somatostatin, it also suppresses LH response to GnRH, decreases splanchnic blood flow and inhibits release of serotonin, gastrin, vasoactive intestinal peptide, secretin, motilin and pancreatic polypeptide. Octreotide substantially reduces growth hormone or IGF-I (somatomedin C) levels in patients with acromegaly. Single doses inhibit gallbladder contractility and decrease bile secretion in healthy volunteers. In clinical trials, the incidence of gallstone or biliary sludge formation was markedly increased. Octreotide also suppresses secretion of thyroid stimulating hormone.

In patients with acromegaly, octreotide reduces growth hormone to within normal ranges in 50% of patients and reduces IGF-I to within normal ranges in 50% to 60% of patients. Since the effects of pituitary irradiation may not become maximal for several years, adjunctive therapy with octreotide to reduce blood levels of growth hormone and IGF-I offers potential benefit before the effects of irradiation are manifested. Improvement in clinical signs and symptoms or reduction in tumor size or rate of growth were not shown in clinical trials.

In patients with vasoactive intestinal peptide tumors, improvement has been noted in the overall condition of these otherwise therapeutically unresponsive patients. Therapy with octreotide results in improvement in electrolyte abnormalities (eg, hypokalemia), often enabling reduction of fluid and electrolyte support. Data are insufficient to determine whether the drug decreases size, rate of growth or development of metastases in patients with these tumors. Octreotide acetate was used in patients ranging in age from 1 month to 83 years without any drug limiting toxicity.

Pharmacokinetics:

Absorption/Distribution – After SC injection, octreotide is absorbed rapidly and completely from the injection site. Peak concentrations of 5.5 ng/ml (100 mcg dose) were reached 0.4 hours after dosing. IV and SC doses are bioequivalent. Peak concentrations and area under the curve values were dose-proportional both after SC or IV single doses of up to 400 mcg and with multiple doses of 200 mcg 3 times daily (600 mcg/day). Clearance was reduced by about 66% suggesting nonlinear kinetics of the drug at daily doses of 600 mcg/day as compared to 150 mcg/day.

The distribution of octreotide from plasma was rapid (alpha half-life = 0.2 hr), the volume of distribution (Vd) was estimated to be 13.6 L and total body clearance was 10 L/hr. In blood, the distribution into the erythrocytes was found to be negligible and about 65% was bound in the plasma in a concentration-independent manner. Binding was mainly to lipoprotein and, to a lesser extent, to albumin.

Metabolism/Excretion – The elimination of octreotide from plasma had an apparent half-life of 1.7 hours compared with 1 to 3 minutes with the natural hormone. The duration of action is variable but extends up to 12 hours depending upon the type of tumor. About 32% of the dose is excreted unchanged in the urine. In elderly patients, dose adjustments may be necessary due to a significant increase in the half-life (46%) and a significant decrease in the clearance (26%) of octreotide.

In patients with acromegaly, the pharmacokinetics differ somewhat from those in healthy volunteers. A mean peak concentration of 2.8 ng/ml (100 mcg dose) was reached in 0.7 hours after SC dosing. The Vd_{ss} was estimated to be 21.6 ± 8.5 L and the total body clearance was increased to 18 L/hr. The mean percent of bound drug was 41.2%. Disposition and elimination half-lives were similar to healthy subjects.

In patients with severe renal failure requiring dialysis, clearance was reduced to about half that found in healthy subjects (from approximately 10 to 4.5 L/hr). The effect of hepatic diseases on the disposition of octreotide is unknown.

Indications:

Acromegaly: To reduce blood levels of growth hormone and IGF-I in acromegaly patients who have had inadequate response to or cannot be treated with surgical resection, pituitary irradiation and bromocriptine at maximally tolerated doses. The goal is to achieve normalization of growth hormone and IGF-I levels.

Carcinoid tumors: Symptomatic treatment of patients with metastatic carcinoid tumors where it suppresses or inhibits associated severe diarrhea and flushing episodes.

Vasoactive intestinal peptide tumors (VIPomas): Treatment of the profuse watery diarrhea associated with VIP-secreting tumors.

OCTREOTIDE ACETATE

Unlabeled uses: Octreotide is effective in treating the following conditions:

GI fistula – To reduce output from GI fistulas. Dosage ranges from 50 to 200 mcg every 8 hours.

Variceal bleeding – Dosage ranges from 25 to 50 mcg/hr via continuous IV infusion. Duration is from 18 hours to 5 days.

Diarrheal states – Since octreotide prolongs intestinal transit time, it is beneficial in relieving diarrhea associated with a variety of conditions including: AIDS-related diarrhea (100 to 500 mcg SC 3 times daily); idiopathic secretory diarrhea; short bowel (ileostomy) syndrome (IV infusion of 25 mcg/hr or SC 50 mcg twice daily); diabetes; pancreatic cholera syndrome; diarrhea due to chemotherapy/radiation therapy in cancer patients (50 to 100 mcg SC 3 times daily for 1 to 3 days).

Pancreatic fistula – To reduce output from pancreatic fistulas. Dosages range from 50 to 200 mcg every 8 hours.

Irritable bowel syndrome – 100 mcg single dose to 125 mcg SC twice daily.

Dumping syndrome – 50 to 150 mcg/day.

Other uses for which octreotide may be beneficial include: Enteric fistula; pancreatitis; pancreatic surgery; glucagonoma; insulinoma; gastrinoma (Zollinger-Ellison syndrome); intestinal obstruction; local radiotherapy; chronic pain management; antineoplastic therapy; decrease insulin requirements in diabetes mellitus; thyrotropin- and TSH-secreting tumors.

Contraindications:

Sensitivity to this drug or any of its components.

Warnings:

Biliary tract effects: Single doses have inhibited gallbladder contractility and decreased bile secretion in healthy volunteers. In clinical trials (primarily patients with acromegaly or psoriasis), the incidence of biliary tract abnormalities was 52% (27% gallstones, 22% sludge without stones, 3% biliary duct dilatation). Incidence of stones or sludge in patients who received the drug for ≥ 12 months was 48%. Among patients treated for ≤ 1 month, < 2% developed gallstones. The incidence of gallstones did not appear related to age, sex or dose. The majority of patients developing gallbladder abnormalities had GI symptoms which were not specific to gallbladder disease. A few patients developed acute cholecystitis, ascending cholangitis, biliary obstruction, cholestatic hepatitis or pancreatitis during therapy or following its withdrawal. One patient developed ascending cholangitis and died.

Renal function impairment: In patients with severe renal failure requiring dialysis, octreotide half-life may be increased, necessitating adjustment of maintenance dose.

Elderly: Dose adjustments may be necessary due to a significant increase in the half-life (46%) and a significant decrease in the clearance (26%) of octreotide.

Pregnancy: Category B. There are no adequate and well controlled studies in pregnant women. Use during pregnancy only if clearly needed.

Lactation: It is not known whether this drug is excreted in breast milk. Exercise caution when octreotide is administered to a nursing woman.

Children: The youngest patient to receive the drug was 1 month old. Doses of 1 to 10 mcg/kg were well tolerated in young patients. A single case of an infant (nesidioblastosis) was complicated by a seizure thought to be independent of octreotide.

Precautions:

Monitoring: Laboratory tests that may be helpful as biochemical markers in determining and following patient response depend on the specific tumor. Based on diagnosis, measurement of the following substances may be useful in monitoring the progress of therapy:

Acromegaly – Growth hormone, IGF-I. Responsiveness to octreotide may be evaluated by determining growth hormone levels at 1 to 4 hour intervals for 8 to 12 hours post dose; alternatively, a single measurement of IGF-I level may be made 2 weeks after drug initiation or dosage change.

Carcinoid – 5-HIAA (urinary 5-hydroxyindole acetic acid), plasma serotonin, plasma Substance P.

VIPoma – VIP (plasma vasoactive intestinal peptide).

Perform baseline and periodic total or free T_4 measurements during chronic use.

Hypo- or hyperglycemia that may occur during therapy is usually mild, but may result in overt diabetes mellitus or necessitate dose changes in insulin or other hypoglycemic agents. Hypo- and hyperglycemia occurred in 3% and 15% of acromegalic patients, respectively. Severe hyperglycemia, subsequent pneumonia and death following initiation of octreotide was reported in one patient with no history of hyperglycemia.

OCTREOTIDE ACETATE

Hypothyroidism: In acromegalic patients, 12% developed biochemical hypothyroidism, only 6% developed goiter and 4% required initiation of thyroid replacement therapy while receiving octreotide. Baseline and periodic assessment of thyroid function (TSH, total or free T_4) is recommended during chronic therapy.

Cardiac effects: In acromegalics, bradycardia (< 50 bpm) developed in 21%; conduction abnormalities and arrhythmias each occurred in 9% of patients during therapy. Other ECG changes observed included QT prolongation, axis shifts, early repolarization, low voltage, R/S transition and early wave progression. These ECG changes are not uncommon in acromegalic patients. Dose adjustments in drugs such as beta blockers that have bradycardia effects may be necessary. In one acromegalic patient with severe CHF, initiation of octreotide resulted in worsening of CHF with improvement when the drug was discontinued. Confirmation of a drug effect was obtained with a positive rechallenge.

Pancreatitis: Several cases of pancreatitis occurred in patients receiving octreotide.

Dietary fat: Dietary fat absorption may be altered in some patients. Perform periodic quantitative 72-hour fecal fat and serum carotene determinations to aid in the assessment of possible drug-induced aggravation of fat malabsorption.

Drug Interactions:

Cyclosporine: A single case of a transplant rejection episode (renal/whole pancreas) in a patient immunosuppressed with cyclosporine was reported. Octreotide used to reduce exocrine secretion and close a fistula in this patient resulted in decreases in blood levels of cyclosporine and may have contributed to the rejection episode.

Drug/Food interactions: Octreotide may alter the absorption of dietary fats in some patients. In addition, depressed vitamin B_{12} levels and abnormal Schilling's tests have been observed in some patients receiving octreotide; monitoring of vitamin B_{12} levels is recommended during chronic therapy.

Adverse Reactions:

Cardiovascular: Sinus bradycardia (21% in acromegalics; see Precautions); conduction abnormalities, arrhythmias (9%; see Precautions); chest pain, shortness of breath, thrombophlebitis, ischemia, hypertensive reaction, CHF, hypertension, palpitations, orthostatic BP decrease, tachycardia (< 1%).

CNS: Headache (6%); dizziness, fatigue, weakness (1% to 4%); depression, anxiety, libido decrease, syncope, tremor, seizure, vertigo, Bell's Palsy, paranoia, pituitary apoplexy, increased intraocular pressure (< 1%).

Dermatologic: Injection site pain (7.5%); flushing, edema, pruritus, hair loss (1% to 4%); rash, cellulitis, petechiae, urticaria (< 1%).

Endocrine: Hyperglycemia, hypoglycemia (15% and 3%, respectively, in acromegalics; 1.5% in others); biochemical hypothyroidism (12% in acromegalics; isolated cases in others). See Precautions.

Galactorrhea, hypoadrenalism, diabetes insipidus, gynecomastia, amenorrhea, polymenorrhea, vaginitis (< 1%).

GI: Diarrhea, loose stools, nausea, abdominal discomfort (30% to 58% acromegalics, 5% to 10% other disorders); frequency was not dose-related, but diarrhea and abdominal discomfort generally resolved more quickly in patients treated with 300 mcg/day than with 750 mcg/day. Vomiting, flatulence, abnormal stools, abdominal distention, constipation (< 10%); hepatitis, jaundice, increase in liver enzymes, GI bleeding, hemorrhoids and appendicitis (< 1%).

GU: Pollakiuria, urinary tract infection (1% to 4%); nephrolithiasis, hematuria (< 1%).

Hematologic: Injection site hematoma, bruise (1% to 4%); anemia, iron deficiency, epistaxis (< 1%).

Musculoskeletal: Backache, joint pain (1% to 4%); arthritis, joint effusion, muscle pain, Raynaud's phenomenon (< 1%).

Respiratory: Cold symptoms (1% to 4%); pneumonia, pulmonary nodule, status asthmaticus (< 1%).

Miscellaneous: Gallbladder abnormalities, especially stones or biliary sludge (frequent with chronic therapy; see Warnings); flu symptoms, fat malabsorption (see Drug Interactions), blurred vision (1% to 4%); otitis, allergic reaction, increased CK, visual disturbance (< 1%); anaphylactoid reactions, including anaphylactic shock (several patients).

Evaluation of 20 patients treated for at least 6 months has failed to demonstrate titers of antibodies exceeding background levels. However, antibody titers to octreotide were subsequently reported in three patients and resulted in prolonged duration of drug action in two patients.

OCTREOTIDE ACETATE

Overdosage:

IV bolus doses of 1 mg (healthy volunteers) or 30 mg IV over 20 minutes and 120 mg IV over 8 hours (research patients) have not resulted in serious ill effects.

Patient Information:

Give careful instruction in sterile SC injection technique to patients and other persons who may administer octreotide.

Administration and Dosage:

Administration: Octreotide may be administered SC or IV. SC injection is the usual route of administration for control of symptoms. Pain with SC use may be reduced by using the smallest volume that will deliver the desired dose. Avoid multiple injections at the same site within short periods of time. Rotate sites in a systematic manner. The initial dosage is usually 50 mcg administered 2 or 3 times daily. Upward dose titration is usually required.

Although not an approved method of administration, continuous subcutaneous infusion (CSI) has been used to administer octreotide. Advantages to CSI include patient convenience, increased compliance, decreased injection site pain, minimization of GI side effects and continuous octreotide serum levels.

Acromegaly: Dosage may be initiated at 50 mcg 3 times daily. This low dose may permit adaptation to adverse GI effects for patients who will require higher doses. IGF-I levels every 2 weeks can be used to guide titration. Alternatively, multiple growth hormone levels at 0 to 8 hours after octreotide administration permit more rapid titration of dose. The goal is to achieve growth hormone levels < 5 ng/ml or IGF-I levels < 1.9 U/ml in males and < 2.2 U/ml in females. The dose most commonly found to be effective is 100 mcg 3 times daily, but some require up to 500 mcg 3 times daily for maximum efficacy. Doses > 300 mcg/day seldom result in additional benefit. If an increase in dose fails to provide additional benefit, reduce the dose. Reevaluate IGF-I or growth hormone levels at 6 month intervals.

Withdraw octreotide yearly for ≈ 4 weeks from patients who have received irradiation to assess disease activity. If growth hormone or IGF-I levels increase and signs and symptoms recur, therapy may be resumed.

Carcinoid tumors: The suggested daily dosage of octreotide during the first 2 weeks of therapy ranges from 100 to 600 mcg/day in 2 to 4 divided doses (mean daily dosage is 300 mcg). In the clinical studies, the median daily maintenance dosage was approximately 450 mcg, but clinical biochemical benefits were obtained in some patients with as little as 50 mcg, while others required doses up to 1500 mcg/day. However, experience with doses > 750 mcg per day is limited.

VIPomas: Daily dosages of 200 to 300 mcg in 2 to 4 divided doses are recommended during the initial 2 weeks of therapy (range, 150 to 750 mcg) to control symptoms of the disease. On an individual basis, dosage may be adjusted to achieve a therapeutic response, but usually doses > 450 mcg/day are not required.

Admixture incompatibility: Although octreotide appears to be physically compatible in total parenteral nutrition (TPN) solutions for 48 hours at room temperature and for 7 days under refrigeration, it is not compatible in TPN solutions because of the formation of a glycosyl octreotide conjugate which may decrease its efficacy.

Admixture compatibility: Octreotide is stable in sterile isotonic saline solutions or sterile solutions of dextrose 5% in water for 24 hours. It may be diluted in volumes of 50 to 200 ml and infused IV over 15 to 30 min or administered by IV push over 3 min. In emergency situations (eg, carcinoid crisis) it may be given by rapid bolus.

Storage/Stability: For prolonged storage, store octreotide amps and multi-dose vials in the refrigerator at 2° to 8° C (36° to 46° F) and protect from light. At room temperature (20° to 30° C; 70° to 86° F), octreotide is stable for 14 days if protected from light. In one study, octreotide was stable in polypropylene syringes for up to 29 days at 3° C (37°F; protected from light) and for up to 22 days at 23° C 73°F; exposed to light). Following refrigeration, the solution can be allowed to come to room temperature prior to administration. Do not warm artificially. After initial use, discard multi-dose vials within 14 days. Open amps just prior to administration and discard the unused portion. Do not use if particulates or discoloration are observed.

Rx	**Sandostatin** (Sandoz)	**Injection:** 0.05 mg/ml	In 1 ml amps.
		0.1 mg/ml	In 1 ml amps.
		0.2 mg/ml	In 5 ml multi-dose vials.
		0.5 mg/ml	In 1 ml amps.
		1 mg/ml	In 5 ml multi-dose vials.

POSTERIOR PITUITARY HORMONES

Actions:

Pharmacology: Posterior pituitary secretions include oxytocin and vasopressin, polypeptides containing eight amino acids. Oxytocin is formed primarily in the paraventricular nuclei and vasopressin in the supraoptic nuclei of the hypothalamus. They are then transported in combination with a carrier protein, neurophysin, to accumulate in nerve endings in the posterior pituitary gland. Under appropriate stimuli, they are released from nerve endings and absorbed into adjacent capillaries.

Vasopressin exhibits its most marked activity on the renal tubular epithelium, where it promotes water resorption of (antidiuretic hormone effect) and smooth muscle contraction throughout the vascular bed (vasopressor effects). Vasoconstriction is marked in portal and splanchnic vessels, somewhat less in peripheral, coronary, cerebral, and pulmonary vessels and slight in intrahepatic vessels. Vasopressin, and to a lesser extent, oxytocin, enhances GI motility and tone.

Neurogenic or central diabetes insipidus is a disorder of water metabolism that results from a partial or complete deficiency in the production and secretion of vasopressin from the neurohypophysis. Nephrogenic or peripheral diabetes insipidus results from an insensitivity of the renal tubules to the action of antidiuretic hormone. Vasopressin and its synthetic analogs are the principal treatment of neurogenic diabetes insipidus, but are ineffective in treating the nephrogenic variant.

Vasopressin is a purified form of the posterior pituitary, having only pressor and antidiuretic hormone (ADH) activity. Vasopressin may be obtained from natural sources or by chemical synthesis. The synthetic derivatives, lypressin and desmopressin, act principally as ADH, possessing little pressor activity, and are relatively free of oxytocic activity. Desmopressin has a longer duration of action.

Posterior Pituitary Hormone Products			
Agent	Indications	Route	Concentration
Vasopressin Derivatives			
Vasopressin	Diabetes insipidus Post-op abdominal distention	Parenteral	20 u/ml
Lypressin	Diabetes insipidus	Nasal spray	0.185 mg/ml
Desmopressin	Diabetes insipidus	Nasal Parenteral	0.1 mg/ml 4 mcg/ml
	Nocturnal enuresis Renal capacity testing	Nasal	0.1 mg/ml
	Hemophilia A von Willebrand's disease (Type I)	Nasal Parenteral	1.5 mg/ml 4 mcg/ml
Oxytocics[1]			
Oxytocin	Initiate/augment labor 2nd trimester abortion Postpartum hemorrhage	Parenteral	10 u/ml
	Initial milk let-down	Nasal	40 u/ml
Ergonovine	Postpartum/postabortal hemorrhage Migraine headache	Oral Parenteral	0.2 mg 0.2 mg/ml
Methylergonovine	Postpartum/postabortal hemorrhage	Oral Parenteral	0.2 mg 0.2 mg/ml

[1] Other agents with oxytocic effects on the uterus used to induce abortion are discussed under Abortifacients.

Pharmacokinetics:

Oxytocin exerts its most marked activity in inducing uterine muscle contraction and inducing contraction of the lacteal glands, which results in milk ejection in lactating women. Uterine motility is controlled by a variety of biochemical and regulatory processes including cAMP, calcium, prostaglandins and oxytocin. The mechanism of oxytocin-facilitated smooth muscle contraction is poorly understood. The sensitivity of the uterus to oxytocin increases gradually during gestation, then increases sharply before parturition.

Naturally derived oxytocin, no longer commercially available, has been replaced by synthetic oxytocin. Oxytocin is most frequently used to induce or improve uterine contractions in labor. Ergot derivatives (ergonovine and methylergonovine) are also used for oxytocic effects on uterine muscle. These agents are most appropriately used to prevent postpartum uterine atony and hemorrhage.

VASOPRESSIN (8-Arginine-Vasopressin)

Refer to the general discussion of these products in the Posterior Pituitary Hormones introduction.

Actions:

Pharmacology: Possesses vasopressor and antidiuretic hormone (ADH) activity.

Pharmacokinetics: Following IM or SC injection, the duration of antidiuretic activity for vasopressin aqueous solution is 2 to 8 hours. Most is metabolized and rapidly destroyed in liver and kidneys. Vasopressin aqueous solution has a plasma half-life of about 10 to 20 minutes. After 4 hours, about 5% of an SC dose is excreted unchanged in urine.

Indications:

Diabetes insipidus: Neurogenic diabetes insipidus.

Abdominal distention/roentgenography: Prevention and treatment of postoperative abdominal distention and in abdominal roentgenography to dispel interfering gas shadows.

Unlabeled uses: Vasopressin infusions (IV or selective intra-arterial) are used to manage bleeding esophageal varices at a dosage of 0.2 units/min initially, increased to 0.4 units/min if bleeding continues. Maximum recommended dose is 0.9 units/min.

Contraindications:

Anaphylaxis or hypersensitivity to vasopressin or its components.

Warnings:

Vascular disease: Use with extreme caution in patients with vascular disease (especially coronary artery disease) since even small doses may precipitate anginal pain; with larger doses, consider the possibility of MI.

Water intoxication: Vasopressin may produce water intoxication. Early signs of drowsiness, listlessness and headaches precede terminal coma and convulsions.

Vasoconstriction/Necrosis: Severe vasoconstriction and local tissue necrosis may result if vasopressin extravasates during IV infusion. Gangrene of the extremities, tongue necrosis and ischemic colitis may occur during treatment of esophageal varices.

Chronic nephritis with nitrogen retention contraindicates use until reasonable nitrogen blood levels have been attained.

Hypersensitivity: Local or systemic allergic reactions may occur in hypersensitive individuals (see Adverse Reactions). Anaphylaxis (cardiac arrest or shock) has been observed shortly after injection. Refer to Management of Acute Hypersensitivity Reactions.

Pregnancy: Category C. It is not known whether vasopressin causes fetal harm when administered to a pregnant woman or affects reproductive capacity. Administer to a pregnant woman only if clearly needed. Doses sufficient for an antidiuretic effect are not likely to produce tonic uterine contractions that could be harmful to the fetus or threaten the continuation of the pregnancy.

Lactation: Exercise caution when giving to a nursing woman.

Precautions:

Monitoring: Electrocardiograms and fluid and electrolyte status determinations are recommended at intervals during therapy.

Special risk patients: Use vasopressin cautiously in the presence of epilepsy, migraine, asthma, heart failure or any state in which a rapid increase in extracellular water may result in further compromise.

Drug Interactions:

Vasopressin Drug Interactions			
Precipitant drug	Object drug*		Description
Carbamazepine	Vasopressin	↑	Carbamazepine, which potentiates ADH, may potentiate the effects of vasopressin.
Chlorpropamide	Vasopressin	↑	Chlorpropamide, which potentiates ADH, may potentiate the effects of vasopressin.

* ↑ = Object drug increased.

Adverse Reactions:

Hypersensitivity: Tremor; sweating; vertigo; cardiac arrest; circumoral pallor; "pounding" in head; abdominal cramps; passage of gas; nausea; vomiting; urticaria and bronchial constriction (see Warnings).

VASOPRESSIN (8-Arginine-Vasopressin)

Overdosage:

Treat water intoxication with water restriction and temporary withdrawal of vasopressin until polyuria occurs. Severe water intoxication may require osmotic diuresis with mannitol, hypertonic dextrose, or urea alone or with furosemide.

Patient Information:

Side effects such as skin blanching, abdominal cramps and nausea may be reduced by taking 1 or 2 glasses of water with the dose. These side effects usually are not serious and will probably disappear within a few minutes.

Administration and Dosage:

May be given IM or SC.

Adults: 5 to 10 units usually elicit full physiologic response. Give IM at 3 or 4 hour intervals as needed. Reduce dosage proportionately for children.

Diabetes insipidus:

Intranasal – The injection solution may be administered intranasally on cotton pledgets, by nasal spray or dropper. Individualize dosage.

Parenteral – 5 to 10 units 2 or 3 times daily as needed.

Abdominal distention: To prevent or relieve postoperative distention, give 5 units initially; increase to 10 units at subsequent injections, if necessary. Give IM at 3 or 4 hour intervals. Reduce dosage proportionately for children. These recommendations also apply to distention complicating pneumonia or other acute toxemias.

Abdominal roentgenography: Administer 2 injections of 10 units each. Give 2 hours and ½ hour, respectively, before films are exposed. An enema may be given prior to first dose.

Rx	**Vasopressin** (American Regent)	**Injection:** 20 pressor units/ml	With 0.5% chlorobutanol. In 0.5, 1 and 10 ml vials.
Rx	**Pitressin Synthetic** (Parke-Davis)		With 0.5% chlorobutanol. In 0.5 and 1 ml amps and vials.

LYPRESSIN (8–Lysine Vasopressin)

Refer to the general discussion of these products in the Posterior Pituitary Hormones introduction.

Actions:

Pharmacology: Lypressin is a synthetic lysine vasopressin analog that possesses antidiuretic activity with little vasopressor or oxytocic effect. The onset of antidiuretic effect is prompt, peaks in 30 to 120 minutes and has a duration of 3 to 8 hours.

Indications:

Diabetes insipidus: For the control or prevention of the symptoms and complications of neurogenic diabetes insipidus (including polydipsia, polyuria and dehydration). Useful in patients who have become unresponsive to other therapy or who experience local or systemic reactions, allergic reactions or other undesirable effects (eg, excessive fluid retention) from preparations of animal origin.

Warnings:

Hypersensitivity: Test patients with known sensitivity to antidiuretic hormones.

Pregnancy: Safety for use during pregnancy is not established. Use only when clearly needed and when potential benefits outweigh potential hazards to the fetus.

Precautions:

Cardiovascular effects: Cardiovascular pressor effects are minimal or absent when administered as a nasal spray in therapeutic doses. Nevertheless, use cautiously when such effects would be undesirable; mild blood pressure elevation has been noted in unanesthetized subjects who received IV lypressin. Large doses intranasally may cause coronary artery constriction; use caution in treating patients with coronary artery disease.

Upper respiratory conditions: Effectiveness may decrease in the presence of nasal congestion, allergic rhinitis and upper respiratory infections because of decreased absorption by the nasal mucosa; larger doses or adjunctive therapy may be required.

LYPRESSIN (8–Lysine Vasopressin)

Drug Interactions:

Lypressin Drug Interactions			
Precipitant drug	Object drug*		Description
Carbamazepine	Lypressin	↑	Carbamazepine, which potentiates ADH, may potentiate the effects of lypressin.
Chlorpropamide	Lypressin	↑	Chlorpropamide, which potentiates ADH, may potentiate the effects of lypressin.

* ↑ = Object drug increased.

Adverse Reactions:

Reactions have been infrequent and mild.

Local: Rhinorrhea; nasal congestion; irritation and pruritus of the nasal passages; nasal ulceration; periorbital edema with itching.

Systemic: Headache; conjunctivitis; heartburn secondary to excessive intranasal use; abdominal cramps and increased bowel movements. Inadvertent inhalation has resulted in substernal tightness, coughing and transient dyspnea. Hypersensitivity manifested by a positive skin test has occurred.

Overdosage:

Overdosage has caused marked, but transient fluid retention.

Patient Information:

Review administration technique with patient. Spray into nostril(s) as directed.

To ensure that a uniform, well-diffused spray is delivered, have the patient hold the bottle upright while in a vertical position with head upright.

Notify physician if drowsiness, listlessness, headache, shortness of breath, heartburn, nausea, abdominal cramps or severe nasal congestion or irritation occurs.

Administration and Dosage:

Administer 1 or 2 sprays to one or both nostrils whenever frequency of urination increases or significant thirst develops. One spray provides approximately 2 Posterior Pituitary (Pressor) Units. The usual dosage for adults and children is 1 or 2 sprays into each nostril 4 times daily. An additional bedtime dose helps eliminate nocturia not controlled with regular daily dosage. For patients requiring more than 2 sprays per nostril every 4 to 6 hours, reduce the time between doses rather than increase the number of sprays at each dose. More than 2 or 3 sprays in each nostril is usually wasted; the unabsorbed excess will drain posteriorly (by way of the nasopharynx) into the digestive tract where it will be inactivated.

The spray permits individualization of dosage necessary to control the symptoms of diabetes insipidus. Patients quickly learn to regulate dosage in accordance with their degree of polyuria and thirst; once determined, daily requirements remain fairly stable for months or years. Dosage has ranged from 1 spray per day at bedtime to 10 sprays into each nostril every 3 to 4 hours. Larger doses may represent greater severity of disease or other phenomena, such as poor nasal absorption. Large doses may also be due to the presence of mixed hypothalamic-hypophyseal and nephrogenic diabetes insipidus, the latter being unresponsive to antidiuretic hormone.

Rx	**Diapid** (Sandoz)	**Nasal Spray:** 0.185 mg lypressin (equivalent to 50 USP Posterior Pituitary [Pressor] Units)/ml	In 8 ml bottles.[1]

[1] With methyl and propyl parabens, sorbitol solution, glycerin and chlorobutanol.

DESMOPRESSIN ACETATE (1-Deamino-8-D-Arginine Vasopressin)

Refer to the general discussion of these products in the Posterior Pituitary Hormones introduction.

Actions:

Pharmacology: A synthetic analog of arginine vasopressin, the naturally occurring human antidiuretic hormone (ADH) provides a prompt onset of action with a long duration. The antidiuretic action is more specific and more prolonged than that of the natural hormone or lypressin. The plasma half-life of lypressin is 17 to 35 minutes. Urine volume is reduced, and urine osmolality is increased.

The change in structure of arginine vasopressin to desmopressin acetate results in less vasopressor activity and decreased action on visceral smooth muscle relative to enhanced antidiuretic activity. Consequently, clinically effective antidiuretic doses are usually below the threshold for effects on vascular or visceral smooth muscle.

Desmopressin produces a dose-related increase in Factor VIII levels. The increase is rapid, becoming evident in ≤ 30 minutes and peaking in 90 to 120 minutes. The Factor VIII-related antigen and ristocetin cofactor activity are also increased to a smaller degree.

Pharmacokinetics:

Injection – Biphasic half-lives of desmopressin acetate are 7.8 and 75.5 minutes for the fast and slow phases, respectively, compared with 2.5 and 14.5 minutes for lysine vasopressin. When administered by injection, desmopressin has an antidiuretic effect ≈ 10 times that of an equivalent dose administered intranasally.

Intranasal – The half-life of the nasal spray is between 3.3 and 3.5 hours, over the range of intranasal doses, 150 to 450 mcg. Plasma concentrations of the nasal spray are maximal at ≈ 40 to 45 minutes after dosing. The bioavailability of the nasal spray when administered by the intranasal route as a 1.5 mg/ml solution is between 3.3% and 4.1%. Plasminogen activator activity increases rapidly after IV infusion, but clinically significant fibrinolysis has not occurred.

Oral – The bioavailability of the tablets is ≈ 5% and 0.15% compared with intranasal and IV desmopressin, respectively. The time to reach maximum plasma levels ranges from 0.9 to 1.5 hours following oral or intranasal administration, respectively. Following administration of tablets, the onset of antidiuretic effect occurs at around 1 hour, and it reaches a maximum at ≈ 4 to 7 hours based on the measurement of increased urine osmolality. The plasma half-life of desmopressin follows a monoexponential time course with $t_{1/2}$ values of 1.5 to 2.5 hours which is independent of dose. Increasing oral doses produces dose-dependent increases in the plasma levels of desmopressin tablets.

Clinical trials: In one study, the tablets and intranasal formulation were compared during an 8–hour dosing interval at steady-state. The doses administered to 36 hydrated (water loaded) healthy male adult volunteers every 8 hours were 0.1, 0.2 and 0.4 mg orally and 0.01 mg intranasally by rhinal tube.

With respect to the mean values of total urine volume decrease and maximum urine osmolality increase from baseline, the 0.4 and 0.2 mg oral dose produced between 95% to 110% and 84% to 99% of pharmacodynamic activity, respectively, when compared with the 0.01 mg intranasal dose.

While both the 0.2 mg and 0.4 mg oral doses are considered pharmacodynamically similar to the 0.01 mg intranasal dose, the pharmacodynamic data on an intersubject basis was highly variable and, therefore, individual dosing is recommended.

In another study in diabetes insipidus patients, the tablet and intranasal formulations were compared over a 12–hour period. Ten fluid-controlled patients < 18 years of age were administered tablet doses of 0.2 and 0.4 mg and intranasal doses of 10 and 20 mcg.

All four dose formulations have a similar, pronounced pharmacodynamic effect on urine volume and urine osmolality. At 2 hours after study drug administration, mean urine volume was 4 ml/min and urine osmolality was > 500 mOsm/kg. Mean plasma osmolality remained relatively constant over the time course recorded (0 to 12 hours).

Indications:

DDAVP:

Primary nocturnal enuresis (intranasal only) – May be used alone or adjunctive to behavioral conditioning or other nonpharmacological intervention. It is effective in some cases that are refractory to conventional therapies.

Central cranial diabetes insipidus (intranasal, oral and parenteral) – ADH replacement therapy in the management of central cranial (neurogenic) diabetes insipidus and for temporary polyuria and polydipsia following head trauma or surgery in the pituitary region. Ineffective for the treatment of nephrogenic diabetes insipidus.

Hemophilia A (intranasal and parenteral) with Factor VIII levels > 5%. Desmopressin will often maintain hemostasis in patients with hemophilia A during

DESMOPRESSIN ACETATE (1-Deamino-8-D-Arginine Vasopressin)

surgery and postoperatively when administered 30 minutes prior to procedure. The drug will also stop bleeding in hemophilia A patients with episodes of spontaneous or trauma-induced injuries such as hemarthroses, IM hematomas or mucosal bleeding.

von Willebrand's disease (Type I) (intranasal and parenteral) – Mild to moderate classic von Willebrand's disease (Type I) with Factor VIII levels > 5%. Hemostasis in these patients can often be maintained during surgery and postoperatively when the drug is administered 30 minutes prior to the procedure. Episodes of spontaneous or trauma-induced injuries such as hemarthroses, IM hematomas or mucosal bleeding can usually be stopped.

Stimate:

Hemophilia A with Factor VIII coagulant activity levels > 5%. Desmopressin will also stop bleeding in patients with hemophilia A with episodes of spontaneous or trauma-induced injuries such as hemarthroses, intramuscular hematomas or mucosal bleeding.

von Willebrand's disease (Type I) – Mild to moderate classic von Willebrand's disease (Type I) with Factor VIII levels > 5%. Desmopressin will also stop bleeding in mild to moderate von Willebrand's disease patients with episodes of spontaneous or trauma-induced injuries such as hemarthroses, intramuscular hematomas, mucosal bleeding or menorrhagia.

Unlabeled uses:

Intranasal – Treatment of chronic autonomic failure (eg, nocturnal polyuria, overnight weight loss, morning postural hypotension).

Contraindications:

Hypersensitivity to desmopressin acetate or its components.

Intranasal delivery may be inappropriate where there is an impaired level of consciousness.

Warnings:

Hemophilia A: Not indicated for treatment of hemophilia A with Factor VIII levels ≤ 5%, for the treatment of hemophilia B or in patients who have Factor VIII antibodies. Some patients with Factor VIII levels between 2% to 5% may be treatable.

von Willebrand's disease: Patients who are least likely to respond are those with severe homozygous von Willebrand's disease with Factor VIII coagulant activity, Factor VIII antigen and von Willebrand's factor (ristocetin cofactor) activities < 1%. Other patients may respond in a variable fashion, depending on the type of molecular defect.

Not indicated for the treatment of severe classic von Willebrand's disease (Type I) and when an abnormal molecular form of Factor VIII antigen is evident.

Do not use for Type IIB von Willebrand's disease; may induce platelet aggregation.

Test dose: Before the initial therapeutic administration of the nasal spray, the physician should establish that the patient shows an appropriate change in the coagulation profile following a test dose of intranasal administration.

Water intoxication: Caution very young and elderly patients to ingest only enough fluid to satisfy thirst to decrease the potential occurrence of water intoxication and hyponatremia. Pay particular attention to the possibility of the rare occurrence of an extreme decrease in plasma osmolality that may result in seizures, that could lead to coma.

Hypersensitivity reactions: Rare severe allergic reactions have been reported with desmopressin. Anaphylaxis has been reported with IV administration but not with intranasal or oral (tablets).

Pregnancy: Category B. Several publications of desmopressin acetate's use in the management of diabetes insipidus during pregnancy are available. However, there are no adequate and well controlled studies in pregnant women. Safety and efficacy for use during pregnancy has not been established. Use only when clearly needed and when the potential benefits outweigh potential hazards to the fetus. Published reports stress that, as opposed to preparations containing the natural hormones, desmopressin in antidiuretic doses has no uterotonic action, but the physician will have to weigh possible therapeutic advantages against possible danger in each case.

Lactation: Safety for use in nursing women has not been established. Patients receiving desmopressin for diabetes insipidus have been reported to breast feed without apparent problems in the infant. A single study in postpartum women showed little, if any, change in breast milk following a 10 mcg intranasal dose. However, there have been no controlled studies in nursing mothers. Exercise caution when administering desmopressin to a nursing woman.

DESMOPRESSIN ACETATE (1-Deamino-8-D-Arginine Vasopressin)

Children: Infants and children require careful fluid intake restriction to prevent possible hyponatremia and water intoxication.

Intranasal desmopressin has been used in children with diabetes insipidus, and the tablets have been used safely in children (≥ 4 years of age) with diabetes insipidus for periods ≤ 44 months. If desmopressin is used in the very young, adjust the dose individually, with attention to the danger of an extreme decrease in plasma osmolality leading to hyponatremia with possible convulsions. Initiate doses at 0.05 ml (intranasal) or 0.05 mg (oral).

Pediatric Use of Desmopressin Acetate	
Indication/Doseform	Safety and effectiveness not proven in children less than age:
Central cranial diabetes insipidus	
Intranasal	Adjust dosage (*DDAVP*)
Oral	4 years
Parenteral	12 years
Hemophilia A	
Intranasal	11 months (*Stimate*)
Oral	Not indicated.
Parenteral	3 months
Primary nocturnal enuresis	
Intranasal	6 years (*DDAVP*)
Oral	Not indicated.
Parenteral	Not indicated.
von Willebrand's disease	
Intranasal	11 months (*Stimate*)
Oral	Not indicated.
Parenteral	3 months

Precautions:

Monitoring:

Diabetes insipidus – Monitor urine volume/osmolality and plasma osmolality.

Hemophilia A – Determine Factor VIII coagulant activity before injecting desmopressin for hemostasis; if the activity is < 5% of normal, do not rely on desmopressin. Other tests to assess patient status include levels of Factor VIII coagulant, Factor VIII antigen and ristocetin cofactor and activated partial thromboplastin time (APTT).

von Willebrand's disease – Assess levels of Factor VIII coagulant, Factor VIII antigen and ristocetin cofactor. Skin bleeding time may also be helpful.

Cardiovascular effects: High intranasal dosage has infrequently produced a slight elevation of blood pressure that disappeared with dosage reduction. This effect has not been observed with single oral doses ≤ 0.6 mg. Use with caution in coronary artery insufficiency or hypertensive cardiovascular disease. Desmopressin injection has infrequently produced changes in blood pressure causing either a slight elevation in blood pressure or a transient fall in blood pressure and a compensatory increase in heart rate. Use the drug with caution in patients with coronary artery insufficiency or hypertensive cardiovascular disease.

Nasal mucosa changes (eg, scarring, edema, discharge, blockage, congestion, severe atrophic rhinitis), cranial surgery (eg, transphenoidal hypophysectomy) and nasal packing compromise intranasal delivery; consider administering IV.

Thrombotic events: There have been rare reports of thrombotic events (thrombosis, acute cerebrovascular thrombosis, acute myocardial infarction) following desmopressin injection in patients predisposed to thrombus formation. No causality has been determined; however, use the drug with caution in these patients.

Decreased response: There are reports of an occasional change in response to intranasal desmopressin with time, usually > 6 months. Some patients may show a decreased responsiveness, others a shortened duration of effect. There is no evidence this effect is because of the development of binding antibodies but it may be because of a local inactivation of the peptide. No lessening of effect has been seen in the 46 patients who were treated with desmopressin tablets for 12 to 44 months and no serum antibodies to desmopressin were detected.

Fluid/Electrolyte imbalance: Use with caution in patients with conditions associated with fluid and electrolyte imbalance, such as cystic fibrosis, because these patients are prone to hyponatremia.

DESMOPRESSIN ACETATE (1-Deamino-8-D-Arginine Vasopressin)

Drug Interactions:

Desmopressin Drug Interactions			
Precipitant drug	Object drug*		Description
Desmopressin	Pressor agents	↑	Although desmopressin pressor activity is very low, use large intranasal doses or parenteral doses as large as 0.3 mcg/kg cautiously with other pressor agents.
Carbamazepine	Desmopressin	↑	Carbamazepine, which potentiates ADH, may potentiate the effects of desmopressin.
Chlorpropamide	Desmopressin	↑	Chlorpropamide, which potentiates ADH, may potentiate the effects of desmopressin.

* ↑ = Object drug increased.

Adverse Reactions:

Intranasal (DDAVP): Adverse reactions that disappear with dosage reduction include: abdominal pain (mild); facial flushing; headache (transient); nasal congestion; nausea; rhinitis. Other adverse reactions include: Asthenia; chills; conjunctivitis; cough; dizziness; epistaxis; eye edema; GI disorder; lacrimation disorder; nosebleed; nostril pain; sore throat; upper respiratory infections.

Intranasal (Stimate): Adverse reactions include: Agitation; balanitis; chest pain; chills; dizziness; dyspepsia; edema; insomnia; itchy or light sensitive eyes; pain; palpitations; somnolence; tachycardia; vomiting; warm feeling.

Parenteral: Adverse reactions that disappear with dosage reduction include: Abdominal pain (mild); facial flushing; headache (transient); nausea; vulval pain. Other adverse reactions include: Anaphylaxis (rare); blood pressure changes; burning pain; edema; erythema (local).

Oral: In long-term clinical studies in which patients with diabetes insipidus were followed for periods ≤ 12 to 44 months of tablet therapy, transient increases in AST ≤ 1.5 times the upper limit of normal occurred. Elevated AST returned to the normal range despite continued use of tablets.

Overdosage:

Symptoms: Abdominal pain, dyspnea, facial flushing, fluid retention, headache and mucous membrane irritation may occur.

Treatment: Reduce the dosage, decrease the frequency of use or withdraw the drug according to the severity of the condition. There is no known specific antidote.

Patient Information:

Patient instructions provided with intranasal product; review administration with patient.

If bleeding is not controlled, contact the physician.

Notify physician if headache, shortness of breath, heartburn, nausea, abdominal cramps or vulval pain occurs.

Intranasal: Inform patients that the bottle accurately delivers 25 or 50 doses. Discard any solution remaining after 25 or 50 doses because the amount delivered thereafter may be substantially less than prescribed. Do not attempt to transfer remaining solution to another bottle.

Administration and Dosage:

Primary nocturnal enuresis: Individualize dosage.

Initial dose (≥ 6 years of age) – 20 mcg (0.2 ml) intranasally at bedtime. Adjustment ≤ 40 mcg is suggested if the patient does not respond. Some patients may respond to 10 mcg and adjustment to that lower dose may be done if the patient has shown a response to 20 mcg. It is recommended that one-half of the dose be administered per nostril. Adequately controlled studies have not been conducted beyond 4 to 8 weeks.

Central cranial diabetes insipidus:

Intranasal – The nasal tube delivery system is supplied with a flexible calibrated plastic tube (rhinyle). Draw solution into the rhinyle. Insert one end of tube into nostril; blow on the other end to deposit solution deep into nasal cavity. The nasal spray pump may also be used.

Adults: 0.1 to 0.4 ml daily, either as a single dose or divided into 2 or 3 doses. Most adults require 0.2 ml daily in 2 divided doses. Adjust morning and evening doses separately for an adequate diurnal rhythm of water turnover.

Children (3 months to 12 years): 0.05 to 0.3 ml daily, either as a single dose or in 2 divided doses.

DESMOPRESSIN ACETATE (1-Deamino-8-D-Arginine Vasopressin)

Parenteral – Administer SC or by direct IV injection.

Adults: 0.5 to 1 ml daily in 2 divided doses, adjusted separately for an adequate diurnal rhythm of water turnover. For patients switching from intranasal to IV, the comparable IV antidiuretic dose is approximately one-tenth the intranasal dose. Estimate response by adequate sleep duration and adequate but not excessive water turnover.

Oral – The dosage must be determined for each individual patient and adjusted according to the diurnal pattern of response. Estimate response by adequate duration of sleep and adequate, not excessive, water turnover. Begin therapy 12 hours after the last intranasal dose for patients previously on intranasal therapy. Observe patients closely during the initial dose titration period and measure appropriate safety parameters to assure adequate response. Monitor patient at regular intervals during therapy to assure adequate antidiuretic response. Implement modifications in dosage regimen as necessary to assure adequate water turnover.

Adults: Begin with 0.05 mg 2 times a day and adjust individually to their optimum therapeutic dose. Separately adjust each dose for an adequate diurnal rhythm of water turnover. Increase or decrease total daily dosage (range, 0.1 to 1.2 mg divided 2 or 3 times a day) as needed to obtain adequate antidiuresis.

Children: Begin dosing with 0.05 mg. Careful fluid intake restrictions in children is required to prevent hyponatremia and water intoxication.

Hemophilia A and von Willebrand's disease (Type I):

Parenteral – Administer 0.3 mcg/kg diluted in sterile physiologic saline; infuse IV slowly over 15 to 30 minutes. In adults and children weighing > 10 kg, use 50 ml diluent; in children weighing ≤ 10 kg, use 10 ml. Monitor blood pressure and pulse during infusion. If used preoperatively, administer 30 minutes prior to the procedure.

Determine the necessity for repeat dose or use of any blood products for hemostasis by laboratory response and patient's clinical condition. Consider the tendency toward tachyphylaxis with repeating dose more than every 48 hours.

Intranasal – Administer by nasal insufflation, 1 spray per nostril, to provide a total dose of 300 mcg. In patients weighing < 50 kg, 150 mcg administered as a single spray provided the expected effect on Factor VIII coagulant activity, Factor VIII ristocetin cofactor activity and skin bleeding time. If used preoperatively, administer 2 hours prior to the scheduled procedure.

The necessity for repeat administration or use of any blood products for hemostasis should be determined by laboratory response as well as the clinical condition of the patient. Consider the tendency toward tachyphylaxis (lessening of response) with repeated administration given more frequently than every 48 hours.

The nasal spray pump only delivers doses of 10 mcg (*DDAVP*) or 150 mcg (*Stimate*). If doses other than these are required, consider nasal tube delivery or injection.

The *Stimate* spray pump must be primed prior to the first use. To prime pump, press down 4 times. Discard the bottle after 25 doses since the amount delivered thereafter per spray may be substantially < 150 mcg of drug.

Storage/Stability:

Intranasal – Refrigerate nasal solution at 2° to 8°C (36° to 46°F). Nasal solution will maintain stability for ≤ 3 weeks when stored at room temperature (22°C; 72°F).

Injection – Store at room temperature between 15° to 30°C (59° to 86°F). Avoid exposure to excessive heat or light.

Rx	**DDAVP** (Rhone-Poulenc Rorer)	**Tablets**: 0.1 mg	Lactose. (DDAVP 01). White. In 100s.
		0.2 mg	Lactose. (DDAVP 02). White. In 100s.
Rx	**DDAVP** (Rhone-Poulenc Rorer)	**Nasal Solution**: 0.1 mg/ml (0.1 mg equals 400 IU arginine vasopressin)	**Nasal spray pump**: 9 mg NaCl/ml. In 2.5 or 5 ml bottle[1] with spray pump (25 or 50 doses of 10 mcg each, respectively).
			Rhinal tube delivery system: 9 mg NaCl/ml. In 2.5 ml vials[1] with applicator tubes.
Rx	**Stimate** (Armour)	**Nasal solution**: 1.5 mg/ml	9 mg NaCl/ml. In 2.5 ml bottle[1] (25 doses of 150 mcg each).
Rx	**DDAVP** (Rhone-Poulenc Rorer)	**Injection**: 4 mcg/ml	9 mg NaCl/ml. In 1 ml amps and 10 ml multiple dose vials.[1]

[1] With 5 mg chlorobutanol per ml.

OXYTOCIN

For complete prescribing information, refer to the Posterior Pituitary Hormones introduction.

Warning:

Important Note: Oxytocin is indicated for the medical rather than the elective induction of labor. Available data and information are inadequate to define the benefit-to-risk considerations in the use of oxytocin for elective induction.

Actions:

Pharmacology: Oxytocin, an endogenous hormone produced in the posterior pituitary gland, has uterine stimulant properties, especially on the gravid uterus, as well as vasopressive and antidiuretic effects. Its exact role in normal labor and medically-induced labor is not fully understood. However, it may act primarily on uterine myofibril activity, thus augmenting the number of contracting myofibrils. The sensitivity of the uterus to oxytocin increases gradually during gestation and increases sharply before parturition.

Oxytocin has weak antidiuretic effects, but has led to fatal water intoxication. It also has a definite but transient relaxing effect on vascular smooth muscle.

Pharmacokinetics: Oxytocin is given parenterally and intranasally; however, the latter may be erratically absorbed. The plasma half-life of synthetic oxytocin is 1 to 6 minutes, but this decreases in late pregnancy and lactation. Following IV administration, uterine response occurs almost immediately and subsides within 1 hour. Uterine response after IM injection is within 3 to 5 minutes and persists for 2 to 3 hours. Steady-state plasma levels and the maximum uterine contractile response are reached in approximately 40 minutes using doses in the therapeutic range. Elimination is through the liver, kidneys and functional mammary gland and by the enzyme oxytocinase.

Indications:

Oxytocin (parenteral):

Antepartum – To initiate or improve uterine contractions to achieve early vaginal delivery, for fetal or maternal reasons, such as Rh problems, maternal diabetes, preeclampsia at or near term, when delivery is in the best interest of mother and fetus, or when membranes are prematurely ruptured and delivery is indicated; stimulation or reinforcement of labor, as in selected cases of uterine inertia; management of inevitable or incomplete abortion. In the first trimester, curettage is generally considered primary therapy. In second trimester abortion, oxytocin infusion is often successful in emptying the uterus. Other means of therapy, however, may be required in such cases.

Postpartum – To produce uterine contractions during the third stage of labor and to control postpartum bleeding or hemorrhage.

Oxytocin (nasal): For initial milk let-down.

Unlabeled uses: Antepartum fetal heart rate testing (oxytocin challenge test); breast engorgement.

Contraindications:

Significant cephalopelvic disproportion; unfavorable fetal positions or presentations which are undeliverable without conversion prior to delivery (eg, transverse lies); in obstetrical emergencies where the benefit-to-risk ratio for either the fetus or the mother favors surgical intervention; cases of fetal distress where delivery is not imminent; prolonged use in uterine inertia or severe toxemia; hypertonic or hyperactive uterine patterns; where adequate uterine activity fails to achieve satisfactory progress; induction or augmentation of labor where vaginal delivery is contraindicated, such as invasive cervical carcinoma, active herpes genitalis, cord presentation or prolapse, total placenta previa and vasa previa; hypersensitivity to the drug.

Oxytocin (nasal) is contraindicated in pregnancy.

Warnings:

When used for induction or stimulation of labor, administer oxytocin only by the IV route. All patients receiving IV oxytocin must be under continuous observation to identify complications. A qualified physician should be immediately available.

Except in unusual circumstances, do not administer oxytocin in the following conditions: Fetal distress; partial placenta previa; prematurity; borderline cephalopelvic disproportion; previous major surgery on the cervix or uterus including cesarean section; overdistention of the uterus; grand multiparity; history of uterine sepsis; traumatic delivery; invasive cervical carcinoma. The decision can only be made by weighing the potential benefits which oxytocin can provide in a given case against rare but definite potential for the drug to produce hypertonicity or tetanic spasm.

OXYTOCIN

Cyclopropane anesthesia may modify oxytocin's cardiovascular effects, producing unexpected results such as hypotension. Concomitant use of oxytocin with cyclopropane anesthesia can cause maternal sinus bradycardia with abnormal atrioventricular rhythms.

Maternal deaths due to hypertensive episodes, subarachnoid hemorrhage, rupture of the uterus, *fetal deaths* due to various causes and *infant brain damage* have been associated with the use of parenteral oxytocic drugs for induction of labor or for augmentation in the first and second stages of labor.

Pregnancy: No known indications for use in the first trimester exist other than in relation to spontaneous or induced abortion. Oxytocin is not expected to present a risk of fetal abnormalities when used as indicated (see Adverse Reactions in the fetus).

Lactation: Oxytocin may be found in small quantities in breast milk. If a postpartum dosage is required to control severe bleeding, nursing should not commence until the day after oxytocin has been discontinued.

Children: Oxytocin is not intended for use in children.

Precautions:

Uterine contractions: When properly administered, oxytocin stimulates uterine contractions similar to those in normal labor. Overstimulation of the uterus can be hazardous to both mother and fetus. Even with proper administration and supervision, hypertonic contractions can occur in a patient whose uterus is hypersensitive to oxytocin.

Water intoxication: Oxytocin has an intrinsic antidiuretic effect, acting to increase water reabsorption from the glomerular filtrate. Consider the possibility of water intoxication, particularly when oxytocin is administered by continuous infusion and the patient is receiving fluids by mouth.

Evaluate pelvic adequacy and maternal and fetal conditions when using oxytocin for induction or reinforcement of already existent labor.

Drug Interactions:

Sympathomimetics: If used concurrently with oxytocic drugs, the pressor effect of the sympathomimetics may be increased, possibly resulting in postpartum hypertension.

Severe hypertension occurred when oxytocin was given 3 to 4 hours following prophylactic administration of a vasoconstrictor in conjunction with caudal block anesthesia.

Adverse Reactions:

Maternal: Anaphylactic reaction; postpartum hemorrhage; cardiac arrhythmia; fatal afibrinogenemia; nausea; vomiting; premature ventricular contractions; increased blood loss; pelvic hematoma. Excessive dosage or hypersensitivity to the drug may result in uterine hypertonicity, spasm, tetanic contraction or rupture of the uterus. Severe water intoxication with convulsions and coma has occurred, associated with a slow oxytocin infusion over a 24 hour period. Maternal death due to oxytocin-induced water intoxication has occurred.

Fetal: Bradycardia, premature ventricular contractions and other arrhythmias, permanent CNS or brain damage and death have been caused by uterine motility. Use of oxytocin in the mother has caused low Apgar scores at 5 minutes, and neonatal jaundice and retinal hemorrhage have occurred.

Overdosage:

Overdosage depends on uterine hyperactivity. Hyperstimulation with hypertonic or tetanic contractions, or a resting tone of ≥ 15 to 20 mm H_2O between contractions can lead to tumultuous labor, uterine rupture, cervical and vaginal lacerations, postpartum hemorrhage, uteroplacental hypoperfusion, and variable deceleration of fetal heart, fetal hypoxia, hypercapnia or death. Water intoxication with convulsions is a serious complication that may occur if large doses (40 to 50 ml/min) are infused for long periods. To treat, discontinue drug, restrict fluid intake, initiate diuresis, administer IV hypertonic saline solution, correct electrolyte imbalance, control convulsions with judicious use of a barbiturate and provide special nursing care for the comatose patient.

OXYTOCIN, PARENTERAL

For complete prescribing information, refer to the Oxytocin monograph.

Administration and Dosage:

Determine dosage by uterine response.

Induction or stimulation of labor:

IV infusion (drip method) – This is the only acceptable method of administration for the induction or stimulation of labor. Accurate control of infusion flow is essential. An infusion pump or other device and frequent monitoring of strength, frequency and duration of contractions, resting uterine tone and fetal heart rate are necessary. If uterine contractions become too powerful, the infusion can be abruptly stopped; oxytocic stimulation of the uterine musculature will soon wane.

Start an IV infusion of non-oxytocin-containing solution. Use physiologic electrolyte solution, except under unusual circumstances.

Dosage: The initial dose should be no more than 1 to 2 mU/min (0.001 to 0.002 units/min). Gradually increase the dose in increments of no more than 1 to 2 mU/min at 15 to 30 minute intervals until a contraction pattern has been established which is similar to normal labor. Maximum doses should rarely exceed 20 mU/minute.

Discontinue the oxytocin infusion immediately in the event of uterine hyperactivity or fetal distress and administer oxygen to the mother, who should be put in a lateral position.

Control of postpartum uterine bleeding:

IV infusion (drip method) – Add 10 to 40 units to a maximum of 40 units to 1000 ml of a nonhydrating diluent and run at a rate necessary to control uterine atony.

IM – Administer 10 units after delivery of the placenta.

Treatment of incomplete of inevitable abortion: IV infusion of 10 units of oxytocin with 500 ml physiologic saline solution, or 5% dextrose in physiologic saline solution infused at a rate of 10 to 20 mU (20 to 40 drops) per minute.

Reconstitution: Add 1 ml (10 units) to 1000 ml of 0.9% aqueous Sodium Chloride or other IV fluid. The solution contains 10 mU/ml (0.01 units/ml). Use a constant infusion pump to accurately control the rate of infusion. Do not exceed 30 units in a 12 hour period due to risk of water intoxication.

IV solution compatibility: At a concentration of 5 U/L, oxytocin is physically compatible with the most commonly used Dextrose, Sodium Chloride and Ringer's solutions, as well as combinations of these solutions.

Oxytocin is rapidly decomposed in the presence of sodium bisulfite.

Rx	**Oxytocin** (Various)	**Injection**: 10 units per ml	In 1 ml amps and 1 and 10 ml vials.
Rx	**Oxytocin** (Wyeth)		In 1 ml Tubex.
Rx	**Pitocin** (Parke-Davis)		In 0.5 and 1 ml amps,[1] 1 ml Steri-Dose syringe[1] and 10 ml Steri-Vial.[1]
Rx	**Syntocinon** (Sandoz)		In 1 ml amps.[2]

[1] With 0.5% chlorobutanol.

[2] With 0.5% chlorobutanol and 0.61% alcohol.

OXYTOCIN, SYNTHETIC, NASAL

For complete prescribing information, refer to the Oxytocin monograph.

Administration and Dosage:

Initial milk let-down: One spray into one or both nostrils 2 to 3 minutes before nursing or pumping of breasts.

Hold the squeeze bottle upright when administering the drug to the nose; the patient should be sitting rather than lying down. If preferred, the solution can be instilled in drop form by inverting the squeeze bottle and exerting gentle pressure.

Rx	**Syntocinon** (Sandoz)	**Nasal Spray**: 40 units/ml	In 2 and 5 ml squeeze bottles.[3]

[3] With glycerin, sorbitol solution, chlorobutanol and methyl and propyl parabens.

ERGONOVINE MALEATE

Refer to the general discussion of these products in the Posterior Pituitary Hormones introduction.

Actions:

Pharmacology: When used after placental delivery, ergonovine increases the strength, duration and frequency of uterine contractions and decreases uterine bleeding. It exerts its effects by acting as a partial agonist or antagonist at α-adrenergic, dopaminergic and tryptaminergic receptors.

Pharmacokinetics: Ergonovine has a rapid onset of action which varies with the route of administration: IV – 40 seconds; IM – 7 to 8 minutes; oral – 10 minutes. Uterine contractions continue for 3 or more hours after injection.

Indications:

Postpartum/Postabortal hemorrhage: Prevention and treatment of postpartum and postabortal hemorrhage due to uterine atony.

Unlabeled uses: Used diagnostically to identify Prinzmetal's angina (variant angina). IV doses during coronary arteriography provoke spontaneous coronary arterial spasms responsible for Prinzmetal's angina, reversible with nitroglycerin. Arrhythmias, ventricular tachycardia and myocardial infarction have been precipitated.

Administered parenterally, ergonovine is generally not as effective as ergotamine in the treatment of migraine headache; however, ergonovine may be more useful than ergotamine when use of ergotamine has caused paresthesias.

Contraindications:

Induction of labor; cases of threatened spontaneous abortion; previous allergic or idiosyncratic reactions to the drug.

Warnings:

Uterine effects: Patients have been injured, and some have died because of the injudicious use of oxytocic agents. Hyperstimulation of the uterus during labor may lead to uterine tetany with marked impairment of the uteroplacental blood flow, uterine rupture, cervical and perineal lacerations, amniotic fluid embolism and trauma to the infant (eg, hypoxia, intracranial hemorrhage).

Calcium deficiency: In some calcium-deficient patients, the uterus may not respond to ergonovine. Responsiveness can be immediately restored by cautious IV injection of calcium salts. Do not give calcium IV to patients receiving digitalis.

Oxytoxic agents must be administered under meticulous observation.

Pregnancy:

Labor and delivery – Because of the high uterine tone produced, ergonovine is not recommended for routine use prior to the delivery of the placenta, unless the surgeon is familiar with the technique described by Davis and others.

Lactation: Ergonovine may lower prolactin levels, which may decrease lactation.

Precautions:

Monitoring: Monitor blood pressure, pulse and uterine response. Note sudden changes in vital signs or frequent periods of uterine relaxation.

Duration: Avoid prolonged use. Discontinue if symptoms of ergotism appear.

Special risk patients: Use cautiously in patients with hypertension, heart disease, venoatrial shunts, mitral-valve stenosis, obliterative vascular disease, sepsis, hepatic or renal impairment.

Vaginal bleeding: Observe the character and amount of vaginal bleeding.

Adverse Reactions:

Cardiovascular: Blood pressure elevation (sometimes extreme) and headache appear in a small percentage of patients; this is most frequently associated with regional anesthesia (caudal or spinal), previous use of a vasoconstrictor and the IV administration of the oxytocic, but it may occur in the absence of these factors. The mechanism of such hypertension is obscure. The elevations are no more frequent with ergonovine than with other oxytocics. They usually subside promptly following 15 mg IV chlorpromazine.

Miscellaneous: Allergic phenomena (including shock); myocardial infarction (rare, associated with postpartom use of ergotrates); ergotism (acute ergotism is described in Overdosage); nausea; vomiting (uncommon).

ERGONOVINE MALEATE

Overdosage:

Symptoms: The principal manifestations of serious overdosage are convulsions (acute) and gangrene (chronic). Acute symptoms include: Nausea, vomiting, diarrhea, rise or fall in blood pressure, weak pulse, dyspnea, loss of consciousness, numbness and coldness of the extremities, tingling, chest pain, gangrene of the fingers and toes, hypercoagulability, confusion, excitement, delirium, hallucinations, convulsions and coma.

Treatment: Delay absorption of ingested drug by giving activated charcoal, then remove by gastric lavage or emesis followed by catharsis. Treat convulsions. Control hypercoagulability by administering heparin, and maintain blood-clotting time at approximately three times normal; give a vasodilator as an antidote. Nitroglycerin (sublingual or IV) is used for coronary vasospasm. Intravenous or intraarterial nitroprusside is the drug of choice for severe vasospasm. Gangrene may require surgical amputation.

Patient Information:

May cause nausea, vomiting, dizziness, increased blood pressure, headache, chest pain or shortness of breath.

Administration and Dosage:

Parenteral: Intended primarily for IM injection. It usually produces a firm contraction of the uterus within a few minutes.

The usual IM (or emergency IV) dose is 0.2 mg. Severe uterine bleeding may require repeated doses, but rarely more than one injection per 2 to 4 hours.

Administration IV produces a quicker response. However, because of the higher incidence of side effects, confine the IV route to emergencies such as excessive uterine bleeding.

Rx	**Ergotrate Maleate** (Bedford Labs)	**Injection:** 0.2 mg per ml	With 0.1% ethyl lactate and 0.25% phenol. In 1 ml vials.

METHYLERGONOVINE MALEATE

Refer to the general discussion of these products in the Posterior Pituitary Hormones introduction.

Actions:

Pharmacology: Methylergonovine increases strength, duration and frequency of uterine contractions and decreases uterine bleeding following placental delivery. It acts directly on the smooth muscle of the uterus and induces a rapid and sustained tetanic uterotonic effect, which shortens the third stage of labor and reduces blood loss.

Pharmacokinetics: The onset of action after IV administration is immediate; after IM administration, 2 to 5 minutes; after oral administration, 5 to 10 minutes.

A 0.2 mg IV injection is rapidly distributed from plasma to peripheral tissues within an α-phase half-life of ≤ 2 to 3 minutes. The β-phase elimination half-life is ≥ 20 to 30 minutes, but clinical effects continue for about 3 hours.

An IM injection of 0.2 mg afforded peak plasma concentrations of < 3 ng/ml at time to reach maximum concentrations of 30 minutes. After 2 hours, total plasma clearance was 120 to 240 ml/min.

After oral administration, bioavailability was reported as 60% with no accumulation after repeated doses. Bioavailability increased to 78% during delivery with parenteral injection.

Excretion is rapid and appears to be partially renal and partially hepatic. Whether the drug is able to penetrate the blood-brain barrier has not been determined.

Indications:

Uterine contractions/bleeding: Routine management after delivery of the placenta; postpartum atony and hemorrhage; subinvolution. Under full obstetric supervision, it may be given in the second stage of labor following delivery of the anterior shoulder.

Contraindications:

Hypertension; toxemia; pregnancy (see Warnings); hypersensitivity.

Warnings:

IV use: This drug should not be routinely administered IV because it may induce sudden hypertension and cerebrovascular accidents. If IV administration is considered essential, give slowly over no less than 60 seconds, with careful blood pressure monitoring.

Pregnancy: Category C. It is not known whether methylergonovine can cause fetal harm or affect reproductive capacity. Use is contraindicated during pregnancy (see Indications).

Labor and delivery – The uterotonic effect of methylergonovine is used after delivery to assist involution and decrease hemorrhage, shortening the third stage of labor. Also use with caution during the second stage of labor. The necessity for manual removal of a retained placenta should occur only rarely with proper technique and adequate allowance of time for its spontaneous separation.

Lactation: Methylergonovine maleate may be given orally for a maximum of 1 week postpartum to control uterine bleeding. Recommended dosage is one 0.2 mg tablet 3 or 4 times daily. At this dosage level, a small quantity of drug appears in breast milk. Adverse effects have not been described, but exercise caution when administering to a nursing woman.

Precautions:

Special risk patients: Exercise caution in the presence of sepsis, obliterative vascular disease, hepatic or renal involvement.

Drug Interactions:

Vasoconstrictors/Ergot alkaloids: Exercise caution during concurrent use with these agents and methylergonovine.

Adverse Reactions:

Hypertension associated in some cases with seizure or headache (most common); hypotension; nausea, vomiting (occasional); transient chest pain, dyspnea, hematuria, thrombophlebitis, water intoxication, hallucinations, leg cramps, dizziness, tinnitus, nasal congestion, diarrhea, diaphoresis, palpitation, foul taste (rare, in order of severity).

METHYLERGONOVINE MALEATE

Overdosage:

Symptoms: Acute overdose may include nausea, vomiting, abdominal pain, numbness, tingling of the extremities and rise in blood pressure. In severe cases, these are followed by hypotension, respiratory depression, hypothermia, convulsions and coma. Because reports of overdosage are infrequent, the lethal dose in humans has not been established. Several cases of accidental injection in newborn infants have been reported, and in such cases 0.2 mg represents an overdose of great magnitude. However, recovery occurred in all but one case following a period of respiratory depression, hypothermia, hypertonicity with jerking movements, and, in one case, a single convulsion.

Also, several children 1 to 3 years of age have accidentally ingested up to ten tablets (2 mg) with no apparent ill effects. A postpartum patient took four tablets (0.8 mg) at one time in error and reported paresthesias and clamminess as her only symptoms.

Treatment: Acute overdosage is symptomatic and includes the usual procedures of inducing emesis, gastric lavage, catharsis and supportive diuresis; maintaining adequate pulmonary ventilation, especially if convulsions or coma develop; correcting hypotension with pressor drugs as needed; controlling convulsions with standard anticonvulsant agents; controlling peripheral vasospasm with warmth to the extremities if needed.

Patient Information:

May cause nausea, vomiting, dizziness, increased blood pressure, headache, ringing in the ears, chest pain or shortness of breath.

Administration and Dosage:

IM: 0.2 mg after delivery of the placenta, after delivery of the anterior shoulder, or during the puerperium. Repeat as required, at intervals of 2 to 4 hours.

IV: (See Warnings). Dosage same as for IM use.

Orally: 0.2 mg 3 or 4 times/day in the puerperium for a maximum of 1 week.

Rx	**Methergine** (Sandoz)	**Injection:** 0.2 mg per ml	With 0.25 mg tartaric acid. In 1 ml ampuls.
		Tablets: 0.2 mg	(Sandoz 78-54). Orchid. Round. Coated. In 100s, 1000s and UD 100s.

RITODRINE HCl

Actions:

Pharmacology: Ritodrine is a β-receptor agonist which exerts a preferential effect on β_2-adrenergic receptors such as those in the uterine smooth muscle. Stimulation of the β_2– receptors inhibits contractility of the uterine smooth muscle through the cycle of adenyl cyclase stimulation, which increases intracellular cyclic adenosine 3′–5′–monophosphate (cAMP); this leads to altering cellular calcium balance that affects smooth muscle contractility. In addition, ritodrine may directly affect the interaction between the actin and myosin of muscle through inhibition of myosin light-chain kinase.

Infusions of 0.05 to 0.3 mg/min IV decrease the intensity and frequency of uterine contractions. These effects are antagonized by β-adrenergic blocking compounds. IV administration induces an immediate dose-related elevation of heart rate (maximum mean increase 19 to 40 bpm) and widening of the pulse pressure. The average increase in systolic blood pressure is 4 mm Hg, and the average decrease in diastolic pressure is 12.3 mm Hg.

During IV infusion, transient elevations of blood glucose, insulin and free fatty acids have been observed. Decreased serum potassium has also been found.

Pharmacokinetics: Following a 60 minute infusion of IV ritodrine, bioavailability is 100% with peak serum levels of 32 to 52 ng/ml. Half-life of the distribution phase is 6 to 9 minutes, 1.7 to 2.6 hours for the second phase and 15 to 17 hours for the elimination phase. At 24 hours, 90% of the drug is eliminated in urine (primarily as metabolites). Protein binding is 32%.The drug crosses the placenta.

Indications:

Preterm labor: Management of preterm labor in suitable patients. Institute therapy as soon as the diagnosis of preterm labor is established and contraindications are ruled out in pregnancies of ≥ 20 weeks gestation.

Contraindications:

Before the 20th week of pregnancy and in those conditions in which continuation of pregnancy is hazardous to the mother or fetus, specifically: Antepartum hemorrhage that demands immediate delivery; eclampsia and severe preeclampsia; intrauterine fetal death; chorioamnionitis; maternal cardiac disease; pulmonary hypertension; maternal hyperthyroidism; uncontrolled maternal diabetes mellitus.

Pre-existing maternal medical conditions that would be seriously affected by the pharmacologic properties of a betamimetic drug including: Hypovolemia; cardiac arrhythmias associated with tachycardia or digitalis intoxication; uncontrolled hypertension; pheochromocytoma; bronchial asthma already treated by betamimetics or steroids.

Hypersensitivity to any component of the product.

Warnings:

Maternal pulmonary edema has been reported in patients treated with ritodrine, sometimes after delivery. It has occurred more often when patients were treated concomitantly with corticosteroids; however, maternal death from this condition has been reported with or without corticosteroids. Closely monitor patients and avoid fluid overload. Fluid loading IV may be aggravated by the use of betamimetics, with or without corticosteroids, and may result in circulatory overload with subsequent pulmonary edema. If pulmonary edema develops, discontinue use and manage edema by conventional means.

Mild to moderate preeclampsia, hypertension or diabetes: Do not administer to patients with these disorders unless the benefits clearly outweigh the risks.

Advanced labor: The safety and efficacy in advanced labor (cervical dilation > 4 cm or effacement > 80%) have not been established.

RITODRINE HCl

Cardiovascular effects: Beta-adrenergic drugs decrease cardiac output, and even in a healthy heart this added myocardial oxygen demand can sometimes lead to myocardial ischemia. Complications may include: Myocardial necrosis, which may result in death; arrhythmia, including premature atrial and ventricular contractions, ventricular tachycardia and bundle branch block; anginal pain with or without ECG changes.

Cardiovascular responses are common and more pronounced during IV administration; monitor these effects, including maternal pulse rate and blood pressure, fetal heart rate and maternal signs and symptoms of pulmonary edema. A persistent tachycardia (> 140 bpm) may be a sign of impending pulmonary edema. Occult cardiac disease may be unmasked with the use of ritodrine. If the patient complains of chest pain or tightness of chest, temporarily discontinue the drug and perform an ECG.

Pregnancy: Category B. There are no adequate and well controlled studies of the drug's effects in pregnant women before 20 weeks gestation; therefore, do not use this drug before the 20th week of pregnancy.

Ritodrine crosses the placenta, but studies of pregnant women from gestation week 20 have not shown increased risk of fetal abnormalities. Follow-up of children for up to 2 years has not shown harmful effects on growth or developmental or functional maturation, but the possibility cannot be excluded. Use only when clearly indicated.

Infants born before 36 weeks gestation make up < 10% of all births, but account for as many as 75% of perinatal deaths and 50% of all neurologically handicapped infants. By delaying or preventing preterm labor, the drug should cause an overall increase in neonatal survival.

Precautions:

Migraine headache: Transient cerebral ischemia associated with β-sympathomimetic therapy has been reported in two patients with migraine headaches.

Chorioamnionitis: When used to manage preterm labor in a patient with premature rupture of membranes, balance benefits of delaying delivery against risk of developing chorioamnionitis.

Intrauterine growth retardation (IUGR): Among low birth weight infants, ≈ 9% may be growth retarded for gestational age. Therefore, consider IUGR in the differential diagnosis of preterm labor, especially when the gestational age is in doubt. The decision to continue or reinitiate administration will depend on an assessment of fetal maturity.

Lab test abnormalities: Administration of ritodrine IV elevates plasma **insulin** and **glucose** and decreases plasma **potassium** concentrations; monitor glucose and electrolyte levels during protracted infusions. Decrease of plasma potassium concentrations is usually transient, returning to normal within 24 hours. Pay special attention to biochemical variables when treating diabetic patients or those receiving potassium-depleting diuretics. Serial hemograms may be helpful as an index of state of hydration.

Baseline ECG should be performed to rule out occult maternal heart disease.

Sulfites: Sulfites may cause serious allergic-type reactions (eg, hives, itching, wheezing, anaphylaxis) in certain susceptible persons. Although the overall incidence of sulfite sensitivity in the general population is probably low, it is seen more frequently in asthmatics or in atopic nonasthmatic persons. Specific products containing sulfites are identified in the product listings.

RITODRINE HCl

Drug Interactions:

Ritodrine Drug Interactions			
Precipitant drug	Object drug*		Description
Atropine	Ritodrine	⬆	Systemic hypertension may be exaggerated with parasympatholytics.
Beta-blockers	Ritodrine	⬇	Beta-adrenergic blockers inhibit the action of ritodrine; avoid coadministration.
Corticosteroids	Ritodrine	⬆	Concomitant use may lead to pulmonary edema (see Warnings).
Diazoxide General anesthetics Magnesium sulfate Meperidine	Ritodrine	⬆	Cardiovascular effects of ritodrine (especially cardiac arrhythmias or hypotension) may be potentiated by concomitant use.
Sympathomimetics	Ritodrine	⬆	The effects of concomitant use may be additive or potentiated. A sufficient time interval should elapse prior to administration of another sympathomimetic drug.

* ⬆ = Object drug increased. ⬇ = Object drug decreased.

Adverse Reactions:

Unwanted effects of ritodrine are usually controllable through dosage adjustment.

Dose-related alterations in maternal and fetal heart rates and in maternal blood pressure (80% to 100%). With a maximum infusion rate of 0.35 mg/min, the maximum maternal and fetal heart rates averaged, respectively, 130 bpm (range, 60 to 180) and 164 bpm (range, 130 to 200). The maximum maternal systolic blood pressures averaged an increase of 12 mm Hg from pretreatment levels. The minimum maternal diastolic blood pressures averaged a decrease of 23 mm Hg from pretreatment levels. In < 1% of patients, persistent maternal tachycardia or decreased diastolic blood pressure required drug withdrawal. Persistent tachycardia (> 140 bpm) may indicate impending pulmonary edema (see Warnings).

Infusion is associated with transient elevation of blood glucose and insulin, which decreases to normal after 48 to 72 hours despite continued infusion. Elevation of free fatty acids and cAMP has been reported. Expect reduced potassium levels.

Palpitations (33%); tremor, nausea, vomiting, headache, erythema (10% to 15%); nervousness, jitteriness, restlessness, emotional upset, anxiety, malaise (5% to 6%); cardiac symptoms including chest pain or tightness (rarely associated with ECG abnormalities) and arrhythmia (ventricular tachycardia), anaphylactic shock, rash, heart murmur, angina pectoris, myocardial ischemia, epigastric distress, ileus, bloating, constipation, diarrhea, dyspnea, hyperventilation, hemolytic icterus, glycosuria, lactic acidosis, sweating, chills, drowsiness, weakness (1% to 3%); impaired liver function (eg, increased transaminase levels, hepatitis; < 1%). Cases of leukopenia or agranulocytosis (in conjunction with IV infusion for > 2 to 3 weeks); leukocyte count returned to normal after cessation of therapy.

Sinus bradycardia may occur upon drug withdrawal.

Miscellaneous:

Neonatal effects infrequently reported are hypoglycemia and ileus. Hypocalcemia and hypotension have been reported in neonates whose mothers were treated with other betamimetic agents.

Overdosage:

Symptoms: Excessive β-adrenergic stimulation including exaggeration of pharmacologic effects, the most prominent being tachycardia (maternal and fetal), palpitations, cardiac arrhythmia, hypotension, dyspnea, nervousness, tremor, nausea and vomiting.

Treatment: Includes usual supportive measures. Refer to General Management of Acute Overdosage. When symptoms occur as a result of IV use, discontinue the drug. Use an appropriate β-blocker as an antidote. Ritodrine is dialyzable.

RITODRINE HCl

Administration and Dosage:

The optimum dose of the drug is determined by a balance of uterine response and unwanted effects. Treat recurrences of unwanted preterm labor with repeated infusion of ritodrine.

Begin as soon as possible after diagnosis. To minimize risks of hypotension, keep patient in the left lateral position during infusion and pay careful attention to hydration. *Avoid circulatory fluid overload.* Frequently monitor maternal uterine contractions, heart rate, blood pressure and fetal heart rate; individualize dosage.

Use a controlled infusion device to adjust flow rate in drops/min. An IV microdrip chamber (60 drops/ml) provides a convenient range of infusion rates.

The initial dose is 0.05 mg/min (0.17 ml/min, or 10 drops/min using a microdrip chamber at the recommended dilution), to be gradually increased by 0.05 mg/min (10 drops/min) every 10 minutes until the desired result is attained. The usual effective dosage is between 0.15 and 0.35 mg/min (30 to 70 drops/min), continued for at least 12 hours after uterine contractions cease. With the recommended dilution, the maximum volume of fluid that might be administered after 12 hours at the highest dose (0.35 mg/min) will be approximately 840 ml.

If other drugs need to be given IV, the use of "piggyback" or another site of IV administration permits continued independent control of the infusion rate of ritodrine.

Preparation of solution: 150 mg ritodrine in 500 ml fluid yields a final concentration of 0.3 mg/ml. When fluid restriction is desirable, a more concentrated solution may be prepared. For IV infusion, dilute with 5% Dextrose Solution. Use promptly after preparation.

Because of the increased probability of pulmonary edema, saline diluents (0.9% Sodium Chloride; Ringer's) and Hartmann's Solution should be reserved for cases where Dextrose Solution is undesirable (eg, diabetes mellitus).

Storage/Stability: Do not use if the solution is discolored or contains any precipitate or particulate matter. Do not use after 48 hours of preparation.

Store at room temperature, below 30°C (86°F). Protect from excessive heat.

Rx	**Ritodrine HCl** (Abbott)	**Injection:** 10 mg per ml	In 5 ml amps.
Rx	**Yutopar** (Astra)		In 5 ml vials and amps.[1]
Rx	**Ritodrine HCl** (Abbott)	**Injection:** 15 mg per ml	In 10 ml flip-top vials.
	Yutopar (Astra)		In 10 ml vials[1] and syringes.[1]
Rx	**Ritodrine HCl in 5% Dextrose** (Abbott)	**Injection:** 0.3 mg per ml	In 500 ml *LifeCare* flexible containers.

[1] With 1 mg sodium metabisulfite, 4.35 mg acetic acid, 2.4 mg sodium hydroxide and 2.9 sodium chloride per ml.

PROSTAGLANDINS

Dinoprostone is also used as an agent for cervical ripening. Refer to the specific monograph for complete information.

Actions:

Pharmacology: Prostaglandins stimulate the myometrium of the gravid uterus to contract in a manner similar to that seen in the term uterus during labor. Mechanism of action has not been determined. The myometrial contractions induced are sufficient to produce uterine evacuation in the majority of cases. Postpartum, the resultant myometrial contractions provide hemostasis at the site of placentation.

These agents also stimulate the smooth muscle of the GI tract; this activity may be responsible for the vomiting or diarrhea that may occur with their use. Large doses of carboprost can elevate blood pressure, probably by contracting the vascular smooth muscle, but this has not been clinically significant with doses used for terminating pregnancy. In contrast, large doses of dinoprostone may lower blood pressure. Body temperature elevation may also occur with both drugs.

Pharmacokinetics:

Carboprost – In two postpartum women treated with a single IM injection of 250 mcg, the mean peak plasma concentration occurred at 15 minutes. With multiple dosing, average peak concentrations were slightly higher following each successive injection but always decreased to levels less than the preceding peak values by 2 hours after each administration.

Six metabolites have been identified. The liver appears to be the primary site for oxidation. Less than 1% of the drug is excreted unchanged in the urine. Urinary excretion of metabolites is rapid and nearly complete within 24 hours following IM administration. About 80% of the dose is excreted in the first 5 to 10 hours and an additional 5% in the next 20 hours.

Indications:

For the termination of pregnancy from the following gestational weeks as calculated from the first day of the last normal menstrual period:

Carboprost – 13 to 20 weeks.

Dinoprostone – 12 to 20 weeks.

Carboprost: Second trimester abortion characterized by failure of expulsion of the fetus during the course of treatment by another method; premature rupture of membranes in intrauterine methods with loss of drug and insufficient or absent uterine activity; requirement of a repeat intrauterine instillation of drug for expulsion of the fetus; inadvertent or spontaneous rupture of membranes in the presence of a previable fetus and absence of adequate activity for expulsion; postpartum hemorrhage due to uterine atony that has not responded to conventional management (prior treatment should include use of IV oxytocin, manipulative techniques such as uterine massage and, unless contraindicated, IM ergot preparations).

Dinoprostone: Evacuation of the uterine content in the management of missed abortion or intrauterine fetal death up to 28 weeks gestational age as calculated from the first day of the last normal menstrual period; management of nonmetastatic gestational trophoblastic disease (benign hydatidiform mole).

Contraindications:

Hypersensitivity to any of these agents; acute pelvic inflammatory disease; active cardiac, pulmonary, renal or hepatic disease.

Warnings:

Recommended dosages: Use only in recommended dosages and only by medical personnel. Use in a hospital that can provide immediate intensive care and acute surgical facilities.

Viable fetus: Prostaglandins are not indicated if the fetus in utero has reached the stage of viability; they are not feticidal agents. They do not appear to directly affect the fetoplacental unit. Therefore, a previable fetus aborted by these agents could exhibit transient life signs.

Pregnancy: Category C. These drugs are embryotoxic in animals and any dose that produces increased uterine tone could put the embryo or fetus at risk. Animal studies suggest that certain prostaglandins may have teratogenic potential. Complete any failed attempts at pregnancy termination with these drugs by some other means.

Precautions:

Special risk patients: Use cautiously in patients with a history of asthma, hypotension or hypertension, cardiovascular, renal or hepatic disease, anemia, jaundice, diabetes, epilepsy or a compromised (scarred) uterus.

PROSTAGLANDINS

Incomplete abortion: Prostaglandin-induced abortion may sometimes be incomplete (incidence with carboprost is about 20%). In such cases, take other measures to ensure complete abortion.

Chorioamnionitis: Use carboprost with caution in patients with chorioamnionitis. During clinical trials, chorioamnionitis was a complication contributing to postpartum uterine atony and hemorrhage in 7% of cases, 3 of which failed to respond to carboprost. This complication during labor may inhibit the uterine response to carboprost, similar to that reported with other oxytocic agents.

Pyrexia: Transient pyrexia due to hypothalamic thermoregulation may be seen. Temperature elevations exceeding 1.1°C (2°F) were observed in ≈ 12% of patients receiving carboprost and 50% of those receiving dinoprostone. Of those experiencing temperature elevation, ≈ 6% had a clinical diagnosis of endometritis. The remaining temperature returned to normal when therapy ended. Force fluids in patients with drug-induced fever and no clinical or bacteriological evidence of intrauterine infection. Other simple empirical measures for temperature reduction are unnecessary because of the transient or self-limiting nature of the drug-induced fever.

Differentiation of postabortion endometritis from drug-induced temperature elevations is difficult; the distinctions are summarized in the following table.

Differentiation of Endometritis vs Prostaglandin-Induced Pyrexia

Parameter	Endometritis pyrexia	Prostaglandin-induced pyrexia
Onset	Typically, on the third day after abortion (≥ 38°C; ≥ 102°F).	Within 1 to 16 hrs. after the first injection of carboprost; within 15 to 45 min. of dinoprostone suppository.
Duration	Untreated pyrexia and infection continue and may give rise to other pelvic infections.	Temperatures return to pretreatment levels after discontinuation of carboprost therapy (within 2 to 6 hours for dinoprostone).
Retention	Products of conception often retained in cervical os or uterine cavity.	Temperature elevation occurs whether or not tissue is retained.
Histology	Endometrium infiltrated with lymphocytes; some areas are necrotic and hemorrhagic.	Endometrial stroma may be edematous and vascular, but not inflamed.
Uterus	Remains boggy with tenderness over the fundus; pain on moving the cervix on bimanual examination.	Uterine involution normal. Uterus is not tender.
Discharge	Foul smelling lochia and leukorrhea.	Lochia normal.
Cervical culture	The culture of pathological organisms from the cervix or uterine cavity after abortion alone does not warrant the diagnosis of septic abortion in the absence of clinical evidence of sepsis. Pathogens have been cultured soon after abortion in patients with no infections. Persistent positive culture with clear clinical signs of infections are significant in the differential diagnosis.	
Blood count	Leukocytosis and differential white cell counts do not distinguish between endometritis and prostaglandin hyperthermia, because total WBCs may increase during infection and transient leukocytosis may also be drug-induced.	

Cervical trauma: Although the incidence of cervical trauma is extremely small, always carefully examine the cervix immediately post-abortion.

Intrauterine fetal death confirmation: When a pregnancy diagnosed as missed abortion is electively interrupted with intravaginal dinoprostone, confirm intrauterine fetal death with a negative pregnancy test for chorionic gonadotropic activity (UCG test or equivalent). When a pregnancy with late fetal intrauterine death is interrupted with intravaginal dinoprostone, first confirm intrauterine fetal death.

Vaginal conditions: Use dinoprostone suppositories with caution in the presence of cervicitis, infected endocervical lesions or acute vaginitis.

Bone effects: High dose animal studies lasting several weeks have shown that prostaglandins of the E and F series can induce proliferation of bone. Such effects have also been noted in neonates who have received prostaglandin E_1 during prolonged treatment. There is no evidence that short-term use can cause similar effects.

GI effects: The pretreatment or concurrent administration of antiemetic and antidiarrheal drugs decreases the incidence of GI effects. Their use is an integral part of the management of patients undergoing abortion.

PROSTAGLANDINS

Increased blood pressure: When used for postpartum hemorrhage, 4% of patients treated with carboprost had a moderate increase in blood pressure. It is not certain whether this hypertension was due to a direct effect of carboprost or a return to a status of pregnancy-associated hypertension manifested by the correction of hypovolemic shock.

Drug Interactions:

Oxytocics: The activity of oxytocic agents may be augmented by the prostaglandins. Concomitant use is not recommended.

Adverse Reactions:

Prostaglandin Adverse Reactions		
Adverse reaction	Carboprost	Dinoprostone
GI		
Vomiting	✓[1]	66%
Diarrhea	✓[1]	40%
Nausea	33%	33%
CNS		
Headache	✓	10%
Flushing	7%	✓
Anxiety/Tension	✓	✓
Hot flashes	✓	✓
Paresthesia	✓	✓
Syncope/Dizziness	✓	✓
Weakness	✓	✓
Cardiovascular		
Arrhythmias	✓	✓
Chest pain/tightness	✓	✓
GU		
Endometritis	✓	✓
Uterine rupture	✓	✓
Uterine/Vaginal pain	✓	✓
Respiratory		
Coughing	✓	✓
Dyspnea/Wheezing	✓	✓
Other		
Chills/Shivering	✓	10%
Backache	✓	✓
Blurred vision	✓	✓
Breast tenderness	✓	✓
Diaphoresis	✓	✓
Eye pain	✓	✓
Muscle cramp/pain	✓	✓
Pyrexia/Fever	✓	✓
Rash	✓	✓
Leg cramps	✓	✓

✓ = Occurs, no incidence reported.

[1] Incidence may be decreased with pretreatment or concurrent use of antiemetics/antidiarrheals.

Other adverse reactions reported (not all clearly drug-related) include the following:

Carboprost: Hiccoughs; drowsiness; dystonia; asthma; injection site pain; tinnitus; sleep disorders; posterior cervical perforation; epigastric pain; thirst; twitching eyelids; gagging; retching; dry throat; choking sensation; thyroid storm; palpitations; vertigo; vasovagal syndrome; dry mouth; hyperventilation; respiratory distress; tachycardia; hematemesis; taste alterations; urinary tract infections; septic shock; torticollis; lethargy; endometritis from UCD; nosebleed; upper respiratory infection; retained placental fragments; shortness of breath; fullness of throat; uterine sacculation; faintness; lightheadedness; hypertension; perforated uterus; nervousness; pulmonary edema.

The most common complications when carboprost was used for abortion requiring additional treatment after hospital discharge were endometritis, retained placental fragments and excessive uterine bleeding (≈ 2%).

Prostaglandins

PROSTAGLANDINS

Dinoprostone: Joint inflammation; arthralgia; myalgia; vaginitis; vulvitis; stiff neck; dehydration; tremor; hearing impairment; urine retention; pharyngitis; laryngitis; skin discoloration; vaginismus; myocardial infarction (patients with a history of cardiovascular disease); transient diastolic blood pressure decreases of > 20 mm Hg (≈10%).

CARBOPROST TROMETHAMINE

For complete prescribing information, see the Prostaglandins group monograph.

Administration and Dosage:

Abortion: For IM use only. Administer an initial dose of 250 mcg (1 ml) by deep IM injection. Give subsequent doses of 250 mcg at 1.5 to 3.5 hour intervals, depending on uterine response. The dose may be increased to 500 mcg if uterine contractility is inadequate after several 250 mcg doses.

An optional test dose of 100 mcg (0.4 ml) may be administered initially.

Do not exceed a 12 mg total dose or continuous administration for > 2 days.

Refractory postpartum uterine bleeding: Give an initial dose of 250 mcg by deep IM injection. The majority of successful cases (73%) responded to single injections. In some cases, multiple dosing at 15 to 90 minute intervals was performed successfully. Do not exceed a total dose of 2 mg (8 doses).

Storage/Stability: Refrigerate at 2° to 8°C (36° to 46°F).

Rx	**Hemabate** (Upjohn)	**Injection:** 250 mcg carboprost and 83 mcg tromethamine per ml	In 1 ml amps.[1]

[1] With 9.45% benzyl alcohol and 9 mg sodium chloride per ml.

DINOPROSTONE (Prostaglandin E_2)

For complete prescribing information, refer to the Prostaglandins group monograph.

Administration and Dosage:

Insert one suppository (20 mg) high into the vagina. The patient should remain supine for 10 minutes following insertion. Administer each subsequent suppository at 3 to 5 hour intervals until abortion occurs. Within the above recommended intervals, determine administration time by abortifacient progress, uterine contractility response and by patient tolerance. Continuous administration for > 2 days is not advisable.

Storage: Store in a freezer not above –20°C (–4°F); bring to room temperature just prior to use.

Unlabeled administration and dosage: Dinoprostone 20 mg suppositories have been used for cervical ripening by compounding into a low-dose gel formula. However, the manufacturer states that the suppository should not be used for extemporaneous preparation of any other dosage form, and that neither the suppository nor any extemporaneous formulation should be used for cervical ripening or any other indication at term pregnancy. Dinoprostone is commercially available as a vaginal insert and gel specifically for cervical ripening; only these products should be used for this purpose (see specific monograph).

Rx	**Prostin E2** (Upjohn)	**Vaginal Suppository:** 20 mg	In containers of 1 each.

DINOPROSTONE (Prostaglandin E_2; PGE_2)

Dinoprostone is also used as an abortifacient. Refer to the Abortifacients monograph.

Actions:

Pharmacology: Dinoprostone is the naturally occurring form of prostaglandin E_2 (PGE_2). In pregnancy, PGE_2 is secreted continuously by the fetal membranes and placenta and plays an important role in the final events leading to the initiation of labor. It is known that PGE_2 stimulates the production of $PGE_2\alpha$ which in turn sensitizes the myometrium to endogenous or exogenously administered oxytocin. Although PGE_2 is capable of initiating uterine contractions and may interact with oxytocin to increase uterine contractility, available evidence indicates that, in the concentrations found during the early part of labor, PGE_2 plays an important role in cervical ripening without affecting uterine contractions. This distinction serves as the basis for considering cervical ripening and induction of labor, usually by the use of oxytocin, as two separate processes.

PGE_2 plays an important role in the complex set of biochemical and structural alterations involved in cervical ripening. Cervical ripening involves a marked relaxation of the cervical smooth muscle fibers of the uterine cervix which must be transformed from a rigid structure to a softened, yielding and dilated configuration to allow passage of the fetus through the birth canal. This process involves activation of the enzyme collagenase, which is responsible for digestion of some of the structural collagen network of the cervix. This is associated with a concomitant increase in the amount of hydrophilic glycosaminoglycan and hyaluronic acid, and a decrease in dermaten sulfate. Failure of the cervix to undergo these natural physiologic changes prior to the onset of effective uterine contractions results in an unfavorable outcome for successful vaginal delivery and may result in fetal compromise. It is estimated that in ≈ 5% of pregnancies the cervix does not ripen normally. In an additional 10% to 11%, labor must be induced for medical or obstetric reasons prior to the time of cervical ripening.

Dinoprostone gel and vaginal insert provide sufficient quantities of PGE_2 to the local receptors to satisfy hormonal requirements. In the majority of patients, these local effects are manifested by changes in the consistency, dilatation and effacement of the cervix. Although some patients experience uterine hyperstimulation as a result of direct PGE_2- or $PGE_2\alpha$-mediated sensitization of the myometrium to oxytocin, systemic effects of PGE_2 are rarely encountered.

Dinoprostone is also capable of stimulating smooth muscle of the GI tract. This activity may be responsible for the vomiting or diarrhea that is occasionally seen when dinoprostone is used for preinduction of cervical ripening.

Large doses can lower blood pressure, probably as a result of its effect on smooth muscle of the vascular system, and can elevate body temperature. However, with the doses used for cervical ripening these effects have not been seen.

Pharmacokinetics: When an unvalidated assay of dinoprostone gel was administered endocervically to women undergoing preinduction ripening, results from measurement of plasma levels of the metabolite 13,14-dihydro-15-keto-PGE_2 (DHK-PGE_2) showed that PGE_2 was relatively rapidly absorbed and the T_{max} was 0.5 to 0.75 hours. Plasma mean C_{max} for gel-treated subjects was 433 vs 137 pg/ml for untreated controls. In those subjects in which a clinical response was observed, mean C_{max} was 484 vs 213 pg/ml in nonresponders and 219 pg/ml in control subjects who had positive clinical progression toward normal labor. These elevated levels in gel-treated subjects appear to be largely a result of absorption of PGE_2 from the gel rather than from endogenous sources.

PGE_2 is completely metabolized. It is extensively metabolized in the lungs (≈ 95% on first pass through pulmonary circulation), and the resulting metabolites are further metabolized in the liver and kidney. The major route of elimination of the products of PGE_2 metabolism is the kidneys. Half-life is estimated to be 2.5 to 5 minutes.

Indications:

Cervical ripening: For initiation or continuation of cervical ripening in pregnant women at or near term with a medical or obstetrical need for labor induction.

Contraindications:

Patients in whom oxytocic drugs are generally contraindicated or where prolonged contractions of the uterus are considered inappropriate, such as: History of cesarean sectionor major uterine surgery; where cephalopelvic disproportion is present; history of difficult labor or traumatic delivery; grand multiparae with ≥ 6 previous term pregnancies; non-vertex presentation; hyperactive or hypertonic uterine patterns; fetal distress where delivery is not imminent; obstetric emergencies where the benefit-to-risk ratio for fetus or mother favors surgical intervention.

Ruptured membranes.

Hypersensitivity to prostaglandinsor constituents of the gel.

Placenta previa or unexplained vaginal bleeding during current pregnancy.

DINOPROSTONE (Prostaglandin E_2; PGE_2)

When vaginal delivery is not indicated such as vasa previa or active herpes genitalia.

Patients already receiving IV oxytocic drugs.

Warnings:

For hospital use only: As with other potent oxytocic agents, use only with strict adherence to recommended dosages. Administer in a hospital that can provide immediate intensive care and acutesurgical facilities.

Feto-pelvic relationships: Carefully evaluate before use (see Contraindications).

Special risk patients: Exercise caution when administering to patients with asthma or history of asthma or glaucoma or raised intraocular pressure.

Renal/Hepatic function impairment: Since dinoprostone gel is extensively metabolized in the lung, liver and kidney, and the major route of elimination is the kidney, use with caution in patients with renal and hepatic dysfunction.

Pregnancy: Category C. Prostaglandin E_2 produced an increase in skeletal anomalies in rats and rabbits. No effect would be expected clinically, when used as indicated, since dinoprostone is embryotoxic in rats and rabbits, and any dose that produces sustained increased uterine tone could put the embryo or fetus at risk (see Precautions).

Precautions:

Monitoring: During use, carefully monitor uterine activity, fetal status and character of the cervix (dilation and effacement) either by auscultation or electronic fetal monitoring to detect possible evidence of undesired responses (eg, hypertonus, sustained uterine contractility, fetal distress). In cases where there is a history of hypertonic uterine contractility or tetanic uterine contractions, continuously monitor uterine activity and the state of the fetus. Consider the possibility of uterine rupture when high-tone myometrial contractions are sustained. If uterine hyperstimulation is encountered or if labor commences, or if there is any evidence of fetal distress or other maternal/fetal adverse reactions, remove the vaginal insert. Also, remove the insert prior to amniotomy.

Degree of effacement:

Gel – Use caution so as not to administer above the level of the internal os. Careful vaginal examination will reveal the degree of effacement which will regulate the size of the shielded endocervical catheter to be used. Use the 20 mm endocervical catheter if no effacement is present, and use the 10 mm catheter if the cervix is 50% effaced. Placement into the extra-amniotic space has been associated with uterine hyperstimulation.

Drug Interactions:

Oxytocics: Dinoprostone gel may augment the activity of other oxytocic agents; their concomitant use is not recommended. For the sequential use of oxytocin following dinoprostone gel administration, a dosing interval of 6 to 12 hours is recommended; a dosing interval of at least 30 minutes is recommended following removal of the dinoprostone insert.

Adverse Reactions:

Dinoprostone is generally well tolerated.

Gel:

Dinoprostone Gel Adverse Reactions (%)		
Adverse reaction	Dinoprostone gel (n = 884)	Control[1] (n = 847)
Maternal		
Uterine contractile abnormality	6.6	4
Any GI effect	5.7	2.6
Back pain	3.1	0
Warm feeling in vagina	1.5	0
Fever	1.4	1.2
Fetal		
Any fetal heart rate abnormality	1.7	14.5
Bradycardia	4.1	3.1
Deceleration		
Late	2.8	2.1
Variable	4.3	3.4
Unspecified	2.1	2.2

[1] Placebo gel or no treatment.

DINOPROSTONE (Prostaglandin E_2; PGE_2)

Amnionitis and intrauterine fetal sepsis have been associated with extra-amniotic intrauterine administration of PGE_2. Uterine rupture has occurred with the use of dinoprostone gel intracervically. Additional events included premature rupture of membranes, fetal depression (1 min Apgar < 7) and fetal acidosis (umbilical artery pH < 7.15).

Insert: The following adverse reactions were reported with the dinoprostone insert: Uterine hyperstimulation without fetal distress (2% to 4.7%); fetal distress without uterine hyperstimulation (2.9% to 3.8%); uterine hyperstimulation with fetal distress (2.8% to 2.9%); fever, nausea, vomiting, diarrhea, abdominal pain (< 1%).

In one study, cases of uterine hyperstimulation reversed within 2 to 13 minutes of product removal; tocolytics were required in 1 of 5 cases. Five minute Apgar scores were ≥ 7 in 98.2% of neonates whose mothers received dinoprostone inserts.

Overdosage:

Overdosage may be expressed by uterine hypercontractility and uterine hypertonus. Because of the transient nature of PGE_2-induced myometrial hyperstimulation, nonspecific, conservative management was found to be effective in the vast majority of the cases (ie, maternal position change and administration of oxygen to the mother). Beta-adrenergic drugs may be used as a treatment of hyperstimulation following the administration of PGE_2 for cervical ripening.

Administration and Dosage:

Gel: Use with caution in handling this product to prevent contact with skin. Wash hands thoroughly with soap and water after administration.

Preparation for use – Bring to room temperature (15° to 30°C; 59° to 86°F) just prior to administration. Do not force the warming process by using a water bath or other source of external heat (eg, microwave oven). Remove the peel-off seal from the end of the syringe, then remove the protective end cap (to serve as plunger extension) and insert the protective end cap into the plunger stopper assembly in the barrel of syringe. Choose the appropriate length shielded catheter (10 or 20 mm) and aseptically remove the sterile shielded catheter from the package. Careful vaginal examination will reveal the degree of effacement which will regulate the size of the shielded endocervical catheter to be used; use the 20 mm endocervical catheter if no effacement is present, and the 10 mm catheter if the cervix is 50% effaced. Firmly attach the catheter hub to the syringe tip as evidenced by a distinct click. Fill the catheter with sterile gel by pushing the plunger assembly to expel air from the catheter prior to administration to the patient.

Proper administration – To properly administer the product, the patient should be in a dorsal position with the cervix visualized using a speculum. Using sterile technique, introduce the gel with the catheter provided into the cervical canal just below the level of the internal os. Administer the contents of the syringe by gentle expulsion and then remove the catheter. Discard the syringe, catheter and any unused package contents after use.

Following administration, the patient should remain in the supine position for at least 15 to 30 minutes to minimize leakage from the cervical canal.

If the desired response is obtained from the starting dose of dinoprostone gel, the recommended interval before giving IV oxytocin is 6 to 12 hours. If there is no cervical/uterine response to the initial dose, repeat dosing may be given. The recommended repeat dose is 0.5 mg with a dosing interval of 6 hours. The need for additional dosing and the interval must be determined by the attending physician based on the course of clinical events. The maximum recommended cumulative dose for a 24 hour period is 1.5 mg (7.5 ml).

DINOPROSTONE (Prostaglandin E_2; PGE_2)

Insert: Dosage of dinoprostone in the insert is 10 mg, designed to be released at ≈ 0.3 mg/hr over a 12 hour period. Remove the insert upon onset of active labor or 12 hours after insertion.

One insert is placed transversely in the posterior fornix of the vagina immediately after removal from the foil package. Insertion does not require sterile conditions. Do not use the insert without its retrieval system. There is no need for previous warming of the insert. A minimal amount of a water-miscible lubricant may be used to assist in insertion of the insert; take care not to permit excess contact or coating with the lubricant and thus prevent optimal swelling and release of dinoprostone from the insert. Have patients remain supine for 2 hours following insertion; thereafter, they may be ambulatory.

Storage/Stability:

Gel – Dinoprostone gel has a shelf life of 24 months when stored under continuous refrigeration (2° to 8°C; 36° to 46°F).

Insert – Store in a freezer between –20° and –10°C (–4° and 14°F). The insert is packed in foil and is stable for a period of 3 years when stored in a freezer.

Rx	**Prepidil** (Upjohn)	**Gel:** 0.5 mg	In 3 g (2.5 ml) syringes[1] with 2 shielded catheters (10 and 20 mm tip).
Rx	**Cervidil** (Forest)	**Vaginal insert:** 10 mg	In 1s.

[1] With 240 mg colloidal silicon dioxide NF and 2760 mg triacetin, USP.

ADRENAL CORTICAL STEROIDS

Cortisol, the major endogenous glucocorticoid produced in the body, is produced and secreted via the hypothalamic-anterior pituitary-adrenocortical (HPA) axis. The adrenal cortex synthesizes and secretes the steroid hormones which include mineralocorticoids (aldosterone), glucocorticoids, and to a minor extent, androgenic hormones. Aldosterone secretion is controlled mainly by potassium and the renin-angiotensin system; physiological regulation of glucocorticoid synthesis and secretion is mediated by corticotropin (ACTH), which is secreted by the anterior pituitary gland. In response to low plasma cortisol levels, ACTH is secreted; high plasma cortisol levels inhibit ACTH secretion. This relationship follows a diurnal pattern. Cholesterol and its esters are converted to pregnenolone by ACTH, which is further converted to cortisol and other intermediary products (eg, androgens). ACTH secretion is also stimulated by hypothalamic corticotropin-releasing factor, which is stimulated by serotonin, dopamine and other neurotransmitters in response to stress (emotional, physical or chemical). ACTH secretion at any given time is influenced by a negative feedback relationship from circulating glucocorticoids and the neural signals associated with stress response and the circadian pattern.

Primary adrenocortical insufficiency (Addison's disease) requires replacement therapy with physiologic doses of both mineralocorticoids and glucocorticoids. Secondary adrenocortical insufficiency due to inadequate ACTH secretion may be treated either with replacement steroid administration or with ACTH. Pharmacologic doses of exogenous glucocorticoids are used for their profound anti-inflammatory effects.

Excessive secretion of glucocorticoids (Cushing's syndrome) is due to excessive ACTH or a primary adrenal source (eg, benign adenoma, carcinoma) and is most effectively treated surgically; however, aminoglutethimide inhibits glucocorticoid synthesis and may be used to suppress excessive adrenal activity.

The agents discussed in this section are listed below:

Adrenocorticotropic hormone (corticotropin or ACTH), secreted by the anterior pituitary, stimulates the adrenal cortex to produce and secrete its natural steroids by activating adenyl cyclase in the cell membranes. ACTH is included in this section since the therapeutic effects of its administration are due to the activity of the liberated adrenal steroids. Adequate adrenal function is necessary for ACTH to elicit a pharmacologic response. *Cosyntropin*, a synthetic analog of ACTH, has similar corticotropic activity, but is devoid of the immunogenic properties of ACTH of porcine origin.

Mineralocorticoids: Fludrocortisone is used for partial replacement therapy in adrenocortical insufficiency and for the treatment of salt-losing adrenogenital syndrome.

Glucocorticoids cause profound and varied metabolic effects in addition to modifying the body's immune response to diverse stimuli. The naturally occurring glucocorticoids and many synthetic steroids have both glucocorticoid and mineralocorticoid activity. Other synthetic steroids have potent glucocorticoid activity without significant mineralocorticoid activity.

Glucocorticoid product listings are included in the following sections:

- Oral and parenteral
- Retention enemas
- Respiratory inhalant
- Intranasal
- Ophthalmic
- Topical

Adrenal steroid inhibitor: Aminoglutethimide inhibits the enzymatic biosynthesis of adrenal steroids. It is useful in suppressing excessive adrenosteroid production in Cushing's syndrome.

CORTICOTROPIN (ACTH)

For complete prescribing information, refer to the Adrenal Cortical Steroids introduction.

Actions:

Pharmacology: Corticotropin (adrenocorticotropic hormone, ACTH) is secreted by the anterior pituitary and stimulates the adrenal cortex to produce and secrete adrenocortical hormones. Adequate adrenal function is necessary for corticotropin to elicit a pharmacological response. ACTH secretion is regulated by a negative feedback mechanism, whereby elevated plasma corticosteroid levels suppress ACTH secretion. Chronic administration of exogenous corticosteroids will decrease ACTH stores and induce morphological changes in the pituitary. In the absence of ACTH stimulation, the adrenal cortex may atrophy.

Cosyntropin is a synthetic peptide corresponding to the amino acid residues 1 to 24 of human ACTH, which exhibits the full corticosteroidogenic activity of natural ACTH. A dose of 0.25 mg cosyntropin is pharmacologically equivalent to 25 units of natural ACTH. Cosyntropin is less allergenic than natural ACTH. Because it is unavailable in a repository form, it is not used therapeutically, only diagnostically.

Pharmacokinetics: ACTH injection has a rapid onset. Plasma half-life is about 15 minutes. After IM or rapid IV administration of 25 units, peak plasma concentrations are usually achieved within 1 hour and begin to decrease after 2 to 4 hours. Repository corticotropin contains ACTH incorporated in a gelatin menstruum designed to delay the absorption rate and increase the period of effectiveness. Corticotropin zinc hydroxide consists of ACTH adsorbed on zinc hydroxide which also delays the absorption rate. Repository corticotropin and corticotropin zinc hydroxide have a slower onset but may sustain effects for up to 3 days.

Indications:

ACTH and cosyntropin: Diagnostic testing of adrenocortical function. Cosyntropin is more potent and less allergenic than the exogenous ACTH preparations.

ACTH: Corticotropin has limited therapeutic value in conditions responsive to corticosteroid therapy; in such cases, corticosteroid therapy is the treatment of choice. Corticotropin may be used in the following disorders:

Endocrine – Nonsuppurative thyroiditis; hypercalcemia associated with cancer.

Nervous system diseases – Acute exacerbations of multiple sclerosis.

Miscellaneous – Tuberculous meningitis with subarachnoid block or impending block when accompanied by antituberculous chemotherapy; trichinosis with neurologic or myocardial involvement; rheumatic, collagen, dermatologic, allergic, ophthalmic, respiratory, hematologic, neoplastic, edematous, and GI diseases in the same manner as the glucocorticoids. Refer to the Glucocorticoids monograph for a listing of specific conditions responsive to therapy.

Unlabeled uses: Treatment of infantile spasms (see Administration and Dosage).

Contraindications:

Scleroderma; osteoporosis; systemic fungal infections; ocular herpes simplex; recent surgery; history of or presence of peptic ulcer; congestive heart failure (CHF); hypertension; sensitivity to porcine proteins. IV administration (except in the treatment of idiopathic thrombocytopenic purpura). IV administration may be used for diagnostic testing of adrenocortical function. Treatment of conditions accompanied by primary adrenocortical insufficiency or adrenocortical hyperfunction.

Warnings:

Do not administer until adrenal responsiveness has been verified with the route of administration (IM or SC) which will be used during treatment. A rise in urinary and plasma corticosteroid values provides direct evidence of a stimulatory effect.

Chronic administration may lead to irreversible adverse effects. ACTH may suppress signs and symptoms of chronic disease without altering the natural course of the disease. Since complications with corticotropin use are dependent on the dose and duration of treatment, a risk to benefit decision must be made in each case.

Prolonged use increases the risk of hypersensitivity reactions and may produce posterior subcapsular cataracts and glaucoma with possible damage to the optic nerve.

Stress: Although the action of ACTH is similar to that of exogenous adrenocortical steroids, the quantity of adrenocorticoid secreted may be variable. In patients who receive prolonged corticotropin therapy, use additional rapidly acting corticosteroids before, during and after an unusually stressful situation.

Infection: ACTH may mask signs of infection including fungal or viral eye infections that may appear during its use. There may be decreased resistance and inability to localize infection. When infection is present, administer appropriate anti-infective therapy.

CORTICOTROPIN (ACTH)

Tuberculosis – Observe patients with latent tuberculosis or tuberculin reactivity who receive ACTH, as reactivation of the disease may occur. During prolonged ACTH therapy, administer chemoprophylaxis.

Immunosuppression: Perform immunization procedures with caution, especially when high doses are administered, because of the possible hazards of neurological complications and lack of antibody response. Immunization with live vaccines is usually contraindicated in patients on ACTH or corticosteroid therapy.

Electrolytes: Corticotropin can elevate blood pressure, cause salt and water retention and increase potassium and calcium excretion. Dietary salt restriction and potassium supplementation may be necessary.

Hypersensitivity: Cosyntropin exhibits slight immunologic activity, does not contain foreign animal protein, and is less risky to use than natural ACTH. Most patients with a history of a previous hypersensitivity reaction to natural ACTH or a preexisting allergic disease will tolerate cosyntropin without incident; however, hypersensitivity reactions are possible. Refer to Management of Acute Hypersensitivity Reactions.

Pregnancy: Category C. ACTH has embryocidal effects. Fetal abnormalities have been observed in animals. Use in pregnancy only when clearly needed and when potential benefits outweigh potential hazards to the fetus. Monitor infants born of mothers who have received substantial doses during pregnancy for signs of hyperadrenalism.

Lactation: It is not known whether this drug is excreted in breast milk. Because of the potential for serious adverse reactions in nursing infants from ACTH, decide whether to discontinue nursing or to discontinue the drug.

Children: Prolonged use of corticotropin in children will inhibit skeletal growth. If use is necessary, give intermittently and carefully observe the child.

Precautions:

Concomitant therapy: Since maximal corticotropin stimulation of the adrenals may be limited during the first few days of treatment, administer a rapidly acting corticosteroid (eg, hydrocortisone) when an immediate therapeutic effect is desirable.

Administer for treatment only when disease is intractable to more conventional therapy; ACTH should be adjunctive and not the sole therapy.

Use the lowest possible dose to control the condition, and when reduction in dosage is possible, it should be gradual.

Sensitivity to porcine proteins: Perform skin testing prior to treatment in patients with suspected sensitivity to porcine proteins. During or following administration, observe for sensitivity reactions.

Adrenocortical insufficiency induced by prolonged ACTH therapy may be minimized by gradual reduction of dosage. Insufficiency may persist for months after therapy discontinuation; therefore, in any situation of stress during that period, reinstitute corticosteroid therapy.

Hypothyroidism and cirrhosis: An enhanced effect of corticotropin may occur.

Multiple sclerosis: Although ACTH may speed the resolution of acute exacerbations of multiple sclerosis, it does not affect the ultimate outcome or natural course of the disease. Relatively high doses of ACTH are necessary to demonstrate a significant effect.

Acute gouty arthritis: Limit treatment of acute gouty arthritis to a few days. Since rebound attacks may occur when corticotropin is discontinued, administer conventional concomitant therapy during corticotropin treatment and for several days after it is stopped.

Mental disturbances: Psychic derangements may appear, ranging from euphoria, insomnia, mood swings, personality changes, and depression to frank psychosis. Existing emotional instability or psychotic tendencies may be aggravated.

Use with caution in patients with diabetes, abscess, pyogenic infections, diverticulitis, renal insufficiency and myasthenia gravis.

Drug abuse and dependence: Although drug dependence does not occur, sudden withdrawal of corticotropin after prolonged use may lead to recurrent symptoms which make it difficult to stop. It may be necessary to taper the dose and increase the injection interval to gradually discontinue the medication.

CORTICOTROPIN (ACTH)

Drug Interactions:

Amphotericin B depletes potassium and may enhance the potassium wasting effect of corticotropin; it may also decrease adrenocortical responsiveness to corticotropin. Closely monitor serum potassium.

Antidiabetic agents: Increased requirements for insulin or oral hypoglycemic agents in diabetes have occurred in patients taking ACTH, due to the intrinsic hyperglycemic activity of glucocorticoids.

Diuretics that deplete potassium may enhance the potassium wasting effect of corticotropin. Closely monitor serum potassium.

Salicylates, indomethacin: Because of its known ulcerogenic effects, use aspirin cautiously in conjunction with corticotropin, especially in hypoprothrombinemia. Corticosteroids may increase the renal clearance of salicylates. Increased serum levels of salicylates and salicylate toxicity may occur when steroid therapy is discontinued.

Drug/Lab test interactions: Corticotropin may decrease I^{131} uptake and may suppress reactions to skin tests. It may affect the method of Brown used for determination of urinary estradiol and estriol, causing falsely decreased concentrations of these estrogens. The drug may also interfere with colorimetric/fluorometric procedures for determination of urinary estrogens causing a falsely decreased concentration of urinary estrogens.

Adverse Reactions:

Infections: Pneumonia, abscess and septic infection, and GI and GU infections (more frequent with higher doses).

Electrolyte Disturbance: Sodium and fluid retention; potassium and calcium loss; hypokalemic alkalosis.

Musculoskeletal: Muscle weakness; steroid myopathy; loss of muscle mass; osteoporosis; vertebral compression fractures; pathologic fracture of long bones; aseptic necrosis of femoral and humeral heads.

GI: Pancreatitis; ulcerative esophagitis; abdominal distention; peptic ulcer with possible perforation and hemorrhage has been associated with steroid therapy (this association has been disputed).

Dermatologic: Impaired wound healing; petechiae and ecchymoses; increased sweating; hyperpigmentation; thin fragile skin; facial erythema; acne; suppression of skin test reactions.

Cardiovascular: Hypertension; CHF; necrotizing angiitis.

CNS: Convulsions; vertigo; headache; increased intracranial pressure with papilledema, pseudotumor cerebri, usually after treatment.

Endocrine: Menstrual irregularities; suppression of growth in children; hirsutism; development of Cushingoid state; manifestations of latent diabetes mellitus; decreased carbohydrate tolerance; increased requirements for insulin or oral hypoglycemic agents in diabetics; secondary adrenocortical and pituitary unresponsiveness, especially during stress.

Ophthalmic: Posterior subcapsular cataracts; increased intraocular pressure; glaucoma with possible damage to optic nerve; exophthalmos.

Metabolic: Negative nitrogen balance due to protein catabolism.

Hypersensitivity: Dizziness; nausea; vomiting; shock; skin reactions.

Miscellaneous: Prolonged use may result in antibody production and subsequent loss of the stimulatory effect of ACTH.

CORTICOTROPIN (ACTH)

Patient Information:

ACTH may mask signs of infection. There may be decreased resistance and inability to localize infection.

Avoid immunizations with live vaccines.

Diabetics may have increased requirements for insulin or oral hypoglycemics.

Notify physician if marked fluid retention, muscle weakness, abdominal pain, seizures, or headache occurs.

Administration and Dosage:

Standard tests for verification of adrenal responsiveness to corticotropin may utilize as much as 80 units as a single injection, or one or more injections of a lesser dosage. Perform verification tests prior to treatment with corticotropins. The test should utilize the route(s) of administration proposed for treatment. Following verification, individualize dosage. Attempt only gradual change in dosage schedules after full drug effects have become apparent.

In the short test (single injection) for the ACTH stimulation test, a normal response is plasma cortisol > 20 mcg/dl on any sample. A blunted response indicates primary or secondary adrenal insufficiency. In the long test (8 hour infusion on 3 consecutive days), an absent or subnormal rise in plasma cortisol and 17-OHCS indicates primary adrenal failure. Plasma cortisol > 20 mcg/dl and a two- to threefold urinary 17-OHCS increase over baseline on day 4 indicates ACTH deficiency.

For diagnostic purposes: 10 to 25 units dissolved in 500 ml of 5% Dextrose Injection infused IV over 8 hours.

The usual IM or SC dose is 20 units 4 times daily. Chronic administration of > 40 units/day may be associated with uncontrollable adverse effects.

When indicated, reduce dosage gradually by increasing the duration between injections or decreasing the quantity of corticotropin injected or both.

Acute exacerbations of multiple sclerosis: 80 to 120 units/day IM for 2 to 3 weeks.

Infantile spasms: 20 to 40 units daily or 80 units every other day IM for 3 months or 1 month after cessation of seizures has been recommended.

Repository corticotropin injection: 40 to 80 units IM or SC every 24 to 72 hours. Inject **corticotropin zinc** preparations deeply into the gluteal muscle only; do not administer SC.

Preparation and storage: Reconstitute powder by dissolving in Sterile Water for Injection or Sodium Chloride Injection so that the individual dose will be contained in 1 to 2 ml of solution. Refrigerate reconstituted solution. Use within 24 hours.

Corticotropin (ACTH)

CORTICOTROPIN INJECTION

For complete prescribing information, refer to the Corticotropin group monograph.

Give IM or SC. May be given IV for diagnostic purposes.

Rx	**Acthar** (Rorer)	**Powder for Injection:** 25 units per vial	In vials.[1]
Rx	**Corticotropin** (Various, eg, Baxter, Schein, Steris)	**Powder for Injection:** 40 units per vial	In vials.
Rx	**ACTH** (Parke-Davis)		In vials.[2]
Rx	**Acthar** (Rorer)		In vials.[3]

[1] With 9 mg hydrolyzed gelatin.
[2] With 5 mg aminoacetic acid.
[3] With 14 mg hydrolyzed gelatin.

REPOSITORY CORTICOTROPIN INJECTION

For complete prescribing information, refer to the Corticotropin group monograph.

Give IM or SC. Not for IV use.

Rx	**H.P. Acthar Gel** (Rorer)	**Repository Injection:** 40 units per ml	In 1 and 5 ml vials.[1]
Rx	**ACTH-80** (Various, eg, Balan, Hauck)	**Repository Injection:** 80 units per ml	In 5 ml vials.
Rx	**H.P. Acthar Gel** (Rorer)		In 1 and 5 ml vials.[1]

[1] With 16% gelatin.

CORTICOTROPIN ZINC HYDROXIDE

For complete prescribing information, refer to the Corticotropin group monograph.

For IM use only.

Rx	**Cortrophin-Zinc** (Organon)	**Repository Injection:** 40 units corticotropin and 2 mg zinc per ml suspension	In 5 ml vials.[1]

[1] With 1% benzyl alcohol.

Corticotropin (ACTH)

COSYNTROPIN

For complete prescribing information, refer to the Corticotropin group monograph.

Administration and Dosage:

Administer IM or IV as a rapid screening test of adrenal function. It may also be given as an IV infusion over 4 to 8 hours to provide a greater stimulus to the adrenal glands. Doses of 0.25 to 0.75 mg have been used and a maximal response noted with the smallest dose. The suggested dose is 0.25 mg dissolved in sterile saline injected IM.

Children (≤ 2 years old): 0.125 mg will often suffice.

IV infusion: Add 0.25 mg cosyntropin to dextrose or saline solutions and give at a rate of approximately 0.04 mg/hour over 6 hours.

For test procedure and interpretation of results, refer to manufacturer's insert.

Rx	**Cortrosyn** (Organon)	**Powder for Injection**: 0.25 mg	In vials[1] with diluent.

[1] With 10 mg mannitol.

Mineralocorticoids

FLUDROCORTISONE ACETATE

For complete prescribing information, refer to the Adrenal Cortical Steroids introduction.

Actions:

Pharmacology: Fludrocortisone is an adrenal cortical steroid with potent mineralocorticoid activity and high glucocorticoid activity (about 15 times as potent as hydrocortisone), but is used only for its mineralocorticoid effects. Because of the similarity of effects, refer to the discussion of Glucocorticoids.

Mechanism – Mineralocorticoids act on the renal distal tubules to enhance the reabsorption of sodium. They increase urinary excretion of both potassium and hydrogen ions. The consequence of these three primary effects together with similar actions on cation transport in other tissues appears to account for the spectrum of physiological activities characteristic of mineralocorticoids.

In small oral doses, fludrocortisone produces marked sodium retention and increased urinary potassium excretion. It also causes a rise in blood pressure, apparently because of these effects on electrolyte levels. In larger doses, fludrocortisone inhibits endogenous adrenal cortical secretion, thymic activity, and pituitary corticotropin excretion, it promotes the deposition of liver glycogen, and, unless protein intake is adequate, it induces negative nitrogen balance.

Pharmacokinetics: Fludrocortisone is readily absorbed from the GI tract with peak concentrations in 1.7 hours. Plasma half-life is approximately 3.5 hours, but biological half-life ranges from 18 to 36 hours.

Indications:

Partial replacement therapy for primary and secondary adrenocortical insufficiency in Addison's disease and for the treatment of salt-losing adrenogenital syndrome.

Unlabeled uses: Fludrocortisone 100 to 400 mcg/day has been used in the management of severe orthostatic hypotension.

Contraindications:

Hypersensitivity to fludrocortisone; systemic fungal infections.

Warnings:

Supplemental measures: Use mineralocorticoid therapy preferably in conjunction with other supplemental measures (eg, glucocorticoids, control of electrolytes, control of infection).

Adrenal insufficiency: To avoid drug-induced adrenal insufficiency, supportive dosage may be required in times of stress (eg, trauma, surgery, severe illness), both during treatment with fludrocortisone and for a year afterwards.

Pregnancy: Category C. Safety for use during pregnancy has not been established. Use only when clearly needed and when the potential benefits outweigh the potential hazards to the fetus. If it is necessary to give steroids during pregnancy, observe the newborn infant for signs of adrenocortical insufficiency and institute appropriate therapy, if necessary.

Lactation: Corticosteroids are found in the breast milk of lactating women. Exercise caution when administering to nursing women.

Children: Safety and efficacy for use in children have not been established. Monitor growth and development of infants and children on prolonged therapy.

Precautions:

Addison's disease: Patients with Addison's disease are more sensitive to the action of the hormone and may exhibit side effects in an exaggerated degree. Closely monitor patients and stop treatment if a significant increase in weight or blood pressure, edema or cardiac enlargement occurs.

Sodium retention and potassium loss are accelerated by a high sodium intake. If edema occurs, restrict dietary sodium. Perform frequent blood electrolyte determinations; potassium supplementation may be necessary.

Infection: Monitor patients for evidence of intercurrent infection. Should this occur, initiate appropriate anti-infective therapy.

Mineralocorticoids

FLUDROCORTISONE ACETATE

Adverse Reactions:

Side effects may occur if dosage is too high or prolonged or if withdrawal is too rapid. Because it possesses glucocorticoid activity, fludrocortisone may cause side effects similar to those of the glucocorticoids (refer to Glucocorticoid section).

Cardiovascular: Edema; hypertension; CHF; enlargement of the heart.

Dermatologic: Bruising; increased sweating; hives or allergic skin rash.

Miscellaneous: Hypokalemic alkalosis.

Overdosage:

Symptoms: Hypertension; edema; hypokalemia; excessive weight gain; increase in heart size.

Treatment: Discontinue the drug; symptoms usually subside within several days. Resume subsequent treatment with reduced doses. Muscular weakness may develop due to excessive potassium loss; treat with potassium supplements. Monitor blood pressure and serum electrolytes regularly.

Patient Information:

Notify physician if dizziness, severe or continuing headaches, swelling of feet or lower legs, or unusual weight gain occurs.

Administration and Dosage:

Addison's disease: The usual dose is 0.1 mg/day (range 0.1 mg 3 times a week to 0.2 mg/day). If transient hypertension develops as a consequence of therapy, reduce the dose to 0.05 mg/day. Administration in conjunction with cortisone (10 to 37.5 mg/day) or hydrocortisone (10 to 30 mg/day) is preferable.

Children and adults – Another recommended dose is 0.05 to 0.1 mg/24 hours.

Infants – A recommended dose is 0.1 to 0.2 mg/24 hours.

Salt-losing adrenogenital syndrome: 0.1 to 0.2 mg/day.

Rx	**Florinef Acetate** (Apothecon)	**Tablets:** 0.1 mg	(429). Pink, scored. Biconvex. In 100s.

GLUCOCORTICOIDS

For complete prescribing information, refer to the Adrenal Cortical Steroids introduction.

Actions:

Pharmacology: The naturally occurring adrenal cortical steroids have both anti-inflammatory (glucocorticoid) and salt-retaining (mineralocorticoid) properties. Glucocorticoids cause profound and varied metabolic effects. In addition, they modify the body's immune responses to diverse stimuli.

These compounds, including hydrocortisone (cortisol) and cortisone, are used as replacement therapy in adrenocortical deficiency states and may be used for their anti-inflammatory effects. The synthetic steroid compounds prednisone, prednisolone and fludrocortisone also have both glucocorticoid and mineralocorticoid activity. Prednisone and prednisolone are used primarily for their glucocorticoid effects.

In addition, a group of synthetic compounds with marked glucocorticoid activity are distinguished by the absence of any significant salt-retaining activity. These include triamcinolone, dexamethasone, methylprednisolone and betamethasone. These agents are used for their potent anti-inflammatory effects.

Pharmacokinetics:

Absorption – Hydrocortisone and most of its congeners are readily absorbed from the GI tract; greatly altered onsets and durations are usually achieved with injections of suspensions and esters.

Distribution – Hydrocortisone is reversibly bound to corticosteroid-binding globulin (CBG or transcortin) and corticosteroid binding albumin (CBA). Exogenous glucocorticoids are bound to these proteins to a significantly lesser degree. In hypoproteinemic or dysproteinemic states, the total endogenous hydrocortisone levels are decreased. Conversely, with increased CBG (pregnancy, estrogen therapy), the total plasma hydrocortisone levels are elevated. These alterations are not of clinical significance because it is the unbound fraction of the hormone that is metabolically active. However, the administration of exogenous glucocorticoids to patients with altered protein binding capacities will result in significant differences in glucocorticoid pharmacological effects.

Metabolism/Excretion – Hydrocortisone is metabolized by the liver, which is the rate-limiting step in its clearance. The metabolism and excretion of the synthetic glucocorticoids generally parallel hydrocortisone. Induction of hepatic enzymes will increase the metabolic clearance of hydrocortisone and the synthetic glucocorticoids. About 1% of its usual daily production, or about 200 mcg unchanged hormone is excreted in urine daily. Renal clearance is increased when plasma levels are increased. Prednisone is inactive and must be metabolized to prednisolone.

The following table summarizes the approximate dosage equivalencies (based on glucocorticoid properties) of the various glucocorticoid preparations and several of their pharmacokinetic parameters. The half-life values refer to the intrinsic activity of each agent; insoluble salts of these drugs are used as repository injections and have sustained effects due to delayed absorption from the injection site.

Glucocorticoid Equivalencies, Potencies and Half-Life

Glucocorticoid	Approximate equivalent dose (mg)	Relative anti-inflammatory (glucocorticoid) potency	Relative mineralocorticoid potency	Half-life Plasma (min)	Half-life Biologic (hrs)
Short-acting					
Cortisone	25	0.8	2	30	8-12
Hydrocortisone	20	1	2	80-118	8-12
Intermediate-acting					
Prednisone	5	4	1	60	18-36
Prednisolone	5	4	1	115-212	18-36
Triamcinolone	4	5	0	200+	18-36
Methylprednisolone	4	5	0	78-188	18-36
Long-acting					
Dexamethasone	0.75	20-30	0	110-210	36-54
Betamethasone	0.6-0.75	20-30	0	300+	36-54

GLUCOCORTICOIDS

Indications:

Endocrine disorders: Primary or secondary adrenal cortical insufficiency (hydrocortisone or cortisone is the drug of choice; synthetic analogs may be used in conjunction with mineralocorticoids; in infancy, mineralocorticoid supplementation is important); congenital adrenal hyperplasia; nonsuppurative thyroiditis; hypercalcemia associated with cancer.

Parenteral – Acute adrenal cortical insufficiency (hydrocortisone or cortisone is drug of choice); preoperatively or in serious trauma or illness with known adrenal insufficiency or when adrenal cortical reserve is doubtful; shock unresponsive to conventional therapy if adrenal cortical insufficiency exists or is suspected.

Rheumatic disorders: Adjunctive therapy for short-term use (acute episode or exacerbation) in: Ankylosing spondylitis; acute and subacute bursitis; acute nonspecific tenosynovitis; acute gouty arthritis; psoriatic arthritis; rheumatoid arthritis, including juvenile (selected cases may require low-dose maintenance therapy); posttraumatic osteoarthritis; synovitis of osteoarthritis; epicondylitis.

Collagen diseases: For exacerbation or maintenance therapy in selected cases of systemic lupus erythematosus, acute rheumatic carditis or systemic dermatomyositis (polymyositis).

Dermatologic diseases: Pemphigus; bullous dermatitis herpetiformis; severe erythema multiforme (Stevens-Johnson syndrome); mycosis fungoides; severe psoriasis; angioedema or urticaria; exfoliative, severe seborrheic, contact or atopic dermatitis.

Allergic states: Control of severe or incapacitating allergic conditions intractable to conventional treatment in serum sickness and drug hypersensitivity reactions.

Parenteral therapy is indicated for urticarial transfusion reactions and acute noninfectious laryngeal edema (epinephrine is the drug of first choice).

Ophthalmic: Severe acute and chronic allergic and inflammatory processes involving the eye and its adnexa such as: Allergic conjunctivitis; keratitis; allergic corneal marginal ulcers; herpes zoster ophthalmicus; iritis and iridocyclitis; chorioretinitis; diffuse posterior uveitis and choroiditis; optic neuritis; sympathetic ophthalmia and anterior segment inflammation.

Respiratory diseases: Symptomatic sarcoidosis; bronchial asthma (including status asthmaticus); Loeffler's syndrome not manageable by other means; berylliosis; fulminating or disseminated pulmonary tuberculosis when accompanied by appropriate antituberculous chemotherapy; aspiration pneumonitis; seasonal or perennial allergic rhinitis.

Hematologic disorders: Idiopathic thrombocytopenic purpura and secondary thrombocytopenia in adults (IV only; IM use is contraindicated); acquired (autoimmune) hemolytic anemia; erythroblastopenia (RBC anemia); congenital (erythroid) hypoplastic anemia.

Neoplastic diseases: For palliative management of leukemias and lymphomas in adults and acute leukemia of childhood.

Edematous states: To induce diuresis or remission of proteinuria in the nephrotic syndrome (without uremia) of the idiopathic type or that due to lupus erythematosus.

GI diseases: To tide the patient over a critical period of the disease in ulcerative colitis, regional enteritis (Crohn's disease) and intractable sprue.

Nervous system: Acute exacerbations of multiple sclerosis (see Precautions).

Miscellaneous: Tuberculous meningitis with subarachnoid block or impending block when accompanied by appropriate antituberculous chemotherapy; in trichinosis with neurologic or myocardial involvement.

Intra-articular or soft tissue administration: Short-term adjunctive therapy (to tide the patient over an acute episode) in synovitis of osteoarthritis; rheumatoid arthritis; acute and subacute bursitis; acute gouty arthritis; epicondylitis; acute nonspecific tenosynovitis; post-traumatic osteoarthritis.

Intralesional administration: Keloids; localized hypertrophic, infiltrated, inflammatory lesions of lichen planus, psoriatic plaques, granuloma annulare, lichen simplex chronicus (neurodermatitis); discoid lupus erythematosus; necrobiosis lipoidica diabeticorum; alopecia areata. May be useful in cystic tumors of an aponeurosis or tendon (ganglia).

Dexamethasone is also indicated for testing of adrenal cortical hyperfunction; cerebral edema associated with primary or metastatic brain tumor, craniotomy or head injury.

Triamcinolone is also indicated for the treatment of pulmonary emphysema where bronchospasm or bronchial edema plays a significant role, and diffuse interstitial pulmonary fibrosis (Hamman-Rich syndrome); in conjunction with diuretic agents to

GLUCOCORTICOIDS

induce a diuresis in refractory congestive heart failure (CHF) and in cirrhosis of the liver with refractory ascites; and for postoperative dental inflammatory reactions.

Unlabeled uses:

Glucocorticoid Unlabeled Uses

Use	Drug/Comment
Acute mountain sickness	Dexamethasone 4 mg q 6 h; prevention or treatment
Antiemetic	Dexamethasone most common, 16 to 20 mg
Bacterial meningitis	Dexamethasone 0.15 mg/kg q 6 h; to decrease incidence of hearing loss
Bronchopulmonary dysplasia in preterm infants	Dexamethasone 0.5 mg/kg, then taper.
COPD	Prednisone 30 to 60 mg/day for 1 to 2 weeks, then taper
Depression, diagnosis of	Dexamethasone 1 mg
Duchenne's muscular dystrophy	Prednisone 0.75 to 1.5 mg/kg/day; to improve strength and function
Graves ophthalmopathy	Prednisone 60 mg/day, taper to 20 mg/day
Hepatitis, severe alcoholic	Methylprednisolone 32 mg/day; to reduce mortality
Hirsutism	Dexamethasone 0.5 to 1 mg/day
Respiratory distress syndrome	Prevention in premature neonates (betamethasone most common); adults, methylprednisolone 30 mg/kg (controversial)
Septic shock	Methylprednisolone 30 mg/kg IV most common (very controversial)
Spinal cord injury, acute	Methylprednisolone IV within 8 hrs of injury; to improve neurologic function
Tuberculous pleurisy	Prednisolone 0.75 mg/kg/day, then taper; concurrently w/antituberculous therapy

Contraindications:

Systemic fungal infections; hypersensitivity to the drug; IM use in idiopathic thrombocytopenic purpura; administration of live virus vaccines (eg, smallpox) in patients receiving immunosuppressive corticosteroid doses (Warnings).

Warnings:

Infections: Corticosteroids may mask signs of infection, and new infections may appear during their use. There may be decreased resistance and inability of the host defense mechanisms to prevent dissemination of the infection. If an infection occurs during therapy, it should be promptly controlled by suitable antimicrobial therapy.

Tuberculosis – Restrict use in active tuberculosis to cases of fulminating or disseminated disease in which the corticosteroid is used for disease management with appropriate chemotherapy. If corticosteroids are indicated in latent tuberculosis or tuberculin reactivity, observe closely; disease reactivation may occur. During prolonged corticosteroid use, these patients should receive chemoprophylaxis.

Fungal – Corticosteroids may exacerbate systemic fungal infections; do not use in such infections, except to control drug reactions due to amphotericin B. Concomitant use of amphotericin B and hydrocortisone has been followed by cardiac enlargement and CHF.

Amebiasis – Corticosteroids may activate latent amebiasis. Rule out amebiasis before giving to a patient who has been in the tropics or has unexplained diarrhea.

Cerebral malaria – A double-blind trial has shown corticosteroid use is associated with prolongation of coma and a higher incidence of pneumonia and GI bleeding.

Hepatitis: Although advocated for use in chronic active hepatitis, corticosteroids may be harmful in chronic active hepatitis positive for hepatitis B surface antigen.

Ocular effects: Prolonged use may produce posterior subcapsular cataracts, glaucoma with possible damage to the optic nerves, and may enhance the establishment of secondary ocular infections due to fungi or viruses. Use cautiously in ocular herpes simplex because of possible corneal perforation.

Fluid and electrolyte balance: Average and large doses of hydrocortisone or cortisone can cause elevation of blood pressure, salt and water retention and increased excretion of potassium. These effects are less likely to occur with the synthetic derivatives except when used in large doses. Dietary salt restriction and potassium supplementation may be necessary. All corticosteroids increase calcium excretion.

Peptic ulcer: The relationship between peptic ulceration and glucocorticoid therapy is unclear. Patients who appear to be at risk are those being treated for nephrotic syndrome or liver disease, or who are comatose postcraniotomy. Other predisposing factors include a total prednisone intake exceeding 1g, a history of ulcer disease, concomitant use of known gastric irritants (as in arthritic patients) and stress. It may be desirable to use prophylactic antacids pending clarification of the relationship.

Immunosuppression: During therapy, do not use live virus vaccines (eg, smallpox). Do not immunize patients who are receiving corticosteroids, especially high doses, because of possible hazards of neurological complications and a lack of antibody response. This does not apply to patients receiving corticosteroids as replacement therapy. Corticosteroids may suppress reactions to skin tests.

Adrenal suppression: Prolonged therapy of pharmacologic doses may lead to hypothalamic-pituitary-adrenal suppression. The degree of adrenal suppression varies with the dosage, relative glucocorticoid activity, biological half-life and duration of glucocorticoid therapy within each individual. Adrenal suppression may be minimized by the use of intermediate-acting glucocorticoids (prednisone, prednisolone, methylprednisolone) on an alternate day schedule (see Administration).

Following prolonged therapy, abrupt discontinuation may result in a withdrawal syndrome without evidence of adrenal insufficiency. To minimize morbidity associated with adrenal insufficiency, discontinue exogenous corticosteroid therapy gradually. During withdrawal therapy, increased supplementation may be necessary during times of stress. Symptoms of adrenal insufficiency as a result of too rapid withdrawal include: Nausea; fatigue; anorexia; dyspnea; hypotension; hypoglycemia; myalgia; fever; malaise; arthralgia; dizziness; desquamation of skin; fainting. Continued supervision after therapy termination is essential; severe disease manifestations may reappear suddenly.

Stress: In patients receiving or recently withdrawn from corticosteroid therapy subjected to unusual stress, increased dosage of rapidly acting corticosteroids is indicated before, during and after stressful situations, except in patients on high-dose therapy. Relative adrenocortical insufficiency may persist for months after therapy ends; in any stress situation occurring during that period, reinstitute therapy. Since mineralocorticoid secretion may be impaired, administer salt or a mineralocorticoid concurrently.

Cardiovascular: Reports suggest an apparent association between corticosteroid use and left ventricular free wall rupture after a recent myocardial infarction. Use with great caution in these patients.

Hypersensitivity: Anaphylactoid reactions have occurred rarely with corticosteroid therapy; take precautionary measures, especially in patients with a history of allergies. Refer to Management of Acute Hypersensitivity Reactions.

Renal function impairment: Edema may occur in the presence of renal disease with a fixed or decreased glomerular filtration rate. Use with caution in renal insufficiency, acute glomerulonephritis and chronic nephritis.

Elderly: Consider the risk/benefit factors of steroid use. Consider lower doses because of body changes caused by aging (ie, diminution of muscle mass and plasma volume). Monitor blood pressure, blood glucose and electrolytes at least every 6 months.

Pregnancy: (Category C - Prednisolone sodium phosphate). Corticosteroids cross the placenta (prednisone has the poorest transport). In animal studies, large doses of cortisol administered early in pregnancy produced cleft palate, stillborn fetuses and decreased fetal size. Chronic maternal ingestion during the first trimester has shown a 1% incidence of cleft palate in humans. If used in pregnancy, or in women of childbearing potential, weigh benefits against the potential hazards to the mother and fetus. Carefully observe infants born of mothers who have received substantial corticosteroid doses during pregnancy for signs of hypoadrenalism.

Lactation: Corticosteroids appear in breast milk and could suppress growth, interfere with endogenous corticosteroid production or cause other unwanted effects in the nursing infant. Advise mothers taking pharmacologic corticosteroid doses not to nurse. However, several studies suggest that amounts excreted in breast milk are negligible with prednisone or prednisolone doses ≤ 20 mg/day or methylprednisolone doses ≤ 8 mg/day, and large doses for short periods may not harm the infant.

GLUCOCORTICOIDS

Alternatives to consider include waiting 3 to 4 hours after the dose before breastfeeding and using prednisolone rather than prednisone (resulting in a lower corticosteroid dose to the infant).

Children: Carefully observe growth and development of infants and children on prolonged corticosteroid therapy. Some of these products contain benzyl alcohol which has been associated with a fatal "gasping syndrome" in premature infants.

Precautions:

Monitoring: Observe patients for weight increase, edema, hypertension, and excessive potassium excretion, as well as for less obvious signs of adrenocortical steroid-induced untoward effects. Monitor for a negative nitrogen balance due to protein catabolism. A liberal protein intake is essential during prolonged therapy. Evaluate blood pressure and body weight, and do routine laboratory studies, including 2 hour postprandial blood glucose and serum potassium and a chest x-ray at regular intervals during prolonged therapy. Upper GI x-rays are desirable in patients with known or suspected peptic ulcer disease or significant dyspepsia or in patients complaining of gastric distress. Observe growth and development of infants and children on prolonged therapy.

Use the lowest possible dose: Make a benefit/risk decision in each individual case as to the size of the dose, duration of treatment and the use of daily or intermittent therapy, since complications of treatment are dependent on these factors.

Use with caution in:

GI – Nonspecific ulcerative colitis if there is a probability of impending perforation, abscess or other pyogenic infection; diverticulitis; fresh intestinal anastomoses; active or latent peptic ulcer (see Warnings).

Cardiovascular – Hypertension; CHF; thromboembolitic tendencies; thrombophlebitis.

Miscellaneous – Osteoporosis; exanthema; Cushing's syndrome; antibiotic-resistant infections; convulsive disorders; metastatic carcinoma; myasthenia gravis; vaccinia; varicella; diabetes mellitus.; hypothyroidism, cirrhosis (enhanced effect of corticosteroids).

Steroid psychosis: Steroid psychosis is characterized by a delirious or toxic psychosis with clouded sensorium. Other symptoms may include euphoria, insomnia, mood swings, personality changes and severe depression. The onset of symptoms usually occurs within 15 to 30 days. Predisposing factors include doses > 40 mg prednisone equivalent, female predominance, and, possibly, a family history of psychiatric illness. A patient history of psychiatric problems does not correlate well with predisposition to steroid-induced psychosis. Incidence appears to correlate with dose. One study of 718 patients treated with prednisone revealed ≤ 40 mg/day = 1.3%; 41 to 80 mg/day = 4.6%; ≥ 80 mg/day = 18.4%. If the steroids cannot be discontinued, psychotropic medication is effective.

Multiple sclerosis: Although corticosteroids are effective in speeding the resolution of acute exacerbations of multiple sclerosis, they do not affect the ultimate outcome or natural history of the disease. Relatively high doses of corticosteroids are necessary to demonstrate a significant effect.

Repository injections: To minimize the likelihood and severity of atrophy, do not inject SC, avoid injection into the deltoid and avoid repeated IM injections into the same site, if possible. Repository injections are not recommended as initial therapy in acute situations.

Local injections: Intra-articular injection may produce systemic and local effects. A marked increase in pain accompanied by local swelling, further restriction of joint motion, fever and malaise is suggestive of septic arthritis. Appropriate examination of any joint fluid present is necessary. If a diagnosis of sepsis is confirmed, institute appropriate antimicrobial therapy. Avoid local injection into an infected site and into unstable joints.

Strongly impress patients with the importance of not overusing joints in which symptomatic benefit has been obtained as long as the inflammatory process remains active. *Frequent intra-articular injection may damage joint tissues.*

Avoid overdistention of the joint capsule and deposition of steroid along the needle track in intra-articular injection, as it may lead to subcutaneous atrophy. While crystals of adrenal steroids in the dermis suppress inflammatory reactions, their presence may cause disintegration of the cellular elements and physiochemical changes in the ground substance of the connective tissue.

The resultant dermal or subdermal changes may form depressions in the skin at the injection site; the degree will vary with the amount of adrenal steroid injection. Regeneration is usually complete within a few months or after all crystals of the adrenal steroid have been absorbed. In order to minimize the incidence of dermal and subdermal atrophy, exercise care not to exceed recommended doses in injections. Make multiple small injections into the area of the lesion whenever possible.

Tartrazine sensitivity: Some of these products contain tartrazine, which may cause allergic-type reactions (including bronchial asthma) in susceptible individuals. Although the incidence of tartrazine sensitivity in the general population is low, it is frequently seen in patients who also have aspirin hypersensitivity. Specific products containing tartrazine are identified in the product listings.

Sulfite sensitivity: Some of these products contain sulfites which may cause severe allergic reactions in certain susceptible individuals, particularly asthmatics. Anaphylactoid and hypersensitivity reactions have occurred. Do not use in patients allergic to sulfites. Products containing sulfites are identified in product listings.

Drug Interactions:

Corticosteroid Drug Interactions

Precipitant drug	Object drug*		Description
Aminoglutethimide	Dexamethasone	⬇	Possible loss of dexamethasone-induced adrenal suppression.
Barbiturates	Corticosteroids	⬇	Decreased pharmacologic effects of the corticosteroid may be observed.
Cholestyramine	Hydrocortisone	⬇	The hydrocortisone AUC may be decreased.
Contraceptives, oral	Corticosteroids	⬆	Corticosteroid half-life and concentration may be increased and clearance decreased.
Ephedrine	Dexamethasone	⬇	A decreased half-life and increased clearance of dexamethasone may occur.
Estrogens	Corticosteroids	⬆	Corticosteroid clearance may be decreased.
Hydantoins	Corticosteroids	⬇	Corticosteroid clearance may be increased, resulting in reduced therapeutic effects.
Ketoconazole	Corticosteroids	⬆	Corticosteroid clearance may be decreased and the AUC increased.
Macrolide antibiotics	Methylprednisolone	⬆	Significant decrease in methylprednisolone clearance has been used to decrease methylprednisolone dose.
Rifampin	Corticosteroids	⬇	Corticosteroid clearance may be increased resulting in decreased therapeutic effects.
Corticosteroids	Anticholinesterases	⬇	Anticholinesterase effects may be antagonized in myasthenia gravis.
Corticosteroids	Anticoagulants, oral	⟷	Anticoagulant dose requirements may be reduced. Conversely, corticosteroids may oppose the anticoagulant action.
Corticosteroids	Cyclosporine	⬆	Although this combination is therapeutically beneficial for organ transplants, toxicity may be enhanced.
Corticosteroids	Digitalis glycosides	⬆	Coadministration may enhance the possibility of digitalis toxicity associated with hypokalemia.
Corticosteroids	Isoniazid	⬇	Isoniazid serum concentrations may be decreased.

Glucocorticoids

GLUCOCORTICOIDS

Corticosteroid Drug Interactions			
Precipitant drug	Object drug*		Description
Corticosteroids	Nondepolarizing muscle relaxants	↔	Corticosteroids may potentiate, counteract or have no effect on the neuromuscular blocking action.
Corticosteroids	Potassium-depleting agents (eg, diuretics)	⬆	Observe patients for hypokalemia.
Corticosteroids	Salicylates	⬇	Corticosteroids will reduce serum salicylate levels and may decrease their effectiveness.
Corticosteroids	Somatrem	⬇	Growth-promoting effect of somatrem may be inhibited.
Corticosteroids	Theophyllines	↔	Alterations in the pharmacologic activity of either agent may occur.

* ⬆ = Object drug increased. ⬇ = Object drug decreased. ↔ = Undetermined effect.

GLUCOCORTICOIDS

Drug/Lab test interactions: **Urine glucose** and **serum cholesterol** levels may increase. Decreased serum levels of **potassium, triiodothyronine (T_3)**, and a minimal decrease of **thyroxine (T_4)** may occur. **Thyroid I^{131}** uptake may be decreased. False-negative results with the **nitroblue-tetrazolium test** for bacterial infection. **Dexamethasone,** given for cerebral edema, may alter the results of a brain scan (decreased uptake of radioactive material).

Adverse Reactions:

Parenteral therapy: Rare instances of blindness associated with intralesional therapy around the face and head; hyperpigmentation or hypopigmentation; subcutaneous and cutaneous atrophy; sterile abscess; Charcot-like arthropathy; burning or tingling, especially in the perineal area (after IV injection); scarring, induration, inflammation, paresthesia, occasional irritation at the injection site or occasional brief increase in joint discomfort; transient or delayed pain or soreness; muscle twitching, ataxia, hiccoughs and nystagmus (low incidence following injection); anaphylactic reactions with or without circulatory collapse; cardiac arrest; bronchospasm; arachnoiditis after intrathecal use; foreign body granulomatous reactions involving the synovium with repeated injections.

Intra-articular – Osteonecrosis; tendon rupture; infection; skin atrophy; postinjection flare; hypersensitivity; facial flushing. Systemic reactions may also occur.

Intraspinal – Meningitis (tuberculous, bacterial, cryptococcal, aseptic, chemical); adhesive arachnoiditis; conus medullaris syndrome.

Electrolyte Disturbance: Sodium and fluid retention; hypokalemia; hypokalemic alkalosis; metabolic alkalosis; hypocalcemia; CHF in susceptible patients; hypotension or shock-like reactions; hypertension (see Warnings).

Musculoskeletal: Muscle weakness; steroid myopathy; muscle mass loss; tendon rupture; osteoporosis; aseptic necrosis of femoral and humeral heads (1% to 37%); spontaneous fractures, including vertebral compression fractures and pathologic fracture of long bones.

Cardiovascular: Thromboembolism or fat embolism; thrombophlebitis; necrotizing angiitis; cardiac arrhythmias or ECG changes due to potassium deficiency; syncopal episodes; aggravation of hypertension; myocardial rupture following recent MI (see Warnings). There are reports of cardiac arrhythmias, fatal arrest or circulatory collapse following the rapid administration of large IV doses of **methylprednisolone** (0.5 to 1 g in < 10 to 120 minutes). See Electrolyte Disturbances.

GI: Pancreatitis; abdominal distension; ulcerative esophagitis; nausea; vomiting; increased appetite and weight gain. Peptic ulcer with perforation and hemorrhage (see Warnings). Perforation of the small and large bowel, particularly in inflammatory bowel disease.

Dermatologic: Impaired wound healing; thin fragile skin; petechiae and ecchymoses; erythema; lupus erythematosus-like lesions; suppression of skin test reactions; subcutaneous fat atrophy; purpura; striae; hirsutism; acneiform eruptions; other cutaneous reactions such as allergic dermatitis; urticaria; angioneurotic edema; perineal irritation.

CNS: Convulsions; increased intracranial pressure with papilledema (pseudotumor cerebri), usually after stopping treatment; vertigo; headache; neuritis/paresthesias; aggravation of pre-existing psychiatric conditions; steroid psychoses (see Precautions).

Endocrine: Amenorrhea, postmenopausal bleeding and other menstrual irregularities; development of Cushingoid state (eg, moonface, buffalo hump, supraclavicular fat pad enlargement, central obesity); suppression of growth in children; secondary adrenocortical and pituitary unresponsiveness, particularly in times of stress (eg, trauma, surgery, illness); increased sweating; decreased carbohydrate tolerance; hyperglycemia; glycosuria; increased insulin or sulfonylurea requirements in diabetics; manifestations of latent diabetes mellitus; negative nitrogen balance due to protein catabolism; hirsutism.

Ophthalmic: Posterior subcapsular cataracts; increased IOP; glaucoma; exophthalmos.

Miscellaneous: Anaphylactoid/hypersensitivity reactions, aggravation/masking of infections (see Warnings); malaise; leukocytosis (including neonates receiving dexamethasone via maternal injection); fatigue; insomnia; increased or decreased motility and number of spermatozoa.

Overdosage:

Symptoms: There are two categories of toxic effects from therapeutic use of glucocorticoids:

GLUCOCORTICOIDS

Acute adrenal insufficiency due to too rapid corticosteroid withdrawal after long-term use resulting in fever, myalgia, arthralgia, malaise, anorexia, nausea, skin desquamation, orthostatic hypotension, dizziness, fainting, dyspnea and hypoglycemia.

Cushingoid changes from continued use of large doses resulting in moonface, central obesity, striae, hirsutism, acne, ecchymoses, hypertension, osteoporosis, myopathy, sexual dysfunction, diabetes, hyperlipidemia, peptic ulcer, increased susceptibility to infection and electrolyte and fluid imbalance. Reports of acute toxicity or death are rare.

Treatment: Recovery of normal adrenal and pituitary function may require up to 9 months. Gradually taper the steroid under the supervision of a physician. Frequent lab tests are necessary. Supplementation is required during periods of stress (eg, illness, surgery, injury). Eventually reduce to the lowest dose that will control the symptoms or discontinue the corticosteroid completely. For large, acute overdoses, treatment includes gastric lavage or emesis and usual supportive measures. Refer to General Management of Acute Overdosage.

Patient Information:

May cause GI upset; take with meals or snacks. Take single daily or alternate day doses in the morning prior to 9 am. Take multiple doses at evenly spaced intervals throughout the day.

Patients on chronic steroid therapy should wear or carry identification to that effect.

Notify physician if unusual weight gain, swelling of the lower extremities, muscle weakness, black tarry stools, vomiting of blood, puffing of the face, menstrual irregularities, prolonged sore throat, fever, cold or infection occurs.

Signs of adrenal insufficiency include fatigue, anorexia, nausea, vomiting, diarrhea, weight loss, weakness, dizziness and low blood sugar. Notify physician promptly if these symptoms occur following dosage reduction or withdrawal of therapy.

High dose or long-term therapy: Avoid abrupt withdrawal of therapy.

Administration and Dosage:

The maximal activity of the adrenal cortex is between 2 and 8 am, and it is minimal between 4 pm and midnight. Exogenous corticosteroids suppress adrenocortical activity the least when given at the time of maximal activity (am). Therefore, administer glucocorticoids in the morning prior to 9 am. When large doses are given, administer antacids between meals to help prevent peptic ulcers.

Initiation of therapy: The initial dosage depends on the specific disease entity being treated. Maintain or adjust the initial dosage until a satisfactory response is noted. If after a reasonable period of time there is a lack of satisfactory clinical response, discontinue the drug and transfer the patient to other appropriate therapy. *It should be emphasized that dosage requirements are variable and must be individualized.* For infants and children, the recommended dosage should be governed by the same considerations rather than by strict adherence to the ratio indicated by age or body weight.

Maintenance therapy: After a favorable response is observed, determine the maintenance dosage by decreasing the initial dosage in small amounts at intervals until the lowest dosage that will maintain an adequate clinical response is reached. Constant monitoring of drug dosage is required. Situations which may make dosage adjustments necessary are changes in the disease process, the patient's individual drug responsiveness, and the effect of patient exposure to stress; in this latter situation it may be necessary to increase the dosage for a period of time consistent with the patient's condition.

Withdrawal of therapy: If, after long-term therapy, the drug is to be stopped, it must be withdrawn gradually. If spontaneous remission occurs in a chronic condition, discontinue treatment gradually. Continued supervision of the patient after discontinuation of corticosteroids is essential, since there may be a sudden reappearance of severe manifestations of the disease.

Alternate day therapy is a dosing regimen in which twice the usual daily dose is administered every other morning. The purpose is to provide the patient requiring long-term treatment with the beneficial effects of corticosteroids while minimizing pituitary-adrenal suppression, the cushingoid state, withdrawal symptoms and growth suppression in children. *The benefits of alternate day therapy are only achieved by using the intermediate-acting agents.*

The rationale for this treatment schedule is based on two major premises: (a) The therapeutic effect of intermediate-acting corticosteroids persists longer than their physical presence and metabolic effects; (b) administration of the corticosteroid every other morning allows for reestablishment of a more normal hypothalamic-

GLUCOCORTICOIDS

pituitary-adrenal (HPA) activity on the off-steroid day. Keep the following in mind when considering alternate day therapy:

1.) Benefits of alternate day therapy do not encourage indiscriminate steroid use.
2.) Alternate day therapy is primarily designed for patients in whom long-term corticosteroid therapy is anticipated.
3.) In less severe disease processes, it may be possible to initiate treatment with alternate day therapy. More severe disease states usually require daily divided high-dose therapy for initial control. Continue initial suppressive dose until satisfactory clinical response is obtained, usually 4 to 10 days in the case of many allergic and collagen diseases. Keep the period of initial suppressive dose as brief as possible, particularly when alternate day therapy is intended. Once control is established, two courses are available: (a) Change to alternate day therapy, then gradually reduce the amount of corticosteroid given every other day or (b) reduce daily corticosteroid dose to the lowest effective level as rapidly as possible, then change over to an alternate day schedule. Theoretically, course (a) may be preferable.
4.) Because of the advantages of alternate day therapy, it may be desirable to try patients on this form of therapy who have been on daily corticosteroids for long periods of time (eg, patients with rheumatoid arthritis). Since these patients may already have a suppressed HPA axis, establishing them on alternate day therapy may be difficult and not always successful; however, it is recommended that such regular attempts be made. It may be helpful to triple or even quadruple the daily maintenance dose and administer this every other day rather than just doubling the daily dose if difficulty is encountered. Once the patient is controlled, attempt to reduce this dose to a minimum.
5.) Long-acting corticosteroids (eg, dexamethasone, betamethasone), due to their prolonged suppressive effect on adrenal activity, are not recommended for alternate day therapy.
6.) It is important to individualize therapy. Complete control of symptoms will not be possible in all patients. An explanation of the benefits of alternate day therapy will help the patient to understand and tolerate the possible flare-up in symptoms which may occur in the latter part of the off-steroid day. Other therapy to relieve symptoms may be added or increased at this time if needed.
7.) In the event of an acute flare-up of the disease process, it may be necessary to return to a full suppressive daily corticosteroid dose for control. Once control is established, alternate day therapy may be reinstituted.

Intra-articular injection: Dose depends on the joint size and varies with the severity of the condition. In chronic cases, injections may be repeated at intervals of 1 to 5 or more weeks depending upon the degree of relief obtained from the initial injection. Injection must be made into the synovial space. Do not inject unstable joints. Repeated intra-articular injection may result in joint instability. X-ray follow-up is suggested in selected cases to detect deterioration.

Suitable sites for injection are the knee, ankle, wrist, elbow, shoulder, hip and phalangeal joints. Since difficulty is frequently encountered in entering the hip joint, avoid any large blood vessels in the area. Joints *not* suitable for injection are those that are anatomically inaccessible and devoid of synovial space such as the spinal joints and the sacroiliac joints. Treatment failures frequently result from failure to enter the joint space; little or no benefit follows injection into surrounding tissue. If failures occur when injections into the synovial spaces are certain, as determined by aspiration of fluid, repeated injections are usually of no benefit. Local therapy does not alter the underlying disease process; whenever possible, employ comprehensive therapy including physiotherapy and orthopedic correction (see Precautions).

Miscellaneous (tendinitis, epicondylitis, ganglion): In the treatment of conditions such as tendinitis or tenosynovitis, inject into the tendon sheath rather than into the substance of the tendon. When treating conditions such as epicondylitis, outline the area of greatest tenderness and infiltrate the drug into the area. For ganglia of the tendon sheaths, inject the drug directly into the cyst. In many cases, a single injection markedly decreases size of the cystic tumor and may effect disappearance. The dose varies with the condition being treated. In recurrent or chronic conditions, repeated injections may be needed.

Injections for local effect in dermatologic conditions: Avoid injection of sufficient material to cause blanching, since this may be followed by a small slough. One to four injections are usually employed. Intervals between injections vary with the type of lesion being treated and duration of improvement produced by initial injection.

Glucocorticoids

CORTISONE

For complete prescribing information, refer to the Glucocorticoids group monograph.

The drug is insoluble in water.

Administration and Dosage:

Initial dosage: 25 to 300 mg/day. In less severe diseases, lower doses may suffice.

Rx	**Cortisone Acetate** (Upjohn)	**Tablets:** 5 mg	(Upjohn 15). White, scored. In 50s.
Rx	**Cortisone Acetate** (Upjohn)	**Tablets:** 10 mg	(Upjohn 23). White, scored. In 100s.
Rx	**Cortisone Acetate** (Various, eg, Bioline, Dixon-Shane, Goldline, Major, Moore, Rugby, Schein)	**Tablets:** 25 mg	In 100s and 500s
Rx	**Cortone Acetate** (Merck)		(MSD 219). White, scored. In 100s.
Rx	**Cortone Acetate** (Merck)	**Injection:** 50 mg/ml	In 10 ml vials.

HYDROCORTISONE (Cortisol)

For complete prescribing information, refer to the Glucocorticoids group monograph.

Cortisol suspension is insoluble in water.

Administration and Dosage:

Initial dosage: 20 to 240 mg/day.

Rx	**Cortef** (Upjohn)	**Tablets:** 5 mg	(Cortef 5). White, scored. In 50s.
Rx	**Hydrocortisone** (Major)	**Tablets:** 10 mg	In 100s.
Rx	**Cortef** (Upjohn)		(Cortef 10). White, scored. In 100s.
Rx	**Hydrocortone** (MSD)		(MSD 619). White, scored. Oval. In 100s.
Rx	**Hydrocortisone** (Various, eg, Major, Moore, Rugby, Schein, URL)	**Tablets:** 20 mg	In 100s.
Rx	**Cortef** (Upjohn)		(Cortef 20). White, scored. In 100s.
Rx	**Hydrocortone** (MSD)		(MSD 625). White, scored. Oval. In 100s.

HYDROCORTISONE CYPIONATE

For complete prescribing information, refer to the Glucocorticoids group monograph.

Administration and Dosage:

Initial dosage: 20 to 240 mg/day.

Rx	**Cortef** (Upjohn)	**Oral Suspension:** 10 mg per 5 ml hydrocortisone (as cypionate)	Sucrose. In 120 ml.

HYDROCORTISONE SODIUM PHOSPHATE

For complete prescribing information, refer to the Glucocorticoids group monograph.

A water soluble salt with a rapid onset but short duration of action.

Administration and Dosage:

Administer by IV, IM or SC injection.

Initial dosage: 15 to 240 mg/day. Usually, ⅓ to ½ the oral dose every 12 hours.

Acute diseases: Doses higher than 240 mg may be required.

Rx	**Hydrocortone Phosphate** (MSD)	**Injection:** 50 mg/ml hydrocortisone (as sodium phosphate) solution	In 2 and 10 ml vials.[1]

[1] With 3.2 mg sodium bisulfite, and 1.5 mg methylparaben and 0.2 mg propylparaben.

Glucocorticoids

HYDROCORTISONE SODIUM SUCCINATE

For complete prescribing information, refer to the Glucocorticoids group monograph.

A water soluble salt which is rapidly active.

Administration and Dosage:

May be administered IV or IM. The initial dose is 100 to 500 mg, and may be repeated at 2, 4 or 6 hour intervals depending on patient response and clinical condition.

Rx	**A-Hydrocort** (Abbott)	**Injection**: 100 mg hydrocortisone (as sodium succinate) per vial	In 2 ml Univials[1] and flip-top vials.
Rx	**Solu-Cortef** (Upjohn)		In vials and 2 ml Act-O-Vials.[1]
Rx	**A-Hydrocort** (Abbott)	**Injection**: 250 mg hydrocortisone (as sodium succinate) per vial	In 2 ml Univials[1] and flip-top vials.
Rx	**Solu-Cortef** (Upjohn)		In 2 ml Act-O-Vials.[1]
Rx	**A-Hydrocort** (Abbott)	**Injection**: 500 mg hydrocortisone (as sodium succinate) per vial	In 4 ml Univials[1] and flip-top vials.
Rx	**Solu-Cortef** (Upjohn)		In 4 ml Act-O-Vials.[1]
Rx	**A-Hydrocort** (Abbott)	**For Injection**: 1000 mg hydrocortisone (as sodium succinate) per vial	In 8 ml Univials[1] and flip-top vials.
Rx	**Solu-Cortef** (Upjohn)		In 8 ml Act-O-Vials.[1]

[1] With benzyl alcohol.

HYDROCORTISONE ACETATE

For complete prescribing information, refer to the Glucocorticoids group monograph.

Hydrocortisone acetate has a slow onset but long duration of action when compared with more soluble preparations. Because of its insolubility, it is suitable for intra-articular, intralesional and soft tissue injection where its anti-inflammatory effects are confined mainly to the area in which it has been injected, although it is capable of producing systemic hormonal effects.

Administration and Dosage:

For intralesional, intra-articular or soft tissue injection only. Not for IV use.

Large joints (eg, knee): 25 mg; occasionally, 37.5 mg.

Small joints (eg, interphalangeal, temporomandibular): 10 to 25 mg.

Tendon sheaths: 5 to 12.5 mg.

Soft tissue infiltration: 25 to 50 mg; occasionally, 75 mg.

Bursae: 25 to 37.5 mg.

Ganglia: 12.5 to 25 mg.

If desired, a local anesthetic may be injected before hydrocortisone acetate or mixed in a syringe and given simultaneously.

If used prior to intra-articular injection of the steroid, inject most of the anesthetic into the soft tissues of the surrounding area and instill a small amount into the joint.

If given together, mix in the injection syringe by drawing the steroid in first, then the anesthetic. In this way, the anesthetic will not be introduced inadvertently into the vial of the steroid. *The mixture must be used immediately and any unused portion discarded.*

Rx	**Hydrocortisone Acetate** (Various, eg, Dixon-Shane, Major, Moore, Rugby, Schein, URL)	**Injection**: 25 mg per ml suspension	In 10 ml vials.
Rx	**Hydrocortone Acetate** (MSD)		In 5 ml vials.[2]
Rx	**Hydrocortisone Acetate** (Various, eg, Major, Moore, Rugby, URL)	**Injection**: 50 mg per ml suspension	In 10 ml vials.
Rx	**Hydrocortone Acetate** (MSD)		In 5 ml vials.[2]

[2] With 4 mg polysorbate 80, 5 mg sodium carboxymethylcellulose and 9 mg benzyl alcohol per ml.

Glucocorticoids

PREDNISONE

For complete prescribing information, refer to the Glucocorticoids group monograph.

Administration and Dosage:

Initial dosage varies from 5 to 60 mg/day. Prednisone is inactive and must be metabolized to prednisolone. This may be impaired in patients with liver disease.

Rx	**Prednisone** (Various, eg, Roxane)	**Tablets**: 1 mg	In 100s, 1000s and UD 100s.
Rx	**Meticorten** (Schering)		Lactose. (KEM or 843). White. In 100s.
Rx	**Orasone** (Solvay)		Lactose. (RR 1). Pink, scored. In 100s and 1000s.
Rx	**Panasol-S** (Seatrace)		Pink, scored. In 100s, 1000s.
Rx	**Deltasone** (Upjohn)	**Tablets**: 2.5 mg	Lactose, sucrose. (Deltasone 2.5). Scored. In 100s.
Rx	**Prednisone** (Various, eg, Barr, Geneva, Goldline, Lannett, Major, Parmed, Rugby)	**Tablets**: 5 mg	In 100s, 500s, 1000s, 5000s and UD 100s.
Rx	**Deltasone** (Upjohn)		Lactose, sucrose. (Deltasone 5). Scored. In 100s, 500s, UD 100s and Dosepak 21s.
Rx	**Orasone** (Solvay)		Lactose. (RR 5). White, scored. In 100s and 1000s.
Rx	**Prednicen-M** (Central)		(131/07). Red. Film coated. In 100s, 1000s and unit pak 21s.
Rx	**Prednisone** (Various, eg, Barr, Geneva, Goldline, Major, Parmed, Rugby)	**Tablets**: 10 mg	In 100s, 500s, 1000s and UD 100s.
Rx	**Deltasone** (Upjohn)		Lactose, sucrose. (Deltasone 10). Scored. In 100s, 500s and UD 100s.
Rx	**Orasone** (Solvay)		Lactose. (RR 10). Blue, scored. In 100s and 1000s.
Rx	**Strerapred DS** (Mayrand)		(MP 0364). White, scored. In Uni-Pak 21s.
Rx	**Prednisone** (Various, eg, Barr, Bioline, Geneva, Goldline, Lannett, Major, Parmed, Rugby)	**Tablets**: 20 mg	In 100s, 500s, 1000s and UD 100s.
Rx	**Deltasone** (Upjohn)		Lactose, sucrose. (Deltasone 20). Scored. In 100s, 500s and UD 100s.
Rx	**Orasone** (Solvay)		Lactose. (RR 20). Yellow, scored. In 100s and 1000s.
Rx	**Prednisone** (Various, eg, Geneva, Major, Rugby)	**Tablets**: 50 mg	In 100s and UD 100s.
Rx	**Deltasone** (Upjohn)		Lactose, sucrose. (Deltasone 500). Scored. In 100s.
Rx	**Orasone** (Solvay)		Lactose. (RR 50). White, scored. Film coated. In 100s.
Rx	**Prednisone** (Roxane)	**Oral Solution**: 5 mg per 5 ml	5% alcohol. Fructose, saccharin. Dye free. In 500 ml and UD 5 ml (40s).

Glucocorticoids

PREDNISONE

Rx	**Prednisone Intensol Concentrate** (Roxane)	**Oral Solution:** 5 mg per ml	30% alcohol. In 30 ml.
Rx	**Liquid Pred** (Muro)	**Syrup:** 5 mg per 5 ml	5% alcohol. Saccharin, sorbitol and sucrose. In 120 and 240 ml.

PREDNISOLONE

For complete prescribing information, refer to the Glucocorticoids group monograph.

Administration and Dosage:

Initial dosage: 5 to 60 mg/day.

Multiple sclerosis: In treatment of acute exacerbations of multiple sclerosis, 200 mg daily for a week followed by 80 mg every other day for 1 month.

Rx	**Prednisolone** (Various, eg, Geneva, Goldline, Major, Moore, Roxane, Rugby, Schein, URL)	**Tablets:** 5 mg	In 100s, 1000s and 5000s.
Rx	**Delta-Cortef** (Upjohn)		Lactose, sucrose. White, scored. In 100s and 500s.
Rx	**Prelone** (Muro)	**Syrup:** 15 mg per 5 ml	5% alcohol. Saccharin, sucrose. Cherry flavor. In 240 ml.

PREDNISOLONE ACETATE

For complete prescribing information, refer to the Glucocorticoids group monograph.

Relatively insoluble.

Administration and Dosage:

Systemic: Not for IV use.

Initial dosage – 4 to 60 mg/day, IM.

Intralesional, intra-articular or soft tissue injection: 4 mg, up to 100 mg.

Multiple sclerosis: 200 mg daily for a week, followed by 80 mg every other day or 4 to 8 mg dexamethasone every other day for 1 month.

Rx	**Prednisolone Acetate** (Various, eg, Rugby, URL)	**Injection:** 25 mg per ml suspension	In 10 and 30 ml vials.
Rx	**Key-Pred 25** (Hyrex)		In 10 and 30 ml vials.
Rx	**Predcor-25** (Hauck)		In 10 ml vials.[1]
Rx	**Prednisolone Acetate** (Various, eg, Geneva Marsam, Goldline, Major, Moore, Rugby, Schein, Steris, URL)	**Injection:** 50 mg per ml suspension	In 10 and 30 ml vials.
Rx	**Key-Pred 50**(Hyrex)		In 10 ml vials.
Rx	**Predalone 50**(Forest)		In 10 ml vials.[1]
Rx	**Predcor-50** (Hauck)		In 10 ml vials.[1]

[1] With polysorbate 80, carboxymethylcellulose and benzyl alcohol.

Glucocorticoids

PREDNISOLONE TEBUTATE

For complete prescribing information, refer to the Glucocorticoids group monograph.

Slightly soluble with a slow onset and prolonged duration of action.

Administration and Dosage:

Intra-articular, intralesional or soft tissue administration:

Large joints (eg, knee) – 20 mg; occasionally, 30 mg. Doses > 40 mg are not recommended.

Small joints (eg, interphalangeal, temporomandibular) - 8 to 10 mg.

Bursae – 20 to 30 mg.

Tendon sheaths – 4 to 10 mg.

Ganglia – 10 to 20 mg.

Rx	**Prednisolone Tebutate** (Major)	**Injection:** 20 mg per ml suspension	In 10 ml vials.
Rx	**Hydeltra-T.B.A.** (MSD)		In 1 and 5 ml vials.[1]
Rx	**Prednisol TBA** (Pasadena)		In 10 ml vials.[1]

[1] With polysorbate 80, sorbitol and benzyl alcohol.

PREDNISOLONE SODIUM PHOSPHATE

For complete prescribing information, refer to the Glucocorticoids group monograph.

Water soluble and rapid acting, but has a short duration of action.

Prednisolone sodium phosphate oral liquid produces a 20% higher peak plasma level of prednisolone which occurs approximately 15 minutes earlier than the peak seen with tablet formulations.

Administration and Dosage:

Parenteral: For IV or IM use.

Initial dosage – 4 to 60 mg/day.

Intra-articular, intralesional or soft tissue administration:

Large joints (eg, knee) – 10 to 20 mg.

Small joints (eg, interphalangeal, temporomandibular) – 4 to 5 mg.

Bursae – 10 to 15 mg.

Tendon sheaths – 2 to 5 mg.

Soft tissue infiltration – 10 to 30 mg.

Ganglia – 5 to 10 mg.

Oral: Initial dosage - 5 to 60 ml (5 to 60 mg base) per day.

Multiple sclerosis (acute exacerbations) – 200 mg daily for a week, followed by 80 mg every other day or 4 to 8 mg dexamethasone every other day for 1 month.

Rx	**Hydeltrasol** (MSD)	**Injection**: 20 mg per ml prednisolone (as sodium phosphate) solution	In 2 and 5 ml vials.[1]
Rx	**Key-Pred-SP** (Hyrex)		In 10 ml vials.[1]
Rx *sf*	**Pediapred** (Fisons)	**Oral Liquid**: 5 mg prednisolone (as sodium phosphate) per 5 ml	Alcohol and dye free. Raspberry flavor. In 120 ml.

[1] With niacinamide, EDTA, phenol and sodium bisulfite.

Glucocorticoids

TRIAMCINOLONE, ORAL

For complete prescribing information, refer to the Glucocorticoids group monograph.

Administration and Dosage:

Initial daily dosage in specific disorders is:

Adrenocortical insufficiency – 4 to 12 mg, in addition to mineralocorticoid therapy.
Rheumatic and dermatological disorders and bronchial asthma – 8 to 16 mg.
Allergic states – 8 to 12 mg.
Ophthalmological diseases – 12 to 40 mg.
Respiratory diseases – 16 to 48 mg.
Hematologic disorders – 16 to 60 mg.
Tuberculous meningitis – 32 to 48 mg.
Acute rheumatic carditis – 20 to 60 mg.
Acute leukemia and lymphoma (adults) – 16 to 40 mg. It may be necessary to give as much as 100 mg/day in leukemia.
Acute leukemia (children): 1 to 2 mg/kg.
Edematous states – 16 to 20 mg (up to 48 mg) until diuresis occurs.
Systemic lupus erythematosus – 20 to 32 mg.

Rx	**Aristocort** (Fujisawa)	**Tablets**: 1 mg	Lactose. (LL A1). Yellow, scored. Oblong, flat. In 50s.
Rx	**Aristocort** (Fujisawa)	**Tablets**: 2 mg	Lactose. (LL A2). Pink, scored. Oblong. In 100s.
Rx	**Triamcinolone** (Various, eg, Dixon-Shane, Moore, Rugby, Schein, URL)	**Tablets**: 4 mg	In 100s and 500s.
Rx	**Aristocort** (Fujisawa)		Lactose. (LL A4). White, scored. Oblong, flat. In 30s, 100s and Aristo-Pak 16s.
Rx	**Atolone** (Major)		White, scored. In 100s and Uni-Pak 16s.
Rx	**Kenacort** (Apothecon)		Lactose. In 100s.
Rx	**Aristocort** (Fujisawa)	**Tablets**: 8 mg	Lactose. (LL A8). Yellow, scored. Oblong, flat. In 50s.
Rx	**Kenacort** (Apothecon)		Lactose, tartrazine. In 50s.
Rx	**Kenacort** (Apothecon)	**Syrup**: 4 mg (as diacetate) per 5 ml	Sucrose. In 120 ml.

TRIAMCINOLONE DIACETATE

For complete prescribing information, refer to the Glucocorticoids group monograph.

Slightly soluble providing a prompt onset of action and a longer duration of effect.

Administration and Dosage:

Systemic: Not for IV use. May be administered IM for initial therapy; however, most clinicians prefer to adjust the dose orally until adequate control is attained. The average dose is 40 mg IM per week. In general, a single parenteral dose 4 to 7 times the oral daily dose controls the patient from 4 to 7 days, up to 3 to 4 weeks.

Intra-articular and intrasynovial: 5 to 40 mg.

Intralesional or sublesional: 5 to 48 mg. Do not use more than 12.5 mg per injection site. The usual average dose is 25 mg per lesion.

Rx	**Aristocort Intralesional** (Fujisawa)	**Injection:** 25 mg per ml suspension	In 5 ml vials.[1]
Rx	**Triamcinolone** (Various, eg, Major, Moore, Rugby, Steris, URL)	**Injection:** 40 mg per ml suspension	In 5 ml vials.
Rx	**Trilone** (Hauck)		In 5 ml vials.
Rx	**Amcort** (Keene)		In 5 ml vials.[1]
Rx	**Aristocort Forte** (Fujisawa)		In 1 and 5 ml vials.[1]
Rx	**Triam Forte** (Hyrex)		In 5 ml vials.
Rx	**Triamolone 40** (Forest)		In 5 ml vials.[1]
Rx	**Tristoject** (Mayrand)		In 5 ml vials.

[1] With polysorbate 80, polyethylene glycol and benzyl alcohol.

TRIAMCINOLONE HEXACETONIDE

For complete prescribing information, refer to the Glucocorticoids group monograph.

Relatively insoluble, slowly absorbed and has a prolonged action.

Administration and Dosage:

Not for IV use.

Intra-articular: 2 to 20 mg average.

Large joints (eg, knee, hip, shoulder) – 10 to 20 mg.

Small joints (eg, interphalangeal, metacarpophalangeal) – 2 to 6 mg.

Intralesional or sublesional: Up to 0.5 mg per square inch of affected area.

Rx	**Aristospan Intralesional** (Fujisawa)	**Injection:** 5 mg per ml suspension	In 5 ml vials.[2]
Rx	**Aristospan Intra-articular** (Fujisawa)	**Injection:** 20 mg per ml suspension	In 1 and 5 ml vials.[2]

[2] With polysorbate 80, sorbitol and benzyl alcohol.

TRIAMCINOLONE ACETONIDE

For complete prescribing information, refer to the Glucocorticoids group monograph.

Relatively insoluble. Has an extended duration which may be permanent or sustained for several weeks.

Administration and Dosage:

Systemic:

Initial IM dose – 2.5 to 60 mg/day. Not for IV use.

Intra-articular or intrabursal administration and for injection into tendon sheaths:

Initial dose – 2.5 to 5 mg for smaller joints and 5 to 15 mg for larger joints. For adults, doses up to 10 mg for smaller areas and up to 40 mg for larger areas are usually sufficient.

Intradermal: Use only 3 mg/ml or 10 mg/ml. Initial dose varies; limit to 1 mg per site.

Clumping results from exposure to freezing temperatures; do not use.

Rx	**Tac-3** (Herbert)	**Injection**: 3 mg per ml suspension	In 5 ml vials.[1]
Rx	**Kenalog-10** (Westwood-Squibb)	**Injection**: 10 mg per ml suspension	In 5 ml vials.[1]
Rx	**Triamcinolone Acetonide** (Various, eg, Bioline, Dixon-Shane, Geneva Marsam, Goldline, Moore, Schein, URL)	**Injection**: 40 mg per ml suspension	In 1 and 5 ml vials.
Rx	**Kenaject-40** (Mayrand)		In 5 ml vials.
Rx	**Kenalog-40** (Westwood-Squibb)		In 1, 5 and 10 ml vials.[1]
Rx	**Tac-40** (Parnell)		In 5 ml vials.
Rx	**Triam-A** (Hyrex)		In 5 ml vials.
Rx	**Triamonide 40** (Forest)		In 5 ml vials.[1]
Rx	**Tri-Kort** (Keene)		In 5 ml vials.[1]
Rx	**Trilog** (Hauck)		In 5 ml vials.[1]

[1] With polysorbate 80, carboxymethlcellulose and benzyl alcohol.

Glucocorticoids

METHYLPREDNISOLONE

For complete prescribing information, refer to the Glucocorticoids group monograph.

Administration and Dosage:

Initial dose: 4 to 48 mg/day; adjust until a satisfactory response is noted. Individualize dosage. Determine maintenance dose by decreasing initial dose in small decrements at appropriate intervals until reaching the lowest effective dose.

Dosepak 21 therapy: Follow manufacturer's directions.

Alternate day therapy (ADT): Twice the usual dose is administered every other morning. The patient on long-term treatment receives the beneficial effects of corticosteroids while minimizing certain undesirable effects. In less severe diseases requiring long-term therapy, treatment may be initiated with ADT.

Rx	**Methylprednisolone** (Various, eg, Geneva, Major, Moore, Parmed, Rugby)	**Tablets:** 4 mg	In 21s and 100s.
Rx	**Methylprednisolone** (Various, eg, Rugby, URL)	**Tablets:** 16 mg	In 50s.
Rx	**Medrol** (Upjohn)	**Tablets:** 2 mg[2]	Pink, scored. Elliptical. In 100s.
		4 mg[2]	White, scored. Elliptical. In 30s, 100s, 500s, UD 100s and Dosepak 21s.
		8 mg[2]	Peach, scored. Elliptical. In 25s.
		16 mg[2]	White, scored. Elliptical. In 50s and ADT Pak 14s.
		24 mg[2]	Tartrazine. Yellow, scored. Elliptical. In 25s.
		32 mg[2]	Peach, scored. Elliptical. In 25s.

[2] With lactose and sucrose.

Glucocorticoids

METHYLPREDNISOLONE SODIUM SUCCINATE

For complete prescribing information, refer to the Glucocorticoids group monograph.

Highly soluble; has rapid effect by IV or IM routes.

Administration and Dosage:

Initial dose: 10 to 40 mg IV, administered over 1 to several minutes. Give subsequent doses IV or IM.

Infants and children : Not less than 0.5mg/kg/24 hours.

For high dose therapy, give 30 mg/kg IV, infused over 10 to 20 minutes. May repeat every 4 to 6 hours, not beyond 48 to 72 hours.

Rx	**Methylprednisolone Sodium Succinate** (Various, eg, Elkins Sinn, Lyphomed)	**Powder for Injection:** 40 mg per vial	In 1 and 3 ml vials.
Rx	**A-Methapred** (Abbott)		In 1 ml Univial.[1]
Rx	**Solu-Medrol** (Upjohn)		In 1 ml Act-O-Vial.[1]
Rx	**Methylprednisolone Sodium Succinate** (Various, eg, Elkins Sinn, Lyphomed)	**Powder for Injection:** 125 mg per vial	In 2 and 5 ml vials.
Rx	**A-Methapred** (Abbott)		In 2 ml Univial.[2]
Rx	**Solu-Medrol** (Upjohn)		In 2 ml Act-O-Vial.[2]
Rx	**Methylprednisolone Sodium Succinate** (Various, eg, Elkins Sinn, Lyphomed)	**Powder for Injection:** 500 mg per vial	In 1, 4 and 20 ml vials.
Rx	**A-Methapred** (Abbott)		In 4 ml Univial and 500 mg ADD-Vantage vials.[3]
Rx	**Solu-Medrol** (Upjohn)		In 8 ml vials and 8 ml vials w/diluent.[3]
Rx	**Methylprednisolone Sodium Succinate** (Various, eg, Elkins Sinn, Lyphomed)	**Powder for Injection:** 1 g per vial	In 1, 8 and 50 ml vials.
Rx	**A-Methapred** (Abbott)		In 8 ml Univial and 500 mg ADD-Vantage vials.[4]
Rx	**Solu-Medrol** (Upjohn)		In 1 g vials, 1 g vials w/diluent and 8 ml Act-O-Vial.[4]
Rx	**Solu-Medrol** (Upjohn)	**Powder for Injection:** 2 g per vial	In 2 g vials w/diluent.

[1] With sodium phosphate anhydrous (1.6 mg monobasic, 17.5 mg dibasic), 25 mg lactose and 9 mg benzyl alcohol.

[2] With sodium phosphate anhydrous (1.6 mg monobasic, 17.4 mg dibasic), ≈ 18 mg benzyl alcohol.

[3] With sodium phosphate anhydrous (6.4 mg monobasic, 69.6 mg dibasic). May contain 36 to 70.2 mg benzyl alcohol.

[4] With sodium phosphate anhydrous (12.8 mg monobasic, 139.2 mg dibasic). May contain 66.8 to 141 mg benzyl alcohol.

[5] With sodium phosphate anhydrous (25.6 mg monobasic, 278 mg dibasic), 273 mg benzyl alcohol.

Glucocorticoids

METHYLPREDNISOLONE ACETATE

For complete prescribing information, refer to the Glucocorticoids group monograph.

Because of its low solubility, methylprednisolone acetate has a sustained effect.

Administration and Dosage:

Systemic: Not for IV use. As a temporary substitute for oral therapy, administer the total daily dose as a single IM injection. For prolonged effect, give a single weekly dose.

Adrenogenital syndrome – A single 40 mg injection IM every 2 weeks.

Rheumatoid arthritis – Weekly IM maintenance dose varies from 40 to 120 mg.

Dermatologic lesions – 40 to 120 mg IM weekly for 1 to 4 weeks. In severe dermatitis (eg, poison ivy), relief may result within 8 to 12 hours of a single dose of 80 to 120 mg IM. In chronic contact dermatitis, repeated injections every 5 to 10 days may be necessary. In seborrheic dermatitis, a weekly dose of 80 mg IM may be adequate.

Asthma and allergic rhinitis – 80 to 120 mg IM.

Intra-articular and soft tissue:

Large joints – 20 to 80 mg.

Medium joints – 10 to 40 mg.

Small joints – 4 to 10 mg.

Ganglion, tendinitis, epicondylitis and bursitis – 4 to 30 mg.

Intralesional: 20 to 60 mg.

Rx	**Methylprednisolone Acetate** (Various, eg, Rugby, Schein)	**Injection:** 20 mg per ml suspension	In 5 and 10 ml vials.
Rx	**Depo-Medrol** (Upjohn)		In 5 ml vials.[1]
Rx	**Methylprednisolone Acetate** (Various, eg, Dixon-Shane, Goldline, Major, Moore, Rugby, Schein, URL)	**Injection:** 40 mg per ml suspension	In 5 and 10 ml vials.
Rx	**Adlone** (UAD)		In 5 ml vials.
Rx	**depMedalone 40** (Forest)		In 5 ml vials.[1]
Rx	**Depoject** (Mayrand)		In 10 ml vials.[1]
Rx	**Depo-Medrol** (Upjohn)		In 1, 5 and 10 ml vials.[1]
Rx	**Depopred-40** (Hyrex)		In 5 and 10 ml vials.
Rx	**Duralone-40** (Hauck)		In 10 ml vials.[1]
Rx	**Medralone 40** (Keene)		In 5 ml vials.[1]
Rx	**M-Prednisol-40** (Pasadena)		In 5 ml vials.
Rx	**Methylprednisolone Acetate** (Various, Dixon-Shane, Goldline, Moore, Rugby, Schein, URL)	**Injection:** 80 mg per ml suspension	In 5 ml vials.
Rx	**Adlone** (UAD)		In 5 ml vials.
Rx	**depMedalone 80** (Forest)		In 5 ml vials.[1]
Rx	**Depoject** (Mayrand)		In 5 ml vials.[1]
Rx	**Depo-Medrol** (Upjohn)		In 1 and 5 ml vials.[1]
Rx	**Depopred-80** (Hyrex)		In 5 ml vials.
Rx	**D-Med 80** (Ortega)		In 5 ml vials.
Rx	**Duralone-80** (Hauck)		In 5 ml vials.[1]
Rx	**Medralone 80** (Keene)		In 5 ml vials.[1]
Rx	**M-Prednisol-80** (Pasadena)		In 5 ml vials.

[1] With polyethylene glycol and myristyl-gamma-picolinium chloride.

Glucocorticoids

DEXAMETHASONE, ORAL

For complete prescribing information, refer to the Glucocorticoids group monograph.

Administration and Dosage:

Initial dosage: 0.75 to 9 mg/day.

In acute, self-limited allergic disorders or acute exacerbations of chronic allergic disorders, the following dosage schedule combining parenteral and oral therapy (0.75 mg tablets) is suggested: Dexamethasone sodium phosphate injection, 4 mg/ml:

First day – 1 or 2 ml IM.
Second day – 4 tablets in 2 divided doses.
Third day – 4 tablets in 2 divided doses.
Fourth day – 2 tablets in 2 divided doses.
Fifth day – 1 tablet.
Sixth day – 1 tablet.
Seventh day – No treatment.
Eighth day – Follow-up visit.

Suppression tests:

For Cushing's syndrome – Give 1 mg at 11 pm. Draw blood for plasma cortisol determination the following day at 8 am. For greater accuracy, give 0.5 mg every 6 hours for 48 hours. Collect 24 hour urine to determine 17-hydroxycorticosteroid excretion.

Test to distinguish Cushing's syndrome due to pituitary ACTH excess from Cushing's syndrome due to other causes – Give 2 mg every 6 hours for 48 hours. Collect 24 hour urine to determine 17-hydroxycorticosteroid excretion.

Unlabeled uses: The dexamethasone suppression test has been used for the detection, diagnosis and management of depression; however, pending further evaluation and research, its value is unproven.

Rx	**Dexamethasone** (Various, eg, Major, Rugby)	**Tablets:** 0.25 mg	In 100s.
Rx	**Decadron** (MSD)		Lactose. (MSD 20). Orange, scored. Pentagonal. In 100s.
Rx	**Dexamethasone** (Various, eg, Bioline, Goldline, Roxane, Rugby)	**Tablets:** 0.5 mg	In 100s.
Rx	**Decadron** (MSD)		Lactose. (MSD 41). Yellow, scored. Pentagonal. In 100s and UD 100s.
Rx	**Dexameth** (Major)		In 100s.
Rx	**Dexone** (Solvay)		Lactose. (RR 3205). Yellow, scored. In 100s, UD 100s.
Rx	**Dexamethasone** (Various, eg, Bioline, Goldline, Parmed, Roxane, Rugby)	**Tablets:** 0.75 mg	In 100s and 1000s.
Rx	**Decadron** (MSD)		Lactose. (MSD 63). Bluish-green, scored. Pentagonal. In 12s, 100s and UD 100s.
Rx	**Dexameth** (Major)		In 100s and Unipak 12s.
Rx	**Dexone** (Solvay)		Lactose. (RR 3210). Green, scored. In 100s, UD 100s.
Rx	**Dexamethasone** (Roxane)	**Tablets:** 1 mg	(54 489). Yellow, scored. In 100s, 1000s and UD 100s.

Glucocorticoids

DEXAMETHASONE, ORAL

Rx	**Dexamethasone** (Various, eg, Bioline, Goldline, Roxane, Rugby)	**Tablets:** 1.5 mg	In 50s and 100s.
Rx	**Decadron** (MSD)		Lactose. (MSD 95). Pink, scored. Pentagonal. In 50s and UD 100s.
Rx	**Dexameth** (Major)		In 100s.
Rx	**Dexone** (Solvay)		Lactose. (RR 3215). Pink, scored. In 100s, UD 100s.
Rx	**Hexadrol** (Organon)		Peach, scored. In 100s.
Rx	**Dexamethasone** (Roxane)	**Tablets:** 2 mg	(54 662). White, scored. In 100s and UD 100s.
Rx	**Dexamethasone** (Various, eg, Bioline, Goldline, Rugby)	**Tablets:** 4 mg	In 50s and 100s.
Rx	**Decadron** (MSD)		Lactose. (MSD 97). White, scored. Pentagonal. In 50s & UD 100s.
Rx	**Dexameth** (Major)		In 100s.
Rx	**Dexone** (Solvay)		Lactose. (RR 3220). White, scored. In 100s, UD 100s.
Rx	**Hexadrol** (Organon)		Green, scored. In 100s.
Rx	**Dexamethasone** (Goldline)	**Tablets:** 6 mg	In 50s and 100s.
Rx	**Decadron** (MSD)		Lactose. (MSD 147). Green, scored. Pentagonal. In 50s and UD 100s.
Rx	**Hexadrol** (Organon)	**Tablets:** Therapeutic Pack	Six 1.5 mg tablets (peach, scored) and eight 0.75 mg tablets (white, scored).
Rx	**Dexamethasone** (Various, eg, Bioline, Geneva, Goldline, Major, PBI, Roxane, Rugby)	**Elixir:** 0.5 mg per 5 ml	In 100, 120, 240 and 500 ml, and UD 5 and 20 ml.
Rx	**Decadron** (MSD)		5% alcohol. Saccharin. In 100 and 237 ml.
Rx	**Hexadrol** (Organon)		5% alcohol. Sorbitol. Cherry flavor. In 120 ml.
Rx *sf*	**Dexamethasone** (Roxane)	**Oral Solution:** 0.5 mg per 5 ml	Dye free. Sorbitol. In 500 ml and UD 5 & 20 ml (100s).
Rx	**Dexamethasone Intensol** (Roxane)	**Oral Solution:** 0.5 mg per 0.5 ml	30% alcohol. In 30 ml w/dropper.

Glucocorticoids

DEXAMETHASONE ACETATE

For complete prescribing information, refer to the Glucocorticoids group monograph.

A long-acting repository preparation with prompt onset of action.

Administration and Dosage:

Not for IV use.

Systemic: 8 to 16 mg IM, may repeat in 1 to 3 weeks.

Intralesional: 0.8 to 1.6 mg.

Intra-articular and soft tissue: 4 to 16 mg; may repeat at 1 to 3 week intervals.

Rx	**Dexamethasone Acetate** (Various, eg, Bioline, Dixon-Shane, Goldline, Major, Moore, Rugby, URL)	**Injection**: 8 mg per ml (as acetate) suspension. Not for IV use.	In 5 ml vials.
Rx	**Dalalone L.A.** (Forest)		In 5 ml vials.[1]
Rx	**Decadron-LA** (MSD)		In 1 and 5 ml vials.[1]
Rx	**Decaject-L.A.** (Mayrand)		In 5 ml vials.
Rx	**Dexasone L.A.** (Hauck)		In 5 ml vials.[1]
Rx	**Dexone LA** (Keene)		In 5 ml vials.[1]
Rx	**Solurex LA** (Hyrex)		In 5 ml vials.
Rx	**Dalalone D.P.** (Forest)	**Injection**: 16 mg/ml (as acetate) suspension. Not for IV or intralesional use.	In 1 and 5 ml vial.[1]

[1] With creatinine, polysorbate 80, carboxymethylcellulose, sodium bisulfite, EDTA, benzyl alcohol.

Glucocorticoids

DEXAMETHASONE SODIUM PHOSPHATE

For complete prescribing information, refer to the Glucocorticoids group monograph.

Has a rapid onset and short duration of action compared to less soluble preparations.

Administration and Dosage:

Systemic:

Initial dosage – 0.5 to 9 mg daily. Usual dose ranges are ⅓ to ½ the oral dose given every 12 hours. However, in certain acute, life-threatening situations, dosages exceeding the usual may be justified and may be in multiples of the oral dosages.

Cerebral edema – In adults, administer an initial IV dose of 10 mg, followed by 4 mg IM every 6 hours until maximum response has been noted. Response is usually noted within 12 to 24 hours. Dosage may be reduced after 2 to 4 days and gradually discontinued over 5 to 7 days. For palliative management of patients with recurrent or inoperable brain tumors, maintenance therapy with either the injection or tablets in a dosage of 2 mg 2 or 3 times daily may be effective.

Unresponsive shock – Reported regimens range from 1 to 6 mg/kg as a single IV injection, to 40 mg initially followed by repeated IV injections every 2 to 6 hours while shock persists.

Intra-articular, intralesional or soft tissue:

Large joints – 2 to 4 mg.
Small joints – 0.8 to 1 mg.
Bursae – 2 to 3 mg.
Tendon sheaths – 0.4 to 1 mg.
Soft tissue infiltration – 2 to 6 mg.
Ganglia – 1 to 2 mg.

Rx	**Dexamethasone Sodium Phosphate** (Various, eg, Bioline, Dixon-Shane, Elkins Sinn, Geneva Marsam, Kendall McGaw, Lyphomed, Major, Moore, Rugby, URL)	**Injection**: 4 mg per ml dexamethasone phosphate (as sodium phosphate) solution	In 1, 5, 10 and 30 ml vials, 1 ml disp. syringe and 1 ml fill in 2 ml vials.
Rx	**Dalalone** (Forest)		In 5 ml vials.[1]
Rx	**Decadron Phosphate** (MSD)		In 1, 5 and 25 ml vials and 2.5 ml syringes.[2]
Rx	**Decaject** (Mayrand)		In 5 and 10 ml vials.
Rx	**Dexasone** (Hauck)		In 5, 10 and 30 ml vials.[3]
Rx	**Dexone** (Keene)		In 5 and 10 ml vials.[1]
Rx	**Hexadrol Phosphate** (Organon)		In 1 and 5 ml vials and 1 ml disp. syringe.[1]
Rx	**Solurex** (Hyrex)		In 5, 10 and 30 ml vials.
Rx	**Dexamethasone Sodium Phosphate** (Various, eg, Elkins-Sinn, Lyphomed, Schein)	**Injection**: 10 mg per ml dexamethasone phosphate (as sodium phosphate) solution	In 1 and 10 ml vials and 1 ml disp. syringe.
Rx	**Hexadrol Phosphate** (Organon)		In 10 ml (IV or IM) vials and 1 ml disp. syringe.[1]
Rx	**Hexadrol Phosphate** (Organon)	**Injection**: 20 mg per ml dexamethasone phosphate (as sodium phosphate solution)	In 5 ml vials (IV).[1]
Rx	**Decadron Phosphate** (MSD)	**Injection**: 24 mg/ml dexamethasone phosphate (as sodium phosphate) solution. For IV use only	In 5 and 10 ml vials.[4]

[1] With sodium sulfite and benzyl alcohol.
[2] With methyl and propyl parabens and sodium bisulfite.
[3] With sodium metabisulfite, EDTA and methyl and propyl parabens.
[4] With EDTA, methyl and propyl parabens and sodium bisulfite.

Glucocorticoids

DEXAMETHASONE SODIUM PHOSPHATE WITH LIDOCAINE HCl

For complete prescribing information, refer to the Glucocorticoids group monograph.

Dexamethasone sodium phosphate provides prompt activity. Lidocaine HCl is a local anesthetic with a rapid onset and a duration of 45 minutes to 1 hour (see Local Anesthetics).Steroid activity usually begins by the time the anesthesia wears off.

Administration and Dosage:

Soft tissue injection: Acute and subacute bursitis: 0.5 to 0.75 ml.

Acute and subacute nonspecific tenosynovitis – 0.1 to 0.25 ml.

Rx	**Decadron w/Xylocaine** (MSD)	**Injection:** 4 mg dexamethasone sodium phosphate and 10 mg lidocaine HCl per ml solution	In 5 ml vials.[1]

[1] With EDTA, parabens and sodium bisulfite.

BETAMETHASONE

For complete prescribing information, refer to the Glucocorticoids group monograph.

Administration and Dosage:

Initial dosage: 0.6 to 7.2 mg/day.

Rx	**Celestone** (Schering)	**Tablets:** 0.6 mg	(Schering BDA or 011). Pink, scored. In 100s and 500s and UD 21s (6 day).
		Syrup: 0.6 mg per 5 ml	< 1% alcohol. Sorbitol, sugar. In 118 ml.

BETAMETHASONE SODIUM PHOSPHATE

For complete prescribing information, refer to the Glucocorticoids group monograph.

Betamethasone phosphate is highly soluble, has a prompt onset and may be given IV.

Administration and Dosage:

Systemic and local: The initial dosage may vary up to 9 mg/day.

Rx	**Betamethasone Sodium Phosphate** (Various, eg, Major, Moore, Rugby, Schein)	**Injection:** 4 mg betamethasone sodium phosphate (equivalent to 3 mg betamethasone alcohol) per ml solution	In 5 ml vials.
Rx	**Celestone Phosphate** (Schering)		In 5 ml vials.[2]
Rx	**Cel-U-Jec** (Hauck)		In 5 ml vials.[2]

[2] With EDTA, phenol and sodium bisulfite.

Glucocorticoids

BETAMETHASONE SODIUM PHOSPHATE AND BETAMETHASONE ACETATE

For complete prescribing information, refer to the Glucocorticoids group monograph.

Betamethasone sodium phosphate provides prompt activity, while betamethasone acetate is only slightly soluble and affords sustained activity.

Administration and Dosage:

Systemic: Not for IV use.

Initial dose – 0.5 to 9 mg/day. Dosage ranges are ⅓ to ½ the oral dose given every 12 hours. In certain acute, life-threatening situations, dosages exceeding the usual may be justified and may be in multiples of oral dosages.

Intrabursal, intra-articular, intradermal and intralesional:

Bursitis, tenosynovitis, peritendinitis – 1 ml.

Rheumatoid arthritis and osteoarthritis – 0.5 to 2 ml.

Very large joints: 1 to 2 ml.

Large joints: 1 ml.

Medium joints: 0.5 to 1 ml.

Small joints: 0.25 to 0.5 ml.

Dermatologic conditions: 0.2 ml/cm^2 intradermally.

Maximum dose – 1 ml/week.

Foot disorders: The following doses are recommended at 3 to 7 day intervals:

Bursitis – Under heloma durum or heloma molle – 0.25 to 0.5 ml. Under calcaneal spur – 0.5 ml. Over hallux rigidus or digiti quinti varus – 0.5 ml.

Tenosynovitis, periostitis of cuboid – 0.5 ml.

Acute gouty arthritis – 0.5 to 1 ml.

Rx	**Betamethasone Sodium Phosphate/Betamethasone Acetate** (Major)	**Injection:** 3 mg betamethasone acetate and 3 mg betamethasone sodium phosphate per ml suspension	In 5 ml vials.
Rx	**Celestone Soluspan** (Schering)		In 5 ml vials.[3]

[3] With EDTA and benzalkonium chloride.

GLUCOCORTICOID RETENTION ENEMAS

For complete prescribing information, refer to the Glucocorticoids group monograph. For information on corticosteroid-containing preparations for anorectal use, refer to the Topicals section.

Actions:

Pharmacology: Hydrocortisone is partially absorbed following rectal administration. Ulcerative colitis patients have absorbed up to 50% of hydrocortisone administered by enema.

Indications:

Adjunctive therapy in the treatment of ulcerative colitis, including ulcerative proctitis, ulcerative proctosigmoiditis and left-sided ulcerative colitis. It has proved useful in some cases involving the transverse and ascending colons.

Contraindications:

Systemic fungal infections; ileocolostomy during immediate or early postoperative period.

Warnings:

If improvement fails to occur within 2 or 3 weeks, discontinue therapy. Symptomatic improvement may be misleading and should not be used as the sole criterion in judging efficacy. Sigmoidoscopic examination and x-ray visualization are essential for adequate monitoring.

Precautions:

Use with caution where there is a probability of impending perforation or abscess; pyogenic infections; intestinal anastomoses; obstruction; extensive fistulas and sinus tracts.

Adverse Reactions:

Local pain or burning; rectal bleeding; apparent exacerbations or sensitivity reactions.

HYDROCORTISONE RETENTION ENEMA

For complete prescribing information, refer to the Glucocorticoid Retention Enemas group monograph.

Administration and Dosage:

Usual course of therapy is 100 mg nightly for 21 days, or until clinical and proctological remission occurs. Clinical symptoms usually subside in 3 to 5 days. Improvement in mucosal appearance may lag behind clinical improvement. Difficult cases may require 2 or 3 months of treatment. If therapy exceeds 21 days, discontinue gradually.

Rx	**Cortenema** (Solvay)	**Retention Enema**: 100 mg per 60 ml unit.[1]

[1] In aqueous solution with carboxypolymethylene, polysorbate 80 and methylparaben.

Glucocorticoids

HYDROCORTISONE ACETATE INTRARECTAL FOAM

For complete prescribing information, refer to the Glucocorticoid Retention Enemas group monograph.

Indications:

Adjunctive therapy in the treatment of ulcerative proctitis of the distal portion of the rectum in patients who cannot retain corticosteroid enemas.

Contraindications:

Obstruction; abscess; perforation; peritonitis; recent intestinal anastomoses; extensive fistulas and sinus tracts.

Warnings:

Because the foam is not expelled, systemic hydrocortisone absorption may be greater than with corticosteroid enema formulations.

If no clinical or proctologic improvement occurs within 2 or 3 weeks, or if the patient's condition worsens, discontinue use.

Administer with caution to patients with severe ulcerative disease because these patients are predisposed to perforation of the bowel wall.

Administration and Dosage:

Usual dose is 1 applicatorful once or twice daily for 2 or 3 weeks, and every second day thereafter. Do not insert any part of the aerosol container into the anus. Satisfactory response usually occurs within 5 to 7 days. Sigmoidoscopy is recommended to judge dosage adjustment, duration of therapy and rate of improvement.

Rx	**Cortifoam** (Schwarz Pharma)	**Aerosol:** 90 mg/applicatorful	In 20 g (14 applications).

AMINOGLUTETHIMIDE

Actions:

Pharmacology: Aminoglutethimide inhibits the enzymatic conversion of cholesterol to Δ^5-pregnenolone, thereby reducing the synthesis of adrenal glucocorticoids, mineralocorticoids, estrogens and androgens. Aminoglutethimide blocks several other steps in steroid synthesis, including the hydroxylations required for the aromatization of androgens to estrogens. A decrease in adrenal secretion of cortisol is followed by an increased secretion of pituitary adrenocorticotropic hormone (ACTH), which will overcome the blockade of adrenocortical steroid synthesis by aminoglutethimide.

Pharmacokinetics: Aminoglutethimide is effectively absorbed orally and is minimally bound to plasma protein. Its half-life is 11 to 16 hours initially, but decreases after 1 to 2 weeks to 5 to 9 hours. Approximately 34% to 54% is excreted unchanged in the urine and 20% to 50% is excreted as the acetylated metabolite (less than one-fifth as active as the parent compound). The acetylation mechanism is genetically controlled.

Clinical trials: Morning levels of plasma cortisol in patients with adrenal carcinoma and ectopic ACTH-producing tumors were reduced on the average to about one half of the pretreatment levels, and in patients with adrenal hyperplasia to about two thirds of the pretreatment levels, during 1 to 3 months of therapy with aminoglutethimide. Data available from the few patients with adrenal adenoma suggest similar reductions in plasma cortisol levels. Measurements of plasma cortisol showed reductions to ≥ 50% of baseline or to normal levels in one third or more of the patients studied, depending on the diagnostic groups and time of measurement.

Indications:

Cushing's syndrome: For the suppression of adrenal function in selected patients with Cushing's syndrome.

Unlabeled uses: Aminoglutethimide has been used successfully in postmenopausal patients with advanced breast carcinoma and in patients with metastatic prostate carcinoma.

Aminoglutethimide was previously marketed as an anticonvulsant, but was withdrawn for that use in 1966.

Contraindications:

Hypersensitivity to glutethimide or aminoglutethimide.

Warnings:

Duration of therapy: Because aminoglutethimide does not affect the underlying disease process, it has been used primarily until more definitive therapy (ie, surgery) can be undertaken, or in cases where such therapy is not appropriate. Only a small number of patients have been treated for > 3 months. A decreased effect or escape from a favorable effect occurs more frequently in pituitary-dependent Cushing's syndrome, probably because of increasing ACTH levels in response to decreasing glucocorticoid levels.

Cortical hypofunction: May cause adrenal cortical hypofunction, especially under conditions of stress such as surgery, trauma or acute illness. Monitor patients carefully and give hydrocortisone and mineralocorticoid supplements as indicated. Do not use dexamethasone. (See Drug Interactions.)

Hypotension: Aminoglutethimide may suppress aldosterone production by the adrenal cortex and may cause orthostatic or persistent hypotension. Monitor blood pressure in all patients at appropriate intervals.

Pregnancy: Category D. Aminoglutethimide can cause fetal harm when administered to pregnant women. In about 5000 patients, two cases of pseudohermaphroditism were reported in female infants whose mothers took aminoglutethimide and concomitant anticonvulsants. Normal pregnancies have also occurred during the administration of the drug. When administered to rats at doses ½ to 3 times the maximum human dose, aminoglutethimide caused a decrease in fetal implantation, and increased fetal deaths, teratogenic effects and pseudohermaphroditism. If this drug must be used during pregnancy, or if the patient becomes pregnant while taking the drug, apprise her of the potential hazard to the fetus.

Lactation: It is not known whether this drug is excreted in breast milk. Decide whether to discontinue nursing or to discontinue the drug, taking into account the importance of the drug to the mother.

Children: Safety and efficacy have not been established.

Precautions:

Monitoring: Hypothyroidism may occur. Make appropriate clinical observations and perform thyroid function studies as indicated. Supplementary thyroid hormone may be required.

AMINOGLUTETHIMIDE

Hematologic abnormalities have been reported. Elevations in AST, alkaline phosphatase and bilirubin have been reported. Perform appropriate clinical observations and regular laboratory studies before and during therapy. Determine serum electrolytes periodically.

Drug Interactions:

Aminoglutethimide Drug Interactions			
Precipitant drug	Object drug*		Description
Aminoglutethimide	Anticoagulants	⬇	Anticoagulant effects may be decreased.
Aminoglutethimide	Dexamethasone	⬇	Possible loss of dexamethasone-induced adrenal suppression. If a corticosteroid is needed, substitute hydrocortisone.
Aminoglutethimide	Digitoxin	⬇	Digitoxin clearance may be increased.
Aminoglutethimide	Medroxyprogesterone	⬇	Medroxyprogesterone serum levels may be decreased.
Aminoglutethimide	Theophyllines	⬇	The action of theophyllines may be reduced.

* ⬇ = Object drug decreased.

Adverse Reactions:

Untoward effects have been reported in ≈ 67% of patients treated for ≥ 4 weeks in Cushing's syndrome. The most frequent effects are: Drowsiness (≈ 33%), morbilliform skin rash (17%), nausea and anorexia (12.5%). These are reversible and often disappear spontaneously within 1 or 2 weeks of continued therapy.

Cardiovascular: Hypotension, occasionally orthostatic (3%); tachycardia (2.5%).

CNS: Headache and dizziness, possibly caused by decreased vascular resistance or orthostasis (5%).

Dermatologic: Rash (17%, often reversible on continued therapy); pruritus (5%). These may be allergic or hypersensitivity reactions. Urticaria has occurred rarely.

Endocrine: Adrenal insufficiency occurred during ≥ 4 weeks of therapy in 3% of patients with Cushing's syndrome. Hypothyroidism, occasionally associated with thyroid enlargement, may be detected early or confirmed by measuring the plasma levels of the thyroid hormones. Masculinization and hirsutism in females and precocious sex development in males have occasionally occurred.

Hematologic: In 4 of 27 patients with adrenal carcinoma who were treated for at least 4 weeks, there were single occurrences of neutropenia, leukopenia (patient received mitotane concomitantly) and pancytopenia. One patient with adrenal hyperplasia showed decreased hemoglobin and hematocrit during treatment. In 1214 non-Cushingoid patients, transient leukopenia was reported once. Coombs-negative hemolytic anemia was reported in one patient. In ≈ 300 patients with nonadrenal malignancy, 4% of cases showed some degree of anemia and two developed pancytopenia. Thrombocytopenia and agranulocytosis have also occurred.

Hepatic: Isolated abnormal liver function tests; suspected hepatotoxicity (< 0.1%); cholestatic jaundice (hypersensitivity mechanism suspected).

Miscellaneous: Vomiting, myalgia (3%). Fever, possibly related to therapy, occurred in several patients on aminoglutethimide for < 4 weeks when given with other drugs.

Overdosage:

Symptoms: Overdosage has caused ataxia, somnolence, lethargy, dizziness, fatigue, coma, hyperventilation, respiratory depression, nausea and vomiting, loss of sodium and water, hyponatremia, hypochloremia, hyperkalemia, hypoglycemia, hypovolemic shock due to dehydration and hypotension. Extreme weakness has been reported with divided doses of 3 g/day. No reports of death following doses estimated as large as 7 g.

The signs and symptoms of acute overdosage with aminoglutethimide may be aggravated or modified if alcohol, hypnotics, tranquilizers or tricyclic antidepressants have been taken at the same time.

Treatment: Gastric lavage and supportive treatment have been employed. Full consciousness following deep coma was regained ≤ 40 hours after ingestion of 3 or 4 g without lavage. No evidence of hematologic, renal or hepatic effects were subsequently found. Consider dialysis in severe intoxication. Treatment includes usual supportive measures. Refer to General Management of Acute Overdosage.

AMINOGLUTETHIMIDE

Patient Information:

May produce drowsiness or dizziness; patients should observe caution while driving or performing other tasks requiring alertness, coordination or physical dexterity.

May cause rash, fainting, weakness or headache; notify physician if pronounced.

Nausea and loss of appetite may occur during the first 2 weeks of therapy; notify physician if these persist or become pronounced.

Administration and Dosage:

Institute treatment in a hospital until a stable dosage regimen is achieved.

Give 250 mg 4 times daily, preferably at 6 hour intervals. Follow adrenal cortical response by careful monitoring of plasma cortisol until the desired level of suppression is achieved. If cortisol suppression is inadequate, dosage may be increased in increments of 250 mg daily at intervals of 1 to 2 weeks to a total daily dose of 2 g.

Dose reduction or temporary discontinuation may be required in the event of adverse responses (ie, extreme drowsiness, severe skin rash or excessively low cortisol levels). If skin rash persists for > 5 to 8 days or becomes severe, discontinue the drug. It may be possible to reinstate therapy at a lower dosage following the disappearance of a mild or moderate rash.

Mineralocorticoid replacement therapy (ie, fludrocortisone) may be necessary. If glucocorticoid replacement therapy is needed, 20 to 30 mg hydrocortisone orally in the morning will replace endogenous secretion.

Rx	**Cytadren** (Ciba)	**Tablets:** 250 mg	(Ciba 24). White, scored. In 100s.

MIGLITOL

Actions:

Pharmacology: Miglitol is an alpha-glucoside inhibitor and desoxynojirimycin derivative that delays the digestion of ingested carbohydrates resulting in a smaller rise in blood glucose concentration following meals. Miglitol reduces levels of glycosylated hemoglobin in patients with Type II (non-insulin-dependent) diabetes mellitus. Systemic nonenzymatic protein glycosylation, as reflected by levels of glycosylated hemoglobin, is a function of average blood glucose concentration over time.

In contrast to sulfonylureas and thiazolidinediones, miglitol does not enhance insulin secretion or increase insulin sensitivity. The antihyperglycemic action of miglitol results from a reversible inhibition of membrane-bound intestinal glucoside hydrolase enzymes. Membrane-bound intestinal glucosidases hydrolyze oligosaccharides and disaccharides to glucose and other monosaccharides in the brush border of the small intestine. In diabetic patients, this enzyme inhibition results in delayed glucose absorption and lowering of postprandial hyperglycemia.

Miglitol has minor inhibitory activity against lactase and, at recommended doses, would not be expected to induce lactose intolerance.

Pharmacokinetics:

Absorption – Absorption of miglitol is saturable at high doses: a dose of 25 mg is completely absorbed, whereas a dose of 100 mg is only 50% to 70% absorbed. For all doses, peak concentrations are reached in 2 to 3 hours.

Distribution – The protein binding of miglitol is negligible (< 4%). Miglitol has a volume of distribution of 0.18 L/kg, consistent with distribution primarily into the extracellular fluid.

Metabolism – Miglitol is not metabolized. No metabolites have been detected in plasma, urine or feces, indicating a lack of either systemic or presystemic metabolism.

Excretion – Miglitol is eliminated by renal excretion as unchanged drug. Following a 25 mg dose, > 95% of the dose is recovered in the urine within 24 hours. At higher doses, the cumulative recovery of drug from urine is somewhat lower because of the incomplete bioavailability. The elimination half-life of miglitol from plasma is ≈ 2 hours.

Renal function impairment: Because miglitol is excreted primarily by the kidneys, accumulation of miglitol is expected in patients with renal impairment. Patients with creatinine clearance < 25 ml/min taking 25 mg 3 times/day exhibited a greater than 2–fold increase in miglitol plasma levels as compared with subjects with creatinine clearance > 60 ml/min. Dosage adjustment to correct the increased plasma concentrations is not feasible because miglitol acts locally. Little information is available on the safety of miglitol in patients with creatinine clearance < 25 ml/min.

Hepatic function impairment: Miglitol pharmacokinetics were not altered in cirrhotic patients. Because miglitol is not metabolized, no influence of hepatic function on the kinetics of miglitol is expected.

Clinical trials:

NIDDM patients on dietary treatment only – Miglitol was evaluated as monotherapy and as combination therapy for 1 year. A statistically significant smaller increase in mean glycosylated hemoglobin (HbA1c) was observed over time in the miglitol 50 mg 3 times/day monotherapy arm compared with placebo. Significant reductions in mean fasting and postprandial plasma glucose levels and in mean postprandial insulin levels were observed in the miglitol-treated patients.

In a 14–week study, there was a significant decrease in HbA1c in patients receiving miglitol 50 mg 3 times/day or 100 mg 3 times/day compared with postprandial plasma glucose and postprandial serum insulin levels.

Patients receiving sulfonylureas – One 14–week study included patients under treatment with maximal doses of sulfonylurea at entry. The mean treatment effects on HbA1c were - 0.82% and - 0.74% for patients receiving a sulfonylurea plus miglitol 50 mg 3 times/day and 100 mg 3 times/day, respectively.

At the end of a 1–year study in which miglitol 25, 50 or 100 mg 3 times/day was added to a maximal dose of glyburide (10 mg twice/day), the mean treatment effects on HbA1c were - 0.3%, - 0.62% and - 0.73%, respectively.

MIGLITOL

Indications:

Non-insulin-dependent diabetes (NIDDM):

Monotherapy adjunct to diet to improve glycemic control in patients with NIDDM whose hyperglycemia cannot be managed with diet alone.

Combination therapy – In combination with a sulfonylurea when diet plus either miglitol or a sulfonylurea alone do not result in adequate glycemic control. The effect of miglitol to enhance glycemic control is additive to that of sulfonylureas when used in combination, presumably because the mechanism of action is different.

Contraindications:

Diabetic ketoacidoses; inflammatory bowel disease; colonic ulceration; partial intestinal obstruction; patients predisposed to intestinal obstruction; chronic intestinal diseases associated with marked disorders of digestion or absorption or with conditions that may deteriorate as a result of increased gas formation in the intestine; hypersensitivity to the drug or any of its components.

Warnings:

GI symptoms are the most common reactions to miglitol. The incidence of diarrhea and abdominal pain tend to diminish considerably with continued treatment (see Adverse Reactions).

Renal function impairment: Plasma concentrations of miglitol in renally impaired volunteers were proportionally increased relative to the degree of renal dysfunction. Long-term clinical trials in diabetic patients with significant renal dysfunction (serum creatinine > 2 mg/dl) have not been conducted. Treatment of these patients with miglitol is not recommended.

Pregnancy: Category B. The safety of miglitol in pregnant women has not been established. There are no adequate and well-controlled studies in pregnant women. Use during pregnancy only if clearly needed.

Lactation: Miglitol is excreted in breast milk to a very small degree. Total excretion into milk accounted for 0.02% of a 100 mg maternal dose. The estimated exposure to a nursing infant is ≈ 0.4% of the maternal dose. Although the levels of miglitol reached in breast milk are exceedingly low, do not administer miglitol to a nursing woman.

Children: Safety and efficacy have not been established.

Precautions:

Monitoring: Monitor therapeutic response to miglitol by periodic blood glucose tests. Measurement of glycosylated hemoglobin levels is recommended for the monitoring of long-term glycemic control.

Hypoglycemia: Because of its mechanism of action, miglitol, when administered alone, should not cause hypoglycemia in the fasted or postprandial state. Sulfonylurea agents may cause hypoglycemia. Because miglitol given in combination with a sulfonylurea will cause a further lowering of blood glucose, it may increase the hypoglycemic potential of the sulfonylurea, although this was not observed in clinical trials. Use oral glucose (dextrose), whose absorption is not delayed by miglitol instead of sucrose (cane sugar) in the treatment of mild-to-moderate hypoglycemia. Sucrose, whose hydrolysis to glucose and fructose is inhibited by miglitol, is unsuitable for the rapid correction of hypoglycemia. Severe hypoglycemia may require the use of either IV glucose infusion or glucagon injection.

Blood glucose control: When diabetic patients are exposed to stress such as fever, trauma, infection or surgery, a temporary loss of control of blood glucose may occur. At such times, temporary insulin therapy may be necessary.

MIGLITOL

Drug Interactions:

Miglitol Drug Interactions			
Precipitant	Object drug*		Description
Miglitol	Digoxin	⬇	Coadministration may reduce the average plasma concentrations of digoxin by 19% to 28%. In one study in diabetic patients under treatment with digoxin, plasma digoxin concentrations of miglitol 100 mg 3 times/day × 14 days were not altered.
Miglitol	Glyburide	⬇	Decreased AUC and C_{max} values for glyburide occurred when coadministered with miglitol. These differences were not statistically significant.
Miglitol	Metformin	⬇	Mean AUC and C_{max} values for metformin were 12% to 13% lower when the volunteers were given miglitol as compared with placebo, but this difference was not statistically significant.
Miglitol	Propranolol	⬇	Miglitol may significantly reduce the bioavailability of propranolol by 40%.
Miglitol	Ranitidine	⬇	Miglitol may significantly reduce the bioavailability of ranitidine by 60%.
Digestive enzymes (eg, amylase, pancreatin)	Miglitol	⬇	Digestive enzyme preparations may reduce the effect of miglitol. Do not take concomitantly.
Intestinal adsorbents (eg, charcoal)	Miglitol	⬇	Intestinal adsorbents may reduce the effect of miglitol. Do not take concomitantly.

* ⬇ = Object drug decreased.

Adverse Reactions:

Dermatologic: Skin rash (4.3%, generally transient).

GI: Flatulence (41.5%); diarrhea (28.7%); abdominal pain (11.7%) (see Warnings).

Lab test abnormalities: Low serum iron (9.2%) usually does not persist in the majority of cases and is not associated with reductions in hemoglobin or changes in other hematologic indices.

Overdosage:

Unlike sulfonylureas or insulin, an overdose of miglitol will not result in hypoglycemia. An overdose may result in transient increases in flatulence, diarrhea and abdominal discomfort. Because of the lack of extra-intestinal effects seen with miglitol, no serious systemic reactions are expected in the event of an overdose.

Patient Information:

Take orally 3 times/day at the start (with the first bite) of each main meal. It is important to continue to adhere to dietary instructions, a regular exercise program and regular testing of urine or blood glucose.

Miglitol itself does not cause hypoglycemia even when administered to patients in the fasted state. Sulfonylurea drugs and insulin can lower blood sugar levels enough to cause symptoms or sometimes life-threatening hypoglycemia. Because miglitol given in combination with a sulfonylurea or insulin will cause a further lowering of blood sugar, it may increase the hypoglycemic potential of these agents. The risk of hypoglycemia, its symptoms and treatment, and conditions that predispose to its development should be well understood by patients and responsible family members. Because miglitol prevents the breakdown of table sugar, have a source of glucose (dextrose, D-glucose) available to treat the symptoms of low blood sugar when taking miglitol in combination with a sulfonylurea or insulin.

MIGLITOL

If side effects occur with miglitol, they usually develop during the first few weeks of therapy. They are most commonly mild-to-moderate dose-related GI effects, such as flatulence, soft stools, diarrhea or abdominal discomfort, and they generally diminish in frequency and intensity with time. Discontinuation of drug usually results in rapid resolution of these GI symptoms.

Administration and Dosage:

In initiating treatment for NIDDM, emphasize diet as the primary form of treatment. Caloric restriction and weight loss are essential in the obese diabetic patient. Proper dietary management alone may be effective in controlling blood glucose and symptoms of hyperglycemia. Also stress the importance of regular physical activity when appropriate. If this treatment program fails to result in adequate glycemic control, consider the use of miglitol. The use of miglitol must be viewed by the physician and patient as a treatment in addition to diet and not as a substitute for diet or as a convenient mechanism for avoiding dietary restraint.

There is no fixed dosage regimen for the management of diabetes mellitus with miglitol. Dosage of miglitol must be individualized on the basis of effectiveness and tolerance while not exceeding the maximum recommended dosage of 100 mg 3 times/day.

Initial dosage: The recommended starting dosage is 25 mg, given orally 3 times/day at the start (with the first bite) of each main meal. However, some patients may benefit by starting at 25 mg once daily to minimize GI adverse effects and gradually increasing the frequency of administration to 3 times/day.

Maintenance dosage: The usual maintenance dose of miglitol is 50 mg 3 times/day although some patients may benefit from increasing the dose to 100 mg 3 times/day. In order to allow adaptation to potential adverse effects, initiate miglitol therapy at a dosage of 25 mg 3 times/day, the lowest effective dosage, and then gradually titrated upward. After 4 to 8 weeks of the 25 mg 3 times/day regimen, increase the dosage to 50 mg 3 times/day for ≈ 3 months. Measure glycosylated hemoglobin at intervals of ≈ 3 months. If, at that time, the glycosylated hemoglobin level is not satisfactory, the dosage may be further increased to 100 mg 3 times/day, the maximum recommended dosage. Pooled data from controlled studies suggest a dose-response for HbA1c and 1–hour postprandial plasma glucose throughout the recommended dosage range. No single study has examined the effect on glycemic control of titrating patients' doses upwards within the same study. If no further reduction in postprandial glucose or glycosylated hemoglobin levels is observed with titration to 100 mg 3 times/day, consider lowering the dose.

Maximum dosage: The maximum recommended dosage of miglitol is 100 mg 3 times/day. In one clinical trial, 200 mg 3 times/day gave additional improved glycemic control but increased the incidence of the GI symptoms.

Combination with sulfonylureas: Sulfonylurea agents may cause hypoglycemia. There was no increased incidence of hypoglycemia in patients who took miglitol in combination with sulfonylurea agents compared with the incidence of hypoglycemia in patients receiving sulfonylureas alone. However, miglitol given in combination with a sulfonylurea will cause a further lowering of blood glucose and may increase the risk of hypoglycemia caused by the additive effects of the two agents. If hypoglycemia occurs, make appropriate adjustments in the dosage of these agents.

Rx	**Glyset** (Bayer)	**Tablets:** 25 mg	(GLYSET 25). In 100s and UD 100s.
		50 mg	(GLYSET 50). In 100s, 1000s and UD 100s.
		100 mg	(GLYSET 100). In 100s, 1000s and UD 100s.

ACARBOSE

Actions:

Pharmacology: Acarbose is an oral alpha-glucosidase inhibitor for use in the management of Type II (non-insulin-dependent) diabetes mellitus (NIDDM). Acarbose is an oligosaccharide obtained from fermentation processes of the microorganism, *Actinoplanes utahensis*. Acarbose is a complex oligosaccharide that delays the digestion of ingested carbohydrates, thereby resulting in a smaller rise in blood glucose concentration following meals. As a consequence of plasma glucose reduction, acarbose reduces levels of glycosylated hemoglobin in patients with NIDDM. Systemic nonenzymatic protein glycosylation, as reflected by levels of glycosylated hemoglobin, is a function of average blood glucose concentration over time.

In contrast to sulfonylureas, acarbose does not enhance insulin secretion. The antihyperglycemic action results from a competitive, reversible inhibition of pancreatic alpha-amylase and membrane-bound intestinal alpha-glucosidase hydrolase enzymes. Pancreatic alpha-amylase hydrolyzes complex starches to oligosaccharides in the lumen of the small intestine while the membrane-bound intestinal alpha-glucosidases hydrolyze oligosaccharides, trisaccharides and disaccharides to glucose and other monosaccharides in the brush border of the small intestine. In diabetic patients, this enzyme inhibition delays glucose absorption and lowers postprandial hyperglycemia.

Because its mechanism of action is different, the effect of acarbose to enhance glycemic control is additive to that of sulfonylureas when used in combination. In addition, acarbose diminishes the insulinotropic and weight-increasing effects of sulfonylureas.

Acarbose has no inhibitory activity against lactose and consequently would not be expected to induce lactose intolerance.

Pharmacokinetics:

Absorption – In a study of six healthy men, < 2% of an oral dose was absorbed as active drug, while ≈ 35% of total radioactivity from a 14C-labeled oral dose was absorbed. An average of 51% of an oral dose was excreted in the feces as unabsorbed drug-related radioactivity within 96 hours of ingestion. Because acarbose acts locally within the GI tract, this low systemic bioavailability of parent compound is therapeutically desired. Following oral dosing of healthy volunteers with 14C-labeled acarbose, peak plasma concentrations of radioactivity were attained 14 to 24 hours after dosing, while peak plasma concentrations of active drug were attained at ≈ 1 hour. The delayed absorption of acarbose-related radioactivity reflects the absorption of metabolites that may be formed by either intestinal bacteria or intestinal enzymatic hydrolysis.

Metabolism – Acarbose is metabolized exclusively within the GI tract, principally by intestinal bacteria, but also by digestive enzymes. A fraction of these metabolites (≈ 34% of the dose) was absorbed and subsequently excreted in the urine. At least 13 metabolites have been identified. The major metabolites have been identified as 4–methylpyrogallol derivatives (ie, sulfate, methyl and glucuronide conjugates). One metabolite (formed by cleavage of a glucose molecule from acarbose) also has alpha-glucosidase inhibitory activity. This metabolite, together with the parent compound recovered from the urine, accounts for < 2% of the total administered dose.

Excretion – The fraction of acarbose that is absorbed as intact drug is almost completely excreted by the kidneys. When acarbose was given IV, 89% of the dose was recovered in the urine as active drug within 48 hours. In contrast, < 2% of an oral dose was recovered in the urine as active (eg, parent compound and active metabolite) drug. This is consistent with the low bioavailability of the parent drug. The plasma elimination half-life of acarbose activity is ≈ 2 hours in healthy volunteers. Consequently, drug accumulation does not occur with 3 times/day dosing.

Special populations: The mean steady-state area under the curve (AUC) and maximum concentrations of acarbose were ≈ 1.5 times higher in elderly compared with young volunteers; however, these differences were not statistically significant. Patients with severe renal impairment (creatinine clearance [Ccr] < 25 ml/min/1.73m^2) attained ≈ 5 times higher peak plasma concentrations of acarbose and 6 times larger AUCs than volunteers with normal renal function.

Clinical trials:

NIDDM patients on dietary treatment only – Results from six controlled, fixed-dose, monotherapy studies of acarbose in the treatment of NIDDM (n = 769) were combined and a weighted average of the difference from placebo in the mean change from baseline in glycosylated hemoglobin (HbA1c) was calculated for each dose level as presented in the following table:

ACARBOSE

Mean Change in HbA1c in Fixed-Dose Acarbose Monotherapy Studies		
Dose of acarbose[1]	No. of patients (n)	Change in HbA1c (%)
25 mg tid	110	-0.44
50 mg tid	131	-0.77
100 mg tid	244	-0.74
200 mg tid[2]	231	-0.86
300 mg tid[2]	53	-1

[1] Acarbose was statistically significantly different from placebo at all doses. Although there were no statistically significant differences among the mean results for doses ranging from 50 to 300 mg tid, some patients may derive benefit from increasing the dosage from 50 to 100 mg tid.

[2] Although studies used a maximum dose of 200 or 300 mg tid, the maximum recommended dose for patients ≤ 60 kg is 50 mg tid; the maximum recommended dose for patients > 60 kg is 100 mg tid.

Results from these six fixed-dose, monotherapy studies were also combined to derive a weighted average of the difference from placebo in mean change from baseline for 1-hour postprandial plasma glucose levels. Acarbose was statistically significantly different from placebo at all doses with respect to effect on 1-hour postprandial plasma glucose. The 300 mg tid regimen was superior to lower doses, but there were no statistically significant differences from 50 to 200 mg tid.

NIDDM patients receiving sulfonylureas – Acarbose was studied as adjunctive therapy to sulfonylureas treatment in three studies. Study 1 involved patients under treatment at entry with diet alone who were subsequently randomized to four treatment groups. At the end of the study, patients in the acarbose plus tolbutamide group showed a mean treatment effect on glycosylated hemoglobin (HbA1c) of –1.78% and were receiving a significantly lower mean daily dose of tolbutamide than patients in the tolbutamide-alone group. Also, the efficacy in the acarbose plus tolbutamide group was significantly better than in the other three treatment groups. Study 2 involved patients taking background treatment with maximum daily doses of sulfonylureas. At the end of this study, the mean effect of the addition of acarbose to maximum sulfonylurea therapy was a change in HbA1c of –0.54%. In addition, there was a significantly greater proportion of patients in the acarbose plus sulfonylurea group who reduced their sulfonlyurea dose vs patients in the placebo plus sulfonylurea group. In study 3, the addition of acarbose to a background treatment of sulfonylurea produced an additional change in mean HbA1c of –0.8%.

Change in HbA1c with Acarbose Therapy				
		HbA1c (%)		
Study	Treatment	Mean baseline[1]	Mean change from baseline	Treatment difference[2]
1	Placebo	9.48	+0.05	-
	Acarbose 200[3] mg tid	9.19	-0.71	-0.76
	Tolbutamide 250-1000 mg tid (mean dose 2.4 g/day)	9.28	-1.22	-1.27
	Acarbose 200[3] mg tid + tolbutamide 250-1000 mg tid (mean dose 1.9 g/day)	8.99	-1.73	-1.78
2	Sulfonylurea + placebo	9.56	+0.24	-
	Sulfonylurea + acarbose 50-300[3] mg tid	9.64	-0.3	-0.54
3	Sulfonylurea + placebo	8	+0.1	-
	Sulfonylurea + acarbose 50-200[3] mg tid	8.1	-0.8	-0.9

[1] Normal range: 4%-6%

[2] The result of subtracting the placebo group average.

[3] Although studies used a maximum dose of 200 or 300 mg tid, the maximum recommended dose for patients ≤ 60 kg is 50 mg tid; the maximum recommended dose for patients > 60 kg is 100 mg tid.

ACARBOSE

Indications:

Hyperglycemia: As monotherapy as an adjunct to diet to lower blood glucose in patients with NIDDM whose hyperglycemia cannot be managed on diet alone.

Acarbose may also be used with a sulfonylurea when diet plus either acarbose or a sulfonylurea do not result in adequate glycemic control. The effect of acarbose to enhance glycemic control is additive to that of sulfonylureas when used in combination, presumably because its mechanism of action is different.

Contraindications:

Hypersensitivity to the drug; diabetic ketoacidosis of cirrhosis; inflammatory bowel disease; colonic ulceration; partial intestinal obstruction or predisposition to intestinal obstruction; chronic intestinal diseases associated with marked disorders of digestion or absorption; conditions that may deteriorate as a result of increased gas formation in the intestine.

Warnings:

Diet/physical activity: In initiating treatment for NIDDM, emphasize diet as the primary form of treatment. Caloric restriction and weight loss are essential in the obese diabetic patient. Proper dietary management alone may be effective in controlling blood glucose and symtoms of hyperglycemia. Also, stress regular physical activity when appropriate. If this treatment program fails to result in adequate glycemic control, consider the use of acarbose. The use of acarbose must be viewed by both the physician and patient as a treatment in addition to diet, and not as a substitute for diet or as a convenient mechanism for avoiding dietary restraint.

Renal function impairment: Plasma concentrations of acarbose in renally impaired volunteers were proportionally increased relative to the degree of renal dysfuntion. Long-term clinical trials in diabetic patients with significant renal dysfunction (serum creatinine > 2 mg/dl) have not been conducted. Therefore, treatment of these patients with acarbose is not recommended.

Carcinogenesis: In rats, acarbose treatment resulted in a significant increase in the incidence of renal tumors (adenomas and adenocarcinomas) and benign Leydig cell tumors. Further studies were performed to separate direct carcinogenic effects of acarbose from indirect effects resulting from the carbohydrate malnutrition induced by the large doses of acarbose employed in the studies. In these studies, the increased incidence of renal tumors found in the original studies did not occur.

Pregnancy: Category B. The safety and efficacy of acarbose in pregnant women has not been established. Use during pregnancy only if clearly needed. Because current information strongly suggests that abnormal blood glucose levels during pregnancy are associated with a higher incidence of congenital anomalies as well as increased neonatal morbidity and mortality, most experts recommend that insulin be used during pregnancy to maintain blood glucose levels as close to normal as possible.

Lactation: A small amount of radioactivity has been found in the milk of lactating rats after administration of radiolabeled acarbose. It is not known whether this drug is excreted in human breast milk. Do not administer to a nursing woman.

Children: Safety and efficacy have not been established.

Precautions:

Monitoring: Monitor therapeutic response to acarbose by periodic blood glucose tests. Measurement of glycosylated hemoglobin levels is recommended for the monitoring of long-term glycemic control.

Acarbose, particularly at doses in excess of 50 mg tid, may give rise to elevations of serum transaminases (see Lab Test Abnormalities) and, in rare instances, hyperbilirubinemia. It is recommended that serum transaminase levels be checked every 3 months during the first year of the treatment with acarbose and periodically thereafter. If elevated transaminases are observed, a reduction in dosage or withdrawal of therapy may be indicated, particularly if the elevations persist.

Hypoglycemia: Because of its mechanism of action, acarbose alone should not cause hypoglycemia in the fasted or postprandial state. Sulfonylurea agents may cause hypoglycemia. Because acarbose given in combination with a sulfonylurea will cause a further lowering of blood glucose, it may increase the hypoglycemic potential of the sulfonylurea. Use oral glucose (dextrose), with which absorption is not inhibited by acarbose, instead of sucrose (cane sugar) in the treatment of mild to moderate hypoglycemia. Sucrose, with which hydrolysis to glucose and fructose is inhibited by acarbose, is unsuitable for the rapid correction of hypoglycemia. Severe hypoglycemia may require the use of either IV glucose infusion or glucagon injection.

Lab test abnormalities:

Elevated serum transaminase levels – In clinical trials, at doses of 50 mg tid and 100 mg tid, the incidence of serum transaminase elevations with acarbose was the

ACARBOSE

same as with placebo. In long-term studies (≤ 12 months, and including acarbose doses up to 300 mg tid), treatment-emergent elevations of serum transaminases (AST or ALT) occurred in 15% of acarbose-treated patients vs 7% with placebo. These serum transaminase elevations appear to be dose-related. At doses > 100 mg tid, the incidence of serum transaminase elevations greater than three times the upper limit of normal was two to three times higher in the acarbose group than in the placebo group. These elevations were asymptomatic, reversible, more common in females and, in general, not associated with other evidence of liver dysfunction.

In international postmarketing experience in > 500,000 patients, 19 cases of serum transaminase elevations > 500 IU/L (12 of which were associated with jaundice) have been reported. Fifteen of these 19 cases received treatment with ≥ 100 mg tid and 13 of 16 patients for whom weight was reported weighed < 60 kg. In the 18 cases where follow-up was recorded, hepatic abnormalities improved or resolved upon discontinuation of acarbose.

Loss of blood glucose control: When diabetic patients are exposed to stress such as fever, trauma, infection or surgery, a temporary loss of control of blood glucose may occur. At such times, temporary insulin therapy may be necessary.

Certain drugs tend to produce hyperglycemia and may lead to loss of blood glucose control. These drugs include the thiazides and other diuretics, corticosteroids, phenothiazines, thyroid products, estrogens, oral contraceptives, phenytoin, nicotinic acid, sympathomimetics, calcium channel blocking drugs and isoniazid. When such drugs are administered to a patient receiving acarbose, closely observe the patient for loss of blood glucose control. When such drugs are withdrawn from a patient receiving acarbose in combination with sulfonylureas or insulin, closely observe patients for any evidence of hypoglycemia.

Drug Interactions:

Acarbose Drug Interactions			
Precipitant drug	Object drug*		Description
Digestive enzymes	Acarbose	⬇	Effect of acarbose may be reduced. Do not use concomitantly.
Intestinal absorbents (eg, charcoal)	Acarbose	⬇	Effect of acarbose may be reduced. Do not use concomitantly.

* ⬇ = Object drug decreased.

Adverse Reactions:

GI: GI symptoms are the most common reaction to acarbose. In trials, the incidences of abdominal pain, diarrhea and flatulence were 21%, 33% and 77%, respectively, with acarbose 50 to 300 mg tid, whereas the corresponding incidences were 9%, 12% and 32% with placebo. Abdominal pain and diarrhea tended to return to pretreatment levels over time, and the frequency and intensity of flatulence tended to abate with time. The increased GI tract symptoms in patients treated with acarbose is a manifestation of the mechansim of action of acarbose and is related to the presence of undigested cabohydrate in the lower GI tract. Rarely, these GI events may be severe and might be confused with paralytic ileus.

Lab test abnormalities: Small reductions in hematocrit occurred more often in acarbose-treated patients than in placebo-treated patients but were not associated with reductions in hemoglobin. Low serum calcium and low plasma vitamin B_6 levels were associated with acarbose therapy but were thought to be either spurious or of no clinical significance. Elevated serum transaminase levels have occurred (see Precautions).

Overdosage:

Unlike sulfonylureas or insulin, an overdose of acarbose will not result in hypoglycemia. An overdose may result in transient increases in flatulence, diarrhea and abdominal discomfort, which shortly subside.

Patient Information:

Tell patients to take acarbose orally three times a day at the start (with the first bite) of main meals. It is important that patients continue to adhere to dietary instructions, a regular exercise program and regular testing of urine or blood glucose.

ACARBOSE

Acarbose does not cause hypoglycemia even when administered in the fasted state. Sulfonylurea drugs and insulin, however, can lower blood sugar levels enough to cause symptoms or sometimes life-threatening hypoglycemia. Because acarbose given in combination with a sulfonylurea or insulin will cause a further lowering of blood sugar, it may increase the hypoglycemic potential of these agents. The risk of hypoglycemia, its symptoms and treatment, and conditions that predispose to its development should be well understood by the patient and family members. Because acarbose prevents the breakdown of table sugar, patients should have a readily available source of glucose (dextrose, D-glucose) to treat symptoms of low blood sugar when taking acarbose in combination with a sulfonylurea or insulin.

If side effects occur, they usually develop during the first few weeks of therapy. They are most commonly mild-to-moderate GI effects, such as flatulence, diarrhea or abdominal discomfort, and generally diminish in frequency and intensity with time.

Administration and Dosage:

Approved by the FDA on September 6, 1995.

There is no fixed dosage regimen for the management of diabetes mellitus with acarbose of any other pharmacologic agent. Dosage of acarbose must be individualized on the basis of both effectiveness and tolerance while not exceeding the maximum recommended dose of 100 mg 3 times daily. Acarbose should be taken three times daily at the start (with the first bite) of each main meal. Start at a low dose, with gradual dose escalation as described below, to both reduce GI side effects and permit identification of the minimum dose required for adequate glycemic control of the patient.

During treatment initiation and dose titration (see below), use 1–hour postprandial plasma glucose to determine the therpapeutic response to acarbose and identify the minimum effective dose for the patient. Thereafter, measure glycosylated hemoglobin at intervals of ≈ 3 months. The therapeutic goal should be to decrease both postprandial plasma glucose and glycosylated hemoglobin levels to normal or near normal by using the lowest effective dose of acarbose, either as monotherapy or in combination with sulfonylureas.

Initial dosage: The recommended starting dosage is 25 mg (half of a 50 mg tablet) given orally three times daily at the start (with the first bite) of each main meal.

Maintenance dosage: Adjust dosage at 4 to 8 week intervals based on 1–hour postprandial glucose levels and on tolerance. After the initial dosage of 25 mg tid, the dosage can be increased to 50 mg tid. Some patients may benefit from further increasing the dosage to 100 mg tid. The maintenance dose ranges from 50 to 100 mg tid. However, because patients with low body weight may be at increased risk for elevated serum transaminases, consider only patients with body weight > 60 kg for dose titration above 50 mg tid. If no further reduction in postprandial glucose or glycosylated hemoglobin levels is observed with titration to 100 mg tid, consider lowering the dose. Once an effective and tolerated dosage has been established, it should be maintained.

Maximum dosage: The maximum recommended dosage for patients ≤ 60 kg is 50 mg tid; for patients > 60 kg, 100 mg tid.

Patients receiving sulfonylureas: Sulfonylurea agents may cause hypoglycemia. Acarbose given in combination with a sulfonylurea will cause a further lowering of blood glucose and may increase the hypoglycemic potential of the sulfonylurea. If hypoglycemia occurs, make appropriate adjustments in the dosage of these agents.

Rx	**Precose** (Bayer)	**Tablets**: 50 mg	(Precose 50). White, scored. In 100s and UD 100s.
		100 mg	(Precose 100). White. In 100s and UD 100s.

Insulin

INSULIN

Actions:

Pharmacology: Insulin, secreted by the beta cells of the pancreas, is the principal hormone required for proper glucose use in normal metabolic processes. It is composed of two amino acid chains, A (acidic) and B (basic), joined together by disulfide linkages. Insulin preparations are commonly extracted from either beef or pork pancreas. Human insulin has minor but significant differences from animal insulin with respect to the amino acid sequence on the B-chain (see below). It is derived from a bio-synthetic process with strains of *E coli* (recombinant DNA; rDNA) or from a semisynthetic process in which pork insulin is enzymatically converted at the B-30 terminal amino acid to human insulin.

Insulin Amino Acids			
	A-Chain		B-Chain
Source	Position 8	Position 10	Position 30
Beef	Alanine	Valine	Alanine
Pork	Threonine	Isoleucine	Alanine
Human	Threonine	Isoleucine	Threonine

Human insulin may have a more rapid onset and shorter duration of action than pork insulin in some patients. However, the bioavailability of the insulins is identical when given SC. The human insulins are slightly less antigenic than either pork or beef insulins. Consider the potential for flocculation with human insulin. Human insulin is also the insulin of choice for patients with insulin allergy, insulin resistance, all pregnant patients with diabetes and any patient who uses insulin intermittently.

Insulin preparations are divided into three categories according to promptness, duration and intensity of action following SC administration: Rapid, intermediate or long-acting.

Crystalline regular insulin is prepared by precipitation in the presence of zinc chloride. Regular insulins available in the US are prepared at neutral pH; this improves stability. Modified forms have been developed to alter the pattern of activity.

PZI – Insulin and zinc react with the basic protein, protamine, to form a protein complex. When injected, it dissolves slowly and insulin is absorbed at a slow but steady rate.

Isophane (NPH) – A modified, crystalline protamine zinc insulin. Its effects are comparable to a mixture of 2 to 3 parts regular insulin and 1 part protamine zinc insulin.

Extended insulin zinc suspension (Ultralente) – Large crystals of insulin with high zinc content are collected and resuspended in a sodium acetate/sodium chloride solution. This relatively insoluble insulin is formed without a modifying protein.

Prompt insulin zinc suspension (Semilente) – Amorphous (noncrystalline) insulin precipitated at a high pH.

Insulin zinc suspension (Lente) – Stable mixture of 70% ultralente and 30% semilente.

Individual response to insulin varies and is affected by diet, exercise, concomitant drug therapy and other factors. Characteristics of various insulins given SC are compared below:

Pharmacokinetics and Compatibility of Various Insulins					
	Insulin Preparations	Onset (hrs)	Peak (hrs)	Duration (hrs)	Compatible mixed with
Rapid-Acting	Insulin Injection (Regular)	½ to 1	6 to 8		All
	Prompt Insulin Zinc Suspension (Semilente)	1 to 1½	5 to 10	12 to 16	Lente
Intermediate-Acting	Isophane Insulin Suspension (NPH)	1 to 1½	4 to 12	24	Regular
	Insulin Zinc Suspension (Lente)	1 to 2½	7 to 15	24	Regular, semilente
Long-Acting	Protamine Zinc Insulin Suspension (PZI)	4 to 8	14 to 24	36	Regular
	Extended Insulin Zinc Suspension (Ultralente)	4 to 8	10 to 30	> 36	Regular, semilente

INSULIN

Purified insulins – The beta cells form insulin from a single-chain precursor, proinsulin. Commercial preparations may contain small amounts of proinsulin and other related molecules due to incomplete conversion of the prohormone. These contaminants may contribute to adverse immunogenic responses including local or systemic allergic reactions, lipodystrophy and antibody formation. Chromatographic purification techniques significantly reduce the amount of proinsulin and other protein contaminants. All commercially available insulins in the US contain no more than 25 parts per million (ppm) proinsulin. "Improved single peak" insulin contains ≤ 20 ppm proinsulin and "purified" insulin contains ≤ 10 ppm proinsulin. Purified pork insulins have ≈ 1 ppm and human insulins (recombinant DNA and semisynthetic) have 0 and 1 ppm, respectively. These three are the least immunogenic insulins available. Internal specifications and the amount of zinc, excess protamine and preservatives vary per manufacturer.

Indications:

Diabetes mellitus type I (insulin-dependent).

Diabetes mellitus type II (non-insulin-dependent) that cannot be properly controlled by diet, exercise and weight reduction.

In hyperkalemia, infusion of glucose and insulin produces a shift of potassium into cells and lowers serum potassium levels.

Insulin injection (regular insulin) may be given IV or IM for rapid effect in severe ketoacidosis or diabetic coma.

Highly purified (single component) and human insulins: Local insulin allergy, immunologic insulin resistance, injection site lipodystrophy; temporary insulin use (ie, surgery, acute stress type II diabetes, gestational diabetes); newly diagnosed diabetics.

Warnings:

Change insulins cautiously and under medical supervision. Changes in purity, strength, brand, type or species source may require dosage adjustment. Teach patients using insulin to self monitor blood glucose levels and keep daily records of results.

Pregnancy may make diabetes management more difficult. Insulin is the drug of choice for diabetes control in pregnancy. Keep patients under close medical supervision. Rigid control of serum glucose and avoidance of ketoacidosis are desired throughout pregnancy. Following delivery, insulin requirements may drop for 24 to 72 hours, rising towards the normal pre-pregnancy dose during the next 6 weeks.

Lactation: Insulin does not pass into breast milk. Breastfeeding may decrease insulin requirements despite the increase in necessary caloric intake.

Precautions:

Insulin resistance occurs rarely. Insulin resistant patients require > 200 units of insulin/day for > 2 days in the absence of ketoacidosis or acute infection. Sometimes, the resistance is due to high levels of IgG antibodies to insulin. Insulin resistance may also occur in obese patients, patients with acanthosis nigricans and patients with insulin receptor defects; insulin resistance during infection may be due to a postreceptor defect. Hyperglycemia may be managed by changing insulin species source (ie, beef or mixed beef-pork to pork or huma insulin). May give corticosteroids if changing the insulin is not effective. Corticosteroids may decrease IgG production or decrease insulin binding to the antibody. Monitor closely for signs of hyperglycemia and for adverse effects of high-dose corticosteroids. Highly concentrated insulin (U-500) may also be given to insulin-resistant patients. Use caution to avoid hypoglycemia. Some Type II patients with insulin resistance have been treated with a combination of glyburide plus insulin (see Administration and Dosage).

Hypoglycemia may result from excessive insulin dose or may be due to: Increased work or exercise without eating; food not being absorbed in the usual manner because of postponement or omission of a meal or in illness with vomiting, fever or diarrhea; when insulin requirements decline.

Eating sugar or a sugar-sweetened product will often correct the condition and prevent more serious symptoms. Commercial products containing 40% glucose are also available; glucagon may be used and IV dextrose may be necessary (see individual monographs). If hypoglycemic symptoms occur, notify a physician promptly.

In acute, usually suicidal overdoses of insulin, successful management has included excision of the injection site.

Symptoms of hypoglycemia are less pronounced with human insulin than with animal-based products. Warn patients using human insulin of this possibility.

INSULIN

Diabetic ketoacidosis, a potentially life-threatening condition, requires prompt diagnosis and treatment. Hyperglucagonemia, hyperglycemia and ketoacidosis may result. Diabetic ketoacidosis may result from stress, illness or insulin omission, or may develop slowly after a long period of insulin control. Treat with fluids, correction of acidosis and hypotension, and low-dose regular insulin IM or IV infusion.

Symptoms of Hypoglycemia vs Ketoacidosis

Reaction	Onset	Urine glucose/ acetone	Symptoms				
			CNS	Respiration	Mouth/GI	Skin	Miscellaneous
Hypoglycemic reaction (insulin reaction)	sudden	0/0	fatigue weakness nervousness confusion headache diplopia convulsions psychoses dizziness unconsciousness	rapid shallow	numb tingling hunger nausea	pallor moist shallow or dry	normal or noncharacteristic pulse eyeballs normal
Ketoacidosis (diabetic coma)	gradual (hours or days)	+/+	drowsiness dim vision	air hunger	thirst acetone breath nausea vomiting abdominal pain loss of appetite	dry flushed	rapid pulse soft eyeballs

Insulin allergy:

Local – Occasionally, redness, swelling and itching at the injection site may develop. This occurs if the injection is not properly made, if the skin is sensitive to the cleansing solution or if the patient is allergic to insulin or insulin additives (ie, preservatives). The condition usually resolves in a few days to a few weeks. A change in the type or species source of insulin may be tried.

Systemic reactions, less common, may present as a rash, shortness of breath, fast pulse, sweating, a drop in blood pressure, anaphylaxis or angioedema and may be life-threatening. Perform a skin test on patients with severe systemic reactions with each new preparation prior to initiating therapy with that preparation.

Lipodystrophy:

Lipoatrophy is the breakdown of adipose tissue at the insulin injection site causing a depression in the skin. It may be the result of an immune response or when less pure insulins are administered. Injection of human or purified pork insulins into the site over a 2 to 4 week period may result in SC fat accumulation.

Lipohypertrophy is the result of repeated insulin injection into the same site. It is the accumulation of SC fat and it may interfere with insulin absorption from the site. This condition may be avoided by rotating the injection site.

Diet: Patients must follow a prescribed diet and exercise regularly. Determine the time, number and amount of individual doses and distribution of food among the meals of the day. Do not change this regimen unless prescribed otherwise.

INSULIN

Drug Interactions:

Decrease Hypoglycemic Effect of Insulin		Increase Hypoglycemic Effect of Insulin	
Contraceptives, oral	Epinephrine	Alcohol	MAO inhibitors
Corticosteroids	Smoking	Anabolic steroids	Phenylbutazone
Dextrothyroxine	Thiazide diuretics	Beta-blockers[1]	Salicylates
Diltiazem	Thyroid hormone	Clofibrate	Sulfinpyrazone
Dobutamine		Fenfluramine	Tetracyclines
		Guanethidine	

[1] Nonselective beta blockers may delay recovery from hypoglycemic episodes and mask their signs/symptoms. Cardioselective agents may be alternatives.

Patient Information:

Use same type and brand syringe to avoid dosage errors. Rotate sites to prevent lipodystrophy. If using "pen-filled" device, follow information for proper use in insert.

Do not change the order of mixing insulins (if applicable) or change the brand, strength, type, species or dose without your physician's knowledge.

Insulin requirements may change in patients who become ill, especially with vomiting or fever. Consult a physician.

See your dentist twice yearly; see an ophthalmologist regularly.

Patient information inserts are available; read and understand all aspects of insulin use. Patients must receive complete instructions about the nature of diabetes. Strict adherence to prescribed diet, exercise program and personal hygiene are essential.

Patients should wear diabetic identification (Medic-Alert) so appropriate treatment can be given if complications occur away from home.

Monitor blood glucose and urine for glucose and ketones as prescribed; monitor blood pressure regularly.

Administration and Dosage:

The number and size of daily doses, time of administration and diet and exercise require continuous medical supervision. Dosage adjustment may be necessary when changing types of insulin, particularly when changing from single-peak to the more purified animal or human insulins.

For insulin suspensions, ensure uniform dispersion by rolling the vial gently between hands. Avoid vigorous shaking that may result in the formation of air bubbles or foam. Regular insulin should be a clear solution.

Administer maintenance doses SC. Rotate administration sites to prevent lipodystrophy. A general rule is to not administer within 1 inch of the same site for 1 month. The rate of absorption is more rapid when the injection is in the abdomen (possibly > 50% faster), followed by the upper arm, thigh and buttocks. Therefore, it may be best to rotate sites within an area rather than rotating areas. Give regular insulin IV or IM in severe ketoacidosis or diabetic coma.

Dosage guidelines: Individualize doses and monitor closely patients with diabetes mellitus; the following dosage guidelines may be considered.

Children and adults – 0.5 to 1 U/kg/day.

Adolescents (during growth spurt) – 0.8 to 1.2 U/kg/day.

Adjust doses to achieve premeal and bedtime blood glucose levels of 80 to 140 mg/dl (children < 5 years of age, 100 to 200 mg/dl).

Storage: Proper storage is critical. Insulin preparations being used are generally stable if stored at room temperature (and not exposed to extreme temperatures or direct sunlight). Discard partially filled bottles if the insulin has not been used for several weeks. Always store extra bottles in the refrigerator; do not freeze.

Insulin prefilled in plastic or glass syringes is stable for 1 week under refrigeration according to one manufacturer. However, there is some documentation that insulin in plastic syringes is stable for at least 14 days. Further studies are needed.

Insulin mixtures: When mixing 2 types of insulin, always draw clear regular insulin into syringe first. Patients stabilized on mixtures should have a consistent response if the mixing is standardized. An unexpected response is most likely when switching from separate injections to use of mixture or vice versa. To avoid dosage error, do not alter order of mixing insulins or change model or brand of syringe or needle. Each different type of insulin used must be of the same concentration (units/ml).

NPH/regular mixtures of insulin are now available from the manufacturer in premixed formulations of 70% NPH and 30% regular. A 50/50 combination will also be available soon. NPH/regular combinations of insulin are stable and are absorbed as if injected separately. In mixtures of regular and lente insulins, binding is detect-

INSULIN

able 5 minutes to 24 hours after mixing. If the regular/lente mixtures are not administered within the first 5 minutes after mixing, the effect of the regular insulin is diminished. The excess zinc binds with the regular and forms a lente type insulin. It is thus critical that mixtures of regular with the lente insulins be mixed and injected immediately.

These mixtures remain stable for 1 month at room temperature or for 3 months under refrigeration. These mixtures can also be stored in prefilled plastic or glass syringes for 1 week to possibly 14 days under refrigeration. Keep filled syringes in a vertical or oblique position with the needle pointing upward to avoid plugging problems. Prior to injection, pull back the plunger, and tip the syringe back and forth and slightly agitate to remix the insulins. Check for normal appearance.

Semilente, ultralente and lente insulins may be mixed in any ratio; they are chemically identical and differ only in size and structure of insulin particles. These mixtures are stable 1 month at room temperature or 3 months under refrigeration.

Insulin adsorption onto plastic IV infusion sets has reportedly removed up to 80% of a dose, but 20% to 30% is more common. Percent adsorbed is inversely proportional to insulin concentration; it takes place within 30 to 60 minutes. Because this phenomenon cannot be accurately predicted, patient monitoring is essential.

Concomitant sulfonylurea therapy: Insulin and oral sulfonylurea coadministration has been used with some success in type II diabetic patients who are difficult to control with diet and sulfonylurea therapy alone. Further study is needed, however.

INSULIN INJECTION

For complete prescribing information, refer to the Insulin group monograph in the Antidiabetic Agents section.

otc	**Regular Iletin** I (Lilly)	**Injection:** 100 units per ml Beef and pork.	In 10 ml bottles.
otc	**Regular Insulin** (Novo Nordisk)	**Injection:** 100 units per ml Pork.	In 10 ml vials.
otc	**Pork Regular Iletin** II (Lilly)	**Injection:** 100 units per ml Purified pork.	In 10 ml bottles.
otc	**Regular Purified Pork Insulin** (Novo Nordisk)		In 10 ml vials.
otc	**Humulin R** (Lilly)	**Injection:** 100 units per ml Human insulin (rDNA).	In 10 ml bottles.
otc	**Novolin R** (Novo Nordisk)		In 10 ml vials.
otc	**Velosulin Human** (Novo Nordisk)	**Injection:** 100 units per ml Human insulin (semisynthetic).	In 10 ml vials.
Rx	**Humalog** (Lilly)	**Injection:** 100 units per ml insulin lispro.	In 10 ml vials or 1.5 ml cartridges.
otc	**Novolin R PenFill** (Novo Nordisk)	**Cartridges:** 100 units per ml Human insulin (rDNA). For use with *NovoPen*	In 1.5 ml.

ISOPHANE INSULIN SUSPENSION (NPH)

For complete prescribing information, refer to the Insulin group monograph in the Antidiabetic Agents section.

Insulin combined with protamine and zinc.

otc	**NPH Iletin** I (Lilly)	**Injection:** 100 units per ml Beef and pork.	In 10 ml bottles.
otc	**NPH Insulin** (Novo Nordisk)	**Injection:** 100 units per ml Beef.	In 10 ml vials.
otc	**NPH-N** (Novo Nordisk)	**Injection:** 100 units per ml Purified pork.	In 10 ml vials.
otc	**Pork NPH Iletin** II (Lilly)		In 10 ml bottles.

Insulin

ISOPHANE INSULIN SUSPENSION (NPH)

otc	**Humulin N** (Lilly)	**Injection:** 100 units per ml Human insulin (rDNA).	In 10 ml bottles.
otc	**Novolin N** (Novo Nordisk)		In 10 ml vials.
otc	**Novolin N PenFill** (Novo Nordisk)	**Cartridges:** 100 units per ml Human insulin (rDNA). For use with *NovoPen*	In 1.5 ml.

ISOPHANE INSULIN SUSPENSION AND INSULIN INJECTION

For complete prescribing information, refer to the Insulin group monograph in the Antidiabetic Agents section.

70% isophane insulin and 30% insulin injection. Provides rapid activity (onset ½ hour) with a duration of up to 24 hours. Maximal effect is within 4 to 8 hours.

otc	**Humulin 70/30** (Lilly)	**Injection:** 100 units per ml Human insulin (rDNA).	In 10 ml bottles.
otc	**Novolin 70/30** (Novo Nordisk)		In 10 ml vials.
otc	**Novolin 70/30 PenFill** (Novo Nordisk)	**Cartridges:** 100 units per ml Human insulin (rDNA). For use with *NovoPen*	In 1.5 ml.

ISOPHANE INSULIN SUSPENSION AND INSULIN INJECTION

For complete prescribing information, refer to the Insulin group monograph in the Antidiabetic Agents section.

50% isophane insulin and 50% insulin injection.

otc	**Humulin 50/50** (Lilly)	**Injection:** 100 units per ml Human Insulin (rDNA).	In 10 ml vials.

INSULIN ZINC SUSPENSION (LENTE)

For complete prescribing information, refer to the Insulin group monograph in the Antidiabetic Agents section.

70% crystalline and 30% amorphous insulin suspension. Has an intermediate duration of activity; duration of effect is approximately 24 hours.

otc	**Lente Iletin I** (Lilly)	**Injection:** 100 units per ml Beef and pork.	In 10 ml bottles.
otc	**Lente Iletin II** (Lilly)	**Injection:** 100 units per ml Purified pork.	In 10 ml bottles.
otc	**Lente L** (Novo Nordisk)		In 10 ml vials.
otc	**Humulin L** (Lilly)	**Injection:** 100 units per ml Human insulin (rDNA).	In 10 ml bottles.
otc	**Novolin L** (Novo Nordisk)		In 10 ml vials.

INSULIN ZINC SUSPENSION, EXTENDED (ULTRALENTE)

For complete prescribing information, refer to the Insulin group monograph in the Antidiabetic Agents section.

Takes effect 4 to 8 hours after injection; activity lasts more than 36 hours.

otc	**Humulin U Ultralente** (Lilly)	**Injection:** 100 units per ml Human insulin (rDNA).	In 10 ml bottles.

High Potency Insulin

INSULIN INJECTION CONCENTRATED

For complete prescribing information, refer to the Insulin group monograph in the Antidiabetic Agents section.

Actions:

Pharmacology:

Insulin resistance – Diabetes can usually be controlled with daily insulin doses of 40 to 60 units or less; however, an occasional patient develops such resistance or becomes so unresponsive to the effect that daily doses of several hundred or even several thousand units are required. Patients who require doses in excess of 300 to 500 units daily usually have impaired insulin receptor function.

Occasionally, the cause of insulin resistance can be found (eg, hemochromatosis, liver cirrhosis, some complicating disease of endocrine glands other than the pancreas, obesity, allergy, infection), but in other cases, no cause can be determined.

Pharmacokinetics: Concentrated insulin injection is not modified by any agent that might prolong its action. It frequently has a duration similar to repository insulin; a single dose demonstrates activity for 24 hours. This has been credited to the high concentration of the preparation.

Indications:

Treatment of diabetic patients with marked insulin resistance (requirements > 200 units/day). A large dose may be administered SC in a reasonable volume.

Contraindications:

Patients with a history of systemic allergic reactions to pork or mixed beef/pork insulin should not receive the product unless they have been successfully desensitized.

Warnings:

Dosage adjustments: Most patients will show a "tolerance" to insulin, so that minor dosage variations will not cause untoward symptoms of insulin shock. It is not possible to identify which patients will require a dosage reduction to avoid hypoglycemia. However, a small number of patients may require dosage adjustments. Adjustment may be needed with the first dose or may be required over a period of several weeks. Symptoms of either hypoglycemia or hyperglycemia may occur.

Insulin shock: Observe extreme caution in the measurement of dosage; inadvertent overdose may result in irreversible insulin shock. Serious consequences may result if not used under constant medical supervision.

Hypersensitivity: Less common than local allergic reactions (see Adverse Reactions), but potentially more serious, is systemic insulin allergy, which may cause generalized urticaria, dyspnea or wheezing and may, on continued use, progress to anaphylaxis. Do not use IV; allergic or anaphylactoid reactions may develop.

If a severe allergic reaction occurs, discontinue the drug and treat the patient with the usual agents (eg, epinephrine, antihistamines, corticosteroids). In such patients, perform a skin test with another insulin preparation before its initiation. Desensitization procedures may permit resumption of insulin administration. Refer to Management of Acute Hypersensitivity Reactions.

High Potency Insulin

INSULIN INJECTION CONCENTRATED

Precautions:

Monitoring: Monitor blood glucose closely and often until dosage is established. Some may require only one dose daily, others may require two or three injections per day.

Insulin resistance: Patients with immunologic insulin resistance to beef insulin (this diagnosis is usually confirmed by the finding of increased serum antibody titers) may require an immediate dosage reduction of 20% to 50% when treated with pork or human insulin. Insulin resistance is frequently self-limited; after several weeks or months of high dosage, responsiveness may be regained and dosage reduced.

Adverse Reactions:

Hypoglycemic reactions may occur. However, secondary hypoglycemic reactions may develop 18 to 24 hours after injection. Consequently, observe patients carefully, and initiate prompt treatment with glucagon injections, glucose by IV injection or gavage.

Hypersensitivity: Erythema, swelling or pruritus may occur at injection sites. Such localized allergic manifestations usually resolve in a few days or weeks (see Warnings).

Administration and Dosage:

Administer SC or IM. Do not inject IV (allergic or anaphylactoid reactions may develop).

Use a tuberculin syringe for dosage measurement. Dosage variations are frequent in the insulin-resistant patient, since the individual is unresponsive to the pharmacologic effect of the insulin. Nevertheless, encourage accuracy of measurement because of the potential danger of the preparations.

Storage: Keep in a cold place, preferably in a refrigerator. Avoid freezing.

Rx	**Regular (Concentrated) Iletin** II U-500 (Lilly)	**Injection**: 500 units per ml purified pork.	In 20 ml vials.[1]

[1] With 0.25% m-cresol and 1.6% glycerin.

SULFONYLUREAS

The sulfonylurea hypoglycemic agents are sulfonamide derivatives, but are devoid of antibacterial activity. These agents are divided into two groups: First generation (acetohexamide, chlorpropamide, tolazamide, tolbutamide) and second generation (glipizide, glyburide). They are used as adjuncts to diet and exercise in the treatment of non-insulin-dependent diabetes mellitus (NIDDM). NIDDM has also been referred to as adult-onset or maturity-onset diabetes, ketosis-resistant diabetes and Type II diabetes.

NIDDM is characterized by insulin resistance and defects in insulin secretion.

Guidelines for oral hypoglycemic therapy in NIDDM patients may include:

- Onset of diabetes at ≥ 40 years of age
- Obese or normal body weight
- Duration of diabetes < 5 years
- Absence of ketoacidosis
- Fasting serum glucose ≤ 200 mg/dl
- Insulin requirement < 40 units/day
- Absence of renal or hepatic dysfunction

Actions:

Pharmacology: The sulfonylurea hypoglycemic agents appear to lower blood glucose by stimulating insulin release from beta cells in the pancreatic islets possibly due to increased intracellular cAMP. These agents are only effective in patients with some capacity for endogenous insulin production. They may improve the binding between insulin and insulin receptors or increase the number of insulin receptors. Hypoglycemic effects seem to be due to improved beta cell sensitivity or extrapancreatic effects (suppression of glucagon release and hepatic glucose production) occurring in the liver, and on insulin sensitivity of peripheral tissues.

Other pharmacologic activity includes: Potentiation of the effect of antidiuretic hormone (ADH); tolazamide, acetohexamide, glyburide and glipizide may produce a mild diuresis; acetohexamide has significant uricosuric activity.

Pharmacokinetics: The sulfonylureas are well absorbed after oral administration. All sulfonylureas except glipizide can be taken with food. Absorption of glipizide is delayed by food; it is more effective when taken about 30 minutes before a meal. Tolazamide is absorbed more slowly than the other sulfonylureas. They are metabolized in the liver to active and inactive metabolites and are excreted primarily in the urine. Glyburide is excreted as metabolites in the bile and urine, approximately 50% by each route. The hypoglycemic effects of sulfonylureas may be prolonged in severe liver disease due to decreased metabolism.

Although the mechanisms of action and maximal hypoglycemic effects are similar, the second and first generation sulfonylureas differ. Second generation compounds possess a more nonpolar or lipophilic side chain. Therapeutically effective doses and serum concentrations of the second generation sulfonylureas are lower, due to their higher intrinsic potency. All sulfonylureas are strongly bound to plasma proteins, primarily albumin. Protein binding of the first generation sulfonylureas is ionic; that of the second generation agents is predominantly nonionic. The clinical therapeutic significance of this difference is unknown; however, because they are bound to albumin by ionic bindings, the first generation agents may be more likely to be displaced by drugs which competitively bind to proteins (eg, warfarin, phenylbutazone). Displacement of sulfonylurea agents from protein would result in greater hypoglycemic response (see Drug Interactions).

Differences exist among the sulfonylureas in the duration of hypoglycemic effects (see following table). Tolbutamide is short-acting because it is rapidly metabolized to an inactive metabolite; it may be useful in patients with kidney disease. The active metabolite of acetohexamide is 2.5 times as potent as the parent compound. Because the metabolite is excreted in the urine, the duration of action of acetohexamide is prolonged in renal disease. Tolazamide has two active metabolites which are less potent than the parent compound. The renal elimination of chlorpropamide may be sensitive to changes in urinary pH; urinary alkalinization increases its excretion in the urine. When the urine pH is < 6, urinary excretion decreases and hepatic metabolism is the primary route of elimination. The half-life of chlorpropamide is prolonged in renal disease.

SULFONYLUREAS

Major Pharmacokinetic Parameters of the Sulfonylureas						
Sulfonylureas	Equivalent doses (mg)	Doses/ day	Serum t½ (hrs)	Onset (hrs)	Duration (hrs)	Metabolism
First generation						
Acetohexamide	500	1-2	6-8 (parent drug + metabolite)	1	12-24	Reduced in liver to potent active metabolite
Chlorpropamide	250	1	36	1	Up to 60	80% metabolized in liver; metabolite activity unknown
Tolazamide	250	1	7	4-6	12-24	Several mildly active metabolites
Tolbutamide	1000	2-3	4.5-6.5	1	6-12	Oxidized in liver to inactive metabolites
Second generation						
Glipizide	10	1-2	2-4	1-1.5	10-16	Liver metabolism to inactive metabolites
Glyburide Nonmicronized	5	1-2	10	2-4	24	Liver metabolism to weakly active metabolites
Micronized	3	1-2	≈ 4	1	24	

Indications:

As an adjunct to diet to lower the blood glucose in patients with non-insulin-dependent diabetes mellitus (Type II) whose hyperglycemia cannot be controlled by diet alone.

Unlabeled uses: **Chlorpropamide** in doses of 200 to 500 mg/day has been used in the treatment of neurogenic diabetes insipidus.

Sulfonylureas have been used as temporary adjuncts to insulin therapy in selected NIDDM patients to improve diabetic control (see Administration and Dosage).

Contraindications:

Hypersensitivity to sulfonylureas; diabetes complicated by ketoacidosis, with or without coma; sole therapy of insulin-dependent (Type I) diabetes mellitus; diabetes when complicated by pregnancy.

Warnings:

The administration of oral hypoglycemic drugs has been associated with increased cardiovascular mortality as compared to treatment with diet alone or diet plus insulin. Despite controversy regarding its interpretation, this warning is based on the study conducted by the University Group Diabetes Program (UGDP). This long-term prospective clinical trial involving 823 patients evaluated the effectiveness of glucose-lowering drugs in preventing or delaying vascular complications in patients with non-insulin-dependent diabetes. (*Diabetes* 1970;19[Suppl 2]:747-830.)

Patients treated for 5 to 8 years with diet plus tolbutamide (1.5 g/day) had a rate of cardiovascular mortality approximately 2.5 times that of patients treated with diet alone. A significant increase in total mortality was not observed. Consider this for other sulfonylureas as well.

Inform the patient of potential risks, advantages and alternative modes of therapy.

Bioavailability: Micronized glyburide 3 mg tablets provide serum concentrations that are *not* bioequivalent to those from the conventional formulation (nonmicronized) 5 mg tablets. Therefore, retitrate patients when transferring patients from any hypoglycemic agent to micronized glyburide.

Renal/Hepatic function impairment: Oral hypoglycemic agents are metabolized in the liver. The drugs and most of their metabolites are excreted by the kidneys. Hepatic impairment may result in inadequate release of glucose in response to hypoglycemia. Renal impairment may cause decreased elimination of sulfonylureas leading to accumulation producing hypoglycemia. Therefore, use these agents with caution in NIDDM patients with renal or hepatic impairment, and monitor renal and liver function frequently.

SULFONYLUREAS

Elderly: Elderly and debilitated patients are particularly susceptible to the hypoglycemic action of the sulfonylureas. Hypoglycemia may be difficult to recognize in the elderly. Use with caution.

Pregnancy: (*Category C. Category B – Glyburide*). Sulfonylureas (except glyburide) are teratogenic in animals. There are no adequate studies in pregnant women. Use only if clearly needed. In general, avoid sulfonylureas in pregnancy; they will not provide good control in patients who cannot be controlled by diet alone.

Because abnormal blood glucose levels during pregnancy may be associated with a higher incidence of congenital abnormalities, insulin is recommended to maintain blood glucose levels as close to normal as possible. However, fetal mortality and major congenital anomalies generally occur 3 to 4 times more often in offspring of diabetic mothers.

Labor and delivery – Prolonged severe hypoglycemia (4 to 10 days) has occurred in neonates born to mothers on a sulfonylurea at the time of delivery. This has been reported more frequently with agents with prolonged half-lives. If used during pregnancy, discontinue at least 2 days to 4 weeks before expected delivery date.

Lactation: Chlorpropamide and tolbutamide are excreted in breast milk. A chlorpropamide breast milk concentration of 5 mcg/ml has been detected following a 500 mg dose (normal peak blood level after 250 mg is 30 mcg/ml). It is not known if other sulfonylureas are excreted in breast milk. Because of the potential for hypoglycemia in nursing infants, decide whether to discontinue nursing or the drug.

Children: Safety and efficacy in children have not been established.

Precautions:

Monitoring: Keep patients under continuous medical supervision. During the initial test period, the patient should communicate with the physician daily, and report at least weekly for the first month for physical examination and evaluation of diabetic control. After the first month, examine at monthly intervals or as indicated. Uncooperative individuals may be unsuitable for treatment with oral agents.

During the transitional period, test the urine for glucose and acetone at least three times daily and have the results reviewed by a physician frequently. Measurement of glycosylated hemoglobin is also useful. It is important that patients be taught to correctly and frequently self-monitor blood glucose.

Hyperglycemia is a major risk factor in the development of diabetic complications. Maintaining blood glucose levels helps prevent the progression of nephropathy, neuropathy and retinopathy. Hyperglycemia is also associated with the risk factors of atherosclerosis.

Diet and exercise remain the primary considerations of diabetic patient management. Caloric restriction and weight loss are essential in the obese diabetic. These drugs are an adjunct to, not a substitute for, dietary regulation. Also, loss of blood glucose control on diet alone may be transient, thus requiring only short-term sulfonylurea therapy. Identify cardiovascular risk factors and take corrective measures where possible.

Hypoglycemia: All sulfonylureas may produce severe hypoglycemia. Proper patient selection, dosage and instructions are important to avoid hypoglycemic episodes. Renal or hepatic insufficiency may elevate drug blood levels and the latter may also diminish gluconeogenic capacity, both of which increase the risk of serious hypoglycemic reactions. Elderly, debilitated or malnourished patients, and those with adrenal or pituitary insufficiency are particularly susceptible to the hypoglycemic action of glucose-lowering drugs. Hypoglycemia may be difficult to recognize in the elderly, and in patients taking β-adrenergic blocking drugs. Hypoglycemia is more likely to occur when caloric intake is deficient, after severe or prolonged exercise, when alcohol is ingested or when more than one glucose-lowering drug is used.

Because of the long half-life of chlorpropamide, patients who become hypoglycemic during therapy require careful supervision of the dose and frequent feedings for at least 3 to 5 days. Hospitalization and IV glucose may be necessary.

Asymptomatic patients: Controlling blood glucose in NIDDM with sulfonylureas has not been definitely established to be effective in preventing the long-term cardiovascular or neural complications of diabetes.

Loss of blood glucose control: When a patient stabilized on any diabetic regimen is exposed to stress such as fever, trauma, infection or surgery, a loss of control may occur. At such times, it may be necessary to discontinue drug and give insulin.

The effectiveness of any oral hypoglycemic in lowering blood glucose to a desired level decreases in many patients over time (secondary failure); this may be due to progression of the severity of the diabetes or to diminished drug responsiveness. Adequately adjust dose and assess adherence to diet before classifying a patient as

SULFONYLUREAS

a secondary failure. Primary failure occurs when the drug is ineffective in a patient when first given. Certain patients who demonstrate an inadequate response or true primary or secondary failure to one sulfonylurea may benefit from a transfer to another sulfonylurea.

Disulfiram-like syndrome: A sulfonylurea-induced facial flushing reaction may occur when some sulfonylureas are administered with alcohol. This syndrome is characterized by facial flushing and occasional breathlessness but without the nausea, vomiting and hypotension seen with a true alcohol-disulfiram reaction. The facial flushing reaction occurs in approximately 33% of NIDDM patients taking chlorpropamide and alcohol. It is uncertain whether glyburide and glipizide can cause the facial flushing reaction.

Syndrome of inappropriate secretion of antidiuretic hormone (SIADH): Water retention and dilutional hyponatremia have occurred after administration of sulfonylureas to NIDDM patients, especially those with congestive heart failure or hepatic cirrhosis. The drugs stimulate antidiuretic hormone (ADH) release, augmenting hypothalamic-pituitary release of ADH. The result is excessive water retention, hyponatremia, low serum osmolality and high urine osmolality.

Glipizide, acetohexamide, tolazamide and glyburide are mildly diuretic.

Drug Interactions:

Sulfonylurea Drug Interactions

Precipitant drug	Object drug*		Description
Androgens Anticoagulants Chloramphenicol Clofibrate Fenfluramine Fluconazole Gemfibrozil Histamine H_2 antagonists Magnesium salts Methyldopa MAO inhibitors Phenylbutazone Probenecid Salicylates Sulfinpyrazone Sulfonamides Tricyclic antidepressants Urinary acidifiers	Sulfonylureas	⬆	The hypoglycemic effect of the sulfonylureas may be enhanced due to various mechanisms (eg, decreased hepatic metabolism, inhibition of renal excretion, displacement from protein binding sites, decreased blood glucose or alteration of carbohydrate metabolism).
Beta blockers Cholestyramine Diazoxide Hydantoins Rifampin Thiazide diuretics Urinary alkalinizers	Sulfonylureas	⬇	The hypoglycemic effect of the sulfonylureas may be decreased due to various mechanisms (eg, increased hepatic metabolism, decreased insulin release, increased renal excretion).
Charcoal	Sulfonylureas	⬇	Charcoal can reduce the absorption of the sulfonylureas; depending on the clinical situation, this will reduce their efficacy or toxicity.
Ethanol	Sulfonylureas	⟷	Ethanol may prolong but not augment glipizide-induced reductions in blood glucose. Chronic ethanol use may decrease the half-life of tolbutamide. Ethanol ingestion by patients taking chlorpropamide may result in a disulfiram-like reaction (see Precautions).
Sulfonylureas	Digitalis glycosides	⬆	Concurrent administration may result in increased digitalis serum levels.

* ⬆ = Object drug increased ⬇ = Object drug decreased ⟷ = Undetermined effect

SULFONYLUREAS

Drug/Lab test interactions: A metabolite of tolbutamide in the urine may give a false-positive reaction for **albumin** if measured by the acidification-after-boiling test, which causes the metabolite to precipitate. There is no interference with the sulfosalicylic acid test.

Drug/Food interactions: Absorption of glipizide is delayed by about 40 minutes when taken with food; the drug is more effective when given approximately 30 minutes before a meal. The other sulfonylureas may be taken with food.

Adverse Reactions:

Hypoglycemia: See Precautions.

Dermatologic: Allergic skin reactions; eczema; pruritus; erythema; urticaria; morbilliform or maculopapular eruptions; lichenoid reactions. These may be transient and may disappear despite continued use of the drug; if skin reactions persist, discontinue the drug. Porphyria cutanea tarda; photosensitivity reactions.

Endocrine: Reactions identical to the syndrome of inappropriate secretion of antidiuretic hormone (SIADH). See Precautions.

GI: GI disturbances (eg, nausea, epigastric fullness, heartburn) are the most common reactions. They tend to be dose-related and may disappear when dosage is reduced. Diarrhea (glipizide); taste alteration (tolbutamide); cholestatic jaundice (rare, discontinue the drug if this occurs).

Hematologic: Leukopenia; thrombocytopenia; aplastic anemia; agranulocytosis; hemolytic anemia; pancytopenia; hepatic porphyria.

Lab test abnormalities: Elevated liver function tests; occasional mild to moderate elevations in BUN and creatinine.

Miscellaneous: Disulfiram-like reactions (see Precautions); weakness; paresthesia; tinnitus; fatigue; dizziness; vertigo; malaise; headache (infrequent).

Overdosage:

Symptoms: Overdosage can produce hypoglycemia. In order of general appearance, the signs and symptoms associated with hypoglycemia include: Tingling of lips and tongue; nausea; diminished cerebral function (lethargy, yawning, confusion, agitation, nervousness); increased sympathetic activity (tachycardia, sweating, tremor, hunger) and ultimately, convulsions, stupor and coma.

Treatment: Treat mild hypoglycemia without loss of consciousness or neurologic findings aggressively with oral glucose and adjustments in drug dosage or meal patterns. Continue close monitoring until the patient is stabilized. Severe hypoglycemic reactions occur infrequently, but require immediate hospitalization. If hypoglycemic coma is suspected, rapidly inject concentrated (50%) dextrose IV. Follow by a continuous infusion of more dilute (10%) dextrose at a rate that will maintain the blood glucose at a level of about 100 mg/dl. Closely monitor for a minimum of 24 to 48 hours since hypoglycemia may recur after apparent clinical recovery. Because of the long half-life of **chlorpropamide**, patients who become hypoglycemic from this drug require close supervision for a minimum of 3 to 5 days.

In one patient with renal failure on hemodialysis, charcoal hemoperfusion shortened the half-life of chlorpropamide following an overdose. Charcoal administration also reduces the absorption of the sulfonylureas and may reduce their toxicity.

Patient Information:

Patients must receive full and complete instructions about the nature of diabetes. Strict adherence to prescribed diet, an exercise program, personal hygiene and avoidance of infection are essential. It is important to teach patients to self-monitor blood glucose.

Do not discontinue medication except on the advice of a physician.

May cause GI upset; may be taken with food. Take glipizide ≈ 30 minutes before a meal to increase effectiveness.

Avoid alcohol (disulfiram reaction and interference with blood sugar control) and salicylates except on professional advice.

Monitor urine for glucose and ketones as prescribed; monitor blood glucose as prescribed.

Notify physician if any of the following occurs:

Hypoglycemia: Fatigue, excessive hunger, profuse sweating, numbness of extremities.

Hyperglycemia: Excessive thirst or urination, urinary glucose or ketones.

Other: Fever, sore throat, rash, unusual bruising or bleeding.

SULFONYLUREAS

Administration and Dosage:

Institution of therapy: Individualize therapy. Selection of an individual agent is influenced by the drug's potency, duration of action, metabolism, adverse reactions and the patient's personal preference.

Short-term administration of sulfonylureas may be sufficient during periods of transient loss of control in patients usually well controlled on diet.

Transfer from other hypoglycemic agents:

Sulfonylureas – When transferring patients from one oral hypoglycemic agent to another, no transitional period and no initial or priming dose is necessary. However, when transferring patients from chlorpropamide, exercise particular care during the first 2 weeks because the prolonged retention of chlorpropamide in the body and subsequent overlapping drug effects may provoke hypoglycemia.

Insulin – During insulin withdrawal period, test blood for glucose and urine for ketones 3 times daily and report results to physician daily. The following may be used as a guide to determine daily insulin requirement.

Insulin Requirement When Instituting Sulfonylurea Therapy

Insulin dose	Insulin requirement
< 20 units	Start directly on oral agent and discontinue insulin abruptly.
20-40 units	Initiate oral therapy with concurrent 25% to 50% reduction in insulin dose. Further reduce insulin as response is observed. With glyburide, insulin may be discontinued immediately.
> 40 units	Initiate oral therapy with concurrent 20% to 50% reduction in insulin dose. Further reduce insulin as response is observed.

Elderly patients may be particularly sensitive to these agents; therefore, start with a lower initial dose before breakfast, and check blood and urine glucose during the first 24 hours of therapy. If control is satisfactory, continue or gradually increase dose. If there is a tendency toward hypoglycemia, reduce dose or discontinue the drug.

Acute complications: During the course of intercurrent complications (eg, ketoacidosis, severe trauma, major surgery, infections, severe diarrhea, nausea, vomiting), supportive therapy with insulin may be necessary. Continue or withdraw sulfonylurea therapy while insulin is used. Insulin is indispensable in managing acute complications; carefully instruct all diabetics in its use.

Combination insulin therapy: Concurrent administration of insulin and an oral sulfonylurea (generally glipizide or glyburide) has been used with some success in Type II diabetic patients who are difficult to control with diet and sulfonylurea therapy alone. One proposed method is referred to as the BIDS system: Bedtime insulin, usually NPH, in combination with a daytime (morning only or morning and evening) sulfonylurea, usually glyburide.

Sulfonylureas

CHLORPROPAMIDE

For complete prescribing information, refer to the Sulfonylureas group monograph in the Antidiabetic Agents section.

Administration and Dosage:

Initial dose: 250 mg/day in the mild to moderately severe, middle-aged, stable diabetic patient; use 100 to 125 mg/day in older patients.

Maintenance therapy: ≤ 100 to 250 mg/day. Severe diabetics may require 500 mg/day. Avoid doses > 750 mg/day.

Rx	**Chlorpropamide** (Various, eg, Geneva, Major, Mylan, Parmed, Rugby)	**Tablets:** 100 mg	In 100s, 250s, 500s, 1000s and UD 100s.
Rx	**Diabinese** (Pfizer)		(393). Blue, scored. D-shaped. In 100s, 500s and UD 100s.
Rx	**Chlorpropamide** (Various, eg, Geneva, Goldline, Major, Mylan, Parmed, Rugby, Schein)	**Tablets:** 250 mg	In 100s, 500s, 1000s and UD 100s.
Rx	**Diabinese** (Pfizer)		(394) Blue, scored. D-shaped. In 100s, 250s, 1000s, UD 100s.

ACETOHEXAMIDE

For complete prescribing information, refer to the Sulfonylureas group monograph in the Antidiabetic Agents section.

Administration and Dosage:

Initial dose: 250 mg to 1.5 g/day. Patients on ≤ 1 g daily can be controlled with once-daily dosage. Those receiving 1.5 g/day usually benefit from twice-daily dosage before morning and evening meals. Doses > 1.5 g/day are not recommended.

Rx	**Acetohexamide** (Various, eg, Raway, Schein)	**Tablets:** 250 mg	In 100s.
Rx	**Dymelor** (Lilly)		White, scored. In 200s.
Rx	**Acetohexamide** (Various, eg, Schein)	**Tablets:** 500 mg	In 100s.
Rx	**Dymelor** (Lilly)		Yellow, scored. In 50s and 200s.

Sulfonylureas

TOLAZAMIDE

For complete prescribing information, refer to the Sulfonylureas group monograph in the Antidiabetic Agents section.

Administration and Dosage:

Initial dose: 100 to 250 mg/day with breakfast or the first main meal. If fasting blood sugar (FBS) is < 200 mg/dl, use 100 mg/day; if FBS is > 200 mg/dl, use 250 mg/day. If patients are malnourished, underweight, elderly or not eating properly, use 100 mg once a day. Adjust dose to response. If > 500 mg/day is required, give in divided doses twice daily. Doses > 1 g/day are not likely to improve control.

Rx	**Tolazamide** (Various, eg, Goldline, Major, Moore, Rugby, UDL, Zenith)	**Tablets:** 100 mg	In 100s, 250s and UD 100s.
Rx	**Tolinase** (Upjohn)		(Tolinase 100). White, scored. In unit-of-use 100s.
Rx	**Tolazamide** (Various, eg, Goldline, Major, Moore, Mylan, Rugby, UDL, Zenith)	**Tablets:** 250 mg	In 100s, 200s, 250s, 500s, 1000s and UD 100s.
Rx	**Tolinase** (Upjohn)		(Tolinase 250). White, scored. In 200s, 1000s, UD 100s and unit-of-use 100s.
Rx	**Tolazamide** (Various, eg, Goldline, Major, Moore, Mylan, Rugby, UDL, Zenith)	**Tablets:** 500 mg	In 100s, 250s, 500s and UD 100s.
Rx	**Tolinase** (Upjohn)		(Tolinase 500). White, scored. In unit-of-use 100s.

TOLBUTAMIDE

For complete prescribing information, refer to the Sulfonylureas group monograph in the Antidiabetic Agents section.

Administration and Dosage:

Initial dose: 1 to 2 g/day. Total dose may be taken in the morning, but divided doses may allow increased GI tolerance.

Maintenance dose: 0.25 to 3 g. A maintenance dose > 2 g/day is seldom required.

Rx	**Tolbutamide** (Various, eg, Goldline, Mylan, Schein, UDL)	**Tablets:** 500 mg	In 100s, 500s, 1000s and UD 100s.
Rx	**Orinase** (Upjohn)		Lactose. (Orinase 500). White, scored. In 200s and unit-of-use 100s.

Sulfonylureas

GLIPIZIDE

For complete prescribing information, refer to the Sulfonylureas group monograph in the Antidiabetic Agents section.

Administration and Dosage:

Give ≈ 30 minutes before a meal to achieve the greatest reduction in postprandial hyperglycemia.

Initial dose: 5 mg, given ≈ 30 minutes before breakfast. Geriatric patients or those with liver disease may be started on 2.5 mg.

Adjust dosage in 2.5 to 5 mg increments, as determined by blood glucose response. Several days should elapse between titration steps. If response to a single dose is not satisfactory, dividing that dose may prove effective. The maximum recommended once-daily dose is 15 mg. The maximum recommended total daily dose is 40 mg.

Maintenance dose: Some patients may be controlled on a once-a-day regimen, while others show better response with divided dosing. Divide total daily doses > 15 mg and give before meals of adequate caloric content. Total daily doses > 30 mg have been safely given on a twice-daily basis to long-term patients.

Rx	**Glipizide** (Various, eg, Mylan, Schein, UDL)	**Tablets:** 5 mg	In 100s, 500s and UD 100s.
Rx	**Glucotrol** (Pfizer)		Lactose. (Pfizer 411). Dye free. White, scored. Diamond shape. In 100s, 500s and UD 100s.
Rx	**Glipizide** (Various, eg, Mylan, Schein, UDL)	**Tablets:** 10 mg	In 100s, 500s and UD 100s.
Rx	**Glucotrol** (Pfizer)		Lactose. (Pfizer 412). Dye free. White, scored. Diamond shape. In 100s, 500s and UD 100s.
Rx	**Glucotrol XL** (Pfizer)	**Tablets, extended release:** 5 mg	White. In 100s and 500s.
		10 mg	White. In 100s and 500s.

GLIMEPIRIDE

For complete prescribing information, refer to the Sulfonylureas group monograph in the Antidiabetic Agents section.

Administration and Dosage:

Approved by the FDA November 30, 1995.

Initial dose: 1 to 2 mg once daily, given with breakfast or the first main meal. Patients sensitive to hypoglycemic drugs should begin at 1 mg once daily; titrate carefully. Maximum starting dose is ≤ 2 mg.

Maintenance dose: 1 to 4 mg once daily. The maximum recommended dose is 8 mg once daily. After a dose of 2 mg is reached, increase dose at increments of ≤ 2 mg at 1 to 2 week intervals based on the patient's blood glucose response.

Combination insulin therapy: The recommended dose is 8 mg once daily with the first main meal with low-dose insulin.

Transfer from other hypoglycemic agents:

Sulfonylureas – When transferring patients to glimepiride, no transition period is necessary (see Sulfonylureas group monograph).

Storage/Stability: Dispense in well-closed containers with safety closures. Store between 15° to 30°C (59° and 86°F).

Rx	**Amaryl** (Hoechst-Roussel)	**Tablets:** 1 mg	Lactose. (Amaryl Hoechst). Pink. Oblong. In 100s and UD 100s.
		2 mg	Lactose. (Amaryl Hoechst). Green. Oblong. In 100s and UD 100s.
		4 mg	Lactose. (Amaryl Hoechst). Blue. Oblong. In 100s and UD 100s.

Sulfonylureas

GLYBURIDE (Glibenclamide)

For complete prescribing information, refer to the Sulfonylureas group monograph in the Antidiabetic Agents section.

Administration and Dosage:

DiaBeta/Micronase:

Initial dose – 2.5 to 5 mg daily, administered with breakfast or the first main meal. For patients who may be more sensitive to hypoglycemic drugs, start at 1.25 mg daily.

Maintenance dose – 1.25 to 20 mg daily. Give as a single dose or in divided doses. Increase in increments of no more than 2.5 mg at weekly intervals based on the patient's blood glucose response. Daily doses > 20 mg are not recommended.

Glynase:

Initial dose – 1.5 to 3 mg/day, administered with breakfast or the first main meal. For patients who may be more sensitive to hypoglycemic drugs, start at 0.75 mg/day.

Maintenance dose – 0.75 to 12 mg/day. Give as a single dose or in divided doses; some patients, particularly those receiving > 6 mg/day, may have a more satisfactory response with twice-daily dosing. Increase in increments of no more than 1.5 mg at weekly intervals based on the patient's blood glucose response. Daily doses > 12 mg are not recommended.

Rx	**Glyburide** (Various, eg, Allscrips, Copley, Coventry, Geneva, Goldline, Rugby, Schein)	**Tablets**: 1.25 mg	In 50s and 100s.
Rx	**DiaBeta** (Hoechst Marion Roussel)		White, scored. Oblong. In 50s.
Rx	**Micronase** (Upjohn)		(Micronase 125). White, scored. In 100s.
Rx	**Micronized Glyburide** (Copley)	**Tablets, micronized:** 1.5 mg	In 100s and UD 100s.
Rx	**Glynase PresTab** (Upjohn)		Lactose. (Glynase 1.5/PT PT). White, scored. Oval. In 100s and UD 100s.
Rx	**Glyburide** (Various, eg, Aligen, Allscrips, Copley, Coventry, Geneva, Goldline, Rugby, Schein)	**Tablets**: 2.5 mg	In 100s, 500s, 1000s and UD 100s.
Rx	**DiaBeta** (Hoechst Marion Roussel)		Pink, scored. Oblong. In 60s, 100s, 500s and UD 100s.
Rx	**Micronase** (Upjohn)		(Micronase 2.5). Pink, scored. In 30s, 60s, 100s and UD 100s.
Rx	**Micronized Glyburide** (Copley)	**Tablets, micronized:** 3 mg	In 100s, 500s, 1000s, and UD 100s.
Rx	**Glynase PresTab** (Upjohn)		Lactose. (Glynase 3/PT PT). Blue, scored. Oval. In 100s, 500s, 1000s and UD 100s.

Sulfonylureas

GLYBURIDE (Glibenclamide)

Rx	**Glyburide** (Various, eg, Aligen, Allscrips, Copley, Coventry, Geneva, Goldline, Rugby, Schein)	**Tablets**: 5 mg	In 100s, 500s, 1000s and UD 100s.
Rx	**DiaBeta** (Hoechst Marion Roussel)		Lt. green, scored. Oblong. In 30s, 60s, 100s, 500s, 1000s and UD 100s.
Rx	**Micronase** (Upjohn)		(Micronase 5). Blue, scored. In 30s, 60s, 90s, 100s, 500s, 1000s and UD 100s.
Rx	**Glynase PresTab** (Upjohn)	**Tablets, micronized**: 6 mg	Lactose. (Glynase 6/PT PT) Yellow. Oval. In 100s and 500s.

Biguanides

METFORMIN HCl

Actions:

Pharmacology: Metformin is an oral antihyperglycemic drug used in the management of non-insulin-dependent diabetes mellitus (NIDDM). It is not chemically or pharmacologically related to the oral sulfonylureas. Metformin improves glucose tolerance in NIDDM subjects, lowering both basal and postprandial plasma glucose. Its pharmacologic mechanisms of action are different from those of sulfonylureas. Metformin decreases hepatic glucose production, decreases intestinal absorption of glucose and improves insulin sensitivity (increases peripheral glucose uptake and utilization). Unlike sulfonylureas, metformin does not produce hypoglycemia in either diabetic or nondiabetic subjects (except in special circumstances; see Precautions) and does not cause hyperinsulinemia. With metformin therapy, insulin secretion remains unchanged while fasting insulin levels and day-long plasma insulin response may actually decrease.

Monotherapy with metformin may be effective in patients who have not responded to sulfonylureas, who have only a partial response to sulfonylureas or who have ceased to respond to sulfonylureas. In such patients, if adequate glycemic control is not attained with metformin monotherapy, the combination of metformin and a sulfonylurea may have a synergistic effect, since both agents act to improve glucose tolerance by different but complementary mechanisms.

The magnitude of the decline in fasting blood glucose concentration following the institution of metformin therapy is proportional to the level of fasting hyperglycemia. Non-insulin-dependent diabetics with higher fasting glucose concentrations will experience greater declines in plasma glucose and glycosylated hemoglobin. Metformin has a modest favorable effect on serum lipids, which are often abnormal in NIDDM patients. In clinical studies, particularly when baseline levels were abnormally elevated, metformin, alone or in combination with a sulfonylurea, lowered mean fasting serum triglycerides, total cholesterol and LDL cholesterol levels and had no adverse effects on other lipid levels.

Summary of Mean Percent Reduction of Major Serum Lipid Variables with Metformin

	Metformin vs placebo (% change from baseline)		Combined metformin/glyburide vs monotherapy (% change from baseline)		
	Metformin (n = 141)	Placebo (n = 145)	Metformin (n = 210)	Metformin/glyburide (n = 213)	Glyburide (n = 209)
Total cholesterol	-5%	1%	-2%	-4%	1%
Total triglycerides	-16%	1%	-3%	-8%	4%
LDL-cholesterol	-8%	1%	-4%	-6%	3%
HDL-cholesterol	2%	-1%	5%	3%	1%

In contrast to sulfonylureas, body weight of individuals on metformin tends to remain stable or may even decrease somewhat.

In summary, metformin-treated patients show significant improvement in all parameters of glycemic control (FPG, PPG and HbA_{1c}), stabilization or decrease in body weight, and a tendency to improve in the lipid profile, particularly when baseline values are abnormally elevated.

Pharmacokinetics:

Absorption/Distribution – The absolute bioavailability of 500 mg metformin given under fasting conditions is ≈ 50% to 60%. Studies using single oral doses of 500 and 1500 mg, and 850 to 2550 mg, indicate that there is a lack of dose proportionality with increasing doses, which is due to decreased absorption rather than an alteration in elimination. Food decreases the extent and slightly delays the absorption of metformin (see Drug Interactions).

The apparent volume of distribution following single oral doses of 850 mg averaged 654 ± 358 L. Metformin is negligibly bound to plasma proteins in contrast to sulfonylureas, which are > 90% protein bound. At usual clinical doses and dosing schedules, steady state plasma concentrations are reached within 24 to 48 hours and are generally < 1 mcg/ml. During controlled clinical trials, maximum metformin plasma levels did not exceed 5 mcg/ml, even at maximum doses.

Biguanides

METFORMIN HCl

Metabolism/Excretion – Metformin is excreted unchanged in the urine and does not undergo hepatic metabolism (no metabolites have been identified in humans) nor biliary excretion. Renal clearance is ≈ 3.5 times greater than creatinine clearance (Ccr) which indicates that tubular secretion is the major route of elimination. Following oral administration, ≈ 90% of the absorbed drug is eliminated via the renal route within the first 24 hours, with a plasma elimination half-life of ≈ 6.2 hours. In blood, the elimination half-life is ≈ 17.6 hours, suggesting that the erythrocyte mass may be a compartment of distribution.

NIDDM subjects: In the presence of normal renal function, there are no differences between single or multiple dose pharmacokinetics of metformin between diabetics and nondiabetics, nor is there any accumulation of metformin in either group at usual clinical doses.

Race: In controlled clinical studies of metformin in patients with NIDDM, the antihyperglycemic effect was comparable in Caucasians (n = 249), African-Americans (n = 51) and Hispanics (n = 24).

Select Metformin Pharmacokinetic Parameters Following Single or Multiple Oral Doses

Subject groups: Metformin dose	C_{max} (mcg/ml)	t_{max} (h)	Renal clearance (ml/min)
Healthy, nondiabetic adults			
500 mg SD[1] (n = 24)	1.03	2.75	600
850 mg SD (n = 74)[2]	1.6	2.64	552
850 mg tid for 19 doses (n = 9)	2.01	1.79	642
Adults with NIDDM			
850 mg SD (n = 23)	1.48	3.32	491
850 mg tid for 19 doses (n = 9)	1.9	2.01	550
Elderly[3], healthy nondiabetic adults			
850 mg SD (n = 12)	2.45	2.71	412
Renal impaired adults: 850 mg SD			
Mild (Ccr 61 to 90 ml/min) (n = 5)	1.86	3.2	384
Moderate (Ccr 31 to 60 ml/min) (n = 4)	4.12	3.75	108
Severe (Ccr 10 to 30 ml/min) (n = 6)	3.93	4.01	130

[1] SD = Single dose.
[2] Combined results (average means) of five studies; mean age 32 years (range, 23 to 59 years).
[3] Elderly subjects, mean age 71 years (range, 65 to 81 years).

Clinical trials: In a double-blind, placebo controlled, multicenter clinical trial involving obese NIDDM patients whose hyperglycemia was not adequately controlled with dietary management alone (baseline fasting plasma glucose [FPG] of ≈ 240 mg/dl), treatment with metformin (up to 2.55 g/day) for 29 weeks resulted in significant mean net reductions in fasting and postprandial plasma glucose (PPG) and HbA_{1c} of 59 mg/dl, 83 mg/dl and 1.8%, respectively, compared to placebo.

A 29-week, double-blind, placebo controlled study of metformin and glyburide, alone and in combination, was conducted in obese NIDDM patients who had failed to achieve adequate glycemic control while on maximum doses of glyburide (baseline FPG of ≈ 250 mg/dl). Patients randomized to continue on glyburide experienced worsening of glycemic control, with mean increases in FPG, PPG and HbA_{1c} of 14 mg/dl, 3 mg/dl and 0.2%, respectively. In contrast, those randomized to metformin (up to 2.5 g/day) did not experience a deterioration in glycemic control, but rather a slight improvement, with mean reductions in FPG, PPG and HbA_{1c} of 1 mg/dl, 6 mg/dl and 0.4%, respectively. The combination of metformin and glyburide was synergistic in reducing FPG, PPG and HbA_{1c} levels by 63 mg/dl, 65 mg/dl and 1.7%, respectively. Compared to results of glyburide treatment alone, the net differences with combination treatment were -77 mg/dl, -68 mg/dl and -1.9%, respectively.

Indications:

Hyperglycemia: As monotherapy, as an adjunct to diet to lower blood glucose in patients with NIDDM whose hyperglycemia cannot be satisfactorily managed on diet alone.

Metformin may be used concomitantly with a sulfonylurea when diet and metformin or a sulfonylurea alone do not result in adequate glycemic control.

Biguanides

METFORMIN HCl

Contraindications:

1. Renal disease or dysfunction (eg, as suggested by serum creatinine levels > 1.5 mg/dl [males], > 1.4 mg/dl [females] or abnormal Ccr) which may also result from conditions such as cardiovascular collapse (shock), acute MI and septicemia.
2. Temporarily withhold metformin in patients undergoing radiologic studies involving parenteral administration of iodinated contrast materials, because use of such products may result in acute alteration of renal function (see Drug Interactions).
3. Hypersensitivity to metformin.
4. Acute or chronic metabolic acidosis, including diabetic ketoacidosis, with or without coma. Treat diabetic ketoacidosis with insulin.

Warnings:

Lactic acidosis: Lactic acidosis is a rare, but serious, metabolic complication that can occur due to metformin accumulation during treatment; when it occurs, it is fatal in ≈ 50% of cases. Lactic acidosis may also occur in association with a number of pathophysiologic conditions, including diabetes mellitus and whenever there is significant tissue hypoperfusion and hypoxemia. Lactic acidosis is characterized by elevated blood lactate levels (> 5 mmol/L), decreased blood pH, electrolyte disturbances with an increased anion gap and an increased lactate/pyruvate ratio. When metformin is implicated as the cause of lactic acidosis, plasma levels > 5 mcg/ml are generally found.

The reported incidence of lactic acidosis in patients receiving metformin is very low (≈ 0.03 cases/1000 patient-years, with ≈ 0.015 fatal cases/1000 patient-years). Reported cases have occurred primarily in diabetic patients with significant renal insufficiency, including both intrinsic renal disease and renal hypoperfusion, often in the setting of multiple concomitant medical/surgical problems and multiple concomitant medications. The risk of lactic acidosis increases with the degree of renal dysfunction and the patient's age. The risk of lactic acidosis may, therefore, be significantly decreased by regular monitoring of renal function in patients taking metformin and by use of the minimum effective dose. In addition, promptly withhold metformin in the presence of any condition associated with hypoxemia or dehydration. Because impaired hepatic function may significantly limit the ability to clear lactate, generally avoid metformin in patients with evidence of hepatic disease. Caution patients against excessive alcohol intake (acute or chronic) since alcohol potentiates the effects of metformin on lactate metabolism. In addition, temporarily discontinue metformin prior to any intravascular radiocontrast study and for any surgical procedure.

The onset of lactic acidosis often is subtle, and accompanied only by nonspecific symptoms such as malaise, myalgias, respiratory distress, increasing somnolence and nonspecific abdominal distress. There may be associated hypothermia, hypotension and resistant bradyarrhythmias with more marked acidosis. The patient and the patient's physician must be aware of the possible importance of such symptoms. Instruct the patient to notify the physician immediately if these symptoms occur. Withdraw metformin until the situation is clarified. Serum electrolytes, ketones, blood glucose and, if indicated, blood pH, lactate levels and even blood metformin levels may be useful. Once a patient is stabilized on any dose level of metformin, GI symptoms, which are common during initiation of therapy, are unlikely to be drug related. Later occurrence of GI symptoms could be due to lactic acidosis or other serious disease.

Levels of fasting venous plasma lactate above the upper limit of normal but < 5 mmol/L in patients taking metformin do not necessarily indicate impending lactic acidosis and may be explainable by other mechanisms, such as poorly controlled diabetes or obesity, vigorous physical activity or technical problems in sample handling.

Suspect lactic acidosis in any diabetic patient with metabolic acidosis lacking evidence of ketoacidosis (ketonuria and ketonemia).

Lactic acidosis is a medical emergency that must be treated in a hospital setting. In a patient with lactic acidosis who is taking metformin, discontinue the drug immediately and promptly institute general supportive measures. Because metformin is dialyzable (with a clearance of up to 170 ml/min under good hemodynamic conditions), prompt hemodialysis is recommended to correct the acidosis and remove the accumulated metformin. Such management often results in prompt reversal of symptoms and recovery.

METFORMIN HCl

Diet: In initiating treatment for NIDDM, emphasize diet as the primary form of treatment. Caloric restriction and weight loss are essential in the obese diabetic patient. Proper dietary management alone may be effective in controlling the blood glucose and symptoms of hyperglycemia. Loss of blood glucose control in diet-managed patients may be transient, thus requiring only short term pharmacologic therapy. Also stress the importance of regular physical activity and identify cardiovascular risk factors and take corrective measures where possible. If this treatment program fails to reduce symptoms or blood glucose, consider the use of metformin alone or metformin plus a sulfonylurea.

Glucose control: If, after a suitable trial of such treatments, glucose control still has not been achieved, give consideration to the use of insulin. Base judgments on regular clinical and laboratory evaluations.

Increased risk of cardiovascular mortality: The administration of oral antidiabetic drugs has been reported to be associated with increased cardiovascular mortality as compared to treatment with diet alone or diet plus insulin. This warning is based on the study conducted by the University Group Diabetes Program (UGDP), a long term prospective clinical trial designed to evaluate the effectiveness of glucose-lowering drugs in preventing or delaying vascular complications in patients with non-insulin-dependent diabetes. The study involved 1027 patients who were randomly assigned to one of five treatment groups (*Diabetes* 1970; 19 [suppl. 2]:747–830; *Diabetes,* 1975; 24 [suppl. 1]: 65–184).

The UGDP reported that patients treated for 5 to 8 years with diet plus a fixed dose of tolbutamide (1.5 g/day) or diet plus a fixed dose of phenformin (100 mg/day), had a rate of cardiovascular mortality ≈ 2.5 times that of patients treated with diet alone, resulting in discontinuation of both these treatments in the UGDP study. Total mortality was increased in both the tolbutamide- and phenformin-treated groups and this increase was statistically significant in the phenformin-treated group. Despite controversy regarding the interpretation of these results, the findings of the UGDP study provide an adequate basis for this warning. Inform the patient of the potential risks and benefits of metformin and alternative modes of therapy.

Although only one drug in the sulfonylurea category (tolbutamide) and one in the biguanide category (phenformin) were included in this study, it is prudent from a safety standpoint to consider that this warning may also apply to other related oral antidiabetic drugs, in view of the similarities in mode of action and chemical structure among the drugs in each category.

Renal/Hepatic function impairment: In subjects with decreased renal function (based on measured Ccr), the plasma and blood half-life of metformin is prolonged and the renal clearance is decreased in proportion to the decrease in Ccr.

Concomitant medication(s) that affect renal function, result in significant hemodynamic change or interfere with the disposition of metformin, such as cationic drugs that are eliminated by renal tubular secretion (See Drug Interactions), should be used with caution.

Since impaired hepatic function has been associated with some cases of lactic acidosis, generally avoid metformin in patients with clinical or laboratory evidence of hepatic disease.

Elderly: Limited data suggest that total plasma clearance is decreased, the half-life is prolonged and C_{max} is increased in healthy elderly subjects compared to healthy young subjects. From these data, it appears that the change in metformin pharmacokinetics with aging is primarily accounted for by a change in renal function. Use with caution as age increases. Use care in dose selection and base on careful and regular monitoring of renal function. Generally, elderly patients should not be titrated to the maximum dose of metformin (see Administration and Dosage).

Pregnancy: Category B. Safety in pregnant women has not been established. Balance any decision to use this drug against the benefits and risks.

Because recent information suggests that abnormal blood glucose levels during pregnancy are associated with a higher incidence of congenital abnormalities, there is a consensus among experts that insulin be used during pregnancy to maintain blood glucose levels as close to normal as possible.

Lactation: Studies in lactating rats show that metformin is excreted into milk and reaches levels comparable to those in plasma. Similar studies have not been conducted in nursing mothers, but exercise caution in such patients, and decide whether to discontinue nursing or to discontinue the drug, taking into account the importance of the drug to the mother.

Children: Safety and efficacy in children have not been established. Studies in maturity-onset diabetes of the young (MODY) have not been conducted.

METFORMIN HCl

Precautions:

Monitoring: Before initiation of therapy and at least annually thereafter, assess renal function and verify as normal. In patients in whom development of renal dysfunction is anticipated, assess renal function more frequently and discontinue the drug if evidence of renal impairment is present.

Evaluate a diabetic patient previously well controlled on metformin who develops laboratory abnormalities or clinical illness (especially vague and poorly defined illness) for evidence of ketoacidosis or lactic acidosis. Evaluation should include serum electrolytes and ketones, blood glucose and, if indicated, blood pH, lactate, pyruvate and metformin levels. If acidosis of either form occurs, metformin must be stopped immediately and other appropriate corrective measures initiated.

Monitor response to all diabetic therapies by periodic measurements of fasting blood glucose and glycosylated hemoglobin levels, with a goal of decreasing these levels toward the normal range. During initial dose titration, fasting glucose can be used to determine the therapeutic response. Thereafter, monitor both glucose and glycosylated hemoglobin. Measurements of glycosylated hemoglobin may be especially useful for evaluating long term control.

Perform initial and periodic monitoring of hematologic parameters (eg, hemoglobin/hematocrit, red blood cell indices) and renal function (serum creatinine) at least on an annual basis. While megaloblastic anemia has rarely been seen with metformin therapy, if this is suspected, exclude vitamin B_{12} deficiency.

Hypoxic states: Cardiovascular collapse (shock), acute CHF, acute MI and other conditions characterized by hypoxemia have been associated with lactic acidosis and may also cause prerenal azotemia. If such events occur, discontinue metformin.

Surgical procedures: Temporarily suspend metformin for surgical procedures (unless minor and not associated with restricted intake of food and fluids). Do not restart until the patient's oral intake has resumed and renal function is normal.

Vitamin B_{12} levels: A decrease to subnormal levels of previously normal serum vitamin B_{12} levels, without clinical manifestations, is observed in ≈ 7% of patients receiving metformin in controlled clinical trials of 29 weeks duration. Such decrease, possibly due to interference with B_{12} absorption from the B_{12}-intrinsic factor complex, is, however, very rarely associated with anemia and appears to be rapidly reversible with discontinuation of metformin or vitamin B_{12} supplementation. Annual measurement of hematologic parameters is advised in patients on metformin and any apparent abnormalities should be appropriately investigated and managed.

Certain individuals with inadequate vitamin B_{12} or calcium intake or absorption appear to be predisposed to developing subnormal vitamin B_{12} levels. In these patients, routine serum vitamin B_{12} measurements at 2 to 3 year intervals may be useful.

Hypoglycemia: Hypoglycemia does not occur in patients receiving metformin alone under usual circumstances, but could occur with deficient caloric intake, strenuous exercise not compensated by caloric supplementation, or during concomitant use with other glucose lowering agents (such as sulfonylureas) or ethanol.

Elderly, debilitated or malnourished patients, and those with adrenal or pituitary insufficiency or alcohol intoxication are particularly susceptible to hypoglycemic effects. Hypoglycemia may be difficult to recognize in the elderly and in people who are taking beta-adrenergic blocking drugs.

Loss of control of blood glucose: When a patient stabilized on any diabetic regimen is exposed to stress such as fever, trauma, infection or surgery, a temporary loss of glycemic control may occur. At such times, it may be necessary to withhold metformin and temporarily administer insulin. Metformin may be reinstituted after the acute episode is resolved.

The effectiveness of oral antidiabetic drugs in lowering blood glucose to a targeted level decreases in many patients over a period of time. This phenomenon, which may be due to progression of the underlying disease or to diminished responsiveness to the drug, is known as secondary failure to distinguish it from primary failure in which the drug is ineffective during initial therapy. Should secondary failure occur with metformin or sulfonylurea monotherapy, combined therapy with metformin and sulfonylurea may result in a response. Should secondary failure occur with combined therapy, it may be necessary to initiate insulin therapy.

Certain drugs tend to produce hyperglycemia and may lead to loss of glycemic control. These drugs include thiazide and other diuretics, corticosteroids, phenothiazines, thyroid products, estrogens, oral contraceptives, phenytoin, nicotinic acid, sympathomimetics, calcium channel blocking drugs and isoniazid. When such drugs are administered to a patient receiving metformin, closely observe the patient to maintain adequate glycemic control.

METFORMIN HCl

Drug Interactions:

Metformin Drug Interactions

Precipitant drug	Object drug*		Description
Metformin	Glyburide	↓	Following coadministration of single doses, decreases in glyburide AUC and C_{max} were observed, but were highly variable. The single-dose nature of this study and the lack of correlation between glyburide blood levels and pharmacodynamic effects makes the clinical significance of this interaction uncertain.
Alcohol	Metformin	↑	Alcohol potentiates the effect of metformin on lactate metabolism. Warn patients against excessive alcohol intake, acute or chronic, while receiving metformin.
Cationic drugs	Metformin	↑	Cationic drugs (eg, amiloride, digoxin, morphine, procainamide, quinidine, quinine, ranitidine, triamterene, trimethoprim, vancomycin) that are eliminated by renal tubular secretion theoretically have the potential for interaction with metformin by competing for common renal tubular transport systems. Although such interactions remain theoretical, careful patient monitoring and dose adjustment of metformin or the interfering drug are recommended in patients who are taking cationic medications that are excreted via the proximal renal tubular secretory system.
Cimetidine	Metformin	↑	Cimetidine caused a 60% increase in peak metformin plasma and whole blood concentrations and a 40% increase in plasma and whole blood AUC.
Furosemide	Metformin	↑	Furosemide increased the metformin plasma and blood C_{max} by 22% and blood AUC by 15%, without any significant change in metformin renal clearance.
Metformin	Furosemide	↓	When administered with metformin, the C_{max} and AUC of furosemide were 31% and 12% smaller, respectively, than when administered alone, and the terminal half-life was decreased by 32%, without any significant change in furosemide renal clearance.
Iodinated contrast material	Metformin	↑	Parenteral contrast studies with iodinated materials can lead to acute renal failure and have been associated with lactic acidosis in patients receiving metformin. Therefore, in patients in whom any such study is planned, withhold metformin for at least 48 hours prior to, and 48 hours subsequent to, the procedure and reinstitute only after renal function has been re-evaluated and found to be normal.
Nifedipine	Metformin	↑	Coadministration increased plasma metformin C_{max} and AUC by 20% and 9%, respectively, and increased the amount excreted in the urine. Nifedipine appears to enhance the absorption of metformin.

* ↑ = Object drug increased. ↓ = Object drug decreased.

Drug/Food interactions: Food decreases the extent and slightly delays the absorption of a single 850 mg dose of metformin as shown by an ≈ 40% lower peak concentration and 25% lower AUC in plasma and a 35 minute prolongation of time to peak plasma concentration compared to the same strength administered under fasting conditions. The clinical relevance of these decreases is unknown.

Adverse Reactions:

GI: Gastrointestinal symptoms (eg, diarrhea, nausea, vomiting, abdominal bloating, flatulence, anorexia) are the most common reactions to metformin and are ≈ 30% more frequent in patients on metformin monotherapy than in placebo-treated patients, particularly during initiation of therapy. These symptoms are generally transient and resolve spontaneously during continued treatment. Occasionally, temporary dose reduction may be useful. In controlled trials, metformin was discontinued due to GI reactions in ≈ 4% of patients.

Biguanides

METFORMIN HCl

Because GI symptoms during therapy initiation appear to be dose-related, they may be decreased by gradual dose escalation and by having patients take metformin with meals.

Because significant diarrhea or vomiting may cause dehydration and prerenal azotemia, under such circumstances, temporarily discontinue metformin.

For patients who have been stabilized on metformin, nonspecific GI symptoms should not be attributed to therapy unless intercurrent illness or lactic acidosis have been excluded.

Hematologic: (See Precautions). During controlled clinical trials of 29 weeks duration, ≈ 9% of patients on metformin monotherapy and 6% of patients on metformin/sulfonylurea therapy developed asymptomatic subnormal serum vitamin B_{12} levels; serum folic acid levels did not decrease significantly. However, only five cases of megaloblastic anemia have been reported with metformin administration and no increased incidence of neuropathy has been observed. Therefore, appropriately monitor serum B_{12} levels or consider periodic parenteral B_{12} supplementation.

Special senses: During initiation of therapy, ≈ 3% of patients may complain of an unpleasant or metallic taste, which usually resolves spontaneously.

Miscellaneous: Lactic acidosis (see Warnings).

Overdosage:

Hypoglycemia has not been seen even with ingestion of up to 85 g of metformin, although lactic acidosis has occurred in such circumstances (see Warnings). Metformin is dialyzable with a clearance of up to 170 ml/min under good hemodynamic conditions. Therefore, hemodialysis may be useful for removal of accumulated drug from patients in whom metformin overdosage is suspected.

Patient Information:

Inform patients of the potential risks and advantages of metformin and of alternative modes of therapy. Also inform them about the importance of adherence to dietary instructions, of a regular exercise program and of regular testing of blood glucose, glycosylated hemoglobin, renal function and hematologic parameters.

Explain the risks of lactic acidosis, its symptoms, and conditions that predispose to its development, as noted in the Warnings section. Advise patients to discontinue metformin immediately and to promptly notify their health practitioner if unexplained hyperventilation, myalgia, malaise, unusual somnolence or other nonspecific symptoms occur. Once a patient is stabilized on metformin, GI symptoms, which are common during initiation of therapy, are unlikely to be drug related. Later occurrence of GI symptoms could be due to lactic acidosis or other serious disease.

Counsel patients against excessive alcohol intake while receiving metformin.

Metformin alone does not usually cause hypoglycemia, although it may occur when metformin is used in conjunction with oral sulfonylureas. When initiating combination therapy, explain the risks of hypoglycemia, its symptoms and treatment, and conditions that predispose to its development.

Administration and Dosage:

Approved by the FDA on December 29, 1994 (1P classification).

There is no fixed dosage regimen for the management of hyperglycemia in diabetes mellitus with metformin or any other pharmacologic agent. Dosage must be individualized on the basis of both effectiveness and tolerance, while not exceeding the maximum recommended daily dose of 2550 mg. Give in divided doses with meals and start at a low dose, with gradual dose escalation as described below, both to reduce GI side effects and to permit identification of the minimum dose required for adequate glycemic control of the patient.

During treatment initiation and dose titration, use fasting plasma glucose to determine therapeutic response to metformin and to identify minimum effective dose. Thereafter, measure glycosylated hemoglobin at intervals of ≈ 3 months. The therapeutic goal should be to decrease both fasting plasma glucose and glycosylated hemoglobin levels to normal or near normal by using the lowest effective dose of metformin, either when used as monotherapy or in combination with a sulfonylurea.

Monitoring of blood glucose and glycosylated hemoglobin will also permit detection of primary failure (inadequate lowering of blood glucose at the maximum recommended dose of medication) and secondary failure (loss of an adequate blood glucose lowering response after an initial period of effectiveness).

Short-term administration may be sufficient during periods of transient loss of control in patients usually well controlled on diet alone.

Biguanides

METFORMIN HCl

Usual starting dose: In general, clinically significant responses are not seen at doses < 1500 mg/day. However, a lower recommended starting dose and gradually increased dosage is advised to minimize GI symptoms.

Metformin 500 mg: The usual starting dose is one 500 mg tablet twice daily, given with the morning and evening meals. Make dosage increases in increments of 500 mg every week, given in divided doses, up to 2500 mg/day. Metformin can be administered twice a day up to 2000 mg/day (eg, 1000 mg twice daily with morning and evening meals). If a 2500 mg daily dose is required, it may be better tolerated given 3 times daily with meals.

Metformin 850 mg: The usual starting dose is one 850 mg tablet daily, given with the morning meal. Make dosage increases in increments of 850 mg every other week, given in divided doses, up to 2550 mg/day. The usual maintenance dose is 850 mg twice daily with the morning and evening meals. When necessary, give patients 850 mg 3 times daily with meals.

Transfer from other antidiabetic therapy: When transferring patients from standard oral hypoglycemic agents other than chlorpropamide to metformin, generally no transition period is necessary. When transferring patients from chlorpropamide, exercise care during the first 2 weeks because of the prolonged retention of chlorpropamide leading to overlapping drug effects and possible hypoglycemia.

Concomitant metformin and oral sulfonylurea therapy: If patients have not responded to 4 weeks of the maximum dose of metformin monotherapy, consider gradual addition of an oral sulfonylurea while continuing metformin at the maximum dose, even if prior primary or secondary failure to a sulfonylurea has occurred. Clinical and pharmacokinetic drug-drug interaction data are available only for metformin plus glyburide. Published clinical information exists for the use of metformin with either chlorpropamide, tolbutamide or glipizide. No published clinical information exists regarding concomitant use of metformin with acetohexamide or tolazamide.

With concomitant metformin and sulfonylurea therapy, the desired control of blood glucose may be obtained by adjusting the dose of each drug. However, make attempts to identify the minimum effective dose of each drug. With concomitant metformin and sulfonylurea therapy, risk of hypoglycemia associated with sulfonylurea therapy continues and may be increased. Take appropriate precautions.

If patients have not satisfactorily responded to 1 to 3 months of concomitant therapy with the maximum doses of metformin and an oral sulfonylurea, consider institution of insulin therapy and discontinuation of these oral agents.

Elderly/Debilitated: Initial and maintenance dosing should be conservative in patients with advanced age because of the potential for decreased renal function in this population. Base any dosage adjustment on a careful assessment of renal function. Generally, elderly patients should not be titrated to the maximum dose.

In debilitated or malnourished patients, the dosing should also be conservative and based on a careful assessment of renal function.

Children: Use is not recommended.

Rx	**Glucophage** (Bristol-Myers Squibb)	**Tablets:** 500 mg	(GL 500). White. Biconvex/cylindrical. Film coated. In 100s.
		850 mg	(GL 850). White. Biconvex/cylindrical. Film coated. In 100s.

Thiazolidinedione

TROGLITAZONE

Actions:

Pharmacology: Troglitazone is a thiazolidinedione antidiabetic agent that lowers blood glucose by improving target cell response to insulin, without increasing pancreatic insulin secretion. It decreases insulin resistance. It has a unique mechanism of action that is dependent on the presence of insulin for activity. Troglitazone decreases hepatic glucose output and increases insulin-dependent glucose disposal in skeletal muscle and possibly liver and adipose tissue. Its mechanism of action is thought to involve binding to nuclear receptors (PPAR) that regulate the transcription of a number of insulin responsive genes critical for the control of glucose and lipid metabolism. Unlike sulfonylureas, troglitazone is not an insulin secretagogue.

Pharmacokinetics:

Absorption – Following daily drug administration, steady-state plasma concentrations of troglitazone are reached within 3 to 5 days.

Troglitazone is absorbed rapidly following oral administration; the time for maximum plasma concentration (T_{max}) occurs within 2 to 3 hours. Food increases the extent of absorption by 30% to 85%; thus, take troglitazone with a meal to enhance systemic drug availability.

Distribution – Mean apparent volume of distribution of troglitazone following multiple-dose administration ranges from 10.5 to 26.5 L/kg of body weight. Troglitazone is extensively bound (> 99%) to serum albumin, [^{14}C]troglitazone partitions into red blood cells (-5% of whole blood radioactivity).

Mean Steady-State Pharmacokinetics of Troglitazone in 21 Healthy Volunteers

Dose (mg/day)	C_{max} (mcg/ml)	AUC (0-24) (mcg•hr/ml)	CL/F[1] (ml/min)
200	0.90	7.4	500
400	1.61	13.4	601
600	2.82	22.1	496

[1] CL/F = Apparent oral clearance.

Metabolism – In six healthy male volunteers given a single 400 mg dose of [^{14}C]troglitazone after 14 days of treatment with 400 mg troglitazone tablets, the major metabolites found in the plasma were the sulfate conjugate (Metabolite 1), followed by the quinone metabolite (Metabolite 3). Only 3.1% of the dose was detected in the urine; this was primarily in the form of the glucuronide conjugate (Metabolite 2), which is present in negligible amounts in the plasma. In both normal volunteers and patients with type II diabetes, steady-state levels of Metabolite 1 are 6 to 7 times that of troglitazone and Metabolite 3.

Troglitazone incubated with expressed human P450 1A1, 1A2, 2A6, 2B6, 2D6, 2E1 and 3A4 in the presence and absence of known inhibitors of these enzymes showed no Metabolite 3 formation above levels in control samples. Incubation of Metabolite 3 with human liver microsomes suggests that it is not subject to further metabolism.

The inhibitory profile of troglitazone against the seven major P450 isozymes was characterized using human liver microsomes. Troglitazone was found to inhibit 3A4, 2C9 and 2C19 by 40% to 67% at a concentration of 11 mcg/ml. Because the highest peak concentrations expected to be achieved on 600 mg/day is in the range of 1 to 3 mcg/ml, inhibition may not be clinically important. The results of in vivo drug interaction studies tend to support this observation (see Drug Interactions); observe caution when troglitazone is used in combination with drugs known to be metabolized by one of these enzymes. The inhibitory characteristics of Metabolite 3 have not been investigated directly.

Excretion – Following oral administration of troglitazone, ≈ 85% is recovered in feces and 3% in urine. Unchanged troglitazone is not recovered in urine following oral administration. Mean plasma elimination half-life of troglitazone ranges from 16 to 34 hours.

Special populations:

Renal function impairment – In patients with various degrees of renal function impairment, the apparent clearance of total and unbound troglitazone and the plasma elimination half-life of troglitazone, Metabolite 1 and Metabolite 3 do not correlate with creatinine clearance. Thus, dose adjustment in patients with renal dysfunction is not necessary.

Thiazolidinedione

TROGLITAZONE

Hepatic function impairment – Troglitazone, Metabolite 1 and Metabolite 3 plasma concentrations in patients with chronic liver disease (Childs-Pugh Grade B or C) were increased by ≈ 30%, 400% and 100%, respectively, compared with those in healthy subjects without hepatic dysfunction. There was no change in plasma protein binding. No adverse events were noted in any group that were attributed to the drug. Nevertheless, use troglitazone with caution in patients with hepatic disease.

Elderly – Steady-state pharmacokinetics of troglitazone, Metabolite 1 and Metabolite 3 in healthy elderly subjects are comparable with those seen in young adults.

Clinical trials: In one 6–month, double-blind, placebo controlled study in insulin-treated type II diabetic patients receiving a mean of 73 (range, 27 to 143) units/day of insulin with a mean baseline HbA_{1C} of 9.42 (range 7.04 to 12.48), troglitazone (200 or 600 mg/day) or placebo was added to the insulin therapy.

Thirty percent of patients treated with 200 mg troglitazone and 57% of patients treated with 600 mg troglitazone had an HbA_{1C} value < 8% at the end of the study compared with 11% of placebo-treated patients. Accompanying this improvement in glycemic control was a significant decrease in exogenous insulin dosage of 15% in the 200 mg troglitazone treatment group and 42% in the 600 mg troglitazone treatment group compared with 1% in the placebo group.

Indications:

Type II diabetes: For use in patients with type II diabetes currently on insulin therapy whose hyperglycemia is inadequately controlled (HbA_{1C} > 8.5%) despite insulin therapy of over 30 units/day given as multiple injections.

Management of type II diabetes should include diet control. Caloric restriction, weight loss and exercise are essential for the proper treatment of the diabetic patient. This is important not only in the primary treatment of type II diabetes, but in maintaining the efficacy of drug therapy. Prior to initiation of troglitazone therapy, investigate secondary causes of poor glycemic control (eg, infection or poor injection technique).

Unlabeled uses: A study showed troglitazone may be beneficial in the productive and metabolic consequences of polycystic ovary syndrome (PCOS) (400 mg/day) and less essential hypertension with NIDDM, but more studies are needed.

Contraindications:

Known hypersensitivity or allergy to troglitazone or any of its components.

Warnings:

Heart Failure: Heart enlargement without microscopic changes has been observed in rodents at exposures exceeding 14 times the AUC of the 400 mg human dose. Serial echocardiographic evaluations in monkeys treated chronically at maximum achievable exposures (3 to 5 times the human exposure at the 400 mg dose) did not reveal changes in heart size or function. In a 2–year echocardiographic clinical study using 600 to 800 mg/day of troglitazone in patients with type II diabetes, no increase in left ventricular mass or decrease in cardiac output was observed. The methodology employed was able to detect a change of ≈ 10% or more in left ventricular mass.

In animal studies, troglitazone treatment was associated with increases of 6% to 15% in plasma volume. In a study of 24 normal volunteers, an increase in plasma volume of 6% to 8% compared with placebo was observed following 6 weeks of troglitazone treatment.

No increased incidence of adverse events potentially related to volume expansion (eg, congestive heart failure) have been observed during controlled clinical trials. However, patients with New York Heart Association (NYHA) Class III and IV cardiac status were not studied during clinical trials. Therefore, caution is advised during the administration of troglitazone to patients with NYHA Class III or IV cardiac status.

Hepatotoxicity: During all clinical studies, a total of 20 troglitazone-treated patients were withdrawn from treatment because of liver function test abnormalities. Two of the 20 patients developed reversible jaundice. Both had liver biopsies that were consistent with an idiosyncratic drug reaction.

Elderly: No differences in effectiveness and safety were observed between ≥ 65 year-old patients and younger patients.

Pregnancy: Category B. Troglitazone was not teratogenic in rats given up to 2000 mg/kg or rabbits given up to 1000 mg/kg during organogenesis. There are no adequate and well-controlled studies in pregnant women. Do not use troglitazone during pregnancy unless the potential benefit justifies the potential risk to the fetus.

Thiazolidinedione

TROGLITAZONE

Because current information strongly suggests that abnormal blood glucose levels during pregnancy are associated with a higher incidence of congenital anomalies as well as increased neonatal morbidity and mortality, most experts recommend that insulin be used during pregnancy to maintain blood glucose levels as close to normal as possible.

Ovulation – In premenopausal anovulatory patients with insulin resistance, troglitazone treatment may result in resumption of ovulation. These patients may be at risk for pregnancy.

Lactation: It is not known whether troglitazone is secreted in breast milk. Troglitazone is secreted in the milk of lactating rats. Do not administer to breastfeeding women.

Children: Safety and efficacy in pediatric patients have not been established.

Precautions:

Type I diabetes: Because of its mechanism of action, troglitazone is active only in the presence of insulin. Therefore, do not use in type I diabetes or for the treatment of diabetic keto-acidosis.

Hypoglycemia: Patients receiving troglitazone in combination with insulin may be at risk for hypoglycemia, and a reduction in the dose of insulin may be necessary. Hypoglycemia has not been observed during the administration of troglitazone as monotherapy and would not be expected based on the mechanism of action.

Hematologic: Across all clinical studies, hemoglobin declined by 3% to 4% in troglitazone-treated patients compared with 1% to 2% in those treated with placebo. White blood cell counts also declined slightly in troglitazone-treated patients compared with those treated with placebo. These changes occurred within the first 4 to 8 weeks of therapy. Levels stabilized and remained unchanged for ≤ 2 years of continuing therapy. These changes may be due to the dilutional effects of increased plasma volume and have not been associated with any significant hematologic clinical effects.

Drug Interactions:

Troglitazone may induce drug metabolism by CYP3A4. Consider this when prescribing other CYP3A4 substrates such as cyclosporine, tacrolimus and some HMG-CoA reductase inhibitors.

Troglitazone Drug Interactions

Precipitant drug	Object drug*		Description
Cholestyramine	Troglitazone	⬇	Concomitant administration of cholestyramine with troglitazone reduces the absorption of troglitazone by ≈ 70%; thus, coadministration of cholestyramine and troglitazone is not recommended.
Troglitazone	Acetaminophen	⬌	Coadministration of acetaminophen and troglitazone does not alter the pharmacokinetics of either drug.
Troglitazone	Contraceptives, oral	⬇	Administration of troglitazone with an oral contraceptive containing ethinyl estradiol and norethindrone reduced the plasma concentrations of both by ≈ 30%. These changes could result in loss of contraception.
Troglitazone	Sulfonylureas (glyburide)	⬆	Coadministration of troglitazone with glyburide does not appear to alter troglitazone or glyburide pharmacokinetics but may further decrease fasting plasma glucose.
Troglitazone	Terfenadine	⬇	Coadministration of troglitazone with terfenadine decreases plasma concentrations of terfenadine and its active metabolite by 50% to 70% and may reduce the effectiveness of terfenadine.
Troglitazone	Warfarin	⬌	Troglitazone has no clinically significant effect on prothrombin time when administered to patients receiving chronic warfarin therapy.

* ⬆ Object drug increased. ⬇ Object drug decreased. ⬌ Undetermined effect.

Drug/Lab test interactions:

Hematologic – Small decreases in hemoglobin, hematocrit, and neutrophil counts (within the normal range) may be related to increased plasma volume observed with troglitazone treatment. Hemoglobin decreases to below the normal range occurred in 5% of troglitazone-treated and 4% of placebo-treated patients.

Thiazolidinedione

TROGLITAZONE

Lipids – Small changes in serum lipids have been observed.

Serum transaminase levels – 2.2% of troglitazone-treated patients had reversible elevations in AST or ALT > 3 times the upper limit of normal, compared with 0.6% of patients receiving placebo. In the population of patients treated with troglitazone, mean and median values for bilirubin, AST, ALT, alkaline phosphatase and GGT were decreased at the final visit compared with baseline, while values for LDH were increased slightly.

Adverse Reactions:

Adverse Events Reported at a Frequency ≥ 5% of Troglitazone-Treated Patients (%)		
Adverse reactions	Placebo n = 492	Troglitazone n = 1450
Infection	22	18
Headache	11	11
Pain	14	10
Accidental injury	6	8
Asthenia	5	6
Dizziness	5	6
Back Pain	4	6
Nausea	4	6
Rhinitis	7	5
Diarrhea	6	5
Urinary tract infection	6	5
Peripheral edema	5	5
Pharyngitis	4	5

Patient Information:

Take troglitazone with meals. If the dose is missed at the usual meal, take it at the next meal. If the dose is missed on one day, do not double the dose the following day.

It is important to adhere to dietary instructions and to have blood glucose and glycosylated hemoglobin tested regularly. During periods of stress such as fever, trauma, infection or surgery, insulin requirements may change, and patients should seek the advice of their physician.

When using combination therapy with insulin, explain the risks of hypoglycemia, its symptoms, treatment and predisposing conditions to patients and their family members.

Administration and Dosage:

Approved January 31, 1997.

Continue the current insulin dose upon initiation of troglitazone therapy. Initiate therapy at 200 mg once daily in patients on insulin therapy. For patients not responding adequately, increase the dose after ≈ 2 to 4 weeks. The usual dose is 400 mg/day. The maximum recommended dose is 600 mg/day. It is recommended that the insulin dose be decreased by 10% to 25% when fasting plasma glucose concentrations decrease to < 120 mg/dl in patients receiving concomitant insulin and troglitazone. Individualize further adjustments based on glucose-lowering response. Take with a meal.

Rx	**Rezulin** (Parke-Davis)	**Tablets:** 200 mg	(PD 352 200). Yellow, oval, film coated. In 30s, 90s and UD 100s.
		400 mg	(PD 353 400). Tan, oval, film coated. In 30s, 90s and UD 100s.

GLUCAGON

Actions:

Pharmacology: Glucagon, a polypeptide hormone produced by the alpha cells of the pancreas, accelerates liver glycogenolysis by stimulating cyclic AMP synthesis and increasing phosphorylase kinase activity. Increased breakdown of glycogen to glucose and inhibition of glycogen synthetase results in blood glucose elevation. Additionally, glucagon stimulates hepatic gluconeogenesis by promoting the uptake of amino acids and converting them to glucose precursors. Lipolysis in the liver and adipose tissue is enhanced (via adenyl cyclase activation), providing free fatty acids and glycerol to further stimulate ketogenesis and gluconeogenesis.

Parenteral administration of glucagon produces relaxation of the smooth muscle of the GI tract. It also decreases gastric and pancreatic secretions in the GI tract and increases myocardial contractility. Administration to comatose hypoglycemic patients (with normal liver glycogen stores) usually produces a return to consciousness within 15 minutes.

Pharmacokinetics: Glucagon is degraded in the liver, kidney and in plasma. Plasma half-life is 3 to 6 minutes.

Indications:

Hypoglycemia: Counteracts severe hypoglycemic reactions in diabetic patients or during insulin shock therapy in psychiatric patients. Glucagon is helpful in hypoglycemia only if liver glycogen is available. It is of little or no help in states of starvation, adrenal insufficiency or chronic hypoglycemia.

In Type I (juvenile diabetics), blood glucose levels do not respond as well as in adult stable diabetics; give supplementary carbohydrates as soon as possible.

Diagnostic aid in the radiologic examination of the stomach, duodenum, small bowel and colon when a hypotonic state is advantageous.

Unlabeled uses: Glucagon has been used in the treatment of propranolol overdose and cardiovascular emergencies.

Contraindications:

Hypersensitivity to glucagon.

Warnings:

Insulinoma/pheochromocytoma: Administer cautiously to patients with a history of insulinoma or pheochromocytoma. In patients with insulinoma, IV glucagon will produce an initial increase in blood glucose, but because of its insulin-releasing effect, it may subsequently cause hypoglycemia. It also stimulates catecholamine release, causing a marked increase in blood pressure in patients with pheochromocytoma.

Pregnancy: Category B. There are no adequate and well controlled studies in pregnant women. Use during pregnancy only if clearly needed.

Lactation: It is not known whether this drug is excreted in breast milk. Exercise caution when administering to a nursing mother.

Precautions:

Hypoglycemia: Although glucagon may be used for emergency treatment of hypoglycemia, notify the physician when hypoglycemic reactions occur so that the insulin dose may be adjusted.

Drug Interactions:

Oral anticoagulants: The hypoprothrombinemic effects may be increased, possibly with bleeding. The interaction may occur after several days of therapy and appears to be dose-related. Monitor prothrombin time and adjust oral anticoagulant dose accordingly.

Adverse Reactions:

Nausea, vomiting (occasional; this may also occur with hypoglycemia); generalized allergic reactions including urticaria, respiratory distress and hypotension.

Overdosage:

There have been no reports of overdosage in humans. Treatment should be symptomatic, primarily for nausea, vomiting and possible hypokalemia.

GLUCAGON

Administration and Dosage:

Patient instructions are provided with product.

Hypoglycemia: 0.5 (children < 20 kg) to 1 mg (adults and children > 20 kg) SC, IM or IV usually produces a response in 5 to 20 minutes. If the response is delayed, administer 1 or 2 additional doses. Arouse the patient as quickly as possible. In view of the deleterious effects of cerebral hypoglycemia, give glucose IV if the patient fails to respond to glucagon.

When the patient responds, give supplemental carbohydrate to restore the liver glycogen and prevent secondary hypoglycemia.

Insulin shock therapy: After 1 hour of coma, inject 0.5 to 1 mg or more, if desired, SC, IM or IV. The patient will usually awaken in 10 to 25 minutes. If no response occurs, repeat the dose. Upon awakening, feed the patient orally, as soon as possible, and follow the usual dietary regimen.

Depending on the duration and depth of coma, parenteral glucose must be considered.

Children/Infants: The following doses have been recommended: Infants, 0.3 mg/kg/dose every 4 hours as needed; children, 0.03 to 0.1 mg/kg/dose, repeated in 20 minutes as needed.

Diagnostic aid: Administer the doses in the following chart for relaxation of the stomach, duodenum and small bowel, depending on the time of onset of action and the duration of effect required. Since the stomach is less sensitive to the effect of glucagon, 0.5 mg IV or 2 mg IM are recommended.

Glucagon Dosing Parameters as a Diagnostic Aid

Dose	Route	Onset (min)	Duration (min)
0.25 to 0.5 mg (0.25-0.5 unit)	IV	1	9-17
1 mg (1 unit)	IM	8-10	12-27
2 mg (2 units)[1]	IV	1	22-25
2 mg (2 units)[1]	IM	4-7	21-32

[1] 2 mg doses produce a higher incidence of nausea and vomiting.

For examination of the colon, administer 2 mg IM approximately 10 minutes prior to initiation of the procedure.

Storage/Stability: Store at room temperature prior to reconstitution. After reconstitution, use immediately. May be kept at 5°C (41°F) for up to 48 hrs, if necessary.

If given in doses > 2 mg, reconstitute with Sterile Water for Injection and use immediately.

Rx	**Glucagon** (Lilly)	**Powder for Injection (lyophilized):** 1 mg (1 unit)	Lactose. In vials with 1 ml diluent.[1]
		10 mg (10 units)	Lactose. In vials with 10 ml diluent.[1]

[1] With 1.6% glycerin and 0.2% phenol.

DIAZOXIDE, ORAL

Parenteral diazoxide is used for hypertensive emergencies. Refer to the monograph in the Cardiovascular section.

Actions:

Pharmacology: Diazoxide is a benzothiadiazine derivative related to the thiazide diuretics. Oral diazoxide produces a prompt dose-related increase in the blood glucose by inhibiting pancreatic insulin release, and also by an extrapancreatic effect. The hyperglycemic effect begins within an hour and generally lasts no more than 8 hours with normal renal function.

Diazoxide decreases sodium chloride and water excretion, resulting in fluid retention. The blood pressure effects are usually not marked with the oral preparation.

Other actions include: Increased pulse rate; increased serum uric acid levels due to decreased excretion; increased serum levels of free fatty acids; decreased para-aminohippuric acid (PAH) clearance with little effect on glomerular filtration rate.

Insulin or tolbutamide reverses diazoxide-induced hyperglycemia.

Pharmacokinetics: Diazoxide is extensively bound (90%) to serum proteins. The plasma half-life is 24 to 36 hours. In four children, the plasma half-life varied from 9.5 to 24 hours. The half-life may be prolonged following overdosage and in patients with impaired renal function. Diazoxide is excreted by the kidneys.

Indications:

Hypoglycemia: Management of hypoglycemia due to hyperinsulinism.

Adults – Inoperable islet cell adenoma or carcinoma, or extrapancreatic malignancy.

Infants and children – Leucine sensitivity, islet cell hyperplasia, nesidioblastosis, extrapancreatic malignancy, islet cell adenoma or adenomatosis. May be used preoperatively as a temporary measure and postoperatively if hypoglycemia persists.

Hypertensive emergency: See monograph in the Cardiovascular section.

Contraindications:

Functional hypoglycemia. Do not use in patients hypersensitive to diazoxide or to other thiazides unless the potential benefits outweigh the possible risks.

Warnings:

Fluid retention in patients with compromised cardiac reserve may precipitate CHF. Fluid retention will respond to conventional diuretic therapy.

Ketoacidosis and nonketotic hyperosmolar coma have occurred with recommended doses, usually during intercurrent illness. Prompt recognition and treatment are essential (see Overdosage), and prolonged surveillance following the acute episode is necessary because of the long half-life. The patient must monitor the urine for glucose and ketones and promptly report abnormal findings and unusual symptoms.

Cataracts: Transient cataracts occurred in association with hyperosmolar coma in an infant and subsided on correction of the hyperosmolarity.

Renal function impairment: Decreased protein binding is seen in patients with renal failure. The higher level of free drug corresponds to an increase in hypotensive effect.

Pregnancy: Category C. Reproduction studies in rats and rabbits have revealed increased fetal resorptions, delayed parturition and fetal skeletal and cardiac anomalies. In animals, the drug causes degeneration of fetal pancreatic beta cells. Since there are no adequate human data, safety for use during pregnancy has not been established. Use only when clearly needed and when the potential benefits outweigh the unknown potential hazards to the fetus.

Diazoxide crosses the placenta. When given to the mother prior to delivery, the drug may produce fetal or neonatal hyperbilirubinemia, thrombocytopenia, altered carbohydrate metabolism or other side effects that have occurred in adults. Alopecia and hypertrichosis lanuginosa have occurred in infants whose mothers received oral diazoxide the last 19 to 60 days of pregnancy.

Labor and delivery – Administration IV during labor may cause cessation of uterine contractions. Oxytocic agents may be required to reinstate labor; use caution.

Precautions:

Monitoring: Observe patients closely when treatment is initiated. Monitor clinical response and blood glucose until the patient's condition has stabilized, usually several days. If not effective after 2 or 3 weeks, discontinue the drug.

Prolonged treatment requires regular monitoring of the urine for glucose and ketones, especially under stress conditions. Monitor blood glucose levels periodically to determine the need for dose adjustment.

Serum uric acid levels might be elevated, particularly in patients with hyperuricemia or a history of gout.

DIAZOXIDE, ORAL

Higher blood levels have been observed with the liquid than with the capsule formulation. Adjust dosage as necessary when changing formulations.

Drug Interactions:

Diazoxide is highly bound to serum protein and may displace other agents resulting in higher blood levels of these substances.

Diazoxide (Oral) Drug Interactions			
Precipitant drug	Object drug*		Description
Diazoxide, oral	Sulfonylureas	⬇	Addition of diazoxide to a patient stabilized on a sulfonylurea could destabilize the patient, resulting in hyperglycemia.
Thiazide diuretics	Diazoxide, oral	⬆	Concomitant administration may potentiate diazoxide's hyperglycemic and hyperuricemic effects. Hypotension may occur.
Diazoxide, oral	Phenytoin	⬇	Concomitant administration may result in a loss of seizure control, possibly due to increased hepatic metabolism of phenytoin
Phenothiazines	Diazoxide, oral	⬆	Concomitant use may cause an increase in the pharmacologic effects of diazoxide. Hyperglycemia may result.

* ⬇ = object drug decreased ⬆ = object drug increased

Drug/Lab test interactions: Increased renin secretion, IgG concentrations and decreased cortisol secretions have occurred. Diazoxide inhibits glucagon-stimulated insulin release and causes a false-negative insulin response to glucagon.

Adverse Reactions:

Sodium and fluid retention is most common in infants and adults; may precipitate CHF in patients with compromised cardiac reserve (see Warnings). Hyperglycemia or glycosuria may require dosage reduction to avoid progression to ketoacidosis or hyperosmolar coma. Diabetic ketoacidosis and hyperosmolar nonketotic coma may develop very rapidly (see Overdosage).

Renal: Increased serum uric acid; azotemia; decreased creatinine clearance; reversible nephrotic syndrome; decreased urinary output; hematuria; albuminuria.

GI: Anorexia; nausea; vomiting; abdominal pain; ileus; diarrhea; transient loss of taste; acute pancreatitis/pancreatic necrosis.

Cardiovascular: Tachycardia; palpitations; occasional hypotension; transient hypertension; chest pain (rare).

Hematologic: Thrombocytopenia with or without purpura may require discontinuation of the drug. Transient neutropenia is not associated with increased susceptibility to infection and ordinarily does not require discontinuance.

Eosinophilia; decreased hemoglobin/hematocrit; excessive bleeding; decreased IgG.

CNS: Headache; weakness; malaise; anxiety; dizziness; insomnia; polyneuritis; paresthesia; extrapyramidal signs.

Ophthalmic: Transient cataracts; subconjunctival hemorrhage; ring scotoma; blurred vision; diplopia; lacrimation.

Dermatologic: Hirsutism of the lanugo type mainly on the forehead, back and limbs, subsides on discontinuation of the drug; skin rash; pruritus; monilial dermatitis; herpes; loss of scalp hair.

Miscellaneous: Gout; advance in bone age; galactorrhea; enlargement of lump in breast; fever; increased AST and alkaline phosphatase.

Overdosage:

Symptoms: Marked hyperglycemia which may be associated with ketoacidosis.

Treatment: Promptly administer insulin and restore fluid and electrolyte balance. Because of the drug's long half-life, symptoms require prolonged surveillance for up to 7 days, until the blood sugar level stabilizes within the normal range. Successful lowering of diazoxide blood levels by peritoneal dialysis and by hemodialysis in two patients has been reported. Treatment includes usual supportive measures. Refer to General Management of Acute Overdosage.

Patient Information:

Monitor urine regularly for glucose and ketones; report abnormalities to physician.

During treatment, advise patient to consult physician regularly and to cooperate with periodic lab test monitoring.

DIAZOXIDE, ORAL

Take the drug on a regular schedule as prescribed. Do not skip doses or take extra doses.

Do not use this drug with other medications unless the physician has been consulted.

Do not allow anyone else to take this medication.

Follow dietary instructions.

Report promptly any adverse effects such as increased urinary frequency, increased thirst or fruity breath odor.

Report pregnancy or discuss plans for pregnancy.

Administration and Dosage:

Individualize dosage. Assure accuracy of dosage in infants and young children.

Adults and children: 3 to 8 mg/kg/day, in 2 or 3 equal doses every 8 or 12 hours. Patients with refractory hypoglycemia may require higher dosages.

Infants and newborns: 8 to 15 mg/kg/day, in 2 or 3 equal doses every 8 or 12 hours.

Storage: Protect suspension from light.

Rx	**Proglycem** (Baker Norton)	**Capsules**: 50 mg	(BMP 6000:). Orange and clear. In 100s.
		Oral Suspension: 50 mg/ml	Chocolate-mint flavor. In 30 ml with calibrated dropper.

GLUCOSE

Refer to parenteral dextrose (d-glucose) which is also used in the treatment of acute hypoglycemia.

Actions:

Pharmacology: Glucose, a monosaccharide, is absorbed from the intestine after administration and then used, distributed and stored by the tissues. Direct absorption takes place, resulting in a rapid increased blood glucose concentration. Therefore, it is effective in small doses; no evidence of toxicity has been reported. Glucose provides 4 calories/gram.

Indications:

Management of hypoglycemia.

Adverse Reactions:

Isolated reports of nausea, which may also occur with hypoglycemia.

Administration and Dosage:

Administer 10 to 20 g orally; repeat in 10 minutes if necessary. Response should occur in 10 minutes.

Glucose is not absorbed from the buccal cavity; it must be swallowed to be effective. While swallowing reflexes may be preserved in the unconscious patient, the lack of normal gag reflexes may lead to aspiration. When possible, use other methods of treating hypoglycemia in unconscious patients.

Children: Do not give to children under 2 years of age, unless directed by a physician.

otc	**Glutose** (Paddock)	**Gel**: Liquid glucose (40% dextrose)	Dye free. In 80 g bottle and 25 g tube.
otc	**Insta-Glucose** (ICN)		Cherry flavor. In UD 30.8 g tubes.
otc	**Insulin Reaction** (Sherwood)		Lime flavor. In UD 25 g tubes.
otc	**Dex4 Glucose** (Can-Am Care)	**Tablets**: Glucose	Lemon, orange, raspberry and grape flavors. In 10s and 50s.
otc	**B-D Glucose** (Becton Dickinson)	**Tablets, chewable**: 5 g	In 36s.

ALGLUCERASE (Glucocerebrosidase-beta-glucosidase)

Actions:

Pharmacology: Alglucerase was approved by the FDA in April 1991. Alglucerase is a modified form of the enzyme beta-glucocerebrosidase used for the treatment of Gaucher's disease; it is prepared by modification of the oligosaccharide chains of human beta-glucocerebrosidase. The modification alters the sugar residues at the nonreducing ends of the oligosaccharide chains of the glycoprotein so that they are predominantly terminated with mannose residues (specifically recognized by carbohydrate receptors on macrophage cells).

Alglucerase is purified from a large pool of human placental tissue collected from selected donors. The risk of viral contamination has been reduced; however, no procedure is totally effective in removing viral infectivity (see Precautions). Each lot of product has been tested and found negative for hepatitis B surface antigen (HBsAg) and for antigens of the human immunodeficiency virus (HIV-1).

Alglucerase catalyzes the hydrolysis of the glycolipid glucocerebroside to glucose and ceramide as part of the normal degradation pathway for membrane lipids. Glucocerebroside is primarily derived from hematological cell turnover.

Gaucher's disease is characterized by a functional deficiency in beta-glucocerebrosidase enzymatic activity and the resultant accumulation of lipid glucocerebroside in tissue macrophages which become engorged and are termed Gaucher's cells. Gaucher's cells are typically found in liver, spleen and bone marrow and, occasionally, in lung, kidney and intestine. Secondary hematologic sequelae include severe anemia and thrombocytopenia in addition to the characteristic progressive hepatosplenomegaly. Skeletal complications, including osteonecrosis and osteopenia with secondary pathological fractures, are a common feature of Gaucher's disease.

Pharmacokinetics: Following an IV infusion of different doses (between 0.6 and 234 U/kg) over a 4 hour period, steady-state enzymatic activity was achieved by 60 minutes. Individual steady-state enzymatic activity and area under the curve of the activity increased linearly with the infused dose (0.6 to 121 U/kg). Following infusion termination, plasma enzymatic activity declined rapidly with elimination half-life ranging between 3.6 and 10.4 minutes. Plasma clearance calculated from plasma enzymatic activity was variable and ranged between 6.34 and 25.39 ml/min/kg, whereas the volume of distribution ranged from 49.4 to 282.1 ml/kg. Within the dosage range of 0.6 and 121 U/kg, elimination half-life, plasma clearance and volume of distribution values appear to be independent of the infused dose.

Clinical trials: Chronic administration of alglucerase in 13 patients with Type 1 Gaucher's disease induced the following effects:

Splenomegaly and hepatomegaly were significantly reduced, presumably by disruption of the lysosomal storage sites and metabolism of glucocerebroside in Gaucher's cells. This effect was demonstrated within 6 months of therapy initiation.

Hematologic deficiencies in hemoglobin, hematocrit, erythrocyte and platelet counts were significantly improved. In most patients, a change in hemoglobin was the first observable effect. In some patients, hemoglobin levels were normalized after 6 months of therapy.

Improved mineralization occurred in four patients after prolonged treatment as a result of a reduction in the osteolytic actions of lipid-laden Gaucher's cells in the marrow.

Cachexia and wasting in children were reduced.

Indications:

Long-term enzyme replacement therapy for patients with a confirmed diagnosis of Type 1 Gaucher's disease who exhibit signs and symptoms severe enough to result in one or more of the following conditions: Moderate-to-severe anemia; thrombocytopenia with bleeding tendency; bone disease; significant hepatomegaly or splenomegaly.

Contraindications:

Hypersensitivity to the product.

Warnings:

Pregnancy: Category C. It is not known whether alglucerase can cause fetal harm when administered to a pregnant woman, or can affect reproductive capacity. Use in pregnancy only if clearly needed.

Lactation: It is not known whether this drug is excreted in breast milk. Exercise caution when administering to a nursing woman.

ALGLUCERASE (Glucocerebrosidase-beta-glucosidase)

Precautions:

Viral infectious agents: Alglucerase is prepared from pooled human placental tissue that may contain the causative agents of some viral diseases. Manufacturing steps have been designed to reduce the risk of transmitting viral infectious agents. These steps have demonstrated in vitro inactivation of a panel of model viruses, including human immunodeficiency virus (HIV-1). The risk of contamination from slowly acting or latent viruses, including the Creutzfeldt-Jacob disease agent, is believed to be remote but has not been tested. Accordingly, assess benefits and risks of treatment with this product prior to use.

Adverse Reactions:

During clinical studies involving 31 patients, 28 adverse experiences occurred that were possibly related to alglucerase. Seven of these were related to the route of administration and included discomfort, burning and swelling at the site of venipuncture. The remaining 21 experiences (of which $\approx$ 75% were reported by 2 patients) consisted of slight fever, chills, abdominal discomfort, nausea or vomiting. None of these events were judged to require medical intervention.

Most patients treated on a chronic basis have not formed detectable antibodies. Six months after therapy initiation, a 72-year-old patient demonstrated a positive response in testing procedures designed to detect antibodies to alglucerase. Close monitoring indicated no diminution of clinical response, and therapy has been continued.

Overdosage:

No obvious toxicity was detected after single doses up to 234 U/kg. There is no experience with higher doses.

Administration and Dosage:

Administer by IV infusion over 1 to 2 hours. Individualize dosage. An initial dosage up to 60 U/kg per infusion may be used. The usual frequency of infusion is once every 2 weeks, but disease severity and patient convenience may dictate administration as often as once every other day or as infrequently as once every 4 weeks. After patient response is well established, dosage may be adjusted downward for maintenance therapy. Dosage can be progressively lowered at intervals of 3 to 6 months while closely monitoring response parameters. Ultrastructural evidence suggests that glucocerebroside lipid storage may respond to doses as low as 1 U/kg.

On the day of use, the appropriate amount of alglucerase for each patient is diluted with normal saline to a final volume not to exceed 100 ml. The use of an in-line particulate filter is recommended for the infusion apparatus.

Relatively low toxicity, combined with the extended time course of response, allows small dosage adjustments to be made occasionally to avoid discarding partially used bottles. Thus, the dosage administered in individual infusions may be slightly increased or decreased to fully utilize each bottle as long as the monthly administered dosage remains substantially unaltered.

Storage/stability: Do not shake; shaking may denature the glycoprotein, rendering it biologically inactive. Store at 4°C (39°F). Do not use any bottles exhibiting particulate matter or discoloration. Do not use after the expiration date on the bottle. Alglucerase does not contain any preservative; after opening, do not store for subsequent use.

Rx	**Ceredase**[1] (Genzyme)	**Injection**: 10 U/ml[2]	In bottles (50 U per bottle with 5 ml fill volume).[3]
		80 U/ml[2]	In bottles (4000 U per bottle with 5 ml fill volume).[3]

[1] Alglucerase will be phased out over time by the manufacturer. This product is being replaced by imiglucerase (see specific monograph).

[2] An international enzyme unit is defined as the amount of enzyme required to hydrolyze 1 micromole of the synthetic substrate.

[3] With 1% albumin (human), 53 mM citrate and 143 mM sodium.

IMIGLUCERASE

Actions:

Pharmacology: Imiglucerase is an analogue of the human enzyme β-glucocerebrosidase, a lysosomal glycoprotein enzyme which catalyzes the hydrolysis of the glycolipid glucocerebroside to glucose and ceramide. Imiglucerase is produced by recombinant DNA technology using mammalian cell culture (Chinese hamster ovary). Purified imiglucerase is a monomeric glycoprotein of 497 amino acids. It differs from placental glucocerebrosidase by one amino acid at position 495 where histidine is substituted for arginine. The modified structures on imiglucerase are somewhat different from those on placental glucocerebrosidase. These mannose-terminated oligosaccharide chains of imiglucerase are specifically recognized by endocytic carbohydrate receptors on macrophages, the cells that accumulate lipid in Gaucher's disease.

Gaucher's disease is characterized by a deficiency of β-glucocerebrosidase activity, resulting in accumulation of glucocerebrosidase in tissue macrophages which become engorged and are typically found in the liver, spleen and bone marrow and occasionally in lung, kidney and intestine. Secondary hematologic sequelae include severe anemia and thrombocytopenia in addition to the characteristic progressive hepatosplenomegaly, skeletal complications, including osteonecrosis and osteopenia, with secondary pathological fractures. Imiglucerase improved anemia and thrombocytopenia, reduced spleen and liver size, and decreased cachexia to a degree similar to that observed with alglucerase.

Pharmacokinetics: During 1 hour IV infusions of four doses (7.5, 15, 30 and 60 U/kg) of imiglucerase, steady-state enzymatic activity was achieved by 30 minutes. Following infusion, plasma enzymatic activity declined rapidly with half-life ranging from 3.6 to 10.4 minutes. Plasma clearance ranged from 9.8 to 20.3 ml/min/kg. The volume of distribution corrected for weight ranged from 0.09 to 0.15 L/kg. These variables do not appear to be influenced by dose or duration of infusion. However, only one or two patients were studied at each dose level and infusion rate. The pharmacokinetics of imiglucerase do not appear to be different from placental-derived alglucerase. In patients who developed IgG antibody to imiglucerase, an apparent effect on serum enzyme levels resulted in diminished volume of distribution and clearance and increased elimination half-life compared to patients without antibody (see Warnings).

Indications:

Gaucher's disease: Long-term enzyme replacement therapy for patients with a confirmed diagnosis of Type 1 Gaucher's disease that results in one or more of the following conditions: Anemia; thrombocytopenia; bone disease; hepatomegaly; splenomegaly.

Contraindications:

Hypersensitivity (carefully re-evaluate treatment if there is significant clinical evidence of hypersensitivity to the product).

Warnings:

Antibodies: During the clinical trials (duration, 9 months), 4 of 25 patients (16%) treated with imiglucerase developed IgG antibodies reactive with imiglucerase. During the same clinical trial, 6 of 15 patients (40%) treated with placental-derived alglucerase developed IgG antibodies to alglucerase, and one of these patients had clinical allergic signs and symptoms resulting in withdrawal from the study. Of those patients treated with imiglucerase, only one patient developed a transient rash. No patients treated with imiglucerase, either initially or after changing over from alglucerase, have exhibited serious symptoms of immediate hypersensitivity, although a risk for such reactions may be present. Approach treatment with caution in patients who have exhibited symptoms of hypersensitivity to the product.

Pregnancy: Category C. It is not known whether imiglucerase can cause fetal harm when administered to a pregnant women, or can affect reproductive capacity. Do not administer during pregnancy except when the indication and need are clear and the potential benefit is judged to substantially justify the risk.

Lactation: It is not known whether this drug is excreted in breast milk. Exercise caution when imiglucerase is administered to a nursing woman.

Adverse Reactions:

During clinical trials with imiglucerase involving 25 patients with Gaucher's disease, the following adverse events were noted: Headache (n = 3); nausea, abdominal discomfort, dizziness, pruritus, rash, mild decrease in blood pressure, decrease in urinary frequency (n = 1). None of these events were judged to be serious or to warrant medical intervention or interruption of therapy. All proved transient and did not recur frequently. Symptoms suggestive of allergic hypersensitivity have been noted in a number of patients treated with alglucerase (see Warnings).

IMIGLUCERASE

Overdosage:

Effects of dosages exceeding 120 U/kg per 4 weeks have not been studied and therefore dosages > 120 U/kg are not recommended.

Administration and Dosage:

Approved by the FDA on March 23, 1994 (1P Classification).

Administered by IV infusion over 1 to 2 hours. Individualize dosage.

Initial dosage may be as little as 2.5 U/kg 3 times a week up to as much as 60 U/kg administered as frequently as once a week or as infrequently as every 4 weeks; 60 U/kg every 2 weeks is the dosage for which the most data are available. Disease severity may dictate that treatment be initiated at a relatively high dose or relatively frequent administration.

Maintenance: After patient response is well established, a reduction in dosage may be attempted for maintenance therapy. Progressive reductions can be made at intervals of 3 to 6 months while carefully monitoring response parameters.

Preparation of solution: On the day of use, after the correct amount of imiglucerase to be administered to the patient has been determined, the appropriate number of vials are each reconstituted with 5.1 ml of Sterile Water for Injection, USP, to give a reconstituted volume of 5.3 ml (40 U/ml). A 5 ml volume is then withdrawn from each vial and pooled with 0.9% Sodium Chloride Injection, USP, to a final volume of 100 to 200 ml. Alternatively the appropriate dose of imiglucerase may be administered such that a rate of no greater than 1 U/ kg/ min is infused. Relatively low toxicity, combined with the extended time course of response, allows small dosage adjustments to be made occasionally to avoid discarding partially used bottles. Thus, the dosage administered in individual infusions may be slightly increased or decreased to fully utilize each vial as long as the monthly administered dosage remains substantially unaltered.

Storage/Stability: Store at 2° to 8°C (36° to 46°F). Any vials exhibiting particulate matter or discoloration should not be used. DO NOT USE imiglucerase after the expiration date on the vial. Since imiglucerase does not contain any preservative, after reconstitution, properly dilute vials and do not store for subsequent use. When diluted to 50 ml, imiglucerase is stable for up to 24 hours when stored at 2° to 8°C (36° to 46°F).

Rx	**Cerezyme** (Genzyme)	**Powder for Injection (lyohilized)**: 212 units (equiv. to a withdrawal dose of 200 units imiglucerase).	Preservative free. In vials[1].

[1] Contains 155 mg mannitol and 70 mg sodium citrate (52 mg trisodium citrate, 18 mg disodium hydrogen citrate) per vial.

Thyroid Hormones

THYROID HORMONES

Preparations: Thyroid hormones include both natural and synthetic derivatives. The natural products, desiccated thyroid and thyroglobulin, are derived from beef or pork. Although these preparations are most economical, standardization by iodine content or bioassay is inexact; synthetic derivatives are generally preferred because of more uniform standardization of potency.

Synthetic derivatives include levothyroxine (T_4), liothyronine (T_3) and liotrix (a 4 to 1 mixture of T_4 and T_3).

Actions:

Pharmacology:

Physiological effects – The mechanisms by which thyroid hormones exert their physiologic action are not well understood. It is believed that most of their effects are exerted through control of DNA transcription and protein synthesis. Their principal effect is to increase metabolic rate of body tissues noted by increases in: Oxygen consumption; respiratory rate; body temperature; cardiac output; heart rate; blood volume; rate of fat, protein and carbohydrate metabolism; enzyme system activity; growth and maturation. Thyroid hormones exert a profound influence on every organ system and are particularly important in CNS development.

Thyroid hormones are also concerned with growth and differentiation of tissues. In deficiency states in the young, there is growth retardation and failure of maturation of the skeletal and other body systems, especially in failure of ossification in the epiphyses and in brain growth and development.

Regulation of thyroid secretion: Thyroid hormone synthesis is controlled by thyrotropin (Thyroid Stimulating Hormone; TSH) secreted by the anterior pituitary. TSH secretion is, in turn, controlled by a feedback mechanism effected by thyroid hormones and thyrotropin releasing hormone (TRH), a tripeptide of hypothalamic origin. Endogenous thyroid hormone secretion is suppressed when exogenous thyroid hormones are given to euthyroid individuals in excess of the normal gland's secretion.

Thyroid administration increases basal metabolic rate. The effect develops slowly, but is prolonged. It begins within 48 hours and reaches a maximum in 8 to 10 days, although full effects of continued use may not be evident for several weeks.

The primary effect of the thyroid hormones is the result of T_3 activity. The normal thyroid gland contains, per gram of gland, approximately 200 mcg of T_4 and 15 mcg of T_3. The ratio of these two hormones in the circulation does not represent the ratio in the thyroid gland, since about 80% of peripheral T_3 comes from monodeiodination of T_4. Peripheral monodeiodination of T_4 also results in the formation of reverse triiodothyronine (rT_3), which is calorigenically inactive. These facts seem to advocate T_4 as the treatment of choice for the hypothyroid patient and to caution against the administration of hormone combinations which, while normalizing thyroxine levels, may produce T_3 levels in the thyrotoxic range.

"Low triiodothyronine syndrome" – The T_3 level is low in the fetus and newborn, in the elderly and in cases of chronic caloric deprivation, hepatic cirrhosis, renal failure, surgical stress and chronic illnesses.

Pharmacokinetics:

Absorption – Absorption of T_4 from the GI tract varies from 48% to 79% of the dose administered; fasting increases absorption; malabsorption syndromes cause excessive fecal loss. In 4 hours, T_3 is 95% absorbed. The hormones in natural preparations are absorbed in a manner similar to the synthetic hormones.

Protein binding: More than 99% of circulating hormones are bound to serum proteins, including thyroid binding globulin (TBg), thyroid binding prealbumin (TBPA) and albumin (TBa), whose capacities and affinities vary for the hormones. The higher affinity of T_4 for both TBg and TBPA as compared to T_3 partially explains the higher serum levels and longer half-life of T_4. Both protein-bound hormones exist in reverse equilibrium with minute amounts of free hormone.

Metabolism – Under normal circumstances, the ratio of T_4 to T_3 released from the thyroid gland is 20:1. Approximately 35% of T_4 is converted in the periphery to T_3. Thus, 80% of T_3 comes from monodeiodination of T_4. Deiodination of T_4 occurs at a number of sites, including liver, kidney and other tissues. The conjugated hormone, in the form of glucuronide or sulfate, is found in the bile and gut where it may complete an enterohepatic circulation. Of T_4 metabolized daily, 85% is deiodinated.

Thyroid Hormones

THYROID HORMONES

Various Pharmacokinetic Parameters of Thyroid Hormones

Hormone	Ratio released from thyroid gland	Biologic potency	Half-life (days)	Protein binding (%)[2]
Levothyroxine (T_4)	20	1	6-7[1]	99+
Liothyronine (T_3)	1	4	≤ 2	99+

[1] 3 to 4 days in hyperthyroidism, 9 to 10 days in myxedema.
[2] Includes TBg, TBPA and TBa.

Indications:

Hypothyroidism: As replacement or supplemental therapy in hypothyroidism of any etiology, except transient hypothyroidism during the recovery phase of subacute thyroiditis. Specific indications include: Cretinism, myxedema, non-toxic goiter and ordinary hypothyroidism; primary hypothyroidism resulting from functional deficiency, primary atrophy, partial or total absence of thyroid gland, or the effects of surgery, radiation or drugs, with or without the presence of goiter; secondary (pituitary) or tertiary (hypothalamic) hypothyroidism.

Pituitary TSH suppressants: In the treatment or prevention of various types of euthyroid goiters, including thyroid nodules, subacute or chronic lymphocytic thyroiditis (Hashimoto's), multinodular goiter and in the management of thyroid cancer.

Thyrotoxicosis: May be used with antithyroid drugs to treat thyrotoxicosis, to prevent goitrogenesis and hypothyroidism and thyrotoxicosis during pregnancy.

Diagnostic use in suppression tests to differentiate suspected hyperthyroidism from euthyroidism.

Unlabeled uses: Thyroid hormones have been used to treat obesity; however, they are ineffective and should not be used for this condition. See Warnings.

Contraindications:

Acute myocardial infarction and thyrotoxicosis uncomplicated by hypothyroidism. However, when hypothyroidism is a complicating or causative factor in myocardial infarction or heart disease, consider the judicious use of small doses of thyroid.

Where hypothyroidism and hypoadrenalism (Addison's disease) coexist, unless treatment of hypoadrenalism with adrenocortical steroids precedes the initiation of thyroid therapy (see Warnings).

Hypersensitivity to active or extraneous constituents.

Warnings:

> *Obesity* has been treated with thyroid hormones. In euthyroid patients, hormonal replacement doses are ineffective for weight reduction. Larger doses may produce serious or even life-threatening toxicity, particularly when given with sympathomimetic amines such as anorexiants.

Infertility: Thyroid hormone therapy is unjustified for the treatment of male or female infertility, unless the condition is accompanied by hypothyroidism.

Cardiovascular disease: Use caution when the integrity of the cardiovascular system, particularly the coronary arteries, is suspect. This includes patients with angina or the elderly, in whom there is a greater likelihood of occult cardiac disease. In these patients, initiate therapy with low doses, ie, 25 to 50 mcg T_4 or its equivalent. When, in such patients, a euthyroid state can only be reached at the expense of an aggravation of the cardiovascular disease, reduce thyroid hormone dosage. The development of chest pain or other worsening of cardiovascular disease requires a decrease in dosage.

Observe patients with coronary artery disease during surgery, since the possibility of precipitating cardiac arrhythmias may be greater in those treated with thyroid hormones.

Endocrine disorders: Thyroid hormone therapy in patients with concomitant diabetes mellitus or insipidus or adrenal insufficiency (Addison's disease) exacerbates the intensity of their symptoms. Appropriate adjustments in the therapy of these concomitant endocrine diseases are required.

Severe and prolonged hypothyroidism can lead to a decreased level of adrenocortical activity commensurate with the lowered metabolic state. When thyroid replacement therapy is administered, the metabolism increases at a greater rate than adrenocortical activity, which can precipitate adrenocortical insufficiency. Therefore,

THYROID HORMONES

supplemental adrenocortical steroids may be necessary. The therapy of myxedema coma requires simultaneous administration of glucocorticoids.

In patients whose hypothyroidism is secondary to hypopituitarism, adrenal insufficiency will probably be present; correct adrenal insufficiency with corticosteroids before administering thyroid hormones.

Morphologic hypogonadism and nephrosis: Rule out prior to initiating therapy.

Myxedema: Patients with myxedema are particularly sensitive to thyroid preparations. Begin treatment with small doses and gradual increments.

Hyperthyroid effects: In rare instances the administration of thyroid hormone may precipitate a hyperthyroid state or may aggravate existing hyperthyroidism.

Pregnancy: Category A. Thyroid hormones do not readily cross the placenta. Clinical experience does not indicate any adverse effect on the fetus when thyroid hormones are administered to a pregnant woman. Do not discontinue thyroid replacement therapy in hypothyroid women during pregnancy.

Lactation: Minimal amounts of thyroid hormones are excreted in breast milk. Thyroid is not associated with serious adverse reactions. However, exercise caution when thyroid is administered to a nursing woman.

Children:

Congenital hypothyroidism – Pregnant women provide little or no thyroid hormone to the fetus. The incidence of congenital hypothyroidism is relatively high (1:4000) and the hypothyroid fetus would not benefit from the small amounts of hormone crossing the placenta. Routine determinations of serum T_4 or TSH are strongly advised in neonates in view of the deleterious effects of thyroid deficiency on growth and development.

Initiate treatment immediately upon diagnosis, and maintain for life, unless transient hypothyroidism is suspected; in this case, therapy may be interrupted for 2 to 8 weeks after the age of 3 years to reassess the condition. Cessation of therapy is justified in patients who have maintained a normal TSH during those 2 to 8 weeks.

In infants, excessive doses of thyroid hormone preparations may produce craniosynostosis.

In children, partial loss of hair may be experienced in the first few months of thyroid therapy; this is usually a transient phenomenon that results in later recovery.

Precautions:

Monitoring: Treatment of patients with thyroid hormones requires the periodic assessment of thyroid status by means of appropriate laboratory tests. The TSH suppression test can be used to test the effectiveness of any thyroid preparation, keeping in mind the relative insensitivity of the infant pituitary to the negative feedback effect of thyroid hormones. Serum T_4 levels can be used to test the effectiveness of all thyroid medications except T_3. When the total serum T_4 is low but TSH is normal, a test specific to assess unbound (free) T_4 levels is warranted. Specific measurements of T_4 and T_3 by competitive protein binding or radioimmunoassay are not influenced by blood levels of organic or inorganic iodine and have essentially replaced older tests (ie, PBI, BEI and T_4 by column). See Administration and Dosage.

Persistent clinical and laboratory evidence of hypothyroidism in spite of adequate dosage replacement indicates poor patient compliance, poor absorption, excessive fecal loss or inactivity of the preparation. Intracellular resistance to thyroid hormone is rare.

Decreased bone density: Long-term levothyroxine therapy has been associated with decreased bone density in the hip and spine in pre- and postmenopausal women. These effects may be avoided by using levothyroxine only after appropriate clinical evaluation, gradually increasing the dose until the appropriate serum level is reached using the minimal dose required and periodically monitoring the patient. It may be beneficial to obtain a basal bone density measurement, then monitor closely for osteoporosis development.

Tartrazine sensitivity: Some of these products contain tartrazine, which may cause allergic-type reactions (including bronchial asthma) in susceptible individuals. Although the incidence of tartrazine sensitivity in the general population is low, it is frequently seen in patients who also have aspirin hypersensitivity. Specific products containing tartrazine are identified in the product listings.

THYROID HORMONES

Drug Interactions:

Thyroid Hormone Drug Interactions			
Precipitant Drug	Object Drug*		Description
Cholestyramine and colestipol	Thyroid hormones	⬇	Loss of efficacy of thyroid hormone and potential hypothyroidism. Administer 4 to 6 hours apart.
Estrogens	Thyroid hormones	⬇	Estrogens increase TBg and may therefore decrease the response to thyroid hormone therapy in patients with a nonfunctioning thyroid gland. This is based on theoretical considerations.
Thyroid hormones	Anticoagulants	⬆	The anticoagulant action is increased; a decreased dose may be necessary.
Thyroid hormones	Beta blockers	⬇	The actions of particular beta blockers may be impaired when the hypothyroid patient is converted to the euthyroid state.
Thyroid hormones	Digitalis glycosides	⬇	Serum digitalis glycoside levels are reduced in hyperthyroidism or when the hypothyroid patient is converted to the euthyroid state. Therapeutic effects of digitalis glycosides may be reduced.
Thyroid hormones	Theophyllines	⬆	Decreased theophylline clearance can be expected in hypothyroid patients; clearance returns to normal when euthyroid state is achieved.

* ⬆ = Object drug increased. ⬇ = Object drug decreased.

Drug/Lab test interactions: Consider changes in TBg concentration when interpreting T_4 and T_3 values. In such cases, measure the unbound (free) hormone. Pregnancy, infectious hepatitis, estrogens and estrogen-containing oral contraceptives increase TBg concentrations. Decreases in TBg concentrations are observed in nephrosis, acromegaly and after androgen or corticosteroid therapy. Familial hyper- or hypothyroxine binding globulinemias have been described. The incidence of TBg deficiency approximates 1 in 9000.

Medicinal or dietary iodine interferes with all in vivo tests of radioiodine uptake, producing low uptakes which may not reflect a true decrease in hormone synthesis.

Thyroid Hormones

THYROID HORMONES

Effects of Drugs on Thyroid Function Tests

Blank space signifies no data ↑ Increased ⇧ Slightly increased ↓ Decreased ⇩ Slightly decreased 0 No effect	Free T_4	Serum T_4	T_3 uptake resin	Free thyroxine index (FTI)	Serum T_3	Serum TSH
p-aminosalicyclic acid		↓		↓		
Aminoglutethimide		↓				↑
Amiodarone	0/↑	↑		↑	↓	↑
Anabolic steroids/androgens	0	↓	↑	0	↓	0
Antithyroid (PTU, methimazole)	0	0	↓	0	↓	0
Asparaginase		↓	↑	0	↓	0
Barbiturates	0	↓	0/⇧	↓	0	0
Carbamazepine	0/↓	↓	0/↑	↓	0/↑	0/↑
Chloral hydrate		↓	0/⇧	0	↓	0
Cholestiramine	0	↓		↓	0/↑	0
Clofibrate	0	↑	↓	0	↑	0
Colestipol	0	↓		↓	0/↑	0/↑
Contraceptives, oral	0	↑	↓	0	↑	0
Corticosteroids	0	↓	↑	0	↓	0/↓
Danazol	0	↓	↑	0	↓	0
Diazepam		↓		⇩		
Estrogens	0	↑	↓	0/⇧	↑	0
Ethionamide		↓				
Fluorouracil		↓	0/⇧	0	↓	0
Heparin (IV)		↓	0/↑	↑	0	
Insulin		↑				
Lithium carbonate		0/↓	0/↓	0/↓	0/↓	0/↑
Methadone		↑	↓	0	↑	0
Mitotane		↓	0/⇧	0	↓	0
Nitroprusside		↓				
Oxyphenbutazone/phenylbutazone		↓	0/⇧	0	↓	0
Perphenazine		↑	↓	↓	↑	
Phenytoin	0/↓	↓	0/⇧	↓	0/↑	0/↑
Propranolol	0	0/↓	0/↑	0/↓	0/↓	0
Resorcinol (excessive topical use)		↓	↓	↓	↓	↑
Salicylates (large doses)	0	↓	0/⇧	0	↓	0
Sulfonylureas		↓	0	0		
Thiazides		0			↑	

THYROID HORMONES

Drug/Food interactions: Fasting increases the absorption of T_4 from the GI tract.

Adverse Reactions:

Adverse reactions other than those indicating hyperthyroidism due to therapeutic overdosage, either initially or during the maintenance period, are rare.

If symptoms of excessive dosage appear, discontinue medication for several days and reinstitute at a lower dosage. Symptoms of overdosage include:

Cardiovascular: Palpitations; tachycardia; arrhythmias; angina pectoris; cardiac arrest.

CNS: Tremors; headache; nervousness; insomnia. Pseudotumor cerebri occurred in two children after initiation of thyroxine for autoimmune thyroiditis.

GI: Diarrhea; vomiting. Gastric intolerance may occur rarely in patients highly sensitive to beef or pork products or corn.

Hypersensitivity: Allergic skin reactions (rare).

Miscellaneous: Weight loss; menstrual irregularities; sweating; heat intolerance; fever.

Overdosage:

These agents rarely result in clinical toxicity.

Chronic excessive dosage may produce signs and symptoms of hyperthyroidism (eg, headache, irritability, nervousness, sweating, tachycardia, increased bowel motility, menstrual irregularities, palpitations, vomiting, psychosis, seizure, fever). Angina pectoris or CHF may be induced or aggravated. Shock may develop. Complications may include cardiac failure and arrhythmias, which could be fatal. Massive overdosage may result in symptoms resembling thyroid storm.

Reduce dosage or temporarily discontinue therapy. Reinstitute treatment at a lower dosage. In healthy individuals, normal hypothalamic-pituitary-thyroid axis function is restored in 6 to 8 weeks after thyroid suppression. Therapeutic regimens are not justified in asymptomatic patients.

Serum T_4 levels do not appear to correlate with the severity of toxicity. Some patients with high T_4 concentrations remain asymptomatic. In five children, T_4 levels were 12.2 to 22.9 mcg/dl (normal 4 to 12 mcg/dl) but the children were asymptomatic. T_4 ingestion also appears to be less toxic than T_3 ingestion, and symptoms may be delayed due to the metabolic conversion time from T_4 to T_3.

Acute massive overdosage: Treatment is aimed at reducing GI absorption of the drug and counteracting central and peripheral effects, mainly those of increased sympathetic activity. Refer to General Management of Acute Overdosage. Cardiac glycosides may be indicated if CHF develops. Control fever, hypoglycemia or fluid loss, if needed. Antiadrenergic agents, particularly propranolol (1 to 3mg IV over 10 minutes or 80 to 160 mg orally per day), have been used to treat increased sympathetic activity. Consider treatment of unrecognized adrenal insufficiency. Acetaminophen may be useful for fever control.

Patient Information:

Replacement therapy is to be taken for life, except in cases of transient hypothyroidism, usually associated with thyroiditis, and in those receiving a trial of the drug.

Take as a single daily dose, preferably before breakfast.

Brand interchange: Do not change from one brand of this drug to another without consulting your pharmacist or physician. Products manufactured by different companies may not be equally effective.

Do not discontinue medication except on advice of a physician.

Notify physician if headache, nervousness, diarrhea, excessive sweating, heat intolerance, chest pain, increased pulse rate, palpitations (symptoms of hyperthyroidism) or any unusual event occurs.

Partial loss of hair may be experienced by children in the first few months of therapy, but this is usually a transient phenomenon that results in later recovery.

Not for use as primary or adjunctive therapy in a weight control program.

If levothyroxine is taken on an empty stomach, absorption is increased.

Administration and Dosage:

Individualize dosage to approximate the deficit in the patient's thyroid secretion. Determine patient response by clinical judgment in conjunction with laboratory findings.

Generally, institute thyroid therapy at relatively low doses and slowly increase in small increments until the desired response is obtained. Administer thyroid as a single daily dose, preferably before breakfast.

Thyroid Hormones

THYROID HORMONES

Treatment of choice for hypothyroidism is T_4 under most circumstances because of its consistent potency, restoration of normal constant serum levels of T_4 and T_3 and its prolonged duration of action. However, it has a slow onset of action and its effects are cumulative over several weeks.

The rapid onset and dissipation of action of T_3, as compared with T_4, have led some clinicians to prefer its use in patients who might be more susceptible to the untoward effects of thyroid medication. However, the wide swings in serum T_3 levels following administration and the possibility of more pronounced cardiovascular side effects tend to offset the stated advantages. If there is a need for rapidly correcting the hypothyroid state, the administration of T_3 is preferable because of its rapid onset and dissipation of action.

T_3 may be preferred to T_4 during radioisotope scanning procedures; induction of hypothyroidism in those cases is more abrupt and can be of shorter duration. It may also be preferred when impaired peripheral conversion of T_4 and T_3 is suspected.

Thyroid cancer: Exogenous thyroid hormone may produce regression of metastases from follicular and papillary carcinoma of the thyroid and is used as ancillary therapy of these conditions with radioactive iodine. Larger doses than used for replacement therapy are required. Medullary thyroid carcinoma is usually unresponsive.

Laboratory tests useful in the diagnosis and evaluation of thyroid function are listed in the following table, indicating the alterations noted in various thyroid disorders.

Laboratory Tests for Diagnosis and Evaluation of Thyroid Function

↑ = Increased ↓ = Decreased N = Normal	Normal	Pregnancy	Primary hypothyroid	Secondary hypothyroid	Hyperthyroid	T_3 thyrotoxicosis	Normal values
Free T_4 (unbound)	N	N	↓	↓	↑	N	
Total T_4	N	↑	↓	↓	↑	N	5-11 mcg/dl
Serum T_3	N	↑	↓	↓	↑	↑	85-185 ng/dl
T_3 resin uptake (RT_3U)	N	↓	↓	↓	↑		25%- 35%
Free thyroxine index (FT_4I)	N	N	↓	↓	↑		1.3 - 4.2
TSH	N	N	↑	↓	N/↓[1]		0.4-4.8 mcU/ml

[1] When tested using the more sensitive immunometric assays.

Thyroid Hormones

THYROID HORMONES

Serum free T_4 and TSH values are usually sufficient to diagnose thyroid status; however, serum TSH is more sensitive. FT_4 appears to be a better indicator of thyroid status than total T_4 since total T_4 levels can vary drastically in the absence of thyroid dysfunction; total T_4 is therefore not reliable and is not an adequate first-line test. Total T_4 may be useful in some special comprehensive situations. All FT_4 immunoassays are 90% to 100% accurate in diagnosing patients with simple thyroid disease. FT_4I is a crude estimate for serum FT_4 and is calculated from the results of total T_4 and the thyroid hormone binding ratio (THBR, formerly T_3 or T_4 uptake). Newer methods for FT_4I have not been fully evaluated. Free T_3 assays have not been fully evaluated at this time but may be a more useful measurement than serum T_3. Serum T_3/FT_3 are adjunctive second-line tests that may be useful in confirming less common forms of hyperthyroidism and diagnosing T_3 thyrotoxicosis, but they should not be used for diagnosing hypothyroidism. In summary, serum TSH by a sensitive immunometric assay is the best general test, followed by FT_4.

Drug effects on thyroid laboratory tests must be considered; see Drug Interactions.

Thyrotropin (TSH) may be utilized to determine subclinical hypothyroidism and to differentiate primary and secondary hypothyroidism. Refer to individual monograph.

Protirelin (thyrotropin releasing hormone) may be useful in the differentiation of primary, secondary and tertiary hypothyroidism. Refer to individual monograph.

Dosage equivalents of thyroid products: In changing from one thyroid product to another, the following dosage equivalents may be used. However, each patient may still require fine dosage adjustments because these equivalents are only estimates.

Dosage Equivalents of Thyroid Products

Preparation	Composition ratio T_4	T_3	Dosage equivalents
Crude hormone			
Thyroid USP	2 to 5	1	60 mg (1 grain)
Thyroglobulin	2.5	1	60 mg
Thyroid Strong	3.1	1	45 mg
Synthetic hormone			
Levothyroxine	1	0	0.05 to 0.06 mg[1]
Liothyronine	0	1	15 to 37.5 mcg
Liotrix	4	1	50 to 60 mcg T_4 and 12.5 to 15 mcg T_3

[1] Previously considered to be 0.1 mg.

Thyroid Hormones

THYROID DESICCATED

For complete prescribing information, refer to the Thyroid Drugs group monograph.

Thyroid USP is composed of desiccated animal thyroid glands. The active thyroid hormones (T_4 and T_3) are available in their natural state and ratio. These preparations are standardized by iodine content; some manufacturers also use biological methods of standardization.

Administration and Dosage:

Optimal dosage is determined by patient's clinical response and laboratory findings.

Hypothyroidism:

Initial dosage – Institute therapy using low doses, with increments that depend on cardiovascular status. Usual starting dose is 30 mg, with increments of 15 mg every 2 to 3 weeks. Use 15 mg/day in patients with long-standing mxyedema, particularly if cardiovascular impairment is suspected. Reduce dosage if angina occurs.

Maintenance dosage – 60 to 120 mg/day; failure to respond to 180 mg doses suggests lack of compliance or malabsorption.

Readjust dosage within the first 4 weeks of therapy after proper clinical and laboratory evaluations.

Thyroid cancer: Larger amounts of thyroid hormone than those used for replacement therapy are required.

Children: Follow recommendations in the following table. In infants with congenital hypothyroidism, institute therapy with full doses as soon as diagnosis is made.

Recommended Pediatric Dosage for Congenital Hypothyroidism

Age	Dose per day (mg)	Daily dose per kg (mg)
0 to 6 mos	15 to 30	4.8 to 6
6 to 12 mos	30 to 45	3.6 to 4.8
1 to 5 yrs	45 to 60	3 to 3.6
6 to 12 yrs	60 to 90	2.4 to 3
> 12 yrs	> 90	1.2 to 1.8

Rx	**Thyroid USP** (Various, eg, Lannett)	**Tablets**: 15 mg (¼ grain)	In 1000s.
Rx	**Armour Thyroid** (Rhone-Poulenc Rorer)		Dextrose. In 100s and 1000s.
Rx	**Thyroid USP** (Various, eg, Major, Rugby, Schein)	**Tablets**: 30 mg (½ grain)	In 1000s.
Rx	**Armour Thyroid** (Rhone-Poulenc Rorer)		Dextrose. In 100s, 1000s, 5000s and UD 100s.
Rx	**Thyroid USP** (Various, eg, Goldline, Major, Moore, Parmed, Rugby, Schein)	**Tablets**: 60 mg (1 grain)	In 100s, 1000s and 5000s.
Rx	**Armour Thyroid** (Rhone-Poulenc Rorer)		Dextrose. In 100s, 1000s, 5000s and UD 100s.
Rx	**Armour Thyroid** (Rhone-Poulenc Rorer)	**Tablets**: 90 mg (1½ grain)	(TJ). In 100s.
Rx	**Thyroid USP** (Various, eg, Goldline, Major, Moore, Parmed, Rugby)	**Tablets**: 120 mg (2 grain)	In 100s, 1000s and 5000s.
Rx	**Armour Thyroid** (Rhone-Poulenc Rorer)		Dextrose. (TF). In 100s, 1000s, 2500s and UD 100s.

Thyroid Hormones

THYROID DESICCATED

Rx	**Thyroid USP** (Various, eg, Major, Parmed, Rugby)	**Tablets**: 180 mg (3 grain)	In 1000s.
Rx	**Armour Thyroid** (Rhone-Poulenc Rorer)		Dextrose. (TG). In 100s and 1000s.
Rx	**Armour Thyroid** (Rhone-Poulenc Rorer)	**Tablets**: 240 mg (4 grain)	Dextrose. (TH). In 100s.
Rx	**Thyroid USP** (Various, eg, Lannett)	**Tablets**: 300 mg (5 grain)	In 500s and 1000s.
Rx	**Armour Thyroid** (Rhone-Poulenc Rorer)		Dextrose. (TI). In 100s.
Rx	**Thyroid Strong** (Jones Medical)	50% stronger than thyroid USP. Each grain is eqivalent to 1½ grains of thyroid USP. **Tablets**: 30 mg (½ grain)	(JMI 686). In 100s and 1000s.
		60 mg (1 grain)	(JMI 674). In 100s and 1000s.
		120 mg (2 grain)	(JMI 675). In 100s and 1000s.
		Tablets, sugar coated: 30 mg (½ grain)	(JMI 626). In 100s.
		60 mg (1 grain)	(JMI 627). In 100s and 1000s.
		120 mg (2 grain)	(JMI 628). In 100s.
		180 mg (3 grain)	(JMI 629). In 100s.
Rx	**Thyrar** (Rhone-Poulenc Rorer)	Bovine thyroid. **Tablets**: 30 mg (½ grain)	In 100s.
		60 mg (1 grain)	In 100s.
		120 mg (2 grain)	In 100s.
Rx	**S-P-T** (Fleming)	Pork thyroid suspended in soybean oil. **Capsules**: 60 mg (1 grain)	Green. In 100s and 1000s.
		120 mg (2 grain)	Brown. In 100s and 1000s.
		180 mg (3 grain)	Red. In 100s and 1000s.
		300 mg (5 grain)	Black. In 100s and 1000s.

THYROGLOBULIN

For complete prescribing information, refer to the Thyroid Hormones group monograph.

Contains T_4 and T_3 in an approximate ratio of 2.5 to 1.

Administration and Dosage:

See Thyroid Desiccated Administration and Dosage.

Not recommended for suppression therapy.

Rx	**Proloid** (Parke-Davis)	**Tablets**: 30 mg (½ grain)	Gray. In 100s.
		60 mg (1 grain)	Gray, scored. In 100s and 1000s.
		90 mg (1½ grain)	Gray. In 100s.
		120 mg (2 grain)	Gray, scored. In 100s.
		180 mg (3 grain)	Gray. In 100s.

Thyroid Hormones

LEVOTHYROXINE SODIUM (T_4; L-thyroxine)

For complete prescribing information, refer to the Thyroid Hormones group monograph.

An active principle of the thyroid gland prepared synthetically in pure crystalline form.

Dosage equivalence: 0.05 to 0.06 mg equals approximately 60 mg (1 grain) thyroid (it was previously considered that 0.1 mg levothyroxine equalled 60 mg thyroid).

Bioavailability: Bioequivalence problems have been documented in the past for levothyroxine products marketed by different manufacturers. Brand interchange is not recommended unless comparative bioavailability data, which provide evidence of therapeutic equivalence, are available. If patients are switched from one product to another, reassess measures of thyroid function and retitrate the levothyroxine dose as necessary.

Administration and Dosage:

Optimal dosage determined by patient's clinical response and laboratory findings.

Hypothyroidism:

Initial dosage – Institute using low doses with increments that depend on cardiovascular status. Usual starting dose is 0.05 mg, with increments of 0.025 mg every 2 to 3 weeks. Use ≤ 0.025 mg/day in patients with long-standing hypothyroidism, particularly if cardiovascular impairment is suspected. Reduce if angina occurs.

Maintenance dosage – Most patients require no more than 0.2 mg/day; failure to respond to 0.3 mg doses suggests lack of compliance or malabsorption. Readjust dosage within the first 4 weeks of therapy after proper evaluations.

IV or IM injection can be substituted for the oral dosage form when oral ingestion is precluded for long periods of time. The initial parenteral dosage should be approximately one-half of the previously established oral dosage.

Myxedema coma: Consider a medical emergency. Levothyroxine may be administered via nasogastric tube, but the IV route is preferred. A starting dose of 0.4 mg given rapidly is usually well tolerated, even in elderly. Sudden administration of large doses is not without cardiovascular risks; therefore, do not undertake IV therapy without weighing alternative risks. Clinical judgment may dictate smaller doses.

The initial dose is followed by daily supplements of 0.1 to 0.2 mg IV. Normal T_4 levels are achieved in 24 hours followed in 3 days by threefold elevation of T_3. Maintain continued daily IV administration of lesser amounts until the patient is fully capable of accepting a daily oral dose.

A daily maintenace dose of 0.05 to 0.1 mg parenterally should suffice to maintain the euthyroid state, once established. Resume oral therapy as soon as the clinical situation has been stabilized and the patient is able to take oral medication.

TSH suppression in thyroid cancer, nodules and euthyroid goiters: Larger amounts of thyroid hormone than those used for replacement therapy are required. This therapy is also used in treating nontoxic solitary nodules and multi-nodular goiters, and to prevent thyroid enlargement in chronic (Hashimoto's) thyroiditis.

Thyroid suppression therapy: 2.6 mcg/kg/day for 7 to 10 days. These doses usually yield normal serum T_4 and T_3 levels and lack of response to TSH.

Children: Follow the recommendations in the following table. In infants with congenital hypothyroidism, institute therapy with full doses as soon as diagnosis is made.

Levothyroxine tablets may be given to infants and children who cannot swallow intact tablets. Crush the proper dose tablet and suspend in a small amount of formula or water. The suspension can be given by spoon or dropper. Do NOT store the suspension for any period of time. The crushed tablet may also be sprinkled over a small amount of food such as cooked cereal or applesauce.

Recommended Pediatric Dosage for Congenital Hypothyroidism

Age	Dose per day (mcg)	Daily dose per kg (mcg)
0 to 6 months	25 to 50	8 to 10
6 to 12 months	50 to 75	6 to 8
1 to 5 years	75 to 100	5 to 6
6 to 12 years	100 to 150	4 to 5
> 12 years	> 150	2 to 3

Alternative suggested doses include: 0 to 1 year, 8 to 10 mcg/kg/day; 1 to 5 years, 4 to 6 mcg/kg/day; > 5 years to adolescence, 3 to 4 mcg/kg/day.

Preparation of injectable solution: Reconstitute by adding 5 ml 0.9% Sodium Chloride Injection, USP or Bacteriostatic Sodium Chloride Injection, USP with Benzyl Alcohol only. Shake the vial to ensure complete mixing. Use immediately after reconstitution. Do not add to other IV fluids. Discard any unused portion.

Thyroid Hormones

LEVOTHYROXINE SODIUM (T_4; L-thyroxine)

Rx	**Levo-T** (Lederle)	**Tablets**: 0.025 mg	In 100s.
Rx	**Levothroid**(Forest)		(LK). Orange. In 100s.
Rx	**Levoxyl** (Daniels)		Orange, oval. In 100s, 1000s and UD 100s.
Rx	**Synthroid** (Knoll)		(Flint 25). Orange, scored. In 100s and 1000s.[1]
Rx	**Eltroxin** (Roberts)	**Tablets** 0.05 mg	Scored. In 100s and 500s.
Rx	**Levo-T** (Lederle)		In 100s and 1000s.
Rx	**Levothroid**(Forest)		(LL). White. In 100s and UD 100s.
Rx	**Levoxyl** (Daniels)		White, oval. In 100s, 1000s and UD 100s.
Rx	**Synthroid** (Knoll)		(Flint 50). White, scored. In 100s, 1000s and UD 100s.[1]
Rx	**Levo-T** (Lederle)	**Tablets**: 0.075 mg	In 100s.
Rx	**Levothroid** (Forest)		(LT). Gray. In 100s.
Rx	**Levoxyl** (Daniels)		Purple, oval. In 100s, 1000s and UD 100s.
Rx	**Synthroid** (Knoll)		(Flint 75). Violet, scored. In 100s, 1000s and UD 100s.[1]
Rx	**Levothroid** (Forest)	**Tablets**: 0.088 mg	Green. In 100s.
Rx	**Levoxyl** (Daniels)		Olive, oval. In 100s, 1000s and UD 100s.
Rx	**Synthroid** (Knoll)		(Flint 88). Olive, scored. In 100s.[1]
Rx	**Eltroxin** (Roberts)	**Tablets**: 0.1 mg	Scored. In 100s and 500s.
Rx	**Levothyroxine Sodium** (Various, eg Lederle)		In 100s, 1000s and UD 100s.
Rx	**Levo-T** (Lederle)		In 100s and 1000s.
Rx	**Levothroid** (Forest)		(LM). Yellow. In 100s and UD 100s.
Rx	**Levoxyl** (Daniels)		Yellow, oval. In 100s, 1000s and UD 100s.
Rx	**Synthroid** (Knoll)		(Flint 100). Yellow, scored. In 100s, 1000s and UD 100s.[1]
Rx	**Levothroid** (Forest)	**Tablets**: 0.112 mg	Rose. In 100s.
Rx	**Levoxyl** (Daniels)		Rose, oval. In 100s, 1000s and UD 100s.
Rx	**Synthroid** (Knoll)		(Flint 112). Rose, scored. In 100s, 1000s and UD 100s[1].
Rx	**Levo-T** (Lederle)	**Tablets**: 0.125 mg	In 100s.
Rx	**Levothroid** (Forest)		(LH). Purple. In 100s.
Rx	**Levoxyl** (Daniels)		Brown, oval. In 100s, 1000s and UD 100s.
Rx	**Synthroid** (Knoll)		(Flint 125). Brown, scored. In 100s, 1000s and UD 100s.[1]
Rx	**Levothroid** (Forest)	**Tablets**: 0.137	Blue. In 100s.
Rx	**Levoxyl** (Daniels)	**Tablets**: 0.137 mg	In 100s, 1000s and UD 100s.

Thyroid Hormones

LEVOTHYROXINE SODIUM (T_4; L-thyroxine)

Rx	**Eltroxin** (Roberts)	**Tablets**: 0.15 mg	Scored. In 100s and 500s.
Rx	**Levothyroxine Sodium** (Various, eg Lederle)		In 100s, 1000s and UD 100s.
Rx	**Levo-T** (Lederle)		In 100s and 1000s.
Rx	**Levothroid** (Forest)		(LN). Blue. In 100s, UD 100s.
Rx	**Levoxyl** (Daniels)		Blue, oval. In 100s, 1000s and UD 100s.
Rx	**Synthroid** (Knoll)		(Flint 150). Blue, scored. In 100s, 1000s and UD 100s.[1]
Rx	**Levothroid** (Forest)	**Tablets**: 0.175 mg	(1¾ LP). Turquoise. In 100s.
Rx	**Levoxyl** (Daniels)		Turquoise, oval. In 100s, 1000s and UD 100s.
Rx	**Synthroid** (Knoll)		(Flint 175). Lilac, scored. In 100s.[1]
Rx	**Eltroxin** (Roberts)	**Tablets**: 0.2 mg	Scored. In 100s and 500s.
Rx	**Levothyroxine Sodium** (Various, eg, Lederle, Major, Moore, Rugby, Schein, URL, Vangard)		In 100s, 1000s and UD 100s.
Rx	**Levo-T** (Lederle)		In 100s and 1000s.
Rx	**Levothroid**(Forest)		(LR). Pink. In 100s and UD 100s.
Rx	**Levoxyl** (Daniels)		Pink, oval. In 100s, 1000s and UD 100s.
Rx	**Synthroid** (Knoll)		(Flint 200). Pink, scored. In 100s, 1000s and UD 100s.[1]
Rx	**Eltroxin** (Roberts)	**Tablets**: 0.3 mg	Scored. In 100s and 500s.
Rx	**Levothyroxine Sodium** (Various, eg, Lederle)		In 100s, 1000s and UD 100s.
Rx	**Levo-T** (Lederle)		In 100s.
Rx	**Levothroid**(Forest)		(LS). Green. In 100s and UD 100s.
Rx	**Levoxyl** (Daniels)		Green, oval. In 100s, 1000s and UD 100s.
Rx	**Synthroid** (Knoll)		(Flint 300). Green, scored. In 100s, 1000s and UD 100s.[1]
Rx	**Levothyroxine** (Various, eg, Loch, Quad, Schein)	**Powder for injection, lyophilized**: 200 mcg per vial	In 6 and 10 ml vials.
Rx	**Levothroid** (Forest)		In 6 ml vials.[2]
Rx	**Levoxine** (Daniels)		In 10 ml vials.[3]
Rx	**Synthroid** (Knoll)		In 10 ml vials.[4]
Rx	**Levothyroxine** (Various, eg, Loch, McGuff, Quad, Schein)	**Powder for injection, lyophilized**: 500 mcg per vial	In vials.
Rx	**Levothroid** (Forest)		In 6 ml vials.[2]
Rx	**Levoxine** (Daniels)		In 10 ml vials.[3]
Rx	**Synthroid** (Knoll)		In 10 ml vials.[4]

[1] With lactose and sugar.
[2] With 15 mg mannitol per vial.
[3] With 10 mg mannitol and 0.7 mg tribasic sodium phosphate hydrous per vial.
[4] With 10 mg mannitol per vial.

Thyroid Hormones

LIOTHYRONINE SODIUM (T_3)

For complete prescribing information, refer to the Thyroid Hormones group monograph.

Liothyronine sodium, a synthetic form of the natural thyroid hormone T_3, has pharmacologic activities of the natural substance. It has a short duration of activity which permits quick dosage adjustment and facilitates control of overdosage. It can be used in patients allergic to desiccated thyroid or thyroid extract derived from pork or beef.

Dosage equivalents: 15 to 37.5 mcg equals $\approx$ 60 mg (1 grain) desiccated thyroid.

Administration and Dosage:

Administer cautiously to patients in whom there is a strong suspicion of thyroid gland autonomy; exogenous hormone effects will be additive to the endogenous source.

Mild hypothyroidism: Starting dose is 25 mcg/day. Daily dosage may then be increased by 12.5 or 25 mcg every 1 or 2 weeks. Usual maintenance dose is 25 to 75 mcg/day. Smaller doses may be fully effective in some patients, while dosages of 100 mcg/day may be required in others.

Congenital hypothyroidism: Starting dose is 5 mcg/day, with a 5 mcg increment every 3 to 4 days until the desired response is achieved. Infants a few months old may require only 20 mcg/day for maintenance. At 1 year of age, 50 mcg/day may be required. Above 3 years, full adult dosage may be necessary.

Simple (nontoxic) goiter: Starting dose is 5 mcg/day. Dosage may be increased every 1 to 2 weeks by 5 or 10 mcg. When 25 mcg/day is reached, dosage may be increased every 1 to 2 weeks by 12.5 or 25 mcg. Usual maintenance dosage is 75 mcg/day.

T_3 suppression test: 75 to 100 mcg daily for 7 days, then repeat I^{131} Thyroid Uptake test. A $\geq$ 50% suppression of uptake indicates a normal thyroid-pituitary axis and thus rules out thyroid gland autonomy.

Myxedema: Starting dose is 5 mcg/day. This may be increased by 5 to 10 mcg/day every 1 to 2 weeks. When 25 mcg/day is reached, dosage may be increased by 12.5 or 25 mcg every 1 or 2 weeks. Usual maintenance dose is 50 to 100 mcg/day.

Myxedema coma/precoma (injection only), usually precipitated in the hypothyroid patient of long standing by intercurrent illness or drugs such as sedatives and anesthetics, is a medical emergency. Direct therapy at the correction of electrolyte disturbances, possible infection or other intercurrent illness in addition to IV liothyronine administration. Simultaneous glucocorticoids are required.

Liothyronine injection is for IV use only; do not give IM or SC. Proper administration of an adequate dose is important in determining clinical outcome. Base initial and subsequent doses on continuous monitoring of patient's clinical status and response. Give $\geq$ 4 hours, and $\leq$ 12 hours, apart. Giving $\geq$ 65 mcg/day initially is associated with lower mortality. There is limited experience with > 100 mcg/day.

An initial IV dose ranging from 25 to 50 mcg is recommended in the emergency treatment of myxedema complications in adults. In patients with known or suspected cardiovascular disease, an initial dose of 10 to 20 mcg is suggested. However, base doses on continuous monitoring of the condition and response to therapy. Exercise caution in adjusting the dose due to the potential of large changes to precipitate adverse cardiovascular events.

Switching to oral therapy – Resume oral therapy as soon as the clinical situation has been stabilized and the patient is able to take oral medication. When switching to tablets, discontinue injection, initiate oral therapy at a low dosage and increase gradually according to response. If oral levothyroxine is used, keep in mind that there is a delay of several days in the onset of action; discontinue IV therapy gradually.

Elderly or children: Start therapy with 5 mcg/day; increase only by 5 mcg increments at the recommended intervals.

Exchange therapy: When switching a patient to T_3 from thyroid, T_4 or thyroglobulin, discontinue the other medication, initiate T_3 at a low dosage and increase gradually according to the patient's response. When selecting a starting dosage, keep in mind that T_3 has a rapid onset of action, and that residual effects of the other thyroid preparation may persist for the first several weeks of therapy.

Storage/Stability-Injection: Store between 2° and 8°C (36° to 46°F).

Rx	**Cytomel** (SK-Beecham)	**Tablets**: 5 mcg	(SKF D14). White. In 100s.
Rx	**Liothyronine Sodium** (Various, eg, Geneva)	**Tablets**: 25 mcg	In 100s.
Rx	**Cytomel** (SK-Beecham)		(SKF D16). In 100s.
Rx	**Cytomel** (SK-Beecham)	**Tablets**: 50 mcg	(SKF D17). In 100s.
Rx	**Triostat** (SK-Beecham)	**Injection**: 10 mcg/ml	In 1 ml vials.[1]

[1] With 6.8% alcohol, 2.19 mg ammonia (as ammonium hydroxide).

Thyroid Hormones

LIOTRIX

For complete prescribing information, refer to the Thyroid Hormones group monograph.

A uniform mixture of synthetic T_4 and T_3 in a 4 to 1 ratio by weight.

Dosage equivalents: As shown in the product listings below, manufacturers differ on approximate equivalents to 1 grain thyroid. In patients previously rendered euthyroid with another thyroid product, each 60 mg liotrix tablet will usually replace 60 mg (1 grain) of desiccated thyroid, 0.05 to 0.06 mg T_4 or 12.5 to 15 mcg T_3.

Administration and Dosage:

Optimal dosage is determined by patient's clinical response and laboratory findings.

Hypothyroidism:

Initial dosage – Institute therapy using low doses, with increments that depend on cardiovascular status. Usual starting dose is 30 mg with 15 mg increments every 2 to 3 weeks. Use 15 mg/day in patients with long-standing hypothyroidism, particularly if cardiovascular impairment is suspected. Reduce dosage if angina occurs.

Maintenance dosage – Most patients require 60 to 120 mg/day; failure to respond to 180 mg doses suggests lack of compliance or malabsorption.

Readjust dosage within the first 4 weeks of therapy after proper clinical and laboratory evaluations.

Thyroid cancer: Larger amounts of thyroid hormone than those used for replacement therapy are required.

Children: Follow recommendations in the following table. In infants with congenital hypothyroidism, institute therapy with full doses as soon as diagnosis is made.

Recommended Pediatric Dosage for Congenital Hypothyroidism

	Tetraiodothyronine (T_4, levothyroxine) sodium	
Age	Dose per day	Daily dose per kg of body weight
0-6 mos	25-50 mcg	8-10 mcg
6-12 mos	50-75 mcg	6-8 mcg
1-5 yrs	75-100 mcg	5-6 mcg
6-12 yrs	100-150 mcg	4-5 mcg
over 12 yrs	over 150 mcg	2-3 mcg

	Product and Distributor	Tablet strength (grain)	Content (mcg) T_4	Content (mcg) T_3	Thyroid equivalent (mg)	How Supplied
Rx	**Thyrolar** (Forest)	¼	12.5	3.1	15	Lactose. (YC). Violet/white. Layered. In 100s.
		½	25	6.25	30	Lactose. (YD). Peach/white. Layered. In 100s.
		1	50	12.5	60	Lactose. (YE). Pink/white. Layered. In 100s.
		2	100	25	120	Lactose. (YF). Green/white. Layered. In 100s.
		3	150	37.5	180	Lactose. (YH). Yellow/white. Layered. In100s.

IODINE PRODUCTS

Actions:

Pharmacology: An adequate intake of iodine is necessary for normal thyroid function and the synthesis of thyroid hormones.

Elemental iodine (from the diet or as medication) is reduced in the GI tract and enters the circulation in the form of iodide, which is actively transported and concentrated by the thyroid gland. Hormone synthesis requires the oxidation of iodide and iodination of tyrosyl residues in thyroglobulin to form iodotyrosine precursors. These precursors undergo a "coupling reaction" to yield the active thyroid hormones T_3 and T_4. High concentrations of iodide greatly influence iodine metabolism by the thyroid gland. Large doses of iodides can inhibit T_4 and T_3 synthesis and rapidly inhibit proteolysis of colloid and the release of T_4 and T_3 into the bloodstream.

The effects of iodides are evident within 24 hours; maximum effects are attained after 10 to 15 days of continuous therapy. If administered chronically, therapeutic effects may persist for up to 6 weeks after the crisis has abated.

Indications:

Used adjunctively with an antithyroid drug in hyperthyroid patients in preparation for thyroidectomy and to treat thyrotoxic crisis or neonatal thyrotoxicosis.

Thyroid blocking in a radiation emergency.

For use of potassium iodide as an expectorant and for other respiratory tract conditions, see the Iodine Products monograph in the Expectorant section.

Unlabeled uses: Potassium iodide (60 mg 3 times daily) has been used effectively in a limited number of patients for Sweet's syndrome (acute febrile neutrophilic dermatosis) in combination with a potent topical steroid, as an alternative to systemic corticosteroids.

Also effective for the treatment of lymphocutaneous sporotrichosis (a dimorphic fungus that typically infects the skin and lymphatic system).

Contraindications:

Hypersensitivity to iodides.

Warnings:

Pregnancy: Category D (potassium iodide). Iodides readily cross the placenta and may cause hypothyroidism and goiter in the fetus or newborn when used long-term or close to term; short-term use (eg, 10 days) may not carry this risk. Administer to pregnant women only if clearly needed.

Lactation: Iodide is excreted in breast milk; however, the significance to the infant is not known. According to the American Academy of Pediatrics, these agents are not contraindicated in breastfeeding.

Drug Interactions:

Lithium carbonate and iodide preparations may have synergistic hypothyroid activity; concomitant use may result in hypothyroidism.

Adverse Reactions:

Possible side effects of potassium iodide include: Skin rashes; swelling of the salivary glands; "iodism" (metallic taste, burning mouth and throat, sore teeth and gums, symptoms of a head cold and sometimes stomach upset and diarrhea); allergic reactions (ie, fever and joint pains, swelling of parts of the face and body and, at times, severe shortness of breath requiring immediate medical attention). Overactivity or underactivity of the thyroid gland or enlargement of the thyroid gland (goiter) may occur rarely.

Overdosage:

Acute poisoning:

Symptoms – Iodine is corrosive, and toxic symptoms are mainly the result of local GI tract irritation. Gastroenteritis, abdominal pain and diarrhea (sometimes bloody) may be seen. Fatalities may occur from circulatory collapse due to shock, corrosive gastritis or asphyxiation from swelling of the glottis or larynx.

Treatment – Gastric lavage with a soluble starch solution (15 g cornstarch or flour in 500 ml water) is recommended for removing iodine from the stomach. A 1% oral solution of sodium thiosulfate is a specific antidote, as it will reduce iodine to iodide. Milk may help relieve gastric irritation. Correct fluid and electrolyte imbalance, and treat shock if necessary.

Chronic poisoning: Discontinue use of iodine or iodides. High sodium chloride intake will speed recovery. For iodism characterized by skin or mucous membrane reactions, give cortisone or equivalent corticosteroid 25 to 100 mg every 6 hours orally until symptoms abate.

IODINE PRODUCTS

Patient Information:

Strong iodine solution: Dilute with water or fruit juice to improve taste.

Discontinue use and notify physician if fever, skin rash, metallic taste, swelling of the throat, burning of the mouth and throat, sore gums and teeth, head cold symptoms, severe GI distress or enlargement of the thyroid gland (goiter) occurs.

Administration and Dosage:

Recommended dietary allowances (RDAs): The RDA for iodine is 150 mcg for adults.

To prepare hyperthyroid patients for thyroidectomy, administer 2 to 6 drops strong iodine solution 3 times daily for 10 days prior to surgery.

For thyroid blocking in a radiation emergency: Use only as directed by state or local public health authorities in the event of a radiation emergency. Take for 10 days unless directed otherwise by state or local public health authorities.

Adults and children (> 1 year) – One tablet (130 mg) daily (crush tablets for small children).

Infants (< 1 year) – ½ crushed tablet (65 mg) daily.

Rx	**Strong Iodine Solution (Lugol's Solution)** (Various, eg, Lannett)	**Solution:** 5% iodine and 10% potassium iodide	In 120 ml, pt and gal.
Rx	**Thyro-Block**[1] (Wallace)	**Tablets:** 130 mg potassium iodide	White, scored. In 14s.

[1] Available only to State and Federal agencies.

ANTITHYROID AGENTS

Actions:

Pharmacology: Propylthiouracil (PTU) and methimazole inhibit the synthesis of thyroid hormones and, thus, are effective in the treatment of hyperthyroidism. They do not inactivate existing thyroxine (T_4) and triiodothyronine (T_3) which are stored in the thyroid or which circulate in the blood, nor do they interfere with the effectiveness of exogenous thyroid hormones. PTU partially inhibits the peripheral conversion of T_4 to T_3.

Both drugs are concentrated in the thyroid gland. Pharmacokinetic data are summarized in the following table:

Various Pharmacokinetic Parameters of Antithyroid Agents						
Antithyroid agent	Bioavailability (%)	Protein binding (%)	Transplacental passage	Breast milk levels (M:P)[1]	Half-life(hrs)	Excreted in urine (%)
Propylthiouracil	80-95	75-80	Low	Low (0.1)	1-2	< 35
Methimazole	80-95	0	High	High (1)	6-13	< 10

[1] Approximate milk:plasma ratio.

Indications:

Hyperthyroidism: Long-term therapy may lead to disease remission. Also used to ameliorate hyperthyroidism in preparation for subtotal thyroidectomy or radioactive iodine therapy.

PTU is also used when thyroidectomy is contraindicated or not advisable.

Unlabeled uses: PTU (300 mg/day) may be useful in reducing the mortality due to alcoholic liver disease by reducing the hepatic hypermetabolic state induced by alcohol.

Contraindications:

Hypersensitivity to antithyroid drugs; nursing mothers (see Warnings).

Warnings:

Agranulocytosis is potentially the most serious side effect of therapy. Instruct patients to report any symptoms of agranulocytosis, such as hay fever, sore throat, skin eruptions, fever, headache or general malaise. In such cases, white blood cell and differential counts should be made to determine whether agranulocytosis has developed. Exercise particular care with patients receiving additional drugs known to cause agranulocytosis. Leukopenia, thrombocytopenia and aplastic anemia (pancytopenia) may also occur. Discontinue the drug in the presence of agranulocytosis, aplastic anemia, hepatitis, fever or exfoliative dermatitis. Monitor the patient's bone marrow function.

One report recommends routine monitoring of the WBC count for at least the first 3 months of therapy, thereby potentially detecting agranulocytosis prior to becoming evident by infection.

Carcinogenesis: Laboratory animals treated with PTU for > 1 year have demonstrated thyroid hyperplasia and carcinoma formation. Such animal findings are seen with continuous suppression of thyroid function by sufficient doses of a variety of antithyroid agents, as well as in dietary iodine deficiency, subtotal thyroidectomy, and implantation of autonomous thyrotropic hormone-secreting pituitary tumors. Pituitary adenomas have also been described.

Pregnancy: Category D. These agents, used judiciously, are effective drugs in hyperthyroidism complicated by pregnancy. Because they readily cross the placenta and can induce goiter and even cretinism in the developing fetus, it is important that a sufficient, but not excessive, dose be given. In many pregnant women, the thyroid dysfunction diminishes as the pregnancy proceeds, thus making a reduction of dose possible. In some instances, these products can be withdrawn 2 or 3 weeks before delivery. PTU can cause fetal harm when administered to a pregnant woman. Approximately 10% will develop neonatal goiter. However, if an antithyroid agent is needed, PTU is preferred because it is less likely than methimazole to cross the placenta and induce fetal/neonatal complications (eg, aplasia cutis).

Lactation: Postpartum patients receiving antithyroid preparations should not nurse their babies. However, if necessary, the preferred drug is PTU.

Children: In several case reports, PTU hepatotoxicity has occurred in pediatric patients. Discontinue the drug immediately if signs and symptoms of hepatic dysfunction develop.

ANTITHYROID AGENTS

Precautions:

Monitoring: Monitor thyroid function tests periodically during therapy. Once clinical evidence of hyperthyroidism has resolved, the finding of an elevated serum TSH indicates that a lower maintenance dose of PTU should be used.

Hemorrhagic effects: Because PTU may cause hypoprothrombinemia and bleeding, monitor prothrombin time during therapy, especially before surgical procedures.

Drug Interactions:

Anticoagulants: The activity of oral anticoagulants may be potentiated by the anti-vitamin K activity attributed to PTU.

Adverse Reactions:

Adverse reactions probably occur in < 1% of patients.

Agranulocytosis is the most serious effect.

CNS: Paresthesias; neuritis; headache; vertigo; drowsiness; neuropathies; CNS stimulation; depression.

Dermatologic: Skin rash; urticaria; pruritis; erythema nodosum; skin pigmentation; exfoliative dermatitis; lupus-like syndrome, including splenomegaly, hepatitis, periarteritis and hypoprothrombinemia and bleeding.

GI: Nausea and vomiting; epigastric distress; loss of taste; sialadenopathy.

Hematologic: Inhibition of myelopoiesis (agranulocytosis, granulocytopenia and thrombocytopenia); aplastic anemia; hypoprothrombinemia; periarteritis. About 10% of patients with untreated hyperthyroidism have leukopenia (WBC count < 4000 per mm^3), often with relative granulocytopenia.

Hepatic: Jaundice (which may persist for several weeks after discontinuance); hepatitis.

Renal: Nephritis.

Miscellaneous: Abnormal hair loss; arthralgia; myalgia; edema; lymphadenopathy; drug fever; interstitial pneumonitis insulin autoimmune syndrome (may result in hypoglycemic coma).

Overdosage:

Symptoms: Nausea; vomiting; epigastric distress; headache; fever; arthralgia; pruritus; edema; pancytopenia. Agranulocytosis is the most serious effect. Rarely, exfoliative dermatitis, hepatitis, neuropathies or CNS stimulation or depression may occur.

Treatment: Protect the patient's airway and support ventilation and perfusion. Meticulously monitor and maintain, within acceptable limits, the patient's vital signs, blood gases, serum electrolytes, etc. Monitor the patient's bone marrow function. Refer to General Management of Acute Overdosage.

Forced diuresis, peritoneal dialysis, hemodialysis or charcoal hemoperfusion have not been established as beneficial for an overdose of propylthiouracil.

Patient Information:

Take at regular intervals around the clock (usually every 8 hours), unless directed otherwise by physician.

Notify physician if fever, sore throat, unusual bleeding or bruising, headache, rash, yellowing of the skin or vomiting occurs.

Administration and Dosage:

In one study, the rate of remission and time to relapse of Grave's disease was significantly increased when antithyroid therapy was given for a prolonged duration (18 months) vs short-term (6 month) treatment. However, the monitoring of thyroid stimulating antibody values may be a useful guide for shortening the duration of treatment in some patients.

One small study reported that single and divided daily doses of methimazole were equally effective in hyperthyroid patients. Traditionally administered in divided doses, it was suggested that a single daily dose would be effective since methimazole is present in the thyroid for 20 hours and is active for 40 hours despite a serum half-life of 6 to 13 hours. Further study is needed.

Antithyroid Agents

PROPYLTHIOURACIL (PTU)

For complete prescribing information, refer to the Antithyroid Agents group monograph.

Administration and Dosage:

Usually administered in 3 equal doses at approximately 8 hour intervals.

Adults:

Initial – 300 mg/day. In patients with severe hyperthyroidism, very large goiters, or both, the initial dosage is usually 400 mg/day; an occasional patient will require 600 to 900 mg/day initially.

Maintenance – Usually, 100 to 150 mg daily.

Children:

6 to 10 years – Initial dose is 50 to 150 mg/day.

≥ 10 years – Initial dose is 150 to 300 mg/day.

Maintenance – Determined by patient response.

Another suggested dosage for children is as follows:

Initial: 5 to 7 mg/kg/day or 150 to 200 mg/m²/day in divided doses every 8 hours.

Maintenance: to the intial dose beginning when the patient is euthyroid.

Rx	**Propylthiouracil** (Various, eg, Barr, Dixon-Shane, Geneva, Major, Rugby, Schein)	**Tablets:** 50 mg	In 100s and 1000s.

METHIMAZOLE

For complete prescribing information, refer to the Antithyroid Agents group monograph.

Administration and Dosage:

Usually administered in 3 equal doses at approximately 8 hour intervals.

Adults:

Initial – 15 mg daily for mild hyperthyroidism, 30 to 40 mg/day for moderately severe hyperthyroidism and 60 mg/day for severe hyperthyroidism.

Maintenance – 5 to 15 mg/day.

Children:

Initial – 0.4 mg/kg daily.

Maintenance – Approximately one-half the initial dose.

Another suggested dosage for children is as follows:

Initial: 0.5 to 0.7 mg/kg/day or 15 to 20 mg/m²/day in 3 divided doses.

Maintenance: to of intial dose beginning when the patient is euthyroid.

Maximum: 30 mg/24 hours.

Rx	**Tapazole** (Lilly)	**Tablets:** 5 mg	(Lilly J94). White, scored. In 100s.
		10 mg	(Lilly J95). White, scored. In 100s.

SODIUM IODIDE I 131

Actions:

Pharmacokinetics: Sodium iodide I 131 is readily absorbed from the GI tract. Following absorption, the iodide is primarily distributed within the extracellular fluid of the body. It is trapped and rapidly converted to protein-bound iodine by the thyroid; it is concentrated, but not protein-bound, by the stomach and salivary glands. It is promptly excreted by the kidneys. About 90% of the local irradiation is caused by beta radiation and 10% by gamma radiation.

Iodine 131 decays by beta and gamma emissions with a physical half-life of 8.04 days. Following oral administration, about 40% of the activity has an effective half-life of 0.34 days and 60% has an effective half-life of 7.61 days. Consult product literature for specific calibration and dosimetry information.

Indications:

Treatment of hyperthyroidism and selected cases of thyroid carcinoma. Palliative effects may be seen in patients with papillary or follicular carcinoma of the thyroid. Thyrotropin may effect stimulation of radioiodide uptake. (Radioiodide will not be taken up by giant cell and spindle cell carcinoma of the thyroid or by amyloid solid carcinomas.)

Contraindications:

Preexisting vomiting and diarrhea; pregnancy (see Warnings).

Warnings:

Patients < 30 years old: Sodium iodide I 131 is not usually used for the treatment of hyperthyroidism in patients < 30 years old unless circumstances preclude other treatment.

Antithyroid Agents

SODIUM IODIDE I 131

Pregnancy: Category X. Sodium iodide I 131 can cause fetal harm when administered to a pregnant woman. Permanent damage to the fetal thyroid can occur. The drug is contraindicated in women who are or may become pregnant. If it is used during pregnancy, or if the patient becomes pregnant while taking this drug, inform her of the potential hazard to the fetus.

Lactation: Since iodine is excreted in breast milk, substitute with formula feedings.

Precautions:

Antithyroid therapy of a severely hyperthyroid patient is usually discontinued for 3 to 4 days before administration of radioiodide.

Drug Interactions:

Stable iodine (any form), thyroid, antithyroid agents: The uptake of iodine 131 will be affected by recent intake of these agents. Question the patient regarding previous medication and procedures involving radiographic contrast media.

Adverse Reactions:

The immediate adverse reactions following treatment of hyperthyroidism are usually mild, but following the larger doses used in thyroid carcinoma, may be much more severe.

Hematologic: Depression of the hematopoietic system (large doses); bone marrow depression; acute leukemia; anemia; blood dyscrasias; leukopenia; thrombocytopenia.

Miscellaneous: Radiation sickness (some degree of nausea and vomiting); chest pain; tachycardia; itching skin; rash; hives; increase in clinical symptoms; acute thyroid crises; severe sialoadenitis; chromosomal abnormalities; death.

Tenderness and swelling of neck, pain on swallowing, sore throat and cough may occur around the third day after treatment and are usually amenable to analgesics.

Temporary thinning of the hair may occur 2 to 3 months after treatment.

Allergic type reactions have been reported infrequently following the administration of iodine-containing radiopharmaceuticals.

Overdosage:

In the treatment of hyperthyroidism, overdosage may result in hypothyroidism, the onset of which may be delayed. Appropriate replacement therapy is recommended if hypothyroidism occurs.

Administration and Dosage:

Measure the dose by a radioactivity calibration system just prior to administration. Consult product literature for specific calibration and dosimetry information.

Hyperthyroidism: The total amount needed to achieve a clinical remission without destruction of the entire thyroid varies widely; the usual dose range is 4 to 10 millicuries (mCi). Toxic nodular goiter and other special situations will require larger doses.

Thyroid carcinoma: Individualize dosage. The usual dose for ablation of normal thyroid tissue is 50 mCi, with subsequent therapeutic doses usually 100 to 150 mCi.

Preparation of oral solution: To prepare stock solution, dilute oral solution with Purified Water, USP containing 0.2% sodium thiosulfate as a reducing agent. Acidic diluents may cause a pH drop below 7.5 and may stimulate volatilization of iodine 131-hydriodic acid.

Rx	**Iodotope** (Squibb Diagnostics)	**Capsules**: Radioactivity range is 8, 15, 30, 50 or 100 mCi per capsule at time of calibration	Blue/buff. In 5s, 10s, 15s and 20s.
		Oral Solution:[1] Radioactivity concentration of 7.05 mCi per ml at time of calibration	In vials containing approximately 7, 14, 28, 70 or 106 mCi at time of calibration.
Rx	**Sodium Iodide I 131 Therapeutic** (Mallinckrodt)	**Capsules**: Radioactivity range is 0.75 to 100 mCi per capsule.	
		Oral Solution: Radioactivity range is 3.5 to 150 mCi per vial.	

[1] With 1 mg EDTA per ml.

CALCITONIN-SALMON

Actions:

Pharmacology: Calcitonins are polypeptide hormones secreted by parafollicular cells of the thyroid in mammals. Calcitonin has a role in the regulation of calcium and bone metabolism and it has direct renal effects and actions on the GI tract. Calcitonin appears essentially identical to mammalian calcitonins, but its potency per mg and duration of action are greater. Single injections of calcitonin transiently inhibit bone resorption. With prolonged use, there is a persistent, smaller decrease in the rate of bone resorption associated with decreased resorptive activity and number of osteoclasts. Osteocytic resorption may also be decreased. Endogenous calcitonin, with parathyroid hormone (PTH), regulates blood calcium. High blood calcium levels increase secretion of calcitonin, which inhibits bone resorption. In healthy adults, administration of exogenous calcitonin only slightly decreases serum calcium.

Paget's disease of bone (osteitis deformans) is characterized by abnormal and accelerated bone formation and resorption in one or more bones. Active Paget's disease involving a large bone mass may increase the urinary hydroxyproline excretion (reflecting breakdown of collagen-containing bone matrix) and serum alkaline phosphatase (reflecting increased bone formation). Calcitonin, presumably by blocking bone resorption, improves the biochemical abnormalities (> 30% reduction). It decreases the rate of bone turnover with a resultant fall in the serum alkaline phosphatase and urinary hydroxyproline excretion in ≈ 66% of patients. These biochemical changes appear to correspond to more normal bone as evidenced by: 1) Radiologic regression of Pagetic lesions; 2) improvement of impaired auditory nerves (infrequent) and other neurologic functions; 3) decreases in abnormally elevated cardiac output. Improvements occur rarely and spontaneously; they cannot be predicted. Some patients with Paget's disease who have good initial biochemical or symptomatic responses later relapse. Explanations are incomplete.

Hypercalcemia – Calcitonin-salmon lowers elevated serum calcium in patients with carcinoma, multiple myeloma or primary hyperparathyroidism (lesser response). Patients with higher serum calcium tend to show a greater reduction. The decrease in calcium occurs about 2 hours after injection and lasts for 6 to 8 hours. Given every 12 hours, the drug lowered calcium for 5 to 8 days. Average reduction of 8 hour post-injection serum calcium was about 9%.

Postmenopausal osteoporosis – Calcitonin, given by the intranasal route, increases spinal bone mass in postmenopausal women with established osteoporosis but not in early postmenopausal women.

Kidney – Calcitonin increases the excretion of filtered phosphate, calcium and sodium by decreasing tubular reabsorption. In some patients, the inhibition of bone resorption is of such magnitude that the consequent reduction of filtered calcium load more than compensates for the decrease in tubular reabsorption of calcium. This decreases rather than increases urinary calcium. Transient increases in sodium and water excretion may occur after the initial injection, but these changes usually return to pretreatment levels with continued therapy.

GI – Short-term administration results in marked transient decreases in the volume and acidity of gastric juice and in the volume of trypsin and amylase content of pancreatic juice. Whether this continues during chronic therapy is not known.

Pharmacokinetics: Animal studies suggest that calcitonin is rapidly converted to smaller inactive fragments, primarily in the kidneys, but also in the blood and peripheral tissues. A small amount of unchanged hormone and its inactive metabolites are excreted in the urine. Peak plasma concentration time for the injection is 16 to 25 minutes. Peak plasma concentration time for the nasal spray is 31 to 39 minutes; the calculated half-life is 43 minutes.

Indications:

Postmenopausal osteoporosis (injection and nasal): Prevention of progressive loss of bone mass. Use nasal formulation only in patients who cannot take estrogen.

Paget's disease of bone (injection only): For patients with moderate to severe Paget's disease characterized by polyostotic involvement with elevated serum alkaline phosphatase and urinary hydroxyproline excretion.

Hypercalcemia (injection only): In early treatment of hypercalcemic emergencies, along with other appropriate agents, use when a rapid decrease in serum calcium is required, until more specific treatment can be accomplished. It may also be added to existing therapeutic regimens for hypercalcemia.

Contraindications:

Clinical allergy to synthetic calcitonin-salmon.

CALCITONIN-SALMON

Warnings:

Antibody formation: Circulating antibodies to calcitonin occur after 2 to 18 months of treatment in about half the treated Paget's disease patients, but calcitonin treatment remained effective in many of these cases. Occasionally, patients with high antibody titers usually will have suffered a biochemical relapse of Paget's disease and are unresponsive to the acute hypocalcemic effects of calcitonin.

Osteogenic sarcoma is known to increase in Paget's disease. Pagetic lesions may appear by x-ray to progress markedly, possibly with some loss of definition of periosteal margins. Evaluate such lesions to differentiate them from osteogenic sarcoma.

Asymptomatic Paget's disease: There is no evidence that prophylactic use is beneficial in asymptomatic patients. Consider treatment in cases in which there is extensive involvement of the skull or spinal cord with the possibility of irreversible neurologic damage. Base treatment on demonstrated effect on Pagetic bone.

Elderly: No unusual adverse events or increased incidence of common adverse events have been noted in patients > 65 years of age receiving the nasal formulation.

Pregnancy: Category C. Calcitonin has decreased fetal birth weights in rabbits when given in doses 14 to 56 times the recommended human dose. Because calcitonin does not cross the placenta, this may be due to metabolic effects of calcitonin on the pregnant animal. There are no studies in pregnant women. Use these agents only if the potential benefits outweigh the unknown hazards to the fetus.

Lactation: Calcitonin inhibits lactation in animals. It is not known whether it is excreted in breast milk. Safety for use during nursing has not been established.

Children: Disorders of bone in children (juvenile Paget's disease) have been reported rarely. No adequate data support usage in children.

Precautions:

Allergy: The possibility of a systemic allergic reaction exists. Refer to Management of Acute Hypersensitivity Reactions. Consider skin testing prior to treatment, particularly for patients with suspected sensitivity. (See Administration and Dosage).

Hypocalcemic tetany could occur with calcitonin, although no cases have been reported. Have parenteral calcium available during the first several doses.

Periodically examine urine sediment of patients on chronic therapy. Coarse granular casts and renal tubular epithelial cell casts were reported in young adult volunteers at bed rest who were given calcitonin to study the effect on immobilization osteoporosis. The urine sediment became normal after calcitonin was stopped.

Nasal examination: Perform a nasal examination prior to the start of treatment and at any time nasal complaints occur.

Adverse Reactions:

Calcitonin Adverse Reactions (Nasal Spray)		
Adverse reaction	Nasal spray (n = 341)	Placebo (n = 131)
Rhinitis	12%	6.9%
Nasal symptoms (eg, irritation, redness, sores)	10%	16%
Back pain	5%	2.3%
Arthralgia	3.8%	5.3%
Epistaxis	3.5%	4.6%
Headache	3.2%	4.6%

Body as a whole: Flu-like symptoms, fatigue (rare).

Cardiovascular: Hypertension, angina pectoris (rare); tachycardia; palpitation; bundle branch block; myocardial infarction.

CNS: Dizziness, paresthesia, depression (rare); insomnia; anxiety; vertigo; migraine; neuralgia; agitation.

Dermatologic: Inflammatory reactions at the injection site (10%); flushing of face or hands (2% to 5%); pruritus of ear lobes; edema of feet; skin rash; skin ulceration; eczema; alopecia; increased sweating.

Endocrine: Goiter; hyperthyroidism.

GI: Nausea with or without vomiting (10%) is most evident when treatment is initiated and tends to decrease with continued use; anorexia; epigastric discomfort; salty taste; flatulence; increased appetite; gastritis; dry mouth; diarrhea, abdominal pain, dyspepsia, constipation (rare).

GU: Cystitis (rare); pyelonephritis; hematuria; renal calculus.

CALCITONIN-SALMON

Hematologic/Lymphatic: Lymphadenopathy, infection (rare); anemia.

Metabolic: Mild tetanic symptoms, asymptomatic mild hypercalcemia (rare); cholelithiasis; thirst; hepatitis; weight increase.

Musculoskeletal: Arthrosis, myalgia (rare); arthritis; polymyalgia rheumatica; stiffness.

Ophthalmic: Abnormal lacrimation, conjunctivitis (rare); blurred vision; vitreous floater.

Respiratory: Sinusitis, upper respiratory tract infection, bronchospasm (rare); pharyngitis; bronchitis; pneumonia; coughing; dyspnea; taste perversion; parosmia.

Miscellaneous: Nocturia; feverish sensation; eye pain; tinnitus; hearing loss; earache; cerebrovascular accident; thrombophlebitis.

Overdosage:

A dose of 1000 IU SC may produce nausea and vomiting as the only adverse effects. Doses of 32 units/kg/day for 1 or 2 days demonstrate no other adverse effects.

Patient Information:

Nasal: Patients should notify their physician if they develop significant nasal irritation.

To activate the pump, hold the bottle upright and depress the two white side arms toward the bottle six times until a faint spray is emitted. The pump is activated once this first faint spray has been emitted. At this point, firmly place the nozzle into the nostril with the head in the upright position, and depress the pump toward the bottle. It is not necessary to reactivate the pump before each daily dose.

Administration and Dosage:

Skin testing: Prepare a dilution at 10 IU/ml by withdrawing 0.05 ml of the 200 IU/ml solution in a tuberculin syringe and filling it to 1 ml with sodium chloride injection. Mix well, discard 0.9 ml and inject intracutaneously 0.1 ml (≈ 1 IU) on the inner aspect of the forearm. Observe the injection site 15 minutes after injection. The appearance of more than mild erythema or wheal constitutes a positive response.

Postmenopausal osteoporosis:

Injection – 100 IU/day SC or IM.

Nasal – 200 IU intranasally every day, alternating nostrils daily. Before the first dose, it is necessary to activate the pump (see Patient Information).

Patients should also receive supplemental calcium carbonate 1.5 g daily and an adequate vitamin D intake (400 units daily). An adequate diet is also essential.

Paget's disease (injection only): Starting dose is 100 IU/day SC (preferred for outpatient self-administration) or IM. Monitor by periodic measurement of serum alkaline phosphatase and 24 hour urinary hydroxyproline and evaluation of symptoms. Normalization of biochemical abnormalities and decreased bone pain is usually seen in the first few months. Improvement of neurologic lesions requires > 1 year.

Doses of 50 IU/day or every other day are usually sufficient to maintain biochemical and clinical improvement. Maintain the higher dose in any patient with serious deformity or neurological involvement.

In any patient with a good response initially who later relapses (clinically or biochemically), investigate for antibody formation (see Warnings).

Hypercalcemia (injection only): Starting dose is 4 IU/kg every 12 hours, SC or IM. If response is not satisfactory after 1 or 2 days, increase to 8 IU/kg every 12 hours. If the response remains unsatisfactory after 2 more days, the dose may be further increased to a maximum of 8 IU/kg every 6 hours. If the volume to be injected exceeds 2 ml, IM injection is preferable and multiple sites of injection should be used.

Storage/Stability:

Injection – Refrigerate between 2° to 6°C (36° to 43°F).

Nasal – Store unopened bottle in the refrigerator between 2° and 8°C. Once the pump has been activated, store at room temperature.

Rx	**Calcimar** (Rhone-Poulenc Rorer)	**Injection:** 200 IU/ml	With phenol. In 2 ml vials.
Rx	**Salmonine** (Lennod)		With phenol. In 2 ml vials.
Rx	**Osteocalcin** (Arcola)		With 5 mg phenol per ml. In 2 ml vials.
Rx	**Miacalcin** (Sandoz)		With phenol. In 2 ml vials.
Rx	**Miacalcin** (Sandoz)	**Nasal spray:** 200 IU/activation (0.09 ml/dose)	8.5 mg sodium chloride. In 2 ml metered dose glass bottle with pump.

BISPHOSPHONATES

Actions:

Pharmacology: Etidronate disodium (EHDP), tiludronate disodium, pamidronate disodium (APD) and alendronate are bisphosphonates that act primarily on bone. Their major pharmacologic action is the inhibition of normal and abnormal bone resorption. Secondarily, etidronate reduces bone formation because formation is coupled to resorption; pamidronate inhibits bone resorption apparently without inhibiting bone formation and mineralization. Alendronate, a highly selective inhibitor of resorption, is a 100– to 500–fold more potent inhibitor of bone resorption. Bone resorption occurs following recruitment, activation and polarization of osteoclasts. Tiludronate disodium appears to inhibit osteoclasts through at least two mechanisms: disruption of the cytoskeletal ring structure, possibly by inhibition of protein-tyrosine-phosphatase, thus leading to detachment of osteoclasts from the bone surface and the inhibition of the osteoclastic proton pump.

Reduction of abnormal bone resorption is responsible for therapeutic benefit in hypercalcemia. Antiresorptive action has been demonstrated under a variety of conditions. The exact mechanism(s) is not fully understood, but may be related to inhibition of hydroxyapatite crystal dissolution or its action on bone resorbing cells. Pamidronate inhibits accelerated bone resorption resulting from osteoclast hyperactivity induced by various tumors in animals. The number of osteoclasts in active bone turnover sites is substantially reduced after etidronate. Etidronate can also inhibit formation and growth of hydroxyapatite crystals and their amorphous precursors at concentrations in excess of those required to inhibit crystal dissolution.

Alendronate – As a result of bone resorption inhibition, asymptomatic reductions in serum calcium and phosphate concentrations are seen after treatment with alendronate. In long-term studies, reductions from baseline in serum calcium (≈ 2%) and phosphate (≈ 4% to 6%) were seen the first month after initiation of 10 mg alendronate, but no further decreases were seen for the 3 year duration of the studies. The reduction in serum phosphate may reflect not only the positive bone mineral balance due to alendronate but also a decrease in renal phosphate reabsorption. Alendronate decreases the rate of bone resorption directly, leading to an indirect decrease in bone formation.

Etidronate does not appear to alter renal tubular reabsorption of calcium, and does not affect hypercalcemia in patients with hyperparathyroidism where increased calcium reabsorption may be a factor in hypercalcemia. Hyperphosphatemia has been observed with etidronate, usually with doses of 10 to 20 mg/kg/day; no adverse effects have been noted, and it is not a contraindication. It is apparently due to drug-related increased phosphate tubular reabsorption by the kidneys. Serum phosphate levels generally return to normal 2 to 4 weeks post-therapy. Hyperphosphatemia occurs less frequently with IV medication in hypercalcemia of malignancy.

Pamidronate therapy has decreased serum phosphate levels, presumably caused by decreased release of phosphate from bone and increased renal excretion as parathyroid hormone levels (usually suppressed in hypercalcemia of malignancy) return towards normal. Phosphate therapy was administered in 30% of patients; levels usually returned to normal within 7 to 10 days. Urinary calcium/creatinine and urinary hydroxyproline/creatinine ratios decrease and usually return to normal or below after treatment. The changes occur within the first week, as do decreases in serum calcium levels.

Tiludronate – In pagetic patients treated with tiludronate 400 mg/day for 3 months, changes in urinary hydroxyproline, a biochemical marker of bone resorption and in serum alkaline phosphatase, a marker of bone formation, indicate a reduction toward normal in the rate of bone turnover. In addition, reduced numbers of osteoclasts by histomorphometric analysis and radiological improvement of lytic lesions indicate that tiludronate can suppress the pagetic disease process.

Hypercalcemia of malignancy is usually related to increased bone resorption due to osteoclastic hyperactivity associated with neoplastic tissue. It occurs in 8% to 20% of patients with malignant disease. Whereas hypercalcemia is more often seen in patients with demonstrable osteolytic, osteoblastic or mixed metastatic tumors in bone, discrete skeletal lesions cannot be demonstrated in at least 30% of patients.

As hypercalcemia of malignancy evolves, the renal tubules develop a diminished capacity to concentrate urine. Resultant polyuria and nocturia decrease the extracellular fluid volume. Thus, the kidney's ability to eliminate excess calcium is compromised. Renal impairment can eventually cause nitrogen retention, acidosis, renal failure and a further decrease in calcium excretion. Infusion of bisphosphonates, by inhibiting excessive bone resorption, interrupts this process. Adequate fluid administration to correct volume deficits is also essential. Salt loading and "high ceiling" or "loop" diuretics promote calcium excretion, because the renal calcium excretion rate is directly related to the sodium excretion rate.

Paget's disease of bone (osteitis deformans) is an idiopathic disease characterized by chronic, focal areas of bone destruction complicated by concurrent excessive bone repair, affecting one or more bones. These changes result in thickened but weakened bones that may fracture or bend under stress. Signs and symptoms may be bone pain, deformity, fractures, neurological disorders resulting from cranial and spinal nerve entrapment and from spinal cord and brain stem compression, increased cardiac output to the involved bone, increased serum alkaline phosphatase levels (reflecting increased bone formation) or urine hydroxyproline excretion (reflecting increased bone resorption). Serum alkaline phosphatase (SAP), the most frequently used biochemical index of disease activity, provides an objective measure of disease severity and response to therapy.

Pharmacokinetics:

Alendronate – There is no evidence that alendronate is metabolized. Relative to an IV reference dose, mean oral bioavailability in women was 0.7% for 5 to 40 mg doses after an overnight fast and 2 hours before a standardized breakfast. Oral bioavailability of the 10 mg tablet in men (0.59%) was similar to that in women (0.78%) given after an overnight fast and 2 hours before breakfast. In 49 postmenopausal women, bioavailability was decreased by ≈ 40% when 10 mg was given either 0.5 or 1 hour before a standardized breakfast when compared with dosing 2 hours before eating. Bioavailability was negligible whether alendronate was given with or up to 2 hours after a standardized breakfast. Concomitant coffee or orange juice reduced bioavailability by ≈ 60%. Mean steady state volume of distribution (exclusive of bone) is ≥ 28 L. Protein binding in plasma is ≈ 78%. After a single IV dose, ≈ 50% was excreted in the urine with little or none recovered in the feces. After a single 10 mg IV dose, renal clearance was 71 ml/min; systemic clearance did not exceed 200 ml/min. Plasma levels fell by > 95% within 6 hours after IV administration. The terminal half-life is estimated to exceed 10 years, probably reflecting alendronate release from the skeleton. Based on the above, it is estimated that after 10 years of 10 mg/day orally, the amount of alendronate released daily from the skeleton is ≈ 25% of that absorbed from the GI tract.

Etidronate is not metabolized. Absorption averages ≈ 1% of an oral dose of 5 mg/kg/day, increasing to ≈ 2.5% at 10 mg/kg/day and 6% at 20 mg/kg/day. Absorption, complete in 2 hours, may be reduced by foods or other preparations containing divalent cations. Most absorbed drug is cleared from the blood in 6 hours. Within 24 hours, about half the absorbed dose is excreted in urine. The remainder is chemically adsorbed to bone, especially to areas of elevated osteogenesis, and is slowly eliminated. Unabsorbed drug is excreted intact in feces.

A large fraction of the infused dose is excreted rapidly and unchanged in the urine. The mean residence time in the exchangeable pool is ≈ 8.7 hours. The mean volume of distribution at steady state in healthy subjects is 1370 ml/kg while the plasma half-life is 6 hours. In these same subjects, nonrenal clearance from the exchangeable pool amounts to 30% to 50% of the infused dose. This nonrenal clearance is caused by uptake by bone; subsequently, the drug is slowly eliminated through bone turnover. The half-life in bone is > 90 days.

Pamidronate – In cancer patients with minimal or no bone involvement who were given a 60 mg IV infusion over 4 or 24 hours, a mean 51% (range, 32% to 80%) was excreted unchanged in urine within 72 hours. Body retention during this period was calculated to be a mean of 49% (range, 20% to 68%) of the dose, or 29.3 mg (12 to 41 mg). The urinary excretion rate profile after 60 mg over 4 hours exhibited biphasic disposition characteristics with an alpha half-life of 1.6 hours and a beta half-life of 27.2 hours. The elimination rate from bone has not been determined.

Pamidronate is not metabolized and is exclusively eliminated by renal excretion. After IV administration in rats, ≈ 50% to 60% was rapidly adsorbed by bone and slowly eliminated by the kidneys. In rats given 10 mg/kg bolus injections, ≈ 30% of the compound was found in the liver shortly after administration and was then redistributed to bone or eliminated by the kidneys over 24 to 48 hours. The drug was rapidly cleared from circulation and taken up mainly by bones, liver, spleen, teeth and tracheal cartilage. Bone uptake occurred preferentially in areas of high bone turnover. The terminal phase of elimination half-life in bone was ≈ 300 days.

Tiludronate – In animals, tiludronic acid undergoes little if any metabolism. In vitro, tiludronic acid is not metabolized in human liver microsomes and hepatocytes.

Relative to IV reference dose, the mean oral bioavailability of tiludronate disodium in healthy male subjects was 6% after an oral dose equivalent to 400 mg tiludronic acid administered after an overnight fast and 4 hours before a standard breakfast. Bioavailability is reduced by food.

After administration of a single dose equivalent to 400 mg tiludronic acid to healthy male subjects, tiludronic acid was rapidly absorbed with peak plasma concentrations of ≈ 3 mg/L occurring within 2 hours. In pagetic patients, after repeated administration of doses equivalent to 400 mg/day tiludronic acid (2 hours before or

2 hours after a meal) for durations of 12 days to 12 weeks, average plasma concentrations of tiludronic acid occurring between 1 and 2 hours after dosing ranged between 1 and 4.6 mg/L.

Clinical trials:

Osteoporosis – Highly significant increases in bone mineral density (BMD) were seen in patients receiving 10 mg/day alendronate. Total body BMD also increased significantly, suggesting that the increases in bone and bone mass of the spine and hip did not occur at the expense of other skeletal sites. Increases in BMD were evident as early as 3 months and continued throughout 3 years of treatment. Thus, alendronate seems to reverse the progression of osteoporosis.

One study found a 48% reduction in the proportion of patients treated with alendronate experiencing ≥ 1 new vertebral fractures (3.2% vs 6.2% with placebo). A reduction in the total number of new vertebral fractures (4.2% vs 11.3%) was also found. Of those patients sustaining any vertebral fracture, alendronate-treated patients experienced less height loss (5.9 vs 23.3 mm) due to a reduction in both number and severity of fractures. After discontinuation, neither further increase in bone mass nor accelerated bone loss rate was seen, indicating that daily treatment is required to maintain the effects of the drug.

Paget's disease –

Alendronate 40 mg once daily for 6 months produced highly significant decreases in serum alkaline phosphatase as well as in urinary markers of bone collagen degradation. As a result of the inhibition of bone resorption, alendronate induced generally mild, transient and asymptomatic decreases in serum calcium and phosphate.

Etidronate slows accelerated bone turnover (resorption and accretion) in pagetic lesions and to a lesser extent, in normal bone. Reduced bone turnover is often accompanied by symptomatic improvement, including reduced bone pain. Incidence of pagetic fractures may decrease, and elevated cardiac output and other vascular disorders improve. In many patients, the disease process will be suppressed at least 1 year following therapy cessation. Etidronate for asymptomatic Paget's disease may be warranted if extensive involvement threatens irreversible neurologic damage, or damage to major joints or major weight-bearing bones.

Alendronate vs etidronate: Efficacy of alendronate 40 mg once daily for 6 months was demonstrated in moderate to severe Paget's disease. At 6 months, suppression of alkaline phosphatase in alendronate-treated patients was significantly greater than that with etidronate. A response occurred in ≈ 85%, 30% and 0% in alendronate, etidronate and placebo-treated patients, respectively.

Pamidronate: In one study, 64 patients with moderate to severe Paget's disease of bone received 5, 15 or 30 mg pamidronate as a single 4–hour infusion on 3 consecutive days, for total doses of 15, 45 and 90 mg. The median maximum percent decreases from baseline in serum alkaline phosphatase and urine hydroxyproline/creatinine ratios were 25%, 41% and 57%, and 25%, 47% and 61% for the 15, 45 and 90 mg groups, respectively. The median time to response (≥ 50% decrease) for serum alkaline phosphatase was ≈ 1 month for the 90 mg group.

Tiludronate vs etidronate: A positive-controlled study was conducted in Europe with treatment groups of 400 mg/day tiliudronate for 3 months with a 3-month treatment-free follow-up, 400 mg/day tiludronate for 6 months and 400 mg/day etidronate for 6 months. The efficacy of tiludronate was primarily assessed by SAP activity after 3 and 6 months.

Six months after the start of dosing, the decrease in SAP levels in patients who ceased dosing after a 3–month course of tiludronate was significantly greater than with 6 months of etidronate 400 mg/day, and was equivalent to levels in patients who completed a 6–month course of tiludronate.

Hypercalcemia of malignancy –

Etidronate: Patients with elevated calcium levels (10.1 to 17.4 mg/dl) were treated simultaneously with daily IV administration over a 3 day period and up to 3000 ml saline and a loop diuretic. In terms of total serum calcium changes, 88% of patients had reductions of serum calcium of ≥ 1 mg/dl. Total serum calcium returned to normal in 63% of patients within 7 days compared to 33% of patients treated with hydration alone. Reductions in urinary calcium excretion, which accompany reductions in excessive bone resorption, became apparent after 24 hours. This was accompanied or followed by maximum decreases in serum calcium which were most frequently observed 72 hours after the first infusion.

When the total serum calcium values were adjusted for serum albumin levels, there was a return of normocalcemia in 24% of etidronate-treated patients and in 7% of patients treated with saline infusion alone. Of patients receiving etidronate, 87% vs 67% of patients on saline had albumin-adjusted serum calcium levels that returned to normal or were reduced by at least 1 mg/dl. Reductions in urinary calcium excretion, which accompany reductions in excessive bone resorption, became apparent after 24 hours. Decreases in serum calcium became maximal on the third day in most patients.

A second 3 day course of IV etidronate was tried in 14 patients who had a recurrence of hypercalcemia following an initial response to a 3 day infusion. All patients showed a decrease in total serum calcium of at least 1 mg/dl. Normalization of total serum calcium occurred in 11 patients.

Continuation of etidronate therapy with oral tablets may maintain clinically acceptable serum calcium levels and prolong normocalcemia.

Pamidronate: Patients who had hypercalcemia of malignancy received either 30, 60 or 90 mg as a single 24 hour IV infusion if their corrected serum calcium levels were ≥ 12 mg/dl after 48 hours of saline hydration. The majority of patients (64%) had decreases in albumin-corrected serum calcium levels by 24 hours after initiation of treatment. Mean-corrected serum calcium levels at days 2 to 7 after treatment initiation were significantly reduced from baseline in all three dosage groups. As a result, by 7 days after initiation of treatment, 40%, 61% and 100% of the patients receiving 30, 60 and 90 mg, respectively, had normal corrected serum calcium levels. Many patients (33% to 53%) in the 60 and 90 mg dosage groups continued to have normal-corrected serum calcium levels, or a partial response (≥ 15% decrease of corrected serum calcium from baseline), at day 14.

Etidronate vs pamidronate: Cancer patients who had corrected serum calcium levels of ≥ 12 mg/dl after at least 24 hours of saline hydration were randomized to receive either 60 mg pamidronate (n = 30) as a single 24 hour IV infusion or 7.5 mg/kg etidronate (n = 35) as a 2 hour IV infusion daily for 3 days. By day 7, 70% of the patients on pamidronate and 41% on etidronate had normal corrected serum calcium levels. When partial responders (≥ 15% decrease of serum calcium from baseline) were included, response rates were 97% for pamidronate and 65% for etidronate. Mean corrected serum calcium for the pamidronate and etidronate groups decreased from baseline values (14.6 and 13.8 mg/dl, respectively) to 10.4 and 11.2 mg/dl, respectively, on day 7. At day 14, 43% on pamidronate and 18% on etidronate still had normal corrected serum calcium levels, or maintenance of a partial response. For responders in pamidronate and etidronate groups, median duration of response was similar (7 and 5 days, respectively). Pamidronate patients had similar response rates in the presence or absence of bone metastases.

Patients (n = 25) with recurrent or refractory hypercalcemia of malignancy were given a second course of 60 mg pamidronate. Of these, 40% showed a complete response and 20% showed a partial response, and these responders had about a 3 mg/dl decrease in mean corrected serum calcium levels 7 days after treatment.

Heterotopic ossification – Etidronate reduces the incidence of clinically important heterotopic bone by ≈ 66%, and retards the progression of immature lesions and reduces the severity by at least 50%. Follow-up data (≥ 9 months) suggest these benefits persist.

Osteolytic bone lesions – Osteolytic bone destruction is a common characteristic of multiple myeloma. Bone destruction can occur as diffuse osteopenia, with radiographic findings similar to those of postmenopausal osteoporosis, or as discrete osteolytic lesions occurring in the axial and appendicular skeleton. Bone disease in multiple myeloma results from the release of soluble factors by myeloma cells that activate osteoclasts to resorb bone.

These bone changes can result in patients having evidence of osteolytic skeletal destruction leading to severe bone pain that requires either radiation therapy or narcotic analgesics (or both) for symptomatic relief. These changes also cause pathologic fractures of bone in both the axial and appendicular skeleton. Axial skeletal fractures of the vertebral bodies may lead to spinal cord compression or collapse with significant neurologic complications. Also, patients may experience episodes of hypercalcemia.

In patients with advanced multiple myeloma (n = 377), 90 mg pamidronate as monthly 4 hour IV for 9 months with antimyeloma therapy resulted in significantly fewer skeletal-related events (SREs; eg, pathologic fractures, radiation therapy to bone, bone surgery and spinal cord compression) vs placebo (24% vs 41%, respectively). Mean skeletal morbidity (number of SREs per year) was significantly greater for placebo; times to the first SRE occurrence, pathologic fracture and radiation were significantly longer for pamidronate. Fewer pamidronate patients suffered pathologic fractures or needed bone radiation; pain also decreased.

Indications:

Alendronate:

Osteoporosis in postmenopausal women – Osteoporosis may be confirmed by the finding of low bone mass or the presence or history of osteoporotic fracture.

BISPHOSPHONATES

Paget's disease of bone – For patients with Paget's disease of bone having alkaline phosphatase at least two times the upper limit of normal, or those who are symptomatic or those at risk for future complications from their disease.

Etidronate:

Paget's disease of bone, symptomatic (oral) – Etidronate arrests or impedes the disease process.

Heterotopic ossification (oral) – Prevention and treatment following total hip replacement or due to spinal injury.

Hypercalcemia of malignancy inadequately managed by dietary modification or oral hydration (parenteral) – Initiate rehydration with saline and "high-ceiling" or "loop" diuretics if indicated to restore urine output. This also increases renal calcium excretion and initiates a reduction in serum calcium. Concurrent therapy with etidronate is recommended as soon as there is a restoration of urine output.

Hypercalcemia of malignancy which persists after adequate hydration has been restored (parenteral) – Patients with and without metastases and with a variety of tumors have been responsive to treatment. Maintain adequate hydration, but avoid overhydration in aged patients and in those with cardiac failure.

Pamidronate:

Paget's disease – Treatment of patients with moderate to severe Paget's disease of bone. The effectiveness of pamidronate was demonstrated in patients with serum alkaline phosphatase ≥ 3 times the upper limit of normal.

Hypercalcemia of malignancy – In conjunction with adequate hydration for the treatment of moderate or severe hypercalcemia associated with malignancy, with or without bone metastases. Patients who have either epidermoid or non-epidermoid tumors respond. Initiate vigorous saline hydration (an integral part of therapy) promptly and attempt to restore urine output to ≈ 2 L/day throughout treatment. Mild or asymptomatic hypercalcemia may be treated with conservative measures (eg, saline hydration, with or without loop diuretics). Hydrate patients adequately throughout treatment, but avoid overhydration, especially in patients who have cardiac failure. Do not use diuretics prior to correction of hypovolemia.

Breast cancer/Multiple myelonoma – In conjunction with standard antineoplastic therapy for the treatment of osteolytic bone metastases of breast cancer and osteolytic lesions of multiple myeloma.

Tiludronate:

Paget's disease – Treatment of Paget's disease of bone (osteitis deformans).

Treatment is indicated in patients with Paget's disease of bone (1) who have a level of serum alkaline phosphatase (SAP) at least twice the upper limit of normal, or (2) who are symptomatic, or (3) who are at risk for future complications of their disease.

Unlabeled uses:

Etidronate has been used to treat postmenopausal osteoporosis (intermittent cyclical therapy of 400 mg/day usually followed by calcium). Spinal bone mass is increased and the incidence of new vertebral fractures is reduced. An NDA has been filed for this indication; however, approval has not been recommended because a follow-up study showed a 50% increase in new vertebral fractures during the third year of treatment. Further study is needed.

Pamidronate may be useful in treating the following conditions: Postmenopausal osteoporosis; hyperparathyroidism; to prevent glucocorticoid-induced osteoporosis; to reduce bone pain in patients with prostatic carcinoma; immobilization-related hypercalcemia.

Contraindications:

Hypersensitivity to bisphosphonates or any component of the products; hypocalcemia (alendronate, see Precautions); Class Dc and higher renal impairment (serum creatinine > 5 mg/dl; etidronate only, see Warnings).

Warnings:

Osteoporosis (alendronate): Consider causes other than estrogen deficiency and aging.

Paget's disease (etidronate): Response may be slow and continue for months after treatment discontinuation. Do not increase dosage prematurely or resume treatment before there is evidence of reactivation of the disease process. Do not initiate retreatment until at least a 90 day drug-free interval.

Renal function impairment:

Alendronate – Although no clinical information is available, it is likely that alendronate elimination via the kidney will be reduced in impaired renal function. Therefore, somewhat greater accumulation of alendronate in bone might be expected in impaired renal function. No dosage adjustment is necessary in mild-to-moderate renal insufficiency (creatinine clearance [Ccr] 35 to 60 ml/min). Alendronate use is not recommended in more severe renal insufficiency (Ccr < 35 ml/min).

BISPHOSPHONATES

Etidronate – Occasional mild-to-moderate renal function abnormalities (elevated BUN or serum creatinine) have occurred when etidronate was given to patients with hypercalcemia of malignancy. These were reversible or remained stable, without worsening, after therapy completion. In some patients with preexisting renal impairment or who had received potentially nephrotoxic drugs, further renal function depression was sometimes seen. Monitor renal function.

Normal renal function is adequate to handle not only the increased fluid load but also the excretion of etidronate itself. In patients with underlying renal disease, use only after a careful assessment of renal status or potential risks and benefits.

Reduction of the etidronate dose, if used at all, may be advisable in Class Cc (Classification of Renal Function Impairment, American Heart Association) renal functional impairment (serum creatinine 2.5 to 4.9 mg/dl). Use only if the potential benefit of hypercalcemia correction will substantially exceed the potential for worsening of renal function. In patients with Class Dc and higher renal functional impairment (serum creatinine > 5 mg/dl), withhold etidronate.

Pamidronate – In animals, nephropathy has been associated with IV (bolus and infusion) pamidronate. In dogs, renal findings such as elevated BUN and creatinine levels, renal tubular necrosis, renal tubular dilation or inflammation, renal toxicity and moribundity/death occurred. In rats, nephrotoxicity was observed and included increased BUN and creatinine levels and tubular degeneration and necrosis. Patients with hypercalcemia who receive an IV infusion of pamidronate should have periodic laboratory and clinical evaluations of renal function.

Pamidronate has not been tested in patients who have Class Dc renal impairment (creatinine > 5 mg/dl) and in few multiple myeloma patients with serum creatinine ≥ 3 mg/dl. Use clinical judgment to determine whether the potential benefit outweighs the potential risk in such patients.

Tiludronate – Tiludronate is not recommended for patients with severe renal failure (creatinine clearance < 30 ml/min). The plasma elimination half-life is longer.

Carcinogenesis/Mutagenesis/Fertility impairment:

Alendronate – Parafollicular cell (thyroid) adenomas were increased in high-dose male rats at doses equivalent to 1 and 3 times the 10 mg human dose.

Pamidronate – In a 104 week carcinogenicity study (daily oral pamidronate administration) in rats, there was a positive dose response relationship for benign adrenal pheochromocytoma in males.

In rats, decreased fertility occurred in first-generation offspring of parents who had received 150 mg/kg oral pamidronate; however, this occurred only when animals were mated with members of the same dose group.

Pregnancy: Category C (alendronate). Decreased postimplantation survivals and decreased body weight gain occurred in normal pups and sites of incomplete fetal ossification occurred in rats with doses from 1 to 9 times the 10 mg human dose. Total and ionized calcium decreased in pregnant rats resulting in delays and failure of delivery. Protracted parturition caused by maternal hypocalcemia occurred in rats at doses of 0.5 times the recommended human dose when rats were treated from before mating through gestation. Maternotoxicity (late pregnancy deaths) occurred in rats treated with alendronate for varying periods of time; these deaths were lessened but not eliminated by treatment cessation. Calcium could not ameliorate hypocalcemia or prevent maternal and neonatal deaths caused by delay in delivery; calcium supplementation IV prevented maternal but not fetal deaths.

There are no studies in pregnant women. Use alendronate during pregnancy only if the potential benefit justifies the risk to the mother and fetus.

Category B (oral etidronate). Etidronate has caused skeletal abnormalities in rats when given at oral dose levels of 300 mg/ml (15 to 60 times the human dose). Other effects on the offspring (including decreased live births) occur at dosages that cause significant toxicity in the parent generation and are 25 to 200 times the human dose. The skeletal effects are thought to be the result of the pharmacological effects of the drug on bone. There are no adequate and well controlled studies in pregnant women. Use only when clearly needed and when potential benefits outweigh potential hazards to the fetus.

Category C (parenteral etidronate and pamidronate). There are no adequate and well controlled studies. Bolus IV pamidronate doses in rats and rabbits produce maternal toxicity and embryo/fetal effects when given during organogenesis at doses of 0.6 to 8.3 times the highest recommended human dose for a single IV infusion. Because pamidronate can cross the placenta and has produced maternal and nonteratogenic embryo/fetal effects in rats and rabbits, do not give to pregnant women.

Category C (tiludronate). Dose-related scoliosis was likely attributable to the pharmacologic properties of tiludronate. Mice and rats have shown maternal toxicity at doses 70 to 10 times the recommended human dose.

BISPHOSPHONATES

Lactation: It is not known whether these drugs are excreted in breast milk. Exercise caution when administering etidronate, tiludronate or pamidronate to a nursing mother. Do not give alendronate to a nursing mother.

Children: Safety and efficacy for use in children have not been established.

Children have been treated with etidronate at doses recommended for adults, to prevent heterotopic ossifications or soft tissue calcifications. A rachitic syndrome has been reported infrequently at doses of ≥ 10 mg/kg/day and for prolonged periods approaching or exceeding a year. The epiphyseal radiologic changes associated with retarded mineralization of new osteoid and cartilage, and occasional symptoms reported, have been reversible when medication is discontinued.

Precautions:

Monitoring: Carefully monitor standard hypercalcemia-related metabolic parameters, such as serum levels of calcium, phosphate, magnesium and potassium following pamidronate initiation. Asymptomatic hypophosphatemia (16%), hypokalemia (7% to 9%), hypomagnesemia (11% to 12%) and hypocalcemia (5% to 12%) have occurred. Also, closely monitor electrolytes, creatinine as well as CBC, differential and hematocrit/hemoglobin. Carefully monitor patients who have preexisting anemia, leukopenia or thrombocytopenia in the first 2 weeks following treatment.

Nutrition: Maintain adequate nutrition, particularly an adequate intake of calcium and vitamin D.

GI disorders: Use caution when using bisphosphonates in patients with active upper GI problems (eg, dysphagia, symptomatic esophageal diseases, gastritis, duodenitis, ulcers). Etidronate therapy has been withheld from patients with enterocolitis because diarrhea is seen in some patients, particularly at higher doses.

Osteoid: Etidronate suppresses bone turnover and may retard mineralization of osteoid laid down during the bone accretion process. These effects are dose- and time-dependent. Osteoid, which may accumulate noticeably at doses of 10 to 20 mg/kg/day, mineralizes normally post-therapy. In patients with fractures, especially of long bones, it may be advisable to delay or interrupt treatment until callus is evident.

Fracture: In Paget's patients, treatment regimens of etidronate exceeding the recommended daily maximum dose of 20 mg/kg or continuous administration for periods > 6 months may be associated with an increased risk of fracture.

Long bones predominantly affected by lytic lesions, particularly in those patients unresponsive to therapy, may be especially prone to fracture. Radiographically and biochemically monitor patients with predominantly lytic lesions to permit termination of etidronate in those patients unresponsive to treatment.

Hormone replacement therapy: Concomitant use with alendronate for osteoporosis in postmenopausal women is not recommended.

Hypocalcemia: In animal studies, administration of etidronate in amounts or at rates in excess of those recommended produced transient hypocalcemia or induced proximal renal tubular damage. In one trial, 18% of patients treated one or more times the recommended dose had serum calcium values below lower limits of normal. When adjusted for reduced serum albumin levels, < 1% of patients were estimated to have hypocalcemic ionized serum calcium levels. No adverse effects have been traced to this hypocalcemia. The hypercalcemia of hyperparathyroidism is refractory to etidronate. It is possible for this disease to coexist in patients with malignancy.

Hypocalcemia (5% to 12%) has occurred with pamidronate therapy. Rare cases of symptomatic hypocalcemia (including tetany) occurred during pamidronate treatment. If hypocalcemia occurs, consider short-term calcium therapy.

Hypocalcemia must be corrected before therapy initiation with alendronate. Other disturbances of mineral metabolism (eg, vitamin D deficiency) should also be effectively treated. Presumably due to the effects of alendronate on increasing bone mineral, small asymptomatic decreases in serum calcium and phosphate may occur, especially in patients with Paget's disease, in whom the pretreatment rate of bone turnover may be greatly elevated. Ensure adequate calcium and vitamin D intake to provide for these enhanced needs.

BISPHOSPHONATES

Drug Interactions:

The patient should wait ≥ 30 minutes after taking alendronate before taking any other drug.

Alendronate Drug Interactions

Precipitant drug	Object drug*		Description
Ranitidine	Alendronate	↑	IV ranitidine doubled alendronate bioavailability. The clinical significance is unknown.
Calcium supplements, antacids	Alendronate, etidronate, tiludronate	↓	Products containing calcium and other multi-valent cations interfere with alendronate and etidronate absorption. The bioavailability of tiludronate is decreased by 60% by some aluminum- or magnesium-containing antacids, when administered 1 hour before tiludronate.
Alendronate	Aspirin	↑	The risk of upper GI adverse effects associated with aspirin increased with alendronate doses > 10 mg/day.
Aspirin	Tiludronate	↓	Aspirin may decrease the bioavailability of tiludronate by up to 50% when taken 2 hours after tiludronate.
Indomethacin	Tiludronate	↑	The bioavailability of tiludronate is increased 2- to 4-fold by indomethacin, but is not significantly altered by coadministration of diclofenac.

* ↑ = Object drug increased. ↓ = Object drug decreased.

Drug/Food interactions: In one study, bioavailability of alendronate was decreased by 40% when 10 mg alendronate was given 0.5 or 1 hour before breakfast vs 2 hours before, and bioavailability was negligible when alendronate was given with or 2 hours after breakfast. Concomitant coffee or orange juice reduced bioavailability by 60%. Take alendronate in the morning ≥ 30 minutes before the first meal, beverage or medication.

Absorption of etidronate may be reduced by foods or other preparations containing divalent cations. Take on an empty stomach 2 hours before a meal.

In single dose studies, bioavailability of tiludronate was reduced by 90% when an oral dose equivalent to 400 mg tiludronic acid was administered with, or 2 hours after, a standard breakfast compared to the same dose administered after an overnight fast and 4 hours before a standard breakfast.

Adverse Reactions:

Alendronate:

Osteoporosis in postmenopausal women – The following adverse reactions occurred with alendronate use:

Flatulence (2.6%); acid regurgitation (2%); esophageal ulcer (1.5%); dysphagia, abdominal distention (1%); gastritis (0.5%). One patient treated with 10 mg/day who had a history of peptic ulcer disease and gastrectomy and was taking concomitant aspirin developed an anastomotic ulcer with mild hemorrhage, which was considered drug-related. Aspirin and alendronate were discontinued and the patient recovered.

Other: Headache (2.6%); musculoskeletal pain (4.1%); rash, erythema (rare).

Paget's disease – In clinical studies in osteoporosis and Paget's disease, patients taking 40 mg/day for 3 to 12 months, the adverse experiences were similar to those in the 10 mg/day osteoporosis study. However, there was an increased incidence of upper GI side effects in the 40 mg/day group (17.7% of the patients taking alendronate vs 10.2% placebo). One case of esophagitis and two cases of gastritis resulted in treatment discontinuation.

Musculoskeletal pain, which also occurs with other bisphosphonates, occurred in approximately 6% of patients treated with 40 mg/day alendronate vs ≈ 1% taking placebo, rarely resulting in discontinuation. Discontinuation caused by any adverse reaction occurred in 6.4% of patients with Paget's disease treated with 40 mg/day alendronate vs 2.4% of placebo-treated patients.

Laboratory test abnormalities – In double-blind, multicenter, controlled studies, asymptomatic, mild and transient decreases in serum calcium and phosphate occurred in ≈ 18% and 10%, respectively, of patients taking alendronate vs ≈ 12% and 3% of those taking placebo. However, the incidence of decreases in serum calcium to < 8 mg/dl (2 mM) and serum phosphate to ≤ 2 mg/dl (0.65 mM) were similar in both treatment groups.

BISPHOSPHONATES

Etidronate: The incidence of GI complaints (diarrhea, nausea) is the same at 5 mg/kg/day as for placebo (about 6.7%). At 10 to 20 mg/kg/day, this may increase to 20% or 30%. These complaints are often alleviated by dividing the total daily dose.

Rare – Hypersensitivity reactions including angioedema, urticaria, rash, pruritus.

Paget's disease – Increased or recurrent bone pain at pagetic sites, or the onset of pain at previously asymptomatic sites has occurred. At 5 mg/kg/day, about 10% (vs 6.7% with placebo) report these phenomena. At higher doses, the incidence rises to about 20%. When the therapy continues, pain resolves in some patients but persists in others. Focal osteomalacia has occurred.

Hypercalcemia of malignancy is frequently associated with abnormal elevations of serum creatinine and BUN which improve in some patients or remain unchanged in most. However, in ≈ 10% of patients, occasional mild to moderate abnormalities in renal function (increases of > 0.5 mg/dl serum creatinine) were observed during or immediately after treatment. The possibility that etidronate contributed to these changes cannot be excluded.

A metallic, altered or loss of taste, which usually disappeared within hours, occurred during or shortly after initiation of etidronate treatment in 5% of patients.

Pamidronate:

Hypercalcemia of malignancy – Transient mild elevation of temperature by at least 1° C was noted 24 to 48 hours after administration in 34% of patients.

Drug-related local soft tissue symptoms (redness, swelling or induration and pain on palpation) at the site of catheter insertion were most common (18%) in patients treated with 90 mg. When all on-therapy events are considered, the rate rises to 41%. Symptomatic treatment resulted in rapid resolution in all patients.

Rare cases of uveitis, iritis, scleritis and episcleritis have occurred including one case of scleritis and one case of uveitis upon separate rechallenges.

Four of 128 patients (3%) had seizures; two had preexisting seizure disorders. None of the seizures were considered to be drug-related.

Other reactions in ≥ 15% of patients are: Fluid overload; generalized/abdominal/bone pain; hypertension; anorexia; constipation; nausea; vomiting; urinary tract infection; anemia; hypokalemia; hypomagnesemia; hypophosphatemia.

Paget's disease – Transient mild elevation of temperature > 1°C above pretreatment baseline was noted within 48 hours after completion of treatment in 21% of patients treated with 90 mg. Drug-related musculoskeletal pain and CNS symptoms (dizziness, headache, paresthesia, increased sweating) were more common with Paget's disease than with hypercalcemia of malignancy (same 90 mg dose).

Other adverse reactions are as follows: Hypertension, arthrosis, bone pain, headache (10%); fever, nausea, back pain (5%).

Osteolytic bone lesions of multiple myeloma – Most adverse reactions may have been related to the underlying disease state or antimyeloma therapy: Fever (31.5%); anemia (29.6%); nausea (26.6%); fatigue (22.7%); upper respiratory infections (23.2%); diarrhea (19.2%); constipation (18.2%); headache (17.7%); dyspnea (16.4%); coughing (15.9%); myalgias (14.8%); arthralgias (6.4%); hypokalemia (5.9%); hypomagnesemia, hypocalcemia (3.4%); hypophosphatemia (1.5%).

Tiludronate: Adverse events associated with tiludronate usually have been mild, and generally have not required discontinuation of therapy. 1.3% of patients receiving 400 mg tiludronate and 5.4% of patients receiving placebo discontinued therapy due to any clinical adverse event.

Paget's disease – The following reactions occurred in ≥ 1% of patients.

CNS: Vertigo, involuntary muscle contractions, anxiety, nervousness.

Dermatologic: Pruritus, increased sweating, Stevens-Johnson type syndrome (rare).

GI: Dry mouth, gastritis.

Miscellaneous: Asthenia, pathological fracture, bronchitis, urinary tract infection, flushing.

BISPHOSPHONATES

Bisphosphonate Adverse Reactions (%)[1]

Adverse reaction	Pamidronate 60 mg over 4 hr (n = 23)	Pamidronate 60 mg over 24 hr (n = 17)	Pamidronate 90 mg over 24 hr (n = 17)	Etidronate (n = 35) 7.5 mg/kg x 3 days	Alendronate (n = 196)[2] 10 mg/day	Tiludronate (n = 75) 400 mg/day
General						
Fever	26	19	18	9	0	0
Pain	0	0	0	0	21.3	0
Infusion site reaction	0	4	18	0	0	0
Fatigue	0	0	12	0	0	≥ 1%
Back pain	0	0	0	0	8	0
Moniliasis	0	0	6	0	0	0
Edema	0	1	0	0	0	0
Fluid overload	0	0	0	6	0	0
Influenza-like symptoms	0	0	0	0	4	0
Accidental injury	0	0	0	0	4	0
Peripheral edema	0	0	0	0	2.7	0
Respiratory						
Rales/Rhinitis	0	0	6	0	0	5.3
Sinusitis	0	0	0	0	0	5.3
URI	0	3	0	0	0	5.3
Dyspnea	0	0	0	3	0	0
Coughing	0	0	0	0	0	2.7
Pharyngitis	0	0	0	0	0	2.7
Cardiovascular						
Atrial fibrillation	0	0	6	0	0	0
Hypertension	0	0	6	0	0	≥ 1%
Syncope	0	0	6	0	0	≥ 1%
Tachycardia	0	0	6	0	0	0
Chest pain	0	0	0	0	2.7	0
Atrial flutter	0	1	0	0	0	0
Cardiac failure	0	1	0	0	0	0
GI						
Nausea	4	0	18	6	3.6	9.3
Anorexia	4	1	12	0	0	≥ 1%
Constipation	4	0	6	3	3.1	≥ 1%
GI hemorrhage	0	0	6	0	0	0
Abdominal pain	0	1	0	0	6.6	≥ 1%
Stomatitis	0	1	0	3	0	0
Diarrhea	0	1	0	0	3.1	9.3
Dyspepsia	4	0	0	0	3.6	5.3
Vomiting	4	0	0	0	1	4
Flatulence	0	0	0	0	0	2.7
CNS						
Headache	0	0	0	0	0	6.7
Somnolence	0	1	6	0	0	≥ 1%
Dizziness	0	0	0	0	0	4
Paresthesia	0	0	0	0	0	4
Insomnia	0	1	0	0	0	≥ 1%
Psychosis	4	0	0	0	0	0
Convulsions	0	0	0	3	0	0
Hemic/Lymphatic						
Anemia	0	0	6	0	0	0
Leukopenia	4	0	0	0	0	0
Neutropenia	0	1	0	0	0	0
Thrombocytopenia	0	1	0	0	0	0
Lab abnormalities						
Hypophosphatemia	0	9	18	3	0	0
Hypokalemia	4	4	18	0	0	0
Hypomagnesemia	4	10	12	3	0	0
Hypocalcemia	0	1	12	0	0	0

BISPHOSPHONATES

Bisphosphonate Adverse Reactions (%)[1]

Adverse reaction	Pamidronate			Etidronate (n = 35)	Alendronate (n = 196)[2]	Tiludronate (n = 75)
	60 mg over 4 hr (n = 23)	60 mg over 24 hr (n = 17)	90 mg over 24 hr (n = 17)	7.5 mg/kg x 3 days	10 mg/day	400 mg/day
Abnormal hepatic function	0	0	0	3	0	0
Musculoskeletal						
Arthralgia	0	0	0	0	0	2.7
Arthrosis	0	0	0	0	0	2.7
Special Senses						
Cataract	0	0	0	0	0	2.7
Conjunctivitis	0	0	0	0	0	2.7
Glaucoma	0	0	0	0	0	2.7
Miscellaneous						
Hypothyroidism	0	0	6	0	0	0
Rash	0	0	0	0	0	2.7
Skin disorder	0	0	0	0	0	2.7
Tooth disorder	0	0	0	0	0	2.7
Dependent edema	0	0	0	0	0	2.7
Hyperparathyroidism	0	0	0	0	0	2.7
Infection	0	0	0	0	0	2.7
Vitamin D deficiency	0	0	0	0	0	2.7
Myalgia	0	1	0	0	0	0
Uremia	4	0	0	0	0	0
Taste perversion	0	0	0	3	0.5	0

[1] Data are pooled from separate studies and are not necessarily comparable.
[2] Alendronate was used for osteoporosis in postmenopausal women in this study.

Overdosage:

Alendronate: Hypocalcemia, hypophosphatemia and upper GI adverse events (eg, upset stomach, heartburn, esophagitis, gastritis or ulcer) may result from overdosage. Consider the administiration of milk or antacids to bind alendronate. Dialysis would not be beneficial.

Etidronate:

Oral –

Symptoms: Clinical experience with etidronate overdosage is extremely limited. Decreases in serum calcium following substantial overdosage may be expected in some patients. Signs and symptoms of hypocalcemia may also occur. In one event, an 18-year-old female who ingested an estimated single dose of 4000 to 6000 mg (67 to 100 mg/kg) was mildly hypocalcemic (7.52 mg/dl) and experienced paresthesia of the fingers. Some patients may develop vomiting and expel the drug.

Treatment: Gastric lavage may remove unabsorbed drug. Standard procedures for treating hypocalcemia, including the administration of calcium IV, would be expected to restore physiologic amounts of ionized calcium and relieve signs and symptoms of hypocalcemia. Such treatment has been effective.

Parenteral – Rapid IV administration of etidronate at doses > 27mg/kg has produced ECG changes and bleeding problems in animals. These abnormalities are probably related to marked or rapid decreases in ionized calcium levels in blood and tissue fluids. They are thought to be due to chelation of calcium by massive amounts of the diphosphonate. These abnormalities have been reversible in animal studies by use of ionizable calcium salts. Similar problems are not expected to occur in humans if treated with etidronate as recommended. Moreover, signs and symptoms of hypocalcemia such as paresthesias and carpopedal spasms have not been reported with either agent. The chelation effects of the diphosphonate, should they occur, should be reversible with IV calcium gluconate.

Administration of IV etidronate at doses and possibly at rates in excess of those recommended has been associated with renal insufficiency.

Pamidronate: There have been several cases of drug maladministration of IV pamidronate in hypercalcemia patients with total doses of 225 to 300 mg given over 2.5 to 4 days. All survived but experienced hypocalcemia requiring IV or oral calcium.

BISPHOSPHONATES

One obese woman (95 kg) who was treated with pamidronate 285 mg/day for 3 days experienced high fever (39.5°C; 102°F), hypotension and transient taste perversion, noted about 6 hours after the first infusion. Fever and hypotension were rapidly corrected with steroids.

Tiludronate: Hypocalcemia is a potential consequence of tiludronate overdose. In one patient with hypercalcemia of malignancy, IV administration of high doses of tiludronate (800 mg/day total dose, 6 mg/kg/day for 2 days) was associated with acute renal failure and death.

Treatment: No specific information is available on the treatment of overdose with tiludronate. Dialysis would not be beneficial. Standard medical practices may be used to manage renal insufficiency or hypocalcemia, if signs of these develop.

Patient Information:

Bisphosphonates may cause GI upset (eg, nausea, diarrhea).

Alendronate: Instruct patients that the expected benefits of alendronate may only be obtained when each tablet is taken with plain water the first thing in the morning and at least 30 minutes before the first food, beverage or medication of the day. Also instruct them that waiting > 30 minutes will improve alendronate absorption. Even dosing with orange juice or coffee markedly reduces the absorption of alendronate.

Instruct patients to take alendronate with a full glass of water (6 to 8 oz; 180 to 240 ml) and not to lie down for at least 30 minutes following administration to facilitate delivery to the stomach and reduce the potential for esophageal irritation.

Instruct patients to take supplemental calcium and vitamin D if dietary intake is inadequate. Consider weight-bearing exercise along with the modification of certain behavioral factors, such as excessive cigarette smoking or alcohol consumption if these factors exist.

Etidronate (oral): Take on an empty stomach 2 hours before meals.

Tiludronate: Take tiludronate with 6 to 8 ounces of plain water. Do not take within 2 hours of food. Maintain adequate vitamin D and calcium intake. Do not take calcium supplements, aspirin and indomethacin within 2 hours before or after tiludronate. Take aluminum- or magnesium-containing antacids, if needed, at least 2 hours after tiludronate.

ETIDRONATE DISODIUM (ORAL)

For complete prescribing information, refer to the Bisphosphonates group monograph.

Administration and Dosage:

Administer as a single dose. However, if GI discomfort occurs, divide the dose. To maximize absorption, avoid the following within 2 hours of dosing:

1) Food, especially items high in calcium, such as milk or milk products.
2) Vitamins with mineral supplements or antacids high in metals (eg, calcium, iron, magnesium or aluminum).

Paget's disease:

Initial treatment – 5 to 10 mg/kg/day (not to exceed 6 months) or 11 to 20 mg/kg/day (not to exceed 3 months). Reserve doses > 10 mg/kg/day for use when lower doses are ineffective, when there is an overriding requirement for suppression of increased bone turnover or when prompt reduction of elevated cardiac output is required. Doses > 20 mg/kg/day are not recommended.

Retreatment – Initiate only after an etidronate-free period of at least 90 days and when there is biochemical, symptomatic or other evidence of active disease process. Monitor patients every 3 to 6 months, although some patients may go drug-free for extended periods. Retreatment regimens are the same as for initial treatment. For most patients, the original dose will be adequate for retreatment. If not, consider increasing the dose within the recommended guidelines.

Heterotopic ossification:

Due to spinal cord injury – 20 mg/kg/day for 2 weeks, followed by 10 mg/kg/day for 10 weeks; total treatment period is 12 weeks. Institute as soon as feasible following the injury, preferably prior to evidence of heterotopic ossification.

Complicating total hip replacement – 20 mg/kg/day for 1 month preoperatively, then 20 mg/kg/day for 3 months postoperatively; total treatment period is 4 months.

Rx	**Didronel** (Procter & Gamble Pharm.)	**Tablets:** 200 mg	(P&G 402). White. In 60s.
		400 mg	(NE 406). White, scored. In 60s.

ETIDRONATE DISODIUM (PARENTERAL)

For complete prescribing information, refer to the Bisphosphonates group monograph.

Administration and Dosage:

Recommended dose is 7.5 mg/kg/day for 3 successive days. This daily dose must be diluted in at least 250 ml of sterile normal saline.

Infusion time: Administer the diluted dose IV over a period of at least 2 hours. Infusion may be added to volumes of fluid > 250 ml when convenient.

Regardless of the volume of solution in which etidronate IV infusion is diluted, slow infusion is important. Observe the minimum infusion time of 2 hours at the recommended dose, or smaller doses. The usual course of treatment is one infusion of 7.5 mg/kg/day on each of 3 consecutive days, but some patients have been treated for up to 7 days. When patients are treated for > 3 days, there may be an increased possibility of hypocalcemia.

Retreatment may be appropriate if hypercalcemia recurs. There should be at least a 7 day interval between courses of treatment. The dose and manner of retreatment is the same as that for initial treatment. Retreatment for > 3 days has not been adequately studied. The safety and efficacy of more than two courses of therapy have not been studied. With renal impairment, dose reduction may be advisable.

Oral editronate may be started on the day after the last infusion. The recommended oral dose for patients who have had hypercalcemia is 20 mg/kg/day for 30 days. If serum calcium levels remain normal or clinically acceptable, treatment may be extended. Use for > 90 days is not adequately studied and is not recommended.

Storage/Stability: Avoid excessive heat (> 40°C; 104°F). The diluted solution stored at room temperature (15° to 30°C; 59° to 86°F) shows no drug loss for 48 hours.

Rx	**Didronel IV** (MGI Pharma)	**Injection:** 300 mg per amp	In 6 ml amps.

PAMIDRONATE DISODIUM

For complete prescribing information, refer to the Bisphosphonates group monograph.

Administration and Dosage:

Approved by the FDA in October 1991.

Hypercalcemia of malignancy: Give consideration to both the severity and the symptoms of hypercalcemia. Vigorous saline hydration alone may be sufficient for treating mild, asymptomatic hypercalcemia. Avoid overhydration in patients who have potential for cardiac failure. In hypercalcemia associated with hematologic malignancies, the use of glucocorticoid therapy may be helpful.

Moderate hypercalcemia – The recommended dose in moderate hypercalcemia (corrected serum calcium of ≈ 12 to 13.5 mg/dl) is 60 to 90 mg. The 60 mg dose is given as an initial, *single-dose*, IV infusion over at least 4 hours. The 90 mg dose must be given as an initial, *single-dose*, IV infusion over 24 hours.

Severe hypercalcemia – Recommended dose (corrected serum calcium > 13.5 mg/dl) is 90 mg, which must be given as an initial *single-dose*, IV infusion over 24 hours.

Retreatment – A limited number of patients have received more than one treatment for hypercalcemia. Retreatment, in patients who show complete or partial response initially, may be carried out if serum calcium does not return to normal or remain normal after initial treatment. Allow a minimum of 7 days to elapse before retreatment to allow for full response to the initial dose. The dose and manner of retreatment are identical to that of the initial therapy.

Osteolytic bone metastases: 90 mg administered over a 2-hour infusion every 3 to 4 weeks.

Paget's disease: The recommended dose in patients with moderate to severe Paget's disease of bone is 30 mg daily, given as a 4 hour infusion on 3 consecutive days for a total dose of 90 mg.

Retreatment – A limited number of patients have received more than one treatment in clinical trials. When clinically indicated, retreat at the dose of initial therapy.

Osteolytic bone lesions of multiple myeloma: The recommended dose is 90 mg given as a 4 hour infusion on a monthly basis. Patients with marked Bence-Jones proteinuria and dehydration should receive adequate hydration prior to pamidronate infusion.

Preparation of solution: Reconstitute by adding 10 ml Sterile Water for Injection to each vial, resulting in a solution of 30, 60 or 90 mg/10 ml. The pH of the reconstituted solution is 6 to 7.4. Allow drug to dissolve completely before withdrawing.

Hypercalcemia of malignancy – Administer as an IV infusion over at least 4 hours for the 60 mg dose and 24 hours for the 90 mg dose. Dilute in 1 L sterile 0.45% or 0.9% NaCl or 5% Dextrose Injection. This infusion solution is stable for up to 24 hours at room temperature.

Paget's disease – Dilute the recommended daily dose of 30 mg in 500 ml sterile 0.45% or 0.9% NaCl or 5% Dextrose Injection and give over a 4 hour period for 3 consecutive days.

Osteolytic bone lesions of multiple myeloma – Dilute the recommended dose of 90 mg in 500 ml of sterile 0.45% or 0.9% of NaCl or 5% Dextrose Injection and give over 4 hours on a monthly basis.

Admixture incompatibility: Do not mix with calcium-containing infusion solutions, such as Ringer's solution and give in a single IV solution and line separate from all other drugs.

Storage/Stability: Pamidronate reconstituted with Sterile Water for Injection may be stored under refrigeration at 2° to 8°C (36° to 46°F) for up to 24 hours.

Rx	**Aredia** (Novartis)	**Powder for Injection, lyophilized**: 30 mg	470 mg mannitol. In vials.
		60 mg	400 mg mannitol. In vials.
		90 mg	375 mg mannitol. In vials.

ALENDRONATE SODIUM

For complete prescribing information, refer to the Bisphosphonates group monograph.

Administration and Dosage:

Approved by the FDA on September 29, 1995 (1P classification).

Alendronate must be taken at least 30 minutes before the first food, beverage or medication of the day with plain water only. Other beverages (including mineral water), food and some medications are likely to reduce the absorption of alendronate. Waiting > 30 minutes before eating will improve the absorption. Waiting < 30 minutes or taking the drug with food, beverages (other than plain water) or other medications will lessen the effect of the drug by decreasing its absorption. To facilitate delivery to the stomach, take with a full glass of water (6 to 8 oz.) and avoid lying down for at least 30 minutes thereafter (see Patient Information).

Patients with osteoporosis or Paget's disease should receive supplemental calcium and vitamin D if dietary intake is inadequate.

Osteoporosis in postmenopausal women: 10 mg once a day. Safety of treatment for > 4 years has not been studied (extension studies are ongoing).

Paget's disease of bone: 40 mg once a day for 6 months.

Retreatment – Relapses during the 12 months following therapy occurred in 9% of patients who responded to treatment. Specific retreatment data are not available, although responses to alendronate were similar in patients who had received prior bisphosphonate therapy and those who had not. Retreatment with alendronate may be considered, following a 6 month post-treatment evaluation period, in patients who have relapsed based on increases in serum alkaline phosphatase, which should be measured periodically. Retreatment may also be considered in those who failed to normalize their serum alkaline phosphatase.

Elderly: No dosage adjustment is necessary.

Renal function impairment: No dosage adjustment is necessary in patients with mild-to-moderate renal insufficiency (creatinine clearance 35 to 60 ml/min). However, alendronate is not recommended for patients with more severe renal insufficiency (creatinine clearance < 35 ml/min) due to lack of experience.

Rx	**Fosamax** (Merck)	**Tablets:** 10 mg	Lactose. (MRK 936 w/ bone image/ Fosamax w/ bone image). White, round. In unit-of-use 30s and 100s and UD 100s.
		40 mg	Lactose. (MRK 212 Fosamax). White, triangular shape. In unit-of-use 30s.

TILUDRONATE SODIUM

For complete prescribing information, refer to the Bisphosphonates group monograph.

Administration and Dosage:

Administer a single 400 mg daily oral dose of tiludronate, taken with 6 to 8 ounces of plain water only for a period of 3 months. Beverages other than plain water (including mineral water), food and some medications (see Drug Interactions) are likely to reduce the absorption of tiludronate. Do not take within 2 hours of food. Take calcium or mineral supplements at least 2 hours before or after tiludronate. Take aluminum- or magnesium-containing antacids at least 2 hours after taking tiludronate. Do not take within 2 hours of indomethacin.

Following therapy, allow an interval of 3 months to assess response. Specific data regarding retreatment are limited, although results from uncontrolled studies indicate favorable biochemical improvement similar to initial tiludronate treatment.

Storage/Stability: Do not remove tablets from the foil strips until they are to be used.

Rx	**Skelid** (Sanofi-Winthrop)	**Tablets:** 240 mg	Lactose. White, round. (S.W 200). In foil strips of 56.

GALLIUM NITRATE

Warning:

Concurrent use of gallium nitrate with other potentially nephrotoxic drugs (eg, aminoglycosides, amphotericin B) may increase the risk for developing severe renal insufficiency in patients with cancer-related hypercalcemia. If use of a potentially nephrotoxic drug is indicated during therapy, discontinue gallium nitrate and continue hydration for several days after administering the potentially nephrotoxic drug. Closely monitor serum creatinine and urine output during and after this period. Discontinue gallium nitrate therapy if the serum creatinine level exceeds 2.5 mg/dl.

Actions:

Pharmacology: Gallium nitrate is a hydrated nitrate salt of the group IIIa element, gallium. Gallium nitrate exerts a hypocalcemic effect by inhibiting calcium resorption from bone, possibly by reducing increased bone turnover. The precise mechanism has not been determined. No cytotoxic effects were observed with bone cells in animals.

Cancer-related hypercalcemia is a common problem in hospitalized patients with malignancy. It may affect 10% to 20% of patients with cancer. Different types of malignancies seem to vary in their propensity to cause hypercalcemia. A higher incidence of hypercalcemia has been observed in patients with non-small-cell lung cancer, breast cancer, multiple myeloma, kidney cancer and cancer of the head and neck. Hypercalcemia of malignancy seems to result from an imbalance between the net resorption of bone and urinary excretion of calcium. Hypercalcemia may produce signs and symptoms including: Anorexia; lethargy; fatigue; nausea; vomiting; constipation; dehydration; renal insufficiency; impaired mental status; coma; cardiac arrest. A rapid rise in serum calcium may cause more severe symptoms for a given level of hypercalcemia.

Pharmacokinetics: Gallium nitrate was infused at a daily dose of 200 mg/m^2 for 5 (n = 2) or 7 (n = 10) consecutive days to 12 cancer patients. Apparent steady state is generally achieved in 24 to 48 hours. The range of average steady-state plasma levels of gallium observed among seven patients was between 1134 and 2399 ng/ml. The average plasma clearance following daily infusion of 200 mg/m^2 for 5 or 7 days was 0.15 L/hr/kg (range: 0.12 to 0.2 L/hr/kg). In one patient who received daily infusion doses of 100, 150 and 200 mg/m^2, the apparent steady-state gallium levels did not increase proportionally with a dose increase. Gallium nitrate is not metabolized either by liver or kidneys and appears to be significantly excreted via kidney.

Clinical trials: A randomized double-blind clinical study comparing gallium nitrate with calcitonin was conducted in patients with a serum calcium concentration (corrected for albumin) ≥ 12 mg/dl following 2 days of hydration. Gallium nitrate was given as a continuous 200 mg/m^2/day IV infusion for 5 days and calcitonin 8 IU/kg IM was given every 6 hours for 5 days. Elevated serum calcium (corrected for albumin) was normalized in 75% (18 of 24) of the patients receiving gallium nitrate and in 27% (7 of 26) of the patients receiving calcitonin. The time-course of effect on serum calcium (corrected for albumin) is summarized in the following table.

Change in Serum Calcium by Gallium Nitrate vs Calcitonin

Time period[1] (hours)	Mean change in serum calcium (mg/dl)[2]	
	Gallium Nitrate	Calcitonin
24	-0.4	-1.6
48	-0.9	-1.4
72	-1.5	-1.1
96	-2.9	-1.1
120	-3.3	-1.3

[1] Time after initiation of therapy in hours.

[2] Serum calcium change from baseline (corrected for albumin).

The median duration of normocalcemia/hypocalcemia was 7.5 days for patients treated with gallium nitrate and 1 day for patients treated with calcitonin. A total of 92% of patients treated with gallium nitrate had a decrease in serum calcium (corrected for albumin) ≥ 2 mg/dl vs 54% of patients treated with calcitonin.

An open-label, non-randomized study was conducted to examine a range of doses and dosing schedules of gallium nitrate for control of cancer-related hypercalcemia. The principal dosing regimens were 100 and 200 mg/m^2/day, administered as continuous IV infusions for 5 days. A 200 mg/m^2/day dose for 5 days normalized elevated serum calcium levels (corrected for albumin) in 83% of patients vs 50% of patients receiving 100 mg/m^2/day for 5 days. A decrease in serum calcium (corrected for albu-

GALLIUM NITRATE

min) ≥ 2 mg/dl was observed in 83% and 94% of patients at dosages of 100 and 200 mg/m^2/day for 5 days, respectively.

Indications:

Cancer-related hypercalcemia (clearly symptomatic) unresponsive to adequate hydration. In patients who have an underlying cancer type that may be sensitive to corticosteroids (eg, hematologic cancers), the use or addition of corticosteroid therapy may be indicated.

In general, patients with a serum calcium (corrected for albumin) < 12 mg/dl would not be expected to be symptomatic. Mild or asymptomatic hypercalcemia may be treated with conservative measures (eg, saline hydration, with or without diuretics). In the treatment of cancer-related hypercalcemia, it is important first to establish adequate hydration, preferably with IV saline, in order to increase the renal excretion of calcium and correct dehydration caused by hypercalcemia.

Contraindications:

Severe renal impairment (serum creatinine > 2.5 mg/dl).

Warnings:

Anemia: The use of very high doses (up to 1400 mg/m^2) has been associated with anemia, and several patients have received red blood cell transfusions. Because of the serious nature of the underlying illness, it is uncertain that the anemia was caused by gallium nitrate.

Renal function impairment: Hypercalcemia in cancer patients is commonly associated with impaired renal function (elevated BUN or serum creatinine). It is strongly recommended that serum creatinine be monitored during therapy. It is important that such patients be adequately hydrated with oral or IV fluids (preferably saline) and that a satisfactory urine output (2 L/day is recommended) be established before beginning therapy. Maintain adequate hydration throughout the treatment period, and avoid overhydration in patients with compromised cardiovascular status. Do not use diuretic therapy prior to correction of hypovolemia. Discontinue gallium nitrate therapy if the serum creatinine level exceeds 2.5 mg/dl.

The use of gallium nitrate in patients with marked renal insufficiency (serum creatinine > 2.5 mg/dl) has not been systematically examined. If therapy is undertaken in patients with moderately impaired renal function (serum creatinine 2 to 2.5 mg/dl), frequently monitor patient's renal status. Discontinue treatment if the serum creatinine level exceeds 2.5 mg/dl.

Pregnancy: Category C. It is not known whether gallium nitrate can cause fetal harm when administered to a pregnant woman or can affect reproductive capacity. Administer to a pregnant woman only if clearly needed.

Lactation: It is not known whether gallium nitrate is excreted in breast milk. Because of the potential for serious adverse reactions in nursing infants, decide whether to discontinue nursing or discontinue the drug, taking into account the importance of the drug to the mother.

Children: The safety and efficacy of gallium nitrate have not been established.

Precautions:

Monitoring: Monitor renal function (serum creatinine and BUN) and serum calcium during gallium nitrate therapy. In addition to baseline assessment, the suggested frequency of calcium and phosphorous determinations is daily and twice weekly, respectively. Discontinue gallium nitrate if the serum creatinine is > 2.5 mg/dl.

Changes in total serum calcium may not accurately reflect changes in the concentration of free-ionized calcium. Measurement of the serum albumin concentration and correction of the total serum calcium concentration may help assess the severity of hypercalcemia in the absence of a direct measurement of free-ionized calcium.

Asymptomatic or mild to moderate hypocalcemia (6.5 to 8 mg/dl, corrected for serum albumin) occurred in ≈ 38% of patients in the controlled clinical trial. One patient exhibited a positive Chvostek's sign. If hypocalcemia occurs, stop gallium nitrate therapy; short-term calcium therapy may be necessary.

GALLIUM NITRATE

Visual and auditory disturbances: A small proportion (< 1%) of patients treated with multiple high doses of gallium nitrate combined with other investigational anticancer drugs, have developed acute optic neuritis. While these patients were critically ill and had received multiple drugs, a reaction to high-dose gallium nitrate is possible. Most patients had full visual recovery; however, at least one case of persistent visual impairment has occurred. One patient with cancer-related hypercalcemia developed a hearing loss following gallium nitrate administration. Because of the patient's underlying condition and concurrent therapies, the relationship of this event to gallium nitrate administration is unclear. Tinnitus and partial loss of auditory acuity have occurred rarely (< 1%) in patients who received high-dose gallium nitrate as anticancer treatment.

Transient hypophosphatemia of mild-to-moderate degree may occur in ≤ 79% of hypercalcemic patients following treatment. In a controlled clinical trial, 33% of patients had at least one serum phosphorous measurement between 1.5 to 2.4 mg/dl, while 46% of patients had at least one serum phosphorous value < 1.5 mg/dl. Patients who develop hypophosphatemia may require oral phosphorous therapy.

Decreased serum bicarbonate, possibly secondary to mild respiratory alkalosis, occurred in 40% to 50% of cancer patients treated with gallium nitrate. The cause was unclear. This effect has been asymptomatic and has not required specific treatment.

Hypotension: A decrease in mean systolic and diastolic blood pressure was observed several days after treatment with gallium nitrate in a controlled clinical trial. The decrease in blood pressure was asymptomatic and did not require specific treatment.

Drug Interactions:

Nephrotoxic drugs (eg, aminoglycosides, amphotericin B): Combined use of gallium nitrate with other potentially nephrotoxic drugs may increase the risk of developing renal insufficiency in patients with cancer-related hypercalcemia (see Warning box).

Adverse Reactions:

Renal: Rise in BUN and creatinine (≈ 12.5%; see Warnings).

Renal toxicity – Two patients receiving gallium nitrate developed acute renal failure, but the relationship of these events to the drug was unclear.

Metabolic: Hypocalcemia, transient hypophosphatemia, decreased serum bicarbonate (see Precautions).

Hematologic: Anemia (See Warnings); leukopenia.

Cardiovascular: Tachycardia; lower extremity edema (causal relationship unknown); hypotension (See Precautions).

Special senses: Acute optic neuritis; visual impairment, decreased hearing (see Precautions).

Respiratory: (Causal relationship unknown). Dyspnea; rales and rhonchi; pleural effusion; pulmonary infiltrates.

GI: (Causal relationship unknown). Nausea or vomiting; diarrhea; constipation.

Miscellaneous: Lethargy; confusion; hypothermia; fever; paresthesia; dreams and hallucinations; skin rash. Because of the serious nature of the underlying condition of these patients, the relationship of these events to therapy with gallium nitrate is unknown.

Overdosage:

Symptoms: Rapid IV infusion of gallium nitrate or use of doses higher than recommended (200 mg/m^2) may cause nausea and vomiting and a substantially increased risk of renal insufficiency.

Treatment: Discontinue further drug administration and monitor serum calcium. Administer vigorous IV hydration, with or without diuretics, for 2 to 3 days. During this time, carefully monitor renal function and urinary output for balanced fluid intake and output.

GALLIUM NITRATE

Administration and Dosage:

Approved by the FDA in January 1991.

Usual dose: 200 mg/m^2 daily for 5 consecutive days. In patients with mild hypercalcemia and few symptoms, a lower dosage of 100 mg/m^2/day for 5 days may be considered. If serum calcium levels are lowered into the normal range in < 5 days, treatment may be discontinued early. Take the patient's acid-base status into consideration while assessing the degree of hypercalcemia. The daily dose must be given as an IV infusion over 24 hours.

Dilute the daily dose, preferably in 1 L 0.9% Sodium Chloride Injection or 5% Dextrose Injection, for administration as an IV infusion over 24 hours. Maintain adequate hydration throughout the treatment period, with careful attention to avoid overhydration in patients with compromised cardiovascular status. Controlled studies have not been undertaken to evaluate the safety and efficacy of retreatment with gallium nitrate.

Storage/Stability: When gallium nitrate is added to either 0.9% Sodium Chloride Injection or 5% Dextrose Injection, it is stable for ≥ 48 hours at room temperature (15° to 30°C; 59° to 86°F) and for 7 days if stored under refrigeration (2° to 8°C; 36° to 46°F). Contains no preservative; discard unused portion. Store vials at 15° to 30°C (59° to 86°F).

Rx	**Ganite** (SoloPak)	**Injection**: 25 mg/ml	Preservative free. In 20 ml flip-top vials.

chapter 4

diuretics and cardiovasculars

THIAZIDES AND RELATED DIURETICS

Actions:

Pharmacology: Thiazide diuretics increase the urinary excretion of sodium and chloride in approximately equivalent amounts. They inhibit reabsorption of sodium and chloride in the cortical thick ascending limb of the loop of Henle and the early distal tubules. Many of these compounds possess some degree of carbonic anhydrase inhibition activity (metolazone has no activity) due to the sulfonamide moiety; however, this is unlikely to be encountered clinically. Other common actions include: Increased potassium and bicarbonate excretion, decreased calcium excretion and uric acid retention. At maximal therapeutic dosages all thiazides are approximately equal in diuretic efficacy, but metolazone may be more effective in patients with impaired renal function. Metolazone and quinethazone (quinazoline derivatives), chlorthalidone (a phthalimidine derivative) and indapamide (an indoline) are included here because of their structural and pharmacological similarities to the thiazides.

The exact antihypertensive mechanism of the thiazides is unknown, although sodium depletion appears to be of primary importance. During initial therapy, cardiac output decreases and extracellular volume diminishes. With chronic therapy, cardiac output normalizes, peripheral vascular resistance falls, and there is a persistent small reduction in extracellular volume.

In hypertensive patients, daily doses of indapamide have no appreciable cardiac inotropic or chronotropic effect, and little or no effect on glomerular filtration rate or renal plasma flow. The drug decreases peripheral resistance, with little or no effect on cardiac output, rate or rhythm. Indapamide had an antihypertensive effect in patients with varying degrees of renal impairment, although in general, diuretic effects declined as renal function decreased.

Pharmacokinetics: The antihypertensive action requires several days to produce effects. Administration for up to 2 to 4 weeks is usually required for optimal therapeutic effect. The duration of the antihypertensive effect of the thiazides is sufficiently long to adequately control blood pressure with a single daily dose. Despite extensive use of diuretics, pharmacokinetic data are limited. It is important to emphasize the lack of relationship between plasma levels and diuretic effect.

Pharmacokinetics of Thiazides and Related Diuretics

Diuretic	Onset (hours)	Peak (hours)	Duration (hours)	Equivalent dose (mg)	Percent absorbed	Half-life (hours)
Bendroflumethiazide	2	4	16 to 12	5	≈ 100	3 to 3.9
Benzthiazide	2	4 to 6	16 to 18	50	nd[1]	nd[1]
Chlorothiazide	2[2]	4[2]	16 to 12	500	10 to 21[3]	0.75 to 2
Chlorthalidone	2 to 3	2 to 6	24 to 72	50	64[3]	40
Hydrochlorothiazide	2	4 to 6	16 to 12	50	65 to 75	5.6 to 14.8
Hydroflumethiazide	2	4	16 to 12	50	50	≈ 17
Indapamide	1 to 2	within 2	up to 36	2.5	93	≈ 14
Methyclothiazide	2	6	24	5	nd[1]	nd[1]
Metolazone[4]	1	2	12 to 24	5	65	nd[1]
Polythiazide	2	6	24 to 48	2	nd[1]	25.7
Quinethazone	2	6	18 to 24	50	nd[1]	nd[1]
Trichlormethiazide	2	6	24	2	nd[1]	2.3 to 7.3

[1] nd = No data.
[2] Following IV use, onset of action is 15 minutes; peak occurs in 30 minutes.
[3] Bioavailability may be dose-dependent.
[4] *Mykrox:* Peak plasma concentrations reached in 2 to 4 hrs, t½ ≈ 14 hrs.

Indications:

Edema: Adjunctive therapy in edema associated with congestive heart failure (CHF), hepatic cirrhosis and corticosteroid and estrogen therapy. Useful in edema due to renal dysfunction (ie, nephrotic syndrome, acute glomerulonephritis, chronic renal failure).

Indapamide alone is indicated for edema associated with CHF.

Metolazone, rapidly acting (Mykrox) has not been evaluated for the treatment of CHF or fluid retention due to renal or hepatic disease, and the correct dosage for these conditions and other edematous states has not been established. Since a safe and effective diuretic dose has not been established, do not use *Mykrox* when diuresis is desired.

Hypertension: As the sole therapeutic agent or to enhance other antihypertensive drugs in more severe forms of hypertension.

THIAZIDES AND RELATED DIURETICS

Unlabeled uses:

Calcium nephrolithiasis – Thiazide diuretics have been used alone and in combination with amiloride or allopurinol to prevent formation and recurrence of calcium nephrolithiasis in hypercalciuric and normal calciuric patients. Thiazides correct hypercalciuria, reduce urinary saturation, enhance inhibitor activity against spontaneous nucleation of both calcium oxalate and brushite, and restore normal parathyroid function and intestinal calcium absorption. Doses of hydrochlorothiazide 50 or 100 mg daily, trichloromethiazide 4 mg/day, chlorthalidone 50 mg/day and indapamide 2.5 mg/day have been used.

Osteoporosis – Thiazide diuretics may be useful in reducing the incidence of osteoporosis in postmenopausal women, either alone or in combination with calcium or estrogen. Further studies are necessary to confirm this use. Although data conflict, use of thiazides in older patients may be associated with a reduced risk of hip fracture.

Diabetes insipidus – Thiazide diuretics reduce urine volume by 30% to 50%. They constitute the mainstay of therapy for nephrogenic diabetes insipidus.

Contraindications:

Anuria; renal decompensation; hypersensitivity to thiazides or related diuretics or sulfonamide-derived drugs; hepatic coma or precoma (**metolazone**).

Warnings:

Parenteral use: Use IV **chlorothiazide** only when patients are unable to take oral medication or in an emergency. In infants and children, IV use is not recommended.

Avoid simultaneous administration of chlorothiazide with whole blood or its derivatives.

Lupus erythematosus exacerbation or activation has occurred.

Hypersensitivity: Hypersensitivity reactions may occur in patients with or without a history of allergy or bronchial asthma; cross-sensitivity with sulfonamides may also occur. Have epinephrine 1:1000 immediately available. Refer to Management of Acute Hypersensitivity Reactions.

Renal function impairment: Use with caution in severe renal disease since these agents may precipitate azotemia. Cumulative effects of the drug may develop in patients with impaired renal function. Monitor renal function periodically. If progressive renal impairment becomes evident, indicated by a rising nonprotein nitrogen (NPN) or BUN, consider withholding or discontinuing therapy. If the patient has a creatinine clearance < 40 to 50 ml/min, a glomerular filtration rate (GFR) < 25 ml/min or is not responsive to thiazides, a loop diuretic may be more effective. **Metolazone** is the only thiazide-like diuretic that may produce diuresis in patients with GFR < 20 ml/min. Indapamide may also be useful in patients with impaired renal function.

Hepatic function impairment: Use with caution since minor alterations of fluid and electrolyte balance may precipitate hepatic coma.

Pregnancy: Category B (chlorothiazide, chlorthalidone, hydrochlorothiazide, indapamide, metolazone); Category C (bendroflumethiazide, benzthiazide, hydroflumethiazide, methyclothiazide, trichlormethiazide). Routine use during normal pregnancy is inappropriate. Diuretics decrease plasma volume and can decrease placental perfusion. Diuretics do not prevent development of toxemia, nor are they useful in the treatment of toxemia.

Thiazides are indicated in pregnancy when edema is due to pathologic causes, just as they are in the absence of pregnancy. Dependent edema in pregnancy, resulting from restriction of venous return by the gravid uterus, is not properly treated by the use of diuretics. In rare instances, hypervolemia during normal pregnancy results in edema that may cause extreme discomfort that is not relieved by rest; a short course of diuretics may provide relief.

Thiazides cross the placental barrier and appear in cord blood. Use only when clearly needed and when potential benefits outweigh the potential hazards to the fetus. These hazards include fetal or neonatal jaundice, thrombocytopenia, hemolytic anemia, electrolyte imbalances and hypoglycemia.

Lactation: Thiazides may appear in breast milk. **Chlorthalidone** has a low milk to plasma ratio of 0.05. Discontinue nursing or the drug taking into account the importance of the drug to the mother.

Children: **Bendroflumethiazide, benzthiazide, chlorthalidone, hydrochlorothiazide, methyclothiazide, metolazone, hydroflumethiazide, trichlormethiazide** , – Safety and efficacy have not been established. **Metolazone** is not recommended for use in children. In infants and children, IV use of **chlorothiazide** has been limited and is generally not recommended.

THIAZIDES AND RELATED DIURETICS

Precautions:

Fluid/electrolyte balance: Perform initial and periodic determinations of serum electrolytes, BUN, uric acid and glucose. Observe patients for clinical signs of fluid or electrolyte imbalance (eg, hyponatremia, hypochloremic alkalosis, hypokalemia, hypomagnesemia, changes in serum and urinary calcium). Serum and urine electrolyte determinations are particularly important in patients vomiting excessively or receiving parenteral fluids, in patients subject to electrolyte imbalance (including those with heart failure, kidney disease and cirrhosis), and in patients on a salt restricted diet. Warning signs of imbalance include: Dry mouth, thirst, weakness, lethargy, drowsiness, restlessness, muscle pains or cramps, confusion, seizures, muscular fatigue, hypotension, oliguria, tachycardia and GI disturbances.

Hypokalemia may develop (with consequent weakness, cramps, cardiac dysrhythmias) during concomitant corticosteroids, ACTH and especially with brisk diuresis, with severe liver disease or cirrhosis, vomiting or diarrhea, or after prolonged therapy. Inadequate oral electrolyte intake also contributes to hypokalemia. Hypokalemia may cause cardiac arrhythmias and sensitize or exaggerate the heart's response to toxic effects of digitalis (eg, increased ventricular irritability). Avoid or treat hypokalemia by using potassium-sparing diuretic, potassium supplements or foods with high potassium content. Hypokalemia is a particular hazard in digitalized patients or patients who have or have had a ventricular arrhythmia; dangerous or fatal arrhythmias may be precipitated. Hypokalemia is dose-related.

Hyponatremia/Hypochloremia – A chloride deficit is generally mild and usually does not require specific treatment, except in extraordinary circumstances (as in liver or renal disease). However, treatment of metabolic or hypochloremic alkalosis may require chloride replacement. Dilutional hyponatremia may occur in edematous patients in hot weather; appropriate therapy is water restriction, rather than salt administration, except in rare life-threatening instances. Thiazide-induced hyponatremia has been associated with death and neurologic damage in elderly patients. CNS manifestations include seizures, coma and extensor-plantar response. Infrequently, severe hyponatremia accompanied by hypokalemia has occurred with recommended **indapamide** doses, primarily in elderly females.

Rarely, the rapid onset of severe hyponatremia or hypokalemia has occurred following initial doses of thiazide and non-thiazide diuretics. When symptoms consistent with electrolyte imbalance appear rapidly, discontinue the drug and initiate supportive measures immediately. Parenteral electrolytes may be required.

Hypomagnesemia – Thiazide diuretics have been shown to increase urinary excretion of magnesium, resulting in hypomagnesemia.

Hypercalcemia – Calcium excretion may be decreased by thiazide diuretics. Thiazides may cause a slight intermittent elevation of serum calcium in the absence of calcium metabolism disorders. Serum calcium levels return to normal upon discontinuation. Pathologic changes in the parathyroid glands with hypercalcemia and hypophosphatemia may occur in a few patients on prolonged thiazide therapy. Marked hypercalcemia may be evidence of hidden hyperparathyroidism. Common complications of hyperparathyroidism such as renal lithiasis, bone resorption and peptic ulceration are not seen. Discontinue thiazides before performing parathyroid function tests.

Hyperuricemia may occur or acute gout may be precipitated in certain patients receiving thiazides, even in those patients without a history of gouty attacks. Hyperuricemia with infrequent gouty attacks may occur in patients with a history of gout. Monitor serum uric acid concentrations periodically during treatment. One report suggests that it is not necessary to lower uric acid levels with pharmacologic measures in patients receiving thiazide diuretics who are without renal damage or history of gout. Serum uric acid increased by an average of 1 mg/dl in patients on **indapamide**.

Glucose tolerance – Hyperglycemia may occur with thiazide diuretics. Insulin or oral hypoglycemic agent dosage requirements in diabetic patients may be altered. Latent diabetes mellitus may become manifest during thiazide diuretic administration; diabetic complications may occur. Monitor serum glucose concentrations (see Drug Interactions). Administration time (ie, morning vs evening) may influence glucose tolerance; in a small study, blood glucose levels were higher when trichlormethiazide was taken in the evening.

Post-sympathectomy: Antihypertensive effects may be enhanced in the postsympathectomy patient.

Lipids: Use thiazides with caution in patients with moderate or high cholesterol concentrations and in patients with elevated triglyceride levels. Thiazides may cause increased concentrations of total serum cholesterol, total triglycerides and LDL (but not HDL) in some patients, although these appear to return to pretreatment levels with long-term therapy. **Indapamide** does not appear to increase serum cholesterol.

THIAZIDES AND RELATED DIURETICS

Photosensitivity: Photosensitization may occur; therefore, caution patients to take protective measures (ie, sunscreens, protective clothing) against exposure to ultraviolet light and/or sunlight until tolerance is determined.

Tartrazine sensitivity: Some of these products contain tartrazine, which may cause allergic–type reactions (including bronchial asthma) in certain susceptible individuals. Although the overall incidence of tartrazine sensitivity in the general population is low, it is frequently seen in patients who also have aspirin hypersensitivity. Specific products containing tartrazine are identified in the product listings.

Drug Interactions:

Thiazides and Related Diuretic Drug Interactions

Precipitant drug	Object drug*		Description
Thiazides	Allopurinol	↑	Concurrent use may increase the incidence of hypersensitivity reactions to allopurinol.
Thiazides	Anesthetics	↑	Effects of these drugs may be potentiated by thiazide administration; dosage adjustments may be required. Monitor and correct fluid and electrolyte imbalance prior to surgery if feasible.
Thiazides	Anticoagulants	↓	Anticoagulant effects may be diminished.
Thiazides	Antigout agents	↓	Since thiazide diuretics may raise blood uric acid levels, dosage adjustment of antigout agents may be necessary.
Thiazides	Antineoplastics	↑	Thiazides may prolong antineoplastic-induced leukopenia.
Thiazides	Calcium salts	↑	Hypercalcemia resulting from renal tubular reabsorption or bone release of calcium may be amplified by exogenous calcium.
Thiazides	Diazoxide	↑	Hyperglycemia, often with symptoms and similar to frank diabetes, may occur.
Thiazides	Digitalis glycosides	↑	Diuretic-induced hypokalemia and hypomagnesemia may precipitate digitalis-induced arrhythmias.
Thiazides	Lithium	↑	Thiazides may induce lithium toxicity by decreasing its renal excretion. However, they have been used together for therapeutic reasons and can be coadministered safely with close lithium level monitoring.
Thiazides	Loop diuretics	↑	Both groups have synergistic effects that may result in profound diuresis and serious electrolyte abnormalities. Certain combinations have been used therapeutically in patients refractory to furosemide (see Administration and Dosage).
Thiazides	Methyldopa	↑	There have been rare occurrences of hemolytic anemia with concomitant use.
Thiazides	Nondepolarizing muscle relaxants	↑	Neuromuscular blocking effects may be increased; respiratory depression may be prolonged.
Thiazides	Sulfonylureas, insulin	↓	Thiazides increase fasting blood glucose and may decrease sulfonylurea hypoglycemia. Hyponatremia may also occur. The dosage may need to be adjusted.
Thiazides	Vitamin D	↑	The biological actions of vitamin D may be enhanced. Hypercalcemia could manifest.
Amphotericin B, corticosteroids	Thiazides	↑	Electrolyte depletion may be intensified, particularly hypokalemia. Monitor potassium levels.
Anticholinergics	Thiazides	↑	Anticholinergics may substantially increase thiazide diuretic absorption.
Bile acid sequestrants (cholestyramine, colestipol)	Thiazides	↓	Bile acid sequestrants bind thiazides and reduce their absorption from the GI tract by up to 85%. Thiazides should be given ≥ 2 hours before the resin.

THIAZIDES AND RELATED DIURETICS

Thiazides and Related Diuretic Drug Interactions			
Precipitant drug	Object drug*		Description
Methenamines	Thiazides	⬇	Possible decreased effectiveness of thiazides due to the alkalinization of urine.
NSAIDs	Thiazides	⬇	Some NSAIDs (particularly indomethacin) may reduce the diuretic, natriuretic and antihypertensive effects of thiazide diuretics. Observe closely to determine if the desired diuretic effects are obtained. Sulindac may enhance the diuretic effect.

* ⬆ = Object drug increased ⬇ = Object drug decreased

Drug/Lab test interactions: Thiazides may decrease serum PBI levels without signs of thyroid disturbance. Thiazides may also cause diagnostic interference of serum electrolyte levels, blood and urine glucose levels (usually only in patients with a predisposition to glucose intolerance), serum bilirubin levels (by displacement from albumin binding), and serum uric acid levels. In uremic patients, serum magnesium levels may be increased. **Bendroflumethiazide** and **trichlormethiazide** may interfere with the **phenolsulfonphthalein test** due to decreased excretion. In the **phentolamine** and **tyramine tests,** bendroflumethiazide may produce false-negative and trichlormethiazide may produce false-positive results.

Adverse Reactions:

Adverse Reactions of Thiazides and Related Diuretics												
Adverse reaction	Bendroflumethiazide	Benzthiazide	Chlorothiazide	Chlorthalidone	Hydrochlorothiazide	Hydroflumethiazide	Indapamide	Methyclothiazide	Metolazone	Polythiazide	Quinethazone	Trichlormethiazide
Cardiovascular												
Hypotension			✓			✓						
Orthostatic hypotension	✓	✓	✓		✓	✓	<5%	✓	<2%[1]	✓	✓	✓
Palpitations							<5%		<2%[2]			✓
CNS												
Dizziness/Lightheadedness	✓	✓	✓	✓	✓	✓	≥5%	✓	10%[2]	✓	✓	✓
Vertigo	✓		✓	✓	✓	✓	<5%	✓	✓[3]	✓	✓	✓
Headache	✓	✓	✓	✓	✓	✓	≥5%	✓	9%[2]	✓	✓	✓
Paresthesias	✓	✓	✓	✓	✓	✓		✓	✓[3]	✓	✓	✓
Xanthopsia	✓	✓	✓	✓	✓	✓		✓		✓	✓	✓
Weakness	✓	✓	✓	✓	✓	✓	≥5%	✓	<2%[2]	✓	✓	✓
Restlessness/Insomnia	✓	✓	✓	✓	✓	✓	<5%	✓	✓[3]	✓	✓	✓
Drowsiness							<5%		✓[3]			✓
Fatigue/Lethargy/Malaise/ Lassitude							≥5%		4%[2]			✓
Anxiety							≥5%		<2%[3]			
Depression							<5%		<2%[2]			✓
Nervousness							≥5%		<2%[3]			
Blurred vision (may be transient)	✓		✓		✓	✓	<5%		✓[3]			
GI												
Anorexia	✓	✓	✓	✓	✓	✓	<5%	✓	✓[3]	✓	✓	✓
Gastric irritation/epigastric distress	✓	✓	✓	✓	✓	✓	<5%	✓		✓	✓	✓
Nausea	✓	✓	✓	✓	✓	✓	<5%	✓	<2%[2]	✓	✓	✓
Vomiting	✓	✓	✓	✓	✓	✓	<5%	✓	<2%[2]	✓	✓	✓
Abdominal pain/cramping/ bloating	✓	✓	✓	✓	✓	✓	<5%	✓	<2%[2]	✓	✓	✓
Diarrhea	✓	✓	✓	✓	✓	✓	<5%	✓	<2%[2]	✓	✓	✓
Constipation	✓	✓	✓	✓	✓	✓	<5%	✓	<2%[2]	✓	✓	✓
Jaundice (intrahepatic/ cholestatic)	✓	✓	✓	✓	✓	✓		✓	✓[3]	✓	✓	✓
Pancreatitis	✓	✓	✓	✓	✓	✓		✓	✓[3]	✓	✓	✓
Sialadenitis	✓	✓	✓	✓	✓	✓		✓				
Hepatitis	✓								✓[3]			
Dry mouth							<5%		<2%[1]			✓

THIAZIDES AND RELATED DIURETICS

Adverse Reactions of Thiazides and Related Diuretics

Adverse reaction	Bendroflumethiazide	Benzthiazide	Chlorothiazide	Chlorthalidone	Hydrochlorothiazide	Hydroflumethiazide	Indapamide	Methyclothiazide	Metolazone	Polythiazide	Quinethazone	Trichlormethiazide
GU												
Nocturia							<5%		<2%[1]			
Impotence/Reduced libido	✓	✓	✓	✓	✓	✓	<5%	✓	<2%[2]	✓	✓	✓
Renal failure/dysfunction			✓		✓							
Interstitial nephritis			✓		✓							
Hematologic:												
Leukopenia	✓	✓	✓	✓	✓	✓		✓	✓[3]	✓	✓	✓
Thrombocytopenia	✓	✓	✓	✓	✓	✓		✓		✓	✓	✓
Agranulocytosis	✓	✓	✓	✓	✓	✓		✓	✓[3]	✓	✓	✓
Aplastic/Hypoplastic anemia	✓	✓	✓	✓	✓	✓		✓	✓[3]	✓	✓	✓
Hemolytic anemia	✓		✓		✓	✓		✓				
Dermatologic												
Purpura	✓	✓	✓	✓	✓	✓		✓	✓[3]	✓	✓	✓
Photosensitivity/Photosensitivity dermatitis	✓	✓	✓	✓	✓	✓		✓	✓[3]	✓	✓	✓
Rash	✓	✓	✓	✓	✓	✓	<5%	✓	<2%[2]	✓	✓	✓
Urticaria	✓	✓	✓	✓	✓	✓		✓	✓[3]	✓	✓	✓
Necrotizing angiitis, vasculitis, cutaneous vasculitis	✓	✓	✓	✓	✓	✓	<5%	✓	✓[2]	✓	✓	✓
Fever	✓		✓		✓	✓		✓				
Anaphylactic reactions	✓		✓		✓[4]	✓		✓				
Pruritus	✓						<5%		<2%[1]			
Alopecia			✓[5]		✓							
Exfoliative dermatitis/toxic epidermal necrolysis	✓		✓[5]	✓	✓							
Erythema multiforme, Stevens-Johnson syndrome			✓[5]		✓			✓				
Metabolic												
Hyperglycemia	✓	✓	✓	✓	✓	✓	<5%	✓	✓[3]	✓	✓	✓
Glycosuria	✓	✓	✓	✓	✓	✓	<5%	✓	✓[3]	✓	✓	✓
Hyperuricemia	✓	✓	✓	✓	✓	✓	<5%	✓		✓[3]		✓
Electrolyte imbalance			✓		✓			✓				
Miscellaneous												
Respiratory distress (including pneumonitis/pulmonary edema)	✓		✓		✓	✓		✓				
Muscle cramp/spasm	✓	✓	✓	✓	✓	✓	≥5%	✓	6%[2]	✓		✓

[1] Rapidly acting doseform only.
[2] Slow acting doseform only.
[3] Percentage of occurrence refers to rapidly acting doseform, however this adverse reaction also occurred with the slow acting doseform.
[4] Possibly with life-threatening anaphylactic shock.
[5] IV doseform.

Whenever adverse reactions are moderate or severe, reducing the thiazide dosage or withdrawing therapy will generally reverse the effect.

Cardiovascular:

Hydrochlorothiazide – Allergic myocarditis.

Indapamide – Premature ventricular contractions, irregular heartbeat (< 5%).

Metolazone, rapidly acting – Chest pain (precordial pain; 3%); cold extremities, edema (< 2%); *slow acting* – Venous thrombosis; chest pain; excessive volume depletion; hemoconcentration.

CNS:

Indapamide – Loss of energy, numbness of extremities, tension, irritability, agitation (> 5%); tingling of extremities (< 5%).

Metolazone, slow acting – Syncope, neuropathy; *rapidly acting* – "weird" feeling, neuropathy (< 2%).

GI: Cholecystitis (possible increased risk in patients with gallstones).

Metolazone, rapidly acting – Bitter taste (< 2%).

THIAZIDES AND RELATED DIURETICS

GU:

Bendroflumethiazide – Allergic glomerulonephritis.
Chlorothiazide IV – Hematuria.
Indapamide – Frequent urination, polyuria (< 5%).

Dermatologic:

Bendroflumethiazide – Ecchymosis.
Indapamide – Hives (< 5%).
Metolazone, rapidly acting – Dry skin (< 2%).
Trichlormethiazide – Lichenoid dermatitis.

Musculoskeletal:

Metolazone – Joint pain; back pain (rapidly acting; < 2%); swelling (slow acting).

Respiratory:

Indapamide – Rhinorrhea (< 5%).
Metolazone, rapidly acting – Cough, epistaxis, sinus congestion, sore throat (< 2%).
Trichlormethiazide – Dyspnea.

Miscellaneous: Neutropenia.

Bendroflumethiazide – Metabolic acidosis in diabetics.
Indapamide – Flushing, weight loss (< 5%).
Methyclothiazide – Inappropriate ADH secretion.
Metolazone, slow acting – Chills; acute gouty attack; *rapidly acting* – Eye itching, tinnitus (< 2%).

Lab test abnormalities: Hypercalcemia; hypokalemia; hyponatremia; hypomagnesemia; hypochloremia; hypochloremic alkalosis; hypophosphatemia; increase in BUN; elevation of creatinine; decreased serum PBI levels.

Clinical hypokalemia occurred in 3% and 7% of patients given **indapamide** 2.5 mg and 5 mg, respectively.

Increases in plasma levels of total cholesterol, triglycerides and LDL cholesterol have been associated with thiazide diuretics (see Precautions).

Fluid/electrolyte imbalance – There are isolated reports of nonedematous individuals developing severe fluid and electrolyte derangements after only brief exposure to normal doses of thiazides. This condition is usually manifested as severe dilutional hyponatremia, hypokalemia and hypochloremia. It may be due to inappropriately increased ADH secretion and appears to be idiosyncratic. Potassium replacement is apparently the most important therapy along with removal of the offending drug.

Overdosage:

Symptoms: Changes due to plasma volume depletion (eg, orthostatic hypotension, dizziness, drowsiness, syncope, electrolyte abnormalities, hemoconcentration, hemodynamic changes); signs of potassium deficiency (eg, confusion, dizziness, muscular weakness, and GI disturbances); nausea; vomiting. In severe instances, hypotension and depressed respiration may occur. Lethargy of varying degrees may progress to coma within a few hours, with minimal depression of respiration and cardiovascular function and without significant serum electrolyte changes or dehydration. GI irritation and hypermotility, temporary BUN elevation, CNS effects, cardiac abnormalities and seizures have also been reported, especially in patients with compromised renal function.

Treatment: Perform gastric lavage or induce emesis; give activated charcoal. Prevent aspiration. Avoid cathartics since electrolyte and fluid loss may be enhanced. GI effects are usually of short duration, but may require symptomatic treatment. Monitor serum electrolyte levels and renal function. Maintain hydration, electrolyte balance, respiration and cardiovascular-renal function. Asymptomatic hyperuricemia usually responds to fluids, but if clinical gout is suspected, indomethacin may be started. Support respiration and cardiac circulation if hypotension and depressed respiration occur. Refer to General Management of Acute Overdosage. Dialysis is unlikely to be effective.

Patient Information:

May cause GI upset; may be taken with food or milk.

Drug will initially increase urination which should subside after a few weeks; take early during the day or as directed.

Notify physician if muscle pain, weakness or cramps, nausea, vomiting, restlessness, excessive thirst, tiredness, drowsiness, increased heart rate or pulse, diarrhea or dizziness occurs.

May cause photosensitivity (sensitivity to sunlight). Avoid prolonged exposure to the sun and other ultraviolet light. Use sunscreens and wear protective clothing until tolerance is determined.

May increase blood sugar levels in diabetics.

THIAZIDES AND RELATED DIURETICS

Do not drink alcohol or take other medications without physician's approval; this includes nonprescription medicines for appetite control, asthma, colds, cough, hay fever or sinus.

Do not interrupt, discontinue or adjust the dose even if feeling well. Follow physician's instructions regarding missed dose.

May cause gout attacks. Contact physician if significant sudden joint pain occurs.

Administration and Dosage:

Edema: Intermittent therapy may be advantageous. With administration every other day, or on a 3 to 5 day per week schedule, electrolyte imbalance is less likely.

Hypertension: Reduce dosage of other agents as soon as thiazides are added to the regimen to prevent excessive hypotension. As blood pressure falls, a further reduction in dosage may be necessary.

Renal impairment: If the patient has a creatinine clearance < 40 to 50 ml/min, a glomerular filtration rate < 25 ml/min or is not responsive to thiazides, a loop diuretic may be more effective. **Metolazone** is the only thiazide-like diuretic that may produce diuresis in patients with GFR < 20 ml/min. Indapamide may also be effective in patients with renal function impairment.

Concomitant administration: Concurrent metolazone and furosemide (and probably other loop diuretics) have been used in the management of patients refractory to furosemide or other diuretics administered alone due to their synergistic effect on diuresis (see Drug Interactions). Metolazone 2.5 to 10 mg is added to the therapy, and the dose is doubled every 24 hours until the desired response is achieved. Decrease the furosemide dose if synergism occurs with the first dose of metolazone. Hydrochlorothiazide (50 mg) may be used and may be safer because of its shorter action. This effect has also been noted with other thiazides in combination with other loop diuretics.

CHLOROTHIAZIDE

For complete prescribing information, refer to the Thiazides and Related Diuretics group monograph.

Administration and Dosage:

Adults:

Edema – 0.5 to 1 g once or twice a day, orally or IV. Reserve IV route for patients unable to take oral medication or for emergency situations.

Many patients with edema respond to intermittent therapy (administration on alternate days or on 3 to 5 days each week). With an intermittent schedule, excessive response and undesirable electrolyte imbalance are less likely to occur.

Hypertension (oral forms only) – Starting dose is 0.5 to 1 g/day as a single or divided dose. Adjust dosage according to the blood pressure response. Rarely, some patients may require up to 2 g/day in divided doses.

Infants and children:

Oral – 22 mg/kg/day (10 mg/lb/day) in 2 doses. Infants < 6 months may require up to 33 mg/kg/day (15 mg/lb/day) in 2 doses.

On this basis, infants up to 2 years of age may be given 125 to 375 mg daily in 2 doses. Children from 2 to 12 years of age may be given 375 mg to 1 g daily in 2 doses.

IV use is not generally recommended.

Preparation of parenteral solution: Add 18 ml of sterile water for injection to the vial to prepare an isotonic solution. Never add < 18 ml. Discard unused solution after 24 hours. The solution is compatible with dextrose or sodium chloride solutions for IV infusion. Avoid simultaneous administration with whole blood or its derivatives. Extravasation must be rigidly avoided. Do not give SC or IM.

Rx	**Chlorothiazide** (Various, eg, Major, Mylan, Parmed)	**Tablets**: 250 mg	In 100s and 250s.
Rx	**Diuril** (Merck)		Lactose. (MSD 214). White, round, scored. In 100s and 1000s.
Rx	**Chlorothiazide** (Various, eg, Goldline, Major, Mylan, Parmed, Schein)	**Tablets**: 500 mg	In 100s, 500s, 1000s and UD 100s.
Rx	**Diurigen** (Goldline)		In 100s and 1000s.
Rx	**Diuril** (Merck)		Lactose. (MSD 432). White, round, scored. In 100s, 1000s, 5000s and UD 100s.
Rx	**Diuril** (Merck)	**Oral Suspension**: 250 mg per 5 ml	0.5% alcohol, saccharin, 0.12% methylparaben, 0.02% propylparaben, 0.1% benzoic acid, sucrose. In 237 ml.
Rx	**Sodium Diuril** (Merck)	**Powder for Injection, lyophilized**: 500 mg (as sodium)	Mannitol 0.25 g, thimerosal 0.4 mg. In 20 vials.

HYDROCHLOROTHIAZIDE

For complete prescribing information, refer to the Thiazides and Related Diuretics group monograph.

Administration and Dosage:

Edema:

Initial – 25 to 200 mg daily for several days, or until dry weight is attained.

Maintenance – 25 to 100 mg daily or intermittently. Refractory patients may require up to 200 mg daily.

Hypertension:

Initial – 50 mg daily as a single or two divided doses. Doses > 50 mg are often associated with marked reductions in serum potassium. Patients usually do not require doses > 50 mg daily when combined with other antihypertensives.

Infants and children – Usual dosage is 2.2 mg/kg (1 mg/lb) daily in two doses. Pediatric patients with hypertension only rarely will benefit from doses > 50 mg daily.

Infants (< 6 months): Up to 3.3 mg/kg (1.5 mg/lb) daily in two doses.

Infants (6 months to 2 years of age): 12.5 to 37.5 mg daily in two doses. Base dosage on body weight.

Children (2 to 12 years of age): 37.5 to 100 mg daily in two doses. Base dosage on body weight.

Rx	**Hydrochlorothiazide** (Various, eg, Geneva, Major, Schein, Zenith)	**Tablets:** 25 mg	In 30s, 100s, 500s, 1000s, 5000s, UD 32s and UD 100s.
Rx	**Esidrix** (Ciba)		Lactose, sucrose. (Ciba 22). Pink, scored. In 100s.
Rx	**HydroDIURIL** (Merck)		Lactose. (MSD 42). Peach, scored. In 100s and 1000s.
Rx	**Hydro-Par** (Parmed)		Peach, scored. In 1000s.
Rx	**Oretic** (Abbott)		Lactose. White. In 100s, 1000s and UD 100s.
Rx	**Hydrochlorothiazide** (Various, eg, Danbury, Geneva, Major, Schein, Zenith)	**Tablets:** 50 mg	In 30s, 100s, 500s, 1000s, 5000s and UD 100s.
Rx	**Esidrix** (Ciba)		Lactose, sucrose. (Ciba 46). Yellow, scored. In 100s and consumer pack 360s and 720s.
Rx	**Ezide** (Econo Med)		In 100s and 1000s.
Rx	**HydroDIURIL** (Merck)		Lactose. (MSD 105). Peach, scored. In 100s, 1000s and 5000s.
Rx	**Hydro-Par** (Parmed)		In 1000s and 5000s.
Rx	**Oretic** (Abbott)		Lactose. White. In 100s, 1000s and UD 100s.
Rx	**Hydrochlorothiazide** (Various, eg, Major, Schein, Zenith)	**Tablets:** 100 mg	In 30s, 100s, 250s, 500s, 1000s and UD 100s.
Rx	**HydroDIURIL** (Merck)		Lactose. (MSD 410). Peach, scored. In 100s.
Rx	**Hydrochlorothiazide** (Roxane)	**Solution:** 50 mg per 5 ml	Saccharin. Mint flavor. In 500 ml.

BENDROFLUMETHIAZIDE

For complete prescribing information, see Thiazides and Related Diuretics group monograph.

Administration and Dosage:

Edema: 5 mg once daily, preferably in the morning. *Initial* - Up to 20 mg once daily or divided into 2 doses. *Maintenance* - 2.5 to 5 mg daily. Intermittent therapy may be advantageous in many patients. By giving the preparation every other day or on a 3 to 5 day per week schedule, electrolyte imbalance is still possible but less likely.

Hypertension: Initial - 5 to 20 mg daily. *Maintenance* - 2.5 to 15 mg/day.

Rx	**Naturetin** (Princeton)	**Tablets:** 5 mg	(606). Green, scored. In 100s.
		10 mg	(618). Orange, scored. In 100s.

METHYCLOTHIAZIDE

For complete prescribing information, see Thiazides and Related Diuretics group monograph.

Administration and Dosage:

Edema (adults): 2.5 to 10 mg once daily. Maximum effective single dose is 10 mg.

Hypertension (adults): 2.5 to 5 mg once daily. If blood pressure control is not satisfactory after 8 to 12 weeks with 5 mg once daily, add another antihypertensive.

Rx	**Methyclothiazide** (Various, eg, Geneva, Schein, Zenith)	**Tablets**: 2.5 mg	In 100s and 1000s.
Rx	**Methyclothiazide** (Various, eg, Geneva, Major, Parmed, Zenith)	**Tablets**: 5 mg	In 100s and 1000s.
Rx	**Aquatensen** (Wallace)		(Wallace 153). Peach, scored. Convex. Rectangular. In 100s, 500s.
Rx	**Enduron** (Abbott)		Salmon. Square. In 100s, 1000s, 5000s and *Abbo-Pac* 100s.

BENZTHIAZIDE

For complete prescribing information, see Thiazides and Related Diuretics group monograph.

Administration and Dosage:

Edema: Initial - 50 to 200 mg daily for several days, or until dry weight is attained. If dosages exceed 100 mg/day, give in 2 doses, following morning and evening meal. *Maintenance* - 50 to 150 mg daily.

Hypertension: Initial - 50 to 100 mg daily. Give in 2 doses of 25 or 50 mg each, after breakfast and after lunch. Continue until a therapeutic drop in blood pressure occurs. *Maintenance* - Individualize dosage; maximal effective dose is 200 mg daily.

Rx	**Exna** (Robins)	**Tablets**: 50 mg	Tartrazine, lactose. (AHR 5449). Yellow, scored. In 100s.

INDAPAMIDE

For complete prescribing information, see Thiazides and Related Diuretics group monograph.

Administration and Dosage:

Edema of congestive heart failure: Adults-2.5 mg as a single daily dose in the morning. If response is not satisfactory after 1 week, increase to 5 mg once daily.

Hypertension:

Adults – 1.25 mg as a single daily dose taken in the morning. If the response to 1.25 mg is not satisfactory after 4 weeks, increase the daily dose to 2.5 mg taken once daily. If the response to 2.5 mg is not satisfactory after 4 weeks, the daily dose may be increased to 5 mg taken once daily, but consider adding another antihypertensive. If the antihypertensive response is insufficient, combine with other antihypertensives. Reduce the usual dose of other agents by 50% during initial combination therapy. Further dosage adjustments may be necessary.

In general, doses ≥5 mg have not provided additional effects on blood pressure or heart failure, but are associated with a greater degree of hypokalemia. There is little experience with doses > 5 mg once daily.

Rx	**Indapamide** (Arcola)	**Tablets**: 2.5 mg	Lactose. (A 3). White. Film coated. In 100s and 1000s.
Rx	**Lozol** (Rhone-Poulenc Rorer)		(R 8). White. Octagonal. Film coated. In 100s, 1000s and UD 100s.
Rx	**Lozol** (Rhone-Poulenc Rorer)	1.25 mg	(R 7). Orange. Octagonal. Film coated. In 100s.

HYDROFLUMETHIAZIDE

For complete prescribing information, refer to the Thiazides and Related Diuretics group monograph.

Administration and Dosage:

Edema:

Initial – 50 mg once or twice a day.

Maintenance – 25 mg to 200 mg daily. Administer in divided doses when dosage exceeds 100 mg daily.

Hypertension:

Initial – 50 mg twice daily.

Maintenance – 50 to 100 mg/day. Do not exceed 200 mg/day.

Rx	**Hydroflumethiazide** (Various, eg, Geneva)	**Tablets:** 50 mg	In 100s.
Rx	**Diucardin** (Wyeth-Ayerst)		(Diucardin 50). White, scored. Oval. In 100s.
Rx	**Saluron** (Apothecon)		In 100s.

TRICHLORMETHIAZIDE

For complete prescribing information, refer to the Thiazides and Related Diuretics group monograph.

Administration and Dosage:

Edema: 2 to 4 mg once daily.

Hypertension: 2 to 4 mg once daily.

In initiating therapy, doses may be given twice daily.

Rx	**Metahydrin** (Hoechst Marion Roussel)	**Tablets:** 2 mg	Tartrazine. (Merrell 62). Pink. In 100s.
Rx	**Naqua** (Schering)		(S AHG or 822). Pink. In 100s.
Rx	**Trichlormethiazide** (Various, eg, Major, Schein)	**Tablets:** 4 mg	In 100s and 1000s.
Rx	**Diurese** (American Urologicals)		In 100s and 1000s.
Rx	**Metahydrin** (Hoechst Marion Roussel)		Tartrazine. (Merrell 63). Aqua. In 100s.
Rx	**Naqua** (Schering)		(S AHH or 547). Aqua. In 100s and 1000s.

POLYTHIAZIDE

For complete prescribing information, refer to the Thiazides and Related Diuretics group monograph.

Administration and Dosage:

Edema: 1 to 4 mg daily.

Hypertension: 2 to 4 mg daily.

Rx	**Renese** (Pfizer)	**Tablets:** 1 mg	White, scored. In 100s.
		2 mg	Yellow, scored. In 100s.
		4 mg	White, scored. In 100s.

QUINETHAZONE

For complete prescribing information, refer to the Thiazides and Related Diuretics group monograph.

Administration and Dosage:

Adults: 50 to 100 mg once daily. Occasionally, 50 mg twice daily; 150 to 200 mg daily may be necessary infrequently.

Rx	**Hydromox** (Lederle)	**Tablets:** 50 mg	(LL H1). White, scored. Flat-faced, beveled. In 100s.

METOLAZONE

For complete prescribing information, refer to the Thiazides and Related Diuretics group monograph.

Administration and Dosage:

Individualize dosage.

Zaroxolyn: Mild to moderate essential hypertension - 2.5 to 5 mg once daily.

Edema of renal disease – 5 to 20 mg once daily.

Edema of cardiac failure – 5 to 20 mg once daily.

Mykrox: Mild to moderate hypertension – 0.5 mg as a single daily dose taken in the morning. If response is inadequate, increase the dose to 1 mg daily.

Do not increase dosage if blood pressure is not controlled with 1 mg. Rather, add another antihypertensive agent with a different mechanism of action.

Brand interchange: The metolazone formulations are not bioequivalent or therapeutically equivalent at the same doses. *Mykrox* is more rapidly and completely bioavailable. Do not interchange brands.

If switching patients currently on *Zaroxolyn* to *Mykrox*, determine the dose by titration starting at 0.5 mg once daily and increasing to 1 mg once daily if needed.

Rx	**Zaroxolyn** (Fisons)	**Tablets:** 2.5 mg	(2 Zaroxolyn). Pink. In 100s, 1000s and UD 100s.
		5 mg	(5 Zaroxolyn). Blue. In 100s, 1000s and UD 100s.
		10 mg	(10 Zaroxolyn). Yellow. In 100s, 1000s and UD 100s.
Rx	**Mykrox** (Fisons)	**Tablets:** 0.5 mg	(MYKROX). White. In 100s.

CHLORTHALIDONE

For complete prescribing information, refer to the Thiazides and Related Diuretics group monograph.

Administration and Dosage:

Individualize dosage. Initiate therapy at lowest possible dose. Give a single dose with food in the morning. Maintenance doses may be lower than initial doses.

Edema: Initiate therapy with 50 to 100 mg (*Thalitone*, 30 to 60 mg) daily, or 100 mg (*Thalitone*, 60 mg) on alternate days. Some patients may require 150 or 200 mg (*Thalitone*, 90 to 120 mg) at these intervals, or 120 mg *Thalitone* daily. Dosages above this level, however, do not usually create a greater response.

Hypertension: Initiate therapy with a single daily dose of 25 mg (*Thalitone*, 15 mg). If response is insufficient after a suitable trial, increase to 50 mg (*Thalitone*, increase from 30 to 50 mg). For additional control, increase dosage to 100 mg once daily (except *Thalitone*) or add a second antihypertensive. Increases in serum uric acid and decreases in serum potassium are dose-related over the 25 to 100 mg/day (*Thalitone*, 15 to 50 mg/day) range.

Note – Doses > 25 mg/day are likely to potentiate potassium excretion, but provide no further benefit in sodium excretion or blood pressure reduction.

Rx	**Thalitone** (Horus Therapeutics)	**Tablets:** 15 mg	Lactose. (HTI/77). White. Kidney shaped. In 100s.
Rx	**Chlorthalidone** (Various, eg, Geneva, Goldline, Major)	**Tablets:** 25 mg	In 100s, 1000s.
Rx	**Hygroton**(RPR)		Lactose. (RPR 22) Peach. Square. In 100s.
Rx	**Thalitone** (Horus Therapeutics)		Lactose. (HTI/76). White, scored. Kidney shape. In 100s.
Rx	**Chlorthalidone** (Various, eg, Geneva, Goldline, Major, Schein)	**Tablets:** 50 mg	In 100s, 250s, and 1000s.
Rx	**Hygroton** (RPR)		Lactose. (RPR 20) Aqua. Square. In 100s.
Rx	**Chlorthalidone** (Various, eg, Major, Goldline, Schein)	**Tablets:** 100 mg	In 100s, 500s and 1000s.
Rx	**Hygroton** (RPR)		(RPR 21) White, scored. In 100s.

LOOP DIURETICS

Warning:
These agents are potent diuretics; excess amounts can lead to a profound diuresis with water and electrolyte depletion. Careful medical supervision is required and dosage must be individualized.

Actions:

Pharmacology: Furosemide and ethacrynic acid inhibit primarily reabsorption of sodium and chloride, not only in proximal and distal tubules, but also the loop of Henle. High efficacy is largely due to unique site of action. Action on distal tubule is independent of any inhibitory effect on carbonic anhydrase or aldosterone.

In contrast, bumetanide is more chloruretic than natriuretic and may have an additional action in the proximal tubule; it does not appear to act on the distal tubule.

Torsemide acts from within the lumen of the thick ascending portion of the loop of Henle, where it inhibits the $Na^+/K^+/2Cl^-$-carrier system; effects in other segments of the nephron have not been demonstrated. Diuretic activity thus correlates better with the rate of drug excretion in urine than with the blood concentration. Torsemide increases the urinary excretion of sodium, chloride, and water, but does not significantly alter glomerular filtration rate, renal plasma flow or acid-base balance.

Because ethacrynic acid inhibits the reabsorption of filtered sodium to a much greater proportion than most other diuretics, it may be effective in many patients with significant degrees of renal insufficiency.

Pharmacokinetics: These agents are metabolized and excreted primarily through the urine. Protein binding of these agents exceeds 90%. Furosemide is metabolized approximately 30% to 40%, and its urinary excretion is 60% to 70%. Significantly more furosemide is excreted in urine after IV injection than after the tablet or oral solution. Recent evidence suggests that furosemide glucuronide is the only, or at least the major, biotransformation product of furosemide.

Oral administration of bumetanide revealed that 81% was excreted in urine, 45% of it as unchanged drug. Bumetanide increases potassium excretion in a dose-related fashion; it also decreases uric acid excretion and increases serum uric acid. Urinary and biliary metabolites are formed by oxidation of the N–butyl side chain. Biliary excretion of bumetanide amounted to only 2% of the administered dose.

Torsemide is cleared from the circulation by both hepatic metabolism (≈ 80% of total clearance) and excretion into the urine (≈ 20% of total clearance). The major metabolite in humans is the carboxylic acid derivative, which is biologically inactive. Two of the lesser metabolites possess some diuretic activity, but for practical purposes metabolism terminates the action of the drug. Most renal clearance occurs via active secretion of the drug by the proximal tubules into tubular urine. Simultaneous food intake delays the time to C_{max} by about 30 minutes, but overall bioavailability and diuretic activity are unchanged.

Pharmacokinetic Parameters of the Loop Diuretics

Diuretic	Bioavailability (%)	Half-life (min)	Onset of action (min)	Peak (min)	Duration (hr)	Dosage (mg)	Relative potency	Doses/day
Furosemide								
Oral	60-64[1]	≈ 120[2]	within 60	60-120[4]	6-8	20-80	1	1-2
IV or IM			within 5[3]	30	2	20-40	1	
Ethacrynic acid								
Oral	≈100	60	within 30	120	6-8	50-100	0.6-0.8	1-2
IV			within 5	15-30	2	50	0.6-0.8	1-2
Bumetanide								
Oral	72-96	60-90[5]	30-60	60-120	4-6	0.5-2	≈ 40	1
IV			within minutes	15-30	0.5-1	0.5-1	≈ 40	1-3
Torsemide								
Oral	≈ 80	210	within 60	60-120	6-8	5-20	2-4	1
IV			within 10	within 60	6-8	5-20	2-4	1

[1] Decreased in uremia and nephrosis.
[2] Prolonged in renal failure, uremia and in neonates.
[3] Somewhat delayed after IM administration.
[4] Decreased in CHF.
[5] Prolonged in renal disease.

LOOP DIURETICS

Indications:

Edema associated with CHF, hepatic cirrhosis and renal disease, including the nephrotic syndrome. Particularly useful when greater diuretic potential is desired.

Parenteral administration is indicated when a rapid onset of diuresis is desired (eg, acute pulmonary edema), when GI absorption is impaired or when oral use is not practical for any reason. As soon as it is practical, replace with oral therapy.

Hypertension (furosemide, oral; torsemide, oral): Alone or in combination with other antihypertensive drugs. Hypertensive patients who are inadequately controlled with thiazides may not be adequately controlled with furosemide alone.

Ethacrynic acid: Ascites: Short-term management of ascites due to malignancy, idiopathic edema and lymphedema.

Congenital heart disease, nephrotic syndrome – Short-term management of hospitalized pediatric patients, other than infants.

Pulmonary edema, acute – Adjunctive therapy.

Unlabeled uses: Ethacrynic acid is being investigated for the treatment of glaucoma; a single injection into the eye may reduce intraocular pressure for a week or more. Further study is needed.

Bumetanide 1 mg may be beneficial in the treatment of adult nocturia; it is not effective in males with prostatic hypertrophy.

Contraindications:

Anuria; hypersensitivity to these compounds or to sulfonylureas; infants (ethacrynic acid); patients with hepatic coma or in states of severe electrolyte depletion until the condition is improved or corrected (bumetanide).

Warnings:

Dehydration: Excessive diuresis may result in dehydration and reduction in blood volume with circulatory collapse and the possibility of vascular thrombosis and embolism, particularly in elderly patients.

Hepatic cirrhosis and ascites: In these patients, sudden alterations of electrolyte balance may precipitate hepatic encephalopathy and coma. Do not institute therapy until the basic condition is improved. Initiate therapy in the hospital with small doses and careful monitoring. Supplemental potassium chloride and, if required, an aldosterone antagonist help to prevent hypokalemia and metabolic alkalosis.

Ototoxicity: Tinnitus, reversible and irreversible hearing impairment, deafness and vertigo with a sense of fullness in the ears have been reported. Deafness is usually reversible and of short duration (1 to 24 hours); however, irreversible hearing impairment has occurred. Usually, ototoxicity is associated with rapid injection, with severe renal impairment, with doses several times the usual dose and with concurrent use with other ototoxic drugs.

Systemic lupus erythematosus may be exacerbated or activated.

Diarrhea: In a few patients, ethacrynic acid has produced severe, watery diarrhea. If this occurs, discontinue the drug and do not readminister.

Because of the amount of sorbitol in the **furosemide** solution vehicle, the possibility of diarrhea, especially in children, exists when higher dosages are given.

Thrombocytopenia – Since there have been rare spontaneous reports of thrombocytopenia with **bumetanide,** observe regularly for possible occurrence.

Hypersensitivity: Patients with known sulfonamide sensitivity may show allergic reactions to **furosemide, torsemide** or **bumetanide**. Bumetanide use following instances of allergic reactions to furosemide suggests a lack of cross-sensitivity. Refer to Management of Acute Hypersensitivity Reactions.

Renal function impairment: If increasing azotemia, oliguria or reversible increases in BUN or creatinine occur during treatment of severe progressive renal disease, discontinue therapy.

If high-dose parenteral **furosemide** therapy is used, controlled IV infusion is advisable. For adults, an infusion rate ≤ 4 mg/min has been used.

Pregnancy: Category B (ethacrynic acid, torsemide); *Category C* (furosemide, bumetanide). There are no adequate and well controlled studies in pregnant women. Use only when clearly needed and when the potential benefits outweigh the potential hazards to the fetus.

Furosemide caused unexplained maternal deaths and abortions in rabbits when 25 to 100 mg/kg (2 to 8 times the maximum recommended human dose) was administered. No pregnant rabbits survived a dose of 100 mg/kg. Data indicate that fetal lethality can preceed maternal deaths. Studies in mice and rabbits showed an increased incidence of fetal hydronephrosis. Since furosemide may increase the incidence of patent ductus arteriosus in preterm infants with respiratory-distress syndrome (see Children), use caution when administering before delivery.

LOOP DIURETICS

Bumetanide appears to be nonteratogenic, but has a slight embryocidal effect in rats when given in doses of 3400 times the maximum human therapeutic dose and in rabbits at doses of 3.4 times the maximum human therapeutic dose. In rabbits, a decrease in litter size and an increase in resorption rate were noted at oral doses 3.4 to 10 times the maximum human therapeutic dose.

Torsemide – Fetal and maternal toxicity (decrease in average body weight, increase in fetal resorption and delayed fetal ossification) occurred in rabbits and rats.

Lactation: **Furosemide** appears in breast milk; such transfer of **ethacrynic acid, torsemide** and **bumetanide** is unknown. Because of the potential for adverse reactions in nursing infants, decide whether to discontinue nursing or to discontinue the drug, taking into account the importance of the drug to the mother.

Children: Safety and efficacy for use of **torsemide** in children, **bumetanide** in children < 18 years old, and **ethacrynic acid** in infants (oral) and children (IV) have not been established.

Furosemide stimulates renal synthesis of prostaglandin E_2 and may increase the incidence of patent ductus arteriosus when given in the first few weeks of life, to premature infants with respiratory-distress syndrome. Renal calcifications (from barely visible on x–ray to staghorn) have occurred in some severely premature infants treated with IV furosemide for edema due to patent ductus arteriosus and hyaline membrane disease. Concurrent use of chlorothiazide has reportedly decreased hypercalciuria and dissolved some calculi.

Precautions:

Monitoring: Observe for blood dyscrasias, liver or kidney damage or idiosyncratic reactions. Perform frequent serum electrolyte, calcium, glucose, uric acid, CO_2, creatinine and BUN determinations during the first few months of therapy and periodically thereafter (see Electrolyte imbalance and Laboratory test abnormalities).

Cardiovascular effects: Too vigorous a diuresis, as evidenced by rapid and excessive weight loss, may induce an acute hypotensive episode. In elderly cardiac patients, avoid rapid contraction of plasma volume and the resultant hemoconcentration to prevent thromboembolic episodes, such as cerebral vascular thromboses and pulmonary emboli.

Electrolyte imbalance may occur, especially in patients receiving high doses with restricted salt intake. Perform periodic determinations of serum electrolytes. Observe patients for signs of fluid or electrolyte imbalance (eg, hyponatremia, hypochloremic alkalosis, hypokalemia, hypomagnesemia, hypocalcemia). Digitalis therapy may exaggerate metabolic effects of hypokalemia with reference to myocardial activity. Serum and urine electrolyte determinations are important in patients who are vomiting excessively, in patients who are receiving parenteral fluids, corticosteroids or ACTH, during brisk diuresis or when cirrhosis is present. Warning signs are dryness of mouth, thirst, anorexia, weakness, lethargy, drowsiness, restlessness, muscle pains or cramps, muscle fatigue, tetany (rarely), hypotension, oliguria, tachycardia, arrhythmia and GI disturbances (eg, nausea/vomiting).

Profound electrolyte and water loss may be avoided by weighing the patient periodically, adjusting dosage, initiating treatment with small doses and using the drugs intermittently. When excessive diuresis occurs, withdraw the drugs until homeostasis is restored. If excessive electrolyte loss occurs, reduce dosage or withdraw the drug temporarily.

Hypokalemia prevention requires particular attention to the following: Patients receiving digitalis and diuretics for CHF, hepatic cirrhosis and ascites; in aldosterone excess with normal renal function; potassium-losing nephropathy; certain diarrheal states; or where hypokalemia is an added risk to the patient (eg, history of ventricular arrhythmias).

Possible drug-related deaths occurred with **ethacrynic acid** in critically ill patients refractory to other diuretics. There are two categories: Patients with severe myocardial disease who received digitalis and developed acute hypokalemia with fatal arrhythmia; or patients with severely decompensated hepatic cirrhosis with ascites, with or without encephalopathy, who had electrolyte imbalances and died because of intensification of the electrolyte defect. Liberalization of salt intake and supplementary potassium are often necessary.

Hypomagnesemia – Loop diuretics increase the urinary excretion of magnesium.

Hypocalcemia – Serum calcium levels may be lowered (rare cases of tetany have occurred).

Gastric hemorrhage: **Ethacrynic acid** may increase the risk of gastric hemorrhage associated with corticosteroid treatment.

Hyperuricemia: Asymptomatic hyperuricemia can occur, and rarely, gout may be precipitated. Reversible elevations of BUN may be seen, usually in association with dehydration, particularly in patients with renal insufficiency. Serum creatinine may also be increased.

Glucose: Increases in blood glucose and alterations in glucose tolerance tests (fasting and 2 hour postprandial sugar) have been observed. Rare cases of precipitation of diabetes mellitus have occurred. Although these effects have not been reported with **bumetanide**, the possibility of an effect on glucose metabolism exists.

Lipids: Increases in LDL and total cholesterol and triglycerides with minor decreases in HDL cholesterol may occur.

Photosensitivity: Photosensitization (photoallergy or phototoxicity) may occur; therefore, caution patients to take protective measures (ie, sunscreens, protective clothing) against exposure to ultraviolet light or sunlight until tolerance is determined.

Drug Interactions:

Loop Diuretic Drug Interactions

Precipitant drug	Object drug*		Description
Loop diuretics	Aminoglycosides	↑	Auditory toxicity appears to be increased with concurrent use. Hearing loss of varying degrees may occur.
Loop diuretics	Anticoagulants	↑	Anticoagulant activity may be enhanced.
Loop diuretics (furosemide)	Beta blockers (propranolol)	↑	Plasma levels of propranolol may be increased.
Loop diuretics	Chloral hydrate	↑	Although rare, transient diaphoresis, hot flashes, hypertension, tachycardia, weakness and nausea may occur with concurrent use.
Loop diuretics	Digitalis glycosides	↑	Diuretic-induced electrolyte disturbances may predispose to digitalis-induced arrhythmias.
Loop diuretics	Lithium	↑	Possible increased plasma lithium levels and toxicity.
Loop diuretics	Nondepolarizing muscle relaxants	↔	The actions of the muscle relaxants may be antagonized or potentiated, perhaps dependent on the loop diuretic dosage.
Loop diuretics	Sulfonylureas	↓	Loop diuretics may decrease glucose tolerance, resulting in hyperglycemia in patients previously well controlled on sulfonylureas.
Loop diuretics	Theophyllines	↔	The actions of theophyllines may be altered, enhanced or inhibited.
Charcoal	Loop diuretics (furosemide)	↓	Charcoal can reduce the absorption of furosemide. Depending on the clinical situation, this will reduce its effectiveness or toxicity.
Cisplatin	Loop diuretics	↑	Additive ototoxicity may occur.
Clofibrate	Loop diuretics (furosemide)	↑	An exaggerated diuretic response may occur.
Hydantoins (phenytoin)	Loop diuretics (furosemide)	↓	Hydantoins may reduce the diuretic effects of furosemide.
NSAIDs	Loop diuretics	↓	Effects of the loop diuretics may be decreased.
Probenecid	Loop diuretics	↓	The actions of the loop diuretics may be reduced.
Salicylates	Loop diuretics	↓	The diuretic response may be impaired in patients with cirrhosis and ascites.
Thiazide diuretics	Loop diuretics	↑	Both groups have synergistic effects that may result in profound diuresis and serious electrolyte abnormalities (see Administration and Dosage).

* ↑ = Object drug increased. ↓ = Object drug decreased. ↔ = Undetermined effect.

Drug/Food interactions: The bioavailability of **furosemide** is decreased and its degree of diuresis reduced when administered with food.

LOOP DIURETICS

Adverse Reactions:

Furosemide:

GI – Anorexia; nausea; vomiting; diarrhea; oral and gastric irritation; cramping; constipation; pancreatitis; jaundice; ischemic hepatitis.

CNS – Vertigo; headache; blurred vision; hearing loss; dizziness; paresthesia; xanthopsia; restlessness; fever.

Hematologic – Anemia; leukopenia; purpura; aplastic anemia; thrombocytopenia; agranulocytosis.

Dermatologic – Photosensitivity; urticaria; pruritus; necrotizing angiitis (vasculitis, cutaneous vasculitis); interstitial nephritis; exfoliative dermatitis; erythema multiforme; rash; occasionally, local irritation and pain with parenteral use.

Cardiovascular – Orthostatic hypotension; thrombophlebitis; chronic aortitis.

Miscellaneous – Glycosuria; muscle spasm; weakness; urinary bladder spasm; hyperuricemia; hyperglycemia.

Ethacrynic acid:

GI – Anorexia; nausea; vomiting; diarrhea; pancreatitis (acute); jaundice; discomfort; pain; sudden watery, profuse diarrhea; GI bleeding; dysphagia.

Hematologic – Severe neutropenia has occurred in a few critically ill patients also receiving agents known to produce this effect. Rare instances of Henoch-Schoenlein purpura have occurred in patients with rheumatic heart disease. Thrombocytopenia; agranulocytosis.

Miscellaneous – Fever; chills; hematuria; apprehension; confusion; fatigue; malaise; acute gout; sense of fullness in the ears; abnormal liver function tests in seriously ill patients on multiple drug therapy that included ethacrynic acid (rare); vertigo; headache; blurred vision; tinnitus; hearing loss (irreversible); rash; occasionally, local irritation and pain have occurred with parenteral use; hyperuricemia; hyperglycemia. Acute symptomatic hypoglycemia with convulsions occurred in two uremic patients who received doses above those recommended.

Bumetanide:

CNS – Asterixis; encephalopathy with preexisting liver disease; impaired hearing; ear discomfort; vertigo; headache; dizziness.

GI – Upset stomach; dry mouth; nausea; vomiting; diarrhea; pain.

GU – Premature ejaculation; difficulty maintaining erection; renal failure.

Musculoskeletal – Weakness; arthritic pain; pain; muscle cramps; fatigue.

Cardiovascular – Hypotension; ECG changes; chest pain.

Miscellaneous – Hives; pruritus; itching; dehydration; sweating; hyperventilation; nipple tenderness; rash; thrombocytopenia.

Lab test abnormalities – Diuresis rarely (≤ 1%) accompanied by changes in LDH, total serum bilirubin, serum proteins, AST, ALT, alkaline phosphatase, cholesterol and creatinine clearance; deviations in hemoglobin, prothrombin time, hematocrit, WBC, platelet counts and differential counts; increases in urinary glucose and protein; hyperuricemia; hypochloremia; hypokalemia; azotemia; hyponatremia; increased serum creatinine; hyperglycemia; variations in phosphorus, CO_2 content, bicarbonate and calcium (see Precautions).

Torsemide:

CNS – Headache (7.3%); dizziness (3.2%); asthenia (2%); insomnia (1.2%); nervousness (1.1%); syncope.

GI – Diarrhea (2%); constipation, nausea (1.8%); dyspepsia (1.6%); edema (1.1%); GI hemorrhage; rectal bleeding.

Cardiovascular – ECG abnormality (2%); sore throat (1.6%); chest pain (1.2%); atrial fibrillation; hypotension; ventricular tachycardia; shunt thrombosis.

Respiratory – Rhinitis (2.8%); cough increase (2%).

Musculoskeletal – arthralgia (1.8%); myalgia (1.6%).

Lab test abnormalities – Hyperglycemia; hyperuricemia; hypokalemia; hypovolemia.

Miscellaneous – Excessive urination (6.7%); rash.

Overdosage:

Symptoms: Acute profound water loss, volume and electrolyte depletion, dehydration, reduction of blood volume, and circulatory collapse with a possibility of vascular thrombosis and embolism. Electrolyte depletion may be manifested by weakness, dizziness, mental confusion, anorexia, lethargy, vomiting and cramps.

Treatment: Replace fluid and electrolyte losses by careful monitoring of the urine and electrolyte output and serum electrolyte levels. Assure adequate drainage in urinary bladder outlet obstruction (such as prostatic hypertrophy). Hemodialysis does not accelerate furosemide or torsemide elimination. Induce emesis or perform gastric lavage. If required, give oxygen or artificial respiration. Treatment includes supportive measures. Refer to General Management of Acute Overdosage.

LOOP DIURETICS

Patient Information:

May cause GI upset; take with food or milk (see Drug Interactions). Torsemide may be given without regard to meals.

Drug will increase urination; take early in the day.

Notify physician if muscle weakness, cramps, nausea or dizziness occurs.

Orthostatic hypotension may occur; get up slowly.

Diabetes mellitus patients: May increase blood glucose levels, affecting urine glucose tests.

Photosensitivity may occur in some patients. Caution patients to take protective measures (ie, sunscreens, protective clothing) against exposure to ultraviolet light or sunlight.

Hypertensive patients should avoid medications that may increase blood pressure, including *otc* products for appetite suppression and cold symptoms.

Administration and Dosage:

Individualize therapy. Reserve parenteral use for when oral medication is not practical or in emergency situations. Replace with oral therapy as soon as practical.

Concomitant administration: Concurrent metolazone and furosemide have been used in the management of patients refractory to furosemide or other diuretics due to their synergistic effect on diuresis. Metolazone 2.5 to 10 mg is added to the therapy, and the dose is doubled every 24 hours until the desired response is achieved. Decrease the furosemide dose if the synergism occurs with the first dose of metolazone. Hydrochlorothiazide (50 mg) may be used and may be safer because of its shorter action. This effect has also been noted with other thiazides in combination with other loop diuretics.

FUROSEMIDE

For complete prescribing information, refer to the Loop Diuretics group monograph.

Administration and Dosage:

Oral:

Edema – 20 to 80 mg/day as a single dose. Ordinarily, prompt diuresis ensues. Depending on response, administer a second dose 6 to 8 hours later. If response is not satisfactory, increase by increments of 20 or 40 mg, no sooner than 6 to 8 hours after previous dose, until desired diuresis occurs. This dose should then be given once or twice daily (eg, at 8 am and 2 pm). Dosage may be titrated up to 600 mg/day in patients with severe edema.

Mobilization of edema may be most efficiently and safely accomplished with an intermittent dosage schedule; the drug is given 2 to 4 consecutive days each week. With doses > 80 mg/day, clinical and laboratory observations are advisable.

Hypertension – 40 mg twice a day; adjust according to response. If the patient does not respond, add other antihypertensive agents. Observe blood pressure changes when used with other antihypertensives, especially during initial therapy. Reduce dosage of other agents by at least 50% as soon as furosemide is added to prevent excessive drop in blood pressure. As blood pressure falls, reduce dose or discontinue other antihypertensives.

Infants and children – 2 mg/kg. If diuresis is unsatisfactory, increase by 1 or 2 mg/kg, no sooner than 6 to 8 hours after previous dose. Doses > 6 mg/kg are not recommended. For maintenance therapy, adjust dose to the minimum effective level. A dose range of 0.5 to 2 mg/kg twice daily has also been recommended.

CHF and chronic renal failure – It has been suggested that doses as high as 2 to 2.5 g/day or more are well tolerated and effective in these patients.

Parenteral:

Edema – Initial dose: 20 to 40 mg IM or IV. Give the IV injection slowly (1 to 2 minutes); ordinarily, prompt diuresis ensues. If needed, another dose may be given in the same manner 2 hours later. The dose may be raised by 20 mg and given no sooner than 2 hours after previous dose, until desired diuretic effect is obtained. This dose should then be given once or twice daily. Administer high-dose parenteral therapy as a controlled infusion at a rate ≤ 4 mg/min.

Acute pulmonary edema – The usual initial dose is 40 mg IV (over 1 to 2 minutes). If response is not satisfactory within 1 hour, increase to 80 mg IV (over 1 to 2 minutes). Additional therapy (eg, digitalis, oxygen) may be given concomitantly.

Infants and children – 1 mg/kg IV or IM given slowly under close supervision. If diuretic response after the initial dose is not satisfactory, increase the dosage by 1 mg/kg, no sooner than 2 hours after previous dose, until desired effect is obtained. Doses > 6 mg/kg are not recommended.

CHF and chronic renal failure – It has been suggested that doses as high as 2 to 2.5 g/day or more are well tolerated and effective in these patients. For IV bolus injections, the maximum should not exceed 1 g/day given over 30 minutes.

FUROSEMIDE

IV incompatibility – Furosemide is a mildly buffered alkaline solution; do not mix with highly acidic solutions of pH < 5.5. Sodium Chloride injection, Lactated Ringer's Injection and 5% Dextrose Injection have been used after pH has been adjusted when necessary. A precipitate formed when furosemide was admixed with gentamicin, netilmicin or milrinone in 5% Dextrose or 0.9% Sodium Chloride, but not with amikacin, kanamycin or tobramycin. Furosemide admixed with cefoperazone sodium in 5% Dextrose is stable for 2 days at 25°C (77°F) and 5 days at 4°C (39°F).

Storage/Stability: Exposure to light may cause slight discoloration; do not dispense discolored tablets or use discolored injection. Store injection and oral solution at room temperature (15° to 30°C; 59° to 86°F)

Rx	**Furosemide** (Various, eg, Danbury, Geneva, Major, Mylan, Parmed, Roxane, Schein, Zenith)	**Tablets:** 20 mg	In 100s, 500s, 1000s and UD 100s.
Rx	**Lasix** (Hoechst Marion Roussel)		Lactose. (Lasix Hoechst). White. Oval. In 100s, 500s, 1000s and UD 100s.
Rx	**Furosemide** (Various, eg, Danbury, Geneva, Major, Mylan, Parmed, Roxane, Schein, Zenith)	**Tablets:** 40 mg	In 60s, 100s, 500s and 1000s and UD 100s.
Rx	**Lasix** (Hoechst Marion Roussel)		Lactose. (Lasix 40). White, scored. In 500s, 1000s, UD 100s and unit-of-use 100s.
Rx	**Furosemide** (Various, eg, Danbury, Geneva, Major, Mylan, Parmed, Roxane, Schein)	**Tablets:** 80 mg	In 100s, 500s, 1000s and UD 100s.
Rx	**Lasix** (Hoechst Marion Roussel)		Lactose. (Lasix 80). White. In 50s, 500s and UD 100s.
Rx	**Furosemide** (Various, eg, Geneva, Roxane)	**Oral Solution:** 10 mg/ml	In 60 and 120 ml.
Rx	**Lasix** (Hoechst Marion Roussel)		11.5% alcohol, sorbitol. Orange flavor. In 60 and 120 ml.
Rx	**Furosemide** (Roxane)	**Oral Solution:** 40 mg/5 ml	Pineapple/peach flavor. In 500 ml and UD 5 & 10 ml.
Rx	**Furosemide** (Various, eg, American Regent, Major, Sanofi-Winthrop)	**Injection:** 10 mg/ml	In 10 ml and 2, 4, and 10 ml single dose vials.
Rx	**Lasix** (Hoechst Marion Roussel)		0.9% benzyl alcohol. In 2, 4 & 10 ml amps, syringes and single-use vials.

BUMETANIDE

For complete prescribing information, refer to the Loop Diuretics group monograph.

Administration and Dosage:

Because cross-sensitivity with furosemide is rare, bumetanide can be substituted at about a 1:40 ratio of bumetanide to furosemide in patients allergic to furosemide.

Oral: 0.5 to 2 mg/day, given as a single dose. If diuretic response is not adequate, give a second or third dose at 4 to 5 hour intervals, up to a maximum daily dose of 10 mg. An intermittent dose schedule, given on alternate days or for 3 to 4 days with rest periods of 1 to 2 days in between, is the safest and most effective method for the continued control of edema. In patients with hepatic failure, keep the dose to a minimum, and if necessary, increase the dose carefully.

Parenteral: Reserve for patients in whom GI absorption may be impaired or in whom oral administration is not practical.

Initially, 0.5 to 1 mg IV or IM. Administer IV over a period of 1 to 2 minutes. If the initial response is insufficient, give a second or third dose at intervals of 2 to 3 hours; do not exceed a daily dosage of 10 mg. End parenteral treatment and start oral treatment as soon as possible.

Renal function impairment: In patients with severe chronic renal insufficiency, a continuous infusion of bumetanide (12 mg over 12 hours) may be more effective and less toxic than intermittent bolus therapy.

Stability: Bumetanide injection with 5% Dextrose in Water, 0.9% Sodium Chloride and Lactated Ringer's solution in glass and plasticized PVC (*Viaflex*) containers have no significant absorption effects or loss due to drug degradation. However, freshly prepare solutions and use within 24 hours.

Rx	**Bumex** (Roche)	**Tablets:** 0.5 mg	Lactose. (Roche Bumex 0.5). Green, scored. In 100s, 500s and UD 100s.
		1 mg	Lactose. (Roche Bumex 1). Yellow, scored. In 100s, 500s and UD 100s.
		2 mg	Lactose. (Roche Bumex 2). Peach, scored. In 100s and UD 100s.
Rx	**Bumex** (Roche)	**Injection:** 0.25 mg per ml	In 2 ml amps[1] and 2, 4, 10 ml vials.[1]
Rx	**Bumetanide** (Various, eg, Bedford, Hoffman-LaRoche, Sanofi Winthrop)		In 2 ml amps, 2, 4 and 10 ml vials and 4 ml fill in 5 ml vials.

[1] With 0.01% EDTA and 1% benzyl alcohol.

ETHACRYNIC ACID

For complete prescribing information, refer to the Loop Diuretics group monograph.

Administration and Dosage:

Oral:

Initial therapy – Give minimally effective dose (usually, 50 to 200 mg daily) on a continuous or intermittent dosage schedule to produce gradual weight loss of 2.2 to 4.4 kg/day (1 to 2 lb/day). Adjust dose in 25 to 50 mg increments. Higher doses, up to 200 mg twice daily, achieved gradually, are most often required in patients with severe, refractory edema.

Children – Initial dose is 25 mg. Make careful increments of 25 mg to achieve maintenance. Dosage for infants has not been established.

Maintenance therapy – Administer intermittently after an effective diuresis is obtained using an alternate daily schedule or more prolonged periods of diuretic therapy interspersed with rest periods. This allows time to correct any electrolyte imbalance and may provide a more efficient diuretic response. The chloruretic effect may cause retention of bicarbonate and metabolic alkalosis. Correct by giving chloride (ammonium chloride or arginine chloride). Do not give ammonium chloride to cirrhotic patients.

Concomitant diuretic therapy – Ethacrynic acid has additive effects when used with other diuretics; therefore, use an initial dose of 25 mg and dose changes of 25 mg increments to avoid electrolyte depletion.

Parenteral: Do not give SC or IM because of local pain and irritation. The usual IV dose for the average adult is 50 mg, or 0.5 to 1 mg/kg. Give slowly through the tubing of a running infusion or by direct IV injection over several minutes. Usually, only one dose is necessary; occasionally, a second dose may be required; use a new injec-

ETHACRYNIC ACID

tion site to avoid thrombophlebitis. A single IV dose, not exceeding 100 mg, has been used. Insufficient pediatric experience precludes recommendation for this age group.

Preparation of solution – Add 50 ml of 5% Dextrose Injection or Sodium Chloride Injection to vial. Dextrose 5% solutions may have a low pH (< 5); the resulting solution may be hazy or opalescent. Use of such a solution is not recommended. Do not mix this solution with whole blood or its derivatives. Discard unused reconstituted solution after 24 hours.

Rx	**Edecrin** (Merck)	**Tablets**: 25 mg	Lactose. (MSD 65). White, scored. Capsule shape. In 100s.
		50 mg	Lactose. (MSD 90). Green, scored. Capsule shape. In 100s.
Rx	**Edecrin Sodium** (Merck)	**Powder for Injection**: 50 mg (as ethacrynate sodium) per vial	In 50 ml vials for reconstitution.[1]

[1] With 62.5 mg mannitol and 0.1 mg thimerosal.

TORSEMIDE

For complete prescribing information, refer to the Loop Diuretics group monograph.

Administration and Dosage:

Approved by the FDA on August 23, 1993.

Torsemide may be given at any time in relation to a meal.

Because of high bioavailability, oral and IV doses are therapeutically equivalent, so patients may be switched to and from the IV form with no change in dose. Administer the IV injection slowly over a period of 2 minutes.

Congestive heart failure: The usual initial dose is 10 or 20 mg once daily oral or IV. If the diuretic response is inadequate, titrate the dose upward by approximately doubling until the desired diuretic response is obtained. Single doses > 200 mg have not been adequately studied.

Chronic renal failure: The usual initial dose is 20 mg once daily oral or IV. If the diuretic response is inadequate, titrate the dose upward by approximately doubling until the desired diuretic response is obtained. Single doses > 200 mg have not been adequately studied.

Hepatic cirrhosis: The usual initial dose is 5 or 10 mg once daily oral or IV, administered together with an aldosterone antagonist or a potassium-sparing diuretic. If the diuretic response is inadequate, titrate the dose upward by approximately doubling until the desired diuretic response is obtained. Single doses > 40 mg have not been adequately studied.

Hypertension: The usual initial dose is 5 mg once daily. If the 5 mg dose does not provide adequate reduction in blood pressure within 4 to 6 weeks, the dose may be increased to 10 mg once daily. If the response to 10 mg is insufficient, add an additional antihypertensive agent to the treatment regimen.

Elderly: Special dosage adjustment is not necessary.

Rx	**Demadex** (Boehringer Mannheim)	**Tablets**: 5 mg	Lactose. (102 5). White, scored. Oval. In UD 100s.
		10 mg	Lactose. (103 10). White, scored. Oval. In UD 100s.
		20 mg	Lactose. (104 20). White, scored. Oval. In UD 100s.
		100 mg	Lactose. (105 100). White, scored. Capsule shape. In UD 100s.
		Injection: 10 mg/ml	In 2 and 5 ml amps.

POTASSIUM-SPARING DIURETICS

Actions:

Pharmacology: In the kidney, potassium is filtered at the glomerulus and then absorbed parallel to sodium throughout the proximal tubule and thick ascending limb of the loop of Henle, so that only minor amounts reach the distal convoluted tubule. As a result, potassium appearing in urine is secreted at the distal tubule and collecting duct. The potassium-sparing diuretics interfere with sodium reabsorption at the distal tubule, thus decreasing potassium secretion. They exert a weak diuretic and antihypertensive effect when used alone. Their major use is to enhance the action and counteract the kaliuretic effect of thiazide and loop diuretics.

Spironolactone, a competitive inhibitor of aldosterone, binds to aldosterone receptors of the distal tubule and prevents the formation of a protein important in sodium transport. The dose of spironolactone required to produce an effect varies according to the amount of aldosterone present. It is effective in both primary and secondary hyperaldosteronism. Spironolactone is effective in lowering systolic and diastolic blood pressure in both primary hyperaldosteronism and essential hypertension, although aldosterone secretion may be normal in benign essential hypertension. In addition, spironolactone interferes with testosterone synthesis and may increase peripheral conversion of testosterone to estradiol. This action may be responsible for endocrine abnormalities occasionally noted with therapy.

Amiloride and *triamterene* not only inhibit sodium reabsorption induced by aldosterone, but they also inhibit basal sodium reabsorption. They are not aldosterone antagonists, but act directly on the renal distal tubule, cortical collecting tubule and collecting duct. They induce a reversal of polarity of the transtubular electrical-potential difference and inhibit active transport of sodium and potassium. Amiloride may inhibit sodium, potassium-ATPase. Amiloride decreases the enhanced urinary excretion of magnesium that occurs when a thiazide or loop diuretic is used alone; it also decreases calcium excretion.

Potassium-Sparing Diuretics: Pharmacological and Pharmacokinetic Properties

Parameters	Amiloride	Spironolactone	Triamterene
Pharmacology			
Tubular site of action	Proximal = distal	Distal	Distal
Mechanism of action	Na^+, K^+–ATPase inhibition; Na^+/H^+ exchange mecha nism inhibition (proximal tubule)	Aldosterone antagonism	Membrane effect
Action:			
Onset (hours)	2	24 to 48	2 to 4
Peak (hours)	6 to 10	48 to 72	6 to 8
Duration (hours)	24	48 to 72	12 to 16
Pharmacokinetics			
Bioavailability	15% to 25%	> 90%	30% to 70%
Protein binding	23%	≥ 98%[1]	50% to 67%
Half-life (hours)	6 to 9	20[2]	3
Active metabolites	none	canrenone	hydroxytriamterene sulfate
Peak plasma levels (hours)	3 to 4	canrenone: 2 to 4[3]	3
Excreted unchanged in urine	≈ 50%[4]	†[4]	≈ 21%
Daily dose (mg)	5 to 20	25 to 400	200 to 300

[1] Canrenone > 98%.
[2] 10 to 35 hours for canrenone.
[3] 40% excreted in stool within 72 hours.
[4] † Metabolites primarily excreted in urine, but also in bile.

AMILORIDE HCl

Refer to the general discussion of these agents in the Potassium-Sparing Diuretics introduction.

Indications:

Adjunctive treatment with thiazide or loop diuretics in congestive heart failure (CHF) or hypertension to: Help restore normal serum potassium in patients who develop hypokalemia on the kaliuretic diuretic; prevent hypokalemia in patients who would be at particular risk if hypokalemia were to develop (eg, digitalized patients or patients with significant cardiac arrhythmias).

Unlabeled uses: Amiloride (10 to 20 mg/day) may be useful in reducing lithium-induced polyuria without increasing lithium levels as is seen with thiazide diuretics.

Aerosolized amiloride (drug dissolved in 0.3% saline delivered by nebulizer) appears to slow the progression of pulmonary function reduction in adults with cystic fibrosis.

Contraindications:

Hypersensitivity to amiloride; serum potassium > 5.5 mEq/L; antikaliuretic therapy or potassium supplementation (see Drug Interactions); renal function impairment (see Warnings); patients receiving spironolactone or triamaterene.

Warnings:

Hyperkalemia: Amiloride may cause hyperkalemia (serum potassium > 5.5 mEq/L) which, if uncorrected, is potentially fatal. Hyperkalemia occurs commonly (about 10%) when amiloride is used alone. This incidence is greater in patients with renal impairment, diabetes mellitus (with or without recognized renal insufficiency) and in the elderly. When amiloride is used concomitantly with a thiazide diuretic in patients without these complications, the risk of hyperkalemia is reduced to about 1% to 2%. Monitor serum potassium carefully, particularly when amiloride is first introduced, at the time of diuretic dosage adjustments and during any illness that could affect renal function.

Symptoms of hyperkalemia include paresthesias, muscular weakness, fatigue, flaccid paralysis of the extremities, bradycardia, shock, and ECG abnormalities. The ECG in hyperkalemia is characterized primarily by tall, peaked T waves or elevations from previous tracings. There may also be lowering of the R wave, increased depth of the S wave, widening or disappearance of the P wave, progressive widening of the QRS complex, prolongation of the PR interval, and ST depression. Mild hyperkalemia is not usually associated with an abnormal ECG.

Treatment discontinue the drug immediately. Monitor ECG and serum potassium levels. If serum potassium exceeds 6.5 mEq/L, take active measures to reduce it, including IV sodium bicarbonate solution or oral or parenteral glucose with rapid-acting insulin. If needed, give sodium polystyrene sulfonate orally or by enema. Persistent hyperkalemia may require dialysis.

Diabetes mellitus: Hyperkalemia has occurred with the use of amiloride, even in patients without evidence of diabetic nephropathy. If possible, avoid use of amiloride in diabetic patients. If it is used, monitor serum electrolytes and renal function frequently. Discontinue use at least 3 days before glucose tolerance testing.

Metabolic or respiratory acidosis: Cautiously institute amiloride in severely ill patients in whom respiratory or metabolic acidosis may occur, such as patients with cardiopulmonary disease or poorly controlled diabetes. Monitor acid-base balance frequently. Shifts in acid-base balance alter the ratio of extracellular/intracellular potassium; the development of acidosis may be associated with rapid increases in serum potassium.

Renal function impairment: Anuria, acute or chronic renal insufficiency and evidence of diabetic nephropathy are contraindications because potassium retention is accentuated and may result in the rapid development of hyperkalemia. Do not give to patients with evidence of renal impairment (BUN > 30 mg/dl or serum creatinine > 1.5 mg/dl) or diabetes mellitus without continuous monitoring of serum electrolytes, creatinine and BUN levels.

Hepatic function impairment: In patients with preexisting severe liver disease, hepatic encephalopathy, manifested by tremors, confusion and coma, and increased jaundice, may occur in association with amiloride. Because amiloride is not metabolized by the liver, drug accumulation is not anticipated in patients with hepatic dysfunction, but accumulation can occur if hepatorenal syndrome develops.

Pregnancy: Category B. There are no adequate and well controlled studies in pregnant women. Safety for use during pregnancy has not been established. Use only when clearly needed and when the potential benefits outweigh the unknown hazards to the fetus. See also discussion of thiazide diuretic use during pregnancy.

AMILORIDE HCl

Lactation: It is not known whether amiloride is excreted in breast milk. In rats, amiloride is excreted in milk in concentrations higher than those found in blood. Because of the potential for serious adverse reactions in nursing infants, decide whether to discontinue nursing or to discontinue the drug, taking into account the importance of the drug to the mother.

Children: Safety and efficacy for use in children have not been established.

Precautions:

Electrolyte imbalance and BUN increases: Hyponatremia and hypochloremia may occur when amiloride is used with other diuretics. Increases in BUN levels usually accompany vigorous fluid elimination, especially when diuretic therapy is used in seriously ill patients, such as those who have hepatic cirrhosis with ascites and metabolic alkalosis, or those with resistant edema. Carefully monitor serum electrolytes and BUN levels.

Drug Interactions:

Amiloride Drug Interactions			
Precipitant drug	Object drug*	Description	
Amiloride	Digoxin	⬇	In six healthy subjects, amiloride increased the renal clearance and decreased the nonrenal clearance of digoxin. It also appeared to decrease the inotropic effect of digoxin.
Amiloride	Potassium preparations	⬆	Concurrent administration may result in severe hyperkalemia, possibly with cardiac arrhythmias or cardiac arrest. Avoid concomitant use.
ACE inhibitors	Amiloride	⬆	Use of ACE inhibitors may result in elevated serum potassium concentration. Concurrent use with amiloride may lead to significant hyperkalemia.
NSAIDs	Amiloride	⬇	NSAIDs may reduce the therapeutic effect of amiloride. Also, since indomethocin may be associated with increased potassium levels, consider this effect when amiloride is used concurrently.

* ⬆ = Object drug increased. ⬇ = Object drug decreased.

Adverse Reactions:

CNS: Headache (3% to 8%); dizziness, encephalopathy (> 1% to < 3%); paresthesia, tremors, vertigo, nervousness, mental confusion, insomnia, decreased libido, depression, somnolence (≤ 1%).

GI: Nausea, anorexia, diarrhea, vomiting (3% to 8%); abdominal pain, gas pain, appetite changes, constipation (> 1% to < 3%); jaundice, GI bleeding, GI disturbance, abdominal fullness, thirst, dry mouth, heartburn, flatulence, dyspepsia (≤ 1%); activation of probable preexisting peptic ulcer; abnormal liver function.

Metabolic: Elevated serum potassium levels > 5.5 mEq/L (> 1% to < 3%).

Musculoskeletal: Weakness, fatigue, muscle cramps (> 1% to < 3%); joint/back/chest pain, neck or shoulder ache, pain of the extremities (≤ 1%).

Respiratory: Cough, dyspnea (> 1% to < 3%); shortness of breath (≤ 1%).

GU: Impotence (> 1% to < 3%); polyuria, dysuria, urinary frequency, bladder spasms (≤ 1%).

Cardiovascular: Angina pectoris, orthostatic hypotension, arrhythmia, palpitations (≤ 1%).

Dermatologic: Skin rash, itching, pruritus, alopecia (≤ 1%).

Special senses: Visual disturbances, nasal congestion, tinnitus, increased intraocular pressure (≤ 1%).

Hematologic: Aplastic anemia; neutropenia.

Overdosage:

Symptoms: The most likely signs are dehydration and electrolyte imbalance.

Treatment: Discontinue therapy and observe patient closely. Induce emesis or perform gastric lavage. Treatment is symptomatic and supportive. Refer to General Management of Acute Overdosage. If hyperkalemia occurs, reduce the serum potassium levels (see Warnings). It is not known whether amiloride is dialyzable.

AMILORIDE HCl

Patient Information:

May cause GI upset; take with food.

Notify physician if any of the following occurs: Muscular weakness, fatigue, muscle cramps.

May cause dizziness, headache or visual disturbances; observe caution while driving or performing other tasks requiring alertness, coordination or physical dexterity.

Avoid large quantities of potassium rich food.

Administration and Dosage:

Administer with food.

Concomitant therapy: Add amiloride 5 mg/day to the usual antihypertensive or diuretic dosage of a kaliuretic diuretic. Increase dosage to 10 mg/day, if necessary; doses > 10 mg are usually not needed. If persistent hypokalemia is documented with 10 mg, increase the dose to 15 mg, then 20 mg, with careful titration of the dose and careful monitoring of electrolytes.

In patients with CHF, potassium loss may decrease after an initial diuresis; reevaluate the need or dosage for amiloride. Maintenance therapy may be intermittent.

Single drug therapy: The starting dose is 5 mg/day. Increase to 10 mg/day, if necessary; doses > 10 mg are usually not needed. If persistent hypokalemia is documented with 10 mg, increase the dose to 15 mg, then 20 mg, with careful monitoring of electrolytes.

Rx	**Midamor** (Merck)	**Tablets:** 5 mg	(MSD 92). Yellow. Diamond shape. In 100s.

SPIRONOLACTONE

Refer to the general discussion of these agents in the Potassium-Sparing Diuretics introduction.

Warning:

Spironolactone has been shown to be a tumorigen in chronic toxicity studies in rats (see Warnings). Use only in those conditions described in the Indications section. Avoid unnecessary use of the drug.

Indications:

Primary hyperaldosteronism: Diagnosis of primary hyperaldosteronism.

Short-term preoperative treatment of patients with primary hyperaldosteronism.

Long-term maintenance therapy for patients with discrete aldosterone-producing adrenal adenomas who are poor operative risks, or who decline surgery.

Long-term maintenance therapy for patients with bilateral micronodular or macronodular adrenal hyperplasia (idiopathic hyperaldosteronism).

Edematous conditions when other therapies are inappropriate or inadequate:

CHF – Management of edema and sodium retention; also indicated with digitalis.

Cirrhosis of the liver accompanied by edema or ascites for maintenance therapy in conjunction with bed rest and the restriction of fluid and sodium.

Nephrotic syndrome.

Essential hypertension, usually in combination with other drugs.

Hypokalemia and the prophylaxis of hypokalemia in patients taking digitalis.

Unlabeled uses: Spironolactone has been used in the treatment of hirsutism (50 to 200 mg/day) due to its antiandrogenic properties. One study suggested that a lower dosage (50 mg twice daily on days 4 through 21 of the menstrual cycle) may help minimize the risk of metrorrhagia that occurs with higher doses.

Symptoms of premenstrual syndrome (PMS) have been relieved at a dosage of 25 mg 4 times daily beginning on day 14 of the menstrual cycle.

The combination of spironolactone (2 mg/kg/day) and testolactone (20 to 40 mg/kg/day) for at least 6 months may be effective for short-term treatment of familial male precocious puberty.

Spironolactone 100 mg/day appears effective in short-term treatment of acne vulgaris.

Contraindications:

Anuria; acute renal insufficiency; significant impairment of renal function; hyperkalemia; patients receiving amiloride or triamterene.

Warnings:

Hyperkalemia: Carefully evaluate patients for possible fluid and electrolyte balance disturbances. Hyperkalemia may occur with impaired renal function or excessive potassium intake and can cause cardiac irregularities which may be fatal. No potassium supplement should ordinarily be given with spironolactone.

Treat hyperkalemia promptly by rapid IV glucose (20% to 50%) and regular insulin, using 0.25 to 0.5 units of insulin/g of glucose. This is a temporary measure to be repeated as required. Treatment of hyperkalemia may also include: IV calcium to antagonize effects on the heart; bicarbonate if patient is acidotic; or sodium polystyrene sulfonate exchange resin to remove potassium. Discontinue spironolactone and restrict potassium intake (including dietary potassium).

Renal function impairment: Use of spironolactone may cause a transient elevation of BUN, especially in patients with preexisting renal impairment. The drug may cause mild acidosis.

SPIRONOLACTONE

Carcinogenesis: Spironolactone was a tumorigen in chronic toxicity studies in rats. At 25 to 250 times the usual human dose, there was a significant dose-related increase in benign adenomas of the thyroid and testes, in malignant mammary tumors and in proliferative changes in the liver. At 500 mg/kg, the effects included hepatocytomegaly, hyperplastic liver nodules and hepatocellular carcinoma. A dose-related (> 20 mg/kg/day) incidence of myelocytic leukemia was observed in rats fed daily doses of potassium canrenoate. In the rat, myelocytic leukemia and hepatic, thyroid, testicular and mammary tumors were observed.

Pregnancy: Spironolactone or its metabolites may cross the placental barrier. Feminization occurs in male rat fetuses. Weigh anticipated benefit against possible hazard to the fetus. See also discussion of thiazide diuretic use during pregnancy.

Lactation: Canrenone, a metabolite of spironolactone, appears in breast milk. The estimated maximum dose to the infant is ≈ 0.2% of the mother's daily dose. Labeling suggests an alternative method of infant feeding when using spironolactone; however, the American Academy of Pediatrics considers the drug to be compatible with breast-feeding.

Precautions:

Hyponatremia may be caused or aggravated by spironolactone, especially in combination with other diuretics. Symptoms include dry mouth, thirst, lethargy, drowsiness.

Gynecomastia may develop and appears to be related to both dosage and duration of therapy. It is normally reversible when therapy is discontinued; however, in rare instances, some breast enlargement may persist.

Reversible hyperchloremic metabolic acidosis, usually in association with hyperkalemia, occurs in some patients with decompensated hepatic cirrhosis, even in the presence of normal renal function.

Drug Interactions:

Spironolactone Drug Interactions

Precipitant drug	Object drug*		Description
Spironolactone	Anticoagulants	↓	The hypoprothrombinemic effect may be decreased.
Spironolactone	Digitalis glycosides	↔	The interaction is complex and difficult to predict. Spironolactone increases the half-life of digoxin and can decrease its clearance. This may result in increased serum digoxin levels and subsequent toxicity. In addition, the drug may attenuate the inotropic action of digoxin. Spironolactone both decreases and increases digitoxin's elimination half-life.
Spironolactone	Mitotane	↓	One patient failed to respond to mitotane while receiving concurrent spironolactone. Mitotane toxicity developed when the drug was discontinued.
Spironolactone	Potassium preparations	↑	Concurrent administration may result in hyperkalemia, possibly with cardiac arrhythmias or cardiac arrest. Avoid concomitant use.
ACE inhibitors	Spironolactone	↑	Use of ACE inhibitors may elevate serum potassium. Concurrent use with spironolactone may lead to significant hyperkalemia.
Salicylates	Spironolactone	↓	The diuretic effect of spironolactone may be decreased by concurrent salicylate use, possibly due to reduced tubular secretion of canrenone; this interaction is dose-dependent. The antihypertensive action does not appear altered.

* ↑ = Object drug increased ↓ = Object drug decreased ↔ = Undetermined effect

Drug/Lab test interactions: Spironolactone and its metabolites can interfere with the radioimmunoassay for measuring **digoxin**, resulting in falsely elevated serum digoxin values.

Drug/Food interactions: The administration of spironolactone with food appears to increase its absorption. In one study, the AUC and maximum serum concentration of spironolactone were significantly increased by food.

Adverse Reactions:

Adverse reactions are usually reversible upon discontinuation of the drug.

GI: Cramping; diarrhea; gastric bleeding; ulceration; gastritis; vomiting.

SPIRONOLACTONE

CNS: Drowsiness; lethargy; headache; mental confusion; ataxia.

Endocrine: Inability to achieve or maintain erection; gynecomastia; irregular menses or amenorrhea; postmenopausal bleeding; hirsutism; deepening of the voice.

Dermatologic: Maculopapular or erythematous cutaneous eruptions; urticaria.

Miscellaneous: Drug fever; hyperchloremic metabolic acidosis in decompensated hepatic cirrhosis; carcinoma of the breast; agranulocytosis.

Patient Information:

May produce drowsiness, lack of coordination and mental confusion; observe caution while driving or performing other tasks requiring alertness, coordination or physical dexterity.

May cause GI cramping, diarrhea, lethargy, thirst, headache, skin rash, menstrual abnormalities, deepening of the voice and breast enlargement in men. Notify physician if these effects occur.

Administration and Dosage:

Spironolactone may be administered in single or divided doses.

Diagnosis of primary hyperaldosteronism: As an initial diagnostic measure to provide presumptive evidence of primary hyperaldosteronism in patients on normal diets, as follows:

Long test – 400 mg/day for 3 to 4 weeks. Correction of hypokalemia and hypertension provides presumptive evidence for diagnosis of primary hyperaldosteronism.

Short test – 400 mg/day for 4 days. If serum potassium increases, but decreases when spironolactone is discontinued, consider a presumptive diagnosis of primary hyperaldosteronism.

Maintenance therapy for hyperaldosteronism: 100 to 400 mg daily in preparation for surgery. For patients unsuitable for surgery, employ the drug for long-term maintenance therapy at lowest possible dose.

SPIRONOLACTONE

Edema:

Adults (CHF, hepatic cirrhosis, nephrotic syndrome) – Initially, 100 mg/day (range, 25 to 200 mg/day). When given as the sole diuretic agent, continue for at least 5 days at the initial dosage level, then adjust to the optimal level. If after 5 days an adequate diuretic response has not occurred, add a second diuretic, which acts more proximally in the renal tubule. Because of the additive effect of spironolactone with such diuretics, an enhanced diuresis usually begins on the first day of combined treatment; combined therapy is indicated when more rapid diuresis is desired. Spironolactone dosage should remain unchanged when other diuretic therapy is added.

Children – 3.3 mg/kg/day (1.5 mg/lb/day) administered in single or divided doses.

Essential hypertension:

Adults – Initially, 50 to 100 mg/day in single or divided doses. May also be combined with diuretics, which act more proximally, and with other antihypertensive agents. Continue treatment for at least 2 weeks since the maximal response may not occur sooner. Individualize dosage.

Children – A dose of 1 to 2 mg/kg twice daily has been recommended.

Hypokalemia: 25 to 100 mg/day. Useful in treating diuretic-induced hypokalemia when oral potassium supplements or other potassium-sparing regimens are considered inappropriate.

Rx	**Spironolactone** (Various, eg, Geneva, Major, Mylan, Parmed)	**Tablets:** 25 mg	In 100s, 250s, 500s and 1000s.
Rx	**Aldactone** (Searle)		(Searle 1001 Aldactone 25). Lt. yellow. Film coated. In 100s, 500s, 1000s, 2500s and UD 100s.
Rx	**Aldactone** (Searle)	**Tablets:** 50 mg	(Searle 1041 Aldactone 50). Lt. orange, scored. Oval. Film coated. In 100s and UD 100s.
Rx	**Aldactone** (Searle)	**Tablets:** 100 mg	(Searle 1031 Aldactone 100). Peach, scored. Film coated. In 100s and UD 100s.

TRIAMTERENE

Refer to the general discussion of these agents in the Potassium-Sparing Diuretics introduction.

Indications:

Edema associated with congestive heart failure (CHF), hepatic cirrhosis and the nephrotic syndrome; steroid-induced edema, idiopathic edema and edema due to secondary hyperaldosteronism.

May be used alone or with other diuretics, either for additive diuretic effect or antikaliuretic (potassium-sparing) effect. It promotes increased diuresis in patients resistant or only partially responsive to other diuretics because of secondary hyperaldosteronism.

Contraindications:

Patients receiving spironolactone or amiloride; anuria; severe hepatic disease; hyperkalemia (see Warnings); hypersensitivity to triamterene; severe or progressive kidney disease or dysfunction, with the possible exception of nephrosis; preexisting elevated serum potassium (impaired renal function, azotemia) or patients who develop hyperkalemia while on triamterene.

Warnings:

Hyperkalemia: Abnormal elevation of serum potassium levels (≥ 5.5 mEq/L) can occur. Hyperkalemia is more likely to occur in patients with renal impairment and diabetes (even without evidence of renal impairment), and in the elderly or severely ill. Since uncorrected hyperkalemia may be fatal, serum potassium levels must be monitored at frequent intervals especially when dosages are changed or with any illness that may influence renal function.

Hyperkalemia rarely occurs in patients with adequate urinary output, but is possible if large doses are used for long periods of time; if it occurs, withdraw triamterene. Normal adult serum potassium range is 3.5 to 5 mEq/L. Treat levels persistently > 6 mEq/L. Neonate levels are higher than adult levels. Serum potassium levels do not necessarily indicate true body potassium concentration. A rise in plasma pH may cause a decrease in plasma potassium concentration and an increase in the intracellular potassium concentration. Patients who receive intensive or prolonged therapy may experience a rebound kaliuresis upon abrupt withdrawal. Gradually withdraw triamterene in such patients.

When triamterene is added to other diuretic therapy, or when patients are switched to triamterene from other diuretics, discontinue potassium supplementation.

If hyperkalemia is present or suspected, obtain an ECG. If the ECG shows no widening of the QRS or arrhythmia in the presence of hyperkalemia, discontinue triamterene and any potassium supplementation and substitute a thiazide alone. Sodium polystyrene sulfonate may be administered to enhance excess potassium excretion. The presence of a widened QRS complex or arrhythmia in association with hyperkalemia requires prompt additional therapy. For tachyarrhythmia, infuse 44 mEq of sodium bicarbonate or 10 ml of 10% calcium gluconate or calcium chloride over several minutes. For asystole, bradycardia or AV block, transvenous pacing is also recommended.

The effect of calcium and sodium bicarbonate is transient. Repeat as required. Remove excess potassium by dialysis or oral or rectal administration of sodium polystyrene sulfonate. Infusion of glucose and insulin are also used to treat hyperkalemia.

The following agents, given with triamterene, may cause hyperkalemia especially in patients with renal insufficiency: Blood from blood bank (may contain up to 30 mEq of potassium per liter of plasma or up to 65 mEq per liter of whole blood when stored for > 10 days); low-salt milk (may contain up to 60 mEq of potassium per liter); potassium-containing medications (such as parenteral penicillin G potassium); salt substitutes (most contain substantial amounts of potassium).

Hypersensitivity: Monitor patients regularly for blood dyscrasias, liver damage or other idiosyncratic reactions.

Renal function impairment: Perform periodic BUN and serum potassium determinations to check kidney function, especially in patients with suspected or confirmed renal insufficiency and in elderly or diabetic patients; diabetic patients with nephropathy are especially prone to develop hyperkalemia.

Hepatic function impairment: Triamterene is extensively metabolized in the liver. One study showed that the clearance of triamterene is markedly decreased in patients with cirrhosis and ascites. However, the overall diuretic response may not be affected.

TRIAMTERENE

Pregnancy: Category B. Triamterene crosses the placental barrier and appears in the cord blood of animals; this may occur in humans. No congenital defects have been noted when used during pregnancy. There are no adequate and well controlled studies in pregnant women. Use only when clearly needed and when the potential benefits outweigh the potential hazards to the fetus. See also discussion of thiazide diuretic use during pregnancy.

Lactation: Triamterene appears in the milk of animals receiving the drug; this may occur in humans. If the drug is essential, the patient should stop nursing.

Children: Safety and efficacy have not been established.

Precautions:

Electrolyte imbalance: In CHF, renal disease or cirrhosis, electrolyte imbalance may be aggravated or caused by diuretics. The use of full doses of a diuretic when salt intake is restricted can result in a low salt syndrome.

Triamterene can cause mild nitrogen retention which is reversible upon withdrawal; this is seldom observed with intermittent therapy.

Renal stones: Triamterene has been found in renal stones with other usual calculus components. Therefore, use cautiously in patients with histories of stone formation.

Hematologic effects: Triamterene is a weak folic acid antagonist. Since cirrhotics with splenomegaly may have marked variations in hematological status, it may contribute to the appearance of megaloblastosis in cases where folic acid stores have been depleted. Perform periodic blood studies in these patients.

Metabolic acidosis: Triamterene may cause decreasing alkali reserve with a possibility of metabolic acidosis.

Diabetes mellitus: Triamterene may raise blood glucose levels for adult-onset diabetes; dosage adjustments of hypoglycemic agents may be necessary. Concurrent use with chlorpropamide may increase the risk of severe hyponatremia.

Photosensitivity: Photosensitization (photoallergy or phototoxicity) is likely to occur; therefore, caution patients to take protective measures (ie, sunscreens, protective clothing) against exposure to ultraviolet light or sunlight until tolerance is determined.

Drug Interactions:

Triamterene Drug Interactions			
Precipitant drug	Object drug*		Description
Triamterene	Amantadine	↑	Amantadine plasma levels may increase and urinary excretion may decrease, possibly increasing the risk for developing adverse effects.
Triamterene	Potassium preparations	↑	Concurrent administration may result in severe hyperkalemia, possibly with cardiac arrhythmias or cardiac arrest. Avoid concomitant use.
ACE inhibitors	Triamterene	↑	Use of ACE inhibitors may elevate serum potassium. Concurrent use with triamterene may lead to significant hyperkalemia.
Cimetidine	Triamterene	↑	Cimetidine may increase the bioavailability and decrease the renal clearance and hydroxylation of triamterene.
Indomethacin	Triamterene	↑	Rapid progress into acute renal failure has occurred with concurrent use. Use this combination only when clearly needed.

* ↑ = Object drug increased

Drug/Lab test interactions: Triamterene and **quinidine** have similar fluorescence spectra; thus, triamterene will interfere with the fluorescent measurement of quinidine serum levels.

TRIAMTERENE

Adverse Reactions:

GI: Diarrhea; nausea; vomiting; jaundice; liver enzyme abnormalities. Nausea can usually be prevented by giving the drug after meals.

Renal: Azotemia; elevated BUN and creatinine. Triamterene has been found in renal stones (see Precautions).

Interstitial nephritis has been reported rarely in patients on a hydrochlorothiazide/triamterene combination and with triamterene alone. Onset was immediate to 10 weeks after initiation of therapy; resolution began upon discontinuation of the drug.

In patients predisposed to gouty arthritis, serum uric acid levels may increase.

Hematologic: Thrombocytopenia; megaloblastic anemia.

Body as a whole: Electrolyte inbalance (see Precautions); hyperkalemia (see Warnings); weakness; fatigue; dizziness; hypokalemia; headache; dry mouth; anaphylaxis; photosensitivity; rash.

Overdosage:

Symptoms: Electrolyte imbalance is the major concern, particularly hyperkalemia (see Warnings). Other symptoms may include nausea, vomiting, other GI disturbances and weakness. Hypotension may occur. Triamterene may induce reversible acute renal failure.

Treatment: Induce immediate evacuation of the stomach through emesis and gastric lavage. Carefully evaluate electrolyte and fluid balance. Dialysis may be of some benefit. Treatment includes usual supportive measures. Refer to General Management of Acute Overdosage.

Patient Information:

May cause GI upset; take after meals.

May cause weakness, headache, nausea, vomiting and dry mouth; notify physician if these become severe or persistent.

Notify physician if fever, sore throat, mouth sores, or unusual bleeding or bruising occurs.

Avoid prolonged exposure to sunlight; photosensitivity may occur.

If single daily dose is prescribed, take in morning to minimize effect of increased frequency of urination on nighttime sleep.

If dose is missed, do not take more than prescribed dose at next dosing interval.

Administration and Dosage:

Individualize dosage.

When used alone, the usual starting dose is 100 mg twice/daily after meals. When combined with other diuretics or antihypertensives, decrease the total daily dosage of each agent initially, and then adjust to the patient's needs. Do not exceed 300 mg/day.

Rx	**Dyrenium** (SmithKline Beecham)	**Capsules:** 50 mg	(Dyrenium 50). Red. In 100s and UD 100s.
		100 mg	(Dyrenium 100). Red. In 100s, 1000s & UD 100s.

CARBONIC ANHYDRASE INHIBITORS

Actions:

Pharmacology: These agents are nonbacteriostatic sulfonamides that inhibit the enzyme carbonic anhydrase. This action reduces the rate of aqueous humor formation, resulting in decreased intraocular pressure (IOP). This action is independent of systemic acid-base balance.

By inhibiting hydrogen ion secretion by the renal tubule, these agents cause increased excretion of sodium, potassium, bicarbonate and water, thus producing an alkaline diuresis. Carbonic anhydrase inhibitors cause some decrease in renal blood flow and glomerular filtration rate. Redistribution of flow to the renal cortex occurs. These changes are mild and unrelated to diuretic activity.

Evidence seems to indicate that acetazolamide has utility as an adjuvant in the treatment of certain dysfunctions of the CNS (eg, epilepsy). Inhibition of carbonic anhydrase in this area appears to retard abnormal, paroxysmal, excessive discharge from CNS neurons.

Pharmacokinetics:

Pharmacokinetics of Carbonic Anhydrase Inhibitors

Carbonic anhydrase inhibitor	IOP Lowering Effects			Relative inhibitor potency
	Onset (hours)	Peak effect (hours)	Duration (hours)	
Dichlorphenamide	within 1	2 to 4	6 to 12	30
Acetazolamide				
Tablets	1 to 1.5	1 to 4	8 to 12	1
Sustained release capsules	2	3 to 6	18 to 24	
Injection (IV)	2 min	15 min	4 to 5	
Methazolamide	2 to 4	6 to 8	10 to 18	†

† Quantitative data not available; reported to be more active than acetazolamide.

Methazolamide – Peak plasma concentrations for the 25, 50 and 100 mg twice daily regimens were 2.5, 5.1 and 10.7 mcg/ml, respectively. Approximately 55% is bound to plasma proteins. The mean steady-state plasma elimination half-life is approximately 14 hours. At steady state approximately 25% of the dose is recovered unchanged in the urine. Renal clearance accounts for 20% to 25% of the total clearance of drug. After repeated dosing,methazolamide accumulates to steady-state concentrations in 7 days.

Indications:

Glaucoma: For adjunctive treatment of chronic simple (open-angle) glaucoma and secondary glaucoma; preoperatively in acute angle-closure glaucoma when delay of surgery is desired to lower IOP.

Acetazolamide:

Tablets, sustained release capsules and injection – For the prevention or amelioration of symptoms associated with acute mountain sickness in climbers attempting rapid ascent and in those who are susceptible to acute mountain sickness despite gradual ascent.

Tablets and injection only – For adjunctive treatment of edema due to CHF, drug-induced edema and centrencephalic epilepsy (petit mal, unlocalized seizures).

Contraindications:

Hypersensitivity to these agents; depressed sodium or potassium serum levels; marked kidney and liver disease or dysfunction; suprarenal gland failure; hyperchloremic acidosis; adrenocortical insufficiency; severe pulmonary obstruction with inability to increase alveolar ventilation since acidosis may be increased (dichlorphenamide); cirrhosis (acetazolamide, methazolamide); long-term use in chronic noncongestive angle-closure glaucoma, since organic closure of the angle may occur while worsening glaucoma is masked by lowered IOP.

Warnings:

Hepatic function impairment: Use of **methazolamide** in this condition could precipitate hepatic coma.

Pregnancy: Category C. Animal studies with some of these drugs have demonstrated teratogenicity (skeletal anomalies). Do not use during pregnancy, especially during the first trimester, unless the potential benefits outweigh the potential hazards.

CARBONIC ANHYDRASE INHIBITORS

Lactation: Safety for use in the nursing mother has not been established. It is not known whether all carbonic anhydrase inhibitors are excreted in breast milk. Acetazolamide appeared in breast milk of a patient taking 500 mg twice/day. However, the infant ingested only 0.06% of the dose, an amount unlikely to cause adverse effects.

Children: Safety and efficacy for use in children have not been established.

Precautions:

Monitoring: Monitor for hematologic reactions common to sulfonamides. Obtain baseline CBC and platelet counts before therapy and at regular intervals during therapy.

Hypokalemia may develop when severe cirrhosis is present, during concomitant use of steroids or ACTH, and with interference with adequate oral electrolyte intake. Hypokalemia can sensitize or exaggerate the response of the heart to the toxic effects of digitalis (eg, increased ventricular irritability). Hypokalemia may be avoided or treated with potassium supplements or foods with a high potassium content.

Dose increases: Increasing the dose of **acetazolamide** does not increase diuresis and may increase drowsiness or paresthesia; it often results in decreased diuresis. However, very large doses have been given with other diuretics to promote diuresis in complete refractory failure.

Pulmonary conditions: Use **dichlorphenamide** with caution in patients with severe degrees of respiratory acidosis. These drugs may precipitate or aggravate acidosis. Use with caution in patients with pulmonary obstruction or emphysema when alveolar ventilation may be impaired.

Cross-sensitivity between antibacterial sulfonamides and sulfonamide derivative diuretics, including acetazolamide and various thiazides, has been reported.

Drug Interactions:

Carbonic Anhydrase Inhibitor (CAI) Drug Interactions			
Precipitant drug	Object drug*		Description
Acetazolamide	Cyclosporine	↑	Increased trough cyclosporine levels with possible nephrotoxicity and neurotoxicity may occur.
Acetazolamide	Primidone	↓	Primidone serum and urine concentrations may be decreased.
CAIs	Salicylates	↑	Concurrent use may result in accumulation and toxicity of the CAI, including CNS depression and metabolic acidosis. Also, CAI-induced acidosis may allow increased CNS penetration by salicylates.
Salicylates	CAIs	↑	
Diflunisal	CAIs	↑	Concurrent use may result in a significant decrease in intraocular pressure; the effect may be less pronounced with methazolamide. Increased side effects may also occur.

* ↑ = Object drug increased ↓ = Object drug decreased

Adverse Reactions:

Sulfonamide-type adverse reactions may occur (see Systemic Sulfonamides monograph in the Anti-infectives section).

GI: Melena; anorexia; nausea; vomiting; constipation; taste alteration; diarrhea.

Renal: Hematuria; glycosuria; urinary frequency; renal colic; renal calculi; crystalluria; polyuria; phosphaturia.

CNS: Convulsions; weakness; malaise; fatigue; nervousness; drowsiness; depression; dizziness; disorientation; confusion; ataxia; tremor; tinnitus; headache; lassitude; flaccid paralysis; paresthesias of the extremities.

Hematologic: Bone marrow depression; thrombocytopenia; thrombocytopenic purpura; hemolytic anemia; leukopenia; pancytopenia; agranulocytosis.

Dermatologic: Urticaria; pruritus; skin eruptions; rash (including erythema multiforme, Stevens-Johnson syndrome, toxic epidermal necrolysis); photosensitivity.

Miscellaneous: Weight loss; fever; acidosis (usually corrected with bicarbonate); decreased/absent libido; impotence; electrolyte imbalance; hepatic insufficiency; transient myopia.

Overdosage:

Symptoms of overdosage or toxicity may include drowsiness, anorexia, nausea, vomiting, dizziness, paresthesias, ataxia, tremor and tinnitus.

CARBONIC ANHYDRASE INHIBITORS

Treatment: In the event of overdosage, induce emesis or perform gastric lavage. The electrolyte disturbance most likely to be encountered from overdosage is hyperchloremic acidosis that may respond to bicarbonate administration. Potassium supplementation may be required. Observe carefully; give supportive treatment.

Patient Information:

If GI upset occurs, take with food.

Avoid prolonged exposure to sunlight or sunlamps; may cause photosensitivity.

May cause drowsiness; observe caution while driving or performing other tasks requiring alertness, coordination or physical dexterity.

Notify physician if sore throat, fever, unusual bleeding or bruising, tingling or tremors in the hands or feet, flank or loin pain, or skin rash occurs.

ACETAZOLAMIDE

For complete prescribing information, see Carbonic Anhydrase Inhibitor monograph.

Administration and Dosage:

Chronic simple (open-angle) glaucoma:

Adults – 250 mg to 1 g/day, usually in divided doses for amounts > 250 mg. Dosage > 1 g daily does not usually increase the effect.

Secondary glaucoma and preoperative treatment of acute congestive (closed-angle) glaucoma:

Adults –

Short-term therapy: 250 mg every 4 hours or 250 mg twice daily.

Acute cases: 500 mg followed by 125 or 250 mg every 4 hours.

IV therapy may be used for rapid relief of increased intraocular pressure. A complementary effect occurs when used with miotics or mydriatics.

Children –

Parenteral: 5 to 10 mg/kg/dose, IM or IV, every 6 hours.

Oral: 10 to 15 mg/kg/day in divided doses, every 6 to 8 hours.

Diuresis in congestive heart failure:

Adults – Initially, 250 to 375 mg (5 mg/kg) once daily in the morning. If, after an initial response, the patient stops losing edema fluid, do not increase the dose; allow for kidney recovery by skipping medication for a day. Best diuretic results occur when given on alternate days, or for 2 days alternating with a day of rest. Failures in therapy may result from overdosage or from too frequent dosages.

Drug-induced edema: Most effective if given every other day or for 2 days alternating with a day of rest.

Adults – 250 to 375 mg once daily for 1 or 2 days.

Children – 5 mg/kg/dose, oral or IV, once daily in the morning.

Epilepsy:

Adults and Children – 8 to 30 mg/kg/day in divided doses. The optimum range is 375 to 1000 mg daily. When given in combination with other anticonvulsants, the starting dose is 250 mg once daily.

It is not clearly known whether the beneficial effects observed in epilepsy are due to direct inhibition of carbonic anhydrase in the CNS or whether they are due to the slight degree of acidosis produced by the divided dosage. The best results to date have been seen in petit mal in children. Good results, however, have been seen in patients, both children and adult, in other types of seizures such as grand mal, mixed seizure patterns, myoclonic jerk patterns.

Acute mountain sickness: 500 to 1000 mg/day, in divided doses of tablets or sustained release capsules. For rapid ascent (ie, in rescue or military operations), use the higher dose (1000 mg). If possible, initiate dosing 24 to 48 hours before ascent and continue for 48 hours while at high altitude, or longer as needed to control symptoms.

Sustained release: May be used twice daily, but is only indicated for use in glaucoma and acute mountain sickness.

Parenteral: Direct IV administration is preferred; IM administration is painful because of the alkaline pH of the solution.

Preparation and storage of parenteral solution: Reconstitute each 500 mg vial with at least 5 ml of Sterile Water for Injection. Reconstituted solutions retain potency for 1 week if refrigerated. However, since this product contains no preservative, use within 24 hours of reconstitution.

Oral liquid dose form: If required, acetazolamide tablets may be crushed and suspended in a cherry, chocolate, raspberry or other sweet syrup. Do not use a vehicle with alcohol or glycerin. Alternatively, one tablet can be submerged in 10 ml of hot water and added to 10 ml of honey or syrup. When prepared in a 70% sorbitol solution with a pH of 4 to 5 and stored in amber glass bottles, the suspension is stable for at least 2 to 3 months at temperatures < 30°C (86°F).

ACETAZOLAMIDE

Rx	**Acetazolamide** (Various, eg, Mutual, URL)	**Tablets**: 125 mg	In 50s, 100s, 250s, 500s and 1000s.
Rx	**Diamox** (Lederle)		(Diamox 125, D1 LL). White, scored. In 100s.
Rx	**Acetazolamide** (Various, eg, Qualitest, Schein, URL)	**Tablets**: 250 mg	In 100s, 500s, 1000s and UD 100s.
Rx	**Dazamide** (Major)		In 100s, 250s, 1000s and UD 100s.
Rx	**Diamox** (Lederle)		(Diamox 250 D2 LL). White, scored. In 100s, 1000s and UD 100s.
Rx	**Diamox Sequels** (Lederle)	**Capsules, sustained release**: 500 mg	(Diamox D3). Orange. In 30s and 100s.
Rx	**Acetazolamide** (Various, eg, Bedford Labs)	**Powder for injection, lyophilized**: 500 mg	In vials.

DICHLORPHENAMIDE

For complete prescribing information, refer to the Carbonic Anhydrase Inhibitor group monograph.

Administration and Dosage:

Glaucoma: Most effective when given with miotics. In acute angle-closure glaucoma, dichlorphenamide may be used with miotics and osmotic agents to rapidly reduce intraocular tension. If quick relief does not occur, surgery may be mandatory.

Adults: Individualize dosage. *Initial dose* - 100 to 200 mg, followed by 100 mg every 12 hours, until the desired response is obtained.

Maintenance dosage - 25 to 50 mg 1 to 3 times daily.

Rx	**Daranide** (Merck)	**Tablets**: 50 mg	Lactose. (MSD 49). Yellow, scored. In 100s.

METHAZOLAMIDE

For complete prescribing information, refer to the Carbonic Anhydrase Inhibitor group monograph.

Administration and Dosage:

Glaucoma: 50 to 100 mg 2 or 3 times daily. May be used with miotic and osmotic agents.

Rx	**Methazolamide** (Various, eg, Mikart)	**Tablets**: 25 mg	In 100s.
Rx	**GlaucTabs** (Akorn)		In 100s.
Rx	**Neptazane** (Lederle)		(N2). White, square. In 100s.
Rx	**Methazolamide** (Various, eg, Mikart)	**Tablets**: 50 mg	In 100s.
Rx	**GlaucTabs** (Akorn)		In 100s.
Rx	**Neptazane** (Lederle)		(LL N1). White, scored. In 100s.

DIURETIC COMBINATIONS

Fixed-dose combination drugs are not indicated for initial therapy of edema or hypertension; they require therapy titrated to the individual patient. If the fixed combination represents the determined dosage, its use may be more convenient in patient management. The treatment of hypertension and edema is not static; reevaluate as conditions in each patient warrant.

The combination of a thiazide and a potassium-sparing diuretic provides additive diuretic activity and antihypertensive effects through different mechanisms of action and also minimizes the potassium depletion characteristics of thiazides.

Triamterene/Hydrochlorothiazide:

Bioavailability: Use caution when changing to another triamterene/hydrochlorothiazide combination product. Combination products are not equivalent.

For complete information concerning the components of the combined diuretic products, consult the appropriate drug monographs in the Diuretics section.

Administration and Dosage:

Dosage for each combination/strength varies. Refer to labeling for specific guidelines.

Amiloride/Hydrochlorothiazide: 1 to 2 tablets daily with meals.

Spironolactone/Hydrochlorothiazide: 25 mg/25 mg – 1 to 8 tablets daily; *50 mg/50 mg* – 1 to 4 tablets daily.

Triamterene/Hydrochlorothiazide: 37.5 mg/25 mg – 1 or 2 tablets/capsules daily; *50 mg/25 mg* – 1 or 2 capsules twice daily after meals; *75 mg/50 mg* – 1 tablet daily.

Rx	**Amiloride/ Hydrochlorothiazide** (Various, eg, Goldline, Warner Chilcott)	**Tablets:** 5 mg amiloride HCl and 50 mg hydrochlorothiazide	In 100s, 500s and 1000s.
Rx	**Moduretic** (Merck)		Lactose. (917). Peach, scored. Diamond shape. In 100s and UD 100s.
Rx	**Spironolactone/ Hydrochlorothiazide** (Various, eg, Danbury, Geneva, Goldline, Major, Mylan, Schein)	**Tablets:** 25 mg spironolactone and 25 mg hydrochlorothiazide	In 100s, 250s, 500s and 1000s.
Rx	**Aldactazide** (Searle)		(Searle 1011 Aldactazide 25). Tan. Film coated. In 100s, 500s, 1000s and UD 100s.
Rx	**Aldactazide** (Searle)	**Tablets:** 50 mg spironolactone and 50 mg hydrochlorothiazide	(Searle 1021 Aldactazide 50). Tan, scored. In 100s and UD 100s.
Rx	**Triamterene/ Hydrochlorothiazide** (Various, eg, Geneva)	**Tablets:** 37.5 mg triamterene and 25 mg hydrochlorothiazide	In 100s, 500s and 1000s.
Rx	**Maxzide-25MG** (Lederle)		(Maxzide LL M9). Lt. green, scored. Bowtie shape. In 100s, UD 100s.
Rx	**Dyazide** (SmithKline Beecham)	**Capsules**: 37.5 mg triamterene and 25 mg hydrochlorothiazide	Lactose. Red and white. In 1000s, unit-of-use 100s and UD 100s.
Rx	**Triamterene/ Hydrochlorothiazide** (Various, eg, Geneva, Goldline, Sidmak, Zenith)	**Capsules**: 50 mg triamterene and 25 mg hydrochlorothiazide	In 100s and 1000s.
Rx	**Triamterene/ Hydrochlorothiazide** (Various, eg, Barr, Danbury, Geneva, Goldline, Major, Parmed, Schein, Warner Chilcott)	**Tablets:** 75 mg triamterene and 50 mg hydrochlorothiazide	In 100s, 250s, 500s and 1000s.
Rx	**Maxzide** (Lederle)		(Maxzide LL M8). Lt. yellow, scored. Bowtie shape. In 100s, 500s, UD 100s.

OSMOTIC DIURETICS

Actions:

Pharmacology: Osmotic agents induce diuresis by elevating the osmolarity of the glomerular filtrate, thereby hindering the tubular reabsorption of water. Excretion of sodium and chloride is increased. These agents are freely filtered at the glomerulus; poorly reabsorbed by the renal tubule; not secreted by the tubule; relatively pharmacologically inert; usually resistant to metabolic alteration (except glycerin). Activity in the kidneys depends on the concentration of osmotically active particles in solution.

The main indication for osmotic diuretics (primarily mannitol) is prophylaxis of acute renal failure in conditions in which glomerular filtration is greatly reduced (ie, severe trauma, cardiovascular operations). By maintaining a flow of dilute urine, damage to the nephron by high concentrations of toxic solute does not occur. They are also employed to reduce intracranial pressure and elevated intraocular pressure. In the eyes, these agents act by creating an osmotic gradient between the plasma and ocular fluids.

Mannitol is the most widely used osmotic diuretic. The other agents include urea, glycerin and isosorbide. For specific approved indications, refer to individual drug monographs.

Pharmacokinetics: **Mannitol** is only slightly metabolized, while the rest is freely filtered by the glomeruli and excreted intact in urine. About 7% is reabsorbed by the renal tubules. Approximately 90% of an injected dose is recovered in urine after 24 hours. In severe renal insufficiency, the rate of mannitol excretion is greatly reduced; retained mannitol may increase extracellular tonicity, expand the extracellular fluid and induce an apparent hyponatremia with increased serum osmolality.

Osmotic Diuretics Pharmacokinetics

Diuretic	Route	Onset (min)	Peak (hrs)	Duration (hrs)	Half-life	Metabolized (%)	Ocular penetration	Distribution
Glycerin	PO	10-30	1-1.5	4-5	30-45 minutes	80	poor	E[1]
Isosorbide	PO	10-30	1-1.5	5-6	5-9.5 hrs	0	good	TBW[2]
Mannitol	IV	30-60	1	6-8	15-100 minutes	7-10	very poor	E[1]
Urea	IV	30-45	1	5-6	-	-	good	TBW[2]

[1] E = extracellular water
[2] TBW = total body water

MANNITOL

Refer to the general discussion of these agents in the Osmotic Diuretics Introduction.

Indications:

Therapeutic: To promote diuresis in the prevention or treatment of the oliguric phase of acute renal failure before irreversible renal failure becomes established.

Reduction of intracranial pressure and treatment of cerebral edema by reducing brain mass.

Reduction of elevated intraocular pressure when the pressure cannot be lowered by other means.

To promote urinary excretion of toxic substances.

Urologic irrigation (2.5% only): Irrigation in transurethral prostatic resection or other transurethral surgical procedures.

Contraindications:

Anuria due to severe renal disease; severe pulmonary congestion or frank pulmonary edema; active intracranial bleeding except during craniotomy; severe dehydration; progressive renal damage or dysfunction after instituting mannitol therapy, including increasing oliguria and azotemia; progressive heart failure or pulmonary congestion after mannitol therapy.

Warnings:

Fluid and electrolyte imbalance: By sustaining diuresis, mannitol may obscure and intensify inadequate hydration or hypovolemia. Excessive loss of water and electrolytes may lead to serious imbalances. Loss of water in excess of electrolytes can cause hypernatremia. Shift of sodium free intracellular fluid into the extracellular compartment following mannitol infusion may lower serum sodium concentration and aggravate preexisting hyponatremia. Also, movement of potassium ions from intracellular to extracellular space may cause hyperkalemia. Electrolyte measurements, including sodium and potassium, are therefore of vital importance in monitoring mannitol infusion.

Renal function impairment: Use a test dose (see Administration and Dosage); try a second test dose if there is an inadequate response, but do not attempt > two.

If urine output continues to decline during infusion, closely review the patient's clinical status and suspend mannitol infusion, if necessary. Accumulation of mannitol may result in overexpansion of the extracellular fluid which may intensify existing or latent CHF.

Osmotic nephrosis, a reversible vacuolization of the tubules of unknown clinical significance, may proceed to severe irreversible nephrosis; monitor renal function closely.

Pregnancy: Category C. It is not known whether mannitol can cause fetal harm when administered to a pregnant woman or can affect reproduction capacity. Give to a pregnant woman only if clearly needed.

Lactation: It is not known whether this drug is excreted in breast milk; exercise caution when administering to a nursing woman.

Children: Safety and efficacy for patients ≤ 12 years of age has not been established.

Precautions:

CHF: Carefully evaluate cardiovascular status before rapid administration of mannitol since sudden expansion of the extracellular fluid may lead to fulminating CHF.

Hypovolemia: By sustaining diuresis, mannitol may obscure and intensify inadequate hydration or hypovolemia.

Pseudoagglutination: Do not give electrolyte free mannitol solutions with blood. If blood is given simultaneously, add at least 20 mEq of sodium chloride to each liter of mannitol solution to avoid pseudoagglutination.

Hemoconcentration: The obligatory diuretic response following rapid infusion of 15%, 20% or 25% mannitol may further aggravate preexisting hemoconcentration.

Adverse Reactions:

Cardiovascular: Edema; thrombophlebitis; hypotension; hypertension; tachycardia; angina-like chest pains; CHF.

CNS: Headache; blurred vision; convulsions; dizziness.

GI: Nausea; vomiting; diarrhea.

Renal: Urinary retention; osmotic nephrosis.

Metabolic: Fluid and electrolyte imbalance; acidosis; electrolyte loss; dehydration.

Miscellaneous: Pulmonary congestion; dry mouth; thirst; rhinitis; local pain; skin necrosis; chills; urticaria; fever.

MANNITOL

Overdosage:

Symptoms: Larger than recommended doses may result in increased electrolyte excretion, particularly sodium, chloride and potassium. Sodium depletion can result in orthostatic tachycardia or hypotension and decreased central venous pressure. Chloride metabolism closely follows that of sodium. Potassium deficit can impair neuromuscular function and cause intestinal dilation and ileus. If urine flow is inadequate, pulmonary edema or water intoxication may occur. Other symptoms include hypotension, polyuria that rapidly converts to oliguria, stupor, convulsions, hyperosmolality, hyponatremia.

Treatment: Discontinue infusion immediately. Institute supportive measures to correct fluid and electrolyte imbalances. Hemodialysis is beneficial to clear mannitol and reduce serum osmolality.

Administration and Dosage:

Administer by IV infusion only. Individualize concentration and rate of administration. The usual adult dose ranges from 20 to 200 g/24 hours; in most instances, an adequate response will be achieved with 50 to 100 g/24 hours. Adjust the administration rate to maintain a urine flow of at least 30 to 50 ml/hour.

Test dose: For patients with marked oliguria or inadequate renal function, give 0.2 g/kg (about 50 ml of a 25% solution, 75 ml of a 20% solution, or 100 ml of a 15% solution) infused over 3 to 5 minutes. If urine flow does not increase, administer a second test dose. If response is inadequate, reevaluate the patient.

Prevention of acute renal failure (oliguria): Adults – 50 to 100 g as a 5% to 25% solution during cardiovascular and other types of surgery.

Treatment of oliguria: Adults – 50 to 100 g of a 15% to 25% solution.

Reduction of intracranial pressure and brain mass: 1.5 to 2 g/kg as a 15% to 25% solution, infused over 30 to 60 minutes, to reduce brain mass before or after neurosurgery. Evaluate the circulatory and renal reserve, fluid and electrolyte balance, body weight, and total input and output before and after mannitol infusion. Reduced cerebrospinal fluid pressure may be observed within 15 minutes after starting infusion.

Reduction of intraocular pressure: 1.5 to 2 g/kg, as a 20% solution (7.5 to 10 ml/kg) or as a 15% solution (10 to 13 ml/kg) over a period as short as 30 minutes. When used preoperatively, administer 1 to 1.5 hours before surgery to achieve maximal effect.

Adjunctive therapy to promote diuresis in intoxications: The concentration depends on the fluid requirement and urinary output of the patient. Give IV fluids and electrolytes to replace losses. If benefits are not seen after 200 g mannitol, discontinue the infusion.

Urologic irrigation: Use 2.5% solution. The use of 2.5% mannitol solution minimizes hemolytic effect of water alone, the entrance of hemolyzed blood into the circulation, and the resulting hemoglobinemia which is considered a major factor in producing serious renal complications.

Dilution of mannitol – Add contents of two 50 ml vials (25% mannitol) to 900 ml sterile water for injection.

Preparation of solution: When exposed to low temperatures, mannitol solution may crystallize. Concentrations > 15% have a greater tendency to crystallize. If crystals are observed, warm the bottle in a hot water bath, a dry heat oven or autoclave, then cool to body temperature or less before administering.

When infusing concentrated mannitol, the administration set should include a filter.

Rx	**Osmitrol** (Baxter)	**Injection:** 5%	In 1000 ml.
		10%	In 500 and 1000 ml.
		15%	In 500 ml.
		20%	In 250 and 500 ml.
Rx	**Mannitol** (Various, eg, American Regent, Astra, IMS, Lyphomed, Pasadena)	**Injection:** 25%	In 50 ml.

UREA

Refer to the general discussion of these agents in the Osmotic Diuretics Introduction.

Indications:

The 30% solution is used to reduce intracranial pressure (in the control of cerebral edema) and intraocular pressure.

Unlabeled uses: Intra-amniotic injection has been used to induce abortion.

Contraindications:

Severely impaired renal function; active intracranial bleeding; marked dehydration; frank liver failure; infusion into veins of the lower extremities of elderly patients (phlebitis and thrombosis of superficial and deep veins may occur).

Warnings:

Electrolyte imbalance: Urea may cause depletion of electrolytes that can result in hyponatremia and hypokalemia.

Extravasation of the solution at the injection site may cause local reactions ranging from mild irritation to tissue necrosis.

Renal function impairment: Administer with caution. Mild elevation of BUN does not preclude its use. Perform frequent laboratory studies; determine if renal function is adequate to eliminate the infused urea and that produced endogenously.

Patients exhibiting a temporary reduction in urine volume are generally able to maintain a satisfactory elimination of urea. However, if diuresis does not follow the injection of urea in such patients within 6 to 12 hours, withdraw the drug pending further evaluation of renal function.

To ensure bladder emptying, use an indwelling urethral catheter in comatose patients.

Hepatic function impairment: Administer with caution in patients with liver impairment, since there may be a significant rise in blood ammonia levels.

Pregnancy: Category C. Safety for use during pregnancy has not been established. Use only when clearly needed and when the potential benefits outweigh the potential hazards to the fetus.

Lactation: It is not known whether this drug is excreted in breast milk. Exercise caution when administering to a nursing mother.

Precautions:

Intracranial bleeding: Arterial oozing has been reported when intracranial surgery is performed on patients following treatment with urea; however, this has not been a significant problem. Do not use in the presence of active intracranial bleeding unless such use is preliminary to prompt surgical intervention to control hemorrhage. Reduction of brain edema induced by urea may result in reactivation of intracranial bleeding.

Rapid IV administration of hypertonic solutions of urea may be associated with hemolysis as well as a direct effect on the cerebral vasomotor centers that may result in increased capillary bleeding. Do not exceed an infusion rate of 4 ml/minute.

Blood loss: Urea may temporarily maintain circulatory volume and blood pressure in spite of considerable blood loss. Consequently, when excessive blood loss occurs within a short period of time, blood replacement should be adequate and simultaneous with the infusion of urea. Do not administer urea through the same administration set that blood is being infused. Hypothermia, when used with urea infusion, may increase the risk of venous thrombosis and hemoglobinuria.

Drug Interactions:

Lithium: Urea may increase the renal excretion of lithium, thereby decreasing its effects.

Adverse Reactions:

No serious reactions have been noted when solutions are infused slowly, provided renal function is not seriously impaired and there is no active intracranial bleeding. If an adverse reaction occurs, discontinue the infusion, evaluate the patient and institute appropriate therapy; save the remainder of the fluid for examination.

The following reactions have occurred: Headaches (similar to those following lumbar puncture); nausea; vomiting; syncope; disorientation; transient agitated confusional state (less frequent); chemical phlebitis and thrombosis near the injection site (infrequent).

Reactions that may occur because of the reconstituted solution or the technique of administration include: Febrile response; infection at the injection site; venous thrombosis or phlebitis extending from the injection site; extravasation; hypervolemia.

UREA

Overdosage:

In the event of overdosage, as reflected by unusually elevated blood urea nitrogen (BUN) levels, discontinue the drug, evaluate the patient and institute corrective measures.

Administration and Dosage:

Administer as a 30% solution by slow IV infusion, at a rate not to exceed 4 ml/minute.

An isosmotic concentration of dextrose or invert sugar is administered with urea to prevent the hemolysis produced by pure solutions of urea.

Do not exceed 120 g/day.

Adults: 1 to 1.5 g/kg (0.45 to 0.68 g/lb).

Children: 0.5 to 1.5 g/kg. In children up to 2 years of age, as little as 0.1 g/kg may be adequate.

Preparation of solution: For 135 ml of a 30% solution of sterile urea, mix the contents of one 40 g vial with 105 ml of 5% or 10% Dextrose Injection or Invert Sugar. Each ml of a 30% solution provides 300 mg of urea. Use fresh solution; discard any unused portion within 24 hours after reconstitution.

Rx	**Ureaphil** (Abbott)	**Injection:** 40 g per 150 ml	In single-dose containers.

GLYCERIN (Glycerol)

Refer to the general discussion of these agents in the Osmotic Diuretics Introduction.

Actions:

Pharmacology: An oral osmotic agent for reducing intraocular pressure. It adds to the tonicity of the blood until metabolized and eliminated by the kidneys. Maximal reduction of intraocular pressure will occur 1 hour after glycerin administration. The effect will last approximately 5 hours.

Indications:

Glaucoma to interrupt acute attacks.

Prior to and after ocular surgery where reduction of intraocular pressure is indicated.

Unlabeled uses: Glycerin has also been given by the IV route (with proper preparation) to lower intraocular and intracranial pressure.

Contraindications:

Well established anuria; severe dehydration; frank or impending acute pulmonary edema; severe cardiac decompensation; hypersensitivity to any of the ingredients.

Warnings:

Route of administration: For oral use only; not for injection.

Pregnancy: Category C. Safety for use during pregnancy has not been established. Use only when clearly needed and when the potential benefits outweigh the potential hazards to the fetus.

Precautions:

Special risk patients: Use cautiously in hypervolemia, confused mental states, congestive heart disease, diabetic patients, severely dehydrated individuals and cardiac, renal or hepatic disease.

Urinary retention: Avoid acute urinary retention in the preoperative period. Continued use may result in weight gain.

Adverse Reactions:

Nausea, vomiting, headache, confusion and disorientation may occur. Severe dehydration, cardiac arrhythmias or hyperosmolar nonketotic coma which can result in death have been reported.

Administration and Dosage:

1 to 2 g/kg, 1 to 1.5 hours prior to surgery.

Rx	**Osmoglyn** (Alcon)	**Solution:** 50% (0.6 g glycerin/ml)	Lime flavor. In 220 ml.

ISOSORBIDE

Refer to the general discussion of these agents in the Osmotic Diuretics Introduction.

Indications:

For the short-term reduction of intraocular pressure prior to and after intraocular surgery.

May be used to interrupt an acute attack of glaucoma. Use where less risk of nausea and vomiting than that posed by other oral hyperosmotic agents is needed.

Contraindications:

Well established anuria; severe dehydration; frank or impending acute pulmonary edema; severe cardiac decompensation; hypersensitivity to any component of this preparation.

Warnings:

Fluid/Electrolyte balance: With repeated doses, maintain adequate fluid and electrolyte balance.

Urinary output: If urinary output continues to decrease, closely review the patient's clinical status. Accumulation may result in overexpansion of the extracellular fluid.

Pregnancy: Category B. There is no adequate information on whether this drug affects fertility in humans or has a teratogenic potential or other adverse fetal effect. Use during pregnancy only if clearly needed.

Precautions:

Repetitive doses: Use repetitive doses with caution, particularly in patients with diseases associated with salt retention. Ensure that the patient's bladder has been emptied prior to surgery.

Adverse Reactions:

Nausea; vomiting; headache; confusion; disorientation; gastric discomfort; thirst; hiccoughs; hypernatremia; hyperosmolarity; rash; irritability; syncope; lethargy; vertigo; dizziness; lightheadedness.

Administration and Dosage:

For oral use only.

Initial dose: 1.5 g/kg (equivalent to 1.5 ml/lb).

Dose range: 1 to 3 g/kg 2 to 4 times a day as indicated.

Palatability may be improved if the medication is poured over cracked ice and sipped.

Rx	**Ismotic** (Alcon)	**Solution:** 45% (100 g per 220 ml)	With 4.6 mEq sodium and 0.9 mEq potassium per 220 ml. Alcohol, saccharin, sorbitol. Vanilla-mint flavor. In 220 ml.

NONPRESCRIPTION DIURETICS

Nonprescription diuretic products are promoted for the alleviation of menstrual discomfort. When taken 5 to 6 days before onset of menses, *otc* diuretics may help relieve symptoms related to water retention. These include: Excess water weight, bloating, swelling, painful breasts, cramps and tension.

The most frequently used *otc* diuretic agents are ammonium chloride and caffeine. These agents are classified as Category I (generally recognized as safe and effective and not misbranded).

AMMONIUM CHLORIDE, an acid-forming salt, has limited value in promoting diuresis (4 to 5 days). Its use in combination with caffeine is effective in water weight reduction. Doses up to 3 g/day may be given in divided doses 3 times daily for up to 6 days. Large doses (4 to 12 g/day) may cause GI symptoms including nausea and vomiting. CNS toxicity including headache, hyperventilation, drowsiness and mental confusion may also occur. Ammonium chloride is contraindicated in patients with impaired renal and liver function; metabolic acidosis may occur.

CAFFEINE, a xanthine derivative, promotes diuresis through inhibition of renal tubular reabsorption of sodium and chloride. Caffeine is effective for relief of premenstrual and menstrual symptoms in doses of 100 to 200 mg every 3 to 4 hours. Doses > 100 mg may cause GI irritation by augmenting gastric secretions. Advise patients that caffeine-containing products taken within 4 hours of bedtime may cause sleeplessness. Consider this when drinking coffee, tea, hot chocolate or colas, and when taking other caffeine-containing products.

Administration and Dosage:

Aqua•Ban: 2 tablets 3 times daily after meals. Take at onset of symptoms for ≤ 6 days.

Aqua•Ban Plus: 1 tablet 3 times daily after meals. Take at onset of symptoms for ≤ 6 days.

otc	**Aqua•Ban** (Thompson Medical)	**Tablets, enteric coated**: 325 mg ammonium chloride, 100 mg caffeine	In 60s.
otc	**Aqua•Ban Plus** (Thompson Medical)	**Tablets, enteric coated**: 650 mg ammonium chloride, 20 mg caffeine, 6 mg iron (as ferrous sulfate)	In 30s.
otc	**Maximum Strength Aqua•Ban** (Thompson Medical)	Tablets: 50 mg pamabrom	Lactose. In 30s.

CARDIAC GLYCOSIDES

The cardiac (or digitalis) glycosides include: Digitoxin, derived from *Digitalis purpurea;* and digoxin, derived from *Digitalis lanata.*

Actions:

Pharmacology: The influence of the digitalis glycosides on the myocardium is dose-related, and involves both a direct action on cardiac muscle and the specialized conduction system, and indirect actions on the cardiovascular system mediated by the autonomic nervous system. These indirect actions involve a vagomimetic action, which is responsible for the depression of the sinoatrial (SA) node and the prolonged conduction to the atrioventricular (AV) node; and also a baroreceptor sensitization which results in increased carotid sinus nerve activity and enhanced sympathetic withdrawal for any given increment in mean arterial pressure.

Direct effects include increasing the force and velocity of myocardial systolic contraction (positive inotropic action), increasing the refractory period of the AV node and increasing total peripheral resistance. In higher doses, digitalis increases sympathetic outflow from the CNS to both cardiac and peripheral sympathetic nerves, which may increase atrial or ventricular rate. This increase in sympathetic activity may be an important factor in digitalis cardiac toxicity. Most of the extracardiac manifestations of digitalis toxicity are also mediated by the CNS.

Mechanism – The cellular basis for the inotropic effects of the digitalis glycosides appears to be inhibition of sodium, potassium-ATPase in the sarcolemmal membrane, which alters excitation-contraction coupling, that process by which chemical energy is converted into mechanical energy when triggered by membrane depolarization. In the myocardium, calcium enters the cell by the slow calcium channel during the action potential, which triggers the release of calcium from intracellular binding sites on the sarcoplasmic reticulum. The digitalis glycosides by inhibiting sodium and potassium-ATPase, make more calcium available to activate the contractile proteins actin and myosin, thereby enhancing the force of myocardial contraction.

Pharmacokinetics:

Absorption – Absorption following oral administration is a function of polarity; digitoxin is well absorbed. Digoxin tablets are absorbed 60% to 80%; the elixir is absorbed 70% to 85% and a solution-filled capsule is 90% to 100%. When oral digoxin is taken after meals, the rate of absorption is slowed but total amount absorbed is usually unchanged. However, when taken with meals high in bran fiber, the amount absorbed may be reduced.

In some patients, orally administered digoxin is converted to cardioinactive reduction products (eg, dihydrodigoxin) by colonic bacteria in the gut thereby reducing its bioavailability. Although inactivation of these bacteria by antibiotics is rapid, serum digoxin concentration will rise at a rate consistent with elimination half-life of digoxin. Magnitude of rise in serum digoxin concentration relates to extent of bacterial inactivation, and may be as much as 2-fold in some cases. This interaction is significantly reduced if digoxin is given as digoxin solution in capsules. Data suggest that one in ten patients treated with digoxin tablets will degrade ≥ 40% of the ingested dose.

Distribution – Cardiac glycosides are widely distributed in tissues; high concentrations are found in the myocardium, skeletal muscle, liver, brain and kidneys. Digoxin crosses both the blood-brain barrier and the placenta. At delivery, serum digoxin concentration in the newborn is similar to the serum level in the mother. Serum digoxin concentrations are not significantly altered by large changes in fat tissue weight, so that distribution space correlates best with lean (ideal) body weight.

Excretion – Digitoxin is inactivated by hepatic degradation, 50% to 80% to inactive metabolites (excreted by the kidneys). About 8% is converted to digoxin; 50% to 75% of digoxin is excreted unchanged by the kidneys,largely as parent drug and active metabolites, which include digitoxigenin, bisdigitoxoside, digoxigenin monodigitoxoside and dihydrodigoxin. In patients with impaired renal function, significant accumulation may occur with digoxin.

Because of the long half-lives of these agents, clinical effects do not fully develop until steady-state plasma levels are achieved. Conversely, several days are required for complete dissipation of effects following therapy discontinuation (ie, 6 to 8 days for digoxin and 3 to 5 weeks for digitoxin). Digoxin is not effectively removed by dialysis, exchange transfusion or during cardiopulmonary bypass, since most is found in tissue rather than circulating in the blood. Digitoxin is not effectively removed by peritoneal or hemodialysis, probably because of its high degree of plasma-protein binding.

CARDIAC GLYCOSIDES

Glycoside serum levels: The relationship of serum digitalis glycoside levels to signs or symptoms of intoxication varies significantly from patient to patient; therefore, the value and limitations of this test must be recognized. It is difficult to establish normal glycoside levels that would accurately define toxicity. Digoxin effect can be expected with steady-state serum concentrations of 1 to 1.5 mg/ml with low risk of toxicity.

Pharmacokinetic Parameters of Digitalis Glycosides

Digitalis glycoside	Route	Onset (minutes)	Peak (hours)	Plasma t½ (hours)	% GI absorption	% Protein binding	Major route of elimination
Digoxin	PO IV	30 - 120 5 - 30	2 - 6 1 - 5	30 - 40[1]	60 - 100	20 - 25	Renal
Digitoxin	PO	60-240	8-12	118-216	90-100	90 - 97	Hepatic, ≈ 32%; Renal (metabolites)

[1] In anuric patients: 100+ hours.

Digitalis Glycoside Serum Levels

Digitalis glycoside	Drug serum levels (ng/ml)	
	Therapeutic	Toxic
Digitoxin	9 to 25	> 35
Digoxin	0.5 to 2.2	> 2.5

Indications:

Congestive heart failure (CHF) all degrees: Increased cardiac output results in diuresis and general amelioration of disturbances characteristic of right heart failure (venous congestion, edema) and left heart failure (dyspnea, orthopnea, cardiac asthma). Digitalis is generally most effective in "low-output" failure and less effective in "high-output" failure (bronchopulmonary insufficiency, arteriovenous fistula, anemia, infection, hyperthyroidism).

Atrial fibrillation, especially when the ventricular rate is elevated. Digitalis rapidly reduces ventricular rates and eliminates the pulse deficit. Palpitation, precordial distress or weakness are relieved and concomitant congestive failure ameliorated. Continue digitalis in doses necessary to maintain the desired ventricular rate, both at rest and in response to exercise and other clinical effects.

Atrial flutter: Digitalis slows the heart; normal sinus rhythm may appear. Often, flutter is converted to atrial fibrillation. Stopping treatment at this point may restore sinus rhythm, especially if the flutter was paroxysmal. It is preferable to continue digitalis if failure ensues or if atrial flutter occurs often (electrical cardioversion is often the treatment of choice for atrial flutter).

Contraindications:

Previous toxic response; ventricular fibrillation; ventricular tachycardia, unless congestive failure supervenes after protracted episode not due to digitalis; presence of digitalis toxicity; beriberi heart disease, hypersensitivity to digoxin; some cases of hypersensitive carotid sinus syndrome. Allergy, though rare, may occur (may not extend to all cardiac glycosides; another may be tried).

Warnings:

Long term use in CHF: The drug is generally continued after heart failure is abolished unless some other known precipitating factor is corrected. Hemodynamic effects can be demonstrated in almost all patients, but corresponding improvement in signs and symptoms of heart failure is not necessarily apparent. In patients in whom digoxin may be difficult to regulate, or in whom risk of toxicity may be great (eg, patients with unstable renal function or whose potassium levels tend to fluctuate), consider a cautious withdrawal of digoxin. If digoxin is discontinued, regularly monitor for clinical evidence of recurrent heart failure.

Obesity: Digitalis alone or with other drugs has been promoted for use in the treatment of obesity. Potentially fatal arrhythmias or other adverse effects make the use of these drugs in treating obesity dangerous and unwarranted.

Digitalis toxicity: Many of the arrhythmias for which digitalis is indicated are identical with those reflecting digitalis intoxication. If digitalis intoxication cannot be excluded, cardiac glycosides should be withheld temporarily, if the clinical situation permits. Determination of drug serum levels may be helpful.

Since symptoms of anorexia, nausea and vomiting may be associated with digitalis intoxication and CHF, a clinical determination of their cause must be made before further administration of the drug.

CARDIAC GLYCOSIDES

When the risk of digitalis intoxication is great, use digoxin, which is a relatively short-acting, rapidly eliminated glycoside. Although intoxication cannot always be prevented by the selection of one glycoside over another, one may be preferred in patients who have fixed disabilities (eg, liver impairment, drug intolerance). Digitoxin can be used in patients with impaired renal function.

Severe carditis: Patients with severe carditis, such as carditis associated with rheumatic fever or viral myocarditis, are especially sensitive to digoxin-induced disturbances in rhythm.

Cardiovascular disease: Electrical conversion of arrhythmias may require reduction of dosage to avoid induction of ventricular arrhythmias. However, consider the consequences of rapid increase in ventricular response to atrial fibrillation if digoxin is withheld 1 to 2 days prior to cardioversion. If digitalis toxicity might exist, delay elective cardioversion. If it is not prudent to delay cardioversion, select a minimal energy level at first and carefully increase to avoid precipitating ventricular arrhythmias.

Exercise great caution when giving digitalis to patients still experiencing effects from previous digitalis preparations.

Patients with incomplete AV block, especially if subject to Stokes-Adams attacks, may develop advanced or complete heart block if given digitalis.

In patients with acute or unstable chronic atrial fibrillation, digitalis may not normalize the ventricular rate even when the serum concentration exceeds the usual therapeutic level. Although these patients may be less sensitive to the toxic effects of digitalis than patients with normal sinus rhythm, do not increase dosage to potentially toxic levels.

Patients with acute myocardial infarction (MI), severe pulmonary disease, severe carditis (eg, carditis associated with rheumatic fever or viral myocarditis) or advanced heart failure may be more sensitive to digitalis and more prone to disturbances of rhythm. If heart failure develops, digitalization may be tried with relatively low doses and cautiously increased until a beneficial effect is obtained. If a therapeutic trial does not result in improvement, discontinue drug. Patients with chronic constrictive pericarditis may fail to respond to digitalis. In addition, slowing of the heart rate by digoxin in some patients may further decrease cardiac output.

Cases of idiopathic hypertrophic subaortic stenosis must be managed with extreme care (outflow obstruction may worsen). Unless cardiac failure is severe, it is doubtful that digitalis should be employed.

In patients with Wolff-Parkinson-White Syndrome and atrial fibrillation, digoxin can enhance transmission of impulses through the accessory pathway. This may result in extremely rapid ventricular rates and even ventricular fibrillation.

In some patients with sinus node disease (ie, sick sinus syndrome), digoxin may worsen sinus bradycardia or sinoatrial block.

Renal function impairment: Renal insufficiency delays excretion of digoxin; adjust dosage in patients with renal disease. Digitoxin may be given in usual doses. Digoxin toxicity also develops more frequently and lasts longer in renal impairment because of decreased digoxin excretion.

The presence of acute glomerulonephritis accompanied by CHF requires extreme care in digitalization. A relatively low total dose, administered in divided doses, and concomitant use of antihypertensive agents has been recommended. Constant ECG monitoring is essential. Discontinue digitalis as soon as possible.

Dialysis (peritoneal and hemodialysis) has little effect on any of these glycosides.

Combined renal and hepatic failure may prolong digoxin elimination more than normally expected.

Hepatic function impairment: Impaired hepatic function does not appear to significantly alter transformation or effects of digoxin; however, reduction in digitoxin dosage may be necessary.

Elderly: Exercise special care in elderly patients because their body mass tends to be small and renal clearance is likely to be reduced.

Pregnancy: Category C. Both digoxin and digitoxin rapidly pass into the fetus in a concentration of 50% to 83% of maternal serum. Maternally administered digoxin has been used to treat fetal tachycardia and CHF; fetal toxicity and neonatal death have been a consequence of maternal overdosage. The dosing and control of digoxin in pregnancy may be less predictable than in nonpregnant patients. It is not known whether cardiac glycosides cause fetal harm when administered to a pregnant woman or affect reproduction capacity. Use only when clearly needed and when the potential benefits outweigh the potential hazards to the fetus.

CARDIAC GLYCOSIDES

Lactation: Digoxin is excreted into breast milk at a milk:plasma ratio of 0.6 to 0.9. The amount the infant receives is very small and no infant adverse effects have been reported. Safety for use in the nursing mother has not been established. It is not known whether **digitoxin** is excreted in breast milk; exercise caution when administering to a nursing woman.

Children: Newborn infants display considerable variability in tolerance. Premature and immature infants are particularly sensitive; dosage must be reduced and digitalization should be even more individualized according to infant's degree of maturity. Digitalis glycosides are an important cause of accidental poisoning in children. Impaired renal function must also be taken into consideration.

Carefully titrate dose. ECG monitoring may be necessary to avoid intoxication.

Precautions:

Electrolyte imbalance:

Potassium – Hypokalemia sensitizes the myocardium to digitalis and may reduce the positive inotropic effect of digitalis. Toxicity may develop even with "normal" serum glycoside levels. Therefore, it is desirable to maintain normal serum potassium levels. Potassium wastage may result from diuretic or corticosteroid therapy, hemodialysis or from suction of GI secretions. It may accompany malnutrition, diarrhea, prolonged vomiting, old age or long-standing CHF. Also, infusion of carbohydrate solution may lower serum potassium by causing an intracellular shift of potassium. In general, avoid rapid changes in serum potassium or other electrolytes; reserve treatment of CHF with IV potassium for special circumstances (see Treatment of Toxicity).

Calcium – Calcium, particularly when administered rapidly IV, may produce serious arrhythmias in digitalized patients. Hypercalcemia from any cause predisposes the patient to digitalis toxicity. However, hypocalcemia can nullify the effects of digoxin; thus, digoxin may be ineffective until serum calcium is restored to normal.

Magnesium – Hypomagnesemia may predispose to digitalis toxicity. If low magnesium levels are detected in a patient receiving digoxin, institute replacement therapy.

Thyroid dysfunction: The plasma levels of cardiac glycosides are inversely related to thyroid status. In myxedema, digitalis requirements are less because excretion rate is decreased. In thyrotoxic patients with heart failure, larger doses of the glycoside may be necessary. Results may not be satisfactory until the hyperthyroidism is corrected.

Atrial arrhythmias associated with hypermetabolic states are particularly resistant to digitalis treatment; avoid toxicity if digitalis is used to treat these arrhythmias. Digoxin requirements are reduced in hypothyroidism; digoxin responses in patients with compensated thyroid disease are normal.

Laboratory tests: Perform periodic determinations of heart rate, electrolytes (especially potassium), ECG and renal function (BUN or serum creatinine). Digoxin may produce false positive ST-T changes in ECG during exercise testing.

Serum digoxin concentrations – It may also be useful to measure glycoside serum concentrations periodically, especially if digitalis intoxication is suspected.

The relationship of serum glycoside levels to signs or symptoms of intoxication varies significantly from patient to patient; therefore, the value and limitations of this test must be recognized. It is difficult to establish normal glycoside levels that would accurately define toxicity.

To allow adequate time for equilibration of digoxin between serum and tissue, sample serum concentrations at least 6 to 8 hours after the last dose. Ideally, sampling for assessment of steady-state concentrations should be done just before the next dose. Interpret the serum concentration data in the overall clinical context; do not use an isolated serum concentration value alone as a basis for increasing or decreasing digoxin dosage.

CARDIAC GLYCOSIDES

Drug Interactions:

Increased digoxin serum levels: The following agents may increase digoxin serum levels via various mechanisms (eg, altered GI flora, increased absorption, decreased clearance), possibly increasing its therapeutic and toxic effects:

Drugs That May Increase Digitalis Serum Levels	
Alprazolam	Hydroxychloroquine
Aminoglycosides, oral[1]	Ibuprofen
Amiodarone	Indomethacin
Anticholinergics	Itraconazole
Benzodiazepines	Nifedipine[3]
Bepridil	Omeprazole
Captopril	Propafenone
Cyclosporine	Propantheline
Diltiazem[2]	Quinidine[2, 3]
Diphenoxylate	Quinine
Erythromycin[1]	Tetracycline[1]
Esmolol	Tolbutamide
Felodipine	Verapamil[2]
Flecainide	

[1] Occurs in < 10% of patients.
[2] Though not as well established, digitoxin data appear similar.
[3] Despite increased levels, positive inotropic effect of digoxin may be diminished.

Decreased digitalis serum levels: The following agents may decrease digitalis serum levels, possibly decreasing therapeutic effects.

DrugsThat May Decrease Digitalis Serum Levels	
Aminoglutethimide	Colestipol
Aminoglycosides, oral	Hydantoins
Aminosalicylic acid	Hypoglycemic agents (oral)
Antacids (aluminum or magnesium salts)	Kaolin/pectin
Antihistamines	Metoclopramide[1]
Antineoplastics, combination (bleomycin, carmustine, cyclophosphamide, cytarabine, doxorubicin, methotrexate, procarbazine, vincristine)[1]	Neomycin
	Penicillamine
	Rifampin
	Sucralfate
Barbiturates	Sulfasalazine
Cholestyramine[1]	

[1] The absorption of the gelatin capsule and elixir formulations of digoxin may not be affected to as great an extent.

Albuterol: Unknown. Possible enhanced skeletal muscle binding of digoxin.

Beta blockers: AV nodal conduction can result in complete heart block.

Disopyramide may alter pharmacologic effects of digoxin, although one study suggests a beneficial pharmacodynamic interaction occurs.

Nondepolarizing muscle relaxants and succinylcholine: When administered with digitalis glycosides, toxicity (cardiac arrhythmias) of either agent may be increased.

Potassium-sparing diuretics: Spironolactone may increase or decrease toxic effects of digitalis glycosides; changes cannot be predicted; monitoring is required. Spironolactone may interfere with some digoxin assays. **Amiloride** may decrease inotropic effects of digoxin; **triamterene** may increase its pharmacologic effects.

Sympathomimetics: Concomitant use with digoxin can increase the risk of cardiac arrhythmias because both enhance ectopic pacemaker activity.

Thiazide and loop diuretics and amphotericin B increase urinary potassium loss; hypokalemia may increase effects and toxicity of digitalis glycosides. Magnesium excretion is increased and possibly sensitizes myocardium to effects of digitalis glycosides. Observe for clinical signs of fluid or electrolyte imbalance; replace electrolytes as appropriate.

Thyroid hormones and thioamines: Thyroid hormones may decrease therapeutic effectiveness of digitalis glycosides; thioamines may increase their therapeutic and toxic effects. Euthyroid patients usually require no dosage adjustment of the digitalis glycoside. However, when converting a patient from hypothyroid or hyperthyroid state to euthyroid state, dosage adjustment may be necessary (see Precautions).

CARDIAC GLYCOSIDES

Drug/Food interactions: When oral digoxin is taken after meals, the rate of absorption is slowed but total amount absorbed is usually unchanged. However, when taken with meals high in bran fiber, the amount absorbed may be reduced.

Adverse Reactions:

The frequency and severity of adverse reactions to digoxin depend on dose and route of administration, and on the patient's underlying disease or concomitant therapy. Overall incidence of adverse reactions is 5% to 20%, with 15% to 20% considered serious (1% to 4% of patients receiving digoxin). Evidence suggests that the incidence of toxicity has decreased since the introduction of serum digoxin assay and improved standardization of digoxin tablets. Cardiac toxicity accounts for about 50%, GI disturbances for about 25% and CNS and other toxicity for about 25% of these adverse reactions.

Anorexia, nausea and vomiting may occur. These effects are central in origin, but following large oral doses, there is also a local emetic action. Abdominal discomfort or pain and diarrhea may also occur. Gynecomastia and allergy (skin rash, eosinophilia, thrombocytopenia and vasculitis), sexual dysfunction and sweating can occur, but are rare.

Overdosage:

Symptoms:

GI – Most common early symptoms are anorexia, nausea, vomiting and diarrhea. However, uncontrolled heart failure may also produce such symptoms. Abdominal discomfort or pain often accompanies GI symptoms. Digitalis toxicity very rarely may cause hemorrhagic necrosis of the intestines.

CNS – Headache, weakness, apathy, drowsiness, visual disturbances (blurred, yellow vision; halo effect), confusion, restlessness, disorientation, seizures, EEG abnormalities, delirium, hallucinations, neuralgia, psychosis.

Cardiac disturbances – Ventricular tachycardia may result from digitalis toxicity. Unifocal or multiform premature ventricular contractions (PVCs), especially in bigeminal or trigeminal patterns, are the most common toxic arrhythmias. Paroxysmal and nonparoxysmal nodal rhythms, AV dissociation, accelerated junctional (nodal) rhythm and PAT with block are also common. Excessive slowing of the pulse is a clinical sign of overdosage. AV block of increasing degree may proceed to complete heart block. Atrial fibrillation can occur following large doses of digitalis. Ventricular fibrillation is the most common cause of death from digitalis poisoning.The ECG is fundamental in determining the presence and nature of these cardiac disturbances. Other ECG changes (PR prolongations, the ST depression) provide no measure of the degree of digitalization.

Alterations in cardiac rate and rhythm occurring in digitalis poisoning may simulate almost any known type of arrhythmia seen clinically. Extrasystoles are probably the most frequent effect. An ECG is necessary to aid in differentiation of arrhythmia due to digitalis poisoning from that due to heart disease. Older patients, particularly those with disease of the coronary arteries and impaired myocardial blood supply, are more susceptible to these untoward effects. Sinus arrhythmia may occur early as a minor toxic effect. Paroxysmal atrial and ventricular tachycardia call for immediate cessation of the drug.

Children – Toxicity differs from the adult in a number of respects. Anorexia, nausea, vomiting, diarrhea, neurologic and visual disturbances are rarely seen as initial signs of digitalis toxicity in children. Visual disturbances (blurred or yellow vision), headache, weakness, apathy and psychosis may occur but may be difficult to recognize in infants and children. Cardiac arrhythmias are more frequent and reliable signs of toxicity. Digoxin in children may produce any arrhythmia. Common manifestations of digitalis toxicity in children include conduction disturbances or supraventricular tachyarrhythmias, such as AV block (Wenckebach), atrial tachycardia with or without block and junctional (nodal) tachycardia. Ventricular arrhythmias such as unifocal or multiform ventricular premature contractions, especially in bigeminal or trigeminal patterns are less common. Ventricular tachycardia may result from digitalis toxicity. Sinus bradycardia may also be a sign of impending digoxin intoxication, especially in infants, even in the absence of first degree heart block. Any arrhythmia or alteration in cardiac conduction that develops in a child taking digoxin should initially be assumed to be a consequence of digoxin intoxication.

Treatment:

Adults – Discontinue digitalis until all signs of toxicity are abolished. This may be all that is necessary if toxic manifestations are not severe and appear after peak effect of the drug.

CARDIAC GLYCOSIDES

Potassium salts are commonly used, particularly if hypokalemia is present. Potassium chloride in divided oral doses totaling 3 to 6 g (40 to 80 mEq) for adults may be given, provided renal function is adequate. When correction of arrhythmia is urgent and serum potassium level is low to normal, give potassium IV in 5% Dextrose Injection. For adults, give a total of 40 to 80 mEq (diluted to a concentration of 40 mEq/500 ml) at a rate ≤ 20 mEq/hour, or slower if limited by pain due to local irritation. Give additional amounts if arrhythmia is uncontrolled and potassium and fluid volume are well tolerated. Monitor the ECG to avoid potassium toxicity (eg, peaking of T waves) and to observe the arrhythmia so that infusion may be stopped when desired effect is achieved. Do not use potassium when severe or complete heart block is due to digitalis and not related to tachycardia. Potassium is contraindicated in the presence of renal failure.

Phenytoin: For atrial and ventricular arrhythmias unresponsive to potassium, administer phenytoin 50 to 100 mg every 5 minutes. The maximum dose should not exceed 600 mg.

Lidocaine: 1 mg/kg over 5 minutes, then infusing 15 to 50 mcg/kg/min to maintain normal cardiac rhythm may be an alternative.

Cholestyramine, colestipol or activated charcoal may be useful in digitalis toxicity by binding the glycoside in the intestine, thus preventing enterohepatic recirculation.

Atropine: Severe sinus bradycardia or a slow ventricular rate due to secondary AV block may be symptomatically treated with atropine (0.01 mg/kg, IV).

Other agents used for the treatment of digitalis toxicity include quinidine, disopyramide, procainamide and propranolol. Other antiarrhythmics appear less successful or more hazardous. In advanced heart block, temporary ventricular pacing may be beneficial.

Countershock: Interruption of life-threatening arrhythmias by direct-current countershock is considered hazardous in digitalis overdosage and should be the last resort. If countershock is required, begin therapy at low voltage levels.

Digoxin immune FAB: A new treatment of digitalis intoxication is digoxin immune FAB (see individual monograph in the Miscellaneous chapter). Given in approximate equimolar quantities as digoxin, it generally reverses all signs and symptoms of toxicity. Improvement usually begins within 30 minutes of administration.

Children – Potassium preparations may be given orally in divided doses totaling 1 to 1.5 mEq/kg. When correction of the arrhythmia is urgent, give ≈ 0.5 mEq/kg/hr of potassium, with careful ECG monitoring. The potassium IV solution should be dilute enough to avoid local irritation; however, take care to avoid IV fluid overload, especially in infants. Digoxin immune FAB may also be used in infants and children.

Patient Information:

Do not discontinue medication without first checking with a physician.

Avoid *otc* antacids, cough, cold, allergy and diet drugs, except on professional advice.

Notify physician if loss of appetite, lower stomach pain, nausea, vomiting, diarrhea, unusual tiredness or weakness, drowsiness, headache, blurred or yellow vision, skin rash or hives, or mental depression occurs.

Administration and Dosage:

Loading doses: The use of initial large loading doses rapidly establishes effective plasma levels, but also increases risks of toxicity because of its narrow toxic-therapeutic ratio. Administration of small daily maintenance doses are then given to replace daily losses due to metabolism and excretion. Without a loading dose, slow digitalization may be achieved within 1 week with digoxin and in 10 to 14 days with digitoxin, with a much lower risk of toxicity than when giving a loading dose. For a rapid effect in acutely ill patients, parenteral administration of digoxin can be used. Use parenterally only when the drug cannot be taken orally or rapid digitalization is urgent.

Maintenance therapy: Maintenance dosage is determined tentatively by the amount necessary to sustain the desired therapeutic effect. Recommended dosages are practical average figures which may require considerable modification as dictated by individual sensitivity or associated conditions. Diminished renal function is the most important factor requiring modification of recommended doses of digoxin.

DIGITOXIN

For complete prescribing information, refer to the Cardiac Glycosides group monograph.

Administration and Dosage:

Loading dose:

Rapid – 0.6 mg initially, followed by 0.4 mg, then 0.2 mg at intervals of 4 to 6 hours.

Slow – 0.2 mg twice daily for a period of 4 days, followed by maintenance dosage.

Maintenance: Ranges from 0.05 to 0.3 mg daily, the most common dose being 0.15 mg daily.

Children: Individualize dosage. Monitor ECG to avoid toxic doses.

Generally, premature and immature infants are particularly sensitive and require a reduced dosage that must be determined by careful adjustment. Divide the total dose into 3, 4 or more portions, with 6 hours or more between doses.

After the neonatal period, the recommended digitalizing dose is as follows –

Under one year of age: 0.045 mg/kg.

One to two years of age: 0.04 mg/kg.

Over two years of age: 0.03 mg/kg (0.75 mg/m^2).

Maintenance dose – Administer one-tenth (10%) of the digitalizing dose.

Rx	**Crystodigin** (Lilly)	**Tablets:** 0.05 mg	Orange, scored. In 100s.
		Tablets: 0.1 mg	Pink, scored. In 100s.

DIGOXIN

For complete prescribing information, refer to the Cardiac Glycosides group monograph.

Administration and Dosage:

Parenteral administration: The IV digitalizing dose is ≈ 20% less than an oral dose. Intramuscular injection offers no advantages and can cause severe pain at injection site; IV administration is preferred. Give injections over 5 minutes or longer, undiluted or diluted with a 4–fold or greater volume of Sterile Water for Injection, 0.9% Sodium Chloride Injection, 5% Dextrose Injection or Lactated Ringer's Injection. Use of less diluent could lead to digoxin precipitation. Use diluted product immediately.

Adults: Rapid digitalization with a loading dose – Peak body digoxin stores of 8 to 12 mcg/kg should provide therapeutic effect. Larger stores (10 to 15 mcg/kg) are often required for control of ventricular rate in patients with atrial flutter or fibrillation. Use conservative projected peak body stores for patients with renal insufficiency (ie, 6 to 10 mcg/kg). Base the loading dose on the projected peak body stores and administer in several portions with roughly half the total given as the first dose. Give additional fractions at 4 to 8 hour intervals IV or orally, with careful assessment of clinical response before each additional dose.

In undigitalized patients, a single initial IV dose of 400 to 600 mcg (0.4 to 0.6 mg) usually produces a detectable effect in 5 to 30 minutes that becomes maximal in 1 to 4 hours. The usual parenteral amount for a 70 kg patient to achieve 8 to 15 mcg/kg peak body stores is 600 to 1000 mcg (0.6 to 1 mg). A single initial oral dose of 500 to 750 mcg (0.5 to 0.75 mg) usually produces a detectable effect in 0.5 to 2 hours that becomes maximal in 2 to 6 hours. The usual oral amount required for a 70 kg patient to achieve 8 to 15 mcg/kg peak body stores is 750 to 1250 mcg (0.75 to 1.25 mg).

Base the maintenance dose upon the percentage of the peak body stores lost each day through elimination. The following formula has wide clinical use:

$$\text{Maintenance dose} = \text{Peak Body Stores (ie, Loading Dose)} \times \frac{\text{\% Daily Loss}}{100}$$

$$\text{\% Daily Loss} = 14 + \text{Ccr}/5.$$

Ccr is creatinine clearance, corrected to 70 kg body weight or 1.73 m^2 body surface area.

Gradual digitalization with a maintenance dose – The following table provides average oral (tablet) daily maintenance dose requirements for patients with heart failure based upon lean body weight and renal function:

DIGOXIN

Usual Digoxin Tablet Daily Maintenance Dose Requirements (mcg) For Estimated Peak Body Stores of 10 mcg/kg[1]

Corrected Ccr (ml/min/70 kg)	Lean Body Weight (kg/lbs) 50/110	60/132	70/154	80/176	90/198	100/220	Number of days before steady-state achieved
0	63[2]	125	125	125	188[3]	188	22
10	125	125	125	188	188	188	19
20	125	125	188	188	188	250	16
30	125	188	188	188	250	250	14
40	125	188	188	250	250	250	13
50	188	188	250	250	250	250	12
60	188	188	250	250	250	375	11
70	188	250	250	250	250	375	10
80	188	250	250	250	375	375	9
90	188	250	250	250	375	500	8
100	250	250	250	375	375	500	7

[1] Example - A patient with an estimated lean body weight of 70 kg and a Ccr of 60 ml/min should be given a 250 mcg (0.25 mg) tablet each day. Steady-state serum concentrations should not be anticipated before 11 days.

[2] ½ of 125 mcg tablet or 125 mcg every other day.

[3] 1½ of 125 mcg tablet.

Usual Digoxin Solution Filled Capsule Daily Maintenance Dose Requirements (mcg) For Estimated Peak Body Stores of 10 mcg/kg

Corrected Ccr (ml/min/70 kg)	Lean Body Weight (kg/lbs) 50/110	60/132	70/154	80/176	90/198	100/220	Number of days before steady-state achieved
0	50	100	100	100	150	150	22
10	100	100	100	150	150	150	19
20	100	100	150	150	150	200	16
30	100	150	150	150	200	200	14
40	100	150	150	200	200	250	13
50	150	150	200	200	250	250	12
60	150	150	200	200	250	300	11
70	150	200	200	250	250	300	10
80	150	200	200	250	300	300	9
90	150	200	250	250	300	350	8
100	200	200	250	300	300	350	7

Infants and children: Individualize dosage. Divided daily dosing is recommended for infants and young children under 10 years of age. Children over 10 require adult dosages in proportion to their body weight.

Rapid digitalization with a loading dose – Digitalizing and daily maintenance doses for each age group are given below. Larger doses are often required for adequate control of ventricular rate in patients with atrial flutter or fibrillation.

Administer loading dose in several portions, give roughly half the total as the first dose. Give additional fractions of total dose at 6 to 8 hr intervals (oral) or 4 to 8 hr intervals (parenteral). Carefully assess clinical response before each additional dose.

DIGOXIN

Usual Digitalizing and Maintenance Dosages with Normal Renal Function Based on Lean Body Weight			
Age	Digitalizing Dose[1] (mcg/kg)		Daily maintenance dose (mcg/kg)
	Oral	IV	
Premature	20-30	15-25	20%-30% of the loading dose[2]
Full term	25-35	20-30	25%-35% of the loading dose[2]
1-24 months	35-60	30-50	
2-5 years	30-40	25-35	
5-10 years	20-35	15-30	
Over 10 years	10-15	8-12	

[1] IV digitalizing doses are 80% of oral digitalizing doses.
[2] Projected or actual digitalizing dose providing desired clinical response.

Gradual digitalization is accomplished by beginning an appropriate maintenance dose. The range of percentages provided above can be used in calculating this dose. *Both the adult and pediatric dosage guidelines provided are based upon average patient response; substantial individual variation can be expected.*

Adjust maintenance dose in previously digitalized patients at steady state in proportion to the ratio of desired vs measured serum concentration (ie, doubling the dose results in doubling the serum concentration).

Lanoxicaps (gelatin capsules) have greater bioavailability than standard tablets. Therefore, the 0.2 mg capsule is equivalent to 0.25 mg tablets; the 0.1 mg capsule is equivalent to 0.125 mg tablets; and the 0.05 mg capsule is equivalent to 0.0625 mg.

Use in the elderly: Since digoxin is eliminated by the kidneys, a decreased clearance may occur in elderly patients with decreased renal function. Therefore, a lower maintenance dose of digoxin may be necessary. Adjust the dose accordingly.

Rx	**Lanoxicaps** (Glaxo Wellcome)	**Capsules:** 0.05 mg	(A2C). In 100s.
		0.1 mg	(B2C). In 30s and 100s.
		0.2 mg	(C2C). In 30s and 100s.
Rx	**Digoxin** (Various, eg Alra, Qualitest, Rugby, Vangard)	**Tablets:** 0.125 mg	In 100s, 1000s and 5000s and UD 100s.
Rx	**Lanoxin** (Glaxo Wellcome)		Lactose. (Lanoxin Y3B). In 30s, 100s, 1000s, 5000s and UD 100s.
Rx	**Digoxin** (Various, eg Alra, Qualitest, Rugby, Vangard)	**Tablets:** 0.25 mg	In 100s and 1000s.
Rx	**Lanoxin** (Glaxo Wellcome)		Lactose. (Lanoxin X3A). In 30s, 100s, 1000s, 5000s and UD 100s.
Rx	**Digoxin** (Various, eg Alra)	**Tablets:** 0.5 mg	In 100s.
Rx	**Lanoxin** (Glaxo Wellcome)		Lactose. (Lanoxin T9A). In 100s.
Rx	**Digoxin**[1] (Various, eg, Bausch & Lomb, Liquipharm, Roxane)	**Elixir, pediatric:** 0.05 mg/ml	In 50 ml and UD 2.5 and 5 ml.
Rx	**Lanoxin** (Glaxo Wellcome)		10% alcohol. Lime flavor. In 60 ml with dropper.
Rx	**Digoxin** (Elkins-Sinn)	**Injection:** 0.25 mg/ml	In 2 ml amps.[2]
Rx	**Digoxin** (Wyeth Ayerst)		In 1 and 2 ml Tubex.[3]
Rx	**Lanoxin** (Glaxo Wellcome)		In 2 ml amps.[3]
Rx	**Lanoxin** (Glaxo Wellcome)	**Injection, pediatric:** 0.1 mg/ml	In 1 ml amps.[3]

[1] May contain 10% alcohol.
[2] With 0.1 ml alcohol and 0.4 ml propylene glycol per ml.
[3] With 40% propylene glycol and 10% alcohol.

AMRINONE LACTATE

Actions:

Pharmacology: Amrinone is a positive inotropic agent with vasodilator activity, different in structure and mode of action from either digitalis glycosides or catecholamines. Its mechanism has not been fully elucidated.

Amrinone is not a beta-adrenergic agonist. It inhibits myocardial cyclic adenosine monophosphate (c-AMP) phosphodiesterase activity and increases cellular levels of c–AMP. It does not inhibit sodium-potassium ATPase activity.

Amrinone reduces afterload and preload by its direct relaxant effect on vascular smooth muscle. In patients with depressed myocardial function, amrinone produces a prompt increase in cardiac output due to its inotropic and vasodilator actions.

Improvement in left ventricular function and relief of congestive heart failure (CHF) in patients with ischemic heart disease have been observed without inducing symptoms or electrocardiographic signs of myocardial ischemia.

Amrinone produces hemodynamic and symptomatic benefits to patients not satisfactorily controlled by conventional therapy with diuretics and cardiac glycosides.

Pharmacokinetics:

Distribution – Amrinone has a volume of distribution of 1.2 liters/kg and a distribution half-life of ≈ 4.6 minutes. It is 10% to 49% protein bound. In CHF patients, after a loading bolus dose, steady-state plasma levels of about 2.4 mcg/ml are maintained by an infusion of 5 to 10 mcg/kg/min. With associated compromised renal and hepatic perfusion, plasma levels may rise.

Metabolism/Excretion – Amrinone is metabolized by conjugative pathways. Mean elimination half-life is ≈ 3.6 hours. In patients with CHF, the mean elimination half-life is ≈ 5.8 hours (range, 3 to 15 hours).

The primary route of excretion is via the urine as both amrinone and metabolites. Approximately 63% of an oral dose is excreted in the urine over 96 hours. Approximately 18% is excreted in the feces in 72 hours. In a 24 hour IV amrinone study, 10% to 40% was excreted unchanged in the urine.

Onset/Duration/Effect: Dose-related maximum increases in cardiac output occur; the peak effect occurs within 10 minutes at all doses. The duration of effect depends upon the dose, lasting ≈ 30 minutes at 0.75 mg/kg and ≈ 2 hours at 3 mg/kg. Increases in cardiac index show a linear relationship to plasma concentration.

Pulmonary capillary wedge pressure (PCWP) and total peripheral resistance show dose-related decreases. At doses up to 3 mg/kg, dose-related decreases in diastolic pressure (up to 13%) have been observed. Mean arterial pressure decreases (9.7%) at a dose of 3 mg/kg. Heart rate is generally unchanged.

Children: Infants and children have a larger volume of distribution and a decreased elimination half-life.

Indications:

Congestive heart failure (CHF): For the short-term management of CHF. Use only in patients who can be closely monitored and who have not responded adequately to digitalis, diuretics or vasodilators. Duration of therapy depends on patient responsiveness.

Contraindications:

Hypersensitivity to amrinone or bisulfites.

Warnings:

Atrial flutter/fibrillation: Amrinone's inotropic effects are additive to those of digitalis. In cases of atrial flutter/fibrillation, amrinone may increase ventricular response rate because of its slight enhancement of atrioventricular (AV) conduction. In these cases, prior treatment with digitalis is recommended.

Hepatotoxicity: If acute marked alterations in liver enzymes occur together with clinical symptoms, discontinue amrinone. If less than marked enzyme alterations occur without clinical symptoms, continue amrinone, reduce dosage or discontinue the drug based on benefit-to-risk considerations.

Hypersensitivity: Hypersensitivity occurred in patients treated for about 2 weeks with oral amrinone (see Adverse Reactions). Consider hypersensitivity reactions in any patient maintained for a prolonged period on amrinone. Refer to Management of Acute Hypersensitivity Reactions.

Carcinogenesis: Dystocia occurred in rats receiving 100 mg/kg/day, resulting in increased numbers of stillbirths, decreased litter size and poor pup survival.

Pregnancy: Category C. Animal studies (15 to 50 mg/kg) are conflicting. There are no adequate and well controlled studies in pregnant women. Use during pregnancy only if the potential benefit justifies the potential risk to the fetus.

Lactation: It is not known whether amrinone is secreted in breast milk. Exercise caution when administering to nursing women.

AMRINONE LACTATE

Children: Safety and efficacy in children have not been established. In a preterm infant, the short-term use of amrinone (5 mcg/kg/min) was effective in the management of the infant's CHF (see Pharmacokinetics).

Precautions:

Aortic or pulmonic valvular disease: Do not use amrinone in patients with severe aortic or pulmonic valvular disease in lieu of surgical relief of the obstruction. It may aggravate outflow tract obstruction in hypertrophic subaortic stenosis.

Arrhythmias, supraventricular and ventricular, have been observed in the very high-risk population treated. While amrinone per se is not arrhythmogenic, the potential for arrhythmia present in CHF itself may be increased by any drug or drug combination.

Thrombocytopenia is more common in patients receiving prolonged therapy. In patients whose platelet counts were not allowed to remain depressed, no bleeding occurred.

Platelet reduction is dose-dependent and appears to be due to a decreased platelet survival time. Bone marrow examinations were normal. There is no evidence of immune response or a platelet-activating factor.

Management of adverse reactions:

Platelet count reductions – Asymptomatic platelet count reduction (to < 150,000/mm^3) may be reversed within 1 week of a decrease in drug dosage. Further, with no change in drug dosage, the count may stabilize at lower than pre-drug levels without any clinical sequelae. Pre-drug platelet counts and frequent platelet counts during therapy are recommended. If a platelet count < 150,000mm^3 occurs, consider the following:

- Maintain total daily dose unchanged.
- Decrease total daily dose.
- Discontinue if risk exceeds the potential benefit.

Acute myocardial infarction: No clinical trials have been carried out in patients in the acute phase of postmyocardial infarction. Therefore, amrinone is not recommended in these cases.

Fluid balance: Patients who have received vigorous diuretic therapy may have insufficient cardiac filling pressure to respond adequately to amrinone; cautious liberalization of fluid and electrolyte intake may be indicated.

Monitoring:

Fluids and electrolytes – Monitor fluid and electrolyte changes and renal function during amrinone therapy; improvement in cardiac output with resultant diuresis may necessitate a reduction in the dose of diuretic. Potassium loss due to excessive diuresis may predispose digitalized patients to arrhythmias. Therefore, correct hypokalemia by potassium supplementation in advance of or during amrinone use.

Blood pressure and heart rate: Monitor blood pressure and heart rate and slow or stop the infusion rate in patients showing excessive decreases in blood pressure.

Central venous pressure (CVP): Monitoring CVP may be valuable in assessing hypotension and fluid balance management. Also, measure urine output and body weight.

Sulfite sensitivity: This product contains sodium metabisulfite, a sulfite that may cause allergic-type reactions (including anaphylactic symptoms and life-threatening or less severe asthmatic episodes) in certain susceptible people. The overall prevalence of sulfite sensitivity in the general population is unknown and probably low. Sulfite sensitivity is seen more frequently in asthmatic people.

Adverse Reactions:

Body as a whole: Thrombocytopenia (< 100,000/mm^3) (2.4%); fever (0.9%); chest pain (0.2%); burning at the injection site (0.2%).

Cardiovascular: Arrhythmia (3%); hypotension (1.3%).

GI: Nausea (1.7%); vomiting (0.9%); abdominal pain, anorexia (0.4%); hepatotoxicity (see Warnings). Should severe or debilitating GI effects occur, reduce dosage or discontinue the drug based on the usual benefit-to-risk considerations.

Hypersensitivity: Pericarditis, pleuritis and ascites (fatal in 1 case), myositis with interstitial shadowing on chest x-ray and elevated sedimentation rate (1 case) and vasculitis with nodular pulmonary densities, hypoxemia and jaundice with oral amrinone (see Warnings).

AMRINONE LACTATE

Overdosage:

A death has occurred with a massive accidental overdose, although the causal relationship is uncertain. Exercise diligence during product preparation and administration.

Amrinone's vasodilator effect may produce hypotension. If this occurs, reduce or discontinue administration. Institute general measures for circulatory support. Refer to Management of Acute Overdosage.

Administration and Dosage:

Administer as supplied or dilute in 0.5% or 0.9% saline solution to a concentration of 1 to 3 mg/ml. Use diluted solutions within 24 hours.

Initial therapy: 0.75 mg/kg IV bolus slowly over 2 to 3 minutes.

Maintenance infusion: 5 to 10 mcg/kg/min.

An additional bolus of 0.75 mg/kg may be given 30 minutes after initiating therapy.

Do not exceed a total daily dose (including loading doses) of 10 mg/kg. A limited number of patients studied at higher doses support a dosage regimen of up to 18 mg/kg/day for shortened durations of therapy.

Adjust rate of administration and duration of therapy according to patient response.

The above dosing regimen creates a plasma concentration of ≈ 3 mcg/ml.

Admixture incompatibilities:

Dextrose solution – A chemical interaction occurs slowly over a 24 hour period when amrinone is mixed directly with dextrose-containing solutions. Therefore, do not dilute with dextrose-containing solutions prior to injection. Amrinone may be injected into a running dextrose infusion through a Y–connector or directly into the tubing where preferable.

Furosemide – When furosemide is injected into an IV line of amrinone infusion, a precipitate immediately forms. Do not administer furosemide in IV lines containing amrinone.

Storage/Stability: Protect ampuls from light. Store at room temperature.

Rx	**Inocor** (Sanofi Winthrop)	**Injection:** 5 mg/ml (as lactate)	In 20 ml amps.[1]

[1] With 0.25 mg/ml sodium metabisulfite.

MILRINONE LACTATE

Actions:

Pharmacology: Milrinone is a member of a new class of bipyridine inotropic/vasodilator agents with phosphodiesterase inhibitor activity. It is a positive inotrope and vasodilator, with little chronotropic activity, different in structure and mode of action from either the digitalis glycosides or catecholamines.

At relevant inotropic and vasorelaxant concentrations, milrinone is a selective inhibitor of peak III cAMP phosphodiesterase isozyme in cardiac and vascular muscle. This inhibitory action is consistent with cAMP-mediated increases in intracellular ionized calcium and contractile force in cardiac muscle, as well as with cAMP-dependent contractile protein phosphorylation and relaxation in vascular muscle. Additional experimental evidence indicates that milrinone is not a beta-adrenergic agonist nor does it inhibit sodium-potassium adenosine triphosphatase activity as do the digitalis glycosides.

In patients with congestive heart failure (CHF) milrinone produces dose-related and plasma drug concentration-related increases in the maximum rate of increase of left ventricular pressure. Milrinone has a direct inotropic effect and direct arterial vasodilator activity. Both the inotropic and vasodilatory effects occur over the therapeutic range of plasma concentrations of 100 to 300 ng/ml. In addition to increasing myocardial contractility, milrinone improves diastolic function as evidenced by improvements in left ventricular diastolic relaxation.

In patients with depressed myocardial function, milrinone produced a prompt increase in cardiac output and decreases in pulmonary capillary wedge pressure and vascular resistance, without a significant increase in heart rate or myocardial oxygen consumption. These hemodynamic improvements were dose and plasma concentration related. Hemodynamic improvement during IV therapy was accompanied by clinical symptomatic improvement. The great majority of patients experience improvements in hemodynamic function within 5 to 15 minutes of the initiation of therapy.

In CHF patients, milrinone (administered as a loading injection followed by a maintenance infusion) produced significant mean initial increases in cardiac index, significant decreases in pulmonary capillary wedge pressure and significant decreases in systemic vascular resistance. The heart rate was generally unchanged. Mean arterial pressure fell by up to 5% at the two lower dose regimens, but by 17% at the highest dose. Patients evaluated for 48 hours maintained improvements in hemodynamic function, with no evidence of diminished response (tachyphylaxis). A smaller number of patients have received infusions for periods up to 72 hours without evidence of tachyphylaxis.

The duration of therapy should depend on patient responsiveness. Patients have been maintained on infusions for up to 5 days.

Milrinone has a favorable inotropic effect in fully digitalized patients without causing signs of glycoside toxicity. Theoretically, in cases of atrial flutter/fibrillation, it is possible that milrinone may increase ventricular response rate because of its slight enhancement of AV node conduction. In these cases, consider digitalis prior to the institution of therapy.

Improvement in left ventricular function in patients with ischemic heart disease has occurred. The improvement has occurred without inducing symptoms or ECG signs of myocardial ischemia.

Pharmacokinetics: The steady-state plasma concentrations after ≈ 6 to 12 hours of unchanging maintenance infusion of 0.5 mcg/kg/min are ≈ 200 ng/ml. Near maximum favorable effects on cardiac output and pulmonary capillary wedge pressure are seen at plasma concentrations in the 150 to 250 ng/ml range. Following IV injections of 12.5 to 125 mcg/kg to CHF patients, milrinone had a volume of distribution of 0.38 L/kg, a mean terminal elimination half-life of 2.3 hours and a clearance of 0.13 L/kg/hr. Following IV infusions of 0.2 to 0.7 mcg/kg/min to CHF patients, the drug had a volume of distribution of about 0.45 L/kg, a mean terminal elimination half-life of 2.4 hours and a clearance of 0.14 L/kg/hr. These pharmacokinetic parameters were not dose-dependent, and the area under the plasma concentration vs time curve following injections was significantly dose-dependent. Milrinone is ≈ 70% bound to plasma protein.

MILRINONE LACTATE

The primary route of excretion is via the urine. The major urinary excretions of orally administered milrinone are milrinone (83%) and its 0-glucuronide metabolite (12%). Elimination in healthy subjects via the urine is rapid, with ≈ 60% recovered within the first 2 hours following dosing and ≈ 90% recovered within the first 8 hours following dosing. The mean renal clearance is ≈ 0.3 L/min, indicative of active secretion.

Clinical trials:

Oral – In a single, multicenter, double-blind trial of the chronic administration of oral milrinone, patients with New York Heart Association (NYHA) class III and IV heart failure and left ventricular ejection fraction of < 35% were randomized to placebo (n = 527) or oral milrinone (40 mg daily, n = 561) and followed for a median of 6 months. Statistically, the oral milrinone treatment group significantly increased all-cause mortality and cardiovascular mortality. This finding in patients on oral milrinone was not apparent during the initial period of chronic treatment (15 days) in either the overall patient population or in the NYHA class IV subgroup.

IV – The acute administration of IV milrinone has been evaluated in clinical trials in > 1600 patients with chronic heart failure, heart failure associated with cardiac surgery and heart failure associated with myocardial infarction. The total number of deaths, either on therapy or shortly thereafter (24 hours) was 15 (< 9%), few of which were thought to be drug-related.

Indications:

Congestive heart failure (CHF): Short-term IV therapy. The majority of experience has been in patients receiving digoxin and diuretics.

Contraindications:

Hypersensitivity to the drug.

Warnings:

Life-threatening arrhythmias were infrequent and, when present, have been associated with certain underlying factors such as pre-existing arrhythmias, metabolic abnormalities (eg, hypokalemia), abnormal digoxin levels and catheter insertion. Supraventricular arrhythmias occurred in 3.8% of the patients; the incidence of both supraventricular and ventricular arrhythmias has not been related to the dose or plasma milrinone concentration.

Elderly: There are no special dosage recommendations for the elderly patient. Patients in all age groups demonstrated clinically and statistically significant responses. No age-related effects on the incidence of adverse reactions have been observed. Controlled pharmacokinetic studies have not disclosed any age-related effects on the distribution and elimination of milrinone.

Pregnancy: Category C. An increased resorption rate was apparent at both 8 and 12 mg/kg/day doses of IV milrinone in pregnant rabbits. There are no adequate and well controlled studies in pregnant women. Use during pregnancy only if the potential benefit justifies the potential risk to the fetus.

Lactation: It is not known whether milrinone is excreted in breast milk. Exercise caution when milrinone is administered to nursing women.

Children: Safety and efficacy have not been established.

Precautions:

Monitoring:

Electrolytes – Carefully monitor fluid and electrolyte changes and renal function during therapy. Improvement in cardiac output with resultant diuresis may necessitate a reduction in the dose of diuretic. Potassium loss due to excessive diuresis may predispose digitalized patients to arrhythmias. Therefore, correct hypokalemia by potassium supplementation in advance of or during use of milrinone.

MILRINONE LACTATE

Blood pressure and heart rate – During therapy monitor blood pressure and heart rate, and slow or stop the rate of infusion in patients showing excessive decreases in blood pressure. If prior vigorous diuretic therapy is suspected to have caused significant decreases in cardiac filling pressure, cautiously administer milrinone with monitoring of blood pressure, heart rate and clinical symptomatology.

Cardiovascular effects:

Obstructive aortic or pulmonic valvular disease – Do not use in patients with severe obstructive aortic or pulmonic valvular disease in lieu of surgical relief of the obstruction. Like other inotropic agents, it may aggravate outflow tract obstruction in hypertrophic subaortic stenosis.

Supraventricular and ventricular arrhythmias have occurred in the high-risk population treated. In some patients, IV and oral milrinone have increased ventricular ectopy, including nonsustained ventricular tachycardia. The potential for arrhythmia, present in CHF itself, may be increased by many drugs or combinations of drugs. Closely monitor patients receiving milrinone during infusion.

Atrial flutter/fibrillation – Milrinone produces a slight shortening of AV node conduction time, indicating a potential for an increased ventricular response rate in patients with atrial flutter/fibrillation which is not controlled with digitalis therapy.

Adverse Reactions:

Cardiovascular: Ventricular arrhythmias (12.1%), including ventricular ectopic activity (8.5%); hypotension (2.9%); nonsustained ventricular tachycardia (2.8%); angina/chest pain (1.2%); sustained ventricular tachycardia (1%); ventricular fibrillation (0.2%).

Miscellaneous: Headaches, usually mild to moderate in severity (2.9%); hypokalemia (0.6%); tremors, thrombocytopenia (0.4%); bronchospasm (rare).

Overdosage:

Doses of milrinone may produce hypotension because of its vasodilator effects. If this occurs, reduce or temporarily discontinue administration of milrinone until the patient's condition stabilizes. No specific antidote is known, but use general measures for circulatory support. Refer to General Management of Acute Overdosage.

Administration and Dosage:

Approved by the FDA in December 1987.

Administer with a loading dose followed by a continuous infusion (maintenance dose) according to the following guidelines. Adjust the infusion rate according to hemodynamic and clinical response. Most patients show an improvement in hemodynamic status as evidenced by increases in cardiac output and reductions in pulmonary capillary wedge pressure.

Milrinone Dosing		
Loading dose 50 mcg/kg: Administer slowly over 10 minutes		
Maintenance dose[1]		
	Infusion rate	Total daily dose (24 hours)
Minimum	0.375 mcg/kg/min	0.59 mg/kg
Standard	0.5 mcg/kg/min	0.77 mg/kg
Maximum	0.75 mcg/kg/min	1.13 mg/kg

[1] Administer as a continuous IV infusion.

MILRINONE LACTATE

Milrinone Rates of Infusion (ml/kg/hr)[1]			
Maintenance dose	Concentration		
Milrinone (mcg/kg/min)	100 mcg/ml[2]	150 mcg/ml[3]	200 mcg/ml[4]
0.375	0.22	0.15	0.11
0.4	0.24	0.16	0.12
0.5	0.3	0.2	0.15
0.6	0.36	0.24	0.18
0.7	0.42	0.28	0.21
0.75	0.45	0.3	0.22

[1] In order to calculate flow rate (ml/hr), multiply infusion delivery rate times patient weight (in kg).
[2] Prepare by adding 180 ml diluent per 20 mg vial (20 ml).
[3] Prepare by adding 113 ml diluent per 20 mg vial (20 ml).
[4] Prepare by adding 80 ml diluent per 20 mg vial (20 ml).

Dilute with 0.45% or 0.9% Sodium Chloride Injection or 5% Dextrose Injection only.

Renal function impairment: Presence of renal impairment significantly increases the terminal elimination half-life of milrinone. Reductions in infusion rate may be necessary. For patients with clinical evidence of renal impairment, use the following table.

Milrinone Infusion Rate in Impaired Renal Function	
Creatinine clearance (ml/min/1.73 m^2)	Infusion rate (mcg/kg/min)
50	0.43
40	0.38
30	0.33
20	0.28
10	0.23
5	0.2

Dosage may be titrated to the maximum hemodynamic effect and should not exceed 1.13 mg/kg/day. Duration of therapy should depend on patient responsiveness.

Admixture incompatibility: There is an immediate chemical interaction which is evidenced by the formation of a precipitate when furosemide is injected into an IV line of an infusion of milrinone.

Storage/Stability: Store at room temperature 15° to 30°C (59° to 86°F).

Rx	**Primacor** (Sanofi Winthrop)	**Injection:** 1 mg/ml[1]	In 10 and 20 ml single-dose vials and 5 ml *Carpuject* sterile cartridge-needle units with *InterLink* system cannula.
		Injection, premixed: 200 mcg/ml in 5% Dextrose Injection[2]	In 100 ml.

[1] With 47 mg anhydrous dextrose.
[2] With 0.282 mg/ml lactic acid.

Antianginal agents include rapid-acting nitrates used to relieve the pain of acute angina and long-acting preparations used for prophylaxis or to decrease the severity of angina pectoris. Dipyridamole, β-adrenergic blocking agents and the calcium channel blockers are also used in the prophylaxis of chronic angina. Refer to individual monographs.

NITRATES

Actions:

Pharmacology: Relaxation of vascular smooth muscle via stimulation of intracellular cyclic guanosine monophosphate production is the principal pharmacologic action of nitrates. Although venous effects predominate, nitroglycerin produces a dose-dependent dilation of both arterial and venous beds. Dilation of the postcapillary vessels, including large veins, promotes peripheral pooling of blood and decreases venous return to the heart, reducing left ventricular end-diastolic pressure (preload). Arteriolar relaxation reduces systemic vascular resistance and arterial pressure (afterload). Myocardial oxygen consumption or demand (as measured by the pressure-rate product, tension-time index and stroke-work index) is decreased by both arterial and venous effects of nitroglycerin, and a more favorable supply-demand ratio is achieved. In coronary circulation, the nitrates redistribute circulating blood flow along collateral channels, improving perfusion to the ischemic myocardium. While the large epicardial coronary arteries are also dilated by nitroglycerin, the extent to which this action contributes to relief of exertional angina is unclear.

Therapeutic doses reduce systolic, diastolic and mean arterial blood pressure. Effective coronary perfusion pressure is usually maintained, but can be compromised if blood pressure falls excessively or increased heart rate decreases diastolic filling time. Elevated central venous and pulmonary capillary wedge pressures (PCWP), pulmonary vascular resistance and systemic vascular resistance are also reduced. Reflex tachycardia may occur, presumably in response to decreased blood pressure. Cardiac index may be increased, decreased or unchanged. Patients with elevated left ventricular filling pressure and systemic vascular resistance values with a depressed cardiac index are likely to have improved cardiac index. When filling pressures and cardiac index are normal, cardiac index may be slightly reduced by nitrates.

Pharmacokinetics:

Doseform, Onset and Duration of Available Nitrates

Nitrates	Dosage form	Onset (minutes)	Duration
Amyl nitrite	Inhalant	0.5	3 to 5 min
Nitroglycerin	IV	1 to 2	3 to 5 min
	Sublingual	1 to 3	30 to 60 min
	Translingual spray	2	30 to 60 min
	Transmucosal tablet	1 to 2	3 to 5 hours[1]
	Oral, sustained release	20 to 45	3 to 8 hours
	Topical ointment	30 to 60	2 to 12 hours[2]
	Transdermal	30 to 60	up to 24 hours[3]
Isosorbide dinitrate	Sublingual	2 to 5	1 to 3 hours
	Oral	20 to 40	4 to 6 hours
	Oral, sustained release	up to 4 hours	6 to 8 hours
Isosorbide mononitrate	Oral	30 to 60	nd

nd = No data.

[1] A significant antianginal effect can persist for 5 hours if the tablet has not completely dissolved by this time.

[2] Depends on total amount used per unit of surface area.

[3] Tolerance may develop after 12 hours (see Precautions and Administration and Dosage).

NITRATES

Nitroglycerin, isosorbide dinitrate and erythrityl tetranitrate are readily absorbed from the sublingual mucosa. Nitroglycerin is also absorbed through the skin. Nitroglycerin ointments and transdermal systems provide a gradual release of the drug which reaches target organs before hepatic inactivation.

Nitroglycerin has a short half-life, estimated at 1 to 4 minutes, resulting in a low plasma concentration after IV infusion. At plasma concentrations between 50 and 500 ng/ml, plasma protein binding of nitroglycerin is approximately 60%.

Nitrates are metabolized in the liver by nitrate reductase. Although less potent as vasodilators, the two active major metabolites, 1,2 and 1,3 dinitroglycerols, have longer plasma half-lives than the parent compound and appear in substantial concentration; therefore, they may be responsible for some of the pharmacologic activity. Dinitrates are further metabolized to inactive mononitrates. Isosorbide dinitrate, however, is metabolized to 2- and 5-mononitrates, which are both active and accumulate more than the parent drug with long-term therapy, and ultimately to glycerol and CO_2. Since isosorbide mononitrate is a major active metabolite of isosorbide dinitrate, and since most of the clinical activity of the dinitrate is attributable to the mononitrate, isosorbide mononitrate is now available as a single entity product.

Extensive first-pass deactivation follows GI absorption. Hepatic reductase activity may be saturated by some oral nitroglycerin doses, resulting in prolonged pharmacologic effects.

Approximately one-third of an inhaled dose of amyl nitrite is excreted in the urine.

Indications:

Acute angina (nitroglycerin-sublingual, transmucosal or translingual spray; isosorbide dinitrate-sublingual; amyl nitrite): For relief of acute anginal episodes; prophylaxis prior to events likely to provoke an attack. Because of the more rapid relief of chest pain with sublingual nitroglycerin, limit the use of sublingual isosorbide dinitrate for aborting an acute anginal attack to patients intolerant or unresponsive to sublingual nitroglycerin.

Angina prophylaxis (nitroglycerin-topical, transdermal, translingual spray, transmucosal and oral sustained release; isosorbide dinitrate; isosorbide mononitrate; erythrityl tetranitrate; pentaerythritol tetranitrate): Prophylaxis and long-term management of recurrent angina.

Nitroglycerin IV: Control of blood pressure in perioperative hypertension associated with surgical procedures, especially cardiovascular procedures, such as endotracheal intubation, anesthesia, skin incision, sternotomy, cardiac bypass and in the immediate postsurgical period.

Congestive heart failure (CHF) associated with acute myocardial infarction (MI); treatment of angina pectoris unresponsive to organic nitrates or β-blockers; production of controlled hypotension during surgical procedures.

Unlabeled uses: Sublingual and topical nitroglycerin and oral nitrates have been used to reduce cardiac workload in patients with acute MI and in CHF.

Nitroglycerin ointment has been used as adjunctive treatment of Raynaud's disease and other peripheral vascular diseases. A synergistic effect (reduced platelet deposition and increased platelet survival) occurred when isosorbide dinitrate (40 mg/day) and prostaglandin E_1 (5 ng/kg/min for 6 hours) were used in patients with peripheral vascular disease. It may also be beneficial as an aid to venous cannulation in children < 1 year of age using a dose of 0.4 to 0.8 mg.

IV nitroglycerin (5 to 100 mcg/min infusion) may be used in the treatment of hypertensive crisis, specifically in patients who have hypertension with angina or MI.

Refer to the following individual drug monographs for FDA labeled indications.

Contraindications:

Hypersensitivity or idiosyncrasy to nitrates; severe anemia; closed angle glaucoma; postural hypotension; early MI (sublingual nitroglycerin); head trauma or cerebral hemorrhage (since these drugs may increase intracranial pressure); allergy to adhesives (transdermal).

Amyl nitrite: Pregnancy (see Warnings).

Nitroglycerin IV: Hypotension or uncorrected hypovolemia, since IV use in such states could produce severe hypotension or shock; inadequate cerebral circulation; increased intracranial pressure; constrictive pericarditis; pericardial tamponade.

Warnings:

MI: Data supporting the use of nitrates during the early days of the acute phase of MI are insufficient to establish safety. In acute MI, use nitrates only under close clinical observation and with hemodynamic monitoring. In general, a long-acting form should not be used because its effects are difficult to terminate rapidly should excessive hypotension or tachycardia develop. The effects of isosorbide mononitrate are difficult to terminate rapidly; avoid use in patients with acute MI or CHF.

Arcing: A cardioverter/defibrillator should not be discharged through a paddle electrode that overlies a transdermal nitroglycerin system. The arcing that may be seen in this situation is harmless in itself, but it may be associated with local current concentration that can cause damage to the paddles and burns to the patient.

Postural hypotension may occur, even with small doses. Transient episodes of dizziness, weakness, syncope or other signs of cerebral ischemia due to postural hypotension may develop following administration, particularly if the patient is standing immobile. Alcohol accentuates this reaction. Use measures which facilitate venous return (eg, head-low posture, deep breathing, movements of the extremities) to hasten recovery. Fatalities have occurred.

Angina: Nitrates may aggravate angina caused by hypertrophic cardiomyopathy.

Nitroglycerin IV: The available preparations differ in concentration or volume per vial or ampul. When switching from one product to another, pay attention to the dilution, dosage and administration instructions. Some of these products contain alcohol and propylene glycol; safety for intracoronary injection has not been established.

Absorption – Nitroglycerin readily migrates into many plastics. To avoid absorption of nitroglycerin into plastic parenteral solution containers, dilute and store only in glass parenteral solution bottles. Since some filters also absorb nitroglycerin, avoid if possible (see IV Administration and Dosage).

Hepatic or renal disease, severe – Use with caution.

Hypotension – Avoid excessive prolonged hypotension, because of possible deleterious effects on the brain, heart, liver and kidney from poor perfusion and the attendant risk of ischemia, thrombosis and altered organ function. Paradoxical bradycardia and increased angina pectoris may accompany nitroglycerin-induced hypotension. Use with caution in subjects who may have volume depletion from diuretics or in those with low systolic blood pressure (eg, < 90 mmHg). Patients with normal or low PCWP are especially sensitive to the hypotensive effects of IV nitroglycerin. A fall in PCWP precedes the onset of arterial hypotension; the PCWP is thus a useful guide to safe titration of the drug.

Alcohol intoxication has developed in patients on high-dose IV nitroglycerin. Consider this complication when administering high doses for prolonged periods.

Sublingual nitroglycerin: Absorption is dependent on salivary secretion. Dry mouth (including drug-induced dry mouth) decreases absorption.

Transdermal nitroglycerin is not for immediate relief of anginal attacks.

Pregnancy: Category C. Safety for use is not established. Use only when clearly needed and when potential benefits outweigh potential hazards to the fetus.

Category X (amyl nitrite). Because it markedly reduces systemic blood pressure and blood flow on the maternal side of the placenta, amyl nitrite can cause harm to the fetus when it is administered to a pregnant woman.

Lactation: It is not known whether nitrates are excreted in breast milk. Exercise caution when administering to a nursing woman.

Because of the potential for serious adverse reactions in nursing infants from **amyl nitrite,** decide whether to discontinue nursing or to discontinue the drug, taking into account the importance of the drug to the mother.

Children: Safety and efficacy for use in children have not been established.

Precautions:

Tolerance to vascular and antianginal effects of nitrates may develop. Several well controlled clinical trials have used exercise testing to assess the antianginal efficacy of continuously delivered nitrates. In the large majority of these trials, active agents were indistinguishable from placebo after 24 hours or less of continuous therapy. Attempts to overcome nitrate tolerance by dose escalation even to doses far in excess of those used acutely, have consistently failed. Only after nitrates had been absent from the body for several hours was their antianginal efficacy restored.

The use of a low-nitrate or nitrate-free period should be part of the therapeutic strategy. Tolerance may be altered with short periods (10 to 12 hours) of nitrate withdrawal. Minimize tolerance by using smallest effective dose, by using pulse therapy (intermittent dosing) or by alternating with other coronary vasodilators. It is generally recommended to take the last daily dose of a short-acting agent no later than 7 pm. Administering short-acting isosorbide dinitrate 2 or 3 times daily instead of 4, sustained-release isosorbide dinitrate once daily or an eccentric regimen of twice daily at 8 am and 2 pm, giving the two daily doses of isosorbide mononitrate 7 hours apart (creating a 17 hour gap between second dose of each day and first dose of next day) or using nitroglycerin transdermal patches for only 12 hours during the day (see Nitroglycerin Transdermal Administration and Dosage), may reduce the possibility of tolerance developing. Although further studies are necessary, administration of acetylcysteine may reverse tolerance to nitroglycerin in patients in whom complete tolerance has developed. Nitrates that appear least likely to be associated with tolerance are the short-acting formulations (eg, sublingual, translingual spray), with the exception of the IV form. The transmucosal formulation also appears to be associated with minimal tolerance.

Controlled clinical trial data suggest that the intermittent use of nitrates is associated with decreased exercise tolerance, in comparison to placebo, during the last part of the nitrate-free interval; the clinical relevance of this observation is unknown, but consider the possibility of increased frequency or severity of angina during the nitrate-free interval. Further investigations of the tolerance phenomenon and best regimen are ongoing. A final evaluation of the effectiveness of the product will be announced by the FDA.

If patients generally experience anginal episodes at night, the use of a beta blocker or calcium channel blocker during this interval may be beneficial. Patients who generally experience anginal episodes during the day do not appear to be at significant risk with a nightly nitrate-poor period.

Glaucoma: Intraocular pressure may be increased; therefore, caution is required in administering to patients with glaucoma.

Excessive dosage may produce severe headache. Lowering the dose and using analgesics will help control the headaches, which diminish or disappear as therapy continues. Discontinue the drug if blurred vision or dry mouth occurs.

Volume depletion/hypotension: Severe hypotension (particularly with upright posture) may occur with even small doses of isosorbide mononitrate. Exercise caution in patients who may be volume depleted or hypotensive for any reason. Hypotension may be accompanied by paradoxical bradycardia and increased angina pectoris.

Withdrawal: In terminating treatment of angina, gradually reduce the dosage to prevent withdrawal reactions.

Drug abuse and dependence: Amyl nitrite is abused for sexual stimulation. The effect of inhalation is almost instantaneous, causing lightheadedness, dizziness and euphoria.

Drug Interactions:

Nitrate Drug Interactions			
Precipitant drug	Object drug*		Description
Alcohol	Nitrates	↑	Severe hypotension and cardiovascular collapse may occur.
Aspirin	Nitrates	↑	Increased nitrate serum concentrations and actions may occur.
Calcium channel blockers	Nitrates	↑	Marked symptomatic orthostatic hypotension may occur. Dosage adjustment of either agent may be necessary.
Dihydroergotamine	Nitrates	↔	Increased bioavailability of dihydroergotamine with resultant increase in mean standing systolic blood pressure, or functional antagonism between these agents, decreasing the antianginal effects.
Nitroglycerin	Heparin	↓	Pharmacologic effects of heparin may be decreased; data conflict.

* ↑ = Object drug increased ↓ = Object drug decreased ↔ = Undetermined effect

Drug/Lab test interactions: Nitrates may interfere with the *Zlatkis-Zak* color reaction causing a false report of decreased serum cholesterol.

Adverse Reactions:

GI: Nausea; vomiting; diarrhea; dyspepsia; involuntary passing of urine and feces; abdominal pain; tenesmus; tooth disorder.

CNS: Headache which may be severe and persistent (up to 50%); apprehension; restlessness; weakness; vertigo; dizziness; agitation; anxiety; confusion; insomnia; nervousness; nightmares; dyscoordination; hypoesthesia; hypokinesia.

Cardiovascular: Tachycardia; retrosternal discomfort; palpitations; hypotension (sometimes with paradoxical bradycardia and increased angina pectoris); syncope; collapse; crescendo angina; rebound hypertension; arrhythmias; atrial fibrillation; premature ventricular contractions; postural hypotension.

NITRATES

Dermatologic: Drug rash or exfoliative dermatitis; cutaneous vasodilation with flushing; crusty skin lesions; pruritus; rash.

Contact dermatitis from **transdermal nitroglycerin** may occur. The transdermal delivery system itself, not the nitroglycerin molecule, may be responsible.

Nitroglycerin ointment may cause topical allergic reactions; erythematous, vesicular and pruritic lesions; anaphylactoid reactions characterized by oral mucosal and conjunctival edema.

Sublingual nitroglycerin tablets may cause a local burning or tingling sensation in the oral cavity at the point of dissolution. Absence of this effect does not indicate loss of potency; some older patients may not experience this effect. The stabilized tablets may be less likely to produce these sensations.

GU: Dysuria; impotence; urinary frequency.

Musculoskeletal: Arthralgia.

Respiratory: Bronchitis; pneumonia; upper respiratory tract infection.

Miscellaneous: Muscle twitching; pallor; perspiration; cold sweat; hemolytic anemia; asthenia; blurred vision; diplopia; edema; malaise; neck stiffness; rigors; increased appetite. Allergic responses, resulting in itching or wheezing and tracheobronchitis have occurred.

Methemoglobinemia: Case reports of clinically significant methemoglobinemia are rare at conventional doses of nitrates. Formation of methemoglobin is dose-related and in the case of genetic abnormalities of hemoglobin that favor methemoglobin formation, even conventional doses of nitrates could produce harmful concentrations of methemoglobin. Treat with high-flow oxygen and administer methylene blue slowly at a dose of 0.2 ml/kg (1 to 2 mg/kg) IV. Refer to the methylene blue monograph in Antidotes Section.

Overdosage:

Symptoms: Toxic effects may result from inhalation of the drug as dust, by ingestion or by excessive absorption through the intact skin or mucous membranes. Prolonged contact will produce skin eruptions. Signs and symptoms result primarily from vasodilation and methemoglobinemia. Manifestations include hypotension, tachycardia, flushing, perspiring skin (later becoming cold and cyanotic), headache, vertigo, palpitations, visual disturbances, diaphoresis, dizziness, syncope, nausea, vomiting (possibly with colic and bloody diarrhea), anorexia, initial hyperpnea, dyspnea and slow breathing, slow pulse (dicrotic and intermittent), heart block, increased intracranial pressure with cerebral symptoms of confusion, moderate fever and paralysis. Tissue hypoxia due to methemoglobinemia can lead to cyanosis, metabolic acidosis, coma, convulsions and death due to cardiovascular collapse.

Treatment: If nitrates were ingested, induce emesis or perform gastric lavage followed by charcoal administration; however, nitrates are usually rapidly and completely absorbed. Keep patient recumbent in shock position and comfortably warm or temporarily terminate the infusion until the patient's condition stabilizes. Gastric lavage may be of use if the medication has only recently been swallowed. Passive movement of the extremities may aid venous return. Administer oxygen and artificial ventilation if necessary. Monitor methemoglobin levels as indicated.

Treat severe hypotension and reflex tachycardia by elevating the legs and administering IV fluids. Since the duration of the hemodynamic effects following IV nitroglycerin administration is quite short, additional corrective measures are usually not required. However, if indicated, consider an IV α-adrenergic agonist (eg, phenylephrine, methoxamine). Treat methemoglobinemia (see Adverse Reactions).

Epinephrine is ineffective in reversing the severe hypotensive events associated with overdosage; epinephrine and related compounds are contraindicated in overdosage.

Patient Information:

Avoid alcohol.

Brand interchange: Do not change from one brand of this drug to another without consulting your pharmacist or physician. Products manufactured by different companies may not be equally effective.

May cause headache, dizziness or flushing. Notify physician if blurred vision, dry mouth or persistent headache occurs. In patients who get headaches, the headaches may be a marker of the drug's activity. Patients should not try to avoid headaches by altering the treatment schedule, since loss of headache may be associated with simultaneous loss of efficacy. Aspirin or acetaminophen may be used for relief.

NITRATES

Take oral nitrates on an empty stomach with a glass of water.

Carefully follow the prescribed schedule of dosing.

Keep tablets and capsules in original container. Keep container closed tightly.

Inhalants: Use when lying down only. Highly flammable; do not use where it might be ignited. Use in a well ventilated room.

Sublingual tablets: Dissolve tablet under tongue; do not swallow. A lack of burning or stinging sensation does not indicate a loss of potency. Use when seated. Take at the first sign of an anginal attack before severe pain develops. If angina is not relieved in 5 minutes, dissolve a second tablet under the tongue. If pain is not relieved within another 5 minutes, dissolve a third tablet. If pain continues or intensifies, notify physician immediately or report to the nearest hospital emergency room.

Translingual spray: Spray onto or under tongue. Do not inhale spray.

Transmucosal tablets: Place under the upper lip or in a buccal pouch (between cheek and gum). Permit to dissolve slowly over a 3 to 5 hour period. Do not chew or swallow tablets. Release of nitroglycerin begins immediately upon contact with the mucosa and will continue until the tablet dissolves. Time to dissolution increases as patients familiarize themselves with the tablet's presence. Rate of dissolution may be increased by touching the tablet with the tongue or drinking hot liquids.

Sustained release nitroglycerin: Swallow whole; do not chew. Not for sublingual use.

Topical ointment: Patient instructions are available with products. Spread a thin layer on skin using applicator or dose-measuring papers; do not use fingers; do not rub or massage. Keep tube tightly closed.

Transdermal nitroglycerin: Patient instructions are available with products. Advise patients that there is enough residual nitroglycerin in discarded patches that they are a potential hazard to children and pets. Use caution when discarding.

ISOSORBIDE MONONITRATE, ORAL

For complete prescribing information, refer to the Nitrates group monograph.

Indications:

Angina pectoris: Prevention of angina pectoris; not to abort acute anginal episodes.

Administration and Dosage:

Approved by the FDA in December 1991.

Tablets: 20 mg twice daily, with the two doses given 7 hours apart. A starting dose of 5 mg (½ tablet of the 10 mg dosing strength) might be appropriate for persons of particularly small stature, but should be increased to at least 10 mg by the second or third day of therapy. Suggested regimen is to give first dose on awakening and second dose 7 hours later. The asymmetric dosing regimen provides a daily nitrate-free interval to minimize the development of tolerance.

Tablets, extended release: Initially, 30 mg (given as ½ of a 60 mg tablet) or 60 mg (one tablet) once daily. After several days, the dosage may be increased to 120 mg (given as two 60 mg tablets) once daily. Rarely 240 mg may be required. Suggested regimen is to give in the morning on arising. Do not crush or chew extended release tablets, and swallow them with a half glassful of liquid.

Rx	**Monoket** (Schwarz Pharma Kremers Urban)	**Tablets**: 10 mg	Lactose. (10 Schwarz 610). White, scored. In 60s, 100s, 180s and UD 100s.
Rx	**ISMO**(Wyeth-Ayerst)	**Tablets**: 20 mg	(ISMO 20W). Orange. Film coated. In 100s, UD 100s.
Rx	**Monoket** (Schwarz Pharma Kremers Urban)		Lactose. (20 Schwarz 620). White, scored. In 60s, 100s, 180s and UD 100s.
Rx	**Imdur** (Key)	**Tablets, extended release**: 30 mg	(Imdur 30 mg). Rose colored. Scored. In 30s,100s and UD 100s.
		Tablets, extended release: 60 mg	(Imdur 60 mg). Yellow, scored. In 30s, 100s and UD 100s.
		Tablets, extended release: 120 mg	(Imdur 120 mg). White. In 30s, 100s and UD 100s.

NITROGLYCERIN, INTRAVENOUS

For complete prescribing information, refer to the Nitrates group monograph.

Indications:

Control of blood pressure in perioperative hypertension, ie, associated with endotracheal intubation, anesthesia, skin incision, sternotomy, cardiac bypass and in the immediate postsurgical period.

Congestive heart failure associated with acute myocardial infarction.

Angina pectoris unresponsive to recommended doses of organic nitrates or β-blockers.

To produce controlled hypotension during surgical procedures.

Administration and Dosage:

Preparation of infusion: Not for direct IV injection. Dilute in D5W or 0.9% NaCl Injection prior to infusion. Do not mix with other drugs. Base infusion concentration on patient's fluid requirements and expected duration of infusion. Preparations differ in concentration or volume per vial. Refer to manufacturers' package literature for dilution recommendations for specific products.

Administration sets: Use only with glass IV bottles and administration set provided. Total amount of nitroglycerin (40% to 80%) in the final diluted solution for infusion could be adsorbed by PVC tubing of IV administration sets in general use. Greater adsorption occurs with low flow rates, high concentrations and long tubing. Although rate of loss is highest during early administration (when flow rates are lowest) the loss is neither constant nor self-limiting; consequently, no simple calculation or correction can convert theoretical infusion rate (based on concentration of solution) to actual delivery rate. Manufacturers have developed non-PVC infusion tubing in which nitroglycerin loss is < 5%. Use IV sets provided by manufacturers or use similar infusion sets.

Infusion pumps may fail to occlude the non-PVC infusion sets completely because non-PVC tubing is less pliable than standard PVC tubing. Excessive flow at low infusion rate settings may result, causing alarms or unregulated gravity flow when the infusion pump is stopped. This could lead to overinfusion of nitroglycerin.

Dosage requirements: Initially, 5 mcg/min delivered through an infusion pump. Titrate to the clinical situation, initially in 5 mcg/min increments with increases every 3 to 5 minutes until some response is noted. If no response occurs at 20 mcg/min, use increments of 10 to 20 mcg/min. Once a partial blood pressure response is observed, reduce the dose and lengthen the interval between increments.

Some patients with normal or low left ventricular filling pressure or PCWP (eg, angina patients without other complications) may be hypersensitive and may respond fully to doses as small as 5 mcg/min. Titrate carefully and monitor closely.

There is no fixed optimum dose. Continuously monitor physiologic parameters (eg, blood pressure, heart rate) and other measurements (eg, PCWP) to achieve correct dose. Maintain adequate blood and coronary perfusion pressures.

Storage: Protect from freezing and light.

Rx	**Tridil** (Faulding)	**Injection**: 0.5 mg per ml	In 10 ml amps.[1]
Rx	**Nitroglycerin** (Various, eg, American Regent, Goldline, Lyphomed, Solopak)	**Injection**: 5 mg per ml	In 5 and 10 ml vials.
Rx	**Nitro-Bid IV** (Hoechst Marion Roussel)		In 1, 5 and 10 ml vials.[2]
Rx	**Tridil** (Faulding)		In 5 & 10 ml amps, 5, 10 & 20[3] ml single use vials &10 ml w/ IV infusion set or infusion pump connector set.
Rx	**Nitroglycerin in 5% Dextrose** (Various, eg, Abbott, Baxter)	**Injection solution**: 25 mg	In 250 ml.
		50 mg	In 250 and 500 ml.
		100 mg	In 250 ml.
		200 mg	In 500 ml.

[1] With 4.5 mg lactose per ml and 10% alcohol.

[2] With 45 mg propylene glycol per ml.

[3] With 30% propylene glycol and 30% alcohol.

AMYL NITRITE

For complete prescribing information, refer to the Nitrates group monograph.

Indications:

Relief of angina pectoris.

Administration and Dosage:

Usual adult dose is 0.3 ml by inhalation, as required.

Crush the capsule and wave under the nose; 1 to 6 inhalations from one capsule are usually sufficient to produce the desired effect. May repeat in 3 to 5 minutes.

Storage: Protect from light. Store in a cool place, 15° to 30°C (59° to 86°F).

Rx	**Amyl Nitrite** (Various, eg, Goldline, Moore)	**Inhalant**: 0.3 ml	In 12s.
Rx	**Amyl Nitrite Aspirols** (Lilly)		In 12s.
Rx	**Amyl Nitrite Vaporole** (B-W)		In 12s.

NITROGLYCERIN, SUBLINGUAL

For complete prescribing information, refer to the Nitrates group monograph.

Indications:

Prophylaxis, treatment and management of angina pectoris.

Administration and Dosage:

Dissolve 1 tablet under tongue or in buccal pouch (between cheek and gum) at first sign of an acute anginal attack. Repeat approximately every 5 minutes until relief is obtained. Take no more than 3 tablets in 15 minutes. If pain continues, notify physician immediately. May be used prophylactically 5 to 10 minutes prior to activities which might precipitate an acute attack.

Storage: Dispense in the original container; store at room temperature. Protect from moisture. The stabilized sublingual tablets are less subject to potency loss than the previous conventional sublingual tablets; Nitrostat carries a 5 year expiration date, under proper storage conditions in the unopened container. Traditionally, unused tablets should be discarded 6 months after the original bottle is opened.

Rx	**Nitrostat** (Parke-Davis)	**Tablets, sublingual**: 0.3 mg (1/200 gr)	In 100s, unit-of-use 100s.
		0.4 mg (1/150 gr)	In 100s, unit-of-use 100s.
		0.6 mg (1/100 gr)	In 100s, unit-of-use 100s.

NITROGLYCERIN, TRANSLINGUAL

For complete prescribing information, refer to the Nitrates group monograph.

Indications:

Acute relief of an attack or prophylaxis of angina pectoris due to coronary artery disease.

Administration and Dosage:

At the onset of attack, spray 1 or 2 metered doses onto or under the tongue. No more than 3 metered doses are recommended within 15 minutes. If chest pain persists, seek prompt medical attention. May use prophylactically 5 to 10 minutes prior to engaging in activities which might precipitate an acute attack. Do not inhale spray.

Rx	**Nitrolingual** (Rhone-Poulenc Rorer)	**Spray**: 0.4 mg per metered dose	In 14.49 g containing 200 metered doses/canister.

NITROGLYCERIN, TRANSMUCOSAL

For complete prescribing information, refer to the Nitrates group monograph.

Indications:

Treatment and prevention of angina pectoris due to coronary artery disease.

Administration and Dosage:

1 mg every 3 to 5 hours during waking hours. Place tablet between lip and gum above incisors, or between cheek and gum.

Rx	**Nitrogard** (Forest)	**Tablets, buccal, controlled release**: 1 mg	(1). Off-white. In 100s and UD 100s.
		2 mg	(2). Off-white. In 100s and UD 100s.
		3 mg	(3). Off-white. In 100s and UD 100s.

NITROGLYCERIN, SUSTAINED RELEASE

For complete prescribing information, refer to the Nitrates group monograph.

Indications:

Prevention of angina pectoris. "Possibly effective" for the management, prophylaxis or treatment of anginal attacks.

Administration and Dosage:

The usual starting dose is 2.5 or 2.6 mg, 3 or 4 times daily. Titrate upward to an effective dose until side effects limit the dose. The dose generally may be increased by 2.5 or 2.6 mg increments 2 to 4 times daily over a period of days or weeks. Doses as high as 26 mg given 4 times daily have been reported effective.

Give the smallest effective dose 2 to 4 times daily. Monitor blood pressure at initiation of therapy or dosage change.

Tolerance may develop. Consider administering on a reduced schedule (once or twice daily). See Precautions.

Capsules must be swallowed; not for chewing or sublingual use.

Rx	**Nitrong** (R-P Rorer)	**Tablets, sustained release:** 2.6 mg	Light green granules. Scored. In 100s.
Rx	**Nitrong** (R-P Rorer)	**Tablets, sustained release:** 6.5 mg	Light orange granules. Scored. In 100s.
Rx	**Nitrong** (R-P Rorer)	**Tablets, sustained release:** 9 mg	Blue granules. Scored. In 60s and 500s.
Rx	**Nitroglycerin** (Various, eg, Dixon-Shane, Geneva Marsam, Goldline, Major, Moore, Purepac, Rugby, Schein, URL, Vitarine)	**Capsules, sustained release:** 2.5 mg	In 60s, 100s and UD 60s and 100s.
Rx	**Nitro-Bid Plateau Caps** (Hoechst Marion Roussel)		Lactose, sucrose. (Marion/1550). Lt. purple/clear, white beads. In 60s, 100s.
Rx	**Nitrocine Timecaps** (Schwarz Pharma Kremers Urban)		Lactose, sucrose. (Kremers Urban 320). Violet/clear, white beads. In 100s.
Rx	**Nitroglyn** (Kenwood)		In 100s.
Rx	**Nitro-Time** (Time-Cap Labs)		Lactose, sucrose. (TCL-1221). Pink/clear. In 60s, 90s and 100s.
Rx	**Nitroglycerin** (Various, eg, Dixon-Shane, Geneva Marsam, Goldline, Major, Moore, Purepac, Rugby, Schein, URL, Vitarine)	**Capsules, sustained release:** 6.5 mg	In 60s, 100s and UD 100s.
Rx	**Nitro-Bid Plateau Caps** (Marion Merrell Dow)		Lactose, sucrose. (Marion/1551). Dk. blue/yellow. In60s and 100s.
Rx	**Nitrocine Timecaps** (Schwarz Pharma Kremers Urban)		Lactose, sucrose. (Kremers Urban 330). Dk. blue/orange. In 100s.
Rx	**Nitroglyn** (Kenwood)		In 100s.
Rx	**Nitro-Time** (Time-Cap Labs)		Lactose, sucrose. (TCL-1222). Blue/yellow. In 60s, 90s and 100s.

NITROGLYCERIN, SUSTAINED RELEASE

Rx	**Nitroglycerin** (Various, eg, Dixon-Shane, Geneva Marsam, Goldline, Major, Moore, Rugby, Schein, URL, Vitarine)	**Capsules, sustained release:** 9 mg	In 30s, 60s, 100s and UD 100s.
Rx	**Nitro-Bid Plateau Caps** (Marion Merrell Dow)		Lactose, sucrose. (Marion/ 1553). Green/yellow. In 60s and 100s.
Rx	**Nitrocine Timecaps** (Schwarz Pharma Kremers Urban)		Lactose, sucrose. (Kremers Urban 340). Clear, white beads. In 100s.
Rx	**Nitroglyn** (Kenwood)		In 100s.
Rx	**Nitro-Time** (Time-Cap Labs)		Lactose, sucrose. (TCL-1223). Green/yellow. In 60s, 90s and 100s.
Rx	**Nitroglyn** (Kenwood)	**Capsules, sustained-release:** 13 mg	In 100s.

NITROGLYCERIN, SUSTAINED RELEASE

For complete prescribing information, refer to the Nitrates group monograph.

Indications:

Prevention of angina pectoris. "Possibly effective" for the management, prophylaxis or treatment of anginal attacks.

Administration and Dosage:

The usual starting dose is 2.5 or 2.6 mg, 3 or 4 times daily. Titrate upward to an effective dose until side effects limit the dose. The dose generally may be increased by 2.5 or 2.6 mg increments 2 to 4 times daily over a period of days or weeks. Doses as high as 26 mg given 4 times daily have been reported effective.

Give the smallest effective dose 2 to 4 times daily. Monitor blood pressure at initiation of therapy or dosage change.

Tolerance may develop. Consider administering on a reduced schedule (once or twice daily). See Precautions.

Capsules must be swallowed; not for chewing or sublingual use.

Rx	**Nitrong** (R-P Rorer)	**Tablets, sustained release:** 2.6 mg	Light green granules. Scored. In 100s.
Rx	**Nitrong** (R-P Rorer)	**Tablets, sustained release:** 6.5 mg	Light orange granules. Scored. In 100s.
Rx	**Nitrong** (R-P Rorer)	**Tablets, sustained release:** 9 mg	Blue granules. Scored. In 60s and 500s.
Rx	**Nitroglycerin** (Various, eg, Dixon-Shane, Geneva Marsam, Goldline, Major, Moore, Purepac, Rugby, Schein, URL, Vitarine)	**Capsules, sustained release:** 2.5 mg	In 60s, 100s and UD 60s and 100s.
Rx	**Nitro-Bid Plateau Caps** (Hoechst Marion Roussel)		Lactose, sucrose. (Marion/ 1550). Lt. purple/clear, white beads. In 60s, 100s.
Rx	**Nitrocine Timecaps** (Schwarz Pharma Kremers Urban)		Lactose, sucrose. (Kremers Urban 320). Violet/ clear, white beads. In 100s.
Rx	**Nitroglyn** (Kenwood)		In 100s.
Rx	**Nitro-Time** (Time-Cap Labs)		Lactose, sucrose. (TCL-1221). Pink/clear. In 60s, 90s and 100s.
Rx	**Nitroglycerin** (Various, eg, Dixon-Shane, Geneva Marsam, Goldline, Major, Moore, Purepac, Rugby, Schein, URL, Vitarine)	**Capsules, sustained release:** 6.5 mg	In 60s, 100s and UD 100s.
Rx	**Nitro-Bid Plateau Caps** (Marion Merrell Dow)		Lactose, sucrose. (Marion/ 1551). Dk. blue/yellow. In60s and 100s.
Rx	**Nitrocine Timecaps** (Schwarz Pharma Kremers Urban)		Lactose, sucrose. (Kremers Urban 330). Dk. blue/ orange. In 100s.
Rx	**Nitroglyn** (Kenwood)		In 100s.
Rx	**Nitro-Time** (Time-Cap Labs)		Lactose, sucrose. (TCL-1222). Blue/yellow. In 60s, 90s and 100s.

NITROGLYCERIN, SUSTAINED RELEASE

Rx	**Nitroglycerin** (Various, eg, Dixon-Shane, Geneva Marsam, Goldline, Major, Moore, Rugby, Schein, URL, Vitarine)	**Capsules, sustained release:** 9 mg	In 30s, 60s, 100s and UD 100s.
Rx	**Nitro-Bid Plateau Caps** (Marion Merrell Dow)		Lactose, sucrose. (Marion/ 1553). Green/yellow. In 60s and 100s.
Rx	**Nitrocine Timecaps** (Schwarz Pharma Kremers Urban)		Lactose, sucrose. (Kremers Urban 340). Clear, white beads. In 100s.
Rx	**Nitroglyn** (Kenwood)		In 100s.
Rx	**Nitro-Time** (Time-Cap Labs)		Lactose, sucrose. (TCL-1223). Green/yellow. In 60s, 90s and 100s.
Rx	**Nitroglyn** (Kenwood)	**Capsules, sustained-release:** 13 mg	In 100s.

NITROGLYCERIN TRANSDERMAL SYSTEMS

For complete prescribing information, refer to the Nitrates group monograph.

Continuously absorbed into systemic circulation from a pad applied to skin.

Nitrate tolerance may be more likely with higher dosages, longer acting products or more frequent dosing. Transdermal systems release nitroglycerin at a constant rate and maintain steady-state plasma concentration; thus, tolerance may occur (see Precautions and Administration and Dosage).

Indications:

Angina: Prevention of angina pectoris due to coronary artery disease.

Administration and Dosage:

Patient instructions for application are provided with products.

Apply once daily to a skin site free of hair and not subject to excessive movement. Do not apply to distal parts of extremities. Avoid areas with cuts or irritations.

Individualize dosage. Titrate dose as needed for optimum effect.

Starting dose: 0.2 to 0.4 mg/hr. Doses between 0.4 and 0.8 mg/hr have shown continued effectiveness for 10 to 12 hours daily for at least 1 month of intermittent administration. Although the minimum nitrate-free interval has not been defined, data show that a nitrate-free interval of 10 to 12 hours is sufficient. Thus, an appropriate dosing schedule would include a daily "patch-on" period of 12 to 14 hours and a "patch-off" period of 10 to 12 hours. Tolerance is a major factor limiting efficacy when the system is used continuously for > 12 hours each day.

These products differ in delivery system mechanism. The most important common denominator is amount of drug released per hour. However, a wide range of patient variability has been seen in bioavailability studies. The skin is a major factor influencing absorption rate; physical exercise and elevated ambient temperatures (eg, sauna) may increase the absorption. Other factors are related to the patient's preference and product differences: Ease of application and removal, adhesiveness, comfort, size and appearance.

	Product/Distributor	Release Rate (mg/hr)	Surface Area (cm^2)	Total NTG Content (mg)	How Supplied
Rx	**Minitran** (3M Pharm.)	0.1	3.3	9	In 33s.
Rx	**Nitro-Dur** (Key)	0.1	5	20	In 30s, 100s, UD 30s and 100s.
Rx	**Transderm-Nitro** (Summit)	0.1	5	12.5	In 30s, UD 30s and 100s.
Rx	**Nitroglycerin Transdermal** (Various, eg, Goldline, Major, Moore, Mylan, Parmed, Schein)	0.2	6 - 10[1]	16 - 62.5[1]	In 30s.
Rx	**Minitran** (3M Pharm.)	0.2	6.7	18	In 33s.
Rx	**Nitrodisc** (Roberts)	0.2	8	16	In 30s and 100s.
Rx	**Nitro-Dur** (Key)	0.2	10	40	In 30s, 100s, UD 30s and 100s.
Rx	**Transderm-Nitro** (Summit)	0.2	10	25	In 30s. UD 30s and 100s.
Rx	**Deponit** (Schwarz Pharma K-U)	0.2	16	16	In 30s and 100s.
Rx	**Nitrodisc** (Roberts)	0.3	12	24	In 30s and 100s.
Rx	**Nitro-Dur** (Key)	0.3	15	60	In 30s, 100s, UD 30s and 100s.
Rx	**Nitroglycerin Transdermal** (Various, eg, Goldline, Major, Moore, Mylan, Parmed, Schein)	0.4	13 - 20[1]	32 - 125[1]	In 30s.
Rx	**Minitran** (3M Pharm.)	0.4	13.3	36	In 33s.
Rx	**Nitrodisc** (Roberts)	0.4	16	32	In 30s and 100s.
Rx	**Nitro-Dur** (Key)	0.4	20	80	In 30s, 100s, UD 30s and 100s.
Rx	**Transderm-Nitro** (Summit)	0.4	20	50	In 30s, UD 30s and 100s.

NITROGLYCERIN TRANSDERMAL SYSTEMS

	Product/Distributor	Release Rate (mg/hr)	Surface Area (cm²)	Total NTG Content (mg)	How Supplied
Rx	**Deponit** (Schwarz Pharma K-U)	0.4	32	32	In 30s and 100s.
Rx	**Nitroglycerine Transdermal** (Various, eg, Goldline, Major, Mylan, Parmed, Rugby)	0.6	20 - 30[1]	75 - 187.5[1]	In 30s.
Rx	**Minitran** (3M Pharm.)	0.6	20	54	In 33s.
Rx	**Nitro-Dur** (Key)	0.6	30	120	In 30s and 100s.
Rx	**Transderm-Nitro** (Summit)	0.6	30	75	In 30s.
Rx	**Nitro-Dur** (Key)	0.8	40	160	In 30s, 100s, UD 30s and 100s.
Rx	**Nitro-Derm** (Reuabuen Inc.)	0.8	40	160	In 30s, 100s, UD 30s and 100s.
Rx	**Transderm-Nitro** (Summit)	0.8	40	100	In 30s and UD 30s.

[1] Various systems have the same release rates but variable surface areas and NTG contents.

NITROGLYCERIN, TOPICAL

For complete prescribing information, refer to the Nitrates group monograph.

Indications:

Angina: Prevention and treatment of angina pectoris due to coronary artery disease.

Administration and Dosage:

Usual therapeutic dose: 1 to 2 inches (25 to 50 mm) every 8 hours, up to 4 to 5 inches (100 to 125 mm) every 4 hours. Start with ½ inch (12.5 mm) every 8 hours; increase by ½ inch with each application to achieve desired effects. The greatest attainable decrease in resting blood pressure not associated with clinical hypotension, especially during orthostasis, indicates optimal dosage.

To apply ointment, use the applicator or dose-measuring paper to spread in a thin uniform layer over at least a 2¼ x 3½ inch area. The ointment may be applied to the chest or back.

One inch (25 mm) of ointment contains ≈ 15 mg nitroglycerin.

Rx	**Nitroglycerin** (Various, eg, Fougera , IDE, Major, Parmed)	**Ointment:** 2% in a lanolin-petrolatum base	In 30 and 60 g tubes.
Rx	**Nitro-Bid** (Hoechst Marion Roussel)		In 20 and 60 g tubes and UD 1 g (100s).
Rx	**Nitrol** (Savage)		In 60 g tube with or without applicator and UD 3 g (50s).

ISOSORBIDE DINITRATE, SUBLINGUAL AND CHEWABLE

For complete prescribing information, refer to the Nitrates group monograph.

Indications:

Angina: Treatment and prevention of angina pectoris.

Administration and Dosage:

Angina pectoris: Usual starting dose is 2.5 to 5 mg for sublingual tablets and 5 mg for chewable tablets. Titrate upward until angina is relieved or side effects limit the dose.

Acute prophylaxis: 5 to 10 mg sublingual or chewable tablets every 2 to 3 hours. Limit use of sublingual or chewable isosorbide dinitrate for aborting an acute anginal attack in patients intolerant of or unresponsive to sublingual nitroglycerin.

Do not crush or chew sublingual tablets; do not crush chewable tablets before administering.

Rx	**Isosorbide Dinitrate** (Various, eg, Major, Moore, Parmed, Rugby, Schein)	**Tablets, sublingual:** 2.5 mg	In 100s, 500s, 1000s and UD 100s.
Rx	**Isordil** (Wyeth-Ayerst)		Lactose. Yellow. In 100s, 500s and Redipak 100s.
Rx	**Sorbitrate** (Zeneca)		(S 853). Lactose. White, scored. In 100s.
Rx	**Isosorbide Dinitrate** (Various, eg, Major, Moore, Parmed, Rugby, Schein, URL)	**Tablets, sublingual:** 5 mg	In 100s, 1000s and UD 100s.
Rx	**Isordil** (Wyeth-Ayerst)		Lactose. Pink. In 100s, 500s and Redipak 100s.
Rx	**Sorbitrate** (Zeneca)		(S 760). Pink. In 100s.
Rx	**Isosorbide DInitrate** (Various, eg, Major)	**Tablets, sublingual:** 10 mg	In 100s and 1000s.
Rx	**Isordil** (Wyeth-Ayerst)		Lactose. White. In 100s.
Rx	**Sorbitrate** (Zeneca)	**Tablets, chewable:** 5 mg	(S 810). Sugar. Green, scored. In 100s and 500s.
Rx	**Sorbitrate** (Zeneca)	**Tablets, chewable:** 10 mg	(S 815). Sugar. Yellow, scored. In 100s.

ISOSORBIDE DINITRATE, ORAL

For complete prescribing information, refer to the Nitrates group monograph.

Indications:

Angina: Treatment and prevention of angina pectoris; not to abort acute anginal episodes.

Administration and Dosage:

Tablets: Initial dose is 5 to 20 mg; maintenance dose is 10 to 40 mg every 6 hours.

Sustained release: The initial dose is 40 mg; maintenance controlled release dose is 40 to 80 mg every 8 to 12 hours. Do not crush or chew these preparations.

Tolerance to these agents may develop. Consider administering the short-acting preparations 2 or 3 times daily (last dose no later than 7 pm) and the sustained release preparations once daily or twice daily at 8 am and 2 pm. See Precautions.

Rx	**Isosorbide Dinitrate** (Various, eg, Geneva, Goldline, Major, Moore, Par, Parmed, Rugby, Schein, UDL, URL)	**Tablets:** 5 mg	In 100s, 1000s and UD 100s.
Rx	**Isordil Titradose** (Wyeth-Ayerst)		Lactose. Pink, scored. In 100s, 500s, 1000s and Redipak 100s.
Rx	**Sorbitrate** (Zeneca)		Lactose. (S 770). Green, scored. Oval. In 100s, 500s and UD 100s.

ISOSORBIDE DINITRATE, ORAL

Rx	**Isosorbide Dinitrate** (Various, eg, Geneva, Goldline, Major, Moore, Par, Parmed, Rugby, Schein, UDL, URL)	**Tablets:** 10 mg	In 100s, 500s, 1000s and UD 100s.
Rx	**Isordil Titradose**(Wyeth-Ayerst)		Lactose. White, scored. In 100s, 500s, 1000s and Redipak 100s.
Rx	**Sorbitrate** (Zeneca)		Lactose. (S 780). Yellow, scored. Oval. In 100s, 500s and UD 100s.
Rx	**Isosorbide Dinitrate** (Various, eg, Geneva, Goldline, Major, Moore, Par, Parmed, Rugby, Schein, UDL, URL)	**Tablets:** 20 mg	In 90s, 100s, 120s, 180s, 240s, 360s, 500s, 1000s and UD 100s.
Rx	**Isordil Titradose** (Wyeth-Ayerst)		Lactose. Green, scored. In 100s, 500s and Redipak 100s.
Rx	**Sorbitrate** (Zeneca)		Lactose. (S 820). Blue, scored. Oval. In 100s and UD 100s.
Rx	**Isosorbide Dinitrate** (Various, eg, Major, Moore, Par, Parmed, Rugby, URL)	**Tablets:** 30 mg	In 100s, 500s, 1000s and UD 100s.
Rx	**Isordil Titradose** (Wyeth-Ayerst)		Lactose. Blue, scored. In 100s, 500s and Redipak 100s.
Rx	**Sorbitrate**(Zeneca)		Lactose. (S 773). White, scored. Oval. In 100s and UD 100s.
Rx	**Isordil Titradose** (Wyeth-Ayerst)	**Tablets:** 40 mg	Lactose. Light green, scored. In 100s and Redipak 100s.
Rx	**Sorbitrate** (Zeneca)		Lactose. (S 774) Light blue, scored. Oval. In 100s and UD 100s.
Rx	**Isosorbide Dinitrate** (Various, eg, Geneva, Goldline, Major, Moore, Parmed, Rugby, Schein, URL)	**Tablets, sustained release:** 40 mg	In 90s, 100s, 250s, 1000s and UD 100s.
Rx	**Isordil Tembids** (Wyeth-Ayerst)		Lactose. Green, scored. In 100s, 500s and 1000s.
Rx	**Dilatrate-SR** (Schwarz Pharma)	**Capsules, sustained release:** 40 mg	Pink/opaque. In 60s and 100s.
Rx	**Isordil Tembids** (Wyeth-Ayerst)		Sugar. Blue/opaque. In 100s and 500s.

ANTIARRHYTHMIC AGENTS

Optimal therapy of cardiac arrhythmias requires documentation, accurate diagnosis and modification of precipitating causes, and if indicated, proper selection and use of antiarrhythmic drugs. Comprehensive information on individual agents is presented in the following monographs.

These drugs are classified according to their effects on the action potential of cardiac cells and their presumed mechanism of action. Although drugs within the same group are similar, that does not imply that another agent within the group would not be more effective or safer in an individual patient.

Group I: Local anesthetics or membrane-stabilizing agents that depress phase 0.

IA (quinidine, procainamide, disopyramide) – Depress phase 0 and prolong the action potential duration.

IB (tocainide, lidocaine, phenytoin, mexiletine) – Depress phase 0 slightly and may shorten the action potential duration. Although arrhythmia is not a labeled indication for *phenytoin,* it is commonly used in treatment of digitalis-induced arrhythmias.

IC (flecainide, encainide, propafenone) – Marked depression of phase 0. Slight effect on repolarization. Profound slowing of conduction. *Encainide* was voluntarily withdrawn from the market, but is still available on a limited basis.

Moricizine is a Group I agent that shares some of the characteristics of the Group IA, B and C agents.

Group II (propranolol, esmolol, acebutolol): Depress phase 4 depolarization.

Group III (bretylium, amiodarone, sotalol): Produce a prolongation of phase 3 (repolarization).

Group IV (verapamil): Depress phase 4 depolarization and lengthen phases 1 and 2 of repolarization.

Digitalis glycosides (digoxin) cause a decrease in maximal diastolic potential and action potential duration and increase the slope of phase 4 depolarization.

Adenosine slows conduction time through the AV node and can interrupt the reentry pathways through the AV node.

Serum drug levels: Some antiarrhythmic drugs (eg, quinidine) can produce toxic effects which can be easily confused with the symptoms for which the drug has been prescribed. Drug serum levels are important in evaluating toxic or subtherapeutic dosage regimens of most antiarrhythmic drugs. They also aid in monitoring active metabolites (eg, procainamide/NAPA), suspected drug interactions and subtherapeutic response due to drug failure, noncompliance, altered clearance or altered absorption.

Proarrhythmic effects: Antiarrhythmic agents may cause new or worsened arrhythmias. Such proarrhythmic effects range from an increase in frequency of PVCs to the development of more severe ventricular tachycardia, ventricular fibrillation or torsade de pointes (ie, tachycardia that is more sustained or more rapid), which may lead to death. It is often not possible to distinguish a proarrhythmic effect from the patient's underlying rhythm disorder. It is therefore essential that each patient be evaluated electrocardiographically and clinically prior to and during therapy to determine whether the response to the drug supports continued treatment.

Cardiac Arrhythmia Suppression Trial: In the National Heart, Lung and Blood Institute's Cardiac Arrhythmia Suppression Trial (CAST), a long-term, multicenter, randomized, double-blind study in patients with asymptomatic non-life-threatening ventricular ectopy who had had a myocardial infarction (MI) > 6 days but < 2 years previously, and who demonstrated mild to moderate left ventricular dysfunction, an excessive mortality or non-fatal cardiac arrest rate was seen in patients treated with encainide or flecainide (56/730) compared with that seen in patients assigned to carefully matched placebo treated groups (22/725). This led to discontinuation of those two arms of the trial. In this study, the average duration of treatment with encainide or flecainide was 10 months.

The moricizine and placebo arms of the trial were continued in CAST II. In this randomized, double-blind trial, patients with asymptomatic non-life-threatening arrhythmias who had had an MI within 4 to 90 days and left ventricular ejection fraction ≤ 0.4 prior to enrollment were evaluated. The average duration of moricizine treatment was 18 months. The study was discontinued because there was no possibility of demonstrating a benefit toward improved survival with moricizine and because of an evolving adverse trend after long-term treatment.

The applicability of these results to other populations (eg, those without recent MI) and to other antiarrhythmic drugs is uncertain, but at present it is prudent (1) to consider any IC agent (especially one documented to provoke new serious arrhythmias) to have a similar risk and (2) to consider the risks of Class IC agents, coupled with the lack of any evidence of improved survival, generally unacceptable in patients without life-threatening ventricular arrhythmias, even if the patients are experiencing unpleasant, but not life-threatening symptoms or signs.

ANTIARRHYTHMIC AGENTS

Pharmacokinetics: The information in the pharmacokinetics table together with clinical data and observation can be a valuable tool. However, the information must be used rationally and the data obtained properly (ie, obtaining and analyzing serum level data) to be effective. See individual monographs for more detailed explanations.

Antiarrhythmic Electrophysiology/Electrocardiogram Effects

Antiarrhythmic		Electrophysiology[1]: Automaticity		Electrophysiology[1]: Conduction velocity			Electrophysiology[1]: Refractory period					ECG changes[1]				
Group	Drug	SA node	Ectopic pacemaker	Atrium	AV node	His-Purkinje	Atrium	AV node	His-Purkinje	Ventricle	Accessory pathways[2]	Heart rate	PR interval	QRS complex	QT_c interval	JT interval
I	Moricizine[3]	0	↓	0	↓	↓	±	0	0	0-↑	↑	0-↑	↑	↑	0	↓
	Quinidine	±	↓	↓	±	↓	↑↑	0-↑[4]	↑↑	↑	↑	±	±	↑	↑	↑
	Procain-amide	±	↓	↓	±	↓	↑	0-↑[4]	↑↑	↑	↑↑	±	±	↑	↑	↑
	Disopyr-amide	±	↓	↓	±	↓	↑↑	0-↑[4]	↑↑	↑	↑	±	±	↑	↑	↑
	Lidocaine	0	↓	—	0	0	0	±	±	±	↑-↓	0	0	0	0-↓	0
	Phenytoin	↓-0	↓	—	0	0	0	±	±	±	—	±	0-↓	0	↓	0
	Tocainide	0-↓	↓	0	0	0	↓	↓	±	↓	↑	0	0	0	0-↓	0
	Mexiletine	↓	↓	0	0	0	0	±	↑	↑	↑	-	0	0	0	0
	Flecainide	↓	↓	↓↓	↓	↓↓	0	0	↑	↑	↑↑	0	↑[5]	↑↑[5]	0-↑[5]	0
	Encainide[6]	0-↓	↓	↓↓	↓	↓↓	0-↑	0-↑	↑	↑	↑↑	0	↑[5]	↑↑[5]	0-↑[5]	0
	Propafenone	0	↓	0	↓	↓	0	↑	↑	↑	↑	0	↑[5]	↑	0-↑[5]	0
II	Propranolol	↓	↓	±	↓	0-↓	±	↑	0	0	0-↑	↓	0-↑	0	0-↓	0
	Esmolol	↓	↓	±	↓	0-	±	↑	0	0	0-↑	↓	0-↑	0	0-↓	0
	Acebutolol	↓	↓	±	↓	0	±	↑	0	0	0-↑	↓	0-↑	0	0-↓	0
III	Bretylium	↑	↑	0	0	0-↑	0	↓-↑[7]	↑	0-↑	±	0	0	0	0	↑
	Amiodarone	↓	↓	↓	↓	↓	↑	↑	↑	↑	↑	↓	↑	↑	↑↑	↑↑
	Sotalol[8]	↓	↓	0	↓	0	↑↑	↑	↑↑	↑↑	↑	↓	↑	0	↑↑	↑↑
IV	Verapamil	↓	↓	0	↓	0	0	↑	0	0	0	↓	↑	0	0	0
—	Digoxin	0-↓	↑	±	↓	0-↓	±	↑	0	↓	↓-↑	↓	↑	0	↓	↓
—	Adenosine	↓	↓	0	↓	0	0	↑	0	0	0	↑	↑	0	0	—

[1] These values assume therapeutic levels.

[2] Accessory pathways occur in Wolff-Parkinson-White syndrome (preexcitation phenomena) and possibly other abnormal conditions.

[3] Does not belong to any of the 3 subclasses (A, B or C), but does have some properties of each.

[4] Retrograde AV node RP↑; antegrade RP not affected.

[5] Dose-related increases.

[6] Withdrawn from the market; however, available on a limited basis.

[7] Due to a complex balance of direct and indirect autonomic effects.

[8] Has both Group II (beta blocking) and III properties; Class III effects are seen at doses > 160 mg.

ANTIARRHYTHMIC AGENTS

Antiarrhythmic Pharmacokinetics

Group		Drug	Onset (hrs) (oral)[1]	Duration (hrs)	Half-life (hrs)	Protein binding (%)	Excreted unchanged (%)	Therapeutic serum level (mcg/ml)	Toxic serum levels (mcg/ml)
I	A	Moricizine	2	10-24	1.5-3.5[2]	95	< 1	Not applicable	—
		Quinidine	0.5	6-8	6-7	80-90	10-50	2-6	> 8
		Procainamide	0.5	3+	2.5-4.7	14-23	40-70	4-8	> 16
		Disopyramide	0.5	6-7	4-10	20-60[3]	40-60	2-8	> 9
	B	Lidocaine	—	0.25[4]	1-2	40-80	< 3	1.5-6	> 7
		Phenytoin	0.5-1	24+	22-36[5]	87-93	< 5	10-20	> 20
		Tocainide	—	—	11-15	10-20	28-55	4-10	> 10
		Mexiletine	—	—	10-12	50-60	10	0.5-2	> 2
	C	Flecainide	—	—	12-27	40	30	0.2-1	> 1
		Encainide[6]	—	—	1-2[7]	75-85	< 5[8]	Not applicable	—
		MODE[9]			6-12	92		wide range	
		ODE[9]			3-4	75-85		0.1-0.3	
		Propafenone	—	—	2-10[10]	97	< 1	0.06-1	
II		Propranolol	0.5	3-5	2-3	90-95	< 1	0.05-0.1	
		Esmolol	< 5 min	very short	0.15	55	< 2	—	
		Acebutolol	—	24-30	3-4	26	15-20	—	
III		Bretylium	—	6-8	5-10	0-8	> 80	0.5-1.5	—
		Amiodarone	1-3 wks[11]	weeks to months	26-107 days	96	negligible	0.5-2.5	> 2.5
		Sotalol	—	—	12	0	100	—	
IV		Verapamil	0.5	6	3-7	90	3-4	0.08-0.3	—
—		Digoxin	0.5-2	24+	30-40	20-25	60	0.5-2 ng/ml	> 2.5 ng/ml
—		Adenosine	(34 sec IV)	1-2 min	< 10 sec	—	0 (enters body pool)	Not applicable	—

[1] Within 1 to 5 minutes with IV use.
[2] Half-life may be reduced in patients after multiple dosing.
[3] Protein binding is concentration-dependent.
[4] Very short after discontinuation of IV infusion.
[5] Half-life increases with increasing dosage.
[6] Withdrawn from the market; however, available on a limited basis.
[7] Half-life 6 to 11 hours in < 10% of patients (poor metabolizers).
[8] > 50% in poor metabolizers.
[9] MODE (3-methoxy-O-demethyl encainide) and ODE (O-demethyl encainide), metabolites more active than encainide on a per mg basis.
[10] Half-life 10 to 32 hours in < 10% of patients (slow metabolizers).
[11] Onset of action may occur in 2 to 3 days.

MORICIZINE HCl

Actions:

Pharmacology: Moricizine is a Class I antiarrhythmic agent with potent local anesthetic activity and myocardial membrane stabilizing effects. It shares some of the characteristics of the IA, B and C agents. Moricizine reduces the fast inward current carried by sodium ions. In isolated dog Purkinje fibers, moricizine shortens Phase 2 and 3 repolarization, resulting in a decreased action potential duration and effective refractory period. A dose-related decrease in the maximum rate of Phase 0 depolarization (V_{max}) occurs without effect on maximum diastolic potential or action potential amplitude. The sinus node and atrial tissue of the dog are not affected.

Although moricizine is chemically related to the neuroleptic phenothiazines, it has no demonstrated central or peripheral dopaminergic activity in animals. Moreover, in patients on chronic moricizine, serum prolactin levels did not increase.

Electrophysiology – In patients with ventricular tachycardia, moricizine 750 and 900 mg/day prolongs AV conduction. Both AV nodal conduction time (AH interval) and His-Purkinje conduction time (HV interval) are prolonged by 10% to 13% and 21% to 26%, respectively. The PR interval is prolonged by 16% to 20% and the QRS by 7% to 18%. Prolongations of 2% to 5% in the corrected QT interval result from widening of the QRS interval, but there is shortening of the JT interval, indicating an absence of significant effect on ventricular repolarization.

Intra-atrial conduction or atrial effective refractory periods are not consistently affected. In patients without sinus node dysfunction, moricizine has minimal effects on sinus cycle length and sinus node recovery time. These effects may be significant in patients with sinus node dysfunction (see Precautions).

Hemodynamics – In patients with impaired left ventricular function, moricizine has minimal effects on measurements of cardiac performance such as cardiac index, stroke volume index, pulmonary capillary wedge pressure, systemic or pulmonary vascular resistance or ejection fraction, either at rest or during exercise. Moricizine is associated with a small, but consistent increase in resting blood pressure and heart rate. In patients with ventricular arrhythmias, exercise tolerance is unaffected. In patients with a history of congestive heart failure (CHF) or angina pectoris, exercise duration and rate-pressure product at maximal exercise are unchanged during moricizine administration. Nonetheless, in some cases, worsened heart failure in patients with severe underlying heart disease has been attributed to moricizine.

The antiarrhythmic and electrophysiologic effects of moricizine are not related in time course or intensity to plasma moricizine concentrations or to the concentrations of any identified metabolite, all of which have short (2 to 3 hours) half-lives. Following single doses of morcizine, there is a prompt prolongation of the PR interval, which becomes normal within 2 hours, consistent with the rapid fall of plasma moricizine. JT interval shortening, however, peaks at about 6 hours and persists for at least 10 hours. Although an effect on ventricular premature depolarizations (VPD) rates is seen within 2 hours after dosing, the full effect is seen after 10 to 14 hours and persists in full, when therapy is terminated, for > 10 hours, after which the effect decays slowly, and is still substantial at 24 hours. This suggests either an unidentified metabolite with an active, long half-life, or a structural or functional "deep compartment" with slow entry from, and release to, the plasma. The following description of parent compound pharmacokinetics is therefore of uncertain relevance to clinical actions.

Pharmacokinetics:

Absorption/Distribution – Following oral administration, moricizine undergoes significant first-pass metabolism resulting in an absolute bioavailability of ≈ 38%. Peak plasma concentrations are usually reached within 0.5 to 2 hours. Administration 30 minutes after a meal delays the rate of absorption, resulting in lower peak plasma concentrations, but the extent of absorption is not altered. Plasma levels are proportional to dose over the recommended therapeutic dose range. The apparent volume of distribution after oral administration is very large (≥ 300 L) and is not significantly related to body weight. Moricizine is ≈ 95% bound to plasma proteins, independent of plasma concentration.

Metabolism/Excretion – Moricizine undergoes extensive biotransformation; < 1% is excreted unchanged in the urine. There are at least 26 metabolites, but no single metabolite has been found to represent as much as 1% of the administered dose, and as stated previously, antiarrhythmic response has relatively slow onset and offset. Two metabolites are pharmacologically active in at least one animal model: Moricizine sulfoxide and phenothiazine-2-carbamic acid ethyl ester sulfoxide. Each of these metabolites represents a small percentage of the administered dose (< 0.6%), is present in lower plasma concentrations than the parent drug, and has a plasma elimination half-life of ≈ 3 hours.

Moricizine induces its own metabolism. Average plasma concentrations in patients decrease with multiple dosing. This decrease in plasma levels of parent drug does not appear to affect clinical outcome for patients on chronic therapy. The plasma half-life is 1.5 to 3.5 hours (most values about 2 hours) following single or multiple oral doses in patients with ventricular ectopy. Approximately 56% is excreted in the feces and 39% is excreted in the urine. Some enterohepatic recycling occurs.

Clinical trials: Moricizine at daily doses of 600 to 900 mg produced a dose-related reduction in the occurrence of frequent VPD and reduced the incidence of nonsustained and sustained ventricular tachycardia (VT). In controlled clinical trials, moricizine had antiarrhythmic activity similar to that of disopyramide, propranolol and quinidine. In programmed electrical stimulation studies (PES), moricizine prevented the induction of sustained ventricular tachycardia in ≈ 25% of patients. Activity of moricizine is maintained during long-term use.

Moricizine is effective in treating ventricular arrhythmias in patients with and without organic heart disease. It may be effective in patients in whom other antiarrhythmics are ineffective, not tolerated or contraindicated.

Arrhythmia exacerbation or "rebound" is not noted following discontinuation of therapy.

Indications:

Treatment of documented ventricular arrhythmias, such as sustained ventricular tachycardia, that are life-threatening. Because of the proarrhythmic effects of moricizine, reserve its use for patients in whom the benefits of treatment outweigh the risks.

Initiate treatment in the hospital.

Unlabeled uses: Moricizine (600 to 900 mg/day) appears effective in treatment of ventricular premature contractions, couplets and nonsustained ventricular tachycardia.

Contraindications:

Pre-existing second- or third-degree AV block; right bundle branch block when associated with left hemiblock (bifascicular block) unless a pacemaker is present; cardiogenic shock; hypersensitivity to the drug.

Warnings:

Mortality: Moricizine was one of three antiarrhythmic drugs included in the National Heart Lung and Blood Institute's Cardiac Arrhythmia Suppression Trial (CAST I), a long-term, multicenter, randomized, double-blind study in patients with asymptomatic non-life-threatening ventricular arrhythmias who had a myocardial infarction (MI) > 6 days, but < 2 years, previously. An excessive mortality or nonfatal cardiac arrest rate was seen in patients treated with both of the Class IC agents included in the trial, which led to discontinuation of those two arms of the trial.

The moricizine and placebo arms of the trial were continued in the NHLBI-sponsored CAST II. In this randomized, double-blind trial, patients with asymptomatic non-life-threatening arrhythmias who had an MI within 4 to 90 days and left ventricular ejection fraction ≤ 0.4 prior to enrollment were evaluated. The average duration of treatment with moricizine in this study was 18 months. The study was discontinued because there was no possibility of demonstrating a benefit toward improved survival with moricizine and because of an evolving adverse trend after long-term treatment.

The applicability of the CAST results to other populations (eg, those without recent MI) is uncertain. Considering the known proarrhythmic properties of moricizine and the lack of evidence of improved survival for any antiarrhythmic drug in patients without life-threatening arrhythmias, it is prudent to reserve the use of moricizine for patients with life-threatening ventricular arrhythmias.

Survival: Antiarrhythmic drugs have not been proven to favorably affect survival or incidence of sudden death.

Proarrhythmic effects: Like other antiarrhythmic drugs, moricizine can provoke new rhythm disturbances or make existing arrhythmias worse. These proarrhythmic effects can range from an increase in the frequency of VPDs to the development of new or more severe ventricular tachycardia (eg, tachycardia that is more sustained or more resistant to conversion to sinus rhythm, with potentially fatal consequences). It is often not possible to distinguish a proarrhythmic effect from the patient's underlying rhythm disorder; therefore, consider the occurrence rates that follow approximations. Note also that drug-induced arrhythmias can generally be identified only when they occur early after starting the drug and when the rhythm can be identified, usually because the patient is being monitored. It is clear from the CAST study that some antiarrhythmic drugs can cause increased sudden death mortality, presumably due to new arrhythmias or asystole that do not appear early after treatment but that represent a sustained increased risk.

MORICIZINE HCl

Domestic pre-marketing trials included 1072 patients given moricizine; 397 had baseline lethal arrhythmias (sustained VT or VF and non-sustained VT with hemodynamic symptoms) and 576 had potentially lethal arrhythmias (increased VPDs or NSVT in patients with known structural heart disease, active ischemia, CHF or an LVEF < 40% or CI < 2 L/min/m^2). In this population there were 40 (3.7%) identified proarrhythmic events, 26 (2.5%) of which were serious, either fatal (6), new hemodynamically significant sustained VT or VF (4), new sustained VT that was not hemodynamically significant (11) or sustained VT that became syncopal/presyncopal when it had not been before (5).

In general, serious proarrhythmic effects were equally common in patients with more and less severe arrhythmias, 2.5% in the patients with baseline lethal arrhythmias vs 2.8% in patients with potentially lethal arrhythmias, although the patients with serious effects were more likely to have a history of sustained VT (38% vs 23%).

Five of the six fatal proarrhythmic events were in patients with baseline lethal arrhythmias; four had prior cardiac arrests. Rates and severity of proarrhythmic events were similar in patients given 600 to 900 mg/day and those given higher doses. Patients with proarrhythmic events were more likely than the overall population to have coronary artery disease (85% vs 67%), history of acute MI (75% vs 53%), CHF (60% vs 43%) and cardiomegaly (55% vs 33%). All of the six proarrhythmic deaths were in patients with coronary artery disease; five of six each had documented acute MI, CHF and cardiomegaly.

In two recent studies, moricizine (400 to 1000 mg/day) was ineffective in patients with refractory sustained ventricular arrhythmias (failed therapy with other class I agents) and carried a considerable risk for life threatening proarrhythmia. In one study, seven of 26 patients (27%) developed proarrhythmia during moricizine loading, and in the other study four of 21 patients (19%) had a probable proarrhythmic response.

Electrolyte disturbances: Hypokalemia, hyperkalemia or hypomagnesemia may alter the effects of Class I antiarrhythmic drugs. Correct electrolyte imbalances before administration of moricizine.

Sick sinus syndrome: Use with extreme caution in patients with sick sinus syndrome since it may cause sinus bradycardia, sinus pause or sinus arrest.

Renal function impairment: Plasma levels of intact moricizine are unchanged in hemodialysis patients, but a significant portion (39%) is metabolized and excreted in the urine. Although no identified active metabolite is known to increase in people with renal failure, metabolites of unrecognized importance could be affected. Administer cautiously. Start patients with significant renal dysfunction on lower doses and monitor for excessive pharmacologic effects, including ECG intervals, before dosage adjustment (see Administration and Dosage).

Hepatic function impairment: Patients with significant liver dysfunction have reduced plasma clearance and an increased half-life of moricizine. Although the precise relationship of moricizine levels to effect is not clear, treat hepatic disease patients with lower doses and closely monitor for excessive pharmacological effects, including ECG intervals, before dosage adjustment. Administer with particular care to patients with severe liver disease, if at all (see Administration and Dosage).

Carcinogenesis: In a 24 month mouse study in which moricizine was administered to provide up to 320 mg/kg/day, ovarian tubular adenomas and granulosa cell tumors were limited to moricizine-treated animals.

In a 24 month study in which moricizine was administered to rats at doses of 25, 50 and 100 mg/kg/day, Zymbal's Gland Carcinoma was observed in one mid-dose and two high-dose males. The rats also showed a dose-related increase in hepatocellular cholangioma in both sexes, along with fatty metamorphosis, possibly due to disruption of hepatic choline utilization for phospholipid biosynthesis.

Pregnancy: Category B. In a study in which rats were dosed with moricizine prior to and during mating, and throughout gestation and lactation, dose levels 3.4 and 6.7 times the maximum recommended human daily dose produced a dose-related decrease in pup and maternal weight gain, possibly related to a larger litter size. In a study in which dosing was begun on day 15 of gestation, moricizine, at a level 6.7 times the maximum recommended human daily dose, produced a retardation in maternal weight gain but no effect on pup growth. There are no adequate and well controlled studies in pregnant women. Use during pregnancy only if clearly needed.

Lactation: Moricizine is excreted in the milk of animals and is present in human breast milk. Because of the potential for serious adverse reactions in nursing infants, decide whether to discontinue nursing or to discontinue the drug, taking into account the importance of the drug to the mother.

Children: Safety and efficacy in children < 18 years of age have not been established.

MORICIZINE HCl

Precautions:

ECG changes/Conduction abnormalities: Moricizine slows AV nodal and intraventricular conduction, producing dose-related increases in PR and QRS intervals. In clinical trials, the average increase in PR interval was 12% and QRS interval was 14%. Although the QTc interval is increased, this is due to QRS prolongation; the JT interval is shortened, indicating absence of significant slowing of ventricular repolarization. The degree of lengthening of PR and QRS intervals does not predict efficacy.

In controlled clinical trials and in open studies, the overall incidence of delayed ventricular conduction, including new bundle branch block pattern, was ≈ 9.4%. In patients without baseline conduction abnormalities, the frequency of second-degree AV block was 0.2% and third-degree AV block did not occur. In patients with baseline conduction abnormalities, the frequencies of second-degree AV block and third-degree AV block were 0.9% and 1.4%, respectively.

Therapy was discontinued in 1.6% of patients due to ECG changes (0.6% due to sinus pause or asystole, 0.2% to AV block, 0.2% to junctional rhythm, 0.4% to intraventricular conduction delay and 0.2% to wide QRS or PR interval).

In patients with pre-existing conduction abnormalities, initiate therapy cautiously. If second- or third-degree AV block occurs, discontinue therapy unless a ventricular pacemaker is in place. When changing the dose or adding concomitant medications which may also affect cardiac conduction, monitor ECG.

Congestive heart failure: Most patients with CHF have tolerated the recommended daily doses without unusual toxicity or change in effect. Pharmacokinetic differences between patients with and without CHF were not apparent (see Hepatic function impairment). In some cases, worsened heart failure has been attributed to moricizine. Carefully watch patients with pre-existing heart failure when therapy is initiated.

Effects on pacemaker threshold: Since the effect of moricizine on the sensing and pacing thresholds of artificial pacemakers has not been sufficiently studied, monitor pacing parameters if moricizine is used.

Drug fever: Three patients developed rechallenge-confirmed drug fever, with one patient experiencing an elevation above 39.5° to 40.6°C (103° to 105°F) with rigors. Fevers occurred at about 2 weeks in two cases, and after 21 weeks in the third. Fevers resolved within 48 hours after discontinuation of moricizine.

Drug Interactions:

Moricizine Drug Interactions			
Precipitant Drug	Object Drug*		Comments
Cimetidine	Moricizine	⬆	1.4 fold increase in moricizine plasma levels, 49% decrease in clearance. Initiate moricizine at low doses (not > 600 mg/day).
Digoxin	Moricizine	⬆	Additive prolongation of the PR interval, but not with a significant increase in the rate of second- or third-degree AV block. Little change in serum digoxin levels or pharmacokinetics.
Propranolol	Moricizine	⬆	Small additive increase in PR interval; no changes in overall ECG intervals.
Moricizine	Theophylline	⬇	Theophylline clearance increased 44% to 66% and plasma half-life decreased 19% to 33% (conventional and sustained-release theophylline).

* ⬆ = Object drug increased ⬇ = Object drug decreased

Drug/Food interactions: Administration of moricizine 30 minutes after a meal delays the rate of absorption, resulting in lower peak plasma concentrations, but the extent of absorption is not altered.

Adverse Reactions:

The most serious adverse reaction reported is proarrhythmia (see Warnings). This occurred in 3.7% of 1072 patients with ventricular arrhythmias who received a wide range of doses under a variety of circumstances. In addition, in controlled clinical trials and in open studies, adverse reactions led to discontinuation of moricizine in 7% of 1105 patients with ventricular and supraventricular arrhythmias, including: Nausea (3.2%); ECG abnormalities (1.6%; principally conduction defects, sinus pause, junctional rhythm or AV block); CHF (1%); dizziness, anxiety, drug fever, urinary retention, blurred vision, GI upset, rash, laboratory abnormalities (0.3% to 0.4%).

MORICIZINE HCl

Other: Sweating, musculoskeletal pain, dry mouth, blurred vision (2% to < 5%); drug fever, hypothermia, temperature intolerance, eye pain, rash, pruritus, dry skin, urticaria, swelling of the lips and tongue, periorbital edema (< 2%).

Two patients developed thrombocytopenia that may have been drug-related. Clinically significant elevations in liver function tests (bilirubin, serum transaminases) and jaundice consistent with hepatitis occurred rarely. Although a cause-and-effect relationship has not been established, caution is advised in patients who develop unexplained signs of hepatic dysfunction; consider discontinuing therapy.

Elderly: Adverse reactions were generally similar in patients > 65 years old (n = 375) and < age 65 (n = 697), although discontinuation of therapy for reasons other than proarrhythmia was more common in older patients (13.9% vs 7.7%). Overall mortality was greater in older patients (9.3% vs 3.9%), but those were not deaths attributed to treatment, and the older patients had more serious underlying heart disease.

Cardiovascular: Palpitations (5.8%); sustained ventricular tachycardia, cardiac chest pain, CHF, cardiac death (2% to < 5%); hypotension, hypertension, syncope, supraventricular arrhythmias (including atrial fibrillations/flutter), cardiac arrest, bradycardia, pulmonary embolism, MI, vasodilation, cerebrovascular events, thrombophlebitis (< 2%).

CNS: Dizziness (15.1%); headache (8%); fatigue (5.9%); hypesthesias, asthenia, nervousness, paresthesias, sleep disorders (2% to < 5%); tremor, anxiety, depression, euphoria, confusion, somnolence, agitation, seizure, coma, abnormal gait, hallucinations, nystagmus, diplopia, speech disorder, akathisia, memory loss, ataxia, abnormal coordination, dyskinesia, vertigo, tinnitus (< 2%).

Dizziness appears to be related to the size of each dose. In a comparison of 900 mg/day given at 450 mg twice daily or 300 mg 3 times daily, > 20% of patients experienced dizziness on the twice daily regimen vs 12% on the 3 times daily regimen.

GU: Urinary retention or frequency, dysuria, urinary incontinence, kidney pain, impotence, decreased libido (< 2%).

Respiratory: Dyspnea (5.7%); hyperventilation, apnea, asthma, pharyngitis, cough, sinusitis (< 2%).

GI: Nausea (9.6%); abdominal pain, dyspepsia, vomiting, diarrhea (2% to < 5%); anorexia, bitter taste, dysphagia, flatulence, ileus (< 2%).

Overdosage:

Symptoms: Emesis; lethargy; coma; syncope; hypotension; conduction disturbances; exacerbation of CHF; MI; sinus arrest; arrhythmias (including junctional bradycardia, ventricular tachycardia, ventricular fibrillation and asystole); respiratory failure. Deaths have occurred after accidental or intentional overdoses of 2250 and 10,000 mg, respectively. Accidental introduction of moricizine into the lungs of monkeys resulted in rapid arrhythmic death.

Treatment: Treatment should be supportive. Hospitalize patients and monitor for cardiac, respiratory and CNS changes. Provide advanced life support systems, including an intracardiac pacing catheter where necessary. Treat acute overdosage with appropriate gastric evacuation, and with special care to avoid aspiration. Refer to General Management of Acute Overdosage.

Patient Information:

Take exactly as prescribed. Dosage changes must be supervised by the physician.

Contact the physician immediately if chest pain or discomfort, pounding in the chest (palpitations), irregular heartbeat or fever occur.

Hospitalization is required when starting on this medication.

MORICIZINE HCl

Administration and Dosage:

Approved by the FDA on June 26, 1990.

Individualize dosage. Clinical, cardiac rhythm monitoring, ECG intervals, exercise testing, or programmed electrical stimulation testing may be used to guide antiarrhythmic response and dosage adjustment. In general, the patients will be at high risk; hospitalize for the initiation of therapy.

Usual adult dosage is between 600 and 900 mg/day, given every 8 hours in three equally divided doses. Within this range, the dosage can be adjusted as tolerated, in increments of 150 mg/day at 3 day intervals, until the desired effect is obtained. Patients with life-threatening arrhythmias who exhibit a beneficial response as judged by objective criteria (eg, Holter monitoring, programmed electrical stimulation, exercise testing) can be maintained on chronic moricizine therapy. As the antiarrhythmic effect of moricizine persists for > 12 hours, some patients whose arrhythmias are well controlled on an every 8 hour regimen may be given the same total daily dose in an every 12 hour regimen to increase convenience and help assure compliance. When higher doses are used, patients may experience more dizziness and nausea on the every 12 hour regimen.

Hepatic or renal function impairment: Start at ≤ 600 mg/day and monitor closely, including measurement of ECG intervals, before dosage adjustment.

Transfer from another antiarrhythmic: Recommendations for transferring patients from another antiarrhythmic to moricizine can be given based on theoretical considerations. Withdraw previous antiarrhythmic therapy for 1 to 2 plasma half-lives before starting moricizine at the recommended dosages. In patients in whom withdrawal of a previous antiarrhythmic is likely to produce life-threatening arrhythmias, hospitalize.

Transferring to Moricizine from Another Antiarrhythmic

Agent transferred from	Start moricizine
Quinidine, disopyramide	6 to 12 hours after last dose
Procainamide	3 to 6 hours after last dose
Encainide, mexiletine, propafenone or tocainide	8 to 12 hours after last dose
Flecainide	12 to 24 hours after last dose

Rx	**Ethmozine** (Roberts)	**Tablets:** 200 mg	Lactose. Light green. Film coated. Oval, convex. In 100s and UD 100s.
		250 mg	Lactose. Light orange. Film coated. Oval, convex. In 100s and UD 100s.
		300 mg	Lactose. Light blue. Film coated. Oval, convex. In 100s and UD 100s.

IBUTILIDE FUMARATE

Warning:

Life-threatening arrhythmias — appropriate treatment environment: Ibutilide can cause potentially fatal arrhythmias, particularly sustained polymorphic ventricular tachycardia, usually in association with QT prolongation (torsades de pointes), but sometimes without documented QT prolongation. In clinical studies, these arrhythmias, which require cardioversion, occurred in 1.7% or treated patients during, or within a number of hours of, use of ibutilide. These arrhythmias can be reversed if treated promptly (see Warnings, Proarrhythmia). It is essential that ibutilide be administered in a setting of continuous ECG monitoring and by personnel trained in identification and treatment of acute ventricular arrthymias, particularly polymorphic ventricular tachycardia. NOTE: Patients with a trial fibrillation of > 2 to 3 days' duration must be adequately anticoagulated, generally for at least 2 weeks.

Choice of patients: Patients with chronic atrial fibrillation have a strong tendency to revert after conversion to sinus rhythm, and treatments to maintain sinus rhythm carry risks. Therefore, carefully select patients to be treated with ibutilide, such that the expected benefits of maintaining sinus rhythm outweigh the immediate resks of ibutilide, and the risks of maintenance therapy, and are likely to offer an advantage compared with alternative management.

Actions:

Pharmacology: Ibutilide is an antiarrhythmic drug with predominantly class III (cardiac action potential prolongation) properties according to the Vaughan Williams Classification. Ibutilide prolongs action potential duration in isolated adult cardiac myocytes and increases both atrial and ventricular refractoriness in vivo, ie, class III electrophysiologic effects. Voltage clamp studies indicate that ibutilide, at nanomolar concentrations, delays repolarization by activation of a slow, inward current (predominantly sodium), rather than by blocking outward potassium currents, which is the mechanism by which most other class III antiarrhythmics act. These effects lead to prolongation of atrial and ventricular action potential duration and refractoriness, the predominant electrophysiologic properties of ibutilide in humans that are thought to be the basis for its antiarrhythmic effect.

Electrophysiology – Ibutilide produces mild slowing of the sinus rate and AV conduction. Ibutilide produces no clinically significant effect on QRS duration at IV doses up to 0.03 mg/kg administered over a 10–minute period. Although there is no established relationship between plasma concentration and antiarrhythmic effect, ibutilide produces dose-related prolongation of the QT interval, which is thought to be associated with its antiarrhythmic activity. (See Warnings for relationship between QTc prolongation and torsades de pointes-type arrhythmias.) In a study in healthy volunteers, IV infusions of ibutilide resulted in prolongation of the QT interval that was directly correlated with ibutilide plasma concentration during and after 10 minute and 8 hour infusions. A steep ibutilide concentration/response (QT prolongation) relationship was shown. The maximum effect was a function of both the dose and the infusion rate.

Hemodynamics – A study of hemodynamic function in patients with ejection fractions both above and below 35% shosed no clinically significant effects on cardiac output, mean pulmonary arterial pressure or pulmonary capillary wedge pressure at doses up to 0.03 mg/kg.

Pharmacokinetics:

Absorption/Distribution – After IV infusion, ibutilide plasma concentrations rapidly decrease in a multiexponential fashion. The pharmacokinetics of ibutilide are highly variable among subjects. Ibutilide has a high systemic plasma clearance that approximates liver blood flow (≈ 29 ml/min/kg), a large steady-state volume of distribution (≈ 11 L/kg) in healthy volunteers and minimal (≈ 40%) protein binding. The drug is cleared rapidly and highly distributed in patients being treated for atrial flutter or atrial fibrillation. The elimination half-life averages about 6 hours (range, 2 to 12 hours). The pharmacokinetics are linear with respect to the dose over the dose range of 0.01 to 0.10 mg/kg. The enantiomers of ibutilide have pharmacokinetic properties similar to each other and to ibutilide.

Metabolism/Excretion – In healthy male volunteers, ≈ 82% of a 0.01 mg/kg dose was excreted in the urine (≈ 7% of the dose as unchanged ibutilide) and the remainder (≈ 19%) was recovered in the feces. Eight metabolites of ibutilide were detected in the urine. These metabolites are thought to be formed primarily by ω-oxidation followed by sequential β-oxidation of the heptyl side chain of ibutilide. Of the eight metabolites, only the ω-hydroxy metabolite possesses class III electrophysiologic properties similar to that of ibutilide in an in vitro isolated rabbit myocardium model. The plasma concentrations of this active metabolite, however, are < 10% that of ibutilide.

Clinical trials: Treatment with IV ibutilide for acute termination of recent onset atrial flutter/fibrillation was eveluated in 466 patients participating in two trials. In one trial, single 10 minute infusions of 0.005 to 0.025 mg/kg were tested in parallel groups. In the second trial, up to two infusions of ibutilide were evaluated — the first 1 mg, the second given 10 minutes after completion of the first infusion, either 0.5 or 1 mg. In a third study, 319 patients with atrial fibrillation or atrial flutter were randomized to receive single, 10 minute IV infusions of either sotalol (1.5 mg/kg) or ibutilide (1 or 2 mg). Among patients with atrial flutter, 53% receiving 1 mg ibutilide and 70% receiving 2 mg ibutilide converted, compared with 18% of those receiving sotalol. In patients with atrial fibrillation, 22% and 43% receiving 1 and 2 mg ibutilide, respectively, converted compared with 10% of patients receiving sotalol.

Conversion of atrial flutter/fibrillation usually (70% of those who converted) occurred within 30 minutes of the start of infusion and was dose related. The latest conversion seen was at 90 minutes after the start of the infusion. Most converted patients remained in normal sinus rhythm for 24 hours.

Overall responses in these patients, defined as termination of arrhythmias for any length of time during or within 1 hour following completed infusion of randomized dose, were in the range of 45% to 50% at doses above 0.0125 mg/kg (vs 2% for placebo). Twenty-four hour responses were similar. For these atrial arrhythmias, ibutilide was more effective in patients with flutter than fibrillation (> 50% vs < 40%).

The number of patients who remained in the converted rhythm at the end of 24 hours were slightly less than those patients who converted intially, but the difference between conversion rates for ibutilide compared with placebo was still statistically significant. In long-term follow-up, ≈ 40% of all patients remained recurrence free, usually with chronic prophylactic treatment, 400 to 500 days after acute treatment, regardless of the method of conversion.

Patients with more recent onset of arrhythmia had a higher rate of conversion. Response rates were 42% and 50% for patients with onset of atrial fibrillation/flutter for < 30 days in the two efficacy studies compared with 16% and 31% in those with more chronic arrhythmias.

Indications:

Atrial fibrillation/flutter: For the rapid conversion of atrial fibrillation or atrial flutter of recent onset to sinus rhythm. Patients with atrial arrhythmias of longer duration are less likely to respond to ibutilide. The effectiveness of ibutilide has not been determined in patients with arrhythmias of > 90 days in duration.

Contraindications:

Hypersensitivity to ibutilide or any of the other product components

Warnings:

Proarrhythmia: Like other antiarrhythmic agents, ibutilide can induce or worsen ventricular arrhythmias in some patients. This may have potentially fatal consequences. Torsades de pointes, a polymorphic ventricular tachycardia that develops in the setting of a prolonged QT interval, may occur because of the effect ibutilide has on cardiac repolarization, but ibutilide can also cause polymorphic VT in the absence of excessive prolongation of the QT interval. In general, with drugs that prolong the QT interval, the risk of torsades de pointes is thought to increase progressively as the QT interval is prolonged and may be worsened with bradycardia, a varying heart rate and hypokalemia.

In clinical trials conducted in patients with atrial fibrillation and atrial flutter, those with QTc intervals > 440 msec were not usually allowed to participate, and serum potassium had to be above 4 mEq/L. Although change in QTc was dose dependent for ibutilide, there was no clear relationship between risk of serious proarrhythmia and dose, possibly due to the small number of events. In clinical trials of IV ibutilide, patients with a history of CHF or low left ventricular ejection fraction appeared to have a higher incidence of sustained polymorphic ventricular tachycardia (VT) than those without such underlying conditions; for sustained polymorphic VT, the rate was 6.2% in patients with a history of CHF and 0.8% without it. There was also a suggestion that women had a higher risk of proarrhythmia, but the sex difference was not observed in all studies and was most prominent for nonsustained VT. The incidence of sustained ventricular arrhythmias was similar in male (1.8%) and female (1.5%) patients, possibly due to the small number of events. Ibutilide is not recommended in patients who have demonstrated polymorphic VT (eg, torsades de pointes).

During clinical trials, 1.7% of patients with atrial flutter or atrial fibrillation treated with ibutilide developed sustained polymorphic VT requiring cardioversion. In these clinical trials, many initial episodes of polymorphic VT occurred after the infusion of ibutilide was stopped but, generally, not more than 40 minutes after the start of the first infusion. There were, however, instances of recurrent polymorphic VT that occurred about 3 hours after the initial infusion. In two cases, the VT degenerated into ventricular fibrillation, requiring immediate defibrillation. Other cases were managed with cardiac pacing and magnesium sulfate infusions. Nonsustained polymorphic VT ocurred in 2.7% of patients, and nonsustained monomorphic VTs occurred in 4.9% of the patients (see Adverse Reactions).

Proarrhythmic events must be anticipated. Skilled personnel and proper equipment, including cardiac monitoring equipment, intracardiac pacing facilities, a cardioverter/defribrillator and medication for treatment of sustained VT, including polymorphic VT, must be available during and after administration of ibutilide. Before treatment, correct hypokalemia and hypomagnesemia to reduce the potential for proarrhythmia. Observe patients with continuous ECG monitoring for at least 4 hours following infusion or until QTc has returned to baseline. Longer monitoring is required if any arrhythmic activity is noted. Management of polymorphic VT includes discontinuation of ibutilide, correction of electrolyte abnormalities, especially potassium and magnesium, and overdrive cardiac pacing, electrical cardioversion or defibrillation. Pharmacologic therapies include magnesium sulfate infusions. Generally avoid treatment with antiarrhythmics.

Renal/Hepatic function impairment: It is unlikely that dosing adjustments would be necessary in patients with compromised renal or hepatic function based on the following considerations: (1) Ibutilide is indicated for rapid IV therapy (duration ≤ 30 min) and is dosed to a known, well-defined pharmacologic action (termination of arrhythmia) or to a maximum of two 10 minute infusions; (2) < 10% of the dose is excreted unchanged in the urine; and (3) drug distribution appears to be one of the primary mechanisms responsible for termination of the pharmacologic effect. Nonetheless, monitor patients with abnormal liver function by telemetry for more that the 4 hour periods generally recommended. In 285 patients with atrial fibrillation or atrial flutter who were treated with ibutilide, the clearance of ibutilide was independent of renal function, as assessed by creatinine clearance (range, 21 to 140 ml/min).

Elderly: The mean age of patients in clinical trials was 65. No age-related differences were observed in pharmacokinetic, efficacy or safety parameters for patients < 65 compared with patients ≥ 65 years of age.

Pregnancy: Category C. Ibutilide administered orally was teratogenic (adactyly, cleft palate, scoliosis) and embryocidal in reproduction studies in rats. Do no administer to a pregnant woman unless clinical benefit outweighs potential risk to the fetus.

Lactation: The excretion of ibutilide into breast milk has not been studied; accordingly, discourage breastfeeding during therapy.

Children: Clinical trials in patients with atrial fibrillation and atrial flutter did not include anyone under the age of 18. Safety and efficacy of ibutilide in children have not been established.

Precautions:

Heart block: Of the nine (1.5%) ibutilide-treated patients with reports of reversible heart block, five had first degree, three had second degree and one had complete heart block.

Drug Interactions:

No specific pharmacokinetic or other formal drug interaction studies were conducted.

Concomitant antiarrhythmics: Class Ia antiarrhythmic drugs (Vaughan Williams Classification), such as disopyramide, quinidine and procainamide, and other class III drugs, such as amiodarone and sotalol, should not be given concomitantly with ibutilide or within 4 hours postinfusion because of their potential to prolont refractoriness. In the clinical trials, class I or other class III antiarrhythmic agents were withheld for at least 5 half-lives prior to ibutilide infusion and for 4 hours after dosing, but thereafter were allowed at the physician's discretion.

Other drugs that prolong the QT interval: The potential for proarrhythmia may increase with the administration of ibutilide to patients who are being treated with drugs that prolong the QT interval, such as phenothiazines, tricyclic and tetracyclic antidepressants and certain antihistamine drugs (H_1 receptor antagonists).

Digoxin: Supraventricular arrhythmias may mask the cardiotoxicity associated with excessive digoxin levels. Therefore, it is advisable to be particularly cautious in patients whose plasma digoxin levels are above or suspected to be above the usual therapeutic range.

Adverse Reactions:

Ibutilide was generally well tolerated in clinical trials. Of the 586 patients with atrial fibrillation or atrial flutter who received ibutilide in phase II/III studies, 149 (25%)

IBUTILIDE FUMARATE

reported medical events related to the cardiovascular system, including sustained polymorphic VT (1.7%) and nonsustained polymorphic VT (2.7%).

Other clinically important adverse events include the following: Nonsustained monomorphic ventricular extrasystoles (5.1%); nonsustained monomorphic VT (4.9%); headache (3.6%); tachycardia/sinus tachycardia/supraventricular tachycardia, nonsustained polymorphic VT (2.7%); hypotension/postural hypotension (2%); bundle branch block (1.9%); sustained polymorphic VT (1.7%); AV block (1.5%); bradycardia/sinus bradycardia, QT segment prolonged, hypertension (1.2%); nausea (> 1%); palpitation (1%); supraventricular extrsystoles (0.9%); nodal arrhythmia (0.7%); congestive heart failure (0.5%); syncope, renal failure (0.3%); idioventricular rhythm, sustained monomorphic VT (0.2%).

Overdosage:

Acute overdose in animals results in CNS toxicity, notably, CNS depression, rapid gasping breathing and convulsions. In clinical trials, four patients were unintentionally overdosed. The largest dose was 3.4 mg administered over 15 minutes. One patient (0.025 mg/kg) developed increased ventricular ectopy and monomorphic ventricular tachycardia, another patient (0.032 mg/kg) developed AV block-3rd degree and nonsustained polymorphic VT and two patients (0.038 and 0.02 mg/kg) had no medical event reports. Based on known pharmacology, the clinical effects of an overdosage with ibutilide could exaggerate the expected prolongation of repolarization seen at usual clinical doses. Treat medical events (eg, proarrhythmia, AV block) that occur after the overdosage with measures appropriate for that condition.

Administration and Dosage:

The recommended dose based on controlled trials is outlined in the table below. Stop ibutilide infusion as soon as the presenting arrhythmia is terminated or in the event of sustained or nonsustained ventricular tachycardia, or marked prolongation of QT or QTc.

Recommended Dose of Ibutilide Injection

Patient weight	Initial infusion (over 10 minutes)	Second Infusion
≥ 60 kg (132 lb)	One vial (1 mg)	If the arrhythmia does not terminate within 10 minutes after the end of the initial infusion, a second 10 minute infusion of equal strength may be administered 10 minutes after completion of the first infusion.
< 60 kg (132 lb)	0.1 ml/kg (0.01 mg/kg)	

In a trial comparing ibutilide and sotalol, 2 mg ibutilide administered as a single infusion to patients weighing > 60 kg was also effective in terminating atrial fibrillation or atrial flutter.

Observe patients with continuous ECG monitoring for at least 4 hours following infusion or until QTc has returned to baseline. Longer monitoring is required if any arrhythmic activity is noted. Skilled personnel and proper equipment, such as a cardioverter/difibrillator and medication for treatment of sustained ventribular tachycardia, including polymorphic ventricular tachycardia, must be available during administration of ibutilide and subsequent monitoring of the patient.

Dilution: Ibutilide may be administered undiluted or diluted in 50 ml diluent. Ibutilide may be added to 0.9% Sodium Chloride Injection or 5% Dextrose Injection before infusion. The contents of one 10 ml vial (0.1 mg/ml) may be added to a 50 ml infusion bag to form an admixture of ≈ 0.017 mg/ml.

Admixture compatibility: The following diluents are compatible with ibutilide (0.1 mg/ml): 5% Dextrose Injection and 0.9% Sodium Chloride Injection. The following IV solution containers are compatible with admixtures of ibutilide (0.1 mg/ml): Polyvinyl choride plastic bags; polyolefin bags.,

Storage/Stability: Admixtures of the product, with approved diluents, are chemically and physically stable for 24 hours at room temperature (15° to 30°C; 59° to 86°F) and for 48 hours at refrigerated temperatures (2°to 8°C; 36° to 46°F).

Rx	**Corvert** (Pharmacia & Upjohn)	**Solution:** 0.1 mg/ml	In 10 ml vials.

QUINIDINE

Refer to the general discussion concerning these products in the Antiarrhythmic Agents group monograph.

Actions:

Pharmacology: Quinidine, a class IA antiarrhythmic, depresses myocardial excitability, conduction velocity and contractility. Therapeutically, it prolongs the effective refractory period and increases conduction time, thereby preventing the reentry phenomenon. In addition, quinidine exerts an indirect anticholinergic effect; it decreases vagal tone and may facilitate conduction in the atrioventricular junction.

Pharmacokinetics:

Absorption/Distribution – ferences in the anhydrous quinidine alkaloid content among the various salts. See table below:

Anhydrous Quinidine Alkaloid Content in Various Salts			
	Quinidine content		
Quinidine salts	Active drug	Absorbed	Time to peak plasma levels (hours)
Quinidine Sulfate	83%	73%	1 to 3[1]
Quinidine Gluconate	62%	70%	3-5
Quinidine Polygalacturonate	80%	—	6

[1] 3 to 5 hours for sustained release form.

Quinidine is rapidly absorbed from the GI tract. Maximum effects of quinidine gluconate occur 30 to 90 minutes after IM administration; onset is more rapid after IV administration. Activity persists for 6 to 8 hours or more. The average therapeutic serum levels are reported to be 2 to 7 mcg/ml. Toxic reactions may occur at levels from 5 to ≥ 8 mcg/ml. Quinidine is 80% to 90% bound to plasma proteins; the unbound fraction may be significantly increased in patients with hepatic insufficiency. Accumulation occurs in most tissues, except the brain. The polygalacturonate salt slows ionization of the drug and protects the GI tract by its demulcent effect.

Metabolism/Excretion – From 60% to 80% of a dose is metabolized via the liver into several metabolites; the primary metabolites are 3-hydroxyquinidine and 2-oxoquinidinone. Whether or not these or other metabolites have antiarrhythmic activity is unclear and controversial. Quinidine is excreted unchanged (10% to 50%) in the urine within 24 hours. The elimination half-life ranges from 4 to 10 hours in healthy patients, with a mean of 6 to 7 hours. Urinary acidification facilitates quinidine elimination, and alkalinization retards it. In patients with cirrhosis, the elimination half-life may be prolonged and the volume of distribution increased. In congestive heart failure (CHF), total clearance and volume of distribution are decreased. In the elderly, the elimination half-life may be increased. The influence of renal dysfunction on the disposition of quinidine is controversial; volume of distribution and renal clearance may be reduced.

Indications:

Oral: Premature atrial, AV junctional and ventricular contractions; paroxysmal atrial (supraventricular) tachycardia; paroxysmal AV junctional rhythm; atrial flutter; paroxysmal and chronic atrial fibrillation; established atrial fibrillation when therapy is appropriate; paroxysmal ventricular tachycardia not associated with complete heart block; maintenance therapy after electrical conversion of atrial fibrillation or flutter.

Parenteral: When oral therapy is not feasible or when rapid therapeutic effect is required.

Quinidine gluconate – Life-threatening *Plasmodium falciparum* malaria: Unless impossible, start therapy in an intensive care setting with continuous ECG monitoring, frequent blood pressure monitoring and periodic monitoring of parasitemia.

Contraindications:

Hypersensitivity or idiosyncrasy to quinidine or other cinchona derivatives manifested by thrombocytopenia, skin eruption or febrile reactions; myasthenia gravis; history of thrombocytopenic purpura associated with quinidine administration; digitalis intoxication manifested by arrhythmias or AV conduction disorders; complete heart block; left bundle branch block or other severe intraventricular conduction defects exhibiting marked QRS widening or bizarre complexes; complete AV block with an AV nodal or idioventricular pacemaker; aberrant ectopic impulses and abnormal rhythms due to escape mechanisms; history of drug-induced torsade de pointes; history of long QT syndrome.

QUINIDINE

Warnings:

Hepatotoxicity (including granulomatous hepatitis) due to quinidine hypersensitivity has occurred. Unexplained fever or elevation of hepatic enzymes, particularly in the early stages of therapy, warrants consideration. Monitor liver function during the first 4 to 8 weeks of therapy. Discontinuing quinidine usually results in toxicity resolution.

Atrial flutter or fibrillation: Reversion to sinus rhythm may be preceded by a progressive reduction in degree of AV block to a 1:1 ratio, which results in an extremely rapid ventricular rate. Prior to use in atrial flutter, pretreat with a digitalis preparation.

Although quinidine reduces recurrences of atrial fibrillation after cardioversion, it may be associated with an increase in mortality.

Cardiotoxicity (eg, increased PR and QT intervals, 50% widening of QRS complex, ventricular tachyarrhythmias, frequent ventricular ectopic beats or tachycardia) dictates immediate discontinuation of quinidine; closely monitor the ECG. Some specialists recommend quinidine therapy be initiated only in hospitalized patients with ECG monitoring. However, this is generally reserved for patients receiving large doses or who are at high risk.

In susceptible individuals (ie, marginally compensated cardiovascular disease), quinidine may produce clinically important depression of cardiac function such as hypotension, bradycardia or heartblock.

Large oral doses may reduce the arterial pressure by means of peripheral vasodilation. Serious hypotension is more likely with parenteral use.

Use quinidine with extreme caution in incomplete AV block, since complete block and asystole may result. The drug may cause unpredictable dysrhythmias in digitalized patients; use with caution in the presence of digitalis intoxication. Use cautiously in patients with partial bundle branch block, severe CHF and hypotensive states due to the depressant effects of quinidine on myocardial contractility and arterial pressure; usefulness of quinidine is limited unless these conditions are due to or aggravated by the arrhythmia. Consider the potential disadvantages and benefits.

Parenteral therapy: The dangers of parenteral use of quinidine are increased in the presence of AV block or absence of atrial activity. Administration is more hazardous in patients with extensive myocardial damage. Use of quinidine in digitalis-induced cardiac arrhythmia is extremely dangerous because the cardiac glycoside may already have caused serious impairment of intracardiac conduction system. Too rapid IV administration of as little as 200 mg may precipitate a fall of 40 to 50 mm Hg in arterial pressure. Inject slowly (see Administration and Dosage).

Syncope occasionally occurs in patients on long-term quinidine therapy, usually resulting from ventricular tachycardia or fibrillation. It is manifested by sudden loss of consciousness and by polymorphic ventricular tachycardia. This syndrome does not appear to be related to dose or plasma levels but occurs more often with prolonged QT intervals. Syncopal episodes frequently terminate spontaneously or respond to treatment, but are sometimes fatal. Torsade de pointes is often the cause.

Renal, hepatic or cardiac insufficiency: Use with caution in renal (especially renal tubular acidosis), cardiac or hepatic insufficiency because of potential toxicity.

Hypersensitivity: Asthma, muscle weakness and infection with fever prior to quinidine administration may mask hypersensitivity reactions to the drug.

Test dose – Administer a single 200 mg tablet of quinidine sulfate or 200 mg IM quinidine gluconate prior to the initiation of treatment to determine whether the patient has an idiosyncrasy to quinidine.

During the first weeks of therapy, although rare, consider hypersensitivity to quinidine including anaphylactoid reactions (eg, angioedema, purpura, acute asthmatic episode, vascular collapse). Refer to Management of Acute Hypersensitivity Reactions.

Pregnancy: Category C. Quinidine crosses the placenta and achieves fetal serum levels similar to maternal levels. Neonatal thrombocytopenia has occurred after maternal use. Safety for use during pregnancy is not established. Use only when clearly needed and when potential benefits outweigh potential hazards to fetus.

Oxytocic properties are reported with quinidine, as with quinine; clinical significance is not known.

Lactation: Safety for use in the nursing mother has not been established. Quinidine is excreted into breast milk with a milk:serum ratio of approximately 0.71. Use caution when quinidine is administered to a nursing woman. The American Academy of Pediatrics considers quinidine to be compatible with breast feeding.

Children: Safety and efficacy have not been established.

QUINIDINE

Precautions:

Monitoring: Perform periodic blood counts and liver and kidney function tests. Discontinue use if blood dyscrasias or signs of hepatic or renal disorders occur. Initiate therapy in the hospital and continuously monitor ECG and check quinidine levels. This is generally done when large doses are used or the patient is at increased risk. Frequently measure arterial blood pressure during IV use; discontinue if blood pressure falls significantly.

Vagolytic effects: Because quinidine has vagolytic activity on the atrium and AV node, administration of cholinergic drugs or use of any other procedure to enhance vagal activity may fail to terminate paroxysmal supraventricular tachycardia.

Potassium balance: The effect of quinidine is enhanced by potassium and reduced if hypokalemia is present. The risk of drug-induced torsade de pointes is increased by concomitant hypokalemia.

Malaria (P falciparum): Dosing schedules known to be effective have been associated with hypotension, increased QRS and corrected QT intervals and cinchonism. Closely monitor ECG and blood pressure.

Drug Interactions:

Quinidine Drug Interactions

Precipitant drug	Object drug*		Description
Amiodarone	Quinidine	↑	Increased quinidine levels may occur with possible production of potentially fatal cardiac dysrhythmias.
Antacids	Quinidine	↑	Certain antacids may increase serum quinidine levels, which may result in toxicity.
Barbiturates	Quinidine	↓	Quinidine serum levels and elimination half-life may be decreased.
Cholinergic drugs	Quinidine	↓	Since quinidine antagonizes the effect of vagal excitation upon the atrium and AV node, concurrent cholinergic agents may result in failure to terminate paroxysmal supraventricular tachycardia.
Cimetidine	Quinidine	↑	Quinidine serum levels may be increased.
Hydantoins	Quinidine	↓	A decrease in the therapeutic effect of quinidine may occur.
Nifedipine	Quinidine	↓	Serum levels and actions of quinidine may be lower than predicted by the dosage.
Rifampin	Quinidine	↓	Increased metabolism of quinidine which may be associated with a reduction in its therapeutic effects.
Sucralfate	Quinidine	↓	Serum quinidine levels may be reduced, decreasing the therapeutic effects.
Urinary alkalinizers	Quinidine	↑	Urinary elimination of quinidine is reduced. Serum quinidine levels may be increased accompanied by increased pharmacologic effects.
Verapamil	Quinidine	↑	Quinidine clearance may be reduced and its half-life prolonged, resulting in hypotension, bradycardia, ventricular tachycardia, AV block and pulmonary edema.
Quinidine	Anticholinergics	↑	Quinidine exhibits a distinct anticholinergic activity in the myocardial tissues. Concurrent use may cause an additive vagolytic effect.
Quinidine	Anticoagulants	↑	Anticoagulation may be potentiated; hemorrhage could occur.
Quinidine	Beta blockers	↑	Effects of metoprolol or propranolol may be increased in "extensive metabolizers."
Quinidine	Cardiac glycosides (digitoxin, digoxin)	↑	Plasma levels of the cardiac glycosides are markedly increased. Pharmacologic effects are increased and toxicity may occur.
Quinidine	Disopyramide	↑	Increased disopyramide levels or decreased quinidine levels may occur.
Disopyramide	Quinidine	↓	

Quinidine Drug Interactions			
Precipitant drug	Object drug*		Description
Quinidine	Nondepolarizing neuromuscular blockers	⬆	Nondepolarizing neuromuscular blocker effects may be enhanced.
Quinidine	Procainamide	⬆	Pharmacologic effects of procainamide may be increased; elevated procainamide and NAPA (major metabolite) plasma levels with toxicity may occur.
Quinidine	Propafenone	⬆	Serum propafenone levels may be increased in rapid extensive metabolizers of the drug (≈ 90% of patients), increasing the pharmacologic effects.
Quinidine	Succinylcholine	⬆	The neuromuscular blockade produced by succinylcholine may be prolonged.
Quinidine	Tricyclic antidepressants	⬆	The clearance of the tricyclic antidepressants may be reduced, possibly resulting in increased pharmacologic effects.

* ⬆ = Object drug increased. ⬇ = Object drug decreased.

Drug/Lab test interactions: **Triamterene** and quinidine have similar fluorescence spectra; thus, triamterene will interfere with the fluorescent measurement of quinidine serum levels.

Adverse Reactions:

Cardiovascular: Widening of QRS complex; cardiac asystole; ventricular ectopy; idioventricular rhythms (including ventricular tachycardia and fibrillation and torsade de pointes in some instances); paradoxical tachycardia; arterial embolism; hypotension; ventricular extrasystoles occurring at the rate of one or more every 6 normal beats; prolonged QT interval; complete AV block; ventricular flutter.

Stop use if any of these occur: Increase of > 25% in duration of QRS complex; disappearance of P waves; restoration of sinus rhythm; decrease in heart rate to 120 bpm in the ECG.

GI: GI effects, the most common reactions seen with quinidine, include: Nausea; vomiting; abdominal pain; diarrhea; anorexia. These may be preceded by fever.

Rarely, oral quinidine has been associated with esophageal disorders, primarily esophagitis.

Hematologic: Acute hemolytic anemia; hypoprothrombinemia; thrombocytopenic purpura; agranulocytosis; drug-induced hypoprothrombinemic hemorrhage in patients on chronic anticoagulant therapy (see Drug Interactions); thrombocytopenia; leukocytosis; shift to left in WBC differential; neutropenia.

CNS: Headache; fever; vertigo; apprehension; excitement; confusion; delirium; syncope; dementia; ataxia; depression.

Ophthalmic: Mydriasis; blurred vision; disturbed color perception; reduced vision field; photophobia; diplopia; night blindness; scotomata; optic neuritis.

Dermatologic: Rash; urticaria; cutaneous flushing with intense pruritus; photosensitivity; eczema; exfoliative eruptions; psoriasis; abnormalities of pigmentation.

Cinchonism: Ringing in the ears; hearing loss; headache; nausea; dizziness; vertigo; lightheadedness; disturbed vision. These may appear after a single dose.

Renal/Hepatic: Lupus nephritis; hepatic toxicity including granulomatous hepatitis; hepatitis.

Lupus erythematosus has occurred. Symptoms include hepatosplenomegaly/lymphadenopathy and a positive antinuclear antibody test. Symptoms resolve after withdrawal of the drug.

Hypersensitivity: Angioedema; acute asthma; vascular collapse; respiratory arrest; hepatic dysfunction including granulomatous hepatitis; hepatic toxicity; purpura; vasculitis. See Warnings.

Body as a whole: Arthralgia; myalgia; increase in serum skeletal muscle creatine phosphokinase; disturbed hearing (tinnitus, decreased auditory acuity).

QUINIDINE

Overdosage:

Severe quinidine intoxication may be associated with depressed mental function, even in hemodynamically stable patients. The patient progresses from lethargy to coma, including respiratory arrest; recurrent generalized motor seizures may occur. The onset of CNS manifestations may be substantially delayed beyond the onset of cardiovascular toxicity; conversely, recovery from coma is often delayed.

Symptoms:

CNS – Lethargy; confusion; coma; respiratory depression or arrest; seizures; headache; parasthesia; vertigo.

GI – Vomiting; abdominal pain; diarrhea; nausea.

Cardiovascular – Tachyarrhythmias (sinus tachycardia, ventricular tachycardia, ventricular fibrillation, torsade de pointes); depressed automaticity and conduction (QRS and QTc prolongation, bundle branch block, sinus bradycardia, sinoatrial block, sinus arrest, AV block, ST depression, T inversion); hypotension (depressed contractility and cardiac output, vasodilation); syncope; heart failure.

Other – Cinchonism; hypokalemia; visual/auditory disturbances; tinnitus; acidosis.

Treatment: If ingestion of quinidine is recent, gastric lavage, emesis or administration of activated charcoal may reduce absorption. Management of overdosage includes: Symptomatic treatment; ECG, blood gases, serum electrolytes and blood pressure monitoring; cardiac pacing if indicated; acidification of the urine. Avoid alkalinization of the urine. Mechanical ventilation and other supportive measures may be required.

IV infusion of ⅙ molar sodium lactate reportedly reduces the cardiotoxic effects of quinidine. Since marked CNS depression may occur even in the presence of convulsions, do not give CNS depressants. Hypotension may be treated, if necessary, with metaraminol or norepinephrine after adequate fluid volume replacement. Tachydysrhythmias should respond to phenytoin or lidocaine. Hemodialysis has been effective in overdosage, but is rarely warranted.

Patient Information:

Do not discontinue therapy unless instructed by physician.

May cause GI upset; take with food.

Notify physician if ringing in the ears, visual disturbances, dizziness, headache, nausea, skin rash or breathing difficulty occurs.

Do not crush or chew sustained release tablets.

Administration and Dosage:

Test dose: Administer a single 200 mg tablet of quinidine sulfate or 200 mg IM quinidine gluconate to determine whether the patient has an idiosyncratic reaction. Continuously monitor ECG when quinidine is used in large doses.

Adjust the dosage to maintain the plasma concentration between 2 to 6 mcg/ml.

Oral:

Premature atrial and ventricular contractions – 200 to 300 mg 3 or 4 times daily.

Paroxysmal supraventricular tachycardias – 400 to 600 mg every 2 or 3 hours until the paroxysm is terminated.

Atrial flutter – Administer quinidine after digitalization. Individualize dosage.

Conversion of atrial fibrillation – 200 mg every 2 or 3 hours for 5 to 8 doses, with subsequent daily increases until sinus rhythm is restored or toxic effects occur. Do not exceed a total daily dose of 3 to 4 g in any regimen. Prior to quinidine administration, control the ventricular rate and CHF (if present) with digoxin.

Maintenance therapy – 200 to 300 mg 3 or 4 times daily. Other patients may require larger doses or more frequent administration than the usually recommended schedule. However, institute such an increased dosage only after careful evaluation of the patient, including ECG and quinidine serum level monitoring.

Sustained release forms – 300 to 600 mg every 8 or 12 hours. Since the rate of absorption from the various sustained release formulations may be markedly different, and since the anhydrous quinidine content is different, do not consider them interchangeable.

Parenteral: The patient must be under close clinical, ECG and blood pressure monitoring, especially during IV administration to detect any change in rate or rhythm. If the patient's condition is not critical, give quinidine gluconate IM. On the other hand, extreme palpitation, dyspnea, vomiting, and a shocklike state in patients with ventricular tachycardia are signs that IV administration may be required as a lifesaving measure when D-C cardioversion is not available.

IM – In the treatment of acute tachycardia, the initial dose is 600 mg quinidine gluconate. Subsequently, 400 mg quinidine gluconate can be repeated as often as every 2 hours. Determine successive doses by the effect of the preceding dose.

QUINIDINE

IV – In about 50% of patients who respond successfully to quinidine, the arrhythmia can be terminated by ≤ 330 mg quinidine gluconate (or its equivalent in other salts); as much as 500 to 750 mg may be required. Inject slowly. Dilute 10 ml (800 mg) of quinidine gluconate injection to 50 ml with 5% Dextrose Injection, USP. Inject the diluted solution slowly at a rate of 1 ml/min for maximum safety.

Quinidine gluconate – P falciparum malaria – Two regimens have been empirically shown to be effective, with or without concomitant exchange transfusions. As soon as practical, institute standard oral antiplasmodial therapy.

1) *Loading,* 15 mg/kg in 250 ml normal saline infused over 4 hours followed by: *Maintenance,* beginning 24 hours after the beginning of the loading dose, 7.5 mg/kg infused over 4 hours, every 8 hours for 7 days or until oral therapy can be instituted.

2) *Loading,* 10 mg/kg in 250 ml normal saline infused over 1 to 2 hours, followed immediately by: *Maintenance,* 0.02 mg/kg/min for up to 72 hours or until parasitemia decreases to < 1% or oral therapy can be instituted.

Children:

The following doses have been suggested –

Oral (quinidine sulfate): 30 mg/kg/24 hours or 900 mg/m^2/24 hours in 5 divided doses.

IV (quinidine gluconate): 2 to 10 mg/kg/dose every 3 to 6 hours as needed; however this route is not recommended.

QUINIDINE SULFATE

For complete prescribing information, refer to the Quinidine group monograph.
Contains 83% anhydrous quinidine alkaloid.

Rx	**Quinidine Sulfate** (Various, eg, Danbury, Goldline, Major, Parmed, Rugby, Schein, Vangard, Warner Chilcott)	**Tablets:** 200 mg	In 90s, 100s, 120s, 200s, 1000s, UD 100s.
Rx	**Quinidine Sulfate** (Various, eg, Danbury, Major, Rugby, Schein)	**Tablets:** 300 mg	In 100s, 500s, 1000s and UD 100s.
Rx	**Quinora** (Key Pharm.)		(Quinora 300). White. Convex. In 100s.
Rx	**Quinidine Sulfate** (Various, eg, Copley)	**Tablets, sustained release:** 300 mg	In 100s, 250s and 1000s.
Rx	**Quinidex Extentabs** (Robins)		Sucrose. (Quinidex AHR). White. Sugar coated. In 100s, 250s and UD 100s.

QUINIDINE GLUCONATE

For complete prescribing information, refer to the Quinidine group monograph.
Contains 62% anhydrous quinidine alkaloid.

Rx	**Quinidine Gluconate** (Various, eg, Geneva, Goldline, Major, Parmed, Rugby, Schein, Warner Chilcott)	**Tablets, sustained release:** 324 mg	In 100s, 250s, 500s, 1000s and UD 100s.
Rx	**Quinaglute Dura-Tabs** (Berlex)		Sugar. White. In 100s, 250s, 500s and UD 100s.
Rx	**Quinalan** (Lannett)		(Q). Off-white, scored. Convex. In 100s, 250s and 500s.
Rx	**Quinidine Gluconate** (Lilly)	**Injection:** 80 mg/ml (50 mg/ml quinidine)	In 10 ml vials.[1]

[1] With 0.005% EDTA and 0.25% phenol.

QUINIDINE POLYGALACTURONATE

For complete prescribing information, refer to the Quinidine group monograph.
Contains 80% anhydrous quinidine alkaloid.

Rx	**Cardioquin** (Purdue Frederick)	**Tablets:** 275 mg (equiv. to 200 mg sulfate)	Lactose. (PF C275). Scored. In 100s and 500s.

PROCAINAMIDE HCL

Refer to the general discussion concerning these products in the Antiarrhythmic Agents group monograph.

> **Warning:**
> The prolonged administration of procainamide often leads to the development of a positive antinuclear antibody (ANA) test, with or without symptoms of a lupus erythematosus-like syndrome. If a positive ANA titer develops, assess the benefit/risk ratio related to continued procainamide therapy.

Actions:

Pharmacology: Procainamide, a class IA antiarrhythmic, increases the effective refractory period of the atria, and to a lesser extent the bundle of His-Purkinje system and ventricles of the heart. It reduces impulse conduction velocity in the atria, His-Purkinje fibers, and ventricular muscle, but has variable effects on the atrioventricular (AV) node, a direct slowing action and a weaker vagolytic effect which may speed AV conduction slightly.

Myocardial excitability is reduced in the atria, Purkinje fibers, papillary muscles, and ventricles by an increase in the threshold for excitation, combined with inhibition of ectopic pacemaker activity by retardation of the slow phase of diastolic depolarization, thus decreasing automaticity especially in ectopic sites. Contractility of the undamaged heart is usually not affected by therapeutic concentrations, although slight reduction of cardiac output may occur, and may be significant in the presence of myocardial damage. Therapeutic levels of procainamide may exert vagolytic effects and produce slight acceleration of heart rate, while high or toxic concentrations may prolong AV conduction time or induce AV block, or even cause abnormal automaticity and spontaneous firing, by unknown mechanisms.

Electrophysiology – The ECG may reflect these effects by showing slight sinus tachycardia (due to the anticholinergic action) and widened QRS complexes and, less regularly, prolonged QT and PR intervals (due to longer systole and slower conduction), as well as some decrease in QRS and T wave amplitude. These direct effects on electrical activity, conduction, responsiveness, excitability and automaticity are characteristic of a group IA antiarrhythmic agent, the prototype for which is quinidine; procainamide effects are very similar. However, procainamide has weaker vagal blocking action than does quinidine, does not induce alpha-adrenergic blockade, and is less depressing to cardiac contractility.

Pharmacokinetics:

Absorption/Distribution – Oral procainamide is resistant to digestive hydrolysis, and the drug is well absorbed from the entire small intestinal surface, but individual patients vary in their completeness of absorption. Following oral administration, plasma levels reach about 50% of peak in 30 minutes, 90% at 1 hour and peak at about 90 to 120 minutes. Following IM injection, absorption into the bloodstream is rapid; plasma levels peak in 15 to 60 minutes, considerably faster than oral administration. IV use can produce therapeutic plasma levels within minutes after an infusion is started. About 15% to 20% is reversibly bound to plasma proteins, and considerable amounts are more slowly and reversibly bound to tissues of the heart, liver, lung and kidney. The apparent volume of distribution eventually reaches about 2 L/kg with a half-life of approximately 5 minutes. While procainamide crosses the blood-brain barrier in the dog, it did not concentrate in the brain at levels higher than in plasma. Plasma esterases are far less active in hydrolysis of procainamide than of procaine.

Metabolism/Excretion – A significant fraction of the circulating procainamide may be metabolized in hepatocytes to N-acetylprocainamide (NAPA), ranging from 16% to 21% of an administered dose in "slow acetylators" to 24% to 33% in "fast acetylators". Since NAPA also has significant antiarrhythmic activity and somewhat slower renal clearance than procainamide, both hepatic acetylation rate capability and renal function, as well as age, have significant effects on the effective biologic half-life of therapeutic action of administered procainamide and the NAPA derivative. The elimination half-life of procainamide is 3 to 4 hours in patients with normal renal function, but reduced creatinine clearance (Ccr) and advancing age each prolong the elimination half-life. Half-life and renal clearance are also reduced in infants. Trace amounts may be excreted in the urine as free and conjugated p-aminobenzoic acid, 30% to 60% as unchanged procainamide, and 6% to 52% as the NAPA derivative. Both procainamide and NAPA are eliminated by active tubular secretion as well as by glomerular filtration. Action of procainamide on the CNS is not prominent, but high plasma concentrations may cause tremors.

PROCAINAMIDE HCL

While therapeutic plasma levels for procainamide have been reported to be 3 to 10 mcg/ml, certain patients such as those with sustained ventricular tachycardia may need higher levels for adequate control. This may justify the increased risk of toxicity (see Overdosage). Where programmed ventricular stimulation has been used to evaluate efficacy of procainamide in preventing recurrent ventricular tachyarrhythmias, higher plasma levels (mean, 13.6 mcg/ml) were found necessary for adequate control. Plasma levels of NAPA that produce arrhythmia suppression range from 10 to 30 mcg/ml. Toxicity may occur with levels > 30 mcg/ml, although there appears to be overlap between the therapeutic and toxic ranges.

Indications:

Treatment of documented ventricular arrhythmias, such as sustained ventricular tachycardia, that are judged to be life-threatening. Because of the proarrhythmic effects, use with lesser arrhythmias is generally not recommended.

Because procainamide has the potential to produce serious hematologic disorders (0.5%), particularly leukopenia or agranulocytosis (sometimes fatal), reserve its use for patients in whom the benefits of treatment clearly outweigh the risks (see Warnings).

Contraindications:

Complete heart block; idiosyncratic hypersensitivity; lupus erythematosus; torsade de pointes (see Warnings).

Warnings:

Blood dyscrasias: Agranulocytosis, bone marrow depression, neutropenia, hypoplastic anemia and thrombocytopenia in patients receiving procainamide have been reported at a rate of approximately 0.5%. Most of these patients received procainamide within the recommended dosage range. Fatalities have occurred (with approximately 20% to 25% mortality in reported cases of agranulocytosis). Since most of these events have been noted during the first 12 weeks of therapy, it is recommended that complete blood counts including white cell, differential and platelet counts be performed at weekly intervals for the first 3 months of therapy, and periodically thereafter. Perform complete blood counts promptly if the patient develops any signs of infection (eg, fever, chills, sore throat, stomatitis), bruising or bleeding. If any of these hematologic disorders are identified, discontinue therapy. Blood counts usually return to normal within 1 month of discontinuation. Use caution in patients with preexisting marrow failure or cytopenia of any type (see Adverse Reactions).

Mortality: In the National Heart, Lung and Blood Institute's Cardiac Arrhythmia Suppression Trial (CAST), a long-term, multicentered, randomized, double-blind study in patients with asymptomatic non-life-threatening ventricular arrhythmias who had had myocardial infarctions (MI) > 6 days but < 2 years previously, an excessive mortality or nonfatal cardiac arrest rate was seen in patients treated with encainide or flecainide (56/730) compared with that seen in patients assigned to matched placebo-treated groups (22/725). The average duration of treatment with encainide or flecainide in this study was 10 months.

The applicability of these results to other populations (eg, those without recent MIs) or to other antiarrhythmic drugs is uncertain, but at present it is prudent to consider any antiarrhythmic agent to have a significant risk in patients with structural heart disease.

Survival: Antiarrhythmic drugs have not been shown to enhance survival in patients with ventricular arrhythmias.

Complete heart block: Do not administer to patients with complete heart block because of its effects in suppressing nodal or ventricular pacemakers and the hazard of asystole. It may be difficult to recognize complete heart block in patients with ventricular tachycardia, but if significant slowing of ventricular rate occurs during treatment without evidence of AV conduction appearing, stop procainamide. In cases of second-degree AV block or various types of hemiblock, avoid or discontinue procainamide because of the possibility of increased severity of block, unless the ventricular rate is controlled by an electrical pacemaker.

Torsade de pointes: In the unusual ventricular arrhythmia called "les torsade de pointes" (twistings of the points), characterized by alternation of one or more ventricular premature beats in the directions of the QRS complexes on ECG in persons with prolonged QT and often enhanced U waves, group IA antiarrhythmic drugs are contraindicated. Administration of procainamide in such cases may aggravate this special type of ventricular extrasystole or tachycardia instead of suppressing it.

PROCAINAMIDE HCL

Lupus erythematosus: An established diagnosis of systemic lupus erythematosus is a contraindication to procainamide therapy, since aggravation of symptoms is highly likely. If the lupus erythematosus-like syndrome develops in a patient with recurrent life-threatening arrhythmias not controlled by other agents, corticosteroid suppressive therapy may be used concomitantly with procainamide. Since the procainamide-induced lupoid syndrome rarely includes the dangerous pathologic renal changes, therapy may not necessarily have to be stopped unless the symptoms of serositis and the possibility of further lupoid effects are of greater risk than the benefit of procainamide in controlling arrhythmias. Patients with rapid acetylation capability are less likely to develop the lupoid syndrome after prolonged procainamide therapy.

Asymptomatic ventricular premature contractions: Avoid treatment of patients with this condition.

Digitalis intoxication: Exercise caution in the use of procainamide in arrhythmias associated with digitalis intoxication. Procainamide can suppress digitalis-induced arrhythmias; however, if there is concomitant marked disturbance of AV conduction, additional depression of conduction and ventricular asystole or fibrillation may result. Therefore, consider use of procainamide only if discontinuation of digitalis, and therapy with potassium, lidocaine or phenytoin, are ineffective.

First-degree heart block: Exercise caution if the patient exhibits or develops first-degree heart block while taking procainamide; dosage reduction is advised in such cases. If the block persists despite dosage reduction, continuation of procainamide must be evaluated on the basis of current benefit vs risk of increased heart block.

Predigitalization for atrial flutter or fibrillation: Cardiovert or digitalize patients with atrial flutter or fibrillation prior to procainamide administration to avoid enhancement of AV conduction which may result in ventricular rate acceleration beyond tolerable limits. Adequate digitalization reduces but does not eliminate the possibility of sudden increase in ventricular rate as the atrial rate is slowed by procainamide in these arrhythmias.

Congestive heart failure (CHF): Use with caution in patients with CHF and in those with acute ischemic heart disease or cardiomyopathy since even slight depression of myocardial contractility may further reduce cardiac output of the damaged heart.

Concurrent antiarrhythmic agents: Concurrent use of procainamide with other group IA antiarrhythmic agents (eg, quinidine, disopyramide) may produce enhanced prolongation of conduction or depression of contractility and hypotension, especially in patients with cardiac decompensation. Reserve such use for patients with serious arrhythmias unresponsive to a single drug and use only if close observation is possible (see Drug Interactions).

Myasthenia gravis: Patients may show worsening of symptoms from procainamide due to its procaine-like effect on diminishing acetylcholine release at skeletal muscle motor nerve endings. Procainamide administration may be hazardous without optimal adjustment of anticholinesterase medications and other precautions. Immediately after initiation of therapy, closely observe patients for muscular weakness if myasthenia gravis is a possibility.

Renal insufficiency may lead to accumulation of high plasma levels from conventional oral doses of procainamide, with effects similar to those of overdosage (see Overdosage), unless dosage is adjusted for the individual patient.

Hypersensitivity: In patients sensitive to procaine or other ester-type local anesthetics, cross-sensitivity to procainamide is unlikely; however, consider the possibility. Do not use procainamide if it produces acute allergic dermatitis, asthma or anaphylactic symptoms.

Pregnancy: Category C. Procainamide crosses the placenta. It is not known whether procainamide can cause fetal harm when administered to a pregnant woman or can affect reproduction capacity. Give to a pregnant woman only if clearly needed.

Lactation: Both procainamide and NAPA are excreted in breast milk and absorbed by the nursing infant. Because of the potential for serious adverse reactions in nursing infants, decide whether to discontinue nursing or the drug, taking into account the importance of the drug to the mother.

Children: Safety and efficacy have not been established. However, see Administration and Dosage.

PROCAINAMIDE HCL

Precautions:

Monitoring: After achieving and maintaining therapeutic plasma concentrations and satisfactory ECG and clinical responses, continue frequent periodic monitoring of vital signs and ECG. If evidence of QRS widening of > 25% or marked prolongation of the QT interval occurs, concern for overdosage is appropriate; reduction in dosage is advisable if a 50% increase occurs. Elevated serum creatinine or urea nitrogen, reduced Ccr or history of renal insufficiency, as well as use in older patients (over age 50), provide grounds to anticipate that less than the usual dosage and longer time intervals between doses may suffice, since the urinary elimination of procainamide and NAPA may be reduced, leading to gradual accumulation beyond normally predicted amounts. If facilities are available for measurement of plasma procainamide and NAPA levels or acetylation capability, individual dose adjustment for optimal therapeutic levels may be easier, but close observation of clinical effectiveness is the most important criterion.

In the longer term, periodic complete blood counts are useful to detect possible idiosyncratic hematologic effects of procainamide on neutrophil, platelet or red cell homeostasis; agranulocytosis may occur occasionally in patients on long-term therapy. A rising titer of serum ANA may precede clinical symptoms of the lupoid syndrome. Laboratory tests such as ECG and serum creatinine or urea nitrogen may be indicated, depending on the clinical situation.

Embolization: In conversion of atrial fibrillation to normal sinus rhythm by any means, dislodgement of mural thrombi may lead to embolization.

Tartrazine sensitivity: Some of these products contain tartrazine which may cause allergic-type reactions (including bronchial asthma) in certain susceptible individuals. Although the overall incidence of tartrazine sensitivity in the general population is low, it is frequently seen in patients who also have aspirin hypersensitivity.

Sulfite sensitivity: Some of these products contain sulfites that may cause allergic-type reactions including anaphylactic symptoms and life-threatening or less severe asthmatic episodes in certain susceptible persons. The overall prevalance of sulfite sensitivity in the general population is unknown and probably low. It is seen more frequently in asthmatic or atopic nonasthmatic persons.

Drug Interactions:

Procainamide Drug Interactions			
Precipitant drug	Object drug*		Description
Beta blockers	Procainamide	↑	Propranolol may increase procainamide serum levels.
Ethanol	Procainamide	↔	The actions of procainamide could be altered, but because the main metabolite (NAPA) is also an antiarrhythmic, specific effects are unclear.
Histamine H_2 antagonists	Procainamide	↑	Cimetidine and ranitidine appear to increase the bioavailability of both procainamide and NAPA.
Quinidine	Procainamide	↑	Pharmacologic effects of procainamide may be increased. Elevated procainamide and NAPA plasma levels with toxicity may occur.
Trimethoprim	Procainamide	↑	Elevated procainamide and NAPA serum levels may occur, possibly resulting in increased pharmacologic effects.
Procainamide	Lidocaine	↑	Additive cardiodepressant action may occur with the potential for conduction abnormalities.
Procainamide	Succinyl-choline	↑	The succinylcholine neuromuscular blockade may be potentiated.

* ↑ = Object drug increased. ↔ = Undetermined effect.

Drug/Lab test interactions: Suprapharmacologic concentrations of lidocaine and meprobamate may inhibit fluorescence of procainamide and NAPA, and propranolol shows a native fluorescence close to the procainamide/NAPA peak wavelengths; therefore, tests that depend on fluorescence measurement may be affected.

Adverse Reactions:

Cardiovascular: Hypotension following oral administration is rare. Hypotension and serious disturbances of cardiorhythm such as ventricular asystole or fibrillation are more common after IV use (see Overdosage and Warnings). Second-degree heart block has occurred in 2 of almost 500 patients taking procainamide orally.

PROCAINAMIDE HCL

Lupus erythematosus: A lupus erythematosus-like syndrome of arthralgia, pleural or abdominal pain, and sometimes arthritis, pleural effusion, pericarditis, fever, chills, myalgia and possibly related hematologic or skin lesions is fairly common after prolonged administration, perhaps more often in patients who are slow acetylators (see Warnings). While some studies have reported the syndrome in < 1 in 500, others have reported it in up to 30% of patients on long-term oral therapy. If discontinuation does not reverse the lupoid symptoms, corticosteroid treatment may be effective.

Hematologic: Neutropenia; thrombocytopenia; hemolytic anemia (rare). Agranulocytosis has occurred after repeated use of procainamide; deaths have occurred (see Warnings).

Dermatologic: Angioneurotic edema; urticaria; pruritus; flushing; maculopapular rash.

GI: Anorexia, nausea, vomiting, abdominal pain, bitter taste, diarrhea (3% to 4%; oral). Hepatomegaly with increased serum aminotransferase activity has occurred after a single oral dose.

CNS: Dizziness; giddiness; weakness; mental depression; psychosis with hallucinations.

Overdosage:

Symptoms: Progressive widening of the QRS complex, prolonged QT and PR intervals, lowering of the R and T waves, as well as increasing AV block, may be seen with doses which are excessive for a given patient. Increased ventricular extrasystoles, or even ventricular tachycardia or fibrillation may occur. After IV administration but seldom after oral therapy, transient high plasma levels may induce hypotension, affecting systolic more than diastolic pressures, especially in hypertensive patients. Such high levels may also produce CNS depression, tremor and even respiratory depression.

Plasma levels > 10 mcg/ml are increasingly associated with toxic findings, which are seen occasionally in the 10 to 12 mcg/ml range, more often in the 12 to 15 mcg/ml range and commonly in patients with plasma levels > 15 mcg/ml. Overdosage symptoms may result following a single 2 g dose, while 3 g may be dangerous, especially if the patient is a slow acetylator and has decreased renal function or underlying organic heart disease.

Treatment: Includes general supportive measures, close observation, monitoring of vital signs and possibly IV pressor agents and mechanical cardiorespiratory support. Refer to General Management of Acute Overdosage. If available, procainamide and NAPA plasma levels may be helpful in assessing the potential degree of toxicity and response to therapy. Both procainamide and NAPA are removed from the circulation by hemodialysis but not peritoneal dialysis. No specific antidote for procainamide is known.

Patient Information:

Close cooperation in adhering to the prescribed dosage schedule is of great importance in safely controlling the cardiac arrhythmia. More medication is not necessarily better and may be dangerous; skipping doses or increasing intervals between doses to suit personal convenience may lead to loss of control of the heart problem, and "making up" missed doses by doubling up later may be hazardous.

The patient should disclose any history of drug sensitivity, especially to procaine, other local anesthetic agents or aspirin, and to report any history of kidney disease, congestive heart failure, myasthenia gravis, liver disease or lupus erythematosus.

The patient should report promptly any symptoms of arthralgia, myalgia, fever, chills, skin rash, easy bruising, sore throat or sore mouth, infections, dark urine or icterus, wheezing, muscular weakness, chest or abdominal pain, palpitations, nausea, vomiting, anorexia, diarrhea, hallucinations, dizziness or depression.

PROCAINAMIDE HCL

Administration and Dosage:

Oral: Oral dosage forms are preferable for less urgent arrhythmias as well as for long-term maintenance after initial parenteral therapy. Individualize dosage based on clinical assessment of the degree of underlying myocardial disease, the patient's age and renal function.

As a general guide, for younger adult patients with normal renal function, an initial total daily oral dose of up to 50 mg/kg may be used, given in divided doses every 3 hours, to maintain therapeutic blood levels. For older patients, especially those > 50 years of age, or for patients with renal, hepatic or cardiac insufficiency, lesser amounts or longer intervals may produce adequate blood levels and decrease the probability of occurrence of dose-related adverse reactions. Administer the total daily dose in divided doses at 3, 4 or 6 hour intervals and adjust according to the patient's response.

Guidelines to Provide up to 50 mg/kg/day Procainamide

Weight		Dose every 3 hours	Dose every 6 hours
lb	kg	(standard formulation)	(sustained release)
88-110	40-50	250 mg	500 mg
132-154	60-70	375 mg	750 mg
176-198	80-90	500 mg	1 g
> 220	> 100	625 mg	1.25 g

[1] Initial dosage schedule guide only, to be adjusted for each patient individually, based on age, cardiorenal function, blood level (if available) and clinical response.

Sustained release products are not recommended for initial therapy. Total dosage (50 mg/kg/day) may be given in divided doses every 6 hours.

Parenteral: Useful for arrhythmias that require immediate suppression and for maintenance of arrhythmia control. IV therapy allows most rapid control of serious arrhythmias, including those following MI; use in circumstances where close observation and monitoring of the patient are possible, such as in hospital or emergency facilities. IM administration is less apt to produce temporary high plasma levels but therapeutic plasma levels are not obtained as rapidly as with IV administration.

IM administration may be used as an alternative to the oral route for patients with less threatening arrhythmias but who are nauseated or vomiting, who are ordered to receive nothing by mouth preoperatively, or who may have malabsorptive problems. An initial daily dose of 50 mg/kg may be estimated. Divide this amount into fractional doses of to to be injected IM every 3 to 6 hours until oral therapy is possible. If > 3 injections are given, assess patient factors such as age and renal function, clinical response and, if available, blood levels of procainamide and NAPA in adjusting further doses for that individual. For treatment of arrhythmias associated with anesthesia or surgery, the suggested dose is 100 to 500 mg by IM injection.

IV –

Dilutions and Rates for IV Infusions of Procainamide

Infusion	Final concentration	Infusion volume[1]	Procainamide to be added	Infusion rate
Initial loading infusion	20 mg/ml	50 ml	1000 mg	1 ml/min (for up to 25 to 30 min)
Maintenance infusion[2]	2 mg/ml	500 ml	1000 mg	1 to 3 ml/min
	or			
	4 mg/ml	250 ml	1000 mg	0.5 to 1.5 ml/min

[1] All infusions should be made up to final volume with 5% Dextrose Injection, USP.

[2] The maintenance infusion rates are calculated to deliver 2 to 6 mg/min depending on body weight, renal elimination rate and steady-state plasma level needed to maintain control of the arrhythmia. The 4 mg/ml maintenance concentration may be preferred if total infused volume must be limited.

PROCAINAMIDE HCL

Cautiously administer the IV injection to avoid a possible hypotensive response. Initial arrhythmia control, under blood pressure and ECG monitoring, may usually be accomplished safely within 30 minutes by either of the two methods that follow:

1) Slowly direct injection into a vein or into tubing of an established infusion line at a rate not to exceed 50 mg/min. It is advisable to dilute either the 100 or the 500 mg/ml concentrations prior to IV injection to facilitate control of dosage rate. Doses of 100 mg may be administered every 5 minutes at this rate until the arrhythmia is suppressed or until 500 mg has been administered, after which it is advisable to wait ≥ 10 minutes to allow for more distribution into tissues before resuming.

2) Alternatively, a loading infusion containing 20 mg/ml (1 g diluted to 50 ml with 5% Dextrose Injection, USP) may be administered at a constant rate of 1 ml/min for 25 to 30 minutes to deliver 500 to 600 mg. Some effects may be seen after infusion of the first 100 or 200 mg; it is unusual to require > 600 mg to achieve satisfactory antiarrhythmic effects.

The maximum advisable dosage to be given either by repeated bolus injections or such loading infusion is 1 g.

To maintain therapeutic levels, a more dilute IV infusion at a concentration of 2 mg/ml is convenient (1 g in 500 ml 5% Dextrose Injection, USP), and may be administered at 1 to 3 ml/min. If daily total fluid intake must be limited, a 4 mg/ml concentration (1 g in 250 ml of 5% Dextrose Injection, USP) administered at 0.5 to 1.5 ml/min will deliver an equivalent 2 to 6 mg/min. Assess the amount needed in a given patient to maintain the therapeutic level principally from the clinical response. This will depend on the patient's weight and age, renal elimination, hepatic acetylation rate and cardiac status, but adjust for each patient based on close observation. A maintenance infusion rate of 50 mcg/kg/min to a person with a normal renal procainamide elimination half-life of 3 hours should to produce a plasma level of approximately 6.5 mcg/ml.

Since the principal route for elimination of procainamide and NAPA is renal excretion, reduced excretion will prolong the half-life of elimination and lower the dose rate needed to maintain therapeutic levels. Advancing age reduces the renal excretion of procainamide and NAPA independently of reductions in Ccr; compared to normal young adults, there is an ≈ 25% reduction at age 50 and a 50% reduction at age 75.

Terminate IV therapy if persistent conduction disturbances or hypotension develop. As soon as the patient's basic cardiac rhythm appears to be stabilized, oral antiarrhythmic maintenance therapy is preferable (if indicated and possible). A period of about 3 to 4 hours (one half-life for renal elimination, ordinarily) should elapse after the last IV dose before administering the first dose of oral procainamide.

Children: The following doses have been suggested.

Oral 15 to 50 mg/kg/day divided every 3 to 6 hours; maximum 4 g/day.

IM – 20 to 30 mg/kg/day divided every 4 to 6 hours; maximum 4 g/day.

IV – Loading dose, 3 to 6 mg/kg/dose over 5 minutes. *Maintenance,* 20 to 80 mcg/kg/min continuous infusion. Maximum 100 mg/dose or 2 g/day.

Rx	**Procainamide HCl** (Rugby)	**Tablets:** 250 mg	In 100s, 120s and 500s.
Rx	**Pronestyl** (Princeton Pharm.)		Tartrazine. (431). Yellow. Filmlok. In 100s.
Rx	**Pronestyl** (Princeton Pharm.)	**Tablets:** 375 mg	Tartrazine. (434). Filmlok. Orange. In 100s.
Rx	**Pronestyl** (Princeton Pharm.)	**Tablets:** 500 mg	Tartrazine. (438). Red. Filmlok. In 100s.
Rx	**Procainamide HCl** (Various, eg, Goldline, Major, Parmed, Rugby, Schein, Zenith)	**Capsules:** 250 mg	In 100s, 250s and 1000s.
Rx	**Pronestyl** (Princeton Pharm.)		Lactose. (758). Yellow. In 100s, 1000s and UD 100s.
Rx	**Procainamide HCl** (Various, eg, Major, Parmed, Rugby, Schein, Zenith)	**Capsules:** 375 mg	In 100s and 1000s.
Rx	**Pronestyl** (Princeton Pharm.)		Lactose. (756). White/orange. In 100s and UD 100s.

PROCAINAMIDE HCL

Rx	**Procainamide HCl** (Various, eg, Major, Parmed, Rugby, Schein, Zenith)	**Capsules:** 500 mg	In 100s, 250s and 1000s.
Rx	**Pronestyl** (Princeton Pharm.)		(757). Yellow/orange. In 100s, 1000s and UD 100s.
Rx	**Procainamide HCl** (Various, eg, Abbott, Elkins Sinn, IMS, Quad, Solopak)	**Injection:** 100 mg/ml	In 10 ml.
Rx	**Pronestyl** (Princeton Pharm.)		In 10 ml vials.[1]
Rx	**Procainamide HCl** (Various, eg, Abbott, Elkins Sinn, IMS, Quad, Sanofi Winthrop, Solopak)	**Injection:** 500 mg/ml	In 2 ml vials and 2 and 4 ml disp. syringes.
Rx	**Pronestyl** (Princeton Pharm.)		In 2 ml vials.[2]
Rx	**Procainamide HCl** (Various, eg, Geneva, Goldline, Major, Parmed, Rugby, Sidmak)	**Tablets, sustained release:** 250 mg	In 100s, 250s, 500s, 1000s and UD 100s.
Rx	**Procainamide HCl** (Various, eg, Geneva, Goldline, Major, Parmed, Rugby, Schein, Sidmak)	**Tablets, sustained release:** 500 mg	In 100s, 250s, 500s and 1000s.
Rx	**Pronestyl-SR** (Princeton Pharm.)		(775). Green-yellow. Biconvex, oval. Filmlok. In 100s.
Rx	**Procainamide HCl** (Various, eg, Geneva, Goldline, Major, Parmed, Rugby, Schein)		In 100s, 250s and 500s.
Rx	**Procanbid** (Parke-Davis)	**Tablets, extended release:** 500 mg	(Procanbid 500). Blue. Eliptical. Film coated. In 60s and UD 100s.
		1000 mg	(Procanbid 1000). Gray. Eliptical. Film coated. In 60s and UD 100s.

[1] With 0.9% benzyl alcohol and ≤ 0.09% sodium bisulfite.
[2] With 0.1% methylparaben and ≤ 0.2% sodium bisulfite.

DISOPYRAMIDE

Refer to the general discussion concerning these products in the Antiarrhythmic Agents group monograph.

Actions:

Pharmacology:

Mechanism of action – Disopyramide is a class IA antiarrhythmic agent pharmacologically similar to, but chemically unrelated to, procainamide and quinidine. It decreases the rate of diastolic depolarization (phase 4), decreases the upstroke velocity (phase 0), increases the action potential duration of normal cardiac cells and prolongs the refractory period (phases 2 and 3). It also decreases the disparity in refractoriness between infarcted and adjacent normally perfused myocardium and does not affect alpha- or beta-adrenergic receptors.

Anticholinergic activity – In vitro anticholinergic activity is approximately 0.06% that of atropine; the usual dose of 150 mg every 6 hours or 300 mg controlled release every 12 hours compares to approximately 0.4 to 0.6 mg of atropine.

Electrophysiology – Disopyramide shortens sinus node recovery time and lengthens atrial and ventricular refractoriness. The effects on AV nodal conduction and refractoriness and sinus node function vary due to a depressant effect that is counteracted by a vagolytic action. The principal metabolite, mono-N-dealkyldisopyramide (MND), exhibits little antiarrhythmic activity, but is 20 to 30 times more anticholinergic than the parent drug. Little effect has been shown on the AV nodal and His-Purkinje conduction times or on QRS duration, but conduction in accessory pathways is prolonged.

Hemodynamics – At recommended oral doses, disopyramide rarely produces significant alterations of blood pressure in patients without congestive heart failure (see Warnings). With IV disopyramide (dosage form not available in US), either increases in systolic/diastolic or decreases in systolic blood pressure have occurred depending on the infusion rate and the patient population. IV disopyramide may cause cardiac depression with an approximate mean 10% reduction of cardiac output, which is more pronounced in patients with cardiac dysfunction.

Pharmacokinetics:

Absorption/Distribution – Following oral administration of immediate release disopyramide, the drug is rapidly and almost completely (approximately 90%) absorbed. Peak plasma levels usually occur within 2 hours. Therapeutic plasma levels of disopyramide are 2 to 4 mcg/ml. Protein binding is concentration-dependent and varies from 50% to 65%; it is difficult to predict the concentration of the free drug when total drug is measured. After the oral administration of 200 mg disopyramide to 10 cardiac patients with borderline to moderate heart failure, the time to peak serum concentration of 2.3 ± 1.5 hours was increased, and the mean peak serum concentration of 4.8 ± 1.6 mcg/ml was higher than in healthy volunteers.

Metabolism/Excretion –

Dialysis: A preliminary report of three patients on long-term hemodialysis revealed a 45% to 72% reduction in disopyramide half-life during dialysis. In contrast, another study in patients on chronic hemodialysis demonstrated little difference in disopyramide half-life without dialysis (16.8 vs 16.1 hours). Resin and charcoal hemoperfusion were effective in rapidly decreasing disopyramide plasma levels in acute overdosage (Overdosage).

About 50% is excreted in the urine as the unchanged drug and 30% as metabolites (20% MND). The plasma concentration of MND is approximately one tenth that of disopyramide. The mean plasma half-life is 6.7 hours (range, 4 to 10 hours). In impaired renal function (creatinine clearance [Ccr] < 40 ml/min), half-life values ranged from 8 to 18 hours. Therefore, decrease the dose in renal failure to avoid drug accumulation (see Administration and Dosage). Altering urinary pH does not affect plasma half-life.

Immediate release vs controlled release: In a crossover study in healthy subjects, the bioavailability of the controlled release form was similar to that from the immediate release capsures. With a single 300 mg oral dose, peak disopyramide plasma concentrations of 3.23 ± 0.75 mcg/ml at 2.5 ± 2.3 hours were obtained with two 150 mg immediate release capsules and 2.22 ± 0.47 mcg/ml at 4.9 ± 1.4 hours with two 150 mg controlled release capsules. The elimination half-life was 8.31 ± 1.83 hours with the immediate release capsules and 11.65 ± 4.72 hours with controlled release capsules. The amount of disopyramide and MND excreted in the urine in 48 hours was 128 and 48 mg, respectively, with the immediate release capsules and 112 and 33 mg, respectively, with controlled release capsules.

Following multiple doses, steady-state plasma levels of between 2 and 4 mcg/ml were attained following either 150 mg every 6 hours with immediate release capsules or 300 mg every 12 hours with controlled release capsules.

Indications:

Treatment of documented ventricular arrhythmias (eg, sustained ventricular tachycardia) considered to be life-threatening.

DISOPYRAMIDE

Unlabeled uses: Disopyramide may be beneficial in the treatment of paroxysmal supraventricular tachycardia.

Contraindications:

Cardiogenic shock; preexisting second- or third-degree AV block (if no pacemaker is present); congenital QT prolongation; sick sinus syndrome; hypersensitivity to disopyramide.

Warnings:

Proarrhythmic effects: Because of the proarrhythmic effects, use with lesser arrhythmias is generally not recommended.

Asymptomatic ventricular premature contractions: Avoid treatment of patients with this condition.

Survival: Antiarrhythmic drugs have not been shown to enhance survival in patients with ventricular arrhythmias.

Negative inotropic properties:

Heart failure/hypotension – May cause or aggravate CHF or produce severe hypotension, especially in patients with depressed systolic function. Do not use in patients with uncompensated or marginally compensated CHF or hypotension unless secondary to cardiac arrhythmia. Treat patients with a history of heart failure with careful attention to the maintenance of cardiac function, including optimal digitalization. If hypotension occurs or CHF worsens, discontinue use; restart at a lower dosage after adequate cardiac compensation has been established.

Do not give a loading dose to patients with myocarditis or other cardiomyopathy; closely monitor initial dosage and subsequent adjustments.

QRS widening (> 25%), although unusual, may occur; discontinue use in such cases.

QT_c prolongation and worsening of the arrhythmia, including ventricular tachycardia and fibrillation, may occur. Patients who have QT prolongation in response to quinidine may be at particular risk. As with other Type IA antiarrhythmics, disopyramide has been associated with torsade de pointes. If QT prolongation > 25% is observed and if ectopy continues, monitor closely and consider discontinuing the drug.

Atrial tachyarrhythmias: Digitalize patients with atrial flutter or fibrillation prior to administration to ensure that enhancement of AV conduction does not increase ventricular rate beyond acceptable limits.

Conduction abnormalities: Use caution in patients with sick sinus syndrome, Wolff-Parkinson-White (WPW) syndrome or bundle branch block.

Heart block: If first degree heart block develops, reduce dosage. If the block persists, drug continuation must depend upon the benefit compared to the risk of higher degrees of heart block. Development of second- or third-degree AV block or unifascicular, bifascicular or trifascicular block requires discontinuation of therapy, unless ventricular rate is controlled by a ventricular pacemaker.

Concomitant antiarrhythmic therapy: Reserve concomitant use of disopyramide with other class IA antiarrhythmics or propranolol for life-threatening arrhythmias unresponsive to a single agent. Such use may produce serious negative inotropic effects or may excessively prolong conduction, particularly in patients with cardiac decompensation.

Hypoglycemia has been reported in rare instances. Monitor blood glucose levels in patients with CHF, chronic malnutrition, hepatic disease and in those taking drugs which could compromise normal glucoregulatory mechanisms in the absence of food (eg, beta-adrenoceptor blockers, alcohol).

Anticholinergic activity: Do not use in patients with urinary retention, glaucoma or myasthenia gravis unless adequate overriding measures are taken. Urinary retention may occur in patients of either sex, but males with benign prostatic hypertrophy are at particular risk. In patients with a family history of glaucoma, measure intraocular pressure before initiating therapy. Use with special care in patients with myasthenia gravis, since disopyramide could precipitate a myasthenic crisis.

Renal function impairment: Reduce dosage in impaired renal function. Carefully monitor ECG for prolongation of PR interval, evidence of QRS widening or other signs of overdosage (see Overdosage). The controlled release form is not recommended for patients with severe renal insufficiency (Ccr ≤ 40 ml/min).

Hepatic function impairment: Hepatic function impairment increases plasma half-life; therefore, reduce dosage in such patients. Carefully monitor the ECG. Patients with cardiac dysfunction have a higher potential for hepatic impairment.

Pregnancy: Category C. Disopyramide was associated with decreased numbers of implantation sites and decreased growth and survival of pups when administered to pregnant rats at 250 mg/kg/day (≥ 20 times the usual daily human dose), a level at which weight gain and food consumption of dams were also reduced. Increased resorption rates were reported in rabbits at 60 mg/kg/day (≥ 5 times the usual daily human dose). At a maternal concentration of 2.3 mg/L disopyramide, the fetal cord concentration is 0.9 mg/L. Well controlled studies have not been performed in pregnant women and experience is limited. Use only when clearly needed and when the potential benefits outweigh the potential hazards to the fetus. Disopyramide has been found in human fetal blood. Disopyramide may stimulate contractions of the pregnant uterus.

Lactation: Disopyramide has been detected in breast milk at a concentration not exceeding that in maternal plasma. Therefore, decide whether to discontinue nursing or to discontinue the drug taking into account the importance of the drug to the mother.

Precautions:

Potassium imbalance: Disopyramide may be ineffective in *hypo*kalemia and its toxic effects may be enhanced in *hyper*kalemia. Correct any potassium deficit before instituting therapy.

Drug Interactions:

Disopyramide Drug Interactions			
Precipitant drug	Object drug*		Description
Antiarrhythmics	Disopyramide	⬆	Other antiarrhythmics (eg, procainamide, lidocaine) have been used with disopyramide; however, widening of the QRS complex or QT prolongation may occur.
Beta blockers	Disopyramide	⬌	This interaction is difficult to predict. Disopyramide clearance may be decreased; other adverse effects (eg, sinus bradycardia, hypotension) may occur. Others report no occurrence of synergistic or additive negative inotropic effects.
Erythromycin	Disopyramide	⬆	Increased disopyramide plasma levels may occur. Arrhythmias and increased QTc intervals have occurred.
Hydantoins	Disopyramide	⬇	Disopyramide serum levels, half-life and bioavailability may be decreased; anticholinergic effects may be enhanced. Effects may persist for several days after hydantoin withdrawal.
Quinidine	Disopyramide	⬆	Concurrent use may result in increased disopyramide serum levels or decreased quinidine levels. This may result in disopyramide toxicity or decreased response to quinidine.
Disopyramide	Quinidine	⬇	
Rifampin	Disopyramide	⬇	Disopyramide serum levels may be decreased.
Disopyramide	Anticoagulants	⬇	Decreased prothrombin time after disopyramide discontinuation may occur. However, this may be due to a hemodynamic effect and not an interaction.
Disopyramide	Digoxin	⬆	Although serum digoxin levels may be increased, a clinically significant interaction appears unlikely. A beneficial interaction has also been suggested.

* ⬆ = Object drug increased. ⬇ = Object drug decreased. ⬌ = Undetermined effect.

Adverse Reactions:

The most serious adverse reactions are hypotension and CHF. The most common reactions are anticholinergic and dose-dependent. These may be transitory, but may be persistent or severe. Urinary retention is the most serious anticholinergic effect.

GU: Urinary retention, frequency and urgency (3% to 9%); impotence (1% to 3%); dysuria, elevated creatinine (< 1%).

Cardiovascular: Hypotension with or without CHF, increased CHF, edema, weight gain, cardiac conduction disturbances, shortness of breath, syncope, chest pain (1% to 3%); AV block (< 1%). There have been reports of severe myocardial depression (with hypotension and an increase in venous pressure) and unexplained severe epigastric pain following standard oral doses.

Hematologic: Decreased hemoglobin, hematocrit (< 1%); thrombocytopenia, reversible agranulocytosis (rare).

CNS: Dizziness, fatigue, headache (3% to 9%); nervousness (1% to 3%); depression, insomnia (< 1%); acute psychosis (rare, prompt reversal when therapy discontinued).

GI: Nausea, pain, bloating, gas (3% to 9%); anorexia, diarrhea, vomiting (1% to 3%); elevated liver enzymes (< 1%); reversible cholestatic jaundice.

Dermatologic: Generalized rash, dermatoses, itching (1% to 3%).

Body as a whole:

Anticholinergic – Dry mouth (32%); urinary hesitancy (14%); constipation (11%); blurred vision, dry nose, eyes and throat (3% to 9%).

Miscellaneous: Muscle weakness, malaise, aches/pain (3% to 9%); hypokalemia, elevated cholesterol and triglycerides (1% to 3%); numbness, tingling, elevated BUN (< 1%); hypoglycemia; fever and respiratory difficulty; gynecomastia (rare); anaphylactoid reactions; lupus erythematosus symptoms (most cases occurred in patients who had been switched to disopyramide from procainamide after developing symptoms).

Overdosage:

Symptoms: Overdose may be followed by apnea, loss of consciousness, cardiac arrhythmias, loss of spontaneous respiration and death. Toxic plasma levels produce excessive widening of the QRS complex and QT interval, worsening of CHF, hypotension, varying conduction disturbances, bradycardia, and finally, asystole. Anticholinergic effects may also be observed.

Treatment: Prompt, vigorous treatment is necessary even in the absence of symptoms. Such treatment may be lifesaving and may include emesis, gastric lavage or a cathartic followed by activated charcoal by mouth or stomach tube.

Administration of isoproterenol, dopamine, cardiac glycosides, diuretics, intra-aortic balloon counterpulsation, mechanical ventilation, hemodialysis or charcoal hemoperfusion may be used. Monitor ECG.

If progressive AV block develops, implement endocardial pacing. In case of impaired renal function, measures to increase the GFR may reduce the toxicity. Altering urinary pH does not affect plasma half-life or the amount of disopyramide excreted in the urine.

Anticholinergic effects can be reversed with neostigmine.

Refer also to General Management of Acute Overdosage.

Patient Information:

May cause dry mouth, difficult urination, dizziness, breathing difficulty, constipation or blurred vision. Notify physician if symptoms persist, but do not discontinue unless instructed to do so by physician.

Do not break or chew sustained release capsules.

Administration and Dosage:

Approved by the FDA in 1977.

Individualize dosage. Initiate treatment in the hospital.

Adults: 400 to 800 mg/day. The recommended dosage for most adults is 600 mg/day. For patients < 50 kg (110 pounds), give 400 mg/day. Divide the total daily dose and administer every 6 hours in the immediate release form or every 12 hours in the controlled release form.

Children: Divide daily dosage and administer equal doses every 6 hours or at intervals according to patient needs. Closely monitor plasma levels and therapeutic response. Hospitalize patients during initial treatment and start dose titration at the lower end of the ranges provided below:

Suggested Total Daily Disopyramide Dosage in Children[1]

Age (years)	Disopyramide (mg/kg/day)
< 1	10 to 30
1 to 4	10 to 20
4 to 12	10 to 15
12 to 18	6 to 15

[1] Prepare a 1 to 10 mg/ml suspension by adding contents of the immediate release capsule to cherry syrup, NF. The resulting suspension, when refrigerated, is stable for 1 month; shake thoroughly before measuring dose. Dispense in an amber glass bottle. Do not use the controlled release form to prepare the solution.

Initial loading dose: For rapid control of ventricular arrhythmia, give an initial loading dose of 300 mg immediate release (200 mg for patients < 50 kg [110 lbs]). Therapeutic effects are attained in 30 minutes to 3 hours. If there is no response or no evidence of toxicity within 6 hours of the loading dose, 200 mg every 6 hours may be administered instead of the usual 150 mg. If there is no response within 48 hours, discontinue the drug or carefully monitor subsequent doses of 250 or 300 mg every 6 hours.

Do not use the controlled release form initially if rapid plasma levels are desired.

Severe refractory ventricular tachycardia: A limited number of patients have tolerated up to 1600 mg/day (400 mg every 6 hours), resulting in plasma levels up to 9 mcg/ml. Hospitalize patients for close evaluation and continuous monitoring.

Cardiomyopathy or possible cardiac decompensation: Do not administer a loading dose, and limit the initial dosage to 100 mg immediate release every 6 to 8 hours. Make subsequent dosage adjustments gradually.

Renal/Hepatic function failure: For patients with moderate renal insufficiency (Ccr > 40 ml/min) or hepatic insufficiency, the recommended dosage is 400 mg/day given in divided doses (either 100 mg every 6 hours for immediate release or 200 mg every 12 hours for controlled release).

In severe renal insufficiency (Ccr ≤ 40 ml/min), the recommended dosage is 100 mg of the immediate release form given at the intervals shown in the table below, with or without an initial loading dose of 150 mg.

Disopyramide Dosage in Renal Impairment

Creatinine clearance (ml/min)	Loading dose (mg)	Dose (mg)	Dosage interval (hours)
40-30	150	100	8
30-15	150	100	12
<15	150	100	24

Transfer to disopyramide: Use the regular maintenance schedule, without a loading dose, 6 to 12 hours after the last dose of quinidine or 3 to 6 hours after the last dose of procainamide. Where withdrawal of quinidine or procainamide is likely to produce life-threatening arrhythmias, consider hospitalization.

When transferring from immediate to controlled release, start maintenance schedule of controlled release 6 hours after the last dose of immediate release.

Rx	**Disopyramide Phosphate** (Various, eg, Barr, Major, Rugby, Schein, Zenith)	**Capsules**: 100 mg (as phosphate)	In 100s, 500s, 1000s and UD 100s.
Rx	**Norpace** (Searle)		Lactose. (Searle 2752 Norpace 100 mg). White and orange. In 100s, 500s, 1000s and UD 100s.
Rx	**Disopyramide Phosphate** (Various, eg, Barr, Major, Rugby, Schein, Zenith)	**Capsules**: 150 mg (as phosphate)	In 100s, 500s, 1000s and UD 100s.
Rx	**Norpace** (Searle)		Lactose. (Searle 2762 Norpace 150 mg). Brown and orange. In 100s, 500s, 1000s and UD 100s.
Rx	**Disopyramide Phosphate** (Various, eg, Ethex, Goldline, Schein)	**Capsules, extended release**: 100 mg (as phosphate)	In 100s.
Rx	**Norpace CR** (Searle)		Sucrose. (Searle 2732 Norpace CR 100 mg). White and light green. In 100s, 500s and UD100s.
Rx	**Disopyramide Phosphate** (Various, eg, Barr, Ethex, Geneva, Goldline, Schein, Warner Chilcott)	**Capsules, extended release**: 150 mg (as phosphate)	In 100s, 500s and UD 100s.
Rx	**Norpace CR** (Searle)		Sucrose. (Searle 2742 Norpace CR 150 mg). Brown and light green. In 100s, 500s and UD 100s.

LIDOCAINE HCl

Refer to the general discussion concerning these products in the Antiarrhythmic Agents group monograph.

Actions:

Pharmacology: Therapeutic concentrations of lidocaine attenuate phase 4 diastolic depolarization, decrease automaticity and cause a decrease or no change in excitability and membrane responsiveness. Action potential duration and effective refractory period (ERP) of Purkinje fibers and ventricular muscle are decreased, while the ratio of ERP to action potential duration is increased. The AV node ERP may increase, decrease or remain unchanged; atrial ERP is unchanged. Lidocaine raises ventricular fibrillation threshold. Lidocaine has little or no effect on autonomic tone.

Clinical electrophysiological studies have demonstrated no change in sinus node recovery time or sinoatrial conduction time. AV nodal conduction time is unchanged or shortened, and His-Purkinje conduction time is unchanged. Lidocaine increases the electrical stimulation threshold of the ventricle during diastole. In therapeutic doses, lidocaine produces no change in myocardial contractility, systolic arterial blood pressure or absolute refractory period.

Pharmacokinetics:

Absorption/Distribution – Lidocaine is ineffective orally; 60% to 70% of an oral dose is metabolized by the liver before reaching the systemic circulation. It is most commonly administered IV with an immediate onset (within minutes) and brief duration (10 to 20 minutes) of action following a bolus dose. Continuous IV infusion of lidocaine (1 to 4 mg/min) is necessary to maintain antiarrhythmic effects. Following IM administration, therapeutic serum levels are achieved in 5 to 15 minutes and may persist for up to 2 hours. Higher and more rapid serum levels are achieved by injection into the deltoid muscle, which is preferred over the gluteus or vastus lateralis. Therapeutic serum levels are 1.5 to 6 mcg/ml; serum levels > 6 to 10 mcg/ml are usually toxic. Lidocaine is about 50% protein bound (concentration dependent).

Metabolism/Excretion – Extensive biotransformation in the liver (≈ 90%) results in at least two active metabolites, monoethylglycinexylidide (MEGX) and glycinexylidide (GX). These metabolites exhibit both antiarrhythmic and convulsant properties. The hepatic extraction ratio is between 62% and 81%. Lidocaine exhibits a biphasic half-life. The distribution phase (half-life ≈ 10 minutes) accounts for the short duration of action following IV bolus administration. The elimination half-life is 1.5 to 2 hours; half-life may be ≥ 3 hours following infusions of > 24 hours. Because of the rapid rate at which lidocaine is metabolized, any condition that alters liver function, including changes in liver blood flow, which could result from severe congestive heart failure (CHF) or shock, may alter lidocaine kinetics. Less than 10% of the parent drug is excreted unchanged in the urine. Renal elimination plays an important role in the elimination of the metabolites. Accumulation of GX in patients with severely impaired renal function on prolonged infusions may contribute to lidocaine toxicity.

Indications:

IV: Acute management of ventricular arrhythmias occurring during cardiac manipulation, such as cardiac surgery or in relation to acute myocardial infarction (MI).

IM: Single doses are justified in the following exceptional circumstances: When ECG equipment is not available to verify the diagnosis but the potential benefits outweigh the possible risks; when facilities for IV administration are not readily available; by the patient in the prehospital phase of suspected acute MI, directed by qualified medical personnel viewing the transmitted ECG.

Unlabeled uses: In pediatric patients with cardiac arrest, < 10% develop ventricular fibrillation, and others develop ventricular tachycardia; the hemodynamically compromised child may develop ventricular couplets or frequent premature ventricular beats. In these cases, lidocaine 1 mg/kg should be administered by the IV, intraosseous or endotracheal route. A second 1 mg/kg dose may be given in 10 to 15 minutes. Start a lidocaine infusion if the second dose is required; a third bolus may be needed in 10 to 15 minutes to maintain therapeutic levels.

Contraindications:

Hypersensitivity to amide local anesthetics; Stokes-Adams syndrome; Wolff-Parkinson-White syndrome; severe degrees of sinoatrial, atrioventricular (AV) or intraventricular block in the absence of an artificial pacemaker.

Warnings:

Survival: Prophylactic single dose lidocaine administered in a monitored environment does not appear to affect mortality in the earliest phase of acute MI, and may harm some patients who are later shown not to have suffered an acute MI.

LIDOCAINE HCl

Constant ECG monitoring is essential for proper administration. Have emergency resuscitative equipment and drugs immediately available to manage adverse reactions involving the cardiovascular, respiratory or central nervous systems.

IV use: Signs of excessive depression of cardiac conductivity, such as sinus node dysfunction, prolongation of PR interval, widening of the QRS complex, and the appearance or aggravation of arrhythmias, should be followed by dosage reduction and, if necessary, prompt cessation of IV infusion.

IM use: May increase creatine phosphokinase (CPK) levels. Use of the enzyme determination without isoenzyme separation, as a diagnostic test for acute MI, may be compromised.

Cardiac effects: Use with caution and in lower doses in patients with CHF, reduced cardiac output, digitalis toxicity accompanied by AV block and in the elderly.

In sinus bradycardia or incomplete heart block, lidocaine administration for the elimination of ventricular ectopy without prior acceleration in heart rate (eg, by atropine, isoproterenol or electric pacing) may promote more frequent and serious ventricular arrhythmias or complete heart block (see Contraindications). Use with caution in patients with hypovolemia and shock, and all forms of heart block.

Acceleration of ventricular rate may occur when administered to patients with atrial flutter or fibrillation.

Hypersensitivity reactions may occur (see Adverse Reactions). Refer to Management of Acute Hypersensitivity Reactions.

Renal/Hepatic function impairment: Lidocaine is metabolized mainly in the liver and excreted by the kidney. Use caution with repeated or prolonged use in liver or renal disease; possible toxic accumulation of lidocaine or its metabolites may occur.

Pregnancy: Category B. Lidocaine readily crosses the placental barrier. However, there are no adequate and well controlled studies in pregnant women; therefore use during pregnancy only when clearly needed.

Lactation: In a single case report, lidocaine was excreted into breast milk at concentrations 40% of serum levels. At this level, an infant might ingest up to 1.5 mg, a very small amount that would not be expected to lead to significant accumulation. However, exercise caution when administering to a nursing woman.

Children: Safety and efficacy have not been established; reduce dosage. The IM autoinjector device is not recommended in children < 50 kg (110 lbs).

Precautions:

Malignant hyperthermia: Amide local anesthetic administration has been associated with acute onset of fulminant hypermetabolism of skeletal muscle known as malignant hyperthermic crisis. Recognition of early unexplained signs of tachycardia, tachypnea, labile blood pressure and metabolic acidosis may precede temperature elevation. Successful outcome depends on early diagnosis, prompt discontinuance of the triggering agent and institution of treatment, including oxygen, supportive measures and IV dantrolene sodium (see individual monograph).

The safety of amide local anesthetics in patients with genetic predisposition of malignant hyperthermia has not been fully assessed; use lidocaine with caution in such patients. In hospitals where triggering agents for malignant hyperthermia are administered, a standard protocol for management should be available.

Drug Interactions:

Lidocaine Drug Interactions

Precipitant drug	Object drug*		Description
Beta blockers	Lidocaine	↑	Increased lidocaine levels may occur, possibly resulting in toxicity.
Cimetidine	Lidocaine	↑	Decreased lidocaine clearance with possible toxicity. Ranitidine, and perhaps other H_2 antagonists, do not appear to interact.
Procainamide	Lidocaine	↑	Additive cardiodepressant action may occur with potential for conduction abnormalities.
Tocainide	Lidocaine	↑	Since these agents are pharmacologically similar, concomitant use may cause an increased incidence of adverse reactions.
Lidocaine	Succinylcholine	↑	Prolongation of neuromuscular blockade may occur.

* ↑ = Object drug increased

LIDOCAINE HCl

Adverse Reactions:

CNS: Lightheadedness; nervousness; drowsiness; dizziness; apprehension; confusion; mood changes; "doom anxiety"; hallucinations; euphoria; tinnitus; blurred or double vision; sensation of heat, cold or numbness; twitching; tremors; convulsions; unconsciousness.

Cardiovascular: Hypotension; bradycardia; cardiovascular collapse, which may lead to cardiac arrest.

Hypersensitivity: Infrequent allergic reactions may occur, characterized by cutaneous lesions, urticaria, edema or anaphylactoid reactions. Skin testing has doubtful value. See Warnings.

Body as a whole: Occasional soreness at the IM injection site; febrile response; infection at the injection site; venous thrombosis or phlebitis extending from the site of injection; extravasation; vomiting; respiratory depression and arrest.

Overdosage:

Symptoms: Lidocaine blood concentrations may correlate with CNS toxicity (see Adverse Reactions). Mild CNS symptoms (drowsiness, dizziness, transient paresthesias) quickly resolve. General guidelines are provided in the table below:

Lidocaine Plasma[1] Concentrations and Effects

Concentration (mcg/ml)	Toxicity[2]
< 1.5	Idiosyncratic
1.5 to 4	Mild CNS and cardiovascular effects
4 to 6	Mild CNS effects common; cardiovascular in those with concomitant disease
6 to 8	Significant risk of CNS and cardiovascular depression
> 8	Seizures, obtundation, hypotension, respiratory depression, decreased cardiac output, coma

[1] Whole blood concentrations may be 10% to 30% lower.

[2] Patients with significant conduction system abnormalities or marginal hemodynamic status may develop apparent toxicity even at very low lidocaine concentrations. Metabolites also can contribute to toxicity even with modest lidocaine plasma concentrations.

Treatment: In the case of severe reaction, discontinue the drug. Institute emergency resuscitative procedures and supportive treatment. For severe convulsions, use small increments of diazepam or an ultra-short-acting barbiturate (thiopental or thiamylal); if those are not available, use a short-acting barbiturate (pentobarbital or secobarbital). If the patient is under anesthesia, succinylcholine may be given IV. Assure a patent airway and adequate ventilation. If circulatory depression occurs, administer vasopressors and, if necessary, institute CPR.

Administration and Dosage:

IM: 300 mg. The deltoid muscle is preferred. Avoid intravascular injection. Use only the 10% solution for IM injection.

The *LidoPen Auto-Injector* unit is for self-administration into the deltoid muscle or anterolateral aspect of thigh. Patient instructions are provided with the product.

Replacement therapy – As soon as possible, change patient to IV lidocaine or to an oral antiarrhythmic preparation for maintenance therapy. However, if necessary, an additional IM injection may be administered after 60 to 90 minutes.

IV: Use only lidocaine injection without preservatives, clearly labeled for IV use. Monitor ECG constantly to avoid potential overdosage and toxicity.

IV bolus is used to establish rapid therapeutic blood levels. Continuous IV infusion is necessary to maintain antiarrhythmic effects. The usual dose is 50 to 100 mg, given at a rate of 25 to 50 mg/minute. If the initial injection does not produce the desired clinical response, give a second bolus dose after 5 minutes. Give no more than 200 to 300 mg/hour.

Reduce loading (bolus) doses in patients with CHF or reduced cardiac output and in the elderly. However, some investigators recommend the usual loading dose be administered and only the maintenance dosage be reduced.

LIDOCAINE HCl

IV continuous infusion is used to maintain therapeutic plasma levels following loading doses in patients in whom arrhythmias tend to recur and who cannot receive oral antiarrhythmic drugs. Administer at a rate of 1 to 4 mg/min (20 to 50 mcg/kg/min). Reduce maintenance doses in patients with heart failure or liver disease, or who are also receiving other drugs known to decrease clearance of lidocaine or decrease liver blood flow (see Drug Interactions) and in patients > 70 years of age. Reassess the rate of infusion as soon as the cardiac rhythm stabilizes or at the earliest signs of toxicity. Change patients to oral antiarrhythmic agents for maintenance therapy as soon as possible. It is rarely necessary to continue IV infusions for prolonged periods. Use a precision volume control IV set for continuous IV infusion.

Children – The American Heart Association's Standards and Guidelines recommend a bolus dose of 1 mg/kg, followed by an infusion of 30 mcg/kg/min. The following dosage has also been suggested:

Loading dose, 1 mg/kg/dose given IV or intratracheally every 5 to 10 min to desired effect, maximum total dose 5 mg/kg; *maintenance,* 20 to 50 mcg/kg/min.

Preparation of infusion – Add 1 or 2 g lidocaine to 1 L of 5% Dextrose in Water to prepare a 0.1% to 0.2% solution; each ml will contain ≈ 1 to 2 mg lidocaine. Therefore, 1 to 4 ml/min (of a 1 mg/ml solution) will provide 1 to 4 mg lidocaine/minute. If fluid restriction is desirable, prepare a more concentrated solution.

Storage/Stability – Stable for 24 hours after dilution in 5% Dextrose in Water.

Rx	**LidoPen Auto-Injector** (Survival Technology)	**Injection:** (for IM administration) 300 mg/3 ml automatic injection device.[1]	
Rx	**Lidocaine HCl for Cardiac Arrhythmias** (Abbott)	**Injection:** (for direct IV administration) 1% (10 mg/ml)	In 5 ml amps, 20, 30 and 50 ml vials and 5 ml *Abboject* syringes.
Rx	**Xylocaine HCl IV for Cardiac Arrhythmias** (Astra)		In 5 ml (50 mg) disp. syringes.
Rx	**Lidocaine HCl for Cardiac Arrhythmias** (Various, eg, Abbott, Lyphomed)	**Injection:** (for direct IV administration) 2% (20 mg/ml)	In 5, 10, 20, 30 and 50 ml vials and 5 ml syringes.
Rx	**Xylocaine HCl IV for Cardiac Arrhythmias** (Astra)		In 5 ml amps and 5 ml disp. syringes.
Rx	**Lidocaine HCl for Cardiac Arrhythmias** (Various, eg, Abbott, Lyphomed)	**Injection:** (for IV admixtures) 4% (40 mg/ml)	In 5 ml amps and 25 and 50 ml vials.
Rx	**Xylocaine HCl IV for Cardiac Arrhythmias** (Astra)		In 25 ml (1 g) and 50 ml (2 g) single dose vials and additive syringes.
Rx	**Lidocaine HCl for Cardiac Arrhythmias** (Abbott)	**Injection:** (for IV admixtures) 10% (100 mg/ml)	In 10 ml additive vials.
Rx	**Lidocaine HCl for Cardiac Arrhythmias** (Abbott)	**Injection:** (for IV admixtures) 20% (200 mg/ml)	In 5 and 10 ml syringes and 10 ml vials.
Rx	**Xylocaine HCl IV for Cardiac Arrhythmias** (Astra)		In 5 ml (1 g) and 10 ml (2 g) additive syringes.
Rx	**Lidocaine HCl in 5% Dextrose** (Various, eg, Baxter, McGaw)	**Injection:** (for IV infusion) 0.2% (2 mg/ml)	In 500 and 1000 ml.
		0.4% (4 mg/ml)	In 250 and 500 ml.
		0.8% (8 mg/ml)	In 250 and 500 ml.

[1] With EDTA and methylparaben.

TOCAINIDE HCl

Refer to the general discussion concerning these products in the Antiarrythmic Agents group monograph.

Warning:

Blood dyscrasias: Agranulocytosis, bone marrow depression, leukopenia, neutropenia, aplastic/hypoplastic anemia, thrombocytopenia and sequelae such as septicemia and septic shock have occurred in patients receiving tocainide, most within the recommended dosage range. Fatalities have occurred (with approximately 25% mortality in reported agranulocytosis cases). Since most of these events have been noted during the first 12 weeks of therapy, perform complete blood counts, including white cell, differential and platelet counts, optimally, at weekly intervals for the first 3 months of therapy, and frequently thereafter. Perform complete blood counts promptly if the patient develops any signs of infection (eg, fever, chills, sore throat, stomatitis), bruising or bleeding. If any of these hematologic disorders is identified, discontinue tocainide and institute appropriate treatment if necessary. Blood counts usually return to normal within 1 month of discontinuation. Use with caution in patients with preexisting bone marrow failure or cytopenia of any type.

Pulmonary fibrosis, interstitial pneumonitis, fibrosing alveolitis, pulmonary edema and pneumonia have occurred in patients receiving tocainide. Many of these events occurred in patients who were seriously ill. Fatalities have occurred. The experiences are usually characterized by bilateral infiltrates on x-ray and are frequently associated with dyspnea and cough. Fever may be present. Instruct patients to promptly report any pulmonary symptoms (eg, exertional dyspnea, cough, wheezing). Chest x-rays are advisable at that time. If these pulmonary disorders develop, discontinue tocainide.

Actions:

Pharmacology: Tocainide, like lidocaine, produces dose-dependent decreases in sodium and potassium conductance, thereby decreasing the excitability of myocardial cells. Most patients who respond to lidocaine also respond to tocainide. Failure to respond to lidocaine usually predicts failure to respond to tocainide, but there are exceptions.

Electrophysiology – Tocainide is a Class IB antiarrhythmic with electrophysiologic properties similar to those of lidocaine. In patients with cardiac disease, tocainide produces no clinically significant changes in sinus nodal function, effective refractory periods or intracardiac conduction times. Tocainide does not prolong QRS duration or QT intervals. Theoretically, it may be useful for ventricular arrhythmias associated with a prolonged QT interval.

Hemodynamics – Tocainide usually produces a small degree of depression of left ventricular function and left ventricular end diastolic pressure. Usually no changes in cardiac output or increasing CHF occur in the well compensated patient. Small significant increases in aortic and pulmonary arterial pressures observed are probably related to small increases in vascular resistance. Used concomitantly with a β-adrenergic blocking drug, tocainide further reduces cardiac index and left ventricular dP/dt and further increases pulmonary wedge pressure.

No clinically significant changes in heart rate, blood pressure or signs of myocardial depression were observed in post-MI patients receiving long-term therapy. Tocainide has been used safely in patients with acute MI and various degrees of CHF. However, a small negative inotropic effect can increase peripheral resistance slightly.

Pharmacokinetics:

Absorption/Distribution – Following oral administration the bioavailability of tocainide approaches 100%; peak serum concentrations are attained in 0.5 to 2 hours. The extent of its bioavailability is unaffected by food. Unlike lidocaine, tocainide undergoes negligible first-pass hepatic degradation. Approximately 10% to 20% is plasma protein bound. The therapeutic range is 4 to 10 mcg/ml.

Metabolism/Excretion – Inactivated via conjugation in the liver. The average plasma half-life is ≈ 15 hours. About 40% is excreted unchanged in urine; alkalinization of urine reduces the percent of drug excreted unchanged, yet acidification causes no alterations. Pharmacokinetics did not differ significantly with MI compared with healthy subjects. Half-life increased in severe renal dysfunction.

Indications:

Treatment of life-threatening ventricular arrhythmias (Warning box).

Unlabeled uses: Tocainide may be beneficial in the treatment of myotonic dystrophy (800 to 1200 mg/day) and trigeminal neuralgia (20 mg/kg/day in 3 divided doses). Further study is needed.

TOCAINIDE HCl

Contraindications:

Hypersensitivity to tocainide or to amide-type local anesthetics; patients with second- or third-degree AV block in the absence of an artificial ventricular pacemaker.

Warnings:

Proarrhythmia: Like other oral antiarrhythmics, tocainide may increase arrhythmias in some patients.

Cardiac effects: Tocainide has not been shown to prevent sudden death in patients with serious ventricular ectopy. It has potentially serious adverse effects, including ability to worsen arrhythmias. Evaluate each patient by ECG and clinically prior to and during therapy to determine if response to tocainide supports continued treatment.

In patients with known heart failure or minimal cardiac reserve, use tocainide with caution because of the potential for aggravating the degree of heart failure.

Use caution when instituting or continuing antiarrhythmic therapy in the presence of signs of increasing depression of cardiac conductivity.

Acceleration of ventricular rate occurs infrequently when tocainide is administered to patients with atrial flutter or fibrillation.

Renal/Hepatic function impairment: In patients with severe liver or kidney disease, the rate of drug elimination may be significantly decreased.

Pregnancy: Category C. Animal studies using higher than recommended doses demonstrated an increase in abortions and stillbirths. There are no adequate and well controlled studies in pregnant women. Use during pregnancy only if the potential benefit justifies the potential risk to the fetus.

Lactation: In one patient receiving tocainide 400 mg every 8 hours, tocainide levels in breast milk were 28 mcg/ml 2 hours after a dose vs serum levels of 9.2 mcg/ml. Because of the potential for serious adverse reactions, decide whether to discontinue nursing or drug, taking into account importance of the drug to the mother.

Children: Safety and efficacy for use in children have not been established.

Precautions:

Hypokalemia: Since antiarrhythmic drugs may be ineffective in patients with hypokalemia, correct potassium deficits if present.

Drug Interactions:

Tocainide Drug Interactions

Precipitant drug	Object drug*		Description
Cimetidine	Tocainide	↓	Tocainide bioavailability and peak concentration may be decreased; ranitidine does not appear to affect tocainide.
Metoprolol	Tocainide	↑	These agents have additive effects on wedge pressure and cardiac index.
Rifampin	Tocainide	↓	Tocainide's elimination half-life, bioavailability may be decreased; oral clearance may be increased.

* ↑ = Object drug increased. ↓ = Object drug decreased.

Adverse Reactions:

Most frequent: Dizziness, vertigo (15.3%); nausea (14.5%); paresthesia (9.2%); tremor (8.4%). These reactions were generally mild, transient, dose-related and reversible with a reduction in dosage, by taking the drug with food or by discontinuation of therapy. Adverse reactions leading to discontinuation of therapy occurred in 21% of patients and were usually related to the CNS or GI system.

TOCAINIDE HCl

Tocainide Adverse Reactions (> 1%)	Controlled studies (%)		Compassionate use (%)
Adverse reaction	Short-term (n = 1358)	Long-term (n = 262)	(n = 1927)
Body as a whole			
Tiredness/drowsiness/fatigue/lethargy/lassitude/sleepiness	1.6	0.8	—
Hot/cold feelings	0.5	1.5	—
Cardiovascular			
Increased ventricular arrhythmias/PVCs	—	—	10.9
CHF/Progression of CHF	—	—	4
Tachycardia	—	—	3.2
Hypotension	3.4	2.7	1.8
Bradycardia	1.8	0.4	1
Palpitations	1.8	0.4	—
Chest pain	1.6	0.4	—
Conduction disorders	1.5	—	1.3
Left ventricular failure	1.4	—	—
GI			
Nausea	15.2	14.5	24.6
Vomiting	8.3	4.6	9
Anorexia	1.2	1.9	11.3
Diarrhea/loose stools	—	3.8	6.8
Musculoskeletal			
Arthritis/arthralgia	—	—	4.7
Myalgia	—	—	1.7
CNS			
Dizziness/vertigo	8	15.3	25.3
Paresthesia	3.5	9.2	9.2
Tremor	2.9	8.4	21.6
Confusion/disorientation/hallucinations	2.1	2.7	11.2
Headache	2.1	4.6	—
Nervousness	1.5	0.4	11.5
Altered mood/awareness	1.5	3.4	11
Incoordination/unsteadiness/walking disturbances	1.2	—	—
Anxiety	1.1	1.5	—
Ataxia	0.2	3	10.8
Skin			
Diaphoresis	5.1	2.3	8.3
Rash/skin lesion	0.4	8.4	12.2
Lupus	—	—	1.6
Special senses			
Blurred vision/visual disturbances	1.3	1.5	10
Tinnitus/hearing loss	0.4	1.5	—
Nystagmus	—	1.1	1.1

Adverse reactions occurring in < 1% include the following:

CNS – Coma; convulsions/seizures; depression; psychosis; agitation; decreased mental acuity; dysarthria; impaired memory; increased stuttering; slurred speech; insomnia; sleep disturbances; local anesthesia; dream abnormalities; myasthenia gravis; malaise.

Dermatologic – Stevens-Johnson syndrome; exfoliative dermatitis; erythema multiforme; urticaria; alopecia; pruritus; pallor/flushed face.

GI – Abdominal pain or discomfort; constipation; stomatitis; dysphagia; dyspepsia; thirst; dry mouth.

Hepatic – Hepatitis; jaundice.

Hematologic – Leukopenia, neutropenia, agranulocytosis, bone marrow depression, hypoplastic/aplastic anemia and thrombocytopenia (0.18%). These hemato-

TOCAINIDE HCl

logic disorders usually manifest during the first 12 weeks of therapy and fatalities have occurred (see Warning box). Hemolytic anemia; anemia; eosinophilia.

Cardiovascular – Ventricular fibrillation; extension of acute MI; cardiogenic shock; angina; AV block; hypertension; increased QRS duration; pericarditis; prolonged QT interval; right bundle branch block; syncope; vaso-vagal episodes; cardiomegaly; sinus arrest; vasculitis; orthostatic hypotension.

Pulmonary – Respiratory arrest; pulmonary edema/embolism; fibrosing alveolitis; pneumonia; interstitial pneumonitis; dyspnea; pleurisy; pulmonary fibrosis (0.11%). Symptoms of pulmonary disorders or x-ray changes usually occurred after 3 to 18 weeks of therapy; fatalities have occurred. See Warning box.

Special Senses – Diplopia; earache; taste perversion/smell perversion.

Body as a whole – Increased ANA; urinary retention; polyuria, increased diuresis; cinchonism; claudication; cold extremities; edema; fever; hiccoughs; muscle cramps; muscle twitching/spasm; neck pain, pain radiating from neck; pressure on shoulder; yawning; pancreatitis; septicemia; septic shock; chills; asthenia.

Lab test abnormalities – Abnormal liver function tests, particularly in early stages of therapy, have occurred. Consider periodic monitoring of liver function.

Overdosage:

Symptoms: The initial and most important signs and symptoms of overdosage are usually related to the CNS. Tremor may indicate that the maximum dose is being approached. Other adverse reactions, such as GI disturbances (see Adverse Reactions), may follow. One patient died after ingesting a large quantity of tocainide; the serum level was 68 mg/L (≈ 7 times the upper recommended therapeutic level). This patient presented with ventricular tachyarrhythmias with coma, indicating that high levels of tocainide may have primary myocardiotoxicity in addition to CNS effects.

Treatment: If convulsions or respiratory depression or arrest develop, immediately assure the patency of the airway and adequacy of ventilation. Gastric lavage and administration of charcoal may be useful. If seizures persist despite ventilatory therapy with oxygen, give small increments of an anticonvulsant IV. Examples of such agents include a benzodiazepine (eg, diazepam), an ultra short-acting barbiturate (eg, thiopental, thiamylal) or a short-acting barbiturate (eg, pentobarbital, secobarbital).

Hemodialysis clearance is approximately equivalent to renal clearance.

Patient Information:

Notify physician if any of the following occurs: Exertional dyspnea, cough, wheezing, tremor, palpitations, rash, easy bruising or bleeding, fever, sore throat, soreness and ulcers in the mouth, or chills.

May cause drowsiness or dizziness. Observe caution while driving or performing other tasks requiring alertness, coordination or physical dexterity.

May cause nausea, vomiting or diarrhea. Notify physician if these become severe.

Administration and Dosage:

Approved by the FDA in 1984.

Individualize dosage. Guide dosage titration by clinical and ECG evaluation. Dose-related adverse effects tend to occur early in treatment, and they usually decrease in severity and frequency with time. These effects may be minimized by taking tocainide with food or by taking smaller, more frequent doses.

Initial dose: 400 mg every 8 hours. Range is 1200 to 1800 mg/day given in 3 divided doses. Doses > 2400 mg/day have been administered infrequently. Patients who tolerate the three times daily regimen may be tried on a twice-daily regimen with careful monitoring.

Some patients, particularly those with renal or hepatic impairment, may be adequately treated with < 1200 mg/day.

Rx	**Tonocard** (Astra Merck)	**Tablets:** 400 mg	(MSD 707). Yellow, scored. Film coated. Oval. In 100s and UD 100s.
		600 mg	(MSD 709). Yellow, scored. Film coated. Oblong. In 100s and UD 100s.

MEXILETINE HCl

Refer to the general discussion concerning these products in the Antiarrhythmic Agents group monograph.

Actions:

Pharmacology:

Mechanism – Like lidocaine, mexiletine inhibits the inward sodium current, thus reducing the rate of rise of the action potential, Phase O. Mexiletine decreases the effective refractory period (ERP) in Purkinje fibers. The decrease in ERP is of lesser magnitude than the decrease in action potential duration (APD), with a resulting increase in ERP/APD ratio.

Electrophysiology – Mexiletine is a local anesthetic and a Class IB antiarrhythmic compound with electrophysiologic properties similar to lidocaine. In patients with normal conduction systems, mexiletine has minimal effect on cardiac impulse generation and propagation. In clinical trials, no development of second- or third-degree AV block was observed. It did not prolong ventricular depolarization (QRS duration) or repolarization (QT intervals). Theoretically, mexiletine may be useful in treating ventricular arrhythmias associated with a prolonged QT interval. In patients with preexisting conduction defects, depression of the sinus rate, prolongation of sinus node recovery time, decreased conduction velocity and increased ERP of the intraventricular conduction system have occasionally been observed.

Among the patients entered into studies, about 30% in each treatment group had a ≥ 70% reduction in PVC count, and about 40% failed to complete the 3 month studies because of adverse effects. Follow-up of patients has demonstrated continued effectiveness in long-term use.

Hemodynamics – Small decreases in cardiac output and increases in systemic vascular resistance have occurred, with no significant negative inotropic effect. Blood pressure and pulse rate remain essentially unchanged. Mild depression of myocardial function has been observed following IV mexiletine (dosage form not available in the US) in patients with cardiac disease.

Pharmacokinetics:

Absorption/Distribution – Mexiletine is well absorbed (≈ 90%) from the GI tract. The absorption rate is reduced in clinical situations in which gastric emptying time is increased. Narcotics, atropine and magnesium-aluminum hydroxide may slow absorption; metoclopramide may accelerate absorption (see Drug Interactions). The first-pass metabolism of mexiletine is low.

Peak blood levels are reached in 2 to 3 hours. The therapeutic range is approximately 0.5 to 2 mcg/ml. An increase in the frequency of CNS adverse effects has been observed when plasma levels exceed 2 mcg/ml. Plasma levels within the therapeutic range can be attained with either 2 or 3 times daily dosing, but peak to trough differences are greater with the twice-daily regimen. It is 50% to 60% bound to plasma protein with a volume of distribution of 5 to 7 L/kg.

Metabolism/Excretion – Mexiletine is metabolized in the liver. The most active minor metabolite is N-methylmexiletine, which is < 20% as potent as mexiletine. The urinary excretion of N-methylmexiletine is < 0.5%.

In healthy subjects, the elimination half-life is 10 to 12 hours. Hepatic impairment prolongs it to a mean of 25 hours. Little change in half-life occurs with reduced renal function. In eight patients with creatinine clearance < 10 ml/min, the mean plasma elimination half-life was 15.7 hours; in seven patients with creatinine clearance between 11 and 40 ml/min, the mean half-life was 13.4 hours.

Approximately 10% is excreted unchanged by the kidney. Urinary acidification accelerates excretion, while alkalinization retards it (see Drug Interactions).

Indications:

Treatment of documented, life-threatening ventricular arrhythmias, such as sustained ventricular tachycardia. Because of the proarrhythmic effects of mexiletine, use with lesser arrhythmias is generally not recommended.

Unlabeled uses: The use of prophylactic mexiletine may significantly reduce the incidence of ventricular tachycardia and other ventricular arrhythmias in the acute phase of myocardial infarction (MI). However, mortality may not be reduced.

Mexiletine (150 mg/day for 3 days, then 300 mg/day for 3 days followed by 10 mg/kg/day) may be beneficial in reducing pain, dysesthesia and paresthesia associated with diabetic neuropathy.

Contraindications:

Cardiogenic shock; preexisting second- or third-degree AV block (if no pacemaker).

Warnings:

Proarrhythmia: Mexiletine can worsen arrhythmias; it is uncommon in patients with less serious arrhythmias (frequent premature beats or nonsustained ventricular tachycardia) but is of greater concern in patients with life-threatening arrhythmias, such as sustained ventricular tachycardia.

MEXILETINE HCl

Survival: Antiarrhythmic drugs have not been shown to enhance survival in patients with ventricular arrhythmias.

Initial therapy: As with other antiarrhythmics, initiate therapy in the hospital.

Mortality: In the National Heart, Lung and Blood Institute's Cardiac Arrhythmia Suppression Trial (CAST), a long-term, multicentered, randomized, double-blind study in patients with asymptomatic non-life-threatening ventricular arrhythmias who had experienced MIs > 6 days but < 2 years previously, an excessive mortality or non-fatal cardiac arrest rate was seen in patients treated with encainide or flecainide (56/730) compared with patients assigned to matched placebo-treated groups (22/725). The average duration of treatment with encainide or flecainide in this study was 10 months.

The applicability of these results to other populations (eg, those without recent MI) or to other antiarrhythmic drugs is uncertain, but at present it is prudent to consider any antiarrhythmic agent to have a significant risk in patients with structural heart disease.

Hepatic function impairment: Since mexiletine is metabolized in the liver, and hepatic impairment prolongs the elimination half-life, carefully monitor patients with liver disease. Observe caution in patients with hepatic dysfunction secondary to CHF.

Pregnancy: Category C. Mexiletine freely crosses the placenta. There are no adequate and well controlled studies in pregnant women. Use during pregnancy only if the potential benefits outweigh the potential hazards to the fetus.

Lactation: Mexiletine appears in breast milk in concentrations similar to or higher than those in plasma. If mexiletine is essential, consider alternative infant feeding.

Children: Safety and efficacy in children have not been established.

Precautions:

Cardiovascular effects: If a ventricular pacemaker is operative, patients with second- or third-degree heart block may be treated with mexiletine if continuously monitored. Some patients with preexisting first-degree AV block were treated with mexiletine; none developed second- or third-degree AV block. Exercise caution in such patients or in patients with preexisting sinus node dysfunction or intraventricular conduction abnormalities.

Use with caution in patients with hypotension and severe CHF.

Hepatic effects: Abnormal liver function tests have been reported, some in the first few weeks of therapy with mexiletine. Most have occurred along with CHF or ischemia; their relationship to mexiletine has not been established.

AST elevation and liver injury – Elevations of AST > 3 times the upper limit of normal occurred in about 1% of both mexiletine-treated and control patients. Approximately 2% of patients in the mexiletine compassionate use program had elevations of AST ≥ 3 times the upper limit of normal. These elevations were frequently associated with CHF, acute MI, blood transfusions and other medications. These elevations were often asymptomatic and transient and usually not associated with elevated bilirubin levels and usually did not require discontinuation of therapy. Marked elevations of AST (> 1000 U/L) were seen before death in four patients with end-stage cardiac disease (severe CHF, cardiogenic shock).

Rare instances of severe liver injury, including hepatic necrosis, have been reported in foreign markets. Carefully evaluate patients in whom an abnormal liver test has occurred, or who have signs or symptoms suggesting liver dysfunction. If persistent or worsening elevation of hepatic enzymes is detected, consider discontinuing therapy.

Hematologic effects: Among 10,867 patients treated with mexiletine in the compassionate use program, marked leukopenia (neutrophils < 1000/mm^3) or agranulocytosis were seen in 0.06%; milder depressions of leukocytes were seen in 0.08% and thrombocytopenia was observed in 0.16%. Many of these patients were seriously ill and were receiving concomitant medications. Rechallenge with mexiletine in several cases was negative. If significant hematologic changes are observed, carefully evaluate the patient and, if warranted, discontinue mexiletine. Blood counts usually return to normal within 1 month of discontinuation.

CNS effects: Convulsions occurred in about 2 of 1000 patients. Of these patients, 28% discontinued therapy. Convulsions occurred in patients with and without a history of seizures. Use with caution in patients with a known seizure disorder.

Urinary pH: Avoid concurrent drugs or diets which may markedly alter urinary pH. Minor fluctuations in urinary pH associated with normal diet do not affect mexiletine excretion. See Drug Interactions.

MEXILETINE HCl

Drug Interactions:

Mexiletine Drug Interactions			
Precipitant drug	Object drug*		Description
Aluminum-Magnesium Hydroxide Atropine Narcotics	Mexiletine	⬇	Mexiletine absorption may be slowed.
Cimetidine	Mexiletine	⬌	Cimetidine may increase or decrease mexiletine plasma levels.
Hydantoins	Mexiletine	⬇	Increased mexiletine clearance leading to lower steady-state plasma levels may occur.
Metoclopramide	Mexiletine	⬆	Mexiletine absorption may be accelerated.
Rifampin	Mexiletine	⬇	Increased mexiletine clearance leading to lower steady-state plasma levels may occur.
Urinary acidifiers	Mexiletine	⬇	Renal clearance of mexiletine is related to urinary pH. In acidic urine, mexiletine clearance may be increased.
Urinary alkalinizers	Mexiletine	⬆	Renal clearance of mexiletine is related to urinary pH. In alkaline urine, mexiletine clearance may be decreased.
Mexiletine	Caffeine	⬇	Clearance of caffeine may be decreased by 50%
Mexiletine	Theophylline	⬆	Serum theophylline levels may be increased; increased pharmacologic and toxic effects may occur.

* ⬆ = Object drug increased ⬇ = Object drug decreased ⬌ = Undetermined effect

Adverse Reactions:

Dosages in controlled studies ranged from 600 to 1200 mg/day; some patients (8%) in the compassionate use program were treated with 1600 to 3200 mg/day. In the controlled trials, the most frequent adverse reactions were upper GI distress (41%), tremor (12.6%), lightheadedness (10.5%) and coordination difficulties (10.2%). These reactions were generally not serious. They were dose-related and were reversible if the dosage was reduced, if the drug was taken with food or antacids or if it was discontinued. However, they still led to therapy discontinuation in 40%.

Cardiovascular: Palpitations (4.3% to 7.5%); chest pain (2.6% to 7.5%); increased ventricular arrhythmias/PVCs (1% to 1.9%); angina/angina-like pain (0.3% to 1.7%); CHF (< 1%); syncope, hypotension (0.6%); bradycardia (0.4%); edema, AV block/conduction disturbances, hot flashes (0.2%); atrial arrhythmias, hypertension, cardiogenic shock (0.1%).

CNS: Dizziness/lightheadedness (18.9% to 26.4%); tremor (13.2%); nervousness (5% to 11.3%); coordination difficulties (≈ 9.7%); changes in sleep habits (≈ 7.5%); headache, blurred vision/visual disturbances (5.7% to 7.5%); paresthesias/numbness (2.4% to 3.8%); weakness (1.9% to 5%); fatigue (1.9% to 3.8%); speech difficulties (2.6%); confusion/clouded sensorium (1.9% to 2.6%); tinnitus (1.9% to 2.4%); depression (2.4%); short-term memory loss (0.9%); hallucinations and other psychological changes, malaise (0.3%); psychosis and convulsions/seizures (0.2%); loss of consciousness (0.06%).

GI: Nausea/vomiting/heartburn (≈ 40%); diarrhea (5.2%); constipation (4%); dry mouth (2.8%); changes in appetite (2.6%); abdominal pain/cramps/discomfort (1.2%); pharyngitis (< 1%); altered taste (0.5%); salivary changes (0.4%); dysphagia (0.2%); oral mucous membrane changes (0.1%); peptic ulcer (0.08%); upper GI bleeding (0.07%); esophageal ulceration (0.01%).

Lab test abnormalities: Abnormal liver function tests (0.5%); positive ANA, thrombocytopenia (0.2%); leukopenia, including neutropenia and agranulocytosis (0.1%); myelofibrosis (0.02%).

Miscellaneous: Rash (3.8% to 4.2%); nonspecific edema (3.8%); dyspnea/respiratory (3.3% to 5.7%); arthralgia (1.7%); fever (1.2%); diaphoresis (0.6%); hair loss, impotence/decreased libido (0.4%); urinary hesitancy/retention (0.2%); hiccoughs, dry skin, laryngeal/pharyngeal changes (0.1%); SLE syndrome (0.04%).

Myelofibrosis was reported in two patients; one was receiving long-term thiotepa therapy and the other had pretreatment myeloid abnormalities.

Exfoliative dermatitis and Stevens-Johnson syndrome have occurred rarely.

MEXILETINE HCl

Overdosage:

Symptoms: Nine cases of mexiletine overdosage have been reported; two were fatal. CNS symptoms almost always precede serious cardiovascular effects.

Symptoms may include dizziness, drowsiness, nausea, hypotension, sinus bradycardia, paresthesia, seizures, intermittent left bundle branch block and temporary asystole. With massive overdoses, coma and respiratory arrest may occur.

Treatment: Includes usual supportive measures. Refer to General Management of Acute Overdosage. Acidification of the urine may be useful. Treatment may include the administration of atropine if hypotension or bradycardia occurs.

Patient Information:

Take medication with food or an antacid.

Adverse effects such as nausea, vomiting, heartburn, diarrhea, constipation, dizziness, tremor, nervousness, coordination difficulties, changes in sleep habits, headache, visual disturbances, tingling/numbness, weakness, ringing in the ears and palpitations/chest pain may occur. Notify physician if they become bothersome.

Notify physician if signs of liver injury or blood cell damage occur, such as unexplained general tiredness, jaundice, fever or sore throat.

Avoid changes in diet that could drastically acidify or alkalinize the urine.

Administration and Dosage:

Approved by the FDA on December 30, 1985.

Individualize dosage. Administer with food or antacids.

Perform clinical and ECG evaluation as needed to determine whether the desired antiarrhythmic effect has been obtained and to guide titration and dose adjustment.

Initial dose: 200 mg every 8 hours when rapid control of arrhythmia is not essential, with a minimum of 2 to 3 days between adjustments. Adjust dose in 50 or 100 mg increments.

Control can be achieved in most patients with 200 to 300 mg given every 8 hours. If satisfactory response is not achieved at 300 mg every 8 hours, and the patient tolerates mexiletine well, try 400 mg every 8 hours. The severity of CNS side effects increases with total daily dose; do not exceed 1200 mg/day.

Renal/hepatic function impairment: In general, patients with renal failure will require the usual doses of mexiletine. Patients with severe liver disease, however, may require lower doses and must be monitored closely. Similarly, marked right-sided CHF can reduce hepatic metabolism and reduce the dose needed.

Loading dose: When rapid control of ventricular arrhythmia is essential, administer an initial loading dose of 400 mg, followed by a 200 mg dose in 8 hours. Onset of therapeutic effect is usually observed within 30 minutes to 2 hours.

MEXILETINE HCl

Twice-daily dosage: If adequate suppression is achieved on a dose of ≤ 300 mg every 8 hours, the same total daily dose may be given in divided doses every 12 hours with monitoring. The dose may be adjusted to a maximum of 450 mg every 12 hours.

Transferring to mexiletine: Based on theoretical considerations, initiate with a 200 mg dose, and titrate to response as described above, 6 to 12 hours after the last dose of quinidine sulfate, 3 to 6 hours after the last dose of procainamide, 6 to 12 hours after the last disopyramide dose or 8 to 12 hours after the last tocainide dose.

Hospitalize patients in whom withdrawal of the previous antiarrhythmic agent is likely to produce life-threatening arrhythmias.

When transferring from lidocaine to mexiletine, stop the lidocaine infusion when the first oral dose of mexiletine is administered. Maintain the IV line until suppression of the arrhythmia appears satisfactory. Consider the similarity of adverse effects of lidocaine and mexiletine and the additive potential.

Rx	**Mexiletine** (Various, eg, Novopharm, Roxane)	**Capsules**: 150 mg	In 100s and UD 100s.
Rx	**Mexitil** (Boehringer Ingelheim)		(BI 66). Red and caramel. In 100s and UD 100s.
Rx	**Mexiletine** (Various, eg, Novopharm, Roxane)	200 mg	In 100s and UD 100s.
Rx	**Mexitil** (Boehringer Ingelheim)		(BI 67). Red. In 100s and UD 100s.
Rx	**Mexiletine** (Various, eg, Novopharm, Roxane)	250 mg	In 100s.
Rx	**Mexitil** (Boehringer Ingelheim)		(BI 68). Red and aqua. In 100s and UD 100s.

ENCAINIDE HCl

Refer to the general discussion concerning these products in the Antiarrhythmic Agents group monograph.

Encainide has been voluntarily withdrawn from the market by the manufacturer because of continuing uncertainty about the implications of the Cardiac Arrhythmia Suppression Trial (CAST). However, the drug will be available on a limited basis for those patients effectively controlled on encainide for life-threatening ventricular arrhythmias, and who according to the patient's physician should not be switched to another agent. The *Enkaid* Continuing Patient Access Program will be available only to those patients who received encainide on or prior to September 16, 1991. For further information, contact Bristol-Myers Squibb at (800) 527-6741.

Actions:

Pharmacology:

Mechanisms of action of the antiarrhythmic effects are unknown but probably are the result of encainide's ability to slow conduction, reduce membrane responsiveness, inhibit automaticity and increase the ratio of the effective refractory period to action potential duration. Encainide produces a differentially greater effect on the ischemic zone as compared with normal cells in the myocardium. This could eliminate the disparity in the electrophysiologic properties between these two zones and eliminate pathways of abnormal impulse conduction, development of boundary currents or sites of abnormal impulse generation.

Electrophysiology – Encainide, a Class IC antiarrhythmic agent, blocks the sodium channel of Purkinje fibers and the myocardium. Its electrophysiologic profile is characterized by a dose-related slowing of phase O depolarization and little effect on either the action potential duration or repolarization.

The electrophysiologic effects are a result of encainide and of two metabolites present in most patients (> 90%) at therapeutic levels. Encainide and its metabolites produce a dose-related decrease in intracardiac conduction in all parts of the heart; with slowing of conduction in the His-Purkinje system and AV node and an increase in the refractoriness in accessory atrioventricular pathways and in the AV node.

Hemodynamics – In oral studies, encainide had no effect on measurements of cardiac performance such as cardiac or stroke volume index, pulmonary capillary wedge pressure or peripheral blood pressure either at rest or during exercise. In noninvasive studies that included both geriatric patients and younger patients with impaired left ventricular function (New York Heart Association Class III & IV), there were no detrimental effects on ejection fractions acutely or after > 12 months of therapy. Doses of 75 to 300 mg/day reduced incidence of premature ventricular complexes by at least 80%, did not adversely affect exercise tolerance, and were well tolerated by those with markedly impaired left ventricular function. In a few instances, however, apparent new or worsened congestive heart failure (CHF) developed.

Pharmacokinetics:

Absorption/Distribution – Absorption after oral administration is nearly complete with peak plasma levels present 30 to 90 minutes after dosing. Encainide and its two active metabolites, O-demethyl encainide (ODE) and 3–methoxy–O–demethyl encainide (MODE), follow a nonlinear pharmacokinetic disposition. Absorption is delayed by food, but the overall bioavailability is not altered.

Encainide and ODE are bound moderately to plasma proteins (75% to 85%), while MODE binding is somewhat greater (92%).

Metabolism/Excretion – There are two major genetically determined patterns of encainide metabolism. In > 90% of patients, the drug is rapidly and extensively metabolized with an elimination half-life of 1 to 2 hours. These patients convert encainide to the two active metabolites, ODE and MODE, that are more active (on a per mg basis) than encainide. These metabolites are eliminated more slowly than encainide, with half-lives of 3 to 4 hours for ODE and 6 to 12 hours for MODE. A major urinary metabolite is ODE, with lesser amounts of encainide and MODE present.

In < 10% of patients, metabolism of encainide is slower and the estimated encainide elimination half-life is 6 to 11 hours. The renal excretion of encainide is a major route of elimination, and little metabolite is present in plasma.

Despite differences in pharmacogenetics, 3 to 5 days are required to achieve steady-state conditions. Recommended dosage regimen is appropriate for all.

Hepatic disease: The clearance of encainide and conversion to active metabolites is reduced, but serum concentrations of ODE and MODE are similar to those in normal patients. There is insufficient experience to determine the need for alteration in the normal dose or dosing interval, but increase doses cautiously.

Renal disease: Clearance is reduced, and plasma levels of active metabolites ODE and MODE are increased in significant renal impairment; reduce dosage.

Indications:

Documented life-threatening arrhythmias (eg, sustained ventricular tachycardia).

ENCAINIDE HCl

Contraindications:

Symptomatic nonsustained ventricular arrhythmias and frequent premature ventricular complexes.

Patients with preexisting second-or third-degree AV block, or with right bundle branch block when associated with left hemiblock (bifascicular block), unless a pacemaker is present to sustain cardiac rhythm should complete heart block occur.

Cardiogenic shock.

Hypersensitivity to encainide.

Warnings:

Proarrhythmia: Encainide can cause new or worsened arrhythmias. Effects range from an increase in frequency of PVCs to the development of more severe ventricular tachycardia. In patients with malignant arrhythmias, it is often difficult to distinguish a spontaneous variation in the patient's underlying rhythm disorder from drug-induced worsening, so the following occurrence rates are approximations:

In clinical trials, about 10% of all patients had proarrhythmic events. About 6% represented new or worsened ventricular tachycardia and were most frequent in patients with history of sustained ventricular tachycardia (12% of such patients), cardiomyopathy (10%), CHF (12%) or sustained ventricular tachycardia with cardiomyopathy or CHF (17%). Incidence of proarrhythmic events in patients without ventricular tachycardia or overt clinical heart disease ranged from 3% to 4%. Proarrhythmia was least common in patients with no known structural heart disease.

Review of deaths in clinical trials indicates about 1% of patients might have died of a possible proarrhythmic effect of encainide; virtually all had a history of ventricular tachycardia. Most had a history of sustained ventricular tachycardia or ventricular fibrillation. Proarrhythmic events were most common during the first week of therapy and were much more common with doses > 200 mg/day. Initiating therapy at 75 mg/day with gradual dose adjustment reduced risk of proarrhythmia.

Congestive heart failure: New or worsened CHF occurred infrequently (< 1%); use cautiously in patients with CHF or congestive cardiomyopathy.

Electrolyte disturbances: Hypo- or hyperkalemia may alter effects of Class I antiarrhythmics. Correct preexisting hypo- or hyperkalemia before use of encainide.

Sick sinus syndrome (bradycardia-tachycardia syndrome): Use only with extreme caution because encainide may cause sinus bradycardia, sinus pause or sinus arrest.

Electrocardiographic changes: Encainide produces dose-related changes in the PR and QRS interval linearly from 30 to 225 mg/day. There is no consistent change in JT. The QTc interval is increased, but only to the extent of the increase in QRS interval.

Encainide-Induced Changes in ECG Intervals[1]

	Total daily dose					
	75 mg		150 mg		200 mg	
	sec	(%)	sec	(%)	sec	(%)
PR	0.02	(12)	0.04	(21)	0.04	(24)
QRS	0.01	(12)	0.02	(23)	0.02	(26)

[1] % change based on mean baseline values: PR = 0.169 and QRS = 0.088 (n = 504).

Unlike the changes in the PR, QRS and QTc intervals observed with the Class IA drugs, the ECG changes induced by encainide are not indications of effectiveness, toxicity or overdosage, nor can they routinely be used to predict efficacy.

Clinically significant changes in cardiac conduction have been observed. Sinus bradycardia, sinus pause or sinus arrest occurred in 1% of the patients and prolongation of QRS interval to ≥ 0.2 sec developed in about 7%. Incidence of second-degree or third-degree AV block was less, 0.5% and 0.2%, respectively.

Renal function impairment: Limited data suggest that reduction in the elimination of encainide and its active metabolites in patients with serum creatinine > 3.5 mg/dl or creatinine clearance < 20 ml/min results in significant accumulation of metabolites and, to a lesser degree, encainide. Initiate therapy with a single daily dose of 25 mg. The dose may be increased to 25 mg twice daily after 7 days, and again to 25 mg, 3 times a day after an additional 7 days. Doses > 150 mg/day are not recommended. Consider reducing dosage if renal function deteriorates significantly.

Hepatic function impairment: Hepatic impairment significantly reduces the elimination rate of encainide. The need for alterations in the dose or dosing interval is uncertain, but it is prudent to increase doses cautiously.

ENCAINIDE HCl

Pregnancy: Category B. There are no adequate and well controlled studies in pregnant women. Use during pregnancy only if clearly needed.

Lactation: Encainide appears in breast milk. However, the potential for serious adverse reactions in nursing infants is unknown. Decide whether to discontinue nursing or to discontinue the drug, taking into account the importance of the drug to the mother.

Children: Safety and efficacy in children < 18 years of age have not been established.

Drug Interactions:

Diuretics/cardiovasculars: Because of possible additive pharmacologic effects, use caution when encainide is used with any other drug that affects cardiac conduction.

Cimetidine increases plasma concentrations of encainide and its metabolites. Although no clinically significant consequences have been reported, use caution when the two drugs are administered simultaneously. If cimetidine is given, reduce encainide dosage.

Adverse Reactions:

Adverse events caused discontinuation in about 7% of patients in clinical trials.

Only 0.4% of patients discontinued therapy due to CHF or related causes. Second-degree or third-degree AV block developed in 0.5% and 0.2%, respectively. Sinus bradycardia, sinus pause or sinus arrest occurred in 1%. There have been rare reports of elevated serum liver enzymes, hepatitis and jaundice, and of elevated blood glucose levels or increased insulin requirements in diabetic patients. If unexplained jaundice or signs of hepatic dysfunction or hyperglycemia occurs, consider discontinuing therapy.

The following table gives the incidence of the most common adverse events during clinical trials involving 749 patients with ventricular arrhythmias and includes all adverse events regardless of relationship to drug therapy. The "Other trials" column includes reports from 2 multicenter trials not reported in dose-response trials.

Incidence (%) of the Most Common Encainide Adverse Reactions at Various Doses

Adverse reaction	Daily doses 75 mg (n = 298)	150 mg (n = 260)	> 200 mg (n = 208)	Other trials (n = 241)
Body as a whole				
Asthenia	4	5	9	6.5 to 14.8
Chest pain	5	2	6	8.5 to 10.2
Death				1.3 to 3.4
Headache	3	5	12	5.7 to 8.5
Upper/Lower extremity pain	< 1	1	2 to 3	2 to 5.7
Pain	< 1	< 1	< 1	
Paresthesia	1	< 1	2	
Cardiovascular				
Congestive heart failure	< 1	1	2	
Palpitations	4	3	8	7.2 to 12.5
Peripheral edema				1.3 to 2.3
PVCs	< 1	< 1	3	
QRS interval prolonged > 0.2 seconds	< 1	3	4	
Syncope	< 1	1	5	
Ventricular tachycardia	3	3	8	
CNS				
Anorexia				1.1 to 2
Dizziness	6	10	18	15.7 to 15.9
Insomnia				2 to 3.4
Nervousness				1.1 to 2
Somnolence				0 to 3.9
Tremor	< 1	< 1	2	
GI				
Abdominal pain	2	2	3	1.1 to 3.3
Constipation	< 1	< 1	2	2.2 to 4.6
Diarrhea	< 1	< 1	2	0 to 9.2
Dry mouth				0 to 3.9
Dyspepsia	< 1	< 1	3	1.3 to 4.5
Nausea	2	2	6	2.3 to 8.5
Vomiting				0.7 to 2.3

ENCAINIDE HCl

Incidence (%) of the Most Common Encainide Adverse Reactions at Various Doses

Adverse reaction	Daily doses 75 mg (n = 298)	150 mg (n = 260)	> 200 mg (n = 208)	Other trials (n = 241)
Respiratory				
Dyspnea	2	5	4	3.9 to 8
Increased cough	< 1	1	2	
Skin and appendages				
Rash	< 1	< 1	4	1.1 to 2
Special senses				
Abnormal/blurred vision	4	8	26	3.4 to 11.1
Taste perversion	1	2	1	
Tinnitus				0 to 3.9

Other events occurring in < 1% of patients include: Malaise; decreased or increased blood pressure; confusion; ataxia; abnormal gait; abnormal sensation; abnormal dreams; diplopia; photophobia; periorbital edema.

Most serious: Provocation or aggravation of ventricular arrhythmias (see Warnings), occurring in about 10% of patients. In some cases, this resulted in sustained ventricular tachycardia or ventricular fibrillation.

Most frequent: Dizziness; blurred or abnormal vision; headache.

Overdosage:

Symptoms: Overdosages have resulted in death. Overdosage may produce excessive widening of the QRS complex and QT interval and AV dissociation. Hypotension, bradycardia and asystole may develop. Conduction disturbances may be observed. Convulsions occurred in one case of intentional overdosage.

Treatment: Provide cardiac monitoring and advanced life support systems. One report suggested that hypertonic sodium bicarbonate may be useful in managing the cardiac toxicity. Treat acute overdosages by gastric lavage followed by activated charcoal and usual supportive measures. Refer to General Management of Acute Overdosage.

Administration and Dosage:

For sustained ventricular tachycardia, initiate therapy in the hospital. Hospitalization is advisable for patients with a high risk of proarrhythmia (ie, symptomatic CHF, cardiomyopathy or nonsustained ventricular tachycardia), depending on their cardiac status and underlying cardiac disease. Also, hospitalize patients at the time of a dose increase to ≥ 200 mg/day.

Individualize dosage.

Initial dose:

Adults – 25 mg every 8 hours. After 3 to 5 days, increase the dosage to 35 mg 3 times a day if necessary. If the desired therapeutic response is not achieved after an additional 3 to 5 days, the dose may be adjusted to 50 mg 3 times a day. Avoid rapid dose escalation.

Hepatic or renal impairment patients may require dose or dosing interval adjustment.

ENCAINIDE HCl

Dosage adjustment: Adjust gradually, allowing 3 to 5 days between dosing increments to achieve steady-state blood levels of encainide and its active metabolites before increasing the dose. Gradual dose adjustments will help prevent the use of higher than necessary doses which may increase the risk of proarrhythmic events.

In an occasional patient with ventricular ectopic activity, the dosage may have to be increased to 50 mg 4 times a day . Higher doses are not normally recommended. However, after careful dose titration has failed, patients with documented life-threatening arrhythmias may be treated with up to 75 mg 4 times a day. Once the desired therapeutic response is achieved, many patients can be maintained on chronic therapy at lower doses.

Patients with malignant arrhythmias who exhibit a beneficial response as judged by objective criteria (eg, Holter monitoring, programmed electrical stimulation, exercise testing) can be maintained on chronic therapy.

Some patients whose arrhythmias are well controlled by dosages of 50 mg 3 times a day or less may be transferred to a 12 hour dosage regimen to increase convenience and compliance. The total daily dose may be given in two equally divided doses at approximately 12 hour intervals; carefully monitor the patient. The maximum single dose is 75 mg.

Loading dose is not recommended. Use of higher initial doses and more rapid dosage adjustments have resulted in an increased incidence of proarrhythmic events, particularly during the first few days of dosing.

Concomitant therapy: Although limited experience with the concomitant use of encainide and IV lidocaine has revealed no adverse effects, no formal studies demonstrate the utility of such combined therapy. Clinical experience on transferring patients to encainide from another antiarrhythmic is also limited. As a general principle, withdraw antiarrhythmic therapy for 2 to 4 plasma half-lives before starting encainide. If withdrawing antiarrhythmic therapy is potentially life-threatening, consider hospitalization. Digoxin/encainide therapy has been administered without adverse effects (see Drug Interactions). No clinical evidence of arrhythmia exacerbation or "rebound" has been noted following discontinuation.

Rx	**Enkaid**[1] (Bristol-Myers Squibb)	**Capsules:** 25 mg	(Enkaid 25 mg Bristol 732). Green and yellow. In 100s and UD 100s.
		35 mg	(Enkaid 35 mg Bristol 734). Green and orange. In 100s and UD 100s.
		50 mg	(Enkaid 50 mg Bristol 735). Green and brown. In 100s and UD 100s.

[1] Voluntarily withdrawn from the market by the manufacturer. Still available on a limited basis through the *Enkaid* Continuing Patient Access Program. For further information contact Bristol-Myers Squibb at (800) 527-6741.

PROPAFENONE HCl

For more information, refer to the Antiarrhythmic Agents group monograph.

Actions:

Pharmacology: Propafenone is a Class IC antiarrhythmic with local anesthetic effects and direct stabilizing action on myocardial membranes. Propafenone's electrophysiological effect manifests itself in reduction of upstroke velocity (Phase 0) of the monophasic action potential. In Purkinje fibers, and to a lesser extent myocardial fibers, propafenone reduces fast inward current carried by sodium ions. Diastolic excitability threshold is increased and effective refractory period prolonged. Propafenone reduces spontaneous automaticity and depresses triggered activity.

Propafenone has beta-sympatholytic activity at about 1/50 the potency of propranolol in animals and a beta-adrenergic blocking potency (per mg) about 1/40 that of propranolol in man. In clinical trials, resting heart rate decreases of about 8% were noted at the higher end of the therapeutic plasma concentration range. At very high concentrations in vitro, propafenone can inhibit the slow inward current carried by calcium but this calcium antagonist effect probably does not contribute to antiarrhythmic efficacy. Propafenone has local anesthetic activity approximately equal to procaine.

Propafenone causes a dose- and concentration-related decrease in rate of single and multiple PVCs and can suppress recurrence of ventricular tachycardia. Based on percent of patients attaining substantial (80% to 90%) suppression of ventricular ectopic activity, it appears trough levels of 0.2 to 1.5 mcg/ml can provide good suppression, with higher concentrations giving a greater rate of good response.

Mean Changes in ECG Intervals Produced by Propafenone[1]

	Total daily dose							
	337.5 mg		450 mg		675 mg		900 mg	
Interval	msec	%	msec	%	msec	%	msec	%
RR	−14.5	−1.8	30.6	3.8	31.5	3.9	41.7	5.1
PR	3.6	2.1	19.1	11.6	28.9	17.8	35.6	21.9
QRS	5.6	6.4	5.5	6.1	7.7	8.4	15.6	17.3
QTc	2.7	0.7	−7.5	−1.8	5	1.2	14.7	3.7

[1] In any individual patient, ECG changes in the table cannot be readily used to predict efficacy or plasma concentration.

Electrophysiology – In electrophysiology studies in patients with ventricular tachycardia, propafenone prolongs atrioventricular (AV) conduction while having little or no effect on sinus node function. Both AV nodal conduction time (AH interval) and His Purkinje conduction time (HV interval) are prolonged. Propafenone has little or no effect on the atrial functional refractory period, but AV nodal functional and effective refractory periods are prolonged. In patients with WPW, propafenone reduces conduction and increases the effective refractory period of the accessory pathway in both directions. Propafenone slows conduction and consequently produces dose-related changes in the PR interval and QRS duration. QTc interval does not change.

Hemodynamics – Sympathetic stimulation may be a vital component supporting circulatory function in patients with congestive heart failure (CHF), and its inhibition by the beta blockade produced by propafenone may in itself aggravate CHF.

Also, like other Class IC antiarrhythmics, propafenone exerts a negative inotropic effect on the myocardium. Cardiac catheterization studies in patients with moderately impaired ventricular function (mean CI = 2.61 L/min/m^2) utilizing IV propafenone infusions (2 mg/kg over 10 min plus 2 mg/min for 30 min) that gave mean plasma levels of 3 mcg/ml (well above the therapeutic range of 0.2 to 1.5 mcg/ml) showed significant increases in pulmonary capillary wedge pressure, systemic and pulmonary vascular resistances and depression of cardiac output and index.

Pharmacokinetics:

Absorption/Distribution – Propafenone is nearly completely absorbed after oral administration with peak plasma levels occurring approximately 3.5 hours after administration in most individuals. It exhibits extensive first-pass metabolism resulting in a dose-dependent and dosage-form-dependent absolute bioavailability (eg, a 150 mg tablet had absolute bioavailability of 3.4%, a 300 mg tablet 10.6% and 300 mg solution 21.4%). Bioavailability increases further at doses above those recommended and with decreased liver function. The clearance of propafenone is reduced and the elimination half-life increased in patients with significant hepatic dysfunction (see Warnings). Propafenone follows a nonlinear pharmacokinetic disposition presumably due to saturation of first-pass hepatic metabolism as the liver is exposed to higher concentrations of propafenone and shows a very high degree of interindividual variability. For example, for a threefold increase in daily dose from 300 to 900 mg/day, there is a tenfold increase in steady-state plasma concentration.

PROPAFENONE HCl

Metabolism/Excretion – There are two genetically determined patterns of propafenone metabolism. In > 90% of patients, the drug is rapidly and extensively metabolized with an elimination half-life of 2 to 10 hours. These patients metabolize propafenone into two active metabolites: 5–hydroxypropafenone and N–depropylpropafenone. In vitro, these metabolites have antiarrhythmic activity comparable to propafenone, but in man they both are usually present in concentrations < 20% of propafenone. Nine additional metabolites have been identified, most in only trace amounts. The saturable hydroxylation pathway is responsible for the nonlinear pharmacokinetic disposition.

In < 10% of patients, propafenone metabolism is slower because the 5–hydroxy metabolite is not formed or is minimally formed. The estimated propafenone elimination half-life ranges from 10 to 32 hours. In these patients, the N–depropyl-propafenone is present in quantities comparable to the levels measured in extensive metabolizers. In slow metabolizers, propafenone pharmacokinetics are linear.

There are significant differences in plasma concentrations of propafenone in slow and extensive metabolizers, the former achieving concentrations 1.5 to 2 times those of the extensive metabolizers at daily doses of 675 to 900 mg/day. At low doses the differences are greater, with slow metabolizers attaining concentrations > 5 times those of extensive metabolizers. Because the difference decreases at high doses and is mitigated by the lack of the active 5–hydroxy metabolite in the slow metabolizers, and because steady-state conditions are achieved after 4 to 5 days of dosing in all patients, the recommended dosing regimen is the same for all patients. Titrate dosage carefully with close attention paid to clinical and ECG evidence of toxicity. In addition, the beta-blocking action of propafenone appears to be enhanced in slow metabolizers.

Indications:

Treatment of documented life-threatening ventricular arrhythmias, such as sustained ventricular tachycardia.

Because of the proarrhythmic effects of propafenone, reserve its use for patients in whom the benefits of treatment outweigh the risks. The use of propafenone is not recommended in patients with less severe ventricular arrhythmias, even if the patients are symptomatic.

Unlabeled uses: Propafenone appears to be effective in the treatment of supraventricular tachycardias including atrial fibrillation and flutter and arrhythmias associated with Wolff-Parkinson-White syndrome.

Contraindications:

Uncontrolled CHF; cardiogenic shock; sinoatrial, AV and intraventricular disorders of impulse generation or conduction (eg, sick sinus node syndrome, AV block) in the absence of an artificial pacemaker; bradycardia; marked hypotension; bronchospastic disorders; manifest electrolyte imbalance; hypersensitivity to the drug.

Warnings:

Mortality: In the National Heart, Lung and Blood Institute's Cardiac Arrhythmia Suppression Trial (CAST), a long-term, multicenter, randomized, double-blind study in patients with asymptomatic non-life-threatening ventricular ectopy who had a myocardial infarction (MI) > 6 days but < 2 years previously, and demonstrated mild to moderate left ventricular dysfunction, an excessive mortality or non-fatal cardiac arrest rate was seen in patients treated with encainide or flecainide (56/730) compared with that seen in patients assigned to carefully matched placebo-treated groups (22/725). The average duration of treatment with encainide or flecainide in this study was 10 months.

The applicability of these results to other populations (eg, those without recent MI) and to other antiarrhythmic drugs is uncertain, but at present it is prudent (1) to consider any IC agent (especially one documented to provoke new serious arrhythmias) to have a similar risk and (2) to consider the risks of Class IC agents, coupled with the lack of any evidence of improved survival, generally unacceptable in patients without life-threatening ventricular arrhythmias, even if the patients are experiencing unpleasant, but not life-threatening symptoms or signs.

Proarrhythmic effects: Propafenone, like other antiarrhythmic agents, may cause new or worsened arrhythmias. Such proarrhythmic effects range from an increase in frequency of PVCs to the development of more severe ventricular tachycardia, ventricular fibrillation or torsade de pointes (ie, tachycardia that is more sustained or more rapid), which may lead to fatal consequences. It is therefore essential that each patient be evaluated electrocardiographically and clinically prior to, and during therapy to determine whether response to propafenone supports continued use.

PROPAFENONE HCl

Overall in clinical trials, 4.7% of all patients had new or worsened ventricular arrhythmia possibly representing a proarrhythmic event. Of the patients who had worsening of VT (4%), 92% had a history of VT or VT/VF, 71% had coronary artery disease and 68% had a prior MI. The incidence of proarrhythmia in patients with less serious or benign arrhythmias, which include patients with an increase in frequency of PVCs, was 1.6%. Although most proarrhythmic events occurred during the first week of therapy, late events also were seen and the CAST study (see Warnings) suggests that an increased risk is present throughout treatment.

Non-life-threatening arrhythmias: Use of propafenone is not recommended in patients with less severe ventricular arrhythmias, even if the patients are symptomatic.

Survival: There is no evidence from controlled trials that the use of propafenone favorably affects survival or the incidence of sudden death.

Nonallergic bronchospasm (eg, chronic bronchitis, emphysema): In general, these patients should not receive propafenone or other agents with beta-adrenergic blocking activity.

Congestive heart failure: New or worsened CHF has occurred in 3.7% of patients; of those, 0.9% were probably or definitely related to propafenone. Of the patients with CHF probably related to propafenone, 80% had preexisting heart failure and 85% had coronary artery disease. CHF attributable to propafenone developed rarely (< 0.2%) in patients who had no previous history of CHF.

As propafenone exerts both beta blockade and a (dose-related) negative inotropic effect on cardiac muscle, patients with CHF should be fully compensated before receiving propafenone. If CHF worsens, discontinue propafenone unless CHF is due to the cardiac arrhythmia and, if indicated, restart at a lower dosage only after adequate cardiac compensation has been established.

Conduction disturbances: Propafenone slows AV conduction and also causes first degree AV block. Average PR interval prolongation and increases in QRS duration are closely correlated with dosage increases and concomitant increases in propafenone plasma concentrations. The incidence of first-, second- and third-degree AV block observed in 2127 patients was 2.5%, 0.6% and 0.2%, respectively. Development of second- or third-degree AV block requires a reduction in dosage or discontinuation of propafenone. Bundle branch block (1.2%) and intraventricular conduction delay (1.1%) have occurred in patients receiving propafenone. Bradycardia has also occurred (1.5%). Experience in patients with sick sinus node syndrome is limited and these patients should not be treated with propafenone.

Effects on pacemaker threshold: Pacing and sensing thresholds of artificial pacemakers may be altered. Monitor and program pacemakers accordingly during therapy.

Hematologic disturbances: One case of agranulocytosis with fever and sepsis occurred. The agranulocytosis appeared after 8 weeks of therapy. Propafenone therapy was stopped, and the white count had normalized by 14 days; the patient recovered. In the course of > 800,000 patient years of exposure during marketing outside the US since 1978, seven additional cases have occurred. Unexplained fever or decrease in white cell count, particularly during the first 3 months of therapy, warrants consideration of possible agranulocytosis/granulocytopenia. Instruct patients to promptly report the development of any signs of infection such as fever, sore throat or chills.

Renal function impairment: A considerable percentage of propafenone metabolites (18.5% to 38% of the dose/48 hours) are excreted in the urine. Administer cautiously to patients with impaired renal function. Carefully monitor for signs of overdosage.

Hepatic function impairment: Propafenone is highly metabolized by the liver; administer cautiously to patients with impaired hepatic function. Severe liver dysfunction increases the bioavailability of propafenone to approximately 70%, compared to 3% to 40% for patients with normal liver function; the mean half-life is approximately 9 hours. The dose of propafenone should be approximately 20% to 30% of the dose given to patients with normal hepatic function. Carefully monitor for excessive pharmacological effects.

Fertility impairment: IV propafenone decreases spermatogenesis in rabbits, dogs and monkeys. These effects were reversible, were not found following oral dosing and were seen only at lethal or sublethal dose levels.

Elderly: Because of the possible increased risk of impaired hepatic or renal function in this age group, use with caution. The effective dose may be lower in these patients.

PROPAFENONE HCl

Pregnancy: Category C. Propafenone is embryotoxic in rabbits and rats when given in doses 10 and 40 times, respectively, the maximum recommended human dose. In a perinatal and postnatal study in rats, propafenone (at ≥ 6 times the maximum recommended human dose) produced dose-dependent increases in maternal and neonatal mortality, decreased maternal and pup body weight gain and reduced neonatal physiological development. There are no adequate and well controlled studies in pregnant women. Use during pregnancy only if the potential benefit justifies the potential risk to the fetus.

Lactation: It is not known whether this drug is excreted in breast milk. Decide whether to discontinue nursing or to discontinue the drug, taking into account the importance of the drug to the mother.

Children: The safety and efficacy of propafenone in children have not been established.

Precautions:

Elevated ANA titers: Positive ANA titers have occurred. They have been reversible upon cessation of treatment and may disappear even with continued therapy. These laboratory findings were usually not associated with clinical symptoms, but there is one case of drug-induced lupus erythematosus (positive rechallenge); it resolved completely upon therapy discontinuation. Carefully evaluate patients who develop an abnormal ANA test and, if persistent or worsening elevation of ANA titers is detected, consider discontinuing therapy.

Renal/hepatic changes: Renal changes have been observed in the rat following 6 months of oral administration of propafenone at doses of 180 and 360 mg/kg/day (12 to 24 times the maximum recommended human dose). Both inflammatory and non-inflammatory changes in the renal tubules with accompanying interstitial nephritis were observed. These lesions were reversible in that they were not found in rats treated at these dosage levels and allowed to recover for 6 weeks. Fatty degenerative changes of the liver were found in rats following chronic administration of propafenone at dose levels 19 times the maximum recommended human dose.

Drug Interactions:

Propafenone Drug Interactions

Precipitant drug	Object drug *		Description
Anesthetics, local	Propafenone	⬆	Concurrent use (ie, during pacemaker implantations, surgery or dental use) may increase the risks of CNS side effects.
Cimetidine	Propafenone	⬆	The maximum propafenone concentration may be increased, possibly resulting in increased pharmacologic effects.
Quinidine	Propafenone	⬆	Serum propafenone levels may be increased in rapid, extensive metabolizers of the drug, possibly increasing the pharmacologic effects.
Rifampin	Propafenone	⬇	Increased propafenone clearance may occur, resulting in decreased plasma levels and a possible loss of therapeutic effect.
Propafenone	Anticoagulants	⬆	Increased warfarin plasma levels and prothrombin time may occur.
Propafenone	Beta blockers	⬆	The plasma levels and pharmacologic effects of beta blockers metabolized by the liver may be increased.
Propafenone	Cyclosporine	⬆	Increased whole blood cyclosporine trough levels and decreased renal function may occur.
Propafenone	Digoxin	⬆	Serum digoxin levels may be increased, resulting in toxicity.

* ⬆ = Object drug increased. ⬇ = Object drug decreased.

Drug/Food interactions: Although food increased the peak blood level and bioavailability of propafenone in a single dose study, food did not change bioavailability significantly during multiple dose administration.

PROPAFENONE HCl

Adverse Reactions:

Propafenone Adverse Reactions (%)							
	Incidence by total daily dose					Incidence vs placebo	
Adverse reaction	450 mg (n = 1430)	600 mg (n = 1337)	≥ 900 mg (n = 1333)	Total incidence (n = 2127)	% of patients who discontinued	Propafenone (n = 247)	Placebo (n = 111)
Cardiovascular:							
Angina	1.7	2.1	3.2	4.6	0.5	1.2	—
Atrial fibrillation	0.7	0.7	0.5	1.2	0.4	—	—
AV block, first degree	0.8	1.2	2.1	2.5	0.3	4.5	0.9
AV block, second degree	—	—	—	—	—	1.2	—
Bradycardia	0.5	0.8	1.1	1.5	0.5	1.2	—
Bundle branch block	0.3	0.7	1	1.2	0.5	1.2	—
Chest pain	0.5	0.7	1.4	1.8	0.2	—	—
CHF	0.8	2.2	2.6	3.7	1.4	—	—
Hypotension	0.1	0.5	1	1.1	0.4	—	—
Intraventricular conduction delay	0.2	0.7	0.9	1.1	0.1	4	—
Palpitations	0.6	1.6	2.6	3.4	0.5	2.4	0.9
Proarrhythmia	2	2.1	2.9	4.7	4.7	1.2	—
PVCs	0.6	0.6	1.1	1.5	0.1	—	—
QRS duration, increased	0.5	0.9	1.7	1.9	0.5	—	—
Syncope	0.8	1.3	1.4	2.2	0.7	—	—
Ventricular tachycardia	1.4	1.6	2.9	3.4	1.2	—	—
CNS:							
Anorexia	0.5	0.7	1.6	1.7	0.4	1.6	0.9
Anxiety	0.7	0.5	0.9	1.5	0.6	2	1.8
Ataxia	0.3	0.6	1.5	1.6	0.2	—	—
Dizziness	3.6	6.6	11	12.5	2.4	6.5	5.4
Drowsiness	0.6	0.5	0.7	1.2	0.2	—	—
Fatigue	1.8	2.8	4.1	6	1	—	—
Headache	1.5	2.5	2.8	4.5	1	4.5	4.5
Insomnia	0.3	1.3	0.7	1.5	0.3	—	—
Loss of balance	—	—	—	—	—	1.2	—
Tremor	0.3	0.8	1.1	1.4	0.3	—	—
GI:							
Abdominal pain/cramps	0.8	0.9	1.1	1.7	0.4	—	—
Constipation	2	4.1	5.3	7.2	0.5	4	—
Diarrhea	0.5	1.6	1.7	2.5	0.6	1.2	0.9
Dry mouth	0.9	1	1.4	2.4	0.2	2	0.9
Dyspepsia	1.3	1.7	2.5	3.4	0.9	—	—
Flatulence	0.3	0.7	0.9	1.2	0.1	1.2	—
Nausea/vomiting	2.4	6.1	8.9	10.7	3.4	2.8	0.9
Unusual taste	2.5	4.9	6.3	8.8	0.7	7.3	0.9
Other:							
Blurred vision	0.6	2.4	3.1	3.8	0.8	2	0.9
Diaphoresis	0.6	0.4	1.1	1.4	0.3	—	—
Dyspnea	2.2	2.3	3.6	5.3	1.6	2	2.7
Edema	0.6	0.4	1	1.4	0.2	—	—
Pain, joints	0.2	0.4	0.9	1	0.1	—	—
Rash	0.6	1.4	1.9	2.6	0.8	—	—
Weakness	0.6	1.6	1.7	2.4	0.7	—	—

PROPAFENONE HCl

Adverse reactions occur most frequently in the GI, cardiovascular and CNS. About 20% of patients discontinued treatment due to adverse reactions. The most common events were dizziness, unusual taste, first-degree AV block, intraventricular conduction delay, nausea or vomiting and constipation. Headache was common, but not increased compared to placebo.

The most common adverse reactions appeared to be dose-related, especially dizziness, nausea or vomiting, unusual taste, constipation and blurred vision. Some less common reactions may also have been dose-related, such as first degree AV block, CHF, dyspepsia and weakness.

In addition to the reactions listed in the table, the following adverse reactions were reported (< 1%) either in clinical trials or in marketing experience (causal relationship not determined).

Cardiovascular: Atrial flutter; AV dissociation; cardiac arrest; flushing; hot flashes; sick sinus syndrome; sinus pause or arrest; supraventricular tachycardia.

CNS: Abnormal dreams, speech or vision; apnea; coma; confusion; depression; memory loss; numbness; paresthesias; psychosis/mania; seizures (0.3%); tinnitus; unusual smell sensation; vertigo.

GI: Cholestasis (0.1%); elevated liver enzymes (alkaline phosphatase, serum transaminases) (0.2%); gastroenteritis, hepatitis (0.03%). A number of patients with liver abnormalities associated with propafenone therapy have been reported in foreign post-marketing experience. Some appeared due to hepatocellular injury, some were cholestatic and some showed a mixed picture.

Hematologic: Agranulocytosis; anemia; bruising; granulocytopenia; increased bleeding time; leukopenia; purpura; thrombocytopenia.

Miscellaneous: Alopecia; eye irritation; hyponatremia/inappropriate ADH secretion; impotence; increased glucose; kidney failure; positive ANA (0.7%); lupus erythematosus; muscle cramps; muscle weakness; nephrotic syndrome; pain; pruritus.

Overdosage:

Symptoms which are usually most severe within 3 hours of ingestion may include hypotension, somnolence, bradycardia, intra-atrial and intraventricular conduction disturbances, and rarely convulsions and high grade ventricular arrhythmias.

Treatment: Defibrillation as well as infusion of dopamine and isoproterenol have been effective in controlling rhythm and blood pressure. Convulsions have been alleviated with IV diazepam. General supportive measures such as ventilatory assistance and cardiopulmonary resuscitation may be necessary. Refer to General Management of Acute Overdosage. Hemodialysis does not appear to alter drug clearance.

Patient Information:

Palpitations, chest pain, blurred or abnormal vision, or difficult breathing may occur. Notify the physician if these become bothersome.

Notify the physician if signs of infection develop such as fever, sore throat, chills or unusual bruising or bleeding.

Be aware of signs of overdosage or toxicity such as hypotension, excessive drowsiness, decreased heart rate or abnormal heartbeat.

Administration and Dosage:

Approved by the FDA in 1989.

Individually titrate on the basis of response and tolerance. Initiate with 150 mg every 8 hours (450 mg/day). Dosage may be increased at a minimum of 3 to 4 day intervals to 225 mg every 8 hours (675 mg/day) and, if necessary, to 300 mg every 8 hours (900 mg/day). The safety and efficacy of dosages exceeding 900 mg/day have not been established. In those patients in whom significant widening of the QRS complex or second- or third-degree AV block occurs, consider dose reduction.

As with other antiarrhythmics, in the elderly or patients with marked previous myocardial damage, increase dose more gradually during initial treatment phase.

Rx	**Rythmol** (Knoll)	**Tablets:** 150 mg	(150). White, scored. Film coated. In 100s and UD 100s.
		225 mg	(225). Tan, scored. Film coated. In 100s and UD 100s.
		300 mg	(300). White, scored. Film coated. In 100s and UD 100s.

FLECAINIDE ACETATE

Refer to the general discussion concerning these products in the Antiarrhythmic Agents group monograph.

Actions:

Pharmacology: Flecainide has local anesthetic activity and belongs to the membrane stabilizing (Class I) group of antiarrhythmic agents; it has electrophysiologic effects characteristic of the IC class of antiarrhythmics.

Electrophysiology – Flecainide produces a dose-related decrease in intracardiac conduction in all parts of the heart, with the greatest effect on the His-Purkinje system (H–V conduction). Effects upon atrioventricular (AV) nodal conduction time and intra-atrial conduction times are less pronounced than those on the ventricle. Significant effects on refractory periods were observed only in the ventricle. Sinus node recovery times (corrected) are somewhat increased; this may be significant in sinus node dysfunction (see Warnings).

Flecainide causes a dose-related and plasma level-related decrease in single and multiple PVCs and can suppress recurrence of ventricular tachycardia. Plasma levels of 0.2 to 1 mcg/ml may be needed to obtain the maximal therapeutic effect; trough plasma levels in patients successfully treated for recurrent ventricular tachycardia were between 0.2 and 1 mcg/ml. Plasma levels > 0.7 to 1 mcg/ml are associated with a higher rate of cardiac adverse experiences (ie, conduction defects or bradycardia). The relationship of plasma levels to proarrhythmic events is not established, but dose reduction appears to lead to a reduced frequency and severity of such events.

Hemodynamics – Flecainide does not usually alter heart rate, although bradycardia and tachycardia have been reported occasionally.

Decreases in ejection fraction, consistent with a negative inotropic effect, have been observed after a single dose of 200 to 250 mg; both increases and decreases in ejection fraction have been encountered during multidose therapy at usual therapeutic doses (see Warnings).

Pharmacokinetics:

Absorption/Distribution – Oral absorption is nearly complete. Peak plasma levels are attained at about 3 hours (range, 1 to 6 hours). Flecainide does not undergo significant first-pass effect. Food or antacids do not affect absorption.

The plasma half-life averages 20 hours (range, 12 to 27 hours) after multiple oral doses. Steady-state levels are approached in 3 to 5 days; once at steady-state, no accumulation occurs during chronic therapy. Over the usual therapeutic range, plasma levels are approximately proportional to dose.

In patients with congestive heart failure (CHF; NYHA class III), the rate of flecainide elimination from plasma (mean half-life, 19 hours) is moderately slower than for healthy subjects (mean half-life, 14 hours).

Plasma protein binding is about 40% and is independent of plasma drug level over the range of 0.015 to about 3.4 mcg/ml.

Metabolism/Excretion – About 30% of a single oral dose (range, 10% to 50%) is excreted in urine unchanged. The two major urinary metabolites are meta-O-dealkylated flecainide (active, but about as potent) and the meta-O-dealkylated lactam (inactive). These two metabolites (primarily conjugated) account for most of the remaining portion of the dose. Several minor metabolites (≤ 3%) are also found in urine; 5% is excreted in feces.

Flecainide elimination depends on renal function. With increasing renal impairment, the extent of unchanged drug in urine is reduced and the half-life is prolonged. There is no simple relationship between creatinine clearance and the rate of flecainide elimination from plasma.

Hemodialysis removes only about 1% of an oral dose as unchanged flecainide.

Indications:

For the prevention of paroxysmal atrial fibrillation/flutter (PAF) associated with disabling symptoms and paroxysmal supraventricular tachycardias (PSVT), including atrioventricular nodal reentrant tachycardia, atrioventricular reentrant tachycardia and other supraventricular tachycardias of unspecified mechanism associated with disabling symptoms in patients without structural heart disease.

Prevention of documented life-threatening ventricular arrhythmias, such as sustained ventricular tachycardia.

Not recommended in patients with less severe ventricular arrhythmias even if the patients are symptomatic (see Warnings). Because of proarrhythmic effects of flecainide (see Warnings), reserve use for patients in whom benefits outweigh risks.

FLECAINIDE ACETATE

Contraindications:

Preexisting second- or third-degree AV block, right bundle branch block when associated with a left hemiblock (bifascicular block), unless a pacemaker is present to sustain the cardiac rhythm if complete heart block occurs; recent myocardial infarction (MI) (see Warnings); presence of cardiogenic shock; hypersensitivity to the drug.

Warnings:

Mortality: Flecainide was included in the National Heart Lung and Blood Institute's Cardiac Arrhythmia Suppression Trial (CAST), a long-term multi-center, randomized, double-blind study in patients with asymptomatic non-life-threatening ventricular arrhythmias who had an MI > 6 days, but < 2 years previously. An excessive mortality or non-fatal cardiac arrest rate was seen in patients treated with flecainide compared with that seen in a carefully matched placebo-treated group. This rate was 16/315 (5.1%) for flecainide and 7/309 (2.3%) for its matched placebo. The average duration of treatment was 10 months.

Ventricular pro-arrhythmic effects in patients with atrial fibrillation/flutter: A review of the world literature revealed reports of 568 patients treated with oral flecainide for paroxysmal atrial fibrillation/flutter (PAF). Ventricular tachycardia was experienced in 0.4% (2/568) of these patients. Of 19 patients in the literature with chronic atrial fibrillation (CAF), 10.5% (2) experienced VT or VF. Flecainide is not recommended for use in patients with chronic atrial fibrillation. Case reports of ventricular proarrhythmic effects in patients treated with flecainide for atrial fibrillation/flutter have included increased PVCs, VT, VF and death.

As with other class I agents, patients treated with flecainide for atrial flutter have been reported with 1:1 atrioventricular conduction due to slowing the atrial rate. A paradoxical increase in the ventricular rate also may occur in patients with atrial fibrillation who receive flecainide. Concomitant negative chronotropic therapy such as digoxin or beta-blockers may lower the risk of this complication.

Survival: As with other antiarrhythmics, there is no evidence that flecainide favorably affects survival or the incidence of sudden death.

Non-life-threatening ventricular arrhythmias: The applicability of the CAST results to other populations (eg, those without recent infarction) is uncertain, but at present it is prudent to consider the risks of Class IC agents, coupled with the lack of any evidence of improved survival, generally unacceptable in patients whose ventricular arrhythmias are not life-threatening, even if the patients are experiencing unpleasant but not life-threatening symptoms or signs.

Proarrhythmic effects: Flecainide can cause new or worsened arrhythmias. Such proarrhythmic effects range from an increase in frequency of PVCs to the development of more severe ventricular tachycardia. Three-fourths of proarrhythmic events were new or worsened ventricular tachyarrhythmias, the remainder being increased frequency of PVCs or new supraventricular arrhythmias.

In patients treated with flecainide for sustained ventricular tachycardia, 80% of proarrhythmic events occurred within 14 days of the onset of therapy. In studies of 225 patients with supraventricular arrhythmia, there were 9 (4%) proarrhythmic events, 8 of them in patients with paroxysmal atrial fibrillation. Of the 9, 7 were exacerbations of supraventricular arrhythmias, while 2 were ventricular arrhythmias, including one fatal case of VT/VF and one wide complex VT, both in patients with paroxysmal atrial fibrillation and known coronary artery disease.

It is uncertain if flecainide's risk of proarrhythmia is exaggerated in patients CAF, high ventricular rate or exercise. Wide complex tachycardia and ventricular fibrillation have been reported in two of 12 CAF patients undergoing maximal exercise tolerance testing. In patients with complex arrhythmias, it is difficult to distinguish a spontaneous variation in the underlying rhythm disorder from drug-induced worsening. As a result, the occurrence rates are approximations.

Among patients treated for sustained ventricular tachycardia (who frequently also had heart failure, a low ejection fraction, a history of MI or cardiac arrest), the incidence of proarrhythmic events was 13% when dosage was initiated at 200 mg/day with slow upward titration, without exceeding 300 mg/day. In patients with *sustained* ventricular tachycardia using a higher initial dose (400 mg/day) the incidence of proarrhythmic events was 26%; moreover, in about 10%, proarrhythmic events were fatal. With lower initial doses, the incidence of fatal proarrhythmic events decreased to 0.5%.

FLECAINIDE ACETATE

The relatively high frequency of proarrhythmic events in patients with sustained ventricular tachycardia and serious underlying heart disease, and the need for titration and monitoring, requires that therapy of patients with sustained ventricular tachycardia be started in the hospital.

Sick sinus syndrome: Use only with extreme caution; the drug may cause sinus bradycardia, sinus pause or sinus arrest. The frequency probably increases with higher trough plasma levels, especially when they exceed 1 mcg/ml.

Heart failure: Flecainide has a negative inotropic effect and may cause or worsen CHF, particularly in patients with cardiomyopathy, preexisting severe heart failure (NYHA functional class III or IV) or low ejection fractions (< 30%). In patients with supraventricular arrhythmias, new or worsened CHF developed in 0.4% of patients. In patients with sustained ventricular tachycardia during a mean duration of 7.9 months of flecainide therapy, 6.3% developed new CHF. In patients with sustained ventricular tachycardia and a history of CHF in a mean duration of 5.4 months of therapy, 25.7% developed worsened CHF. Exacerbation of preexisting CHF occurred more commonly in studies including patients with Class III or IV failure than in studies which excluded such patients. Use cautiously in patients with a history of CHF or myocardial dysfunction. The initial dosage should be no more than 100 mg twice daily; monitor patients carefully. Give close attention to maintenance of cardiac function, including optimal digitalis, diuretic or other therapy. Where CHF has developed or worsened during treatment, the time of onset has ranged from a few hours to several months after starting therapy. Some patients who develop reduced myocardial function while on flecainide can continue with adjustment of digitalis or diuretics; others may require dosage reduction or discontinuation of flecainide. When feasible, monitor plasma flecainide levels. Keep trough plasma levels < 1 mcg/ml.

Cardiac conduction: Flecainide slows cardiac conduction in most patients to produce dose-related increases in PR, QRS and QT intervals.

The PR interval increases an average of 25% (0.04 seconds) and as much as 118%. Approximately one-third of patients may develop new first-degree AV heart block (PR interval ≥ 0.2 seconds). The QRS complex increases an average of 25% (0.02 seconds) and as much as 150%. Many patients develop QRS complexes with a duration of ≥ 0.12 seconds. In one study, 4% of patients developed new bundle branch block. The degree of lengthening of PR and QRS intervals does not predict either efficacy or the development of cardiac adverse effects. In clinical trials, it was unusual for PR intervals to increase to ≥ 0.3 seconds, or for QRS intervals to increase to ≥ 0.18 seconds; thus, use caution and consider dose reductions. The QT interval widens about 8% but most (about 60% to 90%) is due to widening of the QRS duration. The JT interval (QT minus QRS) only widens about 4% on the average. Significant JT prolongation occurs in < 2% of patients. Rare cases of torsade de pointes-type arrhythmias have occurred.

Clinically significant conduction changes have been observed at these rates: Sinus node dysfunction such as sinus pause, sinus arrest and symptomatic bradycardia (1.2%), second-degree AV block (0.5%), and third-degree AV block (0.4%). If second-or third-degree AV block, or right bundle branch block associated with a left hemiblock occurs, discontinue therapy unless a ventricular pacemaker is in place to ensure an adequate ventricular rate.

Electrolyte disturbance: Hypokalemia or hyperkalemia may alter the effects of Class I antiarrhythmic drugs. Correct preexisting hypokalemia or hyperkalemia before administration.

Effects on pacemaker thresholds: Flecainide increases endocardial pacing thresholds and may suppress ventricular escape rhythms. These effects are reversible if flecainide is discontinued. Use with caution in patients with permanent pacemakers or temporary pacing electrodes. Do not administer to patients with existing poor thresholds or nonprogrammable pacemakers unless suitable pacing rescue is available.

Determine the pacing threshold in patients with pacemakers prior to instituting therapy, after 1 week of administration and at regular intervals thereafter. Generally, threshold changes are within the range of multiprogrammable pacemakers, and a doubling of either voltage or pulse width is usually sufficient to regain capture.

Urinary pH alters flecainide elimination; alkalinization (as may occur in rare conditions such as renal tubular acidosis or strict vegetarian diet) decreases, and acidification increases, flecainide renal excretion. These alterations in pH (outside a range of pH 5 to 7) may produce toxic or subtherapeutic plasma levels. See Drug Interactions.

FLECAINIDE ACETATE

Hepatic function impairment: Since flecainide elimination from plasma can be markedly slower in patients with significant hepatic impairment, do not use in such patients unless the potential benefits outweigh the risks. If used, frequent and early plasma level monitoring is required to guide dosage (see Plasma level monitoring in the Administration and Dosage section); make dosage increases very cautiously when plasma levels have plateaued (after > 4 days).

Elderly: From age 20 to 80, plasma levels are only slightly higher with advancing age; flecainide elimination from plasma is somewhat slower in elderly subjects than in younger subjects. Patients up to age 80 and above have been safely treated with usual doses.

Pregnancy: Category C. Flecainide had teratogenic and embryotoxic effects in one breed of rabbit when given in doses up to 35 mg/kg/day. There are no adequate and well controlled studies in pregnant women. Use during pregnancy only if potential benefits outweigh potential hazards to the fetus.

Lactation: Flecainide is excreted in breast milk in concentrations as high as 4 times (with average levels about 2.5 times) corresponding plasma levels; assuming a maternal plasma level at the top of the therapeutic range (1mcg/ml), the calculated daily dose to a nursing infant (assuming about 700 ml breast milk over 24 hours) would be < 3 mg. Because of the drug's potential for serious adverse effects in infants, determine whether to discontinue nursing or discontinue the drug, taking into account the importance of the drug to the mother.

Children: Safety and efficacy for use in children < 18 years of age have not been established.

Based on several studies flecainide appears to be beneficial in treating supraventricular and ventricular arrhythmias in children. Clearance of flecainide is similar to that of adults, but elimination half-life is shorter and volume of distribution is smaller.

Drug Interactions:

Flecainide Drug Interactions			
Precipitant drug	Object drug*		Description
Amiodarone	Flecainide	↑	Flecainide plasma levels may be increased.
Cimetidine	Flecainide	↑	Flecainide bioavailability and total renal excretion may be increased.
Disopyramide	Flecainide	↑	Disopyramide has negative inotropic properties; do not use with flecainide unless benefits outweigh risks.
Propranolol	Flecainide	↑	Flecainide and propranolol levels were increased in healthy subjects. Negative inotropic effects were additive; effects on PR interval were less than additive.
Flecainide	Propranolol	↑	
Smoking	Flecainide	↓	Compared to nonsmokers, smokers have a greater plasma clearance of flecainide. An increased flecainide dose may be necessary.
Urinary acidifiers	Flecainide	↓	Alterations in urinary excretion and plasma elimination of flecainide occur with changes in urinary pH (acidic urine increases elimination and decreases bioavailability; alkaline urine decreases elimination and increases bioavailability). See Warnings.
Urinary alkalinizers	Flecainide	↑	
Verapamil	Flecainide	↑	Verapamil has negative inotropic properties; do not use with flecainide unless benefits outweigh risks.
Flecainide	Digoxin	↑	Digoxin's absorption, peak concentration and bioavailability may be increased.

* ↑ = Object drug increased ↓ = Object drug decreased

Adverse Reactions:

Most frequent: Dizziness (18.9%), including lightheadedness, faintness, unsteadiness and near syncope; dyspnea (10.3%); headache (9.6%); nausea (8.9%); fatigue (7.7%); palpitation (6.1%); chest pain (5.4%); asthenia (4.9%); tremor (4.7%); constipation (4.4%); edema (3.5%); abdominal pain (3.3%).

FLECAINIDE ACETATE

Cardiovascular: New or worsened arrhythmias (see Warnings); episodes of unresuscitatable VT or ventricular fibrillation (cardiac arrest); new or worsened CHF (see Warnings); second-degree (0.5%) or third-degree (0.4%) AV block; sinus bradycardia, sinus pause or sinus arrest (1.2%) (Warnings); tachycardia (1% to 3%); angina pectoris, bradycardia, hypertension, hypotension (< 1%).

In post-MI patients with asymptomatic PVCs and non-sustained ventricular tachycardia, flecainide therapy was associated with a 5.1% rate of death and non-fatal cardiac arrest, compared with a 2.3% rate in a matched placebo group (see Warnings).

CNS: Hypoesthesia, paresthesia, paresis, ataxia, flushing, increased sweating, vertigo, syncope, somnolence, tinnitus, anxiety, insomnia, depression, malaise (1% to 3%); twitching, weakness, convulsions, neuropathy, speech disorder, stupor, amnesia, confusion, euphoria, depersonalization, morbid dreams, apathy (< 1%).

Dermatologic: Rash (1% to 3%); urticaria, exfoliative dermatitis, pruritus, alopecia (< 1%).

GI: Vomiting, diarrhea, dyspepsia, anorexia (1% to 3%); flatulence, change in taste, dry mouth (< 1%).

GU: Impotence, decreased libido, polyuria, urinary retention (< 1%).

Hematologic: Leukopenia, thrombocytopenia (< 1%).

Ophthalmic: Visual disturbances including blurred vision, difficulty in focusing, spots before eyes (15.9%); diplopia (1% to 3%); eye pain/irritation, photophobia, nystagmus (< 1%).

Miscellaneous: Fever (1% to 3%); swollen lips, tongue and mouth, arthralgia, bronchospasm, myalgia (< 1%).

Overdosage:

Symptoms: Animal studies suggest that the following events might occur with overdosage: Lengthening of the PR interval; increase in the QRS duration, QT interval and amplitude of the T wave; reduction in heart rate and myocardial contractility; conduction disturbances; hypotension; death from respiratory failure or asystole.

Treatment should be supportive and may include the following: Removal of unabsorbed drug from the GI tract (charcoal instillation appears to be effective in lowering flecainide plasma concentrations, even after an interval of 90 minutes from ingestion of flecainide); inotropic agents or cardiac stimulants such as dopamine, dobutamine or isoproterenol; mechanical ventilation; circulatory assists such as intra-aortic balloon pumping; transvenous pacing in the event of conduction block. Because of the drug's long plasma half-life (12 to 27 hours) and the possibility of non-linear elimination kinetics at very high doses, these supportive treatments may need to be continued for extended periods of time. Since flecainide elimination is much slower when urine is very alkaline (pH ≥ 8), theoretically, acidification of urine to promote drug excretion may be beneficial in overdose cases with very alkaline urine. There is no evidence that acidification from normal urinary pH increases excretion. Hemodialysis is not effective. Refer to General Management of Acute Overdosage.

Patient Information:

Take as prescribed; serious heart disturbances can result from missing doses, and serious side effects can result from increasing or decreasing doses without supervision.

Administration and Dosage:

Approved by the FDA in 1985.

For patients with sustained ventricular tachycardia, initiate therapy in the hospital and monitor rhythm.

Flecainide has a long half-life (12 to 27 hours). Steady-state plasma levels in normal renal and hepatic function may not be achieved until 3 to 5 days of therapy at a given dose. Therefore, do not increase dosage more frequently than once every 4 days, since optimal effect may not be achieved during the first 2 to 3 days of therapy.

An occasional patient not adequately controlled by (or intolerant of) a dose given at 12 hour intervals may be dosed at 8 hour intervals.

Once the arrhythmia is controlled, it may be possible to reduce the dose, as necessary, to minimize side effects or effects on conduction.

FLECAINIDE ACETATE

PSVT and PAF: The recommended starting dose is 50 mg every 12 hours. Doses may be increased in increments of 50 mg twice daily every 4 days until efficacy is achieved. For PAF patients, a substantial increase in efficacy without a substantial increase in discontinuation for adverse experiences may be achieved by increasing the flecainide dose from 50 to 100 mg twice daily. The maximum recommended dose for patients with paroxysmal supraventricular arrhythmias is 300 mg/day.

Sustained ventricular tachycardia:

Initial dose – 100 mg every 12 hours. Increase in 50 mg increments twice daily every 4 days until effective. Most patients do not require > 150 mg every 12 hours (300 mg/day). Maximum dose is 400 mg/day.

Use of higher initial doses and more rapid dosage adjustments have resulted in an increased incidence of proarrhythmic events and CHF, particularly during the first few days of dosing (see Warnings). Therefore, a loading dose is not recommended.

CHF or MI: Use cautiously in patients with a history of CHF or myocardial dysfunction (see Warnings).

Renal impairment: In severe renal impairment (Ccr ≤ 35 ml/min/1.73 m^2), the initial dosage is 100 mg once daily (or 50 mg twice daily). Frequent plasma level monitoring is required to guide dosage adjustments. In patients with less severe renal disease, initial dosage is 100 mg every 12 hours. Increase dosage cautiously at intervals > 4 days, observing the patient closely for signs of adverse cardiac effects or other toxicity. It may take > 4 days before a new steady-state plasma level is reached following a dosage change. Monitor plasma levels to guide dosage adjustments (see below).

Transfer to flecainide: Theoretically, when transferring patients from another antiarrhythmic to flecainide, allow at least 2 to 4 plasma half-lives to elapse for the drug being discontinued before starting flecainide at the usual dosage. Consider hospitalization of patients in whom withdrawal of a previous antiarrhythmic is likely to produce life-threatening arrhythmias.

Plasma level monitoring: The majority of patients treated successfully had trough plasma levels between 0.2 and 1mcg/ml. The probability of adverse experiences, especially cardiac, may increase with higher trough plasma levels, especially levels > 1 mcg/ml. Monitor trough plasma levels periodically, especially in patients with severe or moderate chronic renal failure or severe hepatic disease and CHF, as drug elimination may be slower.

Rx	**Tambocor** (3M Pharm.)	**Tablets:** 50 mg	(Riker TR 50). White. In 100s and UD 100s.
		100 mg	(Riker TR 100). White, scored. In 100s and UD 100s.
		150 mg	(Riker TR 150). White, scored. Oval. In 100s.

BRETYLIUM TOSYLATE

For more information, refer to the Antiarrhythmic Agents group monograph.

Actions:

Pharmacology: Bretylium tosylate inhibits norepinephrine release by depressing adrenergic nerve terminal excitability, inducing a chemical sympathectomy-like state. Catecholamine stores are not depleted, but the drug causes an early release of norepinephrine from the adrenergic postganglionic nerve terminals. Therefore, transient catecholamine effects on myocardium (tachycardia) and on peripheral vascular resistance (rise in blood pressure) are often seen shortly after use. Subsequently, bretylium blocks the release of norepinephrine in response to neuron stimulation. Peripheral adrenergic blockade causes orthostatic hypotension but has less effect on supine blood pressure. It has a positive inotropic effect on the myocardium.

Electrophysiology – The mechanisms of action are not established. The following actions have been demonstrated in animals: (1) Increase in ventricular fibrillation threshold; (2) increase in action potential duration and effective refractory period without changes in heart rate; (3) little effect on the rate of rise or amplitude of the cardiac action potential (Phase 0) or in resting membrane potential (Phase 4) in normal myocardium. However, when cell injury slows rate of rise, decreases amplitude and lowers resting membrane potential, bretylium transiently restores these parameters toward normal; (4) decrease in disparity in action potential duration between normal and infarcted regions; (5) increase in impulse formation and spontaneous firing rate of pacemaker tissue, and in ventricular conduction velocity.

The restoration of injured myocardial cell electrophysiology toward normal, as well as the increase of the action potential duration and effective refractory period, without changing their ratio, may help suppress reentry of aberrant impulses and decrease induced dispersion of local excitable states.

Hemodynamics – The mild increase in arterial pressure, followed by a modest decrease, remain within normal limits. Pulmonary artery pressure, pulmonary capillary wedge pressure, right atrial pressure, cardiac index, stroke volume index and stroke work index are not significantly changed.

Pharmacokinetics: Peak plasma concentration and peak hypotensive effects are seen within 1 hour of IM administration. However, suppression of premature ventricular beats is not maximal until 6 to 9 hours after dosing, when mean plasma concentration declines to less than one half of peak level. Antifibrillatory effects occur within minutes of an IV injection. Suppression of ventricular tachycardia and other ventricular arrhythmias develops more slowly, usually 20 min to 2 hours after parenteral administration.

The terminal half-life ranges from 6.9 to 8.1 hours. In two patients with creatinine clearances of 1 and 21 ml/min, half-lives were 31.5 and 16 hours, respectively. During dialysis, a twofold increase in clearance occurs. The drug is eliminated intact by the kidneys. Approximately 70% to 80% of an IM dose is excreted in the urine during the first 24 hours, with an additional 10% excreted over the next 3 days.

Indications:

For prophylaxis and therapy of ventricular fibrillation.

In the treatment of life-threatening ventricular arrhythmias (ie, ventricular tachycardia) which have failed to respond to first-line antiarrhythmic agents (eg, lidocaine).

Unlabeled uses: Bretylium is a second-line agent following lidocaine in the protocol for advanced cardiac life support during CPR. For resistant VF and VT (after lidocaine, defibrillation and procainamide failures), give bretylium 5 to 10 mg/kg IV; repeat as needed up to 30 mg/kg; use a bolus every 15 to 30 minutes, infusion 1 to 2 mg/min. For life-threatening arrhythmia use an undiluted infusion of 1 g/250 ml.

Warnings:

Limit use to intensive care units, coronary care units or other facilities with equipment and personnel for constant cardiac and blood pressure monitoring.

Hypotension (postural) occurs regularly in about 50% of patients while they are supine, manifested by dizziness, lightheadedness, vertigo or faintness. Hypotension may occur at doses lower than those needed to suppress arrhythmias. Keep patients supine until tolerance develops. Tolerance occurs unpredictably but may be present after several days. Hypotension with supine systolic pressure > 75 mm Hg need not be treated unless symptomatic. If supine systolic pressure falls below 75 mm Hg, infuse dopamine or norepinephrine to increase blood pressure; use dilute solution and monitor blood pressure closely because pressor effects are enhanced by bretylium. Perform volume expansion with blood or plasma and correct dehydration where appropriate.

Transient hypertension and increased frequency of arrhythmias may occur due to initial release of norepinephrine from adrenergic postganglionic nerve terminals.

BRETYLIUM TOSYLATE

Fixed cardiac output: Avoid use with fixed cardiac output (ie, severe aortic stenosis or severe pulmonary hypertension) since severe hypotension may result from a fall in peripheral resistance without a compensatory increase in cardiac output. If survival is threatened by arrhythmia, the drug may be used, but give vasoconstrictive catecholamines (eg, norepinephrine) promptly if severe hypotension occurs.

Renal function impairment: Since the drug is excreted principally via the kidney, increase the dosage interval in patients with impaired renal function.

Pregnancy: Category C. Reduced uterine blood flow with fetal hypoxia (bradycardia) is a potential risk. It is not known whether bretylium tosylate can cause harm when administered to a pregnant woman or can affect reproduction capacity. Give to a pregnant woman only if clearly needed.

Children: Safety and efficacy for use in children have not been established. It has been administered to a limited number of pediatric patients, but such use has been inadequate to define proper dosage and limitations. See Administration and Dosage.

Drug Interactions:

Bretylium Drug Interactions			
Precipitant drug	Object drug *		Description
Bretylium	Catecholamines	↑	The pressor effects of catecholamines (eg, dopamine, norepinephrine) are enhanced by bretylium. When catecholamines are administered, use dilute solutions and closely monitor blood pressure (see Warnings).
Bretylium	Digoxin	↑	Digitalis toxicity may be aggravated by the initial release of norepinephrine caused by bretylium. When a life-threatening cardiac arrhythmia occurs, use bretylium only if the etiology of the arrhythmia does not appear to be digitalis toxicity and if other antiarrhythmic drugs are not effective. Avoid simultaneous initiation of therapy.

* ↑ = Object drug increased

Adverse Reactions:

Drug relationship not clearly established: Renal dysfunction, diarrhea, abdominal pain, hiccoughs, erythematous macular rash, flushing, hyperthermia, confusion, paranoid psychosis, emotional lability, lethargy, generalized tenderness, anxiety, shortness of breath, diaphoresis, nasal stuffiness, mild conjunctivitis (0.1%).

Cardiovascular: Hypotension and postural hypotension (most frequent; see Warnings); bradycardia, increased premature ventricular contractions, transient hypertension, initial increase in arrhythmias, precipitation of angina, sensation of substernal pressure (0.1% to 0.2%).

GI: Nausea and vomiting, primarily after rapid IV administration (3%).

CNS: Vertigo, dizziness, lightheadedness, syncope (0.7%).

Overdosage:

Symptoms: With life-threatening arrhythmias, underdosing with bretylium probably presents a greater risk to the patient than potential overdosage. However, one case of accidental overdose occurred in which a rapidly injected IV bolus of 30 mg/kg was given instead of an intended 10 mg/kg dose during an episode of ventricular tachycardia. Marked hypertension resulted, followed by protracted refractory hypotension. The patient died 18 hours later in asystole, complicated by renal failure and aspiration pneumonitis. Bretylium serum levels were 8000 ng/ml.

The exaggerated hemodynamic response was attributed to the rapid injection of a very large dose while some effective circulation was still present. Neither the total dose nor the serum levels observed in this patient are in themselves associated with toxicity. Total doses of 30 mg/kg are not unusual and do not cause toxicity when given incrementally during cardio-pulmonary resuscitation procedures. Similarly, patients maintained on chronic bretylium tosylate therapy have had documented serum levels of 12,000 ng/ml. These levels were achieved after sequential dosage increases over time with no apparent ill effects.

Treatment: If bretylium is overdosed and symptoms of toxicity develop, give nitroprusside or consider another short-acting IV antihypertensive agent. Do not use long-acting drugs that might potentiate subsequent hypotensive effects of bretylium. Treat hypotension with appropriate fluid therapy and pressor agents such as dopamine or norepinephrine. Dialysis is probably not useful in treating bretylium overdose.

BRETYLIUM TOSYLATE

Administration and Dosage:

For short-term use only.

Keep patient supine during therapy or closely observe for postural hypotension. The optimal dose has not been determined. Dosages > 40 mg/kg/day have been used without apparent adverse effect. As soon as possible, and when indicated, change patient to an oral antiarrhythmic agent for maintenance therapy.

Immediate life-threatening ventricular arrhythmias: Administer undiluted, 5 mg/kg by rapid IV injection. If ventricular fibrillation persists, increase dosage to 10 mg/kg and repeat as necessary.

Maintenance: For continuous suppression, administer the diluted solution by continuous IV infusion at 1 to 2 mg/minute. Alternatively, infuse the diluted solution at a dosage of 5 to 10 mg/kg over > 8 minutes, every 6 hours.

Other ventricular arrhythmias: IV – Dilute before administration. Administer 5 to 10 mg/kg by IV infusion over > 8 minutes. More rapid infusion may cause nausea and vomiting. Give subsequent doses at 1 to 2 hour intervals if the arrhythmia persists. For maintenance therapy, the same dosage may be administered every 6 hours, or a constant infusion of 1 to 2 mg/min may be given.

IM – 5 to 10 mg/kg undiluted. Do not dilute prior to injection. Give subsequent doses at 1 to 2 hour intervals if the arrhythmia persists. Thereafter, maintain with same dosage every 6 to 8 hours.

Do not give > 5 ml in any one site. Do not inject into or near a major nerve; vary injection sites. Repeated injection into the same site may cause atrophy and necrosis of muscle tissue, fibrosis, vascular degeneration and inflammatory changes.

Children: The following dosages have been suggested.

Acute ventricular fibrillation – 5 mg/kg/dose IV, followed by 10 mg/kg at 15 to 30 minute intervals, maximum total dose 30 mg/kg; *maintenance,* 5 to 10 mg/kg/dose every 6 hours.

Other ventricular arrhythmias – 5 to 10 mg/kg/dose every 6 hours.

Dilution and administration rates for continuous infusion: Dilute bretylium using the following table and administer as a constant infusion of 1 to 2 mg/min.

Administration Rates for Continuous Infusion Maintenance Bretylium Therapy

Preparation				Administration		
Amount of bretylium	Volume of IV fluid[1] (ml)	Final volume (ml)	Final conc. (mg/ml)	Dose (mg/min)	Microdrops per min	ml/hr
500 mg (10 ml)[2]	50[2]	60[2]	8.3[2]	1	7	7
				1.5	11	11
				2	14	14
2 g (40 ml)	500	540	3.7	1	16	16
1 g (20 ml)	250	270	3.7	1.5	24	24
				2	32	32
1 g (20 ml)	500	520	1.9	1	32	32
500 mg (10 ml)	250	260	1.9	1.5	47	47
				2	63	63

[1] May be either Dextrose or Sodium Chloride Injection, USP.
[2] For fluid restricted patients.

IV compatibility: Bretylium is compatible with the following: 5% Dextrose Injection; 5% Dextrose in 0.45% Sodium Chloride; 5% Dextrose in 0.9% Sodium Chloride; 5% Dextrose in Lactated Ringer's; 0.9% Sodium Chloride; 5% Sodium Bicarbonate; 20% Mannitol; ⅙ M Sodium Lactate; Lactated Ringer's; Calcium Chloride (54.4 mEq/L) in 5% Dextrose; Potassium Chloride (40 mEq/L) in 5% Dextrose.

Rx	**Bretylium Tosylate** (Various, eg, Abbott, Astra)	**Injection:** 50 mg/ml	In 10 ml amps, vials and syringes.
Rx	**Bretylol** (DuPont Critical Care)		In 10 ml amps, disp. syringes and 10 and 20 ml single use vials.
Rx	**Bretylium Tosylate in 5% Dextrose** (Various, eg, Abbott, Baxter)	**Injection:** 2 mg/ml (500 mg/vial)	In 250 ml vials.
		4 mg/ml (1000 mg/vial)	In 250 ml vials.

AMIODARONE HCl

Refer to the general discussion concerning these products in the Antiarrhythmic Agents introduction.

Actions:

Pharmacology: Amiodarone has predominantly class III antiarrhythmic effects. This may be due to at least two major properties: A prolongation of the myocardial cell-action potential duration and refractory period, and noncompetitive α- and β-adrenergic inhibition.

There is no well established relationship of plasma concentration to effectiveness, but concentrations much below 1 mg/L are often ineffective and levels > 2.5 mg/L are generally not needed. Plasma concentration measurements can be used to identify patients whose levels are unusually low, and who might benefit from a dose increase, or unusually high, and who might have dosage reduction in the hope of minimizing side effects. Some observations suggest a plasma concentration, dose or dose/duration relationship for side effects such as pulmonary fibrosis, liver enzyme elevations, corneal deposits, facial pigmentation, peripheral neuropathy and GI and CNS effects.

Electrophysiology – Amiodarone increases the cardiac refractory period without influencing resting membrane potential, except in automatic cells where slope of prepotential is reduced, generally reducing automaticity. These electrophysiologic effects are reflected in decreased sinus rate of 15% to 20%, increased PR and QT intervals of about 10%, development of U waves and changes in T wave contour. These changes should not require discontinuation, although amiodarone can cause marked sinus bradycardia or sinus arrest and heart block. On rare occasions, QT prolongation has been associated with worsening of arrhythmia (see Warnings).

Electrophysiologic effects, such as prolongation of QTc, can be seen within hours after a parenteral dose. However, effects on abnormal rhythms are not seen before 2 to 3 days and usually require 1 to 3 weeks, even when a loading dose is used. Time to effect may be shorter when a loading-dose regimen is used.

Hemodynamics – After IV use, amiodarone relaxes vascular smooth muscle, reduces peripheral vascular resistance (afterload) and slightly increases cardiac index. After oral dosing, however, it produces no significant change in left ventricular ejection fraction (LVEF), even in patients with depressed LVEF. After acute IV dosing, it may have a mild negative inotropic effect.

These differences between oral and IV administration suggest that the initial acute effects of IV amiodarone may be predominantly focused on the AV node, causing an intranodal conduction delay and increased nodal refractoriness due to slow channel blockade (class IV activity) and noncompetitive adrenergic antagonism (class II activity).

Pharmacokinetics:

Absorption – Following oral administration, amiodarone is slowly and variably absorbed; bioavailability is ≈ 50% (between 35% and 65%). Maximum plasma concentrations are attained 3 to 7 hours after a single dose. Despite this, the onset of action may occur in 2 to 3 days, but more commonly takes 1 to 3 weeks, even with loading doses. Plasma concentrations with chronic dosing at 100 to 600 mg/day are approximately dose-proportional, with a mean 0.5 mg/L increase for each 100 mg/day. These means, however, include considerable individual variability.

Peak serum concentrations after single 5 mg/kg 15–minute IV infusions in healthy subjects range between 5 and 41 mg/L. Peak concentrations after 10–minute infusions of 150 mg in patients with ventricular fibrillation (VF) or hemodynamically unstable ventricular tachycardia (VT) range between 7 and 26 mg/L. Due to rapid distribution, serum concentrations decline to 10% of peak values within 30 to 45 minutes after the end of the infusion. In clinical trials, after 48 hours of continued infusions (125, 500 or 1000 mg/day) plus supplemental (150 mg) infusions (for recurrent arrhythmias), amiodarone mean serum concentrations between 0.7 to 1.4 mg/L were observed.

Distribution – Amiodarone has a very large but variable volume of distribution, averaging about 60 L/kg, because of extensive accumulation in various sites, especially adipose tissue and highly perfused organs (eg, liver, lung, spleen). One major metabolite, desethylamiodarone (DEA), accumulates to an even greater extent in almost all tissues. The pharmacological activity of this metabolite is not known. During chronic treatment, the plasma ratio of metabolite to parent compound is ≈ 1:1. Amiodarone and its metabolite have a limited transplacental transfer (10% to 50%). They have been detected in breast milk (see Warnings). The drug is highly protein bound (≈ 96%).

Metabolism – Amiodarone is metabolized by the cytochrome P-450 3A (CYP3A) system. The main route of elimination is via hepatic excretion into bile; some enterohepatic recirculation may occur. The drug has a very low plasma clearance with negligible renal excretion; it does not appear necessary to modify dose in patients with renal failure. Neither amiodarone nor its metabolite is dialyzable.

AMIODARONE HCl

Excretion – Following discontinuation of chronic oral therapy, amiodarone has a biphasic elimination with an initial 50% reduction of plasma levels after 2.5 to 10 days. A much slower terminal plasma elimination phase shows a half-life of the parent compound ranging from 26 to 107 days (mean 53 days), with most patients in the 40 to 55 day range. In the absence of a loading dose period, steady-state plasma concentrations would therefore be reached between 130 and 535 days (average 265 days). For the metabolite, mean plasma elimination half-life was ≈ 61 days. The considerable intersubject variation requires attention to individual responses. Antiarrhythmic effects persist for weeks or months after the drug is discontinued. In general, when the drug is resumed after recurrence of arrhythmia, control is established relatively rapid compared to initial response.

Indications:

Ventricular arrhythmias:

Oral – Only for treatment of the following documented life-threatening recurrent ventricular arrhythmias that do not respond to documented adequate doses of other antiarrhythmics or when alternative agents are not tolerated:

1. Recurrent ventricular fibrillation (VF).
2. Recurrent hemodynamically unstable ventricular tachycardia (VT).

Parenteral – Initiation of treatment and prophylaxis of frequently recurring VF and hemodynamically unstable VT in patients refractory to other therapy. It can also be used to treat patients with VT/VF for whom oral amiodarone is indicated, but who are unable to take oral medication.

During or after treatment with IV amiodarone, patients may be transferred to oral amiodarone therapy. Use IV amiodarone for acute treatment until the patient's ventricular arrhythmias are stabilized. Most patients require this therapy for 48 to 96 hours, but IV amiodarone may be given safely for longer periods if necessary.

Unlabeled uses: Amiodarone (600 to 800 mg/day for 7 to 10 days, then 200 to 400 mg/day) appears to be beneficial in the treatment of refractory sustained or paroxysmal atrial fibrillation and paroxysmal supraventricular tachycardia. It also appears useful in symptomatic atrial flutter. Low dose amiodarone (200 mg/day) may produce benefits in left ventricular ejection fraction, exercise tolerance and ventricular arrhythmias in patients with CHF.

Contraindications:

Hypersensitivity to the drug or any of its components.

Oral: Severe sinus-node dysfunction, causing marked sinus bradycardia; second- and third-degree AV block; when episodes of bradycardia have caused syncope (except when used in conjunction with a pacemaker).

Parenteral: Marked sinus bradycardia; second- and third-degree AV block unless a functioning pacemaker is available; cardiogenic shock.

Warnings:

Potentially fatal toxicities with pulmonary toxicity, have occurred with ventricular arrhythmias (≈ 400 mg/day), and symptomless abnormal diffusion capacity has occurred in much higher percentages. Pulmonary toxicity has been fatal ≈ 10% of the time (see Pulmonary toxicity). Hepatic injury is common, but usually mild, and evidenced by abnormal liver enzymes. Overt liver disease can occur, and has been fatal (see Hepatic effects). Amiodarone has made arrhythmia less well tolerated or more difficult to reverse. Significant heart block or sinus bradycardia has been seen (see Cardiac effects). These events should be manageable in the proper clinical setting. Although such events do not appear more frequently with amiodarone than with other agents, effects are prolonged. In patients at high risk of arrhythmic death in whom amiodarone toxicity is an acceptable risk, amiodarone poses major management problems that could be life-threatening in a population at risk of sudden death so that every effort should be made to use alternative agents first.

Hospitalize patients while the loading dose is given; a response generally requires 2 weeks. Absorption and elimination are variable; therefore, maintenance dose selection is difficult. The time at which a life-threatening arrhythmia will recur after discontinuation or dose adjustment is unpredictable, ranging from weeks to months. The patient risk is greatest during this time. Substituting other antiarrhythmics when amiodarone must be stopped is made difficult by the gradually, but unpredictably, changing amiodarone body stores. When amiodarone is ineffective, it still poses the risk of interacting with subsequent treatment.

Survival: There is no evidence that the use of amiodarone favorably affects survival. Refer to the Antiarrhythmic Agents introduction.

AMIODARONE HCl

Pulmonary toxicity:

Oral – Amiodarone may cause a clinical syndrome of cough and progressive dyspnea accompanied by functional, radiographic, gallium scan and pathological data consistent with pulmonary toxicity. The frequency varies from 2% to 17%; fatalities occur in ≈ 10% of cases. However, in patients with life-threatening arrhythmias, discontinuation of amiodarone therapy due to suspected drug-induced pulmonary toxicity should be undertaken with caution, as the most common cause of death in these patients is sudden cardiac death. Therefore, make every effort to rule out other causes of respiratory impairment (eg, CHF with Swan-Ganz catheterization if necessary, respiratory infection, pulmonary embolism, malignancy) before discontinuing amiodarone. In addition, bronchoalveolar lavage, transbronchial lung biopsy or open lung biopsy may be necessary to confirm the diagnosis, especially in those cases where no acceptable alternative therapy is available.

Any new respiratory symptom suggests pulmonary toxicity, therefore repeat and evaluate the history, physical exam, chest x-ray, gallium scan and pulmonary function tests (with diffusion capacity). In some cases, rechallenge at a lower dose has not resulted in return of interstitial/alveolar pneumonitis. A 15% decrease in diffusion capacity has a high sensitivity, but only a moderate specificity for pulmonary toxicity; as the decrease in diffusion capacity approaches 30%, the sensitivity decreases but the specificity increases.

Perform baseline chest x–rays and pulmonary function tests, including diffusion capacity before therapy initiation. Repeat a history, physical exam and chest x-ray every 3 to 6 months.

Pre-existing pulmonary disease does not appear to increase the risk of developing pulmonary toxicity; however, these patients have a poorer prognosis if pulmonary toxicity does develop. Pulmonary toxicity secondary to amiodarone seems to result from either indirect or direct toxicity as represented by hypersensitivity pneumonitis or interstitial/alveolar pneumonitis, respectively.

Hypersensitivity pneumonitis usually appears earlier in the course of therapy, and rechallenging these patients results in a more rapid recurrence of greater severity. Bronchoalveolar lavage is the procedure of choice to confirm this diagnosis which can be made when a T suppressor/cytotoxic (CD8–positive) lymphocytosis is noted. Institute steroid therapy and discontinue amiodarone therapy.

Interstitial/alveolar pneumonitis may result from the release of oxygen radicals or phospholipidosis and is characterized by findings of diffuse alveolar damage, interstitial pneumonitis or fibrosis in lung biopsy specimens. Phospholipidosis (foamy cells, foamy macrophages), due to inhibition of phospholipase, will be present in most cases of amiodarone-induced pulmonary toxicity; however, these changes are also present in ≈ 50% of all patients. Use these cells as markers of therapy, but not as evidence of toxicity. A diagnosis of amiodarone-induced interstitial/alveolar pneumonitis should lead, at a minimum, to dose reduction or, preferably, to withdrawal of amiodarone to establish reversibility, especially if other acceptable antiarrhythmic therapies are available. Where these measures have been instituted, a reduction in symptoms of amiodarone-induced pulmonary toxicity was usually noted within the first week and a clinical improvement was greatest in the first 2 to 3 weeks. Chest x-ray changes usually resolve within 2 to 4 months.

According to some experts, steroids may prove beneficial. Prednisone in doses of 40 to 60 mg/day or equivalent doses of other steroids have been given and tapered over the course of several weeks depending on the condition of the patient. In some cases, rechallenge with amiodarone at a lower dose has not resulted in return of toxicity. Recent reports suggest that the use of lower loading and maintenance doses of amiodarone are associated with a decreased incidence of amiodarone-induced pulmonary toxicity.

If a diagnosis of amiodarone-induced hypersensitivity pneumonitis is made, discontinue amiodarone and institute steroid treatment. If a diagnosis of amiodarone-induced interstitial/alveolar pneumonitis is made, institute steroid therapy and discontinue amiodarone or, at a minimum, reduce dosage. Some cases of amiodarone-induced may resolve following a reduction in amiodarone dosage in conjunction with steroid administration. In some patients, rechallenge at a lower dose has not resulted in return of interstitial/alveolar pneumonitis; however, in some patients (perhaps because of severe alveolar damage), the pulmonary lesions have not been reversible.

AMIODARONE HCl

Parenteral –

ARDS: 2% of patients were reported to have adult respiratory distress syndrome (ARDS) during clinical studies. ARDS is a disorder characterized by bilateral, diffuse pulmonary infiltrates with pulmonary edema and varying degrees of respiratory insufficiency. The clinical and radiographic picture can arise after a variety of lung injuries, such as those resulting from trauma, shock, prolonged cardiopulmonary resuscitation and aspiration pneumonitis, conditions present in many of the patients enrolled in the clinical studies. It is not possible to determine what role, if any, amiodarone IV played in causing or exacerbating the pulmonary disorder in those patients.

Pulmonary fibrosis: Only 1 of > 1000 patients treated with amiodarone IV in clinical studies developed pulmonary fibrosis. In that patient, the condition was diagnosed 3 months after treatment with amiodarone IV, during which time she received oral amiodarone. Pulmonary toxicity is a well recognized complication of long-term amiodarone use.

Cardiac effects:

Proarrhythmia – Amiodarone can cause serious exacerbation of the presenting arrhythmia (2% to 5%), a risk that may be enhanced by concomitant antiarrhythmics. Exacerbation has included new ventricular fibrillation, incessant ventricular tachycardia, increased resistance to cardioversion and polymorphic ventricular tachycardia associated with QT prolongation (torsade de pointes). In addition, amiodarone has caused symptomatic bradycardia, heart block or sinus arrest with suppression of escape foci in 2% to 5% of patients. Drug-related bradycardia occurred in 4% of 1836 patients in clinical trials while they were receiving amiodarone IV for life-threatening VT/VF; it was not dose-related. Treat bradycardia by slowing the infusion rate or discontinuing amiodarone IV. In some patients, inserting a pacemaker is required. Despite such measures, bradycardia was progressive and terminal in one patient during the controlled trials. Treat patients with a known predisposition to bradycardia or AV block with amiodarone IV in a setting where a temporary pacemaker is available.

Hypotension is the most common adverse effect seen with amiodarone IV. In clinical trials, treatment-emergent, drug-related hypotension was reported as an adverse effect in 16% of 1836 patients treated with amiodarone IV. Clinically significant hypotension during infusions was seen most often in the first several hours of treatment and was not dose-related, but appeared to be related to the rate of infusion. Hypotension necessitating alterations in therapy was reported in 3% of patients, with permanent discontinuation required in < 2% of patients. Treat hypotension initially by slowing the infusion; additional standard therapy may be needed, including the following: Vasopressor drugs, positive inotropic agents and volume expansion. Monitor the initial rate of infusion closely and do not exceed that prescribed in Administration and Dosage.

Hepatic effects:

Oral – Elevated hepatic enzyme levels are frequent, and in most cases are asymptomatic. If the increase exceeds 3 times normal, or doubles in a patient with an elevated baseline, consider discontinuation or dosage reduction. When a biopsy has been done, histology has resembled that of alcoholic hepatitis or cirrhosis. Hepatic failure has rarely caused death.

Elevations in liver enzymes (AST and ALT) can occur. Regularly monitor liver enzymes in patients on relatively high maintenance doses. If persistent significant elevations in the liver enzymes or hepatomegaly occur, consider reducing the maintenance dose or discontinuing therapy.

Parenteral – Elevations of blood hepatic enzyme values, ALT, AST and GGT, are seen commonly in patients with immediately life-threatening VT/VF. Interpreting elevated AST activity can be difficult because the values may be elevated in patients who have had recent MI, CHF or multiple electrical defibrillations. Approximately 54% of patients receiving amiodarone IV in clinical studies had baseline liver enzyme elevations and 13% had clinically significant elevations. In 81% of patients with both baseline and on-therapy data available, the liver enzyme elevations either improved during therapy or remained at baseline levels. Baseline abnormalities in hepatic enzymes are not a contraindication to treatment.

Two cases of fatal hepatocellular necrosis after treatment with amiodarone IV have been reported. The patients were treated for atrial arrhythmias with an initial infusion of 1500 mg over 5 hours, a rate much higher than recommended. Both patients developed hepatic and renal failure within 24 hours after the start of amiodarone IV treatment and died on day 14 and day 4, respectively. Because these episodes of hepatic necrosis may have been due to the rapid rate of infusion with possible rate-related hypotension, monitor the initial rate of infusion closely and do not exceed that prescribed in Administration and Dosage.

AMIODARONE HCl

In patients with life-threatening arrhythmias, weigh the potential risk of hepatic injury against the potential benefit of therapy. Monitor carefully for evidence of progressive hepatic injury. Give consideration to reducing the rate of administration or withdrawing amiodarone IV in such cases.

Carcinogenesis/Fertility impairment: Amiodarone caused a statistically significant, dose-related increase in the incidence of thyroid tumors (follicular adenoma or carcinoma) in rats. It also reduced fertility of male and female rats at a dose of 90 mg/kg/day (8 times the highest recommended human maintenance dose).

Elderly: Healthy subjects > 65 years of age show lower clearances of amiodarone than younger subjects (100 vs 150 ml/kg/hr) and an increase in half-life (from 20 to 47 days).

Pregnancy: Category D.

Oral – Oral amiodarone has been embryotoxic (increased fetal resorption and growth retardation) in the rat when given orally at a dose of 200 mg/kg/day (18 times the maximum recommended maintenance dose). Amiodarone can cause fetal harm when administered to a pregnant woman. Amiodarone concentrations in the infant at birth are ≈ 25% of maternal levels, 10% for the metabolite. Although its use is uncommon, there have been a small number of reports of congenital goiter/hypothyroidism and hyperthyroidism. If amiodarone is used during pregnancy or if the patient becomes pregnant while taking amiodarone, apprise the patient of the potential hazard to the fetus. Use only if the potential benefits outweigh the potential hazards to the fetus.

Parenteral – In addition to causing infrequent congenital goiter/hypothyroidism and hyperthyroidism, there has been a variety of adverse effects in animals.

In rabbits, at dosages of 5, 10 or 25 mg/kg/day, maternal deaths occurred in all groups, including controls. Embryotoxicity (as manifested by fewer full-term fetuses and increased resorptions with concomitantly lower litter weights) occurred at dosages of ≥ 10 mg/kg.

In rats, maternal toxicity (as evidenced by reduced weight gain and food consumption) and embryotoxicity (as evidenced by increased resorptions, decreased live litter size, reduced body weights and retarded sternum and metacarpal ossification) were observed in the 100 mg/kg group.

Amiodarone IV should be used during pregnancy only if the potential benefit to the mother justifies the risk to the fetus.

Lactation: Amiodarone is excreted in breast milk. Nursing offspring of lactating rats administered amiodarone are less viable and have reduced body-weight gains. Therefore, when amiodarone therapy is indicated, advise the mother to discontinue nursing.

Children: Safety and efficacy for use in children have not been established. Amiodarone is not recommended in children.

Precautions:

Ophthalmologic effects: Asymptomatic corneal microdeposits appear in virtually all adults treated with amiodarone for > 6 months. They are usually discernible only by slit-lamp examination, but give rise to symptoms such as visual halos or blurred vision in as many as 10% of patients. Corneal microdeposits are reversible upon reduction of dose or drug discontinuation. Asymptomatic microdeposits are not a reason to reduce dose or stop treatment. Some patients develop photophobia and dry eyes. Vision is rarely affected and drug discontinuation is rarely needed.

Thyroid abnormalities: Amiodarone inhibits peripheral conversion of thyroxine (T_4) to triodothyronine (T_3), prompting increased T_4 levels, increased levels of inactive reverse T_3 and decreased levels of T_3. It is also a potential source of large amounts of inorganic iodine. Because of its release of inorganic iodine, or maybe for other reasons, amiodarone can cause hypothyroidism or hyperthyroidism. Monitor thyroid function at baseline and periodically during therapy, particularly in the elderly and in any patient with a history of thyroid nodules, goiter or other thyroid dysfunction. Because of the slow elimination of amiodarone and its metabolites, high plasma iodide levels, altered thyroid function and abnormal thyroid function tests may persist for several weeks or even months following amiodarone withdrawal.

Hypothyroidism has been reported in 2% to 10% of patients. It can be identified by relevant clinical symptoms and particularly by elevated TSH. In some clinically hypothyroid amiodarone-treated patients, free thyroxine index values may be normal. Hypothyroidism is best managed by dose reduction or thyroid hormone supplement. However, therapy must be individualized, and it may be necessary to discontinue amiodarone in some patients.

Hyperthyroidism occurs in about 2% of patients receiving amiodarone, but the incidence may be higher among patients with prior inadequate dietary iodine intake. Amiodarone-induced hyperthyroidism usually poses a greater hazard to the patient than hypothyroidism because of the possibility of arrhythmia breakthrough or aggravation. In fact, if any new signs of arrhythmia appear, consider the possibility of hyperthyroidism. Hyperthyroidism is best identified by relevant clinical symptoms and signs, accompanied usually by abnormally elevated levels of serum T_3 RIA, and further elevations of serum T_4, and a subnormal serum TSH level. Since arrhythmia breakthroughs may accompany amiodarone-induced hyperthyroidism, aggressive medical treatment is indicated, including, if possible, dose reduction or withdrawal of amiodarone. The institution of antithyroid drugs, beta-adrenergic blockers or temporary corticosteroid therapy may be necessary. The action of antithyroid drugs may be especially delayed in amiodarone-induced thyrotoxicosis because of substantial quantities of preformed thyroid hormones stored in the gland. Radioactive iodine therapy is contraindicated because of the low radioiodine uptake associated with amiodarone-induced hyperthyroidism. Experience with thyroid surgery in this setting is extremely limited, and this form of therapy runs the theoretical risk of inducing thyroid storm. Amiodarone-induced hyperthyroidism may be followed by a transient period of hypothyroidism.

Electrolyte disturbances: Antiarrhythmics may be ineffective or arrhythmogenic in patients with hypokalemia; correct potassium or magnesium deficiency before therapy begins as these disorders can exaggerate the degree of QTc prolongation and increase the potential for torsade de pointes. Give special attention to electrolyte and acid-base balance in patients experiencing severe or prolonged diarrhea or in patients receiving concomitant diuretics.

Photosensitivity: Amiodarone has induced photosensitization in about 10% of patients; some protection may be afforded by sun barrier creams or protective clothing. During long-term treatment, a blue-gray discoloration of the exposed skin may occur. The risk may be increased in patients of fair complexion or those with excessive sun exposure and may be related to cumulative dose and duration of therapy. This is slowly and occasionally incompletely reversible on discontinuation of drug but is of cosmetic importance only.

Drug Interactions:

Although only a small number of drug interactions have been formally explored, most of these have shown such an interaction should be anticipated, particularly for drugs with potentially serious toxicity such as other antiarrhythmics. If such drugs are needed, their doses should be reassessed and where appropriate, plasma concentration measured. In view of the long and variable half-life of amiodarone, potential for drug interactions exists not only with concomitant medication but also with drugs given after discontinuation of amiodarone.

The interactions listed in the table occurred with oral administration unless otherwise noted.

Amiodarone Drug Interactions

Precipitant drug	Object drug*		Description
Amiodarone	Anticoagulants	⬆	Hypoprothrombinemic effect of anticoagulants is augmented. Prothrombin time (PT) may increase. Potentiation of anticoagulant response is almost always seen in patients receiving amiodarone and can result in serious or fatal bleeding. A 30% to 50% reduction in dose is typically required. The effect may persist for months after amiodarone discontinuation. Closely monitor PT.
Amiodarone	Beta blockers	⬆	Pharmacologic effects of metoprolol and possibly other beta blockers eliminated by hepatic metabolism may be increased. Since amiodarone has weak beta blocking activity, concomitant use can increase risk of hypotension and bradycardia.
Amiodarone	Calcium blockers	⬆	Amiodarone inhibits AV conduction and decreases myocardial contractility; increased risk of AV block with verapamil or diltiazem or hypotension with any calcium blocker may occur.
Amiodarone	Cyclosporine	⬆	Concomitant use has produced persistently elevated plasma cyclosporine levels resulting in elevated creatinine despite reduction in dose of cyclosporine.
Amiodarone	Dextromethorphan	⬆	Chronic use (> 2 weeks) of oral amiodarone administration impairs metabolism of dextromethorphan.

AMIODARONE HCl

Amiodarone Drug Interactions

Precipitant drug	Object drug*		Description
Amiodarone	Digoxin	↑	Serum levels of digoxin are increased by as much as 70%, perhaps to the point of toxicity.
Amiodarone	Flecainide	↑	Increased flecainide plasma levels may occur.
Amiodarone	Hydantoins	↑	Chronic use (> 2 weeks) of oral amiodarone administration impairs metabolism of phenytoin. Increased hydantoin concentrations with symptoms of toxicity may occur. Also, amiodarone serum levels may be decreased.
Hydantoins	Amiodarone	↓	
Amiodarone	Lidocaine	↑	Sinus bradycardia was seen in a patient receving oral amiodarone who was given lidocaine for local anesthesia. A seizure associated with increased lidocaine concentrations was observed in one patient.
Amiodarone	Methotrexate	↑	Chronic use (> 2 weeks) of oral amiodarone administration impairs metabolism of methotrexate.
Amiodarone	Procainamide	↑	Increased procainamide or NAPA serum levels may occur (55% and 33%, respectively).
Amiodarone	Quinidine	↑	Quinidine serum levels may be increased by 33%, possibly producing potentially fatal cardiac arrhythmias.
Amiodarone	Theophylline	↑	Increased theophylline levels with toxicity may occur. Effects may not be seen for ≥ 1 week of concomitant therapy and may persist for an extended period after amiodarone discontinuation.
Cholestyramine	Amiodarone	↓	Increased enterohepatic elimination of amiodarone and reduced serum levels and half-life may occur.
Cimetidine	Amiodarone	↑	Increased serum amiodarone levels may occur.

* ↑ = Object drug increased ↓ = Object drug decreased.

Drug/Lab test interactions: Amiodarone alters the results of thyroid function tests, causing an increase in serum T_4 and serum reverse T_3 levels and a decline in serum T_3 levels. Despite these biochemical changes, most patients remain clinically euthyroid. (See Precautions).

Adverse Reactions:

Oral: Adverse reactions, very common in virtually all patients treated with amiodarone for ventricular arrhythmias with relatively large doses (≥ 400 mg/day), occur in about 75% of patients and cause discontinuation in 7% to 18%. Most effects appear more frequently with treatment beyond 6 months, though rates appear relatively constant beyond 1 year.

Reactions most frequently requiring discontinuation include: Pulmonary infiltrates or fibrosis, paroxysmal ventricular tachycardia, CHF, elevation of liver enzymes. Other symptoms causing discontinuation less often include: Visual disturbances, solar dermatitis, blue discoloration of skin, hyperthyroidism, hypothyroidism.

Cardiovascular – Cardiovascular reactions, other than exacerbation of arrhythmias (see Warnings), include CHF (3%) and bradycardia. Bradycardia usually responds to dosage reduction but may require a pacemaker. Rarely, CHF requires drug discontinuation. Cardiac conduction abnormalities are infrequent and reversible on discontinuation. The following have also been reported: Cardiac arrhythmias, SA node dysfunction, CHF (1% to 3%); hypotension (< 1%; see Warnings).

CNS – Neurologic problems (20% to 40%) are rarely a reason to stop therapy and may respond to dose reductions. The following have been reported: Malaise, fatigue, tremor/abnormal involuntary movements, lack of coordination, abnormal gait/ataxia, dizziness, paresthesias (4% to 9%); decreased libido, insomnia, headache, sleep disturbances (1% to 3%); peripheral neuropathy.

Dermatologic – Dermatologic reactions occur in about 15% of patients; photosensitivity is most common (10%; see Precautions). Other reactions include: Solar dermatitis (4% to 9%); blue discoloration of skin (see Precautions), rash, spontaneous ecchymosis, alopecia (< 1%).

GI – GI complaints occur in about 25% of patients but rarely require discontinuation of drug. These commonly occur during high-dose administration (eg, loading dose) and usually respond to dose reduction or divided doses. Nausea, vomiting (10% to 33%); constipation, anorexia (4% to 9%); abdominal pain, abnormal taste and smell, abnormal salivation, (1% to 3%).

AMIDARONE HCl

Hepatic – Abnormal liver function tests (4% to 9%; see Warnings); nonspecific hepatic disorders (1% to 3%); hepatitis, cholestatic hepatitis, cirrhosis (rare).

Ophthalmic – Visual disturbances (4% to 9%); optic neuritis (< 1%; see Precautions).

Miscellaneous: Pulmonary inflammation or fibrosis (4% to 9%; see Warnings); hypothyroidism and hyperthyroidism (see Precautions), edema, coagulation abnormalities, flushing (1% to 3%); epididymitis, vasculitis, pseudotumor cerebri, thrombocytopenia (< 1%).

Parenteral: In a total of 1836 patients in controlled and uncontrolled clinical trials, 14% of patients received amiodarone for at least 1 week; 5% received it for at least 2 weeks, 2% received it for at least 3 weeks and 1% received it for > 3 weeks, without an increased incidence of severe adverse reactions.

The most important treatment-emergent adverse effects were hypotension, asystole/cardiac arrest/electromechanical dissociation (EMD), cardiogenic shock, CHF, bradycardia, liver function test abnormalities, VT and AV block. Overall, treatment was discontinued for about 9% of the patients because of adverse effects. The most common adverse effects leading to discontinuation of IV therapy were hypotension (1.6%), asystole/cardiac arrest/EMD (1.2%), VT (1.1%) and cardiogenic shock (1%).

IV Amiodarone Adverse Reactions (%)			
Adverse reaction	Controlled studies (n = 814)	Open label studies (n = 1022)	Total (n = 1836)
Bradycardia	6	4	4.9
Congestive heart failure	2.2	2	2.1
Cardiac arrest	3.5	2.5	2.9
Hypotension	20.2	12	15.6
Ventricular tachycardia	1.8	2.9	2.4
Fever	2.9	1.2	2
Abnormal liver function tests	4.2	2.8	3.4
Nausea	3.5	4.2	3.9

Other adverse reactions include the following:

Cardiovascular – Atrial fibrillation, nodal arrhythmia, prolonged QT interval, sinus bradycardia, VF (< 2%).

GI – Diarrhea, vomiting (< 2%).

Miscellaneous – Abnormal kidney function, lung edema, increased ALT, increased AST, respiratory disorder, shock, Stevens-Johnson syndrome, thrombocytopenia (< 2%).

Overdosage:

Symptoms: There have been a few reported cases of oral overdose in which 3 to 8 g of the drug were taken. There were no deaths or permanent sequelae. The most likely effects of an inadvertent overdose of amiodarone are hypotension, cardiogenic shock, bradycardia, AV block and hepatotoxicity.

Treatment includes usual supportive measures. Refer to General Management of Acute Overdosage. In addition, monitor the patient's cardiac rhythm and blood pressure; if bradycardia occurs, use a β-adrenergic agonist or a pacemaker. Treat hypotension with inadequate tissue perfusion, by using positive inotropic or vasopressor agents. Neither amiodarone nor its metabolite is dialyzable. Cholestyramine may be useful in accelerating the reversal of side effects of amiodarone by enhancing drug elimination; however, it is not known if this is beneficial in an overdose situation.

Administration and Dosage:

Approved by the FDA on December 27, 1985 (oral) and August 3, 1995 (parenteral).

Oral: In order to ensure that an antiarrhythmic effect will be observed without waiting several months, loading doses are required. Individual patient titration is suggested.

Life-threatening ventricular arrhythmias (eg, ventricular fibrillation or hemodynamically unstable ventricular tachycardia) – Closely monitor patient during the loading phase, particularly until risk of recurrent ventricular tachycardia or fibrillation has abated. Because of the serious nature of the arrhythmia and the lack of predictable time course of effect, administer the loading dose in a hospital. Loading doses of 800 to 1600 mg/day are required for 1 to 3 weeks (occasionally longer) until initial therapeutic response occurs. Administer in divided doses with meals for total daily doses of ≥ 1000 mg, or when GI intolerance occurs. If side effects become excessive, reduce the dose. Elimination of recurrence of ventricular fibrillation and

AMIODARONE HCl

tachycardia usually occurs within 1 to 3 weeks, along with reduction in complex and total ventricular ectopic beats.

When starting therapy, attempt to gradually discontinue prior antiarrhythmic drugs (see concurrent antiarrhythmic agents). When adequate arrhythmia control is achieved, or if side effects become prominent, reduce dose to 600 to 800 mg/day for 1 month and then to the maintenance dose, usually 400 mg/day. Some patients may require larger maintenance doses, up to 600 mg/day, and some can be controlled on lower doses. May be administered as a single daily dose, or in patients with severe GI intolerance, as a twice daily dose. In each patient, determine the chronic maintenance dose according to antiarrhythmic effect as assessed by symptoms, Holter recordings or programmed electrical stimulation and by patient tolerance. Plasma concentrations may be helpful in evaluating nonresponsiveness or unexpectedly severe toxicity.

Use the lowest effective dose to prevent the occurrence of side effects. In all instances, be guided by the severity of the patient's arrhythmia and response to therapy. When dosage adjustments are necessary, closely monitor the patient for an extended time because of the long and variable half-life and the difficulty in predicting the time required to attain a new steady-state drug level.

Concurrent antiarrhythmic agents – In general, reserve the combination of amiodarone with other antiarrhythmic therapy for patients with life-threatening arrhythmias who are incompletely responsive to a single agent or incompletely responsive to amiodarone. During transfer to amiodarone, reduce the dose levels of previously administered agents by 30% to 50% several days after the addition of amiodarone when arrhythmia suppression should be beginning. Review the continued need for the other antiarrhythmic agent after the effects of amiodarone have been established and attempt discontinuation. If the treatment is continued, carefully monitor these patients for adverse effects, especially conduction disturbances and exacerbation of tachyarrhythmias, as amiodarone is continued. In amiodarone-treated patients who require additional antiarrhythmic therapy, the initial dose of such agents should be approximately half of the usual recommended dose.

Parenteral: Amiodarone shows considerable interindividual variation in response. Thus, although a starting dose adequate to suppress life-threatening arrhythmias is needed, close monitoring with adjustment of dose as needed is essential. The recommended starting dose of amiodarone IV is about 1000 mg over the first 24 hours of therapy, delivered by the following infusion regimen.

Amiodarone IV Dose Recommendations During the First 24 Hours	
Loading infusions	
First rapid	150 mg over the *first* 10 minutes (15 mg/min). Add 3 ml amiodarone IV (150 mg) to 100 ml D5W (concentration, 1.5 mg/ml). Infuse 100 ml/10 min.
Followed by slow	360 mg over the *next* 6 hours (1 mg/min). Add 18 ml amiodarone IV (900 mg) to 500 ml D5W (concentration, = 1.8 mg/ml).
Maintenance infusion	540 mg over the *remaining* 18 hours (0.5 mg/min). Decrease the rate of the slow loading infusion to 0.5 mg/min.

After the first 24 hours, continue the maintenance infusion rate of 0.5 mg/min (720 mg/24 hrs) utilizing a concentration of 1 to 6 mg/ml (give amiodarone IV concentrations > 2 mg/ml via a central venous catheter). In the event of breakthrough episodes of VF or hemodynamically unstable VT, 150 mg supplemental infusions of amiodarone IV mixed in 100 ml D5W may be given. Administer such infusions over 10 minutes to minimize the potential for hypotension. The rate of the maintenance infusion may be increased to achieve effective arrhythmia suppression.

The first 24 hour dose may be individualized for each patient; however, in controlled clinical trials, mean daily doses > 2100 mg were associated with an increased risk of hypotension. The initial infusion rate should not exceed 30 mg/min.

Based on the experience from clinical studies, a maintenance infusion of up to 0.5 mg/min can be cautiously continued for 2 to 3 weeks regardless of the patient's age, renal function or left ventricular function. There has been limited experience in patients receiving amiodarone IV for > 3 weeks.

The surface properties of solutions containing injectable amiodarone are altered such that the drop size may be reduced. This reduction may lead to underdosage of the patient by up to 30%. If drop counter infusion sets are used, amiodarone must be delivered by a volumetric infusion pump.

Amiodarone IV should, when possible, be administered through a central venous catheter for that purpose. Use an in-line filter during administration.

Amiodarone IV concentrations > 3 mg/ml in D5W have been associated with a high incidence of peripheral vein phlebitis; however, concentrations of ≤ 2.5 mg/ml

AMIODARONE HCl

appear to be less irritating. Therefore, for infusions > 1 hour, amiodarone IV concentrations should not exceed 2 mg/ml unless a central venous catheter is used.

Amiodarone IV infusions exceeding 2 hours must be administered in glass or polyolefin bottles containing D5W.

Amiodarone adsorbs to polyvinyl chloride (PVC) tubing and the clinical trial dose administration schedule was designed to account for this adsorption. All of the clinical trials were conducted using PVC tubing and its use is therefore recommended. The concentrations and rates of infusion provided in Administration and Dosage reflect doses identified in these studies. It is important that the recommended infusion regimen be followed closely.

Amiodarone IV does not need to be protected from light during administration.

Amiodarone Solution Stability

Solution	Concentration (mg/ml)	Container	Comments
5% dextrose in water (D5W)	1 to 6	PVC	Physically compatible, with amiodarone loss < 10% at 2 hours
5% dextrose in water (D5W)	1 to 6	Polyolefin, glass	Physically compatible, with no amiodarone loss at 24 hours

Admixture incompatibility – Amiodarone IV in D5W is incompatible with the drugs shown below.

Amiodarone Y-Site Injection Incompatibility

Drug	Vehicle	Amiodarone Concentration	Comments
Aminophylline	D5W	4 mg/ml	Precipitate
Cefamandole nafate	D5W	4 mg/ml	Precipitate
Cefazolin sodium	D5W	4 mg/ml	Precipitate
Mezlocillin sodium	D5W	4 mg/ml	Precipitate
Heparin sodium	D5W	—	Precipitate
Sodium bicarbonate	D5W	3 mg/ml	Precipitate

IV to oral transition – Patients whose arrhythmias have been suppressed by amiodarone IV may be switched to oral amiodarone. The optimal dose for changing from IV to oral administration will depend on the IV dose already administered, as well as the bioavailability of oral amiodarone. When changing to oral therapy, clinical monitoring is recommended, particularly for elderly patients.

The following table provides suggested doses of oral amiodarone to be initiated after varying durations of IV administration. These recommendations are made on the basis of a comparable total body amount of amiodarone delivered by the IV and oral routes, based on 50% bioavailability of oral amiodarone.

Recommendations for Oral Amiodarone Dosage After IV Infusion

Duration of amiodarone IV infusions[1]	Initial daily dose of oral amiodarone
< 1 week	800 to 1600 mg
1 to 3 weeks	600 to 800 mg
> 3 weeks[2]	400 mg

[1] Assuming a 720 mg/day infusion (0.5 mg/min).
[2] Amiodarone IV is not intended for maintenance treatment.

Storage/Stability: Store at room temperature (≈ 25°C [77°F]). Protect from light.

Rx	**Cordarone** (Wyeth-Ayerst)	**Tablets**: 200 mg	Lactose. (C 200 Wyeth 4188). Pink, scored. Convex. In 60s and UD 100s.
Rx	**Cordarone** (Wyeth-Ayerst)	**Injection**: 50 mg/ml	20.2 mg/ml benzyl alcohol. In 3 ml amps.

ADENOSINE

Refer to the general discussion concerning these products in the Antiarrhythmic Agents group monograph. For information on the relief of vericose veins, refer to the Adenosine Phosphate monograph in the Miscellaneous section.

Actions:

Pharmacology: Adenosine is an endogenous nucleoside occurring in all cells of the body. It is not chemically related to other antiarrhythmic agents. Adenosine slows conduction time through the AV node, can interrupt the re-entry pathways through the AV node and can restore normal sinus rhythm in patients with paroxysmal supraventricular tachycardia (PSVT), including PSVT associated with Wolff-Parkinson-White (W-P-W) syndrome.

The drug is antagonized competitively by methylxanthines such as caffeine and theophylline and potentiated by blockers of nucleoside transport such as dipyridamole (see Drug Interactions). Adenosine is not blocked by atropine.

Hemodynamics – The usual IV bolus dose of 6 or 12 mg will not have systemic hemodynamic effects. When larger doses are given by infusion, adenosine decreases blood pressure by decreasing peripheral resistance.

Pharmacokinetics: IV adenosine is removed from the circulation very rapidly. Following an IV bolus, adenosine is taken up by erythrocytes and vascular endothelial cells. Half-life is estimated to be < 10 seconds. Adenosine enters the body pool and is primarily metabolized to inosine and adenosine monophosphate (AMP).

Clinical trials: In controlled studies, bolus doses of 3, 6, 9 and 12 mg were studied. A cumulative 60% of patients with PSVT had converted to normal sinus rhythm within 1 minute after an IV bolus dose of 6 mg (some converted on 3 mg and failures were given 6 mg), and a cumulative 92% converted after a bolus dose of 12 mg. From 7% to 16% of patients converted after 1 to 4 placebo bolus injections.

Similar results were seen in a variety of patient subsets, including those using or not using digoxin, those with W-P-W syndrome, African Americans, Caucasians and Hispanics.

Indications:

Conversion to sinus rhythm of PSVT, including that associated with accessory bypass tracts (W-P-W syndrome). When clinically advisable, attempt appropriate vagal maneuvers (eg, Valsalva maneuver) prior to use.

Unlabeled uses: Adenosine has been used in the noninvasive assessment of patients with suspected coronary artery disease in conjunction with ^{201}thallium tomography; results are similar to assessment with exercise stress test or IV dipyridamole.

Contraindications:

Second- or third-degree AV block or sick sinus syndrome (except in patients with a functioning artificial pacemaker); atrial flutter, atrial fibrillation and ventricular tachycardia (the drug is not effective in converting these arrhythmias to normal sinus rhythm; see Warnings); hypersensitivity to adenosine.

Warnings:

Heart block: Adenosine decreases conduction through the AV node and may produce a short lasting first-, second- or third-degree heart block. In extreme cases, transient asystole may result (one case has been reported in a patient with atrial flutter who was receiving carbamazepine). Institute appropriate therapy as needed. Patients who develop high-level block on one dose of adenosine should not be given additional doses. Because of the very short half-life, these effects are generally self-limiting.

Arrhythmias: At the time of conversion to normal sinus rhythm, a variety of new rhythms may appear on the ECG. They generally last only a few seconds without intervention and may take the form of premature ventricular contractions, atrial premature contractions, sinus bradycardia, sinus tachycardia, skipped beats and varying degrees of AV nodal block. Such findings were seen in 55% of patients.

Treatment of other arrhythmias: Adenosine is not effective in converting rhythms other than PSVT, such as atrial flutter, atrial fibrillation or ventricular tachycardia to normal sinus rhythm. Use in such patients has not resulted in adverse consequences.

Ventricular response: In the presence of atrial flutter or atrial fibrillation, a transient modest slowing of ventricular response may occur immediately following use.

Hepatic and renal failure: Hepatic and renal failure should have no effect on the activity of a bolus adenosine injection. Since the drug has a direct action, hepatic and renal function are not required for the activation or metabolism of a bolus injection.

Mutagenesis: Adenosine, like other nucleosides at millimolar concentrations present for several doubling times of cells in culture, is known to produce a variety of chromosomal alterations. In rats and mice, adenosine administered intraperitoneally once a day for 5 days at 50, 100 and 150 mg/kg caused decreased spermatogenesis and increased numbers of abnormal sperm, a reflection of the ability of adenosine to produce chromosomal damage.

ADENOSINE

Pregnancy: Category C. As adenosine is a naturally occurring material, widely dispersed throughout the body, no fetal effects would be anticipated. However, because it is not known whether the drug can cause fetal harm when administered to pregnant women, use during pregnancy only if clearly needed.

Precautions:

Asthma: Most patients with asthma who have received IV adenosine have not experienced exacerbation of their asthma. However, inhaled adenosine induces bronchoconstriction in asthmatic patients but not in healthy individuals. Be alert to the possibility of adenosine-induced bronchoconstriction in patients with asthma.

Drug Interactions:

Adenosine Drug Interactions

Precipitant drug	Object drug*		Description
Carbamazepine	Adenosine	↑	Carbamazepine increases the degree of heart block produced by other agents. As the primary effect of adenosine is to decrease conduction through the AV node, higher degrees of heart block may be produced in the presence of carbamazepine.
Dipyridamole	Adenosine	↑	The effects of adenosine are potentiated. Thus, smaller doses of adenosine may be effective in the presence of dipyridamole.
Methylxanthines (eg, caffeine, theophylline)	Adenosine	↓	The effects of adenosine are antagonized. In the presence of methylxanthines, larger doses of adenosine may be required or adenosine may be ineffective.
Adenosine	Digitalis	↑	The use of adenosine with digitalis may rarely be associated with ventricular fibrillation.

* ↑ = Object drug increased ↓= Object drug decreased

Adverse Reactions:

Cardiovascular: Facial flushing (18%); headache (2%); sweating, palpitations, chest pain, hypotension (< 1%); prolonged asystole; ventricular fibrillation, ventricular tachycardia; transient increase in blood pressure (post-market).

CNS: Lightheadedness (2%); dizziness, tingling in arms, numbness (1%); apprehension, blurred vision, burning sensation, heaviness in arms, neck/back pain (< 1%).

GI: Nausea (3%); metallic taste, tightness in throat, pressure in groin (< 1%).

Respiratory: Shortness of breath/dyspnea (12%); chest pressure (7%); hyperventilation, head pressure (< 1%).

Overdosage:

Adverse effects are generally rapidly self-limiting. Individualize treatment of prolonged adverse effects and direct toward the specific effect. Methylxanthines are competitive antagonists of adenosine (see Drug Interactions). Refer to General Management of Acute Overdosage.

Administration and Dosage:

For rapid bolus IV use only. To be certain the solution reaches the systemic circulation, administer either directly into a vein or, if given into an IV line, as proximal as possible and follow with a rapid saline flush.

Initial dose: 6 mg as a rapid IV bolus (administered over a 1 to 2 second period).

Repeat administration: If the first dose does not result in elimination of the supraventricular tachycardia within 1 to 2 minutes, give 12 mg as a rapid IV bolus. Repeat 12 mg dose a second time if required. Doses > 12 mg are not recommended.

Storage/Stability: Store at room temperature (15° to 30°C [59° to 86°F]). Do not refrigerate as crystallization may occur. If this occurs, let crystals warm to room temperature. The solution must be clear at the time of use. Discard unused portion.

Rx	**Adenocard** (Fujisawa)	**Injection:** 3 mg/ml	NaCl 9 mg/ml. Preservative free. In 2 and 5 ml vials.

CALCIUM CHANNEL BLOCKING AGENTS

Warning:

Induction of new serious arrhythmias (bepridil): Bepridil has Class I anti-arrhythmic properties and, like other such drugs, can induce new arrhythmias, including VT/VF. Because it can prolong QT interval, bepridil can cause torsades de pointes type ventricular tachycardia (VT). Because of these properties, reserve for patients in whom other anti-anginals do not offer satisfactory effect.

In US trials, QT and QTc intervals were commonly prolonged by bepridil in a dose-related fashion; increased QT and QTc may be associated with torsades de pointes type VT, seen at least briefly, in ≈ 1% of patients. French marketing experience reports > 100 verified cases of torsades de pointes. While this number, based on total use, represents only 0.01%, the true rate is undoubtedly much higher, as spontaneous reporting systems all suffer from substantial underreporting.

While the safe upper limit of QT is not defined, it is suggested that the interval not be permitted to exceed 0.52 seconds during treatment. If dose reduction does not eliminate the excessive prolongation, stop the drug. If concomitant diuretics are needed, consider low doses and addition or primary use of a potassium-sparing diuretic, and monitor serum potassium.

Bepridil has been associated with the usual range of pro-arrhythmic effects characteristic of Class I anti-arrhythmics (increased premature ventricular contraction rates, new sustained VT, and VT/VF that is more difficult than previously to convert to sinus rhythm). Use in patients with severe arrhythmias (who are most susceptible to certain pro-arrhythmic effects) has been limited, so that risk in these patients is not defined.

In the National Heart, Lung and Blood Institute's Cardiac Arrhythmia Suppression Trial (CAST, a study in patients with asymptomatic non-life-threatening ventricular arrhythmias who had an MI > 6 days but < 2 years previously), an excess mortality/non-fatal cardiac arrest rate was seen in patients treated with encainide or flecainide compared with that seen in patients assigned to matched placebo-treated groups. The applicability of these results to other populations (eg, those without recent MI) or to other anti-arrhythmic drugs is uncertain, but at present it is prudent to consider any drug documented to provoke new serious arrhythmias or worsening of pre-existing arrhythmias as having a similar risk and to avoid their use in the post-infarction period.

Actions:

Pharmacology: In specialized automatic and conducting cells in the heart, calcium is involved in genesis of action potential. In contractile cells of the myocardium, it links excitation to contraction and controls energy storage and use. Systemic and coronary arteries are influenced by movement of calcium across cell membranes of vascular smooth muscle. Contractile processes of cardiac and vascular smooth muscle depend upon movement of extracellular calcium ions into these cells through specific ion channels.

The calcium channel blockers (aka, slow channel blockers, calcium antagonists), share the ability to inhibit movement of calcium ions across the cell membrane. The effects on the cardiovascular system include depression of mechanical contraction of myocardial and smooth muscle, and depression of both impulse formation (automaticity) and conduction velocity. **Bepridil** also inhibits fast sodium inward channels. Calcium channel blockers are classified by structure as follows: Diphenylalkylamines – verapamil; benzothiazepines – diltiazem; dihydropyridines – amlodipine, felodipine, isradipine, nicardipine, nifedipine, nimodipine, nisoldipine.

Although these agents are similar in that they all act on the slow (calcium) channel, they have different degrees of selectivity in their effects on vascular smooth muscle, myocardium or specialized conduction and pacemaker tissues. The resulting clinical effects depend on the direct activity of the drug, reflex physiological responses (primarily β-adrenergic response to vasodilation) and the patient's cardiovascular status. This heterogeneity of the calcium blockers, in part, determines their clinical application and the different side effects produced by each agent.

In animals, **nimodipine** had a greater effect on cerebral arteries than on other arteries, possibly because it is highly lipophilic. While studies show a favorable effect on severity of neurological deficits caused by cerebral vasospasm following subarachnoid hemorrhage (SAH), there is no arteriographic evidence that the drug either prevents or relieves spasm of these arteries. Therefore, the actual mechanism of action is unknown.

Electrophysiology – (see Pharmacology/Pharmacokinetics table): **Verapamil** slows AV conduction and prolongs the ERP within the AV node in a rate-related manner, thus reducing elevated ventricular rate due to atrial flutter or atrial fibrillation. By interrupting reentry at the AV node, verapamil can restore normal sinus rhythm in

CALCIUM CHANNEL BLOCKING AGENTS

patients with paroxysmal supraventricular tachycardias (PSVT), including Wolff-Parkinson-White (W–P–W) syndrome. It can interfere with sinus node impulse generation and induce sinus arrest in patients with sick sinus syndrome. Verapamil may shorten the antegrade ERP of the accessory bypass tracts. It does not alter the normal atrial action potential or intraventricular conduction time, but it depresses amplitude, velocity of depolarization and conduction in depressed atrial fibers.

Patients with supraventricular tachycardia convert to normal sinus rhythm within 10 minutes after IV verapamil (≈ 60% to 80%). About 70% of patients with atrial flutter or fibrillation with a fast ventricular rate respond with a decrease in heart rate of ≥ 20%. Conversion of atrial flutter or fibrillation to sinus rhythm is uncommon (≈ 10%) after verapamil and may reflect the spontaneous conversion rate.

Diltiazem decreases SA and AV conduction in isolated tissues. IV diltiazem in doses of 20 mg prolongs AH conduction time and AV node functional and effective refractory periods by ≈ 20%. Diltiazem-associated prolongation of the AH interval is not more pronounced in patients with first-degree heart block. In patients with sick sinus syndrome, diltiazem significantly prolongs sinus cycle length (≤ 50%).

Hemodynamics – (see Pharmacology/Pharmacokinetics table): These agents dilate the coronary arteries and arterioles, both in normal and ischemic regions, and inhibit coronary artery spasm. This increases myocardial oxygen delivery in patients with vasospastic (Prinzmetal's or variant) angina.

The drugs reduce arterial blood pressure at rest and with exercise by dilating peripheral arterioles and reducing total peripheral resistance (afterload) against which the heart works. This reduces myocardial energy consumption and oxygen requirements and probably accounts for the efficacy in chronic stable angina.

These agents exhibit a negative inotropic effect, but this is clinically rare because of reflex responses to vasodilation. In patients with normal ventricular function, there may be a small increase in cardiac index without major effects on ejection fraction, left ventricular end diastolic pressure or volume (LVEDP or LVEDV). Usual **IV verapamil** doses may slightly increase left ventricular filling pressure. Heart failure may worsen when **verapamil** is used in moderate to severe cardiac dysfunction. When **nifedipine** was administered to patients with decreased ventricular function, increase in ejection fraction and decrease in LVEDP occurred. **Nicardipine** use in normal or moderately abnormal left ventricular function significantly increased ejection fraction and cardiac output with no significant change or a small decrease in LVEDP. Administration of a single dose of **nisoldipine** leads to decreased systemic vascular resistance and blood pressure with a transient increase in heart rate.

CALCIUM CHANNEL BLOCKING AGENTS

Pharmacokinetics:

Calcium Channel Blocking Agents: Pharmacology/Pharmacokinetics

	Parameters	Nifedipine/SR	Verapamil	Diltiazem/SR	Nicardipine	Nisoldipine
Pharmacokinetics	Extent of absorption[1]	90%	90%	80-90%	≈ 100%	nd
	Absolute bioavailability[1]	45-70/86%	20-35%	40-67%	35%	5
	Onset of action – oral (min)	20	30[2]	30-60	20	nd
	Time of peak plasma levels (hrs)	0.5/6	1-2.2	2-3/6-11	0.5-2	6-12
	Protein binding (%)	92-98	83-92	70-80	> 95	> 99
	Therapeutic serum levels (ng/ml)	25-100	80-300	50-200	28-50	nd
	Metabolite	Acid or lactone[3]	Norverapamil[4]	Desacetyl-diltiazem[5]	Glucuronide conjugates	5 major urinary metabolites
	Excreted unchanged in urine (%)	1-2	3-4	2-4	< 1	trace
	Half-life, elimination	2-5	3-7[7]	3.5-6/5-7	2-4	7-12
Electrophysiology	Effective refractory period					
	Atrium	0	0	0	0	0
	AV node	±	↑↑*	↑*	↑↓*	0
	His-Purkinje	0	0	0	↓*	0
	Ventricle	0	0	0	0	0
	Accessory pathway	0	±	na	0	0
	SA node automaticity[8]	0	↓↓*	↓*	0	0
	AV node conduction[8]	±	↓↓↓*	↓↓*	0-↑*	0
	Sinus node recovery time	0	0[9]	0[9]	0	0
ECG Changes	Heart rate	↑*	↑↓*	↓*-0	↑*	±
	QRS complex	0	0	0	0	0
	PR interval	0	↑*	↑*	nd	0
	QT interval	nd	nd	nd	↑*	0
Hemodynamics	Myocardial contractility[8]	↓*	↓↓*	↓*	0	0
	Cardiac output	↑↑*	↑↓*	0-↑*	↑↑*	0
	Peripheral vascular resistance	↓↓↓*	↓↓*	↓*	↓↓↓*	↓↓↓

* ↑↑↑ or ↓↓↓ = pronounced effect; ↑↑ or ↓↓ = moderate effect; ↑ or ↓ = slight effect; ± = negligible effect; nd = no data; na = not applicable;

[1] Although these agents are well absorbed (80% to 90%) following oral administration, they are subject to extensive first-pass effects, resulting in an absolute bioavailability that is considerably less.

[2] Peak therapeutic effects occur within 3 to 5 minutes after IV administration.

[3] Inactive.

[4] Pharmacologic activity 20% of verapamil.

[5] Pharmacologic activity 25% to 50% of diltiazem; plasma levels 10% to 20% of parent drug.

[6] Of 6 metabolites identified, account for > 75%.

[7] 4.5 to 12 hours with multiple dosing; may be prolonged in elderly.

[8] Direct effects may be counteracted by reflex activity.

[9] Prolonged in sick sinus syndrome.

[10] Dose-related.

CALCIUM CHANNEL BLOCKING AGENTS

Calcium Channel Blocking Agents: Pharmacology/Pharmacokinetics						
Nimodipine	Isradipine	Bepridil	Felodipine	Amlodipine	Parameters	
nd	90-95	≈ 100	≈100	nd	Extent of absorption (%)[1]	Pharmacokinetics
13	15-24	59	20	64-90	Absolute bioavailability (%)[1]	
nd	120	60	120-300	nd	Onset of action - oral (min)	
≤1	1.5	2-3	2.5-5	6-12	Time of peak plasma levels (hrs)	
> 95	95	> 99	> 99	93	Protein binding (%)	
nd	nd	1-2	nd	nd	Therapeutic serum levels (ng/ml)	
Unknown[3]	Monoacids and cyclic lactone[6]	4-OH-N-phenyl-bepridil	Six inactive	90% converted to inactive	Metabolite	
< 1	0	±	<0.5	10	Excreted unchanged in urine (%)	
1-2	8	24	11-16	30-50	Half-life, elimination (hrs)	
					Effective refractory period	Electrophysiology
na	0	↑*	0	0	Atrium	
	0	↑*	0	0	AV node	
	0	↑*	0	0	His-Purkinje	
	0	↑*	0	0	Ventricle	
	nd	↑*	0	0	Accessory pathway	
	0	↓*	0	0	SA node automaticity	
	0	↓*	0	0	AV node conduction	
	±	nd	0	0	Sinus node recovery time	
	±	↓*	±	±	Heart rate	ECG Changes
	0	0	0	0	QRS complex	
	0	↑*	0	0	PR interval	
	↑*	↑↑[10]	0	0	QT interval	
	0	↓*	↑*	↑*	Myocardial contractility[8]	Hemodynamics
	↑*	0	↑*	↑*	Cardiac output	
	↓↓↓*	↓*	↓↓↓*	↓↓↓*	Peripheral vascular resistance	

* ↑↑↑ or ↓↓↓ = pronounced effect; ↑↑ or ↓↓ = moderate effect; ↑ or ↓ = slight effect; ± = negligible effect; 0 = no effect; nd = no data; na = not applicable;

[1] Although these agents are well absorbed (80% to 90%) following oral administration, they are subject to extensive first-pass effects, resulting in an absolute bioavailability that is considerably less.

[2] Peak therapeutic effects occur within 3 to 5 minutes after IV administration.

[3] Inactive.

[4] Pharmacologic activity 20% of verapamil.

[5] Pharmacologic activity 25% to 50% of diltiazem; plasma levels 10% to 20% of parent drug.

[6] Of 6 metabolites identified, account for > 75%.

[7] 4.5 to 12 hours with multiple dosing; may be prolonged in elderly.

[8] Direct effects may be counteracted by reflex activity.

[9] Prolonged in sick sinus syndrome.

[10] Dose-related.

CALCIUM CHANNEL BLOCKING AGENTS

Indications:

Calcium Channel Blocking Agents – Summary of Indications

Indications	Amlodipine	Bepridil	Diltiazem	Diltiazem SR	Diltiazem IV	Felodipine	Isradipine	Nicardipine	Nicardipine SR	Nicardipine IV	Nifedipine	Nifedipine SR	Nimodipine	Nisoldipine	Verapamil	Verapamil SR	Verapamil IV
Angina pectoris																	
Vasospastic	✓			✓							✓	✓			✓		
Chronic stable	✓	✓	✓	✓				✓							✓		
Unstable															✓		
Hypertension, essential	✓			✓		✓	✓	✓	✓	✓		✓		✓	✓	✓	
Arrhythmias					✓										✓		
Supraventricular tachyarrhythmias																	✓
Subarachnoid hemorrhage													✓				
Unlabeled uses																	
Migraine headache											✓		✓		✓		
Raynaud's syndrome			✓			✓					✓						
Congestive heart failure						✓		✓			✓						
Cardiomyopathy											✓				✓		

Vasospastic (Prinzmetal's variant) angina (amlodipine, nifedipine, SR nifedipine, oral verapamil, diltiazem): Treatment of spontaneous coronary artery spasm presenting as Prinzmetal's variant angina (resting angina with ST segment elevation during attacks).

Chronic stable (classic effort-associated) angina (amlodipine, nifedipine, SR nifedipine, oral verapamil and diltiazem, nicardipine, bepridil): In patients who cannot tolerate β-adrenergic blockers or nitrates, or who remain symptomatic despite adequate doses of these agents.

Unstable (crescendo, preinfarction) angina (oral verapamil).

Essential hypertension (amlodipine, oral verapamil, SR diltiazem, nicardipine, SR nifedipine, isradipine, felodipine, nisoldipine)

Arrhythmias (oral verapamil, IV diltiazem): In association with digitalis, to control ventricular rate at rest and during stress in chronic atrial flutter or atrial fibrillation (see Warnings).

Also for prophylaxis of repetitive paroxysmal supraventricular tachycardia.

Supraventricular tachyarrhythmias (IV verapamil) including rapid conversion to sinus rhythm of PSVT, including those associated with accessory bypass tracts such as W–P–W and Lown-Ganong-Levine (L–G–L) syndromes.

Also for temporary control of rapid ventricular rate in atrial flutter/fibrillation.

Subarachnoid hemorrhage (nimodipine): Improvement of neurological deficits due to spasm following SAH from ruptured congenital intracranial aneurysms in patients who are in good neurological condition post-ictus (eg, Hunt and Hess Grades I-III). Begin therapy within 96 hours of the SAH and continue for 21 days.

Unlabeled uses:

Nifedipine 10 to 20 mg (children: 10 kg, 2.5 mg; 10 to 20 kg, 5 mg) administered orally, sublingually (squeeze contents under the tongue), chewed (puncture ≈ 10 times, then chew) or rectally has been used to lower blood pressure in hypertensive emergencies. One study indicated that biting the capsule and swallowing the contents results in faster absorption and higher plasma levels compared to SL.

Preliminary studies suggest nifedipine may also be useful for prophylaxis in migraine headache and in the treatment of primary pulmonary hypertension, asthma, preterm labor, severe pregnancy-associated hypertension, esophageal disorders, biliary and renal colic, cardiomyopathy, to reduce progression of coronary artery disease, CHF and Raynaud's syndrome.

Verapamil (oral), 80 to 160 mg 3 times daily, has been used for PSVT. It has also been studied for the prophylaxis of migraine headache (40 to 80 mg 3 or 4 times/day), cluster headache (120 mg twice daily initially) and exercise-induced asthma, for treatment of hypertrophic cardiomyopathy, as alternate therapy in manic depression and for recumbent nocturnal leg cramps (120 mg at bedtime).

Diltiazem has been investigated in the prevention of reinfarction of non-Q-wave myocardial infarction, tardive dyskinesia and Raynaud's syndrome.

Nimodipine appears to be beneficial in patients with common and classic migraine (40 mg 3 times/day) and chronic cluster headache. Development of tolerance in these patients was rare. In one study, nimodipine 30mg every 6 hours starting within 24 hours of the onset of symptoms of an acute ischemic stroke significantly reduced mortality, although this effect was restricted to men; another study did not support these findings.

Nicardipine may be useful in the treatment of congestive heart failure (20 to 40 mg 3 times daily) and in combination with aminocaproic acid for SAH.

Isradipine may be beneficial in the treatment of chronic stable angina.

Contraindications:

Hypersensitivity to the drug; sick sinus syndrome or second- or third-degree AV block except with a functioning pacemaker, hypotension < 90 mm Hg systolic (bepridil, diltiazem and verapamil).

Diltiazem: Acute MI and pulmonary congestion.

Verapamil: Severe left ventricular dysfunction; cardiogenic shock and severe CHF, unless secondary to a supraventricular tachycardia amenable to verapamil therapy and in patients with atrial flutter or atrial fibrillation and an accessory bypass tract.

Verapamil IV – Do not administer concomitantly with IV **β-adrenergic blocking agents** (within a few hours), since both may depress myocardial contractility and AV conduction (see Drug Interactions); ventricular tachycardia, since use in patients with wide-complex ventricular tachycardia (QRS ≥ 0.12 sec) can result in marked hemodynamic deterioration and ventricular fibrillation.

Nicardipine: Advanced aortic stenosis.

Bepridil: History of serious ventricular arrhythmias; uncompensated cardiac insufficiency; congenital QT interval prolongation; use with other drugs that prolong QT interval.

Warnings:

Hypotension, usually modest and well tolerated, may occasionally occur during initial therapy or with dosage increases, and may be more likely in patients taking concomitant β–blockers. Hypotensive episodes may be caused by excess vasodilation induced by **nifedipine** or by direct cardiopressor effects of **verapamil** and **diltiazem.** Nifedipine has the greatest effect on vascular smooth muscle; therefore, incidence of adverse reactions resulting from vasodilation (ie, headache, flushing) is greater. Since **amlodipine**-induced hypotension is gradual in onset, acute hypotension has rarely occurred.

Systolic pressure < 90 mmHg or diastolic pressure < 60 mmHg was seen in 5% to 10% of patients with supraventricular tachycardia and in about 10% of the patients with atrial flutter/fibrillation who were given **IV verapamil.**

Carefully monitor blood pressure during initial administration and titration. Closely observe patients already taking antihypertensives.

Congestive heart failure (CHF) has developed rarely, usually in patients receiving a β-blocker, after beginning **nifedipine.** Patients with tight aortic stenosis may be at greater risk, as the unloading effect would be of less benefit to these patients, due to their fixed impedance to flow across the aortic valve.

Verapamil has a negative inotropic effect which is usually compensated by its afterload reduction (decreased systemic vascular resistance) properties without a net impairment of ventricular performance. In clinical studies with **oral verapamil,** 1.8% developed CHF or pulmonary edema. Avoid verapamil in patients with severe left ventricular dysfunction (ie, ejection fraction < 30%) or moderate to severe symptoms of cardiac failure and in patients with any degree of ventricular dysfunction if they are receiving a β–adrenergic blocker. Control patients with milder ventricular dysfunction, if possible, with digitalis or diuretics before verapamil treatment (see Drug Interactions).

Use **diltiazem, nicardipine, isradipine, felodipine, amlodipine** and **bepridil** with caution in CHF patients.

Cardiac conduction: **IV verapamil** slows AV nodal conduction and SA nodes; it rarely produces second- or third-degree AV block, bradycardia, and in extreme cases, asystole. This is more likely to occur in patients with sick sinus syndrome (which is

CALCIUM CHANNEL BLOCKING AGENTS

more common in older patients). Asystole in patients other than those with sick sinus syndrome is usually of short duration (a few seconds or less), with spontaneous return to AV nodal or normal sinus rhythm. Adverse hemodynamic effects (including severe hypotension) have occurred when verapamil is used in patients with ventricular tachycardia without a supraventricular origin. Caution is warranted; a diagnosis of supraventricular tachycardia should be made before verapamil administration.

Oral verapamil may lead to first-degree AV block and transient bradycardia, sometimes accompanied by nodal escape rhythms. PR-interval prolongation is correlated with verapamil plasma concentrations especially during the early titration phase of therapy. Higher degrees of AV block are infrequent (0.8%). Marked first-degree block or progressive development to second- or third-degree AV block requires dose reduction or discontinuation of verapamil.

Patients with atrial flutter/fibrillation and an accessory AV pathway may develop increased antegrade conduction, producing a very rapid ventricular response after verapamil (or digitalis). Treatment is usually D.C. cardioversion.

Diltiazem prolongs AV node refractory periods without significantly prolonging sinus node recovery time, except in sick sinus syndrome. This may rarely result in abnormally slow heart rates (particularly in sick sinus syndrome) or second- or third-degree AV block (0.48%). Concomitant use with β-adrenergic blockers or digitalis may be additive on cardiac conduction. A patient with Prinzmetal's angina developed periods of asystole (2 to 5 seconds) after 60 mg diltiazem.

Premature ventricular contractions (PVCs): During conversion or marked reduction in ventricular rate, benign complexes of unusual appearance (sometimes resembling PVCs) may occur after **IV verapamil**. Similar complexes of no clinical significance occur during spontaneous conversion of supraventricular tachycardia after D.C. cardioversion and other therapy. Verapamil IV may produce potentially fatal ventricular fibrillation in patients with atrial fibrillation (AF) and W-P-W syndrome. These arrhythmias may respond to cardioversion and stopping the drug. Consider also with oral verapamil.

Hypertrophic cardiomyopathy (IHSS): Serious adverse effects were seen in 120 patients with IHSS (most refractory or intolerant to propranolol) who received oral **verapamil** at doses up to 720 mg/day. Three patients died with pulmonary edema; all had severe left ventricular outflow obstruction and a history of left ventricular dysfunction. Eight had pulmonary edema or severe hypotension; most had abnormally high (> 20 mm Hg) pulmonary wedge pressure and a marked left ventricular outflow obstruction. Coadministration of quinidine preceded the severe hypotension in 3 of the 8 patients (two of whom developed pulmonary edema). Sinus bradycardia occurred in 11%, second-degree AV block in 4% and sinus arrest in 2%. Most adverse effects responded to dose reduction; discontinuation of verapamil was rare.

Antiplatelet effects: Calcium channel blockers, alone and with aspirin, have caused inhibition of platelet function. Episodes of bruising, petechiae and bleeding have occurred.

Nifedipine decreases platelet aggregation in vitro. Limited clinical studies have demonstrated a moderate but statistically significant decrease in platelet aggregation and increase in bleeding time in some patients. This is thought to be a function of inhibition of calcium transport across the platelet membrane.

Withdrawal syndrome: Abrupt withdrawal of calcium channel blockers may cause increased frequency and duration of chest pain. The rebound angina is probably the result of the increased flow of calcium into cells causing coronary arteries to spasm. Gradually taper the dose under medical supervision. Results of other studies do not support the occurrence of a withdrawal syndrome; however, caution is still warranted when discontinuing these agents.

β-blocker withdrawal/nifedipine: Patients recently withdrawn from β-blockers may develop a withdrawal syndrome with increased angina, probably related to increased sensitivity to catecholamines. Initiation of nifedipine will not prevent this occurrence and might exacerbate it by provoking reflex catecholamine release. Taper β-blockers rather than stopping them abruptly before beginning nifedipine.

Nicardipine – Gradually reduce β-blocker dose over 8 to 10 days with coadministration.

Agranulocytosis: In US clinical trials of > 800 patients treated with **bepridil** for up to 5 years, two cases of marked leukopenia and neutropenia were reported. Both patients were diabetic and elderly. One died with overwhelming gram-negative sepsis, itself a possible cause of marked leukopenia. The other recovered rapidly when bepridil was stopped.

Hepatic function impairment: The pharmacokinetics, bioavailability and patient response to **verapamil** and **nifedipine** may be significantly affected by hepatic cirrhosis. With IV verapamil, clearance is greatly reduced, half-life is increased fourfold and volume of distribution is doubled. Peak plasma concentration is higher and occurs earlier; bioavailability is doubled with oral verapamil in cirrhosis. Severe liver dysfunction prolongs **verapamil's** elimination half-life to about 14 to 16 hours; therefore, give ≈ 30% of the normal dose. Bioavailability of nifedipine is increased in hepatic cirrhosis. With IV nifedipine, half-life and volume of distribution are increased and plasma protein binding is decreased. Carefully monitor for abnormal prolongation of the PR interval and other signs of excessive pharmacologic effects.

Since **amlodipine, diltiazem, nicardipine, bepridil, felodipine** and **nimodipine** are extensively metabolized by liver, use with caution in impaired hepatic function or reduced hepatic blood flow. In severe liver disease, elevated nicardipine blood levels (fourfold increase in AUC) and prolonged half-life (19 hrs) occurred; patients on nimodipine had substantially reduced clearance and an approximately doubled maximum drug concentration. Consider decreasing the dose of calcium channel blockers, and monitor drug response (ie, blood pressure, PR interval) in cirrhosis patients.

Renal function impairment: The pharmacokinetics of **diltiazem** and **verapamil** in patients with impaired renal function are similar to the pharmacokinetic profile of patients with normal renal function. However, caution is still advised. About 70% of a dose of **verapamil** is excreted as metabolites in the urine. Administer verapamil cautiously to patients with impaired renal function. Effects of single IV doses should not increase, although duration may be prolonged.

Nifedipine's plasma concentration is slightly increased in patients with renal impairment. One study showed a significant increase in half-life and volume of distribution at steady state with IV nifedipine. Total body clearance remained the same. Hemodialysis and peritoneal dialysis do not significantly affect nifedipine pharmacokinetics. Although nifedipine has been used safely in patients with renal dysfunction and has exerted a beneficial effect in certain cases, rare, reversible elevations in BUN and serum creatinine have occurred in patients with preexisting chronic renal insufficiency. The relationship to therapy is uncertain in most cases.

Nicardipine's mean plasma concentrations, AUC and maximum concentration were approximately twofold higher in patients with mild renal impairment. Doses must be adjusted. However, one study suggested nicardipine can be used without any dosage adjustment in hypertensive patients with advanced chronic renal failure.

Use **bepridil** with caution in patients with serious renal disorders since the metabolites of bepridil are excreted primarily in the urine.

Increased angina: Occasional patients have increased frequency, duration or severity of angina on starting **nifedipine** or **nicardipine** or at the time of dosage increases. The mechanism of this response is not established.

Increased intracranial pressure: **IV verapamil** has increased intracranial pressure in patients with supratentorial tumors at the time of anesthesia induction. Use with caution and perform appropriate monitoring.

Duchenne's muscular dystrophy: **Verapamil** may decrease neuromuscular transmission in patients with Duchenne's muscular dystrophy, and prolong recovery from the neuromuscular blocking agent vecuronium. It may be necessary to decrease dosage of verapamil when administering it to patients with attenuated neuromuscular transmission. IV verapamil can precipitate respiratory muscle failure in these patients; therefore, use with caution.

Carcinogenesis: Rats treated with **nicardipine** showed a dose-dependent increase in thyroid hyperplasia and neoplasia (follicular adenoma carcinoma), possibly linked to a nicardipine-induced reduction in plasma thyroxine levels with a consequent increase in TSH plasma levels. In rats given **nimodipine,** a higher incidence of adenocarcinoma of the uterus and Leydig-cell adenoma of testes occurred. Unilateral follicular adenomas of the thyroid were observed in rats following lifetime high-dose **bepridil**. In rats given **isradipine** or **felodipine,** there were dose-dependent increases in benign Leydig cell tumors and testicular hyperplasia.

Elderly: **Verapamil, nifedipine** and **felodipine** may cause a greater hypotensive effect than that seen in younger patients, probably due to age-related changes in drug disposition. With felodipine, monitor blood pressure closely during dosage adjustment; rarely are doses > 10 mg required.

Pregnancy: Category C. Teratogenic and embryotoxic effects have been demonstrated in small animals, usually at doses higher than the usual human dosage. There are no well controlled studies in pregnant women. Use during pregnancy only when clearly needed and when potential benefits outweigh potential hazards to the fetus.

CALCIUM CHANNEL BLOCKING AGENTS

Diltiazem given at 5 to 10 times the human dose resulted in fetal death and skeletal abnormalities; incidence of stillbirths was increased at ≥ 20 times the human dose.

Verapamil, oral in rats with doses 1.5 and 6 times the human dose was embryocidal and retarded fetal growth and development, probably due to reduced weight gains in dams. Verapamil crosses the placenta and can be detected in umbilical vein blood at delivery.

Nifedipine has been used in severe pregnancy-associated hypertension, and no adverse fetal effects were determined.

Nicardipine was embryocidal in animals at 75 times, but not 25 to 50 times the human dose. However, dystocia, reduced birth weights, reduced neonatal survival and reduced neonatal weight gain occurred at 50 times the human dose.

Nimodipine in animals has resulted in malformations and stunted fetuses at doses of 1 to 10 mg/kg/day, but not at 3 mg/kg/day in one study. Doses of 30 to 100 mg/kg/day resulted in resorption, stunted growth, still births and higher incidences of skeletal variation.

Bepridil, in rats administered doses 37 times the maximum daily recommended dosage, resulted in reduced litter size at birth.

Isradipine produced a significant reduction in maternal weight gain in rats with a dose 150 times the human dose. Decrements in maternal body weight gain and increased fetal resorptions occurred in rabbits following doses 7.5 and 25 times the human dose. Also, reduced maternal body weight gain during late pregnancy in rats was associated with reduced birth weights and decreased peri- and postnatal pup survival.

Felodipine in rabbits at doses 0.4 to 4 times the maximum dosage resulted in digital anomalies (dose-related) in the fetuses, and a prolongation of parturition with difficult labor and increased frequency of fetal and early postnatal deaths occurred in rats. Significant enlargement of the mammary glands also occurred in pregnant rabbits.

Amlodipine significantly decreased litter size (by about 50%) and significantly increased the number of intrauterine deaths (about fivefold) in rats given doses 8 times the maximum human dose for 14 days before mating and throughout mating and gestation. Gestation period and duration of labor is also prolonged.

Lactation: **Verapamil, diltiazem** and **bepridil** are excreted in breast milk. One report suggests that diltiazem concentrations in breast milk may approximate serum levels. Bepridil is estimated to reach about one third the concentration in serum. Significant concentrations of **nicardipine** and **nimodipine** appear in maternal milk of rats. An insignificant amount of **nifedipine** is transferred into breast milk (over 24 hours, < 5% of a dose). It is not known if **isradipine, amlodipine** or **felodipine** are excreted in breast milk. Decide whether to discontinue nursing or discontinue the drug while these agents are being used, taking into account the importance of the drug to the mother.

Children: Safety and efficacy of **diltiazem, bepridil, felodipine, amlodipine** and **isradipine** have not been established.

Controlled studies of **IV verapamil** have not been conducted in pediatric patients, but uncontrolled experience indicates that results of treatment are similar to those in adults. Patients < 6 months of age may not respond to IV verapamil; this resistance may be related to a developmental difference of AV node responsiveness. However, in rare instances, severe hemodynamic side effects have occurred following IV verapamil administration in neonates and infants (see Administration and Dosage).

Precautions:

Acute hepatic injury: In rare instances, symptoms consistent with acute hepatic injury, as well as significant elevations in enzymes such as alkaline phosphatase, CPK, LDH, AST and ALT have occurred with diltiazem and **nifedipine**. These were reversible on drug discontinuation. Drug relationship was uncertain in most cases, but probable in some. These laboratory abnormalities have rarely been associated with clinical symptoms; however, cholestasis with or without jaundice has occurred with **nifedipine**. Rare instances of allergic hepatitis also occurred with **nifedipine**.

Elevations of transaminases with and without concomitant elevations in alkaline phosphatase and bilirubin have occurred with **verapamil**. Elevations have been transient and may disappear with continued verapamil treatment. Several cases of hepatocellular injury related to verapamil have been proven by rechallenge; half of these cases had clinical symptoms (malaise, fever or right upper quadrant pain) in addition to elevations of AST, ALT and alkaline phosphatase. Periodically monitor liver function in patients treated with verapamil.

Isolated cases of elevated LDH, alkaline phosphatase and ALT levels have occurred rarely with **nimodipine**.

CALCIUM CHANNEL BLOCKING AGENTS

Clinically significant transaminase elevations have occurred in approximately 1% of patients receiving **bepridil**; however, no patient became clinically symptomatic or jaundiced, and values returned to normal when the drug was stopped.

Edema, mild to moderate, typically associated with arterial vasodilation and not due to left ventricular dysfunction, occurs in 10% of patients receiving **nifedipine**. It occurs primarily in the lower extremities and usually responds to diuretics. In patients with CHF, differentiate this peripheral edema from the effects of decreasing left ventricular function.

Peripheral edema, generally mild and not associated with generalized fluid retention, may occur with **felodipine** within 2 to 3 weeks of therapy initiation. The incidence is both age- and dose-dependent, with frequency ranging from 10% in patients < 50 years of age taking 5 mg/day to 30% in patients > 60 years of age taking 20 mg/day.

Drug Interactions:

Calcium Channel Blocker Drug Interactions			
Precipitant drug	Object drug*		Description
Barbiturates	Calcium blockers – Felodipine, verapamil	↓	Verapamil and felodipine bioavailability may be decreased.
Calcium salts	Calcium blockers – Verapamil	↓	Clinical effects and toxicities of verapamil may be reversed.
Dantrolene	Calcium blockers – Verapamil	↑	Hyperkalemia and myocardial depression may occur. Consider using a dihy-dropyridine calcium blocker.
Erythromycin	Calcium blockers – Felodipine	↑	Pharmacologic and toxic effects of felodipine may be increased.
Histamine H_2 antagonists	Calcium blockers – Diltiazem, felodipine, nicardipine, nifedipine, verapamil	↑	Cimetidine and ranitidine may increase the bioavailability of diltiazem, felodipine (≈ 50%), nifedipine (small increase or no change with ranitidine) and nicardipine. Cimetidine may increase verapamil's bioavailability, although this has been refuted.
Hydantoins	Calcium blockers – Felodipine, verapamil	↓	Serum felodipine and verapamil levels may be decreased.
Quinidine	Calcium blockers – Verapamil, nifedipine	↑	Hypotension, bradycardia, ventricular tachycardia, AV block and pulmonary edema may occur. Use concomitantly only when no other alternatives exist. Serum quinidine levels may also be decreased by nifedipine.
Calcium blockers – Nifedipine	Quinidine	↓	
Rifampin	Calcium blockers – Verapamil, oral	↓	Loss of clinical effectiveness of oral verapamil may occur; IV verapamil may circumvent the interaction.
Sulfinpyrazone	Calcium blockers – Verapamil	↓	The clearance of verapamil may be increased.
Vitamin D	Calcium blockers – Verapamil	↓	The therapeutic efficacy of verapamil may be reduced.
Calcium blockers – Nifedipine	Anticoagulants	↑	Rare reports of increased prothrombin time.

CALCIUM CHANNEL BLOCKING AGENTS

Calcium Channel Blocker Drug Interactions			
Precipitant drug	Object drug*		Description
Calcium blockers – all	Beta blockers	↑	Although advantageous in some patients, coadministration may also result in increased adverse effects due to depressant effects on myocardial contractility or AV conduction (see Warnings).
Calcium blockers – Diltiazem, verapamil	Carbamazepine	↑	Increased carbamazepine serum levels with possible toxicity may occur. Nifedipine does not appear to interact. Plasma levels of felodipine may be decreased.
Carbamazepine	Calcium blockers – Felodipine	↓	
Calcium blockers – Diltiazem, nicardipine, verapamil	Cyclosporine	↑	Increased cyclosporine levels with possible toxicity may occur. However, verapamil may be nephroprotective when given before cyclosporine. Monitor cyclosporine levels. Nifedipine does not appear to interact.
Calcium blockers - Bepridil, diltiazem, felodipine, nifedipine, verapamil	Digitalis glycosides	↑	Serum digoxin levels may be increased; however, some studies suggest no significant interaction occurs with bepridil, diltiazem or nifedipine. Isradipine and nicardipine do not appear to interact. Verapamil may also increase digitoxin levels.
Calcium blockers - Diltiazem	Encainide	↑	Serum encainide levels may be increased without any change in the levels of the active metabolites.
Calcium blockers – Verapamil	Etomidate	↑	The anesthetic effect of etomidate may be increased with prolonged respiratory depression and apnea.
Calcium blockers – all	Fentanyl	↑	Severe hypotension or increased fluid volume requirements have occurred in patients receiving nifedipine; however, consider for all calcium blockers.
Calcium blockers – Verapamil, diltiazem	Lithium	↔	A reduction in lithium levels causing decreased antimanic control, lithium toxicity and neurotoxic and psychotic symptoms have occurred.
Calcium blockers – Nifedipine	Magnesium sulfate, parenteral	↑	Neuromuscular blockade and hypotension occurred with coadministration.
Calcium blockers – Verapamil	Nondepolarizing muscle relaxants	↑	Muscle relaxant effects may be enhanced, respiratory depression may be prolonged.
Calcium blockers – Verapamil	Prazosin	↑	Prazosin serum concentrations may be increased which may increase the sensitivity to prazosin-induced postural hypotension.
Calcium blockers – Diltiazem, felodipine, nifedipine, verapamil	Theophyllines	↔	The pharmacologic actions of theophyllines may be enhanced, particularly drug intoxication. Theophylline levels may be slightly decreased with felodipine administration, decreasing the effects of theophylline.

* ↑ = Object drug increased. ↓ = Object drug decreased. ↔ = Undetermined effect.

Drug/Food interactions: Food (specifically a low-fat meal) may slow the rate but not extent of **nifedipine** absorption; therefore, it may be administered without regard to meals.

When **nicardipine** was given 1 or 3 hours after a high-fat meal, the mean maximum concentration and AUC were 20% to 30% lower compared to fasting subjects.

Administration of **bepridil** after a meal results in an insignificant delay in time to peak concentration, but neither peak plasma levels nor the extent of absorption was changed.

Administration of **isradipine** with food significantly increases the time to peak by about an hour, but has no effect on the total bioavailability of the drug.

Administration of sustained release **verapamil** with food increases time to reach maximum plasma levels of the parent drug and norverapamil; however, bioavailability is not appreciably affected. May be administered without regard to meals.

Bioavailability of **felodipine** is not affected by food, but increased > twofold when taken with doubly concentrated grapefruit juice vs water or orange juice.

CALCIUM CHANNEL BLOCKING AGENTS

Bioavailability of **amlodipine** is not affected by food.

Adverse Reactions:
Generally not serious; rarely requires discontinuation or dosage adjustment.

	Adverse Reactions of Calcium Channel Blockers (%)									
	Adverse Reactions	Nifedipine	Verapamil Oral (IV)	Diltiazem[1]	Nicardipine	Nimodipine	Bepridil	Isradipine	Felodipine	Amlodipine
Central Nervous System	Dizziness/Light-headedness	4.1-27	3.5 (1.2)	1.5-7	4-6.9	< 1	11.6-27	7.3	5.8	1.1-3.4[2]
	Drowsiness							≤ 1		
	Nervousness	≤ 7		< 1	0.6		7.4-11.6	≤ 1	≤ 1.5	≤ 1
	Sleep disturbances	≤ 2	< 0.5	< 1						
	Psychiatric disturbances (depression, amnesia, paranoia, psychosis, hallucinations)	†	< 1 (†)	< 1	†	1.4	≤ 2	≤ 1	≤ 1.5	≤1
	Blurred vision/Equilibrium disturbances	≤ 2	< 0.5		†		≤ 2	≤ 1		
	Headache	10-23	2.2 (1.2)	2.1-12	6.4-8.2	1.4-4.1	7-13.6	13.7	18.6	7.3
	Weakness/Shakiness/Jitteriness	≤12	< 1	1.2	0.6			1.2		
	Paresthesia	< 3	< 1	< 1	1		2.5	≤ 1	2.5	≤ 1
	Somnolence	< 3	< 1	1.3	1.1-1.4				≤ 1.5	1.3-1.6[3]
	Asthenia	< 3	1.7	2.8-5	4.2-5.8		6.5-14		4.7	1-2
	Insomnia	3		1	0.6		2.7	≤ 1	≤ 1.5	≤1
	Abnormal dreams	≤ 1		< 1	0.4					≤ 1
	Confusion		< 1		†					
	Tinnitus	≤ 1		< 1	†		0-6.5			≤ 1
	Malaise	≤ 1			0.6					≤ 1
	Anxiety	≤1			†		≤ 2		≤ 1.5	≤ 1
	Fatigue/Lethargy							3.9		4.5[2]
	Tremor/Hand tremor			< 1			≤ 9.3			≤ 1
Gastrointestinal	Nausea	3.3-11	2.7 (0.9)	1.6-1.9	1.9-2.2	0.6-1.4	7-26	1.8	1.9	2.9[2]
	Diarrhea	< 3	< 1	< 1		1.7-4.2	0-10.9	1.1	1.6	≤ 1
	Constipation	≤3.3	7.3	1.6	0.6		2.8	≤ 1	1.6	≤ 1
	Hepatitis/Hepatotoxicity	< 0.5	†			< 1				
	Abdominal discomfort/cramps/dyspepsia	≤ 3	< 1 (0.6)	1.3	0.8-1.5	2	≤ 7	1.7	1.8-2.3	1-2
	Dysgeusia	≤ 1		< 1						
	Vomiting	≤ 1		< 1	0.4	< 1		1.1	≤ 1.5	≤ 1
	Dry mouth/Thirst	< 3	< 1	< 1	0.4-1.4		3.4	≤ 1	≤ 1.5	≤ 1
	Flatulence	≤3					≤2		≤ 1.5	≤1

CALCIUM CHANNEL BLOCKING AGENTS

Adverse Reactions of Calcium Channel Blockers (%)

	Adverse Reactions	Nifedipine[1]	Verapamil Oral (IV)	Diltiazem[1]	Nicardipine	Nimodipine	Bepridil	Isradipine	Felodipine	Amlodipine
Cardiovascular	Peripheral edema	10-30	2.1	2.4-9	7.1-8	0.4-1.2	≤ 2	7.2	22.3	1.8-14.6[2]
	Hypotension	≤ 5	2.5 (1.5)	1	< 0.4	1.2-8.1		≤ 1	≤ 1.5	≤1
	Palpitations	≤ 7	< 1	< 1	3.3-4.1	< 1	≤ 6.5	4[2]	1.8	0.7-4.5[2]
	Syncope	≤ 1	< 1	< 1	0.8			≤ 1	≤ 1.5	≤1
	AV block (1°, 2° or 3°)		0.8-1.2	0.6-7.6	< 0.4				≤ 1.5	
	Bradycardia		1.4 (1.2)	1.5-6		0.6-1	≤ 2			≤ 1
	Congestive heart failure	2-6.7	1.8	< 1		< 1		≤ 1		
	Myocardial infarction	4-6.7	< 1		< 0.4			≤ 1	≤ 1.5	
	Arrhythmia (unspecified)	≤ 1		< 1					≤ 1.5	≤ 1
	Pulmonary edema	7	1.8							
	Angina	≤ 1		< 1	5.6			2.4	≤ 1.5	
	Tachycardia	≤ 1	(1)	< 1	0.8-3.4	1	≤ 2	1.5	≤ 1.5	≤ 1
	Abnormal ECG			4.1	0.6	0.6-1.4				
	Ventricular extrasystoles			< 1	†					≤ 0.1
Dermatologic	Dermatitis/Rash	≤ 3	1.2	1-1.5	0.4-1.2	0.6-2.4	≤ 2	1.5	1.5	1-2
	Pruritus/Urticaria	≤ 3	< 1 (†)	< 1		< 1		≤ 1	≤ 1.5	1-2
	Hair loss	≤ 1	< 0.5	†						≤ 0.1
	Photosensitivity	†		< 1						
	Erythema multiforme	†	< 1	†						
	Stevens-Johnson Synd.	†	<1	†						
Hematologic	Anemia	< 0.5				< 1			≤ 1.5	
	Leukopenia	< 0.5		†				≤1		
	Thrombocytopenia	< 0.5				< 1				
	Petechiae/Ecchymosis/ Purpura/Bruising/ Hematoma	< 0.5	< 1	< 1		< 1				≤ 1

CALCIUM CHANNEL BLOCKING AGENTS

Adverse Reactions of Calcium Channel Blockers (%)

	Adverse Reactions	Nifedipine[1]	Verapamil Oral (IV)	Diltiazem[1]	Nicardipine	Nimodipine	Bepridil	Isradipine	Felodipine	Amlodipine
Other	Flushing	< 3-25	< 1	1.7-3	5.6-9.7	1-2.1		2.6	6.4	0.7-4.5[2]
	Nasal or chest congestion/sinusitis/rhinitis	≤ 6	†	<1	†		≤ 2		≤ 1.5	≤ 0.1
	Gingival hyperplasia	≤ 1	†	†					< 0.5	
	Micturition disorder (eg, polyuria, nocturia, dysuria, frequency)	< 3	< 1	1.3	0.4			≤ 1	≤ 1.5	≤ 1
	Sweating	≤ 2	1 (†)			< 1	≤ 2	≤ 1		≤ 1
	Sexual difficulties	≤ 3	< 1	< 1	†		≤ 2	≤ 1	≤ 1.5	1-2
	Shortness of breath/dyspnea/wheezing	≤ 8	1.4	< 1	0.6	1.2	≤ 8.7	1.8	≤ 1.5	1-2
	Muscle cramps/pain/inflammation	≤ 8	< 1			0.2-1.4			≤ 1.9	1-2
	Joint stiffness/pain/arthritis	≤ 3		< 1	†					≤ 1
	Gynecomastia	†	†	†						
	Hyperglycemia	†		< 1						
	Weight gain	≤ 1		< 1						≤ 1
	Epistaxis	≤ 1		< 1					≤ 1.5	≤ 1
	Cough	6					≤ 2	≤ 1	2.9	≤ 0.1
	Anorexia			< 1			≤ 7			≤ 1
	Respiratory infection	≤ 1					2.8		≤ 5.5	

[1] Includes data for sustained release form.
[2] Appears to be dose-related.
[3] Dose-related and higher in females.† Occurs, no incidence reported.

In addition to the adverse effects listed in the table, the following have been reported:

Nifedipine: Giddiness (27%); fever, chills (≤ 3%); facial and periorbital edema, ataxia, hypertonia, hypoesthesia, migraine, gastroesophageal reflux, melena, gout, respiratory disorder, abnormal lacrimation, breast pain, eructation, hematuria (≤ 1%); transient blindness, erythromelalgia (<0.5%); neuromuscular effects (myoclonic dystonia); dysosmia; hypokalemia.

Verapamil: Claudication, hyperkeratosis, spotty menstruation, atrioventricular dissociation, cerebrovascular accident (< 1%); rotary nystagmus; tachyphylaxis, hyperprolactinemia with galactorrhea (one case).

Diltiazem: Gait abnormality, amblyopia, eye irritation, bundle branch block, amnesia (< 1%).

Nicardipine: Infection; allergic reaction; atypical chest pain; peripheral vascular disease; sore throat; hyperkinesia.

Nimodipine: Acne (1%); GI hemorrhage, rebound vasospasm, jaundice, hypertension, hyponatremia, disseminated intravascular coagulation, deep vein thrombosis (< 1%).

Bepridil: Flu syndrome (2%); fever, pain, myalgic asthenia, superinfection, hypertension, vasodilation, ventricular premature contractions, prolonged QT interval (see Warnings), pharyngitis, appetite increase, arthritis, fainting, akathisia, adverse behavior effect, skin irritation, taste change (≤ 2%).

Isradipine: Pollakiuria (1.5%); atrial or ventricular fibrillation, transient ischemic attack, stroke, numbness, throat discomfort, leg/feet cramps (≤ 1%).

Felodipine: Chest pain (2.1%); pharyngitis, rhinorrhea, back pain (1.6%); facial edema, warm sensation, bronchitis, influenza, sneezing, contusion, erythema, irritability (≤ 1.5%).

CALCIUM CHANNEL BLOCKING AGENTS

Amlodipine: Chest pain, peripheral ischemia, hypoesthesia, vertigo, dysphagia, rigors, diplopia, depersonalization, abnormal vision, conjunctivitis, eye pain (≤ 1%); cardiac failure, pulse irregularity, skin discoloration/dryness, twitching, ataxia, hypertonia, migraine, cold/clammy skin, apathy, agitation, amnesia, increased appetite, loose stools, parosmia, taste perversion, abnormal visual accommodation, xerophthalmia (≤ 0.1%).

Lab test abnormalities: Rare, usually transient, but occasionally significant elevations of enzymes such as alkaline phosphatase, CPK, LDH, AST and ALT have occurred with **diltiazem** and **nifedipine** (see Precautions). Positive direct Coombs' test with or without hemolytic anemia has occurred with **nifedipine.** Isolated cases of decreased platelet counts and elevated non-fasting serum glucose, LDH, alkaline phosphatase and ALT have occurred rarely with **nimodipine.** ALT increase has occurred with **bepridil**. Some elevated liver function tests have occurred with **isradipine**.

Overdosage:

Symptoms: Nausea, weakness, dizziness, drowsiness, confusion and slurred speech. Marked and prolonged hypotension and bradycardia, both of which may result in decreased cardiac output. Junctional rhythms and second- or third-degree AV block may be seen. Death has occurred. Toxic diltiazem blood levels in man are not known, but blood levels in excess of 800 g/ml have been associated with toxicity.

Ingestion of 900 to 4800 mg nifedipine SR in two patients resulted in dizziness, palpitations, flushing, nervousness, loss of consciousness, nausea, vomiting, generalized edema and profound hypotension. One patient had sinus bradycardia and varying degrees of AV block. Both patients recovered.

One patient ingested 250 mg amlodipine and was asymptomatic. Another patient ingested 120 mg, underwent gastric lavage and remained normotensive. A third patient took 105 mg and had hypotension (90/50 mm Hg) which normalized following plasma expansion. A 19 month old ingested 30 mg (2 mg/kg) and had no evidence of hypotension but a heart rate of 180bpm. Ipecac was given 3.5 hours after ingestion and no further sequelae were noted.

Treatment: If the patient is seen shortly after oral ingestion, employ emetics or lavage and cathartics. Treatment is supportive. Refer to General Management of Acute Overdosage. Beta-adrenergic agonists and IV calcium have been used effectively. Treat cardiac failure with inotropic agents (isoproterenol, dopamine or dobutamine) and diuretics. Although calcium appears to reverse adverse hemodynamic effects, it may not always reverse electrophysiologic toxicity. Monitor cardiac and respiratory function. In patients with IHSS, use α-adrenergic agents (phenylephrine HCl, metaraminol bitartrate or methoxamine HCl) to maintain blood pressure; avoid isoproterenol and norepinephrine. Monitor cardiac and respiratory function; elevate the extremities. Since these agents are highly protein bound, dialysis is not likely to help. Verapamil cannot be removed by hemodialysis.

Calcium Channel Blocker Overdosage: Treatment Guidelines of Acute Cardiovascular Adverse Reactions

Adverse reaction	Primary treatment[1]	Supportive treatment
Symptomatic hypotension requiring treatment	Dopamine Norepinephrine Metaraminol Isoproterenol Calcium	IV fluids Trendelenburg position
Bradycardia, AV block, asystole	Isoproterenol Norepinephrine Atropine sulfate (0.6 to 1mg) Calcium gluconate (10% solution) Cardiac pacing	IV fluids (slow drip)
Rapid ventricular rate (due to antegrade conduction in flutter/fibrillation with W–P–W or L-G-L syndromes)	D.C. cardioversion Procainamide Lidocaine	IV fluids (slow drip)

[1] Drug therapy is administered intravenously.

Patient Information:

Notify physician if any of the following occur: Irregular heart beat, shortness of breath, swelling of the hands and feet, pronounced dizziness, constipation, nausea or hypotension.

Bepridil: If nausea occurs, take with meals or at bedtime.

CALCIUM CHANNEL BLOCKING AGENTS

Instruct patients on importance of maintaining potassium supplementation or potassium-sparing diuretics, and the need for routine ECGs and serum potassium monitoring.

Nifedipine, sustained release: Swallow whole; do not chew, divide or crush. An empty tablet may appear in the stool; this is no cause for concern.

Felodipine: Swallow whole; do not crush or chew.

Mild gingival hyperplasia has occurred; good dental hygiene decreases its incidence and severity.

Diltiazem (Dilacor XR): Swallow whole; do not open, crush or chew.

NISOLDIPINE

For complete prescribing information, refer to the Calcium Channel Blockers group monograph.

Indications:

Hypertension: Treatment of hypertension, alone or in combination with other antihypertensive agents.

Administration and Dosage:

Approved by the FDA on February 2, 1995.

Administer nisoldipine orally once daily. Administration with a high fat meal can lead to excessive peak drug concentration and should be avoided. Avoid grapefruit products before and after dosing. Nisoldipine is an extended release dosage form; swallow whole, do not bite or divide.

Adjust the dosage to each patient's needs. Initiate therapy with 20 mg orally once daily, then increase by 10 mg per week, or longer intervals, to attain adequate control of blood pressure. The usual maintenance dosage is 20 to 40 mg once daily. Blood pressure response increases over the 10 to 60 mg daily dose range, but adverse event rates also increase. Doses > 60 mg once daily are not recommended. Nisoldipine has been used safely with diuretics, ACE inhibitors and beta-blocking agents.

Elderly/Hepatic function impairment: Patients over age 65 or patients with impaired liver function are expected to develop higher plasma concentrations of nisoldipine. Monitor blood pressure closely during any dosage adjustment. A starting dose not exceeding 10 mg daily is recommended in these patient groups.

Rx	**Sular** (Zeneca)	**Tablets, extended release:** 10 mg	Lactose. (891 Zeneca 10), oyster; (892 Zeneca 20), yellow cream; (893 Zeneca 30), mustard; (894 Zeneca 40), burnt orange. In 100s and UD 100s.
		20 mg	
		30 mg	
		40 mg	

NIFEDIPINE

For complete prescribing information, refer to the Calcium Channel Blockers group monograph.

Indications:

Vasospastic (Prinzmetal's or variant) angina: May also be used when clinical presentation suggests a vasospastic component, but where vasospasm has not been confirmed.

Chronic stable angina (classic effort-associated angina) without vasospasm.

Hypertension (sustained release only).

Administration and Dosage:

Individualize dosage. Excessive doses can result in hypotension.

Initial dosage (capsule): 10 mg 3 times/day. Usual range is 10 to 20 mg 3 times/day. Some patients, especially those with coronary artery spasm, respond only to higher doses, more frequent administration or both. In such patients, 20 to 30 mg 3 or 4 times/day may be effective. Doses > 120 mg/day are rarely necessary. More than 180 mg/day is not recommended.

Titrate throughout 7 to 14 days to assess response to each dose level; monitor blood pressure before proceeding to higher doses. If symptoms warrant, titrate more rapidly but assess frequently based on physical activity level, attack frequency and sublingual nitroglycerin consumption. Increase dose from 10 mg 3 times/day to 20 and then 30 mg 3 times/day throughout 3 days.

In hospitalized patients under close observation, the dose may be increased in 10 mg increments throughout 4 to 6 hours as required to control pain and arrhythmias due to ischemia. A single dose should rarely exceed 30 mg.

NIFEDIPINE

Sustained release:

Procardia XL – 30 or 60 mg once daily. Do not chew or divide tablet. Titrate over a 7 to 14 day period. Titration may proceed more rapidly if the patient is frequently assessed. Titration to doses > 120 mg is not recommended.

Angina patients maintained on the nifedipine capsule formulation may be switched to the sustained release tablet at the nearest equivalent total daily dose. Experience with doses > 90 mg in angina is limited; therefore, use with caution and only when clinically warranted.

Adalat CC – Adjust dosage according to the patient's needs. Administer once daily on an empty stomach. Swallow tablets whole; do not bite, chew or divide. In general, titrate over a 7 to 14 day period starting with 30 mg once daily. Base upward titration on therapeutic efficacy and safety. Usual maintenance dose is 30 to 60 mg once daily. Titration to doses > 90 mg daily is not recommended.

Concomitant drug therapy with β-blockers may be beneficial in chronic stable angina; however, the effects of concurrent treatment cannot be predicted, especially in patients with compromised left ventricular function or cardiac conduction abnormalities. Closely monitor blood pressure since severe hypotension can occur.

Long-acting nitrates may be safely coadministered, but no controlled studies have evaluated the antianginal effectiveness of this combination. Sublingual nitroglycerin may be taken to control acute angina, particularly during titration.

Rx	**Nifedipine** (Various, eg Geneva, Goldline, Moore, Major, Parmed, Purepac, Qualitest, Rugby, Schein, UDL)	**Capsules:** 10 mg	In 100s, 300s and UD100s.
Rx	**Adalat** (Bayer)		(Miles 811). Orange. In 100s, 300s and UD 100s.
Rx	**Procardia** (Pfizer)		Saccharin. (Procardia Pfizer 260). Orange. In 100s, 300s and UD 100s.
Rx	**Nifedipine** (Various, eg, Geneva, Goldline, Moore, Major, Parmed, Purepac, Qualitest, Rugby, Schein, UDL)	**Capsules:** 20 mg	In 100s, 300s and UD 100s.
Rx	**Adalat** (Bayer)		(Miles 821). Orange and light brown. In 100s, 300s and UD 100s.
Rx	**Procardia** (Pfizer)		(Procardia 20 Pfizer 261). Orange & light brown. In 100s, 300s, UD 100s.
Rx	**Adalat CC** (Bayer)	**Tablets, sustained release:** 30 mg	Lactose. (884 Miles 30). Pink. In 100s and 1000s.
Rx	**Procardia XL** (Pfizer)	**Tablets, sustained release:** 30 mg	Rose-pink. Film coated. In 100s, 300s, 5000s, UD 100s.
Rx	**Adalat CC** (Bayer)	**Tablets, sustained release:** 60 mg	Lactose. (885 Miles 60). Salmon. In 100s, 1000s.
Rx	**Procardia XL** (Pfizer)	**Tablets, sustained release:** 60 mg	Rose-pink. Film coated. In 100s, 300s, 5000s, UD 100s.
Rx	**Adalat CC** (Bayer)	**Tablets, sustained release:** 90 mg	Lactose. (886 Miles 90). Dark red. In 100s, 1000s.
Rx	**Procardia XL** (Pfizer)	**Tablets, sustained release:** 90 mg	Rose-pink. Film coated. In 100s.

NICARDIPINE HCl

For complete prescribing information, refer to the Calcium Channel Blockers group monograph.

Indications:

Oral:

Chronic stable (effort-associated) angina (immediate release only) – Use alone or with beta blockers.

NICARDIPINE HCl

Hypertension (immediate and sustained release) – Management of essential hypertension alone or with other antihypertensives. Be aware of the relatively large peak to trough differences in blood pressure (bp) effect.

Parenteral: Short-term treatment of hypertension when oral therapy is not feasible or desirable. For prolonged control of bp, transfer patients to oral medication as soon as possible.

Administration and Dosage:

Approved by the FDA in December 1988.

Oral:

Angina (immediate release only) – Individualize dosage. Usual initial dose is 20 mg 3 times/day (range, 20 to 40 mg 3 times/day). Allow at least 3 days before increasing dose to ensure achievement of steady-state plasma drug concentrations.

Hypertension – Individualize dosage.

Immediate release: Initial dose is 20 mg 3 times daily (range, 20 to 40 mg 3 times daily). The maximum bp lowering effect occurs ≈ 1 to 2 hours after dosing. To assess adequacy of response, measure bp 8 hours after dosing. Because of nicardipine's prominent peak effects, measure bp 1 to 2 hours after dosing, particularly during initiation of therapy. Allow at least 3 days before increasing dose to ensure achievement of steady-state plasma drug concentrations.

Sustained release: Initial dose is 30 mg twice daily. Effective doses have ranged from 30 to 60 mg twice daily. The maximum bp lowering effect at steady state is sustained from 2 to 6 hours after dosing. When initiating therapy or increasing the dose, measure bp 2 to 4 hours after the first dose or dose increase, as well as at the end of a dosing interval.

The total daily dose of immediate release nicardipine may not be a useful guide in judging the effective dose of the sustained release form. Titrate patients currently receiving the immediate release form with the sustained release form starting at their current daily dose of immediate release, then re-examine to assess adequacy of bp control.

Renal impairment – Titrate dose beginning with 20 mg 3 times a day (immediate release) or 30 mg twice daily (sustained release).

Hepatic impairment – Starting dose is 20 mg twice a day (immediate release) with individual titration.

Parenteral: Intended for IV use. Individualize dosage based on severity of hypertension and response of patient during dosing. Monitor bp both during and after the infusion; avoid too rapid or excessive reduction in either systolic or diastolic pressure during parenteral treatment.

Dosage –

Substitute for oral nicardipine: The IV infusion rate required to produce an average plasma concentration equivalent to a given oral dose at steady state is shown in the following table:

Equivalent Nicardipine Doses: Oral vs IV Infusion

Oral dose	Equivalent IV infusion rate
20 mg q 8 hr	0.5 mg/hr
30 mg q 8 hr	1.2 mg/hr
40 mg q 8 hr	2.2 mg/hr

Initiation in a drug free patient: The time course of bp decrease is dependent on the initial rate of infusion and the frequency of dosage adjustment. Administer by slow continuous infusion at a concentration of 0.1 mg/ml. With constant infusion, bp begins to fall within minutes. It reaches about 50% of its ultimate decrease in about 45 minutes and does not reach final steady state for about 50 hours.

When treating acute hypertensive episodes in patients with chronic hypertension, discontinuation of infusion is followed by a 50% offset of action in 30 ± 7 minutes but plasma levels of drug and gradually decreasing antihypertensive effects exist for about 50 hours.

Titration – For gradual reduction in bp, initiate therapy at 50 ml/hr (5 mg/hr). If desired reduction is not achieved at this dose, the infusion rate may be increased by 25 ml/hr (2.5 mg/hr) every 15 minutes up to a maximum of 150 ml/hr (15 mg/hr) until desired reduction of bp is achieved. For more rapid reduction of bp, initiate at 50 ml/hr. If desired reduction is not achieved at this dose, the infusion rate may be increased by 25 ml/hr every 5 minutes up to a maximum of 150 ml/hr until desired reduction of bp is achieved. Following achievement of the bp goal, decrease the infusion rate to 30 ml/hr.

Maintenance – Adjust rate of infusion to maintain desired response.

NICARDIPINE HCl

Conditions requiring infusion adjustment:

Hypotension or tachycardia – If there is concern of impending hypotension or tachycardia, discontinue the infusion. When bp has stabilized, infusion may be restarted at low doses (eg, 30 to 50 ml/hr) and adjusted to maintain desired bp.

Infusion site changes – Continue IV use as long as bp control is needed. Change the infusion site every 12 hours if administered via peripheral vein.

Cardiac/Renal/Hepatic function impairment – Use caution when titrating in patients with CHF or renal or hepatic function impairment.

Transfer to oral antihypertensives: If treatment includes transfer to an oral antihypertensive other than nicardipine, generally initiate therapy upon discontinuation of the infusion. If oral nicardipine is to be used, administer the first dose of a 3 times daily regimen 1 hour prior to discontinuation of the infusion.

Preparation of infusion: Ampules must be diluted before infusion.

Dilution – Administer by slow IV infusion at a concentration of 0.1 mg/ml. Dilute each amp (25 mg) with 240 ml of solution at a concentration of 0.1 mg/ml.

Admixture compatibility – Nicardipine for IV use is compatible and stable in glass or polyvinyl chloride containers for 24 hours at controlled room temperature with the following: Dextrose 5% Injection; Dextrose 5% and Sodium Chloride 0.45% or 0.9% Injection; Dextrose 5% with Potassium 40 mEq; Sodium Chloride 0.45% or 0.9%.

Admixture incompatibility – Nicardipine IV is not compatible with Sodium Bicarbonate 5% Injection or Lactated Ringer's Injection.

Storage/Stability: Store amps at controlled room temperature. Freezing does not adversely affect the product. Avoid exposure to elevated temperature. Protect from light. The diluted solution is stable for 24 hours at room temperature.

Rx	**Cardene** (Syntex)	**Capsules:** 20 mg	(Cardene 20 mg Syntex 2437). White. In 100s and 500s.
Rx	**Nicardipine HCl** (Mylan)		In 90s and 500s.
Rx	**Cardene** (Syntex)	30 mg	(Cardene 30 mg Syntex 2438). Blue. In 100s and 500s.
Rx	**Nicardipine HCl** (Mylan)		In 90s and 500s.
Rx	**Cardene SR** (Syntex)	**Capsules, sustained release:** 30 mg[1]	(Cardene SR 30 mg Syntex 2440). Pink. In 60s and 200s.
		45 mg[1]	(Cardene SR 45 mg Syntex 2441). Powder blue. In 60s and 200s.
		60 mg[1]	(Cardene SR 60 mg Syntex 2442). Blue/white. In 60s, 200s and UD 100s.
Rx	**Cardene I.V.** (Wyeth)	**Injection:** 2.5 mg/ml	In 10 ml amps.[2]

[1] With lactose.
[2] With 48 mg sorbitol.

BEPRIDIL HCl

For complete prescribing information, refer to the Calcium Channel Blockers group monograph.

Indications:

Chronic stable angina (classic effort-associated angina). Because bepridil has caused serious ventricular arrhythmias, including torsade de pointes type ventricular tachycardia, and the occurrence of agranulocytosis associated with its use, reserve for patients failing to respond optimally to, or are intolerant of, other antianginals.

Bepridil may be used alone or with beta blockers or nitrates. An added effect occurs when administered to patients already receiving propranolol.

Administration and Dosage:

Approved by the FDA in December 1990.

Individualize dosage. Usual initial dose is 200 mg/day. After 10 days, dosage may be adjusted upward depending on response. Most patients are maintained at 300 mg. Maximum daily dose is 400 mg; minimum effective dose is 200 mg.

Elderly: Starting dose does not differ from that for younger patients; however, the elderly may require more frequent monitoring.

BEPRIDIL HCl

Rx	**Vascor** (McNeil)	**Tablets:** 200 mg[1]	(Vascor 200). Light blue, scored. Film coated. In 90s and UD 100s.
		300 mg[1]	(Vascor 300). Blue. Film coated. In 90s and UD 100s.
		400 mg[1]	(Vascor 400). Dark blue. Film coated. In 90s and UD 100s.

[1] With lactose.

ISRADIPINE

For complete prescribing information, refer to the Calcium Channel Blockers group monograph.

Indications:

Hypertension: Alone or concurrently with thiazide-type diuretics.

Administration and Dosage:

Approved by the FDA in December 1990.

Individualize dosage. Recommended initial dose is 2.5 mg twice daily. An antihypertensive response usually occurs within 2 to 3 hours; maximal response may require 2 to 4 weeks. If a satisfactory response does not occur after this period, the dose may be adjusted in increments of 5 mg/day at 2 to 4 week intervals up to a maximum of 20 mg/day. However, most patients show no additional response to doses > 10 mg/day, and adverse effects are increased in frequency above 10 mg/day.

Rx	**DynaCirc** (Sandoz)	**Capsules:** 2.5 mg	(DynaCirc 2.5). White. In 60s, 100s and UD 100s.
		5 mg	(DynaCirc 5). Light pink. In 60s, 100s and UD 100s.

NIMODIPINE

For complete prescribing information, refer to the Calcium Channel Blockers group monograph.

Indications:

Subarachnoid hemorrhage (SAH): Improvement of neurological deficits due to spasm following SAH from ruptured congenital intracranial aneurysms in patients who are in good neurological condition post-ictus (eg, Hunt and Hess Grades I-III).

Administration and Dosage:

Approved by the FDA in December 1988.

Commence therapy within 96 hours of the SAH, using 60 mg every 4 hours for 21 consecutive days.

If the capsule cannot be swallowed (eg, time of surgery, unconscious patient), make a hole in both ends of the capsule with an 18 gauge needle and extract the contents into a syringe. Empty the contents into the patient's in situ nasogastric tube and wash down the tube with 30 ml normal saline.

Rx	**Nimotop** (Bayer)	**Capsules, liquid:** 30 mg	(Miles 855). Ivory. In UD 100s.

FELODIPINE

For complete prescribing information, refer to the Calcium Channel Blockers group monograph.

Indications:

Hypertension: Alone or concomitantly with other antihypertensives.

Administration and Dosage:

Approved by the FDA in August 1991.

The recommended starting dose is 5 mg once daily. Depending on the patient's response the dosage can be decreased to 2.5 mg or increased to 10 mg once daily. These adjustments should occur generally at intervals of not less than 2 weeks. The recommended dosage range is 2.5 to 10 mg once daily. In clinical trials, doses >10 mg increased blood pressure response but a large increase in the rate of peripheral edema and other vasodilatory adverse events. Modification of the recommended dosage is usually not required in renal impairment. Because they may develop higher plasma felodipine levels, closely monitor blood pressure in the elderly patients > 65 years old and in impaired hepatic function during dosage adjustment; generally, do not consider doses > 10 mg.

Swallow whole; do not crush or chew.

Rx	**Plendil** (Astra-Merck)	**Tablets, extended release:** 2.5 mg	Lactose. (Plendil 450). Green, convex. In 30s, 100s and UD 100s.
		5 mg	Lactose. (Plendil 451). Light red-brown, convex. In 30s, 100s and UD 100s.
		10 mg	Lactose. (Plendil 452). Red-brown, convex. In 30s, 100s and UD 100s.

AMLODIPINE

For complete prescribing information, refer to the Calcium Channel Blockers group monograph.

Indications:

Hypertension: Alone or in combination with other antihypertensives.

Chronic stable angina: Alone or in combination with other antianginals.

Vasospastic (Prinzmetal's or variant) angina: Confirmed or suspected, alone or in combination with other antianginals.

Administration and Dosage:

Approved by the FDA July 31, 1992.

May be taken without regard to meals.

Hypertension: Individualize dosage. Usual dose is 5 mg once daily. Maximum dose is 10 mg once daily. Small, fragile or elderly patients or patients with hepatic insufficiency may be started on 2.5 mg once daily; this dose may also be used when adding amlodipine to other antihypertensive therapy. In general, titrate over 7 to 14 days; proceed more rapidly if clinically warranted with frequent assessment of the patient.

Angina (chronic stable or vasospastic): 5 to 10 mg, using the lower dose for elderly and patients with hepatic insufficiency. Most patients require 10 mg.

Rx	**Norvasc** (Pfizer)	**Tablets**: 2.5 mg	(Norvasc 2.5). White. Diamond shape. In 100s.
		5 mg	(Norvasc 5). White. Elongated octagon. In 100s and UD 100s.
		10 mg	(Norvasc 10). White. In 100s and UD 100s.

DILTIAZEM HCl

For complete prescribing information, refer to the Calcium Channel Blockers group monograph.

Indications:

Oral: Angina pectoris due to coronary artery spasm.
Chronic stable angina (classic effort-associated angina).
Essential hypertension (sustained release only).

Parenteral: Atrial fibrillation or flutter.
Paroxysmal supraventricular tachycardia.

Administration and Dosage:

Approved by the FDA in 1982.

Oral: Individualize dosage.

Tablets – Start with 30 mg 4 times/day before meals and at bedtime; gradually increase dosage to 180 to 360 mg (given in divided doses 3 or 4 times/day) at 1 to 2 day intervals until optimum response is obtained.

Sustained release –

Cardizem SR: Start with 60 to 120 mg twice daily. Adjust dosage when maximum antihypertensive effect is achieved (usually by 14 days chronic therapy). Optimum dosage range is 240 to 360 mg/day, but some patients may respond to lower doses.

Cardizem CD:

Hypertension – 180 to 240 mg once daily; some patients may respond to lower doses. Maximum antihypertensive effect is usually achieved by 14 days chronic therapy; therefore, adjust dosage accordingly. Usual range is 240 to 360 mg once daily; experience with doses > 360 mg is limited.

Angina – Start with 120 or 180 mg once daily. Some patients may respond to higher doses of up to 480 mg once daily. When necessary, titration may be carried out over a 7 to 14 day period.

Dilacor XR:

Hypertension – 180 to 240 mg once daily; adjust dose as needed. Individual patients, particularly ≥ 60 years of age, may respond to a lower dose of 120 mg. Usual range is 180 to 480 mg once daily. Although current clinical experience with the 540 mg dose is limited, the dose may be increased to 540 mg with little or no increased risk of adverse reactions. Do not exceed 540 mg once daily.

Angina – Adjust dosage to each patient's needs, starting with a dose of 120 mg once daily, which may be titrated to doses of up to 480 mg once daily. When necessary, titration may be carried out over a 7 to 14 day period.

Hypertensive or anginal patients treated with other formulations of diltiazem can safely be switched to *Dilacor XR* at the nearest equivalent total daily dose. Subsequent titration to higher or lower doses may, however, be necessary and should be initiated as clinically indicated.

Administration in the morning on an empty stomach is recommended. Do not open, chew or crush the capsules; swallow whole.

Parenteral:

Direct IV single injections (bolus) – The initial dose is 0.25 mg/kg as a bolus administered over 2 minutes (20 mg is a reasonable dose for the average patient). If response is inadequate, a second dose may be administered after 15 minutes. The second bolus dose should be 0.35 mg/kg administered over 2 minutes (25 mg is a reasonable dose for the average patient). Individualize subsequent IV bolus doses. Dose patients with low body weights on a mg/kg basis. Some patients may respond to an initial dose of 0.15 mg/kg, although duration of action may be shorter.

Continuous IV infusion – For continued reduction of the heart rate (up to 24 hours) in patients with atrial fibrillation or atrial flutter, an IV infusion may be administered. Immediately following bolus administration of 20 mg (0.25 mg/kg) or 25 mg (0.35 mg/kg) and reduction of heart rate, begin an IV infusion. The recommended initial infusion rate is 10 mg/hr. Some patients may maintain response to an initial rate of 5 mg/hr. The infusion rate may be increased in 5 mg/hr increments up to 15 mg/hr as needed, if further reduction in heart rate is required. The infusion may be maintained for up to 24 hours. Therefore, infusion duration longer than 24 hours and infusion rates > 15 mg/hr are not recommended.

Dilution – For continuous IV infusion, aseptically transfer the appropriate quantity (see table) to the desired volume of either Normal Saline, D5W, or D5W/0.45% NaCl. Mix thoroughly. Use within 24 hours. Keep refrigerated until use.

DILTIAZEM HCl

Dilution of Diltiazem Injection

Diluent volume (ml)	Quantity of diltiazem injection	Final concentration (mg/ml)	Dose[1] (mg/hr)	Infusion rate (ml/hr)
100	125 mg (25 ml)	1	10 15	10 15
250	250 mg (50 ml)	0.83	10 15	12 18
500	250 mg (50 ml)	0.45	10 15	22 33

[1] 5 mg/hr may be appropriate for some patients.

Admixture compatibility/incompatibility – Diltiazem is physically compatible and chemically stable in the following parenteral solutions for at least 24 hours when stored in glass or PVC bags at controlled room temperature (15° to 30°C; 59° to 86°F) or refrigerated (2° to 8°C; 36° to 46°F): 5% Dextrose Injection, USP; 0.9% Sodium Chloride Injection, USP; 5% Dextrose and 0.45% Sodium Chloride Injection, USP.

Diltiazem is incompatible when mixed directly with furosemide solution.

Concomitant therapy with β-blockers or digitalis is usually well tolerated, but the effects of coadministration cannot be predicted, especially in patients with left ventricular dysfunction or cardiac conduction abnormalities. Use caution in titrating dosages for impaired renal or hepatic function patients, since dosage requirements are not available.

Sublingual nitroglycerin may be taken as required to abort acute anginal attacks. Diltiazem may be safely used with short-acting and long-acting nitrates, but no controlled studies have evaluated the antianginal efficacy of this combination.

An additive antihypertensive effect occurs when diltiazem is coadministered with other antihypertensives. Adjust the dose of diltiazem or the concomitant antihypertensive accordingly.

Storage/Stability: Store injection under refrigeration at 2° to 8°C (36° to 46°F). Do not freeze. May be stored at room temperature for up to 1 month; destroy after 1 month at room temperature. Discard unused portion of single-use containers.

Rx	**Diltiazem HCl** (Various, eg, Apothecon, Geneva, Goldline, Moore, Lederle, Major, Mylan, Qualitest, Rugby, Schein)	**Tablets:** 30 mg	In 100s, 1000s and unit of issue 30s, 60s, 90s and 120s.
Rx	**Cardizem** (Hoechst Marion Roussel)		(Marion 1771). Green. In 100s, 500s and UD 100s.
Rx	**Diltiazem HCl** (Various, eg, Apothecon, Geneva, Goldline, Moore, Lederle, Major, Mylan, Qualitest, Rugby, Schein)	**Tablets:** 60 mg	In 100s, 500s, 1000s and unit of issue 30s, 60s, 90s and 120s.
Rx	**Cardizem** (Marion Merrell Dow)		(Marion 1772). Yellow, scored. In 90s, 100s, 500s and UD 100s.
Rx	**Diltiazem HCl** (Various, eg, Apothecon, Geneva, Goldline, Moore, Lederle, Major, Mylan, Qualitest, Rugby, Schein)	**Tablets:** 90 mg	In 100s, 500s, 1000s and unit of issue 30s, 60s, 90s and 120s.
Rx	**Cardizem** (Hoechst Marion Roussel)		(Cardizem 90 mg). Green, scored. In 90s, 100s and UD 100s.
Rx	**Diltiazem HCl** (Various, eg, Apothecon, Geneva, Goldline, Moore, Lederle, Major, Mylan, Qualitest, Rugby, Schein)	**Tablets:** 120 mg	In 100s, 500s, 1000s and unit of issue 30s, 60s, 90s and 120s.
Rx	**Cardizem** (Hoechst Marion Roussel)		(Cardizem 120 mg). Yellow, scored. In 100s and UD 100s.

DILTIAZEM HCl

Rx	**Tiamate** (Hoechst Marion Roussel)	**Tablets, extended-release:** 120 mg	Sucrose. (Tiamate 120). Off-white. Capsule shape. Film-coated. In UD 30s.
Rx	**Tiamate** (Hoechst Marion Roussel)	**Tablets, extended-release:** 180 mg	Sucrose. (Tiamate 180). Off-white. Capsule shape. Film-coated. In UD 30s.
Rx	**Tiamate** (Hoechst Marion Roussel)	**Tablets, extended-release:** 240 mg	Sucrose. (Tiamate 240). Off-white. Capsule shape. Film-coated. In UD 30s.
Rx	**Diltiazem HCl Extended Release** (Various, eg, Lemmon, Major)	**Capsules, sustained release:** 60 mg	In 100s.
Rx	**Cardizem SR** (Hoechst Marion Roussel)		(Cardizem SR 60 mg). Ivory and brown. In 100s and UD 100s.
Rx	**Diltiazem HCl Extended Release** (Various, eg, Lemmon, Major)	**Capsules, sustained release:** 90 mg	In 100s.
Rx	**Cardizem SR** (Hoechst Marion Roussel)		(Cardizem SR 90 mg). Gold and brown. In 100s and UD 100s.
Rx	**Diltiazem HCl Extended Release** (Various, eg, Lemmon, Major)	**Capsules, sustained release:** 120 mg	In 100s.
Rx	**Cardizem SR** (Hoechst Marion Roussel)		(Cardizem SR 120 mg). Caramel and brown. In 100s and UD 100s.
Rx	**Cardizem CD** (Hoechst Marion Roussel)	**Capsules, sustained release:** 120 mg	(Cardizem CD 120 mg). Turquoise. In 30s, 90s and UD 100s.
Rx	**Dilacor XR** (Rhone-Poulenc Rorer)	**Capsules, sustained release:** 120 mg	(Dilacor XR 120 mg). Gold/white. In 100s and 1000s.
Rx	**Cardizem CD** (Hoechst Marion Roussel)	**Capsules, sustained release:** 180 mg	Sucrose. (1796 180 mg). Turquoise/blue. In 30s, 90s, 5000s and UD 100s.
Rx	**Dilacor XR** (Rhone-Poulenc Rorer)	**Capsules, sustained release:** 180 mg	(Dilacor XR 180 mg). Orange/white. In 100s and 1000s.
Rx	**Cardizem CD** (Hoechst Marion Roussel)	**Capsules, sustained release:** 240 mg	Sucrose. (1797 240 mg). Blue. In 30s, 90s, 5000s and UD 100s.
Rx	**Dilacor XR** (Rhone-Poulenc Rorer)	**Capsules, sustained release:** 240 mg	(Dilacor XR 240 mg). Brown/white. In 100s and 1000s.
Rx	**Cardizem CD** (Hoechst Marion Roussel)	**Capsules, sustained release:** 300 mg	Sucrose. (1798 300 mg). Gray/blue. In 30s, 90s, 5000s and UD 100s.

DILTIAZEM HCl

Rx	**Tiazac** (Forest	**Capsules, extended release:** 120 mg	(Tiazac-120). Lavender. In 30s and 90s.
		180 mg	(Tiazac-180). White/blue-green. In 30s, 90s and 1000s.
		240 mg	(Tiazac-240). Blue-green/lavender. In 30s, 90s and 1000s.
		300 mg	(Tiazac-300). White/lavender. In 30s, 90s and 1000s.
		360 mg	(Tiazac-360). Blue-green. In 30s and 90s.
Rx	**Cardizem** (Hoechst Marion Roussel)	**Injection:** 25 mg (5 mg/ml)	In 5 ml vials.[1]
Rx	**Diltiazem** (Bedford Labs)		In 5 and 10 ml vials.[2]
Rx	**Cardizem** (Hoechst Marion Roussel)	50 mg (5 mg/ml)	In 10 ml vials.[3]
Rx	**Diltiazem** (Bedford Labs)		In 5 and 10 ml vials.[2]

[1] With 3.75 mg citric acid, 3.25 mg sodium citrate dihydrate and 357 mg sorbitol solution.
[2] With 0.75 mg citric acid, 0.65 mg sdodium citrat dihydrate and 71.4 mg sorbitol solution.
[3] With 7.5 mg citric acid, 6.5 mg sodium citrate dihydrate and 714 mg sorbitol solution.

VERAPAMIL HCl

For complete prescribing information, refer to the Calcium Channel Blockers group monograph.

Indications:

Oral:

Angina – Treatment of vasospastic (Prinzmetal's variant), chronic stable (classic effort-associated) and unstable (crescendo, preinfarction) angina.

Arrhythmias – With digitalis to control ventricular rate at rest and during stress in chronic atrial flutter or fibrillation. May use for prophylaxis of repetitive paroxysmal supraventricular tachycardia (PSVT).

Essential hypertension.

Sustained release – Only for management of essential hypertension.

Parenteral: Supraventricular tachyarrhythmias.

Atrial flutter or fibrillation – Temporary control of rapid ventricular rate.

Administration and Dosage:

If heart failure is not severe or rate-related, use digitalis and diuretics, as appropriate, before verapamil. In moderately severe to severe cardiac dysfunction (PCWP > 20 mm Hg, ejection fraction < 30%), acute worsening of heart failure may occur.

Individualize dosage. Do not exceed 480 mg/day; safety and efficacy are not established. Half-life increases during chronic use; maximum response may be delayed.

Oral:

Angina at rest and chronic stable angina – Usual initial dose is 80 to 120 mg 3 times a day. However, 40 mg 3 times a day may be warranted if patients have increased response to verapamil (eg, decreased hepatic function, elderly). Base upward titration on safety and efficacy evaluated ≈ 8 hours after dosing. Increase dosage daily (eg, unstable angina) or weekly until optimum clinical response is obtained.

Arrhythmias – Dosage range in digitalized patients with chronic atrial fibrillation is 240 to 320 mg/day in divided doses 3 or 4 times/day. Dosage range for prophylaxis of PSVT (non-digitalized patients) is 240 to 480 mg/day in divided doses 3 or 4 times/day. Maximum effects will be apparent during the first 48 hours of therapy.

Essential hypertension – The usual initial monotherapy dose is 80 mg 3 times/day (240 mg/day). Daily dosages of 360 and 480 mg have been used, but there is no evidence that dosages > 360 mg provide added effect. Consider beginning titration at 40 mg 3 times/day in patients who might respond to lower doses, (eg, elderly or people of small stature). Antihypertensive effects are evident within the first week of therapy. Base upward titration on therapeutic efficacy, assessed at the end of the dosing interval.

Sustained release (essential hypertension) – Give with food. Usual daily dose is 240 mg/day in the morning. However, 120 mg/day may be warranted in patients who may have increased response (eg, elderly or people of small stature). Base upward titration on safety and efficacy evaluated ≈ 24 hours after dosing. If adequate response is not obtained, titrate upward to 240 mg/morning and 120 mg/evening, then 240 mg every 12 hours, if needed. When switching from immediate release tablets, total daily dose (in mg) may remain the same. Antihypertensive effects are evident within the first week.

Parenteral (supraventricular tachyarrhythmias): For IV use only. Give as slow IV injection over at least 2 min under continuous ECG and blood pressure monitoring. A small fraction (< 1%) of patients may have life-threatening adverse responses (rapid ventricular rate in atrial flutter/fibrillation, marked hypotension or extreme bradycardia/asystole); monitor initial use of IV verapamil and have resuscitation facilities available. An IV infusion has been used (5 mg/hour); precede the infusion with an IV loading dose.

Initial dose – 5 to 10 mg (0.075 to 0.15 mg/kg) as an IV bolus over 2 minutes.

Repeat dose – 10 mg (0.15 mg/kg) 30 minutes after the first dose if the initial response is not adequate.

Older patients – Give over at least 3 min to minimize risk of untoward drug effects.

Children –

≤ *1 year:* 0.1 to 0.2 mg/kg (usual single dose range, 0.75 to 2 mg) as an IV bolus over 2 minutes (under continuous ECG monitoring).

1 to 15 years: 0.1 to 0.3 mg/kg (usual single dose range, 2 to 5 mg) IV over 2 minutes. Do not exceed 5 mg.

Repeat dose: Repeat above dose 30 minutes after the first dose if the initial response is not adequate (under continuous ECG monitoring). Do not exceed a single dose of 10 mg in patients 1 to 15 years of age.

Incompatibility: A crystalline precipitate immediately forms when verapamil is administered into an infusion line containing 0.45% sodium chloride with sodium bicarbonate. A milky white precipitate forms when verapamil is given by IV push into the same line being used for nafcillin infusion.

For stability reasons this product is not recommended for dilution with sodium lactate injection in polyvinyl chloride bags. Avoid admixing IV verapamil with albumin, amphotericin B, hydralazine HCl, aminophylline and trimethoprim/sulfamethoxazole. Verapamil will precipitate in any solution with a pH above 6.

Storage: Protect IV solution from light. Discard any unused amount of solution.

Rx	**Verapamil HCl** (Various, eg, Geneva, Rugby)	**Tablets**: 40 mg	In 100s.
Rx	**Calan** (Searle)		(Calan 40). Pink. Film coated. In 100s.
Rx	**Isoptin** (Knoll)		Scored. Film coated. In 100s and UD 100s.
Rx	**Verapamil HCl** (Various, eg,Geneva, Rugby)	**Tablets:** 80 mg	In 100s, 250s, 500s, 1000s and UD 100s.
Rx	**Calan** (Searle)		(Calan 80). Peach, scored. Oval. Film coated. In 100s, 500s, 1000s and UD 100s.
Rx	**Isoptin** (Knoll)		(Knoll Isoptin 80). Yellow, scored. Film coated. In 100s, 500s, 1000s and UD 100s.
Rx	**Verapamil HCl** (Various, eg,Geneva, Rugby)	**Tablets:** 120 mg	In 100s, 250s, 500s, 1000s and UD 100s.
Rx	**Calan** (Searle)		(Calan 120). Brown, scored. Oval. Film coated. In 100s, 500s, 1000s and UD 100s.
Rx	**Isoptin** (Knoll)		(Knoll Isoptin 120). White, scored. Film coated. In 100s, 500s, 1000s and UD 100s.
Rx	**Calan SR** (Searle)	**Tablets, sustained release:** 120 mg	(Calan SR 120). Light violet. Oval. Film coated. In 100s and UD 100s.
Rx	**Isoptin SR** (Knoll)		(Knoll 120 SR). Light violet. Oval. Film coated. In 100s and UD 100s.

VERAPAMIL HCl

Rx	**Verapamil HCl SR** (Various, eg, Geneva, Rugby)	**Tablets, sustained release:** 180 mg	In 100s and 500s
Rx	**Calan SR** (Searle)		Light pink, scored. Oval. Film coated. In 100s and UD 100s.
Rx	**Isoptin SR** (Knoll)		(Isoptin SR 180 mg). Light pink, scored. Oval. Film coated. In 100s and UD 100s.
Rx	**Verapamil HCl SR** (Various, eg, Geneva, Rugby)	**Tablets, sustained release:** 240 mg	In 100s and 500s
Rx	**Calan SR**(Searle)		(Calan SR 240). Light green, scored. Capsule shape. Film coated. In 100s, 500s and UD 100s.
Rx	**Isoptin SR** (Knoll)		(Isoptin SR). Light green, scored. Capsule shape. Film coated. In 100s, 500s and UD 100s.
Rx	**Covera-HS** (Searle)	**Tablets, extended release:** 180 mg	(Covera-HS 2011). Lavender. Film-coated. In 30s, 100s and UD 100s.
		240 mg	(Covera-HS 2021). Pale yellow. Film-coated. In 30s, 100s and UD 100s.
Rx	**Verelan** (Lederle)	**Capsules, sustained release**: 120 mg	(Lederle V8 Verelan 120 mg). Yellow. In 100s.
		180 mg	(Lederle V7). Gray/yellow. In 100s.
		240 mg	(Lederle V9 Verelan 240 mg). Blue/yellow. In 100s.
		360 mg	(Lederle V6/Verelan 360 mg) Lavender/yellow. In 100s.
Rx	**Verapamil HCl** (Various, eg, Abbott, SoloPak)	**Injection:** 5 mg/2 ml	In 2 and 4 ml vials, amps and syringes and 4 ml fill in 5 ml vials.
Rx	**Isoptin** (Knoll)		In 2 and 4 ml amps, vials and disp. syringes.

CYCLANDELATE

Actions:

Pharmacology: Cyclandelate is a musculotropic, direct-acting vascular smooth muscle relaxant with no significant adrenergic stimulating or blocking actions. Drug activity measured by pharmacological tests against various types of smooth muscle spasm produced by acetylcholine, histamine and barium chloride, exceeds that of papaverine, particularly with regard to the neurotropic component produced by acetylcholine.

Indications:

"Possibly effective" for adjunctive therapy in intermittent claudication; arteriosclerosis obliterans; thrombophlebitis (to control associated vasospasm and muscular ischemia); nocturnal leg cramps; Raynaud's phenomenon; selected cases of ischemic cerebral vascular disease.

Unlabeled uses: Cyclandelate (1200 to 1600 mg/day) has been used in dementia of cerebrovascular origin, multi-infarct dementia, various memory disorders, migraine prophylaxis, vertigo of circulatory origin, tinnitus and visual disturbances due to chronic cerebrovascular insufficiency and diabetic peripheral polyneuropathy.

Contraindications:

Hypersensitivity to cyclandelate.

Warnings:

Coronary artery/cerebral vascular disease: Use with extreme caution in patients with severe obliterative coronary artery or cerebral vascular disease; these diseased areas may be compromised by vasodilatory effects of the drug elsewhere.

Prolonged bleeding: Although prolongation of bleeding time did not occur with therapeutic dosages, it occurred in animals at very large doses. Consider this hazard when administering cyclandelate to a patient with active bleeding or a bleeding tendency.

Pregnancy: Category C. Safety for use during pregnancy has not been established. Use only when clearly needed and when potential benefits outweigh potential hazards to the fetus.

Lactation: Safety for use in breastfeeding is not established. Use only when clearly needed and when potential benefits outweigh potential hazards to the nursing infant.

Precautions:

Glaucoma: Use with caution in patients with glaucoma.

Adverse Reactions:

GI: Heartburn, pain and eructation (infrequent, mild).

Body as a whole: Mild flushing, headache, feeling of weakness or tachycardia may occur, especially during the first week of administration.

Patient Information:

Take medication with meals or antacids to reduce GI distress.

Administration and Dosage:

Although objective signs of therapeutic benefit may be rapid and dramatic, improvement usually occurs gradually over weeks of therapy. Prolonged use may be necessary. Short-term use is rarely beneficial or permanent.

Initial therapy: 1.2 to 1.6 g/day in divided doses before meals and at bedtime. When a clinical response is noted, decrease dosage in 200 mg decrements until the maintenance dosage is reached.

Maintenance therapy: 400 to 800 mg/day in 2 to 4 divided doses.

Rx	**Cyclandelate** (Various)	**Capsules:** 200 mg	Lactose. In 60s, 100s, 500s, 1000s and UD 100s.
Rx	**Cyclandelate** (Various)	**Capsules:** 400 mg	Lactose. In 60s, 100s, 500s, 1000s and UD 100s.

ISOXSUPRINE HCl

Actions:

Pharmacology: Isoxsuprine is a vasodilator that acts primarily on blood vessels within skeletal muscle. In healthy subjects, resting blood flow in skeletal muscle is increased; cutaneous blood flow is usually not affected. Isoxsuprine is an α-adrenoreceptor antagonist with β-adrenoreceptor stimulating properties; however, vasodilation is not blocked by propranolol. Isoxsuprine may act directly on vascular smooth muscle. The drug also causes cardiac stimulation (increased contractility, heart rate and cardiac output) and uterine relaxation. At high doses, it lowers blood viscosity and inhibits platelet aggregation.

Indications:

"Possibly effective" for relief of symptoms associated with cerebral vascular insufficiency; peripheral vascular disease of arteriosclerosis obliterans, thromboangiitis obliterans (Buerger's disease) and Raynaud's disease.

Unlabeled uses: Isoxsuprine has been used in the treatment of dysmenorrhea and threatened premature labor (see Warnings), but efficacy has not been established.

Contraindications:

Immediately postpartum; in the presence of arterial bleeding.

Warnings:

Rash: If rash appears, discontinue use. A causal relationship is not established.

Pregnancy: Category C. There are no reports of isoxsuprine causing congenital defects. Hypotension, hypocalcemia, hypoglycemia, ileus, tachycardia and death have occurred when cord serum levels are > 10 ng/ml.

Pulmonary edema has been reported in mothers treated with β-stimulants. Isoxsuprine is neither approved nor recommended for use in the treatment of premature labor; more selective agents are available (see the Ritodrine monograph in the Hormones chapter).

Adverse Reactions:

Cardiovascular: Hypotension; tachycardia; chest pain.

GI: Nausea; vomiting; abdominal distress.

Miscellaneous: Dizziness; weakness; severe rash (see Warnings).

Patient Information:

May cause palpitations or skin rash. Notify physician if these symptoms become particularly bothersome.

If dizziness (orthostatic hypotension) occurs, avoid sudden changes in posture.

Administration and Dosage:

10 to 20 mg, 3 or 4 times daily.

Rx	**Isoxsuprine HCl** (Various)	**Tablets:** 10 mg	In 60s, 100s, 500s, 1000s and UD 100s.
Rx	**Vasodilan** (Mead Johnson)		In 100s, 1000s and UD 1000s.
Rx	**Voxsuprine** (Major)		In 100s, 250s, 1000s and UD 100s.
Rx	**Isoxsuprine HCl** (Various)	**Tablets:** 20 mg	In 60s, 100s, 500s, 1000s and UD 100s.
Rx	**Vasodilan** (Mead Johnson)		In 100s and 1000s.
Rx	**Voxsuprine** (Major)		In 100s, 250s, 1000s and UD 100s.

PAPAVERINE HCl

Actions:

Pharmacology: Papaverine directly relaxes the tonus of various smooth muscle, especially when it has been spasmodically contracted. It relaxes the smooth musculature of the larger blood vessels, especially coronary, systemic peripheral and pulmonary arteries. Vasodilation may be related to its ability to inhibit cyclic nucleotide phosphodiesterase, thus increasing levels of intracellular cyclic AMP. During administration, the muscle cell is not paralyzed and still responds to drugs and other stimuli causing contraction. The antispasmodic effect is direct and unrelated to muscle innervation. It has little effect on the CNS, although very large doses tend to produce some sedation and sleepiness. In certain circumstances, mild respiratory stimulation can be observed because of stimulation of carotid and aortic body chemoreceptors.

Possibly because of its direct vasodilating action on cerebral blood vessels, papaverine increases cerebral blood flow and decreases cerebral vascular resistance in healthy subjects; oxygen consumption is unaltered. These effects have been used to explain the reported benefits in cerebral vascular encephalopathy.

Papaverine acts on the heart to depress conduction and irritability and to prolong the refractory period of the myocardium, which provide the basis for its clinical trial in abrogating atrial and ventricualr premature systoles and ominous ventricular arrhythmias. The coronary vasodilator action could be an additional factor of therapeutic value when such rhythms are secondary to insufficiency or occlusion of the coronary arteries.

Pharmacokinetics:

Absorption/Distribution – Oral bioavailability is ≈ 54%. Peak plasma levels occur 1 to 2 hours after a dose.

Metabolism/Excretion – Papaverine is metabolized in the liver. Although estimates of its biologic half-life vary widely, reasonably constant plasma levels can be maintained after 4 days with regular administration at 6–hour intervals. The drug is excreted in the urine in an inactive form.

Indications:

Ischemia: For relief of cerebral and peripheral ischemia associated with arterial spasm and myocardial ischemia complicated by arrhythmias.

Contraindications:

Large doses can depress atrioventricular and intraventricular conduction and thereby produce serious arrhythmias (see Warnings).

Warnings:

Cardiac: Large doses can depress AV and intraventricular conduction and thereby produce serious arrhythmias. When conduction is depressed, it may produce transient ectopy of ventricular origin, either premature beats or paroxysmal tachycardia.

In patients with acute coronary thrombosis, the occurrence of ventricular cardiac arrhythmias is serious and requires measures designed to decrease myocardial irritability.

Hepatic toxicity: Chronic hepatitis, as evidenced by an increase in serum bilirubin and serum glutamic transaminase, has been reported in three cases following long-term papaverine therapy. One patient had jaundice, and another had abnormal liver function on biopsy.

Pregnancy: Category C. Safety for use during pregnancy has not been established. Use only when clearly needed and when the potential benefits outweigh the potential hazards to the fetus.

Lactation: It is not known whether this drug is excreted in breast milk. Safety for use in the nursing mother has not been established.

Children: Safety and efficacy for use in children have not been established.

Precautions:

Glaucoma: Use with caution in patients with glaucoma.

Drug Interactions:

Levodopa: Loss of control of Parkinson's disease may occur, following the introduction of papaverine. Although the mechanism is unknown, papaverine may block dopamine receptors in the striatum.

Adverse Reactions:

Body as a whole: Sweating; flushing of face; skin rash; malaise; hepatic hypersensitivity; chronic hepatitis (see Warnings).

Cardiovascular: Increase in heart rate and depth of respiration; slight increase in blood pressure.

CNS: Vertigo; drowsiness; excessive sedation; headache.

PAPAVERINE HCl

GI: Nausea; abdominal distress; anorexia; constipation; diarrhea.

Overdosage:

Ingestion of > 10 times the usual therapeutic dose has not resulted in untoward effects; however, a single dose of 0.1 to 0.5 g/kg could be fatal to an adult.

Acute poisoning:

Symptoms – Drowsiness, weakness, nystagmus, diplopia, incoordination and lassitude, progressing to coma with cyanosis and respiratory depression.

Treatment – To delay drug absorption, give tap water, milk or activated charcoal; then evacuate stomach contents by gastric lavage or emesis, followed by catharsis. If coma and respiratory depression occur, take appropriate measures. Hemodialysis has been suggested. Maintain blood pressure. Avoid concurrent administration of other depressant drugs.

Chronic poisoning:

Symptoms – Drowsiness, depression, weakness, anxiety, ataxia, headache, blurred vision, gastric upset and pruritic skin rashes characterized by urticaria or erythematous macular eruptions. Any of the formed elements of the blood may be decreased in number.

Treatment – Discontinue medication at the onset of any unusual symptoms or abnormal hematologic findings. Severe hypotension may occur. Recovery should occur, except in patients with aplastic anemia.

Patient Information:

May cause dizziness (hypotension) or drowsiness; use caution when driving or performing other tasks requiring alertness, coordination or physical dexterity. Alcohol may intensify these effects.

May cause flushing, sweating, headache, tiredness, jaundice, skin rash, nausea, anorexia, abdominal distress, constipation or diarrhea. Notify physician if these effects become pronounced.

Administration and Dosage:

150 mg every 12 hours. In difficult cases, increase to 150 mg every 8 hours, or 300 mg every 12 hours.

Rx	**Papaverine HCl** (Various)	**Capsules, timed release:** 150 mg	In 100s and 1000s.
Rx	**Pavabid Plateau Caps** (Hoechst Marion Roussel)		(Marion/1555). In 100s.
Rx	**Pavagen TD** (Rugby)		In 100s, 500s and 1000s.

VASOPRESSORS USED IN SHOCK

Shock is a state of inadequate tissue perfusion. It can be caused by, or cause, a decreased supply of, or an increased demand for, oxygen and nutrients. The imbalance between supply and demand interferes with normal cellular function. Widespread cellular dysfunction can result in death. Inadequate tissue perfusion can occur even if cardiac output, peripheral resistance and other factors which determine blood pressure (eg, blood volume) are normal or elevated. Therefore, hypotension need not be present for the patient to be in shock.

Shock produces various physiologic responses. Some, such as lactic acidosis, occur as a direct result of tissue hypoperfusion. Others, such as catecholamine release, also serve to compensate for the absolute or relative reduction in tissue perfusion. The systemic responses to shock can be beneficial in the early stages and classically consist of an increase in circulating catecholamines, vasodilation and increased vascular permeability. These early responses produce a "hyperdynamic" state which may be referred to as "warm" shock, so named because blood flow to the skin and extremities is still maintained. If left uncorrected, however, these responses become counterproductive, and contribute to the relentless progression of the shock state. Profound vascular decompensation occurs, which is associated with a further loss of blood flow to the vital organs, skin and extremities. Thus, more advanced shock is "cold" shock.

Clinical manifestations of shock are variable and non-specific. In addition, underlying or concurrent disease states, drug therapy and patient age may alter the response to hypoperfusion. Signs and symptoms of shock include:

Skin – Pallor, cyanosis, cold and clammy, sweating

CNS – Agitation, confusion, disorientation, coma

Cardiovascular – Tachycardia, arrhythmias, wide pulse pressure, gallop rhythm, hypotension.

Pulmonary – Tachypnea, pulmonary edema

Renal – Oliguria (<0.5 ml/kg/hr)

Metabolic – Acidosis, hypoglycemia or hyperglycemia.

Causes of shock are varied. Despite the etiology, advanced shock tends to follow a common clinical course. However, identifying the underlying cause may assist in the selection of general supportive therapy and is essential for selecting specific therapy.

Types of shock:

Hypovolemic shock occurs when intravascular volume is reduced by > 15% to 25%. The volume loss can be absolute (eg, hemorrhage, fluid loss due to burns, diarrhea or vomiting, excess diuresis, diabetes) or relative (eg, sequestration of body fluids, capillary leak).

Cardiogenic shock occurs when the heart is unable to deliver an adequate cardiac output to maintain vital organ perfusion. This can be caused by an acute myocardial infarction, sustained ventricular arrhythmias, severe cardiomyopathy or congestive heart failure.

Septic shock occurs as a result of circulatory insufficiency associated with overwhelming infection.

Obstructive shock occurs when obstruction to blood flow results in inadequate tissue perfusion. Massive pulmonary embolism, pericardial tamponade, restrictive pericarditis, and severe cardiac valve dysfunction can reduce blood flow enough to produce shock.

Neurogenic shock is an uncommon form of shock which occurs as a result of blockade of neurohumoral outflow. The neurohumoral blockade may be induced by pharmacologic agents (eg, spinal anesthesia) or by direct injury to the spinal cord.

Other causes of shock include anaphylaxis, hypoglycemia, hypothyroidism and hypoadrenalism (ie, Addison's disease).

Management of shock is aimed at providing basic life support (airway, breathing and circulation) while attempting to correct the underlying cause. Antibiotics, inotropes, hormones (eg, insulin, thyroid) and other agents may be used to treat the underlying disease states in the shock patient. However, initial pharmacologic interventions are primarily aimed at supporting the circulation.

Blood pressure is a function of the peripheral vascular resistance and the cardiac output. Cardiac output is determined by the heart rate and stroke volume. The stroke volume is a function of the contractile state of the heart and the volume of blood in the ventricle available to be pumped out (ie, preload). Manipulation of any of these parameters can produce a change in blood pressure.

VASOPRESSORS USED IN SHOCK

Fluids – Relative or absolute volume depletion occurs in most shock states, especially in the early or "warm" phase in which vasodilation is prominent. Adequate volume repletion is necessary to maintain cardiac output, urine flow, and the integrity of the microcirculation. Attempts to support the circulation with vasopressors or inotropes will be unsuccessful if the intravascular volume is depleted.

The choice of fluids is probably irrelevant in the early stages. Although whole blood might be preferred for the patient with hemorrhagic shock, the delay in availability of blood products often negates any advantage. There is no clear superiority of crystalloids or colloids in emergency fluid resuscitation. Hydroxyethyl starch and the dextrans are also suitable plasma volume expanders.

Vasopressors – Sympathomimetic agents are used in shock to treat hypoperfusion in normovolemic patients and in patients unresponsive to whole blood or plasma volume expanders. These agents increase myocardial contractility, constrict capacitance vessels and dilate resistance vessels. In cardiogenic shock or advanced shock from other causes associated with a low cardiac output, they may be combined with vasodilators (eg, nitroprusside or nitroglycerin) to maintain blood pressure while the vasodilator improves myocardial performance. Nitroprusside is used to reduce preload and afterload and improve cardiac output. Nitroglycerin directly relaxes the venous vasculature and decreases preload.

Pharmacology – Sympathomimetic agents produce α-adrenergic stimulation (vasoconstriction), β_1-adrenergic stimulation (increase myocardial contractility, heart rate, automaticity and AV conduction), and β_2-adrenergic activity (peripheral vasodilation). Dopamine also causes vasodilation of the renal and mesenteric, cerebral and coronary beds by dopaminergic receptor activation. Adrenergic agents are useful in improving hemodynamic status by improving myocardial contractility and increasing heart rate, which results in increased cardiac output. Peripheral resistance is increased by vasoconstriction. Increased cardiac output and increased peripheral resistance increase blood pressure. The relative activity and predominance of these actions result in a number of hemodynamic responses which may affect coronary perfusion, renal perfusion, cardiac output, total peripheral resistance and blood pressure. These actions are summarized in the Sites of Action/Hemodynamic Response table. The actual response of an individual patient will depend largely on clinical status at time of administration.

Other drugs – A number of other drug classes have been used as supportive therapy in shock patients. However, with the exception of vasodilator treatment of cardiogenic shock, none of these treatments appear superior to vasopressor therapy. These drugs include: Opiate antagonists, prostaglandin inhibitors, corticosteroids and thyrotropin-releasing hormone.

Monitoring shock patients and their response to drugs requires special vigilance. Monitor heart rate, blood pressure and ECG continuously. Record urine output and fluid intake frequently. Due to rapid and life-threatening changes that can occur in the hemodynamically unstable patient, optimal drug selection, dose titration and management is probably best achieved with the use of invasive hemodynamic monitoring. Monitoring of central venous pressures via a central venous catheter will provide an estimation of the patient's fluid status by approximating the diastolic pressure of the right ventricle. When warranted, additional hemodynamic data can be obtained through the use of a pulmonary artery catheter (ie, Swan-Ganz). Changes in the pulmonary artery wedge pressure (a measure of left ventricular end diastolic volume), cardiac output and peripheral vascular resistance can be monitored and therapy adjusted accordingly.

Administration should only be via the IV route using a large-bore, free flowing IV in the antecubital vein or a central vein due to unpredictable absorption. Small IVs in the extremities are both unreliable and unsafe for vasopressor administration. Frequent monitoring of the IV sites for extravasation injury is essential when vasopressor agents are being used.

Prolonged, high-dose therapy can produce cyanosis and tissue necrosis of distal extremities. The principle of using the lowest dose which produces an adequate response for the shortest period of time is very important when using these agents.

Plasma volume depletion – Prolonged use of vasopressors may result in plasma volume depletion; this should be corrected by appropriate fluid and electrolyte replacement therapy. If plasma volumes are not corrected, hypotension may recur when these drugs are discontinued. Blood pressure may be maintained at the risk of severe peripheral vasoconstriction with diminution in blood flow and tissue perfusion.

Acidosis lessens the response to vasopressors; therefore, correct acidosis if it exists or develops during the course of vasopressor therapy.

Avoid continuous IV therapy – Acute tolerance develops during continuous IV administration. High concentration/low volume (250 ml) vasopressor solutions administered with the aid of an infusion control device allows for maximum dosing flexibility since fluids and drugs can be regulated independently, and the development of tolerance is minimized.

VASOPRESSORS USED IN SHOCK

Effects of Vasopressors Used in Shock

+++ *pronounced effect*
++ *moderate effect*
+ *slight effect*
0 *no effect*
↑ *increase*
↓ *decrease*

		SITES OF ACTION				HEMODYNAMIC RESPONSE			
		HEART		BLOOD VESSELS					
		Contractility (Inotropic) β_1	SA Node Rate (Chronotropic) β_1	Vasoconstriction α	Vasodilatation β_2	Renal Perfusion	Cardiac Output	tal Peripheral Resistance	Blood Pressure
Inotropic	Isoproterenol	+++	+++	0	+++	↑[1] or ↓[2]	↑	↓	↑[3]↓[4]
	Dobutamine	+++	0 to +[5]	0 to +[5]	+	0	↑	↓	↑
	Dopamine	+++	+ to ++[5]	+ to +++[5]	0 to +[6]	↑[5]	↑	↓[5] or ↑	0 to ↑
Mixed	Epinephrine	+++	+++	+++[5]	++[5]	↓	↑	↓	↑[3]↓[4]
	Norepinephrine	++	++[7]	+++	0	↓	0 or ↓	↑	↑
	Ephedrine	++	++	+	0 to +	↓	↑	↑ or ↓	↑
	Mephentermine	+	+	+	++	↑ or ↓	↑	0 to ↑	↑
Pressors	Metaraminol	+	+	++	0	↓	↓	↑	↑
	Methoxamine	0	0[7]	+++	0	↓	0 or ↓	↑	↑
	Phenylephrine	0	0[7]	+++	0	↓	↓	↑	↑

[1] Cardiogenic or septicemic shock.
[2] Normotensive patient.
[3] Systolic effect.
[4] Diastolic effect.
[5] Effects are dose dependent.
[6] Dilates renal and splanchnic beds via dopaminergic effect at doses < 10 mcg/kg/min.
[7] Decreased heart rate may result from reflex mechanisms.

Common Dilutions and Infusion Rates for Selected Drugs Used in Shock

Drug	Usual Dilution for IV Infusion	Infusion Rate
Isoproterenol	2 mg (10 ml) in 500 ml D5W (4 mcg/ml) or 1 mg (5 ml) in 250 ml D5W	5 mcg/min
Dobutamine	250 mg in 250 to 500 ml NS or D5W (500 to 1000 mcg/ml)	2.5 to 15 mcg/kg/min
Dopamine	200 to 800 mg in 250 to 500 ml NS or D5W (400 to 3200 mcg/ml)	Low dose – 2.5 to 10 mcg/kg/min High dose – 20 to 50 mcg/kg/min
Norepinephrine	4 mg in 250 ml of D5W (16 mcg/ml)	Initial: 8 to 12 mcg/min Maintenance: 2 to 4 mcg/min

ISOPROTERENOL HCl

Refer to the general discussion of these products in the Vasopressors Used in Shock group monograph.

Actions:

Pharmacology: Isoproterenol has $beta_1$ and $beta_2$ adrenergic receptor activity. Primary actions are on the beta receptors of the heart and smooth muscle of the bronchi, skeletal muscle and vasculature and alimentary tract. Isoproterenol relaxes most smooth muscles, with the most pronounced effect on the bronchial and GI smooth muscle. It produces marked relaxation in the smaller bronchi and may even dilate the trachea and main bronchi past the resting diameter.

Hemodynamics – The positive inotropic and chronotropic actions of the drug increase minute blood flow. There is an increase in heart rate, an approximately unchanged stroke volume, and an increase in ejection velocity. The rate of discharge of cardiac pacemakers is increased with isoproterenol injection. Venous return to the heart is increased through a decreased compliance of the venous bed. Systemic resistance and pulmonary vascular resistance are decreased, and there is an increase in coronary and renal blood flow. Systolic blood pressure may increase and diastolic blood pressure may decrease. Mean arterial blood pressure is usually unchanged or reduced. The peripheral and coronary vasodilating effects of the drug may aid tissue perfusion.

Pharmacokinetics: Onset of activity is immediate after IV administration; duration is brief, 1 to 2 hours and < 1 hour, respectively.

Indications:

Hypovolemic and septic shock: As an adjunct to fluid and electrolyte replacement therapy and the use of other drugs and procedures in the treatment of hypovolemic and septic shock, low cardiac output (hypoperfusion) states, congestive heart failure and cardiogenic shock.

Heart block and Adams-Stokes attacks: For mild or transient episodes of heart block that do not require electric shock or pacemaker therapy.

For serious episodes of heart block and Adams-Stokes attacks (except when caused by ventricular tachycardia or fibrillation).

Cardiac arrest: For use in cardiac arrest until electric shock or pacemaker therapy, the treatments of choice, are available

Bronchospasm occurring during anesthesia.

Contraindications:

Tachyarrhythmias; tachycardia or heart block caused by digitalis intoxication; ventricular arrhythmias which require inotropic therapy; angina pectoris.

Warnings:

Cardiogenic shock: Isoproterenol injection, by increasing myocardial oxygen requirements while decreasing effective coronary perfusion, may have a deleterious effect on the injured or failing heart. Its use as the initial agent in treating cardiogenic shock following myocardial infarction is discouraged. However, when a low arterial pressure has been elevated by other means, isoproterenol hydrochloride injection may produce beneficial hemodynamic and metabolic effects.

Heart block: In a few patients, presumably with organic disease of the AV node and its branches, isoproterenol has paradoxically worsened heart block or precipitated Adams-Stokes attacks during normal sinus rhythm or transient heart block.

Pregnancy: Category C. It is not known whether isoproterenol can cause fetal harm when administered to a pregnant woman or can affect reproduction capacity. Use only when needed and when benefits outweigh potential hazards to the fetus.

Lactation: It is not known whether isoproterenol is excreted in breast milk. Exercise caution when administering to a nursing woman.

Precautions:

Hypovolemia: Use is not a substitute for the replacement of blood, plasma, fluids and electrolytes, which should be restored promptly when loss has occurred. Hypovolemia should be corrected by suitable volume expanders before treatment with isoproterenol. Adequate filling of the intravascular compartment by suitable volume expanders is of primary importance in most cases of shock, and should precede the administration of vasoactive drugs. In patients with normal cardiac function, determination of central venous pressure is a reliable guide during volume replacement. If evidence of hypoperfusion persists after adequate volume replacement, give isoproterenol injection. Monitor systemic blood pressure, heart rate, urine flow, ECG; also monitor response to therapy by frequent determination of central venous pressure and blood gases. Closely observe patients in shock during administration.

ISOPROTERENOL HCl

Cardiovascular disorders: Use with caution in patients with coronary artery disease, coronary insufficiency, diabetes or hyperthyroidism and in patients sensitive to sympathomimetic amines.

Cardiac effects: If heart rate exceeds 110 beats/min, it may be advisable to decrease the infusion rate or temporarily discontinue the infusion. Determinations of cardiac output and circulation time may also be helpful. Take appropriate measures to ensure adequate ventilation. Pay careful attention to acid-base balance and to correction of electrolyte disturbances. In cases of shock associated with bacteremia, suitable antimicrobial therapy is, of course, imperative. Doses sufficient to increase heart rate to more than 130 beats/min may induce ventricular arrhythmia. Such increases in heart rate will also tend to increase cardiac work and oxygen requirements which may adversely affect the failing heart or the heart with a significant degree of arteriosclerosis. If precordial distress or anginal-type pain occurs, discontinue the drug immediately.

Sulfite sensitivity: Some of these products contain sulfites which may cause allergic-type reactions including anaphylactic symptoms and life-threatening or less severe asthmatic episodes in certain susceptible persons. The overall prevalence of sulfite sensitivity in the general population is unknown and probably low. Sulfite sensitivity is seen more frequently in asthmatic or atopic nonasthmatic persons.

Drug Interactions:

Isoproterenol Drug Interactions

Precipitant drug	Object drug *		Description
Bretylium	Isoproterenol	↑	Bretylium potentiates the action of vasopressors on adrenergic receptors, possibly resulting in arrhythmias.
Guanethidine	Isoproterenol	↑	Guanethidine may increase the pressor response of the direct-acting vasopressors, possibly resulting in severe hypertension.
Halogenated hydrocarbon anesthetics	Isoproterenol	↑	Halogenated hydrocarbon anesthetics may sensitize the myocardium to the effects of catecholamines. Use of vasopressors may lead to serious arrhythmias; use with caution.
Oxytocic drugs	Isoproterenol	↑	In obstetrics, if vasopressor drugs are used either to correct hypotension or added to the local anesthetic solution, some oxytocic drugs may cause severe persistent hypertension.
Tricyclic antidepressants	Isoproterenol	↑	The pressor response of the direct-acting vasopressors may be potentiated by these agents; use with caution.

* ↑ = Object drug increased.

Adverse Reactions:

Cardiovascular: Tachycardia; palpitations; hypertension; hypotension; ventricular arrhythmias; tachyarrhythmias; precordial distress; angina.

CNS: Flushing of the skin; sweating; mild tremors; nervousness; headache; dizziness; weakness.

GI: Nausea; vomiting.

Overdosage:

Symptoms: Excessive doses in animals or man may result in cardiac enlargement and focal myocarditis. Cases of accidental overdosage are evidenced by tachycardia or other arrhythmias, palpitations, angina, hypotension or hypertension.

Treatment: Reduce rate of administration or discontinue isoproterenol until patient's condition stabilizes. Monitor blood pressure, pulse, respiration and EKG.

Administration and Dosage:

Parenteral: Start isoproterenol 1:50,000 at the lowest recommended dose and gradually increase rate of administration while carefully monitoring the patient.

The usual route of administration is by IV injection or infusion. In an emergency, administer the drug by intracardiac injection. If time is not of utmost importance, initial therapy by IM or SC injection may be used. See Dosage for Adults with Heart Block, Adams-Stokes Attacks and Cardiac Arrest chart below.

There are no well controlled studies in children to establish appropriate dosing; however, the American Heart Association recommends an initial infusion rate of 0.1 mcg/kg/min, with the usual range being 0.1 mcg/kg/min to 1 mcg/kg/min.

ISOPROTERENOL HCl

Dosage for Adults with Heart Block, Adams - Stokes Attacks and Cardiac Arrest			
Route	Dilution	Initial Dose	Subsequent Dose Range
IV injection	Dilute 1 ml of 1:5000 solution (0.2mg) to 10 ml with Sodium Chloride or 5% Dextrose Injection	0.02 to 0.06 mg (1 to 3 ml of diluted solution)	0.01 to 0.2 mg (0.5 to 10 ml of diluted solution)
IV infusion	Dilute 10 ml of 1:5000 solution (2mg) in 500 ml of D5W or dilute 5ml of 1:5000 solution (1 mg) in 250 ml of D5W	5 mcg/min (1.25 ml/min of diluted solution)	
IM	Undiluted 1:5000 solution	0.2 mg (1 ml)	0.02 to 1 mg (0.1 to 5 ml)
SC	Undiluted 1:5000 solution	0.2 mg (1 ml)	0.15 to 0.2 mg (0.75 to 1 ml)
Intracardiac	Undiluted 1:5000 solution	0.02 mg (0.1 ml)	

Storage/Stability: Store at room temperature 15° to 30°C (59° to 86°F). Protect from light. Do not use if solution is pinkish to brownish in color.

Rx	**Isoproterenol** (Various, eg, Abbott)	**Injection**: 1:5000 solution (0.2 mg per ml)[1]	In 5 and 10 ml vials.
Rx	**Isuprel** (Sanofi Winthrop)		In 1 and 5 ml amps.
Rx	**Isuprel** (Sanofi Winthrop)	**Injection**: 1:50,000 (0.02 mg/ml)[1]	In 10 ml w/needle.

[1] With sodium metabisulfite.

DOBUTAMINE

Refer to the general discussion of these products in the Vasopressors Used in Shock group monograph.

Actions:

Pharmacology: Dobutamine is chemically related to dopamine. Its primary activity results from stimulation of the $beta_1$ receptors of the heart while producing comparatively mild chronotropic, hypertensive, arrhythmogenic and vasodilative effects. It has minor $alpha_1$ (vasoconstrictor) and $beta_2$ (vasodilator) effects. It does not cause the release of endogenous norepinephrine, as does dopamine.

Hemodynamics – In patients with depressed cardiac function, both dobutamine and isoproterenol increase the cardiac output to a similar degree. With dobutamine, this increase is usually not accompanied by marked increases in heart rate (although tachycardia is occasionally observed), and the cardiac stroke volume is usually increased. In contrast, isoproterenol increases the cardiac index primarily by increasing the heart rate while stroke volume changes little or declines. Dobutamine produces less increase in heart rate and less decrease in peripheral vascular resistance for a given inotropic effect than does isoproterenol.

Facilitation of atrioventricular conduction has been observed in human electrophysiologic studies and in patients with atrial fibrillation.

Systemic vascular resistance is usually decreased; occasionally, minimal vasoconstriction has been observed.

Pharmacokinetics:

Metabolism/Excretion – routes of metabolism are methylation of the catechol and conjugation. The plasma half-life of dobutamine is two minutes. In urine, the major excretion products are the conjugates of dobutamine and the inactive 3–O–methyl dobutamine.

Onset: The onset of action is within 1 to 2 minutes; however, as much as 10 minutes may be required to obtain the peak effect of a particular infusion rate.

Clinical trials: Most clinical experience with dobutamine is short-term, up to several hours in duration. In the limited number of patients who were studied for 24, 48 and 72 hours, a persistent increase in cardiac output occurred in some, whereas the output of others returned toward baseline values.

Alteration of synaptic concentrations of catecholamines with either reserpine or tricyclic antidepressants does not alter the actions of dobutamine in animals, which indicates that the actions of dobutamine are not dependent on presynaptic mechanisms.

Indications:

Cardiac decompensation: Inotropic support in the short-term treatment of adults with cardiac decompensation due to depressed contractility, resulting either from organic heart disease or from cardiac surgical procedures.

In patients who have atrial fibrillation with rapid ventricular response, use a digitalis preparation prior to instituting therapy with dobutamine.

Unlabeled uses: Doses of dobutamine 2 and 7.75 mcg/kg/min infused for 10 minutes each have been used investigationally in 12 children with congenital heart disease undergoing diagnostic cardiac catheterization. The drug appears effective in augmenting cardiovascular function in children, and no adverse effects were noted.

Contraindications:

Idiopathic hypertrophic subaortic stenosis (IHSS); hypersensitivity to dobutamine.

Warnings:

Increase in heart rate or blood pressure: Dobutamine may cause a marked increase in heart rate or blood pressure, especially systolic pressure. Approximately 10% of patients in clinical studies have had rate increases of 30 beats/min or more, and about 7.5% have had a ≥ 50 mmHg increase in systolic pressure. Usually, reduction of dosage promptly reverses these effects. Because the drug facilitates atrioventricular conduction, patients with atrial fibrillation are at risk of developing rapid ventricular response. Patients with preexisting hypertension appear to face an increased risk of developing an exaggerated pressor response.

Hypotension: Precipitous decreases in blood pressure have occasionally been described in association with dobutamine therapy. Decreasing the dose or discontinuing the infusion typically results in rapid return of blood pressure to baseline values. However, in rare cases, intervention may be required and reversibility may not be immediate.

Ectopic activity: Dobutamine may precipitate or exacerbate ventricular ectopic activity, but it rarely has caused ventricular tachycardia.

Hypersensitivity reactions, including skin rash, pruritus of the scalp, fever, eosinophilia and bronchospasm, may occur occasionally with dobutamine.

DOBUTAMINE

Long-term safety: Infusions of up to 72 hours have revealed no adverse effects other than those seen with infusions of shorter duration.

Pregnancy: Category B. Dobutamine has not been administered to pregnant women; use only when clearly needed and when the potential benefits outweigh the potential hazards to the fetus.

Children: Safety and efficacy for use in children have not been established.

Precautions:

Monitoring: Continuously monitor ECG and blood pressure. Monitor pulmonary wedge pressure and cardiac output whenever possible.

Hypovolemia: Use is not a substitute for the replacement of blood, plasma, fluids and electrolytes, which should be restored promptly when loss has occurred.

Correct hypovolemia with suitable volume expanders before treatment is instituted.

Ineffective in the presence of marked mechanical obstruction, such as severe valvular aortic stenosis.

Usage following acute myocardial infarction: Clinical experience following myocardial infarction has been insufficient to establish the safety of the drug for this use. Any agent that increases contractile force and heart rate may increase the size of an infarction by intensifying ischemia.

Sulfite sensitivity: This product contains sulfites which may cause allergic-type reactions including anaphylactic symptoms and life-threatening or less severe asthmatic episodes in certain susceptible persons. The overall prevalence of sulfite sensitivity in the general population is unknown and probably low. Sulfite sensitivity is seen more frequently in asthmatic or atopic nonasthmatic persons.

Drug Interactions:

Dobutamine Drug Interactions			
Precipitant drug	Object drug*		Description
Bretylium	Dobutamine	⬆	Bretylium may potentiate the action of vasopressors on adrenergic receptors, possibly resulting in arrhythmias.
Guanethidine	Dobutamine	⬆	Guanethidine may increase the pressor response of the direct-acting vasopressors, possibly resulting in severe hypertension.
Halogenated hydrocarbon anesthetics	Dobutamine	⬆	Halogenated hydrocarbon anesthetics may sensitize the myocardium to the effects of catecholamines. Use of vasopressors may lead to serious arrhythmias; use with extreme caution.
Oxytocic drugs	Dobutamine	⬆	In obstetrics, if vasopressor drugs are used either to correct hypotension or added to local anesthetic solutions, some oxytocic drugs may cause severe persistent hypertension.
Tricyclic antidepressants	Dobutamine	⬆	The pressor response of the direct-acting vasopressors may be potentiated by these agents; use with caution.

* ⬆ = Object drug increased.

Adverse Reactions:

Cardiovascular: Increased heart rate, blood pressure, ventricular ectopic activity (see Warnings); hypotension; premature ventricular beats (≈ 5%; dose-related).

Reactions at injection site: Phlebitis has occurred occasionally, and local inflammatory changes have occurred following inadvertent infiltration.

Miscellaneous (uncommon, 1% to 3%): Nausea; headache; anginal pain; nonspecific chest pain; palpitations; shortness of breath.

DOBUTAMINE

Overdosage:

Symptoms: Excessive alteration of blood pressure, anorexia, nausea, vomiting, tremore, anxiety, palpitations, headache, shortness of breath, anginal and nonspecific chest pain, myocardial ischemia, ventricular fibrillation or tachycardia

Treatment: Reduce the rate of administration or temporarily discontinue until condition stabilizes. Establish an airway and ensure oxygenation and ventilation. Initiate resuscitative measures promptly. Severe ventricular tachyarrhythmias may be successfully treated with propranolol or lidocaine.

Administration and Dosage:

Rate of administration: The rate of infusion needed to increase cardiac output usually ranges from 2.5 to 10mcg/kg/min. On rare occasions, infusion rates up to 40mcg/kg/min have been required. A metering device is recommended for controlling the rate of drug administration.

Adjust the rate of administration and the duration of therapy according to patient response, as determined by heart rate, presence of ectopic activity, blood pressure, urine flow, and, whenever possible, measurement of central venous or pulmonary wedge pressure and cardiac output.

Concentrations up to 5000 mcg/ml have been administered (250 mg/50 ml). Determine the final volume administered by the fluid requirements of the patient.

Infusion Rates of Various Dilutions of Dobutamine

Desired Delivery Rate (mcg/kg/min)	Infusion Rate (ml/kg/min)		
	250 mcg/ml	500 mcg/ml	1000 mcg/ml
2.5	0.01	0.005	0.0025
5	0.02	0.01	0.005
7.5	0.03	0.015	0.0075
10	0.04	0.02	0.01
12.5	0.05	0.025	0.0125
15	0.06	0.03	0.015

Admixture incompatibility: Incompatible with alkaline solutions; do not mix with products such as 5% Sodium Bicarbonate Injection. Do not use dobutamine in conjunction with other agents or diluents containing both sodium bisulfite and ethanol. Dobutamine is also physically incompatible with hydrocortisone sodium succinate; cefazolin; cefamandole; neutral cephalothin; penicillin; sodium ethacrynate; sodium heparin.

Admixture compatibility: Dobutamine is compatible when administered through common tubing with dopamine, lidocaine, tobramycin, verapamil, nitroprusside, potassium chloride and protamine sulfate.

Preparation of solution: Reconstituted solution must be further diluted to at least 50 ml prior to administration in 5% Dextrose Injection, 5% Dextrose and 0.45% Sodium Chloride Injection, 5% Dextrose and 0.9% Sodium Chloride Injection, 10% Dextrose Injection, *Isolyte M* with 5% Dextrose Injection, Lactated Ringer's Injection, 5% Dextrose in Lactated Ringer's Injection, *Normosol-M* in D5-W, 20% *Osmitrol* in Water for Injection, 0.9% Sodium Chloride Injection or Sodium Lactate Injection.

Freezing is not recommended due to possible crystallization.

Storage/Stability – Store at room temperature 15°to 30°C (59° to 86°F). After dilution (in glass or Viaflex containers), the solution is stable for 24 hours at room temperature. Use IV solutions within 24 hours.Solutions containing dobutamine may exhibit a pink color that, if present, will increase with time. This color change is due to slight oxidation of the drug, but there is no significant loss of potency during the time periods stated above.

Rx	**Dobutamine HCl** (Various, eg, Abbott, Steris)	**Injection:** 12.5 mg/ml	May contain sulfites. In 20 ml vials.
Rx	**Dobutrex** (Lilly)		In 20 ml vials.[1]

[1] With 0.24 mg sodium bisulfite.

DOPAMINE HCl

Refer to the general discussion of these products in the Vasopressors Used in Shock group monograph.

Actions:

Pharmacology: Dopamine is an endogenous catecholamine and a precursor of norepinephrine. It acts both directly and indirectly (releases norepinephrine stores) on alpha and $beta_1$ receptors and has dopaminergic effects.

$Beta_1$ actions produce an inotropic effect on the myocardium resulting in increased cardiac output. Dopamine causes less increase in myocardial oxygen consumption than isoproterenol and is usually not associated with a tachyarrhythmia. Systolic and pulse pressure usually increases with either no effect or a slight increase in diastolic pressure.

Total peripheral resistance (α effects) at low and intermediate therapeutic doses is usually unchanged. Blood flow to peripheral vascular beds may decrease while mesenteric flow increases. Dopamine dilates the renal and mesenteric vasculature presumptively by activation of a dopaminergic receptor. This action is accompanied by increases in GFR, renal blood flow, and sodium excretion. An increase in urinary output produced by dopamine is usually not associated with a decrease in osmolality of the urine. The dopaminergic effect is overridden by alpha-adrenergic activity at higher doses of dopamine (> 10 mcg/kg/min).

Organ perfusion – Urine flow appears to be one of the better monitoring parameters of vital organ perfusion. Also, observe the patient for signs of reversal of confusion or comatose condition. Loss of pallor, increase in toe temperature or adequacy of nail bed capillary filling may also be used as indices of adequate dosage.

Renal function – When dopamine is given before urine flow has decreased to levels $\approx$ 0.3 ml/minute, prognosis is more favorable. Nevertheless, in oliguric or anuric patients, administration has resulted in an increase in urine flow which has reached normal levels. Dopamine may also increase urine flow in patients whose output is within normal limits, thus reducing preexisting fluid accumulation. Above those optimal doses, urine flow may decrease, necessitating dosage reduction. Coadministration of dopamine and diuretic agents may produce an additive or potentiating effect.

Cardiac output – Increased cardiac output is related to dopamine's direct inotropic effect on the myocardium, and at low or moderate doses appears to be related to a favorable prognosis. Increase in cardiac output has been associated with either static or decreased systemic vascular resistance (SVR). Low or moderate increments in cardiac output is believed to be a reflection of differential effects on specific vascular beds, with increased resistance in peripheral vascular beds (eg, femoral) and concomitant decreases in mesenteric and renal vascular beds. Redistribution of blood flow parallels these changes so that an increase in cardiac output is accompanied by an increase in mesenteric and renal blood flow; often the renal fraction of the total cardiac output has been found to increase. Increase in cardiac output produced by dopamine is not associated with substantial decreases in SVR.

Blood pressure – Manage hypotension due to inadequate cardiac output with low to moderate doses, which have little effect on SVR. At high doses, alpha-adrenergic activity is more prominent and may correct hypotension due to diminished SVR.

Prognosis is better in patients whose blood pressure and urine flow have not undergone extreme deterioration. Administer dopamine as soon as a definite trend toward decreased systolic and diastolic pressure becomes apparent.

Pharmacokinetics:

Absorption/Distribution – Dopamine has an onset of action within 5 minutes, a plasma half-life of $\approx$ 2 minutes and a duration of action of less than 10 minutes. The drug is widely distributed in the body but does not cross the blood-brain barrier.

Metabolism/Excretion – Dopamine is metabolized in the liver, kidney and plasma by MAO and catechol-O-methyltransferase to inactive compounds. About 25% is taken up into specialized neurosecretory vesicles (the adrenergic nerve terminals), where it is hydroxylated to form norepinephrine. About 80% is excreted in the urine within 24 hours, primarily as HVA and its sulfate and glucuronide conjugates and as 3,4-dihydroxy-phenylacetic acid. A small portion is excreted unchanged.

Indications:

Hemodynamic imbalances: Correction of hemodynamic imbalances in shock syndrome due to myocardial infarction, trauma, endotoxic septicemia, open heart surgery, renal failure, and chronic cardiac decompensation as in congestive failure.

Patients most likely to respond adequately are those in whom physiological parameters such as urine flow, myocardial function and blood pressure have not profoundly deteriorated. The shorter the time between onset of signs and symptoms of shock and initiation of therapy with volume correction and dopamine, the better the prognosis.

DOPAMINE HCl

Unlabeled uses: Chronic obstructive pulmonary disease (COPD) (4 mcg/kg/min): congestive heart failure (CHF) (2 to 5 mcg/kg/min); respiratory distress syndrome (RDS) in infants (starting at 5 mcg/kg/min).

Contraindications:

Pheochromocytoma; uncorrected tachyarrhythmias or ventricular fibrillation.

Warnings:

Polyuria: Doses ≤ 3 mcg/kg/min have been shown to improve kidney function.

Pregnancy: Category C. Animal studies have revealed no evidence of teratogenic effects. In one study, administration of dopamine to pregnant rats resulted in a decreased survival rate of the newborn and a potential for cataract formation in the survivors. There are no adequate and well-controlled studies in pregnant women and it is not known if dopamine crosses the placental barrier. The drug may be used in pregnant women when the expected benefits outweigh the potential risk to the fetus.

Lactation: It is not known whether this drug is excreted in breast milk. Because many drugs are excreted in breast milk, exercise caution when administering to a nursing woman.

Children: Safety and efficacy for use in children have not been established. It has been used in a limited number of pediatric patients, but such use has been inadequate to fully define proper dosage and use.

Precautions:

Monitoring: Close monitoring of urine flow, cardiac output, pulmonary wedge pressure and blood pressure during infusion is necessary.

Hypovolemia: Prior to treatment with dopamine, correct hypovolemia with either whole blood or plasma as indicated. Monitoring of central venous pressure or left ventricular filling pressure may be helpful in detecting and treating hypovolemia.

Decreased pulse pressure: If a disproportionate rise in the diastolic pressure (a marked decrease in pulse pressure) is observed in patients receiving dopamine, decrease infusion rate and observe patient carefully for further evidence of predominant vasoconstriction, unless such an effect is desired.

Occlusive vascular disease: Closely monitor patients with a history of occlusive vascular disease (eg, arteriosclerosis, arterial embolism, Raynaud's disease, cold injury, frostbite, diabetic endarteritis, and Buerger's disease) for any changes in color or temperature of the skin of the extremities. If a change occurs and is thought to be the result of compromised circulation to the extremities, weigh the benefits of continued dopamine infusion against the risk of possible necrosis. This condition may be reversed by either decreasing the rate of infusion or discontinuing the drug.

Extravasation: Infuse into a large vein to prevent extravasation. Extravasation may cause necrosis and sloughing of surrounding tissue. Large veins of the antecubital fossa are preferred to veins in the hand or ankle. Monitor the infusion site closely for free flow.

Antidote for extravasation – To prevent sloughing and necrosis in ischemic areas, infiltrate area as soon as possible with 10 to 15 ml 0.9% Sodium Chloride solution containing 5 to 10 mg phentolamine. Use a syringe with a fine hypodermic needle and infiltrate liberally throughout the ischemic area. Sympathetic blockade with phentolamine causes immediate and conspicuous local hyperemic changes if the area is infiltrated within 12 hours.

Discontinuation: When discontinuing the infusion, gradually decrease the dose of dopamine, since sudden cessation may result in marked hypotension.

Sulfite sensitivity: Some of these products contain sulfites that may cause allergic-type reactions including anaphylactic symptoms and life-threatening or less severe asthmatic episodes in certain susceptible persons. The overall prevalence of sulfite sensitivity in the general population is unknown and probably low. It is seen more frequently in asthmatic or atopic nonasthmatic persons.

DOPAMINE HCl

Drug Interactions:

Dopamine Drug Interactions			
Precipitant drug	Object drug*		Description
Dopamine	Guanethidine	↓	The antihypertensive effects of guanethidine may be partially or totally reversed by the mixed-acting sympathomimetics.
Halogenated hydrocarbon anesthetics	Dopamine	↑	Halogenated hydrocarbon anestheticsmay sensitize the myocardium to the effects of catecholamines. Use of vasopressors may lead to serious arrhythmias; use with extreme caution.
Monoamine oxidase (MAO) inhibitors	Dopamine	↑	MAOIs increase the pressor response to dopamine by sixfold to twentyfold. Dopamine is metabolized by MAO, and inhibition of this enzyme prolongs and potentiates the effect of dopamine. This interaction may also occur with furazolidone, an antimicrobial with MAO inhibitor activity. Avoid these combinations; if given inadvertently and hypertension occurs, administer phentolamine.
Oxytocic drugs	Dopamine	↑	In obstetrics, if vasopressor drugs are used either to correct hypotension or are added to the local anesthetic solution, some oxytocics may cause severe persistent hypertension.
Dopamine	Phenytoin	↓	Concomitant infusion of dopamine has been reported to lead to seizures, severe hypotension and bradycardia. If necessary, discontinue phenytoin and provide supportive treatment.
Tricyclic antidepressants	Dopamine	↓	The pressor response of the mixed-acting vasopressors may be decreased by these agents; a higher dose of the sympathomimetic may be necessary.

* ↑ = Object drug increased. ↓ = Object drug decreased.

Adverse Reactions:

Most frequent: Ectopic beats; nausea and vomiting; tachycardia; anginal pain; palpitation; dyspnea; headache; hypotension; vasoconstriction.

Infrequent: Aberrant conduction; bradycardia; piloerection; widened QRS complex; azotemia; elevated pressure.

High doses may cause dilated pupils and ventricular arrhythmia.

Gangrene has occurred when high doses were administered for prolonged periods and in patients with occlusive vascular disease receiving low doses of dopamine. An isolated case of gangrene in a neonate has occurred.

Overdosage:

Symptoms: Accidental overdosage is manifested by excessive blood pressure elevation.

Treatment: Reduce rate of administration or temporarily discontinue until patient's condition is stabilized. Since duration of action is quite short, no additional remedial measures are usually necessary. If these measures fail to stabilize the patient's condition, consider using the short-acting alpha-adrenergic blocking agent, phentolamine.

Administration and Dosage:

This is a potent drug; dilute before use if not prediluted.

Rate of administration: After dilution, administer IV. A metering device is essential for controlling the rate of flow. Titrate each patient to the desired hemodynamic or renal response with dopamine. In titrating to the desired increase in systolic blood pressure, the optimum dosage rate for renal response may be exceeded, thus necessitating a reduction in rate after the hemodynamic condition is stabilized.

Administration at rates > 50 mcg/kg/min have been used safely in advanced circulatory decompensation states.

Suggested regimen: When appropriate, increase blood volume with whole blood or plasma until central venous pressure is 10 to 15 cm water, or pulmonary wedge pressure is 14 to 18 mm Hg.

DOPAMINE HCl

Begin administration of diluted solution at doses of 2 to 5 mcg/kg/min in patients likely to respond to modest increments of cardiac contractility and renal perfusion.

In more seriously ill patients, begin administration of diluted solution at doses of 5 mcg/kg/min and increase gradually using 5 to 10 mcg/kg/min increments, up to a rate of 20 to 50 mcg/kg/min, as needed. If doses in excess of 50 mcg/kg/min are required, check urine output frequently. If urine flow decreases in the absence of hypotension, consider reduction of dosage. More than 50% of patients are satisfactorily maintained on doses less than 20 mcg/kg/min. In patients who do not respond to these doses, additional increments may be employed.

Treatment of all patients requires constant evaluation of therapy in terms of the blood volume, augmentation of cardiac contractility, and distribution of peripheral perfusion. Pay particular attention to diminution of established urine flow rate, increasing tachycardia or development of new dysrhythmias.

As with all potent drugs, take care to avoid inadvertent administration of a bolus of drug.

Preparation of solution: Add 200 to 400 mg dopamine to 250 to 500 ml of one of the following IV solutions: Sodium Chloride Injection, 5% Dextrose Injection, 5% Dextrose and 0.9% Sodium Chloride Injection, 5% Dextrose and 0.45% Sodium Chloride Solution, 5% Dextrose and Lactated Ringer's Solution, Sodium Lactate (1/6 Molar) Injection, Lactated Ringer's Injection.

Admixture incompatibilities – Do not add to 5% Sodium Bicarbonate or other alkaline IV solutions, oxidizing agents or iron salts since the drug is inactivated in alkaline solution.

Storage/Stability – Protect from light. Do not use if solution is discolored. Store at room temperature, 15° to 30°C (59° to 86°F).

Stable for a minimum of 24 hours after dilution; however, dilute just prior to administration.

Rx	**Dopamine HCl** (Various eg, American Regent, Astra, ESI, SoloPak)	**Injection:** 40 mg /ml	In 5 ml amps, 5, 10 and 20 ml vials and 5 and 10 ml syringes.
Rx	**Dopamine HCl** (Abbott)		In 5 ml and 10 ml Pintop vials, Fliptop vials and additive syringes.[2]
Rx	**Intropin** (Faulding)		In 5 ml single dose vials.[3]
Rx	**Dopamine HCl** (Various, eg, American Regent, Astra, ESI, SoloPak)	**Injection:** 80 mg per ml	In 5 ml amps; 5 and 20 ml vials and 10 ml syringes.
Rx	**Dopamine HCl** (Abbott)		In 10 ml[2]
Rx	**Intropin** (Faulding)		In 5 ml (400 mg) amps, single dose vials and Rap-Add additive syringes.[3]
Rx	**Dopamine HCl** (Various)	**Injection:** 160 mg per ml	In 5 ml vials.
Rx	**Intropin** (Faulding)		In 5 ml (800 mg) single dose vials, 5 ml amps and Rap-Add additive syringes.[3]
Rx	**Dopamine HCl in 5% Dextrose** (Abbott)	**Injection:** 80 mg/100 ml (0.8 mg/ml)[1]	In 250 and 500 ml.
		160 mg/100 ml (1.6 mg/ml)[1]	In 250 and 500 ml.
		320 mg/100 ml (3.2 mg/ml)[1]	In 250 ml.

[1] With 50 mg sodium metabisulfite.
[2] With 9 mg sodium metabisulfite.
[3] With 1% sodium metabisulfite.

EPINEPHRINE

Refer to the general discussion of these products in the Vasopressors Used in Shock group monograph.

Actions:

Pharmacology: The actions of epinephrine resemble the effects of stimulation of adrenergic nerves. To a variable degree, it acts on both alpha and beta receptor sites of sympathetic effector cells. At usual doses, its most prominent actions are on the beta receptors of the heart and of vascular and other smooth muscle. However, at high doses, alpha adrenergic effects predominate. When given by rapid IV injection, epinephrine produces a rapid rise in blood pressure (mainly systolic); it produces direct stimulation of cardiac muscle, which increases the strength of ventricular contraction; it increases the heart rate; and it constricts the arterioles in the skin, mucosa and splanchnic areas of circulation.

Epinephrine relaxes the smooth muscle of the bronchi and iris and is a physiologic antagonist of histamine.

The drug also increases both blood sugar and liver glycogenolysis.

Blood pressure – When given by slow IV injection, epinephrine usually produces a moderate rise in systolic and a fall in diastolic pressure. Although some increase in pulse pressure occurs, there is usually no great elevation in mean blood pressure. Accordingly, the compensatory reflex mechanisms that cause a pronounced increase in blood pressure do not antagonize the direct cardiac actions of epinephrine as much as with catecholamines that have a predominant action on alpha receptors.

Total peripheral resistance at usually employed doses decreases by action of epinephrine on beta receptors of the skeletal muscle vasculature, and blood flow is thereby enhanced. Usually, this vasodilator effect predominates so that the modest rise in systolic pressure which follows slow injection or absorption is the result of direct cardiac stimulation and increase in cardiac output. After rapid IV injection or with high infusion rates, total peripheral resistance increases.

Pharmacokinetics: Epinephrine crosses the placenta but not the blood-brain barrier. Intravenous injection produces an immediate and intensified response. Following IV injection, epinephrine disappears rapidly from the blood stream. Given SC or IM, epinephrine has a rapid onset and short duration of action. Subcutaneous administration during asthmatic attacks may produce bronchodilation within 5 to 10 minutes, and maximal effects may occur within 20 minutes.

The drug becomes fixed in the tissues and is rapidly inactivated chiefly by enzymatic transformation to metanephrine or normetanephrine, either of which is subsequently conjugated and excreted in the urine in the form of sulfates and glucuronides. Either sequence results in the formation of 3-methoxy-4-hydroxymandelic acid (vanillyl-mandelic acid; VMA) which is also detectable in the urine.

Epinephrine is rapidly and systematically degraded in the liver and other tissues by the enzymes monoamine oxidase and catechol-O-methyltransferase. Virtually all of an injected dose can be accounted for by urinary excretion of inactive metabolites, including various deaminated and O-methylated metabolites and their sulfated and glucuronidated conjugates. The circulating epinephrine not accounted for by such mechanisms is deactivated by reuptake at synaptic receptor sites.

Indications:

IV: In acute attacks of ventricular standstill, apply physical measures first. When external cardiac compression and attempts to restore the circulation by electrical defibrillation or use of a pacemaker fail, intracardiac puncture and intramyocardial injection of epinephrine may be effective. However, this method of administration should only be employed as a last resort and by personnel skilled in intracardiac injection technique.

Treatment and prophylaxis of cardiac arrest and attacks of transitory atrioventricular (AV) heart block with syncopal seizures (Stokes-Adams syndrome).

Epinephrine is also used as a hemostatic agent, and to treat mucosal congestion of hay fever, rhinitis and acute sinusitis; to relieve bronchial asthmatic paroxysms; in syncope due to complete heart block or carotid sinus hypersensitivity; for symptomatic relief of serum sickness, urticaria and angioneurotic edema; for resuscitation in cardiac arrest following anesthetic accidents; in simple (open angle) glaucoma; for relaxation of uterine musculature and to inhibit uterine contractions; to prolong the action of intraspinal and local anesthetics; acute hypersensitivity (anaphylactoid reactions to drugs, animal serums, insect stings and other allergens); treatment of acute asthmatic attacks to relieve bronchospasm not controlled by inhalation or SC administration of other solutions of the drug.

EPINEPHRINE

Contraindications:

Hypersensitivity to the drug or any component. Narrow-angle (congestive) glaucoma; shock (nonanaphylactic); during general anesthesia with halogenated hydrocarbons or cyclopropane; individuals with cerebral arteriosclerosis or organic brain damage; with local anesthesia of certain areas (eg, fingers, toes) because of the danger of vasoconstriction producing sloughing of tissue; in labor because it may delay the second stage; in cardiac dilatation and coronary insufficiency; to counteract circulatory collapse or hypotension due to phenothiazines, since such agents may reverse the pressor effect of epinephrine, leading to a further lowering of blood pressure.

Warnings:

Use with caution in the following: Elderly patients; cardiovascular disease; hypertension; diabetes; hyperthyroidism; psychoneurotic individuals; bronchial asthma and emphysema with degenerative heart disease; thyrotoxicosis.

Cardiovascular effects: Inadvertently induced high arterial blood pressure may result in angina pectoris (especially when coronary insufficiency is present), or aortic rupture.

Epinephrine may induce potentially serious cardiac arrhythmias in patients not suffering from heart disease. In patients with organic heart disease or who are receiving drugs that sensitize the myocardium, arrhythmias, including fatal ventricular fibrillation may occur. Closely monitor patients. Epinephrine causes changes in the ECG, even in normal patients, including a decrease in amplitude of the T-wave.

Cerebrovascular hemorrhage may occur from overdosage or inadvertent IV injection of epinephrine resulting from the sharp rise in blood pressure.

Injection: Epinephrine solution, alone or in combination with other drugs, must be injected in areas of limited or compromised blood supply only after carefully weighing the potential advantages and risks, including the possibility of vasoconstriction-induced sloughing of tissue. Epinephrine must be administered with great caution and in carefully circumscribed quantities in areas of the body served by end arteries or with otherwise limited blood supply (eg, fingers, toes, nose, ears, genitals, etc) or if peripheral vascular disease is present.

Pulmonary edema may result in fatalities because of the peripheral constriction and cardiac stimulation produced.

Renal function impairment: Initially, epinephrine administered parenterally may produce constriction of renal blood vessels and decrease urine formation.

Pregnancy: Category C. Epinephrine is teratogenic in small animals when given in doses about 25 times the human dose. Epinephrine crosses the placenta. Use during pregnancy may cause anoxia. There are no adequate and well controlled studies in pregnant women. Use during pregnancy only if the potential benefit justifies the potential risk to the fetus.

Labor and delivery – Parenteral administration of epinephrine, if used to support blood pressure during low or other spinal anesthesia for delivery, can cause acceleration of fetal heart rate and should not be used in obstetrics when maternal blood pressure exceeds 130/80 mm Hg. If administered during labor, epinephrine may delay the second stage. If administered in a dosage sufficiently high to reduce uterine contractions, it may cause prolonged uterine atony with hemorrhage.

Lactation: Epinephrine is excreted in breast milk. Because of the potential for serious adverse effects in nursing infants, decide whether to discontinue nursing or to discontinue the drug, taking into account the importance of the drug to the mother.

Children: Administer with caution to infants and children. Syncope has occurred following the administration of epinephrine to asthmatic children.

Precautions:

Fibrillation: Although epinephrine can produce ventricular fibrillation, its actions in restoring electrical activity in asystole and in enhancing defibrillation are well documented. However, use with caution in patients with ventricular fibrillation.

In patients with prefibrillatory rhythm, IV epinephrine must be used with extreme caution because of its excitatory action on the heart. Since the myocardium is sensitized to the drug by many anesthetic agents, epinephrine may convert asystole to ventricular fibrillation if used in the treatment of anesthetic cardiac accidents.

Diabetic patients receiving epinephrine may require an increase in dosage of insulin or oral hypoglycemic agents.

Parkinson's disease: Epinephrine may temporarily increase rigidity and tremor.

Tolerance may occur with prolonged use of epinephrine.

EPINEPHRINE

Psychiatric effects: Epinephrine may induce or aggravate psychomotor agitation, disorientation, impairment of memory, assaultive behavior, panic, hallucinations, suicidal or homicidal tendencies, and schizophrenic-type thought disorder or paranoid delusions.

Hypovolemia: Use is not a substitute for the replacement of blood, plasma, fluids and electrolytes, which should be restored promptly when loss has occurred.

Sulfite sensitivity: Sulfites may cause allergic-type reactions (eg, hives, itching, wheezing, anaphylaxis) in certain susceptible persons. Although the overall prevalence of sulfite sensitivity in the general population is probably low, it is seen more frequently in asthmatics or in atopic nonasthmatic persons. Specific products containing sulfites are identified in the product listings.

Drug Interactions:

Epinephrine Drug Interactions

Precipant drug	Object drug *		Description
Alpha-adrenergic blockers (eg, phentolamine	Epinephrine	↑	The vasoconstricting and hypertensive effects are antagonized by alpha-adrenergic blocking drugs.
Beta-adrenergic blockers, nonspecific	Epinephrine	↓	Concomitant administration may block the beta-adrenergic effects of epinephrine, causing hypertension.
Bretylium	Epinephrine	↑	Bretylium may potentiate the action of vasopressors on adrenergic receptors, possibly resulting in arrhythmias.
Cardiac glycosides	Epinephrine	↑	Cardiac glycosides may sensitize the myocardium to beta-adrenergic stimulation and make cardiac arrhythmias more likely.
Diuretic drugs	Epinephrine'	↓	Diuretic agents may decrease vascular response to pressor durgs such as epinephrine.
Ergot alkaloids and phenothazines	Epinephrine	↓	Ergot alkaloids and phenothiazines may also reverse the pressor effects of epinephrine.
Guanethidine	Epinephrine	↑	Guanethidine may increase the pressor response of the direct-acting vasopressors, possibly resulting in severe hypertension.
Halogenated hydrocarbon anesthetics	Epinephrine	↑	Halogenated hydrocarbon anesthetics may sensitize the myocardium to the effects of catecholamines. Use of vasopressors may lead to serious arrhythmias; use with extreme caution.
Levothyroxine Antihistamines (eg, chlorpheniramine, tripelennamine, diphenhydramine)	Epinephrine	↑	The pressor response of the direct-acting vasopressors may be potentiated by these agents; use with caution.
Oxytocic drugs	Epinephrine	↑	In obstetrics, if vasopressor drugs are used either to correct hypotension or added to the local anesthetic solution, some oxytocic drugs may cause severe persistent hypertension.
Sympathomimetic drugs (eg, isoproterenol)	Epinephrine	↑	Epinephrine should not be administered concomitantly with other sympathomimetic drugs because of possible additive effects and increased toxicity. Combined effects may induce serious cardiac arrhythmias. They may be administered alternately when the preceding effect of other such drugs has subsided.
Tricyclic antidepressants	Epinephrine	↑	The pressor response of the direct-acting vasopressors may be potentiated by these agents; use with caution.

* ↑ = Object drug increased. ↓ = Object drug decreased.

Drug/Lab test interactions: After prolonged use or epinephrine overdosage, elevated serum lactic acid levels with severe metabolic acidosis may occur. Transient elevations of blood glucose may be associated with epinephrine administration.

EPINEPHRINE

Adverse Reactions:

Cardiovascular: Cardiac arrhythmias and excessive rise in blood pressure may occur with therapeutic doses or inadvertent overdosage. Angina may occur in patients with coronary-artery disease.

Transient and minor: Anxiety, headache, fear and palpitations often occur with therapeutic doses, especially in hyperthyroid and hypertensive individuals.

Local: Urticaria, wheal and hemorrhage may occur at the site of injection. Repeated local injections can result in necrosis from vascular constriction at injection sites.

Systemic: Cerebral hemorrhage; hemiplegia; subarachnoid hemorrhage; anginal pain in patients with angina pectoris; anxiety; restlessness; throbbing headache; tremor; weakness; dizziness; pallor; respiratory difficulty; palpitations; apprehensiveness; sweating; occlusion of the central retinal artery; nausea; vomiting; "epinephrine-fastness" with prolonged use; syncope in children.

Overdosage:

Symptoms: Erroneous administration of large doses of epinephrine may lead to precordial distress, vomiting, headache, dyspnea; unusually elevated blood pressure, extremely elevated arterial pressure, which may result in cerebrovascular hemorrhage, particularly in elderly patients; severe peripheral constriction and cardiac stimulation, resulting in pulmonary arterial hypertension and potentially fatal pulmonary edema; and ventricular hypeirritability, which may result in death from ventricular fibrillation.

Epinephrine overdosage can also cause transient bradycardia followed by tachycardia; these may be accompanied by potentially fatal cardiac arrhythmias. Ventricular premature contractions may appear within 1 minute after injection and may be followed by multifocal ventricular tachycardia (prefibrillation rhythm). Subsidence of the ventricular effects may be followed by atrial tachycardia, and occasionally, by atrioventricular block.

The lethal dose is highly variable and appears to depend to a significant extent on patient factors that enhance susceptibility to serious toxicity. Subarachnoid hemorrhage has followed an SC dose of 0.5 mg. While doses of ≤ 10 mg IV have been fatal, survival has followed doses as high as 30 mg IV or 110 mg SC.

Overdosage sometimes results in extreme pallor and coldness of the skin, metabolic acidosis and kidney failure. Take suitable corrective measures.

Treatment: Most toxic effects can be counteracted by injection of an α-adrenergic blocker and a β-adrenergic blocker. In the event of a sharp rise in blood pressure, rapid acting vasodilators such as the nitrites, or α-adrenergic blocking agents can counteract the marked pressor effects. If prolonged hypotension follows, it may be necessary to administer another pressor drug, such as norepinephrine.

If an epinephrine overdose induces pulmonary edema that interferes with respiration, treatment consists of a rapidly acting α-adrenergic blocking drug such as phentolamine or intermittent positive pressure respiration.

Treat cardiac arrhythmias with a β-blocker (eg, propranolol).

Administration and Dosage:

Administer by IV injection or in cardiac arrest by an endotracheal tube or intracardiac injection into the left ventricular chamber.

SC is the preferred route of administration. If given IM, avoid injection into the buttocks.

SC or IM: 0.2 to 1 ml. Start with a small dose and increase if required.

Hypersensitivity reactions: For bronchial asthma and certain allergic manifestations (eg, angioedema, urticaria, serum sickness, anaphylactic shock) use epinephrine SC. The adult IV dose for hypersensitivity reactions or to relieve bronchospasm usually ranges from 0.1 to 0.25 mg injected slowly. Neonates may be given a dose of 0.01 mg/kg body weight; for the infant, 0.05 mg is an adequate initial dose and this may be repeated at 20 to 30 minute intervals in the management of asthma attacks.

Cardiac arrest: 0.5 to 1 mg (5 to 10 ml of 1:10,000 solution) diluted to 10 ml with Sodium Chloride Injection can be administered IV or intracardially to restore myocardial contractility. During a resuscitation effort, administer 0.5 to 1 mg (5 to 10 ml) IV every 5 minutes.

Intracardiac injection should only be administered by personnel well trained in the technique, if there has not been sufficient time to establish an IV route. Follow with external cardiac massage to permit the drug to enter coronary circulation. Use epinephrine secondarily to unsuccessful attempts with physical or electromechanical methods.

The intracardiac dose usually ranges from 0.3 to 0.5 mg (3 to 5 ml of 1:10,000 solution).

EPINEPHRINE

For infiltration of tissue, as with a local anesthetic, the dose of epinephrine is seldom > 1 mg in a concentration of ≤ 1:50,000. To delay absorption of drugs injected into tissue, a concentration of 1:200,000 is usually adequate.

Cardiopulmonary resuscitation for cardiac arrest (Wyeth): IV or intracardiac administration of 1 to 10 ml of a 1:10,000 dilution is recommended. This emergency measure is generally adopted only if other measures (artificial ventilation, internal or external cardiac compression, administration of sodium bicarbonate) have failed. Artificial ventilation and cardiac compression must be continued. Doses of 1 to 10 ml of the 1:10,000 dilution may be repeated every 5 minutes as required. The IV route may be preferred since it need not interrupt cardiac compression.

For ophthalmologic use (for producing conjunctival decongestion, to control hemorrhage, produce mydriasis and reduce intraocular pressure), use a concentration of 1:10,000 (0.1 mg/ml) to 1:1000 (1 mg/ml).

Intraspinal use: Usual dose is 0.2 to 0.4 ml of a 1:1000 solution added to anesthetic spinal fluid mixture (may prolong anesthetic action by limiting absorption).

Endotracheal tube: If IV access is not available, the drug may be injected via the endotracheal tube. Perform 5 rapid insufflations; forcefully expel 10 ml containing 1 mg epinephrine (0.1 mg/ml) directly into the tube; follow with 5 quick insufflations.

Concomitant administration with local anesthetic: Epinephrine 1:200,000 is the usual concentration employed with local anesthetics.

Pediatric dosage in infants and children: The usualy dose if 0.01 mg/kg body weight or 0.3 mg/m² of body surface area (maximum dose, 0.5 mg), administered SC. This dose may be repeated every 4 hours, or more frequently if necessary.

Admixture compatibility: If epinephrine and sodium bicarbonate are to be coadministered, inject individually at separate sites. Epinephrine is unstable in alkaline solution.

Storage/Stability: Store at room temperature 15° to 30°C (59° to 86°F).Protect the solution from light, extreme heat and freezing. Do not remove ampuls or syringes from carton until ready to use. Discard unused portion.

Rx	**Sus-Phrine** (Forest)	**Suspension for Injection:** 1:200 (5 mg/ml)	In 0.3 ml amps or 5 ml multi-dose vials.[1]
Rx	**Epinephrine** (Abbott)	**Solution:** 1:1000 (1 mg/ml as the HCl)	In 1 ml amps[2]
Rx	**Epinephrine HCl** (Elkins-Sinn)		In 1 ml Dosette amps.
Rx	**Epinephrine HCl** (Wyeth-Ayerst)		In 1 ml Tubex.[3]
Rx	**Epinephrine HCl** (Hollister-Stier)		In 2 ml syringe.[2]
Rx	**Adrenalin Chloride** (Parke-Davis)		In 1 ml amps[4] and 30 ml Steri-vials.[3]
Rx	**Epipen** (Center Labs)		In single-dose auto-injectors.[5]
Rx	**Epipen Jr.** (Center Labs)	**Solution:** 1:2000 (0.5 mg/ml as HCl)	In single-dose auto-injectors.[5]
Rx	**Epinephrine** (Various, eg, Astra)	**Solution:** 1:10,000 (0.1 mg/ml)	In 10 ml prefilled syringes.
Rx	**Epinephrine** (Abbott)	**Solution:** 1:10,000 (0.01 mg/ml as HCl)	In 10 ml Abboject and flip-top vials.[6]
Rx	**Epinephrine Pediatric** (Abbott)	**Solution:** 1:100,000 (0.01 mg/ml as HCl)	In 5 ml Abboject.[6]

[1] With 5 mg phenol.
[2] With 0.9 mg sodium metabisulfite per ml.
[3] With not ≤ 5 mg chlorobutanol and 1.5 mg sodium bisulfite per ml.
[4] With ≤ than 0.1% sodium bisulfite.
[5] With 0.5 mg sodium metabisulfite.
[6] With 0.46 mg sodium metabisulfite per ml.

NOREPINEPHRINE (Levarterenol)

Refer to the general discussion of these products in the Vasopressors Used in Shock group monograph.

Actions:

Pharmacology: A powerful peripheral vasoconstrictor acting on both arterial and venous beds (α-adrenergic action) and as a potent inotropic stimulator of the heart (β_1 action). Coronary vasodilation occurs secondary to enhanced myocardial contractility. These actions result in an increase in systemic blood pressure and coronary artery blood flow. Cardiac output will vary in response to systemic hypertension, but is usually increased in hypotension when the blood pressure is raised to an optimal level. Venous return is increased and the heart tends to resume a more normal rate and rhythm than in the hypotensive state.

In hypotension that persists after correction of blood volume deficits, norepinephrine helps raise the blood pressure to an optimal level and establish a more adequate circulation.

Pharmacokinetics: Norepinephrine is ineffective orally; SC absorption is poor. It is rapidly inactivated by catechol-O-methyltransferase and monoamine oxidase. Negligible amounts are normally found in urine. When given by IV infusion, the onset is rapid; duration is 1 to 2 minutes following discontinuation of infusion.

Indications:

Hypotensive states: Restoration of blood pressure in controlling certain acute hypotensive states (eg, pheochromocytomectomy, sympathectomy, poliomyelitis, spinal anesthesia, myocardial infarction (MI), septicemia, blood transfusion, and drug reactions), and as an adjunct in the treatment of cardiac arrest and profound hypotension.

Contraindications:

Do not give to patients who are hypotensive from blood volume deficits, except as an emergency measure to maintain coronary and cerebral artery perfusion until blood volume replacement therapy can be completed. If continuously administered to maintain blood pressure in the absence of blood volume replacement, the following may occur: Severe peripheral and visceral vasoconstriction, decreased renal perfusion and urine output, poor systemic blood flow despite "normal" blood pressure, tissue hypoxia, and lactic acidosis.

Do not give to patients with mesenteric or peripheral vascular thrombosis (because of the risk of increasing ischemia and extending the area of infarction) unless administration is necessary as a life saving procedure.

Use of norepinephrine during cyclopropane and halothane anesthesia is generally considered contraindicated because of the risk of producing ventricular tachycardia or fibrillation. The same type of cardiac arrhythmias may result from use in patients with profound hypoxia or hypercarbia.

Warnings:

Pregnancy: Category C. Animal reproduction studies have not been conducted with norepinephrine. It is also not known whether this drug can cause fetal harm when administered to a pregnant woman or can affect reproduction capacity. Give norepinephrine to a pregnant woman only if clearly needed.

Lactation: It is not known whether this drug is excreted in breast milk. Because many drugs are excreted in breast milk, exercise caution when administering norepinephrine to a nursing woman.

Children: Safety and efficacy in children have not been established.

Precautions:

Hypovolemia: Use is not a substitute for the replacement of blood, plasma, fluids and electrolytes, which should be restored promptly when loss has occurred.

Avoid hypertension: Because of its potency and varying response to pressor substances, dangerously high blood pressure may be produced with overdoses. Monitor the blood pressure every 2 minutes from the time administration is started until the desired blood pressure is obtained, then every 5 minutes if administration is to be continued. Constantly watch flow rate. Never leave patient unattended during infusion. Headache may be a symptom of hypertension due to overdosage.

Infusion site: Whenever possible, infuse into a large vein, particularly an antecubital vein, to minimize necrosis of the overlying skin from prolonged vasoconstriction. The femoral vein may also be an acceptable route of administration. Avoid a catheter tie-in technique, if possible, since the obstruction to blood flow around the tubing may cause stasis and increased local concentration of the drug. Occlusive vascular diseases (ie, atherosclerosis, arteriosclerosis, diabetic endarteritis, Buerger's disease) are more likely to occur in the lower extremity; therefore, avoid the veins of the leg in elderly patients or in those suffering from such disorders.

NOREPINEPHRINE (Levarterenol)

Extravasation: Infuse into a large vein, preferably of the antecubital fossa, to prevent extravasation. Extravasation may cause necrosis and sloughing of surrounding tissue. Monitor the infusion site closely for free flow.

Blanching along the course of the infused vein, sometimes without obvious extravasation, has been attributed to vasa vasorum constriction with increased permeability of the vein wall, permitting some leakage. This may rarely progress to superficial slough, particularly during infusion into leg veins in elderly patients or in those suffering from obliterative vascular disease. Hence, if blanching occurs, consider changing the infusion site at intervals to allow the effects of local vasoconstriction to subside.

Antidote for extravasation – To prevent sloughing and necrosis in ischemic areas, infiltrate area as soon as possible with 10 to 15 ml of saline solution containing 5 to 10 mg of phentolamine. Use a syringe with a fine hypodermic needle and infiltrate liberally throughout the ischemic area. Sympathetic blockade with phentolamine causes immediate and conspicuous local hyperemic changes if the area is infiltrated within 12 hours.

Phentolamine (5 to 10 mg) added directly to the infusion may also be an effective antidote against sloughing should extravasation occur, whereas the systemic vasopressor activity of norepinephrine is not impaired. Sympathetic nerve block has also been suggested.

The incidence of thrombosis in the infused vein and perivenous reactions and necrosis may be reduced if heparin is added to the infusion solution in an amount to supply 100 to 200 units/hour.

Sulfite sensitivity: Sulfites may cause allergic-type reactions (eg, hives, itching, wheezing, anaphylaxis) in certain susceptible persons. Although the overall prevalence of sulfite sensitivity in the general population is probably low, it is more frequent in asthmatics or in atopic nonasthmatic persons. Specific products containing sulfites are identified in the product listings.

Drug Interactions:

Norepinephrine Drug Interactions

Precipitant drug	Object drug*		Description
Bretylium	Norepinephrine	⬆	Bretylium may potentiate the action of vasopressors on adrenergic receptors, possibly resulting in arrhythmias.
Guanethidine	Norepinephrine	⬆	Guanethidine may increase the pressor response of the direct-acting vasopressors, possibly resulting in severe hypertension.
Halogenated hydrocarbon anesthetics	Norepinephrine	⬆	Halogenated hydrocarbon anesthetics may sensitize the myocardium to the effects of catecholamines. Use of vasopressors may lead to serious arrhythmias; use with extreme caution.
Oxytocic drugs	Norepinephrine	⬆	In obstetrics, if vasopressor drugs are used either to correct hypotension or are added to the local anesthetic solution, some oxytocics may cause severe persistent hypertension.
Tricyclic antidepressants	Norepinephrine	⬆	The pressor response of the direct-acting vasopressors may be potentiated by these agents; use with caution.
Monoamine oxidase inhibitors (MAOIs)	Norepinephrine	⬆	Severe, prolonged hypertension may result.⬆

* ⬆ = Object drug increased.

Adverse Reactions:

Cardiovascular: Norepinephrine's therapeutic index is four times that of epinephrine. Bradycardia sometimes occurs, probably as a reflex result of a rise in blood pressure; arrhythmias. Headache may indicate overdosage and extreme hypertension.

CNS: Anxiety; transient headache.

Body as a whole: Ischemic injury due to potent vasoconstrictor action and tissue hypoxia; respiratory difficulty; extravasation necrosis at injection site.

Miscellaneous: Gangrene has been reported in a lower extremity when the drug was infused into an ankle vein.

NOREPINEPHRINE (Levarterenol)

Overdosage:

Symptoms: Overdosage may also result in headache, severe hypertension, reflex bradycardia, marked increase in peripheral resistance and decreased cardiac output. Prolonged administration of any potent vasopressor may result in plasma volume depletion.

Treatment: Correct by appropriate fluid and electrolyte replacement therapy. If plasma volumes are not corrected, hypotension may recur when norepinephrine is discontinued or blood pressure may be maintained at the risk of severe peripheral vasoconstriction with diminution in blood flow and tissue perfusion.

Administration and Dosage:

Restoration of blood pressure in acute hypotensive states: Always correct blood volume depletion as fully as possible before any vasopressor is administered. When, as an emergency measure, intraaortic pressures must be maintained to prevent cerebral or coronary artery ischemia, norepinephrine can be administered before and concurrently with blood volume replacement.

Average IV dosage – Add 4 ml of the solution to 1000 ml of 5% Dextrose Solution (4 mcg base/ml). Avoid a catheter tie-in technique as this promotes stasis. After observing the response to an initial dose of 2 to 3 ml (from 8 to 12 mcg of base) per minute, adjust the rate of flow to establish and maintain a low normal blood pressure (usually 80 to 100 mmHg systolic) sufficient to maintain the circulation to vital organs. In previously hypertensive patients, raise the blood pressure no higher than 40 mmHg below the preexisting systolic pressure. The average maintenance dose ranges from 0.5 to 1 ml (2 to 4 mcg of base) per minute.

Dosage adjustments – Great individual variation in the dose occurs; titrate dosage according to patient response. Occasionally, enormous daily doses (as high as 68 mg base) may be necessary if the patient remains hypotensive, but occult blood volume depletion should always be suspected and corrected when present. Central venous pressure monitoring is usually helpful.

If large fluid volumes are needed at a flow rate involving an excessive dose of the pressor agent per unit of time, use a solution more dilute than 4 mcg/ml. When large fluid volumes are undesirable, a larger concentration may be administered.

Duration of therapy – Continue the infusion until adequate blood pressure and tissue perfusion are maintained without therapy. Reduce infusion gradually, avoiding abrupt withdrawal. In some cases of vascular collapse due to acute MI, treatment was required for up to 6 days.

Adjunctive treatment in cardiac arrest: Usually administered IV during cardiac resuscitation to restore and maintain an adequate blood pressure after an effective heartbeat and ventilation have been established. The powerful β-adrenergic stimulating action is also thought to increase the strength and effectiveness of systolic contractions once they occur.

Diluent: Administer in 5% Dextrose Solution in Distilled Water or 5% Dextrose in Saline Solution. These fluids containing dextrose are protection against significant loss of potency due to oxidation. Administration in saline solution alone is not recommended. If indicated, administer whole blood or plasma separately (for example, by use of a Y–tube and individual flasks if given simultaneously).

Storage/Stability: Store at room temperature. Protect from light.

Rx	**Levophed** (Sanofi Winthrop)	**Injection:** 1 mg (as bitartrate) per ml	In 4 ml ampuls.[1]

[1] Contains ≤ 2 mg metabisulfite.

EPHEDRINE

Refer to the general discussion of these products in the Vasopressors Used in Shock group monograph.

Actions:

Pharmacology: Ephedrine is a potent sympathomimetic that stimulates both alpha and beta receptors and has clinical uses related to both actions. Its peripheral actions, which it owes in part to the release of epinephrine, simulate responses that are obtained when adrenergic nerves are stimulated. These include an increase in blood pressure, stimulation of heart muscle, constriction of arterioles, relaxation of the smooth muscle of the bronchi and GI tract, and dilation of the pupils. In the bladder, relaxation of the detrusor muscle is not prominent, but the tone of the trigone and vesicle sphincter is increased.

CNS – Ephedrine also has a potent effect on the CNS. It stimulates the cerebral cortex and subcortical centers.

Cardiovascular – The cardiovascular responses include moderate tachycardia, unchanged or augmented stroke volume, enhanced cardiac output, variable alterations in peripheral resistance, and, usually, a rise in blood pressure. The action of ephedrine is more prominent on the heart than on the blood vessels. Ephedrine increases the flow of coronary, cerebral and muscle blood.

Metabolic – Hepatic glycogenolysis is increased by ephedrine, but not as much as by epinephrine; usual doses are unlikely to produce hyperglycemia. Ephedrine increases oxygen consumption and metabolic rate, probably by central stimulation.

Myasthenia gravis – Administration of ephedrine produces a real but modest increase in motor power. The exact mechanism by which ephedrine affects skeletal muscle contraction is unknown.

Pharmacokinetics: Ephedrine is rapidly and completely absorbed following parenteral injection. Onset of action by the IM route is more rapid (within 10 to 20 minutes) than by SC injection. Pressor and cardiac responses to ephedrine persist for up to 60 minutes following IM or SC administration of 25 to 50 mg.

Small amounts of ephedrine are slowly metabolized in the liver. The drug and its metabolites are excreted in the urine, mostly as unchanged ephedrine. Rate and percentage of urinary excretion is dependent on urinary pH which is increased by acidification of the urine. Elimination half-life of the drug is ≈ 3 hours when the urine is acidified to a pH of 5 and ≈ 6 hours when urinary pH is 6.3.

Indications:

Hypotensive states: To combat acute hypotensive states, especially those associated with spinal anesthesia; Stokes-Adams syndrome with complete heart block; a CNS stimulant in narcolepsy and depressive states; occasionally, acute bronchospasm. Also used in enuresis and myasthenia gravis.

As a pressor agent in hypotensive states following sympathectomy or following overdosage with ganglionic-blocking agents, antiadrenergic agents, veratrum alkaloids, or other drugs used for lowering blood pressure in the treatment of arterial hypertension.

Contraindications:

Hypersensitivity to the drug; angle closure glaucoma; patients anesthetized with cyclopropane or halothane (these agents may sensitize the heart to the arrhythmic action of sympathomimetic drugs); cases where vasopressor drugs are contraindicated (ie, thyrotoxicosis, diabetes, obstetrics where maternal blood pressure is in excess of 130/80, hypertension and other cardiovascular disorders).

Warnings:

Hypertension: Ephedrine may cause hypertension resulting in intracranial hemorrhage, anginal pain in patients with coronary insufficiency or ischemic heart disease, or potentially fatal arrhythmias in patients with organic heart disease or who are receiving drugs that sensitize the myocardium.

Labor and delivery: Parenteral administration of ephedrine to maintain blood pressure during low or other spinal anesthesia for delivery can cause acceleration of fetal heart rate and should not be used in obstetrics when maternal blood pressure exceeds 130/80 mm Hg. It is not known what effect ephedrine may have on the newborn or on the child's later growth and development when administered to the mother just before or during labor.

Renal function impairment: Initially, parenteral ephedrine may produce constriction of renal blood vessels and decreased urine formation.

Pregnancy: Category C. It is unknown whether ephedrine can cause fetal harm when administered to a pregnant woman or can affect reproduction capacity. Give to a pregnant woman only if clearly needed.

Lactation: Ephedrine is excreted in breast milk. Use by nursing mothers is not recommended.

EPHEDRINE

Precautions:

Administer cautiously to patients with heart disease; coronary insufficiency; cardiac arrhythmias; angina pectoris; diabetes; hyperthyroidism; prostatic hypertrophy; hypertension; unstable vasomotor system or in patients on digitalis.

Prolonged use may produce a syndrome resembling an anxiety state.

Prolonged abuse of ephedrine can lead to symptoms of paranoid schizophrenia (eg, tachycardia, poor nutrition and hygiene, fever, cold sweat and dilated pupils).

Tolerance: Althouth tolerance to ephedrine develops, addiction does not occur. Temporary cessation of medication restores the patient's original response to the drug.

Hypovolemia: Use is not a substitute for the replacement of blood, plasma, fluids and electrolytes, which should be restored promptly when loss has occurred.

Drug Interactions:

Ephedrine Drug Interactions			
Precipitant drug	Object drug *		Description
Ephedrine	Guanethidine	⬇	The antihypertensive effects of guanethidine may be partially or totally reversed by the mixed-acting sympathomimetics.
Halogenated hydrocarbons	Ephedrine	⬆	Halogenated anesthetics may sensitize the myocardium to the effects of catecholamines. Use of vasopressors may lead to serious arrhythmias; use with extreme caution.
Monoamine oxidase inhibitors (MAOIs)	Ephedrine	⬆	MAOIs increase the pressor response to mixed-acting vasopressors. Possible hypertensive crisis and intracranial hemorrhage may occur. This interaction may also occur with **furazolidone,** an antimicrobial with MAO inhibitor activity. Avoid this combination; if given inadvertently and hypertension occurs, administer phentolamine.
Oxytocic drugs	Ephedrine	⬆	In obstetrics, if vasopressor drugs are used either to correct hypotension or added to the local anesthetic solution, some oxytocic drugs may cause severe persistent hypertension.
Tricyclic antidepressants	Ephedrine	⬇	The pressor response of the mixed-acting vasopressors may be decreased; a higher dose of the sympathomimetic may be necessary.

* ⬆ = Object drug increased. ⬇ = Object drug decreased.

Adverse Reactions:

Cardiovascular: Palpitation; tachycardia; precordial pain; cardiac arrhythmias.

CNS: Headache; insomnia; sweating; nervousness; vertigo; confusion; delirium; restlessness; anxiety; tension; tremor; weakness; dizziness; hallucinations.

GI: Nausea; vomiting; anorexia.

GU: Vesical sphincter spasm resulting in difficult and painful urination; urinary retention may develop in males with prostatism.

Miscellaneous: Respiratory difficulty; pallor.

Overdosage:

Symptoms: The principal manifestation of ephedrine poisoning is convulsions. The following have occurred in acute poisoning: Nausea, vomiting, chills, cyanosis, irritability, nervousness, fever, suicidal behavior, tachycardia, dilated pupils, blurred vision, opisthotonos, spasms, convulsions, pulmonary edema, gasping respirations, coma and respiratory failure. Initially, the patient may have marked hypertension, followed later by hypotension accompanied by anuria. Large doses may lead to personality changes, with a psychological craving for the drug. Chronic use of ephedrine can also cause symptoms of tension and anxiety progressing to psychosis.

Treatment: Discontinue the drug. Remove the drug from the stomach by ipecac emesis, followed by activated charcoal or airway protected gastric lavage in depressed or hyperactive patients. If respirations are shallow or cyanosis is present, administer artificial respiration. Vasopressors are contraindicated. In cardiovascular collapse, maintain blood pressure.

For hypertension, 5 mg phentolamine mesylate diluted in saline may be administered slowly IV, or 100 mg may be given orally. Convulsions may be controlled by diazepam or paraldehyde. Cool applications and dexamethasone, 1 mg/kg, administered slowly IV, will control pyrexia.

Administration and Dosage:

May be adminstered SC, IM or slow IV.

Adults: The usual dose is 25 to 50 mg. Absorption by the IM route is more rapid than by SC injection. The IV route may be used if an immediate effect is desired. Also, 5 to 25 mg may be administered slow IV push. Additional doses may be given at 5 to 10 minute intervals.

Pediatric dose: 16.7 mg/m^2 SC or IM every 4 to 6 hours.

Labor: Administer only sufficient dosage to maintain blood pressure at or below 130/80 mmHg.

Acute attacks of asthma: Administer the smallest effective dose (0.25 to 0.5 ml).

Stability and storage: Ephedrine is subject to oxidation. Protect against exposure to light. Do not administer unless solution is clear. Discard unused portion.

Rx	**Ephedrine Sulfate** (Various, eg, UDL)	**Injection:** 50 mg/ml	In 1 ml single-dose vials
Rx	**Ephedrine Sulfate** (Abbott)		Preservative free. In 1 ml single-dose amps.

MEPHENTERMINE SULFATE

Refer to the general discussion of these products in the Vasopressors Used in Shock group monograph.

Actions:

Pharmacology: Mephentermine sulfate is a mixed-acting sympathomimetic amine that acts both directly and indirectly (ie, releases norepinephrine). The increase in blood pressure produced by mephentermine is probably due primarily to an increase in cardiac output resulting from enhanced cardiac contraction; to a lesser degree, an increase in peripheral resistance due to peripheral vasoconstriction may also contribute to the elevation in blood pressure.

Mephentermine is metabolized in the liver by N-demethylation to normephentermine (or phentermine) with subsequent p–hydroxylation to p-hydroxynormephentermine (or p-hydroxyphentermine).

Pharmacokinetics: The duration of action is prolonged. Pressor response is evident 5 to 15 minutes after IM injection and has a duration of 1 to 2 hours. Following IV administration, the pressor response is almost immediate and persists for 15 to 30 minutes after the drug is discontinued.

The excretion rate of the drug and its metaboites is more rapid in an acidic urine and is only slightly influenced by urine output.

Indications:

Hypotension: Treatment of hypotension secondary to ganglionic blockade and that occurring with spinal anesthesia.

Although not recommended as corrective therapy for shock of hypotension secondary to hemorrhage, it may be used as an emergency measure to maintain blood pressure until blood or blood substitutes become available.

Contraindications:

Hypersensitivity to the drug; hypotension induced by chlorpromazine, as the sympathomimetic amines will act to potentiate, rather than correct, the hypotension secondary to the adrenolytic effects of chlorpromazine; in combination with any MAOI (see Drug Interactions).

Warnings:

Cardiovascular disease: Use mephentermine with caution in patients with known cardiovascular disease, and in chronically ill patients, as the drug's action on the cardiovascular system may be profound.

Pregnancy: Category C. Safety for use during pregnancy or in women of childbearing potential has not been established. Use only when clearly needed and when the potential benefits outweigh the potential hazards to the fetus. Mephentermine sulfate may increase uterine contractions especially during the third trimester of pregnancy.

Lactation: Safety for use during nursing has not been established. Use only when the potential benefits outweigh the potential hazards to the nursing infant.

Children: Safety and effectiveness of mephentermine sulfate have not been established.

Precautions:

Hypovolemia: Use is not a substitute for the replacement of blood, plasma, fluids and electrolytes, which should be restored promptly when loss has occurred (ie, during or after surgery).

Hemorrhagic shock: Use with caution in treatment of shock secondary to hemorrhage. For effective emergency treatment, infuse 300 to 600 mg mephentermine in D5W. This will maintain blood pressure until volume replacement is accomplished.

Hyperthyroidism: Increased responsiveness to vasopressor agents may be seen.

Hypertensive patients: Administer with care to known hypertensives.

MEPHENTERMINE SULFATE

Drug Interactions:

Mephentermine Drug Interactions			
Precipitant drug	Object drug*		Description
Mephentermine	Guanethidine Reserpine	⬇	The antihypertensive effects of guanethidine may be partially or totally reversed by the mixed-acting sympathomimetics.
Halogenated hydrocarbon anesthetics	Mephentermine	⬆	Halogenated hydrocarbon anesthetics may sensitize the myocardium to the effects of catecholamines. Use of vasopressors may lead to serious arrhythmias; use with extreme caution.
Monoamine oxidase (MAO) inhibitors	Mephentermine	⬆	MAOIs increase the pressor response to mixed-acting vasopressors. Possible hypertensive crisis and intracranial hemorrhage may occur. This interaction may also occur with **furazolidone**, an antimicrobial with MAO inhibitor activity. Avoid this combination; if given inadvertently and hypertension occurs, administer phentolamine.
Oxytocic drugs	Mephentermine	⬆	In obstetrics, if vasopressor drugs are used either to correct hypotension or are added to the local anesthetic solution, some oxytocics may cause severe persistent hypertension.
Tricyclic antidepressants	Mephentermine	⬇	The pressor response of the mixed-acting vasopressors may be decreased by these agents; a higher dose of the sympathomimetic may be necessary.

* ⬆ = Object drug increased. ⬇ = Object drug decreased.

Adverse Reactions:

Side effects following administration are minimal and result from the central stimulatory effects. Following recommended doses, an occasional patient may display signs of anxiety. Cardiac arrhythmias may be produced and blood pressure may be raised excessively, particularly in patients with heart disease.

Overdosage:

Symptoms: Effects of overdosage are an extension of the pharmacological activity of mephentermine. Cardiac contractility, cardiac output, systolic and diastolic blood pressure are usually raised. Other symptoms include hyperexcitability, prolonged wakefulness, weeping, incoherence, convulsions, flushing, tremor and hallucinations.

Treatment: Therapy of overdosage is symptomatic and supportive. Treat convulsions or cardiac arhythmias promptly if they occur. Because arrhythmias produced by mephentermine sulfate may be due to excessive beta-adrenergic stimulation, consider a beta-blocking agent such as propranolol.

MEPHENTERMINE SULFATE

Administration and Dosage:

Can be administered IM without irritation or abnormal tissue reaction. Injection of an undiluted parenteral solution containing 30 mg/ml, or a continuous infusion of a 1 mg/ml solution in 5% Dextrose in Water, directly into the vein, is the preferable route for treatment of shock. IV administration of undiluted mephentermine does not produce irritation and no untoward reaction will develop should extravasation occur.

Shock and hypotension: Dosage used in treatment of shock and hypotension is based on experimental observation that 0.5 mg/kg produces a positive inotropic action.

Prevention of hypotension attendant to spinal anesthesia: Administer 30 to 45 mg IM 10 to 20 minutes prior to anesthesia, operation or termination of the procedure.

Hypotension following spinal anesthesia: Administer 30 to 45 mg IV in a single injection. Repeat doses of 30 mg as necessary to maintain blood pressure. An immediate response and maintenance of blood pressure can be accomplished by the continuous IV infusion of a 0.1% solution of mephentermine in 5% Dextrose in Water (1 mg/ml). Regulate flow and duration of therapy according to patient response.

Hypotension secondary to spinal anesthesia: Administer an initial dose of 15 mg of mephentermine IV. This dose may be repeated if the response is not adequate.

Treatment of shock following hemorrhage: Although not recommended, the continuous IV infusion of a 0.1% solution of mephentermine in 5% Dextrose in Water may be useful in maintaining blood pressure until whole blood replacement can be accomplished.

Preparation of IV solution: The 0.1% solution can be prepared in the approximate concentration (0.115%) by adding 10 or 20 ml of mephentermine, 30 mg/ml, to 250 or 500 ml of 5% Dextrose in Water, respectively.

Storage/Stability: Store at room temperature, ≈ 25°C (77°F).

Rx	**Wyamine Sulfate** (Wyeth-Ayerst)	**Injection:** 15 mg/ml	Parabens. In 2 and 10 ml.
		30 mg/ml	Parabens. In 10 ml.

METARAMINOL

Refer to the general discussion of these products in the Vasopressors Used in Shock group monograph.

Actions:

Pharmacology: A potent sympathomimetic amine that increases both systolic and diastolic blood pressure, primarily by vasoconstriction; this effect is usually accompanied by a marked reflex bradycardia. Metaraminol has a direct effect on alpha-adrenergic receptors. It does not depend on release of norepinephrine but it has indirect activity. Prolonged infusions can deplete norepinephrine from sympathetic nerve endings. Repeated use may result in an overall diminution of sympathetic activity.

Renal, coronary and cerebral blood flow are a function of perfusion pressure and regional resistance. In most instances of cardiogenic shock, the beneficial effect of sympathomimetic amines is their positive inotropic effect. In patients with insufficient or failing vasoconstriction, there is additional advantage to the peripheral action of metaraminol, but in most patients with shock, vasoconstriction is adequate and any further increase is unnecessary. Therefore, blood flow to vital organs may decrease with metaraminol if regional resistance increases excessively. It increases cardiac output in hypotensive patients.

Metaraminol increases venous tone, causes pulmonary vasoconstriction and elevates pulmonary pressure even when cardiac output is reduced.

Pressor effect is decreased, but not reversed, by alpha-adrenergic blocking agents. When pressor responses are due primarily to vasoconstriction, cardiac stimulation may play a small role. Although uncommon, tachyphylaxis and a fall in blood pressure may occur with repeated use.

Pharmacokinetics: The pressor effect begins 1 to 2 minutes after IV infusion, ≈ 10 minutes after IM injection and 5 to 20 minutes after SC injection. The effect lasts from ≈ 20 minutes to 1 hour.

Indications:

Prevention and treatment of the acute hypotensive state occurring with spinal anesthesia; adjunctive treatment of hypotension due to hemorrhage; reactions to medications; surgical complications; shock associated with brain damage due to trauma or tumor.

"Probably effective" as an adjunct in the treatment of hypotension due to cardiogenic shock or septicemia.

Contraindications:

Use with cyclopropane or halothane anesthesia, unless clinical circumstances demand such use (see Drug Interactions); hypersensitivity to metaraminol.

Warnings:

Cardiac effects: Metaraminol may cause cardiac arrhythmias. This may be particularly dangerous in patients with myocardial infarction or in patients who have received anesthetics that sensitize the heart to catecholamines (ie, cyclopropane, halothane, etc).

Prolonged administration may reduce the venous return and cardiac output and increase the work load of the heart.

Pregnancy: Category C. It is not known whether metaraminol can cause fetal harm when given to a pregnant woman or can affect reproductive capacity. Give metaraminol to a pregnant woman only if clearly needed.

Lactation: It is not known whether this drug is secreted in breast milk. Because many drugs are secreted in breast milk, exercise caution when giving metaraminol to a nursing woman.

Children: Safety and effectiveness in children have not been established.

Precautions:

Use with caution in heart or thyroid disease, hypertension or diabetes.

Hypovolemia: Use is not a substitute for the replacement of blood, plasma, fluids and electrolytes, which should be restored promptly when loss has occurred.

Vasoconstriction: When vasopressor amines are used for long periods, the resulting vasoconstriction may prevent adequate expansion of circulating volume and may perpetuate the shock state. Measurement of central venous pressure is useful in assessment of plasma volume. Therefore, employ blood or plasma volume expanders when circulating volume is decreased.

Hypertension: Avoid excessive blood pressure response. Rapidly induced hypertensive responses have been reported to cause acute pulmonary edema, arrhythmias and cardiac arrest.

Cirrhosis: Treat patients with cirrhosis cautiously and with adequate restoration of electrolytes if diuresis ensues. Fatal ventricular arrhythmia has been reported in one

METARAMINOL

patient with Laennec's cirrhosis while receiving the drug. In several instances, ventricular extrasystoles that appeared during infusion subsided promptly when the rate of infusion was reduced.

Cumulative effects: Because of its prolonged action, a cumulative effect is possible, and with an excessive vasopressor response there may be a prolonged elevation of blood pressure, even with discontinuation. It is important to make frequent assessments of the blood pressure, particularly when administering IV.

Extravasation: Exercise care when selecting the site of administration of this drug, particularly when given by the IV route. The use of larger veins (the antecubital fossa or the thigh) is preferred. Avoid those of the ankle or dorsum of the hand, especially in patients with peripheral vascular disease, diabetes mellitus, Buerger's disease or hypercoagulability states. Extravasation may cause abscess formation, tissue necrosis and sloughing of surrounding tissue. Monitor the infusion site closely for free flow. Discontinue the infusion immediately if infiltration or thrombosis occurs.

Antidote for extravasation – To prevent sloughing and necrosis in ischemic areas, infiltrate area as soon as possible with 10 to 15 ml saline solution containing 5 to 10 mg phentolamine. Use a syringe with a fine hypodermic needle and infiltrate liberally throughout the ischemic area. Sympathetic blockade with phentolamine causes immediate and conspicuous local hyperemic changes if the area is infiltrated within 12 hours.

Malaria: Sympathomimetic amines may provoke a relapse in patients with a history of malaria.

Sulfite sensitivity: Sulfites may cause allergic-type reactions (eg, hives, itching, wheezing, anaphylaxis) in certain susceptible persons. Although the overall prevalence of sulfite sensitivity in the general population is probably low, it is seen more frequently in asthmatics or in atopic nonasthmatic persons. Specific products containing sulfites are identified in the product listings.

Drug Interactions:

Metaraminol Drug Interactions			
Precipitant drug	Object drug*		Description
Metaraminol	Guanethidine	⬇	The antihypertensive effects of guanethidine may be partially or totally reversed by the mixed-acting sympathomimetics.
Digitalis glycosids	Metaraminol	⬆	Use metaraminol with caution in digitalized patients, because the combination of digitalis and sympathomimetic amines may cause ectopic arrhythmias.
Halogenated hydrocarbon anesthetics	Metaraminol	⬆	Halogenated hydrocarbon anesthetics may sensitize the myocardium to the effects of catecholamines. Use of vasopressors may lead to serious arrhythmias; use with extreme caution.
Monoamine oxidase (MAO) inhibitors	Metaraminol	⬆	MAOIs increase the pressor response to mixed-acting vasopressors. Possible hypertensive crisis and intracranial hemorrhage may occur. This interaction may also occur with furazolidone, an antimicrobial with MAO inhibitor activity. Avoid this combination; if given inadvertently and hypertension occurs, administer phentolamine.
Oxytocic drugs	Metaraminol	⬆	If vasopressor drugs are used in obstetrics to correct hypotension or added to the local anesthetic solution, some oxytocic drugs may cause severe persistent hypertension.
Tricyclic antidepressants	Metaraminol	⬇	The pressor response of the mixed-acting vasopressors may be decreased by these agents; a higher dose of the sympathomimetic may be necessary.

* ⬆ = Object drug increased. ⬇ = Object drug decreased.

Adverse Reactions:

Cardiovascular: Sympathomimetic amines may cause sinus or ventricular tachycardia, or other arrhythmias, especially in patients with MI. Hypertension, hypotension following cessation of the drug, cardiac arrhythmias, cardiac arrest and palpitation have occurred.

Miscellaneous: Headache; flushing; sweating; tremors; dizziness; nausea; apprehension; abscess formation; tissue necrosis; sloughing at injection site.

METARAMINOL

Overdosage:

Overdosage with metaraminol may cause convulsions, severe hypertension, headache, constricting sensation in the chest, nausea, vomiting, euphoria, diaphresis, pulmonary edema, tachycardia, bradycardia, sinus arrhythmia, atrial or ventricular arrhythmias, myocardial infarction, cardiac arrest, cerebral hemorrhage or cardiac arrhythmias. Patients with hyperthyroidism or hypertension are particularly sensitive to these effects. An appropriate antiarrhythmic agent may also be required.

Administration and Dosage:

May be given IM, SC or IV. Because the maximum effect is not immediately apparent, allow at least 10 minutes to elapse before increasing the dose. When the vasopressor is discontinued, observe the patient carefully so that therapy can be reinitiated promptly if the blood pressure falls too rapidly. The response to vasopressors may be poor in patients with coexistent shock and acidosis. Established methods of shock management and other measures directed to the specific cause of the shock state should also be employed.

IM or SC injection (prevention of hypotension): The recommended dose is 2 to 10 mg.

IV infusion (adjunctive treatment of hypotension): The recommended dose is 15 to 100 mg in 250 or 500 ml of Sodium Chloride Injection or 5% Dextrose Injection; adjust the rate of infusion to maintain the blood pressure at the desired level. Higher concentrations, 150 to 500 mg in 250 or 500 ml of infusion fluid, have been used. The concentration of drug in the infusion fluid may be adjusted depending on the patient's need for fluid replacement.

Direct IV injection: In severe shock, give by direct IV injection. The suggested dose is 0.5 to 5 mg, followed by an infusion of 15 to 100 mg in 250 to 500 ml of infusion fluid.

Unlabeled route of administration:

Endotracheal tube – If IV access is not available, the drug may be injected via the endotracheal tube. Perform five rapid insufflations; forcefully expel 5mg diluted to a volume of 10 ml into the endotracheal tube; follow with five quick insufflations.

Children: 0.01 mg/kg as a single dose or a solution of 1 mg/25 ml in dextrose or saline.

Admixture compatibility: In addition to Sodium Chloride Injection and 5% Dextrose Injection, the following infusion solutions were found physically and chemically compatible with metaraminol when 5 ml (10 mg/ml) was added to 500 ml of infusion solution: Ringer's Injection, Lactated Ringer's Injection, 5% Dextran in Saline, *Normosol-R* pH 7.4, *Normosol-M* in 5% Dextrose Injection.

Storage/Stability: Avoid storage at temperatures below –20°C (–4°F) and above 40°C (104°F). Infusion solutions should be used within 24 hours.

Rx	**Aramine** (Merck)	**Injection**: 10 mg per ml (1%, as bitartrate)	In 10 ml vials.[1]

[1] With 0.15% methylparaben, 0.02% propylparaben and 0.2% sodium bisulfite.

METHOXAMINE HCl

Refer to the general discussion of these products in the Vasopressors Used in Shock group monograph.

Actions:

Pharmacology: A vasopressor that produces a prompt and prolonged rise in blood pressure by increasing peripheral resistance (α effect). It is especially useful for maintaining blood pressure during operations under spinal anesthesia. It may also be used during general anesthesia.

Provides potent, prolonged pressor action. There is no increase in cardiac rate; occasionally, a decrease in rate develops as the blood pressure increases. This bradycardia is apparently caused by a carotid sinus reflex; this is abolished by atropine.

Pharmacokinetics: Following IV administration of methoxamine in humans, the peak pressor effect occurs within 0.5 to 2 minutes. The duration of the pressor effect following a single IV dose of 2 to 4 mg of methoxamine was 10 to 15 minutes. With administration of 10 to 40 mg methoxamine IM, the peak effect occurs within 15 to 20 minutes, and the duration of action is ≈ 1½ hours.

Indications:

For supporting, restoring or maintaining blood pressure during anesthesia (including cyclopropane anesthesia); for terminating some episodes of supraventricular tachycardia.

Contraindications:

Severe hypertension; hypersensitivity to methoxamine.

Warnings:

Pregnancy: Category C. Methoxamine decreases uterine blood flow, decreases fetal heart rate and adversely affects the fetal acid-base status in pregnant ewes and monkeys at doses comparable to those used in humans. There are no adequate and well controlled studies in pregnant women. There has been one report of a fetal death; the mother received methoxamine concomitantly with several other drugs. A direct causal relationship to methoxamine was not established. Use during pregnancy only if the potential benefit justifies the potential risk to the fetus.

Lactation: It is not known whether methoxamine is excreted in breast milk. Exercise caution when administering methoxamine to a nursing woman.

Children: Safety and efficacy in children have not been established.

Precautions:

Hypovolemia: Use is not a substitute for the replacement of blood, plasma, fluids and electrolytes, which should be restored promptly when loss has occurred.

Extravasation: When infused, large veins of the antecubital fossa are preferred to veins in the hand or ankle to prevent extravasation. Extravasation may cause necrosis and sloughing of surrounding tissue. Monitor the infusion site closely for free flow.

Antidote for extravasation – To prevent sloughing and necrosis in ischemic areas, infiltrate as soon as possible with 10 to 15 ml saline solution containing 5 to 10 mg phentolamine. Use a fine hypodermic needle and infiltrate liberally throughout the ischemic area. Sympathetic blockade with phentolamine causes immediate and conspicuous local hyperemic changes if area is infiltrated within 12 hours.

Use with care in patients with hyperthyroidism, bradycardia, partial heart block, myocardial disease or severe arteriosclerosis.

Sulfite sensitivity: Sulfites may cause allergic-type reactions (eg, hives, itching, wheezing, anaphylaxis) in certain susceptible persons. Although the overall prevalence of sulfite sensitivity in the general population is probably low, it is more frequent in asthmatics or in atopic nonasthmatic persons. Specific products containing sulfites are identified in the product listings.

METHOXAMINE HCl

Drug Interactions:

Methoxamine Drug Interactions			
Precipitant drug	Object drug*		Description
Bretylium	Methoxamine	↑	Bretylium may potentiate the action of vasopressors on adrenergic receptors, possibly resulting in arrhythmias.
Guanethidine	Methoxamine	↑	Guanethidine may increase the pressor response of the direct-acting vasopressors, possibly resulting in severe hypertension.
Halogenated hydrocarbon anesthetics	Methoxamine	↑	Halogenated hydrocarbon anesthetics may sensitize the myocardium to the effects of catecholamines. Use of vasopressors may lead to serious arrhythmias; use with extreme caution.
Oxytocic drugs	Methoxamine	↑	If vasopressors are used in obstetrics to correct hypotension or are added to the local anesthetic solution, some oxytocics may cause severe persistent hypertension.
Tricyclic antidepressants	Methoxamine	↑	The pressor response of the direct-acting vasopressors may be potentiated by these agents; use with caution.

* ↑ = Object drug increased.

Drug/Lab test interactions: Methoxamine may increase plasma cortisol and ACTH levels. Exercise caution when interpreting plasma cortisol and ACTH levels in patients receiving methoxamine.

Adverse Reactions:

Integumentary: Sweating, pilomotor response.

Cardiovascular: Excessive blood pressure elevations particularly with high dosage; fetal bradycardia; ventricular ectopic beats.

GI: Nausea; vomiting (often projectile).

CNS: Headache (often severe); anxiety.

GU: Uterine hypertonus; urinary urgency.

Overdosage:

Symptoms: Undesirably high blood pressure or excessive bradycardia. Clinically significant elevations of blood pressure may be reversed with an α-adrenergic blocking agent (eg, phentolamine). Bradycardia may be abolished with atropine.

Administration and Dosage:

Emergencies: 3 to 5 mg IV injected slowly. IV injection may be supplemented by IM injections to provide a prolonged effect.

Spinal anesthesia – Usual IM dose is 10 to 15 mg shortly before or with spinal anesthesia to prevent hypotension. A 10 mg dose may be adequate at lower levels; 15 to 20 mg may be required at high levels of spinal anesthesia. Repeat doses if necessary, but allow time for the previous dose to act (about 15 minutes).

Correcting a fall in blood pressure – 10 to 15 mg IM, depending on degree of decrease. Where systolic pressure falls below 60 mm Hg or when an emergency exists, give 3 to 5 mg IV. This may be accompanied by 10 to 15 mg IM for prolonged effect.

Pre- and postoperative use (moderate hypotension): 5 to 10 mg IM may be adequate.

Supraventricular tachycardia: Average dose, 10 mg IV injected slowly.

Storage/Stability: Store at 15° to 25°C (59° to 77°F) and protect from light.

Rx	**Vasoxyl** (Glaxo Wellcome)	**Injection**: 20 mg/ml	In 1 ml amps.[1]

[1] With 0.1% potassium metabisulfite.

PHENYLEPHRINE HCl

Refer to the general discussion of these products in the Vasopressors Used in Shock group monograph.

Actions:

Pharmacology: Phenylephrine is a powerful postsynaptic alpha-receptor stimulant with little effect on the beta receptors of the heart.

The predominant actions of phenylephrine are on the cardiovascular system. Parenteral administration causes a rise in systolic and diastolic pressures due to peripheral vasoconstriction. Accompanying the pressor response to phenylephrine is a marked reflex bradycardia that can be blocked by atropine; after atropine, large doses of the drug increase the heart rate only slightly. Cardiac output is slightly decreased, and peripheral resistance is considerably increased. Circulation time is slightly prolonged, and venous pressure is slightly increased; venous constriction is not marked. Most vascular beds are constricted; renal, splanchnic, cutaneous and limb blood flows are reduced, but coronary blood flow is increased. Pulmonary vessels are constricted, and pulmonary arterial pressure is raised.

The drug is a powerful vasoconstrictor with properties similar to those of norepinephrine but almost completely lacking the chronotropic and inotropic actions on the heart. Cardiac irregularities are seen rarely, even with large doses. In contrast to epinephrine and ephedrine, phenylephrine produces longer lasting vasoconstriction, a reflex bradycardia and increases the stroke output, producing no disturbance in the rhythm of the pulse.

In therapeutic doses, it produces little if any stimulation of either the spinal cord or cerebrum. An advantage is that repeated injections produce comparable effects.

Indications:

Treatment of vascular failure in shock, shock-like states, drug-induced hypotension, or hypersensitivity; to overcome paroxysmal supraventricular tachycardia; to prolong spinal anesthesia; as a vasoconstrictor in regional analgesia; to maintain an adequate level of blood pressure during spinal and inhalation anesthesia.

Contraindications:

Hypersensitivity to the drug; severe hypertension; ventricular tachycardia.

Warnings:

Pregnancy: Category C. Safety for use during pregnancy has not been established. Use only when clearly needed and when the potential benefits outweigh the potential hazards to the fetus.

Labor and delivery – If used in conjunction with **oxytocic drugs**, the pressor effect of sympathomimetic pressor amines is potentiated.

Lactation: It is not known whether this drug is excreted in breast milk. Safety for use in the nursing mother has not been established. Because many drugs are excreted in breast milk, exercise caution when administering to a nursing woman.

Precautions:

Use with extreme caution in elderly patients, patients with hyperthyroidism, bradycardia, partial heart block, myocardial disease or severe arteriosclerosis.

Hypovolemia: Use is not a substitute for the replacement of blood, plasma, fluids and electrolytes, which should be restored promptly when loss has occurred.

Extravasation: When infused, large veins of the antecubital fossa are preferred to veins in the hand or ankle to prevent extravasation. Extravasation may cause necrosis and sloughing of surrounding tissue. Monitor the infusion site closely for free flow.

Antidote for extravasation – To prevent sloughing and necrosis in ischemic areas, infiltrate area as soon as possible with 10 to 15 ml saline solution containing 5 to 10 mg phentolamine. Use a syringe with a fine hypodermic needle and infiltrate liberally throughout the ischemic area. Sympathetic blockade with phentolamine causes immediate and conspicuous local hyperemic changes if the area is infiltrated within 12 hours.

Sulfite sensitivity: Sulfites may cause allergic-type reactions (eg, hives, itching, wheezing, anaphylaxis) in certain susceptible persons. Although the overall prevalence of sulfite sensitivity in the general population is probably low, it is seen more frequently in asthmatics or in atopic nonasthmatic persons. Specific products containing sulfites are identified in the product listings.

PHENYLEPHRINE HCl

Drug Interactions:

Phenylephrine Drug Interactions			
Precipitant drug	Object drug *		Description
Bretylium	Phenylephrine	↑	Bretylium may potentiate the action of vasopressors on adrenergic receptors, possibly resulting in arrhythmias.
Guanethidine	Phenylephrine	↑	Guanethidine may increase the pressor response of the direct-acting vasopressors, possibly resulting in severe hypertension.
Halogenated hydrocarbon anesthetics	Phenylephrine	↑	Halogenated hydrocarbon anesthetics may sensitize the myocardium to the effects of catecholamines. Use of vasopressors may lead to serious arrhythmias; use with extreme caution.
Monoamine oxidase inhibitors (MAOIs)	Phenylephrine	↑	MAOIs may significantly enhance the adrenergic effects of phenylephrine, and its pressor response may be increased 2- to 3-fold. Phenylephrine is metabolized by gut and liver MAO. This interaction may also occur with furazolidone, an antimicrobial with MAOI activity. Avoid this combination; if given inadvertently and hypertension occurs, administer phentolamine.
Oxytocic drugs	Phenylephrine	↑	If vasopressors are used in obstetrics to correct hypotension or are added to the local anesthetic solution, some oxytocics may cause severe persistent hypertension.
Tricyclic antidepressants	Phenylephrine	↔	Tricyclic antidepressants have both increased and decreased the sensitivity to IV phenylephrine.

* ↑ = Object drug increased. ↔ = Undetermined effect.

Adverse Reactions:

Headache; reflex bradycardia; excitability; restlessness; arrhythmias (rare).

Overdosage:

Symptoms: Ventricular extrasystoles; short paroxysms of ventricular tachycardia; sensation of fullness in the head; tingling of the extremities.

Treatment: Relieve an excessive elevation of blood pressure by an α-adrenergic blocking agent (ie, phentolamine).

Administration and Dosage:

Inject SC, IM, slow IV or in dilute solution as a continuous IV infusion. In patients with paroxysmal supraventricular tachycardia and, if indicated, in case of emergency, administer directly IV. Adjust dose according to the pressor response.

Phenylephrine Dosage Calculations		
Dose required (mg)	Phenylephrine 1% (ml)	Diluted phenylephrine[1] 0.1% (ml)
0.1	—	0.1
0.2	—	0.2
0.5	—	0.5
1	0.1	—
5	0.5	—
10	1	—

[1] For convenience in intermittent IV administration, dilute 1 ml phenylephrine 1% with 9 ml Sterile Water for Injection, USP.

Mild or moderate hypotension:

SC or IM – 2 to 5 mg (range, 1 to 10 mg). Do not exceed an initial dose of 5 mg. A 5 mg IM dose should raise blood pressure for 1 to 2 hours.

IV – 0.2 mg (range, 0.1 to 0.5 mg). Do not exceed an initial dose of 0.5 mg. Do not repeat injections more often than every 10 to 15 minutes. A 0.5 mg IV dose should elevate the pressure for ≈ 15 minutes.

PHENYLEPHRINE HCl

To prepare a 0.1% solution of phenylephrine (0.1mg/0.1 ml), dilute 1 ml of 1% solution with 9 ml Sterile Water for Injection.

Severe hypotension and shock including drug-related hypotension: Correct blood volume depletion as completely as possible before any vasopressor is administered. When intraaortic pressures must be maintained as an emergency measure to prevent cerebral or coronary artery ischemia, phenylephrine can be administered before and concurrently with blood volume replacement.

Hypotension and occasionally severe shock may result from overdosage or idiosyncratic reactions following administration of certain drugs, especially adrenergic and ganglionic blocking agents, rauwolfia, veratrum alkaloids and phenothiazine derivatives. Patients who receive a phenothiazine as preoperative medication are especially susceptible. As an adjunct in the management of such episodes, phenylephrine is a suitable agent for restoring blood pressure.

Higher initial and maintenance doses are required in patients with persistent or untreated severe hypotension or shock. Hypotension produced by powerful peripheral adrenergic blocking agents (chlorpromazine) or pheochromocytomectomy may also require more intensive therapy.

Continuous infusion: Add 10 mg to 250 or 500 ml of Dextrose Injection or Sodium Chloride Injection (providing a 1:25,000 or 1:50,000 dilution). To raise the blood pressure rapidly, start the infusion at ≈ 100 to 180 mcg/minute (based on 20 drops/ml, this would be 50 to 90 or 100 to 180 drops/minute). When the blood pressure is stabilized (at a low normal level for the individual), a maintenance rate of 40 to 60 mcg/minute usually suffices (based on 20 drops/ml, this would be 20 to 30 or 40 to 60 drops/minute). If the drop size of the infusion system varies from 20 drops/ml, adjust the dose accordingly.

If a prompt initial vasopressor response is not obtained, add additional increments of the drug (≥ 10 mg) to the infusion bottle. Adjust the flow rate until the desired blood pressure level is obtained. (A more potent vasopressor, such as norepinephrine, may be required.) Avoid hypertension. Check blood pressure frequently. Headache or bradycardia may indicate hypertension. Arrhythmias are rare.

Spinal anesthesia:

Hypotension – Administer SC or IM 3 or 4 minutes before injection of the spinal anesthetic. The total requirement for high anesthetic levels is usually 3 mg and, for lower levels, 2 mg. For hypotensive emergencies during spinal anesthesia, phenylephrine may be injected IV beginning with a dose of 0.2 mg. Any subsequent dose should not exceed the previous dose by > 0.1 to 0.2 mg; do not administer > 0.5 mg in a single dose.

Pediatric dose – To combat hypotension during spinal anesthesia in children, administer 0.5 to 1 mg/25 lbs, SC or IM.

Prolongation of spinal anesthesia – The addition of 2 to 5 mg phenylephrine to the anesthetic solution increases the duration of motor block by as much as 50% without an increase in the incidence of complications (eg, nausea, vomiting or blood pressure disturbances).

Vasoconstrictor for regional analgesia: Concentrations about 10 times those of epinephrine are recommended. The optimum strength is 1:20,000 (made by adding 1 mg phenylephrine to every 20 ml of local anesthetic solution). Some pressor responses may be expected when ≥ 2 mg are injected.

Paroxysmal supraventricular tachycardia: Rapid IV injection (within 20 to 30 seconds) is recommended; do not exceed an initial dose of 0.5 mg. Subsequent doses, which are determined by the initial blood pressure response, should not exceed the preceding dose by > 0.1 to 0.2 mg, and should never exceed 1 mg.

Storage/Stability: Protect from light.

Rx	**Phenylephrine HCl** (Various, eg, American Regent)	**Injection**: 1% (10 mg/ml)	In 1 and 5 ml vials.
Rx	**Neo-Synephrine** (Sanofi Winthrop)		In 1 ml Uni-Nest amps.[1]

[1] With sodium bisulfite.

MIDODRINE HCl

Actions:

Pharmacology: Midodrine is a prodrug formed by deglycination. It forms an active metabolite, desglymidodrine, that is an alpha$_1$ agonist, and exerts its actions via activation of the alpha-adrenergic receptors of the arteriolar and venous vasculature, producing an increase in vascular tone and an elevation of blood pressure. Desglymidodrine diffuses poorly across the blood-brain barrier.

Administration of midodrine results in a rise in standing, sitting and supine systolic and diastolic blood pressure in patients with orthostatic hypotension of various etiologies. Standing systolic blood pressure is elevated by ≈ 15 to 30 mmHg at 1 hour after a 10 mg dose of midodrine, with some effect persisting for 2 to 3 hours.

Pharmacokinetics:

Absorption/Distribution – The plasma levels of the prodrug peak after about half an hour and decline with a half-life of ≈ 25 minutes, while the metabolite reaches peak blood concentrations ≈ 1 to 2 hours after a dose of midodrine and has a half-life of ≈ 3 to 4 hours. The absolute bioavailability of midodrine is 93%. Neither midodrine nor desglymidodrine is significantly bound to plasma proteins.

Metabolism – It appears that deglycination of midodrine to desglymidodrine takes place in many tissues, and both compounds are metabolized in part by the liver.

Renal elimination of midodrine is insignificant. The renal clearance of desglymidodrine is 385 ml/min, ≈ 80% by active renal secretion. It is possible that it occurs by the base-secreting pathway responsible for the secretion of other drugs that are bases (see Drug Interactions).

Indications:

Orthostatic hypotension (OH): For the treatment of symptomatic OH. Use only in patients whose lives are considerably impaired despite standard clinical care.

Unlabeled uses: Management of urinary incontinence (2.5 to 5 mg 2 to 3 times a day).

Contraindications:

Severe organic heart disease; acute renal disease; urinary retention; pheochromocytoma; thyrotoxicosis; persistent and excessive supine hypertension (see Warnings).

Warnings:

Supine hypertension is the most potentially serious adverse reaction associated with midodrine. Use of midodrine in such patients is not recommended. Monitor supine and sitting blood pressures in patients beginning maintainence on midodrine.

Supine hypertension can often be controlled by preventing the patient from becoming fully supine (eg, sleeping with the head of the bed elevated).

Renal function impairment: Use midodrine cautiously in patients with urinary retention problems, because desglymidodrine acts on the alpha-adrenergic receptors of the bladder neck.

Desglymidodrine is eliminated via the kidneys, and higher blood levels would be expected in such patients. Use midodrine with caution in patients with renal impairment, with a lower starting dose (see Administration and Dosage). Assess renal function prior to initial use of midodrine.

Hepatic function impairment: Use midodrine with caution in patients with hepatic impairment, as the liver has a role in the metabolism of midodrine.

Pregnancy: Category C. There are no adequate and well controlled studies in pregnant women. Use midodrine during pregnancy only if the potential benefit justifies the potential risk to the fetus.

Lactation: It is not known whether this drug is excreted in breast milk. Because many drugs are excreted in breast milk, exercise caution when administering to a nursing woman.

Children: Safety and effectiveness in pediatric patients have not been established.

Precautions:

Monitoring: Evaluate renal and hepatic function prior to initiating therapy and subsequently, as appropriate.

Monitor blood pressure carefully when midodrine is used concomitantly with other agents that cause vasoconstriction.

Heart rate: A slight slowing of the heart rate may occur after administration of midodrine, primarily due to vagal reflex. If any signs or symptoms suggesting bradycardia occur, discontinue midodrine and re-evaluate.

Visual problems: Use midodrine with caution in orthostatic hypotensive patients who are also diabetic, as well as those with a history of visual problems or who are also taking fludrocortisone acetate (see Drug Interactions).

MIDODRINE HCl

Drug Interactions:

Midodrine Drug Interactions			
Precipitant drug	Object drug*		Description
Midodrine	Cardiac glycosides, psychopharmacologics, beta blockers	⬆	When administered concomitantly with midodrine, cardiac glycosides, psychopharmacologic agents or beta blockers may enhance or precipitate bradycardia, A/V block or arrhythmia (see Precautions).
Midodrine	Alpha-adrenergic agonists	⬆	The use of drugs that stimulate alpha-adrenergic agonists may enhance or potentiate the pressor effects of midodrine.
Midodrine	Steroid therapy (eg, fludrocortisone)	⬆	Reduce the dose of fludrocortisone or decrease the salt intake prior to initiation of treatment with midodrine. Fludrocortisone also causes an increase in intraocular pressure and glaucoma (see Precautions).
Midodrine	Alpha-adrenergic antagonists	⬇	Alpha-adrenergic antagonist agents can antagonize the effects of midodrine.
Metformin, H_2 antagonists, procainamide, triamterene, flecainide, quinidine	Midodrine	⬌	There may be a potential for interactions with these drugs (See Actions).

* ⬆ = Object drug increased. ⬇ = Object drug decreased. ⬌ = Undetermined effect.

Adverse Reactions:

CNS: Paresthesia (18.3%); pain (4.9%).

Dermatologic: Piloerection (13.4%); pruritus (12.2%); rash (2.4%).

Miscellaneous: Dysuria (13.4%); supine hypertension (7.3%); chills (4.9%).

Less frequent: Headache; feeling of pressure/fullness in the head; vasodilation/flushing face; confusion/abnormal thinking; dry mouth; nervousness/anxiety; rash.

Rare: Visual field defect; dizziness; skin hyperesthesia; insomnia; somnolence; erythema multiforme; canker sore; dry skin; dysuria; impaired urination; asthenia; backache; pyrosis; nausea; GI distress; flatulence; leg cramps.

Overdosage:

Symptoms of overdose may include hypertension, piloerection (goosebumps), a sensation of coldness and urinary retention.

There are two reported cases of overdosage with midodrine, both in young males. They ingested between 205 and 250 mg of midodrine and both recovered.

Treatment: Emesis and administration of alpha-sympatholytic drugs (eg, phentolamine). Desglymidodrine is dialyzable.

Administration and Dosage:

Approved by the FDA on September 6, 1996.

The recommended dose of midodrine is 10 mg, 3 times daily. Dosing should take place during the daytime hours when the patient is upright, pursuing daily activities. A suggested dosing schedule of ≈ 4–hour intervals is as follows: Shortly before or upon arising in the morning, midday and late afternoon (not later than 6 pm). Doses may be given in 3–hour intervals, if required, to control symptoms. Do not give midodrine after the evening meal or < 4 hours before bedtime. Because of the risk of supine hypertension, continue midodrine only in patients who appear to attain symptomatic improvement during initial treatment.

Renal function impairment: Starting dose of 2.5 mg (see Warnings).

Rx	**ProAmatine** (Roberts)	**Tablets:** 2.5 mg	(RPC 2.5 003). White, round, scored. In 100s.
		5 mg	(RPC 5 004). Orange, round, scored. In 100s.

BETA-ADRENERGIC BLOCKING AGENTS

Actions:

Pharmacology:

Pharmacologic/Pharmacokinetic Properties of Beta-Adrenergic Blocking Agents

0–none +-low ++-moderate +++-high Drug	Adrenergic receptor blocking activity	Membrane stabilizing activity	Intrinsic sympathomimetic activity	Lipid solubility	Extent of absorption (%)	Absolute oral bioavailability (%)	Half-life (hrs)	Protein binding (%)	Metabolism/ Excretion
Acebutolol	β_1[1]	+	+	Low	90	20-60	3-4	26	Hepatic; renal excretion 30% to 40%; non-renal excretion 50% to 60% (bile; intestinal wall)
Atenolol	β_1[1]	0	0	Low	50	50-60	6-9	16-16	≈ 50% excreted unchanged in feces
Betaxolol	β_1[1]	+	0	Low	≈ 100	89	14-22	≈ 50	Hepatic; > 80% recovered in urine, 15% unchanged
Bisoprolol	β_1[1]	0	0	Low	≥ 90	80	9-12	≈ 30	≈ 50% excreted unchanged in urine, remainder as inactive metabolites; < 2% excreted in feces.
Esmolol	β_1[1]	0	0	Low	na[2]	na[2]	0.15	55	Rapid metabolism by esterases in cytosol of red blood cells
Metoprolol	β_1[1]	0[2]	0	Moderate	95	40-50	3-7	12	Hepatic; renal excretion, < 5% unchanged
Metoprolol, long-acting						77			
Carteolol	β_1 β_2	0	++	Low	80	85	6	23-30	50% to 70% excreted unchanged in urine
Nadolol	β_1 β_2	0	0	Low	30	30-50	20-24	30	Urine, unchanged
Penbutolol	β_1 β_2	0	+	High	≈100	≈100	5	80-98	Hepatic (conjugation, oxidation); renal excretion of metabolites (17% as conjugate)
Pindolol	β_1 β_2	+	+++	Moderate	95	≈100	3-4[3]	40	Urinary excretion of metabolites (60% to 65%) and unchanged drug (35% to 40%)
Propranolol	β_1 β_2	++	0	High	90	30	3-5	90	Hepatic; < 1% excreted unchanged in urine
Propranolol, long-acting						9-18	8-11		
Sotalol	β_1 β_2	0	0	Low	nd	90-100	12	0	Not metabolized; excreted unchanged in urine

BETA-ADRENERGIC BLOCKING AGENTS

Pharmacologic/Pharmacokinetic Properties of Beta-Adrenergic Blocking Agents

0–none +-low ++-moderate +++-high Drug	Adrenergic receptor blocking activity	Membrane stabilizing activity	Intrinsic sympathomimetic activity	Lipid solubility	Extent of absorption (%)	Absolute oral bioavailability (%)	Half-life (hrs)	Protein binding (%)	Metabolism/ Excretion
Timolol	β_1 β_2	0	0	Low to moderate	90	75	4	10	Hepatic; urinary excretion of metabolites and unchanged drug
Labetalol[4]	β_1 β_2 α_1	0	0	Moderate	100	30-40	5.5-8	50	55% to 60% excreted in urine as conjugates or unchanged drug

[1] Inhibits β_2 receptors (bronchial and vascular) at higher doses.
[2] Detectable only at doses much greater than required for beta blockade.
[3] In elderly hypertensive patients with normal renal function, t½ variable: 7 to 15 hours.
[4] See labetalol monograph.
nd = No data.
na = Not applicable (available IV only).

Beta-adrenergic receptor blocking agents compete with beta-adrenergic agonists for available beta receptor sites. Propranolol, nadolol, timolol, penbutolol, carteolol, sotalol and pindolol inhibit both the β_1 receptors (located chiefly in cardiac muscle) and β_2 receptors (located chiefly in the bronchial and vascular musculature), inhibiting the chronotropic, inotropic and vasodilator responses to β-adrenergic stimulation. Metoprolol, acebutolol, bisoprolol, esmolol, betaxolol and atenolol are cardioselective and preferentially inhibit β_1 receptors.

Propranolol and, to a lesser extent, acebutolol, betaxolol and pindolol, exert a quinidine-like (anesthetic) membrane action (membrane stabilizing activity; MSA) which affects cardiac action potential. The other agents do not have MSA and have little direct myocardial depressant activity. MSA was once considered responsible for antiarrhythmic effectiveness of these agents; however, MSA appears to occur only with doses that far exceed those used for arrhythmias. Pindolol, carteolol, penbutolol and acebutolol have intrinsic sympathomimetic activity (ISA) in therapeutic dosage ranges. ISA or partial agonist activity is mediated directly at adrenergic receptor sites and may be blocked by other β antagonists. ISA is manifested by a smaller reduction in resting cardiac output and resting heart rate (4 to 8 bpm) than is seen with drugs lacking ISA; clinical significance has not been evaluated and there is no evidence that exercise cardiac output is less affected by pindolol.

Pharmacokinetics:

Absorption – Systemic bioavailability following oral administration of metoprolol, acebutolol, timolol and propranolol is low because of significant first-pass hepatic metabolism. Pindolol, sotalol and carteolol have no significant first-pass effect; first-pass metabolism of bisoprolol is ≈ 20%. Ingestion with food enhances the bioavailability of propranolol and metoprolol and reduces the absorption of sotalol; this effect is not noted with nadolol, carteolol, pindolol, bisoprolol or betaxolol.

Distribution – There is no simple correlation between dose or plasma level and therapeutic effect; the dose-sensitivity range observed in clinical practice is wide because sympathetic tone varies widely among individuals. There is no reliable test to estimate sympathetic tone or to determine whether total β-blockade has been achieved; proper dosage requires titration. Inhibition of maximal exercise tachycardia is a reasonable index of total β-blockade; isoproterenol sensitivity testing may also be used. There appear to be significant correlations between acebutolol plasma levels and both the reduction in resting heart rate and the percent of β-blockade of exercise-induced tachycardia.

Metoprolol and propranolol readily enter the CNS. Because of their high water solubility, sotalol, acebutolol, carteolol, nadolol and atenolol do not pass the blood-brain barrier; these drugs may have a lower incidence of CNS side effects.

Clinical trials: Clinical response to β-blockade includes slowing of sinus heart rate, depressed AV conduction, decreased cardiac output and reduction of systolic and diastolic blood pressure at rest and on exercise, reduction of both supine and standing blood pressure, inhibition of isoproterenol-induced tachycardia and reduction of reflex orthostatic tachycardia. β-adrenergic receptor blockade is useful in conditions (angina, hypertension) in which, because of pathologic or functional changes, sympathetic activity is detrimental to the patient. Also, in some situations, sympathetic stimulation is vital: In patients with severely damaged hearts, adequate ventricular function is maintained by virtue of sympathetic drive which should be preserved. β-adrenergic blockade may worsen AV block by preventing necessary facilitating effects of sympathetic activity on conduction.

β_2-adrenergic blockade results in passive bronchial constriction by interfering with endogenous adrenergic bronchodilator activity in patients subject to bronchospasm and may also interfere with exogenous bronchodilators. Although **pindolol** does not eliminate sympathetic tone entirely, there is no controlled evidence that it is safer than other agents or is less likely to cause such conditions as heart failure, heart block or bronchospasm.

Hypertension – β-blockers decrease standing and supine blood pressure. They are effective antihypertensives when used alone or with other antihypertensives. Although not established, several mechanisms have been proposed: Competitive antagonism of catecholamines at peripheral (non-CNS) adrenergic neuron sites (especially cardiac) leading to decreased cardiac output; a central effect leading to reduced sympathetic outflow to the periphery; blockade of the beta-adrenergic receptors responsible for renin release from the kidneys. These mechanisms appear less likely for **pindolol** than other β-blockers in view of the modest effect on resting cardiac output and its inconsistent effect on plasma renin activity. Although total peripheral resistance may increase initially, it readjusts to the pretreatment level, or lower, with chronic usage. Effects on plasma volume appear to be minor and somewhat variable. **Propranolol** may cause a small increase in serum potassium concentration when used in the treatment of hypertension.

Angina – May reduce myocardial oxygen requirements by blocking catecholamine-induced increases in heart rate, systolic blood pressure and velocity and extent of myocardial contraction. Oxygen requirements may be increased by increasing left ventricular fiber length, end diastolic pressure and systolic ejection period. Net physiologic effect of β-adrenergic blockade is advantageous and is manifested during exercise by delayed onset of pain and increased work capacity.

Arrhythmias – Antiarrhythmic effects occur in concentrations associated with β-blockade. The significance of the MSA in the treatment of arrhythmias is uncertain. **Propranolol** and **acebutolol** prolong the effective refractory period of the AV node and slow AV conduction.

Myocardial infarction (MI) – The mechanism is unknown, but the protective effect is consistent regardless of age, sex or site of infarction. The effect is clearest in patients with a first infarction who were at high risk of dying, defined as those with one or more of the following characteristics during the acute phase: Transient left ventricular failure; cardiomegaly; new atrial fibrillation or flutter; systolic hypotension or AST levels greater than 4 times the upper normal limit. The incidence of nonfatal reinfarction is also reduced.

Migraine – The mechanism has not been established. Beta-adrenergic receptors have been demonstrated in the pial vessels of the brain.

Antitremor – The specific mechanism has not been established, but β_2 receptors may be involved. A central effect is also possible.

Indications:

Hypertension (except esmolol and sotalol): Used alone as a Step 1 agent or in combination with other drugs, particularly a thiazide diuretic. Not indicated for treatment of hypertensive emergencies.

*Angina pectoris (***nadolol, propranolol, atenolol, metoprolol***):* Long-term management.

*Hypertrophic subaortic stenosis (***propranolol***):* Useful in managing exertional or other stress-induced angina, palpitations and syncope. Improves exercise performance. Efficacy appears due to reduction of elevated outflow pressure gradient which is exacerbated by beta receptor stimulation. Clinical improvement may be temporary.

*Cardiac arrhythmias (***acebutolol, esmolol, propranolol, sotalol***):* Use acebutolol for ventricular premature beats only. Use sotalol for documented life-threatening ventricular arrhythmias, such as sustained ventricular tachycardia.

*Supraventricular arrhythmias (***esmolol, propranolol***)* – Paroxysmal atrial tachycardias, particularly those arrhythmias induced by catecholamines or digitalis or associated with the Wolff-Parkinson-White syndrome (see Warnings); persistent sinus tachycardia which is noncompensatory and impairs the well-being of the patient.

Tachycardias and arrhythmias due to thyrotoxicosis when they cause distress or increased hazard and when immediate effect is necessary as adjunctive, short-term (2 to 4 weeks) therapy. May be used with, but not in place of, specific therapy.

Persistent atrial extrasystoles which impair the well-being of the patient and do not respond to conventional measures. Atrial flutter and fibrillation when ventricular rate cannot be controlled by digitalis alone, or when digitalis is contraindicated.

BETA-ADRENERGIC BLOCKING AGENTS

*Supraventricular tachycardia (***esmolol***)* – Rapid control of ventricular rate in patients with atrial fibrillation or atrial flutter in perioperative, postoperative or other emergent circumstances where short-term control of ventricular rate with a short-acting agent is desirable.

*Sinus tachycardia (***esmolol***)* – Noncompensatory sinus tachycardia where the rapid heart rate requires intervention. Esmolol is not intended for use in chronic settings where transfer to another agent is anticipated.

*Ventricular tachycardias (***propranolol***)* – In ventricular tachycardias, with the exception of those induced by catecholamines or digitalis, propranolol is not the drug of first choice. In critical situations when cardioversion techniques or other drugs are not indicated or are ineffective, propranolol may be considered.

Persistent premature ventricular extrasystoles which impair the well-being of the patient and do not respond to conventional measures.

*Tachyarrhythmias of digitalis intoxication (***propranolol***)*, if persistent following discontinuation of digitalis and correction of electrolyte abnormalities, are usually reversible with oral propranolol. Severe bradycardia may occur. Reserve IV propranolol for life-threatening arrhythmias. Temporary maintenance with oral therapy may be indicated.

*Resistant tachyarrhythmias due to excessive catecholamine action during anesthesia (***propranolol***)* – All general inhalation anesthetics produce some degree of myocardial depression; therefore, use propranolol with extreme caution.

*Myocardial infarction (***propranolol, timolol***):* Indicated in clinically stable patients who have survived the acute phase of an MI to reduce cardiovascular mortality and risk of reinfarction. Initiate treatment within 1 to 4 weeks after infarction.

Metoprolol *and* **atenolol** are also indicated in the treatment of hemodynamically stable patients with definite or suspected acute MI. Treatment can be initiated as soon as the patient's clinical condition allows or within 3 to 10 days of the acute event.

*Pheochromocytoma (***propranolol***):* After primary treatment with an alpha-adrenergic blocking agent has been instituted, propranolol may be useful as adjunctive therapy if the control of tachycardia becomes necessary before or during surgery.

With inoperable or metastatic pheochromocytoma, propranolol may be useful as an adjunct to the management of symptoms due to excessive beta receptor stimulation.

*Migraine (***propranolol, timolol***):* For the prophylaxis of common migraine headache.

*Essential tremor (***propranolol***):* For the management of familial or hereditary essential tremor consisting of involuntary, rhythmic and oscillatory movements. Propranolol causes a reduction in the tremor amplitude but not in the tremor frequency. It is not indicated for the treatment of tremor associated with Parkinsonism.

Unlabeled uses: The agents listed have been evaluated for use in the following conditions:

Alcohol withdrawal syndrome – Atenolol (50 to 100 mg/day) and propranolol.

Aggressive behavior – Metoprolol (200 to 300 mg/day), nadolol (40 to 160 mg/day) and propranolol (80 to 300 mg/day).

Angina pectoris – Carteolol (10 mg/day); bisoprolol (stable angina, 5 to 10 mg/day); esmolol (unstable angina, 2 to 24 mg/min as a continuous infusion).

Antipsychotic-induced akathisia – Nadolol (40 to 80 mg/day), pindolol (5 mg/day), propranolol (20 to 80 mg/day) and metoprolol (> 100 mg/day).

Essential tremor – Metoprolol (50 to 300 mg/day), nadolol (120 to 240 mg/day) and timolol (10 mg/day). Nadolol (20 to 40 mg/day) has also been used to treat lithium-induced tremor, and both nadolol (80 to 320 mg/day) and propranolol (160 mg/day) have been investigated for the treatment of tremors associated with Parkinson's disease.

Migraine prophylaxis – Atenolol (50 to 100 mg/day), metoprolol (50 to 100 mg twice daily) and nadolol (40 to 80 mg/day).

Rebleeding from esophageal varices in cirrhotic patients – Nadolol (40 to 160 mg/day), propranolol (20 to 180 mg twice daily) and atenolol (100 mg/day).

Situational anxiety (eg, stage fright) – Nadolol (20 mg) and propranolol (40 mg); base the timing of administration on the drug's onset of action. Atenolol, timolol and pindolol may also be useful in this condition.

Ventricular arrhythmias – Atenolol (50 to 100 mg/day), metoprolol (200 mg/day), nadolol (10 to 640 mg/day), timolol and pindolol.

In addition, individual agents have been investigated for use in several other conditions:

Atenolol – 50 mg/day, started 72 hours before coronary artery bypass operations, appears effective in reducing the incidence of supraventricular arrhythmias.

Bisoprolol – Supraventricular tachycardias (2.5 to 20 mg/day); PVCs.

Nadolol – A dose of 10 to 20 mg twice daily has significantly reduced intraocular pressure.

BETA-ADRENERGIC BLOCKING AGENTS

Metoprolol – Enhancement of cognitive performance in elderly patients; suppression of atrial ectopy in patients with chronic obstructive pulmonary disease; congestive heart failure (50 to 200 mg/day).

Propranolol – Schizophrenia (300 to 5000 mg/day); acute panic symptoms (40 to 320 mg/day); anxiety (80 to 320 mg/day); intermittent explosive disorder (50 to 1600 mg/day); management of nonvariceal gastric bleeding in portal hypertension (24 to 480 mg/day); thyrotoxicosis symptoms (20 to 40 mg 3 to 4 times daily). Preliminary findings suggest propranolol may be an effective vaginal contraceptive; however, systemic absorption may occur.

Beta-Adrenergic Blocking Agents – Summary of Indications[1]

Indications ✓= labeled x = unlabeled	Acebutolol	Atenolol	Betaxolol	Bisoprolol	Carteolol	Esmolol	Labetalol	Metoprolol[2]	Nadolol	Penbutolol	Pindolol	Propranolol[2]	Sotalol	Timolol
Hypertension	✓	✓	✓	✓	✓		✓	✓	✓	✓	✓	✓		✓
Angina pectoris		✓		x	x	x		✓	✓			✓		
Cardiac arrhythmias														
Supraventricular arrhythmias/ tachycardias		x		x		✓						✓		
Sinus tachycardia						✓								
Ventricular arrhythmias/ tachycardias		x						x	x		x	✓	✓	x
PVCs	✓			x								✓		
Digitalis-induced tachyarrhythmias												✓		
Resistant tachyarrhythmias (during anesthesia)												✓		
Atrial ectopy								x						
Myocardial infarction		✓						✓				✓		✓
Pheochromocytoma							x					✓		
Migraine prophylaxis		x						x	x			✓		✓
Hypertrophic subaortic stenosis												✓		
Tremors														
Essential								x	x			✓		x
Lithium-induced									x					
Parkinsonism									x			x		
Alcohol withdrawal syndrome		x										x		
Aggressive behavior								x	x			x		
Antipsychotic-induced akathisia								x	x		x	x		
Esophageal varices rebleeding		x							x			x		
Anxiety (including situational)		x							x		x	x		x
Enhanced cognitive performance								x						
Schizophrenia/Acute panic												x		
Gastric bleeding in portal hypertension												x		
Vaginal contraceptive												x		
Intraocular pressure reduction									x					
Thyrotoxicosis symptoms[3]												x		
Congestive heart failure[3]								x						

[1] For more detailed information, see preceding Indications and individual monographs.
[2] Includes long-acting formulation.
[3] See Precautions or Warnings

Contraindications:

Sinus bradycardia; greater than first degree heart block; cardiogenic shock; congestive heart failure (CHF) unless secondary to a tachyarrhythmia treatable with β-blockers; overt cardiac failure; hypersensitivity to β-blocking agents.

Acebutolol, carteolol: Persistently severe bradycardia.

Propranolol, nadolol, timolol, penbutolol, carteolol, sotalol and pindolol: Bronchial asthma or bronchospasm, including severe chronic obstructive pulmonary disease.

Metoprolol: Treatment of MI in patients with a heart rate < 45 beats/min; significant heart block greater than first degree (PR interval ≥ 0.24 sec); systolic blood pressure < 100 mm Hg; moderate to severe cardiac failure.

Sotalol: Congenital or acquired long QT syndromes.

Warnings:

Mortality: The National Heart Lung and Blood Institute conducted the Cardiac Arrhythmia Suppression Trial (CAST), a long-term, multicenter, randomized, double-blind study in patients with asymptomatic nonlife-threatening ventricular ectopy who had a myocardial infarction > 6 days but < 2 years previously. An excessive mortality or nonfatal cardiac arrest was seen in patients treated with encainide or flecainide (56/730) compared with that seen in patients assigned to matched placebo-treated groups (22/725) and a similar excess has been seen with moricizine. The average duration of treatment with encainide or flecainide in this study was 10 months.

The applicability of these results to other populations (eg, those without recent MI) and to other than Class I antiarrhythmic agents is uncertain. Sotalol is devoid of Class I effects, and in a large controlled trial in patients with a recent MI who did not necessarily have ventricular arrhythmias, sotalol did not produce increased mortality at doses up to 320 mg/day. On the other hand, in the large post-infarction study using a non-titrated initial dose of 320 mg once daily and in a second small randomized trial in high-risk post-infarction patients treated with high doses (320 mg twice daily), there have been suggestions of an excess of early sudden deaths.

Proarrhythmia: Like other antiarrhythmic agents, **sotalol** can provoke new or worsened ventricular arrhythmias in some patients, including sustained ventricular tachycardia or ventricular fibrillation, with potentially fatal consequences. Because of its effect on cardiac repolarization (QTc interval prolongation), torsade de pointes, a polymorphic ventricular tachycardia with prolongation of the QT interval and a shifting electrical axis, is the most common form of proarrhythmia associated with **sotalol**, occurring in about 4% of high risk (history of sustained VT/VF) patients. The risk of torsade de pointes progressively increases with prolongation of the QT interval, and is worsened also by reduction in heart rate and reduction in serum potassium.

Overall, 4.3% of patients experienced a new or worsened ventricular arrhythmia. Of this 4.3%, there was new or worsened sustained ventricular tachycardia in ≈ 1% of patients and torsade de pointes in 2.4%. Additionally, in ≈ 1% of patients, deaths were considered possibly drug-related and may have been associated with proarrhythmic events. In patients with a history of sustained ventricular tachycardia, the incidence of torsade de pointes was 4% and worsened VT ≈ 1%; in patients with other, less serious, ventricular and supraventricular arrhythmias, the incidence of torsade de pointes was 1% and 1.4%, respectively. Torsade de pointes arrhythmias were dose-related.

In addition to dose and presence of sustained VT, other risk factors for torsade de pointes were gender (females had a higher incidence), excessive prolongation of the QTc interval and history of cardiomegaly or CHF. Patients with sustained ventricular tachycardia and a history of CHF appear to have the highest risk for serious proarrhythmia (7%). Of the patients experiencing torsade de pointes, approximately two-thirds spontaneously reverted to their baseline rhythm. The others were either converted electrically (D/C cardioversion or overdrive pacing) or treated with other drugs. Although **sotalol** therapy was discontinued in most patients experiencing torsade de pointes, 17% were continued on a lower dose. Nonetheless, use with particular caution if the QTc is > 500 msec on-therapy and give serious consideration to reducing the dose or discontinuing therapy when the QTc exceeds 550 msec. Due to the multiple risk factors associated with torsade de pointes, however, exercise caution regardless of the QTc interval.

Proarrhythmic events must be anticipated not only on initiating sotalol therapy, but with every upward dose adjustment. Proarrhythmic events most often occur within 7 days of initiating therapy or of an increase in dose; 75% of serious proarrhythmias (torsade de pointes and worsened VT) occurred within 7 days of initiating therapy, while 60% of such events occurred within 3 days of initiation or a dosage change. Initiating therapy at 80 mg twice daily with gradual upward dose titration and appropriate evaluations for efficacy and safety prior to dose escalation, should reduce the risk of proarrhythmia. Avoiding excessive accumulation of sotalol in patients with diminished renal function, by appropriate dose reduction, should also reduce the risk of proarrhythmia (see Administration and Dosage).

Cardiac failure: Sympathetic stimulation is a vital component supporting circulatory function in CHF, and β-blockade carries the potential hazard of further depressing myocardial contractility and precipitating more severe failure. Administer cautiously in hypertensive patients who have CHF controlled by digitalis and diuretics. β-blockers do not abolish the inotropic action of digitalis on heart muscle. Digitalis and β-blockers both slow AV conduction. If cardiac failure persists, withdraw β-blocker therapy.

Although cardiac failure rarely occurs in properly selected patients, advise patients to consult a physician at the first sign or symptom of impending CHF or unexplained respiratory symptoms.

In patients without a history of cardiac failure, continued myocardial depression can lead to cardiac failure. At the first sign or symptom of impending cardiac failure, fully digitalize patients or treat with diuretics and closely observe the response. If cardiac failure continues, withdraw therapy (gradually, if possible).

BETA-ADRENERGIC BLOCKING AGENTS

Recent studies suggest that in certain patients with CHF, beta-blockers may result in symptomatic and hemodynamic improvements. β_1 selective agents are the drugs of choice; start with a low dose and titrate upward. They should not be used as routine therapy nor for acute heart failure. In these studies, most patients had idiopathic dilated cardiomyopathy. Further study is needed to identify patients most likely to benefit from therapy as well as the appropriate drug.

Wolff-Parkinson-White syndrome: In several cases, the tachycardia was replaced by a severe bradycardia requiring a demand pacemaker after **propranolol** administration with as little as 5 mg.

Abrupt withdrawal: The occurrence of a β-blocker withdrawal syndrome is controversial. However, hypersensitivity to catecholamines has been observed in patients withdrawn from β-blocker therapy. Exacerbation of angina, MI, ventricular arrhythmias and death have occurred after abrupt discontinuation of therapy. When discontinuing chronically administered β-blocking agents, particularly in patients with ischemic heart disease, reduce dosage gradually over 1 to 2 weeks and carefully monitor the patient. If therapy with an alternative β-adrenergic blocker is desired, the patient may be transferred directly to comparable doses of another agent without interrupting β-blocking therapy. If angina markedly worsens or acute coronary insufficiency develops, reinstitute administration promptly, at least temporarily, and employ other measures to manage unstable angina.

Because coronary artery disease may be unrecognized, do not discontinue therapy abruptly, even in patients treated only for hypertension, as abrupt withdrawal may result in transient symptoms (eg, tremulousness, sweating, palpitations, headache, malaise).

It has been suggested that β-adrenergic blockers may be discontinued abruptly during acute MI if indicated since the withdrawal phenomenon is not a major clinical problem in these patients.

Peripheral vascular disease: Treatment with β-antagonists reduces cardiac output and can precipitate or aggravate the symptoms of arterial insufficiency in patients with peripheral or mesenteric vascular disease. Exercise caution with such patients and observe closely for evidence of progression of arterial obstruction.

Nonallergic bronchospasm (eg, chronic bronchitis, emphysema): In general, do not administer β-blockers to patients with bronchospastic diseases. Administer **nadolol, timolol, penbutolol, propranolol, sotalol** and **pindolol** with caution, since they may block bronchodilation produced by endogenous or exogenous catecholamine stimulation of β_2 receptors.

Because of their relative β_1 selectivity, low doses of **metoprolol, acebutolol, bisoprolol** and **atenolol** may be used with caution in patients with bronchospastic disease who do not respond to, or cannot tolerate, other antihypertensive treatment. Since β_1 selectivity is not absolute, use a β_2-stimulating agent. It may be advisable initially to administer in smaller divided doses, instead of larger doses twice daily, to avoid the higher plasma levels associated with the longer dosing interval. **Esmolol** may also be used with caution in patients with asthma if an IV agent is required.

Because it is unknown to what extent β_2-stimulating agents may exacerbate myocardial ischemia and the extent of infarction, β-blockers should not be used prophylactically. If bronchospasm not related to CHF occurs, discontinue β-blockers. A theophylline derivative or a β_2 agonist may be administered cautiously, depending on the clinical condition of the patient. Both theophylline derivatives and β_2 agonists may produce serious cardiac arrhythmias.

Bradycardia:

Metoprolol produces a decrease in sinus heart rate in most patients; this decrease is greatest among patients with high initial heart rates and least among patients with low initial heart rates. Acute MI (particularly inferior infarction) may, in itself, produce significant lowering of the sinus rate. If the sinus rate decreases to < 40 beats/min, particularly if associated with lowered cardiac output, give IV atropine (0.25 to 0.5 mg). If treatment with atropine is not successful, discontinue metoprolol and consider cautious administration of isoproterenol or installation of a cardiac pacemaker.

Pheochromocytoma: It is hazardous to use **propranolol** unless α-adrenergic blocking drugs are already in use, since this would predispose to serious blood pressure elevation. Blocking only the peripheral dilator (β) action of epinephrine leaves its constrictor (α) action unopposed. In the event of hemorrhage or shock, there is a disadvantage in having both β and α blockade; the combination prevents the increase in heart rate and peripheral vasoconstriction needed to maintain blood pressure.

Sinus bradycardia (heart rate < 50 bpm) occurred in 13% of patients receiving **sotalol** in clinical trials, and led to discontinuation in about 3%. Bradycardia itself increases risk of torsade de pointes. Sinus pause, sinus arrest and sinus node dysfunction occur in < 1% of patients. Incidence of 2nd- or 3rd- degree AV block is ≈ 1%.

BETA-ADRENERGIC BLOCKING AGENTS

Electrolyte disturbances: Do not use **sotalol** in patients with hypokalemia or hypomagnesemia prior to correction of imbalance, as these conditions can exaggerate the degree of QT prolongation and increase the potential for torsade de pointes. Give special attention to electrolyte and acid-base balance in patients experiencing severe or prolonged diarrhea or patients receiving concomitant diuretic drugs.

Hypotension: If hypotension (systolic blood pressure ≤ 90 mmHg) occurs, discontinue drug and carefully assess patient's hemodynamic status and extent of myocardial damage. Invasive monitoring of central venous, pulmonary capillary wedge and arterial pressures may be required. Institute fluids, positive inotropic agents, balloon counterpulsation or other appropriate therapy. If hypotension is associated with sinus bradycardia or AV block, direct treatment at reversing these.

In clinical trials, 20% to 50% of patients treated with **esmolol** have had hypotension, generally defined as systolic pressure < 90 mm Hg or diastolic pressure < 50 mm Hg. About 12% of the patients have been symptomatic (mainly diaphoresis or dizziness). Hypotension can occur at any dose, but is dose-related; therefore, doses > 200 mcg/kg/min are not recommended. Closely monitor patients, especially if pretreatment blood pressure is low. Decrease of dose or termination of infusion reverses hypotension, usually within 30 minutes.

Anaphylaxis has occurred and may include symptoms such as profound hypotension, bradycardia with or without AV nodal block, severe sustained bronchospasm, hives and angioedema. Deaths have occurred. Refer to Management of Acute Hypersensitivity Reactions.However, patients have been resistant to conventional therapy, especially epinephrine. Aggressive therapy may be required.

Anesthesia and major surgery: Necessity, or desirability, of withdrawing β-blockers prior to major surgery is controversial. β-blockade impairs the heart's ability to respond to β-adrenergically mediated reflex stimuli. While this might help prevent arrhythmic response, risk of excessive myocardial depression during general anesthesia may be enhanced, and difficulty restarting and maintaining heart beat has occurred. If β-blockers are withdrawn, allow 48 hours between the last dose and anesthesia. If treatment is continued, take particular care when using anesthetics which depress the myocardium, such as ether, cyclopropane and trichlorethylene; use the lowest possible β-blocker doses. Others may recommend withdrawal of β-blockers well before surgery takes place.

In the event of emergency surgery, effects of β-blockers can be reversed by β receptor agonists (eg, isoproterenol, dopamine, dobutamine, norepinephrine).

AV block: **Metoprolol** slows AV conduction and may produce significant first (PR interval ≥ 0.26 sec), second, or third-degree heart block. Acute MI also produces heart block.

If heart block occurs, discontinue metoprolol and give IV atropine (0.25 to 0.5 mg). If treatment with atropine is not successful, consider cautious administration of isoproterenol or installation of a cardiac pacemaker.

Sick sinus syndrome: Use **sotalol** only with extreme caution in patients with sick sinus syndrome associated with symptomatic arrhythmias, because it may cause sinus bradycardia, sinus pauses or sinus arrest.

Renal/Hepatic function impairment: Use with caution. **Timolol's** half-life is essentially unchanged in moderate renal insufficiency; however, marked hypotensive responses have been seen in patients with marked renal impairment undergoing dialysis. Dosage reduction may be necessary in impaired renal or hepatic function.

Because **nadolol, carteolol, sotalol** and **atenolol** are eliminated primarily by kidneys, half-life increases in renal failure; dosage adjustments are necessary (see Administration and Dosage). **Bisoprolol** half-life is increased in patients with creatinine clearance < 40 ml/min and in cirrhosis; adjust dosage. Although **acebutolol** is excreted through GI tract, the active metabolite, diacetolol, is eliminated primarily by kidneys; reduce daily acebutolol dose (see Administration and Dosage). Administer **esmolol** with caution in impaired renal function because its acid metabolite is primarily excreted unchanged by kidneys. Elimination half-life of the acid metabolite was prolonged ten-fold and plasma level was considerably elevated in end-stage renal disease. Poor renal function has only minor effects on **pindolol** clearance, but poor hepatic function may cause pindolol blood levels to increase substantially. Expect **penbutolol** conjugate accumulation upon multiple dosing in renal insufficiency. **Metoprolol's** systemic availability and half-life in renal failure do not differ significantly from those in normal subjects; dosage reduction is usually not needed.

Pregnancy: Category C (**atenolol, labetalol, esmolol, metoprolol, nadolol, timolol, propranolol, penbutolol, carteolol, bisoprolol**). Embryotoxic effects have been demonstrated in animals at doses 5 to 50 times higher than the maximum recommended doses in humans.

Category B (**acebutolol, pindolol, sotalol**) – Acebutolol and its major metabolite, diacetolol, cross the placenta. Neonates of mothers who received acebutolol during pregnancy have reduced birth weight and decreased blood pressure and heart rate. Sotalol crosses the placenta and is found in amniotic fluid; subnormal birth weight has occurred.

Safety for use during pregnancy has not been established. Use only when clearly needed and when the potential benefits outweigh the potential hazards to the fetus.

Although cases of teratogenicity in humans have not been reported, problems have occurred during delivery. These include: Neonatal bradycardia, hypoglycemia and apnea, low Apgar scores, maternal and fetal bradycardia, hypothermia, oliguria, poor peripheral perfusion and small birth weight infants (due to chronic therapy). Some of the effects on the neonate may last up to 72 hours postpartum.

Other studies suggest these agents are relatively safe when used during pregnancy with little risk to the fetus. However, several guidelines have been suggested until further data are available: Avoid use during the first trimester; use the lowest possible dose; discontinue at least 2 to 3 days prior to delivery (if possible); use those agents with β_1 selectivity, intrinsic sympathomimetic activity or α-blocking activity.

Lactation: **Propranolol** is excreted in breast milk but in a concentration too low to have any significant effect. **Pindolol, timolol, sotalol** and **nadolol** are excreted in breast milk. **Acebutolol** and diacetolol (its major metabolite) appear in breast milk with a milk:plasma ratio of 7.1 and 12.2, respectively. **Metoprolol** is excreted in breast milk in very small quantities; an infant consuming 1 L of breast milk would receive a dose of < 1 mg of the drug. **Atenolol** is excreted in breast milk at a ratio of 1.5 to 6.8. In one patient, the peak atenolol milk:plasma ratio was 3.6 and the estimated infant dose (maternal dose, 100 mg/day) was 0.13 mg/feeding (75 ml). Another infant developed cyanosis and two incidences of bradycardia following maternal atenolol ingestion (100 mg/day). Small amounts of **bisoprolol** (< 2% of the dose) are detected in breast milk of rats; it is not known if it is excreted in human breast milk. It is not known if **penbutolol** or **carteolol** are excreted in breast milk. Although adverse effects in the infant have not been demonstrated, in general, nursing should not be undertaken by mothers receiving these drugs.

Children: Safety and efficacy for use in children have not been established.

IV administration of **propranolol** is not recommended in children; however, oral propranolol has been used (see Administration and Dosage).

Precautions:

Diabetes/Hypoglycemia: β-adrenergic blockade may blunt premonitory signs and symptoms (eg, tachycardia, blood pressure changes) of acute hypoglycemia. Nonselective β-blockers may potentiate insulin-induced hypoglycemia. This is less likely with cardioselective agents. **Atenolol** does not potentiate insulin-induced hypoglycemia and, unlike nonselective β-blockers, does not delay recovery of blood glucose to normal levels.

Use with caution in diabetic patients, especially those with labile diabetes. β blockade reduces the release of insulin in response to hyperglycemia; it may be necessary to adjust the dose of antidiabetic drugs.

Thyrotoxicosis: β-adrenergic blockers may mask clinical signs (eg, tachycardia) of developing or continuing hyperthyroidism. Abrupt withdrawal may exacerbate symptoms of hyperthyroidism, including thyroid storm; therefore, monitor closely and withdraw the drug slowly.

In contrast, propranolol may be beneficial in reducing the symptoms of thyrotoxicosis.

Serum lipid concentrations: Although study results conflict, β-blockers may alter serum lipids including an increase in the concentration of total triglycerides, total cholesterol and LDL and VLDL cholesterol, and a decrease in the concentration of HDL cholesterol. Other studies suggest **pindolol** does not significantly alter serum lipid concentrations and **acebutolol** actually lowers total and LDL cholesterol levels; **carteolol** and **bisoprolol** did not significantly alter total cholesterol and triglycerides. Further studies are needed.

Muscle weakness: β-blockade has potentiated muscle weakness consistent with certain myasthenic symptoms (eg, diplopia, ptosis, generalized weakness). **Timolol** rarely increased muscle weakness in some patients with myasthenia gravis or myasthenic symptoms.

BETA-ADRENERGIC BLOCKING AGENTS

Drug Interactions:

Beta-Blocker Drug Interactions			
Precipitant drug	Object drug*		Description
Aluminum salts Barbiturates Calcium salts Cholestyramine Colestipol NSAIDs Penicillins (ampicillin) Rifampin Salicylates Sulfinpyrazone	β-blockers	↓	The bioavailability and plasma levels of certain beta blockers may be decreased by these agents, possibly resulting in a decreased pharmacologic effect.
Calcium blockers	β-blockers	↑	Pharmacologic effects of beta-blockers as well as nifedipine and verapamil may be potentiated. Diltiazem, felodipine and nicardipine may increase the effects of the beta-blockers. Monitor cardiac function and decrease the beta-blocker dose if necessary.
Contraceptives, oral	β-blockers	↑	Bioavailability and plasma levels of certain beta-blockers may be increased.
Ethanol	β-blockers-Propranolol	↔	Pharmacologic and therapeutic effects are difficult to predict. Additive CNS inhibition, increased propranolol levels and increased clearance have all occurred.
Flecainide	β-blockers	↑	The bioavailability of either agent may be increased, possibly increasing the pharmacologic effects.
β-blockers	Flecainide	↑	
Haloperidol	β-blockers-Propranolol	↑	Pharmacologic effects (hypotensive episodes) of both drugs may be increased.
β-blockers-Propranolol	Haloperidol		
H_2 antagonists	β-blockers-Metoprolol, propranolol	↑	Pharmacokinetic parameters of beta-blockers metabolized by cytochrome P-450 may be altered by cimetidine; pharmacodynamic effects may be increased. Although data conflict, ranitidine may increase the bioavailability of metoprolol; other beta-blockers have not been affected.
Hydralazine	β-blockers-Metoprolol, propranolol	↑	Serum levels and, hence, pharmacologic effects of beta-blockers and hydralazine may be enhanced.
β-blockers-Metoprolol, propranolol	Hydralazine		
Loop diuretics	β-blockers-Propranolol	↑	Propranolol plasma levels and cardiovascular effects may be enhanced. Atenolol was not affected.
MAO inhibitors	β-blockers-Metoprolol, nadolol	↑	Bradycardia may develop during concurrent use.
Phenothiazines	β-blockers-Propranolol	↑	Propranolol bioavailability and plasma levels and phenothiazine plasma levels may be increased, possibly resulting in increased effects.
β-blockers-Propranolol	Phenothiazines		
Propafenone	β-blockers-Metoprolol, propranolol	↑	Plasma levels of beta blockers metabolized by the liver may be increased.
Quinidine	β-blockers	↑	Plasma beta-blocker levels may be increased in "extensive metabolizers", possibly resulting in increased effects.
Quinolones-Ciprofloxacin	β-blockers	↑	Bioavailability of beta-blockers metabolized by cytochrome P-450 may be increased.

BETA-ADRENERGIC BLOCKING AGENTS

Beta-Blocker Drug Interactions			
Precipitant drug	Object drug*		Description
Thioamines	β-blockers- Metoprolol, propranolol	⬆	The pharmacokinetics of the beta-blockers may be altered, increasing the pharmacologic effects.
Thyroid hormones	β-blockers- Metoprolol, propranolol	⬇	The actions of certain beta-blockers may be impaired when the hypothyroid patient is converted to the euthyroid state.
β-blockers- Propranolol	Acetaminophen	⬆	Acetaminophen clearance may be decreased.
β-blockers	Anticoagulants	⬆	Propranolol may increase the anticoagulant effect of warfarin.
β-blockers- Metoprolol, propranolol	Benzodiazepines	⬆	Effects of certain benzodiazepines may be increased by lipophilic beta-blockers. Atenolol does not interact.
β-blockers	Clonidine	⬆	Life-threatening and fatal increases in blood pressure have occurred after discontinuation of clonidine in patients receiving a beta-blocker or after simultaneous withdrawal.
β-blockers	Disopyramide	⬌	Difficult to predict; disopyramide clearance may be decreased, adverse effects may occur (eg, sinus bradycardia, hypotension) or there may be no occurrence of synergistic or additive negative inotropic effects.
β-blockers	Epinephrine	⬆	Initial hypertensive episode followed by bradycardia may occur.
β-blockers	Ergot alkaloids	⬆	Peripheral ischemia manifested by cold extremities, possible peripheral gangrene.
β-blockers	Lidocaine	⬆	Increased lidocaine levels may occur, resulting in toxicity.
β-blockers	Nondepolarizing muscle relaxants	⬌	Beta-blockers may potentiate, counteract or have no effect on the actions of the nondepolarizing muscle relaxants.
β-blockers	Prazosin	⬆	Concurrent administration may increase the postural hypotension produced by prazosin.
β-blockers	Sulfonylureas	⬇	Hypoglycemic effects of sulfonylureas may be attenuated.
β-blockers- Nonselective	Theophylline	⬌	Reduced elimination of theophylline may occur. Pharmacologic antagonism can also be expected, thus reducing the effects of one or both agents. Cardioselective agents may be preferred.

* ⬆ = Object drug increased ⬇ = Object drug decreased ⬌ = Undetermined effect

Drug/Lab test interactions: These agents may produce hypoglycemia and interfere with **glucose** or **insulin** tolerance tests. Propranolol may interfere with the glaucoma screening test due to a reduction in intraocular pressure.

Drug/Food interactions: Food enhances the bioavailability of **metoprolol** and **propranolol**; this effect is not noted with **nadolol, bisoprolol** or **pindolol**. The rate of **carteolol** and **penbutolol** absorption is slowed by the presence of food; however, extent of absorption is not appreciably affected. **Sotalol** absorption is reduced approximately 20% by a standard meal.

BETA-ADRENERGIC BLOCKING AGENTS

Adverse Reactions:

Most adverse effects are mild and transient and rarely require withdrawal of therapy.

Hypersensitivity: Pharyngitis; photosensitivity reaction; erythematous rash; fever combined with aching and sore throat; laryngospasm; respiratory distress; angioedema; anaphylaxis (see Warnings).

Cardiovascular: Bradycardia; torsade de pointes and other serious new ventricular arrhythmias (see Warnings); cardiovascular disorder; AICD discharge; development of mitral regurgitation; cardiac reinfarction; total cardiac arrests; nonfatal cardiac arrests; cardiogenic shock; development of ventricular septal defect; chest pain; hypertension; hypotension (including asymptomatic and orthostatic); peripheral ischemia; pallor; flushing; worsening of angina and arterial insufficiency; shortness of breath; peripheral vascular insufficiency (cold extremities, paresthesia of hands); arterial insufficiency usually of Raynaud type; claudication; heart failure; CHF; sinoatrial block; cerebral vascular accident; edema; pulmonary edema; vasodilation; presyncope and syncope; tachycardia (including ventricular); palpitations; worsening of arterial insufficiency; conduction disturbances; first, second and third degree heart block; intensification of AV block; abnormal ECG; bundle branch block plus major axis deviation; supraventricular tachycardia (including atrial fibrillation and flutter).

CNS: Dizziness; vertigo; tiredness/fatigue; headache; mental depression (lassitude, weakness); peripheral neuropathy; paralysis; paresthesias; hypoesthesia; hyperesthesia; lethargy; anxiety; nervousness; diminished concentration/memory; somnolence; restlessness; insomnia; sleep disturbances; nightmares; bizarre or many dreams; sedation; change in behavior; altered consciousness; mood change; emotional lability; slightly clouded sensorium; incoordination; reversible mental depression progressing to catatonia; hallucinations; an acute reversible syndrome characterized by disorientation of time and place, short-term memory loss, emotional lability, decreased performance on neuropsychometrics, slurred speech, tinnitus and lightheadedness; acute mental changes (paranoia, disorientation, combativeness) in the elderly; increase in signs and symptoms of myasthenia gravis.

It has been suggested that the more lipophilic the β-blocker, the higher the CNS penetration and subsequent incidence of adverse CNS effects. These effects may improve or disappear when a less lipophilic agent is substituted.

Endocrine: Hyperglycemia; hypoglycemia; unstable diabetes.

GI: Gastric/epigastric pain; flatulence; gastritis; constipation; nausea; diarrhea; colon problem; dry mouth; vomiting; heartburn; appetite disorder; anorexia; bloating; abdominal discomfort/pain; renal and mesenteric arterial thrombosis; ischemic colitis; retroperitoneal fibrosis; hepatomegaly; acute pancreatitis; dyspepsia; taste distortion; elevated liver enzymes (see Lab test abnormalities); elevated bilirubin.

GU: Sexual dysfunction; impotence or decreased libido; dysuria; nocturia; pollakiuria; urinary retention or frequency; urinary tract infection; cystitis; renal colic; GU disorder; renal failure.

Hematologic: Agranulocytosis; nonthrombocytopenic or thrombocytopenic purpura; bleeding; thrombocytopenia; eosinophilia; leukopenia; pulmonary emboli; hyperlipdemia.

Dermatologic: Rash; pruritus; skin irritation; increased pigmentation; sweating/hyperhidrosis; alopecia (including reversible); dry skin; psoriasis (often reversible); acne; eczema; flushing; exfoliative dermatitis; peripheral skin necrosis; psoriasiform rash or exacerbation of psoriasis; purpura; erythematous rash.

Ophthalmic: Eye irritation/discomfort; visual disturbances; dry/burning eyes; blurred vision; conjunctivitis; ocular pain/pressure; abnormal lacrimation; ptosis; oculomucocutaneous syndrome.

Respiratory: Bronchospasm; dyspnea; cough; bronchial obstruction; rales; wheeziness; nasal stuffiness; pharyngitis; rhonchi; laryngospasm with respiratory distress; asthma; rhinitis; sinusitis; pulmonary problem; upper respiratory tract problem.

Musculoskeletal: Joint pain; arthralgia; muscle cramps/pain; back/neck pain; arthritis; twitching/tremor; localized pain; extremity pain; myalgia.

Miscellaneous: Facial swelling; weight gain; weight loss; decreased exercise tolerance; LE-like reactions; lupus syndrome; Peyronie's disease; Raynaud's phenomenon; speech disorder; rigors; earache; gout; asthenia; malaise; infection; fever; death.

BETA-ADRENERGIC BLOCKING AGENTS

Lab test abnormalities: **Propranolol** may elevate blood urea levels in patients with severe heart disease. **Propranolol** and **metoprolol** may cause elevated serum transaminase, alkaline phosphatase and LDH. **Timolol** may produce slight increases in BUN, serum potassium and serum uric acid, and slight decreases in hemoglobin and hematocrit and HDL cholesterol. Increases in liver function tests have been reported; however, these alterations are not progressive and are not associated with clinical manifestations.

Minor persistent elevations in AST and ALT have occurred in 7% of patients treated with **pindolol**, but progressive elevations were not observed and liver injury has not been reported. Alkaline phosphatase, LDH and uric acid are also elevated on rare occasions. The significance of this is unknown. Elevations of AST and ALT of 1 to 2 times normal have occurred with **bisoprolol** (3.9% to 6.2%). Small increases in uric acid, creatinine, BUN, serum potassium, glucose and phosphorus, and decreases in WBC and platelets have also occurred, although they were generally not of clinical importance. Liver abnormalities (increased AST and ALT) have occurred in a small number of patients receiving **acebutolol**.

The development of antinuclear antibodies (ANA) has been associated with β-blocker therapy. Symptoms of arthralgia and myalgias were infrequent and reversed upon drug discontinuation.

Overdosage:

Symptoms: The patient's underlying disease state may contribute significantly. The main features are bradycardia and hypotension.

Cardiovascular – Bradycardia; hypotension; CHF; cardiogenic shock; intraventricular conduction disturbances; AV block (all degrees); asystole; pulmonary edema, especially in persons with underlying myocardial disease; tachycardia and hypertension (**pindolol**); systemic vascular resistance (**propranolol**).

CNS – Depressed consciousness; coma; seizures; respiratory depression.

Other – Bronchospasm, especially in persons with obstructive pulmonary disease; hypoglycemia; hyperkalemia.

Treatment: Place patients in supine position and raise their legs if necessary to improve blood supply to the brain. Measure blood glucose and serum potassium levels. Continuously monitor blood pressure and ECG. Chest x-rays may demonstrate pulmonary edema. Employ respiratory support, emesis (using syrup of ipecac) or lavage and administer charcoal if necessary. Treatment includes usual supportive measures. See also General Management of Acute Overdosage. Administer IV glucose to treat hypoglycemia. Seizures respond to IV diazepam or, if necessary, phenytoin. **Nadolol** and **atenolol** can be removed by hemodialysis. **Propranolol, labetalol, metoprolol, bisoprolol** and **timolol** are not significantly dialyzable. In determining the duration of corrective therapy, consider their long duration of effect. Treatment of cardiovascular complications includes the following:

Bradycardia – If hemodynamically stable, no specific therapy is indicated. If hypotensive, give atropine 0.6 mg IV or epinephrine. If there is no response to vagal blockade, repeat every 3 minutes to a total of 2 to 3 mg. IV isoproterenol may be given cautiously. Large doses of glucagon (5 to 10 mg IV rapidly over 30 seconds, followed by continuous IV infusion of 5 mg/hr) may increase heart rate, even if atropine and isoproterenol have failed. In refractory cases, transvenous cardiac pacing may be needed.

Ventricular premature contractions are best treated with lidocaine or, if necessary, phenytoin. Avoid quinidine, procainamide and disopyramide; they may further depress myocardial function.

Cardiac failure – Administer a digitalis glycoside, a diuretic and oxygen. In refractory cases, IV aminophylline is suggested. Glucagon may also be useful. In shock resulting from inadequate cardiac contractility, consider dobutamine, dopamine, isoproterenol or glucagon.

Hypotension – Place patient in the Trendelenburg position; treat bradyarrhythmias. Administer IV fluids unless pulmonary edema is present. Administer vasopressors (eg, dopamine, dobutamine, norepinephrine; there is pharmacological evidence that norepinephrine may be the drug of choice) with blood pressure monitoring. In refractory cases, glucagon may be useful. In intractable cardiogenic shock, intra-aortic balloon insertion may be necessary.

Heart block (second or third degree) – Use isoproterenol or transvenous cardiac pacemaker.

Bronchospasm – Administer a β_2 stimulating agent, epinephrine or theophylline derivative.

BETA-ADRENERGIC BLOCKING AGENTS

Patient Information:

Do not discontinue medication abruptly, except on advice of physician. Sudden cessation of therapy may precipitate or exacerbate angina.

Consult pharmacist or physician before using other products which may contain α-adrenergic stimulants (eg, nasal decongestants, otc cold preparations).

Notify physician if symptoms of CHF occur (eg, difficult breathing, especially on exertion or when lying down; night cough; swelling of the extremities).

Notify physician if any of these occur: Slow pulse rate, dizziness, lightheadedness, confusion or depression, skin rash, fever, sore throat or unusual bleeding or bruising.

May produce drowsiness, dizziness, lightheadedness, blurred vision; patient should observe caution while driving or performing other tasks requiring alertness, coordination or physical dexterity.

Diabetics: These agents may mask signs of hypoglycemia or alter blood glucose levels.

Propranolol *and* **metoprolol**: Food may enhance bioavailability; take at the same time each day.

Nadolol, pindolol, acebutolol, atenolol, carteolol, bisoprolol *and* **penbutolol**: May be taken without regard to meals.

Sotalol: Food may reduce absorption. Take on an empty stomach.

ATENOLOL

For complete prescribing information, refer to the Beta-Adrenergic Blocking Agents group monograph.

Indications:

Angina pectoris due to coronary atherosclerosis.

Hypertension: Used alone or with other antihypertensive agents.

Acute myocardial infarction.

Administration and Dosage:

Hypertension (oral):

Initial dosage – 50 mg once daily, used alone or added to a diuretic. The full effect of this dose will usually be seen within 1 to 2 weeks. If an optimal response is not achieved, increase to 100 mg/day. Dosage > 100 mg/day is unlikely to produce any further benefit.

Angina pectoris (oral):

Initial dosage – 50 mg/day. If an optimal response is not achieved within 1 week, increase to 100 mg/day. Some patients may require 200 mg/day for optimal effect.

With once daily dosing, 24 hour control is achieved by giving doses larger than necessary to achieve an immediate maximum effect. The maximum early effect on exercise tolerance occurs with doses of 50 to 100 mg, but the effect at 24 hours is attenuated, averaging about 50% to 75% of that with once daily doses of 200 mg.

Acute myocardial infarction:

IV – Initiate treatment as soon as possible after the patient's arrival in the hospital and after eligibility is established. Begin treatment with 5 mg over 5 minutes followed by another 5 mg IV injection 10 minutes later. Dilutions in Dextrose Injection, Sodium Chloride Injection, or Sodium Chloride and Dextrose Injection may be used. These admixtures are stable for 48 hours if not used immediately.

Oral – In patients who tolerate the full 10 mg IV dose, initiate 50 mg tablets 10 minutes after the last IV dose followed by another 50 mg dose 12 hours later. Thereafter, administer 100 mg once daily or 50 mg twice daily for a further 6 to 9 days or until discharge from the hospital.

If there is any question concerning the use of IV atenolol, eliminate the IV administration and use the tablets at a dosage of 100 mg once daily or 50 mg twice daily for at least 7 days.

ATENOLOL

Renal function impairment: Dosage adjustment is required since atenolol is excreted via the kidneys. No significant accumulation occurs until creatinine clearance falls below 35 ml/min/1.73 m^2. The following maximum dosages are recommended:

Atenolol Dosage Adjustment in Severe Renal Impairment		
Creatinine clearance (ml/min/1.73 m^2)	Elimination half-life (hrs)	Maximum dosage
15-35	16-27	50 mg/day
< 15	> 27	50 mg every other day

Hemodialysis: Give 50 mg after each dialysis; administer under hospital supervision as marked decreases in blood pressure can occur.

Rx	**Atenolol** (Various, eg, Lederle, Rugby)	**Tablets**: 25 mg	In 30s, 60s, 90s, 100s, 120s, 500s and 1000s.
Rx	**Tenormin**(ICI Pharma)		(T 107). White. In 100s.
Rx	**Atenolol** (Various, eg, Apothecon, Danbury, Goldline, IPR, Lederle, Rugby, Schein)	**Tablets**: 50 mg	In 30s, 60s, 90s, 100s, 120s, 500s and 1000s.
Rx	**Tenormin** (ICI Pharma)		(ICI 105). White, scored. In 100s, 1000s, 5000s and UD 100s.
Rx	**Atenolol** (Various, eg, Apothecon, Danbury, Goldline, IPR, Lederle, Rugby, Schein)	**Tablets**: 100 mg	In 30s, 60s, 90s, 100s, 120s, 500s and 1000s.
Rx	**Tenormin** (ICI Pharma)		(ICI 101). White, scored. In 100s and UD 100s.
Rx	**Tenormin** (ICI Pharma)	**Injection**: 5mg/10 ml	In 10 ml amps.

ESMOLOL HCl

For complete prescribing information, refer to the Beta-Adrenergic Blocking Agents group monograph.

Indications:

Supraventricular tachycardia: For rapid control of ventricular rate in patients with atrial fibrillation or atrial flutter in perioperative, postoperative or other emergent circumstances where short-term control of ventricular rate with a short-acting agent is desirable.

Noncompensatory sinus tachycardia when heart rate requires specific intervention.

Administration and Dosage:

Supraventricular tachycardia: 50 to 200 mcg/kg/min; average dose is 100 mcg/kg/min although dosages as low as 25 mcg/kg/min have been adequate. Dosages as high as 300 mcg/kg/min provide little added effect and an increased rate of adverse effects, and are not recommended. Individualize dosage by titration in which each step consists of a loading dose followed by a maintenance dose.

To initiate treatment, administer a loading dose infusion of 500 mcg/kg/min for 1 minute followed by a 4 minute maintenance infusion of 50 mcg/kg/min. If adequate therapeutic effect is not observed within 5 minutes, repeat loading dose and follow with maintenance infusion increased to 100 mcg/kg/min. Continue titration procedure, repeating loading infusion, increasing maintenance infusion by increments of 50 mcg/kg/min (for 4 minutes). As desired heart rate or a safety end-point (eg, lowered blood pressure) is approached, omit loading infusion and reduce incremental dose in maintenance infusion from 50 mcg/kg/min to 25 mcg/kg/min or lower. Also, if desired, increase interval between titration steps from 5 to 10 minutes.

This specific dosage regimen has not been intraoperatively studied. Because of the time required for titration, it may not be optimal for intraoperative use.

Maintenance dosages > 200 mcg/kg/min do not significantly increase benefits. The safety of dosages > 300 mcg/kg/min has not been studied.

In the event of an adverse reaction, reduce dosage or discontinue the drug. If a local infusion site reaction develops, use an alternative site. Avoid butterfly needles.

ESMOLOL HCl

Dosage in Supraventricular Tachycardia						
1 minute loading infusion (mcg/kg/min)	4 minute maintenance infusion (mcg/kg/min)					
500	50	100	150	200	250	300

Suggested Administration for Supraventricular Tachycardia
• Drug dilution: 5 g esmolol in 500 ml diluent = 10 mg/ml

Patient wt lbs	Patient wt kg	Infusion rates (ml/min)	Infusion rates (ml/hr)					
110	50	2.5	15	30	45	60	75	90
121	55	2.75	16.5	33	49.5	66	82.5	99
132	60	3	18	36	54	72	90	108
143	65	3.25	19.5	39	58.5	78	97.5	117
154	70	3.5	21	42	63	84	105	126
165	75	3.75	22.5	45	67.5	90	112.5	135
176	80	4	24	48	72	96	120	144
187	85	4.25	25.5	51	76.5	102	127.5	153
198	90	4.5	27	54	81	108	135	162
209	95	4.75	28.5	57	85.5	114	142.5	171
220	100	5	30	60	90	120	150	180
231	105	5.25	31.5	63	94.5	126	157.5	189
242	110	5.5	33	66	99	132	165	198

Transfer to alternative agents: After achieving adequate heart rate control and stable clinical status, transition to alternative antiarrhythmic agents (eg, propranolol, digoxin, verapamil) may be accomplished. A recommended dosage guideline is propranolol 10 to 20 mg every 4 to 6 hours, digoxin 0.125 to 0.5 mg every 6 hours (orally or IV) or verapamil 80 mg every 6 hours. However, consider labeling instructions for the agent selected.

Reduce the dosage of esmolol as follows: One-half hour after the first dose of the alternative agent, reduce esmolol infusion rate by 50%. Following the second dose of the alternative agent, monitor patient's response and, if satisfactory control is maintained for the first hour, discontinue esmolol infusion.

Withdrawal effects may occur with abrupt withdrawal of β-blockers following chronic use in patients with CAD (see Warnings), but these have not been reported with esmolol. However, use caution when abruptly discontinuing esmolol infusions.

The use of esmolol infusions up to 24 hours has been well documented. Limited data indicate that esmolol is well tolerated up to 48 hours.

The 250 mg/ml strength is concentrated, and is not for direct IV injection; dilute prior to infusion. Do not mix with sodium bicarbonate. Do not mix with other drugs prior to dilution in a suitable IV fluid. The 10 mg/ml vial is ready to use.

Venous irritation and thrombophlebitis are associated more often with infusion concentrations of 20 rather than 10 mg/ml. Avoid concentrations > 10 mg/ml.

Preparation of solution (10 ml amp): Remove 20 ml from a 500 ml bottle of one of the IV fluids listed below (see Compatibility/Stability), and add the contents of two amps (each containing 2.5 g esmolol). This yields a final concentration of 10 mg/ml. The diluted solution is stable for at least 24 hours at room temperature. Esmolol has been well tolerated when administered via a central vein.

Compatibility/Stability: Esmolol, at a final concentration of 10 mg/ml, is compatible with the following solutions and is stable for at least 24 hours at controlled room temperatures or under refrigeration: 5% Dextrose Injection; 5% Dextrose in Lactated Ringer's Injection; 5% Dextrose in Ringer's Injection; 5% Dextrose and 0.9% or 0.45% Sodium Chloride Injection; Lactated Ringer's Injection; Potassium Chloride (40 mEq/L) in 5% Dextrose Injection; 0.9% or 0.45% Sodium Chloride Injection.

Esmolol is NOT compatible with 5% Sodium Bicarbonate Injection.

Rx	**Brevibloc** (Ohmeda)	**Injection:** 10 mg/ml	In 10 ml vials.[1]
		250 mg/ml	In 10 ml amps.[1]

[1] With 25% propylene glycol.

BETAXOLOL HCl

For complete prescribing information, refer to the Beta-Adrenergic Blocking Agents group monograph.

Indications:

Hypertension: Management of hypertension, used alone or concomitantly with other antihypertensive agents, particularly thiazide-type diuretics.

Administration and Dosage:

Initial dose: 10 mg once daily, alone or added to diuretic therapy. The full antihypertensive effect is usually seen within 7 to 14 days; if the desired response is not achieved the dose can be doubled. Increasing the dose > 20 mg has not produced a statistically significant additional hypertensive effect; however, the 40 mg dose is well tolerated. Anticipate an increased effect (reduction) on heart rate with increasing dosage. To discontinue treatment, gradually withdraw betaxolol over 2 weeks.

Elderly: Consider reducing the starting dose to 5 mg.

Rx	**Kerlone** (Searle)	**Tablets:** 10 mg	(Kerlone 10). White, scored. Film coated. In 100s, UD 100s.
		20 mg	(Kerlone 20 β). White. Film coated. In 100s and UD 100s.

PENBUTOLOL SULFATE

For complete prescribing information, refer to the Beta-Adrenergic Blocking Agents group monograph.

Indications:

Hypertension: Treatment of mild to moderate arterial hypertension. Used alone or in combination with other antihypertensive agents.

Administration and Dosage:

Usual starting and maintenance dose, used alone or with other antihypertensive agents (eg, thiazide diuretics) is 20 mg once daily.

Doses of 40 to 80 mg have been well tolerated but have not shown greater antihypertensive effect. Full effect of a 20 or 40 mg dose is seen by the end of 2 weeks. A dose of 10 mg also lowers blood pressure, but the full effect is not seen for 4 to 6 weeks.

Rx	**Levatol** (Schwarz Pharma)	**Tablets:** 20 mg	(RC 22). Yellow, scored. Capsule shape. In 100s.

CARTEOLOL HCl

For complete prescribing information, refer to the Beta-Adrenergic Blocking Agents group monograph.

Indications:

Hypertension: Used alone or in combination with other antihypertensive agents.

Administration and Dosage:

Initial: 2.5 mg as a single daily dose, either alone or with a diuretic. If adequate response is not achieved, gradually increase to 5 and 10 mg as single daily doses. Doses > 10 mg/day are unlikely to produce further benefit, and may decrease response.

Maintenance: 2.5 to 5 mg once daily.

Renal function impairment: Individualize dosage.

Carteolol Dosage Interval in Renal Impairment

Creatinine clearance (ml/min/1.73 m²)	Dosage interval (hrs)
> 60	24
20-60	48
< 20	72

Rx	**Cartrol** (Abbott)	**Tablets:** 2.5 mg	Gray. In 100s.
		5 mg	White. In 100s.

BISOPROLOL FUMARATE

For complete prescribing information, refer to the Beta-Adrenergic Blocking Agents group monograph.

Indications:

Hypertension: Used alone or in combination with other antihypertensive agents.

Administration and Dosage:

Approved by the FDA on July 31, 1992.

Individualize dosage. May be given without regard to meals.

Initial dose: 5 mg once daily. In some patients, 2.5 mg may be appropriate. If the antihypertensive effect of 5 mg is inadequate, the dose may be increased to 10 mg and then, if necessary, to 20 mg once daily.

Renal/Hepatic function impairment: In patient with renal dysfunction (creatinine clearance < 40 ml/min) or hepatic impairment (hepatitis or cirrhosis), use an initial daily dose of 2.5 mg and use caution in dose titration. Since limited data suggest that bisoprolol is not dialyzable, dose adjustment is not necessary in patients undergoing hemodialysis.

Elderly: Dose adjustment is not necessary.

Rx	**Zebeta** (Lederle)	**Tablets:** 5 mg	(B1 LL). Pink, scored. Film coated. Heart shape. Biconvex. In 14s, 30s, 100s, 500s, 1000s, UD 10s.
		10 mg	(B3 LL). White. Film coated. Heart shape. Biconvex. In 14s, 30s, 100s, 500s, 1000s, UD 10s.

PINDOLOL

For complete prescribing information, refer to the Beta-Adrenergic Blocking Agents group monograph.

Indications:

Hypertension: Management of hypertension, used alone or with other antihypertensive agents, particularly with a thiazide-type diuretic.

Administration and Dosage:

Individualize dosage.

Initial dose: 5 mg twice daily, alone or with other antihypertensive agents. The antihypertensive response usually occurs within the first week of treatment. Maximal response, however, may occur within 2 weeks or, occasionally, longer. If a satisfactory reduction in blood pressure does not occur within 3 to 4 weeks, adjust dose in increments of 10 mg/day at 3 to 4 week intervals, to a maximum of 60 mg/day.

Rx	**Pindolol** (Mylan)	**Tablets:** 5 mg	(M 52). White, scored. In 100s and 1000s.
Rx	**Visken** (Sandoz)		(Visken 5V). White. Heart shape. In 100s.
Rx	**Pindolol** (Mylan)	**Tablets:** 10 mg	(M 127). White, scored. In 100s and 1000s.
Rx	**Visken** (Sandoz)		(Visken 10V). White. Heart shape. In 100s.

METOPROLOL

For complete prescribing information, refer to the Beta-Adrenergic Blocking Agents group monograph.

Indications:

Hypertension: Used alone or in combination with other antihypertensive agents.

Angina pectoris.

Myocardial infarction (immediate release tablets and injection).

Administration and Dosage:

Tablets (immediate release) and injection: Individualize dosage; take at the same time each day.

Hypertension –

Initial dosage: 100 mg/day in single or divided doses, used alone or added to a diuretic. The dosage may be increased at weekly (or longer) intervals until optimum blood pressure reduction is achieved. In general, the maximum effect of any given dosage level will be apparent after 1 week of therapy.

Maintenance dose: 100 to 450 mg/day. Dosages > 450 mg/day have not been studied. While once daily dosing is effective and can maintain a reduction in blood pressure throughout the day, lower doses (especially 100 mg) may not maintain a full effect at the end of the 24 hour period; larger or more frequent daily doses may be required. Measure blood pressure near the end of the dosing interval to determine whether satisfactory control is being maintained.

Angina pectoris –

Initial dosage: 100 mg/day in two divided doses. Dosage may be gradually increased at weekly intervals until optimum clinical response is obtained or a pronounced slowing of heart rate occurs. Effective dosage range is 100 to 400 mg/day. Dosages above 400 mg/day have not been studied. If treatment is to be discontinued, reduce dosage gradually over 1 to 2 weeks.

Myocardial infarction (MI) –

Early treatment: During the early phase of definite or suspected acute MI, initiate treatment as soon as possible after the patient's arrival in a coronary care or similar unit immediately after the patient is hemodynamically stable.

Administer 3 IV bolus injections of 5 mg each, at approximately 2 minute intervals. During IV administration, carefully monitor blood pressure, heart rate and ECG.

In patients who tolerate the full IV dose (15 mg), give 50 mg orally every 6 hours 15 minutes after the last IV dose and continue for 48 hours. Thereafter, administer a maintenance dosage of 100 mg twice daily.

In patients who do not tolerate the full IV dose, start with 25 or 50 mg orally every 6 hours (depending on the degree of intolerance) 15 minutes after the last IV dose or as soon as the clinical condition allows. In patients with severe intolerance, discontinue treatment.

Late treatment: Patients with contraindications to early treatment, patients who do not tolerate the full early treatment and patients in whom therapy is delayed for any other reason should be started at 100 mg orally, twice daily, as soon as their clinical condition allows. Continue for at least 3 months. Although the efficacy beyond 3 months has not been conclusively established, data suggest treatment should continue for 1 to 3 years.

Tablets, extended release: The extended release tablets are for once-a-day administration. When switching from immediate release metoprolol tablets to extended release, use the same total daily dose. Individualize dosage; titration may be needed in some patients.

Hypertension – The usual initial dosage is 50 to 100 mg/day in a single dose whether used alone or added to a diuretic. The dosage may be increased at weekly (or longer) intervals until optimum blood pressure reduction is achieved. In general, the maximum effect of any given dosage level will be apparent after 1 week of therapy. Dosages > 400 mg/day have not been studied.

Angina pectoris – Individualize dosage. The usual initial dosage is 100 mg/day in a single dose. The dosage may be gradually increased at weekly intervals until optimum clinical response has been obtained or there is a pronounced slowing of the heart rate. Dosages > 400 mg/day have not been studied. If treatment is to be discontinued, reduce dosage gradually over a period of 1 to 2 weeks.

METOPROLOL

Rx	**Metoprolol Tartrate** (Purepac)	**Tablets:** 50 mg	Lactose. White, scored. Capsule shape. Film coated. In 100s, 1000s, and UD 100s.
Rx	**Lopressor** (Geigy)		(Geigy 51 51). Pink, scored. Capsule shape. In 100s, 1000s, UD 100s and *Gy-Pak* 60s and 100s.
Rx	**Metoprolol Tartrate** (Purepac)	100 mg	Lactose. White, scored. Capsuld shape. Film coated. In 100s, 1000s, and UD 100s.
Rx	**Lopressor** (Geigy)		(Geigy 71 71). Light blue, scored. Capsule shape, biconvex. In 100s, 1000s, UD 100s and *Gy-Pak* 60s and 100s.
Rx	**Toprol XL** (Astra)	**Tablets, extended release:** 50 mg (47.5 mg metoprolol succinate equivalent to 50 mg metoprolol tartrate)	Lactose. (A mo). White, scored. Biconvex. Film coated. In 100s.
		100 mg (95 mg metoprolol succinate equivalent to 100 mg metoprolol tartrate)	Lactose. (A ms). White, scored. Biconvex. Film coated. In 100s.
		200 mg (190 mg metoprolol succinate equivalent to 200 mg metoprolol tartrate)	Lactose. (A my). White, scored. Oval, biconvex. Film coated. In 100s.
Rx	**Metoprolol Tartrate** (Purepac)	**Injection:** 1 mg/ml	In 5 ml amps.
Rx	**Lopressor** (Geigy)		In 5 ml amps.

TIMOLOL MALEATE

For complete prescribing information, refer to the Beta-Adrenergic Blocking Agents group monograph.

Indications:

Hypertension: Used alone or in combination with other antihypertensive agents, especially thiazide-type diuretics.

Myocardial infarction: For clinically stable survivors of acute MI, to reduce cardiovascular mortality and the risk of reinfarction.

Migraine prophylaxis.

Administration and Dosage:

Hypertension:

Initial dosage – 10 mg twice daily used alone or added to a diuretic.

Maintenance dosage – 20 to 40 mg/day. Titrate, depending on blood pressure and heart rate. Increases to a maximum of 60 mg/day divided into 2 doses may be necessary. There should be an interval of at least 7 days between dosage increases.

Myocardial infarction (long-term prophylactic use in patients who have survived the acute phase of an MI): 10 mg twice daily.

Migraine: Initial dosage is 10 mg twice daily. During maintenance therapy the 20 mg daily dosage may be given as a single dose. Total daily dosage may be increased to a maximum of 30 mg in divided doses or decreased to 10 mg once daily depending on clinical response and tolerability. Discontinue if a satisfactory response is not obtained after 6 to 8 weeks of the maximum daily dosage.

Rx	**Timolol Maleate** (Various, eg, Danbury, Geneva, Goldline, Mylan, Schein)	**Tablets:** 5 mg	In 100s.
Rx	**Blocadren** (MSD)		(MSD 59 Blocadren). Light blue. In 100s.
Rx	**Timolol Maleate** (Various, eg, Danbury, Geneva, Goldline, Major, Mylan, Schein)	**Tablets:** 10 mg	In 100s.
Rx	**Blocadren** (MSD)		(MSD 136 Blocadren). Light blue, scored. In 100s and UD 100s.
Rx	**Timolol Maleate** (Various, eg, Danbury, Geneva, Goldline, Major, Mylan, Schein)	**Tablets:** 20 mg	In 100s.
Rx	**Blocadren** (MSD)		(MSD 437 Blocadren). Light blue, scored. In 100s.

SOTALOL HCl

For complete prescribing information, refer to the Beta-Adrenergic Blocking Agents group monograph.

Indications:

Ventricular arrhythmias: Treatment of documented ventricular arrhythmias, such as sustained ventricular tachycardia, that are life-threatening. Because of the proarrhythmic effects, including a 1.5% to 2% rate of torsade de pointes or new VT/VF in patients with either NSVT or supraventricular arrhythmias, its use in patients with less severe arrhythmias, even if the patients are symptomatic, is generally not recommeded. Avoid treatment of patients with asymptomatic ventricular premature contractions.

Administration and Dosage:

Approved by the FDA on October 30, 1992.

The recommended initial dose is 80 mg twice daily. This dose may be increased if necessary, after appropriate evaluation, to 240 or 320 mg/day. In most patients, a therapeutic response is obtained at a total daily dose of 160 to 320 mg/day, given in two or three divided doses. Some patients with life-threatening refractory ventricular arrhythmias may require doses as high as 480 to 640 mg/day; however, only use these doses when the potential benefit outweighs the increased risk of adverse events, in particular proarrhythmia. Because of the long terminal elimination half-life of sotalol, dosing on more than a twice-daily regimen is usually not necessary.

Adjust dosage gradually, allowing 2 to 3 days between dosing increments in order to attain steady-state plasma concentrations, and to allow monitoring of QT intervals. Graded dose adjustment will help prevent the usage of doses which are higher than necessary to control the arrhythmia.

Initiate and increase doses in a hospital with facilities for cardiac rhythm monitoring and assessment. Administer only after appropriate clinical assessment and individualize the dosage for each patient on the basis of therapeutic response and tolerance. Proarrhythmic events can occur not only at initiation of therapy, but also with each upward dosage adjustment.

Renal function impairment: Because sotalol is excreted predominantly in urine and its terminal elimination half-life is prolonged in conditions of renal impairment, modify the dosing interval (when creatinine clearance is < 60 ml/min) according to the following table.

Sotalol Dosing Interval in Renal Impairment	
Creatinine clearance (ml/min)	Dosing interval (hours)
> 60	12
30 - 60	24
10 - 30	36 - 48
< 10	Individualize dose

Since the terminal elimination half-life is increased in patients with renal impairment, a longer duration of dosing is required to reach steady state. Dose escalations in renal impairment should be done after administration of at least 5 to 6 doses at appropriate intervals (see above table).

Transfer to sotalol: Before starting sotalol, generally withdraw previous antiarrhythmic therapy under careful monitoring for a minimum of 2 to 3 plasma half-lives if the patient's clinical condition permits. Treatment has been initiated in some patients receiving IV lidocaine without ill effect. After discontinuation of amiodarone, do not initiate sotalol until the QT interval is normalized.

Rx	**Betapace** (Berlex)	**Tablets:** 80 mg	Lactose. (Betapace Tablets 80 mg). Light blue, scored. Capsule shape. In 100s and UD 100s.
		120 mg	Lactose. (Betapace 120 mg). Light blue. Capsule shape. In 100s and UD 100s.
		160 mg	Lactose. (Betapace Tablets 160 mg). Light blue, scored. Capsule shape. In 100s and UD 100s.
		240 mg	Lactose. (Betapace Tablets 240 mg). Light blue, scored. Capsule shape. In 100s and UD 100s.

ACEBUTOLOL HCl

For complete prescribing information, refer to the Beta-Adrenergic Blocking Agents group monograph.

Indications:

Hypertension: Used alone or in combination with other antihypertensive agents.

Ventricular arrhythmias: Management of ventricular premature beats.

Administration and Dosage:

Hypertension:

Initial dose – 400 mg in uncomplicated mild to moderate hypertension. May be given in a single daily dose, but 200 mg twice daily may be required for adequate control. Optimal response usually occurs with 400 to 800 mg/day (range, 200 to 1200 mg/day given twice daily). The drug may be combined with another antihypertensive agent. As dosage is increased, β_1-selectivity diminishes.

Ventricular arrhythmia:

Initial dose – 400 mg (200 mg twice daily). Increase dosage gradually until optimal response is obtained, usually 600 to 1200 mg/day. To discontinue treatment, gradually reduce dosage over 2 weeks.

Elderly: Since bioavailability increases about twofold, older patients may require lower maintenance doses. Avoid doses > 800 mg/day.

Renal/Hepatic function impairment: Reduce the daily dose by 50% when creatinine clearance is < 50 ml/min/1.73 m^2. Reduce by 75% when it is < 25 ml/min/1.73 m^2. Use cautiously in impaired hepatic function.

Rx	**Acebutolol HCl** (Mylan)	**Capsules:** 200 mg	In 100s.
Rx	**Sectral** (Wyeth-Ayerst)		(Wyeth 4177 Sectral 200). Purple/orange. In 100s and Redipak 100s.
Rx	**Acebutolol HCl** (Mylan)	**Capsules:** 400 mg	In 100s.
	Sectral (Wyeth-Ayerst)		(Wyeth 4179 Sectral 400). Brown/orange. In 100s.

NADOLOL

For complete prescribing information, refer to the Beta-Adrenergic Blocking Agents group monograph.

Indications:

Angina pectoris: Long-term management.

Hypertension: Used alone or in combination with other antihypertensive agents.

Administration and Dosage:

Individualize dosage. May be given without regard to meals.

Angina pectoris:

Initial – 40 mg/day. Gradually increase dosage in 40 to 80 mg increments at 3 to 7 day intervals until optimum clinical response is obtained or there is pronounced slowing of the heart rate.

Maintenance dose – Usual dose is 40 to 80 mg/day. Up to 160 to 240 mg/day may be needed.

The safety and efficacy of dosages exceeding 240 mg/day have not been established. To discontinue, reduce dosage gradually over 1 to 2 weeks.

Hypertension:

Initial – 40 mg once daily, alone or in addition to diuretic therapy. Gradually increase dosage in 40 to 80 mg increments until optimum blood pressure reduction is achieved.

Maintenance dose – Usual dose is 40 to 80 mg once daily. Up to 240 to 320 mg once daily may be needed.

Renal function impairment: Nadolol is excreted principally by the kidneys and, although nonrenal elimination does occur, dosage adjustments are necessary in patients with renal impairment. The following dosage intervals are recommended:

Nadolol Dosage Adjustments in Renal Failures

Creatinine clearance (ml/min/1.73 m²)	Dosage interval (hours)
> 50	24
31-50	24-36
10-30	24-48
< 10	40-60

Rx	Nadolol (Various, eg, Apothecon, Major, Moore, Mylan)	**Tablets:** 20 mg	In 100s and UD 100s.
Rx	**Corgard** (Bristol-Myers Squibb)		(PPP 232). Scored. In 100s and *Unimatic* 100s.
Rx	Nadolol (Various, eg, Apothecon, Major, Moore, Mylan)	**Tablets:** 40 mg	In 100s, 1000s and UD 100s.
Rx	**Corgard** (Bristol-Myers Squibb)		(PPP 207). Scored. In 100s, 1000s and *Unimatic* 100s.
Rx	Nadolol (Various, eg, Apothecon, Major, Moore, Mylan)	**Tablets:** 80 mg	In 100s, 1000s and UD 100s.
Rx	**Corgard** (Bristol-Myers Squibb)		(PPP 241). Scored. In 100s, 1000s and *Unimatic* 100s.
Rx	**Nadolol** (Various, eg, Apothecon)	120 mg	In 100s and 1000s.
Rx	**Corgard** (Bristol-Myers Squibb)		(PPP 208). Scored. In 100s and 1000s.
Rx	**Nadolol** (Various, eg, Apothecon)	160 mg	In 100s.
Rx	**Corgard** (Bristol-Myers Squibb)		(PPP 246). Scored. In 100s.

PROPRANOLOL HCl

For complete prescribing information, refer to the Beta-Adrenergic Blocking Agents group monograph.

Indications:

Cardiac arrhythmias: Supraventricular, ventricular, tachyarrhythmias of digitalis intoxication and resistant tachyarrhythmias due to excessive catecholamine action during anesthesia.

Myocardial infarction.

Hypertrophic subaortic stenosis: Especially for treatment of exertional or other stress-induced angina, palpitations and syncope.

Pheochromocytoma: As adjunctive therapy following primary treatment with an alpha-adrenergic blocker.

Hypertension: Used alone or in combination with other antihypertensive agents.

Migraine prophylaxis.

Angina pectoris due to coronary atherosclerosis.

Essential tremor: Familial or hereditary.

Administration and Dosage:

Propranolol Dosage Based on Indication			
Indication	Initial dosage	Usual range	Maximum daily dose
Arrhythmias		10-30 mg tid-qid (given ac-hs)	
Hypertension	40 mg bid or 80 mg once daily (SR)	120-240 mg/day (given bid-tid) or 120-160 mg once daily (SR)	640 mg
Angina	80-320 mg bid, tid, qid or 80 mg once daily (SR)	160 mg once daily (SR)	320 mg
MI		180-240 mg/day (given tid-qid)	240 mg
IHSS		20-40 mg tid-qid (given ac-hs) or 80-160 mg once daily (SR)	
Pheochromocytoma		60 mg/day × 3 days preoperatively (in divided doses)	
Inoperable tumor		30 mg/day (in divided doses)	
Migraine	80 mg/day once daily (SR) or in divided doses	160-240 mg/day (in divided doses)	
Essential tremor	40 mg bid	120 mg/day	320 mg

Hypertension: The time course of full blood pressure response ranges from a few days to several weeks. While twice daily dosing is effective and can maintain a reduction in blood pressure throughout the day, some patients, especially with lower doses, may experience a modest blood pressure rise toward the end of the 12 hour dosing interval. Evaluate by measuring blood pressure near the end of the dosing interval. If control is inadequate, a larger dose, or 3 times daily dosing may achieve better control.

Angina pectoris: Increased exercise tolerance and reduced ischemic changes in the ECG occur with bid, tid or qid dosing.

Sustained release capsules – Gradually increase initial dosage at 3 to 7 day intervals until optimum response is obtained.

Myocardial infarction: The safety and efficacy of daily dosages > 240 mg for prevention of cardiac mortality have not been established. Higher dosages may be needed to effectively treat coexisting diseases such as angina or hypertension.

Pheochromocytoma: Administer concomitantly with an α-adrenergic blocking agent.

Migraine: Increase dosage gradually to achieve optimum migraine prophylaxis. If a satisfactory response is not obtained within 4 to 6 weeks after reaching the maximum dose, discontinue therapy. Withdraw gradually over several weeks.

Parenteral: Reserve IV use for life-threatening arrhythmias or those occurring under anesthesia.

Usual dose – 1 to 3 mg under careful monitoring (eg, central venous pressure, ECG). Do not exceed 1 mg/min to avoid lowering blood pressure and causing cardiac standstill. Allow time for the drug to reach site of action, particularly when slow circulation is present. If necessary, give a second dose after 2 minutes. Thereafter, do not give additional drug in < 4 hours. Do not give additional propranolol after the desired alteration in rate or rhythm is achieved. Transfer to oral therapy as soon as possible. IV use has not been evaluated adequately in managing hypertensive emergencies.

PROPRANOLOL HCl

Pediatrics: IV use is not recommended; however, an unlabeled dose of 0.01 to 0.1 mg/kg/dose to a maximum of 1 mg/dose by slow push has been used for arrhythmias.

Oral dosage for treating hypertension requires titration, beginning with a 1 mg/kg/day dosage regimen (ie, 0.5 mg/kg twice daily). May be increased at 3 to 5 day intervals to a maximum of 2 mg/kg/day.

The usual pediatric dosage range is 2 to 4 mg/kg/day in two equally divided doses (ie, 1 to 2 mg/kg twice daily). Dosage calculated by weight generally produces plasma levels in a therapeutic range similar to that in adults. Doses based on body surface area are not recommended since they usually result in plasma levels above the mean adult therapeutic range. Do not use doses > 16 mg/kg/day. To discontinue treatment, gradually decrease dose over 1 to 2 weeks. Data on use of sustained release capsules in this age group are too limited to permit adequate directions for use.

Rx	**Propranolol HCl** (Various, eg, Barr, Danbury, Goldline, Lederle, Major, Moore, Mylan, Purepac, Roxane, Schein)	**Tablets:** 10 mg	In 100s, 500s, 1000s and UD 100s.
Rx	**Inderal** (Wyeth-Ayerst)		(I Inderal 10). Orange, scored. Hexagonal. In 100s, 1000s, 5000s and UD 100s.
Rx	**Propranolol HCl** (Various, eg, Barr, Danbury, Goldline, Lederle, Major, Moore, Mylan, Purepac, Roxane, Schein)	**Tablets:** 20 mg	In 100s, 500s, 1000s and UD 100s.
Rx	**Inderal** (Wyeth-Ayerst)		(I Inderal 20). Blue, scored. Hexagonal. In 100s, 1000s, 5000s and UD 100s.
Rx	**Propranolol HCl** (Various, eg, Barr, Danbury, Goldline, Lederle, Major, Moore, Mylan, Purepac, Roxane, Schein)	**Tablets:** 40 mg	In 100s, 500s, 1000s and UD 100s.
Rx	**Inderal** (Wyeth-Ayerst)		(I Inderal 40). Green, scored. Hexagonal. In 100s, 1000s and UD 100s.
Rx	**Propranolol HCl** (Various, eg, Barr, Goldline, Lederle, Major, Moore, Mylan, Purepac, Roxane, Schein)	**Tablets:** 60 mg	In 100s, 500s and UD 100s.
Rx	**Inderal** (Wyeth-Ayerst)		(I Inderal 60). Pink, scored. Hexagonal. In 100s and 1000s.
Rx	**Propranolol HCl** (Various, eg, Barr, Danbury, Goldline, Lederle, Major, Moore, Mylan, Purepac, Roxane, Schein)	**Tablets:** 80 mg	In 100s, 500s, 1000s and UD 100s.
Rx	**Inderal** (Wyeth-Ayerst)		(I Inderal 80). Yellow, scored. Hexagonal. In 100s, 1000s, 5000s and UD 100s.
Rx	**Propranolol HCl** (Various, eg, Qualitest, Sidmak)	**Tablets:** 90 mg	In 100s and 500s.
Rx	**Propranolol HCl** (Various, eg, Goldline, Inwood, Lemmon, Major, Schein)	**Capsules, sustained release:** 60 mg	In 100s, 250s, 500s and 1000s.
Rx	**Inderal LA** (Wyeth-Ayerst)		(Inderal LA 60). White/light blue. In 100s.

PROPRANOLOL HCl

Rx	**Propranolol HCl** (Various, eg, Goldline, Inwood, Lemmon, Major, Moore, Parmed, Schein)	**Capsules, sustained release**: 80 mg	In 100s, 250s, 500s and 1000s.
Rx	**Inderal LA** (Wyeth-Ayerst)		(Inderal LA 80). Light blue. In 100s, 1000s and UD 100s.
Rx	**Propranolol HCl** (Various, eg, Goldline, Inwood, Lemmon, Major, Moore, Schein)	**Capsules, sustained release**: 120 mg	In 100s, 250s, 500s and 1000s.
Rx	**Inderal LA** (Wyeth-Ayerst)		(Inderal LA 120). Two-tone blue. In 100s, 1000s and UD 100s.
Rx	**Propranolol HCl** (Various, eg, Goldline, Inwood, Lemmon, Major, Moore, Schein)	**Capsules, sustained release**: 160 mg	In 100s, 250s, 500s and 1000s.
Rx	**Inderal LA** (Wyeth-Ayerst)		(Inderal LA 160). Dark blue. In 100s, 1000s and UD 100s.
Rx	**Betachron E-R** (Inwood)	**Capsules, extended release**: 60 mg	(IL/3609). Brown/clear. Sucrose. In 100s.
		80 mg	(IL/3610). Blue/clear. Sucrose. In 100s and 250s.
		120 mg	(IL/3611). Blue/clear. Sucrose. In 100s.
		160 mg	(IL/3612). Blue/clear. Sucrose. In 100s.
Rx *sf*	**Propranolol HCl** (Roxane)	**Solution, oral:** 4 mg/ml	Dye free. Strawberry-mint flavor. In 500 ml and UD 5 ml Patient Cups (40s).
		8 mg/ml	Dye free. Strawberry-mint flavor. In 500 ml and UD 5 ml Patient Cups (40s).
Rx *sf*	**Propranolol Intensol** (Roxane)	**Solution, concentrated oral**: 80 mg/ml	Alcohol and dye free. In 30 ml with dropper.
Rx	**Propranolol HCl** (Various, eg, Smith & Nephew SoloPak)	**Injection**: 1 mg/ml	In 1 ml vials.
Rx	**Inderal** (Wyeth-Ayerst)		In 1 ml amps.

sf Sugar free.

LABETALOL HCl

Actions:

Pharmacology: Labetalol combines both selective, competitive postsynaptic α_1-adrenergic blocking and nonselective, competitive β-adrenergic blocking activity. The ratios of α- to β-blockade are ≈ 1:3 and 1:7 after oral and IV use, respectively.

The α- and β-blocking actions decrease blood pressure (BP). Due to α_1-receptor blocking activity, standing BP is lowered more than supine, and symptoms of postural hypotension, including rare instances of syncope, can occur. In dose-related fashion, labetalol blunts increases in exercise-induced BP and heart rate, and in their double product. Pulmonary circulation during exercise is not affected.

Labetalol produces dose-related falls in BP without reflex tachycardia or significant reduction in heart rate. Hemodynamic effects are variable including small, nonsignificant changes in cardiac output and small decreases in total peripheral resistance. Elevated plasma renins are reduced. Doses that controlled hypertension did not affect renal function in patients with mild to severe hypertension and normal renal function.

Although β-adrenergic receptor blockade is useful in angina and hypertension, sympathetic stimulation is vital in some situations. For example, in patients with severely damaged hearts, adequate ventricular function may depend on sympathetic drive. β–blockade may worsen AV block by preventing the necessary facilitating effects of sympathetic activity on conduction. β_2-blockade results in passive bronchial constriction by interfering with endogenous adrenergic bronchodilator activity in patients subject to bronchospasm and may also interfere with exogenous bronchodilators in such patients.

Single oral doses in coronary artery disease patients had no significant effect on sinus rate, intraventricular conduction or QRS duration. AV conduction time may be modestly prolonged. IV doses slightly prolonged AV nodal conduction time and atrial effective refractory period with small heart rate changes. Effects on AV nodal refractoriness were inconsistent.

Pharmacokinetics:

Absorption/Distribution – Oral labetalol is completely absorbed; peak plasma levels occur in 1 to 2 hours. Steady-state plasma levels during repetitive dosing are reached by about the third day. Due to an extensive first-pass effect, absolute bioavailability is 25%; this is increased by food and in the elderly. Protein binding is ≈ 50%. Labetalol is moderately lipid soluble and crosses the placenta.

Metabolism/Excretion – Metabolism is mainly through conjugation to glucuronide metabolites, which are excreted in urine and in feces (via bile). Elimination half-life following oral and IV use is 6 to 8 hours and 5.5 hours, respectively. In decreased hepatic or renal function, elimination half-life is not altered. About 55% to 60% of a dose appears in urine as conjugates or unchanged drug in the first 24 hours. Neither hemodialysis nor peritoneal dialysis removes a significant amount of drug (< 1%).

Onset/Peak/Duration:

Oral – The peak effects of single oral doses occur within 2 to 4 hours. The duration of effect depends upon dose, lasting 8 to 12 hours. The maximum, steady-state BP response upon oral, twice-a-day dosing occurs within 24 to 72 hours.

IV – The maximum effect of each IV injection of labetalol at each dose level occurs within 5 minutes. Following discontinuation of IV therapy, BP rose gradually and progressively, approaching pretreatment baseline values in 16 to 18 hours.

Indications:

Oral: Hypertension, alone or with other agents, especially thiazide and loop diuretics.

Parenteral: For control of blood pressure in severe hypertension.

Unlabeled uses: Labetalol has effectively lowered BP and relieved symptoms in patients with pheochromocytoma; higher IV doses may be required. However, paradoxical hypertensive responses have been reported; therefore, use caution when administering labetalol.

Labetalol has also been used in clonidine withdrawal hypertension.

Contraindications:

Bronchial asthma; overt cardiac failure; greater than first degree heart block; cardiogenic shock; severe bradycardia.

Warnings:

Cardiac failure: Sympathetic stimulation is a vital component supporting circulatory function in congestive heart failure (CHF). β-blockade carries a potential hazard of further depressing myocardial contractility and precipitating more severe failure. Avoid use in overt CHF, although labetalol can be used with caution in patients with a history of heart failure who are well compensated. CHF has been observed in patients receiving labetalol. Labetalol does not abolish the inotropic action of digitalis on heart muscle.

LABETALOL HCl

Patients without history of cardiac failure (latent cardiac insufficiency): Continued depression of myocardium with β-blockers can lead to cardiac failure. At first sign or symptom of impending cardiac failure, fully digitalize or give diuretic; observe closely. If cardiac failure continues, withdraw (gradually, if possible).

Withdrawal: Angina has not been reported upon discontinuation. However, hypersensitivity to catecholamines has been seen in patients withdrawn from β-blockers. Exacerbation of angina and, in some cases, myocardial infarction and ventricular dysrhythmias have occurred after abrupt discontinuation of such therapy. When discontinuing chronic labetalol, particularly in ischemic heart disease, gradually reduce dosage over 1 to 2 weeks and carefully monitor. Do not discontinue abruptly even in patients treated only for hypertension. Even in absence of overt angina, when discontinuation is planned, carefully observe patient and advise to limit physical activity. If angina markedly worsens or acute coronary insufficiency develops, reinstitute promptly, at least temporarily, and take other measures.

Nonallergic bronchospasm (eg, chronic bronchitis and emphysema): Patients with bronchospastic disease should, in general, not receive β-blockers. Labetalol may be used with caution, however, in patients who do not respond to, or cannot tolerate, other antihypertensive agents. Use the smallest effective dose.

Diabetes mellitus and hypoglycemia: β-blockade may prevent the appearance of premonitory signs and symptoms (eg, tachycardia) of acute hypoglycemia. β-blockade also reduces insulin release in response to hyperglycemia; it may be necessary to adjust antidiabetic drug dose.

Major surgery: Withdrawing β-blockers prior to major surgery is controversial. Protracted severe hypotension and difficulty restarting or maintaining heartbeat have been reported with beta-blockers; labetalol has not been evaluated in this setting.

Rapid decreases of BP: Observe caution when reducing severely elevated BP. Although not reported with IV labetalol, adverse reactions, including cerebral infarction, optic nerve infarction, angina and ischemic changes in the ECG have been reported with other agents when severely elevated BP was reduced over several hours to as long as 1 or 2 days. Achieve desired BP lowering over as long a time as possible.

Hepatic function impairment: Use with caution; drug metabolism may be diminished.

Jaundice or hepatic dysfunction has rarely been associated with labetalol. Stop labetalol immediately should a patient develop jaundice or laboratory evidence of liver injury. Both have been reversible on discontinuation of therapy.

Pregnancy: Category C. Teratogenic studies performed in animals at greater than recommended doses produced no fetal malformations. Increased fetal resorptions were seen at doses approximating the recommended human dose. There are no adequate and well controlled studies in pregnant women. Use during pregnancy only if the potential benefits outweigh the potential hazards to the fetus.

Infants of mothers who were treated with labetalol for hypertension during pregnancy did not appear to be adversely affected by the drug.

Labor and delivery – Labetalol did not appear to affect the usual course of labor and delivery when given to pregnant hypertensive patients.

Lactation: Small amounts of labetalol (0.004% of the maternal dose) are excreted in breast milk. Exercise caution when administering to a nursing woman.

Children: Safety and efficacy for use in children have not been established.

Precautions:

Hypotension: Following oral administration, postural hypotension has been transient and is uncommon (2%) when the recommended starting dose and titration increments are closely followed. Symptomatic postural hypotension is most likely to occur 2 to 4 hours after a dose, especially following a large initial dose or upon large changes in dose. It is likely to occur if patients are tilted or allowed to assume the upright position within 3 hours of receiving labetalol injection (incidence 58%). Establish patient's ability to tolerate upright position before permitting ambulation.

Drug Interactions:

Beta-adrenergic agonists: Labetalol can blunt the bronchodilator effect of these drugs in patients with bronchospasm; therefore, greater than the normal dose of β-agonist bronchodilator drugs may be required.

Cimetidine has been shown to increase the bioavailability of oral labetalol.

Glutethimide may decrease the pharmacologic effects of labetalol by inducing microsomal enzymes. This may occur several days after glutethimide discontinuation.

Halothane: Synergistic adverse effects on cardiovascular hemodynamics may occur with concurrent IV labetalol, resulting in significant myocardial depression. During controlled hypotensive anesthesia, do not use high halothane concentrations (≥ 3%). If interaction occurs, reduce halothane dose to rapidly reverse symptoms.

Nitroglycerin: Labetalol blunts reflex tachycardia that nitroglycerin may produce without preventing its hypotensive effect; additional antihypertensive effects may occur.

Drug/Lab test interactions: Presence of a labetalol metabolite in urine may falsely increase urinary catecholamine levels when measured by a nonspecific trihydroxyindole reaction. In screening labetalol patients for pheochromocytoma, use specific radioenzymatic or high performance liquid chromatography assay techniques.

There have been reversible increases of serum transaminases in 4% of patients treated with labetalol and tested, and more rarely, reversible increases in blood urea.

Adverse Reactions:

Labetalol is usually well tolerated. Most adverse effects have been mild and transient. With oral labetalol, most occur early in the course of treatment. Discontinuation was required in 7% of all patients in controlled clinical trials.

Oral:

CNS – Fatigue; headache; drowsiness; paresthesias; rare instances of syncope.

Dermatologic – Rashes such as generalized maculopapular, lichenoid, urticarial; bulous lichen planus; psoriaform; facial erythema; reversible alopecia.

GI – Diarrhea; cholestasis with or without jaundice; reversible increases in serum transaminases.

GU – Ejaculation failure; impotence; priapism; difficulty in micturition; acute urinary bladder retention; Peyronie's disease.

Musculoskeletal – Asthenia; muscle cramps; toxic myopathy.

Respiratory – Dyspnea; bronchospasm.

Miscellaneous – Systemic lupus erythematosus; positive antinuclear factor (ANF); antimitochondrial antibodies; edema; nasal stuffiness; fever; vision abnormality; dry eyes.

Parenteral:

Cardiovascular – Ventricular arrhythmias.

CNS – Hypoesthesia (numbness); somnolence/yawning.

Renal – Transient increases in BUN and serum creatinine, associated with drops in BP, generally in patients with prior renal insufficiency.

Miscellaneous – Pruritus; flushing; wheezing.

Oral and parenteral:

CNS – Dizziness; tingling of scalp/skin; vertigo.

GI – Nausea; vomiting; dyspepsia; taste distortion.

Miscellaneous – Postural hypotension; increased sweating.

Adverse effects not listed above have been reported with other β-adrenergic blockers:

Cardiovascular – Intensification of AV block. See Contraindications.

CNS – Mental depression progressing to catatonia; acute reversible syndrome characterized by disorientation for time/place, short-term memory loss, emotional lability, clouded sensorium and decreased performance on neuropsychometrics.

GI – Mesenteric artery thrombosis; ischemic colitis.

Hematologic – Agranulocytosis; thrombocytopenic/nonthrombocytopenic purpura.

Hypersensitivity – Fever with aching and sore throat; laryngospasm; respiratory distress.

Overdosage:

Symptoms: Excessive hypotension which is posture-sensitive; excessive bradycardia.

Treatment: Institute gastric lavage or induce emesis to remove drug after oral ingestion. Place patient in supine position; raise legs if necessary. Employ these as needed:

Excessive bradycardia – Administer atropine or epinephrine.

Cardiac failure – Administer a digitalis glycoside and a diuretic. Dopamine or dobutamine may also be useful.

Hypotension – Administer vasopressors. Norepinephrine may be drug of choice.

Bronchospasm – Administer epinephrine or an aerosolized β_2-agonist.

Seizures – Administer diazepam.

In severe β-blocker overdose resulting in hypotension or bradycardia, glucagon has been effective in large doses (5 to 10 mg rapidly over 30 seconds, followed by continuous infusion of 5 mg/hr reduce as patient improves).

Neither hemodialysis nor peritoneal dialysis removes a significant amount of labetalol from the general circulation (< 1%).

Patient Information:

Do not discontinue medication except on advice from physician.

Consult physician at any sign of impending cardiac failure.

Transient scalp tingling may occur, especially when treatment is initiated.

LABETALOL HCl

Administration and Dosage:

Oral: Initial dose - Individualize dosage. 100 mg twice daily, alone or added to a diuretic. After 2 or 3 days, using standing BP as an indicator, titrate dosage in increments of 100 mg twice daily, every 2 or 3 days. Full antihypertensive effect is usually seen within first 1 to 3 hours of initial dose or dose increment.

Maintenance dose – 200 to 400 mg twice daily. Patients with severe hypertension may require 1.2 to 2.4 g/day. Should side effects (principally nausea or dizziness) occur with twice daily dosing, the same total daily dose given 3 times/day may improve tolerability. Titration increments should not exceed 200 mg twice/day.

When transferring patients from other antihypertensive drugs, introduce labetalol and progressively decrease the dosage of the existing therapy.

Parenteral: For IV use. Individualize dosage. Keep patients supine during injection. Establish patient's ability to tolerate upright position before permitting ambulation.

Repeated IV injection – Initially, 20 mg (0.25 mg/kg for an 80kg patient) slowly over 2 minutes. Measure supine BP immediately before and at 5 and 10 minutes after injection. Additional injections of 40 or 80 mg can be given at 10 minute intervals until a desired supine BP is achieved or a total of 300 mg has been injected. The maximum effect usually occurs within 5 minutes of each injection.

Slow continuous infusion – Dilute contents with IV fluids listed below. Two methods are – Add 200 mg to 160 ml of IV fluid to prepare 1 mg/ml solution at a rate of 2 ml/min (2 mg/min). Or, add 200 mg to 250ml of an IV fluid to prepare 2 mg/3 ml solution; give at a rate of 3 ml/min (2 mg/min). Adjust infusion rate according to BP response. Use a controlled administration device. Continue infusion until satisfactory response is obtained; then discontinue infusion and start oral labetalol. Effective IV dose range is 50 to 200 mg, up to 300 mg.

Transfer to oral dosing (hospitalized patients): Begin oral dosing when supine diastolic BP begins to rise. Recommended initial dose is 200 mg, then 200 or 400 mg, 6 to 12 hours later, depending on BP response. Thereafter, proceed as follows:

Inpatient Titration Instructions

Regimen	Daily Dose*
200 mg bid	400 mg
400 mg bid	800 mg
800 mg bid	1600 mg
1200 mg bid	2400 mg

* Total daily dose may be given in 3 divided doses.

While in the hospital, the dosage of labetalol may be increased at one day intervals to achieve the desired blood pressure reduction.

IV compatibility: At final concentrations of 1.25 to 3.75mg/ml, labetalol is compatible and stable for 24 hours with the following parenteral solutions: Ringer's; Lactated Ringer's; 5% Dextrose and Ringer's; 5% Lactated Ringer's and 5% Dextrose; 5% Dextrose; 0.9% Sodium Chloride; 5% Dextrose and 0.2% NaCl; 2.5% Dextrose and 0.45% NaCl; 5% Dextrose and 0.9% NaCl; and 5% Dextrose and 0.33% NaCl. Labetalol is NOT compatible with 5% Sodium Bicarbonate Injection.

Storage: Store between 2° and 30°C (36° and 86°F). Protect unit dose boxes from excessive moisture.

Injection: Do not freeze. Protect from light.

Rx	**Normodyne** (Schering)	**Tablets:** 100 mg	(Schering 244 Normodyne 100). Light brown, scored. Film coated. In 100s, 500s, UD 100s.
		200 mg	(Schering 752 Normodyne 200). White, scored. Film coated. In 100s, 500s & UD 100s.
		300 mg	(Schering 438 Normodyne 300). Blue. Film coated. In 100s, 500s, UD 100s.
		Injection: 5 mg/ml[1]	In 20 ml amps, 40 & 60 ml multidose vials.
Rx	**Trandate** (Glaxo Wellcome)	**Tablets:** 100 mg	(Trandate 100 Glaxo). Lt. orange, scored. Film coated. In 100s, 500s, UD 100s.
		200 mg	(Trandate 200 Glaxo). White, scored. Film coated. In 100s, 500s, UD 100s.
		300 mg	(Trandate 300 Glaxo). Peach, scored. Film coated. In 100s, 500s, UD 100s.
		Injection: 5 mg/ml[1]	In 20 and 40 ml multidose vials.

[1] With 0.1 mg EDTA and 0.8 mg methyl and 0.1 mg propyl paraben.

CARVEDILOL

Actions:

Pharmacology: Carvedilol, an antihypertensive agent, is a racemic mixture in which nonselective β-adrenoreceptor blocking activity is present in the S(-) enantiomer and α-adrenergic blocking activity is present in both R(+) and S(-) enantiomers at equal potency. Carvedilol has no intrinsic sympathomimetic activity.

Carvedilol (1) reduces cardiac ouput, (2) reduces exercise- or isoproterenol-induced tachycardia and (3) reduces reflex orthostatic tachycardia. Significant β-blocking effect is usually seen within 1 hour of drug administration. The mechanism by which β-blockade produces an antihypertensive effect has not been established.

Carvedilol also (1) attenuates the pressor effects of phenylephrine, (2) causes vasodilation and (3) reduces peripheral vascular resistance. These effects contribute to the reduction of blood pressure and usually are seen within 30 minutes of drug administration. Due to the α_1-receptor blocking activity of carvedilol, blood pressure is lowered more in the standing than in the supine position and symptoms of postural hypotension (1.8%), including rare instances of syncope, can occur.

When postural hypotension has occurred, it has been transient.

In hypertensive patients with normal renal function, therapeutic doses of carvedilol decreased renal vascular resistance with no change in glomerular filtration rate or renal plasma flow. Changes in excretion of sodium, potassium, uric acid and phosphorus in hypertensive patients with normal renal function were similar after carvedilol and placebo.

Carvedilol has little effect on plasma catecholamines, plasma aldosterone or electrolyte levels, but it does significantly reduce plasma renin activity when given for at least 4 weeks. It also increases levels of atrial natriuretic peptide.

Pharmacokinetics:

Absorption/Distribution – Carvedilol is rapidly and extensively absorbed following oral administration, with absolute bioavailability of ≈ 25% to 35% due to a significant degree of first pass metabolism. Following oral administration, the apparent mean terminal elimination half-life generally ranges from 7 to 10 hours. Plasma concentrations achieved are proportional to the oral dose administered. When administered with food, the rate of absorption is slowed, as evidenced by a delay in the time to reach peak plasma levels, with no significant difference in extent of bioavailability.

Carvedilol is > 98% bound to plasma proteins (primarily albumin). It has a steady-state volume of distribution of ≈ 115 L, indicating substantial distribution into extravascular tissues. Plasma clearance ranges from 500 to 700 ml/min.

Metabolism/Excretion – Carvidilol is extensively metabolized. Following oral administration in healthy volunteers, carvedilol accounted for only about 7% of the total in plasma as measured by area under the curve (AUC). Less than 2% of the dose was excreted unchanged in the urine. Carvedilol is metabolized primarily by aromatic ring oxidation and glucuronidation. The oxidative metabolites are further metabolized by conjugation via glucuronidation and sulfation. The metabolites of carvedilol are excreted primarily via the bile into the feces. Demethylation and hydroxylation at the phenol ring produce three active metabolites with β-receptor blocking activity. Based on preclinical studies, the 4–hydroxyphenyl metabolite is ≈ 13 times more potent than carvedilol for β-blockade.

Compared to carvedilol, the three active metabolites exhibit weak vasodilating activity. Plasma concentrations of the active metabolites are about one-tenth of those observed for carvedilol and have pharmacokinetics similar to the parent.

Carvedilol undergoes stereoselective first-pass metabolism with plasma levels of R(+) carvedilol ≈ 2 to 3 times higher than S(-) carvedilol following oral administration in healthy subjects. The mean apparent terminal elimination half-lives for R(+) carvedilol range from 5 to 9 hours vs 7 to 11 hours for the S(-)enantiomer.

Carvedilol is subject to the effects of genetic polymorphism with poor metabolizers of debrisoquin (a maker for cytochrome P450 2D6) exhibiting 2– to 3–fold higher plasma concentrations of R(+) carvedilol compared to extensive metabolizers. In contrast, plasma levels of S(-) carvedilol are increased only about 20% to 25% in poor metabolizers, indicating this enantiomer is metabolized to a lesser extent by cytochrome P450 2D6 than R(+) carvedilol.

Special populations:

Elderly – Plasma levels of carvedilol average about 50% higher in the elderly compared to young subjects.

Hepatic impairment – Compared to healthy subjects, patients with cirrhotic liver disease exhibit significantly higher concentrations of carvedilol (≈ 4– to 7–fold) following single dose therapy (see Warnings).

Renal insufficiency – Although carvedilol is metabolized primarily by the liver, plasma concentrations of carvedilol have been reported to be increased in patients with renal impairment. Based on mean AUC data, ≈ 40% to 50% higher plasma concentrations of carvedilol were observed in hypertensive patients with moderate to severe renal impairment compared to a control group of hypertensive patients with normal renal function. However, the ranges of AUC values were similar for both groups. Changes in mean peak plasma levels were less pronounced, ≈ 12% to 26% higher in patients with impaired renal function.

Consistent with its high degree of plasma protein-binding, carvedilol does not appear to be cleared significantly by hemodialysis.

Clinical trials:

Hypertension – Carvedilol was studied in two placebo controlled trials that utilized twice daily dosing at total daily doses of 12.5 to 50 mg. At 50 mg/day, carvedilol reduced sitting trough (12–hour) blood pressure by about 9/5.5 mmHg; at 25 mg/day the effect was about 7.5/3.5 mmHg. Heart rate fell by about 7.5 beats per minute at 50 mg/day. In general, as is true for other β-blockers, responses were smaller in African-American than non-African-American patients.

The peak antihypertensive effect occurred 1 to 2 hours after a dose. The dose-related blood pressure response was accompanied by a dose-related increase in adverse effects (see Adverse Reactions).

Indications:

Essential hypertension: Management of essential hypertension. It can be used alone or in combination with other antihypertensive agents, expecially thiazide-type diuretics.

Unlabeled uses: Carvedilol appears to be beneficial in the treatment of the following conditions: Congestive heart failure (12.5 to 50 mg twice daily); angina pectoris (25 to 50 mg twice daily); idiopathic cardiomyopathy (6.25 to 25 mg twice daily.

Contraindications:

Patients with NYHA Class IV decompensated cardiac failure; bronchial asthma (two cases of death from status asthmaticus have been reported in patients receiving single doses of carvedilol) or related bronchospastic conditions; second- or third-degree AV block; cardiogenic shock; severe bradycardia; hypersensitivity to the drug.

Warnings:

Cardiac failure: Sympathetic stimulation is a vital component supporting circulatory function in CHF and β-blockade carries thae potential hazard of further depressing myocardial contractility and precipitating more severe failure. Hypertensive patients who have CHF controlled with digitalis, diuretics or an angiotensin converting enzyme inhibitor should us carvedilol with caution. Both digitalis and carvedilol slow AV conduction

Hepatic injury: Mild hepatocellular injury, confirmed by rechallenge, has occurred rarely with carvedilol therapy. In controlled studies of hypertensive patients, the incidence of liver function abnormalities reported as adverse experiences was 1.1% in patients receiving carvedilol and 0.9% with placebo. One patient receiving carvedilol in a placebo controlled trial withdrew for abnormal hepatic function. Hepatic injury has been reversible and has occurred after short- or long-term therapy with minimal clinical symptomatology. No deaths due to liver function abnormalities have been reported.

At the first symptom/sign of liver dysfunction (eg, pruritus, dark urine, persistent anorexia, jaundice, right upper quadrant tenderness, unexplained flu-like symptoms) perform laboratory testing. If the patient has laboratory evidence of liver injury or jaundice, stop therapy and do not restart.

Peripheral vascular disease: β-blockers can precipitate or aggravate symptoms of arterial insufficiency in patients with peripheral vascular disease. Exercise caution in such individuals.

Anesthesia and major surgery: If carvedilol treatment is to be continued perioperatively, take particular care when anesthetic agents which depress myocardial function (eg, ether, cyclopropane, trichloroethylene) are used. See Overdosage for information on treatment of bradycardia and hypertension.

Diabetes and hypoglycemia: β-blockers may mask some of the manifestations of hypoglycemia, particularly tachycardia. Nonselective β-blockers may potentiate insulin-induced hypoglycemia and delay recovery of serum glucose levels. Caution patients subject to spontaneous hypoglycemia, or diabetic patients receiving insulin or oral hypoglycemic agents about these possibilities and use carvedilol with caution.

Thyrotoxicosis: β-adrenergic blockade may mask clinical signs of hyperthyroidism, such as tachycardia. Abrupt withdrawal of β-blockade may be followed by an exacerbation of the symptoms of hyperthyroidism or may precipitate thyroid storm.

Hepatic function impairment: Use of carvedilol in patients with clinically manifest hepatic impairment is not recommended.

CARVEDILOL

Carcinogenesis/Fertility impairment: Carvedilol was toxic to adult rats (sedation, reduced weight gain) and was associated with a reduced number of successful matings prolonged mating time, significantly fewer corpora lutea and implants per dam, and complete resorption of 18% of the litters.

Elderly: There were no notable differences in efficacy or the incidence of adverse events between older and younger patients. With the exception of dizziness (8.8% in the elderly vs 6% in younger patients), there were no events for which the incidence in the elderly exceeded that in the younger population by > 2%.

Pregnancy: Category C. Studies performed in pregnant rats and rabbits given carvedilol revealed increased post-implantation loss in rats and rabbits. In the rats, there was also a decrease in fetal body weight at the maternally toxic dose of 300 mg/kg/ day, which was accompanied by an elevation in the frequency of fetuses with delayed skeletal development (missing or stunted 13th rib). There are no adequate and well controlled studies in pregnant women. Use during pregnancy only if potential benefit justifies the potential risk to the fetus.

Lactation: It is not known whether this drug is excreted in breast milk. In rats, carvedilol or its metabolites (as well as other β-blockers) cross the placental barrier and are excreted in breast milk. There was increased mortality at one week postpartum in neonates from rats during the last trimester through day 22 of lactation. Because of the potential for serious adverse reactions in nursing infants from β-blockers, especially bradycardia, decide whether to discontinue nursing or to discontinue the drug, taking into account the importance of the drug to the mother. The effects of other α- and β-blocking agents have included perinatal and neonatal distress.

Children: Safety and efficacy in patients < 18 years of age have not been established.

Precautions:

Cardiovascular effects: Since carvedilol has β-blocking activity, it should not be discontinued abruptly, particularly in patients with ischemic heart disease. Instead, discontinue over 1 or 2 weeks.

In clinical trials, varvedilol caused bradycardia in about 2% of patients. If pulse rate drops below 55 beats/min, reduce the dosage.

Postural hypotension occurred in 1.8% and syncope in 0.1% of patients, especially following the initial dose or at the time of dose increase during repeated dosing. Postual hypotension or syncope was a cause for discontinuation of ther apy in 1% of patients.

To decrease the likelihood of syncope or excessive hypotension, always initiate treatment with a 6.25 mg dose. Dosage should then be increased slowly, and the drug should always be taken with food. During initiation of therapy, caution the patient to avoid situations such as driving or hazardous tasks where injury could result should syncope occur.

Anaphylactic reaction: While taking β-blockers, patients with a history of severe anaphylactic reaction to a variety of allergens may be more reactive to repeated challenge, either accidental, diagnostic or therpeutic. Such patients may be unresponsive to the usual doses of epinephrine used to treat allergic reaction.

Bronchospasm, nonallergic (eg, chronic bronchitis, emphysema): Patients with bronchospastic disease should, in general, not receive β-blockers. Carvedilol may be used with caution, however, in patients who do not respond to, or cannot tolerate, other antihypertensive agents. It is prudent, if carvedilol is used, to use the smallest effective dose so that inhibition of endogenous or exogenous β-agonists is minimized.

CARVEDILOL

Drug Interactions:

Carvedilol Drug Interactions

Precipitant Drug	Object drug*		Description
Carvedilol	Antidiabetic agents	↑	Agents with β-blocking properties may enhance the blood sugar-reducing effect of insulin and oral hypoglycemics. Therefore, in patients taking insulin ororal hypoglycemics, regular monitoring of blood glucose is recommended.
Carvedilol	Calcium blockers	↑	Isolated cases of conduction disturbance (rarely with hemodynamic comopromise) have been observed when carvedilol is coadministered with diltiazem. As with other agents with β-blocking properties, if carvedilol is to be administered orally with calcium blockers of the verapamil or diltiazem type, it is recomended that ECG and blood pressure be monitored.
Carvedilol	Clonidine	↑	Concomitant administration of clonidine with agents with β-blocking properties may potentiate blood pressure and heart-rate-lowering effects. When concomitant treatment with agents with β-blocking properties and clonidine is to be terminated, discontinue theβ-blocking agent first. Clonidine therapy can then be discontinued several days later by gradually decreasing the dosage.
Carvedilol	Digoxin	↑	Digoxin concentrations are increased by about 15% during concurrent use. Therefore, increased monitoring of digoxin is recommended when initiating, adjusting or discontinuing carvedilol.
Cimetidine	Carvedilol	↑	Cimetidine increased carvedilol AUC by about 30% but caused no change in C_{max}.
Rifampin	Carvedilol	↓	Rifampin reduced plasma concentration of carvedilol by about 70%.

* ↑ = Object drug increased. ↓ = Object drug decreased.

Drug/Food interactions: When taken with food, rate of absorption is slowed by extent of bioavailability is not affected. Taking with food minimizes the risk of orthostatic hypotension.

Adverse Reactions:

In general, carvedilol is well tolerated at doses up to 50 mg daily. Most adverse events reported during carvedilol therapy were of mild to moderate severity. In clinical trials directly comparing carvedilol monotherapy in doses ≤ 50 mg to placebo, 4.9% of carvedilol patients discontinued for adverse events vs 5.2% of placebo patients. Discontinuations were more common in the carvedilol group for postural hypotension (1% vs 0). The overall incidence of adverse events increased with increasing doses of carvedilol. For individual adverse events this could only be distinguished for dizziness, which increased in frequency from 2% to 5% as total daily dose increased from 6.25 to 50 mg.

Carvedilol Adverse Reactions (%)		
Adverse reaction	Carvedilol (n = 1142)	Placebo (n = 462)
CNS		
Dizziness	6.2	5.4
Somnolence	1.8	1.5
Insomnia	1.6	0.6
GI		
Diarrhea	2.2	1.3
Abdominal pain	1.4	1.3
Cardiovascular		
Bradycardia	2.1	0.2
Postural hypotension	1.8	-
Dependent edema	1.7	1.5
Peripheral edema	1.4	0.4
Respiratory		
Rhinitis	2.1	1.9
Pharyngitis	1.5	0.6
Dyspnea	1.4	0.9
Miscellaneous		
Fatigue	4.3	3.9
Injury	2.9	2.6
Back pain	2.3	1.5
Urinary tract infection	1.8	0.6
Viral infection	1.8	1.3
Hypertriglyceridemia	1.2	0.2
Thrombocytopenia	1.1	0.2

In addition to reactions listed in the table, chest pain, dyspepsia, headach, nausea, pain, sinusitis and upper respiratory tract infection were also reported, but rates were at least as great in placebo treated patients.

The following adverse events were also reported:

Cardiovascular: AV block (see Contraindications), extrasystoles, hypertension, hypotension, palpitations, peripheral ischemia, syncope (> 0.1% to ≤ 1%); angina, arrhythmia, atrial fibrillation, bundle branch block, cardiac failure, myocardial ischemia, cerebrovascular disorder (≤ 0.1%).

CNS: Ataxia, hypesthesia, paresthesia, vertigo, depression, nervousness (> 0.1% to ≤ 1%); migraine, neuralgia, paresis, amnesia, confusion (≤ 0.1%).

Dermatologic: Pruritus, rash (including erythematous, maculopapular and psoriaform) (> 0.1% to ≤ 1%); alopecia (≤ 0.1%).

GI: Bilirubinemia, constipation, flatulence, increased hepatic enzymes (0.2% of patients were discontinued from therapy because of increases in hepatic enzymes [see Warnings]); vomiting (> 0.1% to ≤ 1%).

GU: Male: decreased libido, impotence (> 0.1% to ≤ 1%); albuminuria, hematuria, micturition frequency (> 0.1% to ≤ 1%).

Hematologic: Anemia, leukopenia (> 0.1% to ≤ 1%); increased BUN, decreased HDL, hyperkalemia, hypokalemia, increased NPN, increased alkaline phosphatase, atypical lymphocytes (≤ 0.1%).

Metabolic/Nutritional: Hyperchoesterolemia, hyperglycemia, hyperuricemia (> 0.1% to ≤ 1%); glycosuria, increased weight (≤ 0.1%).

Respiratory: Asthma (see Contraindications), cough (> 0.1% to ≤ 1%); allergy, bronchospasm, respiratory alkalosis, eosinophilia (≤ 0.1%).

Special senses: Abnormal vision, tinnitus (> 0.1% to ≤ 1%); decreased hearing (≤ 0.1%).

Miscellaneous: Asthenia, hot flushes, leg cramp, malaise, dry mouth, sweating increased, myalgia (> 0.1% to ≤ 1%).

CARVEDILOL

Overdosage:

Symptoms: Overdosage may cause severe hypotension, bradycardia, cardiac insufficiency, cardiogenic shock and cardiac arrest. Respiratory problems, bronchospasms, vomiting, lapses of consciousness and generalized seizures may also occur.

Three cases of overdosage have been reported. A 59–year-old male who ingested 200 mg experienced severe chest pain but recovered completely. A 2–year-old child who ingested an unknown quantity suffered no adverse effects following induced vomiting and observation. A 39–year-old female ingested 400 mg with an unknown amount of benzodiazepine. She was hospitalized in a state of stupor and hypotension but recovered completely following supportive measures.

Treatment: Place the patient in a supine position and, where necessary, keep under observation and treat under intensive care conditions. Gastric lavage or pharmacologically induced emesis may be used shortly after ingestion. The following agents may be administered.

For excessive bradycardia – Atropine, 2 mg IV.

To support cardiovascular function – Glucagon, 5 to 10 mg IV rapidly over 30 seconds, followed by a continuous infusion of 5 mg/hr; sympathomimetics (dobutamine, isoprenaline, epinephrine) at doses according to body weight and effect.

If peripheral vasodilation dominates, it may be necessary to administer epinephrine or norepinephrine with continuous monitoring of circulatory conditions. For therapy-resistant bradycardia, perform pacemaker therapy. For bronchospasm, give β-sympathomimetics (as aerosol or IV) or aminophylline IV. In the event of seizures, slow IV injection of diazepam or clonazepam is recommended.

In the event of severe intoxication where there are symptoms of shock, treatment with antidotes must be continued for a sufficiently long period of time consistent with the 7- to 10-hour half-life of carvedilol.

Patient Information:

Do not interrupt or discontinue using carvedilol without a physician's advice.

A drop in blood pressure may be experience when standing, resulting in dizziness and, rarely, fainting. Patients should sit or lie down when these symptoms of lowered blood pressure occur. If experiencing dizziness or faintness, consult a physician about adjusting the dosage. Avoid driving or hazardous tasks if experiencing dizziness or fatigue.

Take with food.

Contact lens wearers may experience decreased lacrimation.

Administration and Dosage:

Approved by the FDA on September 14, 1995.

The recommended starting dose is 6.25 mg twice daily. If this dose is tolerated, using standing systolic pressure measured about 1 hour after dosing as a guide, maintain the dose for 7 to 14 days, and then increase to 12.5 mg twice daily, if needed, based on trough blood pressure, again using standing systolic pressure 1 hour after dosing as a guide for tolerance. This dose should also be maintained for 7 to 14 days and can then be adjusted upward to 25 mg twice daily if tolerated and needed. The full antihypertensive effect of carvedilol is seen within 7 to 14 days. Total daily dose should not exceed 50 mg. Carvedilol should be taken with food to slow the rate of absorption and reduce the incidence of orthostatic effects.

Addition of a diuretic to carvedilol or carvedilol to a diuretic can be expected to produce additive effects and exaggerate the orthostatic component of carvedilol action.

Carvedilol should not be given to patients with severe hepatic impairment (see Warnings).

Rx	**Coreg** (SmithKline Beecham	**Tablets**: 6.25 mg	Lactose. sucrose. (4140 SB). White. Oval, scored. In 30s, 100s and UD 100s.
		12.5 mg	Lactose, sucrose. (4141 SB). White. Oval. In 30s, 100s and UD 100s.
		25 mg	Lactose, sucrose. (4142 SB). White. Oval. In 30s, 100s and UD 100s.

ANTIHYPERTENSIVES

Agents used in hypertension therapy are listed in the following tables:

Pharmacological Effects of Antihypertensive Agents

↑ = increase ⇧ = slight increases 0 = no change ⇩ = slight decrease ↓ = decrease	Onset (min)	Peak effect[1] (hrs)	Duration of action[2] (hrs)	Plasma volume	Plasma renin activity	RBF GFR[3]	Peripheral resistance	Cardiac output	Heart rate	LVH	Total cholesterol	HDL	LDL	Triglycerides
Antiadrenergic Agents – Centrally Acting														
Methyldopa	120	2-6	12-24	↑	⇩/0	⇩/0	↓	⇩/0	⇩/0	↓	0	0	0	0
Clonidine	30-60	2-5	12-24	↑	⇩	⇩/0	↓	⇩/0	↓	↓	0	0	0	0
Guanabenz	60	2-4	6-12	0	↓	0	↓	0	↓	↓	0	0	0	0
Guanfacine		1-4	24	⇩/0	↓		↓	0	⇩	↓	0	0	0	0
Antiadrenergic Agents – Peripherally Acting														
Reserpine	days	6-12	6-24	↑	⇩/0	⇩/0	↑	0/↓	↑					
Guanethidine		6-8	24-48	↑	⇩/0	⇩/0	↓	0/↓	↑					
Guanadrel	30-120	4-6	9-14	↑		0	↑	0	↓					
Doxazosin		2-3								↓	↓	↑	0/↓	↓
Prazosin	120-130	1-3	6-12	0/⇧	⇩/0	0	↓	0/⇧	0/⇧	↓	↓	↑	0/↑	↓
Terazosin	15	1-2	12-24	0	0	0	↑	⇧	⇧	↓	↓	↑	0/↓	↓
Antiadrenergic Agents – Beta-Adrenergic Blockers														
Acebutolol		3-8	24-30				⇩	↓	↓	0/↓	0/↑	↓	↑	0/↑
Atenolol		2-4	24 +	⇩/0	↓	↓/0	0	↓	↓	↓	0/↑	↓	↑	0/↑
Betaxolol								↓	↓		0/↑	↓	↑	0/↑
Bisoprolol								↓	↓		0			0
Carteolol		1-3	24 +					↓	↓		0			0
Metoprolol		1.5	13-19	⇩/0	↓	⇩/0	0/↓	↓	↓	↓	0/↑	↓	↑	0/↑
Nadolol		3-4	17-24	⇩/0	↓	0	0	↓	↓	↓	0/↑	↓	↑	0/↑
Penbutolol		1.5-3	20 +		↓	⇩	0	↓	↓		0	0/↑	0	↑/↓
Pindolol		1	24 +		0	0	↓	⇩	↓	0/↓	0	0/↑	0	↑/↓
Propranolol		2-4	8-12	⇩/0	↓	↓	⇩/0	↓	↓	↓	0	0/↑	0	↑/↓
Timolol		1-3	12	⇩/0	↓		0	↓	↓	↓	0	0/↑	0	↑/↓
Antiadrenergic Agents – Alpha/Beta-Adrenergic Blocker														
Labetalol		2-4	8-12	↑	↓	0/↑	↓	0	↓	↓				
Angiotensin Converting Enzyme (ACE) Inhibitors														
Benazepril	60	0.5-1	24		↑	RBF ↑ GFR 0	↓	0/↑	0	↓	0	0	0	0
Captopril	15-30	0.5-1.5	6-12	⇧	↑	RBF ↑ GFR 0	↓	0/↑	0	↓	0	0	0	0
Enalapril	60	4-6	24	0/⇧	↑	RBF ↑ GFR 0	↓	↑	0	↓	0	0	0	0
Enalaprilat	15	3-4	≈ 6		↑	RBF ↑ GFR 0	↓	↑	0	↓	0	0	0	0
Fosinopril	60	≈ 3	24		↑	RBF ↑ GFR 0	↓	0/↑	0	↓	0	0	0	0
Lisinopril	60	≈ 7	24		↑	RBF ↑ GFR 0	↓	0	0	↓	0	0	0	0
Quinapril	60	1	24		↑	RBF ↑ GFR 0	↓	0/↑	0	↓	0	0	0	0
Ramipril	60-120	1	24		↑	RBF ↑ GFR 0	↓	0/↑	0	↓	0	0	0	0

ANTIHYPERTENSIVES

Pharmacological Effects of Antihypertensive Agents

↑ = increase ⇧ = slight increases 0 = no change ⇩ = slight decrease ↓ = decrease	Onset (min)	Peak effect[1] (hrs)	Duration of action[2] (hrs)	Plasma volume	Plasma renin activity	RBF GFR[3]	Peripheral resistance	Cardiac output	Heart rate	LVH	Total cholesterol	HDL	LDL	Triglycerides
Calcium Channel Blocking Agents														
Amlodipine	gradual	6-12	> 24	0	0	↑	↓↓↓	0	0	↓	0	0	0	0
Diltiazem SR	30-60	6-11					↓	0-↑	↓-0	↓	0	0	0	0
Felodipine	120-300	2.5-5					↓↓↓	↑	↑	↓	0	0	0	0
Isradipine	120	1.5					↓↓↓	↑	↑/↓	↓	0	0	0	0
Nicardipine	20	0.5-2			⇧/↑	⇧	↓	↑	↑	↓	0	0/⇧	0	0
Nifedipine SR	20	6					↓↓↓	↑↑	↑	↓	0	0	0	0
Verapamil	30	1-2.2			0/⇧	0	↓	↑/↓	↑/↓	↓	0	0/⇧	0	0
Diuretics														
Thiazides & deriv.	60-120	4-12	6-72	↓	↑	↓	↓	↓	0	0/??	↑	0	↑	↑
Loop diuretics	within 60	1-2	4-8	↓	↑	↓	↓	↓	0	0/??	↑	0	↑	↑
Amiloride	120	6-10	24	↓	↑	0	↓	↓	0					
Spironolactone	24-48 hr	48-72	48-72	↓	↑	0	↓	0	0					
Triamterene	2-4 hr	6-8	12-16											
Vasodilators														
Hydralazine	45	0.5-2	6-8	↑	↑	↑	↓	↑	↑	↑				
Minoxidil	30	2-3	24-72	↑	↑	0	↓	↑	↑	↑				
Agents For Pheochromocytoma														
Phentolamine	immed.		5-10 min	⇧	↑	↑	↓	0/↑	↑					
Phenoxybenzamine	gradual	2-3	24 +	⇧	↑	↑	↓	↑	↓					
Metyrosine		6 +	2-3 days				↓		↓					
Agents For Hypertensive Emergencies/Urgencies														
Nitroprusside	0.5-1		3-5 min	↑	↑	0	↓	⇩	⇧			NA		
Diazoxide	1-2	5 min	< 12	↑	↑	↑	↓	↑	↑					
Trimethaphan camsylate	1-2		10-15 min	↑	↓	0	↓	↓	↓					
Nitroglycerin (IV)	immed.		transient	0	0		↓	↑	↑					
Captopril[4]				⇧	↑	RBF ↑ GFR 0	↓	0/↑	0					
Enalaprilat[4]					↑	RBF ↑ GFR 0	↓	↑	0					
Hydralazine[4]	10-20		3-6											
Labetalol[4]	5-10		3-6	↑	↓	0/↑	↓	0	↓					
Nicardipine[4]	1-5		3-6		⇧/↑	⇧	↓	↑	↑					
Nifedipine[4]							↓↓↓	↑↑	↑					
Phentolamine[4]	1-2		3-10 min											
Miscellaneous Agents														
Mecamylamine	30-120		6-12+	↑	↓	↓	↓	↓	↑					
Pargyline		4-21 days	3 weeks			↓	↓	0	0					
Tolazoline							↓							

[1] Peak clinical effect following a single oral dose, except where indicated.
[2] Duration of action is frequently dose-dependent.
[3] Renal blood flow and glomerular filtration rate.
[4] Unlabeled use.
[5] NA = Not applicable.

Stepped-Care Antihypertensive Regimen †: Experience in treating essential hypertension (systolic blood pressure [BP] ≥ 140 mm Hg and/or diastolic BP ≥ 90 mm Hg) demonstrates the benefits of pharmacotherapy. Reducing BP decreases cardiovascular mortality and morbidity in patients with hypertension. Antihypertensive therapy protects against stroke, left ventricular hypertrophy, congestive heart failure and progression to more severe hypertension. In addition to drug therapy, lifestyle modifications

† The Fifth-Report of the Joint National Committee on Detection, Evaluation, and Treatment of High Blood Pressure. *Arch Intern Med* 1993;153:154-83.

ANTIHYPERTENSIVES

of adjunctive value include weight reduction, sodium and alcohol restriction, smoking cessation, regular exercise and a diet low in saturated fat.

Hypertension Categories		
Range (mm Hg)		
Systolic	Diastolic	Category[1]
< 130	< 85	Normal BP
130-139	85-89	High normal BP
140-159	90-99	Stage 1 (mild) hypertension
160-179	100-109	Stage 2 (moderate) hypertension
180-209	110-119	Stage 3 (severe) hypertension
≥ 210	≥ 120	Stage 4 (very severe) hypertension

[1] When systolic and diastolic BP fall into different categories, select the higher category to classify the patient's BP (eg, classify 165/95 mm Hg as Stage 2, 170/115 mm Hg as Stage 3). Isolated systolic hypertension is systolic BP ≥ 140 mm Hg and diastolic BP < 90 mm Hg (stage appropriately).

For purposes of risk classification and management, specify presence or absence of target-organ disease and additional risk factors in addition to classifying hypertension stages. For example, classify a diabetic patient with Stage 3 hypertension and left ventricular hypertrophy as "Stage 3 hypertension with target-organ disease (left ventricular hypertrophy) and with one additional risk factor (diabetes)."

The *stepped-care approach* begins with lifestyle modifications. If BP remains ≥ 140/90 mm Hg for 3 to 6 months, start antihypertensive therapy, especially in patients with target-organ disease or other risk factors for cardiovascular disease. Initiate therapy with one agent, increase the dosage gradually, then add or substitute agents with gradual increases in doses until the therapeutic goal is achieved, side effects become intolerable or maximum dosages are reached. Try lifestyle modifications first.

Stepped-Care Approach		
I. Lifestyle modifications	Weight reduction Moderation of alcohol intake Regular physicial activity	Reduction of sodium intake Smoking cessation
II. Inadequate response	Continue lifestyle modifications Initial pharmacological selection[1] 1) Diuretics or beta blockers[2] 2) ACE inhibitors, calcium blockers, $alpha_1$-blockers, alpha-beta blocker[3]	
III. Inadequate response	1) Increase drug dose, or; 2) Substitute another drug, or; 3) Add a second agent from a different class.[4]	
IV. Inadequate response	Add a second or third agent or diuretic if not already prescribed.[4]	

[1] Initial drug therapy is monotherapy for Stage 1 and Stage 2 hypertension.

[2] Preferred because a reduction in morbidity and mortality has been demonstrated.

[3] Equally effective in reducing BP; however, these have not been tested in long-term controlled trials to demonstrate reduction of morbidity and mortality. Reserve for special indications or when preferred agents are unacceptable or ineffective.

[4] Supplemental antihypertensive agents, which include centrally acting $alpha_2$-agonists (clonidine, guanabenz, guanfacine, methyldopa), peripheral-acting adrenergic antagonists (guanadrel, guanethidine, rauwolfia alkaloids) and direct vasodilators (hydralazine, minoxidil), are not routinely well suited for initial monotherapy.

ANTIHYPERTENSIVES

Diuretics – Generally initiate therapy with a thiazide or other oral diuretic. Thiazide-type diuretics are drugs of choice; hydrochlorothiazide or chlorthalidone are generally preferred. Reserve loop diuretics for selected patients. This therapy alone may control many cases of mild hypertension. Diuretics exert an indirect antihypertensive effect by decreasing vascular tone as well as increasing sodium and water excretion. Black people are generally more responsive to diuretics, and these agents are effective in older patients as well. Diuretics are also added or substituted as therapy when blood pressure response to another agent is inadequate. Consider treating diuretic-induced hypokalemia (< 3.5 mEq/L) with potassium supplementation or by adding a potassium-sparing diuretic to therapy.

Beta-adrenergic blocking agents may also be used as initial drug monotherapy. Beta blockers are effective in older patients, but less effective in black people. Beta-adrenergic blocking agents decrease cardiac output without effects on vascular resistance. In addition, they inhibit renin release.

Calcium channel blockers, ACE inhibitors, labetalol and alpha$_1$-blockers may be used as initial monotherapy, although they are not routinely preferred over diuretics and beta blockers. Black people tend to respond better to calcium blockers than ACE inhibitors; labetalol may be more effective in black people than other beta blockers.

Antiadrenergic agents (central and peripheral adrenergic inhibitors) are considered supplemental agents and are used when the initial drug therapy fails to achieve the desired effect. Diuretics are usually continued to provide synergistic effects and to prevent secondary fluid accumulation that may occur with use of antiadrenergic agents alone. Combination therapy may also minimize untoward reactions which are more common at the higher doses necessary when a single drug is used alone.

Decreased adrenergic tone results in reduced cardiac output or decreased peripheral vascular resistance. Methyldopa, guanabenz, guanfacine and clonidine act mainly in the CNS. Although reserpine has been used for years, other agents are preferred. Guanadrel is a peripheral antiadrenergic similar to guanethidine.

Vasodilators are also considered supplemental agents and are not suited for initial monotherapy. A three drug regimen should include agents acting by different mechanisms. Hydralazine and minoxidil have direct vasodilating actions. In order to prevent reflex tachycardia caused by decreased peripheral resistance, these agents are most effective when used with a diuretic and a β-blocker. Minoxidil's undesirable side effects limit its use to severely hypertensive patients who do not respond to minimum doses of a diuretic and two other agents.

ANTIHYPERTENSIVES

Antihypertensive drug withdrawal syndrome may occur after discontinuation of antihypertensives. Patients may experience symptoms associated with catecholamine excess, with or without a rapid rise in blood pressure, including nervousness, agitation, tremors, palpitations, insomnia, headache, sweating, flushing, nausea and vomiting; rarely, malignant hypertension, angina, myocardial infarction and cardiac arrhythmias occur. Most often reported with clonidine, the syndrome also occurs with other agents including centrally acting, peripherally acting and β-blocking drugs. The typical patient is young, has severe hypertension and is taking multiple drugs in high doses for prolonged periods.

To circumvent problems, encourage patient compliance, avoid excessive doses, avoid combining sympatholytics and β-blockers and maintain antihypertensive medication in surgical patients. When discontinuing medication, taper the dose slowly, one drug at a time; use special caution in patients with coronary artery or cerebrovascular disease.

Treatment generally includes reinstitution of therapy, bed rest/sedation and, perhaps, therapy similar to treatment of malignant hypertension.

Step-down therapy – Attempt to decrease the dosage or the number of antihypertensive agents in patients; have them maintain lifestyle modifications. It may be possible to accomplish this in a deliberate, slow, progressive manner if the patient has been effectively controlled for one year and at least four visits.

Patient Information: Consider compliance to weight reduction, sodium and alcohol restriction, discontinuation of smoking, regular exercise and behavior modification.

Do not discontinue medication unless directed by physician; do not discontinue abruptly.

Avoid cough, cold or allergy medications containing sympathomimetics.

If dizziness (orthostatic hypotension) occurs, avoid sudden changes in posture. Taking a hot bath or shower may aggravate the dizziness.

Many of these medications may cause drowsiness, especially during the first days of therapy or when dose is increased. Observe caution while driving or performing other tasks requiring alertness, coordination or physical dexterity.

If dehydration occurs due to nausea, vomiting, diarrhea, etc., the hypotensive effect may be increased. If this occurs, contact the physician; a lower dose may be necessary.

Antiadrenergic Agents — Centrally Acting

METHYLDOPA AND METHYLDOPATE HCl

Refer to the general discussion of these products in the Antihypertensives Introduction.

Actions:

Pharmacology: The mechanism of action of methyldopa has not been conclusively demonstrated, but is probably because of the drug's metabolism to alpha-methyl norepinephrine, which lowers arterial pressure by the stimulation of central inhibitory α-adrenergic receptors, false neurotransmission or reduction of plasma renin activity. Methyldopa causes a net reduction in tissue concentrations of serotonin, dopamine, norepinephrine and epinephrine.

Methyldopa reduces standing blood pressure and supine blood pressure. It usually produces highly effective lowering of supine pressure with infrequent symptomatic postural hypotension. Exercise hypotension and diurnal blood pressure variations rarely occur.

Methyldopate HCl, the ethyl ester of methyldopa HCl, is pharmacologically equal.

Pharmacokinetics:

Absorption/Distribution – Following oral administration, methyldopa is variably and incompletely absorbed. The mean bioavailability is ≈ 50%. Methyldopa crosses the blood-brain barrier and is decarboxylated in the CNS to active alphamethylnoradrenaline. A decrease in blood pressure occurs within 4 to 6 hours following IV or oral administration and lasts 10 to 16 hours or 12 to 24 hours, respectively.

Metabolism – Methyldopa is extensively metabolized. Approximately 17% of a dose of methyldopate HCl appears in plasma as free methyldopa. The elimination half-life of methyldopa is ≈ 1.8 hours. The main metabolite, an inactive O-sulfate conjugate, is formed in intestinal cells. Approximately 70% (oral) and ≈ 49% (IV) of the drug that is absorbed is excreted in the urine as methyldopa and its mono-O-sulfate conjugate. The renal clearance is ≈ 130 ml/min (oral) and ≈ 156 ml/min (IV) in healthy subjects and is diminished in renal insufficiency. The plasma half-life of methyldopa is ≈ 105 minutes. After oral doses, excretion is essentially complete in 36 hours. Blood pressure reduction is pronounced and prolonged in renal failure. Methyldopa is ≈ 8% bound to plasma proteins. The drug is removed by dialysis.

Indications:

Hypertension: Treatment of hypertension.

Hypertensive crises: Methyldopate HCl may be used to initiate treatment of acute hypertensive crises; however, because of its slow onset of action, other agents may be preferred for rapid reduction of blood pressure.

Contraindications:

Active hepatic disease, such as acute hepatitis or active cirrhosis; if previous methyldopa therapy has been associated with liver disorders (see Warnings); coadministration with MAO inhibitors (see Drug Interactions); hypersensitivity to any component of these formulations including sulfites.

Warnings:

Positive Coombs' test/hemolytic anemia: With prolonged therapy, 10% to 20% of patients develop a positive direct Coombs' test, usually between 6 and 12 months of therapy. The lowest incidence reported was at a dosage of ≤ 1 g/day. This is associated rarely with hemolytic anemia, which could lead to potentially fatal complications and is difficult to predict. Prior existence or development of a positive direct Coombs' test is not a contraindication to methyldopa, but if it develops during therapy, determine whether hemolytic anemia exists and whether the positive Coombs' test may be a problem. For example, in addition to a positive direct Coombs' test there is less often a positive indirect Coombs' test that may interfere with cross matching of blood.

Perform baseline and periodic blood counts (hematocrit, hemoglobin or red cell count) to detect hemolytic anemia. A direct Coombs' test may be useful before therapy and at 6 and 12 months later. If Coombs'-positive hemolytic anemia occurs, discontinue methyldopa; anemia usually remits promptly. If not, give corticosteroids and consider other causes. If hemolytic anemia is related to methyldopa, do not reinstitute.

When methyldopa produces a positive Coombs' test alone or with hemolytic anemia, the red cell is usually coated with IgG gamma globulin. The positive Coombs' test may not revert to normal until weeks to months after methyldopa is stopped.

Antiadrenergic Agents — Centrally Acting

METHYLDOPA AND METHYLDOPATE HCl

Blood transfusions: Should the need for transfusion arise in a patient receiving methyldopa, perform both a direct and indirect Coombs' test. In the absence of hemolytic anemia, usually only the direct Coombs' test will be positive. A positive direct Coombs' test alone will not interfere with typing or cross matching. If the indirect Coombs' test is also positive, problems may arise in the major cross-match and the assistance of a hematologist or transfusion expert will be needed.

Hepatic toxicity: Fever has occasionally occurred within the first 3 weeks of therapy, sometimes associated with eosinophilia or abnormalities in one or more liver function tests (eg, alkaline phosphatase, AST, ALT, bilirubin, prothrombin time). Jaundice with or without fever may occur, usually within the first 2 to 3 months of therapy. In some patients, the findings are consistent with cholestasis. Fatal hepatic necrosis has been reported rarely. These hepatic changes may represent hypersensitivity reactions. If fever, abnormalities in liver function tests or jaundice appear, discontinue therapy; temperature and abnormalities in liver function revert to normal when the drug is discontinued. Do not reinstitute methyldopa in such patients.

The incidence of severe cytotoxic injury is < 0.1% to 0.5%.

Hematologic disorders: Rarely, a reversible reduction of the white blood cell (WBC) count with a primary effect on granulocytes has been seen, but promptly returns to normal on discontinuation of the drug. Rare cases of granulocytopenia have been reported. White count returned to normal after drug discontinuation. Reversible thrombocytopenia occurs rarely.

Renal function impairment: The active metabolites of methyldopa accumulate in uremia. Use with caution in patients with renal failure. Prolonged hypotension has been reported.

Hypertension has recurred occasionally after dialysis in patients given methyldopa because the drug is removed by this procedure.

Hepatic function impairment: Use with caution in patients with previous liver disease or dysfunction.

Elderly: Syncope in older patients may be related to an increased sensitivity and advanced arteriosclerotic vascular disease. This may be avoided by lower doses.

Pregnancy: Category B (oral). Category C (IV). Methyldopa crosses the placenta and achieves fetal concentrations similar to the maternal serum. No unusual adverse reactions or obvious teratogenic effects have been reported despite rather wide use during pregnancy. Neonates born to mothers receiving methyldopa have demonstrated a decreased systolic blood pressure of 4 to 5 mmHg for 2 days after delivery, compared with controls.

Safety for use during pregnancy has not been established. Use only when clearly needed and when potential benefits outweigh the potential hazards to the fetus.

Lactation: Methyldopa is excreted in breast milk in small amounts. After 750 to 2000 mg/day, milk levels of free and conjugated methyldopa ranged from 0.1 to 0.9 mcg/ml. The American Academy of Pediatrics considers methyldopa to be compatible with breastfeeding.

Children: See Administration and Dosage.

Precautions:

Monitoring: Perform periodic determinations of hepatic function, particularly during the first 6 to 12 weeks of therapy or when an unexplained fever occurs.

Paradoxical pressor response has been reported with IV methyldopa.

Involuntary choreoathetotic movements have been observed rarely in patients with severe bilateral cerebrovascular disease. Should these occur, discontinue methyldopa therapy.

Sedation, usually transient, may occur during initial therapy or whenever the dose is increased. Therefore, patients should observe caution while driving or performing other tasks requiring alertness, coordination or physical dexterity during these periods.

Urine discoloration: Rarely, when urine is exposed to air after voiding, it may darken because of breakdown of methyldopa or its metabolites.

Sulfite sensitivity: Some of these products contain sulfites that may cause allergic-type reactions including anaphylactic symptoms and life-threatening or less severe asthmatic episodes in certain susceptible persons. The overall prevalence of sulfite sensitivity in the general population is unknown and probably low; it is seen more frequently in asthmatic or atopic nonasthmatic persons.

Antiadrenergic Agents — Centrally Acting

METHYLDOPA AND METHYLDOPATE HCl

Drug Interactions:

Methyldopa Drug Interactions			
Precipitant drug	Object drug*		Description
Methyldopa	Anesthetics	⬆	Reduced doses of anesthetics may be required. Hypotension during anesthesia can be controlled by vasopressors because adrenergic receptors remain sensitive.
Methyldopa	Beta blockers, non-selective (eg, propranolol)	⬆	Non-selective beta blockers and methyldopa may rarely cause paradoxical hypertension.
Methyldopa	Haloperidol	⬆	Methyldopa may potentiate the antipsychotic effects of haloperidol or the combination may produce psychosis.
Levodopa	Methyldopa	⬆	Blood-pressure-lowering effects of methyldopa may be potentiated by levodopa. Central effects of levodopa in Parkinson's disease may be potentiated by methyldopa.
Methyldopa	Levodopa	⬆	
Methyldopa	Lithium	⬆	Lithium toxicity characterized by GI symptoms, polyuria, muscular weakness, lethargy and tremor has been reported following methyldopa coadministration.
Methyldopa	MAO inhibitors	⬆	Metabolites of methyldopa stimulate release of endogenous catecholamines that are usually metabolized by MAO inhibitors, thereby leading to excessive sympathetic stimulation.
Methyldopa	Phenothiazines	⬆	Serious elevations in blood pressure may occur.
Methyldopa	Sympathomimetics	⬆	Methyldopa may potentiate the pressor effects of sympathomimetics and lead to hypertension.
Methyldopa	Tolbutamide	⬆	Tolbutamide metabolism may be impaired by methyldopa, resulting in enhanced hypoglycemic effects.
Barbiturates	Methyldopa	⬇	The actions of methyldopa may be reduced.
Tricyclic antidepressants	Methyldopa	⬇	Reversal or attenuation of the hypotensive effects of methyldopa.

* ⬆ = Object drug increased. ⬇ = Object drug decreased.

Drug/Lab test interactions: Methyldopa may interfere with tests for: Urinary uric acid by phosphotungstic method; serum creatinine by alkaline picrate method; AST by colorimetric methods. Interference with spectrophotometry for AST analysis is not reported.

Because methyldopa causes fluorescence in urine samples at the same wave lengths as catecholamines, falsely high levels of urinary catecholamines may occur and will interfere with the diagnosis of pheochromocytoma. Methyldopa does not interfere with measurement of vanillylmandelic acid (VMA) by methods converting VMA to vanillin.

Adverse Reactions:

Cardiovascular: Bradycardia; prolonged carotid sinus hypersensitivity; aggravation of angina pectoris; congestive heart failure; paradoxical pressor response with IV use; pericarditis; myocarditis; vasculitis; orthostatic hypotension; edema (and weight gain) usually relieved by a diuretic (see Warnings). Discontinue methyldopa if edema progresses or signs of heart failure appear.

CNS: Sedation, usually transient, may occur during initial therapy or whenever the dose is increased; headache, asthenia or weakness (may be early, transient symptoms); dizziness; lightheadedness; symptoms of cerebrovascular insufficiency; paresthesias; parkinsonism; Bell's palsy; decreased mental acuity; involuntary choreoathetotic movements; psychic disturbances including nightmares and reversible mild psychoses or depression.

Dermatologic: Rash; toxic epidermal necrolysis.

METHYLDOPA AND METHYLDOPATE HCl

Endocrine: Breast enlargement; gynecomastia; lactation; hyperprolactinemia; amenorrhea.

GI: Nausea; vomiting; distention; constipation; flatus; diarrhea; colitis; dry mouth; sore or "black" tongue; pancreatitis; sialadenitis.

GU: Impotence; decreased libido.

Hematologic: Positive Coombs' test, hemolytic anemia (see Warnings); bone marrow depression; leukopenia; granulocytopenia; thrombocytopenia; positive tests for antinuclear antibody, lupus erythematosus cells and rheumatoid factor.

Hepatic: Abnormal liver function tests; jaundice; hepatitis, liver disorders (see Warnings).

Hypersensitivity: Fever; lupus-like syndrome.

Miscellaneous: Nasal stuffiness; rise in BUN; arthralgia; myalgia.

Overdosage:

Symptoms: Sedation; acute hypotension; weakness; bradycardia; dizziness; lightheadedness; constipation; distention; flatus; diarrhea; nausea; vomiting and other responses attributable to brain and GI malfunction. Delayed absorption from the gut may delay onset of maximum hypotension.

Treatment: Employ gastric evacuation and general supportive measures when ingestion is recent. When ingestion has been earlier, infusions may be helpful to promote urinary excretion. Otherwise, management includes special attention to cardiac rate and output, blood volume, electrolyte imbalance, paralytic ileus, urinary function and cerebral activity. Refer to General Management of Acute Overdosage. Sympathomimetic drugs (eg, norepinephrine, epinephrine, metaraminol bitartrate) may be indicated. In severe cases consider hemodialysis.

Patient Information:

When urine is exposed to air after voiding, it may darken.

Notify physician of unexplained prolonged general tiredness, fever or jaundice.

Administration and Dosage:

Renal function impairment: Methyldopa is largely excreted by the kidneys; patients with impaired renal function may respond to smaller doses.

Adults: Initial therapy: 250 mg, 2 or 3 times/day in the first 48 hours. Adjust dosage at intervals of ≥ 2 days until an adequate response is achieved. To minimize sedation, increase dosage in the evening. By adjustment of dosage, morning hypotension may be prevented without sacrificing control of afternoon blood pressure.

Maintenance therapy – 500 mg to 2 g daily in 2 to 4 doses.

Concomitant drug therapy – When methyldopa is given with antihypertensives other than thiazides, limit the initial dosage to 500 mg/day in divided doses; when added to a thiazide, the dosage of thiazide need not be changed.

Children: Individualize dosage. Initial oral dosage is based on 10 mg/kg/day in 2 to 4 doses. The maximum daily dosage is 65 mg/kg or 3 g, whichever is less.

Tolerance may occur, usually between the second and third month of therapy. Adding a diuretic or increasing the dosage of methyldopa frequently restores blood pressure control. A thiazide is recommended if therapy was not started with a thiazide or if effective control of blood pressure cannot be maintained on 2 g methyldopa daily.

Discontinuation: Methyldopa has a relatively short duration of action; therefore, withdrawal is followed by return of hypertension, usually within 48 hours. This is not complicated by an overshoot of blood pressure above pretreatment levels.

IV: Add the dose to 100 ml of 5% Dextrose or give in 5% Dextrose in Water in a concentration of 10 mg/ml. Administer over 30 to 60 minutes. When control has been obtained, substitute oral therapy starting with the same parenteral dosage schedule.

Adults – 250 to 500 mg every 6 hours as required (maximum 1 g every 6 hours).

Children – 20 to 40 mg/kg/day in divided doses every 6 hours. The maximum daily dosage is 65 mg/kg or 3 g, whichever is less.

Antiadrenergic Agents — Centrally Acting

METHYLDOPA AND METHYLDOPATE HCl

Rx	**Methyldopa** (Endo, Rugby)	**Tablets:** 125 mg methyldopa	In 100s.
Rx	**Aldomet** (Merck)		(MSD 135). Yellow. Film-coated. In 100s.
Rx	**Methyldopa** (Various, eg Geneva, Lederle, Mylan, Schein)	**Tablets:** 250 mg methyldopa	In 100s, 500s, 1000s and UD 100s.
Rx	**Aldomet** (Merck)		(MSD 401). Yellow. Film-coated. In 100s, 1000s and UD 100s.
Rx	**Methyldopa** (Various, eg Geneva, Lederle, Mylan, Schein)	**Tablets:** 500 mg methyldopa	In 100s, 500s and UD 100s.
Rx	**Aldomet** (Merck)		(MSD 516). Yellow. Film-coated. In 100s, 500s, UD 100s and unit-of-use 100s.
Rx	**Aldomet** (Merck)[1]	**Oral Suspension:** 50 mg methyldopa/ml	1% alcohol. Orange-pineapple flavor. In 473 ml.
Rx	**Methyldopate HCl** (Abbott, American Regent, Raway)	**Injection:** 50 mg methyldopate HCl/ml	In 5 and 10 ml vials.
Rx	**Aldomet** (Merck)		EDTA, parabens, sodium bisulfite. In 5 ml vials.
🍁	**Aldomet** (MSD)	**Tablets:** 125 mg methyldopa	(MSD 135). Yellow. Film-coated. In 100s and 500s.
		250 mg methyldopa	(MSD 401). Yellow. Film-coated. In 100s and 500s.
		500 mg methyldopa	(MSD 516). Yellow. Film-coated. In 100s and 500s.
🍁	**Aldomet** (MSD)	**Injection:** 50 mg methyldopate HCl/ml	EDTA, parabens, sodium bisulfite. In 5 ml ampules.

[1] With 0.2% sodium bisulfite. Avoid light and freezing.

Antiadrenergic Agents — Centrally Acting

CLONIDINE HCl

Refer to the general discussion of these products in the Antihypertensives Introduction.

Injectable clonidine is used for severe pain in cancer patients. For further information, refer to the Clonidine monograph in the Central Analgesics section.

Actions:

Pharmacology: Clonidine, an imidazoline derivative, is a central α-adrenergic stimulant that inhibits sympathetic cardioaccelerator and vasoconstrictor centers. Initially, clonidine stimulates peripheral α-adrenergic receptors producing transient vasoconstriction. Stimulation of α-adrenergic receptors in the brain stem results in reduced sympathetic outflow from the CNS and a decrease in peripheral resistance, renal vascular resistance, heart rate and blood pressure. Renal blood flow and glomerular filtration rate remain essentially unchanged.

Orthostatic effects are mild and infrequent. The drug does not alter normal hemodynamic responses to exercise. Acute studies have demonstrated a moderate reduction (15% to 20%) of cardiac output in the supine position with no change in the peripheral resistance, while at a 45° tilt there is a smaller reduction in cardiac output and a decrease of peripheral resistance. During long-term therapy, cardiac output tends to return to control values while peripheral resistance remains decreased. The coadministration of a diuretic enhances antihypertensive efficacy of clonidine.

Plasma renin activity and excretion of aldosterone and catecholamines is reduced. Clonidine acutely stimulates growth hormone release in children and adults, but does not produce a chronic elevation of growth hormone with long-term use.

Pharmacokinetics: Blood pressure declines within 30 to 60 minutes after an oral dose. The peak plasma level occurs in ≈ 3 to 5 hours with a plasma half-life of 12 to 16 hours and an elimination half-life of 6 to 24 hours. About 50% of the absorbed dose is metabolized in the liver. In patients with impaired renal function, half-life increases up to 41 hours. About 40% to 60% of the absorbed dose is recovered in the urine as unchanged drug in 24 hours.

Transdermal System – The system, a 0.2 mm thick film with four layers, contains a drug reservoir of clonidine, released at an approximately constant rate for 7 days. A microporous polypropylene membrane controls rate of delivery from system to skin.

Therapeutic plasma levels are achieved 2 to 3 days after initial application. Application of a new system at weekly intervals continuously maintains therapeutic plasma concentrations. When system is removed (and not replaced), therapeutic plasma clonidine levels persist for ≈ 8 hours and then decline slowly over several days; blood pressure returns gradually to pretreatment levels.

Indications:

Hypertension: Treatment of hypertension; may be used alone or concomitantly with other antihypertensive agents.

Antiadrenergic Agents — Centrally Acting

CLONIDINE HCl

Unlabeled uses: Clonidine has been evaluated for use in the following conditions:

Clonidine Unlabeled Uses	
Use	Dosage[1]
Alcohol withdrawal	300 to 600 mcg every 6 hours
Atrial fibrillation	75 mcg oral single dose or twice daily; alone or with digoxin
Attention deficit hyperactivity disorder	5 mcg/kg/day for 8 weeks
Constitutional growth delay in children	37.5 to 150 mcg/m²/day
Cyclosporine-associated nephrotoxicity	100 to 200 mcg/day transdermal
Diabetic diarrhea	100 to 600 mcg every 12 hours or 300 mcg/24-hr patch (1 to 2 patches/week)
Gilles de la Tourette's syndrome	150 to 200 mcg/day
Hyperhidrosis	250 mcg 3 to 5 times/day
Hypertensive "urgencies" (diastolic > 120 mm Hg)	Initially 100 to 200 mcg, followed by 50 to 100 mcg every hour to a maximum of 800 mcg
Mania	Unknown
Menopausal flushing	100 to 400 mcg/day or 100 mcg/24-hr patch
Methadone/opiate detoxification	15 to 16 mcg/kg/day
Pheochromocytoma diagnosis (overnight clonidine suppression test)	300 mcg
Postherpetic neuralgia	200 mcg/day
Psychosis in schizophrenic patients	≤ 900 mcg/day
Reduction of allergen-induced inflammatory reactions in patients with extrinsic asthma	150 mcg for 3 days or 75 mcg/1.5 ml saline; inhalation
Restless leg syndrome	100 to 300 mcg/day; up to 900 mcg/day
Smoking cessation facilitation	150 to 400 mcg/day or 200 mcg/24-hour patch
Ulcerative colitis	300 mcg 3 times a day

[1] Dosage given as oral unless otherwise specified.

Contraindications:

Hypersensitivity to clonidine or any component of adhesive layer of transdermal system.

Warnings:

Special risk patients: Use with caution in patients with severe coronary insufficiency, conduction disturbances, recent myocardial infarction (MI) or cerebrovascular disease.

Tolerance may develop, necessitating a re-evaluation of therapy.

Blood pressure control: In rare instances, loss of blood pressure control has been reported in patients using transdermal clonidine.

Defibrillation or cardioversion: Remove the transdermal clonidine systems before attempting defibrillation or cardioversion because of the potential for altered electrical conductivity that may increase the risk of arcing, a phenomenon associated with the use of defibrillators.

Renal function impairment: Use with caution in patients with chronic renal failure.

Pregnancy: Category C. Clonidine crosses the placenta, resulting a in cord:maternal ratio of 0.89 with mean amniotic fluid concentrations of 1.5 ng/ml following a mean maternal dose of 330 mcg/day. Also, the plasma levels in the newborn are approximately half the maternal levels. There are no adequate and well controlled studies in pregnant women. Use clonidine in pregnancy only if clearly needed.

Lactation: Clonidine is excreted in breast milk; following a 150 mcg oral dose, milk concentrations of 1.5 ng/ml may be achieved (milk:plasma ratio 1.5). Clinical significance is unknown. Exercise caution when administering to a nursing woman.

Children: Safety and efficacy for use in children have not been established.

Precautions:

Rebound hypertension: Do not discontinue therapy without consulting a physician (see also Stepped-Care Antihypertensive Regimen section in the Antihypertensives group monograph). Discontinue therapy by reducing the dose gradually over 2 to 4 days to avoid a rapid rise in blood pressure. Abrupt withdrawal of clonidine may result in

CLONIDINE HCl

subjective symptoms such as nervousness, agitation, headache, confusion, tremor and elevated catecholamine concentrations in the plasma, but such occurrences have usually been associated with previous administration of high oral doses (exceeding 1.2 mg/day) or with continuation of concomitant β-blocker therapy. Tachycardia, rebound hypertension, flushing, nausea, vomiting and cardiac arrhythmias have also occurred. The risk may be dose-related and may be increased with multiple drug therapy. Rare instances of hypertensive encephalopathy, cerebrovascular accidents and death have been reported after abrupt cessation of therapy.

If an excessive rise in blood pressure occurs, it can be reversed by resumption of therapy or by IV phentolamine, phenoxybenzamine or prazosin. Direct vasodilators and captopril have also been used. If therapy is to be discontinued in patients receiving β-blockers and clonidine concurrently, discontinue β-blockers several days before the gradual withdrawal of clonidine.

Ophthalmologic effects: Perform periodic eye examinations because retinal degeneration has been noted in animal studies.

Perioperative use: Continue administration of clonidine to within 4 hours of surgery and resume as soon as possible thereafter. Do not interrupt transdermal clonidine during the surgical period. Carefully monitor blood pressure and institute appropriate measures to control it as necessary. If transdermal therapy is started during the perioperative period, note that therapeutic plasma levels are not achieved until 2 to 3 days after initial application.

Sensitization to transdermal clonidine: In patients who have developed localized contact sensitization to transdermal clonidine, substitution of oral clonidine therapy may be associated with development of a generalized skin rash. In patients who develop an allergic reaction to transdermal clonidine that extends beyond the local patch site (such as generalized skin rash, urticaria or angioedema) oral clonidine substitution may elicit a similar reaction.

Drug Interactions:

Clonidine Drug Interactions

Precipitant drug	Object drug*		Description
Clonidine	Levodopa	⬇	The effectiveness of levodopa may be reduced.
Beta-adrenergic blocking agents	Clonidine	⬆	Attenuation or reversal of antihypertensive effect and potentially life-threatening increases in blood pressure.
Prazosin	Clonidine	⬇	The antihypertensive effectiveness of clonidine may be decreased.
Tricyclic antidepressants	Clonidine	⬇	Tricyclic antidepressants may block antihypertensive effects of clonidine and possibly life-threatening elevations in blood pressure may occur.
Verapamil	Clonidine	⬆	Synergistic pharmacologic and toxic effects, possibly causing atrioventricular (AV) block and severe hypotension.

* ⬆ = Object drug increased. ⬇ = Object drug decreased.

Adverse Reactions:

Most common: Dry mouth (40%); drowsiness (33%); dizziness (16%); sedation, constipation (10%).

Cardiovascular: Syncope; congestive heart failure; orthostatic symptoms; palpitations, tachycardia and bradycardia; Raynaud's phenomenon; ECG abnormalities (eg, sinus node arrest) manifested as Wenckebach period or ventricular trigeminy; conduction disturbances, arrhythmias, sinus bradycardia and atrioventricular block (rare).

CNS: Dreams or nightmares; insomnia; hallucinations; delirium; nervousness; agitation; restlessness; anxiety; depression; headache.

Dermatologic: Rash; angioneurotic edema; hives; urticaria; alopecia; pruritus.

Antiadrenergic Agents — Centrally Acting

CLONIDINE HCl

GI: Abdominal pain; anorexia; malaise; nausea; vomiting; mild transient abnormalities in liver function tests; hepatitis; parotitis (rare).

GU: Impotence; decreased sexual activity/loss of libido; nocturia, difficulty in micturition and urinary retention.

Hematologic: Thrombocytopenia (rare).

Metabolic: Weight gain; transient elevation of blood glucose or serum creatine phosphokinase (rare); gynecomastia.

Musculoskeletal: Weakness; fatigue; muscle or joint pain; cramps of the lower limbs.

Miscellaneous: Increased sensitivity to alcohol; dryness, itching or burning of the eyes; dryness of the nasal mucosa; pallor; fever; weakly positive Coombs' test; discontinuation syndrome; blurred vision.

Transdermal system: The most frequent systemic reactions were dry mouth and drowsiness. The following have also been reported:

Cardiovascular – Chest pain; cerebrovascular accident; increases in blood pressure.

CNS – Fatigue; headache; lethargy; sedation; insomnia; nervousness; dizziness; irritability.

Dermatologic – Transient localized skin reactions; pruritus; erythema, allergic contact sensitization and contact dermatitis; localized vesiculation; hyperpigmentation; edema; excoriation; burning; papules; throbbing; blanching; generalized macular rash; maculopapular skin rash; urticaria; angioedema of the face and tongue.

GI – Constipation; nausea; change in taste; dry throat.

GU – Impotence/sexual dysfunction.

Overdosage:

Symptoms: Bradycardia; hypotension; CNS depression; respiratory depression; apnea; hypothermia; miosis; coma; seizures; lethargy; agitation; irritability; vomiting; hypoventilation; reversible cardiac conduction defects; arrhythmias; transient hypertension; profound hypotension; weakness; somnolence; diminished or absent reflexes.

In a patient who ingested 100 mg clonidine, plasma levels were 60 ng/ml (1 hour), 190 ng/ml (1.5 hours), 370 ng/ml (2 hours) and 120 ng/ml (5.5 and 6.5 hours). The patient developed hypertension followed by hypotension, bradycardia, apnea, hallucinations, semicoma and premature ventricular contractions. The patient fully recovered after intensive treatment.

Because children commonly have GI illnesses that lead to vomiting, they may be particularly susceptible to hypertensive episodes resulting from abrupt inability to take medication.

Treatment: Induction of emesis is usually not recommended because of the rapid onset of CNS depression. Establish respiration if necessary, perform gastric lavage and administer activated charcoal. A saline cathartic (magnesium sulfate) will increase the rate of transport through the GI tract. Routine hemodialysis is of limited benefit because a maximum of 5% of circulating clonidine is removed.

Atropine sulfate may be useful for treatment of persistent bradycardia and hypotension with dopamine infusion in addition to IV fluids.

Hypertension has been treated with IV furosemide or diazoxide or α-blocking agents such as phentolamine. Tolazoline, an α-blocker, in IV doses of 10 mg at 30 minute intervals may reverse clonidine's effects if other efforts fail. Naloxone may be a useful adjunct for the management of clonidine-induced respiratory depression, hypotension or coma.

Patient Information:

Advise patients who engage in potentially hazardous activities, such as operating machinery or driving, of a potential sedative effect of clonidine.

Caution patients against interruption of clonidine therapy without a physician's advice.

Antiadrenergic Agents — Centrally Acting

CLONIDINE HCl — ORAL

Administration and Dosage:

Individualize dosage.

Initial dose: 100 mcg twice daily. Elderly patients may benefit from a lower initial dose.

Maintenance dose: Continue increments of 100 mcg/day made at weekly intervals until the desired response is achieved; most common range is 200 to 600 mcg/day given in divided doses. The maximum dose is 2400 mcg/day. Minimize sedative effects by slowly increasing the daily dosage and giving the majority of the daily dose at bedtime.

Children: 50 to 400 mcg orally twice a day.

Unlabeled route of administration: Sublingual clonidine, using a dosage of 200 to 400 mcg/day, may be effective in hypertensive patients unable to take oral medication. The onset occurs within 30 to 60 minutes and blood pressure appears to be maintained on a twice-daily regimen.

Renal function impairment: Adjust dosage according to degree of renal impairment and carefully monitor patients. Because only a minimal amount of clonidine is removed during hemodialysis, there is no need to give supplemental clonidine following dialysis.

Rx	**Clonidine** (Various, eg, Geneva, Mylan, Schein, UDL)	**Tablets:** 0.1 mg	In 100s, 500s, 1000s and UD 100s.
Rx	**Catapres** (Boehringer-Ingelheim)		(BI-6). Tan, scored. In 100s, 1000s and UD 100s.
Rx	**Clonidine** (Various, eg, Geneva, Mylan, Schein, UDL)	**Tablets:** 0.2 mg	In 100s, 500s, 1000s and UD 100s.
Rx	**Catapres** (Boehringer-Ingelheim)		(BI-7). Orange, scored. In 100s, 1000s and UD 100s.
Rx	**Clonidine** (Various, eg, Geneva, Mylan, Schein, UDL)	**Tablets:** 0.3 mg	In 100s and UD 100s.
Rx	**Catapres** (Boehringer-Ingelheim)		(BI-11). Peach, scored. In 100s.
🍁	**Catapres** (Boehringer-Ingelheim)	**Tablets:** 0.1 mg	Lactose. White. In 100s and 500s.
		0.2 mg	Lactose. Orange. In 100s and 500s.

Antiadrenergic Agents — Centrally Acting

CLONIDINE HCl — TRANSDERMAL

Administration and Dosage:

Apply to a hairless area of intact skin on upper arm or torso once every 7 days. Use a different skin site from the previous application. If the system loosens during the 7–day wearing, apply the adhesive overlay directly over the system to ensure good adhesion.

For initial therapy, start with the 0.1 mg system. If, after 1 or 2 weeks, desired blood pressure reduction is not achieved, add another 0.1 mg system or use a larger system. Dosage greater than two 0.3 mg systems usually does not improve efficacy. Note that the antihypertensive effect of the system may not commence until 2 to 3 days after application. Therefore, when substituting the transdermal system in patients on prior antihypertensive therapy, a gradual reduction of prior drug dosage is advised. Previous antihypertensive treatment may have to be continued, particularly in patients with severe hypertension.

	Product/Distributor	Release Rate (mg/24 hr)	Surface Area (cm^2)	Total Clonidine Content (mg)	How Supplied
Rx	**Catapres-TTS-1** (Boehringer-Ingelheim)	0.1	3.5	2.5	Mineral oil. In 12s.
Rx	**Catapres-TTS-2** (Boehringer-Ingelheim)	0.2	7	5	Mineral oil. In 12s.
Rx	**Catapres-TTS-3** (Boehringer-Ingelheim)	0.3	10.5	7.5	Mineral oil. In 4s.

GUANFACINE HCl

Refer to the general discussion of these products in the Antihypertensives Introduction.

Actions:

Pharmacology: Guanfacine is a centrally acting oral antihypertensive with α_2-adrenoreceptor agonist properties. Its principal mechanism of action appears to be stimulation of central α_2-adrenergic receptors. Guanfacine reduces sympathetic nerve impulses from the vasomotor center to the heart and blood vessels, resulting in a decrease in peripheral vascular resistance and a reduction in heart rate.

Hemodynamics – The decrease in blood pressure observed after single dose or long-term oral treatment with guanfacine was accompanied by a significant decrease in peripheral resistance and a slight reduction in heart rate (5 bpm). Cardiac output under conditions of rest or exercise was not altered by guanfacine.

Guanfacine lowered elevated plasma renin activity and plasma catecholamine levels in hypertensive patients, but this does not correlate with individual blood pressure responses. Growth hormone secretion was stimulated with single oral doses of 2 and 4 mg. Long-term use had no effect on growth hormone levels. Guanfacine had no effect on plasma aldosterone. A slight but insignificant decrease in plasma volume occurred after 1 month of guanfacine therapy. There were no changes in mean body weight or electrolytes.

Pharmacokinetics:

Absorption/Distribution – Relative to a 3 mg IV dose, the absolute oral bioavailability of guanfacine is about 80%. Peak plasma concentrations occur from 1 to 4 hours with an average of 2.6 hours after single oral doses or at steady state. The area under the concentration time-curve increases linearly with the dose.

The drug is approximately 70% bound to plasma proteins, independent of drug concentration. The whole body volume of distribution is high (mean, 6.3 L/kg), which suggests a high distribution of drug to the tissues.

Metabolism/Excretion – In individuals with normal renal function, the average elimination half-life is approximately 17 hours (range, 10 to 30 hours). Younger patients tend to have shorter elimination half-lives (13 to 14 hours) while older patients tend to have half-lives at the upper end of the range. Steady-state blood levels were attained within 4 days in most subjects. Guanfacine and its metabolites are excreted primarily in the urine. Approximately 50% (40% to 75%) of the dose is eliminated in the urine as unchanged drug; the remainder is eliminated mostly as conjugates of metabolites produced by oxidative metabolism of the aromatic ring. The guanfacine to creatinine clearance ratio is > 1, suggesting that tubular secretion of drug occurs.

Clinical trials: The dose-response relationship for blood pressure and adverse effects of guanfacine given once daily as monotherapy has been evaluated in patients with mild to moderate hypertension. Patients were randomized to placebo or to 0.5, 1, 2, 3 or 5 mg guanfacine. A positive effect was not observed overall until doses of 2 mg were reached, although responses in caucasian patients were seen at 1 mg; 24 hour effectiveness of 1 to 3 mg doses was documented using 24 hour ambulatory monitoring. While the 5 mg dose added an incremental increase in effectiveness, it caused an unacceptable increase in adverse reactions.

In patients with mild to moderate hypertension receiving a thiazide-type diuretic and guanfacine at bedtime, blood pressure response can persist for 24 hours after a single dose. Observed mean changes from baseline indicate similarity of response for placebo and the 0.5 mg dose. Doses of 1, 2 and 3 mg resulted in decreased blood pressure in the sitting position with no real differences among the three doses.

While most of guanfacine's efficacy was present at 1 mg, adverse reactions at this dose were not clearly distinguishable from those associated with placebo. Adverse reactions were clearly present at 2 and 3 mg (see Adverse Reactions).

In another study of guanfacine and chlorthalidone, a significant decrease in blood pressure was maintained for a full 24 hours after dosing. While there was no significant difference between the 12 and 24 hour blood pressure readings, the fall in blood pressure at 24 hours was numerically smaller, suggesting possible escape of blood pressure in some patients and the need for individualization of therapy.

In a double-blind, randomized trial, either guanfacine or clonidine was given at recommended doses with 25 mg chlorthalidone for 24 weeks and then abruptly discontinued. Results showed equal degrees of blood pressure reduction with the two drugs; there was no tendency for blood pressure to increase despite maintenance of the same daily dose of the two drugs. Signs and symptoms of rebound phenomena were infrequent upon discontinuation of either drug. Abrupt withdrawal of clonidine produced a rapid return of diastolic and, especially, systolic blood pressure to approximately pretreatment levels, with occasional values significantly greater

GUANFACINE HCl

than baseline. Guanfacine withdrawal produced a more gradual increase to pretreatment levels, but also with occasional values significantly greater than baseline.

Indications:

Hypertension: Management of hypertension, alone or in combination with other antihypertensives, especially thiazide-type diuretics.

Unlabeled uses: Guanfacine (0.03 to 1.5 mg/day) may be beneficial in ameliorating withdrawal symptoms in patients discontinuing heroin usage.

In a small study, guanfacine (1 mg/day for 12 weeks) significantly reduced the frequency of migraine headache and reduced nausea and vomiting.

Contraindications:

Hypersensitivity to guanfacine.

Warnings:

Renal function impairment: Guanfacine clearance in patients with varying degrees of renal insufficiency is reduced, but drug plasma levels are only slightly increased compared to patients with normal renal function. Use the low end of the dosing range in patients with renal impairment. Patients on dialysis can be given usual doses of guanfacine, since the drug is poorly dialyzed.

Pregnancy: Category B. Administration to rats and rabbits at doses 200 and 100 times the maximum recommended human dose, respectively, were associated with reduced fetal survival and maternal toxicity. Guanfacine crosses the placenta in rats. There are no adequate and well controlled studies in pregnant women. Use during pregnancy only if clearly needed.

Labor and delivery – Not recommended in the treatment of acute hypertension associated with toxemia of pregnancy.

Lactation: Guanfacine is excreted in breast milk of rats. It is not known whether guanfacine is excreted in human breast milk. Use caution when administering to a nursing mother.

Children: Safety and efficacy in children < 12 years of age have not been demonstrated. Therefore, use in this age group is not recommended.

Precautions:

Special risk patients: Use guanfacine with caution in patients with severe coronary insufficiency, recent myocardial infarction, cerebrovascular disease or chronic renal or hepatic failure.

Sedation: Like other centrally active oral α_2-adrenergic agonists, guanfacine causes sedation or drowsiness, especially when beginning therapy. These symptoms are dose-related. When used with other centrally active depressants (eg, phenothiazines, barbiturates, benzodiazepines), consider the potential for additive sedative effects.

Rebound: Abrupt cessation of therapy with centrally active oral α_2-adrenergic agonists may be associated with increases in plasma and urinary catecholamines, symptoms of nervousness and anxiety and, less commonly, increases in blood pressure to levels significantly greater than those prior to therapy.

The frequency of rebound hypertension is low, but when rebound occurs, it does so after 2 to 4 days, which is delayed compared with clonidine. This is consistent with guanfacine's longer half-life. In most cases, after abrupt withdrawal of guanfacine, blood pressure returns to pretreatment levels slowly (in 2 to 4 days) without ill effects.

Adverse Reactions:

Adverse reactions are similar to those of other central α_2-adrenoreceptor agonists: Dry mouth; sedation (somnolence); weakness (asthenia); dizziness; constipation; impotence. While the reactions are common, most are mild and tend to disappear on continued dosing. The most common reasons for discontinuing therapy with guanfacine, either alone or in combination with chlorthalidone, were as follows: Dry mouth; somnolence; dizziness; fatigue; weakness; constipation; headache; impotence; insomnia; syncope; urinary incontinence; conjunctivitis; paresthesia; dermatitis; confusion; depression; palpitations.

The most commonly observed adverse reactions during guanfacine therapy showed a dose relationship from 0.5 to 3 mg.

Antiadrenergic Agents — Centrally Acting

GUANFACINE HCl

Guanfacine Adverse Reactions (%)					
Adverse reaction	Placebo (n = 59)	0.5 mg (n = 60)	1 mg (n = 61)	2 mg (n = 60)	3 mg (n = 59)
Dry mouth	0	10	10	42	54
Somnolence	8	5	10	13	39
Asthenia	0	2	3	7	3
Dizziness	8	12	2	8	15
Headache	8	13	7	5	3
Impotence	0	0	0	7	3
Constipation	0	2	0	5	15
Fatigue	2	2	5	8	10

In another study of guanfacine in combination with chlorthalidone, the guanfacine dose was adjusted upward to 3 mg/day in 1 mg increments at 3 week intervals (ie, more similar to ordinary clinical use). The most common reactions were: Dry mouth (47%); constipation (16%); fatigue (12%); somnolence (10%); asthenia, dizziness (6%); headache, insomnia (4%).

In the clonidine/guanfacine comparisons, the most common adverse reactions were as follows:

Guanfacine vs Clonidine Adverse Reactions		
Adverse reaction	Guanfacine (n=279)	Clonidine (n = 278)
Dry mouth	30%	37%
Somnolence	21%	35%
Dizziness	11%	8%
Constipation	10%	5%
Fatigue	9%	8%
Headache	4%	4%
Insomnia	4%	3%

Adverse reactions occurring in patients in the three controlled trials with a diuretic and in post-marketing surveillance (monotherapy or with other antihypertensives) were as follows:

Cardiovascular: Bradycardia; palpitations; substernal pain; chest pain; syncope; tachycardia; cardiac fibrillation, CHF, heart block, MI (rare).

CNS: Amnesia; confusion; depression; insomnia; decreased libido; paresthesias; vertigo; agitation; anxiety; malaise; nervousness; tremor.

Dermatologic: Dermatitis; pruritus; purpura; sweating; skin rash with exfoliation; alopecia; rash.

GI: Abdominal pain; diarrhea; dyspepsia; dysphagia; nausea; constipation.

GU: Testicular disorder; urinary incontinence/frequency; impotence; nocturia.

Musculoskeletal: Leg cramps; hypokinesia; arthralgia; leg pain; myalgia.

Special senses: Rhinitis; taste perversion/alterations in taste; tinnitus; conjunctivitis; iritis; vision disturbance; blurred vision.

Miscellaneous: Paresis; dyspnea; abnormal liver function tests; edema; asthenia; acute renal failure, cerebrovascular accident (rare).

Overdosage:

Symptoms: Drowsiness, lethargy, bradycardia and hypotension have been observed. A 25-year-old female intentionally ingested 60 mg guanfacine. She presented with severe drowsiness and bradycardia of 45 bpm. Gastric lavage was performed and an infusion of isoproterenol (0.8 mg in 12 hours) was administered. She recovered quickly and without sequelae.

Treatment: Gastric lavage and supportive therapy, as appropriate. Guanfacine is not dialyzable in clinically significant amounts (2.4%).

Patient Information:

May produce drowsiness or dizziness; observe caution while driving, operating dangerous machinery or performing other tasks requiring alertness, coordination or physical dexterity.

Antiadrenergic Agents — Centrally Acting

GUANFACINE HCl

Warn patients that tolerance for alcohol and other CNS depressants may be diminished.

Advise patients not to discontinue therapy abruptly.

Medication should be taken at bedtime.

Administration and Dosage:

The recommended dose, alone or with other antihypertensives, is 1 mg/day given at bedtime to minimize daytime somnolence.

If 1 mg does not produce a satisfactory result after 3 to 4 weeks of therapy, doses of 2 mg may be given, although most of the drug's effect is seen at 1 mg. The frequency of rebound hypertension is low, but it can occur. When rebound occurs, it does so after 2 to 4 days, which is delayed compared with clonidine HCl. This is consistent with the longer half-life of guanfacine. In most cases, after abrupt withdrawal of guanfacine, blood pressure returns to pretreatment levels slowly (within 2 to 4 days) without ill effects.

Higher daily doses have been used, but adverse reactions increase significantly with doses > 3 mg/day.

Rx	**Tenex** (Robins)	**Tablets:** 1 mg	Lactose. (1 AHR Tenex). Light pink. Diamond shape. In 100s, 500s and *Dis-Co* 100s.
		2 mg	Lactose. (2 AHR Tenex). Yellow. Diamond shape. In 100s.

Antiadrenergic Agents — Centrally Acting

GUANABENZ ACETATE

Refer to the general discussion of these products in the Antihypertensives Introduction.

Actions:

Pharmacology: Guanabenz is an orally active central α_2-adrenergic agonist. Its antihypertensive action appears mediated via stimulation of central α-adrenergic receptors, resulting in decreased sympathetic outflow from the brain.

The acute antihypertensive effect occurs without major changes in peripheral resistance, but its chronic effect appears to be a decrease in peripheral resistance. Blood pressure decreases in both the supine and standing positions without alterations of normal postural mechanisms, so that postural hypotension has not been observed. Guanabenz decreases pulse rate by about five beats per minute. Cardiac output and left ventricular ejection fraction are unchanged during long-term therapy.

During long-term administration, a small decrease in serum cholesterol and total triglycerides occurs without affecting high density lipoprotein.

Plasma norepinephrine, serum dopamine beta-hydroxylase and plasma renin activity decrease during chronic administration.

Pharmacokinetics:

Absorption/Distribution – About 75% of an oral dose is absorbed and metabolized. The onset of action begins within 60 minutes after a single oral dose Peak plasma concentrations of unchanged drug occur between 2 and 5 hours. The effect of meals on the absorption of guanabenz has not been studied.

Metabolism/Excretion – The average half-life is ≈ 6 hours. The effect of a single dose is reduced appreciably 6 to 8 hours after administration, blood pressure approaches baseline values within 12 hours. The site(s) of metabolism have not been determined, but < 1% of unchanged drug is recovered in the urine.

Renal/Hepatic function impairment: The disposition of orally administered guanabenz is altered in patients with alcohol-induced liver disease or renal impairment. Mean plasma concentrations of guanabenz were higher in hepatic impaired patients than in healthy subjects. In renal impaired patients, half-life is prolonged and clearance decreased, especially in patients on hemodialysis. The clinical significance of these findings is unknown.

Clinical trials: With effective control of blood pressure in hypertensive patients, guanabenz has not demonstrated any significant effect on glomerular filtration rate, renal blood flow, body fluid volume or body weight. Similarly, a decrease in blood pressure and a natriuresis (5% to 240% increase in sodium excretion) occurred in hypertensive subjects 24 hours after salt loading following a single oral dose of guanabenz. After 7 consecutive days of administration and effective blood pressure control, no significant change in glomerular filtration rate, renal blood flow or body weight was observed. However, in clinical trials of 6 to 30 months duration, hypertensive patients with effective blood pressure control by guanabenz lost 1 to 4 pounds of body weight. The mechanism of this weight loss has not been established. Tolerance to the antihypertensive effect has not been observed.

Indications:

Hypertension: Treatment of hypertension, alone or with a thiazide diuretic.

Contraindications:

Sensitivity to guanabenz.

Warnings:

Renal/Hepatic function impairment: Use with caution in patients with severe hepatic or renal failure. The disposition of oral guanabenz is altered modestly.

Pregnancy: Category C. Guanabenz may have adverse fetal effects when administered to pregnant women. A teratology study in mice has indicated a possible increase in skeletal abnormalities when guanabenz is given orally at doses of 3 to 6 times maximum recommended human dose. Increased fetal loss has been observed after oral guanabenz administration to pregnant rats (14 mg/kg) and rabbits (20 mg/kg). Rats have shown slightly decreased live-birth indices, decreased fetal survival rate, and decreased pup body weight at oral doses of 6.4 and 9.6 mg/kg. There are no adequate, well controlled studies in pregnant women. Use during pregnancy only if the potential benefit justifies the potential risk to the fetus.

Lactation: No information is available on excretion in breast milk; therefore, do not administer to nursing mothers.

Children: Safety and efficacy for use in children < 12 years of age have not been demonstrated; therefore, use in this age group is not recommended.

Antiadrenergic Agents — Centrally Acting

GUANABENZ ACETATE

Precautions:

Monitoring: Monitor blood pressure carefully in patients with coexisting hypertension and chronic hepatic dysfunction or renal impairment.

Sedation: Guanabenz causes sedation or drowsiness in a large fraction of patients.

Special risk patients: Use with caution in patients with severe coronary insufficiency, recent myocardial infarction or cerebrovascular disease.

Rebound: Sudden cessation of therapy with central α-agonists like guanabenz may rarely result in "overshoot" hypertension and more commonly produces an increase in serum catecholamines and subjective symptomatology.

Laboratory tests: During long-term administration, there is a small decrease in serum cholesterol and total triglycerides; no change in high density lipoprotein occurs.

Rarely, a nonprogressive increase in liver enzymes has been observed, although there is no clinical evidence of hepatic disease.

Drug Interactions:

CNS depressants: When guanabenz is used with centrally active depressants, (eg, phenothiazines, barbiturates and benzodiazepines), consider the potential for additive sedative effects.

Adverse Reactions:

Side effects appear to be dose-related.

Most common (at doses of 16 mg daily): Drowsiness/sedation (20% to 39%; however, the 20% incidence was observed in patients taking 8 mg daily); dry mouth (28% to 38%); dizziness (12% to 17%); weakness (10%); headache (5%).

These effects led to treatment discontinuation ≈ 15% of the time.

Other adverse effects reported, but not distinguishable from placebo effects (≤ 3%):

Cardiovascular – Chest pain; edema; arrhythmias; palpitations; atrioventricular dysfunction, AV block (rare).

CNS – Anxiety; ataxia; depression; sleep disturbances.

Dermatologic – Rash; pruritus.

EENT: Nasal congestion; blurred vision.

GI – Nausea; epigastric pain; diarrhea; vomiting; constipation; abdominal discomfort.

GU – Urinary frequency; disturbances of sexual function.

Musculoskeletal – Aches in extremities; muscle aches.

Miscellaneous – Gynecomastia; taste disorders; dyspnea.

Overdosage:

Symptoms: Overdose has been reported in children. Symptoms included hypotension, somnolence, lethargy, irritability, miosis and bradycardia. Treatment results in complete and uneventful recovery.

Treatment: Institute supportive treatment while the drug is being eliminated from the body and until the patient is no longer symptomatic. Monitor vital signs and fluid balance. Gastric lavage, activated charcoal, ipecac, fluid, pressor agents and atropine have been used successfully to treat guanabenz overdose. Maintain an adequate airway and, if indicated, institute assisted respiration. There are no data regarding dialyzability of guanabenz. Refer to General Management of Acute Overdosage.

Antiadrenergic Agents — Centrally Acting

GUANABENZ ACETATE

Patient Information:

Use caution when operating dangerous machinery or driving motor vehicles until it is determined that drowsiness or dizziness is not manifested from taking guanabenz.

Tolerance for alcohol and other CNS depressants may be diminished.

Advise patients not to discontinue therapy abruptly.

Administration and Dosage:

Initial dose: Individualize dosage.4 mg twice a day, whether used alone or with a thiazide diuretic; increase in increments of 4 to 8 mg/day every 1 to 2 weeks.The maximum dose studied was 32 mg twice daily; doses this high are rarely needed.

Rx	**Guanabenz Acetate** (Various, eg, Copley)	**Tablets**: 4 mg	In 100s and 500s.
Rx	**Wytensin** (Wyeth-Ayerst)		(Wyeth 73/W4). Orange. In 100s, 500s and Redipak 100s.
Rx	**Guanabenz Acetate** (Various, eg, Copley)	8 mg	In 100s and 500s.
Rx	**Wytensin** (Wyeth-Ayerst)		(Wyeth 74/W8). Gray, scored. In 100s.

Antiadrenergic Agents — Peripherally Acting

RESERPINE

Actions:

Pharmacology: Reserpine depletes stores of catecholamine and 5-hydroxytryptamine in many organs, including the brain and adrenal medulla. Most of its pharmacological effects have been attributed to this action. Depletion is slower and less complete in the adrenal medulla than in other tissues. The depression of sympathetic nerve function results in a decreased heart rate and a lowering of arterial blood pressure. The sedative and tranquilizing properties of reserpine are thought to be related to depletion of catecholamine and 5-hydroxytryptamine from the brain.

Pharmacokinetics: Reserpine is characterized by slow onset of action and sustained effects. Both cardiovascular and CNS effects may persist for a period of time following withdrawal of the drug.

Mean maximum plasma levels of 1.54 ng/ml were attained after a median of 3.5 hours in six healthy subjects receiving a single oral 1 mg dose. Bioavailability was $\approx$ 50% of that of a corresponding IV dose. Plasma levels of reserpine after IV administration declined with a mean half-life of 33 hours. Reserpine is extensively bound (96%) to plasma proteins. No definitive studies on the metabolism of reserpine have been made.

Indications:

Hypertension: Mild essential hypertension.

Adjunctive therapy with other antihypertensive agents in more severe forms of hypertension.

Psychotic states: Relief of symptoms in agitated psychotic states (eg, schizophrenia), primarily in those individuals unable to tolerate phenothiazine derivatives or in those who also require antihypertensive medication.

Contraindications:

Hypersensitivity; mental depression or history of mental depression (especially with suicidal tendencies); active peptic ulcer; ulcerative colitis; patients receiving electroconvulsive therapy.

Warnings:

Depression: Exercise extreme caution in treating patients with a history of mental depression. Reserpine may cause mental depression. Recognition of depression may be difficult, because this condition may often be disguised by somatic complaints (masked depression). Discontinue the drug at first signs of depression (eg, despondency, early morning insomnia, loss of appetite, impotence or self-deprecation). Drug-induced depression may persist for several months after drug withdrawal and may be severe enough to result in suicide.

Ulcers: Since reserpine increases GI motility and secretion, use cautiously in patients with a history of peptic ulcer, ulcerative colitis or gallstones (biliary colic may be precipitated).

Cardiovascular effects: Preoperative withdrawal of reserpine does not assure that circulatory instability will not occur. It is important that the anesthesiologist be aware of the patient's drug intake and consider this in the overall management, since hypotension has occurred in patients receiving reserpine. Anticholinergic or adrenergic drugs (eg, metaraminol, norepinephrine) have been employed to treat adverse vagocirculatory effects.

Renal function impairment: Exercise caution when treating hypertensive patients with renal insufficiency, since they adjust poorly to lowered blood pressure levels.

Carcinogenesis: Reserpine is an animal tumorigen, causing an increased incidence of mammary fibroadenomas in female mice, malignant tumors of the seminal vesicles in male mice and malignant adrenal medullary tumors in male rats. The breast neoplasms are thought to be related to reserpine's prolactin-elevating effect. The extent to which these findings indicate a risk to humans is uncertain. Tissue culture experiments show that about 33% of human breast tumors are prolactin-dependent, a factor of considerable importance if the use of the drug is contemplated in a patient with previously detected breast cancer. The possibility of an increased risk of breast cancer in reserpine users has been studied extensively; however, no firm conclusion has emerged. Although a few epidemiologic studies have suggested a slightly increased risk (less than twofold in all studies except one in women who have used reserpine), other studies of generally similar design have not confirmed this.

Pregnancy: Category C. There are no adequate and well controlled studies of reserpine in pregnant women. Reserpine crosses the placental barrier. Increased respiratory tract secretions, nasal congestion, cyanosis and anorexia may occur in neonates of reserpine-treated mothers. Use during pregnancy only if the potential benefit justifies the potential risk to the fetus.

Antiadrenergic Agents — Peripherally Acting

RESERPINE

Lactation: Reserpine is excreted in breast milk. Increased respiratory tract secretions, nasal congestion, cyanosis and anorexia may occur in breastfed infants. Because of the potential for adverse reactions in nursing infants and the potential for tumorigenicity, decide whether to discontinue nursing or to discontinue the drug, taking into account the importance of the drug to the mother.

Children: Safety and efficacy have not been established by means of controlled clinical trials, although there is experience with the use of reserpine in children (see Administration and Dosage). Because of adverse effects such as emotional depression and lability, sedation and stuffy nose, reserpine is not usually recommended as a step-2 drug in the treatment of hypertension in children.

Drug Interactions:

Reserpine Drug Interactions

Precipitant drug	Object drug*		Description
MAO inhibitors	Reserpine	↔	Avoid MAO inhibitors or use with extreme caution.
Tricyclic antidepressants	Reserpine	↓	Concurrent use may decrease the antihypertensive effect of reserpine.
Reserpine	Digitalis glycosides Quinidine	↑	Use reserpine cautiously with digitalis and quinidine, since cardiac arrhythmias have occurred.
Reserpine	Sympatho mimetics, direct-acting	↑	Closely monitor concurrent use of reserpine and direct- or indirect-acting sympathomimetics. The action of direct-acting amines (eg, epinephrine, isoproterenol, phenylephrine, metaraminol) may be prolonged when given to patients taking reserpine. The action of indirect-acting amines (eg, ephedrine, tyramine, amphetamines) is inhibited.
	Sympatho mimetics, indirect-acting	↓	

* ↑ = Object drug increased. ↓ = Object drug decreased. ↔ = Undetermined effect.

Adverse Reactions:

The following adverse reactions are listed in decreasing order of severity, not frequency.

Cardiovascular: Arrhythmias (particularly when used concurrently with digitalis or quinidine); syncope; angina-like symptoms; bradycardia; edema.

CNS: Parkinsonian syndrome and other extrapyramidal tract symptoms (rare); dizziness; headache; paradoxical anxiety; depression; nervousness; nightmares; dull sensorium; drowsiness.

GI: Vomiting; diarrhea; nausea; anorexia; dryness of mouth; hypersecretion.

GU: Pseudolactation; impotence; dysuria; gynecomastia; decreased libido; breast engorgement.

Respiratory: Dyspnea; epistaxis; nasal congestion.

Special senses: Deafness; optic atrophy; glaucoma; uveitis; conjunctival injection.

Miscellaneous: Hypersensitivity reactions: Purpura, rash, pruritus; weight gain; muscular aches.

Antiadrenergic Agents — Peripherally Acting

RESERPINE

Overdosage:

Symptoms: No deaths due to acute poisoning with reserpine have been reported. Highest known doses survived: Children, 1000 mg (age and sex not specified), young children, 200 mg (20-month-old boy). The clinical picture of acute poisoning is characterized chiefly by signs and symptoms due to the reflex parasympathomimetic effect of reserpine.

Impairment of consciousness may occur and may range from drowsiness to coma, depending on the severity of overdosage. Flushing of the skin, conjunctival injection and pupillary constriction are to be expected. Hypotension, hypothermia, central respiratory depression and bradycardia may develop in cases of severe overdosage. Increased salivary secretion, gastric secretion and diarrhea may also occur.

Treatment: There is no specific antidote. Evacuate stomach contents, taking adequate precautions against aspiration and for protection of the airway. Activated charcoal slurry should be instilled.

Treat the effects of reserpine overdosage symptomatically. If hypotension is severe enough to require treatment with a vasopressor, use one having a direct action upon vascular smooth muscle (eg, phenylephrine, norepinephrine, metaraminol). Since reserpine is long-acting, observe the patient carefully for at least 72 hours, and administer treatment as required.

Patient Information:

Inform patients of possible side effects and advise them to take the medication regularly and continuously as directed.

Administration and Dosage:

Hypertension: In the average patient not receiving other antihypertensive agents, the usual initial dosage is 0.5 mg daily for 1 or 2 weeks. For maintenance, reduce to 0.1 to 0.25 mg daily. Use higher dosages cautiously because occurrence of serious mental depression and other side affects may increase considerably.

Psychiatric disorders: The usual initial dosage is 0.5 mg daily, but may range from 0.1 to 1 mg. Adjust dosage upward or downward according to the patient's response.

Children: Reserpine is not recommended for use in children. If it is be used in treating a child, the usual recommended starting dose is 20 mcg/kg daily. The maximum recommended dose is 0.25 mg (total) daily.

Rx	**Reserpine** (Various, eg Eon, Moore, Rugby)	**Tablets:** 0.1 mg	In 100s,1000s and 5000s.
Rx	**Reserpine** (Various, eg Eon, Moore, Rugby, URL)	**Tablets:** 0.25 mg	In 100s, 1000s and 5000s.

Antiadrenergic Agents — Peripherally Acting

GUANETHIDINE MONOSULFATE

Refer to the Antihypertensives Introduction for a general discussion of these products.

> **Warning:**
> Orthostatic hypotension can occur frequently; inform patients about this potential hazard. Fainting spells may occur unless the patient is forewarned to sit or lie down with the onset of dizziness or weakness. Postural hypotension is most marked in the morning and is accentuated by hot weather, alcohol or exercise. Dizziness or weakness may be particularly bothersome during the initial period of dosage adjustment and with postural changes, such as arising in the morning. The potential occurrence of these symptoms may require alteration of previous daily activity. Caution the patient to avoid sudden or prolonged standing or exercise while taking the drug.

Actions:

Pharmacology: Guanethidine inhibits or interferes with the release or distribution of the chemical mediator (presumably norepinephrine) at the sympathetic neuroeffector junction. In contrast to ganglionic blocking agents, the drug suppresses equally the responses mediated by α and β-adrenergic receptors but does not produce parasympathetic blockade. Since sympathetic blockade results in modest decreases in peripheral resistance and cardiac output, guanethidine lowers blood pressure in the supine position. It further reduces blood pressure by decreasing the degree of vasoconstriction which normally results from reflex sympathetic nervous activity on assumption of the upright posture, thus reducing the venous return and cardiac output more. The inhibition of sympathetic venoconstrictive mechanisms results in venous pooling of blood. Therefore, the effect is especially pronounced when the patient is standing. Both the systolic and diastolic pressures are reduced.

Pharmacokinetics: Guanethidine is incompletely absorbed, about 3% to 50% upon oral administration. It is actively transported into adrenergic neurons. Adrenergic blockade occurs with a minimum plasma concentration of 8 ng/ml with doses of 10 to 50 mg/day at steady state. Guanethidine is partially metabolized by the liver to three metabolites (less active than the parent); parent drug and metabolites are excreted primarily in the urine. The drug is eliminated slowly because of extensive tissue binding. Renal clearance is 56 ml/min. Because of its long half-life (4 to 8 days), the drug accumulates slowly. Up to 2 weeks may be required to adequately evaluate the response to daily administration.

Indications:

Moderate and severe hypertension, either alone or as an adjunct.

Renal hypertension, including that secondary to pyelonephritis, renal amyloidosis and renal artery stenosis.

Contraindications:

Known or suspected pheochromocytoma; hypersensitivity to guanethidine; frank congestive heart failure (CHF) not due to hypertension; use of MAO inhibitors (see Drug Interactions).

Warnings:

Potency: This is a potent drug; its use can lead to serious clinical problems.

Orthostatic hypotension can occur frequently. Dizziness or weakness may be particularly bothersome during the initial dosage period and with postural changes. (See warning box.)

Preoperative withdrawal is recommended 2 weeks prior to surgery to reduce the possibility of vascular collapse and cardiac arrest during anesthesia. During emergency surgery, administer preanesthetic and anesthetic agents cautiously in reduced dosages. Have oxygen, atropine, vasopressors and adequate solutions for volume replacement ready for immediate use to counteract vascular collapse. *Use vasopressors only with extreme caution,* since guanethidine augments responsiveness to exogenously administered norepinephrine and vasopressors with respect to blood pressure and their propensity for the production of cardiac arrhythmias.

Antiadrenergic Agents — Peripherally Acting

GUANETHIDINE MONOSULFATE

Fever reduces dosage requirements.

Bronchial asthma patients require special consideration as they are more apt to be hypersensitive to catecholamine depletion and their condition may be aggravated.

Renal function impairment: Use very cautiously in hypertensive patients with renal disease and nitrogen retention or rising BUN levels, since decreased blood pressure may further compromise renal function.

Fertility impairment: Inhibition of ejaculation has occurred. This effect, which is attributable to the sympathetic blockade caused by the drug, is reversible several weeks after discontinuation of the drug. Erectile potency is usually retained.

Pregnancy: Category C. Safety for use during pregnancy has not been established. Use only when clearly needed and when the potential benefits outweigh the potential hazards to the fetus.

Lactation: Guanethidine is excreted in breast milk. Because of the potential for serious adverse reactions in nursing infants, discontinue nursing or discontinue the drug, taking into account the importance of the drug to the mother.

Children: Safety and efficacy for use in children have not been established.

Precautions:

Cumulative effects: The effects of guanethidine are cumulative; initial doses should be small and increased gradually in small increments.

Sodium retention: To minimize sodium retention and compensatory fluid retention, guanethidine is usually used with a thiazide diuretic.

Cardiovascular disease: Use very cautiously in hypertensive patients with coronary disease with insufficiency or recent myocardial infarction, and in cerebral vascular disease, especially with encephalopathy.

Use with great caution in patients with severe cardiac failure, since guanethidine may interfere with the adrenergic compensation in producing circulatory adjustment in patients with CHF. Both digitalis and guanethidine slow the heart rate.

In patients with incipient cardiac decompensation, monitor weight gain or edema, which may be averted by a concomitant thiazide.

Peptic ulcer: Use cautiously in patients with a history of peptic ulcer or other disorders which may be aggravated by a relative increase in parasympathetic tone.

Drug Interactions:

Guanethidine Drug Interactions

Precipitant drug	Object drug*		Description
Anorexiants	Guanethidine	⬇	The hypotensive effects of guanethidine may be reversed.
Haloperidol	Guanethidine	⬇	Haloperidol antagonizes the hypotensive effect of guanethidine.
Methylphenidate	Guanethidine	⬇	Hypotensive effects of guanethidine may be impaired. Arrhythmias were reported in one case.
Minoxidil	Guanethidine	⬆	Administration of minoxidil to patients on guanethidine can result in profound orthostatic effects. Discontinue guanethidine well before minoxidil is begun, if possible. If not possible, hospitalize the patient when starting minoxidil.
MAO inhibitors	Guanethidine	⬇	Discontinue MAOIs at least 1 week before starting guanethidine therapy; the combination may decrease the effects of guanethidine.
Phenothiazines	Guanethidine	⬇	The hypotensive effect of guanethidine is inhibited.
Sympathomimetics	Guanethidine	⬇	The hypotensive effect of guanethidine may be reversed. Also, guanethidine potentiates the effects of the direct-acting sympathomimetics.
Guanethidine	Sympathomimetics	⬆	
Thioxanthenes	Guanethidine	⬇	The hypotensive effect of guanethidine is antagonized.
Tricyclic antidepressants	Guanethidine	⬇	The hypotensive action of guanethidine is inhibited.

* ⬆ = Object drug increased. ⬇ = Object drug decreased.

GUANETHIDINE MONOSULFATE

Adverse Reactions:

Cardiovascular: Bradycardia; fluid retention; edema with occasional development of CHF; angina.

CNS: Dizziness; weakness; lassitude; syncope resulting from either postural or exertional hypotension; fatigue; muscle tremor; mental depression; chest paresthesias; ptosis of the lids; blurred vision.

GI: Nausea; vomiting; dry mouth; parotid tenderness; diarrhea (may be severe and necessitate discontinuance of the medication); increase in bowel movements.

GU: Inhibition of ejaculation (see Warnings); rise in BUN; nocturia; urinary incontinence; priapism, impotence (rare).

Hematologic: Anemia, thrombocytopenia, leukopenia (rare).

Respiratory: Dyspnea; nasal congestion; asthma in susceptible individuals.

Miscellaneous: Myalgia; weight gain; dermatitis; scalp hair loss.

Overdosage:

Symptoms: Postural hypotension and bradycardia are most likely to occur; diarrhea, possibly severe, may also occur. Unconsciousness is unlikely if adequate blood pressure and cerebral perfusion can be maintained.

Treatment: There is no specific antidote. Consider gastric lavage, activated charcoal and laxatives if conditions permit. In previously normotensive patients, treatment has consisted essentially of keeping the patient supine. Homeostatic control usually returns over 72 hours.

In previously hypertensive patients, particularly those with impaired cardiac reserve or other cardiovascular-renal disease, intensive treatment may be required to support vital functions or to control cardiac irregularities. Maintain the supine position if vasopressors are required; guanethidine may increase responsiveness to blood pressure rise and occurrence of cardiac arrhythmias. Administer atropine for sinus bradycardia.

Treat severe or persistent diarrhea symptomatically.

Monitor cardiovascular and renal function for a few days.

Patient Information:

Notify physician of severe diarrhea, frequent dizziness or fainting.

Administration and Dosage:

Ambulatory patients: Begin with 10 mg daily. Increase dosage gradually and do not increase more often than every 5 to 7 days (eg, visit 1, 10 mg/day; visit 2, 20 mg day; visit 3, 30 or 37.5 mg/day; visit 4, 50 mg/day; visit 5 and subsequent, may increase by 12.5 or 25 mg if necessary). Take blood pressure in the supine position, after standing for 10 minutes and immediately after exercise if feasible. Increase dosage only if there has been *no* decrease in standing blood pressure from the previous levels. The average dose is 25 to 50 mg once daily. Reduce dosage in any of the following: Normal supine pressure, excessive orthostatic fall in pressure, severe diarrhea.

Hospitalized patients:

Initial dose – 25 to 50 mg; increase by 25 or 50 mg/day or every other day as indicated. This higher dosage is possible because hospitalized patients can be watched carefully. Unless absolutely impossible, take the standing blood pressure regularly. Do not discharge patients from the hospital until the effect of the drug on the standing blood pressure is known. *Tell patients about the possibility of orthostatic hypotension and warn them not to get out of bed without help during the period of dosage adjustment.*

Loading dose (for severe hypertension) – Guanethidine is given 3 times daily at 6 hour intervals over 1 to 3 days; the nighttime dose is omitted. Once blood pressure is normalized, determine the daily maintenance dosage. Take the standing blood pressure regularly. Do not discharge patients from the hospital until the effect of the drug on the standing blood pressure is known. Advise patients about orthostatic hypotension and warn them not to get out of bed without help during dosage adjustment.

Children:

Initial dose – 0.2 mg/kg/24 hr (6 mg/m^2/24 hr) as a single oral dose.

Increment – 0.2 mg/kg/24 hr every 7 to 10 days.

Maximum – 3 mg/kg/24 hr.

Antiadrenergic Agents — Peripherally Acting

GUANETHIDINE MONOSULFATE

Combination therapy: Thiazide diuretics enhance the effectiveness of guanethidine and may reduce the incidence of edema. When thiazide diuretics are added to the regimen, it is usually necessary to reduce the guanethidine dosage. After control is established, reduce dosage of all drugs to the lowest effective level.

If ganglionic blockers have not been discontinued before guanethidine is started, gradually withdraw them to prevent a spiking blood pressure response during the transfer period.

Rx	**Ismelin** (Ciba)	**Tablets:** 10 mg	(Ciba 49). Yellow, scored. In 100s.	409
		25 mg	(Ciba 103). White, scored. In 100s.	257

GUANADREL SULFATE

For complete prescribing information, refer to the Antihypertensives Introduction.

Actions:

Pharmacology: Guanadrel, structurally and pharmacologically similar to guanethidine, inhibits sympathetic vasoconstriction by inhibiting norepinephrine release from neuronal storage sites in response to nerve stimulation. Depletion of norepinephrine causes a relaxation of vascular smooth muscle which decreases total peripheral resistance and venous return. A hypotensive effect results, greater in the standing than in the supine position by about 10 mm Hg systolic and 3.5 mm Hg diastolic. The drug does not inhibit parasympathetic nerve function nor does it enter the CNS.

Guanadrel begins to decrease blood pressure within 2 hours and produces maximal decreases in 4 to 6 hours. No significant change in cardiac output accompanies the blood pressure decline in normal individuals. Heart rate is also decreased by about 5 beats/minute. Fluid retention occurs, particularly when guanadrel is not accompanied by a diuretic.

Guanadrel causes increased sensitivity to circulating norepinephrine, probably by preventing uptake of norepinephrine by adrenergic neurons. Thus it is dangerous in the presence of excess norepinephrine, eg, pheochromocytoma.

Pharmacokinetics:

Absorption – It is rapidly absorbed after oral administration. Plasma concentrations generally peak 1.5 to 2 hours after ingestion. Protein binding is < 20%.

Metabolism/Excretion – Half-life is about 10 hours, but individual variability is great. Approximately 85% of the drug is eliminated in the urine. Urinary excretion is about 85% complete within 24 hours; about 40% of a dose is excreted unchanged.

Clinical trials: Patients with initial supine blood pressures averaging 160 to 170/105 to 110 mm Hg have decreases in blood pressure of 20 to 25/15 to 20 mm Hg in the standing position. Guanethidine and guanadrel are similar in effectiveness while methyldopa has a larger effect on supine systolic pressure. Side effects of guanadrel and guanethidine are generally similar while methyldopa has more CNS effects (depression, drowsiness) but fewer orthostatic effects and less diarrhea.

Indications:

Treatment of hypertension in patients not responding adequately to a thiazide-type diuretic. Add to a diuretic regimen for optimum blood pressure control.

Contraindications:

Known or suspected pheochromocytoma; concurrently with, or within 1 week of MAOIs; hypersensitivity to guanadrel; frank CHF.

Warnings:

Orthostatic hypotension and its consequences (dizziness and weakness) are frequent. Rarely, fainting upon standing or exercise occurs. Careful instructions to the patient can minimize symptoms; supine blood pressure is not an adequate assessment of guanadrel's effects. Patients with known regional vascular disease (cerebral, coronary) are at particular risk from marked orthostatic hypotension; avoid hypotensive episodes even if this requires a poorer degree of blood pressure control.

Surgery: To reduce the possibility of vascular collapse during anesthesia, discontinue guanadrel 48 to 72 hours before elective surgery. If emergency surgery is required, administer preanesthetic and anesthetic agents cautiously in reduced dosage. Use vasopressors cautiously, as guanadrel can enhance the pressor response and increase arrhythmogenicity.

Asthma: Special care is needed in patients with bronchial asthma, as it may be aggravated by catecholamine depletion and sympathomimetic amines may interfere with the hypotensive effect of guanadrel.

GUANADREL SULFATE

Renal function impairment: As renal function declines, apparent total body clearance, renal and apparent nonrenal clearances decrease, and the terminal elimination half-life is prolonged. Dosage adjustments may be necessary, especially in patients with creatinine clearances (Ccr) < 60 ml/min (see Administration and Dosage).

Fertility impairment: In rats, suppressed libido and reduced fertility were noted at 100 mg/kg/day (12 times the maximum human dose).

Pregnancy: Category B. There are no adequate and well-controlled studies in pregnant women. Use only when clearly needed and when the potential benefits outweigh the potential hazards to the fetus.

Lactation: It is not known if guanadrel is excreted in breast milk. Because of the potential for serious adverse reactions in the nursing infant, decide whether to discontinue nursing or to discontinue the drug, taking into account the importance of the drug to the mother.

Children: Safety and efficacy for use in children have not been established.

Precautions:

Salt and water retention may occur. Patients with CHF have not been studied, but guanadrel could interfere with the adrenergic mechanisms.

Peptic ulcer: Use guanadrel cautiously in patients with a history of peptic ulcer, which could be aggravated by a relative increase in parasympathetic tone.

Drug Interactions:

Drug Interactions

Precipitant drug	Object drug*		Description
Beta blockers	Guanadrel	↑	The effects of guanadrel may be potentiated, causing excessive postural hypotension and bradycardia.
Phenothiazines	Guanadrel	↓	The effects of guanadrel may be reversed.
Sympathomimetics	Guanadrel	↓	The hypotensive effect of guanadrel may be reversed. Also, guanadrel may potentiate the effects of the direct-acting sympathomimetics.
Guanadrel	Sympathomimetics	↑	
Tricyclic antidepressants (TCA)	Guanadrel	↓	TCAs may block the norepinephrine-depleting effect and the blood pressure lowering effect of guanadrel. Use caution with concomitant use. If the TCA is discontinued abruptly, an enhanced effect of guanadrel may occur.
Vasodilators	Guanadrel	↑	Concomitant use may increase the potential for symptomatic orthostatic hypotension and is generally not recommended.

* ↑ = Object drug increased. ↓ = Object drug decreased.

Antiadrenergic Agents — Peripherally Acting

GUANADREL SULFATE

Adverse Reactions:

The following table displays the frequency of side effects which are generally higher during the first 8 weeks of therapy. Approximately 3.6% of patients withdrew from guanadrel therapy because of untoward effects.

Adverse Reactions of Antiadrenergic Drugs (%)

	Adverse reaction	Guanadrel (n = 1544)	Methyldopa (n = 743)	Guanethidine (n = 330)
Cardiovascular/ Respiratory	Shortness of breath on exertion	46	53	49
	Palpitations	30	35	25
	Chest pain	28	37	27
	Coughing	27	36	22
	Shortness of breath at rest	18	22	17
Central nervous system	Fatigue	64	76	57
	Headache	58	69	50
	Faintness (orthostatic/other)	47-49	41-46	45-48
	Drowsiness	45	64	29
	Visual disturbances	29	35	26
	Paresthesias	25	35	16
	Confusion	15	23	11
	Psychological problems	4	5	4
	Depression	2	4	2
	Sleep disorders	2	2	3
	Syncope	< 1	< 1	2
Gastrointestinal	Increased bowel movements	31	28	36
	Gas pain/indigestion	24-32	31-40	19-29
	Constipation	21	29	20
	Anorexia	19	23	18
	Glossitis	8	11	5
	Nausea/vomiting	4	5	4
	Dry mouth, dry throat	2	4	< 1
	Abdominal distress or pain	2	2	2
Genitourinary	Nocturia	48	52	42
	Urination urgency or frequency	34	40	28
	Peripheral edema	29	37	23
	Ejaculation disturbances	18	21	22
	Impotence	5	12	7
	Hematuria	2	4	2
Miscellaneous	Excessive weight gain/loss	42-44	51-54	42
	Aching limbs	43	52	34
	Leg cramps - nighttime	26	33	21
	Leg cramps - daytime	21	26	20
	Backache or neckache	2	1	2
	Joint pain or inflammation	2	2	2

Overdosage:

Symptoms: Marked dizziness and blurred vision related to postural hypotension progressing to syncope on standing. The patient should lie down until these symptoms subside.

Treatment: If excessive hypotension occurs and persists despite conservative treatment, a vasoconstrictor such as phenylephrine may be needed, but use carefully because patients may be hypersensitive to such agents.

Patient Information:

The medication may cause orthostatic hypotension; sit or lie down immediately at the onset of dizziness or weakness to prevent loss of consciousness. Postural hypotension is worst in the morning and upon arising, and may be exaggerated by alcohol, fever, hot weather, prolonged standing or exercise.

Do not take any prescription or over-the-counter medications, especially medications for treatment of colds, allergy or asthma, without physician's or pharmacist's advice.

Antiadrenergic Agents — Peripherally Acting

GUANADREL SULFATE

Administration and Dosage:

Individualize dosage. The usual starting dosage is 10 mg/day, which can be given as 5 mg 2 times daily by breaking the 10 mg tablet. Most patients will require a daily dosage of 20 to 75 mg, usually in twice daily doses. For larger doses, 3 or 4 times daily dosing may be needed. Adjust the dosage weekly or monthly until blood pressure is controlled.

With long-term therapy, some tolerance may occur and the dosage may have to be increased. Because guanadrel has a substantial orthostatic effect, monitor both supine and standing pressures, especially while adjusting dosage.

Renal function impairment: Adjust dosage. for initial therapy, reduce dosage to 5 mg every 24 hours in patients with Ccr 30 to 60 ml/min. For patients with Ccr < 30 ml/min, increase the interval to 48 hours. Cautiously make dosage increases at intervals ≥ 7 days for moderate renal insufficiency and ≥ 14 days for severe insufficiency.

Rx	**Hylorel** (Fisons)	**Tablets**: 10 mg	(Hylorel 10). Light orange, scored. In 100s.
		25 mg	(Hylorel 25). White, scored. In 100s.

Antiadrenergic Agents — Peripherally Acting

ALPHA-1-ADRENERGIC BLOCKERS

Actions:

Pharmacology: Prazosin, terazosin and doxazosin selectively block postsynaptic α_1—adrenergic receptors. These drugs dilate both resistance (arterioles) and capacitance (veins) vessels. Both supine and standing blood pressure are lowered. This effect is most pronounced on the diastolic blood pressure. Terazosin decreases blood pressure gradually within 15 minutes following oral administration. Unlike conventional α-blockers, the antihypertensive actions of prazosin and terazosin are usually not accompanied by reflex tachycardia. With doxazosin, maximum reductions in blood pressure usually occur 2 to 6 hours after dosing and are associated with a small increase in standing heart rate. Tolerance to the antihypertensive effect of these agents has not been observed.

Prazosin does not appear to increase renin release as do the direct-acting vasodilators; a decrease in plasma renin activity has occurred during therapy. Plasma renin activity was unchanged by terazosin.

Use of prazosin as a single antihypertensive agent is limited by its tendency to cause sodium and water retention and increased plasma volume.

In the treatment of benign prostatic hyperplasia (BPH), the reduction in symptoms and improvement in urine flow rates is related to relaxation of smooth muscle produced by blockade of $alpha_1$ adrenoceptors in the bladder neck and prostate. Because there are relatively few $alpha_1$ receptors in the bladder body, terazosin and doxazosin are able to reduce the bladder outlet obstruction without affecting bladder contractility.

Pharmacokinetics: Prazosin is extensively metabolized. The metabolites of prazosin are active. Duration of antihypertensive effect is 10 hours. Elimination is slower in patients with congestive heart failure (CHF) than in normal subjects. The pharmacokinetics may be altered in chronic renal failure (eg, elimination half-life prolonged, protein binding decreased and peak plasma concentrations increased).

Terazosin undergoes minimal hepatic first-pass metabolism; nearly all of the circulating dose is in the form of parent drug. Approximately 10% of an oral dose is excreted as parent drug in the urine, and approximately 20% is excreted in the feces. The remainder is eliminated as metabolites.

Doxazosin is extensively metabolized in the liver, mainly by O-demethylation or hydroxylation. Approximately 4.8% is excreted in the feces as unchanged drug, with only a trace in the urine. Enterohepatic recycling is suggested by secondary peaking of plasma doxazosin concentrations. Although several active metabolites have been identified, their pharmacokinetics have not been characterized. The low plasma concentrations of the known active and inactive metabolites compared to the parent drug indicate that the contribution of even the most potent compound to the antihypertensive efficacy is probably small.

Pharmacokinetics of Alpha-1-Adrenergic Blockers

Parameters	Prazosin	Terazosin	Doxazosin
Oral bioavailability	48% to 68%	90%	65%
Affected by food	No	No	No
Peak plasma level, time	1 to 3 hrs	1 to 2 hrs	2 to 3 hrs
Protein binding	92% to 97%	90% to 94%	98%
Half-life	2 to 3 hrs	9 to 12 hrs	22 hrs
Excretion: Bile/feces	< 90%	60%	63%
Excretion: Urine	< 10%	40%	9%

Clinical trials:

Hypertension – Clinical studies of terazosin used once-daily (the great majority) and twice-daily regimens. Total doses usually ranged from 5 to 20 mg/day in mild (about 77%, diastolic pressure 95 to 105 mm Hg) or moderate (23%, diastolic pressure 105 to 115 mm Hg) hypertension. Blood pressure responses persisted throughout the interval, with the usual supine responses 5 to 10 mm Hg systolic and 3.5 to 8 mm Hg diastolic greater than placebo. The responses in the standing position tended to be somewhat larger, by 1 to 3 mm Hg. The magnitude of the blood pressure responses was similar to prazosin and less than hydrochlorothiazide (in a single study). In measurements 24 hours after dosing, heart rate was unchanged.

ALPHA-1-ADRENERGIC BLOCKERS

Doxazosin has a greater effect on blood pressure and heart rate in the standing position. In placebo controlled studies at doses of 1 to 16 mg given once daily, blood pressure was lowered at 24 hours by about 10/8 mm Hg compared to placebo in the standing position and about 9/5 mm Hg in the supine position.

Benign prostatic hyperplasia (BPH) – In several studies, both symptom scores and peak urine flow rates significantly improved from baseline in patients treated with terazosin from week 2 (or the first clinic visit) and throughout the study duration. Compared to placebo, terazosin significantly improved the symptoms of hesitancy, intermittency, impairment in size and force of urinary stream, sensation of incomplete emptying, terminal dribbling, daytime frequency and nocturia. There is a rapid response, with ≈ 70% of patients experiencing an increase in urinary flow and improvement in symptoms of BPH. Treatment of normotensive men with BPH did not result in a clinically significant blood pressure-lowering effect.

In three studies, doxazosin resulted in statistically significant relief of obstructive and irritative symptoms compared to placebo; improvements in maximum flow rate with doxazosin were 2.3 to 3.3 ml/sec vs 0.1 to 0.7 with placebo. The proportion of patients who responded with a maximum flow rate of ≥ 3 ml/sec was significantly larger with doxazosin (34% to 42%) than placebo (13% to 17%). Doxazosin provides rapid improvement in symptoms and urinary flow rate in 66% to 71% of patients; sustained improvements were seen in patients treated for up to 2 years. Treatment of normotensive men with BPH did not result in a clinically significant blood pressure-lowering effect.

Indications:

Hypertension: For the treatment of hypertension, alone or in combination with other antihypertensive agents.

Benign prostatic hyperplasia (BPH):

Terazosin – Treatment of symptomatic benign prostatic hyperplasia.

Doxazosin – Treatment of both the urinary outflow obstruction and obstructive (hesitation, intermittency, dribbling, weak urinary stream, incomplete emptying of the bladder) and irritative (nocturia, daytime frequency, urgency, burning) symptoms associated with BPH.

Unlabeled uses:

Prazosin – Refractory CHF. It decreases cardiac afterload (left ventricular systolic wall tension) and preload (left ventricular end-diastolic volume or pressure). By reducing aortic impedance and venous return, prazosin helps improve reduced cardiac output and relieve pulmonary congestion. It has produced improvement in the clinical symptoms, exercise tolerance and functional class (NYHA classification) of CHF in short-term studies.

Management of Raynaud's vasospasm.

Treatment of benign prostatic hyperplasia.

Doxazosin – Treatment of CHF with concurrent digoxin and diuretics.

Contraindications:

Hypersensitivity to quinazolines (eg, doxazosin, prazosin, terazosin).

Warnings:

"First-dose" effect: Prazosin, terazosin and doxazosin, like other α-adrenergic blocking agents, can cause marked hypotension (especially postural hypotension) and syncope with sudden loss of consciousness with the first few doses. Anticipate a similar effect if therapy is interrupted for more than a few doses, if dosage is increased rapidly, or if another antihypertensive drug is introduced. Syncope is due to an excessive postural hypotensive effect, although the syncopal episode has occasionally been preceded by severe supraventricular tachycardia with heart rates of 120 to 160 beats per minute.

The "first-dose" phenomenon may be minimized by limiting the initial dose to 1 mg of terazosin or prazosin (given at bedtime) or doxazosin. The 2, 5 and 10 mg terazosin tablets or 2 and 5 mg prazosin capsules or 2, 4 and 8 mg doxazosin tablets are not indicated as initial therapy. Slowly increase dosage of these drugs with increases in dose every 2 weeks. Add additional antihypertensives with caution. Caution patients to avoid situations where injury could result should syncope occur during initiation of therapy. Hypotension may develop in patients also receiving a β-adrenergic blocker.

If syncope occurs, place patient in recumbent position and treat supportively. This effect is self-limiting and in most cases does not recur after the initial period of therapy or during subsequent dosage adjustments. More common than loss of consciousness are dizziness and lightheadedness.

ALPHA-1-ADRENERGIC BLOCKERS

Syncopal episodes have usually occurred within 30 to 90 minutes of the initial dose of prazosin; the incidence is ≈ 1% with an initial dose of ≥ 2 mg. Syncope occurred in about 1% of terazosin patients, was in no case severe or prolonged, and was not necessarily associated with early doses. There is evidence that the orthostatic effect of terazosin is greater, even in chronic use, shortly after dosing. Syncope occurred in 0.7% of doxazosin patients; none of these events were reported at the starting dose of 1 mg and 1.2% occurred at 16 mg/day. Other symptoms of lowered blood pressure, such as dizziness, lightheadedness and palpitations, are more common, occurring in approximately 28% of terazosin patients and up to 23% of doxazosin patients (≈ 2% of doxazosin patients discontinued therapy). This may present an occupational hazard to some patients. Treat these patients with caution and advise them as to what measures to take if symptoms develop.

BPH complications: Long-term effects of terazosin on the incidence of surgery, acute urinary obstruction or other complications of BPH are yet to be determined.

Hepatic function impairment: Administer doxazosin with caution to patients with evidence of impaired hepatic function or to patients receiving drugs known to influence hepatic metabolism.

Fertility impairment: Reduced fertility occurred in male rats treated with doxazosin 20 mg/kg/day (about 75 times the maximum recommended human dose). The effect was reversible within 2 weeks of drug withdrawal. Nine of 39 male rats failed to sire a litter after terazosin 30 to 120 mg/kg/day. Testicular atrophy has also occurred in rats and dogs receiving terazosin or prazosin.

Pregnancy: Category C. A doxazosin dosage of 82 mg/kg/day in rabbits was associated with reduced fetal survival. In rats, maternal doxazosin doses 8 times the human AUC exposure (12 mg/day) delayed postnatal development. Terazosin doses 280 times the maximum recommended human dose in rats resulted in fetal resorptions; increased fetal resorptions, decreased fetal weight and increased number of supernumerary ribs occurred with doses 60 times the maximum recommended human dose. Significantly more rat pups died in the group dosed with terazosin (> 75 times the maximum recommended human dose) vs controls.

There are no adequate and well controlled studies in pregnant women. Safety for use during pregnancy has not been established. Use only when clearly needed and when the potential benefits outweigh the potential hazards to the fetus.

Lactation: Doxazosin accumulates in breast milk of lactating rats following a single 1 mg/kg dose, with a maximum concentration about 20 times greater than the maternal plasma concentration. It is not known whether terazosin is excreted in breast milk. Prazosin is excreted in small amounts in breast milk. Exercise caution when administering these drugs to a nursing woman.

Children: Safety and efficacy for use in children have not been established.

Precautions:

Hemodilution: Small but statistically significant decreases in hematocrit, hemoglobin, white blood cells, total protein and albumin were observed in controlled clinical trials with terazosin. The magnitude of the decreases did not worsen with time. These laboratory findings suggest the possibility of hemodilution.

Leukopenia/Neutropenia: In hypertensive patients receiving doxazosin, mean WBC and neutrophil counts were decreased by 2.4% and 1%, respectively, compared to placebo, a phenomenon seen with other alpha blocking drugs. In BPH patients, the incidence of clinically significant WBC abnormalities was 0.4%. No patients became symptomatic as a result of the low counts. WBCs and neutrophil counts returned to normal after drug discontinuation.

Weight gain: There was a tendency for patients to gain weight during terazosin therapy. In placebo controlled monotherapy trials, male and female patients receiving terazosin gained a mean of 1.7 and 2.2 pounds, respectively, compared to losses of 0.2 and 1.2 pounds, respectively, in the placebo group.

Cholesterol: During controlled clinical studies, patients receiving terazosin monotherapy had a small but statistically significant decrease (3%) in total cholesterol and the combined LDL and VLDL fractions. No significant changes were observed in HDL fraction and triglycerides. Prazosin therapy has also been associated with a decrease in total cholesterol levels and LDL and an increase in HDL. Other studies have shown no change in serum lipids in patients receiving terazosin or prazosin. In clinical trials involving normocholesterolemic patients, doxazosin reduced total serum cholesterol by 2% to 3% and LDL by 4%, and increased HDL to total cholesterol ratio by 4%. The clinical significance is unknown.

Antiadrenergic Agents — Peripherally Acting

ALPHA-1-ADRENERGIC BLOCKERS

Cardiotoxicity: An increased incidence of myocardial necrosis or fibrosis occurred in rats and mice following 6 to 18 months of doxazosin 40 to 80 mg/kg/day. There is no evidence that similar lesions occur in humans.

Prostatic cancer: Carcinoma of the prostate and BPH cause many of the same symptoms and frequently co-exist. Therefore, examine patients thought to have BPH prior to starting terazosin therapy to rule out prostate carcinoma.

Drug Interactions:

Alpha$_1$ Blocker Drug Interactions			
Precipitant drug	Object drug*		Description
Beta blockers	Alpha$_1$ blockers	↑	Beta blockers may enhance the acute postural hypotensive reaction following the first dose of prazosin; terazosin and doxazosin have been combined with beta blockers with no adverse reaction.
Indomethacin	Alpha$_1$ blockers	↓	The antihypertensive action of prazosin may be decreased. No interaction occurred in patients receiving doxazosin and NSAIDs.
Verapamil	Alpha$_1$ blockers	↑	Verapamil appears to increase serum prazosin levels and may increase the sensitivity to prazosin-induced postural hypotension.
Alpha$_1$ blockers	Clonidine	↓	The antihypertensive effect of clonidine may be decreased.

* ↑ = Object drug increased. ↓ = Object drug decreased.

Drug/Lab test interactions: In a study of five patients given prazosin 12 to 24 mg/day for 10 to 14 days, there was an average increase of 42% in the urinary metabolite of norepinephrine and an average increase in urinary VMA of 17%. Therefore, false-positive results may occur in screening tests for pheochromocytoma in patients who are being treated with prazosin. If an elevated VMA is found, discontinue prazosin and retest the patient after a month.

Doxazosin and terazosin do not affect plasma concentrations of prostate specific antigen (PSA) in patients treated for ≤ 3 years (doxazosin) or 2 years (terazosin).

Adverse Reactions:

Alpha-1-Adrenergic Blocker Adverse Reactions (%)[1]					
	Hypertension			BPH	
Adverse Reaction	Prazosin	Terazosin	Doxazosin	Terazosin	Doxazosin
Cardiovascular					
Palpitations	5.3	4.3	2	0.9	1.2
Postural hypotension/hypotension	✓[2]	1.3	0.3 to 1	0.6 to 3.9	0.3 to 1.7
Tachycardia	✓[2]	1.9	0.3		0.9
Arrhythmia, chest pain	no report	1	1 to 2		
Vasodilation	no report	1	no report		
Syncope				0.6	0.5
GI					
Nausea	4.9	4.4	3	1.7	1.5
Vomiting, dry mouth	✓[2]	1	≤ 2		1.4
Diarrhea, constipation	✓[2]	1	1 to 2		2.3
Abdominal discomfort/pain	✓[2]	1	1		1.7 to 2.4
Flatulence	no report	1	1		
Respiratory					
Dyspnea	✓[2]	3.1	1	1.7	2.6
Nasal congestion	✓[2]	5.9	no report	1.9	
Sinusitis	no report	2.6	< 0.5		< 0.5
Bronchitis/cold symptoms/bronchospasm	no report	1	< 0.5		< 0.5
Epistaxis	✓[2]	1	1		
Flu symptoms/increased cough	no report	1	< 0.5	2.4	1.1
Pharyngitis/rhinitis	no report	1	3	1.9	< 0.5

Antiadrenergic Agents — Peripherally Acting

ALPHA-1-ADRENERGIC BLOCKERS

Alpha-1-Adrenergic Blocker Adverse Reactions (%)[1]					
	Hypertension			BPH	
Adverse Reaction	Prazosin	Terazosin	Doxazosin	Terazosin	Doxazosin
Musculoskeletal					
Shoulder/neck/back/extremity pain	no report	1 to 3.5	< 0.5 to 2		< 0.5 to 2
Arthritis, joint/muscle pain, gout, cramps	no report	1	1		< 0.5
Arthralgia/Myalgia	✓[2]	1	1		
Special senses					
Blurred vision	✓[2]	1.6	no report	0.6	
Abnormal vision	no report	1	2	0.6	1.4
Conjunctivitis, reddened sclera/eye pain	✓[2]	1	1		
Tinnitus	✓[2]	1	1		
Vertigo	no report	no report	2	1.4	
CNS					
Depression	✓[2]	< 1	1		
Dizziness	10.3	19.3	19	9.1	15.6
Decreased libido/sexual dysfunction	no report	< 1	2		0.8
Nervousness	✓[2]	2.3	2		
Paresthesia	✓[2]	2.9	1		
Somnolence	no report	5.4	5	3.6	3
Anxiety/Insomnia	no report	1	1		1.1 to 1.2
Asthenia[3]	≈ 7	11.3	1 to 12	7.4	8
Drowsiness	7.6	✓[2]	✓[2]		
Ataxia	no report	no report	1		
Hypertonia	no report	no report	1		
GU					
Impotence	✓[2]	1.2	no report	1.6	1.1
Urinary frequency	✓[2]	1	0		
Urinary tract infection	no report	1	no report	1.3	1.4
Incontinence	✓[2]	no report	1		
Polyuria	no report	no report	2		
Priapism	✓[2]	no report	no report		
Dermatologic					
Pruritus/rash/sweating	✓[2]	1	1		1.1
Alopecia/lichen planus	✓[2]	no report	< 0.5		< 0.5
Miscellaneous					
Headache	7.8	16.2	14	4.9	9.9
Edema	✓[2]	< 1	4		2.7
Peripheral edema	no report	5.5	no report	0.9	
Weight gain	no report	< 1	0.5 to 1	0.5	
Facial edema	no report	1	1		
Fever	✓[2]	1	< 0.5		< 0.5
Flushing	no report	no report	1		

[1] Data are pooled from separate studies and are not necessarily comparable.
[2] Reactions associated with the drug, incidence unknown.
[3] Includes weakness, tiredness, lassitude and fatigue.

Overdosage:

Symptoms: Accidental ingestion of at least 50 mg prazosin in a 2-year-old child produced profound drowsiness and depressed reflexes. No decrease in blood pressure was noted. Recovery was uneventful.

Several cases of doxazosin overdose have been reported (doses ranging from 1 to 40 mg in children and 60 to 70 mg in adults). All children made full recoveries. One adult developed hypotension which responded to fluid therapy. The other adult (with chronic renal failure, epilepsy and depression) died; death was attributed to a

ALPHA-1-ADRENERGIC BLOCKERS

grand mal seizure resulting from hypotension. The most likely manifestation of overdosage would be hypotension.

Treatment: Restore blood pressure and normalize heart rate by keeping the patient supine. Treat shock with volume expanders. If necessary, use vasopressors and monitor and support renal function. These drugs are highly protein bound; dialysis may not be of benefit. Refer to General Management of Acute Overdosage.

Patient Information:

Inform patients of the possibility of syncopal and orthostatic symptoms, especially at the initiation of therapy. Avoid driving or hazardous tasks for 12 to 24 hours after the first dose, after a dosage increase and after interruption of therapy when treatment is resumed. Use caution when rising from a sitting or lying position. If dizziness or palpitations are bothersome, report to the physician so that dose adjustment can be considered.

Drowsiness or somnolence can occur. Use caution when driving or operating heavy machinery.

Prazosin and terazosin: Take the first dose at bedtime.

PRAZOSIN

Indications:

Hypertension: Alone or in combination with other antihypertensive agents such as diuretics or beta blockers.

Administration and Dosage:

Individualize dosage.

Initial dose: 1 mg 2 or 3 times daily. When increasing dosages, give the first dose of each increment at bedtime to reduce syncopal episodes.

Maintenance dose: 6 to 15 mg/day in divided doses. Doses > 20 mg usually do not increase efficacy; however, a few patients may benefit from up to 40 mg/day. After initial adjustment, some patients can be maintained on a twice-daily regimen.

Children: A dose of 0.5 to 7 mg 3 times a day has been suggested.

Concomitant therapy: When adding a diuretic or other antihypertensive agent, reduce dosage to 1 or 2 mg 3 times a day and then retitrate.

Rx	**Prazosin** (Various, eg, Geneva, Goldline, Lederle, Major, Moore, Rugby, Schein, Squibb, Zenith)	**Capsules**: 1 mg	In 30s, 60s, 90s, 100s, 120s, 250s, 500s, 1000s and UD 100s.
Rx	**Minipress** (Pfizer)		(Pfizer 431 Minipress). White. In 250s, 1000s and UD 100s.
Rx	**Prazosin** (Various, eg, Geneva, Goldline, Lederle, Major, Moore, Rugby, Schein, Squibb, Zenith)	**Capsules**: 2 mg	In 30s, 60s, 90s, 100s, 120s, 250s, 500s, 1000s and UD 100s.
Rx	**Minipress** (Pfizer)		(Pfizer 437 Minipress). Pink/white. In 250s, 1000s and UD 100s.
Rx	**Prazosin** (Various, eg, Geneva, Goldline, Lederle, Major, Moore, Rugby, Schein, Squibb, Zenith)	**Capsules**: 5 mg	In 30s, 60s, 90s, 100s, 120s, 250s, 500s, 1000s and UD 100s.
Rx	**Minipress** (Pfizer)		(Pfizer 438 Minipress). Blue/white. In 250s, 500s and UD 100s.

Antiadrenergic Agents — Peripherally Acting

TERAZOSIN

Indications:

Hypertension: Alone or in combination with other antihypertensive agents such as diuretics or beta blockers.

Benign prostatic hyperplasia (BPH): Treatment of symptomatic BPH.

Administration and Dosage:

Hypertension: Adjust dose and the dose interval (12 or 24 hours) individually. The following is a guide.

Initial dose – 1 mg at bedtime for all patients. Do not exceed this dose. Strictly observe this initial dosing regimen to avoid severe hypotensive effects.

Subsequent doses – Slowly increase the dose to achieve the desired blood pressure response. The recommended dose range is 1 to 5 mg daily; however, some patients may benefit from doses as high as 20 mg/day. Doses over 20 mg do not appear to provide further blood pressure effect, and doses over 40 mg have not been studied. Monitor blood pressure at the end of the dosing interval to be sure control is maintained. Measure blood pressure 2 to 3 hours after dosing to see if the maximum and minimum responses are similar, and to evaluate symptoms such as dizziness or palpitations. If response is substantially diminished at 24 hours, consider an increased dose or a twice-daily regimen. If terazosin is discontinued for several days or longer, reinstitute therapy using the initial dosing regimen. In clinical trials, except for the initial dose, the dose was given in the morning.

Benign prostatic hyperplasia:

Initial dose – 1 mg at bedtime is the starting dose for all patients; do not exceed as an initial dose. Closely monitor patients to minimize the risk of severe hypotensive response.

Subsequent doses – Increase the dose in a stepwise fashion to 2, 5 or 10 mg daily to achieve desired improvement of symptoms or flow rates. Doses of 10 mg once daily are generally required for the clinical response; therefore, treatment with 10 mg for a minimum of 4 to 6 weeks may be required to assess whether a beneficial response has been achieved. Some patients may not achieve a clinical response. Although some patients have responded to 20 mg daily, there was an insufficient number of patients to draw definitive conclusions about this dose. There is insufficient data to support the use of doses > 20 mg in patients who do not respond.

Concomitant therapy: Observe caution when terazosin is administered concomitantly with other antihypertensive agents (eg, calcium antagonists) to avoid the possibility of significant hypotension. When adding a diuretic or other antihypertensive agent, dosage reduction and retitration may be necessary.

Rx	**Hytrin** (Abbott)	**Tablets:** 1 mg	(DF). White. In 100s, 500s and UD 100s.
		2 mg	(DH). Orange. In 100s, 500s and UD 100s.
		5 mg	(DJ). Tan. In 100s, 500s and UD 100s.
		10 mg	(DI). Green. In 100s and UD 100s.
		Capsules: 1 mg	Parabens. (HH). Gray. In 100s and UD 100s.
		2 mg	Parabens. (HY). Yellow. In 100s and UD 100s.
		5 mg	Parabens. (HK). Red. In 100s and UD 100s.
		10 mg	Parabens. (HN). Blue. In 100s and UD 100s.

Antiadrenergic Agents — Peripherally Acting

DOXAZOSIN MESYLATE

Indications:

Benign prostatic hyperplasia (BPH): For treatment of both urinary outflow obstruction and obstructive and irritative symptoms associated with BPH; obstructive symptoms (hesitation, intermittency, dribbling, weak urinary stream, incomplete emptying of the bladder) and irritative symptoms (nocturia, daytime frequency, urgency, burning. Doxazosin may be used in all BPH patients whether hypertensive or normotensive.

Hypertension: Alone or in combination with other antihypertensive agents such as diuretics, beta blockers, calcium channel blockers or ACE inhibitors.

Administration and Dosage:

Initial dosage for hypertension or BPH is 1 mg once daily in the a.m. or p.m. This starting dose is intended to minimize the frequency of postural hypotension and first dose syncope associated with doxazosin. Postural effects are most likely to occur between 2 and 6 hours after a dose. Therefore, take blood pressure measurements during this time period after the first dose and with each increase in dose. If doxazosin administration is discontinued for several days, restart therapy using the initial dosing regimen.

Hypertension: Individualize dosage.

Initial dosage – 1 mg once daily. Postural effects are most likely to occur between 2 and 6 hours after a dose; therefore take blood pressure measurements during this time period after the first dose and with each increase.

Maintenance dose – Depending on standing blood pressure response, dosage may be increased to 2 mg and thereafter, if necessary, to 4, 8 and 16 mg to achieve the desired reduction in blood pressure. Increases in dose beyond 4 mg increase the likelihood of excessive postural effects (eg, syncope, postural dizziness/vertigo and postural hypotension). At a titrated dose of 16 mg once daily the frequency of postural effects is about 12% compared to 3% for placebo.

BPH:

Initial dosage – The initial dosage is 1 mg given once daily.

Maintenance dose – Depending on the urodynamics and BPH symptomatology, dosage may then be increased to 2 mg and thereafter to 4 and 8 mg once daily, the maximum recommended dose for BPH. The recommended titration interval is 1 to 2 weeks. Evaluate blood pressure routinely.

Rx	**Cardura** (Roerig)	**Tablets:** 1 mg	White. In 100s.
		2 mg	Yellow. In 100s.
		4 mg	Orange. In 100s.
		8 mg	Green. In 100s.

Vasodilators

HYDRALAZINE HCl

For complete prescribing information, refer to the Antihypertensives Introduction.

Actions:

Pharmacology: Hydralazine exerts a peripheral vasodilating effect through a direct relaxation of vascular smooth muscle. Hydralazine, by altering cellular calcium metabolism, interferes with the calcium movements within the vascular smooth muscle that are responsible for initiating or maintaining the contractile state.

The peripheral vasodilating effect of hydralazine results in decreased arterial blood pressure (diastolic more than systolic); decreased peripheral vascular resistance; and an increased heart rate, stroke volume and cardiac output. The preferential dilation of arterioles, as compared to veins, minimizes postural hypotension and promotes the increase in cardiac output. Hydralazine usually increases the renin activity in plasma, presumably as a result of increased secretion of renin by the renal juxtaglomerular cells in response to reflex sympathetic discharge. This increase in renin activity leads to the production of angiotensin II, which then causes stimulation of aldosterone and consequent sodium reabsorption. The drug also maintains or increases renal and cerebral blood flow. Because of the reflex increases in cardiac function, hydralazine is commonly used in combination with a drug which inhibits sympathetic activity (ie, beta blockers, clonidine, methyldopa).

Pharmacokinetics: Hydralazine is rapidly absorbed after oral use. Half-life is 3 to 7 hours. Protein binding is 87%, and bioavailability is 30% to 50%. Plasma levels vary widely among individuals. Peak plasma concentrations occur 1 to 2 hours after ingestion; duration of action is 6 to 12 hours. Hypotensive effects are seen 10 to 20 minutes after parenteral use and last 2 to 4 hours. Hydralazine is subject to polymorphic acetylation; slow acetylators generally have higher plasma levels of hydralazine and require lower doses to maintain control of blood pressure. Hydralazine undergoes extensive hepatic metabolism; it is excreted in the urine as active drug (12% to 14%) and metabolites.

Indications:

Oral: Essential hypertension, alone or in combination with other agents.

Parenteral: Severe essential hypertension when the drug cannot be given orally or when the need to lower blood pressure is urgent.

Unlabeled uses: Hydralazine in doses up to 800 mg 3 times daily has been effective in reducing afterload in the treatment of congestive heart failure (CHF), severe aortic insufficiency and after valve replacement.

Contraindications:

Hypersensitivity to hydralazine; coronary artery disease; mitral valvular rheumatic heart disease.

Warnings:

Lupus erythematosus: Hydralazine may produce a clinical picture simulating systemic lupus erythematosus (eg, arthralgia, dermatoses, fever, splenomegaly) including glomerulonephritis. Symptoms usually regress when the drug is discontinued, but residual effects have been detected years later. Long-term treatment with steroids may be necessary. Lupus occurs more frequently in "slow acetylators". The syndrome usually occurs after at least 6 months of continuous therapy. Although hydralazine-induced lupus may develop in patients on low doses, the likelihood increases with larger doses and with long duration of therapy. In one study, hydralazine use for 3 years duration resulted in drug-induced lupus in 5.4% of patients on 100 mg/day, 10.4% on 200 mg/day, and no patients on 50 mg/day. It is also more common in women and Caucasians vs men and Blacks, respectively.

Perform complete blood counts and antinuclear antibody (ANA) titer determinations before and during prolonged therapy, even in the asymptomatic patient. These studies are also indicated if the patient develops arthralgia, fever, chest pain, continued malaise or other unexplained signs or symptoms. If the ANA titer reaction is positive, carefully weigh benefits to be derived from hydralazine.

Renal function impairment: In hypertensive patients with normal kidneys who are treated with hydralazine, there is evidence of increased renal blood flow and a maintenance of glomerular filtration rate. Renal function may improve where control values were below normal prior to administration. Use with caution in patients with advanced renal damage.

Vasodilators

HYDRALAZINE HCl

Pregnancy: Category C. Studies in mice indicate that high doses of hydralazine are teratogenic (cleft palate and facial and cranial bone malformations). There are no adequate and well controlled studies in pregnant women. Safety for use during pregnancy has not been established. Use only when the potential benefits outweigh potential hazards to the fetus.

Thrombocytopenia, leukopenia, petechial bleeding and hematomas have been reported in newborns of females taking hydralazine. Symptoms resolved spontaneously within 1 to 3 weeks.

Lactation: Hydralazine is excreted in breast milk. Exercise caution when administering to a nursing woman. Hydralazine is compatible with breastfeeding according to the American Academy of Pediatrics.

Children: Safety and efficacy for use in children have not been established in controlled clinical trials, although there is experience with use in children (see Administration and Dosage).

Precautions:

Cardiovascular: The "hyperdynamic" circulation caused by hydralazine may accentuate specific cardiovascular inadequacies (eg, increased pulmonary artery pressure in patients with mitral valvular disease). It may reduce the pressor responses to epinephrine. Postural hypotension may result from hydralazine but is less common than with ganglionic blocking agents. Use with caution in patients with cerebral vascular accidents.

Coronary artery disease – Myocardial stimulation produced by hydralazine can cause anginal attacks and ECG changes of myocardial ischemia. The drug has been implicated in the production of myocardial infarction. Use with caution in patients with suspected coronary artery disease.

Pulmonary hypertension – Use hydralazine with caution in patients with pulmonary hypertension. Severe hypotension may result. Monitor carefully.

Lipids – Hydralazine may cause some decrease in total cholesterol.

Peripheral neuritis evidenced by paresthesias, numbness and tingling, has been observed. Evidence suggests an antipyridoxine effect; add pyridoxine to the regimen if symptoms develop.

Hematologic effects: Blood dyscrasias consisting of reduction in hemoglobin and red cell count, leukopenia, agranulocytosis and purpura have been reported. If such abnormalities develop, discontinue therapy. Periodic blood counts are advised.

Tartrazine sensitivity: Some of these products contain tartrazine, which may cause allergic-type reactions (including bronchial asthma) in susceptible individuals. Although the incidence of tartrazine sensitivity in the general population is low, it is frequently seen in patients who also have aspirin hypersensitivity. Specific products containing tartrazine are identified in the product listings.

Drug Interactions:

Hydralazine Drug Interactions

Precipitant drug	Object drug*		Description
Beta blockers Metoprolol Propranolol	Hydralazine	↑	Serum levels of either drug may be increased by concurrent use.
Hydralazine	Beta blockers Metoprolol Propranolol	↑	
Indomethacin	Hydralazine	↓	The pharmacologic effects of hydralazine may be decreased.

* ↑ = Object drug increased. ↓ = Object drug decreased.

Drug/Food interactions: Administration with food results in higher plasma hydralazine levels.

Vasodilators

HYDRALAZINE HCl

Adverse Reactions:

Adverse reactions with hydralazine are usually reversible when dosage is reduced. However, it may be necessary to discontinue the drug.

Body as a whole: Headache; anorexia; nausea; vomiting; diarrhea; palpitations; tachycardia; angina pectoris. The incidence of toxic reactions, particularly the LE cell syndrome, is high in the group of patients receiving large doses of hydralazine. (See Warnings.)

Ophthalmic: Lacrimation; conjunctivitis.

CNS: Peripheral neuritis evidenced by paresthesia, numbness and tingling (see Precautions); dizziness; tremors; psychotic reactions characterized by depression, disorientation or anxiety.

Hypersensitivity: Rash; urticaria; pruritus; fever; chills; arthralgia; eosinophilia; hepatitis (rare).

GI: Constipation; paralytic ileus.

Hematologic: Blood dyscrasias, consisting of reduction in hemoglobin and RBC, leukopenia, agranulocytosis and purpura (see Precautions); lymphadenopathy; splenomegaly.

Miscellaneous: Nasal congestion; flushing; edema; muscle cramps; hypotension; paradoxical pressor response; dyspnea; urination difficulty; lupus-like syndrome (see Warnings); hoarseness due to drug-induced lupus.

Overdosage:

No deaths due to acute poisoning have been reported. Highest known dose survived in adults is 10 g orally.

Symptoms: Hypotension, tachycardia, headache and generalized skin flushing. Complications can include myocardial ischemia and subsequent myocardial infarction, cardiac arrhythmias and profound shock.

Treatment: There is no specific antidote. Evacuate gastric contents, prevent aspiration and protect the airway; instill activated charcoal slurry, if possible. These manipulations may have to be omitted or carried out after cardiovascular status has been stabilized, since they might precipitate cardiac arrhythmias or increase the depth of shock.

Cardiovascular support is of primary importance. Treat shock with volume expanders without vasopressors. If necessary, use a vasopressor that is least likely to precipitate or aggravate cardiac arrhythmias. Tachycardia responds to beta blockers. Digitalization may be necessary. Monitor renal function and support as required.

No experience has been reported with extracorporeal or peritoneal dialysis.

Patient Information:

Take with meals.

Notify physician of any unexplained prolonged general tiredness or fever, muscle or joint aching or chest pain.

Administration and Dosage:

The bioavailability of hydralazine tablets is enhanced by the concurrent ingestion of food.

Initiate therapy in gradually increasing dosages; individualize dosage. Start with 10 mg 4 times daily for the first 2 to 4 days, increase to 25 mg 4 times daily for the balance of the first week.

Second and subsequent weeks: Increase dosage to 50 mg 4 times daily.

Maintenance: Adjust dosage to lowest effective level. Twice daily dosage may be adequate. In a few resistant patients, up to 300 mg/day may be required for a significant antihypertensive effect. In such cases, consider a lower dosage of hydralazine combined with a thiazide and/or reserpine or a beta blocker. However, when combining therapy, individual titration is essential to ensure the lowest possible therapeutic dose of each drug.

Children – Initial: 0.75 mg/kg/day in 4 divided doses. Dosage may be increased gradually over the next 3 to 4 weeks to a maximum of 7.5 mg/kg or 200 mg daily.

Vasodilators

HYDRALAZINE HCl

Parenteral: Therapy in the hospitalized patient may be initiated IV or IM. Use parenterally only when the drug cannot be given orally. Usual dose is 20 to 40 mg, repeated as necessary. Certain patients (especially those with marked renal damage) may require a lower dose. Check blood pressure frequently; it may begin to fall within a few minutes after injection; average maximal decrease occurs in 10 to 80 minutes. Where there is a previously existing increased intracranial pressure, lowering the blood pressure may increase cerebral ischemia. Most patients can transfer to the oral form in 24 to 48 hrs.

Children – 0.1 to 0.2 mg/kg/dose every 4 to 6 hours as needed.

Eclampsia – Hydralazine is the drug of choice. A dose of 5 to 10 mg every 20 minutes as an IV bolus has been recommended. If there is no effect after 20 mg, try another agent.

Stability: Use hydralazine injection as quickly as possible after drawing through a needle into a syringe. Hydralazine changes color after contact with a metal filter.

Rx	**Hydralazine** (Various, eg, Camall, Goldline, Major, Rugby, Schein)	**Tablets:** 10 mg	In 100s, 1000s and UD 100s.
Rx	**Apresoline** (Ciba)		Lactose. (Ciba 37). Yellow. In 100s and 1200s.
Rx	**Hydralazine** (Various, eg, Camall, Goldline, Major, Rugby)	**Tablets:** 25 mg	In 100s, 1000s and UD 100s.
Rx	**Apresoline** (Ciba)		(Ciba 39). Blue. In 100s and 1000s.
Rx	**Hydralazine** (Various, eg, Camall, Goldline, Major, Rugby)	**Tablets:** 50 mg	In 100s, 1000s and UD 100s.
Rx	**Apresoline** (Ciba)		Lactose. (Ciba 73). Light blue. In 100s and 1000s.
Rx	**Hydralazine** (Various, eg, Camall, Goldline, Major, Rugby)	**Tablets:** 100 mg	In 100s and 1000s.
Rx	**Apresoline** (Ciba)		Tartrazine. (Ciba 101). Peach. In 100s.
Rx	**Hydralazine** (Solopak)	**Injection:** 20 mg per ml	In 1 ml vials.
Rx	**Apresoline**[1] (Ciba)		In 1 ml amps and vials.

[1] Recently discontinued by manufacturer; however, remaining supply provided for *emergency use only* (ie, *life-threatening* situations where no other therapy is available). Call 1–800–742–2422. Approval of an injectable lyophilized formulation is pending.

Vasodilators

MINOXIDIL

Refer to the Antihypertensives Introduction for a general discussion of these products.

Warning:

Minoxidil may produce serious adverse effects. It can cause pericardial effusion, occasionally progressing to tamponade, and it can exacerbate angina pectoris. Reserve for hypertensive patients who do not respond adequately to maximum therapeutic doses of a diuretic and two other antihypertensive agents.

In experimental animals, minoxidil caused several kinds of myocardial lesions and other adverse cardiac effects (see Warnings).

Administer under close supervision, usually concomitantly with a beta-adrenergic blocking agent, to prevent tachycardia and increased myocardial workload. Usually, it must be given with a diuretic, frequently one acting in the ascending limb of the loop of Henle, to prevent serious fluid accumulation. When first administering minoxidil, hospitalize and monitor patients with malignant hypertension and those already receiving guanethidine (see Drug Interactions) to avoid too rapid or large orthostatic decreases in blood pressure.

Actions:

Pharmacology: Minoxidil is a direct-acting peripheral vasodilator. The exact mechanism of action on the vascular smooth muscle is unknown. It does not interfere with vasomotor reflexes, therefore, it does not produce orthostatic hypotension. The drug does not affect CNS function in man. It appears to block calcium uptake through the cell membrane.

Antihypertensive effects – Minoxidil reduces elevated systolic and diastolic blood pressure by decreasing peripheral vascular resistance. The blood pressure response to minoxidil is dose-related and proportional to the extent of hypertension. In humans, forearm and renal vascular resistance decline; forearm blood flow increases while renal blood flow and glomerular filtration rate (GFR) are preserved.

When used in severely hypertensive patients resistant to other therapy, frequently with an accompanying diuretic and β-adrenergic blocker, minoxidil decreased the blood pressure and reversed encephalopathy and retinopathy. The drug reduced supine diastolic blood pressure by 20 mm Hg, or to $\leq$ 90 mm Hg in $\approx$75% of the patients studied.

Hemodynamics – Because it causes peripheral vasodilation, minoxidil elicits a reduction of peripheral arteriolar resistance. This action, with the associated fall in blood pressure, triggers sympathetic, vagal inhibitory and renal homeostatic mechanisms, including an increase in renin secretion, that leads to increased cardiac rate and output, and salt and water retention. These adverse effects can usually be minimized by coadministration of a diuretic and a β-adrenergic blocking agent or other sympathetic nervous system suppressant.

Pharmacokinetics:

Absorption/Distribution – Minoxidil is at least 90% absorbed from the GI tract. Plasma levels of the parent drug reach a maximum within the first hour and decline rapidly thereafter. Minoxidil is not protein bound; it concentrates in arteriolar smooth muscle.

Onset/Duration: The extent and time course of blood pressure reduction by minoxidil do not correspond closely to its plasma concentration. After an effective single oral dose, blood pressure usually starts to decline within 30 minutes, reaches a minimum between 2 and 3 hours and recovers at a linear rate of about 30% per day. The total duration of effect is $\approx$ 75 hours.

When minoxidil is administered chronically, once or twice a day, the time required to achieve maximum effect on blood pressure is inversely related to the size of the dose. Thus, maximum effect is achieved on 10 mg/day within 7 days, on 20 mg/day within 5 days and on 40 mg/day within 3 days.

Metabolism/Excretion – 90% is metabolized, predominantly by conjugation with glucuronic acid. Metabolites exert much less pharmacologic effect than minoxidil itself; all are excreted principally in the urine. Renal clearance corresponds to the GFR. Minoxidil and its metabolites are hemodialyzable. Average plasma half-life is 4.2 hours.

Vasodilators

MINOXIDIL

Indications:

Severe hypertension that is symptomatic or associated with target organ damage, and is not manageable with maximum therapeutic doses of a diuretic plus two other antihypertensives.

Topical minoxidil is used for the treatment of male pattern baldness (alopecia androgenetica) of the vertex of the scalp (see Minoxidil Topical Solution monograph in the Miscellaneous section). Use of the tablets, in any formulation, to promote hair growth is not an approved use. Effects of extemporaneous formulations and dosages have not been shown to be safe and effective.

Contraindications:

Hypersensitivity to any component of the product; pheochromocytoma (because the drug may stimulate secretion of catecholamines from the tumor through its antihypertensive action); acute myocardial infarction; dissecting aortic aneurysm.

Warnings:

Mild hypertension: Due to potential for serious adverse effects, use in milder degrees of hypertension is not recommended; benefit-risk relationship in such patients is not defined.

Cardiac lesions:

Animal toxicology – Minoxidil has produced cardiac lesions in nonprimate species, including grossly visible hemorrhagic lesions of the atrium, epicardium, endocardium and walls of small arteries and arterioles; necrosis of papillary muscles and subendocardial areas of left ventricle. Cardiac hypertrophy and dilation occurred but was partly reversed by diuretics in monkeys, suggesting increased heart weight may be related to fluid overload. In a 1 year dog study serosanguinous pericardial fluid was noted.

Human toxicology – Autopsies of 150 patients who died from various causes and who had received minoxidil did not reveal right atrial or other hemorrhagic pathology of the kind seen in dogs. Instances of necrotic areas in papillary muscles were seen, but occurred in the presence of known preexisting ischemic heart disease and did not appear different from or more common than lesions in patients never exposed to minoxidil.

ECG changes: Rarely, a large negative amplitude of the T wave may encroach upon the ST segment, but the ST segment is not independently altered. These changes usually disappear with continuance of treatment and revert to the pretreatment state if therapy is discontinued. No symptoms, alterations in blood cell counts or plasma enzyme concentrations, or signs of myocardial damage have been noted. Long-term treatment of patients manifesting such changes has provided no evidence of deteriorating cardiac function. At present, the changes appear to be nonspecific and without identifiable clinical significance.

Fluid and electrolyte balance: Monitor fluid and electrolyte balance and body weight. Give with a diuretic to prevent fluid retention and possible CHF; a loop diuretic is usually required. If used without a diuretic, retention of several hundred mEq salt and corresponding volumes of water can occur in a few days, leading to increased plasma and interstitial fluid volume and local or generalized edema. Diuretics alone, or with restricted salt intake, usually minimize fluid retention, but reversible edema developed in ≈ 10% of nondialysis patients so treated. Ascites has also occurred. Diuretic effectiveness is limited by impaired renal function. Condition of patients with preexisting CHF occasionally deteriorates due to fluid retention, but because of the fall in blood pressure (afterload reduction), more than twice as many improve than worsen.

Refractory fluid retention rarely may require discontinuation of minoxidil. Under close medical supervision, it may be possible to resolve refractory salt retention by discontinuing the drug for 1 or 2 days, and then resuming treatment in conjunction with vigorous diuretic therapy.

Tachycardia: Minoxidil increases heart rate; this can be prevented by concomitant administration of a β-adrenergic blocking drug or other sympathetic nervous system suppressants (eg, clonidine, methyldopa). The ability of β-adrenergic blocking agents to minimize papillary muscle lesions in animals is further reason for such concomitant use.

In addition, angina may worsen or appear for the first time during treatment, probably because of the increased oxygen demands associated with increased heart rate and cardiac output. This can usually be prevented by sympathetic blockade.

MINOXIDIL

Pericardial effusion, occasionally with tamponade, has occurred in about 3% of treated patients not on dialysis, especially those with inadequate or compromised renal function. Many cases were associated with connective tissue disease, the uremic syndrome, CHF or fluid retention, but were instances in which these potential causes of effusion were not present. Observe patients closely for signs of pericardial disorder. Perform echocardiographic studies if suspicion arises. More vigorous diuretic therapy, dialysis, pericardiocentesis or surgery may be required. If the effusion persists, consider drug withdrawal.

Hazard of rapid control of blood pressure: In patients with very severe blood pressure elevation, too rapid control of blood pressure can precipitate syncope, cerebrovascular accidents, MI and ischemia of special sense organs with resulting decrease or loss of vision or hearing. Patients with compromised circulation or cryoglobulinemia may also suffer ischemic episodes of affected organs. Although such events have not been unequivocally associated with minoxidil use, experience is limited.

Hospitalize any patient with malignant hypertension during initial treatment to assure that blood pressure is not falling more rapidly than intended.

Hypersensitivity manifested as a skin rash occurs in < 1% of patients; whether the drug should be discontinued depends on treatment alternatives.

Renal function impairment: Renal failure or dialysis patients may require smaller doses; closely supervise to prevent cardiac failure or exacerbation of renal failure.

Fertility impairment: In rats given one or five times the maximum recommended human dose, there was a dose-dependent reduction in conception rate.

Pregnancy: Category C. Minoxidil reduced conception rate and increased fetal absorption in small animals when administered at 5 times the human dose. There are no adequate and well controlled studies in pregnant women. Use only when clearly needed and when potential benefits outweigh potential hazards to the fetus.

Lactation: Safety for use in the nursing mother has not been established. Minoxidil is excreted in breast milk; do not nurse while taking minoxidil.

Children: Use in children is limited, particularly in infants. The recommendations under Administration and Dosage are only a rough guide; careful titration is essential.

Precautions:

Myocardial infarction: Minoxidil has not been used in patients who have had an MI within the preceding month. A reduction in arterial pressure with the drug might further limit blood flow to the myocardium, although this might be compensated by decreased oxygen demand because of lower blood pressure.

Hypertrichosis: Elongation, thickening and enhanced pigmentation of fine body hair develops within 3 to 6 weeks after starting therapy in approximately 80% of patients. It is usually first noticed on the temples, between the eyebrows, between the hairline and the eyebrows or in the sideburn area of the upper lateral cheek, later extending to the back, arms, legs and scalp. Upon discontinuation of the drug, new hair growth stops, but 1 to 6 months may be required for restoration to pretreatment appearance.

No endocrine abnormalities have been found to explain the abnormal hair growth; thus, it is hypertrichosis without virilism. Inform patients (especially children and women) about this effect before therapy is begun.

Laboratory tests: Repeat tests that are abnormal at initiation of minoxidil therapy (eg, urinalysis, renal function tests, ECG, chest x-ray, echocardiogram) to ascertain whether improvement or deterioration is occurring under therapy. Initially, perform such tests frequently, at 1 to 3 month intervals, and as stabilization occurs, at 6 to 12 month intervals.

Drug Interactions:

Guanethidine: Although minoxidil does not cause orthostatic hypotension, use in patients on guanethidine can result in profound orthostatic effects. If possible, discontinue guanethidine well before minoxidil is instituted. If this is not possible, start minoxidil in the hospital and institutionalize the patient until severe orthostatic effects are no longer present or the patient has learned to avoid activities that provoke them.

MINOXIDIL

Adverse Reactions:

Hypersensitivity: Rashes including bullous eruptions (rare) and Stevens-Johnson syndrome. See Warnings.

Cardiovascular: Pericardial effusion and tamponade (see Warnings). Changes in direction and magnitude of T waves occur (60%) (see Warnings).

Rebound hypertension following gradual withdrawal has occurred in children.

Hematologic: Initially, hematocrit, hemoglobin and erythrocyte count usually fall about 7%, and then recover to pretreatment levels. Thrombocytopenia and leukopenia (WBC < $3000/mm^3$) have been reported rarely.

GI: Nausea; vomiting.

Body as a whole: Temporary edema (7%); breast tenderness (< 1%); fatigue, headache, darkening of the skin.

Hypertrichosis – Elongation, thickening and enhanced pigmentation of fine body hair develops within 3 to 6 weeks after starting therapy in approximately 80% of patients (see Precautions).

Lab test abnormalities: Alkaline phosphatase increased varyingly without other evidence of liver or bone abnormality. Serum creatinine increased an average of 6% and BUN slightly more, but later declined to pretreatment levels.

Overdosage:

Symptoms: Exaggerated hypotension is likely in association with residual sympathetic nervous system blockade from previous therapy (guanethidine-like effects or alpha-adrenergic blockade), which prevents compensatory maintenance of blood pressure.

Treatment: Administer normal saline IV to maintain blood pressure and facilitate urine formation. Avoid sympathomimetics (eg, norepinephrine, epinephrine) with excessive cardiac stimulating action. Phenylephrine, angiotensin II, vasopressin and dopamine reverse hypotension due to minoxidil, but use only in underperfusion of a vital organ.

Radioimmunoassay can determine plasma concentration. However, due to blood level variations, it is difficult to establish a warning level. At 100 mg/day, peak blood levels of 1641 and 2441 ng/ml were seen in two patients, respectively. Regard an increase > 2000 ng/ml as overdosage, unless the patient has taken no more than the maximum dose.

Patient Information:

Patient package insert is available with product.

Minoxidil is usually taken with at least two other antihypertensive medications. Take all medications as prescribed; do not discontinue any except on advice of physician.

Enhanced growth and darkening of fine body hair (≈ 80% of patients) may occur; however, do not stop medication without consulting physician.

Notify physician if any of the following occur: Heart rate of ≥ 20 bpm over normal; rapid weight gain of > 5 pounds (2.3 kg); unusual swelling of extremities, face or abdomen; breathing difficulty, especially when lying down; new or aggravated angina symptoms (chest, arm or shoulder pain); severe indigestion; dizziness, lightheadedness or fainting.

Nausea or vomiting may occur.

Administration and Dosage:

Adults and children (≥ 12 years of age): Initial dosage is 5 mg/day as a single dose. Daily dosage can be increased to 10, 20, then 40 mg in single or divided doses if required. Effective range is usually 10 to 40 mg/day. Maximum dosage is 100 mg/day.

Children: Initial dosage is 0.2 mg/kg/day as a single dose. Dose may be increased in 50% to 100% increments until optimum blood pressure control is achieved. Effective range is usually 0.25 to 1 mg/kg/day. Maximum dosage is 50 mg daily. Experience in children is limited; monitor closely; titrate carefully for optimal effects.

Dose frequency: The magnitude of within-day fluctuation of arterial pressure during therapy is directly proportional to the extent of pressure reduction. If supine diastolic pressure has been reduced < 30 mm Hg, administer the drug only once a day; if reduced > 30 mm Hg, divide the daily dosage into 2 equal parts.

Vasodilators

MINOXIDIL

Dosage adjustment intervals, which must be carefully titrated, should be at least 3 days because the full response to a given dose is not obtained until then. If more rapid management is required, adjustments can be made every 6 hours with careful monitoring.

Concomitant drug therapy:

Diuretics – Use minoxidil with a diuretic in patients relying on renal function for maintaining salt and water balance. Diuretics have been used at the following dosages when starting therapy with minoxidil: Hydrochlorothiazide (50 mg twice daily) or other thiazides at equally effective doses; chlorthalidone (50 to 100 mg once daily); furosemide (40 mg twice daily). If excessive salt and water retention results in a weight gain > 2.3 kg (5 lb), change diuretic therapy to furosemide. In furosemide-treated patients, increase dosage in accordance with their requirements.

Beta-blockers or other sympathetic nervous system suppressants – When therapy is begun, the β-blocker dosage should be equal to 80 to 160 mg/day propranolol in divided doses. If β-blockers are contraindicated, use methyldopa, 250 to 750 mg twice daily; give for at least 24 hours before starting minoxidil due to delay in onset. Clonidine may also be used; usual dosage is 0.1 to 0.2 mg twice daily.

Sympathetic nervous system suppressants may not completely prevent a heart rate increase, but usually prevent tachycardia. Typically, patients receiving a β-blocker prior to minoxidil have bradycardia; expect an increase in heart rate toward normal when minoxidil is added. Simultaneous treatment with minoxidil and a β-blocker or other sympathetic nervous system suppressant causes little change in heart rate, since their opposing cardiac effects usually nullify each other.

Rx	**Minoxidil** (Various eg, IDE, Major, Schein)	**Tablets**: 2.5 mg	In 100s, 500s and 1000s.
Rx	**Loniten** (Upjohn)		(2.5 mg). White, scored. In 100s.
Rx	**Minoxidil** (Various eg, IDE, Major, Schein)	**Tablets**: 10 mg	In 100s, 500s and 1000s.
Rx	**Loniten** (Upjohn)		(10 mg). White, scored. In 100s and 500s.

Angiotensin Converting Enzyme Inhibitors

ACE INHIBITORS

Warning:

Pregnancy: When used in pregnancy during the second and third trimesters, ACE inhibitors can cause injury and even death to the developing fetus. When pregnancy is detected, discontinue the ACE inhibitor as soon as possible (see Warnings). Refer to the general discussion of these products in the Antihypertensives Introduction.

Actions:

Pharmacology: The angiotensin converting enzyme inhibitors (ACEIs) appear to act primarily through suppression of the renin-angiotensin-aldosterone system; however, no consistent correlation has been described between renin levels and drug response.

Synthesized by the kidneys, renin is released into the circulation where it acts on a plasma globulin substrate to produce angiotensin I, a relatively inactive decapeptide. Angiotensin I is then converted by angiotensin converting enzyme (ACE) to angiotensin II, a potent endogenous vasoconstrictor that also stimulates aldosterone secretion from the adrenal cortex, contributing to sodium and fluid retention. These agents prevent the conversion of angiotensin I to angiotensin II by inhibiting ACE; they do not alter pressor responses to other agents. ACEIs may also inhibit local angiotensin II at vascular and renal sites and attenuate the release of catecholamines from adrenergic nerve endings.

Inhibiting ACE results in decreased plasma angiotensin II and increased plasma renin activity (PRA), the latter resulting from loss of negative feedback on renin release caused by reduction in angiotensin II. This leads to decreased aldosterone secretion, resulting in small increases in serum potassium ($\approx$ 0.2 mEq/L with enalapril, 0.07 mmol/L with quinapril), and sodium and fluid loss.

Increased prostaglandin synthesis may also play a role in the antihypertensive action of captopril. Single doses of captopril increase urinary excretion of prostaglandin E_2 and plasma levels of PGE_2 and $PGE_{2\alpha}$ metabolites. The antihypertensive effects persist longer than does demonstrable inhibition of circulating ACE.

The ACEIs produce a reduction of peripheral arterial resistance in hypertensive patients, and either as no change or an increase in cardiac output. Renal blood flow increases, but glomerular filtration rate (GFR) is usually unchanged.

Peak blood pressure reduction is achieved 1 to 6 hours after dosing. Blood pressure reduction may be progressive. To achieve maximal effects, several weeks of therapy may be required. Blood pressure-lowering effects of ACEIs and thiazide-type diuretics are additive, but captopril and β-blockers have a less than additive effect. Standing and supine blood pressures are lowered to about the same extent. Orthostatic effects and tachycardia are infrequent, but may occur in volume- or salt-depleted patients. Abrupt withdrawal is not associated with a rapid increase in blood pressure.

The ACEIs are antihypertensive even in low-renin hypertensives. They are antihypertensive in all races studied, but black hypertensives (usually low-renin hypertensives) show a smaller average response to monotherapy than non-blacks.

In patients with heart failure, captopril, enalapril and quinapril significantly decrease peripheral resistance, blood pressure (afterload), pulmonary capillary wedge pressure (preload), pulmonary vascular resistance and heart size and increase cardiac output and exercise tolerance time. These effects occur after the first dose and persist for the duration of therapy. Quinapril reduces total peripheral resistance and renal vascular resistance with little or no change in heart rate or cardiac index.

Angiotensin Converting Enzyme Inhibitors

ACE INHIBITORS

Pharmacokinetics:

Pharmacokinetics of ACEIs								
					Half-life		Elimination (24 hr)	
ACEI	Onset/ Duration (hrs)	Protein binding	Effect of food on absorption	Active metabolite	Normal renal function	Impaired renal function	Total	Unchanged
Benazepril	1/24	> 95%	none	benazeprilat	10-11[1] hr	prolonged	nd[2]	trace
Captopril	0.25/ dose-related	25%-30%	reduced		< 2 hr	3.5-32 hr	> 95%	40%-50% in urine
Enalapril	1/24	na[3]	none	enalaprilat	1.3 hr	nd[2]	94% urine and feces	54% in urine (40% enalaprilat)
Enalaprilat	0.25/ ≈6	na[3]	na[4]		11 hr	prolonged	nd[2]	> 90% in urine
Fosinopril	1/24	≈ 95%	none	fosinoprilat	12 hr (fosinoprilat IV)	prolonged	50% urine, 50% feces	negligible
Lisinopril	1/24	na[3]	none		12 hr	prolonged	nd[2]	100% in urine
Moexipril	1/24	≈ 50%	reduced	moexiprilat	2-9 hr (moexiprilat)	prolonged	13% urine, 53% feces	1% in urine, 1% in feces
Quinapril	1/24	≈ 97%	reduced	quinaprilat	2 hr (quinaprilat)	prolonged	≈60% urine, ≈37% feces	trace
Ramipril	1 to 2/24	≈ 73% (ramiprilat 56%)	reduced	ramiprilat	13-17 hr (ramiprilat)	prolonged	60% urine, 40% feces	< 2%

[1] Effective t½ of accumulation of metabolite following multiple dosing.
[2] nd – No data.
[3] na – Not applicable.
[4] na – Not applicable; available IV only.

Indications:

Hypertension: The ACEIs are effective alone and in combination with other antihypertensive agents, especially thiazide-type diuretics. Blood pressure-lowering effects of ACEIs and thiazides are approximately additive.

Captopril may be used as initial therapy in patients with normal renal function in whom risk is relatively low. In patients with impaired renal function, particularly those with collagen vascular disease, reserve captopril for patients who develop unacceptable side effects on other drugs or who do not respond to drug combinations.

Enalaprilat is indicated when oral therapy is not practical.

Heart failure:

Captopril – Treatment of CHF, usually in combination with diuretics and digitalis. The presence of digitalis is not required.

Enalapril – Treatment of symptomatic CHF, usually in combination with diuretics and digitalis. In these patients, enalapril improves symptoms, increases survival and decreases the frequency of hospitalization.

Fosinopril/Lisinopril/Quinapril – Adjunctive therapy in the management of CHF in patients not responding adequately to diuretics and digitalis.

Ramipril – For stable patients who have demonstrated clinical signs of CHF within the first few days after sustaining acute MI. In these patients, ramipril decreases the risk of death (principally cardiovascular death) and decreases the risks of failure-related hospitalization and progression to severe/resistant heart failure.

Myocardial infarction:

Lisinopril – Treatment of hemodynamically stable patients within 24 hours of acute myocardial infarction (MI), to improve survival. Patients should receive, as appropriate, the standard recommended treatments such as thrombolytics, aspirin and beta-blockers.

Angiotensin Converting Enzyme Inhibitors

ACE INHIBITORS

Left ventricular dysfunction (LVD):

Captopril – To improve survival following myocardial infarction (MI) in clinically stable patients with LVD manifested as an ejection fraction ≤ 40% and to reduce the incidence of overt heart failure and subsequent hospitalizations for CHF in these patients.

Enalapril – For clinically stable asymptomatic patients with LVD (ejection fraction ≤ 35%); enalapril decreases the rate of development of overt heart failure and decreases the incidence of hospitalization for CHF.

Diabetic nephropathy:

Captopril – Treatment of diabetic nephropathy (proteinuria > 500 mg/day) in patients with type I insulin-dependent diabetes mellitus and retinopathy. Captopril decreases the rate of progression of renal insufficiency and development of serious adverse clinical outcomes (death or need for renal transplantation or dialysis).

Unlabeled uses:

Captopril – Management of hypertensive crises (25 mg initially, 100 mg 90 to 120 minutes later, 200 to 300 mg/day for 2 to 5 days, then adjusted). Sublingual captopril 25 mg has also been used effectively.

Neonatal and childhood hypertension. For neonates, the use of a solution of captopril in water (used immediately) is effective.

Rheumatoid arthritis (75 to 150 mg/day in divided doses).

Diagnosis of anatomic renal artery stenosis ("captopril test").

Hypertension related to scleroderma renal crisis.

Diagnosis of primary aldosteronism.

Idiopathic edema.

Bartter's syndrome (improves potassium metabolism and corrects hypokalemia).

Raynaud's syndrome (symptomatic relief).

Hypertension of Takayasu's disease.

Enalapril – Diabetic nephropathy (reduction of proteinuria, albuminuria and glomerular hypertension). See Warnings.

Childhood hypertension and hypertension related to scleroderma renal crisis.

Enalaprilat – May be used for hypertensive emergencies (1.25 to 5 mg every 6 hours), but the effects are often variable.

Contraindications:

Hypersensitivity to these products (eg, patients with a history of angioedema related to previous treatment with an ACEI).

Warnings:

Neutropenia/Agranulocytosis: Neutropenia (< 1000/mm^3) with myeloid hypoplasia resulted from use of captopril. About half of the neutropenic patients developed systemic or oral cavity infections or other features of agranulocytosis. The risk of neutropenia is dependent on the patient's clinical status.

In hypertension with normal renal function (serum creatinine < 1.6 mg/dl, no collagen vascular disease), neutropenia occurred in one patient of > 8600 exposed.

In patients with some degree of renal failure (serum creatinine ≥ 1.6 mg/dl) but no collagen vascular disease, the risk of neutropenia was about 1 in 500. Daily doses of captopril were relatively high. Concomitant allopurinol and captopril have been associated with neutropenia (see Drug Interactions).

In collagen vascular diseases (eg, systemic lupus erythematosus, scleroderma) and impaired renal function, neutropenia has occurred in 3.7% of patients.

In heart failure, the same risk factors for neutropenia appear present; ≈ ½ of cases had serum creatinine ≥ 1.6 mg/dl, and > 75% were also on procainamide.

Neutropenia has been detected within 3 months after captopril initiation. Bone marrow examinations consistently showed myeloid hypoplasia, frequently accompanied by erythroid hypoplasia and decreased numbers of megakaryocytes (eg, hypoplastic bone marrow and pancytopenia); anemia and thrombocytopenia were sometimes seen.

In general, neutrophils returned to normal ≈ 2 weeks after captopril was discontinued; serious infections were limited to clinically complex patients. About 13% of neutropenia cases were fatal, but almost all were in patients with serious illness having collagen vascular disease, renal failure, heart failure, immunosuppressant therapy or a combination of these factors.

Discontinuation of captopril has generally led to prompt return of the normal WBC count; upon confirmation of neutropenia, withdraw the drug and closely observe the patient.

ACE INHIBITORS

Neutropenia/agranulocytosis has occurred rarely with enalapril or lisinopril and in one patient on quinapril; a causal relationship cannot be excluded. Data are insufficient to show that moexipril, ramipril, quinapril or fosinopril do not cause agranulocytosis at similar rates. Periodically monitor WBC counts.

Anaphylactoid and possibly related reactions: Presumably because ACEIs affect the metabolism of eicosanoids and polypeptides, including endogenous bradykinin, patients receiving ACEIs may be subject to a variety of adverse reactions, some of them serious.

Angioedema has occurred in patients treated with ACEIs. It may occur at any time during treatment, especially following the first dose of enalapril (0.2%), captopril, lisinopril or quinapril (0.1%) or moexipril (< 0.5%). Angioedema of face, extremities, lips, mucous membranes, tongue, glottis or larynx has occurred. In instances where swelling has been confined to the face and lips, the condition has generally resolved without treatment, although antihistamines have been useful in relieving symptoms (enalaprilat). Angioedema associated with laryngeal edema may be fatal. If laryngeal stridor or angioedema of the face, tongue, larynx or glottis occurs and appears likely to cause airway obstruction, discontinue treatment and institute appropriate therapy (eg, epinephrine solution 1:1000 SC) immediately. Use with extreme caution in patients with hereditary angioedema (caused by a deficiency of C1 esterase inhibitor). Patients with a history of angioedema unrelated to ACEI therapy may be at increased risk of angioedema while receiving an ACEI.

Anaphylactoid reactions during desensitization – Two patients undergoing desensitizing treatment with hymenoptera venom while receiving ACEIs sustained life-threatening anaphylactoid reactions. In the same patients, these reactions were avoided when ACEIs were temporarily withheld, but they reappeared upon inadvertent rechallenge.

Anaphylactoid reactions during membrane exposure – Anaphylactoid reactions have been reported in patients dialyzed with high-flux membranes and treated concomitantly with an ACEI. Consider a different type of dialysis membrane or a different class of medication.

Proteinuria: Total urinary proteins > 1 g/day were seen in 0.7% of captopril patients. Nephrotic syndrome occurred in about 20% of these cases. About 90% of affected patients showed evidence of prior renal disease or received relatively high doses of captopril (> 150 mg/day) or both. In most cases, proteinuria cleared within 6 months, regardless of whether captopril was continued. Creatinine and BUN were seldom altered.

Since most cases of proteinuria occur by the eighth month of therapy, estimate urinary protein (dip-stick on first morning urine) prior to therapy and periodically thereafter. However, in patients with diabetic nephropathy, captopril improves renal hemodynamics and associated proteinuria.

Hypotension:

First-dose effect – ACEIs may cause a profound fall in blood pressure following the first dose. Excessive hypotension is rare in hypertensive patients, but is possible with ACEI use in severely salt/volume depleted persons (eg, those treated vigorously with diuretics or patients on dialysis) and in those with CHF; it may be associated with oliguria, progressive azotemia, and rarely with acute renal failure and death. Excessive perspiration, dehydration, vomiting or diarrhea may lead to an excessive fall in blood pressure because of reduction in fluid volume.

In heart failure, where the blood pressure was either normal or low, transient decreases in mean blood pressure > 20% occurred in about half of the patients. Transient hypotension may occur after the first several doses. This effect is usually well tolerated, is asymptomatic or produces brief, mild lightheadedness, although it has been associated with arrhythmia or conduction defects. Hypotension forced drug discontinuation in 3.6% of patients with heart failure.

Start therapy under close medical supervision. Follow patients closely for the first 2 weeks and whenever the dose of ACEI or diuretic is increased. Apply similar considerations to patients with ischemic heart or cerebrovascular disease in whom an excessive fall in blood pressure could result in myocardial infarction or cerebrovascular accident.

Minimize the possibility of hypotension either by discontinuing the diuretic or increasing salt intake approximately 1 week prior to initiating ACEIs, or initiate with small doses. Alternatively, provide medical supervision for at least 2 hours after the initial dose and until blood pressure has stabilized for at least an additional hour.

ACE INHIBITORS

Hypotension is not a reason to discontinue the ACEI. Some decrease in systemic blood pressure is common and desirable in heart failure. The magnitude of the decrease is greatest early in treatment, stabilizes within 1 to 2 weeks, and generally returns to pretreatment levels without a decrease in efficacy within 2 months.

A transient hypotensive response is not a contraindication for further doses of these agents, which usually can be given without difficulty once the blood pressure has stabilized. If excessive hypotension occurs, place patient in supine position and, if necessary, give IV normal saline. A dose reduction or discontinuation of the ACEI or concomitant diuretic may be necessary.

Renal function impairment: Some hypertensive patients with renal disease, particularly those with severe renal artery stenosis, have developed increases in BUN and serum creatinine after reduction of blood pressure (20% of patients with enalapril). Monitor renal function in such patients during the first few weeks of therapy. Dosage reduction or discontinuation of the diuretic may be required. For some patients, it may not be possible to normalize blood pressure and maintain adequate renal perfusion.

About 20% of heart failure patients develop stable elevations of BUN and serum creatinine > 20% above normal or baseline with long-term captopril. Less than 5% of patients, generally those with severe preexisting renal disease, require treatment discontinuation; subsequent improvement probably relies on the severity of underlying renal disease.

In patients with severe CHF whose renal function may depend on the activity of the renin-angiotensin-aldosterone system, treatment with ACEIs may be associated with oliguria or progressive azotemia and, rarely, with acute renal failure or death.

Some hypertensive patients with no apparent preexisting renal vascular disease have developed increases in BUN and serum creatinine; these are usually minor and transient, especially when enalapril, lisinopril or ramipril was given with a diuretic. Dosage reduction of enalapril, lisinopril or ramipril, or discontinuation of the diuretic may be required. However, to confuse the situation, captopril and enalapril have shown renal protective effects in hypertensive patients with some renal dysfunction.

Impaired renal function decreases lisinopril elimination, which is excreted principally through the kidneys, but this decrease becomes clinically important only when the glomerular filtration rate is < 30 ml/min. The elimination half-life of quinaprilat increases as Ccr decreases. Dosage adjustment may be necessary for quinapril, benazepril, ramipril and lisinopril. Impaired renal function decreases total clearance of fosinoprilat and approximately doubles the area under the plasma concentration-time curve (AUC). In general, however, no dosing adjustment is needed.

Hepatic function impairment: Since ramipril and fosinopril are primarily metabolized to their active metabolites, patients with impaired liver function could develop markedly elevated plasma levels of unchanged fosinopril or ramipril. No formal kinetic studies with ramipril have been done in hypertensive patients with impaired liver function. In patients with alcoholic or biliary cirrhosis, the rate, but not extent, of fosinopril hydrolysis was reduced; the total body clearance of fosinoprilat was decreased and AUC approximately doubled. Quinaprilat concentrations are reduced in patients with alcoholic cirrhosis due to impaired deesterification of quinapril.

Hepatic failure – Rarely ACEIs have been associated with a syndrome that starts with cholestatic jaundice and progresses to fulminant hepatic necrosis and (sometimes) death. The mechanism of this syndrome is not understood. Patients receiving ACEIs who develop jaundice or marked elevations of hepatic enzymes should discontinue the ACEI and receive appropriate medical follow-up.

Elderly: Elderly patients may have higher lisinopril blood levels and AUC, and higher peak ramiprilat and quinaprilat levels and AUC than younger patients. This may relate to decreased renal function rather than to age itself. No overall differences in effectiveness or safety were observed between elderly patients receiving fosinopril, moexipril or benazepril and younger patients; however, greater sensitivity of some older individuals cannot be ruled out.

Pregnancy: Category C (first trimester); Category D (second and third trimesters). ACEIs can cause fetal and neonatal morbidity and death when administered to pregnant women. Several dozen cases have been reported in the world literature. When pregnancy is detected, discontinue ACEIs as soon as possible.

ACE INHIBITORS

The use of ACEIs during the second and third trimesters of pregnancy has been associated with fetal and neonatal injury, including hypotension, neonatal skull hypoplasia, anuria, reversible or irreversible renal failure and death. Oligohydramnios has also occurred, presumably resulting from decreased fetal renal function; oligohydramnios in this setting has been associated with fetal limb contractures, craniofacial deformation, and hypoplastic lung development. Prematurity, intrauterine growth retardation and patent ductus arteriosus have also been reported, although it is not clear whether these occurrences were due to the ACEI exposure.

These adverse effects do not appear to have resulted from intrauterine ACEI exposure that has been limited to the first trimester. Mothers whose embryos and fetuses are exposed to ACEIs only during the first trimester should be so informed. Nonetheless, when patients become pregnant, physicians should make every effort to discontinue the use of the ACEI as soon as possible.

Rarely (probably less often than once in every thousand pregnancies), no alternative to ACEIs will be found. In these rare cases, apprise the mother of the potential hazards to the fetus, and perform serial ultrasound examinations to assess the intra-amniotic environment.

If oligohydramnios is observed, discontinue the ACEI unless it is considered lifesaving for the mother. Contraction stress testing (CST), a non-stress test (NST) or biophysical profiling (BPP) may be appropriate, depending on the week of pregnancy. Patients and physicians should be aware, however, that oligohydramnios may not appear until after the fetus has sustained irreversible injury.

Closely observe infants with histories of in utero exposure to ACEIs for hypotension, oliguria and hyperkalemia. If oliguria occurs, direct attention toward support of blood pressure and renal perfusion. Exchange transfusion or dialysis may be required as a means of reversing hypotension or substituting for disordered renal function. Some of these agents may be removed from neonatal circulation by exchange transfusion or dialysis (see Overdosage); however, limited experience has not shown that such removal is central to the treatment of these infants.

Lactation: Ingestion of 20 mg/day fosinopril resulted in detectable fosinoprilat levels in breast milk; do not administer to nursing mothers. Concentrations of captopril in breast milk are approximately 1% of those in maternal blood. Benazepril, enalapril and enalaprilat are detected in breast milk in trace amounts; a newborn would receive < 0.1% of the mg/kg maternal dose of benazepril and benazeprilat. The effect on the nursing infant has not been determined. Exercise caution when these drugs are administered to nursing women. It is not known whether lisinopril, quinapril, moexipril or ramipril is excreted in breast milk; quinapril is excreted to a limited extent in the milk of lactating rats (≤ 5% of plasma concentration). Decide whether to discontinue nursing or discontinue the drug, taking into account the importance of the drug to the mother.

Children: Safety and efficacy have not been established. However, there is limited experience with the use of captopril in children. Dosage, on a weight basis, was comparable to or less than that used in adults. Infants, especially newborns, may be more susceptible to the adverse hemodynamic effects of captopril. Excessive, prolonged and unpredictable decreases in blood pressure and associated complications, including oliguria and seizures, have occurred. Use captopril in children only when other measures for controlling blood pressure have not been effective.

In one study, 11 neonates (five premature) with severe hypertension were effectively treated with captopril 0.01 to 0.5 mg/kg/day. The potency and duration are greater in this age group. Use the lowest possible effective maintenance dose. Other infants, however, have developed neurologic complications following captopril therapy. Caution is warranted.

Precautions:

Hyperkalemia: Elevated serum potassium (> 5.7 mEq/L) was observed in approximately 1% of hypertensive patients given benazepril, enalapril or ramipril, 1.3% of hypertensive patients given moexipril, 2.2% of hypertensive patients given lisinopril, 2.6% of hypertensive patients given fosinopril and 4% of CHF patients given lisinopril. In most cases, these resolved despite continued therapy. Hyperkalemia was a cause of therapy discontinuation in 0.28% of hypertensive patients on enalapril, ≈ 0.1% with lisinopril and fosinopril, no patients on ramipril and 2% of type I diabetics with proteinuria receiving captopril. Risk factors for development of hyperkalemia may include renal insufficiency, diabetes mellitus and concomitant use of agents for treatment of hypokalemia. Hyperkalemia also occurred with captopril.

Valvular stenosis: Theoretically, patients with aortic stenosis might be at risk of decreased coronary perfusion when treated with vasodilators, because they do not develop as much afterload reduction as others.

ACE INHIBITORS

Surgery/Anesthesia: In patients undergoing major surgery or during anesthesia with agents that produce hypotension, ACEIs will block angiotensin II formation secondary to compensatory renin release. Hypotension can be corrected by volume expansion.

Cough: Chronic cough has occurred with the use of all ACEIs, presumably due to the inhibition of the degradation of endogenous bradykinin. Characteristically, the cough is nonproductive, persistent and resolves within 1 to 4 days after therapy discontinuation. Consider ACEI-induced cough as part of the differential diagnosis of cough.

The cough appears to have a higher incidence in women. The incidence of cough, although still reported as 0.5% to 3% by some manufacturers, appears to range from 5% to 25% and has been reported to be as high as 39%, resulting in discontinuation rates as high as 15%. The use of sulindac, diclofenac, indomethacin, nifedipine, cromolyn or nebulized bupivacaine may be effective in managing cough, although this is only based on a small number of patients. Further study is needed.

Drug Interactions:

ACEI Drug Interactions

Precipitant drug	Object drug*		Description
Antacids	ACEIs	⬇	Bioavailability of ACEIs may be decreased. May be more likely with captopril. Separate the administration times by 1 to 2 hours.
Capsaicin	ACEIs	⬆	Capsaicin may cause or exacerbate coughing associated with ACEI treatment and vice versa.
Indomethacin	ACEIs	⬇	Reduced hypotensive effects of ACEIs. More prominent in low-renin or volume-dependent hypertensive patients.
Phenothiazines	ACEIs	⬆	Pharmacologic effects of ACEIs may be increased.
Probenecid	ACEIs – captopril	⬆	Increased captopril blood levels and decreased total clearance have occurred.
Rifampin	ACEIs – enalapril	⬇	Pharmacologic effects of enalapril may be decreased.
ACEIs	Allopurinol	⬆	Higher risk of hypersensitivity reaction possible when these drugs are given concurrently.
ACEIs	Digoxin	⬆	Increased plasma digoxin levels.
ACEIs	Lithium	⬆	Increased serum lithium levels and symptoms of toxicity may occur.
ACEIs	Potassium preparations/ Potassium-sparing diuretics	⬆	Coadministration may result in elevated serum potassium concentrations.
ACEIs – quinapril	Tetracycline	⬇	Tetracycline absorption reduced 28% to 37%, possibly due to the high magnesium content of quinapril tabs.

* ⬆ = Object drug increased. ⬇ = Object drug decreased.

Drug/Lab test interactions: Captopril may cause a false-positive test for *urine acetone*.

Fosinopril may cause a false low measurement of serum digoxin levels with the *Digi-Tab RIA Kit for Digoxin*. Other kits, such as the *Coat-A-Count RIA Kit*, may be used.

Drug/Food interactions: Food significantly reduces the bioavailability of captopril by 30% to 40%. It is not known whether the effects of captopril are significantly affected; administer captopril 1 hour before meals. Food intake reduces the C_{max} and AUC of moexipril by about 70% and 40%, respectively, after a low-fat breakfast and by 80% and 50%, respectively, after a high-fat breakfast; take moexipril in the fasting state. The rate and extent of quinapril absorption are diminished moderately (25% to 30%) when administered during a high-fat meal. The rate, but not extent, of ramipril and fosinopril absorption is reduced by food. Food does not reduce the GI absorption of benazepril, enalapril and lisinopril.

Angiotensin Converting Enzyme Inhibitors

ACE INHIBITORS

Adverse Reactions:

✓ = Reported; no incidence given.	Adverse Reactions Shared by the ACEIs[1] (%)							
Adverse reactions	Benazepril	Captopril	Enalapril	Fosinopril	Lisinopril	Moexipril	Quinapril	Ramipril
Cardiovascular								
Chest pain		1	2.1	≤ 1	1.3	> 1		< 1
Hypotension[2]	0.3	✓	6.7	≤ 1	1.2-5	0.5		0.5
Palpitations	< 1	1	≤ 1	≤ 1	≤ 1	< 1	0.5-1	< 1
Angina pectoris	< 1	0.2-0.3	1.5	≤ 1	≤ 1	< 1	0.5-1	< 1
Cardiac arrest		✓	≤ 1					
Cerebrovascular accident		✓	≤ 1	≤ 1	≤ 1	< 1	0.5-1	
Myocardial infarction		0.2-0.3	≤ 1.2	≤ 1	≤ 1	< 1	0.5-1	< 1
Orthostatic hypotension	≤ 0.4	✓	1.6	1.4	≤ 1	0.5	0.5-1	
Orthostatic effects			1.2-2.2		1.4			
Rhythm disturbances		✓	≤ 1	≤ 1	≤ 1	< 1	0.5-1	
Tachycardia		1	✓		≤ 1		0.5-1	
Peripheral edema	< 1				≤ 1	> 1		
CNS								
Insomnia/ Sleep disturbances	< 1	0.5-2	≤ 1	≤ 1	≤ 1	< 1		< 1
Paresthesias	< 1	0.5-2	≤ 1	≤ 1	0.8			< 1
Headache	5	0.5-2	1.8-5.2	3.2	5.3	> 1	5.6	5.4
Dizziness	3.3	0.5-2	4.3-7.9	1.6	6.3	4.3	3.9	2.2
Fatigue	2.6	0.5-2	1.8-3	1.5	3.3	2.4	2.6	2
Somnolence/Drowsiness		✓	≤ 1		≤ 1	< 1	0.5-1	< 1
Ataxia		✓	≤ 1					
Confusion		✓	≤ 1	≤ 1	≤ 1			
Depression		✓	≤ 1		≤ 1		0.5-1	≤ 1
Malaise		0.5-2			≤ 1	< 1	0.5-1	< 1
Nervousness	< 1	✓	≤ 1		≤ 1	< 1	0.5-1	< 1
Vertigo			1.6	≤ 1	0.1		0.5-1	< 1
Anxiety	<1					< 1		< 1
GI/GU								
Abdominal pain	< 1	0.5-2	1.6	≤ 1	≤ 1	< 1	1	< 1
Vomiting	< 1	0.5-2	1.3	1.2	1.3	< 1	1.4	1.1
Nausea	1.4	0.5-2	1.3-1.4	1.2	2.3	> 1	1.4	1.1
Diarrhea		0.5-2	1.4-2.1	1.5	3.2	3.1		< 1
Dysgeusia		2-4	≤ 1		✓	< 1		< 1
Anorexia		0.5-2	≤ 1		≤ 1			< 1
Constipation	< 1	0.5-2	≤ 1	≤ 1	≤ 1	< 1	0.5-1	< 1
Oliguria		0.1-0.2	≤ 1		≤ 1	< 1		
Dry mouth		0.5-2	≤ 1	≤ 1	≤ 1	< 1	0.5-1	< 1
Dyspepsia		✓	≤ 1		1	> 1		< 1
Glossitis		✓	≤ 1					
Hepatitis		✓[3]	≤ 1	≤ 1	≤ 1	< 1		
Hepatocellular/ Cholestatic jaundice			≤ 1		≤ 1			
Pancreatitis		✓	≤ 1	≤ 1	≤ 1	< 1	0.5-1	
Urinary tract infection	< 1		1.3		≤ 1			
Melena	< 1		≤ 1					

Angiotensin Converting Enzyme Inhibitors

ACE INHIBITORS

Adverse Reactions Shared by the ACEIs[1] (%)								
✓ = Reported; no incidence given.								
Adverse reactions	Benazepril	Captopril	Enalapril	Fosinopril	Lisinopril	Moexipril	Quinapril	Ramipril
Respiratory								
Asthma	< 1	✓	≤ 1	✓	✓		✓	✓
Bronchitis	< 1		1.3		≤ 1			
Bronchospasm	✓	✓	≤ 1	≤ 1	✓	< 1		✓
Cough[4]	1.9-3.4	0.5-2	1.3-2.2	2.2	2.9-4.5	6.1	2	12
Dyspnea	< 1	0.5-2	1.3		1.1	< 1		< 1
Upper respiratory infection			≤ 1			> 1		✓
Sinusitis	< 1			≤ 1	≤ 1	> 1		
Dermatologic								
Alopecia		0.5-2	≤ 1					
Diaphoresis/Increased sweating	< 1		≤ 1	≤ 1	≤ 1	< 1	0.5-1	< 1
Erythema multiforme		✓	≤ 1					
Exfoliative dermatitis		✓	≤ 1				0.5-1	
Flushing	< 1		≤ 1	≤ 1	≤ 1	1.6		
Photosensitivity		✓	✓	≤ 1		< 1	0.5-1	< 1
Pruritus	✓	2	≤ 1		≤ 1	< 1	0.5-1	✓
Rash	✓	4-7	1.3-1.4	≤ 1	1.5	1.6		✓
Stevens-Johnson syndrome		✓	≤ 1					
Urticaria			≤ 1	≤ 1	≤ 1	< 1		
Miscellaneous								
Angioedema[2]	0.5	0.1	0.2	≤ 1	0.1	< 1	0.1	0.3
Impotence	< 1	✓	≤ 1		0.7			< 1
Decreased libido	< 1			≤ 1	≤ 1			
Muscle cramps				≤ 1	≤ 1			0.6
Asthenia	< 1	✓	1.1-1.6		1.3			2
Syncope	0.1	✓	2.2	≤ 1	0.1-1	0.5	0.5-1	< 1
Anemia		✓[5]			✓	< 1		
Blurred vision		✓	≤ 1		≤ 1			
Fever		✓	✓		≤ 1			✓
Myalgia	<1	✓	✓	≤ 1	✓	1.3		< 1
Tinnitus			≤ 1	≤ 1		< 1		< 1
Arthralgia	< 1	✓	✓	≤ 1	✓	< 1		< 1
Arthritis	< 1		✓		✓			< 1
Eosinophilia		✓	✓					
Vasculitis		✓	✓		≤ 1			
Renal[2]	Transient elevation (reversible) of BUN and creatinine may occur, especially in patients with volume depletion or renovascular hypertension. Rapid reduction of long-standing or severely elevated blood pressure may transiently decrease GFR, resulting in transient rises in creatinine and BUN. Small increases in serum potassium concentrations frequently occur, especially in patients with renal impairment. Renal failure has occurred.							

[1] All events; data are pooled from separate studies and are not necessarily comparable. Data included for both hypertension and heart failure indications.
[2] See Warnings or Precautions.
[3] Including rare episodes of necrosis.
[4] See Precautions. Although still reported at 0.5% to 3% by some manufacturers, the incidence appears to range from 5% to 25% and has been reported to be as high as 39%.
[5] Including aplastic or hemolytic.

ACE INHIBITORS

Cardiovascular:

Captopril – Raynaud's syndrome, CHF (0.2% to 0.3%).

Enalapril – Pulmonary embolism and infarction, pulmonary edema, atrial fibrillation, bradycardia (≤ 1%).

Ramipril – Arrhythmia (< 1%).

Fosinopril – Hypertensive crisis, claudication (≤ 1%).

Quinapril – Vasodilation, heart failure, hypertensive crisis (0.5% to 1%); cardiogenic shock (< 0.5%).

CNS:

Enalapril – Peripheral neuropathy (eg, dysesthesia) (0.5% to 1%).

Fosinopril – Memory disturbance, tremor, mood change, drowsiness (≤ 1%).

Lisinopril – Stroke (≤ 1%).

Ramipril – Amnesia, convulsions, hearing loss, neuralgia, neuropathy, tremor, vision disturbances (< 1%).

Moexipril – Mood changes (< 1%).

Dermatologic:

Captopril – Rash, often with pruritus (and sometimes fever, arthralgia and eosinophilia) occurs usually during the first 4 weeks of therapy. The rash is usually maculopapular, rarely urticarial, mild and disappears within a few days of dosage reduction, short-term antihistamine treatment or discontinuation of therapy. Remission may occur even if captopril is continued. Between 7% and 10% of patients with skin rash have shown eosinophilia or positive ANA titers.

Reversible pemphigoid-like lesions; bullous pemphigus; scalded mouth sensation; onycholysis; flushing, pallor (0.2% to 0.5%).

Ramipril – Apparent hypersensitivity reactions (manifested by dermatitis, pruritus or rash with or without fever); purpura (< 1%).

Benazepril – Apparent hypersensitivity reactions (manifested by dermatitis, pruritus or rash).

Enalapril – Pemphigus (0.5% to 1%).

Quinapril – Dermatopolymyositis (< 0.5%).

Moexipril – Apparent hypersensitivity reactions (manifested by urticaria, rash, pemphigus, pruritus, photosensitivity) (< 1%).

Electrolyte Disturbance: Hyperkalemia (see Precautions); hyponatremia (benazepril; captopril, particularly in patients on a low sodium diet or concomitant diuretics).

GI:

Captopril – Gastric irritation, aphthous ulcers, peptic ulcer (0.5% to 2%). Dysgeusia is reversible and usually self-limiting, even with continued therapy (2 to 3 months). Weight loss may be associated with taste loss. Jaundice, cholestasis.

Enalapril – Hepatic failure, ileus, stomatitis (0.5% to 1%).

Fosinopril – Dysphagia, abdominal distention, flatulence, heartburn, appetite/weight change (≤ 1%).

Lisinopril – Flatulence (≤ 1%).

Quinapril – GI hemorrhage (0.5% to 1%).

Ramipril – Abdominal pain occurs, sometimes with enzyme changes suggesting pancreatitis. Dysphagia, gastroenteritis, increased salivation (< 1%).

Moexipril – Appetite/Weight changes (< 1%).

Hematologic:

Captopril – Neutropenia/agranulocytosis (see Warnings); thrombocytopenia; pancytopenia.

Enalapril – Decreased hemoglobin (0.3 g/dl) and hematocrit (1%) occur frequently in hypertensive or CHF patients but are rarely of clinical importance unless another cause of anemia coexists. Discontinuation resulted in < 0.1% of patients. Rarely, bone marrow depression, neutropenia and thrombocytopenia. Hemolytic anemia including hemolysis have occurred in patients with G-6-PD deficiency.

Lisinopril – Decreases in hemoglobin (≈ 0.4 g/dl) and hematocrit (≈ 1.3%) occurred but are rarely of clinical importance in patients without some other cause of anemia. In clinical trials, < 0.1% of patients discontinued therapy due to anemia. Rarely, neutropenia and bone marrow depression.

Ramipril – Decreases in hemoglobin or hematocrit were rare, occurring in 0.4% of patients on ramipril alone and 1.5% of those on ramipril plus a diuretic. Occasional leukopenia, eosinophilia and proteinuria.

Fosinopril – Mean hemoglobin decrease of 0.1 g/dl. Decreases in hemoglobin or hematocrit were usually transient and not associated with symptoms. Occasional neutropenia, leukopenia and eosinophilia.

Benazepril – Decreased hemoglobin (a low value and a decrease of 5 g/dl; rare). Occasional leukopenia, eosinophilia and proteinuria.

Angiotensin Converting Enzyme Inhibitors

ACE INHIBITORS

Quinapril – Agranulocytosis, thrombocytopenia (0.5% to 1%).

Lab test abnormalities: Elevated liver enzymes, serum bilirubin, uric acid and blood glucose; ECG changes (benazepril).

Renal:

Captopril – Proteinuria (1%); renal insufficiency, nephrotic syndrome, polyuria, urinary frequency (0.1% to 0.2%); interstitial nephritis.

Enalapril – Renal dysfunction (≤ 1%).

Lisinopril – Progressive azotemia (≤ 1%).

Quinapril – Worsening renal failure (< 0.5%).

Moexipril – Urinary frequency, renal insufficiency (< 1%).

Miscellaneous: Anaphylactoid reactions have occurred (see Warnings).

Benazepril – Hypertonia, infection (< 1%).

Captopril – Eosinophilic pneumonitis; gynecomastia; myasthenia; rhinitis.

Enalapril – Pneumonia, anosmia, rhinorrhea, sore throat, hoarseness, pulmonary infiltrates, toxic epidermal necrolysis, herpes zoster, conjunctivitis, dry eyes, tearing, hearing loss, myositis (≤ 1%); flank pain, gynecomastia (0.5% to 1%).

Fosinopril – Edema, weakness, sexual dysfunction, gout, lymphadenopathy, musculoskeletal pain, pharyngitis, rhinitis, laryngitis, epistaxis, vision/taste disturbance, eye irritation, renal insufficiency, urinary frequency (≤ 1%).

Lisinopril – Upper respiratory symptoms (3%); pharyngeal pain, back/joint/shoulder pain, nasal congestion, gout, chest discomfort (≤ 1%).

Quinapril – Back pain, amblyopia, pharyngitis, viral infections (0.5% to 1%).

Ramipril – Flu syndrome; edema, epistaxis, weight gain (< 1%).

Moexipril – Flu syndrome (3.1%); pharyngitis (1.8%); pain, rhinitis (≤ 1%).

A symptom complex has occurred and may include: Positive ANA, elevated erythrocyte sedimentation rate, arthralgia, arthritis, myalgia, fever, interstitial nephritis, vasculitis, rash, eosinophilia, serositis, leukocytosis, photosensitivity, other dermatologic manifestations.

Overdosage:

Symptoms: Hypotension is most common. Systolic blood pressures of 95 and 80 mm Hg have occurred following lisinopril and captopril overdoses, respectively.

Treatment: Refer to General Management of Acute Overdosage.The primary concern is correction of hypotension. Volume expansion with an IV infusion of normal saline is the treatment of choice to restore blood pressure.

Captopril, enalaprilat and lisinopril may be removed by hemodialysis. There are inadequate data concerning the efficacy of removing captopril by hemodialysis in neonates and children. Enalaprilat has been removed from neonatal circulation by peritoneal dialysis. Benazeprilat can be removed by dialysis. It is not known if ramipril, moexipril or ramiprilat are removed by hemodialysis. Hemodialysis and peritoneal dialysis have little effect on the elimination of quinapril and quinaprilat. Use caution with concurrent use of ACEIs and polyacrylonitrile (PAN) dialyzers due to the possibility of severe, sudden, sometimes fatal reactions; symptoms may include nausea, abdominal cramps, burning, angioedema and shortness of breath leading rapidly to severe hypotension. Stop the dialysis immediately and treat anaphylactoid reactions.

Patient Information:

Take captopril 1 hour before meals. Take moexipril in the fasting state.

Do not interrupt or discontinue medication without consulting physician.

Notify physician if any of the following occur: Sore throat, fever, swelling of hands or feet, irregular heartbeat, chest pains, signs of angioedema (swelling of face, eyes, lips, tongue, difficulty swallowing or breathing, hoarseness). Excessive perspiration, dehydration, vomiting and diarrhea may lead to a fall in blood pressure.

May cause dizziness, fainting or lightheadedness, especially during the first days of therapy; avoid sudden changes in posture. If actual syncope occurs, discontinue drug until physician has been contacted. Heart failure patients should avoid rapid increases in physical activity.

May cause skin rash or impaired taste perception. Notify physician if these persist.

Do not use salt substitutes containing potassium without consulting a physician.

A persistent dry cough may occur and usually does not subside unless the medication is stopped. If this effect becomes bothersome, consult a physician.

Angiotensin Converting Enzyme Inhibitors

QUINAPRIL HCl

For complete prescribing information, refer to the ACE Inhibitors group monograph.

Indications:

Hypertension: Treating hypertension alone or in combination with thiazide diuretics.

CHF: Adjunctive therapy in the management of CHF when added to conventional therapy including a diuretic or digitalis.

Administration and Dosage:

Approved by the FDA in November 1991.

Hypertension:

Initial dose – 10 mg once daily. Adjust according to blood pressure response at peak (2 to 6 hours) and trough (predose) blood levels. Adjust dosage at intervals of at least 2 weeks.

Maintenance dosage – Most patients require 20, 40 or 80 mg/day as a single dose or in two equally divided doses. In some patients treated with once-daily dosing, the antihypertensive effect may diminish toward the end of the dosing interval. In general, doses of 40 to 80 mg and divided doses give a somewhat greater effect at the end of the dosing interval.

Patients taking diuretics – Symptomatic hypotension may occur following the initial dose of quinapril. To reduce the likelihood of this effect, discontinue the diuretic 2 to 3 days prior to quinapril therapy if possible. If blood pressure is not controlled, resume diuretic therapy. If diuretic cannot be discontinued, use an initial dose of 5 mg quinapril.

Elderly (≥ 65 years old) – 10 mg once daily followed by titration to the optimal response (see above).

Renal function impairment – Initial dose is 10 mg with Ccr > 60 ml/min, 5 mg with Ccr 30 to 60 ml/min and 2.5 mg with Ccr 10 to 30 ml/min.

Patients should subsequently have their dosage titrated (as directed above) to the optimal response.

CHF: Indicated as adjunctive therapy when added to conventional therapy including diuretics or digitalis. The recommended starting dose is 5 mg twice daily. This dose may improve symptoms of heart failure, but increases in exercise duration have generally required higher doses. Therefore, if the initial dose is well tolerated, titrate patients at weekly intervals until an effective dose, usually 20 to 40 mg daily given in 2 equally divided doses, is reached or undesirable hypotension, orthostasis or azotemia prohibit reaching this dose.

Following the initial dose, observe the patient under medical supervision for at least 2 hours for the presence of hypotension or orthostasis and, if present, until blood pressure stabilizes. The appearance of hypotension, orthostasis or azotemia early in dose titration should not preclude further careful dose titration. Consider reducing the dose of concomitant diuretics.

Renal impairment or hyponatremia – Quinapril elimination is dependent on level of renal function. In patients with heart failure and renal impairment, the recommended initial dose is 5 mg with Ccr > 30 ml/min and 2.5 mg with Ccr 10 to 30 ml/min. There are insufficient data for dosage recommendation in patients with Ccr < 10 ml/min.

If the initial dose is well tolerated, quinapril may be given the following day as a twice-daily regimen. In the absence of excessive hypotension or significant deterioration of renal function, the dose may be increased at weekly intervals based on clinical and hemodynamic response.

Rx	**Accupril** (Parke-Davis)	**Tablets**: 5 mg	Lactose. (PD 527 5). Brown, scored. Elliptical. Film coated. In 90s and UD 100s.
		10 mg	Lactose. (PD 530 10). Brown. Triangular. Film coated. In 90s and UD 100s.
		20 mg	Lactose. (PD 532 20). Brown. Film coated. In 90s and UD 100s.
		40 mg	Lactose. (PD 535 40). Brown. Elliptical. Film coated. In 90s.

Angiotensin Converting Enzyme Inhibitors

RAMIPRIL

For complete prescribing information, refer to the ACE Inhibitors group monograph.

Indications:

Hypertension: Treating hypertension alone or in combination with thiazide diuretics.

CHF: For stable patients who have demonstrated clinical signs of CHF within the first few days after sustaining acute MI.

Administration and Dosage:

Approved by the FDA in 1991.

Hypertension:

Initial dose – 2.5 mg once daily in patients not receiving a diuretic. Adjust according to blood pressure response.

Maintenance dosage – 2.5 to 20 mg/day as a single dose or in two equally divided doses. If the antihypertensive effect diminishes at the end of the dosing interval in patients treated once daily, consider twice daily administration or an increase in dosage.

Renal function impairment – 1.25 mg once daily in patients with Ccr of < 40 ml/min/1.73 m^2 (serum creatinine > 2.5 mg/dl). Dosage may be titrated upward until blood pressure is controlled or to a maximum of 5 mg/day.

CHF: Starting dose is 2.5 mg twice daily. A patient who becomes hypotensive at this dose may be switched to 1.25 mg twice daily, but all patients should then be titrated (as tolerated) toward a target dose of 5 mg twice daily.

Renal function impairment – 1.25 mg once daily in patients with Ccr of < 40 ml/min/1.73 m^2 (serum creatinine > 2.5 mg/dl). Dosage may be increased to 1.25 mg twice daily up to a maximum dose of 2.5 mg twice daily depending on clinical response and tolerability.

Patients taking diuretics: Symptomatic hypotension may occur following the initial dose of ramipril. To reduce the likelihood of this effect, discontinue the diuretic 2 to 3 days prior to beginning ramipril if possible. If bp is not controlled, resume diuretic therapy. If diuretic cannot be discontinued, use an initial dose of 1.25 mg ramipril.

Alternative route of administration: Ramipril capsules are usually swallowed whole. However, the capsules may be opened and the contents sprinkled on a small amount of applesauce (≈ 4 oz) or mixed in apple juice or water. The mixture should be consumed in its entirity. Pre-prepared mixtures can be stored for up to 24 hours at room temperature or for up to 48 hours under refrigeration.

Rx	**Altace** (Hoechst Marion Roussel)	**Capsules:** 1.25 mg	Yellow. In 100s and UD 100s.
		2.5 mg	Orange. In 100s and UD 100s.
		5 mg	Red. In 100s and UD 100s.
		10 mg	Blue. In 100s.

CAPTOPRIL

For complete prescribing information, refer to the ACE Inhibitors group monograph.

Indications:

Hypertension: Management of hypertension alone or with thiazide diuretics.

Heart failure: For patients who have not responded adequately to, or cannot be controlled by, conventional diuretic and digitalis therapy. Use with diuretics and digitalis, except when digitalis use is poorly tolerated or otherwise not feasible.

Left ventricular dysfunction after MI: To improve survival following MI in clinically stable patients with LVD manifested as ejection fraction ≤ 40% and to reduce the incidence of overt heart failure and subsequent hospitalizations for CHF in these patients.

Diabetic nephropathy: Treatment of diabetic nephropathy (proteinuria > 500 mg/day) in patients with type I insulin-dependent diabetes mellitus and retinopathy.

Administration and Dosage:

Individualize dosage. Administer 1 hour before meals. If possible, discontinue previous antihypertensive drug regimen 1 week before starting captopril.

Hypertension:

Initial – 25 mg 2 or 3 times/day. If satisfactory blood pressure reduction is not achieved after 1 or 2 weeks, increase to 50 mg 2 or 3 times/day. If blood pressure is not controlled after 1 or 2 weeks at this dose (and patient is not already on a diuretic), add a modest dose of a thiazide diuretic (eg, hydrochlorothiazide 25 mg/day). May increase diuretic dose at 1 to 2 week intervals until its highest usual antihypertensive dose is reached. Concomitant sodium restriction may be beneficial when captopril is used alone.

Angiotensin Converting Enzyme Inhibitors

CAPTOPRIL

If further blood pressure reduction is required, increase to 100 mg captopril 2 or 3 times/day and then, if necessary, to 150 mg 2 or 3 times/day (while continuing diuretic). Usual dose is 25 to 150 mg 2 or 3 times/day. Do not exceed daily dose of 450 mg.

Accelerated or malignant hypertension – When temporary discontinuation of current antihypertensive therapy is not practical, or when prompt titration of blood pressure is indicated, continue diuretic but stop current medication and promptly initiate captopril at 25 mg 2 or 3 times daily under close supervision. Increase dose every 24 hours until a satisfactory response is obtained or the maximum dose is reached. In this regimen, a more potent diuretic (eg, furosemide) may be indicated. Beta blockers may be used with captopril, but the effects are less than additive.

Heart failure: Consider recent diuretic therapy and the possibility of severe salt/volume depletion. In patients with normal or low blood pressure who have been vigorously treated with diuretics and who may be hyponatremic or hypovolemic, a starting dose of 6.25 or 12.5 mg 3 times daily may minimize the magnitude or duration of the hypotensive effect. Titrate to the usual daily dosage within the next several days.

Usual initial dosage is 25 mg 3 times daily. After 50 mg 3 times daily is reached, delay further dosage increases, where possible, for at least 2 weeks to determine if a satisfactory response occurs. Most patients have had a satisfactory clinical improvement at 50 or 100 mg 3 times daily. Do not exceed a daily dose of 450 mg.

LVD after MI: 50 mg 3 times/day is the target maintenance dose. Therapy may be initiated as early as 3 days after an MI. After a single 6.25 mg dose, initiate at 12.5 mg 3 times/day, then increase to 25 mg 3 times/day during the next several days and to a target of 50 mg 3 times daily over the next several weeks as tolerated. Other post-MI therapies (eg, thrombolytics, aspirin, beta blockers) may be used concurrently.

Diabetic nephropathy: Recommended dose for long-term use is 25 mg 3 times daily. Other antihypertensives (eg, diuretics, beta blockers, centrally acting agents, vasodilators) may be used in conjunction with captopril if additional therapy is required to further lower blood pressure.

Angiotensin Converting Enzyme Inhibitors

CAPTOPRIL

Renal impairment: Excretion is reduced in patients with impaired renal function; these patients may respond to smaller or less frequent doses. Accordingly, reduce initial dosage and use smaller increments for titration, which should be quite slow (1 to 2 week intervals). After the desired therapeutic effect is achieved, slowly back-titrate to the minimal effective dose. When diuretic therapy is required, a loop diuretic (eg, furosemide) is preferred in patients with severe renal impairment.

Solution: If a solution form of captopril is desired, the tablets may be utilized for preparation. In one study, the stability of captopril in various solutions (stored in glass bottles) was as follows: Syrup, 7 days at 4° and 22°C (39° and 72°F); distilled water, 7 days at 22°C and 14 days at 4°C; distilled water plus sodium ascorbate, 14 days at 22°C and 56 days at 4°C.

Rx	**Captopril** (Various, eg, Apothecon, Lemmon, Mylan, Royce	**Tablets:** 12.5 mg	In 100s, 1000s, 5000s and UD 100s.
Rx	**Capoten** (Bristol-Myers Squibb)		Lactose. (Squibb 450). White, scored. Oval. In 100s, 1000s and UD 100s.
Rx	**Captopril** (Various, eg, Apothecon, Lemmon, Mylan, Royce	**Tablets:** 25 mg	In 100s, 1000s, 5000s and UD 100s.
Rx	**Capoten** (Bristol-Myers Squibb)		Lactose. (Squibb 452). White, scored. Rounded square. In 100s, 1000s and UD 100s.
Rx	**Captopril** (Various, eg, Apothecon, Lemmon, Mylan, Royce	**Tablets:** 50 mg	In 100s, 1000s and 5000s
Rx	**Capoten** (Bristol-Myers Squibb)		Lactose. (Squibb 482). White, scored. Oval. In 100s, 1000s and UD 100s.
Rx	**Captopril** (Various, eg, Apothecon, Lemmon, Mylan, Royce	**Tablets:** 100 mg	In 100s and 500s.
Rx	**Capoten** (Bristol-Myers Squibb)		Lactose. (Squibb 485). White, scored. Oval. In 100s and UD 100s.

MOEXIPRIL HCL

For complete prescribing information, refer to the ACE Inhibitors group monograph.

Indications:

Hypertension: Treating hypertension, alone or in combination with thiazide diuretics.

Administration and Dosage:

Approved by the FDA on April 19, 1995.

Initial dose: In patients not receiving diuretics, 7.5 mg 1 hour prior to meals once daily. Adjust according to blood pressure response. The antihypertensive effect may diminish towards the end of the dosing interval. If control is not adequate, increase the dose or divide the dosing.

Maintenance dose: 7.5 to 30 mg daily in 1 or 2 divided doses 1 hour before meals.

Patients taking diuretics: Symptomatic hypotension may occur after the initial dose of moexipril. To reduce risk of this effect, discontinue diuretic 2 to 3 days prior to beginning moexipril if possible. If blood pressure is not controlled, resume diuretic therapy. If diuretic cannot be discontinued, use an initial dose of 3.75 mg moexipril.

Renal function impairment: Cautiously use 3.75 mg once daily in patients with Ccr of $\le$ 40 ml/min/1.73 m^2. Dosage may be titrated upward to a maximum of 15 mg/day.

Rx	**Univasc** (Schwarz Pharma)	**Tablets:** 7.5 mg	Lactose. (707 SP 7.5). Pink, scored. Biconvex. In 100s and UD 90s.
		15 mg	Lactose. (715 SP 15). Salmon, scored. Biconvex. In 100s and UD 90s.

Angiotensin Converting Enzyme Inhibitors

FOSINOPRIL SODIUM

For complete prescribing information, refer to the ACE Inhibitors group monograph.

Indications:

Hypertension: Treating hypertension, alone or in combination with thiazide diuretics.

Heart failure: Management of heart failure as adjunctive therapy when added to conventional therapy including diuretics with or without digitalis.

Administration and Dosage:

Approved by the FDA in 1991.

Hypertension:

Initial dose – 10 mg once daily. Adjust according to blood pressure response at peak (2 to 6 hours) and trough (about 24 hours after dosing) blood levels.

Maintenance dosage – Usual range needed to maintain a response is 20 to 40 mg/day, but some patients appear to have a further response to 80 mg. In some patients treated with once-daily dosing, the antihypertensive effect may diminish toward the end of the dosing interval. If trough response is inadequate, consider dividing the daily dose. If blood pressure is not adequately controlled with fosinopril alone, a diuretic may be added.

Patients taking diuretics – Symptomatic hypotension may occur following the initial dose of fosinopril. To reduce the likelihood of this effect, discontinue the diuretic 2 to 3 days prior to beginning fosinopril if possible. If blood pressure is not controlled, resume diuretic therapy. If diuretic cannot be discontinued, use an initial dose of 10 mg fosinopril.

Heart failure: Digitalis is not required for fosinopril to manifest improvements in exercise tolerance and symptoms. Most placebo controlled clinical trial experience has been with both digitalis and diuretics present as background therapy.

The usual starting dose of fosinopril is 10 mg once daily. Following the initial dose, observe the patient under medical supervision for at least 2 hours for the presence of hypotension or orthostasis and, if either is present, until blood pressure stabilizes. An initial dose of 5 mg is preferred in heart failure patients with moderate-to-severe renal failure or in those who have been vigorously diuresed.

Increase dosage over a several week period to a dose that is maximal and tolerated but not exceeding 40 mg once daily. The usual effective dosage range is 20 to 40 mg once daily.

The appearance of hypotension, orthostasis or azotemia early in dose titration should not preclude further careful dose titration. Consider reducing the dose of concomitant diuretic.

Renal function impairment: In impaired renal function, the total body clearance of fosinoprilat is approximately 50% slower than that in normal renal function. Because hepatobiliary elimination partially compensates for diminished renal elimination, the total body clearance of fosinoprilat does not differ appreciably with any degree of renal insufficiency (creatinine clearances < 80 ml/min/1.73 m^2), including end-stage renal failure (creatinine clearance < 10 ml/min/1.73 m^2). This relative constancy of body clearance of active fosinoprilat, resulting from the dual route of elimination, permits use of the usual dose in any degree of renal impairment.

Rx	**Monopril** (Mead Johnson)	**Tablets:** 10 mg	Lactose. (158MJ m). White to off-white. Biconvex, diamond shaped. In 100s and UD 100s.
		20 mg	Lactose. (609MJ m). White to off-white. Oval. In 100s and UD 100s.

Angiotensin Converting Enzyme Inhibitors

BENAZEPRIL HCl

For complete prescribing information, refer to the ACE Inhibitors group monograph.

Indications:

Hypertension: Treating hypertension, alone or in combination with thiazide diuretics.

Administration and Dosage:

Approved by the FDA in June 1991.

Initial dose: 10 mg once daily.

Maintenance dosage: 20 to 40 mg/day as a single dose or two divided doses. The divided regimen is more effective in controlling trough (pre-dosing) blood pressure. Base dosage adjustment on peak (2 to 6 hours after dosing) and trough responses. If a once-daily regimen does not give adequate trough response, consider an increase in dosage or divided administration. A dose of 80 mg gives an increased response, but experience is limited; total daily doses > 80 mg have not been evaluated.

Patients taking diuretics: Symptomatic hypotension may follow the initial dose of benazepril. To reduce this likelihood, discontinue the diuretic 2 to 3 days prior to beginning benazepril therapy. If blood pressure is not controlled, resume diuretic therapy. If the diuretic cannot be discontinued, use an initial dose of 5 mg benazepril.

Renal function impairment: 5 mg once daily in patients with Ccr of < 30 ml/min/1.73 m^2 (serum creatinine > 3 mg/dl). Dosage may be titrated upward until blood pressure is controlled or to a maximum of 40 mg/day.

Rx	**Lotensin** (Ciba)	**Tablets**: 5 mg	Lactose. (Lotensin 5). Light yellow. In 100s and UD 100s.
		10 mg	Lactose. (Lotensin 10). Dark yellow. In 100s and UD 100s.
		20 mg	Lactose. (Lotensin 20). Tan. In 100s and UD 100s.
		40 mg	Lactose. (Lotensin 40). Dark rose. In 100s and UD 100s.

LISINOPRIL

For complete prescribing information, refer to the ACE Inhibitors group monograph.

Indications:

Hypertension: Treating hypertension alone or in combination with thiazide diuretics.

CHF: Adjunctive therapy in the management of CHF in patients not responding adequately to diuretics and digitalis.

Acute myocardial infarction: Treatment of hemodynamically stable patients within 24 hours of acute myocardial infarction, to improve survival. Patients should receive, as appropriate, the standard recommended treatments such as thrombolytics, aspirin and beta blockers.

Administration and Dosage:

Approved by the FDA in 1987.

Hypertension:

Initial therapy – 10 mg once daily in patients with uncomplicated essential hypertension not on diuretic therapy. The usual dosage range is 20 to 40 mg/day as a single daily dose. If blood pressure is not controlled with lisinopril alone, a low dose of a diuretic may be added (eg, 12.5 mg hydrochlorothiazide). After addition of a diuretic, it may be possible to reduce the dose of lisinopril.

Diuretic-treated patients – Symptomatic hypotension may occur occasionally following the initial dose of lisinopril. Discontinue the diuretic, if possible, for 2 to 3 days before beginning therapy with lisinopril to reduce the likelihood of hypotension (see Warnings). If the patient's blood pressure is not controlled with lisinopril alone, resume diuretic therapy as above. If the diuretic cannot be discontinued, use an initial dose of 5 mg under medical supervision for at least 2 hours and until blood pressure has stabilized for at least an additional hour.

Renal function impairment – Initiate lisinopril daily dosage according to the following chart. For hypertension, titrate dosage upward until blood pressure is controlled or to a maximum of 40 mg daily.

Angiotensin Converting Enzyme Inhibitors

LISINOPRIL

Lisinopril Dosage in Renal Impairment

Renal status	Creatinine clearance (ml/min)	Serum creatinine (mg/dl)	Initial dose (mg/day)
Normal function to mild impairment	> 30	≤ 3	10 mg
Moderate to severe impairment	10 to 30	≥ 3	5 mg
Dialysis patients	< 10	—	2.5 mg*

* Adjust dosage or dosing interval depending on the blood pressure response.

CHF:

Initial dose – 5 mg once daily with diuretics and digitalis. When initiating treatment, give under medical observation, especially in patients with low blood pressure (systolic < 100 mmHg). The mean peak blood pressure lowering occurs 6 to 8 hours after dosing. Continue observation until blood pressure is stable. Reduce concomitant diuretic dose, if possible, to help minimize hypovolemia, which may contribute to hypotension. Appearance of hypotension after the initial dose does not preclude subsequent careful dose titration following effective hypotension management. The usual effective dosage range is 5 to 20 mg/day as a single dose. In patients with hyponatremia (serum sodium < 130 mEq/L), initiate dose at 2.5 mg once daily.

Renal failure or hyponatremia – In patients with heart failure who have hyponatremia (serum sodium < 130 mEq/L) or moderate to severe renal impairment (creatinine clearance ≤ 30 ml/min or serum creatinine > 3 mg/dl), therapy with lisinopril should be initiated at a dose of 2.5 mg once a day under close medical supervision.

Acute myocardial infarction: In hemodynamically stable patients within 24 hours of the onset of symptoms of acute MI, the first dose is 5 mg, followed by 5 mg after 24 hours, 10 mg after 48 hours and then 10 mg once daily. Continue dosing for 6 weeks. Patients should receive, as appropriate, the standard recommended treatments such as thrombolytics, aspirin and beta-blockers. Patients with a low systolic blood pressure (≤ 120 mmHg) when treatment is started or during the first 3 days after the infarct should be given a lower 2.5 mg dose. If hypotension occurs (systolic blood pressure ≤ 100 mmHg), a daily maintenance dose of 5 mg may be given with temporary reductions to 2.5 mg if needed. If prolonged hypotension occurs (systolic blood pressure < 90 mmHg for > 1 hour), withdraw lisinopril. For patients who develop symptoms of heart failure, see Administration and Dosage for CHF.

Renal impairment – In acute MI, initiate lisinopril with caution in patients with evidence of renal dysfunction, defined as serum creatinine concentration exceeding 2 mg/dl.

Elderly: In general, blood pressure response and adverse experiences are similar in younger and older patients given similar doses of lisinopril. However, maximum blood levels and area under the plasma concentration-time curve (AUC) are doubled in older patients. Make dosage adjustments with particular caution.

Rx	**Prinivil** (Merck)	**Tablets:** 2.5 mg	(15 MSD). White. In unit-of-use 30s and 100s and UD 100s.
Rx	**Zestril** (Zeneca)		(Zestril 2½ 135). White. Oval. In 100s.
Rx	**Prinivil** (Merck)	**Tablets:** 5 mg	(MSD 19 Prinivil). White, scored. Shield shape. In 1000s, unit-of-use 90s and 100s and UD 100s.
Rx	**Zestril** (Zeneca)		(Zestril 130). Pink, scored. Capsule shape. In 100s, 1000s and UD 100s.
Rx	**Prinivil** (Merck)	**Tablets:** 10 mg	(MSD 106 Prinivil). Light yellow. Shield shape. In 1000s, unit-of-use 30s, 90s and 100s and UD 100s.
Rx	**Zestril** (Zeneca)		(Zestril 10 131). Pink. In 100s, 1000s and UD 100s.

Angiotensin Converting Enzyme Inhibitors

LISINOPRIL

Rx	**Prinivil** (Merck)	**Tablets**: 20 mg	(MSD 207 Prinivil). Peach. Shield shape. In 1000s, unit-of-use 30s, 90s and 100s and UD 100s.
Rx	**Zestril** (Zeneca)		(Zestril 20 132). Red. In 100s, 1000s and UD 100s.
Rx	**Prinivil** (Merck)	**Tablets**: 40 mg	(MSD 237 Prinivil). Red. Shield shape. In unit-of-use 100s.
Rx	**Zestril** (Zeneca)		(Zestril 40 134). Yellow. In 100s.

ENALAPRIL MALEATE

For complete prescribing information, refer to the ACE Inhibitors group monograph.

Administration and Dosage:

Approved by the FDA in 1985.

Oral:

Hypertension –

Patients taking diuretics: Symptomatic hypotension occasionally may occur following the initial dose of enalapril. Discontinue the diuretic, if possible, for 2 to 3 days before beginning enalapril to reduce the likelihood of hypotension. If blood pressure is not controlled with enalapril alone, diuretics may be resumed.

If the diuretic cannot be discontinued, give an initial dose of 2.5 mg. Keep patient under medical supervision for at least 2 hours and until blood pressure has stabilized for at least an additional hour.

Patients not taking diuretics: Initial dose is 5 mg once a day. Adjust dosage according to blood pressure response. The usual dosage range is 10 to 40 mg/day as a single dose or in 2 divided doses. In some patients treated once daily, the antihypertensive effect may diminish toward the end of the dosing interval. In such patients, consider an increase in dosage or twice-daily administration. If blood pressure is not controlled with enalapril alone, a diuretic may be added.

Impaired renal function: Titrate the dosage upward until blood pressure is controlled or until a maximum dose of 40 mg/day is reached. Use initial dose of 5 mg/day in normal renal function and mild impairment (creatinine clearance [Ccr] 30 to 80 ml/min, serum creatinine < 3 mg/dl); 2.5 mg/day in moderate to severe renal impairment (Ccr ≤ 30 ml/min, serum creatinine ≥ 3 mg/dl) and in dialysis patients on dialysis days (adjust dosage on nondialysis days based on blood pressure response).

Heart failure – As adjunctive therapy with diuretics and digitalis, the recommended starting dose is 2.5 mg once or twice daily. After the initial dose, observe the patient for at least 2 hours and until blood pressure has stabilized for at least an additional hour. If possible, reduce the dose of the diuretic; this may diminish the likelihood of hypotension. The appearance of hypotension after the initial dose of enalapril does not preclude subsequent careful dose titration with the drug, following effective management of the hypotension. The usual therapeutic dosing range for the treatment of heart failure is 5 to 20 mg/day given in two divided doses. The maximum daily dose is 40 mg. Once-daily dosing has been effective in a controlled study, but nearly all patients in this study were given 40 mg, the maximum recommended daily dose, and there has been much more experience with twice-daily dosing. In addition, patients in the mortality trial received therapy twice daily. Dosage may be adjusted depending upon clinical or hemodynamic response.

In a placebo controlled study which demonstrated reduced mortality in patients with severe heart failure (NYHA Class IV), patients were treated with 2.5 to 40 mg/day enalapril, almost always administered in two divided doses.

Renal impairment or hyponatremia:

Serum sodium < 130 mEq/L or with serum creatinine > 1.6 mg/dl – Initiate at 2.5 mg/day under close medical supervision. The dose may be increased to 2.5 mg twice daily, then 5 mg twice daily and higher as needed, usually at intervals of ≥ 4 days if, at the time of dosage adjustment, there is not excessive hypotension or significant deterioration of renal function. The maximum daily dose is 40 mg.

Angiotensin Converting Enzyme Inhibitors

ENALAPRIL MALEATE

Asymptomatic left ventricular dysfunction – 2.5 mg twice daily, titrated as tolerated to the targeted daily dose of 20 mg in divided doses. After the initial dose, observe the patient for ≥ 2 hours and until blood pressure has stabilized for at least an additional hour. If possible, reduce the dose of any concomitant diuretic to diminish the likelihood of hypotension. The appearance of hypotension after the initial enalapril dose does not preclude subsequent careful dose titration with the drug, following effective management of the hypotension.

Parenteral (enalaprilat): For IV administration only.

Hypertension – 1.25 mg every 6 hours IV over 5 minutes. A clinical response is usually seen within 15 minutes. Peak effects after the first dose may not occur for up to 4 hours. The peak effects of subsequent doses may exceed those of the first.

No dosage regimen has been clearly shown to be more effective in treating hypertension than 1.25 mg every 6 hours. However, doses as high as 5 mg every 6 hours were well tolerated for up to 36 hours. There is inadequate experience with doses > 20 mg/day. Patients have received enalaprilat for as long as 7 days.

The dose for patients being converted to IV from oral therapy is 1.25 mg every 6 hours. For conversion from IV to oral therapy, the recommended initial dose of tablets is 5 mg/day with subsequent dosage adjustments as necessary.

Patients taking diuretics – Starting dose for hypertension is 0.625 mg IV over 5 minutes. Clinical response is usually seen within 15 minutes. Peak effects after the first dose may not occur for up to 4 hours, although most of the effect is usually apparent within the first hour. If there is inadequate clinical response after 1 hour, repeat the 0.625 mg dose. Give additional doses of 1.25 mg at 6 hour intervals.

For conversion from IV to oral therapy, the recommended initial dose of enalapril maleate tablets for patients who have responded to 0.625 mg enalaprilat every 6 hours is 2.5 mg/day with subsequent dosage adjustment as necessary.

Renal function impairment – Administer 1.25 mg every 6 hours for patients with Ccr > 30 ml/min (serum creatinine < 3 mg/dl). For Ccr ≤ 30 ml/min (serum creatinine ≥ 3 mg/dl), initial dose is 0.625 mg. If there is inadequate clinical response after 1 hour, the 0.625 mg dose may be repeated. May give additional 1.25 mg doses at 6- hour intervals. For dialysis patients, initial dose is 0.625 mg every 6 hours.

For conversion from IV to oral therapy, the recommended initial dose is 5 mg/day for patients with Ccr > 30 ml/min and 2.5 mg/day for patients with Ccr ≤ 30 ml/min. Adjust dosage according to blood pressure response.

Administration – Give as a slow IV infusion, as indicated above, over ≥ 5 min. It may be used as provided or diluted with < 50 ml of a compatible diluent.

Compatibility and stability – Enalaprilat as supplied and mixed with the following IV diluents has been found to maintain full activity for 24 hours at room temperature: 5% Dextrose Injection; 0.9% Sodium Chloride Injection; 0.9% Sodium Chloride Injection in 5% Dextrose; 5% Dextrose in Lactated Ringer's Injection; *Isolyte E.*

Rx	**Vasotec** (Merck)	**Tablets**: 2.5 mg	Lactose. (Vasotec MSD 14). Yellow, scored. In 100s, 1000s, 10,000s, UD 100s and unit-of-use 90s and 180s.
	Vasotec (Frosst)		Lactose. (14 Vasotec). Yellow, scored. In 100s and 500s.
Rx	**Vasotec** (Merck)	5 mg	Lactose. (Vasotec MSD 712). White. In 100s, 1000s, 4000s, 10,000s, UD 100s and unit-of-use 90s and 180s.
	Vasotec (Frosst)		Lactose. (713 Vasotec). White. In 500s.
Rx	**Vasotec** (Merck)	10 mg	Lactose. (Vasotec MSD 713). Salmon. In 100s, 1000s, 4000s, 10,000s, UD 100s and unit-of-use 90s and 180s.
Rx		20 mg	Lactose. (Vasotec MSD 714). Peach. In 100s, 1000s, 10,000s, UD 100s and unit-of-use 90s.
Rx	**Vasotec I.V.** (Merck)	**Injection**: 1.25 mg enalaprilat/ml	9 mg benzyl alcohol. In 1 and 2 ml vials.

Angiotensin Converting Enzyme Inhibitors

TRANDOLAPRIL

For complete prescribing information see the Angiotensin Converting Enzyme Inhibitors group mongraph.

Indications:

Hypertension: Treatment of hypertension. It may be used alone or in combination with other antihypertensive medications such as hydrochlorothiazide.

Administration and Dosage:

The recommended initial dosage of trandolapril for patients not receiving a diuretic is 1 mg/day (2 mg in African–American patients). Adjust dosage according to the blood pressure response. Make dosage adjustments at intervals of ≥ 1 week. Most patients have required dosages of 2 to 4 mg/day. There is little clinical experience with doses > 6 mg.

Patients inadequately treated with once daily dosing at 4 mg may be treated with twice daily dosing. If blood pressure is not adequately controlled with trandolapril monotherapy, a diuretic may be added.

In patients being treated with a diuretic, symptomatic hypotension can occasionally occur following the initial dose of trandolapril. To reduce the likelihood of hypotension, if possible, discontinue the diuretic 2 to 3 days prior to beginning therapy with trandolapril. If blood pressure is not controlled with trandolapril alone, resume diuretic therapy. If the diuretic cannot be discontinued, give an initial dose of 0.5 mg trandolapril with careful medical supervision for several hours until blood pressure has stabilized. Titrate dosage as described above to the optimal response.

Renal/hepatic function impairment: For patients with a creatinine clearance < 30 ml/min or with hepatic cirrhosis, the recommended starting dose, based on clinical and pharmacokinetic data, is 0.5 mg/day. Titrate as described above to the optimal response.

Rx	**Mavik** (Knoll)	**Tablets:** 1 mg	Salmon, scored. (KNOLL 1). In 100s and UD 100s.
		2 mg	Yellow. (KNOLL 2). In 100s and UD 100s.
		4 mg	Rose. (KNOLL 4). In 100s and UD 100s.

ANGIOTENSIN II RECEPTOR ANTAGONISTS

> **Warning:**
> *Pregnancy:* When used in pregnancy during the second and third trimesters, drugs that act directly on the renin-angiotensin system can cause injury and even death to the developing fetus. When pregnancy is detected, discontinue angiotensin II receptor antagonists as soon as possible. See Warnings.

Actions:

Pharmacology: **Losartan** and **valsartan** are angiotensin II receptor (type AT_1) antagonists. Angiotensin II (formed from angiotensin I in a reaction catalyzed by angiotensin converting enzyme [ACE; kininase II]) is a potent vasoconstrictor, the primary vasoactive hormone of the renin-angiotensin system and an important component in the pathophysiology of hypertension. Its effects are vasoconstriction, stimulation of synthesis and release of aldosterone, cardiac stimulation and renal absorption of sodium. Angiotensin II receptor antagonists (AIIRAs) block the vasoconstrictor and aldosterone-secreting effects of angiotensin II by selectively blocking the binding of angiotensin II to the AT_1 receptor found in many tissues (eg, vascular smooth muscle, adrenal gland). There is also an AT_2 receptor found in many tissues, but it is not known to be associated with cardiovascular homeostasis. AIIRAs do not exhibit any partial agonist activity at the AT_1 receptor and have much greater affinity (≈ 1000-fold, losartan; ≈ 20,000-fold, valsartan) for the AT_1 receptor than for the AT_2 receptor. In vitro binding studies indicate that losartan is a reversible, competitive inhibitor of the AT_1 receptor. The active metabolite is 10 to 40 times more potent by weight than losartan and appears to be a reversible, non-competitive inhibitor of the AT_1 receptor. The primary metabolite of valsartan is essentially inactive with an affinity for the AT_1 receptor ≈ 1⁄200 that of valsartan itself.

AIIRAs do not inhibit ACE (kininase II, the enzyme that converts angiotensin I to angiotensin II and degrades bradykinin), nor do they bind to or block other hormone receptors or ion channels known to be important in cardiovascular regulation.

AIIRAs inhibit the pressor effect of angiotensin II (as well as angiotensin I) infusions. Removal of the negative feedback of angiotensin II causes a 2- to 3-fold rise in plasma renin activity and a consequent rise in angiotensin II plasma concentration in hypertensive patients. The resulting increased plasma renin activity and angiotensin II circulating levels are insufficient to alter the effects of AIIRAs on blood pressure. AIIRAs do not affect the response to bradykinin, whereas ACE inhibitors do increase the response. In spite of the decreasing aldosterone secretion, AIIRAs have very little effect on serum potassium.

AIIRAs have no effect on glomerular filtration rate, renal plasma flow, filtration fraction, creatinine clearance (valsartan), renal prostaglandin concentrations (losartan), fasting triglycerides, total cholesterol or HDL-cholesterol (losartan) or fasting glucose concentrations. There was a small uricosuric effect with losartan leading to a minimal decrease in serum uric acid (mean decrease < 0.4 mg/dl) during chronic oral administration.

Pharmacokinetics:

Angiotensin II Antagonist Pharmacokinetics		
Parameters	Losartan (metabolite)	Valsartan
Bioavailability	≈33%	≈ 25%
Food effect (AUC/C_{max})	↓10%	↓40%/↓50%
Plasma bound	98.7% (99.2%)	95%
C_{max}	1 hr (4 hrs)	2 to 4 hrs
Volume of distribution	≈ 34 L (≈ 12 L)	17 L
Converted to metabolite	≈ 14%	≈ 9%
Terminal half-life	≈ 2 hrs (6 to 9 hrs)	≈ 6 hrs[1]
Total plasma clearance	≈ 600 ml/min (≈ 50 ml/min)	≈ 2 L/hr[1]
Renal clearance	≈ 75 ml/min (≈ 25 ml/min)	≈ 0.62 L/hr[1]
Excreted unchanged in the urine	≈ 4% (≈ 6%)	13%
Recovered in the urine	≈ 35%	13%
Recovered in the feces	≈60%	83%

[1] IV dosing.

ANGIOTENSIN II RECEPTOR ANTAGONISTS

AIIRAs do not accumulate in plasma upon repeated once-daily dosing.

Losartan undergoes substantial first-pass metabolism and is converted to an active carboxylic acid metabolite (14% of dose) that is responsible for most of the angiotensin II receptor antagonism. Cytochrome P450 2C9 and 3A4 isozymes are involved in losartan's biotransformation.

Valsartan is metabolized only to a small extent (< 10% of the systemically available dose) and the main metabolite is significantly less potent than valsartan in animal models. The enzyme(s) responsible for valsartan metabolism have not been identified but do seem to be cytochrome P450 isozymes.

AIIRAs are highly bound to serum proteins (≥ 95%), primarily to albumin.

Clinical trials:

Losartan – In four studies of losartan monotherapy (n = 1075) the 10 to 25 mg doses produced some effect at peak (6 hours after dosing) but small and inconsistent trough (24 hour) responses. Doses of 50, 100 and 150 mg once daily gave statistically significant systolic/diastolic mean decreases in blood pressure, compared with placebo in the range of 5.5 to 10.5/3.5 to 7.5 mmHg, with the 150 mg dose giving no greater effect than 50 to 100 mg. Twice daily dosing at 50 to 100 mg/day gave consistently larger trough responses than once-daily dosing at the same total dose. Peak (6 hour) effects were uniformly, but moderately, larger than trough effects, with the trough-to-peak ratio for systolic and diastolic responses 50% to 95% and 60% to 90%, respectively.

Addition of low dose hydrochlorothiazide (12.5 mg) to losartan 50 mg once daily resulted in placebo adjusted blood pressure reductions of 15.5/9.2 mmHg.

African-American patients had notably smaller responses to losartan monotherapy.

The effect of losartan is substantially present within 1 week, but in some studies the maximal effect occurred in 3 to 6 weeks. In long-term follow-up studies (without placebo control) the effect of losartan appeared to be maintained for up to 1 year. There is no apparent rebound effect after abrupt withdrawal of losartan. There was essentially no change in average heart rate in losartan-treated patients in controlled trials.

Valsartan – The 7 studies of valsartan monotherapy included over 2000 patients randomized to various doses of valsartan and ≈ 800 patients randomized to placebo. Doses < 80 mg were not consistently distinguished from those of placebo at trough, but doses of 80, 160 and 320 mg produced dose-related decreases in systolic and diastolic blood pressure, with the difference from placebo of ≈ 6 to 8/3 to 5 mmHg at 80 to 160 mg and 9/6 mmHg at 320 mg. In a controlled trial, the addition of HCTZ to valsartan 80 mg resulted in additional lowering of systolic and diastolic blood pressure by ≈ 6/3 and 12/5 mmHg for 12.5 and 25 mg of HCTZ, respectively, compared with valsartan 80 mg alone.

Patients with an inadequate response to 80 mg once daily were titrated to either 160 mg once daily or 80 mg twice daily, which resulted in a comparable response in both groups.

In controlled trials, the antihypertensive effect of once-daily valsartan 80 mg was similar to that of once-daily enalapril 20 mg or once-daily lisinopril 10 mg.

In a clinical trial, valsartan 80 mg/day was as effective as amlodipine 5 mg/day in the treatment of mild to moderate hypertension.

Indications:

Hypertension: Treatment of hypertension alone or in combination with other antihypertensive agents.

Unlabeled uses: These agents may be beneficial in the treatment of heart failure; however, further studies are needed.

Contraindications:

Hypersensitivity to any component of these products.

Warnings:

Hypotension/Volume- or Salt-depleted patients: In patients who are intravascularly volume-depleted (eg, those treated with diuretics), symptomatic hypotension may occur. Correct these conditions prior to administration. Use a lower starting dose of AIIRAs and monitor closely.

Race: In controlled trials, **losartan** had an effect on blood pressure that was notably less in African-American patients than in non-African-Americans, a finding similar to ACE inhibitors.

Cough: In trials where **valsartan** was compared with an ACE inhibitor with or without placebo, the incidence of dry cough was significantly greater in the ACE inhibitor

ANGIOTENSIN II RECEPTOR ANTAGONISTS

group (7.9%) than in the groups who received valsartan (2.6%) or placebo (1.5%). In patients who had dry cough when previously receiving ACE inhibitors, the incidences of cough in patients who received AIIRAs, HCTZ or lisinopril were ≈ 22.5%, ≈18% and 69% respectively.

There was no significant difference between **losartan** and placebo.

Gender: Plasma concentrations of **losartan** were about twice as high in female hypertensives than male hypertensives, but concentrations of the active metabolite were similar in males and females. No dosage adjustment is necessary.

Renal function impairment:

Losartan – As a consequence of inhibiting the renin-angiotensin-aldosterone system, changes in renal function may be anticipated in susceptible individuals. In patients whose renal function may depend on the activity of the renin-angiotensin-aldosterone system (eg, patients with severe CHF), treatment with ACE inhibitors has been associated with oliguria or progressive azotemia and with acute renal failure or death (rarely). In studies of ACE inhibitors in patients with unilateral or bilateral renal artery stenosis, increases in serum creatinine or BUN have been reported. AIIRAs would be expected to behave similarly. In some patients, these effects were reversible upon discontinuation of therapy. No dosage adjustment is necessary for patients with renal impairment unless they are volume-depleted.

Plasma concentrations of losartan are not altered in patients with creatinine clearance (Ccr) > 30 ml/min. In patients with lower Ccr, AUCs are ≈ 50% greater and they are doubled in hemodialysis patients. Plasma concentrations of the active metabolite are not significantly altered in patients with renal impairment or in hemodialysis patients.

Valsartan – There is no apparent correlation between renal function (measured by Ccr) and exposure (measured by AUC) to valsartan in patients with different degrees of renal impairment. No studies have been performed in patients with severe impairment of renal function (Ccr < 10 ml/min) or patients undergoing dialysis and it is unknown whether valsartan is removed by hemodialysis. In the case of severe renal disease, exercise care with valsartan dosing.

In studies of ACE inhibitors with unilateral or bilateral renal artery stenosis, increases in serum creatinine or BUN have been reported. In a 4–day trial of valsartan in 12 patients with unilateral renal artery stenosis, no significant increases in serum creatinine or BUN were observed. There has been no long-term use of valsartan in patients with unilateral or bilateral renal artery stenosis, but an effect similar to that seen with ACE inhibitors should be anticipated.

Hepatic function impairment:

Losartan – Following administration in patients with mild to moderate alcoholic cirrhosis of the liver, plasma concentrations of losartan and its active metabolite were, respectively, 5 times and ≈ 1.7 times those in young male volunteers. Compared with healthy subjects, the total plasma clearance in patients with hepatic insufficiency was ≈ 50% lower and the oral bioavailability was ≈ 2 times higher. A lower starting dose is recommended for patients with a history of hepatic impairment (see Administration and Dosage).

Valsartan – On average, patients with mild-to-moderate chronic liver disease have twice the exposure (measured by AUC values) to valsartan of healthy volunteers (matched by age, sex and weight). In general, no dosage adjustment is needed in patients with mild-to-moderate liver disease. Care should be exercised, however in this patient population.

Carcinogenesis/Fertility impairment: Female rats given the highest dose (270 mg/kg/day) of **losartan** had a slightly higher incidence of pancreatic acinar adenoma.

Valsartan had no evidence of carcinogenicity (doses 2.5 to 6 times the maximum human dose) or mutagenicity when administered to mice and rats.

The administration of toxic dosage levels of losartan in females was associated with a significant decrease in the number of corpora lutea/female, implants/female and live fetuses/female at C-section. At 100 mg/kg/day only a decrease in the number of corpora lutea/female was observed. Fertility and reproducative performance in male rats were not affected.

Valsartan had no adverse effects on the reproductive performances of male or female rats at oral doses ≤ 200 mg/kg/day (6 times the maximum recommended human dose).

Elderly: No dosage adjustment is necessary when initiating AIIRAs in the elderly. No overall differences in effectiveness or safety of **losartan** were observed between elderly patients and younger patients, but greater sensitivity of some older individuals cannot be ruled out.

ANGIOTENSIN II RECEPTOR ANTAGONISTS

Pregnancy: Category C (first trimester); Category D (second and third trimesters). Drugs that act directly on the renin-angiotensin system can cause fetal and neonatal morbidity and death when administered to pregnant women. Several dozen cases have been reported in patients who were taking ACE inhibitors. When pregnancy is detected, discontinue AIIRAs as soon as possible.

The use of drugs that act directly on the renin-angiotensin system during the second and third trimesters of pregnancy has been associated with fetal and neonatal injury, including hypotension, neonatal skull hypoplasia, anuria, reversible or irreversible renal failure and death. Oligohydramnios has also been reported, presumably resulting from decreased fetal renal function; oligohydramnios, in this setting, has been associated with fetal limb contractures, craniofacial deformation and hypoplastic lung development. Prematurity, intrauterine growth retardation and patent ductus arteriosus have also been reported, although, it is not clear whether these occurrences were caused by exposure to the drug. These adverse effects do not appear to have resulted from intrauterine drug exposure limited to the first trimester.

Mothers whose embryos and fetuses are exposed to an AIIRAs only during the first trimester should be informed. Nonetheless, when patients become pregnant, physicians should have the patient discontinue the use of AIIRAs as soon as possible.

Rarely (probably < 1/1000 pregnancies), no alternative to an AIIRAs will be found. In these rare cases, apprise the mother of the potential hazards to their fetus, and perform serial ultrasound examinations to assess the intra-amniotic environment.

If oligohydramnios is observed, discontinue the drug unless it is considered life-saving for the mother. Contraction stress testing (CST), a non-stress test (NST) or biophysical profiling (BPP) may be appropriate, depending on the week of pregnancy. However, patients and physicians should be aware that oligohydramnios may not appear until after the fetus has sustained irreversible injury.

Closely observe infants with histories of in utero exposure to an AIIRAs for hypotension, oliguria and hyperkalemia. If oliguria occurs, direct attention toward support of blood pressure and renal perfusion. Exchange transfusion or dialysis may be required as means of reversing hypotension or substituting for disordered renal function.

AIIRAs have been shown to produce adverse effects in rat fetuses and neonates, including decreased birth weight, delayed physical and behavioral development, mortality and renal toxicity. Significant levels of **losartan** and its active metabolite were shown to be present in rat fetal plasma during late gestation.

Lactation: AIIRAs were present in rat milk. Because of the potential for adverse effects on the nursing infant, decide whether to discontinue nursing or discontinue the drug, taking into account the importance of the drug to the mother.

Children: Safety and efficacy in patients < 18 years of age have not been established.

Precautions:

Lab test abnormalities:

Liver function tests – Occasional elevations (> 150% in **valsartan** treated patients) of liver enzymes or serum bilirubin have occurred.

Creatinine/Blood urea nitrogen (BUN) – Minor increases in BUN or serum creatinine were observed in < 0.1% of patients with essential hypertension treated with **losartan** alone and in 0.8% of patients taking **valsartan**.

Hemoglobin and hematocrit – Small decreases in hemoglobin and hematocrit occurred frequently in patients treated with **losartan** alone but were rarely of clinical importance. Greater than 20% decreases in hemoglobin and hematocrit were observed in 0.4% and 0.8%, respectively, of **valsartan** patients, vs 0.1% and 0.1% with placebo.

Serum potassium – Greater than 20% increases in serum potassium were observed in 4.4% of **valsartan**-treated patients compared to 2.9% of placebo-treated patients.

ANGIOTENSIN II RECEPTOR ANTAGONISTS

Drug Interactions:

Losartan Drug Interactions			
Precipitant drug	Object drug*		Description
Cimetidine	Losartan	⟷	Coadministration led to an increase of ≈ 18% in AUC of losartan but did not affect the disposition of its active metabolite. The relevance of this reaction is unknown.
Phenobarbital	Losartan	⟷	Coadministration led to a reduction of ≈ 20% in the AUC of losartan and its active metabolite. The clinical relevance of this reaction is unknown.

* ⟷ = Undetermined effect.

In vitro studies show significant inhibition of the formation of the active metabolite of **losartan** by inhibitors of cytochrome P450 3A4 (eg, ketoconazole, troleandomycin) or P450 2C9 (sulfaphenazole) and nearly complete inhibition by the combination of sulfaphenazole and ketoconazole. The pharmacodynamic consequences of concomitant use of losartan and these inhibitors have not been examined.

Drug/Food interactions: A meal slows absorption of AIIRAs and decreases its C_{max} but has only minor effects on **losartan** AUC or on the AUC of the metabolite (≈ 10% decreased). Food decreases **valsartan**'s C_{max} by 50% and its AUC by 40%.

Adverse Reactions:

In general, treatment with **losartan** and **valsartan** was well tolerated. In controlled clinical trials, discontinuation of therapy because of clinical adverse experiences was required in 2.3% of patients treated with losartan or valsartan vs 3.7% and 2%, respectively, of patients given placebo.

Angiotensin II Antagonist Adverse Reactions (%)[1]		
Adverse Reactions	Losartan	Valsartan
CNS		
Dizziness	3.5	>1
Insomnia	1.4	2
Headache	-	>1
Fatigue	-	2
GI		
Diarrhea	2.4	>1
Dyspepsia	1.3	2
Nausea	-	> 1
Abdominal pain	-	2
Musculoskeletal		
Arthralgia	-	> 1
Back pain	1.8	-
Muscle cramp	1.1	-
Myalgia	1	-
Leg pain	1	-
Respiratory		
Upper respiratory infection	7.9	> 1
Cough[2]	3.4	> 1
Nasal congestion	2	-
Sinus disorder	1.5	-
Sinusitis	1	> 1
Pharyngitis	-	> 1
Rhinitis	-	> 1
Miscellaneous		
Viral infection	-	3
Edema	-	> 1

[1] All events. Data are pooled from separate studies and are not necessarily comparable.
[2] See warnings.

ANGIOTENSIN II RECEPTOR ANTAGONISTS

The following adverse events were also reported at a rate of ≥ 1% in losartan patients but were ≤ placebo: Asthenia/fatigue; edema/swelling; chest pain; abdominal pain; nausea; headache; pharyngitis.

In addition to the adverse events above, potentially important events that occurred in at least two patients or other adverse events that occurred in < 1% of patients in clinical studies are listed below. Causal relationship is unknown.

Body as a whole:

Losartan – Facial edema, fever, orthostatic effects, syncope, gout.

Cardiovascular:

Losartan – Angina pectoris, second degree AV block, CVA, hypotension, myocardial infarction, arrhythmias including atrial fibrillation, palpitation, sinus bradycardia, tachycardia, ventricular tachycardia, ventricular fibrillation.

Dermatologic:

Losartan – Alopecia, dermatitis, dry skin, ecchymosis, erythema, flushing, photosensitivity, pruritus, rash, sweating, urticaria; superficial peeling of palms (one patient).

Gastrointestinal:

Losartan – Anorexia, constipation, dental pain, dry mouth, flatulence, gastritis, vomiting.

Genito-urinary:

Losartan – Impotence, nocturia, urinary frequency, urinary tract infection.

Hematologic:

Losartan – Anemia; hemolysis (one patient).

Hypersensitivity:

Losartan – A patient with known hypersensitivity to aspirin and penicillin, when treated with losartan, was withdrawn from study because of swelling of the lips and eyelids and facial rash, reported as angioedema, which returned to normal 5 days after therapy was discontinued.

Musculoskeletal:

Losartan – Arm/hip/knee/shoulder/musculoskeletal pain, joint swelling, stiffness, arthralgia, arthritis, fibromyalgia, muscle weakness.

Psychiatric:

Losartan – Anxiety, anxiety disorder, ataxia, confusion, depression, dream abnormality, hypesthesia, decreased libido, memory impairment, migraine, nervousness, paresthesia, peripheral neuropathy, panic disorder, sleep disorder, somnolence, tremor, vertigo.

Respiratory:

Losartan – Dyspnea, bronchitis, pharyngeal discomfort, epistaxis, rhinitis, respiratory congestion.

Special senses:

Losartan – Blurred vision, burning/stinging in the eye, conjunctivitis, taste perversion, tinnitus, decrease in visual acuity.

Miscellaneous:

Valsartan –

Dyspnea, impotence, palpitations, vertigo.

Overdosage:

Significant lethality was observed in mice and rats after oral administration of 1000 and 2000 mg/kg of **losartan**, respectively, about 44 and 170 times the maximum recommended human dose. The most likely manifestation of overdosage would be hypotension and tachycardia; bradycardia could occur from parasympathetic (vagal) stimulation. If symptomatic hypotension should occur, institute supportive treatment. Refer to General Management of Acute Overdosage. Neither losartan nor its active metabolite can be removed by hemodialysis. It is not known whether **valsartan** or its active metabolite can be removed by hemodialysis.

Patient Information:

Tell patients of childbearing age about the consequences of second- and third-trimester exposure to drugs that act on the renin-angiotensin system, and tell them that these consequences do not appear to have resulted from intrauterine drug exposure that has been limited to the first trimester. Ask these patients to report pregnancies to their physicians as soon as possible.

Angiotensin II Receptor Antagonists

LOSARTAN POTASSIUM

Administration and Dosage:

Approved by the FDA on April 14, 1995.

The usual starting dose is 50 mg once daily, with 25 mg used in patients with possible depletion of intravascular volume (eg, patients treated with diuretics; see Warnings) and patients with a history of hepatic impairment (see Warnings). Losartan can be administered with or without food once or twice daily with total daily doses ranging from 25 to 100 mg.

If the antihypertensive effect measured at trough using once daily dosing is inadequate, a twice daily regimen at the same total daily dose or an increase in dose may give a more satisfactory response.

Losartan may be administered with other antihypertensive agents. If blood pressure is not controlled by losartan alone, a low dose of a diuretic may be added. Hydrochlorothiazide has an additive effect.

Elderly: No initial dosage adjustment is necessary for elderly patients.

Renal function impairment: No initial dosage adjustment is necessary for patients with renal impairment, including patients on dialysis.

Rx	**Cozaar** (Merck)	**Tablets:** 25 mg	Lactose. 2.12 mg potassium. (MRK 951). Lt. green. Teardrop shape. Film coated. In 90s, 100s and UD 100s.
		50 mg	Lactose. 4.24 mg potassium. (MRK 952 Cozaar). Green. Teardrop shape. Film coated. In 30s, 90s, 100s, 1000s and UD 100s.

VALSARTAN

Administration and Dosage:

Approved by the FDA on December 23, 1996.

The recommended starting dose is 80 mg daily, with or without food, when used as monotherapy in patients who are not volume-depleted. Valsartan may be used over a dose range of 80 to 320 mg once daily.

The antihypertensive effect is substantially present ≤ 2 weeks and maximal reduction is generally attained > 4 weeks. If additional antihypertensive effect is required, the dosage may be increased to 160 or 320 mg or a diuretic may be added. Addition of a diuretic has a greater effect than dose increases beyond 80 mg. Valsartan may be administered with other antihypertensive agents.

Elderly: No initial dosage adjustment is necessary for elderly patients.

Hepatic/renal function impairment: While no initial dosage adjustment is necessary in patients with mild to moderate renal of hepatic insufficiency, care should be exercised when dosing patients with hepatic or severe renal function impairment.

Rx	**Diovan** (Ciba-Geigy)	**Capsules:** 80 mg	(CG FZF). Lt. grey/lt. pink opaque. In 100s, 4000s and UD blister 100s.
		160 mg	(CG GOG). Dark grey/lt. pink opaque. In 100s, 4000s and UD blister 100s.

Agents for Pheochromocytoma

PHENTOLAMINE

Refer to the general discussion of these products in the Antihypertensives Introduction.

Actions:

Pharmacology: Phentolamine, an α-adrenergic blocking agent, blocks presynaptic (α_2) and postsynaptic (α_1) α-adrenergic receptors. It is a competitive antagonist of endogenous and exogenous α-active agents. It also acts on both the arterial tree and venous bed. Thus, total peripheral resistance is lowered and venous return to the heart is diminished. Phentolamine also causes cardiac stimulation.

Phentolamine has an immediate onset and a short duration of action.

Indications:

Pheochromocytoma: Prevention or control of hypertensive episodes that may occur in a patient with pheochromocytoma as a result of stress or manipulation during preoperative preparation and surgical excision.

Pharmacological test for pheochromocytoma (not the method of choice – see Warnings).

Prevention and treatment of dermal necrosis and sloughing following IV administration or extravasation of norepinephrine or dopamine.

Unlabeled uses: Phentolamine has been used to treat hypertensive crises secondary to MAO inhibitor/sympathomimetic amine interactions and rebound hypertension on withdrawal of clonidine, propranolol or other antihypertensives. It has also been used in combination with papaverine as an intracavernous injection for impotence.

Contraindications:

Myocardial infarction, coronary insufficiency, angina or other evidence suggestive of coronary artery disease. Hypersensitivity to phentolamine or related compounds.

Warnings:

Myocardial infarction, cerebrovascular spasm and cerebrovascular occlusion have followed phentolamine administration, usually in association with marked hypotensive episodes with shock-like states which occasionally follow parenteral use.

For screening tests in patients with hypertension, the generally available urinary assay of catecholamines or other biochemical assays have largely supplanted phentolamine and other pharmacological tests. None of the chemical or pharmacological tests are infallible in the diagnosis of pheochromocytoma. The phentolamine test is not the procedure of choice; reserve for cases in which additional confirmatory evidence is necessary and consider the risks involved.

Pregnancy and Lactation: Safety for use during pregnancy or lactation has not been established. Use only when clearly needed and when the potential benefits outweigh the potential hazards to the fetus or nursing infant.

Precautions:

Tachycardia and cardiac arrhythmias may occur with phentolamine use. When possible, defer use of cardiac glycosides until cardiac rhythm returns to normal.

Drug Interactions:

Epinephrine and ephedrine: The vasoconstricting and hypertensive effects of these drugs are antagonized by phentolamine.

Adverse Reactions:

Acute and prolonged hypotensive episodes, tachycardia and cardiac arrhythmias.

Weakness; dizziness; flushing; orthostatic hypotension; nasal stuffiness; nausea; vomiting and diarrhea.

Overdosage:

If blood pressure drops to a dangerous level or other evidence of shock occurs, treat vigorously and promptly. Include IV infusion of norepinephrine, titrated to maintain normal blood pressure. Epinephrine is contraindicated because it stimulates both α- and β-receptors; since α-receptors are blocked, the net effect of epinephrine administration is vasodilation and a further drop in blood pressure (epinephrine reversal).

Agents for Pheochromocytoma

PHENTOLAMINE

Administration and Dosage:

Prevention or control of hypertensive episodes in pheochromocytoma: For use in preoperative reduction of elevated blood pressure, inject 5 mg (1 mg for children) IV or IM 1 or 2 hours before surgery. Repeat if necessary. During surgery, administer 5 mg for adults (1 mg for children) IV as indicated to help prevent or control paroxysms of hypertension, tachycardia, respiratory depression, convulsions or other effects of epinephrine intoxication.

Postoperatively, norepinephrine may be given to control hypotension which may follow complete removal of a pheochromocytoma.

Prevention and treatment of dermal necrosis and sloughing following IV administration or extravasation of norepinephrine:: For prevention, add 10 mg to each liter of solution containing norepinephrine. The pressor effect of norepinephrine is not affected. For treatment, inject 5 to 10 mg in 10 ml saline into the area of extravasation within 12 hours. For children, use 0.1 to 0.2 mg/kg up to a maximum of 10 mg.

Diagnosis of pheochromocytoma (phentolamine blocking test): Withhold sedatives, analgesics and all other medication not considered essential for at least 24 hours (preferably 48 to 72 hours) prior to the test. Withhold antihypertensive drugs until blood pressure returns to the untreated, hypertensive level. Do not perform the test on normotensive patients. Keep patient at rest in supine position throughout the test, preferably in a quiet, darkened room. Delay injection until blood pressure is stabilized, as evidenced by blood pressure readings taken every 10 minutes for at least 30 minutes.

IV test – Although a 5 mg test dose (1 mg for children) has been recommended, a 2.5 mg test dose will produce fewer false-positive tests and may minimize dangerous drops in blood pressure in patients with pheochromocytoma. If the 2.5 mg dose is negative, perform a 5 mg test before considering the test negative. Dissolve 5 mg phentolamine mesylate in 1 ml Sterile Water for Injection. Insert the syringe needle into a vein and delay injection until pressor response to venipuncture has subsided. Inject rapidly. Record blood pressure immediately, at 30 second intervals for the first 3 minutes, then at 60 second intervals for the next 7 minutes.

Positive response, suggestive of pheochromocytoma, is indicated by a drop in blood pressure of more than 35 mm Hg systolic and 25 mm Hg diastolic pressure. A typical positive response is a pressure reduction of 60 mm Hg systolic and 25 mm Hg diastolic. Maximal decrease in pressure is usually evident within 2 minutes after injection. Return to preinjection pressure commonly occurs within 15 to 30 minutes, but may return more rapidly. If blood pressure falls to a dangerous level, treat patient as outlined in the Overdosage section. Always confirm a positive response by other diagnostic procedures, preferably the measurement of urinary catecholamines or their metabolites.

Negative response is indicated when the blood pressure is unchanged, elevated or is reduced less than 35 mm Hg systolic and 25 mm Hg diastolic after injection. A negative response may not exclude the diagnosis of pheochromocytoma, especially in patients with paroxysmal hypertension in whom the incidence of false-negative response is high.

IM test – Preparation is the same as for the IV test. Adult dosage is 5 mg IM; for children it is 3 mg. Record blood pressure every 5 minutes for 30 to 45 minutes following IM injection. Positive response is indicated by a drop in blood pressure of 35 mm Hg systolic and 25 mm Hg diastolic or greater within 20 minutes following injection.

Reliability – The test is most reliable in patients with sustained hypertension and least reliable in those with paroxysmal hypertension. False-positive tests may occur in patients with hypertension without pheochromocytoma.

Storage: Store between 15° to 30°C (59° to 86°F). Use reconstituted solution upon preparation; do not store.

Rx	**Regitine** (Ciba Pharm.)	**Injection:** 5 mg (as mesylate) per vial.[1]	In 1 ml vials.

[1] With 25 mg sterile, lyophilized mannitol.

Agents for Pheochromocytoma

PHENOXYBENZAMINE HCl

Refer to the general discussion of these products in the Antihypertensives Introduction.

Actions:

Pharmacology: An irreversible alpha-adrenergic receptor (both pre- and postsynaptic) blocking agent which can produce and maintain "chemical sympathectomy." It increases blood flow to skin, mucosa and abdominal viscera, and lowers supine and standing blood pressures. It has no effect on the parasympathetic system.

Pharmacokinetics: Absorption from the GI tract is incomplete (20% to 30%).

Indications:

Pheochromocytoma, to control episodes of hypertension and sweating. If tachycardia is excessive, it may also be necessary to use a beta-blocker concomitantly.

Unlabeled uses: Phenoxybenzamine (5 to 60 mg/day) has shown efficacy in micturition disorders resulting from neurogenic bladder, functional outlet obstruction and partial prostatic obstruction.

Contraindications:

Conditions where a fall in blood pressure may be undesirable.

Warnings:

Concomitant therapy: Phenoxybenzamine-induced alpha-adrenergic blockade leaves beta-adrenergic receptors unopposed. Compounds that stimulate both types of receptors (ie, epinephrine) may produce an exaggerated hypotensive response and tachycardia.

Carcinogenesis/Mutagenesis: Phenoxybenzamine has shown in vitro mutagenic activity in the Ames test and in the mouse lymphoma assay. In animals, repeated intraperitoneal phenoxybenzamine resulted in peritoneal sarcomas; chronic oral dosing produced malignant GI tract tumors. Clinical significance is not established. Nevertheless, consider these results in determining benefit-to-risk ratio.

Precautions:

Administer with caution to patients with marked cerebral or coronary arteriosclerosis or renal damage. Adrenergic blocking effects may aggravate respiratory infections.

Adverse Reactions:

Nasal congestion, miosis, postural hypotension, tachycardia and inhibition of ejaculation may occur. They vary according to degree of adrenergic blockade, and tend to decrease as therapy continues. GI irritation, drowsiness and fatigue also occur.

Overdosage:

Symptoms: may include postural hypotension resulting in dizziness or fainting; tachycardia, particularly postural; vomiting; lethargy; shock. These are largely due to block of the sympathetic nervous system and of the circulating epinephrine.

Treatment: Discontinue the drug. Treat circulatory failure, if present. In mild overdosage, recumbent position with legs elevated usually restores cerebral circulation. In more severe cases, institute measures to combat shock. Usual pressor agents are not effective. Do not use epinephrine (see Warnings). The patient may have to be kept flat 24 hours or more as drug's effect is prolonged. Leg bandages and an abdominal binder may shorten disability period. May use norepinephrine IV to combat severe hypotension; it primarily stimulates alpha receptors. Although phenoxybenzamine is an alpha-blocker, sufficient norepinephrine will overcome this effect.

Patient Information:

Avoid alcoholic beverages.

If dizziness (postural hypotension) occurs, avoid sudden changes in posture.

Medication may cause nasal congestion and constricted pupils. Inhibition of ejaculation may occur, but generally decreases with continued therapy.

Avoid cough, cold or allergy medications containing sympathomimetics, except on professional recommendation.

Administration and Dosage:

Individualize dosage. Slowly increase small initial doses until the desired effect is obtained or side effects become troublesome. Observe patient before increasing dosage. Increase to a point where symptomatic relief or objective improvement are obtained, but not so high that blockade side effects become troublesome.

Initially, 10 mg twice a day. Increase dosage every other day until optimal dosage is obtained as judged by blood pressure control. Usual dosage range is 20 to 40 mg, 2 or 3 times daily. In children, give 1 to 2 mg/kg/day, divided every 6 to 8 hours.

Rx	**Dibenzyline** (SKF)	**Capsules:** 10 mg.	(SKF E33). Red. In 100s.

Agents for Pheochromocytoma

METYROSINE

Refer to the general discussion of these products in the Antihypertensives Introduction.

Actions:

Pharmacology: Metyrosine inhibits tyrosine hydroxylase, which catalyzes the first transformation in catecholamine biosynthesis, ie, the conversion of tyrosine to dihydroxyphenylalanine (DOPA). Because this is the rate-limiting step, hydroxylase blockade results in decreased endogenous levels of catecholamines, usually measured as decreased urinary excretion of catecholamines and their metabolites.

In patients with pheochromocytoma who produce excessive amounts of norepinephrine and epinephrine, 1 to 4 g/day has reduced catecholamine biosynthesis from about 35% to 80%, as measured by the total excretion of catecholamines and their metabolites (metanephrine and vanillylmandelic acid). The maximum biochemical effect usually occurs within 2 to 3 days; the urinary concentration of catecholamines and their metabolites usually returns to pretreatment levels within 3 to 4 days after discontinuation. In some patients, the total excretion of catecholamines and catecholamine metabolites may be lowered to normal or near normal levels (< 10 mg/24 hours). In most patients treatment duration has been 2 to 8 weeks, but several patients have received metyrosine for periods of 1 to 10 years.

Most patients on metyrosine experience decreased frequency and severity of hypertensive attacks with headache, nausea, sweating and tachycardia. In patients who respond, blood pressure decreases progressively during the first 2 days; after withdrawal, it usually increases gradually to pretreatment values in 2 to 3 days.

Pharmacokinetics: Metyrosine is well absorbed from the GI tract. Approximately 53% to 88% (mean 69%) is recovered in the urine as unchanged drug following maintenance oral dosages of 600 to 4000 mg/24 hours. Less than 1% of administered drug is recovered as catechol metabolites. These metabolites are probably not present in sufficient amounts to contribute to the biochemical effects of metyrosine. The quantities excreted, however, are sufficient to interfere with accurate determination of urinary catecholamines determined by routine techniques.

The plasma half-life over 8 hours after single oral doses was 3.4 to 3.7 hours in three patients.

Indications:

Pheochromocytoma: Preoperative preparation of patients; management when surgery is contraindicated; chronic treatment of malignant pheochromocytoma.

Not recommended for the control of essential hypertension.

Contraindications:

Hypersensitivity to metyrosine.

Warnings:

Maintain fluid volume during and after surgery: When metyrosine is used preoperatively, especially with alpha-adrenergic blocking drugs, maintain adequate intravascular volume intraoperatively (especially after tumor removal) and postoperatively to avoid hypotension and decreased perfusion of vital organs resulting from vasodilatation and expanded volume capacity. After tumor removal, large volumes of plasma may be needed to maintain blood and central venous pressure.

Life-threatening arrhythmias may occur during anesthesia and surgery and may require treatment with a beta-blocker or lidocaine. During surgery, monitor blood pressure and ECG continuously.

Intraoperative effects: While the preoperative use of metyrosine is thought to decrease intraoperative problems with blood pressure control, it does not eliminate the danger of hypertensive crises or arrhythmias during manipulation of the tumor. Phentolamine, an alpha-adrenergic blocking drug, may be needed.

Renal/Hepatic function impairment: Use with caution.

Pregnancy: Category C. Safety for use during pregnancy has not been established. Use only when clearly needed and when the potential benefits outweigh the potential hazards to the fetus.

Lactation: It is not known whether metyrosine is excreted in breast milk. Safety for use in the nursing mother has not been established.

Children: Safety and efficacy for use in children under 12 years of age have not been established.

Precautions:

Long-term use: Human experience is limited and chronic animal studies have not been performed. Therefore, perform laboratory tests periodically in patients requiring prolonged metyrosine use, and observe caution with patients with impaired hepatic or renal function.

Agents for Pheochromocytoma

METYROSINE

Metyrosine crystalluria and urolithiasis have been found in dogs treated at doses similar to those used in humans; crystalluria has also been observed in a few patients. To minimize this risk, maintain sufficient water intake to achieve a daily urine volume of 2000 ml or more, particularly with doses greater than 2 g/day. Routinely examine the urine. Metyrosine will crystallize as needles or rods. If crystalluria occurs, further increase fluid intake; if it persists, reduce dosage or discontinue use.

Drug Interactions:

Phenothiazines or haloperidol: Extrapyramidal effects of these drugs may be potentiated due to inhibition of catecholamine synthesis by metyrosine.

Drug/Lab test interactions: Spurious increases in urinary catecholamines may be observed due to the presence of metyrosine metabolites.

Adverse Reactions:

CNS: Sedation is most common, moderate to severe at low and high dosages. Sedative effects begin within the first 24 hours of therapy, are maximal after 2 to 3 days and tend to wane during the next few days. Sedation usually is not obvious after 1 week unless the dosage is increased, but at dosages greater than 2 g/day, some degree of sedation or fatigue may persist.

In most patients who experience sedation, temporary changes in sleep pattern (insomnia lasting 2 or 3 days; feelings of increased alertness and ambition) occur following drug withdrawal. Even those not experiencing sedation may report symptoms of psychic stimulation when the drug is discontinued.

Headache is reported infrequently.

Extrapyramidal signs Drooling, speech difficulty and tremor (10%), occasionally accompanied by trismus and frank parkinsonism.

Anxiety and psychic disturbances Depression, hallucinations, disorientation and confusion may be dose-dependent and may disappear with dosage reduction.

GI: Diarrhea (10%) may be severe. May need antidiarrheals if drug is continued. Infrequent – Decreased salivation, dry mouth, nausea, vomiting, abdominal pain.

GU: Infrequent-Impotence or failure to ejaculate. Crystalluria, transient dysuria and hematuria.

Body as a whole: Infrequent-Slight breast swelling, galactorrhea, nasal stuffiness, eosinophilia, anemia, thrombocytopenia, thrombocytosis, increased AST, peripheral edema; hypersensitivity reactions such as urticaria and pharyngeal edema (rare).

Overdosage:

Signs of metyrosine overdosage include those central nervous system effects observed in some patients even at low dosages.

At doses exceeding 2 g/day, some degree of sedation or feeling of fatigue may persist. Doses 2 to 4 g/day can result in anxiety or agitated depression, neuromuscular effects (including fine tremor of the hands, gross tremor of the trunk, tightening of the jaw with trismus), diarrhea and decreased salivation with dry mouth.

Reducing dose or discontinuing treatment causes these symptoms to disappear.

Patient Information:

Maintain a daily liberal fluid intake.

Avoid alcohol or other CNS depressants.

May cause drowsiness; use caution while performing tasks requiring alertness.

Notify physician if any of the following occur: Drooling, speech difficulty, tremors, disorientation, diarrhea, painful urination.

Administration and Dosage:

Adults and children over 12: Initial dosage is 250 mg 4 times daily. This may be increased by 250 to 500 mg every day to a maximum of 4 g/day in divided doses. When used for preoperative preparation, give the optimally effective dosage for at least 5 to 7 days (between 2 and 3 g/day); titrate by monitoring clinical symptoms and catecholamine excretion. In hypertensive patients, titrate dosage to achieve normal blood pressure and control of clinical symptoms. In normotensive patients, titrate dosage to reduce urinary metanephrines or vanillylmandelic acid by ≥ 50%.

Use in children under 12 years of age is limited and a dosage schedule cannot be given.

If patients are not adequately controlled by metyrosine, add an alpha-adrenergic blocker (phenoxybenzamine).

Rx	**Demser** (MSD)	**Capsules:** 250 mg	(MSD 690 Demser). Two-tone blue. In 100s.

Agents for Hypertensive Emergencies

NITROPRUSSIDE SODIUM

Refer to the general discussion of these products in the Antihypertensives Introduction.

In addition to the agents listed in this section, parenteral forms of methyldopa and hydralazine are also indicated for use in malignant hypertension.

Warning:

After reconstitution, nitroprusside is not suitable for direct injection. The reconstituted solution must be further diluted in 5% Dextrose Injection before infusion (see Administration and Dosage).

Nitroprusside can cause precipitous decreases in blood pressure (see Administration and Dosage). In patients not properly monitored, these decreases can lead to irreversible ischemic injuries or death. Use only when available equipment and personnel allow blood pressure to be continuously monitored.

Except when used briefly or at low (< 2 mcg/kg/min) infusion rates, nitroprusside injection gives rise to important quantities of cyanide ion, which can reach toxic, potentially lethal levels (see Warnings). The usual dose rate is 0.5 to 10 mcg/kg/min, but infusion at the maximum dose rates should never last > 10 minutes. If blood pressure has not been adequately controlled after 10 minutes of infusion at the maximum rate, terminate administration immediately.

Although acid-base balance and venous oxygen concentration should be monitored and may indicate cyanide toxicity, these laboratory tests provide imperfect guidance.

Actions:

Pharmacology: Nitroprusside is a potent IV antihypertensive agent. The principal pharmacological action of nitroprusside is relaxation of vascular smooth muscle and consequent dilation of peripheral arteries and veins. Other smooth muscle (eg, uterus, duodenum) is not affected. Nitroprusside is more active on veins than on arteries, but this selectivity is much less marked than that of nitroglycerin. Dilation of the veins promotes peripheral pooling of blood and decreases venous return to the heart, thereby reducing left ventricular end-diastolic pressure and pulmonary capillary wedge pressure (preload). Arteriolar relaxation reduces systemic vascular resistance, systolic arterial pressure and mean arterial pressure (afterload). Dilation of the coronary arteries also occurs.

In association with the decrease in blood pressure, nitroprusside administered IV to hypertensive and normotensive patients produces slight increases in heart rate and a variable effect on cardiac output. In hypertensive patients, moderate doses induce renal vasodilation roughly proportional to the decrease in systemic blood pressure, so there is no appreciable change in renal blood flow or glomerular filtration rate.

In normotensive subjects, acute reduction of mean arterial pressure to 60 to 75 mmHg by infusion of nitroprusside caused a significant increase in renin activity. In the same study, 10 renovascular-hypertensive patients given nitroprusside had significant increases in renin release from the involved kidney at mean arterial pressures of 90 to 137 mmHg.

The hypotensive effect of nitroprusside is seen within 1 to 2 minutes after the start of an adequate infusion, and it dissipates almost as rapidly after an infusion is discontinued. The effect is augmented by ganglionic blocking agents and inhaled anesthetics.

Pharmacokinetics: Infused nitroprusside is rapidly distributed to a volume that is approximately coextensive with the extracellular space. The drug is cleared from this volume by intraerythrocytic reaction with hemoglobin (HgB), and nitroprusside's resulting circulatory half-life is about 2 minutes.

The products of the nitroprusside/HgB reaction are cyanmethemoglobin (cyanmetHgB) and cyanide ion (CN^-). Safe use of nitroprusside injection must be guided by knowledge of the further metabolism of these products. The essential features of nitroprusside metabolism are: One molecule of nitroprusside is metabolized by combination with HgB to produce one molecule of cyanmethemoglobin and four CN^- ions; methemoglobin, obtained from HgB, can sequester cyanide as cyanmethemoglobin; thiosulfate reacts with cyanide to produce thiocyanate (SCN^-); thiocyanate is eliminated in the urine; cyanide, not otherwise removed, binds to cytochromes; cyanide is much more toxic than methemoglobin or thiocyanate.

Agents for Hypertensive Emergencies

NITROPRUSSIDE SODIUM

When the Fe^{+++} of cytochromes is bound to cyanide, the cytochromes are unable to participate in oxidative metabolism. In this situation, cells may be able to provide for their energy needs by utilizing anaerobic pathways, but they thereby generate an increasing body burden of lactic acid. Other cells may be unable to utilize these alternate pathways, and they may die hypoxic deaths.

When CN^- is infused or generated within the bloodstream, essentially all of it is bound to methemoglobin until intraerythrocytic methemoglobin has been saturated. At healthy steady state, most people have < 1% of their HgB in the form of methemoglobin. Nitroprusside metabolism can lead to methemoglobin formation (a) through dissociation of cyanmethemeglobin formed in the original reaction of nitroprusside with HgB and (b) by direct oxidation of HgB by the released nitroso group. Relatively large quantities of nitroprusside, however, are required to produce significant methemoglobinemia.

When thiosulfate is supplied only by normal physiologic mechanisms, conversion of CN^- to SCN^- generally proceeds at about 1 mcg/kg/min. This rate of CN^- clearance corresponds to steady-state processing of a nitroprusside infusion of slightly > 2 mcg/kg/min. CN^- accumulates when nitroprusside infusions exceed this rate.

In patients with normal renal function, clearance of SCN^- is primarily renal, with a half-life of about 3 days. In renal failure, the half-life can be doubled or tripled.

Clinical trials: Nitroprusside has a prompt hypotensive effect, at least initially, in all populations. With increasing rates of infusion, nitroprusside lowers blood pressure without an observed limit of effect. The hypotensive effect of nitroprusside is also associated with reduced blood loss in a variety of major surgical procedures.

In patients with acute congestive heart failure and increased peripheral vascular resistance, administration of nitroprusside causes reductions in peripheral resistance, increases in cardiac output and reductions in left ventricular filling pressure.

Many trials have verified the clinical significance of the metabolic pathways described above. In patients receiving unopposed infusions of nitroprusside, cyanide and thiocyanate levels have increased with increasing rates of nitroprusside infusion. Mild to moderate metabolic acidosis has usually accompanied higher cyanide levels, but peak base deficits have lagged behind the peak cyanide levels by ≥ 1 hour.

Progressive tachyphylaxis to the hypotensive effects of nitroprusside has occurred in several trials and numerous case reports. This tachyphylaxis has frequently been attributed to concomitant cyanide toxicity; however, this is unproven and the mechanism of tachyphylaxis to nitroprusside remains unknown.

Indications:

Hypertensive crises: Immediate reduction of blood pressure of patients in hypertensive crises. Administer concomitant longer-acting antihypertensive medication so that the duration of treatment with nitroprusside can be minimized.

Bleeding reduction during surgery: Production of controlled hypotension in order to reduce bleeding during surgery.

Acute congestive heart failure (CHF).

Unlabeled uses: Myocardial infarction with coadministration of dopamine; left ventricular failure with coadministration of oxygen, morphine and a loop diuretic.

Contraindications:

Treatment of compensatory hypertension, where the primary hemodynamic lesion is aortic coarctation or arteriovenous shunting; to produce hypotension during surgery in patients with known inadequate cerebral circulation or in moribund patients (A.S.A. Class 5E) coming to emergency surgery; patients with congenital (Leber's) optic atrophy or with tobacco amblyopia (these rare conditions are probably associated with defective or absent rhodanase and patients with unusually high cyanide/thiocyanate ratios); acute CHF associated with reduced peripheral vascular resistance such as high-output heart failure that may be seen in endotoxic sepsis.

Warnings:

Excessive hypotension: Small transient excesses in the infusion rate of nitroprusside can result in excessive hypotension, sometimes to levels so low as to compromise the perfusion of vital organs. These hemodynamic changes may lead to a variety of associated symptoms (see Adverse Reactions). Nitroprusside-induced hypotension will be self-limited within 1 to 10 minutes after discontinuation of the infusion; during these few minutes, it may be helpful to put the patient into a head-down (Trendelenburg) position to maximize venous return. If hypotension persists more than a few minutes after discontinuation of the infusion, nitroprusside is not the cause, and the true cause must be sought.

Agents for Hypertensive Emergencies

NITROPRUSSIDE SODIUM

Cyanide toxicity: Nitroprusside infusions at rates > 2 mcg/kg/min generate CN^- faster than the body can normally dispose of it. (When sodium thiosulfate is given, the body's capacity for CN^- elimination is greatly increased.) Methemoglobin normally present in the body can buffer a certain amount of CN^-, but the capacity of this system is exhausted by the CN^- produced from about 500 mcg/kg nitroprusside. This amount of nitroprusside is administered in < 1 hour when the drug is administered at 10 mcg/kg/min (the maximum recommended rate). Thereafter, the toxic effects of CN^- may be rapid, serious and even lethal.

The true rates of clinically important cyanide toxicity cannot be assessed from spontaneous reports or published data. Most patients reported to have experienced such toxicity have received relatively prolonged infusions, and the only patients whose deaths have been unequivocally attributed to nitroprusside-induced cyanide toxicity have been patients who had received nitroprusside infusions at rates much greater than those now recommended (30 to 120 mcg/kg/min). Elevated cyanide levels, metabolic acidosis and marked clinical deterioration, however, have occasionally been reported in patients who received infusions at recommended rates for only a few hours and even, in one case, for only 35 minutes. In some of these cases, infusion of sodium thiosulfate caused dramatic clinical improvement, supporting the diagnosis of cyanide toxicity.

Cyanide toxicity may manifest itself as venous hyperoxemia with bright red venous blood, as cells become unable to extract the oxygen delivered to them; metabolic (lactic) acidosis; air hunger; confusion; death. Cyanide toxicity due to causes other than nitroprusside has been associated with angina pectoris and myocardial infarction, ataxia, seizures and stroke, and other diffuse ischemic damage.

Hypertensive patients and patients concomitantly receiving other antihypertensive medications may be more sensitive to the effects of nitroprusside.

Methemoglobinemia: Nitroprusside infusions can cause sequestration of hemoglobin as methemoglobin. The back-conversion process is normally rapid, and clinically significant methemoglobinemia (> 10%) is seen only rarely. Even patients congenitally incapable of back-converting methemoglobin should demonstrate 10% methemoglobinemia only after they have received about 10 mg/kg nitroprusside; a patient receiving nitroprusside at the maximum recommended rate (10 mcg/kg/min) would take > 16 hours to reach this total accumulated dose.

Methemoglobin levels can be measured by most clinical laboratories. Suspect the diagnosis in patients who have received > 10 mg/kg of nitroprusside and who exhibit signs of impaired oxygen delivery despite adequate cardiac output and adequate arterial pO_2. Classically, methemoglobinemic blood is described as chocolate brown, without color change on exposure to air.

When methemoglobinemia is diagnosed, the treatment of choice is 1 to 2 mg/kg of methylene blue, administered IV over several minutes. In patients likely to have substantial amounts of cyanide bound to methemoglobin as cyanmethemoglobin, treatment of methemoglobinemia with methylene blue must be undertaken with extreme caution.

Thiocyanate toxicity: Most of the cyanide produced during metabolism of nitroprusside is eliminated in the form of thiocyanate. When cyanide elimination is accelerated by the co-infusion of thiosulfate, thiocyanate production is increased. Thiocyanate is mildly neurotoxic (eg, tinnitus, miosis, hyperreflexia) at serum levels of 1 mmol/L (60 mg/L). Thiocyanate toxicity is life-threatening when levels are 3 or 4 times higher (200 mg/L).

The steady-state thiocyanate level after prolonged infusions of nitroprusside is increased with increased infusion rate, and the half-time of accumulation is 3 to 4 days. To keep the steady-state thiocyanate level < 1 mmol/L, a prolonged infusion should not be more rapid than 3 mcg/kg/min; in anuric patients, the corresponding limit is just 1 mcg/kg/min. When prolonged infusions are more rapid than these, measure thiocyanate levels daily.

Physiologic maneuvers (eg, those that alter the pH of the urine) are not known to increase the elimination of thiocyanate. Thiocyanate clearance rates during dialysis, on the other hand, can approach the blood flow rate of the dialyzer.

Thiocyanate interferes with iodine uptake by the thyroid.

Hepatic function impairment: Since cyanide is metabolized by hepatic enzymes, it may accumulate in patients with severe liver impairment. Therefore, use with caution in patients with hepatic insufficiency.

Agents for Hypertensive Emergencies

NITROPRUSSIDE SODIUM

Elderly: Use special caution as elderly patients may be more sensitive to the hypotensive effects of the drug.

Pregnancy: Category C. In three studies in pregnant ewes, nitroprusside crossed the placental barrier. Fetal cyanide levels were dose-related to maternal levels of nitroprusside. The metabolic transformation of nitroprusside given to pregnant ewes led to fatal levels of cyanide in the fetuses. The infusion of 25 mcg/kg/min nitroprusside for 1 hour in pregnant ewes resulted in the death of all fetuses. There are no adequate or well controlled studies in pregnant women. It is not known whether nitroprusside can cause fetal harm when administered to a pregnant woman or can affect reproductive capacity. Give to a pregnant woman only if clearly needed.

The effects of administering sodium thiosulfate in pregnancy, either by itself or as a co-infusion with sodium nitroprusside, are completely unknown.

Lactation: It is not known whether nitroprusside and its metabolites are excreted in breast milk. Because of the potential for serious adverse reactions in nursing infants, decide whether to discontinue nursing or to discontinue the drug, taking into account the importance of the drug to the mother.

Children: See Administration and Dosage.

Precautions:

Monitoring: The cyanide-level assay is technically difficult, and cyanide levels in body fluids other than packed red blood cells are difficult to interpret. Cyanide toxicity will lead to lactic acidosis and venous hyperoxemia, but these findings may not be present until ≥ 1 hour after the cyanide capacity of the body's red-cell mass has been exhausted.

Intracranial pressure: Like other vasodilators, nitroprusside can cause increases in intracranial pressure. In patients whose intracranial pressure is already elevated, use only with extreme caution.

Anesthesia: When nitroprusside (or any other vasodilator) is used for controlled hypotension during anesthesia, the patient's capacity to compensate for anemia and hypovolemia may be diminished. If possible, correct pre-existing anemia and hypovolemia prior to administration.

Hypotensive anesthetic techniques may also cause abnormalities of the pulmonary ventilation/perfusion ratio. Patients intolerant of these abnormalities may require a higher fraction of inspired oxygen.

Exercise extreme caution in patients who are especially poor surgical risks (A.S.A. Classes 4 and 4E).

Adverse Reactions:

Rapid blood pressure reduction: Abdominal pain, apprehension, diaphoresis, dizziness, headache, muscle twitching, nausea, palpitations, restlessness, retching and retrosternal discomfort have been noted when the blood pressure was reduced too rapidly. Symptoms quickly disappeared when the infusion was slowed or discontinued, and they did not reappear with a continued (or resumed) slower infusion.

Cardiovascular: Bradycardia; ECG changes; tachycardia.

Hematologic: Decreased platelet aggregation; methemoglobinemia (see Warnings).

Body as a whole: Thiocyanate toxicity (see Warnings); flushing; venous streaking; irritation at the infusion site; rash; hypothyroidism; ileus; increased intracranial pressure (see Precautions).

Overdosage:

Symptoms: Toxicity has occurred at doses well below the recommended maximum infusion rate of 10 mcg/kg/min. Overdosage of nitroprusside can be manifested as excessive hypotension, cyanide toxicity or as thiocyanate toxicity (see Warnings).

The acute IV mean lethal doses (LD_{50}) of nitroprusside in rabbits, dogs, mice and rats are 2.8, 5, 8.4 and 11.2 mg/kg, respectively.

Agents for Hypertensive Emergencies

NITROPRUSSIDE SODIUM

Treatment: Measure cyanide levels and blood gases for venous hyperoxemia or acidosis. Acidosis may not appear until > 1 hour after the appearance of dangerous cyanide levels; do not wait for laboratory tests. Reasonable suspicion of cyanide toxicity is adequate grounds for initiation of treatment.

Treatment of cyanide toxicity consists of: Discontinuing the administration of nitroprusside; providing a buffer for cyanide by using sodium nitrite to convert as much HgB into methemoglobin as the patient can safely tolerate; and then infusing sodium thiosulfate in sufficient quantity to convert the cyanide into thiocyanate.

The medications for treatment are contained in commercially available cyanide antidote kits. Alternatively, discrete stocks of medications can be used. Hemodialysis is ineffective in removal of cyanide, but it will eliminate most thiocyanate.

Cyanide antidote kits contain both amyl nitrite and sodium nitrite for induction of methemoglobinemia. The amyl nitrite is supplied in the form of inhalant ampuls, for use where IV administration of sodium nitrite may be delayed. In a patient who already has a patent IV line, use of amyl nitrite confers no benefit that is not provided by infusion of sodium nitrite.

Nitrite-thiosulfate regimen – Sodium nitrite is available in a 3% solution; inject 4 to 6 mg/kg (about 0.2 ml/kg) over 2 to 4 minutes. This dose converts about 10% of the patient's HgB into methemoglobin; this level of methemoglobinemia is not associated with any important hazard of its own. The nitrite infusion may cause transient vasodilation and hypotension, and this hypotension must, if it occurs, be routinely managed.

Immediately after infusion of the sodium nitrite, infuse sodium thiosulfate. This agent is available in 10% and 25% solutions, and the recommended dose is 150 to 200 mg/kg; a typical adult dose is 50 ml of the 25% solution. Thiosulfate treatment of an acutely cyanide-toxic patient will raise thiocyanate levels, but not to a dangerous degree.

The nitrite-thiosulfate regimen may be repeated, at half the original doses, after 2 hours.

Hydroxocobalamin – No concrete guidelines have been developed for hydroxocobalamin.

Prophylactically during surgery: Doses of 25 mg/hr for 4 hours.

Treatment: A dose of 4 to 5 g of hydroxocobalamin alone, or a combination of 8 g of sodium thiosulfate and 4 g of hydroxocobalamin.

Administration and Dosage:

Reconstitution: Dissolve the contents of a 50 mg vial in 2 to 3 ml Dextrose in Water or Sterile Water for Injection. Depending on the desired concentration, the initially reconstituted solution containing 50 mg must be further diluted in 250 to 1000 ml 5% Dextrose Injection.

Verification of the chemical integrity of the product: Nitroprusside solution can be inactivated by reactions with trace contaminants. The products of these reactions are often blue, green or red, much brighter than the faint brownish color of unreacted nitroprusside. Do not use discolored solutions, or solutions in which particulate matter is visible.

Admixture compatibility: Esmolol and nitroprusside are compatible for at least 24 hours in 5% Dextrose Injection at room temperature and protected from light.

CHF: Nitroprusside can be titrated by increasing the infusion rate until measured cardiac output is no longer increasing, systemic blood pressure cannot be further reduced without compromising the perfusion of vital organs or the maximum recommended infusion rate has been reached, whichever comes earliest.

Avoidance of excessive hypotension: While the average effective rate in adults and children is about 3 mcg/kg/min, some patients will become dangerously hypotensive when they receive nitroprusside at this rate. Therefore, start at a very low rate (0.3 mcg/kg/min), with gradual upward titration every few minutes until the desired effect is achieved or the maximum recommended infusion rate (10 mcg/kg/min) has been reached.

Because nitroprusside's hypotensive effect is very rapid in onset and in dissipation, small variations in infusion rate can lead to wide, undesirable variations in blood pressure. Do not infuse through ordinary IV apparatus regulated only by gravity and mechanical clamps. Use only an infusion pump, preferably a volumetric pump.

Because nitroprusside can induce essentially unlimited blood pressure reduction, the blood pressure of a patient receiving this drug must be continuously monitored, using either a continually reinflated sphygmomanometer or (preferably) an intra-arterial pressure sensor.

Agents for Hypertensive Emergencies

NITROPRUSSIDE SODIUM

Infusion rates: The table below shows the infusion rates for adults and children of various weights corresponding to the recommended initial and maximal doses (0.3 mcg/kg/min and 10 mcg/kg/min, respectively). Some of the listed infusion rates are so slow or so rapid as to be impractical, and these practicalities must be considered when the concentration to be used is selected. Note that when the concentration used in a given patient is changed, the tubing is still filled with a solution at the previous concentration.

Infusion Rates to Achieve Initial (0.3 mcg/kg/min) and Maximal (10 mcg/kg/min) Dosing of Nitroprusside

Patient weight		Nitroprusside concentration					
		200 mcg/ml		100 mcg/ml		50 mcg/ml	
		Infusion rate (ml/hr)		Infusion rate (ml/hr)		Infusion rate (ml/hr)	
kg	lbs	Initial	Maximal	Initial	Maximal	Initial	Maximal
10	22	1	30	2	60	4	120
20	44	2	60	4	120	7	240
30	66	3	90	5	180	11	360
40	88	4	120	7	240	14	480
50	110	5	150	9	300	18	600
60	132	5	180	11	360	22	720
70	154	6	210	13	420	25	840
80	176	7	240	14	480	29	960
90	198	8	270	16	540	32	1080
100	220	9	300	18	600	36	1200

Avoidance of cyanide toxicity: When > 500 mcg/kg nitroprusside is administered faster than 2 mcg/kg/min, cyanide is generated faster than the unaided patient can eliminate it (see Warnings).

Consideration of methemoglobinemia and thiocyanate toxicity: Rare patients receiving > 10 mg/kg of nitroprusside will develop methemoglobinemia; other patients, especially those with impaired renal function, will predictably develop thiocyanate toxicity after prolonged, rapid infusions. Test patients with suggestive findings for these toxicities.

Storage/Stability: Protect the diluted solution from light by promptly wrapping with the supplied opaque sleeve, aluminum foil or other opaque material. It is not necessary to cover the infusion drip chamber or the tubing.

Store at room temperature 15° to 30°C (59° to 86°F).

If properly protected from light, the freshly reconstituted and diluted solution is stable for 24 hours.

Rx	**Sodium Nitroprusside** (Elkins-Sinn)	**Powder for Injection:** 50 mg per vial	In single dose 5 ml vials.
Rx	**Nitropress** (Abbott)		In single dose 2 ml Fliptop Vials.

Agents for Hypertensive Emergencies

DIAZOXIDE, PARENTERAL

Refer to the general discussion of these products in the Antihypertensives Introduction.

Oral diazoxide is used to increase blood glucose levels in hyperinsulinism; see Diazoxide, Oral monograph.

Actions:

Pharmacology: Diazoxide, a nondiuretic antihypertensive, is structurally related to the thiazides. It promptly reduces blood pressure by relaxing smooth muscle in the peripheral arterioles. Increases in heart rate and in cardiac output occur as blood pressure is reduced. Coronary blood flow is maintained. Renal blood flow is increased after an initial decrease. Transient hyperglycemia occurs in the majority of patients treated.

Pharmacokinetics: Diazoxide is extensively bound to serum protein (> 90%) and may therefore displace other highly protein-bound agents. The plasma half-life is 28 ± 8.3 hours. The duration of antihypertensive effect varies, but is generally < 12 hours.

Generally, hypotensive effects begin within 1 min, maximum effects occurring within 2 to 5 min. Blood pressure increases gradually over the next 20 minutes, and then more slowly over the next 3 to 15 hours.

Indications:

Severe hypertension: Emergency reduction of blood pressure, short-term use in severe, nonmalignant and malignant hypertension in hospitalized adults and in acute severe hypertension in hospitalized children when an urgent decrease of diastolic pressure is required. Institute treatment with oral agents as soon as the hypertensive emergency is controlled.

Contraindications:

Treatment of compensatory hypertension, such as that associated with aortic coarctation or arteriovenous shunt; dissecting aortic aneurysm; hypersensitivity to diazoxide, thiazides or to other sulfonamide derivatives.

Warnings:

Myocardial lesions in animals: Diazoxide IV in dogs induces subendocardial necrosis and necrosis of papillary muscles. These lesions, which are also produced by other vasodilators (eg, hydralazine, minoxidil) and catecholamines, are presumed to be related to anoxia from reflex tachycardia and decreased blood pressure.

Rapid decrease in blood pressure: Observe caution when reducing severely elevated blood pressure. Use only the 150 mg minibolus. The 300 mg IV dose of diazoxide is less predictable and less controllable and has been associated with angina and with myocardial and cerebral infarction. Optic nerve infarction was reported when a 100 mm Hg reduction in diastolic pressure occurred over 10 minutes following a single 300 mg bolus. In one prospective trial conducted in patients with severe hypertension and coexistent coronary artery disease, a 50% incidence of ischemic changes in the ECG was observed following single 300 mg bolus injections of diazoxide. Achieve the desired blood pressure over as long a period of time as is compatible with the patient's status. At least several hours and preferably 1 or 2 days is tentatively recommended.

Improved safety with equal efficacy can be achieved by giving diazoxide as a minibolus dose (see Administration and Dosage) until diastolic blood pressure < 100 mm Hg is achieved. If hypotension severe enough to require therapy results, it usually responds to the Trendelenberg maneuver. If necessary, administer sympathomimetics such as dopamine or norepinephrine. Special attention is required in diabetes mellitus and if salt and water retention present serious problems.

Transient hyperglycemia occurs in the majority of patients, but usually requires treatment only in patients with diabetes mellitus; it will respond to the usual management including insulin. Monitor blood glucose levels, especially in patients with diabetes and in those requiring multiple injections of diazoxide. Cataracts have been observed in a few animals receiving repeated daily doses of IV diazoxide.

Fluid and electrolyte balance: Diazoxide causes sodium retention; repeat injections may precipitate edema and CHF. This retention responds to diuretic agents if adequate renal function exists. Coadministered thiazides may potentiate diazoxide's antihypertensive, hyperglycemic and hyperuricemic actions (see Drug Interactions). Increased extracellular fluid volume may cause treatment failure in nonresponsive patients.

Pheochromocytoma: Diazoxide is ineffective against hypertension due to pheochromocytoma.

Pregnancy: Category C. Safety for use is not established. Diazoxide crosses the placenta and appears in cord blood. It reduces fetal or pup survival, and reduces fetal growth in rats, rabbits and dogs at daily doses of 30, 21 or 10 mg/kg, respectively. In rats treated at term, doses of ≥ 10 mg/kg prolonged parturition.

Agents for Hypertensive Emergencies

DIAZOXIDE, PARENTERAL

If given prior to delivery, it may produce fetal or neonatal hyperbilirubinemia, thrombocytopenia, altered carbohydrate metabolism and other adverse reactions.

Labor and delivery – Not for use during pregnancy. IV administration during labor may stop uterine contractions, requiring administration of an oxytocic agent. An episode of maternal hypotension and fetal bradycardia occurred in a patient in labor who received both reserpine and hydralazine prior to administration of diazoxide. Neonatal hyperglycemia following intrapartum administration of diazoxide IV occurred.

Lactation: Information is not available concerning the passage of diazoxide in breast milk. Decide whether to discontinue nursing or to discontinue the drug, taking into account the importance of the drug to the mother.

Precautions:

Monitoring: Diazoxide requires close and frequent blood pressure monitoring; it may cause hypotension requiring treatment with sympathomimetic drugs. Use diazoxide primarily in the hospital and where facilities exist to treat such untoward reactions.

Perform appropriate diagnostic laboratory tests prior to, during and following diazoxide injection. Tests include: Hematologic (hematocrit, hemoglobin, white blood cell and platelet counts); metabolic (glucose, uric acid, total protein, albumin); electrolyte (sodium, potassium) and osmolality; renal function (creatinine, urine-protein); ECG.

Special risk patients: Use with care in patients with impaired cerebral or cardiac circulation, in whom abrupt reductions in blood pressure might be detrimental or in whom mild tachycardia or decreased blood perfusion may be deleterious. Avoid prolonged hypotension so as not to aggravate pre-existing renal failure.

Drug Interactions:

Since diazoxide is highly protein bound, it can be expected to displace other highly protein-bound agents (eg, warfarin), resulting in higher blood levels of these agents.

Diazoxide (Parenteral) Drug Interactions

Precipitant drug	Object drug*		Description
Diazoxide	Hydantoins	↓	Serum hydantoin levels may be decreased, possibly resulting in decreased anticonvulsant action.
Diazoxide	Sulfonylureas	↓	Addition of diazoxide to sulfonylurea therapy could destabilize the patient, resulting in hyperglycemia.
Thiazide diuretics	Diazoxide	↑	Coadministration may potentiate the hyperuricemic and antihypertensive effects of diazoxide.

* ↑ = Object drug increased. ↓ = Object drug decreased.

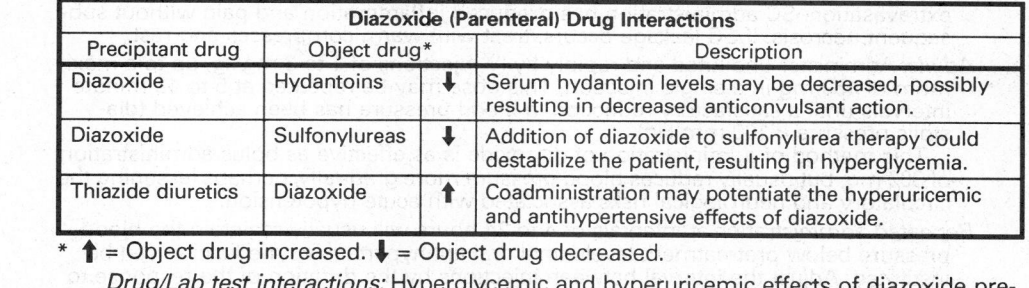

Drug/Lab test interactions: Hyperglycemic and hyperuricemic effects of diazoxide preclude assessment of these metabolic states. Increased renin secretion, IgG concentrations and decreased cortisol secretion have occurred. Diazoxide inhibits glucagon-stimulated insulin release and will cause a false-negative insulin response to glucagon.

Adverse Reactions:

The following adverse reactions were reported with rapid IV bolus administration of 300 mg diazoxide. The currently recommended minibolus dosing regimen may result in similar adverse effects, but with less frequency and severity. The most common adverse reactions were: Hypotension (7%); nausea, vomiting (4%); dizziness, weakness (2%). Additional adverse reactions were as follows:

Cardiovascular: Sodium and water retention after repeated injections, especially important in patients with impaired cardiac reserve; hypotension to shock levels; myocardial ischemia, usually transient and manifested by angina, atrial and ventricular arrhythmias and marked ECG changes, but occasionally leading to myocardial infarction; optic nerve infarction following too rapid decrease in severely elevated blood pressure; supraventricular tachycardia; palpitations; bradycardia; chest discomfort or nonanginal chest tightness.

CNS: Cerebral ischemia, usually transient, but occasionally leading to infarction and manifested by unconsciousness, convulsions, paralysis, confusion or focal neurological deficit such as numbness of the hands; vasodilative phenomena (eg, orthostatic hypotension), sweating, flushing and generalized or localized sensations of warmth; transient neurological findings secondary to alteration in regional blood flow to the brain, such as headache (sometimes throbbing), dizziness, lightheaded-

Agents for Hypertensive Emergencies

DIAZOXIDE, PARENTERAL

ness, sleepiness (also reported as lethargy, somnolence or drowsiness), euphoria or "funny feeling," ringing in the ears and momentary hearing loss; weakness of short duration; apprehension; anxiety; malaise; blurred vision.

GI: Acute pancreatitis (rare); nausea; vomiting; abdominal discomfort; anorexia; alterations in taste; parotid swelling; salivation; dry mouth; ileus; constipation; diarrhea.

Miscellaneous: Hyperglycemia in diabetic patients after repeated injections; hyperosmolar coma in an infant; transient hyperglycemia in nondiabetic patients; transient retention of nitrogenous wastes; respiratory findings secondary to smooth muscle relaxation, such as dyspnea, cough and choking sensation; warmth or pain along injected vein; cellulitis without sloughing or phlebitis at injection site of extravasation; back pain and increased nocturia; lacrimation; hypersensitivity reactions; papilledema induced by plasma volume expansion secondary to the administration of diazoxide in a patient who had received 11 injections (300 mg/dose) over a 22 day period; transient cataract in an infant; hirsutism; decreased libido.

Overdosage:

Overdosage may cause hypotension that can usually be controlled with the Trendelenburg maneuver. If necessary, sympathomimetic agents, such as dopamine or norepinephrine, may be administered. Failure of blood pressure to rise in response to such agents suggests that the hypotension may not have been caused by diazoxide. Excessive hyperglycemia will respond to conventional therapy of hyperglycemia. Diazoxide may be removed from blood by hemodialysis.

Administration and Dosage:

Diazoxide injection was originally recommended for use by bolus administration of 300 mg. However, recent studies have shown that minibolus administration is as effective in reducing blood pressure, and therefore, it is the recommended dosage.

During and immediately following injection, the patient should remain supine. Administer only into a peripheral vein. The dose is given IV in ≤ 30 seconds. Do not give IM, SC or into body cavities. The solution's alkalinity is irritating to tissue; avoid extravasation. SC administration has produced inflammation and pain without subsequent necrosis. If SC leakage occurs, treat with warm compresses and rest.

Adults: Administer undiluted and rapidly by IV injections of 1 to 3 mg/kg, up to a maximum of 150 mg in a single injection. This dose may be repeated at 5 to 15 minute intervals until a satisfactory reduction in blood pressure has been achieved (diastolic pressure < 100 mm Hg).

This method of administration of diazoxide is as effective as bolus administration of 300 mg, but usually reduces blood pressure more gradually, perhaps lessening the circulatory and neurological risks associated with acute hypotension.

Repeated administration at intervals of 4 to 24 hours will usually maintain the blood pressure below pretreatment levels until oral antihypertensive medication can be instituted. Adjust the interval between injections by the duration of the response to each injection. It is usually unnecessary to continue treatment for > 4 to 5 days; do not use for > 10 days.

Monitor the blood pressure closely until it has stabilized. Thereafter, hourly measurements will indicate any unusual response. Further decreases in blood pressure at ≥ 30 minutes after injection may be due to causes other than diazoxide. Have the patient remain recumbent for at least 1 hour after injection. In ambulatory patients, measure the blood pressure with the patient standing before ending surveillance.

Concomitant diuretic therapy: Because repeated administration can lead to sodium and water retention, a diuretic may be necessary for maximal blood pressure reduction and to avoid congestive failure.

Storage/Stability: Protect from light/freezing. Store between 2° to 30°C (36° to 86°F).

Rx	**Hyperstat IV** (Schering)	**Injection:** 15 mg/ml	In 20 ml amps.

Miscellaneous Agents

EPOPROSTENOL SODIUM (PGI_2; PGX; Prostacyclin)

Actions:

Pharmacology: Epoprostenol has two major pharmacological actions: (1) Direct vasodilation of pulmonary and systemic arterial vascular beds, and (2) inhibition of platelet aggregation. In animals, the vasodilatory effects reduce right and left ventricular afterload and increase cardiac output and stroke volume (SV). The effect on heart rate in animals varies with dose. At low doses, there is vagally mediated bradycardia, but at higher doses, epoprostenol causes reflex tachycardia in response to direct vasodilation and hypotension. No major effects on cardiac conduction have been observed. Additional pharmacologic effects in animals are bonchodilation, inhibition of gastric acid secretion and decreased gastric emptying.

Hemodynamics – Acute IV infusion for ≤ 15 minutes in patients with secondary and primary pulmonary hypertension produces dose-related increases in cardiac index (CI) and SV, and dose-related decreases in pulmonary vascular resistance (PVR), total pulmonary resistance (TPR) and mean systemic arterial pressure (mSAP). The effects of epoprostenol on mean pulmonary artery pressure (mPAP) in patients with primary pulmonary hypertension (PPH) were variable and minor.

Pharmacokinetics: Epoprostenol is rapidly hydrolyzed at neutral pH in blood and is also subject to enzymatic degradation.

The in vitro half-life in human blood at 37°C (98°F) and pH 7.4 is ≈ 6 minutes; the in vivo half-life is therefore expected to be ≤ 6 minutes. The in vitro pharmacologic half-life in human plasma, based on inhibition of platelet aggregation, was similar for males and females.

Epoprostenol is metabolized to two primary metabolites: 6–keto-PGF1a (formed by spontaneous degradation) and 6,1 5–diketo-13,14–dihydro-PGF1a (enzymatically formed), both of which have pharmacological activity orders of magnitued less than epoprostenol in animal test systems.

Clinical trials: Exercise capacity, as measured by the 6 minute walk test, improved significantly in patients receiving continuous IV epoprostenol plus standard therapy for 8 or 12 weeks compared with those receiving standard therapy alone. Improvements were apparent the first week of therapy. Increases in exercise capacity were accompanied by significant improvement in dyspnea and fatigue, as measured by the Congestive Heart Failure Questionnaire and the Dyspnea Fatigue Index.

Survival was improved in NYHA functional Class III and Class IV PPH patients treated with epoprostenol for 12 weeks in a multicenter, open, randomized, parallel study. At the end of the treament period, 8 of 40 patients receiving standard therapy alone died, wheras none of the 41 patients receiving epoprostenol died.

Indications:

Pulmonary hypertension: Long-term IV treatment of primary pulmonary hypertension in NYHA Class III and Class IV patients (see Clinical Trials).

Contraindications:

Chronic use in patients with CHF due to severe left ventricular systolic dysfunction; hypersensitivity to the drug or to structurally related compounds.

Warnings:

Reconstitution: Epoprostenol must be reconstituted only as directed using sterile diluent for epoprostenol. Epoprostenol must not be reconstituted or mixed with any other parenteral medications or solutions prior to or during administration.

Abrupt withdrawal: Abrupt withdrawal (including interruptions in drug delivery) or sudden large reductions in dosage may result in symptoms associated with rebound pulmonary hypertension, including dyspnea, dizziness and asthenia. In clinical trials, one Class III PPH patient's death was judged attributable to the interruption of epoprostenol. Avoid abrupt withdrawal.

Pulmonary edema: Some patients with primary pulmonary hypertension have developed pulmonary edema during dose ranging, which may be associated with pulmonary veno-occlusive disease. Epoprostenol should not be used chronically in patients who develop pulmonary edema during dose ranging.

Elderly: In general, dose selection for an elderly patient should be cautions, reflecting the greater frequency of decreased hepatic, renal or cardiac function and of concomitant disease or other drug therapy.

Pregnancy: Category B. There are no adequate and well controlled studies in pregnant women. Use during pregnancy only if clearly needed.

Lactation: It is not known whether this drug is excreted in breast milk. Exercise caution when epoprostenol is administered to a nursing woman.

Children: Safety and efficacy have not been established.

Miscellaneous Agents

EPOPROSTENOL SODIUM (PGI_2; PGX; Prostacyclin)

Precautions:

Diagnosis: Carefully establish the diagnosis of PPH by standard clinical tests to exclude secondary causes of pulmonary hypertension.

Dose ranging: Although dose ranging in clinical trials was performed during right heart catheterization employing a pulmonary artery catheter, in uncontrolled studies, acute dose ranging was performed without cardiac catheterization. Carefully weigh the risk of cardiac catheterization in patients with PPH against the potential benefits. During acute dose ranging, asymptomatic increases in pulmonary artery pressure coincident with increases in cardiac output occurred rarely. In such cases, consider dose reduction, but such an increase does not imply that chronic treatment is contraindicated.

Chronic use of epoprostenol is delivered continuously on an ambulatory basis through a permanent indwelling central venous catheter. Unless contraindicated, administer anticoagulant therapy to PPH patients to reduce the rusk of pulmonary thromboembolism or systemic embolism through a patent foramen ovale. Base the decision to initiate therapy with epoprostenol on the understanding that there is a high likelihood that IV therapy will be needed for prolonged periods, possibly years.

Based on clinical trials, the acute hemodynamic response to epoprostenol did not correlate well with improvement in exercise tolerance of survival during chronic use. Adjust dosage during chronic use at the first sign of recurrence or worsening of symptoms attributable to PPH or the occurrence of adverse events associated with epoprostenol (see Administration and Dosage).

Drug Interactions:

Epoprostenol Drug Interactions			
Precipitant drug	Object drug*		Description
Epoprostenol	Diuretics Vasodilators	⬆	Coadministration could cause additional reductions in blood pressure.
Epoprostenol	Antiplatelet agents Anticoagulants	⬆	Coadministration can increase the risk of bleeding, although this did not occur in clinical trials.

* ⬆ = Object drug increased.

Adverse Reactions:

During clinical trials, adverse reactions were classified as follows: (1) Occurring during acute dose ranging, (2) occurring during chronic dosing and (3) association with the drug delivery system.

Acute dose ranging: During acute dose ranging, epoprostenol was administered in 2 ng/kg/min increments until the patients developed symptomatic intolerance. The adverse reactions that limited further increases in dose were generally related to the major pharmacologic effect of epoprostenol, vasodilation.

Epoprostenol Adverse Reactions (n = 391)	
Adverse reaction	Incidence
Flushing	58
Headache	49
Nausea/Vomiting	32
Hypotension	16
Anxiety, nervousness, agitation	11
Chest pain	11
Dizziness	8
Bradycardia	5
Abdominal pain	5
Musculoskeletal pain	3
Dyspnea	2
Back pain	2
Sweating	1

Miscellaneous Agents

EPOPROSTENOL SODIUM (PGI_2; PGX; Prostacyclin)

Epoprostenol Adverse Reactions (n = 391)	
Adverse reaction	Incidence
Dyspepsia	1
Hypesthesia/Paresthesia	1
Tachycardia	1

Drug delivery system: Local infection (21%); pain at the injection site (13%); sepsis (once); infections (14%). The rate was higher than reported in patients using chronic indwelling central venous catheters to administer parenteral nutrition, but lower than reported in oncology patients using these catheters. Malfunctions in the delivery system resulting in an inadvertent bolus of or a reduction in epoprostenol were associated with symptoms related to excess or insufficient epoprostenol, respectively.

Chronic administration: Interpretation of adverse events is complicated by the clinical features of PPH, which are similar to some of the pharmacologic effects of epoprostenol (eg, dizziness, syncope). Adverse events probably related to the underlying disease include dyspnea, fatigue, chest pain, right ventricular failure and pallor. Several adverse reactions, on the other hand, can clearly be attributed to epoprostenol. These include headache, jaw pain, flushing, diarrhea, nausea and vomiting, flu-like symptoms and anxiety/nervousness. Thrombocytopenia has also been reported. In an effort to separate the adverse effects of the drug from the adverse effects of the underlying disease, the following table lists adverse events that occurred at a rate at least 10% difference in the two groups in controlled trials.

Adverse Reactions Regardless of Attribution Occurring with ≥ 10% Difference Between Epoprostenol and Standard Therapy Alone (%)		
Adverse reaction	Epoprostenol (n = 52)	Standard therapy (n = 54)
Occurrence more common with epoprostenol		
Cardiovascular		
Tachycardia	35	24
Flushing	42	2
GI		
Diarrhea	37	6
Nausea/Vomiting	67	48
Musculoskeletal		
Jaw pain	54	0
Myalgia	44	31
Non-specific musculoskeletal pain	35	15
CNS		
Anxiety/Nervousness/Tremor	21	9
Dizziness	83	70
Headache	83	33
Hypesthesia, hyperesthesia, paresthesia	12	2
Miscellaneous		
Chills/Fever/Sepsis/ Flu-like symptoms	25	11
Occurrence more common with standard therapy		
Cardiovascular		
Heart failure	31	52
Syncope	13	24
Shock	0	13
Respiratory		
Hypoxia	25	37

Miscellaneous Agents

EPOPROSTENOL SODIUM (PGI_2; PGX; Prostacyclin)

Adverse Reactions Regardless of Attribution Occurring With < 10% Difference Between Epoprostenol and Standard Therapy Alone (%)		
Adverse reaction	Epoprostenol (n = 52)	Standard therapy (n = 54)
Cardiovascular		
Angina pectoris	19	20
Arrhythmia	27	20
Bradycardia	15	9
Supraventricular tachycardia	8	0
Pallor	21	30
Cyanosis	31	39
Palpitation	63	61
Cerebrovascular accident	4	0
Hemorrhage	19	11
Hypotension	27	31
Myocardial ischemia	2	6
GI		
Abdominal pain	27	31
Anorexia	25	30
Ascites	12	17
Constipation	6	2
Metabolic		
Edema	60	63
Hypokalemia	6	4
Weight reduction	27	24
Weight gain	6	4
Musculoskeletal		
Arthralgia	6	0
Bone pain	0	4
Chest pain	67	65
CNS		
Confusion	6	11
Convulsion	4	0
Depression	37	44
Insomnia	4	4
Respiratory		
Cough increase	38	46
Dyspnea	90	85
Epistaxis	4	2
Pleural effusion	4	2
Dermatologic		
Pruritus	4	0
Rash	10	13
Sweating	15	20
Special senses		
Amblyopia	8	4
Vision abnormality	4	0
Miscellaneous		
Asthenia	87	81

Overdosage:

Signs and symptoms of excessive doses of epoprostenol during clinical trials are the expected dose-limiting pharmacologic effects of epoprostenol, including flushing, headache, hypotension, tachycardia, nausea, vomiting and diarrhea. Treatment will ordinarily require dose reduction of epoprostenol. One patient vomited and became unconscious with an initially unrecordable blood pressure. Epoprostenol was discontinued and the patient regained consciousness within seconds.

EPOPROSTENOL SODIUM (PGI_2; PGX; Prostacyclin)

Single IV doses (2,703 and 27,027 times the recommended acute phase human dose) were lethal to mice and rats, respectively. Symptoms of acute toxicity were hypoactiviy, ataxia, loss of righting reflex, deep slow breathing and hypothermia.

Patient Information:

Patients receiving epoprostenol should receive the following information: The drug is infused continuously through a permanent indwelling central venous catheter via a small, portable infusion pump. Thus, therapy with epoprostenol requires commitment by the patient to drug reconstitution, drug administration and care of the permanent central venous catheter. Brief interruptions in the delivery of epoprostenol may result in rapid symptomatic deterioration. Base the decision to receive epoprostenol for PPH on the understanding that there is a high likelihood that therapy with epoprostenol will be needed for prolonged periods, possibly years.

Administration and Dosage:

Approved by the FDA on September 10, 1995.

Acute dose ranging: Determine the initial chronic infusion rate of epoprostenol an acute dose-ranging procedure (see Precautions). In clinical trials, the mean maximum dose that did not elicit dose-limiting pharmacologic effects was 8.6 ng/kg/min. (see Adverse Reactions).

Continuous chronic infusion: Administer chronic continous infusion through a central venous catheter. Temporary peripheral IV infusions may be used until central access is established. Initiate chronic infusions at 4 ng/kg/min less than the maximum-tolerated infusion (MTI) rate determined during acute dose ranging. If the MTI rate is < 5 ng/kg/min, start the chronic infusion at one-half the MTI rate. During clinical trials, the mean initial chronic infusion rate was 5 ng/kg/min.

Dosage adjustments:

Increments – Base changes in the chronic infusion rate on persistence, recurrence or worsening of the patient's symptoms of PPH and the occurrence of adverse events due to excessive doses. Expect increases from the initial chronic dose.

Consider increments in dose if symptoms of PPH persist or recur after improving. Increase the infusion by 1 to 2 ng/kg/min increments at intervals sufficient to allow assessment of clinical response; these intervals should be atleast 15 minutes. Observe the patient and monitor standing and supine blood pressure and heart rate for several hours to ensure that the new dose is tolerated.

Decrements – During chronic infusion, the occurrence of dose-related pharmacological events similar to those observed during acute dose ranging may necessitate a decrease in infusion rate, but the adverse event may occasionally resolve without dosage adjustment. Gradually make 2 ng/kg/min decrements every 15 minutes or longer until the dose-limiting effects resolve. Avoid abrupt withdrawal or sudden large reductions in infusion rates.

In patients receiving lung transplants, doses of epoprostenol were tapered after the initiation of cardiopulmonary bypass.

Administration: Epoprostenol is administered by continuous IV infusion via a central venous catheter using an ambulatory infusion pump. During dose-ranging, epoprostenol may be administered peripherally.

The ambulatory infusion pump used to administer epoprostenol should be: (1) Small and light weight, (2) able to adjust infusion rates in 2 ng/kg/min increments, (3) equipped with occlusion, end of infusion and low battery alarms, (4) accurate to ± 6% of the programmed rate and (5) positive pressure driven (continuous or pulsating) with intervals between pulses not exceeding 3 minutes at infusion rates. The reservoir should be made of polyvinyl chloride, polypropylene or glass.

Reconstitution: Important note: Reconstituted solutions of epoprostenol must not be diluted or administered with other parenteral solutions or medications.

To make 100 ml solution with a final concentration of –

3,000 ng/ml: Dissolve contents of one 0.5 mg vial with 5 ml diluent; withdraw 3 ml and add sufficient diluent to make 100 ml.

5,000 ng/ml: Dissolve contents of one 0.5 mg vial with 5 ml diluent; withdraw entire contents and add sufficient diluent to make a total of 100 ml.

10,000 ng/ml: Dissolve contents of two 0.5 mg vials each with 5 ml diluent; withdraw entire contents and add sufficient diluent to make a total of 100 ml.

15,000 ng/ml: Dissolve contents of one 1.5 mg vial with 5 ml diluent; withdraw entire contents and add sufficient diluent to make a total of 100 ml.

Infusion rates may be calculated using the following formula:

$$\text{Infusion rate (ml/hr)} = [\text{Dose (ng/kg/min)} \times \text{Weight (kg)} \times 60] \div \text{final concentration (ng/ml)}$$

EPOPROSTENOL SODIUM (PGI_2; PGX; Prostacyclin)

The following table provides infusion delivery rates for doses ≤ 16 ng/kg/min based on patient weight, drug delivery rate and concentration of the solution to be used. This table may be used to select the most appropriate concentration of epoprostenol that will result in an infusion rate between the minimum and maximum flow rates of the infusion pump and that will allow the desired duration of infusion.

Infusion Rates for Epoprostenol (ml/hr)

	Dose or drug delivery rate (ng/kg/min)							
Patient weight (kg)	2	4	6	8	10	12	14	16
Concentration = 3,000 ng/ml								
10	-	-	1.2	1.6	2	2.4	2.8	3.2
20	-	1.6	2.4	3.2	4	4.8	5.6	6.4
30	1.2	2.4	3.6	4.8	6	7.2	8.4	9.6
40	1.6	3.2	4.8	6.4	8	9.6	11.2	12.8
50	2	4	6	8	10	12	14	16
60	2.4	4.8	7.2	9.6	12	14.4	16.8	19.2
70	2.8	5.6	8.4	11.2	14	16.8	19.6	22.4
80	3.2	6.4	9.6	12.8	16	19.2	22.4	25.6
90	3.6	7.2	10.8	14.4	18	21.6	25.2	28.8
100	4	8	12	16	20	24	28	32
Concentration = 5,000 ng/ml								
10	-	-	-	1	1.2	1.4	1.7	1.9
20	-	1	1.4	1.9	2.4	2.9	3.4	3.8
30	-	1.4	2.2	2.9	3.6	4.3	5	5.8
40	1	1.9	2.9	3.8	4.8	5.8	6.7	7.7
50	1.2	2.4	3.6	4.8	6	7.2	8.4	9.6
60	1.4	2.9	4.3	5.8	7.2	8.6	10.1	11.5
70	1.7	3.4	5	6.7	8.4	10.1	11.8	13.4
80	1.9	3.8	5.8	7.7	9.6	11.5	13.4	15.4
90	2.2	4.3	6.5	8.6	10.8	13	15.1	17.3
100	2.4	4.8	7.2	9.6	12	14.4	16.8	19.2
Concentration = 10,000 ng/ml								
10	-	-	-	-	-	-	-	-
20	-	-	-	1	1.2	1.4	1.7	1.9
30	-	-	1.1	1.4	1.8	2.2	2.5	2.9
40	-	1	1.4	1.9	2.4	2.9	3.4	3.8
50	-	1.2	1.8	2.4	3	3.6	4.2	4.8
60	-	1.4	2.2	2.9	3.6	4.3	5	5.8
70	-	1.7	2.5	3.4	4.2	5	5.9	6.7
80	-	1.9	2.9	3.8	4.8	5.8	6.7	7.7
90	-	2.2	3.2	4.3	5.4	6.5	7.6	8.6
100	-	2.4	3.6	4.8	6	7.2	8.4	9.6
Concentration = 15,000 ng/ml								
10	-	-	-	-	-	-	-	-
20	-	-	-	-	-	-	-	-
30	-	-	-	1	1.2	1.4	1.7	1.9
40	-	-	1	1.3	1.6	1.9	2.2	2.6
50	-	-	1.2	1.6	2	2.4	2.8	3.2
60	-	1	1.4	1.9	2.4	2.9	3.4	3.8
70	-	1.1	1.7	2.2	2.8	3.4	3.9	4.5
80	-	1.3	1.9	2.6	3.2	3.8	4.5	5.1
90	-	1.4	2.2	2.9	3.6	4.3	5	5.8
100	-	1.6	2.4	3.2	4	4.8	5.6	6.4

Miscellaneous Agents

EPOPROSTENOL SODIUM (PGI_2; PGX; Prostacyclin)

Storage/Stability: Store unopened vials at 15° to 25°C (59° to 77°F). Protect from light. Protect reconstituted reconstituted solutions of epoprostenol from light and refrigerate at 2° to 8°C (36° to 46°F) for ≤ 40 hours. Do not freeze. Discard any solution that has been frozen. Discard any solution if it has been refrigerated for > 48 hours.

A single reservoir of reconstituted solution can be administered at room temperature for a duration of 8 hours or it can be used with a cold pouch and administered ≤ 24 hours with the use of two frozen 6–oz gel packs. Insulate solution from temperatures > 25°C (77°F) and < 0°C (32°F). Do not expose to direct sunlight.

Rx	**Flolan** (Glaxo Wellcome)	**Powder for reconstitution:** 0.5 mg	Mannitol, NaCl. In 17 ml.
		1.5 mg	Mannitol, NaCl. In 17 ml.

Miscellaneous Agents

MECAMYLAMINE HCl

Refer to the general discussion of these products in the Antihypertensives Introduction.

Actions:

Pharmacology: Mecamylamine is a potent, oral ganglionic blocker. Although the antihypertensive effect is predominantly orthostatic, the supine blood pressure is also significantly reduced. Because of the many side effects, ganglionic blockers are infrequently used.

Pharmacokinetics: Mecamylamine is almost completely absorbed from the GI tract. It has a gradual onset of action (0.5 to 2 hours) and a long-lasting effect (6 to 12 hours or more). It crosses the placental and the blood-brain barriers. It is slowly excreted unchanged in the urine. The rate of renal elimination is markedly influenced by urinary pH. Alkalinization of urine reduces, and acidification promotes, renal excretion of mecamylamine.

Indications:

Severe hypertension: For moderately severe to severe essential hypertension; uncomplicated malignant hypertension.

Contraindications:

Coronary insufficiency or recent myocardial infarction; uremia (do not treat patients receiving antibiotics and sulfonamides with ganglionic blockers); glaucoma; organic pyloric stenosis; hypersensitivity to mecamylamine; mild, moderate or labile hypertension; uncooperative patients.

Warnings:

CNS effects: Mecamylamine readily penetrates the brain and may produce CNS effects. Tremor, choreiform movements, mental aberrations and convulsions occur rarely, but most often with large doses, especially in patients with cerebral or renal insufficiency.

Discontinuation of therapy: When mecamylamine is suddenly discontinued, hypertension returns. This may occur abruptly and may cause fatal cerebral vascular accidents or acute congestive heart failure. Withdraw drug gradually and substitute other antihypertensive therapy. The effects of mecamylamine can last from hours to days after therapy is discontinued.

Pregnancy: Category C. Mecamylamine crosses the placenta. It is not known whether mecamylamine can cause fetal harm when given to a pregnant woman. Give to a pregnant woman only if clearly needed.

Lactation: Because of the potential for serious adverse reactions in nursing infants, either discontinue nursing or discontinue the drug, taking into account the importance of the drug to the mother.

Precautions:

Renal/Cardiovascular function: Evaluate the patient's condition, particularly renal and cardiovascular function. Give with great discretion, if at all, when renal insufficiency is manifested by a rising or elevated BUN. When renal, cerebral or coronary blood flow is deficient, avoid any additional impairment which might result from hypotension. Use with caution in patients with marked cerebral and coronary arteriosclerosis or after a recent cerebral vascular accident.

Potentiation of effects: The action of mecamylamine may be potentiated by: Excessive heat; fever; infection; hemorrhage; pregnancy; anesthesia; surgery; vigorous exercise; other antihypertensive drugs; alcohol; salt depletion resulting from diminished intake or increased excretion due to diarrhea, vomiting, excessive sweating or diuretics. During therapy, do not restrict sodium intake; if necessary, adjust the dosage.

Urinary retention may occur; use caution in patients with prostatic hypertrophy, bladder neck obstruction and urethral stricture.

Adverse Reactions:

Cardiovascular: Orthostatic dizziness; syncope.

CNS: Weakness; fatigue; sedation; dilated pupils; blurred vision; paresthesia; tremor; choreiform movements; mental aberrations; convulsions.

GI: Anorexia; dry mouth; glossitis; nausea; vomiting; constipation (sometimes preceded by small, frequent, liquid stools); ileus.

Frequent loose bowel movements with abdominal distention and decreased borborygmi may be the first signs of paralytic ileus. Discontinue the drug immediately and take remedial steps.

GU: Decreased libido; impotence; urinary retention.

Respiratory: Interstitial pulmonary edema; fibrosis; postural hypotension.

MECAMYLAMINE HCl

Overdosage:

Symptoms: Signs of overdosage include: Hypotension (which may progress to peripheral vascular collapse); postural hypotension; nausea; vomiting; diarrhea; constipation; paralytic ileus; urinary retention; dizziness; anxiety; dry mouth; mydriasis; blurred vision; palpitations. A rise in intraocular pressure may occur.

Treatment: Pressor amines may be used to counteract excessive hypotension. Since patients treated with ganglionic blockers are more than normally reactive to pressor amines, use small doses to avoid excessive response.

Patient Information:

Take after meals. Use consistent timing of doses in relation to meals.

Notify physician if tremor or signs of ileus occur.

Mecamylamine may cause dizziness, lightheadedness or fainting, especially when rising from a lying or sitting position. This effect may be increased by alcoholic beverages, exercise or hot weather. Arising slowly may alleviate such symptoms.

Administration and Dosage:

Start with 2.5 mg twice daily. Adjust dosage in increments of 2.5 mg at intervals of ≥ 2 days until the desired blood pressure response occurs (a dosage just under that which causes signs of mild postural hypotension).

The average total daily dosage is 25 mg, usually in 3 divided doses. However, as little as 2.5 mg/day may be sufficient. A range of 2 to 4 or more doses may be required in severe cases when smooth control is difficult to obtain. In severe or urgent cases, larger increments at shorter intervals may be needed. Partial tolerance may develop, requiring an increase in dosage.

Administration after meals may cause a more gradual absorption and smoother control of blood pressure. The timing of doses in relation to meals should be consistent. Since blood pressure response is increased in the early morning, give the larger dose at noontime and in the evening. The morning dose should be relatively small or may be omitted.

Blood pressure monitoring: Determine the initial and maintenance dosage by blood pressure readings in the erect position at the time of maximal drug effect, as well as by other signs and symptoms of orthostatic hypertension.

Limit the effective maintenance dose to that which causes slight faintness or dizziness in the erect posture. If the patient or a relative can use a sphygmomanometer or another blood-pressure monitoring device, instructions may be given to reduce or omit a dose if readings fall below a designated level or if faintness or lightheadedness occurs. However, do not institute any changes without consulting a physician.

Close supervision, patient education and critical dosage adjustment are essential to successful therapy.

Concomitant antihypertensive therapy: Reduce the dosage of other agents, as well as that of mecamylamine, to avoid excessive hypotension. However, continue thiazides in usual dosage while decreasing mecamylamine by at least 50%.

Rx	**Inversine** (Merck)	**Tablets:** 2.5 mg	Lactose. (MSD 52). Yellow, scored. In 100s.

Miscellaneous Agents

TOLAZOLINE HCl

Refer to the general discussion of these products in the Antihypertensives Introduction.

Actions:

Pharmacology: Tolazoline is a direct peripheral vasodilator with moderate competitive alpha-adrenergic blocking activity. It decreases peripheral resistance and increases venous capacity. It has the following actions: (1) Sympathomimetic, including cardiac stimulation; (2) parasympathomimetic, including GI tract stimulation that is blocked by atropine; and (3) histamine-like, including stimulation of gastric secretion and peripheral vasodilation. Tolazoline given IV produces vasodilation, primarily due to a direct effect on vascular smooth muscle and cardiac stimulation; blood pressure response depends on the relative contributions of the two effects. Tolazoline usually reduces pulmonary arterial pressure and vascular resistance.

Pharmacokinetics: In neonates, half-life ranges from 3 to 10 hours.

Indications:

Persistent pulmonary hypertension of the newborn ("persistent fetal circulation") when systemic arterial oxygenation cannot be satisfactorily maintained by usual supportive care (supplemental oxygen or mechanical ventilation).

Contraindications:

Hypersensitivity to tolazoline.

Warnings:

Stress ulcers: Gastric secretion is stimulated by tolazoline, which may activate stress ulcers. Through this mechanism, it can produce significant hypochloremic alkalosis. Pretreatment of infants with antacids may prevent GI bleeding.

Hypotension: Observe closely for signs of systemic hypotension. Institute supportive therapy if needed.

Mitral stenosis: May produce either a fall or a rise in pulmonary artery pressure and total pulmonary resistance. Use with caution in suspected mitral stenosis.

Pregnancy: Category C. Safety for use during pregnancy has not been established. Use only when clearly needed and when the potential benefits outweigh the potential hazards to the fetus.

Lactation: It is not known whether this drug is excreted in breast milk. Safety for use in the nursing mother has not been established. Exercise caution when administering to a nursing woman.

Precautions:

Monitoring: Use tolazoline in a highly supervised setting where vital signs, oxygenation, acid-base status and fluid and electrolytes can be monitored and maintained.

Acidosis: The effects of tolazoline on pulmonary vessels may be pH-dependent. Acidosis may decrease the effect.

Drug Interactions:

Epinephrine administration with large doses of tolazoline may cause "epinephrine reversal" (further reduction in blood pressure followed by exaggerated rebound).

Adverse Reactions:

Cardiovascular: Hypotension; tachycardia; cardiac arrhythmias; hypertension; pulmonary hemorrhage.

GI: GI hemorrhage; nausea; vomiting; diarrhea; hepatitis.

Dermatologic: Flushing; increased pilomotor activity with tingling or chilliness; rash.

Hematologic: Thrombocytopenia; leukopenia.

Renal: Edema; oliguria; hematuria.

Overdosage:

Symptoms: Increased pilomotor activity, peripheral vasodilatation and skin flushing, and in rare instances, hypotension and shock.

Treatment: In treating hypotension, place the patient in the Trendelenburg position and administer IV fluids. Do not use epinephrine (see Drug Interactions).

Administration and Dosage:

Initial dose: 1 to 2 mg/kg, via scalp vein over 10 minutes. Follow by an infusion of 1 to 2 mg/kg/hr to significantly increase arterial oxygen. There is very little experience with infusions lasting beyond 36 to 48 hours. Response, if it occurs, can be expected within 30 minutes after the initial dose.

Rx	**Priscoline HCl** (Ciba)	**Injection:** 25 mg per ml	In 4 ml amps.[1]

[1] With 0.65% tartaric acid and 0.65% hydrous sodium citrate.

ANTIHYPERTENSIVE COMBINATIONS

Effective management of many hypertensive patients frequently requires concomitant administration of two or more antihypertensive agents when a single drug does not achieve adequate control. Synergistic effects are achieved by administration of anti hypertensive drugs which act by different mechanisms; therefore, dose-related side effects may be minimized.

The following fixed-combination drugs are not indicated for initial therapy of hypertension. Establish proper therapy by adjusting the dosage of each agent to patient response. Periodically re-evaluate antihypertensive therapy as conditions in each patient warrant. If a fixed combination product represents a satisfactory dosage determined for the patient, its use may be more convenient.

For complete information concerning the components of the antihypertensive combination products, consult the appropriate drug monographs as indicated below:

THIAZIDE and RELATED DIURETICS:
- Bendroflumethiazide
- Chlorothiazide
- Chlorthalidone
- Hydrochlorothiazide
- Hydroflumethiazide
- Methyclothiazide
- Polythiazide
- Trichlormethiazide

BETA-ADRENERGIC BLOCKING AGENTS:
- Atenolol
- Bisoprolol
- Metoprolol
- Nadolol
- Propranolol
- Timolol

ANTIADRENERGIC AGENTS:
- Clonidine
- Guanethidine
- Methyldopa
- Prazosin

RAUWOLFIA DERIVATIVES:
- Deserpidine
- Rauwolfia Serpentina
- Reserpine

ANGIOTENSIN CONVERTING ENZYME INHIBITORS:
- Benazepril
- Captopril
- Enalapril
- Lisinopril

MISCELLANEOUS:
- Hydralazine

ANTIHYPERTENSIVE COMBINATIONS

Refer to the general discussion of these products in the Antihypertensive Combinations Introduction. Content given per capsule or tablet.

	Product and Distributor	Diuretic	Other Content	How Supplied
Rx	**Renese-R Tablets** (Pfizer)	2 mg polythiazide	0.25 mg reserpine	Lactose. (446). Blue, scored. In 100s and 1000s.
Rx	**Regroton Tablets** (Rhone-Poulenc Rorer)	50 mg chlorthalidone	0.25 mg reserpine	Pink. In 100s.
Rx	**Chlorothiazide/Reserpine Tablets** (Various, eg, Mylan)	500 mg chlorothiazide	0.125 mg reserpine	In 100s.
Rx	**Diupres-500 Tablets** (Merck)			Lactose. (MSD 405). Pink. In 100s and 1000s.
Rx	**Chlorothiazide/Reserpine Tablets** (Various, eg, Mylan)	250 mg chlorothiazide	0.125 mg reserpine	In 100s.
Rx	**Chloroserpine Tablets** (Rugby)			In 100s and 1000s.
Rx	**Diupres-250 Tablets** (Merck)			Lactose. (MSD 230). Pink. In 100s and 1000s.
Rx	**Hydrochlorothiazide/Reserpine Tablets** (Various, eg, Schein)	50 mg hydrochlorothiazide	0.125 mg reserpine	In 100s and 1000s.
Rx	**Hydropres-50 Tablets** (Merck)			Lactose. (MSD 127). Green. In 100s and 1000s.
Rx	**Hydro-Serp Tablets** (Rugby)			In 1000s.
Rx	**Hydroserpine #2 Tablets** (Various, eg, Rugby)			In 100s, 250s, 400s and 1000s.

ANTIHYPERTENSIVE COMBINATIONS

	Product and Distributor	Diuretic	Other Content	How Supplied
Rx	**Hydrochlorothiazide/Reserpine Tablets** (Various, eg, Schein)	25 mg hydrochlorothiazide	0.125 mg reserpine	In 100s and 1000s.
Rx	**Hydropres-25 Tablets** (Merck)			Lactose. (MSD 53). Green. In 100s and 1000s.
Rx	**Hydroserpine #1 Tablets** (Various, eg, Rugby)			In 100s and 1000s.
Rx	**Salutensin-Demi**(Roberts)	25 hydroflumethiazide	0.125 mg reserpine	Lactose, sucrose. In 100s and 1000s.
Rx	**Salutensin Tablets** (Roberts)	50 mg hydroflumethiazide	0.125 mg reserpine	Lactose, sucrose. Green. In 100s and 1000s.
Rx	**Demi-Regroton Tablets**(Rhone-Poulenc Rorer)	25 mg chlorthalidone	0.125 mg reserpine	Lactose. White. In 100s.
Rx	**Diutensen-R Tablets** (Wallace)	2.5 mg methyclothiazide	0.1 mg reserpine	White, pink. Mottled. In 100s, 500s and 5000s.
Rx	**Metatensin #4 Tablets** (Hoechst Marion Roussel)	4 mg trichlormethiazide	0.1 mg reserpine	Lactose. (Merrell 65) Lavender. In 100s.
Rx	**Metatensin #2 Tablets** (Hoechst Marion Roussel)	2 mg trichlormethiazide	0.1 mg reserpine	Lactose, tartrazine. (Merrell 64) Yellow. In 100s.
Rx	**Rauwolfia/Bendroflumethiazide Tablets** (Various, eg, Rugby)	4 mg bendroflumethiazide	50 mg powdered rauwolfia serpentina	In 100s.
Rx	**Rauzide Tablets** (B-M Squibb)			In 100s.
Rx	**Enduronyl Forte Tablets** (Abbott)	5 mg methyclothiazide	0.5 mg deserpidine	Lactose. Gray. In 100s and 1000s.
Rx	**Enduronyl Tablets** (Abbott)	5 mg methyclothiazide	0.25 mg deserpidine	Lactose. Yellow. In 100s, 1000s and UD 100s.
Rx	**Hydrap-ES Tablets** (Parmed)	15 mg hydrochlorothiazide	0.1 mg reserpine 25 mg hydralazine HC	(CC124). Salmon pink. In 100s, 500s, 1000s.
Rx	**Marpres Tablets** (Marnel)			Lt. yellow. In 100s and 1000s.
Rx	**Ser-Ap-Es Tablets** (Ciba)			Lactose, sucrose. (Ciba 71). Salmon pink. In 100s and 1000s.
Rx	**Tri-Hydroserpine Tablets** (Rugby)			In 100s and 1000s.
Rx	**Apresazide 100/50 Capsules** (Ciba)	50 mg hydrochlorothiazide	100 mg hydralazine HCl	Parabens. (Apresazide 100/50 Ciba 159). Pink, white. In 100s.
Rx	**Hydrochlorothiazide/Hydralazine Caps** (Various, eg, Major, Moore, Goldline)	50 mg hydrochlorothiazide	50 mg hydralazine HCl	In 100s, 500s and 1000s.
Rx	**Apresazide 50/50 Capsules** (Ciba)			Parabens. (Apresazide 50/50 Ciba 149). Pink, white. In 100s.

ANTIHYPERTENSIVE COMBINATIONS

	Product and Distributor	Diuretic	Other Content	How Supplied
Rx	**Hydrochlorothiazide/Hydralazine Caps** (Various, eg, Major, Moore, Parmed, Goldline)	25 mg hydrochlorothiazide	25 mg hydralazine HCl	In 100s, 500s and 1000s.
Rx	**Apresazide 25/25 Capsules** (Ciba)			Parabens. (Apresazide 25/25 Ciba 139). Lt. blue, white. In 100s.
Rx	**Atenolol/Chlorthalidone Tablets** (Various, eg, Moore, IPR, Goldline)	25 mg chlorthalidone	100 mg atenolol	In 50s, 100s, 250s, 500s and 1000s.
Rx	**Tenoretic 100 Tablets** (Zeneca)			(ICI 117). White, scored. In 100s.
Rx	**Atenolol/Chlorthalidone Tablets** (Various, eg, Moore, Mylan, IPR, Goldline)	25 mg chlorthalidone	50 mg atenolol	In 50s, 100s, 250s, 500s and 1000s.
Rx	**Tenoretic 50 Tablets** (Zeneca)			(ICI 115). White, scored. In 100s.
Rx	**Corzide Tablets 80/5** (Bristol Labs)	5 mg bendroflumethiazide	80 mg nadolol	Lactose. (284). In 100s.
Rx	**Corzide Tablets 40/5** (Bristol Labs)	5 mg bendroflumethiazide	40 mg nadolol	Lactose. (283). In 100s.
Rx	**Ziac Tablets** (Lederle)	6.25 mg hydrochlorothiazide	2.5 mg bisoprolol fumarate	(LL B12). In 30s and 100s.
			5 mg bisoprolol fumarate	(LL B13). In 30s and 100s.
			10 mg bisoprolol fumarate	(LL B14). In 30s.
Rx	**Timolide 10-25 Tablets** (Merck)	25 mg hydrochlorothiazide	10 mg timolol maleate	(Timolide MSD 67). In 100s.
Rx	**Inderide LA 160/50 Capsules** (Wyeth-Ayerst)	50 mg hydrochlorothiazide	160 mg propranolol HCl	Lactose. Long-acting. (Inderide LA 160/50). In 100s.
Rx	**Inderide LA 120/50 Capsules** (Wyeth-Ayerst)	50 mg hydrochlorothiazide	120 mg propranolol HCl	Lactose. Long-acting. (Inderide LA 120/50). In 100s.
Rx	**Inderide LA 80/50 Capsules** (Wyeth-Ayerst)	50 mg hydrochlorothiazide	80 mg propranolol HCl	Lactose. Long-acting. (Inderide LA 80/50). Beige w/gold bands. In 100s.
Rx	**Propranolol/Hydrochlorothiazide Tablets** (Various, eg, Mylan, Major)	25 mg hydrochlorothiazide	80 mg propranolol HCl	In 100s and 1000s.
Rx	**Inderide 80/25 Tablets** (Wyeth-Ayerst)			Lactose. (Inderide 80/25). In 100s.

ANTIHYPERTENSIVE COMBINATIONS

	Product and Distributor	Diuretic	Other Content	How Supplied
Rx	**Propranolol/Hydrochlorothiazide Tablets** (Various, eg, Major, Mylan)	25 mg hydrochlorothiazide	40 mg propranolol HCl	In 100s.
Rx	**Inderide 40/25 Tablets** (Wyeth-Ayerst)			Lactose. (Inderide 40/25). In 100s, 1000s and UD 100s.
Rx	**Methyldopa and Hydrochlorothiazide Tablets** (Various, eg, Major, Rugby, Warner Chilcott)	50 mg hydrochlorothiazide	500 mg methyldopa	In 100s, 250s and 500s.
Rx	**Aldoril D50 Tablets** (Merck)			(MSD 935). White. Oval. Film coated. In 100s.
Rx	**Methyldopa/Hydrochlorothiazide Tablets** (Various, eg, Major, Rugby, Warner Chilcott)	30 mg hydrochlorothiazide	500 mg methyldopa	In 100s, 250s and 500s.
Rx	**Aldoril D30 Tablets** (Merck)			(MSD 694). Salmon. Oval. Film coated. In 100s.
Rx	**Aldoclor-250 Tablets** (Merck)	250 mg chlorothiazide	250 mg methyldopa	(MSD 634). Green. Film coated. In 100s.
Rx	**Aldoclor-150 Tablets** (Merck)	150 mg chlorothiazide	250 mg methyldopa	(MSD 612). Beige. Film coated. In 100s.
Rx	**Methyldopa/Hydrochlorothiazide Tablets** (Various, eg, Goldline, Major, Mylan, Rugby, Warner-Chilcott)	25 mg hydrochlorothiazide	250 mg methyldopa	In 100s, 500s, 1000s and UD 100s.
Rx	**Aldoril-25 Tablets** (Merck)			(MSD 456). White. Film coated. In 100s, 1000s and UD 100s.
Rx	**Methyldopa/Hydrochlorothiazide Tablets** (Various, eg, Goldline, Major, Mylan, Warner Chilcott)	15 mg hydrochlorothiazide	250 mg methyldopa	In 100s, 500s, 1000s and UD 100s.
Rx	**Aldoril-15 Tablets** (Merck)			(MSD 423). Salmon. Film coated. In 100s and 1000s.
Rx	**Lopressor HCT 100/50 Tablets** (Geigy)	50 mg hydrochlorothiazide	100 mg metoprolol tartrate	Lactose, sucrose. (Geigy 73 73). White, yellow, scored. Capsule shape. In 100s.
Rx	**Lopressor HCT 100/25 Tablets** (Geigy)	25 mg hydrochlorothiazide	100 mg metoprolol tartrate	Lactose, sucrose. (Geigy 53 53). White, pink, scored. Capsule shape. In 100s.
Rx	**Lopressor HCT 50/25 Tablets** (Geigy)	25 mg hydrochlorothiazide	50 mg metoprolol tartrate	Lactose, sucrose. (Geigy 35 35). White, blue, scored. Capsule shape. In 100s.
Rx	**Capozide 50/25 Tablets** (B-M Squibb)	25 mg hydrochlorothiazide	50 mg captopril	Peach. Biconvex, oval. In 100s.

ANTIHYPERTENSIVE COMBINATIONS

	Product and Distributor	Diuretic	Other Content	How Supplied
Rx	**Capozide 25/25 Tablets** (B-M Squibb)	25 mg hydrochlorothiazide	25 mg captopril	Peach, scored. Biconvex, square. In 100s.
Rx	**Capozide 50/15 Tablets** (B-M Squibb)	15 mg hydrochlorothiazide	50 mg captopril	White, orange, mottled, scored. Oval. In 100s.
Rx	**Capozide 25/15 Tablets** (B-M Squibb)	15 mg hydrochlorothiazide	25 mg captopril	White, orange, mottled, scored. Biconvex, square. In 100s.
Rx	**Lotensin HCT Tablets 20/25** (Ciba-Geigy))	25 mg hydrochlorothiazide	20 mg benazepril	Lactose. (C-G 75). Red, scored. Oblong. In 100s and *Accu-Pak* 100s.
Rx	**Lotensin HCT Tablets 20/12.5** (Ciba-Geigy)	12.5 mg hydrochlorothiazide	20 mg benazepril	Lactose. (C-G 74). Grayish-violet, scored. Oblong. In 100s and *Accu-Pak* 100s.
Rx	**Lotensin HCT Tablets 10/12.5** (Ciba-Geigy)	12.5 mg hydrochlorothiazide	10 mg benazepril	Lactose. (C-G 72). Lt. pink, scored. Oblong. In 100s and *Accu-Pak* 100s.
Rx	**Lotensin HCT Tablets 5/6.25** (Ciba-Geigy)	6.25 mg hydrochlorothiazide	5 mg benazepril	Lactose. (C-G 57). White, scored. Oblong. In 100s and *Accu-Pak* 100s.
Rx	**Vaseretic 10-25 Tablets** (Merck)	25 mg hydrochlorothiazide	10 mg enalapril maleate	(Vaseretic MSD 720). Red. In 100s.
Rx	**Vaseretic 5-12.5 Tablets** (Merck)	12.5 mg hydrochlorothiazide	5 mg enalapril maleate	Lactose. In unit-of-use 100s.
Rx	**Prinzide 25 Tablets** (Merck)	25 mg hydrochlorothiazide	20 mg lisinopril	(MSD 142 Prinzide). In 30s and 100s.
Rx	**Zestoretic Tablets** (Zeneca)	25 mg hydrochlorothiazide	20 mg lisinopril	(Stuart 145 Zestoretic). Peach. Biconvex. In 100s.
Rx	**Prinzide 12.5 Tablets** (Merck)	12.5 mg hydrochlorothiazide	20 mg lisinopril	(MSD 140 Prinzide). In 30s and 100s.
Rx	**Zestoretic Tablets** (Zeneca)	12.5 mg hydrochlorothiazide	20 mg lisinopril	(Stuart 142 Zestoretic). White. Biconvex. In 100s.
Rx	**Prinzide Tablets** (Merck)	12.5 mg hydrochlorothiazide	10 mg lisinopril	In 30s and 100s.
Rx	**Zestoretic Tablets** (Zeneca)	12.5 mg hydrochlorothiazide	10 mg lisinopril	(Stuart 141). Peach. Biconvex. In 100s.
Rx	**Clonidine HCl/Chlorthalidone Tablets** (Various, eg, Mylan)	15 mg chlorthalidone	0.3 mg clonidine HCl	In 100s.
Rx	**Combipres 0.3 Tablets** (Boehringer Ingelheim)	15 mg chlorthalidone	0.3 mg clonidine HCl	Lactose, parabens. (BI 10). White, scored. Oval. In 100s.

ANTIHYPERTENSIVE COMBINATIONS

	Product and Distributor	Diuretic	Other Content	How Supplied
Rx	**Clonidine HCl/Chlorthalidone Tablets** (Various, eg, Mylan)	15 mg chlorthalidone	0.2 mg clonidine HCl	In 100s, 500s and 1000s.
Rx	**Combipres 0.2 Tablets** (Boehringer Ingelheim)			Lactose, parabens. (BI 9). Blue, scored. Oval. In 100s and 1000s.
Rx	**Clonidine HCl/Chlorthalidone Tablets** (Various, eg, Mylan)	15 mg chlorthalidone	0.1 mg clonidine HCl	In 100s, 500s and 1000s.
Rx	**Combipres 0.1 Tablets** (Boehringer Ingelheim)			Lactose, parabens. (BI 8). Pink, scored. Oval. In 100s and 1000s.
Rx	**Minizide 5 Capsules** (Pfizer)	0.5 mg polythiazide	5 mg prazosin HCl	(436). Blue-green, blue. In 100s.
Rx	**Minizide 2 Capsules** (Pfizer)	0.5 mg polythiazide	2 mg prazosin HCl	(432). Blue-green, pink. In 100s.
Rx	**Minizide 1 Capsules** (Pfizer)	0.5 mg polythiazide	1 mg prazosin HCl	(430). Blue-green. In 100s.
Rx	**Esimil Tablets** (Ciba)	25 mg hydrochlorothiazide	10 mg guanethidine monosulfate	Lactose, sucrose. (Ciba 47). White, scored. In 100s.
rx	**Hyzaar Tablets** (Merck)	12.5 mg hydrochlorothiazide	50 mg losartan potassium, 4.24 mg potassium	Lactose. (MRK 717 Hyzaar). Yellow. Teardrop shape. Film coated. In 30s, 90s, 100s and UD 100s.
Rx	**Lotrel Capsules** (Ciba-Geigy)		2.5 mg amlodipine; 10 mg benazepril HCl	White/gold bands. In 100s.
			5 mg amlodipine; 10 mg benazepril HCl	Lt. brown/white bands. In 100s.
			5 mg amlodipine; 20 mg benazepril HCl	Pink/white bands. In 100s.
Rx	**Teczem Extended-Release Tablets** (Hoechst Marion Roussel)		180 mg diltiazem maleate; 5 mg enalapril maleate	Sucrose. (Teczem 5/180). Gold. Capsule shape. Film-coated. In unit-of-use 100s.
Rx	**Lexxel Extended-Release Tablets** (Astra Merck)		5 mg enalapril maleate; 5 mg felodipine	(Lexxel 1, 5-5). White. Film-coated. in 30s, 100s and UD 100s.

SODIUM POLYSTYRENE SULFONATE

Actions:

Pharmacology: Sodium polystyrene sulfonate is a cation exchange resin used for the reduction of elevated potassium levels. As the resin passes along the intestine, or is retained in the colon after administration by enema, the sodium ions are partially released and are replaced by potassium ions. This action occurs primarily in the large intestine. The efficiency of this process is limited and unpredictable. Although the exchange capacity in vitro approximates 3.1 mEq potassium per gram, in vivo it is approximately 33%, or 1 mEq potassium per gram; however, the range is so large that electrolyte balance must be monitored. Onset of action after oral administration ranges from 2 to 12 hours, and is longer after rectal administration.

Indications:

Hyperkalemia: Treatment of hyperkalemia.

Warnings:

Severe hyperkalemia: Since effective lowering of serum potassium may take hours to days, treatment with this drug alone may be insufficient to rapidly correct severe hyperkalemia associated with states of rapid tissue breakdown (eg, burns, renal failure) or hyperkalemia so marked as to constitute a medical emergency. Consider other definitive measures, including the use of IV calcium to antagonize the effects of hyperkalemia on the heart, IV sodium bicarbonate or glucose and insulin to cause an intracellular shift of potassium, or dialysis.

Hypokalemia: Serious potassium deficiency can occur. Carefully control by frequent serum potassium determinations within each 24 hour period. Since intracellular potassium deficiency is not always reflected by serum potassium levels, determine the level at which treatment should be discontinued based on the patient's clinical condition and ECG. Early clinical signs of severe hypokalemia include irritable confusion and delayed thought processes. It is often associated with a lengthened QT interval, widening, flattening or inversion of the T wave and prominent U waves. Cardiac arrhythmias may occur, such as premature atrial, nodal and ventricular contractions, and supraventricular and ventricular tachycardias. Toxic effects of digitalis are likely to be exaggerated. Severe muscle weakness, at times extending into paralysis, may also occur.

Electrolyte imbalance: Sodium polystyrene sulfonate is not totally selective for potassium, and small amounts of other cations (magnesium and calcium) can also be lost during treatment. Accordingly, monitor patients for all applicable electrolyte disturbances.

Precautions:

Sodium: Use caution when administering to patients who cannot tolerate even a small increase in sodium loads (ie, severe congestive heart failure, severe hypertension, marked edema). One gram contains 100 mg (4.1 mEq) sodium, with about one-third being delivered to the body. Compensatory restriction of sodium intake from other sources may be indicated.

Constipation, if it occurs, is treated with 10 to 20 ml of 70% sorbitol every 2 hours or as needed to produce one or two watery stools daily. This measure also reduces any tendency toward fecal impaction.

Drug Interactions:

Antacids/Laxatives: Systemic alkalosis has occurred after cation exchange resins were administered orally in combination with nonabsorbable cation donating antacids and laxatives (eg, magnesium hydroxide, aluminum carbonate). Do not administer magnesium hydroxide with sodium polystyrene sulfonate. A grand mal seizure has occurred in one patient with chronic hypocalcemia of renal failure who was given sodium polystyrene sulfonate with magnesium hydroxide as a laxative. The simultaneous oral administration of sodium polystyrene sulfonate with these drugs may reduce the resin's potassium exchange capability. The effects of this interaction have only been demonstrated in patients with renal failure.

Adverse Reactions:

GI: Gastric irritation; anorexia, nausea, vomiting and constipation may occur, especially with high doses. Occasionally, diarrhea develops. Large doses in elderly individuals may cause fecal impaction, which may be obviated through use of the resin in enemas. Intestinal obstruction, due to concretions of aluminum hydroxide when used in combination with sodium polystyrene sulfonate, has occurred.

Electrolyte Disturbance: Hypokalemia; hypocalcemia; sodium retention.

SODIUM POLYSTYRENE SULFONATE

Administration and Dosage:

Individualize dosage.

Oral:

Adults – The average dose is 15 to 60 g, best provided by administering 15 g, 1 to 4 times daily.

Children – In smaller children and infants, employ lower doses by using the exchange ratio of 1 mEq potassium per gram of resin as the basis for calculation. A dose of approximately 1 g/kg every 6 hours has been recommended.

Oral suspension (powdered formula): Give each dose as a suspension in water, or for greater palatability, in syrup. The amount of fluid usually ranges from 20 to 100 ml, depending on the dose, or 3 to 4 ml/g resin. Use sorbitol to combat constipation.

Nasogastric tube: The resin may be introduced into the stomach through a plastic tube and, if desired, mixed with a diet appropriate for a patient with renal failure.

A sodium polystyrene sulfonate candy has been used successfully.[1]

Enema: Although less effective, the resin may be given in a daily enema consisting (for adults) of 30 to 50 g every 6 hours. After an initial cleansing enema, insert a soft, large (French 28) rubber tube into the rectum for a distance of about 20 cm, with the tip well into the sigmoid colon, and tape in place. Suspend the resin in the appropriate amount of aqueous vehicle (eg, 100 ml sorbitol or 20% Dextrose in Water) at body temperature and introduce by gravity, while the particles are kept in suspension by stirring. Flush the suspension with 50 or 100 ml of fluid (to make a total fluid of 150 to 200 ml) and then clamp the tube and leave in place. If back leakage occurs, elevate the hips on pillows or assume a knee-chest position temporarily. A somewhat thicker suspension may be used, but take care that no paste is formed, because the latter has a greatly reduced exchange surface and will be ineffective if deposited in the rectal ampulla. Keep the suspension in the sigmoid colon for several hours, if possible. Retention times of at least 30 minutes have been recommended. Then, irrigate the colon with a nonsodium-containing solution at body temperature to remove the resin. Two quarts of flushing solution may be necessary. Drain the returns constantly through a Y-tube connection.

Preparation and storage: Store at 15° to 30°C (59° to 86°F). Dispense in tight containers. Store repackaged product in refrigerator and use within 14 days of repackaging. Freshly prepare suspensions; do not store beyond 24 hours. Do not heat since this may alter the exchange properties of the resin.

Rx	**SPS** (Carolina Medical Products Co.)	**Suspension:** 15 g per 60 ml. Sodium content 1.5 g (65 mEq).	With 21.5 ml sorbitol solution (equivalent to 20 g sorbitol) and 0.3% alcohol per 60 ml, propylene glycol, sodium saccharin and methyl- and propylparabens. Cherry flavor. In 120, 480 ml and UD 60 ml.
Rx	**Sodium Polystyrene Sulfonate** (Roxane)	**Suspension:** 15 g per 60 ml.	With 14.1 g sorbitol and 0.1% alcohol per 60 ml. In 60, 120, 200 and 500 ml.
Rx	**Kayexalate** (Sanofi Winthrop)	**Powder:** Finely powdered sodium polystyrene sulfonate. Sodium content ≈ 100 mg (4.1 mEq) per g.	In 1 lb jars.

[1] Am J Hosp Pharm1978;35:1034-35.

CARDIOPLEGIC SOLUTION

Actions:

Pharmacology: Cardioplegic solution with added sodium bicarbonate, when cooled and instilled into the coronary artery vasculature, causes prompt arrest of cardiac electromechanical activity, combats intracellular ion losses and buffers ischemic acidosis. When used with hypothermia and ischemia, the action may be characterized as cold ischemic potassium-induced cardioplegia. This provides a quiet, relaxed heart and bloodless field of operation. The component electrolytes and their physiologic effects are listed below:

Pharmacokinetics:

Calcium (Ca^{++}) ion maintains integrity of cell membrane to ensure against calcium paradox during reperfusion.

Magnesium (Mg^{++}) ion may help stabilize the myocardial membrane by inhibiting a myosin phosphorylase, which protects adenosine triphosphate (ATP) reserves for postischemic activity. The protective effects of magnesium and potassium are additive.

Potassium (K^{++}) ion causes prompt cessation of mechanical myocardial contractile activity.The immediacy of the arrest thus preserves energy supplies for postischemic contractile activity in diastole.

Chloride (Cl-) and sodium (Na^{+}) ions – Sodium is essential to maintain ionic integrity of myocardial tissue. Chloride ions maintain the electroneutrality of the solution and have no specific role in the production of cardiac arrest.

Bicarbonate (HCO_3-) anion acts as a buffer to render the solution slightly alkaline and compensate for the metabolic acidosis that accompanies ischemia.

Indications:

With ischemia and hypothermia, induces cardiac arrest during open heart surgery.

Contraindications:

Do not administer without the addition of 8.4% Sodium Bicarbonate Injection.

Not for IV injection; only for instillation into cardiac vasculature.

Warnings:

Only those trained to perform open heart surgery should use this solution. It is intended only for use during cardiopulmonary bypass when the coronary circulation is isolated from the systemic circulation.

Right heart venting is recommended. If large volumes of cardioplegic solution are infused and allowed to return to the heart lung machine without any venting from the right heart, plasma magnesium and potassium levels may rise. Development of severe hypotension and metabolic acidosis while on bypass has occurred when large volumes (8 to 10 L) of solution are instilled and allowed to enter the pump and then the systemic circulation.

Pregnancy: Category C. Safety for use during pregnancy has not been established. Use only when clearly needed and when the potential benefits outweigh the potential hazards to the fetus.

Precautions:

Monitor myocardial temperature during surgery to maintain hypothermia.

Continuous ECG monitoring of myocardial activity during the procedure is essential.

Appropriate equipment to defibrillate the heart following cardioplegia and inotropic agents during postoperative recovery should be readily available.

Do not administer unless solution is clear and container is undamaged.

Adverse Reactions:

Potential hazards of open heart surgery include myocardial infarction, ECG abnormalities and arrhythmias, including ventricular fibrillation. Spontaneous recovery may be delayed or absent when circulation is restored. Defibrillation by electric shock may be required to restore normal cardiac function.

Overdosage:

Overzealous instillation may result in unnecessary dilatation of the myocardial vasculature and leakage into the perivascular myocardium, possibly causing tissue edema.

Administration and Dosage:

The following information is a guide:

Following institution of cardiopulmonary bypass at perfusate temperatures of 28° to 30°C, (82° to 86°F) and cross-clamping of the ascending aorta, administer the buffered solution by rapid infusion into the aortic root. The initial rate of infusion may be 300 ml/m^2/minute (about 540 ml/min in a 1.8 meter, 70 kg adult with 1.8 square meters of surface area) given for 2 to 4 minutes. Concurrent external cooling (regional hypothermia of the pericardium) may be accomplished by instilling a refrigerated (4°C) physiologic solution such as *Normosol-R* (balanced electrolyte replacement solution) or Ringer's Injection into the chest cavity. If myocardial electromechanical activity persists or recurs, the solution may be reinfused at a rate of 300 ml/m^2/min for 2 minutes. Repeat every 20 to 30 minutes or sooner if myocardial temperature rises above 15° to 20°C or returning cardiac activity is observed. The regional hypothermia solution around the heart also may be replenished continuously or periodically in order to maintain adequate hypothermia. Suction may be used to remove warmed infusates. An implanted thermistor probe may be used to monitor myocardial temperature.

The volumes of solution instilled into the aortic root may vary depending on the duration or type of open heart surgical procedure.

Preparation of solution: The solution contains no preservatives and is intended only for a single operative procedure. After adjusting pH with sodium bicarbonate, extemporaneous alternative buffering is not recommended. Discard the unused portion.

Add 10 ml (840 mg) of 8.4% Sodium Bicarbonate Injection (10 mEq each of sodium and bicarbonate) to each 1000 ml of the cardioplegic solution just prior to administration to adjust pH to approximately 7.8 when measured at room temperature. Use of any other Sodium Bicarbonate Injection may not achieve this pH due to the varying pH's of Sodium Bicarbonate Injections. Cool the buffered solution with added sodium bicarbonate to 4°C prior to administration and use within 24 hours of mixing.

Admixture incompatibility: Additives may be incompatible. Consult with pharmacist, if possible. When introducing additives, use aseptic technique, mix thoroughly and do not store.

Storage: Store at 25°C (77°F); however, brief exposure up to 40°C (104°F) does not adversely affect the product. Protect from freezing and extreme heat.

Rx	**Plegisol** (Abbott)	**Solution:** 17.6 mg calcium chloride dihydrate, 325.3 mg magnesium chloride hexahydrate, 119.3 mg potassium chloride and 643 mg sodium chloride per 100 ml (approx. 260 mOsm/L)	In single dose 1000 ml flexible plastic container.

SALT SUBSTITUTES

Indications:

Food seasoning to be used as a substitute for salt (NaCl) at the table or in cooking to help regulate dietary sodium intake. Appropriate for persons on low sodium diets (ie, persons whose sodium intake has been restricted for medical reasons).

For normal healthy people. Persons having diabetes, heart or kidney disease or persons receiving medical treatment should consult a physician before using a salt substitute or alternative.

Contraindications:

Hyperkalemia; oliguria; severe kidney disease.

Warnings:

Potassium: Salt substitutes contain a significant amount of potassium and other electrolytes. Excessive use could result in hyperkalemia.

Evaluate the potassium intake of persons receiving potassium-sparing diuretics or potassium supplementation. Use with extreme caution in these patients.

Sodium: Excessive sodium depletion may lead to symptoms such as weakness, nausea and muscle cramps; in severe cases, uremia may follow. On the appearance of early symptoms, liberalize sodium intake.

	Product and Distributor	Contents	Sodium Content[1]		Potassium Content[1]		How Supplied
			mg/5 g	mEq/5 g	mg/5 g	mEq/5 g	
otc	**Adolph's Salt Substitute** (Adolph's)	Potassium chloride, silicon dioxide and tartaric acid	0	0	2480	64	In 99.2 g.
otc	**Morton Salt Substitute** (Morton Salt)	Potassium chloride, fumaric acid, tricalcium phosphate and monocalcium phosphate	< 0.5	< 0.02	2515	64	In 88.6 g.
otc	**Morton Seasoned Salt Substitute** (Morton Salt)	Potassium chloride, spices, sugar, fumaric acid, tricalcium phosphate, monocalcium phosphate	< 1	< 0.04	2165	56	In 85 g.
otc	**Nu-Salt** (Cumberland Pkg.)	Potassium chloride, potassium bitartrate, calcium silicate, natural flavor derived from yeast	0.85	< 0.04	2640	68	In 100 g.

[1] The amounts of sodium and potassium given are approximate values.

EDETATE DISODIUM

> **Warning:**
> Use of this drug is recommended only when the severity of the clinical condition justifies the aggressive measures associated with this type of therapy.

Actions:

Pharmacokinetics: Edetate disodium (EDTA) forms chelates with many divalent and trivalent metals. Because of its affinity for calcium, EDTA will lower serum calcium levels during IV infusion. Slow infusion may cause mobilization of extracirculatory calcium stores. The chelate formed is excreted in the urine. EDTA exerts a negative inotropic effect on the heart.

Additionally, EDTA forms chelates with other polyvalent metals, thus increasing urinary excretion of magnesium, zinc and other trace elements. It does not chelate with potassium, but may reduce the serum level; increased potassium excretion may occur.

Indications:

Hypercalcemia: Emergency treatment of hypercalcemia.

Ventricular arrhythmias: Control of ventricular arrhythmias associated with digitalis toxicity.

Unlabeled uses:

Chelation treatment is not indicated for atherosclerotic vascular diseases. Although it has been advocated for these diseases (eg, coronary artery disease, cerebrovascular disease, peripheral vascular disease) based on the theory of decalcification of atherosclerotic plaques, both the proposed explanations of pathogenesis and mechanism of action are suspect. In addition, EDTA is not innocuous. The medical community generally agrees that chelation therapy is not an acceptable treatment for atherosclerotic vascular diseases.

Contraindications:

Anuria; hypersensitivity to any component of the preparation.

Warnings:

Rapid IV infusion or a high serum concentration of EDTA may cause a precipitous drop in serum calcium and may result in death. Toxicity depends on total dosage and rate of administration. Do not exceed recommended dosage and rates of administration.

Dilution before infusion is necessary because of EDTA's irritant effect on the tissues and because of the danger of serious side effects.

Calcium: The oxalate method of determining serum calcium tends to give low readings in the presence of EDTA; modification (eg, acidifying the sample) or use of a different method may be required for accuracy. The least interference will be noted immediately before a subsequent dose is administered.

Hypokalemia: Use with caution in patients with clinical or subclinical potassium deficiency; monitor serum potassium levels and ECG changes.

Diabetics: Blood sugar and insulin requirements may be lower in insulin-dependent diabetics.

Hypomagnesemia: Consider the possibility of hypomagnesemia during prolonged therapy.

Renal function impairment: Prior to treatment, assess renal excretory function; perform periodic BUN and creatinine determinations and daily urinalysis during treatment.

Pregnancy: Category C. Safety for use during pregnancy has not been established. Use only when clearly needed and when the potential benefits outweigh the potential hazards to the fetus.

Lactation: Safety for use during breastfeeding has not been established.

Precautions:

Monitoring: Because of the possibility of inducing an electrolyte imbalance during treatment, perform appropriate laboratory determinations to evaluate cardiac status. Repeat as often as clinically indicated, particularly in patients with ventricular arrhythmia and those with a history of seizures or intracranial lesions. If clinical evidence suggests any disturbance of liver function during treatment, perform appropriate laboratory determinations; withdraw drug if required.

Postural hypotension: After infusion, have the patient remain supine for a short time because of the possibility of postural hypotension.

EDETATE DISODIUM

Cardiac effects: Consider the possibility of an adverse effect on myocardial contractility when administering the drug to patients with heart disease. Use this drug cautiously in patients with limited cardiac reserve or incipient congestive failure.

Adverse Reactions:

GI: Nausea, vomiting and diarrhea (fairly common).

CNS: Transient circumoral paresthesia, numbness and headache.

Body as a whole: Transient drop in systolic and diastolic blood pressure; thrombophlebitis; febrile reactions; hyperuricemia; anemia; exfoliative dermatitis; other toxic skin and mucous membrane reactions. Nephrotoxicity and damage to the reticuloendothelial system with hemorrhagic tendencies have been reported with excessive dosages.

Overdosage:

Because EDTA may produce a precipitous drop in serum calcium, have an IV calcium salt (such as calcium gluconate) available. Exercise extreme caution in the use of IV calcium in the treatment of tetany, especially in digitalized patients, because the action of the drug and the replacement of calcium ions may produce a reversal of the desired digitalis effect.

Administration and Dosage:

Adults: Administer 50 mg/kg/day to a maximum dose of 3 g in 24 hours. Dissolve dose in 500 ml of 5% Dextrose Injection or 0.9% Sodium Chloride Injection. Infuse over ≥ 3 hours and do not exceed the patient's cardiac reserve. A suggested regimen includes 5 consecutive daily doses followed by 2 days without medication; repeat this regimen as necessary, up to a total of 15 doses.

Children: Administer 40 mg/kg/day (18 mg/lb/day) to a maximum dose of 70 mg/kg/day. Dissolve in a sufficient volume of 5% Dextrose Injection or 0.9% Sodium Chloride Injection to bring the final concentration to not more than 3%. Infuse over ≥ 3 hours; do not exceed the patient's cardiac reserve.

Storage/Stability: Store at room temperature.

Rx	**Edetate Disodium** (Various, eg, McGuff, Schein, Steris)	**Injection:** 150 mg/ml	In 20 ml vials.
Rx	**Disotate** (Forest)		In 20 ml vials.
Rx	**Endrate** (Abbott)		In 20 ml amps.

ANTIHYPERLIPIDEMIC AGENTS

Lowering cholesterol levels can arrest or reverse atherosclerosis in all vascular beds and can significantly decrease the morbidity and mortality associated with atherosclerosis. Each 10% reduction in cholesterol levels is associated with an ≈ 20% to 30% reduction in the incidence of coronary heart disease. Hyperlipidemia, particularly elevated serum cholesterol and low density lipoprotein (LDL) levels, is a risk factor in the development of atherosclerotic cardiovascular disease.

Individually assess potential benefits and risks of therapy. The cornerstone of treatment in primary hyperlipidemia is diet restriction and weight reduction. Limit or eliminate alcohol intake. Use drug therapy in conjunction with diet, and after maximal efforts to control serum lipids by diet alone prove unsatisfactory, when tolerance to or compliance with diet is poor or when hyperlipidemia is severe and risk of complications is high. Treat contributory diseases such as hypothyroidism or diabetes mellitus.

Elevated blood cholesterol levels are a major cause of coronary artery disease. Lowering these levels (specifically, LDL cholesterol) will reduce the risk of heart attacks caused by coronary heart disease (CHD).

Positive risk factors for CHD (other than high LDL) include: Age (men ≥ 45 years of age; women ≥ 55 years of age or women who go through premature menopause without estrogen replacement therapy), history of occlusive peripheral arterial disease, family history of premature CHD, smoking, hypertension (> 140/90 mmHg) or use of antihypertensive medications, low HDL-cholesterol (< 35 mg/dl), obesity (> 30% overweight) and diabetes mellitus. Physical inactivity is not listed but should also be considered.

Negative risk factors include: High HDL-cholesterol (≥ 60 mg/dl); subtract one risk factor if the patient's HDL is at this level. All Americans (except children < 2 years old) should adopt a diet that reduces total dietary fat, decreases intake of saturated fat, increases intake of polyunsaturated fat and reduces daily cholesterol intake to ≤ 250 to 300 mg. The National Cholesterol Education Program Expert Panel on Detection, Evaluation and Treatment of High Blood Cholesterol in Adults has provided guidelines for the treatment of high blood cholesterol in adults ≥ 20 years of age.

Classification of Total and HDL Cholesterol Levels

Level (mg/dl) (mmol/L)	Classification
< 200 (5.2)	desirable
200-239 (5.2 - 6.2)	borderline-high
≥ 240 (6.2)	high
HDL < 35 (0.9)	low

1. Total blood cholesterol < 200 mg/dl: HDL ≥ 35 mg/dl, repeat total cholesterol and HDL measurements within 5 years or with physical exam; provide education on general population eating pattern, physical activity and risk factor education. HDL < 35 mg/dl, do lipoprotein analysis; base further action on LDL levels.
2. Total blood cholesterol 200 to 239 mg/dl: HDL ≥ 35 mg/dl and fewer than two risk factors, provide information on dietary modification, physical activity and risk factor reduction; re-evaluate in 1 to 2 years, repeat total and HDL cholesterol measurements and reinforce nutrition and physical activity education. HDL < 35 mg/dl or two or more risk factors, analyze lipoprotein; base further action on LDL levels.
3. Total blood cholesterol ≥ 240 mg/dl: Analyze lipoprotein; base further action on LDL levels.

Classification of LDL- Cholesterol Levels

Level (mg/dl) (mmol/L)	Classification
< 130 (3.4)	desirable
130 -159 (3.4 - 4.1)	borderline-high
≥ 160 (4.1)	high

1. Level ≥ 160 mg/dl without CHD and with fewer than two risk factors, level ≥ 130 mg/dl without CHD and with two or more risk factors: Dietary treatment.
2. Level ≥ 190 mg/dl without CHD or two other risk factors, or level ≥ 160 mg/dl with CHD or two other risk factors: Drug treatment.

ANTIHYPERLIPIDEMIC AGENTS

Hyperlipidemias: Elevation of serum cholesterol, triglycerides or both is characteristic of hyperlipidemias. Differentiation of the specific biochemical abnormality requires identification of specific lipoprotein fractions in the serum. Lipoproteins transport serum lipids and are identified by their density and electrophoretic mobility. Chylomicrons are the largest and least dense of the lipoproteins, followed in order of increasing density and decreasing size by very low density lipoproteins (VLDL or pre-β), intermediate low density lipoproteins (ILDL or broad-β), low density lipoproteins (LDL or β) and high density lipoproteins (HDL or α). Triglycerides are transported primarily by chylomicrons and VLDL; the predominant cholesterol transporting lipoprotein is LDL.

Elevations and treatment associated with each type of hyperlipidemia follow:

Hyperlipidemias and Their Treatment[1]

Hyperlipidemia type	I	IIa	IIb	III	IV	V
Lipids						
Cholesterol	N-⇧	↑	↑	N-↑	N-⇧	N-↑
Triglycerides	↑	N	↑	N-↑	↑	↑
Lipoproteins						
Chylomicrons	↑	N	N	N	N	↑
VLDL (pre-β)	N-⇧	N-↓	↑	N-⇧	↑	↑
ILDL (broad-β)[2]				↑		
LDL (β)	↓	↑	↑	↑	N-⇩	↓
HDL (α)	↓	N	N	N	N-⇩	↓
Treatment	Diet	Diet HMG-CoA reductase inhibitors Bile acid sequestrants Nicotinic acid Dextrothyroxine	Diet HMG-CoA reductase inhibitors Bile acid sequestrants[3] Gemfibrozil[5] Nicotinic acid Clofibrate[4]	Diet Nicotinic acid Gemfibrozil Clofibrate	Diet Gemfibrozil Nicotinic acid Clofibrate	Diet Gemfibrozil Nicotinic acid[6] Clofibrate

[1] N = normal ↑ = increase ↓ = decrease ⇧ = slight increase ⇩ = slight decrease
[2] An abnormal lipoprotein.
[3] Particularly useful if hypercholesterolemia predominates.
[4] With high serum triglyceride levels and moderately elevated cholesterol.
[5] In patients w/inadequate response to weight loss, bile acid sequestrants, nicotinic acid.
[6] Norethindrone acetate (women) and oxandrolone (men) are effective, but use is not FDA-approved.

The following table summarizes the effects of the various antihyperlipidemic drugs on serum lipids and lipoproteins:

Antihyperlipidemic Drug Effects[1]

Drug	Lipids		Lipoproteins		
	Cholesterol	Triglycerides	VLDL (pre-β)	LDL (β)	HDL
Atorvastatin	↓	↓	↓	↓	↑
Cholestyramine	↓	→↑	→↑	↓	→↑
Clofibrate[2]	↓	↓	↓	→↓	→↑
Colestipol	↓	→↑	↑	↓	→↑
Dextrothyroxine[2]	↓	→	→	↓	→
Fluvastatin	↓	↓	↓	↓	↑
Gemfibrozil	↓	↓	↓	→↓	↑
Lovastatin	↓	↓	↓	↓	↑
Nicotinic Acid	↓	↓	↓	↓	↑
Pravastatin	↓	↓	↓	↓	↑
Simvastatin	↓	↓	↓	↓	↑

[1] ↓ = decrease ↑ = increase → = unchanged
[2] These agents are no longer commonly used as antihyperlipidemics.

ANTIHYPERLIPIDEMIC AGENTS

General considerations:

1.) Define the type of hyperlipoproteinemia and establish baseline serum cholesterol and triglyceride levels.
2.) Institute a trial of diet, weight reduction and physical activity, which are extremely important elements of therapy for high blood cholesterol. Remind patients to restrict their dietary intake of cholesterol and saturated fats and to adhere to prescribed dietary regimens. Drug therapy does not reduce the importance of adhering to diet.
3.) Carefully monitor the patient during treatment, including serum cholesterol and triglyceride levels.
4.) Consider failure of cholesterol level to fall or a significant rise in triglyceride level as indications to discontinue medication.

Dietary treatment: Reducing elevated cholesterol levels and maintaining adequate nutrition is the aim of dietary therapy. Step I and Step II diets are specifically designed to progressively reduce saturated fatty acids and cholesterol intake and promote weight loss in overweight individuals by eliminating excess total calories and increasing physical activity.

Step I – Total fat intake ≤ 30% of calories; saturated fatty acid intake < 8% to 10% of calories; cholesterol intake < 300 mg/day. Measure serum total cholesterol and adherence to diet at 4 to 6 weeks and at 3 months. If cholesterol and LDL level goals are met, monitor quarterly the first year and twice a year thereafter. If response is insufficient, proceed to Step II.

Step II – Saturated fatty acid intake < 7% of calories; cholesterol intake < 200 mg/day. Measure serum total cholesterol and adherence to diet at 4 to 6 weeks and at 3 months. Begin long-term monitoring if goal has been met. Consider drug therapy if goal has not been attained. Carry out intensive diet therapy and counseling for ≥ 6 months before starting drug therapy. Continue dietary treatment during drug treatment.

Drug treatment: Cholestyramine, colestipol and dextrothyroxine are used to lower cholesterol. HMG-CoA reductase inhibitors, gemfibrozil, nicotinic acid and clofibrate are used to lower both cholesterol and triglycerides. Gemfibrozil and clofibrate lower serum triglycerides much more effectively than cholesterol levels. When both cholesterol and triglycerides are elevated, treatment of the hypertriglyceridemia should take precedence. When hypercholesterolemia is treated first, an exacerbation of the hypertriglyceridemia may occur. Serum cholesterol often falls to normal levels without specific therapy following treatment of the hypertriglyceridemia. Clofibrate and dextrothyroxine are no longer commonly used as antihyperlipidemic therapy.

First choice – Drugs of first choice include HMG-CoA reductase inhibitors, gemfibrozil or nicotinic acid. Measure LDL-cholesterol levels at 4 to 6 weeks and at 3 months. The target LDL level for treatment is ≤ 130 mg/dl. If the response is adequate, monitor every 4 months; if inadequate, switch to another agent or use a combination of two drugs. Refer patients who fail to respond to combination therapy to a lipid disorder specialist.

Estrogen replacement therapy can be considered in postmenopausal women with high serum cholesterol, because estrogens lower LDL- and raise HDL- cholesterol levels. Use of these agents may reduce the risk for CHD, but no large studies have confirmed this effect.

Combination therapy – Because drug therapy of different hyperlipoproteinemias involves different mechanisms and pharmacologic actions, consider a combined drug regimen in stubborn cases. However, experience with combination therapy is limited. The coadministration of a bile acid sequestrant with either nicotinic acid or an HMG-CoA reductase inhibitor can lower LDL-cholesterol levels by ≥ 40% to 50%. Use HMG-CoA reductase inhibitors and gemfibrozil concomitantly with caution because of the risks of myopathy, rhabdomyolysis and acute renal failure.

BILE ACID SEQUESTRANTS

Refer to general discussion of these agents in Antihyperlipidemic Agents introduction.

Actions:

Pharmacology: Cholesterol is the major (and probably the sole) precursor of bile acids. During normal digestion, bile acids are secreted via the bile from the liver and gallbladder into the intestines to emulsify the fat and lipid materials in food, thus facilitating absorption. A major portion of the bile acids secreted is reabsorbed from the intestines and returned via the portal circulation to the liver, thus, completing the enterohepatic cycle.

Bile acid sequestering resins bind bile acids in the intestine to form an insoluble complex that is excreted in the feces. This results in a partial removal of bile acids from the enterohepatic circulation, preventing their absorption. Because these agents are anion-exchange resins, the chloride anions of the resin are replaced by other anions. These agents are hydrophilic but insoluble in water. They remain unchanged in the GI tract and are not absorbed.

The increased fecal loss of bile acids leads to increased oxidation of cholesterol to bile acids and a decrease in LDL and serum cholesterol levels. In humans, these drugs increase the hepatic synthesis of cholesterol, but plasma cholesterol levels fall secondary to an increased rate of clearance of cholesterol-rich lipoproteins from the plasma. Serum triglyceride levels may increase.

The fall in LDL concentration is apparent in 4 to 7 days. The decline in serum cholesterol is usually evident by 1 month. When the resins are discontinued, serum cholesterol usually returns to baseline within 1 month. Cholesterol may rise even with continued use; determine serum levels periodically.

When bile secretion is partially blocked, serum bile acid concentration rises. In patients with partial biliary obstruction, reduction of serum bile acid levels by cholestyramine reduces bile acid deposits in the dermal tissues with a resultant decrease in pruritus.

Indications:

Hyperlipoproteinemia: Adjunctive therapy for the reduction of elevated serum cholesterol in patients with primary hypercholesterolemia (elevated LDL) who do not respond adequately to diet.

These agents may lower elevated cholesterol in patients who also have hypertriglyceridemia, but they are not indicated where hypertriglyceridemia is the abnormality of most concern.

Biliary obstruction (cholestyramine only): Relief of pruritus associated with partial biliary obstruction.

Unlabeled uses: **Cholestyramine** in vitro binds the toxin produced by *Clostridium difficile*, the causative organism of antibiotic-induced pseudomembranous colitis, with variable success. It is also effective in bile salt-mediated and postvagotomy diarrhea.

Cholestyramine has been used in the treatment of chlordecone *(Kepone)* pesticide poisoning. By binding chlordecone in the intestine, cholestyramine inhibits its enterohepatic recirculation, increases fecal excretion and accelerates elimination from the body.

Cholestyramine and **colestipol** have been used in the treatment of digitalis toxicity (see Cardiac Glycosides monograph).

Cholestyramine may be useful to treat an overdose with thyroid hormones.

Contraindications:

Hypersensitivity to bile acid sequestering resins or any components of the products; complete biliary obstruction.

Warnings:

Powder: Avoid accidental inhalation or esophageal distress, do not take dry. Mix with fluids.

Calcified material has been observed in the biliary tree and the gall bladder; however, this may be due to liver disease and may not be drug-related. One patient experienced biliary colic on each of three occasions on which he took **cholestyramine**. Another patient, diagnosed as having an acute abdominal symptom complex, showed a "pasty mass" in the transverse colon on x-ray.

Carcinogenesis: The incidence of intestinal tumors in studies was greater in cholestyramine-treated rats than in controls. The total incidence of fatal and nonfatal neoplasms was similar in both treatment groups. Various alimentary system cancers were more prevalent with **cholestyramine**.

Pregnancy: These agents are not absorbed systemically, and fetal harm in pregnancy in recommended doses. Interference with fat-soluble vitamin absorption may be detrimental even with supplementation. **No adverse fetal effects were observed when cholestyramine** was used for the treatment of cholestasis of pregnancy.

Lactation: Exercise caution when administering to a nursing woman. The possible lack of proper vitamin absorption may have an effect on nursing infants.

Children: Dosage schedules have not been established. The effects of long-term administration and effectiveness in maintaining lowered cholesterol levels are unknown.

A 10-month-old baby with biliary atresia had an impaction presumed to be due to **cholestyramine** (9g/day for 3 days). She died of acute intestinal sepsis.

Precautions:

Monitoring: Determine serum cholesterol levels frequently during the first few months of therapy and periodically thereafter. Periodically measure serum triglyceride levels to detect significant changes.

Diet: Before instituting therapy, vigorously attempt to control serum cholesterol by an appropriate dietary regimen and weight reduction.

Contributing diseases: Investigate and treat diseases contributing to increased blood cholesterol before starting therapy (eg, hypothyroidism, diabetes mellitus, nephrotic syndrome, dysproteinemias, obstructive liver disease). Cholesterol reduction should occur during the first month of therapy. Continue therapy to sustain cholesterol reduction. If adequate reduction is not attained, discontinue therapy.

Malabsorption: Because they sequester bile acids, these resins may interfere with normal fat absorption and digestion and may prevent absorption of fat-soluble vitamins such as A, D, E, K and folic acid. With long-term therapy, supplemental vitamins A and D may be given in a water-miscible form or administered parenterally.

Chronic use may increase bleeding tendencies due to hypoprothrombinemia associated with vitamin K deficiency. This usually responds promptly to parenteral vitamin K_1; prevent recurrences by giving oral vitamin K_1.

Reduced folate: Reduction of serum or red cell folate has been reported over long-term administration of **cholestyramine**. Consider supplementation with folic acid.

Hyperchloremic acidosis: These drugs are chloride anion-exchange resins. Prolonged use may cause hyperchloremic acidosis, especially in younger and smaller patients where relative dosage may be higher.

Constipation: These agents may produce or severely worsen preexisting constipation. Fecal impaction may occur and hemorrhoids may be aggravated. Avoid constipation in patients with symptomatic coronary artery disease. Most instances of constipation are mild, transient and controlled with standard treatment. Some patients require decreased dosage or discontinuation of therapy. Predisposing factors are high dose and age > 60 years. A laxative, stool softener or increased fluid and fiber intake may be helpful.

Drug Interactions:

Bile Acid Sequestrant (BAS) Drug Interactions

Precipitant drug	Object drug*		Description
BAS	Anticoagulants	⬇	Cholestyramine may decrease anticoagulant effect.
BAS	Diclofenac	⬇	The AUC and C_{max} of NSAIDS may be reduced.
BAS	Gemfibrozil	⬇	Bioavailability may be reduced by colestipol.
BAS	Iopanoic acid	⬇	Cholestyramine's apparent high affinity for iopanoic aicd caused an abnormal cholecystography.
BAS	Mycophenolate	⬇	≈ 40% decrease in AUC by cholestyramine.
BAS	Piroxicam	⬇	Elimination may be enhanced by cholestyramine.
BAS	Thyroid hormones	⬇	Possible loss of efficacy of thyroid and potential hypothyroidism with concurrent cholestyramine.
BAS	Ursodiol	⬇	Cholestyramine and colestipol may interfere with the action of ursodiol by reducing its absorption.
BAS	Vitamins A, D, E, K	⬇	Malabsorption may occur during administration of bile acid sequestrants (see Precautions).

* ⬇ = Object drug decreased.

BILE ACID SEQUESTRANTS

Binding in the GI tract may delay or reduce the absorption of concomitant oral medication. Take other drugs at least 1 hour before or 4 to 6 hours after these agents. Discontinuation of a resin could pose a hazard if a potentially toxic, significantly bound drug has been titrated to a maintenance level while on the resin.

BAS Drug Interactions (Decreased Serum Levels or GI Absorption)		
Aspirin	Hydrocortisone	Phosphate supplements
Clindamycin	Imipramine	Propranalol
Clofibrate	Methyldopa	Tetracyclines
Digitalis glycosides	Nicotinic acid (niacin)	Thiazide diuretics
Furosemide	Penicillin G	Tolbutamide
Glipizide	Phenytoin	

Adverse Reactions:

GI:

Most common – Constipation at times is severe and is occasionally accompanied by fecal impaction (see Warnings). Hemorrhoids may be aggravated.

Less frequent – Abdominal pain/distention/cramping; GI bleeding; bloating; flatulence; nausea; vomiting; diarrhea; loose stools; indigestion; heartburn; anorexia; steatorrhea; rectal bleeding/pain; black stools; hemorrhoidal bleeding; bleeding duodenal ulcer; peptic ulceration; ulcer attack; GI irritation; dysphagia; dental bleeding; dental caries; hiccoughs; sour taste; pancreatitis; diverticulitis; cholecystitis; cholelithiasis; impaction (rare).

Cardiovascular: Chest pain, angina, tachycardia (infrequent).

CNS: Headache (eg, migraine and sinus); anxiety; vertigo; dizziness; lightheadedness; insomnia; fatigue; tinnitus; syncope; drowsiness; femoral nerve pain; paresthesia.

Hematologic: Increased prothrombin time; ecchymosis; anemia.

Hypersensitivity: Urticaria; dermatitis; asthma; wheezing; rash.

Musculoskeletal: Backache; muscle/joint pains; arthritis.

Renal: Hematuria; dysuria; burnt odor to urine; diuresis.

Miscellaneous: Uveitis; fatigue; weight loss/gain; increased libido; swollen glands; edema; weakness; shortness of breath; swelling of hands/feet.

Bleeding tendencies due to hypoprothrombinemia (vitamin K deficiency); vitamin A (one case of night blindness) and D deficiencies; rash and irritation of the skin, tongue and perianal area; hyperchloremic acidosis in children (see Precautions); osteoporosis; calcified material in biliary tree and gall bladder (see Warnings).

Lab test abnormalities:

Colestipol – Transient, modest elevations of AST, ALT and alkaline phosphatase.

Cholestyramine – Liver function abnormalities.

Overdosage:

The chief potential harm would be GI tract obstruction. Location and degree of obstruction and status of gut motility determine treatment. Overdosage has been reported in a patient taking 150% of the maximum recommended daily dose of **cholestyramine** for several weeks; no ill effects were reported.

Patient Information:

Medication is usually taken before meals.

Do not take the powder in dry form; mix with beverages, highly fluid soups, cereals or pulpy fruits (see Administration and Dosage in individual monographs).

Swallow **colestipol** tablets whole; do not cut, crush or chew.

Medication may interfere with absorption of concomitant drugs. Take other drugs 1 hour before or 4 to 6 hours after **cholestyramine** or **colestipol**. (See Drug Interactions.)

Constipation, flatulence, nausea and heartburn may occur and may disappear with continued therapy. Notify physician if these effects become bothersome or if unusual bleeding (eg, from the gums or rectum) occurs.

Administration and Dosage:

Concomitant therapy: Preliminary evidence suggests that the cholesterol-lowering effects of these agents and an HMG-CoA reductase inhibitor are additive. In addition, this combined effect may be useful in treating severe and refractory forms of hypercholesterolemia. Additive effects on LDL-cholesterol are also seen with combined cholestyramine and nicotinic acid therapy.

Bile Acid Sequestrants

CHOLESTYRAMINE

For complete prescribing information, refer to the Bile Acid Sequestrants group monograph.

Administration and Dosage:

Powder:

Adults – 4 g 1 to 2 times daily. Individualize dosage.

Preparation – Mix the contents of one powder packet or one level scoopful with 60 to 180 ml (2 to 6 fl oz) water or noncarbonated beverage. Do not take in dry form. Always mix with water or other fluids, highly fluid soups or pulpy fruits, such as applesauce or crushed pineapple.

Maintenance – 2 to 4 packets or scoopfuls daily (8 to 16 g anhydrous cholestyramine resin) divided into two doses. Increase dose gradually, with periodic assessment of lipid/lipoprotein levels at intervals of ≥ 4 weeks. The maximum recommended daily dose is 6 packets or scoopfuls. Recommended administration time is at mealtime; may be modified to avoid interference with absorption concomitant medications. Although the recommended dosing schedule is twice daily, cholestyramine may be administered in 1 to 6 doses/day.

Rx	**Questran** (Bristol Labs)	**Powder:** 4 g (as anhydrous resin)/9 g powder	Sucrose. In 378 g cans and 9 g single-dose packets (60s).
Rx	**Questran Light** (Bristol Labs)	**Powder:** 4 g (as anhydrous resin)/5 g powder.	Sucrose, aspartame. In 210 g cans (42 doses) and 5 g packets (60s).
Rx	**Cholestyramine** (Goldline)	**Powder:** 4 g (as anhydrous resin)/5.5 g powder.	Aspartame. In cartons of 42 and 60 single-dose 5.5 g packets.
Rx	**Prevalite** (Upsher-Smith)		Aspartame. In 60 single-dose 5.5 g packets.

COLESTIPOL HCl

For complete prescribing information, refer to the Bile Acid Sequestrants group monograph.

Administration and Dosage:

Granules:

Adults – 5 to 30 g/day given once or in divided doses. The starting dose is 5 g once or twice daily with a daily increment of 5 g at 1 or 2 month intervals.

Preparation – Mix in liquids, soups, cereals or pulpy fruits. Do not take dry. Add the prescribed amount to a glassful (≥ 90 ml) of liquid; stir until completely mixed. Colestipol will not dissolve. May also mix with carbonated beverages slowly stirred in a large glass. Rinse glass with a small amount of additional beverage to ensure that all the medication is taken.

Tablets: 2 to 16 g/day given once or in divided doses. The starting dose is 2 g once or twice daily. Dosage increases of 2 g, once or twice daily, should occur at 1 or 2 month intervals. Periodically assess lipid/lipoprotein levels. If the desired effect is not obtained at recommended dose, consider combined therapy or alternate treatment.

Swallow tablets whole, one at a time; do not cut, chew or crush. The tablets may be taken with plenty of water or other appropriate fluids.

Rx	**Colestid** (Pharmacia & Upjohn)	**Tablets:** 1 g	(U). Yellow. Elliptical. In 120s and 500s.
Rx	**Colestid** (Pharmacia & Upjohn)	**Granules:** 5 g colestipol HCl/7.5 g powder	*Unflavored*: In 300 and 500 g bottles and 5 g packets (30s and 90s). *Flavored*: Aspartame. Orange flavor. In 450 g bottles and 7.5 g packets (60s).

HMG-CoA REDUCTASE INHIBITORS

Refer to the general discussion of these products in the Antihyperlipidemic Agents Introduction.

Actions:

Pharmacology: These agents specifically competitively inhibit 3-hydroxy-3-methylglutaryl-coenzyme A (HMG-CoA) reductase, the enzyme that catalyzes the conversion of HMG-CoA to mevalonate, which is an early rate-limiting step in cholesterol biosynthesis, HMG-CoA reductase inhibitors increase HDL cholesterol and decrease LDL cholesterol (LDL-C), VLDL cholesterol and plasma triglycerides. Epidemiologic investigations have established that cardiovascular morbidity and mortality vary directly with the level of total cholesterol and LDL and inversely with the level of HDL.

The mechanism of the LDL-lowering effect may involve both reduction of VLDL concentration and induction of the LDL receptor, leading to reduced production or increased catabolism of LDL.

These agents are highly effective in reducing total cholesterol and the LDL level in heterozygous familial and non-familial forms of hypercholesterolemia. A marked response was seen within 1 to 2 weeks, and the maximum therapeutic response occurred within 4 to 6 weeks. The response was maintained during therapy. In studies of some agents, single daily doses given in the evening were more effective than in the morning, perhaps because cholesterol is synthesized mainly at night.

Pharmacokinetics:

Pharmacokinetics of HMG-CoA Reductase Inhibitors

	Bioavailability	Excretion	t½ (hrs)	Major metabolites	Protein binding	Effects of renal/hepatic impairment
Fluvastatin	> 90% absorbed; absolute bioavailability 24%; extensive first-pass metabolism(CYP2C)	5% (urine) 90% (feces)	< 1	N-desisopropylpropionic acid (inactive); hydroxylated metabolites (active, do not circulate systemically)	98%	nd
Lovastatin	≈ 35% absorbed; extensive first-pass metabolism (CYP3A); < 5% of oral dose reaches general circulation	10% (urine) 83% (feces)	3-4	Beta-hydroxyacid; 6'–hydroxyderivative; two additional metabolites	> 95%	nd
Pravastatin	34% absorbed; absolute bioavailability 17%; extensive first-pass metabolism; plasma levels may not correlate with efficacy	≈ 20% (urine) 70% (feces)	1.8	Major degradation product: 3α-hydroxy isomeric metabolite	≈ 50%	Mean AUC varied 18-fold in cirrhotic patients and peak values varied 47-fold
Simvastatin	60% to 80% absorbed; extensive first-pass metabolism; < 5% of oral dose reaches general circulation	13% (urine) 60% (feces)	3	Beta-hydroxyacid; 6'–hydroxy, 6'–hydroxymethyl, 6'-exomethylene derivatives	≈ 95%	Higher systemic exposure may occur in hepatic and severe renal insufficiency
Atorvastatin	≈ 12% absolute bioavailability; first pass metabolism (CYP3A4)	< 2% (urine)	14	nd	≥ 98%	Plasma leves not affected by renal disease; markedly increased with chronic alcoholic liver disease.

nd = No data.

Food – Food decreases the rate and extent of drug absorption by ≈ 25% and 9%, respectively. LDL-C reduction is similar whether atorvastatin is given with or without food. Plasma atorvastatin concentrations are lower (≈ 30% for C_{max} and AUC) following evening drug administration compared with morning.

HMG-CoA REDUCTASE INHIBITORS

Clinical trials:

HMG-CoA reductase inhibitors – In multicenter, double-blind studies in patients with familial or non-familial hypercholesterolemia, **lovastatin** (10 to 80 mg), **pravastatin** (10 to 40 mg) and **simvastatin** (5 to 40 mg) consistently and significantly decreased total plasma cholesterol, LDL, total cholesterol/HDL ratio and LDL/HDL ratio. In addition, they increased total HDL and decreased VLDL and plasma triglycerides.**Fluvastatin**(20 to 40 mg) significantly decreased LDL and also decreased total cholesterol, apolipoprotein B and triglycerides and increased HDL.

Combination therapy –

HMG-CoA reductase inhibitor/cholestyramine: **Lovastatin** was compared with cholestyramine in a randomized open parallel study. At all dosage levels tested, **lovastatin** produced a significantly greater reduction of total plasma cholesterol and total cholesterol/HDL ratio when compared with cholestyramine. The increase in HDL was not significantly different when comparing **lovastatin** with cholestyramine.

Simvastatin was compared with cholestyramine in a double-blind parallel study. At all dosage levels, **simvastatin** produced significantly greater reductions in total plasma cholesterol, LDL, VLDL, triglycerides and total cholesterol/HDL ratio. The effect on HDL was not significantly different when comparing **simvastatin** with cholestyramine.

Patients treated with **pravastatin** in combination with cholestyramine had ≥ 50% reductions in LDL. **Pravastatin** attenuated cholestyramine-induced increases in triglyceride levels, which are of unknown clinical significance.

Atherosclerosis – In one trial, **lovastatin** 20 to 80 mg/day significantly slowed the progression of lesions and decreased the proportion of patients categorized with disease progression and with new lesions. In another study, significant slowing of disease was seen, with regression in 23% of patients treated with **lovastatin** vs 11% with placebo. In a third study, **lovastatin** or niacin in combination with a bile acid sequestrant for 2.5 years in hyperlipidemic subjects significantly reduced the frequency of progression and increased the frequency of regression of coronary atherosclerotic lesions compared with diet and, in some cases, low-dose resin.

Pooled events from two studies showed that treatment with pravastatin was associated with a 67% reduction in the event rate of fatal and non-fatal myocardial infarction (MI) (3.8% **pravastatin** vs 11.4% placebo) and 55% for the combined endpoint of non-fatal MI or death from any cause (6.2% **pravastatin** vs 13.8% placebo).

In the Multicenter Anti-Atheroma Study, the effect of therapy with **simvastatin** on atherosclerosis was assessed by quantitative coronary angiography in hypercholesterolemic men and women with coronary heart disease. After 4 years, the groups differed significantly in the proportions of patients categorized with disease progression (23% **simvastatin** vs 33% placebo) and disease regression (18% **simvastatin** vs 12% placebo). In addition, **simvastatin** significantly decreased the proportion of patients with new lesions (13% **simvastatin** vs 24% placebo) and with new total occlusions (5% **simvastatin** vs 11% placebo).

Indications:

Hypercholesterolemia: Adjunct to diet to reduce elevated total and LDL cholesterol levels in primary hypercholesterolemia (Types IIa and IIb) when the response to diet and other nonpharmacological measures alone has been inadequate.

Atherosclerosis (lovastatin/pravastatin): To slow the progression of coronary atherosclerosis in patients with CHD as part of a treatment strategy to lower total-C and LDL-C to target levels; to reduce the risk of acute coronary events.

Coronary heart disease (simvastatin/pravastatin): To reduce the risk of total mortality by reducing coronary death; to reduce the risk of non-fatal myocardial infarction; reduce the risk of undergoing myocardial revascularization procedures.

Unlabeled uses:

Lovastatin may be useful in diabetic dyslipidemia, nephrotic hyperlipidemia, neck artery disease, familial dysbetalipoproteinemia and familial combined hyperlipidemia. Limit such use to high-risk patients not responding to other therapies.

Pravastatin can significantly lower elevated cholesterol levels in: Heterozygous familial hypercholesterolemia; familial combined hyperlipidemia; diabetic dyslipidemia in non-insulin dependent diabetics; hypercholesterolemia secondary to the nephrotic syndrome; homozygous familial hypercholesterolemia in patients not completely devoid of LDL receptors but with reduced LDL receptor activity.

Simvastatin can signficantly lower elevated cholesterol levels in patients with heterozygous familial hypercholesterolemia, familial combined hyperlipidemia, diabetic dyslipidemia in non-insulin dependent diabetics, hyperlipidemia secondary to the

HMG-CoA REDUCTASE INHIBITORS

nephrotic syndrome and homozygous familial hypercholesterolemia in patients with defective, rather than absent, LDL receptors.

Fluvastatin – To slow progression of coronary atherosclerosis in patients with CHD.

Contraindications:

Hypersensitivity to any component of these products; active liver disease or unexplained persistent elevated liver function tests; pregnancy; lactation (see Warnings).

Warnings:

Skeletal muscle effects: Rhabdomyolysis with renal dysfunction secondary to myoglobinuria has occurred with some drugs in this class. Myalgia has occurred with **lovastatin**. Transient, mildly elevated creatine phosphokinase (CPK) levels are commonly seen. In clinical trials of **lovastatin**, ≈ 0.1% to 0.5% of patients developed a myopathy (ie, myalgia or muscle weakness associated with markedly elevated CPK levels). Uncomplicated myalgia has been reported in **atorvastatin**-treated patients. Consider myopathy in conjunction with increases in CPK values > 10 times the upper limit of normal (ULN) in any patient with diffuse myalgias, muscle tenderness, weakness or marked CPK elevation. Advise patients to report promptly unexplained muscle pain, tenderness or weakness, particularly if accompanied by malaise or fever. Discontinue **atorvastatin** therapy if markedly elevated CPK levels occur or myopathy is diagnosed or suspected. Myopathy was reported as possibly due to **pravastatin** in only one patient. In clinical trials with **lovastatin**, severe rhabdomyolysis (rare) has precipitated acute renal failure, especially in cardiac transplant patients on immunosuppressive therapy including cyclosporine or itraconazole. The risk of myopathy is increased when taking these drugs and receiving concomitant therapy with cyclosporine, erythromycin, gemfibrozil or nicotinic acid (see Drug Interactions). In clinical trials, ≈ 30% of patients on concomitant immunosuppressive therapy, including cyclosporine, developed myopathy; the corresponding percentages for gemfibrozil and niacin were ≈ 5% and 2%, respectively. Carefully consider benefits and risks of using **lovastatin** concomitantly with these agents.

In six cardiac transplant patients on both immunosuppressants (including cyclosporine) and **lovastatin** 20 mg/day, average plasma levels of **lovastatin**'s active metabolites were elevated to ≈ 4 times the expected levels. Because of an apparent relationship between increased plasma levels of active metabolites of HMG-CoA reductase inhibitors and myopathy, do not exceed 20 mg/day **lovastatin** or 10 mg/day **simvastatin** in patients on immunosuppressants or itraconazole. Even at this dosage, carefully consider the benefits and risks in immunosuppressed patients.

Myopathy was not observed in small numbers of patients treated with **pravastatin** together with niacin. A small trial of combined therapy with **pravastatin** and gemfibrozil showed a trend toward more frequent CPK elevations and patient withdrawals because of musculoskeletal symptoms compared with placebo, gemfibrozil alone or **pravastatin** alone; myopathy was not reported. One patient developed myopathy when clofibrate was added to a previously well tolerated **pravastatin** regimen; myopathy resolved when clofibrate therapy was stopped. Because the use of fibrates alone may occasionally be associated with myopathy, avoid combined use of HMG-CoA reductase inhibitors and fibrates.

Consider myopathy in any patient with diffuse myalgias, muscle tenderness or weakness, or marked elevation of CPK. Advise patients to report promptly muscle pain, tenderness or weakness, particularly with malaise or fever. Discontinue the drug if markedly elevated CPK levels occur or if myopathy is diagnosed.

Consider temporarily withholding or discontinuing drug therapy in any patient with a risk factor predisposing them to the development of renal failure secondary to rhabdomyolysis, including: Severe acute infection; hypotension; major surgery; trauma; severe metabolic, endocrine or electrolyte disorders; uncontrolled seizures.

Endocrine effects: Although cholesterol is the precursor of all steroid hormones, **lovastatin** has shown no effect on steroidogenesis. **Pravastatin** showed inconsistent results with regard to possible effects on basal steroid hormone levels; **fluvastatin** and **simvastatin** did not reduce basal plasma cortisol concentration or basal plasma testosterone concentration or impair adrenal reserve. Appropriately evaluate patients who display clinical evidence of endocrine dysfunction. Exercise caution when administering HMG-CoA reductase inhibitors with drugs that affect steroid levels or activity.

CNS: In animals, CNS vascular lesions, characterized by perivascular hemorrhage, edema, mononuclear cell infiltration of perivascular spaces and other similar CNS vascular lesions, have been observed with drugs in this class.

Morbidity/Mortality: The effect of HMG-CoA reductase inhibitor-induced changes in lipoprotein levels, including reduction of serum cholesterol, on cardiovascular morbidity or mortality has not been established.**Lovastatin** has enhanced cardiac insufficiency in patients with cardiac disease, but this can be corrected by ubiquinone supplementation.

Hypercholesterolemia, secondary causes: Prior to initiating therapy, exclude secondary causes of hypercholesterolemia (eg, poorly controlled diabetes mellitus, hypothyroidism, nephrotic syndrome, dysproteinemias, obstructive liver disease, other drug therapy, alcoholism) and measure total-C, HDL-C and triglycerides.

Hypersensitivity: An apparent hypersensitivity syndrome has occurred (see Adverse Reactions). Refer to Management of Acute Hypersensitivity Reactions.

Renal function impairment: A single 20 mg dose of **pravastatin** was given to patients with varying degrees of renal impairment. Although no effect on **pravastatin** or its 3α-hydroxy-isomeric metabolite was observed, a small increase in mean AUC values and half-life was seen for the inactive hydroxylation metabolite. Closely monitor patients with renal impairment who are receiving **pravastatin**. Higher systemic exposure of **simvastatin** may occur in severe renal insufficiency.

Hepatic function impairment: Use with caution in patients who consume substantial quantities of alcohol or who have a history of liver disease.

Marked persistent increases (> 3 times ULN) in serum transaminases occurred in 1.1% of **fluvastatin**-treated patients, in 1.9% of adults who received **lovastatin** for ≤ 1 year, in 1.3% of **pravastatin**-treated patients over an average period of 18 months, in 1% of **simvastatin**-treated patients and in 0.7% of **atorvastatin**-treated patients in clinical trials. The incidence of these abnormalities with **atorvastatin** was 0.2%, 0.5%, 0.6% and 2.3% for 10, 20, 40 and 80 mg, respectively. When the drug was interrupted or discontinued, transaminase levels usually fell slowly to pretreatment levels. Increases usually appeared 3 to 12 months after starting **lovastatin** therapy and were not associated with jaundice or other clinical signs or symptoms in **fluvastatin-**,**simvastatin-**,**lovastatin**- and **pravastatin**-treated patients. In **pravastatin**-treated patients, abnormalities did not appear to be related to treatment duration and were not associated with cholestasis.

Pravastatin and **fluvastatin** plasma clearance is decreased but no dose adjustment is needed.

It is recommended that LFTs be performed before the initiation of treatment, at 6 and 12 weeks after initiation of therapy or elevation in dose and periodically (eg, semiannually) thereafter. Liver enzyme changes generally occur in the first 3 months of treatment with **atorvastatin**. Monitor patients who develop increased transaminase levels until the abnormalities resolve. If an increase in ALT or AST > 3 times ULN persist, reduce dose or withdraw **lovastatin** and **atorvastatin**.

Use **atorvastatin** with caution in patients who consume substantial quantities of alcohol and have a history of liver disease. Active liver disease or unexplained persistent transaminase elevations are contraindications to the use of the drug (see Contraindications).

Carcinogenesis/Fertility impairment: In mice, a statistically significant increase in the incidence of hepatocellular carcinomas and adenomas was observed at **lovastatin** doses of 500 mg/kg/day. In addition, an increase in the incidence of papilloma in nonglandular stomach mucosa was seen in mice.

Rats given **pravastatin** doses of 10, 30 or 100 mg/kg showed an increased incidence of hepatocellular carcinomas in males at the highest dose (serum drug levels only 6 to 10 times higher than in humans given 40 mg **pravastatin**). In mice, 10, 30 or 100 mg/kg for 22 months resulted in a significant increase in the incidence of malignant lymphomas in treated females.

In mice receiving **simvastatin** (25, 100 and 400 mg/kg/day), the incidence of liver carcinoma and adenoma and lung adenoma was significantly increased. In female rats receiving simvastatin at levels ≈ 45 times higher than in humans given 40 mg **simvastatin**, there was a statistically significant increase in the incidence of thyroid follicular adenomas.

In rats at **fluvastatin** doses of 6, 9 and 18 to 24 mg/kg/day (≈ 9 to 35 times the mean human drug levels after a 40 mg dose), a low incidence of forestomach squamous papillomas and one forestomach carcinoma was considered to reflect prolonged hyperplasia induced by direct contact exposure to **fluvastatin** rather than to systemic effects. An increased incidence of thyroid follicular cell adenomas and carcinomas occurred in males after 18 to 24 mg/kg/day. In contrast with other HMG-CoA reductase inhibitors, no hepatic adenomas or carcinomas were observed.

Drug-related testicular atrophy, decreased spermatogenesis, spermatocytic degeneration and giant cell formation were seen in dogs given **lovastatin** 20 mg/kg/day and in dogs given **simvastatin** 10 mg/kg/day.

HMG-CoA REDUCTASE INHIBITORS

There was decreased fertility in male rats treated with **simvastatin** 25 mg/kg for 34 weeks. In **simvastatin**-treated humans, there was a small decrease in the mean percentage of vital sperm and a small increase in the mean percentage of abnormal forms; these changes reached statistical significance at week 14. There was no effect on numbers or concentration of motile sperm.

In rats at dose levels of 10, 30 and 100 mg/kg/day of **atorvastatin**, two rare muscle tumors were found in high-dose females. In one, there was a rhabdomyosarcoma and, in another, there was a fibrosarcoma.

A study in mice given 100, 200 or 400 mg/kg/day found a significant increase in liver adenomas in high-dose males and liver carcinomas in high-dose females.

Elderly: For the general patient population, plasma concentrations of **fluvastatin** do not vary either as a function of age or gender, but in patients > 70 years old, the AUC of **lovastatin** and **simvastatin** is increased.**Pravastatin** does not need dosage adjustment. Elderly patients (≥ 65 years old) demonstrated a greater treatment response in respect to LDL-C, total-C and LDL/HDL ratio than patients < 65 years old. The safety and efficacy of **atorvastatin** in patients ≥ 70 years of age were similar to those of patients < 70 years of age.

Pregnancy: Category X. Contraindicated during pregnancy. Skeletal malformations have occurred in animals following **lovastatin** administration. There are no data in pregnant women. However, because HMG-CoA reductase inhibitors can decrease synthesis of cholesterol and possibly other products of the cholesterol biosynthesis pathway, they may cause fetal harm when given to pregnant women. Give to women of childbearing age only if they are highly unlikely to conceive. If a patient becomes pregnant while on the drug, discontinue the drug and apprise her of the potential hazard to the fetus.

Lactation: **Lovastatin** and **atorvastatin** are excreted in the milk of rats; it is not known whether **lovastatin** and **simvastatin** are excreted in breast milk; a small amount of **pravastatin** is excreted in breast milk;**fluvastatin** is present in breast milk in a 2:1 ratio (milk:plasma). Because of the potential for serious adverse reactions in nursing infants, caution women taking these drugs not to nurse their infants.

Children: Safety and efficacy in individuals < 18 years old have not been established; treatment in this age group is not recommended at this time. Because children are not likely to benefit from cholesterol lowering for at least a decade and because experience with this drug is limited, do not use in children.

Precautions:

Monitoring: Perform liver function tests before initiating therapy, at 6 and 12 weeks after initiation of therapy or after dose elevation and periodically thereafter (≈ 6 month intervals). Pay special attention to patients who develop elevated serum transaminase levels. If transaminase levels progress, particularly if they rise to 3 times the upper limit of normal and are persistent, discontinue the drug. Consider liver biopsy if elevations persist beyond drug discontinuation.

Diet: Before instituting therapy, attempt to control hypercholesterolemia with diet, exercise and weight reduction in obese patients. Treat underlying medical problems.

Ophthalmologic effects: There was a high prevalence of baseline lenticular opacities in the patient population included in the early clinical trials with **lovastatin**. During these trials, new opacities appeared in both the **lovastatin** and placebo groups. There was no clinically significant change in visual acuity in the patients who had new opacities reported nor was any patient, including those with opacities noted at baseline, discontinued from therapy because of a decrease in visual acuity.

An interim analysis performed at 2 years in 192 hypercholesterolemic patients in a placebo controlled, parallel, double-blind study found no clinically significant differences between **lovastatin** and placebo groups in the incidence, type or progression of lenticular opacities.

Optic nerve degeneration occurred in dogs given **simvastatin** 180 mg/kg/day.

One study showed newly occurring or worsening posterior subcapsular abnormalities with **fluvastatin** 40 mg/day.

Homozygous familial hypercholesterolemia: **Lovastatin** and **simvastatin** are less effective in patients with rare homozygous familial hypercholesterolemia, possibly because of a decrease in functional LDL receptors. **Lovastatin** appears to increase the risk of elevated serum transaminases (see Warnings) in these patients.

Sleep disturbance: **Lovastatin** and **simvastatin** may interfere with sleep causing insomnia, whereas **pravastatin** does not appear to disturb sleep. However, these uncontrolled studies have been questioned, and further studies are needed.

HMG-CoA REDUCTASE INHIBITORS

Photosensitivity: Photosensitization (photoallergy or phototoxicity) may occur; therefore, caution patients to take protective measures against exposure to ultraviolet or sunlight (ie, sunscreens, protective clothing) until tolerance is determined.

Drug Interactions:

Lovastatin is metabolized by CYP3A; it may interact with CYP3A inhibitors.

Fluvastatin is metabolized by CYP2C; it may interact with CYP2C inhibitors.

HMG-CoA Reductase Inhibitor Drug Interactions

Precipitant drug	Object drug*		Description
Alcohol	Fluvastatin	↑	Daily intake of alcohol 20 g ≥ 2 hours after the evening meal and within 1 hour of fluvastatin 40 mg dose increases fluvastatin AUC by 30% and t_{max} by ≥ 40%.
Antacids	Atorvastatin	↓	Coadministration with **Maalox TC** suspension decreased atorvastatin levels by ≈ 35%; LDL-C reduction was not altered.
Atorvastatin	Oral contraceptives	↑	Coadministration increased AUC for norethindrone and ethinyl estradiol by ≈ 30% and 20%, respectively.
Bile acid sequestrants (BAS)	HMG-CoA reductase inhibitors	↓	A decrease in pravastatin (40% to 50%) and lovastatin bioavailability may occur. Take pravastatin 1 hour before or 4 hours after BAS.
Colestipol	Atorvastatin	↓	Plasma levels of atorvastatin decreased ≈ 25% with coadministration. LDL-C reduction was greater with coadministration than with either drug.
Cyclosporine/ Erythromycin/ Niacin	HMG-CoA reductase inhibitors	↑	Severe myopathy or rhabdomyolysis may occur with concurrent administration.
Cyclosporine	HMG-CoA reductase inhibitors	↑	Coadministration with pravastatin increased the peak pravastatin levels and AUC by 7- and 22-fold, respectively.
Erythromycin	Atorvastatin	↑	Coadministration increased atorvastatin levels by ≈ 40%.
Gemfibrozil	HMG-CoA reductase inhibitors	↑	Severe myopathy or rhabdomyolysis reported with lovastatin. Urinary excretion and protein binding of pravastatin may be decreased. Avoid concurrent use.
HMG-CoA reductase inhibitors	Digoxin	↑	Slight elevation in digoxin levels possible. Concomitant multiple doses of atorvastatin and digoxin increased steady-state digoxin levels by ≈ 20%.
HMG-CoA reductase inhibitors	Warfarin	↑	Anticoagulant effect of warfarin may be increased.
Isradipine	Lovastatin	↓	Isradipine may increase clearance of lovastatin and its metabolites by increasing hepatic blood flow.
Itraconazole	HMG-CoA reductase inhibitors	↑	Coadministration increased HMG-CoA reductase inhibitor levels ≈ 20-fold in normal volunteers; probably due to hepatic enzyme inhibition of competition. Temporarily interrupt HMG-CoA reductase inhibitors if systemic azole antifungals are needed.
Nicotinic Acid/ Propranolol/ Digoxin	Fluvastatin	↓	Decrease in fluvastatin bioavailability may occur with coadministration.
Propranolol	HMG-CoA reductase inhibitors	↓	Decrease in antihyperlipidemic activity.
Rifampin	Fluvastatin	↓	Coadministration may cause a decrease in fluvastatin C_{max}, AUC and plasma clearance.

* ↑ = Object drug increased. ↓ = Object drug decreased.

Drug/Food interactions: Under fasting conditions **lovastatin** levels are about ⅔ of those found when given immediately after meals; take **lovastatin** with meals.

HMG-CoA REDUCTASE INHIBITORS

Food reduces systemic bioavailability of **pravastatin**, but lipid-lowering effects of the drug are similar when taken with, or 1 hour prior to, meals; **pravastatin** may be taken without regard to meals.

Simvastatin levels are similar when administered in a fasting state or with food; **simvastatin** may be taken without regard to meals.

When **fluvastatin** is given with food, even up to 4 hours post prandial, it is completely absorbed, but C_{max} was reduced by 40% to 70%. Because no therapeutic differences were evident, **fluvastatin** may be taken without regard to meals.

Adverse Reactions:

These agents are generally well tolerated; adverse reactions are usually mild and transient.

In placebo controlled trials, 1% of **fluvastatin**-treated patients and 1.7% of **pravastatin**-treated patients discontinued treatment because of adverse events; the most common reasons for discontinuation of pravastatin were asymptomatic serum transaminase increases and mild, non-specific GI complaints.

HMG-CoA Reductase Inhibitor Adverse Reactions (%)[1]

Adverse reaction	Atorvastatin (n = 36)	Fluvastatin (n = 2326)	Lovastatin (n = 613)	Pravastatin (n = 900)	Simvastatin (n = 1583)
GI					
Nausea/Vomiting	—	3.2	1.9 - 4.7	7.3	1.3
Diarrhea	0	4.9	2.6 - 5.5	6.2	1.9
Abdominal pain/Cramps	0	4.9	2 - 5.7	5.4	3.2
Constipation	0	2.6	2 - 4.9	4	2.3
Flatulence	2.8	2.6	3.7 - 6.4	3.3	1.9
Heartburn	—	—	1.6	2.9	—
Dyspepsia	2.8	7.9	1.3 - 3.9	—	1.1
Dysgeusia	—	—	0.8	—	—
Tooth disorder	—	2.1	—	—	—
Acid regurgitation	—	—	0.5 - 1	—	—
Dry mouth	—	—	0.5 - 1	—	—
Musculoskeletal					
Leg pain	—	—	0.5 - 1	—	—
Shoulder pain	—	—	0.5 - 1	—	—
Localized pain	—	—	0.5 - 1	10	—
Myalgia	5.6	5	2.4 - 2.6	2.7	—
Muscle cramps/pain	—	—	0.6 - 1.1	—	—
Back pain	0	5.7	—	—	—
Arthropathy	—	—	—	—	—
Arthritis	—	2.1	—	—	—
Arthralgia	0	4	0.5 - 1	—	—
CNS					
Headache	16.7	8.9	2.6 - 9.3	6.2	3.5
Dizziness	—	2.2	0.7 - 2	3.3	—
Asthenia	0	—	—	—	1.6
Insomnia	—	2.7	0.5 - 1	—	—
Paresthesia	—	—	0.5 - 1	—	—
Respiratory					
Upper respiratory infection	—	16.2	—	—	2.1
Common cold	—	—	—	7	—
Rhinitis	—	4.7	—	4	—
Cough	—	2.4	—	2.6	—
Pharyngitis	0	3.8	—	—	—
Sinusitis	0	2.6	—	—	—
Bronchitis	—	—	—	—	—
Miscellaneous					
Chest pain	—	—	0.5 - 1	3.7	—
Rash/Pruritus	2.8	2.3	0.8 - 5.2	4	—
Cardiac chest pain	—	—	—	4	—
Fatigue	—	2.7	—	3.8	—

HMG-CoA REDUCTASE INHIBITORS

HMG-CoA Reductase Inhibitor Adverse Reactions (%)[1]					
Adverse reaction	Atorvastatin (n = 36)	Fluvastatin (n = 2326)	Lovastatin (n = 613)	Pravastatin (n = 900)	Simvastatin (n = 1583)
Influenza	0	5.1	—	2.4	—
Urinary abnormality	—	—	—	2.4	—
Blurred vision/eye irritation	—	—	1.1 - 1.5	—	—
Allergy	2.8	2.3	—	—	—
Accidental trauma	0	—	—	—	—
Alopecia	—	—	0.5 - 1	—	—
Infection	2.8	—	—	—	—

[1] All events. Data are pooled from separate studies and are not necessarily comparable.

The following adverse effects have also been reported with drugs in this class.

Cardiovascular: Palpitation; vasodilation; syncope; migraine; postural hypotension; phlebitis; arrhythmia.

CNS: Dysfunction of certain cranial nerves (including alteration of taste, impairment of extra-ocular movement, facial paresis); tremor; vertigo; dizziness; memory loss; paresthesia; peripheral neuropathy; peripheral nerve palsy; psychic disturbances; anxiety; insomnia; depression; somnolence; abnormal dreams; emotional lability; incoordination; hyperkinesia; torticollis.

Dermatologic: Pruritus; various skin changes (eg, nodules, discoloration, dryness of skin/mucous membranes, changes in hair/nails); contact dermatitis; alopecia; sweating; acne; urticaria; eczema; seborrhea; skin ulcer.

GI: Pancreatitis; hepatitis, including chronic active hepatitis; cholestatic jaundice; fatty change in liver; cirrhosis; fulminant hepatic necrosis; hepatoma; anorexia; vomiting; gastroenteritis; colitis; gastritis; dry mouth; rectal hemorrhage; esophagitis; eructation; glossitis; mouth ulceration; increased appetite; stomatitis; biliary pain; cheilitis; duodenal ulcer; dysphagia; enteritis; melena; gum hemorrhage; stomach ulcer; tenesmus; ulcerative stomach.

GU: Gynecomastia; loss of libido; erectile dysfunction; cystitis; hematuria; impotence; dysuria; kidney calculus; nocturia; epididymitis; fibrocystic breast; albuminuria; breast enlargement; nephritis; urinary frequency, incontinence, retention and urgency; abnormal ejaculation; vaginal or uterine hemorrhage; metrorrhagia.

Hematologic/Lymphatic: Ecchymosis; anemia; lymphadenopathy; thrombocytopenia; petechiae.

Hypersensitivity: An apparent hypersensitivity syndrome has been reported rarely including one or more of the following features: Anaphylaxis; angioedema; lupus erythematous-like syndrome; polymyalgia rheumatica; vasculitis; purpura; thrombocytopenia; leukopenia; hemolytic anemia; positive anti-nuclear antibody (ANA); erythrocyte sedimentation rate (ESR) increase; eosinophilia; arthritis; arthralgia; urticaria; asthenia; photosensitivity; fever; chills; flushing; malaise; dyspnea; toxic epidermal necrolysis; erythema multiforme (eg, Stevens-Johnson syndrome).

Lab test abnormalities: Increased serum transaminases (AST, ALT), CPK (11% with lovastatin, levels at least twice normal), alkaline phosphatase and bilirubin; γ-glutamyl transpeptidase; thyroid function test abnormalities; liver function test abnormalities.

Metabolic/Nutritional: Hyperglycemia; increased CPK; gout; weight gain; hypoglycemia.

Musculoskeletal: Myopathy; muscle cramps; myalgia; rhabdomyolysis (see Warnings); arthralgias; leg cramps; bursitis; tenosynovitis; myasthenia; tendinous contracture; myositis.

Ophthalmic: Progression of cataracts (lens opacities; see Precautions); ophthalmoplegia.

Respiratory: Pneumonia; dyspnea; asthma; epistaxis.

Special senses: Amblyopia; tinnitus; dry eyes; refraction disorder; eye hemorrhage; deafness; glaucoma; parosmia; taste loss; taste perversion.

Miscellaneous: Face edema; neck rigidity; photosensitivity reaction; generalized edema.

Overdosage:

Five healthy volunteers received up to 200 mg **lovastatin** as a single dose without clinically significant adverse experiences. A few cases of accidental overdosage have been reported; no patients had any specific symptoms, and all recovered without sequelae. The maximum dose taken was 5 to 6 g.

There is no specific treatment for **atorvastatin** overdosage. Because of extensive drug binding to plasma proteins, hemodialysis is not expected to significantly enhance **atorvastatin** clearance.

There has been a single report of two children, one 2 years old and the other 3 years old, either of whom may have possibly ingested **fluvastatin**. The maximum amount that could have been ingested was 80 mg. Vomiting was induced by ipecac in both children and no capsules were noted in their emesis. Neither child experienced any adverse symptoms and both recovered from the incident without problems.

There are two reported cases of **pravastatin** overdose, both of which were asymptomatic and not associated with clinical lab abnormalities.

A few cases of overdosage with **simvastatin** have occurred; no patients had any specific symptoms; all recovered without sequelae. The maximum dose taken was 450 mg.

Treat symptomatically and institute supportive measures as required. The dialyzability of these agents and their metabolites is not known.

Patient Information:

May cause photosensitivity (sensitivity to sunlight). Avoid prolonged exposure to the sun and other ultraviolet light. Use sunscreens and wear protective clothing until tolerance is determined.

Promptly report unexplained muscle pain, tenderness or weakness, especially if accompanied by fever or malaise.

Follow dietary recommendations.

Take **lovastatin** with meals; **fluvastatin, pravastatin** and **simvastatin** may be taken without regard to meals.

LOVASTATIN (Mevinolin)

For complete prescribing information, refer to the HMG-CoA Reductase Inhibitors group monograph.

Administration and Dosage:

Approved by the FDA in 1989.

Place the patient on a standard cholesterol-lowering diet before starting lovastatin and continue on this diet during treatment. Give lovastatin with meals.

Individualize dosage.

Initial dose: 20 mg/day with the evening meal.

Dose range: 10 to 80 mg/day in single or 2 divided doses.

Maximum dose: 80 mg/day. Adjust at intervals of at least 4 weeks.

Monitor cholesterol levels periodically and consider reducing the dosage if cholesterol levels fall below the targeted range.

Immunosuppressive therapy: In patients taking immunosuppressive drugs concomitantly with lovastatin, therapy should begin with 10 mg/day and should not exceed 20 mg/day (see Warnings).

Concomitant therapy: Cholesterol-lowering effects of lovastatin and the bile acid sequestrant, cholestyramine, are additive.

Renal function impairment: In patients with severe renal insufficiency (creatinine clearance < 30 ml/min), use dosage > 20 mg/day with caution.

Rx	**Mevacor** (Merck)	**Tablets**: 10 mg	(MSD 730 MEVACOR). Peach, octagonal. In 60s.
		20 mg	(MSD 731 MEVACOR). Blue, octagonal. In 30s, 60s, 90s, 100s, 180s, 1000s and UD 100s.
		40 mg	(MSD 732 MEVACOR). Green, octagonal. In 60s, 90s and 1000s.
	Mevacor (Merck)	**Tablets**: 20 mg	(MEVACOR 731/731.) Blue, octagonal. In 30s and 500s.
		Tablets: 40 mg	(MEVACOR 732.) Green, octagonal. In 30s and 250s.

SIMVASTATIN

For complete prescribing information, refer to the HMG-CoA Reductase Inhibitors group monograph.

Administration and Dosage:

Approved by the FDA in December 1991.

Place the patient on a standard cholesterol-lowering diet before starting simvastatin and continue on this diet during treatment. May give without regard to meals.

Individualize dosage. Consider reducing dose if cholesterol falls below targeted range.

Initial dose: 5 to 10 mg once daily in the evening.

Elderly: Consider starting dose of 5 mg/day; maximum LDL reductions may be achieved with ≤ 20 mg/day.

Dose range: 5 to 40 mg/day as single dose in the evening. Adjust dose at intervals of at least 4 weeks.

Rx	**Zocor** (Merck)	**Tablets:** 5 mg	Lactose. (MSD 726 ZOCOR). Buff, shield-shaped. In 60s, 90s and UD 100s.
		10 mg	Lactose. (MSD 735 ZOCOR). Peach, shield-shaped. In 60s, 90s, 1000s and UD 100s.
		20 mg	Lactose. (MSD 740 ZOCOR). Tan, shield-shaped. In 60s and 1000s.
		40 mg	Lactose. (MSD 749 ZOCOR). Red, shield-shaped. In 60s.

PRAVASTATIN SODIUM

For complete prescribing information, refer to the HMG-CoA Reductase Inhibitors group monograph.

Administration and Dosage:

Approved by the FDA in October 1991.

Place the patient on a standard cholesterol-lowering diet before starting pravastatin and continue on this diet during treatment. May give without regard to meals.

Individualize dosage.

Initial dose: 10 to 20 mg once daily at bedtime.

Renal/Hepatic function impairment: A starting dose of 10 mg/day at bedtime is recommended.

Elderly: In the elderly, maximum reductions in LDL-cholesterol may be achieved with daily doses of ≤ 20 mg.

Concomitant therapy: In patients taking concomitant immunosuppressive drugs (eg, cyclosporine), start pravastatin at 10 mg once-a-day at bedtime; titrate to higher doses with caution. Most patients treated with this combination received a maximum pravastatin dose of 20 mg/day. (See Warnings.)

Dose range: 10 to 40 mg once daily at bedtime.

Rx	**Pravachol** (Bristol-Myers Squibb)	**Tablets:** 10 mg	(P Pravachol 10). Pink, biconvex, rectangular. In 90s and UD 100s.
		20 mg	(P Pravachol 20). Yellow, biconvex, rectangular. In 90s, 1000s and UD 100s.
		40 mg	(P Pravachol 40). Green, biconvex, rectangular. In 90s and UD 100s.

HMG-CoA Reductase Inhibitors

FLUVASTATIN

For complete prescribing information, refer to the HMG-CoA Reductase Inhibitors group monograph.

Administration and Dosage:

Approved by the FDA on December 31, 1993 (1S Classification).

Place the patient on a standard cholesterol-lowering diet before receiving fluvastatin and continue on this diet during treatment. May be taken without regard to meals, because there are no apparent differences in the lipid-lowering effects of fluvastatin when administered with the evening meal or 4 hours after the evening meal.

Initial dose: 20 to 40 mg once daily at bedtime.

Dose range: 20 to 80 mg/day. Administer the daily regimen of 80 mg in divided doses (eg, 40 mg twice a day) to those whose LDL-cholesterol response is inadequate at 40 mg/day. Because the maximal reductions in LDL-C of a given dose are seen within 4 weeks, perform periodic lipid determinations during this time and adjust the dosage according to the patient's response to therapy and established treatment guidelines. The therapeutic effect is maintained with prolonged administration.

Concomitant therapy: Lipid-lowering effects on total cholesterol and LDL cholesterol are additive when fluvastatin is combined with a bile-acid binding resin or niacin. When administering a bile-acid resin (eg, cholestyramine) and fluvastatin, administer fluvastatin at bedtime, at least 2 hours following the resin to avoid a significant interaction because of drug binding to resin.

Renal function impairment: Because fluvastatin is cleared hepatically with < 6% of the administered dose excreted in the urine, dose adjustments for mild to moderate renal impairment are not necessary. Exercise caution with severe impairment.

Rx	**Lescol** (Sandoz)	**Capsules:** 20 mg	(20 Lescol logo). Brown/ light brown. In 30s and 100s.
		40 mg	(40 Lescol logo). Brown/ gold. In 30s and 100s.

ATORVASTATIN CALCIUM

For complete prescribing information, refer to the HMG-CoA Reductase Inhibitors group monograph.

Administration and Dosage:

Individualize dosage.

Initial dose: 10 mg/day.

Dose range: 10 to 80 mg/day. Atorvastatin can be administered as a single dose at any time of the day, with or without food. Analyze lipid levels within 2 to 4 weeks; adjust the dosage accordingly.

Concomitant therapy: Atorvastatin may be used in combination with a bile acid binding resin for additive effect. Avoid the combination of HMG-CoA reductase inhibitors and fibrates.

Rx	**Lipitor** (Parke-Davis)	**Tablets:** 10 mg	(PD 155 10.) White, elliptical. Film coated. In 90s, 5000s and UD 100s.
		20 mg	(PD 156 20.) White, elliptical. Film coated. In 90s and UD 100s.
		40 mg	(PD 157 40.) White, elliptical. Film coated. In 90s and UD 100s.

DEXTROTHYROXINE SODIUM

Refer to the general discussion of these products in the Antihyperlipidemic Agents Introduction.

Warning:

Obesity: Drugs with thyroid hormone activity have been used to treat obesity. In euthyroid patients, daily hormonal requirement doses are ineffective for weight reduction. Larger doses may produce serious or life-threatening toxicity, particularly when given with sympathomimetic amines used for their anorectic effects.

In a large study involving men who had had a MI, the drug was discontinued because of a trend to increased mortality in dextrothyroxine-treated subjects compared with placebo-treated patients. Even in subjects without known or suspected coronary disease, the potential benefits and risk of using dextrothyroxine should be carefully considered in patients presenting increased risk of coronary disease because of age, sex, obesity, history of smoking, hypertension and other factors increasing the risk of coronary artery disease, such as a positive family history of premature coronary disease.

Actions:

Pharmacology: Dextrothyroxine stimulates the liver to increase catabolism and excretion of cholesterol and its degradation products via the biliary route into the feces. Cholesterol synthesis is not inhibited, and abnormal metabolic end products do not accumulate in the blood. The predominant effect is reduction of serum cholesterol. Elevated β lipoprotein and triglyceride fractions may also be reduced.

Indications:

Reduction of cholesterol: As an adjunct to diet for reduction of elevated serum cholesterol (LDL) in patients with primary hypercholesterolemia (Types IIa and IIb) with no suspected heart disease whose response to diet and other nonpharmacologic measures has been inadequate.

Contraindications:

Euthyroid patients with one or more of the following conditions: Organic heart disease, including angina pectoris; history of MI; history of cardiac arrhythmia, including tachycardia; rheumatic heart disease; history of congestive heart failure; decompensated or borderline compensated cardiac status; hypertension (other than mild, labile systolic hypertension); advanced liver or kidney disease; history of iodism; pregnancy; lactation (see Warnings).

Warnings:

Surgery: Because the possibility of precipitating cardiac arrhythmias during surgery may be greater in patients treated with thyroid hormones, discontinue dextrothyroxine in euthyroid patients at least 2 weeks prior to an elective operation. Observe patients carefully during emergency surgery.

Renal/Hepatic function impairment: When either or both are present, weigh advantages of dextrothyroxine therapy against possible deleterious results.

Pregnancy: Category B. There are no adequate and well-controlled studies in pregnant women. Use during pregnancy only if clearly needed.

Consider the use of a bile acid sequestering resin in women of childbearing age who require drug therapy for hypercholesterolemia.

Lactation: It is not known whether dextrothyroxine is excreted in breast milk. Exercise caution when administering to a nursing woman.

Children: A few children with familial hypercholesterolemia have been treated for ≥ 1 year with no adverse effects on growth. However, continue the drug in children only if a significant serum cholesterol-lowering effect is observed.

Precautions:

Serum thyroxine levels: Increased serum thyroxine levels are evidence of absorption and transport of the drug and should not be interpreted as evidence of hypermetabolism. Therefore, they may not be used for titrating the effective dose. Thyroxine values in the range of 10 to 25 mcg/100 ml in treated patients are common. If signs or symptoms of iodism develop during therapy, discontinue use.

Tartrazine sensitivity: Some of these products contain tartrazine, which may cause allergic-type reactions (including bronchial asthma) in susceptible individuals. Although the incidence of sensitivity is low, it is frequently seen in patients who also have aspirin hypersensitivity. Specific products containing tartrazine are identified in the product listings.

DEXTROTHYROXINE SODIUM

Drug Interactions:

Dextrothyroxine Sodium Drug Interactions

Precipitant drug	Object drug*		Description
Cholestyramine	Dextrothyroxine	↓	Cholestyramine may decrease the GI absorption of dextrothyroxine.
Dextrothyroxine	Antidepressants, tricyclic	↑	Dextrothyroxine given concomitantly may produce CNS stimulation, nervousness, tachycardia and other cardiac arrhythmias.
Dextrothyroxine	Antidiabetic agents	↓	Dextrothyroxine in diabetic patients can increase blood sugar levels with a resultant increase in dosage requirements of hypoglycemic agents.
Dextrothyroxine	Anticoagulants, oral	↑	Dextrothyroxine may potentiate the hypoprothrombinemic effects. Reduce the dosage of anticoagulants when initiating dextrothyroxine therapy and readjust on the basis of prothrombin time; monitor weekly during the first few weeks of therapy. Consider withdrawal of the drug 2 weeks prior to surgery if the use of anticoagulants during surgery is contemplated.
Dextrothyroxine	Beta blockers	↓	Pharmacologic effects may be decreased by dextrothyroxine.
Dextrothyroxine	Digitalis glycosides	↓	Therapeutic effectiveness of digitalis glycosides may be decreased by concurrent dextrothyroxine, with possible exacerbation of cardiac arrhythmias or congestive heart failure. Effects of this interaction may occur up to several days after the discontinuation of dextrothyroxine.
Dextrothyroxine	Thyroid hormones	↑	Consider the dosage when used concomitantly with dextrothyroxine. As with all thyroactive drugs, hypothyroid patients are more sensitive to a given dose of dextrothyroxine than euthyroid patients.

* ↑ = Object drug increased. ↓ = Object drug decreased.

Adverse Reactions:

Side effects are mainly due to increased metabolism and may be minimized by following the recommended dosage schedule. Adverse effects are least commonly seen in euthyroid patients with no signs or symptoms of organic heart disease.

Cardiovascular: Angina pectoris; arrhythmias (extrasystoles, ectopic beats or supraventricular tachycardia); ECG evidence of ischemic myocardial changes; increase in heart size; MIs, both fatal and nonfatal (not unexpected in untreated patients in the age groups studied; drug relationship is unknown).

CNS: Insomnia; nervousness; tremors; headache; tinnitus; dizziness; psychic changes; altered sensorium; paresthesia.

Dermatologic: Hair loss; skin rashes; itching.

GI: Dyspepsia; nausea; vomiting; constipation; diarrhea; decrease in appetite; weight loss; gallstones and cholestatic jaundice (relationship to therapy not established).

Ophthalmic: Visual disturbances; exophthalmos; retinopathy; lid lag.

Miscellaneous: Sweating; flushing; hyperthermia; diuresis; menstrual irregularities; changes in libido; hoarseness; peripheral edema; malaise; tiredness; muscle pain; worsening of peripheral vascular disease.

DEXTROTHYROXINE SODIUM

Overdosage:

Overdosage with dextrothyroxine may result in signs and symptoms of thyrotoxicosis. The dosage at which such symptoms may appear will depend on the previous thyroid status of the patients and their individual sensitivity to the drug.

Treatment: Dextrothyroxine is somewhat protein-bound and would not be expected to be appreciably dialyzable. Treatment of overdosage is similar to that of thyrotoxic storm and may include hydration, sedation and use of beta-adrenergic blocking agents.

Patient Information:

Notify physician of chest pain, palpitations, sweating, diarrhea, headache or skin rash.

Administration and Dosage:

Adults:

Initial dose – 1 to 2 mg/day; increase by 1 to 2 mg at intervals of ≥ 1 month to a maximum of 4 to 8 mg daily.

Maintenance dose – 4 to 8 mg daily.

Children:

Initial dose – 0.05 mg/kg/day; increase in up to 0.05 mg/kg/day increments at monthly intervals to a maximum of 0.4 mg/kg/day or 4 mg/day.

If signs or symptoms of cardiac disease develop during therapy, discontinue use.

Rx	**Choloxin** (Knoll)	**Tablets:** 2 mg	Tartrazine. Yellow, scored. In 100s.
		4 mg	Tartrazine. White, scored. In 100s.

CLOFIBRATE

Refer to the general discussion of these products in the Antihyperlipidemic Agents Introduction.

Actions:

Pharmacology: Clofibrate predominantly lowers serum triglycerides and very low density lipoprotein (VLDL) levels; serum cholesterol and low density lipoproteins (LDL) are lowered less predictably and less effectively.

The mechanism of action is not established; the triglyceride-lowering effect appears to be due to accelerated catabolism of VLDL to LDL and decreased hepatic synthesis of VLDL. Cholesterol formation is inhibited early in the biosynthetic chain, and the excretion of neutral sterols is increased.

Pharmacokinetics:

Absorption/Distribution – Clofibrate is hydrolyzed to chlorophenoxyisobutyric acid (CPIB), the active form of the drug. Peak plasma levels occur within 3 to 6 hours. Plasma protein binding of CPIB is 92% to 97%; it decreases with increasing plasma concentration of CPIB.

Metabolism/Excretion – 40% to 70% of the drug is recovered in the urine as a glucuronide ester of CPIB. The plasma elimination half-life is 15 hours; half-lives of 30 to 110 hours have been reported in patients with renal impairment.

Indications:

Dysbetalipoproteinemia: For primary dysbetalipoproteinemia (type III hyperlipidemia) not responding to diet.

Hyperlipidemia: May be considered for the treatment of adults with very high serum triglyceride levels (types IV and V hyperlipidemia) who present a risk of abdominal pain and pancreatitis and who do not respond to diet. Clofibrate is not useful for the treatment of hypertriglyceridemia of type I hyperlipidemia.

Contraindications:

Clinically significant hepatic or renal dysfunction; primary biliary cirrhosis because clofibrate may raise the already elevated cholesterol in these cases; pregnancy, lactation (see Warnings).

Warnings:

Because of the hepatic tumorigenicity of clofibrate in rodents and the possible increased risk of malignancy and cholelithiasis in humans, use this drug only as indicated; discontinue if significant lipid response is not obtained. No evidence substantiates a beneficial effect from clofibrate on cardiovascular mortality.

Based on studies, consider the following:

1. Clofibrate, in general, causes a relatively modest reduction of serum cholesterol and a somewhat greater reduction of serum triglycerides. In type III hyperlipidemia, however, substantial reductions of both cholesterol and triglycerides can occur.
2. No study shows a convincing reduction in incidence of fatal myocardial infarction.
3. A significantly increased incidence of cholelithiasis has been demonstrated consistently in clofibrate-treated groups. Anticipate an increase in morbidity from this complication and mortality from cholecystectomy during clofibrate treatment.
4. An increase in incidence of noncardiovascular deaths was reported in one study, and another study showed a significant increase in total mortality. An increase in cardiac arrhythmias, intermittent claudication, definite or suspected thromboembolic events and angina was reported in another.
5. Administration of clofibrate (1 to 2 times the human dose) to mice and rats in long-term studies resulted in a higher incidence of benign and malignant liver tumors.

Pregnancy: Category C. Animal studies demonstrate placental transfer of the drug. The drug is metabolized by glucuronide conjugation; because this system is immature in the neonate, accumulation may occur. Strict birth control procedures must be exercised by women of childbearing potential. In patients who plan to become pregnant, withdraw clofibrate several months before conception. Weigh the possible benefits of the drug to the patient against possible hazards to the fetus.

Lactation: Animal studies suggest drug excretion into breast milk; thus, clofibrate is contraindicated in nursing women.

Children: Safety and efficacy for use in children have not been established.

CLOFIBRATE

Precautions:

Monitoring: Perform adequate baseline studies. Obtain serum lipid determinations frequently during the first few months and periodically thereafter. Withdraw the drug after 3 months if response is inadequate. However, in the case of xanthoma tuberosum, use the drug for longer periods (up to 1 year) provided there is a reduction in the size or number of the xanthomata.

Obtain subsequent serum lipid determinations to detect a paradoxical rise in serum cholesterol or triglycerides. Clofibrate will not alter the seasonal variations of serum cholesterol peak elevations in midwinter and late summer and decreases in fall and spring. If the drug is discontinued, maintain the patient on a diet and monitor serum lipids until stabilized; a rise to or above the original baseline value may occur.

Anemia/Leukopenia – Perform complete blood counts periodically because anemia, and, more frequently, leukopenia have been reported in patients taking clofibrate.

Hepatic – During therapy, perform frequent serum transaminase determinations and other liver function tests. Abnormalities are usually reversible when the drug is discontinued. Hepatic biopsies are usually normal. If the hepatic function tests rise steadily or show excessive abnormalities, withdraw the drug. Use with caution in patients with a history of jaundice or hepatic disease.

Cholelithiasis is a possible side effect of clofibrate therapy; perform appropriate diagnostic procedures if signs and symptoms related to biliary disease occur.

Response to therapy: Clofibrate has little effect on the elevated cholesterol levels of most subjects with hypercholesterolemia. A minority of subjects show a more pronounced response. Be selective and confine clofibrate treatment to patients with clearly defined risk because of severe hypercholesterolemia (eg, individuals with familial hypercholesterolemia starting in childhood) who inadequately respond to diet and more effective cholesterol-lowering drugs.

Do not use drug therapy for routine treatment of elevated blood lipids for the prevention of coronary heart disease. Dietary therapy specific for the type of hyperlipidemia is the initial treatment of choice. Excess body weight and alcohol intake may be important factors in hypertriglyceridemia and should be addressed prior to any drug therapy. Physical exercise can be an important ancillary measure. Diagnose and adequately treat contributory diseases such as hypothyroidism or diabetes mellitus. Consider drug therapy only when reasonable attempts have been made to obtain satisfactory results with non-drug methods. If the ultimate decision is to use drugs, instruct the patient that this does not reduce the importance of adhering to diet.

Because clofibrate is associated with certain serious adverse findings reported in two large clinical trials, agents other than clofibrate may be more suitable for a particular patient.

"Flu-like" symptoms (muscular aching, soreness, cramping) may occur; differentiate this from actual viral or bacterial disease.

Various cardiac arrhythmias have occurred with the use of clofibrate.

Peptic ulcer: Use with caution in patients with peptic ulcer because reactivation has been reported; whether this is drug-related is unknown.

Drug Interactions:

Clofibrate Drug Interactions

Precipitant drug	Object drug*		Description
Clofibrate	Anticoagulants, oral	⬆	The hypoprothrombinemic effects of these agents may be increased by concurrent clofibrate. Reduce the dosage of the anticoagulant if necessary to maintain the prothrombin time at the desired level to prevent bleeding complications. Use caution during coadministration; obtain frequent prothrombin determinations until the prothrombin level stabilizes.
Clofibrate	Dantrolene	⬆	Plasma protein binding of dantrolene may be reduced.
Clofibrate	Furosemide	⬆	An exaggerated diuretic response may occur.
Clofibrate	Insulin and Sulfonylureas	⬆	The pharmacologic effects of these agents may be increased by concurrent administration of clofibrate, resulting in hypoglycemia. Monitor blood glucose and reduce the insulin or sulfonylurea dose as necessary.

Clofibrate Drug Interactions			
Precipitant drug	Object drug*		Description
Clofibrate	Ursodiol	⬇	May increase hepatic cholesterol secretion and encourage cholesterol gallstone formation, and hence, may counteract the effectiveness of ursodiol.
Contraceptives, oral	Clofibrate	⬇	Oral contraceptives may increase the elimination of clofibric acid.
Probenecid	Clofibrate	⬆	Probenecid may increase the therapeutic and toxic effects of clofibrate by impairing its renal and metabolic clearance. A lower dose of clofibrate may be necessary.

Adverse Reactions:

GI: Nausea (most common); vomiting; diarrhea; loose stools; dyspepsia; flatulence; bloating; abdominal distress; hepatomegaly (not associated with hepatotoxicity); stomatitis; gastritis; gallstones.

Cardiovascular: Increased or decreased angina, cardiac arrhythmias, swelling and phlebitis at xanthoma site.

Dermatologic: Skin rash; alopecia; dry skin; dry brittle hair; pruritus; allergic reactions, including urticaria.

GU: Impotence; decreased libido; renal dysfunction as evidenced by dysuria, hematuria, proteinuria and decreased urine output. One patient's renal biopsy suggested "allergic reaction."

Hematologic: Leukopenia; anemia; eosinophilia.

Musculoskeletal: Myalgia (muscle cramps, aches, weakness); "flu-like" symptoms; arthralgia.

CNS: Fatigue; weakness; drowsiness; dizziness; headache.

Body as a whole: Weight gain; polyphagia.

Miscellaneous: (Drug relationship not established)-Peptic ulcer; GI hemorrhage; rheumatoid arthritis; tremors; increased perspiration; systemic lupus erythematosus; blurred vision; gynecomastia; thrombocytopenic purpura.

Lab test abnormalities: Increased transaminase (AST and ALT); BSP retention; proteinuria; increased thymol turbidity; increased creatine phosphokinase.

Overdosage:

Institute symptomatic supportive measures. Refer to General Management of Acute Overdosage.

Patient Information:

If GI upset occurs, may be taken with food.

Notify physician if any of the following effects occur: Chest pain; shortness of breath; irregular heartbeat; severe stomach pain with nausea and vomiting; fever and chills or sore throat; blood in the urine; decrease in urination; swelling of lower extremities; weight gain.

Administration and Dosage:

Adults: 2 g daily in divided doses. Some patients may respond to lower dosage.

Maintenance: Same as initial dose.

Rx	**Atromid-S** (Wyeth-Ayerst)	**Capsules:** 500 mg	Orange. Oblong. In 100s.
	Atromid-S (Wyeth-Ayerst)	**Capsules:** 500 mg	(Ayerst.) Orange. Oblong. Parabens. In 100s and 1000s.
		1 g	(Ayerst.) Red. Oblong. Parabens. In 100s.

GEMFIBROZIL

Refer to the general discussion of these products in the Antihyperlipidemic Agents Introduction.

Actions:

Pharmacology: Gemfibrozil is a fibric acid derivative that decreases serum triglycerides and very low density lipoprotein (VLDL) cholesterol, and increases high density lipoprotein (HDL) cholesterol. Modest decreases in total and low density lipoprotein (LDL) cholesterol may be observed, except in Type IV hyperlipoproteinemia patients who often experience a rise in LDL, and in Type IIb patients who experience minimal effects on LDL levels but usually show significant increases in HDL.

Gemfibrozil inhibits peripheral lipolysis and decreases the hepatic extraction of free fatty acids, thus reducing hepatic triglyceride production. Gemfibrozil also inhibits synthesis and increases clearance of VLDL carrier apolipoprotein B, decreasing in VLDL production. The mechanism for increased HDL lvels is unknown.

The drug may, in addition to elevating HDL cholesterol, reduce incorporation of long-chain fatty acids into newly formed triglycerides, accelerate turnover and removal of cholesterol from the liver and increase excretion of cholesterol in the feces.

Pharmacokinetics:

Absorption/Distribution – Gemfibrozil is well absorbed from the GI tract. Peak levels occur in 1 to 2 hours and appear proportional to the dose without accumulating after multiple doses.

Metabolism/Excretion – Gemfibrozil mainly undergoes oxidation to form a hydroxymethyl and a carboxyl metabolite. The plasma half-life is 1.5 hours following multiple doses. Biological half-life is considerably longer, due to enterohepatic circulation and reabsorbtion in the GI tract. Excretion is ≈70% urinary, mostly as the glucuronide conjugate, with < 2% excreted as unchanged drug; 6% is fecal.

Clinical trials: In a 5–year trial , 4081 male patients between the ages of 40 and 55, gemfibrozil therapy were associated with significant reductions in total plasma triglycerides and a significant increase in HDL. Moderate reductions in total plasma cholesterol and LDL were observed for the gemfibrozil treatment group as a whole. The study involved subjects with serum non-HDL-cholesterol of > 200 mg/dl and no previous history of CHD. The gemfibrozil group experienced a 34% reduction in serious coronary events (sudden cardiac deaths plus fatal and nonfatal MIs) compared with placebo. There was a 37% reduction in nonfatal MI. The greatest reduction in the incidence of serious coronary events occurred in Type IIb patients who had elevations of both LDL and total triglycerides. The mean increase in HDL among the Type IIb patients in this study was 12.6%.

Indications:

Hypertriglyceridemia in adult patients (Types IV and V hyperlipidemia) who present a risk of pancreatitis and who do not respond to diet. Consider therapy for those with triglyceride elevations between 1000 and 2000 mg/dl, and who have a history of pancreatitis or of recurrent abdominal pain typical of pancreatitis.

Reducing coronary heart disease risk: Consider gemfibrozil therapy in those Type IIb patients who have low HDL-cholesterol levels in addition to elevated LDL-cholesterol and triglyceride levels and who have not responded to weight loss, dietary therapy, exercise and other pharmacologic agents (eg, bile acid sequestrants, nicotinic acid).

Contraindications:

Hepatic or severe renal dysfunction, including primary biliary cirrhosis; preexisting gallbladder disease (see Warnings); hypersensitivity to gemfibrozil.

Warnings:

Cholelithiasis: Gemfibrozil may increase cholesterol excretion into the bile leading to cholelithiasis. If cholelithiasis is suspected, perform gallbladder studies. Discontinue therapy if gallstones are found.

Skeletal muscle effects: Concomitant therapy with gemfibrozil and lovastatin/simvastatin has been associated with rhabdomyolysis, markedly elevated creatine kinase (CK) levels and myoglobinuria, frequently leading to acute renal failure. In patients who with an unsatisfactory lipid response to either drug alone, any potential benefit of lovastatin/simvastatin and gemfibrozil coadministration does not outweigh the risks of severe myopathy, rhabdomyolysis and acute renal failure (see Drug Interactions).

Myositis – The use of fibrates alone, including gemfibrozil, may occasionally be associated with myositis. Promptly evaluate patients complaining of muscle pain, tenderness or weakness for myositis, including serum CK level determination. Periodic monitoring of CK may not prevent the occurrence of severe myopathy and kidney damage. If myositis is suspected or diagnosed, withdraw therapy.

GEMFIBROZIL

Renal function impairment: There have been reports of worsening renal insufficiency upon the addition of gemfibrozil therapy in individuals with baseline plasma creatinine > 2 mg/dl. In such patients, consider the use of alternative therapy against the risks and benefits of a lower dose of gemfibrozil.

Carcinogenesis/Fertility impairment: Long-term administration of high doses (≈ 1 and 10 times the human dose) of gemfibrozil in rats was associated with an increased incidence of benign liver nodules, liver carcinomas and benign Leydig cell tumors; subcapsular unilateral and bilateral cataracts also occurred. Administration of ≈ 0.6 and 2 times the human dose to male rats for 10 weeks resulted in a dose-related decrease of fertility. This effect was reversed after a drug-free period of ≈ 8 weeks, and it was not transmitted to their offspring.

Pregnancy: Category C. There are no adequate and well controlled studies in pregnant women. Use during pregnancy only when the benefit clearly outweighs the possible risk to the patient or fetus.

Lactation: Due to tumorigenicity potential shown in rats, discontinuation of nursing or drug therapy the drug, should take into account the importance of the drug to the mother.

Children: Safety and efficacy in children have not been established.

Precautions:

Monitoring: Perform adequate pretreatment laboratory studies. Obtain periodic determinations of serum lipids during administration. Withdraw the drug after 3 months if response is inadequate.

Hematologic – Mild hemoglobin, hematocrit and WBC decreases have been observed but have stabilized during long-term administration. Rarely, severe anemia, leukopenia, thrombocytopenia and bone marrow hypoplasia may occur. Perform periodic blood counts during the first 12 months of administration.

Hepatotoxicity – Abnormal elevations of AST, ALT, LDH, bilirubin and alkaline phosphatase have occurred and are usually reversible on drug discontinuation. Perform periodic liver function studies and terminate therapy if abnormalities persist.

Blood glucose – Gemfibrozil has a moderate hyperglycemic effect. Carefully monitor blood glucose levels during therapy.

Estrogen therapy is sometimes associated with massive rises in plasma triglycerides, especially in subjects with familial hypertriglyceridemia. Discontinuation of estrogen may obviate the need for specific drug therapy of hypertriglyceridemia.

Contributory diseases such as hypothyroidism or diabetes mellitus should be adequately treated. Consider the use of drugs only when reasonable attempts have been made to obtain satisfactory results with nondrug methods.

Hazardous tasks: May produce drowsiness (dizziness or blurred vision); patients should observe caution while driving or performing other tasks requiring alertness and physical dexterity.

Drug Interactions:

Gemfibrozil Drug Interactions			
Precipitant drug	Object drug*		Description
Gemfibrozil	HMG-CoA reductase inhibitors	⬆	Rhabdomyolysis has occurred from 3 weeks to several months after with combined gemfibrozil and lovastatin/simvastatin therapy (see Warnings).
Gemfibrozil	Anticoagulants, oral	⬆	Gemfibrozil may enhance the pharmacologic effect of these agents.

* ⬆ = Object drug increased.

Adverse Reactions:

Clofibrate and gemfibrozil have pharmacological similarities; the adverse findings with clofibrate may also apply to gemfibrozil.

GI: Dyspepsia (19.6%); abdominal pain (9.8%); diarrhea (7.2%); nausea/vomiting (2.5%); constipation (1.4%); acute appendicitis (1.2%).

CNS: Fatigue (3.8%); vertigo (1.5%); headache (1.2%); paresthesia; hypesthesia.

Dermatologic: Eczema (1.9%); rash (1.7%).

Cardiovascular: Atrial fibrillation (0.7%).

Special senses: Taste perversion.

Other (drug relationship probable or not established):

Immunologic – Angioedema; laryngeal edema; urticaria; anaphylaxis; lupus-like syndrome; vasculitis.

GEMFIBROZIL

GI – Cholestatic jaundice; pancreatitis; hepatoma; colitis.

CNS – Dizziness; somnolence; peripheral neuritis; decreased libido; depression; headache; confusion; convulsions; syncope.

Cardiovascular – Intracerebral hemorrhage; peripheral vascular disease; extrasystoles.

Special Senses – Blurred vision; retinal edema; cataracts.

Musculoskeletal – Myopathy; myasthenia; myalgia; painful extremities; arthralgia; synovitis; rhabdomyolysis.

Hematologic – Anemia; leukopenia; bone marrow hypoplasia; eosinophilia; thrombocytopenia.

GU – Impotence; decreased male fertility.

Dermatologic – Exfoliative dermatitis; dermatitis; pruritus; alopecia.

Miscellaneous – Weight loss; viral and bacterial infection (common cold, cough and urinary tract infections).

Lab test abnormalities – Liver function abnormalities (increased AST, ALT, LDH, CK, bilirubin, alkaline phosphatase); positive antinuclear antibody; mild decreases in hemoglobin, hematocrit and white blood cells (see Precautions).

Overdosage:

Institute symptomatic supportive measures. Refer to General Management of Acute Overdosage.

Patient Information:

May cause dizziness or blurred vision; patients should observe caution while driving or performing other tasks requiring alertness, coordination or physical dexterity.

Medication may cause abdominal or epigastric pain, diarrhea, nausea or vomiting. Notify physician if these become pronounced.

Administration and Dosage:

Adults: 1200 mg/daily in 2 divided doses, 30 minutes before the morning and evening meals.

Rx	**Lopid** (Parke-Davis)	**Tablets**: 600 mg	White, elliptical, scored. Film coated. In 60s, 500s and UD 100s.
Rx	**Gemfibrozil** (Various, eg, Medirex, Mylan, Purepac, Rugby)		In 60s, 100s, 500s, 600s and 1000s.
🍁	**Lopid** (Parke-Davis)	**Capsule**: 300 mg	Maroon and white. In 100s and 250s.
🍁	**Apo-Gemfibrozil** (Apotex)		(APO 300.) Maroon and white. In 100s and 500s.
🍁	**Novo-Gemfibrozil** (Novopharm)	**Tablets**: 600 mg	White, oval, film coated. In 100s and 500s.
🍁	**Lopid** (Parke-Davis)		(Lopid 600 mg/Parke-Davis.) White, ellipsoidal, film-coated. In 100s and 250s.
🍁	**Apo-Gemfibrozil** (Apotex)		(APO-600.) White, oval, biconvex, film-coated. In 100s and 500s.

NICOTINIC ACID (Niacin)

Refer to the general discussion of these products in the Antihyperlipidemic Agents Introduction.

The following is an abbreviated monograph for nicotinic acid. For complete prescribing information (eg, adverse reactions, a listing of available products), refer to the Niacin monograph in the Nutritionals chapter.

Actions:

Pharmacology: Pharmacologic doses of nicotinic acid reduce serum cholesterol and triglyceride levels in Types II, III, IV and V hyperlipoproteinemia. Triglycerides and very low density lipoproteins (VLDL) are reduced by 20% to 40% in 1 to 4 days. Low density lipoprotein (LDL) reduction may be seen in 5 to 7 days. The effect on LDL concentration is dose-dependent. The maximal effect will be seen in 3 to 5 weeks. The decrease in LDL will be greater if niacin is used with a bile acid-binding resin (40% to 60%). High density lipoproteins (HDL) are increased by 20%. The exact mechanism of action is unknown. It is known that nicotinic acid inhibits lipolysis in adipose tissue, decreases esterification of triglyceride in the liver and increases lipoprotein lipase activity. Niacinamide does NOT have hypolipemic effects.

Sustained-release niacin has been shown to be better than immediate-release niacin at reducing total serum cholesterol and low-density lipoprotein cholesterol while immediate-release niacin has been shown to be better at increasing high-density lipoprotein cholesterol.

Pharmacokinetics: The drug is rapidly absorbed in the intestines. Peak plasma levels are reached in 45 minutes. Urinary recovery of a 3 g dose is 88%.

Indications:

Hyperlipidemia: Adjunctive therapy in patients with significant hyperlipidemia (elevated cholesterol or triglycerides) who do not respond adequately to diet and weight loss.

Contraindications:

Hepatic dysfunction; active peptic ulcer; severe hypotension; hemorrhaging; arterial bleeding.

Warnings:

Hepatotoxicity: Doses > 2 g/day may cause hepatotoxicity. This is more common with the sustained-release formula and may occur within a week to 4 years. Symptoms include: Increased bilirubin, jaundice, nausea, vomiting, ammonia and prolonged prothrombin time. The most severe cases include fulminant hepatic failure, hepatic encephalopathy and liver transplantation. Periodically monitor liver enzymes and uric acid.

Flushing: In patients for whom flushing is distressing or persistent, 300 mg of aspirin given 30 minutes before each scheduled dose of nicotinic acid or slow upward adjustment of dose may help ameliorate this reaction.

Avoid drinking hot liquids with or immediately afterwards because they increase flushing.

Patient Information:

Cutaneous flushing and a sensation of warmth, especially of the face and upper body, may occur. Itching or tingling and headache may also occur. These effects are transient and usually subside with continued therapy.

May cause GI upset; take with meals.

If dizziness occurs, avoid sudden changes in posture.

Administration and Dosage:

Administer dosages of 1 to 2 g, 3 times per day, with or following meals. The usual maximum dose is 8 g/day.

Concomitant therapy: In one study, the triple combination of nicotinic acid, colestipol and lovastatin was more effective in reducing LDL than nicotinic acid in combination with either colestipol or lovastatin.

For complete listing of available products, refer to the Niacin monograph in the Nutritionals chapter.

chapter 5

respiratory drugs

SYMPATHOMIMETICS

Actions:

Pharmacology: These agents are used to produce bronchodilation. They relieve reversible bronchospasm by relaxing the smooth muscles of the bronchioles in conditions associated with asthma, bronchitis, emphysema or bronchiectasis. Bronchodilation may additionally facilitate expectoration. Some agents are also used for other purposes. See monographs for Vasopressors Used in Shock,Nasal Decongestants and Ophthalmic Vasoconstrictors/Mydriatics.

The pharmacologic actions of these agents include: Alpha-adrenergic stimulation (vasoconstriction, nasal decongestion, pressor effects); β_1-adrenergic stimulation (increased myocardial contractility and conduction); and β_2-adrenergic stimulation (bronchial dilation and vasodilation). Beta-adrenergic drugs stimulate adenyl cyclase, the enzyme which catalyzes the formation of cyclic-3'5' adenosine monophosphate (cyclic AMP) from adenosine triphosphate (ATP). The cyclic AMP that is formed mediates the cellular responses.

In addition to the cardiovascular/pulmonary effects, other adrenergic actions include alpha receptor-mediated contraction of GI and urinary sphincters; α and β receptor- mediated lipolysis; and α and β receptor-mediated decrease in GI tone, and changes in renin secretion, uterine relaxation, hepatic glycogenolysis/gluconeogenesis and pancreatic beta cell secretion.

The relative selectivity of action of sympathomimetic agents is the primary determinant of clinical usefulness; it can predict the most likely side effects. The β_2 selective agents provide the greatest benefit with minimal side effects. Direct administration via inhalation provides prompt effects and minimizes systemic activity. These drugs also inhibit histamine release from mast cells, produce vasodilation and increase ciliary motility. Bitolterol functions as a prodrug which must first be hydrolyzed by esterases in tissue and blood to its active moiety, colterol. Isoproterenol is one of the most potent bronchodilators available.

Sympathomimetic Bronchodilators: Pharmacologic Effects and Pharmacokinetic Properties

Sympathomimetic	Adrenergic receptor activity	Route	Onset (minutes)	Duration (hrs)
Albuterol[1]	$\beta_1 < \beta_2$	PO	within 30	4-8
		Inh[2]	within 5	3-8
Bitolterol[1]	$\beta_1 < \beta_2$	Inh	3-4	5 ≥ 8
Isoetharine[1]	$\beta_1 < \beta_2$	Inh[2]	within 5	1-3
Metaproterenol[1]	$\beta_1 < \beta_2$	PO	≈ 30	4
		Inh[2]	5-30	2-6
Pirbuterol[1]	$\beta_1 < \beta_2$	Inh	within 5	5
Salmeterol[1]	$\beta_1 < \beta_2$	Inh	within 20	12
Terbutaline[1]	$\beta_1 < \beta_2$	PO	30	4-8
		SC	5-15	1.5-4
		Inh	5-30	3-6
Isoproterenol	β_1 β_2	SL	≈ 30	1-2
		IV	immediate	< 1
		Inh[2]	2-5	0.5-2
Ethylnorepinephrine	$\alpha < \beta_1$ β_2	SC	5-10	1-2
		IM	5-10	1-2
Ephedrine	α β_1 β_2	PO	within 60	3-5
		SC	> 20	≤ 1
		IM	10-20	≤ 1
		IV	—	—
Epinephrine	α β_1 β_2	SC	5-15	1-4
		IM	—	1-4
		Inh[2]	1-5	1-3

[1] These agents all have minor β_1 activity.

[2] May be administered via aerosol nebulizer, bulb nebulizer or IPPB administration.

SYMPATHOMIMETICS

Indications:

Relief of reversible bronchospasm associated with acute and chronic bronchial asthma, exercise-induced bronchospasm, bronchitis, emphysema, bronchiectasis or other obstructive pulmonary diseases.

According to the National Heart, Lung and Blood Institute, inhaled beta agonists are recommended for mild acute asthma; inhaled or oral beta agonists plus an anti-inflammatory for moderate asthma; and beta agonists plus an oral corticosteroid for severe asthma.

Refer to individual monographs for indications of specific agents.

Contraindications:

Hypersensitivity to any component (allergic reactions are rare); cardiac arrhythmias associated with tachycardia; tachycardia or heart block caused by digitalis intoxication, angina (isoproterenol); narrow angle glaucoma, shock, during general anesthesia with halogenated agents or cyclopropane, organic brain damage (epinephrine).

Warnings:

Special risk patients: Administer with caution to patients with diabetes mellitus, hyperthyroidism, prostatic hypertrophy (ephedrine) or history of seizures; elderly; psychoneurotic individuals, patients with long-standing bronchial asthma and emphysema who have developed degenerative heart disease (epinephrine).

In patients with status asthmaticus and abnormal blood gas tensions, improvement in vital capacity and blood gas tensions may not accompany apparent relief of bronchospasm following isoproterenol. Facilities for administering oxygen and ventilatory assistance are necessary.

Diabetes – Large doses of **IV albuterol** may aggravate preexisting diabetes mellitus and ketoacidosis. Relevance to the use of oral or inhaled albuterol is unknown. Diabetic patients receiving any of these agents may require an increase in dosage of insulin or oral hypoglycemic agents.

Cardiovascular effects: Use with caution in patients with cardiovascular disorders including coronary insufficiency, ischemic heart disease, history of stroke, coronary artery disease, cardiac arrhythmias, CHF and hypertension. These agents may cause toxic symptoms through idiosyncratic response or overdosage. If cardiac rate increases sharply, angina patients may experience anginal pain until the cardiac rate decreases.

Closely monitor patients receiving **epinephrine**. Inadvertently induced high arterial blood pressure may result in angina pectoris, aortic rupture or cerebral hemorrhage. Cardiac arrhythmias develop in some individuals even after therapeutic doses. Epinephrine causes changes in the ECG even in healthy persons, including a decrease in amplitude of the T wave.

Ephedrine may cause hypertension resulting in intracranial hemorrhage. It may induce anginal pain in patients with coronary insufficiency or ischemic heart disease.

Large doses of inhaled or oral **salmeterol** (12 to 20 times the recommended dose) have been associated with clinically significant prolongation of the QTc interval, which has the potential for producing ventricular arrhythmias.

Significant changes in systolic and diastolic blood pressure can occur in some patients after use of any beta-adrenergic aerosol bronchodilator.

Paradoxical bronchospasm: Occasional patients have developed severe paradoxical airway resistance with repeated, excessive use of inhalation preparations; the cause is unknown. Discontinue the drug immediately and institute alternative therapy, since patients may not respond to other therapy until the drug is withdrawn.

Excessive use of inhalants: Deaths have been reported; the exact cause is unknown, but cardiac arrest following an unexpected severe acute asthmatic crisis and subsequent hypoxia is suspected.

Usual dose response: Advise patients to contact a physician if they do not respond to their usual dose of a sympathomimetic amine.

Reduce **epinephrine** dose if bronchial irritation, nervousness, restlessness or sleeplessness occurs. Do not continue to use epinephrine, but seek medical assistance immediately if symptoms are not relieved within 20 min or become worse.

CNS effects: Sympathomimetics may produce CNS stimulation.

Long-term use: Prolonged use of **ephedrine** may produce a syndrome resembling an anxiety state; many patients develop nervousness; a sedative may be needed. After prolonged use or overdosage, elevated serum lactic acid levels with severe metabolic acidosis have occurred, as have transient blood glucose elevations.

SYMPATHOMIMETICS

Acute symptoms: Do not use **salmeterol** to relieve acute asthma symptoms. If the patient's short-acting, inhaled β_2-agonist becomes less effective (eg, the patient needs more inhalations than usual), medical evaluation must be obtained immediately and increasing use of salmeterol in this situation is inappropriate. Do not use salmeterol more frequently than twice daily (morning and evening) at the recommended dose. When prescribing salmeterol, patients must be provided with a short-acting, inhaled β_2-agonist (eg, albuterol) for treatment of symptoms that occur despite regular twice-daily (morning and evening) use of salmeterol.

Asthma may deteriorate acutely over a period of hours or chronically over several days. In this setting, increased use of inhaled, short-acting β_2-agonists is a marker of destabilization of asthma and requires re-evaluation of the patient and consideration of alternative treatment regimens, especially inhaled or systemic corticosteroids. If the patient uses $\geq$ 4 inhalations per day of a short-acting β_2-agonist on a regular basis, or if more than one canister (200 inhalations per canister) is used in an 8-week period, then the patient should see the physician for re-evaluation of treatment.

Use with short-acting β_2-agonists – When patients begin treatment with salmeterol, advise those who have been taking short-acting, inhaled β_2-agonists on a regular daily basis to discontinue their regular daily-dosing regimen and clearly instruct them to use short-acting, inhaled β_2-agonists only for symptomatic relief if they develop asthma symptoms while taking salmeterol.

Morbidity/Mortality: It was previously suggested that an increased risk of death or near death from asthma may be associated with the regular use of inhaled beta agonists. However, a recent meta-analysis was conducted on case-control studies of this possible association. This report determined that the relationship between beta agonist use and death from asthma is of an extremely small magnitude, and may be restricted to the use of these agents via nebulizer. Further study is needed.

Overdosage or inadvertent IV injection of conventional SC **epinephrine** doses may cause severe or fatal hypertension or cerebrovascular hemorrhage resulting from the sharp rise in blood pressure. Fatalities may also occur from pulmonary edema resulting from peripheral constriction and cardiac stimulation. The marked pressor effects may be counteracted by use of rapidly acting vasodilators (eg, nitrites, α-blockers).

Respiratory depression: When compressed oxygen is used as the aerosol propellant, determine the percentage of oxygen by the patient's individual requirements to avoid depression of respiratory drive.

Hypersensitivity (allergic) reactions can occur after administration of **bitolterol, albuterol, metaproterenol, terbutaline, ephedrine, salmeterol** and possibly other bronchodilators. See Management of Acute Hypersensitivity Reactions.

Carcinogenesis: A significant increase in the incidence of leiomyomas of the mesovarium and ovarian cysts has been demonstrated with **albuterol, salmeterol** and **terbutaline** in animal studies. Salmeterol caused a dose-related increase in the incidence of smooth muscle hyperplasia and cystic glandular hyperplasia of the uterus in mice.

Elderly: Lower doses may be required due to increased sympathomimetic sensitivity. Observe special caution when using in elderly patients who have concomitant cardiovascular disease that could be adversely affected by this class of drug. Based on available data, no adjustment of **salmeterol** dosage in geriatric patients is warranted.

Pregnancy: Category B (terbutaline). *Category C* (albuterol, bitolterol, ephedrine, epinephrine, ethylnorepinephrine, isoetharine, isoproterenol, metaproterenol, salmeterol). Several of these agents are teratogenic and embryocidal in animal studies. There is no evidence that these class effects in animals are relevant to use in humans. There are no adequate and well controlled studies in pregnant women. Use only when clearly needed and when potential benefits outweigh potential hazards to the fetus.

Labor and delivery – Use of β_2 active sympathomimetics inhibits uterine contractions (see Terbutaline monograph). Other reactions include increased heart rate, transient hyperglycemia, hypokalemia, cardiac arrhythmias, pulmonary edema, cerebral and myocardial ischemia and increased fetal heart rate and hypoglycemia in the neonate. Although these effects are unlikely with aerosol use, consider the potential for untoward effects.

SYMPATHOMIMETICS

Oral **albuterol** and **terbutaline** have delayed preterm labor. There are no well controlled studies which demonstrate that they stop preterm labor or prevent labor at term. Therefore, use cautiously in pregnant patients when given for relief of bronchospasm to avoid interference with uterine contractility. Maternal death has been reported with terbutaline and other drugs in this class.

Lactation: **Terbutaline** and **epinephrine** are excreted in breast milk. It is not known whether other agents are excreted in breast milk. Decide whether to discontinue nursing or to discontinue the drug, taking into account the drug's importance to the mother.

Children:

Inhalation – Safety and efficacy for use of **bitolterol, pirbuterol, isoetharine, isoproterenol, salmeterol, terbutaline** and **albuterol** in children ≤ 12 years of age (*Ventolin* – < 4 years) have not been established. **Metaproterenol** may be used in children ≥ 6 years of age.

Injection – Parenteral **terbutaline** is not recommended for use in children < 12 years old. Administer **epinephrine** with caution to infants and children. Syncope has occurred following administration to asthmatic children.

Oral – **Metaproterenol** is not recommended for use in children < 6 years old. **Terbutaline** is not recommended for use in children < 12 years old. **Albuterol:** Safety and efficacy have not been established for children < 2 years (syrup), < 6 years (tablets) and < 12 years (tablets, timed release) old.

In children, **ephedrine** is effective in the oral therapy of asthma. Because of its CNS-stimulating effect, it is rarely used alone. This effect is usually countered by an appropriate sedative; however, its rationale has been questioned.

Precautions:

Tolerance may occur with prolonged use of sympathomimetic agents, but temporary cessation of the drug restores its original effectiveness.

Hypokalemia: Decreases in serum potassium levels have occurred, possibly through intracellular shunting which can produce adverse cardiovascular effects. The decrease is usually transient, not requiring supplementation.

Parkinson's disease: Epinephrine may temporarily increase rigidity and tremor.

Parenteral use: Avoid intraneural or intravascular injection of **ethylnorepinephrine**.

Administer **epinephrine** with great caution and in carefully circumscribed quantities in areas of the body served by end arteries or with otherwise limited blood supply (eg, fingers, toes, nose, ears, genitals) or if peripheral vascular disease is present to avoid vasoconstriction-induced tissue sloughing.

Combined therapy: Concomitant use with other sympathomimetic agents is not recommended, as it may lead to deleterious cardiovascular effects. This does not preclude the judicious use of an adrenergic stimulant aerosol bronchodilator in patients receiving tablets. Do not give on a routine basis. If regular coadministration is required, consider alternative therapy.

Patients must be warned not to stop or reduce corticosteroid therapy without medical advice, even if they feel better when they are being treated with β_2 agonists.

Sulfites: Some products contain sulfites that may cause allergic-type reactions including anaphylactic symptoms and life-threatening/less severe asthmatic episodes in susceptible persons. The overall prevalence in the general population is unknown and probably low. It is seen more frequently in asthmatic or atopic nonasthmatic persons.

Drug abuse and dependence: Prolonged abuse of **ephedrine** can lead to symptoms of paranoid schizophrenia. Patients exhibit such signs as tachycardia, poor nutrition and hygiene, fever, cold sweat and dilated pupils. Some measure of tolerance develops, but addiction does not occur. With all sympathomimetic aerosols, cardiac arrest and even death may be associated with abuse.

SYMPATHOMIMETICS

Drug Interactions:

Most interactions listed apply to sympathomimetics when used as vasopressors; however, consider the interaction when using the bronchodilator sympathomimetics.

Sympathomimetic Bronchodilator Drug Interactions			
Precipitant drug	Object drug*		Description
Beta blockers	Epinephrine	↑	An initial hypertensive episode followed by bradycardia may occur.
Furazolidine	Sympathomimetics	↑	The pressor sensitivity to mixed-acting sympathomimetics (eg, ephedrine) may be increased. Direct-acting agents (eg, epinephrine) are not affected.
Guanethidine	Sympathomimetics Direct Mixed	 ↑ ↓	Guanethidine potentiates the effects of the direct-acting sympathomimetics (eg, epinephrine) and inhibits the effects of the mixed-acting agents (eg, ephedrine). Guanethidine hypotensive action may also be reversed.
Sympathomimetics	Guanethidine	↓	
Lithium	Sympathomimetics	↓	The pressor sensitivity of direct-acting sympathomimetics (eg, epinephrine) may be decreased.
Methyldopa	Sympathomimetics	↑	Concurrent administration may result in an increased pressor response.
MAO inhibitors	Sympathomimetics	↑	Coadministration of MAO inhibitors and mixed-acting sympathomimetics (eg, ephedrine) may result in severe headache, hypertension and hyperpyrexia, possibly resulting in hypertensive crisis. Direct-acting agents (eg, epinephrine) interact minimally, if at all.
Oxytocic drugs (eg, ergonovine)	Sympathomimetics	↑	Concurrent administration may result in hypertension.
Rauwolfia alkaloids	Sympathomimetics Direct Mixed	 ↑ ↓	Reserpine potentiates the pressor response of the direct-acting sympathomimetics (eg, epinephrine) which may result in hypertension. The pressor response of the mixed-acting agents (eg, ephedrine) is decreased.
Tricyclic antidepressants (TCAs)	Sympathomimetics Direct Mixed	 ↑ ↓	TCAs potentiate the pressor response of direct-acting sympathomimetics (eg, epinephrine); dysrhythmias have occurred. The pressor response of mixed-acting agents (eg, ephedrine) is decreased.
Albuterol	Digoxin	↓	Digoxin serum levels may be decreased.
Sympathomimetics	Theophylline	↔	Enhanced toxicity, particularly cardiotoxicity, has been noted. Decreased theophylline levels may occur. Ephedrine may cause theophylline toxicity.
Epinephrine	Insulin or oral hypoglycemic agents	↓	Diabetics may require an increased dose of the hypoglycemic agent.

* ↑ = Object drug increased. ↓ = Object drug decreased. ↔ = Undetermined effect.

Drug/Lab test interactions: Isoproterenol causes false elevations of bilirubin as measured in vitro by a sequential multiple analyzer. Isoproterenol inhalation may result in enough absorption of the drug to produce elevated urinary epinephrine values. Although small with standard doses, the effect is likely to increase with larger doses.

SYMPATHOMIMETICS

Adverse Reactions:

Sympathomimetic Bronchodilator Adverse Reactions (%)[1]

	Adverse reaction	Albuterol	Bitolterol	Ephedrine	Epinephrine	Ethylnorepinephrine	Isoetharine	Isoproterenol	Metaproterenol	Pirbuterol	Salmeterol	Terbutaline
Cardiovascular	Palpitations	1-10	1.5-3	✓[2]	7.8-30	✓	✓	5-22	0.3-4	1.3-1.7	1-3	7.8-23
	Tachycardia	1-10	< 1	–	≤ 2.6		–	2-10	< 17	1.3	1-3	1.3-3
	Blood pressure changes/ hypertension	3.1-5			✓	✓	✓	2-5	0.3			< 1
	Chest tightness/pain/discomfort, angina	< 1	< 1		≤ 2.6			✓		1.3		1.5
	PVCs, arrhythmias, skipped beats		0.5	–	✓			1-3		<1		≈ 4
CNS	Tremor	1-20	9-14		16-18		–	< 15	3.3-33	1.3-6	4	5-38
	Dizziness/vertigo	1-7	1-3	–	3.3-7.8	–		1.5-5	1-4	0.6-1.2	≥ 3	1.3-10
	Shakiness/ nervousness/ tension	1-20	1.5-5	–	8.5-31		–	< 15	2.6-14	4.5-7	1-3	5-31
	Weakness	< 2			1.6-2.6		–	✓	1.3	< 1		≤ 1.3
	Drowsiness	< 1			8.2-14			< 5	0.7			5-11.7
	Restlessness	< 1			✓			✓				
	Hyperactivity/ Hyperkinesia, excitement	1-20	< 1					✓		< 1		
	Headache	2-27	≈ 4		3.3-10	–	–	1.5-10	≤ 4	1.3-2	28	7.8-10
	Insomnia	1-3.1	< 1	–	✓		–	1.5		< 1		✓
GI	Nausea/Vomiting	2-15	≤ 3	–	1-11.5	–	–	< 15	< 14	≤ 1.7	1-3	1.3-10
	Heartburn/GI distress/ disorder	≤ 5						5-10	≤ 4		1-4	< 10
	Diarrhea	≤ 1							0.7	< 1.3	1-3	
Respiratory	Dry mouth	< 1							1.3	< 1.3		
	Cough	1-5	4.1					1-5	≤ 4	1.2	7	
	Wheezing	≤ 1.5						1.5				✓
	Dyspnea	1.5	≤ 1		≤ 2			≤ 1.5				≤ 2
	Bronchospasm	1-15.4	≤ 1					≤ 18				✓
	Throat dryness/irritation, pharyngitis	≤ 6	3-5					3.1	≤ 4	< 1	≥ 3	✓
Other	Flushing	< 1	rare		≤ 1.3			✓		< 1		≤ 2.4
	Sweating	< 1		–	✓			✓				≤ 2.4
	Anorexia/ Appetite loss	1			✓					< 1		
	Unusual/bad taste or taste/ smell change	2							0.3	< 1		✓

[1] Data pooled for all routes of administration and all age groups. Data are pooled from separate studies and are not necessarily comparable.

[2] ✓ Reported; no incidence given.

SYMPATHOMIMETICS

Adverse reactions are generally transient, and no cumulative effects have been reported. It is usually not necessary to discontinue treatment; however, in selected cases temporarily reduce dosage. After the reaction has subsided, increase dosage in small increments to optimal dosage. In addition to the table, other adverse reactions are as follows:

Albuterol:

CNS – CNS stimulation; malaise (1.5%); emotional lability, fatigue, nightmares, aggressive behavior (1%); lightheadedness, disturbed sleep, irritability (< 1%).

Respiratory – Bronchitis (1.5% to 4%); nasal congestion (1% to 2%); sputum increase (1.5%); epistaxis (1% to 3%); hoarseness (rare in adults; 2% in children 4 to 12 years old).

Miscellaneous – Increased appetite (3%); muscle cramps (1% to 3%); pallor, conjunctivitis, anorexia, teeth discoloration (1%); dilated pupils, epigastric pain, micturition difficulty, muscle spasm, voice changes (< 1%); urticaria, angioedema, rash, bronchospasm, oropharyngeal edema (rare with inhaled albuterol).

Bitolterol:

Miscellaneous – Lightheadedness (3%). Elevations of AST, decrease in platelets and WBC counts and proteinuria (rare); clinical relevance or relationship unknown. The overall incidence of cardiovascular effects was ≈ 5%.

Ephedrine: Precordial pain; contact dermatitis after topical application.

Parenteral – Vesical sphincter spasm may result in difficult and painful urination; urinary retention may develop in males with prostatism. Confusion, delirium and hallucinations have been reported; excessive doses may cause a sharp rise in blood pressure sufficient to produce cerebral hemorrhage.

Epinephrine: Anxiety, fear, pallor.

Parenteral – Cerebral hemorrhage caused by rapid rises in blood pressure, particularly in elderly patients with cerebrovascular disease. Parenteral use may induce or aggravate psychomotor agitation, disorientation, impairment of memory, assaultive behavior, panic, hallucinations, suicidal or homicidal tendencies, schizophrenic-type thought disorders or paranoid delusions, hemiplegia and subarachnoid and cerebral hemorrhage. Initially, constriction of renal blood vessels and decreased urine formation may occur. Syncope has occurred in children. Patients with Parkinson's disease may experience a temporary increase in rigidity and tremor. Fatal ventricular fibrillation, occlusion of the central retinal artery and shock have occurred. Urticaria, wheal and hemorrhage at injection site; pain at injection site (1.6% to 2.6%). Repeated injections at the same site may result in necrosis from vascular constriction.

Ethylnorepinephrine:

Miscellaneous – Elevated pulse rate.

Isoetharine:

Miscellaneous – Anxiety.

Isoproterenol:

Cardiovascular – Adams-Stokes attacks, cardiac arrest, hypotension, precordial ache/dis- tress. In a few patients, presumably with organic disease of the AV node and its branches, isoproterenol has precipitated Adams-Stokes seizures during normal sinus rhythm or transient heart block.

Respiratory – Bronchitis (5%); sputum increase (1.5%); bronchial edema and inflammation, ECG evidence of coronary insufficiency; paradoxical airway resistance; pulmonary edema.

Miscellaneous – Swelling of the parotid glands with prolonged use.

Metaproterenol:

Respiratory – Asthma exacerbation (1% to 4%); hoarseness, nasal congestion (0.7%).

Miscellaneous – Rash (1.3%); backache, fatigue, skin reaction (0.7%).

Pirbuterol:

CNS – Anxiety, confusion, depression, fatigue, syncope (< 1%).

Dermatologic – Alopecia, edema, pruritus, rash (< 1%); bruising (≤ 1%).

GI – Abdominal pain/cramps, glossitis, stomatitis (< 1%).

Miscellaneous – Hypotension, numbness in extremities, weight gain (< 1%).

Salmeterol:

Respiratory – Upper respiratory tract infection, nasopharyngitis (14%); nasal cavity/sinus disease (6%); sinus headache, lower respiratory tract infection (4%); allergic rhinitis (> 3%); rhinitis, laryngitis, tracheitis/bronchitis (1% to 3%).

SYMPATHOMIMETICS

Musculoskeletal – Joint/back pain, muscle cramp/contraction, myalgia/myositis, muscular soreness (1% to 3%).

Miscellaneous – Giddiness, influenza (> 3%); viral gastroenteritis, urticaria, dental pain, malaise/fatigue, rash/skin eruption, dysmenorrhea (1% to 3%).

Terbutaline:

Miscellaneous – ECG changes such as sinus pause, atrial premature beats, AV block, ventricular premature beats, ST-T-wave depression, T-wave inversion, sinus bradycardia and atrial escape beat with aberrant conduction; increased heart rate; muscle cramps; central stimulation; pain at injection site (0.5% to 2.6%); elevations in liver enzymes and hypersensitivity vasculitis (rare).

Overdosage:

Inhalation: Symptoms - Exaggeration of the effects listed under Adverse Reactions can occur. Seizures, hypokalemia, anginal pain and hypertension may result.

Treatment includes general supportive measures. Sedatives (barbiturates) may be given for restlessness. The judicious use of a cardioselective β-receptor blocker (ie, metoprolol, atenolol) is suggested, bearing in mind the danger of inducing an asthmatic attack. Dialysis is not appropriate.

Systemic: Symptoms - Palpitations; tachycardia; bradycardia; extrasystoles; heart block; chest pain; hypokalemia; elevated blood pressure; fever; chills; cold perspiration; blanching of the skin; nausea; vomiting; mydriasis. Central actions produce insomnia, anxiety and tremor. Delirium, convulsions, collapse and coma may occur.

Treatment – Discontinuation or reduction in dosage will generally control toxicity. Emesis, gastric lavage or charcoal may be useful following overdosage with oral agents. If pronounced, a β-adrenergic blocker (propranolol) may be used, but consider the possibility of aggravation of airway obstruction; phentolamine may be used to block strong α-adrenergic actions. Treatment includes usual supportive measures. Refer to General Management of Acute Overdosage.

Patient Information:

Inhalation: Patient instructions are available with products. Many patients do not use metered-dose inhalers correctly, even after repeated instructions. Do not assume the patient understands the use of inhaled drugs and the proper administration technique. Use verbal instructions as well as an actual demonstration if possible. Repeat instructions at follow-up visits.

Have patient tilt head back and keep the metered dose inhaler mouthpiece ≈ 2 inches (or 2 finger widths) from open mouth or place the mouthpiece between open lips. Spacer devices are also available to aid the patient in proper administration of the drug. The patient should press down on the canister, breathe in slowly, hold breath for at least 10 seconds or as long as comfortable, then exhale. Administer pressurized inhalation during the second half of inspiration as the airways are open wider and the aerosol distribution is more extensive.

Do not exceed recommended dosage; excessive use may lead to adverse effects or loss of effectiveness. Do not stop or adjust the dose.

Do not change brands without consulting the physician or pharmacist.

If more than one inhalation per dose is necessary, wait at least one full minute between inhalations (administer second inhalation at 3 to 5 minutes for isoproterenol and epinephrine, 2 minutes for metaproterenol).

Notify physician of failure to respond to usual dosage or of dizziness or chest pain.

SYMPATHOMIMETICS

Isoproterenol may cause the patient's saliva to turn pinkish-red.

Salmeterol – Shake well before using. Salmeterol is not meant to relieve acute asthmatic symptoms, which should be treated with an inhaled, short-acting bronchodilator. The bronchodilator action usually lasts for at least 12 hours; therefore it should not be used more often than every 12 hours. While using salmeterol, seek medical attention immediately if the short-acting bronchodilator treatment becomes less effective for symptom relief, if more inhalations than usual are needed, or if more than the maximum number of inhalations of short-acting bronchodilator treatment prescribed for a 24-hour period are needed. If the patient uses > 4 inhalations per day of a short-acting beta$_2$-agonist on a regular basis, or if more than one canister (200 inhalations per canister) is used in an 8-week period, then the patient should see the physician for re-evaluation of treatment. When using salmeterol to prevent exercise-induced bronchospasm, administer the dose at least 30 to 60 minutes before exercise.

Oral: Do not exceed prescribed dosage. If GI upset occurs, take with food.

Sublingual tablets (*Isuprel;*) Do not swallow; allow to dissolve under tongue.

May cause nervousness, restlessness, insomnia (especially ephedrine); if these effects continue after reducing dosage, notify physician.

Notify physician if palpitations, tachycardia, chest pain, muscle tremors, dizziness, headache, flushing or difficult urination (ephedrine) occurs, or if breathing difficulty persists.

Sympathomimetics

SALMETEROL

For complete prescribing information, refer to the Sympathomimetic Bronchodilator group monograph.

Indications:

Asthma/Bronchospasm: Long-term, twice-daily (morning and evening) administration in the maintenance treatment of asthma and in the prevention of bronchospasm in patients ≥ 12 years of age with reversible obstructive airway disease, including patients with symptoms of nocturnal asthma, who require regular treatment with inhaled, short-acting $beta_2$-agonists. It should not be used in patients whose asthma can be managed by occasional use of short-acting, inhaled $beta_2$-agonists. Salmeterol may be used with or without concurrent inhaled or systemic corticosteroid therapy.

Exercise-induced bronchospasm: Prevention of exercise-induced bronchospasm in patients ≥ 12 years of age.

Administration and Dosage:

Approved by the FDA on February 4, 1994 (1P classification).

Administer by the orally inhaled route only (see Patient's Instructions for Use).

Asthma/Bronchospasm: For maintenance of bronchodilatation and prevention of symptoms of asthma, including the symptoms of nocturnal asthma, the usual dosage for adults and children ≥ 12 years of age is 2 inhalations (42 mcg) twice daily (morning and evening, approximately 12 hours apart). Adverse effects are more likely to occur with higher doses of salmeterol, and more frequent administration or administration of a larger number of inhalations is not recommended.

To gain full therapeutic benefit, administer twice daily (morning and evening) in the treatment of reversible airway obstruction.

If a previously effective dosage regimen fails to provide the usual response, seek medical advice immediately as this is often a sign of destabilization of asthma. Under these circumstances, reevaluate the therapeutic regimen and consider additional therapeutic options, such as inhaled or systemic corticosteroids. If symptoms arise in the period between doses, use a short-acting, inhaled β_2-agonist for immediate relief.

Prevention of exercise-induced bronchospasm: Two inhalations at least 30 to 60 minutes before exercise protects against exercise-induced bronchospasm in many patients for up to 12 hours. Additional doses of salmeterol should not be used for 12 hours after the administration of this drug. Patients who are receiving salmeterol twice daily (morning and evening) should not use additional salmeterol for prevention of exercise-induced bronchospasm. If this dose is not effective, consider other appropriate therapy for exercise-induced bronchospasm.

Geriatric use: In studies where geriatric patients (≥ 65 years of age, see Precautions) have been treated with salmeterol, efficacy and safety of 42 mcg given twice daily (morning and evening) did not differ from that in younger patients. Consequently, no dosage adjustment is recommended.

Storage/Stability: Store between 2° and 30°C (36° and 86°F). Store canister with nozzle end down. Protect from freezing temperatures and direct sunlight. Do not store at temperatures > 49°C (120°F). As with most inhaled medications in aerosol canisters, the therapeutic effect of this medication may decrease when the canister is cold; for best results, the canister should be at room temperature before use. Shake well before using.

Rx	**Serevent** (Glaxo Wellcome)	**Aerosol:** 25 mcg salmeterol base (as salmeterol xinafoate) per actuation	In 60 (60 actuations) and 13 g canisters and refills (120 actuations).

Sympathomimetics

ALBUTEROL

For complete prescribing information, refer to the Sympathomimetic Bronchodilator group monograph.

Indications:

Relief and prevention of bronchospasm in patients with reversible obstructive airway disease; prevention of exercise-induced bronchospasm.

Unlabeled uses: In a small number of patients on hemodialysis, nebulized albuterol therapy (10 or 20 mg) significantly decreased potassium concentrations and may be useful as an adjunct in serious acute hyperkalemia in hemodialysis patients.

Administration and Dosage:

Inhalation aerosol: Adults and children ≥ 12 years (Ventolin – ≥ 4 years)- 2 inhalations every 4 to 6 hours. In some patients, 1 inhalation every 4 hours may be sufficient. More frequent administration or a larger number of inhalations is not recommended. If previously effective dosage fails to provide relief, seek medical advice immediately. This is often a sign of seriously worsening asthma; reassess therapy.

Prevention of exercise-induced bronchospasm –

Adults and children ≥ 12 years: 2 inhalations 15 minutes prior to exercise.

Inhalation solution: Adults, children ≥ 12 years - 2.5 mg 3 to 4 times/day nebulization. Dilute 0.5 ml 0.5% solution with 2.5 ml sterile normal saline. Deliver over ≈ 5 to 15 min (if needed).

Inhalation capsules: Adults and children ≥ 4 years - Usual dose is 200 mcg inhaled every 4 to 6 hours using a Rotahaler device. Some patients may need 400 mcg every 4 to 6 hours.

Prevention of exercise-induced bronchospasm –

Adults and children ≥ 12 years: 200 mcg inhaled using a Rotahaler inhalation device 15 minutes before exercise.

Tablets: Adults and children ≥ 12 years - Usual starting dosage is 2 or 4 mg 3 or 4 times daily. Do not exceed a total daily dose of 32 mg. Use doses > 4 mg 4 times daily only when the patient fails to respond. If a favorable response does not occur, cautiously increase stepwise, up to a max of 8 mg 4 times daily, as tolerated.

Children 6 to 12 years – Usual starting dosage is 2 mg 3 to 4 times/day. For those who fail to respond to the initial starting dosage, cautiously increase stepwise, but do not exceed 24 mg/day in divided doses.

Elderly patients and those sensitive to β-adrenergic stimulants – Start with 2 mg 3 or 4 times daily. If adequate bronchodilation is not obtained, increase dosage gradually to as much as 8 mg 3 or 4 times daily.

Tablets, extended release: Adults and children ≥ 12 years - Usual starting dosage is 4 or 8 mg every 12 hours. Use doses > 8 mg twice/day only when the patient fails to respond. If a favorable response does not occur with the 4 mg initial dosage, cautiously increase stepwise up to a maximum of 16 mg twice a day. Do not exceed 32 mg/day.

Switching to extended release tablets – Patients maintained on regular release albuterol can be switched to *Proventil Repetabs.* A 4 mg extended release tablet every 12 hours is equivalent to a regular 2 mg tablet every 6 hours. Multiples of this regimen up to the maximum recommended dose also apply.

Syrup: Adults and children > 14 years - Usual dose is 2 or 4 mg 3 or 4 times/day. Give doses > 4 mg 4 times/day only when patient fails to respond. If a favorable response does not occur, cautiously increase, but do not exceed 8 mg 4 times/day.

Children (6 to 14) – Usual starting dose is 2 mg 3 or 4 times/day. If patient does not respond to 2 mg 4 times/day, cautiously increase step-wise. Do not exceed 24 mg/day in divided doses.

Children (2 to 6) – Initiate at 0.1 mg/kg 3 times daily. Do not exceed 2 mg 3 times daily. If the patient does not respond to the initial dose, increase step-wise to 0.2 mg/kg 3 times a day. Do not exceed 4 mg 3 times a day.

Elderly patients and those sensitive to β-adrenergic stimulation: Restrict initial dose to 2 mg 3 or 4 times daily. Individualize dosage thereafter.

Sympathomimetics

ALBUTEROL

Rx	**Albuterol** (Various, eg, Biocraft, Geneva, Goldline, Lederle, Moore, Mutual, Parmed, UDL, URL, Warner Chilcott)	**Tablets:** 2 mg (as sulfate)	In 24s, 100s, 250s, 500s, 1000s and UD 100s.
Rx	**Proventil** (Schering)		Lactose. (Proventil 2 252). White. In 100s and 500s.
Rx	**Ventolin** (Glaxo Wellcome)		Lactose. (Glaxo Ventolin 2). White. In 100s, 500s.
Rx	**Albuterol** (Various, eg, IDE, Major, Moore, Par, Parmed, PBI, Qualitest, Rugby, Schein, URL)	**Tablets:** 4 mg (as sulfate)	In 100s, 250s, 500s, 1000s and UD 100s.
Rx	**Proventil** (Schering)		Lactose. (Proventil 4 573). White. In 100s and 500s.
Rx	**Ventolin** (Glaxo Wellcome)		Lactose. (Glaxo Ventolin 4). White. In 100s, 500s.
Rx	**Proventil Repetabs** (Schering)	**Tablets, extended release:** 4 mg (as sulfate)	Lactose, sugar. (431). White. In 100s, UD 100s.
Rx	**Volmax** (Muro)		(Volmax 4). Blue. Hexagonal. In 100s and 500s.
Rx	**Volmax** (Muro)	**Tablets, extended release:** 8 mg (as sulfate)	(Volmax 8). White. Hexagonal. In 100s and 500s.
Rx	**Albuterol** (Lemmon)	**Syrup:** 2 mg (as sulfate) per 5 ml	Sorbitol. Strawberry flavor. In 480 ml.
Rx	**Proventil** (Schering)		Saccharin. Strawberry flavor. In 480 ml.
Rx	**Ventolin** (Glaxo Wellcome)		Saccharin. Strawberry flavor. In 480 ml.
Rx	**Albuterol** (Various, eg, Dey, Goldline, Warrick)	**Aerosol:** Each actuation delivers 90 mcg albuterol	In 17 g (200 inhalations).
Rx	**Proventil** (Schering)		In 17 g (≈ 200 inhalations).
Rx	**Proventil HFA** (Key)		In 6.7 g (200 inhalations). Contains no chlorofluorocarbons (CFC).
Rx	**Ventolin** (Glaxo Wellcome)		In 17 g (200 inhalations).
Rx	**Airet** (Adams)	**Solution for Inhalation:** 0.083% (as sulfate)	In vials.
Rx	**Albuterol** (Dey)		In UD 3 ml.
Rx	**Proventil** (Schering)		In 3 ml.
Rx	**Ventolin Nebules** (Glaxo Wellcome)		Sulfuric acid. In 3 ml unit dose nebules.
Rx	**Albuterol** (Copley)	**Solution for Inhalation:** 0.5% (as sulfate)	In 20 ml with dropper.
Rx	**Proventil** (Schering)		In 20 ml with dropper.
Rx	**Ventolin** (Glaxo Wellcome)		In 20 ml with dropper.
Rx	**Ventolin Rotacaps** (Glaxo Wellcome)	**Capsules for Inhalation:** 200 mcg microfine (as sulfate)	Lactose. (Ventolin 200 Glaxo). Lt. blue/clear. In UD 24s, 96s w/Rotahaler inhalation device.

METAPROTERENOL SULFATE

For complete prescribing information, refer to the Sympathomimetic Bronchodilator group monograph.

Indications:

For bronchial asthma and reversible bronchospasm; treatment of acute asthmatic attacks in children ≥ 6 years of age (Alupent solution for inhalation *only*).

Administration and Dosage:

Metered dose inhaler: 2 to 3 inhalations every 3 to 4 hours. Do not exceed 12 inhalations/day. Not recommended for children < 12 years of age.

Inhalant solutions: Usually, treatment need not be repeated more often than every 4 hours to relieve acute bronchospasm attacks. In chronic bronchospastic pulmonary diseases, give 3 to 4 times a day. A single dose of nebulized metaproterenol in the treatment of an acute attack of asthma may not completely abort an attack. Not recommended for children < 12 years of age.

Dosage and Dilution for Metaproterenol Inhalant Solutions

Administration	Usual dose	Range	Dilution
Hand bulb nebulizer	10 inhalations	5-15 inhalations	No dilution
IPPB	0.3 ml	0.2-0.3 ml	In ≈ 2.5 ml saline or other diluent

Administer the unit dose vial by oral inhalation using an IPPB device. The usual adult dose is one vial per nebulization treatment. Each 0.4% vial is equivalent to 0.2 ml of the 5% solution diluted to 2.5 ml with normal saline. Each 0.6% vial is equivalent to 0.3 ml of the 5% solution diluted to 2.5 ml with normal saline.

Oral:

Adults and children (> 9 years or > 60 lbs) – 20 mg 3 or 4 times a day.

Children (> 6 to 9 years or < 60 lbs) – 10 mg 3 or 4 times a day.

Children (< 6 years) – Doses of ≈ 1.3 to 2.6 mg/kg/day in divided doses of syrup were well tolerated in 78 children. Tablets are not recommended for this age group.

Storage: Store inhalant solution at 25°C (77°F). Protect from light. Do not use solution if it is brown or darker than slightly yellow, pinkish or if it contains a precipitate.

Rx	**Metaproterenol Sulfate** (Various, eg, Goldline, Major, Moore, Par, Parmed, PBI, Qualitest, Rugby, Schein, URL)	**Tablets:** 10 mg	In 100s and 1000s.
Rx	**Alupent** (Boehringer-Ingelheim)		(BI/74). White, scored. In 100s.[1]
Rx	**Metaproterenol Sulfate** (Various, eg, IDE, Major, Moore, Par, Parmed, PBI)	**Tablets:** 20 mg	In 100s and 1000s.
Rx	**Alupent** (Boehringer-Ingelheim)		(BI/72). White, scored. In 100s.[1]
Rx	**Metaproterenol Sulfate** (Various, eg, Copley, Genetco, Geneva, IDE, Major, Moore)	**Syrup:** 10 mg per 5 ml	In 480 ml.
Rx	**Alupent** (Boehringer-Ingelheim)		Saccharin, sorbitol. Cherry flavor. In 480 ml.
Rx	**Metaprel** (Sandoz)		Saccharin, sorbitol. Cherry flavor. In 480 ml.
Rx	**Prometa** (Muro)		Saccharin, sorbitol. Strawberry flavor. In 480 ml.
Rx	**Alupent** (Boehringer Ingelheim)	**Aerosol:** 75 mg as micronized powder in inert propellant (100 inhalations). Each dose delivers 0.65 mg	In 5 ml inhaler.

Sympathomimetics

METAPROTERENOL SULFATE

Rx	**Alupent** (Boehringer Ingelheim)	**Aerosol:** 150 mg as micronized powder in inert propellant (200 inhalations). Each dose delivers 0.65 mg	In 10 ml inhaler or 10 ml refill.
Rx	**Metaproterenol Sulfate** (Various, eg, Dey, Par)	**Solution for Inhalation:** 0.4%	In 2.5 ml.
Rx	**Alupent** (B-I)		In 2.5 ml UD vials.[2]
Rx	**Arm-a-Med Metaproterenol Sulfate** (Astra)		In 2.5 ml vials.[2]
Rx	**Metaproterenol Sulfate** (Various, eg, Dey, Major, Moore, Par)	**Solution for Inhalation:** 0.6%	In 2.5 ml.
Rx	**Alupent** (B-I)		In 2.5 ml UD vials.[2]
Rx	**Arm-a-Med Metaproterenol Sulfate** (Astra)		In 2.5 ml vials.[2]
Rx	**Metaproterenol Sulfate** (Various, eg, Dey, Goldline, IDE, Moore, PBI, Qualitest, Rugby)	**Solution for Inhalation:** 5%	In 0.3 and 30 ml vials.
Rx	**Alupent** (Boehringer-Ingelheim)		In 10 or 30 ml w/dropper.

[1] Contains lactose.

[2] For use with an IPPB device.

Sympathomimetics

ISOETHARINE HCl

For complete prescribing information, refer to the Sympathomimetic Bronchodilator group monograph.

Indications:

For bronchial asthma and reversible bronchospasm that occurs with bronchitis and emphysema.

Administration and Dosage:

Individualize dosage. Pediatric dosage has not been established.

Isoetharine Doses (Volume) Based on Strength of Solution		
Solution strength	Usual dose (IPPB[1] or oxygen aerosolization[2])	Equivalent isoetharine 1% dose
1%	0.25 to 1 ml (IPPB) or 0.25 to 0.5 ml (0_2 aerosolization) diluted 1:3 with saline or other diluent	same
0.25%	2 ml	0.5 ml
0.2%	1.25 to 2.5 ml	0.25 to 0.5 ml
0.17%	3 ml	0.5 ml
0.167%	3 ml	0.25 to 0.5 ml
0.125%	2 to 4 ml	0.25 to 0.5 ml
0.1%	2.5 to 5 ml	0.25 to 0.5 ml
0.08%	3 ml	0.25 ml
0.062%	4 ml	0.25 ml

[1] Usually an inspiratory flow rate of 15 L/min at a cycling pressure of 15 cm H_2O; may adjust flow rate to 6 to 30 L/min, cycling pressure to 10 to 15 cm H_2O.
[2] When given with oxygen, adjust flow to 4 to 6 L/min over 15 to 20 minutes.

Hand nebulizer: 3 to 7 inhalations undiluted.

Aerosol nebulizer: 1 or 2 inhalations. Occasionally, more may be required; however, wait 1 full minute after the initial dose to be certain another dose is necessary.

Usually, treatment need not be repeated more often than every 4 hours, although in severe cases more frequent administration may be necessary.

Storage/Stability: Do not use if discolored or contains a precipitate. Protect from light.

Rx	**Arm-a-Med Isoetharine HCl** (Astra)	**Solution for inhalation:** 0.062%	In single use 4 ml vials.[1]
Rx	**Isoetharine HCl** (Various, eg, Dey)	**Solution for inhalation:** 0.08%	In 3 ml vials.[2]
Rx	**Isoetharine HCl** (Various, eg, Dey, Roxane)	**Solution for inhalation:** 0.1%	In single use 2.5 and 5 ml vials.
Rx	**Isoetharine HCl** (Roxane)	**Solution for inhalation:** 0.125%	In single use 4 ml vials.[3]
Rx	**Arm-a-Med Isoetharine HCl** (Astra)		In single use 4 ml vials.[1]
Rx	**Isoetharine HCl** (Various, eg, Roxane)	**Solution for inhalation:** 0.167%	In single use 3 ml vials.[3]
Rx	**Arm-a-Med Isoetharine HCl** (Astra)		In single use 3 ml vials.[1]
Rx	**Isoetharine HCl** (Various, eg, Dey)	**Solution for inhalation:** 0.17%	In single use 3 ml vials.[2]
Rx	**Isoetharine HCl** (Various, eg, Roxane)	**Solution for inhalation:** 0.2%	In single use 2.5 ml vials.[3]
Rx	**Arm-a-Med Isoetharine HCl** (Astra)		In single use 2.5 ml vials.[1]
Rx	**Isoetharine HCl** (Various, eg, Dey, Roxane)	**Solution for inhalation:** 0.25%	In single use 2 ml vials.
Rx	**Arm-a-Med Isoetharine HCl** (Astra)		In single use 2 ml vials.[1]

Sympathomimetics

ISOETHARINE HCl

Rx	**Isoetharine HCl** (Various, eg, Dey, Roxane)	**Solution for inhalation:** 1%	In UD 0.25 and 0.5 ml vials.
Rx	**Beta-2** (Nephron)		In 10 and 30 ml with dropper.[4]
Rx	**Bronkosol** (Winthrop)		In 10 and 30 ml.[4]
Rx	**Bronkometer** (Winthrop)	**Aerosol:** 0.61% (as mesylate). Delivers 340 mcg isoetharine per metered dose	In 10 and 15 ml with oral nebulizer (≈ 20 doses/ml).[5]

[1] With sodium metabisulfite and glycerin.
[2] With glycerin and EDTA.
[3] With glycerin, EDTA, sodium sulfite and sodium bisulfite.
[4] With glycerin, sodium bisulfite and parabens.
[5] With saccharin, menthol and alcohol.

TERBUTALINE SULFATE

For complete prescribing information, refer to the Sympathomimetic Bronchodilator group monograph.

Indications:

A bronchodilator for bronchial asthma and for reversible bronchospasm which may occur with bronchitis and emphysema.

Unlabeled uses: Oral and IV terbutaline have successfully inhibited premature labor. Initiate IV use at 10 mcg/minute; titrate upward to a maximum of 80 mcg/minute. Maintain IV dosage at the minimum effective dose for 4 hours. Oral doses of 2.5 mg every 4 to 6 hours have been used as maintenance therapy until term.

Administration and Dosage:

Inhalation:

Adults and children ≥ 12 years – 2 inhalations separated by 60 seconds every 4 to 6 hours. Do not repeat more often than every 4 to 6 hours.

Oral:

Adults and children > 15 years – 5 mg, given at 6 hour intervals, 3 times daily during waking hours. If side effects are pronounced, dose may be reduced to 2.5 mg 3 times daily. Do not exceed 15 mg in 24 hours.

Children (12 to 15 years) – 2.5 mg 3 times daily. Do not exceed 7.5 mg in 24 hours. Not recommended for children < 12 years of age.

Parenteral: Usual dose is 0.25 mg SC into the lateral deltoid area. If significant improvement does not occur in 15 to 30 minutes, administer a second 0.25 mg dose. Do not exceed a total dose of 0.5 mg in 4 hours. If a patient fails to respond to a second 0.25 mg dose within 15 to 30 minutes, consider other therapeutic measures.

Rx	**Brethine** (Geigy)	**Tablets:** 2.5 mg	Lactose. (Geigy 72). White, scored. Oval. In 100s, 1000s, UD 100s and Gy-Pak 100s.
Rx	**Bricanyl** (Hoechst Marion Roussel)		Lactose. (Bricanyl 2). White. In 100s and 1000s.
Rx	**Brethine** (Geigy)	**Tablets:** 5 mg	Lactose. (Geigy 105). White, scored. In 100s, 1000s, UD 100s and Gy-Pak 100s.
Rx	**Bricanyl** (Hoechst Marion Roussel)		Lactose. (Bricanyl 5). White, scored. Square. In 100s and 1000s.
Rx	**Brethaire** (Geigy)	**Aerosol:** 0.2 mg per actuation	In 10.5 g cans (≥ 300 inhalations).
Rx	**Brethine** (Geigy)	**Injection:** 1 mg/ml	In 2 ml amp with 1 ml fill.
Rx	**Bricanyl** (Hoechst Marion Roussel)		In 2 ml amp with 1 ml fill.

Sympathomimetics

ETHYLNOREPINEPHRINE HCl

Complete prescribing information for these products begins in the Sympathomimetics group monograph.

Indications:

A bronchodilator for bronchial asthma and for reversible bronchospasm that may occur with bronchitis and emphysema.

Administration and Dosage:

Adults: The usual dose by SC or IM injection is 0.5 to 1 ml. Depending on severity of the asthmatic attack, smaller doses (0.3 to 0.5 ml) may suffice.

Children: Dosage varies according to age and weight; usual dose is 0.1 to 0.5 ml.

Storage: Protect from light.

Rx	**Bronkephrine** (Winthrop Pharm.)	**Injection:** 2 mg/ml	In 1 ml amps.[1]

[1] With sodium bisulfite.

ISOPROTERENOL

For complete prescribing information, refer to the Sympathomimetic Bronchodilator group monograph.

Indications:

Inhalation: Treatment of bronchospasm associated with acute and chronic bronchial asthma, pulmonary emphysema, bronchitis and bronchiectasis.

Injection: Management of bronchospasm during anesthesia.

Sublingual: Management of patients with bronchopulmonary disease.

Isoproterenol is also used as a vasopressor in shock. Refer to Vasopressors Used in Shock in the Cardiovascular section.

Administration and Dosage:

Inhalation:

Acute bronchial asthma –

Hand bulb nebulizer: In adults and children, administer the 1:200 solution in a dosage of 5 to 15 deep inhalations. In adults, the 1:100 solution may be used if a stronger solution seems indicated. The dose is 3 to 7 deep inhalations. If no relief is evident after 5 to 10 minutes, repeat doses one more time. If acute attack recurs, repeat treatment up to 5 times daily if necessary.

Metered dose inhaler: The usual dose is 1 to 2 inhalations. Start with 1 inhalation. If no relief is evident after 2 to 5 minutes, a second inhalation may be taken. For daily maintenance, use 1 to 2 inhalations 4 to 6 times daily. Do not take more than 2 inhalations at any one time, nor more than 6 inhalations per hour.

Bronchospasm in chronic obstructive lung disease –

Hand bulb nebulizer: Usually 5 to 15 deep inhalations using the 1:200 solution. Some patients with severe attacks may require 3 to 7 inhalations using the 1:100 solution. Do not use at less than 3 to 4 hour intervals.

Nebulization by compressed air or oxygen: 0.5 ml of a 1:200 solution is diluted to 2 to 2.5 ml with appropriate diluent for a concentration of 1:800 to 1:1000. Deliver the solution over 10 to 20 minutes. May repeat up to 5 times daily.

IPPB: 0.5 ml of a 1:200 solution diluted to 2 to 2.5 ml with water or isotonic saline. Deliver over 15 to 20 minutes. May repeat up to 5 times daily.

Metered dose inhaler: 1 or 2 inhalations; repeat at no less than 3 to 4 hour intervals (4 to 6 times daily).

Children – Administration is similar to that of adults, since children's smaller ventilatory exchange capacity automatically provides proportionally smaller aerosol intake. The 1:200 solution is recommended for an acute attack of bronchospasm. Do not use more than 0.25 ml of the 1:200 solution for each 10 to 15 minute programmed treatment.

Injection: For the management of bronchospasm during anesthesia, dilute 1 ml of a 1:5000 solution to 10 ml with Sodium Chloride Injection or 5% Dextrose Injection. Administer an initial dose of 0.01 to 0.02 mg IV and repeat when necessary.

Sublingual: The average adult dose is 10 mg (15 to 20 mg may be required) depending on patient response. However, do not exceed a total of 60 mg/day. For children, the dose is from 5 to 10 mg, not exceeding a total of 30 mg/day.

Allow tablets to disintegrate under the tongue. Do not crush or chew sublingual tablets. Instruct patients not to swallow saliva until absorption has taken place. Do not repeat treatment more often than every 3 or 4 hours, or > 3 times daily.

Sympathomimetics

ISOPROTERENOL

Rx	**Isoproterenol HCl** (Various, eg, Goldline, Moore)	**Solution for inhalation:** 0.25% (1:400)	In 15 ml.
Rx	**Dispos-a-Med Isoproterenol HCl** (Parke-Davis)		In 0.5 ml.[2] (Use only with Dispos-a-vial solutions.)
Rx	**Isoproterenol HCl** (Various, eg, Dey)	**Solution for inhalation:** 0.5% (1:200)	In 0.5 ml single use vials.[3]
Rx	**Dispos-a-Med Isoproterenol HCl** (Parke-Davis)		In 0.5 ml.[2] (Use only with Dispos-a-vial solutions.)
Rx	**Isuprel** (Winthrop Pharm.)		In 10 and 60 ml.[4]
Rx	**Isuprel** (Winthrop Pharm.)	**Solution for inhalation:** 1% (1:100) isoproterenol HCl	In 10 ml.[5]
Rx	**Isoproterenol HCl** (Various, eg, Schein)	**Aerosol:** 0.25% (1:400)	In 15 ml.
Rx	**Isuprel Mistometer** (Winthrop Pharm.)	**Aerosol:** Delivers 131 mcg isoproterenol HCl solution/dose in fine mist	In 10 and 15 ml and 15 ml refill.
Rx	**Medihaler-Iso** (3M)	**Aerosol:** 0.2% isoproterenol sulfate. Delivers 80 mcg/measured dose	In 15 ml (≈ 300 doses) or 22.5 ml (≈ 450 doses) w/adapter and 15 ml refill.
Rx	**Isoproterenol HCl** (Various, eg, Elkins-Sinn)	**Injection:** (1:5000 solution) 0.2 mg/ml	In 5 ml amps.
Rx	**Isuprel** (Winthrop Pharm.)		In 1 and 5 ml amps.[6]

[1] With 2 mg sodium metabisulfite.
[2] With glycerin and sodium bisulfites.
[3] With sodium metabisulfite and parabens.
[4] With cholrobutanol, sodium metabisulfite and glycerin.
[5] With chlorobutanol, sodium metabisulfite and saccharin.
[6] With sodium metabisulfite.

ISOPROTERENOL HCl AND PHENYLEPHRINE BITARTRATE

For complete prescribing information, refer to the Sympathomimetic Bronchodilator group monograph.

Indications:

Treatment of bronchospasm associated with acute and chronic asthma; reversible bronchospasm which may be associated with emphysema or chronic bronchitis.

Administration and Dosage:

Relief of dyspnea: Acute episode, 1 to 2 inhalations. Start with one inhalation; if not relieved in 2 to 5 minutes, administer a second.

Daily maintenance – 1 to 2 inhalations, 4 to 6 times daily. Do not take > 2 inhalations at any one time or > 6 in any 1 hour within 24 hours.

Rx	**Duo-Medihaler** (3M)	**Aerosol:** Each valve actuation releases 0.16 mg isoproterenol HCl and 0.24 mg phenylephrine bitartrate	In 15 ml (≈ 300 metered doses) or 22.5 ml (≈ 450 metered doses) medihalers or 15 and 22.5 ml refills.

Sympathomimetics

BITOLTEROL MESYLATE

For complete prescribing information, refer to the Sympathomimetic Bronchodilator group monograph.

Indications:

Prophylaxis and treatment of bronchial asthma and reversible bronchospasm. May be used with or without concurrent theophylline or steroid therapy.

Administration and Dosage:

Bronchospasm:

Adults and children > 12 years of age – 2 inhalations at an interval of at least 1 to 3 minutes, followed by a third inhalation if needed.

Prevention of bronchospasm: 2 inhalations every 8 hours.

Do not exceed 3 inhalations every 6 hours or 2 inhalations every 4 hours.

Rx	**Tornalate** (Dura)	**Aerosol**: 0.8%. Delivers 0.37 mg/actuation	In 15 ml metered dose inhaler[1] (≥ 300 inhalations) and 15 ml refill.
Rx	**Tornalate** (Dura)	**Solution for Inhalation**: 0.2%	In 10, 30 and 60 ml.[2]

[1] With saccharin, menthol and alcohol.
[2] With 25% alcohol and propylene glycol.

EPINEPHRINE

For complete prescribing information, refer to the Sympathomimetic Bronchodilator group monograph.

Indications:

Inhalation: Temporary relief from acute paroxysms (eg, shortness of breath, tightness of chest, wheezing) of bronchial asthma; postintubation and infectious croup.

MicroNefrin – Chronic obstructive lung disease, chronic bronchitis, broncheolitis, bronchial asthma and other peripheral airway diseases.

Injection: To relieve respiratory distress in bronchial asthma or during acute asthma attacks and for reversible bronchospasm in patients with chronic bronchitis, emphysema and other obstructive pulmonary diseases.

Treatment of hypersensitivity reactions to drugs, sera, insect stings or other allergens, including such symptoms as bronchospasm, urticaria, pruritus, angioneurotic edema, or swelling of the lips, eyelids, tongue and nasal mucosa.

Epinephrine is also used as a vasopressor in shock (refer to Vasopressors Used in Shock in the Cardiovascular section) and for infiltration of tissue to delay absorption of drugs such as local anesthetics.

Administration and Dosage:

Refer to specific product labeling for detailed administration and dosage information.

Inhalation aerosol: Start treatment at the first symptoms of bronchospasm. Individualize dosage. Wait 1 to 5 minutes between inhalations.

Nebulization: Place 8 to 15 drops into the nebulizer reservoir. Place the nebulizer nozzle into the partially opened mouth. Squeeze the bulb 1 to 3 times. Inhale deeply. If relief does not occur within 5 minutes, administer 2 to 3 additional inhalations. Nebulizer use, 4 to 6 times daily, is usually sufficient to maintain comfort.

IPPB – Add 0.5 ml epinephrine to 20 ml water just prior to treatment. Administer for 15 minutes every 3 to 4 hours.

Injection:

Solution (1:1000) – The initial adult: SC or IM dose is 0.3 to 0.5 ml (0.3 to 0.5 mg); repeat every 20 min to 4 hours.

For infants and children: (except premature infants and full-term newborns), give 0.01 ml/kg or 0.3 ml/m^2 (0.01 mg/kg or 0.3 mg/m^2) SC. Do not exceed 0.5 ml (0.5 mg) in a single pediatric dose. Repeat every 20 minutes to 4 hours or more often if necessary.

Suspension (1:200) – For SC use only. Administer subsequent doses only when necessary and not more often than every 6 hours.

Adults – 0.1 to 0.3 ml (0.5 to 1.5 mg) SC.

Infants and children (1 month to 12 years) – 0.005 ml/kg (0.025 mg/kg) SC.

Children ≤ 30 kg – The maximum single dose is 0.15 ml (0.75 mg).

Repeated local injections can result in necrosis at injection sites from vascular constriction. Tolerance can occur with prolonged use.

Storage – Refrigerate the suspension; do not freeze. Do not expose to temperatures > 30°C (86°F). Shake well before using.

Sympathomimetics

EPINEPHRINE

Alkalies and oxidizers (eg, oxygen, chlorine, bromine, iodine, permanganates, chromates, nitrites, salts of reducible metals, especially iron), destroy epinephrine.

Rx	**Adrenalin Chloride** (Parke-Davis)	**Solution for inhalation:** 1:100 solution epinephrine HCl	In 7.5 ml.[1]
otc	**AsthmaNefrin** (Menley & James)	**Solution for inhalation:** 2.25% racepinephrine HCl (equivalent to 1.125% epinephrine base)	In 15 and 30 ml and complete nebulizer.[2]
otc	**microNefrin** (Bird)		In 15 and 30 ml.[3]
otc	**Nephron** (Nephron)		In 7.5 and 15 ml.
otc	**S-2** (Nephron)		In 15 ml.[3]
otc	**Vaponefrin** (Fisons)	**Solution for inhalation:** 2% racepinephrine base (equivalent to 1% epinephrine base)	In 15 and 30 ml.[4]
otc	**AsthmaHaler Mist** (Menley & James)	**Aerosol:** 0.3 mg epinephrine bitartrate (equivalent to 0.16 mg epinephrine base per spray)	Alcohol free. In 15 ml w/adapter or 15 ml refill.
otc	**Bronitin Mist** (Whitehall)		In 15 ml or 15 ml refills.
otc	**Primatene Mist Suspension** (Whitehall)		In 10 ml, 15 ml w/mouthpiece or 15 and 22.5 ml refills.
otc	**Bronkaid Mist** (Sterling Health)[5]	**Aerosol:** 0.5% epinephrine (as nitrate and HCl, equivalent to 0.25 mg epinephrine per spray)	33% alcohol. In 10 ml and 15 ml (≥ 300 doses) w/actuator or 15 and 22.5 ml refills.
otc	**Primatene Mist** (Whitehall)	**Aerosol:** 0.2 mg epinephrine per spray	34% alcohol. In 15 ml w/mouthpiece or 15 and 22.5 ml refills.
Rx	**Epinephrine** (Various, eg, Abbott, American Regent, Elkins-Sinn, IMS, Lyphomed, Wyeth-Ayerst)	**Injection:** 1:1000 (1 mg/ml as HCl) solution	In 1 ml amps.
Rx	**Adrenalin Chloride Solution** (Parke-Davis)		In 1 ml amps[6] and 30 ml Steri-vials.[7]
Rx	**Sus-Phrine** (Forest)	**Injection:** 1:200 (5 mg/ml) suspension	In 0.3 ml amps[8] and 5 ml vials.[8]

[1] With benzethonium chloride and 0.2% sodium bisulfite.
[2] With benzoic acid, chlorobutanol, glycerin and sodium bisulfite.
[3] With sodium bisulfite, potassium metabisulfite, chlorobutanol, benzoic acid and propylene glycol.
[4] With chlorobutanol and sodium metabisulfite.
[5] Sterling Health, 90 Park Ave., New York, NY 10016; (800) 228-0204
[6] With sodium bisulfite.
[7] With sodium bisulfite and chlorobutanol.
[8] With thioglycolic acid, phenol and glycerin.

Sympathomimetics

EPHEDRINE SULFATE

For complete prescribing information, refer to the Sympathomimetic Bronchodilator group monograph.

Actions:

Pharmacology: Ephedrine sulfate is a sympathomimetic alkaloid which stimulates alpha and beta receptors as well as the CNS. It is effective both orally and parenterally. It is longer acting but less potent than epinephrine.

Indications:

Treatment of allergic disorders, such as bronchial asthma, and for local treatment of nasal congestion in acute coryza, vasomotor rhinitis, acute sinusitis and hay fever.

Parenteral ephedrine is sometimes used to relieve acute bronchospasm, but it is less effective than epinephrine for this purpose and has been given as a CNS stimulant in narcolepsy and depressive states.

Ephedrine is also used as a vasopressor in shock. Refer to Vasopressors Used in Shock in the Cardiovascular section.

Administration and Dosage:

Adults: The usual oral dose is 25 to 50 mg, 2 or 3 times a day. The usual parenteral dose is 25 to 50 mg, administered SC, IM or slowly IV.

Children: 3 mg/kg/day or 100 mg/m^2/day divided into 4 to 6 doses by the oral, SC or IV route.

otc	**Ephedrine Sulfate** (Various, eg, Goldline, IDE, Lannett, Major, Moore, Schein, URL, West-Ward)	**Capsules:** 25 mg	In 100s, 500s, 1000s and UD 100s.
Rx	**Ephedrine Sulfate** (Various, eg, Rugby)	**Capsules:** 50 mg	In 1000s.
Rx	**Ephedrine Sulfate** (Lilly)	**Injection:** 25 mg/ml	In 1 ml amps.
Rx	**Ephedrine Sulfate** (Various, eg, Abbott, Lilly, Lyphomed)	**Injection:** 50 mg/ml	In 1 ml amps, 10 ml vials and 10 ml disp. syringes.

PIRBUTEROL ACETATE

For complete prescribing information, refer to the Sympathomimetic Bronchodilator group monograph.

Indications:

Prevention and reversal of bronchospasm in patients with reversible bronchospasm including asthma. Use with or without concurrent theophylline or steroid therapy.

Administration and Dosage:

Adults and children ≥ 12 years of age: 2 inhalations (0.4 mg) repeated every 4 to 6 hours. One inhalation (0.2 mg) may be sufficient for some patients.

Do not exceed a total daily dose of 12 inhalations.

If previously effective dosage regimen fails to provide the usual relief, seek medical advice immediately as this is often a sign of seriously worsening asthma which would require reassessment of therapy.

Rx	**Maxair** (3M Pharm.)	**Aerosol:** Delivers 0.2 mg/actuation	In 25.6 g metered dose inhaler (≥ 300 inhalations).

Diluents

SODIUM CHLORIDE

For complete prescribing information, refer to the Sympathomimetic Bronchodilator group monograph.

Indications:

To dilute bronchodilator solutions for inhalation. Also for tracheal lavage.

otc	**Sodium Chloride 0.45%** (Dey)	**Solution:** 0.45% sodium chloride	Preservative free. In single-use 3 and 5 ml vials.
otc	**Sodium Chloride 0.9%** (Dey)	**Solution:** 0.9% sodium chloride	Preservative free. In 1, 3, 5, 10 & 15 ml Dey-Paks & 3, 5, 10 & 20 ml Dey-Vials.
otc	**Broncho Saline** (Blairex)		In 90 and 240 ml with metered dispensing valve.

XANTHINE DERIVATIVES

Actions:

Pharmacology: The methylxanthines (theophylline, its soluble salts and derivatives) directly relax the smooth muscle of the bronchi and pulmonary blood vessels, stimulate the CNS, induce diuresis, increase gastric acid secretion, reduce lower esophageal sphincter pressure and inhibit uterine contractions. Theophylline is also a central respiratory stimulant. Aminophylline has a potent effect on diaphragmatic contractility in healthy persons and may then be capable of reducing fatigability and thereby improve contractility in patients with chronic obstructive airways disease. The exact mode of action is unclear.

For many years, the proposed main mechanism of action of the xanthines was inhibition of phosphodiesterase, which results in an increase in cyclic adenosine monophosphate (cAMP). However, this effect is negligible at therapeutic concentrations. Other effects that appear to occur at therapeutic concentrations and may collectively play a role in the mechanism of the xanthines include: Inhibition of extracellular adenosine (which causes bronchoconstriction), although it is unlikely that this is a main mechanism; stimulation of endogenous catecholamines, although this also does not appear to be a major mechanism; antagonism of prostaglandins PGE_2 and $PGF_{2}\alpha$; direct effect on mobilization of intracellular calcium resulting in smooth muscle relaxation; beta-adrenergic agonist activity on the airways. None of these mechanisms has been proven.

Pharmacokinetics:

Absorption – Theophylline is well absorbed from oral liquids and uncoated plain tablets; maximal plasma concentrations are reached in 2 hours. Rectal absorption from suppositories is slow and erratic, the oral route is generally preferred. Enteric coated tablets and some sustained release dosage forms may be unreliably absorbed. Food may alter bioavailability and absorption pattern of some sustained release preparations; close monitoring is advised (see Drug Interactions).

Distribution – Average volume of distribution is 0.45 L/kg (range, 0.3 to 0.7 L/kg). Theophylline does not distribute into fatty tissue, but readily crosses the placenta and is excreted into breast milk. Approximately 40% is bound to plasma protein. Therapeutic serum levels generally range from 10 to 20 mcg/ml. Although some bronchodilatory effect occurs at lower concentrations, stabilization of hyperreactive airways is most evident at levels > 10 mcg/ml, and adverse effects are uncommon at levels < 20 mcg/ml. Once a patient is stabilized, serum levels tend to remain constant with the same dosage.

Metabolism/Excretion – Xanthines are biotransformed in the liver (85% to 90%) to 1, 3–dimethyluric acid, 3–methylxanthine and 1–methyluric acid; 3–methylxanthine accumulates in concentrations approximately 25% of those of theophylline.

Excretion is by the kidneys; < 15% of the drug is excreted unchanged. Elimination kinetics vary greatly. Plasma elimination half-life averages about 3 to 15 hours in adult nonsmokers, 4 to 5 hours in adult smokers (1 to 2 packs per day), 1 to 9 hours in children and 20 to 30 hours for premature neonates. In the neonate, theophylline is metabolized partially to caffeine. The premature neonate excretes about 50% unchanged theophylline and may accumulate the caffeine metabolite.

A prolonged half-life may occur in congestive heart failure, liver dysfunction, alcoholism, respiratory infections and patients receiving certain other drugs (see Drug Interactions). Total clearance appears relatively unaffected by renal failure.

Equivalent dose: Because of differing theophylline content, the various salts and derivatives are not equivalent on a weight basis. The table below indicates percentage of anhydrous theophylline and approximate equivalent dose of each compound. Product listings include anhydrous theophylline dosage equivalents.

Theophylline Content and Equivalent Dose of Various Theophylline Salts

Theophylline salts	Theophylline %	Equivalent dose
Theophylline anhydrous	100	100 mg
Theophylline monohydrate	91	110 mg
Aminophylline anhydrous	86	116 mg
Aminophylline dihydrate	79	127 mg
Oxtriphylline	64	156 mg

Dyphylline, a chemical derivative of theophylline, is not a theophylline salt as are the other agents. It is about one-tenth as potent as theophylline. Following oral administration, dyphylline is 68% to 82% bioavailable. Peak plasma concentrations are reached within 1 hour, and its half-life is 2 hours. The minimal effective therapeutic concentration is 12 mcg/ml. It is not metabolized to theophylline and 83% ± 5% is excreted unchanged in the urine.

XANTHINE DERIVATIVES

Indications:

Symptomatic relief or prevention of bronchial asthma and reversible bronchospasm associated with chronic bronchitis and emphysema.

Unlabeled uses: Treatment of apnea and bradycardia of prematurity. Doses of 2 mg/kg/day have been used to maintain serum concentrations between 3 and 5 mcg/ml.

Theophylline 300 mg/day was effective in reducing essential tremor in one study of 20 patients.

Theophylline 10 mg/kg/day may significantly improve pulmonary function and dyspnea in patients with chronic obstructive pulmonary disease.

Contraindications:

Hypersensitivity to any xanthine; peptic ulcer; underlying seizure disorders (unless receiving appropriate anticonvulsant medication).

Aminophylline: Hypersensitivity to ethylenediamine.

Aminophylline rectal suppositories: Irritation or infection of rectum or lower colon.

Warnings:

Status asthmaticus is a medical emergency and is not rapidly responsive to usual doses of conventional bronchodilators. Optimal therapy frequently requires both parenteral medication and close monitoring, preferably in an intensive care setting. Oral theophylline products alone are not appropriate for status asthmaticus.

Toxicity: Excessive doses may cause severe toxicity; monitor serum levels to assure maximum benefit with minimum risk. Incidence of toxicity increases significantly at serum levels > 20 mcg/ml (75% of patients with levels > 25 mcg/ml). Serum levels > 20 mcg/ml are rare after appropriate use of recommended doses. However, if theophylline plasma clearance is reduced for any reason (eg, hepatic impairment; patients > 55 years old, particularly males and those with chronic lung disease; cardiac failure; sustained high fever; infants < 1 year old), even conventional doses may result in increased serum levels and potential toxicity. Frequently, such patients have markedly prolonged levels following drug discontinuation.

Serious side effects such as ventricular arrhythmias, convulsions or even death may appear as the first sign of toxicity without any previous warning. Less serious signs of toxicity (eg, nausea, restlessness) may occur frequently when initiating therapy, but are usually transient; when such signs are persistent during maintenance therapy, they are often associated with serum concentrations > 20 mcg/ml. Serious toxicity is not reliably preceded by less severe side effects.

Cardiac effects: Theophylline may cause dysrhythmias or worsen pre-existing arrhythmias. Any significant change in cardiac rate or rhythm warrants monitoring and further investigation. Many patients who require theophylline may exhibit tachycardia due to underlying disease; the relationship to elevated serum theophylline concentrations may not be appreciated. Ventricular arrhythmias respond to lidocaine.

Pregnancy: Category C. It is not known whether theophylline can cause fetal harm when administered to a pregnant woman or can affect reproduction capacity. Give only if clearly needed. Theophylline has been found in cord serum and crosses the placenta; newborns may have therapeutic serum levels. Apnea has been associated with theophylline withdrawal in a neonate. Theophylline-related human congenital defects or malformations have not been reported.

Lactation: Theophylline distributes readily into breast milk with a milk:plasma ratio of 0.7 and may cause irritability or other signs of toxicity in nursing infants. Decide whether to discontinue nursing or to discontinue the drug, taking into account the importance of the drug to the mother.

Children: Sufficient numbers of infants < 1 year of age have not been studied in clinical trials to support use in this age group; however, there is evidence that the use of dosage recommendations for older infants and young children may result in the development of toxic serum levels. Carefully consider associated benefits and risks in this age group. (See Administration and Dosage and Unlabeled uses.)

Precautions:

Use with caution in: Cardiac disease; hypoxemia; hepatic disease; hypertension; congestive heart failure (CHF); alcoholism; elderly (particularly males); and neonates.

GI effects: Use cautiously in peptic ulcer. Local irritation may occur; centrally mediated GI effects may occur with serum levels > 20 mcg/ml. Reduced lower esophageal pressure may cause reflux, aspiration and worsening of airway obstruction.

Alcohol: The addition of alcohol in liquid formulations is not necessary for absorption and may be potentially harmful.

XANTHINE DERIVATIVES

Drug Interactions:

Agents that Decrease Theophylline Levels		
Aminoglutethimide	Rifampin	Thioamines[3]
Barbiturates	Smoking (cigarettes and marijuana)	Carbamazepine[1]
Charcoal	Sulfinpyrazone	Isoniazid[1]
Hydantoins[2]	Sympathomimetics (β-agonists)	Loop diuretics[1]
Ketoconazole		

Agents that Increase Theophylline Levels		
Allopurinol	Disulfiram	Quinolones
Beta blockers (non-selective)	Ephedrine	Thiabendazole
Calcium channel blockers	Influenza virus vaccine	Thyroid hormones[4]
Cimetidine	Interferon	Carbamazepine[1]
Contraceptives, oral	Macrolides	Isoniazid[1]
Corticosteroids	Mexiletine	Loop diuretics[1]

[1] May increase or decrease theophylline levels.
[2] Decreased hydantoin levels may also occur.
[3] Increased theophylline clearance in hyperthyroid patients.
[4] Decreased theophylline clearance in hypothyroid patients.

Benzodiazepines: The sedative effects of benzodiazepines may be antagonized by theophyllines, although their pharmacokinetics do not appear to be altered. Coadministration may be beneficial in reversing sedation produced by benzodiazepines.

Beta-agonists and theophylline act synergistically in vitro; an additive effect has also been demonstrated in vivo.

Halothane with theophylline has resulted in catecholamine-induced arrhythmias.

Ketamine and theophylline coadministration has resulted in extensor-type seizures.

Lithium plasma levels may be reduced by theophyllines.

Nondepolarizing muscle relaxants: A dose-dependent reversal of neuromuscular blockade by theophyllines may occur.

Probenecid may increase the pharmacologic effects of dyphylline due to decreased dyphylline renal excretion.

Propofol: Theophyllines may antagonize the sedative effects of propofol.

Ranitidine: Case reports suggest that theophylline plasma levels may be increased by ranitidine, possibly increasing pharmacologic and toxic effcts. However, several controlled studies indicate that an interaction does not occur. It appears that if this interaction occurs, it is rare.

Tetracyclines: The incidence of theophylline adverse reactions may possibly be enhanced by concurrent tetracyclines.

Drug/Lab test interactions: Currently available analytical methods for measuring serum theophylline levels are specific, and metabolites and other drugs generally do not affect the results. However, be aware of the specific laboratory method used and whether other factors will interfere with the assay for theophylline.

Drug/Food interactions: Theophylline elimination is increased (half-life shortened) by a low carbohydrate, high protein diet and charcoal broiled beef (due to a high polycyclic carbon content). Conversely, elimination is decreased (prolonged half-life) by a high carbohydrate low protein diet. Food may alter the bioavailability and absorption pattern of certain sustained release preparations. Some sustained release preparations may be subject to rapid release of their contents when taken with food, resulting in toxicity. It appears that consistent administration in the fasting state allows predictability of effects.

Adverse Reactions:

Adverse reactions/toxicity are uncommon at serum theophylline levels < 20 mcg/ml.

Levels > 20 mcg/ml: 75% of patients experience adverse reactions (eg, nausea, vomiting, diarrhea, headache, insomnia, irritability).

Levels > 35 mcg/ml: Hyperglycemia; hypotension; cardiac arrhythmias; tachycardia (> 10 mcg/ml in premature newborns); seizures; brain damage; death.

Other: Fever; flushing; hyperglycemia; inappropriate antidiuretic hormone syndrome; rash; alopecia. Ethylenediamine in aminophylline can cause sensitivity reactions, including exfoliative dermatitis and urticaria.

CNS: Irritability; restlessness; headache; insomnia; reflex hyperexcitability; muscle twitching; convulsions.

GI: Nausea; vomiting; epigastric pain; hematemesis; diarrhea; rectal irritation or bleeding (aminophylline suppositories). Therapeutic doses of theophylline may induce gastroesophageal reflux during sleep or while recumbent, increasing the potential for aspiration which can aggravate bronchospasm.

Cardiovascular: Palpitations; tachycardia; extrasystoles; hypotension; circulatory failure; life-threatening ventricular arrhythmias.

Respiratory: Tachypnea; respiratory arrest.

Renal: Proteinuria; potentiation of diuresis.

Overdosage:

Symptoms: Anorexia; nausea; vomiting; nervousness; insomnia; agitation; irritability; headache; tachycardia; extrasystoles; tachypnea; fasciculation; tonic/clonic convulsions. Convulsions or ventricular arrhythmias may be the first signs of toxicity. Hyperamylasemia, simulating pancreatitis, has also been noted. Other symptoms of intoxication are listed under Adverse Reactions.

Serious adverse effects are rare at serum theophylline concentrations < 20 mcg/ml. Between 20 and 40 mcg/ml, sinus tachycardia and cardiac arrhythmias occur. Above 40 mcg/ml, seizures and cardiorespiratory arrest can occur. However, convulsions and death have been reported at concentrations as low as 25 mcg/ml.

Acute overdosage appears to be better tolerated with the more serious reactions (eg, seizures) occurring with chronic overdosage (levels > 40 mcg/ml), but rarely in the acute situation unless levels exceed 100 mcg/ml. Also, symptoms such as hypokalemia, hypercalcemia, hyperglycemia and decreased serum bicarbonate concentrations occur more frequently with acute overdosage.

Overdosage with sustained release preparations may cause a dramatic increase in serum theophylline concentrations much later (≥ 12 hours) than the increases that occur with other preparations. Early treatment will help but not prevent these delayed elevated levels.

Treatment if seizure has not occurred: Induce vomiting, even if emesis has occurred spontaneously; ipecac syrup is preferred. However, do not induce emesis in patients with impaired consciousness. Take precautions against aspiration, especially in infants and children. If vomiting is unsuccessful or contraindicated, perform gastric lavage (of no value ≥ 1 hour post-ingestion). Administer a cathartic (particularly for sustained-release preparations; sorbitol may be useful) and activated charcoal. Prophylactic phenobarbital may increase the seizure threshold.

If seizure occurs: Establish an airway and administer oxygen. Administer IV diazepam 0.1 to 0.3 mg/kg, up to 10 mg. Monitor vital signs, maintain blood pressure and provide adequate hydration.

Post-seizure coma: Maintain airway and oxygenation. Perform intubation and lavage instead of inducing emesis. Introduce the cathartic and activated charcoal via a large bore gastric lavage tube. Provide full supportive care and adequate hydration while the drug is metabolized. If repeated oral activated charcoal is ineffective, charcoal hemoperfusion may be indicated.

Supportive care: Employ usual supportive measures. Refer to General Management of Acute Overdosage. Do not use stimulants (analeptic agents). Continuously monitor cardiac function. Verapamil has been used to treat atrial arrhythmias; lidocaine or procainamide may be used for ventricular arrhythmias. May need IV fluids to treat dehydration, acid-base imbalance and hypotension; the latter may also be treated with vasopressors. Apnea will require ventilatory support. Treat hyperpyrexia, especially in children, with tepid water sponge baths or a hypothermic blanket.

Monitor theophylline serum level until it falls below 20 mcg/ml because secondary rises of plasma theophylline may occur from redistribution, delayed absorption, etc; this has been reported with sustained release products.

Dialysis: Charcoal hemoperfusion rapidly removes theophylline and may be indicated when the serum concentration is > 60 mcg/ml, even in the absence of obvious toxicity. Forced diuresis, peritoneal dialysis and extracorporeal methods are inadequate. However, hemodialysis appears capable of removing ≈ 36% to 40% of serum theophylline.

"Gastric dialysis" with oral activated charcoal, 20 to 40 g every 4 hours until serum level is < 20 mcg/ml, may shorten half-life and speed removal, regardless of route. Mechanism may include enhancing drug concentration gradient into the GI lumen, a disruption of an enterohepatic recycling process or binding unabsorbed drug.

XANTHINE DERIVATIVES

Patient Information:

If GI upset occurs with liquid or non-sustained release forms, take with food.

Do NOT chew or crush enteric coated or sustained release tablets or capsules.

Take at the same time, with or without food, each day.

Notify physician if nausea, vomiting, insomnia, jitteriness, headache, rash, severe GI pain, restlessness, convulsions or irregular heartbeat occurs.

Avoid large amounts of caffeine-containing beverages, such as tea, coffee, cocoa and cola drinks or large amounts of chocolate; these products may increase side effects.

Brand interchange: Do not change from one brand to another without consulting your pharmacist or physician. Products manufactured by different companies may not be equally effective.

Individual doses are determined by response (decrease in symptoms). Blood levels must be checked regularly to avoid underdosing and overdosing. Do not change the dose of your medication without consulting your physician.

Administration and Dosage:

Parenteral administration: See theophylline and dextrose and aminophylline.

Individualize dosage. Base dosage adjustments on clinical response and improvement in pulmonary function with careful monitoring of serum levels. If possible, monitor serum levels to maintain levels in the therapeutic range of 10 to 20 mcg/ml. Levels > 20 mcg/ml may produce toxicity, and it may even occur with levels between 15 to 20 mcg/ml, particularly when factors known to reduce theophylline clearance are present (see Warnings). Once stabilized on a dosage, serum levels tend to remain constant. Data are available that indicate that the serum theophylline concentrations required to produce maximum physiologic benefit may fluctuate with the degree of bronchospasm present and are variable.

Calculate dosages on the basis of lean body weight, since theophylline does not distribute into fatty tissue. Regardless of salt used, dosages should be equivalent based on anhydrous theophylline content.

Individualize frequency of dosing. With immediate release products, dosing every 6 hours is generally required, especially in children; intervals up to 8 hours may be satisfactory in adults. Some children and adults requiring higher than average doses (those having rapid rates of clearance; eg, half-lives < 6 hours) may be more effectively controlled during chronic therapy with sustained release products. Determine dosage intervals to produce minimal fluctuations between peak and trough serum theophylline concentrations. Consider the absorption profile and the elimination rate. When converting from an immediate release to a sustained release product, the total daily dose should remain the same, and only the dosing interval adjusted.

Acute symptoms requiring rapid theophyllinization in patients not receiving theophylline: To achieve a rapid effect, an initial loading dose is required. Dosage recommendations are for theophylline anhydrous.

Dosage Guidelines for Rapid Theophyllinization[1]		
Patient Group	Oral loading	Maintenance
Children 1 to 9 years	5 mg/kg	4 mg/kg q 6 h
Children 9 to 16 and young adult smokers	5 mg/kg	3 mg/kg q 6 h
Otherwise healthy non-smoking adults	5 mg/kg	3 mg/kg q 8 h
Older patients, patients with cor pulmonale	5 mg/kg	2 mg/kg q 8 h
Patients with congestive heart failure	5 mg/kg	1-2 mg/kg q 12 h

[1] In patients not receiving theophylline.

Infants (preterm to < 1 year):

Theophylline Dosage Guidelines for Infants	
Age	Initial maintenance dose
Premature infants	
≤ 24 days postnatal	1 mg/kg q 12 h
> 24 days postnatal	1.5 mg/kg q 12 h
Infants (6 to 52 weeks)	[(0.2 x age in weeks) = 5] x kg = 24 hr dose in mg
Up to 26 weeks	Divide into q 8 h dosing
26 to 52 weeks	Divide into q 6 h dosing

Guide final dosage by serum concentration after a steady state has been achieved.

XANTHINE DERIVATIVES

Acute symptoms requiring rapid theophyllinization in patients receiving theophylline: Each 0.5 mg/kg theophylline administered as a loading dose will increase the serum theophylline concentration by approximately 1 mcg/ml. Ideally, defer the loading dose if a serum theophylline concentration can be obtained rapidly.

If this is not possible, exercise clinical judgment. When there is sufficient respiratory distress to warrant a small risk, then 2.5 mg/kg of theophylline administered in rapidly absorbed form is likely to increase serum concentration by approximately 5 mcg/ml. If the patient is not experiencing theophylline toxicity, this is unlikely to result in dangerous adverse effects. Maintenance doses are in the Dosage Guidelines table.

Chronic therapy: Slow clinical titration is generally preferred.

Initial dose – 16 mg/kg/24 hours or 400 mg/24 hours, whichever is less, of anhydrous theophylline in divided doses at 6 or 8 hour intervals.

Increasing dose – The above dosage may be increased in approximately 25% increments at 3 day intervals so long as the drug is tolerated or until the maximum dose (indicated below) is reached.

Maximum dose (where the serum concentration is not measured): Do not attempt to maintain any dose that is not tolerated.

Maximum Daily Theophylline Dose Based on Age	
Age	Maximum daily dose[1]
1 to 9 years	24 mg/kg/day
9 to 12 years	20 mg/kg/day
12 to 16 years	18 mg/kg/day
> 16 years	13 mg/kg/day

[1] Not to exceed listed dose or 900 mg, whichever is less.

Exercise caution in younger children who cannot complain of minor side effects. Older adults and those with cor pulmonale, CHF or liver disease may have unusually low dosage requirements; they may experience toxicity at the maximal dosages recommended.

Measurement of serum theophylline concentrations during chronic therapy is recommended. Obtain the serum sample at the time of peak absorption, 1 to 2 hours after administration for immediate release products and 5 to 9 hours after the morning dose for most sustained release formulations. The patient must not miss doses during the previous 48 hours, and dosing intervals must have been reasonably typical during that period of time. The table below provides guidance to dosage adjustments based on serum theophylline level determinations:

Dosage Adjustment After Serum Theophylline Measurement		
If serum theophylline is:		Directions
Too low	5 to 10 mcg/ml	Increase dose by about 25% at 3 day intervals until either the desired clinical response or serum concentration is achieved.[1]
Within desired range	10 to 20 mcg/ml	Maintain dosage if tolerated. Recheck serum theophylline concentration at 6 to 12 month intervals.[2]
Too high	20 to 25 mcg/ml	Decrease doses by about 10%. Recheck serum theophylline concentration after 3 days.[2]
	25 to 30 mcg/ml	Skip next dose and decrease subsequent doses by about 25%. Recheck serum theophylline after 3 days.
	> 30 mcg/ml	Skip next 2 doses and decrease subsequent doses by 50%. Recheck serum theophylline after 3 days.

[1] The total daily dose may need to be administered at more frequent intervals if asthma symptoms occur repeatedly at the end of a dosing interval.

[2] Finer adjustments in dosage may be needed for some patients.

XANTHINE DERIVATIVES

Timed Release Capsules : These dosage forms gradually release the active medication so that the total daily dosage may be administered in 1 to 3 doses divided by 8 to 24 hours, depending on the patient's pharmacokinetic profile, thus reducing the number of daily doses required. In the following timed release capsule product listings, the manufacturer's recommended average dosing intervals are presented in parentheses. Nevertheless, frequency of dosing must be individualized, based on the absorption profile of the drug and the rate of elimination of the drug from the patient. These products are not necessarily interchangeable. If patients are switched from one brand to another, closely monitor their theophylline serum levels; serum concentrations may vary greatly following brand interchange.

THEOPHYLLINE

For complete prescribing information, refer to the Xanthine Derivatives group monograph.

Rx	**Theophylline** (Various, eg, Schein)	**Tablets:** 100 mg	In 100s.
Rx	**Slo-Phyllin** (Rhone-Poulenc Rorer)		Dye free. (WHR 351). White, scored. In 100s & UD 100s.
Rx	**Theolair** (3M Pharmaceuticals)	**Tablets:** 125 mg	(Riker 342). White, scored. In 100s.
Rx	**Theophylline** (Various, eg, Schein)	**Tablets:** 200 mg	In 100s and 500s.
Rx	**Slo-Phyllin** (Rhone-Poulenc Rorer)		Dye free. (WHR 352). White, scored. In 100s & UD 100s.
Rx	**Theolair** (3M Pharmaceuticals)	**Tablets:** 250 mg	(Riker/Theolair 250). White, scored. Capsule shape. In 100s.
Rx	**Theophylline** (Various, eg, Schein)	**Tablets:** 300 mg	In 100s, 500s and 1000s.
Rx	**Quibron-T Dividose** (Roberts)		(BL 512). Ivory. Triple scored. In 100s and 500s.
Rx	**Bronkodyl** (Winthrop)	**Capsules:** 100 mg	Brown and white. In 100s.
Rx	**Elixophyllin** (Forest)		Dye free. (Forest 642). In 100s.
Rx	**Bronkodyl** (Winthrop)	**Capsules:** 200 mg	Green and white. In 100s.
Rx	**Elixophyllin** (Forest)		Dye free. (Forest 643). In 100s and 500s.
Rx	**Aquaphyllin** (Ferndale)	**Syrup:** 80 mg per 15 ml (26.7 mg per 5 ml)	Alcohol free. Dye free. In 120 ml, pt, gal and UD 5, 15 and 30 ml.
Rx sf	**Slo-Phyllin** (Rhone-Poulenc Rorer)		Alcohol free.[1] In pt.
Rx sf	**Theoclear-80** (Central)		Alcohol free. Dye free. Saccharin, sorbitol. Cherry flavor. In pt and gal.
Rx	**Theostat 80** (Laser)		1% alcohol. Sugar. In pt and gal.
Rx	**Accurbron** (Hoechst Marion Roussel)	**Syrup:** 150 mg per 15 ml (50 mg per 5 ml)	7.5% alcohol. Dye free. Saccharin, sorbitol, sugar. In pt.

Xanthine Derivatives

THEOPHYLLINE

Rx	**Theophylline** (Various, eg, Balan, Bar-reNational, Bioline, Geneva, Goldline, Moore, Rugby, Schein, URL)	**Elixir:** 80 mg per 15 ml (26.7 mg per 5 ml)	In pt and gal and UD 15 and 30 ml.
Rx	**Asmalix** (Century)		20% alcohol. In gal.
Rx	**Elixomin** (Cenci)		20% alcohol. Orange raspberry flavor. In pt.
Rx	**Elixophyllin** (Forest)		20% alcohol. Saccharin. Mixed fruit flavor. In pt, qt and gal.
Rx sf	**Lanophyllin** (Lannett)		20% alcohol. In pt and gal.
Rx sf	**Theophylline Oral** (Roxane)	**Solution:** 80 mg per 15 ml (26.7 mg per 5 ml)	0.4% alcohol. Dye free. Saccharin, sorbitol. In 500 ml & UD 15 and 18.75 & 30 ml.
Rx	**Theolair** (3M Pharmaceuticals)		Alcohol free. Sorbitol, sucrose.[1] In pt.
Rx	**Aerolate** (Fleming)	**Capsules, timed release (8 to 12 hours):** III: 65 mg	(III/III). Red and clear. In 100s.
		JR: 130 mg	(JR./JR.). Red and clear. In 100s.
		SR: 260 mg	(SR./SR.). Red and clear. In 100s.
Rx	**Slo-bid Gyrocaps** (Rhone-Poulenc Rorer)	**Capsules, timed release (8 to 12 hours):** 50 mg	Dye free. (50). White/clear. In 100s, 1000s & UD 100s.
		75 mg	Dye free. (75). White and clear. In 100s and UD 100s.
		100 mg	Dye free. (100). Clear. In 100s, 1000s and UD 100s.
		125 mg	Dye free. (125). White. In 100s and UD 100s.
		200 mg	Dye free. (200). White and clear. In 100s, 1000s and UD 100s.
		300 mg	Dye free. (300). White. In 100s, 1000s and UD 100s.
Rx	**Slo-Phyllin Gyrocaps** (Rhone-Poulenc Rorer)	**Capsules, timed release (8 to 12 hours):** 60 mg	Sucrose. (WHR 1354). White. In 100s.
		125 mg	Sucrose. (WHR 1355). Brown. In 100s, 1000s and UD 100s.
		250 mg	Sucrose. (WHR 1356). Purple. In 100s, 1000s and UD 100s.

Xanthine Derivatives

THEOPHYLLINE

Rx	**Theo-24** (Whitby)	**Capsules, timed release (24 hours)**: 100 mg	(Theo-24 100 mg Searle 2832). Gold and clear. In 100s and UD 100s.
		200 mg	(Theo-24 200 mg Searle 2842). Orange and clear. In 100s, 500s and UD 100s.
		300 mg	(Theo-24 300 mg Searle 2852). Red and clear. In 100s, 500s and UD100s.
		Note: Patients receiving once daily doses ≥ 13 mg/kg or ≥ 900 mg (whichever is less) should avoid eating a high-fat-content morning meal or take medication at least 1 hour before eating. If patient cannot comply with this regimen, place on alternative therapy.	
Rx	**Theobid Jr. Duracaps** (Russ)	**Capsules, timed release (12 hours)**: 130 mg	(Theobid 130). Clear. In 60s.
Rx	**Theobid Duracaps** (Russ)	**Capsules, timed release (12 hours)**: 260 mg	(Theobid 260). Clear. In 60s and 500s.
Rx	**Theoclear L.A.** (Central)	**Capsules, timed release (12 hours)**: 130 mg	(130 mg). Clear. In 100s & 1000s.
		260 mg	(260 mg). Clear. In 100s & 1000s.
Rx	**Theophylline** (Various, eg, Lemmon, Major, Mason, Parmed, Schein)	**Capsules, extended release**: 100 mg	In 100s.
		125 mg	In 100s.
		200 mg	In 100s.
		300 mg	In 100s.
Rx	**Theospan-SR** (Laser)	**Capsules, timed release (12 hours)**: 130 mg	Sucrose. (Laser O161 Theospan SR 130). White/clear. In 100s & 1000s.
		260 mg	Sucrose. (Theospan SR 260). White and clear. In 100s and 1000s.
Rx	**Theovent** (Schering)	**Capsules, timed release (12 hours)**: 125 mg	(Schering 402). Green and yellow. In 100s.
		250 mg	(Schering 753). Green and clear. In 100s.
Rx	**Theophylline SR** (Various, eg, Balan, Bioline, Geneva, Goldline, Major, Moore, Purepac, Rugby, Sidmak)	**Tablets, timed release (12 to 24 hours)**: 100 mg	In 100s and 500s.
		200 mg	In 100s, 500s, 1000s, UD 100s.
		300 mg	In 100s, 500s, 1000s, UD 100s.
		450 mg	In 100s.
Rx	**Theophylline Extended-Release** (Sidmak)	**Tablets, extended release (12 to 24 hours)**: 450 mg	Lactose. (SL 518). White, scored. Capsule shape. In 100s, 250s and 500s.
Rx	**Theochron** (Various, eg, Inwood, Lemmon)	**Tablets, extended release (12 to 24 hours)**: 100 mg	In 100s, 500s, 1000s.
		200 mg	In 100s, 500s, 1000s.
		300 mg	In 100s, 500s, 1000s.
Rx	**Quibron-T/SR Dividose** (Roberts)	**Tablets, timed release (8 to 12 hours)**: 300 mg	White. Triple scored. In 100s and 500s.

Xanthine Derivatives

THEOPHYLLINE

Rx	**Respbid** (Boehringer-Ingelheim)	**Tablets, timed release (8 to 12 hours)**: 250 mg	(BI 48). White, scored. In 100s.
		500 mg	(BI 49). White, scored. In 100s.
Rx	**Sustaire** (Pfizer Labs)	**Tablets, sustained release (8 to 12 hours)**: 100 mg	Dye free. Sucrose. Scored. In 100s.
		300 mg	Dye free. Sucrose. Scored. In 100s.
Rx	**Theo-Dur** (Key)	**Tablets, timed release (8 to 24 hours)**: 100 mg	Dye free. (Theo-Dur 100). In 100s, 500s, 1000s, UD 100s.
		200 mg	Dye free. (Theo-Dur 200). In 100s, 500s, 1000s, UD 100s.
		300 mg	Dye free. (Theo-Dur 300). In 100s, 500s, 1000s, UD 100s.
		450 mg	Dye free. (Theo-Dur 450). White, scored. In 100s and UD 100s.
Rx	**Theocron** (Inwood)	**Tablets, timed release (12 to 24 hours)**: 100 mg	Dye free. (IL/3584). White, scored. Convex. In 100s, 500s, 1000s.
		200 mg	Dye free. (IL/3583). White, scored. Oval. In 100s, 500s, 1000s.
		300 mg	Dye free. (IL/3581). White, scored. Capsule shape. In 100s, 500s, 1000s.
Rx	**Theolair-SR** (3M Pharmaceuticals)	**Tablets, timed release (8 to 12 hours)**: 200 mg	(Riker SR 200). White, scored. In 100s and 1000s.
		250 mg	(Riker SR 250). White, scored. In 100s and 250s.
		300 mg	(Riker SR 300). White, scored. Oval. In 100s, 1000s.
		500 mg	(Riker SR 500). White, scored. Capsule shape. In 100s and 250s.
Rx	**Theo-Sav** (Savage)	**Tablets, timed release (8 to 24 hours)**: 100 mg	(S 168). White, scored. In 100s.
		200 mg	(S 169). White, scored. Oval. In 100s, 500s and 1000s.
		300 mg	(S 170). White, scored. Capsule shape. In 100s, 500s and 1000s.
Rx	**Theo-X** (Carnrick)	**Tablets, controlled release (12 to 24 hours)**: 100 mg	Dye free. Lactose. (C 8631). White, scored. In 100s and 500s.
		200 mg	Dye free. Lactose. (C 8632). White, scored. Oval. In 100s, 500s, 1000s.
		300 mg	Dye free. Lactose. (C 8633). White, scored. Capsule shape. In 100s, 500s, 1000s.

Xanthine Derivatives

THEOPHYLLINE

Rx	**T-Phyl** (Purdue Frederick)	**Tablets, timed release (8 to 12 hours)**: 200 mg	(T200). Scored. In 100s.
Rx	**Uni-Dur** (Key)	**Tablets, extended release (24 hours)**: 400 mg	Sugar, lactose. (Uni-Dur 400 mg). Mottled white, scored. Capsule shape. In 100s.
		600 mg	Sugar, lactose. (Uni-Dur 600 mg). Mottled white, scored. Capsule shape. In 100s.
Rx	**Uniphyl** (Purdue Frederick)	**Tablets, timed release (24 hours)**: 400 mg	(PF U400). White, scored. In 100s, 500s, UD 100s.
		600 mg	(PF U600). White, scored. In 100s.

OXTRIPHYLLINE (Choline Theophyllinate) – 64% theophylline

For complete prescribing information, refer to the Xanthine Derivatives group monograph.

Administration and Dosage:

Adults: 4.7 mg/kg every 8 hours.

Children (9 to 16 years) and adult smokers: 4.7 mg/kg every 6 hours.

Children (1 to 9 years): 6.2 mg/kg every 6 hours.

Sustained action: If total daily maintenance dosage is established at approximately 800 or 1200 mg, 1 sustained action tablet every 12 hours may be substituted.

Rx	**Oxtriphylline** (Various, eg, Bolar, Genetco, Goldline, Interstate, Major, Rugby)	**Tablets**: 100 mg (equiv. to 64 mg theophylline)	In 100s and 500s.
Rx	**Choledyl** (Parke-Davis)		Sucrose. (PD 210). Red. Enteric and sugar coated. In 100s.
Rx	**Oxtriphylline** (Various, eg, Balan, Bioline, Bolar, Interstate, Major, Parmed, Rugby)	**Tablets**: 200 mg (equiv. to 127 mg theophylline)	In 100s, 500s and 1000s.
Rx	**Choledyl** (Parke-Davis)		Sucrose. (PD 211). Yellow. Enteric, sugar coated. In 100s, 1000s, UD 100s.
Rx	**Choledyl SA** (Parke-Davis)	**Tablets, sustained action**: 400 mg (equiv. to 254 mg theophylline)	Sugar. Pink. Film coated. In 100s and UD 100s.
		600 mg (equiv. to 382 mg theophylline)	Sugar. Tan. Film coated. In 100s and UD 100s.
Rx	**Oxtriphylline** (Various, eg, Moore, PBI)	**Syrup, pediatric**: 50 mg (equiv. to 32 mg theophylline) per 5 ml	In pt.
Rx	**Choledyl** (Parke-Davis)		Menthol, saccharin, sorbitol, sugar. Vanilla-mint flavor. In 474 ml.
Rx	**Oxtriphylline** (Various, eg, PBI, Schein, UDL)	**Elixir**: 100 mg (equiv. to 64 mg theophylline) per 5 ml	In pt and UD 5 and 10 ml.
Rx	**Choledyl** (Parke-Davis)		20% alcohol. Saccharin, sorbitol, sucrose. In 474 ml.

THEOPHYLLINE AND DEXTROSE

For complete prescribing information, refer to the Xanthine Derivative group monograph.

Administration and Dosage:

Substitute oral therapy for IV theophylline as soon as adequate improvement is achieved.

See also aminophylline for parenteral administration guidelines, noting the difference of theophylline content.

The following may be incompatible when mixed with theophylline in IV fluids: Anileridine; ascorbic acid; chlorpromazine; codeine phosphate; corticotropin; dimenhydrinate; epinephrine HCl; erythromycin gluceptate; hydralazine; hydroxyzine HCl; insulin; levorphanol tartrate; meperidine; methadone; methicillin sodium; morphine sulfate; norepinephrine bitartrate; oxytetracycline; papaverine; penicillin G potassium; phenobarbital sodium; phenytoin sodium; procaine; prochlorperazine maleate; promazine; promethazine; tetracycline; vancomycin; vitamin B complex with C.

Children: Due to marked variation in theophylline metabolism, use this drug only if clearly needed in infants < 6 months of age.

Rx	**Theophylline and 5% Dextrose** (Abbott and Baxter)	**Injection:** 200 mg/container	In 50 ml (4 mg/ml) and 100 ml (2 mg/ml).
		400 mg/container	In 100 ml (4 mg/ml), 250 ml (1.6 mg/ml), 500 ml (0.8 mg/ml) and 1000 ml (0.4 mg/ml).
		800 mg/container	In 250 ml (3.2 mg/ml), 500 ml (1.6 mg/ml) and 1000 ml (0.8 mg/ml).

Xanthine Derivatives

AMINOPHYLLINE (Theophylline Ethylenediamine) – 79% theophylline

For complete prescribing information, refer to the Xanthine Derivative group monograph.

Administration and Dosage:

For oral and rectal dosage refer to the Equivalent Dosage table in Actions and to the Administration section.

For dosage in infants from preterm up to 8-week-old term infants, see Administration section.

IV: The loading dose may be infused into 100 to 200 ml of 5% Dextrose Injection or 0.9% Sodium Chloride Injection. Do not exceed 25 mg/min infusion rate.

Parenteral administration: Inject aminophylline slowly, not more than 25 mg/min, when given IV. Substitute oral therapy for IV aminophylline as soon as adequate improvement is achieved.

Loading dose –

In patients currently not receiving theophylline products: 6 mg/kg.

In patients currently receiving theophylline products: If possible, determine the time, amount, route of administration and form of last dose and defer loading dose if a serum concentration can be rapidly obtained. Each 0.5 mg/kg theophylline (0.6 mg/kg aminophylline) will increase the serum theophylline concentration by approximately 1 mcg/ml. When respiratory distress warrants a small risk, 2.5 mg/kg theophylline (3.1 mg aminophylline IV) increases serum concentration by approximately 5 mcg/ml. If the patient is not experiencing theophylline toxicity, this is unlikely to result in dangerous side effects. The proper time to obtain blood to measure the peak serum level of theophylline after an IV loading dose is 15 to 30 minutes.

Maintenance infusions Administer by a large volume infusion to deliver the desired amount of drug each hour. Aminophylline is compatible with most common IV solutions. Monitor serum theophylline concentrations to accurately maintain therapeutic concentrations and guide dosage adjustments.

Aminophylline Maintenance Infusion Rates (mg/kg/hr)		
Patient Group	First 12 hours	Beyond 12 hours
Neonates to infants < 6 months	Not recommended	
Children 6 months to 9 years	1.2	1
Children ages 9 to 16 and young adult smokers	1	0.8
Otherwise healthy nonsmoking adults	0.7	0.5
Older patients and those with cor pulmonale	0.6	0.3
Patients with CHF, liver disease	0.5	0.1-0.2

Compatibility: Do not mix the following solutions with aminophylline in IV fluids: Anileridine HCl; ascorbic acid; chlorpromazine; codeine phosphate; dimenhydrinate; dobutamine HCl; epinephrine; erythromycin gluceptate; hydralazine; insulin; levorphanol tartrate; meperidine; methadone; methicillin; morphine sulfate; norepinephrine bitartrate; oxytetracycline; penicillin G potassium; phenobarbital; phenytoin; prochlorperazine; promazine; promethazine; tetracycline; vancomycin; verapamil; vitamin B complex with C.

Xanthine Derivatives

AMINOPHYLLINE (Theophylline Ethylenediamine) – 79% theophylline

Rx	**Aminophylline** (Various, eg, Balan, Bioline, Geneva-Marsam, Goldline, Major, Roxane, Rugby, Schein, Searle, URL)	**Tablets**: 100 mg (equiv. to 79 mg theophylline)	Plain or enteric coated. In 100s, 1000s and UD 100s.
Rx	**Aminophylline** (Various, eg, Balan, Bioline, Geneva-Marsam, Goldline, Major, Moore, Roxane, Rugby, Searle, URL)	**Tablets**: 200 mg (equiv. to 158 mg theophylline)	Plain or enteric coated. In 100s, 1000s and UD 100s.
Rx	**Phyllocontin** (Purdue Frederick)	**Tablets, controlled release (12 hours)**: 225 mg (equiv. to 178 mg theophylline)	Scored. In 100s.
Rx	**Aminophylline** (Various, eg, Balan, Barre, Bioline, Major, PBI, Roxane, Rugby, URL)	**Oral Liquid**: 105 mg (equiv. to 90 mg theophylline) per 5 ml	In 240 and 500 ml.
Rx	**Aminophylline** (Various, eg, Abbott, American Regent, Elkins-Sinn, Lyphomed, Moore, Solopak)	**Injection**: 250 mg (equiv. to 197 mg theophylline) per 10 ml For IV use.	In 10 and 20 ml amps & vials & syringes.
Rx	**Aminophylline** (Various, eg, Baxter, Rugby, Schein)	**Suppositories**: 250 mg (equiv. to 197.5 mg theophylline)	In 10s and 25s.
Rx	**Truphylline** (G & W)		In UD 10s and 25s.
Rx	**Aminophylline** (Various, eg, Baxter, Parmed, Rugby, Schein)	**Suppositories**: 500 mg (equiv. to 395 mg theophylline)	In 10s and 25s.
Rx	**Truphylline** (G & W)		In UD 10s, 25s and 50s.

Xanthine Derivatives

DYPHYLLINE (Dihydroxypropyl Theophylline)

For complete prescribing information, refer to the Xanthine Derivatives group monograph.

Dyphylline is a derivative of theophylline; it is not a theophylline salt and is not metabolized to theophylline in vivo. Although dyphylline is 70% theophylline by molecular weight ratio, the amount of dyphylline equivalent to a given amount of theophylline is not known. Dyphylline may result in fewer side effects than theophylline salts, but blood levels and possibly activity are lower. Specific dyphylline serum levels may be used to monitor therapy; serum theophylline levels will NOT measure dyphylline. The minimal effective therapeutic concentration is 12 mcg/ml.

Administration and Dosage:

Oral:

Adults – Up to 15 mg/kg every 6 hours.

IM: (Not for IV administration.)

Adults – 250 to 500 mg injected slowly every 6 hours. Do not exceed 15 mg/kg every 6 hours.

Children – Safety and efficacy have not been established.

Rx	**Dyphylline** (Various, eg, Balan, Major)	**Tablets:** 200 mg	In 100s and 1000s.
Rx	**Dilor** (Savage)		Blue, scored. In 100s, 1000s and UD 100s.
Rx	**Lufyllin** (Wallace)		(Wallace 521). White, scored. Rectangular. In 100s, 1000s, 5000s and UD 100s.
Rx	**Dyphylline** (Various, eg, Balan, Major, URL)	**Tablets:** 400 mg	In 100s and 1000s.
Rx	**Dilor-400** (Savage)		White, scored. In 100s, 1000s and UD 100s.
Rx	**Lufyllin-400** (Wallace)		(Wallace 731). White, scored. Capsule shape. In 100s, 1000s, 2500s and UD 100s.
Rx	**Lufyllin** (Wallace)	**Elixir:** 100 mg per 15 ml (33.3 mg/5 ml)	20% alcohol. White port wine, saccharin. In pt and gal.
Rx	**Dilor** (Savage)	**Elixir:** 160 mg per 15 ml (53.3 mg/5 ml)	18% alcohol. Saccharin, sorbitol, sucrose, parabens. Mint flavor. In pt and gal.
Rx	**Dilor** (Savage)	**Injection:** 250 mg per ml	In 2 ml amps.
Rx	**Lufyllin** (Wallace)		In 2 ml amps.

ZAFIRLUKAST

Actions:

Pharmacology: Zafirlukast is a selective and competitive leukotriene receptor antagonist (LTRA) of leukotriene D_4 and E_4 (LTD_4 and LTE_4), components of slow-reacting substance of anaphylaxis (SRSA). Cysteinyl leukotriene production and receptor occupation have been correlated with the pathophysiology of asthma, including airway edema, smooth muscle constriction and altered cellular activity associated with the inflammatory process, which contribute to the signs and symptoms of asthma.

In vitro studies demonstrated that zafirlukast antagonized the contractile activity of three leukotrienes (LTC_4, LTD_4 and LTE_4) in conducting airway smooth muscle.

Zafirlukast inhibits bronchoconstriction caused by several kinds of inhalational challenges. Pretreatment with single oral doses of zafirlukast inhibited bronchoconstriction caused by sulfur dioxide and cold air in patients with asthma. Pretreatment with single doses of zafirlukast attenuated the early- and late-phase reaction caused by inhalation of various antigens such as grass, cat dander, ragweed and mixed antigens in patients with asthma. Zafirlukast also attenuated the increase in bronchial hyperresponsiveness to inhaled histamine that followed inhaled allergen challenge.

Pharmacokinetics: Zafirlukast is rapidly absorbed following oral administration. Peak plasma concentrations are achieved 3 hours after dosing.

The mean terminal elimination half-life of zafirlukast is ≈ 10 hours in both normal subjects and patients with asthma. Steady-state plasma concentrations of zafirlukast are proportional to the dose and predictable from single-dose pharmacokinetic data.

In the concentration range of 0.25 to 10 mcg/ml, zafirlukast is > 99% bound to plasma proteins, predominantly albumin.

Zafirlukast is extensively metabolized. Urinary excretion accounts for ≈ 10% of the dose and the remainder is excreted in the feces. Unmetabolized zafirlukast is not detected in urine. Liver microsomes that hydroxylate metabolites of zafirlukast are formed through the cytochrome P450 2C9 (CYP2C9) enzyme pathway. Additional in vitro studies utilizing human liver microsomes show that zafirlukast inhibits the cytochrome P450 CYP3A4 and CYP2C9 isoenzymes at concentrations close to the clinically achieved plasma concentrations. The metabolites of zafirlukast found in plasma are at least 90 times less potent as LTD_4 receptor antagonists than zafirlukast in a standard in vitro test of activity.

Elderly – The mean dose (mg/kg) normalized AUC and C_{max} increase and plasma clearance (CL) decreases with increasing age. In patients > 65 years of age, there is an ≈ 2– to 3–fold greater C_{max} and AUC compared to young adult patients.

Hepatic function impairment – In patients with hepatic impairment (biopsy-proven cirrhosis), there is a 50% to 60% greater C_{max} and AUC compared to normal subjects.

Renal function impairment – There are no apparent differences in the pharmacokinetics of zafirlukast between renally impaired patients and normal subjects.

Food – Administration of zafirlukast with food reduced mean bioavailability by ≈ 40%.

Clinical trials: In a study, the effect of zafirlukast on most efficacy parameters was comparable to the active control (1600 mcg inhaled cromolyn sodium four times per day) and superior to placebo at endpoint for decreasing rescue beta-agonist use. Improvement in asthma symptoms occurred within 1 week of initiating treatment with zafirlukast.

Indications:

Asthma: Prophylaxis and chronic treatment of asthma in adults and children ≥ 12 years of age.

Contraindications:

Hypersensitivity to zafirlukast or any of its inactive ingredients.

Warnings:

Acute asthma attacks: Zafirlukast is not indicated for use in the reversal of bronchospasm in acute asthma attacks, including status asthmaticus. Therapy with zafirlukast can be continued during acute exacerbations of asthma.

Infection: An increased proportion of zafirlukast patients > 55 years old reported infections as compared to placebo-treated patients. These infections were mostly mild or moderate in intensity and predominantly affected the respiratory tract. Infections occurred equally in both sexes, were dose-proportional to total milligrams of zafirlukast exposure and were associated with coadministration of inhaled corticosteroids.

ZAFIRLUKAST

Hepatic function impairment: The clearance of zafirlukast is reduced in patients with stable alcoholic cirrhosis such that the C_{max} and AUC are ≈ 50% to 60% greater than those of normal adults.

Carcinogenesis: Male mice given 300 mg/kg/day of zafirlukast had a greater incidence of hepatocellular adenomas as compared to concurrent controls; female mice at this dose showed a greater incidence of whole body histocytic sarcomas. Male and female rats given 2000 mg/kg/day of zafirlukast had a greater incidence of urinary bladder transitional cell papillomas as compared to concurrent controls.

Elderly: The clearance of zafirlukast is reduced in elderly patients (≥ 65 years old), such that C_{max} and AUC are approximately twice those of younger adults.

Pregnancy: Category B. At 2000 mg/kg/day in rats, maternal toxicity and deaths were seen with increased incidence of early fetal resorption. Spontaneous abortions occurred in cynomolgus monkeys at a maternally toxic dose of 2000 mg/kg/day orally. There are no adequate and well controlled trials in pregnant women. Because animal reproduction studies are not always predictive of human response, use zafirlukast during pregnancy only if clearly needed.

Lactation: Zafirlukast is excreted in breast milk. Following repeated 40 mg twice-a-day dosing in healthy women, average steady-state concentrations of zafirlukast in breast milk were 50 ng/ml compared with 255 ng/ml in plasma. Do not administer to nursing women.

Children: The safety and effectiveness of zafirlukast in patients < 12 years of age have not been established.

Precautions:

Hepatotoxicity: Although the frequency of hepatic transaminase elevations was comparable between zafirlukast and placebo-treated patients, a single case of symptomatic hepatitis and hyperbilirubinemia, without other attributable cause, occurred in a patient who had received 40 mg/day of zafirlukast for 100 days. In this patient, the liver enzymes returned to normal within 3 months of stopping zafirlukast.

ZAFIRLUKAST

Drug Interactions:

Due to zafirlukast's inhibition of cytochrome P450 2C9 and 3A4 isoenzymes, use caution with coadministration of drugs known to be metabolized by these isoenzymes.

Zafirlukast Drug Interactions

Precipitant Drug	Object Drug*		Description
Aspirin	Zafirlukast	⬆	Coadministration of zafirlukast with aspirin results in mean increased plasma levels of zafirlukast by ≈ 45%.
Erythromycin	Zafirlukast	⬇	Coadministration of a single dose of zafirlukast with erythromycin to steady state results in decreased mean plasma levels of zafirlukast by ≈ 40% due to a decrease in zafirlukast bioavailability.
Terfenadine	Zafirlukast	⬇	Coadministration of zafirlukast with terfenadine to steady state results in a decrease in the mean C_{max} (-66%) and AUC (-54%) of zafirlukast. No effect of zafirlukast on terfenadine plasma concentrations or ECG parameters (eg, QTc interval) was seen.
Theophylline	Zafirlukast	⬇	Coadministration of zafirlukast at steady state with a single dose of a liquid theophylline preparation results in decreased mean plasma levels of zafirlukast by ≈30%, but no effects on plasma theophylline levels were observed.
Zafirlukast	Warfarin	⬆	Coadministration of zafirlukast with warfarin results in a clinically significant increase in prothrombin time (PT). Closely monitor prothrombin times of patients on oral warfarin anticoagulant therapy and zafirlukast, and adjust anticoagulant dose accordingly.

* ⬆ = Object drug increased. ⬇ = Object drug decreased.

Drug/Food interactions: The bioavailability of zafirlukast may be decreased when taken with food. Take zafirlukast at least 1 hour before or 2 hours after meals.

Adverse Reactions:

CNS: Headache (12.9%); dizziness (1.6%).

GI: Nausea (3.1%); diarrhea (2.8%); abdominal pain (1.8%); vomiting (1.5%).

Miscellaneous: Infection (3.5%; see Warnings); pain (generalized; 1.9%); asthenia (1.8%); accidental injury (1.6%); myalgia, fever (1.6%); back pain, ALT elevation (1.5%); dyspepsia (1.3%).

Overdosage:

No deaths occurred at oral zafirlukast doses of 2000 mg/kg in mice, 2000 mg/kg in rats and 500 mg/kg in dogs.

There is no experience to date with zafirlukast overdose in humans. It is reasonable to employ the usual supportive measures in the event of an overdose.

Patient Information:

Take regularly as prescribed, even during symptom-free periods.

Do not use to treat acute episodes of asthma.

Do not decrease the dose or stop taking any other antiasthma medications unless instructed by a physician.

ZAFIRLUKAST

Nursing women should not take zafirlukast.

Administration and Dosage:

The recommended dose of zafirlukast is 20 mg twice daily in adults and children ≥ 12 years of age. Because food reduces bioavailability of zafirlukast, take at least 1 hour before or 2 hours after meals.

Storage/Stability: Store at controlled room temperature (20° to 25°C; 68° to 77°F). Protect from light and moisture. Dispense in original air-tight container.

Rx	**Accolate** (Zeneca)	**Tablets:** 20 mg	Lactose, povidone. (ZENECA ACCOLATE 20). White. Round, biconvex. Film-coated. In 60s and UD 100s.

ZILEUTON

Actions:

Pharmacology: Zileuton is a specific inhibitor of 5–lipoxygenase and thus inhibits leukotriene (LTB_1, LTC_1, LTD_1 and LTE_1) formation. Both the R(+) and S(–) enantiomers are pharmacologically active as 5–lipoxygenase inhibitors. Leukotrienes are substances that induce numerous biological effects including augmentation of neutrophil and eosinophil migration, neutrophil and monocyte aggregation, leukocyte adhesion, increased capillary permeability and smooth muscle contraction. These effects contribute to inflammation, edema, mucus secretion and bronchoconstriction in the airways of asthmatic patients. Sulfido-peptide leukotrienes (LTC_1, LTD_1, LTE_1, also known as the slow-releasing substances of anaphylaxis) and LTB_4, a chemoattractant for neutrophils and eosinophils, can be measured in a number of biological fluids including bronchoalveolar lavage fluid (BALF) from asthmatic patients. Zileuton inhibits leukotriene-dependent smooth muscle contractions. Pretreatment with zileuton attenuated bronchoconstriction caused by cold air challenge in patients with asthma.

Pharmacokinetics:

Absorption – Zileuton is rapidly absorbed upon oral administration with a mean time to peak plasma concentration (T_{max}) of 1.7 hours and a mean peak level (C_{max}) of 4.98 mcg/ml. The absolute bioavailability of zileuton is unknown. Systemic exposure (mean AUC) following 600 mg zileuton administration is 19.2 mcg•hr/ml. Plasma concentrations of zileuton are proportional to dose, and steady-state levels are predictable from single-dose pharmacokinetic data.

Food: Administration of zileuton with food resulted in a small but statistically significant increase (27%) in zileuton C_{max} without significant changes in the extent of absorption (AUC) or T_{max}. Therefore, zileuton can be administered with or without food.

Distribution – The apparent volume of distribution of zileuton is ≈ 1.2 L/kg. Zileuton is 93% bound to plasma proteins, primarily to albumin, with minor binding to alpha-acid glycoprotein.

Metabolism – Several zileuton metabolites have been identified in plasma and urine. These include two diastereomeric O-glucuronide conjugates (major metabolites) and an N-dehydroxylated metabolite of zileuton. The urinary excretion of the inactive N-dehydroxylated metabolite and unchanged zileuton each accounted for < 0.5% of the dose. Liver microsomes have shown that zileuton and its N-dehydroxylated metabolite can be oxidatively metabolized by the cytochrome P450 isoenzymes 1A2, 2C9 and 3A4 (CYP1A2, CYP2C9 and CYP3A4).

Excretion – Elimination of zileuton is predominantly via metabolism with a mean terminal half-life of 2.5 hours. Apparent oral clearance of zileuton is 7 ml/min/kg. Zileuton activity is primarily because of the parent drug. Orally administered zileuton is well absorbed into the systemic circulation with 94.5% and 2.2% of the dose recovered in urine and feces, respectively.

Elderly: Zileuton pharmacokinetics were similar in healthy elderly subjects (> 65 years) compared with healthy younger adults (18 to 40 years).

Hepatic function impairment: Zileuton is contraindicated in patients with active liver disease (see Contraindications and Precautions).

Renal function impairment: Zileuton pharmacokinetics were similar in healthy subjects and in subjects with mild, moderate and severe renal insufficiency. In subjects with renal failure requiring hemodialysis, pharmacokinetics were not altered by hemodialysis and a very small percentage of the administered zileuton dose (< 0.5%) was removed by hemodialysis. Therefore, dosing adjustment in patients with renal dysfunction or undergoing hemodialysis is not necessary.

Clinical trials: Two double-blind, parallel, placebo controlled, multicenter studies have established the efficacy of zileuton in the treatment of asthma. Three hundred seventy-three patients were enrolled in the 6–month, double-blind phase of Study 1, and 401 patients were enrolled in the 3–month double-blind phase of Study 2. In these studies, the patients were mild-to-moderate asthmatics who had a mean baseline FEV_1 of ≈ 2.3 liters and used inhaled beta-agonists as needed. In each study, patients were randomized to receive zileuton 400 mg four times daily, zileuton 600 mg four times daily or placebo. Only the zileuton 600 mg four times daily dosage regimen was shown to be effective by demonstrating statistically significant improvement across several parameters.

Indications:

Asthma: The prophylaxis and chronic treatment of asthma in adults and children ≥ 12 years of age.

Contraindications:

Active liver disease or transaminase elevations greater than or equal to three times the upper limit of normal (≥ 3×ULN), hypersensitivity to zileuton or any of its inactive ingredients.

ZILEUTON

Warnings:

Hepatotoxicity: Elevations of one or more liver function tests may occur during zileuton therapy. These laboratory abnormalities may progress, remain unchanged or resolve with continued therapy. In a few cases, initial transaminase elevations were first noted after discontinuing treatment, usually within 2 weeks. The ALT test is considered the most sensitive indicator of liver injury. The frequency of ALT elevations (≥ 3×ULN) was ≥ 1.9%.

Sixty-one percent of ALT elevations occurred during the first 2 months of zileuton therapy. After 2 months of treatment, the rate of new ALT elevations ≥ 3×ULN stabilized at a mean of 0.3% per month for patients receiving zileuton plus usual asthma care compared with 0.11% per month for patients receiving usual asthma care alone. Of 61 zileuton plus usual asthma care patients with ALT elevations from 3 to 5×ULN, 32 patients (52%) had ALT values decrease to < 2×ULN while continuing zileuton therapy. Twenty-one of 61 patients (34%) had further increases in ALT levels to ≥ 5×ULN. In patients who discontinued zileuton, elevated ALT levels returned to < 2×ULN in an average of 32 days (range 1 to 111 days). The overall rate of ALT elevation ≥ 3×ULN was 3.2%. One patient developed symptomatic hepatitis with jaundice, which resolved upon discontinuation of therapy. An additional 3 patients with transaminase elevations developed mild hyperbilirubinemia that was < 3×ULN. There was no evidence of hypersensitivity or other alternative etiologies for these findings. In subset analyses, females > 65 years of age appeared to be at an increased risk for ALT elevations. Patients with pre-existing transaminase elevations may also be at an increased risk for ALT elevations.

Acute asthma attacks: Zileuton is not indicated for use in the reversal of bronchospasm in acute asthma attacks, including status asthmaticus. Therapy with zileuton can be continued during acute exacerbations of asthma.

Hematologic: Occurrences of low white blood cell count (≤ 2.8×10^9/L) were observed in 1% of 1678 patients taking zileuton and 0.6% of 1056 patients taking placebo. These findings were transient, and the majority of cases returned toward normal or baseline with continued zileuton therapy. All remaining cases returned toward normal or baseline after discontinuation of zileuton. Similar findings were also noted in a long-term safety surveillance study of 2458 patients treated with zileuton plus usual asthma care versus 489 patients treated only with usual asthma care for ≤ 1 year. The clinical significance of these observations is unknown.

Hepatic function impairment: Because treatment with zileuton may result in increased hepatic transaminases, use with caution in patients who consume substantial quantities of alcohol or have a past history of liver disease.

Carcinogenesis: Increases in the incidence of liver, kidney and vascular tumors in female mice and a trend towards an increase in the incidences of liver tumors in male mice were observed at 450 mg/kg/day.

Pregnancy: Category C. Developmental studies indicated adverse effects (reduced body weight and increased skeletal variations) in rats at an oral dose of 300 mg/kg/day. There are no adequate and well controlled studies in pregnant women. Use zileuton during pregnancy only if the potential benefit justifies the potential risk.

Lactation: Zileuton and its metabolites are excreted in rat milk. It is not known if zileuton is excreted in breast milk. Decide whether to discontinue nursing or to discontinue the drug.

Children: The safety and effectiveness of zileuton in pediatric patients < 12 years of age have not been established.

Precautions:

Monitoring: Evaluate hepatic transaminases at initiation of and during therapy with zileuton. Monitor serum ALT before treatment begins, once-a-month for the first 3 months, every 2 to 3 months for the remainder of the first year and periodically thereafter for patients receiving long-term zileuton therapy. If symptoms of liver dysfunction (right upper quadrant pain, nausea, fatigue, lethargy, pruritus, jaundice or "flu-like" symptoms) develop or transaminase elevations > 5 times the ULN occur, discontinue therapy and follow transaminase levels until normal.

ZILEUTON

Drug Interactions:

Liver microsomes have shown that zileuton and its N-dehydroxylated metabolite can be oxidatively metabolized by the cytochrome P450 isoenzymes 1A2, 2C9 and 3A4. Therefore, use caution when prescribing a medication that inhibits any of these enzymes.

Zileuton Drug Interactions			
Precipitant Drug	Object Drug*		Description
Digoxin Oral Contraceptives Phenytoin Prednisone	Zileuton	⟷	Coadministration have shown no significant interactions.
Zileuton	Propranolol	↑	Coadministration of zileuton and propranolol results in doubling of propranolol AUC and consequent increased beta-blocker activity.
Zileuton	Terfenadine	↑	Administration of multiple doses of terfenadine (60 mg every 12 hours) and zileuton (600 mg every 6 hours) for 7 days resulted in a decrease in clearance of terfenadine by 22% leading to a statistically significant increase in mean AUC and C_{max} of terfenadine of ≈ 35%.
Zileuton	Theophylline	↑	Coadministration of zileuton and theophylline results in, on average, an approximate doubling of serum theophylline concentrations. Reduce theophylline dosage in these patients and monitor serum theophylline concentrations closely.
Zileuton	Warfarin	↑	Coadministration of zileuton and warfarin results in a clinically significant increase in prothrombin time (PT). Monitor PT closely.

* ↑ = Object drug increased ⟷ = Undetermined effect

Adverse Reactions:

Patients Experiencing Adverse Events with Zileuton (%)		
Body System/Event	Zileuton (n = 475)	Placebo (n = 491)
Body as a whole		
Headache	24.6	24
Pain (unspecified)	7.8	5.3
Abdominal pain	4.6	2.4
Asthenia	3.8	2.4
Accidental injury	3.4	2
GI		
Dyspepsia	8.2	2.9
Nausea	5.5	3.7
Miscellaneous		
ALT elevation[1]	12	0.2
Low white blood cell[1]	1	0.6
Myalgia	3.2	2.9
Discontinuation	9.7	8.4

[1] see Warnings

Other adverse events (frequency > 1%): Arthralgia; chest pain; conjunctivitis; constipation; dizziness; fever; flatulence; hypertonia; insomnia; lymphadenopathy; malaise; neck pain/rigidity; nervousness; pruritus; somnolence; urinary tract infection; vaginitis; vomiting.

ZILEUTON

Overdosage:

Human experience of acute overdose with zileuton is limited. A patient in a clinical trial took between 6.6 and 9 g of zileuton in a single dose. Vomiting was induced, and the patient recovered without sequelae. Zileuton is not removed by dialysis. If an overdose occurs, treat the patient symptomatically and institute supportive measures as required. If indicated, achieve elimination of unabsorbed drug by emesis or gastric lavage; observe usual precautions to maintain the airway.

The oral minimum lethal doses in mice and rats were 500 to 1000 and 300 to 1000 mg/kg in various preparations, respectively (providing > 3 and 9 times the systemic exposure achieved at the maximum recommended human daily oral dose, respectively). No deaths occurred, but nephritis was reported in dogs at an oral dose of 1000 mg/kg.

Patient Information:

Inform patients that zileuton is indicated for the chronic treatment of asthma and to take regularly as prescribed even during symptom-free periods.

Zileuton is not a bronchodilator; do not use to treat acute episodes of asthma.

When taking zileuton, do not decrease the dose or stop taking any other antiasthma medications unless instructed by a physician.

While using zileuton, seek medical attention if short-acting bronchodilators are needed more often than usual or if more than the maximum number of inhalations of short-acting bronchodilator treatment prescribed for a 24–hour period are needed.

The most serious side effect of zileuton is elevation of liver enzyme tests. While taking zileuton, patients must have liver enzyme tests monitored on a regular basis.

If patients experience signs or symptoms of liver dysfunction (right upper quadrant pain, nausea, fatigue, lethargy, pruritus, jaundice or "flu-like" symptoms), contact a physician immediately.

Zileuton can interact with other drugs. While taking zileuton, consult a doctor before starting or stopping any prescription or non-prescription medicines.

A patient leaflet is included with the tablets.

Administration and Dosage:

The recommended dosage of zileuton for the symptomatic treatment of patients with asthma is one 600 mg tablet four times a day for a total daily dose of 2400 mg. For ease of administration, zileuton may be taken with meals and at bedtime.

Rx	**Zyflo** (Abbott)	**Tablets**: 600 mg	(ZL 600). White. Ovaloid. Film coated. In 120s.

CORTICOSTEROIDS

For complete prescribing information, refer to the general discussion of Systemic Glucocorticoids.

Warning:

Adrenal insufficiency: Deaths due to adrenal insufficiency have occurred in asthmatic patients during and after transfer from systemic corticosteroids to aerosol steroids. After withdrawal from systemic corticosteroids, several months are required for recovery of hypothalamic-pituitary-adrenal (HPA) function. During this period of HPA suppression, patients may exhibit symptoms of adrenal insufficiency when exposed to trauma, surgery or infections, particularly gastroenteritis. Although aerosolized glucocorticoids may control asthmatic symptoms during these episodes, they do NOT provide the systemic steroid necessary for the treatment of these emergencies.

Stress/Severe asthma attack: During periods of stress or a severe asthmatic attack, patients withdrawn from systemic corticosteroids should resume them (in large doses) immediately and contact physician. Patients should carry a warning card indicating they may need supplementary systemic steroids during such periods.

Actions:

Pharmacology: These agents are synthetic adrenocortical steroids with basic glucocorticoid actions and effects. The mechanism responsible for the potent anti-inflammatory activity and the precise mechanism of action of aerosolized drug in the lung is unknown. Glucocorticoids may decrease number and activity of inflammatory cells, enhance effect of beta-adrenergic drugs on cyclic AMP production, inhibit bronchoconstrictor mechanisms or produce direct smooth muscle relaxation. Inhaler use provides effective local steroid activity with minimal systemic effect.

Pharmacokinetics:

Beclomethasone dipropionate – Systemic absorption occurs rapidly with all routes of administration. There is no evidence of tissue storage of beclomethasone or its metabolites. Lung slices can metabolize beclomethasone dipropionate rapidly to beclomethasone 17-monopropionate, and more slowly to free beclomethasone. The principal route of excretion of drug and metabolites is via feces; < 10% in urine.

Dexamethasone sodium phosphate – Because of the high water solubility of dexamethasone sodium phosphate, the aerosolized particles dissolve readily in bronchial and bronchiolar mucous membrane secretions. On 12 inhalations daily, the patient absorbs ≈ 0.4 to 0.6 mg dexamethasone (≈ 40% to 60% absorption) or 3 to 4 mg or 11 to 16 mg prednisone or hydrocortisone equivalent, respectively.

Triamcinolone acetonide – Studies demonstrate rapid disappearance from the lungs. Peak blood levels occur in 1 to 2 hours. Three metabolites have been identified; the major portion of the dose is eliminated in the feces.

Flunisolide – After inhalation of 1mg flunisolide, systemic availability was 40%. The absorbed flunisolide is rapidly and extensively metabolized during the first pass through the liver. Plasma half-life is approximately 1.8 hours.

Indications:

For control of bronchial asthma in patients requiring chronic treatment with corticosteroids. Such patients include those already receiving systemic corticosteroids, and those inadequately controlled on a nonsteroid regimen in whom steroid therapy has been withheld because of concern over potential adverse effects.

For related corticosteroid-responsive bronchospastic states intractable to adequate trial of conventional therapy.

NOT indicated for relief of asthma which can be controlled by bronchodilators and other nonsteroid medications, in patients who require systemic corticosteroid treatment infrequently, or in the treatment of nonasthmatic bronchitis.

Contraindications:

Primary treatment of status asthmaticus or other acute episodes of asthma when intensive measures are required; hypersensitivity to any ingredient; systemic fungal infections; persistently positive sputum cultures for *Candida albicans.*

Warnings:

Infections: Localized fungal infections with *Candida albicans* or *Aspergillus niger* have occurred in the mouth, pharynx and occasionally in the larynx. Positive cultures for oral *Candida* may be present in up to 75% of patients. The incidence of clinically apparent infection is low, and may require treatment with appropriate antifungal therapy or discontinuance of aerosol steroid treatment.

Acute asthma: These products are not bronchodilators and are not for rapid relief of bronchospasm. Contact a physician immediately when episodes of asthma do not respond to bronchodilators. Patients may require systemic corticosteroids.

There is no evidence that control of asthma can be achieved by administration of inhaled corticosteroids in amounts greater than recommended doses.

Replacement therapy: Transfer from systemic steroid therapy may unmask allergic conditions previously suppressed (eg, rhinitis, conjunctivitis, eczema). During withdrawal from oral steroids, some patients may experience withdrawal symptoms (eg, joint or muscular pain, lassitude, depression) despite maintenance or improvement of respiratory function.

Hypersensitivity reactions have occurred following beclomethasone use (see Adverse Reactions). Refer to Management of Acute Hypersensitivity Reactions.

Pregnancy: (Triamcinolone – Category D. Flunisolide – Category C). Glucocorticoids are teratogenic in rodent species. Findings include cleft palate, internal hydrocephaly and skeletal defects. There are no well controlled studies in pregnant women. Use these agents during pregnancy only if the benefit clearly justifies the potential risk to the fetus. Observe infants born of mothers who received substantial doses during pregnancy for adrenal insufficiency.

Lactation: Glucocorticoids are excreted in breast milk. It is not known whether inhaled corticosteroids are excreted in breast milk, but it is likely. Decide whether to discontinue nursing or to discontinue the drug.

Children: Insufficient information is available to warrant use in children < 6 years old.

Precautions:

Adrenal effects: In responsive patients, inhaled corticosteroids may permit control of asthmatic symptoms without HPA suppression. Since these agents are absorbed and can be systemically active, the beneficial effects in minimizing or preventing HPA dysfunction may be expected only when recommended dosages are not exceeded.

Long-term effects of inhaled glucocorticoids are unknown; although there is no clinical evidence of adverse effects, the local effects on developmental or immunologic processes in the mouth, pharynx, trachea and lung are unknown.

There is no information about effects on pulmonary infection (including active or quiescent tuberculosis), or effects of long-term use on lung or other tissues.

Pulmonary infiltrates with eosinophilia may occur with beclomethasone or flunisolide. This may become manifest due to systemic steroid withdrawal when inhalational agents are used, but a causative role for either agent or vehicle cannot be ruled out.

Dysphonia: A relatively common occurrence, intermittent dysphonia has occurred in ≤ 50% of patients and may be due to laryngeal candidiasis or a bilateral adductor vocal cord deformity induced by the corticosteroid. This symptom may be dose-related.

Coughing and wheezing may be more common with the use of beclomethasone and appears to be due to the dispersant rather than the drug. An alternative agent may diminish these effects. Also, pretreatment with an aerosol bronchodilator is effective in reducing coughing and wheezing in some patients.

Adverse Reactions:

Local: Throat irritation; hoarseness/dysphonia, coughing (see Precautions); dry mouth; rash; wheezing; facial edema. Laryngeal/pharyngeal fungal infections have responded promptly to discontinuation of therapy and institution of antifungal treatment.

Systemic: Suppression of HPA function has occurred in adults who used beclomethasone 1600 mcg/day for 1 month and 4000 mcg/day triamcinolone or recommended doses for 6 to 12 weeks. Deaths due to adrenal insufficiency have occurred during and after transfer from systemic to aerosol corticosteroids. (See Warnings.)

Beclomethasone: Rare cases of immediate and delayed hypersensitivity reactions, including urticaria, angioedema, rash and bronchospasm. See Warnings.

For complete information on the systemic effects of glucocorticoids, the glucocorticoid section of the Adrenal Cortical Steroids group monograph.

Patient Information:

Patient instructions are available with product.

Medication is for preventive therapy only; do NOT use to abort an acute asthmatic attack; use at regularly scheduled intervals as prescribed.

Corticosteroids

CORTICOSTEROIDS

Advise patients receiving bronchodilators (eg, isoproterenol, metaproterenol, epinephrine) by inhalation to use the bronchodilator several minutes before the corticosteroid aerosol to enhance penetration of the steroid into the bronchial tree.

Notify physician if sore throat or sore mouth occurs.

Administration technique: The success of these agents is a function of proper administration technique. Therefore, the following guidelines may be useful: Thoroughly shake the inhaler; take a drink of water to moisten the throat; place the inhaler mouthpiece two finger-widths away from the mouth; tilt head back slightly; while activating the inhaler, take a slow, deep breath for 3 to 5 seconds, hold the breath for ≈ 10 seconds and breathe out slowly; allow at least 1 minute between inhalations (puffs); rinse the mouth with water or mouthwash after each use to help reduce dry mouth and hoarseness.

Administration and Dosage:

Patients receiving concomitant systemic steroids: Transfer to steroid inhalant and subsequent management may be more difficult because of slow HPA function recovery which may last up to 12 months. These agents may be effective and may permit replacement or significant reduction in corticosteroid dosage.

Stabilize the patient's asthma before treatment is started. Initially, use aerosol concurrently with usual maintenance dose of systemic steroid. After approximately 1 week, start gradual withdrawal of the systemic steroid by reducing the daily or alternate daily dose. Make the next reduction after 1 to 2 weeks, depending on response. These decrements should not exceed 2.5 mg prednisone or equivalent. A slow rate of withdrawal cannot be overemphasized.

During withdrawal, some patients may experience symptoms of steroid withdrawal despite maintenance or even improvement of respiratory function. Encourage continuance with the inhaler, but observe for objective signs of adrenal insufficiency. If adrenal insufficiency occurs, increase the systemic steroid dose temporarily and continue further withdrawal more slowly.

During periods of stress or severe asthma attack, transfer patients will require supplementary systemic steroids. See Warnings.

BECLOMETHASONE DIPROPIONATE

Administration and Dosage:

50 mcg released at the valve delivers approximately 42 mcg to the patient.

Adults: 2 inhalations (84 mcg) 3 or 4 times daily. Alternatively, 4 inhalations (168 mcg) given twice daily has been effective in some patients. In patients with severe asthma, start with 12 to 16 inhalations a day and adjust dosage downward according to response. Do not exceed 20 inhalations (840 mcg) daily.

Children: 1 or 2 inhalations (42 to 84 mcg) 3 or 4 times daily according to response. Alternatively, 2 to 4 inhalations (84 to 168 mcg) given twice daily has been effective in some patients. Do not exceed 10 inhalations (420 mcg) daily. Clinical data are insufficient with respect to administration in children < 6 years if age.

Patients not receiving systemic steroids: Follow above directions. In responsive patients, pulmonary function usually improves within 1 to 4 weeks.

Concomitant systemic steroid therapy: See Administration section.

Rx	**Beclovent** (Glaxo Wellcome)	**Aerosol:** Each actuation delivers approx. 42 mcg	In 16.8 g inhaler w/adapter and 16.8 g refill. (200 metered doses per inhaler.)
Rx	**Vanceril** (Schering)		
Rx	**Vanceril Double Strength** (Schering)	**Aerosol:** Each actuation delivers approx. 84 mcg	In 5.4 g inhaler (40 metered doses) and 12.2 g inhaler (120 metered doses).
Rx	**Vancenase Pockethaler** (Schering)	**Nasal inhaler:** Each actuation delivers approx. 42 mcg	In 7 g canisters w/adapter (200 metered doses).

Corticosteroids

DEXAMETHASONE SODIUM PHOSPHATE

Administration and Dosage:

Recommended initial dosage:

Adults – 3 inhalations 3 or 4 times per day; maximum 12 inhalations/day.

Children – 2 inhalations 3 or 4 times per day; maximum 8 inhalations/day.

Concomitant systemic steroid therapy: See Administration section.

Rx	**Dexacort Phosphate in Respihaler** (Adams)	**Aerosol:** Each activation releases dexamethasone sodium phosphate equivalent to approximately 84 mcg dexamethasone	In 12.6 g container.[1] (170 metered doses per inhaler.)

[1] With 2% alcohol.

TRIAMCINOLONE ACETONIDE

Administration and Dosage:

200 mcg released with each actuation delivers approximately 100 mcg to the patient.

Adults: The usual dosage is 2 inhalations (approximately 200 mcg) 3 to 4 times a day. Do not exceed a maximum daily intake of 16 inhalations (1600 mcg). Higher initial doses (12 to 16 inhalations per day) may be advisable in patients with more severe asthma, the dosage then being adjusted downward according to patient response. In some patients, maintenance can be accomplished when the total daily dose is administered twice a day.

Children: The usual dosage is 1 or 2 inhalations (100 to 200 mcg) 3 to 4 times a day. Do not exceed a maximum daily intake of 12 inhalations (1200 mcg). Clinical data are insufficient with respect to use in children < 6 years of age.

Patients not receiving systemic steroids: Follow above directions. In responsive patients, an improvement in pulmonary function is usually apparent within 1 to 2 weeks.

Concomitant systemic steroid therapy: See Administration section.

Rx	**Azmacort** (Rhone-Poulenc Rorer)	**Aerosol:** Each actuation delivers approx. 100 mcg. Contains 60 mg triamcinolone acetonide	In 20 g inhaler w/adapter.[1] (240 metered doses per inhaler.)

FLUNISOLIDE

Administration and Dosage:

Each actuation delivers approximately 250 mcg flunisolide to the patient.

Adults: 2 inhalations (500 mcg) twice daily, morning and evening (total daily dose 1000 mcg). Do not exceed 4 inhalations twice daily (2000 mcg).

Children (6 to 15 years): 2 inhalations twice daily, morning and evening (total daily dose 1000 mcg). Higher doses have not been studied. Safety and efficacy for use in children < 6 years have not been established. With chronic use, monitor children for growth as well as for effects on the HPA axis.

Patients not receiving systemic steroids: In responsive patients, pulmonary function usually improves within 1 to 4 weeks.

Concomitant systemic steroid therapy: See Administration section.

Rx	**AeroBid** (Forest)	**Aerosol:** Each actuation delivers approx. 250 mcg	In 7 g canister with mouthpiece. (100 metered doses per inhaler.)
Rx	**AeroBid-M** (Forest)		In 7 g canister with mouthpiece. (100 metered doses per inhaler.) Menthol flavor.

Mucolytics

ACETYLCYSTEINE (N-Acetylcysteine)

Actions:

Pharmacology: The viscosity of pulmonary mucus secretions depends on the concentration of mucoprotein in the secretory fluid, the presence of disulfide bonds between these macromolecules and, to a lesser extent, DNA. The mucolytic action of acetylcysteine is related to the sulfhydryl group in the molecule, which acts directly to split disulfide linkages between mucoprotein molecular complexes, resulting in depolymerization and a decrease in mucus viscosity. Its action is unaffected by the presence of DNA. The mucolytic activity of acetylcysteine increases with increasing pH. Significant mucolysis occurs between pH 7 and 9.

Acetylcysteine also reduces the extent of liver injury following acetaminophen overdose. It is thought that acetylcysteine protects the liver by maintaining or restoring glutathione levels, or by acting as an alternate substrate for conjugation with, and thus, detoxification of, the reactive metabolite of acetaminophen.

Pharmacokinetics: Following a 200 to 400 mg oral dose, peak plasma concentrations of 0.35 to 4 mg/L are achieved within 1 to 2 hours. Protein binding is ≈ 50% 4 hours post-dose. Volume of distribution is 0.33 to 0.47 L/kg. The terminal half-life of reduced acetylcysteine is 6.25 hours. Approximately 70% of total body clearance is nonrenal.

Indications:

Mucolytic: Adjuvant therapy for abnormal, viscid or inspissated mucus secretions in chronic bronchopulmonary disease (chronic emphysema, emphysema with bronchitis, chronic asthmatic bronchitis, tuberculosis, bronchiectasis, primary amyloidosis of lung).

Acute bronchopulmonary disease (pneumonia, bronchitis, tracheobronchitis).

Pulmonary complications of cystic fibrosis.

Tracheostomy care.

Pulmonary complications associated with surgery.

Use during anesthesia.

Posttraumatic chest conditions.

Atelectasis due to mucus obstruction.

Diagnostic bronchial studies (bronchograms, bronchospirometry, bronchial wedge catheterization).

Antidote: To prevent or lessen hepatic injury which may occur following ingestion of a potentially hepatotoxic quantity of acetaminophen. Initiate treatment as soon as possible after overdose and, in any case, within 24 hours of ingestion.

Unlabeled uses: As an ophthalmic solution to treat keratoconjunctivitis sicca (dry eye). It has been used as an enema to treat bowel obstruction due to meconium ileus or its equivalent.

Contraindications:

Hypersensitivity to acetylcysteine. As an antidote, there are no contraindications.

Warnings:

Bronchial secretions: An increased volume of liquefied bronchial secretions may occur; when cough is inadequate, maintain an open airway by mechanical suction if necessary. When there is a large mechanical block due to a foreign body or local accumulation, clear the airway by endotracheal aspiration, with or without bronchoscopy.

Asthmatics: Carefully observe asthmatics under treatment with acetylcysteine. If bronchospasm progresses, discontinue medication immediately.

Antidotal use:

Allergic effects – Generalized urticaria has been observed rarely. If this or other allergic symptoms appear, discontinue treatment unless it is deemed essential and the allergic symptoms can be otherwise controlled.

Hepatic effects – If encephalopathy due to hepatic failure occurs, discontinue treatment to avoid further administration of nitrogenous substances. No data indicate that acetylcysteine adversely influences hepatic failure, but this is theoretically possible.

Vomiting, occasionally severe and persistent, occurs as a symptom of acute acetaminophen overdose. Treatment with oral acetylcysteine may aggravate this. Evaluate patients at risk of gastric hemorrhage (eg, esophageal varices, peptic ulcers) concerning the risk of upper GI hemorrhage vs the risk of developing hepatic toxicity. Diluting acetylcysteine minimizes its propensity to aggravate vomiting.

Pregnancy: Category B. There are no adequate and well controlled studies in pregnant women. Use only when clearly needed.

Mucolytics

ACETYLCYSTEINE (N-Acetylcysteine)

Lactation: It is not known whether this drug is excreted in breast milk. Exercise caution when administering to a nursing woman.

Precautions:

Disagreeable odor: Administration may initially produce a slight disagreeable odor which soon disappears.

Face mask use: A face mask may cause stickiness on the face after nebulization; remove with water.

Solution color may change in the opened bottle, but does not significantly impair the drug's safety or efficacy.

Continued nebulization of acetylcysteine with a dry gas results in concentration of drug in the nebulizer due to evaporation. Extreme concentration may impede nebulization and drug delivery. Dilute with Sterile Water for Injection as concentration occurs.

Adverse Reactions:

Stomatitis; nausea; vomiting; fever; rhinorrhea; drowsiness; clamminess; chest tightness; bronchoconstriction.

Bronchospasm: Clinically overt acetylcysteine-induced bronchospasm occurs infrequently and unpredictably even in patients with asthmatic bronchitis or bronchitis complicating bronchial asthma.

Acquired sensitization to acetylcysteine has occurred rarely. Sensitization has been confirmed in several inhalation therapists who reported a history of dermal eruptions after frequent and extended exposure to acetylcysteine.

Irritation to the tracheal and bronchial tracts has occurred, and although hemoptysis has occurred in patients receiving acetylcysteine, such findings are not uncommon in patients with bronchopulmonary disease. A causal relationship has not been established.

Antidotal use: Large doses of oral acetylcysteine may result in nausea, vomiting and other GI symptoms. Rash (with or without mild fever), pruritus, angioedema, bronchospasm, tachycardia, hypotension and hypertension have occurred.

Administration and Dosage:

Nebulization (face mask, mouth piece, tracheostomy): 1 to 10 ml of the 20% solution or 2 to 20 ml of the 10% solution every 2 to 6 hours; the dose for most patients is 3 to 5 ml of the 20% solution or 6 to 10 ml of the 10% solution 3 to 4 times a day.

Nebulization (tent, croupette): Very large volumes are required, occasionally up to 300 ml during a treatment period. The dose is the volume of solution that will maintain a very heavy mist in the tent or croupette for the desired period. Administration for intermittent or continuous prolonged periods, including overnight, may be desirable.

Instillation:

Direct – 1 to 2 ml of a 10% to 20% solution as often as every hour.

Tracheostomy – 1 to 2 ml of a 10% to 20% solution every 1 to 4 hours by instillation into the tracheostomy.

May be introduced directly into a particular segment of the bronchopulmonary tree by inserting (under local anesthesia and direct vision) a plastic catheter into the trachea. Instill 2 to 5 ml of the 20% solution by a syringe connected to the catheter.

Percutaneous intratracheal catheter – 1 to 2 ml of the 20% solution or 2 to 4 ml of the 10% solution every 1 to 4 hours by a syringe attached to the catheter.

Diagnostic bronchograms: 2 or 3 administrations of 1 to 2 ml of the 20% solution or 2 to 4 ml of the 10% solution by nebulization or by instillation intratracheally, prior to the procedure.

Preparation of solution: The 20% solution may be diluted with either Sodium Chloride for Injection or Inhalation or Sterile Water for Injection or Inhalation. The 10% solution may be used undiluted. Refrigerate unused, undiluted solution and use within 96 hours.

Equipment compatibility: Certain materials in nebulization equipment react with acetylcysteine, especially certain metals (notably iron and copper) and rubber. Where materials may come into contact with acetylcysteine solution, use parts made of the following materials: Glass, plastic, aluminum, anodized aluminum, chromed metal, tantalum, sterling silver or stainless steel. Silver may become tarnished after exposure, but this is not harmful to the drug action or to the patient.

Mucolytics

ACETYLCYSTEINE (N-Acetylcysteine)

Acetaminophen overdosage: Administer acetylcysteine immediately if ≤ 24 hours have elapsed from the reported time of acetaminophen ingestion. Do not await results of assays for acetaminophen level before initiating treatment. In one study, acetylcysteine administered as long as 36 hours after the acetaminophen overdose was beneficial in some patients. The following procedures are recommended:

1. Empty the stomach promptly by lavage or by inducing emesis with syrup of ipecac. Repeat the ipecac dose if emesis does not occur in 20 minutes.
2. If activated charcoal has been administered, lavage before administering acetylcysteine. Activated charcoal may adsorb acetylcysteine, thereby reducing its effectiveness.
3. Draw blood for acetaminophen plasma assay and for baseline AST, ALT, bilirubin, prothrombin time, creatinine, BUN, blood sugar and electrolytes. If an assay cannot be obtained or if the acetaminophen level is clearly in the toxic range, continue acetylcysteine for the full course of therapy. Monitor hepatic and renal function and electrolyte and fluid balance.
4. Administer a 140 mg/kg loading dose of acetylcysteine.
5. Administer the first maintenance dose (70 mg/kg) 4 hours after the loading dose. Repeat the maintenance dose at 4 hour intervals for a total of 17 doses unless the acetaminophen assay reveals a nontoxic level.
6. If the patient vomits the loading dose or any maintenance dose within 1 hour of administration, repeat that dose.
7. If the patient is persistently unable to retain the orally administered acetylcysteine, administer by duodenal intubation.
8. Repeat AST, ALT, bilirubin, prothrombin time, creatinine, BUN, blood sugar and electrolytes daily if the acetaminophen plasma level is in the potentially toxic range.

Preparation of oral solution – Dilute the 20% solution with cola drinks or other soft drinks to a final concentration of 5% (see Dosage Guide table). If administered via gastric tube or Miller-Abbott tube, water may be used as the diluent. Prepare fresh dilutions and use within 1 hour. Remaining undiluted solutions in opened vials can be refrigerated up to 96 hours.

Acetaminophen assays – The acute ingestion of acetaminophen in quantities of ≥ 150 mg/kg may result in hepatic toxicity. However, the reported history of the quantity of a drug ingested as an overdose is often inaccurate and is not a reliable guide to antidotal therapy. Therefore, determine plasma or serum acetaminophen concentrations as early as possible, but no sooner than 4 hours following an acute overdose to assess the potential risk of hepatotoxicity. If an acetaminophen assay cannot be obtained, assume that the overdose is potentially toxic.

Interpretation of acetaminophen assays (refer to the following nomogram) – When results of the plasma acetaminophen assay are available, refer to the nomogram. Values above the solid line connecting 200 mcg/ml at 4 hours with 50 mcg/ml at 12 hours are associated with a possibility of hepatic toxicity if an antidote is not administered. Do not wait for assay results to begin treatment.

If the plasma level is above the broken line, continue with maintenance doses of acetylcysteine. It is better to err on the safe side; thus, the broken line is plotted 25% below the solid line which defines possible toxicity.

If the plasma level is below the broken line described above, there is minimal risk of hepatic toxicity and acetylcysteine treatment can be discontinued.

Mucolytics

ACETYLCYSTEINE (N-Acetylcysteine)

Estimating potential for hepatotoxicity – The following nomogram estimates the probability that plasma levels in relation to intervals postingestion will result in hepatotoxicity.

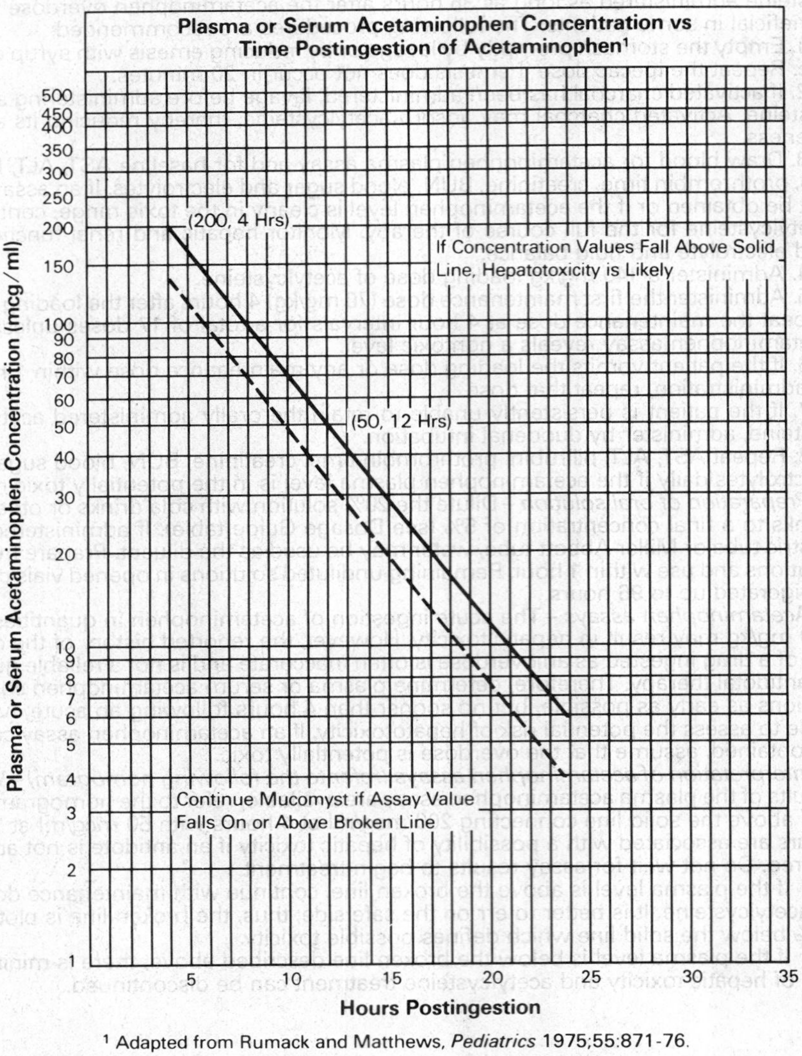

[1] Adapted from Rumack and Matthews, *Pediatrics* 1975;55:871-76.

Mucolytics

ACETYLCYSTEINE (N-Acetylcysteine)

Supportive treatment: Maintain fluid and electrolyte balance. Treat as necessary for hypoglycemia. Administer vitamin K_1 if prothrombin time ratio exceeds 1.5; administer fresh frozen plasma if the prothrombin time ratio exceeds 3. Avoid diuretics and forced diuresis.

Acetylcysteine Dosage Guide and Preparation

Body weight (kg)	Body weight (lb)	Acetylcysteine (g)	20% solution (ml)	Diluent (ml)	5% solution (ml)
Loading dose (140 mg/kg)*					
100-109	220-240	15	75	225	300
90-99	198-218	14	70	210	280
80-89	176-196	13	65	195	260
70-79	154-174	11	55	165	220
60-69	132-152	10	50	150	200
50-59	110-130	8	40	120	160
40-49	88-108	7	35	105	140
30-39	66-86	6	30	90	120
20-29	44-64	4	20	60	80
Maintenance dose (70 mg/kg)*					
(kg)	(lb)				
100-109	220-240	7.5	37	113	150
90-99	198-218	7	35	105	140
80-89	176-196	6.5	33	97	130
70-79	154-174	5.5	28	82	110
60-69	132-152	5	25	75	100
50-59	110-130	4	20	60	80
40-49	88-108	3.5	18	52	70
30-39	66-86	3	15	45	60
20-29	44-64	2	10	30	40

* If patient weighs < 20 kg (usually patients < 6 years of age), calculate the dose. Each ml of 20% solution contains 200 mg acetylcysteine. Add 3 ml of diluent to each ml of 20% solution. Do not decrease the proportion of diluent.

Admixture incompatibility: Tetracycline, chlortetracycline, oxytetracycline, erythromycin lactobionate, amphotericin B and sodium ampicillin are incompatible when mixed in the same solution with acetylcysteine. Administer from separate solutions. Iodized oil, chymotrypsin, trypsin and hydrogen peroxide are also incompatible.

Rx	**Acetylcysteine** (Various, Cetus, Dey, DuPont)	**Solution:** 10% (as sodium)	In 4, 10 and 30 ml vials.[1]
Rx	**Mucomyst** (Apothecon)		In 4, 10 and 30 ml vials.[1]
Rx	**Mucosil-10** (Dey Labs)		In 4, 10 and 30 ml vials.[1]
Rx	**Acetylcysteine** (Various, Cetus, Dey, DuPont)	**Solution:** 20% (as sodium)	In 4, 10, 30 and 100 ml vials.[1]
Rx	**Mucomyst** (Apothecon)		In 4, 10 and 30 ml vials.[1]
Rx	**Mucosil-20** (Dey Labs)		In 4, 10, 30 and 100 ml vials.[1]

[1] May contain EDTA.

Anticholinergics

IPRATROPIUM BROMIDE

Actions:

Pharmacology: Ipratropium for oral inhalation is a synthetic quaternary anticholinergic (parasympatholytic) ammonium compound chemically related to atropine. It appears to inhibit vagally mediated reflexes by antagonizing the action of acetylcholine. Anticholinergics prevent the increases in intracellular concentrations of cyclic guanosine monophosphate (cyclic GMP), which are caused by interaction of acetylcholine with the muscarinic receptor on bronchial smooth muscle.

The bronchodilation following inhalation is primarily a local, site-specific effect. Much of an inhaled dose is swallowed as shown by fecal excretion studies.

Ipratropium has anti-secretory properties and when applied locally, inhibits secretions from the serous and seromucous glands lining the nasal mucosa.

Pharmacokinetics: Ipratropium is poorly absorbed into the systemic circulation from the nasal mucosa. Less than 20% of an 84 mcg per nostril dose is absorbed from the nasal mucosa, but the amount which is systematically absorbed from nasal administration exceeds the amount absorbed from either inhalation solution (2% of a 500 mcg dose) or inhalation aerosol (20% of a 36 mcg mouthpiece dose). Ipratropium is minimally bound (≤ 9% in vitro) to plasma albumin and α_1-acid glycoprotein. It is partially metabolized to inactive ester hydrolysis products. The elimination half-life is about 1.6 hours.

Clinical trials:

Bronchospasm – In controlled 90 day studies in patients with bronchospasm associated with chronic obstructive pulmonary disease (COPD) (chronic bronchitis and emphysema), significant improvements in pulmonary function (FEV_1 and $FEF_{25\%}$ to $_{75\%}$ increases of ≥ 15%) occurred within 15 minutes, reached a peak in 1 to 2 hours and persisted for 3 to 4 hours in most patients and up to 6 hours in some patients. In addition, significant increases in Forced Vital Capacity (FVC) occurred.

Rhinorrhea – In four controlled 4 and 8 week comparisons of ipratropium nasal spray 0.03% (42 mcg per nostril, 2 or 3 times daily), with its vehicle, in patients with allergic or nonallergic perennial rhinitis, there was a statistically significant decrease in the severity and duration of rhinorrhea with ipratropium throughout the entire study period. An effect was seen as early as the first day of therapy. There was no effect of ipratropium nasal spray 0.03% on degree of nasal congestion, sneezing or postnasal drip.

Indications:

Bronchospasm (solution and aerosol): As a bronchodilator for maintenance treatment of bronchospasm associated with COPD, including chronic bronchitis and emphysema.

Rhinorrhea:

Perennial rhinitis (0.03% nasal spray) – Symptomatic relief of rhinorrhea associated with allergic and nonallergic perennial rhinitis in patients ≥ 12 years of age.

Common cold (0.06% nasal spray) – Symptomatic relief of rhinorrhea associated with the common cold in patients ≥ 12 years of age.

Contraindications:

Hypersensitivity to ipratropium, atropine or its derivatives or to soya lecithin or related food products such as soy bean or peanut (inhalation aerosol).

Warnings:

Acute bronchospasm: Use of itratropium as a single agent for relief of bronchospasm in acute COPD exacerbation has not been adequately studied.

Special risk patients: Use with caution in patients with narrow-angle glaucoma, prostatic hypertrophy or bladder neck obstruction.

Hypersensitivity: Immediate hypersensitivity reactions may occur after admininstration of ipratropium bromide, as demonstrated by rare cases of urticaria, angioedema, rash, bronchospasm and oropharyngeal edema.

Pregnancy: Category B. No adequate and well controlled studies have been conducted in pregnant women. Use during pregnancy only if clearly needed.

Lactation: It is not known whether this drug is excreted in breast milk. Although lipid-insoluble quaternary bases pass into breast milk, it is unlikely that ipratropium would reach the infant to an important extent, especially when taken by inhalation. However, exercise caution when administering to a nursing mother.

Children: Safety and efficacy in children < 12 years old have not been established.

Adverse Reactions:

Inhalation aerosol: Cough (≈ 3% to 5.9%); dryness of the oropharynx (≈ 5%); nervousness (3.1%); irritation from aerosol (1.6% to ≈ 3%); dizziness, headache, GI distress,

IPRATROPIUM BROMIDE

dry mouth, exacerbation of symptoms (1% to ≈ 3%); nausea (≈ 1% to 2.8%); palpitation (1.8%); rash (1.2%); blurred vision/difficulty in accommodation, drying of secretions (≈ 1%); urinary difficulty, fatigue, insomnia, hoarseness, tachycardia, paresthesias, drowsiness, coordination difficulty, itching, hives, flushing, alopecia, constipation, tremor, mucosal ulcers (< 1%).

Inhalation solution: Tachycardia, palpitations, eye pain, urinary retention, urinary tract infection, urticaria (< 3%). Headache, mouth dryness and aggravation of COPD symptoms were more common with ≥ 2000 mcg/day.

Ipratropium Inhalation Solution Adverse Reaction (%)[1]					
Adverse Reaction	Ipratropium (500 mcg tid) (n = 219)	Metaproterenol (15 mg tid) (n = 212)	Ipratropium/ Metaproterenol (500 mcg tid/ 15 mg tid) (n =108)	Albuterol (2.5 mg tid) (n = 205)	Ipratropium/ Albuterol (500 mcg tid/ 2.5 mg tid) (n = 100)
Body as a whole					
Headache	6.4	5.2	6.5	6.3	9
Pain	4.1	3.3	0.9	2.9	5
Influenza-like symptoms	3.7	4.7	6.5	0.5	1
Back pain	3.2	1.9	1.9	2.4	0
Chest pain	3.2	4.2	5.6	2	1
Cardiovascular					
Hypertension/Hypertension aggravated	0.9	1.9	0.9	1.5	4
Nervous System					
Dizziness	2.3	3.3	1.9	3.9	4
Insomnia	0.9	0.5	4.6	1	1
Tremor	0.9	7.1	8.3	1	0
Nervousness	0.5	4.7	6.5	1	1
GI					
Mouth dryness	3.2	0	1.9	2	3
Nausea	4.1	3.8	1.9	2.9	2
Constipation	0.9	0	3.7	1	1
Musculoskeletal					
Arthritis	0.9	1.4	0.9	0.5	3
Respiratory (lower)					
Coughing	4.6	8	6.5	5.4	6
Dyspnea	9.6	13.2	16.7	12.7	9
Bronchitis	14.6	24.5	15.7	16.6	20
Bronchospasm	2.3	2.8	4.6	5.4	5
Sputum increased	1.4	1.4	4.6	3.4	0
Respiratory disorder	0	6.1	6.5	2	4
Respiratory (upper)					
Upper respiratory tract infection	13.2	11.3	9.3	12.2	16
Pharyngitis	3.7	4.2	5.6	2.9	4
Rhinitis	2.3	4.2	1.9	2.4	0
Sinusitis	2.3	2.8	0.9	5.4	4

[1] Data are pooled from separate studies and are not necessarily comparable.

Nasal spray (0.03%): Headache, upper respiratory tract infection (9.8%); epistaxis (7% to 9%); pharyngitis (8.1%); nasal dryness (5.1%); miscellaneous nasal symptoms (3.1%); nausea (2.2%); nasal irritation, blood-tinged mucus (2%); dry mouth/throat, dizziness, ocular irritation, blurred vision, conjunctivitis, hoarseness, cough and taste perversion (< 2%).

Nasal spray (0.06%): Epistaxis (8.2%); nasal dryness (4.8%); dry mouth/throat (1.4%); nasal congestion (1.1%); taste perversion, nasal burning, conjunctivitis, coughing, dizziness, hoarseness, palpitation, pharngitis, tachycardia, thirst tinnitus, blurred vision, urinary retention (< 1%).

Anticholinergics

IPRATROPIUM BROMIDE

Allergic-type reactions: Allergic-type reactions such as skin rash, angioedema of the tongue, throat, lips and face, urticaria (including giant urticaria), laryngospasm and anaphylactic reactions have been reported. Many patients had a history of allergies with drugs or food, including soybeans.

Additional anticholinergic reactions reported with ipratropium products included precipitation or worsening of narrow angle glaucoma, urinary retention, prostatic disorders, tachycardia, consipation and bowel obstruction.

Overdosage:

Acute overdosage by inhalation is unlikely.

Patient Information:

Temporary blurred vision, precipitation or worsening of narrow-angle glaucoma or eye pain may result if aerosol is sprayed into eyes or solution comes into direct contact with the eyes. For the solution, use of a nebulizer with mouthpiece rather than face mask may be preferable to reduce the likelihood of the solution reaching the eyes.

Advise patients that the solution can be mixed in the nebulizer with albuterol or metaproterenol if used within 1 hour. Compatibility data are not available with other drugs.

Nasal spray: Initial pump priming requires 7 actuations of the pump. If used regularly as recommended, no further priming is required. If not used for > 24 hours, the pump will require 2 actuations, or if not used for > 7 days, the pump will require 7 actuations to reprime.

Administration and Dosage:

Aerosol: The usual dose is 2 inhalations (36 mcg) 4 times a day. Patients may take additional inhalations as required; however, do not exceed 12 inhalations in 24 hours.

Solution: The usual dose is 500 mcg (1 unit dose vial) administered 3 to 4 times a day by oral nebulization, with doses 6 to 8 hours apart. The solution can be mixed in the nebulizer with albuterol if used within 1 hour.

Nasal spray:

0.03% – The usual dose is 2 sprays (42 mcg) per nostril 2 or 3 times daily (total dose, 168 to 252 mcg/day). Optimum dosage varies.

0.06% – The recommended dose is 2 sprays (84 mcg) per nostril 3 or 4 times daily (total dose, 504 to 672 mcg/day). Optimum dosage varies.

The safety and efficacy of use beyond 4 days on patients with the common cold have not been established.

Concomitant therapy: Ipratropium has been used concomitantly with other durgs, including sympathomimetic bronchodilators, methylxanthines, steroids and cromolyn sodium, commonly used in the treatment of COPD, without adverse drug reactions.

Storage/Stability:

Aerosol – Store below 30°C (86°F); avoid excessive humidity.

Solution – Store between 15° and 30°C (59° and 86°F). Protect from light. Store unused vials in the foil pouch.

Nasal spray – Store tightly closed between 15° and 30°C (59° and 86°F). Avoid freezing.

Rx	**Ipratropium Bromide** (Dey)	**Solution for Inhalation:** 0.02% (500 mcg per vial)	Preservative free. In 25 and 60 unit-dose vials (2.5 ml each).
Rx	**Atrovent** (Boehringer Ingelheim)	**Aerosol:** Each actuation delivers 18 mcg	In 14 g metered dose inhaler w/mouthpiece (200 inhalations).
		Solution for Inhalation: 0.02% (500 mcg per vial)	Preservative free. In 25 unit dose vials per foil pouch.
		Nasal spray: 0.03%. Each spray delivers 21 mcg	In 30 ml bottles with spray pump (345 sprays).
		0.06%. Each spray delivers 42 mcg	In 15 ml bottles with spray pump (165 sprays).

Miscellaneous

CROMOLYN SODIUM (Disodium Cromoglycate)

Actions:

Pharmacology: Cromolyn is an antiasthmatic, antiallergic and mast cell stabilizer. It has no intrinsic bronchodilator, antihistaminic, anticholinergic, vasoconstrictor or anti-inflammatory activity. In animal studies, cromolyn inhibits the degranulation of sensitized and nonsensitized mast cells which occurs after exposure to specific antigens. The drug inhibits the release of histamine and SRS-A (the slow-reacting substance of anaphylaxis, a leukotriene) from the mast cell. Bronchial asthma or rhinitis induced by the inhalation of antigens can be inhibited to varying degrees by cromolyn pretreatment.

Cromolyn acts locally on the lung to which it is directly applied. The Spinhaler (inhalation capsule) route delivers more drug to the lungs compared to nebulization of the solution, but there is no difference in effectiveness.

Pharmacokinetics: After inhalation, about 7% to 8% is absorbed from the lung and is rapidly excreted unchanged in bile and urine. The remainder is either exhaled, or deposited in the oropharynx, swallowed and excreted via the alimentary tract.

Cromolyn is poorly absorbed from the GI tract. No more than 1% of an administered dose is absorbed after oral administration, the remainder being excreted in the feces. Very little absorption of cromolyn was seen after oral administration of 500 mg to each of 12 volunteers. From 0.25% to 0.5% of the administered dose was recovered in the first 24 hours of urinary excretion in 3 subjects. The mean urinary excretion over 24 hours in the remaining 9 subjects was 0.45%.

Clinical trials: Cromolyn solution 20 mg 4 times daily was compared to theophylline alone and to a combination of both drugs in asthmatic children. Cromolyn was at least as effective in controlling the symptoms of chronic asthma as oral theophylline in the 1 to 6 year age group. The combination gave no additional benefits.

Indications:

Severe bronchial asthma (nebulization solution, inhalation capsules, aerosol): Prophylactic management of severe bronchial asthma where the frequency, intensity and predictability of episodes indicate the continued use of symptomatic medication. Such patients must have a significant bronchodilator-reversible component to their airway obstruction as demonstrated by pulmonary function tests.

Improvement ordinarily occurs within the first 4 weeks of administration, manifested by a decrease in the severity of clinical symptoms, or the need for concomitant therapy or both. Long-term use is justified if the drug produces a significant reduction in the severity of symptoms of asthma, permits a significant reduction in, or elimination of, steroid dosage or improves management of those who have intolerable side effects to sympathomimetic agents or methylxanthines.

Prevention of exercise-induced bronchospasm (nebulization solution, capsules, aerosol): Prevention of acute bronchospasm induced by toluene diisocyanate, environmental pollutants and known antigens (aerosol).

Allergic rhinitis (nasal solution): Prevention and treatment of allergic rhinitis.

Mastocytosis (oral): Improves diarrhea, flushing, headaches, vomiting, urticaria, abdominal pain, nausea and itching in some patients.

Unlabeled uses: Oral use is being evaluated in patients with food allergies to prevent GI and systemic reactions and for use in eczema, dermatitis, ulcerations, urticaria pigmentosa, chronic urticaria, hay fever and postexercise bronchospasm.

Contraindications:

Hypersensitivity to cromolyn or to any ingredient contained in these products.

Warnings:

Acute asthma: Cromolyn has no role in the treatment of acute asthma, especially status asthmaticus; it is a prophylactic drug with no benefit for acute situations.

Hypersensitivity: Severe anaphylactic reactions may occur rarely with oral cromolyn. Refer to General Management of Acute Hypersensitivity Reactions.

Renal/Hepatic function impairment: In view of the biliary and renal routes of excretion, decrease the dose or discontinue the drug in these patients

Pregnancy: Category B. Safety for use during pregnancy has not been established. Use only when clearly needed and when the potential benefits outweigh the unknown potential hazards to the fetus. Animal studies have demonstrated adverse fetal effects (increased resorptions, decreased fetal weight) only at very high parenteral doses in combination with high-dose isoproterenol.

Miscellaneous

CROMOLYN SODIUM (Disodium Cromoglycate)

Lactation: Safety for use in the nursing mother has not been established. Exercise caution when the drug is administered to a nursing mother.

Children: Inhalation capsules – Clinical experience in children < 5 years of age is limited due to administration by inhalation. Capsule use is not recommended.

Aerosol – Safety and efficacy in children < 5 years old are not established.

Nebulizer sol – Safety and efficacy in children < 2 years old not established.

Nasal solution – Safety and efficacy in children < 6 years old are not established.

Oral capsule – Animal studies suggest increased risk of toxicity in premature animals when given in doses much higher than clinically recommended. In term infants up to 6 months of age, data suggest the dose not exceed 20 mg/kg/day. Reserve use in children < 2 years for patients with severe disease in which potential benefits clearly outweigh risks.

Precautions:

Bronchospasm: Occasionally, patients experience cough or bronchospasm following inhalation and, at times, may not be able to continue treatment despite prior bronchodilator administration. Very severe bronchospasm has occurred rarely.

Asthma may recur if drug is reduced below recommended dosage or discontinued.

Eosinophilic pneumonia (pulmonary infiltrates with eosinophilia): If this occurs during the course of therapy, discontinue the drug.

Nasal stinging or sneezing may be experienced by some patients following instillation of the nasal solution. This has rarely caused discontinuation of therapy.

Aerosol: Because of the propellants in this preparation, use with caution in patients with coronary artery disease or cardiac arrhythmias.

Drug Interactions:

Isoproterenol and cromolyn sodium: See Pregnancy.

Adverse Reactions:

Inhalation capsules and aerosol:

EENT – Lacrimation; swollen parotid gland.

GU – Dysuria; urinary frequency.

CNS – Dizziness; headache.

Hypersensitivity – Rash; urticaria; angioedema.

Miscellaneous – Joint swelling and pain; nausea.

Causal relationship unknown or rare: Anaphylaxis; anemia; exfoliative dermatitis; hemoptysis; hoarseness; myalgia; nephrosis; periarteric vasculitis; pericarditis; peripheral neuritis; photodermatitis; polymyositis; pulmonary infiltrates with eosinophilia; vertigo; nasal itching, bleeding or burning; sneezing; serum sickness; liver disease.

Adverse effects related to the cromolyn inhalation capsule delivery system are inhalation of gelatin particles, mouthpiece or propeller.

Additional effects reported with the aerosol include: Dry or irritated throat; bad taste; cough; wheezing; substernal burning and myopathy (rare).

Nebulizer solution: Cough; nasal congestion; wheezing; sneezing; nasal itching; epistaxis; nose burning; abdominal pain.

Nasal solution: Sneezing (10%); nasal stinging (5%); nasal burning (4%); nasal irritation (2.5%); headache, bad taste in mouth (2%); epistaxis, postnasal drip, rash (< 1%).

Oral capsules: Most of the adverse events reported in mastocytosis patients have been transient and could represent symptoms of the disease. The most frequently reported adverse events in mastocytosis patients who have received cromolyn during clinical studies were headache and diarrhea. Each occurred in 4 of 87 patients. Pruritis, nausea and myalgia were each reported in 3 patients and abdominal pain, rash and irritability in 2 patients each. One report of malaise was also recorded.

A generally similar profile of adverse events has been reported during studies in other clinical conditions. Additional reports that have been received during the course of these studies and spontaneous reports during foreign marketing include:

CNS – Dizziness; fatigue; paresthesia; migraine; psychosis; anxiety; depression; insomnia; behavior change; hallucinations; postprandial lightheadedness; lethargy.

Dermatologic – Flushing; urticaria/angioedema; skin erythema and burning.

GI – Taste perversion; esophagospasm; flatulence; dysphagia; hepatic function test abnormality; burning mouth and throat.

Miscellaneous – Arthralgia; edema; dyspnea; polycythemia; neutropenia; dysuria; leg stiffness and weakness. These events are infrequent, the majority representing a single report; in many cases, causal relationship to cromolyn is uncertain.

Miscellaneous

CROMOLYN SODIUM (Disodium Cromoglycate)

Overdosage:

No action other than medical observation should be necessary.

Patient Information:

Inhalation or nasal: Do not discontinue therapy abruptly except on advice of physician.

For inhalation use only; do not swallow capsule.

Notify physician if coughing or wheezing occurs.

Patient instructions for use of Spinhaler device and Nasalmatic device accompany each product.

Oral: The effect of therapy depends upon administration at regular intervals as directed.

Take at least one-half hour before meals. Do not mix with fruit juice, milk or foods.

Drink all of the liquid.

Administration and Dosage:

Nebulizer solution and inhalation capsules: Adults and children (≤ 5 years for capsules; ≥ 2 years for nebulizer solution) – Initially, 20 mg inhaled 4 times daily at regular intervals. Carefully instruct patients in the use of the inhaler. The effectiveness of therapy depends upon administration at regular intervals.

Administer solution from a power operated nebulizer having an adequate flow rate and equipped with a suitable face mask. *Hand operated nebulizers are not suitable.*

Introduce cromolyn into the patient's therapeutic regimen when the acute episode has been controlled and the patient is able to inhale adequately.

Prevention of exercise-induced bronchospasm: Inhale one 20 mg capsule or 20 mg of the nebulizer solution no more than 1 hour before anticipated exercise. The drug's protective effect will be stronger the shorter the interval between inhalation and exercise. Repeat inhalation as required for protection during prolonged exercise.

Concomitant corticosteroid treatment and bronchodilators should be continued following the introduction of cromolyn. If the patient improves, attempt to decrease corticosteroid dosage. Even if the steroid-dependent patient fails to improve following cromolyn use, attempt gradual tapering of steroid dosage while maintaining close patient supervision. Consider reinstituting steroid therapy for a patient subjected to significant stress (a severe asthmatic attack, surgery, trauma or severe illness) while being treated or within 1 year (occasionally up to 2 years) after steroid treatment has been terminated, in case of adrenocortical insufficiency. When the inhalation of cromolyn is impaired, a temporary increase in the amount of steroids or other agents may be required.

Cautiously withdraw cromolyn in cases where its use has permitted a reduction in the maintenance dose of steroids as there may be a sudden reappearance of asthma which will require immediate therapy and possible reintroduction of corticosteroids.

Aerosol: For management of bronchial asthma in adults and children ≥ 5 years of age, the usual starting dose is two metered sprays inhaled 4 times daily at regular intervals. Do not exceed this dose. Not all patients will respond to the recommended dose, and a lower dose may provide efficacy in younger patients.

Advise patients with chronic asthma that the effect of therapy is dependent upon its administration at regular intervals, as directed. Introduce therapy into the patient's therapeutic regimen when the acute episode has been controlled, the airway has been cleared and the patient is able to inhale adequately.

For the prevention of acute bronchospasm which follows exercise, exposure to cold dry air or environmental agents, the usual dose is inhalation of two metered dose sprays shortly, (ie, 10 to 15 minutes but not more than 60 minutes), before exposure to the precipitating factor.

Nasal solution:

Adults and children ≥ 6 years – One spray in each nostril 3 to 6 times daily at regular intervals. Clear the nasal passages before administering the spray and inhale through the nose during administration.

Seasonal (pollenotic) rhinitis, and for prevention of rhinitis caused by exposure to other types of specific inhalant allergens – Treatment will be more effective if started prior to contact with the allergen. Continue treatment throughout exposure period.

Perennial allergic rhinitis – Effects of treatment may require 2 to 4 weeks of treatment. Concomitant use of antihistamines or nasal decongestants may be necessary during the initial phase of treatment, but the need for this medication should diminish and may be eliminated when the full benefit of therapy is achieved.

Use with Nasalmatic metered spray device. Replace pump device every 6 months.

Miscellaneous

CROMOLYN SODIUM (Disodium Cromoglycate)

Oral:

Adults – Two capsules 4 times daily, one-half hour before meals and at bedtime.

Children –

Premature to term infants: Not recommended.

Term to 2 years: 20 mg/kg/day in four divided doses. Use of this product in children < 2 years old is not recommended and should be attempted only in those patients with severe incapacitating diseases where benefits clearly outweigh risks.

2 to 12 years: One capsule 4 times daily one-half hour before meals and bedtime.

If satisfactory control of symptoms is not achieved within 2 to 3 weeks, the dosage may be increased but should not exceed 40 mg/kg/day (30 mg/kg/day for children 6 months to 2 years).

The effect of therapy is dependent upon its administration at regular intervals as directed.

Maintenance – Once a therapeutic response has been achieved the dose may be reduced to the minimum required to maintain the patient with a lower degree of symptomatology. To prevent relapses, maintain the dosage.

Administer as a solution in water at least one-half hour before meals after preparation according to the following directions.

1. Open capsule(s) and pour powder contents into one-half glass of hot water.
2. Stir until completely dissolved (clear solution).
3. Add equal quantity of cold water while stirring.
4. Do not mix with fruit juice, milk or foods.
5. Drink all of the liquid.

Each capsule contains a precisely measured dose. The capsules are intentionally oversized to prevent the powder from spilling when the capsule is opened.

Oral capsules are not for inhalation.

Compatibility: Cromolyn **nebulizer solution** is compatible with metaproterenol sulfate, isoproterenol HCl, 0.25% isoetharine HCl, epinephrine HCl, terbutaline sulfate and 20% acetylcysteine solution for at least 1 hour after their admixture.

Storage: Store the **nebulizer solution** below 30°C (86°F); protect from direct light.

Rx	**Cromolyn Sodium** (Dey)	**Inhalation**: 20 mg /2 ml	In UD plastic vials.
		Solution for nebulization: 20 mg/vial	In 2 ml vials.
Rx	**Intal** (Fisons)	**Solution (for nebulizer only)**: 20 mg per amp	In 2 ml amps.
		Aerosol spray: Each actuation delivers 800 mcg	In 8.1 g (≥ 112 metered sprays) and 14.2 g (≥ 200 metered sprays).
otc	**Nasalcrom** (McNeil)	**Nasal Solution**: 40 mg/ml.[1] Each actuation delivers 5.2 mg	In 13 ml (≥ 100 sprays) or 26 ml (200 sprays) metered spray device.
Rx	**Gastrocrom** (Fisons)	**Capsules (Oral)**: 100 mg	In oversized 100s.

[1] With 0.01% benzalkonium chloride and 0.01% EDTA.

Miscellaneous

NEDOCROMIL SODIUM

Actions:

Pharmacology: Nedocromil is an inhaled anti-inflammatory agent for the preventive management of asthma. It inhibits the in vitro activation of, and mediator release from, a variety of inflammatory cell types associated with asthma, including eosinophils, neutrophils, macrophages, mast cells, monocytes and platelets. In vitro, nedocromil inhibits the release of mediators including histamine, leukotriene C_4 and prostaglandin D_2. Similar studies with human bronchoalveolar cells showed inhibition of histamine release from mast cells and beta-glucuronidase release from macrophages.

Nedocromil inhibits the development of early and late bronchoconstriction responses to inhaled antigen. The development of airway hyper-responsiveness to nonspecific bronchoconstrictors was also inhibited. Nedocromil reduced antigen-induced increases in airway, microvasculature leakage when administered IV.

The drug acutely inhibits the bronchoconstrictor response to several kinds of challenge. Pretreatment with single doses inhibited the bronchoconstriction caused by sulfur dioxide, inhaled neurokinin A, various antigens, exercise, cold air, fog and adenosine monophosphate.

Nedocromil has no intrinsic bronchodilator, antihistamine or glucocorticoid activity and when delivered by inhalation at the recommended dose, has no known therapeutic systemic activity.

Pharmacokinetics: Systemic bioavailability is low. In a single-dose study involving 20 healthy subjects who were administered a 3.5 mg dose, the mean AUC was 5 ng•hr/ml and the mean Cmax was 1.6 ng/ml attained about 28 minutes after dosing. The mean half-life was 3.3 hours. Urinary excretion over 12 hours averaged 3.4% of the administered dose, of which ≈ 75% was excreted in the first 6 hours of dosing.

In a multiple dose study, six healthy volunteers received a 3.5 mg single dose followed by 3.5 mg 4 times a day for 7 consecutive days. Accumulation of the drug was not observed. Following single and multiple dose inhalations, urinary excretion accounted for 5.6% and 12% of the drug administered, respectively. After IV administration, urinary excretion was ≈ 70%. The absolute bioavailability was thus 8% for single and 17% for multiple inhaled doses.

Similarly, in a multiple dose study of 12 asthmatic patients, each given a 3.5 mg single dose followed by 3.5 mg 4 times a day for 1 month, both single dose and multiple dose inhalations gave a mean high plasma concentration of 2.8 ng/ml between 5 and 90 minutes, mean AUC of 5.6 ng•hr/ml and a mean terminal half-life of 1.5 hours. The mean 24 hour urinary excretion after either single- or multiple-dose administration represented ≈ 5% of the administered dose.

Nedocromil is ≈ 89% bound to plasma protein over a concentration range of 0.5 to 50 mcg/ml. This binding is reversible. It is not metabolized after IV administration and is excreted unchanged.

Clinical trials: Studies have been conducted both at twice daily and at 4 times daily dosage regimens. Evidence indicates that the 4 times daily regimen has been more effective than the twice daily regimen. A lower dose (2 or 3 times daily) can be considered in patients under good control on the 4 times daily regimen (see Administration and Dosage).

Nedocromil vs placebo – The effectiveness of nedocromil given 4 times daily was examined in a 14 week double-blind, placebo controlled, parallel group trial in 120 patients. To be eligible for entry, the asthmatic patients had to be controlled using only sustained release theophylline (SRT) and beta-agonists. Two weeks after the test therapies were begun, the SRT was discontinued and 4 weeks after that, oral beta-agonists were stopped. Beta-agonist metered dose inhalers could still be used after 6 weeks. Each morning the patient recorded nighttime asthma and before bedtime the patients recorded daytime asthma and cough. Nedocromil was significantly superior to placebo for all measurements. The FEV_1 percentage change relative to baseline also favored nedocromil over placebo throughout the study, with an effect seen first at the 2 week measurement.

This study shows that nedocromil improves symptom control and pulmonary function when it is added to an as-needed inhaled beta-adrenergic bronchodilator regimen and that a beneficial effect could be detected within 2 weeks.

Miscellaneous

NEDOCROMIL SODIUM

Nedocromil vs cromolyn sodium vs placebo – The effectiveness of nedocromil was compared to cromolyn sodium and placebo in an 8 week, double-blind, parallel group trial during which medication was given 4 times daily. Patients (n = 306) were randomized to treatment (103/nedocromil; 104/cromolyn sodium; 99/placebo). All patients were SRT-dependent and this drug was stopped prior to starting the test treatment. Efficacy was assessed on the basis of diary card symptom scores and FEV_1.

This study corroborates the findings of the 14 week study, showing that nedocromil is effective in the management of symptoms and pulmonary function in primarily atopic mild to moderate asthmatics. Both active treatments were significantly better than placebo for the primary efficacy variable (summary symptom score); nedocromil and cromolyn sodium were not significantly different for this parameter. A statistically significant difference favoring cromolyn sodium was, however, seen for nighttime asthma and FEV_1.

In allergic asthmatics who are well controlled on cromolyn sodium, there is no evidence that the substitution of nedocromil for cromolyn sodium would confer additional benefit to the patient. Efficacy with one agent is not known to be predictive of efficacy with the other.

Indications:

Bronchial asthma: Maintenance therapy in the management of patients with mild to moderate bronchial asthma.

Contraindications:

Hypersensitivity to nedocromil or other ingredients in the preparation.

Warnings:

Acute bronchospasm: Nedocromil is not a bronchodilator and, therefore, should not be used for the reversal of acute bronchospasm, particularly status asthmaticus. Ordinarily continue nedocromil during acute exacerbations, unless the patient becomes intolerant to the use of inhaled dosage forms.

Pregnancy: Category B. There are no adequate and well controlled studies in pregnant women. Use during pregnancy only if clearly needed.

Lactation: It is not known whether this drug is excreted in breast milk. Exercise caution when administering to a nursing woman.

Children: Safety and efficacy in children < 12 years of age have not been established.

Precautions:

Coughing/Bronchospasm: Inhaled medications can cause coughing and bronchospasm in some patients. If this should occur with nedocromil, discontinue use and institute alternative therapy as appropriate.

Corticosteroids: If systemic or inhaled steroid therapy is at all reduced, monitor patients carefully. Nedocromil has not been shown to be able to substitute for the total dose of steroids.

Adverse Reactions:

Nedocromil is generally well tolerated. Adverse event information was derived from 5352 patients receiving nedocromil in controlled and open-label clinical trials of 2 to 52 weeks in duration. A total of 3538 patients received 2 inhalations 4 times a day. An additional 1814 patients received 2 inhalations twice daily or some other dose regimen. Seventy-three percent of patients were exposed to study drug for ≥ 8 weeks.

Miscellaneous

NEDOCROMIL SODIUM

Nedocromil Adverse Reactions				
	% Experiencing adverse reaction		% Withdrawing	
Adverse reaction	Nedocromil (n = 2042)	Placebo (n = 1875)	Nedocromil	Placebo
Respiratory				
Coughing	7	7.2	1.4	1.4
Pharyngitis	5.7	5	0.6	0.5
Rhinitis	4.6	3	0.1	0.1
Upper respiratory tract infection	3.9	2.4	0.1	0.1
Sputum increased	1.7	1.4	0.1	0.2
Bronchitis	1.2	1.3	0.1	0.1
Dyspnea	2.8	3.8	0.9	1.3
Bronchospasm	5.4	8.2	1.5	2.3
GI tract				
Nausea	4	2.1	1.3	0.7
Vomiting	1.7	0.9	0.2	0.4
Dyspepsia	1.3	0.6	0.1	0.1
Dry mouth	1	0.9	0.1	0.2
Diarrhea	0.9	0.6	0.1	0
Abdominal pain	1.2	0.5	0.2	0.1
Central/Peripheral nervous system				
Dizziness	0.9	1.2	0.1	0.2
Dysphonia	1	0.6	0.1	0.1
Body as a whole				
Headache	6	4.7	0.5	0.3
Chest pain	4	3.9	0.9	0.6
Fatigue	1.1	0.7	0.2	0.1
Miscellaneous				
Viral infection	2.4	3.4	0.1	0.1
Unpleasant taste	12.6	3.6	2.1	0.4

Other (< 1%): Rash; arthritis; tremor; sensation of warmth. Elevations of ALT (3.3% nedocromil vs 1.7% placebo). The average elevation over placebo was 10 IU with only two patients increasing by > 100 IU and none becoming ill.

One case of pneumonitis with eosinophilia and one case of anaphylaxis have been reported in foreign post-marketing experience.

Overdosage:

Animal studies by several routes of administration (inhalation, oral, IV, SC) have demonstrated little potential for significant toxicity in humans from inhalation of high doses of nedocromil. Head shaking/tremor and salivation were observed in dogs following daily inhalation doses of 5 mg/kg and transient hypotension was detected following daily IV doses of 8 mg/kg. In addition, clonic convulsions were observed in dogs following daily inhalation doses of 20 mg/kg plus SC doses of 20 mg/kg giving peak plasma levels of 7.6 mcg/ml, some three orders of magnitude greater than peak plasma levels (2.5 ng/ml) of the human daily dose. Nedocromil does not pass the blood-brain barrier. Therefore, overdosage is unlikely to result in clinical manifestations requiring more than observation and discontinuation of the drug where appropriate.

Miscellaneous

NEDOCROMIL SODIUM

Patient Information:

An illustrated leaflet for the patient is included in each nedocromil pack.

Nedocromil must be used regularly to achieve benefit, even during symptom-free periods.

Because the therapeutic effect depends on topical application to the lungs, it is essential that patients be properly instructed in the correct method of use (see Patient Instruction leaflet).

Administration and Dosage:

Approved by the FDA on December 30, 1992.

The recommended dosage for symptomatic adults and children (≥ 12 years of age) is 2 inhalations 4 times a day at regular intervals to provide 14 mg/day. Initiate maintenance therapy at the same dose. In patients under good control on 4 times daily dosing (ie, patients whose only medication need is occasional [not more than twice a week] inhaled or oral beta-agonists, and who have no serious exacerbations with respiratory infections), a lower dose can be tried. If use of lower doses is attempted, first reduce to a 3 times daily regimen (10.5 mg/day) then, after several weeks on continued good control, to twice a day (7 mg/day).

Add nedocromil to the patient's existing treatment regimen (eg, bronchodilators). When a clinical response to nedocromil is evident and if the asthma is under good control, an attempt may be made to decrease concomitant medication usage gradually.

Proper inhalational technique is essential (see Patient Instruction leaflet).

Advise patients that the optimal effect of nedocromil therapy depends on its administration at regular intervals, even during symptom-free periods.

Storage: Store between 2° to 30°C (36° to 86°F). Do not freeze.

Rx	**Tilade** (Fisons)	**Aerosol:** 1.75 mg per actuation	In 16.2 g canisters providing at least 112 metered inhalations. With mouthpiece.

Miscellaneous

DORNASE ALFA (Recombinant human deoxyribonuclease; DNase)

Actions:

Pharmacology: Dornase is a highly purified solution of recombinant human deoxyribonuclease I (rhDNase), an enzyme that selectively cleaves DNA. The protein is produced by genetically engineered Chinese Hamster Ovary (CHO) cells containing DNA encoding for the native human protein, deoxyribonuclease I (DNase). The purified glycoprotein contains 260 amino acids with an approximate molecular weight of 37,000 daltons. The primary amino acid sequence is identical to that of the native human enzyme. Dornase is administered by inhalation of an aerosol mist produced by a compressed air driven nebulizer system.

In cystic fibrosis (CF) patients, retention of viscous purulent secretions in the airways contributes both to reduced pulmonary function and to exacerbations of infection. Purulent pulmonary secretions contain very high concentrations of extracellular DNA released by degenerating leukocytes that accumulate in response to infection. In vitro, dornase hydrolyzes the DNA in sputum of CF patients and reduces sputum viscoelasticity.

Pharmacokinetics: When 2.5 mg dornase was administered by inhalation to 18 CF patients, mean sputum concentrations of 3 mcg/ml DNase were measurable within 15 minutes. Mean sputum concentrations declined to an average of 0.6 mcg/ml 2 hours following inhalation. Inhalation of up to 10 mg 3 times daily by four CF patients for 6 consecutive days did not result in a significant elevation of serum concentrations of DNase above normal endogenous levels. After administration of up to 2.5 mg dornase twice daily for 6 months to 321 CF patients, no accumulation of serum DNase was noted.

Clinical trials: In a large, randomized, placebo controlled trial, clinically stable CF patients (≥ 5 years of age) with baseline forced vital capacity (FVC) ≥ 40% of predicted and receiving standard therapies for CF were treated with placebo (n = 325), 2.5 mg dornase once a day (n = 322) or 2.5 mg dornase twice a day (n = 321) for 6 months administered via a nebulizer. Both doses of dornase resulted in significant reductions compared with the placebo group in the number of patients experiencing respiratory tract infections requiring use of parenteral antibiotics. Administration of dornase reduced the relative risk of developing a respiratory tract infection by 27% and 29% for the daily dose and twice daily dose, respectively. The data suggest that the effects of dornase on respiratory tract infections in older patients (> 21 years) may be smaller than in younger patients, and that twice daily dosing may be required in the older patients. Patients with baseline FVC > 85% may also benefit from twice a day dosing. The reduced risk of respiratory infection observed in dornase–treated patients did not directly correlate with improvement in FEV_1 during the initial 2 weeks of therapy.

Within 8 days of the start of treatment with dornase, mean FEV_1 increased 7.9% in those treated once a day and 9% in those treated twice a day compared to the baseline values. The mean FEV_1 observed during long-term therapy increased 5.8% and 5.6% from baseline at the 2.5 mg daily dose level and 2.5 mg twice daily dose level, respectively. Placebo recipients did not show significant mean changes in pulmonary function testing. For patients ≥ 5 years of age with baseline FVC ≥ 40%, administration of dornase decreased the incidence of occurrence of first respiratory tract infection requiring parenteral antibiotics, and improved mean FEV_1 regardless of age or baseline FVC.

Incidence of First Respiratory Tract Infection Requiring Parenteral Antibiotics Following Dornase

	Placebo (n = 325)	2.5 mg once daily (n = 322)	2.5 mg twice daily (n = 321)
Percent of patients infected	43%	34%	33%
Age			
5-20 years	42%	25%	28%
≥ 21 years	44%	48%	39%
Baseline FVC			
40-85% predicted	54%	41%	44%
> 85% predicted	27%	21%	14%

Miscellaneous

DORNASE ALFA (Recombinant human deoxyribonuclease; DNase)

In other studies, dornase did not produce a pulmonary function benefit in short-term usage in patients with FVC < 40% of predicted. Studies are in progress to assess the impact of chronic use on pulmonary function and infection risk in this population. Clinical trials have indicated that dornase therapy can be continued or initiated during an acute respiratory exacerbation. Short-term studies demonstrated that doses in excess of 2.5 mg twice daily did not provide further improvement in FEV_1. Patients who have received the drug on a cyclical regimen (eg, 10 mg twice daily for 14 days, followed by a 14 day washout period) showed rapid improvement in FEV_1 with the initiation of each cycle and a return to baseline with each dornase withdrawal.

Indications:

Cystic fibrosis: Daily administration in conjunction with standard therapies in the management of CF patients to reduce the frequency of respiratory infections requiring parenteral antibiotics and to improve pulmonary function.

Contraindications:

Hypersensitivity to dornase, Chinese Hamster Ovary cell products, or any component of the product.

Warnings:

Pregnancy: Category B. There are no adequate and well controlled studies in pregnant women. Use this drug during pregnancy only if clearly needed.

Lactation: It is not known whether dornase is excreted in breast milk. Exercise caution when administering to a nursing woman.

Children: Safety and efficacy in children < 5 years of age have not been studied.

Precautions:

Administration: Use in conjunction with standard therapies for CF. Safety and efficacy of daily administration have not been demonstrated in patients with FVC < 40% of predicted or for > 12 months.

Drug Interactions:

Clinical trials have indicated that dornase can be effectively and safely used in conjunction with standard CF therapies including oral, inhaled and parenteral antibiotics, bronchodilators, enzyme supplements, vitamins, oral and inhaled corticosteroids and analgesics.

Adverse Reactions:

Patients have been exposed to dornase for up to 12 months in clinical trials. Most adverse events were not more common on dornase than on placebo and probably reflected the sequelae of the underlying lung disease. In most cases, events that were increased were mild, transient in nature, and did not require alterations in dosing. Few patients experienced adverse events resulting in permanent discontinuation from dornase, and the discontinuation rate was similar for placebo (2%) and dornase (3%).

Dornase Adverse Reactions (%)

Adverse Event	Placebo (n=325)	Dornase once daily (n=322)	Dornase twice daily (n=321)
Voice alteration	7	12	16
Pharyngitis	33	36	40
Laryngitis	1	3	4
Rash	7	10	12
Chest pain	16	18	21
Conjunctivitis	2	4	5

Other adverse reactions reported include the following:

Body as a whole: Abdominal pain; asthenia; fever; flu syndrome; malaise; sepsis.

GI: Intestinal obstruction; gall bladder disease; liver disease; pancreatic disease.

Metabolic/Nutritional: Diabetes mellitus; hypoxia; weight loss.

Respiratory: Apnea; bronchiectasis; bronchitis; change in sputum; cough increase; dyspnea; hemoptysis; lung function decrease; nasal polyps; pneumonia; pneumothorax; rhinitis; sinusitis; sputum increase; wheeze.

Miscellaneous

DORNASE ALFA (Recombinant human deoxyribonuclease; DNase)

Miscellaneous:

Death – Causes of death were consistent with progression of CF and included apnea, cardiac arrest, cardiopulmonary arrest, cor pulmonale, heart failure, massive hemoptysis, pneumonia, pneumothorax and respiratory failure.

Allergic reactions – Skin rash and urticaria have been observed, and were mild and transient in nature. Within all studies, a small percentage of patients developed serum antibodies to dornase (2% to 4%). None of these patients developed anaphylaxis, and the clinical significance of serum antibodies to dornase is unknown.

Overdosage:

Cystic fibrosis patients have received up to 20 mg twice daily for up to 6 days and 10 mg twice daily intermittently (2 weeks on/2 weeks off drug) for 168 days. These doses were well tolerated.

Patient Information:

Dornase must be stored in the refrigerator at 2° to 8°C (36° to 46°F) and protected from strong light. Keep refrigerated during transport and do not expose to room temperatures for a total time of 24 hours. Discard the solution if it is cloudy or discolored. Dornase contains no preservative and, once opened, the entire ampule must be used or discarded.

Instruct patients in the proper use and maintenance of the nebulizer and compressor system used in the delivery of the drug. Do not dilute or mix dornase with other drugs in the nebulizer. Mixing of dornase with other drugs could lead to adverse physicochemical or functional changes in dornase or the admixed compound.

Administration and Dosage:

Approved by the FDA on December 30, 1993.

Dosage: The recommended dose for use in most CF patients is one 2.5 mg single-use amp inhaled once daily using a recommended nebulizer. Some patients may benefit from twice daily administration.

Nebulizers: Clinical trials have been performed with the following nebulizers and compressors: The disposable jet nebulizer *Hudson T Up-draft* II and disposable jet nebulizer *Marquest Acorn* II in conjunction with a *Pulmo-Aide* compressor, and the reusable *PARI LC Jet+* nebulizer, in conjunction with the *PARI PRONEB* compressor. Safety and efficacy have been demonstrated only with these recommended nebulizer systems. No clinical data are currently available that support the safety and efficacy of administration of dornase with other nebulizer systems. The patient should follow the manufacturer's instructions on the use and maintenance of the equipment. Do not dilute or mix dornase with other drugs in the nebulizer. Mixing of dornase with other drugs could lead to adverse physicochemical or functional changes in dornase or the admixed compound.

Storage/Stability: Store under refrigeration (2° to 8°C; 36° to 46°F). Protect amps from light. Do not use beyond the expiration date stamped on the amp. Store unused amps in their protective foil pouch under refrigeration.

Rx	**Pulmozyme** (Genentech)	**Solution for inhalation:** 1 mg/ml	Preservative free. With 0.15 mg/ml calcium chloride dihydrate and 8.77 mg/ml sodium chloride. In 2.5 ml amps.

NASAL DECONGESTANTS

Actions:

Pharmacology: Decongestants stimulate α-adrenergic receptors of vascular smooth muscle (vasoconstriction, pressor effects, nasal decongestion), although some retain β-adrenergic properties (eg, ephedrine, pseudoephedrine). Other alpha effects include contraction of the GI and urinary sphincters, mydriasis and decreased pancreatic beta cell secretion. The α-adrenergic effects cause intense vasoconstriction when applied directly to mucous membranes; systemically, the products have similar muted effects and decongestion occurs without drastic changes in blood pressure, vascular redistribution or cardiac stimulation. Constriction in the mucous membranes results in their shrinkage; this promotes drainage, thus improving ventilation and the stuffy feeling.

Decongestants are sympathomimetic amines administered directly to swollen membranes (eg, via spray, drops) or systemically via the oral route. They are used in acute conditions such as hay fever, allergic rhinitis, vasomotor rhinitis, sinusitis and the common cold to relieve membrane congestion.

Oral agents are not as effective as topical products, especially on an immediate basis, but generally have a longer duration of action, cause less local irritation and are not associated with rebound congestion (rhinitis medicamentosa).

Routes, Doses and Strengths of the Nasal Decongestants

	Drug and route	Usual adult dose	Strengths
Arylalkylamines	Phenylpropanolamine Oral	25 mg q 4 hrs; 50 mg q 8 hrs	25 mg, 50 mg
	Oral-SR	75 mg q 12 hrs	75 mg
	Pseudoephedrine Oral	60 mg q 4 to 6 hrs	30 mg, 60 mg, 7.5 mg/0.8 ml, 15 mg/5 ml, 30 mg/5 ml, 30 mg/ml
	Oral-SR	120 mg q 12 hrs	120 mg
	Phenylephrine – Topical	1 to 2 sprays or a few drops q 3 to 4 hrs	0.125%, 0.16%, 0.2%, 0.25%, 0.5%, 1%, 0.5% jelly
	Epinephrine – Topical	Maximum 1 ml/15 min[1]	0.1%
	Ephedrine – Topical	2 to 3 drops q 4 hrs	0.5%, 0.6% jelly
	Desoxyephedrine – Topical	2 inhalations per nostril q 2 h	50 mg inhaler
Imidazolines	Naphazoline – Topical	2 drops q 3 hrs	0.05%
	Oxymetazoline – Topical	2 to 3 sprays twice daily	0.025%, 0.05%
	Tetrahydrozoline – Topical	2 to 4 drops or 3 or 4 sprays q 3 hrs	0.05%, 0.1%
	Xylometazoline – Topical	2 to 3 drops q 8 to 10 hrs	0.05%, 0.1%
Cycloalkylamine	Propylhexedrine – Topical	2 inhalations through each nostril. Use as needed, but avoid excessive use	250 mg inhaler

[1] Refer to manufacturer's directions.

Indications:

Oral: For temporary relief of nasal congestion due to the common cold, hay fever or other upper respiratory allergies, and nasal congestion associated with sinusitis; to promote nasal or sinus drainage; relief of eustachian tube congestion.

Phenylpropanolamine is also used as an anorexiant. Refer to the individual monograph in the Anorexiants section.

Topical: Symptomatic relief of nasal and nasopharyngeal mucosal congestion due to the common cold, sinusitis, hay fever or other upper respiratory allergies.

Adjunctive therapy of middle ear infections by decreasing congestion around the eustachian ostia. Nasal inhalers may relieve ear block and pressure pain in air travel.

NASAL DECONGESTANTS

Contraindications:

Monoamine oxidase inhibitor (MAOI) therapy; hypersensitivity or idiosyncrasy to sympathomimetic amines manifested by insomnia, dizziness, weakness, tremor or arrhythmias.

Oral: Severe hypertension and coronary artery disease.

Phenylpropanolamine, sustained release – Nursing mothers.

Sustained release phenylpropanolamine and pseudoephedrine, naphazoline – Children < 12 years of age.

Topical:

Tetrahydrozoline – 0.1% solution in children < 6 years of age; 0.05% solution in infants < 2 years of age.

Naphazoline – Glaucoma.

Systemic effects are less likely from topical use, but use caution in the conditions listed for oral agents. Adverse reactions are more likely with excessive use, in the elderly and in children.

Warnings:

Special risk patients: Administer with caution to patients with hyperthyroidism, diabetes mellitus, cardiovascular disease, coronary artery disease, ischemic heart disease, increased intraocular pressure or prostatic hypertrophy. Sympathomimetics may cause CNS stimulation and convulsions or cardiovascular collapse with hypotension.

Hypertension: Hypertensive patients should use these products only with medical advice, as they may experience a change in blood pressure because of the added vasoconstriction. Studies suggest pseudoephedrine is the drug of choice and that phenylpropanolamine should be avoided; however, some studies report that lower doses of phenylpropanolamine do not significantly increase blood pressure in normotensive and hypertensive patients. Sustained action preparations may affect the cardiovascular system less.

Excessive use of decongestants may cause systemic effects (eg, nervousness, dizziness, sleeplessness) which are more likely in infants and in the elderly. Habituation and toxic psychosis have followed long-term high-dose therapy.

Rebound congestion (rhinitis medicamentosa) following topical application may occur after the vasoconstriction subsides. Patients may increase the amount of drug and frequency of use, producing toxicity and perpetuating the rebound congestion.

Treatment – A simple but uncomfortable solution is to completely withdraw the topical medication. A more acceptable method is to gradually withdraw therapy by initially discontinuing the medication in one nostril, followed by total withdrawal. Substituting an oral decongestant for a topical one may also be useful.

Elderly: Patients ≥ 60 years of age are more likely to experience adverse reactions to sympathomimetics. Overdosage may cause hallucinations, convulsions, CNS depression and death. Demonstrate safe use of a short-acting sympathomimetic before use of a sustained action formulation in elderly patients.

Pregnancy: (*Category C* — tetrahydrozoline). It is not known whether these agents can cause fetal harm or affect reproduction capacity. Give only when clearly needed. One study reported that oxymetazoline did not affect maternal blood pressure and pulse rates, and therefore is safe in the third trimester of a normal pregnancy.

Lactation: Oral pseudoephedrine and phenylpropanolamine are contraindicated in the nursing mother because of the higher than usual risks to infants from sympathomimetic agents.

Other oral preparations – Consult a physician before using.

Topical – It is not known if these agents are excreted in breast milk. Exercise caution when administering to a nursing woman.

Children: Use in children is product specific. Refer to individual product listings.

Precautions:

Acute use: Use topical decongestants only in acute states and not longer than 3 to 5 days. Use sparingly (especially the imidazolines) in all patients, particularly infants, children and patients with cardiovascular disease.

Stinging sensation: Some individuals may experience a mild, transient stinging sensation after topical application. This often disappears after a few applications.

Sulfite sensitivity: Some of the nasal decongestant products contain sulfites that may cause allergic-type reactions including anaphylactic symptoms and life-threatening or less severe asthmatic episodes in certain susceptible people. The overall prevalence of sulfite sensitivity in the general population is unknown but is probably low. Sulfite sensitivity is seen more frequently in asthmatic than in non-asthmatic people. Products containing sulfites are identified in the product listings.

NASAL DECONGESTANTS

Drug Interactions:

Most interactions listed apply to sympathomimetics when used as vasopressors; however, consider the interaction when using the nasal decongestants.

Nasal Decongestant Drug Interactions			
Precipitant drug	Object drug*		Description
Beta blockers	Epinephrine	↑	An initial hypertensive episode followed by bradycardia may occur.
Furazolidone	Nasal decongestants	↑	The pressor sensitivity to mixed-acting agents (eg, ephedrine) may be increased. Direct-acting agents (eg, epinephrine) are not affected.
Guanethidine	Nasal decongestants Direct Mixed	 ↑ ↓	Guanethidine potentiates the effects of the direct acting agents (eg, epinephrine) and inhibits the effects of the mixed-acting agents (eg, ephedrine). Guanethidine's hypotensive action may also be reversed.
Nasal decongestants	Guanethidine	↓	
Indomethacin	Phenylpropanolamine	↑	Concurrent administration may lead to an increase in blood pressure.
Methyldopa	Nasal decongestants	↑	Concurrent administration may result in an increased pressor response.
MAO inhibitors	Nasal decongestants	↑	Concurrent use of MAOIs and mixed-acting agents (eg, ephedrine) may result in severe headache, hypertension and hyperpyrexia, possibly resulting in hypertensive crisis. Direct-acting agents (eg, epinephrine) interact minimally, if at all.
Phenothiazines	Nasal decongestants	↓	Phenothiazines may antagonize and in some cases reverse the action of the nasal decongestants.
Rauwolfia alkaloids	Nasal decongestants Direct Mixed	 ↑ ↓	Reserpine potentiates the pressor response of direct-acting agents (eg, epinephrine) which may result in hypotension. The pressor response of mixed-acting agents (eg, ephedrine) is decreased.
Tricyclic antidepressants (TCAs)	Nasal decongestants Direct Mixed	 ↑ ↓	TCAs potentiate the pressor response of direct-acting agents (eg, epinephrine); dysrhythmias have occurred. The pressor response of mixed-acting agents (eg, ephedrine) is decreased.
Urinary acidifiers	Nasal decongestants	↓	Acidification of the urine may increase the elimination of the nasal decongestant; therapeutic effects may be decreased. Conversely, urinary alkalinization may decrease the elimination of these agents, possibly increasing therapeutic or toxic effects.
Urinary alkalinizers		↑	
Phenylpropanolamine	Bromocriptine	↑	Possible exacerbation of bromocriptine side effects. Ventricular tachycardia and cardiac dysfunction have occurred.
Phenylpropanolamine	Caffeine	↑	Serum caffeine levels may be increased, possibly increasing pharmacologic and toxic effects.
Nasal decongestants	Theophylline	↔	Enhanced toxicity, particularly cardiotoxicity, has occurred. Decreased theophylline levels may occur. Ephedrine may cause theophylline toxicity.
Epinephrine	Insulin or oral hypoglycemic agents	↓	Diabetics may require an increased dose of the hypoglycemic agent.

* ↑ = Object drug increased ↓ = Object drug decreased ↔ = Undetermined effect.

Adverse Reactions:

Topical use: Burning; stinging; sneezing; dryness; local irritation; rebound congestion.

CNS: Fear; anxiety; tenseness; restlessness; headache; lightheadedness; dizziness; drowsiness; tremor; insomnia; hallucinations; psychological disturbances; prolonged psychosis (paranoia, terror, delusions); convulsions; CNS depression; weakness.

NASAL DECONGESTANTS

Cardiovascular: Arrhythmias and cardiovascular collapse with hypotension; palpitations; tachycardia; transient hypertension; bradycardia.

GI: Nausea; vomiting.

Body as a whole: Pallor; respiratory difficulty; orofacial dystonia; sweating; dysuria; blepharospasm (ocular irritation, tearing, photophobia).

Overdosage:

Symptoms: Somnolence, sedation or coma may occur; sedation may be accompanied by profuse sweating, hypotension or shock. Severe hypertension, bradycardia and rebound hypotension may occur with naphazoline and tetrahydrozoline.

Treatment: Treatment is supportive; in severe cases, IV phentolamine may be used. See General Management of Acute Overdosage.

Tetrahydrozoline – There is no known antidote. The use of stimulants is contraindicated. If respiratory rate drops to ≤ 10, administer oxygen and assist respiration. Monitor blood pressure to prevent hypotensive crisis.

Patient Information:

Patients with hypertension or other cardiovascular diseases, hyperthyroidism, diabetes mellitus or prostatic hypertrophy should use only with medical advice.

Topical: Notify physician of insomnia, dizziness, weakness, tremor, irregular heart beat.

Do not exceed recommended dosage and do not use longer than 3 to 5 days.

Stinging, burning, sneezing, increased nasal discharge or drying of the nasal mucosa may occur.

Do not share container with other patients. Do not allow tip of container to touch the nasal passage. Discard after medication is no longer required.

Proper use – Spray – Keep head upright. Sniff hard for a few minutes after use.

Drops – Recline on a bed and hang your head over the edge; remain in this position for several minutes after using the drops, turning the head from side to side.

Inhalers – Warm in the hand before use. Wipe the inhaler after each use.

Oral: Do not exceed recommended dosage; higher doses may cause nervousness, dizziness or sleeplessness.

If symptoms do not improve within 7 days or are accompanied by a high fever, consult physician before continuing use.

PHENYLPROPANOLAMINE HCl

For complete prescribing information, refer to the Nasal Decongestants group monograph.

Also used as an *otc* anorexiant (see Nonprescription Diet Aids).

Administration and Dosage:

Adults: 25 mg every 4 hours, not to exceed 150 mg/day (or 75 mg sustained release every 12 hours).

Children (6 to 12 years): 12.5 mg every 4 hours. Do not exceed 75 mg/day.

Children (2 to 6 years): 6.25 mg every 4 hours.

otc	**Phenylpropanolamine HCl** (Various, eg, Moore, Rugby, URL)	**Tablets:** 25 mg	In 1000s.
otc	**Propagest** (Reed & Carnrick)		(C). White, scored. Oval. In 100s.
otc	**Phenylpropanolamine HCl** (Various, eg, Moore, Rugby)	**Tablets:** 50 mg	In 1000s.
otc	**Phenylpropanolamine HCl** (Various, eg, Camall)	**Capsules, timed release:** 75 mg	In 100s and 1000s.

PSEUDOEPHEDRINE SULFATE

For complete prescribing information, refer to the Nasal Decongestants group monograph.

Administration and Dosage:

Adults and children 12 years and over: 120 mg every 12 hours.

Do not crush or chew sustained release preparations.

otc	**Afrin** (Schering-Plough)	**Tablets, extended release:** 120 mg (60 mg immediate release/60 mg delayed release)	Butylparaben, lactose, sugar. In 100s.
otc	**Drixoral Non-Drowsy Formula** (Schering-Plough)		Sugar, lactose, parabens. In 20s.

PSEUDOEPHEDRINE HCl (d-Isoephedrine HCl)

For complete prescribing information, refer to the Nasal Decongestants group monograph.

Administration and Dosage:

Adults: 60 mg every 4 to 6 hours (120 mg sustained release every 12 hours). Do not exceed 240 mg in 24 hours.

Children: 30 mg every 4 to 6 hours. Do not exceed 120 mg in 24 hours.

(2 to 5 years) – 15 mg every 4 to 6 hours. Do not exceed 60 mg in 24 hours.

(1 to 2 years) – 7 drops (0.2 ml)/kg every 4 to 6 hours up to 4 doses/day.

(3 to 12 months) – 3 drops/kg every 4 to 6 hours up to 4 doses/day.

otc	**Pseudoephedrine HCl** (Various, eg, Geneva, IDE, Roxane, Rugby, UDL, URL)	**Tablets**: 30 mg	In 24s, 100s, 1000s.
otc	**Congestion Relief** (Schein)		Lactose, sugar. In 24s and 100s.
otc	**Genaphed** (Goldline)		In 24s and 100s.
otc	**Halofed** (Halsey)		In 1000s.
otc	**Pseudo-Gest** (Major)		In 100s.
otc	**Seudotabs** (Parmed)		Sucrose. In 100s.
otc	**Sudafed** (Burroughs Wellcome)		Sucrose. Red. In 24s, 48s, 100s, 1000s.
otc	**Sudex** (Roberts)		In UD 8s and 500s.
otc	**Pseudoephedrine HCl** (Various, eg, Geneva, Goldline, IDE, Roxane, UDL)	**Tablets**: 60 mg	In 100s, 1000s and UD 100s.
otc	**Cenafed** (Century Pharm.)		In 100s and 1000s.
otc	**DeFed-60** (Ferndale)		In 100s and 1000s.
otc	**Dynafed Pseudo** (BDI[1])		In 60s.
otc	**Halofed** (Halsey)		Sugar coated. In100s and 1000s.
otc	**Mini Thin Pseudo** (BDI Pharm)		In 60s.
otc	**Pseudo-Gest** (Major)		In 100s.
otc	**Sudafed** (Glaxo Wellcome)		Sucrose. (Sudafed 60). In 100s.
otc	**Efidac/24** (Ciba)	**Tablets**: 240 mg	In 6s and 12s.
otc	**Sudafed 12 Hour Caplets** (Glaxo Wellcome)	**Tablets, extended release**: 120 mg	(Sudafed 12 Hour). In 10s and 20s.
otc	**Allermed** (Murdock)	**Capsules**: 60 mg	In 30s.
otc	**Sinustop Pro** (Murdock)		In 30s.
Rx	**Novafed** (Hoechst Marion Roussel)	**Capsules, timed release:** 120 mg	Sucrose. (104 or Novafed). Brown, orange. In 100s.
otc	**Dorcol Children's Decongestant** (Sandoz)	**Liquid**: 15 mg per 5 ml	Sucrose, sorbitol. In 120 ml.
otc	**Triaminic AM Decongestant Formula** (Sandoz)		Alcohol and dye free. Sorbitol, sucrose. Orange flavor. In 118 and 237 ml.

PSEUDOEPHEDRINE HCl (d-Isoephedrine HCl)

otc	**Pseudoephedrine HCl** (Various, eg, Cenci, Halsey, Pharmaceutical Associates, Rugby)	**Liquid:** 30 mg per 5 ml	In 120 and 240 ml, pt and gal.
otc	**Decofed Syrup** (Various, eg, Barre-National, Major)		In 118 ml and pt.
otc	**Cenafed Syrup** (Century Pharm.)		Methylparaben. In 120 ml, pt and gal.
otc	**Children's Silfedrine** (Silarx)		In 118 ml.
otc	**Children's Sudafed** (Burroughs Wellcome)		0.1% methylparaben, 0.1% sodium benzoate, sorbitol, sucrose. Raspberry flavor. In 118 ml.
otc	**Children's Congestion Relief** (Tocs Labs)		Methylparaben, sucrose. In 120 ml.
otc	**Pseudo** (Major)		In 118 ml.
otc	**PediaCare Infants' Decongestant** (McNeil)	**Drops:** 7.5 mg per 0.8 ml	Sorbitol, sucrose. Alcohol free. In 15 ml w/dropper.

[1] BDI Pharmaceuticals, Inc., P.O. Box 78610, Indianapolis, IN 46278–0610; (800) 428–2352.

PHENYLEPHRINE HCl

For complete prescribing information, refer to the Nasal Decongestants group monograph.

Administration and Dosage:

Adults: (≥ 12 years old) — 2 to 3 sprays or drops in each nostril. Repeat every 3 to 4 hours (0.25% and 0.5%). The 1% solution should be repeated no more often than every 4 hours. The 0.25% solution is adequate in most cases. However, in resistant cases or if more powerful decongestion is desired, use the 0.5% or 1% solution.

Children (6 to 12 yrs): 0.25% – 2 to 3 sprays or drops in each nostril every 3 to 4 hrs.

Infants (> 6 months old): 0.16% – 1 or 2 drops in each nostril every 3 hours.

otc	**AH-chew D** (WE Pharm)	**Tablets, chewable:** 10 mg	(07). Pink, scored. Bubble gum flavor. In 100s.
otc	**Neo-Synephrine** (Sterling Health)	**Solution:** 0.125%	In 15 ml dropper bottle.[1]
otc	**Alconefrin 12** (PolyMedica)	**Solution:** 0.16%	In 30 ml dropper bottle.[2]
otc	**Phenylephrine HCl** (Various, eg, IDE, Major)	**Solution:** 0.25%	In 480 ml.
otc	**Alconefrin 25** (PolyMedica)		**Drops:** In 30 ml.[2] **Spray:** In 30 ml.[2]
otc	**Neo-Synephrine** (Sterling Health)		**Drops:** In 15 ml.[1] **Spray:** In 15 ml.[1]
otc	**Children's Nostril** (Ciba)		In 15 ml pump spray.[3]
otc	**Rhinall** (Scherer)		**Drops:** In 30 ml.[4] **Spray:** In 40 ml.[4]

PHENYLEPHRINE HCl

otc	**Alconefrin** (PolyMedica)	**Solution**: 0.5%	In 30 ml dropper bottle.[2]
otc	**Neo-Synephrine** (Sterling Health)		**Drops**: In 15 ml.[1] **Spray**: In 15 ml.[1]
otc	**Nostril** (Ciba)		In 15 ml pump spray.[3]
otc	**Sinex** (Richardson-Vicks)		In 15 and 30 ml spray.[5,6]
otc	**Phenylephrine HCl** (Various, eg, Barre, Major, PBI, Rugby, Schein, URL)	**Solution**: 1%	In 30 and 480 ml.
otc	**Neo-Synephrine** (Sterling Health)		**Drops**: In 15 ml.[1] **Spray**: In 15 ml.[1]

[1] With benzalkonium chloride and thimersal.
[2] With benzalkonium chloride and sodium bisulfite.
[3] With benzalkonium chloride and boric acid.
[4] With chlorobutanol, sodium bisulfite and benzalkonium chloride.
[5] With aromatics (eg, menthol, camphor and eucalyptol).
[6] With cetylpyridinium chloride and thimersal.

EPINEPHRINE HCl

For complete prescribing information, refer to the Nasal Decongestants group monograph.

Administration and Dosage:

Adults and children (≥ 6 years): Apply locally as drops or spray, or with a sterile swab, as required. Do not use in children < 6 years of age, except on physician's advice.

otc	**Adrenalin Chloride** (Parke-Davis)	**Solution**: 0.1%	In 30 ml.[1]

[1] With chlorobutanol and sodium bisulfite.

EPHEDRINE

For complete prescribing information, refer to the Nasal Decongestants group monograph.

Administration and Dosage:

Dosage is product-specific; see labeling.

otc	**Pretz-D** (Parnell)	**Spray**: 0.25% ephedrine sulfate	In 15 ml.[1]
otc	**Kondon's Nasal** (Kondon)	**Jelly**: 1% ephedrine alkaloid	In 20 g.

[1] With 3% glycerin, *Mucoprotective Factor* yerba santa, 0.55% sodium chloride, 0.002% phenylmercuric acetate.

NAPHAZOLINE HCl

For complete prescribing information, refer to the Nasal Decongestants group monograph.

Administration and Dosage:

Adults and children (≥ 12 years): 1 or 2 drops or sprays in each nostril as needed, no more than every 6 hours (spray). Do not use in children < 12, unless directed by physician.

otc	**Privine** (Ciba Consumer)	**Drops**: 0.05% solution	In 25 ml w/dropper.[1]
		Spray: 0.05% solution	In 20 and 473 ml.[1]

[1] With benzalkonium chloride and EDTA.

OXYMETAZOLINE HCl

For complete prescribing information, refer to the Nasal Decongestants group monograph.

Administration and Dosage:

Adults and children (≥ 6 years): 2 or 3 sprays or 2 or 3 drops of 0.05% solution in each nostril twice daily, morning and evening or every 10 to 12 hours *(Allerest)*.

Children (2 to 5 years): 2 or 3 drops of 0.025% solution in each nostril twice daily, morning and evening.

otc	**Afrin Children's Nose Drops** (Schering-Plough)	**Solution:** 0.025%	In 20 ml dropper bottle.[2]
otc	**Oxymetazoline HCl** (Various, eg, Ambix, Clay Park, IDE, Moore)	**Solution:** 0.05%	In 15 and 30 ml spray.
otc	**12 Hour Nasal** (Various, eg, Barre-National, URL)		In 15 and 30 ml spray.
otc	**Afrin** (Schering-Plough)		**Drops:** In 20 ml.[2]
			Spray (cherry): In 15 ml.[2]
			Spray (regular): In 15 and 30 ml and 15 ml pump.[2]
			Spray (menthol): In 15 ml.[2,3]
otc	**Afrin Sinus** (Schering-Plough)		Benzyl alcohol. In 15 ml spray.
otc	**Allerest 12 Hour Nasal** (Ciba Cons.)	**Solution:** 0.05%	In 15 ml spray.[1]
otc	**Cheracol Nasal** (Roberts)		In 30 ml spray.[10]
otc	**Chlorphed-LA** (Roberts-Hauck)		In 15 ml spray.[4]
otc	**Dristan 12 Hr Nasal** (Whitehall)		In 15 ml.[5]
otc	**Duramist Plus** (Pfeiffer)		In 15 ml spray.[6]
otc	**Duration** (Schering-Plough)		In 15 and 30 ml spray and 15 ml pump spray.[2]
otc	**4-Way Long Lasting Nasal** (Bristol-Myers)		In 15 ml spray and spray pump.[7]
otc	**Genasal** (Goldline)		In 15 and 30 ml.[4]
otc	**Maximum Strength Nasal Decongestant** (Taro)		In 15 and 30 ml.[11]
otc	**Nasal Relief** (Rugby)		In 30 ml spray.[8]
otc	**Nostrilla** (Ciba Consumer)		In 15 ml pump spray.[9]
otc	**NTZ Long Acting Nasal** (Sterling Health)		**Drops:** In 15 ml.[1]
			Spray: In 15 ml.[1]
otc	**Sinarest 12 Hour** (Ciba Cons.)		In 15 ml spray.[3]
otc	**Vicks Sinex 12-Hour** (Procter & Gamble)		In 15 and 30 ml spray.[3,6]
otc	**Twice-A-Day** (Major)		In 15 and 30 ml.

[1] With benzalkonium chloride and EDTA.
[2] With benzalkonium chloride, glycine, phenylmercuric acetate and sorbitol.
[3] With aromatics (ie, menthol, camphor, eucalyptol).
[4] With phenylmercuric acetate.
[5] With benzalkonium chloride, hydroxypropylmethylcellulose and thimerosol.
[6] With thimerosal.
[7] With benzalkonium chloride, glycerin, sorbitol, EDTA and phenylmercuric acetate.
[8] With phenylmercuric acetate and EDTA.
[9] With benzalkonium chloride, glycine, sorbitol.
[10] With 0.02 mg/ml phenylmercuric acetate, benzalkonium chloride, glycine, sorbitol.
[11] With benzalkonium chloride and phenylmercuric acetate.

TETRAHYDROZOLINE HCl

For complete prescribing information, refer to the Nasal Decongestants group monograph.

Administration and Dosage:

Adults and children (≥ 6 years): 2 to 4 drops of 0.1% solution in each nostril every 3 to 4 hours as needed, or 3 to 4 sprays in each nostril every 4 hours as needed.

Children (2 to 6 years): 2 to 3 drops of 0.05% solution in each nostril every 4 to 6 hours, as necessary. Do not use the 0.1% solution in children < 6 years.

Rx	**Tyzine Pediatric Drops** (Kenwood/Bradley)	**Solution:** 0.05%	In 15 ml.[1]
Rx	**Tyzine** (Kenwood/Bradley)	**Solution:** 0.1%	**Drops:** In 30 ml.[1]
			Spray: In 15 ml.[1]

[1] With benzalkonium chloride and EDTA.

XYLOMETAZOLINE HCl

For complete prescribing information, refer to the Nasal Decongestants group monograph.

Administration and Dosage:

Adults (≥ 12 years): 2 to 3 drops or 2 to 3 sprays (0.1%) in each nostril every 8 to 10 hours.

Children (2 to 12 years): 2 to 3 drops (0.05%) in each nostril every 8 to 10 hours.

otc	**Otrivin Pediatric Nasal Drops** (Ciba Consumer)	**Solution:** 0.05%	In 25 ml dropper bottle.[1]
otc	**Otrivin** (Ciba Consumer)	**Solution:** 0.1%	**Drops:** In 25 ml dropper bottle.[1]
			Spray: In 20 ml.[1]

[1] With benzalkonium chloride and EDTA.

MISCELLANEOUS NASAL DECONGESTANTS

For complete prescribing information, refer to the Nasal Decongestants group monograph.

Rx	**No-Hist** (Dunhall)	**Capsules:** 5 mg phenylephrine HCl, 40 mg phenylpropanolamine HCl, 40 mg pseudoephedrine HCl	Caramel/buff. In 100s.

NASAL DECONGESTANT INHALERS

For complete prescribing information, refer to the Nasal Decongestants group monograph.

Administration and Dosage:

Adults and children (≥ 6 years): 1 to 2 inhalations in each nostril (while blocking the other nostril) not more than every 2 hours. Do not exceed recommended dosage. Do not use propylhexedrine for > 3 days or l-desoxyephedrine for > 7 days. If symptoms persist beyond this time, consult physician.

Abuse: Propylhexedrine has been extracted from inhalers and injected IV as an amphetamine substitute. It has also been ingested by soaking the fibrous interior in hot water. Chronic abuse has caused cardiomyopathy (severe left and right ventricular failure), pulmonary hypertension, foreign body granuloma (emboli), dyspnea and sudden death.

otc	**Benzedrex** (Menley & James)	**Inhaler:** 250 mg propylhexedrine	In single plastic inhalers.[1]
otc	**Vicks Inhaler** (Richardson-Vicks)	**Inhaler:** 50 mg l-desoxyephedrine	In single plastic inhalers.[2]

[1] With menthol and lavender oil.

[2] With bornyl acetate, camphor, lavender oil, menthol.

MISCELLANEOUS NASAL DECONGESTANT COMBINATIONS

For complete prescribing information, refer to the Nasal Decongestants group monograph.

In these combinations: **PHENYLEPHRINE HCl** and **NAPHAZOLINE HCl** are decongestants.

PYRILAMINE MALEATE and **PHENIRAMINE MALEATE** are antihistamines.

otc	**Myci-Spray** (Misemer)	**Solution**: 0.25% phenylephrine HCl, 0.15% pyrilamine maleate	In 20 ml spray.[1]
otc	**Dristan Nasal** (Whitehall)	**Solution**: 0.5% phenylephrine HCl and 0.2% pheniramine maleate	**Spray (regular)**: In 15 and 30 ml.[2]
			Spray (menthol): In 15 and 30 ml.[3]
otc	**4-Way Fast Acting Original** (Bristol-Myers)	**Solution**: 0.5% phenylephrine HCl, 0.05% naphazoline HCl and 0.2% pyrilamine maleate	**Spray (regular)**: In 15 and 30 ml.[4]
			Spray (menthol): In 15 and 30 ml.[5]

[1] With 0.04% cetalkonium chloride.
[2] With alcohol, benzalkonium chloride, eucalyptol, menthol, thimerosal.
[3] With benzalkonium chloride, camphor, eucalyptol, menthol, methyl salicylate, polysorbate 80, thimerosal.
[4] With benzalkonium chloride, thimerosal, poloxamer 188.
[5] With thimerosal, benzalkonium chloride, camphor, eucalyptol, menthol, poloxamer 188, polysorbate 80.

MISCELLANEOUS NASAL PRODUCTS

For complete prescribing information, refer to the Nasal Decongestants group monograph.

To restore moisture and relieve dry, crusted and inflamed nasal membranes due to colds, low humidity, nasal decongestant overuse, allergies, minor nose bleeds, intranasal and endoscopic sinus surgery and other irritations.

otc	**SalineX** (Muro)	**Solution**: 0.4% sodium chloride	**Drops**: In 15 ml.
			Mist: In 50 ml.[6]
otc	**Pretz** (Parnell)	**Solution**: 0.6% sodium chloride	In 15 ml.
otc	**Dristan Saline Spray** (Whitehall)	**Solution**: Sodium chloride	In 15 ml.[8]
otc	**Afrin Moisturizing Saline Mist** (Schering-Plough)	**Solution**: 0.64% sodium chloride	Benzalkonium chloride, EDTA. In 30 ml.
otc	**Ayr Saline** (Ascher)	**Solution**: 0.65% sodium chloride	**Drops**: In 50 ml.[9]
			Mist: In 50 ml.[9]
otc	**Breathe Free** (Thompson)		In 45 ml spray.[10]
otc	**HuMist Nasal Mist** (Scherer)		Alcohol free. In 45 ml spray.[11]
otc	**NaSal** (Sterling Health)		**Drops**: Alcohol free. In 15 ml.
			Spray: Alcohol free. In 15 ml.[9]
otc	**Nasal Moist** (Blairex)		In 45 ml spray.[12]
otc	**Ocean** (Fleming)		In 45 ml and pt.[12]
otc	**SeaMist** (Schein)		In 45 ml spray.[8]
otc	**Pretz Irrigating** (Parnell)	**Solution**: 0.75% sodium chloride	In 237 ml.[13]
otc	**Pretz Moisturizing** (Parnell)	**Drops**: 0.75% sodium chloride	In 50 ml.[13]

[6] With benzalkonium chloride, propylene glycol, polyethylene glycol.
[7] With benzalkonium chloride and 0.002% phenylmercuric acetate.
[8] With benzyl alcohol and benzalkonium chloride.
[9] With thimerosal and benzalkonium chloride.
[10] With benzalkonium chloride.
[11] With chlorobutanol.
[12] With benzyl alcohol.
[13] With 3% glycerin, *Mucoprotective Factor* yerba santa, phenylmercuric acetate.

INTRANASAL STEROIDS

For information on the systemic use of corticosteroids, refer to the Adrenal Cortical Steroids (glucocorticoids) monograph in the Hormones chapter.

Actions:

Pharmacology: These drugs have potent glucocorticoid and weak mineralocorticoid activity. The mechanisms responsible for the anti-inflammatory action of corticosteroids on the nasal mucosa are unknown. However, glucocorticoids have a wide range of inhibitory activities against multiple cell types (eg, mast cells, eosinophils, neutrophils, macrophages, lymphocytes) and mediators (eg, histamine, eicosanoids, leukotrienes, cytokines) involved in allergic and nonallergic/irritant-mediated inflammation. These agents, when administered topically in recommended doses, exert direct local anti-inflammatory effects with minimal systemic effects. Exceeding the recommended dose may result in systemic effects, including hypothalamic-pituitary-adrenal (HPA) function suppression.

Pharmacokinetics: The amount of an intranasal dose that reaches systemic circulation is generally low, and metabolism is rapid.

Indications:

See individual product listings for specific labeled indications.

Contraindications:

Untreated localized infections involving the nasal mucosa; hypersensitivity to the drug or any component of the product.

Warnings:

Systemic corticosteroids: The combined administration of alternate day systemic prednisone with these products may increase the likelihood of HPA suppression. Therefore, use with caution in patients already on alternate day prednisone.

During withdrawal from oral corticosteroids, some patients may experience symptoms (eg, joint or muscular pain, lassitude, depression). Carefully monitor patients previously treated for prolonged periods with systemic corticosteroids and transferred to intranasal steroids to avoid acute adrenal insufficiency in response to stress. This is particularly important in patients who have asthma or other conditions where too rapid a decrease in systemic corticosteroids may cause a severe exacerbation of their symptoms.

Excessive doses/sensitivity: If recommended doses of intranasal beclomethasone are exceeded or if individuals are particularly sensitive or predisposed by virtue of recent systemic steroid therapy, symptoms of hypercorticism may occur, including, very rarely, menstrual irregularities, acneiform lesions and cushingoid features. If such changes occur, discontinue slowly, consistent with accepted procedures for discontinuing oral steroids.

Hypersensitivity: Rare cases of immediate and delayed hypersensitivity reactions, including angioedema and bronchospasm, have occurred. Have epinephrine 1:1000 immediately available. Refer to Management of Acute Hypersensitivity Reactions.

Pregnancy: Category C. In animals, systemic administration of large doses produced teratogenic, fetotoxic and embryocidal effects. Topical administration of recommended doses is unlikely to achieve significant systemic levels; however, use these agents during pregnancy only if the potential benefits outweigh the potential hazards to the fetus.

Carefully observe infants born of mothers who have received substantial doses of corticosteroids during pregnancy for signs of adrenal insufficiency.

Lactation: Advise mothers taking pharmacologic doses not to nurse. **Dexamethasone** appears in breast milk and could suppress growth, interfere with endogenous corticosteroid production or cause other unwanted effects.

Beclomethasone, budesonide, flunisolide, triamcinolone – It is not known whether these drugs are excreted in breast milk. Use caution when administering to nursing women.

Children: Safety and efficacy for use in children < 6 years or < 12 years (**triamcinolone**) have not been established. Use in children < 6 years is not recommended; carefully follow growth and development if prolonged therapy is used.

Precautions:

Infections: Localized infections of the nose and pharynx with *Candida albicans* have developed only rarely. When such an infection occurs, it may require treatment with appropriate local therapy or discontinuation of steroid treatment.

When steroids are used in the presence of infection, use proper anti-infective therapy.

Use with caution in patients with active or quiescent tuberculosis infections of the respiratory tract, or in untreated fungal, bacterial or systemic viral infections or ocular herpes simplex. Avoid exposure to chicken pox or measles.

INTRANASAL STEROIDS

Wound healing: Because of the inhibitory effect of corticosteroids on wound healing in patients who have experienced recent nasal septal ulcers, recurrent epistaxis, nasal surgery or trauma, use nasal steroids with caution until healing has occurred.

Vasoconstrictors: In the presence of excessive nasal mucosa secretion or edema of the nasal mucosa, the drug may fail to reach the site of intended action. In such cases, use a nasal vasoconstrictor during the first 2 to 3 days of therapy.

Systemic effects: Although systemic absorption is low when used in recommended dosage, HPA suppression and other systemic effects may occur, especially with excessive doses.

Long-term treatment: Examine patients periodically over several months or longer for possible changes in the nasal mucosa.

Adverse Reactions:

Most common: Mild nasopharyngeal irritation; nasal irritation (budesonide, 3% to 9%); burning; stinging; dryness; headache.

Other: Lightheadedness; nausea (budesonide, < 1%); epistaxis (budesonide, 3% to 9%) bloody mucus; rebound congestion; bronchial asthma; occasional sneezing attacks (may be more common in children); rhinorrhea; anosmia or reduced sense of smell (budesonide, < 1%); loss of sense of taste/bad taste in mouth (budesonide, < 1%); throat discomfort; ulceration of the nasal mucosa; watery eyes; sore throat; vomiting; immediate and delayed hypersensitivity reactions (Warnings); localized infections of nose and pharynx with *C albicans* (Precautions); wheezing (extremely rare; budesonide, < 1%); nasal septum perforation/mucosal atrophy/necrosis, increased intraocular pressure (extremely rare); signs of adrenal hypercorticism (ie, Cushing's syndrome), especially with overdosage.

Budesonide – Pharyngitis, cough increased (3% to 9%); dry mouth, dyspepsia (> 1%); moniliasis, hoarseness, nasal pain, facial edema, rash, pruritus, herpes simplex, dyspnea, nervousness, alopecia, myalgia, arthralgia (< 1%); contact dermatitis (rare).

Patient Information:

Patient instructions provided with products.

Do not exceed recommended dosage.

May cause irritation and drying of nasal mucosa. Contact physician if symptoms do not improve, if the condition worsens or if sneezing or nasal irritation occurs.

Clear nasal passages of secretions prior to use. If nasal passages are blocked, use a decongestant just before administration to ensure adequate penetration of the spray.

Effects are not immediate. Benefit requires regular use and usually occurs within a few days.

DEXAMETHASONE SODIUM PHOSPHATE

Indications:

Allergic or inflammatory nasal conditions; nasal polyps (excluding polyps originating within the sinuses).

Administration and Dosage:

Adults: 2 sprays (168 mcg) into each nostril 2 or 3 times a day. Maximum daily dose is 12 sprays (1008 mcg).

Children: 1 or 2 sprays (84 to 168 mcg) into each nostril 2 times a day. Maximum daily dose is 8 sprays (672 mcg).

When improvement occurs, reduce dosage. Some patients will be symptom free on 1 spray into each nostril 2 times a day. Do not exceed the recommended dosage. Discontinue therapy as soon as feasible. Reinstitute if symptoms recur.

Rx	**Dexacort Phosphate Turbinaire** (Adams)	**Aerosol:** Each metered spray delivers dexamethasone sodium phosphate equivalent to ≈ 84 mcg dexamethasone (170 sprays per cartridge)	2% alcohol. In 12.6 g with adapter or 12.6 g refill.

FLUNISOLIDE

Indications:

Relief of the symptoms of seasonal or perennial rhinitis when effectiveness of or tolerance to conventional treatment is unsatisfactory.

Administration and Dosage:

Adults: Starting dose is 2 sprays (50 mcg) in each nostril 2 times a day (total dose 200 mcg/day). May increase to 2 sprays in each nostril 3 times a day (total dose 300 mcg/day). Maximum daily dose is 8 sprays in each nostril (400 mcg/day).

Children: Starting dose is 1 spray (25 mcg) in each nostril 3 times a day or 2 sprays (50 mcg) in each nostril 2 times a day (total dose 150 to 200 mcg/day). Maximum daily dose is 4 sprays in each nostril (200 mcg/day).

Improvement in symptoms usually becomes apparent within a few days. However, relief may not occur in some patients for as long as 3 weeks. Do not continue beyond 3 weeks in absence of significant symptomatic improvement.

Maintenance dose: After desired clinical effect is obtained, reduce maintenance dose to smallest amount necessary to control symptoms. Approximately 15% of patients with perennial rhinitis may be maintained on 1 spray in each nostril per day.

Rx	**Nasalide** (Syntex)	**Spray**: Each actuation delivers ≈ 25 mcg flunisolide[1]	In 25 ml bottles (≥ 200 sprays per bottle) with pump unit.
Rx	**Nasarel** (Roche)	**Solution, spray**: 0.025% flunisolide	In 25 ml spray bottle (200 actuations).

[1] With propylene glycol, polyethylene glycol 3350, benzalkonium chloride, EDTA.

BECLOMETHASONE DIPROPIONATE

Indications:

Relief of the symptoms of seasonal or perennial rhinitis in those cases poorly responsive to conventional treatment.

Prevention of recurrence of nasal polyps following surgical removal.

Spray formulations: For nonallergic (vasomotor) rhinitis.

Administration and Dosage:

Adults and children ≥ 12 years: 1 inhalation (42 mcg) in each nostril 2 to 4 times a day (total dose 168 to 336 mcg/day). Patients can often be maintained on a maximum dose of 1 inhalation in each nostril 3 times a day (252 mcg/day).

Children 6 to 12 years of age: 1 inhalation in each nostril 3 times a day (252 mcg/day). Not recommended for children < 6 years of age since safety and efficacy studies have not been conducted in this age group.

Improvement in symptoms usually becomes apparent within a few days. Results from two clinical trials showed significant symptomatic relief within 3 days. Relief may not occur in some patients for as long as 2 weeks. Do not continue therapy beyond 3 weeks in the absence of symptomatic improvement.

Nasal polyps: Treatment may have to be continued for several weeks or more before a therapeutic result can be fully assessed. Recurrence of symptoms due to polyps can occur after stopping treatment, depending on the severity of the disease.

Storage: Therapeutic effect may decrease when aerosol canister is cold. Shake well before using.

Rx	**Beconase Inhalation** (Glaxo Wellcome)	**Aerosol**: Each actuation delivers 42 mcg beclomethasone dipropionate	In 16.8 g canisters (200 metered doses per canister)[1] with adapter or 16.8 g refills.[1]
Rx	**Vancenase Nasal Inhaler** (Schering)		In 16.8 g canisters (200 metered doses per canister)[1] with adapter.
Rx	**Beconase AQ Nasal** (Glaxo Wellcome)	**Spray**: 0.042% beclomethasone dipropionate, monohydrate	In 25 g bottles (≥ 200 metered doses per bottle)[2] with metering atomizing pump and nasal adapter.
Rx	**Vancenase AQ Nasal** (Schering)		In 25 g bottles (≥ 200 metered doses per bottle)[2] with metered pump and nasal adapter.
Rx	**Vancenase AQ Nasal** (Schering)	**Spray**: 0.084% beclomethasone dipropionate, monohydrate	In 19 g[3] (120 actuations) with metered pump.

[1] With propellants.
[2] With benzalkonium chloride and 0.25% w/w phenylethyl alcohol.
[3] With benzalkonium chloride.

TRIAMCINOLONE ACETONIDE

Indications:

Treatment of seasonal and perennial allergic rhinitis symptoms.

Administration and Dosage:

Adults and children > 12 years: Individual patients will experience a variable time to onset and degree of symptom relief. Starting dose is 2 sprays (110 mcg) in each nostril once a day (total dose 220 mcg/day). Assess the effect in 4 to 7 days; some relief can be expected in approximately two-thirds of patients within that time. May increase to 440 mcg/day either as once-a-day dosage or divided up to 4 times a day (ie, twice a day [2 sprays/nostril] or 4 times a day [1 spray/nostril]). The degree of relief does not seem to be significantly different when comparing 2 or 4 times a day dosing with once-a-day dosing. After desired effect is obtained, some patients (≈ 50%) may be maintained on as little as 1 spray in each nostril once a day.

A dose response between 110 and 440 mcg/day is not clearly discernible. In general, the highest dose tends to provide relief sooner. This suggests an alternative approach to starting therapy: Start treatment with 440 mcg (4 sprays/nostril/day), and then, depending on response, decrease the dose by 1 spray per day every 4 to 7 days.

A decrease in symptoms may occur as soon as 12 hours after starting steroid therapy and generally can be expected to occur within a few days of initiating therapy in allergic rhinitis. If improvement is not evident after 2 to 3 weeks, re-evaluate the patient.

Rx	**Nasacort** (Rhone-Poulenc Rorer)	**Spray:** ≈ 55 mcg triamcinolone acetonide per actuation	In 15 mg canisters (100 sprays). In 10 g canisters.
Rx	**Nasacort AQ** (Rhone-Poulenc Rorer)	**Spray pump:** 55 mcg triamcinolone acetonide per actuation	Benzalkonium chloride, EDTA. In aqueous base. In 16.5 g bottles (120 actuations).

BUDESONIDE

Indications:

Management of symptoms of seasonal or perennial allergic rhinitis in adults and children and nonallergic perennial rhinitis in adults.

Administration and Dosage:

Approved by the FDA on February 21, 1994.

Adults and children ≥ 6 years of age: Recommended starting dose is 256 mcg daily, given as either 2 sprays in each nostril in the morning and evening or as 4 sprays in each nostril in the morning. Doses exceeding 256 mcg daily (4 sprays/nostril) are not recommended. After the desired clinical effect has been obtained, reduce the maintenance dose to the smallest amount necessary for control of symptoms; gradually decrease the dose every 2 to 4 weeks as long as desired effect is maintained. If symptoms return, the dose may briefly be increased to the starting dose.

A decrease in symptoms may occur as soon as 24 hours after onset of treatment, but it generally takes 3 to 7 days to reach maximum benefit. If no improvement occurs by the third week of treatment, discontinue therapy.

Children < 6 years of age or with nonallergic perennial rhinitis: Not recommended because adequate numbers of these children have not been studied.

Storage/Stability: Store with valve downwards. Shake well before use. After opening aluminum pouch, use within 6 months. Avoid storage in areas of high humidity.

Rx	**Rhinocort** (Astra)	**Aerosol:** 32 mcg budesonide per actuation	In 7 g canisters (200 sprays).

FLUTICASONE PROPIONATE

Indications:

Management of seasonal and perennial allergic rhinitis in patients ≥ 12 years.

Administration and Dosage:

Approved by the FDA on October 19, 1994.

Adults: Recommended starting dose is 2 sprays (50 mcg each) per nostril once daily (total daily dose, 200 mcg). The same dosage divided into 100 mcg given twice daily (eg, 8:00 am and 8:00 pm) is also effective. After the first few days, dosage may be reduced to 100 mcg (1 spray per nostril) once daily for maintenance therapy. Maximum total daily dosage should not exceed 200 mcg/day.

Adolescents ≥ 12 years of age: Start most adolescents with 100 mcg (1 spray/nostril). Patients not adequately responding to 100 mcg or patients with more severe symptoms may use 200 mcg (2 sprays/nostril). Depending on response, dosage may be decreased to 100 mcg daily. Total daily dosage should not exceed 200 mcg/day.

Children < 12 years of age or patients with nonallergic rhinitis: Use not recommended.

Rx	**Flonase** (Glaxo Wellcome)	**Spray**: 50 mcg fluticasone propionate/ actuation (100 mg)[1]	In 9 g (60 actuations) and 16 g (120 actuations) amber glass bottles.
Rx	**Flovent** (Glaxo Wellcome)	**Spray, aerosol**: 44 mcg fluticasone propionate/ actuation.	In 17.9 g (60 actuations) or 13 g (120 actuations) canisters.
		110 mcg fluticasone propionate/ actuation.	In 13 g (120 actuations) canisters.
		220 mg fluticasone propionate/ actuation.	In 13 g (120 actuations) canisters.

[1] 0.02% w/w benzalkonium chloride, 0.025% w/w phenylethyl alcohol.

ALPHA$_1$-PROTEINASE INHIBITOR (HUMAN)

Actions:

Pharmacology: Alpha$_1$-proteinase inhibitor (alpha$_1$-PI; alpha$_1$-antitrypsin) is a sterile, stable, lyophilized preparation of purified human alpha$_1$-proteinase inhibitor used in patients with panacinar emphysema who have alpha$_1$-antitrypsin deficiency. It is prepared from pooled human plasma of normal donors. Each unit of plasma has been tested and found nonreactive for HIV antibody and hepatitis B surface antigen (HBsAg). See Warnings.

The specific activity of alpha$_1$-proteinase inhibitor is $\geq$ 0.35 mg functional alpha$_1$-PI/mg protein. When reconstituted, alpha$_1$-PI has a concentration of $\geq$ 20 mg/ml, a pH of 6.6 to 7.4, a sodium content of 100 to 210 mEq/L, a chloride content of 60 to 180 mEq/L, a sodium phosphate content of 0.015 to 0.025 M, a polyethylene glycol content of NMT 5 ppm and NMT 0.1% sucrose; contains small amounts of other plasma proteins.

Alpha$_1$-antitrypsin deficiency is a chronic hereditary, usually fatal, autosomal recessive disorder in which a low concentration of alpha$_1$-PI is associated with slowly progressive, severe, panacinar emphysema that most often manifests itself in the third to fourth decades of life. Although the terms "alpha$_1$-proteinase inhibitor" and "alpha$_1$-antitrypsin" are used interchangeably in the scientific literature, the hereditary disorder associated with a reduction in the serum level of alpha$_1$-PI is conventionally referred to as "alpha$_1$-antitrypsin deficiency" while the deficient protein is referred to as "alpha$_1$-proteinase inhibitor".

The pathogenesis is not well understood. It is believed to be due to a chronic biochemical imbalance between elastase (an enzyme capable of degrading elastin tissues, released by inflammatory cells, primarily neutrophils, in the lower respiratory tract) and alpha$_1$-PI (the principal inhibitor of neutrophil elastase). As a result, alveolar structures are unprotected from chronic exposure to elastase resulting in progressive degradation of elastin tissues. The eventual outcome is emphysema. Neonatal hepatitis with cholestatic jaundice appears in $\approx$ 10% of newborns with alpha$_1$-antitrypsin deficiency. In some adults, alpha$_1$-antitrypsin deficiency is complicated by cirrhosis.

Pharmacokinetics: In clinical studies of alpha$_1$-PI in 23 subjects with the PiZZ variant of congenital deficiency of alpha$_1$-antitrypsin deficiency and documented destructive lung disease, the mean in vivo recovery of alpha$_1$-PI was 4.2 mg (immunologic)/dl/mg (functional)/kg administered. Half-life of alpha$_1$-PI in vivo was $\approx$ 4.5 days. Nineteen of the subjects received alpha$_1$-PI replacement therapy, 60 mg/kg, once weekly for up to 26 weeks (avg 24 wks). Blood levels of alpha$_1$-PI were maintained above 80 mg/dl. Within a few weeks, bronchoalveolar lavage studies demonstrated significantly increased levels of alpha$_1$-PI and functional antineutrophil elastase capacity in the epithelial lining fluid of the lower respiratory tract of the lungs.

Indications:

Congenital alpha$_1$-antitrypsin deficiency: For chronic replacement in individuals with clinically demonstrable panacinar emphysema. Only those with early evidence of such disease should be considered for chronic replacement therapy with alpha$_1$-PI. Subjects with the PiMZ or PiMS phenotypes of alpha$_1$-antitrypsin deficiency should not be considered for such treatment as they appear to be at small risk for panacinar emphysema. Only adult subjects have received alpha$_1$-PI to date.

Alpha$_1$-proteinase inhibitor is not indicated for use in patients other than those with PiZZ, PiZ(null) or Pi(null);(null) phenotypes.

Warnings:

Infectious transmission: Alpha$_1$-PI is purified from large pools of fresh human plasma obtained from many paid donors. Although each unit of plasma has been found nonreactive for hepatitis B surface antigen (HBsAg) using an FDA-approved test, the presence of hepatitis viruses in such pools must be assumed.

Alpha$_1$-PI is heat-treated to reduce potential for transmission of infectious agents. No procedure has been totally effective in removing viral infectivity from plasma products. No cases of hepatitis, either hepatitis B or non-A, non-B were recorded in individuals on alpha$_1$-PI. However, all individuals received prophylaxis against hepatitis B.

Pregnancy: Category C. It is not known whether this drug can cause fetal harm when administered to a pregnant woman or can affect reproduction capacity. Use only when clearly needed and when the potential benefits outweigh the potential hazards to the fetus.

Children: Safety and efficacy in children have not been established.

ALPHA$_1$-PROTEINASE INHIBITOR (HUMAN)

Precautions:

Monitoring: The "threshold" level of alpha$_1$-PI in serum believed to provide adequate anti-elastase activity in lungs of individuals with alpha$_1$-antitrypsin deficiency is 80 mg/dl (based on commercial standards for alpha$_1$-PI immunologic assay). However, assays based on commercial standards measure antigenic activity of alpha$_1$-PI whereas labeled potency value is expressed as actual functional activity (ie, actual capacity to neutralize porcine pancreatic elastase). As functional activity may be less than antigenic activity, serum levels determined by commercial immunologic assays may not accurately reflect actual functional alpha$_1$-PI levels. Therefore, although it may help to monitor serum levels using currently available commercial assays of antigenic activity, do not use these results to determine required dosage.

A number of factors could reduce the efficacy of this product or even result in an ill effect, including improper storage and handling of the product, diagnosis, dosage, method of administration and biological differences in patients. It is important that this product be stored properly, that directions be followed carefully, and that the risk of transmitting viruses be carefully weighed before prescribing the product.

Circulatory overload: As with any colloid solution, there will be an increase in plasma volume following IV administration of alpha$_1$-PI. Exercise caution in patients at risk for circulatory overload.

Hepatitis B immunization: In preparation for receiving alpha$_1$-PI, recipients should be immunized against hepatitis B using a licensed Hepatitis B Vaccine. Should it become necessary to treat an individual with alpha$_1$-PI, and time is insufficient for adequate antibody response to vaccination, administer a single dose of Hepatitis B Immune Globulin (Human), 0.06 ml/kg IM, at the time of administration of the initial dose of Hepatitis B Vaccine.

Adverse Reactions:

Delayed fever (maximum temperature rise 38.9°C, resolving spontaneously over 24 hours) occurring up to 12 hours following treatment (0.77%); lightheadedness (0.19%); dizziness (0.19%). Mild transient leukocytosis several hours after infusion also occurred.

Administration and Dosage:

For IV use only. May be given at a rate of 0.08 ml/kg/min or greater.

IV Administration of Alpha$_1$-Proteinase Inhibitor

Body weight (approx lb/kg)	Dosage[1] (mg)	IV administration rate[2] (ml/min)
75/34	2040	2.7
90/41	2460	3.3
105/48	2880	3.8
120/55	3300	4.4
135/61	3660	4.9
150/68	4080	5.5
165/75	4500	6.0
180/82	4920	6.5
195/89	5340	7.1
210/96	5760	7.6
225/102	6120	8.2
240/109	6540	8.7

[1] Based on 60 mg/kg.
[2] Based on 0.08 ml/kg/min.

Dosage: 60 mg/kg once weekly to increase and maintain a level of functional alpha$_1$-PI in the epithelial lining of the lower respiratory tract providing adequate anti-elastase activity in the lungs of individuals with alpha$_1$-antitrypsin deficiency.

Stability: Give within 3 hrs after reconstitution. Give alone without mixing other agents or diluting solutions. If required, alpha$_1$-PI may be diluted with normal saline.

Storage: Refrigerate at 2° to 8°C (35° to 46°F). Avoid freezing. Do not refrigerate after reconstitution. Discard unused solution.

Rx	**Prolastin** (Bayer)	**Injection:** ≥ 20 mg alpha$_1$-PI per ml when reconstituted	Preservative free. In ≈ 500 mg activity/single-dose vial[3] w/20 ml sterile water or ≈ 1000 mg activity/single-dose vial[3] w/40 ml sterile water.

[3] With polyethylene glycol, sucrose and small amounts of other plasma proteins. With total alpha$_1$-PI[3] functional activity in mg stated on the label of each vial.

COLFOSCERIL PALMITATE (Synthetic Lung Surfactant; Dipalmitoylphosphatidylcholine; DPPC)

Actions:

Pharmacology: Surfactant deficiency is an important factor in the development of the neonatal respiratory distress syndrome (RDS). Thus, surfactant replacement therapy early in the course of RDS should ameliorate the disease and improve symptoms. Natural surfactant, a combination of lipids and apoproteins, exhibits not only surface tension reducing properties (conferred by the lipids), but also rapid spreading and adsorption (conferred by the apoproteins). The major fraction of the lipid component of natural surfactant is dipalmitoylphosphatidylcholine (DPPC), which comprises up to 70% of natural surfactant by weight.

Although DPPC reduces surface tension, DPPC alone is ineffective in RDS because it spreads and adsorbs poorly. In colfosceril, which is protein-free, cetyl alcohol acts as the spreading agent for the DPPC on the air-fluid interface. Tyloxapol, a polymeric long-chain repeating alcohol, is a nonionic surfactant which acts to disperse both DPPC and cetyl alcohol. Sodium chloride is added to adjust osmolality.

Pharmacokinetics: Colfosceril is administered directly into the trachea. DPPC can be absorbed from the alveolus into lung tissue where it can be catabolized extensively and reutilized for further phospholipid synthesis and secretion. In the developing rabbit, 90% of alveolar phospholipids are recycled. In premature rabbits, the alveolar half-life of intratracheally administered phosphatidylcholine is approximately 12 hours.

Clinical trials:

Prophylactic treatment – The efficacy of a single dose of colfosceril in prophylactic treatment of infants at risk of developing RDS was examined in three double-blind, placebo controlled studies, one involving 215 infants weighing 500 to 700 g, one involving 385 infants weighing 700 to 1350 g, and one involving 446 infants weighing 700 to 1100 g (see following table). The infants were intubated and placed on mechanical ventilation, and received 5 ml/kg or placebo (air) within 30 minutes of birth.

The efficacy of one vs three doses of colfosceril in prophylactic treatment of infants at risk of developing RDS was examined in a double-blind, placebo controlled study of 823 infants weighing 700 to 1100 g (see following table). The infants were intubated and placed on mechanical ventilation, and received a first 5 ml/kg dose within 30 minutes. Repeat 5 ml/kg doses of colfosceril or placebo (air) were given to all infants who remained on mechanical ventilation at approximately 12 and 24 hours of age.

Prophylactic Colfosceril Treatment - Efficacy Assessment

	Number of doses (birth weight range)							
	Single dose (500 to 700 g)		Single dose (700 to 1350 g)		Single dose (700 to 1100 g)		One vs three doses (700 to 1100 g)	
Parameter	Placebo (n=106)	Colfo-sceril (n=109)	Placebo (n=185)	Colfo-sceril (n=176)	Placebo (n=222)	Colfosceril (n=224)	One dose (n=356)	Three doses (n=360)
Death ≤ day 28	53%	50%	11%	6%	21%	15%	16%	9%
Death through 1 year	59%	60%	14%	11%	30%	20%	17%	12%
Death from RDS	25%	13%	4%	3%	10%	5%	3%	2%
Intact cardiopulmonary survival[1]	29%	25%	69%	78%	65%	68%	74%	78%
Bronchopulmonary dysplasia	43%	44%	23%	18%	19%	21%	8%	12%
RDS incidence	73%	81%	46%	42%	55%	55%	63%	68%

[1] Defined by survival through 28 days of life without bronchopulmonary dysplasia.

Rescue treatment – The efficacy of colfosceril in the rescue treatment of infants with RDS was examined in two double-blind, placebo controlled studies (see following table). One study enrolled 419 infants weighing 700 to 1350 g; the second enrolled 1237 infants weighing ≥ 1250 g. Infants received an initial dose (5 ml/kg) of colfosceril or placebo (air) between 2 and 24 hours of life followed by a second dose (5 ml/kg) approximately 12 hours later to infants who remained on mechanical ventilation.

COLFOSCERIL PALMITATE (Synthetic Lung Surfactant; Dipalmitoylphosphatidylcholine; DPPC)

Rescue Colfosceril Treatment – Efficacy Assessments				
	Number of doses (birth weight range)			
	Two doses (700 to 1350 g)		Two doses (≥ 1250 g)	
Parameter	Placebo (n = 213)	Colfosceril (n = 206)	Placebo (n = 623)	Colfosceril (n = 614)
Death ≤ day 28	23%	11%	7%	4%
Death through 1 year	27%	15%	9%	6%
Death from RDS	10%	3%	3%	1%
Intact cardiopulmonary survival[1]	62%	75%	88%	93%
Bronchopulmonary dysplasia	18%	15%	6%	3%

[1] Defined by survival through 28 days of life without bronchopulmonary dysplasia.

Results – In these six controlled clinical studies, infants in the colfosceril group showed significant improvements in fraction of inspired oxygen (FiO_2) and ventilator settings which persisted for at least 7 days. Pulmonary air leaks were significantly reduced in each study. Five of these studies also showed a significant reduction in death from RDS. Further, overall mortality was reduced for all infants weighing > 700 g. The one vs three dose prophylactic treatment study in 700 to 1100 g infants showed a further reduction in overall mortality with two additional doses. Various forms of pulmonary air leak and use of pancuronium were reduced in infants receiving colfosceril in all six studies. Follow-up data at 1 year adjusted age are available on 1094 of 2470 surviving infants. Growth and development of infants who received colfosceril in this sample were comparable to infants who received placebo.

Indications:

Prophylactic treatment: Infants with birth weights < 1350 g at risk of developing RDS. Infants with birth weights > 1350 g who have evidence of pulmonary immaturity.

Rescue treatment: Infants who have developed RDS.

For *prophylactic* treatment, administer the first dose as soon as possible after birth (see Administration and Dosage).

Infants considered as candidates for *rescue* treatment with colfosceril should be on mechanical ventilation and have a diagnosis of RDS by both of the following criteria:

1.) Respiratory distress not attributable to causes other than RDS, based on clinical and laboratory assessments.

2.) Chest radiographic findings consistent with the diagnosis of RDS.

Warnings:

Intratracheal administration: Administer only by instillation into the trachea (see Administration and Dosage).

The use of colfosceril requires expert clinical care by experienced neonatologists and other clinicians accomplished at neonatal intubation and ventilatory management. Adequate personnel, facilities, equipment and medications are required to optimize perinatal outcome in premature infants.

Instillation of colfosceril should be performed only by trained medical personnel experienced in airway and clinical management of unstable premature infants. Give vigilant clinical attention to all infants prior to, during and after administration.

Pulmonary effects: Colfosceril can rapidly affect oxygenation and lung compliance.

Lung compliance – If chest expansion improves substantially after dosing, reduce peak ventilator inspiratory pressures immediately, without waiting for confirmation of respiratory improvement by blood gas assessment. Failure to reduce inspiratory ventilator pressures rapidly can result in lung overdistention and fatal pulmonary air leak.

Hyperoxia – If the infant becomes pink, and transcutaneous oxygen saturation is in excess of 95%, reduce FiO_2 in small but repeated steps (until saturation is 90% to 95%) without waiting for confirmation of elevated arterial pO_2 by blood gas assessment. Failure to reduce FiO_2 in such instances can result in hyperoxia.

Hypocarbia – If arterial or transcutaneous CO_2 measurements are < 30 torr, reduce the ventilator rate at once. Failure to reduce ventilator rates in such instances can result in marked hypocarbia, which is known to reduce brain blood flow.

COLFOSCERIL PALMITATE (Synthetic Lung Surfactant; Dipalmitoylphosphatidylcholine; DPPC)

Pulmonary hemorrhage: In the single study conducted in infants weighing < 700 g at birth, the incidence of pulmonary hemorrhage was significantly increased in the colfosceril group (10% vs 2% in the placebo group). None of the five studies involving infants with birth weights > 700 g showed a significant increase in pulmonary hemorrhage in the colfosceril group. In an analysis of these five studies, pulmonary hemorrhage was reported for 1% (14/1420) of infants in the placebo group and 2% (27/1411) of infants in the colfosceril group. Fatal pulmonary hemorrhage occurred in three infants, two in the colfosceril group and one in the placebo group. Mortality from all causes among infants who developed pulmonary hemorrhage was 43% in the placebo group and 37% in the colfosceril group.

Pulmonary hemorrhage in both colfosceril and placebo infants was more frequent in infants who were younger, smaller, male or who had a patent ductus arteriosus. Pulmonary hemorrhage typically occurred in the first 2 days of life in both treatment groups.

In > 7700 infants in the open, uncontrolled study, pulmonary hemorrhage occurred in 4%, but fatal pulmonary hemorrhage was reported rarely (0.4%).

In the controlled clinical studies, colfosceril-treated infants who received steroids > 24 hours prior to delivery or indomethacin postnatally had a lower rate of pulmonary hemorrhage than other colfosceril-treated infants. Pay attention to early and aggressive diagnosis and treatment (unless contraindicated) of patent ductus arteriosus during the first 2 days of life (while the ductus arteriosus is often clinically silent). Other potentially protective measures include attempting to decrease FiO_2 preferentially over ventilator pressures during the first 24 to 48 hours after dosing, and attempting to decrease positive end-expiratory pressure (PEEP) minimally for at least 48 hours after dosing.

Mucous plugs: Infants whose ventilation becomes markedly impaired during or shortly after dosing may have mucous plugging of the endotracheal tube, particularly if pulmonary secretions were prominent prior to drug administration. Suctioning of all infants prior to dosing may lessen the chance of mucous plugs obstructing the endotracheal tube. If endotracheal tube obstruction is suspected, and suctioning is unsuccessful in removing the obstruction, replace the blocked endotracheal tube immediately.

Precautions:

Congenital anomalies: In controlled clinical studies, infants known prenatally or postnatally to have major congenital anomalies, or who were suspected of having congenital infection, were excluded from entry. However, these disorders cannot be recognized early in life in all cases, and a few infants with these conditions were entered. The benefits of colfosceril in the affected infants who received the drug appeared to be similar to the benefits observed in infants without anomalies or occult infection.

Prophylactic treatment — Infants < 700 g: In infants weighing 500 to 700 g, a single prophylactic dose of colfosceril significantly improved FiO_2 and ventilator settings, reduced pneumothorax, and reduced death from RDS, but increased pulmonary hemorrhage (see Warnings). Overall mortality did not differ significantly between the placebo and colfosceril groups. Data on multiple doses in infants in this weight class are not yet available. Accordingly, clinicians should carefully evaluate the potential risks and benefits of administration in these infants.

Rescue treatment — Number of doses: A small number of infants with RDS have received more than two doses of colfosceril as rescue treatment. Definitive data on the safety and efficacy of these additional doses are not available.

Adverse Reactions:

Premature birth is associated with a high incidence of morbidity and mortality. Despite significant reductions in overall mortality associated with colfosceril, some infants who received colfosceril developed severe complications and either survived with permanent handicaps or died.

In controlled clinical studies evaluating the safety and efficacy of colfosceril, numerous safety assessments were made. In infants receiving colfosceril, pulmonary hemorrhage, apnea and use of methylxanthines were increased. A number of other adverse events were significantly reduced in the colfosceril group, particularly various forms of pulmonary air leak and use of pancuronium.

COLFOSCERIL PALMITATE (Synthetic Lung Surfactant; Dipalmitoylphosphatidylcholine; DPPC)

Cofosceril Adverse Reactions (%)[1]				
	Prophylactic treatment (1 to 3 doses)		Rescue treatment (2 doses)	
Adverse reaction	Colfosceril (n = 883)	Placebo (n = 878)	Colfosceril (n = 821)	Placebo (n = 835)
Intraventricular hemorrhage				
Overall	27-57	31-51	18-52	23-48
Severe	8-25	9-26	4-9	5-13
Pulmonary air leak				
Overall	11-48	16-52	18-34	30-54
Pneumothorax	6-12	5-23	10-20	20-29
Pneumopericardium	0-4	< 1-2	1-2	1-4
Pneumomediastinum	1-3	2-7	2-4	5-8
Pulmonary interstitial emphysema	7-44	13-43	13-25	24-48
Death	< 1-6	< 1-4	1-3	< 1-7
Patent ductus arteriosus	53-70	49-66	45-57	54-66
Necrotizing enterocolitis	2-13	2-11	2-3	1-3
Pulmonary hemorrhage	4-10	1-4	1	< 1-3
Congenital pneumonia	1-4	1-4	2-3	2
Nosocomial pneumonia	4-15	2-14	2-7	2-5
Non-pulmonary infections	29-39	28-35	13-22	13-19
Sepsis	24-34	23-30	8-17	8-15
Death from sepsis	2-4	1-4	≤ 1	< 1
Meningitis	1-6	1-4	< 1	1
Other infections	3-11	5-10	6-8	5
Major anomalies	1-4	2-7	3-4	3-4
Hypotension	47-77	52-70	39-57	50-62
Hyperbilirubinemia	21-61	20-63	10-19	12-17
Exchange transfusion	1-3	1-4	2-4	1-3
Thrombocytopenia[2]	8-25	9-21	< 1-11	4-10
Persistent fetal circulation	< 1-2	0-1	1-2	1-6
Seizures	2-9	2-11	3-10	6-10
Apnea	33-73	34-76	44-65	37-48
Additional drug therapy required				
Antibiotics	96-99	96-99	98-99	98-100
Anticonvulsants	8-24	9-23	5-17	10-17
Diuretics	37-65	39-64	34-65	45-60
Inotropes	20-40	20-46	16-31	27-36
Methylxanthines	43-82	38-77	53-74	49-62
Pancuronium	11-14	15-22	15-17	33-34
Sedatives	52-71	52-65	64-68	72-76

[1] Data pooled from several birth weight ranges.
[2] Thrombocytopenia requiring platelet transfusion.

Pulmonary hemorrhage: See Warnings.

Abnormal laboratory values are common in critically ill, mechanically ventilated, premature infants. A higher incidence of abnormal laboratory values in the colfosceril group was not reported.

Reflux of colfosceril into the endotracheal tube during dosing has been observed and may be associated with rapid drug administration. If reflux occurs, stop drug administration and, if necessary, increase peak inspiratory pressure on the ventilator by 4 to 5 cm H_2O until the endotracheal tube clears.

Drop in transcutaneous oxygen saturation (> 20%): If transcutaneous oxygen saturation declines during dosing, stop drug administration and, if necessary, increase peak inspiratory pressure on the ventilator by 4 to 5 cm H_2O for 1 to 2 minutes. In addition, increases of FiO_2 may be required for 1 to 2 minutes.

Mucous plugs: See Warnings.

COLFOSCERIL PALMITATE (Synthetic Lung Surfactant; Dipalmitoylphosphatidylcholine; DPPC)

Colfosceril Adverse Reactions During the Open, Uncontrolled Study (%)[1]		
Adverse reaction	Prophylactic treatment (n = 1127)	Rescue treatment (n = 7711)
Reflux of colfosceril	20	31
Drop in O_2 saturation (≥ 20%)	6	22
Rise in O_2 saturation (≥ 10%)	5	6
Drop in transcutaneous pO_2 (≥ 20 mm Hg)	1	8
Rise in transcutaneous pO_2 (≥ 20 mm Hg)	2	5
Drop in transcutaneous pCO_2 (≥ 20 mm Hg)	< 1	1
Rise in transcutaneous pCO_2 (≥ 20 mm Hg)	1	3
Bradycardia (< 60 beats/min)	1	3
Tachycardia (> 200 beats/min)	< 1	< 1
Gagging	1	5
Mucous plugs	< 1	< 1

[1] Infants may have experienced more than one event. Investigators were prohibited from adjusting FiO_2 or ventilator settings during dosing unless significant clinical deterioration occurred.

Administration and Dosage:

Preparation of suspension: Colfosceril is best reconstituted immediately before use because it does not contain antibacterial preservatives. Solutions containing buffers or preservatives should not be used for reconstitution. Do not use Bacteriostatic Water for Injection, USP. Reconstitute each vial with 8 ml of the accompanying diluent (preservative-free Sterile Water for Injection) as follows:

1.) Fill a 10 or 12 ml syringe with 8 ml preservative-free Sterile Water for Injection using an 18 or 19 gauge needle.
2.) Allow the vacuum in the vial to draw the sterile water into the vial.
3.) Aspirate as much as possible of the 8 ml out of the vial into the syringe (while maintaining the vacuum), then suddenly release the syringe plunger.

Repeat Step 3 three or four times to assure adequate mixing of the vial contents. If vacuum is not present, the vial of colfosceril should not be used.

Draw the appropriate dosage volume for the entire dose (5 ml/kg) into syringe from below the froth in the vial (again maintaining vacuum). If the infant weighs < 1600 g, unused suspension will remain in the vial after the entire dose is drawn into syringe. If the infant weighs > 1600 g, at least two vials will be required for each dose.

Reconstituted colfosceril is a milky white suspension with a total volume of 8 ml per vial. If the suspension separates, gently shake or swirl the vial to resuspend the preparation. Inspect the reconstituted product visually for homogeneity immediately before administration; if persistent large flakes or particulates are present, do not use the vial.

Dosage: Accurate determination of weight at birth is the key to accurate dosing.

Prophylactic treatment: Administer the first dose as a single 5 ml/kg dose as soon as possible after birth. Administer second and third doses approximately 12 and 24 hours later to all infants who remain on mechanical ventilation at those times.

Rescue treatment: Administer in two 5 ml/kg doses. Administer the initial dose as soon as possible after the diagnosis of RDS is confirmed. Administer the second dose approximately 12 hours following the first dose, provided the infant remains on mechanical ventilation. A small number of infants with RDS have received more than two doses of colfosceril as rescue treatment. Definitive data on the safety and efficacy of these additional doses are not available (see Precautions).

Use of special endotracheal tube adapter: With each vial of colfosceril, five different-sized endotracheal tube adapters each with a special right-angle Luer-lock sideport are supplied. The adapters are clean but not sterile. Use the adapters as follows:

1.) Select an adapter size that corresponds to the inside diameter of the endotracheal tube.
2.) Insert the adapter into the endotracheal tube with a firm push-twist motion.
3.) Connect the breathing circuit wye to the adapter.
4.) Remove the cap from the sideport on the adapter. Attach the syringe containing drug to the sideport.
5.) After completion of dosing, remove the syringe and recap the sideport.

COLFOSCERIL PALMITATE (Synthetic Lung Surfactant; Dipalmitoylphosphatidylcholine; DPPC)

Administration: Suction the infant prior to administration, but do not suction for 2 hours after colfosceril is administered, except when clinically necessary.

Colfosceril suspension is administered via the sideport on the special endotracheal tube adapter without interrupting mechanical ventilation.

Each dose is administered in two 2.5 ml/kg half-doses. Each half-dose is instilled slowly over 1 to 2 minutes (30 to 50 mechanical breaths) in small bursts timed with inspiration. After the first 2.5 ml/kg half-dose is administered in the midline position, turn the infant's head and torso 45° to the right for 30 seconds while mechanical ventilation is continued. After the infant is returned to midline position, give the second 2.5 ml/kg half-dose in an identical fashion over another 1 to 2 minutes. Then turn the infant's head and torso 45° to the left for 30 seconds while mechanical ventilation is continued, and then turn infant back to the midline position. These maneuvers allow gravity to assist in the lung distribution of colfosceril.

During dosing, monitor heart rate, color, chest expansion, facial expressions, the oximeter and endotracheal tube patency and position. If heart rate slows, the infant becomes dusky or agitated, transcutaneous oxygen saturation falls > 15% or drug backs up in endotracheal tube, slow or halt dosing and, if necessary, turn up peak inspiratory pressure, ventilator rate or FiO_2. However, rapid improvements in lung function may require immediate reductions in peak inspiratory pressure, ventilator rate or FiO_2. (See Warnings and below for additional administration information.)

General guidelines for administration: Administration of colfosceril should not take precedence over clinical assessment and stabilization of critically ill infants.

Intubation: Prior to dosing, ensure that the endotracheal tube tip is in the trachea and not the esophagus or right or left mainstem bronchus. Confirm brisk and symmetrical chest movement with each mechanical inspiration prior to dosing, as well as equal breath sounds in the two axillae. In prophylactic treatment, need not delay dosing for radiographic confirmation of endotracheal tube tip position. In rescue treatment, bedside confirmation tube tip position is usually sufficient, if at least one chest radiograph subsequent to last intubation confirmed proper position. Some lung areas will remain undosed if the tube tip is too low.

Monitoring: Continuous ECG and transcutaneous oxygen saturation monitoring during dosing are essential. In most infants treated prophylactically, initiate such monitoring prior to the first dose of colfosceril. For subsequent prophylactic and all rescue doses, arterial blood pressure monitoring during dosing is also highly desirable. After both prophylactic and rescue dosing, frequent arterial blood gas sampling is required to prevent post-dosing hyperoxia and hypocarbia (see Warnings).

Ventilatory support during dosing: The 5 ml/kg dosage volume may cause transient impairment of gas exchange by physical blockage, particularly in infants on low ventilator settings. As a result, infants may exhibit a drop in oxygen saturation during dosing, especially if on low ventilator settings before dosing. These transient effects are easily overcome by increasing peak inspiratory pressure on the ventilator by 4 to 5 cm H_2O for 1 to 2 min during dosing. May also increase FiO_2 if necessary. In infants particularly fragile or reactive to external stimuli, increase peak inspiratory pressure by 4 to 5 cm H_2O or FiO_2 20% just prior to dosing to minimize any transient deterioration in oxygenation. In virtually all cases it should be possible to return to pre-dose settings within a very short time of dose completion.

Post-Dosing: At the end of dosing, confirm endotracheal tube position by listening for equal breath sounds in the two axillae. Pay attention to chest expansion, color, transcutaneous saturation and arterial blood gases. Some infants on colfosceril and other surfactants have rapid improvements in pulmonary compliance, minute ventilation and gas exchange (see Warnings). Constant bedside attention for at least 30 minutes after dosing and frequent blood gas sampling are absolutely essential. Rapid lung function changes require immediate changes in peak inspiratory pressure, ventilator rate or FiO_2.

Educational material: A videotape on dosing is available from Burroughs Wellcome. This videotape demonstrates techniques for safe administration of colfosceril and should be viewed by health care professionals who will administer the drug.

Storage: Store at 15° to 30°C (59° to 86°F) in a dry place.

Rx	**Exosurf Neonatal** (Glaxo Wellcome)	**Lyophilized Powder for Injection:** 108 mg colfosceril palmitate[1]	In 10 ml vials with 10 ml Sterile Water for Injection and 2.5, 3, 3.5, 4 and 4.5 mm endotracheal tube adapters.

[1] With 12 mg cetyl alcohol and 8 mg tyloxapol. When reconstituted to a total volume of 8 ml per vial, each 1 ml contains 13.5 mg colfosceril, 1.5 mg cetyl alcohol, 1 mg tyloxapol and sodium chloride to provide a 0.1 N concentration.

BERACTANT (Natural Lung Surfactant)

Actions:

Pharmacology: Beractant is a sterile, non-pyrogenic pulmonary surfactant intended for intratracheal use only. It is a natural bovine lung extract containing phospholipids, neutral lipids, fatty acids and surfactant-associated proteins to which colfosceril palmitate (dipalmitoylphosphatidylcholine; DPPC), palmitic acid and tripalmitin are added to standardize the composition and to mimic surface-tension lowering properties of natural lung surfactant. Its protein content consists of two hydrophobic, low molecular weight, surfactant-associated proteins commonly known as SP-B and SP-C. It does not contain the hydrophilic, large molecular weight surfactant-associated protein known as SP-A.

Endogenous pulmonary surfactant lowers surface tension on alveolar surfaces during respiration and stabilizes the alveoli against collapse at resting transpulmonary pressures. Deficiency of pulmonary surfactant causes respiratory distress syndrome (RDS) in premature infants. Beractant replenishes surfactant and restores surface activity to the lungs of these infants.

Beractant reproducibly lowers minimum surface tension to < 8 dynes/cm in vitro, restores pulmonary compliance to excised rat lungs artifically made surfactant-deficient in situ, and improves lung pressure-volume measurements, lung compliance, and oxygenation in premature rabbits and sheep in vivo.

Pharmacokinetics: Beractant is administered directly to the target organ, the lungs, where biophysical effects occur at the alveolar surface. In surfactant-deficient premature rabbits and lambs, alveolar clearance of the lipid components is rapid. Most of the dose becomes lung-associated within hours of administration, and the lipids enter endogenous surfactant pathways of reutilization and recycling. In surfactant-sufficient adult animals, clearance is more rapid than in premature and young animals. There is less reutilization and recycling of surfactant in adult animals.

Clinical trials: Each dose in all studies was 100 mg phospholipids/kg birth weight.

Prevention studies – In infants of 600 to 1250 g birth weight and 23 to 29 weeks estimated gestational age, a dose of beractant was given within 15 minutes of birth to prevent the development of RDS. Up to three additional doses in the first 48 hours, as often as every 6 hours, were given if RDS subsequently developed and infants required mechanical ventilation with an $FiO_2 \geq 0.3$.

Rescue studies – In infants of 600 to 1750 g birth weight with RDS requiring mechanical ventilation and an $FiO_2 \geq 0.4$, the initial dose of beractant was given after RDS developed and before 8 hours of age. Infants could receive up to three additional doses in the first 48 hours, as often as every 6 hours, if they required mechanical ventilation and an $FiO_2 \geq 0.3$.

Prevention/Rescue Studies with Beractant

Parameter	Prevention studies[1]		Rescue studies[1]	
	Beractant (n = 210)	Control (n = 220)	Beractant (n = 402)	Control (n = 396)
Incidence of RDS (%)	27.6 – 28.6	48.3 – 63.5	na	na
Death due to RDS (%)	1.1 – 2.5	10.5 – 19.5	6.4 – 11.6	18.1 – 22.3
Death or BPD due to RDS (%)	27.5 – 48.7	44.2 – 52.8	43.6 – 59.1	63.4 – 66.8
Death due to any cause (%)	7.6 – 16.5[3]	13.7 – 22.8	15.2 – 21.7	26.4 – 28.2
Air leaks[2] (%)	5.9 – 14.5	19.6 – 21.7	11.2 – 11.8	22.2 – 29.5
Pulmonary interstitial emphysema (%)	20.8 – 26.5	33.2 – 40	16.3 – 20.8	34 – 44.4

[1] Data pooled from two studies.
[2] Pneumothorax or pneumopericardium.
[3] In one study, no cause of death in the beractant group was significantly increased; the higher number of deaths in this group was due to the sum of all causes.
na = Not applicable.

Marked improvements in oxygenation may occur within minutes of administration.

Significant improvements in the arterial-alveolar oxygen ratio (a/APO_2), FiO_2 and mean airway pressure (MAP) were sustained for 48 to 72 hours in beractant-treated infants in four single-dose and two multiple-dose rescue studies and in two multiple-dose prevention studies. In the single-dose prevention studies, the FiO_2 improved significantly.

Multiple-dose studies – In 605 (333 treated) of 916 surviving infants, there are trends for decreased cerebral palsy and need for supplemental oxygen in beractant

BERACTANT (Natural Lung Surfactant)

infants. Wheezing at the time of examination tended to be more frequent among beractant infants, although there was no difference in bronchodilator therapy.

Indications:

Prevention and treatment ("rescue") of RDS (hyaline membrane disease) in premature infants. Beractant significantly reduces the incidence of RDS, mortality due to RDS and air leak complications.

Prevention: In premature infants < 1250 g birth weight or with evidence of surfactant deficiency, give beractant as soon as possible, preferably within 15 minutes of birth.

Rescue: To treat infants with RDS confirmed by x-ray and requiring mechanical ventilation, give beractant as soon as possible, preferably by 8 hours of age.

Warnings:

Intratracheal administration: Administer only by instillation into the trachea (see Administration and Dosage).

Oxygenation/lung compliance: Beractant can rapidly affect oxygenation and lung compliance. Therefore, restrict its use to a highly supervised clinical setting with immediate availability of clinicians experienced with intubation, ventilator management and general care of premature infants. Frequently monitor infants receiving beractant with arterial or transcutaneous measurement of systemic oxygen and CO_2.

Transient episodes of bradycardia and decreased oxygen saturation have occurred during dosing. If these occur, stop the dosing procedure and initiate appropriate measures to alleviate the condition. After stabilization, resume the dosing procedure.

Precautions:

Rales and moist breath sounds can occur transiently after administration. Endotracheal suctioning or other remedial action is not necessary unless clear-cut signs of airway obstruction are present.

Nosocomial sepsis: Increased probability of post-treatment nosocomial sepsis in beractant-treated infants was observed in controlled clinical trials. The increased risk for sepsis was not associated with increased mortality among these infants. The causative organisms were similar in treated and control infants.

Adverse Reactions:

The most commonly reported adverse experiences were associated with the dosing procedure. In the multiple-dose controlled clinical trials, transient bradycardia occurred with 11.9% of doses. Oxygen desaturation occurred with 9.8% of doses.

Other reactions during the dosing procedure occurred with < 1% of doses and included: Endotracheal tube reflux; pallor; vasoconstriction; hypotension; endotracheal tube blockage; hypertension; hypocarbia; hypercarbia; apnea. No deaths occurred during the dosing procedure, and all reactions resolved with symptomatic treatment.

The occurrence of concurrent illnesses common in premature infants was evaluated in the controlled trials.

Concurrent Illnesses During Beractant Treatment (%)

Concurrent event	Beractant	Control
Patent ductus arteriosus	46.9	47.1
Intracranial hemorrhage	48.1	45.2
Severe intracranial hemorrhage	24.1	23.3
Pulmonary air leaks	10.9	24.7
Pulmonary interstitial emphysema	20.2	38.4
Necrotizing enterocolitis	6.1	5.3
Apnea	65.4	59.6
Severe apnea	46.1	42.5
Post-treatment sepsis	20.7	16.1
Post-treatment infection	10.2	9.1
Pulmonary hemorrhage	7.2	5.3

When all controlled studies were pooled, there was no difference in intracranial hemorrhage. However, in one of the single-dose rescue studies and one of the multiple-dose prevention studies, the rate of intracranial hemorrhage was significantly higher in beractant patients than control patients (63.3% vs 30.8% and 48.8% vs 34.2%, respectively).

BERACTANT (Natural Lung Surfactant)

Overdosage:

Symptoms: Based on animal data, overdosage might result in acute airway obstruction. Rales and moist breath sounds can transiently occur after beractant is given, and do not indicate overdosage. Endotracheal suctioning or other remedial action is not required unless clear-cut signs of airway obstruction are present.

Treatment: Treatment should be symptomatic and supportive. Refer to General Management of Acute Overdosage.

Administration and Dosage:

For intratracheal administration only.

Marked improvements in oxygenation may occur within minutes of administration of beractant. Therefore, frequent and careful clinical observation and monitoring of systemic oxygenation are essential to avoid hyperoxia.

Dosage: Each dose of beractant is 100 mg of phospholipids/kg birth weight (4 ml/kg). The following table shows the total dosage for a range of birth weights.

Beractant Dosing Chart

Weight (g)	Total dose (ml)	Weight (g)	Total dose (ml)
600-650	2.6	1301-1350	5.4
651-700	2.8	1351-1400	5.6
701-750	3	1401-1450	5.8
751-800	3.2	1451-1500	6
801-850	3.4	1501-1550	6.2
851-900	3.6	1551-1600	6.4
901-950	3.8	1601-1650	6.6
951-1000	4	1651-1700	6.8
1001-1050	4.2	1701-1750	7
1051-1100	4.4	1751-1800	7.2
1101-1150	4.6	1801-1850	7.4
1151-1200	4.8	1851-1900	7.6
1201-1250	5	1901-1950	7.8
1251-1300	5.2	1951-2000	8

Four doses can be administered in the first 48 hours of life; give doses no more frequently than every 6 hours.

Preparation: Inspect visually for discoloration prior to administration. The color of beractant is off-white to light brown. If settling occurs during storage, swirl the vial gently (do not shake) to redisperse. Some foaming at the surface may occur during handling and is inherent in the nature of the product.

Beractant is to be refrigerated (2° to 8°C; 36° to 46°F). Before administration, warm by standing at room temperature for at least 20 minutes or warm in the hand for at least 8 minutes. Artificial warming methods should not be used. If a prevention dose is to be given, begin preparation before the infant's birth.

Unopened, unused vials that have been warmed to room temperature may be returned to the refrigerator within 8 hours of warming and stored for future use. The drug should not be warmed and returned to the refrigerator more than once. Enter each single-use vial of beractant only once. Discard used vials with residual drug. Beractant does not require reconstitution or sonication before use.

Dosing procedures: Beractant is administered intratracheally by instillation through a 5 French end-hole catheter inserted into the infant's endotracheal tube with the tip of the catheter protruding just beyond the end of the endotracheal tube above the infant's carina. Before inserting the catheter through the endotracheal tube, shorten the length of the catheter. Do not instill beractant into a main-stem bronchus.

It is important to ensure homogenous distribution of beractant throughout the lungs. In the controlled clinical trials, each dose was divided into four quarterdoses. Each quarter-dose was administered with the infant in a different position. The sequence of positions was: Head and body inclined slightly down, head turned to the right; head and body inclined slightly down, head turned to the left; head and body inclined slightly up, head turned to the right; head and body inclined slightly up, head turned to the left.

First dose: Determine the total dose based on the infant's birth weight. Slowly withdraw the entire contents of the vial into a plastic syringe through a large-gauge needle (eg, at least 20 gauge). Do not filter beractant and avoid shaking.

Attach the premeasured 5 French end-hole catheter to the syringe. Fill the catheter with beractant and discard any excess through the catheter so that only the total dose to be given remains in the syringe.

BERACTANT (Natural Lung Surfactant)

Before administering beractant, assure proper placement and patency of the endotracheal tube. The endotracheal tube may be suctioned before administering beractant. Allow the infant to stabilize before proceeding with dosing.

Prevention strategy – Weigh, intubate and stabilize the infant. Administer the dose as soon as possible after birth, preferably within 15 minutes. Position the infant appropriately and gently inject the first quarter-dose through the catheter over 2 to 3 seconds.

After administration of the first quarter-dose, remove the catheter from the endotracheal tube. Manually ventilate with a hand-bag with sufficient oxygen to prevent cyanosis, at a rate of 60 breaths/minute, and sufficient positive pressure to provide adequate air exchange and chest wall excursion.

Rescue strategy – Give the first dose as soon as possible after the infant is placed on a ventilator for management of RDS. In the clinical trials, immediately before instilling the first quarter-dose, the infant's ventilator settings were changed to a rate of 60/minute, inspiratory time 0.5 second and FiO_2 1.

Position the infant appropriately and gently inject the first quarter-dose through the catheter over 2 to 3 seconds. After administration of the first quarter-dose, remove the catheter from the endotracheal tube. Return the infant to the mechanical ventilator.

Both strategies – Ventilate the infant for at least 30 seconds or until stable. Reposition the infant for instillation of the next quarter-dose.

Instill the remaining quarter-doses using the same procedures. After instillation of each quarter-dose, remove the catheter and ventilate for at least 30 seconds or until the infant is stabilized. After instillation of the final quarter-dose, remove the catheter without flushing it. Do not suction the infant for 1 hour after dosing unless signs of significant airway obstruction occur.

After completion of the dosing procedure, resume usual ventilator management and clinical care.

Repeat doses: The dosage is also 100 mg phospholipids/kg and is based on the infant's birth weight. The infant should not be reweighed for determination of the dosage.

The need for additional doses is determined by evidence of continuing respiratory distress. Significant reductions in mortality due to RDS were observed in multiple-dose trials. Administer dose no sooner than 6 hours after the preceding dose if the infant remains intubated and requires at least 30% inspired oxygen to maintain a $PaO_2 \leq 80$ torr.

Obtain radiographic confirmation of RDS before administering additional doses to those who received a prevention dose.

Prepare beractant and position the infant for administration of each quarter-dose as previously described. After instillation of each quarter-dose, remove the dosing catheter from the endotracheal tube and ventilate the infant for at least 30 seconds or until stable.

In clinical studies, ventilator settings used to administer repeat doses were different than those used for the first dose. For repeat doses, the FiO_2 was increased by 0.2 or an amount sufficient to prevent cyanosis. The ventilator delivered a rate of 30/minute with an inspiratory time < 1 second. If the infant's pretreatment rate was ≥ 30 it was left unchanged during instillation.

Manual hand-bag ventilation should not be used to administer repeat doses. During the dosing procedure, ventilatory settings may be adjusted at the discretion of the clinician to maintain appropriate oxygenation and ventilation. After completion of the dosing procedure, resume usual ventilator management and clinical care.

Educational material: Review of audiovisual instructional materials describing dosage and administration procedures is recommended before using beractant. Materials are available on request from Ross Laboratories.

Storage: Store unopened vials under refrigeration (2° to 8°C; 36° to 46°F). Protect from light. Store vials in carton until ready for use. Vials are for single use only. Upon opening, discard unused drug.

Rx	**Survanta** (Ross Laboratories)	**Suspension**: 25 mg phospholipids per ml suspended in 0.9% sodium chloride solution.[1]	In single use vials containing 8 ml suspension.

[1] With 0.5 to 1.75 mg triglycerides, 1.4 to 3.5 mg free fatty acids and < 1 mg protein per ml.

ANTIHISTAMINES

Warning:

Astemizole and terfenadine:

QT interval prolongation/ventricular arrhythmias – Rare cases of serious cardiovascular adverse events, including death, cardiac arrest, torsade de pointes and other ventricular arrhythmias, have been observed in the following clinical settings, frequently in association with increased terfenadine and astemizole (including metabolite) levels which lead to electrocardiographic QT prolongation:

1. Overdose including single terfenadine doses as low as 360 mg and astemizole doses as low as 20 to 30 mg/day.
2. Significant hepatic dysfunction
3. Concomitant administration of erythromycin, ketoconazole or itraconazole.

Terfenadine and astemizole are contraindicated in patients taking ketoconazole, itraconazole or erythromycin and in patients with significant hepatic dysfunction.

Do not exceed recommended dose.

In some cases, severe arrhythmias have been preceded by episodes of syncope. Syncope in patients receiving astemizole or terfenadine should lead to discontinuation of treatment and full evaluation of potential arrhythmias, including ECG testing (looking for QT prolongation and ventricular arrhythmias).

Actions:

Pharmacology:

Antihistamines: Dosage and Effects

Antihistamine	Dose[1] (mg)	Dosing interval[2] (hrs)	Sedative effects	Antihistaminic activity	Anticholinergic activity	Antiemetic effects
Ethanolamines						
Carbinoxamine	4 to 8	6 to 8	++	+ to ++	+++	++ to +++
Clemastine	1	12	++	+ to ++	+++	++ to +++
Diphenhydramine	25 to 50	6 to 8	+++	+ to ++	+++	++ to +++
Ethylenediamines						
Pyrilamine	25 to 50	6 to 8	+	+ to ++	±	—
Tripelennamine	25 to 50	4 to 6	++	+ to ++	±	—
Alkylamines						
Brompheniramine	4	4 to 6	+	+++	++	—
Chlorpheniramine	4	4 to 6	+	++	++	—
Dexchlorpheniramine	2	4 to 6	+	+++	++	—
Triprolidine	2.5	4 to 6	+	++ to +++	++	—
Phenothiazines						
Methdilazine	8	6 to 12	+	++ to +++	+++	++++
Promethazine	12.5 to 25	6 to 24	+++	+++	+++	++++
Trimeprazine	2.5	6	++	++ to +++	+++	++++
Piperidines						
Azatadine	1 to 2	12	++	++	++	—
Cyproheptadine	4	8	+	++	++	—
Phenindamine	25	4 to 6	—[3]	++	++	—
Miscellaneous						
Astemizole	10	24	±	++ to +++	±	—
Loratadine	10	24	±	++ to +++	±	—
Terfenadine	60	12	±	++ to +++	±	—

* ++++ = very high, +++ = high, ++ = moderate, + = low, ± = low to none.

[1] Usual single oral adult dose.

[2] For conventional dosage forms.

[3] Stimulation possible.

ANTIHISTAMINES

Antihistamines competitively antagonize histamine at the H_1 receptor site, but do not bind with histamine to inactivate it. Terfenadine and astemizole, the most specific H_1 antagonists available, bind preferentially to peripheral rather than central H_1 receptors. Antihistamines do not block histamine release, antibody production or antigen-antibody interactions. They antagonize in varying degrees most pharmacological effects of histamine. They also have anticholinergic (drying), antipruritic and sedative effects; terfenadine and astemizole have little or no anticholinergic and sedative effects. Antihistamines with predominant sedative effects are used as nonprescription sleep aids (see monograph). Cyproheptadine and azatadine also have antiserotonin activity. Antihistamines with antiemetic effects are useful in management of nausea, vomiting and motion sickness (see Antiemetic/Antivertigo agents). Conversely, GI upset is a frequent side effect of the ethylenediamines.

Although common cold symptoms might be modified by antihistamines, they do not prevent or cure colds, nor do they shorten the course of the disease.

Switching from one class of antihistamine to another may restore responsiveness when a patient becomes refractory to the effects of a particular agent.

Pharmacokinetics:

Pharmacokinetics have not been extensively studied. With a few exceptions, these agents are well absorbed following oral administration use, have an onset of action within 15 to 30 minutes, are maximal within 1 to 2 hours and have a duration of about 4 to 6 hours, although some are much longer acting (see table). Most are metabolized by liver. Antihistamine metabolites and small amounts of unchanged drug are excreted in urine. Small amounts may be excreted in breast milk.

Terfenadine's effects begin in 1 to 2 hrs, reach maximum in 3 to 4 hrs and last in excess of 12 hrs. It reaches peak plasma levels in 2 hrs and has elimination half-life of 20 hrs. It is 97% protein bound. Fecal excretion accounts for 60% of dose, with 40% eliminated via urine. Almost all the dose is eliminated as metabolites.

Astemizole has a slow onset of action, and its effects last up to 24 hours based on once-a-day dosing. It is rapidly absorbed and reaches peak plasma concentrations within 1 hour; its absorption is reduced by 60% when taken with food. Its half-life is biphasic: 20 hours for the distribution phase and 7 to 11 days for the elimination phase. The drug is 96.7% protein bound. Approximately 40% to 50% of the astemizole dose is excreted in the urine by 4 days, with 50% to 70% eliminated via the feces by 14 days. All of the dose is eliminated as metabolites. The principle metabolite may have some antihistaminic activity.

Loratadine's effects begin within 1 to 3 hours, reaching a maximum at 8 to 12 hours and lasting > 24 hours. It is rapidly absorbed and extensively metabolized to an active metabolite (descarboethoxyloratadine). The mean elimination half-life is 8.4 hours for loratadine and 28 hours for the metabolite. Approximately 80% of the dose is equally distributed between urine and feces in the form of metabolic products after 10 days. Loratadine is ≈ 97% protein bound, 73% to 77% for metabolite.

Indications:

Oral: Symptomatic relief of symptoms associated with: Perennial and seasonal allergic rhinitis; vasomotor rhinitis; allergic conjunctivitis; temporary relief of runny nose and sneezing due to the common cold; allergic and non-allergic pruritic symptoms; mild, uncomplicated urticaria and angioedema; amelioration of allergic reactions to blood or plasma; dermatographism; adjunctive therapy in anaphylactic reactions.

Parenteral: Amelioration of allergic reactions to blood or plasma; in anaphylaxis as an adjunct to epinephrine and other measures; for other uncomplicated allergic conditions of the immediate type when oral therapy is not possible.

Unlabeled uses: One study suggested the combination of an H_1 and H_2 antagonist may be useful in patients with chronic idiopathic urticaria who do not adequately respond to an H_1 antagonist alone.

For specific indications refer to the listings for individual agents on the following pages.

Contraindications:

Hypersensitivity to antihistamines; newborn or premature infants (see Warnings); nursing mothers (see Warnings); narrow-angle glaucoma; stenosing peptic ulcer; symptomatic prostatic hypertrophy; asthma attack; bladder neck obstruction; pyloro-duodenal obstruction; monoamine oxidase inhibitor (MAOI) use (see Drug Interactions).

*Phenothiazine antihistamines (***trimeprazine, promethazine** *and* **methdilazine***):* Comatose patients; CNS depression from barbiturates, general anesthetics, tranquilizers, alcohol, narcotics or narcotic analgesics; previous phenothiazine idiosyncrasy, jaundice or bone marrow depression; acutely ill or dehydrated children because there is greater susceptibility to dystonias.

Astemizole/Terfenadine: Significant hepatic dysfunction; concomitant erythromycin, ketoconazole or itraconazole therapy.

ANTIHISTAMINES

Warnings:

Cardiovascular effects: Cases of torsades de pointes have been reported following **terfenadine** use. It is possible that terfenadine, but not its metabolite, has quinidine-like actions that may induce arrhythmias. Be aware of conditions that may inhibit the metabolism of terfenadine such as impaired hepatic function or certain drugs (see Drug Interactions).

Respiratory disease: In general, antihistamines are not recommended to treat *lower* respiratory tract symptoms including asthma, as their anticholinergic (drying) effects may cause thickening of secretions and impair expectoration. However, several reports indicate antihistamines can be safely used in asthmatic patients with severe perennial allergic rhinitis without exacerbating the asthma.

Promethazine may lower the seizure threshold; take this into consideration when administering to persons with known seizure disorders or when giving in combination with narcotics or local anesthetics that may also affect seizure threshold.

Sedatives/CNS depressants: Avoid sedatives and CNS depressants in patients with a history of sleep apnea.

"Ts and Blues": IV injection of oral preparations of **pentazocine** (*Talwin,*Ts) and **tripelennamine** (*PBZ,*Blues) has become a common form of drug abuse, used as a "substitute" for heroin. The tablets are dissolved in tap water, filtered and injected IV.

The most frequent and serious complication of IV "Ts and Blues" addiction is pulmonary disease, due to occlusion of pulmonary arteries and arterioles with unsterile particles of cellulose and talc used as tablet binders. The occlusion leads to granulomatous foreign body reactions, infections, increased pulmonary artery resistance and pulmonary hypertension. Neurologic complications from IV injection of "Ts and Blues" include seizures, strokes and CNS infections. The replacement of oral pentazocine with the combination pentazocine/naloxone *(Talwin Nx)* may decrease this mixture's popularity.

Nonmedical parenteral use of **butorphanol** and **diphenhydramine** has also been reported.

Hypersensitivity reactions may occur, and any of the usual manifestations of drug allergy may develop. Have epinephrine 1:1000 immediately available. Refer to Management of Acute Hypersensitivity Reactions.

Hepatic function impairment: Use caution in patients with cirrhosis or other liver diseases. **Astemizole** and **terfenadine** are contraindicated in patients with significant hepatic dysfunction (see Warning Box). Use a lower initial dose of loratadine (10 mg every other day).

Elderly: Antihistamines are more likely to cause dizziness, excessive sedation, syncope, toxic confusional states and hypotension in elderly patients. Dosage reduction may be required.

The phenothiazine side effects (extrapyramidal signs, especially parkinsonism, akathisia, and persistent dyskinesia) are more prone to develop in the elderly.

Pregnancy: (Category B – chlorpheniramine, dexchlorpheniramine, diphenhydramine, cyproheptadine, clemastine, azatadine, methdilazine, loratadine. Category C – astemizole, brompheniramine, promethazine, carbinoxamine, terfenadine, triprolidine). Safety for use during pregnancy has not been established. Several possible associations with malformations have been found, but significance is unknown. Use only when clearly needed and when the potential benefits outweigh the potential hazards to the fetus. Do not use during the third trimester; newborn and premature infants may have severe reactions (eg, convulsions).

There are reports of jaundice and prolonged extrapyramidal symptoms in infants whose mothers received phenothiazines during pregnancy. Hyperreflexia has been reported in the newborn when a phenothiazine was used during pregnancy. Promethazine, taken within 2 weeks of delivery, may inhibit platelet aggregation in the newborn.

Lactation: Although quantitative determinations of antihistaminic drugs in breast milk have not been reported, qualitative tests have documented the excretion of **diphenhydramine, pyrilamine** and **tripelennamine** in breast milk. **Loratadine** and its metabolite pass easily into breast milk and achieve concentrations that are equivalent to plasma levels with an AUC milk/AUC plasma ratio of 1.17 and 0.85, respectively. Due to the higher risk of adverse effects for infants generally, and for newborns and prematures in particular, antihistamine therapy is contraindicated in nursing mothers.

ANTIHISTAMINES

Children: Antihistamine overdosage may cause hallucinations, convulsions and death. Antihistamines may diminish mental alertness. In the young child, they may produce paradoxical excitation.

Administer IV promethazine with caution. Antiemetics are not recommended for treatment of uncomplicated vomiting in children; limit their use to prolonged vomiting of known etiology. The extrapyramidal symptoms that can occur secondary to IV promethazine administration may be confused with the CNS signs of undiagnosed primary disease (eg, encephalopathy, Reye's syndrome). Hyperreflexia has occurred in a newborn when a phenothiazine was used during pregnancy.

Avoid using **phenothiazines** in children with a history of sleep apnea, a family history of sudden infant death syndrome (SIDS) or hepatic diseases. Avoid use in a child with Reye's syndrome.

Safety and efficacy for use of **promethazine** and **cyproheptadine** in children < 2 years, **methdilazine** in children < 3 years, 4 mg **dexchlorpheniramine** in children < 6 years, and **terfenadine, azatadine, dexchlorpheniramine, loratadine** and **astemizole** in children < 12 years of age have not been established. However, in one study wheals and flares were significantly suppressed following a single terfenadine dose (15 to 60 mg) in 13 children.

Precautions:

Hematologic: Use **promethazine** with caution in bone marrow depression. Leukopenia and agranulocytosis have been reported, usually when used with other toxic agents.

Anticholinergic effects: Antihistamines have varying degrees of atropine-like actions; use with caution in patients with a predisposition to urinary retention, history of bronchial asthma, increased intraocular pressure, hyperthyroidism, cardiovascular disease or hypertension. Antihistamines may thicken bronchial secretions due to anticholinergic (drying) properties and may inhibit expectoration and sinus drainage. Astemizole and terfenadine appear to have less anticholinergic effects.

Phenothiazines: Use phenothiazines with caution in patients with cardiovascular disease, liver dysfunction or ulcer disease. Promethazine has been associated with cholestatic jaundice.

Use cautiously in persons with acute or chronic respiratory impairment, particularly children, since phenothiazines may suppress the cough reflex. If hypotension occurs, epinephrine is not recommended since phenothiazines may reverse its usual pressor effect and cause a paradoxical further lowering of blood pressure. Since these drugs have an antiemetic action, they may obscure signs of intestinal obstruction, brain tumor or overdosage of toxic drugs.

Phenothiazines elevate prolactin levels which persist through chronic administration. Approximately one-third of breast cancers are prolactin-dependent in vitro, an important factor if these drugs are prescribed for a patient with a history of breast cancer. Although galactorrhea, amenorrhea, gynecomastia and impotence have been reported, the clinical significance of elevated serum prolactin levels is unknown.

Discontinue phenothiazines at least 48 hours before myelography and do not resume for at least 24 hours postprocedure. Do not use phenothiazines to control nausea and vomiting before or after myelography.

Parenteral use: Do not give **promethazine** intra-arterially because of possible severe arteriospasm and resultant gangrene. Do not give SC; chemical irritation and necrotic lesions have resulted.

Hazardous tasks: May cause drowsiness and reduce mental alertness; patients should not drive or perform other tasks requiring alertness, coordination or physical dexterity. Astemizole, loratadine and terfenadine appear to cause less sedation. Supervise children who are taking antihistamines when they engage in potentially hazardous activities (eg, bicycle riding).

Photosensitivity: Photosensitization may occur; therefore, caution patients to take protective measures (ie, sunscreens, protective clothing) against exposure to ultraviolet light or sunlight until tolerance is determined.

Sulfite sensitivity: Some of these products contain sulfites, which may cause allergic-type reactions (eg, hives, itching, wheezing, anaphylaxis) in certain susceptible persons. Although the overall prevalence of sulfite sensitivity in the general population is probably low, it is seen more frequently in asthmatics or in atopic nonasthmatic persons. Specific products containing sulfites are identified in the product listings.

ANTIHISTAMINES

Drug Interactions:

Antihistamine Drug Interactions			
Precipitant drug	Object drug*		Description
Azole Antifungals Fluconazole Itraconazole Ketoconazole Miconazole	Antihistamines– Astemizole Terfenadine	↑	Astemizole and terfenadine plasma levels (including metabolite levels) may be increased, which may lead to serious cardiovascular effects (see Warning Box).
Macrolide antibiotics	Antihistamines– Astemizole Terfenadine	↑	Astemizole and terfenadine plasma levels (including metabolite levels) may be increased, which may lead to serious cardiovascular effects (see Warning Box).
MAO inhibitors	Antihistamines	↑	MAOIs may prolong and intensify the anticholinergic effects of the antihistamines. Use with phenothiazine antihistamines may cause hypotension and extrapyramidal reactions. Dexchlorpheniramine may cause severe hypotension when given with an MAOI.
Antihistamines	MAO inhibitors	↑	
Antihistamines	Alcohol, CNS depressants	↑	Additive CNS depressant effects may occur. This may be less likely with astemizole, loratadine, terfenadine.

* ↑ = Object drug increased

See the Antipsychotic Agents monograph for a complete discussion of the drug interactions that relate to the three phenothiazine antihistamines: Promethazine, trimeprazine and methdilazine.

Drug/Lab test interactions: **Diagnostic pregnancy tests** based on immunological reactions between HCG and anti-HCG may result in false-negative or false-positive interpretations in patients on promethazine. Increased **blood glucose** has occurred in promethazine patients.

In patients on phenothiazines, the following have occurred: Increased **serum cholesterol, blood glucose, spinal fluid protein** and **urinary urobilinogen levels;** decreased **protein bound iodine (PBI);** false-positive **urine bilirubin tests;** interference with **urinary ketone determinations, pregnancy tests** and **steroid determinations.**

Discontinue antihistamines about 4 days prior to **skin testing procedures;** these drugs may prevent or diminish otherwise positive reactions to dermal reactivity indicators.

Drug/Food interactions: **Astemizole** absorption is reduced by 60% when taken with food. Take at least 2 hours after a meal, with no food for 1 hour after taking the drug. In a single-dose study, food increased the AUC of **loratadine** by ≈ 40% and the metabolite by ≈ 15%. The time to peak plasma concentration of parent and metabolite was delayed by 1 hour with a meal. Although not expected to be clinically important, take on an empty stomach.

Adverse Reactions:

Allergic reactions: Peripheral, angioneurotic and laryngeal edema; dermatitis; asthma; lupus erythematosus-like syndrome; urticaria drug rash; anaphylactic shock; photosensitivity.

Cardiovascular: Postural hypotension; palpitations; bradycardia; tachycardia; reflex tachycardia; extrasystoles; faintness; increases and decreases in blood pressure; venous thrombosis at injection site following IV promethazine; cardiac arrest; ECG changes, including blunting of T waves and prolongation of the Q-T interval.

CNS:

Most frequent – Drowsiness (often transient); sedation; dizziness; faintness; disturbed coordination.

Other – Fatigue; lassitude; confusion; restlessness; excitation; nervousness; tremor; grand mal seizures; headache; irritability; insomnia; euphoria; paresthesias; blurred vision; oculogyric crisis; torticollis; catatonic-like states; hallucinations; disorientation; tongue protrusion (usually in association with IV administration or excessive dosage); disturbing dreams/nightmares; pseudoschizophrenia; weakness; diplopia; vertigo; tinnitus; acute labyrinthitis; hysteria; neuritis; convulsions; paradoxical excitation, especially in children and in the elderly. Extrapyramidal reactions, including opisthotonos, dystonia, akathisia, dyskinesia and parkinsonism may occur with high doses; these are usually responsive to a reduction in dosage. CNS stimulation is possible with **phenindamine.**

ANTIHISTAMINES

GI:

Most frequent – Epigastric distress (especially ethylenediamines).

Other – Anorexia; increased appetite and weight gain; nausea; vomiting; diarrhea; constipation; change in bowel habits.

GU: Urinary frequency; dysuria; urinary retention; early menses; induced lactation; gynecomastia; inhibition of ejaculation; decreased libido; impotence.

Hematologic: Hemolytic anemia; hypoplastic anemia; aplastic anemia; thrombocytopenia; leukopenia; agranulocytosis; pancytopenia.

Respiratory:

Most frequent – Thickening of bronchial secretions.

Other – Chest tightness; wheezing; nasal stuffiness; dry mouth, nose and throat; sore throat; respiratory depression.

Body as a whole: Tingling, heaviness and weakness of the hands; thrombocytopenic purpura; obstructive jaundice (usually reversible upon drug discontinuation); tissue necrosis following SC administration of IV promethazine; erythema; stomatitis; high or prolonged glucose tolerance curves; glycosuria; elevated spinal fluid proteins; elevation of plasma cholesterol levels; excessive perspiration; chills.

Terfenadine: Alopecia; arrhythmia; visual disturbances; angioedema; skin eruption and itching; bronchospasm; cough; depression; galactorrhea; menstrual disorders (eg, dysmenorrhea); musculoskeletal pain; nightmares; mild or moderate transaminase elevations; torsades de pointes. Terfenadine may cause less drowsiness than **chlorpheniramine** or **clemastine**. Isolated reports of jaundice, cholestatic hepatitis and hepatitis have occurred.

Astemizole: Headache (6.7%); appetite increase (3.9%); weight gain (3.6%, average gain 3.2 kg); nausea (2.5%); nervousness (2.1%); dizziness (2%); diarrhea (1.8%); pharyngitis (1.7%); abdominal pain (1.4%); conjunctivitis, arthralgia (1.2%); angioedema; bronchospasm; depression; edema; epistaxis; myalgia; pruritus. Astemizole caused less drowsiness, fatigue and dry mouth than **chlorpheniramine, clemastine, pheniramine** and **dexchlorpheniramine.**

Loratadine: Altered salivation; asthenia; increased sweating; altered lacrimation; hypoesthesia; thirst; flushing; conjunctivitis; blurred vision; earache; eye pain; back/chest pain; leg cramps; malaise; rigors; fever; aggravated allergy; upper respiratory infection; hyperkinesia; blepharospasm; migraine; dysphonia; flatulence; gastritis; dyspepsia; stomatitis; tooth ache; altered taste; arthralgia; myalgia; anxiety; depression; agitation; paroniria; amnesia; impaired concentration; breast pain; menorrhagia; dysmenorrhea; vaginitis; epistaxis; pharyngitis; dyspnea; coughing; rhinitis; hemoptysis; sinusitis; sneezing; bronchospasm; bronchitis; laryngitis; dry hair; dry skin; pruritus; purpura; urinary discoloration.

Phenothiazine antihistamines infrequently cause typical phenothiazine adverse effects. See the Antipsychotic Agents monograph for a complete discussion of the phenothiazine adverse reactions.

Overdosage:

Symptoms: Effects may vary from mild CNS depression (sedation, apnea, diminished mental alertness) and cardiovascular collapse to stimulation (insomnia, hallucinations, tremors or convulsions), especially in children and geriatric patients. Profound hypotension, respiratory depression, unconsciousness, coma and death may occur, particularly in infants and children. Convulsions rarely occur. The convulsant dose lies near the lethal dose. Convulsions indicate a poor prognosis.

Toxic effects are seen within 30 minutes to 2 hours and result in drowsiness, dizziness, ataxia, tinnitus, blurred vision and hypotension. Anticholinergic effects result in fixed dilated pupils, flushing, dry mouth, hyperthermia (especially likely in children) and fever. GI symptoms may also occur. Hyperpyrexia to 41.8°C (107°F) and acute oral and facial dystonic reactions have been reported.

Children often manifest CNS stimulation and may have hallucinations, toxic psychosis, delirium tremens, excitement, ataxia, incoordination, muscle twitching, athetosis, hyperthermia, cyanosis convulsions and hyperreflexia followed by post-ictal depression and cardiorespiratory arrest. Seizures resistant to therapy may follow and may be preceded by mild depression. A paradoxical reaction has been reported in children receiving single doses of 75 to 125 mg oral **promethazine,** characterized by hyperexcitability and nightmares. CNS stimulation in adults usually manifests as seizures. Marked cerebral irritation, resulting in jerking of muscles and possible convulsions, may be followed by deep stupor. Occasionally, a latent period is followed by respiratory depression, cardiovascular collapse and death.

Less common findings include ECG changes, such as wandering pacemaker, prolonged QT interval and nonspecific ST–T wave changes that disappear quickly. The EEG may show general cerebral dysrhythmia and diffuse delta wave activity that can persist after clinical recovery. Serious ventricular arrhythmias, including torsades de pointes, have occurred following **astemizole** doses of > 200 mg; however, no ill effects have occurred with doses up to 500 mg.

Several cases of **terfenadine** overdosage have occurred. Generally, signs and symptoms were absent or mild (eg, headache, nausea, confusion). However, severe ventricular arrhythmias (torsades de pointes) developed 15 hours after ingestion of 56 tablets (3360 mg) of terfenadine, 14 capsules (7000 mg) of cephalexin and 2 tablets (1200 mg) of ibuprofen. This progressed to ventricular fibrillation that responded well to defibrillation and lidocaine. Therefore, cardiac monitoring for at least 24 hours is recommended along with standard measures to remove any unabsorbed drug.

Single doses as high as ten times (600 mg) the recommended therapeutic dose in adults have been well tolerated.

Treatment: Induce emesis even if emesis has occurred spontaneously, using syrup of ipecac, except with **phenothiazine** antihistamines (see the Antipsychotic Agents monograph for management of phenothiazine overdosage). Following emesis, administer activated charcoal as a slurry with water and a cathartic to minimize absorption. Oral sodium or magnesium sulfate may be given; saline cathartics (eg, milk of magnesia) draw water into the bowel by osmosis and, therefore, are valuable for their action in rapid dilution of bowel content. Correct acidosis and electrolyte imbalances. Do not induce emesis in unconscious patients. If vomiting is unsuccessful, gastric lavage is indicated within 3 hours after ingestion and even later if large amounts of milk or cream were given. Early gastric lavage may be beneficial if **promethazine** has been taken orally. Isotonic or isotonic saline is the lavage of choice, particularly in children. In adults, tap water can be used. Continue therapy directed at reversing the effects of timed-release medication and at supporting the patient for as long as symptoms remain. Treatment includes usual supportive measures. Refer to General Management of Acute Overdosage.

Hypotension is an early sign of impending cardiovascular collapse; treat it vigorously using general supportive measures or specific treatment with a vasopressor (norepinephrine, phenylephrine, dopamine). Avoid epinephrine because it may worsen hypotension. Propranolol can be used for refractory ventricular arrhythmias.

Use only short-acting depressants (eg, diazepam) to treat convulsions; repeat as necessary. IV physostigmine can be used to control centrally mediated convulsions. Avoid analeptics because they may cause convulsions. Note that any depressant effects of **promethazine** are not reversed by naloxone.

Ice packs and cooling sponge baths, not alcohol, can aid in reducing the fever commonly seen in children.

Hemoperfusion may be used in severe cases.

Astemizole and **loratadine** do not appear to be dialyzable. It is not known if **terfenadine** is dialyzable.

Patient Information:

Inform physician of a history of glaucoma, peptic ulcer, urinary retention or pregnancy before starting antihistamine therapy.

May cause nervousness, insomnia and dry mouth.

May cause drowsiness or dizziness (except astemizole, loratadine and terfenadine); patients should observe caution while driving or performing other tasks requiring alertness, coordination or physical dexterity. Avoid alcohol and other CNS depressants (eg, sedatives, hypnotics, tranquilizers).

May cause GI upset; take with food. Take astemizole on an empty stomach, at least 2 hours after or 1 hour before a meal. Take loratadine on an empty stomach.

Avoid prolonged exposure to sunlight; may cause photosensitivity.

Do not crush or chew sustained release preparations.

Astemizole/Terfenadine: Patients should not take these agents if they have hepatic dysfunction or if they are also receiving ketoconazole, itraconazole or erythromycin.

Phenothiazines: Patients should report any involuntary muscle movements or unusual sensitivity to sunlight.

Ethanolamines

DIPHENHYDRAMINE HCl

For complete prescribing information, refer to the Antihistamines group monograph.

Indications:

In addition to the general uses discussed in the group monograph, diphenhydramine is indicated for active and prophylactic treatment of motion sickness; as a nighttime sleep aid; for parkinsonism (including drug-induced) in the elderly intolerant of more potent agents, for mild cases in other age groups and in combination with centrally-acting anticholinergics. As a nonnarcotic cough suppressant; however, only the "syrup" formulations are labeled for this indication.

Administration and Dosage:

Individualize dosage.

Oral: Adults- 25 to 50 mg, every 6 to 8 hours.

Children (over 10 kg) – 12.5 to 25 mg, 3 or 4 times daily or 5 mg/kg/day or 150 mg/m^2/day. Maximum daily dosage is 300 mg.

In motion sickness, give full dosage for prophylactic use; give the first dose 30 minutes before exposure to motion and similar doses before meals and at bedtime for the duration of exposure.

Nighttime sleep aid: Adults: 50 mg at bedtime.

Parenteral: Administer IV or deeply IM.

Adults – 10 to 50 mg; 100 mg if required; maximum daily dosage is 400 mg.

Children – 5 mg/kg/day or 150 mg/m^2/day. Maximum daily dosage is 300 mg divided into 4 doses.

NOTE: The syrup formulations may include ammonium chloride and sodium citrate as expectorants, although there is inadequate evidence of their clinical value. Therapeutic claims for these components have been deleted, although they remain in the product formulation as inactive ingredients.

otc/ Rx[1]	**Diphenhydramine HCl** (Various)		In 20s, 24s, 30s, 100s, 250s, 500s, 1000s and UD 100s.
otc	**Banophen** (Major)		In 100s, 1000s and UD 100s.
Rx	**Benadryl** (Parke-Davis)		(P-D 471). Pink/white. In 100s, 1000s and UD 100s.
otc	**Benadryl 25** (Parke-Davis Consumer)		In 24s and 48s.
otc	**Benadryl Allergy Kapseals** (Glaxo Wellcome		Lactose. In 24s and 48s.
Rx	**Genahist** (Goldline)		In 24s.
otc	**Benadryl Dye-Free Allergy Liqui Gels** (Parke-Davis)	**Capsules, soft gels:** 25 mg diphenhydramine HCl	Sorbitol. In 24s.
otc/ Rx[1]	**Diphenhydramine HCl** (Various)		In 15s, 24s, 30s, 100s, 250s, 500s, 1000s & UD 32s, 100s.
Rx	**Banophen** (Major)		In 100s, 250s, 1000s.
Rx	**Benadryl Kapseals** (Parke-Davis)		(P-D 373). Pink/white. In 100s, 1000s and UD 100s.
otc/ Rx[1]	**Diphenhydramine HCl** (Various)	**Tablets:** 25 mg	In 24s, 30s, 100s and 1000s.
otc	**AllerMax Caplets** (Pfeiffer)		In 24s.
otc	**Banophen Caplets** (Major)		In 24s and 100s.
otc	**Benadryl 25** (Parke-Davis Consumer)		Film coated. In 24s.
otc	**Benadryl Allergy** (Glaxo Wellcome)		In 24s and 100s.
otc	**Diphenhist Captabs** (Rugby)		Capsule shaped. In 100s and UD 24s.
Rx	**Genahist** (Goldline)		In 24s.

Ethanolamines

DIPHENHYDRAMINE HCl

Rx	**Diphenhydramine HCl** (Various)	**Tablets:** 50 mg	In 30s, 50s, 100s and 1000s.
otc	**AllerMax Caplets** (Pfeiffer)		In 24s.
otc	**Dormarex 2** (Republic)		In 16s and 32s.
otc	**Benadryl Allergy** (Glaxo Wellcome)	**Tablets, chewable:** 12.5 mg	Aspartame, 4.2 mg phenylalanine. In 24s.
otc	**Benadryl Dye-Free** (Glaxo Wellcome)	**Liquid:** 6.25 mg/5 ml	Saccharin, sorbitol. Fruit flavor. In 236 ml.
otc	**Benadryl Allergy** (Glaxo Wellcome)	**Liquid:** 12.5 mg/5 ml	Alcohol free. Saccharin, sugar. In 120 and 240 ml.
otc *sf*	**Scot-Tussin Allergy Relief Formula** (Scot-Tussin)		Dye free. Parabens, menthol. In 120 ml.
otc	**Diphenhist** (Rugby)	**Elixir:** 12.5 mg/5 ml	In 120 ml, pt and gal.
otc/ Rx[1]	**Diphenhydramine HCl** (Various)		In 120 ml, pt, gal and UD 5, 10, 20 ml (100s).
otc	**Banophen** (Major)		5.6% alcohol, EDTA, saccharin, sugar. Cherry flavor. In 118 and 240 ml.
otc *sf*	**Belix** (Halsey)		14% alcohol, sorbitol. In 118 ml, pt and gal.
Rx	**Benadryl** (Parke-Davis Consumer)		14% alcohol. In 120 ml, pt, gal and UD 5 ml (100s).
otc	**Diphenhist** (Rugby)		In 120 ml, pt and gal.
otc	**Genahist** (Goldline)		14% alcohol. In 120 ml.
otc	**Phendry** (LuChem)		14% alcohol. In pt and gal.
otc	**Phendry Children's Allergy Medicine** (LuChem)		14% alcohol. In 120 ml.
otc	**Siladryl** (Silarx)		5.6% alcohol. Cherry flavor. In 118 ml.
otc/ Rx[1]	**Diphenhydramine HCl** (Various)	**Syrup:** 12.5 mg per 5 ml	In 4, 120 and 240 ml, pt, gal and UD 5 ml.
otc	**Benylin Cough** (Parke-Davis Consumer)		5% alcohol, saccharin. In 120, 240 ml, pt, gal.
otc	**Bydramine Cough** (Major)		5% alcohol. In 118 ml, pt, gal.
otc	**Diphen Cough** (Pharmaceutical Basics)		In 120 ml, pt and gal.
Rx	**Hydramyn** (LuChem)		5% alcohol. In pt.
Rx	**Tusstat** (Century Pharm.)		5% alcohol. In 120 ml, pt and gal.

Ethanolamines

DIPHENHYDRAMINE HCl

Rx	**Diphenhydramine HCl** (Various, eg, Steris)	**Injection:** 10 mg per ml	In 10 and 30 ml vials.
Rx	**Benadryl** (Parke-Davis)		In 10 and 30 ml Steri-vials.[3]
Rx	**Diphenhydramine HCl** (Various, eg, Steris)	**Injection:** 50 mg per ml	In 1 and 10 ml vials and 1 ml amps.
Rx	**Benadryl** (Parke-Davis)		In 1 ml amps, 10 ml Steri-vials, 1 ml Steri-dose syringe.[3]
Rx	**Ben-Allergin-50** (Dunhall)		In 10 ml vials.[2]
Rx	**Dihydrex** (Kay Pharm.)		In 10 ml vials.[2]
Rx	**Hyrexin-50** (Hyrex)		In 10 ml multi-dose vials.[2]
Rx	**Wehdryl** (Hauck)		In 10 ml vials.[2]

[1] Products are available *otc* or *Rx*, depending on product labeling.
[2] With chlorobutanol.
[3] With benzethonium chloride.

CLEMASTINE FUMARATE

For complete prescribing information, refer to the Antihistamines group monograph.

Administration and Dosage:

Adults and children (over 12): 1.34 mg twice daily to 2.68 mg 3 times daily. Do not exceed 8.04 mg/day. For dermatologic conditions, use 2.68 mg dosage only.

Children (under 12 years): Safety and efficacy for use have not been established.

Rx	**Clemastine Fumarate** (Various, eg, Lemmon, Schein)	**Tablets:** 1.34 mg	In 100s.
otc	**Antihist-1** (Various, eg, Goldline, Major, Rugby)		In 16s.
otc	**Tavist-1** (Sandoz)		(Tavist 1 78/75). White, scored. In 100s.
Rx	**Clemastine Fumarate** (Various, eg, Lemmon, Schein)	**Tablets:** 2.68 mg	In 100s.
Rx	**Tavist** (Sandoz)		(Tavist 78/72). White, scored. In 100s.
Rx	**Clemastine Fumarate** (Various, eg, Barre-National, Copley, Goldline, Major, Moore, Qualitest, Rugby, Schein)	**Syrup:** 0.67 mg (equiv. to 0.5 mg base) per 5 ml	May contain alcohol. In 118 ml.
Rx	**Tavist** (Sandoz)		5.5% alcohol, saccharin and sorbitol. Citrus flavor. In 120 ml.

Ethylenediamines

TRIPELENNAMINE HCl

For complete prescribing information, refer to the Antihistamines group monograph.

Administration and Dosage:

Tablets and elixir:

Adults – 25 to 50 mg every 4 to 6 hours. As little as 25 mg may control symptoms; as much as 600 mg daily may be given in divided doses.

Children and infants – 5 mg/kg/day or 150 mg/m^2/day divided into 4 to 6 doses. Maximum total dose is 300 mg/day.

Sustained release tablets:

Adults – 100 mg in the morning and evening. In difficult cases, 100 mg every 8 hours may be required.

Children – Do not use in children.

Rx	**PBZ** (Geigy)	**Tablets:** 25 mg	(Geigy 111). White, scored. In 100s.
Rx	**Tripelennamine HCl** (Various)	**Tablets:** 50 mg	In 100s and 1000s.
Rx	**PBZ** (Geigy)		(Geigy 117). White, scored. In 100s & 1000s.
Rx	**Pelamine** (Major)		In 1000s.
Rx	**PBZ-SR** (Geigy)	**Tablets, sustained release:** 100 mg	(Geigy 48). Lavender. In 100s.
Rx	**PBZ** (Geigy)	**Elixir:** 37.5 mg tripelennamine citrate (equiv. to 25 mg HCl) per 5 ml	Cinnamon flavor. In 473 ml.

PYRILAMINE MALEATE

For complete prescribing information, refer to the Antihistamines group monograph.

Administration and Dosage:

Adults: 25 to 50 mg, 3 or 4 times daily.

otc	**Pyrilamine Maleate** (Rugby)	**Tablets:** 25 mg	In 1000s.

Alkylamines

CHLORPHENIRAMINE MALEATE

For complete prescribing information, refer to the Antihistamines group monograph.

Administration and Dosage:

Tablets or syrup:

Adults and children over 12 – 4 mg every 4 to 6 hours. Do not exceed 24 mg in 24 hours.

Children (6 to 12) – 2 mg every 4 to 6 hours. Do not exceed 12 mg in 24 hours.

(2 to 6): 1 mg every 4 to 6 hours. Do not exceed 4 mg in 24 hours.

Administration with food delays absorption, but does not affect bioavailability.

Sustained release forms:

Adults (12 years and older) – 8 to 12 mg at bedtime or every 8 to 12 hours during the day. Do not exceed 24 mg in 24 hours.

Children (6 to 12) – 8 mg at bedtime or during the day, as indicated.

(< 6): Not recommended for this age group.

Parenteral: The 10 mg/ml injection is intended for IV, IM or SC administration. The 100 mg/ml injection is intended for IM or SC use only.

Allergic reactions to blood or plasma – 10 to 20 mg as a single dose. The maximum recommended dose is 40 mg per 24 hours.

Anaphylaxis – 10 to 20 mg IV as a single dose.

Uncomplicated allergic conditions – 5 to 20 mg as a single dose.

otc	**Chlo-Amine** (Hollister-Stier)	**Tablets, chewable:** 2 mg	Orange. In 96s.
otc/ Rx[1]	**Chlorpheniramine Maleate** (Various)	**Tablets:** 4 mg	In 24s, 100s, 1000s and UD 24s, 100s and 1000s.
otc	**Aller-chlor** (Rugby)		In 24s, 100s & 1000s.
otc	**Allergy** (Parmed)		In 24s and 100s.
otc	**Chlorate** (Major)		In 24s and 100s.
otc	**Chlor-Trimeton Allergy** (Schering-Plough)		Lactose. In 24s.
otc	**Gen-Allerate** (Goldline)		Lactose. In 24s.
otc	**Pfeiffer's Allergy** (Pfeiffer)		Dye free. In 24s.
Rx	**Phenetron** (Lannett)		In 1000s.
otc	**Chlorpheniramine Maleate** (Various)	**Tablets:** 8 mg	In 100s and 1000s.
otc Rx[1]	**Chlorpheniramine Maleate** (Various)	**Tablets, timed release:** 8 mg	In 100s and 1000s.
otc	**Chlor-Trimeton 8 Hour Allergy** (Schering-Plough)		(Schering CC or 374). Yellow, sugar coated. In 24s, 48s and 100s.
otc/ Rx[1]	**Chlorpheniramine Maleate** (Various)	**Tablets:** 12 mg	In 100s and 1000s.
Rx	**Chlorpheniramine Maleate** (Various)	**Tablets, timed release:** 12 mg	In 100s.
otc	**Chlor-Trimeton 12 Hour Allergy** (Schering-Plough)		(Schering AAE or 009). Sugar coated. Orange. In 12s, 24s and 100s.
otc	**Efidac 24 Chlorphenir-amine** (Ciba)	**Tablets, extended release:** 16 mg	In 6s and 12s.
otc/ Rx[1]	**Chlorpheniramine Maleate** (Various)	**Capsules, timed release:** 8 mg	In 100s, 250s and 1000s.
Rx	**Telachlor** (Major)		In 100s and 1000s.
otc	**Chlorpheniramine Maleate** (Various)	**Capsules:** 12 mg	In 100s.

Alkylamines

CHLORPHENIRAMINE MALEATE

otc/ Rx[1]	**Chlorpheniramine Maleate** (Various)	**Capsules, timed release**: 12 mg	In 100s, 250s and 1000s.
Rx	**Telachlor** (Major)		In 100s, 250s and 1000s.
otc	**Teldrin** (SmithKline Consumer)		In 12s, 24s and 48s.
otc	**Pedia Care Allergy Formula** (McNeil-CPC)	**Liquid**: 1 mg per 5 ml	Alcohol free. Sorbitol, sucrose. Grape flavor. In 120 ml.
otc/ Rx[1]	**Chlorpheniramine Maleate** (Various)	**Syrup**: 2 mg per 5 ml	In 120 ml, pt and gal.
otc	**Aller-Chlor** (Rugby)		In 120 ml, pt and gal.
otc	**Chlor-Trimeton** (Schering)		7% alcohol. In 120 ml.
Rx	**Phenetron** (Lannett)		In pt and gal.
Rx	**Chlorpheniramine Maleate** (Various)	**Injection**: 10 mg per ml	In 30 ml vials.
Rx	**Chlor-Pro 10** (Schein)		In 30 ml vials.[2]
Rx	**Chlor-Trimeton** (Schering)		In 1 ml amps.
Rx	**Chlorpheniramine Maleate** (Various)	**Injection**: 100 mg per ml	In 10 ml vials.
Rx	**Chlor-Pro** (Schein)		In 10 ml vials.[2]

[1] Products are available *otc* or *Rx*, depending on product labeling.
[2] With benzyl alcohol.

DEXCHLORPHENIRAMINE MALEATE

For complete prescribing information, refer to the Antihistamines group monograph.

Administration and Dosage:

Adults: 2 mg every 4 to 6 hours, or 4 to 6 mg timed release tablets at bedtime, or every 8 to 10 hours during the day.

Children:

6 to 11 years – 1 mg every 4 to 6 hours or a 4 mg timed release tablet once daily at bedtime.

2 to 5 years – 0.5 mg every 4 to 6 hours. Do not use timed release form.

Rx	**Polaramine** (Schering)	**Tablets**: 2 mg	(Schering AGT or 820). Red. In 100s.
Rx	**Dexchlorpheniramine Maleate** (Various)	**Tablets, timed release**: 4 mg	In 100s.
Rx	**Dexchlor** (Schein)		In 100s.
Rx	**Poladex** (Major)		In 100s and 1000s.
Rx	**Polaramine** (Schering)		(Schering AGA or 095). Light red. Sugar coated. In 100s.
Rx	**Dexchlorpheniramine Maleate** (Various)	**Tablets, timed release**: 6 mg	In 100s and 1000s.
Rx	**Dexchlor** (Schein)		In 100s and 1000s.
Rx	**Poladex** (Major)		In 100s and 1000s.
Rx	**Polaramine** (Schering)		(Schering AGB or 148). Red. Sugar coated. In 100s and 1000s.
Rx	**Polaramine** (Schering)	**Syrup**: 2 mg/5 ml	6% alcohol. Sorbitol, menthol. Orange flavor. In 480 ml.

Alkylamines

BROMPHENIRAMINE MALEATE

For complete prescribing information, refer to the Antihistamines group monograph.

Administration and Dosage:

Oral: Adults (12 and older) — 4 mg every 4 to 6 hours, or 8 or 12 mg sustained release every 8 to 12 hours. Do not exceed 24 mg in 24 hours.

Children (6 to 12) – 2 mg every 4 to 6 hours. Do not exceed 12 mg in 24 hours. Administer sustained release preparations only as directed by a physician.

Children (< 6 years) – Use only as directed by a physician.

Parenteral: Give IM or SC without dilution. Give IV, either undiluted or diluted 1 to 10 with Sterile Saline for Injection. Administer slowly, preferably to recumbent patient. May add to normal saline, 5% glucose or whole blood for IV use.

Adults – Usual dose, 10 mg (range 5 to 20 mg). Duration of action, 3 to 12 hours; twice daily administration is usually sufficient. Maximum dose is 40 mg/24 hours.

Children (< 12) – 0.5 mg/kg/day or 15 mg/m^2/day, in 3 or 4 divided doses.

otc/ Rx[1]	**Brompheniramine** (Various)	**Tablets**: 4 mg	In 100s and 1000s.
Rx	**Brompheniramine** (Various)	**Tablets**: 8 mg	In 100s and 1000s.
Rx	**Brompheniramine** (Various)	**Tablets**: 12 mg	In 100s.
otc	**Dimetane Extentabs** (Robins)	**Tablets, timed release:** 12 mg	(AHR 1843). Peach. In 12s, 100s and 500s.
otc/ Rx[1]	**Brompheniramine** (Various)	**Elixir**: 2 mg/5 ml	In 120 ml, pt and gal.
otc/ Rx[1]	**Bromphen** (Various)		In 120 ml, pt & gal.
Rx	**Cophene-B** (Dunhall)	**Injection**: 10 mg/ml	In 10 ml vials.[2]
Rx	**Dehist** (Forest)		In 10 ml vials.[2]
Rx	**Nasahist B** (Keene)		In 10 ml vials.[2]
Rx	**ND Stat** (Hyrex)		In 10 ml vials.[2]
Rx	**Sinusol-B** (Kay Pharm.)		In 10 ml vials.[2]

[1] Products are available *otc* or *Rx*, depending on product labeling.
[2] With methyl and propyl parabens.

TRIPROLIDINE HCl

For complete prescribing information, refer to the Antihistamines group monograph.

Administration and Dosage:

Adults (12 and older): 2.5 mg every 4 to 6 hours.

Children (6 to 12 years): 1.25 mg every 4 to 6 hours.

Children < 6: Consult physician.

Do not exceed 4 doses in 24 hours.

Rx	**Triprolidine HCl** (Various)	**Syrup**: 1.25 mg per 5 ml	In 120 ml, pt and gal.
Rx	**Myidyl** (PBI)		In 120 ml, pt, gal.

Phenothiazines

PROMETHAZINE HCl

For complete prescribing information, refer to the Antihistamines group monograph.

Indications:

In addition to uses discussed in the general monograph, promethazine is indicated for: Active and prophylactic treatment of motion sickness; preoperative, postoperative or obstetric sedation; prevention and control of nausea and vomiting associated with anesthesia and surgery; an adjunct to analgesics for control of postoperative pain; sedation and relief of apprehension, and to produce light sleep; antiemetic effect in postoperative patients.

Intravenous: Special surgical situations such as repeated bronchoscopy, ophthalmic surgery, poor risk patients and with reduced amounts of meperidine or other narcotic analgesics as an adjunct to anesthesia and analgesia.

Administration and Dosage:

Oral and Rectal: Tablets and suppositories are not recommended for children less than 2 years of age.

Allergy – Average dose is 25 mg at bedtime. Give 12.5 mg before meals and at bedtime, if necessary. Children may be given 25 mg at bedtime or 6.25 to 12.5 mg 3 times daily. When the oral route is not feasible, use 25 mg suppositories. Repeat dose in 2 hours if necessary, but resume oral therapy when circumstances permit. Promethazine in 25 mg doses will control minor allergic transfusion reactions.

Motion sickness – 25 mg twice daily. Take initial dose ½ to 1 hour before travel; repeat in 8 to 12 hours, if necessary. Thereafter, give 25 mg doses on arising and before the evening meal. For children, 12.5 to 25 mg twice daily, oral or rectal.

Nausea and vomiting – 25 mg orally. Repeat doses of 12.5 to 25 mg, as necessary, at 4 to 6 hour intervals. When oral medication cannot be tolerated, administer parenterally or rectally. For prophylaxis of nausea and vomiting (as during surgery and the postoperative period) the average dose is 25 mg every 4 to 6 hours. For children, adjust the dose to the age and weight of the patient (0.5 mg/lb or 1 mg/kg).

Sedation – Adults: 25 to 50 mg. Children: 12.5 to 25 mg orally or rectally.

Preoperative use – 12.5 to 25 mg for children and 50 mg for adults, given the night before surgery. Children – 0.5 mg/lb (1 mg/kg) in combination with an equal dose of meperidine and the appropriate dose of an atropine-like drug. Adults - 50 mg with an equal amount of meperidine and the required amount of belladonna alkaloid.

Postoperative sedation and adjunctive use with analgesics – 25 to 50 mg in adults and 12.5 to 25 mg in children.

Parenteral: The preferred route is deep IM injection. Proper IV administration is well tolerated, but not without hazard. Injection SC is contraindicated as it may result in tissue necrosis. Do not administer by intra-arterial injection due to the likelihood of arteriospasm and the possibility of resultant gangrene.

Administer promethazine IV in a concentration no greater than 25 mg/ml and at a rate not to exceed 25 mg/minute.

Reduce the dose of barbiturates by at least one-half and the dose of narcotics by one-quarter to one-half when given concomitantly with promethazine.

Adults –

Allergy (including allergic reactions to blood or plasma): 25 mg, repeated within 2 hours if necessary.

Nausea and vomiting: 12.5 to 25 mg, not to be repeated more frequently than every 4 hours. When used for control of postoperative nausea and vomiting, reduce dosage of analgesics and barbiturates accordingly.

Nighttime sedation: 25 to 50 mg.

Preoperative and postoperative use: 25 to 50 mg in adults may be combined with appropriately reduced doses of analgesics and anticholinergics.

Labor: 50 mg in early stages of labor. When labor is established, give 25 to 75 mg IM or IV with a reduced dose of narcotic. Administer amnesic agents as needed. If necessary, give with a reduced dose of analgesic; this may be repeated once or twice, at 4 hour intervals. A maximum total dose in 24 hours is 100 mg.

Children (< 12 years) – Dosage should not exceed one-half the adult dose. As an adjunct to premedication, the dose is 0.5 mg/lb (1 mg/kg) in combination with a narcotic or barbiturate and the appropriate dose of an anticholinergic drug.

Do not use antiemetics in vomiting of unknown etiology.

Phenothiazines

PROMETHAZINE HCl

Rx	**Promethazine HCl** (Various)	**Tablets:** 12.5 mg	In 100s and 1000s.
Rx	**Phenergan** (Wyeth-Ayerst)		Saccharin. (Wyeth 19). Orange, scored. In 100s.
Rx	**Promethazine HCl** (Various)	**Tablets:** 25 mg	In 10s, 20s, 30s, 100s, 1000s and UD 100s.
Rx	**Phenameth** (Major)		In 100s and 1000s.
Rx	**Phenergan** (Wyeth-Ayerst)		Saccharin. (Wyeth 27). White, scored. In 100s and UD 100s.
Rx	**Promethazine HCl** (Various)	**Tablets:** 50 mg	In 100s and 1000s.
Rx	**Phenergan** (Wyeth-Ayerst)		(Wyeth 227). Pink. In 100s.
Rx	**Promethazine HCl** (Various)	**Syrup:** 6.25 mg per 5 ml	In 120 ml, pt, gal and UD 5 ml.
Rx	**Phenergan Plain** (Wyeth-Ayerst)		7% alcohol. Saccharin. In 120, 180 & 240 ml, pt & gal.
Rx	**Prothazine Plain** (Vortech)		7% alcohol. In 118 ml.
Rx	**Promethazine HCl** (Various)	**Syrup:** 25 mg per 5 ml	In 120 ml, pt and gal.
Rx	**Phenergan Fortis** (Wyeth-Ayerst)		1.5% alcohol. Saccharin. In 480 ml.
Rx	**Phenergan** (Wyeth-Ayerst)	**Suppositories:** 12.5 mg	(498). In 12s.
Rx	**Phenergan** (Wyeth-Ayerst)	**Suppositories:** 25 mg	(212). In 12s & UD 25s.
Rx	**Promethazine HCl** (Various)	**Suppositories:** 50 mg	In 12s and 25s.
Rx	**Phenergan** (Wyeth-Ayerst)		(229). In 12s & UD 25s.
Rx	**Promethazine HCl** (Various)	**Injection:** 25 mg per ml	In 1 ml amps and 1 and 10 ml vials.
Rx	**Phenergan** (Wyeth-Ayerst)		In 1 ml amps.[2]
Rx	**Prorex-25** (Hyrex)		In 10 ml vials.[1]
Rx	**Promethazine HCl** (Various, eg, Steris)	**Injection:** 50 mg per ml (For IM use only)	In 1 ml amps and 10 ml vials.
Rx	**Anergan 50** (Forest)		In 10 ml vials.[2]
Rx	**K-Phen-50** (Kay Pharm.)		In 10 ml vials.[2]
Rx	**Pentazine** (Century)		In 10 ml vials.[2]
Rx	**Phenazine 50** (Keene)		In 10 ml vials.[2]
Rx	**Phenergan** (Wyeth-Ayerst)		In 1 ml amps.[2]
Rx	**Phenoject-50** (Mayrand)		In 10 ml vials.[2]
Rx	**Pro-50** (Dunhall)		In 10 ml vials.[2]
Rx	**Prorex-50** (Hyrex)		In 10 ml vials.[2]

[1] With EDTA, benzyl alcohol and sodium metabisulfite.
[2] With EDTA, phenol and sodium metabisulfite.

Phenothiazines

TRIMEPRAZINE

For complete prescribing information, refer to the Antihistamines group monograph.

Administration and Dosage:

Tablets and syrup:

Adults – 2.5 mg 4 times daily.

Children (over 3 years) – 2.5 mg at bedtime or 3 times daily, if needed.

Children (6 months to 3 years) – 1.25 mg at bedtime or 3 times daily, if needed.

Sustained release capsules:

Adults – 5 mg every 12 hours.

Children (≥ 6 years) – 5 mg per day.

Rx	**Temaril** (Herbert Labs)	**Tablets:** 2.5 mg (as tartrate)	(HL T41). Gray. In 100s and UD 100s.
		Spansules (sustained release capsules): 5 mg (as tartrate)	(HL T50). Gray and clear. In 50s.
Rx	**Temaril** (Herbert Labs)	**Syrup:** 2.5 mg per 5 ml (as tartrate)	5.7% alcohol. Saccharin. Raspberry/strawberry flavor. In 120 ml.

METHDILAZINE HCl

For complete prescribing information, refer to the Antihistamines group monograph.

Administration and Dosage:

Adults: 8 mg 2 to 4 times daily.

Children: 4 mg 2 to 4 times daily.

Rx	**Tacaryl** (Westwood-Squibb)	**Tablets, chewable:** 4 mg	(W 7300). Saccharin. Pink. In 100s.
		Tablets: 8 mg	(W 7400). Peach, scored. In 100s.
		Syrup: 4 mg per 5 ml	7.37% alcohol. Menthol. Sorbitol. In pt.

Piperidines

CYPROHEPTADINE HCl

For complete prescribing information, refer to the Antihistamines group monograph.

Indications:

In addition to the general uses discussed in the antihistamine monograph, cyproheptadine is also indicated for cold urticaria.

Unlabeled uses: Cyproheptadine has antihistaminic, anticholinergic, antiserotonin and appetite-stimulating properties. Cyproheptadine has been used with variable success to stimulate appetite in underweight patients and in those with anorexia nervosa. It has also been used to treat vascular cluster headaches.

Administration and Dosage:

Individualize dosage.

Adults: 4 to 20 mg daily. Initiate therapy with 4 mg 3 times daily. A majority of patients require 12 to 16 mg per day and occasionally as much as 32 mg per day. Do not exceed 0.5 mg/kg/day (0.23 mg/lb/day).

Children: Calculate total daily dosage as approximately 0.25 mg/kg (0.11 mg/lb) or 8 mg/m^2.

Children (2 to 7 years) – 2 mg 2 or 3 times daily. Do not exceed 12 mg/day.

Children (7 to 14 years) – 4 mg 2 or 3 times daily. Do not exceed 16 mg/day.

Rx	**Cyproheptadine HCl** (Various, eg, Goldline, Halsey, Major, Moore, Parmed, Rugby, Schein, URL, Zenith)	**Tablets:** 4 mg	In 100s, 500s, 1000s and UD 100s.
Rx	**Periactin** (Merck)		Lactose. (MSD 62). White, scored. In 100s.
Rx	**Cyproheptadine HCl** (Various, eg, Barre-National, Goldline, Moore, Parmed, Rugby, Schein)	**Syrup:** 2 mg per 5 ml	In pt and gal.
Rx	**Periactin** (Merck)		5% alcohol, sucrose, saccharin. In 473 ml.

AZATADINE MALEATE

For complete prescribing information, refer to the Antihistamines group monograph.

Administration and Dosage:

Individualize dosage.

Adults: 1 or 2 mg twice a day.

Children: Not intended for use in children < 12 years old.

Rx	**Optimine** (Schering)	**Tablets:** 1 mg	(Schering 282). White, scored. In 100s.

PHENINDAMINE TARTRATE

For complete prescribing information, refer to the Antihistamines group monograph.

Administration and Dosage:

Adults: 25 mg every 4 to 6 hours. Do not exceed 150 mg in 24 hours.

Children (6 to < 12 Years): 12.5 mg every 4 to 6 hours. Do not exceed 75 mg in 24 hours.

Children (under 6 years): As directed by physician.

otc	**Nolahist** (Carnrick)	**Tablets:** 25 mg	(C 8652). White, scored. In 100s and UD 168s.

Miscellaneous

ASTEMIZOLE

For complete prescribing information, refer to the Antihistamines group monogrpah.

Indications:

For the relief of symptoms associated with seasonal allergic rhinitis and chronic idiopathic urticaria.

Administration and Dosage:

Adults and children ≥ 12 years of age: 10 mg daily. Do not exceed the recommended dose. Advise patients not to increase the dose in an attempt to accelerate the onset of action.

Take on an empty stomach at least 2 hours after a meal. There should be no additional food intake for at least 1 hour post-dosing.

Children 6 to 12 years of age: 5 mg daily.

Hepatic function impairment: Because astemizole is extensively metabolized by the liver, generally avoid use in these patients.

Rx	**Hismanal** (Janssen)	**Tablets:** 10 mg	Lactose, povidone. (Janssen AST/10). White, scored. In 30s and 100s.

LORATADINE

For complete prescribing information, refer to the Antihistamines group monograph.

Indications:

For the relief of nasal and non-nasal symptoms of seasonal allergic rhinitis, and for the management of idiopathic chronic urticaria.

Administration and Dosage:

Adults and children ≥ 12 years of age: 10 mg once daily on an empty stomach.

Children 2 to 12 years of age (weight < 30 kg): 5 mg daily.

Hepatic/Renal function impairment (GFR < 30 ml/min): 10 mg every other day.

Rx	**Claritin** (Schering)	**Tablets:** 10 mg	Lactose. (458/Claritin 10). White to off-white. In 100s and 500s, unit-of-use 14s and 30s and UD 100s.
Rx	**Claritin RediTabs** (Schering)	**Tablets, rapidly disintegrating:** 10 mg	Mannitol. In unit-of-use 30s.
Rx	**Claritin** (Schering)	**Syrup:** 1 mg/ml	Sugar. In 480 ml bottles.

Miscellaneous

TERFENADINE

For complete prescribing information, refer to the Antihistamines group monograph.

Indications:

For the relief of symptoms associated with seasonal allergic rhinitis such as sneezing, rhinorrhea, pruritus and lacrimation.

Administration and Dosage:

Adults and children ≥ 12 years of age: 60 mg twice daily.

Children: The following doses have been suggested:

(6 to 12 years of age) – 30 to 60 mg twice daily.

(3 to 6 years of age) – 15 mg twice daily.

Rx	**Terfenadine** (Goldline)	**Tablets**: 60 mg	In 30s, 100s and 500s.
Rx	**Seldane** (Hoechst Marion Roussel)		Lactose. (Seldane). White. In 100s and 500s.

FEXOFENADINE HCl

For complete prescribing information, refer to the Antihistamines group monograph.

Indications:

For the relief of symptoms associated with seasonal allergic rhinitis in adults and children ≥ 12 years of age. Symptoms treated effectively include sneezing; rhinorrhea; itchy nose, palate and throat; and itchy, watery and red eyes.

Administration and Dosage:

Approved by the FDA on July 25, 1996.

The recommended dose for adults and children ≥ 12 years of age is 60 mg twice daily.

Renal function impairment: 60 mg once daily.

Rx	**Allegra** (Hoechst Marion Roussel)	**Capsules**: 60 mg	Lactose. (1102). White and pink. In 60s, 100s, 500s and UD 100s.

Miscellaneous

CETIRIZINE HCl

For complete prescribing information, refer to the Antihistamines group monograph.

Indications:

Seasonal allergic rhinitis: Relief of symptoms associated with seasonal allergic rhinitis due to allergens such as ragweed, grass and tree pollen in adults and children ≥ 6 years of age. Symptoms treated effectively include sneezing, rhinorrhea, nasal pruritus, ocular pruritus, tearing and redness of the eye.

Perennial allergic rhinitis: Relief of symptoms associated with perennial allergic rhinitis due to allergens such as dust mites, animal dander and molds in adults and children ≥ 6 years of age. Symptoms treated effectively include sneezing, rhinorrhea, post-nasal discharge, nasal pruitus, ocular pruritus and tearing.

Chronic uriticaria: Uncomplicated skin manifestations of chronic idiopathic urticaria in adults and children ≥ 6 years of age. It significantly reduces the occurrence, severity and duration of hives and significantly reduces pruritus.

Administration and Dosage:

Approved by the FDA on December 12, 1995.

The recommended initial dose is 5 or 10 mg/day in adults and children ≥ 6 years of age, depending on symptom severity. Most patients in clinical trials started at 10 mg. Cetirizine is given as a single daily dose, with or without food. The time of administration may be varied to suit individual patient needs.

Renal/Hepatic function impairment: In patients with decreased renal function (creatine clearance 11 to 31 ml/min), hemodialysis patients (creatine clearance < 7 ml/min) and in hepatically impaired patients, 5 mg once daily is recommended.

Rx	**Zyrtec** (Pfizer)	**Tablets:** 5 mg	Lactose, povidone. (Pfizer 550). Dye free, white, film coated. In 100s.
		10 mg	Lactose, povidone. (Pfizer 551). Dye free, white, film coated. In 100s.
Rx	**Zyrtec** (Pfizer)	**Syrup:** 5 mg/5 ml	Fruity banana-grape flavor. Alcohol and dye free. In 120 ml.

AZELASTINE HCl

For complete prescribing information, refer to the Antihistamines group monograph.

Indications:

Seasonal allergic rhinitis: For treatment of symptoms of seasonal allergic rhinitis such as rhinorrhea, sneezing and nasal pruritus in adults and children ≥ 12 years old.

Administration and Dosage:

The recommended dose of azelastine nasal spray in adults and children ≥ 12 years old is 2 sprays per nostril twice daily. Before initial use, replace the child-resistant screw cap on the bottle with the pump unit and prime the delivery system with 4 sprays or until a fine mist appears. When ≥ 3 days have elapsed since the last use, reprime the pump with 2 sprays or until a fine mist appears.

Avoid spraying in the eyes.

Storage/Stability: Store at controlled room temperature 20° to 25°C (68° to 77°F). Protect from freezing.

Rx	**Astelin** (Wallace)	**Spray:** 137 mcg/actuation	Benzalkonium chloride, EDTA. 17 mg (100 actuations) per bottle. In 2s.

Miscellaneous

COMBINED ANTIHISTAMINE PREPARATIONS

For complete prescribing information, refer to the Antihistamines group monograph.

Indications:

Perennial and seasonal allergic rhinitis; vasomotor rhinitis; allergic conjunctivitis due to inhalant allergens and food; mild uncomplicated allergic skin manifestations of urticaria.

Administration and Dosage:

Adults: 10 ml every 4 hours.

Children (6 to 12 years of age): 5 ml every 4 hours.

Children (2 to 6 years of age): 2.5 ml every 4 hours.

Children (< 2 years of age): As directed by physician.

Rx	**Poly-Histine** (Bock)	**Elixir:** 4 mg pheniramine maleate, 4 mg pyrilamine maleate and 4 mg phenyltoloxamine citrate/5 ml	4% alcohol. In 480 ml.

CODEINE

The following is an abbreviated monograph covering the primary considerations in the use of codeine as an antitussive. For complete information on opiates, some having antitussive properties, refer to the Narcotic Agonist Analgesics monograph.

Actions:

Pharmacology: Codeine has good antitussive activity; side effects are infrequent at the usual antitussive dose. The dose required to suppress coughing is lower than the dose required for analgesia.

Pharmacokinetics: Codeine and its salts are well absorbed. Codeine is metabolized primarily in the liver and is excreted primarily in the urine within 24 hours, 5% to 15% as unchanged codeine and the remainder as the products of glucuronide conjugation and metabolites. The plasma half-life of codeine is about 2.9 hours.

Indications:

For suppression of cough induced by chemical or mechanical respiratory tract irritation.

Relief of mild to moderate pain (see Narcotic Agonist Analgesics monograph).

Contraindications:

Hypersensitivity to the drug; premature infants or during labor when delivery of a premature infant is anticipated (see Warnings).

Warnings:

Head injury and increased intracranial pressure: The respiratory depressant effects of the opiates and their capacity to elevate cerebrospinal fluid pressure may be markedly exaggerated in the presence of head injury, intracranial lesions or a preexisting increase in intracranial pressure. Usual oral doses of codeine produce little respiratory depression; however, exercise caution, particularly with larger doses. Furthermore, opiates may produce adverse reactions which may obscure the clinical course of patients with head injuries.

Asthma and other respiratory conditions: Use with extreme caution in patients having an acute asthmatic attack, patients with chronic obstructive pulmonary disease or cor pulmonale, patients having a substantially decreased respiratory reserve and patients with preexisting respiratory depression, hypoxia or hypercapnia. Usual therapeutic doses may decrease respiratory drive while simultaneously increasing airway resistance to the point of apnea. In asthma and pulmonary emphysema, codeine may, due to its drying action on the respiratory mucosa, precipitate insufficiency resulting from increased viscosity of the bronchial secretions and suppression of the cough reflex.

Acute abdominal conditions: Administration of codeine or other opiates may obscure the diagnosis or clinical course in patients with acute abdominal conditions.

Pregnancy: Category C. Dependence has been reported in newborns whose mothers took opiates regularly during pregnancy. Withdrawal signs include irritability, excessive crying, tremors, hyperreflexia, fever, vomiting and diarrhea. Signs usually appear during the first few days of life. Use during pregnancy only if the potential benefits outweigh the potential hazards to the fetus.

Labor and delivery – Opiates cross the placental barrier. The closer to delivery and the larger the dose used, the greater the possibility of respiratory depression in the newborn. Avoid use during labor if a premature infant is anticipated. If the mother has received opiates during labor, closely observe newborn for signs of respiratory depression. Resuscitation and, in severe depression, naloxone may be required. Codeine may also prolong labor.

Lactation: Exercise caution. Some studies have reported detectable amounts of codeine in breast milk. The levels are probably not clinically significant after usual therapeutic dosage. Clinically important amounts may be excreted in breast milk in individuals abusing codeine.

Children: Do not use opiates, including codeine, in premature infants. Opiates cross the immature blood-brain barrier to a greater extent, producing disproportionate respiratory depression. Give opiates to infants and small children only with great caution and carefully monitor dosage. Safety and efficacy of codeine in newborn infants have not been established.

Precautions:

Administer with caution, and reduce the initial dose in patients with acute abdominal conditions, convulsive disorders, significant hepatic or renal impairment, fever, hypothyroidism, Addison's disease, ulcerative colitis, prostatic hypertrophy, urethral stricture, patients with recent GI or urinary tract surgery and in very young, elderly or debilitated patients.

CODEINE

Drug abuse and dependence:

Abuse – The abuse potential of codeine is less than that of heroin or morphine.

Most patients who receive opiates for medical indications do not develop drug-seeking behavior or compulsive drug use. However, give under close supervision to patients with a history of drug abuse or dependence.

Dependence – Psychological dependence, physical dependence and tolerance may occur.

The severity of the abstinence syndrome is related to degree of dependence, abruptness of withdrawal and the drug used. If the syndrome is precipitated by a narcotic antagonist, symptoms appear in a few minutes and are maximal within 30 minutes.

While codeine can partially suppress the symptoms of morphine withdrawal, the codeine withdrawal syndrome (after 1.2 to 1.8 g codeine/day), though similar to that seen with morphine, is less intense. Withdrawal symptoms in patients dependent on codeine include yawning, sweating, lacrimation, rhinorrhea, a restless sleep, dilated pupils, gooseflesh, irritability, tremor, nausea, vomiting and diarrhea. Treatment is primarily symptomatic and supportive, including maintenance of proper fluid and electrolyte balance.

Drug Interactions:

CNS depressants (eg, other opiates, general anesthetics, phenothiazines, tricyclic antidepressants, tranquilizers) and **alcohol**. Use codeine cautiously and in reduced dosage to avoid additive effects when given concomitantly.

Drug/Lab test interactions: Because opiates may increase biliary tract pressure, with resultant increases in plasma amylase or lipase levels, determination of these enzyme levels may be unreliable for 24 hours after an opiate has been given.

Adverse Reactions:

In usual oral antitussive doses, codeine has minimal side effects. Nausea, vomiting, sedation, dizziness and constipation are most common.

Allergic reactions to opiates occur infrequently; pruritus, giant urticaria, angioneurotic edema and laryngeal edema have occurred following IV administration.

CNS: CNS depression, particularly respiratory depression, and to a lesser extent, circulatory depression; respiratory arrest, shock and cardiac arrest, particularly in overdosage or with rapid IV administration. Other effects include: Lightheadedness; dizziness; sedation; euphoria; dysphoria; weakness; headache; hallucinations; disorientation; visual disturbances; convulsions. These effects are more common with larger parenteral doses, in ambulatory patients and in those who are not experiencing severe pain. Some reactions in ambulatory patients may be alleviated by lying down.

GI: Nausea; vomiting; constipation; biliary tract spasm. Patients with ulcerative colitis may experience increased colonic motility or toxic dilation.

Cardiovascular: Tachycardia; bradycardia; palpitation; faintness; syncope; orthostatic hypotension.

GU: Oliguria; urinary retention; antidiuretic effect.

Overdosage:

The lethal oral dose of codeine in an adult is in the range of 0.5 to 1 g. Infants and children are relatively more sensitive to opiates on a body weight basis. Elderly patients are also comparatively intolerant.

For a description of opiate overdosage and treatment, see the Narcotic Agonist Analgesics monograph.Refer also to General Management of Acute Overdosage.

CODEINE

Patient Information:

May impair the mental or physical abilities required for the performance of potentially hazardous tasks. Observe caution while driving or performing other tasks requiring alertness, coordination or physical dexterity.

The concomitant use of alcohol or other CNS depressants, including sedatives, hypnotics, antidepressants, tranquilizers, phenothiazines and antihistamines, may have an additive effect.

May produce orthostatic hypotension (dizziness, lightheadedness when rising quickly from a sitting or lying position) in some ambulatory patients.

Do not take for persistent or chronic cough, such as occurs with smoking, asthma or emphysema; or where cough is accompanied by excessive secretions, except under supervision of physician.

May cause dry mouth or constipation.

May cause GI upset; take with food or milk.

Administration and Dosage:

Adults: 10 to 20 mg every 4 to 6 hours. Maximum 120 mg/day.

Children:

6 to 12 years – 5 to 10 mg every 4 to 6 hours. Maximum 60 mg/day.
2 to 6 years – 2.5 to 5 mg every 4 to 6 hours. Maximum 30 mg/day.

Infants: Do not use in premature infants. Safety and efficacy in newborn infants have not been established.

Codeine is also available in many multi-ingredient respiratory preparations as an antitussive. Refer to the Upper Respiratory Combinations.

c-ii	**Codeine Sulfate** (Various, eg, Halsey, Knoll, Lilly, Roxane)	**Tablets:** 15 mg	In 100s and UD 100s.
		30 mg	In 100s, 1000s and UD 100s.
		60 mg	In 100s and UD 100s.

DEXTROMETHORPHAN HBr

Dextromethorphan is the d–isomer of the codeine analog of levorphanol; it lacks analgesic and addictive properties. Its cough suppressant action is due to a central action on the cough center in the medulla. Dextromethorphan 15 to 30 mg equals 8 to 15 mg codeine as an antitussive.

Indications:

To control nonproductive cough.

Contraindications:

Hypersensitivity to any component.

Warnings:

Do not use for persistent or chronic cough (eg, smoking, asthma, emphysema) or cough accompanied by excessive secretions. Persons with high fever, rash, persistent headache, nausea or vomiting should use only under medical supervision.

Drug Abuse and Dependence: Anecdotal reports of abuse of dextromethorphan-containing cough/cold products has increased, especially among teenagers. The FDA Drug Abuse Advisory Committee states that additional data is needed before determining the abuse and dependency potential of dextromethorphan.

Drug Interactions:

MAO inhibitors: Patients may develop hypotension, hyperpyrexia, nausea, myoclonic leg jerks and coma following coadministration.

Overdosage:

Symptoms:

Adults – Altered sensory perception; ataxia; slurred speech; dysphoria.
Children – Ataxia, respiratory depression; convulsions.

Administration and Dosage:

Liquid, lozenges and syrup: Adults and children (> 12 years of age) — 10 to 30 mg every 4 to 8 hours. Do not exceed 120 mg in 24 hours.

Children (6 to 12 years) – 5 to 10 mg every 4 hours or 15 mg every 6 to 8 hours. Do not exceed 60 mg in 24 hours.

Children (2 to 6 years) – 2.5 to 7.5 mg every 4 to 8 h. Do not exceed 30 mg/day.
Children (< 2 years) – Use only as directed by a physician.

Sustained action liquid: Adults — 60 mg every 12 hours.
Children (6 to 12 years) – 30 mg every 12 hours.
Children (2 to 5 years) – 15 mg every 12 hours.

otc	**Drixoral Cough Liquid Caps** (Schering-Plough)	**Capsules:** 30 mg	Sorbitol. In 10s.
otc sf	**Scot-Tussin DM Cough Chasers** (Scot-Tussin)	**Lozenges:** 2.5 mg	Dye free. Sorbitol. In 20s.
otc	**Children's Hold** (Menley & James)	**Lozenges:** 5 mg	Sucrose, corn syrup. In 10s.
otc	**Hold DM** (Menley & James)		Corn syrup, sucrose. In 10s.
otc	**Robitussin Cough Calmers** (Robins)		Corn syrup, sucrose. (AHR). Square. Cherry flavor. In 16s.
otc	**Sucrets Cough Control** (SK-Beecham)		Corn syrup, sucrose. In 24s.
otc	**Suppress** (Ferndale)	**Lozenges:** 7.5 mg	In 1000s.
otc	**Trocal** (Roberts Med)		In 500s.
otc	**Sucrets 4-Hour Cough** (SK-Beecham)	**Lozenges:** 15 mg	Menthol, sucrose, corn syrup. Wild cherry flavor. In 20s.
otc	**Creo-Terpin** (Lee)	**Liquid:** 10 mg per 15 ml (3.33 mg/5 ml)	Tartrazine, 25% alcohol, creosote, corn syrup, terpin hydrate, saccharin. In 120 ml.
otc	**Pertussin CS** (Pertussin)	**Liquid:** 3.5 mg per 5 ml	Alcohol free. Sorbitol, sucrose. Wild berry flavor. In 120 ml.

DEXTROMETHORPHAN HBr

otc *sf*	**Robitussin Pediatric** (Robins)	**Liquid:** 7.5 mg per 5 ml	Alcohol free. Saccharin, sorbitol. Cherry flavor. In 120 & 240 ml.
otc *sf*	**Benylin Pediatric** (Warner Wellcome)		Alcohol free. Saccharin, sorbitol. Grape flavor. In 118 ml.
otc	**St. Joseph Cough Suppressant** (Schering-–Plough)		Alcohol free. Sucrose. Cherry flavor. In 60 and 120 ml.
otc *sf*	**Benylin Adult** (Glaxo Wellcome)	**Liquid:** 15 mg per 5 ml	Alcohol free. Saccharin, sorbitol. In 118 ml.
otc	**Pertussin ES** (Pertussin)		9.5% alcohol. Sugar, sorbitol. In 120 ml.
otc	**Vicks Dry Hacking Cough** (Procter & Gamble)		10% alcohol. Sugar. In 120 and 240 ml.
otc	**Pediatric Vicks 44d Dry Hacking Cough and Head Congestion** (Procter & Gamble)	**Syrup:** 15 mg per 15 ml (1 mg/ml)	Alcohol free. Sorbitol, sucrose. Cherry flavor. In 120 ml.
otc	**Dextromethorphan** (Various, eg, PBI, Rugby)	**Syrup:** 10 mg per 5 ml	Alcohol. In 120 ml & gal.
otc	**Benylin DM** (Parke-Davis)		5% alcohol. Glucose, menthol, sucrose. In 118 ml.
otc	**Silphen DM** (Silarx)		5% alcohol. In 118 ml.
otc	**Delsym** (Fisons)	**Liquid, sustained action:** Dextromethorphan polistirex equivalent to 30 mg dextromethorphan HBr/5 ml.	Alcohol free. Corn syrup, sucrose. Orange flavor. In 89 ml.

DIPHENHYDRAMINE HCl

Refer to the Antihistamines group monograph for complete prescribing information.

Indications:

For the control of cough due to colds or allergy.

Administration and Dosage:

Adults: 25 mg every 4 hours, not to exceed 150 mg in 24 hours.

Children (6 to 12 years): 12.5 mg every 4 hours, not to exceed 75 mg in 24 hours.

Children (2 to 6 years): 6.25 mg every 4 hours, not to exceed 25 mg in 24 hours.

Note: These formulations may contain ammonium chloride and sodium citrate. Although these ingredients have been used as expectorants, there is inadequate evidence of their clinical value; they have not been approved by the FDA as *otc* expectorants. Products currently on the market have deleted any therapeutic claims for these components. They remain in the product formulation and are listed only as inactive ingredients.

otc/ *Rx*[1]	**Diphenhydramine HCl Cough** (Various, eg, IDE, Major, URL)	**Syrup:** 12.5 mg per 5 ml	In 120 and 240 ml, pt and gal.
otc	**Bydramine** (Major)		5% alcohol. In 118 ml.
otc	**Diphen Cough** (PBI)		Ammonium chloride, sodium citrate, 5% alcohol, sugar, menthol, sorbitol, sucrose. Raspberry flavor. In 120 ml, pt and gal.
otc	**Silphen Cough** (Silarx)		Menthol, sucrose, 5% alcohol. Strawberry flavor. In 118 ml.
Rx	**Tusstat** (Century)		5% alcohol. In 30 and 120 ml, pt and gal.
otc	**Uni-Bent Cough** (URL)		5% alcohol. In 118 ml.

[1] Products are available *otc* or *Rx*, depending on product labeling.

BENZONATATE

Actions:

Pharmacology: Benzonatate is related to tetracaine. It anesthetizes stretch receptors in respiratory passages, lungs and pleura, dampening their activity, and reducing the cough reflex at its source. It has no inhibitory effect on the respiratory center in recommended dosage. Onset of action is 15 to 20 minutes; effects last 3 to 8 hours.

Indications:

Symptomatic relief of cough.

Contraindications:

Hypersensitivity to benzonatate or related compounds (eg, tetracaine).

Warnings:

Pregnancy: Category C. It is not known whether the drug can cause fetal harm or can affect reproduction capacity. Give to a pregnant woman only if clearly needed.

Lactation: It is not known whether this drug is excreted in breast milk. Exercise caution when administering to a nursing woman.

Precautions:

Local anesthesia: Release of benzonatate in the mouth can produce a temporary local anesthesia of the oral mucosa. Swallow the capsules without chewing.

Adverse Reactions:

Sedation; headache; mild dizziness; constipation; nausea; GI upset; pruritus; skin eruptions; nasal congestion; sensation of burning in the eyes; a vague "chilly" sensation; chest numbness; hypersensitivity.

Overdosage:

Symptoms: If capsules are chewed or dissolved in the mouth, oropharyngeal anesthesia will develop rapidly. CNS stimulation may cause restlessness and tremors which may proceed to clonic convulsions followed by profound CNS depression.

Treatment: Includes usual supportive measures. Refer to General Management of Acute Overdosage. Even in the conscious patient, cough and gag reflexes may be so depressed as to necessitate protection against aspiration of gastric contents.

Treat convulsions with IV short-acting barbiturate. Employ intensive support of respiration and cardiovascular-renal function if required. Do not use CNS stimulants.

Patient Information:

Do not chew or break capsules; swallow whole.

Administration and Dosage:

Adults and children (> 10 years): 100 mg 3 times daily, up to 600 mg/day.

Rx	**Benzonatate Softgels** (Various, eg, Schein, Sidmak)	**Capsules:** 100 mg	In 100s and 1000s.
Rx	**Tessalon Perles** (Forest)		Yellow. In 100s and 500s.

DEXTROMETHORPHAN HBr and BENZOCAINE

Administration and Dosage:

Vicks Formula 44:

Adults and children ≥ 12 years – 2 lozenges dissolved in mouth, one at a time, every 4 hours. Do not exceed 12 lozenges in 24 hours.

Children 3 to 12 years – 1 lozenge every 4 hours. Do not exceed 6 in 24 hours.

Children < 3 years – Use only as directed by physician.

Vicks Cough Silencers:

Adults and children ≥ 12 years – 4 lozenges dissolved in mouth, one at a time, every 4 hours. Do not exceed 48 lozenges in 24 hours.

Children 6 to < 12 yrs – 2 to 4 lozenges every 4 hrs. Do not exceed 24 in 24 hrs.

Children 2 to < 6 yrs – 1 to 2 lozenges every 4 hours. Do not exceed 12 in 24 hrs.

Children < 2 – Use only as directed by physician.

Spec-T: Adults and children ≥ 6 years — 1 every 3 hrs. Do not exceed 6 in 24 hrs.

Children < 6 years – Use only as directed.

otc	**Spec-T** (Apothecon)	**Lozenges:** 10 mg dextromethorphan HBr and 10 mg benzocaine	Tartrazine, sucrose, dextrose, glucose. In 10s.
otc	**Cough-X** (Ascher)	Lozenges: 5 mg dextromethorphan and 2 mg benzocaine	Dye free. Menthol-eucalyptus flavor. In 9s.
otc	**Vicks Formula 44 Cough Control Discs** (Richardson-Vicks)	**Lozenges:** 5 mg dextromethorphan HBr and 1.25 mg benzocaine	4.3 mg menthol, sucrose. (F 44). In 24s.
otc	**Vicks Cough Silencers** (Richardson-Vicks)	**Lozenges:** 2.5 mg dextromethorphan HBr, 1 mg benzocaine	Tartrazine, menthol, anethole, corn syrup, sucrose. In 14s.

GUAIFENESIN (Glyceryl Guaiacolate)

Actions:

Pharmacology: Guaifenesin is claimed to enhance the output of respiratory tract fluid by reducing adhesiveness and surface tension facilitating the removal of viscous mucus. As a result, nonproductive coughs become more productive and less frequent. There is a lack of convincing studies to document efficacy.

Indications:

For the symptomatic relief of respiratory conditions characterized by dry, nonproductive cough and in the presence of mucus in the respiratory tract.

Contraindications:

Hypersensitivity to guaifenesin.

Warnings:

Not for persistent cough such as occurs with smoking, asthma or emphysema, or where cough is accompanied by excessive secretions.

Precautions:

Persistent cough may indicate a serious condition. If cough persists for more than 1 week, tends to recur, or is accompanied by high fever, rash or persistent headache, consult physician. Excessive dosage may cause nausea and vomiting.

Drug Interactions:

Drug/Lab test interactions: May cause a color interference with certain laboratory determinations of 5-hydroxyindoleacetic acid (5-HIAA) and vanillylmandelic acid (VMA).

Adverse Reactions:

Nausea, vomiting (most common); dizziness; headache; rash (including urticaria).

Administration and Dosage:

Adults and children (≥ 12): 100 to 400 mg every 4 hours. Do not exceed 2.4 g/day.

Children (6 to 12): 100 to 200 mg every 4 hours. Do not exceed 1.2 g/day.

Children (2 to 6): 50 to 100 mg every 4 hours. Do not exceed 600 mg/day.

otc	**Guaifenesin** (Various, eg, Lederle, Major, Roxane, UDL)	**Syrup:** 100 mg/5 ml	In 120 and 240 ml, pt, gal and UD 5, 10 and 15 ml.
otc	**Guiatuss** (Various, eg, Barre-National, Genetco, Goldline, Moore)		In 120 and 240 ml, pt and gal.
otc	**Anti-Tuss** (Century)		3.5% alcohol. In 120 ml and gal.
otc	**Genatuss** (Goldline)		3.5% alcohol. In 120 ml.
otc	**Glyate** (Geneva)		3.5% alcohol. In 118 & 480 ml.
otc	**Halotussin** (Halsey)		3.5% alcohol. In 120 and 240 ml, pt and gal.
otc	**Mytussin** (PBI)		3.5% alcohol. Sugar, menthol. Raspberry flavor. In 120 ml, pt & gal.
otc	**Robitussin** (Robins Consumer)		3.5% alcohol, glucose, corn syrup, saccharin. In 30, 60, 120 & 240 ml, pt, gal & UD 5, 10 & 15 ml.
otc	**Siltussin** (Silarx)		3.5% alcohol. In 473 ml.
otc sf	**Scot-tussin Expectorant** (Scot-Tussin)		3.5% alcohol, saccharin, menthol, sorbitol. Dye free. In 120 ml, pt and gal.
otc	**Tusibron** (Kenwood/Bradley)		3.5% alcohol. In 118 ml.
otc	**Uni-tussin** (URL)		3.5% alcohol. In 118 ml.
otc sf	**Diabetic Tussin EX** (Health Care Products)	**Liquid:** 100 mg/5 ml	Alcohol and dye free. Saccharin, menthol, methylparaben. In 118 ml.
Rx sf	**Organidin NR** (Wallace)		Alcohol free. Saccharin, sorbitol. In pt and gal. "NR" means "Newly Reformulated."

GUAIFENESIN (Glyceryl Guaiacolate)

otc sf	**Naldecon Senior EX** (Apothecon)	**Liquid**: 200 mg/5 ml	Saccharin, sorbitol. In 118 and 480 ml.
otc	**Breonesin** (Winthrop)	**Capsules**: 200 mg	(Breon). Red. Sugar coated. In 100s.
otc	**GG-Cen** (Central)		Purple/white. In 24s & 100s.
otc sf	**Hytuss 2X** (Hyrex)		(Hyrex). Maroon/white. In 50s, 100s, 1000s.
Rx	**Humibid Sprinkle** (Adams Labs)	**Capsules, sustained release**: 300 mg	(Adams/0018). Green and clear. In 100s.
otc	**Glycotuss** (Pal-Pak)	**Tablets**: 100 mg	White. In 100s and 1000s.
otc sf	**Hytuss** (Hyrex)		Dye free. (HY). White, scored. In 100s and 1000s.
otc	**Gee-Gee** (Jones)	**Tablets**: 200 mg	Green. In 1000s.
otc	**Glytuss** (Mayrand)		White. Film coated. In 100s.
Rx sf	**Organidin NR** (Wallace)		Rose, scored. In 100s.
Rx	**Duratuss-G** (UCB Pharma)	**Tablets**: 1200 mg	(UCB/620). Dye free. White, scored. Capsule shape. Film-coated. In 100s.
Rx	**Guaifenex LA** (Ethex)	**Tablets, extended release**: 600 mg	Lactose. (Ethex/205). White. In 100s.
Rx	**Fenesin** (Dura)		(Dura-009). Lt. blue, scored. In 100s and 600s.
Rx	**Humibid L.A.** (Adams Labs)		(Adams/0012). Green, scored. In 100s and 500s.
Rx	**Liquibid** (Ion)		Dye free. Scored. In 100s.
Rx	**Monafed** (Monarch Pharmaceuticals)		Lactose. (KPI 13). Lt. green, scored. In 100s.
Rx	**Muco-Fen-LA** (Wakefield)		Dye free. In 100s.
Rx	**Pneumomist** (EC Pharm)		(ECR 600). Light pink, scored. In 100s.
Rx	**Respa-GF** (Respa)		In 100s.
Rx	**Sinumist-SR Capsulets** (Hauck)		(048 Hauck Sinumist). Green speckled, scored. In 100s.
Rx	**Touro Ex** (Dartmouth Pharm)	**Caplets, sustained release**: 600 mg	(G 600 Trinity). Light green, scored. In 100s.

TERPIN HYDRATE*

Actions:

Pharmacology: Acts by direct stimulation of respiratory tract secretory glands to increase output of respiratory tract fluid. Recommended dose is insufficient to cause significant mucokinetic effect. Used mainly as a vehicle for cough mixtures.

Indications:

Symptomatic relief of dry, non-productive cough.

Warnings:

Pregnancy: Terpin hydrate contains alcohol, which crosses the placenta. Excessive use may result in congenital abnormalities.

Lactation: Weigh risk to benefit; the alcohol content is excreted in breast milk.

Adverse Reactions:

May cause drowsiness due to the high alcohol content. Observe caution while driving or performing other tasks requiring alertness. Nausea, vomiting or abdominal pain may occur if taken on an empty stomach.

Patient Information:

Drink plenty of liquid; do not exceed recommended dosage; may cause drowsiness.

Administration and Dosage:

85 to 170 mg 3 or 4 times daily. Do not give to children unless directed by physician. Recommended doses for children (given 3 or 4 times a day): 1 to 4 years, 20 mg; 5 to 9 years, 40 mg; 10 to 12 years, 85 mg.

otc	**Terpin Hydrate** (Various)	**Elixir**: 85 mg per 5 ml	≈ 42% alcohol. In 120 ml, pt and gal.

IODINATED GLYCEROL

Administration and Dosage:

Adults: 60 mg 4 times/day.

Children: Up to half the adult dose, based on weight.

Rx	**Iophen** (Rugby)	**Tablets**: 30 mg (15 mg organically bound iodine)	In 100s.
Rx	**Iophen** (Various, eg, Barre-National, Genetco, Geneva, Major, Moore, Rugby)	**Elixir**: 60 mg (30 mg organically bound iodine) per 5 ml	In 120 and 480 ml.
Rx	**Par Glycerol** (Par)		21.75% alcohol, peppermint oil, corn syrup, saccharin. Caramel-mint flavor. In pt.
Rx	**R-Gen** (Goldline)		21.75% alcohol. In pt.
Rx	**Iophen** (Various, eg, Barre-National, Goldline, Major, Moore, Rugby)	**Solution**: 50 mg (25 mg organically bound iodine) per ml	In 30 ml.

* No longer approved for use an an expectorant; product may still be in distribution.

IODINE PRODUCTS

Actions:

Pharmacology: Iodides enhance the secretion of respiratory fluids, thus decreasing the mucus viscosity. In addition, iodides may stimulate breakdown of fibrinoid material in inflammatory exudates. Objective evidence of clinical efficacy is lacking. Because of the potential for adverse effects, other agents are usually preferred.

Pharmacokinetics: Iodide is absorbed as iodinated amino acids and distributed largely extracellularly. It accumulates in the thyroid gland, and its concentration is far greater in gastric and salivary secretions than in extracellular fluids. Most of plasma iodine is in the form of thyroid hormones. The kidney serves as the chief excretory organ.

Indications:

As expectorants in the symptomatic treatment of chronic pulmonary diseases where tenacious mucus complicates the problem, including bronchial asthma, chronic bronchitis, bronchiectasis and pulmonary emphysema. Also used as adjunctive treatment in respiratory tract conditions such as cystic fibrosis, chronic sinusitis and after surgery to help prevent atelectasis.

For other indications for iodine (including use in a radiation emergency), refer to the Iodine Products monograph in the Thyroid Drug section.

Contraindications:

Hypersensitivity to iodides.

Potassium iodide: Impaired renal function; acute bronchitis; hyperthyroidism; Addison's disease; acute dehydration; heat cramps; hyperkalemia; iodism; tuberculosis.

Iodinated glycerol: Pregnancy, newborns, and nursing mothers (see Warnings).

Warnings:

Thyroid disease history: Use with caution or avoid use in these patients.

GI effects: Several reports of nonspecific small bowel lesions (stenosis with or without ulceration) have been associated with the administration of enteric-coated potassium salts. These lesions have caused obstruction, hemorrhage and perforation. Surgery was frequently required, and deaths have occurred. Administer coated potassium-containing formulations only when indicated and discontinue immediately if abdominal pain, distention, nausea, vomiting or GI bleeding occurs.

Hypersensitivity: Occasionally, persons are markedly sensitive to iodides; use care during initial administration. Refer to Management of Acute Hypersensitivity Reactions.

Pregnancy: (Category X – iodinated glycerol; Category D – potassium iodide). The fetal thyroid begins to concentrate iodine in the 12th to 14th week of gestation. Use of inorganic iodides in pregnant women during this period and thereafter has rarely induced fetal goiter (with or without hypothyroidism) with the potential for airway obstruction. Fetal harm, abnormal thyroid function and goiter may occur when potassium iodide is administered to a pregnant woman. Because of the possible development of fetal goiter, if the drug is used during pregnancy or if the patient becomes pregnant during therapy, apprise the patient of the potential hazard.

Lactation: **Potassium iodide** is excreted in breast milk. Use by nursing mothers may cause skin rash and thyroid suppression in the infant. Do not give **iodinated glycerol** to a nursing mother.

Children: Safety and efficacy in children have not been established for **potassium iodide**. **Iodinated glycerol** is contraindicated in newborns.

Precautions:

Hypothyroidism: In some patients, prolonged use of iodides can lead to hypothyroidism. In patients sensitive to iodides and in hyperthyroidism, iodine-induced goiter may occur. Concurrent use of antithyroid drugs may potentiate the hypothyroid effect of iodides.

Cystic fibrosis: Children with this disease appear to have an exaggerated susceptibility to the goitrogenic effect of iodides.

Pulmonary tuberculosis is considered a contraindication to the use of iodides by some authorities; use with caution in such cases and in patients having Addison's disease, cardiac disease, hyperthyroidism, myotonia congenita or renal impairment.

Acne: Iodides may cause a flare-up of adolescent acne.

Dermatitis and other reversible manifestations of iodism have occurred with chronic use of inorganic iodides. If skin rash appears, discontinue use.

IODINE PRODUCTS

Drug Interactions:

Lithium and other antithyroid drugs may potentiate the hypothyroid and goitrogenic effects of these medications if used concurrently.

Potassium-containing medications and potassium-sparing diuretics may result in hyperkalemia and cardiac arrhythmias or cardiac arrest if used with potassium iodide products.

Drug/Lab test interactions: **Thyroid function tests** may be altered by iodide.

Adverse Reactions:

Thyroid adenoma; goiter; myxedema. Hypersensitivity may be manifested by angioneurotic edema, cutaneous and mucosal hemorrhages and symptoms resembling serum sickness, such as fever, arthralgia, lymph node enlargement and eosinophilia.

Other: GI bleeding; confusion; irregular heartbeat; numbness; tingling; pain or weakness in hands or feet; unusual tiredness; weakness or heaviness of legs; fever; swelling of neck or throat; thyroid gland enlargement, acute parotitis (rare).

Chronic iodine poisoning or iodism may occur during prolonged treatment. Symptoms include: Metallic taste; burning of mouth or throat; soreness of the mouth, teeth and gums; ulceration of mucous membranes; increased salivation; coryza; sneezing; swelling of the eyelids. Gastric disturbance, nausea, vomiting, epigastric pain and diarrhea are common. There may be a severe headache, productive cough, pulmonary edema and swelling and tenderness of the salivary glands. Acneiform skin lesions are seen in the seborrheic areas. Severe and sometimes fatal skin eruptions may develop. If iodism appears, withdraw the drug and institute appropriate supportive therapy.

Overdosage:

Acute overdosage with iodinated glycerol is rare; there have been no reports of any serious problems.

Acute toxicity from potassium iodide is also rare. An occasional individual may show marked sensitivity which can occur immediately or hours after administration. Angioedema, laryngeal edema and cutaneous hemorrhages may occur. Symptoms disappear soon after drug discontinuation. Abundant fluid and salt intake helps eliminate iodide. Treat hyperkalemia immediately.

Patient Information:

Discontinue use and notify physician if epigastric pain, skin rash, metallic taste, or nausea and vomiting occurs.

Administration and Dosage:

Adult: Initially, 300 to 1000 mg after meals, 2 or 3 times daily. If tolerated, optimal dose is 1 to 1.5 g 3 times a day.

Children: Half the adult dose of potassium iodide. See individual product inserts for dosage information.

Rx	**Potassium Iodide** (Various, eg, Balan, Barre, Goldline, Harber, Major)	**Solution:** 1 g potassium iodide per ml. *Dose:* 0.3 ml (300 mg) to 0.6 ml (600 mg) 3 or 4 times a day, diluted in water. Do not take more than 12 times a day.	In 30 and 240 ml and pt.
Rx sf	**Potassium Iodide** (Roxane)		In 30 and 240 ml.
Rx	**SSKI** (Upsher-Smith)		In 30 and 240 ml.
Rx	**Pima** (Fleming)	**Syrup:** 325 mg potassium iodide per 5 ml *Dose:* Adults – 5 to 10 ml 3 times daily. Children – 2.5 to 5 ml 3 times daily.	Sugar. Black raspberry flavor. In pt and gal.

RESPIRATORY COMBINATION PRODUCTS

Combination products are frequently used in respiratory conditions. These products present two problems: (1) The patient may not need the components of the product; (2) the patient may need the components, but in different strengths or intervals.

Product Selection Guidelines: When recommending a respiratory combination product, consider the following guidelines.

Patient's data:

Symptoms – Pain, fever, congestion, runny nose, productive/nonproductive cough.

Patient's medical history/health – Age, allergy history, pregnancy, heart disease, hypertension, asthma, bronchitis, glaucoma, hyperthyroidism, diabetes, depression.

Drugs patient is currently taking – Other cold or allergy medications; medications for hypertension, diabetes, etc.

Do not exceed the recommended dosage. Do not take an *otc*product for > 7 days. If symptoms do not improve or are accompanied by fever, consult a physician.

Humidification of room air and adequate fluid intake (6 to 8 glasses/day) are important in treating cold symptoms.

Sulfite/Tartrazine sensitivity: Some of these products contain sulfites or tartrazine, which may cause allergic-type reactions (eg, hives, itching, wheezing, anaphylaxis) in certain susceptible persons. Although overall prevalence of sensitivity in general population is probably low, it is seen more frequently in asthmatics or in atopic nonasthmatic persons (sulfites) or in those with aspirin hypersensitivity (tartrazine).

Sugar free liquid products (sf): The small amount of sugar in usual doses of medication is probably insignificant to the well controlled diabetic. However, consider the effects of alcohol and sympathomimetics in addition to the sugar content.

Sustained release formulations: Products with identical active ingredients are listed together. Due to formulation differences, do not consider them bioequivalent.

Dosage is usually average adult dose. For children, consult package literature or physician.

Groups: These combination products are presented in groups based on the components of their formulations. Products with identical or similar ingredients are listed adjacent to each other, regardless of therapeutic claims, which may differ even for identical formulations. Pediatric preparations (those products intended mainly or exclusively for children) are grouped at the end of each respective section.

Antiasthmatic Combinations contain xanthine derivatives and sympathomimetics for bronchodilation. Many products also contain expectorants to facilitate mobilization of mucus.

- Xanthine Combinations
- Xanthine-Sympathomimetic Combinations

Upper Respiratory Combinations are used primarily for relief of symptoms associated with colds, upper respiratory infections and allergic conditions (eg, acute rhinitis, sinusitis).

- Decongestant Combinations
- Antihistamine and Analgesic Combinations
- Decongestant and Antihistamine Combinations
- Decongestant, Antihistamine and Analgesic Combinations
- Decongestant, Antihistamine and Anticholinergic Combinations

Cough Preparations include an antitussive or expectorant, but may also contain ingredients for relief of associated symptoms.

- Antitussive Combinations
- Expectorant Combinations
- Narcotic Antitussives with Expectorants
- Nonnarcotic Antitussives with Expectorants
- Antitussive and Expectorant Combinations

RESPIRATORY COMBINATION PRODUCTS

Ingredients: An FDA advisory review panel has proposed monographs for all *otc* cold, cough, allergy, bronchodilator and antihistamine products. In addition, the FDA proposes to classify *otc* drugs as "monograph conditions" (old Category I) and "nonmonograph conditions" (old Categories II and III). When using these combination products, consider the prescribing information for each ingredient.

Antihistamines (see individual monograph) are used for symptomatic relief from allergic rhinitis (hay fever) including runny nose, sneezing, itching of the nose or throat, and itchy and watery eyes. The anticholinergic effects of antihistamines may cause a thickening of bronchial secretions; therefore, these agents may be counterproductive in respiratory conditions characterized by congestion. Antihistamines may cause drowsiness.

Xanthines (see individual monograph), primarily theophylline, relieve bronchial spasm by direct action on the bronchial smooth muscle in bronchospastic conditions such as asthma and chronic bronchitis. Product listings include anhydrous theophylline dosage equivalents. Some xanthine-containing combination products are available *otc*, but asthmatic patients should use them only under physician supervision.

Sympathomimetics are used for their α-adrenergic (vasoconstrictor/decongestant) or β_2-adrenergic (bronchodilator) effects.

Decongestants – Used for temporary relief of nasal congestion due to colds or allergy. Given orally, they are less effective than topical nasal decongestants, and they have a potential for systemic side effects. Frequent or prolonged topical use may lead to local irritation and rebound congestion.

Bronchodilators – Ephedrine, common in these combinations, stimulates cardiac (β_1) receptors. Bronchodilation is weaker than with catecholamines; α-adrenergic effects may decrease congestion of mucous membranes. Other β-active agents are effective bronchodilators, but pseudoephedrine is not.

Narcotic antitussives: The antitussive dose is lower than that required for analgesia. Consider general precautions for the use of narcotics, including the potential for abuse, when using these products. See Narcotic Antitussive monograph for complete prescribing information. See also the Narcotic Agonist Analgesics monograph for complete information on the narcotics.

Codeine – 10 to 20 mg every 4 to 6 hours.
Hydrocodone (dihydrocodeinone) – 5 to 10 mg every 6 to 8 hours.
Hydromorphone HCl – 2 mg every 4 hours.

Nonnarcotic antitussives decrease the cough reflex without inducing many of the common characteristics of narcotic preparations.

Dextromethorphan – 10 to 30 mg every 4 to 8 hours.
Diphenhydramine – 25 mg every 4 hours.
Carbetapentane has atropine-like and local anesthetic actions and suppresses cough reflex through selective depression of the medullary cough center.
Dose: 15 to 30 mg, 3 or 4 times daily.
Caramiphen edisylate – A weak anticholinergic and centrally acting antitussive.
Dose:
Adults – 10 to 20 mg every 4 to 6 hours.
Children (6 to 12) – 5 to 10 mg q 4 to 6 h; *(2 to 6)* 2.5 to 5 mg q 4 to 6 h.

RESPIRATORY COMBINATION PRODUCTS

Expectorants: In the FDA's final monograph for *otc* expectorants, guaifenesin (see individual monograph) is the only agent approved for use as an expectorant. Guaifenesin may help loosen phlegm and thin bronchial secretions to rid the bronchial passageways of bothersome mucus, drain bronchial tubes or make coughs more productive. Humidification of room air and adequate fluid intake (6 to 8 glasses/day) are important therapeutic measures as well.

Dose –

Adults: 200 to 400 mg every 4 hours, not to exceed 2400 mg in 24 hours.

Children: Lower dosages are specified on labeling. Consult a physician for children < 2 years of age.

Other ingredients not upgraded by the FDA include: Ammonium chloride, beechwood creosote, benzoin preparations, camphor, eucalyptol/eucalyptus oil, iodines, ipecac syrup, menthol/peppermint oil, pine tar preparations, potassium guaiacolsulfonate, sodium citrate, squill preparations, terpin hydrate preparations, tolu preparations and turpentine oil. Products containing these ingredients must be reformulated.

Analgesics (eg, acetaminophen, aspirin, ibuprofen, sodium salicylate) are frequently included to treat headache, fever, muscle aches, pain. See individual monographs.

Anticholinergics (see individual monograph) are included for their drying effects on mucus secretions. This action may be beneficial in acute rhinorrhea; however, drying of respiratory secretions may lead to thickened mucus and more difficult expectoration. Traditionally, anticholinergics have been avoided in patients with asthma or chronic obstructive pulmonary disease (COPD); however, some patients respond well to these agents. Caution is still advised in this group.

An anticholinergic for oral inhalation is available as a bronchodilator for maintenance of bronchospasm associated with COPD, including chronic bronchitis and emphysema (see Ipratropium monograph).

The FDA has ruled that no anticholinergic product for *otc* use is recognized as safe and effective. Therefore, the products must be reapproved by new drug application (NDA) before November 10, 1986, or be regarded as misbranded (*Federal Register* 1985 Nov 8; 50:46582-87).

Papaverine HCl (see individual monograph) relaxes the smooth muscle of the bronchial tree.

Barbiturates (see individual monograph) are included for sedative effects as "correctives" with xanthines or sympathomimetics which may cause CNS stimulation. The sedative efficacy of low doses (eg, 8 mg phenobarbital) is questionable.

Caffeine (see individual monograph) is included for CNS stimulation to counteract antihistamine depression and to enhance concomitant analgesics.

XANTHINE COMBINATIONS, CAPSULES AND TABLETS

Refer to the general discussion of these products in the Respiratory Combinations Introduction.
Content given per capsule or tablet.

	Product & Distributor	Xanthine[1]	Expectorant	Other	Average Adult Dose	How Supplied
Rx	**Quibron-300 Capsules** (Roberts)	300 mg theophylline	180 mg guaifenesin		16 mg/kg/day or 400 mg theophylline/ day, in divided doses, q 6 to 8 h	(Roberts 068). Yellow and white. In 100s.
Rx	**Bronchial Capsules** (Various, eg, Moore)	150 mg theophylline	90 mg guaifenesin		16 mg/kg/day or 400 mg theophylline/ day, in divided doses, q 6 to 8 h	In 100s and 1000s.
Rx	**Glyceryl-T Capsules** (Rugby)[2]				1 or 2 bid or tid	In 100s.
Rx	**Quibron Capsules** (Roberts)				16 mg/kg/day or 400 mg theophylline/ day, in divided doses, q 6 to 8 h	(Roberts 067). Yellow. In 100s, 1000s and UD 100s.
Rx	**Slo-Phyllin GG Capsules** (Rhone-Poulenc Rorer)				3 mg/kg/day q 6 to 8 h	White. In 100s.
Rx	**Mudrane GG-2 Tablets** (ECR Pharm)	111 mg theophylline	100 mg guaifenesin		1 tid or qid	(GG 9533). Green, mottled. In 100s.

XANTHINE COMBINATIONS, CAPSULES AND TABLETS

	Product & Distributor	Xanthine[1]	Expectorant	Other	Average Adult Dose	How Supplied
Rx	**Dilor-G Tablets** (Savage)	200 mg dyphylline	200 mg guaifenesin		1 tid or qid	In 100s, 1000s and UD 100s.
Rx	**Dyflex-G Tablets** (Econo Med)				1 or 2 qid	In 100s and 1000s.
Rx	**Dyline G.G. Tablets** (Seatrace)				1 tid or qid	(0551 and 0123) Pink, scored. In 100s and 1000s.
Rx	**Lufyllin-GG Tablets** (Wallace)				1 qid	(Wallace 541). Yellow, scored. In 100s, 3000s and UD 100s.

[1] Theophylline content given as anhydrous unless otherwise specified.
[2] Form of theophylline unknown.

XANTHINE COMBINATIONS, LIQUIDS

Refer to the general discussion of these products in the Respiratory Combinations Introduction.

Content given per 15 ml.

	Product & Distributor	Xanthine[1]	Expectorant	Other	Average Adult Dose	How Supplied
Rx	**Theolate Liquid** (Various, eg, Barre-National)	150 mg theophylline	90 mg guaifenesin		15 ml q 6 to 8 h	In 118 ml, pt and gal.
Rx	**Glyceryl-T Liquid** (Rugby)					In 480 ml.
Rx	**Slo-Phyllin GG Syrup** (Rhone-Poulenc Rorer)			Saccharin, sorbitol, sucrose	3 mg theophylline/kg/day q 6 to 8 h	Alcohol and dye free. Lemon-vanilla flavor. In 480 ml.
Rx	**Asbron G Elixir** (Sandoz)	150 mg theophylline (300 mg theophylline sodium glycinate)	100 mg guaifenesin	15% alcohol. Saccharin, sorbitol, sucrose	15 to 30 ml tid or qid	In 480 ml.
Rx	**Synophylate-GG Syrup** (Central)			10% alcohol. Saccharin, sorbitol, sucrose	3 mg theophylline/kg q 8 h	In pt and gal.
Rx *sf*	**Elixophyllin GG Liquid** (Forest)	100 mg theophylline	100 mg guaifenesin	Sorbitol	3 mg theophylline/kg q 8 h	Alcohol and dye free. In 237 and 473 ml.

XANTHINE COMBINATIONS, LIQUIDS

	Product & Distributor	Xanthine[1]	Expectorant	Other	Average Adult Dose	How Supplied
Rx	**Theophylline KI Elixir** (Various, eg, Qualitest)[2]	80 mg theophylline	130 mg potassium iodide		3 mg theophylline/kg q 8 h	In 480 ml and gal.
Rx	**Elixophyllin-KI Elixir** (Forest)			Saccharin, sodium bisulfite, sucrose, anise oil		In 237 ml.
Rx	**Iophylline Elixir** (Various, eg, Major)[2]	120 mg theophylline	30 mg iodinated glycerol		15 to 30 ml tid	In 480 ml.
Rx	**Dilor-G Liquid** (Savage)	300 mg dyphylline	300 mg guaifenesin	Saccharin, sorbitol, sucrose, parabens	5 or 10 ml tid or qid	Alcohol free. Mint flavor. In pt and gal.
Rx	**Dyline-GG Liquid** (Seatrace)	300 mg dyphylline	300 mg guaifenesin	Menthol, parabens, saccharin, sorbitol, sucrose[2]	5 or 10 ml tid or qid	Peppermint flavor. In pt and gal.
Rx	**Dyphylline-GG Elixir** (Various, eg, Barre-National, Goldline, Qualitest, Rugby, Silarx)	100 mg dyphylline	100 mg guaifenesin	17% alcohol. Saccharin, sucrose	30 ml qid	In 473 ml.
Rx	**Lufyllin-GG Elixir** (Wallace)					Wine flavor. In pt and gal.
Rx	**Brondelate Elixir** (Various, eg, Barre-National, CMC, Harber)[2]	192 mg theophylline (300 mg oxtriphylline)	150 mg guaifenesin		10 ml qid	In 480 ml and gal.
Rx	**Oxtriphylline and Guaifenesin Elixir** (Barre-National)			20% alcohol		Cherry flavor. In pt and gal.

[1] Theophylline content given as anhydrous unless otherwise specified.

[2] May contain alcohol.

XANTHINE-SYMPATHOMIMETIC COMBINATIONS, TABLETS

Refer to the general discussion of these products in the Respiratory Combinations Introduction.

Content given per tablet.

	Product & Distributor	Xanthine[1]	Sympathomimetic	Expectorant	Other	Average Adult Dose	How Supplied
otc	**Theodrine Tablets** (Rugby)	120 mg theophylline[2]	22.5 mg ephedrine HCl			1 to 2 q 4 h up to 3 doses/day	In 1000s.
otc	**Tedrigen Tablets** (Goldline)				7.5 mg phenobarbital	1 to 2 q 4 h	In 100s and 1000s.
otc	**Primatene Tablets** (Whitehall)	130 mg theophylline	24 mg ephedrine HCl		7.5 mg phenobarbital	1 q 4 h	In 24s.
Rx	**Hydrophed Tablets** (Rugby)	130 mg theophylline	25 mg ephedrine sulfate		10 mg hydroxyzine HCl	1 bid to qid	In 100s and 1000s.
Rx	**Marax Tablets** (Roerig)						Dye free. Scored. M-shaped. In 100s and 500s.
Rx	**Mudrane GG Tablets** (ECR Pharm)	111 mg theophylline (130 mg aminophylline anhydrous)	16 mg ephedrine HCl	100 mg guaifenesin	8 mg phenobarbital	1 tid or qid	(GG 9551). Yellow, mottled, scored. In 100s.
Rx	**Mudrane Tablets** (ECR Pharm)	111 mg theophylline (130 mg aminophylline anhydrous)	16 mg ephedrine HCl	195 mg potassium iodide	8 mg phenobarbital	1 tid or qid	(9550). Yellow, scored. In 100s.

XANTHINE-SYMPATHOMIMETIC COMBINATIONS, TABLETS

	Product & Distributor	Xanthine[1]	Sympathomimetic	Expectorant	Other	Average Adult Dose	How Supplied
Rx	**Quadrinal Tablets** (Knoll)	65 mg theophylline (130 mg theophylline calcium salicylate)	24 mg ephedrine HCl	320 mg potassium iodide	24 mg phenobarbital	1 tid or qid	(14). White, scored. Biconvex. In 100s.
otc	**Primatene Dual Action Tablets** (Whitehall)	60 mg theophylline	12.5 mg ephedrine HCl	100 mg guaifenesin		2 q 4 h	In 24s.
Rx	**Lufyllin-EPG Tablets** (Wallace)	100 mg dyphylline	16 mg ephedrine HCl	200 mg guaifenesin	16 mg phenobarbital	1 to 2 q 6 h	In 100s.

[1] Theophylline content given as anhydrous unless otherwise specified.
[2] Form of theophylline unknown.

XANTHINE-SYMPATHOMIMETIC COMBINATIONS, LIQUIDS

Refer to the general discussion of these products in the Respiratory Combinations Introduction. Content given per 15 ml.

	Product & Distributor	Xanthine[1]	Sympathomimetic	Expectorant	Other	Average Adult Dose	How Supplied
Rx	**Lufyllin-EPG Elixir** (Wallace)	150 mg dyphylline	24 mg ephedrine HCl	300 mg guaifenesin	5.5% alcohol. 24 mg phenobarbital	10 to 20 ml q 6 h	In 480 ml.

[1] Theophylline content given as anhydrous unless otherwise specified.

PEDIATRIC XANTHINE-SYMPATHOMIMETIC COMBINATIONS

Refer to the general discussion of these products in the Respiratory Combinations Introduction.Content given per 15 ml.

	Product & Distributor	Xanthine[1]	Sympathomimetic	Other	Average Adult Dose	How Supplied
Rx	**Theomax DF Syrup** (Various, eg, Barre-National)	97.5 mg theophylline	18.75 mg ephedrine sulfate	5% alcohol. 7.5 mg hydroxyzine HCl	*Children (> 5 yrs)* - 5 ml tid or qid. *(2 to 5 yrs)* - 2.5 to 5 ml tid or qid	In pt and gal.
Rx	**Marax-DF Syrup** (Roerig)			7.5 mg hydroxyzine HCl, sucrose[2]	*Children (> 5 yrs)* - 5 ml tid or qid. *(2 to 5 yrs)* - 2.5 to 5 ml tid or qid	In pt and gal.

[1] Theophylline content given as anhydrous unless otherwise specified.

DECONGESTANT COMBINATIONS

For complete prescribing information, refer to the Respiratory Combinations Introduction. Content given per capsule, tablet, caplet, packet or lozenge.

	Product & Distributor	Decongestant	Other	Average Adult Dose	How Supplied
otc	**Bayer Select Head Cold Caplets** (Bayer)	30 mg pseudoephedrine HCl	500 mg acetaminophen	2 q 4 to 6 h up to 8/day	In 16s.
otc	**Bayer Select Maximum Strength Sinus Pain Relief Caplets** (Bayer)				In 24s and 50s.
otc	**Dristan Cold Caplets** (Whitehall)				In 20s and 40s.
otc	**Maximum Strength Dynafed Tablets** (BDI[1])				In 36s.
otc	**Max Strength Ornex Caplets** (Menley & James)				(Ornex Max). In 24s and 48s.
otc	**Maximum Strength Sine-Aid Tablets, Caplets and Gelcaps** (McNeil-CPC)				**Tablets and Caplets:** (Sine-Aid). White. In 50s. **Gelcaps:** (Sine-Aid). Red/white. In 20s and 40s.
otc	**Maximum Strength Sinutab Without Drowsiness Tablets and Caplets** (Warner Wellcome)			2 q 6 h	**Tablets:** In 24s. **Caplets:** In 24s and 48s.
otc	**Maximum Strength Sudafed Sinus Tablets and Caplets** (Warner Wellcome)				**Tablets:** In 24s and 48s. **Caplets:** In 24s and 48s.
otc	**Maximum Strength Tylenol Sinus Tablets, Geltabs, Caplets and Gelcaps** (McNeil-CPC)			2 q 4 to 6 h up to 8/day	**Tablets and Caplets:** (Tylenol Sinus). Green. In 24s and 50s. **Gelcaps and Geltabs:** (Tylenol Sinus). Green/white. In 24s and 60s.
otc	**No Drowsiness Sinarest Tablets** (Ciba)			2 q 6 h	In 20s.
otc	**Sine-Off Maximum Strength No Drowsiness Formula Caplets** (SmithKline Beecham)				(Sine-Off). In 24s.
otc	**Sinus Excedrin Extra Strength Tablets and Caplets** (Bristol Myers-Squibb)				In 50s.

DECONGESTANT COMBINATIONS

	Product & Distributor	Decongestant	Other	Average Adult Dose	How Supplied
otc	**Vicks DayQuil Sinus Pressure & Pain Relief Caplets** (Richardson-Vicks)	30 mg pseudoephedrine HCl	500 mg acetaminophen	2 q 6 h	(DQ SP). In 24s.
otc	**Coldrine Tablets** (Roberts Medical)			2 q 6 h	In 1000s and 4-dose boxes.
otc	**No-Drowsiness Allerest Tablets** (Ciba)			2 q 4 to 6 h up to 8/day	In 20s.
otc	**Ornex Caplets** (Menley & James)			2 q 4 h up to 8/day	(Ornex). In 24s and 48s.
otc	**Sinus-Relief Tablets** (Major)				In 24s, 100s and 1000s.
otc	**Allerest No Drowsiness Caplets** (Ciba)		325 mg acetaminophen	2 q 4 to 6 h up to 8/day	In 20s.
otc	**Coldrine Tablets** (Roberts)			2 q 4 h up to 8/day	Sodium metabisulfate. In 1000s, 500s (packets) and 4-dose boxes.
otc	**Ornex No Drowsiness Caplets** (Menley & James)				In 24s 100s and 1000s.
otc	**Sinus-Relief** (Major)			2 q 4 to 6 h up to 8/day	In 24s, 100s and 1000s.
otc	**Sinutab Without Drowsiness Tablets** (Warner Wellcome)			2 q 4 h up to 8/day	In 24s.
otc	**BC Cold-Sinus Powder** (Block)	25 mg phenylpropanolamine HCl	650 mg aspirin, lactose	1 dose q 4 h up to qid	In 6 packets.
otc	**Ursinus Inlay-Tabs** (Sandoz)	30 mg pseudoephedrine HCl	325 mg aspirin, lactose	2 q 4 h up to 8/day	In 24s.
otc	**Dristan Sinus Caplets** (Whitehall)	30 mg pseudoephedrine HCl	200 mg ibuprofen, sucrose	1 to 2 q 4 to 6 h	In 20s, 24s and 40s.
otc	**Advil Cold & Sinus Caplets** (Whitehall)				In 20s, 40s and 75s.
otc	**Dimetapp Sinus Caplets** (Robins)				In 20s and 40s.
otc	**Motrin IB Sinus Caplets** (Upjohn)		200 mg ibuprofen		In 20s and 40s.
otc	**Sine-Aid IB Caplets** (McNeil-CPC)				(Sine-Aid). In 20s.

DECONGESTANT COMBINATIONS

	Product & Distributor	Decongestant	Other	Average Adult Dose	How Supplied
otc	**Alka-Seltzer Plus Sinus Tablets** (McNeil-CPC)	20 mg phenylpropanolamine bitartrate	325 mg aspirin, 8.98 mg phenylalanine		In 20s.
otc	**Rhinocaps Capsules** (Ferndale)	20 mg phenylpropanolamine HCl	162 mg APAP and aspirin	2 q 4 to 6 h up to 6/day	In 100s and 1000s.
otc	**Saleto-D Caplets** (Roberts Medical)	18 mg phenylpropanolamine HCl	240 mg acetaminophen, 120 mg salicylamide, 16 mg caffeine	1 q 4 h	In 50s, 1000s and Sani-Pak 500s.
otc	**Spec-T Sore Throat/Decongestant Lozenges** (Apothecon)	10.5 mg phenylpropanolamine HCl, 5 mg phenylephrine HCl	10 mg benzocaine, tartrazine, dextrose, glucose, sucrose	1 q 3 h up to 6/day	In 10s.

[1] BDI Pharmaceuticals, Inc., P.O. Box 78610, Indianapolis, IN 46278–0610; (800) 428–2352.

PEDIATRIC DECONGESTANT COMBINATIONS

Refer to the general discussion of these products in the Respiratory Combinations Introduction.Content given per tablet.

	Product & Distributor	Decongestant	Other	Average Dose	How Supplied
otc *sf*	**St. Joseph Cold Tablets for Children** (Schering–Plough)	3.125 mg phenylpropanolamine HCl	80 mg acetaminophen	*Children* - 2 to 8 q 4 h up to 4/ day	Chewable. In 30s.

ANTIHISTAMINE AND ANALGESIC COMBINATIONS

For complete prescribing information, refer to the Respiratory Combinations Introduction.

	Product & Distributor	Antihistamine	Analgesic	Other	Average Adult Dose	How Supplied
otc	**Improved Congestant Tablets** (Rugby)	2 mg chlorpheniramine maleate	325 mg acetaminophen	Sucrose, lactose, butyl paraben, sugar	2 q 4 h	In 100s and 1000.
otc	**Coricidin Tablets** (Schering-Plough)					In 100s.
otc	**Tylenol Severe Allergy Caplets** (McNeil)	12.5 mg diphenhydramine HCl	500 mg acetaminophen		2 q 4 to 6 h up to 8/day	In 12s and 24s.
otc	**Aceta-Gesic Tablets** (Rugby)	30 mg phenyltoloxamine citrate	325 mg acetaminophen		1 or 2 q 4 h up to 8/day	In 100s and 1000s.
otc	**Major-gesic Tablets** (Major)					In 100s.
otc	**Percogesic Tablets** (Richardson-Vicks)			Sucrose		(Percogesic). Orange. In 24s, 50s and 90s.
otc	**Phenylgesic Tabs** (Goldline)					In 100s and 1000s.

DECONGESTANTS AND ANTIHISTAMINES, SUSTAINED RELEASE

Refer to the general discussion of these products in the Respiratory Combinations Introduction. Content given per capsule, tablet or caplet.

	Product & Distributor	Decongestant	Antihistamine	Average Adult Dose	Other Content & How Supplied
Rx	**Cophene No. 2 Capsules** (Dunhall)	120 mg pseudo-ephedrine HCl	12 mg chlor-pheniramine maleate	1 q 12 h	In 100s and 500s.
Rx	**ResconCapsules** (Ion)				In 100s.
Rx	**Anamine T.D.Capsules** (Mayrand)	120 mg pseudo-ephedrine HCl	8 mg chlor-pheniramine maleate	1 q 8 to 12 h	In 100s.
Rx	**Brexin L.A. Capsules** (Savage)			1 q 12 h	Red/ clear. In 100s.
Rx	**Chlorafed Timecelles (Capsules)** (Roberts Hauck)				(Dye free). Clear. In 100s.
Rx	**Chlordrine S.R. Capsules** (Rugby)				In 100s.
Rx	**Chlorphedrine SR Capsules** (Goldline)				In 100s.
Rx	**Codimal-L.A. Capsules** (Central)				(40). Clear/red. In 100s and 1000s.
Rx	**Colfed-A Capsules** (Parmed)				In 100s.
Rx	**Duralex Capsules** (American Urologicals)				In 100s and 1000s.
Rx	**Fedahist Timecaps Capsules** (Schwarz Pharma Kremers Urban)				Sucrose. (Kremers Urban 055). Clear. In 100s.
Rx	**Klerist-D Capsules** (Nutripharm)				Dye-free. In 100s and 500s.

DECONGESTANTS AND ANTIHISTAMINES, SUSTAINED RELEASE

	Product & Distributor	Decongestant	Antihistamine	Average Adult Dose	Other Content & How Supplied
Rx	**Kronofed-A Capsules** (Ferndale)	120 mg pseudo-ephedrine HCl	8 mg chlor-pheniramine maleate	1 q 12 h	Dye free. White/clear. In 100s and 500s.
Rx	**N D Clear Capsules** (Seatrace)				Dye free. In 100s and 1000s.
Rx	**Novafed A Capsules** (Hoechst Marion Roussel)				Sucrose. (Novafed A). Red/orange. In 100s.
Rx	**Pseudo-Chlor Capsules** (Various, eg, Geneva, Major, Moore)				In 100s and 250s.
Rx	**Rescon-ED Capsules** (Ion)				In 100s.
Rx	**Chlorpheniramine Maleate/Pseudo-ephedrine HCl Capsules** (Eon)				Sucrose. (E 1304). Dk. blue/clear. In 100s, 250s and 1000s.
Rx	**Deconamine SR Capsules** (Bradley-Kenwood)				Sucrose. Blue and yellow. In 100s and 500s.
Rx	**Time-Hist Capsules** (American)				In 100s.
Rx	**Deconomed SR Capsules** (Iomed)				Sucrose, parabens. In 100s and 500s.
Rx	**Rinade B.I.D. Capsules** (Econo Med)				In 100s.
otc	**Chlor-Trimeton 12 Hour Relief Tablets** (Schering-Plough)	120 mg pseudo-ephedrine sulfate	8 mg chlor-pheniramine maleate	1 q 12 h	Lactose. (LA CTM D). In 12s and 36s.
Rx	**Fedahist Gyrocaps (Capsules)** (Schwarz Pharma Kremers Urban)	65 mg pseudo-ephedrine HCl	10 mg chlor-pheniramine maleate	1 q 12 h	Sucrose. (Kremers Urban 053). White/ yel-low. In 100s.
Rx	**Chlorafed H.S. Timecelles Capsules** (Roberts)	60 mg pseudo-ephedrine HCl	4 mg chlor-pheniramine maleate	1 or 2 q 12 h	Dye free. Sucrose. Clear. In 100s.
Rx	**Codimal-L.A. Half Capsules** (Central)			2 q 12 h	Sucrose. (Central 60/4). Clear. In 100s.

DECONGESTANTS AND ANTIHISTAMINES, SUSTAINED RELEASE

	Product & Distributor	Decongestant	Antihistamine	Average Adult Dose	Other Content & How Supplied
Rx	**Phenylpropanolamine HCl and Chlorpheniramine Maleate Caps** (Various, eg, Geneva, Major)	75 mg phenylpropanolamine HCl	12 mg chlorpheniramine maleate	1 q 12 h	In 50s, 100s and 1000s.
otc	**Allerest Maximum Strength 12 Hour Caplets** (Ciba)				Lactose. (Allerest 12). In 10s.
otc	**Contac Maximum Strength 12 Hour Caplets** (SmithKline Beecham)				Lactose. (Contac). In 10s and 20s.
Rx	**Drize Capsules** (Jones Medical)				Dye free. Sugar. (JMI-405). Clear. In100s.
Rx	**Ornade SpansulesCapsules** (SmithKline Beecham)				Sucrose. (Ornade SKF). Red & natural. In 50s and 500s.
Rx	**Resaid Capsules** (Geneva)				Sucrose, lactose. (GG502). Blue/ clear. In 100s and 1000s.
Rx	**Rhinolar-EX 12 Capsules** (McGregor)				Dye free. Sucrose. In 60s.
otc	**Triaminic-12 Tablets** (Sandoz)				Lactose. In 20s.
Rx	**Dura-Vent/A Capsules** (Dura)	75 mg phenylpropanolamine HCl	10 mg chlorpheniramine maleate	1 q 12 h	Sucrose, parabens. (Dura-Vent/A 51479002). Clear. In 100s.
otc	**Contac 12 Hour Capsules** (SmithKline Beecham)	75 mg phenylpropanolamine HCl	8 mg chlorpheniramine maleate	1 q 12 h	Sucrose, parabens. In 10s and 20s.
otc	**Gencold Capsules** (Goldline)				Sucrose, parabens. In 10s.
Rx	**Rhinolar-EX Capsules** (McGregor)				Dye free. Sucrose. In 60s.
otc	**Cold-Gest Cold Capsules** (Major)				Sucrose, parabens. In 10s and 20s.
otc	**Teldrin 12-Hour Allergy Relief Capsules** (SmithKline Beecham)			1 q 12 h	Sucrose, parabens. In 12s, 24s and 48s.
otc	**Demazin Tablets** (Schering-Plough)	25 mg phenylpropanolamine HCl	4 mg chlorpheniramine maleate	2 q 8 h	Sugar, lactose, butyl paraben. In 24s and 100s.

DECONGESTANTS AND ANTIHISTAMINES, SUSTAINED RELEASE

	Product & Distributor	Decongestant	Antihistamine	Average Adult Dose	Other Content & How Supplied
Rx	**Ed A-Hist Tablets** (Edwards)	20 mg phenylephrine HCl	8 mg chlorpheniramine maleate	1 q 12 h	Tan. In 100s.
Rx	**Prehist Capsules** (Marnel)				In 100s.
Rx	**Allent Capsules** (Ascher)	120 mg pseudoephedrine HCl	12 mg brompheniramine maleate	1 q 12 h	Dye free. (225-480). Clear. In 100s.
Rx	**Bromfed Capsules** (Muro)				Sucrose, parabens. (Bromfed Muro 12-120). Lt. green/clear. In 100s and 500s.
Rx	**Bromfenex Capsules** (Ethex)				Extended release. (Ethex/019). Lt. green/clear. In 100s, 500s.
Rx	**Endafed Capsules** (UAD)				(UAD/Endafed 206). Blue/clear. In 100s.
	IofedCapsules (Iomed)				Extended release. In 100s.
Rx	**ULTRAbrom Capsules** (WE Pharm)				Sucrose. (WE 06). Green/clear. In 100s.
otc	**Bromatapp Tablets** (Copley)	75 mg phenylpropanolamine HCl	12 mg brompheniramine maleate	1 q 12 h	Blue. In 100s.
otc	**Dimaphen Release Tablets** (Major)				Lactose. In 12s.
Rx	**E.N.T. Tablets** (Ion)				In 100s.
otc	**Dimetapp Extentabs Tablets** (Robins)				Sucrose. (Dimetapp AHR). Pale blue. In 12s, 24s, 48s, 100s, 500s and UD 100s.
otc	**Vicks DayQuil Allergy Relief 12 Hour Tablets** (Richardson-Vicks)				Lactose. (A). Blue. In 12s and 24s.

DECONGESTANTS AND ANTIHISTAMINES, SUSTAINED RELEASE

	Product & Distributor	Decongestant	Antihistamine	Average Adult Dose	Other Content & How Supplied
otc	**Cheracol Sinus Tablets** (Roberts)	120 mg pseudo-ephedrine sulfate	6 mg dex-bromphenir-amine maleate	1 q 12 h	Sugar, parabens, sucrose. In 10s.
Rx	**Disobrom Tablets** (Geneva)			1 q am and hs	White. In 100s and 1000s.
Rx	**Dexaphen-S.A. Tablets** (Major)			1 q 12 h	In 100s and 500s.
otc	**Disophrol Chronotabs Tablets** (Schering-Plough)				Sugar, lactose, butylparaben. In 100s.
otc	**Drixoral Cold & Allergy Tablets** (Schering-Plough)				Sugar, lactose, butylparaben. In 10s.
otc	**12-Hour Cold Tablets** (Goldline)				Sugar, sucrose, parabens. In 10s and 20s.
Rx	**Claritin-D Tablets** (Schering-Plough)	120 mg pseudo-ephedrine sulfate	5 mg loratadine		Lactose, butylparaben. (Claritin-D). In 30s and 100s, unit-of-use 10s and 30s and UD 10s and 100s.
Rx	**Claritin-D 24-hour Tablets** (Schering)	240 mg pseudo-ephedrine sulfate	10 mg lorata-dine	1 q 24 h	(Claritin-D 24-hour). White. Film-coated. In 100s and UD 100s.
otc	**Tavist D Tablets** (Sandoz)	75 mg phenylpro-panolamine HCl	1.34 mg clemas-tine fumarate	1 q 12 h	Lactose. In 8s, 16s.
Rx	**Biohist-LA Tablets** (Wakefield)	120 mg pseudo-ephedrine HCl	8 mg carbinox-amine maleate	1 q 12 h	Lactose. In 100s.
Rx	**Carbiset-TR Tablets** (Nutripharm)				Dye free. (512). In 100s.
Rx	**Carbodec TR Tablets** (Rugby)			1 bid	Film coated. In 100s.
Rx	**Rondec-TR Tablets** (Dura)			1 q 12 h	Sugar, lactose. (R 6240). Blue. Film coated. In 100s.
Rx	**Trinalin Repetabs Tablets** (Key)	120 mg pseudo-ephedrine sulfate	1 mg azatadine maleate	1 bid	Sugar, lactose, butylparaben. (Trinalin 703). Coral. Sugar coated. In 100s.
Rx	**Seldane-D Tablets** (Hoechst Marion Roussel)	120 mg pseudo-ephedrine HCl	60 mg terfena-dine	1 q am and hs	Lactose. (Seldane-D). White to off-white. Capsule shape. In 100s.
Rx	**Tanafed Suspension** (Horizon)	75 mg pseudo-ephedrine tannate/5 ml	4.5 mg chlor-pheniramine tannate	10 to 20 ml q 12 h	Methylparaben, saccharin, sucrose. Raspberry flavor. In 20, 118 and 473 ml.

DECONGESTANTS AND ANTIHISTAMINES, SUSTAINED RELEASE

	Product & Distributor	Decongestant	Antihistamine	Average Adult Dose	Other Content & How Supplied
Rx	**Iofed PD Capsules** (Iomed)	60 mg pseudoephedrine HCl	6 mg brompheniramine maleate		Extended release. In 100s.
Rx	**Lodrane LD Capsules** (ECR Pharmaceuticals)			1 or 2 q 12 h	Dye free. (ECR 6006). Clear. In 100s.
Rx	**Respahist Capsules** (Respa)				In 100s.
Rx	**Touro A & H Capsules** (Dartmouth)				(Touro A & H). Orange/clear. In 100s.
Rx	**Comhist LA Capsules** (Roberts)	20 mg phenylephrine HCl	4 mg chlorpheniramine maleate, 50 mg phenyltoloxamine citrate	1 q 8 to 12 h	Sugar. (Roberts Comhist-LA 065). Yellow/clear. In 100s.
Rx	**Nolamine Tablets** (Carnrick)	50 mg phenylpropanolamine HCl	4 mg chlorpheniramine maleate, 24 mg phenindamine tartrate	1 q 8 to 12 h	(C 86204). Pink. In 100s and 250s.
Rx	**Poly-Histine-D Capsules** (Bock)	50 mg phenylpropanolamine HCl	16 mg phenyltoloxamine citrate, 16 mg pyrilamine maleate, 16 mg pheniramine maleate	1 q 8 to 12 h	In 100s.
Rx	**Bromophen T.D. Tablets** (Rugby)	15 mg phenylpropanolamine HCl, 15 mg phenylephrine HCl	12 mg brompheniramine maleate	1 q 8 to 12 h	In 100s and 1000s.
Rx	**Tamine S.R. Tablets** (Geneva)			1 q am and hs or 1 q 8 h	Sugar coated. (GG477). Blue. In 100s and 1000s.

DECONGESTANTS AND ANTIHISTAMINES, SUSTAINED RELEASE

	Product & Distributor	Decongestant	Antihistamine	Average Adult Dose	Other Content & How Supplied
Rx	**Decongestabs Tablets** (Various, eg, Moore, Parmed)	40 mg phenylpropanolamine HCl, 10 mg phenylephrine HCl	5 mg chlorpheniramine maleate, 15 mg phenyltoloxamine citrate	1 tid	In 100s and 1000s.
Rx	**Decongestant Tablets** (Moore)				In 50s, 100s and 1000s.
Rx	**Naldecon Tablets** (Apothecon)				Lactose, sucrose. In 100s and 500s.
Rx	**Nalgest Tablets** (Major)				In 100s and 1000s.
Rx	**Tri-Phen-Chlor Tablets** (Rugby)				In 100s.
Rx	**Uni-Decon Tablets** (URL)				In 100s, 500s and 1000s.
Rx	**Tri-Phen-Mine S.R. Tablets** (Goldline)				In 100s.
Rx	**Vanex Forte Caplets** (Abana)	50 mg phenylpropanolamine HCl, 10 mg phenylephrine HCl	4 mg chlorpheniramine maleate, 25 mg pyrilamine maleate	1 bid or tid	White. In 100s.

PEDIATRIC DECONGESTANTS AND ANTIHISTAMINES, SUSTAINED RELEASE

Refer to the general discussion of these products in the Respiratory Combinations Introduction.Content given per capsule.

	Product & Distributor	Decongestant	Antihistamine	Average Dose	How Supplied
Rx	**Kronofed-A Jr. Capsules** (Ferndale)	60 mg pseudoephedrine HCl	4 mg chlorpheniramine maleate	*Children (6 to 12 years)* - 1 q 12 h	Dye free. White/clear. In 100s and 500s.
Rx	**Dura-Tap/PD Capsules** (Dura)				(51479 007). Blue/clear. In 100s.
Rx	**Rescon JR Capsules** (Ion)				Dye free. In 100s.
Rx	**Atrohist Pediatric Capsules** (Adams)			*Children (6 to 12 years)* - 1 or 2 q 12 h	Sugar. (Adams/ 400). White/yellow. In 100s.
Rx	**Bromfed-PD Capsules** (Muro)	60 mg pseudoephedrine HCl	6 mg brompheniramine maleate	*Children (6 to 12 years)* - 1 q 12 h	Sucrose, parabens, EDTA. (Bromfed-PD Muro 6-60). Green/clear. In 100s and 500s.
Rx	**Bromfenex PD Capsules** (Ethex)				Sucrose. (Ethex/020). In 100s, 500s.
Rx	**Dallergy-JR Capsules** (Laser)				(Dallergy-Jr Laser 176). Maize/clear. In 100s.
Rx	**ULTRAbrom PD Capsules** (WE Pharm)				(WE 04). Purple/clear. In 100s.
Rx	**Poly-Histine-D Ped Caps** (Bock)	25 mg phenylpropanolamine HCl	8 mg phenyltoloxamine citrate, 8 mg pyrilamine maleate, 8 mg pheniramine maleate	*Children (6 to 12 years)* - 1 q 8 to 12 h	(Bock). In 100s.

DECONGESTANTS AND ANTIHISTAMINES, CAPSULES AND TABLETS

Refer to the general discussion of these products in the Respiratory Combinations Introduction.

Content given per capsule or tablet.

	Product & Distributor	Decongestant	Antihistamine	Average Adult Dose	How Supplied
Rx	**Bromfed Tablets** (Muro)	60 mg pseudo-ephedrine HCl	4 mg brom-pheniramine maleate	1 q 4 h	Lactose. (Muro 4060). White, scored. In 100s.
otc	**Co-Pyronil 2 Pulvules** (Dista)	60 mg pseudo-ephedrine HCl	4 mg chlor-pheniramine maleate	1 q 6 h	In 100s.
Rx	**Deconamine Tablets** (Kenwood/Bradley)			1 tid or qid	Dye free. White, scored. In 100s.
otc	**Fedahist Tablets** (Schwarz Pharma)			1 q 4 to 6 h up to 4/day	Lactose. Scored. In 100s.
Rx	**Klerist-D Tablets** (Nutripharm)			1 tid or qid	Dye free. In 24s and 100s.
otc	**Pseudo-Gest Plus Tablets** (Major)			1 q 4 to 6 h up to 4/day	Scored. In 24s, 100s and 200s.
otc	**Sudafed Plus Tablets** (Warner Wellcome)				Lactose. Scored. In 24s and 48s.
otc	**Chlor-Trimeton 4 Hour Relief Tablets** (Schering-Plough)	60 mg pseudo-ephedrine sulfate	4 mg chlor-pheniramine maleate	1 q 4 to 6 h up to 4/day	Lactose. (901). In 24s and 48s.
otc	**Allerest Maximum Strength Tablets** (Ciba)	30 mg pseudo-ephedrine HCl	2 mg chlor-pheniramine maleate	2 q 4 to 6 h up to 8/day	In 24s, 48s and 72s.
Rx	**Semprex-D Capsules** (Glaxo Wellcome)	60 mg pseudo-ephedrine HCl	8 mg acrivastine	1 q 4 to 6 h up to 4/day	Lactose. (Wellcome Semprex-D). Dark green/white. In 100s.
otc	**A.R.M. Caplets** (Menley & James)	25 mg phenylpro-panolamine HCl	4 mg chlor-pheniramine maleate	1 q 4 to 6 h	Lactose. (ARM). In 20s and 40s.
otc	**Triaminic Allergy Tablets** (Sandoz)			1 q 4 h	Methylparaben. In 24s.
otc	**Tri-Nefrin Extra Strength Tablets** (Pfeiffer)			1 q 4 to 6 h	In 24s.
otc	**Chlor-Rest Tablets** (Rugby)	18.7 mg phenyl-propanolamine HCl	2 mg chlor-pheniramine maleate	2 q 4 h up to 8/day	In 100s.

DECONGESTANTS AND ANTIHISTAMINES, CAPSULES AND TABLETS

	Product & Distributor	Decongestant	Antihistamine	Average Adult Dose	How Supplied
otc	**Triaminic Cold Tablets** (Sandoz)	12.5 mg phenylpropanolamine HCl	2 mg chlorpheniramine maleate	2 q 4 h	Methylparaben, lactose. In 24s.
otc	**Histatab Plus Tablets** (Century)	5 mg phenylephrine HCl	2 mg chlorpheniramine maleate	2 initially then 1 q 4 h	In 100s.
otc	**Dimaphen Tablets** (Major)	25 mg phenylpropanolamine HCl	4 mg brompheniramine maleate	1 q 4 h	In 24s.
otc	**Dimetapp Tablets** (Robins)				(AHR 2254). Blue, scored. In 24s.
otc	**Dimetapp 4-Hour Liqui-Gels (Capsules)** (Robins)				Sorbitol. In 12s.
otc	**Maximum Strength Cold & Allergy 4-Hour Liquid Gelcaps (Capsules)** (Goldline)			1 q 4 to 6 h	Sorbitol. In 12s.
otc	**Vicks DayQuil Allergy Relief 4 Hour Tablets** (Richardson-Vicks)			1 q 4 h	(A). Yellow. In 24s.
otc	**Dimetane Decongestant Caplets** (Robins)	10 mg phenylephrine HCl	4 mg brompheniramine maleate	1 q 4 h	(AHR 2117). Light blue, scored. In 24s and 48s.
Rx	**Drixomed Tablets** (Iomed)	120 mg pseudoephedrine sulfate	6 mg dexbrompheniramine maleate	1 q 12 h	In 100s and 500s
otc	**Disophrol Tablets** (Schering-Plough)	60 mg pseudoephedrine sulfate	2 mg dexbrompheniramine maleate	1 q 4 to 6 h up to 4/day	Lactose, sugar. In 100s.
otc	**Banophen Decongestant Capsules** (Major)	60 mg pseudoephedrine HCl	25 mg diphenhydramine HCl	1 q 4 to 6 h up to 4/day	In 24s.
otc	**Benadryl Allergy Decongestant Tablets** (Warner Wellcome)				In 24s.

DECONGESTANTS AND ANTIHISTAMINES, CAPSULES AND TABLETS

	Product & Distributor	Decongestant	Antihistamine	Average Adult Dose	How Supplied
otc	**Actifed AllergyTablets** (Warner Wellcome)	Day: 30 mg pseudoephedrine HCl		2 q 4 to 6 h up to 8/day (total daytime & nighttime)	Lactose. (AA Day). White.
		Night: 30 mg pseudoephedrine HCl	25 mg diphenhydramine HCl	2 hs or 2 q 4 to 6 h up to 8/day	Lactose. (AA Night). Blue. In packs of 24s (daytime) and 8s (nighttime).
Rx	**Carbiset Tablets** (Nutripharm)	60 mg pseudoephedrine HCl	4 mg carbinoxamine maleate	1 qid	Dye free. (510). In 100s and 500s.
Rx	**Carbodec Tablets** (Rugby)				In 100s.
Rx	**Rondec Tablets** (Dura)				Lactose. (R 5726). Orange. Film coated. In 100s and 500s.
Rx	**Hista-Vadrin Tablets** (Scherer)	40 mg phenylpropanolamine HCl, 5 mg phenylephrine HCl	6 mg chlorpheniramine maleate	1 q 6 h	In 100s.
Rx	**Histalet Forte Tablets** (Solvay)	50 mg phenylpropanolamine HCl, 10 mg phenylephrine HCl	4 mg chlorpheniramine maleate, 25 mg pyrilamine maleate	1 bid or tid	Lactose, sugar. (Solvay 1039). White with blue dots, scored. Capsule shape. In 100s and 250s.
Rx	**Comhist Tablets** (Roberts)	10 mg phenylephrine HCl	2 mg chlorpheniramine maleate, 25 mg phenyltoloxamine citrate	1 or 2 tid q 8 h	Sugar. (Comhist 0149 0444). Yellow, scored. In 100s.

DECONGESTANTS AND ANTIHISTAMINES, CAPSULES AND TABLETS

	Product & Distributor	Decongestant	Antihistamine	Average Adult Dose	How Supplied
Rx	**Phenylephrine Tannate, Chlorpheniramine Tannate and Pyrilamine Tannate** (Goldline)	25 mg phenylephrine tannate	8 mg chlorpheniramine tannate, 25 mg pyrilamine tannate		In 100s and 500s.
Rx	**R-Tannate Tablets** (Various, eg, Copley, Schein)			1 or 2 q 12 h	In 100s.
Rx	**Rhinatate Tablets** (Major)				In 100s and 250s.
Rx	**R-Tannamine Tablets** (Qualitest)				In 100s.
Rx	**Rynatan Tablets** (Wallace)				(Wallace 713). Buff, scored. Capsule shape. In 100s, 500s and 2000s.
Rx	**Tanoral Tablets** (Parmed)				In 100s.
Rx	**Triotann Tablets** (Various, eg, Duramed, Invamed)				(INV 234). Buff, scored. Capsule shape. In 100s and 500s.
Rx	**Tritan Tablets** (Eon)				Lactose. (E T7). Tan, scored. Capsule shape. In 100s, 250s and 1000s.
Rx	**Tri-Tannate Tablets** (Rugby)				In 100s and 250s.
Rx[1]	**Pseudoephedrine HCl and Triprolidine HCl Tablets** (Various, eg, UDL, Westward)	60 mg pseudoephedrine HCl	2.5 mg triprolidine HCl	1 q 4 h to 8 h up to 4/day	In 100s, 1000s and UD 100s.
otc	**Actagen Tablets** (Goldline)			1 q 4 to 6 h up to 4/day	In 100s and 1000s.
otc	**Actifed Tablets** (Warner Wellcome)				Sucrose, lactose. In 12s, 24s, 48s and 100s.
otc	**Allercon Tablets** (Parmed)				In 24s, 100s and 1000s.
otc	**Allerfrim Tablets** (Rugby)				(Rugby). Scored. In 24s, 100s and 1000s.
otc	**Aprodine Tablets** (Major)				Sucrose. Scored. In 24s, 100s, 1000s and UD 100s.
otc	**Cenafed Plus Tablets** (Century)				In 100s.
otc	**Genac Tablets** (Goldline)				In 24s and 100s.
otc	**Triposed Tablets** (Halsey)				Lactose. Scored. In 100s and 1000s.

[1] Products available *otc* or *Rx*, depending on product labeling.

DECONGESTANT AND ANTIHISTAMINES, LIQUIDS

For complete prescribing information, refer to the Respiratory Combinations Introduction.
Content given per 5 ml.

	Product & Distributor	Decongestant	Antihistamine	Other	Average Adult Dose	How Supplied
otc	**Rhinosyn Liquid** (Great Southern)	60 mg pseudoephedrine HCl	4 mg chlorphenir-amine maleate	0.45% alcohol, sucrose	5 ml q 4 h	In 120 and 473 ml.
Rx	**Histalet Syrup** (Solvay)	45 mg pseudoephedrine HCl	3 mg chlorphenir-amine maleate	Saccharin, sorbi-tol, sugar, methylparaben	10 ml qid	Alcohol free. Grape flavor. In 473 ml.
Rx sf	**Anamine Syrup** (Mayrand)	30 mg pseudoephedrine HCl	2 mg chlorphenir-amine maleate		10 ml q 4 to 6 h	Alcohol and dye free. In 473 ml.
Rx sf	**Anaplex Liquid** (Medi-Plex)					Alcohol and dye free. In 473 ml.
otc sf	**Chlorafed Liquid** (Roberts)			Parabens, sorbi-tol, saccharin	10 ml q 4 to 6 h up to 40 ml/day	Alcohol and dye free. In 120 and 473 ml.
otc sf	**Hayfebrol Liquid** (Scot-Tussin)			Parabens, men-thol	10 ml q 6 h	Alcohol and dye free. In 118 ml.
otc	**Rhinosyn-PD Liquid** (Great Southern)			1.2% alcohol, sucrose	10 ml q 4 h	In 120 ml.
otc sf	**Ryna Liquid** (Wallace)			Sorbitol	10 ml q 6 h	Alcohol and dye free. In 118 and 473 ml.
otc	**Sudafed Plus Liquid** (Warner Wellcome)			0.1% methyl-paraben, 0.1% sodium benzo-ate, sucrose	10 ml q 4 to 6 h up to 40 ml/day	In 118 ml.
Rx	**Deconamine Syrup** (Kenwood/Bradley)	30 mg d-pseudoephedrine HCl	2 mg chlorphenir-amine maleate	Sorbitol, sucrose	5 to 10 ml tid or qid	Alcohol and dye free. Grape fla-vor. In 473 ml.

DECONGESTANT AND ANTIHISTAMINES, LIQUIDS

	Product & Distributor	Decongestant	Antihistamine	Other	Average Adult Dose	How Supplied
Rx	**Brofed Elixir** (Marnel)	30 mg pseudoephedrine HCl	4 mg brompheniramine maleate	Parabens, saccharin, sorbitol, sucrose, corn syrup, menthol	10 ml tid	Mint. In 473 ml.
otc	**Demazin Syrup** (Schering-Plough)	12.5 mg phenylpropanolamine HCl	2 mg chlorpheniramine maleate	7.5% alcohol, menthol, sugar, parabens	10 ml q 4 to 6 h	In 118 ml.
otc *sf*	**Rescon Liquid** (Ion)				10 ml q 4 h up to 40 ml/day	Alcohol free. In 120 and 473 ml.
otc	**Silaminic Cold Syrup** (Silarx)				10 ml q 4 h	In 118 ml.
otc	**Temazin Cold Syrup** (Trenier Co.)					In 120 ml.
otc	**Thera-Hist Syrup** (Major)			Sorbitol, sucrose	10 ml q 4 h	Alcohol free. In 120 ml.
otc	**Triphenyl Syrup** (Rugby)	6.25 mg phenylpropanolamine HCl	1 mg chlorpheniramine maleate	Sorbitol, sucrose, EDTA	20 ml q 4 h	In 118 ml.
otc	**Genamin Cold Syrup** (Goldline)				20 ml q 4 to 6 h	Alcohol free. In 118 ml.
Rx	**Ed A-Hist Liquid** (Edwards)	10 mg phenylephrine HCl	4 mg chlorpheniramine maleate	5% alcohol	5 ml tid or qid	Grape flavor. In 473 ml.

DECONGESTANT AND ANTIHISTAMINES, LIQUIDS

	Product & Distributor	Decongestant	Antihistamine	Other	Average Adult Dose	How Supplied
otc	**Dallergy-D Syrup** (Laser)	5 mg phenylephrine HCl	2 mg chlorphenir-amine maleate	Sugar	10 ml q 4 h	Alcohol free. Raspberry-vanilla flavor. In 118 ml.
Rx	**Histor-D Syrup** (Roberts Hauck)			2% alcohol	5 to 10 ml q 4 to 6 h	In 473 ml.
otc *sf*	**Novahistine Elixir** (SmithKline—Beecham)			5% alcohol, sor-bitol	10 ml q 4 h	In 118 ml.
otc	**Rolatuss Plain Liquid** (Major)			5% alcohol, sac-charin, glucose, menthol, para-bens	10 ml q 4 to 6 h	In 473 ml.
otc	**Ru-Tuss Liquid** (Boots)					In 473 ml.
otc	**Bromaline Elixir** (Rugby)	12.5 mg phenylpropa-nolamine HCl	2 mg brom-pheniramine maleate	2.3% alcohol, saccharin, sorbi-tol	10 ml q 4 to 6 h	Grape flavor. In 118 ml, 473 ml and gal.
otc *sf*	**Bromanate Elixir** (Barre-National)			Saccharin, sorbi-tol		Alcohol free. Grape flavor. In 118 and 237 ml, 473 ml and gal.
otc *sf*	**Cold & Allergy Elixir** (Goldline)					Alcohol free. Grape flavor. In 118 and 237 ml, 473 ml and gal.

DECONGESTANT AND ANTIHISTAMINES, LIQUIDS

	Product & Distributor	Decongestant	Antihistamine	Other	Average Adult Dose	How Supplied
otc	**Dimaphen Elixir** (Major)	12.5 mg phenylpropanolamine HCl	2 mg brompheniramine maleate	2.3% alcohol, saccharin, sorbitol	10 ml q 4 h 10 ml q 4 h	Grape flavor. In 237 ml.
otc	**Dimetapp Elixir** (Robins)					Alcohol free. Grape flavor. In 120, 240 and 360 ml, 473 ml, gal and UD 5 ml.
otc *sf*	**Genatap Elixir** (Goldline)			Saccharin, sorbitol	10 ml q 4 to 6 h	Alcohol free. Grape flavor. In 118 ml.
otc	**Bromfed Syrup** (Muro)	30 mg pseudoephedrine HCl	2 mg brompheniramine maleate	Saccharin, sorbitol, sucrose, methylparaben	10 ml q 4 to 6 h up to 40 ml/day	Orange-lemon flavor. In 120 and 473 ml.
otc	**Drixoral Syrup** (Schering-Plough)	30 mg pseudoephedrine sulfate	2 mg brompheniramine maleate	Sorbitol, sugar	10 ml q 4 to 6 h up to 40 ml/day	Alcohol free. Cherry flavor. In 118 ml.
otc	**Dimetane Decongestant Elixir** (Robins)	5 mg phenylephrine HCl	2 mg brompheniramine maleate	2.3% alcohol, sorbitol	10 ml q 4 h	Grape flavor. In 120 ml.

DECONGESTANT AND ANTIHISTAMINES, LIQUIDS

	Product & Distributor	Decongestant	Antihistamine	Other	Average Adult Dose	How Supplied
Rx	**Promethazine VC Syrup** (Various, eg, Cenci, Halsey, Major, Qualitest, Rugby, Schein, URL)	5 mg phenylephrine HCl	6.25 mg promethazine HCl		5 ml q 4 to 6 h up to 20 ml	In 120 and 240 ml, 473 ml and gal.
Rx	**Prometh VC Plain Liquid** (Various, eg, Barre-National, Goldline)					In 120 ml, 473 ml and gal.
Rx	**Promethazine VC Plain Syrup** (Goldline)			7% alcohol	5 ml q 4 to 6 h up to 30 ml/day	In 473 ml.
Rx	**Phenergan VC Syrup** (Wyeth-Ayerst)			7% alcohol, saccharin	5 ml q 4 to 6 h	In 118 and 473 ml.
Rx	**Carbodec Syrup** (Rugby)	60 mg pseudoephedrine HCl	4 mg carbinoxamine maleate	Sorbitol, parabens	5 ml qid	Berry flavor. In 473 ml.
Rx	**Carbinoxamine Syrup** (Morton Grove)					Alcohol free. Raspberry, fruit flavors. In 118, 237 and 473 ml.
Rx	**Cardec-S Syrup** (Barre-National)					Fruit flavor. In 473 ml.
Rx *sf*	**Rondec Syrup** (Dura)			Sorbitol, parabens	5 ml qid	Alcohol free. Berry flavor. In 120 ml and 473 ml.

DECONGESTANT AND ANTIHISTAMINES, LIQUIDS

	Product & Distributor	Decongestant	Antihistamine	Other	Average Adult Dose	How Supplied
Rx	**Triprolidine HCl w/Pseudoephedrine HCl Syrup** (Various, eg, Cenci)	30 mg pseudoephedrine HCl	1.25 mg triprolidine HCl		10 ml q 4 to 6 h up to 40 ml/day	In 118 and 237 ml.
otc	**Actagen Syrup** (Goldline)			0.1% methylparaben, sodium benzoate	10 ml q 4 to 6 h up to 40 ml/day	In 118 ml.
otc	**Allerfrim Syrup** (Rugby)	30 mg pseudoephedrine HCl	1.25 mg triprolidine HCl	Sucrose, methylparaben	10 ml q 4 to 6 h up to 40 ml/day	In 118 and 473 ml.
otc	**Allerphed Syrup** (Great Southern)			Saccharin	10 ml q 4 to 6 h up to 40 ml/day	In 118 ml.
otc	**Aprodine Syrup** (Major)			0.1% methylparaben, sorbitol	10 ml q 4 to 6 h up to 40 ml/day	In 120 ml.
otc	**Silafed Syrup** (Silarx)				10 ml q 4 to 6 h up to 40 ml/day	In 120 and 240 ml, 473 ml and gal.
otc	**Triofed Syrup** (Barre-National)			Methylparaben, sucrose	10 ml q 4 to 6 h up to 40 ml/day	In 118 and 473 ml.
otc	**Triposed Syrup** (Halsey)			0.1% methylparaben, sodium benzoate, sucrose	10 ml q 4 to 6 h up to 40 ml/day	In 120 and 240 ml, 473 ml and gal.

UPPER RESPIRATORY COMBINATIONS

DECONGESTANT AND ANTIHISTAMINES, LIQUIDS

	Product & Distributor	Decongestant	Antihistamine	Other	Average Adult Dose	How Supplied
Rx	**Poly-Histine-D Elixir** (Bock)	12.5 mg phenylpropanolamine HCl	4 mg pyrilamine maleate, 4 mg phenyltoloxamine citrate, 4 mg pheniramine maleate	4% alcohol	10 ml q 4 h	In 473 ml.
Rx	**Iohist Elixir** (Iomed)					Cherry flavor. In pints.
Rx	**Liqui-Histine-D Elixir** (Liquipharm)					In 473 ml.
Rx	**Naldelate Syrup** (Various, eg, Barre-National, Moore, Qualitest, URL)	20 mg phenylpropanolamine HCl, 5 mg phenylephrine HCl	2.5 mg chlorpheniramine maleate, 7.5 mg phenyltoloxamine citrate		5 ml q 3 to 4 h up to 20 ml/day	In 473 ml and gal.
Rx *sf*	**Nalgest Syrup** (Major)			Sorbitol	5 ml q 3 to 4 h up to 20 ml/day	Alcohol free. In 473 ml.
Rx	**Naldecon Syrup** (Apothecon)					In 473 ml.
Rx	**Tri-Phen-Chlor Syrup** (Rugby)				5 ml q 4 h up to 20 ml/day	In 473 ml.

PEDIATRIC DECONGESTANTS AND ANTIHISTAMINES

Refer to the general discussion of these products in the Respiratory Combinations Introduction.

Content given per 5 ml liquid, 1 ml drops, packet or tablet.

	Product & Distributor	Decongestant	Antihistamine	Other	Average Dose	How Supplied
otc	**Children's Allerest Tablets** (Ciba)	9.4 mg phenylpropanolamine HCl	1 mg chlorpheniramine maleate	Saccharin, sorbitol	*Children (6 to < 12 yrs)* – 2 q 4 h up to 8/day	Chewable. In 24s.
otc	**Triaminic Syrup** (Sandoz)	6.25 mg phenylpropanolamine HCl	1 mg chlorpheniramine maleate	EDTA, sorbitol, sucrose	*Children (6 to < 12 yrs)* – 10 ml q 4 h	Alcohol free. Orange flavor. In 120 and 240 ml.
otc	**Triaminic Chewable Tablets** (Sandoz)	6.25 mg phenylpropanolamine HCl	0.5 mg chlorpheniramine maleate	Saccharin, sucrose	*Children (6 to < 12 yrs)* – 2 q 4 h	In 24s.
otc	**Dimetapp Cold & Allergy Chewable Tablets** (Robins)	6.25 mg phenylpropanolamine HCl	1 mg brompheniramine maleate	Aspartame, 8 mg phenylalanine, sorbitol	*Children (6 to < 12 yrs)* – 2 q 4 h	Scored. Grape flavor. In 24s.

PEDIATRIC DECONGESTANTS AND ANTIHISTAMINES

	Product & Distributor	Decongestant	Antihistamine	Other	Average Dose	How Supplied
otc sf	**Benadryl Allergy Decongestant Liquid** (Warner-Wellcome)	30 mg pseudoephedrine HCl	12.5 mg diphenhydramine HCl	Saccharin, sorbitol	*Children (6 to < 12 yrs)* – 5 ml q 4 to 6 h up to 20 ml/day	Alcohol free. Grape flavor. In 118 ml.
Rx sf	**Carbinoxamine Drops** (Morton Grove)	25 mg pseudoephedrine HCl per ml	2 mg carbinoxamine maleate per ml	Sorbitol, parabens		Alcohol free. Raspberry, fruit flavors. In 30 ml w/ calibrated dropper.
Rx sf	**Rondec Oral Drops** (Dura)				*Infants* – 0.25 to 1 ml qid	Alcohol free. Berry flavor. In 30 ml.
otc	**Dorcol Children's Cold Formula Liquid** (Sandoz)	15 mg pseudoephedrine HCl	1 mg chlorpheniramine maleate	Sorbitol, sucrose	*Children (6 to < 12 yrs)* – 10 ml q 4 to 6 h up to 40 ml/day	Alcohol free. In 120 ml.
otc	**Pedia Care Cold-Allergy Chewable Tablets** (McNeil-CPC)	15 mg pseudoephedrine HCl	1 mg chlorpheniramine maleate	Aspartame, 8 mg phenylalanine	*Children (12 yrs)* – 4 q 4 to 6 h up to 16/day *(6 to 11 yrs)* – 2 q 4 to 6 h up to 8/day	Scored. Fruit flavor. In 16s.
Rx	**R-Tannate Pediatric Suspension** (Various, eg, Copley, Qualitest, Schein, Warner-C)	5 mg phenylephrine tannate	2 mg chlorpheniramine tannate, 12.5 mg pyrilamine tannate	Methylparaben, saccharin, sucrose	*Children (> 6 yrs)* – 5 to 10 ml q 12 h *(2 to 6 yrs)* – 2.5 to 5 ml q 12 h	In 473 ml.
Rx	**Atrohist Pediatric Suspension** (Adams)					Raspberry flavor. In 118 ml unit-of-use and 473 ml.
Rx	**Rynatan Pediatric Suspension** (Wallace)					Strawberry-currant flavor. In 473 ml.
Rx	**Rynatan-S Pediatric Suspension** (Wallace)					Strawberry-currant flavor. In 120 ml with syringe.
Rx	**Tri-Tannate Pediatric Suspension** (Rugby)					In 473 ml.
Rx	**R-Tannamine Pediatric Suspension** (Qualitest)					In 120 and 473 ml.

PEDIATRIC DECONGESTANTS AND ANTIHISTAMINES

	Product & Distributor	Decongestant	Antihistamine	Other	Average Dose	How Supplied
Rx	**Triaminic Oral Infant Drops** (Sandoz)	20 mg phenylpropanolamine HCl per ml	10 mg pyrilamine maleate, 10 mg pheniramine maleate per ml	Sorbitol, sucrose, saccharin	*Infants* – 1 drop/kg qid	In 15 ml dropper bottle (≈ 24 drops/ml).
Rx	**Naldelate Pediatric Syrup** (Various, eg, Barre-National, Moore, Qualitest, URL)	5 mg phenylpropanolamine HCl, 1.25 mg phenylephrine HCl	0.5 mg chlorpheniramine maleate, 2 mg phenyltoloxamine citrate		*Children (6 to 12 mos)* – 2.5 ml q 3 to 4 h up to 10 ml/day *(1 to 6 yrs)* – 5 ml q 3 to 4 h up to 20 ml/day *(6 to 12 yrs)* – 10 ml q 3 to 4 h up to 40 ml/day	In 120 ml, 473 ml and gal.
Rx	**Naldecon Pediatric Syrup** (Apothecon)			Sorbitol		In 473 ml.
Rx	**Nalgest Pediatric Syrup** (Major)					In 473 ml and gal.
Rx *sf*	**Tri-Phen-Mine Pediatric Syrup** (Goldline)					Alcohol free. In 473 ml.
Rx *sf*	**Tri-Phen-Chlor Pediatric Syrup** (Rugby)			Sorbitol, saccharin		Strawberry flavor. In 118 ml, 473 ml and gal.
Rx	**Naldecon Pediatric Drops** (Apothecon)	5 mg phenylpropanolamine HCl, 1.25 mg phenylephrine HCl per ml	0.5 mg chlorpheniramine maleate, 2 mg phenyltoloxamine citrate per ml	Sorbitol	*Children (3 to 6 mos)* - 0.25 ml q 3 to 4 h *(6 to 12 mos)* - 0.5 ml q 3 to 4 h *(1 to 6 yrs)* - 1 ml q 3 to 4 h up to 4 doses/day	In 30 ml.
Rx	**Nalgest Pediatric Drops** (Major)					In 30 ml.
Rx *sf*	**Tri-Phen-Mine Pediatric Drops** (Goldline)			Sorbitol		Alcohol free. In 30 ml.
Rx	**Tri-Phen-Chlor Pediatric Drops** (Rugby)					In 30 ml with dropper.

DECONGESTANT, ANTIHISTAMINE AND ANALGESIC COMBINATIONS

Refer to the general discussion of these products in the Respiratory Combinations Introduction.

Content given per tablet, capsule or 5 ml.

	Product & Distributor	Decongestant	Antihistamine	Analgesic	Average Adult Dose	How Supplied
Rx	**Phenate Tablets** (Roberts Medical)	40 mg phenylpropanolamine HCl	4 mg chlorpheniramine maleate	325 mg acetaminophen	1 q 6 to 8 h	Timed release. In 100s and 1000s.
otc	**Allerest Sinus Pain Formula Tabs** (Ciba)	30 mg pseudoephedrine HCl	2 mg chlorpheniramine maleate	500 mg acetaminophen	2 q 6 h	In 20s.
otc	**Aspirin-Free Bayer Select Allergy Sinus Caplets** (Sterling Health)					In 16s.
otc	**Maximum Strength Tylenol Allergy Sinus** (McNeil-CPC)					**Caplets:** In 24s and 60s. **Gelcaps:** EDTA, parabens. In 24s and 60s.
otc	**Sinarest Extra Strength Tablets** (Ciba Cons.)					In 24s.
otc	**Sinus Headache & Congestion Tablets** (Rugby)					In 100s and 1000s.
otc	**Allerest Headache Strength Tablets Advanced Formula** (Ciba Cons.)	30 mg pseudoephedrine HCl	2 mg chlorpheniramine maleate	325 mg acetaminophen	2 q 4 to 6 h up to 8/day	In 24s.
otc	**Co-Hist Tablets** (Roberts)				2 q 4 to 6 h	In 500s and 1000s.
otc	**Sinarest Sinus Tablets** (Ciba Cons.)				2 q 4 to 6 h up to 8/day	In 20s, 40s and 80s.
otc	**Alka-Seltzer Plus Cold Liqui-Gels (Capsules)** (Bayer)	30 mg pseudoephedrine HCl	2 mg chlorpheniramine maleate	250 mg acetaminophen	2 q 4 h up to 4 doses/day	Sorbitol. In 12s and 20s.
otc	**Alka-Seltzer Plus Allergy Liqui-Gels (Capsules)** (Bayer)					Sorbitol. In 12s.
otc	**Maximum Strength Dristan Cold Caplets** (Whitehall)	30 mg pseudoephedrine HCl	2 mg brompheniramine maleate	500 mg acetaminophen	2 q 6 h	EDTA. In 16s and 36s.

DECONGESTANT, ANTIHISTAMINE AND ANALGESIC COMBINATIONS

	Product & Distributor	Decongestant	Antihistamine	Analgesic	Average Adult Dose	How Supplied
otc	**Pyrroxate Caplets** (Roberts)	25 mg phenylpropanolamine HCl	4 mg chlorpheniramine maleate	650 mg acetaminophen	1 q 4 h	In 24s and 500s.
otc	**Sinulin Tablets** (Carnrick)				1 q 4 to 6 h	(8666). Peach, scored. In 20s and 100s.
otc	**Triaminicin Cold, Allergy, Sinus Tablets** (Sandoz)				1 q 4 h	Lactose, methylparaben. In 12s.
Rx	**Alumadrine Tablets** (Fleming)	25 mg phenylpropa nolamine HCl	4 mg chlorpheniramine maletae	500 mg acetaminophen	2 initially, then 1 q 4 h	Purple, scored. In 100s and 1000s.
otc	**BC Cold-Sinus-Allergy Powder** (Block)	25 mg phenylpropa nolamine HCl	4 mg chlorpheniramine maleate	650 mg aspirin	1 dose dissolved in water q 4 h up to 4/day	Lactose. In 6 and 24 packets.
otc	**Alka-Seltzer Plus Cold Medicine** (Bayer)	20 mg phenylpropanolamine bitartrate	2 mg chlorpheniramine maleate	325 mg aspirin	2 q 4 h in 120 ml water qid	Aspartame, 14.03 mg phenylalanine. Orange flavor. In 12s, 20s, 36s and 48s.
otc	**Alka-Seltzer Plus Cold Tablets** (Bayer)	24.08 mg phenylpropanolamine bitartrate	2 mg chlorpheniramine maleate	325 mg aspirin	2 q 4 h in 120 ml water qid	In 12s, 20s, 36s and 48s.
otc	**Chlor-Trimeton Allergy-Sinus Caplets** (Schering-Plough)	12.5 mg phenylpropanolamine HCl	2 mg chlorpheniramine maleate	500 mg acetaminophen	2 q 6 h	(CTM Sinus). In 24s.
otc	**Coricidin Maximum Strength Sinus Headache Caplets** (Schering-Plough)					(Coricidin Sinus). In 24s.
otc	**Congestant D Tablets** (Rugby)	12.5 mg phenylpropanolamine HCl	2 mg chlorpheniramine maleate	325 mg acetaminophen	2 q 4 h	In 100s and 1000s.
otc	**Coricidin D Tablets** (Schering-Plough)				2 q 4 h	Sugar, butylparaben. (Schering). In 12s, 24s, 48s and 100s.
otc	**Dapacin Cold Capsules** (Ferndale)				1 or 2 tid or qid	In 100s.
otc	**Duadacin Capsules** (Kenwood/Bradley)				2 q 4 h	In 100s, 1000s and Dispens-A-Pak 1000s. .
otc	**Dimetapp Cold & Flu Caplets** (Robins)	12.5 mg phenylpropanolamine HCl	2 mg brompheniramine maleate	500 mg acetaminophen	2 q 6 h	Parabens. In 24s and 48s.

DECONGESTANT, ANTIHISTAMINE AND ANALGESIC COMBINATIONS

	Product & Distributor	Decongestant	Antihistamine	Analgesic	Average Adult Dose	How Supplied
otc	**Gelpirin-CCF Tablets** (Alra)	12.5 mg phenylpropanolamine HCl	1 mg chlorpheniramine maleate	325 mg acetaminophen, 25 mg guaifenesin	2 q 4 h	White w/blue specks. (G). In 50s.
otc	**Sinapils Tablets** (Pfeiffer)	12.5 mg phenylpropanolamine HCl	2 mg chlorpheniramine maleate	325 mg acetaminophen, 32.5 mg caffeine	2 q 4 to 6 h	In 36s.
otc	**Histosal Tablets** (Ferndale)	20 mg phenylpropanolamine HCl	12.5 mg pyrilamine maleate	324 mg acetaminophen, 30 mg caffeine	1 or 2 q 4 h up to 8/day	In 100s.
Rx	**Norel Plus Capsules** (U.S. Pharmaceutical Corp.)	25 mg phenylpropanolamine HCl	4 mg chlorpheniramine maleate, 25 mg phenyltoloxamine dihydrogen citrate	325 mg acetaminophen	1 q 3 to 4 h up to 6/day	Lactose. (US/US). Yellow and white. In 100s.
otc	**Singlet for Adults Tablets** (SmithKline-Beecham)	60 mg pseudoephedrine HCl	4 mg chlorpheniramine maleate	650 mg acetaminophen	1 q 4 to 6 h up to 4/day	Sucrose. Pink. In 100s.
otc	**Simplet Tablets** (Major)				1 tid or qid	In 100s.
otc	**TheraFlu Flu and Cold Medicine Powder** (Sandoz)				1 packet dissolved in 6 oz hot water q 4 h up to 4/day	Sucrose. Lemon flavor. In 6 and 12 packs.
otc	**Contac Day & Night Allergy/Sinus Caplets** (SmithKline-Beecham)	Day: 60 mg pseudoehpedrine HCl		650 mg acetaminophen	*Day:* 1 q 6 h	(A/SD). White.
		Night: 60 mg pseudoephedrine HCl	50 mg diphenhydramine HCl	650 mg acetaminophen	*Night:* 1 q 6 h	(A/SN). Green. In 20s (15 day; 5 night)

UPPER RESPIRATORY COMBINATIONS

DECONGESTANT, ANTIHISTAMINE AND ANALGESIC COMBINATIONS

	Product & Distributor	Decongestant	Antihistamine	Analgesic	Average Adult Dose	How Supplied
otc	**Comtrex Allergy-Sinus** (Bristol–Myers)	30 mg pseudoephedrine HCl	2 mg chlorphenir-amine maleate	500 mg aceta-minophen	2 q 6 h	**Caplets**: Parabens. (A/S). Green. In 24s and 50s. **Tablets**: Parabens. (Comtrex A/S). Green. In 24s and 50s.
otc	**Sine-Off Sinus Medicine Caplets** (SmithKline-Beecham)					(Sine-Off). In 24s.
otc	**Sinutab Maximum Strength Sinus Allergy** (Warner Well-come)					**Caplets**: In 24s. **Tablets**: In 24s.
otc	**Actifed Sinus Daytime/ NighttimeCaplets or Tablets** (Glaxo Wellcome)	Day: 30 mg pseudo-ephedrine HCl		500 mg aceta-minophen	*Day:* 2 q 6 h	**Daytime**: White (Actifed Day). **Nighttime**: Blue. (Actifed Night). In 24s (18 daytime; 6 nighttime).
		Night: 30 mg pseudo-ephedrine HCl	25 mg diphen-hydramine HCl	500 mg aceta-minophen	*Night:* 2 hs or 2 q 6 h Do Not exceed 8 caplets/day	
otc	**Maximum Strength Tylenol Flu NightTime Gelcaps** (McNeil-CPC)	30 mg pseudoephedrine HCl	2 mg chlorphenir-amine maleate	500 mg aceta-minophen	2 q 6 h	2 hs or 2 q 6 h Parabens, EDTA. In 10s and 20s.
otc	**Benadryl Cold/Flu Tablets** (Warner Wellcome)	30 mg pseudoephedrine HCl	12.5 mg diphen-hydramine HCl	500 mg aceta-minophen	2 q 6 h	In 24s.
otc	**Benadryl Allergy/Sinus Head-ache Caplets** (Warner Well-come)					In 24s.
otc	**Tylenol Flu NightTime Maxi-mum Strength Powder** (McNeil-CPC)	60 mg pseudoephedrine HCl	50 mg diphen-hydramine HCl	1000 mg aceta-minophen, 67 mg phenylala-nine, sucrose	Dissolve in 6 oz hot water q 6 h	Aspartame. Apple cinnamon flavor. In 6s.

DECONGESTANT, ANTIHISTAMINE AND ANALGESIC COMBINATIONS

	Product & Distributor	Decongestant	Antihistamine	Analgesic	Average Adult Dose	How Supplied
otc	**Night-Time Effervescent Cold Tablets** (Goldline)	15 mg phenylpropanolamine HCl	38.33 mg diphenhydramine citrate	325 mg aspirin	Dissolve 2 q 4 to 6 h in 120 ml water up to 8/day	In 20s.
otc	**Codimal** (Central)	30 mg pseudoephedrine HCl	2 mg chlorpheniramine maleate	325 mg acetaminophen	2 q 4 to 6 h	**Capsules:** In 24s, 100s and 1000s. **Tablets:** Film coated. In 24s, 100s and 1000s.
otc	**Kolephrin Caplets** (Pfeiffer)				2 q 4 to 6 h up to 8/day	In 24s and 36s.
otc	**Phenapap Sinus Headache & Congestion Tablets** (Rugby)				2 q 4 h up to 8/day	In 30s, 100s and 1000s.
otc	**Drixoral Cold & Flu Tablets** (Schering-Plough)	60 mg pseudoephedrine sulfate	3 mg dexbrompheniramine maleate	500 mg acetaminophen	2 q 12 h	Extended release. Parabens. (Drixoral C & F). In 12s, 24s and 48s.
otc	**Drixoral Plus Tablets** (Schering-Plough)					Extended release. In 12s and 24s.
otc	**Actifed Plus Caplets and Tablets** (Warner Wellcome)	30 mg pseudoephedrine HCl	1.25 mg triprolidine HCl	500 mg acetaminophen	2 q 6 h	(Actifed Plus). In 20s and 40s.
Rx	**Aclophen Tablets** (Nutripharm)	40 mg phenylephrine HCl	8 mg chlorpheniramine maleate	500 mg acetaminophen	1 tid	Long-acting. Dye free. Capsule shape. In 100s.
otc	**Histagesic Modified Tablets** (Jones Medical)	10 mg phenylephrine HCl	4 mg chlorpheniramine maleate	324 mg acetaminophen	1 q 4 h	Pink, speckled green. In 1000s.
otc	**Decongestant Tablets** (Rugby)	5 mg phenylephrine HCl	2 mg chlorpheniramine maleate	325 mg acetaminophen	2 q 4 h	Lactose. In 50s.
otc	**Dristan Cold Multi-Symptom Formula Tablets** (Whitehall)					In 20s, 40s and 75s.
otc	**Gendecon Tablets** (Goldline)					White and yellow. In 50s.
otc	**ND-Gesic Tablets** (Hyrex)	5 mg phenylephrine HCl	2 mg chlorpheniramine maleate, 12.5 mg pyrilamine maleate	300 mg acetaminophen	2 q 6 h	Orange. In 100s and 1000s.

DECONGESTANT, ANTIHISTAMINE AND ANALGESIC COMBINATIONS

	Product & Distributor	Decongestant	Antihistamine	Analgesic	Average Adult Dose	How Supplied
otc *sf*	**Scot-Tussin Original 5-Action Liquid** (Scot-Tussin)	4.2 mg phenylephrine HCl	13.3 mg pheniramine maleate	83.3 mg Na citrate, 83.3 mg Na salicylate, 25 mg caffeine citrate	5 ml q 3 to 4 h up to qid	Alcohol free. Cherry-strawberry flavor. In 118 ml, 473 ml and gal.
otc	**Scot-Tussin Original 5-Action Cold Formula Syrup** (Scot-Tussin)					Sugar. Alcohol free. In 118 ml, 473 ml and gal.
otc	**Covangesic Tablets** (Wallace)	12.5 mg phenylpropanolamine HCl, 7.5 mg phenylephrine HCl	2 mg chlorpheniramine maleate, 12.5 mg pyrilamine maleate	275 mg acetaminophen	1 q 4 to 6 h up to 4/day	Tartrazine. In 24s.

PEDIATRIC DECONGESTANT, ANTIHISTAMINE AND ANALGESIC COMBINATIONS

Refer to the general discussion of these products in the Respiratory Combinations Introduction.
Content given per tablet or 5 ml.

	Product & Distributor	Decongestant	Antihistamine	Analgesic/Other	Average Dose	How Supplied
otc	**Children's Tylenol Cold Liquid** (McNeil-CPC)	15 mg pseudoephedrine HCl	1 mg chlorpheniramine maleate	160 mg acetaminophen	*Children (6 to 11 yrs)*– 10 ml q 4 to 6 h up to 4/day	Sorbitol, sucrose. Alcohol free. Grape flavor. In 120 ml.
otc	**Children's Tylenol Cold Tablets** (McNeil-CPC)	7.5 mg pseudoephedrine HCl	0.5 mg chlorpheniramine maleate	80 mg acetaminophen	*Children (6 to 11 yrs)*– 4 q 4 to 6 h up to 16/day	Aspartame, sucrose, 4 mg phenylalanine. Chewable. Grape flavor. In 24s.

DECONGESTANT, ANTIHISTAMINE AND ANTICHOLINERGIC COMBINATIONS, SUSTAINED RELEASE

Refer to the general discussion of these products in the Respiratory Combinations Introduction.

	Product & Distributor	Decongestant	Antihistamine	Anticholinergic	Average Adult Dose	Other Content & How Supplied
Rx	**Dallergy Caplets** (Laser)	20 mg phenylephrine HCl	8 mg chlorpheniramine maleate	2.5 mg methscopolamine nitrate	1 q 12 h	(Dallergy 12h) White, scored. In 100s.
Rx	**Dura-Vent/DA Tablets** (Dura)					(Dura DA). Light brown, scored. In 100s.
Rx	**Extendryl S.R. Capsules** (Fleming)					In 100s and 1000s.
Rx	**OMNIhist L.A. Tablets** (WE Pharm)					(WE 02). White, scored. In 100s.
Rx	**Pre-Hist-D** (Marnel)					**Tablets:** (MAR CPM). White, scored. In 100s. **Capsules:** In 100s.
Rx	**Atrohist Plus Tablets** (Adams)	50 mg phenylpropanolamine HCl, 25 mg phenylephrine HCl	8 mg chlorpheniramine maleate	0.19 mg hyoscyamine sulfate, 0.04 mg atropine sulfate, 0.01 mg scopolamine HBr	1 q 12 h	(Adams/024). Lactose. Yellow, scored. In 100s.
Rx	**Deconhist L.A.** (Goldline)					In 100s.
Rx	**Phenchlor S.H.A. Tablets** (Rugby)				1 bid	In 100s and 500s.
Rx	**Stahist Tablets** (Huckaby)					Dye free. (Stahist). White, scored. In 100s.
Rx	**Phenahist-TR Tablets** (T.E. Williams)				1 q 12 h	In 100s.
Rx	**Mescolor Tablets** (Horizon)	120 mg pseudoephedrine HCl	8 mg chlorpheniramine maleate	2.5 mg methscopolamine nitrate	1 q 12 h	(HP 15). Dye free.White, scored. Film coated. In 100s.

PEDIATRIC DECONGESTANT, ANTIHISTAMINE AND ANTICHOLINERGIC COMBINATIONS, SUSTAINED RELEASE

Refer to the general discussion of these products in the Respiratory Combinations Introduction. Content given per capsule.

	Product & Distributor	Decongestant	Antihistamine	Anticholinergic	Average Adult Dose	How Supplied
Rx	**Extendryl JR. Capsules** (Fleming)	10 mg phenylephrine HCl	4 mg chlorpheniramine maleate	1.25 mg methscopolamine nitrate	*Children (6 to 12 yrs)* 1 q 12 h	In 100s and 1000s.

UPPER RESPIRATORY COMBINATIONS

DECONGESTANT, ANTIHISTAMINE AND ANTICHOLINERGIC COMBINATIONS, MISCELLANEOUS

Refer to the general discussion of these products in the Respiratory Combinations Introduction.

Content given per tablet or 5 ml.

	Product & Distributor	Decongestant	Antihistamine	Anticholinergic	Average Adult Dose	How Supplied
Rx	**Dallergy Tablets** (Laser)	10 mg phenylephrine HCl	4 mg chlorphenir-amine maleate	1.25 mg meth-scopolamine nitrate	1 q 4 to 6 h	(Laser Dallergy). Scored. In 100s.
Rx	**D.A.** II (Dura)					(Dura DA II). White. In 100s.
Rx	**AH-chew Tablets** (WE Pharm)	10 mg phenylephrine HCl	2 mg chlorphenir-amine maleate	1.25 mg meth-scopolamine nitrate	1 or 2 q 4 h	Chewable. (WE 03). Scored. Grape flavor. In 100s.
Rx	**D.A. Chew Tabs** (Dura)					(Dura Chew). Orange flavor. Orange. In 100s.
Rx	**Extendryl Chewable Tablets** (Fleming)					Rootbeer flavor. In 100s and 1000s.
Rx	**Extendryl Syrup** (Fleming)				5 or 10 ml q 3 or 4 h qid	Rootbeer flavor. In 473 ml and gal.
Rx	**Dallergy Syrup** (Laser)	10 mg phenylephrine HCl	2 mg chlorphenir-amine maleate	0.625 mg meth-scopolamine nitrate	10 ml q 4 to 6 h	In 473 ml.

ANTITUSSIVE COMBINATIONS, CAPSULES AND TABLETS

For complete prescribing information, refer to the Respiratory Combinations introduction.

Contents given per capsule or tablet.

	Product & Distributor	Decongestant	Antihistamine	Antitussive	Other	Average Adult Dose	How Supplied
c-iii	**Hycodan Tablets** (Du Pont)			5 mg hydrocodone bitartrate	1.5 mg homatropine MBr, lactose	1 q 4 to 6 h	(Hycodan Du Pont). White, scored. In 100s and 500s.
c-iii	**Oncet Capsules** (Wakefield)				500 mg acetamino-phen	1 or 2 q 4 to 6 h	(Wakefield Oncet). White. In 100s.
c-iii	**Tussigon Tablets** (Daniels)				1.5 mg homatropine MBr	1 q 4 to 6 h	Blue, scored. In 100s and 500s.
c-iii	**Nucofed Capsules** (Roberts)	60 mg pseudo-ephedrine HCl		20 mg codeine phosphate	Lactose	1 q 6 h	Green/clear. In 60s.
c-iii	**Hycomine Compound Tablets** (Du Pont)	10 mg phenyleph-rine HCl	2 mg chlorphenir-amine maleate	5 mg hydrocodone bitartrate	250 mg acetamino-phen, 30 mg caffeine	1 q 4 h up to 4/day	Pink, scored. In 100s and 500s.

ANTITUSSIVE COMBINATIONS, CAPSULES AND TABLETS

	Product & Distributor	Decongestant	Antihistamine	Antitussive	Other	Average Adult Dose	How Supplied
Rx	**Ordrine AT Extended-Release Capsules** (Eon)	75 mg phenylpropanolamine HCl		40 mg caramiphen edisylate	Sucrose	1 q 12 h	(E 345). White/ clear. In 50s, 100s and 500s.
Rx	**Rescaps-D S.R. Capsules** (Geneva)						Sustained release. In 100s.
Rx	**Tuss-Allergine Modified T.D. Capsules** (Rugby)						In 100s.
Rx	**Tussogest Extended-Release Capsules** (Major)						Timed release. In 100s, 500s and 1000s.
Rx	**Tuss-Ornade Spansules** (SmithKline Beecham)				Sucrose		Sustained release. (Tuss-Ornade SKF). In 50s and 500s.
otc	**Bayer Select Chest Cold Caplets** (Bayer)			15 mg dextromethorphan HBr	500 mg acetaminophen	2 q 6 h	In 16s.
otc	**Drixoral Cough & Sore Throat Liquid Caps** (Schering-Plough)				325 mg acetaminophen, sorbitol	2 q 6 to 8 h	In 10s.
otc	**Alka-Seltzer Plus Flu & Body Aches Non-Drowsy Liqui-Gels** (Bayer)	30 mg pseudoephedrine HCl		10 mg dextromethorphan HBr	250 mg acetaminophen, sorbitol	2 q 4 h up to 8/day	In 12s.

ANTITUSSIVE COMBINATIONS, CAPSULES AND TABLETS

	Product & Distributor	Decongestant	Antihistamine	Antitussive	Other	Average Adult Dose	How Supplied
otc	**Comtrex Maximum Strength Non-Drowsy Caplets** (Bristol-Myers)	30 mg pseudo-ephedrine HCl		15 mg dextro-methorphan HBr	500 mg acetamino-phen, parabens	2 q 6 h	In 24s.
otc	**Sudafed Severe Cold Caplets & Tabs** (Warner-Wellcome)				500 mg acetamino-phen	2 q 6 h	(Sudafed SCF). In 10s and 20s.
otc	**Thera-Flu Non-Drowsy Formula Maximum Strength Caplets** (Sandoz)				500 mg acetamino-phen, lactose, methyl-paraben		(TheraFlu). In 24s.
otc	**Genapap Cold Caplets & Gel-caps** (Zenith-Goldline)				325 mg acetamino-phen		**Caplets:** In 24s. **Gelcaps:** In 20s.
otc	**Tylenol Cold No Drowsiness Caplets & Gelcaps** (McNeil-CPC)						**Caplets:** White. In 24s and 50s. **Gelcaps:** In 20s and 40s.
otc	**Tylenol Flu Maximum Strength Gelcaps** (McNeil-CPC)				500 mg acetamino-phen, parabens		In 10s and 20s.
otc	**Vicks 44 Non-Drowsy Cold & Cough LiquiCaps** (Richardson-Vicks)	60 mg pseudo-ephedrine HCl		30 mg dextro-methorphan HBr	Sorbitol.	1 q 6 h	(44). Red. In 10s.
otc	**Drixoral Cough & Congestion Liquid Caps** (Schering-Plough)						In 10s.
otc	**Thera-Flu Non-Drowsy Flu, Cold & Cough Maximum Strength Powder** (Sandoz)				1000 mg acetamino-phen, sucrose	1 q 6 h	Lemon flavor. In 6s and 12s.
otc	**Saleto CF Tablets** (Roberts)	12.5 mg phenylpro-panolamine HCl		10 mg dextro-methorphan HBr	325 mg acetamino-phen	2 q 4 h	In UD 8s and 1000s.

ANTITUSSIVE COMBINATIONS, CAPSULES AND TABLETS

	Product & Distributor	Decongestant	Antihistamine	Antitussive	Other	Average Adult Dose	How Supplied
otc	**Triaminicol Multi-Symptom Cough and Cold Tablets** (Sandoz)	12.5 mg phenylpropanolamine HCl	2 mg chlorpheniramine maleate	10 mg dextromethorphan HBr	Lactose, methylparaben	2 q 4 h	In 24s.
otc	**Cold Relief Tablets** (Rugby)				325 mg acetaminophen		In 50s
otc	**Comtrex Liqui-Gels (Capsules)** (Bristol-Myers)				325 mg acetaminophen, sorbitol		(Comtrex). Yellow. In 24s and 50s.
Rx	**Rynatuss Tablets** (Wallace)	10 mg phenylephrine tannate, 10 mg ephedrine tannate	5 mg chlorpheniramine tannate	60 mg carbetapentane tannate		1 or 2 q 12 h	(Wallace 717). Mauve, scored. In 100s.
otc	**Bayer Select Night Time Cold Caplets** (Bayer)	30 mg pseudoephedrine HCl	1.25 mg triprolidine HCl	15 mg dextromethorphan HBr	500 mg acetaminophen	2 hs or q 6 h	In blister-pack 16s.
otc	**Bayer Select Flu Relief Caplets** (Bayer)	30 mg pseudoephedrine HCl	2 mg chlorpheniramine maleate	15 mg dextromethorphan HBr	500 mg acetaminophen	2 q 6 h	In blister-pack 16s.
otc	**Maximum Strength Comtrex Caplets** (Bristol-Myers)				500 mg acetaminophen, parabens		In 24s.
otc	**Co-Apap Tablets** (Various, eg, Rugby)	30 mg pseudoephedrine HCl	2 mg chlorpheniramine maleate	15 mg dextromethorphan HBr	325 mg acetaminophen	2 q 6 h	In 24s, 50s and 1000s.
otc	**Multi-Symptom Tylenol Cold Caplets & Tablets** (McNeil-CPC)						In 24s and 50s.
otc	**Mapap Cold Formula Tablets** (Major)						In 24s.
otc	**Comtrex Maximum Strength Multi-Symptom Cold & Flu Relief Caplets and Tablets** (Bristol-Myers)				500 mg acetaminophen, parabens	2 q 4 h up to 8/day	(Cx). In 24s.

ANTITUSSIVE COMBINATIONS, CAPSULES AND TABLETS

	Product & Distributor	Decongestant	Antihistamine	Antitussive	Other	Average Adult Dose	How Supplied
otc	**Tylenol Multi—Symptom Hot Medication (Powder)** (McNeil-CPC)	60 mg pseudo-ephedrine HCl	4 mg chlorphenir-amine maleate	30 mg dextro-methorphan HBr	650 mg acetamino-phen, aspartame, sucrose, 11 mg phe-nylalanine	1 pack dis-solved in 6 oz hot water q 6 h	Honey lemon flavor. In 6 packs.
otc	**NightTime Thera-Flu Powder** (Sandoz)				1000 mg acetamino-phen, sucrose		Lemon flavor. In 6 packs.
otc	**TheraFlu Flu, Cold & Cough Powder** (Sandoz)	60 mg pseudo-ephedrine HCl	4 mg chlorphenir-amine maleate	20 mg dextro-methorphan HBr	650 mg acetamino-phen, sucrose	1 pack dis-solved in 6 oz water q 4 h up to 4 doses/day	Lemon flavor. In 6 packs.
otc	**Flu, Cold & Cough Medicine Powder** (Major)				500 mg acetamino-phen, sucrose		Lemon flavor. In 6s.
otc	**Contac Day & Night Cold & Flu Caplets** (SmithKline–Beecham)	*Day:* 60 mg pseudo-ephedrine HCl		30 mg dextro-methorphan HBr	650 mg acetamino-phen	*Day:* 1 yellow caplet q 6 h. *Night:* 1 blue caplet q 6 h. ≤4 in any com-bination per day	*Day:* (C-Day). Yellow. *Night:* (C-Night). Blue. In 20s (15 day; 5 night).
		Night: 60 mg pseu-doephedrine HCl	50 mg diphenhydra-mine HCl		650 mg acetamino-phen		
otc	**NyQuil Hot Therapy Powder** (Vicks)	60 mg pseudo-ephedrine HCl	12.5 mg doxylamine succinate	30 mg dextro-methorphan HBr	1000 mg acetamino-phen, sucrose	1 pack dis-solved in 6 oz hot water q 6 h	Honey lemon flavor. In 6 packs.
otc	**Alka-Seltzer Plus NightTime Cold Liqui-Gels** (Bayer)	30 mg pseudo-ephedrine HCl	6.25 mg doxylamine succinate	10 mg dextro-methorphan HBr	250 mg acetamino-phen, sorbitol	2 q 4 h up to 8/day	In 20s.
otc	**Vicks NyQuil LiquiCaps** (Richardson-Vicks)				250 mg acetamino-phen	2 q 4 h up to 8/day	(NyQuil). In 12s and 20s.

ANTITUSSIVE COMBINATIONS, CAPSULES AND TABLETS

	Product & Distributor	Decongestant	Antihistamine	Antitussive	Other	Average Adult Dose	How Supplied
otc	**Vicks 44M Cold, Flu & Cough LiquiCaps** (Proctor & Gamble)	30 mg pseudo-ephedrine HCl	2 mg chlorphenir-amine maleate	10 mg dextro-methorphan HBr	250 mg acetamino-phen	2 q 4 h up to 4/day	(44). Blue. In 12s.
otc	**Alka-Seltzer Plus Cold & Cough Liqui-Gels** (Bayer)				250 mg acetamino-phen, sorbitol	2 q 4 h up to 8/day	In 12s and 20s.
otc	**Genacol Tablets** (Goldline)				325 mg acetamino-phen	2 q 4 h up to 8/day	In 50s.
otc	**Kolephrin/DM Caplets** (Pfeiffer)					2 q 4 to 6 h up to 8/day	In 30s.
otc	**Cold Symptoms Relief Tab-lets** (Major)					2 q 4 h	In 50s.
otc	**Alka-Seltzer Plus Cold & Cough Tablets** (Bayer)	20 mg phenylpro-panolamine bitar-trate	2 mg chlorphenir-amine maleate	10 mg dextro-methorphan HBr	325 mg aspirin, aspartame, 11.2 mg phenylalanine	2 q 4 h up to 8/day	In 12s, 20s and 36s.
otc	**Alka-Seltzer Plus Night-Time Cold Tablets** (Bayer)	20 mg phenylpropa-nolamine bitartrate	6.25 mg doxylamine succinate	15 mg dextro-methorphan HBr	500 mg aspirin, 16.2 mg phenylalanine, aspartame	2 q 4 h dis-solved in 120 ml water up to 8/day	In 12s, 20s and 36s.
otc	**Maximum Strength Comtrex Liqui-Gels (Capsules)** (Bristol-Myers)	12.5 mg phenylpro-panolamine HCl	2 mg chlorphenir-amine maleate	15 mg dextro-methorphan HBr	500 mg acetamino-phen, sorbitol	2 q 6 h	In 24s and 50s.
otc	**Comtrex Max Strength Multi-Symptom Cold & Flu Relief Liqui-Gels (Capsules)** (Bristol-Myers)				500 mg acetamino-phen		(Comtrex LG). In 24s.

Antitussive and Expectorant Combinations

ANTITUSSIVE COMBINATIONS, LIQUIDS

For complete prescribing information, refer to the Respiratory Combinations introduction.

Contents given per 5 ml.

	Product & Distributor	Decongestant	Antihistamine	Antitussive	Other	Average Adult Dose	How Supplied
c-III	**Hydrocodone Compound Syrup** (Various, eg, Goldline, Qualitest, Halsey)			5 mg hydrocodone bitartrate	1.5 mg homatropine MBr	1 q 4 to 6 h	In 473 ml and gal.
c-III	**Hycodan Syrup** (Du Pont)				1.5 mg homatropine MBr, sorbitol, sugar, parabens		Cherry flavor. In 473 ml.
c-III	**Hydromet Syrup** (Barre-National)				1.5 mg homatropine MBr, saccharin, sucrose, methylparaben		Cherry flavor. In 473 ml and gal.
c-III	**Detussin Liquid** (Various, eg, Barre-National, Qualitest)	60 mg pseudoephedrine HCl		5 mg hydrocodone bitartrate	5% alcohol	5 ml qid	In pt and gal.
c-III	**Histussin D** (Bock)						Wild cherry/black raspberry flavor. In 480 ml.
c-III	**Tyrodone** (Major)				5% alcohol		In 473 ml.
c-III *sf*	**Entuss-D Liquid** (Roberts Hauck)	30 mg pseudoephedrine HCl		5 mg hydrocodone bitartrate		5 to 7.5 ml pc and hs (not less than q 4 h)	Alcohol and dye free. In 473 ml.

COUGH PREPARATIONS

Antitussive and Expectorant Combinations

ANTITUSSIVE COMBINATIONS, LIQUIDS

	Product & Distributor	Decongestant	Antihistamine	Antitussive	Other	Average Adult Dose	How Supplied
c-III	**Codamine Syrup** (Various, eg, Barre-National, IDE,Major)	25 mg phenylpropanolamine HCl		5 mg hydrocodone bitartrate		5 ml qid	In 480 ml.
c-III	**Hycomine Syrup** (Du Pont)				Saccharin, sorbitol, parabens	5 ml q 4 h	Cherry flavor. In 473 ml.
c-III	**Hydrocodone PA Syrup** (Morton Grove)						In 473 ml
c-III	**Phenylpropanolamine HCl and Hydrocodone Syrup** (PBI)					5 ml pc and hs ≥ 4 hrs apart	In 480 ml.
otc	**Effective Strength Cough Formula Liquid with Decongestant** (Barre-National)	20 mg pseudoephedrine HCl		10 mg dextromethorphan HBr	10% alcohol, corn syrup, saccharin, sucrose	15 ml q 6 h	Cherry - menthol flavor. In 237 ml.
otc	**Vicks Formula 44D Cough & Decongestant Liquid** (Richardson-Vicks)				10% alcohol, saccharin, sucrose		In 120 and 240 ml.
otc	**Vicks 44D Cough & Head Congestion** (Procter & Gamble)						In 120 and 240 ml.
otc	**Robitussin Maximum Strength Cough & Cold Liquid** (Robins)	30 mg pseudoephedrine HCl		15 mg dextromethorphan HBr	1.4% alcohol, high fructose, corn syrup, saccharin, glucose	10 ml q 6 h	In 240 ml.
c-III	**Nucofed Syrup** (Roberts)	60 mg pseudoephedrine HCl		20 mg codeine phosphate	Sorbitol, sucrose	5 ml q 6 h	Alcohol free. Mint flavor. In 473 ml.

Antitussive and Expectorant Combinations

ANTITUSSIVE COMBINATIONS, LIQUIDS

	Product & Distributor	Decongestant	Antihistamine	Antitussive	Other	Average Adult Dose	How Supplied
otc	**Triaminic-DM Syrup** (Sandoz)	6.25 mg phenylpropanolamine HCl		5 mg dextromethorphan HBr	Sorbitol, sucrose	20 ml q 4 h	Alcohol free. Berry flavor. In 120 and 240 ml.
Rx	**Tuss-Ornade Liquid** (SK-Beecham)	12.5 mg phenylpropanolamine HCl		6.7 mg caramiphen edisylate	5% alcohol, menthol, sorbitol, parabens	10 ml q 4 h	Fruit flavor. In 240 ml.
c-III	**Tussionex Pennkinetic Suspension** (Fisons)		8 mg chlorpheniramine (as polistirex)	10 mg hydrocodone (as polistirex)	Parabens, sucrose, high fructose corn syrup	5 ml q 12 h	Extended release. Alcohol free. In 473 and 900 ml.
c-v	**Bromanyl Syrup** (Various, eg, Barre-National, Harber, Moore, Qualitest, Schein)		12.5 mg bromodiphenhydramine HCl	10 mg codeine phosphate		5 to 10 ml q 4 to 6 h	In 120 ml, pt and gal.
c-v	**Ambenyl Cough Syrup** (Forest)				5% alcohol		In 120 and 480 ml and gal.
c-v	**Amgenal Cough Syrup** (Goldline)						Cherry flavor. In pt.
c-v	**Bromotuss w/Codeine Syrup** (Rugby)						In 120 ml, pt and gal.
c-v	**Bromodiphenhydramine HCl and Codeine Cough Syrup** (Pennex)				6% alcohol		Cherry flavor. In 120 ml, pt and gal.

Antitussive and Expectorant Combinations

ANTITUSSIVE COMBINATIONS, LIQUIDS

	Product & Distributor	Decongestant	Antihistamine	Antitussive	Other	Average Adult Dose	How Supplied
c-v	**Promethazine HCl w/Codeine Liquid** (Various, eg, Century, Geneva, Goldline, Halsey, Major, Qualitest, Schein, URL)		6.25 mg promethazine HCl	10 mg codeine phosphate		5 ml q 4 to 6 h	In 120 ml, pt and gal.
c-v	**Prometh w/ Codeine Syrup** (Various, eg, Barre-National, Goldline, Moore, URL)		6.25 mg promethazine HCl	10 mg codeine phosphate		5 ml q 4 to 6 h	In 120 ml, pt and gal.
c-v	**Pentazine VC w/Codeine Liquid** (Century)						In 118 ml, pt and gal.
c-v	**Phenergan with Codeine Syrup** (Wyeth–Ayerst)				7% alcohol, saccharin		In 118 and 473 ml.
c-v	**Pherazine w/ Codeine Syrup** (Halsey)				7% alcohol, sorbitol, sucrose	5 ml q 4 to 6 h	In 120 ml, pt and gal.
c-v	**Tricodene Cough & Cold Liquid** (Pfeiffer)		12.5 mg pyrilamine maleate	8.2 mg codeine phosphate		10 ml q 6 to 8 h	In 120 ml.
c-III *sf*	**S-T Forte 2 Liquid** (Scot-Tussin)		2 mg chlorpheniramine maleate	2.5 mg hydrocodone bitartrate	99.7% glycerin, menthol, parabens	5 ml tid or qid	Alcohol and dye free. In pt and gal.

Antitussive and Expectorant Combinations

ANTITUSSIVE COMBINATIONS, LIQUIDS

	Product & Distributor	Decongestant	Antihistamine	Antitussive	Other	Average Adult Dose	How Supplied
otc	**Effective Strength Cough Formula Liquid** (Barre-National)		2 mg chlorphenir-maleate	15 mg dextro-methorphan HBr	10% alcohol, corn syrup, sugar, para-bens,saccharin	10 ml q 6 h	In 240 ml.
otc	**Primatuss Cough Mix-ture 4 Liquid** (Rugby)				10 % alcohol, sorbitol, sucrose	10 ml q 8 h	In 118 ml.
otc *sf*	**Scot-Tussin DM Liquid** (Scot-Tussin)					5 ml q 4 h or 10 ml q 6 to 8 h	Alcohol free. In 118 and 236.6 ml, pt and gal.
otc *sf*	**Tricodene Sugar Free Liquid** (Pfeiffer)		2 mg chlorphenir-amine maleate	10 mg dextro-methorphan HBr	Sorbitol	10 ml q 4 to 6 h	In 120 ml.
Rx	**Promethazine DM Liquid** (Various, eg, Geneva, Harber, Major, Moore, Qualitest, Rugby, Schein)		6.25 mg prometha-zine HCl	15 mg dextro-methorphan HBr	Alcohol	5 ml q 4 to 6 h	In 120 ml, pt and gal.
Rx	**Phenameth DM Syrup** (Major)						In 120 ml.
Rx	**Phenergan w/Dextro-methorphan Syrup** (Wyeth-Ayerst)				7% alcohol, saccharin		In 118 and 473 ml.
Rx	**Pherazine DM Syrup** (Halsey)				7% alcohol, sorbitol, sucrose		In 120 ml, pt and gal.
Rx	**Prometh w/Dextro-methorphan Syrup** (Barre-National)				7% alcohol		Lemon-mint flavor. In 118 ml, pt and gal.

ANTITUSSIVE COMBINATIONS, LIQUIDS

	Product & Distributor	Decongestant	Antihistamine	Antitussive	Other	Average Adult Dose	How Supplied
c-III	**ED Tuss HC Liquid** (Edwards)	10 mg phenylephrine HCl	4 mg chlorpheniramine maleate	2.5 mg hydrocodone bitartrate	5% alcohol	5 ml qid	Grape flavor. In 480 ml.
c-III	**Tussanil DH Syrup** (Misemer)						Grape flavor. In 480 ml.
c-III	**ED-TLC Liquid** (Edwards)	5 mg phenylephrine HCl	2 mg chlorpheniramine maleate	1.67 mg hydrocodone bitartrate		10 ml tid or qid	In 473 ml.
c-III	**Endagen-HD Liquid** (Abana)						In 473 ml.
c-III	**Hydrocodone HD** (Morton Grove						In 473 ml.
c-III	**Iodal HD** (Iomed)						In 473 ml.
c-III *sf*	**Para-Hist HD Liquid** (Pharmics)						Alcohol free. In 473 ml.
c-III	**Vanex-HD Liquid** (Abana)						In 473 ml.

Antitussive and Expectorant Combinations

ANTITUSSIVE COMBINATIONS, LIQUIDS

	Product & Distributor	Decongestant	Antihistamine	Antitussive	Other	Average Adult Dose	How Supplied
c-III	**Antuss HD** (Atley)	5 mg phenylephrine HCl	2 mg chlorphenir-amine maleate	2.5 mg hydrocodone bitartrate	Menthol, sucrose		Cherry flavor. In 473 ml.
c-III	**Endal-HD Plus Liquid** (UAD)				Menthol, parabens, sucrose	10 ml q 4 h up to 40 ml/day	Dye and alcohol free. In 473 ml.
c-III	**Histussin HC Syrup** (Bock)						In 120 and 480 ml.
c-III	**Hydrocodone CP Liquid** (Morton Grove)						In 473 ml.
c-III	**Iotussin HCSyrup** (Iomed Labs)						Alcohol free. Fruit flavor. In 473 ml.
c-III sf	**Unituss HC Syrup** (URL)				Saccharin, sorbitol	10 ml q 4 h, up to 40 ml/day	In 473 ml.
c-III sf	**Histinex HCSyrup** (Ethex)	5 mg phenylephrine HCl	2 mg chlorphenir-amine maleate	2 mg hydrocodone bitartrate			Alcohol free. Fruit flavor. In 473 ml.
c-III sf	**Anaplex HD Syrup** (Medi-Plex)	5 mg phenylephrine HCl	2 mg chlorphenir-amine maleate	1.7 mg hydrocodone bitartrate		10 ml tid or qid	Alcohol free. Strawberry flavor. In 120 and 480 ml.
c-III	**Endal-HD Liquid** (UAD)				Menthol, sucrose, parabens	10 ml q 4 h up to 40 ml/day	In 473 ml.
c-III sf	**Chlorgest-HD Liquid** (Great Southern)	5 mg phenylephrine HCl	4 mg chlor-pheniramine maleate	1.67 mg hydro-codone bitartrate		10 ml tid or qid	Alcohol free. In pt and gal.

Antitussive and Expectorant Combinations

ANTITUSSIVE COMBINATIONS, LIQUIDS

	Product & Distributor	Decongestant	Antihistamine	Antitussive	Other	Average Adult Dose	How Supplied
c-III *sf*	**Histinex PV Syrup** (Ethex)	30 mg pseudo-ephedrine HCl	2 mg chlorphenir-amine maleate	2.5 mg hydrocodone bitartrate	Parabens, saccharin, sorbitol	10 ml q 4 to 6 hrs	Alcohol free. Fruit flavor. In 120 and 480 ml.
c-III	**P-V-Tussin Syrup** (Solvay)				5% alcohol, glucose, parabens, saccharin, sorbitol, sucrose	10 ml q 4 to 6 hrs	Banana flavor. In pt and gal.
c-v	**Dihistine DH Liquid** (Various, eg, Barre-National, Goldline, Major)	30 mg pseudo-ephedrine HCl	2 mg chlorphenir-amine maleate	10 mg codeine phosphate	Alcohol	10 ml q 4 to 6 h up to 40 ml/day	In 120 ml, pt and gal.
c-v	**Codehist DH Elixir** (Geneva)				5.7% alcohol	10 ml q 4 h up to 40 ml/day	Grape/honey flavor. In 120 and 480 ml.
c-v	**Decohistine DH Liquid** (Pennex)				5.8% alcohol	5 to 10 ml q 4 to 6 h up to 40 ml/day	Grape/honey flavor. In 120 ml, pt and gal.
c-v	**Novahistine DH Liquid** (SmithKline Beecham)	30 mg pseudo-ephedrine HCl	2 mg chlorphenir-amine maleate	10 mg codeine phosphate	5% alcohol, sugar, saccharin, sorbitol	10 ml q 4 to 6 h up to 40 ml/day	In 120 and 480 ml.
c-v	**Phenhist DH w/ Codeine Liquid** (Rugby)				5% alcohol	10 ml q 4 h up to 40 ml/day	In 120 and 480 ml.
c-v *sf*	**Ryna-C Liquid** (Wallace)				Saccharin, sorbitol	10 ml q 4 to 6 h up to 40 ml/day	Alcohol and dye free. In 118 and 473 ml.

ANTITUSSIVE COMBINATIONS, LIQUIDS

	Product & Distributor	Decongestant	Antihistamine	Antitussive	Other	Average Adult Dose	How Supplied
c-v	**Triacin-C Cough Syrup** (Various, eg, Barre-National, Moore)	30 mg pseudo-ephedrine HCl	1.25 mg triprolidine HCl	10 mg codeine phosphate	Alcohol	10 ml q 4 to 6 h up to 40 ml/day	In 120 ml, pt and gal.
c-v	**Actagen-C Cough Syrup** (Goldline)						In pt and gal.
c-v	**Actifed w/Codeine Cough Syrup** (Glaxo Wellcome)				4.3% alcohol, sorbitol, 0.1%methylparaben, 0.1%sodium benzoate		In 480 ml.
c-v	**Allerfrin w/Codeine Syrup** (Rugby)						In 3840 ml.
c-v	**Aprodine w/Codeine Syrup** (Major)						In pt and gal.
c-v	**Triafed with Codeine Syrup** (Schein)				0.15%methylparaben, 0.1%sodium benzoate		In 473 ml.
c-v	**Trifed-C Cough Syrup** (Geneva)				4.4% alcohol		Raspberry flavor. In 480 ml.

COUGH PREPARATIONS

Antitussive and Expectorant Combinations

ANTITUSSIVE COMBINATIONS, LIQUIDS

	Product & Distributor	Decongestant	Antihistamine	Antitussive	Other	Average Adult Dose	How Supplied
c-v	**Promethazine VC w/ Codeine Liquid** (Various, eg, Geneva, Schein, URL, Warner Chilcott)	5 mg phenylephrine HCl	6.25 mg promethazine HCl	10 mg codeine phosphate	Alcohol	5 ml q 4 to 6 h	In 120 ml, pt and gal.
c-v	**Prometh VC with Codeine Liquid** (Various, eg, Barre-National, Goldline, Warner Chilcott)						In pt and gal.
c-v	**Promethist with Codeine Syrup** (Rahslog Corp)						In 120 ml.
c-v	**Phenergan VC with Codeine Syrup** (Wyeth-Ayerst)				7% alcohol, saccharin		In 118 and 473 ml.
c-v	**Pherazine VC w/ Codeine Syrup** (Halsey)				7% alcohol		Strawberry/orange flavor. In 120 ml, pt and gal.
c-v	**Codimal PH Syrup** (Central)	5 mg phenylephrine HCl	8.33 mg pyrilamine maleate	10 mg codeine phosphate	Menthol, sucrose	5 to 10 ml q 4 to 6 h	In 120 ml, pt and gal.
c-iii	**Codimal DH Syrup** (Central)	5 mg phenylephrine HCl	8.33 mg pyrilamine maleate	1.66 mg hydrocodone bitartrate	Menthol, sucrose	5 to 10 ml q 4 h	Alcohol free. In 120 ml, pt and gal.

Antitussive and Expectorant Combinations

ANTITUSSIVE COMBINATIONS, LIQUIDS

	Product & Distributor	Decongestant	Antihistamine	Antitussive	Other	Average Adult Dose	How Supplied
c-v	**Bromanate DC Cough Syrup** (Various, eg, Barre-National, Goldline, Moore)	12.5 mg phenylpropanolamine HCl	2 mg brompheniramine maleate	10 mg codeine phosphate	Alcohol	10 ml q 4 h	In 120 ml, pt and gal.
c-v	**Bromphen DC w/Codeine Cough Syrup** (Various, eg, Rugby, Schein)						In 120 ml.
c-v	**Brompheniramine DC Cough Syrup** (Geneva)				1.15% alcohol		Raspberry flavor. In 480 ml.
c-v *sf*	**Dimetane-DC Cough Syrup** (Robins)				0.95% alcohol, sorbitol		Raspberry flavor. In pt and gal.
c-v	**Myphetane DC Cough Syrup** (Pennex)				1.2% alcohol		Raspberry flavor. In 118 and 3840 ml.
c-v	**Poly-Histine CS Syrup** (Bock)						Alcohol free. Raspberry/strawberry flavor. In 120 and 480 ml.

Antitussive and Expectorant Combinations

ANTITUSSIVE COMBINATIONS, LIQUIDS

	Product & Distributor	Decongestant	Antihistamine	Antitussive	Other	Average Adult Dose	How Supplied
Rx	**Myphetane DX Cough Syrup** (Pennex)	30 mg pseudo-ephedrine HCl	2 mg brompheniramine maleate	10 mg dextromethorphan HBr	1% alcohol	10 ml q 4 h	In 120 ml, pt and gal.
Rx	**Bromarest DX Cough Syrup** (Warner Chilcott)				0.95% alcohol		Butterscotch flavor. In 480 ml.
Rx	**Bromatane DX Cough Syrup** (Goldline)						Butterscotch flavor. In 480 ml.
Rx	**Bromfed DM Cough Syrup** (Muro)				Saccharin, sorbitol, sucrose, methylparabens		Cherry flavor. In 480 ml.
Rx	**Bromphen DX Cough Syrup** (Rugby)				0.95% alcohol		In 480 ml.
Rx	**Brompheniramine Cough Syrup** (Geneva)						Butterscotch flavor. In 480 ml.
Rx *sf*	**Dimetane-DX Cough Syrup** (Robins)				0.95% alcohol, saccharin, sorbitol		Butterscotch flavor. In pt and gal.

Antitussive and Expectorant Combinations

ANTITUSSIVE COMBINATIONS, LIQUIDS

	Product & Distributor	Decongestant	Antihistamine	Antitussive	Other	Average Adult Dose	How Supplied
Rx	**Cardec DM Syrup** (Various, eg, Barre-National, Goldline, Schein, Moore, URL)	60 mg pseudo-ephedrine HCl	4 mg carbinoxamine maleate	15 mg dextro-methorphan HBr	May also contain alcohol	5 ml qid	In 120 ml, pt and gal.
Rx	**Carbinoxamine Compound Syrup** (Pennex)	60 mg pseudo-ephedrine HCl	4 mg carbinoxamine maleate	15 mg dextro-methorphan HBr	< 0.2% alcohol, sugar, parabens		Grape flavor. In 120 and 480 ml.
Rx	**Carbodec DM Syrup** (Various, eg, Rugby)						In 118 ml, pt and gal.
Rx	**Pseudo-Car DM Syrup** (Geneva)				0.19% alcohol		Grape flavor. In 480 ml.
Rx *sf*	**Rondec-DM Syrup** (Dura)						Alcohol free. In 480 ml.
Rx *sf*	**Tussafed Syrup** (Everett)				Menthol		Alcohol free. Grape flavor. In 120 and 480 ml.
otc *sf*	**Rescon-DM Liquid** (Ion)	30 mg pseudo-ephedrine HCl	2 mg chlorphenir-amine maleate	10 mg dextro-methorphan HBr		10 ml q 4 to 6 h	Alcohol and dye free. In 120 ml.
otc *sf*	**Cerose DM Liquid** (Wyeth-Ayerst)	10 mg phenyl-ephrine HCl	4 mg chlorphenir-amine maleate	15 mg dextro-methorphan HBr	2.4% alcohol, saccharin, EDTA	5 ml qid	In 120 and 480 ml.
otc	**Rhinosyn-DM Liquid** (Great Southern)	30 mg pseudo-ephedrine HCl	2 mg chlorphenir-amine maleate	15 mg dextro-methorphan HBr	1.4% alcohol, sucrose	10 ml q 6 h	In 120 ml.
otc	**Tussar DM Syrup** (Rhone-Poulenc Rorer)				Sucrose, glucose, methylparaben	10 ml q 6 h	Alcohol free. In 473 ml.

COUGH PREPARATIONS

Antitussive and Expectorant Combinations

ANTITUSSIVE COMBINATIONS, LIQUIDS

	Product & Distributor	Decongestant	Antihistamine	Antitussive	Other	Average Adult Dose	How Supplied
otc sf	**Codimal DM Syrup** (Central)	5 mg phenylephrine HCl	8.33 mg pyrilamine maleate	10 mg dextromethorphan HBr	Menthol, saccharin, sorbitol	10 ml q 4 h	Alcohol and dye free. In 120 ml, pt and gal.
Rx	**Histine DM Syrup** (Ethex)	12.5 mg phenylpropanolamine HCl	2 mg brompheniramine maleate	10 mg dextromethorphan HBr	Parabens, saccharin	10 ml q 4 h	Berry flavor. In 120 and 480 ml.
Rx sf	**Iohist DMSyrup** (Iomed)						Alcohol free. Blackberry flavor. In pts.
Rx	**Liqui-Histine DMSyrup** (Liquipharm)						Alcohol free. Black raspberry flavor. In 473 ml.
Rx	**Poly-Histine DM Syrup** (Bock)						Alcohol free. Black raspberry flavor. In 120 and 480 ml.

Antitussive and Expectorant Combinations

ANTITUSSIVE COMBINATIONS, LIQUIDS

	Product & Distributor	Decongestant	Antihistamine	Antitussive	Other	Average Adult Dose	How Supplied
otc	**Kophane Cough & Cold Formula Liquid** (Pfeiffer)	12.5 mg phenylpropanolamine HCl	2 mg chlorpheniramine maleate	10 mg dextromethorphan HBr		10 ml q 4 h	In 120 ml.
otc	**Myminicol Liquid** (Pennex)						Alcohol free. Raspberry-cherry flavor. In 120 ml, pt and gal.
otc	**Threamine DM Syrup** (Barre-National)				Saccharin, sorbitol, sucrose, methylparaben	10 ml q 4 to 6 h	In pt and gal.
otc	**Triaminicol Multi-Symptom Relief Liquid** (Sandoz)				Sorbitol, sucrose		Alcohol free. Cherry flavor. In 120 and 240 ml.
otc	**Tricodene Forte Liquid** (Pfeiffer)	12.5 mg phenylpropanolamine HCl	2 mg chlorpheniramine maleate	10 mg dextromethorphan HBr		10 ml q 4 h	In 120 ml.
otc	**Tricodene NN Liquid** (Pfeiffer)						In 120 ml.
otc	**Triminol Cough Syrup** (Rugby)				Saccharin, sorbitol, sugar		In 118 ml.
otc	**Cheracol Plus Liquid** (Roberts)	8.3 mg phenylpropanolamine HCl	1.3 mg chlorpheniramine maleate	6.7 mg dextromethorphan HBr	8% alcohol, sorbitol, parabens	15 ml q 4 h	In 120 ml.
otc	**Orthoxicol Cough Syrup** (Roberts)						In 60, 120 and 480 ml.

COUGH PREPARATIONS

Antitussive and Expectorant Combinations

ANTITUSSIVE COMBINATIONS, LIQUIDS

	Product & Distributor	Decongestant	Antihistamine	Antitussive	Other	Average Adult Dose	How Supplied
otc	**Dimetapp DM Elixir** (Robins)	12.5 mg phenylpropanolamine HCl	2 mg brompheniramine maleate	10 mg dextromethorphan HBr	Saccharin, sorbitol	10 ml q 4 h	Alcohol free. Grape flavor. In 360 ml.
otc	**Siltapp with Dextromethorphan HBr Cold & CoughElixir** (Silarx)				2.3% alcohol, saccharin, sorbitol.		In 118 ml.
otc	**Vicks NyQuil Multi-Symptom Cold Flu Relief Liquid** (Richardson-Vicks)	10 mg pseudoephedrine HCl	2.1 mg doxylamine succinate	5 mg dextromethorphan HBr	167 mg acetaminophen, 10% alcohol, sucrose		Regular and cherry flavors. In 180, 300 and 420 ml.
otc	**All-Nite Cold Formula Liquid** (Major)	10 mg pseudoephedrine HCl	1.25 mg doxylamine succinate	5 mg dextromethorphan HBr	167 mg acetaminophen, 25% alcohol, sucrose	30 ml hs or 30 ml q 6 h	Mint and cherry flavors. In 180 and 300 ml.

Antitussive and Expectorant Combinations

ANTITUSSIVE COMBINATIONS, LIQUIDS

	Product & Distributor	Decongestant	Antihistamine	Antitussive	Other	Average Adult Dose	How Supplied
otc	**Genite Liquid** (Goldline)	10 mg pseudoephedrine HCl	1.25 mg doxylamine succinate	5 mg dextromethorphan HBr	167 mg acetaminophen, 25% alcohol, tartrazine		Anise flavor. In 177 ml.
otc	**Nite Time Cold Formula Liquid** (Barre–National)				167 mg acetaminophen, 25% alcohol		Licorice and cherry flavors. In 180 and 300 ml.
otc	**NyQuil Nighttime Cold/Flu Medicine Liquid** (Richardson-Vicks)				167 mg acetaminophen, 25% alcohol, sucrose; saccharin (cherry flavor); tartrazine (original flavor)		Original and cherry flavor. In 180, 300 and 420 ml.
otc	**Nytcold Medicine Liquid** (Rugby)				167 mg acetaminophen, 25% alcohol, glucose, saccharin, sucrose		Original and cherry flavors. In 177 ml.
otc	**Contac Severe Cold & Flu Nighttime Liquid** (SK-Beecham)	10 mg pseudoephedrine HCl	0.67 mg chlorpheniramine maleate	5 mg dexromethorphan HBr	167 mg acetaminophen, 18.5% alcohol, saccharin, sorbitol, glucose	30 ml hs or 30 ml q 6 h	In 180 ml.
otc	**Medi-Flu Liquid** (Parke–Davis)				167 mg acetaminophen, 19% alcohol, saccharin, sorbitol, sugar		In 180 ml.
otc	**Robitussin Night Relief Liquid** (Robins)	10 mg pseudoephedrine HCl	8.3 mg pyrilamine maleate	5 mg dextromethorphan HBr	108.3 mg acetaminophen, saccharin, sorbitol	30 ml hs or 30 ml q 6 h	Alcohol free. Cherry flavor. In 300 ml.

COUGH PREPARATIONS

Antitussive and Expectorant Combinations

ANTITUSSIVE COMBINATIONS, LIQUIDS

	Product & Distributor	Decongestant	Antihistamine	Antitussive	Other	Average Adult Dose	How Supplied
otc	**Triaminic AM Cough & Decongestant Formula Liquid** (Sandoz)	15 mg pseudoephedrine HCl		7.5 mg dextromethorphan HBr	sorbitol, sucrose	20 ml q 6 h	Alcohol and dye free. Orange flavor. In 118 and 237 ml.
otc	**Comtrex Liquid** (Bristol-Myers)	10 mg pseudoephedrine HCl	0.67 mg chlorpheniramine maleate	3.3 mg dextromethorphan HBr	108.3 mg acetaminophen, 20% alcohol, sucrose	30 ml q 4 h up to 120 ml/day	Cherry flavor. In 180 ml.
Rx	**Tusquelin Syrup** (Circle)	5 mg phenylpropanolamine, 5 mg phenylephrine HCl	2 mg chlorpheniramine maleate	15 mg dextromethorphan HBr	5% alcohol, 0.17 min fluid-extract ipecac, potassium guaiacolsulfonate	5 or 10 ml qid	In 480 ml.
c-III	**Rolatuss with Hydrocodone Liquid** (Major)	3.3 mg phenylpropanolamine HCl, 5 mg phenylephrine HCl	3.3 mg pyrilamine maleate, 3.3 mg pheniramine maleate	1.7 mg hydrocodone bitartrate		10 ml qid	In 480 ml.
c-III	**Ru-Tuss w/Hydrocodone Liquid** (Boots)				5% alcohol, glucose, menthol, saccharin, sorbitol, parabens	10 ml q 4 to 6 h	In 473 ml.
c-III	**Statuss Green Liquid** (Huckaby)				5% alcohol		In 480 ml.

Antitussive and Expectorant Combinations

ANTITUSSIVE COMBINATIONS, LIQUIDS

	Product & Distributor	Decongestant	Antihistamine	Antitussive	Other	Average Adult Dose	How Supplied
c-v	**T-Koff Liquid** (T.E. Williams)	20 mg phenylpropanolamine HCl, 20 mg phenylephrine HCl	5 mg chlorpheniramine maleate	10 mg codeine phosphate	Menthol, saccharin, sorbitol, sucrose, glucose, parabens	5 ml q 4 to 6 h	Grape flavor. In 480 ml.
otc	**Multi-Symptom Tylenol Cough with Decongestant Liquid** (McNeil)	20 mg pseudoephedrine HCl		10 mg dextromethorphan HBr	200 mg acetaminophen, 5% alcohol, saccharin, sorbitol.	15 ml q 4 to 6 h	Cherry flavor. In 120 ml.
otc	**Multi-Symptom Tylenol Cough Liquid** (McNeil-CPC)			10 mg dextromethorphan HBr	216.7 mg acetaminophen, 5% alcohol	20 ml q 6 to 8 h	In 120 ml.
otc *sf*	**Contac Cough & Sore Throat Liquid** (SK-Beecham)			5 mg dextromethorphan HBr	125 mg acetaminophen, 10% alcohol, saccharin, sorbitol	20 ml q 4 to 6 h up to 80 ml/day	In 120 ml.

Pediatric Antitussive Combinations

PEDIATRIC ANTITUSSIVE COMBINATIONS

Refer to the general discussion of these products in the Respiratory Combinations Introduction. Content given per 5 ml or pack.

	Product & Distributor	Decongestant	Antihistamine	Antitussive	Other	Average Dose	How Supplied
c-iii	**Codamine Pediatric Syrup** (Barre-National)	12.5 mg phenyl-propanolamine HCl		2.5 mg hydro-codone bitartrate		*6 to 12 yrs* – 5 ml q 4 h	In 473 ml.
c-iii	**Hycomine Pediatric Syrup** (Du Pont)				Saccharin, sorbitol, parabens		Cherry flavor. In 480 ml.
c-iii	**Hydrocodone PA Pediatric Syrup** (Morton Grove)						In 473 ml.
otc	**Tricodene Pediatric Cough & Cold Liquid** (Pfeiffer)	12.5 mg phenyl-propanolamine HCl		10 mg dextro-methorphan HBr		*2 to 6 yrs* - 2.5 ml q 4 h *6 to 12 yrs* - 5 ml q 4 h	In 120 ml.
otc	**Snaplets-DM Granules** (Baker Cummins)	6.25 mg phenyl-propanolamine HCl		5 mg dextro-methorphan HBr		*2 to < 6 yrs* – 1 pack q 4 h *6 to < 12 yrs* – 2 packs q 4 h	Taste free. In 30s.
otc	**Robitussin Pediatric Cough & Cold Liquid** (Robins)	15 mg pseudo-ephedrine HCl		7.5 mg dextro-methorphan HBr	Saccharin, sorbitol	*2 to < 6 yrs* - 5 ml q 6 h *6 to < 12 yrs* – 10 ml q 6 h	Alcohol free. Cherry flavor. In 120 ml.
otc	**Triaminic Sore Throat Formula Liquid** (Sandoz)	15 mg pseudo-ephedrine HCl		7.5 mg dextro-methorphan HBr	160 mg aceta-minophen, EDTA, sucrose	*2 to < 6 yrs* - 5 ml q 6 h *6 to < 12 yrs* - 10 ml q 6 h	Alcohol free. Grape flavor. In 240 ml.
otc	**Vicks Pediatric Formula 44d Cough & Decongestant Liquid** (Richardson-Vicks)	10 mg pseudo-ephedrine HCl		5 mg dextro-methorphan HBr	Sorbitol, sucrose	*2 to 5 yrs* - 7.5 ml q 6 h. *6 to 11 yrs* - 15 ml q 6 h	Alcohol free. In 120 ml.

Pediatric Antitussive Combinations

PEDIATRIC ANTITUSSIVE COMBINATIONS

	Product & Distributor	Decongestant	Antihistamine	Antitussive	Other	Average Dose	How Supplied
otc	**Pedia Care NightRest Cough-Cold Liquid** (McNeil-CPC)	15 mg pseudo-ephedrine HCl	1 mg chlorphenir-amine maleate	7.5 mg dextro-methorphan HBr	Sorbitol, corn syrup	*6 to 11 yrs* – 10 ml q 6 to 8 h	Alcohol free. Cherry flavor. In 120 ml.
otc	**Triaminic Nite Light Liquid** (Sandoz)				Sorbitol, sucrose	*6 to < 12 yrs* – 10 ml q 6 h	Alcohol free. Grape flavor. In 120 ml.
otc	**Children's Tylenol Cold Multi Symptom Plus Cough Liquid** (McNeil-CPC)	15 mg pseudo-ephedrine HCl	1 mg chlorphenir-amine maleate	5 mg dextro-methorphan HBr	160 mg aceta-minophen, sorbitol, corn syrup	*6 to 11 yrs* - 10 ml q 4 to 6 h up to 40 ml/day	Alcohol free. Cherry flavor. In 120 ml.
otc	**Pedia Care Cough-Cold Liquid** (McNeil-CPC)				Corn syrup, sorbitol		Alcohol free. Cherry flavor. In 120 ml.
otc	**Pedia Care Cough-Cold Chewable Tablets for Ages 6 - 12** (McNeil-CPC)				Aspartame, 6 mg phenyl-alanine	*6 to 11 yrs* – 2 q 4 to 6 h up to 8/day	Fruit flavor. In 16s.
otc	**Pediatric Cough & Cold Liquid** (Zenith-Goldline)				Sorbitol, sucrose.	*6 to 11 yrs* – 10 ml q 4 to 6 h	Alcohol free. Cherry flavor. In 118 ml.
otc	**Vicks Children's NyQuil Night-time Cold/Cough Liquid** (Richardson-Vicks)	10 mg pseudo-ephedrine HCl	0.67 mg chlor-pheniramine maleate	5 mg dextro-methorphan HBr	Sucrose	*6 to 11 yrs* – 15 ml q 6 h	Alcohol free. Cherry flavor. In 120 and 240 ml.
otc	**Vicks Pediatric Formula 44m Multi-Symptom Cough & Cold-Liquid** (Richardson-Vicks)				Sorbitol, sucrose		Alcohol free. In 120 ml.
otc	**Children's Tylenol Cold Plus Cough Chewable Tablets** (McNeil)	7.5 mg pseudo-ephedrine HCl	0.5 mg chlor-pheniramine maleate	2.5 mg dextro-methorphan HBr	80 mg aceta-minophen	*6 to 11 yrs* – 4 q 4 to 6 h	Cherry flavor. In 24s.
Rx	**Cardec DM Pediatric Syrup** (Schein)	60 mg pseudo–ephedrine HCl	4 mg carbinox-amine maleate	15 mg dextro-methorphan HBr	< 0.6% alco-hol, glucose, menthol, sucrose	2.5 to 5 ml qid	Grape flavor. In 473 ml.
Rx	**Sildec-DM Syrup** (Silarx)						In 473 ml.

Pediatric Antitussive Combinations

PEDIATRIC ANTITUSSIVE COMBINATIONS

	Product & Distributor	Decongestant	Antihistamine	Antitussive	Other	Average Dose	How Supplied
Rx	**Cardec DM Drops** (Various, eg, Barre-National, Goldline, Schein)	25 mg pseudo-ephedrine HCl per ml	2 mg carbinox-amine maleate per ml	4 mg dextro-methorphan HBr per ml	May contain alcohol	*1 to 18 mos* – 0.25 to 1 ml qid	In 30 ml.
Rx	**Carbodec DM Drops** (Rugby)				< 0.6% alcohol	0.25 to 1 ml qid	In 30 ml.
Rx	**Carbinoxamine Compound-Drops** (Pennex)				< 0.2% alco-hol, sugar, parabens	*1 to 18 mos* – 0.25 to 1 ml qid	Grape flavor. In 30 ml.
Rx	**Rondamine-DM Drops** (Major)						In 30 ml.
Rx	**Rondec-DM Drops** (Dura)				Menthol, sor-bitol		Grape flavor. In 30 ml w/dropper.
Rx *sf*	**Sildec-DM Pediatric Drops** (Silarx)						Alcohol free. In 30 ml w/calibrated dropper
Rx	**Tussafed Drops** (Everett)						In 30 ml.
otc	**Snaplets-Multi Granules** (Baker Cummins)	6.25 mg phenylpropa-nolamine HCl	1 mg chlorphenir-amine maleate	5 mg dextro-methorphan HBr		*6 to < 12 yrs* – 2 packs q 4 h	Taste free. In 30s.
otc	**Triaminicol Multi-Symptom Relief Colds with Coughs Liquid** (Sandoz)				Sorbitol, sucrose	*6 to < 12 yrs* - 10 ml q 4 h	Alcohol free. Cherry flavor. In 120 ml.
Rx	**Rentamine Pediatric Suspension** (Major)	5 mg phenylephrine tan-nate, 5 mg ephedrine tannate	4 mg chlorphenir-amine tannate	30 mg carbeta-pentane tannate		*2 to > 6 yrs* – 2.5 to 10 ml q 12 h	In pt.
Rx	**Rynatuss Pediatric Suspension** (Wallace)				Tartrazine, saccharin, sucrose, methyl-paraben	*2 to < 6 yrs* - 2.5 to 5 ml q 12 h *> 6 yrs* - 5 to 10 ml q 12 h	Strawberry-currant flavor. In 240 and 473 ml.
Rx	**Tri-Tannate Plus Pediatric Suspension** (Rugby)				Saccharin, sucrose	*2 to > 6 yrs* - 2.5 to 10 ml q 12 h	In 480 ml.

Expectorant Combinations, Capsules and Tablets

EXPECTORANT COMBINATIONS, CAPSULES AND TABLETS

Refer to the general discussion of these products in the Respiratory Combinations Introduction.

	Product & Distributor	Decongestant	Antihistamine	Expectorant	Average Adult Dose	How Supplied
Rx	**Duratuss Tablets** (Whitby)	120 mg pseudoephedrine HCl		600 mg guaifenesin	1 q 12 h	Dye-free. Long-acting. (Whitby 612). White, scored. Oval. Film coated. In 100s.
Rx	**Entex PSE Tablets** (Procter & Gamble)					Long-acting. Sugar. (Entex PSE NE). Yel-low, scored. In 100s.
Rx	**Guai-Vent/PSE Tablets** (Dura)					Sustained release. In 100s.
Rx	**Guaifenex PSE 120 Tablets** (Ethex)					(Ethex/208). Yellow. Extended release. In 100s.
Rx	**Guaimax-D Tablets** (Central)					Extended release. (Guaimax-D 131 2055). White to off-white, scored. In 100s.
Rx	**Ru-Tuss DE Tablets** (Boots)					Prolonged action. (90). Light blue, scored. Film coated. In 100s.
Rx	**Sudal 120/600** (Atley Pharm)					Sustained release. (SUDAL 120 A P). Film coated. Scored. Yellow, capsule shape. In 100s.
Rx	**Zephrex LA Tablets** (Bock)					Timed release. (Bock Z LA) Orange, scored. Oval. In 100s.

EXPECTORANT COMBINATIONS, CAPSULES AND TABLETS

	Product & Distributor	Decongestant	Antihistamine	Expectorant	Average Adult Dose	How Supplied
Rx	**GP-500 Tablets** (Marnel)	120 mg pseudoephedrine HCl		500 mg guaifenesin	1 bid	In 100s.
Rx	**Nasatab LATablets** (ECR Pharm)				1q 12 h	Long-acting. Dye free. (MX/225). White, scored. Film coated. In 100s.
Rx	**Stamoist E Tablets** (Huckaby)				1 bid	Prolonged action. Dye free. Scored. In 100s.
Rx	**Touro LA Caplet** (Dartmouth)					Long-acting. (DP). White, scored. In 100s.
Rx	**Tuss-LA Tablets** (Hyrex)					Sustained release. (LA/500). White, scored. Capsule shape. In 100s.
Rx	**V-Dec-M Tablets** (Seatrace)					Sustained release. (AM/PM). White, scored. In 12s and 100s.
Rx	**Anatuss LA Tablets** (Mayrand)	120 mg pseudoephedrine HCl		400 mg guaifenesin	1 p 12 h	Long-acting. (M/R). Off-white, scored. Oval. In 100s.
Rx	**Eudal-SR Tablets** (UAD)					Sustained release. (UAD/400). White, scored. In 100s.
Rx	**Histalet X Tablets** (Solvay)					Sugar. (Solvay 1050). White with green dots, scored. In 100s.
Rx	**Touro LA Caplets** (Dartmouth)					Long acting. (DP). In 100s.

EXPECTORANT COMBINATIONS, CAPSULES AND TABLETS

	Product & Distributor	Decongestant	Antihistamine	Expectorant	Average Adult Dose	How Supplied
Rx	**Congess SR. Capsules** (Fleming)	120 mg pseudoephedrine HCl		250 mg guaifenesin	1 q 12 h	Sustained release. Blue/clear. In 100s and 1000s.
Rx	**Guaifed Capsules** (Muro)					Timed release. Sucrose, parabens, EDTA. White/clear. In 100s and 500s.
Rx	**Guaivent Capsules** (Ethex)					Prolonged action. EDTA, parabens, sucrose. (Ethex/016). White/clear. In 100s and 500s.
Rx	**Respaire-120 Capsules** (Laser)				1 q 12 h	Extended release. (Laser 0169). Orange/clear. In 100s.
Rx	**Nasabid Capsules** (Abana)	90 mg pseudoephedrine HCl		250 mg guaifenesin	1 q 12 h	Prolonged action. Sucrose. (Abana 250). Yellow. In 100s.

EXPECTORANT COMBINATIONS, CAPSULES AND TABLETS

	Product & Distributor	Decongestant	Antihistamine	Expectorant	Average Adult Dose	How Supplied
Rx	**Deconsal II Tablets** (Adams)	60 mg pseudoephedrine HCl		600 mg guaifenesin	1 or 2 q 12 h	Sustained release. (Adams/017). Dark blue, scored. In 100s and 500s.
Rx	**Defen-LA Tablets** (Horizon)					Sustained release. (Defen-LA). Dark blue-green, scored. In 100s.
Rx	**Guaifenex PSE 60 Tablets** (Ethex)					Extended release. Lactose. Blue, scored. Capsule shape. In 100s.
Rx	**Iosal II Tablets** (Iomed)					Extended release. In 100s.
Rx	**MED-RxTablets** (Iomed)				14-day regimen of 56 tablets	(ID 122). Lt. blue, scored. In 28s.
Rx	**Respa-1st Tablets** (Respa)				1 bid	Sustained release. In 100s.
Rx	**Syn-Rx Tablets** (Adams)				Pseudoephedrine/guaifenesin tablets: 1 or 2 in morning	Controlled release. Dk. blue. In 28s.
					Guaifenesin-only tablets: 1 or 2, 12 hours after a.m. tablet(s)	Lt. green. In 28s. 14-day treatment regimen of 56 tablets (28 pseudoephedrine/guaifenesin tabs, 28 guaifenesin-only tabs).
Rx	**Sudal 60/500** (Atley Pharm)	60 mg pseudoephedrine HCl		500 mg guaifenesin		Timed release. (SUDAL 60 A P). Film coated. Scored. White, capsule shape. In 100s.

Expectorant Combinations, Capsules and Tablets

EXPECTORANT COMBINATIONS, CAPSULES AND TABLETS

	Product & Distributor	Decongestant	Antihistamine	Expectorant	Average Adult Dose	How Supplied
otc	**Congestac Caplets** (Menley & James)	60 mg pseudoephedrine HCl		400 mg guaifenesin	1 q 4 h up to 4/day	(C). In 24s.
otc	**Guaitab Tablets** (Muro)				1 q 4 to 6 h up to 4/day	Lactose. (Muro 60/400). Purple, layered. Scored. In 100s.
Rx	**Zephrex Tablets** (Bock)				1 q 6 h	(Bock 460). Blue, scored. Oval. Film coated. In 100s.
Rx	**Guaifed-PD Capsules** (Muro)	60 mg pseudoephedrine HCl		300 mg guaifenesin	1 or 2 q 12 h	Prolonged action. Sucrose, parabens, EDTA. (Guaifed-PD Muro 60-300). Blue/clear. In 100s & 500s.
Rx	**Guiavent PD Capsules**(Ethex)					Parabens, sucrose. (Ehtex/015). In 100s, 500s.
Rx	**Sinufed Timecelles (Capsules)** (Roberts/Hauck)					Prolonged action. Green/clear. In 100s.
Rx	**Versacaps Capsules** (Seatrace)					Prolonged action. EDTA, parabens, sucrose. In 100s.
Rx	**Respaire-60 Capsules** (Laser)	60 mg pseudoephedrine HCl		200 mg guaifenesin	2 q 12 h	Extended release. (Laser 0174). Green/clear. In 100s.
Rx	**Congess JR. Capsules** (Fleming)	60 mg pseudoephedrine HCl		125 mg guaifenesin	2 q 12 h	Blue/clear. In 100s and 1000s.
otc	**Robitussin Severe Congestion Liqui-Gels** (Robins)	30 mg pseudoephedrine HCl		200 mg guaifenesin	2 q 4 h up to 8/day	Sorbitol. In 24s.
otc	**Sinutab Non-Drying Capsules** (Glaxo Wellcome)					In 24s.
Rx	**Rymed Capsules** (Edwards)	30 mg pseudoephedrine HCl		250 mg guaifenesin	1 qid	Lactose. (Rymed). Maroon/clear. In 100s.

EXPECTORANT COMBINATIONS, CAPSULES AND TABLETS

	Product & Distributor	Decongestant	Antihistamine	Expectorant	Average Adult Dose	How Supplied
otc	**Glycofed Tablets** (Pal-Pak)	30 mg pseudoephedrine HCl		100 mg guaifenesin	1 or 2 qid	White, scored. In 1000s.
otc	**Bronkaid Dual Action Caplets** (Sterling Health)	25 mg ephedrine HCl		400 mg guaifenesin	1 q 4 h	In 24s.
otc	**Dynafed Asthma Relief Tablets** (BDI[1])	25 mg ephedrine HCl		200 mg guaifenesin	½ to 1 q 4 h	In 60s.
otc	**Mini Thin Asthma Relief Tablets** (BDI Pharm)					In 60s.
otc	**Mini Thin Asthma Relief Tablets** (BDI Pharm)	25 mg ephedrine HCl		100 mg guaifenesin	½ to 1 q 4 h	In 100s.
Rx	**Broncholate Softgels (Capsules)** (Bock)	12.5 mg ephedrine HCl		200 mg guaifenesin	1 or 2 q 4 h	Sorbitol, parabens. In 100s.
Rx	**Liquibid-DTablets** (ION)	40 mg phenylephrine HCl		600 mg guaifenesin		In 100s.
Rx	**Sinupan Capsules** (ION Labs)			200 mg guaifenesin	1 q 12 h	Controlled release. In 100s
Rx	**Endal Tablets** (UAD)	20 mg phenylephrine HCl		300 mg guaifenesin	1 or 2 q 12 h	Timed release. (UAD 204). White. In 100s.
Rx	**Deconsal Sprinkle Capsules** (Adams)	10 mg phenylephrine HCl		300 mg guaifenesin	3 q 12 h	Sustained release. (Adams/019). Blue/clear. In 100s.

EXPECTORANT COMBINATIONS, CAPSULES AND TABLETS

	Product & Distributor	Decongestant	Antihistamine	Expectorant	Average Adult Dose	How Supplied
Rx	**Coldloc-LA Caplets** (Flemming)	75 mg phenylpropanolamine HCl		600 mg guaifenesin	1 q 12 h	Sustained release. (FP/675). White, scored. In 50s and 100s.
Rx	**Dura-Vent Tablets** (Dura)					Prolonged effect. (Dura 7.5/7.5). White, scored. In 100s and 600s.
Rx	**Guaifenex PPA 75 Tablets** (Ethex)					Extended release. Lactose. (Imprex/204). White. Capsule shape. In 100s.
Rx	**Profen LA Tablets** (Wakefield)					Timed release. Dye free. In 100s.
Rx	**SINUvent Tablets** (WE Pharm.)					Long-acting. (WE 01). White, scored. In 100s and 600s.

EXPECTORANT COMBINATIONS, CAPSULES AND TABLETS

	Product & Distributor	Decongestant	Antihistamine	Expectorant	Average Adult Dose	How Supplied
Rx	**Phenylpropanolamine HCl and Guaifenesin Tablets** (Various, eg, Duramed, Schein, Sidmak)	75 mg phenylpropanolamine HCl		400 mg guaifenesin	1 q 12 h	Long-acting. In 100s and 500s.
Rx	**Ami-Tex LA Tablets** (Amide)					Long-acting. In 100s, 500s, 1000s.
Rx	**Entex LA Tablets** (Procter & Gamble)					Sugar. Long-acting. (Entex LA 0149 0436). In 100s and 500s.
Rx	**Guaipax Tabs** (Eon Labs)					Long-acting. In 100s, 500s, 1000s.
Rx	**Exgest LA Tablets** (Carnrick)					Long-acting. (8673 C). White/blue speckled, scored. Oval. In 100s and 500s.
Rx	**Partuss LA Tablets** (Parmed)					Long-acting. In 100s and 500s.
Rx	**Phenylfenesin L.A. Tablets** (Goldline)					Extended release. In 100s.
Rx	**Rymed-TR Caplets** (Edwards)					Long-acting. In 100s.
Rx	**Stamoist LA Tabs** (Huckaby)					Prolonged action. Scored. In 100s.
Rx	**ULR-LA Tablets** (Geneva)					Long-acting. (GG 224). In 100s.

EXPECTORANT COMBINATIONS, CAPSULES AND TABLETS

	Product & Distributor	Decongestant	Antihistamine	Expectorant	Average Adult Dose	How Supplied
Rx	**Dura-Gest Caps** (Dura)	45 mg phenylpropanolamine HCl, 5 mg phenylephrine HCl		200 mg guaifenesin	1 qid (q 6 h)	(Dura-Gest 51479005). In 100s and 500s.
Rx	**Enomine Capsules** (Major)					In 100s and 500s.
Rx	**Entex Capsules** (P & G)					(Entex 0149 0412). In 100s & 500s.
Rx	**NorelCapsules** (US Pharmaceutical)					(US/Norel). Tan/gold. In 100s.
Rx	**Profen II Tablets** (Wakefield)	37.5 mg phenylpropanolamine HCl		600 mg guaifenesin	2 q 12 h	Dye free. In 100s.
otc	**Vicks DayQuil Sinus Pressure & Congestion Relief Caplets** (Procter & Gamble)	25 mg phenylpropanolamine HCl		200 mg guaifenesin	1 q 4 h	(DQ SC). In 12s and 24s.

[1] BDI Pharmaceuticals, Inc., P.O. Box 78610, Indianapolis, IN 46278–0610; (800) 428–2352.

EXPECTORANT COMBINATIONS, LIQUIDS

Refer to the general discussion of these products in the Respiratory Combinations Introduction. Content given per 5 ml.

	Product & Distributor	Decongestant	Antihistamine	Expectorant	Other	Average Adult Dose	How Supplied
Rx	**Broncholate Syrup** (Bock)	6.25 mg ephedrine HCl		100 mg guaifenesin	Saccharin, sucrose	10 to 20 ml q 4 h	In 120 and 480 ml.
Rx	**KIE Syrup** (Laser)	8 mg ephedrine HCl		150 mg potassium iodide		10 to 15 ml q 4 to 6 h	Cherry flavor. In pt and gal.
Rx	**Norisodrine w/Calcium Iodide Syrup** (Abbott)			150 mg anhydrous calcium iodide	3 mg isoproterenol sulfate, 6% alcohol, glucose, sucrose	5 to 10 ml q 4 to 6 h	In 480 ml.
Rx	**Histalet X Syrup** (Solvay)	45 mg pseudoephedrine HCl		200 mg guaifenesin	15% alcohol, fructose, saccharin, sorbitol, sucrose, menthol, methylparaben	10 ml qid	In 473 ml.
otc sf	**Guaifed Syrup** (Muro)	30 mg pseudoephedrine HCl		200 mg guaifenesin	Saccharin, sorbitol, menthol	10 ml q 4 to 6 h up to 40 ml/day	Berry citrus flavor. In 118 and 473 ml.

EXPECTORANT COMBINATIONS, LIQUIDS

	Product & Distributor	Decongestant	Antihistamine	Expectorant	Other	Average Adult Dose	How Supplied
otc	**GuiaCough PE Liquid** (Schein)	30 mg pseudoephedrine HCl		100 mg guaifenesin	1.4% alcohol, corn syrup, methylparaben, saccharin	10 ml q 4 h up to 40 ml/day	In 118 ml.
otc	**Guiatuss PE Syrup** (Barre-National)				1.4% alcohol		In 118 ml.
otc	**Robitussin PE Syrup** (Robins)				1.4% alcohol, high fructose corn syrup, glucose, saccharin		In 120 and 240 ml.
otc	**Rymed Liquid** (Edwards)				1.4% alcohol	10 ml q 4 h	In 480 ml.
otc *sf*	**Fedahist Expectorant Syrup** (Schwarz Pharma KU)	20 mg pseudoephedrine HCl		200 mg guaifenesin	Sorbitol	10 ml q 4 to 6 h	Alcohol free. In 120 ml.

EXPECTORANT COMBINATIONS, LIQUIDS

	Product & Distributor	Decongestant	Antihistamine	Expectorant	Other	Average Adult Dose	How Supplied
otc	**Conex Syrup** (Forest)	12.5 mg phenylpropanolamine HCl		100 mg guaifenesin	0.13% methylparaben, 0.03% propylparaben	5 to 10 ml q 4 h up to 50 ml/day	In 118 ml.
otc	**Genamin Expectorant Liquid** (Goldline)				5% alcohol	10 ml q 4 h	In 120 ml.
otc	**Myminic Expectorant Liquid** (Pennex)				5% alcohol		Fruit punch flavor. In 120 & 240 ml, pt, gal.
otc	**Silaminic Expectorant Liquid** (Silarx)				5% alcohol		In 118 ml.
otc	**Threamine Expectorant Liquid** (Barre-National)				5% alcohol. EDTA, parabens, saccharin, sucrose, sorbitol		Orange spice flavor. In 473 ml.
otc	**Triphenyl Expectorant Liquid** (Rugby)				5% alcohol, saccharin, sorbitol, sucrose		In 118 ml.
otc	**Genamin Expectorant Liquid** (Goldline)	6.25 mg phenylpropanolamine HCl		50 mg guaifenesin	Alcohol free.	20 ml q 4 h	In 118 ml.
otc	**Triaminic Expectorant Liquid** (Sandoz)				EDTA, sorbitol, sucrose		Alcohol free. Citrus flavor. In 120 & 240 ml.

EXPECTORANT COMBINATIONS, LIQUIDS

	Product & Distributor	Decongestant	Antihistamine	Expectorant	Other	Average Adult Dose	How Supplied
Rx	**ColdlocElixir** (Flemming)	20 mg phenylpropanolamine HCl, 5 mg phenylephrine HCl		100 mg guaifenesin	Sorbitol	10 ml q 6 h	Alcohol and dye free. In pt.
Rx	**ContussLiquid** (Parmed)				5% alcohol, saccharin, sorbitol, sucrose	10 ml qid	In 480 ml.
Rx	**Entex Liquid** (Procter & Gamble)					10 ml q 6 h	In 480 ml.
otc	**Guaifenex Liquid** (Ethex)				Parabens, sorbitol		In 118 and 473 ml.
otc	**Sil-TexLiquid** (Silarx)				5% alcohol, saccharin, sorbitol, sucrose	10 ml qid	In 473 ml.
Rx	**Bronkotuss Expectorant Liquid** (Hyrex)	8.2 mg ephedrine sulfate	4 mg chlorpheniramine maleate	100 mg guaifenesin, 1.67 ml hydriodic acid syrup	5% alcohol, dextrose, saccharin, parabens, sucrose	5 ml q 3 to 4 h	Licorice flavor. In pt and gal.
otc	**Rescon-GG Liquid** (Ion)	5 mg phenylephrine HCl		100 mg guaifenesin		10 ml q 4 to 6 h	In 120 ml.
Rx	**Polaramine Expectorant Liquid** (Schering)	20 mg pseudoephedrine sulfate	2 mg dexchlorpheniramine maleate	100 mg guaifenesin	7.2% alcohol, menthol, sorbitol, sugar	5 to 10 ml tid or qid	In 473 ml.

PEDIATRIC EXPECTORANT COMBINATIONS

Refer to the general discussion of these products in the Respiratory Combinations Introduction..

Content given per 5 ml liquid, 1 ml drops or pack.

	Product & Distributor	Decongestant	Antihistamine	Expectorant	Other	Average Dose	How Supplied
otc *sf*	**Naldecon EX Children's Syrup** (Apothecon)	6.25 mg phenylpropanolamine HCl		100 mg guaifenesin	Saccharin, sorbitol	*6 to < 12 yrs* - 10 ml q 4 h *2 to < 6 yrs* - 5 ml q 4 h	Alcohol free. Fruit flavor. In 118 and 480 ml.
otc *sf*	**Pediacon EX Pediatric Drops** (Goldline)	6.25 mg phenylpropanolamine HCl		50 mg guaifenesin		*2 to < 6 yrs* - 1 ml q 4 h	In 30 ml.
otc	**Snaplets-EX Granules** (Baker Cummins)					*6 to < 12 yrs* - 2 packs q 4 h *2 to < 6 yrs* - 1 pack q 4 h	Taste free. In 30s.
otc *sf*	**Naldecon EX Pediatric Drops** (Apothecon)	6.25 mg phenylpropanolamine HCl per ml		50 mg guaifenesin per ml	Saccharin, sorbitol	*2 to < 6 yrs* - 1 ml q 4 h	Alcohol free. Vanilla-raspberry-cherry flavor. In 30 ml with dropper.
otc	**Sildicon-E Pediatric Drops** (Silarx)	6.25 mg phenylpropanolamine HCl		30 mg guaifenesin	0.6% alcohol	*2 to < 6 yrs* - 1 ml q 4 h	In 30 ml.
Rx	**Donatussin Drops** (Laser)	2 mg phenylephrine HCl per ml	1 mg chlorpheniramine maleate per ml	20 mg guaifenesin per ml		*< 3 mos* - 2 to 3 drops per month of age q 4 to 6 h *3 to 6 mos* - 0.3 to 0.6 ml q 4 to 6 h *6 mos to 1 yr* - 0.6 to 1 ml q 4 to 6 h *1 to 2 yrs* - 1 to 2 ml q 4 to 6 h	Peach flavor. In 30 ml with dropper.

PEDIATRIC EXPECTORANT COMBINATIONS

	Product & Distributor	Decongestant	Antihistamine	Expectorant	Other	Average Dose	How Supplied
Rx	**Guiavent PD Capsules** (Ethex)	60 mg pseudoephedrine HCl		300 mg guaifenesin	parabens, sucrose	*6 to 12 years* - 1 q 12 h	(Ethex/015). Blue/clear. In 100s and 500s.
otc	**Fedahist Expectorant Pediatric Drops** (Schwarz Pharma KU)	7.5 mg pseudoephedrine HCl		40 mg guaifenesin	Saccharin, sorbitol		In 30 ml w/dropper.

NARCOTIC ANTITUSSIVES WITH EXPECTORANTS

Refer to the general discussion of these products in the Respiratory Combinations Introduction. Content given per 5 ml.

	Product & Distributor	Antitussive	Expectorant	Other	Average Adult Dose	How Supplied
c-III	**Brontex Tablets** (Procter & Gamble)	10 mg codeine phosphate	300 mg guaifenesin		1 q 4 h	(Brontex). Red. Capsule shape. In 100s.
c-III	**Codeine Phosphate and Guaifenesin Tablets** (Goldline)					In 100s.
c-v	**Guaifenesin and Codeine Phosphate Syrup** (Schein)	10 mg codeine phosphate	100 mg guaifenesin	3.5% alcohol	10 ml q 4 h	Fruit-mint flavor. In 120 ml, pt and gal.
c-v	**Cheracol Cough Syrup** (Roberts)			4.75% alcohol, fructose, sucrose	10 ml q 4 to 6 h	In 60, 120 and 480 ml.
c-v	**Guiatuss AC Syrup** (Various, eg, Barre-National, Goldline, Harber, Mason, Moore)			Alcohol	10 ml q 4 h	In 120 ml, pt and gal.
c-v	**Guiatussin w/Codeine Expectorant Liquid** (Rugby)			3.5% alcohol		In 120 ml, pt and gal.
c-v	**Mytussin AC Cough Syrup** (Pennex)			3.5% alcohol		Fruit flavor. In 120 ml, pt and gal.
c-v	**Robafen AC Cough Syrup** (Major)			3.5% alcohol, sugar, menthol, parabens, sorbitol	5 to 10 ml q 4 to 6 h	In 120 ml, pt and gal.
c-v *sf*	**Robitussin A-C Syrup** (Robins)			3.5% alcohol, saccharin, sorbitol	10 ml q 4 h	In 60 and 120 ml, pt and gal.
c-v	**Tussi-Organidin NR Liquid** (Wallace)			Saccharin, sorbitol.		Raspberry flavor. In pt and gal. "NR" means "Newly Reformulated"
c-v	**Tussi-Organidin-S NR Liquid** (Wallace)					In 30 ml sample or 120 ml unit-of-use container w/10 ml oral syringe. "NR" means "Newly Reformulated"

NARCOTIC ANTITUSSIVES WITH EXPECTORANTS

	Product & Distributor	Antitussive	Expectorant	Other	Average Adult Dose	How Supplied
c-v	**Brontex Liquid** (Procter & Gamble)	2.5 mg codeine phosphate	75 mg guaifenesin	Methylparaben, saccharin, sucrose	20 ml q 4 h	Alcohol free. In 473 ml.
c-v	**Iophen-C Liquid** (Various, eg, Barre-National, Major, Rugby, Schein, URL)	10 mg codeine phosphate	30 mg iodinated glycerol		5 to 10 ml q 4 h	In pt and gal.
c-v	**Iodinated Glycerol and Codeine Phosphate Liquid**(Various, eg, Goldline, Roxane)					In 480 and 500 ml and UD 5 and 10 ml.
c-v	**Calcidrine Syrup** (Abbott)	8.4 mg codeine	152 mg calcium iodide anhydrous	6% alcohol, glucose, sucrose	5 to 10 ml q 4 h	In 480 ml.
c-iii	**Entuss Expectorant Tablets** (Roberts/Hauck)	5 mg hydrocodone bitartrate	300 mg guaifenesin	Lactose	1 to 1.5 qid	(RPC 141). Orange, scored. In 100s.

Narcotic Antitussives with Expectorants

NARCOTIC ANTITUSSIVES WITH EXPECTORANTS

	Product & Distributor	Antitussive	Expectorant	Other	Average Adult Dose	How Supplied
C-III	**Atuss EX** (Atley)	5 mg hydrocodone bitartrate	100 mg guaifenesin	—	5 ml q 4 h pc & hs	
C-III sf	**Codiclear DH Syrup** (Central)					Alcohol and dye free. In 120 and 480 ml.
C-III	**Co-Tuss V Liquid** (Rugby)					In 480 ml.
C-III sf	**HycoClear TussSyrup** (Ethex)					Alcohol and dye free. Fruit flavor. In 118 and 473 ml.
C-III sf	**Hydrocodone GF Syrup** (Morton Grove)					Alcohol and dye free. In 473 ml.
C-III sf	**Pneumotussin HC Syrup** (ECR Pharm)					Alcohol free. Cherry flavor. In 480 ml.
C-III	**Hycotuss Expectorant Syrup** (Du Pont)			10% alcohol, saccharin, sorbitol, sugar, parabens		Butterscotch flavor. In 480 ml.
C-III sf	**Kwelcof Liquid** (Ascher)			Menthol, saccharin, sorbitol		Alcohol and dye free. Fruit flavor. In 480 ml.
C-III sf	**Vicodin Tuss Syrup** (Knoll)			Menthol, saccharin, sorbitol, parabens		Alcohol and dye free. Cherry flavor. In 480 ml.
C-III	**Entuss Expectorant Liquid** (Roberts/Hauck)	5 mg hydrocodone bitartrate	300 mg potassium guaiacolsulfonate	Saccharin, sorbitol	5 to 7.5 ml qid	Alcohol free. Apricot flavor. In 120 and 480 ml.
C-III sf	**Protuss Liquid** (Horizon)					Alcohol free. Grape flavor. In 20, 120 and 480 ml.
C-III	**Marcof Expectorant Syrup** (Marnel)			—		In 480 ml.
C-II	**Dilaudid Cough Syrup** (Knoll)	1 mg hydromorphone HCl	100 mg guaifenesin	5% alcohol, tartrazine	5 ml q 3 to 4 h	Peach flavor. In 480 ml.

Pediatric Narcotic Antitussives with Expectorants Combinations

PEDIATRIC NARCOTIC ANTITUSSIVES WITH EXPECTORANTS COMBINATIONS

Refer to the general discussion of these products beginning in the Respiratory Combinations Introduction.

Content given per 5 ml.

	Product & Distributor	Decongestant	Antihistamine	Antitussive	Expectorant	Average Dose and Other	How Supplied
c-v	**Nucofed Pediatric Expectorant Syrup** (Roberts)	30 mg pseudoephedrine HCl		10 mg codeine phosphate	100 mg guaifenesin	6% alcohol, EDTA, saccharin, sucrose. *2 to < 12 yrs* - 2.5 to 5 ml q 6 h	Strawberry flavor. In 473 ml.
c-v	**Nucotuss Pediatric Expectorant Syrup** (Barre-National)					6% alcohol. *2 to < 12 yrs* - 2.5 to 5 ml q 6 h	Strawberry flavor. In 473 ml.
c-v	**Pediacof Syrup** (Sanofi Winthrop)	2.5 mg phenylephrine HCl	0.75 mg chlorpheniramine maleate	5 mg codeine phosphate	75 mg potassium iodide	0.2% sodium benzoate, 5% alcohol, glucose, saccharin. *6 mos to 12 yrs* - 1.25 to 10 ml q 4 to 6 h	Raspberry flavor. In 480 ml.
c-v	**Pedituss Cough Syrup** (Major)					*6 mos to 12 yrs* - 1.25 to 10 ml q 4 to 6 h	In pt and gal.

NONNARCOTIC ANTITUSSIVES WITH EXPECTORANTS

Refer to the general discussion of these products in the Respiratory Combinations Introduction.

Content given per tablet or 5 ml.

	Product & Distributor	Antitussive	Expectorant	Other	Average Adult Dose	How Supplied
Rx	**Fenesin DM Tablets** (Dura)	30 mg dextromethorphan HBr	600 mg guaifenesin		1 or 2 q 12 h	In 100s.
Rx	**Guaifenex DM Tablets** (Ethex)					Extended release. (Ethex/213). Green, scored. In 100s, 500s and 1000s.
Rx	**Humibid DM Tablets** (Adams)					Sustained release. (Adams/030). Dark green, scored. In 100s.
Rx	**Iobid DM Tablets** (Iomed)					Sustained release. Dark green, scored. In 100s and 500s.
Rx	**Monafed DM Tablets** (Monarch Pharmaceuticals)					Sustained release. (KPI 14). Green, scored. In 100s
Rx	**Muco-Fen-DM Tablets** (Wakefield Pharm)					Timed release. Dye free. Scored. In 100s.
Rx	**Respa-DM Tablets** (Respa)					Sustained release. In 100s.
Rx	**Humibid DM Sprinkle Capsules** (Adams)	15 mg dextromethorphan HBr	300 mg guaifenesin		2 to 4 q 12 h	Sustained release. (Adams/034). Dark green/clear. In 100s.
otc sf	**Scot-Tussin Senior ClearLiquid** (Roberts Med)	15 mg dextromethorphan HBr	200 mg guaifenesin		5 ml q 4 h	Parabens, phenylalanine, menthol, aspartame. Alcohol free. In 118.3 ml.
otc	**Synacol CFTablets** (Roberts Med)				2 q 6 to 8 h	In UD 8s and 500s.

NONNARCOTIC ANTITUSSIVES WITH EXPECTORANTS

	Product & Distributor	Antitussive	Expectorant	Other	Average Adult Dose	How Supplied
otc *sf*	**Clear Tussin 30 Liquid** (Goldline)	15 mg dextromethorphan HBr	100 mg guaifenesin		10 ml q 6 h	Alcohol and dye free. Mint flavor. In 118 ml.
otc	**Guiatussin with Dextromethorphan Liquid** (Rugby)			1.4% alcohol	10 ml q 6 to 8 h	In 480 ml.
otc	**Rhinosyn-DMX Syrup** (Great Southern)				10 ml q 6 h	In 120 ml.
otc *sf*	**Safe Tussin 30 Liquid** (Kramer)					Alcohol and dye free. In 120 ml.
otc	**Tusibron-DM Syrup** (Kenwood/Bradley)				10 ml q 6 to 8 h	In 118 ml.
otc *sf*	**Naldecon Senior DX Liquid** (Apothecon)	10 mg dextromethorphan HBr	200 mg guaifenesin	Saccharin, sorbitol	10 ml q 4 h	Alcohol free. In 118 and 480 ml.
otc	**Phenadex Senior Liquid** (Barre-National)					In 118 ml.
otc	**Tuss-DM Tablets** (Hyrex)				1 or 2 q 4 h	In 100s, 1000s and UD 50s.
otc	**Kolephrin GG/DM Liquid** (Pfeiffer)	10 mg dextromethorphan HBr	150 mg guaifenesin	Glucose, saccharin, sucrose	10 ml q 4 h	Alcohol free. Cherry flavor. In 120 ml.

NONNARCOTIC ANTITUSSIVES WITH EXPECTORANTS

	Product & Distributor	Antitussive	Expectorant	Other	Average Adult Dose	How Supplied
otc	**Cheracol D Cough Liquid** (Roberts)	10 mg dextromethorphan HBr	100 mg guaifenesin	4.75% alcohol, fructose, sucrose	10 ml q 4 h	Cherry flavor. In 120 and 180 ml.
otc *sf*	**Diabetic Tussin DM** (Roberts[1])			Saccharin, methylparaben, menthol		Alcohol and dye free. In 118 ml.
otc	**Extra Action Cough Syrup** (Rugby)			1.4% alcohol, corn syrup, saccharin, sucrose	10 ml q 6 to 8 h	In 120 ml, pt and gal.
otc	**Genatuss DM Syrup** (Goldline)			Sucrose	10 ml q 4 h	Alcohol free. Cherry flavor. In 120 ml.
otc	**Guiatuss-DM Liquid** (Various, eg, Barre-National, Goldline, Mason)					In 120 and 240 ml, pt and gal.
otc	**Glycotuss-dM Tablets** (Pal-Pak)				1 to 2 q 4 h	Yellow. In 100s and 1000s.
otc	**Halotussin-DM Liquid** (Halsey)			Corn syrup, menthol, saccharin, sucrose, parabens	10 ml q 6 to 8 h	Alcohol free. In 120, 240 and 480 ml and gal.
otc *sf*	**Halotussin-DM Sugar Free Liquid** (Halsey)			Saccharin, sorbitol, parabens		Alcohol free. In 120, 240 and 480 ml and gal.
otc	**Mytussin DM Liquid** (Pennex)			1.6% alcohol	10 ml q 4 h	Cherry flavor. In 120 ml, pt and gal.

Nonnarcotic Antitussives with Expectorants

NONNARCOTIC ANTITUSSIVES WITH EXPECTORANTS

	Product & Distributor	Antitussive	Expectorant	Other	Average Adult Dose	How Supplied
otc	**Robafen DM Syrup** (Major)	10 mg dextromethorphan HBr	100 mg guaifenesin	1.4% alcohol, sugar, menthol, sorbitol, parabens	5 to 10 ml q 4 h	In 473 ml.
otc	**Robitussin-DM Liquid** (Robins)			Saccharin, glucose, high fructose corn syrup	10 ml q 4 h	In 120, 240 and 360 ml, pt and gal.
otc	**Siltussin DM Syrup** (Silarx)			Saccharin, sucrose		Alcohol free. In 118 ml.
otc sf	**Tolu-Sed DM Syrup** (Scherer)			10% alcohol	10 ml q 4 h	In 120 ml.
otc	**Tussi-Organidin DM NR Liquid** (Wallace)			Saccharin, sorbitol.		In pt and gal. "NR" means "Newly Reformulated."
otc	**Tussi-Organidin-S DM NR Liquid** (Wallace)					In 30 ml sample or 120 ml unit-of-use container w/ oral syringe. "NR" means "Newly Reformulated."
otc	**Uni-tussin DM Syrup** (URL)			Saccharin, sucrose, methylparaben		Alcohol free. In 118 ml.
otc sf	**Phanatuss Cough Syrup** (Pharmakon Labs)	10 mg dextromethorphan HBr	85 mg glyceryl guaiacolate	Menthol, saccharin, sorbitol, parabens	10 ml q 3 to 4 h	Alcohol free. In 118 and 236 ml.

NONNARCOTIC ANTITUSSIVES WITH EXPECTORANTS

	Product & Distributor	Antitussive	Expectorant	Other	Average Adult Dose	How Supplied
Rx	**Iophen DM Liquid** (Various, eg, Barre-National, Major, Moore, Rugby, Schein)	10 mg dextromethorphan HBr	30 mg iodinated glycerol		5 to 10 ml q 4 h	In 120 ml, pt and gal.
Rx	**Iodinated Glycerol and Dextromethorphan/DM Liquid** (Various, eg, Roxane)					In 500 ml, UD 5 and 10 ml.
Rx sf	**Tusso-DM Liquid** (Everett)					Alcohol free. In 473 ml.
otc	**Vicks 44E Liquid** (Richardson-Vicks)	6.7 mg dextromethorphan HBr	66.7 mg guaifenesin			In 118 and 236 ml.
otc	**Benylin Expectorant Liquid** (Glaxo Wellcome)	5 mg dextromethorphan HBr	100 mg guaifenesin	Saccharin, menthol, sucrose	10 to 20 ml q 4 h	Alcohol free. In 118 and 236 ml.

[1] Health Care Products, 369 Bayview Ave., Amityville, NY 11701; (516) 789–8455.

Pediatric Nonnarcotic Antitussives with Expectorants

PEDIATRIC NONNARCOTIC ANTITUSSIVES WITH EXPECTORANTS

Refer to the general discussion of these products in the Respiratory Combinations Introduction. Content given per 5 ml liquid.

	Product & Distributor	Antitussive	Expectorant	Other	Average Dose	How Supplied
otc	**Children's Formula Cough Syrup** (Pharmakon)	5 mg dextromethorphan HBr	50 mg guaifenesin	Sucrose, corn syrup	*2 to < 12 yrs* – 5 to 10 ml q 6 h	Alcohol free. Grape flavor. In 118 and 236 ml.
otc	**Vicks Pediatric Formula 44E Liquid** (Richardson-Vicks)	3.3 mg dextromethorphan HBr	33.3 mg guaifenesin	Sorbitol, sucrose	*2 to 11 yrs* – 7.5 to 15 ml q 4 h	Alcohol free. In 120 ml with dose cup.

ANTITUSSIVE AND EXPECTORANT COMBINATIONS

Refer to the general discussion of these products in the Respiratory Combinations Introduction. Content given per tablet or 5 ml.

	Product & Distributor	Decongestant	Antitussive	Antihistamine	Expectorant	Adult Dose and Other	How Supplied
c-III	**Atuss-G** (Atley)	10 mg phenylephrine HCl	2 mg hydrocodone bitartrate		100 mg guaifenesin	Sucrose.	Grape flavor. In 480 ml.
c-III	**Donatussin DC Syrup** (Laser)	7.5 mg phenylephrine HCl	2.5 mg hydrocodone bitartrate		50 mg guaifenesin	10 ml q 4 to 6 h	Alcohol free. In 120 and 480 ml.
c-III	**Atuss HD** (Atley)	5 mg phenylephrine HCl	2.5 mg hydrocodone bitartrate	2 mg chlorpheniramine maleate			Alcohol. Cherry flavor. In 480 ml bottles.
Rx	**Atuss DM** (Atley)		15 mg dextromethorphan Hbr	2 mg chlorpheniramine maleate			Sucrose, saccharin. In 480 ml bottles.
c-III	**Deconamine CX Liquid** (Bradley)	60 mg pseudoephedrine HCl	5 mg hydrocodone bitartrate		200 mg guaifenesin	5 ml qid.	In 480 ml.
c-III	**Detussin Expectorant Liquid** (Various, eg, Barre-National, Major, Qualitest, Schein)					5 ml qid. Alcohol	In pt and gal.
c-III	**Cophene XP Liquid** (Dunhall)					5 ml qid. 12.5% alcohol	Fruit flavor. In pt and gal.
c-III	**SRC Expectorant Liquid** (Edwards)					5 ml q 4 to 6 h up to 20 ml/day.	Butterscotch flavor. In 480 ml.
c-III	**Tussafin Expectorant Liquid** (Rugby)					12.5% alcohol, glucose, sorbitol, sucrose, parabens	In 480 ml.

Antitussive and Expectorant Combinations

ANTITUSSIVE AND EXPECTORANT COMBINATIONS

	Product & Distributor	Decongestant	Antitussive	Antihistamine	Expectorant	Adult Dose and Other	How Supplied
c-iii	**Deconamine CX Tablets** (Bradley)	30 mg pseudo-ephedrine HCl	5 mg hydrocodone bitartrate		300 mg guaifenesin	1 to 1.5 up to qid	In 100s.
c-iii	**Entuss-D Tablets** (Roberts/Hauck)						Dye free. In 100s.
c-iii *sf*	**Protuss-D Liquid** (Horizon)	30 mg pseudo-ephedrine HCl	5 mg hydrocodone bitartrate		300 mg potassium guaiacolsulfonate	5 to 7.5 ml q 6 h	Alcohol and dye free. In 120 and 480 ml.
c-iii	**Duratuss HD Elixir** (Whitby)	30 mg pseudo-ephedrine HCl	2.5 mg hydrocodone bitartrate		100 mg guaifenesin	10 ml q 4 to 6 h up to 40 ml/day. 5% alcohol, parabens, glucose, saccharin, sorbitol, sucrose	Fruit-punch flavor. In 473 ml.
c-iii	**Vanex Expectorant Liquid** (Abana)					10 ml q 4 to 6 h. 5% alcohol	In 473 ml.
c-iii	**TussendSyrup** (Monarch)			2 mg chlorphenir-amine maleate		5% alcohol	Banana flavor. In 480 ml.
c-iii	**Nucofed Expectorant Syrup** (Roberts/Hauck)	60 mg pseudo-ephedrine HCl	20 mg codeine phosphate		200 mg guaifenesin	5 ml q 6 h. 12.5% alcohol, saccharin, sucrose	Wintergreen flavor. In 480 ml.
c-iii	**Nucotuss Expectorant Syrup** (Barre-National)					5 ml q 6 h. 12.5% alcohol	Wintergreen flavor. In 473 ml.

ANTITUSSIVE AND EXPECTORANT COMBINATIONS

	Product & Distributor	Decongestant	Antitussive	Antihistamine	Expectorant	Adult Dose and Other	How Supplied
c-v	**Dihistine Expectorant Liquid** (Various, eg, Barre-National, Goldline, Major, Moore)	30 mg pseudo-ephedrine HCl	10 mg codeine phosphate		100 mg guaifenesin	10 ml q 4 h up to 40 ml/day. Alcohol	In 120 and 480 ml.
c-v	**Decongestant Expectorant Liquid** (Schein)					10 ml q 4 h up to 40 ml/day. 7.5% alcohol	Fruit flavor. In 480 ml.
c-v	**Deproist Expectorant with Codeine Liquid** (Geneva)					10 ml q 4 h up to 40 ml/day. 8.2% alcohol	Fruit flavor. In 120 and 480 ml.
c-v	**Guaifenesin and Pseudo-ephedrine HCl and Codeine Phosphate Syrup** (Schein)					10 ml q 4 h up to 40 ml/day. 1.4% alcohol	In 473 ml.
otc	**Guaifenesin DAC** (Cypress)					1.9% alcohol. Saccharin, sorbitol.	In 480 ml.
c-v	**Guiatuss DAC Liquid** (Various, eg, Barre-National, Goldline, Moore, Rugby)					10 ml q 4 h up to 40 ml/day. Alcohol	In 120 and 480 ml.

ANTITUSSIVE AND EXPECTORANT COMBINATIONS

	Product & Distributor	Decongestant	Antitussive	Antihistamine	Expectorant	Adult Dose and Other	How Supplied
c-v *sf*	**Guiatussin DAC Syrup** (Rugby)	30 mg pseudo-ephedrine HCl	10 mg codeine phosphate		100 mg guaifenesin	10 ml q 4 h up to 40 ml/day. 1.6% alcohol, menthol, saccharin, sorbitol	In 480 ml.
c-v	**Isoclor Expectorant Liquid** (Fisons)					10 ml tid or qid. 5% alcohol	In 480 ml.
c-v *sf*	**Mytussin DAC Liquid** (Pennex)					10 ml q 4 h up to 40 ml/day. 1.7% alcohol, menthol saccharin, sorbitol	Strawberry-raspberry flavor. In 120 ml, pt and gal.
c-v	**Novagest Expectorant with Codeine Liquid** (Major)					10 ml q 4 h. 1.4% alcohol	In 120 ml, pt and gal.
c-v	**Novahistine Expectorant Liquid** (SK-Beecham)					10 ml q 4 h up to 40 ml/day. 7.5% alcohol, saccharin, sorbitol, sugar	In 480 ml.
c-v	**Phenhist Expectorant Liquid** (Rugby)					10 ml q 4 h up to 40 ml/day. 7.5% alcohol	In 120 and 480 ml.

ANTITUSSIVE AND EXPECTORANT COMBINATIONS

	Product & Distributor	Decongestant	Antitussive	Antihistamine	Expectorant	Adult Dose and Other	How Supplied
c-v	**Robafen DAC Syrup** (Major)	30 mg pseudo-ephedrine HCl	10 mg codeine phosphate		100 mg guaifenesin	10 ml q 4 h up to 40 ml/day. 1.4% alcohol	In 473 ml.
c-v sf	**Robitussin-DAC Syrup** (Robins)					10 ml q 4 h up to 40 ml/day. 1.9% alcohol, saccharin, sorbitol	In 480 ml.
c-v sf	**Ryna-CX Liquid** (Wallace)					10 ml q 4 to 6 h up to 40 ml/day. Saccharin, sorbitol	Alcohol- and dye free. In 118 and 480 ml.
c-v sf	**Tussar SF Syrup** (Rhone-Poulenc Rorer)					10 ml q 4 h up to 40 ml/day. 2.5% alcohol, saccharin, sorbitol	In 120 and 473 ml.
c-v	**Tussar-2 Syrup** (Rhone-Poulenc Rorer)					10 ml q 4 h up to 40 ml/day. 2.5% alcohol, saccharin, sorbitol, sucrose, methylparaben	In 473 ml.
c-v sf	**Naldecon CX Adult Liquid** (Apothecon)	12.5 mg phenylpropanolamine HCl	10 mg codeine phosphate		200 mg guaifenesin	10 ml q 4 h. Saccharin, glucose	Alcohol free. In 118 and 480 ml.

ANTITUSSIVE AND EXPECTORANT COMBINATIONS

	Product & Distributor	Decongestant	Antitussive	Antihistamine	Expectorant	Adult Dose and Other	How Supplied
c-v *sf*	**Codegest Expectorant Liquid** (Great Southern)	12.5 mg phenylpropanolamine HCl	10 mg codeine phosphate		100 mg guaifenesin	5 to 10 ml tid or qid	Alcohol- and dye free. In pt and gal.
c-v	**Conex w/Codeine Syrup** (Forest)					5 to 10 ml q 4 to 6 h. 0.13% methylparaben, 0.03% propylparaben	In 120 ml.
c-v *sf*	**Endal Expectorant Syrup** (UAD)					5 to 10 ml tid or qid. 5% alcohol. Methyl- and propylparabens, saccharin, sorbitol, thymol	Dye free. In 480 ml.
c-v	**Statuss ExpectorantLiquid** (Huckaby)					5% alcohol, menthol, saccharin, sorbitol	Dye free. In 473 ml.
c-v	**Triaminic Expectorant w/Codeine Liquid** (Sandoz)					10 ml q 4 h. 5% alcohol, sorbitol, sucrose	In 480 ml.
otc	**Tussex Cough Syrup** (Various, eg, Barre-National, Moore, Rugby)	5 mg phenylephrine HCl	10 mg dextromethorphan HBr		100 mg guaifenesin	10 ml q 4 h	In 120 ml.
otc *sf*	**Dexafed Cough Syrup** (Mallard)						Alcohol free. In 118 ml.

ANTITUSSIVE AND EXPECTORANT COMBINATIONS

	Product & Distributor	Decongestant	Antitussive	Antihistamine	Expectorant	Adult Dose and Other	How Supplied
Rx	**MED-Rx DMTablets** (Iomed)	60 mg pseudo-ephedrine HCl			600 mg guaifenesin	14-day regimen of 56 tablets	(ID 122). Lt. blue, scored. In 28s.
			30 mg dextro-methorphan HBr		600 mg guaifenesin		(ID 112) Lt green scored. In 28s.
otc	**Anatuss DM Tablets** (May-rand)	60 mg pseudo-ephedrine HCl	20 mg dextro-methorphan HBr		400 mg guaifenesin	1 q 4 h	(M P 0382). Orange, scored. Oval. In 100s.
otc	**Ambenyl-D Liquid** (Forest)	30 mg pseudo-ephedrine HCl	15 mg dextro-methorphan HBr		100 mg guaifenesin	5 to 10 ml q 4 h. 9.5% alcohol, menthol, methyl-paraben, saccharin, sorbitol, sucrose	In 118 ml.

ANTITUSSIVE AND EXPECTORANT COMBINATIONS

	Product & Distributor	Decongestant	Antitussive	Antihistamine	Expectorant	Adult Dose and Other	How Supplied
otc	**Anatuss DMSyrup** (Mayrand)	30 mg pseudo-ephedrine HCl	10 mg dextro-methorphan HBr		100 mg guaifenesin	10 ml q 4 h.	Cherry flavor. In 480 ml.
otc	**Dimacol Caplets** (Robins)					2 q 4 h up to 8/day. Saccharin, parabens	(Dimacol). In 12s, 24, 100s and 500s.
otc	**Novahistine DMX Liquid** (SmithKline Beecham)					10 ml q 4 h up to 40 ml/day. 10% alcohol, saccharin, sorbitol, sugar	In 120 ml.
otc	**Rhinosyn-X Liquid** (Great Southern)					10 ml q 4 h. 7.5% alcohol, sucrose	In 120 ml.
otc	**Ru-Tuss Expectorant Liquid** (Boots)					10 ml q 4 to 6 h up to 40 ml/day. 10% alcohol, glucose, sorbitol, sucrose, parabens	In 473 ml.
otc	**Sudafed Cold & Cough Liquid Caps** (Burroughs Wellcome)					2 q 4 h up to 8/day. 250 mg acetaminophen, sorbitol	In 10s and 20s.

Antitussive and Expectorant Combinations

ANTITUSSIVE AND EXPECTORANT COMBINATIONS

	Product & Distributor	Decongestant	Antitussive	Antihistamine	Expectorant	Adult Dose and Other	How Supplied
otc	**Guiatuss Cold & Cough Liquid Gel-Caps** (Goldline)	30 mg pseudoephedrine HCl	10 mg dextromethorphan		200 mg guaifenesin	*6 to < 12 yrs* - 1 q 4 h *> 12 yrs* - 2 q 4 h. Sorbitol.	In 12s.
otc	**Robitussin Cold & Cough Liqui-gels** (Robins)					Sorbitol.	In 20s.
otc	**Aspirin-Free Bayer Select Head & Chest Cold Caplets** (Sterling Health)	30 mg pseudoephedrine HCl	10 mg dextromethorphan HBr		100 mg guaifenesin	2 q 4 h up to 8/day. 325 mg acetaminophen	In 16s.
otc	**Vicks DayQuil LiquiCaps** (Richardson-Vicks)					2 q 4 h up to 8/day. 250 mg acetaminophen	(DayQuil). In 12s and 20s.
otc	**Primatuss Cough Mixture 4D Liquid** (Rugby)	20 mg pseudoephedrine HCl	10 mg dextromethorphan HBr		67 mg guaifenesin	15 ml q 6 h. 10% alcohol, corn syrup, sorbitol, sucrose	In 120 ml.
otc	**Cough Formula Comtrex Liquid** (Bristol-Myers)	15 mg pseudoephedrine HCl	7.5 mg dextromethorphan HBr		50 mg guaifenesin	20 ml q 4 h up to 80 ml/day. 125 mg acetaminophen, 20% alcohol, menthol, saccharin, sucrose	Raspberry flavor. In 120 and 240 ml.

ANTITUSSIVE AND EXPECTORANT COMBINATIONS

	Product & Distributor	Decongestant	Antitussive	Antihistamine	Expectorant	Adult Dose and Other	How Supplied
otc sf	**Benylin Multi-Symptom Liquid** (Glaxo Wellcome)	15 mg pseudoephedrine HCl	5 mg dextromethorphan HBr		100 mg guaifenesin	20 ml q 4 h up to 80 ml/day	EDTA, saccharin, sorbitol. Alcohol free. In 118 ml.
otc sf	**Contac Cough & Chest Cold Liquid** (SK-Beecham)				50 mg guaifenesin	20 ml q 4 to 6 h up to 80 ml/day. 125 mg acetaminophen, 10% alcohol, saccharin, sorbitol	In 120 ml.
otc	**Vicks DayQuil Liquid** (Richardson-Vicks)	10 mg pseudoephedrine HCl	3.3 mg dextromethorphan HBr		33.3 mg guaifenesin	30 ml q 4 h up to 120 ml/day. 108.3 mg acetaminophen, saccharin, sucrose	In 180 ml.
otc sf	**Anatuss Syrup** (Mayrand)	25 mg phenylpropanolamine HCl	15 mg dextromethorphan HBr		100 mg guaifenesin	10 ml q 6 h	Alcohol free. In 118.
Rx	**Anatuss Tablets** (Mayrand)					2 q 4 to 6 h up to 8/day. 325 mg acetaminophen	Green. Film coated. In 100s.
c-III	**Tussanil DH Tablets** (Misemer)	25 mg phenylpropanolamine HCl	1.66 mg hydrocodone bitartrate		100 mg guaifenesin	1 to 2 q 4 to 6 h. 300 mg salicylamide	Purple. Capsule shape. In 100s.

COUGH PREPARATIONS

Antitussive and Expectorant Combinations

ANTITUSSIVE AND EXPECTORANT COMBINATIONS

	Product & Distributor	Decongestant	Antitussive	Antihistamine	Expectorant	Adult Dose and Other	How Supplied
c-III	**Statuss Green Liquid** (Huckaby)	3.3 mg phenylpropanolamine HCl, 5 mg phenylephrine HCl,	1.67 mg hydrocodone bitartrate	3.3 mg pheniramine maleate, pyrilamine maleate		5% alcohol, saccharin, parabens, sorbitol, glucose.	In 480 ml.
c-III	**Vetuss HC** (Cypress)	3.3 mg phenylpropanolamine HCl, 5 mg phenylephrine HCl	1.7 mg hydrocodone bitartrate	3.3 mg pheniramine maleate, pyrilamine maleate		5% alcohol.	Strawberry flavored. In 16 oz. bottles.
otc	**Sudafed Cough Syrup** (Burroughs Wellcome)	15 mg pseudoephedrine HCl	5 mg dextromethorphan HBr		100 mg guaifenesin	20 ml q 4 h up to 80 ml/day. 2.4% alcohol, sucrose, saccharin, 0.1% methylparaben	Fruity mint flavor. In 118 and 236 ml.
otc *sf*	**Naldecon DX Adult Liquid** (Apothecon)	12.5 mg phenylpropanolamine HCl	10 mg dextromethorphan HBr		200 mg guaifenesin	10 ml q 4 h. Saccharin, sorbitol	Fruit flavor. Alcohol free. In 118 and 480 ml.
otc	**Naldelate DX Adult Liquid** (Barre-National)						Licorice flavor. In 120 and 480 ml.
otc	**GuiaCough CF Liquid** (Schein)	12.5 mg phenylpropanolamine HC	10 mg dextromethorphan HB		100 mg guaifenesin	10 ml q 4 h. 4.75% alcohol, parabens, saccharin, sorbitol, sucrose	In 118 ml.

ANTITUSSIVE AND EXPECTORANT COMBINATIONS

	Product & Distributor	Decongestant	Antitussive	Antihistamine	Expectorant	Adult Dose and Other	How Supplied
otc	**Guiatuss CF Liquid** (Barre-National)	12.5 mg phenylpropanolamine HC	10 mg dextromethorphan HB		100 mg guaifenesin	10 ml q 4 h. 4.75% alcohol	In 120 ml.
otc	**Robafen CF Liquid** (Major)					10 ml q 4 h	In 118 ml.
otc	**Robitussin-CF Liquid** (Robins)					10 ml q 4 h. 4.75% alcohol, saccharin, sorbitol	In 120, 240, 360 and 480 ml.
otc	**Siltussin-CFLiquid** (Silarx)					10 ml q 4 h. 4.75% alcohol	In 118 ml.
c-v	**Statuss Expectorant Liquid** (Huckaby)					5 -10 ml tid or qid. 5% alcohol.	In 480 ml.
otc sf	**Cough Syrup** (Goldline)	5 mg phenylephrine HCl	10 mg dextromethorphan HBr		100 mg guaifenesin	10 ml q 4 h	Alcohol free. Orange flavor. In 120 ml.
Rx	**Cophene-X Capsules** (Dunhall)	10 mg phenylephrine HCl, 10 mg phenylpropanolamine HCl	20 mg carbetapentane citrate		45 mg potassium guaiacolsulfonate	1 or 2 q 4 to 6 h	Red-orange. In 100s.
c-III	**S-T Forte Syrup and Liquid** (Scot-Tussin)	5 mg phenylpropanolamine HCl, 5 mg phenylephrine HCl	2.5 mg hydrocodone bitartrate	13.33 mg pheniramine maleate	80 mg guaifenesin	5 ml tid or qid. 5% alcohol	**Syrup**: In 120 & 240 ml, pt, gal. **Liquid**: Sugar free. In 120 & 240 ml, pt, gal.

ANTITUSSIVE AND EXPECTORANT COMBINATIONS

	Product & Distributor	Decongestant	Antitussive	Antihistamine	Expectorant	Adult Dose and Other	How Supplied
c-v	**Rolatuss Expectorant Liquid** (Huckaby)	5 mg phenylephrine HCl	9.85 codeine phosphate	2 mg chlorpheniramine maleate	33.3 mg ammonium Cl	5 -10 ml tid or qid. 5% alcohol	In 480 ml.
c-iii	**P-V-Tussin Tablets** (Solvay Pharm.)		5 mg hydrocodone bitartrate	25 mg phenindamine tartrate	200 mg guaifenesin	1 qid pc and hs ≥ q 4 h. Lactose	(Solvay 1088). Peach, scored. In 100s.
otc	**Phanadex Cough Syrup** (Pharmakon)	25 mg phenylpropanolamine HCl	15 mg dextromethorphan HBr	40 mg pyrilamine maleate	100 mg guaifenesin	10 ml q 4 to 6 h up to 80 ml/day. 75 mg K citrate, 35 mg citric acid, sucrose, sugar, parabens	Alcohol free. Grape flavor. In 118 and 236 ml.
Rx	**Donatussin Syrup** (Laser)	10 mg phenylephrine HCl	7.5 mg dextromethorphan HBr	2 mg chlorpheniramine maleate	100 mg guaifenesin	5 ml q 4 to 6 h	In pt and gal.
c-iii	**Triaminic Expectorant DH Liquid** (Sandoz)	12.5 mg phenylpropanolamine HCl	1.67 mg hydrocodone bitartrate	6.25 mg pyrilamine maleate, 6.25 mg pheniramine maleate	100 mg guaifenesin	10 ml q 4 h. 5% alcohol, saccharin, sorbitol, sucrose	In 480 ml.
otc	**Father John's Medicine Plus Liquid** (Oakhurst)	2.5 mg phenylephrine HCl	7.5 mg dextromethorphan HBr	1 mg chlorpheniramine maleate	30 mg glyceryl guaiacolate, 83.3 mg ammonium Cl	5 to 10 ml q 3 to 4 h. Na citrate	Alcohol free. Grape flavor. In 120 ml.
otc	**Quelidrine Cough Syrup** (Abbott)	5 mg phenylephrine HCl, 5 mg ephedrine HCl	10 mg dextromethorphan HBr	2 mg chlorpheniramine maleate	40 mg ammonium Cl, 0.005 ml ipecac fluidextract	5 ml qd to qid. 2% alcohol, glucose, sucrose, parabens	Cherry flavor. In 120 ml.

ANTITUSSIVE AND EXPECTORANT COMBINATIONS

	Product & Distributor	Decongestant	Antitussive	Antihistamine	Expectorant	Adult Dose and Other	How Supplied
c-v	**Tussirex Syrup** (Scot-Tussin)	4.17 mg phenylephrine HCl	10 mg codeine phosphate	13.33 mg pheniramine maleate	83.3 mg sodium citrate	5 ml tid. 83.33 mg sodium salicylate, 25 mg caffeine citrate, 0.17 mg menthol	Alcohol and dye free. In pt and gal.
c-v sf	**Tussirex Sugar Free Liquid** (Scot-Tussin)						Alcohol and dye free. In pt and gal.
otc sf	**Diabetic Tussin Liquid** (Roberts Med)	5 mg phenylephedrine	10 mg dextromethorphan HBr	100 mg guaifenesin			In 120 ml

Pediatric Antitussive and Expectorant Combinations

PEDIATRIC ANTITUSSIVE AND EXPECTORANT COMBINATIONS

Refer to the general discussion of these products in the Respiratory Combinations Introduction.

Content given per 5 ml liquid or 1 ml drops.

	Product & Distributor	Decongestant	Antitussive	Expectorant	Dose	Other	How Supplied
c-v	**Cycofed Pediatric** (Cypress)	30 mg pseudoephedrine HCl	10 mg codeine phosphate	100 mg guaifenesin	*6 to < 12 yrs* - 5 ml q 6 h *2 to < 6 yrs* - 2.5 ml q 6 h	6% alcohol.	Raspberry flavor. In 16 oz. bottles.
c-v	**Deconsal Pediatric Syrup** (Adams)				*6 to < 12 yrs* - 5 ml q 6 h *2 to < 6 yrs* - 2.5 ml q 6 h	6% alcohol, saccharin, sucrose	Orange flavor. In 480 ml.
c-III	**Entuss-D Jr. Liquid** (Roberts/Hauck)	30 mg pseudoephedrine HCl	2.5 mg hydrocodone bitartrate	100 mg guaifenesin	*6 to 12 yrs* – 5 ml q 4 to 6 h up to 20 ml/day	5% alcohol, saccharin, sorbitol, sucrose, glucose, parabens	Tropical fruit punch flavor. In 120 ml & pt.
otc	**Naldecon DX Children's Syrup** (Apothecon)	6.25 mg phenylpropanolamine HCl	5 mg dextromethorphan HBr	100 mg guaifenesin	*6 to < 12 yrs* - 10 ml q 4 h *2 to < 6 yrs* - 5 ml q 4 h	Saccharin	Fruit flavor. In 120 and 480 ml.
otc	**Pediacon DX Children's Syrup** (Goldline)					5% alcohol	In 118 ml.
otc	**Phenadex Children Cough/ Cold Drops** (Barre-National)					5% alcohol	In 118 ml.
otc sf	**Pediacon DX Pediatric Drops** (Goldline)	6.25 mg phenylpropanolamine HCl	5 mg dextromethorphan HBr	50 mg guaifenesin	*2 to < 6 yrs* – 1 ml q 4 h	Saccharin, sorbitol	In 30 ml.
otc sf	**Phenadex Pediatric Cough/ ColdDrops** (Barre-National)						In 30 ml.

Pediatric Antitussive and Expectorant Combinations

PEDIATRIC ANTITUSSIVE AND EXPECTORANT COMBINATIONS

	Product & Distributor	Decongestant	Antitussive	Expectorant	Dose	Other	How Supplied
otc	**Dorcol Children's Cough Syrup** (Sandoz)	15 mg pseudo-ephedrine HCl	5 mg dextro-methorphan HBr	50 mg guai-fenesin	*2 to < 6 yrs* – 5 ml q 4 h up to 20 ml/day *6 to <12 yrs* - 10 ml q 4 h up to 40 ml/day	Sucrose	Alcohol free. In 120 and 240 ml.
otc	**Ipsatol Cough Formula Liquid for Children and Adults** (Kenwood)	9 mg phenylpro-panolamine HCl	10 dextro-methorphan HBr	100 mg guai-fenesin	*2 to < 6 yrs* - 2.5 ml q 4 h *6 to < 12 yrs* - 5 ml q 4 h		Alcohol free. In 118 ml.
otc *sf*	**Naldecon DX Pediatric Drops** (Apothecon)	6.25 mg phenylpro-panolamine HCl per ml	5 mg dextro-methorphan HBr per ml	50 mg guai-fenesin per ml	*2 to < 6 yrs* – 1 ml q 4 h	Saccharin, sorbitol	Alcohol free. Raspberry-strawberry flavor. In 30 ml.

chapter 6

central nervous system

CAFFEINE

Actions:

Pharmacology: Caffeine, a methylxanthine, exerts its pharmacological effects by increasing calcium permeability in sarcoplasmic reticulum, inhibiting phosphodiesterase promoting accumulation of cyclic AMP, and competitively blocking adenosine receptors. It is a potent stimulant of the CNS. It also produces cardiac stimulation, dilatation of coronary and peripheral blood vessels, constriction of cerebral blood vessels, skeletal muscle stimulation, augmentation of gastric acid secretion and diuretic activity. Low concentrations of caffeine produce a small decrease in heart rate; higher concentrations produce tachycardia or premature ventricular contractions.

Because of its CNS stimulating effects and constriction of cerebral blood vessels, caffeine is frequently used as an analgesic adjuvant. In various studies, the addition of ≥ 65 mg per tablet (≤ 600 mg/day) increased the analgesic effects and decreased time to onset of aspirin, acetaminophen and combinations. It also increased absorption of ergot alkaloids.

Tolerance to the cardiovascular, CNS and diuretic effects may develop. Differences in effects of caffeine on various organ systems may be observed in nonusers of caffeine vs habitual consumers. Acute ingestion of caffeine produces increases in systolic blood pressure, plasma catecholamines, plasma renin activity and heart rate; chronic ingestion has little or no effect on these hemodynamic variables, nor is caffeine arrhythmogenic. The amount of caffeine derived from dietary sources is given in the following table:

Caffeine Content from Various Dietary Sources[1]

Dietary source	Range of caffeine content
Coffee – Regular: Brewed	40-180 mg/5 to 8 oz
Instant	30-120 mg/5 to 8 oz
Coffee – Decaffeinated: Brewed	2-5 mg/5 to 8 oz
Instant	1-5 mg/5 to 8 oz
Tea: Brewed	20-110 mg/5 to 8 oz
Instant	25-50 mg/5 to 8 oz
Iced	≈ 70 mg/12 oz
Other: Soft drinks	0-54 mg/12 oz
Cocoa	2-50 mg/5 to 8 oz
Chocolate milk	2-7 mg/5 oz
Milk chocolate	1-15 mg/1 oz
Bakers chocolate	25-35 mg/1 oz

[1] Depending on strength of brew and product.

Pharmacokinetics:

Absorption/Distribution – Caffeine is well absorbed orally (99%). Peak plasma levels of 5 to 25 mcg/ml are achieved 15 to 45 minutes after 250 mg. Protein binding is 15% to 17%. Caffeine readily crosses the blood brain barrier and placenta. Therapeutic plasma concentrations are ≈ 6 to 13 mcg/ml; those > 20 mcg/ml produce adverse effects. The lethal concentration is > 100 mcg/ml.

Metabolism/Excretion – Caffeine is metabolized in the liver; 0.5% to 3.5% is excreted unchanged in the urine. Clearance is decreased in alcoholic liver disease. In the adult, plasma half-life ranges from 3 to 7.5 hours (average 3.5 hours). Half-life is prolonged in pregnancy (up to 18 hours) and with concomitant use of some drugs (see Drug Interactions).

In neonates, caffeine is eliminated almost entirely by excretion of unchanged drug in the urine. Preterm infants at birth exhibit half-lives of 65 to 103 hours; term infants at birth, 82 hours; 3 to 4-month-old infants, 14.4 hours; and 5- to 6-month-old infants, 2.6 hours. In newborns, plasma and cerebrospinal fluid levels are nearly identical.

Indications:

Oral: As an aid in staying awake and restoring mental alertness.

As an adjuvant in analgesic formulations.

Parenteral:

IM – As an analeptic in conjunction with supportive measures to treat respiratory depression associated with overdosage with CNS depressants (eg, narcotic analgesics, alcohol). However, because of questionable benefit and transient action, most authorities believe caffeine and other analeptics should not be used in these conditions and recommend other supportive therapy.

CAFFEINE

Unlabeled uses:

Neonatal apnea – An initial dose of 10 mg/kg caffeine followed by a maintenance dose of 2.5 mg/kg/day. Control is associated with plasma concentrations of 5 to 20 mcg/ml. Do not use products containing sodium benzoate in neonates.

Atopic dermatitis – Topical treatment with 30% caffeine in a hydrophilic base or in a hydrocortisone cream produces improvement in pruritus, erythema, scaling, lichenification, oozing and dermatitis. This may be related to caffeine's property of liberating water from epidermal and subcutaneous tissues, similar to urea.

Headache – To alleviate headaches following spinal puncture (500 mg).

Alcohol – For the treatment of excited or comatose alcoholic patients.

Asthma – Although potentially beneficial at higher doses, caffeine offers no advantage over theophylline.

Orthostatic hypotension due to autonomic failure was attenuated, especially in the postprandial state, by 250 mg caffeine in a small number of patients.

Warnings:

Depression: Too vigorous treatment with parenteral caffeine can produce further depression in the already depressed patient; therefore, do not exceed 1 g as a single dose of caffeine and sodium benzoate.

GI effects: Large quantities of caffeine-containing products may reactivate duodenal ulcers.

Pregnancy: Category C. Safety for use in pregnancy has not been established; pregnant women should consume sparingly or avoid caffeine-containing food and drugs. Caffeine crosses the placenta and achieves fetal blood and tissue levels similar to maternal concentrations. Excessive caffeine intake has been weakly associated with increased fetal loss, low birth weight and premature deliveries; however, when used in moderation there is no association with these effects or congenital malformations. Caffeine causes birth defects in animals.

Lactation: Caffeine appears in the breast milk of nursing mothers. Milk:plasma ratios of 0.5 have been reported. Approximately 1.5 to 3.1 mg of caffeine would be ingested by a nursing infant whose mother had one cup of coffee.

Precautions:

Hyperglycemic effects: Higher blood glucose levels may result from caffeine use.

Drug Interactions:

Caffeine Drug Interactions			
Precipitant drug	Object drug*		Description
Cimetidine Contraceptives, oral Disulfiram Fluoroquinolones ciprofloxacin enoxacin	Caffeine	⬆	Caffeine metabolism may be impaired, resulting in decreased clearance and increased half-life. Excessive CNS effects may occur.
Phenylpropanolamine	Caffeine	⬆	Serum caffeine levels may be increased, resulting in an increase in pharmacologic and toxic effects.
Smoking	Caffeine	⬇	Elimination of caffeine may be enhanced.

* ⬆ = Object drug increased. ⬇ = Object drug decreased.

Drug/Lab test interactions: Caffeine produces false positive elevations of serum urate as measured by the Bittner method. Caffeine also produces slight increases in urine levels of VMA, catecholamines and 5-hydroxyindoleacetic acid. Because high urine levels of VMA or catecholamines may result in false positive diagnosis of pheochromocytoma or neuroblastoma, avoid caffeine intake during tests for these disorders.

Drug/Food interactions: **Coffee** and **tea** consumed with a meal or 1 hour after a meal significantly inhibits the absorption of dietary **iron**. Clinical significance has not been determined.

Adverse Reactions:

CNS: Insomnia; restlessness; excitement; nervousness; tinnitus; scintillating scotoma; muscular tremor; headaches; lightheadedness.

Anxiety neurosis – Large doses of caffeine may produce symptoms mimicking anxiety neurosis (eg, tremulousness, muscle twitching, sensory disturbances, irritability, flushing, tachypnea, palpitations, arrhythmias, GI disturbances, diuresis).

GI: Nausea; vomiting; diarrhea; stomach pain.

CAFFEINE

Cardiovascular: Tachycardia; extrasystoles; palpitations.

GU: Diuresis.

Miscellaneous:

Withdrawal – Headache, anxiety and muscle tension may occur following abrupt cessation of the drug after regular consumption of 500 to 600 mg/day. Symptoms usually start between 12 to 18 hours after the last caffeine ingestion.

Overdosage:

Symptoms: Toxic symptoms can be produced in the adult with ≥ 1 g oral caffeine. Deaths have occurred after the IV and oral administration of caffeine and rectal administration of coffee. The acute lethal dose of caffeine ranges from 5 to 10 g IV or oral.

Adults – Initially, insomnia, dyspnea, mild delirium. Alternating states of consciousness and muscle twitching may appear. Diuresis, arrhythmias and hyperglycemia have occurred. The terminal event is usually seizures.

Infants: Caffeine overdosage has been reported in newborns given a single dose of caffeine, 36 to 94 mg/kg, at birth. Symptoms included hypertonicity alternating with hypotonicity, opisthotonic posturing, coarse tremors, bradycardia, hypotension and severe acidosis. Intracranial hemorrhage has also occurred.

Treatment: Symptomatic and supportive. Gastric lavage followed by activated charcoal may be useful. Control seizures with diazepam or phenobarbital.

Patient Information:

Do not exceed recommended dosage.

Discontinue use if increased or abnormal heart rate, dizziness or palpitations occur.

If fatigue persists or recurs, consult physician.

Not intended for use as a substitute for normal sleep.

Administration and Dosage:

Oral: 100 to 200 mg every 3 to 4 hours, as needed. Not recommended for children.

Timed release – 200 mg every 3 to 4 hours.

An oral solution of caffeine may be prepared as follows – Dissolve 10 g caffeine citrate powder in 250 ml Sterile Water for Irrigation, USP, qs to 500 ml with 2 parts simple syrup to 1 part cherry syrup. Final concentration is 10 mg/ml caffeine base (20 mg/ml caffeine citrate). Stable for at least 3 months.

Parenteral: Sodium benzoate increases caffeine's solubility in aqueous solutions.

Adults – 500 mg (250 mg caffeine) IM (or slow IV injection in emergency respiratory failure) or a maximum single dose of 1 g (500 mg caffeine). The usual and maximum safe dose is 500 mg. Total dose in 24 hours should rarely exceed 2.5 g.

Analeptic use of caffeine is strongly discouraged by most clinicians.

Alternative parenteral formulation – An IV formulation of caffeine may be prepared by one of the two following methods:

1) Dissolve 10 g caffeine citrate powder in 250 ml Sterile Water for Injection, USP, qs to 500 ml, filter, and autoclave. Final concentration is 10 mg/ml caffeine base (20 mg/ml caffeine citrate). Stable for at least 3 months.

2) Dissolve 10 g caffeine powder and 10.94 g citric acid powder in Bacteriostatic Water for Injection, USP, qs to 1 L. Sterilize by filtration.

otc	**Tirend** (SK-Beecham)	**Tablets:** 100 mg	Lactose. Lemon flavor. In 12s, 30s and 60s.
otc	**Quick Pep** (Thompson)	**Tablets:** 150 mg	Dextrose, sucrose. In 32s.
otc	**Vivarin** (SK-Beecham)	**Tablets:** 200 mg	Dextrose. Capsule shape. In 16s, 24s, 40s and 80s.
otc	**NoDoz** (Bristol-Myers)	**Tablets, chewable:** 100 mg	Aspartame, 15 mg phenylalanine. Spearmint flavor. In 12s and 30s.
otc	**Caffedrine** (Thompson)	**Tablets, timed release:** 200 mg anhydrous caffeine	Lactose. Capsule shape. In 20s.
otc	**Caffedrine** (Thompson)	**Capsules, timed release:** 200 mg anhydrous caffeine	Sucrose. (Caffedrine). Clear w/purple band. In 16s.
Rx	**Caffeine and Sodium Benzoate** (Pasadena)	**Injection:** 250 mg per ml (equal parts caffeine and sodium benzoate)	In 2 ml amps.

DOXAPRAM HCl

Actions:

Pharmacology: Doxapram produces respiratory stimulation by activating the peripheral carotid chemoreceptors. The respiratory stimulant action is manifested by an increase in tidal volume associated with a slight increase in respiratory rate. As the dosage is increased, the medullary respiratory centers are stimulated with progressive stimulation of other parts of the brain and spinal cord.

A pressor response due to improved cardiac output rather than peripheral vasoconstriction may occur. If there is no cardiac impairment, the pressor effect is greater in hypovolemic than in normovolemic states. Following administration, an increased release of catecholamines has occurred.

Although opiate-induced respiratory depression is antagonized by doxapram, the analgesia is not affected.

Pharmacokinetics: The onset of respiratory stimulation following the recommended single IV injection usually occurs in 20 to 40 seconds, with peak effect at 1 to 2 minutes. The duration of effect varies from 5 to 12 minutes. Doxapram is rapidly metabolized; metabolites and a small amount of unchanged drug (< 5%) are excreted in the urine. The plasma half-life ranges from 2.4 to 4.1 hours.

Indications:

Postanesthesia: To stimulate respiration in patients with drug-induced postanesthesia respiratory depression or apnea other than that due to muscle relaxants.

With simultaneous administration of oxygen to pharmacologically stimulate deep breathing in the "stir-up" regimen in the postoperative patient.

Drug-induced CNS depression: To stimulate respiration, hasten arousal and encourage return of laryngopharyngeal reflexes in patients with mild to moderate respiratory and CNS depression due to overdosage. Exercise care to prevent vomiting and aspiration.

Controlled ventilation and standard supportive care for respiratory depression due to CNS overdose is safer, more reliable and more effective than doxapram.

Chronic pulmonary disease associated with acute hypercapnia: As a temporary measure in hospitalized patients with acute respiratory insufficiency superimposed on chronic obstructive pulmonary disease. Use for a short period of time (approximately 2 hours) to prevent elevation of arterial CO_2 tension during the administration of oxygen. Do not use in conjunction with mechanical ventilation.

Unlabeled uses: Low dose doxapram (ie, initial dose, 1 to 1.5 mg/kg/hr; maintenance, 0.5 to 2.5 mg/kg/hr) has been used in the treatment of apnea of prematurity when methylxanthines have failed.

Contraindications:

Hypersensitivity to the drug; newborns (product contains benzyl alcohol); epilepsy or other convulsive states; mechanical disorders of ventilation such as mechanical obstruction, muscle paresis, flail chest, pneumothorax, acute bronchial asthma, pulmonary fibrosis or other conditions resulting in restriction of chest wall, muscles of respiration or alveolar expansion; head inury; cerebrovascular accident; significant cardiovascular impairment; severe hypertension.

Warnings:

Postanesthetic use: Doxapram is neither an antagonist to muscle relaxant drugs nor a specific narcotic antagonist. Ensure adequacy of airway and oxygenation prior to use. Administer carefully to patients with hyperthyroidism or pheochromocytoma.

Since narcosis may recur after stimulation with doxapram, maintain close observation until patient has been fully alert for 30 minutes to 1 hour.

Drug-induced CNS and respiratory depression: Doxapram alone may not stimulate adequate spontaneous breathing or provide sufficient arousal in patients who are severely depressed either due to respiratory failure or to CNS depressant drugs. Use as an adjunct to established supportive measures and resuscitative techniques.

Chronic obstructive pulmonary disease: In an attempt to lower pCO_2, do not increase rate of infusion in severely ill patients because of the associated increased work in breathing. Do not use in conjunction with mechanical ventilation.

In some patients, arrhythmias in acute respiratory failure secondary to chronic obstructive pulmonary disease are probably the result of hypoxia. Use with caution in these patients.

Obtain arterial blood gases prior to the initiation of doxapram infusion and oxygen administration, then at least every ½ hour. Doxapram administration does not diminish the need for careful patient monitoring or the need for supplemental oxygen in acute respiratory failure. Discontinue use if the arterial blood gases deteriorate and initiate mechanical ventilation.

Pregnancy: Category B.There are no adequate and well controlled studies in pregnant women. Use during pregnancy only when clearly needed.

DOXAPRAM HCl

Lactation: It is not known whether this drug is excreted in breast milk. Exercise caution when administering to a nursing mother.

Children: Safety and efficacy for use in children < 12 years of age have not been established. The use of benzyl alcohol in newborns has been associated with metabolic, CNS, respiratory, circulatory and renal dysfunction; however, doxapram has been used to treat apnea of prematurity (see Unlabeled uses).

Precautions:

Administration: Avoid extravasation or use of a single injection site over an extended period; thrombophlebitis or local skin irritation may occur. Rapid infusion may result in hemolysis.

Slow administration and careful observation of the patient during and following administration are advisable to ensure that the protective reflexes have been restored and to prevent possible post-hyperventilation hypoventilation. An adequate airway is essential. Employ recommended dosages; do not exceed maximum total dosages. Use the minimum effective dosage to avoid side effects.

Blood pressure increases are generally modest, but significant increases have occurred. Not recommended for use in severe hypertension. If sudden hypotension or dyspnea develops, discontinue use. Monitor blood pressure and deep tendon reflexes to prevent overdosage.

Lowered pCO_2 induced by hyperventilation produces cerebral vasoconstriction and slowing of the cerebral circulation.

Benzyl alcohol: Doxapram contains benzyl alcohol, which has been associated with a fatal "gasping syndrome" in premature infants.

Drug Interactions:

Doxapram Drug Interactions			
Precipitant drug	Object drug*		Description
Doxapram	Anesthetics, inhalation	⬆	Since an increase in epinephrine release has been noted with doxapram, delay initiation of therapy for at least 10 minutes following discontinuance of anesthetics known to sensitize the myocardium to catecholamines.
Doxapram	MAO inhibitors	⬆	Administer cautiously to patients receiving these drugs since an additive pressor effect may occur.
Doxapram	Muscle relaxants	⬇	Doxapram may temporarily mask residual effects of muscle relaxants.
Doxapram	Sympathomimetics	⬆	Administer cautiously to patients receiving these drugs since an additive pressor effect may occur.

* ⬆ = Object drug increased. ⬇ = Object drug decreased.

Adverse Reactions:

Miscellaneous:

Central and autonomic nervous systems – Headache; dizziness; apprehension; disorientation; pupillary dilatation; hyperactivity; convulsions; bilateral Babinski; involuntary movements; muscle spasticity; increased deep tendon reflexes; clonus; pyrexia; flushing; sweating; pruritus and paresthesia such as a feeling of warmth, burning or hot sensation, especially in the area of the genitalia and perineum.

Respiratory: Cough; dyspnea; tachypnea; laryngospasm; bronchospasm; hiccoughs; rebound hypoventilation.

Hematologic: A decrease in hemoglobin, hematocrit or red blood cell count has occurred in postoperative patients. In the presence of preexisting leukopenia, a further decrease in WBC has occurred following anesthesia and treatment with doxapram.

Cardiovascular: Phlebitis; variations in heart rate; lowered T-waves; arrhythmias; chest pain; tightness in chest. A mild to moderate increase in blood pressure is commonly noted and may be of concern in patients with severe cardiovascular diseases (see Precautions).

GI: Nausea; vomiting; diarrhea; desire to defecate.

GU: Urinary retention; spontaneous voiding; elevation of BUN; albuminuria.

DOXAPRAM HCl

Overdosage:

Symptoms: Excessive pressor effect, tachycardia, skeletal muscle hyperactivity and enhanced deep tendon reflexes may be early signs of overdosage. Evaluate blood pressure, pulse rate and deep tendon reflexes periodically and adjust dosage or infusion rate accordingly.

Treatment: There is no specific antidote. Treatment is supportive. Refer to General Management of Acute Overdosage.Convulsive seizures are unlikely at recommended dosages, but short-acting IV barbiturates, oxygen and resuscitative equipment should be available. There is no evidence that doxapram is dialyzable. Due to half-life of doxapram, it is unlikely that dialysis would be appropriate treatment for overdosage.

Administration and Dosage:

Postanesthetic use:

Single IV injection – 0.5 to 1 mg/kg, not to exceed 1.5 mg/kg total as a single injection, or 2 mg/kg total when given as multiple injections at 5 minute intervals.

Infusion – 250 mg doxapram in 250 ml of dextrose or saline solution. Initiate at a rate of approximately 5 mg/min until a satisfactory respiratory response is observed. Maintain at a rate of 1 to 3 mg/min, adjusted to sustain the desired level of respiratory stimulation with minimal side effects. The recommended total dosage is 4 mg/kg, or approximately 300 mg for the average adult.

Management of drug-induced CNS depression:

Intermittent injection – Give priming IV dose of 2 mg/kg (1 mg/lb) and repeat in 5 minutes. Repeat every 1 to 2 hours until patient awakens. Watch for relapse into unconsciousness or development of respiratory depression, since doxapram does not affect the metabolism of CNS depressant drugs.

If relapse occurs, resume 1 to 2 hourly injections until arousal is sustained, or total maximum daily dose (3 g) is given. Allow patient to sleep until 24 hours have elapsed from first injection, using assisted or automatic respiration if necessary.

Repeat procedure the following day until patient breathes spontaneously and sustains desired level of consciousness, or until maximum dosage (3 g) is given. Administer repetitive doses only to patients who have shown response to the initial dose. Failure to respond appropriately indicates the need for neurologic evaluation for a possible CNS source of sustained coma.

Intermittent IV infusion – Give priming dose of 2 mg/kg (1 mg/lb). If patient awakens, watch for relapse; if no response, continue general supportive treatment for 1 to 2 hours and repeat doxapram. If some respiratory stimulation occurs, prepare IV infusion of 250 mg in 250 ml of saline or dextrose solution. Deliver at a rate of 1 to 3 mg/min according to size of patient and depth of coma. Discontinue use at end of 2 hours or if patient begins to awaken.

Continue supportive treatment for 0.5 to 2 hours and repeat steps above. Do not exceed 3 g/day.

Chronic obstructive pulmonary disease associated with acute hypercapnia: Mix 400 mg in 180 ml of IV solution (2 mg/ml). Start infusion at 1 to 2 mg/min (0.5 to 1 ml/min); if indicated, increase to maximum of 3 mg/min. Determine arterial blood gases prior to administration and at least every 30 minutes during the 2 hours of infusion to ensure against development of CO_2 retention and acidosis. Altering oxygen concentration or flow rate may necessitate adjustment in doxapram infusion rate.

Predictable blood gas patterns are more readily established with continuous infusion. If the blood gases deteriorate, discontinue infusion. Additional infusions beyond the maximum 2 hour administration period are not recommended.

Preparation of solution: Doxapram is compatible with 5% and 10% Dextrose in Water or normal saline.

Admixture incompatibility – Admixture of doxapram with alkaline solutions such as 2.5% thiopental sodium, bicarbonate or aminophylline will result in precipitation or gas formation.

Rx	**Doxapram** (Various, eg, Schein, Steris)	**Injection:** 20 mg per ml	Benzyl alcohol. In 20 ml multiple-dose vials.
Rx	**Dopram** (Robins)		0.9% benzyl alcohol. In 20 ml multiple-dose vials.

AMPHETAMINES

Warning:
Amphetamines have a high potential for abuse. Use in weight reduction programs only when alternative therapy has been ineffective. Administration for prolonged periods may lead to drug dependence. Prescribe or dispense sparingly.

Actions:

Pharmacology: Amphetamines are sympathomimetic amines with CNS stimulant activity. CNS effects are mediated by release of norepinephrine from central noradrenergic neurons. At higher doses, dopamine may be released in the mesolimbic system.

Peripheral alpha and beta activity includes elevation of systolic and diastolic blood pressures and weak bronchodilator and respiratory stimulant action. At therapeutic doses, the heart rate may be reflexly slowed; large doses may produce cardiac arrhythmias.

The site of action for appetite suppression is thought to be the lateral hypothalamic feeding center.

Pharmacokinetics:

Absorption/Distribution – Following oral use, amphetamines are completely absorbed within 3 hours. They are widely distributed in the body, with high concentrations in the brain. Therapeutic blood levels of amphetamine range from 5 to 10 mcg/dl.

Metabolism/Excretion – Amphetamine is metabolized in the liver by aromatic hydroxylation, N–dealkylation and deamination. Accumulated hydroxylated metabolites have been implicated in the development of amphetamine psychosis. Urinary excretion of the unchanged drug is pH dependent. Urinary acidification to a pH < 5.6 yields a plasma half-life of 7 to 8 hours; alkalinization increases half-life (range 18.6 to 33.6 hours). For every one unit increase in urinary pH, there is an average 7 hour increase in plasma half-life.

Indications:

Narcolepsy.

Attention deficit disorder with hyperactivity: Indicated as an integral part of a total treatment program which includes other remedial measures (psychological, educational, social) for a stabilizing effect in children with a behavioral syndrome characterized by moderate to severe distractibility, short attention span, hyperactivity, emotional lability and impulsivity. Do not diagnose this syndrome with finality when these symptoms are only of comparatively recent origin. Nonlocalizing (soft) neurological signs, learning disability and abnormal EEG may be present.

Exogenous obesity: As a short-term adjunct in a regimen of weight reduction based on caloric restriction, for patients refractory to alternative therapy (eg, repeated diets, group programs and other drugs). Weigh the limited usefulness against the possible risks inherent in use. Amphetamines have little effect in restricting food intake when overeating is prompted by psychological factors.

Contraindications:

Advanced arteriosclerosis; symptomatic cardiovascular disease; moderate to severe hypertension; hyperthyroidism; hypersensitivity or idiosyncrasy to the sympathomimetic amines; glaucoma; agitated states; history of drug abuse; during or within 14 days following administration of MAO inhibitors (hypertensive crises may result).

Warnings:

Tolerance: When tolerance to the anorectic effect develops, do not exceed recommended dose in an attempt to increase the effect; rather, discontinue the drug.

Drug dependence: Amphetamines have been extensively abused. Tolerance, extreme psychological dependence and severe social disability have occurred. Patients may increase the dosage to many times that recommended. Abrupt cessation following prolonged high dosage results in extreme fatigue, mental depression and changes on the sleep EEG.

Manifestations of chronic intoxication – Severe dermatoses, marked insomnia, irritability, hyperactivity and personality changes. Disorganization of thoughts, poor concentration, visual hallucinations and compulsive behavior often occur. The most severe manifestation of chronic intoxication is psychosis, often clinically indistinguishable from paranoid schizophrenia. This is rare with oral amphetamines.

AMPHETAMINES

Pregnancy: Category C. Safety for use during pregnancy has not been established. Reproduction studies in mammals at many times the human dose have suggested both an embryotoxic and teratogenic potential. Congenital defects associated with amphetamine use include cardiac abnormalities, bifidexencephaly and biliary atresia. There are no adequate and well controlled studies in pregnant women. Use in women who are or who may become pregnant (especially those in the first trimester) only when clearly needed and when the potential benefits outweigh the potential hazards to the fetus.

Infants born to mothers dependent on amphetamines have an increased risk of premature delivery and low birth weight. Also, these infants may experience symptoms of withdrawal as demonstrated by dysphoria, including agitation and significant lassitude.

Lactation: Amphetamines are excreted in breast milk. Advise patients to discontinue nursing while taking amphetamines.

Children: Do not use as anorectic agents in children under 12 years of age.

Amphetamine and dextroamphetamine are not recommended in children under 3 years of age for attention deficit disorder. In psychotic children, amphetamines may exacerbate symptoms of behavior disturbance and thought disorder. Amphetamines may precipitate or exacerbate motor and phonic tics and Tourette's disorder.

Data are inadequate to determine whether chronic administration of amphetamines may be associated with growth inhibition; therefore, monitor growth during treatment.

Long-term effects in children have not been well established.

Precautions:

Hypertension: Use cautiously.

Prescribe or dispense the least amount feasible at one time to minimize the possibility of overdosage.

Potentially hazardous tasks: May cause dizziness. Observe caution while driving or performing other tasks requiring alertness.

Attention deficit disorders: Drug treatment is not indicated in all cases. Amphetamine use should depend on the chronicity and severity of the child's symptoms and appropriateness for his/her age. Use should not depend solely on the presence of one or more of the behavioral characteristics.

When these symptoms are associated with acute stress reactions, amphetamine treatment is usually not indicated.

Tartrazine sensitivity: Some of these products contain tartrazine, which may cause allergic-type reactions (including bronchial asthma) in susceptible individuals. Although the incidence of tartrazine sensitivity in the general population is low, it is frequently seen in patients who also have aspirin hypersensitivity. Specific products containing tartrazine are identified in the product listings.

Drug Interactions:

Guanethidine: Amphetamines may decrease the antihypertensive effectiveness of guanethidine.

Monoamine oxidase (MAO) inhibitors may increase the pressor response to the amphetamines. Possible hypertensive crisis and intracranial hemorrhage may occur. This interaction may also occur with furazolidone, an antimicrobial with MAO inhibitor activity. Avoid this combination; if given inadvertently and hypertension occurs, administer phentolamine.

Tricyclic antidepressants may decrease the effects of the amphetamines. An increased dose may be necessary.

Urinary acidifiers decrease the half-life and shorten the duration of action of amphetamines, possibly decreasing the pharmacologic effects. A higher amphetamine dose may be necessary.

Urinary alkalinizers increase the half-life and prolong the duration of action of amphetamines, possibly increasing the pharmacologic effects and toxic effects (eg, cardiovascular, excessive CNS stimulation). A lower amphetamine dose may be necessary.

Drug/Lab test interactions: Plasma **corticosteroid** levels may be increased. This increase is greatest in the evening. **Urinary steroid** determinations may be altered by amphetamines.

AMPHETAMINES

Adverse Reactions:

Cardiovascular: Palpitations; tachycardia; elevation of blood pressure; reflex decrease in heart rate; arrhythmias (at larger doses).

CNS: Overstimulation; restlessness; dizziness; insomnia; dyskinesia; euphoria; dysphoria; tremor; headache; changes in libido; rarely, psychotic episodes at recommended doses. CNS stimulants have precipitated attacks of Tourette's disorder and have exacerbated motor and phonic tics.

GI: Dry mouth; unpleasant taste; diarrhea; constipation. Anorexia and weight loss may occur as undesirable effects when amphetamines are used other than for their anorectic effect.

Endocrine: Reversible elevations in serum thyroxine (T_4) levels have occurred with heavy amphetamine use.

Body as a whole: Urticaria; impotence.

Overdosage:

Symptoms: The severity of acute amphetamine overdose is roughly correlated with the progression of the following symptoms: Restlessness; irritability; insomnia; tremor; hyperreflexia; rhabdomyolysis; rapid respiration; hyperpyrexia; assaultiveness; hallucinations; panic states; diaphoresis; mydriasis; flushing; hyperactivity; confusion; hypertension or hypotension; extrasystoles; tachypnea; fever; delirium; self-injury; marked hypertension; arrhythmias; convulsions; coma; circulatory collapse; death.

Nausea, vomiting, diarrhea and abdominal cramps may occur. Fatigue and depression usually follow the central stimulation.

Treatment: Treatment is largely symptomatic and includes gastric evacuation, although this is usually ineffective more than 4 hours after ingestion. After emptying the stomach, administer activated charcoal 1 g/kg; follow with a saline cathartic. Acidification of the urine increases amphetamine excretion. Administer fluids until urine flow is 3 to 6 ml/kg/hr; mannitol or furosemide may help. Experience with hemodialysis and peritoneal dialysis is inadequate to permit recommendations.

Maintain patient in a cool room, monitor temperature and minimize external stimulation. Haloperidol may be administered to treat psychotic symptoms. Diazepam or barbiturates may be effective in the treatment of hyperactivity.

If acute, severe hypertension complicates amphetamine overdosage, administration of IV phentolamine has been suggested. However, a gradual drop in blood pressure usually results from sufficient sedation. Chlorpromazine has been useful in decreasing CNS stimulation and sympathomimetic effects. If cardiovascular collapse occurs, treat with fluid replacement; if necessary, administer a vasopressor.

Since much of the long-acting form of medication is coated for gradual release, direct therapy at reversing the effects of the ingested drug and at supporting the patient; continue until overdosage symptoms subside. Use saline cathartics to hasten the evacuation of pellets that have not released medication.

Patient Information:

Take early in the day (especially sustained release dosage forms) to avoid nighttime insomnia.

Do not chew or crush sustained release or long-acting tablets.

Do not increase dosage, except on physician's advice.

May impair ability to drive or perform other tasks requiring alertness. May mask extreme fatigue and cause dizziness.

May cause nervousness, restlessness, insomnia, dizziness, anorexia, dry mouth and GI disturbances. Notify physician if these effects become pronounced.

Administration and Dosage:

Administer at the lowest effective dosage and adjust individually. Avoid late evening doses, particularly with the long-acting form, because of the resulting insomnia.

When treating the attention deficit disorder in children, occasionally interrupt drug administration to determine if there is a recurrence of behavioral symptoms sufficient to require continued therapy.

When used for obesity, intermittent or interrupted courses of therapy may be useful. A 3 to 6 week course of therapy followed by a discontinuation period of half the original treatment length has been suggested.

AMPHETAMINE SULFATE (Racemic Amphetamine Sulfate)

Complete prescribing information for these products begins in the Amphetamines group monograph.

Administration and Dosage:

Narcolepsy: 5 to 60 mg/day in divided doses.

Children (6 to 12 years) – Narcolepsy seldom occurs in children under 12. When it does, initial dose is 5 mg daily; increase in increments of 5 mg at weekly intervals until optimal response is obtained (maximum 60 mg/day).

Adults (12 years and older) – Start with 10 mg daily; raise in increments of 10 mg/day at weekly intervals. If adverse reactions appear (eg, insomnia or anorexia), reduce dose. Long-acting forms may be used for once-a-day dosage. With tablets or elixir, give first dose on awakening; additional doses (1 or 2) at intervals of 4 to 6 hours.

Attention deficit disorder in children:

Not recommended for children under 3 years of age.

Children (3 to 5 years) – 2.5 mg daily; increase in increments of 2.5 mg/day at weekly intervals until optimal response is obtained. Usual range is 0.1 to 0.5 mg/kg/dose every morning.

Children (6 years and older) – 5 mg once or twice daily; increase in increments of 5 mg/day at weekly intervals until optimal response is obtained. Dosage will rarely exceed 40 mg/day. Usual range is 0.1 to 0.5 mg/kg/dose every morning.

Long-acting forms may be used for once-a-day dosage. With tablets or elixir, give first dose on awakening; additional doses (1 or 2) may be given at intervals of 4 to 6 hours.

Exogenous obesity: 5 to 30 mg daily in divided doses of 5 to 10 mg, 30 to 60 minutes before meals. Long-acting form: 10 or 15 mg in the morning. Not recommended for children under 12 years of age.

c-II	**Amphetamine Sulfate** (Lannett)	**Tablets**: 5 mg	In 1000s.
		10 mg	In 1000s.

DEXTROAMPHETAMINE SULFATE

Complete prescribing information for these products begins in the Amphetamines group monograph.

Administration and Dosage:

See amphetamine sulfate.

c-II	**Dextroamphetamine Sulfate** (Various)	**Tablets**: 5 mg	In 500s and 1000s.
c-II	**Dexedrine** (SKF)		Tartrazine. (SKF E19). Orange, scored. In 100s and 1000s.
c-II	**Dextrostat** (Richwood)		Sucrose, lactose, tartrazine. (RP 51). Yellow, scored. In 100s.
c-II	**Dextroamphetamine Sulfate** (Various)	**Tablets**: 10 mg	In 500s and 1000s.
c-II	**Oxydess II** (Vortech)		In 100s.
c-II	**Dexedrine Spansules** (SKF)	**Capsules, sustained release**: 5 mg	Tartrazine. (SKF E12). Natural and brown. In 50s.
c-II	**Dexedrine Spansules** (SKF)	**Capsules, sustained release**: 10 mg	Tartrazine. (SKF E13). Natural and brown. In 50s and 500s.
c-II	**Dextroamphetamine Sulfate** (Various)	**Capsules, sustained release**: 15 mg	In 250s.
c-II	**Dexedrine Spansules** (SKF)		Tartrazine. (SKF E14). Natural and brown. In 50s and 500s.
c-II	**Spancap No. 1** (Vortech)		In 1000s.

METHAMPHETAMINE HCl (Desoxyephedrine HCl)

For complete prescribing information for these products, refer to the Amphetamines general monograph.

Administration and Dosage:

Attention deficit disorder in children: Initially, 5 mg once or twice a day; increase in increments of 5 mg/day at weekly intervals until an optimum response is achieved. Usual effective dose is 20 to 25 mg daily.

Total daily dose may be given as conventional tablets in 2 divided doses, or once daily using the long-acting form. Do not use the long-acting form for initiation of dosage or until the titrated daily dose is equal to or greater than the dosage provided in a long-acting tablet. Where possible, interrupt drug administration to determine if there is a recurrence of behavioral symptoms sufficient to require continued therapy.

Obesity: 5 mg, 30 minutes before each meal.

Long-acting form – 10 to 15 mg in the morning.

Treatment duration should not exceed a few weeks. Do not use in children under 12 years old.

c-II	**Desoxyn** (Abbott)	**Tablets**: 5 mg	White. In 100s.
c-II	**Desoxyn Gradumet** (Abbott)	**Tablets, long-acting:** 5 mg	(MC). White. In 100s.
		10 mg	(ME). Orange. In 100s.
		15 mg	Tartrazine. (MF). Yellow. In 100s.

AMPHETAMINE MIXTURES

For complete prescribing information for these products, refer to the Amphetamines group monograph.

These mixtures contain various salts of amphetamine and dextroamphetamine.

Administration and Dosage:

Refer to Administration and Dosage of Amphetamine Sulfate.

c-II	**Adderall** (Richwood)	**Tablets**: 10 mg (2.5 mg dextroamphetamine sulfate, 2.5 mg dextroamphetamine saccharate, 2.5 mg amphetamine aspartate, 2.5 mg amphetamine sulfate)	Lactose. (OP-32). Blue, scored. In 100s.
		20 mg (5 mg dextroamphetamine sulfate, 5 mg dextroamphetamine saccharate, 5 mg amphetamine aspartate, 5 mg amphetamine sulfate)	Lactose. (OP-33). Orange, scored. In 100s.

ANOREXIANTS

In addition to the nonamphetamine anorexiants included in this section, amphetamines are also used for short-term obesity therapy.

Actions:

Pharmacology: The nonamphetamine anorexiants, commonly known as "anorectics" or "anorexigenics", are indirect-acting sympathomimetic amines. Except for mazindol (an imidazoline), phenmetrazine and phendimetrazine (morpholines), all are phenethylamine (amphetamine-like) analogs, and are pharmacologically similar to the amphetamines.

Although the exact mechanism of action has not been established, it is thought that appetite suppression is produced by a direct stimulant effect on the satiety center in the hypothalamic and limbic regions. Diethylpropion and phentermine act primarily on adrenergic pathways; mazindol acts on both adrenergic and dopaminergic pathways; fenfluramine influences serotonin pathways. Secondary actions include CNS stimulation and blood pressure elevation. Fenfluramine differs from other drugs of this class since it produces CNS depression. Fenfluramine's mechanism of action may be related to brain levels (or turnover rates) of serotonin or to increased glucose utilization.

Pharmacokinetics:

Absorption – After oral administration, the immediate release dosage forms generally exert their effects for 4 to 6 hours, except for mazindol (8 to 15 hours).

Fenfluramine is well absorbed from the GI tract and a maximal anorectic effect generally occurs in 2 to 4 hours.

Distribution – Fenfluramine is widely distributed in body tissues. It is lipid soluble and crosses the blood-brain barrier. Diethylpropion and its active metabolites cross the blood brain barrier and the placenta.

Excretion – Most of the drug and metabolites are excreted via the kidneys. The elimination rate of fenfluramine is pH-dependent; much smaller amounts appear in an alkaline urine than in an acid urine.

The half-life of fenfluramine is about 20 hours compared with 5 hours for amphetamines and from 1.9 to 9.8 hours for phendimetrazine tartrate. Fenfluramine's half-life can be reduced to 11 hours if urinary excretion is rapid and the pH is acidic (< pH 5). Fenfluramine reaches steady-state concentrations in plasma within 3 to 4 days following chronic dosage.

Clinical trials: Short-term clinical trials report greater weight loss in adult obese subjects treated with dietary management and anorexiants vs those treated with diet and placebo. The rate of weight loss is greatest in the first weeks of therapy and decreases in succeeding weeks. The amount of weight loss varies from trial to trial, and appears to be related, in part, to variables other than the drug prescribed, such as the investigator, the population treated and the diet prescribed.

Clinical studies demonstrate that anorexiants with behavior therapy produce better weight loss in obese patients than either therapy alone; however, better weight loss maintenance is achieved with behavior therapy alone.

Factors influencing successful treatment and anorexiant use include: Weight loss during diet alone; eating habits; motivation; personality; obesity characteristics; and adherence to treatment.

Indications:

Exogenous obesity: As a short-term (8 to 12 weeks) adjunct in a regimen of weight reduction based on caloric restriction. Measure the limited usefulness of these agents against their inherent risks.

Unlabeled uses: Preliminary studies suggest fenfluramine may be useful in treating autistic children with elevated serotonin levels. Adverse effects have occurred when used in autistic children without elevated serotonin levels.

Contraindications:

Advanced arteriosclerosis; symptomatic cardiovascular disease; moderate to severe hypertension; hyperthyroidism; known hypersensitivity or idiosyncrasy to sympathomimetic amines; glaucoma; agitated states; history of drug abuse; during or within 14 days following the administration of MAO inhibitors (hypertensive crises may result); coadministration with other CNS stimulants.

Do not administer fenfluramine to alcoholics, since psychiatric symptoms (paranoia, depression, psychosis) have been reported in a few such patients.

Pregnancy: Category X. Benzphetamine HCl is contraindicated during pregnancy (see Warnings).

ANOREXIANTS

Warnings:

Concomitant surgical anesthesia: A fatal cardiac arrest occurred shortly after the induction of anesthesia in a patient who had been taking **fenfluramine** prior to surgery. Fenfluramine may have a catecholamine-depleting effect when administered for prolonged periods; administer potent anesthetics cautiously to patients taking fenfluramine. Full cardiac monitoring and facilities for resuscitative measures are necessary.

Tolerance to the anorectic effects may develop within a few weeks; cross tolerance is almost universal. Discontinue the drug rather than increase the dosage. It has been suggested that therapy may be continued past 12 weeks if the patient continues to lose weight, does not develop dependence or side effects, and does not require an increased dosage. However, patients should be closely monitored and therapy should not exceed 6 months duration.

Drug dependence: These drugs are chemically and pharmacologically related to the amphetamines, and have abuse potential. Intense psychological or physical dependence and severe social dysfunction may be associated with long-term therapy or abuse. If this occurs, gradually reduce the dosage to avoid withdrawal symptoms (eg, extreme fatigue, sleep EEG changes and mental depression). Chronic intoxication is manifested by severe dermatoses, marked insomnia, irritability, hyperactivity and personality changes. Psychosis, often clinically indistinguishable from schizophrenia, is the most severe manifestation.

Fenfluramine's abuse potential appears qualitatively different. Doses of 80 to 400 mg were associated with euphoria, derealization and perceptual changes.

Pregnancy: (Category X - Benzphetamine HCl. Category C – Fenfluramine. Category B - Diethylpropion). Safety for use during pregnancy has not been established. Use in women who are or who may become pregnant (especially those in the first trimester) only when clearly needed and when the potential benefits outweigh the potential hazards to the fetus.

In animal studies with relatively high doses of **mazindol**, neonatal mortality and incidence of rib anomalies were increased; with **phenmetrazine**, conception rate was adversely affected, as well as survival and body weight of pups. Congenital malformations are associated with phenmetrazine use, but a causal relationship has not been proven. **Fenfluramine** produced questionable embryotoxic effects in rats and a reduced conception rate when given in doses 20 times the human dose. Other studies were negative. Animal and clinical studies have not shown a teratogenic potential for **diethylpropion**. Abuse of diethylpropion during pregnancy may result in withdrawal symptoms in the human neonate.

Lactation: Safety for use in the nursing mother has not been established.

Diethylpropion and its metabolites are excreted in breast milk. Exercise caution when administering to a nursing woman.

Children: Not recommended for use in children under 12 years of age.

Precautions:

Potentially hazardous tasks: May produce dizziness, extreme fatigue and depression after abrupt cessation of prolonged high dosage therapy; patients should observe caution while driving or performing other tasks requiring alertness.

Psychological disturbances occurred in patients who received an anorectic agent together with a restrictive diet.

Cardiovascular disease: Use with caution and monitor blood pressure in patients with mild hypertension. Not recommended for patients with symptomatic cardiovascular disease, including arrhythmias.

Pulmonary hypertension occurred in two females taking **fenfluramine** (120 to 160 mg/day) for over 8 months. Symptoms disappeared 3 to 6 weeks after drug discontinuation. In one patient, pulmonary hypertension recurred on rechallenge (80 mg daily for 6 weeks). Advise patients to immediately report any deterioration in exercise tolerance.

Convulsions may increase in some epileptics receiving **diethylpropion**. Dose titration or drug discontinuance may be necessary.

Depression:

Fenfluramine's central effects are mediated by 5-hydroxytryptamine (5-HT) in the brain stem. A rapid reduction in 5-HT in the brain can lead to depression. This commonly occurs immediately following abrupt withdrawal of fenfluramine; therefore, do not discontinue abruptly. Depression may be provoked while the patient is taking fenfluramine or following abrupt withdrawal, especially in those with a history of mental depression. Control symptoms of depression by reinstituting therapy; follow by gradual withdrawal.

ANOREXIANTS

Blood glucose levels: **Mazindol** and **fenfluramine** moderately lower blood glucose levels independent of appetite suppressant effects by increasing glucose uptake in human skeletal muscle.

Tartrazine sensitivity: Some of these products contain tartrazine, which may cause allergic-type reactions (including bronchial asthma) in susceptible individuals. Although the incidence of tartrazine sensitivity in the general population is low, it is frequently seen in patients who also have aspirin hypersensitivity. Specific products containing tartrazine are identified in the product listings.

Drug Interactions:

Guanethidine: Anorexiants may decrease the hypotensive effect of guanethidine.

Insulin and sulfonylureas: Hypoglycemic effects may be increased due to increased skeletal muscle uptake of glucose by fenfluramine. Monitor blood glucose and adjust the insulin or sulfonylurea dose as necessary.

Monoamine oxidase (MAO) inhibitors may increase the pressor response to the anorexiants. Possible hypertensive crisis and intracranial hemorrhage may occur. This interaction may also occur with **furazolidone**, an antimicrobial with MAO inhibitor activity. Avoid this combination; if given inadvertently and hypertension occurs, administer phentolamine.

Tricyclic antidepressants may decrease the effects of the anorexiants. An increased dose may be necessary.

Adverse Reactions:

Cardiovascular: Palpitations; tachycardia; arrhythmias; hypertension or hypotension; fainting; precordial pain; pulmonary hypertension. ECG changes with diethylpropion.

CNS: Overstimulation; nervousness; restlessness; dizziness; insomnia; weakness or fatigue; malaise; anxiety; tension; euphoria; elevated mood; drowsiness; depression; agitation; dysphoria; tremor; dyskinesia; dysarthria; confusion; incoordination; tremor; headache; change in libido; rarely, psychotic episodes. An increase in convulsive episodes occurred in a few epileptics.

Fenfluramine may cause CNS depression, drowsiness and impotence. Withdrawal symptoms (ataxia, tremor, disturbed concentration and memory, loss of sense of reality, visual hallucinations, inverted visual field, depression, suicidal feelings) have been reported following discontinuation of a 1 month course of fenfluramine, 60 mg/day.

GI: Dry mouth; unpleasant taste; nausea; vomiting; abdominal discomfort; diarrhea; constipation; stomach pain.

Hypersensitivity: Urticaria; rash; erythema; burning sensation.

Ophthalmic: Mydriasis; eye irritation; blurred vision.

GU: Dysuria; polyuria; urinary frequency; impotence; menstrual upset. Testicular pain has been reported with **mazindol**.

Hematologic: Bone marrow depression; agranulocytosis; leukopenia.

Miscellaneous: Hair loss; ecchymosis; muscle pain; chest pain; excessive sweating; clamminess; chills; flushing; fever; myalgia; gynecomastia.

Overdosage:

Symptoms:

CNS – Restlessness; tremor; hyperreflexia; rapid respiration; hyperpyrexia; tachypnea; dizziness; confusion; belligerence; assaultiveness; hallucinations; panic states. Depression and fatigue usually follow central stimulation.

Convulsions, coma and death may result.

Cardiovascular – Arrhythmias (tachycardia); hypertension or hypotension; circulatory collapse.

GI – Nausea; vomiting; diarrhea; abdominal cramps.

Fenfluramine –

Frequent: Agitation and drowsiness; confusion; flushing; tremor (or shivering); fever; sweating; abdominal pain; hyperventilation; rotary nystagmus; dilated nonreactive pupils. Reflexes may be either exaggerated or depressed. Tachycardia may be present; blood pressure may be normal or only slightly elevated. Convulsions, coma and ventricular extrasystoles, culminating in ventricular fibrillation and cardiac arrest, may occur at higher dosage; death has occurred.

Doses less than 5 mg/kg are toxic; 5 to 10 mg/kg may produce coma and convulsions. Reported single overdoses have ranged from 300 to 2000 mg; the lowest reported fatal dose was a few hundred milligrams in a small child and the highest reported nonfatal dose was 1800 mg in an adult. Most deaths were due to respiratory failure and cardiac arrest.

ANOREXIANTS

Toxic effects appear within 30 to 60 minutes and may progress rapidly to potentially fatal complications in 1.5 to 4 hours. Symptoms may persist for extended periods depending upon amount ingested.

Treatment: Includes symptomatic and supportive therapy. Refer to Management of Acute Overdosage.

Sedate patient with a barbiturate, maintain respiratory exchange and cardiac monitoring. Chlorpromazine may antagonize the CNS effects when excess CNS stimulation is present. If an anticholinergic drug has been taken recently, administer an antipsychotic without prominent anticholinergic actions (eg, haloperidol). IV phentolamine, a nitrite or a rapidly acting alpha receptor blocking agent may be useful in treating acute, severe hypertension.

Experience with hemodialysis or peritoneal dialysis is inadequate to permit recommendations. Acidification of urine increases excretion.

Fenfluramine – Do not induce emesis because the patient may become unconscious at an early stage. If gastric lavage is not feasible due to trismus, perform endotracheal intubation after administration of muscle relaxants; then induce gastric evacuation. Administer activated charcoal after emesis or lavage. If necessary, institute mechanical respiration, defibrillation or cardioversion. Administer diazepam or phenobarbital for convulsions or muscular hyperactivity; propranolol for extreme tachycardia; lidocaine for ventricular extrasystoles; chlorpromazine for hyperpyrexia. After overdosage, only a small percentage of fenfluramine is excreted in the urine. Forced acid diuresis has been recommended only in extreme cases in which the patient survives the early hours of intoxication but fails to show decisive improvement from other measures.

Since fenfluramine has a slight lowering effect on blood sugar, hypoglycemia may occur; however, this effect has not been reported in clinical overdosage cases.

Patient Information:

May cause insomnia; avoid taking medication late in the day.

Weight reduction requires strict adherence to dietary restriction.

Do not take more frequently than prescribed.

Notify physician if palpitations, nervousness or dizziness occurs.

Medication may cause dry mouth and constipation; notify physician if these become pronounced.

May produce dizziness or blurred vision; observe caution while driving or performing other tasks requiring alertness.

Fenfluramine may cause drowsiness. Avoid concomitant consumption of alcohol.

These drugs should generally be taken on an empty stomach; mazindol may be taken with meals to reduce GI irritation.

Do not crush or chew sustained release products.

Administration and Dosage:

Intermittent or interrupted courses of therapy may be useful in the treatment of obesity. A 3 to 6 week course of therapy followed by a discontinuation period of half the original treatment length has been suggested.

PHENTERMINE HCl

Complete prescribing information begins in the Anorexiants group monograph.

Administration and Dosage:

Take 8 mg 3 times daily, one-half hour before meals, or 15 to 37.5 mg as a single daily dose before breakfast or 10 to 14 hours before retiring.

c-i	**Phentermine HCl** (Various)	**Tablets**: 8 mg (equivalent to 6.4 mg base)	In 100s and 1000s.
c-iv	**Phentrol** (Vortech)		In 100s.
c-iv	**Phentermine HCl** (Various)	**Capsules**: 15 mg (equivalent to 12 mg base)	In 100s and 1000s.
c-iv	**Ionamin** (Medeva)	**Capsules**: 15 mg phentermine resin	(Ionamin 15). Yellow. In 100s and 400s.
c-iv	**Phentermine HCl** (Camall)	**Capsules**: 18.75 mg (equivalent to 15 mg base)	(CC 18.75). Gray and yellow. In 100s, 500s and 1000s.
c-iv	**Phentermine HCl** (Various)	**Tablets**: 30 mg (equivalent to 24 mg base)	In 100s and 1000s.
c-iv	**Phentermine HCl** (Various)	**Capsules**: 30 mg (equivalent to 24 mg base)	In 7s, 30s, 100s and 1000s.
c-iv	**Fastin** (Beecham Labs.)		(Beecham/Fastin). Blue/clear. In 100s, 450s, UD 150s.
c-iv	**Obephen** (Hauck)		Yellow. In 1000s.
c-iv	**OBY-CAP** (Richwood)		Lactose. (RPC-69). Yellow. In 100s and 500s.
c-iv	**Phentrol 2** (Vortech)		In 1000s.
c-iv	**Phentrol 4** (Vortech)		In 1000s.
c-iv	**Phentrol 5** (Vortech)		In 1000s.
c-iv	**Zantryl** (Ion)		In 100s.
c-iv	**Ionamin** (Medeva)	**Capsules**: 30 mg phentermine resin	(Ionamin 30). Yellow. In 100s and 400s.
c-iv	**Phentermine HCl** (Various)	**Tablets**: 37.5 mg (equivalent to 30 mg base)	In 30s, 100s, 500s, 1000s.
c-iv	**Adipex-P** (Lemmon)		(Lemmon 9). Blue and white, scored. In 100s, 400s and 1000s.
c-iv	**Phentermine HCl** (Camall)	**Capsules**: 37.5 mg (equivalent to 30 mg base)	In 100s, 500s and 1000s.
c-iv	**Adipex-P** (Lemmon)		(Adipex-P 37.5). Blue and white. In 100s, 400s and 1000s.
c-iv	**Obe-Nix 30** (Holloway)		In 100s.
c-iv	**Phentermine Resin** (Various)	**Capsules**: 15 mg (as resin complex)	In 100s.
c-iv	**Ionamin** (Pennwalt)		(Ionamin 15). Yellow and gray. In 100s and 400s.
c-iv	**Phentermine Resin** (Various)	**Capsules**: 30 mg (as resin complex)	In 100s and 400s.
c-iv	**Ionamin** (Pennwalt)		(Ionamin 30). Yellow. In 100s and 400s.

BENZPHETAMINE HCl

For complete prescribing information, refer to the Anorexiants group monograph.

Administration and Dosage:

Initiate dosage with 25 to 50 mg once daily; increase according to response. Dosage ranges from 25 to 50 mg, 1 to 3 times daily.

c-III	**Didrex** (Upjohn)	**Tablets**: 25 mg	Sorbitol; tartrazine. (Upjohn 18). Yellow. In 100s.
		50 mg	Sorbitol. (Didrex 50). Peach, scored. In 100s and 500s.

PHENDIMETRAZINE TARTRATE

Complete prescribing information begins in the Anorexiants group monograph.

Administration and Dosage:

Tablets and capsules: 35 mg 2 or 3 times daily, 1 hour before meals.

Sustained release capsules: 105 mg once daily in the morning before breakfast.

c-III	**Phendimetrazine** (Various, eg, Major, Moore, Rugby, URL)	**Tablets**: 35 mg	In 100s and 1000s.
c-III	**Bontril PDM** (Carnrick)		(C 8648). Green, white and yellow layered. Scored. In 100s and 1000s.
c-III	**Plegine** (Ayerst)		(Plegine 35). Scored. In 100s and 1000s.
c-III	**Phendimetrazine Tartrate** (Various, eg, IDE)	**Capsules**: 35 mg	In 1000s.
c-III	**Phendimetrazine Tartrate** (Various, eg, IDE, Hyrex, Rexar)	**Capsules, sustained release**: 105 mg	In 100s, 250s and 500s.
c-III	**Adipost** (Jones)		(225-470). White and clear. In 100s.
c-III	**Bontril Slow-Release** (Carnrick)		(C 8647). Green and yellow. In 100s and 1000s.
c-III	**Dital** (UAD)		In 100s.
c-III	**Dyrexan-OD** (Trimen)		(Trimen/Trimen). Brown and clear. In 100s.
c-III	**Melfiat-105 Unicelles** (Numark)		(RPL 1082). Orange and clear. In 100s.
c-III	**Prelu-2** (Boehringer-Ingelheim)		Celery and green. In 100s.
c-III	**Rexigen Forte** (ION Labs)		(Rexigen Forte). Blue and orange. In 100s.

DIETHYLPROPION HCl

Complete prescribing information begins in the Anorexiants group monograph.

Administration and Dosage:

Tablets: 25 mg 3 times daily, 1 hour before meals, and in midevening if needed to overcome night hunger.

Sustained release tablets: 75 mg once daily, in midmorning.

c-IV	**Diethylpropion HCl** (Various, eg, Goldline, Jones, Moore, Rugby)	**Tablets**: 25 mg	In 100s, 500s and 1000s.
c-IV	**Tenuate** (Hoechst-Marion Roussel)		(Tenuate 25 or Merrell 697). White. In 100s.
c-IV	**Diethylpropion** (Various, eg, Goldline, Major, Qualitest, Rugby, URL)	**Tablets, sustained release**: 75 mg	In 100s, 250s, 500s and 1000s.
c-IV	**Tenuate Dospan** (Hoechst-Marion Roussel)		(Tenuate 75 or Merrell 698). White. In UD 100s and 250s.

MAZINDOL

Complete prescribing information begins in the Anorexiants group monograph.

Administration and Dosage:

Usual dose is 1 mg 3 times daily, 1 hour before meals, or 2 mg once daily, 1 hour before lunch. Initiate therapy at 1 mg once a day and adjust to patient response. Take with meals to avoid GI discomfort.

c-iv	**Mazanor** (Wyeth Ayerst)	**Tablets:** 1 mg	(Wyeth 71). White, scored. In 30s.
c-iv	**Sanorex** (Sandoz)	**Tablets:** 1 mg	(Sanorex 78-71). White. In 100s.
		2 mg	(Sandoz 78-66). White, scored. In 100s.

FENFLURAMINE HCl

Complete prescribing information begins in the Anorexiants group monograph.

Administration and Dosage:

Usual dose: 20 mg 3 times daily, before meals. May increase at weekly intervals by 20 mg daily to a maximum of 40 mg 3 times daily, depending on the degree of effectiveness and side effects. Total dosage should not exceed 120 mg/day.

c-iv	**Pondimin** (Robins)	**Tablets:** 20 mg	(AHR 6447). Orange, scored. In 100s and 500s.

DEXFENFLURAMINE

Actions:

Pharmacology: Defenfluramine, an anti-obesity drug, is a serotonin reuptake inhibitor and releasing agent. The action of dexfenfluramine in treating obesity is primarily via decreased caloric intake associated with increased serotonin levels in brain synapses. In vitro, the drug inhibits serotonin reuptake by axon terminals and causes the release of serotonin from synaptosomes. In animals, the reduced caloric intake and the loss in body weight elicited by dexfenfluramine is associated with release of serotonin from presynaptic axon terminals in the brain, inhibition of neuronal serotonin reuptake and therefore, an increase of serotonin receptor activation. This results in an enhancement of serotoninergic transmission in the centers of feeding behavior located in the ventromedial nucleus of the hypothalmus. In rats, enhanced serotoninergic transmission induced by defenfluramine slectively suppressed appetite for carbohydrates which resulted in reduction of food consumption when the dietary carbohydrate to protein ration was high. Unlike amphetamines and other serotonin-active agonists and antagonists, dexfenfluramine neither enhances nor suppresses dopamine-mediated neuro-transmission.

In clinical trials, dexfenfluramine treatment in conjunction with a reduced calorie diet is associated with a reduction in appetite and may slow gastric emptying. These and other actions may contribute to the reduction in caloric consumption associated with dexfenfluramine. In one clinical trial, dexfenfluramine was shown to preferentially decrease carbohydrate consumption at meals and to manage carbohydrate craving between meals by decreasing the consumption of snack foods with a high carbohydrate content in patients who frequently snack on such foods.

Observational epidemiological studies have established a relationship between obesity and the risks for cardiovascular disease, non-insulin dependent diabetes mellitus (NIDDM), certain forms of cancer, gallstones, certain respiratory disorders and an increase in overall mortality. These studies suggest that weight loss, if maintained, may produce health benefits for some patients with chronic obesity who may also be at risk for other disease.

The long-term effects of dexfenfluramine on the morbidity and mortality associated with obesity have not been established. Some short-term studies have suggested that weight loss with dexfenfluramine may be associated with a reduction in hyperglycemia in obese diabetic patients, a reduction in blood pressure in obese hypertensive patients and improvement in the lipid profile in obese hyperlipidemic patients.

Pharmacokinetics:

Absorption/Distribution – Dexfenfluramine is completely absorbed after oral dosing with a systemic bioavailability of ≈ 68% because of first-pass metabolism by the liver. Following a single 30 mg oral dose, mean peak plasma concentrations ranged between 11 and 41 ng/ml after 1.5 to 8 hours. The average terminal elimination half-life of plasma dexfenfluramine ranged from 17 to 20 hours and the average total body clearance was 691.9 ml/min. Following doses of 15 mcg twice a day for 15 days, mean maximal plasma concentrations ranging from 15 to 92 ng/ml were observed, and steady-state plasma levels were achieved 8 days after the initial dose. The major active metabolite, d-norfenfluramine accumulated to maximal plasma concentrations of ≈ 26 ng/ml, with steady-state plasma levels occurring at ≈ 9 days. The d-norfenfluramine plasma half-life is estimated to be 32 hours. Following administration of single 30, 40, and 60 mg to healthy volunteers, dexfenfluramine C_{max} values of 25, 33 and 51 ng/ml and area-under-the-curve values of 144, 191 and 275 ng•hr/ml, respectively, were found. In a dose-response study of dexfenfluramine involving obese patients treated for 12 weeks, dexfenfluramine C_{min} values of 24 ng/ml at a dose of 15 mg twice daily and 58 ng/ml at a dose of 30 mg twice daily were observed. These data suggest that plasma concentrations of dexfenfluramine increase in proportion to the administered dose.

At a dexfenfluramine plasma concentration of 100 ng/ml, 36% is bound to plasma proteins. Dexfenfluramine is distributed into body tissue in non-obese subjects with a volume of distribution of 839 L.

Metabolism/Excretion – Dexfenfluramine is metabolized in the liver. The first steps in the metabolism are dealkylation, resulting in formation of the active metabolite, d-norfenfluramine and deamination to an inactive hydroxy derivative. In a study of drug metabolism using radiolabeled dexfenfluramine, levo-fenfluramine and d,l-fenfluramine in two healthy subjects, 92% of the administered radioactivity was found in urine and 1% in feces over 6 days. Fenfluramine accounted for 7% to 19% and norfenfluramine accounted for 4% to 11% of the urine radioactivity. Other metabolites (inactive) included 1–(m-trifluoromethylphenyl) — 1,2–propane diol (21% to 38%), m-tri-fluoromethyl benzoic acid (7% to 22%), m-trifluoromethyl hippuric acid (< 1% to 11%) and 1–(m-trifluoro-methylphenyl)-propan-2–ol (2% to 4%).

Clinical trials: Dexfenfluramine has been shown to be effective in reducing excess body weight in obese patients in 16 of 17 trials where all patients were on reduced-calorie

DEXFENFLURAMINE

diets. Dexfenfluramine-treated patients lost statistically significantly more weight on average than those treated with placebo. In these studies, weight loss was evident within 4 weeks of initiating treatment, even in some patients where reduced-calorie diet alone had failed to induce a significant weight loss.

In a one year double-blind, placebo controlled trial of obese patients, dexfenfluramine in conjunction with a reduced-calorie diet produced a significant reduction in weight during the first 4 to 6 months. This response was maintained during continuation of therapy (up to 12 months of treatment). The percentage of patients who achieved various levels of weight loss at 1 year are shown below.

Percentage of Patients Losing Weight at 1 Year: Dexfenfluramine vs Placebo (%)						
	≥ 15% loss		≥ 10% loss		≥ 5% loss	
Patients	Dexfenfluramine	Placebo	Dexfenfluramine	Placebo	Dexfenfluramine	Placebo
Completers[1]	29 (n = 297)	16 (n = 262)	52 (n = 297)	30 (n = 262)	72 (n = 297)	50 (n = 262)
All patients[2]	21 (n = 463)	10 (n = 467)	40 (n = 463)	21 (n = 467)	64 (n = 463)	43 (n = 467)

[1] Data for patients who completed the entire 12 month period trial.

[2] Data for all patients who received study drug and who had any post-baseline measurement for those patients who discontinued treatment before 12 months the last observed data is carried forward through the end of the study and analyzed with data from patients who completed the trial.

Based on another analysis of the study, among all patients who were treated with dexfenfluramine and identified as initial responders (ie, lost at least 4 pounds in the first 4 weeks of therapy), 60% went on to lose ≥ 10% of their initial body weight by the end of 1 year of treatment. Among dexfenfluriamine-treated patients, 78% were identified as initial responders. At the end of the year, the mean weight loss for the initial responders was 22 pounds, while the non-responders had a mean weight loss of 6 pounds.

Among obese patients who had been successful in losing weight by dieting alone (ie, lost at least 10 pounds in the prior year), the addition of dexfenfluramine to the regimen resulted in the further loss of 26% of initial excess weight, while successful dieters who received placebo lost only 7% of initial excess weight.

Indications:

Obesity: Management of obesity including weight loss and a reduced-calorie diet. Dexfenfluramine is recommended for obese patients with an initial body mass index ≥ 30 kg/m^2 or ≥ 27 kg/m^2 in the presence of other risk factors (eg, hypertension, diabetes, hyperlipidemia).

Contraindications:

Diagnosed pulmonary hypertension (see Warnings); patients receiving monamine oxidase inhibitors (see Drug Interactions); hypersensitivity to dexfenfluramine, fenfluramine or related compounds.

Warnings:

Primary pulmonary hypertension: A 2 year international (5 country), case controlled (epidemiological) study identified 95 primary pulmonary hypertension (PPH) cases; 20 of these had been exposed to anorexigens in the past, and 9 of 20 had been exposed to anorexigens for > 3 months. In this study, the use of anorexigens for > 3 months was associated with an increased risk of developing PPH. The increased risk of PPH was concentrated in persons who had used the drugs within the preceding year; there was no significant increase in risk for persons who had taken the drugs for > 1 year ago or for persons who had used these agents for ≤ 3 months. In the general population, the yearly occurrence of PPH is estimated to be about 1 to 2 cases per 1,000,000 persons. Therefore, the case control study indicated an estimated risk associated with the long-term use of anorexigen drugs of about 18 cases per million persons exposed per year. According to the case control study, obesity itself (body mass index ≥ 30 kg/m^2) was also associated with an increase of about 2–fold in the risk of developing PPH.

PPH is a serious condition; the 4 year survival rate has been reported to be 55%.

The initial symptom of pulmonary hypertension is generally dyspnea. Other initial symptoms include: Angina pectoris, syncope or lower extremity edema. Advise patients to report immediately any deterioration in exercise tolerance. Treatment should be discontinued in patients who develop new, unexplained symptoms of dyspnea, angina pectoris, syncope or lower extremity edema. These patients should be evaluated for the etiology of these symptoms and the possible presence of pulmonary hypertension.

Long-term use: The safety and efficacy of dexfenfluramine use for > 1 year have not been determined at this time.

DEXFENFLURAMINE

Diagnosis: Exclude organic causes of obesity (eg, hypothyroidism) before prescribing dexfenfluramine.

Glaucoma: Use with caution in patients with glaucoma.

Elderly: The pharmacokinetics of a single 30 mg dose of dexfenfluramine in eight elderly patients, ranging from 66 to 83 years of age have been examined in one study. The mean maximal plasma concentration was 21.8 ng/ml (range, 9.7 to 33). Time to maximal plasma concentration was about 5 hours (rangs, 3 to 10). Area under the curve to infinity was 615 ng•hr/ml (range 16 to 1205). Mean steady-state plasma concentrations of dexfenfluramine and d-norfenfluramine after 6 months of treatment (15 mg twice daily) to 18 obese patients > 60 years old were 27.3 and 14 ng/ml, respectively, compared to values of 24.1 and 15.6, respectively, in 268 patients < 60 years old. In a cohort of these patients followed through 12 months of treatment (15 mg twice daily), mean steady-state plasma concentrations of dexfenfluramine and d-norfenfluramine in 17 obese patients > 60 years old were 32.9 and 18 ng/ml, respectively, compared to values of 23.9 and 14.4, respectively, in 186 obese patients < 60 years old.

As with all CNS-active medications, exercise caution in treating elderly patients with dexfenfluramine.

Pregnancy: Category C. Dexfenfluramine produced dose-related effects on reproduction and fertility in rats. Administration of dexfenfluramine to female rats at 2.5 and 5 times the human daily dose caused significant reductions in body weight and weight gain throughout pregnancy. The number of placental implantations and fetuses was reduced, there was a reduced number of live young and delayed ossification was seen in the fetuses.

There are no adequate and well controlled studies in pregnant women and its use is not recommended in these patients.

Lactation: Dexfenfluramine is excreted in rat milk. It is not known whether dexfenfluramine is excreted in breast milk. Therefore, do not administer to a nursing woman.

Children: Safety and efficacy in children have not been established.

Precautions:

Drowsiness: Because of dexfenfluramine's potential to produce mild-to-moderate drowsiness, assess the patient's individual response before engaging in activities requiring alertness, coordination or physical dexterity. Dexfenfluramine may potentiate the sedative effects of alcohol or other drugs with CNS action.

Intolerance: If the patient develops any symptoms of intolerance (eg, nausea and vomiting), reduce the dosage or discontinue the drug.

Misuse potential: As with any weight-loss agent, the potential exists for misuse of dexfenfluramine in inappropriate patient populations (eg, patients with anorexia nervosa or bulimia). See recommended prescribing guidelines.

Combination therapy: The safety and efficacy of dexfenfluramine in combination with other weight loss agents have not been studied; therefore, concomitant use is not recommended.

Special risk patients: Weight loss has been associated with a reduction in hyperglycemia in obese diabetic patients, a reduction of blood pressure in obese hypertensive patients, and an improvement in the lipid profile in obese hyperlipidemic patients. Therefore, when dexfenfluramine is used for the management of obesity associated with hypertension, diabetes or dyslipidemia there may be changes in these conditions and the medications used to treat them should be monitored, and adjusted, if necessary.

Drug Interactions:

Dexfenfluramine Drug Interactions			
Precipitant drug	Object drug*		Description
MAO Inhibitors	Dexfenfluramine	↑	In patients receiving nonselective MAOIs (eg, selegiline) in combination with serotoninergic agents (eg, fluoxetine, fluvoxamine, paroxetine, sertraline, venlafaxine), there have been reports of serious, sometimes fatal, reactions. Because dexfenfluramine is an SSRI, do not use concomitantly with an MAOI. At least 14 days should elapse between discontinuation of an MAOI and initiation of dexfenfluramine. At least 3 weeks should elapse between discontinuation of dexfenfluramine and initiaion of an MAOI.

DEXFENFLURAMINE

Dexfenfluramine Drug Interactions			
Precipitant drug	Object drug*		Description
Sumatriptan Dihydroergotamine	Dexfenfluramine	⬆	A rare, but serious, constellation of symptoms termed serotonin syndrome has been reported with the concomitant use of SSRIs and agents for migraine therapy (eg, sumatriptan, dihydroergotamine). The syndrome requires immediate medical attention and may include one or more of the following symptoms: Excitement, hypomania, restlessness, loss of consciousness, confusion, disorientation, anxiety, agitation, motor weakness, myoclonus, tremor, hemiballismus, hyperreflexia, ataxia, dysarthria, incoordination, hypothermia, shivering, pupillary dilation, diaphoresis, emesis and tachycardia.

* ⬆ = Object drug increased.

Drug/Lab test interactions: False-positive urine drug tests for amphetamines by ELISA have been observed for up to 24 hours following a 30 mg dose. In form patients of the possible false-positive laboratory finding when undergoing urine drug screenings. Gas chromatography/mass spectroscopy can distinguish false-positive urine drug tests caused by dexfenfluramine from true-positive drug tests.

Adverse Reactions:

Adverse reactions were generally mild and transient. The most common adverse events resulting in dixcontinuation (7%) included asthenia, insomnia, headache and depression.

Dexfenfluramine Adverse Reactions (%)		
Adverse reaction	Dexfenfluramine (15 mg twice daily) (n = 1159)	Placebo (n = 1138)
Body as a whole		
Headache	16.1	15.5
Asthenia	15.8	10.7
Abdominal pain	6.7	6
Chills	2.9	1.2
Accidental injury	2.8	2.3
Rash	2.3	2.2
Thirst	2.8	1.1
GI		
Diarrhea	17.5	7.3
Vomiting	3.2	2.9
CNS		
Insomnia	19.9	18.6
Dry mouth	12.5	5
Somnolence	7.1	3.4
Dizziness	5.5	4
Depression	4.7	3.6
Vertigo	3.1	1.7
Emotional lability	3.1	2.7
Abnormal dreams	2	1.4
Thinking abnormal	2	1.1
Respiratory		
Pharyngitis	6.1	5.6
Cough increased	3.6	3
Bronchitis	3.4	1.8
GU		
Urinary frequency	2.8	1.1
Polyuria	2.1	1

DEXFENFLURAMINE

Other adverse reactions include the following:

Body as a whole: Infection, flu syndrome, pain, back pain, fever, allergic reaction (> 1%); malaise, neck pain, chest pain, generalized edema, stress, face edema, neoplams, pelvic pain (0.1% to 1%); adenoma, immune system disorder, neck rigidity; suicide attempt (< 0.1%).

Cardiovascular: Hypertension, angina pectoris, palpitation, vasodilation, migraine (> 1%); cardiovascular disorder, tachycardia, postural hypotension, hypotension, peripheral vascular disorder, syncope, arrhythmia, extrasystoles, hemorrhage, thrombophlebitis, varicose vein (0.1% to 1%); heart block, pulmonary embolus, thrombosis (< 0.1%).

CNS: Nervousness, anxiety, increased libido, hypertonia, paresthesia (> 1%); tremor, amnesia, euphoria, decreased libido, incoordination, neuralgia, speech disorder, ataxia, hypokinesia, sleep disorder, abnormal gait, agitation, confusion, depersonalization, diplopia, hostility, hyperesthesia, hyperkinesia, peripheral neuritis (0.1% to 1%); apathy, dementia, hallucinations, hypotonia, neuritis, neurosis, paralysis (< 0.1%).

Dermatologic: Sweating, alopecia, urticaria, pruritus (> 1%); skin disorder, fungal dermatitis, hirsutism, eczema, psoriasis (0.1% to 1%); skin hypertrophy (< 0.1%).

Endocrine: Goiter, diabetes mellitus, thyroid disorder (0.1% to 1%); hypothyroidism (< 0.1%).

GI: Constipation, nausea, dyspepsia, increased appetite, rectal disorder, gastritis, gastroenteritis, flatulence (> 1%); colitis, eructation, gastrointestinal hemorrhage, enteritis, peptic ulcer, hepatitis, hepatomegaly (0.1% to 1%); appendictis, cholelithiasis, fecal incontinence, melena, mouth ulceration, pancreatitis, rectal hemorrhage, sialoadnitis (< 0.1%).

GU: Menstrual disorder, urinary tract infection, nocturia, dysmenorrhea (> 1%); amenorrhea, dysuria, oliguria, albuminuria, breast pain, kidney calculus, kidney pain (0.1% to 1%); spontaneous abortion, threatened abortion, breast neoplasm, endometrial disorder, female lactation, hematuria, impotence, mastitis, nephritis, prostatic disorder, testis disorder, urinary incontinence/retention, uterine hemorrhage (< 0.1%).

Hematologic/Lymphatic: Anemia, lymphedema (0.1% to 1%); coagulation disorder, lymphadenopathy, polycythemia, thrombocythemia (< 0.1%).

Metabolic/Nutritional: Edema, gout, hypoglycemia, hypokalemia (0.1% to 1%); hyperglycemia, hyperkalemia, hyperlipemia, hyperuricemia (< 0.1%).

Musculoskeletal: Arthralgia, myalgia, arthritis (> 1%); leg cramps, joint disorder, bone disorder, tenosynovitis, myasthenia, rheumatoid arthritis (0.1% to 1%); bursitis tetany (< 0.1%).

Respiratory: Rhinitis, sinusitis (> 1%); asthma, dyspnea, epistaxis, laryngitis (0.1% to 1%); apnea, hyperventilation (< 0.1%).

Special senses: Tast perversion, amblyopia (> 1%); abnormal vision, conjunctivitis, eye disorder, glaucoma, tinnitus, vestibular disorder, dry eyes, mydriasis (0.1% to 1%); abnormality of accommodation, anisocoria, lacrimation disorder, miosis, parosmia, retinal disorder (< 0.1%).

Overdosage:

Symptoms: Post-marketing experience in Europe over 10 years in an estimated 10 million patients provided reports of 66 instances of overdose (maximum dose per body mass of 54 mg/kg, maximum total dose of 1800 mg), including eight children ≤ 6 years of age. Three deaths have occurred in association with dexfenfluramine overdosage. One patient with a history of suicide attempts ingested 1800 mg dexfenfluramine and 20 to 30 capsules of clorazepate; one patient was found dead, assumed to have consumed ≈ 1500 mg of dexfenfluramine; the third patient consumed dexfenfluramine (quantity unknown) and several other drugs in an apparent suicide. The exact causes of death were unknown, In 23 other cases of dexfenfluramine overdose, plasma drug levels were determined; the maximum reported plasma drug level for dexfenfluramine was 778 ng/ml (with d-norfenfluramine 37 ng/ml); the maximum d-norfenfluramine level was 371 ng/ml (with dexfenfluramine 483 ng/ml).

Symptoms associated with overdosage consisted mainly of agitation, drowsiness, mydriasis, sweating, shivering, nausea and vomiting.

Treatment: Institute general supportive measures for oral drug overdose. Measures that have been used in dexfenfluramine overdose cases include aspiration of gastric contents, gastric lavage with activated charcoal, osmotic diuresis, forced acid diuresis and careful monitoring of CNS or respiratory depression. The effectiveness of dialysis is not known. Follow patients closely until there is no further evidence of drug-related CNS effects. No specific therapy for dexfenfluramine overdose is known.

DEXFENFLURAMINE

Patient Information:

Inform patients that false-positive urine drug tests for amphetamines have been observed for up to 24 hours following a 30 mg dose. See Drug/Lab Test Interactions.

Administration and Dosage:

Approved by the FDA on April 29, 1996

The usual dosage is 15 mg twice daily with meals. Doses > 30 mg/day are not recommended.

Body mass index (BMI): Below is a chart of Body Mass Index (BMI) based on various heights and weights which may be useful when determining candidates for dexfenfluramine therapy. Patients with BMI values ≥ 30 may be candidates for dexfenfluramine therapy. Patients with BMI values of 27 to 29 may be candidates for dexfenfluramine therapy if they also have a concomitant risk factor (eg, hypertension, diabetes, hyperlipidemia.

BMI is calculated by taking the patient's weight, in kg, divided by the patient's height, in meters, squared. Metric conversions are as follows: Pounds ÷ 2.2 = kg; inches x 0.0254 = meters.

Body Mass Index (BMI; kg/m²)

Weight		Height (feet, inches)					
lbs	kg	5'0"	5'3"	5'6"	5'9"	6'	6'3"
140	64	**27**	25	23	21	19	18
150	69	**29**	**27**	24	22	20	19
160	73	31	**28**	26	24	22	20
170	77	33	30	**28**	25	23	21
180	82	35	32	**29**	**27**	25	23
190	86	37	34	31	**28**	26	24
200	91	39	36	32	30	**27**	25
210	95	41	37	34	31	**29**	26
220	100	43	39	36	33	30	**28**
230	105	45	41	37	34	31	**29**
240	109	47	43	39	36	33	30
250	113	49	44	40	37	34	31

Analysis of numerous variables has indicated that about 60% of patients who lose at least 4 pounds in the first 4 weeks of treatment with dexfenfluramine in combination with a reduced-calorie diet lose at least 10% of their initial body weight by the end of 1 year of treatment. If a patient has not lost at least 4 pounds in the first 4 weeks of treatment, consider reevaluation of therapy which may include discontinualtion of dexfenfluramine.

The safety and efficacy of dexfenfluramine use for > 1 year have not been determined.

Infrequently, symptoms (eg, abdominal pain, anxiety, asthenia, delusion, depression, diarrhea, dizziness, hypertension, insomnia, nausea and vomiting) have occurred within several days following cessation of dexfenfluramine. If such symptoms are noted, clinical judgment should guide the treatment, which may include tapering the dose (15 mg once daily) for 2 weeks prior to complete discontinuation.

c-iv	**Redux** (Wyeth-Ayerst)	**Capsules:** 15 mg	Lactose. (Redux). White. In 60s.

PHENYLPROPANOLAMINE HCl

A sympathomimetic commonly used as a decongestant (see Nasal Decongestants).

Actions:

Pharmacology: Phenylpropanolamine (PPA) is an adrenergic agent similar to ephedrine but causes less CNS stimulation. PPA stimulates both α and β receptors; part of its peripheral action is due to norepinephrine release. Increased blood pressure is due to vasoconstriction (minor) and cardiac stimulation (major).

Pharmacokinetics: Readily absorbed from the GI tract, PPA reaches peak plasma concentrations in 1 to 2 hours and has a half-life of 3 to 4 hours. While small amounts are metabolized in the liver to active hydroxylated metabolites, 80% to 90% is excreted unchanged. Therapeutic serum concentrations are ≈ 60 to 200 ng/ml.

Indications:

Exogenous obesity: As a short-term (8 to 12 weeks) adjunct in a regimen of weight reduction based on caloric restriction.

Unlabeled uses: Mild to moderate stress incontinence in women (50 mg twice/day).

Contraindications:

Cardiovascular disease; hypertension; hyperthyroidism; kidney disease; diabetes; hypersensitivity or idiosyncrasy to sympathomimetic amines; glaucoma; depression; during or within 14 days following administration of MAO inhibitors.

Warnings:

Acute blood pressure elevation may occur. Although usually associated with overdosage, severe hypertensive episodes have been reported with average doses.

Pregnancy: Safety for use has not been established. May constrict uterine vessels and reduce uterine blood flow, producing fetal hypoxia. Some association between use in pregnancy (especially the first trimester) and malformations has been reported. PPA is a common decongestant component of proprietary mixtures of antihistamines and other drugs; it is difficult to separate effects of PPA from other drugs in combination. Use only when potential benefits outweigh potential hazards to the fetus.

Lactation: Safety for use has not been established.

Children: Safety and efficacy for use in children have not been established.

Precautions:

Avoid continuous use for longer than 3 months.

Tartrazine sensitivity: Some of these products contain tartrazine, which may cause allergic-type reactions (including bronchial asthma) in susceptible individuals. Although the incidence of tartrazine sensitivity in the general population is low, it is frequently seen in patients who also have aspirin hypersensitivity. Specific products containing tartrazine are identified in the product listings.

Drug Interactions:

Guanethidine: The hypotensive effect may be decreased by phenylpropanolamine.

Indomethacin: A severe hypertensive episode may occur during coadministration.

Monoamine oxidase (MAO) inhibitors may increase the pressor response to PPA. Hypertensive crisis and intracranial hemorrhage may occur. Interaction may also occur with furazolidone, an antimicrobial with MAO inhibitor activity. Avoid this combination; if given inadvertently and hypertension occurs, give phentolamine.

Adverse Reactions:

Cardiovascular: Palpitations; tachycardia; blood pressure elevation; severe hypertension, hypertensive crisis and possible renal failure (that may include rhabdomyolysis) in previously normotensive patients.

CNS: Restlessness; dizziness; insomnia; headache; bizarre behavior. Serious CNS effects (tremor, increased motor activity, agitation, hallucinations, seizures, stroke and death) have also been reported, probably in abuse situations.

Miscellaneous: Nasal dryness; dry mouth; nausea; dysuria.

Overdosage:

Symptoms:

CNS – Restlessness; tremor; hyperreflexia; tachypnea; confusion; assaultive behavior; hallucinations.

Cardiovascular – Arrhythmias; hypertension.

GI – Nausea; vomiting.

Treatment: Gastric lavage, activated charcoal, seizure control, cardiac monitoring and acidification of urine. Refer to Management of Acute Overdosage.

Patient Information:

Do not exceed recommended dosage. Use in conjunction with a restricted calorie diet.

Discontinue use if rapid pulse, dizziness, nervousness, insomnia or palpitations occur.

PHENYLPROPANOLAMINE HCl

Administration and Dosage:

Immediate release: 25 mg 3 times daily, one-half hour before meals.

Timed release: 75 mg once daily in the morning.

Precision release (16 hours duration): 75 mg after breakfast.

otc	**Phenoxine** (Lannett)	**Tablets:** 25 mg	In 1000s.
otc	**Dexatrim Pre-Meal** (Thompson)	**Capsules, timed release:** 25 mg	In 30s.
otc	**Maximum Strength Dexatrim** (Thompson)	**Tablets, extended release:** 75 mg	(d). Yellow. In 20s.
otc	**Maximum Strength Dex–A–Diet Caplets** (O'Connor)	**Tablets, timed release:** 75 mg	In 24s.
otc	**Phenyldrine** (Rugby)		In 100s.
otc	**Control** (Thompson)	**Capsules, timed release:** 75 mg	In 14s & 28s.
otc	**Maximum Strength Dexatrim** (Thompson)		In 10s, 20s and 40s.
otc	**Unitrol** (Republic Drug)		In 28s.
otc	**Acutrim 16 Hour** (Ciba)	**Tablets, precision release:** 75 mg	In 20s & 40s.
otc	**Acutrim Late Day** (Ciba)		In 20s and 40s.
otc	**Acutrim II, Max.** (Ciba)		In 20s & 40s.
otc	**Spray-U-Thin** (Caprice Greystoke)	**Spray:** 6.58 mg	Sorbitol, saccharin. Chocolate mint, spearmint and cinnamon flavors. In 44 ml (360 sprays).

PHENYLPROPANOLAMINE HCl COMBINATIONS

otc	**Appedrine** (Thompson)	**Tablets:** 25 mg phenylpropanolamine HCl, 5000 IU vitamin A, 400 IU D, 30 IU E, 1.5 mg B_1, 1.7 mg B_2, 20 mg B_3, 10 mg B_5, 2 mg B_6, 6 mcg B_{12}, 60 mg C, 0.4 mg FA, 2 mg Cu, 12 mg Fe, 150 mcg I, 15 mg Zn	In 30s.
otc	**Dexatrim Plus Vitamins** (Thompson)	**Caplets, timed release:** 75 mg phenylpropanolamine, 60 mg vitamin C	Lactose. In 14s/14s and 28s/28s.
		Caplets: 5000 IU vitamin A, 30 IU E, 60 mg C, 25 mg K1, 0.4 mg folic acid, 1.5 mg B_1, 1.7 mg B_2, 20 mg B_3, 2 mg B_6, 6 mcg B_{12}, 400 IU D, 30 mcg biotin, 10 mg B_5, 162 mg Ca, P, I, 18 mg Fe, Mg, Cu, 15 mg Zn, Mn, K, 36.3 mg Cl, Cr, Mo, Se, Ni, Sn, Si, V, B	
otc	**Grapefruit Diet Plan w/Diadax** (O'Connor)	**Tablets, chewable:** 12.5 mg phenylpropanolamine HCl with grapefruit extract	In 42s and 90s.
otc	**Maximum Strength Dexatrim Plus Vitamin C** (Thompson)	**Capsules, timed release:** 75 mg phenylpropanolamine HCl with 180 mg vitamin C	In 20s.
otc	**Grapefruit Diet Plan w/Diadax** (O'Connor)	**Capsules, timed release:** 30 mg phenylpropanolamine HCl and grapefruit extract	Tartrazine. In 20s & 50s.

BENZOCAINE

Indications:

Local anesthetic. Appears to decrease ability to detect degrees of sweetness by taste perception. One factor of overeating is the need to satisfy the sense of taste. Adjunct in a weight reduction regimen based on caloric restriction.

Administration and Dosage:

Take 6 to 15 mg just prior to food consumption. Do not exceed 45 mg/day.

otc	**Diet Ayds** (DEP Corp)	**Candy:** 6 mg	In 48s.
otc	**Slim-Mint** (Thompson)	**Gum:** 6 mg	Lecithin. Tartrazine. In 24s.
otc	**Trocaine** (Roberts)	**Lozenges:** 10 mg	In UD 4s and 500s.

PHENYLPROPANOLAMINE HCl and BENZOCAINE

Administration and Dosage:

One capsule in the morning with a full glass of water.

otc	**Dieutrim T.D.** (Legere)	**Capsules, timed release:** 75 mg phenylpropanolamine, 9 mg benzocaine and 75 mg sodium carboxymethylcellulose	In 100s and 1000s.

NARCOTIC AGONIST ANALGESICS

Actions:

Pharmacology: Narcotic analgesics are classified as agonists, mixed agonist-antagonists, or partial agonists by their activity at opioid receptors. Five major categories of opioid receptors are known: mu (μ), *kappa* (κ), *sigma* (ς), *delta* (δ) and *epsilon* (ε). Actions of the narcotic analgesics now available can be defined by their activity at three specific receptor types: μ, κ and ς.

The μ receptors mediate morphine-like supraspinal analgesia, euphoria and respiratory and physical depression. The κ receptors mediate pentazocine-like spinal analgesia, sedation and miosis. The ς receptors mediate dysphoria, psychotomimetic effects (eg, hallucinations), and respiratory and vasomotor stimulation caused by drugs with antagonist activity.

Morphine-like **narcotic agonists** have activity at the μ and κ receptors, and possibly at the δ. Narcotic agonists include natural opium alkaloids (eg, morphine, codeine), semisynthetic analogs (eg, hydromorphone, oxymorphone, oxycodone) and synthetic compounds (eg, meperidine, levorphanol, methadone).

Mixed *agonist-antagonist* drugs (eg, nalbuphine, pentazocine) have agonist activity at some receptors and antagonist activity at other receptors; also included are the *partial agonists* (eg, butorphanol, buprenorphine).

Narcotic antagonists (eg, naloxone) do not have agonist activity at any of the opioid receptor sites (see individual monographs). Antagonists block the opiate receptor, inhibit pharmacological activity of the agonist and precipitate withdrawal in dependent patients. Opiate receptors in the CNS mediate analgesic activity. Narcotic agonists occupy the same receptors as endogenous opioid peptides (enkephalins or endorphins) and both may alter the central release of neurotransmitters from afferent nerves sensitive to noxious stimuli.

Secondary pharmacological effects – The narcotics have a variety of secondary pharmacological effects, including:

CNS: Euphoria; drowsiness; apathy; mental confusion. Nausea and vomiting are caused by direct stimulation of the emetic chemoreceptors located in the medulla.

Respiratory: Depressant effects first diminish tidal volume, then respiratory rate, due to reduced sensitivity of the respiratory center to carbon dioxide.

Cardiovascular: Peripheral vasodilation, reduced peripheral resistance and inhibition of baroreceptors. Therefore, orthostatic hypotension and fainting may occur.

GI: Inhibiting peristalsis which may induce constipation and Sphincter of Oddi spasm.

Urinary tract: Urinary retention may occur due to increased bladder sphincter tone.

Comparative pharmacology is summarized below. Consider these comparisons as approximations that may vary widely among patients.

Narcotic Agonist Comparative Pharmacology[1]

Drug	Analgesic	Antitussive	Constipation	Respiratory Depression	Sedation	Emesis	Physical Dependence
Phenanthrenes							
Codeine	+	+++	+	+	+	+	+
Hydrocodone	+	+++	nd[2]	+	nd[2]	nd[2]	+
Hydromorphone	++	+++	+	++	+	+	++
Levorphanol	++	++	++	++	++	+	++
Morphine	++	+++	++	++	++	++	++
Oxycodone	++	+++	++	++	++	++	++
Oxymorphone	++	+	++	+++	nd[2]	+++	+++
Phenylpiperidines							
Alfentanil	++	nd[2]	nd[2]	nd[2]	nd[2]	nd[2]	nd[2]
Fentanyl	++	nd[2]	nd[2]	+	nd[2]	+	nd[2]
Meperidine	++	+	+	++	+	nd[2]	++
Sufentanil	+++	nd[2]	nd[2]	nd[2]	nd[2]	nd[2]	nd[2]
Diphenylheptanes							
Methadone	++	++	++	++	+	+	+
Propoxyphene	+	nd[2]	nd[2]	+	+	+	+

[1] Table adapted from Catalano RB. The medical approach to management of pain caused by cancer. *Semin Oncol* 1975;2:379-92 and Reuler JB, et al. The chronic pain syndrome: Misconceptions and management. *Ann Intern Med* 1980;93:588-96.

[2] nd – No data available.

NARCOTIC AGONIST ANALGESICS

Pharmacokinetics: Pharmacokinetic profiles are summarized in the table below using morphine as the standard.

Pharmacokinetics of Narcotic Agonist Analgesics

Drug	Onset (minutes)	Peak (hours)	Duration[1] (hours)	t 1/2 (hours)	Equianalgesic Doses (mg)	
					Parenteral	Other
Alfentanil	immediate	nd[2]	nd[2]	1 to 2[3]	IM 0.4 to 0.8	nd[2]
Codeine	10 to 30	0.5 to 1	4 to 6	3	IM 120 to 130 SC 120	Oral 200[4]
Fentanyl	7 to 8	nd[2]	1 to 2	1.5 to 6	IM 0.1 to 0.2	Transdermal 100 mcg/hr[5]
Hydrocodone	nd[2]	nd[2]	4 to 6	3.3 to 4.5	nd[2]	Oral 5 to 10
Hydromorphone	15 to 30	0.5 to 1	4 to 5	2 to 3	IM 1.3 to 1.5 SC 1 to 1.5	Oral 7.5
Levorphanol	30 to 90	0.5 to 1	6 to 8	12 to 16	IM 2 SC 2	Oral 4
Meperidine	10 to 45	0.5 to 1	2 to 4	3 to 4	IM 75 SC 75 to 100	Oral 300[4]
Methadone	30 to 60	0.5 to 1	4 to 6[6]	15 to 30	IM 10 SC 8 to 10	Oral 10 to 20
Morphine	15 to 60[7]	0.5 to 1	3 to 7	1.5 to 2	IM 10 SC 10	Oral 30 to 60
Oxycodone	15 to 30	1	4 to 6	nd[2]	IM 10 to 15 SC 10 to 15	Oral 30[4]
Oxymorphone	5 to 10	0.5 to 1	3 to 6	nd[2]	IM 1 SC 1 to 1.5	Rectal 5, 10
Propoxyphene (PO)	30 to 60	2 to 2.5	4 to 6	6 to 12	nd[2]	Oral 130[8]
Sufentanil	1.3 to 3[3]	nd[2]	nd[2]	2.5	IM 0.01 to 0.04	nd[2]

[1] After IV administration, peak effects may be more pronounced but duration is shorter. Duration of action may be longer with the oral route.
[2] nd – No data available.
[3] Data based on IV administration.
[4] Starting doses lower (codeine, 30 mg; oxycodone, 5 mg; meperidine, 50 mg).
[5] Recommended starting dose is 25 mcg/hr.
[6] Duration and half-life increase with repeated use due to cumulative effects.
[7] Data based on intrathecal or epidural administration.
[8] Starting doses lower (propoxyphene, 65 to 130 mg).

Administration IV is most reliable and rapid; IM or SC use may delay absorption and peak effect. Many agents undergo a significant first-pass effect. Meperidine is metabolized to normeperidine, a metabolite with significant pharmacologic activity. The half-life of normeperidine is 15 to 30 hours and accumulates with chronic dosing. Accumulation of this metabolite may lead to CNS excitation (eg, tremors, twitches, seizures).

Indications:

Relief of moderate to severe pain; preoperative medication; as analgesic adjuncts during anesthesia; detoxification treatment of narcotic addiction and temporary maintenance treatment of narcotic addiction (methadone only). Also used for their antitussive (see Narcotic Antitussives) and antidiarrheal (see Antidiarrheal Combination Products) effects. Refer to individual product listings for specific indications.

Contraindications:

Hypersensitivity to narcotics; diarrhea caused by poisoning until the toxic material has been eliminated; acute bronchial asthma; upper airway obstruction.

Morphine, epidural or intrathecal: Presence of infection at injection site; anticoagulant therapy; bleeding diathesis; parenterally administered corticosteroids within a 2-week period or other concomitant drug therapy or medical condition that would contraindicate the technique of epidural or intrathecal analgesia.

Levorphanol: Acute alcoholism; bronchial asthma; increased intracranial pressure; respiratory depression; anoxia.

Meperidine: In patients taking monoamine oxidase inhibitors (MAOIs) or in those who have received such agents within 14 days.

NARCOTIC AGONIST ANALGESICS

Hydromorphone injection: In patients not already receiving large amounts of parenteral narcotics; patients with respiratory depression in the absence of resuscitative equipment; status asthmaticus; use as obstetrical analgesia.

Warnings:

Suicide: Do not prescribe **propoxyphene** for patients who are suicidal or addiction-prone. Many of the propoxyphene-related deaths have occurred in patients with previous histories of emotional disturbances or suicide attempts as well as misuse of tranquilizers, alcohol and other CNS-active drugs. Some deaths were accidental, or a consequence of accidental ingestion of excessive quantities of propoxyphene alone or in combination with other drugs. Warn patients not to exceed dosage recommended by physician.

Head injury and increased intracranial pressure: Narcotics may obscure the clinical course of patients with head injuries. The respiratory depressant effects and the capacity to elevate cerebrospinal fluid pressure may be markedly exaggerated in the presence of head injury, brain tumor, other intracranial lesions or a preexisting elevated intracranial pressure. Use with extreme caution and only if deemed essential.

Parenteral therapy: Give by very slow IV injection, preferably as a diluted solution. The patient should be lying down. Rapid IV injection increases the incidence of adverse reactions; respiratory depression, hypotension, apnea, circulatory collapse, cardiac arrest and anaphylactoid reactions have occurred. Do not administer IV unless a narcotic antagonist and facilities for assisted or controlled respiration are available. Use caution when injecting SC or IM in chilled areas or in patients with hypotension or shock, since impaired perfusion may prevent complete absorption; with repeated injections, an excessive amount may be suddenly absorbed if normal circulation is reestablished.

Limit epidural or intrathecal administration of **morphine** to the lumbar area.

Smooth muscle hypertonicity may result in biliary colic, difficulty in urination and possible urinary retention requiring catheterization. Give consideration to inherent risks in urethral catherization (eg, sepsis) when epidural or intrathecal administration is considered, especially in the perioperative period.

Hydrochlorides of opium alkaloids – Do not administer IV.

Asthma and other respiratory conditions: Use with extreme caution in patients with acute asthma, bronchial asthma, chronic obstructive pulmonary disease or cor pulmonale, a substantially decreased respiratory reserve, and with preexisting respiratory depression, hypoxia or hypercapnia. Even therapeutic doses of narcotics may decrease respiratory drive while simultaneously increasing airway resistance to the point of apnea. Reserve use for those whose conditions require endotracheal intubation and respiratory support or control of ventilation.

Hypotensive effect: Narcotic analgesics may cause severe hypotension in individuals whose ability to maintain blood pressure has been compromised by a depleted blood volume, or coadministration of drugs such as phenothiazines or general anesthetics. In ambulatory patients, orthostatic hypotension may occur.

Administer with caution to patients in circulatory shock, since vasodilation produced by the drug may further reduce cardiac output and blood pressure.

Renal/Hepatic function impairment: Renal and hepatic dysfunction may cause a prolonged duration and cumulative effect; smaller doses may be necessary.

Meperidine – In patients with renal dysfunction, normeperidine (an active metabolite of meperidine) may accumulate, resulting in increased CNS adverse reactions.

Pregnancy: Category C. Safety for use during pregnancy has not been established.

The placental transfer of narcotics is rapid. Maternal addiction and neonatal withdrawal occurs following illicit use. Withdrawal symptoms include irritability, excessive crying, yawning, sneezing, increased respiratory rate, tremors, hyperreflexia, fever, vomiting, increased stools and diarrhea. Symptoms usually appear during the first days of life.

Some association between congenital defects and first trimester exposure to **codeine** has been reported. **Alfentanil** and **sufentanil** have an embryocidal effect in rats and rabbits when given in doses 2.5 times the upper human dose for 10 days to over 30 days. **Fentanyl** has been shown to impair fertility and to have an embryocidal effect in rats at doses 0.3 times the upper human dose for 12 days.

Labor – Narcotics cross the placental barrier and can produce depression of respiration and psycho-physiologic effects in the neonate. Resuscitation may be required; have naloxone available. The use of **alfentanyl, sufentanil** and **fentanyl** is not recommended. Do not use **methadone** for obstetrical analgesia. Its long duration of action increases the probability of neonatal respiratory depression. It has also been associated with low infant birth weight and subsequent development of SIDS.

Therapeutic **morphine** and **codeine** doses have increased duration of labor.

NARCOTIC AGONIST ANALGESICS

Lactation: Most of these agents appear in breast milk, but effects on the infant may not be significant. Some recommend waiting 4 to 6 hours after use before nursing.

Methadone enters breast milk in concentrations (range, 0.17 to 5.6 mcg/ml) approaching plasma levels and may prevent withdrawal symptoms in addicted infants. **Meperidine** achieves an average milk:plasma ratio of about 1 (peak milk levels of 0.13 mcg/ml occur 2 hours after a 50 mg IM dose). Significant levels of **alfentanil** were found in breast milk 4 hours after administration of 60 mcg/kg. No detectable levels were found after 28 hours. Use caution when administering alfentanil to nursing women.

Children: Safety and efficacy of **sufentanil** in children < 2 years undergoing cardiovascular surgery have been documented in a limited number of cases. Safety and efficacy of **fentanyl** in children < 2 years is not established. Methemoglobinemia has occurred rarely in premature neonates undergoing emergency anesthesia and surgery including combined use of fentanyl, pancuronium and atropine; cause and effect relationship has not been established. Hypotension has occurred in neonates with respiratory distress syndrome receiving **alfentanil** 20 mcg/kg.

Do not use **oxycodone** in children; **propoxyphene** use is not recommended in children. **Methadone** is not recommended as an analgesic in children; documented clinical experience is insufficient to establish suitable dosage regimens. Safety of **oxymorphone** and **hydromorphone** are not established in children.

Precautions:

Acute abdominal conditions: Narcotics may obscure diagnosis or clinical course.

Special risk patients: Use caution in elderly and debilitated patients and in those suffering from conditions accompanied by hypoxia or hypercapnia when even moderate therapeutic doses may dangerously decrease pulmonary ventilation. Also exercise caution in patients sensitive to CNS depressants, including those with cardiovascular disease; myxedema; convulsive disorders; increased ocular pressure; acute alcoholism; delirium tremens; cerebral arteriosclerosis; ulcerative colitis; fever; decreased respiratory reserve (eg, emphysema, severe obesity); hypothyroidism; kyphoscoliosis; Addison's disease; prostatic hypertrophy; urethral stricture; CNS depression; coma; gallbladder disease; recent GI or GU tract surgery; toxic psychosis.

In obese patients (> 20% above ideal body weight), determine the **alfentanil** and **sufentanil** dosage on the basis of ideal body weight.

Fentanyl *and* **alfentanil** may produce bradycardia which may be treated with atropine. Use caution when administering to patients with bradyarrhythmias.

Supraventricular tachycardias: Use with caution in atrial flutter and other supraventricular tachycardias; vagolytic action may increase the ventricular response rate.

Seizures may be aggravated or may occur in individuals without a history of convulsive disorders if dosage is substantially increased because of tolerance. Observe closely patients with known seizure disorders for **morphine**-induced seizure activity.

Cough reflex is suppressed. Exercise caution when using narcotic analgesics postoperatively and in patients with pulmonary disease.

Tolerance: Some patients develop tolerance to the narcotic analgesic. This may occur after days or months of continuous therapy. The dose generally needs to be increased to obtain adequate analgesia.

Cross-tolerance is not complete. Switching to another narcotic agonist, starting with half the predicted equianalgesic dose, may circumvent the cross-tolerance.

Drug abuse and dependence: Narcotic analgesics have abuse potential. Psychological dependence and physical tolerance/dependence may develop upon repeated use. Most patients who receive opiates for medical reasons do not develop dependence.

Narcotics can lead to physical dependence with prolonged use. Signs are increased tolerance to analgesic effect and complaints, pleas, demands or manipulative actions shortly before next scheduled dose. Treat withdrawal in hospital.

Infants born to mothers physically dependent on narcotics will also be physically dependent and may exhibit respiratory difficulties and withdrawal symptoms.

Acute abstinence syndrome (withdrawal) – Severity is related to the degree of dependence, the abruptness of withdrawal and the drug used. Generally, withdrawal symptoms develop at the time the next dose would ordinarily be given. For heroin and morphine, they gradually increase in intensity, reach a maximum in 36 to 72 hours and subside over 5 to 10 days. In contrast, methadone withdrawal is slower in onset and the patient may not recover for 6 to 7 weeks. Meperidine withdrawal has often run its course within 4 to 5 days. Hydrocodone peaks at 48 to 72 hours. Withdrawal precipitated by narcotic antagonists is manifested by onset of symptoms within minutes and maximum intensity within 30 minutes.

NARCOTIC AGONIST ANALGESICS

Do not use a narcotic antagonist to detect dependence. If a narcotic antagonist must be used for serious respiratory depression in a physically dependent patient, give with extreme care, using one-tenth to one-fifth the usual initial dose.

Symptoms of withdrawal –

Early: Yawning; lacrimation; rhinorrhea; "yen sleep"; sweating.

Intermediate: Mydriasis; piloerection; flushing; tachycardia; twitching; tremor; restlessness; irritability; anxiety; anorexia.

Late: Muscle spasm; fever; nausea; diarrhea; vomiting; severe backache; abdominal and leg pains; abdominal and muscle cramps; hot and cold flashes; insomnia; intestinal spasm; coryza and repetitive sneezing; increase in body temperature, blood pressure, respiratory rate and heart rate; spontaneous orgasm; chills; bone and muscle pain in back and extremities.

Treatment – Primarily symptomatic and supportive; maintain proper fluid and electrolyte balance and administer a tranquilizer to suppress anxiety. Severe withdrawal symptoms may require narcotic replacement. Gradual withdrawal using successively smaller doses will minimize symptoms.

Methadone is not a tranquilizer; patients may react to problems and stresses with the same anxiety symptoms as do others. Do not confuse such symptoms with narcotic abstinence; do not treat anxiety by increasing methadone dose.

During induction of methadone maintenance, patients being withdrawn from heroin may show withdrawal symptoms, to be differentiated from methadone-induced side effects. During prolonged methadone use, side effects gradually disappear over several weeks. However, constipation and sweating often persist.

Hazardous tasks: May produce drowsiness or dizziness; observe caution while driving or performing other tasks requiring alertness or physical dexterity.

Sulfite sensitivity: May cause allergic-type reactions (eg, hives, itching, wheezing, anaphylaxis) in certain susceptible persons. Although the overall prevalence of sulfite sensitivity in the general population is probably low, it is seen more frequently in asthmatics or in atopic nonasthmatic persons. Specific products containing sulfites are identified in the product listings.

Drug Interactions:

Anticoagulants: Propoxyphene may potentiate warfarin's anticoagulant effect.

Barbiturate anesthetics may increase the respiratory and CNS depressive effects of the narcotics due to additive pharmacologic activity.

Carbamazepine: Pharmacologic effects may increase when used with propoxyphene. Monitor serum carbamazepine levels and the patient for symptoms of toxicity.

Chlorpromazine: Although the analgesic effect of narcotics may be potentiated, a higher incidence of toxic effects may occur.

Cimetidine: Case reports have described CNS toxicity (confusion, disorientation, respiratory depression, apnea, seizures) following coadministration with narcotic analgesics; no clear-cut cause and effect relationship was established.

Diazepam may produce cardiovascular depression when given with high doses of fentanyl and alfentanil. Administration prior to or following high doses of alfentanil decreases blood pressure secondary to vasodilation; recovery may be prolonged.

Droperidol/Fentanyl may cause hypotension and decrease pulmonary arterial pressure.

Hydantoins may decrease the pharmacologic effects of meperidine and methadone, possibly due to increased hepatic metabolism of the narcotic.

Monoamine oxidase inhibitors (MAOIs) and furazolidone: Meperidine has precipitated unpredictable, occasionally fatal reactions in those concurrently receiving or those who have received such agents within 14 days. The mechanism may be related to a pre-existing hyperphenylalaninemia. Reactions have included coma, respiratory depression, cyanosis and hypotension; in others, hyperexcitability, convulsions, tachycardia, hyperpyrexia and hypertension have occurred. Use caution.

If a narcotic is needed, perform a sensitivity test. Use hydrocortisone IV or prednisolone for severe reactions; use IV chlorpromazine in those with hypertension and hyperpyrexia. Value of narcotic antagonists for these reactions is unknown.

Nitrous oxide may cause cardiovascular depression w/ high dose sufentanil and fentanyl.

Rifampin may reduce methadone plasma levels, producing withdrawal symptoms. Mechanism may be due to increased methadone hepatic metabolism.

Drug/Lab test interactions: Narcotics may increase biliary tract pressure with resultant increases in plasma **amylase** or **lipase**; therefore, determinations of these levels may be unreliable for 24 hours after narcotic administration.

NARCOTIC AGONIST ANALGESICS

Drug/Food interactions: In one study, morphine oral solution after a high-fat meal increased in morphine's area under the curve 34% vs morphine in the fasting state.

Adverse Reactions:

Major hazards: Respiratory depression; apnea; circulatory depression; respiratory arrest; coma; shock; cardiac arrest.

Most frequent: Lightheadedness; dizziness; sedation; nausea; vomiting; sweating. More prominent in ambulatory patients and in those without severe pain. Use lower doses.

CNS: Euphoria; dysphoria; delirium; insomnia; agitation; anxiety; fear; hallucinations; disorientation; drowsiness; sedation; lethargy; impairment of mental and physical performance; skeletal or uncoordinated movements; coma; mood changes; weakness; headache; mental cloudiness; blurred vision; visual disturbances; diplopia; miosis; tremor; convulsions; psychic dependence; toxic psychoses; depression; increased intracranial pressure; miosis. Injection near a nerve trunk may result in sensory-motor paralysis which is usually transitory.

Choreic movements have been induced by **methadone**. Seizures have occurred following **fentanyl** administration.

GI: Nausea; vomiting; diarrhea; cramps; abdominal pain; taste alterations; dry mouth; anorexia; constipation; biliary tract spasm. Patients with chronic ulcerative colitis may have increased colonic motility; toxic dilatation occurred in acute ulcerative colitis.

Coadministration of anthraquinone laxatives (especially senna compounds) in an approximate dose of 187 mg senna concentrate per 120 mg codeine equivalent may counteract narcotic-induced constipation.

Cardiovascular: Facial flushing; chills; faintness; peripheral circulatory collapse; tachycardia; bradycardia; arrhythmia; palpitations; chest wall rigidity; hypertension; hypotension; orthostatic hypotension; syncope; asystole hypercarbia (**alfentanil**) and phlebitis following IV injection.

GU: Ureteral spasm and spasm of vesical sphincters; urinary retention or hesitancy; oliguria; antidiuretic effect; reduced libido or potency.

Hypersensitivity: Pruritus; urticaria; other skin rashes; diaphoresis; laryngospasm; edema; hemorrhagic urticaria (rare). Wheal and flare over the vein with IV injection may occur. Anaphylactoid reactions have occurred following IV administration. A case of **morphine**-induced thrombocytopenia has occurred.

Miscellaneous: Bronchospasm; depression of cough reflex; interference with thermal regulation; laryngospasm; muscular rigidity; paresthesia; pain at injection site; local tissue irritation and induration following SC injection, particularly when repeated; diaphoresis (**fentanyl**); reversible jaundice (**propoxyphene**); nystagmus (**hydromorphone**). **Sufentanil** may cause erythema, chills and intraoperative muscle movement. Postoperative confusion, blurred vision, shivering and hypercapnia have occurred with **alfentanil**.

Lab test abnormalities: Abnormal liver function tests with **propoxyphene**.

Overdosage:

In general, the shorter the onset and duration of action of opiate, the greater the intensity and rapidity of symptom onset. Infants and children may be relatively more sensitive on a body weight basis. Elderly patients are comparatively intolerant.

Symptoms: In severe overdosage, mainly by the IV route, apnea, circulatory collapse, convulsions, cardiopulmonary arrest and death may occur. The less severely poisoned patient often presents with the triad of CNS depression, miosis and respiratory depression. Serious overdosage is characterized by respiratory depression, extreme somnolence progressing to stupor or coma, constricted pupils, skeletal muscle flaccidity, and cold and clammy skin. Hypotension, bradycardia, hypothermia, pulmonary edema, pneumonia or shock occurs in up to 40% of patients.

Treatment: Give primary attention to adequate respiratory exchange; provide a patent airway and institute assisted or controlled ventilation; if depressed respiration is associated with muscular rigidity, use an IV neuromuscular blocker.

Administer a narcotic antagonist. Since the duration of action of most narcotics exceeds that of the narcotic antagonist, repeat the antagonist to maintain adequate respiration; keep the patient under surveillance. Do not give an antagonist in the absence of clinically significant respiratory or cardiovascular depression. Naloxone is the antagonist of choice (see individual monograph).

NARCOTIC AGONIST ANALGESICS

Employ supportive measures as indicated. Refer to General Management of Acute Overdosage. In cases of oral overdose, absorption of drugs from the gut may be decreased by giving activated charcoal which, in many cases, is more effective than emesis or lavage. Observe the patient for a rise in temperature or pulmonary complications that may require antibiotic therapy.

Forced diuresis, peritoneal dialysis, hemodialysis or charcoal hemoperfusion have not been established as beneficial for a codeine overdosage.

Patient Information:

May cause drowsiness, dizziness or blurring of vision; use caution while driving or performing other tasks requiring alertness.

Avoid alcohol and other CNS depressants.

Notify physician if nausea, vomiting or constipation become prominent.

If GI upset occurs, these agents may be taken with food.

Notify physician if shortness of breath or difficulty in breathing occurs.

Administration and Dosage:

Brompton's Cocktail: Brompton's Cocktail or Mixture is an oral narcotic mixture used for chronic severe pain. The original formula contained heroin or morphine (10 mg), cocaine (10 mg), alcohol, chloroform water and syrup; it was given on schedule as pain prophylaxis, rather than "as needed." Currently, "Brompton's Mixture" designates any alcoholic solution containing morphine and either cocaine or a phenothiazine. A single entity narcotic (usually morphine) can be equally effective. Cocaine apparently does not add to the mixture's effectiveness; methadone has been recommended. Various adjunctive drugs, including aspirin or acetaminophen, tricyclic antidepressants, stimulants (eg, dextroamphetamine) and antihistamines (eg, dimenhydrinate), may be effective when given with a narcotic solution.

The use of Brompton's Cocktail established the value of regular administration of narcotic analgesics for chronic severe pain. Adjunctive drugs may benefit selected patients but "standard" combinations are not advocated.

OPIUM

For complete prescribing information, refer to the Narcotic Agonist Analgesics group monograph.

The activity of opium is primarily due to its morphine content. The major medical use of opium has been for its antiperistaltic activity, particularly in diarrhea. Opium alkaloids (eg, morphine, codeine) have replaced opium in medical use.

Indications:

For all disorders in which the analgesic, sedative-hypnotic narcotic or antidiarrheal effect of an opiate is needed; for relief of severe pain in place of morphine.

C-II	**Pantopon** (Roche)	**Injection**: 20 mg per ml[1] (equiv. to 15 mg morphine). *Dose: Adults* - 5 to 20 mg every 4 to 5 hours IM or SC	In 1 ml amps.
C-II	**Opium Tincture, Deodorized** (Lilly)	**Liquid**: 10%. *Dose: Adults* - 0.6 ml (equiv. to 6 mg morphine) 4 times daily. *Children - Analgesia:* 0.01 to 0.02 ml/kg/dose every 3 to 4 hours. *Diarrhea:* 0.005 to 0.01 ml/kg every 3 to 4 hours.	19% alcohol. In 120 ml and pt.
C-III	**Paregoric** (Various, eg, Balan, Geneva, Goldline, Lilly, Major, Moore, Roxane, Rugby, Schein, URL)	**Liquid (camphorated tincture of opium)**: 2 mg morphine equiv. per 5 ml. *Dose: Adults* - 5 to 10 ml 1 to 4 times daily. *Children* - 0.25 to 0.5 ml/kg 1 to 4 times daily.	With 45% alcohol. In 60 ml, pt, gal and UD 5 ml (40s, 50s and 100s).

[1] With 6% alcohol, 136 mg glycerin and 0.2% parabens.

LEVORPHANOL TARTRATE

For complete prescribing information, refer to the Narcotic Agonist Analgesics group monograph.

Indications:

Relief of moderate to severe pain. Preoperatively to allay apprehension, provide prolonged analgesia, reduce thiopental requirements and shorten recovery time.

Administration and Dosage:

The average adult dose is 2 mg orally or SC; increase to 3 mg, if necessary. It has been given by slow IV injection.

c-II	**Levo-Dromoran** (Roche)	**Injection:** 2 mg per ml	In 1 ml amps[1] and 10 ml vials.[2]
		Tablets: 2 mg	(Roche Levo-Dromoran). White. In 100s.

[1] With 0.2% methyl and propylparabens
[2] With 0.45% phenol.

MORPHINE SULFATE

For complete prescribing information, refer to the Narcotic Agonist Analgesics group monograph.

Morphine is the principal opium alkaloid.

Indications:

Relief of moderate to severe acute and chronic pain. Preoperatively to sedate patient, allay apprehension, facilitate induction of anesthesia, reduce anesthetic dosage.

Unlabeled uses: Dyspnea associated w/acute left ventricular failure, pulmonary edema.

Administration and Dosage:

Morphine sulfate is less potent orally because of first-pass metabolism. Oral administration is ⅓ to ⅙ as effective as parenteral administration.

Oral: 10 to 30 mg every 4 hours or as directed by physician.

Controlled release – 30 mg every 8 to 12 hours or as directed by physician. Do not crush or chew.

Medication may suppress respiration in the elderly, the very ill and those patients with respiratory problems; therefore, lower doses may be required.

SC/IM:

Adults – 10 mg (5 to 20 mg)/70 kg every 4 hours.

Children – 0.1 to 0.2 mg/kg (up to 15 mg) every 4 hours.

IV:

Adults – 2.5 to 15 mg/70 kg in 4 to 5 ml of Water for Injection, administered over 4 to 5 minutes. Rapid IV use increases the incidence of adverse reactions (see Warnings). Do not administer IV unless a narcotic antagonist is immediately available.

Continuous IV infusion – 0.1 to 1 mg/ml in 5% Dextrose in Water by controlled-infusion device; higher concentrations have been used.

Rectal: 10 to 20 mg every 4 hours or as directed by physician.

Epidural:

Adults – Initial injection of 5 mg in the lumbar region may provide satisfactory pain relief for up to 24 hours. If adequate pain relief is not achieved within 1 hour, carefully administer incremental doses of 1 to 2 mg at intervals sufficient to assess effectiveness. Give no more than 10 mg/24 hr.

For continuous infusion, an initial dose of 2 to 4 mg/24 hours is recommended. Further doses of 1 to 2 mg may be given if pain relief is not achieved initially.

Aged or debilitated patients – Administer with extreme caution (see Precautions). Doses < 5 mg may provide satisfactory pain relief for up to 24 hours.

Intrathecal: Adult: Intrathecal dosage is usually 1⁄10 that of epidural dosage. A single injection of 0.2 to 1 mg may provide satisfactory pain relief for up to 24 hours. Caution: This is only 0.4 to 2 ml of the 5 mg/10 ml ampul or 0.2 to 1 ml of the 10 mg/10 ml ampul. Do not inject intrathecally > 2 ml of the 5 mg/10 ml ampul or 1 ml of the 10 mg/10 ml ampul. Use in lumbar area only. Repeated intrathecal injections not recommended. A constant IV infusion of naloxone, 0.6 mg/hr, for 24 hours after intrathecal injection may reduce incidence of potential side effects.

Aged or debilitated – Use extreme caution. Lower dose is usually satisfactory.

Repeat dosage – If pain recurs, consider alternative administration routes, since experience with repeated doses by this route is limited.

Intraventricular: Currently available data indicate that this route of administration is effective in select patients with intractable pain and short life expectancy. One to two doses per day are generally administered.

MORPHINE SULFATE

c-ii	**Morphine Sulfate** (Abbott)	**Injection**: 0.5 mg/ml	In 10 ml amps.
c-ii	**Astramorph PF**[1] (Astra)		In 2, 10 ml amps, 10 ml vials.
c-ii	**Duramorph**[1] (Elkins-Sinn)		In 10 ml amps.
c-ii	**Morphine Sulfate** (Various, eg, Abbott, Baxter)	**Injection**: 1 mg/ml	In 10 ml amps and 30 and 60 ml amps.
c-ii	**Astramorph PF**[1] (Astra)		In 2 and 10 ml amps and 10 ml vials.
c-ii	**Duramorph**[1] (Elkins-Sinn)		In 10 ml amps.
c-ii	**Morphine Sulfate** (Various, eg, Baxter, Winthrop, Wyeth-Ayerst)	**Injection**: 2 mg/ml	In 60 ml vials and 1 and 2 ml disp. syringes.
c-ii	**Morphine Sulfate** (Baxter)	**Injection**: 3 mg/ml	In 50 ml vials.
c-ii	**Morphine Sulfate** (Various, eg, Winthrop, Wyeth-Ayerst)	**Injection**: 4 mg/ml	In 1 and 2 ml disp. syringes.
c-ii	**Morphine Sulfate** (Various, eg, Abbott, Elkins-Sinn)	**Injection**: 5 mg/ml	In 1 and 30 ml vials.
c-ii	**Morphine Sulfate** (Various, eg, Elkins-Sinn, Winthrop, Wyeth-Ayerst)	**Injection**: 8 mg/ml	In 1 ml vials, amps, syringes.
c-ii	**Morphine Sulfate** (Various, eg, Elkins-Sinn, Winthrop, Wyeth-Ayerst)	**Injection**: 10 mg/ml	1 ml vials, amps, 10 ml vials.
c-ii	**Infumorph 200**[1] (Elkins-Sinn)		Preservative free. In 20 ml (200 mg) ampuls.
c-ii	**Morphine Sulfate** (Various, eg, Elkins-Sinn, Lilly)	**Injection**: 15 mg/ml	In 1 ml amps and vials, 20 ml amps and vials.
c-ii	**Morphine Sulfate** (IMS)	**Injection**: 25 mg/ml	In 4, 10, 20 and 40 ml *Select-A-Jet* syringe systems.
c-ii	**Infumorph 500**[1] (Elkins-Sinn)		Preservative free. In 20 ml (500 mg) ampuls.
c-ii	**Morphine Sulfate** (Various, eg, IMS)	**Injection**: 50 mg/ml	In 10, 20 and 40 ml *Select-A-Jet* syringe systems.
c-ii	**Kadian** (Zeneca)	**Capsules, sustained release**: 20 mg	(KADIAN 20 mg). In 60s, 100s, 500s, and UD 100s.
		50 mg	(KADIAN 50 mg). In 60s, 100s, 500s and UD 100s.
		100 mg	(KADIAN 100 mg). In 60s, 100s and UD 100s.
c-ii	**MSIR** (Purdue Frederick)	**Capsules**: 15 mg	Lactose, sucrose. (PF MSIR 15). White/blue. in 50s.
		Capsules: 30 mg	Lactose, sucrose. (PF MSIR 30). Gray/lavender. In 50s.
c-ii	**Morphine Sulfate** (Lilly)	**Soluble Tablets**: 10 mg	In 100s.
		15 mg	In 100s and 500s.
		30 mg	In 100s and 500s.
c-ii	**Morphine Sulfate** (Roxane)	**Tablets**: 15 mg	(54 733). In 100s and UD 100s.
c-ii	**MSIR** (Purdue Frederick)		(PF MI 30). In 50s.
c-ii	**MS Contin** (Purdue Frederick)	**Tablets, controlled release**: 15 mg	(PF M15). Blue. In 100s and UD 100s.

MORPHINE SULFATE

c-II	**Morphine Sulfate** (Roxane)	**Tablets**: 30 mg	(54 2262). In 100s, UD 100s.
c-II	**MSIR** (Purdue Frederick)		(PF MI 30). In 50s.
c-II	**MS Contin** (Purdue Frederick)	**Tablets, controlled release:** 30 mg	In 50s, 100s, 250s, 500s & UD 25s, 100s, 300s.
c-II	**Oramorph SR** (Roxane)		Lactose. White. In 50s, 100s, 250s and UD 100s.
c-II	**MS Contin** (Purdue Frederick)	**Tablets, controlled release:** 60 mg	(PF M 60). Orange. In 100s and UD 25s, 100s, 300s.
c-II	**Oramorph SR** (Roxane)		Lactose. In 100s, UD 25s.
c-II	**MS Contin** (Purdue Frederick)	**Tablets, controlled release:** 100 mg	(PF 100). Gray. In 100s and UD 100s.
c-II	**Oramorph SR** (Roxane)		Lactose. In 100s, UD 25s.
c-II	**MS Contin** (Purdue Frederick)	**Tablets, controlled release:** 200 mg	(PF 100). Green. In 100s and UD 25s.
c-II	**Morphine Sulfate** (Roxane)	**Solution**: 10 mg/5 ml	In 100, 500 ml, UD 5, 10 ml.
c-II	**MS/L** (Richwood)		In 500 ml.
c-II	**MSIR** (Purdue Frederick)		In 120, 500 ml, UD 5 ml.
c-II	**Roxanol Rescudose** (Roxane)	**Solution**: 10 mg/2.5 ml	In UD 2.5 ml.
c-II	**Morphine Sulfate** (Roxane)	**Solution**: 20 mg/5 ml	In 100 and 500 ml.
c-II	**MSIR** (Purdue Frederick)		In 120, 500 ml and UD 5 ml.
c-II	**MSIR** (Purdue Frederick)	**Solution**: 20 mg/ml	In 30 and 120 ml.
c-II	**OMS Concentrate** (Upsher-Smith)		In 30 and 120 ml w/dropper.
c-II	**Roxanol** (Roxane)		In 30 and 120 ml.
c-II	**Roxanol UD** (Roxane)		In UD 1 ml, 1.5 ml vials.
c-II	**MS/L-Concentrate** (Richwood)	**Solution**: 100 mg/5 ml	In 120 ml with calibrated dropper.
c-II	**Roxanol 100** (Roxane)		In 240 ml.
c-II	**Morphine Sulfate** (Various, eg, Nelson, UDL)	**Rectal Suppositories**: 5 mg	In UD 12s and 50s.
c-II	**MS/S** (Richwood)		In 12s.
c-II	**RMS** (Upsher-Smith)		In UD 12s.
c-II	**Roxanol** (Roxane)		In UD 12s.
c-II	**Morphine Sulfate** (Various, eg, Nelson, UDL)	**Rectal Suppositories**: 10 mg	In UD 12s and 50s.
c-II	**MS/S** (Richwood)		In 12s.
c-II	**RMS** (Upsher-Smith)		In UD 12s.
c-II	**Roxanol** (Roxane)		In UD 12s.
c-II	**Morphine Sulfate** (Various, eg, Nelson, UDL)	**Rectal Suppositories**: 20 mg	In UD 12s and 50s.
c-II	**MS/S** (Richwood)		In 12s.
c-II	**RMS** (Upsher-Smith)		In UD 12s.
c-II	**Roxanol** (Roxane)		In UD 12s.
c-II	**Morphine Sulfate** (Various, eg, Nelson, UDL)	**Rectal Suppositories**: 30 mg	In UD 12s and 50s.
c-II	**MS/S** (Richwood)		In 12s.
c-II	**RMS** (Upsher-Smith)		In UD 12s.
c-II	**Roxanol** (Roxane)		In UD 12s.

[1] Preservative free.

HYDROMORPHONE HCl

For complete prescribing information, refer to the Narcotic Agonist Analgesics group monograph.

Indications:

Relief of moderate to severe pain.

Administration and Dosage:

Oral: 2 mg every 4 to 6 hours; ≥ 4 mg every 4 to 6 hours for more severe pain.

Parenteral: 1 to 2 mg SC or IM every 4 to 6 hours as needed. For severe pain, administer 3 to 4 mg every 4 to 6 hours as needed. May be given by slow IV injection over 2 to 5 minutes.

High potency strength should only be given to patients tolerant of other narcotics.

Rectal: 3 mg every 6 to 8 hours.

Children: Safety and efficacy have not been established.

Storage: Protect from light. Refrigerate suppositories.

C-II	**Hydromorphone HCl** (Various, eg, Winthrop, Wyeth-Ayerst)	**Injection**: 1 mg per ml	In 1 ml fill in 2 ml syringe.
C-II	**Dilaudid** (Knoll)		In 1 ml amps.
C-II	**Hydromorphone HCl** (Various, eg, Astra, Elkins-Sinn, Schein, Winthrop, Wyeth-Ayerst)	**Injection**: 2 mg per ml	In 1 and 20 ml vials and 1 ml fill in 2 ml syringe.
C-II	**Dilaudid** (Knoll)		In 1 ml amps and 20 ml vials.[1]
C-II	**Hydromorphone HCl** (Wyeth-Ayerst)	**Injection**: 3 mg per ml	In 1 ml fill in 2 ml syringe.[2]
C-II	**Hydromorphone HCl** (Various, eg, Winthrop, Wyeth-Ayerst)	**Injection**: 4 mg per ml	In 1 ml fill in 2 ml syringe.
C-II	**Dilaudid** (Knoll)		In 1 ml amps.
C-II	**Hydromorphone HCl** (Elkins-Sinn)	**Injection**: 10 mg per ml	In 2 ml vials.
C-II	**Dilaudid-HP** (Knoll)		In 1 and 5 ml amps.
C-II	**Dilaudid-HP** (Knoll)	**Powder for injection, lyophilized**: 250 mg (10 mg per ml after reconstitution)	In single-dose vials.

HYDROMORPHONE HCl

c-II	**HydroStat IR** (Richwood)	**Tablets**: 1 mg	Lactose. (RW/1). Green. In 100s.
c-II	**Hydromorphone HCl** (Roxane)	**Tablets**: 2 mg	(54 743). White. In 100s and UD 100s.
c-II	**Dilaudid** (Knoll)		Orange. In 100s, 500s and UD 100s.
c-II	**HydroStat IR** (Richwood)		Lactose. (RW/2). Orange. In 100s.
c-II	**HydroStat IR** (Richwood)	**Tablets**: 3 mg	Lactose. (RW/3). Pink. In 100s.
c-II	**Hydromorphone HCl** (Roxane)	**Tablets**: 4 mg	(54 609). White. In 100s and UD 100s.
c-II	**Dilaudid** (Knoll)		Yellow. In 100s, 500s and UD 100s.
c-II	**HydroStat IR** (Richwood)		Lactose. (RW/4). Yellow. In 100s.
c-II	**Dilaudid** (Knoll)	**Tablets**: 8 mg	Lactose, sodium bisulfite. (8). White, scored. Triangular. In 100s.
c-II	**Dilaudid-5** (Knoll)	**Liquid**: 5 mg/5 ml	Parabens, sucrose. May contain sodium bisulfite. In pt.
c-II	**Dilaudid** (Knoll)	**Suppositories**: 3 mg	In 6s.

[1] With EDTA and methyl and propyl parabens.
[2] With ≤ 10 mg benzyl alcohol per ml.

METHADONE HCl

For prescribing information, refer to the Narcotic Agonist Analgesics group monograph.

Oral methadone is approximately one-half as potent as parenteral. Oral administration results in a delay of onset, a lower peak and an increased duration of analgesic effect. Duration of effect increases with repeated use due to cumulative effects.

Indications:

For relief of severe pain; detoxification and temporary maintenance treatment of narcotic addiction. Methadone is ineffective for the relief of general anxiety.

Administration and Dosage:

Pain: Adults - 2.5 to 10 mg IM, SC or orally every 3 or 4 hours as necessary. Individualize dosage. For exceptionally severe pain, or in those tolerant of narcotic analgesia, it may be necessary to exceed the usual recommended dosage. Injection IM is preferred for repeated doses; SC use may cause local irritation.

Children – Not for analgesic use, due to insufficient documentation.

Detoxification treatment should not exceed 21 days and may not be repeated earlier than 4 weeks after completion of the preceding course.

Oral administration is preferred. However, if the patient is unable to ingest oral methadone the parenteral form may be used.

Initially, 15 to 20 mg will often suppress withdrawal symptoms. Provide additional methadone if withdrawal symptoms are not suppressed or if symptoms reappear. When patients are physically dependent on high doses, 40 mg/day in single or divided doses is usually an adequate stabilizing dose. Continue stabilization for 2 to 3 days, then gradually decrease the dose on a daily basis or at 2 day intervals. Provide a sufficient amount to keep withdrawal symptoms at a tolerable level. In hospitalized patients, a daily reduction of 20% of total daily dose may be tolerated.

Maintenance treatment: Individualize dosage. Initial dosage should control abstinence symptoms following narcotic withdrawal, but should not cause sedation, respiratory depression or other effects of acute intoxication. If patients have been heavy heroin users up to admission day, they may be given 20 mg methadone 4 to 8 hours after heroin is stopped or 40 mg in a single oral dose. If they enter treatment with little or no narcotic tolerance, initial dosage may be halved. When in doubt, use smaller dose. If abstinence symptoms are distressing, give additional 10 mg doses as needed. Adjust dosage as tolerated and required, up to 120 mg/day.

For a complete description of detoxification and maintenance regulations and dosage protocols, consult a local approved methadone program.

Methadone Maintenance Regulations: Maintenance therapy - If used to treat heroin dependence for > 3 weeks, the procedure passes from treatment of acute withdrawal syndrome (detoxification) to maintenance therapy. Maintenance may be undertaken only by approved methadone programs. This does not preclude maintenance of an addict hospitalized for other conditions.

Distribution – To treat narcotic addiction in detoxification or maintenance programs, methadone may be dispensed only by pharmacies and maintenance programs approved by FDA and designated state authorities according to treatment requirements stipulated in Federal Methadone Regulations (21 CFR 291.505). Failure to abide by these regulations may result in criminal prosecution, seizure of drug, revocation of program approval and injunction precluding program operation.

Methadone, used as an analgesic, may be dispensed in any licensed pharmacy.

C-II	**Dolophine HCl** (Lilly)	**Injection**: 10 mg/ml	In amps & 20 ml vials.[1]
C-II	**Methadone HCl** (Roxane)	**Tablets**: 5 mg	(54 210). White, scored. In 100s and UD 100s.
C-II	**Dolophine HCl** (Lilly)		In 100s.
C-II	**Methadose** (Mallinckrodt)		(METHADOSE 5). White. Scored. In 100s.
C-II	**Methadone HCl** (Roxane)	**Tablets**: 10 mg	(54 142). White, scored. In 100s and UD 100s.
C-II	**Dolophine HCl** (Lilly)		In 100s.
C-II	**Methadose** (Mallickrodt)		(METHADOSE 10). White. Scored. In 100s.
C-II	**Methadone HCl Diskets**[2] (Lilly)	**Dispersible Tablets**: 40 mg	Peach, scored. In 100s.

METHADONE HCl

c-II	**Methadone HCl** (Roxane)	**Oral Solution**: 5 mg/5 ml	8% alcohol. Lemon flavor. In 500 ml and UD 5 ml.
		10 mg/5 ml	Lemon flavor. In 500 ml.
		10 mg/10 ml	Lemon flavor. UD 10 ml.
c-II	**Methadone HCl Intensol** (Roxane)	**Oral Concentrate**: 10 mg/ml	In 30 ml.

[1] With 0.5% chlorobutanol.

[2] For detoxification and maintenance only.

MEPERIDINE HCl

For complete prescribing information, refer to the Narcotic Agonist Analgesics group monograph.

Meperidine HCl is a narcotic analgesic with multiple actions qualitatively similar to those of morphine. Meperidine may produce less intense smooth muscle spasm, and less constipation and depression of the cough reflex than equianalgesic doses of morphine.

Indications:

Oral and parenteral: Relief of moderate to severe pain.

Parenteral: For preoperative medication, support of anesthesia and obstetrical analgesia.

Administration and Dosage:

Relief of pain: Individualize dosage. While SC administration is suitable for occasional use, IM administration is preferred for repeated doses. If IV administration is required, decrease dosage and inject very slowly, preferably using a diluted solution. Meperidine is less effective when administered orally than when given parenterally. Reduce proportionately (usually by 25% to 50%) when administering concomitantly with phenothiazines and other tranquilizers. Take each dose of the syrup in one-half glass of water; if taken undiluted, it may exert a slight topical anesthetic effect on mucous membranes.

Adults – 50 to 150 mg IM, SC or orally every 3 to 4 hours, as necessary.

Children – 1 to 1.8 mg/kg (0.5 to 0.8 mg/lb) IM, SC or orally up to adult dose, every 3 or 4 hours, as necessary.

Preoperative medication:

Adults – 50 to 100 mg IM or SC, 30 to 90 minutes before beginning anesthesia.

Children – 1 to 2 mg/kg (0.5 to 1 mg/lb) IM or SC, up to adult dose, 30 to 90 minutes before beginning anesthesia.

Support of anesthesia: Meperidine may be administered in repeated doses diluted to 10 mg/ml by slow IV injection, or by continuous IV infusion of solution diluted to 1 mg/ml. Individualize dosage.

Obstetrical analgesia: When pains become regular, administer 50 to 100 mg IM or SC; repeat at 1 to 3 hour intervals.

IV admixture:

Incompatibility – Solutions of meperidine and soluble barbiturates, aminophylline, heparin, morphine sulfate, methicillin, phenytoin, sodium bicarbonate, iodide, sulfadiazine and sulfisoxazole are incompatible.

Compatibility – The following IV solutions are compatible with meperidine: 5% Dextrose and Lactated Ringer's; Dextrose-Saline combinations; 2.5%, 5% or 10% Dextrose in Water; Ringer's; Lactated Ringer's; 0.45% or 0.9% Sodium Chloride; ⅙ Molar Sodium Lactate.

c-II	**Meperidine HCl** (Various, eg, Barr, Baxter, Bioline, Goldline, Halsey, Major, Schein, Wyeth-Ayerst)	**Tablets**: 50 mg	In 100s, 250s and 500s.
c-II	**Demerol HCl** (Winthrop)		In 100s, 500s and UD 25s.
c-II	**Meperidine HCl** (Various, eg, Barr, Baxter, Bioline, Goldline, Halsey, Major, Schein)	**Tablets**: 100 mg	In 100s, 500s and 1000s.
c-II	**Demerol HCl** (Winthrop)		In 100s, 500s and UD 25s.
c-II	**Meperidine HCl** (Roxane)	**Syrup**: 50 mg per 5 ml	Sorbitol. In 500 ml.
c-II	**Demerol HCl** (Winthrop)		Glucose and saccharin. Alcohol free. Banana flavor. In pt.
c-II	**Meperidine HCl** (Various, eg, Astra, Wyeth-Ayerst[1])	**Injection**: 50 mg per ml	In 30 ml multi-dose vials.
c-II	**Demerol HCl** (Winthrop)		In 30 ml multi-dose vials.[2]
c-II	**Meperidine HCl** (Various, eg, Astra, Wyeth-Ayerst[1])	**Injection**: 100 mg per ml	In 20 ml multi-dose vials.
c-II	**Demerol HCl** (Winthrop)		In 20 ml multi-dose vials.[2]
c-II	**Meperidine HCl** (IMS)	**Injection**: 10 mg per ml	In 5 and 10 ml single-dose vials.
c-II	**Meperidine HCl** (Abbott)		In single dose 30 ml vials. *For IV infusion only.*

MEPERIDINE HCl

c-ii	**Meperidine HCl** (Elkins-Sinn)	**Injection**: 25 mg per dose	In 1 ml Dosette amps and vials.[1]
c-ii	**Meperidine HCl** (Wyeth-Ayerst)		In 1 ml fill in 2 ml Tubex.
c-ii	**Demerol HCl** (Winthrop)		In 0.5 ml Uni-Nest amps, 0.5 ml Uni-Amps and 2 ml Carpuject.
c-ii	**Meperidine HCl** (Elkins-Sinn)	**Injection**: 50 mg per dose	In 1 ml Dosette amps and vials.[1]
c-ii	**Meperidine HCl** (Wyeth-Ayerst)		In 1 ml fill in 2 ml Tubex.
c-ii	**Demerol HCl** (Winthrop)		In 1 ml Uni-Nest amps, 1 ml Uni-Amps and 2 ml Carpuject.
c-ii	**Meperidine HCl** (Elkins-Sinn)	**Injection**: 75 mg per dose	In 1 ml Dosette amps and vials.[1]
c-ii	**Meperidine HCl** (Wyeth-Ayerst)		In 1 ml fill in 2 ml Tubex.
c-ii	**Demerol HCl** (Winthrop)		In 1.5 ml Uni-Nest amps, 1.5 ml Uni-Amps and 2 ml Carpuject.
c-ii	**Meperidine HCl** (Elkins-Sinn)	**Injection**: 100 mg per dose	In 1 ml Dosette amps and vials.[1]
c-ii	**Meperidine HCl** (Wyeth-Ayerst)		In 1 ml fill in 2 ml Tubex.
c-ii	**Demerol HCl** (Winthrop)		In 1 and 2 ml Uni-Nest amps, 1 and 2 ml Uni-Amps and 1 ml fill in 2 ml Carpuject.

[1] With 1.5 mg sodium metabisulfite and 5 mg phenol per ml.
[2] With 0.1% metacresol.

CODEINE

For complete prescribing information, refer to the Narcotic Agonist Analgesic group monograph.

Codeine is a narcotic analgesic and antitussive that resembles morphine pharmacologically but with milder actions. It is a less potent antitussive than morphine on a weight basis; however, it is widely used as a cough suppressant because of its low incidence of adverse reactions at the usual antitussive dose. Codeine is ⅔ as effective orally as parenterally.

Indications:

Relief of mild to moderate pain and for coughing induced by chemical or mechanical irritation of the respiratory system.

Administration and Dosage:

Analgesic:

Adults – 15 to 60 mg every 4 to 6 hours, orally, IM, IV or SC. Usual dose is 30 mg. Do not exceed 360 mg in 24 hours.

Children (≥ 1 year of age) – 0.5 mg/kg or 15 m^2 of body surface every 4 to 6 hours SC, IM or orally. Do not use IV in children.

Antitussive: (See also Narcotic Antitussive Monograph).

Adults – 10 to 20 mg every 4 to 6 hours. Do not exceed 120 mg in 24 hours.

Children (6 to 12 years) – 5 to 10 mg orally every 4 to 6 hours. Do not exceed 60 mg in 24 hours.

(2 to 6 years): 2.5 to 5 mg orally every 4 to 6 hours. Do not exceed 30 mg in 24 hours.

Storage: Protect from light (injection).

c-II	**Codeine Sulfate** (Various, eg, Lilly, Roxane)	**Tablets:** 15 mg	In 100s and UD 100s.
c-II	**Codeine Sulfate** (Various, eg, Halsey, Knoll, Lilly, Roxane, Wyeth-Ayerst)	**Tablets:** 30 mg	In 25s, 100s, 250s, 1000s and UD 100s.
c-II	**Codeine Sulfate** (Various, eg, Knoll, Lilly, Roxane)	**Tablets:** 60 mg	In 100s, 1000s and UD 100s.
c-II	**Codeine Sulfate** (Lilly)	**Tablets, soluble:** 15 mg	In 100s.
		30 mg	In 100s.
		60 mg	In 100s.
c-II	**Codeine Phosphate** (Various, eg, Elkins-Sinn, Winthrop, Wyeth-Ayerst[1])	**Injection:** 30 mg	In 1 ml vials, 1 and 2 ml syringes and 1 ml Tubex.
c-II	**Codeine Phosphate** (Various, eg, Elkins-Sinn, Winthrop, Wyeth-Ayerst[2])	**Injection:** 60 mg	In 1 ml vials, 1 and 2 ml syringes and 1 ml Tubex.
c-II	**Codeine Phosphate** (Various, eg, Elkins-Sinn)	**Tablets, soluble:** 30 mg	In 100s.
		60 mg	In 100s and 500s.

[1] With ≤ 1.5 mg sodium metabisulfite.
[2] With ≤ 2 mg sodium metabisulfite.

OXYCODONE HCl

For complete prescribing information, refer to the Narcotic Agonist Analgesics group monograph.

Indications:

Relief of moderate to moderately severe pain.

Administration and Dosage:

Adults: 5 mg or 5 ml every 6 hours as needed. Individualize dosage.

Children: Not recommended for use in children.

c-II	**OxyIR** (Purdue Pharma)	**Capsules, immediate-release**: 5 mg	(O-IR/PF5mg). Beige/orange. In 100s.
c-II	**Oxycontin** (Purdue Pharma)	**Tablets, controlled-release**: 10 mg	Lactose. (OC 10). White. Convex. In 100s.
		20 mg	Lactose. (OC 20). Pink. Convex. In 100s.
		40 mg	Lactose. (OC 40). Yellow. Convex. In 100s.
c-II	**Roxicodone** (Roxane)	**Tablets**: 5 mg	(54 582). White, scored. In 100s and UD 100s.
		Oral Solution: 5 mg/5 ml	Sorbitol. Burgundy cherry flavor. In 500 ml.
c-II	**Roxicodone Intensol** (Roxane)	**Solution, concentrate**: 20 mg/ml	In 30 ml w/dropper.

PROPOXYPHENE (Dextropropoxyphene)

Complete prescribing information begins in the Narcotic Agonist Analgesics monograph.

Actions:

Pharmacology: Propoxyphene is a centrally acting narcotic analgesic structurally related to methadone; its analgesic effect resides in the dextrorotatory isomer. Propoxyphene is ½ to ⅔ as potent as codeine. Propoxyphene alone in usual analgesic doses (32 to 65 mg of the hydrochloride or 50 to 100 mg of the napsylate salt), is no more and possibly less effective than 30 to 60 mg codeine or 600 mg aspirin. Propoxyphene combined with other analgesics (eg, codeine, aspirin) is more effective than propoxyphene or other analgesics alone.

Pharmacokinetics:

Absorption/Distribution – Water-soluble hydrochloride (HCl) salt is absorbed more rapidly than the relatively water insoluble napsylate salt; peak plasma concentrations for the HCl are achieved in 2 to 2.5 hours. In equimolar doses (100 mg of napsylate equals 65 mg of HCl), the two salts achieve similar peak plasma concentrations (great intersubject variation). A 65 mg oral dose of propoxyphene HCl achieves peak plasma levels of 0.05 to 0.1 mcg/ml. Bioavailability is reduced to 30% to 70% due to extensive first-pass biotransformation. Approximately 80% of propoxyphene and its metabolites are bound to plasma proteins. Highly lipid soluble, the drug is stored in fatty tissue in large quantities. Propoxyphene crosses the placenta and appears in breast milk.

Metabolism/Excretion – Propoxyphene is metabolized in the liver with a half-life of 6 to 12 hours. The major metabolite, norpropoxyphene, has a half-life of 30 to 36 hours. Propoxyphene is excreted in the urine primarily as metabolites. Norpropoxyphene has substantially less CNS depressant effects than propoxyphene, but a greater local anesthetic effect similar to that of amitriptyline and antiarrhythmic agents, such as lidocaine and quinidine.

Indications:

Relief of mild to moderate pain.

Contraindications:

Hypersensitivity to propoxyphene.

Warnings:

Fatalities: Propoxyphene products in excessive doses, either alone or in combination with other CNS depressants (including alcohol), are a major cause of drug-related deaths. In a survey conducted in 1975, in approximately 20% of the fatal cases, death occurred within the first hour (5% within 15 minutes). Judicious prescribing of propoxyphene is essential for safety. Consider nonnarcotic analgesics for depressed or suicidal patients. Do not prescribe propoxyphene for suicidal or addiction-prone patients. Because of added CNS depressant effects, cautiously prescribe with concomitant sedatives, tranquilizers, muscle relaxants, antidepressants or other CNS depressant drugs. Advise patients of the additive depressant effects of these combinations with alcohol.

Many propoxyphene-related deaths have occurred in patients with histories of emotional disturbances, suicidal ideation or attempts, or misuse of tranquilizers, alcohol and other CNS active drugs. Do not exceed the recommended dosage.

Drug dependence: In higher than recommended doses over long time periods, propoxyphene can produce drug dependence characterized by psychic dependence and, less frequently, physical dependence and tolerance. Propoxyphene will only partially suppress the withdrawal syndrome in individuals physically dependent on other narcotics. Abuse liability is similar to that of codeine.

Renal/Hepatic function impairment: Administer propoxyphene with caution since higher serum concentrations or delayed elimination may occur. Consider reduction of total daily doses for these patients.

Pregnancy: Safety for use during pregnancy has not been established. In 2914 exposures to propoxyphene during pregnancy, 46 (1.6%) possible associations of congenital defects were observed: Clubfoot (18), benign tumors (12), microcephaly (6), ductus arteriosus persistens (5) and cataract (5). Confirmation is required.

Neonatal withdrawal following heavy maternal ingestion has been reported. Use only when the potential benefits outweigh the potential hazards to the fetus.

Lactation: Low levels have been detected in breast milk. No adverse effects have been noted in nursing infants.

Children: Not recommended for use in children.

PROPOXYPHENE (Dextropropoxyphene)

Precautions:

Hazardous tasks: May impair mental or physical abilities required to perform potentially hazardous tasks; observe caution while driving or performing other tasks requiring alertness.

Drug Interactions:

Barbiturate anesthetics may increase respiratory and CNS depressive effects of propoxyphene due to additive pharmacologic activity. The CNS depressant effects are additive.

Carbamazepine: Concomitant administration of propoxyphene may increase carbamazepine levels and produce dizziness, ataxia and nausea.

Charcoal decreases the GI absorption of propoxyphene.

Cigarette smoking may induce liver enzymes responsible for the metabolism of propoxyphene; efficacy is reportedly decreased in smokers. Patients may increase the dosage to obtain adequate pain relief.

Cimetidine: Case reports have described CNS toxicity (confusion, disorientation, respiratory depression, apnea, seizures) following coadministration with narcotic analgesics; no clear-cut cause and effect relationship was established.

Warfarin: Potentiation of the hypoprothrombinemic effect of warfarin by propoxyphene may occur.

Adverse Reactions:

Less than 1% of hospitalized patients taking propoxyphene HCl at recommended doses experience side effects.

The most frequent adverse reactions are: Dizziness; sedation; nausea; vomiting.

Miscellaneous: Constipation; abdominal pain; skin rashes; lightheadedness; headache; weakness; euphoria; dysphoria; minor visual disturbances; abnormal liver function; reversible jaundice (rare).

Overdosage:

Symptoms: The patient is usually somnolent, but may be stuporous or comatose and convulsing. Respiratory depression is characteristic; ventilatory rate or tidal volume is decreased, resulting in cyanosis and hypoxia. Pupils, initially pinpoint, may dilate as hypoxia increases. Cheyne-Stokes respiration and apnea may occur. Blood pressure falls and cardiac performance deteriorates, resulting in pulmonary edema and circulatory collapse, unless corrected promptly. Cardiac arrhythmias and conduction delay may be present. A combined respiratory-metabolic acidosis occurs due to hypercapnia and lactic acid formation. Death may occur.

Treatment: Promptly initiate resuscitative measures. Treatment includes usual supportive measures. Refer to General Management of Acute Overdosage.Induction of emesis may be hazardous; it might coincide with seizures. Naloxone (see individual monograph) will markedly reduce the degree of respiratory depression; administer 0.4 to 2 mg IV promptly, and carefully repeat at 2 to 3 minute intervals, as necessary. Due to the short duration of action of naloxone and the long half-life of propoxyphene and its metabolites, repeated dosages of naloxone may be necessary. Naloxone may also be given by continuous IV infusion. If no response is observed after administration of 10 mg naloxone, question the diagnosis of propoxyphene toxicity.

Monitor blood gases, pH and electrolytes; promptly correct acidosis and electrolyte disturbance. Ventricular fibrillation or cardiac arrest may occur. Respiratory acidosis rapidly subsides as ventilation is restored and carbon dioxide is eliminated, but lactic acidosis may require IV bicarbonate.

Dialysis is of little value.

Patient Information:

May cause drowsiness, dizziness or blurring of vision; use caution while driving or performing other tasks requiring alertness.

Avoid alcohol and other sedative or drowsiness-causing drugs.

May cause nausea, vomiting or constipation; notify physician if these become prominent.

If GI upset occurs, these agents may be taken with food.

Notify physician if shortness of breath or difficulty in breathing occurs.

PROPOXYPHENE (Dextropropoxyphene)

PROPOXYPHENE HCl

Refer to the general discussion of these products in the Propoxyphene group monograph.

Administration and Dosage:

Usual dose: 65 mg every 4 hours as needed. Do not exceed 390 mg per day.

In hepatic or renal impairment, consider reducing total daily dosage.

c-iv	**Propoxyphene HCl** (Various, eg, Balan, Geneva, Goldline, Halsey, Lannett, Lemmon, Moore, Roxane, Rugby, Schein)	**Capsules**: 65 mg	In 20s, 100s, 500s, 1000s and UD 100s.
c-iv	**Darvon Pulvules** (Lilly)		In 100s, 500s and UD 100s and 500s.
c-iv	**Dolene** (Lederle)		(Lederle D36). Pink. In 100s and 500s.

PROPOXYPHENE NAPSYLATE

Complete prescribing information begins in the Narcotic Agonist Analgesics monograph.

Because of differences in molecular weight, 100 mg of propoxyphene napsylate is required to supply propoxyphene equivalent to 65 mg of the HCl. In hepatic or renal impairment, consider reducing total daily dosage.

Administration and Dosage:

Usual dose: 100 mg every 4 hours as needed. Do not exceed 600 mg per day.

Storage: Avoid freezing the suspension.

c-iv	**Darvon-N** (Lilly)	**Tablets**: 100 mg	Buff. In 100s, 500s and UD 100s.
		Suspension: 10 mg/ml	In 480 ml.

OXYMORPHONE HCl

For complete prescribing information, refer to the Narcotic Agonist Analgesics group monograph.

Indications:

Relief of moderate to severe pain.

Parenterally for preoperative medication, support of anesthesia, obstetrical analgesia and for relief of anxiety in patients with dyspnea associated with acute left ventricular failure and pulmonary edema.

Administration and Dosage:

IV: Initially, 0.5 mg.

SC or IM: Initially, 1 to 1.5 mg every 4 to 6 hours, as needed. For analgesia during labor, give 0.5 to 1 mg IM.

Rectal: 5 mg every 4 to 6 hours.

In nondebilitated patients, cautiously increase dose until pain relief is satisfactory.

Safety for use in children < 12 years of age has not been established.

Storage: Refrigerate suppositories.

c-ii	**Numorphan** (DuPont)	**Injection**: 1mg per ml	In 1ml amps.[1]
		1.5 mg per ml	In 1ml amps[1] and 10 ml vials.[1]
		Suppositories: 5 mg	In 6s.

[1] With parabens and 0.1% disodium dithionite.

SUFENTANIL CITRATE

For complete prescribing information, refer to the Narcotic Agonist Analgesics group monograph.

Indications:

Analgesic adjunct at dosages ≤ 8mcg/kg to maintain balanced general anesthesia.

A primary anesthetic agent at dosages ≥ 8mcg/kg to induce and maintain anesthesia with 100% oxygen in patients undergoing major surgical procedures, such as cardiovascular surgery or neurosurgical procedures in the sitting position, to provide favorable myocardial and cerebral oxygen balance or when extended postoperative ventilation is anticipated.

Administration and Dosage:

Individualize dosage. In obese patients (> 20% above ideal total body weight), determine dosage on the basis of lean body weight. Reduce dosage in the elderly or debilitated. Monitor vital signs routinely.

For IV injection.

Adult dosage range: Total dosage:

1 to 2 mcg/kg – Administer with nitrous oxide/oxygen in patients undergoing general surgery ≤ 8 hours in which endotracheal intubation and mechanical ventilation are required. Expected duration of anesthesia is 1 to 2 hours.

Maintenance: 10 to 25 mcg (0.2 to 0.5ml) as needed for surgical stress or lightening of analgesia. Individualize supplemental dosages.

2 to 8 mcg/kg – Administer with nitrous oxide/oxygen in more complicated major surgical procedures. Provides some attenuation of sympathetic reflex activity in response to surgical stimuli, hemodynamic stability and relatively rapid recovery. Expected duration of anesthesia is 2 to 8 hours.

Maintenance: 10 to 50 mcg (0.2 to 1 ml) for stress or lightening of analgesia. Individualize supplemental dosages.

8 to 30 mcg/kg (Anesthetic doses) – Administer with 100% oxygen and a muscle relaxant. Sufentanil produces sleep at dosages ≥ 8 mcg/kg and maintains a deep level of anesthesia without additional agents. At dosages ≤ 25 mcg/kg, catecholamine release is attenuated; 25 to 30 mcg/kg blocks sympathetic responses including catecholamine release. Use high doses in patients undergoing major surgical procedures (eg, cardiovascular surgery and neurosurgery in the sitting position). Postoperative mechanical ventilation and observation are essential due to extended postoperative respiratory depression.

Maintenance: 25 to 50 mcg (0.5 to 1ml) for stress and lightening of anesthesia.

Children (< 12 years of age): For induction and maintenance of anesthesia in children undergoing cardiovascular surgery, a dose of 10 to 25mcg/kg administered with 100% oxygen is recommended. Supplemental dosages of up to 25 to 50 mcg are recommended for maintenance.

C-II	**Sufentanil Citrate** (ESI Lederle)	**Injection:** 50 mcg (as citrate) per ml	In 1, 2 and 5 ml amps.
C-II	**Sufenta**[1] (Janssen)		In 1, 2 and 5 ml amps.

[1] Preservative free.

FENTANYL

For complete prescribing information, refer to the Narcotic Agonist Analgesics group monograph.

Indications:

Pain: For analgesic action of short duration during anesthesia (premedication, induction, maintenance), and in the immediate postoperative period (recovery room) as needed.

For use as a narcotic analgesic supplement in general or regional anesthesia.

For administration with a neuroleptic such as droperidol (see monograph in the General Anesthetics section) as an anesthetic premedication, for induction of anesthesia and as an adjunct in maintenance of general and regional anesthesia.

For use as an anesthetic agent with oxygen in selected high-risk patients (open heart surgery or certain complicated neurological or orthopedic procedures).

Administration and Dosage:

Individualize dosage. Monitor vital signs routinely.

Concomitant anesthesia: Certain forms of conduction anesthesia, such as spinal anesthesia and some peridural anesthetics, can alter respiration by blocking intercostal nerves. Fentanyl can also alter respiration through other mechanisms.

Concomitant narcotic administration: The respiratory depressant effect of fentanyl may persist longer than the analgesic effect. Consider the total dose of all narcotic analgesics used. Use narcotics in reduced doses initially, ¼ to ⅓ those usually recommended.

Premedication: 0.05 to 0.1 mg IM, 30 to 60 minutes prior to surgery.

Adjunct to general anesthesia:

Total low dosage – 0.002 mg/kg in small doses for minor, painful surgical procedures and postoperative pain relief.

Maintenance low dosage – Infrequently needed in minor procedures.

Total moderate dosage – 0.002 to 0.02 mg/kg. In addition to adequate analgesia, some abolition of the stress response should occur. Respiratory depression necessitates artificial ventilation and careful observation of postoperative ventilation.

Maintenance moderate dosage – 0.025 to 0.1 mg IV or IM when movement or changes in vital signs indicate surgical stress or lightening of analgesia.

Total high dosage – 0.02 to 0.05 mg/kg. For "stress free" anesthesia. Use during open heart surgery and complicated neurosurgical and orthopedic procedures where surgery is prolonged and the stress response is detrimental. Inject with nitrous oxide/oxygen to attenuate the stress response. Postoperative ventilation and observation are required.

Maintenance high dosage – Ranging from 0.025 mg to half the initial loading dose. Individualize dosage. Administer when vital signs indicate surgical stress and lightening of analgesia.

Adjunct to regional anesthesia: 0.05 to 0.1 mg IM or slowly IV over 1 to 2 minutes as required.

Postoperatively (recovery room): 0.05 to 0.1 mg IM for the control of pain, tachypnea and emergence delirium; repeat dose in 1 to 2 hours as needed.

Children (2 to 12 years): For induction and maintenance, a reduced dose as low as 2 to 3 mcg/kg is recommended. Safety and efficacy in children < 2 years of age have not been established.

General anesthetic – 0.05 to 0.1 mg/kg with oxygen and a muscle relaxant when attenuation of the responses to surgical stress is especially important. Up to 0.15 mg/kg may be necessary. It has been used for open heart surgery and other major surgical procedures to protect the myocardium from excess oxygen demand and for complicated neurological and orthopedic procedures.

Storage – Protect from light.

c-II	**Fentanyl** (Various, eg, Abbott, Astra, Elkins-Sinn, Sanofi Winthrop)	**Injection**: 0.05 mg base (as citrate) per ml	In 2, 5, 10 and 20 ml amps and 30 and 50 ml vials.
c-II	**Sublimaze** (Janssen)		In 2, 5, 10 & 20 ml amps.

[1] Preservative free.

FENTANYL TRANSDERMAL SYSTEM

For complete prescribing information, refer to the Narcotic Agonist Analgesics group monograph.

Indications:

Pain: Management of chronic pain in patients requiring opioid analgesia.

Not recommended in the management of postoperative pain because it has not been adequately studied in these patients, and because of the interpatient variability in absorption and disposition of fentanyl seen in the controlled clinical trials.

Administration and Dosage:

Individualize dosage. The most important factor to be considered in determining the appropriate dose is the extent of pre-existing opioid tolerance. Reduce initial doses in elderly or debilitated patients.

Application: Apply to non-irritated and non-irradiated skin on a flat surface of the upper torso. Clip (do not shave) hair at the application site prior to system application. If the site of application must be cleansed prior to application of the system, do so with clear water. Do not use soaps, oils, lotions, alcohol or any other agents that might irritate the skin or alter its characteristics. Allow the skin to dry completely prior to system application.

Apply immediately upon removal from the sealed package. Firmly press the transdermal system in place with the palm of the hand for 10 to 20 seconds, making sure the contact is complete, especially around the edges.

Each system may be worn continuously for 72 hours. If analgesia for > 72 hours is required, apply a new system to a different skin site after removal of the previous transdermal system.

Keep out of the reach of children. Fold used systems so that the adhesive side of the system adheres to itself, then flush the system down the toilet immediately upon removal. Dispose of any systems remaining from a prescription as soon as they are no longer needed. Remove unused systems from their pouch and flush down the toilet.

Dose selection: In selecting an initial dose, give attention to 1) the daily dose, potency and characteristics of the opioid the patient has been taking previously (eg, whether it is a pure agonist or mixed agonist-antagonist); 2) the reliability of the relative potency estimates used to calculate the dose needed (potency estimates may vary with the route of administration); 3) the degree of opioid tolerance, if any; 4) the general condition and medical status of the patient. Maintain each patient at the lowest dose providing acceptable pain control. Unless the patient has pre-existing opioid tolerance, use the lowest dose, 25 mcg/hr, as the initial dose.

To convert patients from oral or parenteral opioids to the transdermal system, use the following methodology:

1.) Calculate the previous 24 hour analgesic requirement.
2.) Convert this amount to the equianalgesic oral morphine dose using the table in the Actions section of the Narcotic Agonist Analgesics group monograph.
3.) The following table displays the range of 24 hour oral and IM morphine doses that are approximately equivalent to each transdermal system dose. Use this table to find the calculated 24 hour morphine dose and the corresponding transdermal fentanyl dose. Initiate treatment using the recommended dose and titrate patients upwards until analgesic efficacy is attained. Upwards titration may be done 3 days after the initial dose; thereafter, it may be done no more frequently than every 6 days. For delivery rates in excess of 100 mcg/hr, multiple systems may be used.

FENTANYL TRANSDERMAL SYSTEM

Fentanyl Transdermal Dose Based on Daily Morphine Equivalence Dose[1]		
Oral 24 hour morphine (mg/day)	IM 24 hour morphine (mg/day)	Fentanyl transdermal (mcg/hr)
45-134	8-22	25
135-224	23-37	50
225-314	38-52	75
315-404	53-67	100
405-494	68-82	125
495-584	83-97	150
585-674	98-112	175
675-764	113-127	200
765-854	128-142	225
855-944	143-157	250
945-1034	158-172	275
1035-1124	173-187	300

[1] A 10 mg IM or 60 mg oral dose of morphine every 4 hours for 24 hours (total of 60 mg/day IM or 360 mg/day oral) was considered approximately equivalent to fentanyl transdermal 100 mcg/hr.

The majority of patients are adequately maintained with transdermal fentanyl administered every 72 hours. A small number of patients may require systems to be applied every 48 hours. Because of the increase in serum fentanyl concentration over the first 24 hours following initial system application, the initial evaluation of the maximum analgesic effect cannot be made before 24 hours of wearing. The initial dosage may be increased after 3 days.

During the initial application, patients should use short-acting analgesics for the first 24 hours as needed until analgesic efficacy with the transdermal system is attained. Thereafter, some patients still may require periodic supplemental doses of other short-acting analgesics for breakthrough pain.

Dose titration: The conversion ratio from oral morphine to transdermal fentanyl is conservative, and 50% of patients are likely to require a dose increase after initial application. The initial dosage may be increased after 3 days, based on the daily dose of supplemental analgesics required by the patient in the second or third day of the initial application.

It may take up to 6 days after increasing the dose for the patient to reach equilibrium on the new dose. Therefore, patients should wear a higher dose through 2 applications before any further increase in dosage is made on the basis of the average daily use of a supplemental analgesic.

Base appropriate dosage increments on the daily dose of supplementary opioids, using the ratio of 90 mg/24 hours of oral morphine to a 25 mcg/hr increase in transdermal fentanyl dose.

Discontinuation: Some patients will require a change to other methods of opioid administration when the dose exceeds 300 mcg/hr. To convert patients to another opioid, remove the system and initiate treatment with half the equianalgesic dose of the new opioid 12 to 18 hours later (it takes ≥ 17 hours for the fentanyl serum concentration to fall by 50% after system removal). Titrate the dose of the new analgesic based on the patient's report of pain until adequate analgesia has been attained. For patients requiring discontinuation of opioids, a gradual downward titration is recommended since it is not known at what dose level the opioid may be discontinued without producing the signs and symptoms of abrupt withdrawal.

	Product/Distributor	Dose (mcg/hr)	System size (cm^2)	Fentanyl content (mg)	How Supplied
c-II	**Duragesic-25** (Janssen)	25	10	2.5	In cartons containing 5 individually packaged systems.[2]
c-II	**Duragesic-50**[1] (Janssen)	50	20	5	
c-II	**Duragesic-75**[1] (Janssen)	75	30	7.5	
c-II	**Duragesic-100**[1] (Janssen)	100	40	10	

[1] For use only in opioid tolerant patients.
[2] < 0.2 ml alcohol is released during use.

FENTANYL TRANSMUCOSAL SYSTEM

For complete prescribing information, refer to the Narcotic Agonist Analgesics group monograph.

Warning:

Fentanyl transmucosal contains the potent narcotic fentanyl citrate in a formulation that:

- Carries a risk of hypoventilation with its use that may result in death if not monitored by trained personnel supported by appropriate, immediately available equipment.
- Should only be used as an anesthetic premedication or for inducing conscious sedation prior to a diagnostic or therapeutic procedure in a monitored anesthesia care setting.
- Should only be administered in hospital settings such as the operating room, emergency department, ICU or other monitored anesthesia care settings in hospitals where there is immediate access to life support equipment, oxygen, facilities for endotracheal intubation, IV fluids and opioid antagonists.
- Can only be used safely in patients being monitored by 1) direct visual observation by a health professional whose sole responsibility is observation of the patient and by 2) some means of measuring respiratory function such as pulse oximetry until the patient has completely recovered.
- Should only be administered by persons specifically trained in the use of anesthetic drugs and the management of the respiratory effects of potent opioids, including respiratory and cardiac resuscitation of patients in the age group being treated. Such training must include the establishment and maintenance of a patent airway and assisted ventilation.
- Should only be used by healthcare practitioners instructed in the use of the product by the director of anesthesia of the institution in which the product will be used.
- Is contraindicated for use at any other setting outside a hospital.

Fentanyl transmucosal use is contraindicated in:

- Children who weigh < 10 kg (22 lbs).
- Treatment of acute or chronic pain. The safety of this product for these indications has not been established.
- Doses > 15 mcg/kg in children, and in doses > 5 mcg/kg in adults. Because of the excessive frequency of significant hypoventilation at higher doses, the maximum dose any child or adult should receive is 400 mcg, regardless of weight.

Indications:

Anesthesia: Only indicated for use in a hospital setting 1) as an anesthetic premedication in the operating room setting or 2) to induce conscious sedation prior to a diagnostic or therapeutic procedure in other monitored anesthesia care settings in the hospital.

Administration and Dosage:

Individualize doses based on the status of each patient, the clinical environment and the desired therapeutic effect; reduce dosage in elderly, debilitated or other vulnerable patients.

Some of the factors to be considered in determining an individualized dose are age, body weight, physical status, general condition and medical status, underlying pathological condition, use of other drugs, type of anesthesia to be used and the type and length of the procedure.

Fentanyl transmucosal doses of 5 mcg/kg provide effects similar to usual doses of fentanyl given IM (0.75 to 1.25 mcg/kg). Larger doses have not been shown to increase efficacy. As with all opioids, reduce the dosage in vulnerable patients. The magnitude of the expected effect will vary from mild with doses of 5 mcg/kg to marked with doses of 15 mcg/kg. Adults should not receive doses > 5 mcg/kg (400 mcg), and most children who are not apprehensive at onset may be managed with the same 5 mcg/kg dose. Children apprehensive at onset and some younger children may need doses of 5 to 15 mcg/kg with an attendant increased risk of hypoventilation.

Children: Because of the excessive frequency of significant hypoventilation at higher doses, doses > 15 mcg/kg (maximum dose, 400 mcg) are contraindicated in children.

Selection of dosage strength based on patient weight, with a dose range of 5 to 15 mcg/kg, is recommended. Premedication of children < 40 kg may require doses of 10 to 15 mcg/kg.

FENTANYL TRANSMUCOSAL SYSTEM

Pediatric Fentanyl Transmucosal Dosage Regimen		
Patient weight (kg)	5 to 10 mcg/kg	10 to 15 mcg/kg
<10	contraindicated	contraindicated
10	100 mg	100 mg
15	not available	200 mcg
20	200 mcg	200 or 300 mcg
25	200 mcg	300 mcg
30	300 mcg	300 or 400 mcg
35	300 mcg	400 mcg
≥ 40	400 mcg	use 400 mcg (see Adults)

Adults: Because of the excessive frequency of significant hypoventilation at higher doses, doses > 5 mcg/kg (maximum, 400 mcg) are contraindicated in adults.

Vulnerable patients: Consider selection of a lower dose for vulnerable patients (eg, patients with head injury, cardiovascular or pulmonary disease, hepatic disease, liver dysfunction). If signs of excessive opioid effects appear before the unit is consumed, immediately remove the dosage unit from the patient's mouth.

Elderly: If fentanyl transmucosal is to be used in patients > 65 years old, reduce the dose to 2.5 to 5 mcg/kg. Although studies in the elderly have not been conducted, elderly patients are twice as sensitive to the effects of other forms of fentanyl as the younger population. Like all potent opioid analgesics, fentanyl transmucosal can depress respiration and reduce ventilatory drive to a clinically significant extent.

Administration: Remove the foil overwrap just prior to administration. After the plastic overcap is removed, instruct the patient to place the fentanyl transmucosal unit in the mouth and to suck (not chew) it. Chewed or swallowed fentanyl contributes little to the peak concentration, but is responsible for a prolonged "tail" on the blood level profile as it is slowly absorbed.

Remove the unit using the handle after it is consumed or if the patient has achieved an adequate effect or shows signs of respiratory depression.

Place any remaining portion of the fentanyl transmucosal unit in the plastic overcap and dispose of the unit appropriately as required for Schedule II drugs.

Administration of the unit should begin 20 to 40 minutes prior to the anticipated need of desired effect. Patients typically take 10 to 20 minutes for complete consumption. Peak effect occurs ≈ 20 to 30 minutes after the start of administration. If hypoventilation or some other adverse event occurs before the dosage unit is consumed, immediately remove the unit from the patient's mouth.

The patient should be attended at all times by a healthcare professional skilled in airway management and resuscitative measures. Administer only in monitored settings and by persons specifically trained in the use of anesthetics and the management of the respiratory effects of potent opioids, including maintenance of a patent airway and assisted ventilation. Some means for measuring respiratory function, such as pulse oximetry, is recommended.

Safety and handling: Fentanyl transmucosal is supplied in individually sealed dosage forms that pose no known risk to healthcare providers having incidental dermal contact. Treat accidental dermal exposure by rinsing the affected area with cool water.

Disposal of fentanyl transmucosal: Remove the drug matrix from the handle by grasping it with tissue paper, and separate the drug matrix from the handle using a twisting motion. Then flush the drug matrix down the toilet. If any drug matrix remains on the handle, it may be removed by placing the handle under warm running tap water until the remaining portion of the drug matrix is dissolved. Dispose of the drug-free handle according to institutional protocol. During the disposal process, avoid contact of the drug matrix with the skin, eyes or mucous membranes. Wash hands thoroughly when finished.

Storage/Stability: Protect from freezing and moisture. Do not store above 30°C (86°F). Store in the protective foil pouch until dispensing. Do not use if the foil pouch has been opened.

c-II	**Fentanyl Oralet** (Abbott)	**Lozenges:** 200 mcg	Sucrose, liquid glucose. Raspberry flavor. In 25s with yellow label.
		300 mcg	Sucrose, liquid glucose. Raspberry flavor. In 25s with green label.
		400 mcg	Sucrose, liquid glucose. Raspberry flavor. In 25s with blue label.

ALFENTANIL HCl

Complete prescribing information begins in the Narcotic Agonist Analgesics monograph.

Indications:

Analgesic: Analgesic adjunct given in incremental doses in the maintenance of anesthesia with barbiturate/nitrous oxide/oxygen.

Analgesic administered by continuous infusion with nitrous oxide/oxygen in the maintenance of general anesthesia.

Anesthetic: Primary anesthetic for induction of anesthesia in general surgery when endotracheal intubation and mechanical ventilation are required.

Monitored anesthesia care (MAC): Analgesic component for monitored anesthesia care.

Administration and Dosage:

Individualize dosage. In obese patients (> 20% above ideal total body weight), determine dosage on the basis of lean body weight. Reduce dose in elderly or debilitated patients.

Monitor vital signs routinely.

Children < 12 years of age: Use is not recommended.

Premedication: Individualize the selection of preanesthetic medications.

Neuromuscular blocking agents should be compatible with the patient's condition.

In patients administered anesthetic (induction) dosages, qualified personnel and adequate facilities are essential for the management of intraoperative and postoperative respiratory depression.

Use a tuberculin syringe or equivalent for accuracy in small volumes.

Alfentanil Dosage Range

Indication	≈Duration of Anesthesia	Induction (Initial Dose)	Maintenance (Increments/ Infusion)	Total Dose	Effects
Incremental injection	≤ 30 min	8-20 mcg/kg	3-5 mcg/kg or 0.5-1 mcg/kg/ min	8-40 mcg/ kg	Spontaneous breathing or assisted ventilation when required.
Incremental injection	30-60 min	20-50 mcg/kg	5-15 mcg/kg	up to 75 mcg/kg	Assisted or controlled ventilation required. Attenuation of response to laryngoscopy and intubation.
Anesthetic induction	> 45 min	130-245 mcg/kg	0.5-1.5 mcg/kg/ min or general anesthetic	dependent on duration of procedure	Assisted or controlled ventilation required. Give slowly (over 3 min). Reduce concentration of inhalation agents by 30%-50% for initial hour.
Continuous infusion[1]	> 45 min	50-75 mcg/kg	0.5-3 mcg/kg/ min. Average infusion rate 1-1.5 mcg/ kg/min	dependent on duration of procedure	Assisted or controlled ventilation required. Some attenuation of response to intubation and incision, with intraoperative stability.
MAC	≤ 30 min	3-8 mcg/kg	3-5 mcg/kg every 5-20 min to 1 mcg/kg/min	3-40 mcg/ kg	Assisted or controlled ventilation required.

[1] 0.5-3 mcg/kg/min with nitrous oxide/oxygen in general surgery. Following anesthetic induction dose, reduce infusion rate requirements by 30% to 50% for the first hour of maintenance.

Vital sign changes that indicate response to surgical stress or lightening of anesthesia may be controlled by increasing rate to a max of 4 mcg/kg/min or administering bolus doses of 7 mcg/kg. If changes are not controlled after three bolus doses given over 5 minutes, use a barbiturate, vasodilator or inhalation agent. Always adjust infusion rates downward in the absence of these signs until there is some response to surgical stimulation.

Rather than an increase in infusion rate, administer 7 mcg/kg bolus doses of alfentanil or a potent inhalation agent in response to signs of lightening of anesthesia within the last 15 minutes of surgery. Discontinue infusion at least 10 to 15 minutes prior to the end of surgery.

Admixture compatibility: Physical and chemical compatibilities of alfentanil have been demonstrated in solution (concentration range, 25 to 80 mcg/ml) with Normal Saline, 5% Dextrose in Normal Saline, 5% Dextrose in Water and Lactated Ringers.

c-II	**Alfenta**[1] (Janssen)	**Injection:** 500 mcg (as HCl) per ml	In 2, 5, 10 and 20 ml amps.

[1] Preservative free.

LEVOMETHADYL ACETATE HCl

For complete prescribing information, refer to the Narcotic Agonist Analgesics group monograph.

Warning:

Conditions for distribution and use of levomethadyl (21 CFR 291.505):

Levomethadyl acetate HCl, used for the treatment of narcotic addiction, shall be dispensed only by treatment programs approved by the FDA, the DEA and the designated state authority. Approved treatment programs shall dispense and use levomethadyl in oral form only and according to the treatment requirements stipulated in federal regulations. Failure to abide by these requirements may result in injunction precluding operation of the program, seizure of the drug supply, revocation of the program approval and possible criminal prosecution.

Levomethadyl has no recommended uses outside of the treatment of opiate addiction.

Indications:

Management of opiate dependence.

Administration and Dosage:

Approved by the FDA on July 9, 1993.

Adjust the dose to achieve optimal therapeutic benefit with acceptable adverse opioid effects. Always dilute before administration and mix with diluent prior to dispensing. To avoid confusion between prepared doses of levomethadyl and methadone, use a different color liquid for dilution of each agent.

Dosing schedules: Usually administer 3 times a week, either on Monday, Wednesday and Friday, or on Tuesday, Thursday and Saturday. If withdrawal is a problem during the 72 hour inter-dose interval, the preceding dose may be increased. In some cases, an every-other-day schedule may be appropriate. The usual doses must not be given on consecutive days because of the risk of fatal overdose. No dose mentioned in this section is ever meant to be given as a daily dose.

Induction: The initial dose for street addicts should be 20 to 40 mg. Each subsequent dose, administered at 48 or 72 hour intervals, may be adjusted in increments of 5 to 10 mg until steady state is reached, usually within 1 or 2 weeks.

Patients dependent on methadone may require higher initial doses of levomethadyl. The suggested initial 3 times a week dose for such patients is 1.2 to 1.3 times the daily methadone maintenance dose being replaced. This initial dose should not exceed 120 mg; adjust subsequent doses, administered at 48 or 72 hour intervals, according to clinical response.

Most patients can tolerate the 72 hour inter-dose interval during the induction period. Some patients may require additional intervention. If additional opioids are required, give supplemental methadone in small doses rather than giving levomethadyl on 2 consecutive days. Take-home doses of methadone always pose a risk in this setting and physicians should carefully weigh the potential therapeutic benefit against the risk of diversion.

In some cases, where the degree of tolerance is unknown, patients can be started on methadone to facilitate more rapid titration to an effective dose, then converted to levomethadyl after a few weeks of methadone therapy.

The crossover from methadone to levomethadyl should be accomplished in a single dose; complete transfer to levomethadyl is simpler and preferable to more complex regimens involving escalating doses of levomethadyl and decreasing doses of methadone.

Carefully titrate dosage to the individual; induction too rapid for the patient's level of tolerance may result in overdose. Serious hazards, as seen in association with all narcotic analgesics, are respiratory depression and, to a lesser extent, circulatory depression.

Maintenance: Most patients will be stabilized on doses in the range of 60 to 90 mg 3 times a week. Doses as low as 10 mg and as high as 140 mg 3 times a week have been given in clinical studies.

Supplemental dosing over the 72 hour inter-dose interval (weekend) is rarely needed. For example, if a patient on a Mon/Wed/Fri schedule complains of withdrawal on Sundays, the recommended dosage adjustment is to increase the Friday dose in 5 to 10 mg increments up to 40% over the Mon/Wed dose or to a maximum of 140 mg.

If withdrawal symptoms persist after adjustment of dose, consideration may be given to every-other-day dosing if clinic hours permit. If the clinic is not open 7 days a week and every-other-day dosing is not practical, the patient's schedule may be adjusted so the 72 hour interval occurs during the week and the patient can come to the clinic to receive a supplemental dose of methadone.

LEVOMETHADYL ACETATE HCl

The maximum *total* amount of levomethadyl recommended for any patient is 140-140-140 mg or 130-130-180 mg on a thrice-weekly schedule or 140 mg every other day.

Planned temporary interruption of levomethadyl maintenance: Levomethadyl take-home doses are not permitted by regulation. Thus, several circumstances may cause the planned temporary discontinuation of treatment. Patients eligible for one or more take-home doses of methadone, who are unable to attend the clinic for their next regularly scheduled levomethadyl dose because of illness, personal or family crisis, other hardships, travel or state/federal holidays, may be temporarily transferred directly to methadone.

Patients meeting these criteria may receive one or more methadone doses. Methadone doses should be 80% of the patient's Mon/Wed levomethadyl dose (eg, patients receiving 80-80-100 mg levomethadyl on a Mon/Wed/Fri regimen would be transferred to a daily methadone dose of 64 mg). The first dose of methadone should be ingested no sooner than 48 hours after the last levomethadyl dose. The number of take-home methadone doses should be *two less* than the number of days of expected absence and should not exceed, in any case, the number of take-homes allowed in the methadone regulations.

Upon return to clinic, patients should resume levomethadyl maintenance following the same dosage regimen prior to the temporary interruption (see above). If > 48 hours have elapsed since their last methadone dose, patients should be reinducted on levomethadyl at a dose determined by clinical or toxicological evaluation of the patient by the physician.

Reinduction after an unplanned lapse in dosing:

Following a lapse of one levomethadyl dose – 1) If a patient comes to the clinic to be dosed on the day following a missed scheduled dose (misses Monday, arrives Tuesday), administer the regular Monday dose on Tuesday, with the scheduled Wednesday dose administered on Thursday and the Friday dose given on Saturday. The patient's regular schedule may be resumed the following Monday (misses Wednesday, receives the regular dose on Thursday and Saturday, and returns to the regular Mon/Wed/Fri dosing schedule the next week).

2) If a patient misses one dose and comes to the clinic on the day of the next scheduled dose (misses Monday, arrives Wednesday), the usual dose will be well tolerated in most instances, although a reduced dose may be appropriate in selected cases.

Following a lapse of more than one levomethadyl dose – Restart patients at an initial dose of 50% to 75% of their previous dose, followed by increases of 5 to 10 mg every dosing day (48 or 72 hour intervals) until their previous maintenance dose is achieved. Reinduce patients who have been off levomethadyl treatment for ≥ 1 week.

Transfer from levomethadyl to methadone: Patients maintained on levomethadyl may be transferred directly to methadone. Because of the difference between the two compounds' metabolites and their pharmacological half-lives, it is recommended that methadone be started on a daily dose at 80% of the levomethadyl dose being replaced; the initial methadone dose must be given no sooner than 48 hours after the last levomethadyl dose. Subsequent increases or decreases of 5 to 10 mg in the daily methadone dose may be given to control symptoms of withdrawal or, less likely, symptoms of excessive sedation, in accordance with clinical observations.

Detoxification from levomethadyl: There is limited experience with detoxifying patients from levomethadyl in a systematic manner, and both gradual reduction (5% to 10% a week) and abrupt withdrawal schedules have been used successfully. The decision to discontinue therapy should be made as part of a comprehensive treatment plan.

c-II	**ORLAAM** (BioDevelopment)	**Solution:** 10 mg/ml	With 1.8 mg methylparaben and 0.2 mg propylparaben. In 474 ml.

REMIFENTANIL HCl

Actions:

Pharmacology: Remifentanil is a mu-opioid agonist with rapid onset, peak effect, and short duration of action.

Hemodynamics – In premedicated patients undergoing anesthesia, 1-minute infusions of < 2 mcg/kg of remifentanil cause dose-dependent hypotension and bradycardia, while additional doses > 2 mcg/kg (up to 30 mcg/kg) do not produce any further decreases in heart rate or blood pressure. Peak hemodynamic effects occur within 3 to 5 minutes of a single dose of remifentanil or an infusion rate increase. When appropriate, bradycardia and hypotension can be reversed by reduction of the infusion rate, by the dose of concurrent anesthetics or by the administration of fluids or vasopressors.

Pharmacokinetics:

Distribution – The initial volume of distribution of remifentanil is ≈ 100 ml/kg. Remifentanil subsequently distributes into peripheral tissues with a steady-state volume of distribution of ≈ 350 ml/kg. These two distribution volumes generally correlate with total body weight (except in severely obese patients when they correlate better with ideal body weight [IBW]). Remifentanil is ≈ 70% bound to plasma proteins of which ⅔ is binding to alpha-1-acid-glycoprotein.

Metabolism/Excretion – Remifentanil is rapidly metabolized by hydrolysis of the propanoic acid-methyl ester linkage by nonspecific blood and tissue esterases. Remifentanil is not a substrate for plasma cholinesterase (pseudocholinesterase) and is not appreciably metabolized by the liver or lung.

Remifentanil is an esterase-metabolized opioid that results in the production of the carboxylic acid metabolite. This represents the principal metabolic pathway for remifentanil (> 95%). The carboxylic acid metabolite is essentially inactive and is excreted by the kidneys with an elimination half-life of ≈ 90 minutes.

The clearance of remifentanil is ≈ 40 ml/min/kg. Clearance generally correlates with total body weight (except in severely obese patients when it correlates better with IBW). The high clearance of remifentanil combined with a relatively small volume of distribution produces a short elimination half-life of ≈ 3 to 10 minutes. The duration of action does not increase with prolonged administration.

The pharmacokinetics of remifentanil fit a three-compartment model with a rapid distribution half-life of 1 minute, a slower distribution half-life of 6 minutes and a terminal elimination half-life of 10 to 20 minutes. The effective biological half-life of remifentanil is 3 to 10 minutes.

The analgesic effects of remifentanil are rapid in onset and offset. Its effects and side effects are dose-dependent. Remifentanil in humans has a rapid blood-brain equilibration half-time of 1 minute and a rapid onset of action. The pharmacodynamic effects of remifentanil closely follow the measured blood concentrations, allowing direct correlation between dose, blood levels and response. Blood concentration decreases 50% (in 3 to 6 minutes) after a 1-minute infusion, or after prolonged continuous infusion because of rapid distribution and elimination processes, and is independent of duration of drug administration. Recovery from the effects of remifentanil occurs rapidly (within 5 to 10 minutes). New steady-state concentrations occur within 5 to 10 minutes after changes in infusion rate. When used as a component of an anesthetic technique, remifentanil can be rapidly titrated to the desired depth of anesthesia/analgesia by changing the continuous infusion rate or by administering an IV bolus injection.

Respiration: Remifentanil depresses respiration in a dose-related fashion. The duration of action of remifentanil at a given dose does not increase with longer duration of administration because of lack of drug accumulation.

Spontaneous respiration occurs at blood concentrations of 4 to 5 ng/ml in the absence of other anesthetic agents; for example, after discontinuation of a 0.25 mcg/kg/min infusion of remifentanil, these blood concentrations would be reached in 2 to 4 minutes. In patients undergoing general anesthesia, the rate of respiratory recovery depends upon the concurrent anesthetic, N_2O < propofol < isoflurane.

Muscle rigidity: Skeletal muscle rigidity is related to the dose and speed of administration. Remifentanil may cause chest wall rigidity (inability to ventilate) after single doses of > 1 mcg/kg administered over 30 to 60 seconds or infusion rates > 0.1 mcg/kg/min; peripheral muscle rigidity may occur at lower doses. Administration of doses < 1 mcg/kg may cause chest wall rigidity when given concurrently with a continuous infusion of remifentanil.

Analgesia: Infusions of 0.05 to 0.1 mcg/kg/min, producing blood concentrations of 1 to 3 ng/ml, are typically associated with analgesia with minimal decrease in respiratory rate. Supplemental doses of 0.5 to 1 mcg/kg, incremental increases in infusion rate > 0.05 mcg/kg/min and blood concentrations exceeding 5 ng/ml (typically produced by infusions of 0.2 mcg/kg/min) have been associated with transient and reversible respiratory depression, apnea and muscle rigidity.

Cerebrodynamics: Under isoflurane-nitrous oxide anesthesia ($PaCO_2 < 30$ mmHg), a 1–minute infusion of remifentanil (0.5 or 1 mcg/kg) produced no change in intracranial pressure. Mean arterial pressure and cerebral perfusion decreased as expected with opioids.

Titration to effect: The rapid elimination of remifentanil permits the titration of infusion rate without concern for prolonged duration. In general, every 0.1 mcg/kg/min change in the IV infusion rate will lead to a corresponding 2.5 ng/ml change in blood remifentanil concentration within 5 to 10 minutes. In intubated patients only, a more rapid increase (within 3 to 5 minutes) to a new steady-state can be achieved with a 1 mcg/kg bolus dose in conjunction with an infusion rate increase.

Special populations:

Renal function impairment – The pharmacokinetic profile of remifentanil is not changed in patients with end stage renal disease (creatinine clearance < 10 ml/min). In anephric patients, the half-life of the carboxylic acid metabolite increases from 90 minutes to 30 hours. The metabolite is removed by hemodialysis with a dialysis extraction ratio of ≈ 30%.

Elderly – The pharmacodynamic activity of remifentanil (as measured by the EC_{50} for development of delta waves on the EEG) increases with age. The EC_{50} of remifentanil for this measure was 50% less in patients > 65 years of age when compared with healthy volunteers (25 years of age).

Children – In children 2 to 12 years of age, the blood concentrations of remifentanil after a 1 minute infusion of 5 mcg/kg were similar to those seen in adults receiving the same dose.

Cardiopulmonary bypass (CPB) – Remifentanil clearance is reduced by ≈ 20% during hypothermic CPB.

Clinical trials:

Induction of anesthesia – Remifentanil was administered with isoflurane, propofol or thiopental for the induction of anesthesia. Remifentanil reduced the propofol and thiopental requirements for loss of consciousness. Compared with alfentanil and fentanyl, a higher relative dose of remifentanil resulted in fewer responses to intubation. Overall, hypotension occurred in 5% of patients receiving remifentanil compared with 2% of patients receiving the other opioids.

Recovery – In 2169 patients receiving remifentanil for periods ≤ 16 hours, recovery from anesthesia was rapid, predictable and independent of the duration of the infusion of remifentanil. In the seven controlled, general surgery studies, extubation occurred in a median of 5 minutes in outpatient anesthesia (range: –3 to 17 minutes in 95% of patients) and 10 minutes in inpatient anesthesia (range: 0 to 32 minutes in 95% of patients). Recovery in studies using nitrous oxide or propofol was faster than in those using isoflurane as the concurrent anesthetic. There was no case of remifentanil-induced delayed respiratory depression (occurring > 30 minutes after discontinuation of remifentanil).

Indications:

General anesthesia: An analgesic agent for use during the induction and maintenance of general anesthesia for inpatient and outpatient procedures and for continuation as an analgesic into the immediate postoperative period.

Monitored anesthesia care: An analgesic component of monitored anesthesia care.

Contraindications:

Epidural or intrathecal administration, because of the presence of glycine in the formulation. Hypersensitivity to fentanyl analogs.

Warnings:

Interruption of an infusion of remifentanil will result in rapid offset of effect. Rapid clearance and lack of drug accumulation result in rapid dissipation of respiratory depressant and analgesic effects upon discontinuation of remifentanil at recommended doses. Precede discontinuation of an infusion of remifentanil with the establishment of adequate postoperative analgesia.

IV tubing: Make injections of remifentanil into IV tubing at or close to the venous cannula. Upon discontinuation of remifentanil, clear the IV tubing to prevent the inadvertent administration of remifentanil at a later point in time. Failure to adequately clear the IV tubing to remove residual remifentanil has been associated with the appearance of respiratory depression, apnea and muscle rigidity upon the administration of additional fluids or medications through the same IV tubing.

Respiratory depression in spontaneously breathing patients is generally managed by decreasing the rate of infusion of remifentanil by 50% or by temporarily discontinuing the infusion.

REMIFENTANIL HCl

Skeletal muscle rigidity can be caused by remifentanil and is related to the dose and speed of administration. Remifentanil may cause chest wall rigidity (inability to ventilate) after single doses of > 1 mcg/kg administered over 30 to 60 seconds, or after infusion rates > 0.1 mcg/kg/min. Single doses of < 1 mcg/kg may cause chest wall rigidity when given concurrently with a continuous infusion of remifentanil.

Treat muscle rigidity occurring during the induction of anesthesia by the administration of a neuromuscular blocking agent and the concurrent induction medications.

Muscle rigidity seen during the use of remifentanil in spontaneously breathing patients may be treated by stopping or decreasing the rate of administration of remifentanil. Resolution of muscle rigidity after discontinuing the infusion of remifentanil occurs within minutes. In the case of life-threatening muscle rigidity, a rapid onset neuromuscular blocker or naloxone may be administered.

Obesity: As for all potent opioids, caution is required with use in morbidly obese patients because of alterations in cardiovascular and respiratory physiology.

Long-term use: No data are available on the long-term (> 16 hours) use of remifentanil as an analgesic in ICU patients.

Labor and delivery: Respiratory depression and other opioid effects may occur in newborns whose mothers are given remifentanil shortly before delivery. In a human clinical trial, the average maternal remifentanil concentrations were approximately twice those seen in the fetus. However, in some cases fetal concentrations were similar to those in the mother. The umbilical arterio-venous ratio of remifentanil concentrations was ≈ 30%, suggesting metabolism of remifentanil in the neonate.

Elderly: While the effective biological half-life of remifentanil is unchanged, elderly patients have been shown to be twice as sensitive as the younger population to the pharmacodynamic effects of remifentanil (see Administration and Dosage).

Pregnancy: Category C. There are no adequate and well controlled studies in pregnant women. Use remifentanil during pregnancy only if the potential benefit justifies the potential risk to the fetus.

Lactation: It is not known whether remifentanil is excreted in breast milk. Because fentanyl analogs are excreted in breast milk, exercise caution when administering remifentanil to a nursing woman.

Children: Remifentanil has not been studied in pediatric patients < 2 years of age.

Precautions:

Monitoring: Vital signs and oxygenation must be continually monitored during the administration of remifentanil.

Bradycardia has been reported with remifentanil and is responsive to ephedrine or anticholinergic drugs, such as atropine and glucopyrrolate.

Hypotension has been reported with remifentanil and is responsive to decreases in the administration of remifentanil or to IV fluids or catecholamine (ephedrine, epinephrine, norepinephrine, etc) administration. The elderly are more sensitive to hypotension.

Intraoperative awareness has been reported in patients < 55 years of age when remifentanil has been administered with propofol infusion rates of ≤ 75 mcg/kg/min.

REMIFENTANIL HCl

Adverse Reactions:

Adverse Events Reported in ≥ 1% of Patients in General Anesthesia Studies at the Recommended Doses of Remifentanil			
Adverse event	Induction/Maintenance	Postoperative analgesia	After discontinuation
GI			
Nausea	< 1%	22%	36%
Vomiting	< 1%	8%	16%
CNS			
Shivering	< 1%	5%	5%
Fever	< 1%	< 1%	5%
Dizziness	0	< 1%	3%
Headache	0	< 1%	2%
Agitation	< 1%	1%	< 1%
Cardiovascular			
Hypotension[1]	19%	0	2%
Bradycardia[1]	7%	1%	1%
Tachycardia	< 1%	0	1%
Hypertension	1%	2%	1%
Miscellaneous			
Muscle rigidity[2]	11%[3]	2%	< 1%
Visual disturbance	0	0	3%
Respiratory depression	< 1%	7%	2%
Apnea	0	3%	< 1%
Pruritus	< 1%	2%	2%
Postoperative pain	0	2%	< 1%
Hypoxia	0	< 1%	1%

[1] See Precautions.
[2] See Warnings.
[3] Included in the muscle rigidity incidence is chest wall rigidity (5%). The overall muscle rigidity incidence is < 1% when remifentanil is administered concurrently or after a hypnotic induction agent.

Adverse Reactions Reported in ≥ 1% of Patients in Monitored Anesthesia Care Studies at the Recommended Doses of Remifentanil[1]		
Adverse Event	Remifentanil	Remifentanil + 2 mg midazolam[2]
GI		
Nausea	44%	18%
Vomiting	22%	5%
CNS		
Headache	18%	12%
Shivering	5%	< 1%
Dizziness	5%	5%
Chills	1%	0
Warm sensation	1%	0
Cardiovascular		
Hypotension[3]	4%	0
Bradycardia[3]	4%	0
Dermatologic		
Pruritus	18%	16%
Sweating	6%	0
Pain at study IV site	1%	0
Miscellaneous		
Respiratory depression[1]	3%	< 1%
Muscle rigidity[1]	3%	0
Flushing	1%	0

[1] See Warnings.
[2] With higher midazolam doses, higher incidences of respiratory depression and apnea were observed.
[3] See Precautions.

The following adverse reactions occurred in < 1% of patients:

GI: Constipation; abdominal discomfort; xerostomia; gastroesophageal reflux; dysphagia; diarrhea; heartburn; ileus.

Cardiovascular: Various atrial and ventricular arrhythmias; heart block; ECG change consistent with myocardial ischemia; elevated CPK-MB level; syncope.

Musculoskeletal: Muscle stiffness; musculoskeletal chest pain.

Respiratory: Cough; dyspnea; bronchospasm; laryngospasm; rhonchi; stridor; nasal congestion; pharyngitis; pleural effusion; hiccough(s); pulmonary edema; rales; bronchitis; rhinorrhea.

CNS: Anxiety; involuntary movement; prolonged emergence from anesthesia; tremors; disorientation; dysphoria; nightmare(s); hallucinations; paresthesia; nystigmus; twitch; sleep disorder; seizure; amnesia.

Body as a whole: Decreased body temperature; anaphylactic reaction; delayed recovery from neuromuscular block.

Dermatologic: Rash; urticaria; erythema; pruritus.

GU: Urine retention; oliguria; dysuria; urine incontinence.

Metabolic/Nutritional: Abnormal liver function; hyperglycemia; electrolyte disorders; increased CPK level.

Hematologic/Lymphatic: Anemia; lymphopenia; leukocytosis; thrombocytopenia.

Overdosage:

Symptoms: Apnea, chest-wall rigidity, seizures, hypoxemia, hypotension and bradycardia.

Treatment: In case of overdosage or suspected overdosage, discontinue administration of remifentanil, maintain a patent airway, initiate assisted or controlled ventilation with oxygen and maintain adequate cardiovascular function. If depressed respiration is associated with muscle rigidity, a neuromuscular blocking agent or a mu-opioid antagonist may be required to facilitate assisted or controlled respiration. IV fluids and vasopressors for the treatment of hypotension and other supportive measures may be employed. Glycopyrrolate or atropine may be useful for the treatment of bradycardia or hypotension.

IV administration of an opioid antagonist such as naloxone may be employed as a specific antidote to manage severe respiratory depression or muscle rigidity. Respiratory depression from overdosage with remifentanil is not expected to last longer than the opioid antagonist, naloxone. Reversal of the opioid effects may lead to acute pain and sympathetic hyperactivity.

Administration and Dosage:

Approved by the FDA on July 12, 1996.

For IV use only. Individualize dosage.

Administer continuous infusions of remifentanil only by an infusion device. The injection site should be close to the venous cannula. Clear all IV tubing at the time of discontinuation of infusion.

During general anesthesia: Remifentanil is not recommended as the sole agent in general anesthesia because loss of consciousness cannot be assured and because of a high incidence of apnea, muscle rigidity and tachycardia. Remifentanil is synergistic with other anesthetics and doses of thiopental, propofol, isoflurane and midazolam have been reduced by up to 75% with the coadministration of remifentanil.

Remifentanil Dosing Guidelines - General Anesthesia and Continuing as an Analgesic into the Postoperative Care Unit or Intensive Care Setting

Phase	Continuous IV infusion (mcg/kg/min)	Infusion dose range (mcg/kg/min)	Supplemental IV bolus dose (mcg/kg)
Induction of anesthesia (through intubation)	0.5 to 1[1]	NA[2]	NA[2]
Maintenance of anesthesia with:			
Nitrous oxide (66%)	0.4	0.1 - 2	1
Isoflurane (0.4 to 1.5 MAC)	0.25	0.05 - 2	1
Propofol (100 to 200 mcg/kg/min)	0.25	0.05 - 2	1
Continuation as an analgesic into the immediate postoperative period	0.1	0.025 - 0.2	not recommended

[1] An initial dose of 1 mcg/kg may be administered over 30 to 60 seconds.

[2] No data available.

During induction of anesthesia: Administer at an infusion rate of 0.5 to 1 mcg/kg/min with a hypnotic or volatile agent for the induction of anesthesia. If endotracheal intubation is to occur < 8 minutes after the start of infusion of remifentanil, then an initial dose of 1 mcg/kg may be administered over 30 to 60 seconds.

During maintenance of anesthesia: After endotracheal intubation, decrease the infusion rate of remifentanil in accordance with the dosing guidelines in the table above. Due to the rapid onset and short duration of action of remifentanil, the rate of administration during anesthesia can be titrated upward in 25% to 100% increments or downward in 25% to 50% decrements every 2 to 5 minutes to attain the desired level of mu-opioid effect. In response to light anesthesia or transient episodes of intense surgical stress, supplemental bolus doses of 1 mcg/kg may be administered every 2 to 5 minutes. At infusion rates > 1 mcg/kg/min, consider increases in the concomitant anesthetic agents to increase the depth of anesthesia.

Continuation as an analgesic into the immediate postoperative period under the direct supervision of an anesthesia practitioner: When used as an IV analgesic in the immediate postoperative period, administer remifentanil initially by continuous infusion at a rate of 0.1 mcg/kg/min. The infusion rate may be adjusted every 5 minutes in 0.025 mcg/kg/min increments to balance the patient's level of analgesia and respiratory rate. Infusion rates > 0.2 mcg/kg/min are associated with respiratory depression (respiratory rate < 8 breaths/min).

Guidelines for discontinuation: Upon discontinuation of remifentanil, clear the IV tubing to prevent inadvertent administration at a later time.

Because of the rapid onset of action, no residual opioid activity will be present within 5 to 10 minutes after discontinuation (see Warnings).

Analgesic component of monitored anesthesia care: It is strongly recommended that supplemental oxygen be supplied whenever remifentanil is administered.

REMIFENTANIL HCl

Remifentanil Dosing Guidelines - Monitored Anesthesia Care			
Method	Timing	Remifentanil	Remifentanil + 2 mg midazolam
Single IV dose	Given 90 seconds before local anesthetic	1 mcg/kg over 30 to 60 seconds	0.5 mcg/kg over 30 to 60 seconds
Continuous IV infusion	Beginning 5 minutes before local anesthetic	0.1 mcg/kg/min	0.05 mcg/kg/min
	After local anesthetic	0.05 mcg/kg/min (range: 0.025 to (0.2 mcg/kg/min)	0.025 mcg/kg/min (range: 0.025 to 0.2 mcg/kg/min)

Single dose: A single IV dose of 0.5 to 1 mcg/kg over 30 to 60 seconds may be given 90 seconds before the placement of the local or regional anesthetic block.

Continuous infusion: When used alone as an IV analgesic component of monitored anesthesia care, administer initially by continuous infusion at a rate of 0.1 mcg/kg/min beginning 5 minutes before placement of the local or regional anesthetic block.

Because of the risk for hypoventilation, decrease the infusion rate of remifentanil to 0.05 mcg/kg/min following placement of the block. Thereafter, rate adjustments of 0.025 mcg/kg/min at 5 minute intervals may be used to balance the patient's level of analgesia and respiratory rate. Rates > 0.2 mcg/kg/min are generally associated with repiratory depression (respiratory rates < 8 breaths/min).

Bolus doses of remifentanil administered simultaneously with a continuous infusion of remifentanil to spontaneously breathing patients are not recommended.

Individualization of dosage:

Elderly – Decrease the starting doses of remifentanil by 50% in elderly patients (> 65 years). Cautiously titrate to effect.

Children – The same doses (per kg) as adults are recommended for pediatric patients ≥ 2 years of age.

Obesity – Base the starting dose of remifentanil on ideal body weight (IBW) in obese patients (> 30% over their IBW).

Preanesthetic medication: The need for premedication and the choice of anesthetic agents must be individualized. In clinical studies, patients who received remifentanil frequently received a benzodiazepine premedication.

Admixture compatibility and stability: Remifentanil is stable for 24 hours at room temperature after reconstitution and further dilution to concentrations of 20 to 250 mcg/ml with the following IV fluids: Sterile Water for Injection; 5% Dextrose Injection; 5% Dextrose and 0.9% Sodium Chloride Injection; 0.9% Sodium Chloride Injection; 0.45% Sodium Chloride Injection.

Remifentanil has been shown to be compatible with propofol when coadministered into a running IV administration set.

Storage: Store at 2° to 25°C (36° to 77°F).

Rx	**Ultiva** (Glaxo Wellcome)	**Powder for Injection, lyophilized**	In 3, 5 and 10 ml vials.

NARCOTIC ANALGESIC COMBINATIONS

Components of these combinations include (see individual monographs):

NARCOTIC ANALGESICS: Codeine, hydrocodone bitartrate, dihydrocodeine bitartrate, opium, oxycodone HCl, oxycodone terephthalate, meperidine HCl, propoxyphene HCl, propoxyphene napsylate.

NONNARCOTIC ANALGESICS: Acetaminophen and salicylates.

CAFFEINE, a traditional component of many analgesic formulations, may be beneficial in certain vascular headaches.

BARBITURATES are used for their sedative effects.

PROMETHAZINE HCl (a phenothiazine derivative with antihistaminic properties), used for its sedative effect.

BELLADONNA ALKALOIDS, used as antispasmodics.

Content given per tablet, 5 ml liquid or 1 ml injection.

	Product and Distributor	Narcotic	Acetaminophen	Aspirin	Other Content	Average Adult Dose	How Supplied
c-v	**Acetaminophen w/Codeine Oral Solution**[1] (Various, eg, Moore, Morton Grove, Roxane, Schein)	12 mg codeine phosphate	120 mg			15 ml q 4 h	In 120 ml, pt and gal.
c-v	**Capital w/Codeine Suspension** (Carnrick)						Fruit punch flavor. In 473 ml.
c-v	**Tylenol w/Codeine Elixir** (McNeil)				7% alcohol, saccharin, sucrose		Cherry flavor. In 480 ml.
c-iii	**Acetaminophen w/Codeine Tablets** (Various, eg, Lemmon, Moore, Schein)	15 mg codeine phosphate	300 mg			1 to 4 q 4 h	In 100s and 1000s.
c-iii	**Tylenol w/Codeine No. 2 Tablets** (McNeil)				Sodium metabisulfite		(McNeil Tylenol Codeine 2). White. In 100s and UD 500s.
c-iii	**Phenaphen w/Codeine No. 3 Capsules** (Robins)	30 mg codeine phosphate	325 mg			1 to 2 q 4 h	Black/green. In 100s and 500s.

NARCOTIC ANALGESIC COMBINATIONS

	Product and Distributor	Narcotic	Acetaminophen	Aspirin	Other Content	Average Adult Dose	How Supplied
c-III	**Acetaminophen w/Codeine Tablets** (Various, eg, Lemmon, Moore, Purepac, Roxane, Schein)	30 mg codeine phosphate	300 mg			0.5 to 2 q 4 h	In 100s, 1000s and UD 100s.
c-III	**Aceta w/Codeine Tablets** (Century)					1 tid	In 100s and 1000s.
c-III	**Tylenol w/Codeine No. 3 Tablets** (McNeil)				Sodium metabisulfite	0.5 to 2 q 4 h	(McNeil Tylenol Codeine 3). White. In 100s, 500s, 1000s and UD 500s.
c-III	**Acetaminophen w/Codeine Tabs** (Various, eg, Lemmon, Moore, Purepac, Schein)	60 mg codeine phosphate	300 mg			1 q 4 h	In 100s, 500s, 1000s.
c-III	**Tylenol w/Codeine No. 4 Tablets** (McNeil)				Sodium metabisulfite		(McNeil Tylenol Codeine 4). White. In 100s, 500s, and UD 500s.
c-III	**Phenaphen w/Codeine No. 4 Capsules** (Robins)	60 mg codeine phosphate	325 mg			1 q 4 h	Lactose. Green/white. In 100s and 500s.

NARCOTIC ANALGESIC COMBINATIONS

	Product and Distributor	Narcotic	Acetaminophen	Aspirin	Other Content	Average Adult Dose	How Supplied
c-III	**Aspirin w/Codeine No. 3 Tablets** (Various, eg, Goldline, Major, Moore, Schein, URL, Zenith)	30 mg codeine phosphate		325 mg		1 or 2 q 4 h	In 100s and 1000s.
c-III	**Empirin w/Codeine No. 3 Tablets** (Glaxo Wellcome)						(Empirin 3). White. In 100s, 500s, 1000s and *Dispenserpak* 25s.
c-III	**Aspirin w/Codeine No. 4 Tablets** (Various, eg, Goldline, Major, Moore, Rugby, Schein, URL, Zenith)	60 mg codeine phosphate		325 mg		1 q 4 h	In 100s, 500s and 1000s.
c-III	**Empirin w/Codeine No. 4 Tablets** (Burroughs Wellcome)						(Empirin 4). White. In 100s, 500s and *Dispenserpak* 25s.
c-III	**Fioricet w/Codeine Capsules** (Sandoz)	30 mg codeine phosphate	325 mg		40 mg caffeine, 50 mg butalbital	1 or 2 q 4 h up to 6/day	(Fioricet codeine). Dark blue/gray. In 100s and *ControlPak* 25s.
c-III	**Fiorinal w/Codeine Capsules** (Sandoz)	30 mg codeine phosphate		325 mg	40 mg caffeine, 50 mg butalbital	1 or 2 q 4 h up to 6/day	(F-C Sandoz 78-107). Blue/yellow. In 100s and *Control-Pak* 25s.
c-III	**Lortab Elixir** (Whitby)	2.5 mg hydrocodone bitartrate	167 mg		7% alcohol, saccharin, sorbitol, sucrose, parabens	15 ml q 4 to 6 h up to 6/day	Tropical fruit punch flavor. In 473 ml.

NARCOTIC ANALGESIC COMBINATIONS

	Product and Distributor	Narcotic	Acetaminophen	Aspirin	Other Content	Average Adult Dose	How Supplied
c-iii	**Lortab 2.5/500 Tablets** (Whitby)	2.5 mg hydrocodone bitartrate	500 mg		Sucrose	1 or 2 q 4 to 6 h up to 8/day	(Whitby/901). White/pink specks. In 100s and 500s.
c-iii	**Hydrocodone Bitartrate & Acetaminophen Caps** (Various, eg, Goldline, Rugby)	5 mg hydrocodone bitartrate	500 mg			1 or 2 q 4 to 6 h up to 8/day	In 100s and 500s.
c-iii	**Hydrocodone Bitartrate and Acetaminophen Tablets** (Various, eg, Geneva, Goldline, Moore, Rugby, Watson)						In 100s and 500s.
c-iii	**Bancap HC Capsules** (Forest)						(Forest 610A). Yellow/orange. In 100s and 500s.
c-iii	**Ceta-Plus Capsules** (Seatrace)						(Seatrace). White. In 100s.
c-iii	**Co-Gesic Tablets** (Central)						(500-5) White, scored. Oval. In 100s and 500s.
c-iii	**Duocet Tablets** (Mason)						In 100s.
c-iii	**Dolacet Capsules** (Roberts Hauck)						(Dolacet Capsules Hauck 256). Black/red. In 100s.
c-iii	**Hydrocet Capsules** (Carnrick)						(C 8657). Blue/white. In 100s.

NARCOTIC ANALGESIC COMBINATIONS

	Product and Distributor	Narcotic	Acetaminophen	Aspirin	Other Content	Average Adult Dose	How Supplied
c-iii	**Hydrogesic Capsules** (Edwards)	5 mg hydrocodone bitartrate	500 mg			1 or 2 q 4 to 6 h up to 8/day	In 100s.
c-iii	**Hy-Phen Tablets** (B.F. Ascher)						(225-450). White, scored. Capsule shape. In 100s.
c-iii	**Margesic H Capsules** (Marnel)						(Margesic H). Gray/lavender. In 100s.
c-iii	**Medipain 5 Capsules** (Medi-Plex)						(MX 405). White. In 100s.
c-iii	**Lorcet Tablets** (UAD)						(MIA/108). White, scored. Capsule shape. In 500s.
c-iii	**Lorcet-HD Capsules** (UAD)						(1120). Maroon. In 100s.
c-iii	**Lortab 5/500 Tablets** (Whitby)				Sugar		White w/blue specks, scored. Capsule shape. In 100s, 500s and UD 100s.
c-iii	**Anexsia 5/500 Tablets** (Mallinckrodt)						(BMP 207). White, scored. In 100s.
c-iii	**Panacet 5/500 Tablets** (ECR Pharm)						(ECR 0141). White, scored. Oval. In 100s.

NARCOTIC ANALGESIC COMBINATIONS

	Product and Distributor	Narcotic	Acetaminophen	Aspirin	Other Content	Average Adult Dose	How Supplied
c-iii	**Stagesic Capsules** (Huckaby)	5 mg hydrocodone bitartrate	500 mg		Parabens	1 or 2 q 4 to 6 h up to 8/day	(Stagesic). White. In 100s.
c-iii	**T-Gesic Capsules** (T.E. Williams)						(T-Gesic/TEW). White. In 100s.
c-iii	**Vicodin Tablets** (Knoll)						(Vicodin). White, scored. Capsule shape. In 100s, 500s and UD 100s.
c-iii	**Zydone Capsules** (DuPont)						(DuPont Zydone). White. In 100s.
c-iii	**Lortab 7.5/500 Tablets** (Whitby)	7.5 mg hydrocodone bitartrate	500 mg		Sucrose	1 q 4 to 6 h	(Whitby/903). White w/green specks, scored. Capsule shape. In 100s, 500s and UD 100s.
c-iii	**Hydrocodone with Acetaminophen Tablets** (Various, eg, Watson, Warner-Chilcott)						In 100s and 500s.

NARCOTIC ANALGESIC COMBINATIONS

	Product and Distributor	Narcotic	Acetaminophen	Aspirin	Other Content	Average Adult Dose	How Supplied
c-III	**Anexsia 7.5/650 Tablets** (Mallinckrodt)	7.5 mg hydrocodone bitartrate	650 mg			1 q 4 to 6 h	(BMP 188). Peach, scored. Capsule shape. In 100s.
c-III	**Lorcet Plus Tablets** (UAD)						(U 201). White, scored. Capsule shape. In 100s, 500s and UD 100s.
c-III	**Hydrocodone Bitartrate/ Acetaminophen Caplets** (Various, eg, King Pharm)						In 100s and 500s.
c-III	**Vicodin ES Tablets** (Knoll)	7.5 mg hydrocodone bitartrate	750 mg			1 q 4 to 6 h up to 5/day	(Vicodin ES). White, scored. Oval. In 100s and UD 100s.
c-III	**Lortab 10/500 Tablets** (UCB Pharma)	10 mg hydrocodone	500 mg				(UCB/910). Pink. Capsule shape. In 100s and 500s.

NARCOTIC ANALGESIC COMBINATIONS

	Product and Distributor	Narcotic	Acetaminophen	Aspirin	Other Content	Average Adult Dose	How Supplied
c-iii	**Lorcet 10/650 Tablets** (UAD)	10 mg hydrocodone bitartrate	650 mg			1 q 4 to 6 h	(UAD 6350). Light blue, scored. Capsule shape. In 20s, 100s and UD 100s.
c-iii	**Anexsia 10/660** (Mallinkrodt)	10 mg hydrocodone bitartrate	660 mg				(KPI 3). White, scored. Capsule shape. In 100s and 1000s.
c-iii	**Vicodin HP** (Knoll)						(Vicodin HP). White, scored. Oval. In 100s.
c-iii	**Alor 5/500** (Atley)	5 mg hydrocodone bitartrate		500 mg			(AP Alor). In 100s.
c-iii	**Azdone Tablets** (Central)					1 or 2 q 4 to 6 h up to 8/day	(21). Pink, scored. Oval. In 100s and 1000s.
c-iii	**Damason-P Tablets** (Mason)						(M D-P). Pink, mottled. In 100s, 500s and 1000s.
c-iii	**Lortab ASA Tablets** (Whitby)					1 or 2 q 4 to 6 h	Pink, scored. In 100s.
c-iii	**Panasal 5/500 Tablets** (E.C. Robins)					1 or 2 q 4 to 6 h up to 8/day	(ECR 0131). Pink, mottled, scored. In 100s.

NARCOTIC ANALGESIC COMBINATIONS

	Product and Distributor	Narcotic	Acetaminophen	Aspirin	Other Content	Average Adult Dose	How Supplied
c-III	**DHC Plus Capsules** (Purdue Frederick)	16 mg dihydro-codeine bitartrate	356.4 mg		30 mg caffeine	2 q 4 h	(Purdue). Light aqua. In 100s.
c-III	**Synalgos-DC Capsules** (Wyeth-Ayerst)	16 mg dihydro-codeine bitartrate		356.4 mg	30 mg caffeine	2 q 4 h	(Wyeth 4191). Blue/gray. In 100s and 500s.
c-II	**Acetaminophen with Oxy-codone Tablets** (Various, eg, Halsey, Goldline, Major, Schein)	5 mg oxycodone HCl	325 mg			1 q 6 h	In 100s, 500s 1000s and UD 25s.
c-II	**Percocet Tablets** (DuPont)	5 mg oxycodone HCl	325 mg			1 q 6 h	(Percocet DuPont). In 100s, 500s and UD 100s.
c-II	**Roxicet Tablets** (Roxane)						(54 543). White, scored. In 100s, 500s and UD 100s.
c-II	**Roxicet Oral Solution** (Roxane)				0.4% alcohol, EDTA, saccharin, sucrose	5 ml q 6 h	In 500 ml and UD 5 ml.

NARCOTIC ANALGESIC COMBINATIONS

	Product and Distributor	Narcotic	Acetaminophen	Aspirin	Other Content	Average Adult Dose	How Supplied
c-ii	**Oxycodone with Acetaminophen Capsules** (Various, eg, Goldline, Halsey, Major, Schein)	5 mg oxycodone HCl	500 mg			1 q 6 h	In 100s, 500s, 1000s and UD 25s.
c-ii	**Roxicet 5/500 Caplets** (Roxane)						(54 730). White, scored. In 100s and UD 100s.
c-ii	**Roxilox Capsules** (Roxane)						(HD532). In 100s.
c-ii	**Tylox Capsules** (McNeil)				Sodium metabisulfite		(Tylox McNeil). Red. In 100s and UD 100s.
c-ii	**Percodan-Demi Tablets** (DuPont)	2.25 mg oxycodone HCl and 0.19 mg oxycodone terephthalate		325 mg		1 or 2 q 6 h	White, scored. In 100s.
c-ii	**Oxycodone with Aspirin Tablets** (Various, eg, Goldline, Major)	4.5 mg oxycodone HCl and 0.38 mg oxycodone terephthalate		325 mg		1 q 6 h	In 100s, 500s, 1000s and UD 25s.
c-ii	**Percodan Tablets** (DuPont)						Yellow, scored. In 100s, 500s, 1000s and UD 250s.
c-ii	**Roxiprin Tablets** (Roxane)						(54 902). White, scored. In 100s, 1000s and UD 100s.

NARCOTIC ANALGESIC COMBINATIONS

	Product and Distributor	Narcotic	Acetaminophen	Aspirin	Other Content	Average Adult Dose	How Supplied
c-II	**Mepergan Injection** (Wyeth-Ayerst)	25 mg meperidine HCl			25 mg promethazine HCl, 0.1 mg EDTA, 0.04 mg CaCl, ≤ 0.75 mg sodium formaldehyde sulfoxylate, 0.25 mg sodium metabisulfite, 5 mg phenol	1 to 2 ml q 3 to 4 h	In 2 ml *Tubex* and 10 ml vials.
c-II	**Mepergan Fortis Capsules** (Wyeth-Ayerst)	50 mg meperidine HCl			25 mg promethazine HCl, lactose	1 q 4 to 6 h	(Wyeth 261). Maroon. In 100s.
c-IV	**Propoxyphene Napsylate and Acetaminophen Tablets** (Various, eg, Major, Moore, Rugby)	50 mg propoxyphene napsylate	325 mg			2 q 4 h	In 100s, 500s, 550s, 1000s and UD 100s.
c-IV	**Darvocet-N 50 Tablets** (Lilly)	50 mg propoxyphene napsylate	325 mg			2 q 4 h	Orange. In *RxPak* 100s, 500s and UD 100s.

NARCOTIC ANALGESIC COMBINATIONS

	Product and Distributor	Narcotic	Acetaminophen	Aspirin	Other Content	Average Adult Dose	How Supplied
c-iv	**Propoxyphene Napsylate and Acetaminophen Tablets** (Various, eg, Geneva, Goldline, Lemmon, Major, Moore, Mylan, Rugby, Zenith)	100 mg propoxyphene napsylate	650 mg			1 q 4 h	In 30s, 50s, 100s, 500s, 1000s and UD 100s.
c-iv	**Darvocet-N 100 Tablets** (Lilly)						Orange. In *RxPak* 100s, 500s, UD 100s, UD 500s and RN 500s.
c-iv	**Propacet 100 Tablets** (Lemmon)						(Propacet). White. Film coated. In 100s and 500s.
c-iv	**Propoxyphene HCl w/Acetaminophen Tablets** (Various, eg, Moore, Mylan, Rugby)	65 mg propoxyphene HCl	650 mg			1 q 4 h	In 500s.
c-iv	**Wygesic Tablets** (Wyeth-Ayerst)	65 mg propoxyphene HCl	650 mg			1 q 4 h	(Wyeth 85). Green. Film coated. Capsule shape. In 100s, 500s and *Redipak* 100s.
c-iv	**Propoxyphene HCl Compound Capsules** (Various, eg, Goldline, Lemmon, Moore, Mylan, Schein)	65 mg propoxyphene HCl		389 mg	32.4 mg caffeine	1 q 4 h	In 100s and 500s.
c-iv	**Darvon Compound-65 Pulvules** (Lilly)						Red/gray. In 500s and *RxPak* 100s.

NARCOTIC ANALGESIC COMBINATIONS

	Product and Distributor	Narcotic	Acetaminophen	Aspirin	Other Content	Average Adult Dose	How Supplied
c-II	**B & O Supprettes No. 15A Suppositories** (PolyMedica)	30 mg powdered opium			16.2 mg powdered belladonna extract. Polyethylene glycol/ Polysorbate 60 base	1 or 2/day	Scored. In 12s.
c-II	**Opium and Belladonna Suppositories** (Wyeth-Ayerst)	60 mg powdered opium			15 mg belladonna extract. Cocoa butter base	1 or 2/day	In 20s.
c-II	**B & O Supprettes No. 16A Suppositories** (PolyMedica)				16.2 mg powdered belladonna extract. Polyethylene glycol/ Polysorbate 60 base	1 or 2/day	Scored. In 12s.

[1] May contain alcohol.

NARCOTIC AGONIST-ANTAGONIST ANALGESICS

Narcotic agonist-antagonist analgesics compete with other substances at the mu (μ) receptor. The μ receptors mediate morphine-like supraspinal analgesia, euphoria and respiratory and physical depression. Refer to the Narcotic Agonist Analgesic introduction for further information on the action of the narcotics in general.There are two types of narcotic agonist-antagonists: 1) Drugs which are antagonists at the μ receptor and are agonists at other receptors (ie, pentazocine), 2) Partial agonists (ie, buprenorphine) which have limited agonist activity at the μ receptor.

The narcotic agonist-antagonist analgesics are potent analgesic agents with a lower abuse potential than pure narcotic agonists. Because of their narcotic antagonist activity, these agents may precipitate withdrawal symptoms in those with opiate dependence.

Narcotic Agonist-Antagonist Pharmacokinetics

Agonist/Antagonist		Onset (min)	Peak (min)	Duration (hrs)	$t^1/_2$ (hrs)	Equivalent Dose[1] (mg)	Relative Antagonist Activity
Buprenorphine	IM	15	60	6	2.2-3.5	0.3	Equipotent with Naloxone
	IV[2]						
Butorphanol	IM	<10	30-60	3-4	2.5-4	2-3	30x Pentazocine or $^1/_{40}$ Naloxone
Dezocine	IM	≤ 30	30-150	2-4[3]	nd	10	Greater than Pentazocine
	IV	≤ 15			2.4[4]		
Nalbuphine	IM	< 15[5]	60	3-6	5	10	10x Pentazocine
	IV	12-30[2]	30				
Pentazocine	IM	15-20[2]	15-601	3	2.2-3.5	30	Weak
	IV	12-30[2]	nd				
	Oral	15-30[2]	60-180				

[1] Parenteral dose equivalent to 10 mg morphine.
[2] Time to onset and peak effect shorter.
[3] Dose related.
[4] For 10 or 20 mg dose; 1.7 hr for 5 mg dose.
[5] Also for subcutaneous administration.
* nd – no data

DEZOCINE

Actions:

Pharmacology: Dezocine is a strong synthetic opioid agonist-antagonist parenteral analgesic of the aminotetralin series. Its analgesic potency, onset and duration of action in the relief of postoperative pain are comparable to morphine.

Pharmacokinetics:

Absorption/Distribution – Dezocine is completely and rapidly absorbed following IM injection in healthy volunteers, with an average peak serum concentration of 19 ng/ml (range, 10 to 38 ng/ml) occurring between 10 and 90 minutes after a 10 mg IM injection. Following a 10 mg IV infusion over 5 minutes, the average terminal half-life of dezocine is 2.4 hours (range, 1.2 to 7.4 hours). The average volume of distribution is 10.1 L/kg (range, 4.7 to 20.1 L/kg), and the average total body clearance is 3.3 L/hr/kg (range, 1.7 to 7.2 L/hr/kg). There is evidence of nonlinear (dose-dependent) pharmacokinetics at doses > 10 mg: In a study where 5, 10 and 20 mg IV doses of dezocine were given (n = 12), dose-proportional serum levels were observed after 5 and 10 mg injections, but the area under the serum concentration-time curve for the 20 mg dose was about 25% greater, and the total body clearance was about 20% lower when compared to the 5 and 10 mg doses. The pharmacokinetics of dezocine following chronic administration (steady-state pharmacokinetics) are predicted to yield serum levels for 5 and 15 mg IM doses given every 4 hours of 6 to 9 ng/ml and 240 to 310 ng/ml, respectively. Pain relief in patients with postoperative pain is clinically evident when steady-state serum levels exceed 5 to 9 ng/ml. The side effects listed in Adverse Reactions were observed in patients whose average peak levels were < 45 ng/ml. Peak analgesic effect lags peak serum levels by 20 to 60 minutes.

Metabolism/Excretion – Approximately two-thirds of a dose is recovered in the urine with about 1% being excreted as unchanged dezocine and the remainder as the glucuronide conjugate.

Mean (Range) Pharmacokinetic Parameters of Dezocine in Healthy Volunteers

Route/Parameter	Dose: 5 mg (n = 12)	10 mg (n = 36)	20 mg (n = 12)
Intravenous			
Clearance (L/hr/kg)	3.52 (2.1-6.2)	3.33 (1.7-7.2)	2.76 (1.7-4.1)
Volume of distribution (L/kg)	10.7 (6.4-15.5)	10.1 (4.7-20.1)	8.8 (5.8-13.5)
Half-life (hr)	1.7 (0.6-4.4)	2.4 (1.2-7.4)	2.4 (1.4-5.2)
Intramuscular		(n = 24)	
Bioavailability		100%	
Peak plasma concentration (ng/ml)		10-38	
Time-to-peak plasma concentration (min)		10-90	

Hepatic insufficiency did not alter total body clearance in one study of 7 patients with cirrhosis. The volume of distribution and consequently the half-life, however, were increased by 30% to 50% relative to healthy volunteers following a 10 mg IV dose.

Use cautiously with reduced doses in patients with renal dysfunction because the primary elimination of dezocine is through the urine as a glucuronide.

Narcotic antagonist activity: Dezocine is a mixed opioid agonist-antagonist analgesic. Its opioid antagonist activity is less than that of nalorphine but greater than that of pentazocine when measured by antagonism of morphine-induced narcosis in rats.

Effect on respiration: Decozine and morphine produce a similar degree of respiratory depression when given in the usual analgesic doses. The effect is dose-dependent and may be reversed by naloxone. As the dose of dezocine is increased, there appears to be an upper limit to the magnitude of the respiratory depression produced by the drug in both animals and healthy human volunteers. Dezocine, like other mixed agonist-antagonist analgesics, may offer increased safety over pure agonist drugs such as morphine.

Cardiovascular effects: Dezocine is not associated with significant changes in mean systemic artery pressure, mean pulmonary artery pressure, pulmonary capillary wedge pressure, cardiac output, stroke index and left ventricular stroke work index.

DEZOCINE

Clinical trials:

Postoperative analgesia – The analgesic efficacy of dezocine was investigated in randomized controlled clinical trials in postoperative general surgical pain (orthopedic, gynecologic, abdominal). The studies were primarily double-blind, single-dose, parallel trials in which IV doses of 2.5 to 10 mg (85 to 160 patients per treatment group) or IM doses of 5 to 20 mg (39 to 221 patients per treatment group) was compared to 5 to 10 mg of morphine or 1 mg of IV butorphanol in patients with moderate-to-severe pain.

The onset of analgesic action was similar for dezocine, morphine and butorphanol, occurring within 15 minutes of IV and 30 minutes of IM administration of the drug. Doses of 10 mg IM produced analgesia similar to that produced by 10 mg of IM morphine while 5 mg IV was equivalent to 1 mg of IV butorphanol.

The peak analgesic effect and duration of analgesia were comparable for both routes of administration. Half of the patients remedicated within 2 hours after 5 mg of dezocine or 1 mg of butorphanol IV, 3 hours after 10 mg of dezocine or morphine IM and 4 hours after 15 mg of dezocine IM.

Pain relief was proportional to the dose of dezocine for single doses < 20 mg. Some data suggest that the maximally effective dose of dezocine in postoperative pain may be 15 mg due to dezocine's mixed agonist-antagonist pharmacology.

Chronic pain states – Data has been gathered in trials of burn patients (n = 16) and cancer pain (n = 88). The daily dose for most patients has ranged between 20 and 60 mg/day, although doses as large as 90 to 140 mg/day have been used. Dezocine has not been adequately studied in the management of chronic pain. It is not recommended for use in patients who may have developed significant tolerance to opioid drugs from long-term use because of the risk of precipitating acute withdrawal symptoms.

Indications:

Management of pain when the use of an opioid analgesic is appropriate.

Contraindications:

Hypersensitivity to the drug.

Warnings:

Drug dependence/abuse: Because of its opioid antagonist properties, dezocine is not recommended for patients physically dependent on narcotics. Patients who have recently taken substantial amounts of narcotics may experience withdrawal symptoms. Because of the difficulty in assessing dependence in patients who have previously received substantial amounts of narcotics, use caution in the administration of dezocine to such patients. To avoid precipitating an acute narcotic abstinence reaction, allow a sufficient period of withdrawal from opioids before administering dezocine.

Use of dezocine in combination with alcohol or other CNS depressant drugs will result in increased risk to the patient. Use with caution in individuals with active drug or alcohol addiction who are not in a medically controlled environment. Self-administration of any strong opioid may increase the relapse rate in populations recovering from addiction in abstinence-based recovery programs.

Dezocine has shown no evidence of abuse in clinical use during drug development. Mixed opioid agonist-antagonists of this type generally have less potential for abuse than pure agonists such as morphine or meperidine, but all such drugs have abuse potential, especially in those individuals with a history of opioid drug abuse or dependence.

Renal/Hepatic function impairment: Dezocine undergoes extensive hepatic metabolism and renal excretion of the glucuronide metabolite (see Pharmacokinetics). Give cautiously with reduced doses to patients with hepatic or renal dysfunction.

Elderly: Like all strong, mixed opioid agonist-antagonist analgesics, dezocine can depress respiration and reduce ventilatory drive to a clinically significant extent. It also can alter mental status or induce delirium in elderly patients. Dezocine has not undergone sufficient clinical testing in the geriatric population to assess its relative risk compared to other opioid analgesics, but reduce the initial dose of all drugs of this class in the geriatric patient and individualize subsequent doses.

DEZOCINE

Pregnancy: Category C. Dezocine caused a dose-related suppression of body weight and food consumption of the parental generation in rats receiving either IV or IM doses. Pup body weight was suppressed in a dose-related fashion. There are no adequate and well controlled studies in pregnant women. Use during pregnancy only if the potential benefit justifies the potential risk to the fetus.

Labor and delivery – Safety to the mother and fetus after dezocine administration during labor is unknown. Use in labor and delivery only when its use is essential to the welfare of the mother and infant.

Lactation: The use of dezocine in nursing mothers is not recommended since it is not known whether this drug is excreted in breast milk.

Children: Safety and efficacy in patients < 18 years old have not been established.

Precautions:

Head injury and increased intracranial pressure: Although there is no clinical experience in patients with head injury, the possible respiratory depressant effect and the potential of strong analgesics to elevate cerebrospinal fluid pressure (resulting from vasodilation following CO_2 retention) may be markedly exaggerated in the presence of head injury, intracranial lesions, or a preexisting increase in intracranial pressure. Strong analgesics can produce effects that may obscure the clinical course of patients with head injuries. Use only when essential and with extreme caution.

Chronic obstructive pulmonary disease: Because strong opioids cause some respiratory depression, administer only with caution and in low doses to patients with preexisting respiratory depression (eg, from other medication, uremia, severe infection), severely limited respiratory reserve, bronchial asthma, obstructive respiratory conditions or cyanosis. Respiratory depression induced by dezocine can be reversed by naloxone.

Biliary surgery: Although there is no evidence that dezocine alters the tonic pressure within the common bile duct, therapeutic doses of other opioid analgesics can significantly increase pressure within the common bile duct. Therefore, use with caution in such settings.

Ambulatory patients: Strong opioid analgesics impair the mental or physical abilities required for the performance of potentially dangerous tasks such as driving a car or operating machinery. Patients who have been given dezocine should not drive or operate dangerous machinery until the effects of the drug are no longer present.

Sulfite sensitivity: This product contains sodium metabisulfite, a sulfite that may cause allergic-type reactions including anaphylactic symptoms and life-threatening or less severe asthmatic episodes in certain susceptible people. The overall prevalence of sulfite sensitivity in the general population is unknown and probably low. Sulfite sensitivity is seen more frequently in asthmatic than in nonasthmatic people.

Drug Interactions:

CNS depressants: Opioid analgesics, general anesthetics, sedatives, tranquilizers, hypnotics or other CNS depressants (including alcohol) administered concomitantly with dezocine may have an additive effect. When such combined therapy is contemplated, reduce the dose of one or both agents.

Adverse Reactions:

A total of 2192 patients have received dezocine on an acute or chronic basis in the initial clinical trials. In nearly all cases, the type and incidence of side effects were those expected of a strong analgesic, and no unforeseen or unusual toxicity occurred. There is, as yet, limited information on the use of dezocine for periods longer than 48 to 72 hours, but there was no evidence of hepatic, hematologic or renal toxicity in 73 patients who received the drug for > 7 days.

Body as a whole: Sweating, chills, flushing, low hemoglobin, edema (< 1%).

Cardiovascular: Hypotension, heart or pulse irregularity, hypertension, chest pain, pallor, thrombophlebitis (< 1%).

GI: Nausea, vomiting (3% to 9%); dry mouth, constipation, diarrhea, abdominal pain/distress/disorder (< 1%); increased alkaline phosphatase and AST (< 1%, causal relationship unknown).

DEZOCINE

Musculoskeletal: Cramps/aching/pain (< 1%).

CNS: Sedation (3% to 9%); dizziness/vertigo (1% to 3%); anxiety, confusion, crying, delusions, sleep disturbance, headache, delirium, depression (< 1%).

Respiratory: Respiratory depression, respiratory symptoms, atelectasis (< 1%); hiccups (< 1%, causal relationship unknown).

Dermatologic: Injection site reactions (3% to 9%); pruritus, rash, erythema (< 1%).

Special senses: Diplopia, slurred speech, blurred vision (< 1%); congestion in ears, tinnitus (< 1%, causal relationship unknown).

GU: Urinary frequency, hesitancy and retention (< 1%).

Overdosage:

Symptoms: Based on preclinical pharmacology, overdosage will produce acute respiratory depression, cardiovascular compromise and delirium. The largest dose of dezocine given to nontolerant healthy volunteers without toxicity has been 30 mg/70 kg.

Treatment: Administer naloxone IV. Evaluate the respiratory and cardiac status of the patient constantly and institute appropriate supportive measures, such as oxygen, IV fluids, vasopressors and assisted or controlled respiration. Refer to General Management of Acute Overdosage.

Administration and Dosage:

Adults:

IM – Single dose of 5 to 20 mg (usual, 10 mg). Adjust dosage according to the patient's weight, age, severity of pain, physical status and other medications that the patient may be receiving. Repeat every 3 to 6 hours as necessary.

Maximum dose – 20 mg; probable upper limit of 120 mg/day. There is insufficient information regarding the risk of chronic use of dezocine to establish limits for the maximum recommended duration of treatment with the drug.

IV – 2.5 to 10 mg repeated every 2 to 4 hours. The usual initial IV dose is 5 mg.

SC – Not recommended. Repeated injection of dezocine at a single site has been associated with subcutaneous inflammation, vascular irritation and venous thrombosis in animals. The significance for patients is unknown, although injection site reactions occurred in 4% of patients treated with dezocine in clinical trials.

Children: Not recommended for patients < 18 years old.

Storage: Store at room temperature and protect from light. Do not use if the solution contains a precipitate.

Rx	**Dalgan** (Astra)	**Injection:** 5 mg/ml	In 2 ml[1] single-dose vials and 2 ml[1] Tubex syringes.
		10 mg/ml	In 2 ml[1] single-dose vials, 10 ml multiple-dose vials and 2 ml[1] Tubex syringes.
		15 mg/ml	In 2 ml[1] single-dose vials and 2 ml[1] Tubex syringes.

[1] 1 ml fill in 2 ml.

PENTAZOCINE

> **Warning:**
> *Talwin Nx* is intended for oral use only. Severe, potentially lethal reactions (eg, pulmonary emboli, vascular occlusion, ulceration and abscesses, withdrawal symptoms in narcotic-dependent individuals) may result from misuse of this drug by injection or in combination with other substances.

Actions:

Pharmacology: Pentazocine, a potent analgesic, weakly antagonizes the effects of morphine, meperidine and other opiates at the μ-opioid receptor. Pentazocine, presumed to exert its agonistic actions at the kappa (κ) and sigma (&b.sigma;) opioid receptors, may precipitate withdrawal symptoms in patients taking narcotic analgesics regularly. In addition, it produces incomplete reversal of cardiovascular, respiratory and behavioral depression induced by morphine and meperidine. Pentazocine also has sedative activity. Parenterally, 30 mg is usually as effective as 10 mg morphine or 75 to 100 mg meperidine. Orally, a 50 mg dose is equivalent to 60 mg codeine.

Talwin NX tablets, which contain naloxone, produce analgesic effects when administered orally because naloxone has poor bioavailability. Injected IV (an unintended use), naloxone will block the pharmacologic effects of pentazocine, producing withdrawal symptoms in opioid-dependent individuals.

Pharmacokinetics: Pentazocine is well absorbed from the GI tract and from SC and IM sites. However, it undergoes extensive first-pass hepatic metabolism. Oral bioavailability is < 20%, and was increased threefold in cirrhotic patients. Concentrations in plasma coincide closely with onset, intensity and duration of analgesia. Pentazocine passes into fetal circulation. It is excreted via the kidney, < 5% unchanged.

Indications:

Oral and parenteral: Relief of moderate to severe pain.

Parenteral: For preoperative or preanesthetic medication; supplement to surgical anesthesia.

Contraindications:

Hypersensitivity to pentazocine, naloxone (in *Talwin NX*) or any product component.

Warnings:

Drug dependence: Exercise special care in prescribing to emotionally unstable patients and to those with history of drug abuse; closely supervise when therapy exceeds 4 or 5 days. Psychological and physical dependence have occurred in such patients and, rarely, in patients without history of drug abuse. Abrupt discontinuation after extended use has resulted in withdrawal symptoms. If more than minor difficulty is encountered, reinstitute parenteral pentazocine with gradual withdrawal. Avoid substituting methadone or other narcotics in pentazocine abstinence syndrome.

"Ts and Blues": Injection IV of oral preparations of **pentazocine** (*Talwin,* "Ts") and **tripelennamine** (PBZ, "Blues"), an H_1-blocking antihistamine has become a common form of drug abuse. The combination is used as a "substitute" for heroin. The tablets are dissolved in tap water, filtered and injected IV.

The most frequent and serious complication of IV "Ts and Blues" addiction is pulmonary disease, due to occlusion of pulmonary arteries and arterioles with unsterile particles of cellulose and talc used as tablet binders. The occlusion leads to granulomatous foreign body reactions, infections, increased pulmonary artery resistance and pulmonary hypertension. Neurologic complications from IV injection of "Ts and Blues" include seizures, strokes and CNS infections. The replacement of oral pentazocine with the pentazocine/naloxone combination may decrease the popularity of this mixture. A few cases of abuse involving pentazocine/naloxone combination and tripelennamine have been reported, however.

Tissue damage: Severe sclerosis of skin, subcutaneous tissues and underlying muscle has occurred at injection sites following multiple doses of pentazocine lactate. Rotate injection sites; IM may be tolerated better than SC.

Head injury and increased intracranial pressure: Pentazocine can produce effects which may obscure the clinical course of head injury patients. The potential for elevating cerebrospinal fluid pressure may be attributed to CO_2 retention due to the respiratory depressant effects of the drug. These effects may be exaggerated in the presence of head injury, other intracranial lesions or a preexisting increase in intracranial pressure. Use with extreme caution and only if essential.

Myocardial infarction (MI): Exercise caution in the IV use of pentazocine for patients with acute MI accompanied by hypertension or left ventricular failure. Pentazocine IV elevates systemic and pulmonary arterial pressure, systemic vascular resistance and left ventricular end-diastolic pressure, causing increased cardiac workload. Use the oral form with caution in MI patients who have nausea or vomiting.

PENTAZOCINE

Acute CNS manifestations: Patients receiving therapeutic doses have experienced hallucinations (usually visual), disorientation and confusion which have cleared spontaneously. If the drug is reinstituted, acute CNS manifestations may recur.

Seizures have occurred with the use of pentazocine.

Renal/Hepatic function impairment: The drug is metabolized in liver and excreted by kidney; administer with caution to patients with such impairment. Extensive liver disease predisposes to greater side effects (eg, marked apprehension, anxiety, dizziness, drowsiness), and may be the result of decreased drug metabolism.

Pregnancy: Category C. Pentazocine rapidly crosses the placenta with cord blood levels 40% to 70% of maternal serum levels. Chronic maternal ingestion of pentazocine may result in neonatal withdrawal symptoms. Mothers addicted to "Ts and Blues" have lower birth weight infants who have problems similar to infants born of other narcotic addicted mothers. Safe use during pregnancy has not been established. Administer only when the benefits outweigh the hazards.

Labor – Patients receiving pentazocine during labor have experienced no adverse effects other than those that occur with commonly used analgesics. Use with caution in women delivering premature infants.

Lactation: Safety for use in the nursing mother has not been established.

Children: Safety and efficacy in children < 12 years old have not been established.

Precautions:

Respiratory conditions: Use caution and low dosage in patients with respiratory depression (eg, from other medication, uremia, severe infection), severely limited respiratory reserve, severe bronchial asthma, obstructive respiratory conditions, cyanosis.

Biliary tract pressure elevation generally occurs for varying periods following narcotic use. However, some evidence suggests pentazocine causes little or no elevation in biliary tract pressures. Clinical significance of these findings is unknown.

Patients receiving narcotics: Pentazocine is a mild narcotic antagonist. Some patients previously given narcotics, including methadone for the daily treatment of narcotic dependence, have experienced withdrawal symptoms after receiving pentazocine.

Hazardous tasks: May produce sedation, dizziness and occasional euphoria; observe caution while driving or performing other tasks requiring alertness, coordination or physical dexterity.

Sulfite sensitivity: May cause allergic-type reactions (eg, hives, itching, wheezing, anaphylaxis) in certain susceptible persons. Although the overall prevalence of sulfite sensitivity in the general population is probably low, it is seen more frequently in asthmatics or in atopic nonasthmatic persons.

Drug Interactions:

Alcohol: Due to the potential for increased CNS depressant effects, use cautiously in patients currently receiving pentazocine.

Barbiturate anesthetics may increase the respiratory and CNS depression of pentazocine because of additive pharmacologic activity.

Adverse Reactions:

Most common: Nausea; dizziness or lightheadedness; vomiting; euphoria.

GI: Constipation; cramps; abdominal distress; anorexia; diarrhea; dry mouth; taste alteration.

CNS: Sedation; headache; weakness or faintness; depression; disturbed dreams; insomnia; syncope; hallucinations; tremor; irritability; excitement; tinnitus; disorientation; confusion (see Warnings).

Ophthalmic: Blurred vision; focusing difficulty; nystagmus; diplopia; miosis.

Hypersensitivity: Edema of the face; sweating; anaphylactic reaction; rash; urticaria.

Dermatologic: Soft tissue induration; nodules; cutaneous depression; ulceration (sloughing); severe sclerosis of the skin, subcutaneous tissues and, rarely, underlying muscle at the injection site; diaphoresis; stinging on injection; flushed skin; dermatitis; pruritus; toxic epidermal necrolysis.

Cardiovascular: Hypotension; decrease in blood pressure; tachycardia; circulatory depression; shock; hypertension.

Respiratory: Respiratory depression; dyspnea; transient apnea in newborns whose mothers received parenteral pentazocine during labor.

Hematologic: Depression of white blood cells (especially granulocytes), usually reversible; moderate transient eosinophilia.

Miscellaneous: Urinary retention; paresthesia; chills; neuromuscular and psychiatric muscle tremors; alterations in rate or strength of uterine contractions during labor (parenteral form).

PENTAZOCINE

Overdosage:

Symptoms: The clinical picture of overdosage has not been well defined. High doses produce marked respiratory depression, increased blood pressure and tachycardia.

Treatment: Employ oxygen, IV fluids, vasopressors and other supportive measures, as indicated. Consider assisted or controlled ventilation. For respiratory depression, parenteral naloxone is a specific and effective antagonist (see individual monograph).

Refer to General Management of Acute Overdosage.

Patient Information:

May cause drowsiness; observe caution while driving or performing other tasks requiring alertness, coordination or physical dexterity.

Avoid alcohol and other CNS depressants.

Notify physician if skin rash, confusion or disorientation occurs.

Administration and Dosage:

Oral:

Adults – Initially, 50 mg every 3 or 4 hours; increase to 100 mg if necessary. Do not exceed a total daily dosage of 600 mg. When anti-inflammatory or antipyretic effects are desired in addition to analgesia, aspirin can be administered concomitantly.

Children (< 12 years old) – Clinical experience is limited; use is not recommended.

Pentazocine tablets are intended for oral use only. Severe, potentially lethal reactions may result from misuse by injection or when combined with other substances. Oral pentazocine tablets contain 0.5 mg naloxone, a narcotic antagonist, to aid in elimination of the abuse potential.

Parenteral:

Adults – 30 mg IM, SC or IV; may repeat every 3 to 4 hours. Doses in excess of 30 mg IV or 60 mg IM or SC are not recommended. Do not exceed a total daily dosage of 360 mg.

Use SC only when necessary; severe tissue damage is possible at injection sites. When frequent injections are needed, administer IM, constantly rotating injection sites.

Patients in labor – A single 30 mg IM dose is most common. A 20 mg IV dose, given 2 or 3 times at 2 to 3 hour intervals, has resulted in adequate pain relief when contractions become regular.

Children (< 12 years old) – Clinical experience is limited; use is not recommended.

Admixture incompatibility – Do not mix pentazocine in the same syringe with soluble barbiturates because precipitation will occur.

c-iv	**Talwin** (Sanofi Winthrop)	**Injection:** 30 mg (as lactate) per ml	In 10 ml vials[1], 1, 1.5 and 2 ml Uni-Amps, 1 and 2 ml Uni-Nest amps and 1, 1.5 and 2 ml fill in 2 ml Carpuject.[2]
Rx	**Pentazocine and Naloxone HCl** (Royce)	**Tablets:** 50 mg (as HCl) and 0.5 mg naloxone HCl	In 100s, 500s and 1000s.
c-iv	**Talwin NX** (Sanofi Winthrop)		(T51). Yellow, scored. Oblong. In 100s and UD 250s.

[1] With 2 mg acetone sodium bisulfite and 1 mg methylparaben per ml.
[2] With 1 mg acetone sodium bisulfite.

PENTAZOCINE COMBINATIONS

For complete prescribing information, refer to the Pentazocine monograph.

Administration and Dosage:

Adults:

Pentazocine and aspirin – 2 tablets 3 or 4 times daily.

Pentazocine and acetaminophen – 1 tablet every 4 hours, up to 6 tablets per day.

Children: Not recommended for children < 12 years old.

c-iv	**Talwin Compound Caplets** (Sanofi Winthrop)	**Tablets:** 12.5 mg (as HCl) and 325 mg aspirin	White. In 100s.
c-iv	**Talacen Caplets** (Sanofi Winthrop)	**Tablets:** 25 mg (as HCl) and 650 mg acetaminophen	Sodium metabisulfite. (Winthrop T37). Blue, scored. In 100s and UD 250s.

BUTORPHANOL TARTRATE

Actions:

Pharmacology: Butorphanol is a potent analgesic with both narcotic agonist and antagonist effects. The analgesic potency on a weight basis appears to be 3.5 to 7 times that of morphine, 30 to 40 times that of meperidine and 20 times that of pentazocine. The exact mechanism of action is unknown. Narcotic antagonist analgesics may exert their analgesic effect via a CNS mechanism, perhaps subcortical, in the limbic system.

Narcotic antagonist activity – Butorphanol's narcotic antagonist activity is approximately 30 times that of pentazocine and 1/40 that of naloxone.

Effect on respiration – A parenteral dose of 2 to 3 mg butorphanol produces analgesia and respiratory depression approximately equal to that of 10 mg morphine or 80 mg meperidine. However, butorphanol appears to have a ceiling effect at 30 to 60 mcg/kg in the degree of respiratory depression produced; it is reversible by naloxone.

Cardiovascular effects – Hemodynamic changes after IV administration, similar to those seen with pentazocine, include increased pulmonary artery pressure, pulmonary wedge pressure, left ventricular end-diastolic pressure, systemic arterial pressure, pulmonary vascular resistance and increased cardiac workload.

Pharmacokinetics:

Butorphanol Pharmacokinetics Based on Route of Administration

Parameter	IV	IM	Nasal
Onset (min)	rapid	10-15	within 15
Peak (hrs)	0.5-1	0.5-1	1-2
Duration (hrs)	3-4	3-4	4-5
Half-life (hrs)	2.1-8.8	—	2.9-9.2
AUC (hr • ng/ml)	4.4-13	—	0.3-10.3

Butorphanol is extensively metabolized in the liver. The major metabolite is hydroxybutorphanol; norbutorphanol is produced in small amounts. The elimination half-life of hydroxybutorphanol may be greater than the parent compound. Elimination occurs in the urine (70% to 80%) and feces (≈ 15%). In the urine, ≈ 5% is excreted unchanged, 49% as hydroxybutorphanol and < 5% as norbutorphanol. Elimination half-life is increased in the elderly and in patients with decreased creatinine clearance. Protein binding is ≈ 80%.

Indications:

Parenteral/Nasal: Management of pain (including postoperative analgesia).

In clinical trials, nasal butorphanol was effective in the treatment of migraine headache pain.

Parenteral: For preoperative or preanesthetic medication; to supplement balanced anesthesia; for relief of pain during labor.

Contraindications:

Hypersensitivity to butorphanol or any components of the products.

Warnings:

Physically dependent narcotic patients should not receive butorphanol prior to detoxification; it may precipitate withdrawal. However, there is some controversy whether butorphanol can induce withdrawal in opioid-dependent patients based on its relative action/inaction at various opiate receptors; specifically, whether it has antagonistic action at the μ receptor.

Drug dependence: Although butorphanol has low physical dependence liability, exercise care in administering to emotionally unstable patients and to those prone to drug misuse and abuse. Abuse has been reported, sometimes in combination with diphenhydramine. A distinct withdrawal syndrome developed upon discontinuation of the drug.

Head injury and increased intracranial pressure: Butorphanol, like other potent analgesics, may elevate cerebrospinal fluid pressure; use in cases of head injury can produce effects (eg, miosis) which may obscure the clinical course of these patients. Use with extreme caution and only if essential.

Cardiovascular disease: Butorphanol increases the cardiac workload; limit its use in acute myocardial infarction or in ventricular dysfunction or coronary insufficiency to those situations where the benefits outweigh the risk.

Severe hypertension has occurred rarely. Discontinue butorphanol and treat the hypertension. Naltrexone has also been effective.

BUTORPHANOL TARTRATE

Renal/Hepatic function impairment: The drug is metabolized in the liver and excreted by the kidneys; increase the dosage interval (see Administration and Dosage).

Elderly: The mean half-life of butorphanol is increased by 25% (to > 6 hours) in patients > 65 years of age. Elderly patients may be more sensitive to its side effects, especially dizziness.

Pregnancy: Category C. Safety for use during pregnancy prior to 37 weeks of gestation has not been established. Prolonged use during gestation may result in neonatal withdrawal. At term, butorphanol rapidly crosses the placenta. Use only when clearly needed and when potential benefits outweigh potential hazards to the fetus.

Labor and delivery – Butorphanol injection may be used during labor (see Administration and Dosage). Reports of infant respiratory distress/apnea following butorphanol use during labor have been associated with administration of a dose ≤ 2 hours prior to delivery, use of multiple doses, use with additional analgesic or sedative drugs or use in preterm pregnancies. In 119 patients, 1 mg IV during labor was associated with transient (10 to 90 minutes) sinusoidal fetal heart rate patterns but was not associated with adverse neonatal outcomes. Use with caution in the presence of an abnormal fetal heart rate pattern.

Nasal spray is not recommended during labor/delivery.

Lactation: Butorphanol appears in breast milk following the injectable route; assume the drug will appear in breast milk following the nasal route as well. The amount an infant would receive is probably clinically insignificant (estimated at 4 mcg/L of milk using 2 mg IM 4 times daily).

Children: Safety and efficacy for use in children < 18 years of age have not been established. Not recommended for use in this age group.

Precautions:

Respiratory conditions: Butorphanol causes some respiratory depression. Administer with caution and in low dosage to patients with respiratory depression, severely limited respiratory reserve, bronchial asthma, obstructive respiratory conditions or cyanosis.

Hazardous tasks: May cause dizziness or drowsiness; observe caution while driving or performing other tasks requiring alertness, coordination or physical dexterity.

Drug Interactions:

Barbiturate anesthetics may increase the respiratory and CNS depression of butorphanol because of additive pharmacologic activity.

Adverse Reactions:

Parenteral/Nasal:

Cardiovascular – Hypotension (< 1%).

GI – Nausea/Vomiting (13%); dry mouth (3% to 9%); stomach pain (≥ 1%).

CNS – Somnolence (43%); dizziness (19%); confusion (3% to 9%); anxiety, euphoria, floating feeling, nervousness, paresthesia (≥ 1%); abnormal dreams, agitation, dysphoria, hallucinations, hostility, drug dependence (< 1%).

Dermatologic – Sweating/Clammy (3% to 9%); pruritus (≥ 1%); rash/hives (< 1%).

Miscellaneous – Asthenia/Lethargy, headache (3% to 9%); blurred vision, sensation of heat (≥ 1%); impaired urination (< 1%).

Nasal:

Cardiovascular – Vasodilation (3% to 9%); palpitations (≥ 1%); hypertension (< 1%).

GI – Anorexia, constipation (3% to 9%).

CNS – Insomnia (11%); tremor (≥ 1%); convulsion, delusions, depression (< 1%).

Respiratory – Nasal congestion (13%); dyspnea, epistaxis, nasal irritation, pharyngitis, rhinitis, sinus congestion, upper respiratory infection (3% to 9%); bronchitis, cough, sinusitis (≥ 1%); apnea, shallow breathing (< 1%).

Special Senses – Tinnitus, unpleasant taste (3% to 9%); ear pain (≥ 1%).

Miscellaneous – Edema (< 1%).

Overdosage:

Symptoms: Overdosage could produce some respiratory depression and variable cardiovascular and CNS effects.

Treatment: Immediate treatment for suspected overdosage is IV naloxone (see individual monograph). Constantly evaluate the respiratory and cardiac status. Institute appropriate supportive measures (eg, oxygen, IV fluids, vasopressors, assisted or controlled respiration). Refer to General Management of Acute Overdosage.

BUTORPHANOL TARTRATE

Patient Information:

May cause drowsiness; observe caution while driving or performing other tasks requiring alertness, coordination or physical dexterity.

Do not use alcohol or other CNS depressant drugs concurrently.

Instruct patients on the proper use of the nasal spray.

Administration and Dosage:

Pain:

IV – 1 mg (dosage range, 0.5 to 2 mg) repeated every 3 to 4 hours as necessary.

IM – 2 mg (dosage range, 1 to 4 mg) every 3 to 4 hours as necessary in patients who will be able to remain recumbent. Do not exceed single doses of 4 mg.

Nasal – 1 mg (1 spray in one nostril). If adequate pain relief is not achieved within 60 to 90 minutes, an additional 1 mg dose may be given. The initial 2 dose sequence may be repeated in 3 to 4 hours as needed. Depending on the pain severity, an initial 2 mg dose (1 spray in each nostril) may be used in patients who will be able to remain recumbent. Do not give additional 2 mg doses for 3 to 4 hours.

Preoperative/Preanesthetic use: Individualize dosage. Usual dose is 2 mg IM 60 to 90 minutes before surgery.

Balanced anesthesia: 2 mg IV shortly before induction or 0.5 to 1 mg IV in increments during anesthesia. The increment may be up to 0.06 mg/kg depending on previous drugs administered. The total dose will vary, but patients seldom require < 4 mg or > 12.5 mg.

Labor: 1 to 2 mg IV or IM in patients at full term in early labor; repeat after 4 hours.

Children: Not recommended in children < 18 years of age.

Elderly:

Parenteral – Use one-half the usual dose at twice the usual interval. Base subsequent doses and intervals on patient response.

Nasal – 1 mg initially. Allow 90 to 120 minutes to elapse before deciding whether a second 1 mg dose is needed.

Renal/Hepatic function impairment: Increase the initial dosage interval to 6 to 8 hours. Determine subsequent doses by patient response.

Rx	**Stadol** (Mead Johnson)	**Injection:** (1 mg of tartrate salt is equal to 0.68mg base)	
		1 mg per ml	In 1 ml vials.
		2 mg per ml	In 1, 2 and 10[1] ml vials.
Rx	**Stadol NS** (Mead Johnson)	**Nasal spray:** 10 mg/ml	In 2.5 ml metered dose spray pump. Delivers an average of 14 to 15 doses.[2]

[1] With 0.1 mg/ml benzethonium chloride.

[2] If not used for ≥ 48 hours, the unit must be reprimed. With repriming before each dose, the unit will deliver ≈ 8 to 10 doses.

NALBUPHINE HCl

Actions:

Pharmacology: Nalbuphine, a potent analgesic with narcotic agonist and antagonist actions, has a chemical structure similar to phenanthrene derivatives, oxymorphone and naloxone. Its analgesic potency is essentially equivalent to that of morphine and about 3 times that of pantozocine on a milligram basis. Unlike the other agonist-antagonists, nalbuphine does not significantly increase pulmonary artery pressure or systemic vascular resistance or cardiac work.

Pharmacokinetics: Onset of action occurs within 2 to 3 minutes after IV administration, and in < 15 minutes following SC or IM injection. Nalbuphine is metabolized in the liver; plasma half-life is 5 hours. The duration of analgesic activity ranges from 3 to 6 hours. Aproximately 7% is excreted unchanged in the urine.

The narcotic antagonist activity of nalbuphine is 10 times that of pentazocine.

Indications:

Relief of moderate to severe pain.

For preoperative analgesia, as a supplemental to balanced analgesia, to surgical and post-surgical anesthesia and for obstetrical analgesia during labor and delivery.

Contraindications:

Hypersensitivity to nalbuphine.

Warnings:

Drug dependence: Nalbuphine's low abuse potential is less than codeine and propoxyphene. Psychological and physical dependence and tolerance may follow nalbuphine abuse. Cautiously prescribe to emotionally unstable patients or to individuals with a history of narcotic abuse.

Abrupt discontinuation after prolonged use has been followed by symptoms of narcotic withdrawal.

Head injury and increased intracranial pressure: The possible respiratory depressant effects and the potential of potent analgesics to elevate cerebrospinal fluid pressure may be markedly exaggerated in the presence of head injury, intracranial lesions or a preexisting increase in intracranial pressure. Potent analgesics can produce effects which may obscure the clinical course of patients with head injuries. Therefore, use with extreme caution and only if deemed essential.

Renal/Hepatic function impairment: The drug is metaboilized in the liver and excreted by the kidneys; patients with renal or liver dysfunction may overreact to customary doses. Therefore, use with caution and administer in reduced amounts.

Pregnancy: Safe use in pregnancy has not been established. Prolonged use during pregnancy could result in neonatal withdrawal. Administer to pregnant women only when the potential benefits outweigh the possible hazards.

Labor and delivery: May produce respiratory depression in the neonate. Use with caution in women delivering premature infants.

Children: Clinical experience not available; not recommended in patients < 18 years old.

Precautions:

Respiratory depression: At the usual adult dose of 10 mg/70 kg, nabuphine causes respiratory depression approximately equal to that produced by equal doses of morphine. However, in contrast to morphine, nalbuphine exhibits a ceiling effect; increases in dosage beyond 30 mg produce no further respiratory depression. Respiratory depression induced by nalbuphine can be reversed by naloxone. Administer with caution at low doses to patients with impaired respiration (eg, from other medication, uremia, bronchial asthma, severe infection, cyanosis or respiratory obstructions).

Myocardial infarction: Use with caution in patients with myocardial infarction who have nausea or vomiting.

Biliary tract surgery: Use with caution in patients about to undergo biliary tract surgery since it may cause spasm of the sphincter of Oddi.

Potentially hazardous tasks: May produce drowsiness. Observe caution while driving or performing other tasks requiring alertness, coordination or physical dexterity.

Sulfite sensitivity: May cause allergic-type reactions (eg, hives, itching, wheezing, anaphylaxis) in certain susceptible persons. Although the overall prevalence of sulfite sensitivity in the general population is probably low, it is seen more frequently in asthmatics or in atopic nonasthmatic persons. Specific products containing sulfites are identified in the product listings.

Drug Interactions:

Barbiturate anesthetics may increase the respiratory and CNS depression of nalbuphine because of additive pharmacologic activity.

NALBUPHINE HCl

Adverse Reactions:

Most frequent: Sedation (36%).

Less frequent: Sweaty/clammy feeling (9%); nausea/vomiting (6%); dizziness/vertigo (5%); dry mouth (4%); headache (3%).

Other adverse reactions (≤ 1%):

Cardiovascular: Hypertension; hypotension; bradycardia; tachycardia, pulmonary edema.

CNS: Nervousness; depression; restlessness; crying; floating feeling; hostility; unusual dreams; confusion; faintness; hallucinations; euphoria; dysphoria; feeling of heaviness; numbness; tingling; unreality. The incidence of psychotomimetic effects (unreality, depersonalization, delusions, dysphoria, hallucinations) is less than with pentazocine.

Dermatologic: Itching; burning; urticaria.

GI: Cramps; dyspepsia; bitter taste.

Respiratory: Respiratory depression; dyspnea; asthma.

Miscellaneous: Speech difficulty; urinary urgency; blurred vision; flushing; warmth.

Overdosage:

Symptoms: The administration of single doses of 72 mg nalbuphine SC to eight normal subjects resulted primarily in symptoms of sleepiness and mild dysphoria.

Treatment: The immediate IV administration of naloxone is a specific antidote (see individual monograph). Treatment includes usual supportive measures. Refer to General Management of Acute Overdosage.

Patient Information:

May cause drowsiness; observe caution while driving or performing other tasks requiring alertness.

Administration and Dosage:

Adults: Usual dose is 10 mg/70 kg administered SC, IM or IV every 3 to 6 hours as necessary. Individualize dosage. In nontolerant individuals, the recommended single maximum dose is 20 mg, with a maximum total daily dose of 160 mg.

Patients dependent of narcotics may experience withdrawal symptoms upon the administration of nalbuphine. If unduly troublesome, control by slow IV administration of small increments of morphine until relief occurs. If the previous analgesic was morphine, meperidine, codeine or another narcotic with similar duration of activity, administer ¼ the anticipated nalbuphine dose initially. Observe for signs of withdrawal. If untoward symptoms do not occur, progressively increase doses at appropriate intervals until analgesia is obtained.

Rx	**Nalbuphine HCl** (Various, eg, Astra, Bioline, DuPont Critical Care, Goldline, Lyphomed, Moore, Quad, Rugby, Schein, VHA Supply)	**Injection**: 10 mg per ml	In 1 and 10 ml vials.
Rx	**Nubain** (DuPont)		In 1ml amps[2] and 10 ml vials.
Rx	**Nalbuphine HCl** (Various, eg, Astra, Bioline, DuPont Critical Care, Goldline, Lyphomed, Moore, Quad, Rugby, Schein, VHA Supply)	**Injection**: 20 mg per ml[1]	In 1 and 10 ml vials.
Rx	**Nubain** (DuPont)		In 1ml amps,[2] 10 ml vials and 1 ml disp. syringe.

[1] With 0.1% sodium metabisulfite and methyl and propyl parabens.
[2] This size also available as sulfite/paraben-free.

BUPRENORPHINE HCl

Actions:

Pharmacology: Buprenorphine is a semisynthetic centrally-acting opioid analgesic derived from thebaine; a 0.3 mg dose is approximately equivalent to 10 mg morphine in analgesic effects. Buprenorphine exerts its analgesic effect via high affinity binding of CNS opiate receptors. It has a high affinity for the μ receptors and dissociates from them slowly, which may contribute to its long duration of action and low physical dependence.

Its narcotic antagonist activity is approximately equipotent to naloxone.

Cardiovascular – Buprenorphine may cause a decrease or, rarely, an increase in pulse rate and blood pressure in some patients.

Respiratory effects – A therapeutic dose of 0.3 mg buprenorphine can decrease respiratory rate similarly to an equianalgesic dose of morphine (10 mg).

Pharmacokinetics: Onset of analgesic effect occurs 15 minutes after IM injection, peaks in about 1 hour, and persists up to 6 hours. When given IV, the time to onset and peak is shortened.

Plasma protein binding is about 96%. Buprenorphine is metabolized by the liver and its clearance is related to hepatic blood flow. Terminal half-life is 2 to 3 hours. The drug is excreted predominantly in the feces as free buprenorphine with traces of the N–dealkyl metabolite.

Indications:

Relief of moderate to severe pain.

Contraindications:

Hypersensitivity to buprenorphine.

Warnings:

Narcotic-dependent patients: Because of the narcotic antagonist activity of buprenorphine, use in physically dependent individuals may result in withdrawal effects. Buprenorphine, a partial agonist, has opioid properties which may lead to psychic dependence due to a euphoric component of the drug. Direct dependence studies have shown little physical dependence when the drug is withdrawn. The drug may not be substituted in acutely dependent narcotic addicts due to its antagonist component.

Respiratory effects: There have been occasional reports of clinically significant respiratory depression associated with buprenorphine. Use with caution in patients with compromised respiratory function and those given other respiratory depressants. In such cases, reduce the dose by one half. The use of assisted or controlled ventilation may be necessary.

Head injury/increased intracranial pressure: Buprenorphine may elevate cerebrospinal fluid (CSF) pressure; use with caution in head injury, intracranial lesions and other states where CSF pressure may be increased. Buprenorphine can produce miosis and changes in consciousness levels which may interfere with patient evaluation.

Hepatic function impairment: Buprenorphine is metabolized by the liver; the activity may be altered in those individuals with impaired hepatic function.

Pregnancy: Category C. In animals, buprenorphine produced mild post-implantation losses and early fetal deaths at 10 and 100 times the human dose. In rabbits, buprenorphine produced a dose-related trend for extra rib formation at 1000 times the human dose.

There are no adequate and well controlled studies in pregnant women. Use only if the potential benefits outweigh the potential hazards to the fetus.

Labor and delivery – Safety and efficacy have not been established.

Lactation: It is not known whether buprenorphine is excreted in breast milk. Exercise caution when administering to a nursing mother.

Children: Safety and efficacy for use in children have not been established.

Precautions:

Use with caution in the following: Elderly or debilitated; severe impairment of hepatic, pulmonary or renal function; myxedema or hypothyroidism; adrenal cortical insufficiency (eg, Addison's disease); CNS depression or coma; toxic psychoses; prostatic hypertrophy or urethral stricture; acute alcoholism; delirium tremens or kyphoscoliosis. Naloxone may not be effective in reversing respiratory depression.

Biliary tract dysfunction: Buprenorphine increases intracholedochal pressure to a similar degree as other opiates; administer with caution.

Potentially hazardous tasks: May cause dizziness or drowsiness; observe caution while driving or performing other tasks requiring alertness.

BUPRENORPHINE HCl

Drug Interactions:

Barbiturate anesthetics may increase the respiratory and CNS depression of buprenorphine because of additive pharmacologic activity.

Diazepam: Respiratory and cardiovascular collapse was reported in a patient who received therapeutic doses of buprenorphine and this drug.

Adverse Reactions:

CNS: Sedation (66%); dizziness/vertigo (5% to 10%); headache (1% to 5%); confusion, dreaming, psychosis, euphoria, weakness/fatigue, nervousness, slurred speech, paresthesia, depression (< 1%); malaise, hallucinations, depersonalization, coma, tremor (infrequent); dysphoria/agitation, convulsions/lack of muscle coordination (rare).

Cardiovascular: Hypotension (1% to 5%); hypertension, tachycardia, bradycardia, Wenckebach block (< 1%).

GI: Nausea/vomiting (1% to 5%); constipation, dry mouth (< 1%); dyspepsia, flatulence (infrequent); loss of appetite, diarrhea (rare).

Respiratory: Hypoventilation (1% to 5%); dyspnea, cyanosis (< 1%); apnea (infrequent).

Ophthalmic: Miosis (1% to 5%); blurred vision, diplopia, conjunctivitis, visual abnormalities (< 1%); amblyopia (infrequent).

Dermatologic: Sweating (1% to 5%); pruritus, injection site reaction (< 1%); rash, pallor (infrequent); urticaria (rare).

Miscellaneous: Urinary retention; flushing/warmth; chills/cold; tinnitus.

Overdosage:

Symptoms: Although the antagonist activity of buprenorphine may become manifest at doses somewhat above the recommended therapeutic range, doses in the recommended therapeutic range may produce clinically significant respiratory depression in certain circumstances (see Warnings).

Treatment: Carefully monitor cardiac and respiratory status. Establish a patent airway and institute assisted or controlled ventilation. Employ oxygen, IV fluids, vasopressors and other supportive measures as indicated. Refer to General Management of Acute Overdosage. The primary management of overdose is mechanical assistance of respiration. Naloxone may be of value in managing overdose; doxapram has also been used.

Patient Information:

May cause dizziness or drowsiness; observe caution while driving or performing other tasks requiring alertness.

Do not exceed prescribed dosage. Avoid alcohol and benzodiazepines.

Administration and Dosage:

Patients ≥ 13 years of age: 0.3 mg IM or slow IV, every 6 hours, as needed. Repeat once (up to 0.3 mg) if required, 30 to 60 minutes after initial dosage, giving consideration to previous dose pharmacokinetics; use thereafter only as needed. In high-risk patients (eg, elderly, debilitated, presence of respiratory disease) or in patients where other CNS depressants are present, such as in the immediate postoperative period, reduce dose by approximately one-half. Exercise extra caution with the IV route of administration, particularly with the initial dose.

Occasionally, it may be necessary to give up to 0.6 mg. Data are insufficient to recommend single IM doses > 0.6 mg for long-term use.

IV compatibility: Buprenorphine is compatible with: Isotonic saline, Lactated Ringer's Solution, 5% Dextrose and 0.9% Saline, 5% Dextrose, scopolamine HBr, haloperidol, glycopyrrolate, droperidol and hydroxyzine HCl.

IV incompatibility: Buprenorphine is incompatible with diazepam and lorazepam.

Storage: Avoid excessive heat (> 40°C or 104°F) and light.

c-v	**Buprenex** (Reckitt & Colman)	**Injection:** 0.324 mg (equiv. to 0.3 mg buprenorphine) per ml	In 1 ml amps.[1]

[1] With 50 mg anhydrous dextrose.

METHOTRIMEPRAZINE

This agent acts by central mechanisms and is therefore distinct from the salicylates and othernonsteroidal anti-inflammatory agents which act peripherally.

Actions:

Pharmacology: A phenothiazine derivative and potent CNS depressant which produces suppression of sensory impulses, reduction of motor activity, sedation and tranquilization. Methotrimeprazine raises the pain threshold and produces amnesia. It also has antihistaminic, anticholinergic and antiadrenergic effects.

It produces an analgesic effect comparable to morphine and meperidine with a marked sedative effect. Respiratory depression in the patient or in the newborn during or following preanesthetic or obstetrical use occurs infrequently. The drug does not appear to affect the cough reflex. Its use has not been reported to result in addiction, dependence or withdrawal symptoms even with large doses or with prolonged administration.

Pharmacokinetics: Peak plasma concentrations occur 30 to 90 minutes after injection. Maximum analgesic effect usually occurs within 20 to 40 minutes after IM injection and is maintained for about 4 hours. Methotrimeprazine is metabolized into sulfoxides and glucuronic conjugates and largely excreted in the urine as such. Elimination half-life is 15 to 30 hours. Small amounts of unchanged drug are excreted in the feces and in the urine (1%). Elimination into the urine usually continues for several days after IM administration is discontinued.

Indications:

Relief of moderate to marked pain in nonambulatory patients.

For obstetrical analgesia and sedation where respiratory depression is to be avoided.

Preanesthetic for producing sedation, somnolence and relief of apprehension and anxiety.

Contraindications:

Concurrent administration with antihypertensive agents including MAO inhibitors; history of phenothiazine hypersensitivity; presence of overdosage of CNS depressants or comatose states; severe myocardial, renal or hepatic disease; clinically significant hypotension; patients <12 years of age.

Warnings:

Following administration, orthostatic hypotension, sedation, fainting or dizziness may occur. Avoid or carefully supervise ambulation for at least 6 hours following the initial dose. Once this effect is tolerated, it will usually be maintained unless more than several days elapse between subsequent doses. Therapy with vasopressors has been required very rarely. Phenylephrine and methoxamine are suitable vasopressors; however, do not use epinephrine since a paradoxical decrease in blood pressure may result. Reserve norepinephrine for hypotension not reversed by other vasopressors.

Elderly: Elderly and debilitated patients with heart disease are more sensitive to phenothiazine effects. Therefore, give a low initial dose and individualize dosage thereafter. Monitor pulse, blood pressure and general circulatory status until dosage requirements and response are stabilized.

Pregnancy: Use with caution in women of childbearing potential and during early pregnancy. There is no evidence of adverse developmental effects when administered during late pregnancy and labor.

Children: Do not use in children < 12 years of age since safety and efficacy have not been established.

Precautions:

Prolonged administration for > 30 days is usually unnecessary, and is only advised when narcotic drugs are contraindicated or in terminal illnesses. When long-term use is anticipated, perform periodic blood counts and liver function studies.

Sulfite sensitivity: May cause allergic-type reactions (eg, hives, itching, wheezing, anaphylaxis) in certain susceptible persons. Although the overall prevalence of sulfite sensitivity in the general population is probably low, it is seen more frequently in asthmatics or in atopic nonasthmatic persons.

Drug Interactions:

CNS depressant drugs (eg, **narcotics, barbiturates, general anesthetics**) exert CNS additive effects. Individualize each drug regimen.

Atropine, scopolamine and succinylcholine: Use cautiously. Tachycardia and fall in blood pressure may occur, and undesirable CNS effects such as stimulation, delirium and extrapyramidal symptoms may be aggravated.

METHOTRIMEPRAZINE

Adverse Reactions:

Most of these effects have occurred only with long-term, high dosage administration. Some of these effects have been reported in users of methotrimeprazine whose dosages were not within the recommended range.

Cardiovascular: The most important side effects are associated with orthostatic hypotension, and include fainting or syncope and weakness. Avoid by keeping the patient supine for about 6 to 12 hours after injection. Blood pressure (usually within physiological range) often drops, beginning within 10 to 20 minutes following IM injection, and may last 4 to 6 hours (up to 12 hours); it usually diminishes or disappears with continued or intermittent administration. Occasionally, fall in blood pressure may be profound and may require immediate restorative measures.

CNS: Disorientation; dizziness; excessive sedation; weakness; slurring of speech.

GI: Abdominal discomfort; nausea; vomiting.

GU: Difficult urination; rarely, uterine inertia.

Hypersensitivity: Local inflammation; swelling.

Hematologic: Agranulocytosis with long-term, high dosage.

Hepatic: Jaundice with long-term, high dosage.

Miscellaneous: Chills; dry mouth; nasal congestion; pain at injection site.

Refer to the Antipsychotic Agents group monograph for a complete discussion of adverse effects related to use of phenothiazines.

Administration and Dosage:

Administer by deep IM injection into a large muscle mass. Rotate injection sites. Do not administer SC, as local irritation may occur. Do not administer IV.

Analgesia (adult): 10 to 20 mg (0.5 to 1 ml) IM every 4 to 6 hours as required (range, 5 to 40 mg [0.5 to 2 ml] at intervals of 1 to 24 hours). A flexible dosage schedule and initial dose of 10 mg are advisable until individual patient response and tolerance have been determined.

Elderly: Initial dose of 5 to 10 mg (0.25 to 0.5 ml). Gradually increase subsequent doses if needed.

Analgesia for acute or intractable pain: Initially, 10 to 20 mg, with adjustment of subsequent doses every 4 to 6 hours for pain relief.

Obstetrical analgesia: During labor, an initial dose of 15 to 20 mg may be repeated or adjusted as needed.

Preanesthetic medication: Administer 2 to 20 mg 45 minutes to 3 hours before surgery. A dose of 10 mg is often satisfactory, and 15 to 20 mg may be used for more sedation. Atropine sulfate or scopolamine HBr may be used concurrently in lower than usual doses.

Postoperative analgesia: In the immediate postoperative period, give an initial dose of 2.5 to 7.5 mg, as residual effects of anesthetic agents and other medications may be additive. Administer at intervals of 4 to 6 hours as needed. Supervise ambulation.

IV admixture incompatibilities: May be given IM in the same syringe with either atropine sulfate or scopolamine HBr. Do NOT mix in the same syringe with other drugs.

Rx	**Levoprome** (Lederle)	**Injection:** 20 mg (as HCl) per ml	With 0.9% benzyl alcohol, 0.065% EDTA and 0.3% sodium metabisulfite. In 10 ml vials.

TRAMADOL HCl

Actions:

Pharmacology: Tramadol is a centrally acting synthetic analgesic compound that is not derived from natural sources nor is it chemically related to opiates. Although its mode of action is not completely understood, from animal tests at least two complementary mechanisms appear applicable: Binding to μ-opioid receptors and inhibition of reuptake of norepinephrine and serotonin. Tramadol opioid activity derives from low affinity binding of the parent compound to μ-opioid receptors and higher affinity binding of the M1 metabolite. In animal models, M1 is up to 6 times more potent than tramadol in producing analgesia and 200 times more potent in μ-opioid binding. The contribution to human analgesia of tramadol relative to M1 is unknown.

Tramadol-induced antinociception is only partially antagonized by the opiate antagonist naloxone in animal tests. In addition, tramadol inhibits reuptake of norepinephrine and serotonin in vitro, as have some other opioid analgesics. These latter mechanisms may contribute independently to the overall analgesic profile of tramadol. Onset of analgesia is evident within 1 hour after administration and reaches a peak in ≈ 2 to 3 hours. Peak plasma concentrations are reached about 2 hours after administration, which correlates closely with the time to peak pain relief.

Apart from analgesia, tramadol may produce a constellation of symptoms (including dizziness, somnolence, nausea, constipation, sweating and pruritus) similar to that of an opioid. However, tramadol causes significantly less respiratory depression than morphine. In contrast to morphine, tramadol has not been shown to cause histamine release. At therapeutic doses, tramadol has no effect on heart rate, left-ventricular function or cardiac index. Orthostatic changes in blood pressure have been observed.

Pharmacokinetics:

Absorption – Tramadol is rapidly and almost completely absorbed after oral administration. The mean absolute bioavailability of a 100 mg oral dose is ≈ 75%. Administration with food does not significantly affect its rate or extent of absorption; therefore, it can be administered without regard to meals. The mean peak plasma concentration is 308 ± 78 ng/ml and occurs at ≈ 2 hours after a single 100 mg oral dose in healthy subjects. At this dose, the mean peak plasma concentration of the active mono-*O*-desmethyl metabolite (racemic M1) is 55 ± 20 ng/ml and occurs ≈ 3 hours post-dose. The separate [+]- and [-]-enantiomers of tramadol generally follow a parallel time course in plasma after a single 100 mg oral dose. Following a 100 mg dose, the maximum plasma concentrations of the [-]-enantiomer are somewhat lower than those of the [+]-enantiomer (148 ± 33 vs 168 ± 36 ng/ml, respectively). The [-]-M1 enantiomer is present at slightly higher plasma concentrations than the [+]-M1 enantiomer (35 ± 10 vs 26 ± 13 ng/ml, respectively).

Steady state is achieved after 2 days of a 100 mg four times daily dosing regimen (maximum plasma concentration was 592 ± 177 ng/ml). The plasma half-life of tramadol, following single and multiple dosing, was 6 and 7 hours, respectively. This increase in half-life upon multiple dosing is not considered to be clinically significant or to warrant dosage adjustment for chronic use.

Distribution – The volume of distribution was 2.6 and 2.9 L/kg in male and female subjects, respectively, following a 100 mg IV dose. Binding to human plasma proteins is ≈ 20% and appears to be independent of concentration up to 10 mcg/ml. Although not confirmed in humans, tramadol crosses the blood-brain barrier in rats.

Metabolism – Tramadol is extensively metabolized after oral administration. Approximately 30% of the dose is excreted in the urine as unchanged drug, whereas 60% of the dose is excreted as metabolites. The remainder is excreted either as unidentified or as unextractable metabolites. The major metabolic pathways appear to be *N*- and *O*-demethylation and glucuronidation or sulfation in the liver. Only one metabolite, M1, is pharmacologically active. Production of M1 is dependent on the CYP2D6 isoenzyme of cytochrome P-450.

Excretion – The mean terminal plasma elimination half-lives of racemic tramadol and racemic M1 are 6.3 ± 1.4 and 7.4 ± 1.4 hours, respectively. The plasma elimination half-life of tramadol increased from ≈ 6 to 7 hours upon multiple dosing.

Renal function impairment results in a decreased rate and extent of excretion of tramadol and its active metabolite M1. In patients with creatinine clearances of < 30 ml/min, adjustment of the dosing regimen is recommended (see Administration and Dosage). The total amount of tramadol and M1 removed during a dialysis period is < 7% of the administered dose.

TRAMADOL HCl

Hepatic function impairment: Metabolism of tramadol and M1 is reduced in patients with advanced cirrhosis of the liver, resulting in a larger area under the serum concentration vs time curve for tramadol and longer tramadol and M1 elimination half-lives (13 and 19 hours, respectively). In cirrhotic patients, adjustment of the dosing regimen is recommended (see Administration and Dosage).

Elderly: Healthy elderly subjects aged 65 to 75 years have plasma tramadol concentrations and elimination half-lives comparable to those observed in healthy subjects < 65 years of age. In subjects > 75 years of age, maximum serum concentrations are slightly elevated (208 vs 162 mg/ml) and the elimination half-life is slightly prolonged (7 vs 6 hours) compared to subjects 65 to 75 years of age. Adjustment of the daily dose is recommended for patients > 75 years of age (see Administration and Dosage).

Gender: The absolute bioavailability of tramadol was 73% in males and 79% in females. The plasma clearance was 6.4 ml/min/kg in males and 5.7 in females following a 1 mg IV dose. Following a single oral dose, and after adjusting for body weight, females had a 12% higher peak tramadol concentration and a 35% higher area under the concentration-time curve compared to males. This difference may not be of any clinical significance.

Clinical trials: Tramadol hydrochloride has been given in single oral doses of 50, 75, 100, 150 and 200 mg to patients with pain following surgical procedures (orthopedic, gynecological, cesarean section) and pain following oral surgery (extraction of impacted molars).

Following oral surgery, pain relief was demonstrated in some patients at single doses of 50 and 75 mg. A dose of 100 mg tended to provide analgesia superior to codeine sulfate 60 mg, but it was not as effective as the combination of aspirin 650 mg/codeine phosphate 60 mg. In single-dose models of pain following surgical procedures, 150 mg provided analgesia generally comparable to the combination of acetaminophen 650 mg/propoxyphene napsylate 100 mg.

Patients with chronic conditions such as low back pain, cancer, neuropathic pain and orthopedic and joint conditions entered a double-blind phase of 1 to 3 months. Average daily doses of ≈ 250 mg tramadol in divided doses produced analgesia comparable with five doses of acetaminophen 300 mg/codeine phosphate 30 mg daily, five doses of aspirin 325 mg/codeine phosphate 30 mg daily, and with two to three doses of acetaminophen 500 mg/oxycodone HCl 5 mg daily.

Indications:

Pain: Management of moderate to moderately severe pain.

Contraindications:

Hypersensitivity to tramadol; acute intoxication with alcohol, hypnotics, centrally acting analgesics, opioids or psychotropic drugs.

Warnings:

Seizure: Tramadol causes seizures in animals, and a few seizures have been reported in humans receiving excessive single oral doses (700 mg) or large IV doses (300 mg). Administration of tramadol may enhance the seizure risk in patients taking MAO inhibitors, neuroleptics, other drugs that reduce the seizure threshold, patients with epilepsy or patients otherwise at increased risk for seizure.

Concomitant CNS depressants: Use with caution and in reduced dosages when administering to patients receiving CNS depressants such as alcohol, opioids, anesthetic agents, phenothiazines, tranquilizers or sedative hypnotics.

Concomitant MAO inhibitors: Use with great caution in patients taking MAO inhibitors, since tramadol inhibits the uptake of norepinephrine and serotonin.

Renal/hepatic function impairment: Impaired renal function results in a decreased rate and extent of excretion of tramadol and its active metabolite, M1. In patients with creatinine clearances < 30 ml/min, dosing reduction is recommended (see Administration and Dosage).

Metabolism of tramadol and M1 is reduced in patients with advanced cirrhosis of the liver. In cirrhotic patients, dosing reduction is recommended (see Administration and Dosage).

With the prolonged half-life in these conditions, achievement of steady state is delayed, so that it may take several days for elevated plasma concentrations to develop.

Elderly: In subjects > 75 years of age, serum concentrations are slightly elevated and the elimination half-life is slightly prolonged. The aged also can be expected to vary more widely in their ability to tolerate adverse drug effects. Daily doses > 300 mg are not recommended in patients > 75 years of age (see Administration and Dosage).

TRAMADOL HCl

Pregnancy: Category C. Tramadol is embryotoxic and fetotoxic in mice, rats and rabbits at maternally toxic doses 3 to 15 times the maximum human dose or higher. Embryo and fetal toxicity consisted primarily of decreased fetal weights, skeletal ossification and increased supernumerary ribs at maternally toxic dose levels. Transient delays in developmental or behavioral parameters were also seen in pups from rat dams allowed to deliver.

In peri- and post-natal studies in rats, progeny of dams receiving oral (gavage) dose levels of ≥ 50 mg/kg had decreased weights, and pup survival was decreased early in lactation at 80 mg/kg (6 to 10 times the maximum human dose). Maternal toxicity was observed at all dose levels, but effects on progeny were evident only at higher dose levels where maternal toxicity was more severe.

Do not use in pregnant women prior to or during labor unless the potential benefits outweigh the risks. Safe use in pregnancy has not been established. Tramadol has been shown to cross the placenta. The mean ratio of serum tramadol in the umbilical veins compared to maternal veins was 0.83 for 40 women given tramadol during labor. There are no adequate and well controlled studies in pregnant women. Use during pregnancy only if the potential benefit justifies the risk to the fetus.

Lactation: Tramadol is not recommended for obstetrical preoperative medication or for post-delivery analgesia in nursing mothers because its safety in infants and newborns has not been studied. Following a single IV 100 mg dose, the cumulative excretion in breast milk within 16 hours post-dose was 100 mcg of tramadol (0.1% of the maternal dose) and 27 mcg of M1.

Children: Not recommended in children because safety and efficacy in patients < 16 years of age have not been established.

Precautions:

Respiratory depression: When large doses of tramadol are administered with anesthetic medications or alcohol, respiratory depression may result. Cases of intraoperative respiratory depression, usually with large IV doses of tramadol and with concurrent administration of respiratory depressants, have been reported in foreign experience. Such cases should be treated as overdoses (see Overdosage). Administer cautiously in patients at risk for respiratory depression.

Increased intracranial pressure or head trauma: Use with caution in patients with increased intracranial pressure or head injury. Pupillary changes (miosis) from tramadol may obscure the existence, extent or course of intracranial pathology. Clinicians should also maintain a high index of suspicion for adverse drug reactions when evaluating altered mental status in these patients if they are receiving tramadol.

Acute abdominal conditions: Tramadol may complicate the clinical assessment of patients with acute abdominal conditions.

Opioid dependence: Tramadol is not recommended for patients who are dependent on opioids. Patients who have recently taken substantial amounts of opioids may experience withdrawal symptoms. Because of the difficulty in assessing dependence in patients who have previously received substantial amounts of opioid medication, use caution in the administration of tramadol to such patients.

Drug abuse and dependence: Although tramadol can produce drug dependence of the μ-opioid type (like codeine or dextropropoxyphene) and potentially may be abused, there has been little evidence of abuse in foreign clinical experience. In clinical trials, tramadol produced effects similar to an opioid, and at supratherapeutic doses was recognized as an opioid in subjective/behavioral studies. Tolerance development has been reported to be relatively mild and withdrawal, when present, is not considered to be as severe as that produced by other opioids. Part of tramadol's activity is believed to be derived from its active metabolite, which is responsible for some delay in onset of activity and some extension of the duration of μ-opioid activity. Delayed μ-opioid activity is believed to reduce a drug's abuse liability.

An assay for tramadol is not included in routine urine screens for drugs of abuse.

TRAMADOL HCl

Drug Interactions:

Tramadol Drug Interactions

Precipitant drug	Object drug*		Description
Carbamazepine	Tramadol	⬇	Concomitant administration causes a significant increase in tramadol metabolism, presumably through metabolic induction by carbamazepine. Patients receiving chronic carbamazepine doses of up to 800 mg daily may require up to twice the recommended dose of tramadol.
MAO inhibitors	Tramadol	⬆	Use concurrently with caution as tramadol inhibits norepinephrine and serotonin reuptake.
Quinidine	Tramadol	⬌	Tramadol is metabolized to M1 by the CYP2D6 P-450 isoenzyme. Quinidine is a selective inhibitor of that isoenzyme. Therefore, concomitant use results in increased concentrations of tramadol and reduced concentrations of M1. The clinical consequences of this effect have not been fully investigated.

* ⬇ = Object drug decreased. ⬆ = Object drug increased. ⬌ = Undetermined effect.

Drug/Food interactions: Food does not affect rate or extent of absorption; tramadol can be administered without regard to meals.

Adverse Reactions:

Cumulative Incidence of Tramadol Adverse Reactions (%)

Adverse reaction	Up to 7 days	Up to 30 days	Up to 90 days
Dizziness/Vertigo	26	31	33
Nausea	24	34	40
Constipation	24	38	46
Headache	18	26	32
Somnolence	16	23	25
Vomiting	9	13	17
Pruritus	8	10	11
CNS stimulation [1]	7	11	14
Asthenia	6	11	12
Sweating	6	7	9
Dyspepsia	5	9	13
Dry mouth	5	9	10
Diarrhea	5	6	10

[1] CNS stimulation is a composite of nervousness, anxiety, agitation, tremor, spasticity, euphoria, emotional lability and hallucinations.

Body as a whole: Malaise (1% to < 5%); allergic reaction, accidental injury, weight loss (< 1%); suicidal tendency.

Cardiovascular: Vasodilation (1% to < 5%); syncope, orthostatic hypotension, tachycardia (< 1%); abnormal ECG; hypertension; myocardial ischemia; palpitations.

CNS: Anxiety, confusion, coordination disturbance, euphoria, nervousness, sleep disorder (1% to < 5%); seizure (see Warnings), paresthesia, cognitive dysfunction, hallucinations, tremor, amnesia, difficulty in concentration, abnormal gait (< 1%); migraine.

GI: Abdominal pain, anorexia, flatulence (1% to < 5%); GI bleeding; hepatitis; stomatitis.

Dermatologic: Rash (1% to < 5%); urticaria, vesicles (< 1%).

Special senses: Visual disturbance (1% to < 5%); dysgeusia (< 1%); cataracts; deafness; tinnitus.

GU: Urinary retention/frequency, menopausal symptoms (1% to < 5%); dysuria, menstrual disorder (< 1%).

Lab test abnormalities: Creatinine increase; elevated liver enzymes; hemoglobin decrease; proteinuria.

Miscellaneous: Hypertonia (1% to < 5%); dyspnea (< 1%).

TRAMADOL HCl

Overdosage:

Symptoms: Few cases of overdose with tramadol have been reported. Estimates of ingested doses in foreign fatalities have been in the range of 3 to 5 g. A 3 g intentional overdose in a patient in the clinical studies produced emesis and no sequelae. The lowest dose reported to be associated with fatality was possibly between 500 and 1000 mg in a 40 kg woman, but details of the case are not completely known. Serious potential consequences of overdosage are respiratory depression and seizure.

Treatment: Naloxone will reverse some symptoms caused by overdosage with tramadol, therefore general supportive treatment is recommended (see General Management of Acute Overdosage). Give primary attention to the assurance of adequate respiratory exchange. Hemodialysis is not expected to be helpful because it removes only a small percentage of the administered dose. Convulsions occurring in mice following the administration of toxic doses of tramadol could be suppressed with barbiturates or benzodiazepines but were increased with naloxone. Naloxone did not change the lethality of an overdose in mice.

Patient Information:

Tramadol may impair mental or physical abilities or coordination required for the performance of potentially hazardous tasks such as driving a car or operating machinery.

Administration and Dosage:

Approved by the FDA on March 3, 1995 (1S classification).

For the treatment of painful conditions, 50 to 100 mg can be administered orally as needed for relief every 4 to 6 hours, not to exceed 400 mg/day. For moderate pain, 50 mg may be adequate as the initial dose, and for more severe pain, 100 mg is usually more effective as the initial dose.

Elderly: Available data do not suggest that a dosage adjustment is necessary in elderly patients 65 to 75 years of age unless they also have renal or hepatic impairment. For elderly patients > 75 years old, administer < 300 mg/day in divided doses as above.

Renal function impairment: In all patients with creatinine clearance < 30 ml/min, it is recommended that the dosing interval be increased to 12 hours, with a maximum daily dose of 200 mg. Because only 7% of an administered dose is removed by hemodialysis, dialysis patients can receive their regular dose on the day of dialysis.

Hepatic function impairment: The recommended dose for patients with cirrhosis is 50 mg every 12 hours.

Rx	**Ultram** (Ortho-McNeil)	**Tablets**: 50 mg	Lactose. (McNeil 659). White. Film coated. Capsule shape. In 100s and UD 100s.

CLONIDINE HCL

Clonidine is also used orally as an antihypertensive. For further information, refer to the Clonidine monograph in the Antihypertensives section.

Warning:

Epidural clonidine is not recommended for obstetrical, post-partum or peri-operative pain management. The risk of hemodynamic instability, especially hypotension and bradycardia, from epidural clonidine may be unacceptable in these patients. However, in a rare obstetrical, post-partum or peri-operative patient, potential benefits may outweigh the possible risks.

Clonidine injection is a centrally-acting analgesic solution for use in continuous epidural infusion devices.

Clonidine is an imidazole derivative and exists as a mesomeric compound.

Actions:

Pharmacology: Epidurally administered clonidine produces dose-dependent analgesia not antagonized by opiate antagonists. The analgesia is limited to the body regions innervated by the spinal segments where analgesic concentrations of clonidine are present. Clonidine is thought to produce analgesia at presynaptic and postjunctional alpha-2-adrenoceptors in the spinal cord by preventing pain signal transmission to the brain.

Pharmacokinetics:

Distribution – Following a 10 minute IV infusion of 300 mcg clonidine to five male volunteers, plasma clonidine levels showed an initial rapid distribution phase (mean half–life of 11 minutes), followed by a slower elimination phase (half–life of 9 hours) over 24 hours. Clonidine's total body clearance (CL) was 219 ml/min.

Following a 700 mcg clonidine epidural dose given over five minutes to four male and five female volunteers, peak clonidine plasma levels (4.4 ng/ml) were obtained in 19 minutes. Following sample collection for 24 hours, the plasma elimination half-life was determined to be 22 hours. CL was 190 ml/min. In cerebral spinal fluid (CSF), peak clonidine levels (418 ng/ml) were achieved in 26 minutes. The clonidine CSF elimination half-life was 1.3 hours when samples were collected for 6 hours. Compared with men, women had a lower mean plasma clearance, longer mean plasma half-life and higher mean peak level of clonidine in both plasma and CSF.

In cancer patients who received 14 days of clonidine epidural infusion (rate = 30 mcg/hr) plus morphine by patient-controlled analgesia (PCA), steady-state clonidine plasma concentrations of 2.2 and 2.4 ng/ml were obtained on dosing days 7 and 14, respectively. CL was 279 and 272 ml/min on these days. CSF concentrations were not determined in these patients.

Clonidine is highly lipid soluble and readily distributes into extravascular sites, including the central nervous system. Clonidine's volume of distribution is 2.1 L/kg. The binding of clonidine to plasma protein is primarily to albumin and varies between 20% and 40% in vitro. Epidurally administered clonidine readily partitions into plasma via the epidural veins and attains systemic concentrations (0.5 to 2.0 ng/ml) that are associated with a hypotensive effect mediated by the central nervous system.

Metabolism – Clonidine metabolism follows minor pathways with the major metabolite p-hydroxyclonidine present at < 10% of the concentration of unchanged drug in the urine.

Excretion – Following an IV dose of clonidine, 72% of the administered dose was excreted within 96 hours in urine, of which 40% to 50% was unchanged clonidine. Renal clearance for clonidine was determined to be 133 ml/min.

Renal function impairment: In a study in which clonidine was given to subjects with varying degrees of kidney function, elimination half-lives varied (17.5 to 41 hours) as a function of creatinine clearance. In subjects undergoing hemodialysis, only 5% of body clonidine stores was removed.

Clinical trials: In a double-blind, randomized study of cancer patients with severe intractable pain below the C4 dermatome not controlled by morphine, 38 patients were randomized to an epidural infusion of clonidine plus epidural morphine, and 47 subjects received epidural placebo plus epidural morphine. Successful analgesia, defined as a decrease in either morphine use or Visual Analog Score (VAS) pain, was significantly more common with epidural clonidine than placebo (45% vs 21%).

Indications:

Severe pain: Clonidine is indicated in combination with opiates for the treatment of severe pain in cancer patients that is not adequately relieved by opioid analgesics alone. Epidural clonidine is more likely to be effective in patients with neuropathic pain than somatic or visceral pain.

CLONIDINE HCL

Contraindications:

Patients with a history of sensitivity or allergic reactions to clonidine; in the presence of an injection site infection; in patients on anticoagulant therapy; patients with a bleeding diathesis; administration above the C4 dermatome because there are no adequate safety data to support such use.

Warnings:

Postoperative or obstetrical analgesia: Epidural clonidine is not recommended for obstetrical, post-partum or peri-operative pain management. The risk of hemodynamic instability, especially hypotension and bradycardia, from epidural clonidine may be unacceptable in these patients.

Hypotension: Because severe hypotension may follow clonidine administration, use with caution in all patients. It is not recommended in most patients with severe cardiovascular disease or in those who are otherwise hemodynamically unstable. Balance the benefit of administration in these patients against the potential risks resulting from hypotension.

Monitor vital signs frequently, especially during the first few days of epidural clonidine therapy. When clonidine is infused into the upper thoracic spinal segments, more pronounced decreases in blood pressure may be seen.

Clonidine decreases sympathetic outflow from the central nervous system resulting in decreases in peripheral resistance, renal vascular resistance, heart rate and blood pressure. However, in the absence of profound hypotension, renal blood flow and glomerular filtration rate remain essentially unchanged.

Most episodes of hypotension occur within the first 4 days after beginning epidural clonidine. However, hypotensive episodes may occur throughout the trial duration. There was a tendency for these episodes to occur more commonly in women and in those with higher serum clonidine levels. Patients experiencing hypotension also tended to weigh less than those who did not experience hypotension. The hypotension usually responded to IV fluids and, if necessary, parenteral ephedrine. Severe hypotension may occur even if IV fluid pretreatment is given.

Withdrawal: Sudden cessation of clonidine treatment, regardless of the route of administration, has, in some cases, resulted in symptoms such as nervousness, agitation, headache and tremor, accompanied or followed by a rapid rise in blood pressure. The likelihood of such reactions appears to be greater after administration of higher doses or with concomitant beta-blocker treatment. Special caution is therefore advised in these situations. Rare instances of hypertensive encephalopathy, cerebrovascular accidents and death have been reported after abrupt clonidine withdrawal. Patients with a history of hypertension or other underlying cardiovascular conditions may be at particular risk of the consequences of abrupt discontinuation of clonidine.

When discontinuing therapy with epidural clonidine, the physician should reduce the dose gradually over 2 to 4 days to avoid withdrawal symptoms.

An excessive rise in blood pressure following discontinuation of epidural clonidine can be treated by administration of clonidine or by IV phentolamine. If therapy is to be discontinued in patients receiving a beta-blocker and clonidine concurrently, discontinue the beta-blocker several days before the gradual discontinuation of epidural clonidine.

Catheter-related infection: Implantable epidural catheters are associated with a risk of catheter-related infections, including meningitis and epidural abscess. Eighteen percent of subjects discontinued this study as a result of catheter-related problems (infections, accidental dislodging, etc), and one subject developed meningitis, possibly as a result of a catheter-related infection. Evaluation of fever in a patient receiving epidural clonidine should include the possibility of a catheter-related infection such as meningitis or epidural abscess.

Renal function impairment: Adjust dosage according to the degree of renal impairment, and monitor patients carefully. Because only a minimal amount of clonidine is removed during routine hemodialysis, there is no need to give supplemental clonidine following dialysis.

Pregnancy: Category C. Clonidine readily crosses the placenta and its concentrations are equal in maternal and umbilical cord plasma; amniotic fluid concentrations can be four times those found in serum. There are no adequate and well controlled studies in pregnant women during early gestation when organ formation takes place. Use epidural clonidine during pregnancy only if the potential benefits justify the potential risk to the fetus.

Labor and delivery – Clonidine during labor has demonstrated no apparent adverse effects on the infant at the time of delivery. However, these studies did not monitor the infants for hemodynamic effects in the days following delivery. There are no adequate controlled clinical trials evaluating the safety, efficacy and dosing of clonidine in obstetrical settings. Because maternal perfusion of the placenta is critically dependent on blood pressure, use of clonidine as an analgesic during labor and delivery is not indicated.

Lactation: Concentrations of clonidine in human breast milk are approximately twice those found in maternal plasma. Exercise caution when clonidine is administered to a nursing woman.

Children: Restrict the use of clonidine to pediatric patients with severe intractable pain from malignancy that is unresponsive to epidural or spinal opiates or other more conventional analgesic techniques. Select the starting dose on a per kilogram basis (0.5 mcg/kg/hour) and cautiously adjust based on the clinical response.

Precautions:

Monitoring: Closely monitor patients receiving epidural clonidine from a continuous infusion device for the first few days to assess their response.

Cardiac effects: Clonidine frequently causes decreases in heart rate. Symptomatic bradycardia can be treated with atropine. Rarely, atrioventricular block greater than first degree has been reported. Clonidine does not alter the hemodynamic response to exercise but may mask the increase in heart rate associated with hypovolemia.

Respiratory depression and sedation: Clonidine administration may result in sedation through the activation of alpha-adrenoceptors in the brainstem. High clonidine doses cause sedation and ventilatory abnormalities that are usually mild. Tolerance to these effects can develop with chronic administration. These effects have been reported with bolus doses.

Depression has been seen in a small percentage of patients treated with oral or transdermal clonidine. Depression commonly occurs in cancer patients and may be exacerbated by clonidine treatment. Monitor for the signs and symptoms of depression, especially in patients with a known history of affective disorders.

Pain: Clonidine is most effective in well-localized, "neuropathic" pain that is characterized as electrical, burning or shooting in nature and is localized to a dermatomal or peripheral nerve distribution. It may be less effective or ineffective in the treatment of pain that is diffuse, poorly localized or visceral in origin.

Hazardous tasks: May produce drowsiness; patients should observe caution while driving or performing other tasks requiring alertness or physical dexterity.

Drug Interactions:

Clonidine Drug Interactions

Precipitant drug	Object drug*		Description
Beta blockers	Clonidine	↑	Beta blockers may exacerbate the hypertensive response seen with clonidine withdrawal. Also, because of the potential for additive effects such as bradycardia and AV block, use caution in patients receiving clonidine with agents known to affect sinus node function or AV nodal conduction (eg, digitalis, calcium channel blockers and beta-blockers).
Fluphenazine	Clonidine	↑	There is one reported case of a patient with acute delirium associated with the simultaneous use of fluphenazine and oral clonidine. Symptoms resolved when clonidine was withdrawn and recurred when the patient was rechallenged with clonidine.
Narcotic analgesics	Clonidine	↑	Narcotic analgesics may potentiate the hypotensive effects of clonidine.
Tricyclic antidepressants	Clonidine	↓	Tricyclic antidepressants may antagonize the hypotensive effects of clonidine. The effects of tricyclic antidepressants on clonidine's analgesic actions are not known.
Clonidine	Alcohol/ barbiturates	↑	Clonidine may potentiate the CNS-depressive effect of alcohol, barbiturates or other sedating drugs.
Clonidine	Local anesthetics	↑	Epidural clonidine may prolong the duration of pharmacologic effects of epidural local anesthetics, including sensory and motor blockade.

* ↑ = Object drug increased. ↓ = Object drug decreased.

CLONIDINE HCL

Adverse Reactions:

The following adverse events may be related to administration of either clonidine or morphine.

Clonidine Adverse Reactions		
Adverse Events	Clonidine (%)	Placebo (%)
Total number of patients who experienced at least one adverse event	97.4	80.5
Hypotension	44.8	10.6
Postural hypotension	31.6	0
Dry mouth	13.2	8.5
Nausea	13.2	21.3
Somnolence	13.2	21.3
Dizziness	13.2	4.3
Confusion	13.2	10.6
Vomiting	10.5	14.9
Nausea/vomiting	7.9	2.1
Sweating	5.3	0
Anxiety	11	2
Chest pain	5.3	0
Hallucination	5.3	2.1
Tinnitus	5.3	0
Constipation	6	4.3
Tachycardia	2.6	4.3
Hypoventilation	2.6	4.3
Urinary tract infection	22	nd[1]
Dyspnea	6	nd
Infection	6	nd
Asthenia	5	nd
Hyperaesthesia	5	nd
Pain	5	nd
Skin ulcer	5	nd
Decreased heart rate	†[2]	nd
Rebound hypertension	11	nd

[1] nd = No data.
[2] † = Occurs, but the incidence is unknown.

The following adverse reactions have also been reported with the use of any dosage form of clonidine. In many cases patients were receiving concomitant medication and a causal relationship has not been established. For more adverse reactions, refer to the oral clonidine monograph in the antihypertensives section.

CNS: Cerebrovascular accidents, other behavioral changes (rare).

GI: Hepatitis, parotitis, ileus and pseudo-obstruction, abdominal pain (rare).

Metabolic: Transient elevation of serum phosphatase (rare).

Miscellaneous: Thrombocytopenia, syncope, blurred vision (rare); withdrawal syndrome (1%).

Overdosage:

The largest overdose reported to date involved a 28-year-old white male who ingested 100 mg clonidine powder. This patient developed hypertension followed by hypotension, bradycardia, apnea, hallucinations, semicoma and premature ventricular contractions. The patient fully recovered after intensive treatment. Plasma clonidine levels were 60 ng/ml after 1 hour, 190 ng/ml after 1.5 hours, 370 ng/ml after 2 hours and 120 ng/ml after 5.5 and 6.5 hours. In mice and rats, the oral LD50 of clonidine is 206 and 465 mg/kg, respectively.

Symptoms: Hypertension may develop early and may be followed by hypotension, bradycardia, respiratory depression, hypothermia, drowsiness, decreased or absent reflexes, irritability and miosis. With large oral overdoses, reversible cardiac conduction defects or arrhythmias, apnea, coma and seizures have been reported. As little as 100 mcg of oral clonidine has produced signs of toxicity in pediatric patients.

Treatment: There is no specific antidote for clonidine overdosage. Supportive care may include atropine sulfate for bradycardia, IV fluids or vasopressor agents for hypotension. Hypertension associated with overdosage has been treated with IV furosemide, diazoxide or alpha-blocking agents such as phentolamine. Naloxone may be a useful adjunct in the treatment of clonidine-induced respiratory depression, hypotension or coma; monitor blood pressure because the administration of naloxone has occasionally resulted in paradoxical hypertension. Tolazoline administration has yielded inconsistent results and is not recommended as first-line therapy. Dialysis is not likely to significantly enhance clonidine elimination.

Patient Information:

Warn patients of the risks of rebound hypertension. Patients should not discontinue clonidine except under the supervision of a physician. Patients should notify their physician immediately if clonidine administration is inadvertently interrupted for any reason.

Advise patients who engage in potentially hazardous activities, such as operating machinery or driving, of the potential sedative and hypotensive effects of epidural clonidine.

Inform patients that sedative effects may be increased by CNS-depressing drugs and that opiates may increase hypotensive effects.

Administration and Dosage:

The recommended starting dose of clonidine for continuous epidural infusion is 30 mcg/hr. Although dosage may be titrated up or down depending on pain relief and occurrence of adverse events, experience with dosage rates > 40 mcg/hr is limited.

Clonidine must not be used with a preservative.

Storage/Stability: Store at controlled room temperature 15° to 30°C (59° to 86°F). Discard unused portion.

Rx	**Duraclon** (Fujisawa)	**Injection:** 100 mcg/ml	Preservative-free. In 10 ml vials.

ACETAMINOPHEN (N-Acetyl-P-Aminophenol, APAP)

Actions:

Pharmacology: Acetaminophen (APAP) is the active metabolite of phenacetin and acetanilid.

The site and mechanism of the analgesic effect is unclear. APAP reduces fever by a direct action on the hypothalamic heat-regulating centers, which increases dissipation of body heat (via vasodilation and sweating). The action of endogenous pyrogen on heat-regulating centers is inhibited. APAP is almost as potent as aspirin in inhibiting prostaglandin synthetase in the CNS, but its peripheral inhibition of prostaglandin synthesis is minimal, which may account for its lack of clinically significant antirheumatic or anti-inflammatory effects.

Generally, antipyretic and analgesic effects of APAP and aspirin are comparable. Aspirin is clearly superior to APAP for pain of inflammatory origin. APAP does not inhibit platelet aggregation, affect prothrombin response or produce GI ulceration.

Pharmacokinetics:

Absorption of acetaminophen is rapid and almost complete from the GI tract. Peak plasma concentrations occur within 0.5 to 2 hours, with slightly faster absorption of liquid preparations. With overdosage, absorption is complete in 4 hours.

Distribution – Serum protein binding varies from 20% to 50% at toxic concentrations.

Metabolism/Excretion – The half-life in plasma is ≈ 2 hours. Acetaminophen is relatively uniformly distributed throughout most body fluids. Binding of the drug to plasma proteins is variable; only 20% to 50% may be bound at the concentrations encountered during acute intoxication. Ninety percent to 100% of the drug is recovered in the urine within the first day, primarily after hepatic conjugation with glucuronic acid (≈ 60%), sulfuric acid (≈ 35%) or cysteine (≈ 3%); small amounts of hydroxylated and deacetylated metabolites also have been detected.

Acetaminophen is extensively metabolized and excreted in urine primarily as inactive glucuronate and sulfate conjugates (94%). About 4% is metabolized via cytochrome P–450 oxidase to a toxic metabolite normally detoxified by preferential conjugation with cellular glutathione and excreted in urine as conjugates of cysteine and mercapturic acid. When APAP is used chronically or taken acutely in large doses, glutathione stores are depleted and hepatic necrosis may occur; 2% is excreted unchanged. Half-life is slightly prolonged in neonates and in cirrhotics.

Indications:

An analgesic-antipyretic in the presence of aspirin allergy, patients with blood coagulation disorders who are being treated with oral anticoagulants, bleeding diatheses (eg, hemophilia), upper GI disease (eg, ulcer, gastritis, hiatal hernia) and gouty arthritis; a variety of arthritic and rheumatic conditions involving musculoskeletal pain, as well as in other painful disorders; headache; pain associated with earache, teething, tonsillectomy, menstruation; toothache; diseases accompanied by discomfort and fever such as the common cold, "flu" and other bacterial or viral infections.

Unlabeled uses: Prophylactic APAP use in children receiving DTP vaccination appears to decrease incidence of fever and injection site pain. A dose immediately following vaccination and every 4 to 6 hours thereafter for 48 to 72 hours is suggested.

Contraindications:

Hypersensitivity to acetaminophen.

Warnings:

Dosage: Do not exceed recommended dosage.

Hepatotoxicity and severe hepatic failure occurred in chronic alcoholics following therapeutic doses. The hepatotoxicity is believed to be caused by induction of hepatic microsomal enzymes resulting in an increase in toxic metabolites, or by the reduced amount of glutathione responsible for conjugating toxic metabolites. A safe dose for a chronic alcohol abuser has not been determined. Caution chronic alcoholics to limit acetaminophen intake to ≤ 2 g/day.

Hypersensitivity: If a sensitivity reaction occurs, discontinue use.

Pregnancy: Category B. Acetaminophen crosses the placenta. It is routinely used during all stages of pregnancy; when used in therapeutic doses, it appears safe for short-term use. Continuous high daily dosage probably caused severe anemia in a mother, and the neonate had fatal kidney disease. Although there is no evidence of a relationship between acetaminophen ingestion and congenital malformations, three cases of congenital hip dislocation may have been associated with acetaminophen.

Lactation: Acetaminophen is excreted in breast milk in low concentrations with reported milk:plasma ratios of 0.91 to 1.42 at 1 and 12 hours, respectively. No adverse effects in nursing infants were reported.

Children: Consult physician for use > 5 days (children), > 10 days (adults) or > 3 days for fever (adults and children).

ACETAMINOPHEN (N-Acetyl-P-Aminophenol, APAP)

Precautions:

Severe or recurrent pain or high or continued fever may indicate serious illness. If pain persists for > 5 days or if redness or swelling is present, consult physician.

Drug Interactions:

The potential hepatotoxicity of APAP may be increased by large doses or long-term administration of the following agents because of hepatic microsomal enzyme induction. The therapeutic effects of APAP may also be decreased.

Barbiturates
Carbamazepine
Hydantoins
Isoniazid
Rifampin
Sulfinpyrazone

Acetaminophen Drug Interactions

Precipitant drug	Object drug*		Description
Alcohol, ethyl	APAP	⬆	Hepatotoxicity has occurred in chronic alcoholics following various dose levels (moderate to excessive) of acetaminophen.
Anticholinergics	APAP	⬇	The onset of acetaminophen effect may be delayed or decreased slightly, but the ultimate pharmacological effect is not significantly affected by anticholinergics.
Beta blockers, propranolol	APAP	⬆	Propranolol appears to inhibit the enzyme systems responsible for the glucuronidation and oxidation of acetaminophen. Therefore, the pharmacologic effects of acetaminophen may be increased.
Charcoal, activated	APAP	⬇	Reduces acetaminophen absorption when administered as soon as possible after overdose.
Contraceptives, oral	APAP	⬇	Increase in glucuronidation resulting in increased plasma clearance and a decreased half-life of acetaminophen.
Probenecid	APAP	⬆	Probenecid may increase the therapeutic effectiveness of acetaminophen slightly.
APAP	Lamotrigine	⬇	Serum lamotrigine concentrations may be reduced, producing a decrease in therapeutic effects.
APAP	Loop diuretics	⬇	The effects of the loop diuretic may be decreased because APAP may decrease renal prostaglandin excretion and decrease plasma renin activity.
APAP	Zidovudine	⬇	The pharmacologic effects of zidovudine may be decreased because of enhanced nonhepatic or renal clearance of zidovudine.

* ⬆ = Object drug increased. ⬇ = Object drug decreased.

Drug/Lab test interactions: Acetaminophen may interfere with home blood glucose measurement systems; decreases of > 20% in mean glucose values may be noted. This effect appears to be drug, concentration and system dependent.

Adverse Reactions:

Hematologic: Hemolytic anemia; neutropenia; leukopenia; pancytopenia; thrombocytopenia.

Hypersensitivity: Skin eruptions; urticarial and erythematous skin reactions; fever.

Miscellaneous: Hypoglycemic coma; jaundice.

Overdosage:

Symptoms: Acute poisoning may be manifested by nausea, vomiting, drowsiness, confusion, liver tenderness, low blood pressure, cardiac arrhythmias, jaundice and acute hepatic and renal failure. These occur within the first 24 hours and may persist for ≥ 1 week. Death has occurred because of liver necrosis. Acute renal failure may also occur. However, there are often no specific early symptoms or signs.

The course of APAP poisoning is divided into four stages (postingestion time):

Stage I: (12-24 hours) – Nausea, vomiting, diaphoresis, anorexia;

Stage 2: (24-48 hours) – Clinically improved; AST, ALT, bilirubin and prothrombin levels begin to rise;

Stage 3: (72-96 hours) – Peak hepatotoxicity; AST of 20,000 not unusual;

Stage 4: (7-8 days) – Recovery.

Hepatotoxicity may result. The minimal toxic dose is 10 g (140 mg/kg), but liver damage has occurred with a single 5.85 g dose; ≥ 20 to 25 g are potentially fatal. Children appear less susceptible to toxicity than adults because they have less capac-

ACETAMINOPHEN (N-Acetyl-P-Aminophenol, APAP)

ity for glucuronidation metabolism. Initial signs of toxicity may include nausea, vomiting, anorexia, malaise, diaphoresis, abdominal pain and diarrhea. Hepatotoxicity usually is not apparent for 48 to 72 hours. If an acute dose of ≥ 150 mg/kg was ingested, or if the dose cannot be determined, obtain a serum acetaminophen assay after 4 hours following ingestion. If in the toxic range, obtain liver function studies and repeat at 24-hour intervals. Hepatic failure may lead to encephalopathy, coma and death.

Plasma acetaminophen levels > 300 mcg/ml at 4 hours postingestion were associated with hepatic damage in 90% of patients; minimal hepatic damage is anticipated if plasma levels at 4 hours are < 120 mcg/ml or < 30 mcg/ml at 12 hours after ingestion.

Chronic excessive use (> 4 g/day) eventually may lead to transient hepatotoxicity. The kidneys may undergo tubular necrosis; the myocardium may be damaged.

Treatment: Perform gastric lavage in all cases, preferably within 4 hours of ingestion.

Refer also to General Management of Acute Overdosage.

Oral **N–acetylcysteine** is a specific antidote for APAP toxicity. Administration IV can cause anaphylaxis. If patient vomits within 1 hour of administration of **N–acetylcysteine,** repeat the dose. Refer to the Acetylcysteine monograph in the Respiratory Drugs chapter for complete prescribing information and for a specific nomogram to guide treatment.

Patient Information:

Severe or recurrent pain or high or continued fever may indicate serious illness. If pain persists for > 5 days or if redness or swelling is present, consult physician.

Do not exceed the recommended dosage. Consult physician for use > 5 days (children), > 10 days (adults) or > 3 days for fever (adults and children).

Administration and Dosage:

Oral:

Adults – 325 to 650 mg every 4 to 6 hrs, or 1 g 3 to 4 times/day. Do not exceed 4 g/day.

Children – May repeat doses every 4 hours; do not exceed 5 doses in 24 hours.

Acetaminophen Dosage for Children

Age	Dosage (mg)	Age	Dosage (mg)
0-3 months	40	6-8 years	320
4-11 months	80	9-10 years	400
1-< 2 years	120	11 years	480
2-3 years	160	12-14 years	640
4-5 years	240	> 14 years	650

A 10 to 15 mg/kg/dose schedule has also been recommended.

Suppositories:

Adults – 650 mg every 4 to 6 hrs. Give no more than 4 g in 24 hours.

Children –

(3 to 11 months): 80 mg every 6 hours.
(1 to 3 years): 80 mg every 4 hours.
(3 to 6 years): 120 to 125 mg every 4 to 6 hours. Give ≤ 720 mg in 24 hrs.
(6 to 12 years): 325 mg every 4 to 6 hours. Give ≤ 2.6 g in 24 hours.

Storage/Stability: Store suppositories below 27°C (80°F) or refrigerate. Store tablets and oral solutions at 15° to 30°C (59° to 86°F).

otc	**Feverall, Infants** (Upsher-Smith)	**Suppositories:** 80 mg	In 6s.
otc	**Acetaminophen** (Various, eg, Goldline, Moore, Rugby, Schein)	**Suppositories:** 120 mg	In 12s.
otc	**Acetaminophen Uniserts** (Upsher-Smith)		In 12s.
otc	**Acephen** (G & W Labs)		In 6s, 12s and UD 12s, 50s and 100s.
otc	**Feverall, Children's** (Upsher-Smith)		In 6s.
🍁	**Abenol 120 mg** (SmithKline Beecham)		In 4s and 12s.

ACETAMINOPHEN (N-Acetyl-P-Aminophenol, APAP)

otc	**Neopap** (PolyMedica)	**Suppositories**: 125 mg	In 12s.
otc	**Acetaminophen** (Harber)	**Suppositories**: 300 mg	In 12s.
otc	**Acetaminophen** (Various, eg, Rugby)	**Suppositories**: 325 mg	In 12s.
otc	**Acetaminophen Uniserts** (Upsher-Smith)		In 12s.
otc	**Acephen** (G & W Labs)		In 6s, 12s, 50s and 100s.
otc	**Feverall, Junior Strength** (Upsher-Smith)		In 6s.
🍁	**Abenol 325 mg** (SmithKline Beecham)		In 4s and 12s.
otc	**Acetaminophen** (Various, eg, Goldline, Moore, Rugby)	**Suppositories**: 650 mg	In 12s.
otc	**Acetaminophen Uniserts** (Upsher-Smith)		In 12s.
otc	**Acephen** (G & W Labs)		In 12s, 500s and UD 50s and 100s.
🍁	**Abenol 650 mg** (SmithKline Beecham)		In 4s and 12s.
otc	**Acetaminophen** (Various, eg, Moore, Rugby, Schein)	**Tablets, chewable**: 80 mg	In 30s, and 100s.
otc	**Apacet** (Parmed)		In 30s.
otc	**Genapap, Children's** (Goldline)		Fruit flavor. Saccharin free. In 30s.
otc *sf*	**Panadol, Children's** (SmithKline Beecham)		(P.) Scored. Fruit flavor. In 30s.
otc	**Tempra 3** (Mead Johnson Nutritional)		In 30s.
otc	**Tylenol, Children's** (McNeil-CPC)		(Tylenol) Scored. Fruit, bubble gum or grape flavor. In 30s, 48s and 96s.
🍁	**Tylenol Chewable Tablets Fruit** (McNeil Consumer)		In 24s.
otc	**Tylenol Junior Strength** (McNeil-CPC)	**Tablets**: 160 mg	Aspartame (6 mg phenylalanine). Grape and fruit flavors. In 24s.
otc	**Tempra** (Mead-Johnson Nutritional)		Chewable. In 30s.
🍁	**Tylenol Junior Strength Chewable Tablets Fruit** (McNeil Consumer)		In 20s.

ACETAMINOPHEN (N-Acetyl-P-Aminophenol, APAP)

otc	**Acetaminophen** (Various, eg, Geneva, Moore, Roxane, Rugby, Schein)	**Tablets**: 325 mg	In 50s, 100s, 1000s and UD 100s.
otc	**Aceta** (Century)		In 100s and 1000s.
otc	**Aspirin Free Pain Relief** (Hudson)		In 100s.
otc	**Genapap** (Goldline)		In 100s.
otc	**Fem-Etts** (Roberts)		With 25 mg pamabrom. In UD 8s and 500s.
otc	**Genebs** (Goldline)		In 100s.
otc	**Mapap Regular Strength** (Major)		Scored. In 100s, 1000s and UD 100s.
otc	**Maranox** (C.S. Dent)		In 8s.
otc	**Meda Tab** (Circle)		In 100s.
otc	**Tapanol Regular Strength** (Circle)		In 100s and 250s.
otc	**Tylenol Caplets** (McNeil-CPC)		In 24s, 50s and 100s.
otc	**Tylenol Regular Strength Tablets** (McNeil-CPC)		In 24s, 50s, 100s and 200s.
🍁	**Tylenol Tablets 325 mg** (McNeil Consumer)		In 24s, 50s, 100s and 200s.
otc	**Acetaminophen** (Various, eg, Geneva, Moore)	**Tablets**: 500 mg	In 100s, 1000s and UD 100s.
otc	**Aceta** (Century)		In 100s and 1000s.
otc	**Aspirin Free Pain Relief** (Hudson)		In 50s ansd 100s.
otc	**Aspirin Free Anacin Maximum Strength** (Whitehall)		In 60s.
otc	**Genapap Extra Strength** (Goldline)		In 60s and 100s
otc	**Genebs Extra Strength** (Goldline)		In 100s.
otc	**Mapap Extra Strength** (Major)		In 30s, 60s, 100s, 200s, 1000s and UD 100s.
otc	**Panadol** (SmithKline Beecham)		(P 500.) In 30s and 60s.
otc	**Redutemp** (Inter. Ethical Labs)		In 60s.
otc	**Tapanol Extra Strength** (Republic)		In 100s.
otc	**Tylenol Extra Strength** (McNeil-CPC)		In 100s.
🍁	**Tylenol Tablets 500 mg** (McNeil Consumer)		In 10s, 24s, 50s and 100s.
otc	**Acetaminophen** (Roxane)	**Tablets**: 650 mg	In 1000s and UD 100s.
otc *sf*	**Panadol, Junior Strength** (Sterling Health)	**Caplets**: 160 mg	In 30s.

ACETAMINOPHEN (N-Acetyl-P-Aminophenol, APAP)

otc	**Arthritis Foundation Pain Reliever Aspirin Free** (McNeil-CPC)	**Caplets**: 500 mg	In 50s.
otc	**Aspirin Free Pain Relief** (Hudson)		In 100s.
otc	**Aspirin Free Anacin Maximum Strength** (Whitehall)		(AF Anacin.) In 100s.
otc	**Genapap Extra Strength** (Goldline)		In 50s and 100s.
otc	**Genebs Extra Strength** (Goldline)		In 100s.
otc	**Panadol** (SmithKline Beecham)		(P 500.) In 24s.
otc	**Tapanol Extra Strength** (Republic)		In 50s, 100s and 175s.
otc	**Tylenol Extended Relief** (McNeil-CPC)	**Caplets**: 650 mg	(Tylenol ER.) In 100s.
otc	**Aspirin Free Anacin Maximum Strength** (Whitehall)	**Gelcaps**: 500 mg	(AF Anacin.) In 100s.
otc	**Tapanol Extra Strength** (Republic[1])		In 100s and 175s.
otc	**Tylenol Extra Strength** (McNeil-CPC)		Gelatin coated. In 24s, 50s and 100s.
otc	**Dapacin** (Ferndale)	**Capsules**: 325 mg	In 1000s.
otc	**Acetaminophen** (Various, eg, Moore)	**Capsules**: 500 mg	In 50s, 100s and 1000s.
otc	**Meda Cap** (Circle)		In 100s.
otc	**Feverall, Children's** (Upsher-Smith)	**Capsules, sprinkle**: 80 mg	In 20s.
otc	**Feverall, Junior Strength** (Upsher-Smith)	**Capsules, sprinkle**: 160 mg	In 20s.
otc	**Silapap, Children's** (Silarx)	**Elixir**: 80 mg/2.5 ml	Alcohol free. In 237 ml.
otc	**Ridenol** (R.I.D.)	**Elixir**: 80 mg/5 ml	In 120 ml.
otc	**Acetaminophen** (Various, eg, Pharm. Assoc. Inc)	**Elixir**: 120 mg/5 ml	In UD 27 ml (100s).
otc	**Aceta** (Century)		In 120 ml and gal.
otc	**Oraphen-PD** (Great Southern)		In 120 ml.
otc	**Acetaminophen** (Various, eg, Goldline, Major, Rugby, Schein)	**Elixir**: 160 mg/5 ml	In 118 and 120 ml, pt and gal.
otc	**Genapap, Children's** (Goldline)		In 120 ml.
otc	**Mapap, Children's** (Major)		Alcohol free. Grape and cherry flavors. In 120 ml.
otc	**Tylenol, Children's** (McNeil-CPC)		Alcohol free. Sorbitol, sucrose, butylparaben, corn syrup. Cherry flavor. In 60 and 120 ml.

ACETAMINOPHEN (N-Acetyl-P-Aminophenol, APAP)

otc	**Acetaminophen** (Various, eg, Roxane, UDL Labs)	**Liquid:** 160 mg/5 ml	In 120 and 500 ml and UD 100s.
otc	**Halenol, Children's** (Halsey)		In 120, 240 and 480 ml and gal.
otc sf	**Panadol, Children's** (SmithKline Beecham)		Alcohol free. Saccharin, sorbitol. Fruit flavor. In 59 and 118 ml.
otc	**Tempra 2 Syrup** (Mead Johnson Nutritional)		In 120 ml.
otc	**Acetaminophen** (Various, eg, Goldline)	**Liquid:** 500 mg/15 ml	In 237 ml.
otc	**Tylenol Extra Strength** (McNeil-CPC)		7% alcohol. Sorbitol, sucrose. Mint flavor. In 240 ml with dosage cup.
otc	**Liquiprin Drops for Children** (Menley & James)	**Solution:** 80 mg/1.66 ml	Alcohol free. Berry flavor. In 30 ml with dropper.
otc	**Acetaminophen Drops** (Various, eg, Bioline, Moore, Schein)	**Solution:** 100 mg/ml	In 15 ml.
otc	**Apacet** (Parmed)		In 15 ml.
otc	**Genapap, Infants' Drops** (Goldline)		Alcohol free. Fruit flavor. In 15 ml w/0.8 ml dropper.
otc	**Mapap Infant Drops** (Major)		Alcohol free. Fruit flavor. In 15 and 30 ml.
otc sf	**Panadol, Infants' Drops** (SmithKline Beecham)		Alcohol free. Saccharin. Fruit flavor. In 14.8 ml with 0.8 ml dropper.
otc	**Silapap, Infants** (Silarx)		Alcohol free. Fruit flavor. In 15 ml with dropper.
otc	**Tempra 1** (Mead Johnson Nutritional)		In 15 ml.
otc	**Tylenol, Infants' Drops** (McNeil-CPC)		Alcohol free. Saccharin, butylparaben, corn syrup, sorbitol. Fruit and grape flavors. In 7.5 ml and in 30 ml w/0.8 ml dropper.
otc	**Uni-Ace** (United Research Laboratories)		Alcohol free. Fruit flavor. In 15 ml with dropper.
🍁	**Tylenol Infants' Suspension Drops** (McNeil Consumer)	**Suspension:** 80 mg/ml	In 15 and 24 ml
🍁	**Tylenol Children's Suspension** (McNeil Consumer)	**Suspension:** 32 mg/ml	Grape and cherry flavors. In 100 ml
🍁	**Tempra Children's Syrup** (Mead Johnson Nutritional)	**Syrup:** 16 mg/ml	In 100 ml.

[1] Republic Drug Company can be reached at P.O. Box 807; Buffalo, NY 14207; Telephone: 800–828–7444.

ACETAMINOPHEN, BUFFERED

For complete prescribing information, refer to the Acetaminophen group monograph.

otc	**Bromo Seltzer** (Warner-Lambert)	**Effervescent Granules:** 325 mg w/2.781 g sodium bicarbonate & 2.224 g citric acid/dose measure	With 761 mg sodium. In 78.75, 127.5 and 270 g and UD 48s.

SALICYLATES

The salicylates have analgesic, antipyretic and anti-inflammatory effects. Aspirin and other salicylic acid derivatives are hydrolyzed to salicylic acid. Salicylamide and diflunisal are structurally related, but are not true salicylates since they are not hydrolyzed to salicylic acid.

Warning:
Children and teenagers should not use salicylates for chickenpox or flu symptoms before a doctor is consulted about Reye's syndrome, a rare but serious illness.

Actions:

Pharmacology: Salicylates have analgesic, antipyretic, anti-inflammatory and antirheumatic effects. The pharmacological effects of these agents are qualitatively similar. Salicylates lower elevated body temperature through vasodilation of peripheral vessels, thus enhancing dissipation of excess heat. The anti-inflammatory and analgesic activity may be mediated through inhibition of the prostaglandin synthetase enzyme complex.

Aspirin differs from the other agents in this group in that it more potently inhibits prostaglandin synthesis, has greater anti-inflammatory effects and irreversibly inhibits platelet aggregation. The aspirin molecule's acetyl group is believed to account for these differences. Aspirin inhibits prostaglandin production by acetylating cyclo-oxygenase, the initial enzyme in the prostaglandin biosynthesis pathway.

Irreversible inhibition of platelet aggregation (aspirin) – Single analgesic aspirin doses prolong bleeding time. Acetylation of platelet cyclo-oxygenase prevents synthesis of thromboxane A_2, a prostaglandin derivative, which is a potent vasoconstrictor and inducer of platelet aggregation and platelet release reaction. Aspirin (no other salicylates) inhibits platelet aggregation for the life of the platelet (7–10 days).

Aspirin has shown some success as an antiplatelet agent in patients with thromboembolic disease. Low doses of aspirin inhibit platelet aggregation and may be more effective than higher doses. Larger doses inhibit cyclo-oxygenase in arterial walls, interfering with prostacyclin production, a potent vasodilator and inhibitor of platelet aggregation. Combinations of dipyridamole or sulfinpyrazone with aspirin have been recommended for antithrombotic action for prophylaxis in various high risk situations (ie, coronary bypass graft patency and total hip replacement).

Myocardial infarction (MI) – Aspirin use in MI patients was associated with an ≈ 20% reduction in risk of subsequent death and nonfatal reinfarction, a median absolute decrease of 3% from the 12% to 22% event rates with placebo. Daily aspirin dosage in post-MI studies was 300 mg in one and 900 to 1500 mg in five. In aspirin-treated unstable angina patients (325 mg/day), reduction in risk was about 50%, a reduction in event rate of 5% from the 10% rate with placebo over the 12 week study.

In the Aspirin Myocardial Infarction Study (AMIS) trial, 1 g per day was associated with small increases in systolic BP (average, 1.5 to 2.1 mm Hg) and diastolic BP (0.5 to 0.6 mm Hg). Uric acid levels and BUN increased by < 1 mg%.

In the Second International Study of Infarct Survival (ISIS-2) trial, patients who received a combination of aspirin (160 mg/day) and streptokinase after the onset of suspected acute MI had significantly fewer reinfarctions, strokes and deaths than those patients who received placebo. Also, the combination was significantly better than either drug alone; their separate effects on vascular deaths appeared additive.

Other pharmacological actions – Inhibition of prothrombin synthesis and prolonged prothrombin time are clinically significant only after large doses (≥ 6 g/day). Doses > 3 to 5 g/day have a uricosuric effect; low doses (< 2 g/day) decrease uric acid secretion.

Pharmacokinetics:

Absorption/Distribution – Salicylates are rapidly and completely absorbed after oral use. Bioavailability is dependent on the dosage form, presence of food, gastric emptying time, gastric pH, presence of antacids or buffering agents and particle size. Bioavailability of some enteric coated products may be erratic. Food slows the absorption of salicylates. Absorption from rectal suppositories is slower, resulting in lower salicylate levels. Aspirin is partially hydrolyzed to salicylic acid during absorption and is distributed to all body tissues and fluids, including fetal tissues, breast milk and CNS. Highest concentrations are found in plasma, liver, renal cortex, heart and lungs. Protein binding of salicylates is concentration-dependent. At low therapeutic concentrations (100 mcg/ml), ≈ 90% is bound; at higher plasma concentrations (400 mcg/ml), 76% is bound. Signs of salicylism (eg, tinnitus) occur at serum levels > 200 mcg/ml; severe toxic effects may occur at levels > 400 mcg/ml (see Adverse Reactions).

SALICYLATES

Metabolism/Excretion – Salicylic acid is eliminated by renal excretion and by oxidation and conjugation of metabolites. Aspirin has a half-life of ≈ 15 to 20 min. Salicylic acid has a half-life of 2 to 3 hrs at low doses; at higher doses, it may exceed 20 hrs. In therapeutic anti-inflammatory doses, half-life ranges from 6 to 12 hrs. Plasma salicylate levels increase disproportionately as dosage is increased. Elimination is determined by zero order kinetics. Renal excretion of unchanged drug depends upon urine pH. As urinary pH changes from 5 to 8, renal clearance of free ionized salicylate increases from 2% to 3% of amount excreted to > 80%.

Indications:

Mild to moderate pain; fever; various inflammatory conditions such as rheumatic fever, rheumatoid arthritis and osteoarthritis.

Aspirin, for reducing the risk of recurrent transient ischemic attacks (TIAs) or stroke in men who have had transient ischemia of the brain due to fibrin platelet emboli. It has not been effective in women and is of no benefit for completed strokes.

Aspirin, to reduce the risk of death or nonfatal myocardial infarction (MI) in patients with previous infarction or unstable angina pectoris.

Unlabeled uses: Possible effect of long-term aspirin-like analgesics to prevent cataract formation is being studied. Dipyridamole is often added to aspirin to prevent MI and stroke, but data do not show improved antithrombotic aspirin efficacy during coadministration. Low-dose aspirin may help prevent toxemia of pregnancy and may be beneficial in pregnant women with inadequate uteroplacental blood flow (eg, systemic lupus erythematosus). Further studies are needed. See Warnings.

Contraindications:

Hypersensitivity to salicylates or nonsteroidal anti-inflammatory drugs (NSAIDs). Use extreme caution in patients with history of adverse reactions to salicylates. Cross-sensitivity may exist between aspirin and other NSAIDs which inhibit prostaglandin synthesis, and aspirin and tartrazine. Aspirin cross-sensitivity does not appear to occur with sodium salicylate, salicylamide or choline salicylate. Aspirin hypersensitivity is more prevalent in those with asthma, nasal polyposis, chronic urticaria.

In hemophilia, bleeding ulcers and hemorrhagic states.

Magnesium salicylate in advanced chronic renal insufficiency due to Mg retention.

Warnings:

Reye's syndrome:

Salicylate association – Use of salicylates, particularly aspirin, in children or teenagers with influenza or chickenpox may be associated with development of Reye's syndrome. This rare, acute, life-threatening condition is characterized by vomiting, lethargy and belligerence that may progress to delirium and coma. Mortality rate is 20% to 30%; permanent brain damage has been reported in survivors.

A causal relationship is controversial, but CDC, FDA, American Academy of Pediatrics' Committee on Infectious Diseases and Surgeon General advise against salicylate use in children and teens with influenza or chickenpox. (See Warning Box.)

Otic effects: Discontinue use if dizziness, ringing in ears (tinnitus) or impaired hearing occurs. Tinnitus probably represents blood salicylic acid levels reaching or exceeding the upper limit of the therapeutic range. It is a helpful guide to dose titration. Temporary hearing loss disappears gradually upon discontinuation of the drug.

Use in surgical patients: Avoid aspirin, if possible, for 1 week prior to surgery because of the possibility of postoperative bleeding.

Hypersensitivity: Aspirin intolerance, manifested by acute bronchospasm, generalized urticaria/angioedema, severe rhinitis or shock occurs in 4% to 19% of asthmatics. Symptoms occur within 3 hours after ingestion. The aspirin triad consists of the association of asthma, nasal polyps and aspirin intolerance. Have epinephrine 1:1000 immediately available. Refer to Management of Acute Hypersensitivity Reactions.

Foods may contribute to a reaction. Some foods with 6 mg/100 g salicylate include curry powder, paprika, licorice, Benedictine liqueur, prunes, raisins, tea, gherkins. A typical American diet contains 10 to 200 mg/day salicylate.

Desensitization has been successfully induced and maintained. Perform in hospital; generally maintain with one aspirin/day. Any NSAID can maintain desensitization. However, if maintenance is interrupted, sensitivity will reappear (2 to 5 days).

Hepatic function impairment: Use caution in liver damage, preexisting hypoprothrombinemia and vitamin K deficiency. Reversible hepatic encephalopathy occurred in a chronic alcoholic with cirrhosis who took ASA 5 g/day for osteoarthritis. Aspirin-induced hepatotoxicity occurred after therapeutic doses for rheumatoid arthritis.

Salicylic Acid Derivatives

SALICYLATES

Pregnancy: Category D (aspirin); Category C (salsalate, magnesium salicylate). Aspirin may produce adverse maternal effects: Anemia, ante- or postpartum hemorrhage, prolonged gestation and labor. Salicylates readily cross placenta. By inhibiting prostaglandin synthesis, salicylates may cause constriction of ductus arteriosus, and, possibly, other untoward fetal effects. Maternal aspirin use during later stages of pregnancy may cause adverse fetal effects: Low birth weight, increased incidence of intracranial hemorrhage in premature infants, stillbirths, neonatal death. Salicylates may be teratogens. Avoid use during pregnancy, especially in third trimester.

Lactation: Salicylates are excreted in breast milk in low concentrations, producing peak milk levels ranging from 1.1 to 10 mcg/ml. Adverse effects on platelet function in the nursing infant have not been reported, but are a potential risk.

Children: Safety and efficacy of **magnesium salicylate** or **salsalate** have not been established. Administration of **aspirin** to children (including teenagers) with acute febrile illness has been associated with the development of Reye's syndrome. Dehydrated febrile children appear more prone to salicylate intoxication.

Precautions:

Renal effects: Use with caution in chronic renal insufficiency; aspirin may cause a transient decrease in renal function, and may aggravate chronic kidney diseases (rare).

In patients with renal impairment, take precautions when administering **magnesium salicylate**. Discontinue other drugs containing magnesium and monitor serum magnesium levels if dosage levels of magnesium salicylate are high.

GI effects: Use caution in those intolerant to salicylate because of GI irritation, and in gastric ulcers, peptic ulcer, mild diabetes, gout, erosive gastritis or bleeding tendencies. **Salsalate** and **choline salicylate** may cause less GI irritation than aspirin.

Although fecal blood loss is less with enteric coated aspirin than with uncoated, give enteric coated aspirin with caution to patients with GI distress, ulcer or bleeding problems. Occult GI bleeding occurs in many patients but is not correlated with gastric distress. The amount of blood lost is usually clinically insignificant (average, 2.5 ml), but with prolonged use, it may result in iron deficiency anemia. Patients developing peptic ulcers while taking salicylates for rheumatic disease have healed during treatment with cimetidine and antacids despite continued salicylate use. In addition, although acute aspirin use results in mucosal lesions, only 20% to 25% of those on chronic aspirin for rheumatism develop mucosal injury.

Hematologic effects: Aspirin interferes with hemostasis. Avoid use if patients have severe anemia, history of blood coagulation defects, or take anticoagulants (see Drug Interactions).

Long-term therapy: To avoid potentially toxic concentrations, warn patients on long-term therapy not to take other salicylates (nonprescription analgesics, etc).

Periodically monitor plasma salicylic acid concentrations during long-term treatment to aid maintenance of therapeutic levels (100 to 300 mcg/ml). Toxic manifestations are not usually seen until concentrations exceed 300 mcg/ml. Monitor urinary pH regularly; sudden acidification, as from pH 6.5 to 5.5, can double the plasma level, resulting in toxicity.

Salicylism may require dosage adjustment.

Controlled release aspirin, because of its relatively long onset of action, is not recommended for antipyresis or short-term analgesia. Not recommended in children > 12; contraindicated in all children with fever accompanied by dehydration.

Drug Interactions:

Drugs affecting aspirin:

Activated charcoal – Coadministration decreases aspirin absorption, depending on charcoal dose and interval between ingestion. May be useful (see Overdosage).

Ammonium chloride, ascorbic acid or methionine – Urinary acidifiers decrease salicylate excretion.

Antacids and urinary alkalinizers may decrease the pharmacologic effects of salicylates. Urinary alkalinization increases the renal excretion of salicylic acid due to decreased tubular reabsorption of un-ionized drug. The magnitude of the antacid interaction depends on the agent, dose and pretreatment urine pH.

Carbonic anhydrase inhibitors – Salicylate intoxication has occurred after coadministration of these agents. However, salicylic acid renal elimination may be increased if urine is kept alkaline. Conversely, salicylates may displace acetazolamide from protein binding sites resulting in toxicity. Further study is needed.

Corticosteroids increase salicylate clearance and decrease serum levels.

Nizatidine – Increased serum salicylate levels have occurred in patients receiving high dose aspirin (3.9 g/day) and concurrent nizatidine.

Salicylic Acid Derivatives

SALICYLATES

Drugs affected by aspirin:

Alcohol – The risk of GI ulceration increases when salicylates are given concomitantly. Ingestion of alcohol during salicylate therapy may also prolong bleeding time.

Angiotensin converting enzyme inhibitors – Antihypertensive effectiveness of these agents may be decreased by concurrent salicylate administration, possibly due to prostaglandin inhibition. Consider discontinuing salicylates if problems occur.

Anticoagulants, oral – Therapeutic aspirin has an additive hypoprothrombinemic effect. Impaired platelet function may prolong bleeding time. Use caution.

Beta-adrenergic blockers may have their antihypertensive action blunted by concurrent salicylate administration, possibly due to prostaglandin inhibition. Consider discontinuing salicylates if problems occur.

Heparin – Aspirin can increase bleeding risk in heparin anticoagulated patients.

Loop diuretics may be less effective when given with salicylates in patients with compromised renal function or with cirrhosis with ascites; however, data conflict.

Methotrexate – Salicylates increase drug levels causing toxicity by interfering with protein binding and renal elimination of the antimetabolite.

Nitroglycerin, when taken with aspirin, may result in unexpected hypotension. Data are limited. If hypotension occurs, reduce the nitroglycerin dose.

NSAIDs – Aspirin may decrease NSAID serum concentrations. Concomitant use offers no advantage and may significantly increase incidence of GI effects.

Probenecid and sulfinpyrazone – Salicylates antagonize the uricosuric effect. While salicylates in large doses (> 3 g/day) have a uricosuric effect, smaller amounts may reduce the uricosuric effect of these agents.

Spironolactone – Salicylates may inhibit the diuretic effects; antihypertensive action does not appear altered. Effects depend on the dose of spironolactone.

Sulfonylureas and exogenous insulin – Salicylates in doses greater than 2 g/day have a hypoglycemic action, perhaps by altering pancreatic beta cell function. They may potentiate the glucose lowering effect of these drugs.

Valproic acid – Aspirin displaces the drug from its protein binding sites and may decrease its total body clearance, thus increasing the pharmacological effects.

Drug/Lab test interactions: Salicylates compete with thyroid hormone for binding sites on thyroid binding pre-albumin and possibly thyroid binding globulin resulting in increases in **protein bound iodine (PBI)**. Salicylates probably do not interfere with T_3 resin uptake.

Serum uric acid levels are elevated by salicylate levels < 10 mg/dl and decreased by levels > 10 mg/dl. Combined **phenylbutazone** and salicylates decrease uric acid excretion and may increase serum uric acid by an average of 2 mg/dl.

Salicylates in moderate to large (anti-inflammatory) doses cause false-negative readings for **urine glucose** by the glucose oxidase method and false-positive readings by the copper reduction method.

Salicylates in the urine interfere with **5–HIAA** determinations by fluorescent methods, but not by the nitrosonaphthol colorimetric method.

Salicylates in the urine interact with **urinary ketone** determinations by the ferric chloride (Gerhardt) method producing a reddish color.

Large doses may decrease urinary excretion of **PSP (phenolsulfonphthalein)**.

Salicylates in the urine result in falsely elevated **VMA (vanillylmandelic acid)** with most tests, but falsely decrease VMA determinations by the Pisano method.

Adverse Reactions:

GI: Nausea, dyspepsia (5% to 25%), heartburn, epigastric discomfort, anorexia, acute reversible hepatotoxicity, massive GI bleeding and occult blood loss may occur. Aspirin may potentiate peptic ulcer.

Chronic aspirin use may cause a persistent iron deficiency anemia.

Dermatologic: Hives, rashes and angioedema may occur, especially in patients suffering from chronic urticaria.

Hepatic: High aspirin doses reportedly produced reversible hepatic dysfunction.

Hematologic: Prolongation of bleeding time, leukopenia, thrombocytopenia, purpura, decreased plasma iron concentration, shortened erythrocyte survival time.

Miscellaneous: Fever, thirst, dimness of vision.

Allergic and anaphylactic reactions were noted when hypersensitive individuals took aspirin. Fatal anaphylactic shock, while not common, has been reported.

Aspirin intolerance, manifested by exacerbation of bronchospasm and rhinitis, may occur in patients with a history of nasal polyps, asthma or rhinitis. The mechanism of this intolerance may be the result of aspirin-induced shunting of prostaglandin synthesis to the lipoxygenase pathway and liberation of leukotrienes, ie, slow-reacting substance of anaphylaxis.

Salicylic Acid Derivatives

SALICYLATES

Mild "salicylism" may occur after repeated use of large doses and consists of dizziness, tinnitus (manifested as musical perceptions in one patient), difficulty hearing, nausea, vomiting, diarrhea, mental confusion, CNS depression, headache, sweating, hyperventilation and lassitude. Salicylate serum concentrations correlate with pharmacological actions and adverse effects observed. See table below:

Serum Salicylate: Clinical Correlations		
Serum Salicylate Concentration (mcg/ml)	Desired Effects	Adverse Effects/ Intoxication
≈100	Antiplatelet Antipyresis Analgesia	GI intolerance and bleeding, hypersensitivity, hemostatic defects
150-300	Anti-inflammatory	Mild salicylism
250-400	Treatment of rheumatic fever	Nausea/vomiting, hyperventilation, salicylism, flushing, sweating, thirst, headache, diarrhea and tachycardia
> 400-500		Respiratory alkalosis, hemorrhage, excitement, confusion, asterixis, pulmonary edema, convulsions, tetany, metabolic acidosis, fever, coma, cardiovascular collapse, renal and respiratory failure

Overdosage:

Symptoms:

Acute lethal dose (approximate) –

Adults: 10 to 30 g.

Children: 4 g.

Respiratory alkalosis is seen initially in acute salicylate ingestions. Hyperpnea and tachypnea occur as a result of increased CO_2 production and a direct stimulatory effect of salicylate on the respiratory center. Other symptoms may include nausea, vomiting, hypokalemia, tinnitus, neurologic abnormalities (eg, disorientation, irritability, hallucinations, lethargy, stupor, coma, seizures), dehydration, hyperthermia, hyperventilation, hyperactivity, thrombocytopenia, platelet dysfunction, hypoprothrombinemia, increased capillary fragility and other hematologic abnormalities. Symptoms may progress quickly to depression, coma, respiratory failure and collapse. Although blood glucose is usually normal or slightly elevated, hypoglycemia may occur with chronic toxicity or in late acute toxicity. A mixed respiratory alkalosis and metabolic acidosis may also develop.

Chronic salicylate toxicity may occur when > 100 mg/kg/day is ingested for 2 or more days. It is more difficult to recognize and is associated with increaed morbidity and mortality. Compared to acute poisoning, hyperventilation, dehydration, systemic acidosis and severe CNS manifestations occur more frequently.

Treatment: Initial treatment includes induction of emesis or gastric lavage to remove any unabsorbed drug from the stomach. Activated charcoal diminishes salicylate absorption, most effectively if given within 2 hours after ingestion. Monitor salicylate levels, acid-base and fluid and electrolyte balance. Further therapy is largely supportive. Refer to General Management of Acute Overdosage.Reduce hyperthermia; treat severe convulsions with diazepam. Forced alkaline diuresis will enhance renal excretion of salicylates. Hemodialysis is very efficient in eliminating salicylate, but use only in patients who are severely poisoned, and in those with noncardiogenic pulmonary edema, severe CNS symptoms, renal failure, acidosis refractory to conservative therapy or clinical deterioration despite other therapies. Rarely, IV vitamin K may be indicated to correct hypoprothrombinemia.

Patient Information:

May cause GI upset; take with food or after meals.

Do not crush or chew sustained release preparations.

Take with a full glass of water (240 ml) to reduce the risk of lodging medication in the esophagus.

Patients allergic to tartrazine dye should avoid **aspirin**.

Notify physician if ringing in ears or persistent GI pain occurs.

Do not use **aspirin** if it has a strong vinegar-like odor.

Salicylic Acid Derivatives

ASPIRIN (Acetylsalicylic Acid; ASA)

For complete prescribing information, refer to the Salicylates group monograph.

Administration and Dosage:

Minor aches and pains: 325 to 650 mg every 4 hours as needed. Some extra strength (500 mg) products suggest 500 mg every 3 hours or 1000 mg every 6 hours.

Arthritis, other rheumatic conditions (eg, osteoarthritis): 3.2 to 6 g/day in divided doses.

Juvenile rheumatoid arthritis – 60 to 110 mg/kg/day in divided doses (every 6 to 8 hours). When starting at lower doses (eg, 60 mg/kg/day), may increase by 20 mg/kg/day after 5 to 7 days, followed by 10 mg/kg/day after another 5 to 7 days.

Maintain a serum salicylate level of 150 to 300 mcg/ml.

Acute rheumatic fever:

Adults – 5 to 8 g/day, initially.

Children – 100 mg/kg/day for 2 weeks, then 75 mg/kg/day for 4 to 6 weeks.

Therapeutic salicylate level is 150 to 300 mcg/ml.

Transient ischemic attacks in men: 1300 mg/day in divided doses (650 mg 2 times daily, or 325 mg 4 times daily). One study indicated that a dose of 300 mg/day is as effective as the larger dose and may be associated with fewer side effects.

Myocardial infarction prophylaxis: 300 or 325 mg/day. This use applies to solid oral doseforms (buffered and plain) and to buffered aspirin in solution.

Children:

Analgesic/antipyretic dosage – 10 to 15 mg/kg/dose every 4 hours (see table), up to 60 to 80 mg/kg/day. Do not use in children or teenagers with chickenpox or flu symptoms due to the possibility of Reye's syndrome (see Warnings). Dosage recommendations by age and weight are as follows:

Recommended Aspirin Dosage in Children

Age (years)	Weight lbs	Weight kg	Dosage (mg every 4 hours)	No. of 81 mg tablets (every 4 hours)	No. of 325 mg tablets (every 4 hours)
2-3	24-35	10.6-15.9	162	2	½
4-5	36-47	16-21.4	243	3	
6-8	48-59	21.5-26.8	324	4	1
9-10	60-71	26.9-32.3	405	5	
11	72-95	32.4-43.2	486	6	1½
12-14	≥ 96	≥ 43.3	648	8	2

Kawasaki disease (mucocutaneous lymph node syndrome) – For acute febrile period, 80 to 180 mg/kg/day; very high doses may be needed to achieve therapeutic levels. After the fever resolves, dosage may be adjusted to 10 mg/kg/day.

otc	**Bayer Children's Aspirin** (Glenbrook)	**Tablets, chewable:** 81 mg	Saccharin. Orange flavor. In 36s.
otc	**St. Joseph Adult Chewable Aspirin** (Schering-Plough)		Saccharin. Orange flavor. In 36s.
otc	**½ Halfprin** (Kramer)	**Tablets, enteric coated:** 165 mg	Red. In 60s and 200s.
otc	**Ecotrin Adult Low Strength** (SmithKline Beecham)	81 mg	Yellow. In 36s.
otc	**Halfprin 81** (Kramer)		In 90s.
otc	**Aspergum** (Schering-Plough)	**Gum tablets:** 227.5 mg	Chewable. Glucose, saccharin, sugar. Orange or cherry flavor. In 16s, 40s.

Salicylic Acid Derivatives

ASPIRIN (Acetylsalicylic Acid; ASA)

otc	**Aspirin** (Various, eg, Major, Moore, Parmed, Rugby, URL, Warner-C)	**Tablets:** 325 mg	In 100s, 200s, 250s, 500s and 1000s.
otc	**Genuine Bayer Aspirin Tablets and Caplets** (Glenbrook)		**Tablets:** Film coated. In 12s, 24s, 50s, 100s, 200s and 300s.
			Caplets: Film coated. In 50s, 100s and 200s.
otc	**Empirin** (Burroughs Wellcome)	**Tablets:** 325 mg	(Tabloid brand). White. In 50s, 100s and 250s.
otc	**Genprin** (Goldline)		White. In 100s.
otc	**Aspirin** (URL)	**Tablets:** 500 mg	In 100s.
otc	**Arthritis Foundation Pain Reliever** (McNeil-PPC)		In 50s.
otc	**Maximum Bayer Aspirin Tablets and Caplets** (Glenbrook)		**Tablets:** Film coated. In 30s, 60s and 100s.
			Caplets: Film coated. In 30s and 60s.
otc	**Norwich Extra-Strength** (Procter & Gamble)		In 150s.
otc	**Aspirin** (Various, eg, Geneva, Major, Moore, Parmed, Rugby, URL)	**Tablets, enteric coated:** 325 mg	In 30s, 60s, 90s, 100s, 1000s and UD 100s.
otc	**Ecotrin Tablets and Caplets** (SmithKline Beecham)		**Tablets:** (Ecotrin Reg). In 100s, 250s and 1000s.
			Caplets: (Ecotrin Reg). In 100s.
otc	**Regular Strength Bayer Enteric Coated Caplets** (Sterling Health)		Delayed release. In 50s and 100s.
otc	**Ecotrin Maximum Strength Tablets and Caplets** (SmithKline Beecham)	**Tablets, enteric coated:** 500 mg	**Tablets:** (Ecotrin Max). In 60s and 150s.
			Caplets: (Ecotrin Max). In 60s.
otc	**Extra Strength Bayer Enteric 500 Aspirin** (Sterling Health)		(Bayer 500). In 60s.
otc	**Aspirin** (Various, eg, Goldline, Moore, Rugby)	**Tablets, enteric coated:** 650 mg	In 100s and 1000s.
Rx	**Aspirin** (Rugby)	**Tablets, enteric coated:** 975 mg	In 100s.
Rx	**Easprin** (Parke-Davis)		Delayed release. (P-D 490). In 100s.
otc	**Extended Release Bayer 8-Hour Caplets** (Bayer)	**Tablets, extended release:** 650 mg	White, scored. In 50s.
Rx	**ZORprin** (Boots)	**Tablets, controlled release:** 800 mg	(BA57). White. Elongated. In 100s.
otc	**Bayer Low Adult Strength** (Sterling Health)	**Tablets, enteric coated:** 81 mg	Delayed release. Lactose. In 120s.
otc	**Aspirin** (Various, eg, Goldline, Moore, Rugby, URL)	**Suppositories**[1]: 120 mg	In 12s.
		200 mg	In 12s.
		300 mg	In 12s.
		600 mg	In 12s and 100s.

[1] Refrigerate

Salicylic Acid Derivatives

ASPIRIN (Acetylsalicylic Acid; ASA), BUFFERED

Complete prescribing information for these products begins in the Salicylates monograph.

The addition of small amounts of antacids may decrease GI irritation and increase the dissolution and absorption rates of these products.

otc	**Tri-Buffered Bufferin Tablets and Caplets** (Bristol Myers Squibb)	**Tablets:** 325 mg with caldium carbonate, magnesium oxide and magnesium carbonate	**Tablets:** (B). White. In 12s, 36s, 60s, 100s, 200s, 275s, 1000s.
			Caplets: (B). White. scored. In 36s, 60s and 100s.
otc	**Buffered Aspirin** (Various, eg, Geneva, Goldline, Major, Moore, Rugby, UDL, URL)	**Tablets:** 325 mg with buffers	In 100s, 500s, 1000s and UD 100s and 200s.
otc	**Bayer Buffered Aspirin** (Sterling Health)		(Bayer Buffered). In 100s.
otc	**Buffex** (Roberts Med)	**Tablets:** 325 mg with aluminum glycinate and magnesium carbonate	In 1000s and Sani-Pak 1000s.
otc	**Adprin-B** (Pfeiffer)	**Tablets, coated:** 325 mg with calcium carbonate, magnesium carbonate and magnesium oxide	In 130s.
otc	**Gennin** (Goldline)		In 100s.
otc	**Asprimox** (Invamed)	**Tablets, coated:** 325 mg with 50 mg magnesium hydroxide, 50 mg aluminum hydroxide and calcium carbonate	In 100s and 500s.
otc	**Magnaprin** (Rugby)		Film coated. In 100s and 500s.
otc	**Regular Strength Ascriptin** (Rhone Poulenc Rorer)		In 60s.
otc	**Ascriptin A/D** (Rorer)	**Tablets, coated:** 325 mg with 75 mg magnesium hydroxide, 75 mg aluminum hydroxide and calcium carbonate	Capsule shape. In 225s.
otc	**Asprimox Extra Protection for Arthritis Pain**(Invamed)		In 100s and 500s.
otc	**Magnaprin Arthritis Strength Captabs** (Rugby)		Capsule shape. In 100s and 500s.
otc	**Bufferin** (Bristol-Myers)	**Tablets, coated:** 325 mg with 158 mg calcium carbonate, 63 mg magnesium oxide and 34 mg magnesium carbonate	**Tablets:** (B). In 12s, 36s, 60s, 100s, 200s and UD 150s.
			Caplets: (B/B). Coated, scored. In 36s, 60s and 100s.
otc	**Extra Strength Adprin-B** (Pfeiffer)	**Tablets, coated:** 500 mg with calcium carbonate, magnesium carbonate and magnesium oxide	In 130s.
otc	**Extra Strength Bayer Plus Caplets** (Sterling Health)	**Tablets:** 500 mg with calcium carbonate, magnesium carbonate and magnesium oxide	In 30s and 60s.
otc	**Ascriptin Extra Strength** (Rhone-Poulenc Rorer)	**Tablets, coated:** 500 mg with 80 mg magnesium hydroxide, 80 mg aluminum hydroxide and calcium carbonate	Capsule shape. In 50s.

Salicylic Acid Derivatives

ASPIRIN (Acetylsalicylic Acid; ASA), BUFFERED

otc	**Cama Arthritis Pain Reliever** (Sandoz)	**Tablets:** 500 mg with 150 mg magnesium oxide and 125 mg aluminum hydroxide	(Dorsey Cama 500). Methylparaben. White w/salmon inlay. In 100s.
otc	**Arthritis Pain Formula** (Whitehall)	**Tablets:** 500 mg with 100 mg magnesium hydroxide and 27 mg aluminum hydroxide	Capsule shape. In 40s, 100s and 175s.
otc	**Alka-Seltzer with Aspirin** (Miles Inc)	**Tablets, effervescent:** 325 mg with 1.9 g sodium bicarbonate and 1 g citric acid per dry tablet, 567 mg sodium/tablet	In 12s, 24s, 36s, 72s, 96s and 100s.
otc	**Alka-Seltzer with Aspirin (Flavored)** (Miles Inc)	**Tablets, effervescent:** 325 mg with 1.7 g sodium bicarbonate and 1.2 g citric acid per dry tablet, 506 mg sodium/tablet	Saccharin and flavoring. In 12s, 24s and 36s.
otc	**Alka-Seltzer Extra Strength with Aspirin** (Miles)	**Tablet, effervescent:** 500 mg with 1.9 g sodium bicarbonate and 1 g citric acid	In 12s and 24s.

SALSALATE (Salicylsalicyclic Acid)

Complete prescribing information for these products begins in the Salicylates monograph.

After absorption, the drug is partially hydrolyzed into two molecules of salicylic acid. Insoluble in gastric secretions, it is not absorbed until it reaches the small intestine.

Administration and Dosage:

Usual adult dose is 3000 mg/day given in divided doses.

Rx	**Amigesic** (Amide)	**Capsules:** 500 mg	White and green. In 100s and 500s.
Rx	**Disalcid** (3M)		(Riker Disalcid). Aqua and white. In 100s.
Rx	**Salsalate** (Various, eg, Geneva, Goldline, Major, Moore, Rugby, Schein, URL, Vitarine)	**Tablets:** 500 mg	In 100s, 500s and UD 100s.
Rx	**Amigesic** (Amide)		Yellow or blue. Film coated. In 100s and 500s.
Rx	**Argesic-SA** (Econo Med)		In 100s.
Rx	**Disalcid** (3M)		(Riker Disalcid). Aqua, scored. Film coated. In 100s, 500s and UD 100s.
Rx	**Salflex** (Carnrick)		Dye free. (C 8671). White. Film coated. In 100s.
Rx	**Salsitab** (Upsher-Smith)		(500). Blue. Film coated. In 100s, 500s and UD 100s.

Salicylic Acid Derivatives

SALSALATE (Salicylsalicyclic Acid)

Rx	**Salsalate** (Various, eg, Copley, Geneva, Goldline, Major, Moore, Rugby, Schein, URL, Vitarine)	**Tablets:** 750 mg	In 100s, 500s and UD 100s.
Rx	**Amigesic Caplets** (Amide)		Yellow or blue, scored. Film coated, Capsule shaped. In 100s and 500s.
Rx	**Artha-G** (T.E. Williams)		(Artha-G). Lavender, scored. In 120s.
Rx	**Disalcid** (3M)		(Riker Disalcid 750). Aqua, scored. Film coated. In 100s, 500s and UD 100s.
Rx	**Marthritic** (Marnel)		In 100s.
Rx	**Mono-Gesic** (Central)		(Central 750 mg). Pink, scored. Film coated. In 100s and 500s.
Rx	**Salsitab** (Upsher-Smith)		(750). Blue, scored. Film coated. In 100s, 500s and UD 100s.
Rx	**Salflex** (Carnrick)		Dye free. (C 8672). White, scored. Film coated. In 100s and 500s.

Salicylic Acid Derivatives

SODIUM SALICYLATE

Complete prescribing information for these products begins in the Salicylates monograph.

Less effective than an equal dose of aspirin in reducing pain or fever. Patients hypersensitive to aspirin may be able to tolerate sodium salicylate. Platelets are not affected; however, prothrombin time is increased. Each gram contains 6.25 mEq sodium.

Administration and Dosage:

325 to 650 mg every 4 hours.

otc	**Sodium Salicylate** (Various, eg, Moore, Rugby)	**Tablets, enteric coated:** 325 mg	In 100s.
otc	**Sodium Salicylate** (Various, eg, Moore, Rugby)	**Tablets, enteric coated:** 650 mg	In 100s, 500s and 1000s.

SODIUM THIOSALICYLATE

Complete prescribing information for these products begins in the Salicylates monograph.

Administration and Dosage:

Intramuscular administration is preferred.

Acute gout: 100 mg every 3 to 4 hrs for 2 days, then 100 mg/day until asymptomatic.

Muscular pain, musculoskeletal disturbances: 50 to 100 mg/day or on alternate days.

Rheumatic fever: 100 to 150 mg every 4 to 8 hours for 3 days, then reduce to 100 mg twice daily. Continue until patient is asymptomatic.

Rx	**Sodium Thiosalicylate** (Various)	**Injection:** 50 mg per ml	In 30 ml vials and 2 ml amps.
Rx	**Rexolate** (Hyrex)		In 30 ml vials.

[1] With 2% benzyl alcohol.

CHOLINE SALICYLATE

Complete prescribing information for these products begins in the Salicylates monograph.

Has fewer GI side effects than aspirin.

Administration and Dosage:

Adults and children (over 12 years): 870 mg every 3 to 4 hours; maximum 6 times/day. Rheumatoid arthritis patients may start with 5 to 10 ml, up to 4 times/day.

otc	**Arthropan** (Purdue Frederick)	**Liquid:** 870 mg per 5 ml	Menthol. Mint flavor. In 240 and 480 ml.

Salicylic Acid Derivatives

MAGNESIUM SALICYLATE

Complete prescribing information for these products begins in the Salicylates monograph.

A sodium free salicylate derivative that may have a low incidence of GI upset. The product labeling and dosage are expressed as magnesium salicylate anhydrous. The possibility of magnesium toxicity exists in persons with renal insufficiency.

Administration and Dosage:

Usual dose is 650 mg every 4 hours or 1090 mg, 3 times a day. May increase to 3.6 to 4.8 g/day in 3 or 4 divided doses.

Safety and efficacy for use in children have not been established.

otc	**Original Doan's** (Ciba Consumer)	**Caplets**: 325 mg	In 24s and 48s.
otc	**Backache Maximum Strength Relief** (B-M Squibb)	**Caplets**: 467 mg (as tetrahydrate)	Film coated. In 24s and 50s.
otc	**Extra Strength Doan's** (Ciba Consumer)	**Caplets**: 500 mg	In 24s and 48s.
otc	**Bayer Select Maximum Strength Backache** (Sterling Health)	**Caplets**: 580 mg (as tetrahydrate)	In 24s and 50s.
otc	**Momentum Muscular Backache Formula** (Whitehall)	**Caplets**: 580 mg (as tetrahydrate, equivalent to 467 mg magnesium salicylate anhydrous)	(MSM). In 48s.
Rx	**Magan** (Adria)	**Tablets**: 545 mg	(Adria 412). Pink. In 100s and 500s.
Rx	**Mobidin** (Ascher)	**Tablets**: 600 mg	(0310). Yellow, scored. In 100s and 500s.

SALICYLATE COMBINATIONS

Complete prescribing information for these products begins in the Salicylates monograph.

Rx	**Choline Magnesium Trisalicylate** (Sidmak)	**Tablets**: 500 mg salicylate (as 293 mg choline salicylate and 362 mg Mg salicylate)	(SL 528). Yellow, scored. In 100s and 500s.
Rx	**Trilisate** (Purdue Frederick)		(PF/T500). Pink, scored. In 100s and UD 100s.
Rx	**Choline Magnesium Trisalicylate** (Sidmak)	**Tablets**: 750 mg salicylate (as 440 mg choline salicylate and 544 mg Mg salicylate)	(SL 529). Blue, scored. Film coated. Capsule shape. In 100s and 500s.
Rx	**Trilisate** (Purdue Frederick)		(PF/T750). White, scored. In 100s, UD 100s.
Rx	**Choline MagnesiumTrisalicylate** (Sidmak)	**Tablets**: 1000 mg salicylate (as 587 mg choline salicylate, 725 mg Mg salicylate)	(SL 530). Pink, scored. In 100s and 500s.
Rx	**Trilisate**(Purdue Frederick)		(PF/T1000). Red, scored. Film coated. In 60s.
Rx	**Trilisate** (Purdue Frederick)	**Liquid**: 500 mg salicylate (as 293 mg choline salicylate and 362 mg Mg salicylate) per 5 ml	Cherry-cordial flavor. In 237 ml.

Salicylic Acid Derivatives

DIFLUNISAL

Actions:

Pharmacology: Diflunisal, a salicylic acid derivative, is a nonsteroidal, peripherally-acting, nonnarcotic analgesic with anti-inflammatory and antipyretic properties. Chemically, it differs from aspirin and is not metabolized to salicylic acid. Its mechanisms are unknown. Diflunisal is a prostaglandin synthetase inhibitor.

Pharmacokinetics:

Absorption/Distribution – Diflunisal is rapidly and completely absorbed following oral administration; peak plasma concentrations occur between 2 to 3 hours, producing significant analgesia within 1 hour and maximum analgesia within 2 to 3 hours. The first dose tends to have a slower onset of pain relief than other drugs achieving comparable peak effects. Time required to achieve steady-state increases with dosage, from 3 to 4 days with 125 mg twice daily to 7 to 9 days with 500 mg twice daily, because of its long half-life and nonlinear pharmacokinetics. An initial loading dose shortens the time to reach steady-state levels; 2 to 3 days of observation are necessary for evaluating changes in treatment regimens if a loading dose is not used. More than 99% is bound to plasma proteins.

Metabolism – Concentration-dependent pharmacokinetics prevail; doubling the dosage more than doubles drug accumulation. The plasma half-life of diflunisal is 8 to 12 hours; it increases in renal impairment. The drug is excreted in the urine as glucuronide conjugates which account for about 90% of the dose. Less than 5% is recovered in the feces.

Clinical trials: Diflunisal 500 mg is comparable in analgesic efficacy but produces longer lasting responses than aspirin 650 mg, acetaminophen 600 to 650 mg and acetaminophen 650 mg with propoxyphene napsylate 100 mg. Diflunisal 1 g is comparable in analgesic efficacy to acetaminophen 600 mg with codeine 60 mg. Patients treated with diflunisal generally continue to have a good analgesic effect 8 to 12 hours after dosing.

Osteoarthritis – Diflunisal 500 or 750 mg daily was as effective as aspirin 2 or 3 g daily, and produced a lower overall incidence of GI disturbances, dizziness, edema and tinnitus.

Rheumatoid arthritis – In controlled clinical trials, diflunisal's effectiveness was established for both acute exacerbations and long-term management of rheumatoid arthritis. Activity was demonstrated by clinical improvement in the signs and symptoms of disease activity.

Diflunisal has been compared to aspirin in several controlled trials. Diflunisal dosages of 500 mg to 1 g daily have been comparable to aspirin dosages of 2 to 4 g daily for 8 to 12 weeks (up to 52 weeks in open-label extensions). Patients also generally experienced less GI effects, tinnitus, hearing loss and dyspepsia with diflunisal.

In two double-blind multicenter studies of 12 weeks' duration, diflunisal 500 or 750 mg daily was compared to ibuprofen 1.6 or 2.4 g daily or naproxen 750 mg daily; they were comparable in effectiveness and tolerability. The naproxen study was extended to 48 weeks on an open-label basis; diflunisal continued to be effective and generally well tolerated.

In patients with rheumatoid arthritis, diflunisal and gold salts may be used in combination at their usual dosage levels. The combination does not alter the course of the underlying disease but usually results in additional symptomatic relief.

Antipyretic activity – Diflunisal is not recommended for use as an antipyretic agent. In single 250, 500 or 750 mg doses, the drug produced measurable, but not clinically useful, decreases in temperature in patients with fever; however, it may mask fever in some patients, particularly with chronic or high doses.

Uricosuric effect – An increase in the renal clearance of uric acid and a decrease in serum uric acid occurred with diflunisal doses of 500 or 750 mg daily. Patients on long-term diflunisal therapy, 500 mg or 1 g daily, showed prompt and consistent reduction in mean serum uric acid levels, as much as 1.4 mg%. It is not known whether diflunisal interferes with the activity of other uricosuric agents.

Effect on platelet function – As an inhibitor of prostaglandin synthetase, diflunisal has a dose-related effect on platelet function and bleeding time. At 2 g daily, diflunisal inhibits platelet function. In contrast to aspirin, these effects were reversible because of the absence of the acetyl group. Bleeding time was only slightly increased at 1g daily; at 2 g daily, a greater increase occurred.

Effect on fecal blood loss was not significantly different from placebo at a dose of 1 g daily. Diflunisal 2 g daily caused a statistically significant increase in fecal blood loss, but only one-half that associated with aspirin 2.6 g daily.

Salicylic Acid Derivatives

DIFLUNISAL

Indications:

Acute or long-term symptomatic treatment of mild to moderate pain, rheumatoid arthritis and osteoarthritis.

Contraindications:

Hypersensitivity to diflunisal.

Patients in whom acute asthmatic attacks, urticaria or rhinitis are precipitated by aspirin or other nonsteroidal anti-inflammatory drugs.

Warnings:

Peptic ulceration and GI bleeding have been reported. Fatalities occurred rarely. In patients with active GI bleeding or an active peptic ulcer, weigh the benefits of therapy against possible hazards; institute an appropriate ulcer treatment regimen and monitor progress. When administered to patients with a history of GI disease, monitor closely.

Renal function impairment: Since diflunisal is eliminated primarily by the kidneys, monitor patients with significant renal impairment; use a lower daily dosage.

Pregnancy: Category C. Safety for use during pregnancy has not been established. Use during the first two trimesters only if the potential benefits outweigh the unknown potential hazards to the fetus. Because of the known effect of this drug class on the fetal cardiovascular system (closure of ductus arteriosus), use during the third trimester is not recommended.

Lactation: Diflunisal is excreted in breast milk in concentrations 2% to 7% of that in plasma. Because of the potential for adverse reactions in nursing infants, discontinue either nursing or the drug.

Children: Use in children below 12 years of age is not recommended. Safety and efficacy in infants and children have not been established.

Precautions:

Platelet function and bleeding time are inhibited by diflunisal at higher doses.

Ophthalmologic effects have been reported with these agents; perform ophthalmologic studies in patients who develop eye complaints during treatment.

Peripheral edema has been observed. Use with caution in patients with compromised cardiac function, hypertension or other conditions predisposing to fluid retention.

Acetylsalicylic acid has been associated with Reye's syndrome. Since diflunisal is a salicylic acid derivative, the possibility of its association with Reye's syndrome cannot be excluded.

Laboratory tests: Borderline elevations of *liver tests* may occur in up to 15% of patients. These abnormalities may progress, may remain essentially unchanged or may be transient with continued therapy. Meaningful (3 times the upper limit of normal) elevations of ALT or AST occurred in less than 1% of patients.

A patient with signs or symptoms suggesting liver dysfunction, or with an abnormal liver test, should be evaluated for evidence of development of more severe hepatic reactions. Severe hepatic reactions, including jaundice, have occurred with diflunisal and other NSAIDs. Although such reactions are rare, if abnormal liver tests persist or worsen, if clinical signs and symptoms consistent with liver disease develop, or if systemic manifestations occur (eg, eosinophilia, rash), discontinue drug; liver reactions can be fatal.

Drug Interactions:

Acetaminophen: Administration of diflunisal resulted in ≈ 50% increased acetaminophen plasma levels. Acetaminophen had no effect on diflunisal plasma levels.

Anticoagulants, oral: Coadministration of diflunisal may increase hypoprothrombinemic effects of anticoagulants. Diflunisal competitively displaces coumarins from protein-binding sites. Monitor prothrombin time during and for several days after coadministration. Adjust dosage of oral anticoagulants as required.

Hydrochlorothiazide: Coadministration of diflunisal resulted in significantly increased plasma levels of hydrochlorothiazide. Diflunisal decreased the hyperuricemic effects of hydrochlorothiazide.

Indomethacin: Administration of diflunisal decreased renal clearance and significantly increased plasma levels of indomethacin. The combined use has also been associated with fatal GI hemorrhage.

Sulindac: Administration of diflunisal resulted in lowering of the plasma levels of the active sulindac sulfide metabolite by approximately one-third.

DIFLUNISAL

Adverse Reactions:

Listed below are adverse reactions reported in 1314 patients who received long-term treatment (24 to 96 weeks). In general, the adverse reactions listed below were 2 to 14 times less frequent in 1113 patients who received short-term treatment.

Incidence < 1% to 9% (causal relationship known):

GI – Nausea, dyspepsia, GI pain, diarrhea (3% to 9%); vomiting, constipation, flatulence (1% to 3%); peptic ulcer, GI bleeding/perforation, anorexia, eructation, cholestasis, jaundice (sometimes with fever), gastritis, hepatitis, abnormal liver function tests (< 1%).

GU – Dysuria, renal impairment (including renal failure), interstitial nephritis, hematuria, proteinuria (< 1%).

CNS – Headache (3% to 9%); dizziness, somnolence, insomnia (1% to 3%); vertigo, nervousness, depression, hallucinations, confusion, disorientation, lightheadedness, paresthesias (< 1%).

Hypersensitivity –

(< 1%): Acute anaphylactic reaction with bronchospasm. A potentially life-threatening apparent hypersensitivity syndrome was reported. This multisystem syndrome includes constitutional symptoms (fever, chills) and cutaneous findings. It may involve major organs (changes in liver function, jaundice, leukopenia, thrombocytopenia, eosinophilia, renal impairment including renal failure) and less specific findings (adenitis, arthralgia, arthritis, malaise, anorexia, disorientation).

Dermatologic – Rash (3% to 9%); pruritus, sweating, dry mucous membranes, stomatitis, erythema multiforme, Stevens-Johnson syndrome, toxic epidermal necrolysis, exfoliative dermatitis, photosensitivity, urticaria (< 1%).

Miscellaneous – Fatigue/tiredness, tinnitus (1% to 3%); asthenia, edema, thrombocytopenia, agranulocytosis (rare), transient visual disturbances including blurred vision (< 1%).

Incidence < 1% (causal relationship unknown):

Miscellaneous – Dyspnea; muscle cramps; palpitations; syncope; chest pain.

Overdosage:

Symptoms: Cases of overdosage have occurred and deaths have been reported. Most patients recovered without permanent sequelae. The most common signs and symptoms were drowsiness, vomiting, nausea, diarrhea, hyperventilation, tachycardia, sweating, tinnitus, disorientation, stupor and coma. Diminished urine output and cardiorespiratory arrest have also been reported.

The lowest fatal dosage was 15 g without any other drugs. In a mixed drug overdose, ingestion of 7.5 g diflunisal resulted in death.

Treatment: Treatment is symptomatic and supportive. Empty the stomach by inducing vomiting or by gastric lavage. Refer to General Management of Acute Overdosage .Because of high degree of protein binding, hemodialysis may not be effective.

Patient Information:

May cause GI upset; may be taken with water, milk or meals.

Do not take **aspirin** or **acetaminophen** with diflunisal, except on professional advice.

Swallow tablets whole; do not crush or chew.

Administration and Dosage:

Mild to moderate pain: Initially, 1 g, followed by 500 mg every 8 to 12 hours. A lower dosage may be appropriate; for example, 500 mg initially, followed by 250 mg every 8 to 12 hours.

Osteoarthritis/rheumatoid arthritis: 500 mg to 1 g daily in 2 divided doses. Individualize dosage. Do not exceed maintenance doses higher than 1.5 g daily.

Rx	**Diflunisal** (Various, eg, Lemmon, West Point Pharma)	**Tablets**: 250 mg	In 100s, 500s and unit-of-use 60s.
Rx	**Dolobid** (MSD)		(MSD 675). Peach. Film coated. In unit-of-use 60s and UD 100s.
Rx	**Diflunisal** (Various, eg, Lemmon, West Point Pharma)	**Tablets**: 500 mg	In 100s, 500s and unit-of-use 60s.
Rx	**Dolobid** (MSD)		(MSD 697). In UD 100s and unit-of-use 60s.

NONNARCOTIC ANALGESIC COMBINATIONS

Components of these combinations include (see individual monographs):

NONNARCOTIC ANALGESICS: Acetaminophen, salicylates, salsalate, salicylamide.

BARBITURATES, MEPROBAMATE and *ANTIHISTAMINES* are used for their sedative effects.

ANTACIDS are used to minimize gastric upset from salicylates.

CAFFEINE, a traditional component of many analgesic formulations, may be beneficial in certain vascular headaches.

BELLADONNA ALKALOIDS are used as antispasmodics.

PAMABROM is used as a diuretic.

AMINOBENZOATE retards the conjugation of salicylic acid and prolongs the action of salicylates.

Other components listed, but not contributing to the analgesic properties of these products include: Calcium gluconate.

Dose: The average adult dose is 1 or 2 capsules or tablets or 1 powder packet, every 2 to 6 hours as needed for pain.

Content given per capsule or tablet.

	Product and Distributor	Acetaminophen	Aspirin	Other Analgesics	Caffeine	Other Content	How Supplied
otc sf	**Saleto Tablets** (Roberts Med)	115 mg	210 mg	65 mg salicylamide	16 mg		Pink. In 50s, 100s, 1000s, sani-pak 1000s.
otc	**Gelpirin Tablets** (Alra)	125 mg	240 mg		32 mg		Buffered. In 100s, 1000s.
otc	**Supac Tablets** (Mission)	160 mg	230 mg		33 mg	60 mg calcium gluconate	In 100s.
otc	**Buffets II Tablets** (JMI)	162 mg	227 mg		32.4 mg	50 mg aluminum hydroxide	In 1000s.
otc	**Vanquish Caplets** (Sterling Health)	194 mg	227 mg		33 mg	Magnesium hydroxide, aluminum hydroxide	(Vanquish). In 30s, 60s and 100s.
otc	**Pain Reliever Tabs** (Rugby)	250 mg	250 mg		65 mg		In 100s and 1000s.

NONNARCOTIC ANALGESIC COMBINATIONS

	Product and Distributor	Acetaminophen	Aspirin	Other Analgesics	Caffeine	Other Content	How Supplied
otc	**Extra Strength Excedrin Caplets, Tablets** and **Geltabs** (Bristol-Myers)	250 mg	250 mg		65 mg		**Caplets**: In 24s, 50s and 80s. **Tablets**: (E). White. In 12s, 30s, 60s, 100s, 165s & 225s. **Geltabs**: In 20s and 40s.
otc	**Maximum Pain Relief Pamprin Caplets** (Chattem)	250 mg				250 mg magnesium salicylate, 25 mg pamabrom	In 16s and 32s.
otc *sf*	**Maximum Strength Arthriten** (Alva-Amco)				32.5 mg	250 mg magnesium salicylate, buffered with magnesium carbonate, magnesium oxide, calcium carbonate.	In 40s.
otc	**Goody's Extra Strength Headache Powders** (Goody)	260 mg	520 mg				In 2s, 6s, 24s and 50s.
otc	**Menoplex Tablets** (Fiske)	325 mg				30 mg phenyltoloxamine citrate	In 20s.
otc	**Midol Regular Strength Multi-Symptom Caplets** (Sterling Health)					12.5 mg pyrilamine maleate	In 32s.
otc	**Teen Midol Caplets** (Sterling Health)	400 mg				25 mg pamabrom	In 16s and 32s.

NONNARCOTIC ANALGESIC COMBINATIONS

	Product and Distributor	Acetaminophen	Aspirin	Other Analgesics	Caffeine	Other Content	How Supplied
otc	**Aspirin Free Excedrin Caplets** and **Geltabs** (Bristol-Myers)	500 mg			65 mg		**Caplets**: Saccharin. In 24s, 50s and 100s. **Geltabs**: In 20s, 40s and 80s.
otc	**Bayer Select Maximum Strength Headache Caplets** (Sterling Health)						In 36s.
otc	**Midol Maximum Strength Multi-Symptom Menstrual Caplets** and **Gelcaps** (Sterling Health)				60 mg	15 mg pyrilamine maleate	**Caplets**: In 8s, 16s and 32s. **Gelcaps**: (Midol). In 12s and 24s.
otc	**Prēmsyn PMS Caplets** (Chattem)					25 mg pamabrom, 15 mg pyrilamine maleate	In 20s and 40s.
otc	**Aspirin Free Excedrin Dual Caplets** (Bristol-Myers)					111 mg calcium carbonate, 64 mg magnesium carbonate, 30 mg magnesium oxide	Saccharin. Film coated. In 100s.
otc	**Lurline PMS Tablets** (Fielding)					25 mg pamabrom, 50 mg pyridoxine	In 24s and 50s.
otc	**Multi-Symptom Pamprin Caplets** and **Tablets** (Chattem)					25 mg pamabrom, 15 mg pyrilamine maleate	**Caplets**: In 24s and 48s. **Tablets**: In 12s, 24s and 48s.

NONNARCOTIC ANALGESIC COMBINATIONS

	Product and Distributor	Acetaminophen	Aspirin	Other Analgesics	Caffeine	Other Content	How Supplied
otc	**Extra Strength Tylenol Headache Plus Caplets** (McNeil-CPC)	500 mg				250 mg calcium carbonate	In 24s, 50s and 100s.
otc	**Maxiumum Strength Midol PMSCaplets** and **Gelcaps** (Sterling Health)					25 mg pamabrom, 15 mg pyrilamine maleate	**Caplets**: In 8s, 16s and 32s. **Gelcaps**: In 12s and 24s.
otc	**Bayer Select Maximum Strength Menstrual Caplets** (Sterling Health)					25 mg pamabrom	In 24s and 50s.
otc	**BC Tablets** (Block)		325 mg	95 mg salicylamide	16 mg		In 4s, 50s and 100s.
c-iv	**EquagesicTablets** (Wyeth)		325 mg			200 mg meprobamate	(Wyeth 91). Pink/yellow, scored. In 100s and UD100s.
c-iv	**Micrainin Tablets** (Wallace)						In 100s.
otc	**Anacin Caplets** and **Tablets** (Whitehall)		400 mg		32 mg		**Caplets**: In 30s, 50s and 100s. **Tablets**: White. In 12s, 30s, 50s, 100s and 200s.
otc	**Gensan Tablets** (Goldline)						In 100s.
otc	**CopeTablets** (Mentholatum)		421 mg		32 mg	50 mg magnesium hydroxide, 25 mg aluminum hydroxide	In 36s and 60s.

NONNARCOTIC ANALGESIC COMBINATIONS

	Product and Distributor	Acetaminophen	Aspirin	Other Analgesics	Caffeine	Other Content	How Supplied
otc	**Anacin Maximum Strength Tablets** (Whitehall)		500 mg		32 mg		(500, A-3). White. In 12s, 20s, 24s, 40s, 72s, 75s, and 150s.
otc	**Momentum Caplets** (Whitehall)		500 mg			15 mg phenyltoloxaminecitrate	(M). White. In 24s and 48s.
otc	**BC Powder** (Block)		650 mg	145 mg salicylamide			In 2s, 6s, 24s and 50s.
otc	**Arthritis Strength BC Powder** (Block)		742 mg	222 mg salicylamide	36 mg		In 6s, 24s and 50s.
otc	**Pabalate Enteric Coated Tablets** (Robins)			300 mg sodium salicylate		300 mg sodium amiobenzoate	(AHR 5816). Yellow. In 100s and 500s.
otc	**Mobigesic Tablets** (Ascher)			325 mg magnesium salicylate		30 mg phenyltoloxamine citrate	In 18s, 50s and 100s.
Rx	**Magsal Tablets** (U.S. Pharm)			600 mg magnesium salicylate		25 mg phenyltoloxamine dihydrogen citrate	Green, oval. In 100s.

NONNARCOTIC ANALGESICS WITH BARBITURATES

For complete prescribing information, refer to the Nonnarcotic Analgesic Combinations group monograph.

Administration and Dosage:

Adults: 1 or 2 every 4 hours, as needed.

Rx	**Butalbital, Acetaminophen and Caffeine Tablets** (Various, eg, Balan, Geneva, Goldline, Halsey, Major, Moore, Parmed, Qualitest, Schein)	**Tablets:** 325 mg acetaminophen, 40 mg caffeine, 50 mg butalbital	In 100s and 500s.
Rx	**Esgic** (Forest)		(Forest 630). White, scored. In 100s, 500s.
Rx	**Fioricet** (Sandoz)		(S Fioricet). Light blue. In 100s, 500s and UD 100s.
Rx	**Fiorpap** (Creighton)		(275 Cp). Light blue. In 100s and 500s.
Rx	**Isocet** (Rugby)		In 100s.
Rx	**Repan** (Everett)		(Everett 162). White. In 100s.
Rx	**Amaphen** (Trimen)	**Capsules:** 325 mg acetaminophen, 40 mg caffeine, 50 mg butalbital	(Trimen/Trimen). White/pink. In 100s.
Rx	**Anoquan** (Roberts Med)		In 100s and 1000s.
Rx	**Butace** (American Urologicals)		(AUI). Clear. In 100s.
Rx	**Endolor** (Keene)		(Keene 7777). Pink and white. In 100s.
Rx	**Esgic** (Forest)		(Forest 631). White. In 100s.
Rx	**Femcet** (Russ Pharmaceuticals)		(Russ/702). Lavender. In 100s.
Rx	**Margesic** (Marnel)		In 100s.
Rx	**Medigesic** (U.S. Pharm.)		(US-US). Gray and maroon. In 100s.
Rx	**Repan** (Everett)		(Everett). Clear. In 100s.
Rx	**Tencet** (Hauck)		(244-03). Dark/Lt blue. In 100s, 1000s.
Rx	**Triad** (UAD)		In 100s.
Rx	**Two-Dyne** (Hyrex)		(Hyrex/Hyrex) Red. In 100s and 1000s.
Rx	**Phrenilin** (Carnrick)	**Tablets:** 325 mg acetaminophen, 50 mg butalbital	(C 8650). Violet, scored. In 100s.
Rx	**Triaprin** (Dunhall)	**Capsules:** 325 mg acetaminophen, 50 mg butalbital	(Dunhall 2811). Orange and white. In 100s and 500s.
Rx	**Esgic-Plus** (Forest)	**Tablets:** 500 mg acetaminophen, 40 mg caffeine, 50 mg butalbital	(Forest 678). White, scored. Capsule shape. In 100s, 500s.

Nonnarcotic Analgesics with Barbiturates

NONNARCOTIC ANALGESICS WITH BARBITURATES

Rx	**Prominol** (MCR American Pharm)	**Tablets:** 650 mg acetaminophen, 50 mg butalbital	In 100s.
Rx	**Repan CF** (Everett)		(Everett 166). Blue, scored. Capsule shape. In 100s.
Rx	**Sedapap-10** (Mayrand)		(M/R). White, scored. In 100s.
Rx	**Bucet** (UAD)	**Capsules:** 650 mg acetaminophen, 50 mg butalbital	In 100s.
Rx	**Phrenilin Forte** (Carnrick)		(C 8656). Amethyst. In 100s.
Rx	**Tencon** (Inter. Ethical Labs)		(Tencon). Gray. In 100s.
Rx	**Axocet** (Savage)	**Capsules:** 850 mg acetaminophen, 50 mg butalbital	Opaque grey. In 100s.
c-iii	**Butalbital, Aspirin and Caffeine Tablets** (Various, eg, Gen-King, Goldline, Halsey, Harber, Pharmafair, Scripts, Towne Paulsen, VHA Supply, Veratex, West-Ward)	**Tablets:** 325 mg aspirin, 40 mg caffeine, 50 mg butalbital	In 20s, 100s, 1000s and UD 100s.
c-iii	**Butalbital Compound** (Various, eg, Dixon-Shane, General, Lemmon, Parmed, Purepac, Schein, Texas Drug, Zenith)		In 15s, 30s, 100s, 500s and 1000s.
c-iii	**Fiorgen PF** (Goldline)		White. In 100s and 1000s.
c-iii	**Fiorinal** (Sandoz)		(Fiorinal/Sandoz). White. In 100s, 1000s and UD 100s.
c-iii	**Isollyl Improved** (Rugby)		In 100s and 1000s.
c-iii	**Lanorinal** (Lannett)		(0527/1043). White. In 1000s.
c-iii	**Marnal** (Vortech)		In 100s.

Nonnarcotic Analgesics with Barbiturates

NONNARCOTIC ANALGESICS WITH BARBITURATES

c-iii	**Butalbital, Aspirin and Caffeine Capsules** (Various, eg, Dixon-Shane, Harber, Regal)	Capsules: 325 mg aspirin, 40 mg caffeine, 50 mg butalbital	In 100s and 1000s.
c-iii	**Butalbital Compound** (Various, eg, Parmed, Purepac, Qualitest, Redi-Med)		In 24s, 30s, 100s and 1000s.
c-iii	**Fiorinal** (Sandoz)		(Fiorinal 78-103). Two-tone green. In 100s, 500s & UD 25s.
c-iii	**Isollyl Improved** (Rugby)		In 100s and 1000s.
c-iii	**Lanorinal** (Lannett)		(0527/1552). Green/Lt green. In 100s & 1000s.
c-iii	**Marnal** (Vortech)		In 100s and 1000s.
Rx	**Axotal** (Adria)	**Tablets**: 650 mg aspirin, 50 mg butalbital	(Adria 130). White. In 100s and 500s.

NONSTEROIDAL ANTI-INFLAMMATORY AGENTS

Clinically, there are no clear guidelines to assist in selecting the most appropriate agent. Base selection on clinical experience, patient convenience, side effects and cost.

Actions:

Pharmacology: Nonsteroidal anti-inflammatory drugs (NSAIDs) have analgesic and antipyretic activities. Exact mode of action is not known. Major mechanism is believed to be inhibition of cyclooxygenase activity and prostaglandin synthesis. Other mechanisms may exist as well, such as inhibition of lipoxygenase, leukotriene synthesis, lysosomal enzyme release, neutrophil aggregation and various cell-membrane functions. They may also suppress rheumatoid factor production.

Although most NSAIDs are primarily used for anti-inflammatory effects, they are effective analgesics and useful for relief of mild to moderate pain (eg, post-extraction dental pain, postsurgical episiotomy pain, soft tissue athletic injuries, primary dysmenorrhea). They do not alter the course of the underlying disease.

Pharmacokinetics:

Absorption/Distribution – NSAIDs are rapidly and almost completely absorbed; naproxen sodium is used as an analgesic because it is more rapidly absorbed. In general, food delays absorption but does not significantly affect total amount absorbed. Administer with meals to minimize GI effects. Some NSAIDs can be given with an aluminum and magnesium hydroxide antacid, which does not affect absorption. All NSAIDs are highly protein bound (> 90%). Since diclofenac is enteric coated, its time to peak levels are delayed despite its relatively short half-life.

Metabolism/Excretion – Elimination of the NSAIDs depends largely on hepatic biotransformation. Excretion is via the kidney, primarily as metabolites. Sulindac and nabumetone are inactive prodrugs converted by the liver to active metabolites.

Pharmacokinetic Parameters / Maximum Dosage Recommendations of NSAIDS

NSAID	Time to peak levels (hrs)[1]	Half-life (hrs)	Analgesic action: Onset (hrs)	Analgesic action: Duration (hrs)	Antirheumatic action: Onset (days)	Antirheumatic action: Peak (weeks)	Maximum recommended daily dose (mg)
Propionic acids							
Fenoprofen	1 to 2	2 to 3	—	—	2	2 to 3	3200
Flurbiprofen	1.5	5.7	—	—	—	—	300
Ibuprofen	1 to 2	1.8 to 2.5	0.5	4 to 6	within 7	1 to 2	3200
Ketoprofen	0.5 to 2	2 to 4	—	—	—	—	300
Naproxen	2 to 4	12 to 15	1	up to 7	within 14	2 to 4	1500
Naproxen sodium	1 to 2	12 to 13	1	up to 7	within 14	2 to 4	1375
Oxaprozin	3 to 5	42 to 50	—	—	within 7	—	1800 mg
Acetic acids							
Diclofenac sodium	2 to 3	1 to 2	—	—	—	—	200
Etodolac	1 to 2	7.3	0.5	4 to 12	—	—	1200
Indomethacin	1 to 2 SR: 2 to 4	4.5 SR: 4.5 to 6	0.5	4 to 6	within 7	1 to 2	200 SR: 150
Ketorolac	0.5 to 1	2.4 to 8.6	IM: 10 min	IM: up to 6	—	—	IM: 120[2] Oral: 40
Nabumetone[3]	2.5 to 4	22.5 to 30[4]	—	—	—	—	2000
Sulindac	2 to 4	7.8 (16.4)[4]	—	—	within 7	2 to 3	400
Tolmetin	0.5 to 1	1 to 1.5	—	—	within 7	1 to 2	2000
Fenamates (anthranilic acids)							
Meclofenamate	0.5 to 1	2 (3.3)[5]	—	—	few days	2 to 3	400
Mefenamic acid	2 to 4	2 to 4	—	—	—	—	1000
Oxicams							
Piroxicam	3 to 5	30 to 86	1	48 to 72	7 to 12	2 to 3	20

[1] Food decreases the rate of absorption and may delay the time to peak levels.
[2] 150 mg on the first day.
[3] The active metabolite of nabumetone is an acetic acid.
[4] Half-life of active metabolite.
[5] Half-life with multiple doses.

NONSTEROIDAL ANTI-INFLAMMATORY AGENTS

Clinical trials: In rheumatoid arthritis and osteoarthritis, NSAIDs are comparable to aspirin in controlling signs and symptoms, and some agents may be associated with a significant reduction in milder GI side effects. However, long-term use of oral ketorolac 10 mg is associated with more GI tract adverse effects than aspirin 650 mg 4 times a day. NSAIDs may be well tolerated in some who experience GI side effects with aspirin, but carefully follow such patients for signs and symptoms of ulceration and bleeding. Information is insufficient to further differentiate these agents on the basis of side effects.

Rheumatoid arthritis – Anti-inflammatory activity is shown by reduced joint swelling, pain, duration of morning stiffness and disease activity, increased mobility and by enhanced functional capacity (demonstrated by an increase in grip strength, delay in time to onset of fatigue and a decrease in time to walk 50 feet).

Osteoarthritis – Improvement is demonstrated by reduced tenderness with pressure, pain in motion and at rest, night pain, stiffness and swelling, overall disease activity, by increased range of motion, and other symptoms of allergic or anaphylactoid reactions.

Acute gouty arthritis, ankylosing spondylitis – Relief of pain, reduced fever, swelling, redness and tenderness, and increased range of motion have occurred.

Dysmenorrhea – Excess prostaglandins may produce uterine hyperactivity. These agents reduce elevated prostaglandin levels in menstrual fluid and reduce resting and active intrauterine pressure, as well as frequency of uterine contractions. Probable mechanism of action is to inhibit prostaglandin synthesis rather than provide analgesia.

Indications:

NSAIDs: Summary of Indications

Indications (✓ -Labeled X- Unlabeled)	Diclofenac	Etodolac	Fenoprofen	Flurbiprofen	Ibuprofen	Indomethacin/SR	Ketoprofen	Ketorolac	Meclofenamate	Mefenamic acid	Nabumetone	Naproxen/Naproxen Sod.	Oxaprozin	Piroxicam	Sulindac	Tolmetin
Rheumatoid arthritis	✓	X	✓	✓	✓	✓	✓		✓		✓	✓	✓	✓	✓	✓
Osteoarthritis	✓	✓	✓	✓	✓	✓	✓		✓		✓	✓	✓	✓	✓	✓
Ankylosing spondylitis	✓	X		X		✓						✓			✓	
Mild to moderate pain	X	✓	✓	X	✓		✓	✓	✓	✓[1]		✓				
Primary dysmenorrhea				X	✓	X	✓			✓		✓		X		
Juvenile rheumatoid arthritis	X		X		X		X					✓/		X	X	✓
Tendinitis		X		X		✓						✓			✓	
Bursitis		X		X		✓						✓			✓	
Acute painful shoulder	X	X		X		✓										
Acute gout		X		X		✓/						✓			✓	
Fever					✓							X				
Sunburn	X		X	X	X	X[2]	X		X	X		X		X	X	X
Migraine																
Abortive (acute attack)				X					X	X		/X				
Prophylactic			X			X/	X					X				
Menstrual			X				X		X	X		X				
Cluster headache						X/										
Polyhydramnios						X/										
Acne vulgaris, resistant					X[3]											
Menorrhagia									X							
Premenstrual syndrome										X		/X				
Cystoid macular edema						X[4]										
Closure of persistent patent ductus arteriosus						X[5]										

[1] If therapy will be ≤ 1 week.
[2] Topical indomethacin may prevent and treat sunburn.
[3] With tetracycline.
[4] Topical eye drops 0.5% to 1%.
[5] Indomethacin IV approved for this indication (see Agents for Patent Ductus Arteriosus).

Rheumatoid arthritis (except etodolac, ketorolac and mefenamic acid) and osteoarthritis (except ketorolac and mefenamic acid): Relief of signs and symptoms; treatment of acute flares and exacerbation; long-term management.

Concomitant therapy with other second-line drugs (eg, gold salts) demonstrates additional therapeutic benefit. Whether they can be used with partially effective doses of corticosteroids for a "steroid-sparing" effect and result in greater improvement is not established.

NONSTEROIDAL ANTI-INFLAMMATORY AGENTS

Use with salicylates is not recommended; greater benefit is not achieved, and the potential for adverse reactions is increased. The use of aspirin with NSAIDs may cause a decrease in blood levels of the nonaspirin drug.

Juvenile rheumatoid arthritis (tolmetin, naproxen)

Mild to moderate pain (**etodolac, fenoprofen, ibuprofen, ketoprofen, ketorolac, meclofenamate, mefenamic acid, naproxen, naproxen sodium, nabumetone**): Post-extraction dental pain, postsurgical episiotomy pain and soft tissue athletic injuries.

Primary dysmenorrhea (ibuprofen, ketoprofen, mefenamic acid, naproxen, naproxen sodium)

Unlabeled uses: Selected NSAIDs have been used in the treatment of juvenile rheumatoid arthritis, symptomatic treatment of sunburn and for various migraine headaches. For other uses, refer to the Summary of Indications table.

Contraindications:

NSAID hypersensitivity: Because of potential cross-sensitivity to other NSAIDs, do not give these agents to patients in whom aspirin, iodides or other NSAIDs have induced symptoms of asthma, rhinitis, urticaria, nasal polyps, angioedema, bronchospasm and other symptoms of allergic or anaphylactoid reactions.

Fenoprofen or mefenamic acid: Preexisting renal disease.

Mefenamic acid: Active ulceration or chronic inflammation of either the upper or lower GI tract.

Indomethacin suppositories: History of proctitis or recent rectal bleeding.

Warnings:

GI effects: Serious GI toxicity such as bleeding, ulceration and perforation can occur at any time, with or without warning symptoms, in patients treated chronically with NSAID therapy. Although minor upper GI problems (eg, dyspepsia) are common, usually developing early in therapy, remain alert for ulceration and bleeding in patients treated chronically with NSAIDs even in the absence of previous GI tract symptoms. In patients observed in clinical trials of several months to 2 years duration, symptomatic upper GI ulcers, gross bleeding or perforation occurred in approximately 1% of patients treated for 3 to 6 months, and in about 2% to 4% of patients treated for 1 year; in patients receiving nabumetone, the incidence of peptic ulcers was 0.3% at 3 to 6 months, 0.5% at 1 year and 0.8% at 2 years. Inform patients about the signs or symptoms of serious GI toxicity and what steps to take if they occur.

Studies have not identified any subset of patients not at risk of developing peptic ulceration and bleeding. Except for a history of serious GI events and other risk factors associated with peptic ulcer disease (eg, alcoholism, smoking) no factors (eg, age, sex) are associated with increased risk. Elderly or debilitated patients seem to tolerate ulceration or bleeding less than other individuals and account for most spontaneous reports of fatal GI events. Studies are inconclusive concerning the relative risk of NSAIDs in causing such reactions. High dose NSAIDs probably carry a greater risk of these reactions, although controlled clinical trials generally do not show this. In considering the use of relatively large doses (within the recommended dosage range), sufficient benefit should offset the potential increased risk of GI toxicity.

In patients with active peptic ulcer and active rheumatoid arthritis, attempt to treat the arthritis with nonulcerogenic drugs.

Do not give **indomethacin** or **sulindac** to patients with active GI lesions or a history of recurrent GI lesions, unless the very high risk is warranted and patients can be monitored very closely. To reduce GI effects, give NSAIDs after meals, with food or with antacids (does not apply to enteric-coated **diclofenac**).

If diarrhea occurs with **mefenamic acid** or **meclofenamate**, reduce dosage or temporarily discontinue use. Some patients may be unable to tolerate further therapy with these agents.

CNS effects: **Indomethacin** may aggravate depression or other psychiatric disturbances, epilepsy and parkinsonism; use with considerable caution. If severe CNS adverse reactions develop, discontinue the drug. Some of these agents may also cause headaches (highest incidence with fenoprofen, indomethacin and ketorolac). If headache persists despite dosage reduction, discontinue use.

Renal effects: Acute renal insufficiency, interstitial nephritis, hyperkalemia, hyponatremia and renal papillary necrosis may occur.

NONSTEROIDAL ANTI-INFLAMMATORY AGENTS

Acute renal insufficiency – Patients with preexisting renal disease or compromised renal perfusion are at greatest risk. A form of renal toxicity seen in patients with prerenal conditions leads to reduced renal blood flow or blood volume. NSAID use may cause a dose-dependent reduction in prostaglandin formation and precipitate renal decompensation. Patients at greatest risk are the elderly, premature infants, those with heart failure, renal or hepatic dysfunction, SLE, chronic glomerulonephritis and on diuretics. Recovery usually follows discontinuation.

Interstitial nephritis has occurred with increased frequency in patients receiving NSAIDs and may be due to altered prostaglandin metabolism.

GU tract problems have occurred in patients taking **fenoprofen**, most frequently, dysuria, cystitis, hematuria, interstitial nephritis and nephrotic syndrome. This may be preceded by fever, rash, arthralgia, oliguria and azotemia, and may progress to anuria. Rapid recovery followed early recognition and drug withdrawal.

Hyperkalemia with a sudden decrease in renal function has occurred in patients with mild renal insufficiency receiving NSAIDs; degree of hyperkalemia was greater than expected. Significant hyperkalemia has occurred in patients with normal renal function. This is probably due to suppression of renal prostaglandin biosynthesis.

Hyponatremia – Sodium retention, possibly leading to edema, may occur, probably due to suppression of renal prostaglandin synthesis or a direct effect on capillary permeability.

Papillary necrosis (chronic renal injury) – Irreversible renal injury in the form of papillary necrosis has occurred in association with some NSAIDs; however, a cause and effect relationship has not been firmly established.

Hypersensitivity: A potentially fatal apparent hypersensitivity syndrome has occurred with **sulindac**; this syndrome may include constitutional symptoms, cutaneous findings, involvement of major organs or other less specific findings. Severe hypersensitivity reactions with fever, rashes, abdominal pain, headache, nausea, vomiting, signs of liver damage and meningitis have occurred in **ibuprofen** patients, especially those with systemic lupus erythematosus (SLE) or other collagen diseases.

Anaphylactoid reactions have occurred in patients with aspirin hypersensitivity and in patients who discontinued **tolmetin**, then restarted it. These reactions appear to occur more often with tolmetin than other NSAIDs not structurally related, but data conflict. Refer to Management of Acute Hypersensitivity Reactions.

Renal function impairment: NSAID metabolites are eliminated primarily by kidneys; use with caution. Assess renal function before and during therapy. Monitor serum creatinine or creatinine clearance. Reduce dosage to avoid excessive accumulation.

Hepatic function impairment: Naproxen may exhibit an increase in unbound fraction and a reduced clearance of free drug in cirrhotic liver patients, suggesting an increased potential for toxicity in this group; may need to reduce dose. Also, sulindac AUC may increase in patients with cirrhosis due to altered sulfide formation/metabolism. Disposition of total and free etodolac is not altered in patients with compensated hepatic cirrhosis. Effects of hepatic disease on other NSAIDs is unknown. Use caution in patients with impaired hepatic function or history of liver disease.

Elderly: Age appears to increase the possibility of adverse reactions to NSAIDs. The risk of serious ulcer disease is increased in elderly patients (> 65 years of age) taking NSAIDs; this risk appears to increase with dose. Use with greater care and begin with reduced dosages. In **nabumetone**-treated patients, no differences in overall efficacy and safety were observed between older and younger patients. **Ketorolac** is cleared more slowly by the elderly; use caution and reduce dosage.

Pregnancy:

Category B (ketoprofen, naproxen, flurbiprofen, diclofenac). Category C (etodolac, ketorolac, mefenamic acid, nabumetone, oxaprozin, tolmetin) – Safety for use during pregnancy has not been established; use is not recommended. There are no adequate, well controlled studies in pregnant women. An increased incidence of dystocia, increased post-implantation loss and delayed parturition occurred in animals. Agents that inhibit prostaglandin synthesis may cause closure of the ductus arteriosus and other untoward effects to the fetus. GI tract toxicity increased in pregnant women in the last trimester. Some NSAIDs may prolong pregnancy if given before onset of labor. Avoid during pregnancy, especially in the third trimester.

Lactation: Most NSAIDs are excreted in breast milk. **Naproxen** appears at ≈ 1% of maternal serum concentration. In 10 healthy women, recovery of **flurbiprofen** in breast milk accounted for 0.05% (range, 0.03% to 0.07%) of a 100 mg dose; average peak concentration in milk was 0.09 mcg/ml. **Ibuprofen** was not detected in breast milk of 12 women who had ingested 400 mg every 6 hrs over 24 hrs. **Ketorolac** was detected in breast milk at a maximum milk-to-plasma ratio of 0.037. In general, do not use in nursing mothers because of effects on infant's cardiovascular system.

NONSTEROIDAL ANTI-INFLAMMATORY AGENTS

Children: **Mefenamic acid** and **meclofenamate** are not recommended in children < 14 years old. **Indomethacin's** safety is not established in children; not recommended in children ≤ 14 years old, except in circumstances that warrant the risk. When using in children ≥ 2 years old, closely monitor liver function. Hepatotoxicity, including fatalities, has occurred in children with juvenile rheumatoid arthritis. Suggested starting dose is 2 mg/kg/day in divided doses. Do not exceed 4 mg/kg/day or 150 to 200 mg/day, whichever is less. As symptoms subside, reduce dosage or discontinue drug. For use of IV indomethacin in premature infants, see Agents for Patent Ductus Arteriosus.**Tolmetin** and **naproxen** are the only agents labeled for juvenile rheumatoid arthritis, although studies are being conducted with other agents. Safety and efficacy of tolmetin in infants < 2 years old are not established. Safety and efficacy of other NSAIDs in children are not established.

Precautions:

Monitoring: Serious GI tract ulceration and bleeding can occur without warning. Follow chronically treated patients for signs and symptoms of ulceration and bleeding; inform them of the importance of this follow-up (see Warnings).

Functional Class IV rheumatoid arthritis patients (incapacitated, largely or wholly bedridden, confined to wheelchair): Safety and efficacy are not established.

Steroid dosage: If reduced or eliminated during therapy, reduce slowly and observe patient closely for evidence of adverse effects, including adrenal insufficiency and exacerbation of symptoms (see Adrenal Cortical Steroids, Glucocorticoids).

Platelet aggregation: NSAIDs can inhibit platelet aggregation; the effect is quantitatively less and of shorter duration than that seen with aspirin. These agents prolong bleeding time (within normal range) in healthy subjects. This may be exaggerated in patients with underlying hemostatic defects; use with caution in persons with intrinsic coagulation defects and in those on anticoagulant therapy.

Hematologic effects: Decreased hemoglobin or hematocrit levels have rarely required discontinuation. If anemia is suspected in patients on long-term therapy, determine hemoglobin and hematocrit values. Frequently determine hemoglobin values in patients with initial values ≤ 10 g/dl who are to receive long-term therapy.

Low white blood cell counts occur rarely, are transient and usually return to normal while therapy continues. Persistent leukopenia, granulocytopenia or thrombocytopenia warrants further evaluation and may require discontinuing the drug.

Postoperative hematomas and other signs of wound bleeding have occurred with perioperative IM use of **ketorolac**. Exercise caution when administering pre- or intraoperatively and when administering perioperatively if strict hemostasis is critical.

Cardiovascular effects: May cause fluid retention and peripheral edema. Use caution in compromised cardiac function, hypertension or other conditions predisposing to fluid retention. Agents may be associated with significant deterioration of circulatory hemodynamics in severe heart failure and hyponatremia, presumably due to inhibition of prostaglandin-dependent compensatory mechanisms.

Ophthalmologic effects: Perform ophthalmological studies in patients who develop eye complaints during therapy. Effects include blurred or diminished vision, scotomata, changes in color vision, corneal deposits and retinal disturbances, including maculas. Discontinue therapy if ocular changes are noted. Blurred vision may be significant and warrants thorough examination, including central visual fields and color vision testing. These changes may be asymptomatic; perform periodic examinations in patients on prolonged therapy.

Infection: NSAIDs may mask the usual signs of infection. Use with extra care in the presence of existing controlled infection.

Hepatic effects: Borderline liver function test elevations may occur in ≈ 15% of patients and may progress, remain essentially unchanged or become transient with continued therapy. Meaningful (3 times upper limit of normal) AST or ALT elevations occurred in < 1% of patients. If symptoms or signs suggesting liver dysfunction, or an abnormal test occurs, evaluate for more severe hepatic reactions. Severe reactions, including jaundice and fatal hepatitis, are rare. Discontinue treatment if abnormal tests persist or worsen, if clinical signs and symptoms consistent with liver disease develop or if systemic manifestations occur (eg, eosinophilia, rash).

Pancreatitis has occurred in patients receiving **sulindac**. If pancreatitis is suspected, discontinue drug, start supportive therapy and monitor closely. Check for other causes of pancreatitis as well as for conditions that mimic pancreatitis.

Auditory effects: Perform periodic auditory function tests during chronic **fenoprofen** therapy in patients with impaired hearing.

Dermatologic effects: Promptly discontinue **mefenamic acid** if rash occurs.

Concomitant therapy: Do not use **naproxen sodium** and **naproxen** concomitantly; both drugs circulate as naproxen anion.

NONSTEROIDAL ANTI-INFLAMMATORY AGENTS

Photosensitivity may occur; caution patients to take protective measures (ie, sunscreens, protective clothing) against UV or sunlight until tolerance is determined.

Drug Interactions:

NSAID Drug Interactions			
Precipitant drug	Object drug*		Description
NSAIDs	Anticoagulants	↑	Coadministration may prolong prothrombin time (PT). Also consider the effects NSAIDs have on platelet function and gastric mucosa. Monitor PT and patients closely, and instruct patients to watch for signs and symptoms of bleeding.
NSAIDs	ACE inhibitors	↓	Antihypertensive effects of captopril may be blunted or completely abolished by indomethacin.
NSAIDs	Beta blockers	↓	The antihypertensive effect of the beta blockers may be impaired. Sulindac and naproxen did not affect atenolol.
NSAIDs	Cyclosporine	↑	Nephrotoxicity of both agents may be increased.
NSAIDs	Digoxin	↑	Ibuprofen and indomethacin may increase digoxin serum levels.
NSAIDs	Dipyridamole	↑	Indomethacin and dipyridamole coadministration may augment water retention.
NSAIDs	Hydantoins	↑	Serum phenytoin levels may be increased, resulting in an increase in pharmacologic and toxic effects of phenytoin.
NSAIDs	Lithium	↑	Serum lithium levels may be increased; however, sulindac has no effect or may decrease lithium levels.
NSAIDs	Loop diuretics	↓	Effects of the loop diuretics may be decreased.
NSAIDs	Methotrexate	↑	The risks of methotrexate toxicity (eg, stomatitis, bone marrow suppression, nephrotoxicity) may be increased.
NSAIDs	Penicillamine	↑	Indomethacin may increase the bioavailability of penicillamine.
NSAIDs	Sympathomimetics	↑	Indomethacin and phenylpropanolamine coadministration may result in increased blood pressure.
NSAIDs	Thiazide diuretics	↓	Decreased antihypertensive and diuretic action of thiazides may occur with concurrent indomethacin. Naproxen has also been implicated. Sulindac may enhance the effects of thiazides.
Cimetidine	NSAIDs	↔	NSAID plasma concentrations may be increased or decreased by cimetidine; some studies report no effect. Also, indomethacin and sulindac have increased ranitidine and cimetidine bioavailability.
Probenecid	NSAIDs	↑	Probenecid may increase the concentrations and possibly the toxicity of the NSAIDs.
Salicylates	NSAIDs	↓	Plasma concentrations of NSAIDs may be decreased by salicylates. Avoid concurrent use since it offers no therapeutic advantage and may significantly increase the incidence of GI effects. Use of salicylates resulted in decreased binding of ketorolac (twofold increase of free drug).
DMSO	Sulindac	↓	DMSO may decrease the formation of the active metabolite of sulindac, possibly resulting in a decreased therapeutic effect. Also, topical DMSO with sulindac has resulted in severe peripheral neuropathy.

* ↑ = Object drug increased ↓ = Object drug decreased ↔ = Undetermined effect

NONSTEROIDAL ANTI-INFLAMMATORY AGENTS

Drug/Lab test interactions: **Naproxen** use may result in increased urinary values for 17-ketogenic steroids because of an interaction between naproxen or its metabolites with m–dinitro-benzene used in this assay. Although 17-hydroxycorticosteroid measurements (Porter-Silber test) do not appear to be artificially altered, temporarily discontinue naproxen therapy 72 hours before **adrenal function tests** are performed.

Naproxen may interfere with some urinary assays of 5-hydroxy indoleacetic acid.

Tolmetin metabolites in urine give positive tests for **proteinuria** using acid precipitation tests (eg, sulfosalicylic acid). Use commercially available dye-impregnated reagent strips.

Mefenamic acid – A false-positive reaction for urinary bile, using the **diazo tablet test,** may result. If biliuria is suspected, use other procedures (ie, the Harrison spot test).

Fenoprofen – Amerlex-M kit assay values of total and free triiodothyronine in patients on fenoprofen have been reported as falsely elevated on the basis of a chemical cross-reaction that directly interferes with the assay. Thyroid stimulating hormone, total thyroxine and thyrotropin releasing hormone response are not affected.

NSAIDs, by decreasing platelet adhesion and aggregation, can prolong bleeding time approximately 3 to 4 minutes.

Drug/Food interactions: Administration of **tolmetin** with milk had no effect on peak plasma tolmetin concentration, but decreased total tolmetin bioavailability by 16%. When tolmetin was taken immediately after a meal, peak plasma concentrations were reduced by 50%, while total bioavailability was again decreased by 16%. Peak concentration of **etodolac** is reduced by approximately one-half and the time to peak is increased by 1.4 to 3.8 hours following administration with food; however, the extent of absorption is not affected. Food may reduce the rate of absorption of **oxaprozin,** but the extent is unchanged.

Adverse Reactions:

GI: (see Warnings) Common GI adverse reactions are listed in the table below:

Common NSAID GI Adverse Reactions (%)

GI adverse reactions	Diclofenac	Etodolac	Fenoprofen	Flurbiprofen	Ibuprofen	Indomethacin	Ketoprofen	Ketorolac	Meclofenamate	Mefenamic acid	Nabumetone	Naproxen	Oxaproxen	Piroxicam	Sulindac	Tolmetin
Nausea (with or without vomiting)	3-9	3-9	3-9	3-9	3-9	3-9	>3	12	11	†	3-9	3-9	3-9	3-9	3-9	11
Vomiting	<1	1-3	3-9	1-3			>1	< 3			1-3	< 1	< 3	< 1		3-9
Diarrhea	3-9	3-9		3-9	<3	<3	>3	3-9	10-33	5	14	<3	3-9	1-3	3-9	3-9
Constipation	3-9	1-3	3-9	1-3	<3	<3	>3	< 3	1-3	†	3-9	3-9	3-9	1-3	3-9	<3
Abdominal distress/cramps/pain	3-9	3-9	<3	3-9	<3	<3	>3	13	3-9	†	12	3-9	< 3	1-3	10	3-9
Dyspepsia	3-9	10	3-9	3-9	3-9	3-9	11.5	12			13	3-9	3-9	3-9	3-9	3-9
Flatulence	1-3	3-9	<3	1-3	<3	<1	>3	< 3	3-9	†	3-9		< 3	1-3	1-3	3-9
Anorexia		< 1	<3			<1	>1		1-3	†	< 1		< 3	< 3	1-3	1-3
Stomatitis	<1	< 1		<1		<1	>1	< 3	1-3		1-3	<3	< 1	1-3	<1	<1

† Occurs, no incidence reported.

Ulcer – Gastric or duodenal ulcer with bleeding or perforation; intestinal ulceration associated with stenosis and obstruction; ulcerative stomatitis or colitis; gingival ulcer; rectal irritation, mucosal inflammation or necrosis with bleeding (**indomethacin** suppositories).

Bleeding – Occult blood in the stool; GI bleeding with or without peptic ulcer; melena; perforation and hemorrhage of esophagus, stomach, duodenum or small or large intestine; hematemesis; rectal bleeding.

Hepatic – Cholestatic hepatitis; jaundice; toxic hepatitis and jaundice with some fatalities; abnormal liver function tests; elevated liver enzymes.

Pancreatitis – See Precautions.

NONSTEROIDAL ANTI-INFLAMMATORY AGENTS

Other – Gastritis; gastroenteritis; proctitis; paralytic ileus; eructation; salivation; glossitis; dry mouth; icterus; pyrosis; sore or dry mucous membranes; colitis.

CNS: Dizziness (3% to 9%; **flurbiprofen** and **diclofenac** 1% to 3%); headache (see Warnings; **ketorolac** 17%; **fenoprofen** 15%; **indomethacin** 11%; **diclofenac, flurbiprofen, meclofenamate, nabumetone, naproxen** and **tolmetin** 3% to 9%; **ketoprofen** > 3%); somnolence/drowsiness (**fenoprofen** 15%; **naproxen** 3% to 9%; **oxaprozin** < 3%); lightheadedness; vertigo; nervousness; excitation; paresthesia; peripheral neuropathy; tremor; convulsions; aggravation of epilepsy and parkinsonism; myalgia; muscle weakness; asthenia; somnolence; malaise; fatigue; insomnia; confusion; inability to concentrate; depression; emotional lability; psychic disturbances, including psychotic episodes; hallucinations; depersonalization; migraine; aseptic meningitis with fever and coma; akathisia; syncope; amnesia; coma; anxiety; mental confusion; involuntary muscle movements; dyspnea; muzziness; sleep disturbance.

Cardiovascular: Congestive heart failure; exacerbation of angiitis; hypotension; hypertension; palpitations; arrhythmias; tachycardia; vasodilation; peripheral edema and fluid retention (see Precautions); chest pain; sinus bradycardia; peripheral vascular disease.

Renal: Hematuria; cystitis; urinary tract infection; azotemia; nocturia; proteinuria; elevated BUN; increased serum creatinine; decreased creatinine clearance; polyuria; dysuria; urinary frequency; pyuria; oliguria; anuria; renal insufficiency, including renal failure; acute renal failure in patients with impaired renal function; renal papillary necrosis; nephrosis; nephrotic syndrome; glomerular and interstitial nephritis; urinary casts. (See Warnings.)

Hematologic: Neutropenia; eosinophilia; leukopenia; pancytopenia; thrombocytopenia; agranulocytosis; granulocytopenia; aplastic anemia; hemolytic anemia; decreases in hemoglobin and hematocrit; anemia secondary to obvious or occult bleeding; hypocoagulability; epistaxis; menometrorrhagia; menorrhagia; hemorrhage; bruising; bone marrow depression; mild hepatic toxicity (see Precautions).

Cases of autoimmune hemolytic anemia are associated with continuous use of **mefenamic acid** for 12 months or longer. In such cases, Coombs test results are positive with evidence of both accelerated RBC production and destruction. The process is reversible upon drug discontinuation.

Special senses: Visual disturbances; blurred vision; photophobia; amblyopia; scotomata; swollen, dry or irritated eyes; corneal deposits; retinal degeneration; retinal hemorrhage and pigmentation change; conjunctivitis; iritis; reversible loss of color vision (see Precautions); hearing disturbances or loss (see Precautions); deafness; ear pain; change in taste (metallic or bitter); diplopia; optic neuritis; cataracts; tinnitus; parosmia.

Hypersensitivity: Asthma; anaphylaxis; acute respiratory distress; rapid fall in blood pressure resembling a shock-like state; angioedema; dyspnea; angiitis. (See Warnings.)

Respiratory: Dyspnea; hemoptysis; pharyngitis; bronchospasm; laryngeal edema; rhinitis; shortness of breath; eosinophilic pneumonitis; pulmonary infiltrates (**naproxen**).

Dermatologic: Rash; erythema; urticaria; desquamation; vesiculobullous eruptions; cutaneous vasculitis; toxic epidermal necrolysis; exfoliative dermatitis; erythema multiforme; Stevens-Johnson syndrome; erythema nodosum; angioneurotic edema; ecchymosis; petechiae; purpura; alopecia; pruritus; eczema; skin discoloration; hyperpigmentation; onycholysis; photosensitivity (see Precautions); skin irritation; peeling. Rash/dermatitis, including maculopapular type (3% to 9%; **ibuprofen, sulindac** and **meclofenamate**).

Metabolic: Decreased or increased appetite; weight decrease or increase (3% to 9% with **tolmetin**); glycosuria; hyperglycemia; hypoglycemia; hyperkalemia; hyponatremia; flushing or sweating; menstrual disorders; impotence; vaginal bleeding; diabetes mellitus.

Miscellaneous: Thirst; pyrexia (fever and chills); sweating; breast changes; gynecomastia; muscle cramps; facial edema; serum sickness; pain; aseptic meningitis.

Causal relationship unknown: Aphthous ulceration of buccal mucosa; fever; pseudotumor cerebri; disorientation; dysphoria; dream abnormalities; trigeminal neuralgia; libido changes; personality changes; pulmonary edema; ECG changes; atrial fibrillation; supraventricular tachycardia; myocardial infarction; burning tongue; lupus erythematosus; acute tubulopathy; Henoch-Schönlein vasculitis; acidosis; mastodynia; lymphadenopathy; septicemia; shock; leukemia; vesicular exanthema; nail disorders; aphasia; impaired consciousness; nystagmus; cerebrovascular accident;

NONSTEROIDAL ANTI-INFLAMMATORY AGENTS

blepharitis; renal calculi; lens opacities; puffy or twitching eyelids; respiratory infections; bronchitis; sinusitis; pulmonary thromboembolism; hematuria; leukorrhea; renal calculus.

Overdosage:

Symptoms may include: Drowsiness; dizziness; mental confusion; disorientation; lethargy; paresthesia; numbness; vomiting; gastric irritation; nausea; abdominal pain; intense headache; tinnitus; sweating; convulsions; blurred vision; elevations in serum creatinine and BUN; acute renal failure, coma, grand mal seizures and muscle twitching (mefenamic acid); hypotension and tachycardia (acute ingestion of **fenoprofen**); stupor, coma, diminished urine output and hypotension (**sulindac**; deaths have occurred); metabolic acidosis (acute **ibuprofen** overdosage); acute renal failure (**diclofenac** 2.5 g).

Treatment includes general supportive measures. Refer to General Management of Acute Overdosage. Because these agents are acidic and are excreted in the urine, it is theoretically beneficial to administer alkali and induce diuresis. NSAIDs are strongly bound to plasma proteins; hemodialysis and peritoneal dialysis may be of little value.

Ketoprofen is dialyzable; hemodialysis may be useful to remove circulating drug and to assist in renal failure.

Meclofenamate – Dialysis may be required to correct serious azotemia or electrolyte imbalance.

Patient Information:

Side effects of NSAIDs can cause discomfort and, rarely, more serious side effects such as GI bleeding which may result in hospitalization and even fatalities. NSAIDs are often essential in the management of arthritis and have a major role in treating pain, but they also may be commonly employed for less serious conditions. Apprise patients of potential risks.

Avoid aspirin and alcoholic beverages while taking medication.

If GI upset occurs, take with food, milk or antacids. For GI upset with tolmetin, use antacids other than sodium bicarbonate; bioavailability is affected by food and milk. If GI symptoms persist, notify physician.

May cause drowsiness, dizziness or blurred vision; patients should observe caution while driving or performing other tasks requiring alertness.

Notify physician if skin rash, itching, visual disturbances, weight gain, edema, black stools or persistent headache occurs.

Mefenamic acid and meclofenamate: If rash, diarrhea or other digestive problems occur, discontinue use and consult a physician.

Ibuprofen (otc use): Do not take for > 3 days for fever, or 10 days for pain. If these symptoms persist, worsen or if new symptoms develop, contact a physician.

FLURBIPROFEN

For complete prescribing information, refer to the NSAIDs group monograph.

Flurbiprofen was approved by the FDA in November 1988.

Indications:

Acute or long-term treatment of the signs and symptoms of rheumatoid arthritis and osteoarthritis.

Administration and Dosage:

Rheumatoid arthritis and osteoarthritis: Initial recommended total daily dose is 200 to 300 mg; administer in divided doses 2, 3 or 4 times daily. Most experience with rheumatoid arthritis has been with dosage 3 or 4 times per day. The largest recommended single dose in a multiple-dose daily regimen is 100 mg. Tailor the dose to each patient according to the severity of the symptoms and the response to therapy.

Although a few patients have received higher doses, doses > 300 mg per day are not recommended until more clinical experience is obtained.

Rx	**Flurbiprofen** (Various, eg, Mylan, UDL)	**Tablets:** 50 mg	In 100s and 500s.
Rx	**Ansaid** (Upjohn)		(Ansaid 50 mg). White. In 100s, 500s and UD 100s.
Rx	**Flurbiprofen** (Various, eg, Mylan, UDL)	**Tablets:** 100 mg	In 100s and 500s.
Rx	**Ansaid** (Upjohn)		(Ansaid 100 mg). Blue. In 100s, 500s and UD 100s.

FENOPROFEN CALCUIM

For complete prescribing information, refer to the NSAIDs group monograph.

Indications:

Relief of the signs and symptoms of rheumatoid arthritis and osteoarthritis (in acute flares and exacerbations and long-term management); relief of mild to moderate pain.

Administration and Dosage:

Do not exceed 3.2 g/day. If GI upset occurs, take with meals or milk.

Rheumatoid arthritis and osteoarthritis: 300 to 600 mg 3 or 4 times daily. Individualize dosage. Improvement may occur in a few days, but 2 to 3 weeks may be required.

Mild to moderate pain: 200 mg every 4 to 6 hours, as needed.

Rx	**Fenoprofen** (Various, eg, Dixon-Shane, Geneva, Halsey, Major, Par, Parmed, Qualitest, Rugby)	**Capsules:** 200 mg	In 100s.
Rx	**Nalfon Pulvules** (Dista)		(H76). White/ocher. In Rx pak 100s.
Rx	**Fenoprofen** (Various, eg, Dixon-Shane, Major, Par, Parmed, Rugby, Warner Chilcott)	**Capsules:** 300 mg	In 100s.
Rx	**Nalfon Pulvules** (Dista)		(H77). Yellow & ocher. In 500s, Rx pak 100s.
Rx	**Fenoprofen** (Various, eg, Dixon-Shane, Geneva, Major, Rugby, Schein, Warner Chilcott, Zenith)	**Tablets:** 600 mg	In 100s and 500s,

NABUMETONE

For complete prescribing information, refer to the NSAIDs group monograph.

Indications:

For acute and chronic treatment of signs and symptoms of osteoarthritis and rheumatoid arthritis.

Administration and Dosage:

Nabumetone was approved in December 1991.

Recommended starting dose is 1000 mg as a single dose with or without food. Some patients may obtain more symptomatic relief from 1500 to 2000 mg/day. Nabumetone can be given either once or twice daily. Dosages > 2000 mg/day have not been studied. Use the lowest effective dose for chronic treatment.

Rx	**Relafen** (SmithKline-Beecham)	**Tablets:** 500 mg	(Relafen 500). White. Film coated. Oval shape. In 100s, 500s and UD 100s.
		750 mg	(Relafen 750). Beige. Film coated. Oval shape. In 100s, 500s and UD 100s.

IBUPROFEN

For complete prescribing information, refer to the NSAIDs group monograph.

Indications:

Relief of signs and symptoms of rheumatoid arthritis and osteoarthritis; relief of mild to moderate pain; treatment of primary dysmenorrhea; reduction of fever.

Administration and Dosage:

Approved by the FDA in 1974.

Adults: Do not exceed 3.2 g/day. If GI upset occurs, take with meals or milk.

Rheumatoid arthritis and osteoarthritis – Individualize dosage. 1.2 to 3.2 g/day (300 mg 4 times daily or 400, 600 or 800 mg 3 or 4 times daily). In chronic conditions, therapeutic response sometimes occurs in a few days to a week, but most often within 2 weeks. Rheumatoid arthritis patients seem to require higher doses than osteoarthritis patients.

Mild to moderate pain – 400 mg every 4 to 6 hours, as necessary.

Primary dysmenorrhea – 400 mg every 4 hours, as necessary.

OTC use (minor aches and pains, dysmenorrhea, fever reduction) – 200 mg every 4 to 6 hours while symptoms persist. If pain or fever do not respond to 200 mg, 400 mg may be used. Do not exceed 1.2 g in 24 hours. Do not take for pain for > 10 days or for fever for > 3 days, unless directed by physician.

Children:

Juvenile arthritis – Usual dose is 30 to 70 mg/kg/day in 3 or 4 divided doses; 20 mg/kg/day may be adequate for milder disease.

Fever reduction (6 months to 12 years old) – Adjust dosage on the basis of the initial temperature level. If baseline temperature is ≤ 39.2°C (102.5°F), recommended dose is 5 mg/kg; if baseline temperature is > 39.2°C (102.5°F), recommended dose is 10 mg/kg. Duration of fever reduction is generally 6 to 8 hours. Maximum daily dose is 40 mg/kg.

IBUPROFEN

Rx	**Junior Strength Advil** (Whitehall-Robins)	**Tablets**: 100 mg	Coated. Sucrose. In 24s.
Rx	**Motrin** (McNeil)		(M 100). White. Scored. Capsule shape. Film coated. In 100s.
otc	**Ibuprofen** (Various, eg, Geneva, Major, Rugby, Parmed, UDL)	**Tablets**: 200 mg	In 50s, 100s, 250s.
otc	**Advil** (Whitehall)		**Tablets**: Sucrose. In 4s, 8s, 24s, 50s, 100s, 165s and 250s.
			Caplets: Parabens. In 24s, 50s, 100s, 165s and 250s
otc	**Arthritis Foundation** (McNeil-CPC)		In 50s and 100s.
otc	**Bayer Select Pain Relief Formula Caplets** (Bayer)		In 36s and 50s.
otc	**Genpril** (Goldline)		**Tablets**: Lactose. White. Film coated. In 50s and 100s.
			Caplets: Lactose. White. Capsule shape. Film coated. In 100s.
otc	**Haltran** (Roberts)		(Haltran). In 30s.
otc	**Ibuprin** (Thompson Med.)		In 50s and 100s.
otc	**Ibuprohm** (Ohm Labs)		**Tablets and Caplets**: In 24s, 50s, 100s, 165s, 250s, 500s and 1000s.
otc	**Menadol** (Rugby)		In 50s, 100s and 1000s.
otc	**Midol IB** (Bayer)		In 24s and 50s.
otc	**Motrin IB** (Upjohn)		**Tablets**: In 24s, 50s, 100s, 130s and 165s.
			Caplets: In 24s, 50s, 100s, 130s and 165s.
			Gelcaps: Parabens. In 24s and 50s.
otc	**Nuprin** (Bristol-Myers Squibb)	**Tablets**: 200 mg	**Tablets**: Yellow. In 24s, 50s and 100s.
			Caplets: Yellow. In 24s, 50s and 100s.
otc	**Saleto-200** (Roberts Med)		In 1000s and UD 500s.
Rx	**Ibuprofen** (Various, eg, Major, Qualitest)	**Tablets**: 300 mg	In 50s, 100s and 500s.
Rx	**Motrin** (Upjohn)		(Motrin 300 mg). White. In 500s and unit-of-use 60s.

IBUPROFEN

Rx	**Ibuprofen** (Various, eg, Geneva, Mylan, Parmed, Qualitest, Rugby, Schein, Vangard, Warner Chilcott)	**Tablets**: 400 mg	In 50s, 100s and 500s.
Rx	**IBU** (Knoll)		(Ibu 400). White. Film coated. In 100s and 500s.
Rx	**Ibuprohm** (Ohm Labs)		Red. In 50s, 100s, 500s and 1000s.
Rx	**Motrin** (Upjohn)		Lactose. (Motrin 400 mg). White. In 500s, UD 100s and unit-of-use 100s and 120s.
Rx	**Saleto-400** (Roberts Med)		In 100s and 500s.
Rx	**Ibuprofen** (Various, eg, Geneva, Major, Mylan, Parmed, Qualitest, Rugby, Schein, Warner Chilcott)	**Tablets**: 600 mg	In 50s, 100s and 500s.
Rx	**IBU** (Knoll)		(Ibu 600). White. Film coated. In 100s and 500s.
Rx	**Motrin** (Upjohn)		Lactose. (Motrin 600 mg). White. Elliptical. In 500s, UD 100s and unit-of-use 90s and 100s.
Rx	**Saleto-600** (Roberts Med)		In 100s and 500s.
Rx	**Ibuprofen** (Various, eg, Geneva, Parmed, Qualitest, Rugby, Schein, Warner Chilcott)	**Tablets**: 800 mg	In 12s, 15s, 21s, 30s, 40s, 50s, 60s, 100s, 360s, 500s and UD 100s.
Rx	**IBU** (Knoll)		(Ibu 800). White. Film coated. In 100s and 500s.
Rx	**Motrin** (Upjohn)		Lactose. (Motrin 800 mg). White. Elliptical. In 500s, UD 100s and unit-of-use 90s and 100s.
Rx	**Saleto-800** (Roberts Med)		In 100s and 500s.
Rx	**Motrin** (McNeil)	**Tablets, chewable**: 50 mg	(Motrin 50). Orange, scored. Citrus flavor. In 100s.
Rx	**Motrin** (McNeil)	**Tablets, chewable**: 100 mg	(Motrin 100). Orange, scored. Citrus flavor. In 100s.
Rx	**Motrin, Junior Strength** (McNeil)		Aspartame, 6 mg phenylalanine. Orange flavor. In 24s.
Rx	**Children's Advil** (Wyeth-Ayerst)	**Suspension**: 100 mg/5 ml	Sorbitol, sucrose, EDTA. Fruit flavor. In 119 and 473 ml.
otc	**Children's Motrin** (McNeil-CPC)		Sucrose. Berry flavor. In 60 and 120 ml.
Rx	**Ibuprofen** (Various, eg, UDL)		In UD 50s.
Rx	**Motrin** (McNeil)		Sucrose. Berry flavor. In 120 and 480 ml.
Rx	**Children's Motrin** (McNeil)	**Oral Drops**: 40 mg/ml	Sorbitol, sucrose. Berry flavor. In 15 ml.

KETOPROFEN

For complete prescribing information, refer to the NSAIDs group monograph.

Indications:

Capsules: Acute or long-term treatment of the signs and symptoms of rheumatoid arthritis and osteoarthritis; mild to moderate pain; primary dysmenorrhea.

Capsules, extended release: Treatment of the signs and symptoms of rheumatoid arthritis and osteoarthritis.

OTC: Temporary relief of minor aches and pains associated with common cold, headache, toothache, muscular aches, backache, minor pain of arthritis, menstrual cramps and reduction of fever.

Administration and Dosage:

Individualize dosage. May be taken with antacids, food or milk to minimize adverse GI effects.

Rheumatoid arthritis and osteoarthritis: Do not exceed 300 mg/day.

Daily dose – 150 to 300 mg divided into 3 or 4 doses.

Starting dose – 75 mg 3 times/day or 50 mg 4 times/day. Reduce initial dose to ½ to ⅓ in elderly or debilitated patients or those with impaired renal function.

If minor side effects appear, they may disappear at a lower dose that may still have an adequate therapeutic effect. If well tolerated but not optimally effective, dosage may be increased. Individuals may show better response to 300 mg daily compared to 200 mg, although in well controlled clinical trials, patients on 300 mg did not show greater mean effectiveness. They did show an increased frequency of upper- and lower-GI distress and headaches. Women had an increased frequency of these adverse effects compared to men. When treating patients with 300 mg/day, observe sufficient increased clinical benefit to offset potential increased risk.

Extended release – 200 mg once daily.

Mild to moderate pain, primary dysmenorrhea: 25 to 50 mg every 6 to 8 hours as needed. Give smaller dosages initially to smaller patients, the elderly and those with renal or liver disease. Doses > 50 mg may be given, but doses > 75 mg do not display added therapeutic effects. Administer high doses with caution and closely observe patient response. Do not exceed 300 mg/day.

Hepatic function impairment: For patients with alcoholic cirrhosis, no significant changes in the kinetic disposition of ketoprofen capsules were observed relative to age-matched normal subjects (see Warnings).

Hypoalbuminemia/Renal function impairment: Hypoalbuminemia/reduced renal function increase fraction of free drug (biologically active form), patients with both conditions may be at greater risk of adverse effects. Give lower doses and closely monitor.

OTC:

Adults – 12.5 mg with a full glass of liquid every 4 to 6 hours. If pain or fever persists after 1 hour, follow with 12.5 mg. With experience, some patients may find an initial dose of 25 mg will give better relief. Do not exceed 25 mg in a 4 to 6 hour period or 75 mg in a 24 hour period. Use the smallest effective dose.

Children – Do not give to those < 16 years of age unless directed by physician.

otc	**Orudis KT** (Whitehall-Robins)	**Tablets:** 12.5 mg	Tartrazine, sugar. In 24s and 50s.
otc	**Actron Caplets** (Bayer)		Lactose. In 24s.
Rx	**Ketoprofen** (Various, eg, Biocraft)	**Capsules:** 25 mg	In 100s.
Rx	**Orudis** (Wyeth-Ayerst)		Lactose. (Wyeth 4186 Orudis 25). Dark green and red. In 100s.
Rx	**Ketoprofen** (Various, eg, Biocraft, Qualitest, Schein)	**Capsules:** 50 mg	In 100s.
Rx	**Orudis** (Wyeth-Ayerst)		Lactose. (Wyeth 4181 Orudis 50). Dark green and light green. In 100s.
Rx	**Ketoprofen** (Various, eg, Biocraft, Qualitest, Schein)	**Capsules:** 75 mg	In 100s and 500s.
Rx	**Orudis** (Wyeth-Ayerst)		Lactose. (Wyeth 4187 Orudis 75). Dark green and white. In 100s, 500s and *Redipak* 100s.

KETOPROFEN

Rx	**Oruvail** (Wyeth-Ayerst)	**Capsules, extended release**: 100 mg	Sucrose. (Oruvail 100). Pink/dark green. In 100s and *Redipak* 100s.
		150 mg	Sucrose. (Oruvail 150). Pink/light green. In 100s and *Redipak* 100s.
		200 mg	Sucrose. (Oruvail 200). Pink/White. In 100s and *Redipak* 100s.

PIROXICAM

For complete prescribing information, refer to the NSAIDs group monograph.

Indications:

Arthritis: For acute or long-term use in relief of signs and symptoms of osteoarthritis and rheumatoid arthritis.

Administration and Dosage:

Initiate and maintain at a single daily dose of 20 mg. May divide daily dose. Although therapeutic effects are evident early in treatment, increase in response progresses over several weeks. Do not assess effect of therapy for 2 weeks.

Children: Dosage recommendations and indications for use in children have not been established.

Rx	**Piroxicam** (Various, eg, Goldline, Moore, Mylan, Par, Qualitest, Roxane, Rugby, Schein, Schiapparelli Searle, Zenith)	**Capsules:** 10 mg	In 100s, 500s and 1000s.
Rx	**Feldene** (Pfizer)		Lactose. Blue/maroon. In 100s.
Rx	**Piroxicam** (Various, eg, Goldline, Moore, Mylan, Par, Qualitest, Roxane, Rugby, Schiapparelli Searle, URL, Zenith)	**Capsules:** 20 mg	In 100s, 500s and 1000s.
Rx	**Feldene** (Pfizer)		Lactose. Maroon. In 100s, 500s and UD 100s.

NAPROXEN

For complete prescribing information, refer to the NSAIDs group monograph.

Indications:

Rx: Relief of mild to moderate pain; treatment of primary dysmenorrhea, rheumatoid arthritis, osteoarthritis, ankylosing spondylitis, tendinitis, bursitis, acute gout.

Delayed release – Delayed release naproxen is not recommended for initial treatment of acute pain because absorption is delayed compared with other naproxen formulations.

Naproxen (not naproxen sodium) – Juvenile arthritis.

OTC: Temporary relief of minor aches and pains associated with the common cold, headache, toothache, muscular aches, backache, minor pain of arthritis, pain of menstrual cramps and reduction of fever.

Administration and Dosage:

Rx: Do not exceed 1.25 g naproxen (1.375 g naproxen sodium) per day.

Rheumatoid arthritis, osteoarthritis, ankylosing spondylitis, pain, dysmenorrhea, acute tendinitis and bursitis –

Naproxen: 250 to 500 mg twice/day. May increase to 1.5 g/day for limited periods. Symptomatic improvement in arthritis usually begins within 2 weeks. However, if improvement does not occur within 2 weeks, consider an additional 2 week trial.

Delayed release naproxen (EC-Naprosyn): 375 to 500 mg twice/day. Do not break, crush or chew tablets.

Controlled release (Naprelan): 750 mg or 1000 mg once daily. Individualize dosage. Do not exceed 1000 mg/day.

Naproxen sodium: 275 to 550 mg twice daily. May increase to 1.65 g for limited periods.

Morning and evening doses do not have to be equal, and use of the drug more frequently than twice daily is not necessary. Symptomatic arthritis improvement usually begins in 2 weeks; if no improvement is seen, consider a trial for 2 more weeks.

Juvenile arthritis –

Naproxen: Total daily dose is ≈ 10 mg/kg in 2 divided doses.

Suspension – Use the following as a guide:

Naproxen Suspension: Children's Dose	
Child's weight	Dose
13 kg (29 lb)	2.5 ml (0.5 tsp) bid
25 kg (55 lb)	5 ml (1 tsp) bid
38 kg (84 lb)	7.5 ml (1.5 tsp) bid

Acute gout –

Naproxen: 750 mg, followed by 250 mg every 8 hours until the attack subsides.

Naproxen sodium: 825 mg, then 275 mg every 8 hours until attack subsides.

Controlled release (Naprelan): 1000 to 1500 mg once daily on the first day followed by 1000 mg once daily until the attack has subsided.

Mild to moderate pain; primary dysmenorrhea; acute tendinitis and bursitis –

Naproxen: 500 mg, followed by 250 mg every 6 to 8 hours. Do not exceed a 1.25 g total daily dose.

Naproxen sodium: 550 mg, followed by 275 mg every 6 to 8 hours. Do not exceed a 1.375 g total daily dose.

Controlled release (Naprelan): 1000 once daily. For patients requiring greater analgesic benefit, 1500 mg/day may be used for a limited period.

Children – Safety and efficacy in children < 2 years of age have not been established.

OTC:

Adults – 200 mg with a full glass of liquid every 8 to 12 hours while symptoms persist. With experience, some patients may find an initial dose of 400 mg followed by 200 mg 12 hours later, if necessary, will give better relief. Do not exceed 600 mg in 24 hours unless otherwise directed. Use the smallest effective dose.

Elderly (> 65 years of age) – Do not take > 200 mg every 12 hours.

Children – Do not give to children < 12 years of age except under the advice and supervision of a physician.

NAPROXEN

otc	**Naproxen Sodium** (Goldline)	**Tablets:** 200 mg (220 mg naproxen sodium)	In 24s.
otc	**Aleve** (Procter & Gamble)		Capsule or hexagonal shape. In 24s, 50s and 100s.
Rx	**Naproxen Sodium** (Various, eg, Hamilton, Purepac, Qualitest, Roxane, Zenith)	**Tablets:** 250 mg (275 mg naproxen sodium)	In 100s, 500s, 1000s and UD 100s.
Rx	**Anaprox** (Syntex)		(Syntex 274). 1 mEq (25 mg) sodium. Lactose. Lt blue. Oval. Film coated. In 100s and 500s.
Rx	**Naproxen Sodium** (Various, eg, Hamilton, Purepac, Qualitest, Roxane)	**Tablets:** 500 mg (550 mg naproxen sodium)	In 100s, 500s, 1000s and UD 100s.
Rx	**Anaprox DS** (Syntex)		(Syntex/Anaprox DS). 2 mEq (50 mg) sodium. Dark blue. Capsule shape. Film coated. In 100s, 500s and UD 100s.
Rx	**Naproxen** (Various, eg, Goldline, Lederle, Moore, Purepac, Qualitest, Roxane)	**Tablets:** 250 mg	In 100s, 500s, 1000s and UD 100s.
Rx	**Naprosyn** (Syntex)		(Naprosyn 250). Yellow. In 100s and 500s.
Rx	**Naproxen** (Various, eg, Goldline, Lederle, Moore, Mylan, Purepac, Qualitest, Roxane)	**Tablets:** 375 mg	In 100s, 500s, 1000s and UD 100s.
Rx	**Naprosyn** (Syntex)		(Naprosyn 375). Peach. In 100s and 500s.
Rx	**Naproxen** (Various, eg, Goldline, Lederle, Moore, Purepac, Qualitest, Roxane)	**Tablets:** 500 mg	In 100s, 500s, 1000s and UD 100s.
Rx	**Naprosyn** (Syntex)		(Naprosyn 500). Yellow. In 100s and 500s.
Rx	**Napron X** (Nilor Pharm)		(Napron 500). Yellow. In 100s, 500s and UD 100s.
Rx	**EC-Naprosyn** (Syntex)	**Tablets, delayed release:** 375 mg	(EC-Naprosyn 375). White. Capsule shape. Enteric coated. In 100s.
		500 mg	(EC-Naprosyn 500). White. Capsule shape. Enteric coated. In 100s.
Rx	**Naprelan** (Wyeth Ayerst)	**Tablets, controlled release:** 375 mg (421.5 mg naproxen sodium)	(W901). White. Capsule shape. In 100s.
		500 mg (550 mg naproxen sodium)	(W902). White. Capsule shape. In 75s.
Rx	**Naprosyn** (Syntex)	**Suspension:** 125 mg/5 ml	Sorbitol, sucrose, parabens. Orange-pineapple flavor. In 474 ml.
Rx	**Naproxen** (Roxane)		Methylparaben, sorbitol, sucrose. Pineapple-orange flavor. In 5 and 500 ml and UD 10 and 20 ml.

INDOMETHACIN

For complete prescribing information, refer to the NSAIDs group monograph. For information on parenteral indomethacin, see Agents for Patent Ductus Arteriosus.

Indomethacin cannot be considered a simple analgesic and should not be used in conditions other than those recommended under Indications.

Indications:

For active stages of moderate to severe rheumatoid arthritis (including acute flares of chronic disease); moderate to severe ankylosing spondylitis; moderate to severe osteoarthritis; acute painful shoulder (bursitis/tendinitis); acute gouty arthritis.

Sustained release dosage form is not indicated for acute gouty arthritis.

Unlabeled uses: Indomethacin has been used for pharmacologic closure of persistent patent ductus arteriosus in premature infants as an alternative to surgical ligation. Clinical closure of ductus has occurred within 24 to 30 hours without untoward effects in majority of neonates given single doses of 0.3 mg/kg or ≥ 1 dose of 0.1 mg/kg via retention enema or orogastric tube. Parenteral indomethacin is indicated for this use. See monograph in Agents for Patent Ductus Arteriosus section.

Indomethacin suppresses uterine activity by inhibiting prostaglandin synthesis and has been used to prevent premature labor. Prolonged maternal administration of indomethacin for this purpose could result in prenatal ductus arteriosus closure and increased neonatal morbidity; *avoid this use.*

Topical indomethacin as eye drops in 0.5% and 1% concentrations has been used to treat cystoid macular edema.

Administration and Dosage:

Adverse reactions appear to correlate with the dose in most patients. Determine the smallest effective dosage. Always give capsules or oral suspension with food, immediately after meals or with antacids to reduce gastric irritation.

Moderate to severe rheumatoid arthritis (including acute flares of chronic disease), ankylosing spondylitis and osteoarthritis: 25 mg 2 or 3 times daily. If well tolerated, increase daily dose by 25 or 50 mg (if required by continuing symptoms) at weekly intervals until satisfactory response is obtained or until total daily dose of 150 to 200 mg is reached. Doses above this generally do not increase effectiveness.

In patients who have persistent night pain or morning stiffness, giving a large portion, up to a maximum of 100 mg of the total daily dose at bedtime, may help to relieve pain. The total daily dose should not exceed 200 mg.

In acute flares of chronic rheumatoid arthritis, it may be necessary to increase dosage by 25 or 50 mg daily. If minor adverse effects develop, reduce dosage rapidly to tolerated dose; observe patient closely. If severe adverse reactions occur, discontinue. After acute phase of disease is controlled, attempt to reduce daily dose repeatedly until patient receives smallest effective dose or drug is discontinued.

Acute painful shoulder (bursitis or tendinitis): 75 to 150 mg daily in 3 or 4 divided doses. Discontinue the drug after inflammation has been controlled for several days. Usual course of therapy is 7 to 14 days.

Acute gouty arthritis: 50 mg 3 times daily until pain is tolerable, then rapidly reduce the dose to complete cessation of the drug. Definite relief of pain usually occurs within 2 to 4 hours. Tenderness and heat usually subside in 24 to 36 hours, and swelling gradually disappears in 3 to 5 days. Do not use sustained release form.

Sustained release form: Do not crush. The 75 mg sustained release capsule can be taken once a day as an alternative to 25 mg capsule 3 times daily. There will be significant differences between the regimens in indomethacin blood levels, especially after 12 hrs. One 75 mg sustained release capsule twice daily can be substituted for 50 mg capsule 3 times daily. Do not use sustained release form in acute gouty arthritis.

Children: Effectiveness in children ≤ 14 years of age has not been established.

Storage:

Oral suspension and suppositories – Store below 30°C (86°F). Protect oral suspension from freezing.

INDOMETHACIN

Rx	**Indomethacin** (Various, eg, Geneva, Goldline, Lederle, Lemmon, Major, Moore, Purepac, Rugby, Schein, URL)	**Capsules**: 25 mg	In 60s, 100s, 500s, 1000s and UD 100s.
Rx	**Indocin** (Merck)		Lactose, lecithin. (MSD 25). Blue and white. In 100s, 1000s, UD 100s and unit-of-use 100s.
Rx	**Indomethacin** (Various, eg, Geneva, Goldline, Lederle, Lemmon, Major, Moore, Purepac, Rugby, Schein, URL)	**Capsules**: 50 mg	In 23s, 72s, 100s, 250s, 500s and UD 100s.
Rx	**Indocin** (Merck)		Lactose, lecithin. (MSD 50). Blue/white. In 100s and UD 100s.
Rx	**Indomethacin SR** (Various, eg, Geneva, Goldline, Lemmon, Moore, Rugby, Schein, URL, Warner Chilcott)	**Capsules, sustained release**: 75 mg	In 60s and 100s.
Rx	**Indochron E-R** (Inwood)		Sucrose, parabens. (IL-3607). Lavender/Clear. In 60s and 100s.
Rx	**Indocin SR** (Merck)		(MSD 693). Blue and clear. In unit-of-use 30s and 60s.
Rx	**Indomethacin** (Roxane)	**Oral Suspension**: 25 mg per 5 ml	Fruit mint flavor. In 500 ml.
Rx	**Indocin** (Merck)		1% alcohol, sorbitol. Pineapple coconut mint flavor. In 237 ml.
Rx	**Indocin** (Merck)	**Suppositories**: 50 mg	White. In 30s.

SULINDAC

For complete prescribing information, refer to the NSAIDs group monograph.

Indications:

For acute or long-term use in the relief of signs and symptoms of the following: Osteoarthritis; rheumatoid arthritis; ankylosing spondylitis; acute painful shoulder (acute subacromial bursitis/supraspinatus tendinitis); acute gouty arthritis.

Administration and Dosage:

Administer twice a day with food. The usual maximum dosage is 400 mg/day. Dosages above 400 mg/day are not recommended.

Osteoarthritis, rheumatoid arthritis and ankylosing spondylitis: Initial dosage is 150 mg twice a day. Individualize dosage.

Response occurs within 1 week in about half of patients with osteoarthritis, ankylosing spondylitis and rheumatoid arthritis. Others may require longer to respond.

Acute painful shoulder (acute subacromial bursitis/supraspinatus tendinitis); acute gouty arthritis: 200 mg twice/day. After satisfactory response, reduce dosage accordingly.

In acute painful shoulder, therapy for 7 to 14 days is usually adequate. In acute gouty arthritis, therapy for 7 days is usually adequate.

Children: Safety and efficacy have not been established.

Rx	**Sulindac** (Various, eg, Danbury, Dixon-Shane, Major, Parmed, Schein, UDL, Warner Chilcott)	**Tablets:** 150 mg	In 60s, 100s, 500s and UD 100s.
Rx	**Clinoril** (MSD)		(MSD 941). Yellow. Hexagonal. In 100s, UD 100s and unit-of-use 60s and 100s.
Rx	**Sulindac** (Various, eg, Major, Schein, UDL, Warner Chilcott)	**Tablets:** 200 mg	In 60s, 100s and 500s.
Rx	**Clinoril** (MSD)		(MSD 942). Yellow, scored. Hexagonal. In 100s, UD 100s & unit-of-use 60s and 100s.

TOLMETIN SODIUM

For complete prescribing information, refer to the NSAIDs group monograph.

Indications:

Treatment of acute flares and long-term management of rheumatoid arthritis and osteoarthritis; treatment of juvenile rheumatoid arthritis.

Administration and Dosage:

Expect therapeutic response in a few days to a week. Anticipate progressive improvement during succeeding weeks of therapy. If GI symptoms occur, give with antacids other than sodium bicarbonate; bioavailability is affected by food or milk.

Adults:

Rheumatoid arthritis and osteoarthritis – Initially, 400 mg 3 times/day; preferably include dose on arising and at bedtime. Control is usually achieved at doses of 600 to 1800 mg/day generally in 3 divided doses. Doses > 1800 mg/day have not been studied and are not recommended.

Children:

(≥ 2 yrs) – Initially, 20 mg/kg/day in 3 or 4 divided doses. When control is achieved, usual dose ranges from 15 to 30 mg/kg/day. Doses > 30 mg/kg/day have not been studied and are not recommended.

Rx	**Tolmetin Sodium** (Various, eg, Mutual, URL)	**Tablets**: 200 mg tolmetin (as sodium)	In 100s.
Rx	**Tolectin 200** (McNeil Pharm.)		18 mg sodium. (McNeil Tolectin 200). White, scored. In 100s.
Rx	**Tolmetin Sodium** (Various, eg, Mutual, URL)	**Tablets**: 600 mg tolmetin (as sodium)	In 100s, 500s and 1000s.
Rx	**Tolectin 600**(McNeil Pharm.)		54 mg sodium. (McNeil Tolectin 600). Orange. Film coated. In 100s and 500s.
Rx	**Tolmetin Sodium** (Various, eg, Mutual, URL)	**Capsules**: 400 mg tolmetin (as sodium)	In 100s, 500s and 1000s.
Rx	**Tolectin DS** (McNeil Pharm.)		36 mg sodium. (McNeil Tolectin DS). Orange. In 100s, 500s and UD 100s.

MECLOFENAMATE SODIUM

For complete prescribing information, refer to the NSAIDs group monograph.

Indications:

Relief of mild to moderate pain; treatment of primary dysmenorrhea; treatment of idiopathic heavy menstrual blood loss; acute and chronic rheumatoid arthritis and osteoarthritis: Use requires careful assessment of benefit/risk ratio.

Administration and Dosage:

Mild to moderate pain: 50 mg every 4 to 6 hours. Doses of 100 mg may be required for optimal pain relief. Do not exceed daily dosage of 400 mg.

Excessive menstrual blood loss and primary dysmenorrhea: 100 mg 3 times daily for up to 6 days, starting at the onset of menstrual flow.

Rheumatoid arthritis and osteoarthritis:

Usual dosage – 200 to 400 mg per day in 3 or 4 equal doses.

Initial dosage – Initiate at lower dosage; increase as needed to improve response. Individualize dosage. Do not exceed 400 mg/day. Improvement may occur in a few days; optimum benefit may not occur for 2 to 3 weeks.

Dosage adjustment – After satisfactory response is achieved, adjust as required. A lower dosage may suffice for long-term use. May give with meals or milk. If intolerance occurs, reduce dosage. Discontinue if severe adverse reactions occur.

Functional Class IV – Safety and efficacy not established in these patients.

Children: Safety and efficacy in children < 14 years of age are not established.

Rx	**Meclofenamate** (Various, eg, Bolar, Geneva, Goldline, Lederle, Lemmon, Major, Moore, PBI, Purepac, Rugby)	**Capsules:**[1] 50 mg	In 100s, 250s, 500s and UD 100s.
Rx	**Meclomen** (Parke-Davis)		Lactose. In 100s, UD 100s.
Rx	**Meclofenamate** (Various, eg, Bolar, Geneva , Goldline, Lederle, Lemmon, Major, Moore, PBI, Purepac, Rugby)	**Capsules:**[1] 100 mg	In 100s, 250s, 500s and UD 100s.
Rx	**Meclomen** (Parke-Davis)		Lactose. In 100s, 500s, UD 100s.

[1] Meclofenamic acid equivalent, as meclofenamate sodium.

MEFENAMIC ACID

For complete prescribing information, refer to the NSAIDs group monograph.

Indications:

Relief of moderate pain if therapy will be ≤ 1 week; primary dysmenorrhea.

Administration and Dosage:

Acute pain:

Adults (> 14 yrs) – 500 mg, then 250 mg every 6 hours, as needed, usually not to exceed 1 week. Give with food.

Primary dysmenorrhea: 500 mg, then 250 mg every 6 hours. Start with onset of bleeding and associated symptoms. Should not be necessary for > 2 to 3 days.

Children: Safety and efficacy in children < 14 years have not been established.

Rx	**Ponstel** (Parke-Davis)	**Capsules:** 250 mg	In 100s.

ETODOLAC

For complete prescribing information, refer to the NSAIDs group monograph.

Indications:

Acute and long-term use in the management of signs and symptoms of osteoarthritis; management of pain.

Administration and Dosage:

Osteoarthritis: Initially 800 to 1200 mg/day in divided doses, followed by adjustment in the range of 600 to 1200 mg/day in divided doses (400 mg 2 or 3 times/day; 300 mg 2, 3 or 4 times/day; 200 mg 3 or 4 times/day). Do not exceed 1200 mg/day.

Patients ≤ 60 kg – Do not exceed 20 mg/kg.

Analgesia: Acute pain – 200 to 400 mg every 6 to 8 hrs. Do not exceed 1200 mg/day.

Patients ≤ 60 kg – Do not exceed 20 mg/kg.

Rx	**Etodolac** (Zenith Goldline)	**Tablets:** 400 mg	Lactose, polyethylene glycol, povidone. In 100s, 500s and 1000s.
Rx	**Lodine** (Wyeth-Ayerst)		Lactose. (LODINE 400). Yellow-orange. Oval. Film coated. In 100s and UD 100s.
Rx	**Lodine XL** (Wyeth-Ayerst)	**Tablets, extended release:** 400 mg	Lactose. (LODINE XL 400). Orange-red. Capsular-oval shape. Biconvex. Film coated. In 100s and UD 100s.
		600 mg	Lactose. (Lodine XL 600). Lt. gray. Capsular-oval shape. Biconvex. Film-coated. In 100s and UD 100s.
Rx	**Lodine** (Wyeth-Ayerst)	**Capsules:** 200 mg	Lactose. (Lodine 200). Two-tone gray w/red bands. In 100s, UD 100s.
		300 mg	Lactose. (Lodine 300). Lt. gray w/red bands. In 100s and UD 100s.

KETOROLAC TROMETHAMINE

For complete prescribing information, refer to the NSAIDs group monograph.

Warning:

Ketorolac is indicated for the short-term (up to 5 days) management of moderately severe acute pain that requires analgesia at the opioid level. It is not indicated for minor or chronic painful conditions. Ketorolac is a potent NSAID analgesic, and its administration carries many risks. The resulting NSAID-related adverse events can be serious in certain patients for whom ketorolac is indicated, especially when the drug is used inappropriately. Increasing the dose beyond the label recommendations will not provide better efficacy but will result in increasing the risk of developing serious adverse events.

GI effects: Ketorolac can cause peptic ulcers, GI bleeding or perforation. Therefore, it is contraindicated in patients with active peptic ulcer disease, recent GI bleeding or perforation, or a history of peptic ulcer disease or GI bleeding.

Renal effects: Ketorolac is contraindicated in patients with advanced renal impairment and in patients at risk for renal failure due to volume depletion.

Risk of bleeding: Ketorolac inhibits platelet function and is therefore contraindicated in patients with suspected or confirmed cerebrovascular bleeding, hemorrhagic diathesis, incomplete hemostasis and those at high risk of bleeding.

Ketorolac is contraindicated as prophylactic analgesia before any major surgery and is contraindicated intra-operatively when hemostasis is critical because of the increased risk of bleeding.

Hypersensitivity: Hypersensitivity reactions, ranging from bronchospasm to anaphylactic shock, have occurred, and appropriate counteractive measures must be available when administering the first dose of ketorolac. Ketorolac is contraindicated in patients with previously demonstrated hypersensitivity to ketorolac tromethamine or allergic manifestations to aspirin or other NSAIDs.

Intrathecal or epidural administration: Ketorolac is contraindicated for intrathecal or epidural administration due to its alcohol content.

Labor, delivery and lactation: Use in labor and delivery is contraindicated because ketorolac may adversely affect fetal circulation and inhibit uterine contractions. Use in nursing mothers is contraindicated because of the potential adverse effects of prostaglandin-inhibiting drugs on neonates.

Concomitant use with NSAIDs: Ketorolac is contraindicated in patients currently receiving aspirin or other NSAIDs because of the cumulative risk of inducing serious NSAID-related side effects.

Administration and dosage: Ketorolac (oral) is indicated only as continuation therapy to ketorolac IV/IM; the combined duration of use of IV/IM and oral is not to exceed 5 days because of the increased risk of serious adverse events. The recommended total daily oral dose (maximum, 40 mg) is significantly lower than for IV/IM (maximum 120 mg). (See Administration and Dosage and Transition from IV/IM to oral)

Special populations: Adjust dosage for patients ≥ 65 years old, for patients < 50 kg (110 lbs) or for body weight (see Administration and Dosage) and for patients with moderately elevated serum creatinine. IV/IM doses are not to exceed 60 mg/day in these patients.

Indications:

Moderately severe, acute pain: Short-term (≤ 5 days) management of moderately severe, acute pain that requires analgesia at the opioid level, usually in a postoperative setting. Therapy should always be initiated with IV/IM, and oral is to be used only as continuation treatment, if necessary. Combined use of IV/IM and oral is not to exceed 5 days of use because of the potential of increasing the frequency and severity of adverse reactions associated with the recommended doses. Switch patients to alternative analgesics as soon as possible. Ketorolac therapy is not to exceed 5 days.

KETOROLAC TROMETHAMINE

Ketorolac IV/IM has been used concomitantly with morphine and meperidine, and has shown an opioid-sparing effect. For breakthrough pain, it is recommended to supplement the lower end of the IV/IM dosage range with low doses of narcotics as needed, unless otherwise contraindicated. Ketorolac and narcotics should not be administered in the same syringe (see Administration and Dosage).

Administration and Dosage:

Approved by the FDA in November 1989.

The combined duration of ketorolac IV/IM and oral is not to exceed 5 days. Oral use is only indicated as continuation therapy to IV/IM.

IV/IM: Ketorolac IV/IM may be used as a single or multiple dose, on a regular or as needed schedule for the management of moderately severe, acute pain that requires analgesia at the opioid level, usually postoperatively. Correct hypovolemia prior to administration. Switch patients to alternative analgesics as soon as possible. Ketorolac therapy is not to exceed 5 days.

When administering IM/IV, the IV bolus must be given over no less than 15 seconds. Give IM administration slowly and deeply into the muscle. The analgesic effect begins in 30 minutes with maximum effect in 1 to 2 hours after IV or IM dosing. Duration of analgesic effect is usually 4 to 6 hours.

Single-dose treatment – Limit the following regimen to single administration use only:

IM dosing:

< 65 years old – One 60 mg dose.

≥ 65 years old, renal impairment or weight < 50 kg (110 lbs) – One 30 mg dose.

IV dosing:

< 65 years old – One 30 mg dose.

≥ 65 years old, renal impairment or weight < 50 kg (110 lbs) – One 15 mg dose.

Multiple-dose treatment –

< 65 years old: The recommended dose is 30 mg every 6 hours. The maximum daily dose should not exceed 120 mg.

≥ 65 years old, renal impairment (see Warnings) or weight < 50 kg (110 lbs): The recommended dose is 15 mg every 6 hours. The maximum daily dose for these populations should not exceed 60 mg.

For breakthrough pain, do not increase the dose or the frequency of ketorolac. Consider supplementing these regimens with low doses of opioids as needed unless otherwise contraindicated.

Admixture incompatibility – Do not mix IV/IM ketorolac in a small volume (eg, in a syringe) with morphine sulfate, meperidine HCl, promethazine HCl or hydroxyzine HCl; this will result in precipitation of ketorolac from solution.

Oral: Indicated only as continuation therapy to ketorolac IV/IM for the management of moderately severe, acute pain that requires analgesia at the opioid level.

Transition from IV/IM to oral – The recommended oral dose is as follows:

< 65 years old: 20 mg as a first oral dose for patients who received 60 mg IM single dose, 30 mg IV single dose or 30 mg multiple dose IV/IM followed by 10 mg every 4 to 6 hours, not to exceed 40 mg/24 hours.

> 65 years old, renal impairment or weight < 50 kg (110 lb): 10 mg as a first oral dose for patients who received a 30 mg IM single dose, 15 mg IV single dose or 15 mg multiple dose IV/IM followed by 10 mg every 4 to 6 hours, not to exceed 40 mg/24 hours.

Shortening the recommended dosing intervals may result in increased frequency and severity of adverse reactions.

Storage:

Injection – Protect from light.

Rx	**Ketorolac Tromethamine** (Ethex)	**Tablets:** 10 mg	Lactose. (Ethex 301). White. Film coated. In 100s.
Rx	**Toradol** (Syntex)		Lactose. (Toradol Syntex). White. Film coated. In 100s.
Rx	**Toradol** (Syntex)	**Injection:** 15 mg/ml	In 1 ml *Tubex* syringes.[1]
		30 mg/ml	In 1[2] and 2[3] ml *Tubex* syringes.

[1] With 10% alcohol and 6.68 mg sodium chloride in sterile water.
[2] With 10% alcohol and 4.35 mg sodium chloride in sterile water.
[3] For IM use only. With 10% alcohol and 8.7 mg sodium chloride in sterile water.

DICLOFENAC

For complete prescribing information, refer to the NSAIDs group monograph.

Indications:

Acute and chronic treatment of the signs and symptoms of rheumatoid arthritis, osteoarthritis and ankylosing spondylitis.

Diclofenac potassium: Management of pain and primary dysmenorrhea when prompt pain relief is desired.

Administration and Dosage:

Osteoarthritis: 100 to 150 mg/day in divided doses (50 mg twice daily or 3 times daily [diclofenac sodium or potassium] or 75 mg twice daily [diclofenac sodium]). Dosages > 150 mg/day have not been studied.

Rheumatoid arthritis: 150 to 200 mg/day in divided doses (50 mg 3 times daily or 4 times daily [diclofenac sodium or potassium] or 75 mg twice daily [diclofenac sodium]). Dosages > 225 mg/day are not recommended.

Ankylosing spondylitis: 100 to 125 mg/day as 25 mg 4 times daily, with an extra 25 mg dose at bedtime, if necessary. Dosages > 125 mg/day have not been studied.

Analgesia and primary dysmenorrhea (diclofenac potassium only): Recommended starting dose is 50 mg 3 times daily. In some patients, an initial dose of 100 mg followed by 50 mg doses will provide better relief. After the first day, when the maximum recommended dose may be 200 mg, the total daily dose should generally not exceed 150 mg.

Rx	**Cataflam** (Geigy)	**Tablets**: 50 mg (as potassium)	Sucrose. (Cataflam 50). Lt brown. Biconvex. In 100s and UD 100s.
Rx	**Diclofenac Sodium** (Roxane)	**Tablets, delayed release (enteric coated):** 25 mg (as sodium)	In 60s, 100s and UD 100s.
Rx	**Voltaren** (Geigy)		(Voltaren 25). Yellow. In 60s, 100s and UD 100s.
Rx	**Diclofenac Sodium** (Roxane)	**Tablets, delayed release (enteric coated)**: 50 mg (as sodium)	In 60s, 100s, 1000s and UD 100s.
Rx	**Voltaren** (Geigy)		(Voltaren 50). Lt brown. In 60s, 100s, 1000s and UD 100s.
Rx	**Diclofenac Sodium** (Roxane)	**Tablets, delayed release (enteric coated)**: 75 mg (as sodium)	In 60s, 100s, 1000s and UD 100s.
Rx	**Voltaren** (Geigy)		(Voltaren 75). White. In 60s, 100s, 1000s and UD 100s.
Rx	**Voltaren-XR** (Geigy)	**Tablets, extended release:** 100 mg (as sodium)	Sucrose. (Voltaren-XR 100). Light pink. Biconvex. In 100s and UD 100s.

OXAPROZIN

For complete prescribing information, refer to the NSAIDs group monograph.

Indications:

Acute and long-term use in the management of signs and symptoms of osteoarthritis and rheumatoid arthritis.

Administration and Dosage:

Approved by the FDA on October 29, 1992.

Rheumatoid arthritis: 1200 mg once a day. Both smaller and larger doses may be required in individual patients.

Regardless of the indication, individualize the dosage to the lowest effective dose to minimize adverse effects.

Osteoarthritis: 1200 mg once a day. For patients of low body weight or with milder disease, an initial dosage of 600 mg once a day may be appropriate.

Maximum dose: 1800 mg/day (or 26 mg/kg, whichever is lower) in divided doses.

Rx	**Daypro** (Searle)	**Caplets**: 600 mg	(Daypro 1381). White, scored. Capsule shape. Film coated. In 100s and UD 100s.

ANTIRHEUMATIC AGENTS

Therapeutic alternatives in the treatment of rheumatoid arthritis and related conditions include a diverse array of agents ranging from aspirin and similarly acting nonsteroidal anti-inflammatory agents (NSAIDs), to the slow-acting and possibly disease modifying agents such as gold compounds and penicillamine. Because of their toxicity, the slow-acting agents are generally reserved for progressive diseases unresponsive to more conservative therapy. Drugs and groups of drugs useful in the treatment of rheumatoid arthritis are listed below (refer to individual monographs).

Anti-inflammatory Agents:

GLUCOCORTICOIDS provide dramatic anti-inflammatory effects by inhibiting the initiation of inflammatory reactions. However, because of the consequences of prolonged therapy, use chronically only in patients with uncontrollable rheumatoid arthritis who fail to respond to other measures. Short-term therapy can be used in acute flares until other agents have a chance to act.

SALICYLATES – Aspirin, the most widely used NSAID, is generally considered the drug of first choice for rheumatoid arthritis. Adequate analgesia is usually achieved with 3 g/day of aspirin; 3 to 6 g/day are usually required for significant anti-inflammatory effects. At maximum doses, aspirin is as effective as any of the other NSAIDs. Gastrointestinal intolerance is the most common side effect. Other salicylate derivatives may offer the advantage of fewer GI complaints without interfering with platelet aggregation at recommended doses; however, when comparing anti-inflammatory agents, nonaspirin salicylates have not been proven as effective as aspirin.

NONSTEROIDAL ANTI-INFLAMMATORY DRUGS (NSAIDS) have essentially the same therapeutic benefits as aspirin. With the exception of indomethacin, the NSAIDS may offer the advantage of a lower incidence of GI side effects.

Slow-Acting Antirheumatic Agents:

HYDROXYCHLOROQUINE SULFATE, an antimalarial agent, may be effective in moderate to severe rheumatoid arthritis unresponsive to conventional treatment. Up to 6 months may be required for a clinical response. Side effects are frequent.

GOLD COMPOUNDS are quite effective in the treatment of actively progressing rheumatoid arthritis. Prolonged therapy is required. Serious side effects may require discontinuation of therapy.

PENICILLAMINE is used in severe rheumatoid arthritis unresponsive to conventional therapy. Response to therapy is slow (2 to 3 months); adverse effects may be severe.

AZATHIOPRINE and *CYCLOSPORINE* are immunosuppressive agents used in the treatment of severe, active and erosive disease not responsive to conventional therapy.

METHOTREXATE is used in severe, active, classical or definite rheumatoid arthritis unresponsive to other therapy.

CAPTOPRIL has been used investigationally to treat severe rheumatoid arthritis.

HYDROXYCHLOROQUINE SULFATE

Hydroxychloroquine sulfate is also indicated for treatment of acute attacks and suppression of malaria. Refer to the monograph in the Anti-infectives section.

Actions:

Pharmacology: A 4-aminoquinoline compound with antimalarial actions similar to those of chloroquine. In the treatment of acute or chronic rheumatoid arthritis, clinical improvement is slow; it is not a first-line drug. Potential toxicity limits its use. The precise mechanism of action is not known, but appears to involve suppression of formation of antigens responsible for hypersensitivity reactions which cause symptoms to develop.

Pharmacokinetics: Hydroxychloroquine is readily absorbed from the GI tract; peak plasma concentrations occur in 1 to 3 hours. The drug concentrates in the liver, spleen, kidney, heart, lung and brain. About 50% of the unchanged drug is excreted in the urine. Renal excretion is increased by acidification and decreased by alkalinization of the urine.

Indications:

Systemic lupus erythematosus: Treatment of chronic discoid and systemic lupus erythematosus (SLE).

Rheumatoid arthritis: Treatment of acute or chronic rheumatoid arthritis.

Use in patients who have not responded satisfactorily to drugs with less potential for serious side effects.

Malaria: Refer to the monograph in the Anti-infectives section.

Contraindications:

Retinal or visual field changes attributable to any 4-aminoquinoline compound; hypersensitivity to 4-aminoquinoline compounds; long-term therapy in children.

Warnings:

Psoriasis: Use in patients with psoriasis may precipitate a severe attack. Porphyria may be exacerbated. Do not use unless benefit to patient outweighs possible hazard.

Ophthalmic effects: Irreversible retinal damage has been observed in some patients who had received long-term or high dosage 4-aminoquinoline therapy for discoid and SLE or rheumatoid arthritis. When prolonged therapy is contemplated, perform initial (baseline) and periodic (every 3 months) ophthalmologic examinations (including visual acuity, expert slit-lamp, funduscopic and visual field tests). If there is any indication of abnormality in the visual acuity, visual field or retinal macular areas (such as pigmentary changes, loss of foveal reflex) or any visual symptoms (such as light flashes and streaks) not fully explainable by difficulties of accommodation or corneal opacities, discontinue drug immediately and observe patient for possible progression (see Adverse Reactions).

Retinal changes (and visual disturbances) may progress even after cessation of therapy.

Chloroquine retinopathy – Methods recommended for early diagnosis of "chloroquine retinopathy" consist of (1) funduscopic examination of macula for fine pigmentary disturbances or loss of the foveal reflex and (2) examination of central visual field with a small red test object for pericentral or paracentral scotoma or determination of retinal thresholds to red. Regard unexplained visual symptoms (ie, light flashes or streaks) as possible manifestations of retinopathy.

Muscular weakness: Examine patients on long-term therapy periodically, and test knee and ankle reflexes to detect evidence of muscular weakness. If weakness occurs, discontinue drug.

Rheumatoid arthritis: In rheumatoid arthritis, discontinue if objective improvement does not occur within 6 months. Safety for use in juvenile arthritis has not been established.

Renal/Hepatic function impairment: Use with caution.

Pregnancy: Avoid use during pregnancy. Chloroquine administered IV to pregnant mice rapidly crossed the placenta, accumulated selectively in the melanin structures of the fetal eyes and was retained in the ocular tissues for 5 months after the drug was eliminated from the rest of the body.

Lactation: A very low concentration of hydroxychloroquine appeared in the breast milk of a patient following doses of 200 mg twice daily over 48 hours.

Children: Children are especially sensitive to 4-aminoquinolines. A number of fatalities have been reported following ingestion of chloroquine in small doses (0.75 g or 1 g in one 3-year-old).

Safe use of the drug in treating juvenile rheumatoid arthritis is limited; however, its use may be warranted in some cases. See Administration and Dosage.

HYDROXYCHLOROQUINE SULFATE

Precautions:

Monitoring: Perform periodic blood cell counts during prolonged therapy. If a severe blood disorder appears, consider discontinuation. Use caution in G–6–PD deficiency.

Alcoholism: Use with caution in patients with alcoholism.

Dermatologic reactions may occur; exercise care when given to any patient receiving a drug with significant tendency to produce dermatitis.

Toxic symptoms: If serious toxic symptoms occur, administer ammonium chloride (8 g daily in divided doses for adults) 3 or 4 days a week for several months after therapy has been stopped; acidification of the urine increases renal excretion by 20% to 90%. Exercise caution in metabolic acidosis.

Drug Interactions:

Digoxin: Concurrent administration of hydroxychloroquine and digoxin has been reported to increase serum digoxin levels. Monitor digoxin levels.

Adverse Reactions:

The following have occurred with one or more of the 4-aminoquinoline compounds.

CNS: Irritability; nervousness; emotional changes; nightmares; psychosis; headache; dizziness; vertigo; tinnitus; nystagmus; nerve deafness; convulsions; ataxia.

Ophthalmic:

Ciliary body – See Warnings. Disturbance of accommodation with blurred vision. This reaction is dose-related and reversible with cessation of therapy.

Cornea – Transient edema; punctate to lineal opacities; decreased corneal sensitivity. The corneal changes, with or without accompanying symptoms (blurred vision, halos around lights, photophobia), are fairly common, but reversible. Corneal deposits may appear as early as 3 weeks following initiation of therapy. The incidence of corneal changes and visual side effects appears to be considerably lower with hydroxychloroquine than with chloroquine.

Retina – Edema; atrophy; abnormal pigmentation (mild pigment stippling to a "bull's eye" appearance); loss of foveal reflex; increased macular recovery time following exposure to a bright light (photo-stress test); elevated retinal threshold to red light in macular, paramacular and peripheral retinal areas.

Other fundus changes – Optic disc pallor and atrophy; attenuation of retinal arterioles; fine granular pigmentary disturbances in the peripheral retina; prominent choroidal patterns in advanced stage.

Visual field defects – Pericentral or paracentral scotoma; central scotoma with decreased visual acuity; rarely, field constriction.

Retinopathy – The most common visual symptoms attributed to the retinopathy are: Reading and seeing difficulties (words, letters or parts of objects missing); photophobia; blurred distance vision; missing or blacked out areas in the central or peripheral visual field; light flashes and streaks. Retinopathy appears to be dose-related and has occurred within several months (rarely) to several years of daily therapy; a few cases have been reported several years after drug was discontinued.

Patients with retinal changes may have visual symptoms or may be asymptomatic (with or without visual field changes). Rarely, scotomatous vision or field defects may occur without obvious retinal change. Retinopathy may progress even after the drug is discontinued. In a number of patients, early retinopathy (macular pigmentation sometimes with central field defects) diminished or regressed completely after therapy was discontinued. Paracentral scotoma to red targets ("premaculopathy") is indicative of early retinal dysfunction which is usually reversible with cessation of therapy.

A small number of cases of retinal changes have occurred in patients who received only hydroxychloroquine. These usually consisted of alteration in retinal pigmentation which was detected on periodic ophthalmologic examination; visual field defects were also present in some. A case of delayed retinopathy has been reported with vision loss starting 1 year after the drug was discontinued.

Dermatologic: Bleaching of hair; alopecia; pruritus; skin and mucosal pigmentation; skin eruptions (urticarial, morbilliform, lichenoid, maculopapular, purpuric, erythema annulare centrifugum and exfoliative dermatitis); precipitation of nonlight-sensitive psoriasis.

Hematologic: Aplastic anemia; agranulocytosis; leukopenia; thrombocytopenia; (hemolysis in individuals with G-6-PD deficiency).

GI: Anorexia; nausea; vomiting; diarrhea; abdominal cramps.

Musculoskeletal: Extraocular muscle palsies; skeletal muscle weakness; absent or hypoactive deep tendon reflexes.

Miscellaneous: Weight loss; lassitude; exacerbation or precipitation of porphyria.

HYDROXYCHLOROQUINE SULFATE

Overdosage:

Symptoms: Toxic symptoms may occur within 30 minutes and consist of headache, drowsiness, visual disturbances, cardiovascular collapse and convulsions, followed by sudden and early respiratory and cardiac arrest. ECG may reveal atrial standstill, nodal rhythm, prolonged intraventricular conduction time and progressive bradycardia leading to ventricular fibrillation or arrest. Rarely, these symptoms occur with lower doses in hypersensitive patients.

Treatment is symptomatic and must be prompt, with immediate evacuation of the stomach by emesis or gastric lavage. Treatment includes usual supportive measures. Refer to General Management of Acute Overdosage. Activated charcoal, in a dose not less than 5 times the estimated dose ingested, may inhibit further intestinal absorption if introduced by stomach tube after lavage within 30 minutes after ingestion. Control convulsions before attempting gastric lavage. If due to cerebral stimulation, attempt cautious administration of an ultrashort-acting barbiturate; if due to anoxia, correct with oxygen, artificial respiration or, in shock with hypotension, use vasopressor therapy. Perform tracheal intubation or tracheostomy followed by gastric lavage if necessary. Exchange transfusions have been used to reduce the level of drug in the blood. Closely observe, for at least 6 hours, patients surviving the acute phase who are asymptomatic. Fluids may be forced. Sufficient ammonium chloride (8 g daily in divided doses for adults) administered for a few days will acidify the urine and help promote urinary excretion.

Patient Information:

May cause GI upset; take with food or milk.

Notify physician if any of the following occur: Blurring or other vision changes; ringing in the ears or hearing loss; fever, sore throat or unusual bleeding or bruising; unusual pigmentation (blue-black) of the skin; muscle weakness; bleaching or loss of hair; mood or mental changes.

Administration and Dosage:

Rheumatoid arthritis:

Initial dosage (adults) – 400 to 600 mg daily, taken with a meal or a glass of milk. Side effects rarely require temporary reduction. Later (usually from 5 to 10 days), dose may gradually be increased to optimum response level, often without return of side effects.

Maintenance dosage (adults) – When a good response is obtained (usually in 4 to 12 weeks), reduce dosage by 50% and continue at a level of 200 to 400 mg daily. Incidence of retinopathy is higher when this dose is exceeded.

The compound is cumulative and requires several weeks to exert therapeutic effects; minor side effects may occur early. Maximum effects may not be obtained for several months. If objective improvement (reduced joint swelling, increased mobility) does not occur within 6 months, discontinue the drug. Safe use of hydroxychloroquine to treat juvenile rheumatoid arthritis has not been established.

Should relapse occur after medication is withdrawn, resume therapy or continue on an intermittent schedule if there are no ocular contraindications.

Corticosteroids and salicylates may be used in conjunction with this compound; generally they can be gradually decreased or eliminated after hydroxychloroquine has been used for several weeks. When gradual reduction of steroid dosage is indicated, reduce (every 4 to 5 days) dose of cortisone by no more than 5 to 15 mg; hydrocortisone from 5 to 10 mg; prednisolone and prednisone from 1 to 2.5 mg; methylprednisolone and triamcinolone from 1 to 2 mg; or dexamethasone from 0.25 to 0.5 mg.

Children: Although experience with hydroxychloroquine in children for rheumatoid arthritis or lupus erythematosus is limited, its use may be warranted in some cases. A dose of 3 to 5 mg/kg/day, up to a maximum of 400 mg/day (given once or twice daily) has been recommended. Do not exceed a dose of 7 mg/kg/day.

Lupus erythematosus: Initially, 400 mg once or twice daily in adults, continued for several weeks or months, depending on response. For prolonged maintenance therapy, a smaller dose (200 to 400 mg daily) will frequently suffice. The incidence of retinopathy has reportedly been higher when maintenance dose is exceeded.

Rx	**Plaquenil Sulfate** (Sanofi Winthrop)	**Tablets:** 200 mg (equivalent to 155 mg base).	(P61). Scored. In 100s.

GOLD COMPOUNDS

Warning:

Signs of gold toxicity include: Fall in hemoglobin, leukopenia < 4000 WBC/mm^3, granulocytes < 1500/mm^3, platelets < 100,000 to 150,000/mm^3, proteinuria, hematuria, pruritus, rash, stomatitis or persistent diarrhea. Review recommended laboratory work results before instituting therapy and before each injection or written prescription for oral gold. See patient before each injection to determine presence or absence of adverse reactions; some of these can be severe or even fatal. Physicians planning to use gold compounds should be experienced with chrysotherapy and thoroughly familiar with both toxicity and benefits of gold.

Explain the possibility of adverse reactions to patients before starting therapy.

Advise patients to report promptly any toxicity symptoms (see Patient Information).

Actions:

Pharmacology: Gold suppresses or prevents, but does not cure, arthritis and synovitis. It is taken up by macrophages, resulting in inhibition of phagocytosis and possibly, lysosomal enzyme activity. Gold decreases concentrations of rheumatoid factor and immunoglobulins. The exact mode of action in rheumatoid arthritis is unknown; however, gold compounds may decrease synovial inflammation and retard cartilage and bone destruction. No substantial evidence exists that gold induces remission of rheumatoid arthritis.

Therapeutic effects from gold compounds occur slowly. Early improvement, often limited to reduction in morning stiffness, may begin after 6 to 8 weeks of treatment with gold sodium thiomalate, but beneficial effects may not be observed until after months of therapy. Therapeutic effects from auranofin may be seen after 3 to 4 months of treatment, but in some patients, not before 6 months.

Pharmacokinetics: Due to differences in administration routes (IM vs oral), dosage regimens (weekly vs daily) and actual quantity of gold administered to the patient, expect differences in the pharmacokinetic parameters of injectable and oral gold.

Parenteral gold compounds are water soluble. Aurothioglucose is an oily suspension; suspension results in delayed IM absorption. Both are similar in biologic and pharmacokinetic behavior.

After initial injection, serum level of gold rises sharply and declines over the next week. Peak levels of aqueous preparations are higher and decline faster than oily preparations. After a standard weekly dose, considerable individual variation in levels of gold has been found. Small amounts are found in the serum for months after discontinuation.

Although parenteral gold is widely distributed in body tissues, highest concentrations occur in the reticuloendothelial system and in adrenal and renal cortices. Binding of gold to red blood cells from injectable gold compounds is lower compared to auranofin-derived gold. Blood to synovial fluid ratios are similar, ≈ 1.7:1, and synovial fluid levels are ≈ 50% of the blood concentrations. No correlation between blood-gold concentrations and safety or efficacy has been established.

Major pharmacokinetic differences are summarized below:

Pharmacokinetics of Auranofin and Injectable Gold Compounds

Drug	Gold content (%)	% Absorbed	Time to peak (hrs)	Mean steady-state plasma levels (mcg/ml)	Protein binding (%)	Plasma half-life (days)	% Excreted in urine	% Excreted in feces
Auranofin	29	25 (15-33)	1-2	0.2-1	60	26 (21-31)	60[1]	85-95
Aurothioglucose	50	nd	4-6	1-5	95-99	3-27 (single dose) 14-40 (3rd dose)	70	30
Gold sodium thiomalate			2-6			up to 168 (11th dose)		

[1] 60% of the absorbed gold (15% of administered dose). nd – No data.

GOLD COMPOUNDS

Indications:

Rheumatoid arthritis:

Parenteral – Active early rheumatoid arthritis, both adult and juvenile types (cases not adequately controlled by other anti-inflammatory agents or conservative measures). Use only as one part of therapy program; alone, it is not a complete treatment.

Oral – Management of adults with active classical or definite rheumatoid arthritis (ARA criteria) with insufficient therapeutic response to or intolerant of an adequate trial of full doses of one or more NSAIDs. Add auranofin to baseline program; include non-drug therapies.

Unlabeled uses: Alternative or adjuvant to corticosteroids in treatment of pemphigus. For psoriatic arthritis in patients who do not tolerate or respond to NSAIDs.

Contraindications:

Parenteral: Hypersensitivity to any component; uncontrolled diabetes mellitus; severe debilitation; renal disease; hepatic dysfunction or history of infectious hepatitis; marked hypertension; uncontrolled CHF; systemic lupus erythematosus; agranulocytosis or hemorrhagic diathesis; blood dyscrasias; patients recently radiated; those with severe toxicity from previous exposure to gold or other heavy metals; urticaria; eczema; colitis; pregnancy (see Warnings).

Oral: A history of any of the following gold-induced disorders: Anaphylactic reactions, necrotizing enterocolitis, pulmonary fibrosis, exfoliative dermatitis, bone marrow aplasia or other severe hematologic disorders; pregnancy (see Warnings).

Warnings:

Active disease: When cartilage and bone damage has already occurred, gold cannot reverse structural damage to joints caused by previous disease. The greatest potential benefit occurs in patients with active synovitis, particularly in its early stage.

Thrombocytopenia has occurred in 1% to 3% of patients treated with auranofin, some of whom developed bleeding. It appears peripheral in origin and is usually reversible upon withdrawal. Onset is not related to duration of therapy; its course may be rapid. Monitor platelet counts at least monthly, however, if a precipitous decline in platelets or a platelet count < 100,000/mm^3 occurs or if signs and symptoms of thrombocytopenia (eg, purpura, ecchymoses or petechiae) occur, immediately withdraw auranofin and other therapies; obtain additional platelet counts. Do not reinstate auranofin unless thrombocytopenia resolves and studies show that it was not due to gold therapy.

Special risk patients: Control diabetes mellitus or CHF before gold therapy begins.

Extreme caution is indicated in patients with any of the following: History of blood dyscrasias such as agranulocytopenia or anemia caused by drug sensitivity; allergy or hypersensitivity to medications; skin rash; previous kidney or liver disease; marked hypertension; compromised cerebral or cardiovascular circulation.

Weigh the potential benefits of using auranofin in patients with inflammatory bowel disease, skin rash or history of bone marrow depression against potential risks of gold toxicity on compromised organ systems and the difficulty in quickly detecting and correctly attributing the toxic effect.

Immediate effects following injection, or at any time during therapy, include: Anaphylactic shock, syncope, bradycardia, thickening of the tongue, difficulty swallowing or breathing and angioneurotic edema. These effects may occur immediately after injection or as late as 10 minutes after injection. If such effects occur, discontinue treatment.

Renal/Hepatic function impairment: Weigh the potential benefits of using auranofin in patients with progressive renal disease or significant hepatocellular disease against potential risks of gold toxicity on compromised organ systems and the difficulty in quickly detecting and correctly attributing the toxic effect.

Carcinogenesis: Renal adenomas developed in rats receiving injectable gold at doses higher and more frequent than recommended human doses. Sarcomas at the injection site occurred in some rats.

Studies demonstrated a significant increase in the frequency of renal tubular cell karyomegaly and cytomegaly, renal adenoma and malignant renal epithelial tumors in animals treated with auranofin and gold sodium thiomalate.

Elderly: Tolerance to gold usually decreases with advancing age.

GOLD COMPOUNDS

Pregnancy: Category C. Gold crosses the placenta. The placenta showed gold deposits; smaller amounts were detected in fetal liver and kidneys.

Gold therapy is usually contraindicated in pregnant patients. Warn the patient about the hazards of becoming pregnant while on gold therapy. Rheumatoid arthritis frequently improves when a patient becomes pregnant. Do not superimpose the potential nephrotoxicity of gold on the increased renal burden which normally occurs in pregnancy. Discontinue therapy upon recognition of pregnancy, if possible. Consider slow excretion of gold and its persistence in body tissues after discontinuing treatment when a woman receiving gold plans to become pregnant.

Animals – Gold sodium thiomalate was teratogenic during the organogenic period in small animals when given in doses 140 to 175 times the usual human dose. Auranofin showed impaired food intake, decreased maternal and fetal weights, and increased resorptions, abortions and congenital abnormalities, mainly abdominal defects (eg, gastroschisis, umbilical hernia).

There are no adequate, well controlled studies in pregnant women. Use only when benefits outweigh potential hazards to the fetus.

Lactation: Injectable gold is excreted in breast milk. Following auranofin administration, gold is excreted in the milk of rodents; human data are not available. Trace amounts appear in the serum and red blood cells of nursing offspring. This may cause rashes, nephritis, hepatitis and hematologic aberrations in nursing infants. Decide whether to discontinue nursing or to discontinue parenteral gold, taking into account the importance of the drug to the mother. Nursing during auranofin therapy is not recommended. Consider the slow excretion and persistence of gold in the mother even after therapy is discontinued.

Children: Safety and efficacy for use of aurothioglucose in children < 6 years of age have not been established. Auranofin is not recommended for use in children; safety and efficacy have not been established (however, see Administration and Dosage).

Precautions:

Monitoring: Before instituting treatment, rule out pregnancy; perform CBC with differential, platelet, hemoglobin, WBC and erythrocyte counts, urinalysis and renal and liver function tests. Perform urinalysis for protein and sediment changes prior to each injection. Perform CBC, including platelet estimation, before every second injection (every 2 weeks) throughout treatment. Purpura or ecchymoses always require a platelet count. Inquire regarding pruritus, rash, sore mouth, metallic taste and indigestion before each injection. Observe patient at least 15 minutes after each injection. For patients on auranofin, monitor CBC with differential, platelet count and urinalysis at least monthly.

Rapid reduction of hemoglobin, granulocytes < 1500/mm^3, leukopenia < 4000 WBC/mm^3, eosinophilia > 5%, platelets < 100,000 to 150,000/mm^3, albuminuria, hematuria, rash, dermatitis, pruritus, skin eruption, stomatitis, persistent diarrhea, jaundice or petechiae are signs of possible gold toxicity. Do not give additional therapy unless further studies show these abnormalities to be caused by conditions other than gold toxicity. Monitor patients with GI symptoms for GI bleeding (auranofin).

Proteinuria:

Auranofin – Proteinuria has developed in 3% to 9% of auranofin patients. If clinically significant proteinuria or microscopic hematuria is found, immediately stop auranofin and other therapies with the potential to cause proteinuria or microscopic hematuria.

Aurothioglucose – Patients with HLA-D locus histocompatibility antigens DRw2 and DRw3 may have a genetic predisposition to develop certain toxic reactions, such as proteinuria, during treatment with gold or D–penicillamine. Use aurothioglucose with caution in patients with compromised cardiovascular or cerebral circulation.

Concomitant antirheumatic therapy: Use of salicylates, NSAIDs and systemic corticosteroids may be continued when parenteral gold therapy is instituted. After improvement begins, slowly discontinue analgesics and NSAIDs as symptoms permit. Do not use penicillamine with gold salts.

Non-vasomotor post-injection reaction: Arthralgia may occur for a day or two after injection; it usually subsides after the first few injections. The mechanism of the transient increase in rheumatic symptoms after gold injection is unknown. These reactions are usually mild, but occasionally may be so severe that treatment is stopped prematurely.

GOLD COMPOUNDS

Drug Interactions:

Phenytoin: One report suggests coadministration with auranofin may increase phenytoin blood levels.

Adverse Reactions:

Adverse reactions to gold therapy may occur during treatment or many months after discontinuation. Incidence of toxic reactions is apparently unrelated to gold plasma levels, but may relate to cumulative body content of gold. Higher than conventional dosages may increase occurrence and severity of toxicity. Adverse reactions are most frequent when cumulative dose is 400 to 800 mg (gold sodium thiomalate) or 300 to 500 mg (aurothioglucose). Auranofin appears to cause fewer adverse reactions than injectable gold; however, therapeutic efficacy may also be less.

Adverse Reactions of Oral vs Parenteral Gold (%)

Adverse reaction	Auranofin (oral gold) (n = 445)	Injectable gold (n = 445)
Diarrhea	42.5	13
Rash	26	39
Stomatitis	13	18
Anemia	3.1	2.7
Elevated liver function tests	1.9	1.7
Leukopenia	1.3	2.2
Proteinuria	0.9	5.4
Thrombocytopenia	0.9	2.2
Pulmonary	0.2	0.2

Dermatologic: Dermatitis is the most common reaction to injectable gold and second most common to auranofin. Any eruption, especially pruritic, is considered to be a reaction until proven otherwise. Rash, urticaria (auranofin, 1 to 3%) and angioedema (auranofin, < 0.1%) may occur. Pruritus (auranofin, 17%) often exists before dermatitis, and is a warning of reaction. Erythema, and occasionally more severe reactions, such as papular, vesicular and exfoliative dermatitis leading to alopecia and nail shedding, may occur. Chrysiasis (gray-to-blue pigmentation caused by gold deposits in tissues) has occurred, especially on photoexposed areas. Gold dermatitis may be aggravated by exposure to sunlight or an actinic rash may develop.

Renal: Gold may produce a nephrotic syndrome or glomerulitis with proteinuria and hematuria; these are usually relatively mild and subside completely if recognized early and treatment is discontinued. They may become severe and chronic if treatment continues after onset. Acute renal failure secondary to acute tubular necrosis, acute nephritis or degeneration of proximal tubular epithelium may occur; perform regular urinalysis and discontinue treatment immediately if proteinuria or hematuria develop. Hematuria (1% to 3%) and proteinuria (3% to 9%) occur with auranofin.

Hematologic:

Auranofin – Thrombocytopenia (with or without purpura), leukopenia, eosinophilia, anemia (1% to 3%); neutropenia (0.1% to 1%); agranulocytosis, pancytopenia, hypoplastic anemia, aplastic anemia, pure red cell aplasia (< 0.1%).

Granulocytopenia; panmyelopathy; hemorrhagic diathesis. Constantly monitor patients throughout treatment for blood dyscrasias of the formed elements of the blood (see Warnings and Precautions). Though rare, these reactions have potentially serious consequences. These reactions may occur separately or in combination at any time during treatment.

Hepatic: Elevated liver enzymes (auranofin 1% to 3%), jaundice (auranofin < 0.1%) with or without cholestasis, hepatitis with jaundice, toxic hepatitis, intrahepatic cholestasis.

GI:

Auranofin – Diarrhea/loose stools (50%), generally manageable by reducing the dose (eg, from 6 to 3 mg/day), and only 6% need permanent drug discontinuation; abdominal pain (14%); nausea (10%); anorexia, flatulence, dyspepsia (3% to 9%); constipation, dysgeusia (1% to 3%); GI bleeding, melena, positive stool for occult blood (0.1% to 1%); ulcerative enterocolitis (can be severe or fatal), dysphagia (< 0.1%).

Aurothioglucose – Nausea, vomiting, anorexia, abdominal cramps, ulcerative enterocolitis (can be severe or fatal), colitis (rare).

GOLD COMPOUNDS

CNS: Confusion; hallucinations; seizures.

Miscellaneous: Iritis, corneal ulcers and gold deposits in ocular tissues (gold sodium thiomalate rare). These include deposits in the lens or cornea unassociated clinically with eye disorders or visual impairment (auranofin incidence < 0.1%). Acute yellow atrophy; encephalitis; immunological destruction of the synovia; EEG abnormalities; peripheral neuropathy (auranofin < 0.1%) with and without fasciculations or neuritis; partial or complete hair loss (auranofin 1% to 3%); fever; headache (aurothioglucose rare); sensorimotor effects (including Guillain-Barre syndrome) and elevated spinal fluid protein have occurred (gold sodium thiomalate rare).

Mucous membranes: Stomatitis, the second most common adverse reaction with injectable gold, is also seen with auranofin (13%). It may be manifested by shallow ulcers on buccal membranes, on borders of tongue and on palate or in pharynx and may be the only adverse reaction or occur with dermatitis. Diffuse glossitis or gingivitis may develop. Metallic taste may precede these reactions. Careful oral hygiene is important. Inflammation of upper respiratory tract, pharyngitis, gastritis, colitis, tracheitis, vaginitis and rarely, conjunctivitis (auranofin 3% to 9%) have been reported. Glossitis (auranofin 1% to 3%), gingivitis (auranofin 0.1% to 1%) and thickening of the tongue have occurred.

Pulmonary injury may be shown by gold bronchitis, interstitial pneumonitis (auranofin < 0.1%) or fibrosis, fever and partial or complete hair loss.

Nitritoid and allergic (parenteral): Reactions of the "nitritoid type" may resemble anaphylactoid effects. Flushing, fainting, dizziness and sweating are most frequent. Other symptoms may include nausea, vomiting, malaise, headache and weakness.

Management of adverse reactions: Discontinue immediately if toxic reactions occur. Minor complications (ie, localized dermatitis, mild stomatitis, slight proteinuria) generally require no other therapy and resolve spontaneously with therapy suspension. For mild reactions, it may be sufficient to briefly stop use and then resume with smaller doses. Moderately severe skin and mucous membrane reactions often benefit from topical corticosteroids, oral antihistamines and anesthetic lotions.

If stomatitis or dermatitis become severe or more generalized, systemic corticosteroids (generally, 10 to 40 mg prednisone daily in divided doses) may provide symptomatic relief.

For serious renal, hematologic, pulmonary and enterocolitic complications, use high doses of systemic corticosteroids (40 to 100 mg prednisone daily in divided doses). The duration of corticosteroid treatment varies. Larger doses and a longer treatment period may be required than for dermatologic reactions. Often this treatment may be required for many months because of the slow elimination of gold from the body. Therapy may also be required for months when adverse effects are unusually severe or progressive.

In high-dose gold patients whose serious adverse reactions do not improve with high-dose corticosteroids, or who develop significant steroid-related adverse reactions, a chelating agent may be given to enhance gold excretion (eg, dimercaprol, penicillamine). Monitor patients given dimercaprol carefully; untoward reactions may occur. Corticosteroids and a chelating agent may be coadministered. Adjunctive use of an anabolic steroid with other drugs (eg, dimercaprol, penicillamine, corticosteroids) may contribute to recovery of bone marrow deficiency.

Do not reinstitute after severe or idiosyncratic reactions – After resolution of mild reactions, reduced doses may be given. If test dose of 5 mg is well tolerated, give progressively larger doses (5 to 10 mg increments) at weekly to monthly intervals until 25 to 50 mg is reached.

Overdosage:

Symptoms: Overdosage from too rapid increases in dosing are manifested by rapid appearance of toxic reactions, particularly renal damage (eg, hematuria, proteinuria), and hematologic effects (eg, thrombocytopenia, granulocytopenia). Other toxic effects include fever, nausea, vomiting, diarrhea and skin disorders (eg, papulovesicular lesions, urticaria and exfoliative dermatitis, all with severe pruritus).

Auranofin overdosage experience is limited. A 50-year-old female took 27 mg daily for 10 days and developed encephalopathy and peripheral neuropathy. Auranofin was discontinued and she eventually recovered.

GOLD COMPOUNDS

Treatment: Promptly discontinue; give dimercaprol. Use specific supportive therapy for renal/hematologic complications. Refer to General Management of Acute Overdosage.Chelating agents are used with injectable gold; consider their use also for auranofin overdosage. In acute overdosage, immediately induce emesis or perform gastric lavage with supportive therapy.

Patient Information:

Patient package insert is available with auranofin.

Notify physician of the following: Itching, rash, sore mouth, indigestion, metallic taste, easy bruising or nosebleed.

Increased joint pain may continue 1 or 2 days after an injection and usually subsides after the first few injections.

Chrysiasis (gray-to-blue pigmentation) may occur, especially on photoexposed areas. Minimize exposure to sunlight or artificial ultraviolet light.

Observe careful oral hygiene in conjunction with therapy.

Warn women of childbearing potential of the risks of using gold therapy during pregnancy.

AURANOFIN

For complete prescribing information, refer to the Gold Compounds group monograph.

Contains 29% gold.

Administration and Dosage:

Adults: 6 mg daily, either as 3 mg twice daily or 6 mg once daily. Initiating dosages > 6 mg/day is not recommended; it is associated with increased incidence of diarrhea. If response is inadequate after 6 months, an increase to 9 mg/day (3 mg 3 times/day) may be tolerated. If response remains inadequate after 3 months of 9 mg/day, discontinue. Safety at doses > 9 mg/day has not been studied.

Transfer from injectable gold – Discontinue the injectable agent and start auranofin with 6 mg daily. At 6 months, control of disease activity of patients transferred to auranofin and those maintained on the injectable agent was not different.

Children: The following doses have been recommended.

Initial – 0.1 mg/kg/day.
Maintenance – 0.15 mg/kg/day.
Maximum dose – 0.2 mg/kg/day.

Rx	**Ridaura** (SmithKline-Beecham)	**Capsules:** 3 mg	(Ridaura SKF). Tan and brown. In 60s.

AUROTHIOGLUCOSE

For complete prescribing information, refer to the Gold Compounds group monograph.

Contains approximately 50% gold.

Administration and Dosage:

Administer only by IM injection, preferably intragluteally, using an 18 gauge, 1½ inch needle. For obese patients, an 18-gauge, 2 inch needle may be used.

Adults:

Weekly injections – First dose, 10 mg; second and third doses, 25 mg; fourth and subsequent doses, 50 mg. Continue the 50 mg dose at weekly intervals until 0.8 to 1 g has been given. If the patient has improved and has no signs of toxicity, continue the 50 mg dose many months longer, at 3 to 4 week intervals. A weekly dose above 50 mg is usually unnecessary and contraindicated; tend toward lower dosage. A 25 mg dose may be the dose of choice. If no improvement is demonstrated after a total administration of 1 g, reevaluate the necessity of gold therapy.

Children (6 to 12 years): One-fourth the adult dose, governed by body weight, not to exceed 25 mg per dose. Patient should remain recumbent ≈ 10 minutes after injection. Observe patient at least 15 minutes after each injection.

Rx	**Solganal** (Schering)	**Injection Suspension:** 50 mg/ml[1]	In 10 ml vials.

[1] In sesame oil with 2% aluminum monostearate and 1 mg propylparaben.

Gold Compounds

GOLD SODIUM THIOMALATE

For complete prescribing information, refer to the Gold Compounds group monograph.

Contains approximately 50% gold.

Administration and Dosage:

Administer only by IM injection, preferably intragluteally. Have patient remain recumbent for approximately 10 minutes after injection.

Adults: For the average size adult, the following dosage schedule is recommended:

Weekly injections – 1st injection, 10 mg; 2nd injection, 25 mg; 3rd and subsequent injections, 25 to 50 mg until major clinical improvement or toxicity occurs, or until the cumulative dose reaches 1 g. If significant clinical improvement occurs before a cumulative dose of 1 g has been administered, the dose may be decreased or the interval between injections increased as with maintenance therapy.

Maintenance – 25 to 50 mg every other week for 2 to 20 weeks. If the clinical course remains stable, give 25 to 50 mg every third and subsequently every fourth week indefinitely. Some patients may require maintenance intervals of 1 to 3 weeks. Should arthritis exacerbate during maintenance, resume weekly injections temporarily until disease activity is suppressed.

Should a patient fail to improve during initial therapy (cumulative dose of 1 g), several options are available: Discontinue the drug, continue the same dose (25 to 50 mg) for approximately 10 additional weeks or increase the dose by increments of 10 mg every 1 to 4 weeks, not to exceed 100 mg in a single injection.

If significant clinical improvement occurs using the second or third option, initiate the maintenance schedule described above. If there is no significant improvement or if toxicity occurs, discontinue therapy. The higher the individual dose, the greater the risk of toxicity. Base selection of these options on several factors, including the physician's experience with gold therapy, the course of the patient's condition, the choice of alternative treatments and patient availability for close supervision.

Children: The pediatric dose is proportional to the adult dose on a weight basis. After the initial test dose of 10 mg, give 1 mg/kg, not to exceed 50 mg for a single injection. Otherwise, adult guidelines apply.

Other doses recommended are as follows: Initial, 0.25 mg/kg/dose (one dose); incremental dose increases of 0.25 mg/kg/dose may be used, increasing with each weekly dose; maintenance dose is 1 mg/kg/dose weekly for a total of 20 doses, then every 2 to 4 weeks, using the longest interval consistent with remission.

Storage/Stability: Do not use if material has darkened. Color should not exceed pale yellow.

Rx	**Aurolate** (Pasadena)	**Injection:** 50 mg/ml[1]	In 2 and 10 ml vials.
Rx	**Gold Sodium Thiomalate** (King)		In 10 ml vials.
Rx	**Myochrysine** (Merck)		In 1 ml amps and 10 ml vials.

[1] With 0.5% benzyl alcohol.

METHOTREXATE (Amethopterin; MTX)

This is an abbreviated monograph. For complete prescribing information and use of methotrexate as an antineoplastic agent, see Methotrexate Antimetabolite monograph.

Warning:

Severe reactions: Because of the possibility of severe toxic reactions, fully inform patient of the risks involved and assure constant supervision.

Deaths have occurred with the use of methotrexate.

In rheumatoid arthritis treatment, restrict use to patients with severe, recalcitrant, disabling disease, which is not adequately responsive to other forms of therapy, and only after established diagnosis and appropriate consultation.

Pregnancy: Fetal death or congenital anomalies have occurred; do not use in women of childbearing potential unless benefits outweigh possible risks. Pregnant rheumatoid arthritis patients should not receive methotrexate.

Periodic monitoring for toxicity, including CBC with differential and platelet counts, and liver and renal function tests is mandatory. Periodic liver biopsies may be indicated in some situations. Monitor patients at increased risk for impaired methotrexate elimination (eg, renal dysfunction, pleural effusions or ascites) more frequently.

Liver: MTX causes hepatotoxicity, fibrosis and cirrhosis, but generally only after prolonged use. Acutely, liver enzyme elevations are frequent, usually transient and asymptomatic, and also do not appear predictive of subsequent hepatic disease. Liver biopsy after sustained use often shows histologic changes, and fibrosis and cirrhosis have been reported; these latter lesions often are not preceded by symptoms or abnormal liver function tests.

MTX-induced lung disease, a potentially dangerous lesion, may occur acutely at any time during therapy and has been reported at doses as low as 7.5 mg/week. It is not always fully reversible. Pulmonary symptoms (especially a dry, nonproductive cough) may require treatment interruption and careful investigation.

Marked bone marrow depression may occur, with resultant anemia, leukopenia or thrombocytopenia.

Unexpectedly severe (sometimes fatal) marrow suppression and GI toxicity have been reported with coadministration of methotrexate (usually in high dosage) and some NSAIDs.

GI: Diarrhea and ulcerative stomatitis require interruption of therapy; hemorrhagic enteritis and death from intestinal perforation may occur.

Renal use: Use MTX in patients with impaired renal function with extreme caution, and at reduced dosages, because renal dysfunction will prolong elimination.

Actions:

Clinical trials: The mechanism of action in rheumatoid arthritis is unknown; it may affect immune function. Two reports describe in vitro MTX inhibition of DNA precursor uptake by stimulated mononuclear cells and another (in animals) describes partial correction by MTX of spleen cell hyporesponsiveness and suppressed interleukin–2 production. Other laboratories, however, have been unable to demonstrate similar effects. Clarification of its effect on immune activity and its relation to rheumatoid immunopathogenesis await further studies.

In patients with rheumatoid arthritis, effects of MTX on articular swelling and tenderness can be seen as early as 3 to 6 weeks. Although MTX clearly ameliorates symptoms of inflammation (pain, swelling, stiffness), there is no evidence that it induces remission of rheumatoid arthritis nor has a beneficial effect been demonstrated on bone erosions and other radiologic changes which result in impaired joint use, functional disability and deformity.

Most studies of MTX in patients with rheumatoid arthritis are relatively short term (3 to 6 months). Limited data from long-term studies indicate that an initial clinical improvement is maintained for at least 2 years with continued therapy.

METHOTREXATE (Amethopterin; MTX)

Indications:

Severe, active, classical or definite rheumatoid arthritis (ARA criteria) in selected adults who have had an insufficient therapeutic response to, or are intolerant of, an adequate trial of first line therapy including full dose NSAIDs and usually a trial of at least one or more disease-modifying antirheumatic drugs.

Contraindications:

Pregnant and lactating patients (see Warnings); alcoholism, alcoholic liver disease or other chronic liver disease; overt or laboratory evidence of immunodeficiency syndromes; preexisting blood dyscrasias, such as bone marrow hypoplasia, leukopenia, thrombocytopenia or significant anemia; hypersensitivity to MTX.

Warnings:

Pregnancy: Category X. MTX can cause fetal death or teratogenic effects when administered to a pregnant woman and is contraindicated in pregnant patients with rheumatoid arthritis. Women of childbearing potential should not be started on MTX until pregnancy is excluded and should be fully counseled on the serious risk to the fetus should they become pregnant while undergoing treatment. Avoid pregnancy if either partner is receiving MTX: During and for a minimum of 3 months after therapy for male patients, and during and for at least one ovulatory cycle after therapy for female patients.

Lactation: Because of the potential for serious adverse reactions from MTX in breast fed infants, it is contraindicated in nursing mothers.

Children: Safety and efficacy in children have not been established other than in cancer chemotherapy.

Precautions:

Monitoring: Monitor hematology at least monthly, and liver and renal function every 1 to 3 months during therapy. During initial or changing doses, or periods of increased risk of elevated MTX blood levels (eg, dehydration), more frequent monitoring may be indicated. Stop MTX immediately if there is a significant drop in blood counts.

Aspirin, NSAIDs or low dose steroids may be continued, although the possibility of increased toxicity with concomitant use of NSAIDs including salicylates has not been fully explored. Studies of MTX in patients with rheumatoid arthritis have usually included concomitant NSAIDs, without apparent problems. Note, however, that doses used in rheumatoid arthritis (7.5 to 15 mg/week) are somewhat lower than those used in psoriasis; larger doses could lead to unexpected toxicity.

Physicians and pharmacists should emphasize that the dose is taken weekly. Mistaken daily use has led to fatal toxicity. Encourage patients to read the Patient Instructions in the Dose Pack. Do not write or refill prescriptions on a PRN basis.

Adverse Reactions:

Elevated liver function tests (15%); nausea/vomiting (10%); thrombocytopenia (platelet count < 100,000/mm^3); stomatitis (3% to 10%); rash/pruritus/dermatitis, diarrhea, alopecia, leukopenia (WBC < 3000/mm^3), pancytopenia, dizziness (1% to 3%).

Other less common reactions included: Decreased hematocrit; headache; upper respiratory infection; anorexia; arthralgias; chest pain; coughing; dysuria; eye discomfort; epistaxis; fever; infection; sweating; tinnitus; vaginal discharge.

Administration and Dosage:

Initial therapy may be instituted with the MTX 2.5 mg tablet dose pack, designated to initiate therapy with a 7.5 mg weekly dose. The dose pack is not recommended for titration to higher weekly doses, if they are necessary. Individualize dose. An initial test dose may be given prior to the regular dosing schedule to detect any extreme sensitivity to adverse effects. Maximal myelosuppression usually occurs in 7 to 10 days.

Recommended Starting Dosage Schedules: Single oral doses of 7.5 mg/week or divided oral dosages of 2.5 mg at 12 hour intervals for 3 doses given as a course once weekly.

Dosages in each schedule may be adjusted gradually to achieve an optimal response, but not ordinarily to exceed a total weekly dose of 20 mg. Limited experience shows a significant increase in the incidence and severity of serious toxic reactions, especially bone marrow suppression, at doses greater than 20 mg/week. Once response has been achieved, reduce each schedule, if possible, to the lowest possible effective dose.

Therapeutic response usually begins within 3 to 6 weeks and the patient may continue to improve for another 12 weeks or more.

Optimal duration of therapy is unknown. Limited data indicate that initial clinical improvement is maintained at least 2 years with continued therapy. When MTX is

METHOTREXATE (Amethopterin; MTX)

discontinued, the arthritis usually worsens within 3 to 6 weeks.

Rx	**Rheumatrex Dose Pack**[1] (Lederle)	**Tablets:** 2.5 mg (as sodium)	(LL/M1). Yellow, scored. 4 cards, each w/ 2, 3, 4, 5 or 6 tablets, ie, 5, 7.5, 10, 12.5 or 15 mg/week.
Rx	**Methotrexate** (Immunex)		Lactose. (LL/M1). Yellow, scored. In 100s.

[1] Patient package insert is available with product.

In addition to the agents in this section, sulindac and indomethacin (see Nonsteroidal Anti-inflammatory Agents monograph) and phenylbutazone and oxyphenbutazone (see individual monographs) are indicated for the treatment of gout.

Uricosurics

PROBENECID

Actions:

Pharmacology: A uricosuric and renal tubular blocking agent, probenecid inhibits the tubular reabsorption of urate, thus increasing the urinary excretion of uric acid and decreasing serum uric acid levels. Effective uricosuria reduces the miscible urate pool, retards urate deposition and promotes reabsorption of urate deposits.

Probenecid is most useful in gouty arthritis patients with reduced urinary excretion of uric acid (< 800 mg/day) on an unrestricted diet. Allopurinol is more appropriate for patients with excessive uric acid synthesis as indicated by > 800 mg uric acid through urinary excretion daily on a purine-free diet.

Probenecid also inhibits the tubular secretion of most penicillins and cephalosporins and usually increases plasma levels by any route the antibiotic is given. A 2- to 4-fold plasma elevation has been demonstrated.

Pharmacokinetics: Probenecid is well absorbed after oral administration and produces peak plasma concentrations in 2 to 4 hours. It is highly protein bound (85% to 95%) to plasma albumin. The half-life is dose-dependent and varies from < 5 to > 8 hours. Probenecid is hydroxylated to active metabolites and is excreted in the urine primarily in metabolite form.

Indications:

Treatment of hyperuricemia associated with gout and gouty arthritis.

Prolongation of plasma levels of antibiotics: Adjuvant to therapy with penicillins or cephalosporins, for elevation and prolongation of plasma levels of the antibiotic.

Contraindications:

Hypersensitivity to probenecid; children < 2 years of age; blood dyscrasias or uric acid kidney stones. Do not start therapy until an acute gouty attack has subsided.

Warnings:

Exacerbation of gout following therapy with probenecid may occur; in such cases, colchicine or other appropriate therapy is advisable.

Salicylates: Use of salicylates is contraindicated in patients on probenecid therapy. Salicylates antagonize probenecid's uricosuric action.

Sulfa drug allergy: Probenecid is a sulfonamide; patients with a history of allergy to sulfa drugs may react to probenecid. Use with caution.

Hypersensitivity: Rarely, severe allergic reactions and anaphylaxis have occurred. Most of these occur within several hours after readministration following prior use of the drug. The appearance of hypersensitivity reactions requires therapy cessation. Refer to Management of Acute Hypersensitivity Reactions.

Renal function impairment: Dosage requirements may be increased in renal impairment. Probenecid may not be effective in chronic renal insufficiency, particularly when the glomerular filtration rate is ≤ 30 ml/minute. Probenecid is not recommended in conjunction with a penicillin in the presence of known renal impairment

Pregnancy: Category B. Probenecid crosses the placenta and appears in cord blood. It has been used during pregnancy without producing adverse effects in the fetus or in the infant. Use only when clearly needed and when potential benefits outweigh potential hazards to the fetus.

Children: Do not use in children < 2 years of age.

Precautions:

Alkalinization of urine: Hematuria, renal colic, costovertebral pain and formation of urate stones associated with use in gouty patients may be prevented by alkalization of urine and liberal fluid intake; monitor acid-base balance. See Administration and Dosage.

Peptic ulcer history: Use with caution.

Uricosurics

PROBENECID

Drug Interactions:

Probenecid Drug Interactions			
Precipitant drug	Object drug*		Description
Probenecid	Acyclovir	⬆	Decreased acyclovir renal clearance and increased bioavailability following IV use may occur.
Probenecid	Allopurinol	⬆	A beneficial interaction; coadministration may increase the uric acid lowering effect.
Probenecid	Barbiturates	⬆	The anesthesia produced by thiopental may be extended or achieved at lower doses.
Probenecid	Benzodiazepines	⬆	A more rapid onset or more prolonged benzodiazepine effect may occur.
Probenecid	Clofibrate	⬆	Accumulation of clofibric acid (active metabolite of clofibrate) may occur, leading to higher steady-state serum concentrations.
Probenecid	Dapsone	⬆	Possible accumulation of dapsone and its metabolites.
Probenecid	Dyphylline	⬆	Increased half-life and decreased clearance of dyphylline may occur. This may be beneficial in extending the dyphylline dosing interval.
Probenecid	Methotrexate	⬆	Methotrexate's plasma levels, therapeutic effects and toxicity may be enhanced.
Probenecid	NSAIDs	⬆	NSAID plasma levels may be increased; toxicity may be enhanced.
Probenecid	Pantothenic acid	⬆	Renal transport of pantothenic acid may be inhibited; plasma levels may increase.
Probenecid	Penicillamine	⬆	Pharmacologic effects of penicillamine may be attenuated.
Probenecid	Rifampin	⬆	Renal transport of rifampin may be inhibited; plasma levels may increase.
Probenecid	Sulfonamides	⬆	Renal transport of sulfonamides may be inhibited; plasma levels may increase.
Probenecid	Sulfonylureas	⬆	Half-life of sulfonylureas may be increased.
Probenecid	Zidovudine	⬆	Increased zidovudine bioavailability may occur; cutaneous eruptions accompanied by systemic symptoms including malaise, myalgia or fever have occurred.
Salicylates	Probenecid	⬇	Coadministration may inhibit the uricosuric action of either drug alone.

* ⬆ = Object drug increased. ⬇ = Object drug decreased.

Drug/Lab test interactions: A reducing substance may appear in the urine during therapy. Although this disappears with discontinuation, a false diagnosis of glycosuria may be made. Confirm suspected glycosuria by using a test specific for glucose.

A falsely high determination of **theophylline** has occurred in vitro using the Schack and Waxler technique when therapeutic concentrations of theophylline and probenecid were added to human plasma.

Probenecid may inhibit the renal excretion of: **Phenolsulfonphthalein (PSP), 17–ketosteroids** and **sulfobromophthalein (BSP)**.

Adverse Reactions:

Headache; anorexia; nausea; vomiting; urinary frequency; hypersensitivity reactions (including anaphylaxis, dermatitis, pruritus and fever; see Warnings); sore gums; flushing; dizziness; anemia; hemolytic anemia (possibly related to G-6-PD deficiency); nephrotic syndrome; hepatic necrosis; aplastic anemia; exacerbation of gout; uric acid stones with or without hematuria; renal colic or costovertebral pain.

Patient Information:

Avoid taking aspirin or other salicylates that antagonize the effects of probenecid.

May cause GI upset; may be taken with food or antacids. If nausea, vomiting or loss of appetite persists, notify physician.

Uricosurics

PROBENECID

Drink plenty of water, at least 6 to 8 full (8 oz) glasses daily, to prevent development of kidney stones.

Administration and Dosage:

Gout: Do not start therapy until an acute gouty attack has subsided. However, if an acute attack is precipitated during therapy, probenecid may be continued. Give full therapeutic doses of colchicine or other appropriate therapy to control the acute attack.

Adults – 0.25 g twice daily for 1 week, followed by 0.5 g twice daily thereafter. Gastric intolerance may indicate overdosage and may be reduced by decreasing dosage.

Renal function impairment – Some degree of renal impairment may be present in patients with gout. A daily dosage of 1 g may be adequate. However, if necessary, the daily dosage may be increased by 0.5 g increments every 4 weeks within tolerance (usually ≤ 2 g/day) if symptoms of gouty arthritis are not controlled or the 24-hour urate excretion is not ≤ 700 mg. Probenecid may not be effective in chronic renal insufficiency, particularly when the glomerular filtration rate is ≤ 30 ml/min.

Urinary alkalinization – Urates tend to crystallize out of an acid urine; therefore, a liberal fluid intake is recommended, as well as sufficient sodium bicarbonate (3 to 7.5 g/day) or potassium citrate (7.5 g/day) to maintain an alkaline urine; continue alkalization until the serum uric acid level returns to normal limits and tophaceous deposits disappear. Thereafter, urinary alkalization and the restriction of purine-producing foods may be relaxed.

Maintenance therapy – Continue the dosage that maintains normal serum uric acid levels. When there have been no acute attacks for ≥ 6 months and serum uric acid levels have remained within normal limits, decrease the daily dosage by 0.5 g every 6 months. Do not reduce the maintenance dosage to the point where serum uric acid levels increase.

Penicillin or cephalosporin therapy: The phenolsulfonphthalein excretion test (PSP) may be used to determine the effectiveness of probenecid in retarding penicillin excretion and maintaining therapeutic levels. The renal clearance of PSP is reduced to ⅕ the normal rate when dosage of probenecid is adequate.

Adults – 2 g/day in divided doses. Reduce dosage in older patients in whom renal impairment may be present. Not recommended in conjunction with penicillin or a cephalosporin in the presence of known renal impairment.

Children (2 to 14 yrs) – Initial dose 25 mg/kg or 0.7 g/m^2 body surface. Maintenance dose 40 mg/kg/day or 1.2 g/m^2 body surface divided into 4 doses. For children weighing > 50 kg (110 lbs), use the adult dosage. Do not use in children < 2 years of age.

Gonorrhea (uncomplicated) – Give probenecid as a single 1 g dose immediately before or with 4.8 million units penicillin G procaine, aqueous, divided into at least two doses.

Neurosyphilis – Aqueous procaine penicillin G, 2.4 million units/day IM plus probenecid 500 mg orally 4 times daily, both for 10 to 14 days†.

Pelvic inflammatory disease (PID) – Cefoxitin 2 g IM plus probenecid, 1 g orally in a single dose concurrently.

Rx	**Probenecid** (Various, eg, Geneva, Goldline, Moore, Parmed, Purepac, Schein, URL)	**Tablets:** 0.5 g	In 100s and 1000s.
	Benemid (MSD)		(MSD 501). White. In 100s.
	Benuryl (ICN)		(ICN B11). White, scored. In 100s and 500s.

† CDC 1993 Sexually Transmitted Diseases Treatment Guidlines. *Morbidity and Mortality Weekly Report* 1993 Sept 24;42 (No. RR-14).

SULFINPYRAZONE

Actions:

Pharmacology: Sulfinpyrazone, a pyrazolidine derivative, is a potent uricosuric agent that inhibits renal tubular reabsorption of uric acid, thereby reducing elevated blood uric acid levels and causing a slow depletion of urate deposits from around joints and in other tissues. It also exhibits antithrombotic and platelet inhibitory effects but lacks anti-inflammatory and analgesic properties of its congener, phenylbutazone. It reduces renal tubular secretion of organic anions (eg, antibiotics, sulfonamides) and displaces other anions bound extensively to plasma proteins (eg, tolbutamide, warfarin, phenytoin). Sulfinpyrazone is not intended for relief of an acute attack of gout.

Sulfinpyrazone competitively inhibits platelet prostaglandin synthesis, which prevents platelet aggregation.

Pharmacokinetics: Sulfinpyrazone is well absorbed after oral administration; 98% to 99% is bound to plasma proteins. The plasma half-life is ≈ 4 hours after IV administration. Approximately 50% of the orally administered dose appears in the urine after 24 hours: 90% as unchanged drug and 10% as it's active metabolite, N^1-p-hydroxyphenol.

Indications:

Gouty arthritis: Treatment of chronic and intermittent gouty arthritis.

Unlabeled uses: Sulfinpyrazone may decrease the incidence of sudden cardiac death when given to patients 1 to 6 months post-myocardial infarction 300 mg 4 times daily; Sulfinpyrazone may decrease the frequency of systemic embolism in patients with rheumatic mitral stenosis.

A placebo controlled study of 186 patients with rheumatic mitral stenosis suggested that sulfinpyrazone may decrease the frequency of systemic embolism.

Contraindications:

Active peptic ulcer or symptoms of GI inflammation or ulceration; hypersensitivity to phenylbutazone or other pyrazoles; blood dyscrasias.

Warnings:

Secondary hyperuricemia: Do not use sulfinpyrazone to control hyperuricemia secondary to the treatment of malignant disease.

Renal function impairment: Periodically assess renal function. Renal failure has occurred, but a cause and effect relationship has not always been clearly established.

Pregnancy: Use only when clearly needed and when the potential benefits outweigh the potential hazards to the fetus.

Precautions:

Monitoring: Keep patients under close medical supervision; perform periodic blood counts.

Healed peptic ulcer: Administer with care.

Alkalinization of urine: Because it is a potent uricosuric, sulfinpyrazone may precipitate acute gouty arthritis, urolithiasis and renal colic, especially in initial stages of therapy. Adequate fluid intake and alkalinization of the urine are recommended.

Uricosurics

SULFINPYRAZONE

Drug Interactions:

Sulfinpyrazone Drug Interactions			
Precipitant drug	Object drug*		Description
Sulfinpyrazone	Acetaminophen	↔	Risk of acetaminophen hepatotoxicity may be increased. Also, therapeutic effects of acetaminophen may be reduced.
Sulfinpyrazone	Anticoagulants, oral	↑	The anticoagulant activity of warfarin will likely be enhanced; hemorrhage could occur.
Sulfinpyrazone	Theophylline	↓	Plasma theophylline clearance may be increased, thus lowering plasma levels.
Sulfinpyrazone	Tolbutamide	↑	Decreased clearance and increased half-life of tolbutamide may occur; hypoglycemia may result. Glyburide was not affected in one study.
Sulfinpyrazone	Verapamil	↓	Increased clearance and decreased bioavailability of verapamil may occur.
Niacin	Sulfinpyrazone	↓	Sulfinpyrazone's uricosuric effect may be reduced.
Salicylates	Sulfinpyrazone	↓	Sulfinpyrazone's uricosuric effect may be suppressed.

* ↑ = Object drug increased. ↓ = Object drug decreased. ↔ = Undetermined effect.

Adverse Reactions:

Most frequent: Upper GI disturbances. Administer with food, milk or antacids; despite this precaution, the drug may aggravate or reactivate peptic ulcer.

Less frequent: Rash (in most instances did not necessitate discontinuing therapy); rare blood dyscrasias (eg, anemia, leukopenia, agranulocytosis, thrombocytopenia, aplastic anemia); bronchoconstriction in patients with aspirin-induced asthma.

Overdosage:

Symptoms: Nausea; vomiting; diarrhea; epigastric pain; ataxia; labored respiration; convulsions; coma. Possible symptoms seen after overdosage with other pyrazolidine derivatives: Anemia; jaundice; ulceration.

Treatment: No specific antidote. Treatment includes usual supportive measures. Refer to General Management of Acute Overdosage.

Patient Information:

May cause GI upset; take with food, milk or antacids.

Avoid aspirin and other products containing salicylates that may antagonize the action of sulfinpyrazone.

Drink at least 10 to 12 glasses (8 ounces each) of fluid daily.

Treatment should continue without interruption even during acute exacerbations.

Uricosurics

SULFINPYRAZONE

Administration and Dosage:

Initial: 200 to 400 mg daily in two divided doses, with meals or milk, gradually increasing when necessary to full maintenance dosage in 1 week.

Maintenance: 400 mg daily in two divided doses; may increase to 800 mg daily or reduce to as low as 200 mg daily after the blood urate level has been controlled. Continue treatment without interruption even in the presence of acute exacerbations, which can be concomitantly treated with phenylbutazone or colchicine. Patients previously controlled with other uricosuric therapy may be transferred to sulfinpyrazone at full maintenance dosage.

Rx	**Sulfinpyrazone** (Various, eg, Barr, Goldline, Major, Rugby, Schein)	**Tablets:** 100 mg	In 100s and 500s.
Rx	**Anturane** (Ciba)		(Ciba 41). White, scored. In 100s.
Rx	**Sulfinpyrazone** (Various, eg, Barr, Goldline, Major, Rugby, Schein, Zenith)	**Capsules:** 200 mg	In 100s, 500s and 1000s.
Rx	**Anturane** (Ciba)		(Anturane 200 Ciba 168). Green. In 100s.

ALLOPURINOL

Actions:

Pharmacology: Allopurinol inhibits xanthine oxidase, the enzyme responsible for the conversion of hypoxanthine and xanthine to uric acid. Allopurinol is metabolized to oxipurinol (alloxanthine), which is also an inhibitor of xanthine oxidase. Allopurinol acts on purine catabolism, reducing the production of uric acid, without disrupting the biosynthesis of vital purines.

Reutilization of both hypoxanthine and xanthine for nucleotide and nucleic acid synthesis is markedly enhanced when their oxidation is inhibited by allopurinol. However, this does not disrupt normal nucleic acid anabolism because feedback inhibition is an integral part of purine biosynthesis. The serum concentration of hypoxanthine plus xanthine in patients receiving allopurinol for hyperuricemia usually ranges from 0.3 to 0.4 mg/dl compared with a normal level of ≈ 0.15 mg/dl. A maximum of 0.9 mg/dl of these oxypurines has been reported when the serum urate was lowered to < 2 mg/dl by high doses of allopurinol. These values are far below the saturation levels, at which point their precipitation would occur (> 7 mg/dl).

Administration generally results in a fall in both serum and urinary uric acid within 2 to 3 days. The magnitude of this decrease is dose-dependent. One week or more of treatment may be required before the full effects of the drug are manifested; likewise, uric acid may return to pretreatment levels slowly following cessation of therapy. This reflects primarily the accumulation and slow clearance of oxipurinol. In some patients, a dramatic fall in urinary uric acid excretion may not occur, particularly in those with severe tophaceous gout. This may be caused by the mobilization of urate from tissue deposits as the serum uric acid level begins to fall.

Pharmacokinetics: Allopurinol is ≈ 90% absorbed from the GI tract. Peak plasma levels occur at 1.5 hours and 4.5 hours for allopurinol and oxipurinol, respectively. After a single 300 mg dose, maximum plasma levels of ≈ 3 mcg/ml of allopurinol and 6.5 mcg/ml of oxipurinol are produced.

Allopurinol has a plasma half-life of ≈1 to 2 hours. However, oxipurinol has a plasma half-life of ≈ 15 hours. Therefore, effective xanthine oxidase inhibition is maintained for 24 hours with single daily doses. Allopurinol is cleared essentially by glomerular filtration; oxipurinol is reabsorbed in the kidney tubules in a manner similar to the reabsorption of uric acid. Approximately 20% is excreted in the feces.

The clearance of oxipurinol is increased by uricosuric drugs, and as a consequence, the addition of a uricosuric may reduce the degree of xanthine oxidase inhibition by oxipurinol and increase the urinary uric acid excretion. Some patients may benefit from combined therapy and may achieve minimum serum uric acid levels, provided the total urinary uric acid load does not exceed the competence of the patient's renal function.

Indications:

Gout: Management of signs and symptoms of primary or secondary gout (acute attacks, tophi, joint destruction, uric acid lithiasis or nephropathy).

Malignancies: Management of patients with leukemia, lymphoma and malignancies receiving therapy that causes elevations of serum and urinary uric acid. Discontinue allopurinol when the potential for overproduction of uric acid is no longer present.

Calcium oxalate calculi: Management of patients with recurrent calcium oxalate calculi whose daily uric acid excretion exceeds 800 mg/day (males) or 750 mg/day (females). Carefully assess therapy initially and periodically to determine that treatment is beneficial and that the benefits outweigh the risks.

Unlabeled uses: Allopurinol mouthwash (20 mg in 3% methylcellulose; 1 mg/ml) has been used successfully to prevent fluorouracil-induced stomatitis; 600 mg/day ameliorated the granulocyte suppressant effect of fluorouracil.

ALLOPURINOL

Recent studies suggest a role for allopurinol in the prevention of ischemic reperfusion tissue damage; to reduce the incidence of perioperative mortality and postoperative arrhythmias in coronary artery bypass surgery patients (300 mg 12 hours and 1 hour before surgery); to reduce relapse rates of *H. pylori*-induced duodenal ulcers and treatment of hematemesis from NSAID-induced erosive gastritis (50 mg four times daily); to alleviate pain related to acute pancreatitis (50 mg 4 times/day, rectally); to ex vivo preservation and function of organs for liver and kidney transplantation by supplementing preservation solutions with allopurinol; and to reduce rejection episodes in adult cadaver renal transplant recipients by adding low-dose allopurinol 25 mg on alternate days to a triple immunosuppressive regimen of azathioprine/cyclosporine/prednisolone. Allopurinol 20 mg/kg for 15 days has been used successfully against *Leishmania* in the treatment of American cutaneous leishmaniasis and against *Trypanosoma cruzi*; for Chagas' disease (600 to 900 mg/day for 60 days); and as an alternative for patients with epileptic seizures refractory to standard therapy (150 mg/day for children < 20 kg, otherwise 300 mg/day).

Contraindications:

Do not restart patients who have developed a severe reaction to the drug.

Warnings:

Asymptomatic hyperuricemia: This drug is not innocuous. Do not use to treat asymptomatic hyperuricemia.

Skin rash, usually maculopapular, sometimes scaly or exfoliative, is most common. Incidence of skin rash may be increased in renal disorders. Skin reactions can be severe and sometimes fatal; therefore, discontinue therapy at the first sign of rash. The most severe reactions also include: Fever; chills; arthralgias; cholestatic jaundice; eosinophilia; mild leukocytosis; leukopenia.

Hepatotoxicity: A few cases of reversible clinical hepatotoxicity have occurred; in some patients, asymptomatic rises in serum alkaline phosphatase or serum transaminase levels have been observed. If anorexia, weight loss or pruritis develop in patients on allopurinol, evaluation of liver function should be part of their diagnostic workup. Perform periodic liver function tests during early stages of therapy, particularly in patients with preexisting liver disease.

Hypersensitivity: Discontinue at first appearance of skin rash or other signs of allergic reactions. In some instances, rash may be followed by more severe hypersensitivity reactions such as exfoliative, urticarial or purpuric lesions, or Stevens-Johnson syndrome (erythema multiforme exudativum), generalized vasculitis, irreversible hepatotoxicity and rarely, death. Refer to Management of Acute Hypersensitivity Reactions.

Renal function impairment: Some patients with preexisting renal disease or poor urate clearance have increased BUN during allopurinol administration. Although the mechanism has not been established, patients with impaired renal function require less drug and careful observation during the early stages of treatment; reduce dosage or discontinue therapy if increased abnormalities in renal function appear and persist.

In patients with severely impaired renal function or decreased urate clearance, the plasma half-life of oxipurinol is greatly prolonged (See Administration and Dosage).

Renal failure in association with allopurinol has been observed among patients with hyperuricemia secondary to neoplastic diseases. Concurrent conditions such as multiple myeloma and congestive myocardial disease were present. Renal failure is also frequently associated with gouty nephropathy and rarely with allopurinol-associated hypersensitivity reactions. Albuminuria has occurred among patients who developed clinical gout following chronic glomerulonephritis and chronic pyelonephritis.

Pregnancy: Category C. There are no adequate and well controlled studies in pregnant women. Use only when clearly needed.

Lactation: Allopurinol and oxipurinol have been found in breast milk. Exercise caution when administering to a nursing woman.

Children: Allopurinol is rarely indicated for use in children, with the exception of those with hyperuricemia secondary to malignancy or in certain rare inborn errors of purine metabolism.

ALLOPURINOL

Precautions:

Monitoring: Periodically determine liver and kidney function especially during the first few months of therapy. Perform BUN, serum creatinine or creatinine clearance and reassess the patient's dosage.

Acute attacks of gout have increased during the early stages of allopurinol administration, even when normal or subnormal serum uric acid levels have been attained; in general, give maintenance doses of colchicine prophylactically when allopurinol is begun. The attacks usually become shorter and less severe after several months of therapy. A possible explanation for these episodes may be the mobilization of urates from tissue deposits, which causes fluctuations in the serum uric acid level. Even with adequate therapy, it may require several months to deplete the uric acid pool sufficiently to control acute episodes.

Fluid intake sufficient to yield a daily urinary output of ≥ 2 L and the maintenance of a neutral or slightly alkaline urine are desirable to avoid the theoretic possibility of formation of xanthine calculi under the influence of allopurinol therapy and to help prevent renal precipitation of urates in patients receiving concomitant uricosurics.

Drowsiness has occurred occasionally. Patients should observe caution while driving or performing other tasks requiring alertness, coordination or physical dexterity.

Bone marrow depression has occurred in patients receiving allopurinol, most of whom received concomitant drugs with the potential for causing this reaction. This has occurred as early as 6 weeks to 6 years after the initiation of therapy. Rarely, a patient may develop varying degrees of bone marrow depression, affecting one or more cell lines, while receiving allopurinol alone.

Drug Interactions:

Allopurinol Drug Interactions

Precipitant drug	Object drug*		Description
Allopurinol	Ampicillin	↑	The rate of ampicillin-induced skin rash appears much higher with allopurinol coadministration than with either drug alone.
Allopurinol	Anticoagulants, oral	↑	Data are conflicting. The anticoagulant action of some agents may be enhanced, but probably not that of warfarin.
Allopurinol	Cyclophosphamide	↑	Myelosuppressive effects of cyclophosphamide may be enhanced, possibly increasing the risk of bleeding or infection.
Allopurinol	Theophyllines	↑	Theophylline clearance may be decreased with large allopurinol doses (600 mg/day) leading to increased plasma theophylline levels and possible toxicity.
Allopurinol	Thiopurines	↑	Clinically significant increases in pharmacologic and toxic effects of oral thiopurines have occurred.
ACE Inhibitors	Allopurinol	↑	There is possibly a higher risk of hypersensitivity reaction when these agents are coadministered than when each drug is administered alone.
Aluminum salts	Allopurinol	↓	Pharmacologic effects of allopurinol may be decreased.
Thiazide diuretics	Allopurinol	↑	Coadministration may increase the incidence of hypersensitivity reactions to allopurinol.
Uricosuric agents	Allopurinol	↓	Uricosuric agents that increase the excretion of urate are also likely to increase the excretion of oxipurinol and thus lower the degree of inhibition of xanthine oxidase.

* ↑ = Object drug increased. ↓ = Object drug decreased.

ALLOPURINOL

Adverse Reactions:

CNS: Headache; peripheral neuropathy; neuritis; paresthesia; somnolence.

Dermatologic: Skin rash (See Warnings); vesicular bullous dermatitis; eczematoid dermatitis; pruritus; urticaria; onycholysis; *lichen planus*; Stevens-Johnson syndrome (erythema multiforme exudativum); purpura; toxic epidermal necrolysis (Lyell's syndrome).

GI: Nausea; vomiting; diarrhea; intermittent abdominal pain; gastritis; dyspepsia.

Hematologic: Leukopenia; leukocytosis; eosinophilia; thrombocytopenia.

Hepatic: Increased alkaline phosphatase, AST and ALT; hepatomegaly; cholestatic jaundice; granulomatous hepatitis; hepatic necrosis.

Miscellaneous: Arthralgia; acute attacks of gout; ecchymosis; fever; myopathy; epistaxis; taste loss or perversion; renal failure; uremia; alopecia; hypersensitivity vasculitis; necrotizing angitis.

The following have occurred in < 1% of patients; causal relationship is unknown:

Cardiovascular – Pericarditis; peripheral vascular disease; thrombophlebitis; bradycardia; vasodilation.

CNS – Optic neuritis; confusion; dizziness; vertigo; foot drop; depression; amnesia; tinnitis; asthenia; insomnia; malaise.

Dermatologic – Furunculosis; facial edema; sweating; skin edema.

Endocrine – Infertility, gynecomastia (male); hypercalcemia.

GI – Hemorrhagic pancreatitis; GI bleeding; stomatitis; salivary gland swelling; hyperlipidemia; tongue edema; anorexia.

GU – Nephritis; impotence; primary hematuria; albuminuria.

Hematologic – Eosinophilic fibrohistiocytic lesion of bone marrow; prothrombin decrease; reticulocytosis; lymphadenopathy; lymphocytosis; hemolytic and aplastic anemia; agranulocytosis; pancytopenia; anemia.

Ophthalmic – Macular retinitis; iritis; conjunctivitis; amblyopia; cataracts.

Respiratory – Bronchospasm; asthma; pharyngitis; rhinitis.

Miscellaneous – Myalgia; decrease in libido.

Overdosage:

Both allopurinol and oxipurinol are dialyzable; however, the usefulness of hemodialysis or peritoneal dialysis in the management of allopurinol overdose is unknown.

Patient Information:

Allopurinol is better tolerated if taken with food or milk. A fluid intake, sufficient to yield a daily urinary output of ≥ 2 L and the maintenance of a neutral or, preferably, slightly alkaline urine are desirable. Drink ≥ 10 to 12 (8 oz.) glasses of fluids per day.

May produce drowsiness; observe caution while driving or performing other tasks requiring alertness, coordination or physical dexterity.

Notify physician if skin rash, painful urination, blood in the urine, irritation of the eyes or swelling of the lips and mouth occurs.

Remind patients to continue drug therapy prescribed for gouty attacks since optimal benefit may be delayed for 2 to 6 weeks.

Urinary acidification with large doses of vitamin C may increase the possibility of kidney stone formation.

Administration and Dosage:

Control of gout and hyperuricemia: The average dose is 200 to 300 mg/day for mild gout and 400 to 600 mg/day for moderately severe tophaceous gout. Divide doses that are > 300 mg. The minimum effective dose is 100 to 200 mg daily; the maximum recommended dose is 800 mg/day.

Children (6 to 10 years of age) – In secondary hyperuricemia associated with malignancy, give 300 mg daily; those < 6 years old are generally given 150 mg/day. Evaluate response after ≈ 48 hours of therapy and adjust dosage if necessary.

Another suggested dose is 1 mg/kg/day divided every 6 hours, to a maximum of 600 mg/day. After 48 hours of treatment, titrate dose according to serum uric acid levels.

ALLOPURINOL

Prevention of uric acid nephropathy during vigorous therapy of neoplastic disease: 600 to 800 mg daily for 2 to 3 days with a high fluid intake. Similar considerations govern dosage regulation for maintenance purposes in secondary hyperuricemia.

To reduce the possibility of flare-up of acute gouty attacks: Start with 100 mg daily and increase at weekly intervals by 100 mg (without exceeding the maximum recommended dosage) until a serum uric acid level of ≤ 6 mg/dl is attained.

Serum uric acid levels: Normal serum urate levels are usually achieved in 1 to 3 weeks. The upper limit of normal is ≈ 7 mg/dl for men and postmenopausal women and 6 mg/dl for premenopausal women. Do not rely on a single reading because estimation of uric acid may be difficult. By selecting the appropriate dose and using uricosuric agents in certain patients, it is possible to reduce the serum uric acid level to normal and, if desired, to hold it as low as 2 to 3 mg/dl indefinitely.

Renal function impairment: Accumulation of allopurinol and its metabolites can occur in renal failure; consequently, reduce the dose. With a creatinine clearance (Ccr) of 10 to 20 ml/min, 200 mg/day is suitable. When the Ccr is < 10 ml/min, do not exceed 100 mg/day. With extreme renal impairment (Ccr < 3 ml/min) the interval between doses may also need to be increased. The correct dosage is best determined by using the serum uric acid level as an index.

Suggested Allopurinol doses	
Ccr (ml/min)	Dose
60	200 mg/day
40	15 mg/day
20	100 mg/day
10	100 mg on alternate days
< 10	100 mg 3 times/week

Concomitant therapy: In patients treated with colchicine or anti-inflammatory agents, continue therapy while adjusting the allopurinol dosage until a normal serum uric acid level and freedom from acute attacks have been maintained for several months.

Replacement therapy: In transferring a patient from a uricosuric agent to allopurinol, gradually reduce the dose of the uricosuric agent over several weeks and gradually increase the dose of allopurinol until a normal serum uric acid level is maintained.

Recurrent calcium oxalate stones: For hyperuricosuric patients, 200 to 300 mg/day in single or divided doses. Adjust dose up or down depending upon the resultant control of the hyperuricosuria based upon subsequent 24- hour urinary urate determinations. Patients may also benefit from dietary changes such as reduction of animal protein, sodium, refined sugars, oxalate-rich foods and excessive calcium intake as well as increase in oral fluids and dietary fiber.

Storage/Stability: Store at 15° to 25°C (59° to 77°F) in a dry place.

Rx	**Allopurinol** (Various, eg, Boots, Geneva, Major, Mylan, Parmed, Vangard)	**Tablets**: 100 mg	In 100s, 500s, 1000s and UD 100s.
✱	**Purinol** (Horner)		White. Lactose. In 100s and 500s.
Rx	**Zyloprim** (Glaxo Wellcome)		Lactose. (Zyloprim 100). White, scored. In 100s.
Rx	**Allopurinol** (Various, eg, Boots, Geneva, Major, Mylan, Parmed, Vangard)	**Tablets**: 300 mg	In 100s, 500s, 1000s and UD 100s.
✱	**Purinol** (Horner)		Salmon-colored. Lactose. In 100s and 500s.
Rx	**Zyloprim** (Glaxo Wellcome)		Lactose. (Zyloprim 300). Peach, scored. In 100s and 500s.

COLCHICINE

Actions:

Pharmacology: The exact mechanism of action of colchicine in gout is unknown. It is involved in leukocyte migration inhibition; reduction of lactic acid production by leukocytes that results in a decreased deposition of uric acid; interference with kinin formation; and reduction of phagocytosis with inflammatory response abatement.

Colchicine apparently exerts its effect by reducing the inflammatory response to the deposited crystals and also by diminishing phagocytosis. Colchicine directly diminishes lactic acid production by leukocytes and diminishes phagocytosis and thereby interrupting the cycle of urate crystal deposition and inflammatory response that sustains the acute attack. The oxidation of glucose in phagocytizing as well as in nonphagocytizing leukocytes in vitro is suppressed by colchicine.

Although it relieves pain in acute attacks, colchicine is not an analgesic. It is not a uricosuric and will not prevent the progression of gout to chronic gouty arthritis. Its prophylactic, suppressive effect helps reduce the incidence of acute attacks and relieves the patient's occasional residual pain and mild discomfort.

Colchicine can produce a temporary leukopenia, followed by leukocytosis.

Pharmacokinetics: Colchicine is rapidly absorbed after oral administration and is deacetylated primarily by the liver. It undergoes enterohepatic recirculation with large amounts of drug and metabolites present in bile and intestinal secretions. Peak plasma levels occur in 0.5 to 2 hours; plasma half-life is 10 to 60 minutes. Colchicine concentrates in leukocytes with leukocyte half-life values of ≤ 46 hours and detectable drug levels in urine and leukocytes for ≤ 10 days. High concentrations are also found in the kidney, liver and spleen. Colchicine is moderately plasma protein bound (≈ 50%); volume of distribution is 1 to 3 L/kg. Excretion occurs primarily by biliary and renal routes; 10% to 20% is eliminated unchanged in urine.

Indications:

Gout: Relieves pain of acute attacks, especially if adequate doses are given early in the attack. Many therapists use colchicine as interval therapy to prevent acute attacks. Recommended for regular prophylactic use between attacks and is often effective in aborting an attack when taken at the first sign of articular discomfort.

Colchicine IV is used when rapid response is desired or GI side effects interfere with oral use. Occasionally, it is effective when the oral preparation is not. After the acute attack has subsided, the patient can usually be given oral colchicine.

Unlabeled uses: Currently has orphan drug designation for arresting the progression of neurologic disability caused by chronic progressive multiple sclerosis.

Familial Mediterranean fever (1 to 3 mg/day); to lessen frequency and severity of acute febrile episodes and to prevent amyloidosis.

Hepatic cirrhosis (1 mg/day for 5 days a week).

Primary biliary cirrhosis (0.6 mg twice daily). Further study is needed.

Adjunctive treatment of primary amyloidosis (0.5 mg once or twice daily).

Treatment of Behçet's disease (0.5 to 1.5 mg/day).

Pseudogout caused by chondrocalcinosis (0.6 mg twice daily).

Refractory idiopathic thrombocytopenic purpura (1.2 to 1.8 mg/day ≥ 2 weeks).

Skin manifestations of scleroderma (progressive systemic sclerosis; 1 mg/day).

Various dermatologic disorders including: Psoriasis (0.02 mg/kg/day); palmoplantar pustulosis (0.5 to 1 mg/day); dermatitis herpetiformis (0.6 mg 2 or 3 times daily); pyoderma gangrenosum associated with Crohn's disease (1 mg/day).

Contraindications:

Hypersensitivity to colchicine; serious GI, renal, hepatic or cardiac disorders; blood dyscrasias.

Warnings:

Renal/Hepatic function impairment: Increased colchicine toxicity may occur. IV colchicine is not recommended in patients with severe renal/hepatic dysfunction.

Fertility impairment: Colchicine arrests cell division in animals and plants. It has adversely affected spermatogenesis in humans and in some animal species.

Elderly: Administer colchicine with great caution to elderly and debilitated patients.

Pregnancy: Category C (Parenteral – Category D). Colchicine can cause fetal harm when administered to a pregnant woman. Use only when clearly needed and when the potential benefits outweigh the potential hazards to the fetus.

Lactation: It is not known whether this drug is excreted in breast milk. Exercise caution when administering colchicine to a nursing woman.

Children: Safety and efficacy for use in children have not been established.

Precautions:

Monitoring: Perform periodic blood counts in patients receiving long-term therapy.

COLCHICINE

GI effects: Vomiting, diarrhea, abdominal pain and nausea may occur, especially with maximum doses. These may be particularly troublesome with peptic ulcer or spastic colon. At toxic doses, colchicine may cause severe diarrhea, generalized vascular damage and renal damage with hematuria and oliguria. GI symptoms may occur with IV therapy, usually large doses. To avoid more serious toxicity, discontinue use when these symptoms appear, regardless of whether joint pain has been relieved.

Thrombophlebitis rarely occurs at the site of IV injection.

Myopathy and neuropathy: Colchicine myoneuropathy commonly causes weakness in patients on standard therapy who have elevated plasma levels because of altered renal function. It is often unrecognized and misdiagnosed as polymyositis or uremic neuropathy. Proximal weakness and elevated serum creatine kinase are generally present and resolve in 3 to 4 weeks following drug withdrawal.

Malabsorption of vitamin B_{12}: Colchicine induces reversible malabsorption of vitamin B_{12}, apparently by altering the function of ileal mucosa.

Drug Interactions:

Drug/Lab test interactions: Decreased **thrombocyte** values may be obtained. Colchicine may cause false-positive results when testing **urine** for **RBC** or **hemoglobin**.

Adverse Reactions:

Bone marrow depression with aplastic anemia; agranulocytosis or thrombocytopenia (long-term therapy); peripheral neuritis; purpura; myopathy (see Precautions); loss of hair; reversible azoospermia; dermatoses; hypersensitivity; vomiting, diarrhea, abdominal pain, nausea (see Precautions).

Lab test abnormalities: Elevated alkaline phosphatase and AST.

Overdosage:

Symptoms: There is usually a latent period of several hours between overdosage and symptom onset. The lethal dose is estimated to be 65 mg; however, deaths have occurred with as little as 7 mg IV, although higher doses have reportedly not been fatal. Cumulative IV doses > 4 mg have resulted in organ failure and death.

The first symptoms to appear are nausea, vomiting, abdominal pain and diarrhea. Fluid extravasation may lead to shock. Myocardial injury may be accompanied by ST-segment elevation, decreased contractility and profound shock. Muscle weakness or paralysis may occur and progress to respiratory failure. Hepatocellular damage, renal failure and lung parenchymal infiltrates may occur and, by the fifth day after overdose, leukopenia, thrombocytopenia and coagulopathy may also occur. If the patient survives, alopecia and stomatitis may occur. There is no clear separation of nontoxic, toxic and lethal doses. Diarrhea may be bloody suggesting hemorrhagic gastroenteritis. Burning sensations in throat, stomach and skin may occur. Extensive vascular damage may result in shock. Hematuria and oliguria may indicate kidney damage. Muscular weakness is marked, and an ascending paralysis of the CNS may develop. The patient usually remains conscious; however, delirium and convulsions may occur. Death may result from respiratory depression.

Treatment: Begin with gastric lavage (if too much time has not elapsed) and measures to prevent shock. Recent studies support the use of hemodialysis or peritoneal dialysis. Atropine and morphine may relieve abdominal pain. Respiratory assistance may be needed. Refer to General Management of Acute Overdosage.

Patient Information:

Notify physician if skin rash, sore throat, fever, unusual bleeding, bruising, tiredness, weakness, numbness or tingling occurs.

Discontinue medication as soon as gout pain is relieved or at the first sign of nausea, vomiting, stomach pain or diarrhea. If symptoms persist, notify physician.

Administration and Dosage:

Oral:

Acute gouty arthritis – Begin at the first warning of an acute attack. Usual initial dose is 1 to 1.2 mg; follow with 0.5 to 1.2 mg every 1 to 2 hours, until pain is relieved or nausea, vomiting or diarrhea occurs. (Opiates may be needed to control diarrhea.) After one or more attacks, a patient can often judge his requirement accurately enough to stop before the "diarrheal dose."

The total amount of colchicine needed to control pain and inflammation during an acute attack is 4 to 8 mg. Articular pain and swelling typically abate ≤ 12 hours and are usually gone in 24 to 48 hours. Wait 3 days before initiating a second course to minimize the possibility of cumulative toxicity.

If ACTH is used to treat a gouty arthritis attack, give colchicine ≥ 1 mg/day, and continue for a few days after ACTH is withdrawn.

Prophylaxis during intercritical periods – To reduce the frequency and severity of paroxysms, administer continuously. If patients have < 1 attack/year, the usual dose

COLCHICINE

is 0.5 to 0.6 mg/day for 3 or 4 days a week; if > 1 attack/year, the usual dose is 0.5 to 0.6 mg/day. Severe cases may require 1 to 1.8 mg/day.

Prophylaxis in patients undergoing surgery – In patients with gout, an attack may be precipitated by even a minor surgical procedure. Administer 0.5 or 0.6 mg 3 times/day for 3 days before and 3 days after surgery.

Parenteral: For IV use only. Severe local irritation occurs if given SC or IM. If leakage into surrounding tissue or outside the vein should occur, considerable irritation and possible tissue damage may follow. There is no specific antidote. Local application of heat or cold and the use of analgesics may afford relief.

Administer for 2 to 5 minutes. Do not dilute with 5% Dextrose in Water. If a decrease in concentration of colchicine is required, use 0.9% Sodium Chloride Injection, which does not contain a bacteriostatic agent. Do not use turbid solutions.

Treatment of acute gouty arthritis – Average initial dose is 2 mg. This may be followed by 0.5 mg every 6 hours until a satisfactory response is achieved. Do not exceed a total dosage of 4 mg for a 24-hour period. Do not exceed a total dosage of 4 mg for one course of treatment. Some clinicians recommend a single IV dose of 3 mg, while others recommend ≤ 1 mg IV for the initial dose followed by 0.5 mg once or twice daily if needed.

If pain recurs, it may be necessary to give 1 to 2 mg/day for several days; however, do not give more colchicine by any route for ≤ 7 days after a full course of IV therapy (4 mg). Transfer to oral colchicine with a dose similar to that given IV.

Prophylaxis or maintenance of recurrent or chronic gouty arthritis – 0.5 to 1 mg once or twice daily. Oral colchicine is preferable, usually in conjunction with a uricosuric agent.

Rx	**Colchicine** (Abbott)	**Tablets**: 0.5 mg (1/120 gr)	Sugar, sucrose. Sugar coated. In 100s.
Rx	**Colchicine** (Various, eg, West-ward)	**Tablets**: 0.6 mg (1/100 gr)	Lactose. In 100s, 250s, 1000s and UD 100s.
Rx	**Colchicine** (Lilly)	**Injection**: 1 mg (1/60 gr)	In 2 ml amps.

PROBENECID AND COLCHICINE COMBINATIONS

For prescribing information, refer to individual probenecid and colchicine monographs.

Indications:

Treatment of chronic gouty arthritis complicated by frequent, recurrent acute attacks.

Administration and Dosage:

Do not initiate therapy until an acute gouty attack has subsided. If an acute attack is precipitated during therapy, administer additional colchicine or other appropriate therapy to control the attack; do not alter the dose of probenecid.

Initial dosage: 1 tablet daily for 1 week, followed by 1 tablet twice daily. Gastric intolerance may indicate overdose; correct by decreasing dosage.

Fluid intake and urinary alkalinization: Maintain a liberal fluid intake and sufficient sodium bicarbonate (3 to 7.5 g daily) or potassium citrate (7.5 g daily) to maintain an alkaline urine. Alkalinize the urine until serum urate levels return to normal (maximum normal level in males: 6 mg/dl; in females: 5 mg/dl), and tophaceous deposits disappear (eg, when urinary excretion of urates is at a high level). Thereafter, urine alkalinization and the restriction of purine-producing foods may be relaxed.

Maintenance therapy: Continue therapy at the dosage needed to maintain normal serum urate levels. When there have been no acute attacks for ≥ 6 months and serum urate levels have remained normal, decrease daily dosage by 1 tablet every 6 months. Do not reduce to the point where serum urate levels begin to rise.

Renal function impairment: Some degree of renal impairment may be present in patients with gout. A daily dose of 2 tablets may be adequate for control. Increase the dose by 1 tablet every 4 weeks within tolerance (usually not ≥ 4 tablets/day) if symptoms of gouty arthritis are not controlled or the 24–hour urate excretion is not ≤ 700 mg. Probenecid may not be effective in chronic renal insufficiency, particularly when the glomerular filtration rate is ≤ 30 ml/min.

Rx	**Probenecid w/ Colchicine** (Various, eg, Rugby)	**Tablets** 500 mg probenecid /0.5 mg colchicine	In 100s and 1000s.
Rx	**Col-Probenecid** (Various, eg, URL)		In 100s.

In addition to the agents on the following pages, propranolol and timolol are indicated for migraine prophylaxis (see Beta-Adrenergic Blocking Agents monograph).

SUMATRIPTAN SUCCINATE

Actions:

Pharmacology: Sumatriptan, a selective agonist for a vascular 5-hydroxytryptamine$_1$ (serotonin) receptor subtype (probably a member of the 5-HT$_1$D family), has no significant affinity or pharmacological activity at 5-HT$_2$ or 5-HT$_3$ receptor subtypes or at alpha$_1$-, alpha$_2$- or beta-adrenergic, dopamine$_1$, dopamine$_2$, muscarinic or benzodiazepine receptors. The vascular 5-HT$_1$ receptor subtype to which sumatriptan binds selectively and through which it presumably exerts its antimigrainous effect is present on cranial arteries in dogs and primates, on the human basilar artery and in vasculature of the isolated human dura mater. In these tissues, sumatriptan activates this receptor to cause vasoconstriction, an action in humans correlating with the relief of migraine. In dogs, sumatriptan selectively reduces carotid arterial blood flow with little or no effect on arterial blood pressure or total peripheral resistance. In cats, sumatriptan selectively constricts carotid arteriovenous anastomoses with little effect on blood flow or resistance in cerebral or extracerebral tissues.

Physiologic responses –

Blood pressure (BP): Transient increases in systolic and diastolic BP may be observed after sumatriptan administration. In a study of hypertensive migraineurs with documented diastolic BP of ≥ 95 mmHg on two occasions during a migraine-free period, administration of 6 mg SC caused transient (usually < 1 hour) elevations of BP. Mean peak systolic and diastolic BP were both 6 mmHg above baseline; peak increases were usually within 30 minutes of injection. In controlled studies of migraine patients receiving 4 to 8 mg sumatriptan, clinically significant increases or decreases in BP were present in ≤ 1% of patients; identical results were observed with placebo. In elderly patients (age, 67 to 79 years) receiving a single dose of oral sumatriptan, statistically significant increases in mean peak systolic BP of up to 14 mmHg occurred over the first 3 hours; there was some evidence of increasing effect with dose. However, younger patients (age, 19 to 37 years) had no change in systolic BP. Diastolic BP increased between 2 and 6 mmHg in both groups of patients. No consistent effect on BP has been observed.

Peripheral (small) arteries: In healthy volunteers, after 8 mg, the mean toe-arm pressure gradient fell by 6.6 mmHg systolic during the first 2 hours postdose. The maximum decrease in systolic toe-arm gradient occurred at 1 hour postdose and returned to baseline values (a mean decrease of 8.3 mmHg) by 4 hours. These changes are interpreted as being slight and not indicating a clinically significant risk of peripheral vasospasm.

Heart rate: Overall, there was a mean decrease of 4 bpm associated with sumatriptan injection in two large studies; while not of clinical significance, it is possible that this was associated with relief of migraine.

Pharmacokinetics:

Injection – Following a 6 mg SC injection into the deltoid area in nine males, systemic clearance was 1194 ml/min, distribution half-life was 15 minutes, terminal half-life was 115 minutes and volume of distribution central compartment was 50 L. Of this dose, 22% was excreted in the urine as unchanged sumatriptan and 38% as the indole acetic acid metabolite. After a single 6 mg SC manual injection into the deltoid area in 18 healthy males, the maximum serum concentration (C_{max}) was 74 ng/ml and the time to peak concentration (T_{max}) was 12 minutes after injection (range, 5 to 20 minutes). In this study, the same dose injected SC in the thigh gave a C_{max} of 61 ng/ml by manual injection vs 52 ng/ml by autoinjector techniques. The T_{max} or amount absorbed were not significantly altered by either the site or technique of injection. The bioavailability via SC injection to 18 healthy male subjects was 97% of that obtained following IV injection.

Oral – Sumatriptan is rapidly absorbed after oral administration, with low absolute bioavailability (≈ 15%), primarily because of presystemic metabolism and partly because of incomplete absorption. Mean maximum concentration (C_{max}) following a 100 mg dose is 51 ng/ml vs 75 ng/ml following a 6 mg SC dose. C_{max} is similar during a migraine attack and during a migraine-free period, but the T_{max} is slightly later during the attack (≈ 2.5 vs 2 hours). The apparent volume of distribution is 2.4 L/kg. Elimination half-life is ≈ 2.5 hours. Sumatriptan is largely renally excreted (≈ 60%) with ≈ 40% found in the feces. Most excreted in the urine is the major metabolite, indole acetic acid (IAA), which is inactive, or the IAA glucuronide. Only 3% is recovered as unchanged drug.

Hepatic function impairment: The liver plays an important role in the presystemic clearance of orally administered sumatriptan. Accordingly, the bioavailability may be markedly increased in patients with liver disease (see Warnings).

Protein binding is low, ≈ 14% to 21%. In vitro, sumatriptan appears to be metabolized by monoamine oxidase (MAO), predominantly the A isoenzyme. The use of an

SUMATRIPTAN SUCCINATE

MAO-A inhibitor may increase sumatriptan's bioavailability (see Drug Interactions). The pharmacokinetics of sumatriptan in healthy elderly were similar to those in healthy younger subjects.

Clinical trials:

Injection – In clinical trials, onset of relief began as early as 10 minutes following a 6 mg injection. Smaller doses may also prove effective, although the proportion of patients obtaining adequate relief is decreased, and the latency to that relief is greater. In two clinical trials in 1104 migraine patients with moderate and severe migraine pain, the onset of relief was rapid (< 10 minutes). Headache relief, as evidenced by a reduction in pain from severe or moderately severe to mild or no headache, was achieved in 70% of the patients within 1 hour of single 6 mg SC doses. Headache relief was achieved in ≈ 82% of patients within 2 hours, and 65% of all patients were pain-free within 2 hours.

Sumatriptan Injection Efficacy Data[1] (%)

Parameters	One hour data		Two hour data	
	Placebo	Sumatriptan 6 mg	Placebo[2]	Sumatriptan 6 mg[3]
Patients with pain relief (grade 0/1)	18-26	70	31-39	81-82
Patients with no pain	5-13	48-49	11-19	63-65
Patients without nausea	48-50	73	56-63	81-82
Patients without photophobia	23-25	56-58	31-35	71-72
Patients with little or no clinical disability[4]	34	76	42-49	84-85

[1] Data pooled from 2 separate studies.

[2] Includes patients that may have received an additional placebo injection 1 hour after the initial injection.

[3] Includes patients that may have received an additional 6 mg sumatriptan injection 1 hour after the initial injection.

[4] A successful outcome in terms of clinical disability was defined prospectively as able to work mildly impaired or able to work and function normally.

Sumatriptan Injection Dose Response Relationship for Efficacy

Sumatriptan dose (mg)	Patients with relief[1] at 10 minutes (%)	Patients with relief[1] at 30 minutes (%)	Patients with relief[1] at 1 hour (%)	Patients with relief[1] at 2 hours (%)	Adverse events incidence (%)
Placebo	5	15	24	21	55
1	10	40	43	40	63
2	7	23	57	43	63
3	17	47	57	60	77
4	13	37	50	57	80
6	10	63	73	70	83
8	23	57	80	83	93

[1] Relief is defined as the reduction of moderate or severe pain to no or mild pain after dosing without use of rescue medication.

Sumatriptan also relieved photophobia, phonophobia (sound sensitivity) and nausea and vomiting associated with migraine attacks. Similar efficacy was seen when patients self-administered sumatriptan using an autoinjector.

Oral – In two studies, patients with migraine attacks experiencing moderate or severe pain were given 25, 50 and 100 mg single doses of sumatriptan. Onset of relief (no or mild pain) was seen as early as 1 to 1.5 hours after all three doses. There was no evidence of a dose response for pain and other measures of effectiveness. At 2 hours, ≈ 54% (range, 50% to 57%) of patients on any dose had achieved relief vs 17% to 26% with placebo. By 4 hours postdosing, response rates in drug-treated patients were ≈ 71% (range, 65% to 78%) vs 19% to 38% with placebo. Sumatriptan also relieved nausea and photophobia associated with migraine attacks.

SUMATRIPTAN SUCCINATE

Oral Sumatriptan Dose Response Relationship for Efficacy[1] (%)				
Parameters	Placebo	Sumatriptan 25 mg	Sumatriptan 50 mg	Sumatriptan 100 mg
	Two hour data			
Patients with pain relief (grade 0/1)	17-26	52	50-54	56-57
Patients with no pain	6-8	21	16-17	23-24
Patients with meaningful relief[2]	21-34	54-59	54-55	56-57
Patients without nausea	40-57	56-67	61-68	65-72
Patients without photophobia	13-22	29-41	26-37	39-44
Patients with little or no clinical disability[3]	28-35	58	52-60	59-67
	Four hour data			
Patients with pain relief (grade 0/1)	19-38	65-70	68-72	71-78
Patients with no pain	11-15	35-45	32-41	41-52
Patients with meaningful relief[2]	26-45	69-71	71-72	79-83
Patients without nausea	45-60	73-76	70-79	83-91
Patients without photophobia	28-40	62-69	65-66	65-71
Patients with little or no clinical disability[3]	23-40	68-73	70-71	71-83

[1] Data pooled from 2 separate studies.
[2] Meaningful relief is a patient assessment of when they felt onset of relief of headache pain.
[3] A successful outcome in terms of clinical disability was defined prospectively as ability to work mildly impaired or ability to work and function normally.

The efficacy of sumatriptan is unaffected by whether or not migraine is associated with aura, duration of attack, gender or age of the patient, relationship to menses or concomitant use of common migraine prophylactic drugs (eg, beta blockers, calcium blockers, tricyclic antidepressants).

Indications:

Migraine: Acute treatment of migraine attacks with or without aura and the acute treatment of cluster headache episodes.

Contraindications:

IV use (because of its potential to cause coronary vasospasm); patients with ischemic heart disease (angina pectoris, history of MI or documented silent ischemia) or patients with Prinzmetal's angina; patients with symptoms or signs consistent with ischemic heart disease; patients with uncontrolled hypertension (because it can cause increases in blood pressure, usually small); with concurrent ergotamine-containing preparations or concurrent MAO inhibitor therapy (or within 2 weeks of discontinuing an MAOI; see Drug Interactions); hypersensitivity to sumatriptan; management of hemiplegic or basilar migraine.

Warnings:

Migraine diagnosis: Use oral sumatriptan only where a clear diagnosis of migraine has been established. Do not administer to patients with basilar or hemiplegic migraine. Before treating headaches in patients not previously diagnosed as migraineurs and in migraineurs with atypical symptoms, take care to exclude other potentially serious neurological conditions.

Cardiac events/Coronary constriction: Serious coronary events, including some that have been fatal, following sumatriptan have occurred but are extremely rare. Although it is not clear how many of these can be attributed to sumatriptan, because of their potential to cause coronary vasospasm, do not give to patients in whom unrecognized coronary artery disease (CAD) is likely without a prior evaluation for underlying cardiovascular disease. Such patients include postmenopausal women, males > 40 years of age and patients with other risk factors for CAD such as hypertension, hypercholesterolemia, obesity, diabetes, smokers and strong family history of CAD. Following a satisfactory cardiovascular assessment, it is recommended that the first dose be given in the physician's office for patients with underlying risk factors for CAD unless they have previously received sumatriptan. If symptoms consistent with angina occur, carry out ECG evaluation to look for ischemic changes.

Sumatriptan may cause coronary vasospasm in patients with a history of CAD, who are known to be more susceptible to coronary artery vasospasm, and, rarely, in patients without history suggestive of CAD. In clinical trials, 8 of > 1900 patients receiving SC sumatriptan and 2 of 6348 receiving the oral form sustained clinical events during or shortly after receiving sumatriptan that may have reflected coronary vasospasm. Six of these eight SC patients had ECG changes consistent with transient ischemia, but without symptoms or signs. Of the eight patients, four had some findings suggestive of CAD prior to treatment. None of these adverse events with either doseform was associated with a serious clinical outcome.

There have been rare reports of serious or life-threatening arrhythmias, including atrial fibrillation, ventricular fibrillation, ventricular tachycardia and MI, as well as marked ischemic ST elevations associated with sumatriptan. In addition, there have been rare, but more frequent, reports of chest and arm discomfort thought to represent angina pectoris.

Fatalities: In extensive worldwide postmarketing experience, deaths have been reported following the use of sumatriptan. In most cases, these have occurred well after sumatriptan use (eg, ≥ 3 hours postdose) and probably reflect underlying disease and spontaneous events.

However, there have been several fatalities that occurred within a few hours after sumatriptan's use. The specific contribution of sumatriptan to most of these deaths cannot be determined, but in one case, a 41–year-old woman with a 6–day history of unilateral headache, uncertain history of cardiovascular disease with known risk factors (positive family history, postmenopausal woman, smoking) and a history of asthma and codeine allergy, experienced nausea, vomiting, a sense of warmth, chest pressure and sweating within 7 minutes of dosing. This was followed by hypotension at ≈ 30 minutes and ventricular tachycardia/fibrillation leading to death. In other cases, death was attributed to myocardial infarction occurring hours after drug administration.

Deaths attributed to strokes, cerebral hemorrhage and other cerebrovascular events have also been reported in patients treated with sumatriptan. In many cases, it appears possible that the cerebrovascular events were primary; sumatriptan having been administered in the incorrect belief that the symptoms experienced were migrainous in origin when they were not. Accordingly, it is important to advise patients not to administer sumatriptan if a headache being experienced is atypical.

Hypersensitivity: Hypersensitivity reactions have occurred on rare occasions, and severe anaphylaxis/anaphylactoid reactions have occurred. Such reactions can be life-threatening or fatal. Refer to Management of Acute Hypersensitivity Reactions.

Renal/Hepatic function impairment: Administer with caution to patients with diseases that may alter the absorption, metabolism or excretion of drugs. The liver plays an important role in the presystemic clearance of orally administered sumatriptan. Accordingly, the bioavailability may be markedly increased in patients with liver disease. In a small study of hepatically impaired patients, there was an ≈ 70% increase in AUC and C_{max} and a T_{max} 40 minutes earlier vs healthy subjects.

Fertility impairment: In male and female rats dosed daily with oral sumatriptan prior to and throughout mating, there was a treatment-related decrease in fertility secondary to a decrease in mating in animals treated with 50 and 500 mg/kg/day.

Elderly: Pharmacokinetic disposition of sumatriptan in the elderly is similar to that seen in younger adults.

Pregnancy: Category C. In rats and rabbits, sumatriptan is associated with embryolethality, fetal abnormalities and pup mortality. There are no adequate and well controlled studies in pregnant women. Use during pregnancy only if the potential benefit justifies the potential risk to the fetus.

Lactation: Sumatriptan is excreted in breast milk. Therefore, exercise caution when administering to a nursing woman.

Children: Safety and efficacy have not been established.

Precautions:

Chest, jaw or neck tightness is relatively common after sumatriptan administration, and atypical sensations over the precordium (tightness, pressure, heaviness) have occurred, but these have only rarely been associated with ischemic ECG changes.

Blood pressure changes: Sumatriptan injection may cause mild, transient elevation of blood pressure and peripheral vascular resistance (see Pharmacology).

Seizures: There have been rare reports of seizures following sumatriptan use.

SUMATRIPTAN SUCCINATE

Binding to melanin-containing tissues: Because sumatriptan binds to melanin, it could accumulate in melanin-rich tissues (such as the eye) over time, raising the possibility that toxicity in these tissues could occur after extended use. Be aware of the possibility of long-term ophthalmologic effects.

Corneal opacities: Sumatriptan causes corneal opacities and defects in dogs, raising the possibility that these changes may occur in humans. Be aware of the possibility of these changes.

Drug Interactions:

Sumatriptan Drug Interactions			
Precipitant drug	Object drug*		Description
MAO-A inhibitors	Sumatriptan	↑	MAOIs can markedly increase sumatriptan systemic exposure and affect its elimination. In one study, a marked increase in sumatriptan AUC and half-life occurred. The effect may be greater with the oral doseform. No effect was seen with selegiline, an MAO-B inhibitor. Do not use concurrently or within 2 weeks of discontinuing the MAOI.
Ergot-containing drugs	Sumatriptan	↑	Ergot-containing drugs have caused prolonged vasospastic reactions. Because there is a theoretical basis that these effects may be additive, avoid concurrent use within 24 hours of each other.

* ↑ = Object drug increased.

Drug/Food interactions: Food has no significant effect on oral sumatriptan bioavailability, but slightly delays the T_{max} by about 30 min.

Adverse Reactions:

Injection: In clinical trials of SC sumatriptan, up to 3.5% of patients withdrew for reasons related to adverse events.

Sumatriptan Injection Adverse Reactions (%)

Adverse reaction	Sumatriptan 6 mg SC (n = 547)	Placebo (n = 370)	Adverse reaction	Sumatriptan 6 mg SC (n = 547)	Placebo (n = 370)
Atypical sensations	42	9.2	*Musculoskeletal*		
Tingling	13.5	3	Weakness	4.9	0.3
Warm/Hot sensation	10.8	3.5	Neck pain/stiffness	4.8	0.5
Burning sensation	7.5	0.3	Myalgia	1.8	0.5
Feeling of heaviness	7.3	1.1	Muscle cramp(s)	1.1	0
Pressure sensation	7.1	1.6	*Chest discomfort*	4.5	1.4
Feeling of tightness	5.1	0.3	Tightness in chest	2.7	0.5
Numbness	4.6	2.2	Pressure in chest	1.8	0.3
Feeling strange	2.2	0.3	*Ear, nose and throat*		
Tight feeling in head	2.2	0.3	Throat discomfort	3.3	0.5
Cold sensation	1.1	0.5	Nasal cavity/sinus discomfort	2.2	0.3
Neurological					
Dizziness/vertigo	11.9	4.3	*Miscellaneous*		
Drowsiness/sedation	2.7	2.2	Injection site reaction	58.7	23.8
Headache	2.2	0.3	Flushing	6.6	2.4
Anxiety	1.1	0.5	Discomfort of mouth/ tongue	4.9	4.6
Malaise/fatigue	1.1	0.8			
GI			Jaw discomfort	1.8	0
Abdominal discomfort	1.3	0.8	Sweating	1.6	1.1
Dysphagia	1.1	0	Vision alterations	1.1	0

Cardiovascular: Hypertension, hypotension, bradycardia, tachycardia, palpitations, pulsating sensations, various transient ECG changes (non-specific ST or T wave changes, prolongation of PR or QTc intervals, sinus arrhythmia, nonsustained ventricular premature beats, isolated junctional ectopic beats, atrial ectopic beats, delayed activation of the right ventricle), syncope (0.1% to 1%); pallor, arrhythmia, abnormal pulse, vasodilation, Raynaud's syndrome (< 0.1%).

SUMATRIPTAN SUCCINATE

Serious or life-threatening arrhythmias, including atrial fibrillation, ventricular fibrillation, ventricular tachycardia, MI and marked ischemic ST elevations have been associated with sumatriptan. More often, there has been chest discomfort that appeared to represent angina pectoris.

Metabolic: Thirst (0.1% to 1%); polydipsia, dehydration (< 0.1%).

GI: Gastroesophageal reflux, diarrhea, disturbances of liver function tests (0.1% to 1%); peptic ulcer, retching, flatulence/eructation, gallstones (< 0.1%).

Musculoskeletal: Various joint disturbances (pain, stiffness, swelling, ache) (0.1% to 1%); muscle stiffness, need to flex calf muscles, backache, muscle tiredness, swelling of the extremities (< 0.1%).

CNS: Mental confusion, euphoria, agitation, relaxation, chills, sensation of lightness, tremor, shivering, taste disturbances, prickling sensations, paresthesia, stinging sensations, headaches, facial pain, photophobia, lacrimation (0.1% to 1%); transient hemiplegia, hysteria, globus hystericus, intoxication, depression, myoclonia, monoplegia/diplegia, sleep disturbance, difficulties in concentration, smell disturbances, hyperesthesia, dysesthesia, simultaneous hot and cold sensations, tickling sensations, dysarthria, yawning, reduced appetite, hunger, dystonia (< 0.1%).

Respiratory: Dyspnea (0.1% to 1%); influenza, diseases of the lower respiratory tract, hiccoughs (< 0.1%).

Dermatologic: Erythema, pruritus, skin rashes, eruptions (0.1% to 1%); skin tenderness (< 0.1%).

GU: Dysuria, urinary frequency, dysmenorrhea, renal calculus (< 0.1%).

Miscellaneous: Miscellaneous laboratory abnormalities (including minor disturbances in liver function tests), "serotonin agonist effect," hypersensitivity to various agents, eye irritation (0.1% to 1%); fever (< 0.1%).

Postmarketing experience – Episodes of Prinzmetal's variant angina; MI; acute renal failure; seizure; CVA; dysphasia; subarachnoid hemorrhage; arrhythmias (atrial fibrillation, ventricular fibrillation and ventricular tachycardia).

Oral:

Oral Sumatriptan Adverse Reactions (%)

Adverse reaction	Placebo (n = 112)	Sumatriptan 25 mg (n = 114)	Sumatriptan 50 mg (n = 108)	Sumatriptan 100 mg (n = 112)
Atypical sensations				
Feeling of heaviness	< 1	< 1	< 1	2
Feeling of tightness	0	< 1	2	2
Pressure sensation	0	< 1	2	2
Tingling	4	8	4	5
Warm/Hot sensation	< 1	2	3	3
Cardiovascular				
Flushing	< 1	0	4	2
Palpitations	< 1	0	< 1	2
Special senses				
Nasal discomfort	4	5	5	7
Eye(s) irritation	0	0	0	2
Visual disturbance	< 1	0	< 1	3
Miscellaneous				
Weakness	0	2	< 1	2
Agitation	0	0	0	2
Dysuria	< 1	0	0	2

Other adverse reactions include the following:

Cardiovascular: Chest discomfort/pressure/heaviness/tightness (≥ 1%); arrhythmia, ECG changes, hypertension, hypotension, pallor, pulsating sensations, tachycardia (0.1% to 1%); angina, atherosclerosis, bradycardia, cerebral ischemia, cerebrovascular lesion, heart block, peripheral cyanosis, thrombosis, transient myocardial ischemia, vasodilation (< 0.1%).

Special senses: Throat symptoms (≥ 1%); hearing disturbances, smell disturbance, otalgia (0.1% to 1%); feeling of fullness in ear, disorders of sclera, mydriasis (< 0.1%).

Endocrine: Thirst (0.1% to 1%); elevated TSH levels, galactorrhea, hyperglycemia, hypoglycemia, hypothyroidism, polydipsia, weight gain/loss (< 0.1%).

SUMATRIPTAN SUCCINATE

GI: Diarrhea, gastric symptoms (≥ 1%); constipation, dysphagia, gastroesophageal reflux (0.1% to 1%); GI bleeding, hematemesis, melena, peptic ulcer (< 0.1%); abdominal/mouth/tongue discomfort; taste disturbance; nausea/vomiting.

Musculoskeletal: Myalgia (≥ 1%); muscle cramps (0.1% to 1%); tetany (< 0.1%); neck stiffness.

CNS: Phonophobia, photophobia (≥ 1%); confusion, depression, difficulty concentrating, dysarthria, euphoria, facial pain, heat sensitivity, incoordination, lacrimation, monoplegia, sleep disturbance, shivering, syncope, tremor (0.1% to 1%); aggressiveness, apathy, bradylogia, cluster headache, convulsions, decreased appetite, drug abuse, dystonic reaction, facial paralysis, hallucinations, hunger, hyperesthesia, hysteria, increased alertness, memory disturbance, neuralgia, paralysis, personality change, phobia, radiculopathy, rigidity, suicide, twitching (< 0.1%); anxiety; headache; drowsiness/sedation; dizziness/vertigo; malaise/fatigue.

Respiratory: Dyspnea (≥ 1%); asthma (0.1% to 1%); hiccoughs (< 0.1%).

Dermatologic: Sweating (≥ 1%); erythema, pruritus, rash, skin tenderness (0.1% to 1%); dry/scaly skin, tightness/wrinkling of skin (< 0.1%).

GU: Breast tenderness, dysmenorrhea, increased urination, intermenstrual bleeding (0.1% to 1%); nipple discharge, abortion, hematuria (< 0.1%).

Miscellaneous: Hypersensitivity (including rash, urticaria, pruritus, erythema, shortness of breath; see Warnings), burning sensation, numbness, paresthesia (≥ 1%); tight feeling in head, cough, fever, fluid retention, overdose (0.1% to 1%); dysesthesia, hot/cold sensation, anemia, edema, hematoma, lymphadenopathy, speech/voice disturbance (< 0.1%).

Postmarketing experience: Acute renal failure; angioneurotic edema; cardiomyopathy; cerebrovascular accident; cyanosis; deafness; death; disturbances of liver function tests; exacerbation of sunburn; hepatic impairment; intraocular disorders; ischemic optic neuropathy; pancytopenia; panic disorder; periorbital edema; photosensitivity; pulmonary embolism; retinal artery occlusion; shock; subarachnoid hemorrhage; temporal arteritis; thrombocytopenia; xerostomia.

Overdosage:

Symptoms: Patients and volunteers have received single injections from 8 to 12 mg and oral doses of 140 to 300 mg without significant adverse effects. Coronary vasospasm was observed after IV administration. Overdoses would be expected to possibly cause convulsions, tremor, inactivity, erythema of the extremities, reduced respiratory rate, cyanosis, ataxia, mydriasis, injection site reactions (desquamation, hair loss and scab formation) and paralysis.

Treatment: The elimination half-life of sumatriptan is ≈ 2 to 2.5 hours; therefore, continue monitoring of patients after overdose while symptoms or signs persist, and for at least 10 hours. It is unknown what effect hemodialysis or peritoneal dialysis has on the serum concentrations of sumatriptan.

Patient Information:

Patient information leaflet is provided for patients.

Injection: Although written instructions are supplied with the autoinjector, instruct patients who are advised to self-administer sumatriptan in medically unsupervised situations on the proper use of the product prior to doing so for the first time. Before using the autoinjector, see the enclosed instruction pamphlet on loading your autoinjector and discarding the empty syringes.

For adults, the usual dose is a single injection given just below the skin. Administer as soon as migraine symptoms appear, but it may be given at any time during an attack. A second injection may be given if your symptoms of migraine come back. Do not use > 2 injections in any 24 hours and allow at least 1 hour between each dose.

You may experience pain or redness at the site of injection, but this usually lasts < 1 hour.

Oral: Take a single dose with fluids as soon as symptoms of migraine appear; a second dose may be taken if symptoms return, but no sooner than 2 hours following the first dose. For a given attack, if you have no response to the first tablet, do not take a second tablet without first consulting with your doctor. Do not take > 300 mg in any 24–hour period.

If you have risk factors for heart disease (eg, high blood pressure, high cholesterol, obesity, diabetes, smoking, strong family history of heart disease, are postmenopausal or a male > 40 years of age) tell your physician.

Sumatriptan is intended to relieve your migraine, but not to prevent or reduce the number of attacks you experience. Use only to treat an actual migraine attack.

SUMATRIPTAN SUCCINATE

Do not use sumatriptan if you are pregnant, think you might be pregnant, are trying to become pregnant or are not using adequate contraception, unless you have discussed this with your physician.

If you experience pain or tightness in the chest or throat when using sumatriptan, then discuss it with your physician before using any more sumatriptan. If the chest pain is severe or does not go away, call your physician immediately.

If wheeziness; heart throbbing; swelling of eyelids, face or lips; or a skin rash, skin lumps or hives occur, then tell your physician immediately. Do not take any more sumatriptan unless your physician tells you to do so.

If you develop feelings of tingling, heat, flushing (redness of face lasting a short time), heaviness, pressure, drowsiness, dizziness, tiredness or sickness, tell your physician of these symptoms at your next visit.

Administration and Dosage:

Approved by the FDA on December 28, 1992.

Injection: The maximum single adult dose is 6 mg injected SC. Controlled clinical trials have failed to show that clear benefit is associated with the administration of a second 6 mg dose in patients who have failed to respond to a first injection.

The maximum recommended dose that may be given in 24 hours is two 6 mg injections separated by at least 1 hour. Although the recommended dose is 6 mg, if side effects are dose limiting, then lower doses may be used. In patients receiving doses < 6 mg, use only the single-dose vial dosage form. An autoinjection device is available for use with 6 mg prefilled syringes to facilitate self-administration in patients in whom this dose is deemed necessary.

Oral: Recommended adult dose is 25 mg taken with fluids; maximum recommended single dose is 100 mg. There is no evidence that an initial dose of 100 mg provides substantially greater relief than 25 mg.

If a satisfactory response has not been obtained at 2 hours, a second dose of up to 100 mg may be given. Efficacy of this second dose has not been examined. If headache returns, additional doses may be taken at intervals of at least 2 hours up to a daily maximum of 300 mg. If headache returns following an initial treatment with the injection, additional doses of single tablets (up to 200 mg/day) may be given with an interval of at least 2 hours between tablet doses.

Maximum dose in a 24–hour period to patients with migraine headaches has been 300 mg, given as either a single 300 mg dose or as three 100 mg single doses at intervals of no less than every 2 hours. There is no evidence that these higher doses afford greater relief.

Sumatriptan is equally effective at whatever stage of the attack they are administered, although it is advisable to take as early as possible after the onset of a migraine attack.

Storage/Stability:

Injection – Protect from light.

Rx	**Imitrex** (Glaxo Wellcome)	**Tablets**: 25 mg	Lactose. (I 25). White. Round. Film-coated. In 9s.
		50 mg	Lactose. (Imitrex 50). White. Capsule shape. Film-coated. In 9s.
Rx	**Imitrex** (Glaxo Wellcome)	**Injection**: 12 mg/ml	Sodium chloride 7 mg/ml. In 6 mg single-dose vials (0.5 ml in 2 ml) and *STATdose System* kit[1] (2 unit-of-use syringes, 1 *STATdose* Pen and instructions for use).
🍁	**Imitrex** (Glaxo Wellcome)	**Tablets**: 50 mg	Lactose. (Imitrex 50). White. Capsule shape. Film-coated. In 9s.
		100 mg	Lactose. (100). Capsule shape. Pink. Film-coated. In 6s.
🍁	**Imitrex** (Glaxo Wellcome)	**Injection**: 12 mg/ml	Sodium chloride 7 mg/ml. In 6 mg single-dose vials (0.5 ml in 2 ml) and *STATdose System* kit[1] (2 unit-of-use syringes, 1 *STATdose* Pen and instructions for use).

[1] Injection cartridge pack containing 2 prefilled syringe cartridges for refill of *STATdose System* only.

METHYSERGIDE MALEATE

Warning:
Retroperitoneal fibrosis, pleuropulmonary fibrosis and fibrotic thickening of cardiac valves may occur in patients receiving long-term methysergide therapy. Reserve this drug for prophylaxis in patients whose vascular headaches are frequent or severe and uncontrollable and who are under close medical supervision.

Actions:
Pharmacology: Methysergide is a semisynthetic ergot derivative. It has no intrinsic vasoconstrictor properties and its mechanism of action has not been established. It inhibits or blocks the effects of serotonin, a substance which may be involved in the mechanism of vascular headaches. Serotonin has been described as a central neurohumoral agent or chemical mediator and also as a "headache substance" acting directly or indirectly to lower pain threshold. Serotonin is also a potent vasoconstrictor. Plasma serotonin levels are elevated during the preheadache phase of classical migraine and decreased during an attack. Without serotonin, the extracranial arteries are dilated and distended, resulting in headache. Methysergide may displace serotonin on receptor pressor sites of the walls of cranial arteries during a migraine attack, preserving the vasoconstriction afforded by serotonin.

Methysergide is a peripheral antagonist of serotonin, competitively blocking the serotonin receptor in the blood vessel. It also inhibits histamine release from mast cells and stabilizes platelets against spontaneous or induced release of serotonin. Centrally, methysergide may act as a serotonin agonist, especially in the midbrain. It has very weak uterotonic and emetic actions.

Allow 1 to 2 days for the protective effects to develop; following termination, 1 to 2 days are required before the effects subside.

Indications:
Vascular headache:
Prevention or reduction of intensity and frequency in patients suffering from one or more severe vascular headaches per week or from vascular headaches that are so severe that preventive therapy is indicated, regardless of the frequency of the attack.

Prophylaxis of vascular headache. Not for management of acute attacks.

Contraindications:
Pregnancy (see Warnings); peripheral vascular disease; severe arteriosclerosis; severe hypertension; coronary artery disease; phlebitis or cellulitis of the lower limbs; pulmonary disease; collagen diseases or fibrotic processes; impaired liver or renal function; valvular heart disease; debilitated states; serious infections.

Warnings:
Prolonged therapy: With long-term, uninterrupted administration, retroperitoneal fibrosis or related conditions (pleuropulmonary fibrosis and cardiovascular disorders with murmurs or vascular bruits) have occurred. Continuous administration should not exceed 6 months. There must be a drug-free interval of 3 to 4 weeks after each 6-month treatment course. Reduce dosage gradually during the last 2 to 3 weeks of each treatment course to avoid "headache rebound."

Retroperitoneal fibrosis, a nonspecific fibrotic process, is usually confined to the retroperitoneal connective tissue above the pelvic brim and may present clinically with one or more symptoms such as general malaise, fatigue, weight loss, backache, low grade fever (elevated sedimentation rate), urinary obstruction (girdle or flank pain, dysuria, polyuria, oliguria, elevated BUN) or vascular insufficiency of the lower limbs (leg pain, Leriche syndrome, edema of legs, thrombophlebitis). The most useful diagnostic procedure is IV pyelography. Typical deviation and obstruction of one or both ureters may be observed.

Pleuropulmonary fibrosis, a similar nonspecific fibrotic process limited to pleural and immediately subjacent pulmonary tissues, usually presents with dyspnea, chest tightness/pain, pleural friction rubs and pleural effusion. Confirm by chest x-ray.

Cardiac fibrosis – Nonrheumatic fibrotic thickenings of the aortic root and of the aortic and mitral valves usually present clinically with cardiac murmurs and dyspnea.

Other fibrotic complications – Fibrotic plaques simulating Peyronie's disease.

Supervise and regularly examine patients for developing fibrotic or vascular complications. The manifestations of retroperitoneal fibrosis, pleuropulmonary fibrosis and vascular shutdown have shown a high incidence of regression once methysergide is withdrawn. Cardiac murmurs, which may indicate endocardial fibrosis, have shown varying degrees of regression, with complete disappearance in some and persistence in others.

METHYSERGIDE MALEATE

Pregnancy: Contraindicated in pregnancy due to oxytocic properties.

Lactation: Ergot derivatives in the milk of nursing mothers have caused symptoms of ergotism (eg, vomiting, diarrhea) in the infant.

Children: Not recommended for use in children.

Precautions:

Tartrazine sensitivity: This product contains tartrazine, which may cause allergic-type reactions (including bronchial asthma) in susceptible individuals. Although the incidence of tartrazine sensitivity in the general population is low, it is frequently seen in patients who also have aspirin hypersensitivity.

Drug Interactions:

Beta blockers and concurent methysergide therapy may result in peripheral ischemia manifested by cold extremities with possible peripheral gangrene.

Adverse Reactions:

Adverse reactions occur in up to 30% to 50% of patients.

Fibrosis: See Warnings.

Cardiovascular: Encroachment of retroperitoneal fibrosis on the aorta, inferior vena cava and their common iliac branches may cause vascular insufficiency of the lower limbs.

Intrinsic vasoconstriction of large and small arteries, involving one or more vessels or vessel segments, may occur at any stage of therapy. Depending on the vessel, this complication may present with chest pain, abdominal pain or cold, numb, painful extremities with or without paresthesias and diminished or absent pulses. Progression to ischemic tissue damage is rare.

Postural hypotension and tachycardia have also been observed.

GI: Nausea, vomiting, diarrhea, heartburn and abdominal pain tend to appear early and can frequently be obviated by gradual introduction of the medication and by administration with meals. Constipation and elevation of gastric hydrochloric acid have occurred.

CNS: Insomnia; drowsiness; mild euphoria; dizziness; ataxia; weakness; lightheadedness; hyperesthesia; unworldly feelings (described as "dissociation" or "hallucinatory experiences"). Some symptoms may be unrelated to the drug.

Dermatologic: Facial flush, telangiectasia, nonspecific rashes (rare); increased hair loss (usually abates despite continued therapy).

Edema – Peripheral edema, and more rarely, localized brawny edema. Dependent edema has responded to lowered doses, salt restriction or diuretics.

Hematologic: Neutropenia; eosinophilia.

Miscellaneous: Arthralgia; myalgia; weight gain.

Patient Information:

May cause GI upset; take with food or milk.

Caution patients regarding their caloric intake.

May cause drowsiness; use caution when driving or performing other tasks requiring alertness, coordination or physical dexterity.

Continuous administration should not exceed 6 months. There must be a drug free interval of 3 to 4 weeks after each 6 month course of treatment. Do not stop taking suddenly; reduce dosage gradually during the last 2 to 3 weeks of each treatment course to avoid "headache rebound".

Notify physician of cold, numb or painful extremities, leg cramps when walking, girdle, flank or chest pain, painful urination or shortness of breath.

Administration and Dosage:

Adults: 4 to 8 mg daily; take with meals. There must be a drug free interval of 3 to 4 weeks after every 6 month course of treatment. If, after a 3 week trial period, efficacy has not been demonstrated, continued administration is unlikely to be beneficial.

Rx	**Sansert** (Sandoz)	**Tablets:** 2 mg	Tartrazine, lactose, sucrose. (Sandoz 78-58). In 100s.

ERGOTAMINE DERIVATIVES

Actions:

Pharmacology: Ergotamine has partial agonist or antagonist activity against tryptaminergic, dopaminergic and alpha-adrenergic receptors, depending upon their site; it is a highly active uterine stimulant. It constricts peripheral and cranial blood vessels and depresses central vasomotor centers.

Ergotamine reduces extracranial blood flow, causes a decline in the amplitude of pulsation in the cranial arteries and decreases hyperperfusion of the basilar artery territory. It does not reduce cerebral hemispheric blood flow. It may inhibit receptor reuptake of norepinephrine at sympathetic nerve endings, increasing the vasoconstrictive action. Ergotamine is a potent emetic that stimulates the chemoreceptor trigger zone. Small doses increase force and frequency of uterine contractions; larger doses increase resting uterine tone. The gravid uterus is more sensitive to these effects.

Dihydroergotamine, a hydrogenated derivative of ergotamine, differs mainly in its degree of activity. It has less vasoconstrictive action than ergotamine, is 12 times less active as an emetic and has less oxytocic effect.

Pharmacokinetics:

Absorption/Distribution – GI absorption of ergotamine is incomplete and erratic; following oral administration, peak blood levels are reached in about 2 hours. Absorption by inhalation of the aerosol preparation appears rapid and complete. Absorption across the buccal mucosa is extremely poor. For patients who cannot tolerate or retain oral ergotamine, rectal suppositories may be beneficial (ergotamine is only available as a rectal dosage form in combination with other agents). Caffeine administered concurrently increases absorption rate and peak plasma levels of ergotamine; caffeine/ergotamine combination products are listed under Migraine Combinations.

Onset of action occurs in 15 to 30 minutes following IM administration of dihydroergotamine and persists for 3 to 4 hours. Repeat dosage at 1 hour intervals; up to 3 hours may be required to obtain maximal effect.

Metabolism/Excretion – Ergotamine is metabolized by the liver; 90% of the metabolites are excreted in the bile. Unmetabolized drug is erratically secreted in saliva, and only trace amounts of unmetabolized drug are excreted in the feces and urine. Although plasma half-life is about 2 hours, ergotamine has long-lasting effects which may be due to tissue storage.

Clinical trials: Ergotamine effectively controls up to 70% of acute migraine attacks; thus, it is specific for this syndrome. Ergotamine constricts both arteries and veins. In doses used in vascular headaches, it usually produces only small increases in blood pressure, but it increases peripheral resistance and decreases blood flow in various organs.

Indications:

To abort or prevent vascular headaches such as migraine, migraine variant and cluster headache (histaminic cephalalgia).

Dihydroergotamine is used when rapid control is desired or when other routes of administration are not feasible.

Contraindications:

Pregnancy, women who may become pregnant (ergotamine's powerful uterine stimulant actions may cause fetal harm; see Warnings); hypersensitivity to ergot alkaloids; peripheral vascular disease (eg, thromboangiitis obliterans, leutic arteritis, severe arteriosclerosis, thrombophlebitis, Raynaud's disease); hepatic or renal impairment; severe pruritus; coronary artery disease; hypertension; sepsis; malnutrition.

Warnings:

Pregnancy: Category X. Although no specific teratogenic effects have been found, the fetus suffers if ergotamine is given to the mother. Retarded fetal growth, increased intrauterine death and resorption occurred in animals, possibly resulting from drug-induced uterine motility and increased vasoconstriction in the placental vascular bed.

Lactation: Ergotamine is secreted into breast milk and has caused symptoms of ergotism (eg, vomiting, diarrhea) in the infant. Exercise caution when administering to a nursing woman. Excessive dosing or prolonged administration may inhibit lactation.

Children: Safety and efficacy for use in children have not been established.

ERGOTAMINE DERIVATIVES

Precautions:

Avoid prolonged administration or excessive dosage because of the danger of ergotism and gangrene.

Drug abuse and dependence: Patients who take ergotamine for extended periods of time may become dependent upon it and require progressively increasing doses for relief of vascular headaches and for prevention of dysphoric effects which follow withdrawal.

Drug Interactions:

Ergot Alkaloid Drug Interactions			
Precipitant drug	Object drug*		Description
Beta blockers	Ergot alkaloids	↑	Peripheral ischemia manifested by cold extremities, possible peripheral gangrene.
Macrolides	Ergot alkaloids	↑	Acute ergotism manifested as peripheral ischemia has occurred.
Dihydroergotamine	Nitrates	↓	Functional antagonism between these agents, decreasing the antianginal effects. Also, increased bioavailability of oral dihydroergotamine (dosage form not available in US) with resultant increase in mean standing systolic blood pressure.
Ergot alkaloids	Vasodilators	↑	The pressor effects of concurrent use can combine to cause dangerous hypertension.

* ↑ = Object drug increased. ↓ = Object drug decreased.

Adverse Reactions:

Side effects usually do not necessitate interruption of therapy; however, serious toxicity may occur (see Overdosage). Nausea and vomiting occur in up to 10% of patients and may be relieved by atropine or phenothiazine antiemetics.

Miscellaneous: Numbness and tingling of fingers and toes; muscle pain in the extremities; pulselessness; weakness in the legs; precordial distress and pain; transient tachycardia or bradycardia; localized edema; itching.

Large doses raise arterial pressure, produce coronary vasoconstriction and slow the heart by both a direct action and a vagal effect. Ergotamine has oxytocic and spasmolytic properties.

Overdosage:

Symptoms: Some cases of ergotamine poisoning have occurred in patients who have taken < 5 mg. Usually, however, toxicity is seen at doses in excess of about 15 mg in 24 hours or 40 mg in a few days. Overdosage causes nausea, vomiting, weakness of the legs, pain in limb muscles, numbness and tingling of fingers and toes, precordial pain, tachycardia or bradycardia, hypertension or hypotension, and localized edema and itching with signs and symptoms of ischemia due to vasoconstriction of peripheral arteries and arterioles. The feet and hands become cold, pale and numb. Muscle pain occurs while walking and later at rest also. Gangrene may ensue. Confusion, depression, drowsiness and convulsions are occasional signs of ergotamine toxicity. Overdosage is particularly likely to occur in patients with sepsis or impaired renal or hepatic function. Patients with peripheral vascular disease are especially at risk of developing peripheral ischemia following treatment with ergotamine.

Treatment: Treatment consists of the withdrawal of the drug followed by symptomatic measures including attempts to maintain an adequate circulation in the affected parts. Anticoagulant drugs, low molecular weight dextran and potent vasodilator drugs may all be beneficial. IV infusion of sodium nitroprusside has been successful. Vasodilators must be used with special care in the presence of hypotension. Ergotamine is dialyzable.

ERGOTAMINE DERIVATIVES

Patient Information:

A patient package insert is available with these products.

Initiate therapy at first sign of attack. Do *NOT* exceed recommended dosage.

Notify physician if any of the following occurs: Irregular heart beat, nausea, vomiting, numbness or tingling of fingers or toes, or pain or weakness of extremities.

Administration and Dosage:

Sublingual: Initiate therapy as soon as possible after the first symptoms of an attack. Place 1 tablet under the tongue; take subsequent doses at 30 minute intervals if necessary. Do not exceed 3 tablets/24 hours. Do not exceed 10 mg/week.

Inhalation: Start with 1 inhalation; repeat if not relieved in 5 minutes. Space additional inhalations at least 5 minutes apart. Do not exceed 6 inhalations in 24 hours or 15 inhalations/week.

ERGOTAMINE TARTRATE

For complete prescribing information, refer to the Ergotamine Derivatives group monograph.

Rx	**Ergomar** (Lotus)	**Tablets, sublingual:** 2 mg	Lactose, peppermint oil, saccharin. (LB2). Green. In 20s.
Rx	**Ergostat** (Parke-Davis)		Lactose, saccharin. (P-D 111). Orange. In UD 24s.

DIHYDROERGOTAMINE MESYLATE

For complete prescribing information, refer to the Ergotamine Derivatives group monograph.

Administration and Dosage:

IM: Inject 1 mg at first sign of headache; repeat at 1 hour intervals to a total of 3 mg. For optimal results, adjust the dose for several headaches to determine the minimal effective dose; use this dose at the onset of subsequent attacks.

IV: Where more rapid effect is desired, administer IV to a maximum of 2 mg. Do not exceed 6 mg/week.

Rx	**D.H.E. 45** (Sandoz)	**Injection:** 1 mg per ml	In 1 ml amps.[1]

[1] With methanesulfonic acid, 6.1% alcohol and 15% glycerin.

ISOMETHEPTENE MUCATE/DICHLORALPHENAZONE/ACETAMINOPHEN

Actions:

Pharmacology: Isometheptene mucate is an unsaturated aliphatic amine with sympathomimetic properties. It acts by constricting dilated cranial and cerebral arterioles, thus reducing the stimuli that lead to vascular headaches.

Pharmacokinetics: Dichloralphenazone, a mild sedative, reduces the patient's emotional reaction to the pain of both vascular and tension headaches.

Acetaminophen raises the threshold to painful stimuli, thus exerting an analgesic effect against all types of headaches. Refer to individual monograph.

Indications:

For relief of tension and vascular headaches.

Based on a review of this drug (isometheptene mucate) by the National Academy of Sciences-National Research Council or other information, FDA has classified the other indication as "possibly" effective in the treatment of migraine headache. Final classification of the less-than-effective indication requires further investigation.

Contraindications:

Glaucoma; severe cases of renal disease; hypertension; organic heart disease; hepatic disease; MAO inhibitor therapy (see Drug Interactions).

Precautions:

Observe caution in hypertension, peripheral vascular disease and after recent cardiovascular attacks.

Drug Interactions:

MAO inhibitors: Since isometheptene has sympathomimetic properties, concurrent use may result in severe headache, hypertension and hyperpyrexia, possibly resulting in hypertensive crisis.

Adverse Reactions:

Transient dizziness and skin rash may appear in hypersensitive patients; this can usually be eliminated by reducing the dose.

Administration and Dosage:

Migraine headache: Usual dosage is 2 capsules at once followed by 1 capsule every hour until relieved, up to 5 capsules within a 12 hour period.

Tension headache: Usual dosage is 1 or 2 capsules every 4 hours, up to 8 capsules per day.

Rx	**Isometheptene/ Dichloralphenazone/ Acetaminophen** (Various, eg, Goldline, URL)	**Capsules:** 65 mg isometheptene mucate, 100 mg dichloralphenazone, 325 mg APAP	In 100s.
Rx	**Isocom** (Nutripharm)		In 50s, 100s and 250s.
Rx	**Isopap** (Geneva Marsam)		Red/white. In 100s.
Rx	**Midchlor** (Schein)		In 100s.
Rx	**Midrin** (Carnrick)		(C 86120). Red with pink band. In 50s and 100s.
Rx	**Migratine** (Major)		In 100s and 250s.

MIGRAINE COMBINATIONS

For complete information on these ingredients, refer to the individual monographs.

Ingredients:

ERGOTAMINE TARTRATE is used for its specific action against migraine.

CAFFEINE, a cranial vasoconstrictor, is added to ergotamine to enhance vasoconstrictive effects. It may enhance the absorption of ergotamine.

BARBITURATES are used for sedation.

BELLADONNA ALKALOIDS are used for their anticholinergic and antiemetic effects in individuals experiencing excessive nausea and vomiting during attacks.

	Product & Distributor	Ergotamine tartrate	Caffeine	Other Content	Dosage	How Supplied
Rx	**Cafergot Tablets** (Sandoz)	1 mg	100 mg		2 tablets at first sign of an attack; follow with 1 tablet every hour, if needed. Maximum dose is 6 tablets/attack. Do not exceed 10 tablets/week.	(Cafergot). Pink. In 90s and 250s.
Rx	**Ercaf Tablets** (Geneva Marsam)					Beige. In 100s.
Rx	**Wigraine Tablets** (Organon)					Lactose. (Organon 542). White. In foil strip 20s and 100s.
Rx	**Cafatine-PB Tablets** (Major)	1 mg	100 mg	0.125 mg l-alkaloids of belladonna, 30 mg sodium pentobarbital	2 tablets at first sign of an attack; follow with 1 tablet every hour, if needed. Maximum dose is 6 tablets/attack. Do not exceed 10 tablets/week.	In 90s.
Rx	**Cafatine Supps** (Major)	2 mg	100 mg		Maximum dose is 2/attack.	In 12s.
Rx	**Cafergot Supps** (Sandoz)			Cocoa butter		(Cafergot Suppository 78-33 Sandoz) In 12s.
Rx	**Cafetrate Supps** (Schein)					In 12s.
Rx	**Wigraine Supps** (Organon)	2 mg	100 mg	21.5 mg tartaric acid	Maximum dose is 2/attack.	In 12s.

ANTIEMETIC/ANTIVERTIGO AGENTS

Actions:

Pharmacology: Drug-induced vomiting (eg, drugs, radiation, metabolic disorders) is generally stimulated through the chemoreceptor trigger zone (CTZ), which in turn stimulates the vomiting center (VC) in the brain. Nausea of motion sickness is initiated by stimulation of labyrinthine mechanism of the ear, which sends impulses to CTZ. VC may also be stimulated directly (by GI irritation, motion sickness, vestibular neuritis, etc). Increased activity of central neurotransmitters, dopamine in CTZ or acetylcholine in VC appears to be a major mediator for inducing vomiting.

Patients undergoing cancer chemotherapy often experience nausea and vomiting so intolerable that they may refuse further treatment. Some antineoplastic agents are more emetogenic than others. Prophylaxis with an antiemetic drug before the patient receives chemotherapy and treatment afterward may enable the patient to overcome this unpleasant side effect and continue a potentially curative protocol.

Vertigo is a feeling of whirling or rotation accompanied by involuntary swaying, weakness and lightheadedness. Motion sickness, a functional disorder, is caused by repetitive angular, linear or vertical motion. Both of these conditions are characterized by pallor, sweating, hyperventilation, nausea and vomiting.

The drugs that are effective as antiemetics are the **antidopaminergic** agents (phenothiazines, metoclopramide) which are especially effective for drug-induced emesis. **Anticholinergic agents** (antihistamines, trimethobenzamide, scopolamine) may be more appropriate in motion sickness, labyrinthine disorders, etc. Other agents, whose mechanisms are not known or that may act differently (eg, hydroxyzine, corticosteroids, cannabinoids), are effective in various types of emesis.

The following table indicates manufacturers' recommended uses for agents in this group. Several of these are indicated for uses other than as antiemetic/antivertigo agents. For a full discussion, see individual drug monographs.

Recommended Uses for Antiemetic/Antivertigo Agents

		Indications		
	Drug	Nausea and Vomiting	Motion Sickness	Vertigo
ANTIDOPAMINERGICS				
Phenothiazines	Chlorpromazine[1]	✓		
	Triflupromazine	✓		
	Perphenazine[1]	✓		
	Prochlorperazine	✓		
	Promethazine	✓	✓	
	Thiethylperazine	✓		
Other	Metoclopramide	✓		
ANTICHOLINERGICS				
Antihistamines	Cyclizine	✓	✓	
	Meclizine	✓	✓	✓[2]
	Buclizine	✓	✓	
	Diphenhydramine		✓	
	Dimenhydrinate	✓	✓	✓
Other	Trimethobenzamide	✓		
	Scopolamine		✓	
MISCELLANEOUS				
Miscellaneous	Diphenidol	✓		✓
	Benzquinamide	✓		
	Phosphorated Carbohydrate Solution	✓		
	Hydroxyzine HCl	✓[3]		
	Corticosteroids	✓[3]		
	Cannabinoids	✓		

[1] Also indicated for relief of intractable hiccoughs.
[2] Classified "possibly effective" by the FDA.
[3] This is an *unlabeled* use.

ANTIEMETIC/ANTIVERTIGO AGENTS

Warnings:

Children: Not recommended for uncomplicated vomiting in children; limit use to prolonged vomiting of known etiology for three principal reasons:

1. Although there is no confirmatory evidence, centrally-acting antiemetics may contribute, in combination with viral illnesses (a possible cause of vomiting in children), to the development of Reye's syndrome, a potentially fatal acute childhood encephalopathy. This syndrome follows a nonspecific febrile illness, and is characterized by an abrupt onset of persistent, severe vomiting, lethargy, irrational behavior, visceral fatty degeneration (especially involving the liver), progressive encephalopathy leading to coma, convulsions and death.

2. The extrapyramidal symptoms that can occur secondary to some drugs may be confused with the CNS signs of an undiagnosed primary disease responsible for the vomiting, eg, Reye's syndrome or other encephalopathy.

3. Drugs with hepatotoxic potential may unfavorably alter the course of Reye's syndrome. Avoid such drugs in children whose signs and symptoms (vomiting) could represent Reye's syndrome. It should also be noted that salicylates and acetaminophen are hepatotoxic at large doses. Although it is not known whether at usual doses they would represent a hazard in patients with the underlying hepatic disorder of Reye's syndrome, these drugs, too, should be avoided in children whose signs and symptoms could represent Reye's syndrome, unless alternative methods of controlling fever are not successful.

Children with acute illnesses (eg, chickenpox, CNS infections, measles, gastroenteritis) or dehydration seem to be much more susceptible to neuromuscular reactions, particularly dystonias, than are adults. In such patients, use antiemetics only under close supervision. Do not use dimenhydrinate in children under 2 years of age unless directed by a doctor.

Severe emesis should not be treated with an antiemetic drug alone; where possible, establish cause of vomiting. Direct primary emphasis toward restoration of body fluids and electrolyte balance, and relief of fever and causative disease process. Avoid overhydration which may result in cerebral edema. Antiemetic effects may impede diagnosis of such conditions as brain tumors, intestinal obstruction and appendicitis, and may obscure signs of toxicity from overdosage of other drugs.

Precautions:

Tartrazine sensitivity: Some of these products contain tartrazine, which may cause allergic-type reactions (including bronchial asthma) in susceptible individuals. Although the incidence of sensitivity is low, it is frequently seen in patients who also have aspirin hypersensitivity. Specific products containing tartrazine are identified in the product listings.

Sulfite sensitivity: Some of these products contain sulfites which may cause allergic-type reactions (eg, hives, itching, wheezing, anaphylaxis) in certain susceptible persons. Although the overall prevalence of sulfite sensitivity in the general population is probably low, it is seen more frequently in asthmatics or in atopic nonasthmatic persons. Specific products containing sulfites are identified in the product listings.

Patient Information:

These agents may cause drowsiness; patients should observe caution while driving or performing other tasks requiring alertness.

Avoid alcohol and other CNS depressants.

Antidopaminergics

CHLORPROMAZINE HCl

This is an abbreviated monograph. Complete prescribing information begins in the Antipsychotic Agents group monograph.

Indications:

Control of nausea and vomiting; relief of intractable hiccoughs

Administration and Dosage:

Individualize dosage.

Adults:

Nausea and vomiting –

Oral: 10 to 25 mg every 4 to 6 hours, as needed; increase if necessary.

Rectal: 50 to 100 mg every 6 to 8 hours, as needed.

IM: 25 mg. If no hypotension occurs, give 25 to 50 mg every 3 to 4 hours, as needed, until vomiting stops. Then switch to oral dosage.

Intractable hiccoughs: Orally, 25 to 50 mg 3 or 4 times daily. If symptoms persist for 2 to 3 days, give 25 to 50 mg IM. Should symptoms persist, use slow IV infusion with patient flat in bed. Administer 25 to 50 mg in 500 to 1000 ml of saline. Monitor blood pressure.

Children:

Nausea and vomiting – Do not use in children under 6 months of age except where potentially lifesaving. Do not use in conditions for which specific children's dosages have not been established. The activity following IM use may last 12 hours.

Oral: 0.25 mg/lb (0.55 mg/kg) every 4 to 6 hours, as needed.

Rectal: 0.5 mg/lb (1.1 mg/kg) every 6 to 8 hours, as needed.

IM: 0.25 mg/lb (0.55 mg/kg) every 6 to 8 hours, as needed.

Maximum IM dosage: Children up to 5 years of age — 40 mg/day.

Children 5 to 12 years of age — 75 mg/day, except in severe cases.

PERPHENAZINE

This is an abbreviated monograph. For complete prescribing information, refer to the Antipsychotic Agents group monograph.

Indications:

Control of severe nausea and vomiting in adults; relief of intractable hiccoughs.

Administration and Dosage:

Oral: 8 to 16 mg daily in divided doses; occasionally, 24 mg may be necessary. Early dosage reduction is desirable.

IM: Give to seated or recumbent patient; observe patient for a short period afterward.

Adults – 5 mg repeated every 6 hours as necessary. Do not exceed 15 mg in ambulatory or 30 mg in hospitalized patients. For severe conditions, an initial dose of 10 mg may be given. Place patients on oral therapy as soon as possible, usually within 24 hours. In general, reserve higher dosages for hospitalized.

Children (> 12) – The lowest adult dose (5 mg). Pediatric dose not established.

IV: Use only when necessary to control severe vomiting, intractable hiccoughs or acute conditions such as violent retching during surgery. Limit use to recumbent hospitalized adults in doses not exceeding 5 mg. Give as a diluted solution by either fractional injection or slow drip infusion. In the surgical patient, slow infusion is preferred. When administered in divided doses, dilute of 0.5 mg/ml (1 ml mixed with 9 ml saline solution) and give not more than 1 mg per injection at not less than 1 to 2 minute intervals. Discontinue as soon as symptoms are controlled. Do not exceed 5 mg. Hypotensive and extrapyramidal side effects may occur. IV norepinephtine may alleviate hypotension.

Storage/Stability:

Concentrate – Protect from light. Store between 2° and 30°C (36° and 86°F). Store in carton until contents are used. Shake well.

Injection – Protect from light. Slight yellow discoloration will not alter potency or efficacy; if markedly discolored, discard. Store in carton until used.

Antidopaminergics

PERPHENAZINE

Rx	**Trilafon** (Schering)	**Tablets:** 2 mg	(Schering ADH or 705). Gray. In 100s and 500s.
		Tablets: 4 mg	(Schering ADK or 940). Gray. In 100s and 500s.
		Tablets: 8 mg	(Schering ADJ or 313). Gray. In 100s and 500s.
		Tablets: 16 mg	(Schering ADM or 077). Gray. In 100s and 500s.
		Concentrate: 16 mg/5 ml	Alcohol. Sorbitol. In 118 ml w/dropper.
		Injection: 5 mg/ml	In 1 ml amps.[1]

[1] With sodium bisulfite.

Antidopaminergics

TRIFLUPROMAZINE HCl

Refer to the general discussion of these products in the Antiemetic/Antivertigo Agents monograph.

This is an abbreviated monograph. For complete prescribing information refer to the Antipsychotic Agents monograph.

Indications:

Control of severe nausea and vomiting.

Administration and Dosage:

Adults:

IM (range) – 5 to 15 mg repeated every 4 hours, up to 60 mg maximum daily dose. Elderly or debilitated: 2.5 mg; maximum daily dose, 15 mg.

IV (range) – 1 mg, up to 3 mg total daily dose.

Children (over 2½ years of age): Individualize dosage. Do not administer IV.

IM – 0.2 to 0.25 mg/kg; maximum 10 mg/day. The duration of activity following IM administration may last up to 12 hours.

Rx	**Vesprin** (Princeton)	**Injection:** 10 mg per ml	In 10 ml multi-dose vials.[1]
		20 mg per ml	In 1 ml multi-dose vials.[1]

[1] With 1.5 benzyl alcohol.

PROCHLORPERAZINE

This is an abbreviated monograph. For complete prescribing information, refer to the Antipsychotic Agents group monograph.

Indications:

Control of severe nausea and vomiting.

Administration and Dosage:

Do not crush or chew sustained release preparations.

Individualize dosage.

Do not use in pediatric surgery.

Adults:

Control of severe nausea and vomiting –

Oral: Usually, 5 to 10 mg, 3 or 4 times daily; 15 mg (sustained release) on arising; 10 mg (sustained release) every 12 hours.

Rectal: 25 mg twice daily.

IM: Initially, 5 to 10 mg. If necessary, repeat every 3 or 4 hours. Do not exceed 40 mg/day.

SC: Do not administer SC because of local irritation.

Adult surgery:

Control of severe nausea and vomiting – Total parenteral dosage should not exceed 40 mg/day. Hypotension may occur if the drug is given IV or by infusion.

IM – 5 to 10 mg, 1 to 2 hours before induction of anesthesia (may repeat once in 30 minutes), or to control acute symptoms during and after surgery (may repeat once).

IV injection – 5 to 10 mg, 15 to 30 minutes before induction of anesthesia, or to control acute symptoms during or after sugery. Repeat once if necessary. Prochlorperazine may be administered either undiluted or diluted in isotonic solution, but do not exceed 10 mg in a single dose of the drug. Do not exceed 5 mg/ml/min. Do not use bolus injection.

IV infusion – 20 mg/L of isotonic solution. Do not dilute in less than 1 L of isotonic solution. Add to IV infusion 15 to 30 minutes before induction.

In one study, a dosage of 30 or 40 mg prochlorperazine in 100 ml normal saline was significantly superior to a 10 mg dose in treating cisplatin-induced emesis; toxicity was only moderate.

Children (over 20 pounds or 2 years of age):

Control of severe nausea and vomiting –

Oral or rectal: More than one days therapy is seldom necessary.

20 to 29 lbs (9.1 to 13.2 kg) — 2.5 mg 1 or 2 times/day (not to exceed 7.5 mg/day).

30 to 39 lbs (13.6 to 17.7 kg) — 2.5 mg 2 or 3 times/day (not to exceed 10 mg/day).

40 to 85 lbs (18.2 to 38.6 kg) — 2.5 mg 3 times/day or 5 mg twice daily (not to exceed 15 mg/day).

IM: 0.06 mg/lb (0.132 mg/kg). Give by deep IM injection. Control is usually obtained with one dose. Duration of action may be 12 hours. Subsequent doses may be given if necessary.

Antidopaminergics

PROCHLORPERAZINE

Rx	**Prochlorperazine** (Various)	**Tablets (as maleate):** 5 mg	In 12s, 30s, 100s, 1000s and UD 100s.
Rx	**Compazine** (SKF)		(SKF C66). Yellow-green. In 100s, 1000s and UD 100s.
Rx	**Prochlorperazine** (Various)	**Tablets (as maleate):** 10 mg	In 20s, 30s, 100s, 1000s and UD 32s and 100s.
Rx	**Compazine** (SKF)		(SKF C67). Yellow-green. In 100s, 1000s and UD 100s.
Rx	**Prochlorperazine** (Various)	**Tablets (as maleate):** 25 mg	In 100s, 1000s and UD 100s.
Rx	**Compazine** (SKF)		(SKF C69). Yellow-green. In 100s and 1000s.
Rx	**Compazine** (SKF)	**Spansules (sustained release capsules as maleate):** 10 mg	(SKF C44). Black/clear. In 50s, 500s & UD 100s.
		15 mg	(SKF C46). Black/clear. In 50s, 500s & UD 100s.
		30 mg	(SKF C47). Black/clear. In 50s, 500s & UD 100s.
Rx	**Compazine** (SKF)	**Suppositories:** 2.5 mg	In 12s.
		5 mg	In 12s.
		25 mg	In 12s.
Rx	**Prochlorperazine** (G & W Labs)		Coconut oil, palm kernel oil. In 12s.
Rx	**Compazine** (SKF)	**Syrup (as edisylate):** 5 mg per 5 ml	Fruit flavor. In 120 ml.
Rx	**Prochlorperazine** (Various)	**Injection:** 5 mg per ml	In 10 ml vials.
Rx	**Prochlorperazine** (Wyeth-Ayerst)	**Injection (as edisylate):** 5 mg per ml	In 2 ml amps and 2 and 10 ml vials.
Rx	**Compazine** (SKF)		In 2 ml amps[1], 2 ml disp. syringes[2] and 10 ml multi-dose vials.[2]

[1] With sodium saccharin and benzyl alcohol.
[2] With sodium sulfite and sodium bisulfite.

Antidopaminergics

PROMETHAZINE

Refer to the general discussion of these products beginning in the Antiemetic/Antivertigo monograph.

This is an abbreviated monograph. For complete information see Antihistamines.

Indications:

Oral or rectal: Active and prophylactic treatment of motion sickness; prevention and control of nausea and vomiting associated with anesthesia and surgery; antiemetic in postoperative patients.

Parenteral: Treatment of motion sickness; prevention and control of nausea and vomiting associated with anesthesia and surgery.

Administration and Dosage:

Oral and rectal:

Motion sickness – The average adult dose is 25 mg twice daily. Take the initial dose ½ to 1 hour before travel, and repeat 8 to 12 hours later, if necessary. On succeeding days, administer 25 mg on arising and again before the evening meal. For children, administer 12.5 to 25 mg twice daily.

Nausea and vomiting – The average dose for active therapy in children or adults is 25 mg. Repeat as necessary in doses of 12.5 to 25 mg at 4 to 6 hour intervals.

Children: 0.25 to 0.5 mg/kg every 4 to 6 hours rectally, as needed. Do not use in children < 2 yrs. Adjust dose based on age, weight and severity of condition.

Parenteral: Administer preferably by deep IM injection. Proper IV administration is well tolerated, but hazardous. When used IV, give in a concentration no greater than 25 mg/ml, and at a rate not to exceed 25 mg/min; it is preferable to inject through an appropriate site in tubing of an IV infusion set.

Motion sickness – 12.5 to 25 mg; may repeat as necessary 3 or 4 times a day.

Nausea and vomiting – 12.5 to 25 mg; do not repeat more frequently than every 4 hours. For postoperative nausea and vomiting, administer IM or IV and reduce dosage of analgesics and barbiturates accordingly.

In children < 12 years, do not exceed ½ the adult dose. As an adjunct to premedication, use 0.5 mg/lb (1.1 mg/kg) with an equal dose of narcotic or barbiturate and the appropriate dose of an atropine-like drug. Do not use in premature infants or neonates or in vomiting of unknown etiology in children.

Inadvertent intra-arterial injection can result in gangrene of the affected extremity. Subcutaneous injection is contraindicated as it may result in tissue necrosis.

For complete listing of promethazine products refer to Antihistamine Product Pages.

Antidopaminergics

THIETHYLPERAZINE MALEATE

Refer to the general discussion of these products in the Antiemetic/Antivertigo Agents monograph.

This is an abbreviated monograph. For complete information, see Antipsychotics.

Actions:

Pharmacology: Mechanism unknown. Animal experiments suggest a direct action on both the chemoreceptor trigger zone (CTZ) and the vomiting center (VC).

Indications:

Relief of nausea and vomiting.

Contraindications:

Severe CNS depression; comatose states; hypersensitivity to phenothiazines; IV administration; pregnancy.

Administration and Dosage:

Do not use IV (may cause severe hypotension). Use of this drug has not been studied following intracardiac or intracranial surgery.

When used for nausea or vomiting associated with anesthesia and surgery, administer by deep IM injection at, or shortly before, termination of anesthesia.

Adults:

Oral and Rectal – 10 to 30 mg daily in divided doses.

IM – 2 ml, 1 to 3 times daily.

Children: Dosage not determined. Not recommended in children < 12 years old.

Storage: Store suppositories below 25°C (77°F) in a tight container (eg, sealed foil).

Rx	**Norzine** (Purdue Frederick)	**Tablets:** 10 mg	Tartrazine. Sorbitol. In 100s.
Rx	**Torecan** (Roxane)		Tartrazine. Sorbitol. In 100s.
Rx	**Norzine** (Purdue Frederick)	**Suppositories:** 10 mg	In 12s.
Rx	**Torecan** (Roxane)		In 12s.
Rx	**Norzine** (Purdue Frederick)	**Injection:** 5 mg per ml	In 2 ml amps.[1]
Rx	**Torecan** (Roxane)		In 2 ml amps.[1]

[1] With ascorbic acid, sodium metabisulfite and sorbitol.

Antidopaminergics

METOCLOPRAMIDE

Refer to the general discussion of these products beginning in the Antiemetic/Antivertigo monograph.

This is an abbreviated monograph. For complete prescribing information refer to the GI Stimulants monograph.

Indications:

Parenteral: Prevention of nausea and vomiting associated with emetogenic cancer chemotherapy.

Unlabeled uses: Studies have indicated some potential value of metoclopramide (10 mg orally or IV 30 minutes before each meal and at bedtime) in nausea and vomiting of a variety of etiologies (uncontrolled studies report 80% to 90% efficacy), including emesis during pregnancy and labor (5 to 10 mg orally or 5 to 20 mg IV or IM, 3 times a day).

Administration and Dosage:

Prevention of chemotherapy-induced emesis: For doses in excess of 10 mg, dilute injection in 50 ml of a parenteral solution (Dextrose 5% in Water, Sodium Chloride Injection, Dextrose 5% in 0.45% Sodium Chloride, Ringer's or Lactated Ringer's Injection). Infuse slowly IV over not less than 15 minutes, 30 minutes before beginning cancer chemotherapy; repeat every 2 hours for 2 doses, then every 3 hours for 3 doses.

The initial 2 doses should be 2 mg/kg if highly emetogenic drugs such as cisplatin or dacarbazine are used alone or in combination. For less emetogenic regimens, 1 mg/kg/dose may be adequate.

If extrapyramidal symptoms occur, administer 50 mg diphenhydramine IM.

Rx *sf*	**Reglan** (Robins)	**Syrup**: 5 mg/5 ml (as monohydrochloride monohydrate)	In pt and UD 10 ml (100s).
Rx	**Metoclopramide HCl** (Quad)	**Injection**: 5 mg/ml (as monohydrochloride monohydrate)	In 2, 10, 30, 50 and 100 ml vials.
Rx	**Reglan** (Robins)		In 2 and 10 ml amps and 2, 10 and 30 ml vials.
Rx	**Reglan** (Robins)	**Tablets**: 5 mg metoclopramide HCl	In 100s.
Rx	**Metoclopramide** (Various)	**Tablets**: 10 mg (as monohydrochloride monohydrate)	In 100s, 500s, 1000s and UD 100s.
Rx	**Clopra** (Quantum)		(QPL/217). White, scored. In 100s, 500s and 1000s.
Rx	**Maxolon** (Beecham)		(BMP 192). Blue, scored. In 100s.
Rx	**Octamide** (Adria)		(Adria 230). In 100s and 500s.
Rx	**Reclomide** (Major)		In 100s, 500s, 1000s and UD 100s.
Rx	**Reglan** (Robins)		(Reglan AHR 10). Pink, scored. In 100s, 500s and UD 100s.

Anticholinergics

CYCLIZINE AND MECLIZINE

Refer to the general discussion of these products in the Antiemetic/Antivertigo Agents group monograph.

Actions:

Pharmacology: Cyclizine and meclizine have antiemetic, anticholinergic and antihistaminic properties. They reduce the sensitivity of the labyrinthine apparatus. The action may be mediated through nerve pathways to the vomiting center (VC) from the chemoreceptor trigger zone (CTZ), peripheral nerve pathways, the VC or other CNS centers.

Cyclizine and meclizine have an onset of action of 30 to 60 minutes, depending on dosage; their duration of action is 4 to 6 hours and 12 to 24 hours, respectively.

Indications:

Prevention and treatment of nausea, vomiting and dizziness of motion sickness.

Meclizine is "possibly effective" for the management of vertigo associated with diseases affecting the vestibular system.

Contraindications:

Hypersensitivity to cyclizine or meclizine.

Warnings:

Pregnancy: Category B. Cyclizine and meclizine have been teratogenic in rodents, but large scale human studies have not demonstrated adverse fetal effects. Use only when clearly needed and when the potential benefits outweigh the potential hazards to the fetus. It has been suggested that, based on available data, meclizine presents the lowest risk of teratogenicity and is the drug of first choice in treating nausea and vomiting during pregnancy.

Lactation: Safety for use in the nursing mother has not been established.

Children: Safety and efficacy for use in children have not been established. Not recommended for use in children under 12 years of age.

Precautions:

Hazardous tasks: May produce drowsiness; patients should observe caution while driving or performing other tasks requiring alertness.

Because of the anticholinergic action of these agents, use with caution and with appropriate monitoring in patients with glaucoma, obstructive disease of the GI or GU tract and in elderly males with possible prostatic hypertrophy. These drugs may have a hypotensive action, which may be confusing or dangerous in postoperative patients.

May have additive effects with alcohol and other CNS depressants (eg, hypnotics, sedatives, tranquilizers, antianxiety agents); use with caution.

Adverse Reactions:

CNS: Drowsiness; restlessness; excitation; nervousness; insomnia; euphoria; blurred vision; diplopia; vertigo; tinnitus; auditory and visual hallucinations (particularly when dosage recommendations are exceeded).

Dermatologic: Urticaria; rash.

GI: Dry mouth; anorexia; nausea; vomiting; diarrhea; constipation; cholestatic jaundice (cyclizine).

GU: Urinary frequency; difficult urination; urinary retention.

Cardiovascular: Hypotension; palpitations; tachycardia.

Miscellaneous: Dry nose and throat.

Overdosage:

Symptoms: Moderate overdosage may cause hyperexcitability alternating with drowsiness. Massive overdosage may cause convulsions, hallucinations and respiratory paralysis.

Treatment: includes appropriate supportive and symptomatic treatment. Refer to General Management of Acute Overdosage. Consider dialysis.

Caution – Do not use morphine or other respiratory depressants.

Anticholinergics

CYCLIZINE

For complete prescribing information, refer to the Antiemetic/Antivertigo Agents group monograph.

Administration and Dosage:

Oral:

Adults – 50 mg taken ½ hour before departure; repeat every 4 to 6 hours. Do not exceed 200 mg daily.

Children (6 to 12 years of age) – 25 mg, up to 3 times daily.

Parenteral: For IM use only.

Adults – 50 mg every 4 to 6 hours, as necessary.

Not recommended for use in children.

otc	**Marezine** (Himmel)	**Tablets**: 50 mg (as HCl)	(Marezine T4A). Scored. In 12s and 100s.

MECLIZINE

For complete prescribing information, refer to the Antiemetic/Antivertigo Agents group monograph.

Administration and Dosage:

Motion sickness: Take an initial dose of 25 to 50 mg, 1 hour prior to travel. May repeat dose every 24 hours for the duration of the journey.

Vertigo: 25 to 100 mg daily in divided doses.

Rx	**Meclizine HCl** (Various)	**Tablets**: 12.5 mg	In 30s, 60s, 100s, 500s, 1000s and UD 100s.
Rx	**Antivert** (Roerig)		(Antivert 210). In 100s, 1000s and UD100s.
Rx	**Antrizine** (Major)		In 100s, 500s and 1000s.
otc/ Rx[1]	**Meclizine HCl** (Various)	**Tablets**: 25 mg	In 12s, 20s, 30s, 60s, 100s, 500s, 1000s and UD32s and 100s.
Rx	**Antivert/25** (Roerig)		(Antivert 211). In 100s, 1000s and UD100s.
Rx	**Antrizine** (Major)		In 100s, 500s, 1000s and UD100s.
otc	**Dramamine** II (Upjohn)		Lactose. In 8s.
Rx	**Ru-Vert-M** (Solvay)		(RPL 7025). Red. Film coated. In 100s.
otc/ Rx[1]	**Meclizine HCl** (Various)	**Tablets, chewable**: 25 mg	In 20s, 30s, 60s, 100s, 1000s and UD 100s.
otc	**Bonine** (Leeming)		In 8s.
otc	**Dizmiss** (JMI Canton)		Pink. In 1000s.
Rx	**Meclizine HCl** (Various)	**Tablets**: 50 mg	In 100s.
Rx	**Antivert/50** (Roerig)		(Antivert 214). Scored. In100s.
Rx	**Antrizine** (Major)		In 100s.
Rx	**Meni-D** (Seatrace)	**Capsules**: 25 mg	(Meni-D 1-4X Day). Light blue and clear. In 100s.
otc	**Vergon** (Marnel)	**Capsules**: 30 mg	In 100s.

[1] Products are available *otc* or *Rx*, depending on product labeling.

Anticholinergics

BUCLIZINE HCl

Refer to the general discussion of these products beginning in the Antiemetic/Antivertigo monograph.

Actions:

Pharmacology: Acts centrally to suppress nausea and vomiting.

Indications:

For the control of nausea, vomiting and dizziness of motion sickness.

Contraindications:

Hypersensitivity to buclizine HCl; pregnancy (see Warnings).

Warnings:

Pregnancy: When administered to the pregnant rat at doses above the human therapeutic range, buclizine induced fetal abnormalities. Clinical data are not adequate to establish safety in early pregnancy.

Children: Safety and efficacy for use in children have not been established.

Precautions:

Tartrazine sensitivity: This product contains tartrazine, which may cause an allergic-type reaction (including bronchial asthma) in susceptible individuals. Although the incidence of tartrazine sensitivity in the general population is low, it is frequently seen in patients who also have aspirin hypersensitivity.

Adverse Reactions:

Drowsiness, dry mouth, headache and jitteriness.

Administration and Dosage:

Tablets can be taken without swallowing water. Place tablet in mouth and allow to dissolve, or chew or swallow whole.

Adults: A 50 mg dose usually alleviates nausea. In severe cases, 150 mg/day may be taken. Usual maintenance dose is 50 mg, 2 times daily. In prevention of motion sickness, take 50 mg at least hour before beginning travel. For extended travel, a second 50 mg dose may be taken after 4 to 6 hours.

Rx	**Bucladin-S Softabs** (Stuart)	**Tablets:** 50 mg	Tartrazine. (Stuart 864). Yellow, scored. In 100s.

DIPHENHYDRAMINE

For complete prescribing information and product availability, see Antihistamines group monograph.

Indications:

Treatment and prophylaxis (oral only) of motion sickness.

Administration and Dosage:

Individualize dosage.

Oral: Adults – 25 to 50 mg 3 or 4 times daily.

Children > 20 lbs (9.1kg) – 12.5 to 25 mg 3 or 4 times daily (5 mg/kg/24 hrs, or 150 mg/m^2/24 hours. Do not exceed 300 mg.

Give first dose 30 minutes before exposure to motion and repeat before meals and upon retiring for the duration of journey.

Parenteral: For use only when the oral form is impractical.

Adults – 10 to 50 mg IV or deep IM; 100 mg if required. Maximum daily dosage is 400 mg.

Children – 5 mg/kg/24 hrs or 150 mg/m^2/24 hrs, in 4 divided doses, IV or deep IM. Maximum daily dosage is 300 mg.

For a complete listing of diphenhydramine HCl products refer to the Antihistamine monograph's product pages.

Anticholinergics

DIMENHYDRINATE

Refer to the general discussion of these products beginning in the Antiemetic/Antivertigo monograph.

Actions:

Pharmacology: Dimenhydrinate consists of equimolar proportions of diphenhydramine and chlorotheophylline.

Pharmacokinetics: Dimenhydrinate has a depressant action on hyperstimulated labyrinthine function. The precise mode of action is not known. The antiemetic effects are believed to be due to the diphenhydramine, an antihistamine also used as an antiemetic agent.

Indications:

For the prevention and treatment of nausea, vomiting, dizziness or vertigo of motion sickness.

Contraindications:

Neonates; patients hypersensitive to dimenhydrinate or its components.

Note: Most IV products contain benzyl alcohol, which has been associated with a fatal "Gasping Syndrome" in premature infants and low birth weight infants.

Warnings:

Pregnancy: Category B. Safety for use during pregnancy has not been established. Use only when clearly needed and when the potential benefits outweigh the potential hazards to the fetus.

Lactation: Small amounts of dimenhydrinate are excreted in breast milk. Because of the potential for adverse reactions in nursing infants, decide whether to discontinue nursing or to discontinue the drug, taking into account the importance of the drug to the mother.

Children: For infants and children especially, an overdose of antihistamines may cause hallucinations, convulsions or death. Mental alertness may be diminished. In the young child, dimenhydrinate may produce excitation. Do not give to children under 2 years of age unless directed by a physician.

Precautions:

Use with caution in conditions which might be aggravated by anticholinergic therapy (eg, prostatic hypertrophy, stenosing peptic ulcer, pyloroduodenal obstruction, bladder neck obstruction, narrow angle glaucoma, bronchial asthma, cardiac arrhythmias, etc).

Drug Interactions:

Concomitant use of **alcohol** or other **CNS depressants** with dimenhydrinate may have an additive effect.

Antibiotics: Use caution when given in conjunction with certain antibiotics that may cause ototoxicity; dimenhydrinate is capable of masking ototoxic symptoms, and irreversible damage may result.

Adverse Reactions:

CNS: Drowsiness is most common. Confusion; nervousness; restlessness; headache; insomnia (especially in children); tingling, heaviness and weakness of hands; vertigo; dizziness; lassitude; excitation.

GI: Nausea; vomiting; diarrhea; epigastric distress; constipation; anorexia.

Ophthalmic: Blurring of vision; diplopia.

Cardiovascular: Palpitations, hypotension, tachycardia.

Miscellaneous: Anaphylaxis; photosensitivity; urticaria; drug rash; hemolytic anemia; difficult or painful urination; nasal stuffiness; tightness of chest; wheezing; thickening of bronchial secretions; dryness of mouth, nose and throat.

Overdosage:

Symptoms: Drowsiness is the usual side effect. Convulsions, coma and respiratory depression may occur with massive overdosage.

Treatment: No specific antidote is known. If respiratory depression occurs, initiate mechanically assisted respiration and administer oxygen. Treat convulsions with appropriate doses of diazepam. Give phenobarbital (5 to 6 mg/kg) to control convulsions in children. Refer to General Management of Acute Overdosage.

Anticholinergics

DIMENHYDRINATE

Administration and Dosage:

Adults:

Oral – 50 to 100 mg every 4 to 6 hours. Do not exceed 400 mg in 24 hours.

IM – 50 mg, as needed.

IV – 50 mg in 10 ml Sodium Chloride Injection given over 2 minutes. Do not inject intra-arterially.

Children:

Oral (6 to 12 years) – 25 to 50 mg every 6 to 8 hours; do not exceed 150 mg in 24 hours.

Oral (2 to 6 years) – Up to 12.5 to 25 mg every 6 to 8 hours; do not exceed 75 mg in 24 hours.

IM – 1.25 mg/kg or 37.5 mg/m^2 4 times daily; do not exceed 300 mg daily.

Children (under 2 years): Only on advice of a physician.

otc	**Dimenhydrinate** (Various)	**Tablets**: 50 mg	In 12s, 100s, 300s, 500s, 1000s and UD 100s.
otc	**Calm-X** (Republic Drug)		In 16s.
Rx	**Dimetabs** (Jones Medical)		In 1000s.
otc	**Dramamine** (Upjohn)		(1701). White, scored. In UD 100s.
otc	**Marmine** (Vortech)		In 1000s.
otc	**Triptone Caplets** (Commerce)		Long acting. Scored. In 12s.
otc	**Dramamine** (Upjohn)	**Tablets, chewable**: 50 mg	Tartrazine. Aspartame, sorbitol. Orange, scored. Orange flavor. In 8s and 24s.
Rx	**Nico-Vert** (Edwards)	**Capsules**: 50 mg	In 100s.
otc	**Tega-Vert** (Ortega)		In 100s and 1000s.
Rx	**Dimenhydrinate** (Various, eg, Steris)	**Injection**: 50 mg per ml	In 1 and 10 ml vials and 1 ml amps.
Rx	**Dinate** (Seatrace)		In 10 ml vials.[1]
Rx	**Dramamine** (Upjohn)		In 1 ml amps[1] & 5 ml vials.[1]
Rx	**Dramanate** (Pasadena)		In 10 ml vials.[1]
Rx	**Dramilin** (Kay Pharm.)		In 10 ml vials.[1]
Rx	**Dymenate** (Keene)		In 10 ml vials.[1]
Rx	**Hydrate** (Hyrex)		In 10 ml vials.[1]
Rx	**Marmine** (Vortech)		In 10 ml vials.[1]
otc	**Dimenhydrinate** (Various)	**Liquid**: 12.5 mg per 4 ml	In pt and gal.
otc	**Dramamine** (Upjohn)		5% alcohol. Cherry flavor. In 90 ml.
otc	**Children's Dramamine** (Upjohn)	**Liquid**: 12.5 mg per 5 ml	5% alcohol, sucrose. Cherry flavor. In 120 ml.
Rx	**Dramamine** (Upjohn)	**Liquid**: 15.62 mg per 5 ml	In 480 ml.

[1] In benzyl alcohol and propylene glycol.

Anticholinergics

TRIMETHOBENZAMIDE HCl

Refer to the general discussion of these products beginning in the Antiemetic/Antivertigo monograph.

Actions:

Pharmacokinetics: Mechanism is obscure, but may be mediated through the chemoreceptor trigger zone; direct impulses to vomiting center are not inhibited.

Indications:

Control of nausea and vomiting.

Contraindications:

Hypersensitivity to trimethobenzamide, benzocaine or similar local anesthetics; parenteral use in children; suppositories in premature infants or neonates.

Warnings:

Pregnancy: Safety for use has not been established. Use only when clearly needed and when the potential benefits outweigh the potential hazards to the fetus.

Lactation: Safety for use in the nursing mother has not been established.

Precautions:

Encephalitides, gastroenteritis, dehydration, electrolyte imbalance (especially in children and the elderly or debilitated) and CNS reactions have occurred when used during acute febrile illness.

Exercise caution when giving the drug with alcohol and other CNS-acting agents such as phenothiazines, barbiturates and belladonna derivatives.

Adverse Reactions:

Hypersensitivity reactions; parkinson-like symptoms; hypotension or pain following IM injection; blood dyscrasias; blurred vision; coma; convulsions; depression; diarrhea; disorientation; dizziness; drowsiness; headache; jaundice; muscle cramps; opisthotonos; allergic-type skin reactions. If these occur, discontinue use. While these usually disappear spontaneously, symptomatic treatment may be indicated.

Administration and Dosage:

Oral: Adults - 250 mg, 3 or 4 times daily.

Children (30 to 90 lbs; 13.6 to 40.9 kg) – 100 to 200 mg, 3 or 4 times daily.

Rectal: Adults - 200 mg, 3 or 4 times daily.

Children (30 to 90 lbs; 13.6 to 40.9 kg) – 100 to 200 mg, 3 or 4 times daily.

(< 30 lbs) – 100 mg, 3 or 4 times daily. Do not use in premature or newborn infants.

Injection: For IM use only. *Adults* - 200 mg 3 or 4 times/day. Pain, stinging, burning, redness and swelling may develop at injection site.

Rx	**Tigan** (Roberts)	**Capsules:** 100 mg	(Tigan 100 mg). In 100s.
Rx	**Trimazide** (Major)		In 100s.
Rx	**Trimethobenzamide** (Various)	**Capsules:** 250 mg	In 100s and 500s.
Rx	**Tigan**(Roberts)		(Tigan 250 mg). Blue. In 100s.
Rx	**Trimethobenzamide** (Various)	**Pediatric Suppositories:** 100 mg	In 10s.
Rx	**Pediatric Triban** (Great Southern)		In 10s.[1]
Rx	**Tebamide** (G&W Labs)		In 10s.[1]
Rx	**T-Gen** (Goldline)		In 10s.[1]
Rx	**Tigan** (Roberts)		In 10s.[1]
Rx	**Trimazide** (Major)		In 10s.
Rx	**Trimethobenzamide** (Various)	**Suppositories:** 200 mg	In 10s and 50s.
Rx	**Tebamide** (G&W)		In 10s[1] and 50s.[1]
Rx	**T-Gen** (Goldline)		In 10s[1] and 50s.[1]
Rx	**Tigan** (Roberts)		In 10s[1]and 50s.[1]
Rx	**Triban** (Great Southern)		In 10s[1] and 50s[1].
Rx	**Trimazide** (Major)		In 10s.

Anticholinergics

TRIMETHOBENZAMIDE HCl

Rx	**Trimethobenzamide HCl** (Various)	**Injection**: 100 mg per ml	In 2 ml amps and 20 ml vials.
Rx	**Arrestin** (Vortech)		In 20 ml vials.[2]
Rx	**Ticon** (Hauck)		In 20 ml vials.[2]
Rx	**Tigan** (Roberts)		In 2 ml amps[3], 20 ml vials[2] and 2 ml syringe.[4]

[1] With 2% benzocaine.
[2] With phenol.
[3] With methyl and propyl parabens.
[4] With phenol and EDTA.

SCOPOLAMINE, TRANSDERMAL

Refer to the general discussion of these products beginning in the Antiemetic/Antivertigo group monograph.

Actions:

Pharmacology: In addition to its systemic anticholinergic effects, scopolamine is effective in motion sickness. Refer to the Gastrointestinal Anticholinergic/Antispasmodics monograph.

Scopolamine is a belladonna alkaloid with well-known pharmacological properties. The drug has a long history of oral and parenteral use for central anticholinergic activity, including prophylaxis of motion sickness. The mechanism of action of scopolamine in the CNS is not definitely known but may include anticholinergic effects. The ability of scopolamine to prevent motion-induced nausea is believed to be associated with inhibition of vestibular input to the CNS, which results in inhibition of the vomiting reflex. In addition, scopolamine may have a direct action on the vomiting center within the reticular formation of the brain stem.

Pharmacokinetics: The transdermal system is a 0.2 mm thick film with four layers. It is 2.5 cm^2 in area and contains 1.5 mg scopolamine which is gradually released from an adhesive matrix of mineral oil and polyisobutylene following application to the postauricular skin. An initial priming dose released from the system's adhesive layer saturates the skin binding site for scopolamine and rapidly brings the plasma concentration to the required steady-state level. A continuous controlled release of scopolamine flows from the drug reservoir through the rate controlling membrane to maintain a constant plasma level. Antiemetic protection is produced within several hours following application behind the ear.

Clinical trials: In clinical studies at sea or in a controlled motion environment, there was a 75% reduction in incidence of motion-induced nausea and vomiting. The system provided significantly greater protection than did oral dimenhydrinate.

Indications:

Prevention of nausea and vomiting associated with motion sickness in adults.

Contraindications:

Hypersensitivity to scopolamine or any component of the product; glaucoma.

Warnings:

Potentially alarming idiosyncratic reactions may occur with therapeutic doses.

Pregnancy: Category C. Studies in rabbits at plasma levels ≈ 100 times those achieved in humans using a transdermal system revealed a marginal embryotoxic effect. Use in pregnancy only if potential benefits justify potential risk to fetus.

Lactation: It is not known whether scopolamine is excreted in breast milk. Exercise caution when administering to a nursing woman.

Children: Safety and efficacy have not been established. Children are particularly susceptible to the side effects of belladonna alkaloids. Do not use the transdermal system in children.

Precautions:

Use with caution in patients with pyloric obstruction, urinary bladder neck obstruction and in patients suspected of having intestinal obstruction. Use with special caution in the elderly or in individuals with impaired metabolic, liver or kidney functions because of the increased likelihood of CNS effects.

Potentially hazardous tasks: May produce drowsiness, disorientation and confusion. Warn patients against engaging in activities that require mental alertness, such as driving a motor vehicle or operating dangerous machinery.

Anticholinergics

SCOPOLAMINE, TRANSDERMAL

In patients taking drugs which cause CNS effects, including alcohol, use scopolamine with care.

Drug withdrawal: Dizziness, nausea, vomiting, headache and disturbances of equilibrium have been reported in a few patients following discontinuation of the use of the transdermal system. This occurred most often in patients who used the system for more than 3 days.

Adverse Reactions:

Most common: Dry mouth (67%); drowsiness (< 17%); transient impairment of eye accommodation including blurred vision and dilation of the pupils. Unilateral fixed and dilated pupil has been reported, apparently from accidentally touching one eye after manipulation of the patch.

Infrequent: Disorientation; memory disturbances; dizziness; restlessness; hallucinations; confusion; difficulty urinating; rashes or erythema; acute narrow-angle glaucoma; dry, itchy or red eyes.

Overdosage:

Disorientation, memory disturbances, dizziness, restlessness, hallucinations or confusion. Remove the system immediately if these symptoms occur. Initiate appropriate parasympathomimetic therapy if symptoms are severe. Refer to General Management of Acute Overdosage.

For information on overdosage with other dose forms, refer to the GI Anticholinergics/Antispasmodics monograph.

Patient Information:

Patient package insert is available with the transdermal product.

Medication may cause dry mouth. May produce drowsiness or blurred vision; patients should observe caution while driving or performing other tasks requiring alertness. If eye pain, blurred vision, dizziness or rapid pulse occurs, discontinue use and consult physician.

Wash hands thoroughly after handling the transdermal disc. Temporary dilation of the pupils and blurred vision may occur if scopolamine comes in contact with the eyes.

Administration and Dosage:

Initiation of therapy: Apply one system to the postauricular skin (ie, behind the ear) at least 4 hours before the antiemetic effect is required. Scopolamine 0.5 mg will be delivered over 3 days. Wear only one disc at a time.

Handling: After applying the disc on dry skin behind the ear, wash hands thoroughly with soap and water, then dry them. Discard the removed disc and wash the hands and application site thoroughly with soap and water to prevent any traces of scopolamine from coming into direct contact with the eyes.

Continuation of therapy: If the disc is displaced, discard it and place a fresh one on the hairless area behind the other ear. If therapy is required for longer than 3 days, discard the first disc and place a fresh one on the hairless area behind the other ear.

Rx	**Transderm-Scop** (Ciba)	**Transdermal Therapeutic System:** 1.5 mg scopolamine (delivers 0.5 mg scopolamine in vivo over 3 days)	(4345). In 4 unit blister packs.

Miscellaneous

DIPHENIDOL

Refer to the general discussion beginning in the Antiemetics/Antivertigo monograph.

Warning:

May cause hallucinations, disorientation or confusion. Limit use to patients who are hospitalized or under comparable continuous, professional supervision. Carefully weigh benefits against risks and consider alternate therapies.

Actions:

Pharmacology: Diphenidol exerts a specific antivertigo effect on the vestibular apparatus to control vertigo, and inhibits the chemoreceptor trigger zone (CTZ) to control nausea and vomiting.

Indications:

Peripheral (labyrinthine) vertigo and associated nausea and vomiting; Meniere's disease and middle and inner ear surgery (labyrinthitis).

Control of nausea and vomiting in postoperative states, malignant neoplasms and labyrinthine disturbances.

Contraindications:

Hypersensitivity to diphenidol; anuria (since approximately 90% of the drug is excreted in the urine, accumulation could occur); nausea and vomiting of pregnancy.

Warnings:

CNS effects: The incidence of auditory and visual hallucinations, disorientation and confusion appears to be < 0.5%, or approximately one in 350 patients. The reaction usually occurs within 3 days of starting the drug and subsides spontaneously, usually within 3 days after discontinuation. If such a reaction occurs, discontinue the drug.

Pregnancy: Safety for use during pregnancy has not been established. Use only when clearly needed and when the potential benefits outweigh the potential hazards to the fetus. Do not use diphenidol for nausea and vomiting of pregnancy.

Lactation: Safety for use is not established. Weigh benefits against hazards.

Children: Diphenidol is not recommended for use in children < 50 pounds.

Precautions:

The antiemetic action may mask signs of drug overdose or may obscure diagnosis of conditions such as intestinal obstruction and brain tumor.

Diphenidol has a weak peripheral anticholinergic effect; use with care in patients with glaucoma, obstructive lesions of the GI and GU tracts such as stenosing peptic ulcer, prostatic hypertrophy, pyloric and duodenal obstruction and organic cardiospasm.

Tartrazine sensitivity: This product contains tartrazine, which may cause allergic-type reactions (including bronchial asthma) in susceptible individuals. Although the incidence of tartrazine sensitivity in the general population is low, it is frequently seen in patients who also have aspirin hypersensitivity.

Adverse Reactions:

CNS: Auditory and visual hallucinations; disorientation; confusion; drowsiness; overstimulation; depression; sleep disturbance; blurred vision. Rarely: Slight dizziness, malaise, headache.

Cardiovascular: Slight, transient lowering of blood pressure.

GI: Dry mouth; nausea; indigestion; heartburn (rare).

Miscellaneous: Skin rash; mild jaundice (relationship not established).

Overdosage:

Treatment includes usual supportive measures. Refer to General Management of Acute Overdosage. Early gastric lavage may be indicated, depending on the amount of overdose and symptoms.

Administration and Dosage:

Adults: For vertigo or nausea and vomiting. The usual dose is 25 mg every 4 hours. Some patients may require 50 mg.

Children: For nausea and vomiting only. Usual dose is 0.4 mg/lb (0.88 mg/kg). For children 50 to 100 lbs, give 25 mg. Do not give more often than every 4 hrs. However, if symptoms persist after first dose, repeat after 1 hr. Thereafter, give every 4 hours, as needed. Do not exceed 2.5 mg/lb (5.5 mg/kg) in 24 hrs.

Rx	**Vontrol** (SKB)	**Tablets:** 25 mg (as HCl)	Tartrazine. In 100s.

Miscellaneous

DRONABINOL

Refer to the general discussion of these products beginning in the Antiemetic/Antivertigo Agents monograph.

Actions:

Pharmacology: Dronabinol is the principal psychoactive substance present in Cannabis sativa L (marijuana). Nontherapeutic effects of dronabinol are identical to those of marijuana and other centrally active cannabinoids (see Warnings). The mechanism of action is unknown.

Cannabinoids have complex CNS effects, including central sympathomimetic activity. Cannabinoid receptors have been discovered in neural tissues. These receptors may play a role in mediating the effects of dronabinol. Patients may experience mood changes (eg, euphoria, detachment, depression, anxiety, panic, paranoia), decrements in cognitive performance and memory, a decreased ability to control drives and impulses, and alterations of reality (eg, distortions in perception of objects and sense of time, hallucinations). These latter phenomena are more common with larger doses; however, a full blown picture of psychosis (psychotic organic brain syndrome) may occur in patients receiving doses in the lower portion of the therapeutic range.

Dronabinol, within or slightly above the recommended dose range, increases heart rate and conjunctival injection. Blood pressure effects are inconsistent, but occasional subjects experience orthostatic hypotension or fainting upon standing. In one study, a slight but consistent decrease in oral temperature was recorded.

Pharmacokinetics:

Absorption/Distribution – Following oral administration, dronabinol is almost completely absorbed (90% to 95%). It has a systemic bioavailability of 10% to 20%, an onset of action of ≈ 0.5 to 1 hour and peak effect at 2 to 4 hours. Duration for psychoactive effects is 4 to 6 hours, but the appetite stimulant effect may continue for ≥ 24 hours after administration. Dronabinol has a large apparent volume of distribution, approximately 10 L/kg, because of its lipid solubility. The plasma protein binding of dronabinol and its metabolites is approximately 97%.

Metabolism/Excretion – Dronabinol undergoes extensive first-pass hepatic metabolism, primarily by microsomal hydroxylation, yielding both active and inactive metabolites. Dronabinol and its principal active metabolite, 11-OH-delta-9-THC, are present in ≈ equal concentrations in plasma. Concentrations of both parent drug and metabolite peak at ≈ 2 to 4 hours after oral dosing and decline over several days.

Biliary excretion is major route of elimination. Within 72 hours after oral administration, ≈ 50% of dose is recovered in feces; 10% to 15% appears in urine. Less than 5% is excreted unchanged in urine. Low levels of dronabinol metabolites have been detected for > 5 weeks in the urine and feces following a single dose. The elimination phase of dronabinol exhibits biphasic kinetics with an alpha half-life of 4 hours and a terminal half-life of 25 to 36 hours. Extended use at recommended doses may cause accumulation of toxic amounts of dronabinol and metabolites.

Clinical trials:

Appetite stimulation – The initial dosage of dronabinol in all patients was 5 mg/day, given in doses of 2.5 mg 1 hour before lunch and 1 hour before supper. Early morning administration appeared to be associated with an increased frequency of adverse experiences, as compared to dosing later in the day. Side effects (eg, feeling high, dizziness, confusion, somnolence) occurred in 18% of patients at this dosage level; the dosage was reduced to 2.5 mg/day, administered as a single dose at supper or bedtime. Compared to placebo, dronabinol treatment resulted in a statistically significant improvement in appetite as measured by visual analog scale. Trends toward improved body weight and mood, and decreases in nausea were also seen. After completing the 6 week study, patients were allowed to continue treatment with dronabinol in which there was a sustained improvement in appetite.

Antiemetic – Dronabinol treatment of chemotherapy-induced emesis was evaluated in patients with cancer who received a total of 750 courses of treatment of various malignancies. The antiemetic efficacy was greatest in patients receiving cytotoxic therapy with MOPP for Hodgkin's and non-Hodgkin's lymphomas. Dosages ranged from 2.5 to 40 mg/day, administered in equally divided doses every 4 to 6 hours (four times daily). Escalating the dose > 7 mg/m^2 increased the frequency of adverse experiences, with no additional antiemetic benefit.

Combination antiemetic therapy with dronabinol and a phenothiazine (eg, prochlorperazine) may result in synergistic or additive antiemetic effects and attenuate the toxicities associated with each of the agents.

Miscellaneous

DRONABINOL

Indications:

Antiemetic: Treatment of nausea and vomiting associated with cancer chemotherapy in patients not responding adequately to conventional antiemetic treatment.

Appetite stimulation: Treating anorexia associated with weight loss in AIDS patients.

Contraindications:

Hypersensitivity to dronabinol, marijuana or sesame oil.

Warnings:

Tolerance: Following 12 days of dronabinol, tolerance to the cardiovascular and subjective effects developed at doses up to 210 mg/day. An initial tachycardia induced by dronabinol was replaced successively by normal sinus rhythm and then bradycardia. A fall in supine blood pressure, made worse by standing, was also observed initially. Within days, these effects disappeared, indicating development of tolerance. Tachyphylaxis and tolerance did not, however, appear to develop to the appetite stimulant effect. In AIDS patients, the appetite stimulant effect was sustained for up to 5 months at doses of 2.5 to 20 mg/day.

Patient supervision: Because of individual variation, determine clinically the period of patient supervision required. Closely observe patients within an inpatient setting, if possible. This is especially important during treatment of patients with no prior experience with cannabis or dronabinol. However, even patients experienced with these agents may have serious untoward responses not predicted by prior uneventful exposures. Closely observe any patient who has a psychotic experience with dronabinol until the mental state returns to normal. Do not give additional doses until the patient has been examined and the circumstances evaluated. If the situation warrants it, give a lower dose under very close supervision.

Fertility impairment: In rats, dronabinol doses of 30 to 150 mg/m^2 (0.3 to 1.5 times maximum recommended human dose in cancer patients and 2 to 10 times in AIDS patients) reduced ventral prostate, seminal vesicle and epididymal weights and caused a decrease in seminal fluid volume. Decreases in spermatogenesis, number of developing germ cells and number of Leydig cells in the testis were also observed.

Elderly: Use caution because the elderly are generally more sensitive to the psychoactive effects. In antiemetic studies, no difference in tolerance or efficacy was apparent in patients > 55 years old.

Pregnancy: Category B. In mice and rats, dronabinol decreased maternal weight gain and number of viable pups and increased fetal mortality and early resorptions. The effects were dose-dependent and less apparent at lower doses. There are no adequate and well controlled studies in pregnant women. Use during pregnancy only if clearly needed.

Lactation: Dronabinol is concentrated and excreted in breast milk, and is absorbed by the nursing baby. Because the effects on the infant of chronic exposure to the drug and its metabolites are unknown, nursing mothers should not use dronabinol.

Children: Not recommended for AIDS-related anorexia in children because it has not been studied in this population. Dosage for chemotherapy-induced emesis is the same as in adults. Use caution in children because of the psychoactive effects.

Precautions:

Hypertension or heart disease: Use with caution since dronabinol may cause a general increase in central sympathomimetic activity.

Psychiatric patients: In manic, depressive or schizophrenic patients, symptoms of these disease states may be exacerbated by the use of cannabinoids.

Drug abuse and dependence: Dronabinol is highly abusable. Limit prescriptions to the amount necessary for a single cycle of chemotherapy.

It is not known what proportion of individuals exposed chronically to these drugs will develop either psychological or physical dependence. Long-term use of cannabinoids has been associated with disorders of motivation, judgment and cognition. It is not clear if this is a manifestation of the underlying personalities of chronic users of this class of drugs, or if cannabinoids are directly responsible.

A withdrawal syndrome consisting of irritability, insomnia and restlessness was observed in some subjects within 12 hours following abrupt withdrawal of dronabinol. The syndrome reached its peak intensity at 24 hours when subjects exhibited hot flashes, sweating, rhinorrhea, loose stools, hiccoughs and anorexia. The syndrome was essentially complete within 96 hours. EEG changes following discontinuation were consistent with a withdrawal syndrome. Several subjects reported impressions of disturbed sleep for several weeks after discontinuing high doses.

Miscellaneous

DRONABINOL

Hazardous tasks: Because of its profound effects on mental status, warn patients not to drive, operate complex machinery or engage in any activity requiring sound judgment and unimpaired coordination while receiving treatment. Effects may persist for a variable and unpredictable period of time. Dronabinol is highly lipid soluble, and its metabolites may persist in tissues, including plasma, for days.

Drug Interactions:

Some of the following drug interactions occurred following the use of marijuana. Although dronabinol has not been specifically cited in these instances, consider the possibility of a similar interaction.

Cannabinoid Drug Interactions			
Precipitant drug	Object drug*		Description
Dronabinol	Amphetamines Cocaine Sympathomimetics	↑	Additive hypertension, tachycardia, possibly cardiotoxicity.
Dronabinol	Anticholinergics Antihistamines	↑	Additive or super-additive tachycardia, drowsiness.
Dronabinol	Antidepressants, tricyclic	↑	Additive tachycardia, hypertension, drowsiness.
Dronabinol	Alcohol Sedatives Hypnotics Psychomimetics	↑	Additive or synergistic CNS effects. Also, clearance of barbiturates may be decreased possibly due to inhibition of metabolism.
Cannabinoids	Disulfiram	↑	A reversible hypomanic reaction occurred in a patient who smoked marijuana; confirmed by rechallenge.
Cannabinoids	Fluoxetine	↑	A patient with depression and bulimia became hypomanic after smoking marijuana; symptoms resolved after 4 days.
Cannabinoids	Theophylline	↓	Increased theophylline metabolism reported with marijuana smoking.

* ↑ = Object drug increased. ↓ = Object drug decreased.

Adverse Reactions:

Cardiovascular: Palpitations, tachycardia, vasodilation (> 1%); conjunctivitis, hypotension (0.3% to 1%).

GI: Nausea, vomiting (3% to 10%); diarrhea (0.3% to 1%); fecal incontinence, anorexia, hepatic enzyme elevation (< 1%).

CNS: Euphoria (3% to 24%); dizziness, paranoid reaction, somnolence (3% to 10%); asthenia, amnesia, ataxia, confusion, depersonalization, hallucination, abnormal thinking (> 1%); depression, emotional lability, nightmares, speech difficulties, headache, anxiety/nervousness, tremors (< 1%).

Special senses: Vision difficulties (> 1%); tinnitus (< 1%).

Dermatologic: Flushing (0.3% to 1%); sweating (< 1%).

Respiratory: Cough, rhinitis, sinusitis (< 1%).

Musculoskeletal: Myalgias (< 1%).

Overdosage:

Symptoms:

Mild intoxication – Drowsiness, euphoria, heightened sensory awareness, altered time perception, reddened conjunctiva, dry mouth and tachycardia.

Moderate intoxication – Memory impairment, depersonalization, mood alteration, urinary retention and reduced bowel motility.

Severe intoxication – Decreased motor coordination, lethargy, slurred speech and postural hypotension.

Apprehensive patients may experience panic reactions, and seizures may occur in patients with existing seizure disorders.

Miscellaneous

DRONABINOL

The estimated lethal human dose of IV dronabinol is 30 mg/kg. Significant CNS symptoms in antiemetic studies followed oral doses of 0.4 mg/kg.

Treatment: Manage potentially serious oral ingestion, if recent, with gut decontamination. In unconscious patients with a secure airway, instill activated charcoal via a nasogastric tube. A saline cathartic or sorbitol may be added to the first dose of activated charcoal. Place patients experiencing depressive, hallucinatory or psychotic reactions in a quiet area and offer reassurance. Benzodiazepines (5 to 10 mg oral diazepam) may be used for treatment of extreme agitation. Hypotension usually responds to Trendelenburg position and IV fluids. Pressors are rarely required. Refer to General Management of Acute Overdosage.

Patient Information:

Avoid alcohol and barbiturates.

May cause dizziness or drowsiness; do not drive or perform hazardous tasks requiring alertness, coordination or physical dexterity.

Apprise patients of possible changes in mood and other adverse behavioral effects of the drug so they will not panic in the event of such manifestations.

Patients should remain under the supervision of a responsible adult.

Administration and Dosage:

Antiemetic: Initially, give 5 mg/m² 1 to 3 hours prior to the administration of chemotherapy, then every 2 to 4 hours after chemotherapy is given, for a total of 4 to 6 doses/day. If the 5 mg/m² dose is ineffective and there are no significant side effects, increase the dose by 2.5 mg/m² increments to a maximum of 15 mg/m² per dose. However, use caution, as the incidence of disturbing psychiatric symptoms increases significantly at this maximum dose. Administration with phenothiazines (eg, prochlorperazine) may improve efficacy (vs either drug alone) without additional toxicity.

Appetite stimulation: Initially, give 2.5 mg twice a day before lunch and supper. For patients who cannot tolerate 5 mg/day, reduce dosage to 2.5 mg/day as a single evening or bedtime dose. When adverse reactions are absent or minimal and further therapeutic effect is desired, increase to 2.5 mg before lunch and 5 mg before supper (or 5 mg at lunch and 5 mg after supper). Although most patients respond to 2.5 mg twice daily, 10 mg twice daily has been tolerated in ≈ 50% of patients. The dosage may be increased to a maximum of 20 mg/day in divided doses. Use caution in escalating the dosage because of the increased frequency of dose-related adverse reactions at higher dosages.

C-II	Marinol (Roxane)	**Gelatin Capsules**[1]: 2.5 mg	(RL). White. In 25s, 60s and 100s.
		5 mg	(RL). Brown. In 25s and 100s.
		10 mg	(RL). Orange. In 25s and 60s.

[1] In sesame oil.

5–HT_3 RECEPTOR ANTAGONISTS

Actions:

Pharmacology: Selective 5-hydroxytryptamine$_3$ (5-HT_3) receptor antagonists are antinauseant and antiemetic agents with little or no affinity for other serotonin receptors, alpha- or beta-adrenergic, dopamine-D_2, histamine-H_1, benzodiazepine, picrotoxin or opioid receptors.

Chemotherapy-induced vomiting – Serotonin receptors of the 5-HT_3 type are located peripherally on vagal nerve terminals and centrally in the chemoreceptor trigger zone. During chemotherapy, mucosal enterochromaffin cells from the small intestine release serotonin, which stimulates the 5–HT_3 receptors. This evokes vagal afferent discharge, inducing vomiting.

5–HT_3 antagonists have little effect on blood pressure, heart rate or ECG. No evidence of an effect on plasma prolactin or aldosterone concentrations has been found. **Ondansetron** has no effect on esophageal and gastric motility, lower esophageal sphincter pressure or small intestinal transit time, cardiac output and stroke volume. Multi-day administration of ondansetron and oral **granisetron** have been shown to slow colonic transit.

Pharmacokinetics:

5-HT_3 Antagonist Pharmacokinetics

	mean C_{max} (ng/ml)	mean t½ (hr)	mean Cl (L/hr/kg)	mean V_d (L/kg)
IV				
Ondansetron (single 0.15 mg/kg dose)				
Adults	104	4.1	0.35	NA[2]
Elderly[1]	170	5.5	0.262	NA[2]
Cancer/Surgery	NA[2]	3.5	NA[2]	NA[2]
Granisetron (single 40 mcg/kg dose)				
Adults	64	5	0.79	3
Elderly[3]	57	7.5	0.44	4
Cancer patients	84	9	0.38	3
PO				
Ondansetron (single 8 mg dose)				
Adults, male (female)	25 (47)	3.6 (4.2)	0.3935 (0.3045)	NA[2]
Elderly[1], male (female)	37 (46)	4.5 (6)	0.277 (0.249)	NA[2]
Granisetron				
Adults (single 1 mg dose)	3.6	6	0.41	4
Cancer patients (1 mg BID × 7 days)	6	NA[2]	0.52	NA[2]

[1] ≥ 75 years old.
[2] NA = not available.
[3] ≥ 65 years old.

Plasma protein binding is 65% for **granisetron** and 70% to 76% for **ondansetron**. Both drugs also distribute into erythrocytes.

Clinical trials:

Granisetron vs chlorpromazine – Granisetron injection 40 mcg/kg was compared with the combination of chlorpromazine (50 to 200 mg/24 hrs) and dexamethasone (12 mg) in patients treated with moderately emetogenic chemotherapy, including primarily carboplatin, cisplatin and cyclophosphamide. Granisetron was superior to the chlorpromazine regimen in preventing nausea and vomiting.

5–HT$_3$ RECEPTOR ANTAGONISTS

Prevention of Chemotherapy-Induced Nausea and Vomiting: Granisetron vs Chlorpromazine		
Parameter	Granisetron (n = 133)	Chlorpromazine[1] (n = 133)
Response over 24 hours		
Complete response[2]	68%	47%
No vomiting	73%	53%
No more than mild nausea	77%	59%

[1] Patients also received 12 mg dexamethasone.
[2] No vomiting and no moderate or severe nausea.

In other studies of moderately emetogenic chemotherapy, no significant difference in efficacy was found between granisetron doses of 40 and 160 mcg/kg doses.

Ondansetron vs metoclopramide – Ondansetron injection was compared with metoclopramide in a single-blind trial in 307 patients on cisplatin ≥ 100 mg/m^2 with or without other chemotherapy agents. Patients received the first dose of ondansetron or metoclopramide 30 minutes before cisplatin. Two additional ondansetron doses were administered 4 and 8 hours later, or five additional metoclopramide doses were administered 2, 4, 7, 10 and 13 hours later. Cisplatin was given over ≤ 3 hours. Episodes of vomiting and retching were tabulated over the 24 hours after cisplatin.

Ondansetron vs Metoclopramide - Prevention of Emesis Induced by Cisplatin (≥ 100 mg/m^2) Single-day Therapy[1]		
Parameters	Ondansetron (n = 136) 0.15 mg/kg x 3	Metoclopramide (n = 138) 2 mg/kg x 6
Treatment Response		
0 emetic episodes	40%	30%
1 to 2 emetic episodes	25%	22%
3 to 5 emetic episodes	14%	13%
> 5 emetic episodes/rescued	21%	36%
Median # of emetic episodes	1	2
Median time to first emetic episode (hours)	20.5	4.3
Global satisfaction with control of nausea and vomiting (0-100)[2]	85	63
Acute dystonic reactions	0	8
Akathisia	0	10

[1] In addition to cisplatin, 68% of patients received other chemotherapy agents, including cyclophosphamide, etoposide and fluorouracil.
[2] Visual analog scale assessment: 0 = not at all satisfied, 100 = totally satisfied.

Indications:

Antiemetic: Prevention of nausea and vomiting associated with initial and repeat courses of emetogenic cancer therapy, including high-dose cisplatin; prevention of postoperative nausea or vomiting (ondansetron); prevention of nausea and vomiting associated with radiotherapy in patients receiving either total body irradiation, single high-dose fraction or daily fractions to the abdomen (oral ondansetron).

Unlabeled uses:

Granisetron – Acute nausea and vomiting following surgery (1 to 3 mg IV).

Contraindications:

Hypersensitivity to the drug or components of the product.

Warnings:

Routine prophylaxis is not recommended for patients in whom there is little expectation that nausea or vomiting will occur postoperatively. In patients where nausea or vomiting must be avoided postoperatively, IV **ondansetron** is recommended even where the incidence of postoperative nausea or vomiting is low. For patients who have postoperative nausea or vomiting, ondansetron may be given to prevent further episodes.

Peristalsis: **Ondansetron** does not stimulate gastric or intestinal peristalsis. Do not use instead of nasogastric suction. Use in abdominal surgery may mask a progressive ileus or gastric distension.

5–HT_3 RECEPTOR ANTAGONISTS

Hypersensitivity: Rare cases of hypersensitivity reactions, sometimes severe (eg, anaphylaxis, bronchospasm, shortness of breath, hypotension, shock, angioedema, urticaria), have occurred. Refer to Management of Acute Hypersensitivity Reactions.

Carcinogenesis/Mutagenesis: Rats were treated orally with **granisetron** 1, 5 or 50 mg/kg/day (16, 81 and 405 times the recommended human clinical dose). There was a statistically significant increase in the incidence of hepatocellular carcinomas and adenomas. Treatment with granisetron 100 mg/kg/day (1622 times the recommended human dose) produced hepatocellular adenomas in male and female rats.

Granisetron produced a significant increase in UDS in HeLa cells in vitro and a significantly increased incidence of cells with polyploidy in an in vitro human lymphocyte chromosomal aberration test.

Elderly: Dosage adjustment is not needed in patients > 65 years of age. Prevention of nausea and vomiting in elderly patients was no different than in younger age groups.

Pregnancy: Category B. There are no adequate and well controlled studies in pregnant women. Use during pregnancy only if the potential benefit justifies the potential risk to the fetus.

Lactation: **Ondansetron** is excreted in the breast milk of rats. It is not known whether 5-HT_3 antagonists are excreted in human breast milk. Exercise caution when 5-HT_3 antagonists are administered to a nursing woman.

Children:

Granisetron – Safety and efficacy of the injection in children < 2 years of age have not been established; see Administration and Dosage for use in children 2 to 16 years of age. Safety and efficacy of the oral doseform in children have not been established.

Ondansetron – Little information is available about dosage in children ≤ 3 years of age. See Administration and Dosage for use in children 4 to 18 years of age.

Drug Interactions:

Because 5–HT_3 antagonists are metabolized by hepatic cytochrome P-450 enzymes, inducers or inhibitors of these enzymes may change the clearance and, hence, the half-life of 5-HT_3 antagonists. However, on the basis of available data, no dosage adjustment is recommended for patients on these drugs.

Drug/Food interactions:

Granisetron – When a single dose of oral granisetron 10 mg was administered with food, AUC was decreased by 5% and C_{max} increased by 30% in non-fasted healthy volunteers.

Ondansetron – The extent of absorption of oral ondansetron is significantly increased (≈ 17%) by food but is not believed to be clinically relevant. C_{max} and T_{max} are not significantly affected.

Adverse Reactions:

5-HT_3 Receptor Antagonist Adverse Reactions[1]

Adverse Event	Ondansetron (%)	Granisetron (%)
CNS		
Anxiety/Agitation	6	
Dizziness	7	
Drowsiness/Sedation	8	-
Headache	9 to 27[2,3]	14 to 21
Malaise/Fatigue	9 to 13	-
GI		
Abdominal pain	3[2]	6
Constipation	6 to 9	18
Diarrhea	6	8
Xerostomia	2	-
Miscellaneous		
Asthenia	-	14
Cold sensation	2	-
Fever/Pyrexia	2 to 8	-
Gynecological disorder	7	-

5–HT_3 RECEPTOR ANTAGONISTS

5-HT_3 Receptor Antagonist Adverse Reactions[1]		
Adverse Event	Ondansetron (%)	Granisetron (%)
Hypoxia	9	-
Injection site reaction	4	-
Paresthesia	2	-
Pruritus	2 to 5	-
Urinary retention	5	-
Weakness[1]	2	-

[1] Greater than placebo or comparator regardless of route of administration or indication. Data from separate studies; not necessarily comparable.
[2] More common with PO tid vs bid dosing.
[3] More common with IV single high-dose.

CNS:

Ondansetron – Extrapyramidal syndrome (6%); grand mal seizures (rare).

Granisetron – CNS stimulation; Somnolence (3% to 5%); insomnia (<2% to 3%); extrapyramidal syndrome (rare).

Cardiovascular:

Ondansetron – Arrhythmias (6%); hypotension (3% to 5%); chest pain (2%); angina, syncope (rare).

Granisetron – Hypertension (2%); angina, arrhythmias, syncope (rare).

GI:

Granisetron – Nausea (15%); vomiting (9%); decreased appetite (5%); taste disorder (2%).

Miscellaneous:

Ondansetron – Wound problem (28%); musculoskeletal pain (10%); shivers (7%); postoperative CO_2-related pain (2%); bronchospasm, hypersensitivity, hypokalemia, transient blurred vision (rare).

Granisetron – Leukopenia (11%); shivers (5%); anemia (4%); alopecia, thrombocytopenia (3%); hypersensitivity (rare).

Overdosage:

Symptoms: "Sudden blindness" (amaurosis) of a 2 to 3 minute duration plus severe constipation occurred in one patient who was given a single 72 mg IV dose of **ondansetron**. Hypotension and faintness occurred in a patient who took 48 mg of ondansetron orally. Following the infusion of a 32 mg dose of ondansetron over only a 4 minute period, a vasovagal episode with transient second degree heart block was observed. In all instances, the events completely resolved. Individual doses as large as 145 mg and total daily dosages (three doses) as large as 252 mg have been administered IV without significant adverse events. Overdosage of up to 38.5 mg **granisetron** injection has been reported without symptoms or with only the occurrence of a slight headache.

Treatment: Manage patients with appropriate supportive therapy. Refer to General Management of Acute Overdosage.

ONDANSETRON HCl

For complete prescribing information, refer to the 5–HT$_3$ Receptor Antagonists Agents group monograph.

Administration and Dosage:

Prevention of nausea/vomiting associated with cancer chemotherapy:

IV – Dilute in 50 ml of 5% Dextrose or 0.9% NaCl Injection before administration. Do not mix with solutions for which compatibility has not been established; in particular, this applies to alkaline solutions because a precipitate may form.

The recommended IV dosage is three 0.15 mg/kg doses or a single 32 mg dose. With the 3 dose regimen, the first dose is infused over 15 minutes beginning 30 minutes before the start of emetogenic chemotherapy. Subsequent doses are administered 4 and 8 hours after the first dose. The single 32 mg dose is infused over 15 minutes, beginning 30 minutes before the start of emetogenic chemotherapy.

Children: On the basis of the limited available information, the dosage in children 4 to 18 years of age should be three 0.15 mg/kg doses (see above). Little information is available about dosage in children ≤ 2 years of age.

Oral – Recommended dose is 8 mg twice daily. Administer the first dose 30 minutes before the start of emetogenic chemotherapy, with a subsequent dose 8 hours after the first dose. Administer 8 mg twice a day (every 12 hours) for 1 to 2 days after completion of chemotherapy.

Children: For patients ≥ 12 years of age, dosage is the same as for adults; for children 4 to 11 years, give 4 mg 3 times/day. Give the first dose 30 minutes before chemotherapy, with subsequent doses 4 and 8 hours after the first dose. Give 4 mg 3 times/day (every 8 hours) for 1 to 2 days after completion of chemotherapy.

Elderly: No dosage adjustment is necessary.

Prevention of nausea/vomiting associated with radiotherapy (oral): 8 mg 3 times/day.

Total body irradiation – 8 mg 1 to 2 hours before each fraction of radiotherapy administered each day.

Single high-dose fraction radiotherapy to the abdomen – 8 mg 1 to 2 hours before radiotherapy, with subsequent doses every 8 hours after the first dose for 1 to 2 days after completion of radiotherapy.

Daily fractionated radiotherapy to the abdomen – 8 mg 1 to 2 hours before radiotherapy, with subsequent doses every 8 hours after the first dose for each day radiotherapy is given.

Children – There is no experience in children for this indication.

Elderly – No dosage adjustment is necessary.

Prevention of postoperative nausea or vomiting:

IV – Immediately before induction of anesthesia, or postoperatively if the patient experiences nausea or vomiting occurring shortly after surgery, administer 4 mg IV undiluted over ≥ 30 seconds, preferably over 2 to 5 minutes. Repeat dosing for patients who continue to experience nausea or vomiting postoperatively has not been studied.

Oral – 16 mg given as a single dose 1 hour before induction of anesthesia.

Children – Patients 2 to 12 years of age weighing ≤ 40 kg may receive 0.1 mg/kg IV, give a single 4 mg dose for those weighing > 40 kg. Administer over ≥ 30 seconds, preferably over 2 to 5 minutes. There is no experience in children with the use of tablets for this indication.

Elderly: No dosage adjustment is necessary.

Hepatic function impairment: Do not exceed an 8 mg oral dose. For IV use, a single maximum daily dose of 8 mg infused over 15 minutes beginning 30 minutes before the start of emetogenic chemotherapy is recommended.

Admixture compatibility: Ondansetron 0.03 and 0.3 mg/ml has been reported to be stable in a TPN admixture (333 ml of 15% amino acids, 500 ml of 70% dextrose, 400 ml of 20% lipids, common therapeutic doses of vitamins and minerals) at 24°C for ≥ 48 hours. Ondansetron and dexamethasone sodium phosphate in 5% Dextrose Injection or 0.9% Sodium Chloride Injection were stable for ≤ 24 hours when stored at room temperature (23° to 25°C) in PVC bags or glass bottles. Admixtures containing lorazepam, ondansetron and dexamethasone sodium phosphate in 5% Dextrose Injection were stable for ≤ 24 hours at room temperature when stored in glass bottles. Stability of an ondansetron/cisplatin continuous IV infusion combination has been reported to be ≥ 8 days when stored under refrigeration (2° to 8°C) for ≥ 24 hours. Admixtures of 0.9% Sodium Chloride Injection, ondansetron 0.1 and 1 mg/ml *plus morphine* sulfate 1 mg/ml or hydromorphone HCl 0.5 mg/ml are compatible and stable for ≥ 7 days at 32°C and for at least 31 days at 4°C and 22°C. Ondansetron 0.05 mg/ml and cyclophosphamide 0.3 mg/ml were stable in 5% Dextrose Injection or 0.9% Sodium Chloride Injection for 4 days at 23°C to 25°C or for 8 days at 4°C.

5–HT_3 Receptor Antagonists

ONDANSETRON HCl

Y-site compatibility: Ranitidine 0.5 or 2 mg/ml may be administered through a Y-injection port with ondansetron 0.03, 0.1 or 0.3 mg/ml for ≤ 4 hours. Ondansetron with fluconazole, aztreonam, ceftazidime or cefazolin are compatible for 4 hours under simulated Y-site conditions.

Storage/Stability: Ondansetron IV is stable at room temperature under normal lighting conditions for 48 hours after dilution with the following IV fluids: 0.9% Sodium Chloride Injection; 5% Dextrose Injection; 5% Dextrose and 0.9% Sodium Chloride Injection; 5% Dextrose and 0.45% Sodium Chloride Injection; 3% Sodium Chloride Injection.

When stored in polypropylene syringes, ondansetron 2 mg/ml undiluted, or concentrations of 0.25, 0.5 or 1 mg/ml is reported to be stable for 3 months at -20°C, 14 days at 4°C and 48 hours at 22° to 25°C.

Suppositories: Add pulverized ondansetron tablet powder into the melted fatty acid base and mix thoroughly. Pour the melt continuously into the suppository molds until all are filled. Store in light-resistant containers under refrigeration. Stability has been reported to be ≥ 30 days.

Solution: Ondansetron tablets may be compounded extemporaneously with Cherry Syrup, USP; Syrpalta; Ora Sweet and Ora Sweet Sugar-Free to contain ondansetron 0.8 mg/ml (4 mg/5 ml). It is stable for 42 days at 4°C.

Rx	**Zofran** (Glaxo Wellcome)	**Tablets**: 4 mg	Lactose. (Zofran 4). White, oval. Film coated. In 30s, UD 100s and 1 x 3 daily UD pack.
		8 mg	Lactose. (Zofran 8). Yellow, oval. Film coated. In 30s, UD 100s and 1 x 3 daily UD pack.
Rx	**Zofran** (Glaxo Wellcome)	**Injection**: 2 mg/ml	1.2 mg methylparaben, 0.15 mg propylparaben. In 2 ml single-dose vials and 20 ml multi-dose vials.
		32 mg/50 ml (premixed)	Preservative free. With 2500 mg dextrose, 26 mg citric acid and 11.5 mg sodium citrate. In 50 ml single-dose containers (6s).

GRANISETRON HCl

For complete prescribing information, refer to the 5–HT_3 Receptor Antagonist Agents group monograph.

Administration and Dosage:

Approved by the FDA on December 29, 1993 (1S classification).

IV: The recommended dosage is 10 mcg/kg infused IV over 5 minutes, given within 30 minutes before initiation of chemotherapy and only on day(s) of chemotherapy.

Children – The recommended dose in children 2 to 16 years of age is 10 mcg/kg. Children < 2 years of age have not been studied.

Elderly/Renal/Hepatic function impairment – No dosage adjustment is needed.

Infusion preparation – Dilute granisetron in 0.9% Sodium Chloride or 5% Dextrose to a total volume of 20 to 50 ml.

Admixture incompatibility – Do not mix granisetron injection in solution with other drugs.

Storage/Stability – Prepare the IV infusion of granisetron at the time of administration. However, granisetron is stable for ≥ 24 hours when diluted in 0.9% Sodium Chloride or 5% Dextrose and stored at room temperature under normal lighting conditions. Do not freeze vials. Protect from light.

Oral: 1 mg twice daily. Give the first dose ≤ 1 hour before chemotherapy and the second dose 12 hours after the first, only on the day(s) chemotherapy is given. Continued treatment while not on chemotherapy has not been found to be useful.

Children – Data not available.

Elderly/Renal/Hepatic function impairment – No dosage adjustment is needed.

Rx	**Kytril** (SmithKline Beecham)	**Tablets**: 1 mg (1.12 mg as HCl)	Lactose. (K1). White, biconvex. Triangular. Film-coated. In 20s and unit-of-use 2s.
		Injection: 1 mg/ml (1.12 mg/ml as HCl)	Preservative free. In 1 ml single-use vials.

PHOSPHORATED CARBOHYDRATE SOLUTION

Refer to the general discussion beginning in the Antiemetics/Antivertigo monograph.

Actions:

Pharmacology: Hyperosmolar carbohydrate solutions with phosphoric acid relieve nausea and vomiting by a direct local action on the wall of the GI tract that reduces smooth muscle contraction and delays gastric emptying time in direct proportion to the amount used.

The data available do not appear sufficient to document effectiveness.

Indications:

Antiemetic: Symptomatic relief of nausea and vomiting.

Precautions:

Nausea may signal a serious condition. If symptoms are not relieved or recur often, consult a physician.

Diabetic patients should avoid these preparations because they contain significant amounts of carbohydrates.

Hereditary fructose intolerance: Individuals with this condition should avoid these preparations.

Adverse Reactions:

Large doses of fructose can cause abdominal pain and diarrhea.

Administration and Dosage:

Do not dilute. Do not take oral fluids immediately before the dose or for at least 15 minutes after the dose.

Epidemic and other functional vomiting or nausea and vomiting due to psychogenic factors:

Infants and children – 5 or 10 ml at 15-minute intervals until vomiting ceases. Do not take for more than 1 hour (5 doses).

Adults – 15 or 30 ml in same manner. If first dose is rejected, resume same dosage schedule in 5 minutes.

Regurgitation in infants: 5 or 10 ml, 10 to 15 minutes before each feeding; in refractory cases, 10 or 15 ml, 30 minutes before feeding.

Morning sickness: 15 to 30 ml on arising; repeat every 3 hours or when nausea threatens.

Motion sickness and nausea and vomiting due to drug therapy or inhalation anesthesia: 5 ml doses for young children; 15 ml doses for older children and adults.

otc	**Emetrol** (Pharmacia & Upjohn)	**Solution:** Fructose, dextrose and orthophosphoric acid with controlled hydrogen ion concentration	Lemon-mint or cherry flavor. In 120, 240 and 480 ml.
otc	**Nausetrol** (Various)		In 120 ml, pt and gal.
otc	**Nausea Relief** (Goldline)	**Solution:** 1.87 g dextrose, 1.87 g levulose, 21.5 mg phosphoric acid	Methylparaben. In 118 ml.
otc	**Emecheck** (Savage)	**Liquid:** 21.5 mg phosphoric acid, glucose, fructose per 5 ml	Methylparaben. Cherry flavor. In 118 ml.

MEPROBAMATE

Actions:

Pharmacology: Meprobamate, an antianxiety agent, is a carbamate derivative that has selective effects at multiple sites in the CNS, including the thalamus and limbic system. It also appears to inhibit multineuronal spinal reflexes. Meprobamate is mildly tranquilizing, and has some anticonvulsant and muscle relaxant properties.

Pharmacokinetics:

Absorption/Distribution – Meprobamate is well absorbed from the GI tract; peak plasma concentrations are reached within 1 to 3 hours. During chronic administration of sedative doses, concentrations in blood range between 5 and 20 mcg/ml. Plasma protein binding is approximately 15%.

Metabolism/Excretion – The liver metabolizes 80% to 92% of the drug; the remainder is excreted unchanged in the urine. Following a single dose, the plasma half-life ranges from 6 to 17 hours, but during chronic administration, may be as long as 24 to 48 hours. Meprobamate can induce some hepatic microsomal enzymes, but it is not known whether it induces its own metabolism. Excretion is mainly renal (90%), with < 10% appearing in feces.

Indications:

Management of anxiety disorders or short-term relief of the symptoms of anxiety. Anxiety or tension associated with the stress of everyday life usually does not require treatment with an anxiolytic.

Effectiveness in long-term use (> 4 months) has not been assessed by systematic clinical studies. Periodically reassess usefulness of the drug for the individual patient.

Contraindications:

Acute intermittent porphyria; allergic or idiosyncratic reactions to meprobamate or related compounds (eg, carisoprodol).

Warnings:

Drug dependence: Physical and psychological dependence and abuse may occur. Avoid prolonged use, especially in alcoholics and addiction prone persons. Consider possibility of suicide attempts. Carefully supervise dose and amounts prescribed; dispense least amount of drug feasible at any one time.

Abrupt discontinuation after prolonged and excessive use may precipitate a recurrence of pre-existing symptoms or withdrawal syndrome characterized by anxiety, anorexia, insomnia, vomiting, ataxia, tremors, muscle twitching, confusional states and hallucinations. Generalized seizures occur in about 10% of cases and are more likely to occur in persons with CNS damage or preexistent or latent convulsive disorders. Onset of withdrawal symptoms usually occurs within 12 to 48 hours after drug discontinuation; symptoms usually cease in the next 12 to 48 hours.

When excessive dosage has continued for weeks or months, reduce gradually over a period of 1 or 2 weeks rather than stopping abruptly. Alternatively, a short-acting barbiturate may be substituted and then gradually withdrawn.

Hypersensitivity: Usually seen between the first to fourth dose in patients having no previous exposure to the drug. In case of allergic or idiosyncratic reactions, discontinue the drug and initiate approprate symptomatic therapy, which may include epinephrine, antihistamines and in severe cases, corticosteroids. In evaluating possible allergic reactions, also consider allergy to excipients. See Adverse Reactions. Refer to Management of Acute Hypersensitivity Reactions.

Renal function impairment: Use with caution to avoid accumulation, since meprobamate is metabolized in the liver and excreted by the kidney.

Elderly: To avoid oversedation, use lowest effective dose.

Pregnancy: Meprobamate passes the placental barrier. It is present in umbilical cord blood, at or near maternal plasma levels. An increased risk of congenital malformations is associated with its use during the first trimester of pregnancy. Since few indications exist for this drug in the pregnant woman, use with extreme caution, if at all, during pregnancy. Consider the possibility that a woman of childbearing potential may be pregnant at the time of institution of therapy.

Lactation: Meprobamate is excreted into breast milk at concentrations 2 to 4 times that of maternal plasma. The effect of this amount of drug on the nursing infant is unknown.

Children: Do not administer to children < 6 years of age since there is a lack of documented evidence of safety and efficacy. The 600 mg tablet is not intended for use in children.

Precautions:

Epilepsy: May precipitate seizures in epileptic patients.

Hazardous tasks: May produce drowsiness, dizziness or blurred vision; patients should observe caution while driving or performing other tasks requiring alertness.

MEPROBAMATE

Drug Interactions:

Alcohol: Acute ingestion may result in a decreased clearance of meprobamate through inhibition of hepatic metabolic systems; enhanced CNS depressant effects may occur. Tolerance may occur with chronic alcohol ingestion, presumably due to enhanced metabolic capacity.

CNS depressants (eg, barbiturates, narcotics): Anticipate additive CNS depressant effects.

Adverse Reactions:

CNS: Drowsiness; ataxia; dizziness; slurred speech; headache; vertigo; weakness; impairment of visual accommodation; euphoria; overstimulation; paradoxical excitement; fast EEG activity.

GI: Nausea; vomiting; diarrhea.

Cardiovascular: Palpitations; tachycardia; various arrhythmias; transient ECG changes; syncope and hypotensive crises (including one fatality).

Miscellaneous:

Allergic or idiosyncratic – Usually seen between the first to fourth dose in patients having no previous exposure to the drug.

Milder reactions are characterized by an itchy, urticarial or erythematous maculopapular rash which may be generalized or confined to the groin. Other reactions have included leukopenia, acute nonthrombocytopenic purpura, petechiae, ecchymoses, eosinophilia, peripheral edema, adenopathy, fever, fixed drug eruption with cross reaction to carisoprodol.

More severe, rare hypersensitivity reactions include hyperpyrexia, chills, angioneurotic edema, bronchospasm, oliguria, anuria, anaphylaxis, erythema multiforme, exfoliative dermatitis, stomatitis and proctitis. Stevens-Johnson syndrome and bullous dermatitis have also occurred, including one fatal case of the latter after administration of meprobamate in combination with prednisolone (see Warnings).

Other – Exacerbation of porphyric symptoms; paresthesias.

Hematologic: Agranulocytosis and aplastic anemia (rarely fatal) have occurred, but no causal relationship has been established. Rarely, thrombocytopenic purpura.

Overdosage:

Symptoms: Acute intoxication produces drowsiness, lethargy, stupor, ataxia, coma, shock, vasomotor and respiratory collapse and death. Cardiovascular disturbances include arrhythmias, tachycardia, bradycardia and reduced venous return. Profound and persistent hypotension occurs and can appear unexpectedly in mildly comatose patients. Excessive oronasal secretion or relaxation of the pharyngeal wall may cause airway obstruction problems. The following data represent the usual ranges:

Acute simple overdose (meprobamate alone) – Death has occurred with ingestion of as little as 12 g and survival with as much as 40 g.

Blood levels – 0.5 to 3 mg/dl – Therapeutic range.

3 to 10 mg/dl – Mild to moderate overdosage; stupor, light coma.

10 to 20 mg/dl – Deeper coma requiring intensive therapy; some fatalities.

> 20 mg/dl – > 50% fatalities.

Acute combined overdose with other psychotropic drugs, other CNS depressants or alcohol renders the above values useless as a prognostic indicator.

Treatment: Since meprobamate is rapidly absorbed, gastric lavage (or emesis in a conscious patient) may be of value only if carried out shortly after ingestion. Ingestion of large amounts may form drug conglomerates in the stomach; continue gastric lavage. Gastroscopy may be indicated. Relapse and death after initial recovery have been attributed to incomplete gastric emptying and delayed absorption. Frequent measurements of vital signs cannot be overemphasized.

Provide symptomatic and supportive treatment. Hypotension may appear rapidly and become persistent unless blood volume is expanded. Avoid fluid overload; fatal pulmonary edema has occurred. Provide respiratory assistance when needed. Exercise care in the treatment of convulsions because of the combined effect of agents on CNS depression. Refer to General Management of Acute Overdosage.

If the patient's condition deteriorates despite assisted respiration, try forced diuresis and pressor agents, then institute hemodialysis. Meprobamate is dialyzable. Hemoperfusion (resin or charcoal) is more effective than hemodialysis. The half-life during hemoperfusion may be reduced more than threefold.

Patient Information:

Advise patients that if they become pregnant during therapy or intend to become pregnant, they should consult with their physician about use of the drug.

May cause drowsiness, dizziness or blurred vision; use caution while driving or performing other tasks requiring alertness.

Avoid alcohol and other CNS depressants while taking this drug.

MEPROBAMATE

Notify physician if skin rash, sore throat or fever occurs.

Do not crush or chew tablets and sustained release capsules.

Administration and Dosage:

Adults: 1.2 to 1.6 g/day in 3 to 4 divided doses; do not exceed 2.4 g/day.

Sustained release – 400 to 800 mg in the morning and at bedtime.

Children: 100 to 200 mg 2 or 3 times daily.

Sustained release – 200 mg in the morning and at bedtime.

c-iv	**Meprobamate** (Various, eg, Balan, Dixon-Shane, Geneva, Goldline, Lannett, Major, Moore, Rugby, Schein, Spencer Mead)	**Tablets:** 200 mg	In 20s, 100s and 1000s.
c-iv	**Equanil** (Wyeth-Ayerst)		(Wyeth 2). White. In 100s.
c-iv	**Miltown** (Wallace)		(Wallace 37 1101). White. Sugar coated. In 100s.
c-iv	**Meprobamate** (Various, eg, Balan, Dixon-Shane, Geneva, Goldline, Lannett, Major, Moore, Rugby, Schein, Spencer Mead)	**Tablets:** 400 mg	In 20s, 100s, 500s, 1000s and UD 100s.
c-iv	**Equanil** (Wyeth-Ayerst)		(Wyeth 1). White, scored. In 100s and 500s.
c-iv	**Miltown** (Wallace)		(Wallace 37 1001). White, scored. In 100s, 500s and 1000s.
c-iv	**Neuramate** (Halsey)		In 100s and 1000s.
c-iv	**Miltown 600** (Wallace)	**Tablets:** 600 mg	(Wallace 600 37 1601). White. Capsule shape. In 100s.
c-iv	**Meprospan** (Wallace)	**Capsules, sustained release:** 200 mg	(Wallace 200 37-1401). Yellow. In 100s.
c-iv	**Meprospan** (Wallace)	**Capsules, sustained release:** 400 mg	(Wallace 400 37-1301). Blue. In 100s.

BENZODIAZEPINES

Actions:

Pharmacology: Benzodiazepines appear to potentiate the effects of gamma-aminobutyrate (GABA) (ie, they facilitate inhibitory GABA neurotransmission) and other inhibitory transmitters by binding to specific benzodiazepine receptor sites. Recent evidence suggest there are at least two benzodiazepine receptors, BZ_1 and BZ_2. BZ_1 is thought to be associated with sleep mechanisms; BZ_2 with memory, motor, sensory and cognitive functions. The activity of the benzodiazepines may involve the following sites: Spinal cord (muscle relaxation); brain stem (anticonvulsant properties); cerebellum (ataxia); limbic and cortical areas (emotional behavior). Anxiolytic effects are distinct from nonspecific consequences of CNS depression (ie, sedation and motor impairment). A distinctive feature of the benzodiazepines is the wide margin of safety between therapeutic and toxic doses. Ataxia and sedation occur only at doses beyond those needed for anxiolytic effects.

Clonazepam suppresses the spike and wave discharge in petit mal seizures and decreases frequency, amplitude, duration and spread of discharge in minor motor seizures.

Pharmacokinetics:

Absorption – The major determinant of the onset and intensity of action of a single oral dose of a benzodiazepine is the rate of absorption from the GI tract. Benzodiazepines are readily absorbed following oral administration.

IM administration of chlordiazepoxide and diazepam results in slow erratic absorption and lower peak plasma levels than oral or IV administration. However, IM administration of diazepam into the deltoid muscle is more likely to be rapid and complete. Lorazepam IM is rapidly and completely absorbed.

Distribution – The highly lipid soluble benzodiazepines are widely distributed in the body tissues and highly bound to plasma proteins (70% to 99%). The duration of action is related to their lipid solubility. Highly lipophilic drugs, like diazepam, are rapidly taken into the brain and then rapidly redistributed throughout the body.

Metabolism – The effect of lipid solubility on duration of action is complicated by hepatic biotransformation to active metabolites. The benzophenone metabolite of alprazolam is inactive, while alpha-hydroxy-alprazolam is approximately one-half as active as the parent compound; both metabolites have the same half-life as alprazolam. Other benzodiazepines have active metabolites with very long half-lives; cumulative effects occur with chronic administration. Desmethyldiazepam is an active metabolite common to many of these agents (eg, clorazepate, halazepam, prazepam, diazepam); clorazepate is hydrolyzed in the stomach and absorbed as desmethyldiazepam. Chlordiazepoxide has several active intermediate metabolites. Five metabolites of clonazepam have been identified. Biotransformation of clonazepam is by oxidative hydroxylation and reduction.

Since hepatic biotransformation is the predominant route for benzodiazepine metabolism, the disposition of these drugs may be impaired in patients with chronic liver disease. Oxazepam and lorazepam are metabolized to inactive compounds and therefore have relatively short half-lives and duration of activity. Because of their simple one-step inactivation, oxazepam or lorazepam may be preferred in patients with liver disease and in the elderly. Sustained clinical effects require multiple daily doses; significant accumulation does not occur. The other agents with prolonged half-lives may be administered as a single daily dose at bedtime. The elimination half-life of diazepam and desmethyldiazepam is prolonged in obese patients; total metabolic clearance does not change.

Benzodiazepine Metabolic Pathways

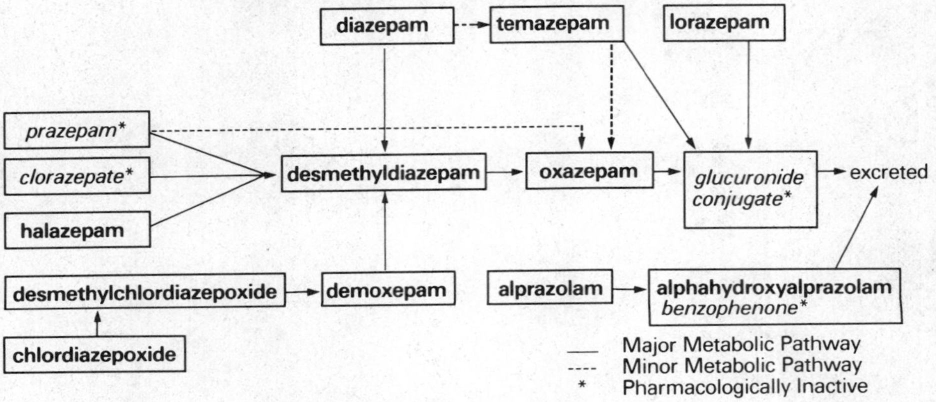

BENZODIAZEPINES

Excretion – Most of the benzodiazepines are excreted almost entirely in the urine and in the form of oxidized and glucuronide-conjugated metabolites.

There is little clinical evidence to suggest that one benzodiazepine is more effective than another. The major differences are reflected in their pharmacokinetic profiles and relative costs. The following table summarizes the major pharmacokinetic variables of these agents:

Benzodiazepine Pharmacokinetics

Drug	Dosage Range (mg/day)[1]	Peak Plasma Level (hrs)[1]	Elimination t½ (hrs)	Metabolites	Speed of Onset[1]	Protein Binding
Alprazolam	0.75-4	1-2	6.3-26.9	Alpha-hydroxy-alprazolam; Benzophenone	intermediate	80%
Chlordiazepoxide	15-100	0.5-4	5-30	Desmethylchlordiazepoxide[2]; Demoxepam; Desmethyldiazepam	intermediate	96%
Clonazepam	1.5-20	1-2	18-50	Inactive 7–amino or 7–acetyl-amino derivatives[2]	intermediate	97%
Clorazepate	15-60	1-2	40-50	Desmethyl-diazepam	fast	97%-98%[3]
Diazepam	4-40	0.5-2	20-80	Desmethyl-diazepam[2]; nordiazepam	very fast	98%
Halazepam	60-160	1-3	14	Desmethyl-diazepam[2]; 3-hydroxy-halazepam	slow	97%
Lorazepam	2-4	2-4	10-20	Inactive glucuronide conjugate	intermediate	85%
Oxazepam	30-120	2-4	5-20	Inactive glucuronide conjugate	slow	87%

[1] Oral administration.
[2] Major metabolite.
[3] Nordiazepam (active metabolite).

Indications:

Anxiety: For the management of anxiety disorders or for the short-term relief of the symptoms of anxiety. Anxiety or tension associated with the stress of everyday life usually does not require treatment with an antianxiety agent.

Consult individual drug monographs for specific indications.

In addition to use as antianxiety agents, some benzodiazepines are also useful as hypnotics, anticonvulsants and muscle relaxants. Midazolam, an injectable short-acting benzodiazepine, is used for induction of general anesthesia, preoperative sedation, conscious sedation for diagnostic procedures and to supplement nitrous oxide and oxygen for short surgical procedures (see individual monograph).

Unlabeled uses: Management of irritable bowel syndrome (chlordiazepoxide, diazepam, clorazepate, lorazepam, oxazepam, prazepam, alprazolam); panic attacks (alprazolam, diazepam); depression (alprazolam); premenstrual syndrome (alprazolam); status epilepticus, chemotherapy-induced nausea and vomiting, acute alcohol withdrawal syndrome, psychogenic catatonia (lorazepam injection); chronic insomnia (lorazepam).

Contraindications:

Hypersensitivity to benzodiazepines; psychoses; acute narrow-angle glaucoma (may be used in patients with open-angle glaucoma and appropriate therapy); patients with clinical or biochemical evidence of significant liver disease (clonazepam); intra-

BENZODIAZEPINES

arterial use (lorazepam injection); children < 6 months; lactation (diazepam); coadministration with ketoconazole and itraconazole due to inhibition of cytochrome P450 3A (see Warnings).

Warnings:

Psychiatric disorders: These agents are not intended for use in patients with a primary depressive disorder or psychosis, nor in those psychiatric disorders in which anxiety is not a prominent feature.

Long-term use (> 4 months): Effectiveness has not been assessed by systematic clinical studies. Periodically reassess the usefulness of the drug for the individual patient.

Dependence: Prolonged use of therapeutic doses can lead to dependence. Withdrawal syndrome has occurred after as little as 4 to 6 weeks treatment. It is more likely if the drug is short-acting (eg, alprazolam), taken regularly for > 3 months and abruptly discontinued.

After rapid decrease of dosage or abrupt discontinuation, withdrawal seizures were reported in **alprazolam** patients.

Onset is within 1 to 10 days; duration of reaction may be 5 days to ≥ to a month depending on agent, dose, etc. Symptoms generally begin with anxiety-like manifestations; the following may occur in ≥ 50% of cases: Increased anxiety; sensory disturbances (paresthesias, hypercusis, photophobia, hypersomnia, metallic taste); concentration difficulties; fatigue; anorexia; dizziness; vomiting; insomnia; confusion; headache; muscle tension/cramps; tremor; dysphoria; muscle twitching; "psychosis"; paranoid delusions; hallucinations; memory impairment; seizures (grand mal).

Abrupt withdrawal of **clonazepam**, particularly in those patients on long-term, high dose therapy, may precipitate status epilepticus. While clonazepam is being gradually withdrawn, the simultaneous substitution of another anticonvulsant may be indicated. Other symptoms include vomiting, diarrhea and sweating.

When discontinuing therapy in patients who have used these agents for prolonged periods, decrease dosage gradually over 4 to 8 weeks to avoid the possibility of withdrawal symptoms, especially in patients with a history of seizures or epilepsy, regardless of their concomitant anticonvulsant drug therapy. Patients on short-acting benzodiazepines may be switched to longer-acting drugs (eg, diazepam) which produce a gradual decrease in drug concentration and decrease the chance of withdrawal symptoms. Clonidine, propranolol and carbamazepine have been used as adjuncts in the treatment of benzodiazepine withdrawal symptoms.

Parenteral administration: Parenteral (IM or IV) therapy is indicated primarily in acute states. Keep patients under observation, preferably in bed, for ≤ 3 hours.

Do not inject intra-arterially; may produce arteriospasm resulting in gangrene which may require amputation.

Administer parenterally with extreme care (particularly IV) to elderly, very ill and those with limited pulmonary reserve. Because of possible apnea or cardiac arrest, resuscitative facilities should be available. Not recommended for obstetric use. Do not administer to patients in shock, coma or in acute alcohol intoxication.

Hypotension or muscular weakness is possible, particularly when benzodiazepines are used with narcotics, barbiturates or alcohol.

Renal function impairment: Observe usual precautions in the presence of impaired renal or hepatic function to avoid accumulation of these agents. **Lorazepam** injection is not recommended in these patients. Metabolites of **clonazepam** are excreted by the kidneys; to avoid excess accumulation, exercise caution in patients with impaired renal function. Also, clonazepam is contraindicated in patients with significant liver disease.

Elderly: The initial dose should be small and dosage increments made gradually, in accordance with the response of the patient, to preclude ataxia or excessive sedation. Hypotension is rare; however, use with caution if cardiac complications may result from a drop in blood pressure.

Pregnancy: Category D (No category designation for **clonazepam**). Benzodiazepines and their metabolites freely cross the placenta and accumulate in the fetal circulation. An increased risk of congenital malformations associated with the use of minor tranquilizers during the first trimester of pregnancy has been suggested. Malformations reported include cleft lip or palate. Recent studies suggest diazepam use in the first trimester does not cause an increased risk of this. Because use of these drugs is rarely a matter of urgency, avoid them during this period. Consider the possibility that a woman of childbearing potential may be pregnant at the time of institution of therapy. Advise patients that if they become pregnant, or plan to become pregnant, they should discuss the desirability of discontinuing the drug.

BENZODIAZEPINES

Labor and delivery – Benzodiazepines have been found in maternal and cord blood, indicating placental transfer of drug. Therefore, benzodiazepines are not recommended for obstetrical use.

Neonatal withdrawal consisting of severe tremulousness and irritability has been attributed to maternal ingestion of benzodiazepines as well as neonatal flaccidity and respiratory problems. Use during labor has resulted in a "floppy infant" syndrome, manifested by hypotonia, lethargy and sucking difficulties.

Prolonged CNS depression has been observed in neonates, apparently due to inability to biotransform **diazepam** into inactive metabolites.

Lactation: Benzodiazepines are excreted in breast milk (**lorazepam** not known). Since neonates metabolize benzodiazepines more slowly than adults, accumulation of the drug and its metabolites to toxic levels is possible. Chronic **diazepam** use in nursing mothers reportedly caused infants to become lethargic and to lose weight; do not give to nursing mothers.

Children: The initial dose should be small and dosage increments made gradually, in accordance with the response of the patient, to preclude ataxia or excessive sedation. Hypotension is rare; however, use with caution if cardiac complications may result from a drop in blood pressure.

Chlordiazepoxide is not recommended in children < 6 years (oral) or 12 years (injectable).

Halazepam, prazepam, alprazolam: Safety and efficacy for use in patients < 18 years old have not been established.

Lorazepam: Do not use in patients < 18 years old (injection); safety and efficacy for use in patients < 12 years old are not established (oral).

Clorazepate: Not recommended for use in patients < 9 years old.

Diazepam: Not for use in children < 6 months old (oral); safety and efficacy have not been established in the neonate (≤ 30 days old; injectable).

Precautions:

Monitoring: Because of isolated reports of neutropenia and jaundice, perform periodic blood counts and liver function tests during long-term therapy. There have been reports of abnormal liver and kidney function tests and of decrease in hematocrit.

Suicide: In those patients in whom depression accompanies anxiety, suicidal tendencies may be present, and protective measures may be required. Dispense the least amount of drug feasible to the patient.

Paradoxical reactions: Excitement, stimulation and acute rage have occurred in psychiatric patients and hyperactive aggressive children. These reactions may be secondary to relief of anxiety and usually appear in the first 2 weeks of therapy. Acute hyperexcited states, anxiety, hallucinations, increased muscle spasticity, insomnia and sleep disturbances have also occurred. Should these occur, discontinue the drug. Minor EEG changes, usually low voltage fast activity, have been observed during and after therapy and are of no known significance. Anger, hostility and episodes of mania and hypomania have been reported with **alprazolam**.

Multiple seizure type: When used in patients in whom several different types of seizure disorders coexist, **clonazepam** may increase the incidence or precipitate the onset of generalized tonic-clonic (grand mal) seizures. This may require the addition of other anticonvulsants or an increase in their dosage.

Diazepam – If use in patients with seizure disorders results in an increase in the frequency or severity of grand mal seizures, there may be a need to increase the dosage of standard anticonvulsant medication.

Chronic respiratory disease: **Clonazepam** may produce an increase in salivation. Use with caution in patients if increased salivation causes respiratory difficulty. Due to possibility of respiratory depression, use with caution in such patients.

Hazardous tasks: May produce drowsiness or dizziness; observe caution while driving or performing other tasks requiring alertness.

Tartrazine sensitivity: Some of these products contain tartrazine, which may cause allergic-type reactions (including bronchial asthma) in susceptible individuals. Although the incidence of tartrazine sensitivity in the general population is low, it is frequently seen in patients who also have aspirin hypersensitivity. Specific products containing tartrazine are identified in the product listings.

BENZODIAZEPINES

Drug Interactions:

The elimination of benzodiazepines that undergo oxidative hepatic metabolism (alprazolam, chlordiazepoxide, clorazepate, diazepam, halazepam, prazepam) may be decreased by the following drugs due to inhibition of hepatic metabolism. Pharmacologic effects of these benzodiazepines may be increased and excessive sedation/impaired psychomotor function may occur.

cimetidine	**isoniazid**	**propoxyphene**
contraceptives, oral	**ketoconazole**	**propranolol**
disulfiram	**metoprolol**	**valproic acid**
fluoxetine		

Alcohol and other CNS depressants (eg, barbiturates, narcotics): Increased CNS effects (eg, impaired psychomotor function, sedation) may occur.

Antacids may alter the rate but generally not the extent of GI absorption. Staggering administration times may help avoid possible interaction.

Contraceptives, oral: The clearance rate of benzodiazepines that undergo glucuronidation (lorazepam, oxazepam) may be increased.

Digoxin's serum concentrations may be increased. Toxicity characterized by GI and neuropsychiatric symptoms and cardiac arrhythmias may occur. Monitor digoxin serum levels.

Levodopa's antiparkinson efficacy may be decreased by coadministration of benzodiazepines.

Neuromuscular blocking agents: Benzodiazepines may potentiate, counteract or have no effect on the actions of these agents.

Phenytoin serum concentrations may be increased, resulting in toxicity, but data are conflicting. Phenytoin may increase oxazepam clearance.

Probenecid may interfere with benzodiazepine conjugation in the liver, possibly resulting in a more rapid onset or prolonged effect.

Ranitidine may reduce the GI absorption of diazepam.

Rifampin: The oxidative metabolism of benzodiazepines may be increased due to microsomal enzyme induction. Pharmacologic effects of some benzodiazepines may be decreased.

Scopolamine, used concomitantly with parenteral lorazepam, may increase the incidence of sedation, hallucinations and irrational behavior.

Theophyllines may antagonize the sedative effects of the benzodiazepines.

Adverse Reactions:

Discontinuation of therapy due to undesirable effects is rare. Transient mild drowsiness is commonly seen in the first few days of therapy. Drowsiness, ataxia and confusion have occurred, especially in the elderly and debilitated. If persistent, reduce dosage. Ataxia is rare with oxazepam and does not appear to be specifically related to dose or age. Other adverse reactions less frequently reported include:

CNS: Sedation and sleepiness; depression; lethargy; apathy; fatigue; hypoactivity; lightheadedness; memory impairment; disorientation; anterograde amnesia; restlessness; confusion; crying; sobbing; delirium; headache; slurred speech; aphonia; dysarthria; stupor; seizures; coma; syncope; rigidity; tremor; dystonia; vertigo; dizziness; euphoria; nervousness; irritability; difficulty in concentration; agitation; inability to perform complex mental functions; akathisia; hemiparesis; hypotonia; unsteadiness; ataxia; incoordination; weakness; vivid dreams; psychomotor retardation; "glassy-eyed" appearance; extrapyramidal symptoms; paradoxical reactions (see Precautions).

Psychiatric: Behavior problems; hysteria; psychosis; suicidal tendencies.

GI: Constipation; diarrhea; dry mouth; coated tongue; sore gums; nausea; anorexia; change in appetite; vomiting; difficulty in swallowing; increased salivation; gastritis.

GU: Incontinence; changes in libido; urinary retention; menstrual irregularities.

Cardiovascular: Bradycardia; tachycardia; cardiovascular collapse; hypertension; hypotension; palpitations; edema; phlebitis and thrombosis at IV sites. Decrease in systolic blood pressure has been observed.

Ophthalmic: Visual disturbances; diplopia; nystagmus.

Respiratory: Respiratory disturbances; nasal congestion.

BENZODIAZEPINES

Dermatologic: Urticaria; pruritus; skin rash, including morbilliform, urticarial and maculopapular; dermatitis; hair loss; hirsutism; ankle and facial edema.

Body as a whole: Depressed hearing; auditory disturbances; hiccoughs; fever; diaphoresis; paresthesias; muscular disturbance; gynecomastia; galactorrhea; elevations of LDH, alkaline phosphatase, ALT and AST; hepatic dysfunction (including hepatitis and jaundice); leukopenia; blood dyscrasias including agranulocytosis; anemia; thrombocytopenia; eosinophilia; increase or decrease in body weight; dehydration; lymphadenopathy; joint pain; pain, burning and redness following IM injection. Partial airway obstruction has occurred and is believed to be due to excessive sedation at time of procedure (lorazepam injection).

Overdosage:

There are no well documented fatal overdoses resulting from oral ingestion of benzodiazepines alone. Most fatalities implicate benzodiazepines only as a component in multiple drug ingestions.

Symptoms: Mild symptoms include drowsiness, confusion, somnolence, impaired coordination, diminished reflexes and lethargy. These agents rarely cause significant respiratory or circulatory depression, particularly when they are the sole agents ingested. Serious symptoms may include ataxia, hypotonia, hypotension, hypnosis, stages one to three coma, and rarely, death. Consider multiple drug ingestion.

Unlike oral ingestions, IV administration of diazepam is associated with 1.7% incidence of life-threatening reactions, including hypotension and respiratory or cardiac arrest.

Treatment: Induce vomiting if it has not occurred spontaneously. Employ general supportive measures, along with immediate gastric lavage or ipecac. Follow with activated charcoal administration and a saline cathartic. Monitor respiration, pulse and blood pressure. Administer IV fluids and maintain an adequate airway. Treat hypotension with norepinephrine or metaraminol. With normal kidney function, forced diuresis with osmotic diuretics, IV fluids and electrolytes may accelerate elimination of benzodiazepines. Dialysis is of limited value; however, in more critical situations, renal dialysis and exchange blood transfusions may be indicated. Refer to General Management of Acute Overdosage.

Infusion of 0.5 to 4 mg of physostigmine IV at the rate of 1 mg/minute may reverse symptoms suggestive of central anticholinergic overdose (eg, confusion, memory disturbance, visual disturbances, hallucinations, delirium); however, weigh the hazards associated with the use of physostigmine (eg, induction of seizures) against its possible clinical benefit.

There have been occasional reports of excitation in patients following overdosage with chlordiazepoxide; if this occurs, do not give barbiturates.

Patient Information:

May cause drowsiness; avoid driving or other tasks requiring alertness.

Avoid alcohol or other CNS depressants.

May be taken with food or water if stomach upset occurs.

Patients on long-term or high dosage therapy may experience withdrawal symptoms on abrupt cessation of therapy; do not discontinue therapy abruptly or change dosage except on advice of physician.

Concomitant ingestion with antacids may alter the rate of absorption of these drugs (documented with **diazepam** and **chlordiazepoxide**).

Clonazepam, clorazepate *and* **diazepam:** Patient should carry identification (Medic Alert) indicating medication usage and epilepsy.

OXAZEPAM

Complete prescribing information begins in the Benzodiazepines group monograph.

Indications:

For the management of anxiety disorders or for the short-term relief of the symptoms of anxiety. Anxiety associated with depression is also responsive to oxazepam.

For the management of anxiety, tension, agitation and irritability in older patients.

Alcoholics with acute tremulousness, inebriation or with anxiety associated with alcohol withdrawal are responsive to therapy.

Administration and Dosage:

Individualize dosage.

Mild to moderate anxiety, with associated tension, irritability, agitation or related symptoms of functional origin or secondary to organic disease: 10 to 15 mg 3 or 4 times daily.

Severe anxiety syndromes, agitation or anxiety associated with depression: 15 to 30 mg 3 or 4 times daily.

Older patients with anxiety, tension, irritability and agitation: Initial dosage is 10 mg 3 times daily. If necessary, increase cautiously to 15 mg 3 or 4 times daily.

Alcoholics with acute inebriation, tremulousness or anxiety on withdrawal: 15 to 30 mg 3 or 4 times daily.

Children (6 to 12 years): Dosage is not established.

c-iv	**Oxazepam** (Various)	**Capsules:** 10 mg	In 100s, 250s, 500s, 1000s.
c-iv	**Serax** (Wyeth-Ayerst)		(Wyeth 51). Pink and white. In 100s, 500s and Redipak 25s and 100s.
c-iv	**Oxazepam** (Various)	**Capsules:** 15 mg	In 100s, 500s, 1000s and UD 100s.
c-iv	**Serax** (Wyeth-Ayerst)		(Wyeth 6). Red and white. In 100s, 500s and Redipak 25s and 100s.
c-iv	**Oxazepam** (Various)	**Capsules:** 30 mg	In 100s, 250s, 500s, 1000s and UD 100s.
c-iv	**Serax** (Wyeth-Ayerst)		(Wyeth 52). Maroon and white. In 100s, 500s and Redipak 25s and 100s.
c-iv	**Oxazepam** (Various)	**Tablets:** 15 mg	In 100s, 500s and 1000s.
c-iv	**Serax** (Wyeth-Ayerst)		Tartrazine. (Wyeth 317). Yellow. In100s.

PRAZEPAM

Complete prescribing information begins in the Benzodiazepines group monograph.

Indications:

Management of anxiety disorders; short-term relief of the symptoms of anxiety.

Administration and Dosage:

Individualize dosage.

The usual dose is 30 mg/day administered in divided doses. Adjust dosage gradually within the range of 20 to 60 mg/day in accordance with the response of the patient.

Elderly: Initiate treatment at 10 to 15 mg/day in divided doses.

May also be administered as a single daily dose at bedtime. The starting dose is 20 mg/night. Adjust dosage to maximize the antianxiety effect with a minimum of daytime drowsiness. The optimum dose ranges from 20 to 40 mg.

c-iv	**Prazepam** (Various, eg, Goldline, Major, Moore, Parmed, Rugby, Schein, URL)	**Capsules:** 5 mg	In 100s and 500s.
		10 mg	In 100s and 500s.
c-iv	**Prazepam** (Various, eg, Geneva, PBI)	**Tablets:** 5 mg	In 100s and 500s.
c-iv	**Prazepam** (Various, eg, Geneva, PBI)	**Tablets:** 10 mg	In 100s and 500s.

Benzodiazepines

LORAZEPAM

Complete prescribing information begins in the Benzodiazepines group monograph.

Indications:

For the management of anxiety disorders or for the short-term relief of the symptoms of anxiety or anxiety associated with depressive symptoms.

Parenteral: In adults for preanesthetic medication, producing sedation, relief of anxiety and a decreased ability to recall events related to surgery.

Unlabeled uses: Lorazepam injection may help manage status epilepticus, chemotherapy-induced nausea and vomiting, acute alcohol withdrawal syndrome and psychogenic catatonia. Oral lorazepam appears useful for chronic insomnia.

Lorazepam given sublingually is absorbed more rapidly than after oral administration and compares favorably to IM administration.

Administration and Dosage:

Individualize dosage. Increase dosage gradually to minimize adverse effects. When higher dosage is indicated, increase the evening dose before the daytime doses.

Oral: 2 to 6 mg/day (varies from 1 to 10 mg/day) given in divided doses; take the largest dose before bedtime.

Anxiety – Initial dose, 2 to 3 mg/day given 2 or 3 times daily.

Insomnia due to anxiety or transient situational stress – 2 to 4 mg at bedtime.

Elderly or debilitated patients – Initial dose, 1 to 2 mg/day in divided doses; adjust as needed and tolerated.

IM: 0.05 mg/kg up to a maximum of 4 mg. For optimum effect, administer at least 2 hours before operative procedure. Inject undiluted, deep into the muscle mass.

IV: Initial dose is 2 mg total or 0.044 mg/kg (0.02 mg/lb), whichever is smaller. This will sedate most adults; ordinarily, do not exceed in patients > 50 years old. If a greater lack of recall would be beneficial, doses as high as 0.05 mg/kg up to a total of 4 mg may be given. For optimum effect, give 15 to 20 minutes before the procedure.

Immediately prior to IV use, dilute with an equal volume of compatible solution (Sterile Water for Injection, Sodium Chloride Injection or 5% Dextrose Injection). Inject directly into a vein or into tubing of an existing IV infusion. Do not exceed 2 mg/min. Have equipment to maintain a patent airway available.

Children (< 18 years): Due to insufficient data, parenteral use is not recommended.

Storage and stability: Do not use if solution is discolored or contains a precipitate. Protect from light; refrigerate solution.

c-iv	**Lorazepam** (Various, eg, Elkins-Sinn, Lederle, Major, Rugby, Squibb Mark, Warner-C)	**Tablets:** 0.5 mg	In 30s, 100s, 250s, 500s, 1000s and UD 100s and 32s.
c-iv	**Ativan** (Wyeth-Ayerst)		Lactose. (A Wyeth 81). White. Five sided. In 100s, 500s, Redipak 250s, 100s.
c-iv	**Lorazepam** (Various, eg, Elkins-Sinn, Geneva, Goldline, Lederle, Major, Moore, Rugby, Squibb Mark, Warner-C)	**Tablets:** 1 mg	In 20s, 30s, 100s, 500s, 1000s and UD 100s and 32s.
c-iv	**Ativan** (Wyeth-Ayerst)		Lactose. (A Wyeth 64). White, scored. Five sided. In 100s, 500s, 1000s & Redipak 100s and 250s.
c-iv	**Lorazepam** (Various, eg, Elkins-Sinn, Lederle, Major, Rugby, Squibb Mark, Warner-C)	**Tablets:** 2 mg	In 20s, 30s, 100s, 250s, 500s, 1000s and UD 100s.
c-iv	**Ativan** (Wyeth-Ayerst)		Lactose. (A Wyeth 65). White, scored. In 100s, 500s, 1000s & Redipak 100s & 250s.
c-iv	**Lorazepam Intensol** (Roxane)	**Concentrated oral solution:** 2 mg/ml	Alcohol and dye free. In 30 ml with dropper.

Benzodiazepines

LORAZEPAM

c-iv	**Lorazepam** (Various, eg, Sanofi Winthrop, Schein, Steris)	**Injection**: 2 mg/ml	In 1 ml fill in 2 ml and 10 ml multi-dose vials.
c-iv	**Ativan** (Wyeth-Ayerst)		In 10 ml multi-dose vials[1] and 1 ml fill in 2 ml Tubex.[1]
c-iv	**Lorazepam** (Various, eg, Sanofi Winthrop, Schein, Steris)	**Injection**: 4 mg/ml	In 1 ml fill in 2 ml and 10 ml multi-dose vials.
c-iv	**Ativan** (Wyeth-Ayerst)		In 10 ml multi-dose vials[1] and 1 ml fill in 2 ml Tubex.[1]

[1] With PEG 400, propylene glycol, 2% benzyl alcohol.

Benzodiazepines

ALPRAZOLAM

Complete prescribing information begins in the Benzodiazpines monograph.

Indications:

For the management of anxiety disorders or for the short-term relief of the symptoms of anxiety. Anxiety associated with depression is also responsive.

Treatment of panic disorder, with or without agoraphobia.

Unlabeled uses: Treatment of agoraphobia with social phobia (2 to 8 mg/day); depression; premenstrual syndrome (0.25 mg 3 times a day).

Alprazolam given sublingually is absorbed as rapidly as after oral administration; completeness of absorption is comparable.

Administration and Dosage:

Individualize dosage. Increase cautiously to avoid adverse effects. Reduce gradually when terminating or decreasing daily dose. Decrease by not > 0.5 mg every 3 days.

Anxiety disorders: Initial dose is 0.25 to 0.5 mg 3 times/day. Titrate to max total dose of 4 mg/day in divided doses. If side effects occur with starting dose, decrease dose.

Elderly or debilitated patients: 0.25 mg, given 2 or 3 times daily. Gradually increase if needed and tolerated.

Panic disorder: Initial dose is 0.5 mg 3 times daily. Depending on response, increase dose at intervals of 3 to 4 days in increments of no more than 1 mg/day.

Successful treatment has required doses > 4 mg/day; in controlled studies, doses in the range of 1 to 10 mg/day were used.

c-iv	**Alprazolam** (Various, eg, Geneva, Lederle, Major, Moore, Purepac, Roxane, Rugby, Schein, URL)	**Tablets:** 0.25 mg	In 30s, 100s, 500s, 1000s & UD 100S.
c-iv	**Xanax** (Upjohn)		Lactose. (Xanax 29). White, scored. Oval. In 100s, 500s, UD 100s, Visipak 100s and unit-of-issue 30s and 90s.
c-iv	**Alprazolam** (Various, eg, Geneva, Lederle, Major, Moore, Purepac, Roxane, Rugby, Schein, URL)	**Tablets:** 0.5 mg	In 30s, 100s, 500s 1000s & UD 100s.
c-iv	**Xanax** (Upjohn)		Lactose. (Xanax 55). Peach, scored. Oval. In 100s, 500s, UD 100s, Visipak 100s and unit-of-issue 30s and 90s.
c-iv	**Alprazolam** (Various, eg, Geneva, Lederle, Major, Moore, Purepac, Roxane, Rugby, Schein, URL)	**Tablets:** 1 mg	In 30s, 100s, 500s 1000s & UD 100s.
c-iv	**Xanax** (Upjohn)		Lactose. (Xanax 90). Blue, scored. Oval. In 30s, 90s, 100s, 500s, UD 100s.
c-iv	**Alprazolam** (Various, eg, Geneva, Lederle, Major, Moore, Purepac, Roxane, Rugby, Schein, URL)	**Tablets:** 2 mg	In 100s and 500s.
c-iv	**Xanax** (Upjohn)		Lactose. White, multi-scored. Oblong. In 100s, 500s, UD 100s, Visipak 100s.
c-iv	**Alprazolam** (Roxane)	**Oral Solution:** 0.5 mg/5 ml	Sorbitol Saccharin. Fruit-mint flavor. In 500 ml, UD 2.5, 5 and 10 ml.
		Intensol Solution: 1 mg/ml	Flavorless. In 30 ml with calibrated dropper.

Benzodiazepines

CHLORDIAZEPOXIDE

Complete prescribing information begins in the Benzodiazepines monograph.

Indications:

Management of anxiety disorders or for short-term relief of anxiety symptoms; for symptoms of acute alcohol withdrawal; preoperative apprehension and anxiety.

Administration and Dosage:

Oral: Individualize dosage.

Mild to moderate anxiety – 5 or 10 mg 3 or 4 times daily.

Severe anxiety – 20 or 25 mg 3 or 4 times daily.

Geriatric patients or patients with debilitating disease – 5 mg 2 to 4 times daily.

Preoperative apprehension and anxiety – On days preceding surgery, 5 to 10 mg 3 or 4 times daily.

Acute alcohol withdrawal – 50 to 100 mg; repeat as needed (up to 300 mg/day). Parenteral form usually used initially. Reduce to maintenance levels.

Children – Initially, 5 mg 2 to 4 times daily. (May be increased in some children to 10 mg 2 or 3 times daily.) Not recommended in children under 6 years of age.

A dosage of 0.5 mg/kg/day every 6 to 8 hours in children > 6 years of age has also been recommended.

Parenteral: Use lower doses (25 to 50 mg) for elderly or debilitated patients and for older children. A dosage of 0.5 mg/kg/day every 6 to 8 hours IM in children > 12 years of age has also been recommended. Acute symptoms may be rapidly controlled by parenteral administration; subsequent treatment, if necessary, may be given orally. While 300 mg may be given during a 6 hour period, do not exceed this dose in any 24 hour period. Not recommended in children < 12 years of age.

Acute alcohol withdrawal – 50 to 100 mg IM or IV initially; repeat in 2 to 4 hours if necessary.

Acute or severe anxiety – 50 to 100 mg IM or IV initially; then 25 to 50 mg 3 or 4 times daily if necessary.

Preoperative apprehension/anxiety – 50 to 100 mg IM 1 hour prior to surgery.

Preparation and administration of injections: Prepare solution immediately before administration. Discard any unused portion.

IM – Reconstitute solutions for IM injection only with the special diluent provided. Do not use diluent if it is opalescent or hazy. Solutions made with physiological saline or Sterile Water for Injection should not be given IM because of the pain on injection. Give deep IM injection slowly into the upper outer quadrant of the gluteus muscle. Although this preparation has been given IV without untoward effects, such administration is not recommended because air bubbles form on the surface of the solution.

IV – When rapid action is mandatory, administer IV. Add 5 ml of sterile physiological saline or Sterile Water for Injection to contents of amp (100 mg). Agitate gently until thoroughly dissolved. Give injection slowly over 1 minute.

Benzodiazepines

CHLORDIAZEPOXIDE

c-iv	**Chlordiazepoxide HCl** (Various, eg, Balan, Barr, Geneva, Goldline, Lannett, Lederle, Major, Moore, Rugby, Schein)	**Capsules:** 5 mg (as HCl)	In 20s, 100s, 500s, 1000s and UD 100s.
c-iv	**Librium** (Roche)		Green and yellow. In 100s, 500s, UD 100s and reverse number 100s (4x25s).
c-iv	**Chlordiazepoxide HCl** (Various, eg, Balan, Barr, Geneva, Goldline, Lannett, Lederle, Major, Moore, Rugby, Schein)	**Capsules:** 10 mg (as HCl)	In 20s, 100s, 500s, 1000s and UD 100s.
c-iv	**Librium** (Roche)		Green and black. In 100s, 500s, UD 100s and reverse number 100s (4x25s).
c-iv	**Mitran** (Hauck)		Green and black. In 100s and 500s.
c-iv	**Reposans-10** (Wesley)		In 1000s.
c-iv	**Chlordiazepoxide HCl** (Various, eg, Balan, Barr, Geneva, Goldline, Lannett, Lederle, Major, Moore, Rugby, Schein)	**Capsules:** 25 mg (as HCl)	In 20s, 100s, 500s, 1000s and UD 100s.
c-iv	**Librium** (Roche)		Green and white. In 100s, 500s, UD 100s and reverse number 100s (4x25s).
c-iv	**Libritabs** (Roche)	**Tablets:** 5 mg	(Libritabs 5 Roche). Green, scored. Film coated. In 100s.
		10 mg	(Libritabs 10 Roche). Green, scored. Film coated. In 100s.
c-iv	**Librium** (Roche)	**Powder for Injection:** 100 mg (as HCl) per amp	In 5 ml amp with 2 ml amp of IM diluent.[1]

[1] With 1.5% benzyl alcohol, polysorbate 80, 20% propylene glycol, maleic acid, sodium hydroxide.

DIAZEPAM

Complete prescribing information begins in the Benzodiazepines monograph.

Indications:

Anxiety: For the management of anxiety disorders or for the short-term relief of the symptoms of anxiety.

Acute alcohol withdrawal: May be useful in symptomatic relief of acute agitation, tremor, impending or acute delirium tremens and hallucinosis.

Muscle relaxant: As an adjunct for the relief of skeletal muscle spasm due to reflex spasm due to local pathology (eg, inflammation of muscles or joints, or secondary to trauma); spasticity caused by upper motor neuron disorders (eg, cerebral palsy and paraplegia); athetosis; stiff-man syndrome. Used parenterally in the treatment of tetanus.

Anticonvulsant: Parenteral diazepam is a useful adjunct in status epilepticus and severe recurrent convulsive seizures. Oral diazepam may be used adjunctively in convulsive disorders.

Preoperative: Used parenterally for relief of anxiety and tension in patients undergoing surgical procedures; IV prior to cardioversion for the relief of anxiety and tension and to diminish patient's recall; and as an adjunct prior to endoscopic procedures for apprehension, anxiety or acute stress reactions and to diminish patient's recall.

Unlabeled uses: Diazepam has been effective in the treatment of panic attacks.

Administration and Dosage:

Oral: Individualize dosage. Increase dosage cautiously to avoid adverse effects.

Benzodiazepines

DIAZEPAM

Management of anxiety disorders and relief of symptoms of anxiety (depending upon severity of symptoms) – 2 to 10 mg 2 to 4 times daily.

Acute alcohol withdrawal – 10 mg 3 or 4 times during first 24 hours; reduce to 5 mg 3 or 4 times daily, as needed.

Adjunct in skeletal muscle spasm – 2 to 10 mg 3 or 4 times daily.

Adjunct in convulsive disorders – 2 to 10 mg 2 to 4 times daily.

Elderly patients or in the presence of debilitating disease – 2 to 2.5 mg 1 or 2 times daily initially; increase gradually as needed and tolerated.

Children – 1 to 2.5 mg 3 or 4 times daily initially; increase gradually as needed and tolerated. Not for use in children under 6 months. For sedation or muscle relaxation, a dosage of 0.12 to 0.8 mg/kg/24 hours divided 3 to 4 times a day has been recommended.

Oral, sustained release: Individualize dosage. Do not crush or chew sustained release formula.

Whenever oral diazepam 5 mg 3 times a day would be considered appropriate dosage, one 15 mg sustained release capsule daily may be used.

Sustained release capsules (15 mg) are recommended for elderly or debilitated patients and children only when it has been determined that 5 mg oral diazepam 3 times a day is the optimal daily dose. Oral diazepam is not recommended for children under 6 months of age.

Management of anxiety disorders and relief of symptoms of anxiety – 15 to 30 mg/day, depending upon severity of symptoms.

Adjunct in skeletal muscle spasm – 15 to 30 mg/day.

Oral, solution: Dosage same as oral tablets.

Intensol – The *Intensol* is a concentrated oral solution as compared to standard oral liquid medications. It is recommended that the *Intensol* be mixed with liquid or semisolid food such as water, juices, soda or soda-like beverages, applesauce and puddings.

Use only the calibrated dropper provided with the product. Draw into the dropper the amount prescribed for a single dose. Then squeeze the dropper contents into a liquid or semi-solid food. Stir the liquid or food gently for a few seconds. The entire amount of the mixture should be consumed immediately. Do not store for future use.

Parenteral: Individualize dosage.

Older children and adults – 2 to 20 mg IM or IV, depending on the indication and its severity. In some conditions (eg, tetanus) larger doses may be required. In acute conditions, the injection may be repeated within 1 hour, although an interval of 3 to 4 hours is usually satisfactory. Use lower doses (2 to 5 mg) and more gradual increases in dosage for elderly and debilitated patients and when other sedatives are administered.

IV – When used IV, observe the following procedures to reduce the possibility of venous thrombosis, phlebitis, local irritation, swelling, and rarely, vascular impairment: Inject slowly, at most 5 mg (1 ml) per minute; do not use small veins (ie, dorsum of hand or wrist); avoid intra-arterial administration or extravasation. Do not mix or dilute with other solutions or drugs in syringe or infusion flask. If not feasible to administer directly IV, inject slowly through infusion tubing as close as possible to the vein insertion. Because of the possibility of precipitation of diazepam in IV fluids and the instability of the drug in plastic (PVC) bags and infusion tubing, IV infusion of diazepam is not recommended. Glass, polypropylene, polyethylene or polyolefin solution bottles and infusion tubing have been used with negligible loss of diazepam. Once acute symptoms are controlled with injectable diazepam, place patient on oral therapy.

Children – To obtain maximum clinical effect with minimum amount of drug and to reduce the risk of hazardous side effects such as apnea or prolonged periods of somnolence, administer slowly over 3 minutes. Do not exceed 0.25 mg/kg. After an interval of 15 to 30 minutes, the initial dose can be repeated. If relief of symptoms is not obtained after a third dose, appropriate adjunctive therapy is recommended. When IV use is indicated, facilities for respiratory assistance should be readily available.

Moderate anxiety disorders and symptoms of anxiety – 2 to 5 mg IM or IV. Repeat in 3 to 4 hours if necessary.

Severe anxiety disorders and symptoms of anxiety – 5 to 10 mg IM or IV. Repeat in 3 to 4 hours if necessary.

Acute alcohol withdrawal – 10 mg IM or IV initially; then 5 to 10 mg in 3 to 4 hours if necessary.

Benzodiazepines

DIAZEPAM

Endoscopic procedures –

IV: Titrate dosage to desired sedative response, such as slurring of speech. Administer slowly just prior to procedure. Reduce narcotic dosage by at least one-third, and in some cases, they may be omitted; 10 mg or less is usually adequate; up to 20 mg may be used, especially when concomitant narcotics are omitted.

IM: 5 to 10 mg 30 minutes prior to procedure if IV route cannot be used.

Muscle spasm – 5 to 10 mg IM or IV initially; then 5 to 10 mg in 3 to 4 hours if necessary. Tetanus may require larger doses.

Status epilepticus and severe recurrent convulsive seizures – The IV route is preferred; administer slowly. Use the IM route if IV administration is impossible. Administer 5 to 10 mg initially; repeat if necessary at 10 to 15 minute intervals up to a maximum dose of 30 mg. If necessary, repeat therapy in 2 to 4 hours. A dose of 0.2 to 0.5 mg/kg every 15 to 30 minutes for 2 to 3 doses (maximum dose, 30 mg) has been recommended. Exercise extreme caution in patients with chronic lung disease or unstable cardiovascular status. Although seizures may be controlled promptly, many patients experience a return to seizure activity, presumably due to the short-lived effect of IV diazepam; be prepared to readminister the drug. Diazepam is not recommended for maintenance. Once seizures are controlled, consider other agents for long-term control.

Infants (over 30 days of age) and children (under 5 years) – Inject 0.2 to 0.5 mg slowly every 2 to 5 minutes up to a maximum of 5 mg; 0.2 to 0.5 mg/kg/dose every 15 to 30 minutes for 2 to 3 doses (maximum dose 5 mg) has also been recommended.

Children (5 years or older) – Inject 1 mg every 2 to 5 minutes up to a maximum of 10 mg. Repeat in 2 to 4 hours if necessary. EEG monitoring of seizure may be helpful. A dose of 0.2 to 0.5 mg/kg/dose every 15 to 30 minutes for 2 to 3 doses (maximum dose, 10 mg) has also been recommended.

Neonates – 0.5 to 1 mg/kg/dose every 15 to 30 minutes for 2 to 3 doses has been suggested.

Preoperative medication – 10 mg IM before surgery. If atropine, scopolamine or other premedications are desired, administer in separate syringes.

Cardioversion – 5 to 15 mg IV, 5 to 10 minutes prior to procedure.

Tetanus – Infants (over 30 days of age) – 1 to 2 mg IM or IV slowly, repeated every 3 to 4 hours as necessary.

Children (5 years or older: 5 to 10 mg repeated every 3 to 4 hours may be required.

Sedation or muscle relaxation –

Children: 0.04 to 0.2 mg/kg/dose every 2 to 4 hours, maximum of 0.6 mg/kg within an 8 hour period.

Adults: 2 to 10 mg/dose every 3 to 4 hours as needed.

c-iv	**Diazepam** (Roxane)	**Oral Solution**: 5 mg per 5 ml	Wintergreen-spice flavor. In 500 ml and 5 and 10 mg patient cups.
c-iv	**Diazepam Intensol** (Roxane)	**Oral Solution**: 5 mg per ml	In 30 ml with dropper.
c-iv	**Diazepam** (Various, eg, Elkins-Sinn, Geneva, Goldline, Lederle, Lemmon, Major, Roxane, Squibb Mark, Warner Chilcott, Zenith)	**Tablets**: 2 mg	In 30s, 100s, 500s, 1000s, 2500s and UD 32s, 100s and 500s.
c-iv	**Valium** (Roche)		(Roche 2 Valium). White, scored. In 100s, 500s, UD 100s and RN 500s.
c-iv	**Diazepam** (Various, eg, Elkins-Sinn, Geneva, Goldline, Lederle, Lemmon, Major, Roxane, Squibb Mark, Warner Chilcott, Zenith)	**Tablets**: 5 mg	In 15s, 30s, 100s, 500s, 720s, 1000s, 1080s, 2500s and UD 32s and 100s.
c-iv	**Valium**(Roche)		(Roche 5 Valium). Yellow, scored. In 100s, 500s, UD 100s and RN 500s.

Benzodiazepines

DIAZEPAM

c-iv	**Diazepam** (Various, eg, Elkins-Sinn, Geneva, Goldline, Lederle, Lemmon, Major, Roxane, Squibb Mark, Warner Chilcott, Zenith)	**Tablets:** 10 mg	In 15s, 30s, 100s, 500s, 720s, 1000s, 1080s and UD 100s.
c-iv	**Valium** (Roche)		(Roche 10 Valium). Blue, scored. In 100s, 500s, UD 100s and RN 500s.
c-iv	**Diazepam** (Various, eg, Baxter, Elkins-Sinn, Goldline, Lederle, Lemmon, Lyphomed, Moore, Rugby, Schein, Warner Chilcott)	**Injection:** 5 mg per ml	In 2 ml amps & 1, 2 and 10 ml vials & 2 ml disposable syringes.
c-iv	**Valium** (Roche)		In 2 ml amps, 10 ml vials and 2 ml Tel-E-Ject.[1]
c-iv	**Zetran** (Hauck)		In 10 ml vials.[1]
c-iv	**Dizac** (Ohmeda)	**Injection, emulsified:** 5 mg per ml	Preservative free. In 3 ml single-dose vials.

[1] With 40% propylene glycol, 10% ethyl alcohol, 5% sodium benzoate, benzoic acid and 1.5% benzyl alcohol.

Benzodiazepines

CLORAZEPATE DIPOTASSIUM

Complete prescribing information begins in the Benzodiazepines monograph.

Indications:

For management of anxiety disorders or short-term relief of symptoms of anxiety.

For the symptomatic relief of acute alcohol withdrawal.

As adjunctive therapy in the management of partial seizures (see Anticonvulsants section).

Administration and Dosage:

Symptomatic relief of anxiety: 30 mg/day in divided doses. Adjust gradually within the range of 15 to 60 mg/day.

Elderly or debilitated patients: initiate treatment at a dose of 7.5 to 15 mg/day. Lower doses may be indicated.

May also be administered as a single daily dose at bedtime; the initial dose is 15 mg. After the initial dose, the patient may require adjustment of subsequent dosage. Drowsiness may occur at the initiation of treatment and with dosage increments.

Maintenance therapy – Give the 22.5 mg tablet in a single daily dose as an alternate dosage form for patients stabilized on 7.5 mg 3 times/day. Do not use to initiate therapy.

The 11.25 mg tablet may be administered as a single dose every 24 hours.

Symptomatic relief of acute alcohol withdrawal: Day 1 – 30 mg initially; followed by 30 to 60 mg in divided doses.

Day 2 – 45 to 90 mg in divided doses.
Day 3 – 22.5 to 45 mg in divided doses.
Day 4 – 15 to 30 mg in divided doses.

Thereafter, gradually reduce the dose to 7.5 to 15 mg daily. Discontinue drug as soon as patient's condition is stable.

The maximum recommended total daily dose is 90 mg. Avoid excessive reductions in the total amount of drug administered on successive days.

c-iv	**Clorazepate Dipotassium** (Various, eg, American Therapeutics, Geneva, Lederle, Martec, Moore, PBI, Rugby, Squibb Mark, URL)	**Capsules:** 3.75 mg	In 100s, 500s, 1000s and UD 100s.
c-iv	**Clorazepate Dipotassium** (Various, eg, American Therapeutics, Geneva, Lederle, Martec, Moore, PBI, Rugby, Squibb Mark, URL)	**Capsules:** 7.5 mg	In 100s, 500s and 1000s.
c-iv	**Clorazepate Dipotassium** (Various, eg, American Therapeutics, Geneva, Lederle, Martec, Moore, PBI, Rugby, Squibb Mark, URL)	**Capsules:** 15 mg	In 100s, 500s and 1000s.

Benzodiazepines

CLORAZEPATE DIPOTASSIUM

c-iv	**Clorazepate Dipotassium** (Various, eg, American Therapeutics, Bioline, Goldline, Lederle, Major, Moore, Rugby, Schein, Squibb Mark, Warner Chilcott)	**Tablets:** 3.75 mg	In 100s, 500s, 1000s and UD 100s.
c-iv	**Gen-Xene** (Alra)		(Alra GX). Gray, scored. In 30s, 100s, 500s and UD 100s.
c-iv	**Tranxene** (Abbott)		(TL). Blue, scored. In 100s, 500s and UD 100s.
c-iv	**Clorazepate Dipotassium** (Various, eg, American Therapeutics, Bioline, Goldline, Lederle, Major, Moore, Rugby, Schein, Squibb Mark, Warner Chilcott)	**Tablets:** 7.5 mg	In 20s, 100s, 500s, 1000s and UD 100s and 500s.
c-iv	**Gen-Xene** (Alra)		(Alra GT). Yellow, scored. In 30s, 100s, 500s and UD 100s.
c-iv	**Tranxene** (Abbott)		(TM). Peach, scored. In 100s, 500s and UD 100s.
c-iv	**Clorazepate Dipotassium** (Various, eg, American Therapeutics, Bioline, Goldline, Lederle, Major, Moore, Rugby, Schein, Squibb Mark, Warner Chilcott)	**Tablets:** 15 mg	In 100s, 500s, 1000s and UD 100s.
c-iv	**Gen-Xene** (Alra)		(Alra GN). Green, scored. In 30s, 100s, 500s and UD 100s.
c-iv	**Tranxene** (Abbott)		(TN). Lavender, scored. In 100s, 500s and UD 100s.
c-iv	**Tranxene-SD Half Strength** (Abbott)	**Tablets, single dose:** 11.25 mg	(TX). Blue. In 100s.
c-iv	**Tranxene-SD** (Abbott)	**Tablets, single dose:** 22.5 mg	(TY). Tan. In 100s.

Miscellaneous Agents

BUSPIRONE HCl

Actions:

Pharmacology: Buspirone HCl is an azaspirodecanedione agent not chemically or pharmacologically related to the benzodiazepines, barbiturates or other sedative/anxiolytic drugs. Mechanism of action is unknown. Buspirone differs from benzodiazepines in that it does not exert anticonvulsant or muscle relaxant effects. It also lacks prominent sedative effects associated with more typical anxiolytics. In vitro, buspirone has a high affinity for serotonin ($5\text{-}HT_1A$) receptors; it has no significant affinity for benzodiazepine receptors and does not affect GABA bindings. Buspirone has moderate affinity for brain D_2-dopamine receptors and appears to act as a presynaptic dopamine agonist. It also increases norepinephrine metabolism in the locus ceruleus.

Pharmacokinetics:

Absorption – Buspirone is rapidly absorbed and undergoes extensive first-pass metabolism. Following oral administration, plasma concentrations of unchanged buspirone are very low and variable between subjects. Peak plasma levels of 1 to 6 ng/ml have been observed 40 to 90 minutes after single oral doses of 20 mg. The single dose bioavailability of unchanged buspirone from a tablet is about 90% of an equivalent dose of solution, but there is large variability.

Administration with food may decrease the rate of absorption, but it may increase the bioavailability by decreasing the first-pass metabolism. In one study, the AUC doubled when a 20 mg oral dose was administered with food.

Distribution – Approximately 95% of buspirone is plasma protein bound, but other highly bound drugs (eg, phenytoin, propranolol, warfarin) are not displaced in vitro; however, buspirone does displace digoxin.

Metabolism – Buspirone is metabolized primarily by oxidation, producing several hydroxylated derivatives and a pharmacologically active metabolite, 1-pyrimidinyl piperazine (1-PP). Blood samples from humans chronically exposed to buspirone do not exhibit high levels of 1-PP.

Excretion – In a single dose study, 29% to 63% of the dose was excreted in the urine within 24 hours, primarily as metabolites; fecal excretion accounted for 18% to 38% of the dose. The average elimination half-life of unchanged buspirone after single doses of 10 to 40 mg is about 2 to 3 hours (range, 2 to 11 hours).

A multiple dose study suggests that buspirone has nonlinear pharmacokinetics. Thus, dose increases and repeated dosing may lead to somewhat higher blood levels of unchanged buspirone than would be predicted from results of single dose studies.

Clinical trials: Although buspirone is for the short-term treatment of anxiety, there is no evidence that the effects differ when the drug is used in "longer-term" therapy, ie, > 4 weeks. In studies of patients receiving buspirone for up to 1 year, the dosage remained consistently near 20 mg, with efficacy maintained and no increase in side effects over time. No withdrawal syndrome or other significant adverse reactions were reported upon abrupt discontinuation after 1 year of therapy.

Patients on buspirone often show improvement within 7 to 10 days. However, as with many psychotropic drugs, optimal therapeutic results are generally achieved after 3 to 4 weeks of treatment. During initial stages of therapy, look for subtle improvement in anxious symptoms, interpersonal skills and overall patient functioning. Because the drug is not associated with the prominent sedative effects characteristic of benzodiazepines, advise patients of the need to adhere to the therapeutic regimen.

Indications:

Management of anxiety disorders or short-term relief of symptoms of anxiety.

Unlabeled uses: Buspirone 25 mg/day may be useful in decreasing the symptoms (eg, aches, pains, fatigue, cramps, irritability) of premenstrual syndrome.

Contraindications:

Hypersensitivity to buspirone HCl.

Warnings:

Buspirone has no established antipsychotic activity; it should not be employed in lieu of appropriate antipsychotic treatment.

Miscellaneous Agents

BUSPIRONE HCl

Physical and psychological dependence: Buspirone has shown no potential for abuse or diversion and there is no evidence that it causes tolerance or physical or psychological dependence. However, it is difficult to predict from experiments the extent to which a CNS active drug will be misused, diverted or abused once marketed. Consequently, carefully evaluate patients for a history of drug abuse and follow such patients closely, observing them for signs of misuse or abuse (eg, tolerance, drug-seeking behavior).

Renal/Hepatic function impairment: Since buspirone is metabolized by the liver and excreted by the kidneys, do not use in patients with severe hepatic or renal impairment.

Elderly: Buspirone has not been systematically evaluated in older patients; however, several hundred elderly patients have participated in clinical studies and no unusual adverse age-related phenomena have been identified.

Pregnancy: Category B. Adequate and well controlled studies have not been performed in pregnant women. Use during pregnancy only if clearly needed.

Lactation: The extent of the excretion in breast milk of buspirone or its metabolites is not known. In rats, however, buspirone and its metabolites are excreted in milk. Avoid administration to nursing women, if possible.

Children: Safety and efficacy for use in children < 18 years are not known.

Precautions:

Monitoring: Effectiveness for more than 3 to 4 weeks has not been demonstrated in controlled trials. However, patients have been treated for several months without ill effect. If used for extended periods, periodically reassess the usefulness of the drug.

Interference with cognitive and motor performance: Buspirone is less sedating than other anxiolytics and does not produce significant functional impairment. However, its CNS effect may not be predictable. Therefore, caution patients about driving or using complex machinery until they are certain that buspirone does not affect them adversely.

Withdrawal reactions: Buspirone does not exhibit cross-tolerance with benzodiazepines and other sedative/hypnotic drugs. It will not block the withdrawal syndrome often seen with cessation of therapy with these drugs. Therefore, withdraw patients from their prior treatment gradually before starting buspirone, especially patients who have been using a CNS depressant chronically. Rebound or withdrawal symptoms may occur over varying time periods, depending in part on the type of drug and its effective elimination half-life.

Dopamine receptor binding: Buspirone can bind to central dopamine receptors; a question has been raised about its potential to cause acute and chronic changes in dopamine-mediated neurological function (eg, dystonia, pseudoparkinsonism, akathisia, tardive dyskinesia). Clinical experience in controlled trials has failed to identify any significant neuroleptic-like activity; however, a syndrome of restlessness has appeared shortly after initiation of treatment in a small fraction of buspirone-treated patients. The syndrome may be explained in several ways. For example, buspirone may increase central noradrenergic activity. Alternatively, the effect may be attributable to dopaminergic effects (ie, may represent akathisia).

Drug Interactions:

Alcohol: Formal studies of the interaction of buspirone with alcohol indicate that buspirone does not increase alcohol-induced impairment in motor and mental performance, but it is prudent to avoid concomitant use.

Haloperidol and buspirone coadministration may result in increased serum haloperidol concentrations.

Monoamine oxidase inhibitors (MAOIs): There have been reports of elevated blood pressure when buspirone was added to a regimen including an MAOI. Therefore, do not use concomitantly.

Trazodone: One report suggests that concomitant use may have caused threefold to sixfold elevations of ALT in a few patients. In a similar study attempting to replicate this finding, no interactive effect on hepatic transaminases was identified.

Drug/Food interactions: Administration with food may decrease buspirone's rate of absorption, but food may increase its bioavailability by decreasing first-pass metabolism. In one study, the AUC doubled when a 20mg oral dose was given with food.

Miscellaneous Agents

BUSPIRONE HCl

Adverse Reactions:

Approximately 10% of the 2200 patients in premarketing trials in anxiety disorders lasting 3 to 4 weeks discontinued treatment due to adverse events which included: CNS disturbances (3.4%), primarily dizziness, insomnia, nervousness, drowsiness and lightheadedness; GI disturbances (1.2%), primarily nausea; miscellaneous disturbances (1.1%), primarily headache and fatigue. In addition, 3.4% of patients had multiple complaints, none of which were primary.

Adverse Reactions of Buspirone HCl vs Placebo (%)

Adverse Reaction	Buspirone (n = 477)	Placebo (n = 464)
CNS		
Dizziness	12	3
Drowsiness	10	9
Nervousness	5	1
Insomnia	3	3
Lightheadedness	3	< 1
Decreased concentration	2	2
Excitement	2	< 1
Anger/Hostility	2	< 1
Confusion	2	< 1
Depression	2	2
GI		
Nausea	8	5
Dry mouth	3	4
Abdominal/Gastric distress	2	2
Diarrhea	2	< 1
Constipation	1	2
Vomiting	1	2
Neurological		
Numbness	2	< 1
Paresthesia	1	< 1
Incoordination	1	< 1
Tremor	1	< 1
Miscellaneous		
Headache	6	3
Fatigue	4	4
Weakness	2	< 1
Blurred vision	2	< 1
Tachycardia/Palpitations	1	1
Sweating/Clamminess	1	< 1
Musculoskeletal aches/Pains	1	< 1
Skin rash	1	< 1

Most common: Dizziness; nausea; headache; nervousness; lightheadedness; excitement.

Cardiovascular: Nonspecific chest pain (≥ 1%); syncope, hypotension, hypertension (0.1% to 1%); cerebrovascular accident, congestive heart failure, myocardial infarction, cardiomyopathy, bradycardia (< 0.1%).

CNS: Dream disturbances (≥ 1%); depersonalization, dysphoria, noise intolerance, euphoria, akathisia, fearfulness, loss of interest, disassociative reaction, hallucinations, suicidal ideation, seizures (0.1% to 1%); feelings of claustrophobia, cold intolerance, stupor and slurred speech, psychosis (< 0.1%).

Endocrine: Galactorrhea, thyroid abnormality (< 0.1%).

GI: Flatulence, anorexia, increased appetite, salivation, irritable colon, rectal bleeding (0.1% to 1%); burning of the tongue (< 0.1%).

GU: Urinary frequency, urinary hesitancy, menstrual irregularity, spotting and dysuria (0.1% to 1%); amenorrhea, pelvic inflammatory disease, enuresis, nocturia (< 0.1%).

Musculoskeletal: Muscle cramps, muscle spasms, rigid/stiff muscles, arthralgias (0.1% to 1%).

Miscellaneous Agents

BUSPIRONE HCl

Sexual function: Decreased or increased libido (0.1% to 1%); delayed ejaculation, impotence (< 0.1%).

Neurological: Involuntary movements, slowed reaction time (0.1% to 1%); muscle weakness (< 0.1%).

EENT: Tinnitus, sore throat, nasal congestion (≥ 1%); redness and itching of the eyes, altered taste, altered smell, conjunctivitis (0.1% to 1%); inner ear abnormality, eye pain, photophobia, pressure on eyes (< 0.1%).

Respiratory: Hyperventilation, shortness of breath, chest congestion (0.1% to 1%); epistaxis (< 0.1%).

Dermatologic: Edema, pruritus, flushing, easy bruising, hair loss, dry skin, facial edema, blisters (0.1% to 1%); acne, thinning of nails (< 0.1%).

Body as a whole: Weight gain, fever, roaring sensation in the head, weight loss, malaise (0.1% to 1%); alcohol abuse, bleeding disturbance, loss of voice, hiccoughs (< 0.1%).

Lab test abnormalities: Increases in hepatic aminotransferases (AST, ALT) (0.1% to 1%); eosinophilia, leukopenia, thrombocytopenia (< 0.1%).

Overdosage:

Symptoms: Doses as high as 375 mg/day were administered to healthy male volunteers. As this dose was approached, the following symptoms were observed: Nausea, vomiting, dizziness, drowsiness, miosis and gastric distress. No deaths have been reported.

Treatment: No specific antidote is known. Use general symptomatic and supportive measures along with immediate gastric lavage. Refer to General Management of Acute Overdosage. Dialyzability of buspirone has not been determined.

Patient Information:

Inform physician if any chronic abnormal movements occur (eg, motor restlessness, involuntary repetitive movements of facial or neck muscles).

May cause drowsiness and dizziness. Use caution while driving or performing other tasks requiring alertness. Avoid alcohol and use other CNS depressants with caution.

Inform physician if you are pregnant, become pregnant or are planning to become pregnant while taking buspirone or if you are breast-feeding.

Optimum results are generally achieved after 3 to 4 weeks of treatment. Some improvement will be seen in 7 to 10 days.

Administration and Dosage:

Initial dose: 15 mg daily (5 mg 3 times a day).

To achieve an optimal therapeutic response, increase the dosage 5 mg/day, at intervals of 2 to 3 days, as needed. Do not exceed 60 mg/day. Divided doses of 20 to 30 mg/day have been commonly used.

Rx	**BuSpar** (Mead Johnson Pharm.)	**Tablets:** 5 mg	Lactose. (MJ 5 mg BuSpar). White, scored. Ovoid-rectangular. In 100s, 500s and UD100s.
		10 mg	Lactose. (MJ 10 mg BuSpar). White, scored. Ovoid-rectangular. In 100s, 500s and UD 100s.

Miscellaneous Agents

HYDROXYZINE

Actions:

Pharmacology: Hydroxyzine is a piperazine antihistamine. It is not a cortical depressant; its action may be due to suppressing activity in subcortical areas of CNS.

Primary skeletal muscle relaxation has been demonstrated experimentally. Bronchodilator activity, antihistaminic and analgesic effects have been confirmed clinically. Hydroxyzine has antispasmodic properties, apparently mediated through interference with the mechanism that responds to spasmogenic agents such as serotonin, acetylcholine and histamine. An antiemetic effect has been demonstrated. Hydroxyzine in therapeutic dosage does not increase gastric secretion or acidity and in most cases provides mild antisecretory activity.

Pharmacokinetics: Oral hydroxyzine is rapidly absorbed from the GI tract; clinical effects are usually noted within 15 to 30 minutes after administration. Following a single 100 mg oral dose, peak levels of 82 ng/ml were reached in ≈ 3 hours. Mean elimination half-life is 3 hours; half-life may be longer in elderly patients. Hydroxyzine is mainly metabolized by the liver.

Indications:

Symptomatic relief of anxiety and tension associated with psychoneurosis and as an adjunct in organic disease states in which anxiety is manifest.

The efficacy of hydroxyzine as an antianxiety agent for long-term use (> 4 months) has not been assessed; periodically reevaluate its usefulness.

Management of pruritus due to allergic conditions such as chronic urticaria, atopic and contact dermatoses and in histamine-mediated pruritus.

As a sedative when used as premedication and following general anesthesia.

IM only: For the acutely disturbed or hysterical patient; the acute or chronic alcoholic with anxiety withdrawal symptoms or delirium tremens; as pre- and postoperative and pre- and postpartum adjunctive medication to permit reduction in narcotic dosage, allay anxiety and control emesis; adjunctive therapy in asthma.

Contraindications:

Hypersensitivity to hydroxyzine; early pregnancy, lactation (Warnings).

Hydroxyzine injection is for IM use only. Do not inject SC, IV or intra-arterially. Tissue necrosis has been associated with SC or intra-arterial injection; hemolysis has occurred following IV administration.

Warnings:

Hypersensitivity reactions have occurred (Adverse Reactions). Refer to Management of Acute Hypersensitivity Reactions.

Pregnancy: Clinical data in humans are inadequate to establish safety in early pregnancy. In doses substantially above the human therapeutic range, hydroxyzine has induced fetal abnormalities in animals. Do not use in pregnancy.

Lactation: It is not known whether this drug is excreted in breast milk; therefore, do not give hydroxyzine to nursing mothers.

Precautions:

Potentially hazardous tasks: May produce drowsiness; patients should observe caution while driving or performing other tasks requiring alertness.

IM use: Inject well within the body of a relatively large muscle. In adults, the preferred site is the upper outer quadrant of the buttock or the midlateral thigh. In children, inject into the midlateral muscles of the thigh. In infants and small children, use the periphery of the upper outer quadrant of the gluteal region only when necessary, such as in burn patients, in order to minimize the possibility of sciatic nerve damage.

Use the deltoid area only if well developed, and then only with caution to avoid radial nerve injury. Do not inject into the lower and mid-third of the upper arm.

Drug Interactions:

CNS depressants (eg, narcotics, barbiturates): Consider the potentiating action when used with hydroxyzine. When CNS depressants are given concomitantly with hydroxyzine, reduce their dosage by 50%. Cardiac arrest has occurred (rare).

Adverse Reactions:

Dry mouth; drowsiness is usually transitory and may disappear after a few days of continued therapy or upon dosage reduction; involuntary motor activity, including rare instances of tremor and convulsions, usually with higher than recommended dosage; hypersensitivity reactions (wheezing, dyspnea, chest tightness) have occurred (Warnings).

Miscellaneous Agents

HYDROXYZINE

Overdosage:

Symptoms: The most common manifestation is oversedation. As in management of any overdosage, consider that multiple agents may have been ingested.

Treatment: Induce vomiting if it has not occurred spontaneously. Immediate gastric lavage is also recommended. General supportive care is indicated; frequently monitor vital signs and observe the patient. Control hypotension with IV fluids and norepinephrine or metaraminol. Do not use epinephrine; hydroxyzine counteracts its pressor action. There is no specific antidote. It is doubtful that hemodialysis would be of value. Refer also to General Management of Acute Overdosage.

Patient Information:

May produce drowsiness; patients should observe caution while driving or performing other tasks requiring alertness. Avoid alcoholic beverages and other CNS depressants; they may intensify this effect.

Administration and Dosage:

Start patients on IM therapy when indicated. Maintain on oral therapy whenever practicable. Adjust dosage according to patient's response.

Oral:

Symptomatic relief of anxiety – Adults: 50 to 100mg 4 times/day. Children (> 6): 50 to 100 mg/day in divided doses. Children (< 6): 50 mg/day in divided doses.

Management of pruritus – Adults: 25 mg 3 or 4 times daily. Children (> 6): 50 to 100 mg/day in divided doses. Children (< 6): 50 mg/day in divided doses.

Sedative (as premedication and following general anesthesia) – Adults: 50 to 100 mg. Children: 0.6 mg/kg.

IM:

For adult psychiatric and emotional emergencies, including acute alcoholism – 50 to 100 mg immediately and every 4 to 6 hours as needed.

Nausea and vomiting – Adults: 25 to 100 mg. Children: 1.1 mg/kg (0.5 mg/lb).

Pre- and postoperative adjunctive medication – Adults: 25 to 100 mg. Children: 1.1 mg/kg (0.5 mg/lb).

Pre- and postpartum adjunctive therapy – 25 to 100 mg.

Rx	**Hydroxyzine HCl** (Various, eg, Baxter, Geneva, Goldline, Lannett, Lederle, Major, Moore, PBI, Rugby, Schein)	**Tablets:** 10 mg (as HCl)	In 20s, 30s, 50s, 100s, 250s, 500s, 1000s and UD 32s and 100s.
Rx	**Atarax** (Roerig)		Orange. In 100s, 500s, UD 100s.
Rx	**Hydroxyzine HCl** (Various, eg, Baxter, Geneva, Goldline, Lannett, Lederle, Major, Moore, PBI, Rugby, Schein)	**Tablets:** 25 mg (as HCl)	In 12s, 15s, 20s, 24s, 30s, 40s, 50s, 60s, 100s, 250s, 500s, 1000s and UD 32s and 100s.
Rx	**Anxanil** (Econo Med)		(ANX). Lt. green, scored. Film coated. In 100s, 500s.
Rx	**Atarax**(Roerig)		Green. In 100s, 500s and UD 100s.
Rx	**Hydroxyzine HCl** (Various, eg, Baxter, Geneva, Goldline, Lannett, Major, Moore, PBI, Rugby, Schein, Spencer Mead)	**Tablets:** 50 mg (as HCl)	In 30s and 100s.
Rx	**Atarax** (Roerig)		Yellow. In 100s, 500s and UD100s.
Rx	**Atarax 100** (Roerig)	**Tablets:** 100 mg (as HCl)	Red. In 100s and UD100s.

Miscellaneous Agents

HYDROXYZINE

Rx	**Hydroxyzine HCl** (Various, eg, Baxter, Geneva, Goldline, Major, Moore, PBI, Rugby, Schein, UDL, Warner-C)	**Syrup:** 10 mg per 5 ml (as HCl)	In 16 and 120 ml, pt, gal and UD 5, 12.5 and 25 ml.
Rx	**Atarax** (Roerig)		Sucrose and menthol. 0.5% alcohol. In 480 ml.
Rx	**Hydroxyzine Pamoate** (Various, eg, Baxter, Geneva, Goldline, Lannett, Major, Moore, Rugby, Schein, Spencer Mead, Zenith)	**Capsules:** 25 mg (as pamoate equivalent to HCl)	In 12s, 20s, 50s, 100s, 500s, 1000s and UD 32s and 100s.
Rx	**Vistaril** (Pfizer)		Two-tone green. In100s, 500s and UD 100s.
Rx	**Hydroxyzine Pamoate** (Various, eg, Baxter, Geneva, Goldline, Lannett, Major, Moore, Rugby, Schein, Spencer Mead, Zenith)	**Capsules:** 50 mg (as pamoate equivalent to HCl)	In 12s, 20s, 100s, 500s, 1000s and UD 32s and 100s.
Rx	**Vistaril** (Pfizer)		Green and white. In 100s, 500s and UD100s.
Rx	**Hydroxyzine Pamoate** (Various, eg, Barr, Baxter, Goldline, Lannett, Major, Moore, Rugby, Spencer Mead, URL)	**Capsules:** 100 mg (as pamoate equivalent to HCl)	In 100s, 500s, 1000s and UD 100s.
Rx	**Vistaril** (Pfizer)		Green/gray. In 100s, 500s, UD100s.
Rx	**Vistaril** (Pfizer)	**Oral Suspension:** 25 mg per 5 ml (as pamoate equiv. to HCl)	Sorbitol. Lemon flavor. In 120 and 480 ml.
Rx	**Hydroxyzine HCl** (Various, eg, American Regent, Balan, Goldline, Lyphomed, Major, Moore, Rugby, Schein, Solopak, Steris)	**Injection:** 25 mg/ml (as HCl)	In 2 ml syringes and 1 and 10 ml vials.
Rx	**Hydroxyzine HCl** (Elkins-Sinn)		In 1 ml Dosette vials.
Rx	**Hydroxyzine HCl** (Winthrop Pharm.)		In 1 ml fill in 2 ml Carpuject syringe.[1]
Rx	**Vistaril** (Roerig)		In 10 ml vials.[1]

Miscellaneous Agents

HYDROXYZINE

Rx	**Hydroxyzine HCl** (Various, eg, Balan, Bioline, Goldline, Lyphomed, Major, Moore, Rugby, Schein, Solopak, Steris)	**Injection:** 50 mg/ml (as HCl)	In 2 ml amps, 1 and 2 ml syringes and 1, 2 and 10 ml vials.
Rx	**Hydroxyzine HCl** (Elkins-Sinn)		In 1 and 2 ml Dosette vials and 10 ml vials.[1]
Rx	**Hydroxyzine HCl** (Winthrop Pharm.)		In 1 and 2 ml fill in 2 ml Carpuject syringes.[1]
Rx	**Hyzine-50** (Hyrex)		In 10 ml vials.[1]
Rx	**Quiess** (Forest)		In 10 ml vials.[1]
Rx	**Vistacon** (Hauck)		In 10 ml vials.[1]
Rx	**Vistaquel 50** (Pasadena)		In 10 ml vials.[1]
Rx	**Vistaril** (Roerig)		In 10 ml vials[1], 1 & 2 ml UD vials.[1]
Rx	**Vistazine 50** (Keene)		In 10 ml vials.[1]

[1] With benzyl alcohol

DOXEPIN HCl

Doxepin is a tricyclic antidepressant which also has antianxiety effects. The following is an abbreviated monograph for doxepin. For complete prescribing information, refer to the Tricyclic Antidepressants monograph.

Indications:

For the treatment of psychoneurotic patients with depression or anxiety; depression or anxiety associated with alcoholism or organic disease; psychotic depressive disorders with associated anxiety including involutional depression and manic-depressive disorders.

The target symptoms of psychoneurosis that respond to doxepin include anxiety, tension, depression, somatic symptoms and concerns, insomnia, guilt, lack of energy, fear apprehension and worry.

Administration and Dosage:

Individualize dosage.

The total daily dosage may be given on a divided or once-a-day dosage schedule. If the once-a-day schedule is employed, the maximum recommended dose is 150 mg/day, given at bedtime.

Not recommended for use in children < 12 years old.

Mild to moderate severity: Start with 75 mg/day. The optimum dose range is 75 to 150 mg/day.

More severely ill: Gradual increase to 300 mg/day may be necessary. Additional therapeutic effect is rarely obtained by exceeding a dose of 300 mg/day.

Very mild symptoms or emotional symptoms accompanying organic disease: Some of these patients have been controlled on doses as low as 25 to 50 mg/day.

Dilute oral concentrate with 120 ml of liquid (eg, water, milk and some fruit juices) just prior to administration; not compatible with a number of carbonated beverages. For patients on methadone maintenance taking oral doxepin, mix the concentrate with methadone and lemonade, orange juice, water, sugar water or powdered fruit drink. *Do not mix with grape juice.* Preparation and storage of bulk dilutions are not recommended.

Miscellaneous Agents

DOXEPIN HCl

Rx	**Doxepin HCl** (Various, eg, Balan, Baxter, Elkins Sinn, Geneva, Goldline, Lederle, Major, Moore, Rugby, Schein)	**Capsules:** 10 mg	In 100s, 500s, 1000s and UD 100s.
Rx	**Sinequan** (Roerig)		In 100s, 1000s and UD 100s.
Rx	**Doxepin HCl** (Various, eg, Balan, Baxter, Bioline, Elkins Sinn, Geneva, Goldline, Major, Moore, Rugby, Schein)	**Capsules:** 25 mg	In 30s, 50s, 100s, 360s, 500s, 1000s and UD 100s.
Rx	**Sinequan** (Roerig)		In 100s, 1000s, 5000s and UD 100s & unit-of-use 90s.
Rx	**Doxepin HCl** (Various, eg, Balan, Baxter, Elkins Sinn, Geneva, Goldline, Lederle, Major, Moore, Rugby, Schein)	**Capsules:** 50 mg	In 30s, 100s, 360s, 500s, 1000s and UD 100s.
Rx	**Sinequan** (Roerig)		In 100s, 1000s, 5000s and UD 100s & unit-of-use 90s.
Rx	**Doxepin HCl** (Various, eg, Balan, Baxter, Elkins Sinn, Geneva, Goldline, Lederle, Major, Moore, Rugby, Schein)	**Capsules:** 75 mg	In 30s, 100s, 500s, 1000s and UD 100s.
Rx	**Sinequan** (Roerig)		In 100s, 1000s, UD 100s.
Rx	**Doxepin HCl** (Various, eg, Balan, Baxter, Bioline, Geneva, Goldline, Lederle, Major, Moore, Rugby, Schein)	**Capsules:** 100 mg	In 100s, 500s, 1000s and UD 100s.
Rx	**Sinequan** (Roerig)		In 100s, 1000s, UD 100s.
Rx	**Doxepin HCl** (Various, eg, Balan, Bioline, Dixon-Shane, Goldline, Lederle, Major, Martec, Par, Rugby)	**Capsules:** 150 mg	In 50s, 100s and 500s and UD 100s.
Rx	**Sinequan** (Roerig)		In 50s, 500s and UD 100s.
Rx	**Doxepin HCl** (Various, eg, Balan, Bioline, Geneva, Goldline, Harber, PBI, Rugby, Schein, Warner-C)	**Oral Concentrate:** 10mg/ml	In 120 ml.
Rx	**Sinequan Concentrate** (Roerig)		In 120 ml.

CHLORMEZANONE

Actions:

Pharmacology: Chlormezanone improves the emotional state by allaying mild anxiety, usually without impairing clarity of consciousness. The mechanism of action is unknown.

Pharmacokinetics: The relief of symptoms is often apparent 15 to 30 minutes after administration and may last 6 hours or longer. Peak plasma concentrations are attained within 1 to 2 hours; mean elimination half-life is 24 hours.

Indications:

Treatment of mild anxiety and tension states.

The effectiveness of chlormezanone in long-term use (> 4 months) has not been assessed by clinical studies. Periodically reassess the usefulness of the drug for the individual patient.

Contraindications:

Hypersensitivity to chlormezanone.

Miscellaneous Agents

CHLORMEZANONE

Warnings:

Pregnancy and lactation: Safety for use during pregnancy or lactation has not been established. Use only when clearly needed and when the potential benefits outweigh the potential hazards to the fetus.

Precautions:

Hazardous tasks: Should drowsiness occur, reduce dose; patients should observe caution while driving or performing other tasks requiring alertness.

Drug Interactions:

Alcohol or other CNS depressants (eg, barbiturates, narcotics): Possible additive CNS effects may occur when taken with chlormezanone.

Adverse Reactions:

Drug rash; dizziness; flushing; nausea; drowsiness; depression; edema; inability to void; dry mouth; weakness; excitement; tremor; confusion; headache. Rare instances of erythema multiform, Stevens-Johnson syndrome and toxic epidermal necrolysis have occurred. Discontinue medication or adjust as the case demands. Cholestatic jaundice has occurred rarely, but was reversible upon discontinuance.

Overdosage:

Two patients ingested 7 g and 9 g; one patient became sleepy and vomited, the other was comatose with depressed reflexes. Neither exhibited disturbances of respiratory, renal or hepatic function. Both made uneventful recoveries. Five hours after ingesting 11 g of chlormezanone, a third patient alternated between periods of coma and excitement. He also experienced anticholinergic effects.

Patient Information:

This drug may impair the mental or physical abilities required for the performance of potentially hazardous tasks such as driving or operating machinery.

Avoid alcohol while taking this drug.

Notify physician if skin rash, sore throat or fever occurs.

Administration and Dosage:

Adults: 200 mg 3 or 4 times daily; in some patients 100 mg may suffice.

Children: 50 to 100 mg 3 or 4 times daily.

Since the effect of CNS acting drugs varies, treatment, particularly in children, should begin with the lowest dosage possible which may be increased as needed.

Rx	**Trancopal Caplets** (Winthrop Pharm.)	**Tablets:** 100 mg	Saccharin. Peach, scored. In 100s.
		200 mg	Saccharin. Green, scored. In 100s and 1000s.

ANTIDEPRESSANTS

Drugs with clinically useful antidepressant effects include the tricyclic antidepressants (TCAs), maprotiline, trazodone, bupropion, venlafaxine, nefazodone, selective serotonin reuptake inhibitors (SSRIs) and the monoamine oxidase inhibitors (MAOIs). The antidepressant agents all appear effective in the treatment of depression. "Major depressive episode" implies a prominent and relatively persistent (nearly every day for at least 2 weeks) depressed or dysphoric mood that usually interferes with daily functioning, and includes at least five of the following nine symptoms: Depressed mood; markedly diminished interest or pleasure in all, or almost all activities; significant weight loss or gain when not dieting, or decrease or increase in appetite; insomnia or hypersomnia; psychomotor agitation or retardation; fatigue or loss of energy; feelings of worthlessness, or excessive or inappropriate guilt; diminished ability to think or concentrate, or indecisiveness; recurrent thoughts of death, suicidal ideation or suicide attempt.

Mechanism of action: Effective antidepressant activity has traditionally been associated with the "biogenic amine hypothesis of depression." The theory is that depression is due to reduced functional activity of one or more of the endogenous monoamines (norepinephrine, serotonin) in the brain. It was believed that certain types of depression were caused by brain neurotransmitter deficiency and that antidepressants relieved depression by inhibiting the reuptake of serotonin and norepinephrine, thereby correcting this deficiency and facilitating neurotransmission. This explanation is now being questioned for several reasons. First, several antidepressant agents lack any apparent effect on neurotransmitter reuptake. More importantly, the blockade of neurotransmitter reuptake occurs within minutes to hours of antidepressant drug initiation while the antidepressant effects usually take 1 to 4 weeks to become manifest.

The emphasis of research has shifted from acute reuptake effects to the slower adaptive changes in norepinephrine and serotonin receptor systems induced by chronic antidepressant therapy. Postsynaptic receptors participate in nerve impulse neurotransmission while the presynaptic receptors regulate neurotransmitter release and reuptake, an important mechanism of neurotransmitter inactivation. Long-term antidepressant treatment produces complex changes in the sensitivities of both presynaptic and postsynaptic receptor sites. The available antidepressant agents may increase the sensitivity of postsynaptic alpha (α_1) adrenergic and serotonin receptors and may decrease the sensitivity of presynaptic receptor sites. The net effect is the correction (re-regulation) of an abnormal receptor-neurotransmitter relationship. Clinically, this re-regulatory action speeds up the patient's natural recovery process from the depressive episode by normalizing neurotransmission efficacy.

Drug selection: The non-MAOIs are used much more frequently than the MAOIs mainly because of the perception that MAOIs are less effective than the non-MAOI antidepressants and the risk of hypertensive crisis from ingesting foods containing tyramine or from drug interaction (eg, sympathomimetics) with the MAOIs. However, when MAOIs are used in therapeutic doses, they are probably equally effective to non-MAOIs for the treatment of depression. In general, MAOIs are used for atypical depression.

Base antidepressant drug selection on the patient's history of drug response (if any), the specific drug's side effect profile relative to patient medical conditions and other factors, and clinician familiarity with specific antidepressants. Nortriptyline and desipramine are preferred TCAs in a patient without a history of favorable response to a specific antidepressant because they cause less sedation and have less anticholinergic activity than tertiary TCAs such as amitriptyline and, in the case of nortriptyline, are less likely to cause orthostatic hypotension. Trazodone has less anticholinergic activity than TCAs and causes fewer problems than TCAs when taken in overdose. SSRIs generally lack the adverse reactions (eg, sedation, anticholinergic effects) associated with TCAs, cause few cardiovascular side effects (including orthostasis), are associated with weight loss rather than weight gain as is the case with TCAs, and cause fewer problems than TCAs when taken in overdose. However, they do not have a faster amount of action, and their use is associated with other side effects such as headache, nervousness and insomnia. Fluoxetine and paroxetine are recommended to be taken in the morning; sertraline can be taken morning or evening, and fluvoxamine is recommended to be taken at bedtime. Use maprotiline and bupropion only when other antidepressants have not proven effective. In cases of mild depression, drug therapy and psychotherapy appear to be equally effective.

As a general guideline, continue treatment for 9 months after remission in patients who experience their first episode of depression; following a second episode, continue treatment for 5 years after remission; with a third episode, treat indefinitely.

ANTIDEPRESSANTS

Actions: The following table summarizes some of the important pharmacologic and pharmacokinetic data of these agents.

Antidepressant Pharmacologic and Pharmacokinetic Parameters

0 -none + -slight ++ -moderate +++ -high ++++ -very high +++++ -highest	Major side effects			Amine uptake blocking activity					
	Anticholinergic	Sedation	Orthostatic hypotension	Norepinephrine	Serotonin	Half-life (hours)	Therapeutic plasma level (ng/ml)	Time to reach steady state (days)	Dose range (mg/day)
Tricyclics - Tertiary Amines									
Amitriptyline	++++	++++	++	++	++++	31-46	110-250[1]	4-10	50-300
Clomipramine	+++	+++	++	++	+++++	19-37	80-100	7-14	25-250
Doxepin	++	+++	++	+	++	8-24	100-200[1]	2-8	25-300
Imipramine	++	++	+++	++[2]	++++	11-25	200-350[1]	2-5	30-300
Trimipramine	++	+++	++	+	+	7-30	180[1]	2-6	50-300
Tricyclics - Secondary Amines									
Amoxapine[3]	+++	++	+	+++	++	8[4]	200-500	2-7	50-600
Desipramine	+	+	+	++++	++	12-24	125-300	2-11	25-300
Nortriptyline	++	++	+	++	+++	18-44	50-150	4-19	30-100
Protriptyline	+++	+	+	++++	++	67-89	100-200	14-19	15-60
Phenethylamine									
Venlafaxine	0	0	0	+++	+++	5-11[1]	-	3-4	75-375
Tetracyclic									
Maprotiline	++	++	+	+++	0/+	21-25	200-300[1]	6-10	50-225
Triazolopyridine									
Trazodone	+	++	++	0	+++	4-9	800-1600	3-7	150-600
Aminoketone									
Bupropion[5]	++	++	+	0/+	0/+	8-24	-	1.5-5	200-450
Selective Serotonin Reuptake Inhibitors									
Fluoxetine	0/+	0/+	0/+	0/+	+++++	2-9 days[1]	-	2-4 weeks	20-80
Paroxetine	0	0/+	0	0/+	+++++	10-24	-	7-14	10-50
Sertraline	0	0/+	0	0/+	+++++	1-4[1]	-	7	50-200
Fluvoxamine	0/+	0/+	0	0/+	+++++	15.6	-	3-8 hours	50-300
Monoamine Oxidase Inhibitors									
Tranylcypromine	+	+	0	-	-	2.4-2.8	-	-	30-60
Phenelzine	+	+	+	-	-	-	-	-	45-90
Miscellaneous									
Nefazodone	0/+	++	+	0/+	+++++	2-4	-	4-5	200-600

[1] Parent compound plus active metabolite.
[2] Via desipramine, the major metabolite.
[3] Also blocks dopamine receptors.
[4] 30 hours for major metabolite 8-hydroxyamoxapine.
[5] Inhibits dopamine uptake.

TRICYCLIC COMPOUNDS

Maprotiline, a tetracyclic antidepressant, is included in this monograph because of pharmacologic and therapeutic similarities to the tricyclic agents.

Actions:

Pharmacology: The tricyclic antidepressants (TCAs), structurally related to the phenothiazine antipsychotic agents, possess three major pharmacologic actions in varying degrees: Blocking of the amine pump, sedation, and peripheral and central anticholinergic action. In contrast to phenothiazines, which act on dopamine receptors, TCAs inhibit reuptake of norepinephrine or serotonin (5-hydroxytryptamine, 5-HT) at the presynaptic neuron. Amoxapine, a metabolite of loxapine, retains some of the postsynaptic dopamine receptor-blocking action of neuroleptics.

Amine uptake inhibition – The amine hypothesis of depression proposes a relationship between depression and levels of CNS bioamines at postsynaptic adrenergic receptors in the brain. TCAs can be characterized by their ability to inhibit presynaptic reuptake of norepinephrine and serotonin (see table in introduction).

Although amine pump blockade may be immediate, antidepressant response can take days to weeks.

Other pharmacological effects – Inhibition of histamine and acetylcholine activity. Clinical effects, in addition to antidepressant effects, include sedation, anticholinergic effects, mild peripheral vasodilator effects and possible "quinidine-like" actions.

Pharmacokinetics:

Absorption/Distribution – Although the TCAs are well absorbed from the GI tract with peak plasma concentrations occurring in 2 to 4 hours, they undergo a significant first-pass effect. They are highly bound (> 90%) to plasma proteins, are lipid soluble and are widely distributed in tissues, including the CNS. Although there is a suggested therapeutic range for many of the TCAs (see table in introduction), the association between plasma levels and therapeutic effect has not been adequately defined. Wide interpatient variation in steady-state plasma levels at a given dosage is due primarily to differences in the rate of metabolism or first-pass effect. Effective dosage levels vary greatly and must be individualized.

Metabolism/Excretion – Metabolism of TCAs occurs in the liver by demethylation, hydroxylation and glucuronidation, and it varies for each patient. Some intermediate active metabolites include:

Amitriptyline ➡ nortriptyline
Amoxapine ➡ 7 hydroxy and 8 hydroxyamoxapine
Clomipramine ➡ desmethylclomipramine
Doxepin ➡ desmethyldoxepin
Imipramine ➡ desipramine

The TCAs are partially secreted into the hepatobiliary circulation and stomach and are reabsorbed and excreted in the urine.

Because of the long half-life, a single daily dose may be given. Up to 2 to 4 weeks may be required to achieve maximal clinical response.

Indications:

Relief of symptoms of depression (except clomipramine).

Agents with significant sedative action may be useful in depression associated with anxiety and sleep disturbances.

Doxepin: Anxiety.

Imipramine: Treatment of enuresis in children ≥ 6 years of age.

Clomipramine: Only for treatment of Obsessive-Compulsive Disorder (OCD).

Unlabeled uses: Chronic pain (migraine, chronic tension headache, diabetic neuropathy, tic douloureux, cancer pain, peripheral neuropathy with pain, postherpetic neuralgia, arthritic pain): Amitriptyline (50 to 100 mg/day); doxepin (50 to 300 mg/day); imipramine (75 to 150 mg/day); clomipramine.

Pathologic laughing and weeping secondary to forebrain disease – Amitriptyline (25 to 75 mg).

Obstructive sleep apnea – Protriptyline.

Peptic ulcer disease – Trimipramine; doxepin.

Facilitation of cocaine withdrawal – Desipramine (50 to 200 mg/day).

Panic disorder – Imipramine; clomipramine; nortriptyline (25 to 75 mg/day). Other antidepressants may also be used.

Eating disorders (effective in bulimia nervosa) – Imipramine; desipramine; amitriptyline.

Premenstrual depression – Nortriptyline (50 to 125 mg/day).

Dermatologic disorders (chronic urticaria and angioedema, nocturnal pruritis in atopic eczema) – Doxepin (10 to 30 mg/day); trimipramine (50 mg/day); nortriptyline (75 mg/day).

TRICYCLIC COMPOUNDS

Contraindications:

Prior sensitivity to any tricyclic drug. Not recommended for use during the acute recovery phase following myocardial infarction. Concomitant use of monoamine oxidase inhibitors (MAOIs) is generally contraindicated (see Drug Interactions).

Doxepin: Patients with glaucoma or a tendency to urinary retention.

Maprotiline: Patients with known or suspected seizure disorder.

Warnings:

Tardive dyskinesia, a syndrome consisting of potentially irreversible, involuntary, dyskinetic movements may develop in patients treated with neuroleptics (eg, antipsychotics). **Amoxapine** is not an antipsychotic, but it has substantive neuroleptic activity. Although the syndrome appears most often among the elderly, especially elderly women, it is impossible to determine which patients will develop the syndrome. Whether neuroleptic drugs differ in their potential to cause tardive dyskinesia is unknown. For a more complete discussion of tardive dyskinesia, see the Antipsychotic Agents group monograph.

Neuroleptic malignant syndrome (NMS) is a potentially fatal condition reported in association with antipsychotic drugs and with **amoxapine**. Clinical manifestations of NMS are hyperpyrexia, muscle rigidity, altered mental status and evidence of autonomic instability (irregular pulse or blood pressure, tachycardia, diaphoresis and cardiac arrhythmias). The management of NMS should include: (1) Immediate discontinuation of antipsychotic drugs, amoxapine and other drugs not essential to concurrent therapy, (2) intensive symptomatic treatment and medical monitoring, and (3) treatment of any concomitant serious medical problems for which specific treatments are available. There is no general agreement about specific pharmacological treatment regimens for uncomplicated NMS.

Once the NMS is resolved, use a different antidepressant drug if the patient continues to require antidepressant treatment.

Hyperthermia has occurred with **clomipramine;** most cases occurred when it was used with other drugs (eg, neuroleptics) and may be examples of an NMS.

Seizure disorders: Because TCAs lower the seizure threshold, use with caution in patients with a history of seizures. However, seizures have occurred both in patients with and without a history of seizure disorders. **Maprotiline** is associated with seizure occurrence in overdose and with therapeutic doses. Seizure was identified as the most significant risk of **clomipramine** use in premarket evaluation.

Anticholinergic effects: Use with caution in patients with a history of urinary retention, urethral or ureteral spasm; angle-closure glaucoma or increased intraocular pressure. In angle-closure glaucoma, even average doses may precipitate an attack. In occasional susceptible patients or in those receiving anticholinergics (including antiparkinson agents), the atropine-like effects may become more pronounced (eg, paralytic ileus). See table in introduction for relative anticholinergic actions.

Cardiovascular disorders: Use with extreme caution in patients with cardiovascular disorders (eg, severe coronary heart disease with ECG abnormalities, progressive heart failure, conduction disturbances, angina pectoris, paroxysmal tachycardia). In high doses, TCAs may produce arrhythmias, sinus tachycardia and prolong conduction time. Tachycardia may increase the frequency and severity of anginal attacks in the patient with coronary artery disease. Tachycardia and postural hypotension may occur more frequently with **protriptyline**. Orthostatic hypotension may occur in patients with decreased left ventricular performance (LVP). Myocardial infarction and stroke have occurred.

Hyperthyroid patients or those receiving thyroid medication require close supervision because of the possibility of cardiovascular toxicity, including arrhythmias.

Psychiatric patients: Schizophrenic or paranoid patients may exhibit a worsening of psychosis with TCA therapy, and manic-depressive patients may experience a shift to a hypomanic or manic phase; this may also occur when switching antidepressants and withdrawing them. In overactive or agitated patients, increased anxiety or agitation may occur. Paranoid delusions, with or without associated hostility, may be exaggerated. Reduction of TCA dosage and concomitant antipsychotic therapy may be necessary.

The possibility of suicide in depressedpatients remains during treatment and until significant remission occurs. Patients should not have easy access to large quantities of the drug; *prescribe small quantities of TCAs.*

TRICYCLIC COMPOUNDS

Renal/Hepatic function impairment: Use with caution and in reduced doses in patients with hepatic impairment; metabolism may be impaired, leading to drug accumulation. Use with caution in patients with significantly impaired renal function.

Pregnancy: (Category C - Amoxapine, trimipramine; Category B - Imipramine, maprotiline). Clinical experience is limited. These agents have demonstrated teratogenicity and embryotoxicity in dosages greater than maximum human doses. There have been clinical reports of congenital malformations associated with **imipramine.** Limb reduction anomalies have been reported with **amitriptyline**and **nortriptyline** and neonatal withdrawal symptoms have been seen with **clomipramine, desipramine** and **imipramine.** All are isolated reports.

Safety for use during pregnancy has not been established; use only when clearly needed and when the potential benefits outweigh the potential hazards to the fetus.

Lactation: These agents are excreted into breast milk in low concentrations (approximate milk:plasma ratio of 0.4 to 1.5). Exercise caution when using in a nursing woman. At steady state, concentrations of **maprotiline** in milk correspond closely to concentrations in whole blood. Clinical effects of exposure are not known.

Children: Not recommended for patients < 12 years of age. Safety and efficacy not established for **amoxapine** in children < 16, **maprotiline** in children < 18 or **trazodone** or **clomipramine** in children < 10 years old. Safety and efficacy are not established in the pediatric age group for **trimipramine, nortriptyline** and **protriptyline**.

Do not exceed 2.5 mg/kg/day of **imipramine**. ECG changes of unknown significance have occurred in pediatric patients with doses twice this amount. Effectiveness of imipramine in children for conditions other than nocturnal enuresis has not been established.

Precautions:

Monitoring: Perform baseline and periodic leukocyte and differential counts and liver function studies. Fever or sore throat may signal serious neutrophil depression; discontinue therapy if there is evidence of pathological neutropenia.

Monitor ECG prior to initiation of large doses of TCAs and at appropriate intervals thereafter. Patients with cardiovascular disease require cardiac surveillance at all dosage levels. Elderly patients and patients with cardiac disease or a history of cardiac disease are at special risk of developing cardiac abnormalities with TCAs.

Electroconvulsive therapy with TCAs may increase the hazards of therapy.

Elective surgery: Discontinue therapy for as long as possible before elective surgery.

Elevated and lowered blood sugar levels have occurred.

Sexual dysfuntion was markedly increased in male patients with OCD taking clomipramine (42% ejaculatory failure, 20% impotence) compared to placebo.

Weight changes: Weight gain occurred in 18% of patients receiving **clomipramine**. Some patients had weight gain in excess of 25% of their initial body weight.

Hazardous tasks: May impair mental or physical abilities required for the performance of potentially hazardous tasks; patients should observe caution while driving or performing other tasks requiring alertness, coordination or dexterity.

Photosensitivity: Photosensitization (photoallergy or phototoxicity) may occur; therefore, caution patients to take protective measures (ie, sunscreens, protective clothing) against exposure to ultraviolet light or sunlight until tolerance is determined.

Tartrazine sensitivity: Some of these products contain tartrazine, which may cause allergic type reactions (including bronchial asthma) in susceptible individuals. Although the incidence of tartrazine sensitivity in the general population is low, it is frequently seen in patients who also have aspirin hypersensitivity. Specific products containing tartrazine are identified in the product listings.

Sulfite sensitivity: Some of the injectable antidepressant products contain sulfites that may cause allergic-type reactions including anaphylactic symptoms and life-threatening or less severe asthmatic episodes in certain susceptible people. The overall prevalence of sulfite sensitivity in the general population is unknown but is probably low. Sulfite sensitivity is seen more frequently in asthmatic than in nonasthmatic people. Products containing sulfites are identified in the product listings.

Drug Interactions:

Anticholinergics: The anticholinergic effects may be enhanced by the coadministration of certain TCAs.

Barbiturates may lower serum levels of TCAs; central and respiratory depressant effects may be additive.

Charcoal can prevent TCA absorption, thereby reducing their effectiveness or toxicity.

TRICYCLIC COMPOUNDS

Cimetidine has increased serum TCA concentrations. Anticholinergic symptoms (eg, severe dry mouth, urinary retention, blurred vision) have been associated with elevated TCA serum levels when cimetidine therapy is initiated. Additionally, higher than expected TCA levels have occurred when they are begun in patients already taking cimetidine. Ranitidine may be an alternative.

Clonidine: Dangerous elevation in blood pressure and hypertensive crisis have occurred in patients receiving concurrent TCAs. Avoid coadministration.

Dicumarol: TCAs may increase the half-life or bioavailability of dicumarol, possibly resulting in increased anticoagulation effects.

Disulfiram and TCA coadministration may result in acute organic brain syndrome. The bioavailability of the antidepressant may also be increased.

Fluoxetine may increase the pharmacologic and toxic effects of TCAs; symptoms may persist for several weeks after the discontinuation of fluoxetine.

Guanethidine: TCAs may antagonize guanethidine's antihypertensive action by inhibiting uptake into adrenergic neurons. Avoid this combination when possible; if concurrent therapy is required, monitor blood pressure. At up to 150 mg/day, may give doxepin with guanethidine without reducing antihypertensive effect.

Haloperidol may increase serum concentrations of TCAs; a tonic-clonic seizure occurred in one patient.

Levodopa absorption may be delayed and its bioavailability decreased by TCAs. Hypertensive episodes have also occurred.

MAOIs should not be given with or immediately following TCAs. Such combinations can produce seizures, sweating, coma, hyperexcitability, hyperthermia, tachycardia, tachypnea, headache, mydriasis, flushing, confusion, hypotension, disseminated intravascular coagulation and death. At least 7 to 10 days should elapse between MAOI discontinuation and TCA institution. Some TCAs have been used safely and successfully with MAOIs. Initiate TCA cautiously with gradual dosage increase until achieving optimum response. **Furazolidone** may interact similarly with TCAs.

Oral contraceptives inhibit the hepatic metabolism of TCAs and may increase their plasma levels. **Estrogens** may increase or decrease the pharmacologic effect of TCAs depending on the estrogen dose.

Phenothiazines may increase serum TCA levels by inhibiting hepatic metabolism.

Smoking may increase the metabolic biotransformation of TCAs.

Adverse Reactions:

Sedation and anticholinergic effects are reported most frequently. Tolerance to these effects develops, but side effects may be minimized by starting with a low dose and then gradually increasing the dose.

Cardiovascular: Orthostatic hypotension; hypertension; syncope; tachycardia; palpitations; myocardial infarction; arrhythmias; heart block; precipitation of CHF; stroke; ECG changes (most frequently with toxic doses); hypertensive episodes during surgery **(desipramine)**.

Hematologic: Bone marrow depression including agranulocytosis; eosinophilia; purpura; thrombocytopenia; leukopenia; anemia **(clomipramine)**.

CNS: Confusion (especially in the elderly); disturbed concentration; hallucinations, disorientation; decrease in memory; feelings of unreality; delusions; anxiety; nervousness; restlessness; agitation; panic; insomnia; nightmares; hypomania; mania; exacerbation of psychosis; drowsiness; dizziness; weakness; fatigue; headache; depression, hypertonia, sleep disorder, psychosomatic disorder, yawning, abnormal dreaming, migraine, depersonalization, irritability, emotional lability, aggressive reaction **(clomipramine)**.

Numbness; tingling; paresthesias of extremities; incoordination; motor hyperactivity; akathisia; ataxia; tremors; peripheral neuropathy; tardive dyskinesia **(amoxapine)**; extrapyramidal symptoms; seizures; alterations in EEG patterns; myoclonus, twitching, paresis, asthenia **(clomipramine)**.

Other: Nasal congestion; excessive appetite; weight gain or loss; increased perspiration; hyperthermia; flushing; chills; alopecia; tooth disorder, abnormal skin odor, chest pain, fever, halitosis, thirst, myalgia, back pain, arthralgia, muscle weakness **(clomipramine)**.

Anticholinergic: Dry mouth, rare associated sublingual adenitis; blurred vision; disturbance of accommodation, increased intraocular pressure, mydriasis; constipation; paralytic ileus; urinary retention; delayed micturition; urinary tract dilation.

TRICYCLIC COMPOUNDS

Withdrawal symptoms: Although not indicative of addiction, abrupt cessation after prolonged therapy may produce nausea, headache, vertigo, nightmares, malaise. Gradual dosage reduction may produce, within 2 weeks, transient symptoms including irritability, restlessness, dreams and sleep disturbance. Rarely mania or hypomania occurred within 2 to 7 days following cessation of chronic therapy.

Enuretic children: Consider adverse reactions reported with adult use. Most common are nervousness, sleep disorders, tiredness and mild GI disturbances. These usually disappear with continued therapy or dosage reduction. Other reported reactions include: Constipation; convulsions; anxiety; emotional instability; syncope; collapse. Do not exceed 2.5 mg/kg/day of **imipramine**.

Hypersensitivity: Skin rash; pruritus; vasculitis; petechiae, urticaria; photosensitization; itching; edema (general or of face and tongue); drug fever; dermatitis, acne, dry skin **(clomipramine)**.

GI: Nausea and vomiting; anorexia; epigastric distress; diarrhea; flatulence; dysphagia; peculiar taste in mouth; increased salivation; stomatitis; glossitis; parotid swelling; abdominal cramps; pancreatitis; black tongue; dyspepsia, esophagitis, eructation **(clomipramine)**.

Hepatic: Rarely, hepatitis and jaundice. Elevation in transaminase; changes in alkaline phosphatase.

Endocrine: Gynecomastia and testicular swelling in the male; breast enlargement, menstrual irregularity and galactorrhea in the female; increased or decreased libido; painful ejaculation; impotence; nocturia; urinary frequency; urinary tract infection, dysuria, cystitis, dysmenorrhea, lactation (nonpuerperal), vaginitis, leukorrhea, breast pain, amenorrhea, ejaculation failure **(clomipramine)**.

Elevation or depression of blood sugar levels; elevation of prolactin levels; inappropriate ADH secretion.

Respiratory: Pharyngitis, rhinitis, sinusitis, coughing, bronchospasm, epistaxis, dyspnea, laryngitis **(clomipramine)**.

Special senses: Speech blockage; dysarthria; tinnitus; abnormal lacrimation; conjunctivitis, anisocoria, blepharospasm, otitis media, occular allergy, vestibular disorder **(clomipramine)**.

Overdosage:

Children are reportedly more sensitive than adults to acute overdose. Consider any overdose in infants or young children serious and potentially fatal.

Symptoms:

CNS – Early signs include confusion, agitation and hallucinations. Seizures are common, especially with **maprotiline** and **amoxapine**, and may begin within 12 hours after ingestion. Status epilepticus may develoPhysical examination may reveal clonus, choreoathetosis, hyperactive reflexes and a positive Babinski's sign. The patient may rapidly succumb to coma. Overdoses with amoxapine are particularly characterized by CNS toxicity. Maprotiline is associated with a high incidence of seizures (often with QRS intervals > 0.1 sec).

Anticholinergic – Flushing; dry mouth; dilated pupils; hyperpyrexia.

Cardiovascular – TCAs exert cardiotoxicity due to anticholinergic activity and quinidine-like effect that depresses myocardial contractility, heart rate and coronary blood flow. Arrhythmias include tachycardia, intraventricular blocks and complete AV block. With up to 20 mg/kg, re-entry ventricular arrhythmias, premature ventricular contractions, ventricular tachycardia or fibrillation may occur. Sudden cardiac arrest has been reported. Pulmonary edema and hypotension are common.

Renal – Renal failure may develop 2 to 5 days after toxic overdosage of **amoxapine** in patients who may appear otherwise recovered; acute tubular necrosis with rhabdomyolysis and myoglobinuria is most common. This probably occurs in < 5% of overdose cases, and is typical in those who have experienced multiple seizures.

Treatment: Hospitalize and closely observe with ECG monitoring, even when the amount ingested is thought to be small or the initial degree of intoxication appears slight to moderate. Blood and urine levels are unreliable indicators for clinical management. Monitor patients with ECG abnormalities continuously for at least 3 to 5 days; observe closely until well after cardiac status returns to normal. A prolonged QRS interval may indicate the patient to be at higher risk for developing seizures, arrhythmias or hypotension. Relapses may occur after apparent recovery.

Maintain adequate respiratory exchange. Do not use respiratory stimulants. Use normal or half-normal saline to avoid water intoxication, especially in children. Instillation of activated charcoal slurry may help reduce absorption. Refer to General Management of Acute Overdosage.

TRICYCLIC COMPOUNDS

Treat cardiovascular effects aggressively. Sodium bicarbonate (hypertonic, 1 M) by IV infusion has effectively treated cardiac dysrhythmias and hypotension. It is usually given 0.5 to 2 mEq/kg IV bolus, followed by an IV infusion to maintain the blood at pH 7.5. If hypotension does not respond to sodium bicarbonate, fluid expansion and vasopressors (eg, dopamine) may be required; if cardiac dysrhythmias do not respond, lidocaine, or phenytoin may be used. Isoproterenol may be help control bradyarrhythmias and torsade de pointes ventricular tachycardia while overdrive pacing is being established. Propranolol (0.1 mg/kg IV, up to 0.25 mg IV bolus) is used for life-threatening ventricular arrhythmias in children. Quinidine, procainamide, disopyramide and atropine are contraindicated for TCA overdose.

Treat shock and metabolic acidosis with supportive measures (eg, IV fluids, bicarbonate, oxygen, corticosteroids). Digitalis may increase conduction abnormalities and further irritate an already sensitized myocardium. If CHF necessitates rapid digitalization, exercise care. Closely monitor cardiac function for at least 5 days. Support renal function.

Minimize external stimulation (darken the room) to prevent seizures. If anticonvulsants are necessary, phenytoin or diazepam may be useful. With **amoxapine**, seizures may appear precipitously in otherwise relatively asymptomatic patients. Consider prophylactic anticonvulsants. Control hyperpyrexia by any available external means, including ice packs and cooling sponge baths, if necessary.

Hemodialysis, peritoneal dialysis, exchange transfusions and forced diuresis have generally been ineffective because of the rapid fixation of TCAs in the tissues.

Patient Information:

Before using, tell your doctor and pharmacist (1) if you have other medical conditions; (2) what other medications you are currently taking; (3) if you have ever had an unusual or allergic reaction to any tricyclic antidepressant or maprotiline; (4) if you are pregnant or may become pregnant and (5) if you are breast-feeding.

Discontinue drug and get emergency help if any of the following occur: Seizures; difficult or fast breathing; fever with increased sweating; high or low blood pressure; loss of bladder control; severe muscle stiffness; unusual tiredness or weakness.

Warn male patients receiving **clomipramine** of high incidence of sexual dysfunction.

Do not discontinue therapy or take other drugs without consent of physician. Abrupt discontinuation of therapy may cause nausea, headache and malaise.

May cause drowsiness, dizziness or blurred vision; use caution when driving or performing other tasks requiring alertness, coordination or dexterity. Avoid alcohol and other CNS depressant drugs.

Avoid prolonged exposure to sunlight or sunlamps; photosensitivity may occur.

Administration and Dosage:

If minor side effects develop, reduce dosage. Discontinue treatment promptly if serious adverse effects or allergic manifestations occur.

Plasma levels: Determination of plasma levels may be useful in identifying patients who appear to have toxic effects and may have excessively high levels, or those in whom lack of absorption or noncompliance is suspected. Make adjustments in dosage according to patient's clinical response and not based on plasma levels.

Adolescent, elderly and outpatients: Lower dosages are recommended. Initiate therapy at a low dosage and increase gradually, noting the clinical response and any evidence of intolerance. Maintain initial dose of **maprotiline** for 2 weeks. Following remission, maintenance medication may be required for a longer time. Continue maintenance therapy 3 months or longer to decrease the possibility of relapse.

Single daily dose: A single daily dose may be used for maintenance therapy. A single daily dose at bedtime is convenient, will minimize daytime side effects (sedation and anticholinergic effects), and the sedative effect at bedtime may be beneficial in patients with sleep disorders. Because of increased risk of cardiovascular and other complications, the elderly may not tolerate single daily dosages. **Protriptyline** may have a mild stimulant effect; it is generally not given as a single bedtime dose.

Tricyclic/MAOI combined use is traditionally contraindicated because of the potential serious adverse reactions (see Drug Interactions). Such combinations may offer significant advantages in patients refractory to more conservative therapy. In conservative dosages, with observance of MAOI dietary restrictions, and under close medical observation, combined therapy has been safe. At least 7 to 10 days should elapse between MAOI discontinuation and TCA institution.

Specific dosage guidelines for individual agents are included in the product listings.

Tricyclic Compounds

AMITRIPTYLINE HCl

For complete prescribing information, refer to the Tricyclic Compounds group monograph.

Administration and Dosage:

Outpatients: 75 mg/day in divided doses. May increase to 150 mg/day. Make increases preferably in late afternoon or at bedtime. A sedative effect may be apparent before the antidepressant effect is noted. An adequate therapeutic effect may take as long as 30 days to develop.

Alternatively, initiate therapy with 50 to 100 mg at bedtime. Increase by 25 to 50 mg as necessary, to a total of 150 mg/day.

Hospitalized patients may require 100 mg/day initially. Gradually increase to 200 to 300 mg, if necessary.

Adolescent and elderly patients: 10 mg 3 times a day with 20 mg at bedtime may be satisfactory in adolescent and elderly patients who cannot tolerate higher dosages.

Maintenance: 40 to 100 mg/day. Total daily dosage may be given in a single dose, preferably at bedtime. When patient has satisfactorily improved, reduce dosage to lowest effective amount. Continue 3 months or longer to lessen the possibility of relapse.

IM: Do not administer IV. Initially, 20 to 30 mg IM, 4 times a day. The effects may be more rapid with IM than with oral administration. When used for initial therapy in patients unable or unwilling to take tablets, the tablets should replace the injection as soon as possible.

Children: Not recommended for children < 12 years of age.

Rx	**Amitriptyline HCl** (Various, eg, Geneva, Mutual, Purepac, Sidmak)	**Tablets**: 10 mg	In 100s and 1000s.
Rx	**Elavil** (Zeneca)		(Elavil 40). Blue. Film coated. In 100s and 1000s.
Rx	**Amitriptyline HCl** (Various, eg, Geneva, Mutual, Purepac, Sidmak)	**Tablets**: 25 mg	In 100s and 1000s.
Rx	**Elavil** (Zeneca)		(Elavil 45). Yellow. Film coated. In 100s, 1000s, 5000s and UD 100s.
Rx	**Amitriptyline HCl** (Various, eg, Geneva, Mutual, Purepac, Goldline, Sidmak)	**Tablets**: 50 mg	In 100s and 1000s.
Rx	**Elavil** (Zeneca)		(Elavil 41). Beige. Film coated. In 100s, 1000s and UD 100s.
Rx	**Amitriptyline HCl** (Various, eg, Geneva, Mutual, Purepac, Sidmak)	**Tablets**: 75 mg	In 100s and 1000s.
Rx	**Elavil** (Zeneca)		(Elavil 42). Orange. Film coated. In 100s.
Rx	**Amitriptyline HCl** (Various, eg, Geneva, Mutual, Purepac, Sidmak)	**Tablets**: 100 mg	In 100s and 500s.
Rx	**Elavil** (Zeneca)		(Elavil 43). Mauve. Film coated. In 100s.

Tricyclic Compounds

AMITRIPTYLINE HCl

Rx	**Amitriptyline HCl** (Various, eg, Geneva, Mutual, Sidmak)	**Tablets**: 150 mg	In 100s and 1000s.
Rx	**Elavil** (Zeneca)		(Elavil 47). Blue. Capsule shape. Film coated. In 30s and 100s.
Rx	**Elavil** (Zeneca)	**Injection**: 10 mg/ml	In 10 ml vials. [1]

[1] With dextrose and parabens.

NORTRIPTYLINE HCl

For complete prescribing information, refer to the Tricyclic Compounds group monograph.

Administration and Dosage:

Not recommended for use in children.

Adults: 25 mg 3 or 4 times daily; begin at a low level and increase as required. Doses > 150 mg/day are not recommended.

Elderly and adolescent patients: 30 to 50 mg daily in divided doses.

Storage/Stability: Store at controlled room temperature 15° to 30°C (59° to 86°F).

Rx	**Nortriptyline HCl** (Various, eg, Lemmon, Rugby)	**Capsules**: 10 mg	In 100s, 500s and 1000s.
Rx	**Aventyl Pulvules** (Lilly)		White/yellow. In 100s, 500s and UD 100s.
Rx	**Pamelor** (Sandoz)		(Pamelor 10 mg Sandoz). In 100s and UD 100s.
Rx	**Nortriptyline HCl**(Various, eg, Lemmon, Rugby)	**Capsules**: 25 mg	In 100s, 500s and 1000s.
Rx	**Aventyl Pulvules** (Lilly)		White/yellow. In 100s, 500s and UD 100s.
Rx	**Pamelor** (Sandoz)		(Pamelor 25 mg Sandoz). In 100s, 500s and UD 100s.
Rx	**Nortriptyline HCl** (Various, eg, Lemmon, Rugby)	**Capsules**: 50 mg	In 100s, 500s and 1000s.
Rx	**Pamelor** (Sandoz)		(Pamelor 50 mg Sandoz). In 100s and UD 100s.
Rx	**Nortriptyline HCl** (Various, eg, Lemmon, Rugby)	**Capsules**: 75 mg	In 100s, 500s and 1000s.
Rx	**Pamelor** (Sandoz)		(Pamelor 75 mg Sandoz). In 100s.
Rx	**Aventyl** (Lilly)	**Solution**: 10 mg/5 ml	In pt.
Rx	**Pamelor** (Sandoz)		4% alcohol, sorbitol. In pt.

IMIPRAMINE HCl

For complete prescribing information, refer to the Tricyclic Compounds group monograph.

Administration and Dosage:

Depression: Use parenteral administration for starting therapy only in patients unable or unwilling to use oral medication. Do not administer IV. Initially, up to 100 mg/day IM in divided doses. The oral form should replace the parenteral as soon as possible.

Hospitalized patients – Initially, 100 to 150 mg/day orally in divided doses; gradually increase to 200 mg/day, as required. If no response occurs after 2 weeks, increase to 250 to 300 mg/day. Administer the total daily dosage once daily at bedtime.

Outpatients – Initially, 75 mg/day, increased to 150 mg/day. Do not exceed 200 mg/day. Give once daily, preferably at bedtime.

Maintenance:50 to 150 mg/day.

Children – 1.5 mg/kg/day in 3 divided doses has been recommended, with increments of 1 to 1.5 mg/kg/day every 3 to 5 days. Maximum dose is 5 mg/kg/day.

Adolescent and geriatric patients – Initially, 30 to 40 mg/day orally; it is generally not necessary to exceed 100 mg/day.

Childhood enuresis (≥ 5 years of age): Initially, 25 mg/day 1 hour before bedtime. If no satisfactory response in 1 week, increase up to 50 mg/night if < 12 years of age; up to 75 mg/night if > 12 years of age. A dose > 75 mg/day does not enhance efficacy-and increases side effects. Do not exceed 2.5 mg/kg/day. Dosage of 10 to 25 mg/day was recommended, with increments of 10 to 25 mg/dose at 1 to 2 week intervals. In early night bedwetters, it may be more effective given earlier and in divided amounts (25 mg midafternoon and bedtime). Institute a drug-free period after an adequate trial with favorable response. Gradually tapering dosage may reduce tendency to relapse. Children who relapse after discontinuation do not always respond to a subsequent course.

Rx	**Imipramine HCl** (Various, eg, Biocraft, Geneva, Mutual, Par)	**Tablets:** 10 mg	In 50s, 100s, 250s, 500s, 1000s and UD 20s and 100s.
Rx	**Tofranil** (Geigy)		(Geigy 32). Coral. Sugar coated. Trianglular In 100s.
Rx	**Imipramine HCl** (Various, eg, Biocraft, Geneva, Mutual, Par)	**Tablets:** 25 mg	In 50s, 100s, 250s, 500s, 1000s and UD 20s and 100s.
Rx	**Tofranil** (Geigy)		(Geigy 140). Coral. Sugar coated. In 100s, 1000s and *Gy-Pak* 100s.
Rx	**Imipramine HCl** (Various, eg, Biocraft, Geneva, Mutual, Par)	**Tablets:** 50 mg	In 50s, 100s, 250s, 500s, 1000s and UD 20s and 100s.
Rx	**Tofranil** (Geigy)		(Geigy 136). Coral. Sugar coated. In 100s, 1000s and *Gy-Pak* 100s.
Rx	**Tofranil** (Geigy)	**Injection:** 25 mg/2 ml	In 2 ml amps.[1]

[1] With ascorbic acid, sodium bisulfite and anhydrous sodium sulfite.

IMIPRAMINE PAMOATE

For complete prescribing information, refer to the Tricyclic Compounds group monograph.

Rx	**Tofranil-PM** (Geigy)	**Capsules:**[2] 75 mg	(Geigy 20). Coral. In 30s, 100s and UD 100s.
		100 mg	(Geigy 40). Dark yellow/coral. In 30s and 100s.
		125 mg	(Geigy 45). Ivory/coral. In 30s and 100s.
		150 mg	(Geigy 22). Coral. In 30s and 100s.

[2] Strengths are expressed as imipramine HCl equivalent.

Tricyclic Compounds

DOXEPIN HCl

For complete prescribing information, refer to the Tricyclic Compounds group monograph.

Administration and Dosage:

Not recommended for use in children < 12 years old.

Mild to moderate anxiety or depression: Initially, 75 mg/day. Individualize dosage. Usual optimum dosage is 75 to 150 mg/day. Alternatively, the total daily dosage, up to 150 mg, may be given at bedtime.

Mild symptomatology or emotional symptoms accompanying organic disease: 25 to 50 mg/day is often effective.

More severe anxiety or depression: Higher doses (eg, 50 mg 3 times per day) may be required; if necessary, gradually increase to 300 mg/day. Additional effectiveness is rarely obtained by exceeding 300 mg/day.

Although optimal antidepressant response may not be evident for 2 to 3 weeks, antianxiety activity is rapidly apparent.

Dilute oral concentrate with ≈ 120 ml of water, milk or fruit juice just prior to administration. Do not prepare or store bulk dilutions.

Storage/Stability: Store at controlled room temperature of 15° to 30°C (59° to 86°F).

Rx	**Doxepin HCl** (Various, eg, Geneva, Major, Mylan, Par, Royce, Rugby)	**Capsules:** 10 mg	In 100s, 500s, 1000s and UD 100s.
Rx	**Sinequan** (Roerig)		In 100s and 1000s.
Rx	**Doxepin HCl** (Various, eg, Geneva, Major, Mylan, Par, Royce, Rugby)	**Capsules:** 25 mg	In 100s, 500s, 1000s and UD 100s.
Rx	**Sinequan** (Roerig)		In 100s, 1000s and 5000s.
Rx	**Doxepin HCl** (Various, eg, Geneva, Mylan, Par, Royce, Rugby)	**Capsules:** 50 mg	In 100s, 500s, 1000s and UD 100s.
Rx	**Sinequan** (Roerig)		In 100s, 1000s and 5000s.
Rx	**Doxepin HCl** (Various, eg, Geneva, Major, Mylan, Par, Rugby)	**Capsules:** 75 mg	In 100s, 500s, 1000s and UD 100s.
Rx	**Sinequan** (Roerig)		In 100s and 1000s.
Rx	**Doxepin HCl** (Various, eg, Geneva, Major, Mylan, Par, Rugby, Schein)	**Capsules:** 100 mg	In 100s, 500s, 1000s and UD 100s.
Rx	**Sinequan** (Roerig)		In 100s and 1000s.
Rx	**Doxepin HCl** (Various, eg, Major, Par, Rugby)	**Capsules:** 150 mg	In 50s, 100s, 500s and 1000s.
Rx	**Sinequan** (Roerig)		In 50s and 500s.
Rx	**Doxepin HCl** (Various, eg, Copley)	**Oral Concentrate:** 10 mg/ml	In 120 ml.
Rx	**Sinequan** (Roerig)		In 120 ml.

Tricyclic Compounds

TRIMIPRAMINE MALEATE

For complete prescribing information, refer to the Tricyclic Compounds group monograph.

Administration and Dosage:

Not recommended for use in children.

Adult outpatients: Initially, 75 mg/day in divided doses; increase to 150 mg/day. Do not exceed 200 mg/day. The total dosage requirement may be given at bedtime.

Adult hospitalized patients: Initially, 100 mg/day in divided doses, increase gradually in a few days to 200 mg/day depending upon individual response and tolerance. If improvement does not occur in 2 to 3 weeks, increase to a maximum dose of 250 to 300 mg/day.

Adolescent and elderly patients: Initially, 50 mg/day, with gradual increments up to 100 mg/day.

Maintenance medication may be required at the lowest dose that will maintain remission (range, 50 to 150 mg/day). Administer as a single bedtime dose. To minimize relapse, continue maintenance therapy for ≈ 3 months.

Storage/Stability: Store at room temperature, ≈ 25°C (77°F).

Rx	**Surmontil** (Wyeth-Ayerst)	**Capsules**: 25 mg	(Wyeth 4132). Blue/yellow. In 100s.
		50 mg	(Wyeth 4133). Blue/orange. In 100s.
		100 mg	(Wyeth 4158). Blue/white. In 100s.

AMOXAPINE

For complete prescribing information, refer to the Tricyclic Compounds group monograph.

Administration and Dosage:

Amoxapine is not recommended for patients < 16 years old.

Usual effective dosage is 200 to 300 mg/day. Three weeks is an adequate trial period providing dosage has reached 300 mg/day (or a lower level of tolerance) for at least 2 weeks. If no response is seen at 300 mg, increase dosage, depending upon tolerance, to 400 mg/day. Hospitalized patients refractory to antidepressant therapy and who have no history of convulsive seizures may have dosage cautiously increased up to 600 mg/day in divided doses.

Adults: Initially, 50 mg 2 or 3 times daily. Depending upon tolerance, increase dosage to 100 mg 2 or 3 times daily by the end of the first week. Initial dosage of 300 mg/day may cause sedation during the first few days of therapy. Increase above 300 mg/day only if 300 mg/day has been ineffective for at least 2 weeks. Once an effective dosage is established, the drug may be given in a single bedtime dose (not to exceed 300 mg). If the total daily dosage exceeds 300 mg, give in divided doses.

Elderly patients: Initially, 25 mg 2 or 3 times a day. If tolerated, dosage may be increased by the end of the first week to 50 mg 2 or 3 times a day. Although 100 to 150 mg/day may be adequate for many elderly patients, some may require higher dosage; carefully increase up to 300 mg/day.

Maintenance dosage is the lowest dose that will maintain remission. If symptoms reappear, increase dosage to the earlier level until they are controlled.

Storage/Stability: Store at controlled room temperature, 15° to 30°C (59° to 86°F).

Rx	**Amoxapine** (Various, eg, Geneva, Watson)	**Tablets**: 25 mg	In 30s, 100s and 1000s.
Rx	**Asendin** (Lederle)		(LL 25 A13). White, scored. Heptagonal. In 100s.
Rx	**Amoxapine** (Various, eg, Geneva, Watson)	**Tablets**: 50 mg	In 30s, 100s, 500s and 1000s.
Rx	**Asendin** (Lederle)		(LL 50 A15). Orange, scored. Heptagonal. In 100s, 500s and UD 100s.

Tricyclic Compounds

AMOXAPINE

Rx	**Amoxapine** (Various, eg, Geneva, Watson)	**Tablets:** 100 mg	In 30s, 100s and 1000s.
Rx	**Asendin** (Lederle)		(LL 100 A17). Blue, scored. Heptagonal. In 100s and UD 100s.
Rx	**Amoxapine** (Various, eg, Geneva, Watson)	**Tablets:** 150 mg	In 30s, 100s and 1000s.
Rx	**Asendin** (Lederle)		(LL 150 A18). Peach, scored. Heptagonal. In 30s.

DESIPRAMINE HCl

For complete prescribing information, refer to the Tricyclic Compounds group monograph.

Administration and Dosage:

Not recommended for use in children < 12 years of age.

Initial therapy may be given in divided doses or as a single daily dose. Maintenance therapy may be administered once daily. Continue a lower maintenance dosage for at least 2 months after a satisfactory response has been achieved.

Adults: 100 to 200 mg/day. In more severely ill patients, gradually increase to 300 mg/day, if necessary. Do not exceed 300 mg/day. Doses as high as 300 mg should generally be initiated in hospitals. Maintain continued therapy at the optimal dosage level during the active phase of depression. In cases of relapse because of premature drug withdrawal, a prompt response may be obtained by immediate resumption of treatment. Clinical symptoms of intolerance (eg, drowsiness, dizziness and postural hypotension) require dosage reduction.

Geriatrics and adolescents: 25 to 100 mg/day. Dosages > 150 mg/day are not recommended.

Storage/Stability: Store at room temperature, preferably below 30°C (86°F). Protect from excessive heat.

Rx	**Desipramine HCl** (Various, eg, Geneva)	**Tablets:** 10 mg	In 100s and 1000s.
Rx	**Norpramin**(Hoechst-Marion Roussel)		(68-7). Blue. Coated. In 100s.
Rx	**Desipramine HCl** (Various, eg, Geneva, Rugby, Sidmak)	**Tablets:** 25 mg	In 100s, 500s, 1000s and UD 100s.
Rx	**Norpramin**(Hoechst-Marion Roussel)		(Norpramin 25). Yellow. Coated. In 100s and UD 100s.
Rx	**Desipramine HCl** (Various, eg, Eon, Geneva, Rugby)	**Tablets:** 50 mg	In 30s, 100s, 500s, 1000s and UD 100s.
Rx	**Norpramin** (Hoechst-Marion Roussel)		(Norpramin 50). Green. Coated. In 100s and UD 100s.
Rx	**Desipramine HCl** (Various, eg, Eon, Geneva, Rugby)	**Tablets:** 75 mg	In 100s, 1000s and UD 100s.
Rx	**Norpramin** (Hoechst-Marion Roussel)		(Norpramin 75) Orange. Coated. In 100s.
Rx	**Desipramine HCl** (Various, eg, Geneva, Rugby)	**Tablets:** 100 mg	In 100s, 500s and 1000s.
Rx	**Norpramin** (Hoechst-Marion Roussel)		(Norpramin 100). Peach. Coated. In 100s.
Rx	**Desipramine HCl** (Various, eg, Geneva)	**Tablets:** 150 mg	In 50s and 1000s.
Rx	**Norpramin** (Hoechst-Marion Roussel)		(Norpramin 150). White. Coated. In 50s.

Tricyclic Compounds

PROTRIPTYLINE HCl

For complete prescribing information, refer to the Tricyclic Compounds group monograph.

Administration and Dosage:

Not recommended for use in children.

Adults: 15 to 40 mg/day divided into 3 or 4 doses. May increase to 60 mg/day. Dosages > 60 mg/day are not recommended. Make any increases in the morning dose.

Adolescent and elderly patients: Initially, 5 mg 3 times/day; increase gradually, if necessary. In elderly, monitor cardiovascular system closely if dose exceeds 20 mg/day.

Maintenance: When satisfactory improvement has been reached, reduce dosage to the smallest amount that will maintain relief of symptoms.

Rx	**Protriptyline HCl** (Sidmak)	**Tablets:** 5 mg	(SL 523). Orange. Oblong. Film coated. In 100s and 1000s.
		10 mg	(SL 524). Yellow. Oblong. Film coated. In 100s and 1000s.
Rx	**Vivactil** (Merck)	**Tablets:** 5 mg	(MSD 26). Orange. Oval. Film coated. In 100s.
		10 mg	(MSD 47). Yellow. Oval. Film coated. In 100s and UD 100s.

CLOMIPRAMINE HCl

For complete prescribing information, refer to the Tricyclic Compounds group monograph.

Indications:

Obsessive-compulsive disorder (OCD): Treatment of obsessions and compulsions in patients with OCD. The obsessions or compulsions must cause marked distress, be time-consuming or significantly interfere with social or occupational functioning, in order to meet the DSM-III-R (circa 1989) diagnosis of OCD.

Administration and Dosage:

Initial:

Adults – Initiate at 25 mg daily and gradually increase, as tolerated, to ≈ 100 mg during the first 2 weeks. Administer in divided doses with meals to reduce GI side effects. Thereafter, the dosage may be increased gradually over the next several weeks to a maximum of 250 mg/day. After titration, the total daily dose may be given once daily at bedtime to minimize daytime sedation.

Children and adolescents – Initiate at 25 mg daily and gradually increase during the first 2 weeks, as tolerated, to a daily maximum of 3 mg/kg or 100 mg, whichever is smaller. Administer in divided doses with meals to reduce GI side effects. Thereafter, the dosage may be increased to a daily maximum of 3 mg/kg or 200 mg, whichever is smaller. After titration, the total daily dose may be given once daily at bedtime to minimize daytime sedation.

Maintenance:

Adults, adolescents and children – The efficacy of clomipramine after 10 weeks has not been documented in controlled trials. However, patients have continued therapy in double-blind studies for up to 1 year without loss of benefit. Adjust the dosage to maintain the patient on the lowest effective dosage and periodically reassess the patient to determine the need for treatment.

Storage/Stability: Do not store above 30°C (86°F). Protect from moisture.

Rx	**Anafranil** (Ciba)	**Capsules:** 25 mg	(Anafranil 25 mg). Ivory and melon yellow. In 100s and UD 100s.
		50 mg	(Anafranil 50 mg). Ivory and aqua blue. In 100s and UD 100s.
		75 mg	(Anafranil 75 mg). Ivory and yellow. In 100s and UD 100s.

TETRACYCLIC COMPOUNDS

Actions:

Pharmacology: The mechanism of action is unknown. Tetracyclics enhance central noradrenergic and serotonergic activity. They act as antagonists at central presynaptic α_2 adrenergic inhibitory autoreceptors and heteroreceptors, an action that is postulated to result in an increase in central noradrenergic and serotonergic activity.

Mirtazapine is a potent antagonist of 5-HT_2 and 5-HT_3 receptors. It does not have significant affinity for the 5-HT_{1A} and 5-HT_{1B} receptors. It is a potent antagonist of histamine (H_1) receptors, a property that may explain its prominent sedative effects. It is also a moderate antagonist at muscarinic receptors, a property that may explain the relatively low incidence of anticholinergic side effects.

Pharmacokinetics:

Maprotiline – The mean time to peak is 12 hours. The elimination half-life averages 61 hours. Steady-state levels measured prior to the morning dose on a one-dosage regimen demonstrated an average minimum concentration of 238 ng/ml and 95% confidence limits of 181 to 295 ng/ml.

Mirtazapine is rapidly and completely absorbed following oral administration and has a half-life of ≈ 20 to 40 hours. Peak plasma concentrations are reached within ≈ 2 hours following an oral dose. The presence of food in the stomach has a minimal effect on both the rate and extent of absorption and does not require a dosage adjustment. Steady-state plasma levels of mirtazapine are attained within 5 days. Mirtazapine is ≈ 85% bound to plasma protein.

Metabolism/Excretion: Mirtazapine is extensively metabolized after oral administration. Major pathways of biotransformation are demethylation and hydroxylation followed by glucuronide conjugation. In vitro, cytochrome enzymes 2D6 and 1A2 are involved in the formation of the 8-hydroxy metabolite of mirtazapine, whereas cytochrome 3A is considered to be responsible for the formation of the N–desmethyl and N-oxide metabolites. Mirtazapine has an absolute bioavailability of ≈ 50%. It is eliminated predominantly via urine (75%) with 15% in feces. Several unconjugated metabolites possess pharmacological activity but are present in the plasma at very low levels. The (-) enantiomer has an elimination half-life that is approximately twice as long as the (+) enantiomer and, therefore, achieves plasma levels that are ≈ 3 times as high.

Plasma levels are linearly related to dose over a dose range of 15 to 80 mg. The mean elimination half-life of mirtazapine after oral administration ranges from ≈ 20 to 40 hours, with females of all ages exhibiting significantly longer elimination half-lives than males (37 hours vs 26 hours).

Indications:

Depression: Treatment of depression.

Contraindications:

Hypersensitivity to maprotiline or mirtazapine; coadministration with monamine oxidase inhibitors (MAOIs).

Maprotiline: Known or suspected seizure disorders.

Warnings:

Anticholinergic properties: Maprotiline should be administered with caution in patients with increased intraocular pressure, history of urinary retention or history of narrow-angle glaucoma because of the drug's anticholinergic properties.

CNS: Maprotiline may enhance the response to alcohol, barbiturates and other CNS depressants, requiring appropriate caution during administration.

Monamine oxidase inhibitors (MAOIs): Do not give tetracyclics with MAOIs. Allow a minimum of 14 days to elapse after discontinuation of MAOIs before starting a tetracyclic.

Seizures are rare. The risk of seizues may be increased when tetracyclics are taken concomitantly with phenothiazines, when the dosage of benzodiazepines is rapidly tapered in patients receiving tetracyclics or when the recommended dosage of the tetracyclic is exceeded. While a cause and effect relationship has not been established, the risk of seizures in patients treated with tetracyclics may be reduced by:

- Initiating therapy at a low dosage.
- Maintaining the initial dosage for 2 weeks before raising it gradually in small increments as necessary.
- Keeping the dosage at the minimally effective level during maintenance therapy.

TETRACYCLIC COMPOUNDS

Cardiovascular: Use with caution in patients with a history of myocardial infarction and angina because of the possibilty of conduction defects, arrhythmia, myocardial infarction, strokes and tachycardia. Use with caution in patients predisposed to hypotension.

Electroshock therapy: Avoid concurrent administration of maprotiline with electroshock therapy because of the lack of experience in this area.

Agranulocytosis: In clinical trials, two patients treated with mirtazapine developed agranulocytosis (absolute neutrophil count [ANC] < 500/mm^3 with associated signs and symptoms, eg, fever, infection) and a third patient developed severe neutropenia (ANC < 500/mm^3 without any associated symptoms). For these three patients, onset of severe neutropenia was detected on days 61, 9 and 14 of treatment, respectively. All three patients recovered after mirtazapine was stopped. If a patient develops a sore throat, fever, stomatitis or other signs of infection, along with a low WBC count, discontinue treatment with the tetracyclic and monitor the patient closely.

Hepatic function impairment: Following a single 15 mg dose, the oral clearance decreased by ≈ 30% in hepatically impaired patients. Use mirtazapine with caution in patients with impaired hepatic function.

Renal function impairment: Following a single 15 mg dose, patients with moderate (glomerular filtration rate [GFR] = 11 to 39 ml/min/1.73m^2) and severe (GFR < 10 ml/min/1.73m^2) renal impairment had reductions in mean oral clearance of ≈ 30% and 50%, respectively, compared with healthy subjects.

Carcinogenesis: There was an increased incidence of hepatocellular adenoma and carcinoma in male mice at high doses and an increase in thyroid follicular adenoma/cystandenoma and carcinoma in male rats at high doses. Hepatocellular adenoma increased in female rats with mid and high doses with mirtazapine. Maprotiline did not show any drug or dose related occurrence of carcinogenesis in rats.

Elderly: Following administration of 20 mg/day for 7 days to subjects 25 to 74 years of age, oral clearance was reduced in the elderly compared with the younger subjects. The differences were most striking in males, with a 40% lower clearance in elderly males compared with younger males, while the clearance in elderly females was only 10% lower compared with younger females. Caution is indicated in administering mirtazapine to elderly patients.

Pregnancy:

Maprotiline – Category B. There are no adequate and well controlled studies in pregnant women. Use this drug during pregnancy only if clearly needed.

Mirtazapine – Category C. Use during pregnancy only if clearly needed.

Lactation:

Maprotiline is excreted in breast milk. At steady state, the concentration in milk corresponds closely to the concentrations in whole blood. Exercise caution when maprotiline is administered to a nursing woman.

Mirtazapine – It is not known if mirtazapine is excreted in breast milk. Use caution when mirtazapine is administered to nursing women.

Children: Safety and efficacy in children have not been established.

Precautions:

Somnolence was reported in 54% of patients treated with mirtazapine. Somnolence resulted in discontinuation of treatment for 10.4% of treated patients. It is unclear whether or not tolerance deveolps to the somnolent effects. Because mirtazapine has potentially significant effects on performance, caution patients about engaging in activities requiring alertness until they have been able to assess the drug's effect on their psychomotor performance.

Dizziness was reported in 7% of patients treated with mirtazapine. It is unclear whether or not tolerance develops to the dizziness.

Increased appetite/Weight gain: Appetite increase was reported in 17% of patients treated with mirtazapine. In some trials, weight gain of ≥ 7% of body weight was reported in 7.5% of patients treated. Of patients receiving mirtazapine, 8% discontinued because of weight gain.

Cholesterol/Triglycerides: Nonfasting cholesterol increases to ≥ 20% above the upper limits of normal were observed in 15% of patients treated with mirtazapine. In some cases, nonfasting triglyceride increases to ≥ 500 mg/dl were observed in 6% of patients treated with mirtazapine, compared with 3% for placebo and 3% for amitriptyline.

TETRACYCLIC COMPOUNDS

Mania/Hypomania occured in ≈ 0.2% of patients receiving mirtazapine. Although the incidence of mania/hypomania was very low during treatent with mirtazapine, use carefully in patients with a history of mania/hypomania.

Suicidal ideation is inherent in depression and may persist until significant remission occurs. As with any patient receiving antidepressants, closely supervise high-risk patients during initial drug therapy. Hypomanic or manic episodes have been known to occur rarely.

Transaminase elevations: Clinically significant ALT elevations (≥ 3 times the upper limit of the normal range) were observed in 2% of patients exposed to mirtazapine. Most of these patients with ALT increases did not develop signs or symptoms associated with compromised liver function. While some patients were discontinued for the ALT increases, in other cases, the enzyme levels returned to normal despite continued mirtazapine treatment.

Orthostatic hypotension: Mirtazapine was associated with significant orthostatic hypotension in clinical trials with healthy volunteers. Orthostatic hypotension was infrequently observed in clinical trials with depressed patients.

Drug Interactions:

The metabolism and pharmacokinetics of tetracyclics may be affected by the induction or inhibition of drug-metabolizing enzymes.

Tetracyclic Drug Interactions

Precipitant drug	Object drug*		Description
Maprotiline	Anticholinergics	⬆	Additive atropine-like effects may occur.
Maprotiline	Guanethidine	⬇	Maprotiline may block the pharmacologic effects of guanethidine or similar drugs.
Maprotiline	Phenothiazines	⬆	The risk of seizures may be increased with concomitant use (see Warnings).
Thyroid hormones	Maprotiline	⬆	Use caution when administering maprotiline to hyperthyroid patients or those on thyroid medication because of the possibility of enhanced potential for cardiovascular toxicity of maprotiline.
Mirtazapine	Alcohol	⬆	Concomitant administration has a minimal effect on plasma levels of mirtazapine. However, the impairment of cognitive and motor skills produced by mirtazapine are additive with those produced by alcohol.
Mirtazapine	Diazepam	⬆	Concomitant administration has a minimal effect on plasma levels of mirtazapine. However, the impairment of motor skills produced by mirtazapine is additive with those caused by diazepam.

⬆ = Object drug increased. ⬇ = Object drug decreased.

TETRACYCLIC COMPOUNDS

Adverse Reactions:

Adverse Reactions: Maprotiline vs Mirtazapine (%)

Adverse reactions	Maprotiline	Mirtazapine
Body as a whole		
Asthenia	-	8
Back pain	-	2
Flu syndrome	-	5
GI		
Dry mouth	22	25
Constipation	8	13
Increased appetite	-	17
Nausea	2	1.5
Vomiting	rare	1
Metabolic/Nutritional		
Edema	rare	1
Peripheral edema	-	2
Weight gain	rare	12
Weight loss	rare	< 1
Musculoskeletal		
Myalgia		2
Cardiovascular		
Hypertension	rare	1
Hypotension	rare	< 1
CNS		
Abnormal dreams	rare	4
Agitation	2	1
Anxiety	3	1
Ataxia	rare	< 1
Confusion	rare	2
Dizziness	8	7
Drowsiness	18	-
Extrapyramidal symptoms	rare	< 1
Hallucinations	rare	< 1
Headache	4	-
Insomnia	2	-
Mania	rare	< 1
Nervousness	6	-
Somnolence	-	54
Abnormal thinking		3
Tremor	3	2
Weakness and fatigue	4	-
Dermatologic		
Alopecia	rare	< 1
Pruritus	rare	1
Rash	rare	1
Respiratory		
Dyspnea		1
GU		
Urinary frequency	rare	2
Miscellaneous		
Altered liver function	rare	< 1
Blurred vision	4	

Maprotiline:

Cardiovascular – Tachycardia, palpitation, arrhythmia, heart block, syncope (rare).

CNS – Disorientation, delusions, restlessness, hypomania, exacerbation of psychosis, decrease in memory, feelings of unreality, numbness, tingling, motor hyperactivity, akathisia, seizures, EEG alterations, tinnitus, dysarthria (rare).

Dermatologic – Petechiae, photosensitization, drug fever (rare).

Endocrine – Increased or decreased libido, impotence, elevation or depression of blood sugar levels (rare).

GI – Accomodation disturbances, epigastric distress, diarrhea, bitter taste, abdominal cramps, dysphagia (rare).

Miscellaneous – Jaundice, mydriasis, urinary retention and delayed micturition, excessive perspiration, flushing, increased salivation, nasal congestion (rare).

Mirtazapine:

Body as a whole – Malaise, abdominal pain, acute abdominal syndrome (1%); chills, fever, face edema, ulcer, photosensitivity reaction, neck rigidity, neck pain, enlarged abdomen (< 1%); cellulitis, substernal chest pain substernal (rare).

Cardiovascular – Vasodilatation (1%); angina pectoris, myocardial infarction, bradycardia, ventricular extrasystoles, syncope, migraine (< 1%); atrial arrhythmia, bigeminy, vascular headache, pulmonary embolus, cerebral ischemia, cardiomegaly, phlebitis, left heart failure (rare).

CNS – Hypesthesia, apathy, depression, hypokinesia, vertigo, twitching, amnesia, hyperkinesia, paresthesia (1%); delirium, delusions, depersonalization, dyskinesia, increased libido, abnormal coordination, dysarthria, neurosis, dystonia, hostility, increased reflexes, emotional lability, euphoria, paranoid reaction (< 1%); aphasia, nystagmus akathisia, stupor, dementia, diplopia, drug dependence, paralysis, grand mal convulsion, hypotonia, myoclonus, psychotic depression, withdrawal syndrome (rare).

Dermatologic – Acne exfoliative dermatitis, dry skin, herpes simplex (< 1%); urticaria, herpes zoster, skin hypertrophy, seborrhea, skin ulcer (rare).

Endocrine – Goiter, hypothyroidism (rare).

GI – Anorexia (1%); eructation, glossitis, cholecystitis, gum hemorrhage, stomatitis, colitis (< 1%); tongue discoloration, ulcerative stomatitis, salivary gland enlargement, increased salivation, intestinal obstruction, pancreatitis, aphthous stomatitis, cirrhosis of the liver, gastritis, gastroenteritis, oral moniliasis, tongue edema (rare).

GU – Urinary tract infection (1%); kidney calculus, cystitis, dysuria, urinary incontinence, urinary retention, vaginitis, hematuria, breast pain, amenorrhea, dysmenorrhea, leukorrhea, impotence (< 1%); polyuria, urethritis, metrorrhagia, menorrhagia, abnormal ejaculation, breast engorgement, breast enlargement, urinary urgency (rare).

Hematologic/Lymphatic – Lymphadenopathy, leukopenia, petechiae, anemia, thrombocytopenia, lymphocytosis, pancytopenia (rare).

Metabolic/Nutritional – Thirst (1%); dehydration (< 1%); gout, AST increased, healing abnormal, acid phosphatase increased, ALT increased, diabetes mellitus (rare).

Musculoskeletal – Myasthenia, arthralgia (1%); arthritis, tenosynovitis (< 1%); pathological fracture, osteoporosis fracture, bone pain, myositis, tendon rupture, arthrosis, bursitis (rare).

Respiratory – Cough increased, sinusitis (1%); epistaxis, bronchitis, asthma, pneumonia (< 1%); asphyxia, laryngitis, pneumothorax, hiccough (rare).

Special Senses – Eye pain, abnormality of accommodation, conjunctivitis, deafness, keratoconjunctivitis, lacrimation disorder, glaucoma, hyperacusis, ear pain (< 1%); blepharitis, partial transitory deafness, otitis media, taste loss, parosmia (rare).

Overdosage:

Maprotiline:

Symptoms – Critical manifestations of overdose include cardiac dysrhythmias, severe hypotension, convulsions and CNS depression, including coma. Changes in the ECG, particularly in QRS axis or width, are clinically significant indicators of toxicity. Other clinical manifestations include drowsiness, tachycardia, ataxia, vomiting, cyanosis, shock, restlessness, agitation, hyperpyrexia, muscle rigidity, athetoid movements and mydriasis. Because CHF has been seen with overdosages of tricyclic antidepressants, consider CHF with maprotiline overdosage as well.

Management – Obtain an ECG and immediately initiate cardiac monitoring. Protect the patient's airway, establish an IV line and initiate gastric decontamination. A minimum of 8 hours of observation with cardiac monitoring and observation for signs of CNS or respiratory depression, hypotension, cardiac dysrhythmias or conduction blocks and seizures is necessary. If signs of toxicity occur at any time during this period, extended monitoring is required. There are case reports of patients succumbing to fatal dysrhythmias late after tricyclic overdose; these patients had clinical evidence of significant poisoning prior to death and most received inadequate GI decontamination. Monitoring of plasma drug levels should not guide management of the patient.

GI decontamination: All patients suspected of overdose should receive GI decontamination. This should include large volume gastric lavage followed by activated charcoal. Emesis is contraindicated.

Cardiovascular: A maximal limb-lead QRS duration of ≥ 0.10 seconds may be the best indication of the severity of the overdose. Serum alkalinization, to a pH of 7.45 to 7.55 using IV sodium bicarbonate and hyperventilation (as needed), should be instituted for patients with dysrhythmias or QRS widening. A pH > 7.60 or a Pco_2 < 20 mmHg is undesirable. Dysrhythmias unresponsive to sodium bicarbonate therapy/hyperventilation may respond to lidocaine, bretylium or phenytoin. Type 1A and 1C antiarrhythmics are generally contraindicated (eg, quinidine, disopyramide, procainamide).

In rare instances, hemoperfusion may be beneficial in acute refractory cardiovascular instability in patients with acute toxicity. However, hemodialysis, peritoneal dialysis, exchange transfusions and forced diuresis generally have been ineffective.

CNS: In patients with CNS depression, early intubation is advised because of the potential for abrupt deterioration. Control seizures with benzodiazepines, or if these are ineffective, other anticonvulsants (eg, phenobarbital, phenytoin). Physostigmine is not recommended except to treat life-threatening symptoms that have been unresponsive to other therapies, and then only in consultation with a poison control center.

Mirtazapine: There is very limited experience with mirtazapine overdose. In premarketing clinical studies, there were eight reports of mirtazapine overdose alone or in combination with other pharmacological agents. The only drug-overdose death reported while taking mirtazapine was in combination with amitriptyline and chlorprothixene. All other premarketing overdose cases resulted in full recovery. Signs and symptoms reported in association with overdose included disorientation, drowsiness,

TETRACYCLIC COMPOUNDS

impaired memory and tachycardia. There were no reports of ECG abnormalities, coma or convulsions following overdose with mirtazapine alone.

Patient Information:

Warn patients who are to receive tetracyclics about the risk of developing agranulocytosis. Advise patients to contact their physician if they experience any indication of infection such as fever, chills, sore throat, mucous membrane ulceration or other possible signs of infection. Pay particular attention to any flu-like complaints or other symptoms that might suggest infection.

Tetracyclics may impair judgement, thinking and, particularly, motor skills, because of their prominent sedative effect. The drowsiness associated with mirtazapine use may impair a patient's ability to drive, use machines or perform tasks that require alertness, coordination or physical dexterity. Thus, caution patients about engaging in hazardous activities until they are reasonably certain that tetracyclic therapy does not adversely affect their ability to engage in such activities.

Advise patients to inform their physician if they are taking, or intend to take, any prescription or *otc* drugs because there is a potential for tetracyclics to interact with other drugs.

The impairment of cognitive and motor skills produced by tetracyclics has been shown to be additive with those produced by alcohol. Accordingly, advise patients to avoid alcohol while taking tetracyclics.

Advise patients to notify their physician if they become pregnant or intend to become pregnant or are breast-feeding during tetracyclic therapy.

Tetracyclic Compounds

MAPROTILINE HCl

For complete prescribing information, refer to the Tetracyclic Compounds group monograph.

Indications:

Depression: For the treatment of depressive illness in patients with depressive neurosis (dysthymic disorder) and manic-depressive illness, depressed type (major depressive disorder). Also effective for the relief of anxiety associated with depression.

Administration and Dosage:

May be given as a single daily dose or in divided doses. Therapeutic effects are sometimes seen within 3 to 7 days, although 2 to 3 weeks are usually necessary.

Initial adult dosage: An initial dose of 75 mg/day is suggested for outpatients with mild to moderate depression. In some patients, especially the elderly, an initial dose of 25 mg/day may be used. Because of the long half-life of maprotiline, maintain initial dosage for 2 weeks. The dosage may then be increased gradually in 25 mg increments, as required and tolerated. Most patients respond to a dose of 150 mg/day, but doses as high as 225 mg/day may be required.

Severe depression: Give hospitalized patients an initial daily dose of 100 to 150 mg, which may be gradually increased, as required and tolerated. Most hospitalized patients with moderate to severe depression respond to a daily dosage of 150 mg, although dosages as high as 225 mg may be required. Do not exceed 225 mg/day.

Maintenance: Keep dosage during prolonged maintenance therapy at the lowest effective level. Dosage may be reduced to 75 to 150 mg/day with adjustment depending on therapeutic response.

Elderly: In general, lower doses are recommended for patients > 60 years of age. Doses of 50 to 75 mg/day are satisfactory as maintenance therapy for elderly patients who do not tolerate higher amounts.

Storage/Stability: Do not store above 30°C (86°F).

Rx	**Maprotiline HCl** (Various, eg, Major, Rugby, URL, Watson)	**Tablets**: 25 mg	In 30s, 100s and 500s.
Rx	**Ludiomil** (Ciba)		(Ciba 110). Dark orange, scored. Oval. Coated. In 100s.
Rx	**Maprotiline HCl** (Various, eg, Major, Rugby, URL, Watson)	**Tablets**: 50 mg	In 30s, 100s and 500s.
Rx	**Ludiomil** (Ciba)		(Ciba 26). Dark orange, scored. Coated. In 100s.
Rx	**Maprotiline HCl** (Various, eg, Major, URL, Watson)	**Tablets**: 75 mg	In 30s, 100s and 500s.
Rx	**Ludiomil** (Ciba)		(Ciba 135). White, scored. Oval. Coated. In 100s.

Tetracyclic Compounds

MIRTAZAPINE

For complete prescribing information, refer to the Tetracyclic Compounds group monograph.

Indications:

Depression: Treatment of depression.

Administration and Dosage:

Initial treatment: The recommended starting dose for mirtazapine is 15 mg/day administered in a single dose, preferably in the evening prior to sleep.

Maintenance/Extended treatment: Treatment for acute episodes of depression should continue for 6 months.

Switching to or from a monoamine oxidase inhibitor (MAOI): At least 14 days should elapse between discontinuation of an MAOI and initiation of therapy with mirtazapine. In addition, allow at least 14 days after stopping mirtazapine before starting an MAOI.

Rx	**Remeron** (Organon)	**Tablets:** 15 mg	(Organon TZ3). Yellow, scored. Oval. Coated. In 30s and UD 100s.
		30 mg	(Organon TZ5). Red-brown, scored. Oval. Coated. In 30s and UD 100s.

TRAZODONE HCl

Actions:

Pharmacology: The mechanism of antidepressant action in humans is not fully understood. Trazodone is not a monoamine oxidase inhibitor and, unlike amphetamine-type drugs, does not stimulate the CNS. In animals, it selectively inhibits serotonin uptake by brain synaptosomes and potentiates the behavioral changes induced by the serotonin precursor, 5-hydroxytryptophan.

Cardiac conduction effects in the anesthetized dog are qualitatively dissimilar and quantitatively less pronounced than those seen with tricyclic antidepressants.

Pharmacokinetics:

Absorption/Distribution – Trazodone is well absorbed after oral administration without selective localization in any tissue. When taken shortly after ingestion of food, there may be a slight increase in the amount of drug absorbed, a decrease in maximum concentration and a lengthening in the time to maximum concentration. Peak plasma levels occur in approximately 1 hour when taken on an empty stomach or in 2 hours when taken with food.

Metabolism/Excretion – Trazodone is extensively metabolized in the liver; < 1% is excreted unchanged in the urine and feces. Elimination is biphasic, with a half-life of 3 to 6 hours (mean, 4.4) and 5 to 9 hours (mean, 7 to 8), respectively, and is unaffected by food. Since the clearance of trazodone from the body is sufficiently variable, in some subjects it may accumulate in the plasma. The clearance of trazodone may be reduced in elderly male patients.

Onset of action: For those who responded to trazodone, one-third of the inpatients and one-half of the outpatients had a significant therapeutic response by the end of the first week of treatment. Three-fourths of all responders demonstrated a significant therapeutic effect by the end of the second week. One-fourth of responders required 2 to 4 weeks for a significant therapeutic response.

Indications:

Treatment of depression.

Unlabeled uses: Trazodone 50 mg twice daily and tryptophan 500 mg twice daily have been successful in the treatment of aggressive behavior. Dose adjustments were made until therapeutic response was achieved or unacceptable adverse effects developed. A dosage of 300 mg/day may also be useful for treatment of patients with panic disorder or agoraphobia with panic attacks.

Trazodone has also been used to treat cocaine withdrawal.

Contraindications:

Hypersensitivity to trazodone.

Warnings:

Preexisting cardiac disease: Not recommended for use during the initial recovery phase of myocardial infarction. Clinical studies and post-marketing reports in patients with preexisting cardiac disease indicate that trazodone may be arrhythmogenic in some patients. Arrhythmias identified include isolated PVCs, ventricular couplets and short episodes (3 to 4 beats) of ventricular tachycardia. Closely monitor patients with preexisting cardiac disease, particularly for cardiac arrhythmias.

Priapism has been reported in patients receiving trazodone. Patients with prolonged or inappropriate penile erection should discontinue use immediately and consult a physician. Injection of norepinephrine, epinephrine or dopamine may be successful in treating priapism. In approximately one-third of the cases reported, surgical intervention was required and, in a portion of these cases, permanent impairment of erectile function or impotence resulted.

Pregnancy: Category C. Trazodone has caused increased fetal resorption and congenital anomalies in the rat and rabbit fetus when given at approximately 15 to 50 times the maximum human dose. There are no adequate and well controlled studies in pregnant women. Use during pregnancy only if the potential benefit justifies the potential risk to the fetus.

Lactation: Trazodone and its metabolites have been found in the milk of rats, suggesting that the drug may be excreted in breast milk. Exercise caution when administering to a nursing mother.

Children: Safety and efficacy for use in children < 18 years of age are not established.

Precautions:

Suicide: The possibility of suicide in seriously depressed patients is inherent in the illness and may persist until significant remission occurs. Therefore, write prescriptions for the smallest number of tablets consistent with good patient management.

Hypotension, including orthostatic hypotension and syncope, has occurred.

Electroconvulsive therapy: Avoid concurrent administration with electroconvulsive therapy because of the absence of experience in this area.

TRAZODONE HCl

Potentially hazardous tasks: May produce drowsiness, dizziness or blurred vision; patients should observe caution while driving or performing other tasks requiring alertness, coordination or dexterity.

Laboratory tests: Occasional low white blood cell and neutrophil counts have been noted, but were not considered clinically significant; however, discontinue the drug in any patient whose white blood cell count or absolute neutrophil count falls below normal levels. White blood cell and differential counts are recommended for patients who develop fever and sore throat (or other signs of infection) during therapy.

Drug Interactions:

Alcohol, barbiturates and other CNS depressants: Trazodone may enhance the CNS depressant response to these agents.

Digoxin serum levels were increased in a patient receiving concurrent trazodone.

Monoamine oxidase inhibitors: It is not known whether interactions will occur. If MAOIs are discontinued shortly before, or are to be given concomitantly with trazodone, initiate therapy cautiously.

Phenytoin serum levels were increased in a patient receiving trazodone.

Warfarin: In a single case report, trazodone coadministration with warfarin decreased prothrombin time and partial thromboplastin time. The hypoprothrombinemic effect of warfarin may be decreased.

Adverse Reactions:

Hypersensitivity: Skin conditions, edema (> 1%); allergic reaction; purpuric and maculopapular eruptions; rash; pruritis; urticaria.

Renal: Hematuria; delayed urine flow; increased urinary frequency; urinary incontinence/retention.

Miscellaneous: Decreased appetite, sweating, clamminess, head (full/heavy), weight gain or loss, malaise, nasal/sinus congestion (> 1%); increased appetite; apnea; alopecia; edema; leukonychia; unexplained death.

Ophthalmic: Tinnitus, blurred vision, red eyes (tired/itching), (> 1%); diplopia.

Cardiovascular: Hypertension, hypotension, shortness of breath, syncope, tachycardia, palpitations (> 1%); chest pain; myocardial infarction; ventricular ectopic activity including ventricular tachycardia; vasodilation; conduction block; orthostatic hypotension; bradycardia; cardiac arrest; atrial fibrillation; arrhythmias. Occasional sinus bradycardia has occurred in long-term studies (see Warnings).

CNS: Anger, hostility, nightmares/vivid dreams, confusion, disorientation, decreased concentration, dizziness, lightheadedness, drowsiness, excitement, fatigue, headache, insomnia, impaired memory, nervousness, incoordination, paresthesia, tremors (> 1%); hallucinations; psychosis; vertigo; hypomania; mania; impaired speech; akathisia; numbness; delusions; agitation; weakness; grand mal seizures; extrapyramidal symptoms; tardive dyskinesia; stupor.

Endocrine: Decreased libido (> 1%); increased libido; impotence; priapism; retrograde ejaculation; early menses; missed periods; breast enlargement and engorgement; lactation.

GI: Abdominal/gastric disorder, bad taste in mouth, dry mouth, nausea, vomiting, diarrhea, constipation (> 1%); flatulence; hypersalivation; inappropriate ADH syndrome.

Hematologic: Anemia; hemolytic anemia; methemoglobinemia.

Hepatic: Liver enzyme alterations; intrahepatic cholestasis; hyperbilirubinemia; jaundice.

Musculoskeletal: Musculoskeletal aches and pains (> 1%); muscle twitches; ataxia.

Overdosage:

Symptoms: Death from overdose has occurred in patients ingesting trazodone and other drugs concurrently (ie, alcohol, alcohol plus chloral hydrate plus diazepam, amobarbital, chlordiazepoxide or meprobamate).

The most severe reactions reported with overdose of trazodone alone have been priapism, respiratory arrest, seizures and ECG changes. Overdosage may cause an increase in incidence or severity of any of the reported adverse reactions.

Clinical manifestations of overdose may include any of those listed in Adverse Reactions, with drowsiness and vomiting reported most frequently.

Treatment: There is no specific antidote. Treatment should be symptomatic and supportive for hypotension or excessive sedation. Patients suspected of having taken an overdose should have their stomachs emptied by gastric lavage. Forced diuresis may be useful in elimination of the drug. Refer to General Management of Acute Overdosage.

TRAZODONE HCl

Patient Information:

Take with food.

May produce drowsiness or dizziness; patients should observe caution while driving or performing other tasks requiring alertness, coordination or dexterity.

Notify physician of dizziness, lightheadedness, fainting or blood in urine.

Male patients with prolonged, inappropriate and painful erections should immediately discontinue the drug and consult their physician.

Medication may cause dry mouth, irregular heartbeat, shortness of breath, nausea and vomiting; notify physician if these become pronounced.

Avoid alcohol and other depressant drugs.

Administration and Dosage:

Initiate dosage at a low level and increase gradually. Drowsiness may require the administration of a major portion of the daily dose at bedtime or a reduced dosage. Take shortly after a meal or light snack. Symptomatic relief may be seen during the first week, with optimal effects typically evident within 2 weeks. Approximately 25% of those who respond to therapy require 2 to 4 weeks of drug administration.

Adults: An initial dose is 150 mg/day. This may be increased by 50 mg/day every 3 to 4 days. The maximum dose for outpatients usually should not exceed 400 mg/day in divided doses. Inpatients or more severely depressed subjects may be given up to, but not in excess of, 600 mg/day in divided doses.

Maintenance: Keep dosage at the lowest effective level. Once an adequate response has been achieved, dosage may be gradually reduced with subsequent adjustment depending on response.

Rx	**Trazodone HCl** (Various, eg, Balan, Elkins-Sinn, Geneva, Goldline, Lederle, Moore, Rugby, Schein, Squibb Mark, Warner-C)	**Tablets:** 50 mg	In 30s, 100s, 250s, 500s, 1000s and UD 100s.
Rx	**Desyrel** (Mead Johnson Pharm.)		(MJ 775 Desyrel). Orange, scored. Film coated. In 100s, 1000s and UD 100s.
Rx	**Trazodone HCl** (Various, eg, Balan, Elkins-Sinn, Geneva, Goldline, Lederle, Moore, Rugby, Schein, Squibb Mark, Warner-C)	**Tablets:** 100 mg	In 30s, 100s, 250s, 500s, 1000s and UD 100s.
Rx	**Desyrel** (Mead Johnson Pharm.)		(MJ 776 Desyrel). White, scored. Film coated. In 100s, 1000s and UD 100s.
Rx	**Trazodone HCl** (Various, eg, Balan, Bioline, Dixon-Shane, Goldline, Lederle, Major, Moore, Rugby, Schein, Warner-C)	**Tablets:** 150 mg	In 30s, 100s, 250s, 500s and 1000s.
Rx	**Desyrel Dividose** (Mead Johnson Pharm.)		(MJ 778 50). Orange, triple scored. In 100s and 500s.
Rx	**Desyrel Dividose** (Mead Johnson Pharm.)	**Tablets:** 300 mg	(MJ 796 100). Yellow. Triple scored. In 100s.

BUPROPION HCl

Actions:

Pharmacology: Bupropion, an antidepressant of the aminoketone class, is chemically unrelated to other available antidepressant agents. Its structure closely resembles that of diethylpropion; it is related to phenylethylamines. The neurochemical mechanism of the antidepressant effect of bupropion is not known. Bupropion does not inhibit monoamine oxidase. Compared to classical tricyclic antidepressants, it is a weak blocker of the neuronal uptake of serotonin and norepinephrine; it also inhibits the neuronal reuptake of dopamine to some extent.

Bupropion produces the following dose-related CNS stimulant effects in animals: Increased locomotor activity, increased rates of responding in various schedule-controlled operant behavior tasks, and induction of mild stereotyped behavior.

Pharmacokinetics:

Absorption/Distribution – Following oral administration, peak plasma concentrations are usually achieved within 2 hours, followed by a biphasic decline. The average half-life of the second (post-distributional) phase is 14 hours (range, 8 to 24 hours). Six hours after a single dose, plasma concentrations are ≈ 30% of peak concentrations. Plasma concentrations are dose-proportional following single doses of 100 to 250 mg; however, it is not known if the proportionality between dose and plasma level is maintained in chronic use. It appears likely that only a small portion of any orally administered dose reaches the systemic circulation intact. The absolute bioavailability of bupropion in rats and dogs is 5% to 20%. Bupropion is ≥ 80% bound to human albumin at plasma concentrations up to 800 micromolar (200 mcg/ml).

Metabolism/Excretion – Following oral administration of 200 mg bupropion, 87% and 10% of the dose were recovered in the urine and feces, respectively; the fraction excreted unchanged was only 0.5%.

Several of the metabolites of bupropion are pharmacologically active, but their potency and toxicity relative to bupropion have not been fully characterized. However, because of their longer elimination half-lives, the plasma concentrations of at least two of the known metabolites will be much higher than the plasma concentration of bupropion, especially in long-term use. This is of potential clinical importance because conditions altering metabolic capacity (eg, liver disease, congestive heart failure, age, concomitant medications) or elimination may influence the degree and extent of accumulation of these active metabolites.

Bupropion induces its own metabolism in animal species following subchronic administration. If induction also occurs in humans, the relative contribution of bupropion and its metabolites to the clinical effects may be changed in chronic use.

Plasma and urinary metabolites so far identified include biotransformation products formed via reduction of the carbonyl group or hydroxylation of the tert-butyl group of bupropion. Four basic metabolites have been identified: The erythro- and threo-amino alcohols, the erythro-amino diol and a morpholinol metabolite. The morpholinol metabolite appears in the systemic circulation almost as rapidly as the parent drug following a single oral dose. Its peak level is 3 times the peak level of the parent drug; it has a half-life of 24 hours, and its area under the curve is about 15 times that of bupropion. The threo-amino alcohol metabolite has a plasma concentration-time profile similar to that of the morpholinol metabolite. The erythro-amino alcohol and the erythro-amino diol metabolites generally cannot be detected in the systemic circulation following a single oral dose of the parent drug. The morpholinol and the threo-amino alcohol metabolites are half as potent as bupropion in animal tests.

During a chronic dosing study in 14 depressed patients with left ventricular dysfunction, there was substantial interpatient variability (two- to five-fold) in trough steady-state concentrations of bupropion and the morpholinol and threo-amino alcohol metabolites. In addition, steady-state plasma concentrations of these metabolites were 10 to 100 times those of the parent drug.

The elimination of the major metabolites may be affected by reduced renal or hepatic function because they are moderately polar compounds and are likely to undergo conjugation in the liver prior to urinary excretion. Half-lives of the metabolites are prolonged by cirrhosis and the metabolites accumulate to levels 2 to 3 times those in healthy individuals.

Indications:

Depression treatment: Effectiveness of bupropion in long-term use (> 6 weeks) has not been evaluated. Therefore, periodically reevaluate long-term usefulness of the drug.

BUPROPION HCl

Contraindications:

Hypersensitivity to the drug; seizure disorder; current or prior diagnosis of bulimia or anorexia nervosa (because of a higher incidence of seizures noted in such patients treated with bupropion); concurrent administration of a monoamine oxidase inhibitor (MAOI; at least 14 days should elapse between discontinuation of an MAOI and initiation of treatment with bupropion).

Warnings:

Seizures: Bupropion is associated with seizures in ≈ 0.4% of patients treated at doses up to 450 mg/day. This incidence of seizures may exceed that of other marketed antidepressants by as much as fourfold. The estimated seizure incidence increases almost tenfold between 450 and 600 mg/day, which is twice the usually required daily dose (300 mg) and one and one-third the maximum recommended daily dose (450 mg). Given the wide variability among individuals and their capacity to metabolize and eliminate drugs, this disproportionate increase in seizure incidence with dose incrementation calls for caution in dosing.

The risk of seizure appears strongly associated with dose and the presence of predisposing factors. A significant predisposing factor (eg, history of head trauma or prior seizure, CNS tumor, concomitant medications that lower seizure threshold) was present in approximately 50% of patients experiencing a seizure. Sudden and large increments in dose may also increase risk. While many seizures occurred early in the course of treatment, some seizures occurred after several weeks at fixed dose.

Recommendations for reducing seizure risk: (1) The total daily dose does not exceed 450 mg, (2) the daily dose is administered 3 times daily, with each single dose not to exceed 150 mg to avoid high peak concentrations of bupropion or its metabolites, and (3) the rate of incrementation of dose is very gradual.

Use extreme caution when: (1) Administered to patients with a history of seizure, cranial trauma, or other predisposition toward seizure, or (2) prescribed with other agents (eg, antipsychotics, other antidepressants) or treatment regimens (eg, abrupt discontinuation of a benzodiazepine) that lower seizure threshold.

Hepatotoxicity: In animals receiving large doses of bupropion chronically, there was an increased incidence of hepatic hyperplastic nodules, hepatocellular hypertrophy and histologic changes with laboratory tests that suggested mild hepatocellular injury. Although scattered abnormalities in liver function tests were detected in patients participating in clinical trials, there is no clinical evidence that bupropion is hepatotoxic in humans.

Renal/Hepatic function impairment: Because bupropion and its metabolites are almost completely excreted through the kidney and metabolites are likely to undergo conjugation in the liver, initiate treatment of patients with renal or hepatic impairment at reduced dosage; bupropion and its metabolites may accumulate. Closely monitor for possible toxic effects of elevated blood and tissue levels of drug and metabolites.

Carcinogenesis: In rats there was an increase in nodular proliferative lesions of the liver at doses of 100 to 300 mg/kg/day.

Bupropion produced a borderline positive response in some strains in the Ames bacterial mutagenicity test. A high oral dose (300, but not 100 or 200 mg/kg) produced a low incidence of chromosomal aberrations in rats. The relevance of these results to human exposure is unknown.

Pregnancy: Category B. There are no adequate and well controlled studies in pregnant women. Use during pregnancy only if clearly needed.

Lactation: Because of the potential for serious adverse reactions in nursing infants, decide whether to discontinue nursing or to discontinue the drug, taking into account the importance of the drug to the mother.

Children: The safety and efficacy in individuals < 18 years old have not been established.

BUPROPION HCl

Precautions:

Drug abuse/dependence: Studies in healthy volunteers, in subjects with a history of multiple drug abuse, and in depressed patients showed some increase in motor activity and agitation/excitement. In individuals experienced with drugs of abuse, a single dose of 400 mg produced mild amphetamine-like activity as compared to placebo. Studies in rodents have shown that bupropion exhibits some pharmacologic actions common to psychostimulants.

Evidence from single dose studies suggests that the recommended daily dosage of bupropion when administered in divided doses is not likely to be especially reinforcing to amphetamine or stimulant abusers. However, higher doses, not tested because of the risk of seizure, may modestly attract those who abuse stimulant drugs.

CNS symptoms: A substantial proportion of patients experience some degree of increased restlessness, agitation, anxiety and insomnia, especially shortly after initiation of treatment. Symptoms were sometimes of sufficient magnitude to require treatment with sedative/hypnotic drugs. In approximately 2% of patients, symptoms were sufficiently severe to require discontinuation.

Neuropsychiatric phenomena: Patients have shown a variety of neuropsychiatric signs and symptoms including delusions, hallucinations, psychotic episodes, confusion and paranoia. In several cases, neuropsychiatric phenomena abated upon dose reduction or withdrawal of treatment.

Activation of psychosis or mania: Antidepressants can precipitate manic episodes in Bipolar Manic Depressive patients during the depressed phase of their illness and may activate latent psychosis in other susceptible patients.

Altered appetite and weight: A weight loss of > 5 pounds occurred in 28% of patients. This incidence is approximately double that seen in comparable patients treated with tricyclic antidepressants or placebo. Furthermore, 34.5% of patients receiving tricyclic antidepressants gained weight, vs only 9.4% of bupropion patients. Consequently, if weight loss is a major presenting sign of a patient's depressive illness, consider the anorectic or weight reducing potential.

Suicide: The possibility of a suicide attempt is inherent in depression and may persist until significant remission occurs. Accordingly, write prescriptions for the smallest number of tablets consistent with good patient management.

Heart disease: Exercise care in patients with a recent history of myocardial infarction or unstable heart disease.

Drug Interactions:

Bupropion may be an inducer of drug metabolizing enzymes. Exercise care when administering drugs known to affect hepatic drug metabolizing enzyme systems.

Use caution during coadministration of bupropion and agents that lower seizure threshold. Use low initial dosing and small gradual dose increases.

Bupropion Drug Interactions

Precipitant drug	Object drug*		Description
Bupropion	Levodopa	↑	There is a higher incidence of adverse experiences with concurrent use of these agents. Use small initial doses and small gradual dose increases of bupropion.
MAOIs	Bupropion	↑	Animal data demonstrate bupropion's acute toxicity is enhanced by phenelzine. At least 14 days should elapse between discontinuation of an MAOI and initiation of bupropion.

* ↑ = Object drug increased.

BUPROPION HCl

Adverse Reactions:

Bupropion Adverse Reactions (%)					
Adverse reaction	Bupropion (n = 323)	Placebo (n = 185)	Adverse reaction	Bupropion (n = 323)	Placebo (n = 185)
GI			*Special senses*		
Constipation	26	17.3	Auditory disturbance	14.6	10.3
Weight loss	23.2	23.2	Blurred vision	5.3	3.2
Nausea/Vomiting	22.9	18.9	Gustatory disturbance	3.1	1.1
Anorexia	18.3	18.4	*Cardiovascular*		
Weight gain	13.6	22.7	Dizziness	22.3	16.2
Diarrhea	6.8	8.6	Tachycardia	10.8	8.6
Appetite increase	3.7	2.2	Cardiac arrythmias	5.3	4.3
Dyspepsia	3.1	2.2	Hypertension	4.3	1.6
GU			Palpitations	3.7	2.2
Menstrual complaints	4.7	1.1	Hypotension	2.5	2.2
Impotence	3.4	3.1	Syncope	1.2	0.5
Urinary frequency	2.5	2.2	*Dermatologic*		
Urinary retention	1.9	2.2	Rash	8	6.5
Neurologic			Pruritus	2.2	0
Dry mouth	27.6	18.4	*Neuropsychiatric*		
Headache/migraine	25.7	22.2	Agitation	31.9	22.2
Excessive sweating	22.3	14.6	Confusion	8.4	4.9
Tremor	21.1	7.6	Hostility	5.6	3.8
Sedation	19.8	19.5	Disturbed concentration	3.1	3.8
Insomnia	18.6	15.7	Decreased libido	3.1	1.6
Akinesia/Bradykinesia	8	8.6	Anxiety	3.1	1.1
Sensory disturbance	4	3.2	Delusions	1.2	1.1
Impaired sleep quality	4	1.6	Euphoria	1.2	0.5
Increased salivary flow	3.4	3.8	*Other*		
Muscle spasms	1.9	3.2	Upper respiratory complaints	5	11.4
Cutaneous temperature disturbance	1.9	1.6	Fatigue	5	8.6
Pseudoparkinsonism	1.5	1.6	Arthritis	3.1	2.7
Akathisia	1.5	1.1	Fever/chills	1.2	0.5

Discontinuation: Adverse reactions caused discontinuation in approximately 10% of 2400 patients and volunteers. The more common events causing discontinuation include: Neuropsychiatric disturbances, primarily agitation and abnormalities in mental status (3%); GI disturbances, primarily nausea and vomiting (2.1%); neurological disturbances, primarily seizures, headaches and sleep disturbances (1.7%); dermatologic problems, primarily rashes (1.4%). Many of these events occurred at doses that exceeded the recommended daily dose.

Other adverse reactions include the following:

GI – Stomatitis (1%); toothache, bruxism, gum irritation, oral edema, dysphagia, thirst disturbance, liver damage/jaundice (0.1% to 1%); glossitis, rectal complaints, colitis, GI bleeding, stomach ulcer, intestinal perforation (< 0.1%); esophagitis; hepatitis.

CNS – See Warnings; Ataxia/incoordination, seizure, myoclonus, dyskinesia, dystonia (1%); mydriasis, vertigo, dysarthria (0.1% to 1%); EEG abnormality, abnormal neurological exam, impaired attention, sciatica, aphasia (< 0.1%); coma; delirium; dream abnormalities; paresthesia; unmasking of tardive dyskinesia.

Cardiovascular – Edema (1%); ECG abnormalities (premature beats and nonspecific ST-T changes), chest pain, shortness of breath/dyspnea (0.1% to 1%); pallor, phlebitis, flushing, myocardial infarction (< 0.1%); orthostatic hypotension; third degree heart block.

Dermatologic – Rashes (1%); alopecia, dry skin (0.1% to 1%); acne, hair color change, hirsutism (< 0.1%); Stevens-Johnson syndrome; angioedema; exfoliative dermatitis; urticaria.

Endocrine – Gynecomastia (0.1% to 1%); glycosuria, hormone level change (< 0.1%); SIADH.

GU – Nocturia (1%); vaginal irritation, testicular swelling, urinary tract infection, painful erection, retarded ejaculation (0.1% to 1%); dysuria, enuresis, urinary incontinence, menopause, ovarian disorder, pelvic infection, cystitis, dyspareunia, painful ejaculation (< 0.1%).

Hematologic – Anemia, pancytopenia, lymphadenopathy (< 0.1%); ecchymosis; leukocytosis; leukopenia.

Psychiatric – see Precautions; mania/hypomania, increased libido, hallucinations, decreased sexual function, depression (1%); memory impairment, depersonalization, psychosis, dysphoria, mood instability, paranoia, formal thought disorder, frigidity (0.1% to 1%); suicidal ideation (< 0.1%).

Respiratory – Bronchitis, shortness of breath/dyspnea (0.1% to 1%); epistaxis, rate or rhythm disorder, pneumonia, pulmonary embolism (< 0.1%).

Special Senses – Visual disturbance (0.1% to 1%); diplopia (< 0.1%); tinnitus.

Musculoskeletal – Arthralgia; myalgia; muscle rigidity/fever/rhabdomyolysis.

Miscellaneous – Flu-like symptoms (1%); nonspecific pain (0.1% to 1%); body odor, surgically related pain, infection, medication reaction, musculoskeletal chest pain, overdose (< 0.1%).

Overdosage:

Thirteen overdoses occurred during clinical trials; 12 patients ingested 850 to 4200 mg and recovered without significant sequelae. Another patient who ingested 9000 mg bupropion and 300 mg tranylcypromine experienced a grand mal seizure and recovered without further sequelae. Since product release, overdoses up to 17,500 mg have occurred. Seizure was reported in ≈ 33% of all cases. Other serious reactions included hallucinations, loss of consciousness and tachycardia. Although most paients recovered without sequelae, deaths have been reported rarely in patients ingesting massive doses; multiple uncontrolled seizures, bradycardia, cardiac failure and cardiac arrest prior to death were reported in these patients.

Treatment: Hospitalize. If the patient is conscious, induce vomiting with syrup of ipecac, administer activated charcoal every 6 hours during the first 12 hours after ingestion and obtain baseline laboratory values; perform ECG and EEG monitoring for the next 48 hours. Provide adequate fluid intake. If the patient is stuporous, comatose, or convulsing, perform airway intubation prior to undertaking gastric lavage. Although there is little clinical experience, lavage is likely to be of benefit within the first 12 hours after ingestion since absorption of the drug may not yet be complete. Refer to General Management of Acute Overdosage.

Because diffusion of bupropion from tissue to plasma may be slow, dialysis may be of minimal benefit several hours after overdose. Treat seizures with IV benzodiazepines and other supportive measures.

Patient Information:

Take in equally divided doses 3 or 4 times a day to minimize the risk of seizure.

May impair ability to perform tasks requiring judgment or motor and cognitive skills; patients should refrain from driving an automobile or operating complex, hazardous machinery until they are reasonably certain the drug does not adversely affect their performance.

Use and cessation of use of alcohol may alter the seizure threshold; therefore, minimize the consumption of alcohol and, if possible, avoid completely.

Administration and Dosage:

General: It is particularly important to administer bupropion in a manner most likely to minimize the risk of seizure (see Warnings). Do not exceed dose increases of 100 mg/day in a 3 day period. Gradual escalation of dosage is also important to minimize agitation, motor restlessness and insomnia often seen during the initial days of treatment. If necessary, these effects may be managed by temporary reduction of dose or the short-term administration of an intermediate to long-acting sedative/hypnotic. A sedative/hypnotic is not usually required beyond the first week of treatment. Insomnia may also be minimized by avoiding bedtime doses. If distressing, untoward effects supervene, stop dose escalation.

No single dose of bupropion should exceed 150 mg. Administer 3 times daily, preferably with at least 6 hours between successive doses.

Adults: 300 mg/day, given 3 times daily. Begin dosing at 200 mg/day, given as 100 mg twice daily. Based on clinical response, this dose may be increased to 300 mg/day, given as 100 mg 3 times daily no sooner than 3 days after beginning therapy (see table below).

BUPROPION HCl

Bupropion Dosage Regimen					
			Number of Tablets		
Treatment Day	Total Daily Dose	Tablet Strength	Morning	Midday	Evening
1	200 mg	100 mg	1	0	1
4	300 mg	100 mg	1	1	1

Increasing the dosage above 300 mg/day: As with other antidepressants, the full antidepressant effect of bupropion may not be evident until 4 weeks of treatment or longer. An increase in dosage, up to a maximum of 450 mg/day, given in divided doses of not more than 150 mg each, may be considered for patients in whom no clinical improvement is noted after several weeks of treatment at 300 mg/day. Dosing above 300 mg/day may be accomplished using the 75 or 100 mg tablets. The 100 mg tablets must be administered 4 times daily with at least 4 hours between successive doses in order not to exceed the limit of 150 mg in a single dose. Discontinue in patients who do not demonstrate an adequate response after an appropriate period of 450 mg/day.

Maintenance: Use the lowest dose that maintains remission. Although it is not known how long the patient should remain on bupropion, acute episodes of depression generally require several months or longer of treatment.

Rx	**Wellbutrin** (Glaxo Wellcome)	**Tablets:** 75 mg	(Wellbutrin 75). Yellow-gold. Biconvex. In 100s.
		100 mg	(Wellbutrin 100). Red. Biconvex. In 100s.
Rx	**Wellbutrin SR** (Glaxo Wellcome)	**Tablets, sustained-release:** 100 mg	(Wellbutrin SR 100). Blue. Round, biconvex. Film-coated. In 60s.
		Tablets, sustained-release: 150 mg	(Wellbutrin SR 150). Purple. Round, biconvex. Film-coated. In 60s.

VENLAFAXINE

Actions:

Pharmacology: Venlafaxine is chemically unrelated to tricyclic, tetracyclic or other available antidepressant agents. The mechanism of action is believed to be associated with its potentiation of neurotransmitter activity in the CNS. Venlafaxine and its active metabolite, O-desmethylvenlafaxine (ODV), are potent inhibitors of neuronal serotonin and norepinephrine reuptake and weak inhibitors of dopamine reuptake. Venlafaxine and ODV have no significant affinity for muscarinic, histaminergic or alpha-1 adrenergic receptors in vitro, and they do not possess monoamine oxidase (MAO) inhibitory activity.

Pharmacokinetics: Venlafaxine is well absorbed (at least 92%) and extensively metabolized in the liver. ODV is the only major active metabolite. Approximately 87% of a dose is recovered in the urine within 48 hours as either unchanged venlafaxine (5%), unconjugated ODV (29%), conjugated ODV (26%) or other minor inactive metabolites (27%). Renal elimination of venlafaxine and its metabolites is the primary route of excretion. The relative bioavailability from a tablet was 100% when compared to an oral solution. Food has no significant effect on the absorption of venlafaxine.

The degree of binding of venlafaxine to plasma is 25% to 29% at concentrations ranging from 2.5 to 2215 ng/ml. The degree of ODV binding to plasma is 30% ± 12% at concentrations ranging from 100 to 500 ng/ml. Protein-binding-induced drug interactions with venlafaxine are not expected.

Steady-state concentrations of both venlafaxine and ODV in plasma were attained within 3 days of multiple-dose therapy. Plasma clearance, elimination half-life and steady-state volume of distribution were unaltered after multiple dosing. Mean steady-state plasma clearance of venlafaxine and ODV is 1.3 ± 0.6 and 0.4 ± 0.2 L/hr/kg, respectively; elimination half-life is 5 ± 2 and 11 ± 2 hours, respectively; and steady-state volume of distribution is 7.5 ± 3.7 and 5.7 ± 1.8 L/kg, respectively. When equal daily doses of venlafaxine were administered as either 2 or 3 times daily regimens, the drug exposure (AUC) and fluctuation in plasma levels of venlafaxine and ODV were comparable following both regimens.

Hepatic disease – In nine patients with hepatic cirrhosis, the pharmacokinetic disposition of both venlafaxine and ODV was significantly altered after oral administration. Venlafaxine and ODV elimination half-life was prolonged by about 30% and 60%, and clearance decreased by about 50% and 30%, respectively, in cirrhotic patients compared to healthy subjects. A large degree of intersubject variability was noted. Three patients with more severe cirrhosis had a more substantial decrease in venlafaxine clearance (about 90%) compared to healthy subjects. Dosage adjustment is necessary in these patients (see Administration and Dosage).

Renal disease – Venlafaxine elimination half-life after oral administration was prolonged by about 50% and clearance was reduced by about 24% in renally impaired patients (GFR, 10 to 70 ml/min), compared to healthy subjects. In dialysis patients, venlafaxine elimination half-life was prolonged by about 180% and clearance was reduced by about 57% compared to healthy subjects. Similarly, ODV elimination half-life was prolonged by about 40% although clearance was unchanged in patients with renal impairment. In dialysis patients, ODV elimination half-life was prolonged by about 142% and clearance was reduced by about 56% compared to healthy subjects. A large degree of intersubject variability was noted. Dosage adjustment is necessary in these patients (see Administration and Dosage).

Indications:

Treatment of depression.

Warnings:

MAO inhibitors: In patients receiving antidepressants with pharmacological properties similar to venlafaxine in combination with an MAOI, there have been reports of serious, sometimes fatal, reactions. For a selective serotonin reuptake inhibitor, these reactions have included hyperthermia, rigidity, myoclonus, autonomic instability with possible rapid fluctuations of vital signs and mental status changes that include extreme agitation progressing to delirium and coma. Some cases presented with features resembling neuroleptic malignant syndrome.

Severe hyperthermia and seizures, sometimes fatal, have been reported in association with the combined use of tricyclic antidepressants and MAOIs. These reactions have also been reported in patients who have recently discontinued these drugs and have been started on an MAOI. The effects of combined use of venlafaxine and MAOIs have not been evaluated. Therefore, because venlafaxine is an inhibitor of both norepinephrine and serotonin reuptake, it is recommended that venlafaxine not be used in combination with an MAOI, or within 14 days of discontinuing treatment with an MAOI. Based on the half-life of venlafaxine, allow at least 7 days after stopping venlafaxine before starting an MAOI.

Sustained hypertension: Venlafaxine treatment is associated with sustained increases in blood pressure. In a study comparing three fixed doses of venlafaxine (75, 225 and 375 mg/day) and placebo, a mean increase in supine diastolic blood pressure (SDBP) of 7.2 mm Hg was seen in the 375 mg/day group at week 6 compared to essentially no changes in the 75 and 225 mg/day groups and a mean decrease in SDBP of 2.2 mm Hg in the placebo group. There is a dose-dependent increase in the incidence of sustained hypertension for venlafaxine.

Probability of Sustained Elevation in SDBP with Venlafaxine

Venlafaxine	Incidence of sustained elevation in SDBP
< 100 mg/day	3%
101-200 mg/day	5%
201-300 mg/day	7%
> 300 mg/day	13%
Placebo	2%

An analysis of patients with sustained hypertension and the 19 patients who were discontinued from treatment because of hypertension revealed that most of the blood pressure increases were in a modest range (10 to 15 mm Hg, SDBP). Nevertheless, sustained increases of this magnitude could have adverse consequences. Therefore, it is recommended that patients receiving venlafaxine have regular monitoring of blood pressure. For patients who experience a sustained increase in blood pressure, consider either dose reduction or discontinuation.

Renal/Hepatic function impairment: Use with caution. In patients with renal impairment (GFR, 10 to 70 ml/min) or cirrhosis of the liver, the clearances of venlafaxine and its active metabolite were decreased, thus prolonging the elimination half-lives. A lower dose may be necessary (see Administration and Dosage).

Elderly: No overall differences in effectiveness, safety or response were observed between elderly and younger patients. However, greater sensitivity of some older individuals cannot be ruled out.

Pregnancy: Category C. In rats there was a decrease in pup weight, an increase in stillborn pups and an increase in pup deaths during the first 5 days of lactation, when dosing began during pregnancy and continued until weaning. These effects occurred at 10 times (mg/kg) the maximum human daily dose. There are no adequate and well controlled studies in pregnant women. Use during pregnancy only if clearly needed.

Lactation: It is not known whether venlafaxine or its metabolites are excreted in breast milk. Exercise caution when administering to a nursing woman.

Children: Safety and efficacy in patients < 18 years old have not been established.

Precautions:

Monitoring: There are no specific laboratory tests recommended.

Long-term use: The effectiveness of venlafaxine in long-term use (ie, > 4 to 6 weeks) has not been evaluated. Therefore, periodically re-evaluate the long-term usefulness of the drug for the individual patient.

Anxiety and insomnia: Anxiety, nervousness and insomnia were more commonly reported for venlafaxine-treated patients (6%, 13% and 18%, respectively) vs placebo (3%, 6% and 10%, respectively), and led to drug discontinuation in 2%, 2% and 3%, respectively.

Appetite/Weight changes: Anorexia was more commonly reported for venlafaxine-treated (11%) patients than placebo (2%). A dose-dependent weight loss was often noted in patients treated for several weeks. Significant weight loss, especially in underweight depressed patients, may be an undesirable result of treatment. A loss of ≥ 5% of body weight occurred in 6% of patients treated with venlafaxine compared with 1% with placebo and 3% with another antidepressant. However, discontinuation for weight loss associated with venlafaxine was uncommon (0.1%).

Mania/Hypomania: Hypomania or mania occurred in 0.5% of patients treated with venlafaxine. Activation of mania/hypomania has also been reported in a small proportion of patients with major affective disorder who were treated with other marketed antidepressants. As with all antidepressants, use venlafaxine cautiously in patients with a history of mania.

VENLAFAXINE

Seizures were reported in 0.26% of venlafaxine-treated patients. Most seizures occurred in patients receiving doses of ≤ 150 mg/day. Use venlafaxine cautiously in patients with a history of seizures. Discontinue use in any patient who develops seizures.

Suicide: The possibility of a suicide attempt is inherent in depression and may persist until significant remission occurs. Close supervision of high-risk patients should accompany initial therapy. Write prescriptions for the smallest quantity of tablets consistent with good patient management in order to reduce the risk of overdose.

Concomitant illness: Caution is advised in administering venlafaxine to patients with diseases or conditions that could affect hemodynamic responses or metabolism.

Cardiac patients: Venlafaxine has not been evaluated in patients with a recent history of myocardial infarction or unstable heart disease. Evaluation of the ECGs for patients who received venlafaxine in 4- to 6 week double-blind, placebo controlled trials, however, showed that the incidence of trial-emergent conduction abnormalities did not differ from that with placebo. The mean heart rate in venlafaxine-treated patients was increased relative to baseline by about 4 beats per minute.

Drug abuse and dependence: There was no indication of drug-seeking behavior in the clinical trials. However, it is not possible to predict on the basis of premarketing experience the extent to which a CNS active drug will be misused, diverted or abused once marketed. Consequently, carefully evaluate patients for history of drug abuse and follow such patients closely, observing them for signs of misuse or abuse of venlafaxine (eg, development of tolerance, incrementation of dose, drug-seeking behavior).

Drug Interactions:

Venlafaxine is metabolized to its active metabolite, ODV, by cytochrome $P\text{–}450IID_6$. Therefore, the potential exists for a drug interaction between venlafaxine and drugs that inhibit this isoenzyme. Drugs that reduce the metabolism of venlafaxine to ODV could potentially increase the plasma concentrations of venlafaxine and lower the concentrations of the active metabolite.

Venlafaxine Drug Interactions

Precipitant drug	Object drug*		Description
Cimetidine	Venlafaxine	⬆	Concomitant use resulted in inhibition of first-pass metabolism of venlafaxine in 18 healthy subjects. Oral clearance was reduced by about 43%, and AUC and C_{max} were increased by about 60%. However, cimetidine had no apparent effect on ODV. Consequently, the overall pharmacological activity is expected to increase only slightly.
MAOIs	Venlafaxine	⬆	Serious, sometimes fatal reactions may occur, including hyperthermia, rigidity, myoclonus, autonomic instability with possible rapid fluctuation of vital signs, and mental status changes that include extreme agitation and coma (see Warnings).

* ⬆ = Object drug increased.

Adverse Reactions:

In various studies, 19% of venlafaxine patients discontinued treatment due to an adverse reaction. The more common events associated with discontinuation included: Nausea (6%); somnolence, insomnia, dizziness, abnormal ejaculation, headache (3%); nervousness, dry mouth, anxiety, asthenia, sweating (2%).

VENLAFAXINE

Venlafaxine Adverse Reactions (%)

Adverse reaction	Venlafaxine (n = 1033)	Placebo (n = 609)	Adverse reaction	Venlafaxine (n = 1033)	Placebo (n = 609)
Special senses			*Body as a whole*		
Blurred vision	6	2	Headache	25	24
Taste perversion	2	—	Asthenia	12	6
Tinnitus	2	—	Infection	6	5
Mydriasis	2	—	Chills	3	—
Cardiovascular			Chest pain	2	1
Vasodilation	4	3	Trauma	2	1
Increased blood pressure/ hypertension	2	—	Weight loss	1	—
Tachycardia	2	—	Yawn	3	—
Postural hypotension	1	—	*Dermatologic*		
CNS			Sweating	12	3
Somnolence	23	9	Rash	3	2
Dry mouth	22	11	Pruritus	1	—
Dizziness	19	7	*GI*		
Insomnia	18	10	Nausea	37	11
Nervousness	13	6	Constipation	15	7
Anxiety	6	3	Anorexia	11	2
Tremor	5	1	Diarrhea	8	7
Abnormal dreams	4	3	Vomiting	6	2
Hypertonia	3	2	Dyspepsia	5	4
Paresthesia	3	2	Flatulence	3	2
Decreased libido	2	—	*GU*		
Agitation	2	—	Abnormal ejaculation/orgasm	12	—
Confusion	2	1	Impotence	6	—
Abnormal thinking	2	1	Urinary frequency	3	2
Depersonalization	1	—	Impaired urination	2	—
Depression	1	—	Orgasm disturbance	2	—
Urinary retention	1	—	Menstrual disorder	1	—
Twitching	1	—			

Venlafaxine Adverse Reactions (%): Dose Comparison

Adverse reaction	Placebo (n = 92)	Venlafaxine (mg/day) 75 (n = 89)	225 (n = 89)	375 (n = 88)
Body as a whole				
Abdominal pain	3.3	3.4	2.2	8
Asthenia	3.3	16.9	14.6	14.8
Chills	1.1	2.2	5.6	6.8
Infection	2.2	2.2	5.6	2.3
Cardiovascular				
Hypertension	1.1	1.1	2.2	4.5
Vasodilation	0	4.5	5.6	2.3
GI				
Anorexia	2.2	14.6	13.5	17
Dyspepsia	2.2	6.7	6.7	4.5
Nausea	14.1	32.6	38.2	58
Vomiting	1.1	7.9	3.4	6.8

Venlafaxine Adverse Reactions (%): Dose Comparison				
		Venlafaxine (mg/day)		
Adverse reaction	Placebo (n = 92)	75 (n = 89)	225 (n = 89)	375 (n = 88)
CNS				
Agitation	0	1.1	2.2	4.5
Anxiety	4.3	11.2	4.5	2.3
Dizziness	4.3	19.1	22.5	23.9
Insomnia	9.8	22.5	20.2	13.6
Libido decreased	1.1	2.2	1.1	5.7
Nervousness	4.3	21.3	13.5	12.5
Somnolence	4.3	16.9	18	26.1
Tremor	0	1.1	2.2	10.2
GU				
Abnormal ejaculation/ orgasm	0	4.5	2.2	12.5
Impotence	0	5.8	2.1	3.6
(Number of men)	(n = 63)	(n = 50)	(n = 48)	(n = 58)
Miscellaneous				
Yawn	0	4.5	5.6	8
Sweating	5.4	6.7	12.4	19.3
Abnormality of accommodation	0	9.1	7.9	5.6

Over a 6 week period there was evidence of adaptation to some adverse events with continued therapy (eg, dizziness, nausea), but less to other effects (eg, abnormal ejaculation, dry mouth).

Other adverse reactions that occurred are as follows:

Body as a whole – Accidental injury, malaise, neck pain (1%); enlarged abdomen, allergic reaction, cyst, facial edema, generalized edema, hangover effect, hernia, intentional injury, moniliasis, neck rigidity, overdose, substernal chest pain, pelvic pain, photosensitivity reaction, suicide attempt (0.1% to 1%); appendicitis, body odor, carcinoma, cellulitis, halitosis, ulcer, withdrawal syndrome (< 0.1%).

Cardiovascular – Migraine (1%); angina pectoris, extrasystoles, hypotension, peripheral vascular disorder (mainly cold feet or hands), syncope, thrombophlebitis (0.1% to 1%); arrhythmia, first-degree AV block, bradycardia, bundle branch block, mitral valve disorder, mucocutaneous hemorrhage, sinus bradycardia, varicose vein (< 0.1%).

Venlafaxine treatment was associated with a mean increase in pulse rate of ≈3 bpm, compared to no change for placebo. It was associated with mean increases in diastolic blood pressure ranging from 0.7 to 2.5 mm Hg averaged over all dose groups vs 0.9 to 3.8 mm Hg for placebo. However, there is a dose dependency for blood pressure increase (see Warnings).

In an analysis of ECGs obtained in 769 patients treated with venlafaxine and 450 patients treated with placebo, the only statistically significant difference observed was for heart rate (mean increase from baseline of 4 bpm for venlafaxine).

GI – Dysphagia, eructation (1%); colitis, tongue edema, esophagitis, gastritis, gastroenteritis, gingivitis, glossitis, rectal hemorrhage, hemorrhoids, melena, stomatitis, stomach ulcer, mouth ulceration (0.1% to 1%); cheilitis, cholecystitis, cholelithiasis, hematemesis, gum hemorrhage, hepatitis, ileitis, jaundice, oral moniliasis, intestinal obstruction, proctitis, increased salivation, soft stools, tongue discoloration, esophageal ulcer, peptic ulcer syndrome (< 0.1%).

Endocrine – Goiter, hyperthyroidism, hypothyroidism (< 0.1%).

Hematologic/Lymphatic – Ecchymosis (1%); anemia, leukocytosis, leukopenia, lymphadenopathy, lymphocytosis, thrombocythemia, thrombocytopenia, WBC abnormal (0.1% to 1%); basophilia, cyanosis, eosinophilia, erythrocytes abnormal (< 0.1%).

VENLAFAXINE

Metabolic/Nutritional – Peripheral edema, weight gain (1%); alkaline phosphatase/creatinine increased, diabetes mellitus, edema, glycosuria, hypercholesteremia, hyperglycemia, hyperlipemia, hyperuricemia, hypoglycemia, hypokalemia, AST increased, thirst (0.1% to 1%); alcohol intolerance, bilirubinemia, BUN increased, gout, hemochromatosis, hyperkalemia, hyperphosphatemia, hypoglycemic reaction, hyponatremia, hypophosphatemia, hypoproteinemia, ALT increased, uremia (< 0.1%).

Musculoskeletal – Arthritis, arthrosis, bone pain, bone spurs, bursitis, joint disorder, myasthenia, tenosynovitis (0.1% to 1%); osteoporosis (< 0.1%).

CNS – Emotional lability, trismus, vertigo (1%); apathy, ataxia, circumoral paresthesia, CNS stimulation, euphoria, hallucinations, hostility, hyperesthesia, hyperkinesia, hypertonia, hypotonia, incoordination, increased libido, myoclonus, neuralgia, neuropathy, paranoid reaction, psychosis, psychotic depression, sleep disturbance, abnormal speech, stupor, torticollis (0.1% to 1%); akathisia, akinesia, alcohol abuse, aphasia, bradykinesia, cerebrovascular accident, loss of consciousness, delusions, dementia, dystonia, hypokinesia, neuritis, nystagmus, reflexes increased (< 0.1%).

Respiratory – Bronchitis, dyspnea (1%); asthma, chest congestion, epistaxis, hyperventilation, laryngismus, laryngitis, pneumonia, voice alteration (0.1% to 1%); atelectasis, hemoptysis, hypoxia, pleurisy, pulmonary embolus, sleep apnea, sputum increased (< 0.1%).

Dermatologic – Acne, alopecia, brittle nails, contact dermatitis, dry skin, herpes simplex, herpes zoster, maculopapular rash, urticaria (0.1% to 1%); skin atrophy, exfoliative dermatitis, fungal dermatitis, lichenoid dermatitis, hair discoloration, eczema, furunculosis, hirsutism, skin hypertrophy, leukoderma, psoriasis, pustular rash, vesiculobullous rash (< 0.1%).

Special Senses – Abnormal vision, ear pain (1%); cataract, conjunctivitis, corneal lesion, diplopia, dry eyes, exophthalmos, eye pain, otitis media, parosmia, photophobia, subconjunctival hemorrhage, taste loss, visual field defect (0.1% to 1%); blepharitis, chromatopsia, conjunctival edema, deafness, glaucoma, hyperacusis, keratitis, labyrinthitis, miosis, papilledema, decreased pupillary reflex, scleritis (< 0.1%).

GU – Anorgasmia, dysuria, hematuria, metrorrhagia, urination impaired, vaginitis (1%); albuminuria, amenorrhea, kidney calculus, cystitis, leukorrhea, menorrhagia, nocturia, bladder pain, breast pain, kidney pain, polyuria, prostatitis, pyelonephritis, pyuria, urinary incontinence, urinary urgency, uterine fibroids enlarged, uterine hemorrhage, vaginal hemorrhage, vaginal moniliasis (0.1% to 1%); abortion, breast engorgement, breast enlargement, calcium crystalluria, female lactation, hypomenorrhea, menopause, prolonged erection, uterine spasm (< 0.1%).

Lab test abnormalities – Patients treated with venlafaxine had mean serum cholesterol increases from baseline of 3 mg/dl).

Overdosage:

Symptoms: There were 14 reports of acute overdose with venlafaxine, either alone or in combination with other drugs or alcohol. The majority of the reports involved ingestions in which the total dose of venlafaxine taken was estimated to be no more than several-fold higher than the usual therapeutic dose. The three patients who took the highest doses were estimated to have ingested ≈ 6.75 , 2.75 and 2.5 g. The resultant peak plasma levels of venlafaxine for the latter two patients were 6.24 and 2.35 mcg/ml, respectively, and the peak plasma levels of ODV were 3.37 and 1.3 mcg/ml, respectively. All 14 patients recovered without sequelae. Most patients reported no symptoms. Among the remaining patients, somnolence was most commonly reported. The patient who ingested 2.75 g was observed to have two generalized convulsions and a prolongation of QT_c to 500 msec compared to 405 msec at baseline. Mild sinus tachycardia was reported in two of the other patients.

Treatment: Treatment should consist of those general measures employed in the management of overdosage with any antidepressant. Ensure an adequate airway, oxygenation and ventilation. Monitoring of cardiac rhythm and vital signs is recommended. General supportive and symptomatic measures are also recommended. Refer to General Management of Acute Overdosage. Consider use of activated charcoal, induction of emesis or gastric lavage. Due to the large volume of distribution of venlafaxine, forced diuresis, dialysis, hemoperfusion and exchange transfusion are unlikely to be of benefit. No specific antidotes are known.

Patient Information:

Caution patients about operating hazardous machinery, including automobiles, until they are reasonably certain that venlafaxine therapy does not adversely affect their ability to engage in such activities.

VENLAFAXINE

Advise patients to notify their physician if they become pregnant or intend to become pregnant during therapy, and to notify their physician if they are breastfeeding.

Advise patients to inform their physician or pharmacist if they are taking, or plan to take, any prescription or over-the-counter drugs, since there is a potential for interactions.

Advise patients to avoid alcohol while taking venlafaxine.

Advise patients to notify their physician if they develop a rash, hives or a related allergic phenomenon.

Administration and Dosage:

Approved by the FDA on December 28, 1993.

Initial treatment: The recommended starting dose is 75 mg/day, administered in 2 or 3 divided doses, taken with food. Depending on tolerability and the need for further clinical effect, the dose may be increased to 150 mg/day. If needed, further increase the dose up to 225 mg/day. When increasing the dose, make increments of up to 75 mg/day at intervals of ≥ 4 days. In outpatient settings there was no evidence of usefulness of doses > 225 mg day for moderately depressed patients, but more severely depressed inpatients responded to a mean dose of 350 mg/day. Certain patients, including more severely depressed patients, may therefore respond more to higher doses, up to a maximum of 375 mg/day, generally in 3 divided doses.

Hepatic function impairment: Given the decrease in clearance and increase in elimination half-life for both venlafaxine and ODV that is observed in patients with hepatic cirrhosis compared to healthy subjects, it is recommended that the total daily dose be reduced by 50% in patients with moderate hepatic impairment. Since there was much individual variability in clearance between patients with cirrhosis, it may be necessary to reduce the dose even more than 50%, and individualization of dosing may be desirable in some patients.

Renal function impairment: Given the decrease in clearance for venlafaxine and the increase in elimination half-life for both venlafaxine and ODV that is observed in patients with renal impairment (GFR, 10 to 70 ml/min) compared to healthy patients, it is recommended that the total daily dose be reduced by 25% in patients with mild to moderate renal impairment. It is recommended that the total daily dose be reduced by 50% and the dose be withheld until the dialysis treatment is completed (4 hrs) in patients undergoing hemodialysis. Since there was much individual variability in clearance between patients with renal impairment, individualization of dosing may be desirable in some patients.

Elderly: No dose adjustment is recommended for elderly patients on the basis of age. As with any antidepressant, however, exercise caution in treating the elderly. When individualizing the dosage, take extra care when increasing the dose.

Maintenance/Continuation/Extended treatment: It is not known how long a patient should continue to be treated with venlafaxine. It is generally agreed that acute episodes of major depression require several months or longer of sustained pharmacologic therapy. Whether the dose of antidepressant needed to induce remission is identical to the dose needed to maintain or sustain euthymia is unknown.

Discontinuing venlafaxine: When discontinuing venlafaxine after > 1 week of therapy, it is generally recommended that the dose be tapered to minimize the risk of discontinuation symptoms. Patients who have received venlafaxine for ≥ 6 weeks should have their dose tapered gradually over a 2 week period.

Switching patients to or from an MAO inhibitor: At least 14 days should elapse between discontinuation of an MAOI and initiation of therapy with venlafaxine. In addition, allow at least 7 days after stopping venlafaxine before starting an MAOI.

Rx	**Effexor** (Wyeth-Ayerst)	**Tablets**: 25 mg	Lactose. (25 W 701). Peach, scored. Shield shape. In 100s, *Redipak* 100s.
		37.5 mg	Lactose. (37.5 W 781). Peach, scored. Shield shape. In 100s, *Redipak* 100s.
		50 mg	Lactose. (50 W 703). Peach, scored. Shield shape. In 100s, *Redipak* 100s.
		75 mg	Lactose. (75 W 704). Peach, scored. Shield shape. In 100s, *Redipak* 100s.
		100 mg	Lactose. (100 W 705). Peach, scored. Shield shape. In 100s, *Redipak* 100s.

NEFAZODONE HCl

Actions:

Pharmacology: Nefazodone is an antidepressant with a chemical structure unrelated to selective serotonin reuptake inhibitors, tricyclics, tetracyclics or monoamine oxidase inhibitors (MAOIs). The mechanism of action of nefazodone, as with other antidepressants, is unknown. Nefazodone inhibits neuronal uptake of serotonin and norepinephrine.

Nefazodone occupies central 5-HT_2 receptors and acts as an antagonist at this receptor. Nefazodone antagonizes alpha$_1$-adrenergic receptors, a property which may be associated with postural hypotension. In vitro, nefazodone had no significant affinity for the following receptors: Alpha$_2$ and beta-adrenergic, 5-HT_{1A}, cholinergic, dopaminergic or benzodiazepine.

Pharmacokinetics:

Absorption/Distribution – Nefazodone is rapidly and completely absorbed, but is subject to extensive metabolism so that its absolute bioavailability is low (about 20%) and variable. Food delays absorption of nefazodone and decreases the bioavailability by ≈ 20%. Peak plasma concentrations occur at about 1 hour. Half-life is 2 to 4 hours. Nefazodone is widely distributed in body tissues, including the CNS. Volume of distribution ranges from 0.22 to 0.87 L/kg.

Both nefazodone and its pharmacologically similar metabolite, hydroxynefazodone, exhibit nonlinear kinetics for both dose and time, with AUC and C_{max} increasing more than proportionally with dose increases and more than expected upon multiple dosing over time, compared to single dosing. Data suggests extensive and greater than predicted accumulation of nefazodone and its hydroxy metabolite with multiple dosing. Steady-state plasma nefazodone and metabolite concentrations are attained within 4 to 5 days of initiation of twice daily dosing or upon dose increase or decrease.

Metabolism/Excretion – Nefazodone is extensively metabolized after oral administration by n-dealkylation and aliphatic and aromatic hydroxylation, and < 1% is excreted unchanged in urine. Three metabolites identified in plasma include hydroxynefazodone (HO-NEF), meta-chlorophenylpiperazine (mCPP) and a triazoledione metabolite. The AUC (expressed as a multiple of the AUC for nefazodone dosed at 100 mg twice daily) and elimination half-lives (hr), respectively, for these three metabolites were as follows: HO-NEF, 0.4 and 1.5 to 4; mCPP, 0.07 and 4 to 8; triazole-dione, 4 and 18.

HO-NEF possesses a pharmacological profile qualitatively and quantitatively similar to that of nefazodone. mCPP has some similarities to nefazodone, but also has agonist activity at some serotonergic receptor subtypes. The pharmacological profile of the triazole-dione metabolite has not yet been well characterized. In addition to the above compounds, several other metabolites were present in plasma but have not been tested for pharmacological activity.

The mean half-life of nefazodone ranged between 11 and 24 hours. Approximately 55% was detected in urine and about 20% to 30% in feces. Nefazodone is extensively (> 99%) bound to human plasma proteins in vitro; nefazodone did not alter the in vitro protein binding of chlorpromazine, desipramine, diazepam, phenytoin, lidocaine, prazosin, propranolol, verapamil or warfarin. There was a 5% decrease in the protein binding of haloperidol; this is probably of no clinical significance.

Renal function impairment (creatinine clearances ranging from 7 to 60 ml/min/1.73 m^2) had no effect on steady-state nefazodone plasma concentrations.

Liver function impairment: In a multiple-dose study of patients with liver cirrhosis, the AUC values for nefazodone and HO-NEF at steady state were ≈ 25% greater than those observed in healthy volunteers.

Age/Gender effects: After single doses of 300 mg, C_{max} and AUC for nefazodone and hydroxynefazodone were up to twice as high in the older patients. With multiple doses, however, differences were much smaller (10% to 20%). A similar result was seen for gender, with a higher C_{max} and AUC in women after single doses but no difference after multiple doses. Initiate treatment with nefazodone at half the usual dose in elderly patients, especially women (see Administration and Dosage); the therapeutic dose range is similar in younger and older patients.

Indications:

Depression: Treatment of depression.

Contraindications:

Coadministration with terfenadine or astemizole (see Warnings and Drug Interactions); hypersensitivity to nefazodone or other phenylpiperazine antidepressants.

NEFAZODONE HCl

Warnings:

Long-term use: The effectiveness of nefazodone in long-term use (ie, for more than 6 to 8 weeks) has not been systematically evaluated. Therefore, periodically reevaluate the long-term usefulness of the drug for the individual patient.

MAO inhibitors: In patients receiving antidepressants with pharmacological properties similar to nefazodone in combination with an MAOI, there have been reports of serious, sometimes fatal, reactions. For a selective serotonin reuptake inhibitor, these reactions have included hyperthermia, rigidity, myoclonus, autonomic instability with possible rapid fluctuations of vital signs and mental status changes that include extreme agitation progressing to delirium and coma. Some cases presented with features resembling neuroleptic malignant syndrome. Severe hyperthermia and seizures, sometimes fatal, have occurred with the combined use of tricyclic antidepressants and MAOIs. These reactions have also been reported in patients who have recently discontinued these drugs and have been started on an MAOI.

Although the effects of combined use of nefazodone and MAOIs have not been evaluated, because nefazodone is an inhibitor of both serotonin and norepinephrine reuptake, it is recommended that nefazodone not be used in combination with an MAOI, or within 14 days of discontinuing treatment with an MAOI. Allow at least 1 week after stopping nefazodone before starting an MAOI.

Antihistamines, nonsedating: Terfenadine and astemizole are both metabolized by the cytochrome P450IIIA4 isozyme; inhibitors of IIIA4 can block the metabolism of terfenadine and astemizole, resulting in increased plasma concentrations of a parent drug which are associated with QT prolongation and with rare cases of serious cardiovascular adverse events, including death, due principally to ventricular tachycardia of the torsade de pointes type. In vitro, nefazodone inhibits IIIA4. Consequently, it is recommended that nefazodone not be used in combination with either terfenadine or astemizole (see Contraindications and Drug Interactions).

Fertility impairment: A fertility study in rats showed a slight decrease in fertility at 200 mg/kg/day (approximately three times the maximum human daily dose).

Elderly: Initiate treatment at half the usual dose, but titration upward should take place over the same range as in younger patients (see Administration and Dosage). Observe the usual precautions in elderly patients who have concomitant medical illnesses or who are receiving concomitant drugs.

Pregnancy: Category C. Increased early pup mortality was seen in rats at a dose approximately five times the maximum human dose and decreased pup weights were seen at this and lower doses, when dosing began during pregnancy and continued until weaning. There are no adequate and well controlled studies in pregnant women. Use during pregnancy only if the potential benefit justifies the potential risk to the fetus.

Lactation: It is not known whether nefazodone or its metabolites are excreted in breast milk. Exercise caution when nefazodone is administered to a nursing woman.

Children: Safety and efficacy in individuals < 18 years old have not been established.

Precautions:

Postural hypotension: Studies revealed that 5.1% of nefazodone patients compared to 2.5% of placebo patients met criteria for a potentially important decrease in blood pressure at some time during treatment (systolic blood pressure ≤ 90 mm Hg and a change from baseline of ≥ 20 mm Hg). While there was no difference in the proportion of nefazodone and placebo patients having adverse events characterized as syncope (nefazodone, 0.2%; placebo, 0.3%), the rates for adverse events characterized as postural hypotension were as follows: Nefazodone (2.8%), tricyclic antidepressants (10.9%), SSRIs (1.1%) and placebo (0.8%). Use nefazodone with caution in patients with known cardiovascular or cerebrovascular disease that could be exacerbated by hypotension (eg, history of MI, angina, ischemic stroke) and conditions that would predispose patients to hypotension (eg, dehydration, hypovolemia, treatment with antihypertensive medication).

Mania/hypomania: Hypomania or mania occurred in 0.3% of nefazodone-treated unipolar patients, compared to 0.3% of tricyclic and 0.4% of placebo-treated patients. In patients classified as bipolar the rate of manic episodes was 1.6% for nefazodone, 5.1% for the combined tricyclic-treated groups and 0% for placebo-treated patients. Activation of mania/hypomania is a known risk in a small proportion of patients with major affective disorder treated with other marketed antidepressants. As with all antidepressants, use nefazodone cautiously in patients with a history of mania.

Suicide: The possibility of a suicide attempt is inherent in depression and may persist until significant remission occurs. Closely supervise high-risk patients during initial therapy. Write prescriptions for the smallest quantity of nefazodone consistent with good patient management to reduce the risk of overdose.

Seizures: A recurrence of a petit mal seizure was observed in a patient receiving nefazodone who had a history of such seizures. One nonstudy participant took 2000 to 3000 mg nefazodone with methocarbamol and alcohol; this person reportedly experienced a convulsion (type not documented).

Priapism: While priapism did not occur during premarketing experience with nefazodone, priapism has been reported with a structurally related drug, trazodone. If patients present with prolonged or inappropriate erections, they should discontinue therapy immediately and consult their physicians. If the condition persists for > 24 hours, consult a urologist to determine appropriate management.

Bradycardia: Sinus bradycardia (eg, heart rate ≤ 50 bpm and a decrease of at least 15 bpm from baseline) was observed in 1.5% of nefazodone patients (0.4% with placebo). Treat patients with a recent MI or unstable heart disease with caution.

Hepatic cirrhosis: In patients with cirrhosis of the liver, the AUC values of nefazodone and its metabolite HO-NEF were increased by ≈ 25%.

Drug abuse and dependence: Premarketing clinical experience with nefazodone did not reveal any tendency for a withdrawal syndrome or any drug-seeking behavior. However, carefully evaluate patients for a history of drug abuse and follow such patients closely, observing them for signs of misuse or abuse of nefazodone.

Drug Interactions:

Potential interaction with drugs that inhibit or are metabolized by cytochrome P450 (IIIA4 and IID6) isozymes: In vitro, nefazodone is an inhibitor of cytochrome P450IIIA4. This is consistent with the interaction observed between nefazodone and triazolam and alprazolam, drugs metabolized by this isozyme. Consequently, caution is indicated in the combined use of nefazodone with any drugs known to be metabolized by the IIIA4 isozyme (in particular, terfenadine or astemizole).

Nefazodone and its metabolites in vitro are extremely weak inhibitors of P450IID6. Thus, it is not likely that nefazodone will decrease the metabolic clearance of drugs metabolized by this isozyme.

Drugs highly bound to plasma protein: Because nefazodone is highly bound to plasma protein, administration to a patient taking another drug that is highly protein bound may cause increased free concentrations of the other drug, potentially resulting in adverse events. Conversely, adverse effects could result from displacement of nefazodone by other highly bound drugs.

Nefazodone Drug Interactions			
Precipitant drug	Object drug*		Description
MAOIs	Nefazodone	↑	Serious, sometimes fatal reactions may occur, including hyperthermia, rigidity, myoclonus and mental status changes that include extreme agitation and coma (see Warnings).
Nefazodone	Antihistamines, nonsedating	↑	Plasma levels of astemizole and terfenadine may be increased, resulting in QT prolongation or torsade de pointes, sometimes fatal (see Warnings). Do not use concurrently.
Nefazodone	Benzodiazepines	↑	Substantial and clinically important increases in plasma concentrations of alprazolam and triazolam have occurred. Lorazepam was not affected.
Nefazodone	Digoxin	↑	In one study, C_{max}, C_{min} and AUC of digoxin were increased by 29%, 27% and 15%, respectively. Plasma level monitoring for digoxin is recommended.
Nefazodone	Haloperidol	↑	Haloperidol apparent clearance decreased by 35% with no significant increase in peak plasma concentrations or time to peak.
Nefazodone	Propranolol	↓	Coadministration resulted in 30% and 14% reductions in C_{max} and AUC of propranolol, respectively, and a 14% reduction in C_{max} for the metabolite, 4-hydroxypropranolol. C_{max}, C_{min} and AUC of the nefazodone metabolite m-chlorophenylpiperazine were increased by 23%, 54% and 28%, respectively.

* ↑ = Object drug increased. ↓ = Object drug decreased.

NEFAZODONE HCl

Adverse Reactions:

Approximately 16% of the 3496 patients who received nefazodone in worldwide premarketing clinical trials discontinued treatment due to an adverse experience. The more common events in clinical trials associated with discontinuation included: Nausea (3.5%); dizziness (1.9%); insomnia (1.5%); asthenia (1.3%); agitation (1.2%).

Nefazodone Adverse Reactions (%)

Adverse reaction	Nefazodone (n = 393)	Placebo (n = 394)
GI		
Dry mouth	25	13
Nausea	22	12
Constipation	14	8
Dyspepsia	9	7
Diarrhea	8	7
Increased appetite	5	3
Nausea and vomiting	2	1
Special senses		
Blurred vision	9	3
Abnormal vision (scotoma, visual trails)	7	1
Tinnitus	2	1
Taste perversion	2	1
Visual field defect	2	0
Cardiovascular		
Postural hypotension	4	1
Hypotension	2	1
Respiratory		
Pharyngitis	6	5
Cough increased	3	1
Metabolic		
Peripheral edema	3	2
Thirst	1	< 1
GU		
Urinary frequency	2	1
Urinary tract infection	2	1
Urinary retention	2	1
Vaginitis (incidence adjusted for gender)	2	1
Breast pain (incidence adjusted for gender)	1	< 1

Adverse reaction	Nefazodone (n = 393)	Placebo (n = 394)
CNS		
Somnolence	25	14
Dizziness	17	5
Insomnia	11	9
Lightheadedness	10	3
Confusion	7	2
Memory impairment	4	2
Paresthesia	4	2
Vasodilation (flushing, feeling warm)	4	2
Abnormal dreams	3	2
Concentration decreased	3	1
Ataxia	2	0
Incoordination	2	1
Psychomotor retardation	2	1
Tremor	2	1
Hypertonia	1	0
Libido decreased	1	< 1
Body as a whole		
Headache	36	33
Asthenia	11	5
Infection	8	6
Flu syndrome	3	2
Chills	2	1
Fever	2	1
Neck rigidity	1	0
Arthralgia	1	< 1
Dermatological		
Pruritus	2	1
Rash	2	1

Dose Dependency of Nefazodone Adverse Reactions (%)

Adverse reaction	Nefazodone 300 to 600 mg/day (n = 209)	Nefazodone ≤ 300 mg/day (n = 211)	Placebo (n = 212)
GI			
Nausea	23	14	12
Constipation	17	10	9
CNS			
Somnolence	28	16	13
Dizziness	22	11	4
Confusion	8	2	1
Special senses			
Abnormal vision	10	0	2
Blurred vision	9	3	2
Tinnitus	3	0	1

NEFAZODONE HCl

Body as a whole: Allergic reaction, malaise, photosensitivity reaction, face edema, hangover effect, abdomen enlarged, hernia, pelvic pain, halitosis (0.1% to 1%); cellulitis (< 0.1%).

Cardiovascular: Sinus bradycardia (1.5%); tachycardia, hypertension, syncope, ventricular extrasystoles, angina pectoris (0.1% to 1%); AV block, CHF, hemorrhage, pallor, varicose vein (< 0.1%).

Dermatologic: Dry skin, acne, alopecia, urticaria, maculopapular rash, vesiculobullous rash, eczema (0.1% to 1%).

GI: Gastroenteritis (1%); eructation, periodontal abscess, abnormal liver function tests, gingivitis, colitis, gastritis, mouth ulceration, stomatitis, esophagitis, peptic ulcer, rectal hemorrhage (0.1% to 1%); glossitis, hepatitis, dysphagia, GI hemorrhage, oral moniliasis, ulcerative colitis (< 0.1%).

Hematologic/Lymphatic: Decrease in hematocrit (2.8%); ecchymosis, anemia, leukopenia, lymphadenopathy (0.1% to 1%).

Metabolic/Nutritional: Weight loss, gout, dehydration, lactic dehydrogenase increased, AST and ALT increased (0.1% to 1%); hypercholesterolemia, hypoglycemia (< 0.1%).

Musculoskeletal: Arthritis, tenosynovitis, muscle stiffness, bursitis (0.1% to 1%); tendinous contracture (< 0.1%).

CNS: Vertigo, twitching, depersonalization, hallucinations, suicide thoughts/attempt, apathy, euphoria, hostility, abnormal gait, thinking abnormal, attention decreased, derealization, neuralgia, paranoid reaction, dysarthria, increased libido, suicide, myoclonus (0.1% to 1%); hyperkinesia, increased salivation, cerebrovascular accident, hyperesthesia, hypotonia, ptosis, neuroleptic malignant syndrome (< 0.1%).

Respiratory: Dyspnea, bronchitis (1%); asthma, pneumonia, laryngitis, voice alteration, epistaxis, hiccup (0.1% to 1%); hyperventilation, yawn (< 0.1%).

Special senses: Eye pain (1%); dry eye, ear pain, abnormality of accommodation, diplopia, conjunctivitis, mydriasis, keratoconjunctivitis, hyperacusis, photophobia (0.1% to 1%); deafness, glaucoma, night blindness, taste loss (< 0.1%).

GU: Impotence (1%); cystitis, urinary urgency, metrorrhagia, amenorrhea, polyuria, vaginal hemorrhage, breast enlargement, menorrhagia, urinary incontinence, abnormal ejaculation, hematuria, nocturia, kidney calculus (0.1% to 1%); uterine fibroids enlarged, uterine hemorrhage, anorgasmia, oliguria (< 0.1%).

Overdosage:

Symptoms: In premarketing clinical studies, there were seven reports of nefazodone overdose alone or in combination with other pharmacological agents. The amount of nefazodone ingested ranged from 1000 to 11,200 mg. Commonly reported symptoms included nausea, vomiting and somnolence. None of the patients died.

Treatment: Overdosage may cause an increase in incidence or severity of any of the reported adverse reactions (see Adverse Reactions). There is no specific antidote for nefazodone. Treatment should be symptomatic and supportive in the case of hypotension or excessive sedation. Any patient suspected of having taken an overdose should have the stomach emptied by gastric lavage. Refer to General Management of Acute Overdosage.

Patient Information:

Several weeks of treatment may be required to obtain the full antidepressant effect. Once improvement is noted, it is important for patients to continue drug treatment as directed.

Caution patients about operating hazardous machinery, including automobiles, until they are reasonably certain that nefazodone therapy does not adversely affect their ability to engage in such activities. Avoid alcohol while taking nefazodone.

Advise patients to notify their physician if they become pregnant or intend to become pregnant during therapy or if they are breastfeeding an infant.

Advise patients to inform their physician or pharmacist if they are taking, or plan to take, any prescription or over-the-counter drugs, since there is a potential for interactions. Significant caution is indicated if nefazodone is to be used in combination with either alprazolam or triazolam and concomitant use with astemizole or terfenadine is contraindicated (see Warnings).

Advise patients to notify their physician if they develop a rash, hives, or a related allergic phenomenon.

NEFAZODONE HCl

Administration and Dosage:

Approved by the FDA on December 22, 1994 (1S classification).

Initial treatment: Recommended starting dose is 200 mg/day, administered in two divided doses. In clinical trials, the effective dose range was generally 300 to 600 mg/day. Consequently, most patients, depending on tolerability and the need for further clinical effect, should have their dose increased. Increase doses in increments of 100 to 200 mg/day, again on a twice daily schedule, at intervals of ≥ 1 week. Several weeks of treatment may be required to obtain a full antidepressant response.

Elderly/Debilitated patients: The recommended initial dose is 100 mg/day on a twice daily schedule. These patients often have reduced nefazodone clearance or increased sensitivity to the side effects of CNS-active drugs. It may also be appropriate to modify the rate of subsequent dose titration. As steady-state plasma levels do not change with age, the final target dose based on a careful assessment of the patient's clinical response may be similar in healthy younger and older patients.

Maintenance/Continuation/Extended treatment: There is no evidence to indicate how long the depressed patient should be treated with nefazodone. It is generally agreed, however, that pharmacological treatment for acute episodes of depression should continue for ≥ 6 months. Whether the dose of antidepressant needed to induce remission is identical to the dose needed to maintain euthymia is unknown. In clinical trials, > 250 patients were treated for ≥ 1 year.

Switching to or from an MAOI: At least 14 days should elapse between discontinuation of an MAOI and initiation of therapy with nefazodone. In addition, allow at least 7 days after stopping nefazodone before starting an MAOI.

Rx	**Serzone** (Bristol-Myers Squibb)	**Tablets:** 100 mg	(BMS 100 mg). White, scored. In 60s and 100s.
		150 mg	(BMS 150 mg). Peach, scored. In 60s and 100s.
		200 mg	(BMS 200 mg). Lt. yellow. In 60s and 100s.
		250 mg	(BMS 250 mg). White. In 60s.

SELECTIVE SEROTONIN REUPTAKE INHIBITORS

Actions:

Pharmacology: Selective serotonin reuptake inhibitors (SSRIs) are oral antidepressant agents chemically unrelated to the tricyclic, tetracyclic or other available antidepressants. The antidepressant action of the SSRIs is presumed to be linked to their inhibition of CNS neuronal uptake of serotonin (5HT). Studies in humans and in vitro studies have demonstrated that fluoxetine (and its active metabolite norfluoxetine), fluvoxamine, paroxetine and sertraline are potent and selective inhibitors of neuronal serotonin reuptake, and they also have a weak effect on norepinephrine and dopamine neuronal reuptake. SSRIs have little affinity for muscarinic, GABA, benzodiazepine, $alpha_1$, $alpha_2$, beta-adrenergic, dopamine (D_2), 5-HT_1, 5-HT_2 and histamine (H_1) receptors; antagonism of muscarinic, histaminergic and $alpha_1$-adrenergic receptors has been associated with various anticholinergic, sedative and cardiovascular effects for other psychotropic drugs.The chronic administration of sertraline in animals was found to down-regulate brain norepinephrine receptors, as has been observed with other clinically effective antidepressants.

Pharmacokinetics:

SSRI Pharmacokinetics							
SSRIs	Time to peak plasma concentration (hr)	Peak plasma concentration (ng/ml)	Half-life (hrs)	Protein binding (%)	Time to reach steady state (days)	Primary route of elimination	Bioavailability (%)
Fluoxetine	6-8	15-55	1 to 384[1]	≈ 94.5	28-35	hepatic	94
Fluvoxamine	3-8	88-546	13.6-15.6	77- 80	≈ 7	renal	53
Paroxetine	5.2	61.7	21	93-95	≈10	64% renal, 36% hepatic	100
Sertraline	4.5-8.4	20-55	26-104[1]	98	7	40%-45% renal, 40%-45% hepatic	nd

[1] t½ includes the active metabolite.
nd = no data

Elderly – A study of **fluvoxamine** 50 to 100 mg in elderly subjects (66 to 73 years) found that the mean maximum plasma concentration was 40% higher compared to subjects aged 19 to 35 years. The elimination half-life was also delayed. AUC and C_{max} were also affected. In a multi-dose study of **paroxetine** in the elderly at daily doses of 20, 30 and 40 mg, C_{min} concentrations were ≈ 70% to 80% greater than the respective C_{min} concentrations in nonelderly subjects. Therefore, reduce the initial dosage of paroxetine in the elderly (see Administration and Dosage). **Sertraline** plasma clearance in a group of 16 (8 male, 8 female) elderly patients treated for 14 days at a dose of 100 mg/day was ≈ 40% lower than in a similarly studied group of younger (25 to 32 years old) individuals. Steady state, therefore, should be achieved after 2 to 3 weeks in older patients. The same study showed a decreased clearance of desmethylsertraline in older males but not in older females.

Indications:

Obsessive-Compulsive Disorder (OCD): Treatment of obsessions and compulsions in patients with OCD, as defined in the DSM-III-R (obsessions and compulsions cause marked distress, are time-consuming, or significantly interfere with functioning).

Depression: Fluoxetine, paroxetine, sertraline -Treatment of depression.

Bulimia Nervosa: Fluoxetine –Treatment of binge-eating and vomiting behaviors in patients with moderate to severe bulimia nervosa.

Unlabeled uses: Fluoxetine-Alcoholism (40 to 80 mg/day); anorexia nervosa (20 to 80 mg/day); attention-deficit hyperactivity disorder (20 to 60 mg/day); bipolar II affective disorder (20 to 80 mg/day); borderline personality disorder (5 to 80 mg/day); cataplexy and narcolepsy (20 to 40 mg/day); kleptomania (60 to 80 mg/day); migraine, chronic daily headaches and tension-type headache (20 mg every other day to 40 mg/day); obesity (20 to 60 mg/day) (see Precautions); posttraumatic stress disorder (10 to 80 mg/day); premenstrual syndrome (20 mg/day); recurrent syncope (20 mg/day); schizophrenia (20 to 60 mg/day); Tourette's syndrome (20 to 40 mg/day); trichotillomania (20 to 80 mg/day); levodopa-induced dyskinesia (40 mg/day); social phobia (10 to 60 mg/day).

Fluvoxamine is being investigated in the treatment of depression.

SELECTIVE SEROTONIN REUPTAKE INHIBITORS

Paroxetine – Diabetic neuropathy (10 to 60 mg/day); headaches (10 to 50 mg/day); premature ejaculation (20 mg/day).

Contraindications:

Hypersensitivity to SSRIs; in combination with an MAO inhibitor, or within 14 days of discontinuing an MAOI (see Drug Interactions); coadministration of **fluvoxamine** with astemizole, cisapride or terfenadine (see Drug Interactions).

Warnings:

Long-term use: The effectiveness of long-term use of SSRIs (> 5 to 10 weeks for depression [**sertraline** >12 weeks]) (>13 weeks for OCD with **fluoxetine**) has not been systematically evaluated, except for **paroxetine** (the efficacy of paroxetine in maintaining an antidepressant response for up to 1 year was demonstrated in a placebo controlled trial). Therefore, periodically reevaluate the SSRIs used for extended periods to determine long-term usefulness of the drug for the individual patient.

MAO inhibitors: In patients receiving an SSRI in combination with an MAOI, serious, sometimes fatal, reactions have occurred including hyperthermia, rigidity, myoclonus, autonomic instability with possible rapid fluctuations of vital signs, and mental status changes that include extreme agitation progressing to delirium and coma. These reactions have also occurred in patients who have recently discontinued an SSRI and have been started on an MAOI. Some cases presented with features resembling neuroleptic malignant syndrome. While there are no human data showing such an interaction with **paroxetine**, limited animal data suggest that the drugs may act synergistically to elevate blood pressure and evoke behavioral excitation. Therefore, it is recommended that SSRIs not be used in combination with an MAOI or within 14 days of discontinuing treatment with an MAOI. Allow at least 2 weeks after stopping the SSRIs before starting an MAOI; allow at least 5 weeks after stopping fluoxetine before starting an MAOI. (see Drug Interactions).

Altered platelet function or abnormal results from laboratory studies in patients taking **fluoxetine, paroxetine** or **sertraline** have occured. There have been reports of abnormal bleeding in several patients; it is unclear whether the SSRIs had a causative role.

Rash and accompanying events: Approximately 4% of patients taking **fluoxetine** have developed a rash or urticaria; ≈ 33% were withdrawn from treatment. Clinical findings reported in association with rash include: Fever, leukocytosis, arthralgias, edema, carpal tunnel syndrome, respiratory distress, lymphadenopathy, proteinuria and mild transaminase elevation. Most patients improved promptly with discontinuation of fluoxetine or adjunctive treatment with antihistamines or steroids; all patients recovered completely. Two patients treated with fluoxetine developed a serious cutaneous systemic illness. Neither had an unequivocal diagnosis, but one had a leukocytoclastic vasculitis; the other had a severe desquamating syndrome that was considered to be vasculitis or erythema multiforme. Other patients have had systemic syndromes suggestive of serum sickness.

Systemic events, possibly related to vasculitis, have developed in patients with rash. Although rare, these events may be serious, involving lung, kidney or liver. Death has been associated with the events. Anaphylactoid events, including bronchospasm, angioedema and urticaria, alone and in combination, have occurred with fluoxetine. Pulmonary events, including inflammatory processes of varying histopathology or fibrosis, have occurred rarely. These events have occurred with dyspnea as the only preceding symptom. It is unknown whether the association of rash and other events constitutes a true fluoxetine-induced syndrome. No patient sustained lasting injury. Though almost 66% of patients developing a rash continued to take fluoxetine without any consequences, discontinue if rash appears.

Renal function impairment: In single-dose studies, kinetics of **fluoxetine** and norfluoxetine were similar among all levels of impaired renal function, including anephric patients on chronic hemodialysis. However, with chronic use, additional accumulation of fluoxetine or its metabolites may occur with severely impaired renal function; use a lower or less frequent dose.

Increased plasma concentrations of **paroxetine** occur in subjects with renal and hepatic impairment. Reduce the initial dosage of paroxetine in patients with severe renal impairment; upward titration, if necessary, should be at increased intervals (see Administration and Dosage).

Since **sertraline** is extensively metabolized by the liver, excretion of unchanged drug in the urine is a minor route of elimination. However, use with caution in patients with severe renal impairment.

Hepatic function impairment: SSRIs are extensively metabolized by the liver. Use with caution in patients with severe liver impairment. The elimination half-life of

SELECTIVE SEROTONIN REUPTAKE INHIBITORS

fluoxetine was prolonged in a study of cirrhotic patients, with a mean of 7.6 days; norfluoxetine elimination was also delayed, with a mean duration of 12 days. **Fluvoxamine** clearance was decreased by 30%; slowly titrate fluvoxamine during initiation of treatment. **Paroxetine** levels increased ≈ 2-fold. The clearance of **sertraline** is decreased in mild, stable cirrhotics. Give a lower or less frequent dose in patients with severe hepatic dysfunction; upward titration, if necessary, should be at increased intervals. (See Administration and Dosage.)

Carcinogenesis: In mice and rats given **paroxetine** at 2 to 4 times the maximum recommended human dose (MRHD) for depression on a mg/m^2 basis, there was a significantly greater number of male rats with reticulum cell sarcomas and a significantly increased linear trend across dose groups for the occurrence of lymphoreticular tumors in male rats. There was a dose-related increase in the incidence of liver adenomas in male mice receiving **sertraline** at 10 to 40 mg/kg (0.25 to 1 times the MRHD on a mg/m^2 basis). Liver adenomas have a variable rate of spontaneous occurrence in the CD-1 mouse and are of unknown significance to humans. There was an increase in follicular adenomas of the thyroid in female rats receiving sertraline at 40 mg/kg; this was not accompanied by thyroid hyperplasia. While there was an increase in uterine adenocarcinomas in rats receiving sertraline at 10 to 40 mg/kg compared to placebo controls, this effect was not clearly drug-related.

Fertility impairment: A decrease in fertility was seen with **sertraline** in one of two rat studies at a dose of 80 mg/kg (4 times the MRHD on a mg/m^2 basis).

Elderly: The disposition of single doses of **fluoxetine** in healthy elderly subjects (≥ 65 years of age) did not differ significantly from that in younger normal subjects. However, data are insufficient to rule out possible age-related differences during chronic use. Clearance of **fluvoxamine** is decreased by ≈ 50% in elderly patients. In clinical trials, 17% of **paroxetine**-treated patients were > 65 years of age. Pharmacokinetic studies revealed a decreased clearance in the elderly, and a lower starting dose is recommended; there was, however, no overall difference in the adverse event profile between elderly and younger patients, and efficacy was similar. Several hundred elderly patients have participated in clinical studies with **sertraline**. The pattern of adverse reactions in the elderly was similar to that in younger patients. However, sertraline plasma clearance may be lower (see Pharmacokinetics).

Pregnancy: Category B (fluoxetine); Category C (paroxetine, sertraline, fluvoxamine). There are no adequate and well controlled studies in pregnant women. Use during pregnancy only if clearly needed. In a study involving 228 women who had received fluoxetine during pregnancy, 5.5% of the women who took fluoxetine in the first trimester delivered with major structural anomalies. Also, the rate of prematurity was significantly higher when the fetus was exposed to fluoxetine late in the pregnancy (14.3%) versus early in the pregnancy (4.1%). At doses 0.5 to 4 times the maximum recommended human mg/kg dose, **sertraline** was associated with delayed ossification in fetuses of rats and rabbits. The decrease in pup survival was most probably due to in utero exposure to sertraline. In rats, **fluvoxamine** increased pup mortality at birth and decreased postnatal pup weight and survival.

Lactation: **Fluoxetine, fluvoxamine** and **paroxetine** are excreted in breast milk. It is not known whether **sertraline** or its metabolites are excreted in breast milk. In one breast milk sample, the concentration of fluoxetine plus norfluoxetine was 70.4 ng/ml; the mother's plasma concentration was 295 ng/ml. No adverse effects were noted in the infant. Exercise caution when SSRIs are administered to a nursing woman.

Children: Safety and efficacy in children (< 18 years of age) have not been established.

Precautions:

Anxiety, nervousness and insomnia occurred in 3% to 33% of patients treated with an SSRI.

Altered appetite and weight: Significant weight loss, especially in underweight depressed patients, has occurred. Approximately 3% to ≈ 9% of patients treated with an SSRI experienced anorexia, although this side effect was not reported with **paroxetine**-treated patients. A weight loss of > 5% occurred in 13% of **fluoxetine**-treated patients compared to 4% of placebo and 3% of tricyclic antidepressant-treated patients. Significant weight loss may be an undesirable result of treatment for some patients, but on average, patients in controlled trials treated with paroxetine or **sertraline** had a minimal 1 to 2 pound weight loss vs smaller changes with placebo. However, only rarely have the SSRIs been discontinued because of weight loss or anorexia (see Adverse Reactions).

Activation of mania/hypomania occurred infrequently in ≈ 0.1% to 2.2% of patients taking SSRIs (**fluoxetine,** ≈ 1%; **fluvoxamine,** ≈ 1%; ≈ **paroxetine** 1% in unipolar patients, 2.2% in bipolar patients; **sertraline** ≈ 0.4%). Paroxetine-treated patients with bipolar depression had a lower rate of manic episodes (2.2%) compared to active controls (11.6%). Activation of mania/hypomania has also occurred in a small proportion of patients with Major Affective Disorder treated with other antidepressants. Use cautiously in patients with a history of mania.

Seizures have occurred with **fluoxetine** (0.2%), **fluvoxamine** (0.2%), **paroxetine** (0.1%) and **sertraline** (0.2%). Sertraline has not been evaluated in patients with a seizure disorder. These percentages appear similar to the rate associated with other antidepressants. Use with care in patients with history of seizures.

Suicide: The possibility of a suicide attempt is inherent in depression and may persist until significant remission occurs. Close supervision of high-risk patients should accompany initial drug therapy. Write prescriptions for the smallest quantity of tablets or capsules in order to reduce the risk of overdose.

Dose changes: The long elimination half-life of **fluoxetine** and norfluoxetine means that changes in dose will not be fully reflected in plasma for several weeks, affecting titration to final dose and withdrawal from treatment.

Concomitant illness: Clinical experience is limited. Use caution in patients with diseases or conditions that could affect metabolism or hemodynamic responses.

Electroconvulsive therapy (ECT): There are no clinical studies establishing the benefit of the combined use of ECT and SSRIs. Rare prolonged seizure in patients on **fluoxetine** has occurred.

Hyponatremia: Several cases of **fluoxetine, sertraline** and **paroxetine**-induced hyponatremia (some with serum sodium < 110 mmol/L) have occurred. The hyponatremia appeared to be reversible when fluoxetine, sertraline or paroxetine were discontinued. Although these cases were complex with varying possible etiologies, some were possibly due to the syndrome of inappropriate antidiuretic hormone secretion (SIADH). The majority of these occurrences have been in older patients and in patients taking diuretics or who were otherwise volume-depleted.

Diabetes: **Fluoxetine** may alter glycemic control. Hypoglycemia has occurred during therapy, and hyperglycemia has developed following discontinuation of the drug. The dosage of insulin or oral hypoglycemia may need to be adjusted when fluoxetine is started or discontinued.

Uricosuric effect: **Sertraline** is associated with a mean decrease in serum uric acid of ≈ 7%. The clinical significance of this weak uricosuric effect is unknown, and there have been no reports of acute renal failure with sertraline.

Drug abuse and dependence: Premarketing clinical experience did not reveal any tendency for a withdrawal syndrome or any drug-seeking behavior. There have been 2 cases of men without a history of major psychiatric disorder developing severe behavioural symptoms when **paroxetine** was withdrawn. It is not possible to predict on the basis of this limited experience the extent to which a CNS active drug will be misused, diverted or abused once marketed. Consequently, before starting an SSRI, carefully evaluate patients for history of drug abuse and follow such patients closely, observing them for signs of misuse or abuse.

Hazardous tasks: SSRIs may cause dizziness or drowsiness. Patients should be instructed to observe caution while driving or performing tasks requiring alertness, coordination or physical dexterity.

Photosensitivity: Photosensitization may occur; therefore, caution patients to take protective measures (eg, sunscreens, protective clothing) against exposure to ultraviolet light or sunlight until tolerance is determined.

Drug Interactions:

Drugs highly bound to plasma protein: Because SSRIs are highly bound to plasma protein, administration to a patient taking another drug that is highly protein-bound may cause increased free concentrations of the other drug, potentially resulting in adverse events. Conversely, adverse effects could result from displacement of SSRIs by other highly bound drugs.

Microsomal enzyme induction: Concomitant use of SSRIs with drugs metabolized by cytochrome $P450IID_6$ may require lower doses than usually prescribed for either SSRIs or the other drug because SSRIs may significantly inhibit the activity of this isozyme. In most patients (> 90%), this isozyme is saturated early during dosing. Therefore, coadministration of paroxetine with other drugs that are metabolized by this isozyme (eg, certain antidepressants, phenothiazines, Type IC antiarrhythmics) or drugs that inhibit this enzyme (eg, quinidine) should be approached with caution. **Fluvoxamine** is a relatively weak inhibitor of this isozyme. However, in vitro the drug

SELECTIVE SEROTONIN REUPTAKE INHIBITORS

inhibits the IA_2 and IIC_9 isozymes, which are involved in the metabolism of warfarin, theophylline, propranolol and alprazolam.

Sertraline induced hepatic microsomal enzymes minimally in clinical studies.

SSRI Drug Interactions

Precipitant drug	Object drug*		Description
Cimetidine	SSRIs Paroxetine Sertraline	↑	Cimetidine increased steady-state paroxetine concentrations by ≈ 50%. Cimetidine increases sertraline AUC (50%), Cmax (24%) and half-life (26%).
Dextromethorphan	SSRIs Fluoxetine	↑	Hallucinations have occurred during concurrent use.
MAO inhibitors	SSRIs	↑	Serious, sometimes fatal, reactions have occurred in patients receiving SSRIs in combination with an MAOI and in patients who have recently discontinued the SSRI and are then started on an MAOI (see Warnings).
Phenobarbital	SSRIs Paroxetine	↓	Phenobarbital decreased the AUC and half-life of paroxetine by 25% and 38%, respectively.
Phenytoin	SSRIs Paroxetine	↓	Phenytoin reduced the AUC and half-life of paroxetine by 50% and 35%, respectively. Also, paroxetine reduced the AUC of phenytoin by 12%, and fluoxetine may increase hydantoin levels.
SSRIs Paroxetine Fluoxetine	Phenytoin	↔	
Smoking	SSRIs Fluvoxamine	↓	Smokers had a 25% increase in the metabolism of fluvoxamine.
L-tryptophan	SSRIs Fluoxetine Fluvoxamine Paroxetine	↑	Concurrent use with fluoxetine or paroxetine may produce symptoms related to both central toxicity (eg, headache, sweating, dizziness, agitation, restlessness) and peripheral toxicity (GI: eg, nausea, vomiting).
SSRIs	Alcohol	↔	Although potentiation of impairment of mental and motor skills caused by alcohol has not occurred, concurrent use is not recommended in depressed patients.
SSRIs	Antidepressants, tricyclic	↑	Plasma TCA levels may be increased.
SSRIs Fluvoxamine	Antihistamines, nonsedating	↑	Plasma levels of astemizole and terfenadine may be increased, resulting in QT prolongation or torsades de pointes, sometimes fatal. Do not use concurrently.
SSRIs Fluvoxamine Sertraline Fluoxetine	Benzodiazepines	↑	Clearance of benzodiazepines metabolized by hepatic oxidation may be decreased; those metabolized by glucuronidation are unlikely to be affected. Coadministration of alprazolam and fluoxetine has resulted in increased alprazolam levels and decreased psychomoter performance.
SSRIs Fluvoxamine	Beta blockers	↑	Minimal propranolol levels have increased 5-fold; a slight potentiation of propranolol-induced reduction in heart rate and exercise diastolic pressure has occurred. Bradycardia and hypotension occurred with metoprolol. Atenolol levels were not affected.
SSRIs Fluoxetine	Buspirone	↓	Effects of buspirone may be decreased. Paradoxical worsening of OCD has occurred.
SSRIs Fluoxetine Fluvoxamine	Carbamazepine	↑	Serum carbamazepine levels may be increased, possibly resulting in toxicity.
SSRIs Fluvoxamine Fluoxetine	Clozapine	↑	Elevated serum clozapine levels have occurred.

SELECTIVE SEROTONIN REUPTAKE INHIBITORS

SSRI Drug Interactions

Precipitant drug	Object drug*		Description
SSRIs Fluvoxamine	Diltiazem	↑	Bradycardia has occurred with concurrent use.
SSRIs Fluoxetine	Cyclosporine	↑	An elevated cyclosporine trough was reported in a 59-year-old patient during concomitant administration.
SSRIs Paroxetine	Digoxin	↓	Paroxetine decreased the AUC of digoxin by 15%.
SSRIs Fluvoxamine Fluoxetine	Haloperidol	↑	Serum concentrations of haloperidol may be increased; recall memory and attentional functions test may be delayed.
SSRIs Fluoxetine Sertraline Fluvoxamine	Lithium	↑↓	Lithium levels may be increased or decreased by fluoxetine with possible neurotoxicity. In healthy volunteers, sertraline did not affect lithium levels. It is recommended that plasma lithium levels be monitored following initiation of sertraline. Lithium may enhance the serotonergic effects of fluvoxamine.
Lithium	SSRIs Fluvoxamine	↑	
SSRIs Fluvoxamine	Methadone	↑	Significantly increased methadone (plasma level: dose) ratios have occurred. One patient developed opioid intoxication, another had opioid withdrawal symptoms with fluvoxamine discontinuation.
SSRIs Fluoxetine	Phentermine	↑	Eight days after stopping fluoxetine, a patient took phentermine and developed hyperstimulation.
SSRIs Fluoxetine	Pimozide	↑	A single case report has suggested possible additive effects of pimozide and fluoxetine leading to bradycardia.
SSRIs Paroxetine	Procyclidine	↑	Paroxetine increased the AUC, C_{max} and C_{min} of procyclidine by 35%, 37% and 67%, respectively. Reduce procyclidine dose if anticholinergic effects occur.
SSRIs Fluvoxamine	Sumatriptan	↑	Weakness, hyperreflexia and incoordination have occured with coadministration.
SSRIs Fluvoxamine Paroxetine	Theophylline	↑	Clearance of theophylline may be decreased by 3-fold; reduce dosage. Elevated theophylline levels have occured with paroxetine.
SSRIs Sertraline	Tolbutamide	↑	In one study sertraline significantly decreased the clearance of tolbutamide (16%). Clinical significance is unknown.
SSRIs	Warfarin	↑	A pharmacodynamic interaction (increased bleeding diathesis with unaltered prothrombin time [PT]) may occur with paroxetine or fluoxetine. Concurrent administration of sertraline and warfarin has resulted in an 8% increase in PT and delayed PT normalization. Fluvoxamine increased warfarin plasma levels by 98%; PT was prolonged. Monitor PT.

* ↑ = Object drug increased. ↓ = Object drug decreased. ↔ = Undetermined effect.

Drug/Food interactions: In one study following a single dose of **sertraline** with and without food, sertraline AUC was slightly increased and C_{max} was 25% greater. Time to reach peak plasma level decreased from 8 hours post dosing to 5.5 hours.

Food does not appear to affect systemic bioavailability of **fluoxetine** although it may delay absorption. **Fluvoxamine** bioavailability is not affected by food. Thus, fluoxetine and fluvoxamine may be given with or without food.

Adverse Reactions:

Discontinuation of treatment: In clinical trials, 15% of fluoxetine patients, 20% of paroxetine patients, 10% to 15% of sertraline patients and 22% of fluvoxamine patients discontinued treatment due to an adverse event.

SELECTIVE SEROTONIN REUPTAKE INHIBITORS

SSRIs Adverse Reactions (%) (≥ 1% in at least one agent)				
Adverse reaction	Fluoxetine	Fluvoxamine	Paroxetine	Sertraline
Body as a whole				
Headache	21	22	18	20
Asthenia	12	14	15	1
Infection, viral or bacterial	3.4	—	—	—
Pain, limb	1.6	—	—	—
Fever	2	—	—	2
Allergy/allergic reaction	1.2	0.1-1	0.1-1	—
Influenza/Flu syndrome	5	3	—	—
Chills	≥ 1	2	2	1.6
Back pain	2	—	3	2
Accidental injury	4	≥ 1	—	—
Surgical procedure	3	—	—	—
Allergic reaction	3	—	—	—
Malaise	0.1-1	≥ 1	>1	—
Pain	—	—	—	3
Cardiovascular				
Palpitations	2	3	3	4
Hot flushes	1.8	—	—	2.2
Vasodilatation	3	3	3	—
Postural hypotension	—	≥ 1	—	—
Hypertension	1	≥ 1	1	—
Syncope	—	≥ 1	1	—
Tachycardia	—	≥ 1	1	—
Chest pain	1.3	—	3	3
CNS				
Insomnia	20	21	13	16
Somnolence	13	22	23	13
Nervousness	13	12	5	3
Anxiety	13	5	5	3
Dizziness	10	11	13	12
Tremor	10	5	8	11
Depression	—	2	1	—
Libido decreased/ sexual dysfunction	4	2	3	2(female) 16 (male)
Myoclonus/twitching	0.1-1	≥ 1	3	1.4
Agitation	≥ 1	2	5	6
Paresthesia	—	—	4	3
Hypertonia	0.1-1	2	—	1
CNS stimulation	0.1-1	2	1	—
Confusion	1	—	1	1
Drowsiness	11.6	—	—	—
Fatigue /Malaise	4.2	≥ 1	—	11
Sedation	1.9	—	—	—
Sensation disturbances	1.7	—	—	—
Lightheadedness	1.6	—	—	—
Concentration, decreased	1.5	—	3	—
Drugged feeling	—	—	2	—
Amnesia	1	≥ 1	2	—
Emotional lability	1	0.1-1	1	—
Vertigo	—	0.1-1	1	—
Hypoesthesia	—	—	—	2
Apathy	—	≥ 1	—	—
Hypo-/Hyperkinesia	—	≥ 1	—	—
Manic reaction	—	≥ 1	—	—
Psychotic reaction	—	≥ 1	—	—
Abnormal dreams	5	—	4	0.1-1

SELECTIVE SEROTONIN REUPTAKE INHIBITORS

SSRIs Adverse Reactions (%) (≥ 1% in at least one agent)				
Adverse reaction	Fluoxetine	Fluvoxamine	Paroxetine	Sertraline
Abnormal thinking	4	—	0.1-1	0.1-1
Sleep disorder	3	—	—	—
Depersonalization	0.1-1	0.1-1	3	3
Nightmares	—	—	0.1-1	2
Miscellaneous				
Weight loss	2	≥ 1	1	0.1-1
Weight gain	1	≥ 1	1	3
Edema	—	≥ 1	1	0.1-1
Lymphadenopathy	2	—	—	—
GI				
Nausea	23	40	26	26
Vomiting	3	5	—	4
Diarrhea/loose stools	12	11	12	18
Dyspepsia	8	10	2	6
Dry mouth	10	14	18	16
Anorexia	11	6	6	3
Constipation	4.5	10	14	8
Abdominal pain	3.4		4	
Flatulence	3	4	4	4
Gastroenteritis	1	0.1-1	< 0.1	< 0.1
Increased appetite	≥ 1		3	3
Tooth disorder/caries	—	3	< 0.1	—
Oropharynx disorder	—		2	—
Dysphagia	—	2	—	—
Liver transaminases elevated	—	≥ 1	—	—
GI disorder	6	—	—	—
Melena	2	—	—	—
Musculoskeletal				
Pain, joint	1.2	—	—	—
Pain, muscle	1.2	—	—	—
Myalgia	5	—	2	1.7
Myasthenia	Rare	—	1	—
Myopathy	Rare	—	2	—
Arthralgia	3	0.1-1	0.1-1	0.1-1
Respiratory				
Upper respiratory infection	7.6	9	—	—
Pharyngitis	5	—	—	4
Nasal congestion	2.6	—	—	—
Headache, sinus	2.3	—	—	—
Sinusitis	2.1	≥ 1	—	—
Cough	1.6	≥ 1	1	—
Dyspnea	1.4	2	—	—
Bronchitis	≥ 1	0.1-1	—	—
Rhinitis	≥ 1	—	3	2
Yawn	3	2	4	2
Respiratory disorder	—	—	5.9	—
Dermatologic				
Sweating, excessive	8	7	11	8
Rash	4	—	2	2
Pruritus	3	—	1	0.1 to 1
Acne	2	0.1-1	0.1-1	0.1-1
Special senses				
Vision disturbances/ blurred vision	3	—	4	4

SELECTIVE SEROTONIN REUPTAKE INHIBITORS

SSRIs Adverse Reactions (%) (≥ 1% in at least one agent)				
Adverse reaction	Fluoxetine	Fluvoxamine	Paroxetine	Sertraline
Taste perversion/change	1	3	2	3
Tinnitus	1	—	0.1-1	1.4
Amblyopia	3	3	—	—
GU				
Menstruation, painful	2.6	—	—	0.1-1
Sexual dysfunction/ impotence/anorgasmia	1.9	2	6.5	16
Urinary frequency	1	3	3	2
Urinary tract infection	1.2	0.1-1	2	—
Abnormal ejaculation	—	8	13	17
Male genital disorders, others	—	—	10	—
Urination disorder/ retention	—	1	3	Rare
Female genital disorders	—	—	2	—
Menstrual disorder	—	0.1-1	0.1-1	1
Anorgasmia	0.1-1	2	—	—

Dose dependency of adverse reactions: A comparison of adverse event rates in a fixed-dose study comparing **paroxetine** 10, 20, 30 and 40 mg/day with placebo revealed a clear dose dependency for some of the more common adverse events associated with paroxetine use.

Adverse Reactions by Indications of Fluoxetine						
	Depression		OCD		Bulimia	
Adverse Reaction	Fluoxetine	Placebo	Fluoxetine	Placebo	Fluoxetine	Placebo
Body as a Whole						
Asthenia	9	5	15	11	21	9
Flu syndrome	3	4	10	7	8	3
Cardiovascular						
Vasodilatation	3	2	5	—	2	1
GI						
Nausea	21	9	26	13	29	11
Anorexia	11	2	17	10	8	4
Dry mouth	10	7	12	3	9	6
Dyspepsia	7	5	10	4	10	6
CNS						
Insomnia	16	9	28	22	33	13
Anxiety	12	7	14	7	15	9
Nervousness	14	9	14	15	11	5
Somnolence	13	6	17	7	13	5
Tremor	10	3	9	1	13	1
Libido decreased	3	—	11	2	5	1
Abnormal dreams	1	1	5	2	5	3
Respiratory System						
Pharyngitis	3	3	11	9	10	5
Sinusitis	1	4	5	2	6	4
Yawn	—	—	7	—	11	—
Dermatologic						
Sweating	8	3	7	—	8	3
Rash	4	3	6	3	4	4
GU						
Impotence	2	—	—	—	7	—
Abnormal ejaculation	—	—	7	—	7	—

Adaptation to certain adverse events: Over a 4 to 6 week period, there was evidence of adaptation to some adverse events with continued therapy (eg, nausea, dizziness), but less to other effects (eg, dry mouth, somnolence, asthenia).

SELECTIVE SEROTONIN REUPTAKE INHIBITORS

Body as a whole:

Fluoxetine – Cyst, intentional overdose, suicide attempt, facial edema, hangover effect, jaw pain, neck pain, neck rigidity, pelvic pain (0.1% to 1%); abdomen enlarged, abdominal syndrome acute, intentional injury, neuroleptic malignant syndrome, photosensitivity reaction, cellulitis, hydrocephalus, hypothermia, LE syndrome, moniliasis, serum sickness (< 0.1%).

Fluvoxamine – Neck pain/rigidity, overdose, suicide attempt (0.1% to 1%); cyst, pelvic pain, sudden death (< 0.1%).

Paroxetine – Carcinoma, facial edema, moniliasis, neck pain (0.1% to 1%); abscess, adrenergic syndrome, cellulitis, neck rigidity, pelvic pain, peritonitis, ulcer (< 0.1%).

Cardiovascular:

Fluoxetine – Congestive heart failure (1%); angina pectoris, arrhythmia, hemorrhage, hypotension, migraine, postural hypotension, syncope, tachycardia (0.1% to 1%); first degree AV block, atrial fibrillation cerebral embolism, cerebrovascular accident, extrasystoles, heart arrest, heart block, pallor, peripheral vascular disorder, phlebitis, shock, thrombosis, vasospasm, ventricular extrasystoles, ventricular fibrillation, bradycardia, bundle branch block, cerebral ischemia, myocardial infarct, thrombophlebitis, vascular headache, ventricular arrhythmia (< 0.1%).

Fluvoxamine – Angina pectoris, bradycardia, cardiomyopathy, cardiovascular disease, cold extremities, conduction delay, heart failure, MI, pallor, pulse irregular, ST segment changes (0.1% to 1%); AV block, CVA, CAD, embolus, pericarditis, phlebitis, pulmonary infarction, supraventricular extrasystoles (< 0.1%).

Paroxetine – Bradycardia, conduction abnormalities, ECG abnormal, hypotension, hematoma, migraine, peripheral vascular disorder (0.1% to 1%); angina pectoris, arrhythmia, atrial fibrillation, bundle branch block, cerebral ischemia, cerebrovascular accident, CHF, heart block, low cardiac output, MI, myocardial ischemia, pallor, phlebitis, pulmonary embolus, supraventricular/ventricular extrasystoles, thrombophlebitis, thrombosis, varicose vein, vascular headache (< 0.1%).

Sertraline – Postural dizziness, hypertension, hypotension, postural hypotension, edema (dependent, periorbital, peripheral), peripheral ischemia, syncope, tachycardia (0.1% to 1%); precordial/substernal chest pain, aggravated hypertension, myocardial infarction, varicose veins (< 0.1%).

CNS:

Fluoxetine – Sleep disorder (1%); neurosis, personality disorder, abnormal gait, acute brain syndrome, akathisia, amnesia, apathy, ataxia, buccoglossal syndrome, convulsions, delusions, depersonalization, emotional lability, euphoria, hallucinations, hostility, hyperkinesia, hypoesthesia, incoordination, libido increased, manic reaction, neuralgia, neuropathy, paranoid reaction, psychosis, vertigo (0.1% to 1%); abnormal EEG, delusions, foot drop, hyperesthesia, neuritis, reflexes increased, antisocial reaction, chronic brain syndrome, circumoral paresthesia, CNS depression, coma, dysarthria, dystonia, extrapyramidal syndrome, hypertonia, hysteria, myoclonus, nystagmus, paralysis, decreased reflexes, stupor, torticollis, tardive dyskinesia (< 0.1%).

Fluvoxamine – Agoraphobia, akathisia, ataxia, CNS depression, convulsion, delirium, delusion, drug dependence, dyskinesia, dystonia, euphoria, extrapyramidal syndrome, gait unsteady, hallucinations, hemiplegia, hostility, hypersomnia, hypochondriasis, hypotonia, hysteria, incoordination, increased salivation, increased libido, neuralgia, paralysis, paranoid reaction, phobia, psychosis, sleep disorder, stupor, twitching (0.1% to 1%); akinesia, coma, fibrillations, mutism, obsessions, reflexes decreased, slurred speech, tardive dyskinesia, torticollis, trismus, withdrawal syndrome (< 0.1%).

Paroxetine – Akinesia, alcohol abuse, aphasia, ataxia, convulsions, CNS stimulation, hallucinations, hyperkinesia, hypertonia, incoordination, hostility, hypesthesia, neurosis, lack of emotion, manic reaction (0.1% to 1%); abnormal EEG, abnormal gait, antisocial reaction, choreoathetosis, delirium, cumoral paresthesias, extrapyramidal syndrome, grand mal convulsion, peripheral neuritis, reflexes decreased, trismus, delusions, diplopia, drug dependence, dysarthria, dyskinesia, dystonia, euphoria, fasciculations, hyperalgesia, hypokinesia, hysteria, libido increased, manic-depressive reaction, meningitis, myelitis, neuralgia, neuropathy, nystagmus, paralysis, paranoid reaction, psychosis, psychotic depression, reflexes increased, stupor, withdrawal syndrome (< 0.01%).

Sertraline – Mydriasis, flushing, ataxia, abnormal coordination, abnormal gait, hyperesthesia, hyperkinesia, hypokinesia, migraine, nystagmus, vertigo, aggressive reaction, amnesia, apathy, delusion, depression, aggravated depression, emotional lability, euphoria, hallucination, neurosis, paranoid reaction, suicide ideation/attempt

SELECTIVE SEROTONIN REUPTAKE INHIBITORS

(0.1% to 1%); local anesthesia, coma, convulsions, dyskinesia, dysphonia, hyporeflexia, hypotonia, ptosis, hysteria, somnambulism, withdrawal syndrome (< 0.1%).

GI:

Fluoxetine – Aphthous stomatitis, dysphagia, eructation, esophagitis, gastritis, gingivitis, glossitis, abnormal liver function tests, gum hemorrhage, melena, stomatitis, thirst (0.1% to 1%); bloody diarrhea, cholecystitis, cholelithiasis, colitis, duodenal ulcer, enteritis, fecal incontinence, hematemesis, hepatitis, biliary pain, esophageal ulcer, GI hemorrhage, hemorrhage of colon, intestinal obtruction, liver fatty deposit, pancreatitis, peptic ulcer, rectal hemorrhage, hepatomegaly, hyperchlorhydria, increased salivation, jaundice, liver tenderness, mouth ulceration, salivary gland enlargement, stomach ulcer, tongue discoloration, tongue edema (< 0.1%).

Fluvoxamine – Colitis, gastritis, eructation, esophagitis, GI hemorrhage, GI ulcer, gingivitis, glossitis, hemorrhoids, melena, rectal hemorrhage, stomatitis, (0.1% to 1%); biliary pain, cholecystitis, cholelithiasis, fecal incontinence, hematemesis, intestinal obstruction, jaundice (< 0.1%).

Paroxetine – Bruxism, colitis, dysphagia, eructation, gastritis, glossitis, increased salivation, abnormal liver function tests, mouth ulceration, rectal hemorrhage (0.1% to 1%); aphthous stomatitis, bloody diarrhea, bulimia, cholelithiasis, duodenitis, enteritis, esophagitis, fecal impaction/incontinence, gingivitis, gum hemorrhage, hematemesis, hepatitis, ileus, intestinal obstruction, jaundice, melena, peptic ulcer, salivary gland enlargement, stomach ulcer, stomatitis, tongue discoloration, tongue edema, ulcerative stomatitis, tooth malformation (< 0.1%).

Sertraline – Increased saliva, teeth grinding, dysphagia, eructation (0.1% to 1%); diverticulitis, fecal incontinence, gastritis, glossitis, gum hyperplasia, hemorrhoids, hiccup, melena, hemorrhagic peptic ulcer, proctitis, stomatitis, ulcerative stomatitis, tenesmus, tongue edema/ulceration, aphthous stomatitis (< 0.1%).

Musculoskeletal:

Fluoxetine – Arthritis, bone pain, bursitis, tenosynovitis, twitching (0.1% to 1%); bone necrosis, chondrodystrophy, muscle hemorrhage, myositis, osteoporosis, pathological fracture, osteomyelitis, arthrosis, rheumatoid arthritis (< 0.1%).

Fluvoxamine – Arthritis, bursitis, generalized muscle spasm, myasthenia, tendinous contracture, tenosynovitis (0.1% to 1%); arthrosis, myopathy, pathological fracture (< 0.1%).

Paroxetine – Arthritis (0.1% to 1%); arthrosis, bursitis, myositis, osteoporosis, tetany, generalized spasm, tenosynovitis (< 0.1%).

Sertraline – Arthrosis, dystonia, muscle cramps/weakness (0.1% to 1%); hernia (< 0.1%).

Respiratory:

Fluoxetine – Asthma, epistaxis, hiccups, hyperventilation, atelectasis, cough decreased, emphysema, hypoventilation, pneumothorax, stridor, pneumonia (0.1% to 1%); apnea, hemoptysis, hypoxia, laryngeal edema, lung edema, lung fibrosis/alveolitis, pleural effusion (< 0.1%).

Fluvoxamine – Asthma, epistaxis, hoarseness, hyperventilation (0.1% to 1%); apnea, congestion of upper airway, hemoptysis, hiccups, laryngismus, obstructive pulmonary disease, pneumonia (< 0.1%).

Paroxetine – Asthma, bronchitis, dyspnea, epistaxis, hyperventilation, pneumonia, respiratory flu, voice alterations, sinusitis (0.1% to 1%); emphysema, hemoptysis, lung fibrosis, pulmonary edema, hiccups, sputum increased (< 0.1%).

Sertraline – Bronchospasm, coughing, dyspnea, epistaxis (0.1% to 1%); bradypnea, hyperventilation, sinusitis, stridor (< 0.1%).

Dermatologic:

Fluoxetine – Alopecia, contact dermatitis, dry skin, herpes simplex, maculopapular rash, skin discoloration, skin ulcer, urticaria (0.1% to 1%); eczema, erythema multiforme, fungal dermatitis, herpes zoster, hirsutism, psoriasis, furunculosis, petechial rash, purpuric rash, pustular rash, seborrhea, skin hypertrophy, subcutaneous nodule; vesiculobullous rash (< 0.1%).

Fluvoxamine – Alopecia, dry skin, eczema, exfoliative dermatitis, furunculosis, photosensitivity, seborrhea, skin discoloration, urticaria (0.1% to 1%).

Paroxetine – Alopecia, dry skin, ecchymosis, eczema, furunculosis, urticaria (0.1% to 1%); angioedema, contact dermatitis, erythema nodosum, maculopapular rash, photosensitivity, skin discoloration, skin melanoma, erytherma multiforme, fungal dermatitis, herpes simplex, herpes zoster, hirsutism seborrhea, skin hypertrophy, skin ulcer, vesiculobullous rash (< 0.1%).

Sertraline – Alopecia, face edema, erythematous rash, maculopapular rash, dry skin, cold/clammy skin (0.1% to 1%); bullous eruption, dermatitis, erythema multi-

SELECTIVE SEROTONIN REUPTAKE INHIBITORS

forme, abnormal hair texture, hypertrichosis, photosensitivity, follicular rash, pruritus, skin discoloration, abnormal skin odor, urticaria, pallor (< 0.1%).

Special senses:

Fluoxetine – Amblyopia, conjunctivitis, ear pain, eye pain, mydriasis, photophobia, tinnitus (0.1% to 1%); blepharitis, cataract, corneal lesion, deafness, diplopia, eye hemorrhage, glaucoma, iritis, ptosis, exophthalmos, hyperacusis, parosmia, dry eyes, scleritis, visual field defect, strabismus, taste loss (< 0.1%).

Fluvoxamine – Accommodation abnormal, conjunctivitis, deafness, diplopia, dry eyes, ear pain, eye pain, mydriasis, otitis media, parosmia, photophobia, taste loss, visual field defect (0.1% to 1%); corneal ulcer, retinal detachment (< 0.1%).

Paroxetine – Abnormality of accommodation, conjunctivitis, visual field defect, ear pain, eye pain, mydriasis, otitis media (0.1% to 1%); amblyopia, cataract, conjunctival edema, blepharitis, deafness, keratoconjunctivitis, night blindness, parosmia, ptosis, retinal hemorrhage, corneal ulcer, exophthalmos, eye hemorrhage, glaucoma, hyperacusis, otitis externa, photophobia, anisocoria (< 0.1%).

Sertraline – Abnormal accommodation, conjunctivitis, diplopia, earache, eye pain, xerophthalmia (0.1% to 1%); abnormal lacrimation, photophobia, visual field defect, anisocoria (< 0.1%).

GU:

Fluoxetine – Nocturia, polyuria, abnormal ejaculation, amenorrhea, breast pain, cystitis, dysuria, fibrocystic breast, leukorrhea, menopause, menorrhagia, ovarian disorder, urinary incontinence/retention/urgency, urination impaired, vaginitis (0.1% to 1%); abortion, albuminuria, breast enlargement, dyspareunia, epididymitis, female lactation, hematuria, hypomenorrhea, kidney calculus, metrorrhagia, orchitis, polyuria, pyelonephritis, salpingitis, urethral pain, urethritis, urinary tract disorder, urolithiasis, uterine spasm, glycosuria, kidney pain, oliguria, priapism, uterine fibroids enlarged, vaginal/uterine hemorrhage (< 0.1%).

Fluvoxamine – Anuria, breast pain, cystitis, dysuria, female lactation, hematuria, menopause, menorrhagia, metrorrhagia, nocturia, polyuria, premenstrual syndrome, urinary incontinence, urinary urgency, urination impaired, vaginal hemorrhage, vaginitis (0.1% to 1%); kidney calculus, hematospermia, oliguria (< 0.1%).

Paroxetine – Abortion, amenorrhea, breast pain, cystitis, dysmenorrhea, dysuria, menorrhagia, nocturia, polyuria, urethritis, urinary incontinence/retention/urgency, vaginitis (0.1% to 1%); breast atrophy/carcinoma/neoplasm, female lactation, breast enlargement, epididymitis, fibrocystic breast, kidney pain, leukorrhea, metrorrhagia, pyuria, urethritis, uterine spasm, urolith, vaginal hemorrhage, hematuria, kidney calculus, kidney function abnormal, mastitis, nephritis, oliguria, prostatic carcinoma, vaginal moniliasis (< 0.1%).

Sertraline – Dysuria, nocturia, polyuria, urinary incontinence (0.1% to 1%); oliguria, renal pain, urinary retention, amenorrhea, balanoposthitis, breast enlargement, female breast pain, leukorrhea, menorrhagia, atrophic vaginitis, galactorrhea (< 0.1%).

Miscellaneous:

Fluoxetine – Anemia, generalized edema, hypoglycemia, hypothyroidism, lymphadenopathy, ecchymosis, hypochromic anemia, lymphedema, thrombocytopenia, peripheral edema, weight gain (0.1% to 1.0%); bleeding time increased, blood dyscrasia, dehydration, goiter, gout, hypercholesterolemia, hyperglycemia, hyperlipemia, hyperthyroidism, hypoglycemic reaction, hypokalemia, hyponatremia, iron deficiency anemia, hyperkalemia, leukopenia, lymphocytosis, petechia, alcohol intolerance, purpura, sedimentation rate increased, diabetic acidosis, diabetes mellitus, thrombocythemia (< 0.1%).

Fluvoxamine – Hypothyroidism, anemia, ecchymosis, leukocytosis, lymphadenopathy, thrombocytopenia, dehydration, hypercholesterolemia (0.1% to 1%); goiter, leukopenia, purpura, diabetes mellitus, hyperglycemia, hyperlipidemia, hypoglycemia, hypokalemia, lactate dehydrogenase increased (< 0.1%).

Paroxetine – Anemia, leukopenia, lymphadenopathy, purpura, hyperglycemia, peripheral edema, thirst (0.1% to 1%); abnormal erythrocytes, basophilia, hypochromic anemia, eosinophilia, iron deficiency anemia, lymphocytosis, thrombocythemia, BUN increased, creatinine phosphokinase increased, hypercalcemia, hyperkalemia, hyperphosphatemia, ketosis, lactic dehydrogenase increased, gamma globulins increased, leukocytosis, lymphedema, abnormal lymphocytes, lymphocytosis, microcytic/normocytic anemia, monocytosis, alkaline phosphatase increased, bilirubinemia, dehydration, gout, hypercholesteremia, hypocalcemia, hypoglycemia, hypokalemia, hyponatremia, AST/ALT increased, diabetes mellitus, hyperthyroidism, hypothyroidism, thyroiditis (< 0.1%).

SELECTIVE SEROTONIN REUPTAKE INHIBITORS

Sertraline – Malaise, asthenia, rigors, lymphadenopathy, purpura (0.1% to 1%); abdomen enlarged, halitosis, otitis media, anemia, anterior chamber eye hemorrhage, dehydration, hypercholesterolemia, hypoglycemia, exophthalmos, gynecomastia (< 0.1%).

Lab test abnormalities:

Fluoxetine – Alkaline phosphatase increased, BUN increased, creatine phosphokinase increased, hyperuricemia, hypocalcemia, ALT increased (< 0.1 %).

Sertraline – Asymptomatic elevations in serum transaminases (AST or ALT) have occurred infrequently (≈ 0.8%) in association with sertraline administration. These hepatic enzyme elevations usually occurred within the first 1 to 9 weeks of drug treatment and promptly diminished upon drug discontinuation.

Sertraline therapy was associated with small mean increases in total cholesterol (≈ 3%) and triglycerides (≈ 5%) and a small mean decrease in serum uric acid (≈ 7%) of no apparent clinical importance.

Overdosage:

Symptoms:

Fluoxetine – There have been two deaths among ≈ 38 reports of acute overdose with fluoxetine, either alone or in combination with other drugs or alcohol. One death involved a combined overdose with ≈ 1.8 g fluoxetine and an undetermined amount of maprotiline. Plasma concentrations of fluoxetine and maprotiline were 4.57 mg/L and 4.18 mg/L, respectively. A second death involved three drugs yielding plasma concentrations as follows: Fluoxetine, 1.93 mg/L; norfluoxetine, 1.1 mg/L; codeine, 1.8 mg/L; temazepam 3.8 mg/L.

One other patient who reportedly took 3 g of fluoxetine experienced two grand mal seizures that remitted spontaneously without specific anticonvulsant treatment. The actual amount of drug absorbed may have been less due to vomiting.

Nausea and vomiting were prominent in overdoses involving higher fluoxetine doses. Other symptoms of overdose include agitation, restlessness, hypomania and other signs of CNS excitation.

Fluvoxamine – Of 354 cases of overdose, there were 19 deaths. The highest reported overdose was 10,000 mg (equivalent to 1 to 3 months dosage); the patient fully recovered with no sequelae. Common symptoms include drowsiness, vomiting, diarrhea and dizziness; other signs include coma, tachycardia, bradycardia, hypotension, ECG abnormalities, liver function abnormalities and convulsions.

Paroxetine – Overdose with paroxetine (up to 2000 mg) alone and in combination with other drugs has been reported. Signs and symptoms of overdose with paroxetine include nausea, vomiting, sedation, dizziness, sweating and facial flush. There are no reports of coma or convulsions following overdosage with paroxetine alone. A fatal outcome has been reported rarely when paroxetine was taken in combination with other agents, or when taken alone.

Sertraline – Symptons of overdose with sertraline alone included somnolence, nausea, vomiting, tachycardia, ECG changes, anxiety and dilated pupils.

Treatment: There are no specific antidotes. Establish and maintain an airway, ensure adequate oxygenation and ventilation. Activated charcoal, which may be used with sorbitol, may be as or more effective than emesis or lavage.

Monitor cardiac and vital signs along with general symptomatic and supportive measures. SSRI-induced seizures that fail to respond spontaneously may respond to diazepam.

Due to the large volume of distribution of SSRIs, forced diuresis, dialysis, hemoperfusion and exchange transfusion are unlikely to be of benefit.

Treatment includes usual supportive measures. Refer to General Management of Acute Overdosage.

SELECTIVE SEROTONIN REUPTAKE INHIBITORS

Patient Information:

Hazardous tasks: SSRIs may cause dizziness or drowsiness. Patient should observe caution while driving or performing other tasks requiring alertness, coordination or physical dexterity.

Concomitant medication: Consult physician or pharmacist before taking concomitant *otc* physical or prescription drugs (see Drug Interactions). Avoid alcohol or other depressant medications.

Pregnancy or lactation: Notify physician of pregnancy, of intent to become pregnant or if breastfeeding.

Rash: Notify physician if rash or hives develop.

Completing course of therapy: While patients may notice improvement in therapy in 1 to 4 weeks, advise patients to continue therapy as directed.

Photosensitivity: May cause photosensitivity (sensitivity to sunlight). Avoid prolonged exposure to the sun and other ultraviolet light. Use sunscreens and wear protective clothing until tolerance is determined.

Selective Serotonin Reuptake Inhibitors

SERTRALINE HCl

For complete prescribing information, refer to the SSRIs group monograph.

Indications:

Depression: Treatment of depression.

Obsessive-Compulsive Disorder (OCD): Treatment of obsessions and compulsions in patients with OCD, as defined in the DSM-III-R.

Administration and Dosage:

Approved by the FDA in December 1991.

Initial treatment: 50 mg once daily, either in the morning or evening. While a relationship between dose and antidepressant effect has not been established, patients were dosed in a range of 50 to 200 mg/day in the clinical trials. Consequently, patients not responding to a 50 mg dose may benefit from dose increases up to a maximum of 200 mg/day. Given the 24 hour elimination half-life of sertraline, dose changes should not occur at intervals of < 1 week.

Hepatic/Renal function impairment: Give a lower or less frequent dosage in patients with hepatic or renal impairment.

Maintenance/Continuation/Extended treatment: There is evidence to suggest that depressed patients responding during an initial 8 week treatment phase will continue to benefit during an additional 8 weeks of treatment. While there are insufficient data regarding any benefits from treatment beyond 16 weeks, it is generally agreed among expert psychopharmacologists that acute episodes of depression require several months or longer of sustained pharmacological therapy. Whether the dose of antidepressant needed to induce remission is identical to the dose needed to maintain or sustain euthymia is unknown.

Rx	**Zoloft** (Roerig)	50 mg	(Zoloft 50 mg). Lt. blue, scored. Capsule shape. Film coated. In 100s, 500s and 100 UD.
		100 mg	(Zoloft 100 mg). Lt. yellow, scored. Capsule shape. Film coated. In 100s, 500s and 100 UD.
🍁	**Zoloft** (Pfizer)	**Capsules**: 25 mg	Yellow. In 100s.
		50 mg	White/yellow. In 100s and 250s.
		100 mg	Orange. In 100s and 250s.

PAROXETINE HCl

For complete prescribing information, refer to the SSRIs group monograph.

Indications:

Depression: Treatment of depression.

Obsessive-Compulsive Disorder (OCD): Treatment of obsessions and compulsions in patients with OCD, as defined in the DSM-III-R.

Panic Disorder: Treatment of panic disorder, with or without agoraphobia, as defined in DSM-IV.

Unlabeled uses: Diabetic neuropathy (10 to 60 mg/day); headaches (10 to 50 mg/day); premature ejaculation (20 mg/day).

Administration and Dosage:

Approved by the FDA on December 29, 1992.

Depression:

Initial dose – 20 mg/day. Administer as a single daily dose, usually in the morning. Usual range is 20 to 50 mg/day. As with all antidepressants, the full antidepressant effect may be delayed. Some patients not responding to a 20 mg dose may benefit from dose increases, in 10 mg/day increments, up to a maximum of 50 mg/day. Dose changes should occur at intervals ≥ 1 week.

Maintenance therapy – It is generally agreed that acute episodes of depression require several months or longer of sustained pharmacologic therapy. Whether the dose of an antidepressant needed to induce remission is identical to the dose needed to maintain or sustain euthymia is unknown. Efficacy has been maintained for periods of up to 1 year with doses that averaged about 30 mg.

OCD:

Initial – 40 mg/day. Administer as a single daily dose, usually in the morning. Start with 20 mg/day and may be increased in 10 mg/day increments. Dose changes

Selective Serotonin Reuptake Inhibitors

PAROXETINE HCl

should occur at intervals of at least 1 week. Usual range is 20 to 60 mg/day. The maximum dosage should not exceed 60 mg/day.

Maintenance therapy – Patients have been continued on therapy for 6 months without loss of benefit. However, make dosage adjustments to maintain the patient on the lowest effective dosage, and periodically reassess the patient to determine the need for treatment.

Panic Disorder:

Initial – 40 mg/day. Administer as a single daily dose, usually in the morning. Start with 10 mg/day and may be increased in 10 mg/day increments. Dose changes should occur at intervals of at least 1 week. Usual range is 10 to 60 mg/day. The maximum dosage shoould not exceed 60 mg/day.

Maintenance therapy – Long-term maintenance of efficacy has been demonstrated for 3 months. Make dosage adjustments to maintain the patient on the lowest effective dosage, and reassess the patient periodically to determine the need for continued treatment.

Elderly or debilitated or patients with severe renal or hepatic impairment: The recommended initial dose is 10 mg/day. Increases may be made if indicated. Dosage should not exceed 40 mg/day.

Rx	**Paxil** (SmithKline Beecham)	**Tablets:** 10 mg	(Paxil 10). Yellow. Oval. Film coated. In 30s.
		20 mg	(Paxil 20). Pink, scored. Oval. Film coated. In 30s, 100s and UD 100s.
		30 mg	(Paxil 30). Blue. Oval. Film coated. In 30s.
		40 mg	(Paxil 40). Green. Oval. Film coated. In 30s.
🍁	**Paxil** (SmithKline Beecham)	**Tablets:** 20 mg	(Paxil 20). Pink, scored. Oval. Film coated. In 100s.
		30 mg	(Paxil 30). Blue. Oval. Film coated. In 30s.

FLUOXETINE HCl

For complete prescribing information, refer to the SSRIs group monograph.

Indications:

Depression: Treatment of depression.

Obsessive-Compulsive Disorder (OCD): Treatment of obsessions and compulsions in patients with OCD, as defined in the DSM-III-R.

Bulimia Nervosa: Treatment of binge-eating and vomiting behaviors in patients with moderate to severe bulimia nervosa.

Unlabeled uses: Alcoholism (40 to 80 mg/day); anorexia nervosa (20 to 80 mg/day); attention-deficit hyperactivity disorder (20 to 60 mg/day); bipolar II affective disorder (20 to 80 mg/day); borderline personality disorder (5 to 80 mg/day); cataplexy and narcolepsy (20 to 40 mg/day); kleptomania (60 to 80 mg/day); migraine, chronic daily headaches and tension-type headache (20 mg every other day to 40 mg/day); obesity (20 to 60 mg/day) (see Precautions); posttraumatic stress disorder (10 to 80 mg/day); premenstrual syndrome (20 mg/day); recurrent syncope (20 mg/day); schizophrenia (20 to 60 mg/day); Tourette's syndrome (20 to 40 mg/day); trichotillomania (20 to 80 mg/day); levodopa-induced dyskinesia (40 mg/day); social phobia (10 to 60 mg/day).

Administration and Dosage:

Depression:

Initial – 20 mg/day in the morning. Consider a dose increase after several weeks if no clinical improvement is observed. Administer doses > 20 mg/day on a once (morning) or twice (eg, morning and noon) daily schedule. Do not exceed a maximum dose of 80 mg/day.

The full antidepressant effect may be delayed until ≥ 4 weeks of treatment.

Maintenance – Optimal duration of fluoxetine therapy remains speculative. Acute episodes of depression generally require several months or longer of sustained pharmacologic therapy. Whether the dose of antidepressant needed to induce remission is identical to the dose needed to maintain or sustain euthymia is unknown.

OCD:

Initial – 20 mg/day in the morning. Consider a dose increase after several weeks if insufficient clinical improvement is observed. Administer doses > 20 mg/day on a

Selective Serotonin Reuptake Inhibitors

FLUOXETINE HCl

once (morning) or twice (morning and noon) daily schedule. A dose range of 20 to 60 mg/day is recommended; however, doses of up to 80 mg/day have been well tolerated. Do not exceed 80 mg/day.

The full therapeutic effect may be delayed until ≥ 5 weeks of treatment.

Maintenance – Patients have been continued on therapy for an additional 6 months without loss of benefit. However, make dosage adjustments to maintain the patient on the lowest effective dosage, and periodically reassess the patient to determine the need for treatment.

Bulimia Nervosa:

Initial – The recommended dose is 60 mg/day, administered in the morning. For some patients it may be advisable to titrate up to this target dose over several days. Fluoxetine doses > 60 mg/day have not been systematically studied in patients with bulimia.

Maintenance – Patients have been continued on therapy for an additional 6 months without loss of benefit. However, make dosage adjustments to maintain the patient on the lowest effective dosage, and periodically reassess the patient to determine the need for treatment.

Renal/Hepatic function impairment: Use a lower or less frequent dosage.

Special risk patients: Consider a lower or less frequent dosage for patients, such as the elderly, or those with concurrent disease or on multiple medications.

Rx	**Prozac** (Dista)	**Pulvules**: 10 mg	Green/green. In 100s, 2000s and UD 31s.
		20 mg	Green/off-white. In 30s, 100s, 2000s, UD 31s and 100s.
		Liquid: 20 mg/5 ml	0.23% alcohol, sucrose. Mint flavor. In 120 ml.
🍁	**Prozac** (Lilly)	**Capsules**: 10 mg	Green/gray. In 100s.
		20 mg	Green/white. In 100s.
		Liquid: 20 mg/5 ml	Sucrose. Mint flavor. In 120 ml.

FLUVOXAMINE MALEATE

For complete prescribing information, refer to the SSRIs group monograph.

Indications:

Obsessive-Compulsive Disorder (OCD): Treatment of obsessions and compulsions in patients with OCD, as defined in the DSM-III-R.

Unlabeled uses: Fluvoxamine is being investigated in the treatment of depression.

Administration and Dosage:

Approved by the FDA on December 5, 1994 (1S classification).

Initial therapy: Recommended starting dose is 50 mg as a single bedtime dose. In trials, patients were titrated within a range of 100 to 300 mg/day. Increase dose in 50 mg increments every 4 to 7 days, as tolerated, until maximum therapeutic benefit is achieved, not to exceed 300 mg/day. It is advisable to give total daily doses > 100 mg in two divided doses; if doses are unequal, give larger dose at bedtime.

Maintenance therapy: Although efficacy has not been documented > 10 weeks in controlled trials, OCD is a chronic condition; it is reasonable to consider continuation for a responding patient. Adjust dose to maintain patient on lowest effective dosage. Periodically reassess patient to determine need for continued treatment.

Elderly/Hepatic function impairment: These patients have been observed to have decreased fluvoxamine clearance. It may be appropriate to modify initial dose and subsequent titration.

Rx	**Luvox** (Solvay)	**Tablets**: 50 mg	(Solvay 4205). Yellow, scored. Elliptical. Film coated. In 100s, 1000s and UD 100s.
		100 mg	(Solvay 4210). Beige, scored. Elliptical. Film coated. In 100s, 1000s and UD 100s.

MONOAMINE OXIDASE INHIBITORS

Actions:

Pharmacology: Monoamine oxidase is a complex enzyme system, widely distributed throughout the body, which is responsible for the metabolic decomposition of biogenic amines, thus terminating their activity. Drugs that inhibit this enzyme system (MAOIs) cause an increase in the concentration of endogenous epinephrine, norepinephrine and serotonin (5HT) in storage sites throughout the nervous system. The increase in the concentration of monoamines in the CNS is the basis for the antidepressant activity of these agents.

Tranylcypromine is a non-hydrazine MAOI. It has a rapid onset of activity.

Drugs that have MAOI activity cause a wide range of clinical effects and have the potential for serious interactions with other substances. Clinicians and patients should be fully aware of the potential hazards associated with their use.

Pharmacokinetics: MAOIs are well absorbed orally. The clinical effects of phenelzine may continue for up to 2 weeks after discontinuation of therapy. When tranylcypromine is withdrawn, MAO activity is recovered in 3 to 5 days (possibly up to 10 days), although the drug is excreted in 24 hours.

Indications:

Depression: In general, the MAOIs appear to be indicated in patients with atypical (exogenous) depression, and in some patients unresponsive to other antidepressive therapy. They are rarely a drug of first choice.

For indications of specific agents, see individual product listings.

Unlabeled uses: MAOIs have shown promise in the treatment of bulimia (having characteristics of atypical depression). Phenelzine (15 mg on alternate days to 90 mg/day) has been investigated in the treatment of cocaine addiction; careful supervision is required. Anecdotal cases and small studies indicate beneficial effects of phenelzine in patients with night terrors (30 mg twice daily); post-traumatic stress disorder (60 to 75 mg/day); some migraines resistant to other therapies (15 mg three times daily); likewise, with tranylcypromine in Binswanger's encephalopathy (40 mg/day); seasonal affective disorder (≈ 30 mg/day); and subjective symptoms in multiple sclerosis patients (10 to 120 mg/day). MAOIs have also been used in the treatment of panic disorder with associated agoraphobia and globus hystericus syndrome.

Contraindications:

Hypersensitivity to these agents; pheochromocytoma; congestive heart failure; a history of liver disease or abnormal liver function tests; severe impairment of renal function; confirmed or suspected cerebrovascular defect; cardiovascular disease; hypertension; history of headache; coadministration with guanethidine.

Refer also to the Drug Interactions section.

Warnings:

Hypertensive crises: The most serious reactions involve changes in blood pressure; it is inadvisable to use these drugs in elderly or debilitated patients or in the presence of hypertension, cardiovascular or cerebrovascular disease.

Hypertensive crises have sometimes been fatal. These crises usually occur within several hours after ingestion of a contraindicated substance and are characterized by some or all of the following symptoms: Occipital headache which may radiate frontally; palpitation; neck stiffness or soreness; nausea; vomiting; sweating (sometimes with fever or cold, clammy skin); dilated pupils; photophobia. Either tachycardia or bradycardia may be present and can be associated with constricting chest pain.

Note – Intracranial bleeding (sometimes fatal) has been reported in association with the paradoxical increase in blood pressure.

Monitor blood pressure frequently to detect evidence of any pressor response. Do not place full reliance on blood pressure readings, but observe patient frequently.

Discontinue therapy immediately if palpitations or frequent headaches occur. These signs may be prodromal of a hypertensive crisis.

Treatment – If a hypertensive crisis occurs, discontinue these drugs immediately and institute therapy to lower blood pressure. Do not use parenteral reserpine. Headaches tend to abate as blood pressure is lowered. Administer alpha-adrenergic blocking agents such as phentolamine 5 mg IV slowly to avoid producing an excessive hypotensive effect. Manage fever by means of external cooling.

MONOAMINE OXIDASE INHIBITORS

Warning to the patient – Warn all patients against eating foods with high tyramine or tryptophan content (see table) and for 2 weeks after discontinuing MAOIs. Any high protein food that is aged or undergoes breakdown by putrefaction process to improve flavor is suspect of being able to produce a hypertensive crisis in patients taking MAOIs. Also warn patients against drinking alcoholic beverages and against self-medication with certain proprietary agents such as cold, hay fever or weight reduction preparations containing sympathomimetic amines while undergoing therapy. Instruct patients not to consume excessive amounts of caffeine in any form and to report promptly the occurrence of headache or other unusual symptoms.

Tyramine-Containing Foods[1]		
Cheese/Dairy Products		
American, processed Blue[2] Boursault[2] Brick, natural Brie	Camembert[2] Cheddar[2] Emmenthaler[2] Gruyere Mozzarella Parmesan	Romano Roquefort Sour cream Stilton[2] Swiss[2] Yogurt
Meat/Fish		
Beef or chicken liver,[2] other meats, fish (unrefrigerated, fermented) Meats prepared with tenderizer	Fermented sausages (bologna, pepperoni, salami, summer sausage)[2] Game meat[2] Meat extracts	Caviar Dried fish (salted herring) Herring, pickled, spoiled[2] Shrimp paste
Alcoholic Beverages (Undistilled)		
Beer and ale (imports, some nonalcoholic)	Red wine (especially Chianti)[2]	Sherry[2] Vermouth[2] Distilled spirits
Fruit/Vegetables		
Avocados (especially overripe) Yeast extracts (Marmite, etc.)[2]	Bananas Figs, canned (overripe) Raisins Sauerkraut[2]	Soy sauce Miso soup Bean curd
Foods Containing Other Vasopressors		
Fava beans (overripe) – dopa[2]	Caffeine (eg, coffee, tea, colas)	Chocolate – phenylethylamine Ginseng

[1] Tyramine contents are not predictable and may vary. The amounts of tyramine are estimated from low to very high.

[2] Contains high to very high amounts of tyramine.

Suicidal risks: In patients who may be suicidal risks, no single form of treatment, such as MAOIs, electroconvulsive or other therapy should be relied upon as a sole therapeutic measure. Strict supervision and, preferably, hospitalization are advised.

Concomitant antidepressants: In patients receiving a selective serotonin reuptake inhibitor (SSRI) in combination with an MAOI, there have been reports of serious, sometimes fatal, reactions including hyperthermia, rigidity, myoclonus, autonomic instability with possible rapid fluctuations of vital signs, and mental status changes that include extreme agitation progressing to delirium and coma. These reactions have also occurred in patients who have recently discontinued that drug and have been started on a MAOI. Some cases presented with features resembling neuroleptic malignant syndrome. It is recommended that SSRIs not be used in combination with a MAOI, or within 14 days of a MAOI. Allow at least 2 weeks after stopping the SSRIs before starting a MAOI (see Drug Interactions). Allow at least 5 weeks after stopping fluoxetine before starting a MAOI.

Do not administer MAOIs with or immediately following tricyclic antidepressants (TCAs). Such combinations can produce seizures, sweating, coma, hyperexcitability, hyperthermia, tachycardia, tachypnea, headache, mydriasis, flushing, confusion, hypotension, disseminated intravascular coagulation and death. Allow at least 14 days to elapse between the discontinuation of the MAOIs and the institution of a TCA. Some TCAs have been used safely and successfully in combination with MAOIs.

MONOAMINE OXIDASE INHIBITORS

Withdrawal may be associated with nausea, vomiting and malaise. An uncommon withdrawal syndrome following abrupt withdrawal of MAOIs has been infrequently reported. Signs and symptoms of this syndrome generally commence 24 to 72 hours after drug discontinuation and may range from vivid nightmares with agitation to frank psychosis and convulsions. This syndrome generally responds to reinstitution of low-dose MAOI therapy followed by cautious downward titration and discontinuation.

Coexisting symptoms: **Tranylcypromine** may aggravate coexisting symptoms in depression, such as anxiety and agitation.

Renal function impairment: Observe caution in patients with impaired renal function because there is a possibility of cumulative effects in such patients.

Carcinogenesis: **Phenelzine,** like other hydrazine derivatives, has induced pulmonary and vascular tumors in an uncontrolled lifetime study in mice.

Elderly: Older patients may suffer more morbidity than younger patients during and following an episode of hypertension or malignant hyperthermia with MAOI use. Older patients have less compensatory reserve to cope with any serious adverse reactions. Therefore, use **tranylcypromine** with caution in the elderly.

Pregnancy: Category C. Safety for use during pregnancy has not been established. Use during pregnancy or in women of childbearing age only when clearly needed and when the potential benefits outweigh the potential hazards to the fetus.

Doses of **phenelzine** in pregnant mice well exceeding the maximum recommended human dose have caused a significant decrease in the number of viable offspring per mouse. The growth of dogs and rats has been retarded by doses exceeding the maximum human dose. **Tranylcypromine** passes through the placental barrier of animals into the fetus.

Lactation: Safety for use during lactation has not been established. **Tranylcypromine** is excreted in breast milk. Because of the potential for serious adverse effects in the nursing infant, decide whether to discontinue nursing or the drug, taking into account the importance of the drug to the mother.

Children: Not recommended for patients < 16 years of age.

Precautions:

Hypotension: Follow all patients for symptoms of postural hypotension. Hypotensive side effects have occurred in hypertensive as well as normal and hypotensive patients. Blood pressure usually returns to pretreatment levels rapidly when the drug is discontinued or the dosage is reduced.

At doses > 30 mg/day, postural hypotension is a major side effect and may result in syncope. Make dosage increases more gradually in patients showing a tendency toward hypotension at the beginning of therapy. Postural hypotension may be relieved by the patient lying down until blood pressure returns to normal.

Hypomania: Hypomania has been the most common severe psychiatric side effect reported. This has been largely limited to patients in whom disorders characterized by hyperkinetic symptoms coexist with, but are obscured by, depressive affect; hypomania usually appeared as depression improved. If agitation is present, it may be increased with MAOIs. Hypomania and agitation have also occurred at higher than recommended doses or following long-term therapy.

These drugs may cause excessive stimulation in agitated or schizophrenic patients; in manic-depressive states, it may result in a swing from a depressive to a manic phase.

Diabetes: There is conflicting evidence as to whether MAOIs affect glucose metabolism or potentiate hypoglycemic agents. Consider this if used in diabetics.

Epilepsy: The effect of MAOIs on the convulsive threshold may vary; take adequate precautions when treating epileptic patients.

Hepatotoxicity: It is difficult to differentiate most cases of drug-induced hepatocellular jaundice from viral hepatitis; they are histopathologically, biochemically and clinically indistinguishable. Although the reaction is rare, watch for hepatic complications. Perform periodic liver function tests, such as bilirubins, alkaline phosphatase or transaminases during therapy; discontinue at the first sign of hepatic dysfunction or jaundice.

Myocardial ischemia: MAOIs may suppress anginal pain that would otherwise serve as a warning of myocardial ischemia.

Hyperthyroid patients: Use **tranylcypromine** cautiously because of increased sensitivity to pressor amines.

MONOAMINE OXIDASE INHIBITORS

Switching MAOIs: In several case reports, hypertensive crisis, cerebral hemorrhage and death have possibly resulted from switching from one MAOI to another without a waiting period. However, in other patients no adverse reactions occurred. Nevertheless, a waiting period of 10 to 14 days is recommended when switching from one MAOI to another.

Drug abuse and dependence: There have been reports of drug dependency in patients using doses of **tranylcypromine** significantly in excess of the therapeutic range. Some of these patients had a history of previous substance abuse. The following withdrawal symptoms have been reported: Restlessness; anxiety; depression; confusion; hallucinations; headaches; weakness; diarrhea.

Drug Interactions:

MAOI Drug Interactions

Precipitant drug	Object drug*		Description
Dibenzazepine-related entities	MAOIs	↑	Do not administer MAOIs together or in rapid succession with other MAOIs or with dibenzazepine-related entities. Hypertensive crises or severe convulsive seizures may occur in patients receiving such combinations.
Disulfiram	Tranylcypromine	↑	There has been one report of coadministration resulting in delirium, agitation, disorientation, visual hallucinations, nystagmus and a subcomatose state.
Methylphenidate	MAOIs	↑	Coadministration may cause a hypertensive crisis.
Metrizamide	MAOIs	↑	Discontinue MAOIs at least 48 hours before myelography and do not resume for at least 24 hours postprocedure due to the decrease of the seizure threshold.
MAOIs	Anesthetics	↑	Although it has been suggested to discontinue MAOIs at least 1 to 2 weeks prior to elective surgery due to the risk of adverse cardiovascular effects, recent data suggest that MAOIs may be continued through surgery as long as precautions are undertaken to avoid sympathetic stimulation.
MAOIs	Antidepressants	↑	Do not administer MAOIs together with or immediately following venlafaxine, TCAs or SSRIs (see Warnings). There have been reports of serious, sometimes fatal, reactions (including hyperthermia, rigidity, myoclonus, autonomic instability with possible fluctuations of vital signs, and mental status changes that include extreme agitation progressing to delirium and coma). Some TCAs have been used safely and successfully in combination with MAOIs. Use cyclobenzaprine, which is structurally related to TCAs, with caution.
MAOIs	Antidiabetic agents	↑	MAOIs may potentiate the hypoglycemic response to insulin or sulfonylureas and delay recovery from hypoglycemia.
MAOIs	Barbiturates	↑	MAOIs potentiate hexobarbital hypnosis in animals. Therefore, give barbiturates at a reduced dose with MAOIs.
MAOIs	Beta blockers	↑	Bradycardia may develop during concurrent use of certain MAOIs and beta blockers.
MAOIs	Dextromethorphan	↑	Hyperpyrexia, hypotension and death have been associated with this combination. However, lack of adequate patient data makes it difficult to draw conclusions; additional documentation is needed.
MAOIs	Guanethidine	↓	MAOIs may inhibit the hypotensive effects of guanethidine.
MAOIs	Levodopa	↑	Hypertensive reactions occur if levodopa is given to patients receiving MAOIs.

MONOAMINE OXIDASE INHIBITORS

MAOI Drug Interactions			
Precipitant drug	Object drug*		Description
MAOIs	Meperidine	↑	Coadministration may result in agitation, seizures, diaphoresis and fever, and progress to coma, apnea and death. Adverse reactions are possible weeks after MAOI withdrawal. Avoid this combination; administer other narcotic analgesics with caution.
MAOIs	Methyldopa	↑	Coadministration may cause loss of blood pressure control or signs of central stimulation (eg, excitation, hallucinations).
MAOIs	Rauwolfia alkaloids	↑	MAOIs inhibit the destruction of serotonin and norepinephrine, which are believed to be released from tissue stores by rauwolfia alkaloids. Exercise caution when rauwolfia is used concomitantly with MAOIs.
MAOIs Sulfonamide	Sulfonamide MAOIs	↑	Coadministration may cause sulfonamide or MAOI toxicity.
MAOIs	Sumatriptan	↑	Systemic exposure to sumatriptan may be increased, producing toxicity.
MAOIs	Sympathomimetics	↑	The MAOIs' potentiation of indirect- or mixed-acting sympathomimetic substances, including anorexiants, may result in severe headache, hypertension and hyperpyrexia, possibly resulting in hypertensive crisis; avoid coadministration. Direct-acting agents appear to interact minimally, if at all (see Warnings).
MAOIs	Thiazide diuretics	↑	Exaggerated hypotensive effects may result from concurrent use.
MAOIs	L-Tryptophan	↑	Coadministration may result in hyperreflexia, confusion, disorientation, shivering, myoclonic jerks, agitation, amnesia, delirium, hypomanic signs, ataxia, ocular oscillations, Babinski signs.

* ↑ = Object drug increased. ↓ = Object drug decreased.

Drug/Food interactions: Warn all patients against eating foods with a high **tyramine** content. Hypertensive crisis may result. (See Warnings.)

Adverse Reactions:

Common:

Cardiovascular – Orthostatic hypotension, associated in some patients with falling; disturbances in cardiac rate and rhythm.

CNS – Dizziness; vertigo; headache; hyperreflexia; tremors; muscle twitching; mania; hypomania (see Precautions); confusion; memory impairment; sleep disturbances including hypersomnia and insomnia; weakness; myoclonic movements; fatigue; drowsiness; restlessness; overstimulation including increased anxiety, agitation and manic symptoms.

GI – Constipation; nausea; diarrhea; abdominal pain.

Miscellaneous – Edema; dry mouth; elevated serum transaminases; anorexia; weight changes; weight gain; sexual disturbances.

Less common:

CNS – Akathisia; jitteriness; euphoria; neuritis; palilalia; chills; convulsions; paresthesia .

Cardiovascular – Palpitations; tachycardia.

GU – Dysuria; urinary retention.

Hematologic – Hematologic changes including anemia, agranulocytosis, thrombocytopenia.

Ophthalmic – Glaucoma; nystagmus; blurred vision.

Miscellaneous – Sweating; skin rash; hypernatremia; hypermetabolic syndrome.

Rare:

CNS – Convulsions; ataxia; coma; hallucinations with high dosages; acute anxiety reaction; precipitation of schizophrenia; toxic delirium; manic reaction; headaches without blood pressure elevation; muscle spasm; myoclonic jerks; numbness.

GU – Impaired water excretion compatible with the syndrome of inappropriate secretion of antidiuretic hormone (SIADH).

MONOAMINE OXIDASE INHIBITORS

Hepatic – Reversible jaundice; hepatitis; fatal progressive necrotizing hepatocellular damage.

Metabolic – Hypermetabolic syndrome which may include, but is not limited to, hyperpyrexia, tachycardia, tachypnea, muscular rigidity, elevated CK levels, metabolic acidosis, hypoxia, coma and may resemble an overdose.

Miscellaneous – Edema of the glottis; transient respiratory and cardiovascular depression following ECT; leukopenia; lupus-like syndrome; fever associated with increased muscle tone; tinnitus; localized scleroderma, cystic acne flare-up, ataxia, akinesia, disorientation, urinary frequency or incontinence, urticaria, fissuring in corner of mouth (tranylcypromine).

Overdosage:

Depending on the amount of overdosage, a mixed clinical picture may develop involving signs and symptoms of the CNS, cardiovascular stimulation or depression. Signs and symptoms may be absent or minimal during the initial 12 hour period following ingestion and may develop slowly thereafter, reaching a maximum in 24 to 48 hours. Some symptoms may persist for 8 to 14 days. Immediate hospitalization, with continuous patient monitoring throughout this period, is essential.

Symptoms: Early symptoms of MAOI toxicity include: Excitement; irritability; hyperactivity; anxiety; hypotension; vascular collapse; insomnia; restlessness; dizziness; faintness; weakness; drowsiness; hallucinations; trismus; flushing; sweating; tachypnea; tachycardia; movement disorders including grimacing, opisthotonus, rigidity, clonic movements and muscular fasciculation; severe headache. In serious cases, coma, convulsions, hypertension with severe headache, acidosis, precordial pain, respiratory depression and failure, hyperpyrexia, diaphoresis, cool and clammy skin, cardiorespiratory arrest, incoherence, agitation, mental confusion, extreme dizziness, shock and death may occur. Rare instances have been reported in which hypertension was accompanied by twitching or myoclonic fibrillation of skeletal muscles with hyperpyrexia, sometimes progressing to generalized rigidity and coma.

Treatment: Induce emesis or gastric lavage with instillation of charcoal slurry in early poisoning; protect the airway against aspiration. Support respiration by appropriate measures, including management of the airway, use of supplemental oxygen and mechanical ventilatory assistance, as required. Refer to General Management of Acute Overdosage.

Cardiovascular complications include hypertension and hypotension; hence, any cardiovascular agent must be administered cautiously and blood pressure monitored frequently. Severe hypertension may be treated with an alpha-adrenergic blocker (eg, phentolamine, phenoxybenzamine). Beta-blocking agents are not necessarily contraindicated and may be useful for tachycardia, tachypnea and hyperpyrexia; however, more data are needed.Treat hypotension and vascular collapse with IV fluids and, if necessary, titrate blood pressure with an IV infusion of a dilute pressor agent. Adrenergic agents may produce a markedly increased pressor response.

CNS stimulation, including convulsions, may be treated with diazepam given slowly IV. Avoid phenothiazine derivatives and CNS stimulants. Monitor body temperature closely. Intensive management of hyperpyrexia may be required. Maintenance of fluid and electrolyte balance is essential.

Hemodialysis, peritoneal dialysis and charcoal hemoperfusion may be of value in massive overdosage, but sufficient data are not available to recommend their routine use. External cooling is recommended if hyperpyrexia occurs. Barbiturates have been reported to help relieve myoclonic reactions.

The pathophysiologic effects of massive overdosage may persist for several days; recovery may be expected within 3 to 4 days. Continue treatment for several days until homeostasis is restored. Liver function studies are recommended during the 4 to 6 weeks after recovery. It is not known if tranylcypromine is dialyzable.

Patient Information:

Do not discontinue this medication or adjust dosage except on the advice of a physician. Consult physician before taking any other medication, including *otc* items.

Avoid tyramine-containing foods and certain *otc* drug products (see Warnings).

May cause drowsiness or blurred vision; use with caution when driving or performing other tasks requiring alertness, coordination or physical dexterity.

Dizziness, weakness or fainting may occur when arising from a sitting position.

Effects may be delayed a few weeks. Take as directed. Avoid alcohol and tryptophan.

Notify physician if severe headache, palpitation or tachycardia, a sense of constriction in the throat or chest, sweating, dizziness, neck stiffness, nausea or vomiting or other unusual symptoms occur.

Monoamine Oxidase Inhibitors

PHENELZINE

For complete prescribing information, refer to the MAOIs group monograph.

Indications:

Depression: Effective in depressed patients clinically characterized as "atypical", "nonendogenous" or "neurotic". These patients often have mixed anxiety and depression and phobic or hypochondriacal features. There is less conclusive evidence of usefulness in severely depressed patients with endogenous features.

Phenelzine sulfate is rarely the first antidepressant drug used. Rather, it is more suitable for use in treatment-resistant patients.

Administration and Dosage:

Initial dose: 15 mg 3 times/day.

Early phase treatment: Increase dosage to at least 60 mg/day at a fairly rapid pace consistent with patient tolerance. It may be necessary to increase dosage up to 90 mg/day to obtain sufficient MAO inhibition. Many patients do not show a clinical response until treatment at 60 mg has been continued for at least 4 weeks.

Maintenance dose: After maximum benefit is achieved, reduce dosage slowly over several weeks. Maintenance dose may be as low as 15 mg/day or every other day; continue for as long as required.

Rx	**Nardil** (Parke-Davis)	**Tablets:** 15 mg (as sulfate)	Sucrose. (P-D 270). Orange. Biconvex. Sugar coated. In 100s.
🍁	**Nardil** (Parke-Davis)	**Tablets:** 15 mg (as sulfate)	Sucrose. Orange. Biconvex. Sugar coated. In 100s and 500s.

TRANYLCYPROMINE

For complete prescribing information, refer to the MAOIs group monograph.

Indications:

Depression: Effective for use with adult outpatients with reactive depression (a Major Depressive Episode without Melancholia according to DSM III diagnosis). Efficacy for use in endogenous depression has not been established.

Administration and Dosage:

Individualize dosage. Improvement should be seen within 48 hours to 3 weeks after starting therapy. The usual effective dosage is 30 mg/day in divided doses. If there is no improvement after 2 weeks, increase dosage in 10 mg/day increments at intervals of 1 to 3 weeks. Dosage range may be extended to a maximum of 60 mg/day from the usual 30 mg/day. Gradually withdraw tranylcypromine.

Rx	**Parnate** (SmithKline Beecham)	**Tablets:** 10 mg (as sulfate)	Lactose. (Parnate SKF). Red. Film coated. In 100s.
🍁	**Parnate** (SmithKline Beecham)	**Tablets:** 10 mg (as sulfate)	Sucrose. (SKF N71). Red. Biconvex. Sugar coated. In 100s.

ANTIPSYCHOTIC AGENTS

The discussion below applies to antipsychotics as a therapeutic class. Due to pharmacological similarities, consider all information when using these drugs. Reserpine, not discussed in this section, was previously used as an antipsychotic. Lithium, pimozide, clozapine and risperidone are discussed separately (see individual monographs).

Actions:

Pharmacology:

Select Dosage and Pharmacologic Parameters of Antipsychotics							
Incidence of Side Effects: +++ = High, ++ = Moderate, + = Low; Antipsychotic agent	Approx. equiv. dose (mg)	Adult daily dosage range (mg)	Sedation	Extrapyramidal symptoms	Anticholinergic effects	Orthostatic hypotension	Therapeutic plasma concentration (ng/ml)
Phenothiazines: Aliphatic							
Chlorpromazine	100	30-800	+++	++	++	+++	30-500
Promazine	200	40-1200	++	++	+++	++	
Triflupromazine	25	60-150	+++	++	+++	++	
Phenothiazines: Piperidine							
Thioridazine	100	150-800	+++	+	+++	+++	
Mesoridazine	50	30-400	+++	+	+++	++	
Phenothiazines: Piperazine							
Acetophenazine	20	60-120	++	+++	+	+	
Perphenazine	10	12-64	+	+++	+	+	0.8-1.2
Prochlorperazine	15	15-150	++	+++	+	+	
Fluphenazine	2	0.5-40	+	+++	+	+	0.13-2.8
Trifluoperazine	5	2-40	+	+++	+	+	
Thioxanthenes							
Chlorprothixene	100	75-600	+++	++	++	++	
Thiothixene	4	8-30	+	+++	+	+	2-57
Butyrophenone							
Haloperidol	2	1-15	+	+++	+	+	5-20
Dihydroindolone							
Molindone	10	15-225	+	+++	+	+	
Dibenzoxazepine							
Loxapine	15	20-250	++	+++	+	++	
Dibenzodiazepine							
Clozapine	50	300-900	+++	+	+++	+++	
Benzisoxazole							
Risperidone		4-16	+	0/+	+	+	
Diphenylbutylpiperidine							
Pimozide	0.3-0.5	1-10	++	+++	++	+	

The phenothiazines are subdivided into three groups, based on side chain substitution at position 10 of the chemical structure: Aliphatic, piperidine and piperazine. Aliphatics cause more sedation, hypotension, dermatitis and convulsions and fewer extrapyramidal side effects (EPS). Piperazines cause more EPS and less sedation, hypotension and lens opacities. Piperidines cause more retinal toxicity, ejaculatory disturbances and ECG effects and the fewest EPS. Though chemically distinct, these agents share many pharmacological and clinical properties.

The exact mode of action is not fully understood. Antipsychotics block postsynaptic dopamine receptors in the basal ganglia, hypothalamus, limbic system, brain stem and medulla. Inhibition or alteration of dopamine release, an increased neuronal cell firing rate in the midbrain and an increased turnover rate of dopamine in the forebrain have been noted. These observations support the theory that antipsychotics interfere with dopamine, but do not prove that dopaminolytic activity is sufficient for antipsychotic efficacy. The phenothiazines appear to act at both D_1 and D_2 receptors, whereas haloperidol appears to act primarily at D_2 receptors.

The phenothiazines are believed to depress various components of the reticular activating system which is involved in the control of basal metabolism and body temperature, wakefulness, vasomotor tone, emesis and hormonal balance. In addition, the drugs exert anticholinergic and alpha-adrenergic blocking effects.

ANTIPSYCHOTIC AGENTS

The term "neuroleptic," a synonym for antipsychotic agent, refers to effects of these agents that differ from classical CNS depressants. They diminish conditional behavioral responses, selectively dampen neurophysiologic effects of peripheral stimuli on the forebrain and have limited ability to induce generalized sedation. These drugs cause lack of initiative and interest in the environment, little display of emotion and limited affect and neurological (ie, EPS and parkinsonian) effects.

Pharmacokinetics:

Absorption – Oral absorption tends to be erratic and variable. Peak plasma levels are seen 2 to 4 hours after oral use. Oral liquid forms are most predictably absorbed. Conventional tablets are preferred over sustained release forms which are usually more expensive and not necessary due to long duration of action of these agents. IM use provides 4 to 10 times more active drug than oral doses.

Distribution – These agents are widely distributed in tissues; CNS concentrations exceed those in plasma. They are highly bound to plasma proteins (91% to 99%). Because they are highly lipophilic, the antipsychotics and metabolites accumulate in the brain, lungs and other tissues with high blood supply. They are stored in these tissues and may be found in urine for up to 6 months after the last dose.

Metabolism – Extensive biotransformation occurs in the liver. Numerous active metabolites, which persist for prolonged periods, have important side effects and contribute to the biological activity of the parent drug.

Excretion – One-half of the excretion of these agents occurs via the kidneys and the other half occurs through enterohepatic circulation. Elimination half-lives range from 10 to 20 hours. Less than 1% is excreted as unchanged drug.

Clinical trials: There is little evidence of clinical differences in efficacy among these agents (except clozapine) when used in equitherapeutic dosages; however, a patient who fails to respond to one agent may respond to another and agents are not necessarily interchangeable. Clozapine is used for severely ill schizophrenic patients who fail to respond adequately to standard antipsychotic treatment.

The principal differences between antipsychotic agents are the type and severity of side effects which include: Sedation, extrapyramidal effects, anticholinergic effects and antiadrenergic effects (orthostatic hypotension). Clozapine also differs in its effects on various dopamine-mediated behaviors. Changing agents may minimize undesirable or intolerable side effects (refer to table). Coadministration of two or more antipsychotics does not improve clinical response and may increase the potential for adverse effects.

In chronic therapy, full clinical effects may not be achieved for ≥ 6 weeks. Approximately 4 to 7 days are required to achieve steady-state plasma levels; therefore, do not make more than weekly dosage adjustments in chronic therapy.

Since plasma concentrations of antipsychotics are highly variable from patient to patient, plasma monitoring of these agents may not be useful for determining therapeutic response. Plus, therapeutic levels are only available for a small number of these agents. However, monitoring may help decrease the incidence of toxicity since plasma levels are relatively stable in each individual.

Indications:

Management of psychotic disorders.

Some of these agents are used as antiemetics (refer to Antiemetic/Antivertigo Agents).

Refer to individual product listings for approved indications.

Unlabeled uses: Chlorpromazine and haloperidol are effective in the treatment of phencyclidine (PCP) psychosis; coadministration of ascorbic acid with haloperidol may be more effective than haloperidol alone.

IV or IM chlorpromazine may be beneficial for migraine headaches; IV prochlorperazine may be effective in treating severe vascular or tension headaches.

Neuroleptics appear useful for the treatment of Tourette's syndrome; switching from one agent to another may occasionally be necessary. Haloperidol (approved for Tourette's) and nicotine polacrilex gum coadministration resulted in improvement of symptoms in two children. Further study is needed.

Neuroleptics are effective in control of acute agitation in the elderly; use lowest dose for shortest duration possible. May also be useful in treating some symptoms of dementia including agitation, hyperactivity, hallucinations, suspiciousness, hostility and uncooperativeness; however, they do not improve memory loss and may impair cognitive function.

Other potential uses include treatment of: Huntington's chorea (chlorpromazine, fluphenazine, haloperidol); hemiballismus (perphenazine, haloperidol); chorea associated with rheumatic fever or SLE, spasmodic torticollis and Meige's syndrome (haloperidol).

ANTIPSYCHOTIC AGENTS

Contraindications:

Comatose or severely depressed states; hypersensitivity (cross sensitivity between phenothiazines may occur); presence of large amounts of other CNS depressants; bone marrow depression; blood dyscrasias; circulatory collapse (thioxanthenes); subcortical brain damage; Parkinson's disease (haloperidol); liver damage; cerebral arteriosclerosis; coronary artery disease; severe hypotension or hypertension; pediatric surgery (prochlorperazine).

Warnings:

Tardive dyskinesia (TD), a syndrome consisting of potentially irreversible, involuntary dyskinetic movements, may develop in patients treated with neuroleptic drugs. Although prevalence of TD appears highest among the elderly, especially women, it is impossible to rely upon prevalence estimates to predict, at the inception of neuroleptic treatment, which patients are likely to develop the syndrome. Whether neuroleptic drugs differ in their potential to cause TD is unknown. Both the risk of developing TD and the likelihood that it will become irreversible are increased as duration of treatment and total cumulative dose administered increase. However, the syndrome can develop, although much less commonly, after relatively brief treatment periods at low doses. Anticholinergic agents may worsen these effects.

There is no known treatment for established cases of TD, although it may remit, partially or completely, if neuroleptics are withdrawn. Neuroleptic treatment itself, however, may suppress (or partially suppress) signs and symptoms TD, possibly masking the underlying disease process. The effect of symptomatic suppression on the long-term course of the syndrome is unknown.

Given these considerations, prescribe neuroleptics in a manner most likely to minimize the occurrence of tardive dyskinesia. In general, reserve chronic neuroleptic treatment for patients who suffer from a chronic illness that responds to neuroleptic drugs and for whom alternative, equally effective, but potentially less harmful treatments are not available or appropriate. In patients who require chronic treatment, use the smallest dose and the shortest duration of treatment producing a satisfactory clinical response. Periodically reassess the need for continued treatment.

If signs and symptoms of TD appear, consider drug discontinuation. However, some patients may require treatment despite the presence of the syndrome.

Neuroleptic malignant syndrome (NMS) is a rare idiosyncratic combination of EPS, hyperthermia and autonomic disturbance. Onset may be hours to months after drug initiation, but once started, proceeds rapidly over 24 to 72 hours. It is most commonly associated with **haloperidol** and depot **fluphenazines**, but has occurred with **thiothixene** and **thioridazine** and may occur with other agents. NMS is potentially fatal, and requires intensive symptomatic treatment and immediate discontinuation of neuroleptic treatment. Treatment of choice is not yet established, but dantrolene may be beneficial (see individual monograph). Rechallenge with a neuroleptic may result in an 80% recurrence of NMS; however, some success has occurred by using a low-potency agent and gradually increasing dose. See Adverse Reactions.

CNS effects: These agents may impair mental or physical abilities, especially during the first few days. Drowsiness may occur during the first or second week, after which it generally disappears. If troublesome, lower the dosage. Caution patients against activities requiring alertness (eg, operating vehicles or machinery). Use cautiously in depressed patients. Use caution in agitated states with depression, (particularly if a suicidal tendency is recognized). When **haloperidol** is used for mania in cyclic disorders, a rapid mood swing to depression may occur.

Antiemetic effects: Drugs with antiemetic effect can obscure signs of toxicity of other drugs, or mask symptoms of disease (eg, brain tumor, intestinal obstruction, Reye's syndrome). They can suppress the cough reflex; aspiration of vomitus is possible.

Pulmonary: Cases of bronchopneumonia (some fatal) have followed the use of antipsychotic agents. Lethargy and decreased sensation of thirst due to central inhibition may lead to dehydration, hemoconcentration and reduced pulmonary ventilation. If the above signs appear, especially in the elderly, institute remedial therapy promptly.

Use with caution in respiratory impairment due to acute pulmonary infections or chronic respiratory disorders, such as severe asthma or emphysema. "Silent pneumonias" may develop in patients treated with phenothiazines.

Decreased serum cholesterol occurs. **Chlorpromazine** may raise plasma cholesterol.

Cardiovascular: Use with caution in patients with cardiovascular disease or mitral insufficiency. Increased pulse rates occur in most patients. One result of therapy may be an increase in mental and physical activity. For example, a few patients with angina pectoris have complained of increased pain while taking **trifluoperazine**. Therefore, withdraw the drug from angina patients if an unfavorable response is noted.

Hypertension – Pulse rates have increased in most patients receiving antipsychotics. Rebound hypertension may occur in pheochromocytoma patients.

ANTIPSYCHOTIC AGENTS

Hypotension – Carefully watch patients who are undergoing surgery, and who are on large doses of phenothiazines, for hypotensive phenomena. It may be necessary to reduce amounts of anesthetics or CNS depressants. The hypotensive effects may occur after the first injection of the antipsychotic, occasionally after subsequent injections, and rarely after the first oral dose. Recovery is usually spontaneous and symptoms disappear within 0.5 to 2 hours. If hypotension occurs, place the patient in a recumbent position. Females appear to have a greater tendency to orthostatic hypotension. Patients with hypovolemia have increased sensitivity to the hypotensive effects of these agents. Volume replacement, when needed, should precede use of vasopressors. If a vasopressor is indicated, use phenylephrine or norepinephrine. Avoid using epinephrine in drug-induced hypotension (see Drug Interactions).

Ophthalmic: Use with caution in patients with a history of glaucoma. The anticholinergic effects may precipitate angle closure in susceptible patients. During prolonged therapy, ocular changes may occur; these include particle deposition in the cornea and lens, progressing in more severe cases to star-shaped lenticular opacities.

Pigmentary retinopathy occurs most frequently in patients receiving **thioridazine** dosages > 1 g/day. Pigmentary retinopathy is characterized by diminution of visual acuity, brownish coloring of vision, impairment of night vision and pigment deposits on the fundus. Ophthalmological (slit lamp) evaluation is recommended. Discontinue use if retinal changes occur.

Seizure disorders: These drugs can lower the convulsive threshold and may precipitate seizures. Petit mal and grand mal seizures have occurred, particularly in patients with EEG abnormalities or a history of such disorders. Use cautiously in patients with a history of epilepsy and only when absolutely necessary. These drugs may be used concomitantly with anticonvulsants; maintain an adequate anticonvulsant dosage (see Adverse Reactions). In animals, **molindone** does not lower the seizure threshold to the degree noted with more sedating agents. However, convulsive seizures have occurred in humans.

Adynamic ileus occasionally occurs with phenothiazine therapy and, if severe, can result in complications and death.

Sudden death: Previous brain damage or seizures may be predisposing factors; avoid high doses in known seizure patients. Several patients have shown sudden flare-ups of psychotic behavior patterns shortly before death. In some cases, death was apparently due to cardiac arrest; in others, asphyxia was due to failure of the cough reflex. Autopsy findings usually reveal acute fulminating pneumonia or pneumonitis, aspiration of gastric contents or intramyocardial lesions. In some patients, cause could not be determined. Phenothiazine use in infants < 1 year may be a factor in sudden infant death syndrome (SIDS).

Hepatic effects: Jaundice usually occurs between the second and fourth weeks of treatment and is regarded as a hypersensitivity reaction. The clinical picture resembles infectious hepatitis with laboratory features of obstructive jaundice. It is usually reversible; however, chronic jaundice and biliary stasis have occurred. If fever with flu-like symptoms occurs, perform liver function tests. If tests are positive, discontinue treatment. Withhold exploratory laparotomy until extrahepatic obstruction is confirmed. Because of the possibility of liver damage, periodically monitor hepatic function. AST and ALT elevation has occurred with **loxapine**.

Renal function impairment: Administer cautiously to those with diminished renal function. Monitor renal function in long-term therapy; lower the dose or discontinue if BUN becomes abnormal.

Hepatic function impairment: Use with caution in patients with impaired hepatic function. Patients with a history of hepatic encephalopathy due to cirrhosis have increased sensitivity to the CNS effects of antipsychotic drugs (ie, impaired cerebration and abnormal slowing of the EEG).

There is no conclusive evidence that preexisting liver disease makes patients more susceptible to jaundice. Alcoholics with cirrhosis have been successfully treated with chlorpromazine without complications. Nevertheless, use cautiously in patients with liver disease. Patients who have experienced jaundice with a phenothiazine should not, if possible, be reexposed.

Carcinogenesis: Neuroleptic drugs (except promazine) elevate prolactin levels which persist during chronic use. Tissue culture experiments indicate ≈⅓ of human breast cancers are prolactin-dependent in vitro, a factor of potential importance if use of these drugs is contemplated in a patient with previously detected breast cancer. Although disturbances such as galactorrhea, amenorrhea, gynecomastia and impotence have occurred, clinical significance of elevated serum prolactin levels is unknown for most patients. An increase in mammary neoplasms has occurred in rodents after chronic neuroleptic use. Studies, however, have not shown an association between chronic use of these drugs and mammary tumorigenesis.

ANTIPSYCHOTIC AGENTS

Mutagenesis: Chromosomal aberrations in spermatocytes and abnormal sperm has occurred in rodents.

Elderly: Dosages in the lower range are sufficient for most elderly patients. Since these patients appear more susceptible to various cardiovascular and neuromuscular reactions, observe patients closely. Monitor response and adjust dosage accordingly. Increase dosage gradually in elderly patients.

Pregnancy: Safety for use during pregnancy has not been established. Use only when clearly needed and when potential benefits outweigh potential hazards to the fetus.

Phenothiazines readily cross the placenta; however, most studies have found them safe for both mother and fetus if used occasionally in low doses. Isolated reports of multiple congenital anomalies are offset by numerous studies showing no correlation of drug and defect. These drugs are apparently nonteratogenic. However, use near term may cause maternal hypotension and adverse neonatal effects (extrapyramidal syndrome, hyperreflexia/hyporeflexia, jaundice).

Animal studies show a potential for embryotoxicity and increased neonatal mortality. Tests in offspring of drug-treated rodents demonstrate decreased performance. The possibility of permanent neurological damage cannot be excluded.

Lactation: **Chlorpromazine** and **haloperidol** have been detected in breast milk. Although few cases are documented, a milk:plasma ratio of 0.5 to 0.7 or less is reported, representing a milk drug level of 290 ng/ml and 2 to 23.5 ng/ml, respectively. Safety for use in the nursing mother has not been established.

Children: In general, these products are not recommended for children < 12 years old. Loxapine is not recommended in children < 16 years old. (See individual product listings for agents that may be used in children.) Children with acute illnesses (eg, chickenpox, CNS infections, measles, gastroenteritis) or dehydration appear much more susceptible to neuromuscular reactions, particularly dystonias, than adults.

Extrapyramidal symptoms can occur and be confused with CNS signs of an undiagnosed primary disease responsible for the vomiting (eg, Reye's syndrome or other encephalopathy). Avoid antipsychotics and other potential hepatotoxins in children and adolescents whose signs and symptoms suggest Reye's syndrome.

Although limited data suggest the risk of SIDS may be increased by phenothiazine use in predisposed infants, epidemiological studies do not implicate the drug as a potential causative factor. Nevertheless, consider the risk:benefit ratio in infants.

Precautions:

Concomitant conditions: Use with caution in patients: Exposed to extreme heat or phosphorus insecticides; in a state of alcohol withdrawal; with dermatoses or other allergic reactions to phenothiazine derivatives because of the possibility of cross-sensitivity; who have exhibited idiosyncrasy to other centrally-acting drugs.

Hematologic: Various blood dyscrasias have occurred (see Adverse Reactions). If sore throat or other sign of infection occurs, or if white cell and differential counts indicate cellular depression, stop treatment and institute an antibiotic and other suitable therapy. A single case of transient granulocytopenia has been associated with **mesoridazine**.

Myelography: Discontinue phenothiazines at least 48 hours before myelography due to the possibility of seizures; do not resume therapy for at least 24 hours postprocedure. Do not use phenothiazines to control nausea and vomiting occurring before or after myelography.

Thyroid: Severe neurotoxicity (rigidity, inability to walk or talk) may occur in patients with thyrotoxicosis who are also receiving antipsychotics.

Hyperpyrexia: A significant, not otherwise explained rise in body temperature may indicate intolerance to antipsychotics. Discontinue in this case (see Adverse Reactions).

ECT: Reserve concurrent use with electroconvulsive treatment for those patients for whom it is essential; the hazards may be increased.

Abrupt withdrawal: These drugs are not known to cause psychic dependence and do not produce tolerance or addiction. However, following abrupt withdrawal of high dose therapy, symptoms such as gastritis, nausea, vomiting, dizziness, headache, tachycardia, insomnia and tremulousness have occurred. Onset of symptoms occurred in 2 to 4 days and subsided in 1 to 2 weeks. To lessen the likelihood of adverse reactions related to cumulative drug effects, periodically determine whether the maintenance dosage could be lowered or drug therapy discontinued. These symptoms can be reduced by gradual reduction of the dosage (one suggestion is 10% to 25% every 2 weeks) or by continuing antiparkinson agents for several weeks after the antipsychotic is withdrawn.

Suicide possibility in depressed patients remains during treatment and until significant remission occurs. This type of patient should not have access to large quantities of the drug.

ANTIPSYCHOTIC AGENTS

Cutaneous pigmentation changes/photosensitivity: Rare instances of skin pigmentation have occurred, primarily in females on long-term, high dose therapy. These changes, restricted to exposed areas of the skin, range from almost imperceptible darkening to a slate gray color, sometimes with a violet hue. Pigmentation may fade following drug discontinuation. Photosensitization may occur; caution patients against exposure to ultraviolet light or undue exposure to sunlight during phenothiazine therapy. These effects occur most commonly with **chlorpromazine** (3%) and have not been seen with **molindone** therapy.

Tartrazine sensitivity: Some of these products contain tartrazine, which may cause allergic-type reactions (including bronchial asthma) in susceptible individuals. Although the incidence of tartrazine sensitivity in the general population is low, it is frequently seen in patients who also have aspirin hypersensitivity. Specific products containing tartrazine are identified in the product listings.

Sulfite sensitivity: Some of these products contain sulfites that may cause allergic-type reactions including anaphylactic symptoms and life-threatening or less severe asthmatic episodes in certain susceptible persons. The overall prevalence of sulfite sensitivity in the general population is unknown and probably low. It is seen more frequently in asthmatic or atopic nonasthmatic persons.

Drug Interactions:

Alcohol and phenothiazine coadministration may result in additive CNS depression. Extrapyramidal reactions may also occur.

Aluminum salts may impair the GI absorption of the phenothiazines, possibly reducing its therapeutic effect. Administer the antacid at least 1 hour before or 2 hours after the phenothiazine.

Anorexiants and phenothiazine coadministration may diminish the pharmacologic effects of amphetamines and congeners.

Anticholinergics may reduce the pharmacologic/therapeutic actions of the phenothiazines. An increase in the incidence of anticholinergic side effects has occurred. Worsening of schizophrenic symptoms, decreased haloperidol serum concentrations and development of tardive dyskinesia may occur with anticholinergic coadministration.

Barbiturates may reduce phenothiazine or haloperidol plasma levels, possibly resulting in decreased pharmacologic effects. Barbiturate plasma levels may also be decreased by phenothiazines.

Barbiturate anesthetics: Preanesthesia administration of phenothiazines may raise the frequency and severity of neuromuscular excitation and hypotension in patients who receive barbiturate anesthesia. The significance of this interaction is variable depending on the specific agents used.

Bromocriptine effectiveness may be inhibited by phenothiazine coadministration.

Carbamazepine may decrease haloperidol serum concentrations, decreasing its therapeutic effects.

Charcoal can prevent the absorption of phenothiazines. Depending on the clinical situation, this will reduce the effectiveness or toxicity of the phenothiazine.

Epinephrine, norepinephrine: Chlorpromazine decreases the pressor effect of norepinephrine and eliminates bradycardia. In addition, chlorpromazine antagonizes the peripheral vasoconstrictive effects of epinephrine and in some instances reverses its action.

Fluoxetine: A patient developed severe extrapyramidal reactions during haloperidol coadministration.

Guanethidine: The hypotensive action of guanethidine may be inhibited by phenothiazines, haloperidol and possibly by thioxanthenes.

Lithium and phenothiazine or haloperidol coadministration may induce disorientation, unconsciousness and extrapyramidal symptoms.

Meperidine and phenothiazine coadministration may result in excessive sedation and hypotension.

Methyldopa may potentiate the antipsychotic effects of haloperidol or the combination may produce psychosis. Serious elevations in blood pressure occurred in a patient receiving concurrent methyldopa and trifluoperazine.

Metrizamide: The possibility of seizure may be increased during subarachnoid injection of metrizamide in patients maintained on a phenothiazine.

Phenytoin: An increase or decrease in phenytoin serum levels may occur; in two patients, thioridazine levels were decreased by concurrent phenytoin. Haloperidol serum concentrations may also be decreased.

ANTIPSYCHOTIC AGENTS

Propranolol and phenothiazine coadministration may result in increased plasma levels of both drugs. A hypotensive episode occurred in a patient receiving haloperidol and propranolol.

Tricyclic antidepressant serum concentrations may be increased by phenothiazine or haloperidol coadministration.

Valproic acid clearance may be decreased and half-life and trough levels increased in patients receiving chlorpromazine.

Drug/Lab test interactions: An increase in **cephalin flocculation** sometimes accompanied by alterations in other **liver function tests** has occurred in patients receiving fluphenazine enanthate who have had no clinical evidence of liver damage.

Phenothiazines may discolor the urine pink to red-brown.

False-positive **pregnancy tests** have occurred, but are less likely to occur when a serum test is used.

An increase in **protein bound iodine**, not attributable to an increase in thyroxine, has been noted.

Adverse Reactions:

Sudden death has occasionally been reported. See Warnings.

Neuroleptic malignant syndrome (NMS) or syndrome malin is a rare (0.5% to 1%) idiosyncratic combination of extrapyramidal symptoms, hyperthermia and autonomic disturbance; fatalities (20%) are usually caused by respiratory failure. Symptoms include: Hyperpyrexia; muscle rigidity; altered mental status (including catatonic signs); evidence of autonomic instability (irregular pulse or blood pressure); elevated CPK; myoglobinuria (rhabdomyolysis); acute renal failure; tachycardia; diaphoresis; cardiac arrhythmias. See Warnings.

Tardive dyskinesia: (See Warnings.) Symptoms are persistent and in some patients irreversible. The syndrome is characterized by rhythmical involuntary movements of the tongue, face, mouth or jaw (eg, protrusion of tongue, puffing of cheeks, puckering of mouth, chewing movements). Sometimes these may be accompanied by involuntary movements of extremities. In rare instances, these involuntary movements of the extremities are the only manifestations of tardive dyskinesia. A variant of tardive dyskinesia, tardive dystonia, has also been described.

Adverse behavioral effects: Exacerbation of psychotic symptoms including hallucinations; catatonic-like states; lethargy; restlessness; hyperactivity; agitation; nocturnal confusion; toxic confusional states; bizarre dreams; depression; euphoria; excitement; paranoid reactions.

Other CNS effects: Cerebral edema; headache; weakness; tremor; staggering gait; twitching; tension; jitteriness; akinesia; ataxia; fatigue; slurring; abnormal cerebrospinal fluid proteins; insomnia; vertigo; drowsiness (80%, usually lasts 1 week).

The *epileptogenic* effects (< 1%) are generally increased with the more sedative agents, ie, aliphatic phenothiazines > thioxanthenes = butyrophenones > piperidines > piperazines, although this may vary depending on the individual agent within the group. High doses, sudden dose changes, gross brain damage or history of epilepsy increase the likelihood of EEG changes or seizures.

Autonomic: Dry mouth; nasal congestion; nausea; vomiting; paresthesia; anorexia; pallor; flushed facies; salivation; perspiration; constipation; obstipation; fecal impaction; diarrhea; atonic colon; adynamic or paralytic ileus (see Warnings); urinary retention, frequency or incontinence; bladder paralysis; polyuria; enuresis; priapism; ejaculation inhibition; male impotence (not reported with **molindone**).

Heatstroke/Hyperpyrexia induced by neuroleptics has occurred. They may act in several ways including disrupting the hypothalamic thermoregulator center, alpha-adrenergic blockade and autonomic mechanisms. Use caution in patients predisposed to heat-related illness. Mild fever may occur after large IM doses.

Hepatic: Jaundice usually occurs between the second and fourth weeks of therapy and is regarded as a hypersensitivity reaction. See Warnings.

Hematologic: Eosinophilia; leukopenia; leukocytosis; anemia; tendency toward lymphomonocytosis; thrombocytopenia; granulocytopenia; aplastic anemia; hemolytic anemia; thrombocytopenic or nonthrombocytopenic purpura; pancytopenia.

Agranulocytosis – Most cases occurred between therapy weeks 4 and 10. Watch for sudden appearance of sore mouth, gums, throat or other signs of infection. If white cell count and differential show significant cellular depression, discontinue use. A slightly lowered white count alone is not an indication to discontinue drug.

Cardiovascular: Hypotension; postural hypotension; hypertension; tachycardia (especially with rapid increase in dosage); bradycardia; cardiac arrest; circulatory collapse; syncope; lightheadedness; faintness; dizziness. The hypotensive effect may occasionally produce a shock-like condition.

ANTIPSYCHOTIC AGENTS

The phenothiazines are direct myocardial depressants and may induce cardiomegaly, congestive heart failure and refractory arrhythmias, some fatal. Quinidine-like ECG changes (increased QT interval, ST depression and changes in AV conduction) and a variety of nonspecific ECG changes may occur. These are usually reversible and their relationship to myocardial damage has not been confirmed.

Cardiovascular effects are generally attributable to the piperidine phenothiazines > aliphatic > piperazines (see table).

Hypersensitivity: Urticarial (5%), maculopapular hypersensitivity reactions; pruritus; angioneurotic edema; dry skin; seborrhea; papillary hypertrophy of the tongue; erythema; photosensitivity (see Precautions); eczema; asthma; laryngeal edema; anaphylactoid reactions; rashes, including acneiform; hair loss; exfoliative dermatitis. Contact dermatitis can result from administering phenothiazine liquids.

Endocrine: Lactation and moderate breast engorgement in females; galactorrhea; syndrome of inappropriate ADH secretion; mastalgia; amenorrhea; menstrual irregularities; gynecomastia in males on large doses; changes in libido; hyperglycemia or hypoglycemia; hyponatremia; glycosuria; raised plasma cholesterol levels; pituitary tumor correlated with hyperprolactinemia. Resumption of menses in previously amenorrheic women has been reported with **molindone**. Initially, heavy menses may occur.

Ophthalmic: (See Warnings.) Glaucoma; photophobia; blurred vision; miosis; mydriasis; ptosis; star-shaped lenticular opacities; epithelial keratopathies; pigmentary retinopathy. Eye lesions may regress after drug withdrawal. Lens opacities and pigmentary retinopathy have not occurred with **molindone**.

Respiratory: Laryngospasm; bronchospasm; increased depth of respiration; dyspnea.

Miscellaneous: Enlarged parotid glands; increases in appetite and weight (excessive weight gain has not occurred with **molindone**); polyphagia; dyspepsia; peripheral or facial edema; suppression of cough reflex (with potential for aspiration or asphyxia); polydipsia; systemic lupus erythematosus-like syndrome.

Extrapyramidal: These are usually dose-related and take three forms: Pseudoparkinsonism (4% to 40%); akathisia (7% to 20%); dystonias (2% to 50%).

Management of extrapyramidal symptoms includes use of a barbiturate, antipsychotic dosage reduction and anticholinergic-type antiparkinson agents. Prophylactic anticholinergic medication is controversial. Parenteral diphenhydramine, 50 mg (2 mg/kg, to a maximum of 50 mg for children), or parenteral benztropine, 2 mg, will ameliorate the acute dystonic reaction within 2 to 5 minutes when given IV or within 30 to 60 minutes when given IM. Employ supportive measures, such as maintaining a clear airway and adequate hydration. Anticholinergics are often ineffective for akathisia; benzodiazepines, propranolol and clonidine have been used.

Pseudoparkinsonism symptoms may include mask-like facies, drooling, tremors, pillrolling motion, cogwheel rigidity and shuffling gait. In most cases, these symptoms are readily controlled with antiparkinson agent therapy of a few weeks to 2 or 3 months. After this time, evaluate patients to determine their need for continued treatment. (Note: Levodopa has not been effective in neuroleptic-induced pseudoparkinsonism.) Occasionally, dosage reduction or psychotropic discontinuation is necessary. Patients < 40 years of age may be more susceptible to the parkinsonian effects of haloperidol.

Dystonias include: Neck muscle spasms; extensor rigidity of back muscles; hyperreflexia; carpopedal spasm; trismus; torticollis; retrocollis; opisthotonos; oculogyric crises; aching and numbness of limbs; protrusion, discoloration, aching and rounding of the tongue; tonic spasm of masticatory muscles; tight feeling in the throat; dysphagia; dyskinesia; akathisia. These usually subside within 24 to 48 hours after drug discontinuation.

Akathisia is a condition of constant motor restlessness and may include feelings of muscle quivering, an inability to sit still and an urge to constantly move about. This can occur early in treatment or after several months of therapy. Patients between 30 and 60 years of age are more susceptible to akathisia.

Overdosage:

Symptoms: Primarily, CNS depression to the point of somnolence, deep sleep from which patient can be aroused or coma. Hypotension and extrapyramidal symptoms may occur. Hypertension instead of hypotension occurred in a 2-year-old with an accidental overdose of **haloperidol** and in an adult following **thioridazine** overdose. Other manifestations include: Agitation; restlessness; convulsions; fever; hypothermia; hyperthermia; coma; autonomic reactions; ECG changes; cardiac arrhythmias.

ANTIPSYCHOTIC AGENTS

Treatment: Includes usual supportive measures. Refer to General Management of Acute Overdosage. Emetics are unlikely to be of value due to antiemetic effects of these drugs; emesis induction may result in a dystonic reaction of the head or neck that could result in aspiration of vomitus. Treat extrapyramidal symptoms with antiparkinson drugs, barbiturates or diphenhydramine (see Adverse Reactions).

If hypotension occurs, initiate the standard measures for managing circulatory shock, including volume replacement. If a vasoconstrictor is desired, use norepinephrine or phenylephrine. Do not administer epinephrine (see Drug Interactions).

Phenytoin, 1 mg/kg IV, not to exceed 50 mg/min, with ECG control may be used for ventricular arrhythmias; may repeat every 5 minutes, up to 10 mg/kg.

Control convulsions or hyperactivity with pentobarbital or diazepam.

Limited experience indicates that these drugs are not dialyzable.

Sustained release formulations – Direct therapy at reversing the effects of ingested drug and supporting the patient for as long as overdosage symptoms remain. Saline cathartics are useful for hastening evacuation of pellets that have not already released medication.

Patient Information:

Because some patients exposed chronically to neuroleptics will develop tardive dyskinesia, inform all patients in whom chronic use is contemplated, if possible, about this risk. The decision to inform patients or their guardians must obviously take into account the clinical circumstances and the patient's competence to understand the information. See Warnings.

May cause drowsiness; use caution while driving or performing other tasks requiring alertness. Avoid alcohol and other CNS depressants due to possible additive effects and hypotension.

Liquid concentrates: Avoid skin contact (contact dermatitis may occur). Liquid concentrates are light sensitive; keep in amber or opaque bottles, protect from light. Solutions are most conveniently used when diluted in fruit juices or other liquids. Use immediately after dilution. See individual products for specific guidelines.

Phenothiazines: Avoid prolonged exposure to sunlight or use sunscreens conscientiously; photosensitivity may occur.

May discolor the urine pink or reddish-brown.

If dizziness or fainting occurs, avoid sudden changes in posture and use caution when climbing stairs, etc (more common during first week of therapy).

Use caution in hot weather. These drugs may increase susceptibility to heat stroke.

Notify physician if sore throat, fever, skin rash, weakness, tremors, impaired vision or jaundice occurs.

Other agents: Notify physician if impaired vision, tremors, involuntary muscle twitching or jaundice occurs.

Administration and Dosage:

Although divided daily dosages are recommended for initiation of therapy, once-daily dosing may be used during chronic therapy because of the long-acting effects of these agents. Administration at bedtime may be preferred to minimize the effects of sedation and orthostatic hypotension.

Individualize dosage. The milligram for milligram potency relationship among all dosage forms has not been precisely established. Increase dosage until symptoms are controlled. Increase dosage gradually in elderly, debilitated or emaciated patients. In continued therapy, gradually reduce dosage to the lowest effective maintenance level after symptoms have been controlled. Increase parenteral dosage only if hypotension has not occurred.

Elderly patients: Institute doses at ¼ to ⅓ that recommended for younger adults and increase more gradually.

Combative patients or those who have other serious manifestations of acute psychosis: Repeat parenteral administration every 1 to 4 hours until the desired effects are obtained or until cardiac arrhythmias or rhythm changes, hypotension or other disturbing side effects emerge.

Maintenance therapy can be administered as a single daily bedtime dose.

Oral liquid concentrates are light sensitive; dispense in amber or opaque bottles and protect from light. These solutions are most conveniently administered by dilution in fruit juices or other liquids. Administer these solutions immediately after dilution.

Bioequivalence: Bioavailability differences between solid oral dosage forms and suppositories marketed by different manufacturers have been documented for various phenothiazines. Brand interchange is not recommended unless comparative bioavailability data which provide evidence of therapeutic equivalence are available.

Thienbenzodiazepine

OLANZAPINE

Actions:

Pharmacology: Olanzapine, a thienbenzodiazepine antipsychotic, is a selective monoaminergic antagonist with high affinity binding to the following receptors: Serotonin $5HT_{2A/2C}$, dopamine D_{1-4}, muscarinic M_{1-5}, histamine H_1 and adrenergic alpha$_1$ receptors. Olanzapine binds weakly to $GABA_A$, BZD and beta adrenergic receptors.

The mechanism of action of olanzapine is unknown. However, it has been proposed that this drug's antipsychotic activity is mediated through a combination of dopamine and serotonin type 2 ($5HT_2$) antagonism. Antagonism at receptors other than dopamine and $5HT_2$ with similar receptor affinities may explain some of the other therapeutic and side effects of olanzapine. Olanzapine's antagonism of muscarinic M_{1-5} receptors may explain its anticholinergic effects, with somnolence and orthostatic hypotension resulting from antagonism of histaminic H_1 and alpha$_1$ adrenergic receptors, respectively.

Pharmacokinetics:

Absorption/Distribution – Olanzapine is well absorbed and reaches peak concentrations in ≈ 6 hours following an oral dose. It is eliminated extensively by first pass metabolism, with ≈ 40% of the dose metabolized before reaching the systemic circulation. Food does not affect the rate or extent of olanzapine absorption.

Olanzapine displays linear kinetics over the clinical dosing range. Its half-life ranges from 21 to 54 hours (mean, 30 hr), and apparent plasma clearance ranges from 12 to 47 L/hr (mean, 25 L/hr).

Administration of olanzapine once daily leads to steady-state concentrations in about 1 week that are approximately twice the concentrations after single doses.

Olanzapine is extensively distributed throughout the body, with a volume of distribution of ≈ 1000 L. It is 93% bound to plasma proteins over the concentration range of 7 to 1100 ng/ml, binding primarily to albumin and alpha$_1$-acid glycoprotein.

Metabolism/Excretion – Following a single oral dose of olanzapine, 7% of the dose of olanzapine was recovered in the urine as unchanged drug, indicating that olanzapine is highly metabolized. Approximately 57% and 30% of the dose was recovered in the urine and feces, respectively. In the plasma, olanzapine accounted for only 12% of the AUC for total radioactivity, indicating significant exposure to metabolites. After multiple dosing, the major circulating metabolites were the 10–N-glucuronide, present at steady state at 44% of the concentration of olanzapine, and 4'-N-desmethyl olanzapine, present at steady state at 31% of the concentration of olanzapine. Both metabolites lack pharmacological activity at the concentrations observed.

Direct glucuronidation and cytochrome P450 (CYP) mediated oxidation are the primary metabolic pathways for olanzapine. In vitro studies suggest that CYPs 1A2 and 2D6, and the flavin-containing monooxygenase system are involved in olanzapine oxidation. CYP2D6 mediated oxidation appears to be a minor metabolic pathway in vivo, because the clearance of olanzapine is not reduced in subjects who are deficient in this enzyme.

Renal function impairment: Because olanzapine is highly metabolized before excretion and only 7% of the drug is excreted unchanged, renal dysfunction alone is unlikely to have a major impact on the pharmacokinetics of olanzapine. The pharmacokinetic characteristics of olanzapine were similar in patients with severe renal impairment and in normal subjects, indicating that dosage adjustment based upon the degree of renal impairment is not required. In addition, olanzapine is not removed by dialysis. The effect of renal impairment on metabolite elimination has not been studied.

Hepatic function impairment: The presence of hepatic impairment may be expected to reduce the clearance of olanzapine.

Elderly: The mean elimination half-life of olanzapine may be ≈ 1.5 times greater in elderly (> 65 years of age) than in non-elderly subjects (≤ 65 years of age). Use caution in dosing the elderly (see Administration and Dosage).

Gender: Clearance of olanzapine is ≈ 30% lower in women than in men. There were, however, no apparent differences between men and women in effectiveness or adverse effects. Dosage modifications based on gender should not be needed.

Smoking: Olanzapine clearance is ≈ 40% higher in smokers than in non-smokers, although dosage modifications are not routinely recommended.

Race: No specific pharmacokinetic study was conducted to investigate the effects of race. A cross-study comparison between data obtained in Japan and data obtained in the US suggests that exposure to olanzapine may be ≈ 2–fold greater in the Japanese when equivalent doses are administered. Dosage modifications for race are not recommended.

Thienbenzodiazepine

OLANZAPINE

Combined effects: The combined effects of age, smoking and gender could lead to substantial pharmacokinetic differences in populations. Dosing modifications may be necessary in patients who exhibit a combination of factors that may result in slower metabolism of olanzapine (see Administration and Dosage).

Clinical trials: In a 6–week, placebo controlled trial (n = 253) involving 3 fixed-dose ranges of olanzapine (≈ 5 mg/day, 10 mg/day and 15 mg/day) on a once-daily schedule, the two highest olanzapine dose groups (actual mean doses of 12 and 16 mg/day, respectively) were superior to placebo on Brief Psychiatric Rating Scale (BPRS) total score, BPRS psychosis cluster and Clinical Global Impression (CGI) severity score; the highest olanzapine dose group was superior to placebo on the Scale for Assessing Negative Symptoms (SANS). There was no clear advantage for the high dose group over the medium dose group.

Examination of population subsets (race and gender) did not reveal any differential responsiveness on the basis of these subgroupings.

Indications:

Psychotic disorders: Management of the manifestations of psychotic disorders.

Contraindications:

Hypersensitivity to the product.

Warnings:

Neuroleptic Malignant Syndrome (NMS): A potentially fatal symptom complex sometimes referred to as Neuroleptic Malignant Syndrome (NMS) has been reported in association with administration of antipsychotic drugs. Clinical manifestations of NMS are hyperpyrexia, muscle rigidity, altered mental status and evidence of autonomic instability (irregular pulse or blood pressure, tachycardia, diaphoresis and cardiac dysrhythmia). Additional signs may include elevated creatinine phosphokinase, myoglobinuria (rhabdomyolysis) and acute renal failure.

The diagnostic evaluation of patients with this syndrome is complicated. In arriving at a diagnosis, it is important to exclude cases where the clinical presentation includes both serious medical illness (eg, pneumonia, systemic infection, etc) and untreated or inadequately treated extrapyramidal signs and symptoms (EPS). Other important considerations in the differential diagnosis include central anticholinergic toxicity, heat stroke, drug fever and primary central nervous system pathology.

The management of NMS should include: 1) Immediate discontinuation of antipsychotic drugs and other drugs not essential to concurrent therapy; 2) intensive symptomatic treatment and medical monitoring; and 3) treatment of any concomitant serious medical problems for which specific treatments are available. There is no general agreement about specific pharmacological treatment regimens for NMS.

If a patient requires antipsychotic drug treatment after recovery from NMS, carefully consider the potential reintroduction of drug therapy. Monitor the patient, because recurrences of NMS have been reported.

Tardive dyskinesia may develop in patients treated with antipsychotic drugs. Prescribe olanzapine in a manner that is most likely to minimize the occurrence of tardive dyskinesia. Chronic antipsychotic treatment should generally be reserved for patients (1) who suffer from a chronic illness that is known to respond to antipsychotic drugs and (2) for whom alternative, equally effective but potentially less harmful treatments are not available or appropriate. In patients who do require chronic treatment, seek the smallest dose and the shortest duration of treatment that produces a satisfactory clinical response. Periodically reassess the need for continued treatment.

If the signs and symptoms of tardive dyskinesia appear in a patient on olanzapine, consider discontinuation of the drug. However, some patients may require treatment with olanzapine despite the presence of the syndrome.

Tachycardia: Olanzapine use was associated with a mean increase in heart rate of 2.4 beats per minute compared with no change among placebo patients. This slight tendency to tachycardia may be related to olanzapine's potential for inducing orthostatic changes (see Precautions).

Hepatic function impairment: Use caution in patients with signs and symptoms of hepatic impairment, in patients with pre-existing conditions associated with limited hepatic functional reserve, and in patients who are being treated with potentially hepatotoxic drugs.

Carcinogenesis: The incidence of liver hemangiomas and hemangiosarcomas was significantly increased in female mice dosed at 8 mg/kg/day. These tumors were not increased in female mice dosed at 10 or 30 mg/kg/day. There was a high incidence of early mortality in male mice dosed at 30 mg/kg/day, requiring the dose to be adjusted to 20 mg/kg/day for the remainder of the study. The incidence of mammary gland

OLANZAPINE

adenomas and adenocarcinomas was significantly increased in female mice dosed at ≥ 2 mg/kg/day and in female rats dosed at ≥ 4 mg/kg/day. Antipsychotic drugs have been shown to chronically elevate prolactin levels in rodents. Serum prolactin levels were not measured during the olanzapine carcinogenicity studies; however, measurements during subchronic toxicity studies showed that olanzapine elevated serum prolactin levels up to 4–fold in rats at the same doses used in the carcinogenicity study. An increase in mammary gland neoplasms has been found in rodents after chronic administration of other antipsychotic drugs and is considered to be prolactin mediated.

Elderly: In general, there was no indication of any different tolerability of olanzapine in the elderly compared with younger adults. Nevertheless, the presence of factors that might decrease pharmacokinetic clearance or increase the pharmacodynamic response to olanzapine should lead to consideration of a lower starting dose (see Administration and Dosage).

Pregnancy: Category C. Seven pregnancies were observed during clinical trials with olanzapine, including 2 resulting in normal births, 1 resulting in neonatal death due to cardiovascular defect, 3 therapeutic abortions and 1 spontaneous abortion. There are no adequate and well controlled trials with olanzapine in pregnant women. Because animal reproduction studies are not always predictive of human response, use this drug during pregnancy only if the potential benefit justifies the potential risk to the fetus. Advise patients to notify their physician if they become pregnant or intend to become pregnant during therapy with olanzapine.

Lactation: Olanzapine was excreted in the milk of treated rats. It is not known if olanzapine is excreted in breast milk. Advise patients not to breastfeed an infant if they are taking olanzapine.

Children: Safety and effectiveness in pediatric patients < 18 years of age have not been established.

Precautions:

Monitoring: Periodic assessment of transaminases is recommended in patients with significant hepatic disease.

Orthostatic hypotension: Olanzapine may induce orthostatic hypotension associated with dizziness, tachycardia, and in some patients, syncope, especially during the initial dose-titration period, probably reflecting its $alpha_1$-adrenergic antagonistic properties. Syncope was reported in 0.6% of olanzapine-treated patients. The risk of orthostatic hypotension and syncope may be minimized by initiating therapy with 5 mg once daily (see Administration and Dosage). Consider a more gradual titration to the target dose if hypotension occurs. Use olanzapine with caution in patients with known cardiovascular disease (history of myocardial infarction or ischemia, heart failure or conduction abnormalities), cerebrovascular disease and conditions which would predispose patients to hypotension (dehydration, hypovolemia and treatment with antihypertensive medications).

Seizures: Seizures occurred in 0.9% of olanzapine-treated patients. There were confounding factors that may have contributed to the occurrence of seizures in many of these cases. Use olanzapine with caution in patients with a history of seizures or with conditions that potentially lower the seizure threshold (eg, Alzheimer's dementia). Conditions that lower the seizure threshold may be more prevalent in a population of > 65 years of age.

Hyperprolactinemia: As with other drugs that antagonize dopamine D_2 receptors, olanzapine elevates prolactin levels and a modest elevation persists during chronic administration. Experiments indicate that approximately one-third of human breast cancers are prolactin-dependent in vitro, a factor of potential importance if the prescription of these drugs is contemplated in a patient with previously detected breast cancer of this type. As is common with compounds that increase prolactin release, an increase in mammary gland neoplasia was observed in the olanzapine carcinogenicity studies conducted in mice and rats. However, neither clinical studies nor epidemiologic studies have shown an association between chronic administration of this class of drugs and tumorigenesis in humans; the available evidence is considered too limited to be conclusive.

Transaminase elevations: Clinically significant ALT elevations (≥ 3 times the upper limit of the normal range) were observed in 2% of patients. No patients experienced jaundice. In two patients, liver enzymes decreased toward normal despite continued treatment and in two others, enzymes decreased upon discontinuation of olanzapine. In two patients, one, seropositive for hepatitis C, had persistent enzyme eleva-

Thienbenzodiazepine

OLANZAPINE

tion for 4 months after discontinuation, and the other had insufficient follow-up to determine if enzymes normalized.

About 1% of patients discontinued treatment due to transaminase increases. Periodic assessment of transaminases is recommended in patients with significant hepatic disease.

Potential for cognitive and motor impairment: Somnolence was a commonly reported adverse event associated with olanzapine treatment, occurring in 26% of olanzapine patients. This adverse event was also dose related. Somnolence led to discontinuation in 0.4% of patients.

Because olanzapine has the potential to impair judgment, thinking or motor skills, caution patients about operating hazardous machinery, including automobiles, until they are reasonably certain that olanzapine therapy does not affect them adversely.

Body temperature regulation: Disruption of the body's ability to reduce core body temperature has been attributed to antipsychotic agents. Appropriate care is advised when prescribing olanzapine for patients who will be experiencing conditions which may contribute to an elevation in core body temperature (eg, exercising strenuously, exposure to extreme heat, receiving concomitant medication with anticholinergic activity or being subject to dehydration).

Dysphagia: Esophageal dysmotility and aspiration have been associated with antipsychotic drug use. Two subjects in a study of olanzapine in Alzheimer's dementia died from aspiration pneumonia. One of these patients had experienced dysphagia prior to the development of aspiration pneumonia. Aspiration pneumonia is a common cause of morbidity and mortality in patients with advanced Alzheimer's dementia. Use cautiously in patients at risk for aspiration pneumonia.

Suicide: The possibility of a suicide attempt is inherent in schizophrenia, and close supervision of high-risk patients should accompany drug therapy. Write prescriptions for olanzapine for the smallest quantity of tablets consistent with good patient management in order to reduce the risk of overdose.

Anticholinergic effects: Olanzapine exhibits in vitro muscarinic receptor affinity. In premarketing clinical trials, olanzapine was associated with constipation, dry mouth and tachycardia, all adverse events possibly related to cholinergic antagonism. Such adverse events were not often the basis for discontinuations from olanzapine, but caution should be used in patients with clinically significant prostatic hypertrophy, narrow-angle glaucoma or a history of paralytic ileus.

Drug Interactions:

Agents that induce CYP1A2 or glucuronyl transferase enzymes, such as omeprazole and rifampin, may cause an increase in olanzapine clearance. Inhibitors of CYP1A2 (eg, fluvoxamine) could potentially inhibit olanzapine elimination. Because olanzapine is metabolized by multiple enzyme systems, inhibition of a single enzyme may not appreciably decrease olanzapine clearance.

Thienbenzodiazepine

OLANZAPINE

Olanzapine Drug Interactions			
Precipitant drug	Object drug*		Description
Carbamazepine	Olanzapine	⬇	Carbamazepine therapy causes an ≈ 50% increase in the clearance of olanzapine. This increase is likely due to the fact that carbamazepine is a potent inducer of CYP1A2 activity. Higher daily doses of carbamazepine may cause an even greater increase in olanzapine clearance.
Olanzapine	Antihypertensive agents	⬆	Because of its potential for inducing hypotension, olanzapine may enhance the effects of certain antihypertensive agents.
Olanzapine	CNS acting drugs (eg, alcohol)	⬆	Due to the primary CNS effects of olanzapine, use caution when olanzapine is taken in combination with other centrally acting drugs and alcohol.
Olanzapine	Levodopa and dopamine agonists	⬇	Olanzapine may antagonize the effects of levodopa and dopamine agonists.

* ⬆ = Object drug increased. ⬇ = Object drug decreased.

Adverse Reactions:

Olanzapine Adverse Events		
Body system/Adverse event	Olanzapine (%; n = 248)	Placebo (%; n = 118)
Body as a whole		
Headache	17	15
Fever	5	3
Abdominal pain	4	2
Back pain	4	3
Chest pain	4	2
Neck rigidity	2	1
Intentional injury	1	0
Cardiovascular system		
Postural hypotension	5	2
Tachycardia	4	1
Hypotension	2	1
GI		
Constipation	9	3
Dry mouth	7	4
Increased appetite	2	1
Metabolic and nutritional		
Weight gain	6	1
Peripheral edema	2	0
Lower extremity edema	1	0
Musculoskeletal		
Joint pain	5	3
Extremity pain (other than joint)	4	3
Twitching	2	1
CNS		
Somnolence	26	15
Agitation	23	17
Insomnia	20	19
Nervousness	16	14

Thienbenzodiazepine

OLANZAPINE

Olanzapine Adverse Events		
Body system/Adverse event	Olanzapine (%; n = 248)	Placebo (%; n = 118)
Hostility	15	14
Dizziness	11	4
Anxiety	9	8
Personality disorder[1]	8	4
Akathisia	5	1
Hypertonia	4	3
Tremor	4	3
Amnesia	2	0
Articulation impairment	2	0
Euphoria	2	0
Stuttering	2	0
Respiratory system		
Rhinitis	10	6
Cough increased	5	3
Pharyngitis	5	3
Dermatologic		
Vesiculobullous rash	2	1
Special senses		
Amblyopia	5	4
Blepharitis	2	1
Corneal lesion	1	0
GU		
Premenstrual syndrome	2	0

[1] Personality disorder is the COSTART term for designating non-aggressive objectionable behavior.

Body as a whole: Flu syndrome, suicide attempt (1%); chills, chills and fever, face edema, hangover effect, malaise, moniliasis, neck pain, pelvic pain, photosensitivity reaction (≤ 1%); abdomen enlarged, sudden death (rare).

Cardiovascular: Cerebrovascular accident, hemorrhage, migraine, palpitation, vasodilation, ventricular extrasystoles (≤ 1%); heart arrest (rare).

GI: Increased salivation, nausea and vomiting, thirst (1%); aphthous stomatitis, dysphagia, eructation, esophagitis, fecal incontinence, flatulence, gastritis, gastroenteritis, gingivitis, glossitis, hepatitis, melena, mouth ulceration, oral moniliasis, periodontal abscess, rectal hemorrhage, stomatitis, tongue edema (≤ 1%); enteritis, esophageal ulcer, tongue discoloration (rare).

Endocrine: Diabetes mellitus, goiter (≤ 1%); diabetic acidosis (rare).

Hematologic/Lymphatic: Cyanosis, leukocytosis, lymphadenopathy, thrombocythemia (≤ 1%).

Metabolic/Nutritional: Weight gain (5.6%); weight loss (1%); alkaline phosphatase increased, bilirubinemia, dehydration, hyperglycemia, hyperkalemia, hyperuricemia, hypoglycemia, hypokalemia, hyponatremia, ketosis, water intoxication (≤ 1%); hypercholesteremia, hyperlipidemia (rare).

Musculoskeletal: Arthritis, back and hip pain, bursitis, leg cramps, myasthenia, rheumatoid arthritis (≤ 1%); bone pain, myopathy (rare).

CNS: Tardive dyskinesia (1%); abnormal gait, alcohol misuse, antisocial reaction, ataxia, CNS stimulation, coma, delirium, depersonalization, hypesthesia, hypotonia, incoordination, libido decreased, obsessive compulsive symptoms, phobias, somatization, stimulant misuse, stupor, vertigo, withdrawal syndrome (≤ 1%); facial paralysis, neuralgia, nystagmus, subarachnoid hemorrhage (rare).

Respiratory: Dyspnea (1%); apnea, asthma, epistaxis, hemoptysis, hyperventilation, voice alteration (≤ 1%); laryngitis (rare).

Dermatologic: Alopecia, contact dermatitis, dry skin, eczema, hirsutism, seborrhea, skin ulcer, urticaria (≤ 1%); maculopapular rash, skin discoloration (rare).

Special senses: Cataract, deafness, diplopia, dry eyes, ear pain, eye hemorrhage, eye inflammation, eye pain, ocular muscle abnormality, taste perversion, tinnitus (≤ 1%); abnormality of accommodation, glaucoma, keratoconjunctivitis, macular hypopigmentation, mydriasis, pigment deposits lens (rare).

GU: Hematuria, metrorrhagia, urinary incontinence, urinary tract infection (1%); abnormal ejaculation, amenorrhea, breast pain, cystitis, decreased menstruation, dysuria, increased menstruation, female lactation, impotence, menorrhagia, polyuria, pyuria, urinary retention, urinary frequency, urination impaired, uterine fibroids enlarged (≤ 1%); albuminuria (rare).

Lab test abnormalities: An assessment of the premarketing experience for olanzapine revealed an association with asymptomatic increases in AST, ALT and GGT. Olanzapine administration was also associated with increases in serum prolactin, with an asymptomatic elevation of the eosinophil in 0.3% of patients, and with an increase in CPK.

Overdosage:

Human experience: Accidental or intentional acute overdosage of olanzapine was identified in 67 patients. In the patient taking the largest identified amount, 300 mg, the only symptoms reported were drowsiness and slurred speech. In the limited number of patients who were evaluated in hospitals, including the patient taking 300 mg, there were no observations indicating an adverse change in laboratory analytes or ECG. Vital signs were usually within normal limits following overdoses.

Treatment: In case of acute overdosage, establish and maintain an airway and ensure adequate oxygenation and ventilation. Consider gastric lavage (after intubation, if patient is unconscious) and administration of activated charcoal together with a laxative. The possibility of obtundation, seizures or dystonic reaction of the head and neck following overdose may create a risk of aspiration with induced emesis. Cardiovascular monitoring should commence immediately and should include continuous electrocardiographic monitoring to detect possible arrhythmias.

There is no specific antidote to olanzapine. Therefore, initiate appropriate supportive measures. Treat hypotension and circulatory collapse with appropriate measures such as IV fluids or sympathomimetic agents. Do not use epinephrine, dopamine or other sympathomimetics with beta-agonist activity, because beta stimulation may worsen hypotension in the setting of olanzapine-induced alpha blockade. Close medical supervision and monitoring should continue until the patient recovers (refer to Management of Acute Overdosage).

Patient Information:

Orthostatic hypotension: Advise patients of the risk of orthostatic hypotension, especially during the period of initial dose titration and in association with the use of concomitant drugs that may potentiate the orthostatic effect of olanzapine (eg, diazepam or alcohol).

Cognitive and motor performance: Olanzapine has the potential to impair judgment, thinking or motor skills. Caution patients about operating hazardous machinery, including automobiles, until the effects of olanzapine are known.

Pregnancy: Advise patients to notify their physician if they become pregnant or intend to become pregnant during therapy.

Lactation: Advise patients not to breastfeed an infant if they are taking olanzapine.

Concomitant medication: Advise patients to inform their physician if they are taking, or plan to take, any prescription or over-the-counter drugs, because there is a potential for interactions.

Alcohol: Avoid alcohol while taking olanzapine.

Heat exposure and dehydration: Avoid overheating and dehydration.

Administration and Dosage:

Usual dose: Administer olanzapine on a once-a-day schedule without regard to meals, generally beginning with 5 to 10 mg initially, with a target dose of 10 mg/day within several days. Further dosage adjustments, if indicated, should generally occur at intervals of not < 1 week, because steady state for olanzapine would not be achieved for ≈ 1 week in the typical patient. When dosage adjustments are necessary, dose increments/decrements of 5 mg once daily are recommended.

Antipsychotic efficacy was demonstrated in a dose range of 10 to 15 mg/day in the clinical trials. However, increases in efficacy were not demonstrated in doses above 10 mg/day. An increase to a dose greater than the target dose of 10 mg/day is recommended only after clinical assessment. The safety of doses > 20 mg/day has not been evaluated in clinical trials.

Thienbenzodiazepine

OLANZAPINE

Dosing in special populations: The recommended starting dose is 5 mg in patients who are debilitated, who have a predisposition to hypotensive reactions, who otherwise exhibit a combination of factors that may result in slower metabolism of olanzapine (eg, nonsmoking female patients ≥ 65 years of age), or who may be more pharmacodynamically sensitive to olanzapine.

When indicated, use caution with dose escalation.

Maintenance treatment: While there is no body of evidence available to answer the question of how long the patient treated with olanzapine should remain on it, the effectiveness of maintenance treatment is well established for many other antipsychotic drugs. It is recommended that responding patients be continued on olanzapine, but at the lowest dose needed to maintain remission. Periodically reassess patients to determine the need for maintenance treatment.

Storage/Stability: Store at controlled room temperature, 20° to 25°C (68° to 77°F). Protect from light and moisture.

Rx	**Zyprexa** (Eli Lilly)	**Tablets:** 5 mg	Lactose. (LILLY 4115). White, round. Film coated. In 60s and UD 100s.
		7.5 mg	Lactose. (LILLY 4116). White, round. Film coated. In 60s and UD 100s.
		10 mg	Lactose. (LILLY 4117). White, round. Film coated. In 60s and UD 100s.

Phenothiazine Derivatives

CHLORPROMAZINE HCl

Complete prescribing information begins in the Antipsychotic Agents group monograph.

Indications:

Management of manifestations of psychotic disorders; control of the manifestations of the manic type of manic depressive illness; relief of restlessness and apprehension prior to surgery; an adjunct in treatment of tetanus; treatment of acute intermittent porphyria.

Treatment of severe behavioral problems in children marked by combativeness or explosive hyperexcitable behavior (out of proportion to immediate provocations), and in the short-term treatment of hyperactive children who show excessive motor activity with accompanying conduct disorders consisting of some or all of the following symptoms: Impulsivity, difficulty sustaining attention, aggressivity, mood lability and poor frustration tolerance.

Also indicated for the control of nausea and vomiting and relief of intractable hiccoughs (see Antiemetic/Antivertigo Agents).

Unlabeled uses: Treatment of phencyclidine (PCP) psychosis; treatment of migraine headaches (IV or IM).

Administration and Dosage:

Adults:

Concentrate – Add desired dosage to ≥ 60 ml of diluent just prior to administration. Suggested vehicles are tomato or fruit juice, milk, simple syrup, orange syrup, carbonated beverages, coffee, tea or water. Semisolid foods (eg, soups, puddings) may also be used.

Sustained release capsules – Do not crush or chew. Swallow whole.

Injection – Do not inject SC. Inject IM slowly, deep into upper outer quadrant of buttock. Because of possible hypotensive effects, reserve for bedfast patients or for acute ambulatory cases, and keep patient recumbent for at least hour after injection. If irritation is a problem, dilute injection with saline or 2% procaine; do not mix with other agents in the syringe. Avoid injecting undiluted into vein. Use the IV route only for severe hiccoughs, surgery and tetanus.

Because of the possibility of contact dermatitis, avoid getting solution on hands or clothing.

Outpatients – For prompt control of severe symptoms 25 mg IM; if necessary, repeat in 1 hour. Give subsequent oral doses of 25 to 50 mg 3 times daily.

The usual initial oral dose is 10 mg 3 or 4 times daily or 25 mg 2 or 3 times daily. For more serious cases, give 25 mg 3 times/day. After 1 or 2 days, increase daily dosage by 20 to 50 mg semiweekly, until patient becomes calm and cooperative. Maximum improvement may not be seen for weeks or even months. Continue optimum dosage for 2 weeks, then gradually reduce to maintenance level; 200 mg per day is not unusual. Some patients require higher dosages (eg, 800 mg per day is not uncommon in discharged mental patients).

Surgery –

Preoperative: 25 to 50 mg orally 2 to 3 hours before surgery or 12.5 to 25 mg IM 1 to 2 hours before surgery.

Intraoperative (to control acute nausea and vomiting):

IM – 12.5 mg. Repeat in hour if necessary and if no hypotension occurs.

IV – 2 mg per fractional injection at 2 minute intervals. Do not exceed 25 mg (dilute to 1 mg/ml with saline).

Acute intermittent porphyria – 25 to 50 mg orally or 25 mg IM 3 or 4 times daily until patient can take oral therapy.

Tetanus – 25 to 50 mg IM 3 or 4 times daily, usually with barbiturates. For IV use, 25 to 50 mg diluted to at least 1 mg/ml and administered at a rate of 1 mg/minute.

Psychiatry, hospitalized patients (acutely manic or disturbed) – IM – 25 mg initially. If necessary, give an additional 25 to 50 mg injection in 1 hour. Increase gradually over several days (up to 400 mg every 4 to 6 hours in severe cases) until patient is controlled. Patient usually becomes quiet and cooperative within 24 to 48 hours. Substitute oral dosage and increase until the patient is calm; 500 mg/day is usually sufficient. While gradual increases to 2000 mg or more/day may be necessary, little therapeutic gain is achieved by exceeding 1000 mg/day for extended periods.

Psychiatry, hospitalized patients (less acutely disturbed) –

Oral: 25 mg 3 times daily. Increase gradually until effective dose is reached, usually 400 mg/day.

Phenothiazine Derivatives

CHLORPROMAZINE HCl

Children: Chlorpromazine should generally not be used in children < 6 months old except where potentially lifesaving. It should not be used in conditions for which specific children's dosages have not been established.

Psychiatric outpatients –

Oral: 0.5 mg/kg (0.25 mg/lb) every 4 to 6 hours, as needed.

Rectal: 1 mg/kg (0.5 mg/lb) every 6 to 8 hours, as needed.

IM: 0.5 mg/kg (0.25 mg/lb) every 6 to 8 hours, as needed.

Surgery –

Preoperative: 0.5 mg/kg (0.25 mg/lb) orally 2 to 3 hours before operation or 0.5 mg/kg (0.25 mg/lb) IM 1 to 2 hours before operation.

Intraoperative (administer only to control acute nausea and vomiting):

IM – 0.25 mg/kg (0.125 mg/lb); repeat in hour if needed, and if no hypotension occurs.

IV – 1 mg per fractional injection at 2 minute intervals; do not exceed IM dosage. Always dilute to 1 mg/ml with saline.

Psychiatry: Hospitalized patients –

Oral: Start with low doses and increase gradually. In severe behavior disorders or psychotic conditions, 50 to 100 mg daily, or in older children, 200 mg or more daily may be necessary. There is little evidence that improvement in severely disturbed mentally retarded patients is enhanced by doses > 500 mg/day.

IM: Up to 5 years: Do not exceed 40 mg/day. *5 to 12 years old* –Do not exceed 75 mg/day, except in unmanageable cases.

Tetanus (IM or IV) – 0.5 mg/kg (0.25 mg/lb) every 6 to 8 hours. When given IV, dilute to at least 1 mg/ml and administer at a rate of 1 mg per 2 minutes. In children up to 23 kg (50 lbs), do not exceed 40 mg daily; 23 to 45 kg (50 to 100 lbs), do not exceed 75 mg/day, except in severe cases.

Concentrate – Slight yellowing will not alter potency. Discard if markedly discolored.

Admixture compatibility – A mixture of chlorpromazine, hydroxyzine and meperidine in the same glass or plastic syringe is stable for 1 year when stored at refrigeration (4°C; 39°F) or room temperature (25°C; 77°F). The combination was unstable at higher temperatures.

A precipitate or discoloration may occur when chlorpromazine is admixed with morphine, meperidine or other products preserved with cresols.

Rx	**Chlorpromazine HCl** (Various, eg, Balan, Geneva, Goldline, Lannett, Major, Moore, Parmed, Purepac, Rugby, Schein)	**Tablets:** 10 mg	In 100s, 1000s and UD 100s.
Rx	**Thorazine** (SKF)		(SKF T73). Orange. In 100s, 1000s and UD 100s.
Rx	**Chlorpromazine HCl** (Various, eg, Balan, Geneva, Goldline, Lederle, Major, Moore, Parmed, Purepac, Rugby, Schein)	**Tablets:** 25 mg	In 100s, 1000s and UD 100s.
Rx	**Thorazine** (SKF)		(SKF T74). Orange. In 100s, 1000s and UD 100s.
Rx	**Chlorpromazine HCl** (Various, eg, Balan, Geneva, Goldline, Lederle, Major, Moore, Parmed, Purepac, Rugby, Schein)	**Tablets:** 50 mg	In 100s, 1000s and UD 100s.
Rx	**Thorazine** (SKF)		(SKF T76). Orange. In 100s, 1000s and UD 100s.

Phenothiazine Derivatives

CHLORPROMAZINE HCl

Rx	**Chlorpromazine HCl** (Various, eg, Balan, Geneva, Goldline, Lederle, Major, Moore, Parmed, Purepac, Rugby, Schein)	**Tablets:** 100 mg	In 100s, 1000s and UD 100s.
Rx	**Thorazine** (SKF)		(SKF T77). Orange. In 100s, 1000s and UD 100s.
Rx	**Chlorpromazine HCl** (Various, eg, Balan, Geneva, Goldline, Lederle, Major, Moore, Parmed, Purepac, Rugby, Schein)	**Tablets:** 200 mg	In 100s, 1000s and UD 100s.
Rx	**Thorazine** (SKF)		(SKF T79). Orange. In 100s, 1000s and UD 100s.
Rx	**Thorazine Spansules** (SKF)	**Capsules, sustained release:** 30 mg	(SKF T63). Orange/natural. In 50s, 500s and UD 100s.
		75 mg	(SKF T64). Orange/natural. In 50s, 500s and UD 100s.
		150 mg	(SKF T66). Orange/natural. In 50s, 500s and UD 100s.
		200 mg	(SKF T67). Orange/natural. In 50s, 500s and UD 100s.
		300 mg	(SKF T69). In 50s and UD 100s.
Rx	**Chlorpromazine HCl** (Geneva)	**Syrup:** 10 mg per 5 ml	Wintergreen flavor. In 120 ml.
Rx	**Thorazine** (SKF)		Sucrose. Orange-custard flavor. In 120 ml.
Rx	**Chlorpromazine HCl** (Various, eg, Balan, Geneva, Harber, Moore, PBI, RID, Raway, Roxane, Warner Chilcott)	**Concentrate:** 30 mg per ml	In 120 ml.
Rx	**Thorazine** (SKF)		In 120 ml
Rx	**Chlorpromazine HCl** (Various, eg, Balan, Geneva, Harber, Lederle, Moore, PBI, Raway, Roxane, Schein, Warner Chilcott)	**Concentrate:** 100 mg per ml	In 60 and 240 ml.
Rx	**Thorazine** (SKF)		Saccharin. Custard flavor. In 240 ml.
Rx	**Thorazine** (SKF)	**Suppositories (as base):** 25 mg	(T70). In 12s.
		100 mg	(T71). In 12s.
Rx	**Chlorpromazine HCl** (Various, eg, Balan, Elkins-Sinn, Geneva, Goldline, Lannett, Major, Moore, Parmed, Rugby, Schein)	**Injection:** 25 mg per ml	In 1 & 2 ml amps and 10 ml vials.
Rx	**Ormazine** (Hauck)		In 10 ml vials.[1]
Rx	**Thorazine** (SKF)		In 1 and 2 ml amps[2] and 10 ml vials.[3]

[1] With sodium metabisulfite, sodium sulfite and 2% benzyl alcohol.
[2] With sodium bisulfite and sodium sulfite.
[3] With sodium bisulfite, sodium sulfite and 2% benzyl alcohol.

Phenothiazine Derivatives

PROMAZINE HCl

Complete prescribing information begins in the Antipsychotic Agents group monograph.

Indications:

Management of the manifestations of psychotic disorders.

Administration and Dosage:

Reserve parenteral administration for bedfast patients, although acute states in ambulatory patients may also be treated by IM injection, provided proper precautions are taken to eliminate the possibility of postural hypotension.

Injection IM is preferred. Give IM injections deep into large muscle masses (eg, gluteal region).

IV administration is not recommended. Do not give intra-arterially.

Adults: Dosage for acute or chronic mental disease varies with the severity of condition.

In the management of severely agitated patients, administer initial doses of 50 to 150 mg IM, depending on the degree of excitation. In general, these doses are sufficient, but if the desired calming effect is not apparent within 30 minutes, may give additional doses up to a total of 300 mg. Once control is obtained, administer orally. The oral or IM dose is 10 to 200 mg at 4 to 6 hour intervals. In less severe disturbances, adjust dosage downward. Maintenance dosage may range from 10 to 200 mg given at 4 to 6 hour intervals.

The degree of CNS depression induced by promazine has not been great; however, in the acutely inebriated patient the initial dose should not exceed 50 mg, to avoid potentiation of the depressant effect of alcohol.

Do not exceed a total daily dose of 1000 mg, since higher doses have not yielded greater results.

Children (> 12 years of age): In acute episodes of chronic psychotic disease, 10 to 25 mg may be given every 4 to 6 hours.

Rx	**Sparine** (Wyeth-Ayerst)	**Tablets:** 25 mg	(Wyeth 29). Yellow. In 50s.
		50 mg	(Wyeth 28). Orange. In 50s.
		100 mg	(Wyeth 200). Pink. In 50s.
Rx	**Promazine HCl** (Various, eg, General Injectables, Schein)	**Injection:** 25 mg per ml	In 10 ml vials.
Rx	**Promazine HCl** (Various, eg, Balan, Baxter, General Injectables, Pasadena, Rugby, Schein, Steris, Veratex, Vita-Rx)	**Injection:** 50 mg per ml	In 10 ml vials.
Rx	**Prozine-50** (Hauck)		In 10 ml vials.
Rx	**Sparine** (Wyeth-Ayerst)		In 2 and 10 ml vials and 1 ml Tubex.[1]

[1] With EDTA and sodium metabisulfite.

TRIFLUPROMAZINE HCl

Complete prescribing information begins in the Antipsychotic Agents group monograph.

Indications:

Management of manifestations of psychotic disorders (excluding psychotic depressive reactions).

Also indicated for the control of severe nausea and vomiting (see Antiemetic/Antivertigo Agents).

Administration and Dosage:

Psychotic disorders: 60 mg IM, up to a maximum of 150 mg/day.

Children – The recommended IM dosage range is 0.2 to 0.25 mg/kg (0.1 to 0.125 mg/lb), up to a maximum total dose of 10 mg/day. Do not administer to children < 2 years of age.

Rx	**Vesprin** (Princeton)	**Injection:** 10 mg per ml	In 10 ml vials.[2]
		20 mg per ml	In 1 ml vials.[2]

[2] With 1.5% benzyl alcohol.

Phenothiazine Derivatives

THIORIDAZINE HCl

Complete prescribing information begins in the Antipsychotic Agents group monograph.

Indications:

Management of manifestations of psychotic disorders and short-term treatment of moderate to marked depression with variable degrees of anxiety in adults.

Treatment of multiple symptoms such as agitation, anxiety, depressed mood, tension, sleep disturbances and fears in the geriatric patient.

Treatment of severe behavioral problems in children marked by combativeness or explosive hyperexcitable behavior (out of proportion to immediate provocations), and in the short-term treatment of hyperactive children who show excessive motor activity with accompanying conduct disorders consisting of some or all of the following symptoms: Impulsivity, difficulty sustaining attention, aggressivity, mood lability and poor frustration tolerance.

Administration and Dosage:

Psychotic manifestations: Usual initial dose is 50 to 100 mg 3 times daily; increase gradually to a maximum of 800 mg/day, if necessary, to control symptoms; then reduce gradually to the minimum maintenance dose. Total daily dosage ranges from 200 to 800 mg divided into 2 to 4 doses.

Short-term treatment of moderate to marked depression with variable degrees of anxiety, and treatment of multiple symptoms such as agitation, anxiety, depressed mood, tension, sleep disturbances and fears in geriatric patients: Usual initial dose is 25 mg 3 times daily. Dosage ranges from 10 mg 2 to 4 times daily in milder cases, to 50 mg 3 or 4 times daily for more severely disturbed patients. Total daily dosage ranges from 20 to 200 mg.

Children: Not recommended for children < 2 years of age. For children aged 2 to 12, the dosage ranges from 0.5 mg to a maximum of 3 mg/kg/day.

Moderate disorders – 10 mg 2 or 3 times daily is the usual starting dose.

Hospitalized, severely disturbed or psychotic children – 25 mg 2 or 3 times daily.

Concentrate may be administered in distilled or acidified tap water or suitable juices.

Rx	**Thioridazine HCl** (Various, eg, Balan, Geneva, Goldline, Lederle, Major, Moore, Roxane, Rugby, Schein, Warner Chilcott)	**Tablets:** 10 mg	In 100s, 500s, 1000s and UD 100s.
Rx	**Mellaril** (Sandoz)		(78-2). Chartreuse. In 100s, 1000s & UD 100s.
Rx	**Thioridazine HCl** (Various, eg, Balan, Bioline, Bolar, Dixon-Shane, Geneva, Goldline, Major, Moore, Parmed, Schein)	**Tablets:** 15 mg	In 100s, 500s, 1000s and UD 100s.
Rx	**Mellaril** (Sandoz)		(78-8). Pink. In 100s, 1000s & UD 100s.
Rx	**Thioridazine HCl** (Various, eg, Balan, Geneva, Goldline, Lederle, Major, Moore, Roxane, Rugby, Schein, Warner Chilcott)	**Tablets:** 25 mg	In 100s, 500s, 1000s and UD 100s.
Rx	**Mellaril** (Sandoz)		(Mellaril 25). Tan. In 100s, 1000s & UD 100s.
Rx	**Thioridazine HCl** (Various, eg, Balan, Geneva, Goldline, Lederle, Major, Moore, Roxane, Rugby, Schein, Warner Chilcott)	**Tablets:** 50 mg	In 100s, 500s, 1000s and UD 100s.
Rx	**Mellaril** (Sandoz)		(Mellaril 50). White. In 100s, 1000s & UD 100s.

Phenothiazine Derivatives

THIORIDAZINE HCl

Rx	**Thioridazine HCl** (Various, eg, Balan, Geneva, Goldline, Lederle, Major, Moore, Roxane, Rugby, Schein, Warner Chilcott)	**Tablets:** 100 mg	In 100s, 500s, 1000s and UD 100s.
Rx	**Mellaril** (Sandoz)		(Mellaril 100). Green. In 100s, 1000s and UD 100s.
Rx	**Thioridazine HCl** (Various, eg, Balan, Barr, Bioline, Bolar, Geneva, Goldline, Major, Parmed, Rugby, Schein)	**Tablets:** 150 mg	In 100s, 500s, 1000s and UD 100s.
Rx	**Mellaril** (Sandoz)		(Mellaril 150). Yellow. In 100s & 1000s.
Rx	**Thioridazine HCl** (Various, eg, Balan, Bioline, Geneva, Goldline, Major, Moore, Parmed, Purepac, Rugby, Schein)	**Tablets:** 200 mg	In 100s, 500s, 1000s and UD 100s.
Rx	**Mellaril** (Sandoz)		(Mellaril 200). Pink. In 100s, 1000s and UD 100s.
Rx	**Thioridazine HCl** (Various, eg, Balan, Geneva, Goldline, Harber, Major, Moore, PBI, Rugby, Schein, Warner Chilcott)	**Concentrate:** 30 mg per ml	In 120 ml.
Rx	**Thioridazine HCl Intensol** (Roxane)		In 120 ml w/dropper.
Rx	**Thioridazine HCl** (Various, eg, Balan, Geneva, Harber, Major, Moore, PBI, Rugby, Schein, Warner Chilcott, Xactdose)	**Concentrate:** 100 mg per ml	In 120 ml and 3.4ml (UD 100s).
Rx	**Thioridazine HCl Intensol** (Roxane)		In 120 ml w/dropper.
Rx	**Mellaril** (Sandoz)	**Concentrate:** 30 mg per ml	3% alcohol. In 118 ml w/dropper.
		100 mg per ml	4.2% alcohol. In 118 ml w/dropper.
Rx	**Mellaril-S** (Sandoz)	**Suspension:** 25 mg per 5 ml	Buttermint flavor. In pt.
		100 mg per 5 ml	Buttermint flavor. In pt.

Phenothiazine Derivatives

MESORIDAZINE

Complete prescribing information begins in the Antipsychotic Agents group monograph.

Indications:

Schizophrenia: Reduces the severity of emotional withdrawal, conceptual disorganization, anxiety, tension, hallucinatory behavior, suspiciousness and blunted affect.

Behavioral problems in mental deficiency and chronic brain syndrome: Reduces hyperactivity and uncooperativeness associated with mental deficiency and chronic brain syndrome.

Alcoholism (acute and chronic): Ameliorates anxiety, tension, depression, nausea and vomiting in acute and chronic alcoholics without producing hepatic dysfunction or hindering the functional recovery of the impaired liver.

Psychoneurotic manifestations: Reduces the symptoms of anxiety and tension and prevalent symptoms often associated with neurotic components of many disorders. It also benefits personality disorders in general.

Administration and Dosage:

Mesoridazine Dosage Guidelines

Disease state	Initial oral dose	Optimum total dosage range (mg/day)
Schizophrenia	50 mg tid	100-400
Behavior problems in mental deficiency and chronic brain syndrome	25 mg tid	175-300
Alcoholism	25 mg bid	150-200
Psychoneurotic manifestations	10 mg tid	130-150

IM administration: For most patients, 25 mg initially. May repeat dose in 30 to 60 minutes, if necessary. The usual optimum dosage range is 25 to 200 mg/day.

Concentrate may be diluted just prior to administration with distilled water, acidified tap water, orange or grape juice. Do not prepare and store bulk dilutions.

Rx	**Serentil** (Boehringer Ingelheim)	**Tablets:** (as besylate) 10 mg	In 100s.
		25 mg	In 100s.
		50 mg	In 100s.
		100 mg	In 100s.
sf		**Concentrate:** (as besylate) 25 mg/ml	0.61% alcohol. In 118 ml w/dropper.
		Injection: (as besylate) 25 mg/ml	In 1 ml amps.[1]

[1] With EDTA.

TRIFLUOPERAZINE HCl

Complete prescribing information begins in the Antipsychotic Agents group monograph.

Indications:

Management of manifestations of psychotic disorders; short-term treatment of nonpsychotic anxiety (not the drug of choice in most patients).

Administration and Dosage:

Individualize dosage. Increase dosage more gradually in debilitated or emaciated patients. When maximum response is achieved, reduce dosage gradually to a maintenance level. Patients may be controlled with once or twice daily administration.

Psychotic disorders: 2 to 5 mg orally twice daily. (Start small or emaciated patients on the lower dosage.) Most patients will show optimum response with 15 or 20 mg/day, although a few may require ≥ 40 mg/day. Optimum therapeutic dosage levels should be reached within 2 or 3 days.

IM (for prompt control of severe symptoms): 1 to 2 mg by deep injection every 4 to 6 hours, as needed. More than 6 mg/24 hours is rarely necessary.

Only in very exceptional cases should IM dosage exceed 10 mg/24 hours. Do not give injections at less than 4 hour intervals because of a possible cumulative effect. Equivalent oral dosage may be substituted once symptoms are controlled.

Children: Adjust dosage to the weight of the child and severity of symptoms. These dosages are for children, aged 6 ro 12, who are hospitalized or under close supervision.

Oral – Initial dose is 1 mg once or twice daily. While it is usually not necessary to exceed 15 mg/day, older children with severe symptoms may require higher doses.

Phenothiazine Derivatives

TRIFLUOPERAZINE HCl

IM – There has been little experience in children. However, it it is necessary to achieve rapid control of severe symptoms, administer 1 mg once or twice a day.

Elderly patients: Usually, lower dosages are sufficient. The elderly appear more susceptible to hypotension and neuromuscular reactions; observe closely and increase dosage gradually.

Treatment of nonpsychotic anxiety: 1 or 2 mg twice daily. Do not administer > 6 mg per day or for > 12 weeks.

Concentrate: For institutional use only. Use in severe neuropsychiatric conditions when oral medication is preferred and other oral forms are impractical. Add dose to 60 ml or more of diluent just prior to administration. Vehicles suggested for dilution are: Tomato or fruit juice, milk, simple syrup, orange syrup, carbonated beverages, coffee, tea or water. Semisolid foods (soup, puddings, etc) may also be used.

Rx	**Trifluoperazine** (Various, eg, Balan, Geneva, Goldline, Major, Moore, Parmed, Rugby, Schein, Warner-C, Zenith)	**Tablets:** 1 mg	In 100s, 500s, 1000s & UD 100s.
Rx	**Stelazine** (SKF)		(SKF S03). Blue. Film coated. In 100s, 1000s and UD 100s.
Rx	**Trifluoperazine** (Various, eg, Balan, Geneva, Goldline, Major, Moore, Parmed, Rugby, Schein, Warner-C, Zenith)	**Tablets:** 2 mg	In 100s, 500s, 1000s and UD 100s and 1000s.
Rx	**Stelazine** (SKF)		(SKF S04). Blue. Film coated. In 100s, 1000s and UD 100s.
Rx	**Trifluoperazine** (Various, eg, Balan, Geneva, Goldline, Major, Moore, Parmed, Rugby, Schein, Warner-C, Zenith)	**Tablets:** 5 mg	In 100s, 500s, 1000s and UD 100s.
Rx	**Stelazine** (SKF)		(SKF S06). Blue. Film coated. In 100s, 1000s and UD 100s.
Rx	**Trifluoperazine** (Various, eg, Balan, Geneva, Goldline, Major, Moore, Parmed, Rugby, Schein, Warner-C, Zenith)	**Tablets:** 10 mg	In 100s, 500s, 1000s & UD 100s.
Rx	**Stelazine** (SKF)		(SKF S07). Blue. Film coated. In 100s, 1000s and UD 100s.
Rx	**Trifluoperazine** (Various, eg, Geneva, Harber, Moore, PBI, Raway, UDL, Warner-C)	**Concentrate:** 10 mg per ml	In 60 ml.
Rx	**Stelazine** (SKF)		Sucrose. Banana-vanilla flavor. In 60 ml w/dropper.[1]
Rx	**Trifluoperazine** (Quad)	**Injection:** 2 mg/ml	In 10 ml vials.
Rx	**Stelazine** (SKF)		In 10 ml vials.[2]

[1] With sodium bisulfite.

[2] With sodium saccharin and 0.75% benzyl alcohol.

Phenothiazine Derivatives

PERPHENAZINE

Complete prescribing information begins in the Antipsychotic Agents group monograph.

Indications:

Management of manifestations of psychotic disorders.

IV only: To control severe nausea and vomiting and intractable hiccoughs (see Antiemetic/Antivertigo Agents).

Administration and Dosage:

Oral: Moderately disturbed nonhospitalized patients: 4 to 8 mg 3 times/day; reduce as soon as possible to minimum effective dosage.

Hospitalized patients – 8 to 16 mg 2 to 4 times/day; avoid dosages > 64 mg/day.

IM: Use when rapid effect and prompt control are required or when oral administration is not feasible. Administer by deep IM injection to a seated or recumbent patient; observe patient for a short period after administration. Therapeutic effect usually occurs in 10 minutes and is maximal in 1 to 2 hours. The average duration of effect is 6 hours, occasionally, 12 to 24 hours.

Initial dose – 5 mg every 6 hours. The total daily dosage should not exceed 15 mg in ambulatory patients or 30 mg in hospitalized patients. Initiate oral therapy as soon as possible, generally within 24 hours. However, patients have been maintained on parenteral therapy for several months. Use equal or higher dosage when the patient is transferred to oral therapy after receiving the injection.

Psychotic conditions – While 5 mg IM has a definite tranquilizing effect, it may be necessary to use 10 mg to initiate therapy in severely agitated states. Most patients are controlled and oral therapy can be instituted within a maximum of 24 to 48 hours. Acute conditions (hysteria, panic reaction) often respond well to a single dose, whereas in chronic conditions, several injections may be required.

Children: Pediatric dosage has not been established. Children > 12 years of age may receive the lowest limit of the adult dosage.

Elderly: Administer one-third to one-half the adult dose.

Concentrate: Dilute only with water, saline, homogenized milk, carbonated orange drink and pineapple, apricot, prune, orange, tomato and grapefruit juices. Do NOT mix with beverages containing caffeine (coffee, cola), tannics (tea) or pectinates (apple juice), since physical incompatibility may result. Use approximately 60 ml diluent for each 16 mg (5 ml) concentrate. Store between 2°C and 30°C (36°F and 86°F).

Rx	**Perphenazine** (Various, eg, Geneva, Goldline, Lemmon, Major, Moore, Rugby, URL, Zenith)	**Tablets:** 2 mg	In 100s and 500s.
Rx	**Trilafon** (Schering)		(Schering ADH or 705). Gray. In 100s and 500s.
Rx	**Perphenazine** (Various, eg, Geneva, Goldline, Lemmon, Major, Moore, Rugby, URL, Zenith)	**Tablets:** 4 mg	In 100s and 500s.
Rx	**Trilafon** (Schering)		(Schering ADK or 940). Gray. In 100s and 500s.
Rx	**Perphenazine** (Various, eg, Geneva, Goldline, Lemmon, Major, Moore, Rugby, URL, Zenith)	**Tablets:** 8 mg	In 100s, 250s and 500s.
Rx	**Trilafon** (Schering)		(Schering ADJ or 313). Gray. In 100s and 500s.
Rx	**Perphenazine** (Various, eg, Geneva, Goldline, Lemmon, Major, Moore, Rugby, URL, Zenith)	**Tablets:** 16 mg	In 100s and 500s.
Rx	**Trilafon** (Schering)		(Schering ADM or 077). Gray. In 100s and 500s.
Rx	**Trilafon** (Schering)	**Concentrate:** 16 mg/5 ml	Alcohol. Sorbitol. In 118 ml w/dropper.
		Injection: 5 mg/ml	In 1 ml amps.[1]

[1] With sodium bisulfite.

Phenothiazine Derivatives

ACETOPHENAZINE MALEATE

Complete prescribing information begins in the Antipsychotic Agents group monograph.

Indications:

Management of manifestations of psychotic disorders.

Administration and Dosage:

20 mg 3 times daily. In patients who have difficulty sleeping, take the last tablet 1 hour before bedtime. Total dosage range is 40 to 80 mg/day.

Hospitalized patients: Optimum dosage is 80 to 120 mg/day in divided doses. Certain hospitalized patients with severe schizophrenia have received doses as high as 400 to 600 mg/day.

Rx	**Tindal** (Schering)	**Tablets**: 20 mg	(BBA or 968). Salmon. Sugar coated. In 100s.

PROCHLORPERAZINE

Complete prescribing information begins in the Antipsychotic Agents group monograph.

Indications:

Management of manifestations of psychotic disorders. Short-term treatment of generalized nonpsychotic anxiety; however, prochlorperazine is not the drug of choice for this indication.

To control severe nausea and vomiting (see Antiemetic/Antivertigo Agents).

Administration and Dosage:

Adults: Administration SC is not advisable because of local irritation. Individualize dosage. Begin with the lowest recommended dosage.

Elderly: Lower doses are sufficient for most elderly patients. Since they appear more susceptible to hypotension and neuromuscular reactions, observe patients closely. Monitor response and adjust dosage accordingly; increase dosage gradually.

Nonpsychotic anxiety:

Oral – 5 mg 3 or 4 times daily; 15 mg (sustained release) on arising, or 10 mg (sustained release) every 12 hours. Do not administer > 20 mg/day or for > 12 weeks.

Psychiatry: Although response ordinarily is seen within 1 to 2 days, longer treatment is usually required before maximal improvement is observed.

Oral – In mild conditions, give 5 or 10 mg 3 or 4 times daily. In moderate to severe conditions, for hospitalized or adequately supervised patients, give 10 mg 3 or 4 times daily. Increase dosage gradually until symptoms are controlled or side effects become bothersome. When dosage is increased by small increments every 2 or 3 days, side effects either do not occur or are easily controlled. Some patients respond to 50 to 75 mg/day. In more severe disturbances, optimum dosage is 100 to 150 mg/day.

IM – For immediate control of severely disturbed adults, inject an initial dose of 10 to 20 mg deeply into the upper outer quadrant of the buttock. Many patients respond shortly after the first injection. If necessary, repeat every 2 to 4 hours (or in resistant cases, every hour) to gain control. More than 3 or 4 doses are seldom necessary. After control is achieved, switch patient to the oral drug at the same dosage level or higher. If prolonged parenteral therapy is needed, give 10 to 20 mg every 4 to 6 hours.

Children: Do not use in children < 20 lbs (9.1 kg) or < 2 years of age. Do not use in pediatric surgery. Children seem more prone to develop extrapyramidal reactions, even on moderate doses. Use the lowest effective dose. Occasionally, the patient may react to the drug with signs of restlessness and excitement; if this occurs, do not administer additional doses. Use with caution in children with acute illnesses or dehydration. Do not use in conditions for which children's dosages are not established.

Oral or rectal –

Children 2 to 12 years: 2.5 mg 2 or 3 times daily. Do not give > 10 mg on first day. Increase dosage according to patient response.

Children 2 to 5 years: Do not exceed 20 mg total daily dose. Children 6 to 12 years – Do not exceed 25 mg total daily dose.

IM –

Children < 12 years: 0.03 mg/kg (0.06 mg/lb) by deep IM injection. After control is achieved, usually after 1 dose, switch to oral form at same dosage level or higher.

Compatibility – Do not mix prochlorperazine injection with other agents in the syringe. Do not dilute with any diluent containing parabens as a preservative.

Phenothiazine Derivatives

PROCHLORPERAZINE

Rx	**Prochlorperazine** (Various, eg, Balan, Bioline, Bolar, Geneva, Goldline, Major, Moore, Parmed, Rugby, Schein)	**Tablets (as maleate)**: 5 mg	In 30s, 100s, 1000s and UD 100s.
Rx	**Compazine** (SKF)		Sucrose. (SKF C66). Yellow-green. In 100s, 1000s and UD 100s.
Rx	**Prochlorperazine** (Various, eg, Balan, Bioline, Bolar, Geneva, Goldline, Major, Moore, Parmed, Rugby, Schein)	**Tablets (as maleate)**: 10 mg	In 30s, 100s, 1000s and UD 100s.
Rx	**Compazine** (SKF)	**Tablets (as maleate)**: 10 mg	Sucrose. (SKF C67). Yellow-green. In 100s, 1000s and UD 100s.
Rx	**Prochlorperazine** (Various, eg, Balan, Bolar, Geneva, Gen-King, Harber, Major, Moore, Parmed, Raway, Rugby)	**Tablets (as maleate)**: 25 mg	In 100s, 1000s and UD 100s.
Rx	**Compazine** (SKF)		Sucrose. (SKF C69). Yellow-green. In 100s and 1000s.
Rx	**Compazine** (SKF)	**Spansules (sustained release capsules as maleate)**: 10 mg	Benzyl alcohol, sucrose. (SKF C44). Black/natural. In 50s, 500s & UD 100s.
		15 mg	Benzyl alcohol, sucrose. (SKF C46). Black/natural. In 50s, 500s & UD 100s.
		30 mg	Benzyl alcohol, sucrose. (SKF C47). Black/natural. In 50s, 500s & UD 100s.
Rx	**Compazine** (SKF)	**Suppositories**: 2.5 mg	In 12s.
		5 mg	In 12s.
		25 mg	In 12s.
Rx	**Compazine** (SKF)	**Syrup (as edisylate)**: 5 mg per 5 ml	Sucrose. Fruit flavor. In 120 ml.
Rx	**Prochlorperazine** (Various, eg, Dixon-Shane, Elkins-Sinn, Goldline, Rugby, Schein, Squibb Marsam)	**Injection (as edisylate)**: 5 mg per ml	In 2 ml amps and 10 ml vials.
Rx	**Prochlorperazine** (Wyeth-Ayerst)		In 1 and 2 ml Tubex.[1]
Rx	**Compazine** (SKF)		In 2 ml amps[2], 2 ml syringes[1] and 2 and 10 ml vials.[1]

[1] With sodium saccharin and benzyl alcohol.
[2] With sodium sulfite and sodium bisulfite.

Phenothiazine Derivatives

FLUPHENAZINE HCl

Complete prescribing information begins in the Antipsychotic Agents group monograph.

Indications:

Management of manifestations of psychotic disorders.

Administration and Dosage:

Individualize dosage. The oral dose is approximately 2 to 3 times the parenteral dose. Institute treatment with a low initial dosage; increase as necessary. Therapeutic effect is often achieved with doses < 20 mg/day. However, daily doses up to 40 mg may be needed. Acutely ill patients may respond to lower doses and may require a rapid dosage increase. Elderly, debilitated and adolescent patients may respond to low dosages. Outpatients should receive smaller doses than hospitalized patients.

Administration IM is useful when patients are unable or unwilling to take oral therapy. When symptoms are controlled, oral maintenance therapy can be instituted, often with single daily doses. Continued treatment, oral if possible, is needed to achieve maximum therapeutic benefits; further dosage adjustments may be necessary.

Oral:

Adults – Initially 0.5 to 10 mg/day in divided doses administered at 6 to 8 hour intervals. In general, a daily dose in excess of 3 mg is rarely necessary. Use doses in excess of 20 mg with caution. When symptoms are controlled, reduce dosage gradually to daily maintenance doses of 1 to 5 mg, often given as a single daily dose.

Geriatric patients: Starting dose is 1 to 2.5 mg/day, adjusted according to response.

IM: The average starting dose is 1.25 mg IM. The initial total daily dosage may range from 2.5 to 10 mg, divided and given at 6 to 8 hour intervals. In general, the parenteral dose is approximately ⅓ to ½ the oral dose. Institute treatment with a low initial dosage and increase, if necessary, until desired clinical effects are achieved. Use dosages exceeding 10 mg/day IM with caution.

For psychotic patients stabilized on a fixed daily dosage of fluphenazine HCl tablets or liquid, conversion from oral therapy to the long-acting injectable fluphenazine decanoate may be indicated.

Concentrate: Suitable for administration only with the following diluents: Water, saline, *Seven-Up,* homogenized milk, carbonated orange beverage, and pineapple, apricot, prune, orange, *V-8,* tomato and grapefruit juices. Do NOT mix with beverages containing caffeine (coffee, cola), tannics (tea) or pectinates (apple juice), since physical incompatibility may result.

Storage: Store concentrate between 2° and 30°C (36° and 86°F). Avoid freezing.

Rx	**Fluphenazine HCl** (Various, eg, Geneva, Goldline, Major, Moore, Rugby, Schein, URL, Warner-C)	**Tablets**: 1 mg	In 50s, 100s, 500s, 1000s and UD 100s.
Rx	**Prolixin** (Princeton)		(863). In 50s, 100s, 500s and UD 100s.
Rx	**Fluphenazine HCl** (Various, eg, Geneva, Goldline, Major, Moore, Rugby, Schein, URL, Warner-C)	**Tablets**: 2.5 mg	In 50s, 100s, 500s and UD 100s.
Rx	**Permitil** (Schering)		(WDR or 442). Orange, scored. Oval. In 100s.
Rx	**Prolixin** (Princeton)		Tartrazine. (864). In 50s, 100s, 500s and UD 100s.
Rx	**Fluphenazine HCl** (Various, eg, Geneva, Goldline, Major, Moore, Rugby, Schein, URL, Warner-C)	**Tablets**: 5 mg	In 50s, 100s, 500s and UD 100s.
Rx	**Permitil** (Schering)		(WFF or 550). Purple-pink, scored. Oval. In 100s.
Rx	**Prolixin** (Princeton)		Tartrazine. (877). In 50s, 100s and UD 100s.

Phenothiazine Derivatives

FLUPHENAZINE HCl

Rx	**Fluphenazine HCl** (Various, eg, Geneva, Goldline, Major, Moore, Rugby, Schein, URL, Warner-C)	**Tablets:** 10 mg	In 50s, 100s, 500s and UD 100s.
Rx	**Permitil** (Schering)		(WFG or 316). Red, scored. Oval. In 1000s.
Rx	**Prolixin** (Princeton)		Tartrazine. (956). In 50s, 100s, 500s and UD 100s.
Rx	**Prolixin** (Princeton)	**Elixir:** 2.5 mg per 5 ml	14% alcohol, sucrose. In 60 ml w/dropper, 473 ml.
Rx	**Permitil** (Schering)	**Concentrate:** 5 mg per ml	1% alcohol. In 118 ml w/dropper.
Rx	**Prolixin** (Princeton)		14% alcohol. In 120 ml w/dropper.
Rx	**Fluphenazine HCl** (Quad)	**Injection:** 2.5 mg per ml	In 10 ml vials.
Rx	**Prolixin** (Princeton)		In 10 ml vials.[1]

[1] With methyl and propyl parabens.

FLUPHENAZINE ENANTHATE AND DECANOATE

Complete prescribing information begins in the Antipsychotic Agents group monograph.

Actions:

Pharmacokinetics: The esterification of fluphenazine markedly prolongs the duration of effects without unduly attenuating its beneficial action.

Selected Fluphenazine Pharmacokinetics Parameters

Fluphenazine Ester	Peak Plasma Level (days)	Half-life (days)		Onset of Action (days)	Duration (weeks)
		Single-dose	Multiple-dose		
Enanthate	2 to 3	3.5 to 4.1		1 to 3	1 to 3
Decanoate	1 to 2	6.8 to 9.6	14.3	1 to 3	≥ 4

Indications:

Management of patients requiring prolonged parenteral neuroleptic therapy (eg, chronic schizophrenics).

Administration and Dosage:

Administer IM or SC. Initiate with 12.5 to 25 mg. Determine subsequent injections and dosage interval in accordance with patient response. Do not exceed 100 mg. If doses > 50 mg are needed, increase succeeding doses cautiously in 12.5 mg increments.

In one study, significantly more injection site leakage occurred after IM administration compared to SC use; consider this possibility with nonresponders to IM therapy.

Initially, treat patients who have never taken phenothiazines with a shorter-acting form of the drug before administering the enanthate or decanoate. This helps to determine the response to fluphenazine and to establish appropriate dosage. The equivalent dosage of fluphenazine HCl to the longer-acting forms is not known; exercise caution when switching from shorter-acting forms to the enanthate.

No precise formula can be given to convert to use of fluphenazine decanoate. However, in a controlled multicenter study, 20 mg fluphenazine HCl daily was equivalent to 25 mg decanoate every 3 weeks. This is an approximate conversion ratio of 0.5 ml (12.5 mg) decanoate every 3 weeks for every 10 mg fluphenazine HCl daily.

Severely agitated patients: Treat initially with a rapid-acting phenothiazine such as fluphenazine HCl injection. When acute symptoms have subsided, administer 25 mg of the enanthate or decanoate; adjust subsequent dosage as necessary.

"Poor risk" patients (known phenothiazine hypersensitivity or with disorders predisposing to undue reactions): Initiate cautiously oral or parenteral HCl. When appropriate dosage is established, give equivalent dose of enanthate or decanoate.

Rx	**Prolixin Enanthate** (Princeton)	**Injection:** 25 mg/ml[2]	In 5 ml vials.
Rx	**Fluphenazine Decanoate** (Quad)	**Injection:** 25 mg/ml[2]	In 5 ml vials.
Rx	**Prolixin Decanoate** (Princeton)		In 5 ml vials, 1 ml Unimatic syringes.

[2] In sesame oil with benzyl alcohol.

Thioxanthene Derivatives

THIOXANTHENE DERIVATIVES

Indications:

Management of manifestations of psychotic disorders.

THIOTHIXENE

Complete prescribing information begins in the Antipsychotic Agents group monograph.

Administration and Dosage:

Not recommended in children < 12 years of age.

Oral: Mild conditions - Initially 2 mg 3 times daily. If indicated, an increase to 15 mg/day is often effective.

Severe conditions – Initially 5 mg twice/day. Optimal is 20 to 30 mg/day. If indicated, 60 mg/day is often effective. Exceeding 60 mg/day rarely increases response.

IM: 4 mg 2 to 4 times daily. Most patients are controlled on 16 to 20 mg/day (maximum 30 mg/day). Used for more rapid control and treatment of acute behavior and when oral administration is impractical. Institute oral medication as soon as feasible. May need to adjust dosage when changing from IM to oral forms.

Preparation and storage: Reconstitute powder for injection with 2.2 ml Sterile Water for Injection; may then store at room temperature for 48 hours before discarding. The IM solution is stable for 12 months at room temperature.

Rx	**Thiothixene** (Various, eg, Geneva, Major, Moore, Parmed, Rugby, Schein)	**Capsules:** 1 mg	In 100s.
Rx	**Navane** (Roerig)		(Navane Roerig 571). In 100s and UD100s.
Rx	**Thiothixene** (Various, eg, Danbury, Geneva, Goldline, Major, Moore, Parmed, Rugby, Schein)	**Capsules:** 2 mg	In 100s and 500s.
Rx	**Navane** (Roerig)		(Navane Roerig 572). In 100s, 1000s and UD100s.
Rx	**Thiothixene** (Various, eg, Danbury, Geneva, Goldline, Major, Moore, Parmed, Rugby)	**Capsules:** 5 mg	In 100s, 500s and 1000s.
Rx	**Navane** (Roerig)		(Navane Roerig 573). In 100s, 1000s and UD100s.
Rx	**Thiothixene** (Various, eg, Danbury, Geneva, Goldline, Major, Moore, Parmed, Rugby, Schein)	**Capsules:** 10 mg	In 100s and 500s.
Rx	**Navane** (Roerig)		(Navane Roerig 574). In 100s, 1000s and UD100s.

Thioxanthene Derivatives

THIOTHIXENE

Rx	**Thiothixene** (Various, eg, Geneva, Goldline, Major, Moore, Parmed, Rugby, Schein)	**Capsules**: 20 mg	In 100s.
Rx	**Navane** (Roerig)		(Navane Roerig 577). In 100s, 500s and UD 100s.
Rx	**Thiothixene** (Various, eg, Barre-National, Goldline, Lemmon, Major, Rugby, Schein, Warner-C)	**Concentrate**: 5 mg (as HCl) per ml	In 30 and 120 ml.
Rx	**Thiothixene HCl Intensol** (Roxane)		Alcohol free. EDTA. In 30 and 120 ml with dropper.
Rx	**Navane** (Roerig)		7% alcohol, sorbitol. Fruit flavor. In 30, 120 ml w/dropper.
Rx	**Navane** (Roerig)	**IM Solution**: 2 mg (as HCl) per ml	In 2 ml vials.[1]
		Powder for Injection: 5 mg (as HCl) per ml when reconstituted	In 2 ml vials.[2]

[1] With 5% dextrose, 0.9% benzyl alcohol, 0.02% propyl gallate.
[2] With 59.6 mg mannitol per ml.

Butyrophenone

HALOPERIDOL

Complete prescribing information begins in the Antipsychotic Agents group monograph.

Actions:

Pharmacokinetics: An antipsychotic agent with pharmacologic effects similar to piperazine phenothiazines.

Dosage adjustment is unnecessary in renal failure; however, hypotension and excessive sedation may occur. Dialysis is ineffective in treating overdosage.

Selected Pharmacokinetics of Haloperidol

Route	Absorption %	Time to peak concentration	Half-life (hours)	Protein binding	Metabolism	Excretion
Oral	60	3 to 5 hours	24 (12-38)[1]	90%-92%	Liver 1% excreted unchanged	40% urine 15% bile
IM	75[2]	20 min	21 (13-36)[1]			
Decanoate		4 to 11 days (average, 6)	3 weeks			
IV[3]	100	immediate	14 (10-19)[1]			

[1] Range.
[2] Within 30 minutes.
[3] Not an approved route of administration.

Indications:

Psychotic disorder management.

Tourette's disorder in children and adults for the control of tics and vocal utterances.

Severe behavioral problems in children with combative, explosive hyperexcitability which cannot be accounted for by immediate provocation.

Hyperactive children (short-term treatment) who show excessive motor activity with accompanying conduct disorders consisting of impulsivity, difficulty sustaining attention, aggression, mood lability or poor frustration tolerance.

Prolonged parenteral neuroleptic therapy (eg, chronic schizophrenia): Haloperidol decanoate is a long-acting parenteral antipsychotic for patients requiring such therapy.

Unlabeled uses: Haloperidol is an effective antiemetic in small doses. Haloperidol has been given IV for acute psychiatric situations at 2 to 25 mg, approximately every 30 or more minutes, at a rate of 5 mg/minute. It is effective in the treatment of phencyclidine (PCP) psychosis (possibly more effective with concurrent ascorbic acid). In two children, use of nicotine polacrilex gum and haloperidol resulted in improvement of symptoms of Tourette's syndrome.

Administration and Dosage:

Individualize dosage. Children, debilitated or geriatric patients and those with a history of adverse reactions to neuroleptic drugs may require less haloperidol; optimal response is usually obtained with more gradual dosage adjustments and at lower dosage levels.

Adults: Initial dosage range: Moderate symptoms or geriatric or debilitated patients: 0.5 to 2 mg 2 or 3 times daily; severe symptoms or chronic or resistant patients: 3 to 5 mg 2 or 3 times daily. To achieve prompt control, higher doses may be required.

Patients who remain severely disturbed or inadequately controlled may require dosage adjustment. Daily dosages up to 100 mg may be necessary. Infrequently, doses > 100 mg have been used for severely resistant patients; however, safety of prolonged administration of such doses has not been demonstrated.

Children: Do not use in children < 3 years of age. Initial dose is 0.5 mg/day. If required, increase in 0.5 mg increments each 5 to 7 days until therapeutic effect is obtained. Total dose may be divided and given 2 or 3 times daily. The dose in this age group has not been well established.

Psychotic disorders – 0.05 to 0.15 mg/kg/day.

Nonpsychotic behavior disorders; Tourette's disorder: 0.05 to 0.075 mg/kg/day.

Severely disturbed psychotic children may require higher doses.

In severely disturbed, nonpsychotic children or in hyperactive children with conduct disorders, short-term administration may suffice. There is little evidence that behavior improvement is further enhanced by dosages > 6 mg/day.

Other suggested doses for children 3 to 6 years old include: Agitation and hyperkinesia – 0.01 to 0.03 mg/kg/day orally; infantile autism – 0.5 to 4 mg/day.

Butyrophenone

HALOPERIDOL

Maintenance dosage – Upon achieving a satisfactory therapeutic response, gradually reduce dosage to the lowest effective maintenance level.

IM administration – 2 to 5mg for prompt control of the acutely agitated patient with moderately severe to very severe symptoms. Depending on response, administer subsequent doses as often as every 60 minutes, although 4 to 8 hour intervals may be satisfactory.

The safety and efficacy of IM administration in children have not been established.

The oral form should replace the injectable as soon as feasible. For an approximation of the total daily dose required, use the parenteral dose administered in the preceding 24 hours; carefully monitor the patient for the first several days. Give the first oral dose within 12 to 24 hours following the last parenteral dose.

Haloperidol decanoate injection: Administer by deep IM injection. A 21 gauge needle is recommended. The maximum volume per injection site should not exceed 3 ml. The recommended interval between doses is 4 weeks. Do not administer IV.

Intended for use in chronic psychotic patients who require prolonged parenteral antipsychotic therapy. These patients should be previously stabilized on antipsychotic medication before considering a conversion to haloperidol decanoate. Furthermore, it is recommended that patients being considered for haloperidol decanoate therapy have been treated with, and tolerate well, short-acting haloperidol in order to exclude the possibility of an unexpected adverse sensitivity to haloperidol. Close clinical supervision is required during the initial period of dose adjustment in order to minimize the risk of overdosage or reappearance of psychotic symptoms before the next injection. During dose adjustment or episodes of exacerbation of psychotic symptoms, haloperidol decanoate therapy can be supplemented with short-acting forms of haloperidol.

Express the dose in terms of its haloperidol content. Base the starting dose of haloperidol decanoate on the patient's clinical history, physical condition and response to previous antipsychotic therapy. The preferred approach to determining the minimum effective dose is to begin with lower initial doses and to adjust the dose upward as needed. For patients previously maintained on low doses of antipsychotics (eg, up to the equivalent of 10 mg/day oral haloperidol), it is recommended that the initial dose of haloperidol decanoate be 10 to 15 times the previous daily dose in oral haloperidol equivalents; limited clinical experience suggests that lower initial doses may be adequate. The initial dose of haloperidol decanoate should not exceed 100 mg regardless of previous antipsychotic dose requirements. Haloperidol decanoate has been effectively administered at monthly intervals in several clinical studies. However, variation in patient response may dictate a need for adjustment of the dosing interval as well as the dose.

Elderly/Debilitated: Lower initial doses and more gradual adjustment are recommended. Clinical experience with haloperidol decanoate at doses > 300 mg per month has been limited.

Butyrophenone

HALOPERIDOL

Rx	**Haloperidol** (Various, eg, Geneva, Goldline, Major, Moore, Roxane, Rugby, Schein)	**Tablets**: 0.5mg	In 100s, 500s, 1000s and UD 100s.
Rx	**Haldol** (McNeil-CPC)		(Haldol/McNeil). White, scored. In 100s and UD 100s.
Rx	**Haloperidol** (Various, eg, Geneva, Goldline, Major, Moore, Roxane, Rugby, Schein)	**Tablets**: 1mg	In 100s, 500s, 1000s and UD 100s.
Rx	**Haldol** (McNeil-CPC)		Tartrazine. (1 Haldol/ McNeil). Yellow, scored. In 100s and UD 100s.
Rx	**Haloperidol** (Various, eg, Geneva, Goldline, Major, Moore, Roxane, Rugby, Schiapparelli Searle)	**Tablets**: 2 mg	In100s, 500s, 1000s and UD 100s.
Rx	**Haldol** (McNeil-CPC)		(2 Haldol/McNeil). Pink, scored. In 100s and UD 100s.
Rx	**Haloperidol** (Various, eg, Geneva, Goldline, Major, Moore, Roxane, Rugby, Schein)	**Tablets**: 5 mg	In 100s, 500s, 1000s and UD 100s.
Rx	**Haldol** (McNeil-CPC)		Tartrazine. (5 Haldol/ McNeil). Green, scored. In 100s and UD 100s.
Rx	**Haloperidol** (Various, eg, Geneva, Goldline, Major, Moore, Roxane, Rugby, Schein)	**Tablets**: 10 mg	In 100s, 500s and UD 100s.
Rx	**Haldol** (McNeil-CPC)		Tartrazine. (10 Haldol/ McNeil). Aqua, scored. In 100s.
Rx	**Haloperidol** (Various, eg, Geneva, Goldline, Major, Roxane, Rugby, Schein)	**Tablets**: 20 mg	In 100s and UD 100s.
Rx	**Haldol** (McNeil-CPC)		(20 Haldol/McNeil). Salmon, scored. In 100s.
Rx	**Haloperidol** (Various, eg, Geneva, Goldline, Major, Roxane, Rugby, Schein)	**Concentrate**: 2 mg (as lactate) per ml	In 15 and 120 ml and 5 and 10 ml UD 100s.
Rx	**Haldol** (McNeil-CPC)		In 15, 120 and 240 ml.
Rx	**Haloperidol** (Various, eg, Lyphomed, Quad, Raway, Xactdose)	**Injection**: 5mg (as lactate) per ml	In 1 ml amps, syringes and vials and 2, 2.5 and 10 ml vials.
Rx	**Haldol** (McNeil-CPC)		In 1ml amps,[1] 10 ml vials[1] and 1 ml disp. syringes[1].
Rx	**Haldol Decanoate 50** (McNeil-CPC)	**Injection**: 50 mg (as 70.5 mg decanoate)/ml	In 1ml amps[2] and 5 ml vials[2].
Rx	**Haldol Decanoate 100** (McNeil-CPC)	**Injection**: 100 mg (as 141.04 mg decanoate)/ml	In 1ml amps[2] and 5 ml vials[2].

[1] With methyl and propyl parabens.
[2] In sesame oil with 1.2% benzyl alcohol.

Dihydroindolone

MOLINDONE HCl

Complete prescribing information begins in the Antipsychotic Agents group monograph.

Actions:

Pharmacology: Molindone is structurally unrelated to the phenothiazines, butyrophenones or thioxanthenes, but it resembles the piperazine phenothiazines in its clinical action.

Pharmacokinetics: Molindone is rapidly absorbed and metabolized. Unmetabolized drug reaches peak blood levels at 1.5 hours. Effects from a single oral dose persist for 24 to 36 hours. Less than 2% to 3% is excreted unmetabolized in urine and feces.

Indications:

Management of manifestations of psychotic disorders.

Administration and Dosage:

Initial dosage: 50 to 75 mg/day, increased to 100 mg/day in 3 or 4 days. Individualize dosage; patients with severe symptoms may require up to 225 mg/day.

Start elderly and debilitated patients on lower dosage.

Maintenance therapy:

Mild – 5 to 15 mg 3 or 4 times daily;
Moderate – 10 to 25 mg 3 or 4 times daily;
Severe – 225 mg/day may be required.

Tablets contain calcium sulfate as an excipient; calcium ions may interfere with the absorption of drugs such as phenytoin sodium or tetracyclines.

Rx	**Moban** (DuPont)	**Tablets:** 5 mg	Orange. In 100s.
		10 mg	Lavender. In 100s.
		25 mg	Green. In 100s.
		50 mg	Blue. In 100s.
		100 mg	Tan. In 100s.
		Concentrate: 20 mg/ml[1]	Alcohol, sorbitol. Cherry flavor. In 120 ml.

[1] With parabens and sodium metabisulfite.

Dibenzoxapine

LOXAPINE

Complete prescribing information begins in the Antipsychotic Agents group monograph.

Actions:

Pharmacology: Loxapine is chemically distinct from thioxanthenes, butyrophenones and phenothiazines. No advantages over other antipsychotics are established.

Pharmacokinetics: Loxapine is metabolized extensively and is excreted within the first 24 hours. Metabolites are excreted in the urine as conjugates and in the feces unconjugated. Signs of sedation are usually seen within 20 to 30 minutes after administration, are most pronounced within 1.5 to 3 hours and last approximately 12 hours.

Indications:

Management of the manifestations of psychotic disorders.

Administration and Dosage:

Oral: Individualize dosage. Administer in divided doses, 2 to 4 times daily.

Initial – 10 mg twice daily. In severely disturbed patients, up to 50 mg/day may be desirable. Increase dosage fairly rapidly over the first 7 to 10 days until symptoms are controlled. Usual range is 60 to 100 mg/day. Dosage > 250 mg/day not recommended.

Maintenance – Reduce dosage to the lowest level compatible with control of symptoms; usual range is 20 to 60 mg/day.

Mix concentrate with orange or grapefruit juice shortly before administration.

IM: For prompt symptomatic control in the acutely agitated patient and in patients whose symptoms render oral medication temporarily impractical.

Administer IM (not IV) in 12.5 to 50 mg doses at intervals of 4 to 6 hours or longer. Many patients respond satisfactorily to twice daily dosage. Individualize dosage. Once control is achieved, institute oral medication, usually within 5 days.

Rx	**Loxapine Succinate** (Various, eg, Bristol-Myers Squibb, Geneva, Goldline, Major, Moore, Parmed, Schein, Warner Chilcott)	**Capsules** (as succinate): 5 mg	In 100s.
Rx	**Loxitane** (Lederle)		(Lederle L1 5 mg). Green. In 100s and UD 100s.
Rx	**Loxapine Succinate** (Various, eg, Bristol-Myers Squibb, Geneva, Goldline, Major, Moore, Parmed, Schein, Warner Chilcott)	**Capsules** (as succinate): 10 mg	In 100s.
Rx	**Loxitane** (Lederle)		(Lederle L2 10 mg). Green and yellow. In 100s, 1000s and UD 100s.
Rx	**Loxapine Succinate** (Various, eg, Bristol-Myers Squibb, Geneva, Goldline, Major, Moore, Parmed, Schein, Warner Chilcott)	**Capsules** (as succinate): 25 mg	In 100s.
Rx	**Loxitane** (Lederle)		(Lederle L3 25 mg). Two-tone green. In 100s, 1000s and UD 100s.
Rx	**Loxapine Succinate** (Various, eg, Bristol-Myers Squibb, Geneva, Goldline, Major, Moore, Parmed, Schein, Warner-C)	**Capsules** (as succinate): 50 mg	In 100s.
Rx	**Loxitane** (Lederle)		(Lederle L4 50 mg). Green and blue. In 100s, 1000s and UD 100s.
Rx	**Loxitane C** (Lederle)	**Concentrate** (as HCl): 25 mg per ml	In 120 ml with dropper.
Rx	**Loxitane IM** (Lederle)	**Injection** (as HCl): 50 mg per ml	In 1ml amps and 10 ml vials.[1]

[1] With 5% polysorbate 80 and 70% propylene glycol.

CLOZAPINE

Warning:
Because of the significant risk of agranulocytosis, a potentially life-threatening adverse event (see below), reserve clozapine for use in the treatment of severely ill schizophrenic patients who fail to show an acceptable response to adequate courses of standard antipsychotic drug treatment, either because of insufficient effectiveness or the inability to achieve an effective dose due to intolerable adverse effects from those drugs. Consequently, before initiating treatment with clozapine, it is strongly recommended that a patient be given at least two trials, each with a different standard antipsychotic drug product, at an adequate dose and for an adequate duration. Patients who are being treated with clozapine must have a baseline white blood cell (WBC) and differential count before initiation of treatment, and a WBC count every week throughout treatment and for 4 weeks after the discontinuation of clozapine.

Actions:

Pharmacology: Clozapine, a tricyclic dibenzodiazepine derivative, is classified as an "atypical" antipsychotic drug because its profile of binding to dopamine receptors and its effects on various dopamine mediated behaviors differ from those exhibited by more typical antipsychotic drug products. In particular, although clozapine does interfere with the binding of dopamine at both D-1 and D-2 receptors, it does not induce catalepsy nor inhibit apomorphine-induced stereotypy. This evidence, consistent with the view that clozapine is preferentially more active at limbic than at striatal dopamine receptors, may explain clozapine's relative freedom from extrapyramidal side effects. Clozapine also acts as an antagonist at adrenergic, cholinergic, histaminergic and serotonergic receptors. In contrast to more typical antipsychotic drugs, clozapine therapy produces little or no prolactin elevation.

As is true of more typical antipsychotic drugs, clozapine increases delta and theta activity and slows dominant alpha frequencies of the EEG. Enhanced synchronization occurs, and sharp wave activity and spike and wave complexes may also develop. Patients rarely may report intensification of dream activity. REM sleep was increased to 85% of the total sleep time. In these patients, the onset of REM sleep occurred almost immediately after falling asleep.

Pharmacokinetics:

Absorption/Distribution – Clozapine tablets (25 and 100 mg) are equally bioavailable relative to a clozapine solution. Following a dosage of 100 mg twice daily, the average steady-state peak plasma concentration was 319 ng/ml (range: 102 to 771 ng/ml), occurring at an average of 2.5 hours (range: 1 to 6 hours) after dosing. The average minimum concentration at steady state was 122 ng/ml (range: 41 to 343 ng/ml) after 100 mg twice daily dosing. Food does not appear to affect the systemic bioavailability of clozapine; thus clozapine may be administered with or without food.

Clozapine is approximately 95% bound to serum proteins. The interaction between clozapine and other highly protein-bound drugs has not been fully evaluated but may be important (see Drug Interactions).

Metabolism/Excretion – Clozapine is almost completely metabolized prior to excretion and only trace amounts of unchanged drug are detected in the urine and feces. Approximately 50% of the administered dose is excreted in the urine and 30% in the feces as demethylated, hydroxylated and N–oxide derivatives. The desmethyl metabolite has only limited activity, while the hydroxylated and N–oxide derivatives are inactive.

The mean elimination half-life of clozapine after a single 75 mg dose was 8 hours (range: 4 to 12 hours), compared to a mean elimination half-life of 12 hours (range: 4 to 66 hours) after achieving steady state with 100 mg twice daily dosing. In comparisons of single and multiple dose administration of clozapine, the elimination half-life increased significantly after multiple dosing relative to that after single dose administration, suggesting concentration dependent pharmacokinetics. However, at steady state, linearly dose-proportional changes with respect to area under the curve, peak and minimum clozapine plasma concentrations were observed after administration of 37.5, 75 and 150 mg twice daily.

Indications:
Management of severely ill schizophrenic patients who fail to respond adequately to standard antipsychotic drug treatment.

Contraindications:
Myeloproliferative disorders; history of clozapine-induced agranulocytosis or severe granulocytopenia; simultaneous administration with other agents having a well-

CLOZAPINE

known potential to suppress bone marrow function; severe CNS depression or comatose states from any cause.

Warnings:

Agranulocytosis, defined as a granulocyte count of < 500/mm^3, occurs in association with clozapine use at a cumulative incidence at 1 year of approximately 1.3%, based on 15 cases out of 1743 patients exposed to clozapine during clinical testing. All of these cases occurred when the need for close monitoring of WBC counts was already recognized. This reaction could prove fatal if not detected early and therapy interrupted. While no fatalities have been associated with these agranulocytosis cases, and all cases have recovered fully, the sample is too small to reliably estimate the case fatality rate. Of the 112 cases of agranulocytosis reported worldwide in association with clozapine use as of December 31, 1986, 35% were fatal. However, few of these deaths occurred since 1977, when knowledge of clozapine-induced agranulocytosis became more widespread, and close monitoring of WBC counts more widely practiced.

Patients must have a blood sample drawn for a WBC count before initiation of treatment with clozapine, and must have subsequent WBC counts done at least weekly for the duration of therapy, as well as for 4 weeks thereafter. The distribution of clozapine is contingent upon performance of the required blood tests.

Clozapine Therapy Guidelines Based on WBC and Granulocyte Count

WBC Count (mm^3)	Granulocyte Count (mm^3)	Guidelines
< 3500, or history of myeloproliferative disorder, or previous clozapine-induced agranulocytosis or granulocytopenia		Do not initiate treatment.
< 3500, or > 3500 with a substantial drop from baseline, following initiation of treatment		Repeat WBC and differential counts. Symptoms of infection: Lethargy, weakness, fever, sore throat.
3000 to 3500 on subsequent counts	> 1500	Perform twice weekly WBC and differential counts.
< 3000	< 1500	Interrupt therapy, monitor for flu-like symptoms or other symptoms of infection. May resume therapy if no signs of infection develop, WBC count > 3000 and granulocyte count > 1500. However, continue twice weekly WBC and differential counts until WBC returns to 3500.
< 2000	<1000	Consider bone marrow aspiration to ascertain granulopoietic status. If granulopoiesis is deficient, consider protective isolation. If infection develops, perform cultures and institute antibiotics. Do *not rechallenge with clozapine since agranulocytosis may develop with a shorter latency.*

Except for evidence of significant bone marrow suppression during initial clozapine therapy, there are no established risk factors for the development of agranulocytosis. However, a disproportionate number of the US cases of agranulocytosis occurred in patients of Jewish background compared to the overall proportion of such patients exposed during clozapine's domestic development. Most of the US cases occurred with 4 to 10 weeks of exposure, but neither dose nor duration is a reliable predictor. No patient characteristics have been clearly linked to the development of agranulocytosis in association with clozapine use, but agranulocytosis associated with other antipsychotic drugs has been reported to occur with a greater frequency in women, the elderly and in patients who are cachectic or have serious underlying medical illness; such patients may also be at particular risk with clozapine.

To reduce the risk of agranulocytosis developing undetected, clozapine will be dispensed only within the clozapine Patient Management System.

Seizure occurs in association with clozapine use at a cumulative incidence at 1 year of approximately 5%, based on 61 of 1743 patients exposed to clozapine during its clinical testing (ie, a crude rate of 3.5%). Dose appears to be an important predictor of seizure, with a greater likelihood of seizure at the higher clozapine doses used.

Use caution when administering to patients with history of seizures or other predisposing factors. Advise patients not to engage in any activity where sudden loss of consciousness could cause serious risk to themselves or others, (eg, operation of complex machinery, driving an an automobile, swimming, climbing).

Cardiovascular disease: Use clozapine with caution; carefully observe the recommendation for gradual titration of dose.

Orthostatic hypotension can occur, especially during initial titration in association with rapid dose escalation, and may represent a continuing risk in some patients.

Tachycardia, which may be sustained, has also been observed in approximately 25% of patients, with patients having an average increase in pulse rate of 10 to 15 bpm. The sustained tachycardia is not simply a reflex response to hypotension, and is present in all positions monitored.

Either tachycardia or hypotension may pose a serious risk for an individual with compromised cardiovascular function.

ECG Changes: A minority of patients experience ECG repolarization changes similar to those seen with other antipsychotic drugs, including S-T segment depression and flattening or inversion of T waves, which all normalize after discontinuation of clozapine. The clinical significance is unclear. However, several patients have experienced significant cardiac events, including ischemic changes, myocardial infarction, nonfatal arrhythmias and sudden unexplained death. Causality assessment was difficult in many of these cases because of serious preexisting cardiac disease and plausible alternative causes. Rare instances of sudden, unexplained death have been reported in psychiatric patients, with or without associated antipsychotic drug treatment, and the relationship of these events to antipsychotic drug use is unknown.

Neuroleptic Malignant Syndrome (NMS), a potentially fatal symptom complex has occurred in association with antipsychotic drugs. Clinical manifestations of NMS are hyperpyrexia, muscle rigidity, altered mental status and evidence of autonomic instability (irregular pulse or blood pressure, tachycardia, diaphoresis and cardiac dysrhythmias).

Management of NMS should include 1) immediate discontinuation of antipsychotic drugs and other drugs not essential to concurrent therapy, 2) intensive symptomatic treatment and medical monitoring, and 3) treatment of any concomitant serious medical problems for which specific treatments are available. There is no general agreement about specific pharmacological treatment regimens for uncomplicated NMS.

If a patient requires antipsychotic drug treatment after recovery from NMS, the potential reintroduction of drug therapy should be carefully considered. The patient should be carefully monitored, since recurrences of NMS have been reported.

No cases of NMS have been attributed to clozapine alone. However, there have been several reported cases of NMS in patients treated concomitantly with lithium or other CNS-active agents.

Tardive dyskinesia, a syndrome consisting of potentially irreversible, involuntary, dyskinetic movements may develop in patients treated with antipsychotic drugs. Although the prevalence of the syndrome appears to be highest among the elderly, especially elderly women, it is impossible to predict which patients are likely to develop the syndrome. There have been no confirmed cases of tardive dyskinesia developing in association with clozapine use. Nevertheless, it cannot yet be concluded, without more extended experience, that clozapine is incapable of inducing this syndrome. Prescribe clozapine in a manner that is most likely to minimize the occurrence of tardive dyskinesia. If signs and symptoms of tardive dyskinesia appear in a patient on clozapine, consider drug discontinuation. However, some patients may require treatment with clozapine despite the presence of the syndrome.

Both the risk of developing the syndrome and the likelihood that it will become irreversible are believed to increase as the duration of treatment and the total cumulative dose of antipsychotic drugs administered to the patient increase. However, the syndrome can develop, although much less commonly, after relatively brief treatment periods at low doses. There is no known treatment, although the syndrome may remit, partially or completely, if antipsychotic drug treatment is withdrawn. Antipsychotic drug treatment itself, however, may suppress (or partially suppress) the signs and symptoms of the syndrome and thereby may possibly mask the underlying process. The effect that symptom suppression has upon the long-term course of the syndrome is unknown.

CLOZAPINE

Pregnancy: Category B. There are no adequate or well controlled studies in pregnant women. Use during pregnancy only if clearly needed.

Lactation: Animal studies suggest that clozapine may be excreted in breast milk and have an effect on the nursing infant. Therefore, women on clozapine should not nurse.

Children: Safety and efficacy in children < 16 years old have not been established.

Precautions:

Fever: Patients may experience transient temperature elevations > 100.4°F (38°C), with the peak incidence within the first 3 weeks of treatment. While this fever is generally benign and self-limiting, it may necessitate discontinuing patients from treatment. On occasion, there may be an associated increase or decrease in WBC count. Carefully evaluate patients with fever to rule out the possibility of an underlying infectious process or the development of agranulocytosis. In the presence of high fever, the possibility of NMS must be considered (see Warnings).

Anticholinergic effects of clozapine are very potent; exercise great care in using this drug in the presence of prostatic enlargement or narrow angle glaucoma.

Interference with cognitive and motor performance: Because of initial sedation, clozapine may impair mental or physical abilities, especially during the first few days of therapy. Carefully adhere to the recommendations for gradual dose escalation, and caution patients about activities requiring alertness.

Concomitant illness: Clinical experience is limited. Nevertheless, caution is advisable in using clozapine in patients with hepatic, renal or cardiac disease.

Drug Interactions:

Anticholinergics: The anticholinergic effects may be potentiated by clozapine.

Antihypertensives: The hypotensive effects may be potentiated by clozapine.

CNS drugs: Given the primary CNS effects of clozapine, caution is advised in using it concomitantly with other CNS-active drugs.

Agents that suppress bone marrow function: Mechanism of clozapine in agranulocytosis is unknown; nonetheless, consider the possibility that causative factors may interact synergistically to increase the risk or severity of bone marrow suppression. Do not use with other agents that suppress bone marrow function.

Protein binding: Because clozapine is highly bound to serum protein, the administration of clozapine to a patient taking another drug which is highly bound to protein (eg, warfarin, digoxin) may cause an increase in plasma concentrations of these drugs, potentially resulting in adverse effects. Conversely, adverse effects may result from displacement of protein-bound clozapine by other highly bound drugs.

Adverse Reactions:

Of 1080 patients who received clozapine in premarketing clinical trials, 16% discontinued treatment due to an adverse event which included:

CNS: Drowsiness/sedation; seizures; dizziness/syncope.

Cardiovascular: Tachycardia; hypotension; ECG changes.

GI: Nausea/vomiting.

Hematologic: Leukopenia/granulocytopenia/agranulocytosis.

Miscellaneous: Fever.

The following table lists adverse events that occurred at a frequency of ≥ 1% among patients who participated in clinical trials:

CLOZAPINE

Clozapine Adverse Reactions (n = 842)

Adverse Reaction	(%)	Adverse Reaction	(%)
CNS		*Cardiovascular*	
Drowsiness/sedation	39	Tachycardia	25
Dizziness/vertigo	19	Hypotension	9
Headache	7	Hypertension	4
Tremor	6	Chest pain/angina	1
Syncope	6	ECG change/cardiac abnormality	1
Disturbed sleep/nightmares	4	*GI*	
Restlessness	4	Constipation	14
Hypokinesia/akinesia	4	Nausea	5
Agitation	4	Abdominal discomfort/ heartburn	4
Seizures (convulsions)	3	Nausea/vomiting	3
Rigidity	3	Diarrhea	2
Akathisia	3	Liver test abnormality	1
Confusion	3	Anorexia	1
Fatigue	2	*Musculoskeletal*	
Insomnia	2	Muscle weakness	1
Hyperkinesia	1	Pain (back, neck, legs)	1
Weakness	1	Muscle spasm	1
Lethargy	1	Muscle pain, ache	1
Ataxia	1	*Respiratory*	
Slurred speech	1	Throat discomfort	1
Depression	1	Dyspnea, shortness of breath	1
Epileptiform movements /Myoclonic jerks	1	Nasal congestion	1
Anxiety	1	*Hemic/Lymphatic*	
Autonomic Nervous System		Leukopenia/decreased WBC/neutropenia	3
Salivation	31	Agranulocytosis	1
Sweating	6	Eosinophilia	1
Dry mouth	6	*Miscellaneous*	
Visual disturbances	5	Fever	5
GU		Weight gain	4
Urinary abnormalities	2	Rash	2
Incontinence	1	Tongue numb/sore	1
Abnormal ejaculation	1		
Urinary urgency/frequency	1		
Urinary retention	1		

Overdosage:

Symptoms:

Most common – Altered states of consciousness, including drowsiness, delirium and coma; tachycardia; hypotension; respiratory depression; hypersalivation. Seizures have occurred in a minority of reported cases. Fatal overdoses have been reported with clozapine, generally at doses > 2.5 g. There have also been reports of patients recovering from overdoses well in excess of 4g.

Treatment: Establish and maintain an airway; ensure adequate oxygenation and ventilation. Activated charcoal, which may be used with sorbitol, may be as or more effective than emesis or lavage. Monitoring cardiac and vital signs is recommended along with general symptomatic and supportive measures. Continue additional surveillance for several days because of the risk of delayed effects. Avoid epinephrine and derivatives when treating hypotension, and quinidine and procainamide when treating cardiac arrhythmia. Refer to General Management of Acute Overdosage.

Forced diuresis, dialysis, hemoperfusion and exchange transfusion are unlikely to be of benefit.

CLOZAPINE

Patient Information:

Warn patients about the significant risk of developing agranulocytosis. Inform them that weekly blood tests are required to monitor for the occurrence of agranulocytosis, and that clozapine tablets will be made available only through a special program designed to ensure the required blood monitoring. Advise patients to report immediately the appearance of lethargy, weakness, fever, sore throat, malaise, mucous membrane ulceration or other possible signs of infection. Pay particular attention to "flu-like" complaints or other symptoms that might suggest infection.

Inform patients of the significant risk of seizure during clozapine treatment, and advise them to avoid driving and any other potentially hazardous activity.

Advise patients of the risk of orthostatic hypotension, especially during the period of initial dose titration.

Patients should notify their physician if they are taking, or plan to take, any prescription or over-the-counter drugs or alcohol.

Patients should notify their physician if they become pregnant or intend to become pregnant during therapy.

Patients should not breast feed an infant if they are taking clozapine.

Administration and Dosage:

Initial: 25 mg once or twice daily, and then continued with daily dosage increments of 25 to 50 mg/day, if well tolerated, to achieve a target dose of 300 to 450 mg/day by the end of 2 weeks. Make subsequent dosage increments no more than once or twice weekly, in increments not to exceed 100 mg. Cautious titration and a divided dosage schedule are necessary to minimize the risks of hypotension, seizure and sedation.

In a multicenter study, patients were titrated during the first 2 weeks up to a maximum dose of 500 mg/day, on a 3 times daily basis, and were then dosed in a total daily dose range of 100 to 900 mg/day, on a 3 times daily basis thereafter, with clinical response and adverse effects as guides to correct dosing.

Dose adjustment: Continue daily dosing on a divided basis to an effective and tolerable dose level. While many patients may respond adequately at doses between 300 to 600 mg/day, it may be necessary to raise the dose to the 600 to 900 mg/day range. Do not exceed 900 mg/day. The mean and median clozapine doses are approximately 600 mg/day.

Because of the possibility of increased adverse reactions at higher doses, particularly seizures, give patients adequate time to respond to a given dose level before escalation to a higher dose.

Because of the significant risk of agranulocytosis and seizure, events which both present a continuing risk over time, avoid the extended treatment of patients failing to show an acceptable level of clinical response.

Maintenance: Continue clozapine at the lowest level needed to maintain remission. Periodically reassess patients to determine the need for maintenance treatment.

Discontinuation: In the event of planned termination of clozapine therapy, gradual reduction in dose is recommended over a 1 to 2 week period. However, should a patient's medical condition require abrupt discontinuation (eg, leukopenia), carefully observe the patient for the recurrence of psychotic symptoms.

Reinitiation of treatment: Follow the original dosage build-up guidelines. However, certain additional precautions seem prudent. Reexposure of a patient might enhance the risk of an untoward event's occurrence and increase its severity. Patients discontinued for WBC counts < 2000 per mm^3 or a granulocyte count < 1000 per mm^3 must not be restarted on clozapine. (See Warnings.)

Clozapine is available only through the *Clozaril* Patient Management System, a program that combines WBC testing, patient monitoring, pharmacy, and drug distribution services, all linked to compliance with required safety monitoring. Do not dispense more than a 1 week supply.

Rx	**Clozaril** (Sandoz)	**Tablets:** 25 mg 100 mg	(Clozaril 25 or 100). Yellow. In UD 100s. Also in total daily dose packages, each containing 1 week's worth of medication and containing various combinations of 25 and 100 mg tablets; in 150, 200, 250, 300, 400, 500 and 600 mg/day.

Benzisoxazole

RISPERIDONE

Actions:

Pharmacology: Risperidone is an antipsychotic agent belonging to the benzisoxazole derivatives class. The mechanism of action is unknown. However, antipsychotic activity may be mediated through a combination of dopamine (D_2 and serotonin $5HT_2$) antagonism. Antagonism at receptors other than D_2 and $5HT_2$ may explain some of the other effects of risperidone. Risperidone is a selective monoaminergic antagonist that also has high affinity for the α_1, α_2 and H_1 histaminergic receptors. Risperidone antagonizes other receptors, but with lower potency. It has low to moderate affinity for the serotonin $5HT_{1C}$, $5HT_{1D}$ and $5HT_{1A}$ receptors, weak affinity for the dopamine D_1 and haloperidol-sensitive sigma site, and no affinity for cholinergic, muscarinic or β_1 and β_2 adrenergic receptors.

Pharmacokinetics: Risperidone is well absorbed. It is extensively metabolized in the liver to a major active metabolite, 9-hydroxyrisperidone, which appears approximately equi-effective with risperidone with respect to receptor binding activity and some effects in animals. Consequently, the clinical effect of the drug likely results from the combined concentrations of risperidone plus 9-hydroxyrisperidone. Plasma concentrations of risperidone and 9-hydroxyrisperidone are dose-proportional over the dosing range of 1 to 16 mg daily. The relative oral bioavailability of risperidone from a tablet was 94% when compared to a solution. Food does not affect either the rate or extent of absorption; thus risperidone can be given with or without meals. The absolute oral bioavailability of risperidone is 70%.

The enzyme catalyzing hydroxylation of risperidone to 9-hydroxyrisperidone is cytochrome $P450IID_6$, which is subject to genetic polymorphism (about 6% to 8% of caucasians, and a very low percent of Asians, have little or no activity and are "poor metabolizers") and to inhibition by a variety of substrates and some non-substrates, notably quinidine. Extensive metabolizers convert risperidone rapidly into 9-hydroxyrisperidone, while poor metabolizers convert it much more slowly. Extensive metabolizers, therefore, have lower risperidone and higher 9-hydroxyrisperidone concentrations than poor metabolizers. Following oral administration, mean peak plasma concentrations occurred at about 1 hour. Peak 9-hydroxyrisperidone occurred at about 3 and 17 hours (extensive and poor metabolizers, respectively.) The apparent half-life of risperidone and 9-hydroxyrisperidone was 3 and 21 hours in extensive metabolizers and 20 and 30 hours in poor metabolizers, respectively. Steady-state concentrations of risperidone are reached in 1 day in extensive metabolizers and would be expected to reach steady state in about 5 days in poor metabolizers. Steady-state concentrations of 9-hydroxyrisperidone are reached in 5 to 6 days (extensive metabolizers). The pharmacokinetics of the sum of risperidone and 9-hydroxyrisperidone, after single and multiple doses, were similar in extensive and poor metabolizers, with an overall mean elimination half-life of about 20 hours.

The plasma protein binding of risperidone and 9-hydroxyrisperidone was about 90% and 77%, respectively. High therapeutic concentrations of sulfamethazine, warfarin and carbamazepine caused only a slight increase in the free fraction of risperidone and 9-hydroxyrisperidone, changes of unknown clinical significance.

Renal impairment – In patients with moderate to severe renal disease, clearance of the sum of risperidone and its active metabolite decreased by 60% compared to young healthy subjects. Reduce doses in patients with renal disease (see Administration and Dosage).

Hepatic impairment – While the pharmacokinetics of risperidone in subjects with liver disease were comparable to those in young healthy subjects, the mean free fraction of risperidone in plasma was increased by about 35% because of the diminished concentration of both albumin and α_1-acid glycoprotein. Reduce doses in patients with liver disease (see Administration and Dosage).

Elderly – In healthy elderly subjects, renal clearance of both risperidone and 9-hydroxyrisperidone was decreased, and elimination half-lives were prolonged compared to young healthy subjects. Modify dosing accordingly in elderly patients (see Administration and Dosage).

Indications:

Management of the manifestations of psychotic disorders.

Contraindications:

Hypersensitivity to risperidone.

Warnings:

Long-term use: The effectiveness of risperidone in long-term use (eg, > 6 to 8 weeks) has not been systematically evaluated. Therefore, periodically re-evaluate the long-term usefulness of the drug for the individual patient.

Benzisoxazole

RISPERIDONE

Neuroleptic malignant syndrome (NMS): A potentially fatal symptom complex sometimes referred to as NMS has occurred with antipsychotic drugs. Clinical manifestations of NMS are hyperpyrexia, muscle rigidity, altered mental status and evidence of autonomic instability (eg, irregular pulse or blood pressure, tachycardia, diaphoresis, cardiac dysrhythmia). Additional signs may include elevated creatinine phosphokinase, myoglobinuria (rhabdomyolysis) and acute renal failure.

The management of NMS should include: 1) Immediate discontinuation of antipsychotic drugs and other drugs not essential to concurrent therapy; 2) intensive symptomatic treatment and medical monitoring; and 3) treatment of any concomitant serious medical problems for which specific treatments are available. There is no general agreement about specific pharmacological treatment regimens for uncomplicated NMS. If a patient requires antipsychotic drug treatment after recovery from NMS, carefully consider the potential reintroduction of drug therapy. Carefully monitor the patient since recurrences of NMS have been reported.

Tardive dyskinesia: A syndrome of potentially irreversible, involuntary, dyskinetic movements may develop in patients treated with antipsychotic drugs. Although the prevalence of the syndrome appears to be highest among the elderly, especially elderly women, it is impossible to predict which patients are likely to develop the syndrome. Whether antipsychotic drug products differ in their potential to cause tardive dyskinesia is unknown. The risk of developing tardive dyskinesia and the likelihood that it will become irreversible are believed to increase as the duration of treatment and the total cumulative dose of antipsychotic drugs administered to the patient increase. However, the syndrome can develop after relatively brief treatment periods at low doses.

There is no known treatment for established cases of tardive dyskinesia, although the syndrome may remit, partially or completely, if treatment is withdrawn. Antipsychotic treatment, itself, however, may suppress (or partially suppress) the signs and symptoms of the syndrome and thereby may possibly mask the underlying process. The effect that symptomatic suppression has upon the long-term course of the syndrome is unknown.

Prescribe risperidone in a manner that is most likely to minimize the occurrence of tardive dyskinesia. Generally reserve chronic treatment for patients who suffer from a chronic illness that (1) is known to respond to antipsychotic drugs, and (2) for whom alternative, equally effective, but potentially less harmful treatments are not available or appropriate. In patients who do require chronic treatment, seek the smallest dose and the shortest duration of treatment producing a satisfactory clinical response. Periodically reassess the need for continued treatment. If signs and symptoms of tardive dyskinesia appear, consider drug discontinuation. However, some patients may require treatment with risperidone despite the presence of the syndrome.

Cardiac effects:

Proarrhythmic effects – Risperidone or 9-hydroxyrisperidone appear to lengthen the QT interval in some patients, even at 12 to 16 mg/day, well above the recommended dose. Other drugs that prolong the QT interval have been associated with the occurrence of torsade de pointes, a life-threatening arrhythmia. Bradycardia, electrolyte imbalance, concomitant use with other drugs that prolong QT or the presence of congenital prolongation in QT can increase the risk.

Orthostatic hypotension – Risperidone may induce orthostatic hypotension associated with dizziness, tachycardia, and in some patients, syncope, especially during the initial dose-titration period, probably reflecting its alpha-adrenergic antagonistic properties. Syncope was reported in 0.2%. Risk may be minimized by limiting the initial dose to 1 mg twice daily in healthy adults and 0.5 mg twice daily in the elderly and patients with renal or hepatic impairment (see Administration and Dosage). Consider a dose reduction if hypotension occurs. Use with particular caution in patients with known cardiovascular disease (history of MI or ischemia, heart failure or conduction abnormalities), cerebrovascular disease and conditions which would predispose patients to hypotension (eg, dehydration, hypovolemia, treatment with antihypertensives).

Cardiac patients – Eight of ≈ 380 patients taking risperidone whose baseline QT_c interval was < 450 msec were observed to have QT_c intervals > 450 msec during treatment; no such prolongations were seen in the placebo group. There were three such episodes in the ≈ 125 patients who received haloperidol. Because of the risks of orthostatic hypotension and QT prolongation, observe caution in cardiac patients.

RISPERIDONE

Renal/Hepatic function impairment: Increased plasma concentrations of risperidone and 9-hydroxyrisperidone occur in patients with severe renal impairment (creatinine clearance < 30 ml/min/1.73 m^2), and an increase in the free fraction of risperidone is seen in patients with severe hepatic impairment. Use a lower starting dose in such patients (see Administration and Dosage).

Carcinogenesis/Fertility impairment: Risperidone was administered to mice and rats at doses of 0.63, 2.5 and 10 mg/kg for 18 or 25 months (equivalent to 2.4, 9.4 and 37.5 times the maximum human dose [16 mg/day] on a mg/kg basis). There were statistically significant increases in pituitary gland adenomas, endocrine pancreas adenomas and mammary gland adenocarcinomas. Risperidone elevated serum prolactin levels five- to sixfold. An increase in mammary, pituitary, and endocrine pancreas neoplasms has been found in rodents after chronic administration of other antipsychotic drugs and is considered to be prolactin mediated. The relevance for human risk of the findings of prolactin-mediated endocrine tumors in rodents is unknown (see Hyperprolactinemia).

Risperidone (0.16 to 5 mg/kg) impaired mating, but not fertility, in rats at doses of 0.1 to 3 times the maximum recommended human dose on a mg/m^2 basis. The effect appeared to be in females. In a study in dogs, sperm motility and concentration were decreased at doses of 0.6 to 10 times the human dose on a mg/m^2 basis. Dose-related decreases were also noted in serum testosterone. Serum testosterone and sperm parameters partially recovered but remained decreased after treatment was discontinued.

Elderly: In general, a lower starting dose is recommended for an elderly patient, reflecting a decreased pharmacokinetic clearance as well as a greater frequency of decreased hepatic, renal or cardiac function, and a greater tendency to postural hypotension (see Administration and Dosage).

Pregnancy: Category C. In rats there was an increase in pup deaths during the first 4 days of lactation at doses of 0.1 to 3 times the human dose on a mg/m^2 basis, and an increase in stillborn rat pups at a dose 1.5 times higher than the human dose. Placental transfer of risperidone occurs in rat pups. There are no adequate and well controlled studies in pregnant women. However, there was one report of a case of agenesis of the corpus callosum in an infant exposed to risperidone in utero. Use during pregnancy only if the potential benefit justifies the potential risk to the fetus.

Lactation: It is not known whether risperidone is excreted in breast milk. In animal studies, risperidone and 9-hydroxyrisperidone were excreted in breast milk. Therefore, women receiving risperidone should not breastfeed.

Children: Safety and efficacy in children have not been established.

Precautions:

Monitoring: No specific laboratory tests are recommended.

Seizures occurred in 0.3% of patients, two in association with hyponatremia. Use cautiously in patients with a history of seizures.

Hyperprolactinemia: As with other drugs that antagonize dopamine D_2 receptors, risperidone elevates prolactin levels and the elevation persists during chronic administration. Approximately 33% of human breast cancers are prolactin-dependent in vitro, a factor of potential importance if use of these drugs is contemplated in a patient with previously detected breast cancer. Although disturbances such as galactorrhea, amenorrhea, gynecomastia and impotence have occurred with prolactin-elevating compounds, the clinical significance of elevated serum prolactin levels is unknown for most patients. As is common with compounds which increase prolactin release, an increase in pituitary gland, mammary gland and pancreatic islet cell hyperplasia or neoplasia was observed in the carcinogenicity studies conducted in mice and rats (see Warnings).

Cognitive/Motor impairment: Somnolence was a commonly reported adverse event. This reaction is dose-related; 41% of the high-dose patients (16 mg/day) reported somnolence vs 16% with placebo. Since risperidone has the potential to impair judgment, thinking or motor skills, caution patients about operating hazardous machinery, including automobiles, until they are reasonably certain that risperidone therapy does not affect them adversely.

Priapism: A single case of priapism was reported in a 50-year-old patient receiving risperidone. This event occurred after 11 months of treatment with risperidone alone, and required surgical intervention. Other drugs with alpha-adrenergic blocking effects have been reported to induce priapism, and it is possible that risperidone may share this capacity.

Benzisoxazole

RISPERIDONE

Thrombotic thrombocytopenic purpura (TTP): A single case of TTP was reported in a 28 year-old female patient receiving risperidone. She experienced jaundice, fever and bruising, but eventually recovered after receiving plasmapheresis.

Antiemetic effect: Risperidone has an antiemetic effect in animals which may also occur in humans, and may mask signs and symptoms of overdosage with certain drugs or of conditions such as intestinal obstruction, Reye's syndrome and brain tumor.

Body temperature regulation: Disruption of body temperature regulation has been attributed to other antipsychotic agents. Caution is advised when prescribing for patients who will be exposed to extreme heat.

Suicide: The possibility of a suicide attempt is inherent in schizophrenia, and close supervision of high-risk patients should accompany drug therapy. Write prescription for the smallest quantity of tablets consistent with good patient management, in order to reduce the risk of overdose.

Drug abuse and dependence: Evaluate patients for a history of drug abuse, and observe such patients closely for signs of risperidone misuse or abuse (eg, development of tolerance, increases in dose, drug-seeking behavior).

Photosensitivity: Photosensitization may occur; therefore, caution patients to take protective measures (ie, sunscreens, protective clothing) against exposure to ultraviolet light or sunlight until tolerance is determined.

Drug Interactions:

Drug interactions that reduce the metabolism of risperidone to 9-hydroxyrisperidone may increase risperidone plasma concentrations and lower the concentrations of 9-hydroxyrisperidone. Risperidone is metabolized by cytochrome P–450IID$_6$, an enzyme that can be inhibited by a variety of other drugs. In vitro, drugs metabolized by other P–450 isozymes are only weak inhibitors of risperidone metabolism.

Risperidone Drug Interactions

Precipitant drug	Object drug*		Description
Risperidone	Levodopa	⬇	Risperidone may antagonize the effects of levodopa and dopamine agonists.
Carbamazepine	Risperidone	⬇	Chronic administration of carbamazepine with risperidone may increase the clearance of risperidone.
Clozapine	Risperidone	⬆	Chronic administration of clozapine with risperidone may decrease the clearance of risperidone.

* ⬆ = Object drug increased. ⬇ = Object drug decreased.

Adverse Reactions:

Approximately 9% percent of patients discontinued treatment due to an adverse event vs 7% on placebo and 10% on active control drugs. The more common events (≥ 0.3%) associated with discontinuation included: Extrapyramidal symptoms; dizziness; hyperkinesia; somnolence; nausea. Suicide attempt was associated with discontinuation in 1.2% of risperidone-treated patients compared to 0.6% with placebo, but given the almost 40-fold greater exposure time in risperidone compared to placebo, it is unlikely that suicide attempt is a risperidone-related adverse event (see Precautions).

Risperidone Adverse Reactions (%)

Adverse Reaction	Risperidone ≤ 10 mg/day (n = 324)	Risperidone 16 mg/day (n = 77)	Placebo (n =142)
Psychiatric			
Insomnia	26	23	19
Agitation	22	26	20
Anxiety	12	20	9
Somnolence	3	8	1
Aggressive reaction	1	3	1
CNS			
Extrapyramidal symptoms[1]	17	34	16
Headache	14	12	12
Dizziness	4	7	1

Benzisoxazole

RISPERIDONE

Risperidone Adverse Reactions (%)

	Risperidone		
Adverse Reaction	≤ 10 mg/day (n = 324)	16 mg/day (n = 77)	Placebo (n = 142)
GI			
Constipation	7	13	3
Nausea	6	4	3
Dyspepsia	5	10	4
Vomiting	5	7	4
Abdominal pain	4	1	0
Saliva increased	2	0	1
Toothache	2	0	0
Respiratory			
Rhinitis	10	8	4
Coughing	3	3	1
Upper respiratory infection	3	3	1
Sinusitis	2	1	1
Pharyngitis	2	3	0
Dyspnea	1	0	0
Body as a whole			
Tachycardia	3	5	0
Arthralgia	2	3	0
Back pain	2	0	1
Chest pain	2	3	1
Fever	2	3	0
Abnormal vision	2	1	1
Dermatologic			
Rash	2	5	1
Dry skin	2	4	0
Seborrhea	1	0	0

[1] Includes tremor, dystonia, hypokinesia, hypertonia, hyperkinesia, oculogyric crisis, ataxia, abnormal gait, involuntary muscle contractions, hyporeflexia and extrapyramidal disorders.

Other adverse reactions observed during the premarketing evaluation of risperidone included the following:

Body as a whole – Fatigue (1%); edema, rigors, malaise, influenza-like symptoms (0.1% to 1%); pallor, enlarged abdomen, allergic reaction, ascites, sarcoidosis, flushing (< 0.1%).

Psychiatric – Increased dream activity, diminished sexual desire, nervousness (1%); impaired concentration, depression, apathy, catatonic reaction, euphoria, increased libido, amnesia (0.1% to 1%); emotional lability, nightmares, delirium, withdrawal syndrome, yawning (< 0.1%).

CNS – Increased sleep duration (1%); dysarthria, vertigo, stupor, paraesthesia, confusion (0.1% to 1%); aphasia, cholinergic syndrome, hypoesthesia, tongue paralysis, leg cramps, torticollis, hypotonia, coma, migraine, hyperreflexia, choreoathetosis (< 0.1%).

GI – Anorexia, reduced salivation (1%); flatulence, diarrhea, increased appetite, stomatitis, melena, dysphagia, hemorrhoids, gastritis (0.1% to 1%); fecal incontinence, eructation, gastroesophageal reflux, gastroenteritis, esophagitis, tongue discoloration, cholelithiasis, tongue edema, diverticulitis, gingivitis, discolored feces, GI hemorrhage, hematemesis (< 0.1%).

Respiratory – Hyperventilation, bronchospasm, pneumonia, stridor (0.1% to 1%); asthma, increased sputum, aspiration (< 0.1%).

Dermatologic – Photosensitivity (see Precautions), increased pigmentation (1%); increased/decreased sweating, acne, alopecia, hyperkeratosis, pruritus, skin exfoliation (0.1% to 1%); bullous eruption, skin ulceration, aggravated psoriasis, furunculosis, verruca, dermatitis lichenoid, hypertrichosis, genital pruritus, urticaria (< 0.1%).

Cardiovascular – Palpitation, hypertension, hypotension, AV block, MI (0.1% to 1%); ventricular tachycardia, angina pectoris, premature atrial contractions, T-wave inversions, ventricular extrasystoles, ST depression, myocarditis (< 0.1%).

RISPERIDONE

Ophthalmic – Abnormal accommodation, xerophthalmia (0.1% to 1%); diplopia, eye pain, blepharitis, photopsia, photophobia, abnormal lacrimation (< 0.1%).

Metabolic/Nutritional – Hyponatremia, weight increase, creatine phosphokinase increase, thirst, weight decrease, diabetes mellitis (0.1% to 1%); decreased serum iron, cachexia, dehydration, hypokalemia, hypoproteinemia, hypertriglyceridemia, hyperuricemia, hypoglycemia (< 0.1%).

Renal – Polyuria/polydipsia (1%); urinary incontinence, hematuria, dysuria (0.1% to 1%); urinary retention, cystitis, renal insufficiency (< 0.1%).

Musculoskeletal – Myalgia (0.1% to 1%); arthrosis, synostosis, bursitis, arthritis, skeletal pain (< 0.1%).

GU – Menorrhagia, orgastic dysfunction, dry vagina, erectile dysfunction (1%); nonpuerperal lactation, amenorrhea, female breast pain, leukorrhea, mastitis, dysmenorrhea, female perineal pain, intermenstrual bleeding, vaginal hemorrhage, ejaculation failure (0.1% to 1%).

Hepatic – Increased AST and ALT (0.1% to 1%); hepatic failure, cholestatic hepatitis, cholecystitis, cholethiasis, hepatitis, hepatocellular damage (< 0.1%).

Hematologic – Epistaxis, purpura, anemia, hypochromic anemia (0.1% to 1%); hemorrhage, superficial phlebitis, thrombophlebitis, thrombocytopenia, normocytic anemia, leukocytosis, lymphadenopathy, leukopenia, Pelger-Huet anomaly (< 0.1%).

Special Senses – Tinnitus, hyperacusis, decreased hearing, bitter taste (< 0.1%).

Endocrine – Gynecomastia, male breast pain, antidiuretic hormone disorder (< 0.1%).

Miscellaneous –

Vital sign changes: Risperidone is associated with orthostatic hypotension and tachycardia (see Precautions).

Weight changes: There was a statistically greater incidence of weight gain for risperidone (18%) compared to placebo (9%).

Laboratory changes: Risperidone administration was associated with increases in serum prolactin (see Precautions).

ECG changes: Risperidone may be associated with ECG changes (see Warnings).

Overdosage:

Symptoms: In eight reports, with estimated doses ranging from 20 to 300 mg, no fatalities occurred. In general, reported signs and symptoms were those resulting from an exaggeration of the drug's known pharmacological effects (eg, drowsiness, sedation, tachycardia, hypotension, extrapyramidal symptoms). One case (240 mg) was associated with hyponatremia, hypokalemia, prolonged QT and widened QRS. Another case (36 mg) was associated with a seizure.

Treatment: In case of acute overdosage, establish and maintain an airway and ensure adequate oxygenation and ventilation. Consider gastric lavage and administration of activated charcoal together with a laxative. Commence cardiovascular monitoring immediately, including continuous ECG monitoring to detect possible arrhythmias. If antiarrhythmic therapy is administered, disopyramide, procainamide and quinidine carry a theoretical hazard of QT-prolonging effects that might be additive to those of risperidone. Similarly, it is reasonable to expect that the alpha-blocking properties of bretylium might be additive to those of risperidone, resulting in problematic hypotension.

There is no specific antidote to risperidone. Therefore, institute appropriate supportive measures. Treat hypotension and circulatory collapse with appropriate measures such as IV fluids or sympathomimetic agents (epinephrine and dopamine should not be used, since beta stimulation may worsen hypotension in the setting of risperidone-induced alpha blockade). In cases of severe extrapyramidal symptoms, administer anticholinergic medication.

Patient Information:

Advise patients of the risk of orthostatic hypotension, especially during the period of initial dose titration.

Since risperidone has the potential to impair judgment, thinking or motor skills, caution patients about operating hazardous machinery, including automobiles. Advise patients to avoid alcohol while taking risperidone.

Advise patients to notify their physician if they become pregnant or intend to become pregnant during therapy, and not to breastfeed if they are taking risperidone.

Benzisoxazole

RISPERIDONE

Advise patients to inform their physician if they are taking, or plan to take, any prescription or over-the-counter drugs, since there is a potential for drug interactions.

Photosensitivity may occur. Avoid exposure to ultraviolet light or sunlight. Use sunscreen and protective clothing until tolerance is determined.

Administration and Dosage:

Approved by the FDA on December 29, 1993.

Usual initial dose: Administer on a twice-daily schedule, generally beginning with 1 mg twice daily, with increases in increments of 1 mg twice daily on the second and third day, as tolerated, to a target dose of 3 mg twice daily by the third day. Further dosage adjustments, if indicated, should generally occur at intervals of ≥ 1 week, since steady state for the active metabolite would not be achieved for ≈ 1 week in the typical patient. When dosage adjustments are necessary, small dose increments/decrements of 1 mg twice daily are recommended.

Antipsychotic efficacy was demonstrated in a dose range of 4 to 16 mg/day; however, maximal effect was generally seen in a range of 4 to 6 mg/day. Doses > 6 mg/day were not demonstrated to be more efficacious than lower doses, were associated with more extrapyramidal symptoms and other adverse effects, and are not generally recommended. Safety of doses > 16 mg/day has not been evaluated.

Special populations: The recommended initial dose is 0.5 mg twice daily in patients who are elderly or debilitated, patients with severe renal or hepatic impairment, and patients either predisposed to hypotension or for whom hypotension would pose a risk. Use dosage increases in these patients in increments of 0.5 mg twice daily. Dosage increases above 1.5 mg twice daily should generally occur at intervals of ≥ 1 week. Elderly or debilitated patients, and patients with renal impairment, may have less ability to eliminate risperidone than other adults. Patients with impaired hepatic function may have increases in the free fraction of risperidone, possibly resulting in an enhanced effect.

Maintenance therapy: It is recommended that responding patients be continued on risperidone, but at the lowest dose needed to maintain remission. Periodically reassess patients to determine the need for maintenance treatment.

Reinitiation of treatment: When restarting patients who have had an interval off risperidone, follow the initial 3-day dose titration schedule.

Switching from other antipsychotics: When switching from other antipsychotics to risperidone, immediate discontinuation of the previous antipsychotic treatment upon initiation of risperidone therapy is recommended when medically appropriate. In all cases, minimize the period of overlapping antipsychotic administration. When switching patients from depot antipsychotic, initiate risperidone therapy in place of the next scheduled injection. Periodically reevaluate the need for continuing existing EPS medications.

Rx	**Risperdal** (Janssen)	**Tablets:** 1 mg	(Janssen R 1). White. In 60s and blister pack 100s.
		2 mg	(Janssen R 2). Orange. In 60s and blister pack 100s.
		3 mg	(Janssen R 3). Yellow. In 60s and blister pack 100s.
		4 mg	(Janssen R 4). Green. In 60s and blister pack 100s.
Rx	**Risperdal** (Janssen)	**Oral solution:** 1 mg/ml	Mix with 3-4 oz of water, coffee, orange juice or lowfat milk. Not compatible with cola or tea. In 100 ml w/calibrated pipette.

Diphenylbutylpiperidine

PIMOZIDE

Actions:

Pharmacology: Pimozide is a neuroleptic which blocks CNS dopaminergic receptors. It has no effect on norepinephrine receptors. Its ability to suppress motor and phonic tics in Tourette's Disorder is thought to be a function of its dopaminergic blocking activity.

Pharmacokinetics: More than 50% of a dose of pimozide is absorbed after oral administration. Peak serum levels occur 6 to 8 hours (range 4 to 12 hours) after dosing. There are few correlations between plasma levels and clinical findings. Pimozide is extensively metabolized in the liver; mean elimination half-life in schizophrenic patients is approximately 55 hours. Two major metabolites with undetermined neuroleptic activity have been identified. The major route of elimination is via the kidney; 38% to 45% of the dose is recovered in the urine, mostly as metabolites.

Indications:

For the suppression of severely compromising motor and phonic tics in patients with Tourette's Disorder who have failed to respond satisfactorily to standard treatment.

Contraindications:

Treatment of simple tics or tics other than those associated with Tourette's Disorder.

Drug-induced motor and phonic tics (eg, pemoline, methylphenidate, amphetamines) until it is determined whether the tics are caused by drugs or Tourette's Disorder.

Patients with congenital long QT syndrome or history of cardiac arrhythmias.

Administration with other drugs that prolong the QT interval.

Severe toxic CNS depression or comatose states from any cause.

Hypersensitivity to pimozide. It is not known whether cross-sensitivity exists among anti-psychotics. Use pimozide with caution in patients hypersensitive to other anti-psychotics.

Warnings:

Persistent tardive dyskinesia may appear on long-term therapy or after drug therapy has been discontinued. The risk appears to be greater in elderly patients on high-dose therapy, especially females. The symptoms are persistent, and in some patients appear irreversible. The risk of developing tardive dyskinesia and the likelihood that it will become irreversible are believed to increase as treatment duration and total cumulative dose increase. However, the syndrome can develop after relatively brief treatment periods at low doses. The syndrome is characterized by rhythmical involuntary movements of tongue, face, mouth or jaw (eg, protrusion of tongue, puffing of cheeks, puckering of mouth, chewing movements), sometimes accompanied by involuntary movements of extremities. Fine vermicular movement of the tongue may be an early sign of the syndrome; if the medication is stopped at this time, the syndrome may not develop. There is no known treatment for established cases of tardive dyskinesia, although the syndrome may remit, partially or completely, if antipsychotics are withdrawn. However, antipsychotic drugs may suppress (or partially suppress) signs and symptoms of the syndrome, possibly masking the underlying process. The effect of symptomatic suppression on the long-term course of the syndrome is unknown.

Given these considerations, administer antipsychotics with caution to minimize occurrence of tardive dyskinesia. Reserve chronic antipsychotic treatment for patients who suffer from a chronic illness that is known to respond to antipsychotic drugs, and for whom alternative, equieffective, but potentially less harmful treatments are not available or appropriate. In patients requiring chronic treatment, use the smallest dose and the shortest duration of treatment producing a satisfactory clinical response.

Prolongation of QT interval: Sudden death has occurred in conditions other than Tourette's Disorder in patients receiving dosages of ≈ 1 mg/kg. Sudden, unexpected deaths and grand mal seizure have occurred at doses above 20 mg/day. One possible mechanism is prolongation of the QT interval predisposing patients to ventricular arrhythmias. Perform an ECG before treatment is initiated and periodically thereafter, especially during dose adjustment. If the QT interval is prolonged beyond a limit of 0.47 seconds (children) or 0.52 seconds (adults), or more than 25% above the patient's original baseline, stop further dose increase and consider a lower dose.

Tumorigenicity: Pimozide may be tumorigenic. In mice, pimozide produced a dose-related increase in pituitary and mammary tumors. The significance is not known. Consider this effect, especially in young patients and when chronic use is anticipated.

Diphenylbutylpiperidine

PIMOZIDE

Neuroleptic malignant syndrome (NMS) is a potentially fatal symptom complex that has been associated with antipsychotic drugs. Clinical manifestations are hyperpyrexia, muscle rigidity, altered mental status (including catatonic signs) and evidence of autonomic instability (irregular pulse or blood pressure, tachycardia, diaphoresis, cardiac dysrhythmias). Additional signs may include elevated creatinine phosphokinase, myoglobinuria (rhabdomyolysis) and acute renal failure.

Management should include immediate discontinuation of antipsychotic drugs and other drugs not essential to concurrent therapy, intensive symptomatic treatment and medical monitoring, and treatment of any concomitant serious medical problems for which specific treatments are available. There is no general agreement about treatment regimens for uncomplicated NMS.

If a patient requires antipsychotic drug treatment after recovery from NMS, carefully consider the potential reintroduction of drug therapy. Monitor the patient carefully, since recurrences of NMS have been reported.

Pregnancy: Category C. Studies in rats and rabbits in doses up to 8 times the maximum human dose did not reveal evidence of teratogenicity. In rats, this dose resulted in decreased pregnancies and in retarded fetal development. In rabbits, maternal toxicity, mortality, decreased weight gain and embryotoxicity were dose-related. Administer pimozide to a pregnant woman only if the potential benefits clearly outweigh the potential risks.

Lactation: It is not known whether pimozide is excreted in breast milk. Because of the potential for tumorigenicity and unknown cardiovascular effects in the infant, decide whether to discontinue nursing or to discontinue the drug, taking into account the importance of the drug to the mother.

Children: Although Tourette's Disorder often has its onset between the ages of 2 and 15 years, the use of pimozide in patients less than 12 years is limited. Pimozide is not recommended for any childhood condition other than Tourette's Disorder.

Precautions:

Hypokalemia has been associated with ventricular arrhythmias. Correct potassium insufficiency secondary to diuretics, diarrhea or any other cause before initiating therapy; maintain normal potassium during therapy.

Anticholinergic side effects are produced by pimozide; use with caution in individuals whose conditions may be aggravated by anticholinergic activity.

Hepatic or renal function impairment: Use with caution since pimozide is metabolized by the liver and excreted by the kidney.

Hazardous tasks: May produce drowsiness or blurred vision; patients should observe caution while driving or performing other tasks requiring alertness.

Drug Interactions:

Anticonvulsants: Administer pimozide with caution to patients receiving these drugs; pimozide may lower the convulsive threshold.

Phenothiazines, tricyclic antidepressants or antiarrhythmic agents: Avoid concomitant administration. Pimozide prolongs the QT interval; anticipate an additive effect on QT interval if administered with other drugs that prolong the QT interval.

CNS depressants, including **analgesics, sedatives, anxiolytics** and **alcohol:** Pimozide may be capable of potentiating the effects of these drugs.

Adverse Reactions:

Extrapyramidal reactions have been reported frequently, often during the first few days of treatment, involving Parkinson-like symptoms which were usually mild to moderately severe and, in most cases, reversible. Other types of neuromuscular reactions (motor restlessness, dystonia, akathisia, hyperreflexia, opisthotonos, oculogyric crises) have been reported far less frequently. Generally, the occurrence and severity are dose-related since they occur at relatively high doses and disappear or become less severe when the dose is reduced. Administration of antiparkinson drugs may be required. Persistent extrapyramidal reactions may require the drug to be discontinued.

Withdrawal emergent neurological signs: Some patients on maintenance treatment experience transient dyskinetic signs after abrupt withdrawal. This may be indistinguishable from the syndrome of persistent tardive dyskinesia except for duration. It is not known whether gradual withdrawal of neuroleptic drugs will reduce the rate of occurrence, but it seems reasonable to gradually withdraw use of pimozide.

Persistent tardive dyskinesia may be associated with pimozide (See Warnings).

Neuroleptic malignant syndrome has occurred. (See Warnings).

Diphenylbutylpiperidine

PIMOZIDE

ECG changes: Prolongation of the QT interval; flattening, notching and inversion of the T-wave; appearance of U-waves. Sudden, unexpected deaths and grand mal seizure have occurred at doses > 20 mg/day. (See Warnings).

Special senses: Visual disturbance; taste change; sensitivity of eyes to light; decreased accommodation; blurred vision; spots before eyes; cataracts.

GU: Impotence; nocturia; urinary frequency.

Cardiovascular/respiratory: Postural hypotension; hypotension; hypertension; tachycardia; palpitations; chest pain.

Hyperpyrexia has been reported with other neuroleptic drugs.

GI: Dry mouth; diarrhea; constipation; thirst; appetite increase; belching; increased salivation; nausea; vomiting; anorexia; GI distress.

Musculoskeletal: Muscle tightness; muscle cramps; asthenia; stooped posture.

CNS: Headache; drowsiness; sedation; insomnia; rigidity; speech disorder; handwriting change; akinesia; dizziness; tremor; fainting; dyskinesia; akathesia. Depression; excitement; nervousness; adverse behavior effect; parkinsonism.

Dermatologic: Rash; sweating; skin irritation.

Miscellaneous: Weight gain; weight loss; periorbital edema; loss of libido; menstrual disorder; breast secretions.

Overdosage:

Symptoms: ECG abnormalities; severe extrapyramidal reactions; hypotension; coma with respiratory depression.

Treatment: Perform gastric lavage, establish a patent airway and, if necessary, institute mechanically-assisted respiration. Continue ECG monitoring until the parameters are within the normal range. Treat hypotension and circulatory collapse with IV fluids, plasma or concentrated albumin, and vasopressor agents such as norepinephrine. Do not use epinephrine. In case of severe extrapyramidal reactions, administer antiparkinson medication. Observe patients for at least 4 days.

Patient Information:

May cause drowsiness; use caution while driving or performing other tasks requiring alertness.

Inform patient of the risks of developing tardive dyskinesia with chronic use.

Do not exceed prescribed dose. Sudden, unexpected deaths have occurred in patients taking high doses of pimozide for conditions other than Tourette's Disorder.

Administration and Dosage:

Introduce the drug slowly and gradually. Perform ECG at baseline and periodically thereafter, especially during dosage adjustment.

Initial dose: 1 to 2 mg/day in divided doses. Thereafter, increase dose every other day.

Maintenance dose: < 0.2 mg/kg/day or 10 mg/day, whichever is less. Do not exceed 0.2 mg/kg/day or 10 mg/day.

Gradual withdrawal: Periodically attempt to reduce dosage to see if tics persist. Increases of tic intensity and frequency may represent a transient, withdrawal-related phenomenon rather than a return of symptoms. Allow 1 or 2 weeks to elapse before concluding that an increase in tic manifestations is due to the underlying disease rather than drug withdrawal.

Rx	**Orap** (Lemmon)	**Tablets:** 2 mg	(Lemmon Orap 2). White, scored. In 100s.

Antimanic Agent

LITHIUM

> **Warning:**
> Toxicity is closely related to serum lithium levels and can occur at therapeutic doses. Facilities for serum lithium determinations are required to monitor therapy.

Actions:

Pharmacology: Lithium alters sodium transport in nerve and muscle cells, and effects a shift toward intraneuronal catecholamine metabolism. The specific mechanism in mania is unknown, but it affects neurotransmitters associated with affective disorders (norepinephrine and serotonin). Its antimanic effects may be the result of increases in norepinephrine reuptake and increased serotonin receptor sensitivity.

Lithium also affects distribution of sodium, calcium and magnesium ions. The contribution of these effects to its antimanic qualities is uncertain.

Pharmacokinetics:

Absorption/Distribution – Lithium is readily absorbed from the GI tract. Absorption is not significantly impaired by food. Peak serum levels occur in 1 to 4 hours and absorption is complete within 8 hours. Slow-release preparations have a slower and more variable absorption rate. Onset of action is slow (5 to 14 days); therefore, there is no advantage to parenteral use. Until the desired therapeutic effect is attained, maintain a steady-state serum level of 0.8 to 1.4 mEq/L, then slowly decrease the lithium dose to a maintenance level. The therapeutic serum level range is from 0.4 to 1 mEq/L. Dose-related adverse effects are not usually serious at serum levels maintained < 1.5 mEq/L. Significant adverse reactions and toxicity occur at serum levels > 2 mEq/L.

Distribution approximates total body water. Lithium is not protein bound. Although distribution across the blood-brain barrier is slow, the cerebrospinal fluid lithium level is about 40% of the plasma concentration.

Excretion – About 95% of the lithium dose is eliminated by the kidney. Renal clearance is 20% of creatinine clearance (15 to 30ml/min). It varies with the age and renal status of the patient. In the elderly, and in patients with renal impairment, clearance will be low; in younger patients, it will be higher. The average elimination half-life is 24 hours (range, 17 to 36 hours); steady state is reached in 5 to 7 days.

In the kidneys, 80% of lithium is reabsorbed. Lithium and sodium compete for reabsorption in the proximal renal tubule. During periods of sodium depletion (eg, dehydration, diuretic use), the kidney will try to conserve sodium and lithium by reabsorbing > 80% from the proximal tubule. The increased reabsorption causes the lithium serum level to rise, possibly leading to toxicity. Sodium loading will cause increased lithium excretion and the serum levels will decrease.

Indications:

For the treatment of manic episodes of manic-depressive illness. Maintenance therapy prevents or diminishes the frequency and intensity of subsequent manic episodes in those manic-depressive patients with a history of mania.

Unlabeled uses: Lithium carbonate (300 to 1000 mg/day) has improved the neutrophil count in patients with cancer chemotherapy-induced neutropenia, in children with chronic neutropenia, and in AIDS patients receiving zidovudine.

Lithium has also been used successfully in the prophylaxis of cluster headache; premenstrual tension; bulimia; alcoholism (especially if patient has a concomitant affective disorder such as depression); syndrome of inappropriate secretion of ADH; tardive dyskinesia; hyperthyroidism; postpartum affective psychosis; corticosteroid-induced psychosis.

A topical lithium succinate preparation has been studied in the treatment of seborrheic dermatitis and genital herpes.

Warnings:

High-risk patients: The risk of lithium toxicity is very high in patients with significant renal or cardiovascular disease, severe debilitation, dehydration or sodium depletion, or in patients receiving diuretics. Undertake treatment with extreme caution. Daily serum lithium determinations are recommended until the serum level and the clinical condition of the patient are stabilized; hospitalization is necessary.

Encephalopathic syndrome (characterized by weakness, lethargy, fever, tremulousness, confusion, extrapyramidal symptoms, leukocytosis, elevated serum enzymes, BUN and FBS) has occurred in a few patients given lithium plus a neuroleptic. In some instances, irreversible brain damage occurred. Monitor closely for evidence of neurologic toxicity; discontinue treatment if such signs appear. This syndrome may be similar to or the same as neuroleptic malignant syndrome.

Antimanic Agent

LITHIUM

Renal function impairment: Morphologic changes with glomerular and interstitial fibrosis and nephron atrophy have occurred in patients on chronic lithium therapy (up to 10% to 20%) and in manic-depressive patients never exposed to lithium. The relationship between such changes and renal function has not been established.

Acquired nephrogenic diabetes insipidus unresponsive to vasopressin has been associated with chronic lithium administration. Polydipsia and polyuria occur frequently. The mechanism is thought to be the decreased response of the renal tubules to the antidiuretic hormone causing decreased reabsorption of water. Impairment of the concentrating ability of the kidneys is reversed when lithium therapy is discontinued. Management may involve decreasing the dose, discontinuing lithium, or the cautious use of a thiazide diuretic or amiloride. Monitor the patient's renal status.

Elderly: The decreased rate of excretion in the elderly contributes to a high incidence of toxic effects. Use lower doses and more frequent monitoring.

Pregnancy: Category D. Lithium crosses the placenta; serum concentration is equal in the mother and fetus. Lithium may cause fetal harm when given to a pregnant woman. Data from lithium birth registries suggest an increase in cardiac and other anomalies, especially Ebstein's anomaly. If the patient becomes pregnant while taking lithium, apprise her of the potential risk to the fetus.

Lithium toxicity in the newborn has included cyanosis, hypotonia, GI bleeding, cardiomegaly, bradycardia, thyroid depression, ECG abnormalities and diabetes insipidus. Most of these are self-limiting, resolving in 1 to 2 weeks, and corresponding to prolonged neonatal elimination of lithium and a half-life of 68 to 96 hours. Do not use in pregnancy, especially during the first trimester, unless the potential benefits outweigh potential hazards.

Lactation: Lithium is excreted in breast milk at about a 40% concentration of maternal serum. Milk and infant serum levels are approximately equal. Do not nurse during lithium therapy, except in unusual instances where the potential benefits to the mother outweigh possible hazards to the infant.

Children: Safety and efficacy for use in children < 12 years old have not been established. A report of a transient syndrome of acute dystonia and hyperreflexia was reported in a 15 kg child who ingested 300 mg lithium carbonate.

Precautions:

Concomitant infection with elevated temperature may necessitate a temporary reduction or cessation of medication.

Potentially hazardous tasks: Observe caution while driving or performing other tasks requiring alertness.

Tolerance of lithium is greater during the acute manic phase and decreases when manic symptoms subside.

Hypothyroidism may occur with long-term lithium administration (5% to 15%). Patients may develop enlargement of the thyroid gland and increased thyroid-stimulating hormone (TSH) levels (30%). Lithium-induced hypothyroidism may be treated with thyroid hormone replacement therapy. Hyperthyroidism occurs occasionally.

Sodium depletion: Lithium decreases renal sodium reabsorption, which could lead to sodium depletion (see Actions). Therefore, the patient must maintain a normal diet (including salt) and an adequate fluid intake (2500 to 3000 ml), at least during the initial stabilization period. Decreased tolerance to lithium may ensue from protracted sweating or diarrhea; if this occurs, administer supplemental fluid and salt.

Parameters to monitor: Perform the following laboratory tests prior to and periodically during lithium therapy: Serum creatinine; complete blood count (lithium may induce a benign leukocytosis, 10,000 to 18,000 WBC/mm^3); urinalysis; sodium and potassium; fasting glucose; electrocardiogram; and thyroid function tests. Check lithium serum levels twice weekly until dosage is stabilized. Once steady state has been reached, monitor the level weekly. Once the patient is on maintenance therapy, the level may be checked every 2 to 3 months. Monitor the elderly on maintenance therapy more frequently. Direct physical exams and history toward detection of cardiovascular, renal or organic brain disease.

Tartrazine sensitivity: Some of these products contain tartrazine, which may cause allergic-type reactions (including bronchial asthma) in susceptible individuals. Although the incidence of tartrazine sensitivity in the general population is low, it is frequently seen in patients who also have aspirin hypersensitivity. Specific products containing tartrazine are identified in the product listings.

Antimanic Agent

LITHIUM

Drug Interactions:

Lithium Drug Interactions			
Precipitant Drug	Object Drug*		Description
Acetazolamide	Lithium	↓	Increased renal excretion of lithium
Carbamazepine	Lithium	↑	Increased neurotoxic effects despite therapeutic serum levels and normal dosage range
Fluoxetine	Lithium	↑	Increased lithium serum levels; mechanism unknown
Haloperidol	Lithium	↑	Increased neurotoxic effects despite therapeutic serum levels and normal dosage range
Loop diuretics	Lithium	↑	Increased lithium serum levels; mechanism unknown
Methyldopa	Lithium	↑	Increased neurotoxic effects with or without increased lithium serum levels
NSAIDS	Lithium	↑	Decreased renal clearance of lithium possibly due to inhibition of renal prostaglandin synthesis
Osmotic diuretics (urea)	Lithium	↓	Increased renal excretion of lithium
Theophyllines	Lithium	↓	Increased renal excretion of lithium
Thiazide diuretics	Lithium	↑	Increased lithium serum levels due to decreased renal lithium clearance
Urinary alkalinizers	Lithium	↓	Enhanced renal lithium clearance
Verapamil	Lithium	↔	Both a reduction in lithium levels and lithium toxicity have occurred
Lithium	Iodide salts	↑	Synergistic action to more readily produce hypothyroidism
Lithium	Neuromuscular blocking agents	↑	Neuromuscular blocking effects may be increased; profound and severe respiratory depression may occur
Lithium	Phenothiazines	↔	Neurotoxicity, decreased phenothiazine concentrations or increased lithium concentrations may occur
Lithium	Sympathomimetics	↓	The pressor sensitivity of the sympathomimetic may be decreased.
Lithium	Tricyclic antidepressants	↑	Pharmacologic effects of the tricyclic may be increased

* ↑ = Object drug increased ↓ = Object drug decreased ↔ = Undetermined effect

Adverse Reactions:

Adverse reactions are seldom encountered at serum lithium levels < 1.5 mEq/L, except in the occasional patient sensitive to lithium. Mild to moderate toxic reactions may occur at levels from 1.5 to 2.5 mEq/L, and moderate to severe reactions may be seen at levels from 2 to 2.5 mEq/L, depending upon individual response. See Overdosage.

Fine hand tremor, polyuria and mild thirst may occur during initial therapy for the acute manic phase, and may persist throughout treatment. Transient and mild nausea and general discomfort may also appear during the first few days of administration. These side effects are an inconvenience rather than a disabling condition, and usually subside with continued treatment or a temporary reduction or cessation of dosage. If persistent, a cessation of dosage is indicated.

Reactions related to serum levels by organ system (see also Overdosage):

Cardiovascular – Arrhythmia; hypotension; peripheral circulatory collapse; bradycardia; sinus node dysfunction with severe bradycardia (which may result in syncope).

ECG changes: Reversible flattening, isoelectricity or inversion of T–waves.

Neuromuscular: Tremor; muscle hyperirritability (fasciculations, twitching, clonic movements); ataxia; choreo-athetotic movements; hyperactive deep tendon reflexes.

Neurological: Pseudotumor cerebri (increased intracranial pressure and papilledema) has been reported. If undetected, this condition may result in enlargement of the blind spot, constriction of visual fields and eventual blindness due to optic atrophy. Discontinue lithium, if clinically possible, if this syndrome occurs.

LITHIUM

Thyroid: Euthyroid goiter or hypothyroidism (including myxedema) accompanied by lower T_3 and T_4. Iodine 131 uptake may be elevated. (See Precautions.) Paradoxically, rare cases of hyperthyroidism have occurred.

EEG changes: Diffuse slowing; widening of frequency spectrum; potentiation; disorganization of background rhythm.

CNS – Blackout spells; epileptiform seizures; slurred speech; dizziness; vertigo; incontinence of urine or feces; somnolence; psychomotor retardation; restlessness; confusion; stupor; coma; acute dystonia; downbeat nystagmus; blurred vision; startled response; hypertonicity; slowed intellectual functioning; hallucinations; poor memory; tongue movements; tics; tinnitus; cog wheel rigidity.

GI – Anorexia; nausea; vomiting; diarrhea; dry mouth; gastritis; salivary gland swelling; abdominal pain; excessive salivation; flatulence; indigestion.

GU – Albuminuria; oliguria; polyuria; glycosuria; decreased creatinine clearance; symptoms of nephrogenic diabetes.

Dermatologic – Drying and thinning of hair; anesthesia of skin; chronic folliculitis; xerosis cutis; alopecia; exacerbation of psoriasis; acne; angioedema.

Miscellaneous – Fatigue; lethargy; sleepiness; dehydration; weight loss; transient scotomata; impotence/sexual dysfunction; dysgeusia/taste distortion; tightness in chest; hypercalcemia; hyperparathyroidism; salty taste; thirst; swollen lips; swollen, painful joints; fever; polyarthralgia; dental caries.

Reactions unrelated to dosage: Transient EEG and ECG changes; leukocytosis; headache; diffuse nontoxic goiter with or without hypothyroidism; transient hyperglycemia; generalized pruritis with or without rash; cutaneous ulcers; albuminuria; worsening of organic brain syndromes; excessive weight gain; edematous swelling of ankles or wrists; thirst or polyuria, sometimes resembling diabetes insipidus; metallic taste.

The development of painful discoloration of fingers and toes and coldness of the extremities within 1 day of the starting of treatment of lithium has occurred. The mechanism through which these symptoms (resembling Raynaud's Syndrome) developed is not known. Recovery followed discontinuance.

Overdosage:

Symptoms: Lithium toxicity – Toxic lithium levels are close to therapeutic. The likelihood of toxicity increases with increasing serum lithium levels. Serum lithium levels > 1.5 mEq/L carry a greater risk than lower levels. Do not permit levels to exceed 2 mEq/L during the acute treatment phase. Discontinue the drug if early toxic symptoms occur.

Lithium levels < 2 mEq/L – Diarrhea; vomiting; nausea; drowsiness; muscular weakness; lack of coordination. May be early signs of toxicity.

Lithium levels 2 to 3 mEq/L: Giddiness; ataxia; blurred vision; tinnitus; vertigo; increasing confusion; slurred speech; blackouts; fasciculations; myoclonic twitching or movement of entire limbs; choreoathetoid movements; urinary or fecal incontinence; agitation or manic-like behavior; hyperreflexia; hypertonia; dysarthria.

Lithium levels > 3 mEq/L may produce a complex clinical picture involving multiple organs and organ systems including: Seizures (generalized and focal); arrhythmias; hypotension; peripheral vascular collapse; stupor; muscle group twitching; spasticity; coma.

Treatment: Early symptoms of toxicity can usually be treated by dosage reduction or cessation and resumption of the treatment at a lower dose after 24 to 48 hours. In severe cases, first eliminate the ion from the patient. Treatment is essentially the same as that used in barbiturate toxicity: Gastric lavage; correction of fluid and electrolyte imbalance including the use of normal saline; regulation of kidney function. Charcoal is of no value. Urea, mannitol and aminophylline all produce significant increases in lithium excretion. Infection prophylaxis, chest x–rays, preservation of respiration and monitoring of thyroid status are essential. Hemodialysis effectively and rapidly lowers serum lithium levels in the severely toxic patient (generally, levels > 3.5 to 4 mEq/L); however, in some circumstances it may be indicated for patients with lower lithium levels. Refer to General Management of Acute Overdosage.

Patient Information:

Take immediately after meals or with food or milk to avoid stomach upset.

Stop medication and contact physician if signs of overdose or toxicity occur, such as diarrhea, vomiting, unsteady walking, tremor, drowsiness or muscle weakness.

Antimanic Agent

LITHIUM

May cause drowsiness. Use caution while driving or performing other tasks requiring alertness.

Drink 8 to 12 glasses of water or other liquid every day while on this drug. Maintain a regular diet (including salt). Contact physician if fever or diarrhea develops.

Administration and Dosage:

Individualize dosage according to both serum levels and clinical response.

Serum lithium levels: Draw blood samples immediately prior to the next dose (8 to 12 hours after the previous dose) when lithium concentrations are relatively stable. Do not rely on serum levels alone.

Acute mania: Optimal patient response is usually established and maintained with 600 mg 3 times daily or 900 mg twice daily for the slow release form. Such doses normally produce an effective serum lithium level ranging between 1 and 1.5 mEq/L.

Determine serum levels twice weekly during the acute phase, and until the serum level and clinical condition of the patient have been stabilized.

Long-term use: The desirable serum levels are 0.6 to 1.2 mEq/L. Dosage will vary, but 300 mg 3 to 4 times/day will usually maintain this level. Monitor serum levels in uncomplicated cases on maintenance therapy during remission every 2 to 3 months.

Rx	**Lithium Carbonate** (Roxane)	**Capsules**: 150 mg lithium carbonate (4.06 mEq lithium)	(54 213). White. In 100s, 1000s and UD 100s.
Rx	**Lithium Carbonate** (Various, eg, Dixon-Shane, Geneva, Goldline, Major, Moore, Roxane, Rugby, Schein, URL)	**Capsules**: 300 mg lithium carbonate (8.12 mEq lithium)	In 100s, 1000s and UD 100s.
Rx	**Eskalith** (SKF)		(Eskalith SKF). Yellow and gray. In 100s and 500s.
Rx	**Lithonate** (Solvay)		(RR 7512). Peach. In 100s, 1000s, UD 100s.
Rx	**Lithium Carbonate** (Roxane)	**Capsules**: 600 mg lithium carbonate (16.24 mEq lithium)	(54 702). White and flesh. In100s, 1000s and UD 100s.
Rx	**Lithium Carbonate** (Various, eg, Harber, International Labs, RID, Roxane)	**Tablets**: 300 mg lithium carbonate (8.12 mEq lithium)	In 100s, 1000s and UD 100s.
Rx	**Eskalith** (SK-Beecham)		(SKF J09). Gray, scored. In 100s.
Rx	**Lithane** (Bayer)		Tartrazine. (Miles 951). Green, scored. In 100s.
Rx	**Lithotabs** (Solvay)		(RR 7516). White, scored. Film coated. In 100s, 1000s & UD 100s.
Rx	**Lithobid** (Ciba)	**Tablets, slow release**: 300 mg lithium carbonate (8.12 mEq lithium)	(Ciba 65). Peach. Film coated. In 100s, 1000s and UD 100s.
Rx	**Eskalith CR** (SK-Beecham)	**Tablets, controlled release**: 450 mg lithium carbonate (12.18 mEq lithium)	(SKF J10). Buff, scored. In100s.
Rx	**Lithium Citrate** (Various, eg, Geneva, Major, PBI, Raway, Roxane, Schein, Xactdose)	**Syrup**: 8 mEq lithium (as citrate equivalent to 300 mg lithium carbonate) per 5 ml	In 480 and 500 ml and UD 5 and 10 ml.

TACRINE HCl (Tetrahydroaminoacridine; THA)

Actions:

Pharmacology: Tacrine is a centrally acting reversible cholinesterase inhibitor, commonly referred to as THA. Although widespread degeneration of multiple CNS neuronal systems eventually occurs, early pathological changes in Alzheimer's disease involve, in a relatively selective manner, cholinergic neuronal pathways that project from the basal forebrain to the cerebral cortex and hippocampus. The resulting deficiency of cortical acetylcholine is believed to account for some of the clinical manifestations of mild to moderate dementia. Tacrine presumably acts by elevating acetylcholine concentrations in the cerebral cortex by slowing the degradation of acetylcholine released by still intact cholinergic neurons. If this theoretical mechanism of action is correct, tacrine's effects may lessen as the disease process advances and fewer cholinergic neurons remain functionally intact. There is no evidence that tacrine alters the course of the underlying dementing process.

Pharmacokinetics:

Absorption – Tacrine is rapidly absorbed after oral administration. Maximal plasma concentrations occur within 1 to 2 hours. Absolute bioavailability of tacrine is ≈ 17%. Food reduces tacrine bioavailability by ≈ 30% to 40%; however, food has no effect if tacrine is administered at least 1 hour before meals. The effect of achlorhydria on absorption is unknown.

Distribution – Mean volume of distribution of tacrine is ≈ 349 L. Tacrine is ≈ 55% bound to plasma proteins. The extent and degree of distribution within various body compartments has not been systematically studied; however, 336 hours after the administration of a single radiolabeled dose, ≈ 25% was not recovered, suggesting the possibility that tacrine or one or more of its metabolites may be retained.

Metabolism – Tacrine is extensively metabolized by the cytochrome P450 system to multiple metabolites, not all of which have been identified. The vast majority of radiolabeled species present in the plasma following a single dose of radiolabeled tacrine are unidentified (eg, only 5% of radioactivity in plasma has been identified [tacrine and 3–hydroxylated metabolites; 1–, 2– and 4-hydroxytacrine]). Cytochrome P450 IA2 is the principal isozyme involved in metabolism. These findings are consistent with the observation that tacrine or one of its metabolites inhibits the metabolism of theophylline (see Drug Interactions). Following aromatic ring hydroxylation, tacrine metabolites undergo glucuronidation.

Excretion – Tacrine undergoes first-pass metabolism, the extent of which depends on the dose administered. Because the enzyme system involved can be saturated at relatively low doses, a larger fraction of a high dose of tacrine will escape first-pass elimination than a smaller dose. Elimination of tacrine from the plasma is not dose-dependent. The elimination half-life is ≈ 2 to 4 hours. Following initiation of therapy or a change in daily dose, steady-state plasma concentrations will be attained within 24 to 36 hours.

Special populations:

Age – There is no clinically relevant influence of age (50 to 84 years) on tacrine clearance.

Gender – Average tacrine plasma concentrations are ≈ 50% higher in females than in males. This is not explained by differences in body surface area or elimination half-life. The difference is probably because of higher systemic availability after oral dosing and may reflect the known lower activity of cytochrome P450 IA2 in women.

Smoking – Mean plasma tacrine concentrations in current smokers are ≈⅓ the concentrations in nonsmokers.

Renal function impairment – Renal disease does not appear to affect the clearance of tacrine.

Hepatic function impairment – Although studies in patients with liver disease have not been done, it is likely that functional hepatic impairment will reduce the clearance of tacrine and its metabolites.

TACRINE HCl (Tetrahydroaminoacridine; THA)

Clinical trials: In the following studies, outcomes during treatment with tacrine and placebo were assessed on two primary measures: (1) The cognitive subscale of the Alzheimer's Disease Assessment Scale (ADAS cog) and (2) a clinician's rated clinical global impression of change. The ADAS cog is a multi-item test battery administered by a psychometrician that examines aspects of memory, attention, praxis, reason and language. The worst possible score is 70. Healthy elderly adults may score as low as 0 or 1 unit, but individuals judged not to be demented can score higher. The mean score of patients entering each study was ≈ 28 units (range, 7 to 62). The ADAS cog score is reported to deteriorate at a rate of about 6 to 10 units per year for untreated patients at this stage of dementia. The clinician's global assessments used in the two studies relied on a clinician's judgment about the overall clinical change observed in patients over the course of the study. Although the conditions for obtaining the clinical assessment differed in each study, the global assessment was rated on a 7-point scale in both studies. A rating of 4 represents no change; lower ratings indicate improvement from baseline and higher ratings, deterioration.

Twelve-week study – In one study of 12 weeks duration, patients were randomized to sequences that provided a comparison among placebo, 20, 40 and 80 mg/day by study's end. Statistically significant drug-placebo differences were detected on both primary outcome measures for the group titrated to 80 mg/day. Estimates of the size of the treatment effect varied between 2 and 4 ADAS cog units. The placebo vs 80 mg/day comparison also achieved statistical significance on the clinician's global impression of change with a 0.3 to 0.4 unit mean difference.

Thirty week study – The second study was 30 weeks long. Patients (n = 663) were randomized to four treatment sequences (placebo and three drug groups) that called for the daily dose of tacrine to be increased at 6-week intervals, starting with a 40 mg/day dose. By study's end, a comparison among placebo, 80, 120 and 160 mg/day was possible. Patients in the 160 mg group received this dose for the final 12 weeks; the 120 mg group received that dose for 18 weeks. The study showed statistically significant drug-placebo differences for the 80 and 120 mg/day groups at 18 weeks and for the 120 and 160 mg/day groups at 30 weeks on both the ADAS cog and a clinician's assessment of global change. All analyses confirmed the effectiveness of tacrine, although the estimated mean treatment effect was different in each analysis.

Indications:

Alzheimer's disease: Treatment of mild to moderate dementia of the Alzheimer's type.

Contraindications:

Hypersensitivity to tacrine or acridine derivatives; patients previously treated with tacrine who developed treatment-associated jaundice confirmed by elevated total bilirubin > 3 mg/dl.

Warnings:

Anesthesia: Tacrine is likely to exaggerate succinylcholine-type muscle relaxation during anesthesia.

Cardiovascular: Because of its cholinomimetic action, tacrine may have vagotonic effects on the heart rate (eg, bradycardia). This action may be particularly important to patients with conduction abnormalities, bradyarrhythmia or a "sick sinus syndrome."

GI: Tacrine is an inhibitor of cholinesterase and may be expected to increase gastric acid secretion because of increased cholinergic activity. Therefore, closely monitor patients at increased risk for developing ulcers (eg, those with a history of ulcer disease or those receiving concurrent NSAIDs) for symptoms of active or occult GI bleeding. Tacrine can cause nausea, vomiting and loose stools at recommended doses.

TACRINE HCl (Tetrahydroaminoacridine; THA)

Hepatotoxicity: Prescribe with care in patients with current evidence or history of abnormal liver function indicated by significant abnormalities in serum transaminase (ALT, AST), bilirubin and gamma-glutamyl transpeptidase (GGT) levels. The use of tacrine in patients without a prior history of liver disease is commonly associated with serum aminotransferase elevations, some to levels ordinarily considered to indicate clinically important hepatic injury. If tacrine is promptly withdrawn following detection of these elevations, clinically evident signs and symptoms of liver injury are rare. Long-term follow-up of patients who experience transaminase elevations, however, is limited; it is, therefore, impossible to exclude with certainty the possibility of chronic sequelae.

One of > 8000 patients exposed to tacrine in clinical studies and the treatment IND program had documented elevated bilirubin (5.3 x upper limit of normal [ULN]) and jaundice with transaminase levels (AST) nearly 20 x ULN. A dosing regimen employing a more rapid escalation of the daily dose of tacrine may be associated with more serious clinical events.

Cumulative Incidence of ALT Elevations with Tacrine			
Maximum ALT	Males (n = 229)	Females (n = 250)	Total (n = 479)
Within normal limits	53%	40%	46%
> ULN	47%	60%	54%
> 2 x ULN	34%	42%	38%
> 3 x ULN	25%	32%	29%
> 10 x ULN	5%	8%	6%
> 20 x ULN	1%	2%	2%

Experience in 2446 patients who participated in all clinical trials, including the 30–week study, indicates ≈ 50% of patients treated with tacrine can be expected to have at least 1 ALT level above ULN; ≈ 25% of patients are likely to develop elevations > 3 x ULN and ≈ 7% of patients may develop elevations > 10 x ULN. Data collected from the treatment IND program were consistent with those obtained during clinical studies and showed 3% of 5665 patients experiencing an ALT elevation > 10 x ULN. In clinical trials where transaminases were monitored weekly, the median time to onset of the first ALT elevation above ULN was ≈ 6 weeks, with maximum ALT occurring 1 week later, even in instances when treatment was stopped. Under the conditions of forced slow upwards dose titration (increases of 40 mg/day every 6 weeks) employed in clinical studies, 95% of transaminase elevations > 3 x ULN occurred within the first 18 weeks of therapy, and 99% of the 10-fold elevations occurred by the 12th week on ≤ 80 mg. Note, however, that for most patients ALT was monitored weekly and tacrine was stopped when liver enzymes exceeded 3 x ULN. With less frequent monitoring or the less stringent discontinuation criteria, it is possible that marked elevations might be more common. It must also be appreciated that experience with prolonged exposure to the high dose (160 mg/day) is limited. In all cases, transaminase levels returned to within normal limits upon discontinuation of treatment or following dosage reduction, usually within 4 to 6 weeks. This relatively benign experience may be the consequence of careful laboratory monitoring that facilitated the discontinuation of patients early on after the onset of their transaminase elevations. Consequently, frequent monitoring of serum transaminase levels is recommended.

Liver biopsy results in seven patients who received tacrine revealed hepatocellular necrosis in six patients, and granulomatous changes in the seventh. In all cases, liver function tests returned to normal with no evidence of persisting hepatic dysfunction.

TACRINE HCl (Tetrahydroaminoacridine; THA)

Among the 866 patients assigned to tacrine in the 12– and 30–week studies, 212 were withdrawn because they developed transaminase elevations > 3 x ULN. Of these patients, 145 were subsequently rechallenged. During their initial exposure to tacrine, 20 of these 145 had experienced initial elevations > 10 x ULN, while the remainder had experienced elevations between 3 and 10 x ULN. Upon rechallenge with an initial dose of 40 mg/day, only 48 (33%) of the 145 patients developed transaminase elevations > 3 × ULN. Of these patients, 44 had elevations that were between 3 and 10 x ULN and 4 had elevations that were > 10 x ULN. The mean time to onset of elevations occurred earlier on rechallenge than on initial exposure (22 vs 48 days). Of the 145 patients rechallenged, 127 (88%) were able to continue treatment, and 91 of these 127 patients titrated to doses higher than those associated with the initial transaminase elevation.

The incidence of transaminase elevations is higher among females. There are no other known predictors of the risk of hepatocellular injury.

Monitoring – Monitor serum transaminase levels (specifically ALT) every other week for at least the first 16 weeks following initiation of treatment, after which monitoring may be decreased to monthly for 2 months and every 3 months thereafter. Resume weekly monitoring for a minimum of 6 weeks. Repeat a full monitoring sequence in the event that a patient suspends treatment with tacrine for > 4 weeks. If transaminase elevations occur, modify the dose (see Administration and Dosage).

Rechallenge – Patients with clinical jaundice confirmed by a significant elevation in total bilirubin (> 3 mg/dl) or those exhibiting clinical signs or symptoms of hypersensitivity in association with transaminase elevations should permanently discontinue tacrine and not be rechallenged. Patients who are required to discontinue treatment because of transaminase elevations may be rechallenged once transaminase levels return to within normal limits (see Administration and Dosage). Rechallenge of patients with transaminase elevations < 10 x ULN has not resulted in serious liver injury. However, because experience in the rechallenge of patients who had elevations > 10 x ULN is limited, the risks associated with the rechallenge of these patients are not well characterized. Use careful, frequent (weekly) monitoring of serum ALT when rechallenging such patients. If rechallenged, give patients an initial dose of 40 mg/day (10 mg 4 times daily) and monitor transaminase levels weekly. If, after 6 weeks on 40 mg/day, the patient is tolerating the dosage with no unacceptable elevations in transaminases, resume recommended dose titration and transaminase monitoring.

Liver biopsy is not indicated in cases of uncomplicated transaminase elevation.

GU: Cholinomimetics may cause bladder outflow obstruction.

Neurological conditions:

Seizures – Cholinomimetics are believed to have some potential to cause generalized convulsions; seizure activity may, however, also be a manifestation of Alzheimer's disease.

Worsening of cognitive function has been reported following abrupt discontinuation of tacrine or after a large reduction in total daily dose (≥ 80 mg/day).

Pulmonary conditions: Because of its cholinomimetic action, use tacrine with care in patients with a history of asthma.

Carcinogenesis/Mutagenesis: Tacrine was mutagenic to bacteria in the Ames test. Unscheduled DNA synthesis was induced in rat and mouse hepatocytes in vitro. Results of cytogenetic (chromosomal aberration) studies were equivocal. Overall, the results of these tests, along with the fact that tacrine belongs to a chemical class (acridines) containing some members that are animal carcinogens, suggest that tacrine may be carcinogenic.

Pregnancy: Category C. It is not known whether tacrine can cause fetal harm when administered to a pregnant woman or can affect reproductive capacity.

Lactation: It is not known whether this drug is excreted in breast milk.

Children: There are no adequate and well controlled trials to document the safety and efficacy of tacrine in any dementing illness occurring in children.

TACRINE HCl (Tetrahydroaminoacridine; THA)

Precautions:

Monitoring: Monitor serum transaminase levels (specifically ALT) every other week for at least the first 16 weeks following initiation of treatment, after which monitoring may be decreased to monthly for 2 months and every 3 months, thereafter. Resume weekly monitoring for a minumum of 6 weeks. Repeat a full monitoring sequence in the event that a patient suspends treatment with tacrine for > 4 weeks. If transaminase elevations occur, modify the dose (see Warnings and Administration and Dosage).

Hematology: An absolute neutrophil count (ANC) < 500/mcl occurred in four patients who received tacrine during the course of clinical trials. Three of the four patients had concurrent medical conditions commonly associated with a low ANC; two of these patients remained on tacrine. The fourth patient, who had a history of hypersensitivity (penicillin allergy), withdrew from the study as a result of a rash and also developed an ANC < 500/mcl, which returned to normal; this patient was not rechallenged and, therefore, the role played by tacrine in this reaction is unknown. Six patients had an ANC ≤ 1500/mcl, associated with an elevation of ALT. The total clinical experience in > 8000 patients does not indicate a clear association between tacrine treatment and serious white blood cell abnormalities.

Drug Interactions:

Tacrine is primarily eliminated by hepatic metabolism via cytochrome P450 drug metabolizing enzymes. Drug interactions may occur when it is given concurrently with agents, such as theophylline, that undergo extensive metabolism via cytochrome P450 IA2.

Tacrine Drug Interactions

Precipitant drug	Object drug*		Description
Tacrine	Anticholinergics	⬇	Because of its mechanism of action, tacrine has the potential to interfere with the activity of anticholinergic medications.
Tacrine	Cholinomimetics Cholinesterase inhibitors	⬆	A synergistic effect is expected when tacrine is given concurrently with succinylcholine, cholinesterase inhibitors or cholinergic agonists, such as bethanechol.
Tacrine	Theophylline	⬆	Coadministration increased theophylline elimination half-life and average plasma concentrations by ≈ 2-fold. Therefore, monitoring of plasma theophylline concentrations and appropriate reduction of theophylline dose are recommended.
Cimetidine	Tacrine	⬆	Cimetidine increased the C_{max} and AUC of tacrine by ≈ 54% and 64%, respectively.

* ⬆ = Object drug increased. ⬇ = Object drug decreased.

Drug/Food interactions: Taking tacrine with meals can reduce plasma levels ≈ 30% to 40%; take between meals whenever possible.

Adverse Reactions:

Transaminase elevations were the most common reason for withdrawals during treatment (8% of all tacrine-treated patients). Apart from withdrawals because of transaminase elevations, 9% withdrew for adverse events. Other adverse events that most frequently led to the withdrawal of tacrine-treated patients in clinical trials were nausea/vomiting (1.5%), agitation (0.9%), rash (0.7%), anorexia (0.7%) and confusion (0.5%).

The most common adverse events were elevated transaminases, nausea, vomiting, diarrhea, dyspepsia, myalgia, anorexia and ataxia. Of these events, nausea, vomiting, diarrhea, dyspepsia and anorexia appeared to be dose-dependent.

TACRINE HCl (Tetrahydroaminoacridine; THA)

Tacrine Adverse Reactions (%)					
Adverse reaction	Tacrine (n = 634)	Placebo (n = 342)	Adverse reaction	Tacrine (n = 634)	Placebo (n = 342)
Body as a whole			*Psychiatric*		
Headache	11	15	Agitation	7	9
Fatigue	4	3	Depression	4	4
Chest pain	4	5	Abnormal thinking	3	4
Weight decrease	3	1	Anxiety	3	2
Back pain	2	4	Hallucination	2	4
Asthenia	2	2	Hostility	2	2
GI			*Respiratory*		
Nausea/Vomiting	28	9	Rhinitis	8	6
Diarrhea	16	5	Upper respiratory infection	3	3
Dyspepsia	9	6	Coughing	3	5
Anorexia	9	3	*Dermatologic*		
Abdominal pain	8	7	Rash	7	5
Flatulence	4	2	Facial/Skin flushing	3	<1
Constipation	4	2	*GU*		
CNS			Urination frequency	3	4
Dizziness	12	11	Urinary tract infection	3	6
Confusion	7	7	Urinary incontinence	3	3
Ataxia	6	4	*Miscellaneous*		
Insomnia	6	5	Elevated transaminase	29	2
Somnolence	4	3	Purpura	2	2
Tremor	2	<1	Myalgia	9	5

Body as a whole: Chill, fever, malaise, peripheral edema (1%); facial edema, dehydration, weight increase, cachexia, generalized edema, lipoma (0.1% to 1%); heat exhaustion, sepsis, cholinergic crisis, death (< 0.1%).

Cardiovascular: Hypotension, hypertension (1%); heart failure, myocardial infarction, angina pectoris, cerebrovascular accident, transient ischemic attack, phlebitis, venous insufficiency, abdominal aortic aneurysm, atrial fibrillation or flutter, palpitation, tachycardia, bradycardia, pulmonary embolus, migraine, hypercholesterolemia (0.1% to 1%); heart arrest, premature atrial contractions, A-V block, bundle branch block (< 0.1%).

CNS: Convulsions, vertigo, syncope, hyperkinesia, paresthesia (1%); abnormal dreaming, dysarthria, aphasia, amnesia, wandering, twitching, hypesthesia, delirium, paralysis, bradykinesia, movement disorder, cogwheel rigidity, paresis, neuritis, hemiplegia, Parkinson's disease, neuropathy, extrapyramidal syndrome, decreased/absent reflexes (0.1% to 1%); tardive dyskinesia, dysesthesia, dystonia, encephalitis, coma, apraxia, oculogyric crisis, akathisia, oral facial dyskinesia, Bell's palsy (< 0.1%).

Dermatologic: Increased sweating (1%); acne, alopecia, dermatitis, eczema, dry skin, herpes zoster, psoriasis, cellulitis, cyst, furunculosis, herpes simplex, hyperkeratosis, basal cell carcinoma, skin cancer (0.1% to 1%); desquamation, seborrhea, squamous cell carcinoma, skin ulcer, skin necrosis, melanoma (< 0.1%).

Endocrine: Diabetes (0.1% to 1%); hyperthyroid, hypothyroid (< 0.1%).

GI: Glossitis, gingivitis, dry mouth or throat, stomatitis, increased salivation, dysphagia, esophagitis, gastritis, gastroenteritis, GI hemorrhage, stomach ulcer, hiatal hernia, hemorrhoids, bloody stools, diverticulitis, fecal impaction, fecal incontinence, rectal hemorrhage, cholelithiasis, cholecystitis, increased appetite (0.1% to 1%); duodenal ulcer, bowel obstruction (< 0.1%).

GU: Hematuria, renal stone, kidney infection, glycosuria, dysuria, polyuria, nocturia, pyuria, cystitis, urinary retention, urination urgency, vaginal hemorrhage, pruritus (genital), breast pain, impotence, prostate cancer (0.1% to 1%); bladder tumor, renal tumor, renal failure, urinary obstruction, breast cancer, ovarian carcinoma, epididymitis (< 0.1%).

Hematologic/Lymphatic: Anemia, lymphadenopathy (0.1% to 1%); leukopenia, thrombocytopenia, hemolysis, pancytopenia (< 0.1%).

Musculoskeletal: Fracture, arthralgia, arthritis, hypertonia (1%); osteoporosis, tendinitis, bursitis, gout (0.1% to 1%); myopathy (< 0.1%).

Psychiatric: Nervousness (1%); apathy, increased libido, paranoia, neurosis (0.1% to 1%); suicidal, psychosis, hysteria (< 0.1%).

TACRINE HCl (Tetrahydroaminoacridine; THA)

Respiratory: Pharyngitis, sinusitis, bronchitis, pneumonia, dyspnea (1%); epistaxis, chest congestion, asthma, hyperventilation, lower respiratory infection (0.1% to 1%); hemoptysis, lung edema, lung cancer, acute epiglottitis (< 0.1%).

Special senses: Conjunctivitis (1%); cataract, dry eyes, eye pain, visual field defect, diplopia, amblyopia, glaucoma, hordeolum, deafness, earache, tinnitus, inner ear infection, otitis media, unusual taste (0.1% to 1%); vision loss, ptosis, blepharitis, labyrinthitis, inner ear disturbance (< 0.1%).

Overdosage:

Symptoms: Overdosage with cholinesterase inhibitors can cause a cholinergic crisis characterized by severe nausea, vomiting, salivation, sweating, bradycardia, hypotension, collapse and convulsions. Increasing muscle weakness is a possibility and may result in death if respiratory muscles are involved.

The estimated median lethal dose of tacrine following a single oral dose in rats is 40 mg/kg or ≈ 12 times the maximum recommended human dose of 160 mg/day. Dose-related signs of cholinergic stimulation were observed in animals and included vomiting, diarrhea, salivation, lacrimation, ataxia, convulsions, tremor and stereotypic head and body movements.

Treatment: As in any case of overdose, use general supportive measures. Refer to General Management of Acute Overdosage. Tertiary anticholinergics, such as atropine, may be used as an antidote for tacrine overdosage. IV atropine sulfate titrated to effect is recommended (initial dose of 1 to 2 mg IV with subsequent doses based on clinical response). Atypical increases in blood pressure and heart rate have been reported with other cholinomimetics when coadministered with quaternary anticholinergics such as glycopyrrolate.

It is not known whether tacrine or its metabolites can be eliminated by dialysis (hemodialysis, peritoneal dialysis or hemofiltration).

Patient Information:

Advise patients and caregivers that the effect of tacrine therapy is thought to depend on its administration at regular intervals, as directed. Take between meals whenever possible; however, it may be taken with meals to avoid GI upset.

Advise the caregiver about the possibility of adverse effects. Two types should be distinguished: (1) Those occuring in close temporal association with the initiation of treatment or an increase in dose (eg, nausea, vomiting, loose stools, diarrhea); and (2) those with a delayed onset (eg, rash, jaundice, changes in the color of stool [black, very dark or light, eg, acholic]).

Encourage patients and caregivers to inform the physician about the emergence of new events or any increase in the severity of existing adverse clinical events.

Advise caregivers that abrupt discontinuation or a large reduction in total daily dose (≥ 80 mg/day) may cause a decline in cognitive function and behavioral disturbances. Unsupervised increases in the dose of tacrine may also have serious consequences. Changes in dose should not be undertaken in the absence of direct instruction of a physician.

Administration and Dosage:

Approved by the FDA on September 9, 1993.

The rate of dose escalation may be slowed if a patient is intolerant to the recommended titration schedule. It is not advisable, however, to accelerate the dose incrementation plan. Following initiation of therapy, or any dosage increase, observe patients carefully for adverse effects. Take between meals whenever possible; however, if minor GI upset occurs, take with meals to improve tolerability. Taking tacrine with meals can be expected to reduce plasma levels ≈ 30% to 40%.

Initiation of treatment: The initial dose of tacrine is 40 mg/day (10 mg 4 times daily). Maintain this dose for ≥ 6 weeks with weekly monitoring of transaminase levels. It is important that the dose not be increased during this period because of the potential for delayed onset of transaminase elevations.

Dose titration: Following 6 weeks of treatment at 40 mg/day, increase the dose to 80 mg/day (20 mg 4 times daily), providing there are no significant transaminase elevations and the patient is tolerating treatment. Titrate patients to higher doses (120 and 160 mg/day in divided doses on a 4 times daily schedule) at 6 week intervals on the basis of tolerance.

TACRINE HCl (Tetrahydroaminoacridine; THA)

Dose adjustment: Monitor serum transaminase levels (specifically ALT) every other week for at least the first 16 weeks following initiation of treatment, after which monitoring may be decreased to monthly for 2 months and every 3 months thereafter.

A full monitoring and dose titration sequence must be repeated in the event that a patient suspends treatment with tacrine for > 4 weeks. If transaminase elevations occur, modify the dose according to the following table.

Recommended Tacrine Dose and Monitoring Regimen Modification in Response to Transaminase Elevations

Transaminase levels	Treatment and monitoring regimen
≤ 2 x ULN	Continue treatment and monitoring according to recommended titration and monitoring schedule.
> 2 to ≤ 3 x ULN	Continue treatment according to recommended titration. Monitor transaminase levels weekly until levels return to normal limits.
> 3 to ≤ 5 x ULN	Reduce the daily dose by 40 mg/day. Resume dose titration and every other week monitoring when transaminases return to within normal limits.
> 5 x ULN	Stop treatment. Monitor transaminase levels until within normal limits (see Rechallenge section).

Experience is limited in patients with ALT > 10 x ULN. The risk of rechallenge must be considered against demonstrated clinical benefit. Patients with clinical jaundice confirmed by a significant elevation in total bilirubin (> 3 mg/dl) should permanently discontinue tacrine and not be rechallenged.

Rechallenge: Patients who are required to discontinue treatment because of transaminase elevations may be rechallenged once transaminase levels return to within normal limits. Rechallenge of patients exposed to transaminase elevations < 10 x ULN has not resulted in serious liver injury. However, because experience in the rechallenge of patients who had elevations > 10 x ULN is limited, the risks associated with the rechallenge of these patients are not well characterized. Carefully and frequently (weekly) monitor serum ALT when rechallenging such patients. If rechallenged, give patients an initial dose of 40 mg/day (10 mg 4 times daily) and monitor transaminase levels weekly. If, after 6 weeks on 40 mg/day, the patient is tolerating the dosage with no unacceptable elevations in transaminases, recommended dose titration and transaminase monitoring may be resumed.

Storage/Stability: Store at controlled room temperature 15° to 30°C (59° to 86°F) away from moisture.

Rx	**Cognex** (Parke-Davis)	**Capsules**: 10 mg	Lactose. (Cognex 10). Yellow/dark green. In 120s and UD 100s.
		20 mg	Lactose. (Cognex 20). Yellow/light blue. In 120s and UD 100s.
		30 mg	Lactose. (Cognex 30). Yellow/orange. In 120s and UD 100s.
		40 mg	Lactose. (Cognex 40). Yellow/lavender. In 120s and UD 100s.

DONEPEZIL HCl

Actions:

Pharmacology: Donepezil is postulated to exert its therapeutic effect by enhancing cholinergic function. Deficiency of cholinergic neurotransmission may be the cause of Alzheimer's disease. This increase in cholinergic function is accomplished by increasing the concentration of acetylcholine through reversible inhibition of its hydrolysis by acetylcholinesterase (AChE). If this proposed mechanism of action is correct, donepezil's effect may lessen as the disease process advances and fewer cholinergic neurons remain functionally intact. There is no evidence that donepezil alters the course of the underlying dementing process.

Pharmacokinetics:

Absorption – Donepezil is well absorbed with a relative oral bioavailability of 100% and reaches peak plasma concentrations in 3 to 4 hours. Pharmacokinetics are linear over a dose range of 1 to 10 mg given once daily. Neither food nor time of administration (morning vs evening dose) influences the rate or extent of absorption.

Distribution – Following multiple dose administration, donepezil accumulates in plasma by 4- to 7-fold and steady-state is reached within 15 days. The steady-state volume of distribution is 12 L/kg. Donepezil is ≈ 96% bound to human plasma proteins, mainly to albumins (≈ 75%) and $alpha_1$–acid glycoprotein (≈ 21%) over the concentration range of 2 to 1000 ng/ml.

Metabolism – Donepezil is both excreted in the urine intact and extensively metabolized to four major metabolites, two of which are known to be active and a number of minor metabolites, not all of which have been identified. Donepezil is metabolized by CYP 450 isoenzyme 2D6 and 3A4 and undergoes glucuronidation. Following administration of donepezil, plasma radioactivity was present primarily as intact donepezil (53%) and as 6-O-desmethyl donepezil (11%), which has been reported to inhibit AChE to the same extent as donepezil in vitro and was found in plasma at concentrations equal to ≈ 20% of donepezil.

Excretion – The elimination half-life of donepezil is ≈ 70 hours and the mean apparent plasma clearance is 0.13 L/hr/kg.

Approximately 57% and 15% of the total dose was recovered in urine and feces, respectively, over a period of 10 days, while 28% remained unrecovered, with ≈ 17% of the donepezil dose recovered in the urine as unchanged drug.

Special Populations:

Hepatic function impairment – In a study of 10 patients with stable alcoholic cirrhosis, the clearance of donepezil was decreased by 20% relative to 10 healthy age- and sex-matched subjects.

Renal function impairment – In a study of 4 patients with moderate to severe renal impairment (Cl_{cr} < 22 ml/min/1.72 m^2), the clearance of donepezil did not differ from age- and sex-matched subjects.

Clinical trials:

Thirty-week study – In a 30–week study, 473 patients were randomized to receive single daily doses of placebo or 5 or 10 mg/day of donepezil. The study was divided into a 24–week, double-blind active treatment phase followed by a 6–week single-blind placebo washout period.

Effects on the Alzheimer's Disease Assessment Scale (ADAS cog): After 24 weeks of treatment, the mean differences in the ADAS cog change scores for the donepezil-treated patients compared with the patients on placebo were 2.8 and 3.1 units for the 5 mg/day and 10 mg/day treatments, respectively. These differences were statistically significant.

Following 6 weeks of placebo washout, scores on the ADAS cog for both donepezil treatment groups were indistinguishable from those patients who had received only placebo for 30 weeks. This suggests that the beneficial effects of donepezil abate over 6 weeks following discontinuation of treatment and do not represent a change in the underlying disease. There is no evidence of a rebound effect 6 weeks after abrupt discontinuation.

Effects on the Clinician's Interview Based Impression of Change (CIBIC-Plus): The mean drug-placebo differences for these groups of patients were 0.35 units and 0.39 units for 5 mg/day and 10 mg/day of donepezil, respectively. These differences were statistically significant. There was no statistically significant difference between the two active treatments.

Fifteen-week study – In a 15–week study, patients were randomized to receive single daily doses of placebo or 5 or 10 mg/day of donepezil for 12 weeks, followed by a 3–week placebo washout period.

DONEPEZIL HCl

Effects on the ADAS cog: After 12 weeks of treatment, the differences in mean ADAS cog change scores were 2.7 and 3 units each, for the 5 and 10 mg/day donepezil treatment groups, respectively. These differences were statistically significant.

Following 3 weeks of placebo washout, scores on the ADAS cog for both donepezil treatment groups increased, indicating that discontinuation of donepezil resulted in a loss of its treatment effect. The duration of this placebo washout period was not sufficient to characterize the rate of loss of the treatment effect, but, the 30–week study demonstrated that treatment effects associated with the use of donepezil abate within 6 weeks of treatment discontinuation.

Effects on the CIBIC-Plus: The differences in mean scores for donepezil-treated patients, compared with the patients on placebo at week 12, were 0.36 units and 0.38 units for the 5 mg/day and 10 mg/day treatment groups, respectively. These differences were statistically significant.

Indications:

Alzheimer's disease: The treatment of mild to moderate dementia of the Alzheimer's type.

Contraindications:

Hypersensitivity to donepezil or to piperidine derivatives.

Warnings:

Anesthesia: Donepezil, as a cholinesterase inhibitor, is likely to exaggerate succinylcholine-type muscle relaxation during anesthesia.

Cardiovascular: Because of their pharmacological action, cholinesterase inhibitors may have vagotonic effects on heart rate (eg, bradycardia). The potential for this action may be particularly important to patients with "sick sinus syndrome" or other supraventricular cardiac conduction conditions. Syncopal episodes have been reported in association with the use of donepezil.

GI: Through their primary action, cholinesterase inhibitors may be expected to increase gastric acid secretion because of increased cholinergic activity. Therefore, monitor patients closely for symptoms of active or occult GI bleeding, especially those at increased risk for developing ulcers, eg, those with a history of ulcer disease or those receiving concurrent nonsteroidal anti-inflammatory drugs (NSAIDs). Clinical studies of donepezil have shown no increase, relative to placebo, in the incidence of either peptic ulcer disease or GI bleeding.

Donepezil, as a predictable consequence of its pharmacological properties, has been shown to produce diarrhea, nausea and vomiting. These effects, when they occur, appear more frequently with the 10 mg/day dose than with the 5 mg/day dose. In most cases, these effects have been mild and transient, sometimes lasting 1 to 3 weeks, and have resolved during continued use of donepezil.

GU: Although not observed in clinical trials, cholinomimetics may cause bladder outflow obstruction.

Seizures: Cholinomimetics are believed to have some potential to cause generalized convulsions. However, seizure activity also may be a manifestation of Alzheimer's disease.

Pulmonary: Because of their cholinomimetic actions, prescribe cholinesterase inhibitors with care for patients with a history of asthma or obstructive pulmonary disease.

Pregnancy: Category C. In a study in which pregnant rats were given up to 10 mg/kg/day from day 17 of gestation through day 20 post partum, there was a slight increase in still births and a slight decrease in pup survival through day 4 post partum at this dose. There are no adequate or well controlled studies in pregnant women. Use donepezil during pregnancy only if the potential benefit justifies the potential risk to the fetus.

Lactation: It is not known whether donepezil is excreted in breast milk.

Children: There are no adequate and well controlled trials to document the safety and efficacy of donepezil in any illness occurring in children.

DONEPEZIL HCl

Drug Interactions:

Inducers of CYP 2D6 and CYP 3A4 could increase the rate of elimination of donepezil.

Donepezil Drug Interactions			
Precipitant drug	Object drug*		Description
Donepezil	Anticholinergics	↓	Because of their mechanism of action, cholinesterase inhibitors have the potential to interfere with the activity of anticholinergic medications.
Donepezil	Cholinomimetics/cholinesterase inhibitors	↑	A synergistic effect may be expected when cholinesterase inhibitors are given concurrently with succinylcholine, similar neuromuscular blocking agents or cholinergic agonists such as bethanechol.
Donepezil	NSAIDs	↑	Donepezil increases gastric acid secretions due to increased cholinergic activity. Therefore, monitor for active or occult GI bleeding.
Donepezil	Furosemide Digoxin Warfarin	↔	Donepezil at concentrations of 0.3 to 10 mcg/ml did not affect the binding of furosemide, digoxin and warfarin to albumin.
Donepezil	Theophylline Cimetidine Warfarin Digoxin	↔	No significant effects on the pharmacokinetics of these drugs have been observed.
Ketoconazole Quinidine	Donepezil	↑	Inhibitors of CYP 450, 3A4 and 2D6, inhibit donepezil metabolism in vitro. Whether there is a clinical effect of these inhibitors is not known.

* ↑ = Object drug increased. ↓ = Object drug decreased. ↔ = Undetermined effect.

Adverse Reactions:

Adverse Events Reported for Donepezil (%)		
Adverse event	Donepezil (n = 747)	Placebo (n = 355)
Body as a whole		
Headache	10	9
Pain, various locations	9	8
Accident	7	6
Fatigue	5	3
GI[1]		
Nausea[2]	11	6
Diarrhea[2]	10	5
Vomiting[3]	5	3
Anorexia	4	2
Musculoskeletal		
Muscle cramps	6	2
Arthritis	2	1
CNS		
Insomnia	9	6
Dizziness	8	6
Depression	3	< 1
Abnormal dreams	3	0
Somnolence	2	< 1

Adverse Events Reported for Donepezil (%)		
Adverse event	Donepezil (n = 747)	Placebo (n = 355)
Miscellaneous		
Syncope	2	1
Ecchymosis	4	3
Weight decrease	3	1
Frequent urination	2	1

[1] See Warnings.
[2] 1% to 3% discontinued because of adverse reactions.
[3] 1% to 2% discontinued because of adverse reactions.

Other adverse reactions include:

Body as a whole: Influenza, chest pain, toothache (1%); fever, facial edema, periorbital edema, hernia, hiatal hernia, abscess, cellulitis, chills, generalized coldness, head fullness, head pressure, listlessness (≤ 1%).

Cardiovascular: Hypertension, vasodilation, atrial fibrillation, hot flashes, hypotension (1%); angina pectoris, postural hypotension, myocardial infarction, AV block (first degree), congestive heart failure, arteritis, bradycardia (see Warnings), peripheral vascular disease, supraventricular tachycardia, deep vein thrombosis (≤ 1%).

Dermatologic: Diaphoresis, urticaria, pruritus (1%); dermatitis, erythema, skin discoloration, hyperkeratosis, alopecia, fungal dermatitis, herpes zoster, nevus, hirsutism, skin striae, night sweats, skin ulcer (≤ 1%).

Endocrine: Diabetes mellitus, goiter (≤ 1%).

GI: Fecal incontinence, GI bleeding (see Warnings), bloating, epigastric pain (1%); eructation, gingivitis, increased appetite, flatulence, periodontal abscess, cholelithiasis, diverticulitis, drooling, dry mouth, fever sore, gastritis, irritable colon, coated tongue, tongue edema, epigastric distress, gastroenteritis, increased transaminases, hemorrhoids, ileus, increased thirst, jaundice, melena, polydypsia, duodenal ulcer, stomach ulcer (≤ 1%).

GU: Urinary incontinence (see Warnings), nocturia (1%); dysuria, hematuria, urinary urgency, metrorrhagia, cystitis, enuresis, prostate hypertrophy, pyelonephritis, inability to empty bladder, breast fibroadenosis, fibrocystic breast, mastitis, pyuria, renal failure, vaginitis (≤ 1%).

Hematologic/Lymphatic: Anemia, thrombocythemia, thrombocytopenia, eosinophilia, erythrocytopenia (≤ 1%).

Metabolic/Nutritional: Dehydration (1%); gout, hypokalemia, increased creatine kinase, hyperglycemia, weight increase, increased lactate dehydrogenase (≤ 1%).

Musculoskeletal: Bone fracture (1%); muscle weakness, muscle fasciculation (≤ 1%).

Respiratory: Dyspnea, sore throat, bronchitis (1%); epistaxis, postnasal drip, pneumonia, hyperventilation, pulmonary congestion, wheezing, hypoxia, pharyngitis, pleurisy, pulmonary collapse, sleep apnea, snoring (≤ 1%).

Special senses: Cataract, eye irritation, vision blurred (1%); dry eyes, glaucoma, earache, tinnitus, blepharitis, decreased hearing, retinal hemorrhage, otitis externa, otitis media, bad taste, conjunctival hemorrhage, ear buzzing, motion sickness, spots before eyes (≤ 1%).

DONEPEZIL HCl

Overdosage:

Symptoms: Overdosage with cholinesterase inhibitors can result in cholinergic crisis characterized by severe nausea, vomiting, salivation, sweating, bradycardia, hypotension, respiratory depression, collapse and convulsions. Increasing muscle weakness is a possibility and may result in death if respiratory muscles are involved.

Treatment: As in any case of overdose, use general supportive measures. Tertiary anticholinergics such as atropine may be used as an antidote for donepezil overdosage. Intravenous atropine sulfate titrated to effect is recommended: An initial dose of 1 to 2 mg IV with subsequent doses based upon clinical response. Atypical responses in blood pressure and heart rate have been reported with other cholinomimetics when co-administered with quarternary anticholinergics such as glycopyrrolate. It is not known whether donepezil or its metabolites can be removed by dialysis (hemodialysis, peritoneal dialysis or hemofiltration).

Administration and Dosage:

The dosages of donepezil are 5 and 10 mg once per day.

The higher dose of 10 mg did not provide a statistically significant clinical benefit greater than that of 5 mg. There is a suggestion, however, based upon order of group mean scores and dose trend analyses of data, that a daily dose of 10 mg donepezil might provide additional benefit for some patients. Do not increase to 10 mg until patients have been on a daily dose of 5 mg for 4 to 6 weeks.

Take donepezil in the evening, just prior to retiring.

Donepezil may be taken with or without food.

Storage/Stability: Store at controlled room temperature, 15° to 30°C (59° to 86°F).

Rx	**Aricept** (Eisai/Pfizer)	**Tablets:** 5 mg	White. (5/E 245). In 30s and UD blister pack 100s.
		10 mg	Yellow. (10/E 246). In 30s and UD blister pack 100s.

METHYLPHENIDATE HCl

Actions:

Pharmacology: A mild CNS stimulant with actions similar to the amphetamines. The exact mechanism of action is not fully understood.

Pharmacokinetics: Methylphenidate is rapidly and well absorbed from the GI tract. Peak plasma levels occur in children in 4.7 hours for the sustained release (SR) tablets and 1.9 hours for the regular tablets. Plasma half-life ranges from 1 to 3 hours, but pharmacologic effects persist for 4 to 6 hours. About 80% of a dose is metabolized to ritalinic acid and excreted in urine. In adult patients who received SR tablets, plasma concentrations of methylphenidate's major metabolite appear to be greater in females than in males. SR tablets are more slowly but as extensively absorbed as regular tablets. Relative bioavailability of SR tablets compared with the regular tablet was 105% in children and 101% in adults. In children, an average of 67% of a dose was excreted vs 86% in adults.

Indications:

Attention deficit disorders: As part of a total treatment program in children with a behavioral syndrome characterized by moderate to severe distractibility, short attention span, hyperactivity, emotional lability and impulsivity.

Stimulants are not for the child who exhibits symptoms secondary to environmental factors or primary psychiatric disorders, including psychosis. When symptoms are associated with acute stress reactions, methylphenidate is usually not indicated.

Narcolepsy.

Unlabeled uses: Some success has been reported in the treatment of depression in elderly, cancer and post-stroke patients.

Has been used with variable success in treating anesthesia-related hiccups.

Contraindications:

Marked anxiety, tension and agitation because the drug may aggravate these symptoms; hypersensitivity to methylphenidate; glaucoma; motor tics or a family history or diagnosis of Tourette's syndrome; severe depression of either exogenous or endogenous origin; for the prevention or treatment of normal fatigue states.

Warnings:

Seizure disorders: Methylphenidate may lower the convulsive threshold in patients with history of seizures, with prior EEG abnormalities in absence of seizures and, very rarely, in the absence of history of seizures and no prior EEG evidence of seizures. Safe concomitant use with anticonvulsants has not been established. If seizures occur, discontinue the drug.

Hypertension: Use cautiously; monitor blood pressure in all patients, especially those with hypertension.

Visual disturbances have been encountered rarely. Difficulties with accommodation and blurring of vision have been reported.

Carcinogenesis: In a lifetime carcinogenicity study of mice, methylphenidate caused an increase in hepatocellular adenomas and, in males only, an increase in hepatoblastomas, at a daily dose of $\approx$ 60 mg/kg/day.

Pregnancy: Category C. Use in women of childbearing age only when clearly needed and when potential benefits outweigh potential hazards to the fetus. In the small numbers of patients reported who received methylphenidate during their pregnancy, no evidence of increased malformation rate was found.

Lactation: Safety for use in the nursing mother has not been established.

Children: Do not use in children < 6 years old because safety and efficacy have not been established. In psychotic children, the drug may exacerbate symptoms of behavior disturbance and thought disorder. Precipitation of Tourette's syndrome has been reported following the initiation of methylphenidate therapy.

Safety and efficacy of long-term use in children are not established. Although a causal relationship has not been established, suppression of growth (eg, weight gain or height) has been reported with long-term use of stimulants in children. Carefully monitor patients on long-term therapy.

Precautions:

Monitoring: Perform periodic CBC, differential and platelet counts during prolonged therapy.

Agitation: Patients with an element of agitation may react adversely; discontinue therapy if necessary.

Prescribing: Drug treatment is not indicated in all cases of this behavioral syndrome; consider only in light of the complete history and evaluation of the child. The decision to prescribe methylphenidate should depend on the physician's assessment of the chronicity and severity of the child's symptoms and their appropriateness for

METHYLPHENIDATE HCl

his or her age. Prescription should not depend solely on the presence of one or more of the behavioral characteristics.

Acute stress: When symptoms are associated with acute stress reactions, treatment with methylphenidate is usually not indicated.

Drug abuse and dependence: Give cautiously to emotionally unstable patients, such as those with a history of drug dependence or alcoholism, because such patients may increase dosage on their own initiative.

Chronic abuse can lead to marked tolerance and psychic dependence with abnormal behavior. Frank psychotic episodes can occur, especially with parenteral abuse. Carefully supervise drug withdrawal because severe depression as well as the effects of chronic overactivity can be unmasked. Long-term follow-up may be required.

Drug Interactions:

Methylphenidate Drug Interactions

Precipitant drug	Object drug*		Description
Methylphenidate	Guanethidine	⬇	Antihypertensive effect of guanethidine may be decreased by concurrent methylphenidate. This interaction may be dose-dependent. Avoid this combination when possible.
Methylphenidate	Phenytoin	⬆	Serum phenytoin levels may be increased, resulting in an increase in the pharmacologic and toxic effects of phenytoin.
Methylphenidate	Tricyclic antidepressants	⬆	Coadministration may cause increased serum concentration of tricyclic antidepressants.
Monamine oxidase inhibitors (MAOIs)	Methylphenidate	⬆	Pharmacologic effects of methylphenidate may be increased by concurrent use of these agents. Headache, GI symptoms and hypertension may occur. The effects may occur up to several weeks after discontinuation of the MAOIs. If hypertension occurs, administer phentolamine.

* ⬇ = Object drug decreased. ⬆ = Object drug increased.

Adverse Reactions:

Hypersensitivity: Skin rash; urticaria; fever; arthralgia; exfoliative dermatitis; erythema multiforme with necrotizing vasculitis; thrombocytopenic purpura.

CNS: Dizziness; headache; dyskinesia; drowsiness; Tourette's syndrome (rare); toxic psychosis.

Cardiovascular: Blood pressure and pulse changes, increased and decreased; tachycardia; angina; cardiac arrhythmias; palpitations.

GI: Anorexia; nausea; abdominal pain; weight loss during prolonged therapy.

Miscellaneous:

Most common – Nervousness and insomnia, usually controlled by reducing dosage and omitting the drug in the afternoon or evening.

Other (causal relationship not established) – Leukopenia; anemia; scalp hair loss; abnormal liver function, ranging from transaminase elevation to hepatic coma; cerebral arteritis or occlusion; transient depressed mood; fixed drug eruption (rare).

Children – Loss of appetite, abdominal pain, weight loss during prolonged therapy, insomnia and tachycardia may occur more frequently; however, any of the other adverse reactions listed above may also occur.

Overdosage:

Symptoms: Symptoms result principally from CNS overstimulation and excessive sympathomimetic effects and include: Vomiting; agitation; tremors; hyperreflexia; muscle twitching; convulsions (may be followed by coma); euphoria; confusion; hallucinations; delirium; sweating; flushing; headache; hyperpyrexia; tachycardia; palpitations; cardiac arrhythmias; hypertension; mydriasis; dry mucous membranes.

Treatment: Treatment consists of supportive measures. Protect the patient against self-injury and against external stimuli that would aggravate overstimulation. If signs and symptoms are not too severe and the patient is conscious, evacuate gastric contents by emesis or gastric lavage. In severe intoxication, use a carefully titrated dosage of a short-acting barbiturate before gastric lavage. Other measures to detoxify the gut include administration of activated charcoal and a cathartic. Maintain adequate circulation and respiratory exchange; external cooling procedures may be

METHYLPHENIDATE HCl

required for hyperpyrexia. Efficacy of peritoneal dialysis or extracorporeal hemodialysis has not been established.

Patient Information:

Take last daily dose early in the evening (prior to 6 p.m.) to avoid insomnia. It is often recommended that methylphenidate be taken 30 to 45 minutes before meals.

May mask symptoms of fatigue, impair physical coordination or produce dizziness or drowsiness. Use caution while driving or performing other tasks requiring alertness.

Notify physician of nervousness, insomnia, palpitations, vomiting, fever or skin rash.

Do not crush or chew SR medication.

Administration and Dosage:

Adults: Individualize dosage. Administer in divided doses 2 or 3 times daily, preferably 30 to 45 minutes before meals. Average dose is 20 to 30 mg/day. Dosage ranges from 10 to 15 mg/day up to 40 to 60 mg/day. In patients who are unable to sleep if medication is taken late in the day, take the last dose before 6 p.m.

Children (≥ 6): Start with small doses (eg, 5 mg before breakfast and lunch) with gradual increments of 5 to 10 mg weekly. Daily dosage > 60 mg is not recommended. If improvement is not observed after dosage adjustment over 1 month, discontinue use. If paradoxical aggravation of symptoms or other adverse effects occurs, reduce dosage or discontinue the drug.

Discontinue periodically to assess condition. Improvement may be sustained when the drug is either temporarily or permanently discontinued. Drug treatment should not be indefinite and usually may be discontinued after puberty.

All patients: SR tablets have a duration of ≈ 8 hours and may be used in place of regular tablets when the 8-hour dosage of the SR tablets corresponds to the titrated 8-hour dosage of the regular tablets. SR tablets must be swallowed whole, never crushed or chewed.

Storage/Stability: Do not store > 30°C (86°F). Protect from moisture. Dispense in a tight, light-resistant container.

c-II	**Methylphenidate HCl** (Various, eg, Goldline, Major, Parmed, Purepac, Qualitest, Rugby, Schein)	**Tablets:** 5 mg	In 100s and 1000s.
c-II	**Ritalin** (Ciba-Geigy)		Lactose. (CIBA 7). Yellow. In 100s.
c-II	**Methylphenidate HCl** (Various, eg, Goldline, Major, Parmed, Purepac, Qualitest, Rugby, Schein)	**Tablets:** 10 mg	In 100s and 1000s.
c-II	**Ritalin** (Ciba-Geigy)		Lactose. (CIBA 3). Pale green, scored. In 100s.
c-II	**Methylphenidate HCl** (Various, eg, Goldline, Major, Parmed, Purepac, Qualitest, Rugby, Schein)	**Tablets:** 20 mg	In 100s and 1000s.
c-II	**Ritalin** (Ciba-Geigy)		Lactose. (CIBA 34). Pale yellow, scored. In 100s.
c-II	**Methylphenidate** (Various, eg, Goldline, Major, Parmed, Purepac, Qualitest, Rugby, Schein)	**Tablets, sustained release:** 20 mg	In 100s.
c-II	**Ritalin-SR** (Ciba-Geigy)		Lactose. Dye free. (CIBA 16). White. In 100s.

PEMOLINE

Actions:

Pharmacology: Pemoline is a CNS stimulant. Although structurally dissimilar from the amphetamines and methylphenidate, it has pharmacologic activity similar to that of other stimulants but with minimal sympathomimetic effects. Although the exact mechanism of action is unknown, pemoline may act through dopaminergic mechanisms.

Pharmacokinetics: Pemoline is rapidly absorbed from the GI tract. Approximately 50% is protein bound. Peak serum levels occur within 2 to 4 hours after ingestion of a single dose. The serum half-life is approximately 12 hours; however, in two studies of 35 children 5 to 12 years of age, the mean half-life ranged from 7 to 8.6 hours. Steady state is reached in approximately 2 to 3 days. Pemoline is metabolized by the liver and is primarily excreted by the kidneys. Approximately 50% is excreted unchanged and only minor fractions are present as metabolites. The drug is widely distributed throughout body tissues, including the brain.

Pemoline has a gradual onset of action. Using the recommended schedule of dosage titration, significant clinical benefit may not be evident until the third or fourth week of drug administration.

Indications:

Attention deficit disorder: As part of a total treatment program in children with a behavioral syndrome characterized by moderate to severe distractibility, short attention span, hyperactivity, emotional lability and impulsivity.

Unlabeled uses: Pemoline 50 to 200 mg/day in two divided doses has been used in the treatment of narcolepsy and excessive daytime sleepiness.

Contraindications:

Known hypersensitivity or idiosyncrasy to pemoline; hepatic insufficiency.

Warnings:

Renal function impairment: Administer with caution to patients with significantly impaired renal function.

Pregnancy: Category B. There are no adequate and well controlled studies in pregnant women. Use pemoline during pregnancy only if clearly needed. Studies in rats have shown an increased incidence of stillbirths and cannibalization when pemoline was administered at a dose of 37.5 mg/kg/day. Postnatal survival was reduced at doses of 18.75 and 37.5 mg/kg/day.

Lactation: It is not known whether pemoline is excreted in breast milk. Exercise caution when administering pemoline to a nursing woman.

Children: Safety and efficacy in children under 6 years of age have not been established.

In psychotic children, administration may exacerbate symptoms of behavior disturbance and thought disorder. CNS stimulants, including pemoline, can precipitate motor and phonic tics and Tourette's syndrome. Therefore, clinical evaluation for tics and Tourette's syndrome in children and their families should precede use of stimulants.

Chronic administration may be associated with growth inhibition; therefore, monitor growth during treatment. Long-term effects in children have not been well established.

Treatment is not indicated in all cases of attention deficit disorder with hyperactivity; consider therapy only in light of complete history and evaluation of the child. The decision to prescribe pemoline should depend on the assessment of the chronicity and severity of the child's symptoms and their appropriateness for his or her age, and not depend solely on the presence of one or more of the behavioral characteristics.

Precautions:

Hepatic effects: Perform liver function tests prior to and periodically during therapy. Discontinue use if abnormalities are revealed and confirmed by follow-up tests (see Adverse Reactions).

Drug abuse and dependence: The pharmacologic similarity of pemoline to other psychostimulants with known dependence liability suggests that psychological or physical dependence might occur. There have been isolated reports of transient psychotic symptoms occurring in adults following the long-term misuse of excessive oral doses. Give with caution to emotionally unstable patients who may increase the dosage on their own initiative.

PEMOLINE

Adverse Reactions:

Mild adverse reactions early in treatment often remit with continuing therapy.

If adverse reactions are significant or protracted, reduce dosage or discontinue drug.

Body as a whole:

Most frequent – Insomnia usually occurs early in therapy prior to optimum therapeutic response; it is often transient or responds to dosage reduction.

CNS: Dyskinetic movements of tongue, lips, face and extremities; Tourette's syndrome; abnormal oculomotor function (eg, nystagmus and oculogyric crisis); convulsive seizures; increased irritability; mild depression; dizziness; headache; drowsiness; hallucinations.

GI: Anorexia with weight loss may occur during the first weeks. In most cases it is transient; weight gain usually resumes within 3 to 6 months. Stomachache; nausea.

GU: A case of elevated acid phosphatase in association with prostatic enlargement occurred in a 63-year-old male who received pemoline for sleepiness. The acid phosphatase normalized with discontinuation of pemoline and was again elevated with rechallenge.

Hepatic: Hepatic dysfunction including elevated liver enzymes, hepatitis and jaundice has occurred. Elevated liver enzymes are not rare and appear reversible upon drug discontinuance. Most patients with elevated liver enzymes were asymptomatic. Although no causal relationship has been established, two hepatic-related fatalities occurred in patients taking pemoline.

Miscellaneous: Skin rashes; growth suppression with long-term use of stimulants in children; aplastic anemia (rare).

Overdosage:

Symptoms of acute overdosage result principally from CNS overstimulation and excessive sympathomimetic effects and include: Vomiting; agitation; tremors; hyperreflexia; muscle twitching; convulsions (may be followed by coma); euphoria; confusion; hallucinations; delirium; sweating; flushing; headache; hyperpyrexia; tachycardia; hypertension; mydriasis.

Other – Overactivity, irregular respiration, increased salivation, intermittent tongue protrusion, generalized hyperreflexia and severe choreoathetosis with rhabdomyolysis have occurred.

Treatment consists of appropriate supportive measures. Protect the patient against self-injury and external stimuli that would aggravate overstimulation already present. If symptoms are not too severe and the patient is conscious, gastric contents may be evacuated. Chlorpromazine is reported useful in decreasing CNS stimulation and sympathomimetic effects.

Efficacy of peritoneal dialysis or extracorporeal hemodialysis for pemoline overdosage is not established.

Patient Information:

Take daily dose in the morning.

If dizziness occurs, use caution when performing tasks requiring alertness.

Notify physician if insomnia occurs and continues.

Administration and Dosage:

Administer as a single dose each morning. Recommended starting dose is 37.5 mg/day. Gradually increase at 1 week intervals using increments of 18.75 mg until desired response is obtained. Mean effective doses range from 56.25 to 75 mg/day. Maximum recommended dose is 112.5 mg/day.

Clinical improvement is gradual; significant benefit may not be evident until week 3 or 4 of administration.

Interrupt drug administration occasionally to determine if there is a recurrence of behavioral symptoms sufficient to require continued therapy.

c-iv	**Cylert** (Abbott)	**Tablets:** 18.75 mg	(TH). White, scored. In 100s.
		37.5 mg	(TI). Orange, scored. In 100s.
		75 mg	(TJ). Tan, scored. In 100s.
		Tablets, chewable: 37.5 mg	(TK). Orange, scored. In 100s.

AMPHETAMINES

Amphetamine, dextroamphetamine and methamphetamine are also indicated for attention deficit disorders in children, as part of a total treatment program.

For complete prescribing information on the amphetamines for this and other uses, consult the general amphetamine monograph.

Psychotherapeutic Combinations

MEPROBAMATE AND BENACTYZINE HCl

Actions:

Pharmacology: In the following combination:

MEPROBAMATE is used for its antianxiety effect. (For complete prescribing information refer to the general Antianxiety Agent monograph.)

BENACTYZINE HCl is a mild antidepressant and anticholinergic agent which in animals reduces the autonomic response to emotion-provoking stress.

Indications:

"Possibly effective" in the management of depression, both acute (reactive) and chronic. Useful in the less severe depressions and where the depression is accompanied by anxiety, insomnia, agitation or rumination. Also useful for managing depression and associated anxiety accompanying or related to organic illnesses. Final classification of this indication requires further investigation.

Contraindications:

Acute intermittent porphyria; glaucoma; allergic or idiosyncratic reactions to meprobamate, benactyzine or related compounds.

Precautions:

Tartrazine sensitivity: This product contains tartrazine, which may cause an allergic-type reaction (including bronchial asthma) in susceptible individuals. Although incidence of sensitivity is low, it is frequently seen in patients with aspirin hypersensitivity.

Adverse Reactions:

Nausea, dry mouth and other GI symptoms; syncope; severe nervousness and loss of power of concentration (one case each).

The following side effects, which have occurred after administration of the components alone, have either occurred or might occur when the combination is taken.

Benactyzine hydrochloride (particularly in high dosage): Dizziness; thought-blocking; depersonalization; aggravation of anxiety; disturbance of sleep patterns; a subjective feeling of muscle relaxation; blurred vision; dry mouth; failure of visual accommodation; gastric distress; allergic response; ataxia; euphoria.

Meprobamate:

CNS – Drowsiness; ataxia; dizziness; slurred speech; headache, vertigo; weakness; paresthesias; impairment of visual accommodation; euphoria; overstimulation; paradoxical excitement; fast EEG activity.

GI – Nausea; vomiting; diarrhea.

Cardiovascular – Palpitations; tachycardia; arrhythmias; transient ECG changes; syncope; hypotensive crises (including one fatal case).

Hypersensitivity – Reactions are usually seen within the first to fourth dose in patients having no previous contact with the drug. Milder reactions are characterized by an itchy, urticarial, or erythematous maculopapular rash which may be generalized or confined to the groin. Other reactions include: Leukopenia; acute nonthrombocytopenic purpura; petechiae; ecchymoses; eosinophilia; peripheral edema; adenopathy; fever; fixed drug eruption with cross reaction to carisoprodol.

More severe hypersensitivity reactions (rare): Hyperpyrexia; chills; angioneurotic edema; bronchospasm; oliguria; anuria; anaphylaxis; erythema multiforme; exfoliative dermatitis; stomatitis; proctitis; Stevens-Johnson syndrome; bullous dermatitis, including one fatal case following meprobamate with prednisolone.

Treatment: In case of allergic or idiosyncratic reactions to meprobamate, discontinue the drug and initiate appropriate symptomatic therapy, which may include epinephrine, antihistamines, and in severe cases corticosteroids. In evaluating possible allergic reactions, also consider allergy to excipients.

Hematologic – Agranulocytosis and aplastic anemia (rarely fatal, no causal relationship established); thrombocytopenic purpura (rare).

Miscellaneous – Exacerbation of porphyric symptoms.

Administration and Dosage:

Adults: One tablet 3 or 4 times daily. May gradually increase to a maximum of 6 tablets daily. Gradually reduce dosage to maintenance level when relief is achieved. Doses above 6 tablets daily are not recommended, although higher doses have been used to control depression and in chronic psychotic patients.

Children: Not intended for use in children.

c-iv	**Deprol** (Wallace)	**Tablets**: 400 mg meprobamate, 1 mg benactyzine HCl	Tartrazine. Light pink, scored. In 100s and 500s.

Psychotherapeutic Combinations

CHLORDIAZEPOXIDE AND AMITRIPTYLINE

Consider the prescribing information for chlordiazepoxide in the Antianxiety Agents monograph and amitriptyline in the Antidepressants monograph.

Indications:

Treatment of moderate to severe depression associated with moderate to severe anxiety. The therapeutic response to this combination has occurred earlier and with fewer treatment failures than when either ingredient is used alone. Symptoms likely to respond in the first week of treatment include: Insomnia; feelings of guilt or worthlessness; agitation; psychic and somatic anxiety; suicidal ideation; anorexia.

Contraindications:

Hypersensitivity to either benzodiazepines or tricyclic antidepressants; concomitant monoamine oxidase inhibitors (MAOIs; see Drug Interactions); during the acute recovery phase following myocardial infarction.

Drug Interactions:

MAOIs: Hyperpyretic crises, severe convulsions and deaths have occurred in patients receiving a tricyclic antidepressant and an MAOI simultaneously. When it is desired to replace an MAOI with this combination, allow a minimum of 14 days to elapse after the former is discontinued. Cautiously initiate this combination with a gradual increase in dosage until optimum response is achieved.

Patient Information:

May cause drowsiness or dizziness; use caution while driving or performing other tasks requiring alertness.

Avoid alcohol and other CNS depressants.

Consult a physician before either increasing the dose or abruptly discontinuing the drug.

Administration and Dosage:

Initially, administer 10 mg chlordiazepoxide with 25 mg amitriptyline 3 or 4 times daily in divided doses; increase to 6 times daily, as required. Some patients respond to smaller doses and can be maintained on 2 tablets daily.

After a satisfactory response is obtained, reduce dosage to smallest amount needed. The larger portion of the total daily dose may be taken at bedtime. In some patients, a single dose at bedtime may be sufficient. In general, lower dosages are recommended for elderly patients.

C-IV	**Chlordiazepoxide and Amitriptyline** (Various, eg, Geneva, Goldline, Lederle, Lemmon, Major, Moore, Par, Rugby, Schein)	**Tablets:** 5 mg chlordiazepoxide and 12.5 mg amitriptyline	In 100s and 500s.
C-IV	**Chlordiazepoxide and Amitriptyline** (Various, eg, Geneva, Goldline, Lederle, Lemmon, Major, Moore, Par, Rugby, Schein)	**Tablets:** 10 mg chlordiazepoxide and 25 mg amitriptyline	In 100s and 500s.
C-IV	**Limbitrol DS 10-25** (Roche)		(Limbitrol DS). White. Film coated. In 100s, 500s, unit-of-use 50s and UD 100s.

Psychotherapeutic Combinations

PERPHENAZINE AND AMITRIPTYLINE HCl

Consider the prescribing information for perphenazine in the Antipsychotic Agents monograph and amitriptyline in the Antidepressants monograph.

Indications:

Treatment of moderate to severe anxiety or agitation and depressed mood; patients with depression in whom anxiety or agitation are moderate or severe; patients with anxiety and depression associated with chronic physical disease; patients in whom depression and anxiety cannot be clearly differentiated; schizophrenic patients who have associated symptoms of depression.

Many patients presenting symptoms such as agitation, anxiety, insomnia, psychomotor retardation, functional somatic complaints, tiredness, loss of interest and anorexia have responded well to this combination.

Patient Information:

May cause drowsiness or dizziness, and response to alcohol and other CNS depressants may be enhanced. Use caution while driving or performing other tasks requiring alertness.

Administration and Dosage:

Initially, 2 to 4 mg perphenazine with 10 to 50 mg amitriptyline, 3 or 4 times daily. After a satisfactory response is noted, reduce to smallest amount necessary to obtain relief. Not recommended for use in children.

Rx	**Perphenazine/ Amitriptyline** (Various, eg, Bolar, Geneva, Goldline, Lemmon, Par, Rugby, Schein, Zenith)	**Tablets:** 2 mg perphenazine and 10 mg amitriptyline	In 21s, 100s, 500s and 1000s.
Rx	**Etrafon 2-10** (Schering)		(Schering ANA or 287). Yellow. In 100s, 500s, UD 100s.
Rx	**Triavil 2-10** (MSD)		(MSD 914). Blue. Film coated. In 100s, 500s, UD 100s.
Rx	**Perphenazine/ Amitriptyline** (Various, eg, Bolar, Geneva, Goldline, Lemmon, Par, Rugby, Schein, Zenith)	**Tablets:** 2 mg perphenazine and 25 mg amitriptyline	In 100s, 500s and 1000s.
Rx	**Etrafon** (Schering)		(Schering ANC or 598). Pink. Sugar coated. In 100s, 500s, UD 100s.
Rx	**Triavil 2-25**(MSD)		(MSD 921). Orange. Film coated. In 100s, 500s, UD 100s.
Rx	**Perphenazine/ Amitriptyline** (Various, eg, Bolar, Geneva, Goldline, Lemmon, Par, Rugby, Schein, Zenith)	**Tablets:** 4 mg perphenazine and 10 mg amitriptyline	In 100s, 250s, 500s and 1000s.
Rx	**Etrafon-A** (Schering)		(Schering ANB or 119). Orange. In 100s, 500s, UD 100s.
Rx	**Triavil 4-10**(MSD)		(MSD 934). Salmon. Film coated. In 100s, 500s, UD 100s.

Psychotherapeutic Combinations

PERPHENAZINE AND AMITRIPTYLINE HCl

Rx	**Perphenazine/ Amitriptyline** (Various, eg, Bolar, Geneva, Goldline, Lemmon, Par, Rugby, Schein, Zenith)	**Tablets:** 4 mg perphenazine and 25 mg amitriptyline	In 100s, 500s, 800s and 1000s.
Rx	**Etrafon-Forte** (Schering)		(Schering ANE or 720). Red. Sugar coated. In 100s, 500s, UD 100s.
Rx	**Triavil 4-25** (MSD)		(MSD 946). Yellow. Film coated. In 100s, 500s, UD 100s.
Rx	**Perphenazine/ Amitriptyline** (Various, eg, Bolar, Geneva, Goldline, Lemmon, Par, Rugby, Schein, Zenith)	**Tablets:** 4 mg perphenazine and 50 mg amitriptyline	In 100s and 250s.
Rx	**Triavil 4-50** (MSD)		(MSD 517). Orange. Film coated. In 60s, 100s, UD 100s.

ERGOLOID MESYLATES (Dihydrogenated Ergot Alkaloids, Dihydroergotoxine)

Actions:

Pharmacology: Ergoloid mesylates contain equal proportions of dihydroergocornine mesylate, dihydroergocristine mesylate and dihydroergocryptine mesylate.

The mechanism by which ergoloid mesylates produce mental effects is unknown. There is no conclusive evidence they directly affect cerebral arteriosclerosis or cerebrovascular insufficiency. Formerly, it was believed this drug caused cerebral vasodilation by alpha-adrenergic blockade; recent evidence suggests it may act primarily to increase brain metabolism, possibly increasing cerebral blood flow. It does not possess the vasoconstrictor properties of the natural ergot alkaloids.

Pharmacokinetics: Ergoloid mesylates are rapidly absorbed from the GI tract; peak plasma concentrations are achieved within 0.6 to 3 hours. The drug undergoes rapid first-pass biotransformation in the liver. Systemic bioavailability is approximately 6% to 25%. The liquid capsule has a 12% greater bioavailability than the oral tablet. The mean half-life of unchanged ergoloid in plasma is about 2.6 to 5.1 hours.

Clinical trials: In efficacy studies, modest but statistically significant changes were observed at the end of 12 weeks in the following parameters: Mental alertness, confusion, recent memory, orientation, emotional lability, self-care, depression, anxiety/fears, cooperation, sociability, appetite, dizziness, fatigue, bothersomeness and an overall impression of clinical status.

Indications:

Age-related mental capacity decline: Individuals over 60 years of age who manifest signs and symptoms of an idiopathic decline in mental capacity (ie, cognitive and interpersonal skills, mood, self-care, apparent motivation). Patients who respond suffer from some process related to aging or have some underlying dementing condition (ie, primary progressive dementia; Alzheimer's dementia; senile onset; multi-infarct dementia).

Contraindications:

Hypersensitivity to ergoloid mesylates.

Acute or chronic psychosis, regardless of etiology.

Precautions:

Before prescribing ergoloid mesylates, exclude the possibility that the patient's signs and symptoms arise from a potentially reversible and treatable condition. Exclude delirium and dementiform illness secondary to systemic disease, primary neurological disease or primary disturbance of mood.

Periodically reassess the diagnosis and the benefit of current therapy to the patient.

Do not chew or crush sublingual tablets.

Adverse Reactions:

Sublingual irritation; transient nausea; GI disturbances.

Patient Information:

May cause transient nausea and GI disturbances.

Allow sublingual tablets to completely dissolve under tongue.

Administration and Dosage:

The usual starting dose is 1 mg 3 times daily. Alleviation of symptoms is usually gradual; results may not be observed for 3 to 4 weeks. Doses up to 4.5 to 12 mg/day have been used. Up to 6 months of treatment may be necessary to determine efficacy, using doses of at least 6 mg/day.

ERGOLOID MESYLATES (Dihydrogenated Ergot Alkaloids, Dihydroergotoxine)

Rx	**Ergoloid Mesylates** (Various, eg, Bioline, Bolar, Dixon-Shane, Geneva, Goldline, Lederle, Major, Moore, Parmed, Qualitest)	**Tablets, sublingual:** 0.5 mg	In 100s, 500s, 1000s and UD 100s.
Rx	**Gerimal** (Rugby)		(Rugby 3859). White. In 100s, 500s and 1000s.
Rx	**Hydergine** (Sandoz)		(S Hydergine 0.5). White. In 100s and 1000s.
Rx	**Ergoloid Mesylates** (Various, eg, Cenci, Martec, R.I.D.)	**Tablets, oral:** 0.5 mg	In 100s and 1000s.
Rx	**Ergoloid Mesylates** (Various, eg, Bioline, Bolar, Dixon-Shane, Geneva, Goldline, Major, Moore, Parmed, Qualitest, Zenith)	**Tablets, sublingual:** 1 mg	In 100s, 500s, 1000s and UD 100s.
Rx	**Gerimal** (Rugby)		(Rugby 3857). White. In 100s, 500s and 1000s.
Rx	**Hydergine** (Sandoz)		(Hydergine 78-77). White. In 100s and 1000s.
Rx	**Ergoloid Mesylates** (Various, eg, Bioline, Bolar, Dixon-Shane, Geneva, Goldline, Lederle, Major, Moore, Parmed, Qualitest)	**Tablets, oral:** 1 mg	In 60s, 100s, 500s, 1000s and UD 32s, 100s and 1000s.
Rx	**Gerimal** (Rugby)		(Rugby 3856). White. In 100s, 500s and 1000s.
Rx	**Hydergine** (Sandoz)		(S Hydergine 1). White. In 100s, 500s and UD 100s and 500s.
Rx	**Hydergine LC** (Sandoz)	**Capsules, liquid:** 1 mg	(S Hydergine LC 1 mg). Off-white. In 100s, 500s and UD 100s and 500s.
Rx	**Hydergine** (Sandoz)	**Liquid:** 1 mg per ml	30% alcohol. In 100 ml with dropper.

SEDATIVE/HYPNOTICS, NONBARBITURATES

The following is a general discussion of nonbarbiturate sedative/hypnotics.

To facilitate comparison, the products are divided into two groups: The miscellaneous nonbarbiturates and the benzodiazepines. Although sedative doses can be given, these agents are primarily intended to be hypnotics (agents that produce drowsiness and facilitate sleep). Agents intended primarily for sedation or tranquilization are discussed in other parts of this chapter.

In the table below, some pharmacokinetic properties of the nonbarbiturate sedative/hypnotics are compared. Do not use this table to predict exact duration of effect, but use as a guide in drug selection.

Nonbarbiturate Sedative/Hypnotics Pharmacokinetic Parameters

Drug	Adult oral dose		Onset (min)	Duration of action (hrs)	Half-life (hrs)	Protein binding (%)	Urinary excretion, unchanged (%)
	Hypnotic	Sedative					
Miscellaneous nonbarbiturates							
Acetylcarbromal	nd	250-500 mg bid or tid	nd	nd	nd	nd	nd
Chloral hydrate	0.5-1 g	250 mg tid pc	30	nd	7-10[1]	35-41	nd
Ethchlorvynol	500 mg	100-200 mg bid or tid	15-60	5	10-20[2]	nd	40[3]
Glutethimide	250-500 mg	nd	30	4-8	10-12	50	< 2
Methyprylon	200-400 mg	50-100 mg up to qid	45	5-8	13-61	60	< 1
Paraldehyde	10-30 ml	5-10 ml	10-15	8-12	3.4-9.8	nd	small
Propiomazine	nd	10-20 mg	nd	nd	nd	nd	nd
Zolpidem	10 mg	na	nd	nd	≈ 2.5	92.5	0
Benzodiazepines							
Estazolam	1-2 mg	na	nd	nd	10-24	93	< 5
Flurazepam	15-30 mg	na	17	7-8	150-100[4]	97	< 1[4]
Quazepam	15 mg	na	nd	nd	25-41	> 95	trace
Temazepam	15-30 mg	na	nd	nd	10-17	98	1.5
Triazolam	0.125-0.5 mg	na	nd	nd	1.5-5.5	90	2

na – Not applicable. nd = No data.

[1] Trichloroethanol, the principal metabolite.

[2] In acute use, half-life of the distribution phase (1 to 3 hours) is more appropriate.

[3] Free and conjugated forms of the major metabolite, secondary alcohol of ethchlorvynol.

[4] Active metabolite, desalkylflurazepam.

Imidazopyridines

ZOLPIDEM TARTRATE

Actions:

Pharmacology: Zolpidem is a non-benzodiazepine hypnotic of the imidazopyridine class. Subunit modulation of the GABA receptor chloride channel macromolecular complex is hypothesized to be responsible for sedative, anticonvulsant, anxiolytic and myorelaxant drug properties. The major modulatory site of the GABA receptor complex is located on its alpha subunit and is referred to as the benzodiazepine (BZ) or omega receptor. At least three subtypes of the omega receptor have been identified. While zolpidem is a hypnotic agent with a chemical structure unrelated to benzodiazepines, barbiturates or other drugs with known hypnotic properties, it interacts with a GABA-BZ receptor complex and shares some of the pharmacological properties of the benzodiazepines. In contrast to the benzodiazepines, which non-selectively bind to and activate all three omega receptor subtypes, zolpidem in vitro binds the $omega_1$ receptor preferentially. This selective binding of zolpidem on the $omega_1$ receptor is not absolute, but it may explain the relative absence of myorelaxant and anticonvulsant effects in animal studies as well as the preservation of deep sleep (stage 3 through 4) in human studies of zolpidem at hypnotic doses.

Pharmacokinetics: The pharmacokinetic profile is characterized by rapid absorption from the GI tract and a short elimination half-life in healthy subjects. In a single-dose crossover study in 45 healthy subjects administered 5 and 10mg, the mean peak concentrations (C_{max}) were 59 (range, 29 to 113) and 121 (range, 58 to 272)ng/ml, respectively, occurring at a mean time (T_{max}) of 1.6 hours for both. The mean elimination half-life was 2.6 (range, 1.4 to 4.5) and 2.5 (range, 1.4 to 3.8) hours for the 5 and 10mg tablets, respectively. Zolpidem is converted to inactive metabolites that are eliminated primarily by renal excretion. Total protein binding was 92.5% and remained constant, independent of concentration between 40 and 790 ng/ml. Zolpidem did not accumulate in young adults following 20 mg/night for 2 weeks.

The half-life, bioavailability and C_{max} of zolpidem are increased in elderly patients and patients with hepatic function impairment (see Warnings). Food decreases the bioavailability and C_{max} of zolpidem (see Drug Interactions).

In patients with end stage renal failure, zolpidem was not hemodialyzable. No accumulation of unchanged drug appeared after 14 or 21 days. Zolpidem pharmacokinetics were not significantly different in renally impaired patients; therefore, no dosage adjustment is necessary in patients with compromised renal function. However, as a general precaution, closely monitor these patients.

Clinical trials:

Transient insomnia – Healthy adults experiencing transient insomnia during the first night in a sleep laboratory were evaluated in a double-blind, parallel-group, single-night trial comparing 2 doses of zolpidem (7.5 and 10 mg) and placebo. Both doses were superior to placebo on objective (polysomnographic) measures of sleep latency, sleep duration and number of awakenings.

Chronic insomnia – Adult outpatients with chronic insomnia were evaluated in a double-blind, parallel group, 5 week trial comparing 2 doses of zolpidem tartrate (10 and 15 mg) and placebo. On objective (polysomnographic) measures of sleep latency and sleep efficiency, zolpidem 15 mg was superior to placebo for all 5 weeks; zolpidem 10 mg was superior to placebo on sleep latency for the first 4 weeks and on sleep efficiency for weeks 2 and 4. Zolpidem was comparable to placebo on number of awakenings at both doses studied. Another group was evaluated in a double-blind, parallel-group, 4 week trial comparing 2 doses of zolpidem (10 and 15 mg) and placebo. Zolpidem 10 mg was superior to placebo on a subjective measure of sleep latency for all 4 weeks, and on subjective measures of total sleep time, number of awakenings, and sleep quality for the first treatment week. Zolpidem 15 mg was superior to placebo on a subjective measure of sleep latency for the first 3 weeks, on a subjective measure of total sleep time for the first week, and on number of awakenings and sleep quality for the first 2 weeks.

Next-day residual effects – There was no evidence of residual next-day effects seen with zolpidem in several studies utilizing the Multiple Sleep Latency Test (MSLT), the Digit Symbol Substitution Test (DSST) and patient ratings of alertness. In one study involving elderly patients, there was a small but statistically significant decrease in one measure of performance, the DSST, but no impairment was seen in the MSLT.

Rebound effects – There was no objective (polysomnographic) evidence of rebound insomnia at recommended doses in studies evaluating sleep on the nights following discontinuation of zolpidem. There was subjective evidence of impaired sleep in the elderly on the first post-treatment night at doses above the recommended elderly dose of 5 mg.

Imidazopyridines

ZOLPIDEM TARTRATE

Memory impairment – Two small studies utilizing objective measures of memory yielded little evidence for memory impairment following zolpidem. There was subjective evidence from adverse event data for anterograde amnesia occurring in association with the administration of zolpidem predominantly at doses > 10 mg.

Effects on sleep stages – In studies that measured the percentage of sleep time spent in each sleep stage, zolpidem generally preserves sleep stages. Sleep time spent in stage 3 to 4 (deep sleep) was found comparable to placebo with only inconsistent, minor changes in REM (paradoxical) sleep at the recommended dose.

Indications:

Insomnia: Short-term treatment.

Warnings:

Duration of therapy: Generally limit hypnotics to 7 to 10 days of use; re-evaluate the patient if they are to be taken for > 2 to 3 weeks. Do not prescribe in quantities exceeding a 1 month supply.

Psychiatric/physical disorder: Since sleep disturbances may be the presenting manifestation of a physical or psychiatric disorder, initiate symptomatic treatment of insomnia only after a careful evaluation of the patient. The failure of insomnia to remit after 7 to 10 days of treatment may indicate the presence of a primary psychiatric or medical illness which should be evaluated. Worsening of insomnia or the emergence of new thinking or behavior abnormalities may be the consequence of an unrecognized psychiatric or physical disorder. Such findings have emerged during the course of treatment with sedative/hypnotic drugs, including zolpidem. Because some of the important adverse effects of zolpidem appear to be dose-related, it is important to use the smallest possible effective dose, especially in the elderly.

A variety of abnormal thinking and behavior changes have occurred in association with the use of sedative/hypnotics. Some of these changes may be characterized by decreased inhibition (eg, aggressiveness and extroversion that seem out of character), similar to effects produced by alcohol and other CNS depressants. Other reported behavior changes have included bizarre behavior, agitation, hallucinations and depersonalization. Amnesia and other neuropsychiatric symptoms may occur unpredictably. In primarily depressed patients, worsening of depression, including suicidal thinking, has occurred with sedative/hypnotics.

It can rarely be determined with certainty whether a particular instance of the abnormal behaviors listed above are drug-induced, spontaneous in origin, or a result of an underlying psychiatric or physical disorder. Nonetheless, the emergence of any new behavioral sign or symptom of concern requires careful and immediate evaluation.

Abrupt discontinuation: Following the rapid dose decrease or abrupt discontinuation of sedative/hypnotics, signs and symptoms similar to those associated with withdrawal from other CNS-depressant drugs have occurred (see Precautions).

CNS-depressant effects: Zolpidem, like other sedative/hypnotic drugs, has CNS-depressant effects. Due to the rapid onset of action, only ingest immediately prior to going to bed. Caution patients against engaging in hazardous occupations requiring complete mental alertness, motor coordination or physical dexterity after ingesting the drug (ie, operating machinery or driving a motor vehicle), including potential impairment of the performance of such activities that may occur the day following ingestion of zolpidem. Zolpidem had additive effects when combined with alcohol; therefore, do not take with alcohol. Also caution patients about possible combined effects with other CNS-depressant drugs. Dosage adjustments may be necessary when zolpidem is administered with such agents because of the potentially additive effects.

Hepatic function impairment: The pharmacokinetics of zolpidem in eight patients with chronic hepatic insufficiency were compared to results in healthy subjects. Following a single 20 mg dose, mean C_{max} and area under the concentration-time curve (AUC) were found to be 2 times (250 vs 499 ng/ml) and 5 times (788 vs 4203 ng•hr/ml) higher, respectively, in the hepatically compromised patients; T_{max} did not change. The mean half-life in cirrhotic patients of 9.9 hrs (range, 4.1 to 25.8 hrs) was greater than that observed in healthy subjects of 2.2 hrs (range, 1.6 to 2.4 hrs). Modify dosing accordingly in patients with hepatic insufficiency (see Administration and Dosage).

ZOLPIDEM TARTRATE

Carcinogenesis/Fertility impairment: Zolpidem was administered to rats and mice for 2 years at dosages of 4, 18 and 80 mg/kg/day (26 to 876 times the maximum recommended human dose on a mg/kg basis). Renal liposarcomas were seen in 4/100 rats (3 males, 1 female) receiving 80 mg/kg/day and a renal lipoma was observed in one male rat at the 18mg/kg/day dose. Incidence rates of lipoma and liposarcoma for zolpidem were comparable to those seen in historical controls and the tumor findings are thought to be a spontaneous occurrence.

In a rat reproduction study, 100 mg/kg zolpidem resulted in irregular estrus cycles and prolonged precoital intervals, but there was no effect on male or female fertility after daily oral doses of 4 to 100mg.

Elderly: Closely monitor these patients. Impaired motor or cognitive performance after repeated exposure or unusual sensitivity to sedative/hypnotic drugs is a concern in the treatment of elderly or debilitated patients. Therefore, the recommended dosage is 5 mg in such patients (see Administration and Dosage) to decrease the possibility of side effects. This recommendation is based on several studies in which the mean C_{max}, half-life and AUC were significantly increased when compared to results in young adults. In one study of eight elderly subjects (> 70 years of age), the means for C_{max}, half-life and AUC significantly increased by 50% (255 vs 384 ng/ml), 32% (2.2 vs 2.9 hrs) and 64% (955 vs 1562 ng•hr/ml), respectively, compared to younger adults (20 to 40 years of age) following a single 20 mg dose. Zolpidem did not accumulate in elderly subjects following nightly oral dosing of 10 mg for 1 week.

Pregnancy: Category B. In rats, adverse maternal and fetal effects occurred at 20 and 100 mg/kg and included dose-related maternal lethargy and ataxia, and a dose-related trend to incomplete ossification of fetal skull bones. Underossification of various fetal bones indicates a delay in maturation and is often seen in rats treated with sedative/hypnotic drugs. In rabbits, dose-related maternal sedation and decreased weight gain occurred at all doses tested. At the high dose, 16 mg/kg, there was an increase in postimplantation fetal loss and underossification of sternebrae in viable fetuses. These fetal findings in rabbits are often secondary to reductions in maternal weight gain.

There are no adequate and well controlled studies in pregnant women. Use during pregnancy only if clearly needed. Children born of mothers taking sedative/hypnotic drugs may be at some risk for withdrawal symptoms from the drug during the postnatal period. In addition, neonatal flaccidity has been reported in infants born of mothers who received sedative/hypnotic drugs during pregnancy.

Lactation: Studies in lactating mothers indicate that the half-life of zolpidem is similar to that in young healthy volunteers (2.6 hrs). Between 0.004% and 0.019% of the total administered dose is excreted into breast milk, but the effect of zolpidem on the infant is unknown. In a rat study, zolpidem inhibited the secretion of milk. The use of zolpidem in nursing mothers is not recommended.

Children: Safety and efficacy in children < 18 years of age have not been established.

Precautions:

Respiratory depression: Although preliminary studies did not reveal respiratory depressant effects at hypnotic doses in healthy individuals, observe caution if zolpidem is prescribed to patients with compromised respiratory function, since sedative/hypnotics have the capacity to depress respiratory drive.

Renal function impairment: Data in end stage renal failure patients repeatedly treated with zolpidem did not demonstrate drug accumulation or alterations in pharmacokinetic parameters. No dosage adjustment in renally impaired patients is required; however, closely monitor these patients (see Pharmacokinetics).

Depression: As with other sedative/hypnotic drugs, administer zolpidem with caution to patients exhibiting signs or symptoms of depression. Suicidal tendencies may be present in such patients and protective measures may be required. Intentional overdosage is more common in this group of patients; therefore, prescribe the least amount of drug that is feasible for the patient at any one time.

ZOLPIDEM TARTRATE

Drug abuse and dependence: Studies of abuse potential in former drug abusers found that the effects of single doses of zolpidem 40 mg were similar, but not identical, to diazepam 20 mg, while zolpidem 10 mg was difficult to distinguish from placebo.

Sedative/hypnotics have produced withdrawal signs and symptoms following abrupt discontinuation. These reported symptoms range from mild dysphoria and insomnia to a withdrawal syndrome that may include abdominal and muscle cramps, vomiting, sweating, tremors and convulsions. Zolpidem does not reveal any clear evidence for withdrawal syndrome. Nevertheless, the following adverse events included in DSM-III-R criteria for uncomplicated sedative/hypnotic withdrawal were reported during US clinical trials with zolpidem following placebo substitution and occurred within 48 hours following last zolpidem treatment: Fatigue, nausea, flushing, lightheadedness, uncontrolled crying, emesis, stomach cramps, panic attack, nervousness, abdominal discomfort (≤ 1%).

Because individuals with a history of addiction to, or abuse of, drugs or alcohol are at risk of habituation and dependence, they should be under careful surveillance when receiving zolpidem or any other hypnotic.

Drug Interactions:

Drug/Food interactions: A study of 30 healthy volunteers compared the pharmacokinetics of zolpidem 10 mg when administered while fasting or 20 minutes after a meal. With food, mean AUC and C_{max} were decreased by 15% and 25%, respectively, while mean T_{max} was prolonged by 60% (from 1.4 to 2.2 hours). The half-life remained unchanged. For faster sleep onset, do not administer with or immediately after a meal.

Adverse Reactions:

Approximately 4% to 6% of patients who received zolpidem at all doses discontinued treatment because of an adverse clinical event. Events most commonly associated with discontinuation were daytime drowsiness (0.5% to 1.6%), amnesia (0.6%), dizziness (0.4% to 0.6%), headache (0.5% to 0.6%), nausea (0.6%) and vomiting (0.5%).

During short-term treatment (up to 10 nights) at doses up to 10 mg, the most commonly observed adverse events were as follows: Drowsiness (2%), dizziness (1%) and diarrhea (1%). During longer term treatment (28 to 35 nights) with doses up to 10 mg, the most commonly observed adverse events were dizziness (5%) and drugged feelings (3%).

Zolpidem Adverse Reactions (Short-Term Trials[1]) (%)

Adverse reaction	Zolpidem (≤ 10mg) (n = 685)	Placebo (n = 473)
Central and peripheral nervous system		
Headache	7	6
Drowsiness	2	—
Dizziness	1	—
GI		
Nausea	2	3
Diarrhea	1	—
Musculoskeletal		
Myalgia	1	2

[1] From a pool of 11 placebo controlled trials.

Imidazopyridines

ZOLPIDEM TARTRATE

Zolipidem Adverse Reactions (Long-Term Trials[1]) (%)		
Adverse reaction	Zolpidem (≤ 10 mg) (n =152)	Placebo (n = 161)
Body as a whole		
Allergy	4	1
Back pain	3	2
Influenza-like symptoms	2	—
Chest pain	1	—
Fatigue	1	2
Central and peripheral nervous system		
Headache	19	22
Drowsiness	8	5
Dizziness	5	1
Lethargy	3	1
Drugged feeling	3	—
Lightheaded	2	1
Depression	2	1
Abnormal dreams	1	—
Amnesia	1	—
Anxiety	1	1
Nervousness	1	3
Sleep disorder	1	—
GI		
Nausea	6	6
Dyspepsia	5	6
Diarrhea	3	2
Abdominal pain	2	2
Constipation	2	1
Anorexia	1	1
Vomiting	1	1
Musculoskeletal		
Myalgia	7	7
Arthralgia	4	4
Respiratory		
Upper respiratory infection	5	6
Sinusitis	4	2
Pharyngitis	3	1
Rhinitis	1	3
Other		
Rash	2	1
Urinary tract infection	2	2
Palpitation	2	—
Dry mouth	3	1
Infection	1	1

[1] Treatment of chronic insomnia for 28 to 35 nights.

Other adverse reactions reported with zolpidem are as follows:

Body as a whole: Asthenia, edema, falling, fever, malaise, trauma (0.1% to 1%); allergic reaction, allergy aggravated, abdominal body sensation, anaphylactic shock, face edema, hot flashes, increased ESR, pain, restless legs, rigors, tolerance increased, weight decrease (< 0.1%);menstrual disorder, vaginitis (0.1% to 1%); breast fibroadenosis/neoplasm/pain (< 0.1%).

Immunologic – Abscess, herpes simplex/zoster, otitis externa/media (< 0.1%).

Cardiovascular: Cerebrovascular disorder, hypertension, tachycardia (0.1% to 1%); arrhythmia, arteritis, circulatory failure, extrasystoles, hypertension, aggravated myocardial infarction, phlebitis, pulmonary embolism, pulmonary edema, varicose veins, ventricular tachycardia (< 0.1%).

Hematologic/Lymphatic: Anemia, hyperhemoglobinemia, leukopenia, lymphadenopathy, macrocytic anemia, purpura (0.1%).

Imidazopyridines

ZOLPIDEM TARTRATE

CNS: Ataxia, confusion, euphoria, insomnia, vertigo (> 1%); agitation, decreased cognition, detachment, difficulty concentrating, dysarthria, emotional lability, hallucination, hypoesthesia, migraine, paresthesia, sleeping (after daytime dosing), stupor, tremor (0.1% to 1%); abnormal thinking, aggressive reaction, appetite increased, decreased libido, delusion, dementia, depersonalization, dysphasia, feeling strange, hypotonia, hysteria, illusion, intoxicated feeling, leg cramps, manic reaction, neuralgia, neuritis, neuropathy, neurosis, panic attacks, paresis, personality disorder, somnambulism, suicide attempts, tetany, yawning (< 0.1%).

Autonomic nervous system – Increased sweating, pallor, postural hypotension (0.1% to 1%); altered saliva, flushing, glaucoma, hypotension, impotence, syncope, tenesmus (< 0.1%).

GI: Constipation, dysphagia, flatulence, gastroenteritis, hiccup (0.1% to 1%); enteritis, eructation, esophagospasm, gastritis, hemorrhoids, intestinal obstruction, rectal hemorrhage, tooth caries (< 0.1%).

Hepatic: Increased ALT (0.1% to 1%); abnormal hepatic function, bilirubinemia, increased AST (< 0.1%).

Metabolic/Nutritional: Hyperglycemia (0.1% to 1%); gout, hypercholesterolemia, hyperlipidemia, increased BUN, periorbital edema, thirst, weight decrease (< 0.1%).

Musculoskeletal: Arthritis (0.1% to 1%); arthrosis, muscle weakness, sciatica, tendinitis (< 0.1%).

Respiratory: Bronchitis, coughing, dyspnea (0.1% to 1%); bronchospasm, epistaxis, hypoxia, laryngitis, pneumonia (< 0.1%).

Dermatologic: Acne, bullous eruption, dermatitis, furunculosis, injection-site inflammation, photosensitivity reaction, urticaria (< 0.1%).

Special senses: Diplopia, vision abnormal (> 1%); eye irritation/pain, scleritis, taste perversion, tinnitus (0.1% to 1%); corneal ulceration, abnormal lacrimation, photopsia (< 0.1%).

GU: Cystitis, urinary incontinence (0.1% to 1%); acute renal failure, dysuria, micturition frequency, polyuria, pyelonephritis, renal pain, urinary retention (< 0.1%).

Reproductive: Menstrual disorder, vaginitis (0.1% to 1%); breast fibroadenosis/neoplasm/pain (< 0.1%).

Overdosage:

Symptoms: In reports of overdose with zolpidem alone, impairment of consciousness has ranged from somnolence to light coma. There was one case each of cardiovascular and respiratory compromise. Individuals have fully recovered from zolpidem overdoses up to 400 mg (40 times the maximum recommended dose). Overdose cases involving multiple CNS depressant agents, including zolpidem, have resulted in more severe symptomatology, including fatal outcomes.

Treatment: Employ general symptomatic and supportive measures along with immediate gastric lavage where appropriate. Administer IV fluids as needed. Refer to General Management of Acute Overdosage. Flumazenil may be useful; in one study it reversed the sedative/hypnotic effects of zolpidem; however, no significant alterations in zolpidem pharmacokinetics were found. Monitor hypotension and CNS depression; treat with appropriate medical intervention. Withhold sedating drugs following overdosage, even if excitation occurs. The value of dialysis in treating overdosage is not determined; hemodialysis studies in patients with renal failure receiving therapeutic doses have demonstrated that zolpidem is not dialyzable.

Patient Information:

May cause drowsiness; use caution when performing tasks requiring alertness, coordination or physical dexterity. Avoid alcohol and other CNS depressants while taking this drug.

Imidazopyridines

ZOLPIDEM TARTRATE

Administration and Dosage:

Adults: Individualize dosage. Usual dose is 10 mg immediately before bedtime. Downward dosage adjustment may be necessary when given with agents having known CNS depressant effects because of the potentially additive effects.

Elderly or debilitated patients may be especially sensitive to the effects of zolpidem. Patients with hepatic insufficiency do not clear the drug as rapidly as healthy individuals. An initial 5 mg dose is recommended in these patients.

Maximum dose: The total dose should not exceed 10 mg.

c-IV	**Ambien** (Searle)	**Tablets:** 5 mg	Lactose. (AMB 5 5401). Pink. Film coated. In 100s, 500s and UD 100s.
		10 mg	Lactose. (AMB 10 5421). White. Film coated. In 100s, 500s and UD 100s.

PARALDEHYDE

Actions:

Pharmacology: Paraldehyde, a polymer of acetaldehyde, is a colorless, bitter tasting liquid with a strong, unpleasant odor; it produces nonspecific, reversible depression of the CNS. With usual therapeutic doses, paraldehyde has little effect on respiration and blood pressure; large doses may cause respiratory depression and hypotension. It has generally been replaced by safer and more effective agents.

Pharmacokinetics:

Absorption/Distribution – The drug is rapidly absorbed after oral administration. Peak serum concentrations are attained 30 to 60 minutes following oral use. Paraldehyde acts rapidly, producing sleep within 10 to 15 minutes after a therapeutic dose; sleep lasts about 8 to 12 hours.

Metabolism/Excretion – Plasma half-life ranges from 3.4 to 9.8 hours. Approximately 70% to 80% of the drug is metabolized in the liver, 11% to 28% is exhaled unchanged via the lungs and a negligible amount is excreted in the urine. In hepatic disease, elimination rate is decreased and more drug is excreted through the lungs.

Indications:

Sedative and hypnotic. Also used to quiet the patient and to produce sleep in delirium tremens and in other psychiatric states characterized by excitement.

Contraindications:

Bronchopulmonary disease (excretion of the drug by the lungs); hepatic insufficiency (metabolized by the liver); gastroenteritis (especially if ulceration is present).

Warnings:

Mucous membrane irritation: Paraldehyde is irritating to mucous membranes and must be well diluted. Esophagitis, hemorrhagic gastritis and proctitis have occurred.

Hepatic function impairment: Patients with liver dysfunction may be more susceptible to effects of paraldehyde.

Pregnancy: Category C. Paraldehyde crosses the placenta and appears in the fetal circulation. It is not known whether the drug can cause fetal harm. Use during pregnancy only if potential benefits outweigh potential hazards to the fetus.

Labor – Use during labor may cause respiratory depression in the neonate.

Lactation: Problems in the nursing infant have not been documented; however, consider the risk-benefit.

Children: Safety and efficacy for use in children have not been established.

Precautions:

Strong, unpleasant breath: Although medically insignificant, paraldehyde has a strong odor that is imparted to the exhaled air for as long as 24 hours after ingestion. The patient is often unaware of the odor.

May be habit forming; avoid sudden withdrawal after chronic use.

Drug Interactions:

Disulfiram inhibits acetaldehyde dehydrogenase. Avoid concomitant use.

Adverse Reactions:

Prolonged use may result in addiction resembling alcoholism. Withdrawal may produce delirium tremens and vivid hallucinations. Several cases of metabolic acidosis have occurred in association with paraldehyde addiction, although the etiology is uncertain. Prolonged use may produce yellowing of eyes or skin (hepatitis).

Miscellaneous: Strong, unpleasant breath may occur (see Precautions).

PARALDEHYDE

Overdosage:

Symptoms: Death has occurred following 25 ml orally or 12 ml rectally. The hallmark of toxicity is metabolic acidosis; treat with IV sodium bicarbonate or sodium lactate. Clinical features are: Unconsciousness; coma; rapid, labored respirations; pulmonary hemorrhage; edema; irritation of the throat, stomach and rectum (enema); nausea; vomiting; esophagitis; hemorrhagic gastritis; hepatitis; renal damage; agitation; pseudoketosis; hyperacetaldehydemia; right heart dilation.

Treatment: Intensive support therapy is paramount. Support respiratory function, treat acidosis and protect the liver. Gastric lavage is inappropriate since the drug is rapidly absorbed after administration. Hemodialysis or peritoneal dialysis may be required to treat acidosis and to support renal function.

Patient Information:

May cause GI upset; take with food or mix with milk or iced fruit juice to improve taste.

Avoid alcohol and other sedatives while taking this drug.

May cause drowsiness; use caution while driving or performing tasks requiring alertness.

Do not use paraldehyde in any plastic container; do not dispense with a plastic spoon or syringe.

Discard any unused paraldehyde after opening bottle.

Do not use if liquid has a brownish color or a strong vinegar odor.

Administration and Dosage:

Hypnosis:

Adults –

Oral: 4 to 8 ml in milk or iced fruit juice to mask the taste and odor.

Delirium tremens: 10 to 35 ml may be necessary.

Rectal: Dissolve in oil as a retention enema. Mix 10 to 20 ml with 1 or 2 parts of olive oil or isotonic sodium chloride solution to avoid rectal irritation.

Children – 0.3 ml/kg orally or rectally.

Sedation:

Adults – 5 to 10 ml orally or rectally.

Children – 0.15 ml/kg orally or rectally

Stability and storage: Upon exposure to light and air, paraldehyde decomposes to acetaldehyde and oxidizes to acetic acid. Do not use if liquid has a brownish color or sharp odor of acetic acid. Keep away from heat, open flame or sparks. Paraldehyde solidifies at approximately 12°C (54°F) and must be liquefied before use. Do not store in direct sunlight or expose to temperatures above 25°C (77°F). Keep product covered in box until use. Discard unused portion. Do not use paraldehyde from a container that has been opened for longer than 24 hours.

c-iv	**Paral** (Forest)	**Liquid (Oral, Rectal)**	In 30 ml.
c-iv	**Paraldehyde** (Various, eg, J.T. Baker, Spectrum)	**Liquid (Oral, Rectal):** 1g per ml	In 30 ml.

CHLORAL HYDRATE

Actions:

Pharmacology: The mechanism of action by which the CNS is affected is not known. Hypnotic dosage produces mild cerebral depression and quiet, deep sleep. In therapeutic doses, chloral hydrate has little effect on respiration, blood pressure and reflexes. "Hangover" is less common than with most barbiturates and some benzodiazepines. It has generally been replaced by safer and more effective agents.

Pharmacokinetics: Chloral hydrate is readily absorbed and metabolized to trichloroethanol, the principal active metabolite. Trichloroethanol has a plasma half-life of 7 to 10 hours; plasma protein binding is 35% to 41%. The drug is converted in the liver and kidney to trichloroacetic acid and excreted in the urine and bile. Although inactive, trichloroacetic acid is 71% to 88% protein bound and can displace other acidic drugs from plasma protein binding sites.

Indications:

Nocturnal sedation; preoperative sedation to lessen anxiety and induce sleep without depressing respiration or cough reflex; in postoperative care and control of pain as an adjunct to opiates and analgesics; preventing or suppressing alcohol withdrawal symptoms (rectal).

Chloral hydrate is effective as a hypnotic only for short-term use; it loses much of its effectiveness for inducing and maintaining sleep after 2 weeks of use.

Contraindications:

Marked hepatic or renal impairment; severe cardiac disease; gastritis; hypersensitivity or idiosyncrasy to chloral derivatives.

Warnings:

Pregnancy: Category C. Safety for use during pregnancy has not been established. Chloral hydrate crosses the placenta; chronic use during pregnancy may cause withdrawal symptoms in the neonate. Congenital defects have not been reported. Use only when clearly needed and when potential benefits outweigh potential hazards to the fetus.

Lactation: Chloral hydrate is excreted in breast milk; use by nursing mothers may cause sedation in the infant.

Precautions:

Potentially hazardous tasks: May produce drowsiness; patients should observe caution while driving or performing other tasks requiring alertness.

Cardiac disease: Continued use of therapeutic doses does not have a deleterious effect on the heart. However, do not use large doses in patients with severe cardiac disease.

GI conditions: Avoid use in patients with esophagitis, gastritis or gastric or duodenal ulcers.

Acute intermittent porphyria attacks may be precipitated by chloral hydrate; use with caution in susceptible patients.

Drug dependency: Abuse: May be habit forming. Exercise caution in administering to patients prone to addiction. Slurred speech, incoordination, tremulousness and nystagmus should arouse suspicion. Drowsiness, lethargy and hangover are frequently observed from excessive drug intake.

Dependence – Prolonged use of large doses may result in psychic and physical dependence. Tolerance and psychologic dependence may develop by the second week of continued administration. Chloral hydrate addicts may take huge doses of the drug (up to 12 g nightly). Sudden withdrawal may result in CNS excitation with tremor, anxiety, hallucinations or even delirium, which may be fatal. Gastritis, skin eruptions and parenchymatous renal injury may also occur. Undertake withdrawal in a hospital using supportive therapy similar to that used for barbiturate withdrawal.

Skin/mucous membrane irritation: Chloral derivatives irritate the skin and mucous membranes; gastric necrosis has occurred following intoxicating doses.

Tartrazine sensitivity: Some of these products contain tartrazine, which may cause allergic-type reactions (including bronchial asthma) in susceptible individuals. Although the incidence of tartrazine sensitivity in the general population is low, it is frequently seen in patients who also have aspirin hypersensitivity. Specific products containing tartrazine are identified in the product listings.

CHLORAL HYDRATE

Drug Interactions:

Alcohol may have synergistic effects with chloral hydrate. With alcohol, there is mutual inhibition of metabolism in addition to the combined depressant effect. Disulfiram-like reactions (eg, increased respiration and pulse rate, flushing), although rare, have occurred. Avoid concomitant use.

Anticoagulants, oral: Hypoprothrombinemic effects may occur by displacement from protein binding sites. However, this effect is usually small and fleeting. Monitor prothrombin levels and adjust coumarin dose accordingly.

CNS depressants (eg, barbiturates, narcotics) may have additive CNS effects with chloral hydrate coadministration.

Furosemide: Administration of chloral hydrate followed by IV furosemide may result in sweating, hot flashes, tachycardia, hypertension, weakness and nausea.

Hydantoins: The elimination of phenytoin may be increased by concurrent chloral hydrate, possibly reducing its effectiveness.

Drug/Lab test interactions: Chloral hydrate may interfere with the **copper sulfate test** for glycosuria (confirm suspected glycosuria by a glucose oxidase test), **fluorometric tests** for urine catecholamines (do not administer medication for 48 hours preceding the test) or **urinary 17-hydroxycorticosteroid determinations** (when using the Reddy, Jenkins and Thorn procedure).

Adverse Reactions:

CNS: Somnambulism, disorientation, incoherence, paranoid behavior (occasional); excitement, delirium, drowsiness, staggering gait, ataxia, lightheadedness, vertigo, dizziness, nightmares, malaise, mental confusion, headache, hallucinations (rare).

Hematologic: Leukopenia, eosinophilia (occasional).

Dermatologic: Allergic skin rashes including hives, erythema, eczematoid dermatitis, urticaria, scarlatiniform exanthems (occasional).

GI: Gastric irritation; nausea and vomiting (occasional); flatulence; diarrhea; unpleasant taste in mouth.

Miscellaneous: Hangover, idiosyncratic syndrome, ketonuria (rare).

Overdosage:

Symptoms: Stupor; coma; pinpoint pupils; hypotension; slow or rapid and shallow respiration; hypothermia; areflexia; muscle flaccidity.

Corrosive action – Nausea; vomiting; esophagitis; gastritis; hemorrhagic gastritis; gastric necrosis; enteritis.

Organ damage – Hepatic damage (jaundice); renal damage (albuminuria); cardiac damage (ventricular and atrial arrhythmias).

Doses > 2 g may produce symptoms of toxicity. The toxic oral dose of chloral hydrate for adults is approximately 5 to 10 g; however, death has occurred following doses of 1.25 and 3 g; some patients have survived after taking 36 g.

Treatment: Perform gastric lavage or induce vomiting to empty the stomach. Activated charcoal may prevent drug absorption. Treatment includes usual supportive measures. Refer to General Management of Acute Overdosage. Hemoperfusion and hemodialysis are effective, but peritoneal dialysis is not useful. Hemodialysis is reported to promote the clearance of trichloroethanol.

Patient Information:

May cause GI upset. Take capsules with a full glass of water or fruit juice; swallow capsules whole – do not chew. Dilute syrup in a half glass of water or fruit juice.

May cause drowsiness; use caution when performing tasks requiring alertness. Avoid alcohol and other CNS depressants.

May be habit forming; do not discontinue the drug abruptly.

CHLORAL HYDRATE

Administration and Dosage:

Take capsules with a full glass of liquid. Administer syrup in glass of water, fruit juice or ginger ale.

Adults: Single doses or daily dosage should not exceed 2 g.

Hypnotic – 500 mg to 1 g 15 to 30 minutes before bedtime or 30 minutes before surgery.

Sedative – 250 mg 3 times daily after meals.

Children:

Hypnotic – 50 mg/kg/day, up to 1 g per single dose. May be given in divided doses.

Sedative – 25 mg/kg/day, up to 500 mg per single dose. May be given in divided doses.

Dental sedation – Higher doses than those suggested by the manufacturer are generally used. Doses of 75 mg/kg, supplemented by nitrous oxide may provide better sedation than the lower dose with no change in the vital signs or adverse effects.

c-iv	**Chloral Hydrate** (Various, eg, Balan, Dixon-Shane, Goldline, Lannett, Major, Moore, Roxane, Rugby, Schein, URL)	**Capsules**: 500 mg	In 100s, 500s, 1000s and UD100s.
c-iv	**Chloral Hydrate** (Various, eg, Pharmaceutical Assoc., Roxane)	**Syrup**: 250 mg per 5 ml	In UD 10 ml (40s and 100s).
c-iv	**Chloral Hydrate** (Various, eg, Balan, Dixon-Shane, Geneva, Lannett, Major, Roxane, Rugby, Schein, UDL, URL)	**Syrup**: 500 mg per 5 ml	In pt, gal and UD 5 ml (100s) and 10 ml (40s and 100s).
c-iv	**Aquachloral Supprettes** (Polymedica)	**Suppositories**: 324 mg	Tartrazine. In 12s.
c-iv	**Chloral Hydrate** (G & W)	**Suppositories**: 500 mg	In UD 100s.
c-iv	**Aquachloral Supprettes** (Polymedica)	**Suppositories**: 648 mg	In 12s.

Ureides

ACETYLCARBROMAL

Actions:

Pharmacology: Acetylcarbromal is a short-acting CNS depressant used as a daytime sedative and as a hypnotic. It releases free bromide which may lead to bromide intoxication. It is metabolized to urea and is readily eliminated. It has generally been replaced by safer, more effective products.

Indications:

Anxiety states; emotional stress; menopausal syndrome; premenstrual tension; insomnia; preoperative or pre-examination sedation; fears and psychogenic complications of organic illness; spastic colitis; postoperative and posttraumatic sedation.

Contraindications:

Sensitivity to bromides.

Warnings:

May be habit forming. Should not be used chronically.

Lactation: Bromides are excreted in breast milk and may cause drowsiness and symptoms of brominism in the nursing infant.

Adverse Reactions:

Large doses may cause drowsiness.

Overdosage:

Symptoms: Poisoning with the ureides occurs more often with chronic use than with acute ingestion. Brominism occurs with accumulation of the bromide ion and its displacement of chloride in body fluids. Symptoms related to the CNS, skin, exocrine glands and the GI tract include narcosis, respiratory depression, mental disturbances, impaired thought and memory, dizziness, irritability, dermatitis, conjunctivitis, headache, constipation and gastric distress. Bromide intoxication occurs when serum levels exceed 9 mEq/L.

Treatment: Treat mild to moderate poisoning by gastric lavage and forced diuresis. Chloride loading with sodium chloride (at least 6 g/day) or ammonium chloride is also useful. Use dialysis when salt loading is contraindicated, when diuresis is not achieved or when serum bromide levels exceed 20 mEq/L. Charcoal hemoperfusion may be effective. Refer also to General Management of Acute Overdosage.

Patient Information:

May cause drowsiness; use caution while driving or performing other tasks requiring alertness.

Avoid alcohol and other CNS depressants.

Administration and Dosage:

Adults: 250 to 500 mg 2 or 3 times daily.

Children: Administer proportionately less, according to age and weight.

Rx	**Paxarel** (Circle)	**Tablets:** 250 mg	In 100s.

Piperidine Derivatives

GLUTETHIMIDE

Actions:

Pharmacology: Produces CNS depression similar to the barbiturates. Glutethimide exhibits pronounced anticholinergic activity, which is manifested by mydriasis, inhibition of salivary secretions and decreased intestinal motility. It suppresses REM sleep and is associated with REM rebound. It has generally been replaced by safer and more effective agents.

Pharmacokinetics:

Absorption/Distribution – It is erraticallly absorbed from the GI tract. Following single oral doses of 500 mg, the peak plasma concentration occurs from 1 to 6 hours after administration. The average plasma half-life is 10 to 12 hours. About 50% of the drug is bound to plasma proteins. Glutethimide stimulates hepatic microsomal enzymes.

Metabolism/Excretion – Glutethimide is a racemate; both isomers are hydroxylated and then conjugated with glucuronic acid. The glucuronides pass into the enterohepatic circulation and are excreted in the urine (< 2% unchanged).

Indications:

For short-term relief of insomnia (3 to 7 days). Not indicated for chronic administration. Should insomnia persist, a drug free interval of 1 or more weeks should elapse before retreatment is considered. Attempt to find alternative nondrug therapy in chronic insomnia.

Contraindications:

Hypersensitivity to glutethimide; porphyria.

Warnings:

Physical and psychological dependence occur; carefully evaluate patients before prescribing glutethimide. Ordinarily, an amount adequate for 1 week is sufficient, then reevaluate the patient. Withdrawal symptoms include nausea, abdominal discomfort, tremors, convulsions and delirium. In the presence of dependence, reduce dosage gradually.

Pregnancy: Category C. It is not known whether glutethimide can cause fetal harm or can affect reproduction capacity. Give to a pregnant woman only if clearly needed. Newborn infants of mothers dependent on glutethimide may exhibit withdrawal symptoms.

Lactation: Because of the potential for serious adverse reactions in nursing infants, decide whether to discontinue nursing or to discontinue the drug, taking into account the importance of the drug to the mother.

Children: Safety and efficacy have not been established. Use is not recommended.

Precautions:

Hazardous tasks: May produce drowsiness; observe caution while driving or performing other tasks requiring alertness.

Drug Interactions:

Alcohol and CNS depressants (eg, barbiturates, narcotics): Additive CNS effects may occur when used concomitantly with glutethimide.

Anticoagulants, oral: Glutethimide induces hepatic microsomal enzymes, resulting in increased metabolism of the anticoagulant and possibly a decreased anticoagulant response.

Charcoal may prevent the GI absorption of glutethimide. Depending on the clinical situation, this will reduce the toxicity or effectiveness of glutethimide.

Adverse Reactions:

Clinical studies revealed the following effects: Skin rash (8.6%); nausea (2.7%); hangover (1.1%); drowsiness (1%). When a generalized skin rash occurs, withdraw the drug. The rash usually clears spontaneously, a few days after withdrawal.

The following occurred in < 1% of patients: Vertigo; headache; depression; dizziness; ataxia; confusion; edema; indigestion; lightheadedness; nocturnal diaphoresis; vomiting; dry mouth; euphoria; impaired memory; slurred speech; tinnitus.

Rare: Paradoxical excitation; blurred vision; acute hypersensitivity; porphyria; blood dyscrasia such as thrombocytopenic purpura, aplastic anemia and leukopenia.

GLUTETHIMIDE

Overdosage:

Acute overdosage: The lethal dose ranges from 10 to 20 g; patients have died from 5 g and other patients have recovered from single doses as high as 35 g. A single oral dose of 5 g usually produces severe intoxication. A plasma level of 3 mg/dl is indicative of severe poisoning. A lower level does not preclude the possibility of severe poisoning because of sequestration of the drug in body fat depots and in the GI tract. Serial plasma level determinations are mandatory for proper patient evaluation.

Symptoms are dose-dependent and indistinguishable from barbiturate intoxication. The degree of CNS depression often fluctuates, possibly due to irregular absorption of the drug or accumulation of an active toxic metabolite. Symptoms include: CNS depression, including coma (profound and prolonged in severe intoxication); hypothermia, which may be followed by fever; depressed or lost deep tendon reflexes; depression or absence of corneal and pupillary reflexes; dilation of pupils; depressed or absent response to painful stimuli; inadequate ventilation (even with relatively normal respiratory rate), sometimes with cyanosis; sudden apnea, especially with manipulation such as gastric lavage or endotracheal intubation; diminished or absent peristalsis. Severe hypotension unresponsive to volume expansion, tonic muscular spasms, twitching and convulsions may occur.

Treatment – Maintenance of a patent airway with assisted ventilation; monitoring of vital signs and level of consciousness; continuous ECG to detect arrhythmias; maintenance of blood pressure with plasma volume expanders and, if essential, pressor drugs.

Gastric lavage: Induce vomiting only if the patient is fully conscious. Institute gastric lavage in all cases, regardless of elapsed time since ingestion. Lavage with a 1:1 mixture of castor oil and water. Leave 50 ml of castor oil in the stomach as a cathartic. Delay absorption by giving activated charcoal in water. Follow up as soon as possible with production of emesis or gastric lavage.

Intestinal lavage is used to remove unabsorbed drug (100 to 250 ml of 20% to 40% sorbitol or mannitol).

Urinary output: If coma is prolonged, monitor and maintain urine output while preventing overhydration which might contribute to pulmonary or cerebral edema.

Dialysis/hemoperfusion: Consider in Grade III or Grade IV coma, when renal shutdown or impaired renal function are manifest, and in life-threatening situations complicated by pulmonary edema, heart failure, circulatory collapse, significant liver disease, major metabolic disturbance or uremia.

Use of pure food grade soybean oil as the dialysate enhances removal of glutethimide by hemodialysis. While aqueous hemodialysis is less effective for glutethimide than for readily water-soluble compounds, glutethimide blood levels may decline more rapidly with hemodialysis, and the duration of coma may be shortened; efficacy of the procedure, however, is controversial. Peritoneal dialysis is of minimal value.

Charcoal hemoperfusion has been simpler and more effective than hemodialysis. Similarly, a microcapsule artificial kidney has been developed using activated charcoal granules. Resin hemoperfusion with an Amberlite XAD-2 column has shown exceptionally high clearance capabilities in glutethimide intoxication and has been clinically superior to hemodialysis.

Lipid storage: Glutethimide is highly lipid soluble; it rapidly accumulates in lipoid tissue. As the drug is removed from the bloodstream by any technique, it is gradually released from fat storage back into the bloodstream. Even after substantial quantities of the drug have been extracted, this blood-level rebound can cause coma to persist or recur. Continue drug extraction techniques for at least 2 hours after the patient regains consciousness.

Piperidine Derivatives

GLUTETHIMIDE

Chronic overdosage:

Symptoms – Impairment of memory and ability to concentrate; impaired gait; ataxia; tremors; hyporeflexia; slurring of speech. Abrupt discontinuation after chronic overdosage frequently causes withdrawal reactions including: Nervousness; anxiety; grand mal seizures; abdominal cramping; chills; numbness of extremities; dysphagia.

Treatment – Gradual, stepwise reduction of dosage over a period of days or weeks. If withdrawal reactions occur, readminister glutethimide, or substitute pentobarbital and subsequently withdraw gradually.

Patient Information:

May decrease alertness or physical ability. Use caution when driving or performing tasks requiring alertness.

Avoid alcohol and other CNS depressants.

Administration and Dosage:

Individualize dosage. Not recommended for children.

Adults: Usual adult dose is 250 to 500 mg at bedtime.

For elderly or debilitated patients, initial daily dosage should not exceed 500 mg at bedtime, to avoid oversedation.

c-II	**Glutethimide** (Halsey)	**Tablets:** 250 mg	(HD 564). White, scored. In 100s.

Tertiary Acetylenic Alcohols

ETHCHLORVYNOL

Actions:

Pharmacology: Ethchlorvynol has sedative-hypnotic, anticonvulsant and muscle relaxant properties. It produces EEG patterns similar to those produced by barbiturates. It has generally been replaced by safer and more effective agents.

Pharmacokinetics:

Absorption/Distribution – Rapidly absorbed from GI tract; peak plasma concentrations occur within 2 hours after a single oral fasting dose. Maximum blood concentrations occur in 1 to 1.5 hours; ≈ 90% of the drug is destroyed in the liver. There is extensive tissue concentration, particularly in adipose tissue.

Metabolism/Excretion – Within 24 hours, 33% of a single 500 mg dose is excreted in the urine, mostly as metabolites. The free and conjugated forms of the major metabolite, the secondary alcohol of ethchlorvynol, in the urine accounts for about 40% of the dose. The parent compound and its metabolites undergo extensive enterohepatic recirculation. Plasma half-life of parent compound is 10 to 20 hrs.

Onset/Duration: The usual hypnotic dose induces sleep within 15 to 60 minutes. The duration of effect is about 5 hours.

Indications:

Short-term hypnotic therapy for periods up to 1 week in the management of insomnia. If retreatment becomes necessary after drug free intervals of 1 or more weeks, undertake only upon further evaluation of the patient.

Unlabeled uses: A sedative dose for ethchlorvynol is 100 to 200 mg 2 or 3 times daily.

Contraindications:

Hypersensitivity to ethchlorvynol; porphyria.

Warnings:

Psychological and physical dependence: Use with caution in mentally depressed patients, with or without suicidal tendencies, and to those with psychological potential for drug dependence. Prescribe least amount of drug that is practical. Prolonged use may result in tolerance and psychological and physical dependence.

Intoxication symptoms have been reported with the prolonged use of doses as low as 1 g/day. Signs and symptoms may include incoordination, tremors, ataxia, confusion, slurred speech, hyperreflexia, diplopia and generalized muscle weakness. Toxic amblyopia, scotoma, nystagmus and peripheral neuropathy have also occurred; these symptoms are usually reversible.

Withdrawal symptoms similar to those seen during barbiturate and alcohol withdrawal follow abrupt discontinuance after prolonged use. Symptoms can appear as late as 9 days after sudden drug withdrawal and may include: Convulsions; delirium; schizoid reaction; perceptual distortions; memory loss; ataxia; insomnia; slurring of speech; unusual anxiety; irritability; agitation; tremors; anorexia; nausea; vomiting; weakness; dizziness; sweating; muscle twitching; weight loss.

Withdrawal management – Readminister drug to approximately the same level of intoxication that existed before the abrupt discontinuance. Phenobarbital may be substituted for ethchlorvynol. Make a gradual, stepwise reduction of dosage over a period of days or weeks. In addition, a phenothiazine may be used for patients who exhibit psychotic symptoms during withdrawal. Hospitalize or closely observe the patient and give general supportive care as indicated.

Elderly or debilitated patients should receive the smallest effective dose.

Renal/Hepatic function impairment: Use with caution in these patients.

Pregnancy: Category C. The drug is associated with a high percentage of stillbirths and a low survival rate of progeny in rats given 40mg/kg/day. Ethchlorvynol crosses the placental barrier. Not recommended for use during the first and second trimesters of pregnancy. Use during the third trimester of pregnancy may produce CNS depression and transient withdrawal symptoms in the newborn (eg, episodic jitteriness, hyperactivity, restlessness, irritability disturbed sleep, hunger). Use during pregnancy only if the potential benefit justifies the potential risk to the fetus.

Lactation: It is not known whether this drug is excreted in breast milk. Because of the potential for serious adverse reactions in the infant, decide whether to discontinue nursing or the drug, taking into account importance of the drug to the mother.

Children: Safety and efficacy are not been determined; use is not recommended.

Precautions:

CNS effects: Patients who exhibit unpredictable behavior or paradoxical restlessness or excitement in response to barbiturates or alcohol may react in this manner to ethchlorvynol. Do not use for the management of insomnia in the presence of pain, unless insomnia persists after pain is controlled with analgesics.

Tertiary Acetylenic Alcohols

ETHCHLORVYNOL

Hazardous tasks: May cause dizziness; observe caution while driving or performing other tasks requiring alertness.

Tartrazine sensitivity: Some of these products contain tartrazine, which may cause allergic-type reactions (including bronchial asthma) in susceptible individuals. Although the incidence of tartrazine sensitivity in the general population is low, it is frequently seen in patients who also have aspirin hypersensitivity.

Drug Interactions:

Alcohol or other CNS depressants (eg, barbiturates, narcotics): Exaggerated depressant effects will occur when used concomitantly with ethchlorvynol.

Anticoagulants, oral: Ethchlorvynol may decrease the hypoprothrombinemic effect of the anti-coagulant. Dosage adjustment may be required at initiation and discontinuation of therapy. Alternatively, consider the use of a benzodiazepine in place of ethchlorvynol.

Adverse Reactions:

Reactions within each category are given in decreasing order of severity.

GI: Vomiting; gastric upset; nausea; aftertaste.

CNS: Dizziness; facial numbness. Transient giddiness and ataxia have occurred when absorption of the drug is especially rapid.

Hematologic: Thrombocytopenia; fatal immune thrombocytopenia (one case).

Hypersensitivity: Cholestatic jaundice; urticaria; rash.

Body as a whole: Blurred vision; hypotension; mild "hangover."

Idiosyncratic (occasional) – Syncope without marked hypotension; mild stimulation; marked excitement; hysteria; prolonged hypnosis; profound muscular weakness.

Overdosage:

Symptoms: Acute intoxication is characterized by prolonged deep coma, severe respiratory depression, hypothermia, hypotension and relative bradycardia. Nystagmus and pancytopenia have been reported. Death has occurred following ingestion of 6 g; however, patients have survived overdoses of 50 g and more with intensive care. Fatal blood concentrations range from 20 to 50 mcg/ml. Because large amounts are taken up by adipose tissue, the blood concentration is an unreliable parameter.

Treatment: Perform immediate gastric evacuation. In the unconscious patient, precede gastric lavage by tracheal intubation with a cuffed tube. Supportive care is essential. Place emphasis on pulmonary care and monitoring of blood gases. Hemoperfusion using the Amberlite column technique (XAD-4 resin) has been the most effective method of managing acute overdose. Hemodialysis and peritoneal dialysis (aqueous and oil dialysates) are of some value. Hemoperfusion with charcoal has been effective. Forced diuresis with maintenance of a high urinary output is also of value. Refer to General Management of Acute Overdosage.

Patient Information:

May cause drowsiness, dizziness or blurred vision; observe caution while driving or performing other tasks requiring alertness.

Avoid alcohol and other CNS depressants. Do not exceed prescribed dosage.

Symptoms of giddiness, ataxia or GI upset may be reduced if drug is taken with food.

Administration and Dosage:

Hypnotic: Usual adult dose is 500 mg at bedtime; 750 mg may be required for patients whose response to 500 mg is inadequate, or for patients being changed from barbiturates or nonbarbiturate hypnotics. Give the smallest effective dose to elderly or debilitated patients. Do not prescribe for > 1 week.

Severe insomnia: Up to 1000 mg may be given as a single bedtime dose.

Supplemental dose in insomnia characterized by untimely awakening during early morning hours. Administer 200 mg to reinstitute sleep in patients who awaken after the original bedtime dose of 500 or 750 mg.

c-iv	**Placidyl** (Abbott)	**Capsules:** 200 mg	Red. In 100s.
		500 mg	Red. In 100s, 500s and Abbo-Pac 100s.
		750 mg[1]	(KN). Green. In 100s and Abbo-Pac 100s.

[1] Contains tartrazine.

PROPIOMAZINE HCl

Actions:

Pharmacology: This phenothiazine compound with sedative, antiemetic and antihistaminic properties is a potent premedicant, with a short duration of action.

Pharmacokinetics: Following IM administration, peak serum concentrations are reached in 1 to 3 hours; mean bioavailability is 60%. Mean elimination half-lives reported in five healthy volunteers after IV and IM doses of 20 mg each were 7.7 ± 3.9 hours and 10.8 ± 1.9 hours, respectively.

Indications:

Sedative: Relief of restlessness and apprehension, preoperatively or during surgery.

Analgesic adjunct: Relief of restlessness and apprehension during labor.

Contraindications:

Intra-arterial injection: Arterial/arteriolar spasm with local circulation impairment may occur.

Warnings:

Pregnancy: Safety for use during the first trimester has not been established.

Precautions:

Neuroleptic malignant syndrome (NMS), a potentially fatal symptom complex, has occurred in association with antipsychotic drugs, which may include propiomazine. See Antipsychotic agents for a more complete discussion.

Thrombophlebitis: Inject IV only into vessels previously undamaged by multiple injections or trauma. Do not allow extravasation, since chemical irritation may be severe.

Hazardous tasks: May produce drowsiness, dizziness; use caution while performing tasks requiring alertness.

Drug Interactions:

CNS depressants: Propiomazine enhances the CNS effects. Eliminate or reduce the dose of **barbiturates** by at least in the presence of propiomazine. Reduce the doses of **meperidine, morphine** and other **analgesic depressants** by ¼ to ½.

Adverse Reactions:

Body as a whole: Autonomic reactions are rare. Dry mouth may occur (usually desirable in patients undergoing anesthesia).

Neuroleptic malignant syndrome has occurred (see Warnings).

Cardiovascular: Moderate elevation in blood pressure (desirable in many cases) and hypotension (rare). Tachycardia has also occurred.

Norepinephrine appears to be most suitable if a vasopressor must be administered to patients receiving propiomazine. The pressor response to epinephrine is usually reduced and may even be reversed in the presence of propiomazine.

Administration and Dosage:

Adults: Administer IV or IM.

Preoperative medication – 20 mg propiomazine with 50 mg meperidine. Although 20 mg propiomazine is sufficient for most patients, some will require as much as 40 mg for adequate sedation. Belladonna alkaloids may be added as required.

Surgical sedation with local, nerve block or spinal anesthesia – 10 to 20 mg.

Obstetrics – 20 mg will provide sedation and relieve apprehension in early stages of labor. Some patients may require up to 40 mg. When labor is definitely established, give 20 to 40 mg propiomazine with 25 to 75 mg meperidine (average dose, 50 mg). Use mnesic agents as required. If average doses of propiomazine and meperidine are used, it is seldom necessary to repeat medication during normal labor. May repeat additional doses at 3 hour intervals. Neither prolongation of labor nor significant maternal or fetal depression has been observed.

Children: Use as a sedative the night before surgery and for preanesthetic and postoperative medication. In children under 27 kg (60 lb), calculate dosage on the basis of 0.55 to 1.1 mg/kg (0.25 to 0.5 mg/lb). The higher dosage recommendation should be necessary only in the extremely nervous, excitable child.

Satisfactory results were obtained with the following dosage schedule:

Propiomazine HCl Pediatric Dosage

Age (yrs)	Single Dosage
2 to 42	10 mg
4 to 62	15 mg
6 to 12	25 mg

Stability: Do not use if solution is cloudy or contains a precipitate.

Rx	**Largon** (Wyeth-Ayerst)	**Injection:** 20 mg per ml	In 1 ml amps.

BENZODIAZEPINES

For information on benzodiazepines used as antianxiety agents, refer to the group monograph in the Antianxiety Agents section.

Actions:

Pharmacology: Estazolam, flurazepam, quazepam, temazepam and triazolam are benzodiazepine derivatives useful as hypnotics. Benzodiazepines are believed to potentiate gamma aminobutyric acid (GABA) neuronal inhibition. The sedative and anticonvulsant actions involve GABA receptors located in the limbic, neocortical and mesencephalic reticular systems.

At least two benzodiazepine receptor subtypes have been identified in the brain, BZ_1 and BZ_2. BZ_1 is thought to be associated with sleep mechanisms; BZ_2 with memory, motor, sensory and cognitive functions. Quazepam and its active metabolite 2-oxoquazepam have a high affinity for BZ_1 receptors; this selectivity is not seen with estazolam, flurazepam, temazepam and triazolam. It is possible this selectivity of quazepam facilitates GABA transmission; however, further study is needed to determine the clinical significance of this receptor sensitivity.

Benzodiazepines generally decrease sleep latency, the number of awakenings and the time spent in stage 0 (awake stage). Flurazepam, quazepam and temazepam decrease stage 1 (descending drowsiness). Stage 2 (unequivocal sleep) is increased by all benzodiazepines, and most benzodiazepines shorten stages 3 and 4 (slow wave sleep). Temazepam has prolonged stage 3 and shortened stage 4 in neurotic patients or patients with depression. All but flurazepam prolong REM latency. REM sleep is usually shortened, but with temazepam or low-dose flurazepam, this may not be the case. The result of benzodiazepine administration is an increase in total sleep time.

If benzodiazepines are discontinued after 3 or 4 weeks of continued use, the patient may experience REM rebound; however, REM rebound with flurazepam, quazepam and possibly estazolam is slight.

Pharmacokinetics:

Absorption – These agents are rapidly and completely absorbed within 1 to 3 hours of oral administration. All have high lipid:water distribution coefficients in the non-ionized form. Times to peak plasma concentration range from 0.5 to 2 hours for parent compounds. The major active metabolite of flurazepam reaches peak plasma levels in ≈ 10 hours.

Distribution – Plasma protein binding ranges from 70% to 99% with free-drug concentrations closely approximating CSF levels. IV and rapidly absorbed oral benzodiazepines are rapidly taken into the brain and other highly perfused organs. Redistribution, favoring lipophilic compounds, follows and can greatly influence the duration of CNS effects. They also cross the placenta and are secreted into breast milk.

Metabolism – Benzodiazepines are extensively metabolized in the liver. Biotransformation to active metabolites is an important factor in product selection especially in the elderly or patients with severe liver disease. Flurazepam is biotransformed to an active metabolite, N-desalkylflurazepam, which has a half-life ranging from 47 to 100 hours. Quazepam is extensively metabolized to 2-oxoquazepam, an active metabolite; 2-oxoquazepam is further biotransformed to N-desalkyl-2-oxoquazepam, which is identical to N-desalkylflurazepam and is therefore also active. Temazepam, estazolam and triazolam do not form active long-acting metabolites.

Select Benzodiazepine (Hypnotic) Pharmacokinetic Parameters

Drug	Usual adult oral dose (mg)	Time to peak plasma levels (hrs)	Half-life (hrs)	Protein binding (%)	Urinary excretion, unchanged (%)
Estazolam	1-2	2	8-28	93	< 5
Flurazepam	15-30	0.5-1 (7.6-13.6)[1]	2-3 (47-100)[1]	97	< 1
Quazepam	7.5-15	2 (1-2)	41 (47-100)[1]	> 95	trace
Temazepam	15-30	1.2-1.6	3.5-18.4 (9-15)	96	0.2
Triazolam	0.125-0.5	1-2	1.5-5.5	78-89	2

[1] N-desalkylflurazepam, active metabolite.

BENZODIAZEPINES

Indications:

Insomnia characterized by difficulty in falling asleep, frequent nocturnal awakenings or early morning awakening. Can be used for recurring insomnia or poor sleeping habits and in acute or chronic medical situations requiring restful sleep.

Insomnia is often transient and intermittent; therefore, prolonged administration is generally not recommended. Because insomnia may be a symptom of other disorders, consider the possibility that the complaint may be related to a condition for which there is more specific treatment.

Contraindications:

Hypersensitivity to other benzodiazepines; pregnancy (see Warnings); established or suspected sleep apnea (quazepam).

Concurrent use with ketoconazole, itraconazole and nefazodone, medications that significantly impair the oxidative metabolism of **triazolam** mediated by cytochrome P450 3A (CYP3A).

Warnings:

Anterograde amnesia of varying severity and paradoxical reactions have occurred following therapeutic doses of **triazolam**. Although these effects generally occurred with a 0.5 mg dose, they have also been reported with 0.125 and 0.25 mg doses. These effect may occur with some other benzodiazepines, but data suggest that they may occur at a higher rate with triazolam.

Cases of "traveler's amnesia" have been reported by individuals who have taken **triazolam** to induce sleep while traveling. In some of these cases, insufficient time was allowed for the sleep period prior to awakening and before beginning activity. Also, the concomitant use of alcohol may have been a factor in some cases.

Renal/Hepatic function impairment: Observe usual precautions under these conditions; the potential for excessive sedation or impaired coordination exists.

Abnormal liver function tests as well as blood dyscrasias have been reported with benzodiazepines.

Elderly: The risk of developing oversedation, dizziness, confusion or ataxia increases substantially with larger doses of benzodiazepines in elderly and debilitated patients. Initiate with lowest effective dose.

Pregnancy: Category X (estazolam, quazepam, temazepam, triazolam). Flurazepam is contraindicated in pregnancy.

Teratogenic potential – Benzodiazepines may cause fetal damage when administered during pregnancy. An increased risk of congenital malformations associated with the use of diazepam and chlordiazepoxide during the first trimester of pregnancy has been suggested. Transplacental distribution results in neonatal CNS depression following ingestion of therapeutic doses of a benzodiazepine hypnotic during the last weeks of pregnancy.

Reproduction studies with **temazepam** in animals demonstrated an increased nursling mortality, increased fetal resorptions and increased occurrence of rudimentary ribs. Exencephaly and fusion or asymmetry of the ribs occurred without dose relationship.

Warn the patient of the potential risk to the fetus if there is a likelihood of the patient becoming pregnant while receiving benzodiazepines. Instruct patients to discontinue the drug prior to becoming pregnant. Consider the possibility that a woman of childbearing potential may be pregnant at the time of therapy institution.

Nonteratogenic effects – A child born to a mother taking benzodiazepines may be at some risk of withdrawal symptoms during the postnatal period. Neonatal flaccidity has occurred in an infant whose mother had been receiving benzodiazepines.

A neonate whose mother received 30 mg **flurazepam** nightly for insomnia during the 10 days prior to delivery appeared hypotonic and inactive during the first 4 days of life. Serum levels of N–desalkylflurazepam in the infant indicated transplacental circulation.

Lactation: Safety for use in the nursing mother has not been established. Benzodiazepines are excreted in breast milk. One study showed only 0.11% of quazepam and its metabolites were excreted in breast milk 48 hours after administration. Animal studies indicate that **triazolam, estazolam** and their metabolites are secreted in milk. Therefore, administration to nursing mothers is not recommended.

Children:

Flurazepam – Not for use in children < 15 years of age.

Estazolam, quazepam, temazepam, triazolam – Not for use in children < 18 years of age.

BENZODIAZEPINES

Precautions:

Monitoring: When triazolam or estazolam treatment is protracted, obtain periodic blood counts, urinalysis and blood chemistry analyses. Minor EEG changes, usually low-voltage fast activity, are of no known significance.

Depression: Administer with caution in severely depressed patients or in those in whom there is evidence of latent depression or suicidal tendencies. Signs or symptoms of depression may be intensified by hypnotic drugs. Protective measures may be required. Intentional overdosage is more common in these patients, and the least amount of drug that is feasible should be available to the patient at any one time.

Rebound sleep disorder, which is characterized by recurrence of insomnia to levels worse than before treatment began, may occur following abrupt withdrawal of triazolam, usually during the first 1 to 3 nights. Gradual rather than abrupt discontinuation of the drug may help avoid this syndrome. Rebound insomnia appears to be less likely after withdrawal of agents with intermediate or long half-lives (eg, estazolam, flurazepam, quazepam).

Disturbed nocturnal sleep may occur for the first or second night after discontinuing use.

Early morning insomnia, or early morning awakenings, appears to be more common with the use of short half-life agents (temazepam, triazolam) than agents with intermediate or long half-lives (estazolam, flurazepam, quazepam). However, daytime sleepiness appears to be more prevalent with the long half-life agents.

Respiratory depression and sleep apnea: Observe caution. In patients with compromised respiratory function, respiratory depression and sleep apnea have occurred. Estazolam may cause dose-related respiratory depression that is ordinarily not clinically relevant at recommended doses in patients with normal respiratory function. However, patients with compromised respiratory function may be at risk; therefore, monitor appropriately. Benzodiazepines have the capacity to depress respiratory drive, although there are insufficient data to characterize the relative potency of these agents in depressing respiratory drive at clinically recommended doses.

Drug abuse and dependence: Withdrawal symptoms following abrupt discontinuation of benzodiazepines have occurred in patients receiving excessive doses over extended periods of time. Symptoms are similar to those noted with barbiturates and alcohol following abrupt discontinuance and range from mild dysphoria to abdominal and muscle cramps, vomiting, sweating, tremor and convulsions.

Milder withdrawal symptoms infrequently occur following abrupt discontinuance of higher therapeutic levels of benzodiazepines taken continuously for several months. Exercise caution in administering to individuals known to be addiction-prone or those who may increase the dosage on their own initiative. Limit repeated prescriptions without adequate medical supervision.

Gradual withdrawal is the preferred course for any patient taking benzodiazepines for a prolonged period. Patients with a history of seizures, regardless of their concomitant anti-seizure therapy, should not be withdrawn abruptly from benzodiazepines.

Hazardous tasks: Observe caution while driving or performing tasks requiring alertness. Be aware of potential impairment of the performance of such activities the day following ingestion.

Amnesia, paradoxical reactions (eg, excitement, agitation) and other adverse behavioral effects may occur unpredictably.

BENZODIAZEPINES

Drug Interactions:

Benzodiazepine (Hypnotic) Drug Interactions			
Precipitant drug	Object drug*		Description
Alcohol/CNS depressants	Benzodiazepines	↑	Additive CNS depressant effects. Potential for this interaction continues for several days following flurazepam withdrawal.
Cimetidine	Benzodiazepines (metabolized by oxidation)	↑	The hepatic metabolism of the benzodiazepines may be inhibited, their half-life prolonged and their clearance decreased, possibly resulting in increased pharmacologic and CNS depressant effects. Temazepam, metabolized by glucuronidation, would probably not interact; however, its half-life may be decreased by oral contraceptive agents.
Contraceptives, oral			
Disulfiram			
Isoniazid			
Probenecid	Benzodiazepines	↑	More rapid onset or more prolonged benzodiazepine effect.
Rifampin	Benzodiazepines (metabolized by oxidation)	↓	Increased clearance and decreased half-life of benzodiazepines may occur. Temazepam would probably not interact.
Smoking	Benzodiazepines	↓	Benzodiazepine clearance is increased in cigarette smokers, probably due to enzyme induction.
Theophyllines	Benzodiazepines	↓	Benzodiazepine pharmacologic effects may be antagonized.
Macrolides	Triazolam	↑	Bioavailability of triazolam may be increased.
Benzodiazepines	Digoxin	↑	Digoxin serum levels and toxicity may increase.
Benzodiazepines	Neuromuscular blocking agents (nondepolarizing)	↔	Benzodiazepines may potentiate, counteract or have no effect on these agents.
Benzodiazepines	Phenytoin	↑	Phenytoin serum levels may be increased, resulting in toxicity, but data are conflicting.

* ↑ = Object drug increased. ↓ = Object drug decreased. ↔ = Undetermined effect.

Adverse Reactions:

CNS: Headache; nervousness; talkativeness; apprehension; irritability; confusion; euphoria; relaxed feeling; weakness; tremor; lack of concentration; coordination disorders; confusional states/memory impairment; depression; dreaming/nightmares; insomnia; paresthesia; restlessness; tiredness; dysesthesia. Hallucinations, horizontal nystagmus and paradoxical reactions, including excitement, stimulation and hyperactivity were rare. Dizziness, drowsiness, lightheadedness, staggering, ataxia, falling, particularly in elderly or debilitated patients. Severe sedation, lethargy, disorientation and coma are probably indicative of drug intolerance or overdosage.

GI: Heartburn; nausea; vomiting; diarrhea; constipation; GI pain; anorexia; taste alterations; dry mouth; excessive salivation (rare); death from hepatic failure in a patient also receiving diuretics; jaundice; glossitis, stomatitis (triazolam).

Cardiovascular: Palpitations; chest pains; tachycardia; hypotension (rare).

Dermatologic: Dermatitis/allergy; sweating, flushes, pruritus, skin rash (rare).

Miscellaneous: Body/joint pain; tinnitus; GU complaints; cramps/pain; congestion. Leukopenia, granulocytopenia, blurred vision, burning eyes, faintness, difficulty in focusing, visual disturbances, shortness of breath, apnea, slurred speech (rare).

Lab test abnormalities: Elevated AST, ALT, total and direct bilirubin and alkaline phosphatase with **flurazepam**.

Estazolam: Other adverse reactions reported only for estazolam include the following:

CNS – Somnolence (42%); asthenia (11%); hypokinesia (8%); hangover (3%); abnormal thinking (2%); anxiety (1%); agitation, amnesia, apathy, emotional lability, hostility, seizure, sleep disorder, stupor, twitch (0.1% to 1%); ataxia, decreased libido, decreased reflexes, neuritis (< 0.1%).

GI – Dyspepsia (2%); decreased/increased appetite, flatulence, gastritis (0.1% to 1%); enterocolitis, melena, mouth ulceration (< 0.1%).

Cardiovascular – Arrhythmia, syncope (< 0.1%).

Dermatologic – Urticaria (0.1% to 1%); acne, dry skin, photosensitivity (< 0.1%).

Respiratory – Cold symptoms (3%); pharyngitis (1%); asthma, cough, dyspnea, rhinitis, sinusitis (0.1% to 1%); epistaxis, hyperventilation, laryngitis (< 0.1%).

Special Senses – Ear pain, eye irritation/pain/swelling, photophobia (0.1% to 1%); decreased hearing, diplopia, nystagmus, scotomata (< 0.1%).

GU – Frequent urination, menstrual cramps, urinary hesitancy/urgency, vaginal discharge/itching (0.1% to 1%); hematuria, nocturia, oliguria, penile discharge, urinary incontinence (< 0.1%).

Miscellaneous – Lower extremity/back/abdominal pain (1% to 3%); stiffness (1%); allergic reaction, chills, fever, neck/upper extremity pain, thirst, arthritis, muscle spasm, myalgia (0.1% to 1%); edema, jaw pain, swollen breast, thyroid nodule, purpura, swollen lymph nodes, agranulocytosis, increased AST, weight gain/loss, arthralgia (< 0.1%).

Overdosage:

Symptoms: Somnolence; confusion with reduced or absent reflexes; respiratory depression; apnea; hypotension; impaired coordination; slurred speech; seizures; ultimately, coma. Death has occurred with overdoses of benzodiazepines alone and with alcohol.

Treatment: If excitation occurs, do not use barbiturates. Consider the possibility that multiple agents may have been ingested. Monitor respiration, pulse and blood pressure. Employ general supportive measures. Administer IV fluids and maintain an adequate airway. Perform gastric lavage. Refer to General Management of Acute Overdosage. Hemodialysis and forced diuresis are of little value.

Use of IV pressor agents may be necessary to treat hypotension. Administer IV fluids to encourage diuresis.

Patient Information:

Avoid alcohol and other CNS depressants. Do not exceed prescribed dosage.

Do not discontinue medication abruptly after prolonged therapy.

Advise patients that they may experience disturbed nocturnal sleep for the first or second night after discontinuing the drug.

May cause drowsiness or dizziness; observe caution while driving or performing other tasks requiring alertness.

Inform your physician if you are planning to become pregnant, if you are pregnant, or if you become pregnant while taking this medicine.

Triazolam: Advise patients not to take triazolam in circumstances where a full night's sleep and clearance of the drug from the body are not possible before they would again need to be active and functional.

ESTAZOLAM

For complete prescribing information, refer to the Benzodiazepines group monograph.

Administration and Dosage:

Adults: 1 mg at bedtime; however, some patients may need a 2 mg dose.

Elderly: If healthy, 1 mg at bedtime; initiate increases with particular care.

Debilitated or small elderly patients: Consider a starting dose of 0.5 mg, although this is only marginally effective in the overall elderly population.

c-iv	**ProSom** (Abbott)	**Tablets:** 1 mg	Lactose. White, scored. In 100s and UD 100s.
		2 mg	Lactose. Coral, scored. In 100s and UD 100s.

Benzodiazepine Compounds

FLURAZEPAM HCl

For complete prescribing information, refer to the Benzodiazepines group monograph.

Administration and Dosage:

Individualize dosage.

Adults: 30 mg before bedtime. In some patients, 15 mg may suffice.

Elderly or debilitated: Initiate with 15 mg until individual response is determined.

c-iv	**Flurazepam** (Various, eg, Goldline, Major, Moore, PBI, Rugby, Schein, Warner Chilcott)	**Capsules:** 15 mg	In 100s and 100s.
c-iv	**Dalmane** (Roche)		Orange/ivory. In 100s, 500s, Reverse number pack 100s, UD 100s.
c-iv	**Flurazepam** (Various, eg, Goldline, Major, Moore, PBI, Rugby, Schein, Warner Chilcott)	**Capsules:** 30 mg	In 100s and 100s.
c-iv	**Dalmane** (Roche)		Red/ivory. In 100s, 500s, Reverse number pack 100s, UD 100s.

TEMAZEPAM

For complete prescribing information, refer to the Benzodiazepines group monograph.

Administration and Dosage:

Adults: Individualize dosage. Give 15 to 30 mg before bedtime.

Elderly or debilitated: Initiate with 15 mg until individual response is determined.

c-iv	**Restoril**(Sandoz)	**Capsules:** 7.5 mg	Lactose. (Restoril 7.5 mg For Sleep). Blue/pink. In 100s, ControlPak 25s, UD 100s.
c-iv	**Temazepam** (Various, eg, Goldline, Lederle, Major, Moore, PBI, Rugby, Warner Chilcott)	**Capsules:** 15 mg	In 100s, 500s and UD 100s
c-iv	**Restoril** (Sandoz)		(Restoril 15 mg). Maroon/pink. In 100s, 500s, Control Pack 25s, Sando Pak 100s.
c-iv	**Temazepam** (Various, eg, Goldline, Major, Moore, PBI, Rugby, Warner-Chilcott)	**Capsules:** 30 mg	In 100s, 500s and UD 100s.
c-iv	**Restoril** (Sandoz)		(Restoril 30 mg). Maroon/blue. In 100s, 500s, Control Pak 25s, Sando Pak 100s.

Benzodiazepine Compounds

TRIAZOLAM

For complete prescribing information, refer to the Benzodiazepines group monograph.

Administration and Dosage:

Adults: 0.125 to 0.5 mg before bedtime.

Elderly or debilitated: 0.125 to 0.25 mg. Initiate with 0.125 mg until individual response is determined.

c-iv	**Triazolam** (Various, eg, Geneva, Goldline, Par, Roxane, Schein)	**Tablets:** 0.125 mg	In 10s, 100s, 500s and UD 100s.
c-iv	**Halcion** (Upjohn)		(0.125 Halcion 10). White. In 100s, 500s, UD 100s, Visipak 100s.
c-iv	**Triazolam** (Various, eg, Geneva, Goldline, Par, Roxane, Schein)	**Tablets:** 0.25 mg	In 10s, 100s, 500s and UD 100s.
c-iv	**Halcion** (Upjohn)		(0.25 Halcion 17). Blue, scored. In 100s, 500s, UD 100s, Visipak 100s.

QUAZEPAM

For complete prescribing information, refer to the Benzodiazepines group monograph.

Administration and Dosage:

Adults: Initiate at 15 mg until individual responses are determined; may reduce to 7.5 mg in some patients.

Elderly or debilitated: Attempt to reduce nightly dosage after the first 1 or 2 nights.

c-iv	**Doral** (Wallace)	**Tablets:** 7.5 mg	(7.5 Doral). Capsule shaped, light orange w/white speckles. In 100s, 500s, UD 100s.
		15 mg	(15 Doral). Capsule shaped, light orange w/white speckles. In 100s, 500s, UD 100s.

NONPRESCRIPTION SLEEP AIDS

For complete prescribing information for the antihistamines and for a complete listing of diphenhydramine HCl products, refer to the Antihistamines monograph in the Respiratory Drugs section.

Actions:

Pharmacology: These products contain antihistamines which act on the CNS, producing prominent sedative effects.

Indications:

Aid in the relief of insomnia.

Traditionally, products containing analgesics have been used for relief of insomnia due to minor pain.

Contraindications:

Asthma, glaucoma or prostate gland enlargement, except under a physician's advice.

Warnings:

Prolonged insomnia: Not for use > 2 weeks. If insomnia persists for > 2 weeks, consult a physician; it may be a symptom of a serious underlying illness.

Pregnancy: Consult a physician before using these products. **Doxylamine** should not be taken by pregnant women.

Lactation: **Doxylamine** should not be taken by a nursing woman.

Children: Do not use in children < 12 years of age.

Precautions:

Hazardous tasks: May cause drowsiness; observe caution while driving or performing other tasks requiring alertness, coordination or physical dexterity.

Adverse Reactions:

Occasional anticholinergic effects may occur with doxylamine.

Overdosage:

Antihistamine overdosage reactions may vary from CNS depression to stimulation. See the Antihistamines monograph for a more complete description of reactions.

Patient Information:

Avoid alcoholic beverages while taking this product. Do not take this product if you are taking sedatives or tranquilizers without first consulting the physician.

May cause drowsiness; observe caution while driving or performing other tasks requiring alertness, coordination or physical dexterity.

Do not use if you have asthma, glaucoma, emphysema, chronic pulmonary disease, shortness of breath, difficulty in breathing or difficulty in urination due to prostate enlargement unless directed by the physician.

Administration and Dosage:

Administer 25 mg doxylamine or 50 mg diphenhydramine HCl (76 mg diphenhydramine citrate) before bedtime.

otc	**Unisom Nighttime Sleep-Aid** (Pfizer)	**Tablets:** 25 mg doxylamine succinate	Blue, scored. Oval. In 8s, 16s, 32s, 48s.
otc	**Dormin Caplets** (Randob)	**Tablets:** 25 mg diphenhydramine HCl	In 32s.
otc	**Miles Nervine Caplets** (Miles)		(Nervine). In 12s and 30s.
otc	**Nytol** (Block)		Lactose. (N). In 16s, 32s and 72s.
otc	**Sleep-eze 3** (Whitehall)		In 12s and 24s.
otc	**Sleepwell 2-nite** (Rugby)		Sucrose. In 72s.
otc	**Sominex** (SK-Beecham)		(S). In 16s, 32s and 72s.

NONPRESCRIPTION SLEEP AIDS

otc	**Extra Strength Tylenol PM** (McNeil-CPC)	**Tablets**: 25 mg diphenhydramine, 500 mg acetaminophen	**Tablets**: In 24s, 50s. **Caplets**: (Tylenol PM). In 24s and 50s.
otc	**Aspirin Free Anacin P.M. Caplets** (Robins)		Film coated. In 20s.
otc	**Bayer Select Maximum Strength Night Time Pain Relief Caplets** (Sterling Health)		In 24s and 50s.
	Sominex Pain Relief (SK-Beecham)		In 16s and 32s.
otc	**Extra Strength Doan's P.M. Caplets** (Ciba)	**Tablets**: 25 mg diphenhydramine HCl, 500 mg magnesium salicylate	In 20s.
otc	**Bufferin AF Nite Time Caplets** (B-M Squibb)	**Tablets**: 38 mg diphenhydramine citrate, 500 mg acetaminophen	Parabens. Light blue. In 24s and 50s.
otc	**Excedrin P.M.** (B-M Squibb)		**Tablets**: Propylparaben. (PM). In 10s, 30s, 50s and 80s. **Caplets**: Parabens. (Excedrin P.M.). Light blue. In 30s and 50s.
otc	**Unisom with Pain Relief** (Pfizer)	**Tablets**: 50 mg diphenhydramine HCl, 650 mg acetaminophen	In 16s.
otc	**Diphenhydramine HCl** (Rugby)	**Tablets**: 50 mg diphenhydramine HCl	Blue. In 50s.
otc	**Compoz Nighttime Sleep Aid** (Medtech)		Lactose. In 12s and 24s.
otc	**40 Winks** (Roberts Med)		In 30s.
otc	**Maximum Strength Nytol** (Block)		Lactose. (N). In 8s and 16s.
otc	**Sominex Caplets** (SK-Beecham)		In 8s, 16s and 32s.
otc	**Twilite Caplets** (Pfeiffer)		Lactose. In 20s.
otc	**Excedrin PM Liquigels** (Bristol-Myers)	**Capsules**: 25 mg diphenhydramine HCl, 500 mg acetaminophen	Sorbitol. In 20s and 40s.
otc	**Extra Strength Tylenol PMGelcaps** (McNeil-CPC)		EDTA, propylparaben. In 20s and 40s.
otc	**Compoz Gel Caps** (Medtech)	**Capsules**: 25 mg diphenhydramine HCl	In 16s.
otc	**Dormin** (Randob)		Lactose. In 32s and 72s.
otc	**Maximum Strength Sleepinal Capsules and Soft Gels** (Thompson)	**Capsules**: 50 mg diphenhydramine HCl	**Capsules**: Lactose. In 16s. **Soft Gels**: Sorbitol. (Sleepinal). In 16s.
otc	**Maximum Strength Unisom SleepGels** (Pfizer)		Sorbitol. In 8s.

NONPRESCRIPTION SLEEP AIDS

otc	**Midol PM** (Sterling Health)	**Caplets**: 25 mg diphenhydramine HCl, 500 mg acetaminophen	In 16s.
otc	**Legatrin PM** (Columbia)	**Caplets**: 50 mg diphenhydramine HCl, 500 mg acetaminophen	In 30s and 50s.
otc	**Nighttime Pamprin** (Chattem)	**Powder**: 50 mg diphenhydramine HCl, 650 mg acetaminophen	Sugar. Apple cinnamon and hot chocolate flavors. In 4s.
otc	**Excedrin P.M.** (B-M Squibb)	**Liquid**: 1000 mg acetaminophen 50 mg diphengydramine HCL/30 ml.	Sucrose, 10% alcohol. Wildberry flavor. In 180 ml.

SEDATIVES AND HYPNOTICS, BARBITURATES

The following general discussion of the barbiturates refers to their use as sedative-hypnotic agents and as anticonvulsants. In addition, barbiturates are discussed under General Anesthetics, Barbiturates.

Actions:

Pharmacology: Barbiturates can produce all levels of CNS mood alteration from excitation to mild sedation, hypnosis and deep coma. In sufficiently high therapeutic doses, barbiturates induce anesthesia. Overdosage can produce death.

These agents depress the sensory cortex, decrease motor activity, alter cerebellar function and produce drowsiness, sedation and hypnosis.

Barbiturates have little analgesic action at subanesthetic doses and may increase the reaction to painful stimuli. All barbiturates exhibit anticonvulsant activity in anesthetic doses. However, only phenobarbital and mephobarbital are effective as oral anticonvulsants in subhypnotic doses.

Barbiturates are respiratory depressants; the degree of respiratory depression is dose-dependent. With hypnotic doses, respiratory depression is similar to that which occurs during physiologic sleep and is accompanied by a slight decrease in blood pressure and heart rate.

Pharmacokinetics:

Absorption – Barbiturates are absorbed in varying degrees following oral, rectal or parenteral administration. The salts are more rapidly absorbed than the acids. The rate of absorption is increased if the sodium salt is ingested as a dilute solution or taken on an empty stomach.

Onset of action for oral or rectal administration varies from 20 to 60 minutes. For IM administration, onset is slightly faster than the oral route. Following IV administration, onset ranges from almost immediate for pentobarbital sodium and secobarbital to 5 minutes for phenobarbital sodium. Maximal CNS depression may not occur for ≥ 15 minutes after IV administration of phenobarbital sodium.

Duration of action varies and is related to dose and to the rate at which the barbiturates are redistributed throughout the body. In the following table, the barbiturates are classified according to their duration of action. Do not use this classification to predict the exact duration of effect, but use as a guide in drug selection.

Pharmacokinetics of Sedatives and Hypnotic Barbiturates

		Half-Life (hrs)		Oral dosage range (mg)		Onset	Duration
	Barbiturate	Range	Mean	Sedative[1]	Hypnotic	(minutes)	(hours)
Long-Acting	Phenobarbital	53 – 118	79	30 – 120	100 – 320	30 – ≥ 60	10 – 16
	Mephobarbital	11 – 67	34	32 – 200	—		
Intermediate	Amobarbital[2]	16 – 40	25	—	—	45 – 60	6 – 8
	Aprobarbital	14 – 34	24	120	40 – 160		
	Butabarbital	66 – 140	100	45 – 120	50 – 100		
Short-Acting	Secobarbital	15 – 40	28	—	100	10 – 15	3 – 4
	Pentobarbital	15 – 50	†[3]	40 – 120	100		

[1] Total daily dose; administered in 2 to 4 divided doses.

[2] Available as injection only.

[3] May follow dose-dependent kinetics. Mean t½ is 50 hrs for 50 mg and 22 hrs for 100 mg.

Distribution – Barbiturates are weak acids that are rapidly distributed to all tissues and fluids with high concentrations in the brain, liver and kidneys. Lipid solubility of the barbiturates is the dominant factor in their distribution. The more lipid soluble the barbiturate, the more rapidly it penetrates body tissue. Barbiturates are bound to plasma and tissue proteins; the degree of binding increases directly as a function of lipid solubility.

Phenobarbital has the lowest lipid solubility, plasma binding and brain protein binding, the longest delay in onset of activity and the longest duration of action. Secobarbital has the highest lipid solubility, plasma protein binding and brain protein binding, the shortest delay in onset of activity and the shortest duration of action.

SEDATIVES AND HYPNOTICS, BARBITURATES

Excretion – Barbiturates are metabolized primarily by the hepatic microsomal enzyme system, and the metabolic products are excreted in the urine, and less commonly, in the feces. Approximately 25% to 50% of a phenobarbital dose and 13% to 24% of an aprobarbital dose is eliminated unchanged in the urine, whereas the amount of other barbiturates excreted unchanged in the urine is negligible. The excretion of unmetabolized barbiturate is one feature that distinguishes the long-acting agents. The inactive metabolites of the barbiturates are excreted as conjugates of glucuronic acid.

Clinical trials: Barbiturate-induced sleep reduces the amount of time spent in the rapid eye movement (REM) phase of sleep or dreaming stage. Also, Stages III and IV sleep are decreased. Following abrupt cessation of barbiturates used regularly, patients may experience markedly increased dreaming, nightmares or insomnia.

Secobarbital and pentobarbital lose most of their effectiveness for inducing and maintaining sleep by the end of 2 weeks of continued drug administration, even with the use of multiple doses. Other barbiturates might also be expected to lose their effectiveness for inducing and maintaining sleep after about 2 weeks. However, definitions of tolerance vary; these two barbiturates have been given for weeks to months for chronic sedation with little tolerance developing, although decreased effects on sleep stages occur. In addition, the chronic disruption of the normal sleep pattern may make sleep less satisfying; therefore, dosages may be increased possibly resulting in enhanced tolerance. The short, intermediate and, to a lesser degree, long-acting barbiturates have been widely prescribed for treating insomnia. Although the clinical literature abounds with claims that the short-acting agents are superior for producing sleep, while the intermediate-acting compounds are more effective in maintaining sleep, controlled studies have failed to demonstrate these differential effects.

Mephobarbital has a relatively mild hypnotic effect, but exerts strong sedative effects. When used as a sedative, patients usually become more calm, cheerful and better adjusted to surroundings without clouding of mental faculties. It reportedly produces less sedation than phenobarbital.

Indications:

The following indications apply to most barbiturates. For specific indications, to the individual monographs.

Sedation: Although traditionally used as nonspecific CNS depressants for daytime sedation, the barbiturates have generally been replaced by the benzodiazepines.

Hypnotic: Short-term treatment of insomnia, since barbiturates appear to lose their effectiveness in sleep induction and maintenance after 2 weeks. If insomnia persists, seek alternative therapy (including nondrug) for chronic insomnia.

Preanesthetic: Used as preanesthetic sedatives.

Anticonvulsant (**mephobarbital, phenobarbital**): Treatment of partial and generalized tonic-clonic and cortical focal seizures.

Acute convulsive episodes: Emergency control of certain acute convulsive episodes (eg, those associated with status epilepticus, cholera, eclampsia, meningitis, tetanus and toxic reactions to strychnine or local anesthetics).

Contraindications:

Barbiturate sensitivity; manifest or latent porphyria; marked impairment of liver function; severe respiratory disease when dyspnea or obstruction is evident; nephritic patients; patients with respiratory disease where dyspnea or obstruction is present; intra-arterial administration (consequences vary from transient pain to gangrene); SC administration (produces tissue irritation ranging from tenderness and redness to necrosis); previous addiction to the sedative/hypnotic group (ordinary doses may be ineffective and may contribute to further addiction).

Warnings:

Habit forming: Tolerance or psychological and physical dependence may occur with continued use (see Drug abuse and dependence in the Precautions section). Administer with caution, if at all, to patients who are mentally depressed, have suicidal tendencies or a history of drug abuse (eg, alcoholics, opiate abusers, other sedative-hypnotic and amphetamine abusers). Limit prescribing and dispensing to the amount required for the interval until the next appointment.

IV administration: Too rapid administration may cause respiratory depression, apnea, laryngospasm or vasodilation with fall in blood pressure. Parenteral solutions of barbiturates are highly alkaline. Therefore, use extreme care to avoid perivascular extravasation or intra-arterial injection. Extravascular injection may cause local tissue damage with subsequent necrosis; consequences of intra-arterial injection may vary from transient pain to gangrene of the limb. Any complaint of pain in the limb warrants stopping the injection.

SEDATIVES AND HYPNOTICS, BARBITURATES

Phenobarbital sodium may be administered IM or IV as an anticonvulsant for emergency use. When administered IV, it may require ≥ 15 minutes before reaching peak concentrations in the brain. Therefore, injecting phenobarbital sodium until the convulsions stop may cause the brain level to exceed that required to control the convulsions and may lead to severe barbiturate-induced depression.

Pain: Exercise caution when administering to patients with acute or chronic pain, because paradoxical excitement could be induced or important symptoms could be masked. However, the use of barbiturates as sedatives in postoperative surgery and as adjuncts to cancer chemotherapy is well established.

Seizure disorders: Status epilepticus may result from abrupt discontinuation, even when administered in small daily doses in the treatment of epilepsy.

Effects on vitamin D: Barbiturates may increase vitamin D requirements, possibly by increasing the metabolism of vitamin D via enzyme induction. Rickets and osteomalacia have been reported rarely following prolonged use of barbiturates.

Renal function impairment: Barbiturates are excreted either partially or completely unchanged in the urine and are contraindicated in patients with impaired renal function.

Hepatic function impairment: Barbiturates are metabolized primarily by hepatic microsomal enzymes. Administer with caution and initially in reduced doses. Do not use in patients showing premonitory signs of hepatic coma.

Elderly: May produce marked excitement, depression and confusion. In some persons, barbiturates repeatedly produce excitement rather than depression.

Pregnancy: Category D. Barbiturates can cause fetal damage when administered to a pregnant woman. Studies suggest a connection between maternal consumption of barbiturates and a higher incidence of fetal abnormalities. If this drug is used during pregnancy, or if the patient becomes pregnant while taking this drug, apprise her of the potential hazards to the fetus.

Barbiturates readily cross the placental barrier and are distributed throughout fetal tissues. Fetal blood levels approach maternal blood levels following parenteral use.

Withdrawal symptoms occur in infants born to mothers who receive barbiturates throughout the last trimester of pregnancy. Reports include the acute withdrawal syndrome of seizures and hyperirritability from birth to a delayed onset of up to 14 days.

Anticonvulsant use – Because of the strong possibility of precipitating status epilepticus with attendant hypoxia and risk to both mother and unborn child, do not discontinue anticonvulsants when used to prevent major seizures. However, consider discontinuing anticonvulsants prior to and during pregnancy when the nature, frequency and severity of the seizures do not pose a serious threat to the patient. It is not known whether even minor seizures constitute some risk to the embryo or fetus.

Maternal ingestion of anticonvulsants, particularly barbiturates, may be associated with a neonatal coagulation defect that may cause bleeding, usually within 24 hours of birth. The defect is characterized by decreased levels of vitamin K-dependent clotting factors, and prolongation of prothrombin time, partial thromboplastin time or both. Give prophylactic vitamin K to the mother 1 month prior to and during delivery, and to the infant immediately after birth.

Labor and delivery – Hypnotic doses do not appear to significantly impair uterine activity during labor. Full anesthetic doses decrease the force and frequency of uterine contractions. Administration to the mother during labor may result in respiratory depression in the newborn; premature infants are particularly susceptible. If barbiturates are used during labor and delivery, have resuscitation equipment available.

Lactation: Exercise caution when administering to the nursing mother, since small amounts are excreted in breast milk. Drowsiness in the nursing infant has been reported.

Children: In some persons, especially children, barbiturates repeatedly produce excitement rather than depression. Barbiturates may produce irritability, excitability, inappropriate tearfulness and aggression in children. Hyperkinetic states may also be induced and are primarily related to a specific drug sensitivity. Cognitive deficits have been associated with phenobarbital use for complicated febrile seizures in children. Safety and efficacy of amobarbital (children < 6 years of age) and aprobarbital have not been established.

SEDATIVES AND HYPNOTICS, BARBITURATES

Precautions:

Monitoring: During prolonged therapy, perform periodic laboratory evaluation of organ systems, including hematopoietic, renal and hepatic systems.

Special risk patients: Untoward reactions may occur in the presence of fever, hyperthyroidism, diabetes mellitus and severe anemia. Use with caution.

Use **mephobarbital** with caution in patients with myasthenia gravis and myxedema.

Drug abuse and dependence: Barbiturates may be habit forming. Tolerance, psychological dependence and physical dependence may occur, especially following prolonged use of high doses. Doses in excess of 400 mg/day pentobarbital or secobarbital for ≈ 90 days are likely to produce some degree of physical dependence. A dose of 600 to 800 mg taken for at least 35 days is sufficient to produce withdrawal seizures. The average daily dose for the barbiturate addict is usually about 1.5 g. As tolerance develops, the amount needed to maintain the same level of intoxication increases; tolerance to a fatal dosage, however, does not increase more than two-fold. As this occurs, the margin between an intoxicating dosage and fatal dosage becomes smaller.

Intoxication – Symptoms of acute intoxication include unsteady gait, slurred speech and sustained nystagmus. Mental signs of chronic intoxication include confusion, poor judgment, irritability, insomnia and somatic complaints. If an individual appears to be intoxicated with alcohol to a degree that is radically disproportionate to the amount of alcohol in his/her blood, suspect the use of barbiturates. The lethal dose of a barbiturate is far less if alcohol is also ingested.

Dependence – Symptoms are similar to those of chronic alcoholism and include: A strong desire or need to continue taking the drug; tendency to increase the dose; psychic dependence on the effects of the drug related to subjective and individual appreciation of those effects; and physical dependence on the effects of the drug requiring its presence for maintenance of homeostasis resulting in a definite, characteristic and self-limited abstinence syndrome when the drug is withdrawn.

Withdrawal symptoms can be severe and may cause death.

Minor symptoms: These may appear 8 to 12 hours after the last dose of a barbiturate and usually appear in the following order: Anxiety, muscle twitching, tremor of hands and fingers, progressive weakness, dizziness, distortion in visual perception, nausea, vomiting, insomnia and orthostatic hypotension.

Major symptoms: Convulsions and delirium may occur within 16 hours and last up to 5 days after abrupt cessation of these drugs. Intensity of withdrawal symptoms gradually declines in ≈ 15 days.

Treatment of dependence consists of cautious and gradual withdrawal of the drug which takes an extended period of time.

One method involves substituting 30 mg phenobarbital for each 100 to 200 mg dose of barbiturate the patient has been taking. The total daily amount of phenobarbital is administered in 3 to 4 divided doses, not to exceed 600 mg/day. Should signs of withdrawal occur on the first day of treatment, administer an IM loading dose of 100 to 200 mg phenobarbital in addition to the oral dose. After stabilization on phenobarbital, decrease the total daily dose by 30 mg/day as long as withdrawal is proceeding smoothly. A modification of this regimen involves initiating treatment at the patient's regular dosage level and decreasing the daily dosage by 10%, if tolerated. Severely dependent individuals may generally be withdrawn over 2 to 3 weeks.

Infants physically dependent on barbiturates may be given phenobarbital 3 to 10 mg/ kg/day. After withdrawal symptoms (eg, hyperactivity, disturbed sleep, tremors, hyperreflexia) are relieved, gradually decrease the dosage of phenobarbital; completely withdraw over 2 weeks.

Tartrazine sensitivity: Some of these products contain tartrazine, which may cause allergic-type reactions (including bronchial asthma) in susceptible individuals. Although the incidence of tartrazine sensitivity in the general population is low, it is frequently seen in patients who also have aspirin hypersensitivity. Specific products containing tartrazine are identified in the product listings.

SEDATIVES AND HYPNOTICS, BARBITURATES

Drug Interactions:

Most reports of clinically significant drug interactions occurring with the barbiturates have involved phenobarbital.

Sedative/Hypnotic Barbiturate Drug Interactions			
Precipitant drug	Object drug*		Description
Alcohol	Barbiturates	↑	Concomitant use may produce additive CNS effects and death.
Charcoal	Barbiturates	↓	Charcoal can reduce the absorption of barbiturates. Depending on the clinical situation, this will reduce their efficacy or toxicity.
Chloramphenicol	Barbiturates	↓	Chloramphenicol may inhibit phenobarbital metabolism. Barbiturates may enhance chloramphenicol metabolism.
Barbiturates	Chloramphenicol	↑	
MAO inhibitors	Barbiturates	↑	MAOIs may enhance the sedative effects of barbiturates.
Rifampin	Barbiturates	↓	Rifampin induces hepatic microsomal enzymes and may decrease the effectiveness of barbiturates.
Valproic acid	Barbiturates	↑	Valproic acid appears to decrease barbiturate metabolism, resulting in an increased effect.
Barbiturates	Acetaminophen	↑	Risk of increased hepatotoxicity may exist with large or chronic barbiturate doses.
Barbiturates	Anticoagulants	↓	Barbiturates can increase metabolism of anticoagulants resulting in a decreased response. Patients stabilized on anticoagulants may require dosage adjustments if barbiturates are added to or withdrawn from their regimen.
Barbiturates	Beta blockers	↓	Pharmacokinetic parameters of certain β-blockers (metoprolol and propranolol) may be altered by barbiturates. Timolol does not appear to be affected.
Barbiturates	Carbamazepine	↓	Decreased serum carbamazepine levels may occur.
Barbiturates	Clonazepam	↓	Increased clonazepam clearance may occur, which can lead to lower steady-state levels and loss of efficacy.
Barbiturates	Contraceptives, oral	↓	Decreased contraceptive effect may occur due to induction of microsomal enzymes. Menstrual irregularities (spotting, breakthrough bleeding) or pregnancy may occur. An alternate form of birth control is suggested.
Barbiturates	Corticosteroids	↓	Barbiturates may enhance corticosteroid metabolism through the induction of hepatic microsomal enzymes.
Barbiturates	Digitoxin	↓	Barbiturates may increase digitoxin metabolism.
Barbiturates	Doxorubicin	↓	Total doxorubicin plasma clearance may be increased.
Barbiturates	Doxycycline	↓	Phenobarbital decreases doxycycline's half-life and serum levels, which may persist for 2 weeks after barbiturate therapy is discontinued.
Barbiturates	Felodipine	↓	Felodipine plasma levels and bioavailability may be reduced.
Barbiturates	Fenoprofen	↓	Fenoprofen bioavailability may be decreased.
Barbiturates	Griseofulvin	↓	Phenobarbital appears to interfere with the absorption of oral griseofulvin, thus decreasing its blood level; however, the effect on therapeutic response has not been established.
Barbiturates	Hydantoins	↔	The effect of barbiturates on metabolism is unpredictable; monitor hydantoin and barbiturate blood levels frequently if these drugs are given concurrently.

SEDATIVES AND HYPNOTICS, BARBITURATES

Sedative/Hypnotic Barbiturate Drug Interactions			
Precipitant drug	Object drug*		Description
Barbiturates	Methoxy-flurane	↑	Enhanced renal toxicity may occur.
Barbiturates	Metronidazole	↓	Barbiturates may decrease the antimicrobial effectiveness of metronidazole.
Barbiturates	Narcotics	↔	Methadone actions may be reduced. CNS depressant effects of meperidine may be prolonged.
Barbiturates	Phenmetra-zine	↓	The effects of phenmetrazine are decreased by amobarbital.
Barbiturates	Phenylbuta-zone	↓	The elimination half-life of phenylbutazone may be reduced.
Barbiturates	Quinidine	↓	Phenobarbital may significantly reduce the serum levels and half-life of quinidine.
Barbiturates	Theophylline	↓	Barbiturates decrease theophylline levels, possibly resulting in decreased effects.
Barbiturates	Verapamil	↓	The clearance of verapamil may be increased and its bioavailability decreased.

* ↓=Object drug decreased, ↑=Object drug increased, ↔=Undetermined effect.

Adverse Reactions:

The following adverse reactions and their incidence were from observations of hospitalized patients. Because such patients may be less aware of milder adverse effects of barbiturates, the incidence may be higher in fully ambulatory patients.

CNS: Somnolence (1% to 3%); agitation, confusion, hyperkinesia, ataxia, CNS depression, nightmares, nervousness, psychiatric disturbance, hallucinations, insomnia, anxiety, dizziness, abnormal thinking, headache, fever (especially with chronic phenobarbital use) (< 1%); vertigo; lethargy; residual sedation (hangover effect); drowsiness.

Emotional disturbances and phobias may be accentuated with phenobarbital use. In some persons, barbiturates repeatedly produce excitement rather than depression; the patient may appear to be inebriated. Irritability and hyperactivity can occur in children.

Barbiturates, when given in the presence of pain, may cause restlessness, excitement and even delirium. Rarely, the use of barbiturates results in localized or diffuse myalgic, neuralgic or arthritic pain, especially in psychoneurotic patients with insomnia. The pain may appear in paroxysms, is most intense in the early morning hours and is most frequently located in the region of the neck, shoulder girdle and upper limbs. Symptoms may last for days after the drug is discontinued.

Respiratory: Hypoventilation, apnea (< 1%); circulatory collapse; respiratory depression.

Cardiovascular: Bradycardia, hypotension, syncope (< 1%).

GI: Nausea, vomiting, constipation (<1%); liver damage, particularly with chronic phenobarbital use (< 1%).

Hypersensitivity: Skin rashes, angioedema (particularly following chronic phenobarbital use) (< 1%); exfoliative dermatitis (eg, Stevens-Johnson syndrome and toxic epidermal necrolysis) may be caused by phenobarbital and may be fatal (rare).

Acquired hypersensitivity to barbiturates consists chiefly in allergic reactions that occur especially in persons who tend to have asthma, urticaria, angioedema and similar conditions. Hypersensitivity reactions in this category include localized swelling, particularly of the eyelids, cheeks or lips, and erythematous dermatitis. The skin eruption may be associated with fever, delirium and marked degenerative changes in the liver and other parenchymatous organs.

Local: Inadvertent intra-arterial injection may produce arterial spasm with resultant thrombosis and gangrene of an extremity. Reactions range from transient pain to severe tissue necrosis and neurological deficit. Injection SC may produce tissue necrosis, pain, tenderness and redness. Injection into or near peripheral nerves may result in permanent neurological deficit. Thrombophlebitis after IV use and pain at IM injection site have been reported.

Hematologic: Megaloblastic anemia (rarely, following chronic phenobarbital use).

SEDATIVES AND HYPNOTICS, BARBITURATES

Overdosage:

The toxic dose of barbiturates varies considerably. In general, an oral dose of 1 g produces serious poisoning in an adult. Death commonly occurs after 2 to 10 g of ingested barbiturate.

Symptoms: Onset of symptoms may not occur until several hours after ingestion. Acute barbiturate overdosage is manifested by CNS and respiratory depression which may progress to Cheyne-Stokes respiration, areflexia, constriction of the pupils to a slight degree (though in severe poisoning they may show paralytic dilation), nystagmus, ataxia, oliguria, tachycardia, hypotension, lowered body temperature and coma. Typical shock syndrome (eg, apnea, circulatory collapse, respiratory arrest, death) may occur.

In extreme overdose, all electrical activity in the brain may cease, in which case a "flat" EEG normally equated with clinical death cannot be accepted. This effect is fully reversible unless hypoxic damage occurs. Consider the possibility of barbiturate intoxication even in situations that appear to involve trauma.

Complications such as pneumonia, pulmonary edema, cardiac arrhythmias, congestive heart failure and renal failure may occur. Uremia may increase sensitivity to barbiturates if renal function is impaired. Include hypoglycemia, head trauma, cerebrovascular accidents, convulsive states and diabetic coma in differential diagnosis.

Treatment: Treatment is mainly supportive. Maintain an adequate airway, with assisted respiration and oxygen administration, as necessary. Monitor vital signs and fluid balance. Refer to General Management of Acute Overdosage.

If the patient is conscious and has not lost the gag reflex, emesis may be induced with ipecac. Take care to prevent pulmonary aspiration of vomitus. After completion of vomiting, administer 30 g activated charcoal in a glass of water. Nasogastric administration of multiple doses of activated charcoal has been successful in accelerating the elimination of phenobarbital from the body. If emesis is contraindicated, perform gastric lavage with a cuffed endotracheal tube in place with the patient in the face down position. Activated charcoal may be left in the emptied stomach and a saline cathartic administered.

Administer fluid and other standard treatments for shock, if needed. If renal function is normal, forced diuresis may aid in the elimination of the barbiturate. However, diuresis and peritoneal dialysis are of little value. Alkalinization of the urine increases renal excretion of some barbiturates, especially phenobarbital, aprobarbital and mephobarbital (which is metabolized to phenobarbital).

Hemodialysis and hemoperfusion may be used in severe barbiturate intoxication or if the patient is anuric or in shock. Patient should be rolled from side to side every 30 minutes.

Patient Information:

Do not increase the dose of the drug without consulting a physician.

Barbiturates may impair mental or physical abilities required for the performance of potentially hazardous tasks (eg, driving, operating machinery).

Alcohol should not be consumed while taking barbiturates. Concurrent use of barbiturates with other CNS depressants (eg, alcohol, narcotics, tranquilizers and antihistamines) may result in additional CNS depressant effects.

Notify physician if any of the following occurs: Fever; sore throat; mouth sores; easy bruising or bleeding; tiny broken blood vessels under the skin.

Use as an aid to sleep is limited; do not use > 2 weeks.

SEDATIVES AND HYPNOTICS, BARBITURATES

Administration and Dosage:

Individualize dosage; consider patient's age, weight and condition. Use parenteral routes only when oral administration is impossible or impractical.

IM injection of the sodium salts should be made deeply into a large muscle. Do not exceed 5 ml at any one site because of possible tissue irritation. Monitor patient's vital signs.

IV: Restrict to conditions in which other routes are not feasible, either because the patient is unconscious (as in cerebral hemorrhage, eclampsia or status epilepticus), or because the patient resists (as in delirium), or because prompt action is imperative. Slow IV injection is essential; observe patients carefully during administration. Maintain blood pressure, respiration and cardiac function, monitor vital signs and have equipment for resuscitation and artificial ventilation available.

Rectal administration: Rectally administered barbiturates are absorbed from the colon and are used occasionally in infants for prolonged convulsive states, or when oral or parenteral administration may be undesirable. If the rectal form is not available, the soluble sodium salt may be incorporated in a retention enema.

Elderly: Reduce dosage because these patients may be more sensitive to barbiturates.

Hepatic/Renal function impairment: Reduce dosage.

Long-Acting

PHENOBARBITAL

For complete prescribing information, refer to the Barbiturates group monograph.

Indications:

Oral: Sedative; hypnotic (short-term treatment of insomnia since it appears to lose its effectiveness after 2 weeks); anticonvulsant (treatment of partial and generalized tonic-clonic and cortical focal seizures); emergency control of certain acute convulsive episodes (eg, those associated with status epilepticus, eclampsia, tetanus and toxic reactions to strychnine or local anesthetics).

Parenteral: Sedative; hypnotic (short-term treatment of insomnia since it appears to lose its effectiveness after 2 weeks); preanesthetic; anticonvulsant (treatment of generalized tonic-clonic and cortical focal seizures); emergency control of acute convulsions (eg, tetanus, eclampsia, status epilepticus).

Administration and Dosage:

Individualize dosage. Factors of consideration are age, weight and condition.

Anticonvulsant: In infants and children, a loading dose of 15 to 20 mg/kg produces blood levels of ≈ 20 mcg/ml shortly after administration. To achieve therapeutic blood levels (10 to 25 mcg/ml), higher dosages per kilogram are generally necessary compared to adults.

Oral:

Adults –

Sedation: 30 to 120 mg/day in 2 to 3 divided doses. A single dose of 30 to 120 mg may be given at intervals; frequency is determined by response. It is generally considered that no more than 400 mg should be given during a 24 hour period.

Hypnotic: 100 to 200 mg.

Anticonvulsant: 60 to 100 mg/day.

Children –

Anticonvulsant: 3 to 6 mg/kg/day.

Sedation: 8 to 32 mg.

Hypnotic: Determined by age and weight.

Parenteral: Observe the effect of large doses. Use only when oral use is impossible or impractical.

Adults –

Sedation: 30 to 120 mg/day IM or IV in 2 to 3 divided doses.

Preoperative sedation: 100 to 200 mg, IM only, 60 to 90 min before surgery.

Hypnotic: 100 to 320 mg IM or IV.

Acute convulsions: 200 to 320 mg IM or IV, repeated in 6 hours as necessary.

Children –

Preoperative sedation: 1 to 3 mg/kg IM or IV.

Anticonvulsant: 4 to 6 mg/kg/day for 7 to 10 days to blood level of 10 to 15 mcg/ml, or 10 to 15 mg/kg/day, IV or IM.

Status epilepticus: 15 to 20 mg/kg IV over 10 to 15 minutes. It is imperative to achieve therapeutic levels as rapidly as possible. When given IV, it may require ≥ 15 minutes to attain peak levels in the brain. If injected continuously until convulsions stop, the brain concentration would continue to rise and could exceed that required to control seizures. Since a barbiturate-induced depression may occur, it is important to use the minimal amount required and to wait for the anticonvulsant effect to develop before giving a second dose.

IM – Administer deep IM into one of the large muscles (gluteus maximus, vastus lateralis) or other areas where there is little risk of encountering a nerve trunk or a major artery. Injection into or near peripheral nerves may result in permanent neurological deficit.

IV – Restrict IV use to conditions in which other routes are not feasible, either because the patient is unconscious (as in cerebral hemorrhage, eclampsia or status epilepticus) or because of resistance (as in delirium) or because prompt action is imperative.

No average IV dose reliably produces similar effects in all patients. Possibility of overdose and respiratory depression is remote with slow injection of fractional doses. Observe physical signs closely. Onset of action is usually within 5 minutes of IV use.

In convulsive states, minimize dosage to avoid compounding the depression which may follow convulsions. The injection must be made slowly.

Any vein may be used; administer preferably into a larger vein (to minimize the possibility of thrombosis). Avoid administration into varicose veins, because circulation is retarded. Inadvertent injection into or adjacent to an artery may result in gangrene requiring amputation of an extremity or a portion thereof. Careful technique, including aspiration, is necessary to avoid inadvertent intra-arterial injection.

Long-Acting

PHENOBARBITAL

Elderly/Debilitated: Reduce dosage; these patients may be more sensitive to the drug.

Hepatic/Renal function impairment: Reduce dosage.

c-iv	**Phenobarbital** (Various, eg, Harber, Lilly, Major, Moore, PBI, Parmed, Roxane, Rugby, Schein, Warner Chilcott)	**Tablets:** 15 mg	In 100s, 1000s, 5000s and UD 100s.
c-iv	**Solfoton** (ECR Pharm.)	**Tablets:** 16 mg	In 100s and 500s.
c-iv	**Bellatal** (Richwood)	**Tablets:** 16.2 mg	Lactose. 0.1037 mg hyoscyamine sulfate, 0.0194 mg atropine sulfate, 0.0065 mg scopolamine hydrobormide. (0478/5477. White, scored. In 100s and 500s.
c-iv	**Phenobarbital** (Various, eg, Goldline, Harber, Lilly, Major, Moore, PBI, Parmed, Roxane, Rugby, Warner Chilcott)	**Tablets:** 30 mg	In 100s, 1000s and 5000s and UD 100s.
c-iv	**Phenobarbital** (Various, eg, Century, Harber, Lilly, Moore, PBI, Parmed, Roxane, Schein, Warner Chilcott)	**Tablets:** 60 mg	In 100s, 1000s and UD 100s.
c-iv	**Phenobarbital** (Various, eg, Century, Harber, Lilly, Roxane, Schein)	**Tablets:** 100 mg	In 100s and 1000s.
c-iv	**Solfoton** (ECR Pharm.)	**Capsules:** 16 mg	In 100s and 500s.
c-iv	**Phenobarbital** (Pharmaceutical Associates)	**Elixir:** 15 mg per 5 ml	13.5% alcohol. Fruit flavor. In pt and UD 5, 10 and 20 ml.
c-iv	**Phenobarbital** (Various, eg, Barre-National, Century, Goldline, Halsey, Harber, Lilly, Roxane, Rugby, Schein)	**Elixir:** 20 mg per 5 ml	Alcohol. In pt, gal, UD 5 ml and UD 7.5 ml.
c-iv	**Phenobarbital Sodium** (Wyeth-Ayerst)	**Injection:** 30 mg/ml	In 1 ml Tubex.
c-iv	**Phenobarbital Sodium** (Wyeth-Ayerst)	**Injection:** 60 mg/ml	In 1 ml Tubex.
c-iv	**Phenobarbital Sodium** (Wyeth-Ayerst)	**Injection:** 65 mg/ml	In 1 ml vials.
c-iv	**Phenobarbital Sodium** (Various, eg, Elkins-Sinn, Wyeth-Ayerst)	**Injection:** 130 mg/ml	In 1 ml Tubex and 1 ml vials.
c-iv	**Luminal Sodium** (Sanofi Winthrop)		In 1 ml amps.[1]

[1] With 10% alcohol and 67.8% propylene glycol.

Long-Acting

MEPHOBARBITAL

For complete prescribing information, refer to the Barbiturates group monograph.

Indications:

Sedative for the relief of anxiety, tension and apprehension; anticonvulsant for the treatment of grand mal and petit mal epilepsy.

Administration and Dosage:

Sedative:

Adults – 32 to 100 mg 3 or 4 times a day. Optimum dose is 50 mg 3 or 4 times/day.

Children – 16 to 32 mg 3 or 4 times per day.

Epilepsy:

Adults – Average dose is 400 to 600 mg daily.

Children (< 5 years of age) – 16 to 32 mg 3 or 4 times per day.

Children (> 5 years of age) – 32 to 64 mg 3 or 4 times per day.

Take at bedtime if seizures generally occur at night, and during the day if attacks are diurnal. Start treatment with a small dose and gradually increase over 4 or 5 days until optimum dosage is determined.

Replacement therapy: Start with a small dose and gradually increase over 4 or 5 days until optimum dose is determined. If the patient has been taking another antiepileptic drug, gradually reduce the dosage of the other drug as the doses of mephobarbital are increased, to guard against the temporary marked attacks that may occur when treatment for epilepsy is changed abruptly. Similarly, when the dose is to be lowered to a maintenance level or to be discontinued, reduce the amount gradually over 4 or 5 days.

Combination drug therapy: May be used in combination with phenobarbital, in alternating courses or concurrently. When the two are used at the same time, the dose should be about one-half the amount of each used alone. The average daily dose for an adult is from 50 to 100 mg phenobarbital and from 200 to 300 mg mephobarbital. May also be used with phenytoin. When used concurrently, a reduced dose of phenytoin is advisable, but the full dose of mephobarbital may be given. Satisfactory results have been obtained with an average daily dose of 230 mg phenytoin plus about 600 mg mephobarbital.

Elderly/Debilitated: Reduce dosage since these patients may be more sensitive to the drug.

Hepatic/Renal function impairment: Reduce dosage.

c-iv	**Mebaral** (Sanofi Winthrop)	**Tablets:** 32 mg	(M 705). In 250s.
		50 mg	(M 715). In 250s.
		100 mg	(M 725). In 250s.

Intermediate-Acting

AMOBARBITAL SODIUM

For complete prescribing information, refer to the Barbiturates group monograph.

Indications:

Sedation; hypnotic (short-term treatment of insomnia since it appears to lose its effectiveness after 2 weeks); preanesthetic.

Administration and Dosage:

Individualize dosage. The maximum single dose for an adult is 1 g.

Sedative: The usual adult dosage is 30 to 50 mg, 2 or 3 times per day.

Hypnotic: The usual adult dose is 65 to 200 mg.

IM: Do not inject a volume > 5 ml IM, regardless of drug concentration, at any one site because of possible tissue irritation. The average IM dose ranges from 65 to 500 mg. Solutions of 20% may be used so that a small volume can contain a large dose. Inject deeply into a large muscle, such as the gluteus maximus. Superficial IM or SC injections may be painful and may produce sterile abscesses or sloughs.

IV: Restrict IV use to conditions in which other routes are not feasible, either because the patient is unconscious, resists, or because prompt action is imperative. Slow injection is essential. Monitor patients carefully. Do not exceed the rate of 50 mg/min. Ordinarily, 65 to 500 mg may be given to a child 6 to 12 years of age. The final dosage is determined to a great extent by the patient's reaction to the slow administration of the drug.

Preparation of solution: Add Sterile Water for Injection to the vial and rotate to facilitate solution of the powder. Do not shake the vial.

Stability: Do not use a solution which is not absolutely clear after 5 minutes. Amobarbital sodium hydrolyzes in solution or upon exposure to air. No more than 30 minutes should elapse from the time the vial is opened until contents are injected.

Elderly/Debilitated: Reduce dosage since these patients may be more sensitive to the drug.

Hepatic/renal function impairment: Reduce dosage.

c-II	**Amytal Sodium** (Lilly)	**Powder for Injection**	In 250 mg vials.
			In 500 mg vials.

APROBARBITAL

For complete prescribing information, refer to the Barbiturates group monograph.

Indications:

Short-term sedation and sleep induction.

Administration and Dosage:

Sedative: 40 mg, 3 times per day.

Mild insomnia: 40 to 80 mg before retiring.

Pronounced insomnia: 80 to 160 mg before retiring.

Elderly/Debilitated: Reduce dosage since these patients may be more sensitive to the drug.

Hepatic/Renal function impairment: Reduce dosage.

c-III	**Alurate** (Roche)	**Elixir:** 40 mg per 5 ml	20% alcohol, saccharin, sorbitol, sucrose. In pt.

Intermediate-Acting

BUTABARBITAL SODIUM

For complete prescribing information, refer to the Barbiturates group monograph.

Indications:

Sedative or hypnotic. Barbiturates appear to lose their effectiveness for sleep induction and maintenance after 2 weeks.

Administration and Dosage:

Adults:

Daytime sedation – 15 to 30 mg, 3 or 4 times daily.

Bedtime hypnotic – 50 to 100 mg.

Preoperative sedation – 50 to 100 mg, 60 to 90 minutes before surgery.

Children:

Preoperative sedation – 2 to 6 mg/kg; maximum 100 mg.

Elderly/Debilitated: Reduce dosage; these patients may be more sensitive to the drug.

Hepatic/Renal function impairment: Reduce dosage.

c-III	**Butabarbital Sodium** (Various)	**Tablets:** 15 mg	In 1000s.
c-III	**Butisol Sodium** (Wallace)		(Butisol Sodium 37 112). Lavender, scored. In 100s and 1000s.
c-III	**Butabarbital Sodium** (Various, eg, Major)	**Tablets:** 30 mg	In 100s and 1000s.
c-III	**Butisol Sodium** (Wallace)		Tartrazine. (Butisol Sodium 37 113). Green, scored. In 100s and 1000s.
c-III	**Butisol Sodium** (Wallace)	**Tablets:** 50 mg	Tartrazine. (Butisol Sodium 37 114). Orange, scored. In 100s.
c-III	**Butisol Sodium** (Wallace)	**Tablets:** 100 mg	(Butisol Sodium 37 115). Pink, scored. In 100s.
c-III	**Butabarbital Sodium** (Various, eg, Barre-National, Harber, Major, Rugby)	**Elixir:** 30 mg per 5 ml	In pt.
c-III	**Butisol Sodium** (Wallace)		7% alcohol, tartrazine, saccharin. In pt and gal.

Short-Acting

SECOBARBITAL SODIUM

For complete prescribing information, refer to the Barbiturates group monograph.

Indications:

Oral: Hypnotic (short-term treatment of insomnia since it appears to lose its effectiveness after 2 weeks); preanesthetic.

Parenteral: For intermittent use as a sedative, hypnotic or preanesthetic.

Administration and Dosage:

Oral:

Adults –

Preoperative sedation: 200 to 300 mg 1 to 2 hours before surgery.

Bedtime hypnotic: 100 mg.

Children – For preoperative sedation, 2 to 6 mg/kg (max. 100 mg).

Parenteral: Adjust dosage on basis of age, weight and patient's condition.

IM – Inject deeply into a large muscle mass. Inject no more than 250 mg (5 ml) into any one site because of possible tissue irritation. Monitor patient's vital signs after injection.

IV – Restrict IV use to conditions in which other routes are not feasible, including unconsciousness, resistance or because prompt action is imperative.

Adults –

Hypnotic: Usual dose is 100 to 200 mg IM or 50 to 250 mg IV.

Properative sedation: For light sedation, 1 mg/kg (0.5 to 0.75 mg/lb) IM, 10 to 15 minutes before procedure.

For children, the IM dose is 4 to 5 mg/kg.

Dentistry: In patients who are to receive nerve blocks, 100 to 150 mg IV.

Children –

Preoperative sedation: 4 to 5 mg/kg IM.

Status epilepticus: 15 to 20 mg/kg IV over to to 15 minutes.

Stability and storage – Refrigerate; protect from light. Do not use if solution contains a precipitate.

Elderly/debilitated: Reduce dosage; these patients may be more sensitive to the drug.

Hepatic/Renal function impairment: Reduce dosage.

c-II	**Secobarbital Sodium** (Various, eg, Halsey)	**Capsules:** 100 mg	In 100s, 500s and 1000s.
c-II	**Seconal Sodium Pulvules** (Lilly)		(F40). Orange. In 100s and UD 100s.
c-II	**Secobarbital Sodium** (Wyeth-Ayerst)	**Injection:** 50 mg per ml	In 2 ml Tubex.[1]

[1] With 50% polyethylene glycol and not more than 2.5 mg phenol.

PENTOBARBITAL SODIUM

For complete prescribing information, refer to the Barbiturates group monograph.

Indications:

Oral: Sedative; hypnotic (short-term treatment of insomnia, since it appears to lose its effectiveness after 2 weeks); preanesthetic.

Rectal: Sedation (when oral or parenteral administration may be undesirable); hypnotic (short-term treatment of insomnia, since it appears to lose its effectiveness after 2 weeks).

Parenteral: Sedative; hypnotic (short-term treatment of insomnia since it appears to lose its effectiveness after 2 weeks); preanesthetic; anticonvulsant, in anesthetic doses, for the emergency control of certain acute convulsive episodes (eg, those associated with status epilepticus, eclampsia, meningitis, tetanus and toxic reactions to strychnine or local anesthetics).

Administration and Dosage:

Oral:

Adults –

Sedation: 20 mg 3 or 4 times per day.

Hypnotic: 100 mg at bedtime.

Children –

Sedation: 2 to 6 mg/kg/day, depending on age, weight and degree of sedation desired.

Hypnotic: Base dosage on age and weight.

Preanesthetic: 2 to 6 mg/kg/day (max. 100 mg), depending on age, weight and desired degree of sedation.

Short-Acting

PENTOBARBITAL SODIUM

Rectal: Do not divide suppositories.

Adults – 120 to 200 mg.

Children –

12 to 14 years (36.4 to 50 kg; 80 to 110 lbs): 60 or 120 mg.

5 to 12 years (18.2 to 36.4 kg; 40 to 80 lbs): 60 mg.

1 to 4 years (9 to 18.2 kg; 20 to 40 lbs): 30 or 60 mg.

2 months to 1 year (4.5 to 9 kg; 10 to 20 lbs): 30 mg.

Parenteral: Pentobarbital solutions are highly alkaline. Therefore, exercise extreme care to avoid perivascular extravasation or intra-arterial injection.

IV – Restrict IV use to conditions in which other routes are not feasible, including patient unconsciousness (as in cerebral hemorrhage, eclampsia or status epilepticus), because of resistance (as in delirium), or because prompt action is imperative. Slow IV injection is essential; carefully observe patients during administration. The rate of IV injection should not exceed 50 mg/min. No average IV dose can be relied upon to produce similar effects in different patients. The possibility of overdose and respiratory depression is remote when the drug is injected slowly in fractional doses. The clinical response is the basis for dosage determination, although the patient's weight and age may influence the total amount of the drug required. Watch the physical signs closely to accurately obtain and maintain the desired degree of sedation.

Initially administer 100 mg in the 70 kg adult. Reduce dosage proportionally for pediatric or debilitated patients. At least 1 minute is necessary to determine the full effect. If needed, additional small increments of the drug may be given to a total of 200 to 500 mg for healthy adults.

In convulsive states, keep dosages to a minimum to avoid compounding the depression which may follow convulsions. Inject slowly with regard to the time required for the drug to penetrate the blood-brain barrier.

IM – Inject deeply into a large muscle mass. Do not exceed a volume of 5 ml at any one site because of possible tissue irritation.

Calculate dosage on basis of age, weight and the patient's condition. The usual adult dosage is 150 to 200 mg; children's dosage frequently ranges from 2 to 6 mg/kg as a single IM injection, not to exceed 100 mg.

Stability – Do not use if solution is discolored or contains a precipitate.

Elderly/Debilitated: Reduce dosage; these patients may be more sensitive to the drug.

Hepatic/Renal function impairment: Reduce dosage.

c-ii	**Nembutal Sodium** (Abbott)	**Capsules:** 50 mg	Lactose. Orange and clear. In 100s.
c-ii	**Pentobarbital Sodium** (Various)	**Capsules:** 100 mg	In 1000s.
c-ii	**Nembutal Sodium** (Abbott)		Tartrazine. Yellow. In 100s, 500s and *Abbo-Pac* 100s.
c-iii	**Nembutal Sodium** (Abbott)	**Suppositories:** 30 mg	In 12s.
		60 mg	In 12s.
		120 mg	In 12s.
		200 mg	In 12s.
c-ii	**Pentobarbital Sodium** (Wyeth-Ayerst)	**Injection:** 50 mg per ml	In 2 ml Tubex.[1]
c-ii	**Nembutal Sodium Solution** (Abbott)		In 2 ml amps and 20 and 50 ml vials.[1]

[1] With propylene glycol and 10% alcohol.

Oral Combinations

ORAL COMBINATIONS

Combined barbiturate products are promoted to provide a more balanced effect through the combination of those with differing rates of action and dissipation.

Consider the information given for Barbiturates (see group monograph) when using these products.

c-II	**Tuinal 100 mg Pulvules** (Lilly)	**Capsules**: 50 mg amobarbital sodium and 50 mg secobarbital sodium	Blue and orange. In 100s.
c-II	**Tuinal 200 mg Pulvules** (Lilly)	**Capsules**: 100 mg amobarbital sodium and 100 mg secobarbital sodium	Blue and orange. In 100s.

BARBITURATES

Actions:

Pharmacology: The ultrashort-acting barbiturates, thiopental, thiamylal and methohexital, depress the CNS to produce hypnosis and anesthesia without analgesia. Methohexital does not possess muscle relaxant properties. These drugs are frequently used to provide hypnosis during balanced anesthesia with other agents for muscle relaxation and analgesia.

Biotransformation products of thiopental are pharmacologically inactive and mostly excreted in the urine.

Pharmacokinetics: The rapid onset and brief duration of action of these drugs is a function of their high lipid solubility. They quickly cross the blood-brain barrier, but are rapidly redistributed from the brain to other body tissues, first to highly perfused visceral organs (liver, kidneys, heart) and muscle, and later to fatty tissues.

Administered IV as the sodium salts, these agents produce anesthesia within 1 minute. Recovery after a small dose is rapid, with somnolence and retrograde amnesia. Muscle relaxation occurs at the onset of anesthesia. The duration of anesthetic activity following a single IV dose is 20 to 30 minutes for thiopental and thiamylal, and somewhat shorter for methohexital. Thiopental is readily absorbed by the rectal route when administered as a suspension; onset of action usually occurs within 8 to 10 minutes. Thiopental IV produces hypnosis within 30 to 40 seconds following administration. Repeated doses or continuous infusion of these agents causes accumulation. Slow release of the drug from lipoidal storage sites results in prolonged anesthesia, somnolence and respiratory and circulatory depression. The plasma half-life is 3 to 8 hours.

Indications:

Induction of anesthesia; supplementation of other anesthetic agents; IV anesthesia for short surgical procedures with minimal painful stimuli; induction of a hypnotic state.

Thiopental (IV): Control of convulsive states and in neurosurgical patients with increased intracranial pressure if adequate ventilation is provided.

Thiopental (rectal suspension): Used when preanesthetic sedation or basal narcosis by the rectal route is desired. It may be employed as the sole agent in selected brief, minor procedures where muscular relaxation and analgesia are not required.

Contraindications:

Absolute: Latent or manifest porphyria; hypersensitivity to barbiturates; absence of suitable veins for IV administration.

Relative: Severe cardiovascular disease; hypotension or shock; conditions in which hypnotic effects may be prolonged or potentiated (excessive premedication, Addison's disease, hepatic or renal dysfunction, myxedema, increased blood urea and severe anemia); increased intracranial pressure; asthma; myasthenia gravis; status asthmaticus (thiopental).

If barbiturates are used in conditions involving relative contraindications, reduce dosage and administer slowly.

Rectal suspension: Patients who are to undergo rectal surgery; presence of inflammatory, ulcerative, bleeding or neoplastic lesions of the lower bowel; patients with acute asthmatic attacks, and variegate or acute intermittent porphyria.

Warnings:

Status asthmaticus: Use **methohexital** and **thiamylal** with extreme caution in patients with status asthmaticus.

Repeated or continuous infusion may cause cumulative effects resulting in prolonged somnolence and respiratory and circulatory depression. Resuscitative and endotracheal intubation equipment and oxygen should be immediately available. Maintain patency of the airway at all times.

Pregnancy: Category C (thiopental); Category B (methohexital). Safety for use during pregnancy has not been established. Use only when clearly needed and when the potential benefits outweigh the potential hazards to the fetus.

Thiopental readily crosses the placental barrier.

Methohexital has been used in cesarean section delivery, but because of its solubility and lack of protein binding, it readily and rapidly traverses the placenta.

Lactation: Small amounts of **thiopental** may appear in breast milk following administration of large doses. Exercise caution when administering barbiturates to a nursing woman.

Children:

Methohexital – Safety and efficacy in children have not been established.

BARBITURATES

Precautions:

Special risk patients: Respiratory depression, apnea or hypotension may occur due to individual variations in tolerance or to the physical status of the patient. Exercise caution in debilitated patients, or those with impaired function of respiratory, circulatory, cardiac, renal, hepatic or endocrine systems.

Extravascular injection may cause pain, swelling, ulceration and necrosis. Intra-arterial injection is dangerous and may produce gangrene of an extremity.

Rectal dose: If evacuation of the instilled rectal dose occurs, assess the effects of any retained portion before administering a repeat dose.

Drug abuse and dependence: May be habit-forming.

Drug Interactions:

Barbiturate Drug Interactions			
Precipitant Drug	Object Drug*		Description
Narcotics	Barbiturate anesthetics	⬆	The barbiturate dose required to induce anesthesia may be reduced. Apnea may be more common with this combination.
Phenothiazines	Barbiturate anesthetics	⬆	Preanesthetic use of phenothiazines may raise the frequency and severity of neuromuscular excitation and hypotension in patients who receive barbiturate anesthesia.
Probenecid	Barbiturate anesthetics	⬆	The anesthesia produced by the barbiturate may be extended or achieved at lower doses.
Sulfisoxazole	Barbiturate anesthetics	⬆	Sulfisoxazole may enhance the anesthetic effects of the barbiturate.

* ⬆ = Object drug increased.

Drug/Lab test interactions: BSP and liver function studies may be influenced by administration of a single dose of barbiturates.

Adverse Reactions:

Cardiovascular: Circulatory depression; thrombophlebitis; hypotension; peripheral vascular collapse; convulsions in association with cardiorespiratory arrest; myocardial depression; cardiac arrhythmias.

Respiratory: Respiratory depression including apnea; dyspnea; rhinitis; laryngospasm; bronchospasm; sneezing; coughing.

CNS: Emergence delirium; headache; restlessness; anxiety; seizures; prolonged somnolence and recovery.

GI: Nausea; emesis; abdominal pain. Rectal irritation; diarrhea; cramping; rectal bleeding (rectal administration).

Local: Pain or nerve injury at injection site.

Hypersensitivity:

Acute allergic reactions – Erythema; pruritus; urticaria; anaphylactic reaction.

Miscellaneous: Salivation; hiccups skin rashes; skeletal muscle hyperactivity; shivering.

Rarely, immune hemolytic anemia with renal failure and radial nerve palsy have occurred.

Overdosage:

Symptoms: Overdosage may occur from too rapid or repeated injections. Too rapid injection may be followed by an alarming fall in blood pressure, even to shock levels. Apnea, occasional laryngospasm, coughing and other respiratory difficulties with excessive or too rapid injections may occur.

Treatment: In the event of suspected or apparent overdosage, discontinue the drug, maintain or establish a patent airway (intubate if necessary) and administer oxygen with assisted ventilation if necessary. The lethal dose of barbiturates varies and cannot be stated with certainty. Lethal blood levels may be as low as 1 mg/dl for short-acting barbiturates; less if other depressant drugs or alcohol are also present.

Barbiturates

THIOPENTAL SODIUM

For complete prescribing information refer to the Barbiturate Anesthetics group monograph.

Administration and Dosage:

Parenteral: Administer IV only. Individual response is so varied that there can be no fixed dosage. Titrate against patient requirement as governed by age, sex and body weight.

Test dose – Inject a small test dose of 25 to 75 mg to assess tolerance or unusual sensitivity. Observe patient reaction for ≥ 60 seconds.

Anesthesia – Moderately slow induction can be accomplished in the average adult by injection of 50 to 75 mg (2 to 3 ml of a 2.5% solution) at intervals of 20 to 40 seconds, depending on patient response. Once anesthesia is established, additional injections of 25 to 50 mg can be administered whenever the patient moves. Slow injection is recommended to minimize respiratory depression and the possibility of overdosage.

When used for induction in balanced anesthesia with a skeletal muscle relaxant and an inhalation agent, the total dose can be estimated and then injected in two to four fractional doses. With this technique, brief periods of apnea may occur, which may require assisted or controlled pulmonary ventilation. As an initial dose, 210 to 280 mg (3 to 4 mg/kg) is usually required for rapid induction in the average adult (70 kg).

When used as the sole anesthetic agent, the desired level of anesthesia can be maintained by injection of small repeated doses as needed or by using a continuous IV drip in a 0.2% or 0.4% concentration.

Convulsive states following anesthesia (inhalation or local) or other causes – Administer 75 to 125 mg (3 to 5 ml of a 2.5% solution) as soon as possible after the convulsion begins. Convulsions following the use of a local anesthetic may require 125 to 250 mg, given over a 10–minute period.

Neurosurgical patients with increased intracranial pressure – Administer intermittent bolus injections of 1.5 to 3.5 mg/kg to reduce intra-operative elevations of intracranial pressure, if adequate ventilation is provided.

Psychiatric disorders – For narcoanalysis and narcosynthesis, premedication with an anticholinergic agent may precede administration of thiopental. After a test dose, thiopental is injected at a slow rate of 100 mg/min (4 ml/min of a 2.5% solution) with the patient counting backwards from 100.

Alternative thiopental may be administered by rapid IV drip using a 0.2% concentration in 5% Dextrose in Water. The rate of administration should not exceed 50 ml/min.

Preparation of parenteral solution: Use one of the following diluents: Sterile Water for Injection; 0.9% Sodium Chloride Injection; 5% Dextrose Injection. A 2% or 2.5% solution is most commonly used for intermittent injections, although concentrations vary between 2% and 5%. A 3.4% concentration in Sterile Water for Injection is isotonic. Do not use concentrations < 2% in Sterile Water for Injection because they cause hemolysis.

Use concentrations of 0.2% or 0.4% for continuous IV administration. Prepare them with 5% Dextrose Injection, 0.9% Sodium Chloride Injection or Normosol-R.

Admixture incompatibility: The most stable solutions are those in water or in isotonic saline, refrigerated and tightly stoppered. Do not mix solutions of succinylcholine, tubocurarine or other drugs that have an acid pH with thiopental solutions.

Storage/Stability: Freshly prepare parenteral solutions and use promptly; discard unused portions after 24 hours.

Barbiturates

THIOPENTAL SODIUM

c-III	**Thiopental Sodium** (IMS)	**Powder for Injection:** 2% (20 mg/ml)	In 400 mg *Min-I-Mix* vials with *Min-I-Mix* injector.
c-III	**Pentothal** (Abbott)		In 1, 2.5 and 5 g kits, 400 mg Ready-to-Mix syringes and 400 mg Ready-to-Mix *LifeShield* syringes.
c-III	**Thiopental Sodium** (Gensia, IMS)	**Powder for Injection:** 2.5% (25 mg/ml)	In 250 and 500 mg *Min-I-Mix* vials with *Min-I-Mix* and 500 mg, 1, 2.5, 5 and 10 g kits.
c-III	**Pentothal** (Abbott)		In 1, 2.5, 5 g and 500 mg kits, 250 and 500 mg Ready-to-Mix syringes and 250 and 500 mg Ready-to-Mix *LifeShield* syringes.

METHOHEXITAL SODIUM

For complete prescribing information, refer to the Barbiturate Anesthetics group monograph.

Administration and Dosage:

Pre-anesthetic medication is generally advisable. Any of the recognized pre-anesthetic medications may be used, but the phenothiazines are less satisfactory than the combination of an opiate and a belladonna derivative.

Individualize dosage. Administer IV in a concentration ≤ 1%. Higher concentrations markedly increase the incidence of muscular movements and irregularities in respiration and blood pressure.

Induction: The dose for induction of anesthesia may range from 50 to 120 mg or more, but averages ≈ 70 mg. Give a 1% solution at ≈ 1 ml/5 seconds. The induction dose usually provides anesthesia for 5 to 7 minutes. Usual dosage in adults ranges from 1 to 1.5 mg/kg.

Maintenance of anesthesia may be accomplished by intermittent injections of the 1% solution or by continuous IV drip of a 0.2% solution. Intermittent injections of ≈ 20 to 40 mg (2 to 4 ml of a 1% solution) may be given as required, usually every 4 to 7 minutes. For continuous drip, the average rate of administration is ≈ 3 ml of a 0.2% solution/min (1 drop/sec). Individualize the rate of flow for each patient. For longer surgical procedures, gradual reduction in the rate of administration is recommended.

Admixture compatibility/incompatibility: Do not use bacteriostatic diluents; Sterile Water for Injection is preferred. The 5% Dextrose Injection or 0.9% Sodium Chloride Injection may be used. (Not compatible with Lactated Ringer's Injection). Do not mix methohexital in the same syringe or administer simultaneously during IV infusion through the same needle with acid solutions, such as atropine sulfate, metocurine iodide and succinylcholine chloride (alteration of pH may cause free barbituric acid to be precipitated).

Reconstitution – When the first dilution is made, the solution in the vial will be yellow. When further diluted to make a 1% solution, it must be clear and colorless, or should not be used.

Preparation of 1% Methohexital Solutions	
Vial	Amount diluent (ml)
500 mg	50 ml
2.5 g	250 ml
5.0 g	500 ml

Continuous drip anesthesia: Prepare a 0.2% solution by adding 500 mg to 250 ml diluent. For this dilution, use 5% Dextrose or Isotonic (0.9%) Sodium Chloride instead of distilled water to avoid extreme hypotonicity.

Storage/Stability: Reconstituted solutions are chemically stable at room temperature for 24 hours. Store vials at room temperature.

c-IV	**Brevital Sodium** (Lilly)	**Powder for Injection:** 500 mg	In 50 ml vials with and without diluent.
		2.5 g	In 20 ml vials.
		5 g	In 30 ml vials.
🍁	**Brietal Sodium** (Lilly)	**Powder for Injection:** 10 mg/ml	Preservative-free. In 500 mg/50 ml vials.

KETAMINE HCl

Warning:

Emergence reactions occur in ≈ 12% of patients. The incidence is least in young (≤ 15 years old) and elderly (> 65 years old) patients. Also less frequent with IM use.

Psychological manifestations – Severity varies between pleasant dream-like states, vivid imagery, hallucinations and emergence delirium sometimes accompanied by confusion, excitement and irrational behavior. The duration is ordinarily a few hours; however, recurrences have been seen up to 24 hours postoperatively. No residual psychological effects are known.

The incidence may be reduced by using lower dosages with IV diazepam. These reactions may be reduced if verbal, tactile and visual patient stimulation is minimized during recovery. This does not preclude monitoring vital signs.

Management – To terminate a severe emergence reaction, a small hypnotic dose of a short-acting or ultrashort-acting barbiturate may be required.

When used on an outpatient basis, do not release patient until recovery from anesthesia is complete. Patients should be accompanied by an adult.

Actions:

Pharmacology: Ketamine is a rapid-acting general anesthetic producing an anesthetic state characterized by profound analgesia, normal pharyngeal-laryngeal reflexes, normal or slightly enhanced skeletal muscle tone, cardiovascular and respiratory stimulation and occasionally, a transient and minimal respiratory depression. A patent airway is maintained partly by virtue of unimpaired pharyngeal and laryngeal reflexes.

The anesthetic state produced by ketamine has been termed "dissociative anesthesia" in that it appears to selectively interrupt association pathways of the brain before producing somatesthetic sensory blockade. It may selectively depress the thalamoneocortical system before significantly obtunding the more ancient cerebral centers and pathways (reticular-activating and limbic systems).

Pharmacokinetics: Following IV administration, the ketamine concentration has an initial slope (α-phase) lasting ≈ 45 minutes with a half-life of 10 to 15 minutes, corresponding to anesthetic effect. Anesthetic action is terminated by redistribution from CNS and by hepatic biotransformation. The major metabolite is ≈ ⅓ as active as ketamine. The β-phase half-life of ketamine is 2.5 hours.

Elevation of blood pressure begins shortly after injection, reaches a maximum in minutes and returns to pre-anesthetic values within 15 minutes. The systolic and diastolic blood pressure peaks from 10% to 50% above pre-anesthetic levels.

An IV dose of 2 mg/kg usually produces surgical anesthesia within 30 seconds after injection, lasting 5 to 10 minutes. Additional increments can be administered IV or IM to maintain anesthesia without significant cumulative effects.

IM doses of 9 to 13 mg/kg usually produce surgical anesthesia within 3 to 4 minutes and last ≈ 12 to 25 minutes.

Indications:

Diagnostic/Surgical procedures: Sole anesthetic agent for diagnostic and surgical procedures that do not require skeletal muscle relaxation. Ketamine is best suited for short procedures, but it can be used with additional doses for longer procedures.

Anesthesia: For induction of anesthesia prior to administration of other general anesthetics.

Supplement: Used to supplement low-potency agents, such as nitrous oxide.

Contraindications:

Patients in whom a significant elevation of blood pressure would be a serious hazard; hypersensitivity to the drug.

Warnings:

Cardiac effects: Monitor cardiac function continuously during the procedure in patients with hypertension or cardiac decompensation.

Respiratory effects: Respiratory depression may occur with overdosage or too rapid a rate of administration, in which case employ supportive ventilation. Mechanical support of respiration is preferred to administration of analeptics.

Tonic-clonic movements: Purposeless and tonic-clonic movements of extremities may occur during the course of anesthesia. These movements do not imply a light plane and are not indicative of the need for additional doses of the anesthetic.

Emergence reactions and psychological manifestation: See Warning Box.

Pregnancy: Category C. Safety for use during pregnancy, including obstetrics, has not been established; use is not recommended.

KETAMINE HCl

Precautions:

Respiratory surgery/diagnostic procedures: Do not use in surgery or diagnostic procedures of the pharynx, larynx or bronchial tree. Do not administer ketamine alone because pharyngeal and laryngeal reflexes are usually active. Muscle relaxants, with proper attention to respiration, may be required.

Vomiting: Vomiting has been reported following administration. Laryngeal-pharyngeal reflexes may offer some airway protection, however the possibility of aspiration must be considered because protective reflexes may also be diminished by supplementary anesthetics and muscle relaxants.

Visceral pain: In surgical procedures involving visceral pain pathways, supplement with an agent that obtunds visceral pain.

Preoperative preparation: Give atropine, scopolamine or another drying agent at an appropriate interval prior to induction.

Alcohol: Use with caution in chronic alcoholics and acutely alcohol intoxicated patients.

Resuscitative equipment should be ready for use.

Cerebrospinal fluid pressure increase has been reported following administration.

Hazardous tasks: Warn patients not to drive, operate hazardous machinery or engage in hazardous activities for 24 hours or more after anesthesia.

Drug Interactions:

Ketamine Drug Interactions			
Precipitant Drug	Object Drug*		Description
Ketamine	Nondepolarizing muscle relaxants	↑	Ketamine may increase the neuromuscular effects resulting in prolonged respiratory depression.
Ketamine	Thiopental	↓	The hypnotic effect of thiopental may be antagonized.
Barbiturates/Narcotics	Ketamine	↑	Prolonged recovery time may occur if used with ketamine.
Halothane	Ketamine	↓	Cardiac output, blood pressure and pulse rate may be decreased. Halothane blocks the cardiovascular stimulatory effects of ketamine. Closely monitor cardiac function if ketamine and halothane are used together.
Theophyllines	Ketamine	↔	Unpredictable extensor-type seizures have been reported with coadministration.
Thyroid hormones	Ketamine	↑	Concurrent use may produce hypertension and tachycardia.

↑ = Object drug increased. ↓ = Object drug decreased. ↔ = Undetermined effect.

Adverse Reactions:

Cardiovascular: Elevated blood pressure and pulse rate (frequent); hypotension; bradycardia; arrhythmia.

Respiratory: Although respiration is frequently stimulated, severe depression of respiration or apnea may occur following rapid IV administration of high doses. Laryngospasm and other forms of airway obstruction have occurred.

Ophthalmic: Diplopia; nystagmus; slight elevation in intraocular pressure.

Psychiatric: (See Warning Box).

GI: Anorexia; nausea; vomiting.

CNS: Enhanced skeletal muscle tone manifested by tonic and clonic movements, sometimes resembling seizures.

Body as a whole: Local pain and exanthema at the injection site (infrequent); transient erythema or morbilliform rash.

KETAMINE HCl

Overdosage:

Respiratory depression may occur with overdosage or too rapid administration rate; employ supportive ventilation. Mechanical support of respiration is preferred to analeptic use.

Administration and Dosage:

Individualize dosage.

Induction:

IV route – Administer over 60 seconds. Initial dose ranges from 1 to 4.5 mg/kg. The average amount to produce 5 to 10 minutes of surgical anesthesia is 2 mg/kg.

Alternatively, in adults, 1 to 2 mg/kg administered at a rate of 0.5 mg/kg/min may be used for induction of anesthesia. In addition, diazepam may be given in 2 to 5 mg doses (total: ≤ 15 mg IV), in a separate syringe over 60 seconds. This may reduce incidence of psychological manifestations during emergence.

Administer slowly (over 60 seconds). More rapid administration may result in respiratory depression and enhanced pressor response.

Note: Do not inject 100 mg/ml concentration IV without proper dilution. Dilute with equal volume Sterile Water for Injection, Normal Saline or 5% Dextrose in Water.

IM route – Initial dose ranges from 6.5 to 13 mg/kg. A dose of 10 mg/kg will usually produce 12 to 25 minutes of surgical anesthesia.

Maintenance: Increments of one-half to the full induction dose may be repeated as needed for maintenance of anesthesia. The larger the total dose administered, the longer the time to complete recovery.

Adults induced with ketamine augmented with IV diazepam may be maintained on ketamine given by slow microdrip infusion at 0.1 to 0.5 mg/minute, augmented with 2 to 5 mg IV diazepam, given as needed. Often, ≤ 20 mg of IV diazepam total for combined induction and maintenance will suffice. The incidence of psychological manifestations during emergence may be reduced.

Dilution – To prepare a dilute solution containing 1 mg/ml, transfer 10 ml (50 mg/ml vial) or 5 ml (100 mg/ml vial) to 500 ml of 5% Dextrose Injection or Sodium Chloride (0.9%) Injection and mix well.

Vials of 10 mg/ml are not recommended for dilution.

If fluid restriction is required, add ketamine to a 250 ml infusion, as described above, to provide a 2 mg/ml concentration.

Admixture incompatibility – Barbiturates and ketamine are incompatible (precipitate); do not inject from same syringe. Do not mix ketamine and diazepam in syringe or infusion flask.

Ketamine is clinically compatible with the commonly used general and local anesthetic agents when an adequate respiratory exchange is maintained.

Storage/Stability: Store between 15° to 30°C (59° to 86°F). Protect from light.

Rx	**Ketalar** (Parke-Davis)	**Injection:** Ketamine base (as HCl): 10 mg/ml	In 20 ml vials.[1]
		50 mg/ml	In 10 ml vials.[1]
		100 mg/ml	In 5 ml vials.[1]
🍁	**Ketalar** (Parke-Davis)	**Injection:** Ketamine base (as HCl): 10 mg/ml	In 20 ml vials.[1]
		50 mg/ml	In 10 ml vials.[1]

[1] With benzethonium chloride.

ETOMIDATE

Actions:

Pharmacology: Etomidate, a nonbarbiturate hypnotic without analgesic activity, has fewer cardiovascular depressant effects than thiopental sodium. Up to 0.6 mg/kg in patients with severe cardiovascular disease has little or no effect on myocardial metabolism, cardiac output, peripheral circulation or pulmonary circulation. Hemodynamic effects are qualitatively similar to those of thiopental sodium. Etomidate lowers cerebral blood flow and cerebral oxygen consumption. It will usually lower intracranial pressure slightly and intraocular pressure moderately.

Pharmacokinetics: Injection IV produces hypnosis rapidly, usually within 1 minute. Duration is usually 3 to 5 minutes. Immediate recovery period will usually be shortened in adults by ≈ 0.1 mg IV fentanyl, 1 or 2 min before induction of anesthesia, probably because less etomidate is generally required. Protein binding, primarily to albumin, is ≈ 76%. Etomidate is rapidly metabolized in the liver. Plasma levels of unchanged drug decrease rapidly up to 30 minutes following injection and thereafter more slowly with a half-life of ≈ 75 minutes. Approximately 75% of the dose is excreted in the urine, mostly as metabolite (80%).

Indications:

Anesthesia: Induction of general anesthesia.

Supplementation of subpotent anesthetic agents, such as nitrous oxide in oxygen, during maintenance of anesthesia for short operative procedures.

Unlabeled uses: Etomidate has been used for prolonged sedation of critically ill patients or ventilator-dependent patients; however, this use has been associated with increased risks, including acute adrenal insufficiency and increased mortality.

Contraindications:

Hypersensitivity to etomidate.

Warnings:

Corticosteroid replacement: Although no changes in vital signs or increased mortality have been reported with etomidate-induced reduced plasma cortisol levels, consider exogenous corticosteroid replacement in patients undergoing severe stress.

Myoclonus: Prior IV narcotic or benzodiazepine administration may reduce the incidence of these involuntary muscle movements.

Renal/Hepatic function impairment: Limited pharmacokinetic data in patients with cirrhosis and esophageal varices suggest that the volume of distribution and elimination half-life of etomidate are approximately double that seen in healthy subjects.

Pregnancy: Category C. Etomidate has embryocidal effects in rats when given in doses 1 and 4 times the human dose and has caused maternal toxicity in rats and rabbits. Use only when clearly needed and when the potential benefits outweigh the unknown potential hazards to the fetus. Use in labor and delivery is not recommended.

Lactation: Some etomidate is excreted in breast milk. Use caution when administering to a nursing mother.

Children: Safety and efficacy for use in children < 10 years of age have not been established. Use is not recommended.

Drug Interactions:

Verapamil: The anesthetic effect of etomidate may be increased with prolonged respiratory depression and apnea.

Adverse Reactions:

Most frequent: Transient skeletal muscle movements (32%) classified as myoclonic in the majority of cases (74%; see Warnings); transient venous pain (20%); tonic movements (10%); eye movements (9%); averting movements (7%).

Cardiovascular: Hypertension; hypotension; tachycardia; bradycardia; arrhythmias.

Miscellaneous: Hyperventilation; hypoventilation; apnea of short duration (5 to 90 seconds with spontaneous recovery); laryngospasm; hiccoughs; snoring; postoperative nausea or vomiting following induction of anesthesia.

Administration and Dosage:

Induction of anesthesia: For IV use only. Adults and children > 10 years old, 0.2 to 0.6 mg/kg. Usual dose is 0.3 mg/kg, injected over 30 to 60 seconds.

Concomitant anesthesia – Smaller increments may be given to adults during short operative procedures to supplement subpotent anesthetic agents. Compatible with commonly used preanesthetic medication.

Rx	**Amidate** (Abbott)	**Injection:** 2 mg/ml	In 10, 20 ml amps, 20 ml *Abboject.*

MIDAZOLAM HCl

Benzodiazepine compounds used as antianxiety agents appear under the Antianxiety Agents monograph.

Warning:

Midazolam IV has been associated with respiratory depression and respiratory arrest. In some cases, where this was not recognized promptly and treated effectively, death or hypoxic encephalopathy resulted. Use midazolam IV only in hospital or ambulatory care settings, including physicians' offices, that provide for continuous monitoring of respiratory and cardiac function. Assure immediate availability of resuscitative drugs and equipment and personnel trained in their use. (See Warnings.)

The initial IV dose for conscious sedation may be as little as 1 mg, but should not exceed 2.5 mg in a normal healthy adult. Lower doses are necessary for older (> 60 years) or debilitated patients and in patients receiving concomitant narcotics or other CNS depressants. Never give the initial dose and all subsequent doses as a bolus; administer over at least 2 minutes and allow an additional 2 or more minutes to fully evaluate sedative effect. Use of 1 mg/ml formulation or dilution of 1 mg/ml or 5 mg/ml formulation is recommended to facilitate slower injection. See Administration and Dosage for complete dosing information.

Actions:

Pharmacology: Midazolam is a short-acting benzodiazepine CNS depressant.

In patients without intracranial lesions, induction is associated with a moderate decrease in cerebrospinal fluid pressure, similar to thiopental. Preliminary data in intracranial surgical patients with normal intracranial pressure but decreased compliance show comparable elevations of intracranial pressure with midazolam and with thiopental during intubation.

Induction doses depress the ventilatory response to carbon dioxide stimulation for 15 minutes or more beyond the duration of ventilatory depression following administration of thiopental. Impairment of ventilatory response is more marked in patients with chronic obstructive pulmonary disease (COPD). Sedation with IV midazolam does not adversely affect the mechanics of respiration; total lung capacity and peak expiratory flow decrease significantly, but static compliance and maximum expiratory flow at 50% of awake total lung capacity (V_{max}) increase.

Induction is associated with a slight to moderate decrease in mean arterial pressure, cardiac output, stroke volume and systemic vascular resistance. Slow heart rates (less than 65/minute), particularly in patients taking propranolol for angina, tend to rise slightly; faster heart rates (eg, 85/minute) tend to slow slightly.

Pharmacokinetics:

Absorption/Distribution – The mean absolute bioavailability following IM use is > 90% with mean peak plasma concentrations (C_{max}) of 90 ng/ml occuring within 30 minutes. C_{max} and time to peak (T_{max}) for the 1–hydroxy metabolite following the IM dose were 8 ng/ml and 1 hour, respectively. Midazolam has a large volume of distribution (Vd) of 1 to 3.1 L/kg. Peak concentrations of midazolam as well as 1-hydroxymethyl midazolam after IM administration are about one-half of those achieved after equivalent IV doses. The concentration of midazolam is 10- to 30-fold greater than that of 1–hydroxymethyl midazolam after single IV administration. Midazolam can accumulate in peripheral tissues with continuous infusion. Maintain the lowest effective midazolam infusion rate to reduce effects of accumulation.

Midazolam is ≈ 97% plasma protein bound, primarily to albumin. It crosses the placenta and enters fetal circulation.

Metabolism/Excretion – Elimination of the parent drug takes place via hepatic metabolism of midazolam to hydroxylated metabolites that are conjugated and excreted in the urine. Midazolam IV has an elimination half-life of 1.8 to 6.4 hours and a plasma clearance (Cl) of 0.25 to 0.54 L/hr/kg; < 0.5% of the dose is excreted in the urine intact. The biotransformation of midazolam is mediated by cytochrome P450–3A4. 1–hydroxy-midazolam accounts for 60% to 70% of biotransformation while 4–hydroxy-midazolam constitutes ≤ 5%. 1–hydroxy-midazolam is at least as potent as the parent compound and may contribute to the net pharmacologic activity of midazolam. The affinities of 1– and 4–hydroxy-midazolam for the benzodiazepine receptor are ≈ 20% and 7%, respectively, relative to midazolam. Midazolam follows linear kinetics at IV doses of 0.15 to 0.3 mg/kg but clearance is successively reduced by ≈ 30% at doses of 0.45 to 0.6 mg/kg indicating non-linear kinetics in this dose range.

Onset/Duration: Onset of IM sedation in adults is 15 minutes; peak sedation, 30 to 60 minutes. Sedative effects in the pediatric population begin within 5 minutes and peak at 15 to 30 minutes depending upon the dose administered.

MIDAZOLAM HCl

Sedation after IV injection was achieved within 3 to 5 minutes. The time of onset is affected by total dose administered and the concurrent administration of narcotic premedication. In endoscopy patients, 71% had no recall of introduction of the endoscope; 82% had no recall of endoscope withdrawal.

When given IV, anesthesia induction occurs in ≈1.5 minutes when narcotic premedication is given and in 2 to 2.5 minutes without narcotic or with sedative premedication. Some memory impairment was noted in 90% of patients. Midazolam does not delay awakening from general anesthesia, which usually occurs within 2 hours but may take up to 6 hours.

Plasma concentration-effect relationship: At plasma concentrations > 100 ng/ml there is ≥ 50% probability that patients will be sedated but respond to verbal commands (sedation score = 3). At 200 ng/ml there is ≥ 50% probability that patients will be asleep but respond to glabellar tap (sedation score = 4).

Congestive heart failure (CHF): Patients with CHF have a 2–fold increase in the elimination half-life, a 25% decrease in the plasma clearance and a 40% increase in volume of distribution.

Renal function impairment: There was a 2-fold increase in clearance and volume of distribution in patients with chronic renal failure. Midazolam clearance may be reduced (1.9 vs 2.8 ml/min/kg) and the half-life prolonged (7.6 vs 13 hr) in acute renal failure (ARF) patients. The renal clearance of the 1–hydroxy-midazolam glucuronide was prolonged in the ARF patients (4 vs 136 ml/min) and the half-life was prolonged (12 hr vs > 25 hr). Plasma levels accumulated to ≈ 10 times that of the parent drug.

Hepatic function impairment: The mean half-life of midazolam is increased 2.5–fold in alcoholic patients. Clearance is reduced by 50% and the Vd increased by 20%.

Pediatrics: In pediatric patients, weight-normalized clearance is similar or higher (0.19 to 0.8 L/hr/kg) than in adults and the terminal elimination half-life (0.78 to 3.3 hours) is similar to or shorter than in adults. In seriously ill neonates, the terminal elimination half-life of midazolam is substantially prolonged (6.5 to 12 hours) and the clearance reduced (0.07 to 0.12 L/hr/kg).

Obesity: The mean half-life is greater in obese patients (5.9 vs 2.3 hours) because of an increase of ≈ 50% in the Vd, corrected for total body weight. Clearance is not significantly affected.

Elderly: Plasma half-life is ≈ 2–fold higher in the elderly. The mean Vd based on total body weight increases consistently between 15% to 100% and mean Cl is decreased ≈ 25%.

Indications:

Preoperative sedation (IV and IM): Preoperative sedation, anxiolysis and amnesia.

Sedation/Anesthesia (IV): Sedation, anxiolysis and amnesia prior to or during short diagnostic, therapeutic or endoscopic procedures, either alone or with other CNS depressants; for induction of general anesthesia before administration of other anesthetic agents; to supplement nitrous oxide and oxygen (balanced anesthesia); infusion for sedation of intubated and mechanically ventilated patients as a component of anesthesia or during treatment in a critical care setting.

Unlabeled uses: Treatment of epileptic seizures (10 to 15 mg); alternative for the termination of refractory status epilepticus.

Contraindications:

Hypersensitivity to benzodiazepines; acute narrow-angle glaucoma (use in open-angle glaucoma only if patients are receiving appropriate therapy).

Warnings:

Respiratory depression: Prior to IV administration in any dose, ensure the immediate availability of oxygen, resuscitative equipment and skilled personnel for the maintenance of a patent airway and support of ventilation. Continuously monitor patients for early signs of underventilation or apnea, which can lead to hypoxia/cardiac arrest. Continue to monitor vital signs during recovery period. Because midazolam IV depresses respiration and because opioid agonists and other sedatives can add to this depression, administer midazolam as an induction agent only by a person trained in general anesthesia. The immediate availability of specific reversal agents (eg, flumazenil) is highly recommended. Use in conscious sedation only when a person skilled in early detection of underventilation, maintaining a patent airway and supporting ventilation is present. Titrate slowly when used for sedation, anxiolysis and amnesia, do not administer midazolam by rapid or single bolus IV administration.

Serious cardiorespiratory adverse events have occurred, including respiratory depression, airway obstruction, desaturation, apnea, respiratory arrest or cardiac arrest, sometimes resulting in death or permanent neurologic injury. There have been rare reports of hypotensive episodes requiring treatment during or after diagnostic or surgical manipulations in patients who received midazolam. Hypotension may occur more frequently in conscious sedation patients premedicated with a narcotic. Adverse hemodynamic events have been reported in pediatric patients with cardiovascular instability.

Improper dosing: Reactions such as agitation, involuntary movements (including tonic/clonic movements and muscle tremor), hyperactivity and combativeness have been reported. These reactions may be caused by inadequate or excessive dosing or improper administration of midazolam; however, consider cerebral hypoxia or true paradoxical reactions. Should such reactions occur, evaluate response to each dose of midazolam and all other drugs, including local anesthetics, before proceeding.

Neonates – Reversal of such responses with flumazenil has been reported in pediatric patients. Avoid rapid injection in the neonatal population. IV injection (< 2 minutes) has been associated with severe hypotension in neonates, particularly when the patient has also received fentanyl. Severe hypotension has also been observed in neonates receiving a continuous infusion of midazolam who then receive a rapid IV injection of fentanyl. Seizures have been reported in several neonates following rapid IV administration. The neonate has reduced or immature organ function and is also vulnerable to profound or prolonged respiratory effects of midazolam.

Ophthalmic: Measurements of intraocular pressure in patients without eye disease show a moderate lowering following induction with midazolam.

Do not administer to patients in shock or coma, or in acute alcohol intoxication with depression of vital signs. Exercise particular care in use of midazolam IV in patients with uncompensated acute illnesses, such as severe fluid or electrolyte disturbances.

Intra-arterial injection hazards are unknown; therefore, take extreme precautions against unintended intra-arterial injection. Avoid extravasation.

Abrupt withdrawal: Withdrawal symptoms (convulsions, hallucinations, tremor, abdominal and muscle cramps, vomiting and sweating) may occur following abrupt discontinuation of benzodiazepines, including midazolam. Abdominal distension, nausea, vomiting and tachycardia are prominent symptoms of withdrawal in infants. Severe withdrawal symptoms are usually limited to patients receiving excessive doses over an extended period of time. Milder withdrawal symptoms (eg, dysphoria and insomnia) generally follow abrupt discontinuance of benzodiazepines taken therapeutically for several months. After extended therapy, avoid abrupt discontinuation and gradually taper dosage.

Higher risk surgical patients, elderly or debilitated patients require lower dosages for induction of anesthesia, whether premedicated or not. Patients with COPD are unusually sensitive to the respiratory depressant effect of midazolam. Patients with chronic renal failure and patients with CHF eliminate midazolam more slowly. Because elderly patients frequently have inefficient function of one or more organ systems, and because dosage requirements decrease with age, reduce initial dosage of midazolam and consider possibility of profound or prolonged effect.

With concomitant CNS depressant medication, decrease IV doses by 50% for elderly and debilitated patients. These patients will probably take longer to recover completely after induction of anesthesia.

Renal function impairment: Patients with renal impairment may have longer elimination half-lives for midazolam and its metabolites, which may result in slower recovery.

Carcinogenesis: In mice given 80 mg/kg/day of midazolam for 2 years, there was a marked increase in the incidence of hepatic tumors in female mice, and a small but statistically significant increase in benign thyroid follicular cell tumors in male mice.

Pregnancy: Category D. An increased risk of congenital malformations is associated with the use of benzodiazepine drugs. If this drug is used during pregnancy, apprise the patient of the potential hazard to the fetus.

Labor and delivery – Following IM administration of 0.05 mg/kg, both venous and umbilical arterial serum concentrations were lower than maternal concentrations.

Because midazolam is transferred transplacentally and because other benzodiazepines given in the last weeks of pregnancy have resulted in neonatal CNS depression, midazolam is not recommended for obstetrical use.

Lactation: Midazolam is excreted in breast milk. Exercise caution when administering to a nursing mother.

Children: As a group, pediatric patients generally require higher dosages of midazolam (mg/kg) than do adults. Younger (< 6 years old) pediatric patients may require higher dosages (mg/kg) than older pediatric patients and may require closer monitoring. In obese pediatric patients, calculate the dose based on ideal body weight. The neo-

MIDAZOLAM HCl

nate has reduced or immature organ function and is also vulnerable to profound or prolonged respiratory effects of midazolam.

Precautions:

Intracranial pressure/circulatory side effects: Midazolam does not protect against the increase in intracranial pressure or circulatory effects associated with endotracheal intubation under light general anesthesia.

Hazardous tasks: No patient should operate hazardous machinery or a motor vehicle until the effects of the drug, such as drowsiness, have subsided or until the day after anesthesia and surgery, whichever is longer.

Drug Interactions:

Caution is advised when midazolam is administered concomitantly with drugs that are known to inhibit the P450–3A4 enzyme system such as cimetidine, erythromycin, diltiazem, verapamil, ketaconazole and itraconazole. These drug interactions may result in prolonged sedation caused by a decrease in plasma clearance of midazolam.

Midazolam Drug Interactions

Precipitant drug	Object drug*		Description
Midazolam	Anesthetics, inhalation	⬆	Inhalation anesthetics may need to be reduced if midazolam is used as an induction agent. IV administration decreases minimum alveolar concentration (MAC) of halothane required for general anesthesia. This correlates with midazolam dosage.
Midazolam	CNS depressants	⬆	Barbiturates, alcohol or other CNS depressants may increase risk of hypoventilation, airway obstruction, desaturation or apnea and contribute to prolonged effect with midazolam. Narcotic premedication also depresses ventilatory response to carbon dioxide stimulation.
Midazolam	Narcotic analgesics	⬆	Narcotics, secobarbital and droperidol used as premedications accentuate midazolam's hypnotic effect. Adjust midazolam dosage according to the premedication used. Hypotension occurs more frequently with IV midazolam and meperidine in conscious sedation. Severe hypotension has been reported with concomitant administration of fentanyl.
Midazolam	Propofol	⬆	The pharmacologic effects of propofol may be increased.
Midazolam	Thiopental	⬆	A moderate reduction in induction dosage requirements (≈ 15%) has been noted following use of IM midazolam for premedication.
Azole antifungal agents	Midazolam	⬆	Serum concentrations of certain benzodiazepines may be increased and prolonged, producing enhanced CNS depression and prolonged effects.
Cimetidine	Midazolam	⬆	Serum levels of some benzodiazepines may be increased. Certain actions, especially sedation, may be enhanced.

Midazolam Drug Interactions			
Precipitant drug	Object drug*		Description
Contraceptives, oral	Midazolam	⬆	Coadministration of combination oral contraceptives and benzodiazepines that undergo oxidation may result in a prolongation of benzodiazepine half-life.
Ethanol	Midazolam	⬆	Increased CNS effects with acute ethanol ingestion. Tolerance may occur with chronic ethanol use.
Fluvoxamine	Midazolam	⬆	Reduced clearance, prolonged half-life and increased serum concentrations of certain benzodiazepines may occur. Sedation or ataxia may be increased.
Indinavir	Midazolam	⬆	Possibly prolonged sedation and respiratory depression.
Rifamycins	Midazolam	⬇	The pharmacokinetic parameters of benzodiazepines may be altered (eg, increase in drug and metabolite clearance and decrease in elimination half-life).
Ritonavir	Midazolam	⬆	Possibly severe sedation and respiratory depression.
Theophyllines	Midazolam	⬇	The sedative effects of benzodiazepines may be antagonized by theophyllines.
Valproic acid	Midazolam	⬆	Pharmacokinetic parameters of benzodiazepines may be increased. Liver metabolism of some benzodiazepines may be decreased.
Verapamil	Midazolam	⬆	Effects of certain benzodiazepines may be increased, producing increased CNS depression and prolonged effects.

* ⬆ = Object drug increased. ⬇ = Object drug decreased. ⟷ = Undetermined effect.

Adverse Reactions:

See Warnings concerning serious cardiorespiratory events and paradoxical reactions.

Fluctuations in vital signs are most frequent and include decreased tidal volume or respiratory rate decrease (IV – 23.3%; IM – 10.8%); apnea (IV – 15.4%); variations in blood pressure and pulse rate..

IM: Headache (1.3%); pain at injection site (3.7%); induration and redness (0.5%), muscle stiffness (0.3%).

IV: The following were observed mainly following IV administration:

Respiratory – Coughing (1.3%); laryngospasm, bronchospasm, dyspnea, hyperventilation, wheezing, shallow respirations, airway obstruction, tachypnea (< 1%).

Cardiovascular – Bigeminy, premature ventricular contractions, vasovagal episode, bradycardia, tachycardia, nodal rhythm (< 1%).

GI: Hiccoughs (3.9%); nausea (2.8%); vomiting (2.6%); acid taste, excessive salivation, retching (< 1%).

CNS: Oversedation (1.6%); headache (1.5%); drowsiness (1.2%); retrograde amnesia, euphoria, confusion, argumentativeness, nervousness, agitation, anxiety, grogginess, restlessness, emergence delirium, prolonged emergence from anesthesia, dreaming during emergence, insomnia, nightmares, tonic/clonic movements, involuntary or athetoid movements, ataxia, dizziness, dysphoria, slurred speech, dysphonia, paresthesia (< 1%).

MIDAZOLAM HCl

Special senses: Blurred vision, diplopia, nystagmus, pinpoint pupils, cyclic eyelid movements, visual disturbance, difficulty focusing, blocked ears, loss of balance (< 1%).

Dermatologic: Hives, hive-like elevation at injection site, swelling or feeling of burning, warmth or coldness at injection site, rash, pruritus (< 1%).

Miscellaneous: Tenderness at injection site (5.6%); pain during injection (5%); redness (2.6%); induration (1.7%); phlebitis (0.4%); yawning, lethargy, chills, weakness, toothache, faint feeling, hematoma (< 1%).

Children: Desaturation (4.6%); apnea (2.8%); hypotension (2.7%); paradoxical reactions (2%); hiccough (1.2%); seizure-like activity (1.1%); nystagmus (1.1%).

Overdosage:

Symptoms are similar to other benzodiazepines; sedation, somnolence, confusion, impaired coordination and reflexes, coma and untoward effects on vital signs.

Treatment: Monitor respiration, pulse rate and blood pressure and employ supportive measures. Maintain a patent airway and support ventilation. Start an IV infusion. Treat hypotension with IV fluid therapy, repositioning, judicious use of vasopressors and other appropriate measures. The value of peritoneal dialysis, forced diuresis or hemodialysis is unknown.

Flumazenil, a specific benzodiazepine-receptor antagonist, is indicated for the complete or partial reversal of the sedative effects of benzodiazepines and may be used in situations when an overdose with a benzodiazepine is known or suspected (see the Flumazenil monograph in the Antidotes section). Flumazenil is intended as an adjunct to, not as a substitute for, proper management of benzodiazepine overdose. Monitor patients treated with flumazenil for resedation, respiratory depression and other residual benzodiazepine effects for an appropriate period after treatment. Flumazenil will only reverse benzodiazepine-induced effects but will not reverse the effects of other concomitant medications. Refer to General Management of Acute Overdosage.

Patient Information:

Inform physician about any alcohol consumption and other medicine being taken, especially blood pressure medication and antibiotics, including non-prescription drugs. Alcohol has an increased effect when consumed with benzodiazepines; therefore, exercise caution regarding simultaneous ingestion of alcohol during benzodiazepine treatment.

Inform the physician if pregnant, planning to become pregnant or breastfeeding.

Patients receiving continuous infusion of midazolam in critical care settings over an extended period of time may experience symptoms of withdrawal following abrupt discontinuation.

Administration and Dosage:

Administer IV or IM only.

Individualize dosage. Midazolam is a potent sedative agent which requires slow administration. Midazolam is 3 to 4 times as potent per mg as diazepam. Because serious and life-threatening cardiorespiratory events have been reported, make provisions for monitoring, detection and correction of these reactions for every patient, regardless of age or health status. Excessive doses or rapid or single bolus IV doses may result in respiratory depression or arrest. (See Warnings.)

Elderly or debilitated patients: In general, lower doses are required. Adjust the IV dosage according to the type and amount of premedication used.

Preoperative sedation anxiolysis and amnesia (IM): Inject deep in a large muscle mass. 0.07 to 0.08 mg/kg (≈ 5 mg for an average adult) up to 1 hour before surgery. For patients > 60 years of age, debilitated, chronically ill or receiving concomitant CNS depressants, the dose must be individualized and reduced. Onset is in 15 minutes, peaking at 30 to 60 minutes. Atropine or scopolamine and reduced narcotic doses may be coadministered.

Sedation, anxiolysis or amnesia for procedures (IV): Use midazolam either alone or with a narcotic. For peroral procedures, use an appropriate topical anesthetic. For bronchoscopic procedures, use narcotic premedication.

Use 1 mg/ml to facilitate slower injection. Dilute the 1 and 5 mg/ml formulations with 0.9% sodium chloride or 5% dextrose in water. Individualize dosage. Do not give by rapid or single bolus IV. Response will vary with age, physical status and concomitant medications, but may also vary independent of these factors. (See Warnings.)

Healthy adults < 60 years of age – Titrate slowly to the desired effect (eg, the initiation of slurred speech). Some patients may respond to as little as 1 mg. Give no more than 2.5 mg over at least 2 minutes. Wait an additional 2 or more minutes to fully evaluate the sedative effect. If further titration is necessary, use small increments to the appropriate level of sedation. Wait an additional 2 or more minutes after each increment to fully evaluate sedative effect. A total dose > 5 mg is usually not necessary.

If narcotic premedication or other CNS depressants are used, patients will require ≈ 30% less midazolam than unpremedicated patients.

Patients ≥ 60 years of age, debilitated or chronically ill patients – The danger of underventilation or apnea is greater and the peak effect may take longer in these patients; reduce increments and slow the rate of injection.

Titrate slowly to desired effect (eg, initiation of slurred speech). Some patients may respond to as little as 1 mg. Give ≤ 1.5 mg over ≥ 2 minutes. Wait an additional 2 or more minutes to fully evaluate sedative effect. If additional titration is needed, give at a rate of no more than 1 mg over 2 minutes, waiting an additional 2 or more minutes each time to fully evaluate sedative effect. Total doses > 3.5 mg are not usually necessary.

If CNS depressant premedications are used in these patients, they will require at least 50% less midazolam than healthy young unpremedicated patients.

Maintenance – Give in increments of 25% of the dose used to first reach the sedative endpoint, only by slow titration, especially in the elderly/chronically ill/debilitated. Give only if thorough evaluation clearly indicates need for additional sedation.

Induction of general anesthesia, before use of other anesthetics (IV): Individual response is variable, particularly when a narcotic premedication is not used. Titrate dosage to desired clinical effect according to patient's age and clinical status. When midazolam is used before other IV agents for induction of anesthesia, the initial dose of each agent may be significantly reduced, at times as low as 25% of the usual initial dose of the individual agents.

Unpremedicated patients – An average adult < 55 years of age will initially require 0.3 to 0.35 mg/kg over 20 to 30 seconds, allowing 2 minutes for effect. If needed to complete induction, use increments of ≈ 25% of initial dose; may complete induction with volatile liquid inhalational anesthetics. Up to 0.6 mg/kg total dose may be used, but may prolong recovery.

Unpremedicated patients > 55 years of age or with severe systemic disease or other debilitation may require less midazolam. For patients > 55 years of age, an initial dose is 0.3 mg/kg. For patients with severe systemic disease or other debilitation, an initial dose of 0.2 to 0.25 mg/kg will usually suffice; in some cases, as little as 0.15 mg/kg.

Premedicated patients – Give 0.15 to 0.35 mg/kg. In average adults < 55 years of age , give 0.25 mg/kg over 20 to 30 seconds and allow 2 minutes for effect. Use 0.2 mg/kg for good risk (ASA I & II) surgical patients > 55 years of age. In patients with severe systemic disease or debilitation, 0.15 mg/kg may suffice.

Narcotic premedication used during clinical trials included fentanyl (1.5 to 2 mcg/kg IV, given 5 minutes before induction), morphine (individualized, up to 0.15 mg/kg IM) or meperidine (individualized, up to 1 mg/kg IM). Sedative premedications were hydroxyzine pamoate (100 mg orally) and sodium secobarbital (200 mg orally). Except for IV fentanyl, give all other premedications ≈ 1 hr before midazolam.

Maintenance of anesthesia (IV) for short surgical procedures, as a component of balanced anesthesia. Give incremental injections of ≈ 25% of the induction dose in response to signs of lightening of anesthesia and repeat as necessary.

Continuous infusion: Dilute 5 mg/ml to a concentration of 0.5 mg/ml with 0.9% Sodium Chloride or 5% Dextrose in Water.

Usual adult dose – If a loading dose is necessary to rapidly initiate sedation, 0.01 to 0.05 mg/kg (≈ 0.5 to 4 mg for a typical adult) may be given slowly or infused over several minutes. This dose may be repeated at 10 to 15 minute intervals until adequate sedation is achieved. For maintenance of sedation, the usual initial infusion rate is 0.02 to 0.1 mg/kg/hr (1 to 7 mg/hr). Higher loading or maintenance infusion rates may occasionally be required in some patients. Use the lowest recommended doses in patients with residual effects from anesthetic drugs or in those concurrently receiving other sedatives or opioids.

Individual response to midazolam is variable. Titrate the infusion rate to the desired level of sedation. Perform assessment of sedation at regular intervals and adjust the midazolam infusion rate up or down by 25% to 50% of the initial infusion rate to assure adequate titration of sedation level. Larger adjustments or even a small incremental dose may be necessary if rapid changes in the level of sedation are indicated. In addition, decrease the infusion rate by 10% to 25% every few hours to find the minimum effective infusion rate. Finding the minimum effective infusion rate decreases the potential accumulation of midazolam and provides for the most rapid recovery once the infusion is terminated. Patients who exhibit agitation, hypertension or tachycardia in response to noxious stimulation, but who are oth-

MIDAZOLAM HCl

erwise adequately sedated, may benefit from concurrent administration of an opioid analgesic. Addition of an opioid will generally reduce the minimum effective midazolam infusion rate.

Pediatric (non-neonatal): To initiate sedation, an IV loading dose of 0.05 to 0.2 mg/kg administered over at least 2 to 3 minutes can be used to establish the desired clinical effect in patients whose trachea is intubated. This loading dose may be followed by a continuous IV infusion to maintain the effect. Assisted ventilation is recommended for pediatric patients who are receiving other CNS depressant medications such as pioids. Initiate continuous IV infusions of midazolam at a rate of 0.06 to 0.12 mg/kg/hr (1 to 2 mcg/kg/min). The rate of infusion can be increased or decreased (generally by 25% of the initial or subsequent infusion rate) as required, or supplemental IV doses of midazolam can be administered to increase or maintain the desired effect. Frequent assessment at regular intervals using standard pain/sedation scale is recommended.

Hemodynamically compromised patients – When initiating an infusion with midazolam in hemodynamically compromised patients, titrate the usual loading dose of midazolam in small increments and monitor the patient for hemodynamic instability (eg, hypotension). Monitor respiratory rate and oxygen saturation carefully.

Neonatal: In intubated preterm and term neonates, initiate continuous IV infusions of midazolam at a rate of 0.03 mg/kg/hr (0.5 mcg/kg/min) in neonates < 32 weeks of age and 0.06 mg/kg/hr (1 mcg/kg/min) in neonates > 32 weeks of age. Do not use IV loading doses in neonates; rather the infusion may be run more rapidly for the first several hours to establish therapeutic plasma levels. Frequently reassess the rate of infusion, particularly after the first 24 hours, so as to administer the lowest possible effective dose and reduce the potential for drug accumulation. This is particularly important because of the potential for adverse effects related to metabolism of the benzyl alcohol.

Children:

Sedation, anxiolysis or amnesia (IM) – Sedation after IM midazolam is age- and dose-dependent; higher doses may result in deeper and more prolonged sedation. Doses of 0.1 to 0.15 mg/kg are usually effective and do not prolong emergence from general anesthesia. For more anxious patients, doses up to 0.5 mg/kg have been used. Although not systemically studied, the total dose usually does not exceed 10 mg. If midazolam is given with an opioid, the initial dose of each must be reduced.

Sedation, anxiolysis or amnesia (IV) – Administer the initial dose of midazolam over 2 to 3 minutes. Because midazolam is water soluble, it takes approximately three times longer than diazepam to achieve peak EEG effects; therefore one must wait an additional 2 to 3 minutes to fully evaluate the sedative effect before initiating a procedure or repeating a dose. If further sedation is necessary, continue to titrate with small increments until the appropriate level of sedation is achieved. If other medications capable of depressing the CNS are coadministered, consider the peak effect of those concomitant medications and adjust the dose of midazolam.

< 6 months old – Pediatric patients < 6 months old are particularly vulnerable to airway obstruction and hypoventilation; therefore titration with small increments to clinical effect and careful monitoring are essential.

6 months to 5 years old – Initial dose 0.05 to 0.1 mg/kg. A total dose up to 0.6 mg/kg may be necessary to reach the desired endpoint but usually does not exceed 6 mg. Prolonged sedation and risk of hypoventilation may occur with higher doses.

6 to 12 years old – Initial dose 0.025 to 0.05 mg/kg; total dose up to 0.4 mg/kg may be needed to reach the desired endpoint but usually does not exceed 10 mg. Prolonged sedation and risk of hypoventilation may be associated with higher doses.

12 to 16 years old – Dose as adults.

Compatibility: May be mixed in same syringe with: Morphine; meperidine; atropine; scopolamine. Midazolam, at a concentration of 0.5 mg/ml, is compatible with 5% Dextrose in Water and 0.9% Sodium Chloride for up to 24 hours and Lactated Ringer's solution for up to 4 hours.

Storage/Stability: Store at 15° to 30°C (59° to 86°F).

c-iv	**Versed** (Roche)	**Injection:** 1 mg (as HCl) per ml[1]	In 2, 5 and 10 ml vials.
		5 mg (as HCl) per ml[1]	In 1, 2, 5 and 10 ml vials, 2 ml *Tel-E-Ject* syringes.
	Versed (Roche)	**Injection:** 1 mg (as HCl) per ml[1]	In 2, 5 and 10 ml vials.
		5 mg (as HCl) per ml[1]	In 1, 2 and 10 ml vials.

[1] With 1% benzyl alcohol and EDTA.

PROPOFOL

Actions:

Pharmacology: Propofol is an IV sedative hypnotic agent for induction and maintenance of anesthesia or sedation. IV injection of a therapeutic dose produces hypnosis rapidly and smoothly with minimal excitation, usually within 40 seconds from the start of an injection. As with other rapidly acting IV anesthetic agents, the half-time of blood-brain equilibration is approximately 1 to 3 minutes, and this accounts for the rapid induction of anesthesia. Propofol blood concentrations required for maintenance of anesthesia have not been completely characterized. When nitrous oxide, oxygen and propofol are used for maintenance of general anesthesia, supplementation with analgesics (eg, narcotics) is generally required; neuromuscular blocking agents may also be required. (See Administration and Dosage.)

Pharmacodynamic properties of propofol depend on the therapeutic blood propofol concentrations. Steady-state concentrations are generally proportional to infusion rates, especially within an individual patient. Undesirable side effects such as cardiorespiratory depression are likely to occur at higher blood levels which result from bolus dosing or rapid increase in infusion rate. Allow an adequate interval (3 to 5 min) between clinical dosage adjustments in order to assess drug effects.

Propofol Therapeutic Range in Various Anesthetic Techniques

Technique	Range (mcg/ml)
Monitored anesthesia care sedation	0.5 to 1
Light ICU sedation	0.5 to 1
Deep ICU sedation	1 to 1.5
Light general anesthesia, with nitrous oxide	3 to 5
Deep general anesthesia, with nitrous oxide	4 to 7
TIVA[1], propofol/opioid/oxygen	4 to 7
TIVA[1], propofol/oxygen	8 to 16

[1] TIVA = total IV anesthesia.

Induction of anesthesia with propofol is frequently associated with apnea. In 1573 adult patients given propofol (2 to 2.5 mg/kg), apnea lasted 0 to 30 sec in 7%, 30 to 60 sec in 24%, and > 60 sec in 12%. In 213 children 3 to 12 years of age, the values were 12%, 10% and 5%, respectively. During maintenance, propofol (0.1 to 0.2 mg/kg/min) causes a decrease in ventilation usually associated with an increase in arterial carbon dioxide tension which may be marked depending on the rate of administration and other concurrent agents (eg, narcotics, sedatives).

In humans and animals, propofol does not suppress the adrenal response to ACTH. Preliminary findings in patients with normal intraocular pressure indicate that propofol anesthesia produces a decrease in intraocular pressure which may be associated with a concomitant decrease in systemic vascular resistance. Animal studies and limited experience in susceptible patients have not indicated any propensity of propofol to induce malignant hyperthermia. Propofol is rarely associated with elevation of plasma histamine levels and does not cause signs of histamine release.

If anesthesia is continued by infusion of propofol, endotracheal intubation and surgical stimulation may return arterial pressure towards normal. However, cardiac output may remain depressed. In comparative clinical studies, hemodynamic effects of propofol during induction are generally more pronounced than with traditional IV induction agents.

Insufficient data are available regarding the cardiovascular effects of propofol when used for induction or maintenance of anesthesia in elderly, hypotensive, debilitated patients, patients with severe cardiac disease (ejection fraction < 50%) or other ASA III/IV patients. However, limited information suggests that these patients may have more profound adverse cardiovascular responses. If propofol is used in these patients, it is recommended that a lower induction dose and a slower maintenance rate of administration be used. (See Administration and Dosage.)

Hemodynamics – The hemodynamic effects of propofol injection during induction of anesthesia vary. If spontaneous ventilation is maintained, major cardiovascular effects are arterial hypotension (sometimes > 30% decrease) with little or no change in heart rate and no appreciable decrease in cardiac output. If ventilation is assisted or controlled (positive pressure ventilation), degree and incidence of decrease in cardiac output are accentuated. Addition of a potent opioid (eg, fentanyl) as a premedicant further decreases cardiac output and respiratory drive.

Pharmacokinetics: Propofol is chiefly eliminated by hepatic conjugation to inactive metabolites which are excreted by the kidney. A glucuronide conjugate accounts for about 50% of the administered dose. Propofol has a high metabolic clearance that ranges from 1.6 to 3.4 L/min in healthy 70 kg adults. As a consequence of its high lipid solubility, it has a volume of distribution approaching 60 L/kg. The terminal half-life is 1 to 3 days, reflecting the extensive tissue uptake.

Following an IV bolus dose, plasma levels initially decline rapidly due to both high metabolic clearance and rapid drug distribution into tissues. Distribution accounts for about half of this decline following a bolus of propofol. With longer infusions, the return to the plasma of the drug accumulated in the tissues causes plasma levels to fall more slowly. Plasma levels fall to about 50% of peak levels in about 5 minutes following a 1 hour infusion and in about 7 minutes following a 10 hour infusion. Titration of infusion to clinical response in MAC or ICU sedation corresponds to a plasma level of about 1 mcg/ml. A fall in plasma level of about 50% (to 0.5 mcg/ml) generally corresponds to patient awakening.

The large contribution of distribution (about 50%) to the fall of propofol plasma levels following brief infusions means that after very long infusions (at steady state), about half the initial rate will maintain the same plasma levels. Thus, titration to clinical response and daily wake up assessments are important during use of propofol infusion for ICU sedation, especially infusions of long duration.

Adults – Clearance ranges from 23 to 50 ml/kg/min. It is chiefly eliminated by hepatic conjugation to inactive metabolites which are excreted by kidney. A glucuronide conjugate accounts for about 50% of dose. Steady-state volume of distribution approaches 60 L/kg. Terminal half-life after a 10 day infusion is 1 to 3 days.

Elderly – With increasing age, the dose needed to achieve a defined anesthetic endpoint (dose requirement) decreases. This does not appear to be an age related change. With increasing age, higher peak plasma levels occur, which can explain the decreased dose requirement. These higher levels can predispose patients to cardiorespiratory effects including hypotension, apnea, airway obstruction or oxygen desaturation. Lower doses are thus recommended in the elderly.

Children – In children undergoing general surgeries lasting ≈ 1 to 2 hours, the elimination half-life is 250 to 400 minutes, steady-state volume of distribution is 7 to 10 L/kg and clearance is ≈ 35 ml/kg/min. The observed differences between children and adults in terms of elimination phase and distributional volume are related to the much longer duration of propofol administration in adults.

Organ failure – Propofol pharmacokinetics do not appear to be different in patients with chronic hepatic cirrhosis or chronic renal impairment compared to adults with normal hepatic and renal function.

Indications:

Induction or maintenance of anesthesia as part of a balanced anesthetic technique for inpatient and outpatient surgery in adults and children ≥ 3 years of age. Propofol can be used to initiate and maintain monitored anesthesia care (MAC) sedation during diagnostic procedures in adults, and it may also be used for MAC sedation in conjunction with local/regional anesthesia in patients undergoing surgical procedures.

Continuous sedation and control of stress responses in intubated or respiratory-controlled adult patients in Intensive Care Units (ICU).

Contraindications:

When general anesthesia or sedation are contraindicated; hypersensitivity to propofol or components of the product.

Warnings:

Administration: Only persons trained in the administration of general anesthesia should administer propofol. Facilities for maintenance of a patent airway, artificial ventilation, and oxygen enrichment and circulatory resuscitation must be immediately available. For sedation of intubated, mechanically ventilated patients in the ICU, administer only by persons skilled in the management of critically ill patients and trained in cardiovascular resuscitation and airway management.

Blood/plasma coadministration: Do not coadminister through the same IV catheter with blood or plasma because compatibility has not been established. In vitro, aggregates of the globular component of the emulsion vehicle have occurred with blood/plasma/serum from humans and animals.

Aseptic technique: Always maintain strict aseptic techniques during handling since propofol is a single-use parenteral product and contains no antimicrobial preservatives. The vehicle is capable of supporting rapid growth of microorganisms. Failure to follow aseptic handling procedures may result in microbial contamination causing fever, infection/sepsis or other adverse consequences which could lead to life-threatening illness.

Anaphylaxis: Rarely, features of anaphylaxis, which may include bronchospasm, erythema and hypotension, have occurred after the administration of propofol, although the use of other drugs in most instances makes the relationship to propofol unclear.

Elderly: Use a lower induction dose and a slower maintenance rate of administration. See Special Risk Patients in Precautions.

Pregnancy: Category B. Propofol crosses the placenta. Propofol causes maternal deaths in rats and rabbits and decreased pup survival during the lactating period in animals treated with 15 mg/kg/day (or 6 times the recommended human induction dose). The pharmacological activity (anesthesia) of the drug on the mother is probably responsible for the adverse effects seen in the offspring. There are, however, no adequate and well controlled studies in pregnant women. Use during pregnancy only if clearly needed.

Labor and delivery – Not recommended for obstetrics, including cesarean section deliveries. Propofol crosses the placenta and may be associated with neonatal depression.

Lactation: Not recommended for use in nursing mothers because propofol is excreted in breast milk and the effects of oral absorption of small amounts of propofol are not known.

Children: Not recommended for use in children < 3 years of age or for ICU or MAC sedation in children because safety and efficacy have not been established. Although no causal relationship has been established, serious adverse events (including fatalities) have been reported in children given propofol for ICU sedation. These events were seen most often in children with respiratory tract infections given doses in excess of those recommended for adults.

Precautions:

Special risk patients: Use a lower induction dose and a slower maintenance rate of administration in elderly, debilitated and ASA III or IV patients (see Administration and Dosage). Continuously monitor patients for early signs of significant hypotension or bradycardia. Treatment may include increasing the rate of IV fluid, elevation of lower extremities, use of pressor agents or administration of atropine. Apnea often occurs during induction and may persist for > 60 seconds. Ventilatory support may be required. Because propofol is an emulsion, use caution in patients with lipid metabolism disorders (eg, primary hyperlipoproteinemia, diabetic hyperlipidemia, pancreatitis).

Discharge of patient: Satisfy the clinical criteria for discharge from the recovery/day surgery area established for each institution before discharge of the patient from the care of the anesthesiologist.

Epilepsy: When administered to an epileptic patient, there may be a risk of convulsion during the recovery phase.

Transient local pain may occur during IV injection, which may be reduced by prior injection of IV lidocaine (1 ml of a 1% solution). Venous sequelae (phlebitis or thrombosis) have occurred rarely (< 1%). In two well controlled clinical studies using dedicated IV catheters, no instances of venous sequelae were reported up to 14 days following induction. Pain can be minimized if the larger veins of the forearm or antecubital fossa are used. Accidental clinical extravasation and intentional injection into SC or perivascular tissues of animals caused minimal tissue reaction. Intra-arterial injection in animals did not induce local tissue effects. One accidental intra-arterial injection has been reported in a patient, and other than pain, there were no major sequelae.

Perioperative myoclonia, rarely including convulsions and opisthotonus, has occurred.

Pulmonary edema has been reported rarely with propofol use, although a causal relationship is not known.

Cardiovascular effects: Propofol has no vagolytic activity and has been associated with reports of bradycardia, occasionally profound, or asystole. Consider the IV administration of anticholinergic agents to modify potential increases in vagal tone due to concomitant agents (eg, succinylcholine) or surgical stimuli. There have been rare reports of cardiac arrest. Monitor patients for early signs of significant hypotension or cardiovascular depression, which may be profound. These effects are responsive to discontinuation of propofol, IV fluid administration or vasopressor therapy.

Hyperlipidemia: Since propofol is formulated in an oil-in-water emulsion, elevations in serum triglycerides may occur when it is administered for extended periods of time. Monitor patients at risk of hyperlipidemia for increases in serum triglycerides or serum turbidity. Adjust if fat is being inadequately cleared from the body. A reduction in the quantity of concurrently administered lipids is indicated to compensate for the amount of lipid infused as part of the formulation; 1 ml of propofol contains approximately 0.1 g of fat (1.1 kcal).

PROPOFOL

Neurosurgical anesthesia: When propofol is used in patients with increased intracranial pressure (ICP) or impaired cerebral circulation, avoid significant decreases in mean arterial pressure because of the resultant decreases in cerebral perfusion pressure. To avoid significant hypotension and decreases in cerebral perfusion pressure, utilize an infusion or slow bolus of ≈ 20 mg every 10 seconds instead of rapid and large boluses. Slower injection titrated to clinical responses will generally result in reduced induction dosage requirements (1 to 2 mg/kg). When increases ICP is suspected, hyperventilation and hypocarbia should accompany use of propofol.

Drug abuse and dependence: Rare cases of self-administration of propofol by healthcare professionals have been reported. Manage propofol to prevent the risk of diversion.

Drug Interactions:

CNS depressants (eg, hypnotics/sedatives, inhalational anesthetics, narcotics) can increase the CNS depression induced by propofol. Morphine premedication with nitrous oxide decreases the necessary propofol maintenance infusion rate and therapeutic blood concentrations when compared to non-narcotic (eg, lorazepam) premedication. In addition, the induction dose requirements of propofol may be reduced in patients with IM or IV premedication, particularly with narcotics alone or in combination with sedatives. These agents may increase the anesthetic effects of propofol and may also result in more pronounced decreases in systolic, diastolic and mean arterial pressures and cardiac output.

Adverse Reactions:

CNS: Amorous behavior, hypotonia, hallucinations, neuropathy, opisthotonos.

Miscellaneous: Asthenia, myocardial ischemia, conjunctival hyperemia, nystagmus.

Anesthesia/MAC sedation:

Body as a whole – Awareness, extremities pain, fever, increased drug effect, neck rigidity/stiffness, chest/trunk pain (< 1%).

CNS – Movement (3% to 10%); hypertonia/dystonia, paresthesia, abnormal dreams, agitation, anxiety, bucking/jerking/thrashing, chills/shivering, clonic/myoclonic movement, combativeness, confusion, delirium, depression, dizziness, emotional lability, euphoria, fatigue, headache, hysteria, insomnia, moaning, rigidity, seizures, somnolence, tremor, twitching (< 1%).

Cardiovascular – Hypotension (3% to 10%); bradycardia (> 1%); bleeding, premature atrial contractions, syncope, arrhythmia, atrial fibrillation, AV heartblock, bigeminy, bundle branch block, cardiac arrest, abnormal ECG, edema, extrasystole, heart block, hypertension, myocardial infarction, PVCs, ST segment depression, supraventricular tachycardia, tachycardia, ventricular fibrillation (< 1%).

GI – Hypersalivation, cramping, diarrhea, dry mouth, enlarged parotid, nausea, swallowing, vomiting (< 1%).

Respiratory – Apnea (> 1%); bronchospasm, burning in throat, wheezing, cough, dyspnea, hiccough, hypoventilation, hyperventilation, hypoxia, laryngospasm, pharyngitis, sneezing, tachypnea, upper airway obstruction (< 1%).

Dermatologic – Rash (> 1%); flushing, pruritus, diaphoresis, urticaria (< 1%).

Special Senses – Amblyopia, diplopia, ear pain, eye pain, taste perversion, tinnitus (< 1%).

GU – Abnormal urine, oliguria, urine retention (< 1%).

Local – Burning/stinging or pain (17.6%); hives/itching, phlebitis, redness/discoloration (< 1%).

Miscellaneous – Myalgia, coagulation disorder, leukocytosis, hyperkalemia, hyperlipidemia (< 1%).

ICU sedation:

Body as a whole – Fever, sepsis, trunk pain, weakness, rash (< 1%).

CNS – Agitation, chills/shivering, intracranial hypertension, seizures, somnolence, abnormal thinking (< 1%).

Cardiovascular – Hypotension (26%); bradycardia, decreased cardiac output (> 1%); arrhythmia, atrial fibrillation, bigeminy, cardiac arrest, extrasystole, ventricular tachycardia (< 1%).

Metabolic/Nutritional – Hyperlipidemia (3% to 10%); increased BUN, creatinine and osmolality, dehydration, hyperglycemia, metabolic acidosis (< 1%).

Respiratory – Respiratory acidosis during weaning (3% to 10%); decreased lung function, hypoxia (< 1%).

Miscellaneous – Ileus, abnormal liver function, green urine, kidney failure (< 1%).

Children: Generally, the adverse reaction profile in children 3 to 12 years of age is similar to adults. The following reactions have occurred: Hypotension, movement (17%); burning/stinging or pain (10%); hypertension (8%); rash (5%); apnea.

PROPOFOL

Overdosage:

If accidental overdosage occurs, discontinue propofol immediately. Overdosage is likely to cause cardiorespiratory depression. Treat respiratory depression by artificial ventilation with oxygen. Cardiovascular depression may require raising the patient's legs, increasing the flow rate of IV fluids and administering pressor agents or anticholinergic agents. Refer to General Management of Acute Overdosage.

Patient Information:

Performance of activities requiring mental alertness, coordination or physical dexterity may be impaired for some time after general anesthesia or sedation.

Administration and Dosage:

Anesthesia: Individualize dosage. Propofol blood concentrations at steady state are generally proportional to infusion rates, especially within an individual patient. Undesirable effects such as cardiorespiratory depression are likely to occur at higher blood levels which result from bolus dosing or rapid increase in the infusion rate. An adequate interval (3 to 5 minutes) must be allowed between clinical dosage adjustments in order to assess drug effects.

Other drugs that cause CNS depression (eg, hypnotics/sedatives, inhalational anesthetics, opioids) can increase CNS depression induced by propofol. Morphine premedication (0.15 mg/kg) with nitrous oxide 67% in oxygen decreases the necessary propofol injection maintenance infusion rate and therapeutic blood concentrations when compared to non-narcotic (eg, lorazepam) premedication.

For minor surgical procedures (ie, body surface) 60% to 70% nitrous oxide can be combined with a variable rate infusion to provide satisfactory anesthesia. With more stimulating surgical procedures (ie, intra-abdominal), consider supplementation with analgesics to provide a satisfactory anesthetic and recovery profile. When supplementation with nitrous oxide is not provided, increase administration rate(s) of propofol or opioids in order to provide adequate anesthesia.

Always titrate infusion rates downward in the absence of clinical signs of light anesthesia until a mild response to surgical stimulation can be perceived in order to avoid the administration of unnecessarily high doses of propofol at rates higher than are clinically necessary. Generally, achieve infusion rates of 50 to 100 mcg/kg/min during maintenance in order to optimize recovery times.

Intermittent bolus – Increments of 25 to 50 mg (2.5 to 5 ml) may be administered with nitrous oxide in patients undergoing general surgery. Administer the incremental boluses when changes in vital signs indicate a response to surgical stimulation or light anesthesia.

In the elderly, do not use rapid bolus doses as this will increase cardiorespiratory effects including hypotension, apnea, airway obstruction or oxygen desaturation.

Monitored anesthesia care (MAC) sedation: Individualize rates of administration and titrate to clinical response. In most patients the rates of administration will be approximately 25% of those used for maintenance of general anesthesia.

During initiation of MAC sedation, slow infusion or slow injection techniques are preferable over rapid bolus administration. During maintenance of MAC sedation, a variable rate infusion is preferable over intermittent bolus dose administration. In the elderly, debilitated and ASA III or IV patients, rapid (single or repeated) bolus dose administration should not be used for MAC sedation (see Warnings.) The rate of administration should be over 3 to 5 minutes and reduce the dosage to approximately 80% of the adult dosage in these patients according to their condition, response and changes in vital signs.

Initiation – Utilize either an infusion or a slow injection method while closely monitoring cardiorespiratory function. With the infusion method, initiate sedation by infusing 100 to 150 mcg/kg/min (6 to 9 mg/kg/hr) for a period of 3 to 5 minutes and titrate to the desired level of sedation while closely monitoring respiratory function. With the slow injection method for initiation, patients will require ≈ 0.5 mg/kg administered over 3 to 5 minutes and titrated to clinical responses. When administered slowly over 3 to 5 minutes, most patients will be adequately sedated and the peak drug effect can be achieved while minimizing undesirable cardiorespiratory effects occurring at high plasma levels.

Maintenance – A variable rate infusion method is preferable over an intermittent bolus dose method. With the variable rate infusion method, patients will generally require maintenance rates of 25 to 75 mcg/kg/min (1.5 to 4.5 mg/kg/hr) during the first 10 to 15 minutes of sedation maintenance. Subsequently decrease infusion over time to 25 to 50 mcg/kg/min and adjust to clinical response. In titrating to clinical effect, allow approximately 2 minutes for onset of peak drug effect.

Always titrate downward in the absence of clinical signs of light sedation until mild responses to stimulation are obtained in order to avoid sedative administration at rates higher than are clinically necessary.

If intermittent bolus method is used, 10 or 20 mg (1 or 2 ml) increments can be given and titrated to desired level of sedation. There is the potential for respiratory depression, transient increases in sedation depth or prolongation of recovery.

Can be the sole agent for maintenance of MAC sedation during surgical/diagnostic procedures, supplemented with opioids or benzodiazepines, which increase sedative and respiratory effects and may also result in a slower recovery profile.

ICU sedation: For intubated, mechanically ventilated adult patients, initiate slowly with a continuous infusion to titrate to desired clinical effect and minimize hypotension.

In clinical studies, the mean infusion maintenance rate for all patients was 27 mcg/kg/min. The maintenance infusion rates required to maintain adequate sedation ranged from 0.3 to 130 mcg/kg/min. The infusion rate was lower in patients > 55 years of age (≈ 20 mcg/kg/min) compared to patients < 55 years of age (≈ 38 mcg/kg/min). In these studies, morphine or fentanyl was used as needed for analgesia.

Most adult ICU patients recovering from the effects of general anesthesia or deep sedation will require maintenance rates of 5 to 50 mcg/kg/min (0.3 to 3 mg/kg/hr) individualized and titrated to clinical response. With medical ICU patients or patients who have recovered from the effect of general anesthesia or deep sedation, the rate of administration of ≥ 50 mcg/kg/min may be required to achieve adequate sedation. These higher rates may increase the likelihood of hypotension.

Although there are reports of reduced analgesic requirements, most patients received opioids for analgesia during maintenance of ICU sedation. Some patients also received benzodiazepines or neuromuscular blocking agents. During long term maintenance of sedation, some ICU patients were awakened once or twice every 24 hours for assessment of neurologic or respiratory function.

Avoid discontinuation prior to weaning or for daily wake up assessments. This may result in rapid awakening with associated anxiety, agitation and resistance to mechanical ventilation. Adjust to maintain light sedation through these processes.

Propofol Dosage Guidelines

Indication	Administration and dosage
Anesthesia Induction	Individualize dosage. *Adults (< 55 years of age):* ≈ 40 mg every 10 sec until induction onset (2 to 2.5 mg/kg). *Elderly, debilitated or ASA* III *or* IV *patients:* ≈ 20 mg every 10 seconds until induction onset (1 to 1.5 mg/kg). *Neurosurgical patients:* 20 mg every 10 seconds until induction onset (1 to 2 mg/kg). *Children (≥ 3 years of age):* 2.5 to 3.5 mg/kg over 20 to 30 seconds.
Maintenance Infusion	*Variable rate infusion:* Titrate to the desired clinical effect. *Adults (< 55 years of age):* Generally 100 to 200 mcg/kg/min (6 to 12 mg/kg/hr). *Elderly, debilitated or ASA* III *or* IV *patients:* Generally 50 to 100 mcg/kg/min (3 to 6 mg/kg/hr). *Neurosurgical patients:* 100 to 200 mcg/kg/min (6 to 12 mg/kg/hr). *Children (≥ 3 years of age):* 125 to 300 mcg/kg/min (7.5 to 18 mg/kg/hr).
Maintenance Intermittent bolus	*Adults:* 25 to 50 mg increments, as needed.
MAC sedation Initiation	Individualize dosage. *Adults (< 55 years of age):* Slow infusion or slow injection techniques are preferable over a rapid bolus. Most require an infusion of 100 to 150 mcg/kg/min (6 to 9 mg/kg/hr) or a slow injection of 0.5 mg/kg, both over 3 to 5 min, followed immediately by a maintenance infusion. *Elderly debilitated, or ASA* III *or* IV *patients:* Most require dosages similar to adults, but must be given as a slow infusion or slow injection and not as a rapid bolus.

Propofol Dosage Guidelines	
Indication	Administration and dosage
Maintenance	Titrate dosage and rate to clinical effects. *Adults (< 55 years of age):* A variable rate infusion is preferable over an intermittent bolus. Most require an infusion of 25 to 75 mcg/kg/min (1.5 to 4.5 mg/kg/hr) or incremental bolus doses of 10 or 20 mg. *Elderly, debilitated or ASA* III *or* IV *patients:* Most require a 20% reduction of the adult dose. A rapid (single or repeated) bolus dose should not be used.
ICU sedation	Individualize dosage and rate of infusion. Most require an infusion of 5 mcg/kg/min (0.3 mg/kg/hr) for at least 5 minutes. Subsequent increments of 5 to 10 mcg/kg/min (0.3 to 0.6 mg/kg/hr) over 5 to 10 minutes may be used until desired level of sedation is achieved. Maintenance rates of 5 to 50 mcg/kg/min (0.3 to 3 mg/kg/hr) or higher may be required. Wake up and assessment of CNS function should be carried out daily throughout maintenance to determine the minimum dose required for sedation.

Concomitant therapy: Propofol has been used with a variety of agents commonly used in anesthesia such as atropine, scopolamine, glycopyrrolate, diazepam, depolarizing and nondepolarizing muscle relaxants and narcotic analgesics, as well as with inhalational and regional anesthetic agents. (See also Drug Interactions.)

Admixture compatibility and stability: Propofol should not be mixed with other therapeutic agents prior to administration.

Dilution prior to administration: Only dilute with 5% Dextrose Injection, USP and do not dilute to a concentration < 2 mg/ml because it is an emulsion. In diluted form it is more stable when in contact with glass than with plastic (95% potency after 2 hours of running infusion in plastic).

Administration with other fluids: Compatibility of propofol with the coadministration of blood/serum/plasma has not been established. (See Warnings.) Propofol is compatible with the following IV fluids when administered into a running IV catheter: 5% Dextrose Injection, USP; Lactated Ringer's Injection, USP; Lactated Ringer's and 5% Dextrose Injection; 5% Dextrose and 0.45% Sodium Chloride Injection, USP; 5% Dextrose and 0.2% Sodium Chloride Injection, USP.

Storage/Stability: Do not use if there is evidence of separation of the phases of the emulsion.

Discard any unused portions of propofol or solutions containing propofol at the end of the anesthetic procedure or at 6 hours, whichever occurs sooner; for ICU sedation discard after 12 hours (if administered directly from the vial) or 6 hours (if transferred to a syringe or other container).

Store below 22°C (72°F). Do not store below 4°C (40°F). Refrigeration is not recommended. Protect from light. Shake well before use.

Propofol undergoes oxidative degradation in the presence of oxygen, and is therefore packaged under nitrogen to eliminate this degradation path.

Rx	**Diprivan** (Zeneca)	**Injection:** 10 mg/ml	In 20 ml amps and 50 and 100 ml infusion vials.[1]

[1] With 100 mg/ml soybean oil, 22.5 mg/ml glycerol and 12 mg/ml egg lecithin.

DROPERIDOL

Actions:

Pharmacology: Droperidol, a butyrophenone derivative, produces marked tranquilization, sedation and an antiemetic effect. It also produces mild alpha-adrenergic blockade, peripheral vascular dilatation and reduction of the pressor effect of epinephrine, resulting in hypotension and decreased peripheral vascular resistance. It may decrease pulmonary arterial pressure (particularly if it is abnormally high). It may reduce the incidence of epinephrine-induced arrhythmias, but it does not prevent other cardiac arrhythmias.

Pharmacokinetics: The onset of action occurs in 3 to 10 minutes following IV or IM administration. The full effect may not be apparent for 30 minutes. The duration of the sedative and tranquilizing effect is generally 2 to 4 hours. Alteration of consciousness may persist as long as 12 hours. Droperidol is metabolized in the liver and is excreted in the urine and feces. Approximately 1% is excreted unchanged in the urine. Terminal half-life averages 2.2 hours.

Indications:

To produce tranquilization and reduce the incidence of nausea and vomiting in surgical and diagnostic procedures.

Premedication, induction and as an adjunct in the maintenance of general and regional anesthesia.

Neuroleptanalgesia, in which droperidol is given concurrently with a narcotic analgesic (eg, fentanyl), to aid in producing tranquility and decreasing anxiety and pain.

Unlabeled uses: Droperidol has been used as an IV antiemetic in cancer chemotherapy.

Contraindications:

Hypersensitivity to droperidol.

Warnings:

Concomitant narcotic analgesic therapy: If administered with a narcotic analgesic such as fentanyl, be familiar with the special properties of each drug, particularly the widely differing durations of action. In addition, when such a combination is used, have resuscitative equipment and a narcotic antagonist readily available to manage apnea.

Renal/Hepatic function impairment: Administer with caution because of the importance of these organs in the metabolism and excretion of drugs.

Elderly: Reduce the initial dose of droperidol. Consider the effect of the initial dose in determining incremental doses.

Pregnancy: Category C. There are no adequate and well controlled studies in pregnant women. Use only when clearly needed or when the potential benefit justifies the potential risk to the fetus. Droperidol administered IV has caused a slight increase in newborn rat mortality at 4.4 times the upper human dose. Following IM administration, increased mortality of the offspring at 1.8 times the upper human dose is attributed to CNS depression in the dams.

Labor and delivery – Droperidol has been used to promote analgesia for cesarean section patients without respiratory effects in the neonate. Placental transfer is slow. The drug has been used as a continuous IV infusion for hyperemesis gravidarum during the 2nd and 3rd trimesters without apparent fetal harm.

Lactation: It is not known whether droperidol is excreted in breast milk. Exercise caution when administering to a nursing mother.

Children: Safety and efficacy for use in children < 2 years of age have not been established.

Precautions:

Hypotension: If hypotension occurs, consider the possibility of hypovolemia and manage with appropriate parenteral fluid therapy. Reposition patient to improve venous return to the heart when operative conditions permit. In spinal and peridural anesthesia, tilting the patient into a head-down position may result in a higher level of anesthesia than desired, and impair venous return to the heart. Exercise care in moving and positioning patients because of the possibility of orthostatic hypotension. If volume expansion with fluids plus other countermeasures do not correct the hypotension, use pressor agents other than epinephrine. Epinephrine may paradoxically decrease the blood pressure in patients treated with droperidol due to the α-adrenergic blocking action of droperidol. Droperidol may also decrease pulmonary arterial pressure.

EEG: When the EEG is used for postoperative monitoring, the EEG pattern may slowly return to normal.

DROPERIDOL

Drug Interactions:

Anesthesia: Certain forms of conduction anesthesia (eg, spinal anesthesia, some peridural anesthetics) can cause peripheral vasodilation and hypotension because of sympathetic blockade. Droperidol can alter circulation through other mechanisms.

CNS depressants (eg, antidepressants, barbiturates) have additive or potentiating CNS effects with droperidol; thus, droperidol dose will be less than usual. Likewise, following the droperidol, reduce the dose of other CNS depressants.

Adverse Reactions:

Most common: Postoperative drowsiness. Mild to moderate hypotension and occasionally tachycardia usually subside without treatment. If hypotension is severe or persists, consider hypovolemia and manage with appropriate parenteral therapy.

Extrapyramidal symptoms (dystonia, akathisia and oculogyric crisis) occur in about 1% of patients. Restlessness, hyperactivity and anxiety which can be the result of inadequate dosage or a part of the symptom complex of akathisia may occur. When these occur, they can usually be controlled with antiparkinson agents.

Respiratory depression: When droperidol is used with a narcotic analgesic such as fentanyl, respiratory depression, apnea and muscular rigidity can occur; if these remain untreated, respiratory arrest could occur.

Elevated blood pressure, with or without preexisting hypertension, occurred after droperidol with fentanyl or other parenteral analgesics. This may be due to unexplained alterations in sympathetic activity following large doses; it is also frequently attributed to anesthetic or surgical stimulation during light anesthesia.

Other: Dizziness; chills or shivering; laryngospasm; bronchospasm; postoperative hallucinatory episodes (sometimes associated with transient mental depression).

Overdosage:

Symptoms: Extension of pharmacologic actions (eg, sedation, hypotension).

Treatment: In the presence of hypoventilation or apnea, administer oxygen and assist or control respiration as indicated. Maintain a patent airway. Observe the patient for 24 hours; maintain body warmth and fluid intake. If hypotension occurs and is severe or persists, consider hypovolemia and manage with parenteral fluid therapy. Refer to General Management of Acute Overdosage.

Administration and Dosage:

Individualize dosage. Monitor vital signs routinely.

Adults:

Premedication – 2.5 to 10 mg IM 30 to 60 minutes preoperatively.

Adjunct to general anesthesia –

Induction: 2.5 mg/9 to 11 kg (20 to 25 lb) usually IV with an analgesic or general anesthetic. Smaller doses may be adequate. Titrate total amount.

Maintenance: 1.25 to 2.5 mg (usually IV).

If fentanyl plus droperidol (*Innovar*) is given with droperidol, consider the amount of droperidol in the injection when calculating recommended dose.

Use without a general anesthetic in diagnostic procedures – 2.5 to 10 mg IM 30 to 60 minutes before the procedure. Additional 1.25 to 2.5 mg amounts may be administered (usually IV). When droperidol is used in procedures such as bronchoscopy, appropriate topical anesthesia is still necessary.

Adjunct to regional anesthesia – 2.5 to 5 mg IM or slowly IV.

Children (2 to 12 years) – For premedication or induction of anesthesia, reduced dose as low as 1 to 1.5 mg/9 to 11 kg (20 to 25 lb) is recommended.

Stability: Stable in 5% Dextrose Injection, 0.9% Sodium Chloride Injection and Lactated Ringers' Injection for 7 to 10 days in glass bottles and for 7 days in polyvinyl chloride bags (only for the 5% Dextrose Injection and 0.9% Sodium Chloride Injection) all at a concentration of 20 mcg/ml (1 mg/50 ml).

Admixtures: Droperidol in a concentration of 2.5 mg/ml is physically compatible for at least 15 minutes with the following admixed in a syringe: Atropine sulfate, butorphanol tartrate, chlorpromazine HCl, diphenhydramine HCl, fentanyl citrate, glycopyrrolate, hydroxyzine HCl, meperidine HCl, morphine sulfate, perphenazine, promazine HCl, promethazine HCl, scopolamine HBr. Precipitation occurs if mixed with barbiturates.

Rx	**Droperidol** (Various, eg, American Regent Labs, Astra, DuPont, Lyphomed, Solopak)	**Injection:** 2.5 mg/ml	In 2, 5 and 10 ml vials.
Rx	**Inapsine** (Janssen Pharm.)		In 1, 2, 5 ml amps, 10 ml vials.[1]

[1] With methyl and propyl parabens.

FENTANYL CITRATE AND DROPERIDOL

Actions:

Pharmacology: A combination containing a narcotic analgesic, fentanyl, and a neuroleptic (major tranquilizer), droperidol (see individual monographs). The combined effect, sometimes referred to as neuroleptanalgesia, is characterized by general quiescence, reduced motor activity and profound analgesia; complete loss of consciousness usually does not occur from use of this combination alone.

Indications:

To produce tranquilization and analgesia for surgical and diagnostic procedures. It may be used as an anesthetic premedication, for the induction of anesthesia and as an adjunct in the maintenance of general and regional anesthesia.

Administration and Dosage:

Varies depending on application and patient. Consult package literature.

c-II	**Fentanyl Citrate and Droperidol** (Astra)	**Injection:** 0.05 mg fentanyl (as citrate) and 2.5 mg droperidol per ml	In 2 and 5 ml amps and vials.
c-II	**Innovar** (Janssen)	**Injection:** 0.05 mg fentanyl (as citrate) and 2.5 mg droperidol per ml	In 2 and 5 ml amps.

ATROPINE SULFATE AND MEPERIDINE HCl

Actions:

Pharmacology: A combination containing a belladonna alkaloid, atropine, and a synthetic narcotic analgesic, meperidine (see individual monographs).

Indications:

For preoperative sedation and antisecretory effect.

Administration and Dosage:

Administer the appropriate dose, IM 30 to 90 minutes prior to beginning anesthesia.

c-II	**Atropine and Demerol** (Sanofi Winthrop)	**Injection:** 0.4 mg atropine sulfate and 50 mg meperidine HCl per ml[1]	In 1 ml fill in 2 ml Carpuject.
		0.4 mg atropine sulfate and 75 mg meperidine HCl per ml[1]	In 1 ml fill in 2 ml Carpuject.

[1] With 1.5 mg sodium metabisulfite, 5 mg phenol.

ATROPINE SULFATE AND MORPHINE SULFATE

Actions:

Pharmacology: A combination containing a belladonna alkaloid, atropine, and a narcotic analgesic, morphine (see individual monographs).

Indications:

For preoperative sedation and antisecretory effect.

Administration and Dosage:

Give 0.25 to 2 ml SC, IM or IV as condition demands.

c-II	**Morphine and Atropine Sulfates** (SK-Beecham)	**Injection:** 0.4 mg atropine sulfate and 16 mg morphine sulfate per ml[2]	In 30 ml vials.

[2] With 0.5% chlorobutanol.

Gases

GASES

The information on General Anesthetic Gases is not intended to supply complete information on actions, uses, cautions and contraindications. Recommended uses and product availability are given. Consult detailed literature before using. These agents should be administered only by those with appropriate training and experience.

NITROUS OXIDE (N_2O)

The most commonly used anesthetic gas, nitrous oxide is a weak anesthetic usually used in combination with other anesthetics. It does not cause skeletal muscle relaxation. The chief danger in the use of nitrous oxide is hypoxia; at least 20% oxygen should be used. An increased risk of renal and hepatic diseases and peripheral neuropathy has been reported in dental personnel who work in areas where nitrous oxide is used.

The gas can diffuse into air-containing cavities faster than nitrogen can leave, causing potentially dangerous pressure accumulation (eg, middle ear abnormalities, bowel obstruction, pneumothorax). Nitrous oxide also oxidizes and inactivates vitamin B_{12}, thus affecting some enzymes. This action may be linked to observations of adversely affected hematological, immune, neurological and reproductive systems.

In high concentrations, nitrous oxide may cause vomiting, respiratory depression and death. A primary advantage of nitrous oxide is that it is nonexplosive.

Abuse and dependence have been documented, with speculation that interaction with the endogeneous opioid system may be involved.

Malignant hyperthermia may be triggered by most of the potent, fat-soluble, inhalational anesthetics and by many skeletal muscle relaxants, especially when used as prophylaxis and treatment.

Supplied in blue cylinders.

CYCLOPROPANE

An anesthetic gas with a rapid onset of action. May be used for analgesia and induction and maintenance of anesthesia. Produces skeletal muscle relaxation in full anesthetic doses. Administer in a closed system with oxygen. Disadvantages include difficulty in detection of planes of anesthesia, occasional laryngospasm and cardiac arrhythmia. Postanesthetic nausea, vomiting and headache are frequent.

Malignant hyperthermia may be triggered by most of the potent, fat-soluble, inhalational anesthetics and by many skeletal muscle relaxants, especially when used as prophylaxis and treatment.

Caution: Cyclopropane/oxygen mixtures are flammable and EXPLOSIVE. Due to this undesirable property, ethylene is rarely used.

Supplied in orange cylinders.

ETHYLENE

An anesthetic gas with rapid onset and recovery. Provides adequate analgesia but has poor muscle relaxation properties. Must be administered in high (80%) concentrations with oxygen (20%). Advantages include minimal bronchospasm and laryngospasm and minimal postanesthetic vomiting. Ethylene is nontoxic; hypoxia is the primary complication.

Caution: Ethylene/oxygen mixtures are flammable and EXPLOSIVE. Due to this undesirable property, ethylene is rarely used.

Supplied in red cylinders.

Volatile Liquids

VOLATILE LIQUIDS

The information on General Anesthetic Volatile Liquids is not intended to supply complete information on actions, uses, cautions and contraindications. Recommended uses and product availability are given. Consult detailed literature before using. Should be administered only by those with appropriate training and experience.

Malignant hyperthermia may be triggered by most of the potent, fat-soluble, inhalational anesthetics and by many skeletal muscle relaxants, especially when used concurrently. Monitor the patient closely; dantrolene (see individual monograph) has been used as prophylaxis and treatment.

HALOTHANE

Actions:

Pharmacology: An inhalation anesthetic. Induction and recovery are rapid and depth of anesthesia can be rapidly altered. Halothane is not an irritant to the respiratory tract, and no increase in salivary or bronchial secretions ordinarily occurs. Pharyngeal and laryngeal reflexes are rapidly obtunded. It causes bronchodilation. Hypoxia, acidosis or apnea may develop during deep anesthesia. It sensitizes the myocardium to the action of epinephrine and norepinephrine; the combination may cause serious cardiac arrhythmias. Halothane produces moderate muscular relaxation. Muscle relaxants are used as adjuncts to maintain lighter levels of anesthesia.

Indications:

Induction and maintenance of general anesthesia.

Warnings:

Hepatic function impairment: Halothane administration has been associated with hepatic dysfunction. There may be two types: One characterized by increased serum enzyme levels (20% to 25% of patients) and the other, fulminant hepatic failure (1 in 7000 to 1 in 30,000). Patients at particular risk appear to be middle-aged obese females with previous closely spaced halothane administration.

Administration and Dosage:

Halothane may be administered by the nonrebreathing technique, partial rebreathing or closed technique. The induction dose varies. The maintenance concentration varies from 0.5% to 1.5%. May be administered with either oxygen or a mixture of oxygen and nitrous oxide.

Rx	**Halothane** (Abbott)	In 250 ml.[1]
Rx	**Fluothane** (Wyeth-Ayerst)	In 125 and 250 ml.[2]

[1] With 0.01% thymol.
[2] With 0.01% thymol and up to 0.00025% ammonia.

Volatile Liquids

METHOXYFLURANE

Actions:

Pharmacology: Provides anesthesia or analgesia. After surgical anesthesia, analgesia and drowsiness may persist after consciousness has returned. This may reduce the need for narcotics in the immediate postoperative period.

When used alone in safe concentration, it will not produce appreciable skeletal muscle relaxation; use a muscle relaxant as an adjunct. Bronchiolar constriction or laryngeal spasm is not ordinarily provoked.

Indications:

Usually used in combination with oxygen and nitrous oxide, to provide anesthesia for surgical procedures in which the total duration of administration is anticipated to be ≤ 4 hours, and in which methoxyflurane is not to be used in concentrations that will provide skeletal muscle relaxation.

May be used alone or in combination with oxygen and nitrous oxide for analgesia in obstetrics and in minor surgical procedures.

Warnings:

Renal function impairment: May cause renal failure or damage due to release of the fluoride ion.

Administration and Dosage:

Analgesia and anesthesia: 0.3% to 0.8%.

Induction: Up to 2%.

Maintenance: 0.1% to 2% is adequate for maintenance when administered in a carrier gas flow of oxygen and at least 50% nitrous oxide.

Rx	**Penthrane** (Abbott)	In 15 and 125 ml.[1]

[1] With 0.01% butylated hydroxytoluene.

Volatile Liquids

ENFLURANE

Actions:

Pharmacokinetics: An inhalation anesthetic. Induction and recovery from anesthesia are rapid. There is mild stimulus to salivation or tracheobronchial secretions. Pharyngeal and laryngeal reflexes are readily obtunded. The level of anesthesia changes rapidly. Reduces ventilation as depth of anesthesia increases. High $PaCO_2$ levels can be obtained at deeper levels of anesthesia if ventilation is not supported. Provokes a sigh response reminiscent of that seen with diethyl ether.

Progressive increases in depth of anesthesia produce increasing hypotension. Heart rate remains relatively constant without significant bradycardia; cardiac rhythm remains stable and is unaffected by carbon dioxide elevation in arterial blood.

Muscle relaxation may be adequate for intra-abdominal operations at normal levels of anesthesia. If greater relaxation is necessary, muscle relaxants may be used.

Indications:

Induction and maintenance of general anesthesia. Provides analgesia for vaginal delivery. Also used to supplement other general anesthetic agents during delivery by cesarean section.

Warnings:

Renal function impairment: May cause renal failure or may damage already impaired kidneys due to release of fluoride ion.

Administration and Dosage:

Induction: 2% to 4.5% produces anesthesia in 7 to 10 minutes.

Maintenance: Surgical levels of anesthesia may be maintained with 0.5% to 3% concentrations. Maintenance concentration should not exceed 3%.

Rx	**Enflurane** (Abbott)	In 125 and 250 ml.
Rx	**Ethrane** (Ohmeda)	In 125 and 250 ml.

ISOFLURANE

Actions:

Pharmacokinetics: Induction and recovery from isoflurane anesthesia are rapid. Its mild pungency limits the rate of induction, although excessive salivation or tracheobronchial secretions do not appear to be stimulated. Pharyngeal and laryngeal reflexes are readily obtunded. The level of anesthesia changes rapidly; it is a profound respiratory depressant. Monitor respiration closely and support when necessary. As the dose is increased, tidal volume decreases and respiratory rate is unchanged. This depression is partially reversed by surgical stimulation.

Blood pressure decreases with induction of anesthesia, progresses with increasing depth, but returns toward normal with surgical stimulation. Progressive increases in depth of anesthesia produce decreases in blood pressure. Nitrous oxide diminishes the concentration of isoflurane required and may reduce the arterial hypotension seen with isoflurane alone. With controlled ventilation and normal $PaCO_2$, cardiac output is maintained through an increase in heart rate which compensates for a reduction in stroke volume. The hypercapnia attending isoflurane anesthesia further increases heart rate and raises cardiac output above awake levels. Isoflurane does not sensitize the myocardium to exogenously administered epinephrine.

Muscle relaxation is adequate for intra-abdominal operations at normal levels of anesthesia. Complete muscle paralysis is attained with small doses of muscle relaxants.

Indications:

Induction and maintenance of general anesthesia.

Administration and Dosage:

Induction: Inspired concentrations of 1.5% to 3% isoflurane usually produce surgical anesthesia in 7 to 10 minutes.

Maintenance: Surgical levels of anesthesia may be sustained with a 1% to 2.5% concentration when nitrous oxide is used concomitantly.

Rx	**Isoflurane** (Abbott)	In 100 ml.
Rx	**Forane** (Anaquest)	In 100 ml.

Volatile Liquids

DESFLURANE

Actions:

Pharmacology: Desflurane is a volatile liquid inhalation anesthetic minimally biotransformed in the liver. Less than 0.02% of the desflurane absorbed can be recovered as urinary metabolites (compared to 0.2% for isoflurane). Minimum alveolar concentration (MAC) of desflurane in oxygen for a 25-year-old adult is 7.3%. The MAC of desflurane decreases with increasing age and with addition of depressants such as opioids or benzodiazepines. Changes in the clinical effects of desflurane rapidly follow changes in the inspired concentration.

Although desflurane can be used in adults for the inhalation induction of anesthesia via mask, it produces a high incidence of respiratory irritation (coughing, breathholding, apnea, increased secretions, laryngospasm).

Do not use desflurane as the sole agent for anesthetic induction in patients with coronary artery disease or any patients where increases in heart rate or blood pressure are undesirable. If desflurane is to be used in patients with coronary artery disease, use in combination with other medications for induction of anesthesia, preferably IV opioids and hypnotics.

Desflurane is not recommended for induction of general anesthesia in infants or children because of a high incidence of moderate to severe laryngospasm, coughing, breathholding and secretions.

Indications:

Anesthesia: An inhalation agent for induction or maintenance of anesthesia for inpatient and outpatient surgery in adults.

Warnings:

Children: Desflurane is not recommended for induction of anesthesia in children because of a high incidence of moderate to severe upper airway adverse events. After induction of anesthesia with agents other than desflurane, and tracheal intubation, desflurane is indicated for maintenance of anesthesia in infants and children.

Administration and Dosage:

Approved by the FDA on September 18, 1992.

Deliver desflurane from a vaporizer specifically designed and designated for use with desflurane. The administration of general anesthesia must be individualized based on the patient's response.

Preanesthetic medication: Issues such as whether or not to premedicate and the choice of premedicant(s) must be individualized. In clinical studies, patients scheduled to be anesthetized with desflurane frequently received IV preanesthetic medication, such as opioids or benzodiazepines.

Induction: In adults, a frequent starting concentration was 3%, increased in 0.5% to 1% increments every 2 to 3 breaths. End-tidal concentrations of 4% to 11% desflurane, with and without N_2O, produced anesthesia within 2 to 4 minutes.

After induction in adults with an IV drug such as thiopental or propofol, desflurane can be started at approximately 0.5 to 1 MAC, whether the carrier gas is O_2 or N_2O/O_2.

Maintenance: Surgical levels of anesthesia in adults may be maintained with concentrations of 2.5% to 8.5% with or without the concomitant use of nitrous oxide. In children, surgical levels of anesthesia may be maintained with concentrations of 5.2% to 10% with or without the concomitant use of nitrous oxide.

During the maintenance of anesthesia, increasing concentrations produce dose-dependent decreases in blood pressure. Excessive decreases in blood pressure may be due to depth of anesthesia and in such instances may be corrected by decreasing the inspired concentration of desflurane.

Concentrations of desflurane exceeding 1 MAC may increase heart rate. Thus, with this drug an increased heart rate may not serve reliably as a sign of inadequate anesthesia. The use of desflurane decreases the required doses of neuromuscular blocking agents.

Rx	**Suprane** (Ohmeda)	In 240 ml.

Volatile Liquids

SEVOFLURANE

Actions:

Pharmacology: Sevoflurane is an inhalational anesthetic. Minimum alveolar concentration (MAC) of sevoflurane in oxygen for a 40-year-old adult is 2.1%. The MAC of sevoflurane decreases with age.

Alveolar concentration/inspired concentration (F_A/F_1) of sevoflurane was compared with F_A/F_1 data of other halogenated anesthetics in healthy volunteers. When all data were normalized to isoflurane, the uptake and distribution of sevoflurane was faster than isoflurane and halothane, but slower than desflurane.

The low solubility of sevoflurane facilitates rapid elimination via the lungs. In healthy volunteers, rate of elimination was similar compared with desflurane but faster compared with halothane or isoflurane.

Sevoflurane is a dose-related cardiac depressant. It does not produce increases in heart rate at doses < 2 MAC.

Indications:

Anesthesia: Induction and maintenance of general anesthesia in adult and pediatric patients for inpatient and outpatient surgery.

Administration and Dosage:

Approved by the FDA on June 7, 1995 (1S classification).

The concentration of sevoflurane being delivered from a vaporizer should be known. This may be accomplished by using a vaporizer calibrated specifically for sevoflurane. Administration of general anesthesia must be individualized based on patient response.

Preanesthetic medication: No specific premedication is either indicated or contraindicated. The decision as to whether or not to premedicate and choice of premedication is left to the discretion of the anesthesiologist.

Induction: Sevoflurane has a nonpungent odor and does not cause respiratory irritability; it is suitable for mask induction in pediatrics and adults.

Maintenance: Surgical levels of anesthesia can usually be obtained with concentrations of 0.5% to 3% with or without the concomitant use of nitrous oxide. Sevoflurane can be administered with any type of anesthesia circuit.

Rx	**Ultane** (Abbott)	In 250 ml.

ANTICONVULSANTS

Anticonvulsant drugs include a variety of agents, all possessing the ability to depress abnormal neuronal discharges in the CNS, thus inhibiting seizure activity. Because of differences in pharmacology, therapeutic use and adverse reaction potential, these agents are discussed in groups as follows:

Barbiturates	**Oxazolidinediones**
Hydantoins	**Benzodiazepines**
Succinimides	**Miscellaneous**

Warnings:

Pregnancy: Reports suggest an association between use of anticonvulsant drugs by women with epilepsy and an elevated incidence of birth defects in children born to these women. Data are more extensive with respect to phenytoin and phenobarbital; other reports indicate a possible similar association with other anticonvulsants. Other factors (eg, genetics or the seizure disorder *per se*) may also contribute to the higher incidence of birth defects. The great majority of mothers receiving anticonvulsant medication deliver normal infants.

Do not discontinue anticonvulsant drugs in patients in whom the drug is administered to prevent major seizures because of the strong possibility of precipitating status epilepticus with attendant hypoxia and risk to both the mother and the unborn child. Consider discontinuation of anticonvulsants prior to and during pregnancy when the nature, frequency and severity of the seizures do not pose a serious threat to the patient. It is not known whether even minor seizures constitute some risk to the developing embryo or fetus.

An increase in seizure frequency during pregnancy occurs in a high proportion of patients because of altered phenytoin absorption or metabolism. Periodic measurement of serum phenytoin levels is particularly valuable in the management of pregnant epileptic patients as a guide to an appropriate adjustment of dosage. However, postpartum restoration of the original dosage will probably be indicated.

Reports suggest that maternal ingestion of anticonvulsant drugs, particularly barbiturates and hydantoins, is associated with a neonatal coagulation defect that may cause bleeding during the early (usually within 24 hours of birth) neonatal period. The defect is characterized by decreased levels of vitamin K-dependent clotting factors, and prolongation of either the prothrombin time or the partial thromboplastin time, or both. It has been suggested that prophylactic vitamin K be given to the mother 1 month prior to and during delivery, and to the infant immediately after birth.

In addition to the reports of increased incidence of congenital malformations, such as cleft lip/palate and heart malformations in children of women receiving phenytoin and other antiepileptic drugs, there have been more recent reports of a fetal hydantoin syndrome. This consists of prenatal growth deficiency, microcephaly and mental deficiency in children born to mothers who have received phenytoin, barbiturates, alcohol or trimethadione. However, these features are all interrelated and are frequently associated with intrauterine growth retardation from other causes.

There have been isolated reports of malignancies, including neuroblastoma, in children whose mothers received phenytoin during pregnancy.

Seizures may be classified based on their clinical form. The following is based on the International Classification of Epileptic Seizures*:

1.) Partial seizures (generally involve one hemisphere of the brain at onset)
   - a.) Simple (consciousness not impaired)
     1. With motor symptoms (Jacksonian, adversive)
     2. With somatosensory or other special sensory symptoms
     3. With autonomic symptoms
     4. With psychic symptoms
   - b.) Complex (consciousness impaired)
     1. Simple partial onset followed by impaired consciousness
     2. Impaired consciousness at onset
   - c.) Secondarily generalized
     1. Simple partial seizures evolving to generalized tonic-clonic seizures
     2. Complex partial seizures evolving to generalized tonic-clonic seizures
     3. Simple partial seizures evolving to complex partial seizures, then to generalized tonic-clonic seizures.

* Commission on Classification and Terminology of the International League Against Epilepsy. *Epilepsia* 1981;22:489-501 and 1989;30:389-99.

ANTICONVULSANTS

2.) Generalized seizures (involve both hemispheres of the brain at onset, consciousness usually impaired)
   a.) Absence
      1. Typical
      2. Atypical
   b.) Myoclonic
   c.) Clonic
   d.) Tonic
   e.) Tonic-clonic
   f.) Atonic
3.) Localization-related (focal)
   a.) Idiopathic
      1. Benign focal epilepsy of childhood
   b.) Symptomatic
      1. Chronic progressive epilepsia partialis continua
      2. Temporal-lobe
      3. Extratemporal
4.) Generalized epilepsy
   a.) Idiopathic
      1. Benign neonatal convulsions
      2. Childhood absence
      3. Juvenile myoclonic
      4. Other
   b.) Cryptogenic or symptomatic
      1. West syndrome (infantile spasms)
      2. Early myoclonic encephalopathy
      3. Lennox-Gastaut syndrome
      4. Progressive myoclonic epilepsy
5.) Special syndromes
   a.) Febrile seizures
6.) Unclassified

Withdrawal of anticonvulsants: A long-term prospective study suggests that epileptic adults may remain seizure-free if their anticonvulsant is withdrawn following at least 2 years of a single therapy regimen. Approximately one-third of patients relapsed following withdrawal of the anticonvulsants.

Predictors of relapse include: Seizure type (highest relapse rates occurred with complex partial seizures with secondary generalization and generalized seizures).

Number of seizures (higher risk with > 100 seizures before control).

Number of drugs (highest rate with patients taking two or three drugs).

Treatment duration (longer duration of drug treatment resulted in higher relapse rate).

EEG classification (lower relapse rate with less severe EEG abnormalities).

Type of drug (higher relapse rate following withdrawal of valproic acid).

ANTICONVULSANTS

Anticonvulsants: Indications and Pharmacokinetics

	Drug	Labeled indications	Protein binding (%)	Metabolism/ Excretion	t½ (hrs)	Therapeutic serum levels (mcg/ml)
Barbiturates	Phenobarbital[1] (PB)	Status epilepticus Cortical focal Tonic-clonic	40-60	Liver; 25% eliminated unchanged in urine	53-140	15-40
Hydantoins	Phenytoin	Tonic-clonic Psychomotor Status epilepticus	≈ 90	Liver; renal excretion. < 5% excreted unchanged	Dose-dependent[2]	5-20
	Mephenytoin	Tonic-clonic Psychomotor Focal Jacksonian	nd	Liver	95 (active metabolite)	nd
	Ethotoin	Tonic-clonic Psychomotor	nd	Liver; renal excretion of metabolites	3-9[3]	15-50
Succinimides	Ethosuximide	Absence	0	Liver; 25% excreted unchanged in urine	30 (children 7-9 yrs) 40-60 (adults)	40-100
	Methsuximide	Absence	nd	Liver; < 1% excreted unchanged in urine	< 2 (40, active metabolite)	nd
	Phensuximide	Absence	nd	Urine, bile	8 (active metabolite)	nd
Oxazolidinediones	Paramethadione	Absence	nd	Demethylated to active metabolite; excreted in urine	nd	nd
	Trimethadione	Absence	0	Demethylated to dimethadione; 3% excreted unchanged	6-13 days (dimethadione)	≥700 (dimethadione)
Benzodiazepines	Clonazepam	Absence Myoclonic Akinetic	50-85	5 metabolites identified; urine is major excretion route	18-60	20-80 ng/ml
	Clorazepate	Partial[4]	97	Hydrolyzed in stomach to desmethyldiazepam (active); metabolized in liver, renally excreted	30-100	nd
	Diazepam	Status epilepticus[4] Convulsive disorders, all forms[4]	97-99	Liver, active metabolites	20-50	nd

ANTICONVULSANTS

	Drug	Labeled indications	Protein binding (%)	Metabolism/ Excretion	t½ (hrs)	Therapeutic serum levels (mcg/ml)
Miscellaneous	Lamotrigine	Partial (adults)	≈ 55	Glucuronic acid conjugation to inactive metabolites; 94% excreted in urine, 2% in feces.	≈33[5]	nd
	Primidone	Tonic-clonic Psychomotor Focal	20-25	Metabolized to PB and PEMA, both active	5-15 (primidone) 10-18 (PEMA) 53-140 (PB)	5-12 (primidone) 15-40 (PB)
	Valproic acid	Absence	80-94	Liver; excreted in urine	5-20	50-150
	Carbamazepine	Tonic-clonic Mixed Psychomotor	≈75	Liver to active 10, 11–epoxide. 72% excreted in urine, 28% in feces	18-54 (initial) 10-20[5] ≈ 6 (10, 11-epoxide)	4-12
	Phenacemide	Severe mixed psychomotor	nd	Liver	nd	nd
	Felbamate[6]	Partial (adults) Partial/generalized assoc. with Lennox-Gastaut syndrome (children)	22-25	40% to 50% unchanged in urine, 40% as unidentified metabolites and conjugates	20-23	nd[7]
	Gabapentin	Partial (adults) with and without secondary generalization	< 3	Not appreciably metabolized; excreted in urine unchanged	5-7	nd

Table title: Anticonvulsants: Indications and Pharmacokinetics

[1] Other barbiturates are also used as anticonvulsants. See Sedatives/Hypnotics section.
[2] Exhibits dose-dependent, nonlinear pharmacokinetics.
[3] Below 8 mcg/ml; > 8 mcg/ml, t½ not defined due to dose-dependent, nonlinear pharmacokinetics.
[4] Recommended for adjunctive use.
[5] Undergoes autoinduction. Half-life after repeated doses.
[6] Because of cases of aplastic anemia, it has been recommended that the use of this drug be discontinued unless, in the judgment of the physician, continued therapy is warranted. Refer to the specific monograph.
[7] Value of monitoring blood levels not established.

HYDANTOINS

Actions:

Pharmacology: The primary site of action of the hydantoins appears to be the motor cortex, where the spread of seizure activity is inhibited. Possibly by promoting sodium efflux from neurons, hydantoins tend to stabilize the threshold against hyperexcitability caused by excessive stimulation or environmental changes capable of reducing membrane sodium gradient. This includes the reduction of post-tetanic potentiation at synapses. Loss of posttetanic potentiation prevents cortical seizure foci from detonating adjacent cortical areas. Hydantoins reduce the maximal activity of brain stem centers responsible for the tonic phase of grand mal seizures.

Phenytoin is available as phenytoin acid (chewable tablets, suspension) or phenytoin sodium (capsules, injection); phenytoin sodium contains 92% phenytoin.

Pharmacokinetics:

Absorption/Distribution – Phenytoin is slowly absorbed from the small intestine. Rate and extent of absorption varies and is dependent on the product formulation. Bioavailability may differ among products of different manufacturers. Oral phenytoin sodium extended reaches peak plasma levels in 12 hours; phenytoin sodium prompt peaks within 1.5 to 3 hours. Administration IM results in precipitation of phenytoin at the injection site, resulting in slow and erratic absorption, which may continue for up to 5 days or more; 50% to 75% of an IM dose is absorbed within 24 hours. Plasma levels vary and are significantly lower than those achieved with an equal oral dose. Plasma protein binding is 87% to 93% and is lower in uremic patients and neonates. Volume of distribution averages 0.6 L/kg.

Phenytoin's therapeutic plasma concentration is 10 to 20 mcg/ml, although many patients achieve complete seizure control at lower serum concentrations. At plasma concentrations > 20 mcg/ml, far-lateral nystagmus may occur and at concentrations > 30 and 40 mcg/ml, ataxia and gross mental changes are usually seen.

Metabolism/Excretion – Phenytoin is metabolized in the liver to inactive hydroxylated metabolites and excreted in the urine by tubular secretion. The metabolism of phenytoin is capacity-limited and shows saturability. The major metabolite is 5–(p–hydroxyphenyl)-5–phenylhydantoin (p–HPPH); 1% to 5% is excreted unchanged. Because the elimination of p–HPPH glucuronide is rate-limited by its formation from phenytoin, measurement of the metabolite in urine can be used to assess the rate of phenytoin metabolism, patient compliance or bioavailability. Elimination is exponential (first-order) at plasma concentrations < 10 mcg/ml, and plasma half-life ranges from 6 to 24 hours. Dose-dependent elimination is apparent at higher concentrations, and half-life increases; values of 20 to 60 hours may be found at therapeutic levels. A genetically determined limitation in ability to metabolize phenytoin has occurred. Good correlation is generally seen between total phenytoin plasma concentration and therapeutic effects. Serum level monitoring is essential.

Ethotoin is fairly rapidly absorbed. The drug exhibits saturable metabolism with respect to the formation of N–deethyl and p–hydroxyl-ethotoin, the major metabolites. The drug is apparently biotransformed by the liver. Where plasma concentrations are below about 8 mcg/ml, the elimination half-life of ethotoin is in the range of 3 to 9 hours. Experience suggests that therapeutic plasma concentrations fall in the range of 15 to 50 mcg/ml.

Indications:

Control of grand mal and psychomotor seizures.

Phenytoin: To prevent and treat seizures occurring during or following neurosurgery.

Parenteral – For the control of status epilepticus of the grand mal type.

Mephenytoin: For patients refractory to less toxic anticonvulsants; focal and Jacksonian seizures.

Unlabeled uses: Phenytoin is useful as an antiarrhythmic agent, particularly in cardiac glycoside-induced arrhythmias. (Oral loading dose = 14 mg/kg; oral maintenance = 200 to 400 mg/day. IV loading dose = 50 mg every 5 minutes to total dose of 1 g; IV maintenance dose = 200 to 400 mg/day.) Pharmacokinetic, electrophysiologic and ECG effects of phenytoin are summarized in the Antiarrhythmic Agents monograph.

Phenytoin has been used as an alternative to magnesium sulfate for severe preeclampsia (15 mg/kg IV, given as 10 mg/kg initially and 5 mg/kg 2 hours later).

Phenytoin has been used in the treatment of trigeminal neuralgia (tic douloureux), recessive dystrophic epidermolysis bullosa and junctional epidermolysis bullosa.

Contraindications:

Hypersensitivity to hydantoins.

Ethotoin: Hepatic abnormalities or hematologic disorders.

Phenytoin: Because of its effect on ventricular automaticity, do not use phenytoin in sinus bradycardia, sino-atrial block, second and third degree AV block or in patients with Adams-Stokes syndrome.

HYDANTOINS

Warnings:

Abrupt withdrawal in epileptic patients may precipitate status epilepticus. Reduce dosage, discontinue or substitute other anticonvulsant medication gradually.

Other seizures: Hydantoins are not indicated in seizures due to hypoglycemia or other metabolic causes. Perform appropriate diagnostic procedures.

Mephenytoin: Use only if safer anticonvulsants have failed after an adequate trial.

Phenytoin: Use with caution in hypotension and severe myocardial insufficiency.

Hepatic function impairment: Biotransformation of hydantoins occurs in the liver; elderly patients or those with impaired liver function or severe illness may show early signs of toxicity. Discontinue drug if hepatic dysfunction occurs.

Induced abnormalities – Phenytoin-induced hepatitis is one of the more commonly reported hypersensitivity syndromes.

Pregnancy: Refer to information for use during pregnancy in the Anticonvulsants introduction. If megaloblastic anemia occurs during gestation, consider folic acid therapy.

Lactation: These drugs are excreted in breast milk. Because of the potential for serious adverse reactions in nursing infants, decide whether to discontinue nursing or to discontinue the drug.

Precautions:

Hematologic effects: Perform blood counts and urinalyses when therapy is begun and at monthly intervals for several months thereafter. Blood dyscrasias have occurred. Avoid use in combination with other drugs known to adversely affect the hematopoietic system. Be alert for general malaise, sore throat, fever, mucous membrane bleeding, glandular swelling, petechiae, epistaxis, easy bruising, cutaneous reactions and other symptoms indicative of blood dyscrasias. Signs of marked depression of the blood count indicate the need for drug withdrawal.

Some evidence suggests that hydantoins may interfere with folic acid metabolism, precipitating megaloblastic anemia.

Dermatologic effects: Discontinue these drugs if a skin rash appears. If the rash is exfoliative, purpuric or bullous, do not resume use. If the rash is milder (measles-like or scarlatiniform), resume therapy after the rash has completely disappeared. If rash recurs upon reinstitution of therapy, further medication is contraindicated.

Lymph node hyperplasia has been associated with hydantoins, and may represent a hypersensitivity reaction. Rarely, this may progress to frank malignant lymphoma. If lymph node enlargement occurs, attempt to substitute another anticonvulsant drug or drug combination.

Differentiate lymphadenopathy from other lymph gland pathology. Lymphadenopathy which simulates Hodgkin's disease has been observed. If a lymphoma-like syndrome develops, withdraw the drug and observe the patient closely for regression of signs and symptoms before resuming treatment.

Monoclonal gammopathy and multiple myeloma have occurred during prolonged phenytoin therapy.

Hypersensitivity: In the event of an allergic or hypersensitivity reaction, rapid substitution of alternative therapy may be necessary. Alternative therapy should be an anticonvulsant not belonging to the hydantoin chemical class. Phenytoin hypersensitivity reactions are not typical; they may present as one of many different syndromes (eg, lymphoma, hepatitis, Stevens-Johnson syndrome) and may include such symptoms as fever, rash, arthralgias or lymphadenopathy.

Hyperglycemia, resulting from the drug's inhibitory effect on insulin release, has occurred. Hydantoins may also raise blood sugar levels in hyperglycemic persons.

Cardiovascular: Death from cardiac arrest has occurred after too-rapid IV administration, sometimes preceded by marked QRS widening. Observe the patient closely when the drug is administered IV when possible SA node depression exists. Administer cautiously in the presence of advanced AV block. Do not exceed an IV infusion rate of 50 mg/minute.

Grand mal and petit mal seizures: Drugs that control grand mal seizures are not effective for petit mal seizures. Therefore, if both conditions are present, combined drug therapy is needed.

Slow metabolism: A small percentage of individuals treated with hydantoins metabolize the drug slowly. Slow metabolism may be due to limited enzyme availability and lack of induction. It appears to be genetically determined. Metabolism of phenytoin is dose-dependent.

Osteomalacia has been associated with phenytoin therapy.

Acute intermittent porphyria: Administer hydantoins cautiously to patients with acute intermittent porphyria.

HYDANTOINS

Drug Interactions:

The following drug interactions have occurred with the use of phenytoin; however, they may occur when using any of the hydantoins.

Increased pharmacologic effects of hydantoins may occur when the following drugs are administered concurrently. Mechanisms of these interactions may include:

Hydantoin Drug Interactions: Increased Hydantoin Effects			
Inhibit metabolism		Displace anticonvulsant	Unknown
Amiodarone	Metronidazole	Salicylates[1]	Chlorpheniramine
Benzodiazepines	Miconazole	Tricyclic antidepressants	Ibuprofen
Chloramphenicol	Omeprazole	Valproic acid[2]	Phenothiazines
Cimetidine	Phenacemide		
Disulfiram	Phenylbutazone		
Ethanol (acute ingestion)	Succinimides		
	Sulfonamides		
Fluconazole	Trimethoprim		
Isoniazid	Valproic acid[2]		

[1] **Salicylates** displace phenytoin from its plasma protein binding sites in a dose-dependent manner; no significant change occurs in the free phenytoin level.

[2] **Valproic acid** affects phenytoin disposition in different ways. Displacement of phenytoin from plasma proteins increases the free fraction and decreases total phenytoin levels; the concentration of unbound phenytoin is not significantly altered. Increased levels may result from inhibition of phenytoin metabolism. Conversely, phenytoin increases metabolism of valproic acid.

Decreased pharmacologic effects of hydantoins may occur when the following drugs are administered concurrently. Mechanisms of these interactions may include:

Hydantoin Drug Interactions: Decreased Hydantoin Effects		
Increase metabolism	Decrease absorption	Unknown
Barbiturates[3]	Antacids	Antineoplastics
Carbamazepine[4]	Charcoal	Folic acid[5]
Diazoxide	Sucralfate	Influenza virus vaccine[6]
Ethanol		Loxapine
(chronic ingestion)		Nitrofurantoin
Rifampin		Pyridoxine
Theophylline		

[3] **Barbiturates** effect on phenytoin is variable and unpredictable. Addition of phenytoin generally increases phenobarbital serum concentrations. Individual monitoring is needed, especially when starting or stopping either drug.

[4] **Carbamazepine's** effect on phenytoin is variable. Carbamazepine serum levels may also be decreased.

[5] See also Drug/Food interactions.

[6] **Influenza virus vaccine** may increase, decrease, or have no effect on total serum phenytoin concentrations.

Phenytoin may decrease the pharmacologic effects of the following drugs:

Hydantoin Drug Interactions: Decreased Effects of Other Drugs		
Increased metabolism by phenytoin		Other
Acetaminophen[7]	Haloperidol	Cyclosporine
Amiodarone	Methadone	Dopamine
Carbamazepine	Metyrapone[8]	Furosemide
Cardiac glycosides	Mexiletine	Levodopa
Corticosteroids	Oral contraceptives	Levonorgestrel
Dicumarol	Quinidine	Mebendazole
Disopyramide	Theophylline	Nondepolarizing muscle relaxants
Doxycycline	Valproic acid	Phenothiazines
Estrogens		Sulfonylureas

[7] **Acetaminophen** Although the therapeutic effects of acetaminophen may be reduced by concomitant phenytoin use, the potential hepatotoxicity of acetaminophen may be increased, especially with chronic phenytoin use.

[8] See also Drug/Lab test interactions.

HYDANTOINS

Clonazepam: Plasma levels of clonazepam or phenytoin may be decreased with concomitant use, or phenytoin toxicity may occur.

Corticosteroid use may mask systemic manifestations of phenytoin hypersensitivity reactions.

Dopamine: Five critically ill patients requiring dopamine to maintain blood pressure developed severe hypotension when IV phenytoin was administered.

Lithium toxicity may be increased by coadministration of phenytoin. Marked neurologic symptoms were reported despite normal serum levels of lithium.

Meperidine's analgesic effectiveness may be decreased, while the toxic effects could be increased by phenytoin. The hepatic metabolism of meperidine is increased, but the formation of normeperidine, a potentially toxic metabolite, is increased.

Primidone's pharmacologic effects may be increased by phenytoin administration; toxicity has occurred. The metabolic conversion of primidone to phenobarbital and phenylethylmalonamide (PEMA) may also be increased. Monitor serum concentrations of primidone and primidone metabolites following alterations in hydantoin therapy.

Warfarin may be displaced by phenytoin; in one report, a patient died of bleeding complications.

Drug/Lab test interactions: Phenytoin may interfere with the **metyrapone** and the 1 mg **dexamethasone** tests. Discontinuing hydantoins prior to metyrapone testing would be ideal, but not practical; consider doubling the oral metyrapone dose.

Drug/Food interactions: Several case reports and single-dose studies suggest that enteral nutritional therapy may decrease phenytoin concentrations; however, this has not been substantiated. Monitor phenytoin concentrations. Consider giving phenytoin 2 hours before and after the enteral feeding, or stopping the enteral therapy for 2 hours before and after phenytoin administration.

Long-term phenytoin therapy may result in folate deficiency, possibly progressing to megaloblastic anemia (rare).

Adverse Reactions:

CNS: (most common): Nystagmus; ataxia; dysarthria; slurred speech; mental confusion; dizziness; insomnia; transient nervousness; motor twitchings; diplopia; fatigue; irritability; drowsiness; depression; numbness; tremor; headache. These side effects may disappear by reducing dosage. Psychotic disturbances and increased seizures have occurred, but a definite causal relationship is uncertain. Choreoathetosis following IV phenytoin infusion has occurred.

Cardiovascular: Phenytoin IV–Cardiovascular collapse; CNS depression; hypotension (when the drug is administered rapidly IV). Rate of administration is very important; do not exceed 50 mg/minute. Severe cardiotoxic reactions and fatalities have occurred with atrial and ventricular conduction depression and ventricular fibrillation, most commonly in elderly or gravely ill patients.

GI: Nausea; vomiting; diarrhea; constipation. Administration of the drug with or immediately after meals may help prevent GI discomfort.

Gingival hyperplasia occurs frequently with phenytoin; incidence may be reduced by good oral hygiene, including gum massage, frequent brushing and appropriate dental care.

Connective tissue system: Coarsening of the facial features; enlargement of the lips; Peyronie's disease.

Hepatic: Toxic hepatitis and liver damage may occur and rarely can be fatal. Hypersensitivity reactions with hepatic involvement include hepatocellular degeneration and fatal hepatocellular necrosis. Hepatitis, jaundice and nephrosis have been reported, but a definite cause and effect relationship has not been established. Warnings.

Dermatologic: manifestations sometimes accompanied by fever have included scarlatiniform, morbilliform, maculopapular, urticarial and nonspecific rashes; a morbilliform rash is the most common. Rashes are more frequent in children and young adults. Serious forms which may be fatal include bullous, exfoliative or purpuric dermatitis, lupus erythematosus syndrome, Stevens-Johnson syndrome and toxic epidermal necrolysis. Hirsutism and alopecia have occurred.

HYDANTOINS

Hematologic: complications, some fatal, include thrombocytopenia, leukopenia, granulocytopenia, agranulocytosis and pancytopenia. Macrocytosis and megaloblastic anemia usually respond to folic acid therapy. Eosinophilia; monocytosis; leukocytosis; simple anemia; hemolytic anemia; aplastic anemia.

Connective tissue system: Coarsening of the facial features; enlargement of the lips; Peyronie's disease.

Body as a whole: Polyarthropathy; hyperglycemia; weight gain; chest pain; edema; IgA depression; fever; photophobia; conjunctivitis; gynecomastia; periarteritis nodosa; pulmonary fibrosis; soft tissue injury at the injection site with and without extravasation of IV phenytoin; lymph node hyperplasia (see Precautions).

Lab test abnormalities: Phenytoin may decrease serum thyroxine and free thyroxine concentrations. Although these decreases are generally not associated with clinical hypothyroidism, some patients may develop goiter or hypothyroidism.

Overdosage:

Symptoms: The lethal dose in adults is estimated to be 2 to 5 g. Initial symptoms are nystagmus, ataxia and dysarthria; the patient may then become comatose and hypotensive, with pupils unresponsive. At plasma concentrations > 20 mcg/ml, far-lateral nystagmus may occur and at concentrations > 30 mcg/ml, ataxia is usually seen. Significantly diminished mental capacity occurs at levels > 40mcg/ml. Death is due to respiratory and circulatory depression.

Treatment: Treatment is nonspecific; there is no known antidote. Refer to General Management of Acute Overdosage. Consider hemodialysis, since phenytoin is not completely bound to plasma proteins. Total exchange transfusion has been utilized in the treatment of severe intoxication in children.

Patient Information:

Take medication with food to reduce GI upset.

Phenytoin suspension must be thoroughly shaken immediately prior to use.

Do not discontinue medication abruptly or change dosage, except on advice of physician.

Maintain good oral hygiene (regular brushing and flossing) while taking phenytoin. Inform dentist of medication usage.

Patients should carry identification (Medic Alert) indicating medication usage and epilepsy.

May cause drowsiness, dizziness or blurred vision; alcohol may intensify these effects. Observe caution while driving or performing other tasks requiring alertness, coordination or physical dexterity. Notify physician if drowsiness, slurred speech or impaired coordination (ataxia) occurs.

Do not use capsules which are discolored.

Diabetic patients: Monitor urine sugar regularly and report any abnormalities to physician.

Notify physician if any of the following occurs: Skin rash; severe nausea or vomiting; swollen glands; bleeding, swollen or tender gums; yellowish discoloration of the skin or eyes; joint pain; unexplained fever; sore throat; unusual bleeding or bruising; persistent headache; malaise; any indication of an infection or bleeding tendency; pregnancy.

Hydantoins

PHENYTOIN SODIUM, PARENTERAL

For complete prescribing information, refer to the Hydantoins group monograph.

Administration and Dosage:

Phenytoin sodium contains 92% phenytoin.

IV administration: The addition of phenytoin solution to an IV infusion is not recommended due to lack of solubility and resultant precipitation.

Inject parenteral phenytoin slowly and directly into a large vein through a large-gauge needle or IV catheter.

Do not exceed an IV infusion rate of 50 mg/minute in adults or 1 to 3 mg/kg/minute in neonates. There is a relatively small margin between full therapeutic effect and minimally toxic doses. Monitor ECG and blood pressure continuously. In status epilepticus, the IV route is preferred because of the delay in absorption with IM administration.

Follow each IV injection with an injection of sterile saline through the same needle or IV catheter to avoid local venous irritation due to alkalinity of the solution. Avoid continuous infusion.

Soft tissue irritation and injury, with and without extravasation of IV phenytoin, have occurred at the injection site.

Although not recommended, some studies indicate that an IV infusion of phenytoin may be feasible if proper precautions are observed, such as a suitable vehicle (eg, Sodium Chloride 0.9% or Lactated Ringer's injection), appropriate concentration, preparing the infusion shortly before administration and using an inline filter.

IM administration: Avoid the IM route due to erratic absorption of phenytoin and pain and muscle damage at the injection site. When IM administration is required for a patient previously stabilized orally, compensating dosage adjustments are necessary to maintain therapeutic plasma levels; an IM dose 50% greater than the oral dose is necessary. When returned to oral administration, reduce the dose by 50% of the original oral dose for 1 week to prevent excessive plasma levels due to sustained release from IM tissue sites. Determine serum drug levels when possible drug interactions are suspected.

If the patient requires > 1 week of IM therapy, consider alternative routes (eg, gastric intubation), using oral preparations. For periods < 1 week, the patient shifted back from IM administration should receive ½ the original oral dose for the same period of time the patient received IM therapy. Monitor plasma levels.

Status epilepticus: In adults, administer loading dose of 10 to 15 mg/kg slowly. Follow by maintenance doses of 100 mg orally or IV every 6 to 8 hours. For neonates and children, oral absorption of phenytoin is unreliable; IV loading dose is 15 to 20 mg/kg in divided doses of 5 to 10 mg/kg. If administration does not terminate the seizure, consider the use of other anticonvulsants, IV barbiturates, general anesthesia or other measures.

Neurosurgery (prophylactic dosage): 100 to 200 mg IM at ≈ 4 hour intervals during surgery and the postoperative period.

Storage of solution: The solution is suitable for use as long as it remains free of haziness and precipitate. Upon refrigeration or freezing, a precipitate might form; this will dissolve again after the solution is allowed to stand at room temperature. The solution is still suitable for use. Use only a clear solution. A faint yellow color may develop, but has no effect on the potency of the solution.

Rx	**Phenytoin Sodium** (Elkins-Sinn)	**Injection:** 50 mg /ml (46 mg phenytoin)[1]	In 2 and 5 ml Dosette amps, 2 ml Dosette vials and 5 ml vials.
Rx	**Phenytoin Sodium** (SoloPak)		In 2 and 5 ml fill in vials.
Rx	**Dilantin** (Parke-Davis)		In 2 ml Steri-Dose syringes, 2 and 5 ml Steri-Vials.

[1] With propylene glycol and alcohol.

Hydantoins

PHENYTOIN and PHENYTOIN SODIUM, ORAL

For complete prescribing information, refer to the Hydantoins group monograph.

Administration and Dosage:

Phenytoin sodium contains 92% phenytoin.

Individualize dosage. Determine serum levels for optimal dosage adjustments; the clinically effective serum level is usually in the range of 10 to 20 mcg/ml.

Monitor serum concentrations and exercise care when switching a patient from the sodium salt to the free acid form or vice versa. The free acid form of phenytoin is used in the *Dilantin Infatabs* and *Dilantin-125* suspension, as opposed to the sodium salt in the other products. Because there is an ≈ 8% increase in drug content with the free acid form, dosage adjustment and serum monitoring may be necessary.

Loading dose: Some authorities have advocated use of an oral loading dose of phenytoin in adults who require rapid steady-state serum levels and where IV administration is not desirable. Reserve this dosing regimen for patients in a clinic or hospital setting where phenytoin serum levels can be monitored. Patients with a history of renal or liver disease should not receive the oral loading regimen.

Initially, 1 g of phenytoin capsules is divided into 3 doses (400 mg, 300 mg, 300 mg) and administered at intervals of 2 hours. Normal maintenance dosage is then instituted 24 hours after the loading dose, with frequent serum level determinations.

Adults who have received no previous treatment may be started on 100 mg (125 mg suspension) 3 times daily; individualize dosage. Satisfactory maintenance dosage - 300 to 400 mg/day. An increase to 600 mg/day (625 mg/day suspension) may be necessary.

Pediatric: Initially, 5 mg/kg/day in 2 or 3 equally divided doses with subsequent dosage individualized to a maximum of 300 mg/day. Daily maintenance dosage - 4 to 8 mg/kg. Children over 6 years may require the minimum adult dose (300 mg/day). If the daily dosage cannot be divided equally, the larger dose should be given before retiring.

Single daily dosage: In adults, if seizure control is established with divided doses of three 100 mg extended phenytoin sodium capsules daily, once-a-day dosage with 300 mg may be considered. Once-a-day dosage offers convenience to the patient or to nursing personnel for institutionalized patients; it may improve compliance and it is intended to be used only for patients requiring this amount of drug daily. Caution patients not to miss a dose. Only extended phenytoin sodium capsules are recommended once-a-day.

Bioavailability: Because of potential bioavailability differences between products, brand interchange is not recommended. Dosage adjustments may be required when switching from the extended to the prompt products.

PHENYTOIN

For complete prescribing information, refer to the Hydantoins group monograph.

Not for once-a-day dosing.

Rx	**Dilantin Infatab** (Parke-Davis)	**Tablets, chewable:** 50 mg	Saccharin, sucrose. Yellow, scored. Triangular. In 100s and UD 100s.
Rx	**Dilantin-125** (Parke-Davis)	**Oral Suspension:** 125 mg per 5 ml	≤ 0.6% alcohol, sucrose. Orange-vanilla flavor. In 240 ml.

PHENYTOIN SODIUM, PROMPT

For complete prescribing information, refer to the Hydantoins group monograph.

Not for once-a-day dosing.

Dissolution rate: Not < 85% in 30 minutes.

Rx	**Phenytoin Sodium** (Various, eg, Major, Parmed, Zenith)	**Capsules:** 100 mg (92 mg phenytoin)	In 100s, 1000s and UD 100s.

Hydantoins

PHENYTOIN SODIUM, EXTENDED

For complete prescribing information, refer to the Hydantoins group monograph.

Administration and Dosage:

May be used for once-a-day dosing.

Rx	**Phenytoin Sodium** (Various, eg, Goldline, Major)	**Capsules**: 100 mg (92 mg phenytoin)	Clear. In 100s and 1000s.
Rx	**Dilantin Kapseals** (Parke-Davis)	**Capsules**: 30 mg (27.6 mg phenytoin)	Lactose, sucrose. Transparent w/pink band. In 100s.
		100 mg (92 mg phenytoin)	Lactose, sucrose. Transparent w/orange band. In 100s, 1000s and UD 100s.

MEPHENYTOIN

For complete prescribing information, refer to the Hydantoins group monograph.

Administration and Dosage:

Individualize dosage. Start with 50 or 100 mg/day during the first week and thereafter increase the daily dose by 50 or 100 mg at weekly intervals. No dose should be increased until it has been taken for at least 1 week.

Adults: The average dose ranges from 200 to 600 mg/day. In some instances, as much as 800 mg/day or more may be required to obtain full seizure control.

Children usually require from 100 to 400 mg/day.

Replacement therapy: The recommended dosage of mephenytoin is 50 or 100 mg daily during the first week. Gradually increase the daily dose of mephenytoin at weekly intervals while gradually reducing that of the drug being discontinued over 3 to 6 weeks. If seizures are not completely controlled with the dose so attained, increase the daily dose by 1 tablet weekly, to the point of maximum effect. If the patient has also been receiving phenobarbital, continue it until the transition is completed, at which time gradual withdrawal of the phenobarbital may be attempted.

Rx	**Mesantoin** (Sandoz)	**Tablets**: 100 mg	Lactose, sucrose. (78/52). Pink, scored. In 100s.

ETHOTOIN

For complete prescribing information, refer to the Hydantoins group monograph.

Administration and Dosage:

Administer in 4 to 6 divided doses daily. Take after food; space doses as evenly as practicable. Initial dosage should be conservative.

Adults: The initial daily dose should be ≤ 1 g, with subsequent gradual dosage increases over several days. The usual adult maintenance dose is 2 to 3 g/day; < 2 g/day is ineffective in most adults.

Pediatric: Dosage depends upon the age and weight of the patient. Initial dose should not exceed 750 mg/day. The usual maintenance dose in children ranges from 500 mg to 1 g/day, although occasionally 2 g or rarely 3 g daily may be necessary.

Replacement therapy: Reduce the dosage of the other drug gradually as that of ethotoin is increased. Ethotoin may eventually replace the other drug, or the optimal dosage of both anticonvulsants may be established.

Concomitant anticonvulsant therapy: Ethotoin is compatible with all commonly employed anticonvulsant medications with the possible exception of phenacemide. In grand mal seizures, concomitant use with phenobarbital may be beneficial. It may be used in combination with drugs such as trimethadione or paramethadione, as an adjunct in those patients with petit mal associated with grand mal seizures.

Rx	**Peganone** (Abbott)	**Tablets**: 250 mg	Lactose. White, scored. In 100s.
		500 mg	Lactose. White, scored. In 100s.

Hydantoins

FOSPHENYTOIN SODIUM

Administration and Dosage:

The dose, concentration in dosing solutions and infusion rate of IV fosphenytoin is expressed as phenytoin sodium equivalents (PE) to avoid the need to perform molecular weight-based adjustments when converting between fosphenytoin and phenytoin sodium doses. Prescribe and dispense fosphenytoin in phenytoin sodium equivalent units (PE). Fosphenytoin has important differences in administration from those for parenteral phenytoin sodium.

Dilute fosphenytoin in 5% Dextrose or 0.9% Saline Solution for Injection to a concentration ranging from 1.5 to 25 mg PE/ml.

Status epilepticus: The loading dose 15 to 20 mg PE/kg administered at 100 to 150 mg PE/min.

Because the full antiepileptic effect of phenytoin, whether given as fosphenytoin or parenteral phenytoin, is not immediate, other measures, including concomitant administration of an IV benzodiazepine, will usually be necessary for control of status epilepticus.

Nonemergent and maintenance dosing:

Loading dose – 10 to 20 mg PE/kg given IV or IM.

Maintenance dose – 4 to 6 mg PE/kg/day.

Because of the risk of hypotension, administer at a rate of ≤ 150 mg PE/min.

Continuously monitor the electrocardiogram, blood pressure and respiratory function and observe the patient throughout the period of maximal serum phenytoin concentrations, ≈ 10 to 20 min after the end of the infusion.

Renal/Hepatic function impairment: Due to an increased fraction of unbound phenytoin in patients with renal or hepatic disease, or in those with hypoalbuminemia, interpret total phenytoin plasma concentrations with caution. Unbound phenytoin concentrations may be more useful in these patients. After IV administration, fosphenytoin clearance to phenytoin may be increased without a similar increase in phenytoin clearance. This has the potential to increase the frequency and severity of adverse events.

Elderly: Age does not have a significant impact on the pharmacokinetics of fosphenytoin following administration. Phenytoin clearance is decreased slightly in elderly patients and lower or less frequent dosing may be required.

Storage/Stability: Refrigerate at 2° to 8°C (36° to 46°F). Do not store at room temperature for more than 48 hours.

Rx	**Cerebyx** (Parke-Davis)	**Injection**: 150 mg (100 mg phenytoin sodium)	In 2 ml vials.
		750 mg (500 mg phenytoin sodium)	In 10 ml vials.

SUCCINIMIDES

Actions:

Pharmacology: Succinimides suppress the paroxysmal three cycle per second spike and wave activity associated with lapses of consciousness common in absence (petit mal) seizures. The frequency of epileptiform attacks is reduced, apparently by motor cortex depression and elevation of the threshold of the CNS to convulsive stimuli.

Pharmacokinetics:

Absorption/Distribution – These agents are readily absorbed from the GI tract. Peak serum levels of ethosuximide are achieved in 3 to 7 hours; peak levels of methsuximide and phensuximide are reached in 1 to 4 hours. Therapeutic serum concentrations of ethosuximide range from 40 to 100 mcg/ml.

Metabolism/Excretion – Ethosuximide is extensively metabolized to inactive metabolites; approximately 20% is excreted unchanged via the kidneys. The plasma half-life is 30 hours in children and 60 hours in adults. Less than 1% of a dose of methsuximide is recovered unchanged in urine; plasma half-lives range from 2.6 to 4 hours. Phensuximide is excreted in urine and in bile; half-life is approximately 4 hours.

Indications:

Control of absence (petit mal) seizures.

Methsuximide: For petit mal seizures when refractory to other drugs.

Contraindications:

Hypersensitivity to succinimides.

Warnings:

Hematologic effects: Blood dyscrasias, some fatal, have occurred; therefore, perform periodic blood counts. Should signs or symptoms of infection (eg, sore throat, fever) develop, consider blood counts at that point.

Lupus: Cases of systemic lupus erythematosus have occurred.

Renal/Hepatic function impairment: Succinimides have produced morphological and functional changes in animal liver. Abnormal liver and renal function have been reported in humans. For this reason, administer with extreme caution to patients with known liver or renal disease. Perform periodic urinalyses and liver function studies for all patients receiving these drugs.

Pregnancy: Refer to information for use during pregnancy in the Anticonvulsant introduction.

Precautions:

Grand mal seizures: Succinimides, when used alone in mixed types of epilepsy, may increase the frequency of grand mal seizures in some patients.

Dosage changes/other medication: It is important to proceed slowly when increasing or decreasing dosage, and when adding or eliminating other medication. Abrupt withdrawal of anticonvulsant medication may precipitate absence (petit mal) status.

Acute intermittent porphyria: Use phensuximide with caution.

Drug Interactions:

Succinimide Drug Interactions			
Precipitant drug	Object drug*		Description
Succinimides	Hydantoins	⬆	Serum hydantoin levels may be increased.
Succinimides	Primidone	⬇	Lower primidone and phenobarbital levels may occur.
Valproic acid	Succinimides	⟷	Both increases and decreases in succinimide levels have occurred.

* ⬆ = Object drug increased ⬇ = Object drug decreased ⟷ = Undetermined effect

Adverse Reactions:

The following have been reported with one or more of the succinimides:

GI: (frequent): Nausea; vomiting; vague gastric upset; cramps; anorexia; diarrhea; weight loss; epigastric and abdominal pain; constipation.

Hematologic: Eosinophilia; granulocytopenia; leukopenia; agranulocytosis; monocytosis; pancytopenia, with or without bone marrow suppression.

Miscellaneous: Periorbital edema; hyperemia; muscle weakness; swelling of the tongue; gum hypertrophy.

SUCCINIMIDES

CNS: Drowsiness; ataxia; dizziness; irritability; nervousness; headache; blurred vision; myopia; photophobia; hiccoughs; euphoria; dream-like state; lethargy; hyperactivity; fatigue; insomnia. Drowsiness, ataxia and dizziness are the most frequent methsuximide side effects.

Psychiatric: Confusion; instability; mental slowness; depression; hypochondriacal behavior; sleep disturbances; night terrors; aggressiveness; inability to concentrate. These effects may be noted particularly in patients who have previously exhibited psychological abnormalities. There have been rare reports of paranoid psychosis, suicidal behavior, auditory hallucinations, increased libido and increased state of depression.

Dermatologic: Pruritus; urticaria; Stevens-Johnson syndrome; pruritic erythematous rashes; skin eruptions; erythema multiforme; systemic lupus erythematosus; alopecia; hirsutism.

GU: Urinary frequency, renal damage, hematuria (**phensuximide**); vaginal bleeding; microscopic hematuria.

Overdosage:

The therapeutic range of ethosuximide serum levels is 40 to 100 mcg/ml, although levels as high as 150 mcg/ml have occurred without signs of toxicity. Methsuximide levels > 40 mcg/ml have caused toxicity; coma has been seen at levels of 150 mcg/ml.

Symptoms:

Acute overdosage – Confusion; sleepiness; unsteadiness; flaccid muscles; coma with slow, shallow respiration; hypotension; cyanosis; hypo- or hyperthermia; absent reflexes; nausea; vomiting; CNS depression including coma with respiratory depression.

Chronic overdosage – Skin rash; confusion; ataxia; dizziness; drowsiness; hangover; depression; irritability; poor judgment; periorbital edema; proteinuria; hepatic dysfunction; fatal bone marrow aplasia; delayed onset of coma; nausea; vomiting; muscular weakness; hematuria; casts; nephrosis.

Treatment: includes usual supportive measures. Refer to General Management of Acute Overdosage. Charcoal hemoperfusion may be indicated. Hemodialysis may be useful for ethosuximide. Forced diuresis and exchange transfusions are ineffective.

Patient Information:

If GI upset occurs, take with food or milk.

Do not discontinue medication abruptly or change dosage, except on advice of physician.

Patients should carry identification (Medic Alert) indicating medication usage and epilepsy.

May cause drowsiness, dizziness or blurred vision; alcohol may exacerbate these effects. Use caution while driving or performing other tasks requiring alertness, coordination or physical dexterity.

Notify physician if any of the following occurs: Skin rash, joint pain, unexplained fever, sore throat, unusual bleeding or bruising, drowsiness, dizziness, blurred vision or pregnancy.

Phensuximide may discolor the urine pink, red or red-brown. This is not harmful.

Succinimides

ETHOSUXIMIDE

For complete prescribing information, refer to the Succinimides group monograph.

Administration and Dosage:

Children (3 to 6 years of age): Initial dose – 250 mg/day.

Children and adults (≥ 6 years if age): 500 mg/day.

Maintenance therapy: Individualize dosage. Increase by small increments. One method is to increase the daily dose by 250 mg every 4 to 7 days until control is achieved with minimal side effects. Administer dosages exceeding 1.5 g/day in divided doses only under strict supervision. The optimal dose for most children is 20 mg/kg/day.

Concomitant therapy: May be administered in combination with other anticonvulsants when other forms of epilepsy coexist with absence (petit mal) seizures.

Rx	**Zarontin** (Parke-Davis)	**Capsules:** 250 mg	Sorbitol. In 100s.
Rx	**Ethosuximide** (Copley)	**Syrup:** 250 mg per 5 ml	Saccharin, sucrose. Raspberry flavor. In 483 ml.
Rx	**Zarontin** (Parke-Davis)		Raspberry flavor. Saccharin, sucrose. In pt.

METHSUXIMIDE

For complete prescribing information, refer to the Succinimides group monograph.

Administration and Dosage:

Determine optimum dosage by trial. A suggested schedule is 300 mg/day for the first week. If required, increase at weekly intervals by 300 mg/day for 3 weeks, up to a dosage of 1.2 g/day. Individualize therapy according to patient response. The 150 mg capsule facilitates pediatric administration.

Concomitant therapy: May be administered in combination with other anticonvulsants when other forms of epilepsy coexist with absence (petit mal) seizures.

Rx	**Celontin Kapseals** (Parke-Davis)	**Capsules, Half Strength:** 150 mg	In 100s.
		Capsules: 300 mg	In 100s.

PHENSUXIMIDE

For complete prescribing information, refer to the Succinimides group monograph.

Administration and Dosage:

Administer 500 to 1000 mg 2 or 3 times daily. Individualize dosage. The total dosage, regardless of age, may vary between 1 and 3 g/day (average, 1.5 g).

Concomitant therapy: May be administered in combination with other anticonvulsants when other forms of epilepsy coexist with absence (petit mal) seizures.

Rx	**Milontin Kapseals** (Parke-Davis)	**Capsules:** 500 mg	In 100s.

OXAZOLIDINEDIONES

> **Warning:**
> Because of their potential to produce fetal malformations and serious side effects, use these agents only when other less toxic drugs have been found ineffective in controlling petit mal seizures.

Actions:

Pharmacology: Unlike hydantoins and anticonvulsant barbiturates, neither drug modifies maximal seizure pattern in humans receiving electroconvulsive therapy. These agents have a sedative effect which may increase to ataxia with excessive doses.

Pharmacokinetics: Readily absorbed from the GI tract. Demethylated by liver microsomes to an active metabolite, dimethadione, which is slowly excreted by kidneys. About 3% of a daily trimethadione dose is recovered in urine unchanged. Almost no unmetabolized paramethadione is excreted. Trimethadione has a plasma half-life of 16 to 24 hours; dimethadione's is 6 to 13 days. While no definite therapeutic trimethadione levels have been determined, patients with petit mal attacks are usually controlled by serum dimethadione levels ≥ 700 mcg/ml.

Indications:

For the control of absence (petit mal) seizures refractory to treatment with other drugs.

Contraindications:

Hypersensitivity to oxazolidinediones.

Warnings:

Side effects: May cause serious side effects. Strict medical supervision of the patient is mandatory, especially during the initial year of therapy.

Pregnancy: Category D. Refer to the Anticonvulsant introduction.

Lactation: It is not known whether these drugs are excreted in breast milk. Decide whether to discontinue nursing or to discontinue the drug, taking into account the importance of the drug to the mother.

Precautions:

Lupus: Manifestations of systemic lupus erythematosus have been associated with the use of the oxazolidinediones. Lymphadenopathies simulating malignant lymphoma have also occurred. Lupus-like manifestations or lymph node enlargement are indications for drug withdrawal. Signs and symptoms may disappear after discontinuation of therapy, and specific treatment may be unnecessary.

Withdrawal: Abrupt discontinuation of paramethadione or trimethadione may precipitate absence (petit mal) status. Withdraw gradually unless serious adverse effects dictate otherwise. If this occurs, another anticonvulsant may be substituted.

Dermatologic effects: Withdraw these agents promptly if skin rash appears, because of the possibility of exfoliative dermatitis or severe erythema multiforme. Even a minor acneiform or morbilliform rash should be allowed to clear completely before treatment is resumed; reinstitute therapy cautiously.

Hepatic effects: Perform liver function tests prior to initiating therapy and at monthly intervals thereafter. Hepatitis has been associated rarely with oxazolidinediones. Jaundice or other signs of liver dysfunction are an indication for drug withdrawal. These agents should ordinarily not be used in severe hepatic impairment.

Renal effects: Perform urinalysis prior to therapy and at monthly intervals. Fatal nephrosis has occurred. If persistent or increasing proteinuria, or any other significant renal abnormality occurs, withdraw the drug. Oxazolidinediones should ordinarily not be used in patients with severe renal dysfunction.

Ophthalmic effects: Hemeralopia has occurred with the use of these agents; this appears to be an effect on the neural layers of the retina, and usually can be reversed by a reduction in dosage. Scotomata are an indication for withdrawal of the drug. Use caution when treating patients who have diseases of the retina or optic nerve.

Hematologic effects: Perform a complete blood count prior to initiating therapy and monthly thereafter. If marked depression of blood count occurs, withdraw drug. If no abnormality appears within 12 months, may extend interval between blood counts. A moderate degree of neutropenia, with or without corresponding drop in leukocyte count, is not uncommon. Therapy need not be withdrawn unless neutrophil count is ≤ 2500; perform more frequent blood examinations when the count is < 3000. Leukopenia, eosinophilia, thrombocytopenia, pancytopenia, agranulocytosis, hypoplastic anemia and fatal aplastic anemia have also occurred.

These agents are not ordinarily used in patients with severe blood dyscrasias.

CNS effects: May cause drowsiness or blurred vision. Observe caution while driving or performing other tasks requiring alertness, coordination or physical dexterity.

OXAZOLIDINEDIONES

Myasthenia gravis-like syndrome has been associated with the chronic use of the oxazolidinediones. If symptoms suggest this condition, withdraw the drug.

Porphyria: Use trimethadione with caution in patients with acute intermittent porphyria.

Photosensitivity: Photosensitization may occur; therefore, caution patients to take protective measures (ie, sunscreens, protective clothing) against exposure to ultraviolet light or sunlight until tolerance is determined.

Tartrazine sensitivity: Paramethadione 300 mg capsules contain tartrazine, which may cause allergic-type reactions (including bronchial asthma) in susceptible individuals. Although the incidence of tartrazine sensitivity in the general population is low, it is frequently seen in patients who also have aspirin hypersensitivity.

Adverse Reactions:

Renal: Fatal nephrosis; proteinuria.

Hematologic: Fatal aplastic anemia; hypoplastic anemia; pancytopenia; agranulocytosis; leukopenia; neutropenia; thrombocytopenia; eosinophilia; retinal and petechial hemorrhages; vaginal bleeding; epistaxis; bleeding gums.

Dermatologic: Acneiform or morbilliform skin rash that may progress to severe forms of erythema multiforme or to exfoliative dermatitis; hair loss.

CNS: Myasthenia gravis-like syndrome (see Precautions); precipitation of tonic-clonic (grand mal) seizures; vertigo; personality changes; increased irritability; drowsiness; headache; paresthesias; fatigue; malaise; insomnia; diplopia; hemeralopia; photophobia. Drowsiness usually subsides with continued therapy; if it persists, a reduction in dosage is indicated.

GI: Vomiting; abdominal pain; gastric distress; nausea; anorexia; weight loss; hiccups.

Miscellaneous: Hepatitis (rare); lupus erythematosus and lymphadenopathies simulating malignant lymphoma; pruritus associated with lymphadenopathy and hepatosplenomegaly in hypersensitive individuals; changes in blood pressure.

Overdosage:

Symptoms: Nausea; drowsiness; dizziness; ataxia; visual disturbances. Coma may follow massive overdosage.

Treatment: Gastric evacuation by induced emesis, lavage or both, should be done immediately. General supportive care, including frequent monitoring of the vital signs is required. Refer to General Management of Acute Overdosage. Alkalinization of urine has increased the renal excretion of the active metabolite of both drugs. Monitor blood counts and hepatic and renal function following recovery.

Patient Information:

If GI upset occurs, may be taken with food.

Photosensitivity may occur. Avoid exposure to ultraviolet light or sunlight. Use sunscreen and protective clothing until tolerance is determined.

Do not discontinue abruptly or change dosage except on advice of physician.

Carry identification (Medic Alert) indicating medication usage and epilepsy.

Medication may cause sensitivity to bright light.

May cause drowsiness or blurred vision; observe caution while driving or performing other tasks requiring alertness, coordination or physical dexterity.

Notify physician if any of the following occur: Visual disturbances, excessive drowsiness or dizziness, sore throat, fever, skin rash, pregnancy, malaise, easy bruising, petechiae, epistaxis, or anything indicative of infection or bleeding tendency.

Administration and Dosage:

Adults: 900 mg to 2.4 g/day in 3 or 4 equally divided doses (300 to 600 mg 3 or 4 times daily). Initially, give 900 mg daily; increase this by 300 mg at weekly intervals until therapeutic results are seen or until toxic symptoms appear. Adjust maintenance dosage to the minimum required to maintain control.

Children: 300 to 900 mg/day in 3 or 4 equally divided doses.

TRIMETHADIONE

For complete prescribing information, refer to the Oxazolidinediones group monograph.

Rx	**Tridione** (Abbott)	**Dulcets (Tablets, chewable):** 150 mg	Sucrose. White. In 100s.
		Capsules: 300 mg	White. In 100s.

Benzodiazepines

CLONAZEPAM

For complete prescribing information, refer to the Benzodiazepine monograph in the Antianxiety Agents section.

Indications:

Used alone or as adjunctive treatment of the Lennox-Gastaut syndrome (petit mal variant), akinetic and myoclonic seizures. It may be useful in patients with absence (petit mal) seizures who have failed to respond to succinimides.

Up to 30% of patients have shown a loss of anticonvulsant activity, often within 3 months of administration; dosage adjustment may reestablish efficacy.

Unlabeled uses: Periodic leg movements during sleep (0.5 to 2 mg/night).
Parkinsonian (hypokinetic) dysarthria (0.25 to 0.5 mg/day).
Acute manic episodes of bipolar affective disorder (0.75 to 16 mg/day).
Multifocal tic disorders (1.5 to 12 mg/day).
Adjunct in the treatment of schizophrenia (0.5 to 2 mg/day).
Neuralgias (deafferentation pain syndromes; 2 to 4 mg/day).

Administration and Dosage:

Adults: Initial dose should not exceed 1.5 mg/day in 3 divided doses. Increase in increments of 0.5 to 1 mg every 3 days until seizures are adequately controlled or until side effects preclude any further increase. Individualize maintenance dosage. Maximum recommended dosage is 20 mg/day.

Infants and children (up to 10 years or 30 kg): To minimize drowsiness, the initial dose should be between 0.01 to 0.03 mg/kg/day, not to exceed 0.05 mg/kg/day, given in 2 or 3 divided doses. Increase dosage by not more than 0.25 to 0.5 mg every third day until a daily maintenance dose of 0.1 to 0.2 mg/kg has been reached, unless seizures are controlled or side effects preclude further increase. When possible, divide the daily dose into 3 equal doses. If doses are not equally divided, give the largest dose at bedtime.

Therapeutic serum concentrations of clonazepam are 20 to 80 ng/ml.

Multiple anticonvulsant use may result in an increase of depressant effects. Consider this before adding clonazepam to an existing anticonvulsant regimen.

c-IV	**Clonazepam** (Lemmon)	**Tablets:** 0.5 mg	In 100s.
c-IV	**Klonopin** (Roche)		(1/2 Klonopin/Roche). Lactose. Orange, scored. In 100s.
c-IV	**Clonazepam** (Lemmon)	1 mg	In 100s.
c-IV	**Klonopin** (Roche)		(1 Klonopin/Roche). Lactose. Blue, scored. In 100s.
c-IV	**Clonazepam** (Lemmon)	2 mg	In 100s.
c-IV	**Klonopin** (Roche)		(2 Klonopin/Roche). Lactose. White, scored. In 100s.

Benzodiazepines

CLORAZEPATE DIPOTASSIUM

For complete prescribing information, refer to the Benzodiazepine monograph in the Antianxiety Agents section.

Indications:

Partial seizures: As adjunctive therapy in the management of partial seizures.

Alcohol withdrawal: Symptomatic relief of anxiety and for the symptomatic relief of acute alcohol withdrawal (see monograph in the Antianxiety Agents section).

Administration and Dosage:

To minimize drowsiness, do not exceed recommended initial dosages and increments.

Adults and children (> 12 years): The maximum initial dose is 7.5 mg 3 times daily. Increase dosage by no more than 7.5 mg every week and do not exceed 90 mg/day.

Children: Maximum initial dose is 7.5 mg 2 times/day. Increase by ≤ 7.5 mg every week; do not exceed 60 mg/day. Not recommended in patients < 9 years old.

c-iv	**Clorazepate** (Various, eg, Barre-National, Geneva, Goldline, Major, Moore, Mylan, Parmed, Rugby, Schein)	**Tablets:** 3.75 mg	In 100s and 500s.
c-iv	**Gen-Xene** (Alra)		(Alra GX). Gray, scored. In 30s, 100s, 500s and UD 100s.
c-iv	**Tranxene-T** (Abbott)		(TL). Blue, scored. Six sided. In 100s, 500s and UD 100s.
c-iv	**Clorazepate** (Various, eg, Barre-National, Geneva, Goldline, Major, Moore, Mylan, Parmed, Rugby, Schein)	**Tablets:** 7.5 mg	In 100s and 500s.
c-iv	**Gen-Xene** (Alra)		(Alra GT). Yellow, scored. In 30s, 100s, 500s and UD 100s.
c-iv	**Tranxene-T** (Abbott)		(TM). Peach, scored. Six sided. In 100s, 500s and UD 100s.
c-iv	**Tranxene-SD** (Abbott)	**Tablets:** 11.25 mg	Lactose. Blue. In 100s.
c-iv	**Clorazepate** (Various, eg, Barre-National, Geneva, Goldline, Major, Moore, Mylan, Parmed, Rugby, Schein)	**Tablets:** 15 mg	In 100s and 500s.
c-iv	**Gen-Xene** (Alra)		(Alra GN). Green, scored. In 30s, 100s, 500s and UD 100s.
c-iv	**Tranxene-T** (Abbott)		(TN). Lavender, scored. Six sided. In 100s, 500s and UD 100s.
c-iv	**Tranxene-SD** (Abbott)	**Tablets:** 22.5 mg	Lactose. Tan. In 100s.

Benzodiazepines

DIAZEPAM

For complete prescribing information, refer to the Benzodiazepine monograph in the Antianxiety Agents section.

Indications:

Oral: May be used adjunctively in convulsive disorders; it is not proven useful as sole therapy. When used as an adjunct in convulsive disorders, the possibility of an increase in frequency or severity of grand mal seizure may require an increase in the dosage of standard anticonvulsant medication. Abrupt diazepam withdrawal in such cases may also be associated with a temporary increase in frequency or severity of seizures.

Parenteral: Adjunct in status epilepticus and severe recurrent convulsive seizures.

Diazepam is also used as a muscle relaxant (see individual monograph in the Skeletal Muscle Relaxants section), as an antianxiety agent and in acute alcohol withdrawal (see group monograph in Antianxiety Agents section).

Administration and Dosage:

Individualize dosage. Some patients may require higher doses than those given below. In such cases, increase dosage cautiously to avoid adverse effects. Use lower doses and slowly increase the dose in elderly or debilitated patients and when other sedative drugs are administered.

Oral (tablets, oral solution and Intensol): Adults – 2 to 10 mg 2 to 4 times daily.

Elederly or debilitated patients – 2 to 2.5 mg once or twice daily initially. Limit dosage to the smallest effective amount to preclude the development of ataxia or oversedation.

Children – Not for use in children < 6 months of age. Give 1 to 2.5 mg 3 or 4 times daily initially; increase gradually as needed and tolerated.

Oral, sustained release: Adults – 15 to 30 mg once daily.

Intensol preparation: Mix with liquid or semi-solid food such as water, juices, soda or soda-like beverages, applesauce and puddings. Consume the entire amount immediately. Do not store.

Parenteral: Although seizures may be brought under control promptly, a significant proportion of patients experience a return to seizure activity due to short-lived effect of IV diazepam. Be prepared to readminister. Not recommended for maintenance; once seizures are controlled, administer agents indicated for long-term seizure control.

Tonic status epilepticus has been precipitated in patients treated with IV diazepam for petit mal status or petit mal variant status.

Use extreme care in administering IV diazepam to the elderly, to very ill patients and to those with limited pulmonary reserve; apnea or cardiac arrest may occur.

To reduce possibility of venous thrombosis, phlebitis, swelling, local irritation and rarely, vascular impairment. Inject IV slowly (at least 1 min for each 5 mg). Do not use small veins (eg, dorsum of hand or wrist); avoid intra-arterial use and extravasation.

Do not mix or dilute with other solutions or drugs in syringe or infusion flask. If it is not feasible to administer directly IV, it may be injected slowly through the infusion tubing as close as possible to the vein insertion. Diazepam interacts with plastic containers and administration sets, significantly decreasing availability of drug delivered.

The IV route is preferred in the convulsing patient. However, if IV administration is impossible, the IM route may be used. Inject deeply. IM administration results in low or erratic plasma levels.

Adults – 5 to 10 mg initially. May be repeated at 10 to 15 minute intervals up to a maximum dose of 30 mg if necessary. Therapy may be repeated in 2 to 4 hours; however, residual active metabolites may persist. Exercise extreme caution in individuals with chronic lung disease or unstable cardiovascular status.

Children ≥ 5 years – 1 mg every 2 to 5 minutes up to a maximum of 10 mg. Repeat in 2 to 4 hours if necessary. EEG monitoring of the seizure may be helpful.

Infants > 30 days of age and children < 5 years – 0.2 to 0.5 mg slowly every 2 to 5 minutes up to a maximum of 5 mg.

Safety and efficacy of parenteral diazepam has not been established in the neonate (≤ 30 days of age). Prolonged CNS depression has been observed in neonates, apparently due to inability to biotransform diazepam into inactive metabolites. In pediatric use, give slowly over a 3 minute period at a dosage not to exceed 0.25 mg/kg. After an interval of 15 to 30 minutes, the initial dosage can be repeated. If relief of symptoms is not obtained after a third administration, other therapy is recommended. Have facilities for respiratory assistance readily available.

Benzodiazepines

DIAZEPAM

c-iv	**Diazepam** (Various, eg, Lederle, Mylan, Purepac, Rugby, Schein, Zenith-Goldline)	**Tablets:** 2 mg	In 100s, 500s and 1000s.
c-iv	**Valium** (Roche)		(Roche 2 Valium). White, scored. Round with cut out V. In 100s, 500s and UD 100s.
c-iv	**Diazepam** (Various, eg, Lederle, Mylan, Purepac, Rugby, Schein, Zenith-Goldline)	**Tablets:** 5 mg	In 100s, 500s and 1000s.
c-iv	**Valium** (Roche)		(Roche 5 Valium). Yellow, scored. Round with cut out V. In 100s, 500s and UD 100s.
c-iv	**Diazepam** (Various, eg, Lederle, Mylan, Purepac, Rugby, Schein, Zenith-Goldline)	**Tablets:** 10 mg	In 100s, 500s and 1000s.
c-iv	**Valium** (Roche)		(Roche 10 Valium). Blue, scored. Round with cut out V. In 100s, 500s and UD 100s.
c-iv	**Diazepam** (Roxane)	**Solution:** 1 mg/ml	Orange. Wintergreen-spice flavor. In 500 ml and UD 5 and 10 ml.
c-iv	**Diazepam Intensol** (Roxane)	**Solution (Intensol):** 5 mg/ml	In 30 ml w/dropper.
c-iv	**Diazepam** (Elkins-Sinn, Sanofi-Winthrop, Steris, Zenith-Goldline)	**Injection:** 5 mg/ml	In 2 ml amps, 1 and 2 ml cartridges, 1 and 2 ml syringes and 1, 2 and 10 ml vials.
c-iv	**Valium** (Roche)		In 40% propylene glycol and 10% ethyl alcohol with 5% sodium benzoate, benzoic acid and 1.5% benzyl alcohol. In 2 ml amps, 10 ml vials and 2 ml *Tel-E-Ject* disp. syringes.
c-iv	**Dizac** (Ohmeda)	**Injection, emulsified:** 5 mg/ml	Preservative free. In 3 ml single-dose vials.
🍁	**Valium Roche Oral** (Roche)	**Tablets:** 5 mg	Lactose. (ROCHE 5). Yellow. Cylindrical. In 100s and 1000s.
		10 mg	Lactose. (ROCHE 10). Light blue. Cylindrical. In 100s.
🍁	**Diazemuls** (Pharmacia & Upjohn)	**Injection, emulsified:** 5 mg/ml	Preservative free. In 2 ml ampules.

Miscellaneous

LAMOTRIGINE

Warning:

Severe, potentially life-threatening rashes have been reported in association with the use of lamotrigine. These reports, occurring in approximately one in every thousand adults, have included Stevens-Johnson syndrome (SJS) and, rarely, toxic epidermal necrolysis (TEN). Rare deaths have been reported, but their numbers are too few to permit a precise estimate of the rate.

The incidence of severe, potentially life-threatening rash in pediatric patients, however, is very much higher than that reported in adults; specifically, reports from clinical trials suggest as many as 1 in 50 to 1 in 100 pediatric patients develop a potentially life-threatening rash. It bears emphasis, accordingly, that lamotrigine is not approved for use in patients below the age of 16 (see Indications).

Other than age, no factors have been identified that are known to predict the risk of occurrence or the severity of rash associated with lamotrigine. It is suggested, yet to be proven, that the risk of rash may also be increased by 1) coadministration of lamotrigine with valproic acid (VPA), 2) exceeding the recommended initial dose of lamotrigine or 3) exceeding the recommended dose escalation for lamotrigine. However, cases have been reported in the absence of these factors.

Nearly all cases of life-threatening rashes associated with lamotrigine have occurred within 2 to 8 weeks of treatment initiation. However, isolated cases have been reported after prolonged treatment (eg, 6 months). Accordingly, duration of therapy cannot be relied upon as a means to predict the potential risk heralded by the first appearance of a rash.

Although benign rashes also occur with lamotrigine, it is not possible to predict reliably which rashes will prove to be life-threatening. Accordingly, discontinue lamotrigine at the first sign of rash, unless the rash is clearly not drug-related. Discontinuation of treatment may not prevent a rash from becoming life-threatening or permanently disabling or disfiguring.

Actions:

Pharmacology: Lamotrigine, an anti-epileptic drug (AED) of the phenyltriazine class, is chemically unrelated to existing AEDs. The precise mechanism(s) by which lamotrigine exerts its anticonvulsant action are unknown. In animals, lamotrigine prevented seizure spread in the maximum electroshock and pentylenetetrazol tests and prevented seizures in the visually and electrically evoked after-discharge tests for anti-epileptic activity. One proposed mechanism involves an effect on sodium channels. In vitro studies suggest that it inhibits voltage-sensitive sodium channels thereby stabilizing neuronal membranes and consequently modulating presynaptic transmitter release of excitatory amino acids (eg, glutamate, aspartate).

Lamotrigine has a weak inhibitory effect on the serotonin 5-HT_3 receptor. It does not exhibit high affinity binding to the following neurotransmitter receptors: Adenosine α_1 and α_2, adrenergic α_1, α_2 and β; dopamine D_1 and D_2; γ-aminobutyric acid (GABA) A and B; histamine H_1; kappa opioid; muscarinic acetylcholine; serotonin 5-HT_2. Studies have failed to detect an effect of lamotrigine on dihydropyridine-sensitive calcium channels. It had weak effects at sigma opioid receptors. It did not inhibit the uptake of norepinephrine, dopamine, serotonin or aspartic acid.

Lamotrigine binds to melanin-containing tissues (eg, eye, pigmented skin). It has been found in the uveal tract up to 52 weeks after a single dose in rodents.

In dogs, lamotrigine is extensively metabolized to a 2-N-methyl metabolite. This metabolite causes dose-dependent prolongations of the PR interval, widening of the QRS complex and, at higher doses, complete AV conduction block. Similar cardiovascular effects are not anticipated in humans because only trace amounts of the 2-N-methyl metabolite (< 0.6% of the dose) have been found in human urine. However, plasma concentrations of this metabolite could be increased in patients with a reduced capacity to glucuronidate lamotrigine (eg, liver disease).

In vitro, lamotrigine inhibits dihydrofolate reductase, the enzyme that catalyzes reduction of dihydrofolate to tetrahydrofolate. Inhibition of this enzyme may interfere with biosynthesis of nucleic acids and proteins. When lamotrigine was given to pregnant rats during organogenesis, fetal, placental and maternal folate concentrations were reduced. Significantly reduced concentrations of folate are associated with teratogenesis (see Pregnancy). Folate concentrations were reduced in male rats given repeated oral doses of lamotrigine. Reduced concentrations were partially returned to normal when supplemented with folinic acid.

Miscellaneous

LAMOTRIGINE

Pharmacokinetics:

Absorption/Distribution – Lamotrigine is rapidly and completely absorbed after oral administration with negligible first-pass metabolism (absolute bioavailability is 98%). The bioavailability is not affected by food. Peak plasma concentrations occur anywhere from 1.4 to 4.8 hours following drug administration and are dose-related. Lamotrigine is ≈ 55% bound to human plasma proteins.

Estimates of the mean apparent volume of distribution (Vd) of lamotrigine following oral administration ranged from 0.9 to 1.3 L/kg. Vd is independent of dose and is similar following single and multiple doses in patients with epilepsy and in healthy volunteers.

Metabolism/Excretion – Lamotrigine is metabolized predominantly by glucuronic acid conjugation; the major metabolite is an inactive 2-N-glucuronide conjugate. Lamotrigine was recovered in the urine (94%) and in the feces (2%). The urine contained unchanged lamotrigine (10%).

Following multiple administrations (150 mg twice a day) to healthy volunteers taking no other medications, lamotrigine induced its own metabolism resulting in a 25% decrease in half-life and a 37% increase in plasma clearance at steady state compared with values obtained in the same volunteers following a single dose. Evidence suggests that self-induction by lamotrigine may not occur when given as add-on therapy in patients receiving enzyme-inducing AEDs.

The clearance of lamotrigine is affected by the coadministration of anti-epileptic drugs. Lamotrigine is eliminated more rapidly in patients who have been taking hepatic enzyme-inducing anti-epileptic drugs. Valproic acid, however, actually decreases the clearance of lamotrigine (eg, more than doubles the elimination half-life of lamotrigine). If lamotrigine is administered to a patient receiving valproic acid, give lamotrigine at reduced dosage, less than half the dose used in patients not receiving valproic acid (see Drug Interactions and Administration and Dosage).

The apparent oral clearance of lamotrigine was 25% lower in noncaucasians than caucasians but was not affected by gender.

Renal function impairment: Twelve volunteers with chronic renal failure (mean creatinine clearance, 13 ml/min; range 6 to 23) and another six individuals undergoing hemodialysis were each given a single 100 mg dose of lamotrigine. The mean plasma half-lives determined in the study were 42.9 hours (chronic renal failure), 13 hours (during hemodialysis) and 57.4 hours (between hemodialysis) compared with 26.2 hours in healthy volunteers. On average, ≈ 20% (range, 5.6 to 35.1) of the amount present in the body was eliminated during a 4–hour hemodialysis session.

Miscellaneous

LAMOTRIGINE

Various Lamotrigine Pharmacokinetic Parameters: Adult Epilepsy Patients or Healthy Volunteers			
Population	Time of maximum plasma concentration (hrs)	Elimination half-life (hrs)	Plasma clearance (ml/min/kg)
Patients taking enzyme-inducing AEDs[1]:			
Single-dose lamotrigine (n = 24)	2.3	14.4	1.1
Multiple-dose lamotrigine (n = 17)	2	12.6	1.21
Patients taking enzyme-inducing AEDs + valproic acid:			
Single-dose lamotrigine (n = 25)	3.8	27.2	0.53
Patients taking valproic acid only:			
Single-dose lamotrigine (n = 4)	4.8	58.8	0.28
Healthy volunteers taking valproic acid:			
Single-dose lamotrigine (n = 6)	1.8	48.3	0.3
Multiple-dose lamotrigine (n = 18)	1.9	70.3	0.18
Healthy volunteers taking no other medications:			
Single-dose lamotrigine (n = 179)	2.2	32.8	0.44
Multiple-dose lamotrigine (n = 36)	1.7	25.4	0.58

[1] Examples of enzyme-inducing anti-epileptic drugs are carbamazepine, phenobarbital, phenytoin and primidone.

Clinical trials:

Concomitant AED therapy – In a trial consisting of a 24–week treatment period, patients (n = 216) could not be on more than two other anticonvulsants, and valproic acid was not allowed. Patients were randomized to receive placebo, a target dose of 300 mg/day lamotrigine or a target dose of 500 mg/day lamotrigine. The median reductions in the frequency of all partial seizures relative to baseline were 8% in patients receiving placebo, 20% in patients receiving 300 mg/day lamotrigine and 36% in patients receiving 500 mg/day lamotrigine. The seizure frequency reduction was statistically significant in the 500 mg/day group compared with the placebo group but not in the 300 mg/day group.

In a trial consisting of two 14–week treatment periods, patients (n = 98) could not be on more than two other anticonvulsants, and valproic acid was not allowed. The target dose of lamotrigine was 400 mg/day. When the first 12 weeks of treatment periods were analyzed, median change in seizure frequency was a 25% reduction on lamotrigine vs placebo.

A third study consisted of two 12-week treatment periods. Patients (n = 41) could not be on more than two other anticonvulsants. Thirteen patients were on concomitant valproic acid; these patients received 150 mg/day of lamotrigine. The 28 other patients had a target dose of 300 mg/day of lamotrigine. The median change in seizure frequency was a 26% reduction on lamotrigine compared with placebo.

Indications:

Epilepsy: Adjunctive therapy in the treatment of partial seizures in adults with epilepsy.

Unlabeled uses: Lamotrigine may be useful in adults with generalized tonic-clonic, absence, atypical absence and myoclonic seizures.

Lamotrigine may be beneficial in infants and children with Lennox-Gastaut syndrome.

Contraindications:

Hypersensitivity to the drug or its components.

Warnings:

Dermatologic: See Warning Box. Use caution, especially in pediatric patients.

Miscellaneous

LAMOTRIGINE

Approximately 10% of lamotrigine-exposed individuals develop a rash. However, not all cases of rash can be attributed to lamotrigine (5% of patients exposed to placebo developed a rash). Typically, rash occurs in the first 2 to 8 weeks of treatment initiation. The incidence of rash appears to be increased among patients being treated with a multi-drug regimen that includes valproate and enzyme-inducing AEDS. When valproate and lamotrigine are used as a two-drug combination, the incidence of rash is even higher.

Lamotrigine-associated rashes do not appear to have unique identifying features. Maculopapular or erythematous eruptions occur. Rarely, more serious rashes with systemic involvement occur. A benign initial appearance of a rash cannot predict an entirely benign outcome.

Prior to initiation of treatment, instruct patients that rash may occur, that it may herald a serious medical event and that, should it occur, it must be reported promptly to their physician. Promptly evaluate whether treatment withdrawal is necessary. If treatment continues in the face of rash, close monitoring is essential.

Serious rash leading to hospitalization – Rash resulting in hospitalization occurred in 0.3% of the ≈ 3400 subjects who participated in clinical trials. No fatalities occurred among these individuals, but rash has been associated with a fatal outcome in reports from post-marketing experience. Among the rashes leading to hospitalization were Stevens-Johnson syndrome, toxic epidermal necrolysis, angioedema and a rash associated with a number of the following systemic manifestations: Fever, lymphadenopathy, facial swelling, hematologic and hepatologic abnormalities.

There is evidence that the inclusion of valproate in a multi-drug regimen increases the risk of serious, potentially life-threatening rash. Specifically, of 584 patients administered lamotrigine with valproate in clinical trials, 1% were hospitalized in association with rash. In contrast, 0.16% of 2398 patients and volunteers given lamotrigine in the absence of valproate were hospitalized.

Pure red cell aplasia (PRCA): A case of PRCA was reported in a 32-year-old male with a history of beta-thalassemia. The patient had a microcytic anemia (hemoglobin 11 g/dl) that was stable while receiving carbamazepine but had become more severe in the 3 months after lamotrigine was added. A bone marrow aspirate revealed markedly decreased erythropoiesis but normal granulopoiesis and thrombopoiesis. Erythropoiesis resumed after discontinuation of lamotrigine and transfusions of packed red cells. Although PRCA is known to occur in patients with hemoglobinopathies, it is not known if beta-thalassemia is a specific risk factor for the development of PRCA.

Sudden unexplained death in epilepsy (SUDEP): During premarketing development, 20 sudden and unexplained deaths were recorded among 4700 patients with epilepsy (5747 patient-years of exposure). Some of these could represent seizure-related deaths in which the seizure was not observed (eg, at night). This represents an incidence of 0.0035 deaths per patient-year. Although this rate exceeds that expected in a healthy population matched for age and sex, it is within the range of estimates for the incidence of SUDEP in patients not receiving lamotrigine (ranging from 0.0005 for the general population of patients with epilepsy, to 0.004 for a recently studied clinical trial population similar to that in the clinical development program for lamotrigine, to 0.005 for patients with refractory epilepsy). Consequently, whether these figures are reassuring or suggest concern depends on the comparability of the populations and the accuracy of the estimates provided. Probably most reassuring is the similarity of estimated SUDEP rates in patients receiving lamotrigine and those receiving another anti-epileptic drug that underwent clinical testing in a similar population at about the same time. Importantly, that drug is chemically unrelated to lamotrigine. This evidence suggests, although it certainly does not prove, that the high SUDEP rates reflect population rates, not a drug effect.

Withdrawal seizures: As a rule, do not abruptly discontinue AEDs because of the possibility of increasing seizure frequency. Unless safety concerns require a more rapid withdrawal, taper the dose of lamotrigine over a period of at least 2 weeks (see Administration and Dosage).

Status epilepticus: Valid estimates of the incidence of treatment-emergent status epilepticus among lamotrigine-treated patients are difficult to obtain. At a minimum, 7 of 2343 adult patients had episodes that could unequivocally be described as status epilepticus. In addition, variably defined episodes of seizure exacerbation (eg, seizure clusters, seizure flurries) were reported.

Organ failure: Fatalities associated with multi-organ failure and various degrees of hepatic failure have been reported in five patients of 7000 exposed during premar-

Miscellaneous

LAMOTRIGINE

keting development. These cases occurred in association with other serious events (eg, status epilepticus, overwhelming sepsis) making it impossible to identify the initiating cause.

Renal/Hepatic function impairment: A study in patients with severe chronic renal failure (mean creatinine clearance, 13 ml/min) not receiving other AEDs indicated that the elimination half-life of unchanged lamotrigine is prolonged relative to individuals with normal renal function. Use with caution in these patients, generally using a reduced maintenance dose for patients with significant impairment.

Hepatic metabolism to the glucuronide followed by renal excretion is the principal route of elimination of lamotrigine. The use of lamotrigine in patients with impaired liver function may be associated with risks.

Elderly: The pharmacokinetics of lamotrigine in elderly volunteers were similar to those of young healthy volunteers.

Pregnancy: Category C. Maternal toxicity and secondary fetal toxicity were seen in mice and rats at doses up to 1.2 times the highest usual human maintenance dose (eg, 500 mg/day). Although lamotrigine was not found to be teratogenic, it decreases fetal folate concentrations in rats, an effect known to be associated with teratogenesis in animals and humans. There are no adequate and well controlled studies in pregnant women. Use during pregnancy only if the potential benefit justifies the potential risk to the fetus. Refer to Warnings in the Anticonvulsants introduction.

Pregnancy Exposure Registry – To monitor fetal outcomes of pregnant women exposed to lamotrigine, Glaxo Wellcome maintains a Lamotrigine Pregnancy Registry. Physicians can register patients by calling (888) 233-2334.

Lactation: Preliminary data indicate that lamotrigine passes into breast milk. Because the effects on the infant exposed to lamotrigine by this route are unknown, breastfeeding while taking lamotrigine is not recommended.

Children: Safety and efficacy in children < 16 years of age have not been established.

Precautions:

Monitoring: The value of monitoring plasma concentrations of lamotrigine has not been established. Because of the possible pharmacokinetic interactions between lamotrigine and other AEDs being taken concomitantly (see Drug Interactions), monitoring of the plasma levels of lamotrigine and concomitant AEDs may be indicated, particularly during dosage adjustments. In general, exercise clinical judgment regarding monitoring of plasma levels of lamotrigine and other AEDs.

Special risk patients: Caution is advised when using lamotrigine in patients with diseases or conditions that could affect metabolism or elimination of the drug, such as renal or hepatic function impairment (see Warnings) or cardiac function impairment.

Melanin-containing tissues: Because lamotrigine binds to melanin, it could accumulate in melanin-rich tissues over time. This raises the possibility that lamotrigine may cause toxicity in these tissues after extended use. Accordingly, although there are no specific recommendations for periodic ophthalmological monitoring, be aware of the possibility of long-term ophthalmologic effects.

Photosensitivity: Photosensitization (photoallergy or phototoxicity) may occur; therefore, caution patients to take protective measures against exposure to ultraviolet or sunlight (ie, sunscreens, protective clothing) until tolerance is determined.

Drug Interactions:

Lamotrigine Drug Interactions			
Precipitant drug	Object drug*		Description
Acetaminophen	Lamotrigine	⬇	Serum lamotrigine concentrations may be reduced, producing a decrease in therapeutic effects.
Carbamazepine	Lamotrigine	⬇	Lamotrigine concentration is decreased by ≈ 40%. Carbamazepine epoxide levels may be increased.
Lamotrigine	Carbamazepine	⬆	
Folate inhibitors	Lamotrigine	⬆	Lamotrigine is an inhibitor of dihydrofolate reductase. Be aware of this action when prescribing or dispensing other medications that inhibit folate metabolism.
Phenobarbital Primidone	Lamotrigine	⬇	Lamotrigine concentration is decreased by ≈ 40%.

Miscellaneous

LAMOTRIGINE

Lamotrigine Drug Interactions

Precipitant drug	Object drug*		Description
Phenytoin	Lamotrigine	↓	Lamotrigine concentration is decreased by 45% to 54%. Lamotrigine has no appreciable effect on steady-state phenytoin plasma concentration.
Lamotrigine	Phenytoin	↔	
Valproic acid	Lamotrigine	↑	Lamotrigine concentration is increased by 2-fold, and valproic acid concentration is decreased by 25%.
Lamotrigine	Valproic acid	↓	

* ↑ = Object drug increased. ↓ = Object drug decreased. ↔ = Undetermined effect.

Adverse Reactions:

The most commonly observed adverse experiences associated with the use of lamotrigine in combination with other anti-epileptic drugs were: Dizziness, diplopia, ataxia, blurred vision, nausea and vomiting (dose-related) and somnolence, headache and rash. Dizziness, diplopia, ataxia and blurred vision occurred more commonly in patients receiving carbamazepine with lamotrigine than in patients receiving other enzyme-inducing AEDs with lamotrigine. Clinical data suggest a higher incidence of rash, including serious rash, in patients receiving concomitant valproic acid than in patients not receiving valproic acid (see Warnings).

Approximately 10% of the 3501 individuals who received lamotrigine in premarketing clinical trials discontinued treatment because of an adverse experience. The adverse events most commonly associated with discontinuation were: Rash (4%), dizziness and headache (1.3%).

Miscellaneous

LAMOTRIGINE

Lamotrigine Adverse Reactions (%)

Adverse reaction	Lamotrigine (n = 711)	Placebo (n = 419)
Body as a whole		
Headache	29.1	19.1
Accidental injury	9.1	8.6
Flu syndrome	7	5.5
Fever	5.5	3.6
Abdominal pain	5.2	3.6
Infection	4.4	4.1
Neck pain	2.4	1.2
Malaise	2.3	1.9
Seizure exacerbation	2.3	0.5
Chills	1.3	0.5
Cardiovascular		
Hot flashes	1.3	0
Palpitations	1	0.5
GI		
Nausea	18.6	9.5
Vomiting	9.4	4.3
Diarrhea	6.3	4.1
Dyspepsia	5.3	2.1
Constipation	4.1	3.1
Tooth disorder	3.2	1.7
Anorexia	1.8	1.4
Dry mouth	1	0.2
Musculoskeletal		
Arthralgia	2	0.2
Joint disorder	1.3	1
Myasthenia	1.3	0
CNS		
Dizziness	38.4	13.4
Ataxia	21.7	5.5
Somnolence	14.2	6.9
Incoordination	6	2.1
Insomnia	5.6	1.9
Tremor	4.4	1.4
Depression	4.2	2.6

Adverse reaction	Lamotrigine (n = 711)	Placebo (n = 419)
Anxiety	3.8	2.6
Convulsion	3.2	1.2
Irritability	3	1.9
Speech disorder	2.5	0.2
Memory decreased	2.4	1.9
Confusion	1.8	1.7
Concentration disturbance	1.7	0.7
Sleep disorder	1.4	0.5
Emotional lability	1.3	0.2
Vertigo	1.1	0.2
Mind racing	1	0.5
Nystagmus	1	0.5
Dysarthria	1	0.2
Muscle spasm	1	0.2
Respiratory		
Rhinitis	13.6	9.3
Pharyngitis	9.8	8.8
Cough increased	7.5	5.7
Dyspnea	1.1	0.2
Dermatologic		
Rash	10	5
Pruritus	3.1	1.7
Alopecia	1.3	1.2
Acne	1.3	0.5
Special senses		
Diplopia	27.6	6.7
Blurred vision	15.5	4.5
Vision abnormality	3.4	1
Ear pain	1.8	1.7
Tinnitus	1.1	1
GU	(n = 365)	(n = 207)
Dysmenorrhea	6.6	6.3
Vaginitis	4.1	0.5
Amenorrhea	1.9	0.5

Other events that occurred in > 1% of patients, but equally or more frequently in the placebo group included: Asthenia; back pain; chest pain; flatulence; menstrual disorder; mylagia; paresthesia; respiratory disorder; urinary tract infection.

Other adverse reactions: Lamotrigine has been administered to 3501 individuals during all clinical trials, only some of which were placebo controlled. All reported events are included except those already listed in the previous table.

Body as a whole: Facial edema, halitosis (0.1% to 1%); abdomen enlarged, photosensitivity, suicide attempt (< 0.1%).

Cardiovascular: Flushing, migraine, syncope, tachycardia, vasodilation (0.1% to 1%); angina pectoris, atrial fibrillation, deep thrombophlebitis, hemorrhage, hypertension, myocardial infarction, postural hypotension (< 0.1%).

Dermatologic: Dry skin, eczema, erythema, hirsutism, maculopapular rash, sweating, urticaria (0.1% to 1%); angioedema, fungal dermatitis, herpes zoster, leukoderma, petechial rash, pustular rash, seborrhea, skin discoloration, Stevens-Johnson syndrome, vesiculobullous rash (< 0.1%).

GI: Dysphagia, gingivitis, gum hyperplasia, increased appetite, increased salivation, abnormal liver function tests, mouth ulceration, stomatitis, thirst (0.1% to 1%); eructation, gastritis, GI hemorrhage, glossitis, gum hemorrhage, hemorrhagic colitis, hepatitis, stomach ulcer, tongue edema (< 0.1%).

Endocrine: Goiter, hyperthyroidism (< 0.1%).

Miscellaneous

LAMOTRIGINE

Hematologic/Lymphatic: Anemia, ecchymosis, leukocytosis, leukopenia, lymphadenopathy, petechia (0.1% to 1%); allergic reactions, eosinophilia, fibrin decrease, iron deficiency anemia, thrombocytopenia (< 0.1%).

Metabolic/Nutritional: Weight gain (1%); alkaline phosphatase increase, peripheral edema, weight loss (0.1% to 1%); alcohol intolerance, hyperglycemia (< 0.1%).

Musculoskeletal: Twitching (0.1% to 1%); arthritis, bursitis, leg cramps, tendinous contracture, pathological fracture (< 0.1%).

CNS: Amnesia, nervousness, abnormal thinking (1%); abnormal dreams, abnormal gait, agitation, akathisia, aphasia, CNS depression, depersonalization, dyskinesia, dysphoria, euphoria, faintness, hallucinations, hostility, hyperkinesia, hypesthesia, myoclonus, panic attack, paranoid reaction, personality disorder, psychosis, stupor (0.1% to 1%); apathy, cerebrovascular accident, cerebellar syndrome, cerebral sinus thrombosis, choreoathetosis, CNS stimulation, delirium, delusions, dystonia, grand mal convulsions, hemiplegia, hyperalgesia, hyperesthesia, hypertonia, hypokinesia, hypomania, hypotonia, libido decreased/increased, manic depression reaction, movement disorder, neuralgia, neurosis, paralysis, suicidal ideation (< 0.1%).

Respiratory: Epistaxis, hyperventilation (0.1% to 1%); bronchospasm, hiccough, pneumonia (< 0.1%).

Special senses: Abnormality of accommodation, conjunctivitis, oscillopsia, photophobia, taste perversion (0.1% to 1%); deafness, dry eyes, lacrimation disorder, parosmia, ptosis, strabismus, taste loss (< 0.1%).

GU: Female lactation, hematuria, polyuria, urinary frequency/incontinence, vaginal moniliasis (0.1% to 1%); abnormal ejaculation, acute kidney failure, breast pain, breast abscess, cystitis, dysuria, breast neoplasm, creatinine increase, epididymitis, impotence, kidney pain, menorrhagia, urine abnormality, urinary retention (< 0.1%).

The following adverse experiences have been reported in patients receiving marketed lamotrigine in other countries and from worldwide non-controlled investigational use. A causal relationship is unknown: Aplastic anemia, apnea, disseminated intravascular coagulation, erythema multiforme, esophagitis, hematemesis, hemolytic anemia, hypersensitivity reaction, multi-organ failure, neutropenia, pancreatitis, pancytopenia and progressive immunosuppression.

Overdosage:

Symptoms: The highest known overdoses were in two women who each ingested doses > 4000 mg. The plasma concentration of lamotrigine in one woman was 52 mcg/ml 4 hours after ingestion (a value more than 10 times greater than that seen in clinical trials). She became comatose and remained comatose for 8 to 12 hours; no ECG abnormalities were detected. The other patient had dizziness, headache and somnolence. Both women recovered without sequelae.

Treatment: There are no specific antidotes for lamotrigine. Following a suspected overdose, hospitalization of the patient is advised. General supportive care is indicated, including frequent monitoring of vital signs and close observation of the patient. If indicated, induce emesis or perform gastric lavage. Observe usual precautions to protect the airway. Keep in mind that lamotrigine is rapidly absorbed. It is uncertain whether hemodialysis is an effective means of removing lamotrigine from the blood. In six renal failure patients, ≈ 20% of the amount of lamotrigine in the body was removed during 4 hours of hemodialysis.

Patient Information:

Advise patients to notify their physician immediately if they develop a skin rash or if they acutely develop any worsening of seizure control while taking lamotrigine.

Advise patients that lamotrigine may cause dizziness, somnolence and other symptoms and signs of CNS depression. Patients should observe caution while driving or performing other tasks requiring alertness, coordination or physical dexterity.

Advise patients to notify their physician if they become pregnant or intend to become pregnant during therapy, if they intend to breastfeed or are breastfeeding an infant.

Photosensitization (photoallergy or phototoxicity) may occur; therefore, caution patients to take protective measures against exposure to ultraviolet or sunlight (ie, sunscreens, protective clothing) until tolerance is determined.

Administration and Dosage:

Approved by the FDA December 27, 1994 (1P classification).

Adults (> 16 years of age): Recommended as add-on therapy in patients > 16 years of age. Safety and efficacy in patients < 16 years of age have not been established.

Miscellaneous

LAMOTRIGINE

Patients receiving enzyme-inducing AEDs but not valproate: The initial dose in patients not taking valproic acid is 50 mg once a day for 2 weeks, followed by 100 mg/day given in 2 divided doses for 2 weeks. Thereafter, the usual maintenance dose is 300 to 500 mg/day given in 2 divided doses (see table).

Patients receiving valproic acid as one component of a combination regimen also including enzyme-inducing AEDs: The initial dose is 25 mg every other day for 2 weeks, followed by 25 mg once a day for 2 weeks. Because the clearance of lamotrigine is decreased by ≈ 50% in the presence of valproate, the daily dose of lamotrigine should be ≤ 150 mg/day administered on a twice daily schedule (see table).

Lamotrigine Dose Recommendations (mg/day) for Adults (> 16 years of age)

Lamotrigine plus:	Weeks 1 and 2	Weeks 3 and 4	Usual maintenance dose
Enzyme-inducing AEDs and *no* valproic acid	50 mg (once a day)	100 mg (two divided doses)	300 to 500 mg/day (two divided doses). Escalate dose by 100 mg/day every week.
Enzyme-inducing AEDs *plus* valproic acid	25 mg (every other day)	25 mg (once a day)	100 to 150 mg/day (two divided doses). Escalate dose by 25 to 50 mg/day every 1 to 2 weeks.

In patients receiving multidrug regimens employing enzyme-inducing AEDs without valproic acid, maintenance doses of lamotrigine as high as 700 mg/day have been used. In patients receiving multidrug regimens using enzyme-inducing AEDs with valproic acid, maintenance doses of lamotrigine ≤ 200 mg/day have been used. The advantage of using doses above those recommended in the table above has not been established.

The efficacy of add-on lamotrigine in patients taking valproic acid alone has not been evaluated in controlled trials although it has been used in some patients. Consequently, an effective and safe dosing recommendation for the use of lamotrigine and valproic acid as a two-drug regimen cannot be offered. If this regimen is used, note that blood concentrations of lamotrigine appear to be twice those associated with the use of lamotrigine in a regimen containing enzyme-inducing AEDs and valproic acid.

Renal function impairment: Base initial doses on the patient's AED regimen (see above); reduced maintenance doses may be effective for patients with significant renal function impairment. Use with caution in these patients.

Discontinuation strategy: For patients receiving lamotrigine in combination with other AEDs, consider a reevaluation for all AEDs in the regimen if a change in seizure control or an appearance or worsening of adverse experiences is observed.

If a decision is made to discontinue therapy with lamotrigine, a stepwise reduction of dose over ≥ 2 weeks (≈ 50%/week) is recommended unless safety concerns require a more rapid withdrawal (see Precautions).

Discontinuing an enzyme-inducing AED should prolong the half-life of lamotrigine; discontinuing valproic acid should shorten the half-life of lamotrigine.

Target plasma levels: A therapeutic plasma concentration range has not been established for lamotrigine. Base dosing of lamotrigine on therapeutic response.

Rx	**Lamictal**[1] (Glaxo Wellcome)	**Tablets**: 25 mg	Lactose. (Lamictal 25). White, scored. Shield shape. In 100s.
		100 mg	Lactose. (Lamictal 100). Peach, scored. Shield shape. In 100s.
		150 mg	Lactose. (Lamictal 150). Cream, scored. Shield shape. In 60s.
		200 mg	Lactose. (Lamictal 200). Blue, scored. Shield shape. In 60s.

[1] Also available in Canada as Lamictal; strengths and package sizes may vary.

Miscellaneous

TOPIRAMATE

Actions:

Pharmacology: Topiramate is a sulfamate-substituted monosaccharide with a broad spectrum of anti-epileptic activity. The precise mechanism by which topiramate exerts its antiseizure effect is unknown; however, electrophysiological and biochemical studies of the effects of topiramate on cultured neurons have revealed three properties that may contribute to topiramate's anti-epileptic efficacy. First, action potentials elicited repetitively by a sustained depolarization of the neurons are blocked by topiramate in a time-dependent manner, suggestive of a state-dependent sodium channel blocking action. Second, topiramate increases the frequency at which γ-aminobutyrate (GABA) activates $GABA_A$ receptors and enhances the ability of GABA to induce a flux of chloride ions into neurons, suggesting that topiramate potentiates the activity of this inhibitory neurotransmitter. Third, topiramate antagonizes the ability of kainate to activate the kainate/AMPA (α-amino-3-hydroxy-5-methylisoxazole-4-propionic acid; non-NMDA) subtype of excitatory amino acid (glutamate) receptor but has no apparent effect on the activity of N-methyl-D-aspartate (NMDA) at the NMDA receptor subtype.

Topiramate inhibits some isoenzymes of carbonic anhydrase (CA-II; CA-IV). This pharmacologic effect is generally weaker than that of acetazolamide and is not thought to be a major contributing factor to topiramate's anti-epileptic activity.

Pharmacokinetics:

Absorption – Absorption of topiramate is rapid, with peak plasma concentrations occurring at ≈ 2 hours following a 400 mg oral dose. The relative bioavailability of topiramate from the tablet formulation is ≈ 80% compared with a solution. The bioavailability of topiramate is not affected by food.

Distribution – Pharmacokinetics of topiramate are linear with dose proportional increases in plasma concentration over dose range studies (200 to 800 mg/day). Mean plasma elimination half-life is 21 hours after single or multiple doses.

Steady-state is reached in ≈ 4 days in patients with normal renal function. Topiramate is 13% to 17% bound to human plasma proteins over the concentration range of 1 to 250 mcg/ml.

Metabolism/Excretion – Topiramate is not extensively metabolized and is primarily eliminated unchanged in the urine (≈ 70% of an administered dose). Six metabolites have been identified in humans, none of which constitutes > 5% of an administered dose. The metabolites are formed via hydroxylation, hydrolysis and glucuronidation. There is evidence of renal tubular reabsorption of topiramate. The mean plasma elimination half-life is 18.7 to 23 hours. Overall, plasma clearance is ≈ 20 to 30 ml/min following oral administration.

Special populations:

Hemodialysis – Topiramate is cleared by hemodialysis. Using a high efficiency, counterflow, single pass-dialysate hemodialysis procedure, topiramate dialysis clearance was 120 ml/min with blood flow through the dialyzer at 400 ml/min. This high clearance (compared with 20 to 30 ml/min total oral clearance in healthy adults) will remove a clinically significant amount of topiramate from the patient over the hemodialysis treatment period. Therefore, a dose adjustment may be required (see Dosage and Administration).

Renal function impairment – The clearance of topiramate was reduced by 42% in moderately renally-impaired subjects (creatinine clearance [Ccr] 30 to 69 ml/min/1.73 m^2) and by 54% in severely renally-impaired subjects (Ccr < 30 ml/min/1.73 m^2) compared with normal renal function subjects (Ccr > 70 ml/min/1.73 m^2). Because topiramate is presumed to undergo significant tubular reabsorption, it is uncertain whether this experience can be generalized to all situations of renal impairment. It is conceivable that some forms of renal disease could differentially affect glomerular filtration rate and tubular reabsorption resulting in a clearance of topiramate not predicted by Ccr. However, one-half the usual dose is recommended in patients with moderate or severe renal impairment.

Hepatic function impairment – In hepatically-impaired subjects, topiramate clearance may be decreased; the underlying mechanism is not well understood.

Children – Pharmacokinetics of topiramate were evaluated in patients 4 to 17 years of age receiving one or two other anti-epileptic drugs. Clearance was independent of dose. Although the relationship between age and clearance among patients of pediatric age has not been systematically evaluated, it appears that the weight adjusted clearance of topiramate is higher in pediatric patients than in adults.

Clinical trials: Following randomization, patients began the double-blind phase of treatment. Patients received active drug beginning at 100 mg/day; the dose was then increased weekly or every other week by increments of 100 or 200 mg/day until the

TOPIRAMATE

assigned dose was reached, unless intolerance prevented increases. After titration, patients entered an 8- or 12-week stabilization period.

In all add-on trials, the reduction in seizure rate from baseline during the entire double-blind phase was measured. Responder rate (fraction of patients with at least a 50% reduction) was also measured. The median percent reductions in seizure rates ranged from –20.6% to 11.6%, and the responder rates ranged from 0 to 18%.

Indications:

Partial onset seizures: Adjunctive therapy for partial onset seizure treatment in adults.

Contraindications:

A history of hypersensitivity to any component of this product.

Warnings:

Withdraw antiepileptic drugs, including topiramate, gradually to minimize the potential of increased seizure frequency.

CNS-related adverse events: Adverse events most often associated with the use of topiramate were CNS-related. The most significant of these can be classified into two general categories: 1) Psychomotor slowing, difficulty with concentration and speech or language problems, in particular, word-finding difficulties and 2) somnolence or fatigue. Additional nonspecific CNS effects occasionally observed with topiramate as add-on therapy include dizziness or imbalance, confusion, memory problems and exacerbation of mood disturbances (eg, irritability and depression).

Reports of psychomotor slowing, speech and language problems and difficulty with concentration and attention were common. Although in some cases these events were mild to moderate, they at times led to withdrawal from treatment. The incidence of psychomotor slowing is only marginally dose-related, but both language problems and difficulty with concentration or attention clearly increased in frequency with increasing dosage.

Somnolence and fatigue were the most frequently reported adverse events during clinical trials with topiramate. These events were generally mild to moderate and occurred early in therapy. While the incidence of somnolence does not appear to be dose-related, fatigue increases at dosages > 400 mg/day.

Renal function impairment: The major route of elimination of unchanged topiramate and its metabolites is via the kidney. Dosage adjustment may be required (see Dosage and Administration).

Hepatic function impairment: In hepatically-impaired patients, administer topiramate with caution because the clearance of topiramate may be decreased.

Carcinogenesis: An increase in urinary bladder tumors was observed in mice given topiramate (20, 75 and 300 mg/kg).

Elderly: In clinical trials, 2% of patients were > 60. No age-related difference in effectiveness or adverse effects were seen. There were no pharmacokinetic differences related to age alone, but consider age-associated renal function abnormalities.

Pregnancy: Category C. Topiramate has demonstrated selective developmental toxicity, including teratogenicity, in animal studies. There are no studies using topiramate in pregnant women. Use topiramate during prengancy only if the potential benefit outweighs the potential risk to the fetus.

Labor and delivery – The effect of topiramate on labor and delivery is unknown.

Lactation: Topiramate is excreted in the milk of lactating rats. It is not known if topiramate is excreted in breast milk. Weigh the potential benefit to the mother against the potential risk to the infant.

Children: Safety and effectiveness in children have not been established. Topiramate's pharmacokinetic profile was studied in patients 4 to 17 years of age.

Precautions:

Kidney stones: A total of 32/2086 (1.5%) patients exposed to topiramate during its development reported the occurrence of kidney stones; an incidence ≈ 2 to 4 times that expected in a similar, untreated population. As in the general population, the incidence of stone formation among topiramate-treated patients was higher in men.

An explanation for the association of topiramate and kidney stones may lie in the fact that topiramate is a weak carbonic anhydrase inhibitor. Carbonic anhydrase inhibitors (eg, acetazolamide or dichlorphenamide) promote stone formation by reducing urinary citrate excretion and by increasing urinary pH. The concomitant use of topiramate with other carbonic anhydrase inhibitors may create a physiological environment that increases the risk of kidney stone formation and should be avoided.

TOPIRAMATE

Increased fluid intake increases urinary output, lowering substance concentration involved in stone formation. Hydration is recommended to reduce new stone formation.

Paresthesia, an effect associated with the use of other carbonic anhydrase inhibitors, appears to be a common effect of topiramate.

Drug Interactions:

Topiramate has demonstrated inhibitory effect on the cytochrome $P4502C_{meph}$.

Antiepileptic Drug (AED) Interactions with Topiramate

AED Co-administered	AED concentration	Topiramate concentration
Phenytoin	NC* or 25% increase[1]	48% decrease
Carbamazepine (CBZ)	NC	40% decrease
CBZ epoxide[2]	NC	NE**
Valproic acid	11% decrease	14% decrease
Phenobarbital	NC	NE
Primidone	NC	NE

[1] Plasma concentration increased 25% in some patients, generally those on a twice daily dosing regimen of phenytoin.
[2] Is not administered but is an active metabolite of carbamazepine.
* NC = < 10% change in plasma concentration. ** NE = Not evaluated.

Topiramate Drug Interactions

Precipitant Drug	Object Drug*		Description
Topiramate	Alcohol; CNS depressants	↑	Use topiramate with extreme caution because of the potential to cause CNS depression, as well as other cognitive or neuropsychiatric adverse events.
Topiramate	Carbonic anhydrase inhibitors	↑	Concomitant use may increase the risk of renal stone formation and should be avoided (see Precautions).
Topiramate	Contraceptives, oral	↓	The mean total exposure to the estrogenic component decreased by 18%, 21% and 30% at daily doses of 200, 400 and 800 mg/day, respectively. Efficacy of oral contraceptives may be compromised.
Topiramate	Digoxin	↓	Serum digoxin AUC is decreased by 12% with concomitant topiramate administration. The clinical relevance of this observation has not been established.

* ↑ Object drug increased. ↓ Object drug increased.

Adverse Reactions:

Approximately 28% of epilepsy patients who received topiramate dosages of 200 to 1600 mg/day in clinical studies discontinued treatment because of the following: Psychomotor slowing (4.1%); difficulty with memory, fatigue (3.3%); confusion, somnolence (3.2%); difficulty with concentration/attention, anorexia (2.9%); depression, dizziness (2.6%); weight decrease (2.5%); nervousness, ataxia (2.2%); paresthesia, language problems (2%).

Topiramate Adverse Reactions (%)[1]

		Topiramate dosage (mg/day)	
Body system/Adverse event[2]	Placebo	200-400	600-1000
Body as a whole			
Asthenia	1.1	8	4.5
Back pain	4	6.2	2
Chest pain	2.3	4.4	2
Influenza-like symptoms	2.9	3.5	3.2
Leg pain	2.3	3.5	2.4
Hot flushes	1.7	2.7	0.8
Body odor	0	1.8	0
Edema	1.1	1.8	1.2
Rigors	0	1.8	0.4

Miscellaneous

TOPIRAMATE

Topiramate Adverse Reactions (%)[1]			
		Topiramate dosage (mg/day)	
Body system/Adverse event[2]	Placebo	200-400	600-1000
CNS			
Somnolence	10.3	30.1	25.9
Dizziness	14.4	28.3	32.4
Ataxia	6.9	21.2	17
Psychomotor slowing	2.3	16.8	25.1
Speech disorders/Related speech problems	2.9	16.8	13.8
Nervousness	7.5	15.9	20.6
Nystagmus	11.5	15	15
Paresthesia	3.4	15	14.6
Difficulty with memory	2.9	12.4	12.6
Tremor	6.3	10.6	13.8
Confusion	5.2	9.7	15
Difficulty with concentration/ attention	1.1	8	15.4
Depression	6.3	8	13.4
Language problems	0.6	6.2	11.7
Coordination abnormal	1.7	5.3	3.6
Agitation	1.7	4.4	4
Mood problems	1.7	3.5	10.1
Aggressive reaction	0.6	2.7	4
Hypoesthesia	1.1	2.7	0.8
Apathy	0	1.8	4.5
Emotional lability	1.1	1.8	2.4
Depersonalization	0.6	1.8	1.6
Dermatologic			
Rash	4	4.4	3.2
Pruritus	1.1	1.8	3.2
Sweating increased	0	1.8	0.4
GI			
Nausea	6.3	11.5	13.8
Dyspepsia	5.2	8	5.7
Anorexia	4	5.3	11.3
Abdominal pain	2.9	5.3	7.3
Constipation	0.6	5.3	3.2
Dry mouth	1.1	2.7	3.2
Gingivitis	0	1.8	0.4
GU			
Breast pain	0	8.3	0
Dysmenorrhea	2.6	8.3	0
Menstrual disorder	0	4.2	0
Hematuria	0.6	1.8	0.8
Respiratory			
Upper respiratory infection	11.5	12.4	12.1
Pharyngitis	2.9	7.1	2.8
Sinusitis	4	4.4	4
Dyspnea	1.1	1.8	3.2
Special Senses			
Diplopia	6.3	14.2	14.6
Vision abnormal	2.9	14.2	10.5
Eye pain	1.1	1.8	2

Miscellaneous

TOPIRAMATE

Topiramate Adverse Reactions (%)[1]			
		Topiramate dosage (mg/day)	
Body system/Adverse event[2]	Placebo	200-400	600-1000
Miscellaneous			
Weight decrease	2.3	7.1	12.6
Leukopenia	0.6	2.7	1.6
Hearing decreased	1.1	1.8	1.6
Myalgia	1.1	1.8	1.2
Epistaxis	1.1	1.8	0.8

[1] Patients in these add-on trials were receiving 1 to 2 concomitant antiepileptic drugs in addition to topiramate or placebo.
[2] See Warnings.

Incidence (%) of Dose-Related Adverse Events From Five Placebo Controlled, Add-On Trials				
	Placebo	Topiramate dosage (mg/day)		
Adverse event	(n = 174)	200 (n = 45)	400 (n = 68)	600-1000 (n = 247)
Fatigue	14.4	11.1	11.8	30.8
Nervousness	7.5	13.3	17.6	20.6
Difficulty with concentration/attention	1.1	6.7	8.8	15.4
Confusion	5.2	8.9	10.3	15
Depression	6.3	8.9	7.4	13.4
Anorexia	4	4.4	5.9	11.3
Language problems	0.6	2.2	8.8	11.7
Anxiety	5.2	2.2	2.9	9.3
Mood problems	1.7	0	5.9	10.1
Cognitive problems NOS	0.6	0	0	4
Weight decrease	2.3	4.4	8.8	12.6
Tremor	6.3	13.3	8.8	13.8

Other adverse events that occurred in > 1% of patients treated with 200 to 400 mg of topiramate in placebo controlled trials but with equal or greater frequency in the placebo group were: Fatigue, headache, injury, anxiety, rash, pain, aggravated convulsions, coughing, gastroenteritis, rhinitis, back pain, hot flushes, bronchitis, abnormal gait, involuntary muscle contractions and epistaxis.

Body as a whole: Fatigue, fever, malaise (≥ 1%); syncope, halitosis, enlarged abdomen (0.1% to 1%); alcohol intolerance, substernal chest pain, sudden death (< 0.1%).

Cardiovascular: Palpitation (≥ 1%); hypertension, hypotension, postural hypotension, AV block, bradycardia, bundle branch block, angina pectoris (0.1% to 1%); arrhythmia, atrial arrhythmia, atrial fibrillation (< 0.1%).

CNS: Hypokinesia, vertigo, stupor, grand mal convulsions, hyperkinesia, hypertonia, insomnia, personality disorder, impotence, hallucination, euphoria, psychosis, decreased libido, suicide attempt (≥ 1%); leg cramps, hyporeflexia, neuropathy, migraine, apraxia, hyperesthesia, dyskinesia, hyperreflexia, dysphonia, scotoma, ptosis, dystonia, visual field defect, coma, encephalopathy, fecal incontinence, upper-motor neuron lesion, paranoid reaction, delusion, paranoia, delirium, abnormal dreaming, neurosis (0.1% to 1%); cerebellar syndrome, abnormal EEG, tongue paralysis, increased libido, manic reaction (< 0.1%).

Dermatologic: Acne, alopecia (≥ 1%); dermatitis, nail disorder, folliculitis, dry skin, urticaria, skin discoloration, eczema, photosensitivity reaction, erythematous rash, seborrhea, decreased sweating, abnormal hair texture (0.1% to 1%); chloasma(< 0.1%).

GI: Diarrhea, vomiting, flatulence, gastroenteritis (≥ 1%); gum hyperplasia, hemorrhoids, increased appetite, tooth caries, stomatitis, dysphagia, melena, gastritis, saliva increased, hiccough, gastroesophageal reflux, tongue edema, esophagitis (0.1% to 1%); eructation (< 0.1%).

GU: Intermenstrual bleeding, leukorrhea, menorrhagia, vaginitis, amenorrhea, urinary tract infection, micturition frequency, urinary incontinence, dysuria, renal calculus (≥ 1%); ejaculation disorder, breast discharge, urinary retention, facial edema, renal pain, nocturia, albuminuria, polyuria, oliguria (0.1% to 1%).

Hematologic: Anemia (≥ 1%); lymphadenopathy, eosinophilia, lymphopenia, granulocytopenia, lymphocytosis (0.1% to 1%); marrow depression, pancytopenia (< 0.1%).

Miscellaneous

TOPIRAMATE

Hepatic: ALT increased, AST increased, gall bladder disorder (0.1% to 1%); gamma-GT increased (< 0.1%).

Metabolic/Nutritional: Weight increase (≥ 1%); thirst, hypokalemia, increased alkaline phosphatase, dehydration, hypocalcemia, hyperlipemia, acidosis, hyperglycemia, creatinine increased, hyperchloremia, xerophthalmia (0.1% to 1%); diabetes mellitus, hypernatremia, abnormal serum folate, hyponatremia, hypocholesterolemia, hypoglycemia, hypophosphatemia (< 0.1%).

Musculoskeletal: Arthralgia, muscle weakness (≥ 1%); arthrosis, osteoporosis (≤ 1%).

Respiratory: Coughing, bronchitis (≥ 1%); asthma, bronchospasm (0.1% to 1%); laryngismus (< 0.1%).

Special senses: Taste perversion, tinnitus, conjunctivitis (≥ 1%); taste loss, parosmia, abnormal accommodation, photophobia, abnormal lacrimation, strabismus, color blindness, myopia, mydriasis (0.1% to 1%); earache, hyperacusis, cataract, corneal opacity, iritis (< 0.1%).

Miscellaneous: Vasodilation, goiter, basal cell carcinoma, thrombocythemia, gingival bleeding, purpura, thrombocytopenia, pulmonary embolism, flushing, DVT (0.1% to 1%); thyroid disorder, polycythemia, vasospasm, phlebitis (< 0.1%)

Overdosage:

In acute topiramate overdose, if the ingestion is recent, empty the stomach immediately by lavage or by induction of emesis. Activated charcoal has not been shown to adsorb topiramate in vitro. Therefore, its use in overdosage is not recommended. Treatment should be appropriately supportive. Hemodialysis is an effective means of removing topiramate from the body. However, in the few cases of acute overdosage reported, hemodialysis has not been necessary.

Patient Information:

Instruct patients, particularly those with predisposing factors, to maintain an adequate fluid intake in order to minimize the risk of renal stone formation.

Warn patients about the potential for somnolence, dizziness, confusion and difficulty concentrating; and advise them not to drive or operate machinery until they have gained sufficient experience with topiramate to gauge whether it adversely affects their mental or motor performance.

Administration and Dosage:

Approved December 24, 1996.

The recommended total daily dose of topiramate as adjunctive therapy is 400 mg/day in 2 divided doses. Effects of 200 mg/day are inconsistent and less effective than 400 mg/day. Initiate therapy at 50 mg/day followed by titration to an effective dose. Doses > 400 mg/day (600, 800 and 1000 mg/day) have not been shown to improve responses. Doses > 1600 mg/day have not been studied.

Recommended Titration Rate for Topiramate

Week	AM dose (mg)	PM dose (mg)
1	none	50
2	50	50
3	50	100
4	100	100
5	100	150
6	150	150
7	150	200
8	200	200

It is not necessary to monitor topiramate plasma concentrations to optimize topiramate therapy. On occasion, the addition of topiramate to phenytoin may require an adjustment of the dose of phenytoin to achieve optimal clinical outcome. The addition or withdrawal of phenytoin or carbamazepine during adjunctive therapy with topiramate may require adjustment of the dose of topiramate.

Because of the bitter taste, do not break tablets.

Topiramate can be taken without regard to meals.

Renal function impairment: In renally impaired subjects (creatinine clearance < 70 ml/min/1.73 m^2), one half of the usual adult dose is recommended. Such patients will require a longer time to reach steady-state at each dose.

Hemodialysis: Topiramate is cleared by hemodialysis 4 to 6 times faster than a normal individual; a prolonged period of dialysis may cause topiramate levels to fall

Miscellaneous

TOPIRAMATE

below that required to maintain an anti-seizure effect. To avoid rapid drops in topiramate plasma concentration during hemodialysis, a supplemental dose of topiramate may be required. The actual adjustment should take into account 1) the duration of the dialysis period, 2) the clearance rate of the dialysis system being used and 3) the effective renal clearance of topiramate in the patient being dialyzed.

Rx	**Topamax** (Ortho-McNeil)	**Tablets**: 25 mg	(TOP 25). White, coated. In 60s.
		100 mg	(TOPAMAX 100). Yellow, coated. In 60s.
		200 mg	(TOPAMAX 200). Salmon, coated. In 60s.

Miscellaneous

PRIMIDONE

Actions:

Pharmacology: Primidone raises electroshock or chemoshock seizure thresholds or alters seizure patterns in animals. Mechanism of antiepileptic action is unknown.

Primidone and its two metabolites, phenobarbital and phenylethylmalonamide (PEMA), have anticonvulsant activity. In addition, PEMA potentiates the activity of phenobarbital in animals.

Pharmacokinetics:

Absorption/Distribution – Primidone is readily absorbed from the GI tract. Peak serum concentrations occur in 3 hours (range, 0.5 to 9 hrs) after the initial oral dose and later with continuous use. Peak serum concentrations of PEMA occur after 7 to 8 hours. Phenobarbital appears in plasma after several days of continuous therapy. Protein binding of primidone and PEMA is negligible; phenobarbital is ≈ 50% protein bound. Monitoring of primidone therapy should include plasma level determinations of primidone and phenobarbital. Therapeutic plasma concentrations are 5 to 12 mcg/ml for primidone and 15 to 40 mcg/ml for phenobarbital.

Metabolism/Excretion – PEMA is the major metabolite and is less active than primidone. Phenobarbital formation ranges from 15% to 25%. The plasma half-life of primidone is 5 to 15 hours. PEMA and phenobarbital have longer half-lives (10 to 18 hrs and 53 to 140 hrs, respectively) and accumulate with chronic use. About 40% of primidone is excreted unchanged in the urine. The remainder of the drug is excreted as unconjugated PEMA and as phenobarbital and its metabolites.

For further information, refer to the Barbiturates monograph.

Indications:

Epilepsy: For control of grand mal, psychomotor or focal epileptic seizures, either alone or with other anticonvulsants. It may control grand mal seizures refractory to other anticonvulsants.

Unlabeled uses: Benign familial tremor (essential tremor, 750 mg/day).

Contraindications:

Porphyria; hypersensitivity to phenobarbital.

Warnings:

Status epilepticus: Abrupt withdrawal of antiepileptic medication may precipitate *status epilepticus.*

Therapeutic efficacy of a dosage regimen takes several weeks to assess.

Pregnancy: The effects of primidone in pregnancy is unknown (see Warnings in the Anticonvulsants introduction).

Lactation: Primidone appears in breast milk in substantial quantities. It is suggested that undue somnolence and drowsiness in nursing newborns of primidone-treated mothers be taken as an indication to discontinue nursing.

Precautions:

Monitoring: Because therapy generally extends over prolonged periods, perform complete blood counts and a sequential multiple analysis test every 6 months.

Hazardous tasks: Patients should use caution while driving or performing other tasks requiring alertness, coordination or physical dexterity.

Drug Interactions:

Primidone Drug Interactions

Precipitant drug	Object drug*		Description
Acetazolamide	Primidone	⬇	Coadministration may decrease primidone concentrations.
Carbamazepine	Primidone	⬇	Coadministration may result in lower primidone and phenobarbital concentrations and higher carbamazepine concentrations.
Primidone	Carbamazepine	⬆	
Hydantoins	Primidone	⬆	Primidone, phenobarbital and PEMA concentrations may be increased.
Isoniazid	Primidone	⬆	Primidone concentrations may be increased.
Nicotinamide	Primidone	⬆	The clearance rate of primidone may be decreased.
Succinimides	Primidone	⬇	Coadministration may result in lower primidone and phenobarbital concentrations.

* ⬆ = Object drug increased ⬇ = Object drug decreased

Miscellaneous

PRIMIDONE

Adverse Reactions:

CNS: Ataxia and vertigo (these tend to disappear with continued therapy or with reduction of initial dosage); fatigue; hyperirritability; emotional disturbances; diplopia; nystagmus; drowsiness; personality deterioration with mood changes and paranoia.

GI: Nausea; anorexia; vomiting.

Hematologic: Megaloblastic anemia may occur as a rare idiosyncrasy and responds to folic acid without necessity of discontinuing medication. Thrombocytopenia has also occurred.

Miscellaneous: Impotence; morbilliform and maculopapular skin eruptions. Eight cases of crystalluria have been reported following primidone overdose.

Patient Information:

Drowsiness, dizziness or muscular incoordination may occur initially, but these symptoms usually disappear with continued therapy. Observe caution while driving or performing other tasks requiring alertness, coordination or physical dexterity.

If GI upset occurs, take with food.

Do not discontinue medication abruptly or change dosage, except on advice of physician.

Notify physician if skin rash or fever occurs or if patient becomes pregnant.

Patients should carry identification (Medic Alert) indicating medication usage and epilepsy.

Oral suspension: Shake well before using.

Administration and Dosage:

Individualize dosage.

Adults and children (> 8 years of age): Patients who have received no previous treatment may be started on primidone according to the following regimen:

Days 1 to 3 – 100 to 125 mg at bedtime.
Days 4 to 6 – 100 to 125 mg twice daily.
Days 7 to 9 – 100 to 125 mg 3 times daily.
Day 10 – maintenance – 250 mg 3 to 4 times daily. If required, increase dose to 250 mg 5 to 6 times daily, but do not exceed doses of 500 mg 4 times daily (2 g/day).

Children (< 8 years): The following regimen may be used to initiate therapy:

Days 1 to 3 – 50 mg at bedtime.
Days 4 to 6 – 50 mg twice daily.
Days 7 to 9 – 100 mg twice daily.
Day 10 – maintenance – 125 to 250 mg 3 times daily, or 10 to 25 mg/kg/day in divided doses.

Patients already receiving other anticonvulsants: Start primidone at 100 to 125 mg at bedtime and gradually increase to maintenance level as the other drug is gradually decreased. Continue this regimen until satisfactory dosage level is achieved for the combination or the other drug is completely withdrawn. When therapy with primidone alone is the objective, the transition should not be completed in < 2 weeks.

Bioequivalence problems have been documented for primidone products marketed by different manufacturers. Brand interchange is not recommended unless comparative bioavailability data are available.

Rx	**Mysoline** (Wyeth-Ayerst)	**Tablets:** 50 mg	Lactose. (Mysoline 50). White, scored. Square. In 100s and 500s.
Rx	**Primidone** (Various, eg, Goldline, Major, Moore, Rugby, Schein, URL)	**Tablets:** 250 mg	In 100s, 500s, 1000s and UD 100s.
Rx	**Mysoline** (Wyeth-Ayerst)		Lactose. (Mysoline 250). Yellow, scored. Square. In 100s, 1000s and UD 100s.
Rx	**Mysoline** (Wyeth-Ayerst)	**Oral Suspension:** 250 mg per 5 ml	Saccharin. In 240 ml.

Miscellaneous

VALPROIC ACID and DERIVATIVES

This group includes valproic acid, sodium valproate (the sodium salt) and divalproex sodium, a stable coordination compound containing equal proportions of valproic acid and sodium valproate. Regardless of form, dosage is expressed as valproic acid equivalents.

Warning:

Hepatic failure resulting in fatalities has occurred in patients receiving valproic acid and its derivatives. Children < 2 years of age are at a considerably increased risk of developing fatal hepatotoxicity, especially those on multiple anticonvulsants, those with congenital metabolic disorders, those with severe seizure disorders accompanied by mental retardation and those with organic brain disease. In this patient group, use with extreme caution and as a sole agent. Weigh benefits of seizure control against risks. Above this age group, the incidence of fatal hepatotoxicity decreases considerably in progressively older patient groups. These incidents usually have occurred during the first 6 months of treatment. Serious or fatal hepatotoxicity may be preceded by nonspecific symptoms such as loss of seizure control, malaise, weakness, lethargy, facial edema, anorexia, jaundice and vomiting. Monitor patients closely for appearance of these symptoms. Perform liver function tests prior to therapy and at frequent intervals thereafter, especially during the first 6 months; however, serum biochemistry tests may not be abnormal. Also perform a careful interim medical history and physical examination.

Actions:

Pharmacology: Valproic acid is chemically unrelated to other drugs used to treat seizure disorders. Although the mechanism of action is not established, its activity may be related to increased brain levels of gamma-aminobutyric acid (GABA). This may also account for its prolactin-lowering effects. Valproate may also inhibit an enzyme responsible for the catabolism of GABA, potentiate postsynaptic GABA responses, affect the potassium channel or have a direct membrane-stabilizing effect.

Pharmacokinetics:

Absorption – Valproic acid is rapidly absorbed orally. Absorption of enteric coated divalproex is delayed 1 hour; thereafter, the enteric coated form is uniformly and reliably absorbed. Peak serum levels occur ≈ 1 to 4 hours after a single oral dose. Absorption is more rapid from the syrup (sodium valproate), with peak levels reached in 15 minutes to 2 hours. A slight delay in absorption occurs when administered with meals, but this does not affect the bioavailability. Peak levels after IV administration of valproate sodium occur at the end of the 1 hour infusion. Because the kinetics of unbound valproate are linear, bioequivalence between IV valproate sodium and oral divalproex sodium up to the maximum recommended dose of 60 mg/kg/day can be assumed.

Equivalent doses of intravenous and oral products deliver equivalent quantities of valproate ion systemically. Although the rate of valproate ion absorption may vary with the formulation administered, conditions of use and the method of administration, these differences should be of minor clinical importance under the steady state conditions achieved in chronic use in the treatment of epilepsy. Whether or not rate of absorption influences the efficacy of valproate as an antimanic agent is unknown.

Distribution – Valproate is rapidly distributed and is highly bound (90%) to plasma proteins, primarily albumin. Increases in dose may decrease protein binding. Significantly reduced plasma protein binding has occurred in renal insufficiency, cirrhosis and acute viral hepatitis. Although optimum serum levels have not been clearly defined, a therapeutic range of 50 to 100 mcg/ml is suggested. Valproate concentrates in fetal cord blood with a cord-blood:maternal-plasma ratio of total valproate (bound and unbound) of 1.4 to 2.4. CSF levels are approximately equal to the concentration of free drug in the blood (≈ 10% of total concentration).

Metabolism/Excretion – Primarily metabolized in liver and excreted as glucuronide. Elimination of valproate and its metabolites occurs principally in urine. Very little unmetabolized drug is excreted in urine and feces.

Mean plasma clearance for total valproate is 0.56 L/hr/1.73 m^2; volume of distribution is 11 L/1.73 m^2. The serum half-life is in the range of 6 to 16 hours. Half-lives in the lower part of the range are usually found in patients taking other antiepileptic drugs; concomitant primidone, phenytoin, phenobarbital or carbamazepine decreases half-life to an average of 9 hours. Half-life in children < 10 days of age ranges from 10 to 67 hours compared with a range of 7 to 13 hours in children > 2 months and up to 18 hours in patients with cirrhosis or acute hepatitis.

Miscellaneous

VALPROIC ACID and DERIVATIVES

Indications:

Epilepsy: For use as sole and adjunctive therapy in the treatment of simple and complex absence seizures and adjunctively in patients with multiple seizure types that include absence seizures; as monotherapy and adjunctive therapy in the treatment of patients with complex partial seizures that occur either in isolation or in association with other types of seizures (divalproex sodium, valproate sodium injection).

Valproate sodium injection is indicated as an intravenous alternative in patients for whom oral administration of valproate products is temporarily not feasible.

Mania (divalproex sodium delayed release tablets): Manic episodes associated with bipolar disorder.

Migraine (divalproex sodium delayed release tablets): As prophylaxis of migraine headaches.

Unlabeled uses: May be effective alone or in combination in the treatment of atypical absence, myoclonic and grand mal seizures, and possibly effective against atonic, elementary partial and infantile spasm seizures. It may also be effective in patients with intractable status epilepticus who have not responded to other therapies (adults: 200 to 1200 mg every 6 hours rectally with phenytoin and phenobarbital; children: 15 to 20 mg/kg). To prevent recurrent febrile seizures in children; minor incontinence after ileoanal anastomosis (subchronic administration); management of anxiety disorders/panic attacks.

Contraindications:

Hepatic disease/dysfunction (see Warnings); hypersensitivity to valproic acid.

Warnings:

Acute head injuries: A study evaluating the effect of IV valproate in the prevention of post-traumatic seizures in patients with acute head injuries found a higher incidence of death in valproate treatment groups compared to the IV phenytoin treatment group (13% vs 8.5%, respectively). Until further information is available, it seems prudent not to use valproate sodium injection in patients with acute head trauma for the prophylaxis of post-traumatic seizures.

Hepatotoxicity: See Warning Box. Use caution in patients who have a history of hepatic disease.

Discontinue immediately in the presence of significant hepatic dysfunction, suspected or apparent. In some cases, hepatic dysfunction has progressed in spite of drug discontinuation. The frequency of adverse effects (particularly elevated liver enzymes and thrombocytopenia) may be dose-related.

Long-term use: Safety and effectiveness for long-term use in mania (> 3 weeks) have not been systematically evaluated in clinical trials. Continually re-evaluate the drug's usefulness if used for extended periods.

Discontinuation: Do not abruptly discontinue in patients in whom the drug is administered to prevent major seizures because of the strong possibility of precipitating status epilepticus with attendant hypoxia and threat to life.

Carcinogenesis: Increased incidences of subcutaneous fibrosarcomas and benign pulmonary adenomas have occurred in male rodents given up to 3 times the human dose for 2 years. The significance of these findings for humans is unknown.

Fertility impairment: Chronic toxicity studies in animals demonstrated reduced spermatogenesis and testicular atrophy.

Elderly: A reduced starting dose will be required (see Administration and Dosage).

Pregnancy: Category D. The incidence of neural tube defects in the fetus may be increased in mothers receiving valproic acid during the first trimester. The CDC estimates the risk of valproic acid-exposed women having children with spina bifida to be ≈ 1% to 2%. This risk is similar to that for nonepileptic women who have had children with neural tube defects (anencephaly and spina bifida).

Administer antiepileptic drugs to women of child-bearing potential only if they are clearly shown to be essential in the management of their seizures; even minor seizures may pose some hazard to the developing embryo or fetus. Do not abruptly discontinue antiepileptic drugs administered to prevent major seizures because of the strong possibility of precipitating status epilepticus with attendant hypoxia and threat to life.

Lactation: Concentrations of valproic acid in breast milk are 1% to 10% of serum concentrations. It is not known what effect this would have on a nursing infant. Exercise caution when administering to a nursing woman.

Children: See Warning Box. The safety and efficacy of divalproex sodium for the treatment of acute mania has not been studied in individuals < 18 years of age.

Miscellaneous

VALPROIC ACID and DERIVATIVES

Migraine – The safety and effectiveness of divalproex sodium for the prophylaxis of migraines has not been studied in individuals < 16 years of age.

Precautions:

Hematologic effects: Thrombocytopenia, inhibition of the secondary phase of platelet aggregation and abnormal coagulation parameters have occurred. The probability of thrombocytopenia increases significantly at total trough valporate plasma concentrations > 110 mcg/ml in females and 135 mcg/ml in males. Determine platelet counts and bleeding time before initiating therapy, at periodic intervals and prior to surgery. Hemorrhage, bruising or a hemostasis/coagulation disorder is an indication for reduction of dosage or withdrawal of therapy.

Hyperammonemia, with or without lethargy or coma, may occur in the absence of abnormal liver function tests. If elevation occurs, discontinue the drug. Valproate increased renal ammonium production and inhibited urea synthesis in several patients. Combined effect of these two actions may contribute to hepatotoxicity. Asymptomatic elevations of ammonia are more common and, when present, require more frequent monitoring; consider discontinuation of therapy.

Suicidal ideation may be a manifestation of certain psychiatric disorders and may persist until a significant remission of symptoms occurs. Closely supervise high-risk patients during initial drug therapy.

Hazardous tasks: Patients should use caution while driving or performing other tasks requiring alertness, coordination or physical dexterity.

Drug Interactions:

Valproic Acid Drug Interactions

Precipitant drug	Object drug *		Description
Charcoal	Valproic acid	↓	Valproic acid absorption is decreased.
Chlorpromazine	Valproic acid	↑	Valproate $t_{1/2}$ and trough levels may increase, clearance may decrease.
Cimetidine	Valproic acid	↑	Small but potentially significant decrease in valproate clearance and increase in $t_{1/2}$.
Erythromycin	Valproic acid	↑	Erythromycin may increase serum valproic acid concentrations, producing valproic acid toxicity.
Felbamate	Valproic acid	↑	Coadministration revealed a 35% increase in mean peak valproate levels.
Rifampin	Valproic acid	↓	In one study, rifampin increased the oral clearance of valproate by 40%.
Salicylates (eg, aspirin)	Valproic acid	↑	In pediatric patients, protein binding and metabolism of valproate decreased; valproate free fraction was increased. Use caution if coadministered.
Valproic acid	Carbamazepine	↑	Variable changes in carbamazepine concentrations with increased levels of the active metabolite or decreased valproic acid levels with possible loss of seizure control may occur.
Carbamazepine	Valproic acid	↓	
Valproic acid	Clonazepam	↔	Concomitant use may induce absence status in patients with a history of absence type seizures.
Valproic acid	CNS depressants	↑	Concurrent use may result in an increase in CNS effects, with or without increased plasma levels of the object drug.
Valproic acid	Diazepam	↑	Valproate displaces diazepam from its plasma albumin binding sites and inhibits its metabolism.
Valproic acid	Ethosuximide	↑	Valproate inhibits ethosuximide metabolism; monitor plasma levels of both drugs, especially in the presence of other anticonvulsants.
Valproic acid	Lamotrigine	↑	Valproic acid serum levels may be decreased while lamotrigine levels may be increased. Reduce lamotrigine dosage.
Lamotrigine	Valproic acid	↓	
Valproic acid	Phenobarbital	↑	Valproate inhibits phenobarital metabolism; phenobarbital can increase valproate clearance.
Phenobarbital	Valproic acid	↓	

Miscellaneous

VALPROIC ACID and DERIVATIVES

Valproic Acid Drug Interactions			
Precipitant drug	Object drug *		Description
Valproic acid	Phenytoin	↑	Increased action of phenytoin, even at therapeutic levels, or increased metabolism of valproic acid with decreased pharmacologic effects may occur.
Phenytoin	Valproic acid	↓	
Valproic acid	Tolbutamide	↔	The unbound fraction of tolbutamide may be increased from 20% to 50%. The clinical relevance of this displacement is unknown.
Valproic acid	Warfarin	↑	The potential exists for valproate to displace warfarin from protein binding sites. Monitor coagulation tests.
Valproic acid	Zidovudine	↑	Zidovudine clearance was decreased in HIV seropositive patients.

* ↑ = Object drug increased. ↓ = Object drug decreased. ↔ = Undetermined effect.

Drug/Lab test interactions: Valproic acid is partially eliminated in the urine as a keto-metabolite which may lead to a false interpretation of the **urine ketone test**. There have been reports of altered **thyroid function tests** associated with valproic acid. The clinical significance is unknown.

Drug/Food interactions: A slight delay in the absorption of valproic acid may occur when administered with meals, but this does not affect the bioavailability.

Adverse Reactions:

Epilepsy:

GI – Nausea; vomiting; indigestion; diarrhea; abdominal cramps; constipation; anorexia with weight loss; increased appetite with weight gain. Use of delayed release divalproex sodium may reduce GI side effects in some patients.

CNS – Sedation has occurred (alone and in combination) and usually disappears upon reduction of other anticonvulsant medication. Tremor (may be dose-related); hallucinations; ataxia; headache; nystagmus; diplopia; asterixis; "spots before eyes"; dysarthria; dizziness; confusion; hypesthesia; vertigo; incoordination; coma (rare, alone or in conjunction with phenobarbital); encephalopathy with fever (rare, developed shortly after introduction of valproate monotherapy without evidence of hepatic dysfunction or inappropriate plasma levels); reversible cerebral atrophy and dementia (several reports).

Psychiatric – Emotional upset; depression; psychosis; aggression; hyperactivity; behavioral deterioration.

Dermatologic – Transient hair loss; skin rash; petechiae; erythema multiforme; photosensitivity; generalized pruritis, Stevens-Johnson syndrome; toxic epidermal necrolysis (rare, two fatal cases).

Hematologic – Valproic acid inhibits the secondary phase of platelet aggregation; this may be reflected in altered bleeding time. Thrombocytopenia; bruising; hematoma formation; epistaxis; frank hemorrhage; relative lymphocytosis; macrocytosis; hypofibrinogenemia; leukopenia; eosinophilia; anemia; bone marrow suppression; bone marrow toxicity suggestive of a myelodysplastic syndrome; pancytopenia; aplastic anemia; acute intermittent porphyria.

Hepatic – Minor elevations of AST, ALT and LDH (frequent, dose-related); increases in serum bilirubin and abnormal changes in other liver function tests (occasionally); severe hepatotoxicity; death. (See Warning Box and Warnings.)

Endocrine – Irregular menses; secondary amenorrhea; abnormal thyroid function tests; parotid gland swelling; breast enlargement; galactorrhea.

Metabolic – Hyperammonemia (see Precautions); hyponatremia; inappropriate ADH secretion; Fanconi's syndrome (rare and seen primarily in children); hyperglycinemia associated with a fatal outcome in a patient with preexistent nonketotic hyperglycinemia; hypocarnitinemia.

Body as a whole – Extremity edema; weakness; acute pancreatitis (including rare fatal cases); lupus erythematosus; fever; enuresis; urinary tract infection; hearing loss; ear pain; bone pain; cough increased; pneumonia; otitis media; bradycardia; cutaneous vasculitis; injection site pain, injection site reaction (≈ 2.5%); injection site inflammation (rare).

Mania: Nausea (22%); somnolence (19%); dizziness, vomiting (12%); accidental injury (11%); asthenia (10%); abdominal pain, dyspepsia (9%); rash (6%).

The following additional adverse events were reported (> 1% to 5%).

Body as a whole – Chest pain; chills; chills and fever; cyst; fever; infection; neck pain; neck rigidity.

Miscellaneous

VALPROIC ACID and DERIVATIVES

Cardiovascular – Hypertension; hypotension; palpitations; postural hypotension; tachycardia; vascular anomaly; vasodilation.

GI – Anorexia; fecal incontinence; flatulence; gastroenteritis; glossitis; periodontal abscess.

Hematologic/Lymphatic – Ecchymosis.

Metabolic/Nutritional – Edema; peripheral edema.

Musculoskeletal – Arthralgia; arthrosis; leg cramps; twitching.

CNS – Abnormal dreams; abnormal gait; agitation; ataxia; catatonic reaction; confusion; depression; diplopia; dysarthria; hallucinations; hypertonia; hypokinesia; insomnia; paresthesia; reflexes increased; tardive dyskinesia; thinking abnormalities; vertigo.

Respiratory – Dyspnea; rhinitis.

Dermatologic – Alopecia; discoid lupus erythematosis; dry skin; furunculosis; maculopapular rash; seborrhea.

Special Senses – Abnormal vision; amblyopia; conjunctivitis; deafness; dry eyes; ear disorder; ear pain; eye pain; tinnitus.

GU – Dysmenorrhea; dysuria; urinary incontinence.

Overdosage:

Symptoms: Overdosage may result in somnolence, heart block and deep coma. Motor restlessness, visual hallucinations, asterixis and death have also occurred. A patient has recovered with a valproate serum concentration > 2000 mcg/ml.

Treatment: Valproic acid is absorbed very rapidly; efficacy of gastric lavage varies with time since ingestion. Use general supportive measures and carefully maintain adequate urinary output. Hemodialysis and hemoperfusion have been used. See General Management of Acute Overdosage. Naloxone has reversed CNS depressant effects. It could theoretically reverse anticonvulsant effects; use caution.

Patient Information:

If GI upset occurs, take with food.

Do not chew tablets or capsules; swallow whole to avoid irritation of mouth and throat.

Patients should use caution while driving or performing other tasks requiring alertness, coordination or physical dexterity.

Diabetic patients: Medication may interfere with urine tests for ketones.

Administration and Dosage:

Oral products: Bedtime administration may minimize effects of CNS depression. GI irritation may be minimized by taking with food or by slowly increasing the dose. Delayed-release divalproex sodium may reduce the incidence of irritative GI effects.

Sprinkle capsules: May swallow whole or open capsule and sprinkle entire contents on a small amount (teaspoonful) of soft food such as applesauce or pudding. Swallow drug/food mixture immediately; do not chew. Do not store for future use.

Injection: For intravenous use only. Administer as a 60 minute infusion (≤ 20 mg/min) with the same frequency as the oral products. Rapid infusion of valproate has been associated with an increase in adverse events. Use of valproate sodium injection for periods of > 14 days has not been studied. Switch patients to oral valproate products as soon as it is clinically feasible.

Younger children, especially those receiving enzyme-inducing drugs, will require larger maintenance doses to attain targeted valproic acid concentrations.

Elderly: Due to a decrease in unbound clearance of valproate, reduce the starting dose; base therapeutic dose on clinical response.

Dose-related adverse reactions: Because the frequency of adverse effects (particularly elevated liver enzymes and thrombocytopenia) may be dose-related, weigh the benefit of improved therapeutic effect with higher doses against the possibility of a greater incidence of adverse reactions.

Epilepsy:

Complex partial seizures (monotherapy) – Adults and children ≥ 10 years of age.

10 to 15 mg/kg/day; increase by 5 to 10 mg/kg/week until seizures are controlled or side effects preclude further increases. The maximum recommended dosage is 60 mg/kg/day. If the total daily dose is > 250 mg, give in divided doses.

Therapeutic serum levels for most patients will range from 50 to 100 mcg/ml; however, a good correlation has not been established between daily dose, serum level and therapeutic effect.

Conversion to monotherapy – Concomitant antiepilepsy drug (AED) dosage can ordinarily be reduced by ≈ 25% every 2 weeks. This reduction may be started at initiation of therapy or delayed by 1 to 2 weeks if there is a concern that seizures are

Miscellaneous

VALPROIC ACID and DERIVATIVES

likely to occur with a reduction. The speed and duration of withdrawal of the concomitant AED can be highly variable; monitor patients closely during this period for increased seizure frequency.

Adjunctive therapy – Divalproex sodium may be added to the patient's regimen at a dosage of 10 to 15 mg/kg/day. The dosage may be increased by 5 to 10 mg/kg/week to achieve optimal clinical response. Ordinarily, optimal clinical response is achieved at daily doses < 60 mg/kg/day.

Simple and complex absence seizures – The recommended initial dose is 15 mg/kg/day, increasing at 1 week intervals by 5 to 10 mg/kg/day until seizures are controlled or side effects preclude further increase. The maximum recommended dosage is 60 mg/kg/day. If the total daily dose is > 250 mg, give in divided doses.

Conversion from valproic acid to divalproex sodium – In patients previously receiving valproic acid, initiate divalproex sodium at the same total daily dose and dosing schedule. After the patient is stabilized on divalproex sodium, administration 2 or 3 times daily may be used in selected patients.

Conversion from oral products to injection – When switching from oral products, the total daily dose of valproate sodium injection should be equivalent to the total daily dose of the oral product. Closely monitor patients receiving doses near the maximum recommended daily dose of 60 mg/kg/day, particularly those not receiving enzyme-inducing drugs. If the total daily dose exceeds 250 mg, give in a divided regimen. The equivalence between injectable and oral valproate products at steady state was only evaluated in an every-6-hour regimen. If given less frequently (eg, 2 or 3 times a day), trough levels might fall below those of an oral dosage form given via the same regimen; closely monitor trough plasma levels.

Conversion to generic – A breakthrough seizure was reported in a patient converting from brand name to generic valproic acid capsules after 3 seizure-free years.

Mania (divalproex sodium delayed release tablets): 750 mg daily in divided doses; increase as rapidly as possible to achieve the lowest therapeutic dose that produces the desired clinical effect. Maximum recommended dosage is 60 mg/kg/day.

Migraine (divalproex sodium delayed release tablets): 250 mg orally twice daily. Some patients may benefit from doses up to 1000 mg/day. There is no evidence that higher doses lead to greater efficacy.

Compatibility and stability: Valproate sodium injection was found to be physically compatible and chemically stable in dextrose (5%) injection, sodium chloride (0.9%) injection and lactated ringer's injection for at least 24 hours when stored in glass or polyvinyl chloride (PVC). Store vials at controlled room temperature 15° to 30°C (59° to 86°F). Discard unused portion of container.

Rx	**Valproic Acid** (Various, eg, Goldline, Moore, Rugby, Sidmark, Solvay)	**Capsules:** 250 mg (valproic acid)	In 100s, 250s and 500s.
Rx	**Depakene** (Abbott)		Parabens. Orange. In 100s and UD 100s.
Rx	**Valproic Acid** (Various, eg, Goldline, Moore, Morton Grove, Rugby)	**Syrup:** 250 mg (as sodium valproate)/5 ml	In 480 ml.
Rx	**Depakene** (Abbott)		Parabens, sorbitol, sucrose. In 480 ml.
Rx	**Depakote** (Abbott)	**Tablets, delayed release:** 125 mg (as divalproex sodium)	Salmon pink. In 100s and UD 100s.
		250 mg (as divalproex sodium)	Peach. In 100s, 500s and UD 100s.
		500 mg (as divalproex sodium)	Lavender. In 100s, 500s and UD 100s.
Rx	**Depakote** (Abbott)	**Capsules, sprinkle:** 125 mg (as divalproex sodium)	White/blue. In 100s and UD 100s.
Rx	**Depacon** (Abbott)	**Injection:** 5 ml (as valproate sodium)	Single-dose vials. In trays of 10.

Miscellaneous

CARBAMAZEPINE

Warning:
Aplastic anemia and agranulocytosis have been reported in association with carbamazepine therapy. The risk of developing these reactions is 5 to 8 times greater than in the general population. However, the overall risk of these reactions in the untreated general population is low, approximately six and two patients per one million per year for agranulocytosis and aplastic anemia, respectively. Although reports of transient or persistent decreased platelet or white blood cell counts are not uncommon in association with the use of carbamazepine, data are not available to estimate accurately their incidence or outcome. However, the vast majority of the cases of leukopenia have not progressed to the more serious conditions of aplastic anemia or agranulocytosis. Because of the very low incidence of agranulocytosis and aplastic anemia, the vast majority of minor hematologic changes observed in monitoring of patients on carbamazepine are unlikely to signal the occurrence of either abnormality. Nonetheless, obtain complete pretreatment hematological testing as a baseline. If a patient in the course of treatment exhibits low or decreased white blood cell or platelet counts, monitor the patient closely. Consider discontinuation of the drug if any evidence of significant bone marrow depression develops.

Actions:

Pharmacology: Carbamazepine is an iminostilbene derivative chemically related to the tricyclic antidepressants and unrelated to other anticonvulsants or agents used to control the pain of trigeminal neuralgia. Its mechanism of action is unknown. It appears to act by reducing polysynaptic responses and blocking post-tetanic potentiation.

Pharmacokinetics:

Absorption/Distribution – Carbamazepine is adequately absorbed, with peak serum levels achieved 4 to 5 hours following administration. Both the suspension and tablet deliver equivalent amounts of drug to the systemic circulation; however, the suspension is absorbed somewhat faster than the tablet (serum levels peak in ≈ 1.5 hours). Following a twice-daily dosage regimen, the suspension has higher peak levels and lower trough levels than those obtained from the tablet formulation for the same dosage regimen. However, the suspension given three times daily affords steady-state plasma levels comparable to the tablets given twice daily when administered at the same total daily dose. Plasma levels are variable and may range from 0.5 to 25 mcg/ml, with no apparent relationship to the daily intake of the drug. Usual adult therapeutic levels are between 4 and 12 mcg/ml. Carbamazepine is 76% bound to plasma proteins. The CSF/serum ratio is 0.22, similar to 22% unbound carbamazepine in serum. Transplacental passage of carbamazepine is rapid (30 to 60 minutes); the drug accumulates in fetal tissues, with higher levels found in liver and kidney than in brain and lungs.

Metabolism/Excretion – Carbamazepine is metabolized in the liver to the 10,11–epoxide, which also has anticonvulsant activity. It may induce its own metabolism. Initial half-life ranges from 25 to 65 hours, and decreases to 12 to 17 hours with repeated doses. The half-life of the metabolite is somewhat shorter than that of the parent drug's.

After administration, 72% of a dose is found in urine and 28% in feces. Urinary products are composed largely of hydroxylated and conjugated metabolites, with only 3% unchanged carbamazepine.

Indications:

Epilepsy: Partial seizures with complex symptoms (psychomotor, temporal lobe). Patients with these seizures appear to show greatest improvement. Generalized tonic-clonic seizures (grand mal); mixed seizure patterns or other partial or generalized seizures.

Trigeminal neuralgia: Treatment of pain associated with true trigeminal neuralgia. Beneficial results have also been reported in glossopharyngeal neuralgia.

Unlabeled uses: Certain psychiatric disorders, including bipolar disorders, unipolar depression, schizoaffective illness, resistant schizophrenia, dyscontrol syndrome associated with limbic system dysfunction, intermittent explosive disorder, post-traumatic stress disorder and atypical psychosis.

Management of alcohol, cocaine and benzodiazepine withdrawal.

Restless legs syndrome (100 to 300 mg at bedtime).

Although carbamazepine has been used for cranial diabetes insipidus, it is generally ineffective.

CARBAMAZEPINE

Nonhereditary chorea in children (15 to 25 mg/kg/day).

Contraindications:

History of bone marrow depression; hypersensitivity to carbamazepine and tricyclic antidepressants; concomitant use of monoamine oxidase (MAO) inhibitors. Discontinue MAO inhibitors for a minimum of 14 days before carbamazepine administration.

Warnings:

Minor pain: This drug is not a simple analgesic. Do not use for the relief of minor aches or pains.

Hematologic: Patients with a history of adverse hematologic reaction to any drug may be particularly at risk.

Glaucoma: Carbamazepine has shown mild anticholinergic activity; therefore, use with caution in patients with increased intraocular pressure.

CNS effects: Because of the drug's relationship to other tricyclic compounds, the possibility of activating latent psychosis, confusion or agitation in elderly patients exists.

Carcinogenesis: Carbamazepine administered to rats for 2 years at doses of 25 to 250 mg/kg/day resulted in a dose-related increase in the incidence of hepatocellular tumors in females and benign interstitial cell adenomas in the testes of males. The significance of these findings to humans is unknown.

Pregnancy: Category C. Adverse effects have been observed in animal studies.

Use only when clearly needed and when the potential benefits outweigh the unknown potential hazards to the fetus. For information on use during pregnancy, refer to the Anticonvulsants introduction.

Lactation: Concentration of carbamazepine in breast milk is approximately 60% of the maternal plasma concentration. Because of the potential for serious adverse reactions, decide whether to discontinue nursing or to discontinue the drug, taking into account the importance of the drug to the mother.

Children: Safety and efficacy for use in children < 6 years of age have not been established.

Precautions:

Monitoring: Perform baseline liver function tests and periodic evaluations. Discontinue drug immediately if liver dysfunction occurs. Obtain baseline and periodic eye examinations (slit lamp, funduscopy and tonometry), urinalysis and BUN determinations.

Monitoring of blood levels may be particularly useful in cases of dramatic increase in seizure frequency, for verification of compliance and in determining the cause of toxicity when more than one medication is being used.

Obtain complete pretreatment hematological testing as a baseline. Repeat these tests at monthly intervals during the first 2 months and thereafter obtain yearly or every other year CBC, white cell differential and platelet count.

Absence seizures (petit mal) do not appear to be controlled by carbamazepine. Use with caution in patients with a mixed seizure disorder that includes atypical absence seizures because carbamazepine has been associated with increased frequency of generalized convulsions in these patients.

Special risk patients: Prescribe carbamazepine only after benefit-to-risk appraisal in patients with a history of: Cardiac, hepatic or renal damage; adverse hematologic reaction to other drugs; interrupted courses of therapy with the drug.

Hazardous tasks: May produce drowsiness, dizziness or blurred vision; patients should observe caution while driving or performing other tasks requiring alertness, coordination or physical dexterity.

Miscellaneous

CARBAMAZEPINE

Drug Interactions:

Precipitant drug	Object drug*		Description
Cimetidine Danazol Diltiazem Isoniazid Macrolides (except azithromycin) Propoxyphene Verapamil	Carbamazepine	↑	These agents may inhibit the hepatic metabolism of carbamazepine; resultant elevated carbamazepine levels may result in toxicity (eg, nausea, vomiting, somnolence, nystagmus, ataxia and other cerebellar symptoms). Conversely, carbamazepine may increase the risk of isoniazid-induced hepatotoxicity.
Antihistamines, nonsedating	Carbamazepine	↑	Terfenadine may increase carbamazepine levels.
Barbiturates Primidone	Carbamazepine	↓	The concurrent use may lower carbamazepine levels. No loss of seizure control has been reported with the addition of phenobarbital, because the anticonvulsant action is probably additive with carbamazepine. In addition, studies indicate that the active metabolite of primidone (phenobarbital) may be increased by carbamazepine.
Carbamazepine	Primidone	↑	
Charcoal	Carbamazepine	↓	Charcoal may decrease the GI absorption of carbamazepine. See Overdosage.
Felbamate	Carbamazepine	↓	Serum levels of either agent may be decreased.
Carbamazepine	Felbamate	↓	
Hydantoins	Carbamazepine	↓	Both increased and decreased hydantoin plasma levels as well as decreased carbamazepine plasma levels have occurred during coadministration.
Carbamazepine	Hydantoins	⟷	
SSRIs Fluoxetine Fluvoxamine	Carbamazepine	↑	Carbamazepine levels may be increased, producing possible toxicity.
Theophylline	Carbamazepine	↓	Carbamazepine levels may be decreased. Theophylline levels may be increased or decreased.
Carbamazepine	Theophylline	⟷	
Tricyclic antidepressants	Carbamazepine	↑	Carbamazepine levels may be increased; TCA levels may be decreased.
Carbamazepine	Tricyclic antidepressants	↓	
Valproic acid	Carbamazepine	↑	Valproic acid plasma levels may be decreased by carbamazepine. However, valproic acid may prolong carbamazepine's half-life, decrease its protein binding and increase the plasma ratio of carbamazepine 10,11-epoxide/carbamazepine. Clinical effects are difficult to predict.
Carbamazepine	Valproic acid	↓	
Carbamazepine	Acetaminophen	↓	Carbamazepine may increase the metabolism of acetaminophen, increasing the risk of acetaminophen-induced hepatotoxicity or decreasing its analgesic/antipyretic effectiveness.
Carbamazepine	Anticoagulants	↓	Carbamazepine may increase the metabolism of these agents due to induction of hepatic microsomal enzyme induction. Hypoprothrombinemic effect of the anticoagulants may be decreased.
Carbamazepine	Contraceptives, oral	↓	Decrease in OC effectiveness, possibly leading to unintended pregnancy.
Carbamazepine	Doxycycline	↓	Doxycycline half-life may be reduced when coadministered with carbamazepine.

Miscellaneous

CARBAMAZEPINE

Drug Interactions			
Precipitant drug	Object drug*		Description
Carbamazepine	Haloperidol	⬇	Haloperidol serum levels and efficacy may be decreased by carbamazepine.
Carbamazepine	Lithium	⬆	Increased CNS toxicity may occur during concomitant carbamazepine therapy.
Carbamazepine	Nondepolarizing neuromuscular blockers	⬇	Carbamazepine may cause resistance to, or reversal of, the neuromuscular blocking effects of these agents.
Carbamazepine	Posterior pituitary hormones	⬆	Carbamazepine, which potentiates ADH, may potentiate the antidiuretic effects of vasopressin, lypressin or desmopressin.
Carbamazepine	Succinimides	⬇	Plasma levels of these agents may be reduced by carbamazepine due to induction of hepatic microsomal enzymes, although there may be no loss of seizure control because the anticonvulsant action is probably additive.

* ⬆ = Object drug increased. ⬇ = Object drug decreased. ⟷ = Undetermined effect.

Drug/Lab test interactions:

Thyroid function tests show decreased values with carbamazepine.

Adverse Reactions:

If adverse reactions are so severe that the drug must be discontinued, abrupt discontinuation in a responsive epileptic patient may lead to seizures or status epilepticus.

Most frequent: Dizziness; drowsiness; unsteadiness; nausea; vomiting. To minimize such reactions, initiate therapy at low doses.

Hematologic: Aplastic anemia; leukopenia; agranulocytosis; eosinophilia; leukocytosis; thrombocytopenia; pancytopenia; bone marrow depression, acute intermittent porphyria. (See Warning Box).

Pulmonary: Pulmonary hypersensitivity characterized by fever, dyspnea, pneumonitis or pneumonia.

Hepatic: Abnormal liver function tests; cholestatic/hepatocellular jaundice; hepatitis.

GU: Urinary frequency; acute urinary retention; oliguria with hypertension; renal failure; azotemia; impotence; albuminuria; glycosuria; elevated BUN; microscopic deposits in urine.

CNS: Dizziness; drowsiness; disturbances of coordination; confusion; headache; fatigue; blurred vision; visual hallucinations; speech disturbances; abnormal involuntary movements; peripheral neuritis and paresthesias; depression with agitation; talkativeness; tinnitus; hyperacusis; behavioral changes in children; paralysis and other symptoms of cerebral arterial insufficiency.

Dermatologic: Pruritic and erythematous rashes; urticaria; Stevens-Johnson syndrome; photosensitivity reactions; alterations in pigmentation; exfoliative dermatitis; alopecia; diaphoresis; erythema multiforme and nodosum; purpura; aggravation of disseminated lupus erythematosus and toxic epidermal necrolysis (Lyell's syndrome). Discontinuation of therapy may be necessary.

GI: Nausea; vomiting; gastric distress; abdominal pain; diarrhea; constipation; anorexia; dryness of mouth or pharynx; glossitis and stomatitis.

Cardiovascular: Congestive heart failure; aggravation of hypertension; hypotension; syncope and collapse; edema; primary thrombophlebitis; recurrence of thrombophlebitis; aggravation of coronary artery disease; arrhythmias, AV block; adenopathy or lymphadenopathy. Some cardiovascular complications have resulted in fatalities.

Ophthalmic: Transient diplopia and oculomotor disturbances; nystagmus; scattered, punctate cortical lens opacities; conjunctivitis.

Musculoskeletal: Aching joints and muscles; leg cramps.

Metabolic: Fever and chills; inappropriate antidiuretic hormone secretion syndrome (SIADH).

Miscellaneous

CARBAMAZEPINE

Overdosage:

Toxic doses:

Lowest known lethal dose –

Adults: > 60 g (39-year-old man).

Highest known doses survived –

Adults: 30 g (31-year-old woman).

Children: 10 g (6-year-old boy).

Small children: 5 g (3-year-old girl).

Symptoms and signs first appear after 1 to 3 hours. Neuromuscular disturbances are the most prominent. Cardiovascular disorders are generally mild, and severe cardiac complications occur only when very high doses (> 60 g) have been ingested.

Respiration – Irregular breathing; respiratory depression.

Cardiovascular – Tachycardia; hypotension or hypertension; shock; conduction disorders.

CNS – Impaired consciousness ranging to deep coma; convulsions, especially in small children; motor restlessness; muscular twitching; tremor; athetoid movements; opisthotonos; ataxia; drowsiness; dizziness; mydriasis; nystagmus; adiadochokinesia; ballism; psychomotor disturbances; dysmetria; initial hyperreflexia followed by hyporeflexia; EEG may show dysrhythmias.

GI/GU – Nausea; vomiting; anuria or oliguria; urinary retention.

Laboratory findings: Isolated instances of overdosage have included leukocytosis, reduced leukocyte count, glycosuria and acetonuria.

Treatment: The prognosis in cases of severe poisoning is dependent upon prompt elimination of the drug. Even when more than 4 hours have elapsed following ingestion of the drug, irrigate the stomach repeatedly, especially if the patient has also consumed alcohol. There is no specific antidote. Refer to General Management of Acute Overdosage. Charcoal administration is effective in increasing the total body clearance of carbamazepine. The recommended dosage is 50 to 100 g initially followed by a rate of ≥ 12.5 g/hour, preferably via a nasogastric tube; continue until the patient is symptom free.

Dialysis is indicated only in severe poisoning associated with renal failure. Replacement transfusion is indicated in severe poisoning in small children.

In treating convulsions, diazepam or barbiturates may aggravate respiratory depression (especially in children), hypotension and coma. Do not use barbiturates if MAO inhibitors have also been taken by the patient either in overdosage or in recent therapy (within 1 week).

Monitor respiration, ECG, blood pressure, body temperature, pupillary reflexes and kidney and bladder function for several days.

Treatment of blood count abnormalities – If evidence of significant bone marrow depression develops: Discontinue drug; perform daily CBC, platelet and reticulocyte counts; perform bone marrow aspiration and trephine biopsy immediately and repeat with sufficient frequency to monitor recovery. Fully developed aplastic anemia requires intensive monitoring and therapy; seek specialized consultation.

Special periodic studies might be helpful as follows: White cell and platelet antibodies; ^{59}Fe – ferrokinetic studies; peripheral blood cell typing; cytogenetic studies on marrow and peripheral blood; bone marrow cultures for colony-forming units; hemoglobin electrophoresis for A_2 and F hemoglobin; serum folic acid; B_{12} levels.

Patient Information:

May produce drowsiness, dizziness or blurred vision; patients should observe caution while driving or performing other tasks requiring alertness, coordination or physical dexterity.

Notify physician if any of the following occurs: Unusual bleeding or bruising, jaundice, abdominal pain, impotence, CNS disturbances, edema, fever, chills, sore throat or ulcers in the mouth.

May cause GI upset; take with food.

Administration and Dosage:

Individualize dosage. A low initial daily dosage with gradual increase is advised. As soon as adequate control is achieved, reduce dosage gradually to the minimum effective level. Take with meals.

Miscellaneous

CARBAMAZEPINE

Epilepsy:

Adults and children (> 12 years of age) –

Initial dose is 200 mg twice daily (100 mg 4 times daily of suspension). Increase at weekly intervals by up to 200 mg/day using a 3 or 4 times per day regimen until the best response is obtained. Do not exceed 1000 mg/day in children 12 to 15 years or 1200 mg/day in patients > 15 years. In rare instances, doses up to 1600 mg/day have been used in adults.

Maintenance: Adjust to minimum effective level, usually 800 to 1200 mg daily.

Children (6 to 12 years) –

Initial dose is 100 mg twice daily (50 mg 4 times daily of suspension). Increase at weekly intervals gradually by adding 100 mg/day using a 3 or 4 times per day regimen until the best response is obtained. Do not exceed 1000 mg daily. May also be calculated on basis of 20 to 30 mg/kg/day, in divided doses 3 or 4 times a day.

Maintenance: Adjust to minimum effective level, usually 400 to 800 mg daily.

Combination therapy – When added to existing anticonvulsant therapy, do so gradually while other anticonvulsants are maintained or gradually decreased, except phenytoin, which may have to be increased.

Trigeminal neuralgia:

Initial – 100 mg twice daily on the first day (50 mg 4 times daily of suspension). May increase by up to 200 mg/day using 100 mg increments every 12 hours (50 mg 4 times daily of suspension) as needed. Do not exceed 1200 mg daily.

Maintenance – Control of pain can usually be maintained with 400 to 800 mg daily (range 200 to 1200 mg/day). Attempt to reduce the dose to the minimum effective level or to discontinue the drug at least once every 3 months.

Rx	**Carbamazepine** (Various, eg, Lemmon, Moore, Schein, Warner-Chilcott)	**Tablets, chewable:** 100 mg	In 100s.
Rx	**Tegretol** (Ciba-Geigy)		(Tegretol 52). Sucrose. Pink, red-speckled, scored. In 100s and UD 100s.
Rx	**Carbamazepine** (Various, eg, Goldline, Lederle, Lemmon, Major, Moore, Purepac, Rugby, Schein, Vangard, Warner-Chilcott)	**Tablets:** 200 mg	In 30s, 100s, 500s, 1000s and UD 100s.
Rx	**Atretol** (Athena Neurosciences)		(A 554). Lactose. White, scored. In 100s.
Rx	**Epitol** (Lemmon)		(Epitol 93). White, scored. In 100s, 500s, 1000s and UD 100s.
Rx	**Depitol** (Kavon)		White, scored. In 100s, 500s, 1000s and UD 100s.
Rx	**Tegretol** (Ciba-Geigy)		(Tegretol 27). Pink, scored. Capsule-shaped. In 100s, 1000s and UD 100s.
Rx	**Tegretol-XR** (Ciba-Geigy)	**Tablets, extended release:** 100 mg	Mannitol. (T 100 mg). Yellow. In 100s and UD 100s.
		200 mg	Mannitol. (T 200 mg). Pink. In 100s and UD 100s.
		400 mg	Mannitol (T 400 mg). Brown. In 100s and UD 100s.
Rx	**Tegretol** (Ciba-Geigy)	**Suspension:** 100 mg/5 ml	Sorbitol, sucrose. Citrus/vanilla flavor. In 450 ml.

Miscellaneous

FELBAMATE

Warning:

There have been reports of 21 cases (including 3 deaths) of aplastic anemia (pancytopenia in the presence of a bone marrow largely depleted of myeloid and erythroid precursors) in association with the use of felbamate. Time to onset in these cases from time of treatment initiation ranged from 5 to 30 weeks; mean time to onset was 128 days. How long the risk persists and whether its magnitude changes with time are not known. Aplastic anemia is a rare, frequently fatal, form of acquired bone marrow failure, occurring at an estimated rate of 2 to 5 cases per million persons per year. The case fatality rate varies with severity and cause.

The 21 cases represent a great increase over the expected rate. The absolute rate may be higher than the 1 in 5000 observed to date because 1) drug-induced aplastic anemia is typically delayed in onset, occurring weeks to months after treatment initiation and 2) post-marketing surveillance typically captures only a fraction of incident cases. The risk may actually be closer to 1 in 2000.

It is recommended that the use of felbamate be suspended unless, in the judgment of the physician, the patient's well-being is judged to be so dependent on continued treatment that abrupt withdrawal is deemed to pose an even greater risk. Patients should not discontinue the drug on their own. While it might appear prudent to perform frequent CBCs in patients while continuing therapy, there is no evidence that such monitoring will provide early detection of marrow suppression before aplastic anemia occurs.

In addition to aplastic anemia, eight cases of acute liver failure have occurred, including four deaths, in association with the use of felbamate. One of the four survivors received a liver transplant. The number of cases reported greatly exceeds the number that is expected based on the annual incidence of acute liver failure in the US (about 2000 per year). In several cases there were nonspecific premonitory signs, but in others the patients were already in frank liver failure at the time the illness was detected. Time between initiation of treatment and diagnosis of these cases ranged from 14 to 257 days.

At a minimum, evaluate patients prior to treatment initiation for evidence of pre-existing liver damage; avoid use in patients with pre-existing liver pathology. Once treatment is initiated, monitor ALT, AST and bilirubin on a weekly basis. Immediately withdraw the drug in patients who develop lab findings indicating liver injury, although it is not known if treatment withdrawal reduces the risk of subsequent damage.

An FDA advisory committee has recommended that felbamate be used as a second-line therapy only. For further information, contact Wallace Labs at 800–526–3840.

Actions:

Pharmacology: Felbamate is an oral antiepileptic agent. The mechanism by which it exerts its anticonvulsant activity is unknown, but in animals, felbamate has properties in common with other anticonvulsants. Felbamate is effective in mice and rats in the maximal electroshock test, the subcutaneous pentylenetetrazol seizure test and the subcutaneous picrotoxin seizure test. Felbamate also exhibits anticonvulsant activity against seizures induced by intracerebroventricular administration of glutamate in rats and N-methyl-D,L-aspartic acid in mice. Protection against maximal electroshock-induced seizures suggests that felbamate may reduce seizure spread, an effect possibly predictive of efficacy in generalized tonic-clonic or partial seizures. Protection against pentylenetetrazol-induced seizures suggests that felbamate may increase seizure threshold, an effect considered to be predictive of potential efficacy in absence seizures.

Receptor-binding studies in vitro indicate that felbamate has weak inhibitory effects on GABA-receptor binding and benzodiazepine receptor binding, and is devoid of activity at the MK-801 receptor binding site of the NMDA receptor-ionophore complex. However, felbamate interacts as an antagonist at the strychnine-insensitive glycine recognition site of the NMDA receptor-ionophore complex.

In adults, there is no effect of felbamate on blood pressure. Small but statistically significant mean increases in heart rate were seen during adjunctive therapy and monotherapy; however, these mean increases of up to 5 bpm were not clinically significant. In children, no clinically relevant changes in blood pressure or heart rate were seen during adjunctive therapy or monotherapy.

Miscellaneous

FELBAMATE

The only change in vital signs was a mean decrease in respiratory rate of approximately 1 respiration per minute during adjunctive therapy in children. In adults, statistically significant mean reductions in body weight were observed during monotherapy and adjunctive therapy. In children, there were mean decreases in body weight during adjunctive therapy and mono-therapy; however, these mean changes were not statistically significant. These mean reductions in adults and children were approximately 5% of the mean weights at baseline.

Pharmacokinetics:

Absorption/Distribution – Felbamate is well absorbed after oral administration. Over 90% of a 1000 mg dose was found in the urine. Pharmacokinetic parameters of the tablet and suspension are similar. There was no effect of food on tablet absorption; the effect of food on suspension absorption has not been evaluated.

Metabolism/Excretion – Following oral administration, felbamate is the predominant plasma species (about 90%). About 40% to 50% of absorbed dose appears unchanged in urine and an additional 40% is present as unidentified metabolites and conjugates. About 15% is present as parahydroxyfelbamate, 2-hydroxyfelbamate and felbamate monocarbamate, none of which have significant anticonvulsant activity. Binding to plasma protein was independent of concentrations between 10 and 310 mcg/ml. Binding ranged from 22% to 25%, mostly to albumin.

Felbamate is excreted with a terminal half-life of 20 to 23 hours, which is unaltered after multiple doses. Clearance after a single 1200 mg dose is 26 ± 3 ml/hr/kg; after multiple daily doses of 3600 mg, it is 30 ± 8 ml/hr/kg. The apparent volume of distribution was 756 ± 82 ml/kg after a 1200 mg dose. Felbamate C_{max} and AUC are proportionate to dose. C_{min} (trough) blood levels are also dose-proportional. Multiple daily doses of 1200, 2400 and 3600 mg gave C_{min} values of 30 ± 5, 55 ± 8 and 83 ± 21 mcg/ml, respectively (n = 10). Felbamate gave dose-proportional steady-state peak plasma concentrations in children ages 4 to 12 over a range of 15, 30 and 45 mg/kg/day with peak concentrations of 17, 32 and 49 mcg/ml, respectively. Plasma concentrations in males and females given felbamate have been similar.

Indications:

Partial seizures: Monotherapy and adjunctive therapy in the treatment of partial seizures with and without generalization in adults with epilepsy.

Lennox-Gastaut syndrome: Adjunctive therapy in the treatment of partial and generalized seizures associated with Lennox-Gastaut syndrome in children.

An FDA advisory committee has recommended that felbamate be used as second-line therapy only.

Contraindications:

Hypersensitivity to felbamate or ingredients of the product. Use cautiously in those who have demonstrated hypersensitivity reactions to other carbamates.

Warnings:

Aplastic anemia: There have been reports of 21 cases of aplastic anemia (including 3 deaths) in association with the use of felbamate. See Warning box.

Hepatic failure: There have been eight cases of acute liver failure (including four deaths) in association with the use of felbamate. See Warning box.

Discontinuation: Antiepileptic drugs should not be suddenly discontinued because of the possibility of increasing seizure frequency. See Administration and Dosage.

FELBAMATE

Carcinogenesis: In mice and rats, there was a statistically significant increase in hepatic cell adenomas in high-dose male and female mice (1200 mg/kg) and in high-dose female rats (100 mg/kg). Hepatic hypertrophy was significantly increased in a dose-related manner in mice. There was a statistically significant increase in benign interstitial cell tumors of the testes in male rats receiving high-dose felbamate.

As a result of the synthesis process, felbamate could contain small amounts of two known animal carcinogens, the genotoxic compound ethyl carbamate (urethane) and the nongenotoxic compound methyl carbamate. It is theoretically possible that a 50 kg patient receiving 3600 mg of felbamate could be exposed to up to 0.72 mcg urethane and 1800 mcg methyl carbamate. These daily doses are ≈ 1/35,000 (urethane) and 1/5500 (methyl carbamate) on a mg/kg basis of the dose levels carcinogenic in rodents. Any presence of these two compounds in felbamate used in the lifetime carcinogenicity studies was inadequate to cause tumors.

Elderly: Clinical experience has not identified differences in responses between the elderly and younger patients. In general, dosage selection for an elderly patient should be cautious, usually starting at the low end of the dosing range, reflecting the greater frequency of decreased hepatic, renal or cardiac function and of concomitant disease or other drug therapy.

Pregnancy: Category C. Placental transfer of felbamate occurs in rat pups. The no-effect dose for rat pup mortality was 6.9 times the human dose on a mg/kg basis. There are no studies in pregnant women. Use during pregnancy only if clearly needed.

Lactation: Felbamate has been detected in breast milk. The effect on the nursing infant is unknown. In rats, there was a decrease in pup weight and an increase in pup deaths during lactation.

Children: Safety and efficacy in children, other than those with Lennox-Gastaut syndrome, have not been established.

Precautions:

Monitoring: Clinical trials data indicate that routine monitoring of clinical laboratory parameters is not necessary for the safe use of felbamate. The value of monitoring blood levels has not been established. Because of the effect of felbamate on the plasma levels of other AEDs being taken concomitantly, monitoring of the plasma concentrations of these AEDs may be indicated. In general, exercise clinical judgment regarding monitoring of other laboratory parameters.

Photosensitivity: Photosensitization (photoallergy or phototoxicity) may occur; therefore, caution patients to take protective measures against exposure to ultraviolet light or sunlight (ie, sunscreens, protective clothing) until tolerance is determined.

Drug Interactions:

Felbamate Drug Interactions

Precipitant drug	Object drug*		Description
Felbamate	Phenytoin	⬆	Felbamate causes an increase in steady-state phenytoin levels. C_{min} increases were dose-related. To maintain phenytoin levels and achieve felbamate dosages of 3600 mg/day, a 40% dose reduction of phenytoin was necessary. In contrast, phenytoin causes a doubling of felbamate clearance, resulting in an ≈ 45% decrease in steady-state levels.
Phenytoin	Felbamate	⬇	
Felbamate	Carbamazepine	⬇	Felbamate causes a decrease in steady-state carbamazepine levels and an increase in steady-state carbamazepine epoxide (metabolite) levels. Carbamazepine C_{min} decreases were dose-related, as were the epoxide C_{min} increases. In addition, carbamazepine causes an ≈ 50% increase in felbamate clearance, resulting in an ≈ 40% decrease in steady-state trough levels.
Carbamazepine	Felbamate	⬇	
Felbamate	Valproic acid	⬆	Felbamate causes an increase in steady-state valproic acid levels. C_{min} increases were dose-related. Valproic acid does not appear to affect felbamate levels.

* ⬆ = Object drug increased; ⬇ = Object drug decreased.

Miscellaneous

FELBAMATE

Adverse Reactions:

Felbamate Adverse Reactions (%)						
	Adults				Children	
	Monotherapy		Adjunctive therapy		Lennox-Gastaut	
Adverse reaction	Felbamate (n=58)	Valproate (n=50)	Felbamate (n=114)	Placebo (n=43)	Felbamate (n=31)	Placebo (n=27)
Body as a whole						
Fatigue	6.9	4	16.8	7	9.7	3.7
Weight decrease	3.4	0	—	—	6.5	0
Facial edema	3.4	0	—	—	—	—
Fever	—	—	2.6	4.7	22.6	11.1
Chest pain	—	—	2.6	0	—	—
Pain	—	—	—	—	6.5	0
CNS						
Insomnia	8.6	4	17.5	7	16.1	14.8
Headache	6.9	18	36.8	9.3	6.5	18.5
Anxiety	5.2	2	5.3	4.7	—	—
Somnolence	—	—	19.3	7	48.4	11.1
Dizziness	—	—	18.4	14	—	—
Nervousness	—	—	7	2.3	16.1	18.5
Tremor	—	—	6.1	2.3	—	—
Abnormal gait	—	—	5.3	0	9.7	0
Depression	—	—	5.3	0	—	—
Paresthesia	—	—	3.5	2.3	—	—
Ataxia	—	—	3.5	0	6.5	3.7
Dry mouth	—	—	2.6	0	—	—
Stupor	—	—	2.6	0	—	—
Thinking abnormal	—	—	—	—	6.5	3.7
Emotional lability	—	—	—	—	6.5	0
Miosis	—	—	—	—	6.5	0
Dermatologic						
Acne	3.4	0	—	—	—	—
Rash	3.4	0	3.5	4.7	9.7	7.4
GI						
Dyspepsia	8.6	2	12.3	7	6.5	3.7
Vomiting	8.6	2	16.7	4.7	38.7	14.8
Constipation	6.9	2	11.4	2.3	12.9	0
Diarrhea	5.2	0	5.3	2.3	—	—
ALT increased	5.2	2	3.5	0	—	—
Nausea	—	—	34.2	2.3	6.5	0
Anorexia	—	—	19.3	2.3	54.8	14.8
Abdominal pain	—	—	5.3	0	—	—
Hiccups	—	—	—	—	9.7	3.7
Respiratory						
Upper respiratory tract infection	8.6	4	5.3	7	45.2	25.9
Rhinitis	6.9	0	—	—	—	—
Sinusitis	—	—	3.5	0	—	—
Pharyngitis	—	—	2.6	0	9.7	3.7
Coughing	—	—	—	—	6.5	0
Special senses						
Diplopia	3.4	4	6.1	0	—	—
Otitis media	3.4	0	—	—	9.7	0
Taste perversion	—	—	6.1	0	—	—
Vision abnormal	—	—	5.3	2.3	—	—

Miscellaneous

FELBAMATE

Felbamate Adverse Reactions (%)						
	Adults				Children	
	Monotherapy		Adjunctive therapy		Lennox-Gastaut	
	Felbamate	Valproate	Felbamate	Placebo	Felbamate	Placebo
Adverse reaction	(n=58)	(n=50)	(n=114)	(n=43)	(n=31)	(n=27)
GU						
Urinary incontinence	—	—	—	—	6.5	7.4
Intramenstrual bleeding	3.4	0	—	—	—	—
UTI	3.4	2	—	—	—	—
Hematologic						
Purpura	—	—	—	—	12.9	7.4
Leukopenia	—	—	—	—	6.5	0
Miscellaneous						
Hypophosphatemia	3.4	0	—	—	—	—
Myalgia	—	—	2.6	0	—	—

Miscellaneous: Weight increase, asthenia, malaise, influenza-like symptoms (1%); dystonia (0.1% to 1%); anaphylactoid reaction, substernal chest pain, photosensitivity, allergic reaction (< 0.1%).

Cardiovascular: Palpitation, tachycardia (1%); supraventricular tachycardia (< 0.1%).

CNS: Agitation, psychological disturbance, aggressive reaction (1%); hallucination, euphoria, suicide attempt, migraine (0.1% to 1%).

GI: AST increased (1%); esophagitis, appetite increased (0.1% to 1%); GGT elevated (< 0.1%).

Hematologic: Lymphadenopathy, leukopenia, leukocytosis, thrombocytopenia, granulocytopenia (0.1% to 1%); positive antinuclear factor test, qualitative platelet disorder, agranulocytosis (< 0.1%).

Metabolic/Nutritional: Hypokalemia, hyponatremia, LDH increased, alkaline phosphatase increased, hypophosphatemia (0.1% to 1%); creatine phosphokinase increased (< 0.1%).

Dermatologic: Pruritus (1%); urticaria, bullous eruption (0.1% to 1%); buccal mucous membrane swelling, Stevens-Johnson syndrome (< 0.1%).

Overdosage:

Symptoms: Four subjects inadvertently received felbamate as adjunctive therapy in dosages ranging from 5400 to 7200 mg/day for 6 to 51 days. One subject who received 5400 mg/day as monotherapy for 1 week reported no adverse experiences. Another subject attempted suicide by ingesting 12,000 mg in a 12 hour period. The only adverse experiences reported were mild gastric distress and a resting heart rate of 100 bpm. No serious adverse reactions have been reported.

Treatment: Employ general supportive measures if overdosage occurs. Refer to General Management of Acute Overdosage. It is not known if felbamate is dialyzable.

Patient Information:

Instruct patients to take felbamate only as prescribed. Instruct patients to store this medication in its tightly closed container at room temperature away from excessive heat, direct sunlight or moisture and away from children.

Avoid prolonged exposure to sunlight or sunlamps; may cause photosensitivity.

Administration and Dosage:

Approved by the FDA on July 29, 1993.

Discontinuation of therapy: Because of reports of aplastic anemia in association with felbamate, it has been recommended to discontinue use of the drug unless the physician decides that withdrawal would pose an even greater risk to the patient (see Warning box).

Patients should not discontinue the drug on their own. If the decision is made to discontinue therapy, felbamate may be discontinued by reducing the dosage by one-third increments every 4 to 5 days. As with any antiepileptic, abrupt discontinuation may result in an increase in seizure frequency; however, if it is necessary to discontinue felbamate abruptly, it may be stopped without tapering as long as the patient is covered by adequate dosages of other antiepileptics.

Miscellaneous

FELBAMATE

The following prescribing information is applicable to those physicians who opt to continue the use of felbamate in select patients.

Felbamate is used as monotherapy and adjunctive therapy in adults and as adjunctive therapy in children. When the drug is added to or substituted for existing antiepileptic drugs (AEDs), it is necessary to reduce the dosage of those AEDs in the range of 20% to 30% to minimize side effects.

Adults (≥ 14 years of age): Most of the patients received 3600 mg/day in clinical trials.

Monotherapy (initial therapy) – Felbamate has not been systematically evaluated as initial monotherapy. Initiate at 1200 mg/day in divided doses 3 or 4 times daily. Titrate previously untreated patients under close clinical supervision, increasing the dosage in 600 mg increments every 2 weeks to 2400 mg/day based on clinical response and thereafter to 3600 mg/day if clinically indicated.

Conversion to monotherapy – Initiate at 1200 mg/day in divided doses 3 or 4 times daily. Reduce the dosage of concomitant AEDs by one-third at initiation of felbamate therapy. At week 2, increase the felbamate dosage to 2400 mg/day while reducing the dosage of other AEDs up to an additional one-third of their original dosage. At week 3, increase the felbamate dosage up to 3600 mg/day and continue to reduce the dosage of other AEDs as clinically indicated.

Adjunctive therapy – Add felbamate at 1200 mg/day in divided doses 3 or 4 times daily while reducing present AEDs by 20% in order to control plasma concentrations of concurrent phenytoin, valproic acid and carbamazepine (and its metabolites). Further reductions of the concomitant AED dosage may be necessary to minimize side effects due to drug interactions. Increase the dosage of felbamate by 1200 mg/day increments at weekly intervals to 3600 mg/day. Most side effects seen during adjunctive therapy resolve as the dosage of concomitant AEDs is decreased.

Felbamate/Concomitant AED Dosage (Adults): Adjunctive Therapy

Drugs	Week 1	Week 2	Week 3
Dosage reduction of concomitant AEDs	Reduce original dose by 20% to 33%[1]	Reduce original dose by up to an additional 33%[1]	Reduce as clinically indicated
Felbamate dosage	1200 mg/day initial dose	2400 mg/day therapeutic dosage range	3600 mg/day therapeutic dosage range

[1] See Adjunctive Therapy and Conversion to Monotherapy sections.

While the previous conversion guidelines may result in a felbamate 3600 mg/day dose within 3 weeks, in some patients titration to 3600 mg/day has been achieved in as little as 3 days with appropriate adjustment of other AEDs.

Children with Lennox-Gastaut syndrome (ages 2 to 14 years):

Adjunctive therapy – Add felbamate at 15 mg/kg/day in divided doses 3 or 4 times daily while reducing present AEDs by 20% in order to control plasma levels of concurrent phenytoin, valproic acid and carbamazepine (and its metabolites). Further reductions of the concomitant AED dosage may be necessary to minimize side effects due to drug interactions. Increase the dosage of felbamate by 15 mg/kg/day increments at weekly intervals to 45 mg/kg/day. Most side effects seen during adjunctive therapy resolve as the dosage of concomitant AEDs is decreased.

Storage/Stability:

Suspension – Shake well before using.

Rx	**Felbatol**[1] (Wallace Labs)	**Tablets**: 400 mg	Lactose. (Wallace 0430). Yellow, scored. Capsule shape. In 100s and UD 100s.
		600 mg	Lactose. (Wallace 0431). Peach, scored. Capsule shape. In 100s and UD 100s.
		Suspension : 600 mg/5 ml	Sorbitol, parabens, saccharin. In 240 and 960 ml.

[1] It has been recommended that use of this drug be discontinued unless, in the judgment of the physician, continued therapy is warranted. See Warning box. For further information contact Wallace Labs at (609) 655–6474.

Miscellaneous

GABAPENTIN

Actions:

Pharmacology: Gabapentin is an oral antiepileptic agent. The mechanism by which it exerts its anticonvulsant action is unknown, but in animals it has properties in common with other anticonvulsants. Gabapentin exhibits anti-seizure activity in mice and rats in both the maximal electroshock and pentylenetetrazole seizure models and other preclinical models (eg, strains with genetic epilepsy). The relevance of these models to human epilepsy is not known.

Gabapentin is structurally related to the neurotransmitter gamma-aminobutyric acid (GABA) but it does not interact with GABA receptors, it is not converted metabolically into GABA or a GABA agonist, and it is not an inhibitor of GABA uptake or degradation. Gabapentin does not exhibit affinity for a number of other common receptor sites. In vitro studies have revealed a gabapentin binding site in areas of rat brain including neocortex and hippocampus. The identity and function of this binding site remain to be elucidated.

All pharmacological actions following gabapentin administration are due to the activity of the parent compound; gabapentin is not appreciably metabolized.

Pharmacokinetics:

Absorption – Gabapentin bioavailability is not dose-proportional (ie, as dose is increased, bioavailability decreases). A 400 mg dose, for example, is about 25% less bioavailable than a 100 mg dose. Over the recommended dose range of 300 to 600 mg 3 times daily, however, the differences in bioavailability are not large, and bioavailability is about 60%. Food has no effect on the rate and extent of absorption.

Distribution – Gabapentin circulates largely unbound (< 3%) to plasma protein. The apparent volume of distribution after 1 mg IV administration is 58 ± 6 L. In patients with epilepsy, steady-state predose (C_{min}) concentrations of gabapentin in cerebrospinal fluid (CSF) were ≈ 20% of the corresponding plasma concentrations.

Metabolism/Excretion – Gabapentin is eliminated from the systemic circulation by renal excretion as unchanged drug; it is not appreciably metabolized.

Gabapentin elimination half-life is 5 to 7 hours and is unaltered by dose or following multiple dosing. Elimination rate constant, plasma clearance and renal clearance are directly proportional to creatinine clearance (Ccr; see Special Populations). In elderly patients and in patients with impaired renal function, gabapentin plasma clearance is reduced. Gabapentin can be removed from plasma by hemodialysis.

Special populations:

Renal insufficiency – Subjects (n = 60) with renal insufficiency were administered single 400 mg oral doses. The mean half-life ranged from about 6.5 hours (patients with Ccr > 60 ml/min) to 52 hours (Ccr < 30 ml/min) and renal clearance from about 90 ml/min (> 60 ml/min group) to about 10 ml/min (< 30 ml/min). Mean plasma clearance decreased from ≈ 190 to 20 ml/min. Dosage adustment in patients with compromised renal function is necessary (see Administration and Dosage).

Hemodialysis – In a study in anuric subjects (n = 11), the apparent elimination half-life of gabapentin on nondialysis days was about 132 hours; dialysis 3 times a week (4 hours duration) lowered the apparent half-life of gabapentin by about 60%, from 132 to 51 hours. Hemodialysis thus has a significant effect on gabapentin elimination in anuric subjects. Dosage adjustment in patients undergoing hemodialysis is necessary (see Administration and Dosage).

Age – The effect of age was studied in subjects 20 to 80 years of age. Apparent oral clearance of gabapentin decreased as age increased, from about 225 ml/min in those < 30 years of age to about 125 ml/min in those > 70 years of age. Renal clearance also declined with age; however, the decline in the renal clearance of gabapentin with age can largely be explained by the decline in renal function. Reduction of gabapentin dose may be required in patients who have age-related compromised renal function. (See Administration and Dosage).

Clinical trials: The effectiveness of gabapentin as adjunctive therapy was established in three multicenter placebo controlled, double-blind, parallel-group clinical trials in 705 adults with refractory partial seizures. The patients had a history of at least 4 partial seizures per month in spite of receiving one or more antiepileptic drugs at therapeutic levels. In patients continuing to have at least 2 (or 4 in some studies) seizures per month, gabapentin or placebo was then added on to the existing therapy during a 12 week treatment period. Effectiveness was assessed primarily on the basis of the percent of patients with a ≥ 50% reduction in seizure frequency from baseline to treatment (the "responder rate") and a derived measure called response ratio. Response ratio is distributed within the range -1 to +1. A zero value indicates no change while complete elimination of seizures would give a value of - 1; increased seizure rates would give positive values. A response ratio of -0.33 corresponds to a 50% reduction in seizure frequency.

Miscellaneous

GABAPENTIN

One study compared gabapentin 1200 mg/day 3 times daily with placebo. Responder rate was 23% (14/61) in the gabapentin group and 9% (6/66) in the placebo group. Response ratio was also better in the gabapentin group (-0.199) than in the placebo group (-0.044).

A second study compared primarily 1200 mg/day gabapentin (n = 101) divided 3 times daily with placebo (n = 98). Additional smaller gabapentin dosage groups (600 mg/day, n = 53; 1800 mg/day, n = 54) were also studied for information regarding dose response. Responder rate was higher in the gabapentin 600, 1200 and 1800 mg/day groups (17%, 16% and 26%, respectively) than in the placebo group (8%). Response ratio was better in the gabapentin 1200 mg/day group (-0.103) than in the placebo group (-0.022). A better response was seen in the gabapentin 600 mg/day group (-0.105) and 1800 mg/day group (-0.222) than in the 1200 mg/day group.

A third study compared gabapentin 900 mg/day divided 3 times daily (n = 111) and placebo (n = 109). An additional gabapentin 1200 mg/day dosage group (n = 52) provided dose-response data. A statistically significant difference in responder rate was seen in the gabapentin 900 mg/day group (22%) compared to that in the placebo group (10%). Response ratio was also statistically significantly superior in the gabapentin 900 mg/day group (-0.119) compared to that in the placebo group (-0.027), as was response ratio in 1200 mg/day gabapentin (-0.184) compared to placebo.

Analyses were also performed in each study to examine the effect of gabapentin on preventing secondarily generalized tonic-clonic seizures. Patients who experienced a secondarily generalized tonic-clonic seizure in either the baseline or in the treatment period in all three placebo controlled studies were included in these analyses. There were several response ratio comparisons that showed a statistically significant advantage for gabapentin compared to placebo and favorable trends for almost all comparisons.

Analysis of responder rate using combined data from all three studies and all doses (n = 162, gabapentin; n = 89, placebo) also showed a significant advantage for gabapentin over placebo in reducing the frequency of secondarily generalized tonic-clonic seizures.

In two of the three controlled studies, more than one dose of gabapentin was used. Within each study the results did not show a consistently increased response to dose. However, looking across studies, a trend toward increasing efficacy with increasing dose is evident.

Indications:

Adjunctive therapy in the treatment of partial seizures with and without secondary generalization in adults with epilepsy.

Contraindications:

Hypersensitivity to the drug or its ingredients.

Warnings:

Withdrawal-precipitated seizure: Antiepileptic drugs should not be abruptly discontinued because of the possibility of increasing seizure frequency.

Status epilepticus: In the placebo controlled studies, the incidence of status epilepticus in patients receiving gabapentin was 0.6% vs 0.5% with placebo. Among the 2074 patients treated with gabapentin across all studies, 31 (1.5%) had status epilepticus. Of these, 14 patients had no prior history of status epilepticus either before treatment or while on other medications. Because adequate historical data are not available, it is impossible to say whether or not treatment with gabapentin is associated with a higher or lower rate of status epilepticus than would be expected to occur in a similar population not treated with gabapentin.

Sudden and unexplained deaths: During the course of premarketing development of gabapentin, eight sudden and unexplained deaths were recorded among 2203 patients. Some of these could represent seizure-related deaths in which the seizure was not observed (eg, at night). This represents an incidence of 0.0038 deaths per patient-year. Although this rate exceeds that expected in a healthy population matched for age and sex, it is within the range of estimates for the incidence of sudden unexplained deaths in patients with epilepsy not receiving gabapentin.

Carcinogenesis: An unexpectedly high incidence of pancreatic acinar adenocarcinomas was identified in male, but not female, rats. The clinical significance of this finding is unknown. Clinical experience during gabapentin's premarketing development provides no direct means to assess its potential for inducing tumors in humans. In clinical studies comprising 2085 patient-years of exposure, new tumors were reported in 10 patients, and pre-existing tumors worsened in 11 patients during or up to 2 years following discontinuation of gabapentin.

Miscellaneous

GABAPENTIN

Elderly: No systematic studies in geriatric patients have been conducted. Adverse clinical events reported among 59 gabapentin-exposed patients over age 65 did not differ in kind from those reported for younger individuals. The small number of older individuals evaluated, however, limits the strength of any conclusions reached about the influence, if any, of age on the kind and incidence of adverse events or laboratory abnormality associated with the use of gabapentin. Because gabapentin is eliminated primarily by renal excretion, adjust the dose of gabapentin for elderly patients with compromised renal function (see Administration and Dosage). Creatinine clearance is difficult to measure in outpatients and serum creatinine may be reduced in the elderly because of decreased muscle mass.

Pregnancy: Category C. Gabapentin is fetotoxic in rodents, causing delayed ossification of several bones in the skull, vertebrae, forelimbs and hindlimbs. These effects occurred when pregnant mice received oral doses of 1000 or 3000 mg/kg/day during the period of organogenesis, or approximately 1 to 4 times the maximum dose of 3600 mg/day.

When rats were dosed prior to and during mating, and throughout gestation, pups from all dose groups (500, 1000 and 2000 mg/kg/day) were affected. These doses are equivalent to less than ≈ 1 to 5 times the maximum human dose. There was an increased incidence of hydroureter or hydronephrosis in rats. The doses at which the effects occurred are ≈ 1 to 5 times the maximum human dose of 3600 mg/day.

In rabbits, an increased incidence of postimplantation fetal loss occurred in dams exposed to 60, 300 and 1500 mg/kg/day, or less than ≈ 1/4 to 8 times the maximum human dose.

There are no adequate and well controlled studies in pregnant women. Use during pregnancy only if the potential benefit justifies the potential risk to the fetus.

Lactation: It is not known if gabapentin is excreted in breast milk, and the effect on the nursing infant is unknown. However, use in women who are nursing only if the benefits clearly outweigh the risks.

Children: Safety and efficacy in children < 12 years of age have not been established.

Precautions:

Monitoring: Clinical trials data do not indicate that routine monitoring of clinical laboratory parameters is necessary for the safe use of gabapentin. The value of monitoring blood concentrations has not been established. Gabapentin may be used in combination with other antiepileptic drugs without concern for alteration of the blood concentrations of gabapentin or of other antiepileptic drugs.

Drug Interactions:

Gabapentin is not appreciably metabolized nor does it interfere with the metabolism of commonly coadministered anti-epileptic drugs.

Gabapentin Drug Interactions

Precipitant drug	Object drug*		Description
Antacids	Gabapentin	⬇	Antacids reduced the bioavailability of gabapentin by about 20%. This decrease in bioavailability was about 5% when gabapentin was given 2 hours after the antacid. It is recommended that gabapentin be taken at least 2 hours following antacid administration.
Cimetidine	Gabapentin	⬆	The mean apparent oral clearance of gabapentin fell by 14% and Ccr fell by 10%. Thus cimetidine seemed to alter the renal excretion of both gabapentin and creatinine. This small decrease in gabapentin excretion is not expected to be of clinical importance.
Gabapentin	Contraceptives, oral	⬆	The C_{max} of norethindrone was 13% higher when coadministered with gabapentin; this interaction is not expected to be of clinical importance.

* ⬆ = Object drug increased. ⬇ = Object drug decreased.

Drug/Lab test interactions: Because false positive readings were reported with the *Ames N-Multistix SG* dipstick test for urinary protein when gabapentin was added to other antiepileptic drugs, the more specific sulfosalicylic acid precipitation procedure is recommended to determine the presence of urine protein.

Miscellaneous

GABAPENTIN

Adverse Reactions:

The most commonly observed adverse events associated with the use of gabapentin in combination with other antiepileptic drugs, not seen at an equivalent frequency among placebo-treated patients, were somnolence, dizziness, ataxia, fatigue and nystagmus. Approximately 7% of the 2074 individuals who received gabapentin in premarketing clinical trials discontinued treatment because of adverse events. The adverse events most commonly associated with withdrawal were somnolence (1.2%), ataxia (0.8%), fatigue (0.6%), nausea or vomiting (0.6%) and dizziness (0.6%).

Gabapentin Adverse Reactions (%)

Body System/ Adverse Event	Gabapentin[1] (n=543)	Placebo[1] (n=378)	Body System/ Adverse Event	Gabapentin[1] (n=543)	Placebo[1] (n=378)
Body as a whole			*CNS*		
Fatigue	11	5	Somnolence	19.3	8.7
Weight increase	2.9	1.6	Dizziness	17.1	6.9
Back pain	1.8	0.5	Ataxia	12.5	5.6
Peripheral edema	1.7	0.5	Nystagmus	8.3	4
GI			Tremor	6.8	3.2
Dyspepsia	2.2	0.5	Nervousness	2.4	1.9
Dryness of mouth/ throat	1.7	0.5	Dysarthria	2.4	0.5
Constipation	1.5	0.8	Amnesia	2.2	0
Dental abnormalities	1.5	0.3	Depression	1.8	1.1
Increased appetite	1.1	0.8	Abnormal thinking	1.7	1.3
Musculoskeletal			Twitching	1.3	0.5
Myalgia	2	1.9	Abnormal coordination	1.1	0.3
Fracture	1.1	0.8	*Dermatologic*		
Respiratory			Pruritus	1.3	0.5
Rhinitis	4.1	3.7	Abrasion	1.3	0
Pharyngitis	2.8	1.6	*Miscellaneous*		
Coughing	1.8	1.3	Impotence	1.5	1.1
Special senses			Leukopenia	1.1	0.5
Diplopia	5.9	1.9	WBC decreased	1.1	0.5
Amblyopia[2]	4.2	1.1	Vasodilation	1.1	0.3

[1] Plus background antiepileptic drug therapy.
[2] Amblyopia was often described as blurred vision.

Other events in > 1% of patients but equally or more frequent in the placebo group included: Headache; viral infection; fever, nausea or vomiting; abdominal pain; diarrhea; convulsions; confusion; insomnia; emotional lability; rash; acne.

Among the treatment-emergent adverse events occurring at an incidence of at least 10% of gabapentin-treated patients, somnolence and ataxia appeared to exhibit a positive dose-response relationship.

Body as a whole: Asthenia, malaise, facial edema (1%); allergy, generalized edema, weight decrease, chill (0.1% to 1%); strange feelings, lassitude, alcohol intolerance, hangover effect (< 0.1%).

Cardiovascular: Hypertension (1%); hypotension, angina pectoris, peripheral vascular disorder, palpitation, tachycardia, migraine, murmur (0.1% to 1%); atrial fibrillation, heart failure, thrombophlebitis, deep thrombophlebitis, myocardial infarction, cerebrovascular accident, pulmonary thrombosis, ventricular extrasystoles, bradycardia, premature atrial contraction, pericardial rub, heart block, pulmonary embolus, hyperlipidemia, hypercholesterolemia, pericardial effusion, pericarditis (< 0.1%).

GI: Anorexia, flatulence, gingivitis (1%); glossitis, gum hemorrhage, thirst, stomatitis, increased salivation, gastroenteritis, hemorrhoids, bloody stools, fecal incontinence, hepatomegaly (0.1% to 1%); dysphagia, eructation, pancreatitis, peptic ulcer, colitis, blisters in mouth, tooth discoloration, perleche, salivary gland enlarged, lip hemorrhage, esophagitis, hiatal hernia, hematemesis, proctitis, irritable bowel syndrome, rectal hemorrhage, esophageal spasm (< 0.1%).

Miscellaneous

GABAPENTIN

Endocrine: Hyperthyroid, hypothyroid, goiter, hypoestrogen, ovarian failure, epididymitis, swollen testicle, cushingoid appearance (< 0.1%).

Hematologic/Lymphatic: Purpura (1%; most often described as bruises resulting from physical trauma); anemia, thrombocytopenia, lymphadenopathy (0.1% to 1%); WBC count increased, lymphocytosis, non-Hodgkin's lymphoma, bleeding time increased (< 0.1%).

Musculoskeletal: Arthralgia (1%); tendinitis, arthritis, joint stiffness/swelling, positive Romberg test (0.1% to 1%); costochondritis, osteoporosis, bursitis, contracture (< 0.1%).

CNS: Vertigo, hyperkinesia, paresthesia, decreased/absent/increased reflexes, anxiety, hostility (1%); CNS tumors, syncope, abnormal dreaming, aphasia, hypesthesia, intracranial hemorrhage, hypotonia, dysesthesia, paresis, dystonia, hemiplegia, facial paralysis, stupor, cerebellar dysfunction, positive Babinski sign, decreased position sense, subdural hematoma, apathy, hallucination, decrease or loss of libido, agitation, paranoia, depersonalization, euphoria, feeling high, doped-up sensation, suicidal, psychosis (0.1% to 1%); choreoathetosis, orofacial dyskinesia, encephalo pathy, nerve palsy, personality disorder, increased libido, subdued temperament, apraxia, fine motor control disorder, meningismus, local myoclonus, hyperesthesia, hypokinesia, mania, neurosis, hysteria, antisocial reaction, suicide gesture (< 0.1%).

Respiratory: Pneumonia (1%); epistaxis, dyspnea, apnea (0.1% to 1%); mucositis, aspiration pneumonia, hyperventilation, hiccup, laryngitis, nasal obstruction, snoring, bronchospasm, hypoventilation, lung edema (< 0.1%).

Dermatologic: Alopecia, eczema, dry skin, increased sweating, urticaria, hirsutism, seborrhea, cyst, herpes simplex (0.1% to 1%); herpes zoster, skin discoloration, skin papules. photosensitive reaction, leg ulcer, scalp seborrhea, psoriasis, desquamation, maceration, skin nodules, subcutaneous nodule, melanosis, skin necrosis, local swelling (< 0.1%).

GU: Hematuria, dysuria, urination frequency, cystitis, urinary retention/incontinence, vaginal hemorrhage, amenorrhea, dysmenorrhea, menorrhagia, breast cancer, unable to climax, ejaculation abnormal (0.1% to 1%); kidney pain, leukorrhea, genital pruritus, renal stone, acute renal failure, anuria, glycosuria, nephrosis, nocturia, pyuria, urination urgency, vaginal pain, breast pain, testicle pain (< 0.1%).

Special senses: Abnormal vision (1%); cataract, conjunctivitis, dry eyes, eye pain, visual field defect, photophobia, bilateral or unilateral ptosis, eye hemorrhage, hordeolum, hearing loss, earache, tinnitus, inner ear infection, otitis, taste loss, unusual taste, eye twitching, ear fullness (0.1% to 1%); eye itching, abnormal accommodation, perforated ear drum, sensitivity to noise, eye focusing problem, watery eyes, retinopathy, glaucoma, iritis, corneal disorders, lacrimal dysfunction, degenerative eye changes, blindness, retinal degeneration, miosis, chorioretinitis, strabismus, eustachian tube dysfunction, labyrinthitis, otitis externa, odd smell (< 0.1%).

Overdosage:

Symptoms: A lethal dose of gabapentin was not identified in mice and rats receiving single oral doses as high as 8000 mg/kg. Signs of acute toxicity in animals included ataxia, labored breathing, ptosis, sedation, hypoactivity or excitation. Acute oral overdoses of gabapentin up to 49 g have been reported. In these cases, double vision, slurred speech, drowsiness, lethargy and diarrhea were observed. All patients recovered with supportive care.

Treatment: Gabapentin can be removed by hemodialysis. Although hemodialysis has not been performed in the few overdose cases reported, it may be indicated by the patient's clinical state or in patients with significant renal impairment.

Patient Information:

Instruct patients to take gabapentin only as prescribed.

Advise patients that gabapentin may cause dizziness, somnolence and other symptoms and signs of CNS depression. Accordingly, advise them to neither drive a car nor operate other complex machinery until they have gained sufficient experience on gabapentin to gauge whether or not it affects their mental or motor performance adversely.

Miscellaneous

GABAPENTIN

Administration and Dosage:

Approved by the FDA on December 30, 1993.

Recommended for add-on therapy in patients > 12 years of age, taken with or without food.

The effective dose is 900 to 1800 mg/day in divided doses (3 times a day). Titration to an effective dose can take place rapidly, over a few days, giving 300 mg on day 1, 300 mg twice a day on day 2 and 300 mg 3 times a day on day 3. To minimize potential side effects, especially somnolence, dizziness, fatigue and ataxia, the first dose on day 1 may be administered at bedtime. If necessary, the dose may be increased by using 300 or 400 mg 3 times a day up to 1800 mg/day. Dosages up to 2400 to 3600 mg/day bave been well tolerated. The maximum time between doses in the 3 times daily schedule should not exceed 12 hours.

It is not necessary to monitor gabapentin plasma concentrations to optimize therapy. Further, because there are no significant pharmacokinetic interactions with other commonly used anti-epileptic drugs, the addition of gabapentin does not alter the plasma levels of these drugs appreciably.

If gabapentin is discontinued or an alternate anticonvulsant medication is added to the therapy, this should be done gradually over a minimum of 1 week.

Renal function impairment:

Gabapentin Dosage Based on Renal Function

Creatinine clearance (ml/min)	Total daily dose (mg/day)	Dose regimen (mg)
> 60	1200	400 tid
30 to 60	600	300 bid
15 to 30	300	300 qd
< 15	150	300 qod[1]
Hemodialysis	—	200 to 300[2]

[1] Every other day.

[2] Loading dose of 300 to 400 mg in patients who have never received gabapentin, then 200 to 300 mg gabapentin following each 4 hours of hemodialysis.

Rx	**Neurontin** (Parke-Davis)	**Capsules:** 100 mg	Lactose. (PD Neurontin/ 100 mg). White. In 100s and UD 50s.
		300 mg	Lactose. (PD Neurontin/ 300 mg). Yellow. In 100s and UD 50s.
		400 mg	Lactose. (PD Neurontin/ 400 mg). Orange. In 100s and UD 50s.

Miscellaneous

PHENACEMIDE

Actions:

Pharmacology: In animals, phenacemide in doses well below those causing neurological signs elevates the threshold for minimal electroshock convulsions and abolishes the tonic phase of maximal electroshock seizures. It prevents or modifies seizures induced by pentylenetetrazol or other convulsants.

Pharmacokinetics: Phenacemide is well absorbed from the intestine and is degraded by the liver.

Indications:

Severe epilepsy, particularly mixed forms of complex partial (psychomotor) seizures refractory to other drugs.

Warnings:

Toxicity: Phenacemide can produce serious side effects as well as direct organ toxicity. Do not administer unless other available anticonvulsants are ineffective in controlling seizures.

Behavioral effects: Exercise extreme caution in treating patients who have previously shown personality disorders. It may be advisable to hospitalize such patients during the first week of treatment. Personality changes, including suicide attempts and the occurrence of psychoses requiring hospitalization, have been reported during therapy. Apprise the patient and the family of these possibilities so that they can watch for changes in the patient's behavior, such as decreased interest in surroundings, depression or aggressiveness. Withdraw the drug if severe or exacerbated personality changes occur.

Hematologic effects: Perform complete blood counts before instituting therapy, and at monthly intervals thereafter. If no abnormality appears within 12 months, the interval between blood counts may be extended. Blood changes have been reported with leukopenia (leukocyte count ≤ 4,000 per mm^3) the most commonly observed effect. However, aplastic anemia and death have occurred in association with phenacemide therapy. Instruct the patient to report immediately any symptoms indicative of a developing blood dyscrasia such as malaise, sore throat or fever. Marked depression of blood count is an indication for drug withdrawal.

Renal effects: Nephritis has occasionally occurred; examine urine at regular intervals. Abnormal urinary findings are an indication for discontinuing therapy.

Hypersensitivity: Administer with caution to patients with a history of allergy, particularly in association with other anticonvulsants. Discontinue at the first sign of a skin rash or other allergic manifestation.

Hepatic function impairment: Perform liver function tests before and during therapy. Use with caution in patients with a history of previous liver dysfunction. Death attributable to liver damage during therapy has been reported. If jaundice or other signs of hepatitis appear, discontinue use.

Pregnancy: Category D. Phenacemide can cause fetal harm when administered to a pregnant woman. If phenacemide is used during pregnancy, or if the patient becomes pregnant while taking this drug, the patient should be apprised of the potential hazard to the fetus. Refer to the Pregnancy section in the Anticonvulsants Introduction.

Lactation: It is not known whether this drug is excreted in human milk. Because of the potential for serious adverse reactions, decide whether to discontinue nursing or to discontinue the drug, taking into account the importance of the drug to the mother.

Children: Safety and efficacy for use in children < 5 years of age have not been established.

Drug Interactions:

Hydantoins: Serum hydantoin levels and half-life may be increased by phenacemide.

Adverse Reactions:

GI: GI disturbances (8%) including anorexia (5%) and weight loss (< 1%).

CNS: Drowsiness (4%); headache (2%); insomnia (1%); dizziness, paresthesias (< 1%).

Renal: Abnormal urinary findings (including a rise in serum creatinine), nephritis (≤1%).

Miscellaneous: Psychic changes (17%); skin rash (5%); hepatitis (including fatalities), blood dyscrasias (primarily leukopenia) including fatal aplastic anemia (2%); fatigue, fever, muscle pain, palpitations (< 1%).

Miscellaneous

PHENACEMIDE

Overdosage:

Symptoms: Excitement or mania, followed by drowsiness, ataxia and coma. In one case of acute overdosage, dizziness was followed by coma which lasted about 24 hours.

Treatment: Induce emesis; consider gastric lavage as an alternative or adjunct. General supportive measures will be necessary. Refer to General Management of Acute Overdosage. Evaluate liver and kidney function, mental state and the blood-forming organs following recovery.

Patient Information:

Notify physician if jaundice, abdominal pain, pale stools, darkened urine, fever, sore throat, mouth sores, unusual bleeding or bruising, loss of appetite, or skin rash occurs.

May produce drowsiness or dizziness; patients should observe caution while driving or performing other tasks requiring alertness, coordination or physical dexterity.

Administration and Dosage:

Phenacemide may produce serious toxic effects; therefore, keep the dosage at the minimum amount necessary to achieve an adequate therapeutic effect.

Adults: The usual starting dose is 1.5 g/day, administered in 3 divided doses of 500 mg each. After the first week, if seizures are not controlled and the drug is well tolerated, an additional 500 mg may be taken upon arising. In the third week, if necessary, the dosage may be further increased by another 500 mg at bedtime.

Satisfactory results have been noted in some patients on an initial dose of 250 mg 3 times daily. The effective total daily dose usually ranges from 2 to 3 g, up to 5 g.

Children (5 to 10 years): Give approximately ½ the adult dose at the same intervals as for adults.

Concomitant anticonvulsant therapy: May be administered alone or in conjunction with other anticonvulsants. However, exercise extreme caution if other anticonvulsants cause toxic effects similar to phenacemide.

Replacement therapy: When phenacemide is to replace other anticonvulsant medication, withdraw the latter gradually as the dosage of phenacemide is increased to maintain seizure control.

Rx	**Phenurone** (Abbott)	**Tablets:** 500 mg	White, grooved. In 100s.

Miscellaneous

MAGNESIUM SULFATE

Actions:

Pharmacology: Magnesium prevents or controls convulsions by blocking neuromuscular transmission and decreasing the amount of acetylcholine liberated at the end plate by the motor nerve impulse. Magnesium has a CNS depressant effect. Normal plasma magnesium levels range from 1.5 to 3 mEq/L.

One gram of magnesium sulfate provides 8.12 mEq of magnesium.

Pharmacokinetics: With IV use, the onset of anticonvulsant action is immediate and lasts about 30 minutes. With IM use, onset occurs in 1 hour and persists for 3 to 4 hours. Effective anticonvulsant serum levels range from 2.5 or 3 to 7.5 mEq/L. Magnesium is excreted by the kidney.

Indications:

Seizure prevention and control in severe pre-eclampsia or eclampsia without producing deleterious CNS depression in the mother or infant, and in convulsions associated with abnormally low levels of plasma magnesium as a contributing factor.

Acute nephritis in children to control hypertension, encephalopathy and convulsions.

Hypomagnesemia: Magnesium deficiency, prevention and correction in total parenteral nutrition (see the monograph in the IV Nutritional Therapy section).

Unlabeled uses: Magnesium has demonstrated some effectiveness as an agent to inhibit premature labor (tocolytic); however, it is not a first-line agent. It also appears to be beneficial when added to ritodrine therapy, although efficacy has been questioned and an increase in adverse reactions has been observed.

In asthmatic patients who respond poorly to β-agonists, IV magnesium sulfate (1.2 g) may be a beneficial adjunct for treatment of acute exacerbations of moderate to severe asthma.

The use of IV magnesium sulfate appears to be effective in reducing early mortality in patients with acute myocardial infarction when given as soon as possible after the MI and continued for 24 to 48 hours.

Contraindications:

Do not give in toxemia of pregnancy during the 2 hours preceding delivery.

Warnings:

IV use in eclampsia is reserved for immediate control of life-threatening convulsions.

Renal function impairment: Because magnesium is excreted by the kidneys, parenteral use in the presence of renal insufficiency may lead to magnesium intoxication. Use with caution.

Pregnancy: Category A. Magnesium sulfate has not been shown to increase the risk of fetal abnormalities if administered during all trimesters. The possibility of fetal harm appears remote; however, use only if clearly needed.

When administered by continuous IV infusion (especially for > 24 hours preceding delivery) to control convulsions in toxemic mothers, the newborn may show signs of magnesium toxicity, including neuromuscular or respiratory depression. Hypermagnesemia in the newborn may require resuscitation and assisted ventilation via endotracheal intubation or intermittent positive pressure ventilation as well as IV calcium.

Precautions:

Monitoring: Monitor serum magnesium levels and clinical status to avoid overdosage. See Overdosage for serum level/toxicity relationships.

Urine output: Maintain at a level of 100 ml every 4 hours.

Drug Interactions:

Neuromuscular blockers: Magnesium sulfate potentiates the neuromuscular blockade produced by tubocurarine, vecuronium and succinylcholine.

Adverse Reactions:

Miscellaneous:

Magnesium intoxication is the usual cause of adverse effects which include: Flushing, sweating, hypotension, depressed reflexes, flaccid paralysis, hypothermia, circulatory collapse, cardiac and CNS depression proceeding to respiratory paralysis.

Hypocalcemia with signs of tetany secondary to magnesium sulfate therapy for eclampsia has occurred.

Miscellaneous

MAGNESIUM SULFATE

Overdosage:

Symptoms: Sharp drop in blood pressure and respiratory paralysis. ECG changes reported include increased PR interval, increased QRS complex and prolonged QT interval. Heart block and asystole may occur.

An approximate correlation of magnesium toxicity versus serum level is presented in the table.

Effects of Magnesium Toxicity vs Serum Level

Serum level (mEq/L)	Effect
1.5 to 3	Normal serum concentration
4 to 7	"Therapeutic" level for preeclampsia/ eclampsia/convulsions
7 to 10	Loss of deep tendon reflexes, hypotension, narcosis
13 to 15	Respiratory paralysis
> 15	Cardiac conduction affected[1]
> 25	Cardiac arrest

[1] PR interval lengthening, QRS widening, prolonged QT interval dysrhythmias.

Treatment: Provide artificial ventilation until a calcium salt can be injected IV to antagonize the effects of magnesium. A dose of 5 to 10 mEq calcium will usually reverse the respiratory depression and heart block. Peritoneal dialysis or hemodialysis is also effective.

Administration and Dosage:

Individualize dosage. Monitor the patient's clinical status to avoid toxicity. Discontinue as soon as the desired effect is obtained. Repeat doses are dependent on continuing presence of the patellar reflex and adequate respiratory function.

IM: 4 to 5 g of a 50% solution every 4 hours as necessary.

IV: 4 g of a 10% to 20% solution, not exceeding 1.5 ml/min of a 10% solution.

IV infusion: 4 to 5 g in 250 ml of 5% Dextrose or Sodium Chloride, not exceeding 3 ml/min.

Pediatric: IM - 20 to 40 mg/kg in a 20% solution; repeat as necessary.

Rx	**Magnesium Sulfate** (Various, eg, Abbott, American Regent, Pasadena)	**Injection:** 12.5% (1 mEq/ml)	In 8 ml vials.
		50% (4 mEq/ml)	In 2 and 10 ml amps, 10, 20 and 50 ml vials and 5 and 10 ml disp. syringes and 2 ml fill in 5 ml vials.

Miscellaneous

ACETAZOLAMIDE

This is an abbreviated monograph. For complete prescribing information, refer to the Carbonic Anhydrase Inhibitors group monograph.

Actions:

Pharmacology: Acetazolamide has been used as an adjuvant in the treatment of certain CNS dysfunctions (eg, epilepsy). Inhibition of carbonic anhydrase in this area appears to retard abnormal, paroxysmal, excessive discharge from CNS neurons. The mechanism of this anticonvulsant action is not fully understood. Beneficial effects may be related to direct inhibition of carbonic anhydrase, or due to acidosis produced by therapy.

Indications:

Centrencephalic epilepsies (petit mal, unlocalized seizures): The best results have been in petit mal seizures in children. Good results, however, have been seen in both children and adults with other seizure disorders.

Contraindications:

Known allergy or hypersensitivity to sulfonamides; depressed sodium or potassium serum levels; marked kidney and liver disease or dysfunction; suprarenal gland failure; hyperchloremic acidosis.

The sustained release dosage form is not recommended for use as an anticonvulsant.

Administration and Dosage:

Epilepsy: 8 to 30 mg/kg/day in divided doses. Optimum range is 375 to 1000 mg daily.

Concomitant anticonvulsant therapy: When given in combination with other anticonvulsants, the starting dose is 250 mg/day. Increase to levels as indicated above.

Replacement therapy: The change from other medication to acetazolamide should be gradual.

Parenteral: Direct IV administration is preferred because IM administration is painful, due to the alkaline pH of the solution.

Preparation and storage of parenteral solution: Reconstitute each 500 mg vial with at least 5 ml Sterile Water for Injection. Reconstituted solutions retain potency for 1 week if refrigerated; however, since this product contains no preservative, use within 24 hours of reconstitution.

Oral suspension: A 25 mg/ml suspension compounded from 250 mg tablets (with 70% sorbitol in a suspension vehicle of magnesium aluminum silicate, carboxymethylcellulose sodium, sweeteners, flavoring, preservatives, humectants and pH adjusters) was stable for at least 79 days at 5°, 22° and 30°C (41°, 72° and 86°F). Store in amber glass bottles at pH 4 to 5.

Rx	**Acetazolamide** (Various, eg, Moore, Mutual, URL)	**Tablets**: 125 mg	In 100s.
Rx	**Diamox** (Lederle)		(LL D1/Diamox 125). White, scored. In 100s.
Rx	**Acetazolamide** (Various, eg, IDE, Major, Moore, Mutual, Parmed, Qualitest, Schein, UDL, URL)	**Tablets**: 250 mg	In 100s, 1000s and UD 100s.
Rx	**Diamox** (Lederle)		(LL D2/Diamox 250). White, scored. In 100s, 1000s and UD 100s.
Rx	**Diamox** (Lederle)	**Injection**: 500 mg per vial	In 500 mg vials.
Rx	**Acetazolamide** (Various, eg, Bedford Labs)	**Powder for injection, lyophilized**: 500 mg (as sodium)	In vials.

Nondepolarizing Neuromuscular Blockers, Curare Preparations

CURARE PREPARATIONS

Actions:

Pharmacology: Curare preparations block nerve impulses to skeletal muscles at the myoneural junction. This is a nondepolarizing (competitive) neuromuscular blockade. **Metocurine iodide** may not produce the autonomic ganglionic blockade seen with other nondepolarizing muscle relaxants. Metocurine iodide reaches the neuromuscular junction more rapidly than does tubocurarine and is approximately twice as potent.

Repeated doses may have a cumulative effect. The duration of action and degree of muscle relaxation are altered by dehydration, body temperature changes, hypocalcemia, excess magnesium, acid-base imbalance or by some carcinomas. Since these drugs are excreted by the kidneys, severe renal disease, conditions associated with poor renal perfusion (shock states) or hypotension may result in a more prolonged action.

Coadministered general anesthetics, certain antibiotics, abnormal states (eg, acidosis), electrolyte imbalance and neuromuscular disease may potentiate activity of these drugs.

Curare preparations do not affect consciousness or cerebration, and do not relieve pain.

Pharmacokinetics: Following IV infusion, onset of flaccid paralysis occurs within a few minutes. Maximum relaxation occurs within a mean time of ≈ 6 minutes following IV use. Maximal effects persist for 35 to 60 minutes and effective muscle paralysis may persist for 25 to 90 minutes. Complete recovery may require several hours.

Tubocurarine – Approximately 50% is bound in plasma. First phase half-life is < 5 minutes, second phase half-life ranges from 7 to 40 minutes. Third phase half-life is 2 ± 1.1 hours; approximately 30% to 43% is excreted unchanged in the urine. Tubocurarine is also excreted to a lesser extent (up to 11%) in the bile. Approximately 1% undergoes hepatic metabolism (N-demethylation); the metabolite is excreted in bile.

Metocurine – Half-life is 3.6 hours with approximately 50% of the drug excreted unchanged in the urine and approximately 35% bound to plasma globulins.

Indications:

Adjunct to anesthesia to induce skeletal muscle relaxation; to reduce the intensity of muscle contractions in pharmacologically or electrically induced convulsions; to facilitate management of patients undergoing mechanical ventilation.

Tubocurarine is used as a diagnostic agent for myasthenia gravis when the results of tests with neostigmine or edrophonium are inconclusive.

Contraindications:

Allergic reaction or hypersensitivity to these drugs.

Tubocurarine: Patients in whom histamine release is a definite hazard.

Metocurine iodide: Patients sensitive to it or to its iodide content.

Warnings:

Respiratory effects: These drugs may cause respiratory depression and should be used only by those experienced in artificial respiration and administration of oxygen under positive pressure. Facilities for these procedures (including intubation of the trachea and availability of antagonistic agents for reversing nondepolarizing block) should be immediately available. Prolonged apnea may result from overdosage.

Rapid IV injection may produce histamine release with resultant decreased respiratory capacity due to bronchospasm and paralysis of the respiratory muscles. Hypotension may occur due to ganglionic blockade, or it may be a complication of positive pressure respiration. Histamine release with **metocurine** occurs less frequently and is related to dosage and rapidity of administration; cardiovascular effects (eg, changes in the pulse rate, hypotension) are less than those with equipotent doses of tubocurarine and gallamine.

Myasthenia gravis: Use with extreme caution in patients with known myasthenia gravis since prolonged respiratory paralysis may occur. A peripheral nerve stimulator may be valuable in assessing the effects of administration.

Elderly: Dosage requirements and recovery times may be increased.

Nondepolarizing Neuromuscular Blockers, Curare Preparations

CURARE PREPARATIONS

Pregnancy: Category C. Safety for use during pregnancy has not been established. There are no adequate and well controlled studies in pregnant women. Use in women of childbearing potential, especially during early pregnancy, only when clearly needed and when the potential benefits outweigh the potential hazards to the fetus.

Metocurine passes the placental barrier; 6 minutes following IV injection in the mother, fetal plasma concentration is ≈ one-tenth the maternal level.

Tubocurarine in prolonged doses (used in management of tetanus in a patient during early pregnancy), may be associated with fetal contractures. Following a total dose of ≈1.3 g tubocurarine chloride injected IV and IM over 10 days to a 10 to 12 week pregnant woman suffering from severe generalized tetanus, the infant was born at term with joint contractures. The condition was attributed to immobilization of the fetus at the time of joint formation.

Placental transfer and fetal distribution of tubocurarine has been reported. When given during delivery, blood levels in the newborn are directly related to maternal dose and time interval between injection and delivery. Although most infants do not grossly manifest drug effect following delivery, myoneural block has been reported in the newborn following repeated doses of tubocurarine to the mother (245mg total) for prolonged management of eclampsia.

Lactation: It is not known whether these drugs are excreted in breast milk. Exercise caution when administering to a nursing woman.

Children: Metocurine is twice as potent as tubocurarine in children, but the recovery rate is the same. There may be a slight increase in heart rate, but no change in blood pressure or ECG. Doses calculated on the basis of body weight or body surface area may be applicable.

Premature infants and neonates may be more sensitive to these drugs. Infants and children exhibit the same widely variable responses as do adults.

Doses based on body weight appear to be suitable for children (as for adults) whereas doses based on body surface area are more accurate for premature infants and neonates. Incremental doses of 0.25 mg may constitute a useful practical titration to obtain satisfactory conditions in infants and neonates.

Reduce dosage in event of prematurity, acidosis, hypothermia or halothane use.

Precautions:

Concomitant conditions: Use with caution in patients with respiratory depression or with impaired cardiovascular, renal, hepatic, pulmonary or endocrine function. Hypotension can follow rapid injection or the administration of large doses. The action of the drug may be altered by electrolyte imbalance (hypokalemia potentiates the paralysis), body temperature, some carcinomas, dehydration and renal disease.

Histamine release: Use with caution in patients in whom a sudden increase of histamine release is a definite hazard.

Drug accumulation: Tubocurarine accumulates and may be present for several hours after the effects are not clinically apparent. Keep this in mind should a patient require successive doses or a second anesthesia after having previously received this drug.

Sulfite sensitivity: Some of these products may contain sulfites which may cause allergic-type reactions (eg, hives, itching, wheezing, anaphylaxis) in certain susceptible persons. Although the overall prevalence of sulfite sensitivity in the general population is probably low, it is seen more frequently in asthmatics or in atopic nonasthmatic persons. Specific products containing sulfites are identified in the product listings.

Nondepolarizing Neuromuscular Blockers, Curare Preparations

CURARE PREPARATIONS

Drug Interactions:

Nondepolarizing Neuromuscular Blocker (NNB) Drug Interactions (Curare Preparations)

Precipitant drug	Object drug*		Description
Aminoglycosides	NNBs	↑	The action of the NNBs may be enhanced. The more significant event would be protracted respiratory depression.
Benzodiazepines	NNBs	↔	Benzodiazepines may potentiate, counteract or have no effect on actions of NNBs.
Beta blockers	NNBs	↔	Beta blockers may potentiate, counteract or have no effect on actions of NNBs.
Carbamazepine	NNBs	↓	NNBs may have shorter than expected duration or be less effective.
Lincosamides (clindamycin, lincomycin)	NNBs	↑	Actions of the NNBs may be enhanced, possibly resulting in profound and severe respiratory depression.
Corticosteroids	NNBs	↓	Actions of the NNBs may be decreased.
Inhalation anesthetics	NNBs	↑	Inhalation anesthetics potentiate the actions of the NNBs.
Hydantoins	NNBs	↓	NNBs may have a shorter than expected duration or be less effective.
Ketamine	NNBs	↑	Actions of the NNBs may be enhanced, possibly resulting in profound and severe respiratory depression.
Lithium	NNBs	↑	Prolonged recovery time from NNBs may occur, possibly resulting in profound and severe respiratory depression.
Loop diuretics	NNBs	↔	Actions of NNBs may be potentiated or antagonized, perhaps dependent on dosage.
Magnesium sulfate	NNBs	↑	Actions of the NNBs may be potentiated possibly resulting in profound and severe respiratory depression.
Nitrates	NNBs	↑	Actions of the NNBs may be potentiated, possibly resulting in profound and severe respiratory depression.
Piperacillin	NNBs	↑	Actions of the NNBs may be potentiated, possibly producing protracted respiratory depression.
Polypeptide antibiotics	NNBs	↑	Neuromuscular blockade may be enhanced.
Quinine derivatives	NNBs	↑	NNB effects may be enhanced.
Ranitidine	NNBs	↓	Ranitidine may induce profound resistance to the effects of the NNBs.
Theophyllines	NNBs	↓	A dose-dependent reversal of neuromuscular blockade may occur.
Thiazide diuretics	NNBs	↑	NNB effects may be enhanced; respiratory depression may be prolonged.
Thiopurines	NNBs	↓	NNB actions may be decreased or reversed.
Trimethaphan	NNBs	↑	Prolonged apnea may occur.
Verapamil	NNBs	↑	NNB effects may be enhanced; respiratory depression may be prolonged.

* ↓ = Object drug decreased ↑ = Object drug increased ↔ = Undetermined effect

Nondepolarizing Neuromuscular Blockers, Curare Preparations

CURARE PREPARATIONS

Drug/Lab test interactions: In patients with tetanus, continuous administration of tubocurarine in large doses results in production of a factor that interferes with detection of catecholamines in urine when assayed fluorimetrically.

Adverse Reactions:

Most frequent: Prolongation of the drugs' pharmacologic action. Profound and prolonged muscle relaxation with consequent respiratory depression to the point of apnea.

Rare: Hypersensitivity, isolated cases of allergic or anaphylactoid type reactions, idiosyncrasy, interference with physical signs of anesthesia, circulatory depression, ganglionic blockade and histamine release can occur.

Metocurine: Allergic or hypersensitivity reactions to the drug or its iodide content and histamine release when large doses are administered rapidly. Signs of histamine release include erythema, edema, skin rash, flushing, tachycardia, hypotension, bronchospasm and circulatory collapse.

Cardiovascular: Cardiac arrhythmias, cardiac arrest, bradycardia and hypotension. Premature children and neonates may experience a higher frequency of these reactions.

GI: Excessive salivation during very light anesthesia (particularly in the absence of anticholinergic premedication).

Overdosage:

Symptoms: Extended skeletal muscle weakness, decreased respiratory reserve, low tidal volume, prolonged apnea, cardiovascular collapse and sudden release of histamine. Sufficiently excessive doses of nondepolarizing muscle relaxants have no antidote.

Treatment: A peripheral nerve stimulator may be used to assess the degree of residual neuromuscular blockade. For residual neuromuscular blockade with respiratory paralysis or inadequate ventilation, maintain airway and administer manual or mechanical ventilation.

Determine derangements of blood pressure, electrolyte imbalance or circulating blood volume and correct by appropriate fluid and electrolyte therapy.

Hypotension – Determine the etiology. When it is due to ganglionic blockade, treat with fluid and vasopressors which act at the adrenergic receptors.

Apnea – Treat apnea or prolonged curarization with controlled respiration. Edrophonium, pyridostigmine or neostigmine may antagonize the skeletal muscle relaxant action. Accompany or precede neostigmine or pyridostigmine injection by an injection of atropine sulfate or its equivalent to minimize muscarinic cholinergic side effects, notably excessive secretions and bradycardia. Take care to avoid underventilation. The optimum time to administer the antagonist is when the patient is being hyperventilated and the carbon dioxide level of the blood is low. The effects of IV neostigmine last from 30 to 90 minutes; the effects of edrophonium usually dissipate within 5 minutes. Pyridostigmine injected IV produces full recovery in 15 minutes; some patients may require 30 minutes or more. The antagonists are merely adjuncts.

Satisfactory reversal can be judged by return of skeletal muscle tone and respiration; may use a peripheral nerve stimulator to monitor restoration of twitch height. Duration of action of a nondepolarizing neuromuscular blocking agent may exceed that of the antagonist, observe carefully for evidence of recurrent neuromuscular blockade.

Nondepolarizing Neuromuscular Blockers, Curare Preparations

CURARE PREPARATIONS

TUBOCURARINE CHLORIDE

Complete prescribing information begins in the Curare Preparations group monograph.

Administration and Dosage:

Administer IV as a sustained injection over 1 to 1.5 minutes. May also give IM. Rate of injection influences amount given. Although rapid injection may be dangerous, curarization can be accomplished with a smaller dose if given more rapidly.

Administer in incremental doses until desired level of relaxation is achieved.

Individualize dosage. Calculate estimated dosage on the basis of 0.1 to 0.2 mg/kg (amount anticipated to produce limb paresis). If inhalation anesthetics known to enhance the action of curariform drugs are used, or if renal function is compromised, reduce initial tubocurarine dose and note response as a guide to incremental doses.

For general reference, effective doses for a 70 kg adult are ≈ 0.1 to 0.2 mg/kg for paresis of limb musculature, 0.4 to 0.5 mg/kg for abdominal relaxation, and 0.5 to 0.6 mg/kg for endotracheal intubation. In prolonged procedures, repeat incremental doses in 40 to 60 minutes as required. As a precaution, reduce the initial dose to 20 units below the calculated amount.

The following doses are for average patients (70 kg) without altered sensitivity.

Surgery: In an average weight patient, give 40 to 60 units IV when incision is made, and 20 to 30 units in 3 to 5 min if required. For long operations, use supplemental doses of 20 units as required. Calculate on the basis of 0.5 units/lb (1.1 units/kg).

Electroshock therapy: Give just before therapy to reduce severity of convulsions and to prevent fractures. Observe closely until consciousness is regained in case respiratory failure develops. Give 0.5 units/lb (1.1 units/kg) IV slowly as a sustained 1 to 1.5 min injection. Rapid administration is dangerous. Initial dose is 20 units less than this.

Diagnosis of myasthenia gravis: With small doses, a profound exaggeration of this syndrome occurs. The IV dose is 1/15 to 1/5 of the average electroshock therapy dose. Terminate the test within 2 or 3 minutes by IV injection of neostigmine; exaggeration of myasthenia symptoms may be dangerous.

Children: Induction and maintenance in neonates, 0.3 mg/kg; 0.6 mg/kg in children.

Drug incompatibilities: Because of the high pH of barbiturates, a precipitate will form when tubocurarine is combined with such agents as methohexital and thiopental. Give from separate syringes to assure more uniform and predictable results.

Trimethaphan camsylate in solution with tubocurarine at a concentration of 1 g and 60 mg, respectively, per liter of 5% dextrose in water, develops a haze in 3 hours.

Storage: Avoid excessive heat. Do not use if more than a faint color develops.

Rx	**Tubocurarine** (Abbott)	**Injection:** 3 mg (20 units) per ml	In 20 ml vials and 5 ml syringes.[1]
Rx	**Tubocurarine** (Lilly)		In 10 ml vials.[2]
Rx	**Tubocurarine** (Apothecon)		In 10 and 20 ml vials.[3]

[1] With 9 mg benzyl alcohol and 1 mg sodium metabisulfite.
[2] With 0.5% chlorobutanol and 0.1% sodium bisulfite.
[3] With 9 mg benzyl alcohol and 1 mg sodium bisulfite

Nondepolarizing Neuromuscular Blockers, Curare Preparations

METOCURINE IODIDE

Complete prescribing information begins in the Curare Preparations group monograph.

Administration and Dosage:

Administer IV as a sustained injection over 30 to 60 seconds. Do not give IM.

Surgery: Type anesthetic used and nature of surgical procedure influences amount of drug required. Doses of 0.2 to 0.4 mg/kg are satisfactory for endotracheal intubation. Relaxation following initial dose is effective for 25 to 90 minutes (avg. 60 min). Supplement doses (avg. 0.5 to 1 mg) as indicated for surgical relaxation.

Use of strong anesthetics that potentiate effect of neuromuscular blocking drugs reduces requirement for metocurine. Reduce incremental doses by ≈ ⅓ to ½.

Electroshock therapy: 1.75 to 5.5 mg. For initial treatment, give slowly IV as a sustained injection until a head-drop response ensues. After dosage is established, complete subsequent injections in 15 to 50 seconds. Average doses range from 2 to 3 mg.

Drug incompatibilities: Metocurine is unstable in alkaline solutions. When combined with barbiturate solutions, precipitation may occur. Do not administer solutions of barbiturates, meperidine or morphine sulfate from the same syringe.

Rx	**Metocurine Iodide** (Quad)	**Injection:** 2 mg per ml	In 20 ml vials.[1]
Rx	**Metubine Iodide** (Lilly)		In 20 ml vials.[1]

[1] With 0.5% phenol.

Nondepolarizing Neuromuscular Blockers

MIVACURIUM CHLORIDE

Actions:

Pharmacology: Mivacurium is a short-acting, nondepolarizing skeletal muscle relaxant for IV administration. Mivacurium binds competitively to cholinergic receptors on the motor end-plate to antagonize the action of acetylcholine, resulting in a block of neuromuscular transmission. This action is antagonized by acetylcholinesterase inhibitors, such as neostigmine.

Pharmacodynamics – The time to maximum neuromuscular block is similar to intermediate-acting agents (eg, atracurium). The clinically effective duration of action of the stereoisomers in mivacurium is one-third to one-half that of intermediate-acting agents and 2 to 2.5 times that of succinylcholine.

The average ED_{95} (dose required to produce 95% suppression of the adductor pollicis muscle twitch response to ulnar nerve stimulation) of mivacurium is 0.07mg/kg (range, 0.06 to 0.09) in adults receiving opioid/nitrous oxide/oxygen anesthesia. The pharmacodynamics of doses of mivacurium ≥ ED_{95} administered over 5 to 15 seconds during opioid/nitrous oxide/oxygen anesthesia are summarized in the following table. The mean time for spontaneous recovery of the twitch response from 25% to 75% of control amplitude is about 6 minutes (range, 3 to 9) following an initial dose of 0.15mg/kg, and 7 to 8 minutes (range, 4 to 24) following initial doses of 0.2 or 0.25 mg/kg.

Pharmacodynamic Dose Response to Mivacurium During Opioid/Nitrous Oxide/Oxygen Anesthesia[1]

Initial dose (mg/kg)	Time to maximum block (min)	Time to Spontaneous Recovery: 5% recovery (min)	25% recovery[2] (min)	95% recovery[3] (min)	T_4/T_1 ratio ≥ 75%[3] (min)
Adults					
0.07 to 0.1 (n = 47)	4.9 (2-7.6)	11 (7-19)	13 (8-24)	21 (10-36)	21 (10-36)
0.15 (n = 50)	3.3 (1.5-8.8)	13 (6-31)	16 (9-38)	26 (16-41)	26 (15-45)
0.2 (n = 50)	2.5 (1.2-6)	16 (10-29)	20 (10-36)	31 (15-51)	34 (19-56)
0.25 (n = 48)	2.3 (1-4.8)	19 (11-29)	23 (14-38)	34 (22-64)	43 (26-75)
Children 2 to 12 years					
0.11 to 0.12 (n = 17)	2.8 (1.2-4.6)	5 (3-9)	7 (4-10)	—	—
0.2 (n = 18)	1.9 (1.3-3.3)	7 (3-12)	10 (6-15)	19 (14-26)	16 (12-23)
0.25 (n = 9)	1.6 (1-2.2)	7 (4-9)	9 (5-12)	—	—

[1] Values shown are medians of means (range).
[2] Clinically effective duration of neuromuscular block.
[3] Data available for as few as 40% of adults in specific dose groups and for 22% of children in the 0.2 mg/kg dose group due to administration of reversal agents or additional doses of mivacurium prior to 95% recovery or T_4/T_1 ratio recovery to ≥ 75%.

Volatile anesthetics may decrease the dosing requirement for mivacurium and prolong the duration of action; the magnitude of these effects may be increased as the concentration of the volatile agent is increased. Isoflurane and enflurane may decrease the effective dose of mivacurium by as much as 25%, and may prolong the clinically effective duration of action and decrease the average infusion requirement by as much as 35% to 40%. Halothane has little or no effect on the ED_{50} of mivacurium, but may prolong the duration of action and decrease the average infusion requirement by as much as 20% (see Administration and Dosage).

Administration over 60 seconds does not alter the time to maximum neuromuscular block or the duration of action. The duration of action of the stereoisomers of mivacurium may be prolonged in patients with reduced plasma cholinesterase (pseudocholinesterase) activity (see Precautions and Administration and Dosage).

Nondepolarizing Neuromuscular Blockers

MIVACURIUM CHLORIDE

Interpatient variability in duration of action occurs. However, analysis of data from 224 diverse patients in clinical studies indicated that approximately 90% of the patients had clinically effective durations of block within 8 minutes of the median duration predicted from the dose-response data. Variations in plasma cholinesterase activity were not associated with clinically significant effects or duration. The variability in duration, however, was greater in patients with plasma cholinesterase activity at or slightly below the lower limit of the normal range.

A dose of 0.15 mg/kg (2 x ED_{95}) administered during the induction of anesthesia produced generally good-to-excellent conditions for tracheal intubation in 2.5 minutes. Doses of 0.2 and 0.25 mg/kg (3 and 3.5 x ED_{95}) yielded similar conditions in 2 minutes.

Repeated administration of maintenance doses or continuous infusion for up to 2.5 hours is not associated with development of tachyphylaxis or cumulative neuromuscular blocking effects in ASA Physical Status I-II patients. Spontaneous recovery of neuromuscular function after infusion is independent of the duration of infusion and comparable to recovery reported for single doses.

The neuromuscular block produced by the stereoisomers in mivacurium is readily antagonized by anticholinesterase agents. The more profound the neuromuscular block at the time of reversal, the longer the time and the greater the dose of anticholinesterase agent required for recovery of neuromuscular function.

Children: In children 2 to 12 years, mivacurium has a higher ED_{95} (0.1mg/kg), faster onset, and shorter duration of action than in adults. The mean time for spontaneous recovery of the twitch response from 25% to 75% of control amplitude is about 5 minutes (n = 4) following an initial dose of 0.2 mg/kg. Recovery following reversal is faster in children than in adults.

Hemodynamics – Administration of doses up to and including 0.15mg/kg (2 x ED_{95}) over 5 to 15 seconds to ASA Physical Status I-II patients during opioid/nitrous oxide/oxygen anesthesia is associated with minimal change in mean arterial blood pressure (MAP) or heart rate.

Higher doses of ≥ 0.2 mg/kg (≥ 3 x ED_{95}) may be associated with transient decreases in MAP and increases in heart rate in some patients. These decreases in MAP are usually maximal within 1 to 3 minutes following the dose, typically resolved without treatment in an additional 1 to 3 minutes, and are usually associated with increases in plasma histamine concentration. Decreases in MAP can be minimized by administering mivacurium over 30 or 60 seconds.

Analysis of 426 patients in clinical studies receiving initial doses ≤ 0.3mg/kg (2 times the recommended intubating dose) during anesthesia showed that high initial doses and a rapid rate of injection contributed to a greater probability of experiencing a decrease of ≥ 30% in MAP after administration. Obese patients also had a greater probability of experiencing a decrease of ≥ 30% in MAP when dosed on the basis of actual body weight, thereby receiving a larger dose than if dosed on the basis of ideal body weight.

Children experience minimal changes in MAP or heart rate after doses ≤ 0.2 mg/kg over 5 to 15 seconds, but higher doses (≥ 0.25 mg/kg) may be associated with transient decreases in MAP.

Pharmacokinetics:

Metabolism/Excretion – Enzymatic hydrolysis by plasma cholinesterase is the primary mechanism for inactivation of mivacurium and yields a quaternary alcohol and a quaternary monoester metabolite. Renal and biliary excretion of unchanged mivacurium are minor elimination pathways; urine and bile are important elimination pathways for the two metabolites. Each metabolite is unlikely to produce clinically significant neuromuscular, autonomic or cardiovascular effects.

The following table describes the results from a study of 9 adult patients receiving an infusion of mivacurium at 5 mcg/kg/min for 60 minutes followed by 10 mcg/kg/min for 60 minutes. Mivacurium is a mixture of isomers which do not interconvert in vivo. The two more potent isomers, *cis-trans* (36% of the mixture) and *trans-trans* (57% of the mixture), have very high clearances that exceed cardiac output reflecting the extensive metabolism by plasma cholinesterase. The volume of distribution is relatively small, reflecting limited tissue distribution secondary to the polarity and large molecular weight of mivacurium. The combination of high metabolic clearance and low distribution volume results in the short elimination half-life of approximately 2 minutes for the two active isomers. The pharmacokinetics of the *cis-trans* and *trans-trans* isomers are dose-proportional. The *cis-cis* isomer (6% of the mixture) has approximately one-tenth the neuromuscular blocking potency of the *trans-trans* and *cis-trans* isomers in cats and data suggest that it produces minimal (< 5%) neuromuscular block during a 2 hour infusion.

Nondepolarizing Neuromuscular Blockers

MIVACURIUM CHLORIDE

Stereoisomer Pharmacokinetic Parameters of Mivacurium in ASA Physical Status I-II Adult Patients (n = 9)[1]			
Parameter	*trans-trans* isomer	*cis-trans* isomer	*cis-cis* isomer
Elimination half-life (min)	2.3 (1.4-3.6)	2.1 (0.8-4.8)	55 (32-102)
Volume of distribution (L/kg)	0.15 (0.06-0.24)	0.27 (0.08-0.56)	0.31 (0.18-0.46)
Plasma clearance (ml/min/kg)	53 (32-105)	99 (52-230)	4.2 (2.4-5.4)

[1] Values shown are mean (range).

Special populations: Preliminary evidence indicates that reduced clearance of one or more isomers is responsible for the longer duration of action of mivacurium seen in patients with end-stage kidney or liver disease. The data did not provide a pharmacokinetic explanation for the 15% to 20% longer duration of block seen in the elderly.

Indications:

As an adjunct to general anesthesia, to facilitate tracheal intubation and to provide skeletal muscle relaxation during surgery or mechanical ventilation.

Contraindications:

Allergic hypersensitivity to mivacurium or other benzylisoquinolinium agents, as manifested by reactions such as urticaria, severe respiratory distress or hypotension; use of multi-dose vials in patients with allergy to benzyl alcohol.

Warnings:

Administration: Administer in carefully adjusted dosage by or under the supervision of experienced clinicians who are familiar with the drug's actions and the possible complications of its use. The drug should not be administered unless personnel and facilities for resuscitation and life support (tracheal intubation, artificial ventilation, oxygen therapy), and an antagonist of mivacurium are immediately available. Use a peripheral nerve stimulator to measure neuromuscular function during administration in order to monitor drug effect.

Conscious patients: Mivacurium has no known effect on consciousness, pain threshold, or cerebration. To avoid distress to the patient, neuromuscular block should not be induced before unconsciousness.

Renal function impairment: The clinically effective duration of action of 0.15 mg/kg mivacurium was about 1.5 times longer in patients with end-stage kidney disease, presumably due to reduced clearance of one or more isomers.

Hepatic function impairment: The clinically effective duration of action of 0.15 mg/kg mivacurium was 3 times longer in patients with end-stage liver disease than in healthy patients and is likely related to the markedly decreased plasma cholinesterase activity (30% of healthy patient values) which could decrease the clearance of one or more isomers.

Elderly: Mivacurium was safely administered during clinical trials to 64 elderly patients (≥ 65 years of age), including 31 patients with significant cardiovascular disease. The duration of neuromuscular block may be slightly longer in elderly patients than in young adult patients.

Pregnancy: Category C. There are no adequate and well controlled studies in pregnant women. Use during pregnancy only if the potential benefit justifies the potential risk to the fetus.

Lactation: It is not known whether mivacurium or any of the stereoisomers are excreted in breast milk. Exercise caution following administration to a nursing woman.

Children: Mivacurium has not been studied in children < 2 years of age (see Administration and Dosage for use in children 2 to 12 years of age). In children 2 to 12 years of age, mivacurium has a faster onset, a shorter duration, and recovery following reversal is faster compared to adults (see Pharmacodynamics).

MIVACURIUM CHLORIDE

Precautions:

Histamine release: Although mivacurium is not a potent histamine releaser, the possibility of substantial histamine release must be considered. Release of histamine is related to the dose and speed of injection.

Exercise caution in administering mivacurium to patients with clinically significant cardiovascular disease and patients with any history suggesting a greater sensitivity to the release of histamine or related mediators (eg, asthma). In such patients, use an initial dose of ≤ 0.15 mg/kg, administered over 60 seconds; maintain adequate hydration and carefully monitor hemodynamic status.

Obese patients may be more likely to experience clinically significant transient decreases in MAP than non-obese patients when the dose is based on actual rather than ideal body weight. Determine the initial dose using the patient's ideal body weight.

Bradycardia: Recommended doses have no clinically significant effects on heart rate; therefore, mivacurium will not counteract the bradycardia produced by many anesthetic agents or by vagal stimulation.

Neuromuscular diseases: Neuromuscular blocking agents may have a profound effect in patients with neuromuscular diseases (eg, myasthenia gravis and the myasthenic syndrome). In these and other conditions in which prolonged neuromuscular block is a possibility (eg, carcinomatosis), the use of a peripheral nerve stimulator and a dose of ≤ 0.015 to 0.02 mg/kg is recommended.

Burn patients: Mivacurium has not been studied, but resistance to nondepolarizing neuromuscular blocking agents may develop in patients with burns depending upon the time elapsed since the injury and the size of the burn. Patients with burns may have reduced plasma cholinesterase activity which may offset this resistance.

Acid-base or serum electrolyte abnormalities may potentiate or antagonize the action of neuromuscular blocking agents; their action may be enhanced by magnesium salts administered for the management of toxemia of pregnancy.

Reduced plasma cholinesterase activity: Mivacurium is metabolized by plasma cholinesterase. Prolonged neuromuscular block following administration of mivacurium must be considered in patients with reduced plasma cholinesterase (pseudocholinesterase) activity. Plasma cholinesterase activity may be diminished in the presence of genetic abnormalities of plasma cholinesterase (eg, patients heterozygous or homozygous for the atypical plasma cholinesterase gene), pregnancy, liver or kidney disease, malignant tumors, infections, burns, anemia, decompensated heart disease, peptic ulcer or myxedema. Plasma cholinesterase activity may also be diminished by chronic administration of oral contraceptives, glucocorticoids, or certain MAO inhibitors and by irreversible inhibitors of plasma cholinesterase (eg, organophosphate insecticides, echothiophate, certain antineoplastic drugs).

Mivacurium has been used safely in patients heterozygous for the atypical plasma cholinesterase gene. At doses of 0.1 to 0.2 mg/kg, the clinically effective duration of action was 8 to 11 minutes longer in patients heterozygous for the atypical gene than in genotypically normal patients.

As with succinylcholine, patients homozygous for the atypical plasma cholinesterase gene (1 in 2500 patients) are extremely sensitive to the neuromuscular blocking effect of mivacurium. In three such adult patients, a small dose of 0.03 mg/kg (approximately the ED_{10-20} in genotypically normal patients) produced complete neuromuscular block for 26 to 128 minutes. Once spontaneous recovery had begun, neuromuscular block in these patients was antagonized with conventional doses of neostigmine. One adult patient, who was homozygous for the atypical plasma cholinesterase gene, received a dose of 0.18 mg/kg and exhibited complete neuromuscular block for about 4 hours. The patient was extubated after 8 hours; reversal was not attempted. Use with great caution, if at all, in patients known to be or suspected of being homozygous for the atypical plasma cholinesterase gene.

Drug Interactions:

Mivacurium can be expected to interact similarly to other nondepolarizing neuromuscular blockers. Refer to the Nondepolarizing Neuromuscular Blockers – Curare Preparations monograph.

MIVACURIUM CHLORIDE

Adverse Reactions:

Prolonged neuromuscular block was reported in 3 of 2074 patients. The most common adverse experience was transient, dose-dependent cutaneous flushing about the face, neck or chest, most frequently after the initial dose in about 20% of adult patients who received 0.15 mg/kg over 5 to 15 seconds. Flushing typically began within 1 to 2 minutes after the dose and lasted for 3 to 5 minutes. Of 60 patients who experienced flushing after 0.15 mg/kg, one patient also experienced mild hypotension that was not treated, and one patient experienced moderate wheezing that was successfully treated.

Cardiovascular: Flushing (15%); tachycardia, bradycardia, cardiac arrhythmia, phlebitis (<1%).

Respiratory: Bronchospasm, wheezing, hypoxemia (< 1%).

Dermatologic: Rash, urticaria, erythema, injection site reaction (< 1%).

Hypotension: 1% to 2% of healthy adults given ≥ 0.2 mg/kg over 5 to 15 seconds and 2% to 4% of cardiac surgery patients given ≥ 0.2 mg/kg over 60 seconds were treated for decreases in blood pressure associated with the administration of mivacurium.

Other: Prolonged drug effect, dizziness, muscle spasms (< 1%).

Overdosage:

Overdosage with neuromuscular blocking agents may result in neuromuscular block beyond the time needed for surgery and anesthesia. The primary treatment is maintenance of a patent airway and controlled ventilation until recovery of normal neuromuscular function is ensured. Once evidence of recovery from neuromuscular block is observed, further recovery may be facilitated by administration of an anticholinesterase agent (eg, neostigmine, edrophonium) in conjunction with an appropriate anticholinergic agent. Overdosage may increase the risk of hemodynamic side effects, especially decreases in blood pressure. If needed, cardiovascular support may be provided by proper positioning of the patient, fluid administration, or vasopressor agent administration.

Antagonism of neuromuscular block: Antagonists (such as neostigmine) should not be administered when complete neuromuscular block is evident or suspected. Use a peripheral nerve stimulator to evaluate recovery and antagonism of neuromuscular block. Administration of 0.03 to 0.064 mg/kg neostigmine or 0.5 mg/kg edrophonium at ≈ 10% recovery from neuromuscular block produced 95% recovery of the muscle twitch response and a T_4/T_1 ratio ≥ 75% in about 10 minutes. The times from 25% recovery of the muscle twitch response to T_4/T_1 ratio ≥ 75% following these doses of antagonists averaged about 7 to 9 minutes. In comparison, average times for spontaneous recovery from 25% to T_4/T_1 ≥ 75% were 12 to 13 minutes. Evaluate patients receiving antagonists for adequate clinical evidence of antagonism (eg, 5 second head lift and grip strength). Ventilation must be supported until no longer required.

Antagonism may be delayed in the presence of debilitation, carcinomatosis, and the concomitant use of certain broad-spectrum antibiotics, anesthetic agents and other drugs which enhance neuromuscular block or cause respiratory depression. Management is the same as that of prolonged neuromuscular block.

Administration and Dosage:

Approved by the FDA on January 22, 1992.

Administer IV only. Individualize doses. Factors that may warrant dosage adjustment include but may not be limited to: The presence of significant kidney, liver or cardiovascular disease, obesity (patients weighing ≥ 30% more than ideal body weight for height), asthma, reduction in plasma cholinesterase activity and the presence of inhalational anesthetic agents. The use of a peripheral nerve stimulator will permit the most advantageous use of mivacurium, minimize the possibility of overdosage or underdosage, and assist in the evaluation of recovery.

Renal or hepatic impairment: 0.15 mg/kg for facilitation of tracheal intubation. However, the clinically effective duration of block produced by this dose is about 1.5 times longer in patients with end-stage kidney disease and about 3 times longer in patients with end-stage liver disease. Decrease infusion rates by as much as 50% in these patients depending on the degree of renal or hepatic impairment.

Nondepolarizing Neuromuscular Blockers

MIVACURIUM CHLORIDE

Reduced plasma cholinesterase activity: Use with great caution, if at all, in patients known or suspected of being homozygous for the atypical plasma cholinesterase gene (see Warnings). Doses of 0.03 mg/kg produced complete neuromuscular block for 26 to 128 minutes in three such patients; thus initial doses > 0.03 mg/kg are not recommended in homozygous patients. Infusions of mivacurium are not recommended in homozygous patients.

Mivacurium has been used safely in patients heterozygous for the atypical plasma cholinesterase gene and in genotypically normal patients with reduced plasma cholinesterase activity. After recommended intubating doses, the clinically effective duration of block in heterozygous patients may be approximately 10 minutes longer. Use lower infusion rates in these patients.

Drugs or conditions causing potentiation of or resistance to neuromuscular block: Cachectic or debilitated patients, patients with neuromuscular diseases or carcinomatosis. In these or other patients in whom potentiation of neuromuscular block or difficulty with reversal may be anticipated, decrease initial dose. A test dose of ≤ 0.015 to 0.02 mg/kg (lower end of the dose-response curve) is recommended.

The neuromuscular blocking action of mivacurium is potentiated by isoflurane or enflurane anesthesia. The initial dose of 0.15 mg/kg may be used for intubation prior to the administration of these agents. If mivacurium is first administered after establishment of stable-state isoflurane or enflurane anesthesia, reduce the initial dose by as much as 25%, and reduce the infusion rate by as much as 35% to 40%. A greater potentiation of the neuromuscular blocking action may be expected with higher concentrations of enflurane or isoflurane. The use of halothane requires no adjustment of the initial dose of mivacurium but may prolong the duration of action and decrease the average infusion rate by as much as 20%.

When mivacurium is administered to patients receiving certain antibiotics, magnesium salts, lithium, local anesthetics, procainamide and quinidine, longer durations of neuromuscular block may be expected and infusion requirements may be lower.

Burns: While patients with burns develop resistance to nondepolarizing neuromuscular blocking agents, they may also have reduced plasma cholinesterase activity. Consequently a test dose of not more than 0.015 to 0.02 mg/kg is recommended, followed by additional dosing guided by the use of a neuromuscular block monitor.

Cardiovascular disease: In patients with clinically significant cardiovascular disease, use an initial dose of ≤ 0.15 mg/kg, administered over 60 seconds.

Obesity (patients weighing ≥ 30% more than their ideal body weight [IBW]): Determine the initial dose using the patient's IBW, according to the following formulas

Men: IBW in kg = (106 + [6 x inches in height above 5 feet])/2.2

Women: IBW in kg = (100 + [5 x inches in height above 5 feet])/2.2

Allergy and sensitivity: In patients with any history suggestive of a greater sensitivity to the release of histamine or related mediators (eg, asthma), use an initial dose of ≤ 0.15 mg/kg, administered over 60 seconds.

Adults:

Initial doses – 0.15 mg/kg administered over 5 to 15 seconds for facilitation of tracheal intubation for most patients. When administered as a component of a thiopental/opioid/nitrous oxide/oxygen induction-intubation technique, 0.15 mg/kg (2 x ED_{95}) produces generally good-to-excellent conditions for tracheal intubation in 2.5 minutes. Lower doses may result in a longer time for development of satisfactory intubation conditions. Administration of doses ≥ 0.2 mg/kg is associated with the development of transient decreases in blood pressure in some patients.

Clinically effective neuromuscular block may last for 15 to 20 minutes (range, 9 to 38) and spontaneous recovery may be 95% complete in 25 to 30 minutes (range, 16 to 41) following 0.15 mg/kg administered to patients receiving opioid/nitrous oxide/oxygen anesthesia. Maintenance dosing is generally required approximately 15 minutes after an initial dose of 0.15 mg/kg during opioid/nitrous oxide/oxygen anesthesia. Maintenance doses of 0.1 mg/kg each provide approximately 15 minutes of additional clinically effective block. For shorter or longer durations of action, smaller or larger maintenance doses may be administered.

Nondepolarizing Neuromuscular Blockers

MIVACURIUM CHLORIDE

Continuous infusion may be used to maintain neuromuscular block. Upon early evidence of spontaneous recovery from an initial dose, an initial infusion rate of 9 to 10 mcg/kg/min is recommended. If continuous infusion is initiated simultaneously with the administration of an initial dose, use a lower initial infusion rate (eg, 4 mcg/kg/min). In either case, adjust the initial infusion rate according to the response to peripheral nerve stimulation and to clinical criteria. On average, an infusion rate of 6 to 7 mcg/kg/min (range, 1 to 15) will maintain neuromuscular block within the range of 89% to 99% for extended periods in adults receiving opioid/nitrous oxide/oxygen anesthesia. Consider reduction of the infusion rate by up to 35% to 40% when mivacurium is administered during stable-state conditions of isoflurane or enflurane anesthesia.

Children:

Initial doses – Dosage requirements on a mg/kg basis are higher in children, and onset and recovery of neuromuscular block occur more rapidly. The recommended dose for facilitating tracheal intubation in children 2 to 12 years of age is 0.2 mg/kg administered over 5 to 15 seconds. When administered during stable opioid/nitrous oxide/oxygen anesthesia, 0.2 mg/kg produces maximum neuromuscular block in an average of 1.9 minutes (range, 1.3 to 3.3) and clinically effective block for 10 minutes (range, 6 to 15). Maintenance doses are generally required more frequently in children than in adults. Administration of mivacurium doses above the recommended range (> 0.2 mg/kg) is associated with transient decreases in MAP in some children.

Continuous infusion – Children require higher mivacurium infusion rates. During opioid/nitrous oxide/oxygen anesthesia, the infusion rate required to maintain 89% to 99% neuromuscular block averages 14 mcg/kg/min (range, 5 to 31). The principles for infusion in adults are also applicable to children (see above).

Infusion rate tables: For adults and children, the amount of infusion solution required per hour depends upon the clinical requirements of the patient, the concentration of mivacurium in the infusion solution and the patient's weight. Consider the contribution of the infusion solution to the fluid requirements of the patient. The following tables provide guidelines for delivery in ml/hr (equivalent to microdrops/min when 60 microdrops = 1 ml) of mivacurium premixed infusion (0.5 mg/ml) and of mivacurium injection (2 mg/ml).

Infusion Rates for Maintenance of Neuromuscular Block During Opioid/Nitrous Oxide/Oxygen Anesthesia Using Mivacurium Premixed Infusion (0.5 mg/ml)

Patient weight (kg)	Drug delivery rate (mcg/kg/min)									
	4	5	6	7	8	10	14	16	18	20
	Infusion delivery rate (ml/hr)									
10	5	6	7	8	10	12	17	19	22	24
15	7	9	11	13	14	18	25	29	32	36
20	10	12	15	17	19	24	34	38	43	48
25	12	15	18	21	24	30	42	48	54	60
35	17	21	26	29	34	42	59	67	76	84
50	24	30	36	42	48	60	84	96	108	120
60	29	36	43	50	58	72	101	115	130	144
70	34	42	50	59	67	84	118	134	151	168
80	39	48	58	67	77	96	134	154	173	192
90	44	54	65	76	86	108	151	173	194	216
100	48	60	72	84	96	120	168	192	216	240

Nondepolarizing Neuromuscular Blockers

MIVACURIUM CHLORIDE

Infusion Rates for Maintenance of Neuromuscular Block During Opioid/Nitrous Oxide/Oxygen Anesthesia Using Mivacurium Injection (2 mg/ml)

Patient weight (kg)	Drug delivery rate (mcg/kg/min)									
	4	5	6	7	8	10	14	16	18	20
	Infusion delivery rate (ml/hr)									
10	1.2	1.5	1.8	2.1	2.4	3	4.2	4.8	5.4	6
15	1.8	2.3	2.7	3.2	3.6	4.5	6.3	7.2	8.1	9
20	2.4	3	3.6	4.2	4.8	6	8.4	9.6	10.8	12
25	3	3.8	4.5	5.3	6	7.5	10.5	12	13.5	15
35	4.2	5.3	6.3	7.4	8.4	10.5	14.7	16.8	18.9	21
50	6	7.5	9	10.5	12	15	21	24	27	30
60	7.2	9	10.8	12.6	14.4	18	25.2	28.8	32.4	36
70	8.4	10.5	12.6	14.7	16.8	21	29.4	33.6	37.8	42
80	9.6	12	14.4	16.8	19.2	24	33.6	38.4	43.2	48
90	10.8	13.5	16.2	18.9	21.6	27	37.8	43.2	48.6	54
100	12	15	18	21	24	30	42	48	54	60

Mivacurium premixed infusion in flexible plastic containers:

Caution – Do not introduce additives into this solution. Do not administer unless solution is clear and container is undamaged. Mivacurium premixed infusion is intended for single patient use only. Discard the unused portion.

Warning – Do not use flexible plastic container in series connections.

Mivacurium injection compatibility and admixtures:

Y-site administration – Mivacurium may not be compatible with alkaline solutions having a pH > 8.5 (eg, barbiturate solutions).

Mivacurium is compatible with: 5% Dextrose Injection, USP; 0.9% Sodium Chloride Injection, USP; 5% Dextrose and 0.9% Sodium Chloride Injection, USP; Lactated Ringer's Injection, USP; 5% Dextrose in Lactated Ringer's Injection; sufentanil; alfentanil; fentanyl; midazolam; droperidol.

Dilution stability: Mivacurium diluted to 0.5 mg/ml in 5% Dextrose Injection, USP, 5% Dextrose and 0.9% Sodium Chloride Injection, USP, 0.9% Sodium Chloride Injection, USP, Lactated Ringer's Injection, USP or 5% Dextrose in Lactated Ringer's Injection is physically and chemically stable when stored in PVC (polyvinyl chloride) bags at 5° to 25°C (41° to 77°F) for up to 24 hours. Prepare admixtures of mivacurium for single patient use only and use within 24 hours of preparation. Discard the unused portion of diluted mivacurium after each use.

Storage: Store injection and premixed infusion at room temperature of 15° to 25°C (59° to 77°F). Avoid exposure to direct ultraviolet light. Do not freeze. Avoid excessive heat.

Rx	**Mivacron** (Glaxo Wellcome)	**Injection:** 0.5 mg/ml	Premixed infusion in 5% Dextrose Injection, USP in 50 ml (100 ml unit) flexible plastic containers.
		2 mg/ml	In 5 and 10 ml single use vials in Water for Injection.

ROCURONIUM BROMIDE

Actions:

Pharmacology: Rocuronium injection is a nondepolarizing neuromuscular blocking agent with a rapid to intermediate onset (depending on dose) and intermediate duration. It acts by competing for cholinergic receptors at the motor end-plate. This action is antagonized by acetylcholinesterase inhibitors such as neostigmine and edrophonium.

Intubating Conditions in Patients with Intubations Initiated at 60 to 70 seconds

Rocuronium dose (mg/kg; administered over 5 sec)	Patients with excellent or good intubating conditions[1]	Time to completion of intubation (min; median)
Adults 18-64 yrs		
0.45 (n = 43)	86%	1.6
0.6 (n = 51)	96%	1.6
Pediatric 3 mo-1 yr		
0.6 (n = 18)	100%	1
Pediatric 1-12 yrs		
0.6 (n = 12)	100%	1

[1] Excellent intubating conditions = jaw relaxed, vocal cords apart and immobile, no diaphragmatic movement; good intubating conditions = same as excellent but with some diaphragmatic movement.

Time to Onset and Clinical Duration Following Initial (Intubating) Dose (Median)

Rocuronium dose (mg/kg; administered over 5 sec)	Time to ≥ 80% block (min)	Time to maximum block (min)	Clinical duration (min)
Adults 18-64 yrs			
0.45 (n = 50)	1.3	3	22
0.6 (n = 142)	1	1.8	31
0.9 (n = 20)	1.1	1.4	58
1.2 (n = 18)	0.7	1	67
Elderly ≥ 65 yrs			
0.6 (n = 31)	2.3	3.7	46
0.9 (n = 5)	2	2.5	62
1.2 (n = 7)	1	1.3	94
Pediatric 3 mo-1 yr			
0.6 (n = 17)	-	0.8	41
0.8 (n = 9)	-	0.7	40
Pediatric 1-12 yrs			
0.6 (n = 27)	0.8	1	26
0.8 (n = 18)	-	0.5	30

There were no reports of less than satisfactory clinical recovery of neuromuscular function.

The neuromuscular blocking action of rocuronium may be enhanced in the presence of potent inhalation anesthetics.

Hemodynamics – There were no dose-related effects on the incidence of changes from baseline (≥ 30%) in mean arterial blood pressure (MAP) or heart rate associated with rocuronium over the dose range of 0.12 to 1.2 mg/kg within 5 min after rocuronium administration and prior to intubation. Increases or decreases in MAP were observed in 2% to 5% of geriatric and other adult patients and in about 1% of pediatric patients. Heart rate changes (≥ 30%) occurred in ≤ 2% of geriatric and other adult patients. Tachycardia (≥ 30%) occurred in 12 of 127 children. Laryngoscopy and tracheal intubation following rocuronium administration were accompanied by transient tachycardia (≥ 30% increases) in about 33% of adult patients under opioid/nitrous oxide/oxygen anesthesia. Animal studies have indicated that the ratio of vagal:neuromuscular block following rocuronium administration is less than vecuronium but greater than pancuronium. The tachycardia observed in some patients may result from this vagal blocking activity.

Histamine release – Clinically significant concentrations of plasma histamine occurred in 1 of 88 patients. Clinical signs of histamine release (eg, flushing, rash, bronchospasm) associated with the administration of rocuronium were reported in 9 of 1137 (0.8%) patients.

Nondepolarizing Neuromuscular Blockers

ROCURONIUM BROMIDE

Pharmacokinetics: Following IV administration, rocuronium plasma levels follow a three compartment open model. The rapid distribution half-life is 1 to 2 min and the slower distribution half-life is 14 to 18 min. Rocuronium is ≈ 30% bound to plasma proteins. In geriatric and other adult surgical patients undergoing either opioid/nitrous oxide/oxygen or inhalational anesthesia the observed pharmacokinetic profile was essentially unchanged.

Rocuronium Pharmacokinetic Parameters					
Parameters	Adults (n = 22; ages 27 to 58 yrs)	Elderly (n = 20; ≥ 65 yrs)	Normal renal/ hepatic function (n = 10)	Renal transplant patients (n = 10)	Hepatic dysfunction patients (n = 9)
Clearance (L/kg/hr)	0.25	0.21	0.16	0.13	0.13
Volume of distribution at steady state (L/kg)	0.25	0.22	0.26	0.34	0.53
Half-life β elimination (hrs)	1.4	1.5	2.4	2.4	4.3

In animals, rocuronium is eliminated primarily by the liver. The rocuronium analog 17-desacetyl-rocuronium, a metabolite, has been rarely observed in the plasma or urine of humans administered single doses of 0.5 to 1 mg/kg with or without a subsequent infusion (for up to 12 hrs). In the cat, 17-desacetyl-rocuronium has approximately one-twentieth the neuromuscular blocking potency of rocuronium.

In general, patients undergoing cadaver kidney transplant have a small reduction in clearance which is offset pharmacokinetically by a corresponding increase in volume, such that the net effect is an unchanged plasma half-life. Patients with demonstrated liver cirrhosis have a marked increase in their volume of distribution resulting in a plasma half-life approximately twice that of patients with normal hepatic function.

The net result of these findings is that subjects with renal failure have clinical durations that are similar to but somewhat more variable than the duration that one would expect in subjects with normal renal function. Hepatically impaired patients, due to the large increase in volume, may demonstrate clinical durations approaching 1.5 times that of subjects with normal hepatic function. In both populations, individualize the dose to the needs of the patient.

Tissue redistribution accounts for most (about 80%) of the initial amount of rocuronium administered. As tissue compartments fill with continued dosing (4 to 8 hours), less drug is redistributed away from the site of action and, for an infusion-only dose, the rate to maintain neuromuscular blockade falls to about 20% of the initial infusion rate. The use of a loading dose and a smaller infusion rate reduces the need for adjustment of dose.

Children –

Rocuronium Pharmacokinetics in Children			
	Patient age range		
Parameters	3 to < 12 mo (n = 6)	1 to < 3 yrs (n = 5)	3 to < 8 yrs (n = 7)
Clearance (L/kg/hr)	0.35	0.32	0.44
Volume of distribution at steady state (L/kg)	0.3	0.26	0.21
Half-life β elimination (hrs)	1.3	1.1	0.8

Indications:

For inpatients and outpatients as an adjunct to general anesthesia to facilitate both rapid sequence and routine tracheal intubation, and to provide skeletal muscle relaxation during surgery or mechanical ventilation.

Contraindications:

Hypersensitivity to rocuronium.

ROCURONIUM BROMIDE

Warnings:

Administration: Administer in carefully adjusted dosages by or under the supervision of experienced clinicians familiar with the drug's actions and the possible complications of its use. The drug should not be administered unless facilities for intubation, artificial respiration, oxygen therapy and an antagonist are immediately available. It is recommended that clinicians administering neuromuscular blocking agents such as rocuronium use a peripheral nerve stimulator to monitor drug response, need for additional relaxant and adequacy of spontaneous recovery or antagonism.

Recuronium has no known effect on consciousness, pain threshold or cerebration. Therefore, its administration must be accompanied by adequate anesthesia or sedation.

Myasthenia gravis: In patients with myasthenia grains or myasthenic (Eaton-Lambert) syndrome, small doses of nondepolarizing neuromuscular blocking agents may have profound effects. In such patients, a peripheral nerve stimulator and use of a small test dose may be of value in monitoring the response to administration of muscle relaxants.

Pulmonary hypertension: Rocuronium may be associated with increased pulmonary vascular resistance; therefore, caution is appropriate in patients with pulmonary hypertension or valvular heart disease.

Burns: Patients with burns are known to develop resistance to nondepolarizing neuromuscular blocking agents, probably due to up-regulation of post-synaptic skeletal muscle cholinergic receptors.

Renal function impairment: Due to the limited role of the kidney in the excretion of rocuronium, usual dosing guidelines should be adequate. The mean clinical duration of 54 ± 22 min was not considered prolonged compared to 46 ± 12 min in normal patients; however, there was substantial variation (range, 22 to 90 min).

Hepatic function impairment: Since rocuronium is primarily excreted by the liver, use with caution in patients with clinically significant hepatic disease. Duration of 60 min (range, 35 to 166) was moderately prolonged in patients with significant hepatic disease compared to 42 min in patients with normal hepatic function. The median recovery time of 53 min was also prolonged in patients with cirrhosis compared to 20 min in patients with normal hepatic function. Four of eight patients with cirrhosis did not achieve complete block. These findings are consistent with the increase in volume of distribution at steady state observed in patients with significant hepatic disease. If used for rapid sequence induction in patients with ascites, an increased initial dosage may be necessary to assure complete block. Duration will be prolonged in these cases.

Elderly: Rocuronium was evaluated in 55 geriatric patients (ages, 65 to 80 years). Doses of 0.6 mg/kg provided excellent to good intubating conditions in a median time of 2.3 min (range, 1 to 8). Recovery times from 25% to 75% after these doses were not prolonged in geriatric patients compared to other adult patients.

Pregnancy: Category B. There are no adequate and well controlled studies in pregnant women. Use during pregnancy only if the potential benefit justifies the potential risk to the fetus. Rocuronium is not recommended for rapid sequence induction in cesarean section patients.

Children: The use of rocuronium in children < 3 months of age has not been studied. See Administration and Dosage for use in infants and children 3 months to 12 years of age.

Precautions:

Tolerance: As with other nondepolarizing neuromuscular blocking drugs, apparent tolerance to rocuronium may develop rarely during chronic administration in the ICU. While the mechanism for development of this resistance is not known, receptor up-regulation may be a contributing factor. It is strongly recommended that neuromuscular transmission be monitored continuously during administration and recovery with the help of a nerve stimulator. Additional doses of rocuronium or any other neuromuscular blocking agent should not be given until there is a definite response (one twitch of the train-of-four) to nerve stimulation. Prolonged paralysis or skeletal muscle weakness may be noted during initial attempts to wean patients who have chronically received neuromuscular blocking drugs in the ICU from the ventilator. Therefore, use in this setting if the specific advantages of the drug outweigh the risk.

Nondepolarizing Neuromuscular Blockers

ROCURONIUM BROMIDE

Malignant hyperthermia (MH): Malignant hyperthermia has not been reported with the administration of rocuronium. Because rocuronium is always used with other agents, and the occurrence of MH during anesthesia is possible even in the absence of known triggering agents, be familiar with early signs, confirmatory diagnosis and treatment of MH prior to the start of any anesthetic.

Onset time: Conditions associated with slower circulation time (eg, cardiovascular disease, advanced age) may be associated with a delay in onset time. Because higher doses of rocuronium produce a longer duration of action, the initial dosage should usually not be increased in these patients to reduce onset time; instead, when feasible, allow more time for the drug to achieve onset of effect.

Electrolyte imbalance: Rocuronium-induced neuromuscular blockade was modified by alkalosis and acidosis in animals. Both respiratory and metabolic acidosis prolonged the recovery time. The potency of rocuronium was significantly enhanced in metabolic acidosis and alkalosis, but was reduced in respiratory alkalosis. In addition, experience with other drugs has suggested that acute (eg, diarrhea) or chronic (eg, adrenocortical insufficiency) electrolyte imbalance may alter neuromuscular blockade. Since electrolyte imbalance and acid-base imbalance are usually mixed, either enhancement or inhibition may occur.

Extravasation: In animals, rocuronium was well tolerated following IV, intra-arterial and perivenous administration with only a slight irritation of surrounding tissues observed after perivenous administration. In humans, if extravasation occurs it may be associated with signs or symptoms of local irritation; terminate the injection or infusion immediately and restart in another vein.

Drug Interactions:

Rocuronium can be expected to interact similarly to other nondepolarizing neuromuscular blockers. Refer to the Nondepolarizing Neuromuscular Blockers, Curare Preparations monograph.

Adverse Reactions:

Cardiovascular: Arrhythmia, abnormal ECG, tachycardia (< 1%).

GI: Nausea, vomiting (< 1%).

Respiratory: Asthma (bronchospasm, wheezing, rhonchi), hiccup (< 1%).

Dermatologic: Rash, injection site edema, pruritus (< 1%).

Miscellaneous: Transient hypotension and hypertension (2%).

Overdosage:

No cases of significant accidental or intentional overdose with rocuronium have been reported. Overdosage with neuromuscular blocking agents may result in neuromuscular block beyond the time needed for surgery and anesthesia. The primary treatment is maintenance of a patent airway and controlled ventilation until recovery of normal neuromuscular function is assured. Once evidence of recovery from neuromuscular block is observed, further recovery may be facilitated by administration of an anticholinesterase agent (eg, neostigmine, edrophonium) in conjunction with an appropriate anticholinergic agent.

Antagonism of neuromuscular blockade: Antagonists (such as neostigmine) should not be administered prior to the demonstration of some spontaneous recovery from neuromuscular blockade. The use of a nerve stimulator to document recovery and antagonism of neuromuscular blockade is recommended.

Evaluate patients for adequate clinical evidence of antagonism (eg, 5 sec head lift, adequate phonation, ventilation, upper airway maintenance). Ventilation must be supported until no longer required.

Antagonism may be delayed in the presence of debilitation, carcinomatosis, and concomitant use of certain broad spectrum antibiotics, anesthetic agents or other drugs that enhance neuromuscular blockade or separately cause respiratory depression. Under such circumstances the management is the same as that of prolonged neuromuscular blockade.

ROCURONIUM BROMIDE

Administration and Dosage:

Approved by the FDA on March 17, 1994.

For IV use only. Consider individualization of dosage in each case.

The following dosage information is intended to serve as an initial guide to clinicians familiar with other neuromuscular blocking agents to acquire experience with rocuronium. The monitoring of twitch response is recommended to evaluate recovery from rocuronium and decrease the hazards of overdosage if additional doses are administered. It is recommended that clinicians administering neuromuscular blocking agents such as rocuronium use a peripheral nerve stimulator to monitor drug response, determine the need for additional relaxant and adequacy of spontaneous recovery or antagonism.

Rapid sequence intubation: In appropriately premedicated and adequately anesthetized patients, 0.6 to 1.2 mg/kg will provide excellent or good intubating conditions in most patients in < 2 minutes.

Dose for tracheal intubation: The recommended initial dose regardless of anesthetic technique is 0.6 mg/kg. Neuromuscular block sufficient for intubation (≥ 80% block) is attained in a median time of 1 min (range, 0.4 to 6) and most patients have intubation completed within 2 min. Maximum blockade is achieved in most patients in < 3 min. This dose may be expected to provide 31 min (range, 15 to 85) of clinical relaxation under opioid/nitrous oxide/oxygen anesthesia. Under halothane, isoflurane and enflurane anesthesia, expect some extension of the period of clinical relaxation.

A lower dose (0.45 mg/kg) may be used. Neuromuscular block sufficient for intubation (≥ 80% block) is attained in a median time of 1.3 min (range, 0.8 to 6.2) and most patients have intubation completed within 2 min. Maximum blockade is achieved in most patients in < 4 minutes. This dose may be expected to provide 22 min (range, 12 to 31) of clinical relaxation under opioid/nitrous oxide/oxygen anesthesia. Patients receiving this low dose of 0.45 mg/kg who achieve < 90% block (about 16% of these patients) may have a more rapid time to 25% recovery (12 to 15 min).

Should there be reason for the selection of a larger bolus dose in individual patients, initial doses of 0.9 or 1.2 mg/kg can be given during surgery under opioid/nitrous oxide/oxygen anesthesia without adverse effects to the cardiovascular system. These doses will provide ≥ 80% block in most patients in < 2 min, with maximum blockade occurring in most patients in < 3 min. Doses of 0.9 and 1.2 mg/kg may be expected to provide 58 (range, 27 to 111) and 67 min (range, 38 to 160), respectively, of clinical relaxation under opioid/nitrous oxide/oxygen anesthesia.

Maintenance: Maintenance doses of 0.1, 0.15 and 0.2 mg/kg, administered at 25% recovery of control T_1 (defined as 3 twitches of train-of-four), provide a median of 12 (range, 2 to 31), 17 (range, 6 to 50) and 24 min (range, 7 to 69) of clinical duration under opioid/nitrous oxide/oxygen anesthesia. In all cases, guide dosing based on the clinical duration following initial dose or prior maintenance dose and do not administer until recovery of neuromuscular function is evident. A clinically insignificant cumulation of effect with repetitive maintenance dosing has been observed.

Continuous infusion: Initiate infusion at an initial rate of 0.01 to 0.012 mg/kg/min only after early evidence of spontaneous recovery from an intubating dose. Due to rapid redistribution and the associated rapid spontaneous recovery, initiation of the infusion after substantial return of neuromuscular function (>10% of control T_1), may necessitate additional bolus doses to maintain adequate block for surgery.

Upon reaching the desired level of neuromuscular block, the infusion must be individualized for each patient. Adjust the rate of administration according to the patient's twitch response as monitored with the use of a peripheral nerve stimulator. In clinical trials, infusion rates have ranged from 0.004 to 0.016 mg/kg/min.

Inhalation anesthetics, particularly enflurane and isoflurane, may enhance the neuromuscular blocking action of nondepolarizing muscle relaxants. In the presence of steady-state concentrations of enflurane or isoflurane, it may be necessary to reduce the rate of infusion by 30% to 50% at 45 to 60 min after the intubating dose.

Spontaneous recovery and reversal of neuromuscular blockade following discontinuation of rocuronium may be expected to proceed at rates comparable to that following comparable total doses administered by repetitive bolus injections.

Infusion solutions can be prepared by mixing rocuronium with an appropriate infusion solution such as 5% dextrose in water or Lactated Ringer's (see Admixture compatibility). Discard unused portions of infusion solutions.

Nondepolarizing Neuromuscular Blockers

ROCURONIUM BROMIDE

Children: Initial doses of 0.6 mg/kg in children under halothane anesthesia produce excellent to good intubating conditions within 1 min. The median time to maximum block was 1 min (range, 0.5 to 3.3). This dose will provide a median time of clinical relaxation of 41 min (range, 24 to 68) in 3 months to 1 year-old children and 27 min (range, 17 to 41) in 1 to 12 year-old children. Maintenance doses of 0.075 to 0.125 mg/kg, administered upon return of T_1 to 25% of control, provide clinical relaxation for 7 to 10 min.

Spontaneous recovery proceeds at approximately the same rate in children 3 months to 1 year as in adults, but is more rapid in children 1 to 12 years than adults. A continuous infusion initiated at a rate of 0.012 mg/kg/min upon return of T_1 to 10% of control (one twitch present in the train-of-four), may also be used to maintain neuromuscular blockade in children. The infusion must be individualized for each patient. Adjust the rate of administration according to the patient's twitch response as monitored with the use of a peripheral nerve stimulator. Spontaneous recovery and reversal of neuromuscular blockade following discontinuation of rocuronium may be expected to proceed at rates comparable to that following similar total exposure to single bolus doses.

Obesity: Pharmacodynamics of rocuronium are not different between obese and nonobese patients when dosed based upon their actual body weight.

Elderly: Geriatric patients (≥ 65 years) exhibited a slightly prolonged median clinical duration of 46 (range, 22 to 73), 62 (range, 49 to 75), and 94 min (range, 64 to 138) under opioid/nitrous oxide/oxygen anesthesia following doses of 0.6, 0.9 and 1.2 mg/kg, respectively. Maintenance doses of 0.1 and 0.15 mg/kg administered at 25% recovery of T_1, provide approximately 13 and 33 min of clinical duration under opioid/nitrous oxide/oxygen anesthesia. The median rate of spontaneous recovery of T_1 from 25% to 75% in geriatric patients is 17 min (range, 7 to 56) which is not different from that in other adults.

Admixture compatibility: Rocuronium is compatible in solution with 0.9% NaCl solution, sterile water for injection, 5% dextrose in water, Lactated Ringer's and 5% dextrose in saline. Use within 24 hours of mixing with these solutions.

Admixture incompatability: Rocuronium, which has an acid pH, should not be mixed with alkaline solutions (eg, barbiturates) in the same syringe or administered simultaneously during IV infusion through the same needle.

Storage/Stability: Store under refrigeration, 2° to 8°C (36° to 46°F). Do not freeze. Upon removal from refrigeration to room temperature storage conditions (25°C; 77°F), use within 30 days.

Rx	**Zemuron** (Organon)	**Injection:** 10 mg/ml	In 5 ml vials.

PANCURONIUM BROMIDE

Warning:
Administer in carefully adjusted dosage only by, or under the supervision of, experienced clinicians. Do not administer unless reversal agents and facilities for intubation, artificial respiration and oxygen therapy are immediately available. Be prepared to assist or control respiration.

Actions:

Pharmacology: Pancuronium, a nondepolarizing neuromuscular blocking agent, possesses all of the characteristic pharmacological actions on the myoneural junction. It is ≈ 5 times as potent as d-tubocurarine chloride and ≈ ⅓ less potent than vecuronium.

Pancuronium has little effect on the circulatory system, except for a moderate rise in heart rate, mean arterial pressure and cardiac output; systemic vascular resistance is not changed significantly and central venous pressure may fall slightly. The heart rate rise is inversely related to the rate immediately before administration of pancuronium, is blocked by prior administration of atropine and appears unrelated to the concentration of halothane or dose of pancuronium. Histamine release rarely occurs.

Pharmacokinetics: The ED_{95} (dose required to produce 95% suppression of the muscle twitch response) is ≈ 0.05 mg/kg under balanced anesthesia and 0.03 mg/kg under halothane anesthesia. These doses produce effective skeletal muscle relaxation (as judged by time from maximum effect to 25% recovery of control twitch height) for ≈ 22 minutes. Recovery to 90% of control twitch height usually occurs in ≈ 65 minutes. The intubating dose of 0.1 mg/kg (balanced anesthesia) will effectively abolish twitch response within ≈ 4 minutes; time from injection to 25% recovery from this dose is ≈ 100 minutes. Supplemental incremental doses following the initial dose slightly increase the magnitude of blockade and significantly increase the duration of blockade.

The elimination half-life of pancuronium ranges between 89 to 161 minutes. The volume of distribution ranges from 241 to 280 ml/kg, and plasma clearance is ≈ 1.1 to 1.9 ml/min/kg. Approximately 40% of the total dose of pancuronium has been recovered in urine as unchanged pancuronium and its metabolites while ≈ 11% has been recovered in bile. As much as 25% of an injected dose may be recovered as 3-hydroxy metabolite, which is half as potent a blocking agent as pancuronium. Less than 5% of the injected dose is recovered as 17–hydroxy metabolite and 3.17–dihydroxy metabolite, which have been judged to be ≈ 50 times less potent than pancuronium.

Pancuronium exhibits strong binding to gamma globulin and moderate binding to albumin. Approximately 87% is bound to plasma protein.

Renal failure – The elimination half-life is doubled and the plasma clearance is reduced by ≈ 60%. The volume of distribution is variable and, in some cases, elevated. The rate of recovery of neuromuscular blockade, as determined by peripheral nerve stimulation is variable and sometimes very much slower than normal.

Hepatic function impairment – In patients with cirrhosis, the volume of distribution is increased by ≈ 50%, the plasma clearance is decreased by ≈ 22% and the elimination half-life is doubled. Similar results were noted in patients with biliary obstruction, except that plasma clearance was less than half the normal rate. The initial dose to achieve adequate relaxation may thus be high in patients with hepatic or biliary tract dysfunction, while the duration of action is greater than usual.

Indications:

Adjunct to anesthesia to induce skeletal muscle relaxation; to facilitate the management of patients undergoing mechanical ventilation; to facilitate tracheal intubation.

Contraindications:

Hypersensitivity to pancuronium.

Warnings:

Myasthenia gravis: In patients with myasthenia gravis or the myasthenic (Eaton-Lambert) syndrome, small doses of pancuronium may have profound effects. In such patients, a peripheral nerve stimulator and use of a small test dose may be of value in monitoring the response to administration of muscle relaxants.

Renal/Hepatic/Pulmonary function impairment: Although it has been used successfully in pre-existing pulmonary, hepatic or renal disease, exercise caution in these situations, especially in renal disease, because a major portion of pancuronium is excreted unchanged in the urine. (See Actions.)

Pregnancy: Category C. Safety for use during pregnancy has not been established. Do not use during early pregnancy, unless the potential benefits outweigh the unknown potential hazards to the fetus.

May be used in cesarean section, but reversal of pancuronium may be unsatisfactory in patients receiving magnesium sulfate for preeclampsia, because magnesium salts enhance neuromuscular blockade. Dosage should usually be reduced. Interval between use of pancuronium and delivery should be reasonably short to avoid clinically significant placental transfer.

Children: Dose response and, with the exception of neonates, dosage requirements in children are the same as for adults. Neonates are especially sensitive to nondepolarizing neuromuscular blocking agents during the first month of life.

The prolonged use in neonates undergoing mechanical ventilation has been associated in rare cases with severe skeletal muscle weakness that may be first noted during attempts to wean such patients from the ventilator; these patients usually receive other drugs such as antibiotics which may enhance neuromuscular blockade. Microscopic changes consistent with disuse atrophy have been noted at autopsy. Although a cause-and-effect relationship has not been established, the benefit-to-risk ratio must be considered when there is a need for neuromuscular blockade to facilitate long-term mechanical ventilation of neonates.

Rare cases of unexplained, clinically significant methemoglobinemia have been reported in premature neonates undergoing emergency anesthesia and surgery that included combined use of pancuronium, fentanyl and atropine. A direct cause-and-effect relationship has not been established.

Nondepolarizing Neuromuscular Blockers

PANCURONIUM BROMIDE

Precautions:

Benzyl alcohol, contained in some of these products as a preservative, has been associated with a fatal "gasping syndrome" in premature infants.

Altered circulation time: Conditions associated with slower circulation time (cardiovascular disease, old age and edematous states resulting in increased volume of distribution) may contribute to a delay in onset time; dosage should not be increased.

Hepatic or biliary tract disease: The doubled elimination half-life and reduced plasma clearance determined in patients with hepatic or biliary tract disease, as well as limited data showing that recovery time is prolonged an average of 65% in patients with biliary tract obstruction, suggest that prolongation of neuromuscular blockade may occur. At the same time, these conditions are characterized by an ≈ 50% increase in volume of distribution of pancuronium, suggesting that the total initial dose to achieve adequate relaxation may be high in some cases. The possibility of slower onset, higher total dosage and prolongation of neuromuscular blockade must be considered when pancuronium is used in these patients.

Long-term use: In rare cases, long-term use of neuromuscular blocking drugs to facilitate mechanical ventilation may be associated with prolonged paralysis or skeletal muscle weakness that may first be noted during attempts to wean such patients from the ventilator. Typically, such patients receive other drugs such as broad spectrum antibiotics, narcotics or steroids and may have electrolyte imbalance and diseases that lead to electrolyte imbalance, hypoxic episodes of varying duration, acid-base imbalance and extreme debilitation, any of which may enhance the actions of a neuromuscular blocking agent. Additionally, patients immobilized for extended periods frequently develop symptoms consistent with disuse muscle atrophy. Therefore, when there is a need for long-term mechanical ventilation, the benefits-to-risk ratio of neuromuscular blockade must be considered.

Severe obesity or neuromuscular disease: Patients with severe obesity or neuromuscular disease may pose airway or ventilatory problems requiring special care before, during and after the use of neuromuscular blocking agents such as pancuronium.

Pancuronium has no known effect on consciousness, the pain threshold or cerebration. Administration should be accompanied by adequate anesthesia.

Electrolyte imbalance and diseases that lead to electrolyte imbalance, such as adrenal cortical insufficiency, alter neuromuscular blockade. Depending on the nature of the imbalance, either enhancement or inhibition may be expected.

Nondepolarizing Neuromuscular Blockers

PANCURONIUM BROMIDE

Drug Interactions:

Pancuronium Bromide Drug Interactions			
Precipitant drug	Object drug*		Description
Antibiotics (eg, aminoglycosides, tetracyclines, bacitracin, polymyxin B, clindamycin, lincomycin, colistin and sodium colistimethate)	Pancuronium	↑	Parenteral/intraperitoneal administration of high doses of certain antibiotics may produce neuromuscular block on its own. If these agents are used preoperatively or in conjunction with pancuronium during surgery, unexpected prolongation of neuromuscular block is a possibility.
Azathioprine	Pancuronium	↓	Azathioprine may cause reversal of neuromuscular blocking effects of pancuronium.
Inhalational anesthetics (eg, halothane, enflurane, isoflurane)	Pancuronium	↑	Use of these drugs with pancuronium will enhance neuromuscular blockade. Potentiation is most prominent with use of enflurane and isoflurane.
Magnesium sulfate	Pancuronium	↑	When administered for the management of toxemia of pregnancy, may enhance neuromuscular blockade of pancuronium.
Metocurine/ Tubocurarine	Pancuronium	↑	The combination of pancuronium and either metocurine or tubocurarine appears to be synergistic; however, the duration of blockade is not prolonged.
Pancuronium	Halothane/ Tricyclic antidepressants	↑	Patients receiving chronic tricyclic antidepressant therapy who are anesthetized with halothane should have pancuronium administered with caution because severe ventricular arrhythmias may result from the combination. The severity of arrhythmias appears, in part, related to the dose of pancuronium.
Quinidine	Pancuronium	↑	Quinidine, injected during recovery from use of other muscle relaxants, suggests that recurrent paralysis may occur. Consider this possibility for pancuronium bromide injection.
Succinylcholine	Pancuronium	↑	Prior administration, such as that used for endotracheal intubation, enhances the relaxant effect of pancuronium and its duration of action. If succinylcholine is used before pancuronium, delay administration of pancuronium until the effects of succinylcholine begin to subside. If a small dose of pancuronium is given at least 3 minutes prior to the administration of succinylcholine to reduce the incidence of and intensity of succinylcholine-induced fasciculations, this dose may induce a degree of neuromuscular block sufficient to cause respiratory depression in some patients.

* ↑ = Object drug increased. ↓ = Object drug decreased.

Adverse Reactions:

Neuromuscular: The most frequent reactions are an extension of pharmacological actions beyond the time period needed for surgery and anesthesia. This varies from skeletal muscle weakness to profound and prolonged skeletal muscle relaxation, resulting in respiratory insufficiency or apnea. Inadequate reversal of the neuromuscular blockade by anticholinesterases has also occurred. Manage adverse reactions by manual or mechanical ventilation until there is adequate recovery.

Hypersensitivity reactions (rare), eg, bronchospasm, flushing, redness, hypotension, tachycardia and other reactions are possibly mediated by histamine release.

Cardiovascular: Increase in heart rate, arterial pressure and cardiac output; decrease in venous pressure (see Actions).

GI: Salivation during light anesthesia, especially with no anticholinergic premedication.

Dermatologic: Transient rash (occasional).

Nondepolarizing Neuromuscular Blockers

PANCURONIUM BROMIDE

Overdosage:

Management of prolonged neuromuscular blockade: Residual neuromuscular blockade beyond the time needed for surgery and anesthesia may occur, manifested by skeletal muscle weakness, decreased respiratory reserve, low tidal volume or apnea. May use peripheral nerve stimulator to assess degree of residual neuromuscular blockade. Primary treatment is manual or mechanical ventilation and maintenance of a patent airway until complete recovery of normal respiration is assured.

Pyridostigmine bromide, neostigmine or edrophonium, in conjunction with atropine or glycopyrrolate, will usually antagonize the action of pancuronium. Judge satisfactory reversal by adequacy of skeletal muscle tone and respiration. Failure of prompt reversal (within 30 minutes) may occur in the presence of extreme debilitation and carcinomatosis and with concomitant use of certain broad spectrum antibiotics or anesthetic agents and adjuncts that enhance neuromuscular blockade or cause respiratory depression of their own. Under such circumstances, the management is the same as that of prolonged neuromuscular blockade; support ventilation by artificial means until the patient has resumed respiratory control.

Administration and Dosage:

For IV use only. Individualize dosage.

Concomitant therapy: Because potent inhalation agents or prior administration of succinylcholine enhance the intensity and duration of blockade of pancuronium, consider these factors when determining initial and incremental dosage.

Adults: Initial IV dosage is 0.04 to 0.1 mg/kg. Later, use incremental doses starting at 0.01 mg/kg. These increments slightly increase the magnitude of the blockade and significantly increase the duration of blockade because a significant number of myoneural junctions are still blocked when there is clinical need for more drug.

Skeletal muscle relaxation for endotracheal intubation – Bolus dose of 0.06 to 0.1 mg/kg. Conditions satisfactory for intubation usually occur in 2 to 3 min.

Cesarean section – The dosage to provide relaxation for intubation and operation and the dosage to provide relaxation following use of succinylcholine for intubation (see Drug Interactions) are the same as for general surgical procedures.

Children: With the exception of neonates, dosage requirements are the same as for adults. Neonates are especially sensitive to this drug class during the first month of life. Give a test dose of 0.02 mg/kg to assess responsiveness.

Admixture compatibility: Pancuronium is compatible in solution with 0.9% Sodium Chloride Injection, 5% Dextrose Injection, 5% Dextrose and Sodium Chloride and Lactated Ringer's Injection.

Storage/Stability: Refrigerate at 2° to 8°C (36° to 46°F) to maintain potency for 18 months. If stored at 18° to 22°C (65° to 72°F), potency is maintained for 6 months.

Mixed with compatible solutions in glass or plastic containers, pancuronium will remain stable for 48 hours with no alteration in potency or pH.

Rx	**Pancuronium Bromide** (Various, eg, Astra, Elkins-Sinn)	**Injection:** 1 mg/ml	In 10 ml vials.
Rx	**Pavulon** (Organon)		In 10 ml vials.[1]
Rx	**Pancuronium Bromide** (Various, eg, Astra, Elkins-Sinn)	**Injection:** 2 mg/ml	In 2 and 5 ml vials, amps and syringes.
Rx	**Pavulon** (Organon)		In 2 and 5 ml amps.[1]

[1] With benzyl alcohol.

Nondepolarizing Neuromuscular Blockers

ATRACURIUM BESYLATE

> **Warning:**
> Atracurium should be used only by those skilled in airway management and respiratory support. Equipment and personnel must be immediately available for endotracheal intubation and support of ventilation, including use of positive pressure oxygen. Adequacy of respiration must be assured through assisted or controlled ventilation. Have anticholinesterase reversal agents immediately available.

Actions:

Pharmacology: Atracurium, a nondepolarizing skeletal muscle relaxant, antagonizes the neurotransmitter action of acetylcholine by binding competitively with cholinergic receptor sites on the motor end-plate.

Atracurium is a less potent histamine releaser than d-tubocurarine or metocurine. Histamine release is minimal with initial doses up to 0.5 mg/kg, and hemodynamic changes are minimal within the recommended dose range. A moderate histamine release and significant fall in blood pressure have occurred following 0.6 mg/kg. The effects were generally short-lived and manageable.

Pharmacokinetics: Essentially linear within the range of 0.3 to 0.6 mg/kg.

Onset, peak and duration of action – The time to onset of paralysis decreases and the duration of maximum effect increases with increasing doses. The duration of neuromuscular blockade is ≈ ⅓ to ½ that of d-tubocurarine, metocurine and pancuronium at initially equipotent doses.

The ED_{95} (dose required to produce 95% suppression of the muscle twitch response with balanced anesthesia) has averaged 0.23 mg/kg (0.11 to 0.26 mg/kg). An initial dose of 0.4 to 0.5 mg/kg generally produces maximum neuromuscular blockade within 3 to 5 minutes of injection, with good or excellent intubation conditions within 2 to 2.5 minutes in most patients. Recovery from neuromuscular blockade (under balanced anesthesia) begins ≈ 20 to 35 minutes after injection; recovery to 25% of control is achieved ≈ 35 to 45 minutes after injection, and recovery is usually 95% complete ≈ 60 to 70 minutes after injection.

Repeated administration of maintenance doses has no cumulative effect on the duration of neuromuscular blockade if recovery is allowed to begin prior to repeat dosing. After the initial dose, the first maintenance dose (0.08 to 0.1 mg/kg) is generally required within 20 to 45 minutes, and subsequent doses are required at ≈ 15 to 25 minute intervals.

Recovery proceeds more rapidly than recovery from d-tubocurarine, metocurine and pancuronium. Regardless of dose, the time from start of recovery to complete (95%) recovery is ≈ 30 minutes under balanced anesthesia and ≈ 40 minutes under halothane, enflurane or isoflurane anesthesia. Repeated doses have no cumulative effect on recovery rate.

Excretion – The elimination half-life is ≈ 20 minutes. The duration of neuromuscular blockade does not correlate with plasma pseudocholinesterase levels and is not altered by the absence of renal function. Atracurium is inactivated in plasma via two nonoxidative pathways. Some placental transfer occurs.

Indications:

As an adjunct to general anesthesia to facilitate endotracheal intubation; to relax skeletal muscle during surgery or mechanical ventilation.

Contraindications:

Hypersensitivity to atracurium besylate.

Warnings:

Anesthesia: Atracurium has no known effect on consciousness, pain threshold or cerebration. Use only with adequate anesthesia.

Elderly: No differences have been identified in effectiveness, safety or dosage requirements.

Pregnancy: Category C. There are no adequate and well controlled studies in pregnant women. Use during pregnancy only if the potential benefits outweigh the potential hazards to the fetus.

Labor and delivery – Atracurium (0.3 mg/kg) has been administered to 26 pregnant women during delivery by cesarean section. No harmful effects occurred in any of the newborn infants, although small amounts crossed the placental barrier. Consider the possibility of respiratory depression in the newborn.

ATRACURIUM BESYLATE

It is not known whether muscle relaxants given during vaginal delivery have immediate or delayed adverse effects on the fetus or increase the likelihood that resuscitation of the newborn will be necessary. The possibility of forceps delivery may increase.

Lactation: It is not known whether this drug is excreted in breast milk. Safety for use in the nursing mother has not been established.

Children: Safety and efficacy for children < 1 month old are not established.

Precautions:

Histamine release: Exercise caution, especially when substantial histamine release would be hazardous (eg, patients with clinically significant cardiovascular disease, severe anaphylactoid reactions or asthma). The recommended initial dose is lower (0.3 to 0.4 mg/kg); administer slowly or in divided doses over 1 minute.

Benzyl alcohol: This product contains benzyl alcohol, which has been associated with a fatal "gasping syndrome" in premature infants.

Bradycardia during anesthesia may be more common with atracurium than with other muscle relaxants because atracurium has no clinically significant effects on heart rate. It will not counteract bradycardia or vagal stimulation.

Usage in neuromuscular diseases in which potentiation of nondepolarizing agents has been noted (eg, myasthenia gravis, Eaton-Lambert syndrome) may cause profound effects. The use of a peripheral nerve stimulator is especially important for assessing neuromuscular blockade in these patients. Take similar precautions in patients with severe electrolyte disorders or carcinomatosis.

Malignant hyperthermia (MH): Halogenated anesthetic agents and succinylcholine are recognized as the principal pharmacologic triggering agents in MH-susceptible patients; however, because MH can develop in the absence of established triggering agents, the clinician should be prepared to recognize and treat MH in any patient scheduled for general anesthesia. Reports of MH have been rare in cases in which atracurium has been used.

Long-term use: Average infusion rates of 11 to 13 mcg/kg/min (range: 4.5 to 29.5) were required to achieve adequate neuromuscular block. These data suggest that there is wide interpatient variability in dosage requirements. Dosage requirements may decrease or increase with time. Following discontinuation of infusion of atracurium, spontaneous recovery of four twitches in a train-of-four occurred in an average of ≈ 30 minutes (range: 15 to 75 min) and spontaneous recovery to a train-of-four ratio > 75% (the ratio of the height of the fourth to the first twitch in a train-of-four) occurred in an average of ≈ 60 minutes (range: 32 to 108 min).

When atracurium is used in the ICU, it is recommended that neuromuscular transmission be monitored continuously during administration with the help of a nerve stimulator. Do not give additional doses of atracurium or any other neuromuscular blocking agent before there is a definite response to T_1 (first twitch). If no response is elicited, discontinue infusion administration until a response returns.

ATRACURIUM BESYLATE

Drug Interactions:

Atracurium Drug Interactions

Precipitant drug	Object drug*		Description
Diuretics	Atracurium	↑	The neuromuscular blocking effects of atracurium may be increased by thiazide diuretics. Hypokalemia enhances the neuromuscular blockade, possibly by hyperpolarizing the end-plate membrane, increasing resistance to depolarization.
General anesthetics (enflurane, isoflurane, halothane) Antibiotics (eg, aminoglycosides, polypeptide antibiotics) Lithium Verapamil Trimethaphan Procainamide Quinidine	Atracurium	↑	These medications may enhance the neuromuscular blocking action of atracurium. Neuromuscular blockade was prolonged 20% by halothane and 35% by enflurane and isoflurane.
Magnesium sulfate	Atracurium	↑	When administered for the management of toxemia of pregnancy, may enhance neuromuscular blockade of pancuronium. However, in one patient, reversal of neuromuscular blockade was not affected by magnesium sulfate.
Other muscle relaxants	Atracurium	↔	If administered during the same procedure, consider the possibility of a synergistic or antagonist effect.
Phenytoin Theophylline	Atracurium	↓	Phenytoin and theophylline may cause resistance to, or reversal of, the neuromuscular blocking action of atracurium.
Succinylcholine	Atracurium	↑	Succinylcholine does not enhance duration, but quickens onset and may increase depth of atracurium-induced neuromuscular blockade.
Acetylcholinesterase inhibitors (eg, neostigmine, edrophonium and pyridostigmine)	Atracurium	↓	Antagonism is inhibited and neuromuscular block is reversed by acetylcholinesterase inhibitors.
Corticosteroids	Atracurium	↑	Prolonged weakness may occur.

* ↑ = Object drug increased. ↓ = Object drug decreased. ↔ = Undetermined effect.

Adverse Reactions:

The following adverse reactions are among those reported most frequently, but data are insufficient to estimate incidence.

Hypersensitivity: Allergic reactions (anaphylactic or anaphylactoid responses), rarely severe.

Dermatologic: Rash, urticaria, reaction at injection site.

Musculoskeletal: Inadequate block, prolonged block.

Cardiovascular: Hypotension, vasodilatation (flushing), tachycardia, bradycardia.

Respiratory: Dyspnea, bronchospasm, laryngospasm.

Nondepolarizing Neuromuscular Blockers

ATRACURIUM BESYLATE

Atracurium Adverse Reactions				
	Initial dose (mg/kg)			
Adverse reaction	0 - 0.3 (n = 485)	0.31 - 0.5[1] (n = 366)	≥ 0.6 (n = 24)	Total (n = 875)
Skin flush	1%	8.7%	9.2%	5%
Erythema	0.6%	0.5%	0%	0.6%
Itching	0.4%	0%	0%	0.2%
Wheezing/Bronchial secretions	0.2%	0.3%	0%	0.2%
Hives	0.2%	0%	0%	0.1%
Vital sign change[2] (≥ 30%)	(n = 365)	(n = 144)	(n = 21)	(n = 530)
Mean arterial pressure				
Increase	1.9%	2.8%	0%	2.1%
Decrease	1.1%	2.1%	14.3%	1.9%
Heart rate				
Increase	1.6%	2.8%	4.8%	2.1%
Decrease	0.8%	0%	0%	0.6%

[1] Recommended range for most patients.
[2] Clinical trials (n = 530) patients without cardiovascular disease.

Overdosage:
Excessive doses produce enhanced pharmacological effects. Overdosage may increase risk of histamine release and cardiovascular effects, especially hypotension. Provide cardiovascular support as needed. Ensure airway and ventilation. Longer neuromuscular blockade may occur. Use an anticholinesterase reversing agent (eg, neostigmine, edrophonium, pyridostigmine) with an anticholinergic such as atropine or glycopyrrolate.

Administration and Dosage:
To avoid patient distress, do not administer before unconsciousness has been induced.

Administer IV. IM use may result in tissue irritation.

Use a peripheral nerve stimulator to monitor twitch suppression and recovery.

Adjust the rate of administration according to patient response as determined by peripheral nerve stimulation.

Bolus doses for intubation and maintenance of neuromuscular blockade:

Initial adult dose – 0.4 to 0.5 mg/kg (1.7 to 2.2 times ED_{95}) IV bolus. Expect good conditions for nonemergency intubation in 2 to 2.5 minutes in most patients; maximum neuromuscular blockade is achieved ≈ 3 to 5 minutes after injection.

Maintaining neuromuscular blockade during prolonged surgical procedures – 0.08 to 0.1 mg/kg. The first maintenance dose is generally required 20 to 45 minutes after initial injection. Give maintenance doses at regular intervals, every 15 to 25 minutes under balanced anesthesia, slightly longer under isoflurane or enflurane. Higher doses (up to 0.2 mg/kg) permit maintenance dosing at longer intervals.

Histamine release – Initially, 0.3 to 0.4 mg/kg given slowly or in divided doses over 1 minute (see Precautions).

Neuromuscular disease, severe electrolyte disorders or carcinomatosis – Consider dosage reductions in which potentiation of neuromuscular blockade or difficulties with reversal have been demonstrated. There has been no clinical experience in these patients and no specific dosage adjustments. No dosage adjustments are required for patients with renal diseases.

Following use of succinylcholine for intubation under balanced anesthesia – Initially, 0.3 to 0.4 mg/kg. Further reductions may be desirable with the use of potent inhalational anesthetics. Permit the patient to recover from the effects of succinylcholine prior to atracurium administration. Data are insufficient to recommend specific initial doses following administration of succinylcholine in infants and children.

Pediatrics – No dosage adjustments required for patients ≥ 2 years old. An initial dose of 0.3 to 0.4 mg/kg is recommended for infants (1 month to 2 years old) under halothane anesthesia. More frequent maintenance doses may be required.

Use by infusion: After administration of an initial bolus dose of 0.3 to 0.5 mg/kg, give a diluted solution by continuous infusion for maintenance of neuromuscular blockade during extended surgical procedures. Long-term use in the ICU has not been studied sufficiently to support dosage recommendations. Accuracy is best achieved using a precision infusion device.

Nondepolarizing Neuromuscular Blockers

ATRACURIUM BESYLATE

Initiate infusion only after early evidence of spontaneous recovery from the bolus dose. An initial infusion rate of 9 to 10 mcg/kg/min may be required to rapidly counteract the spontaneous recovery of neuromuscular function. Thereafter, a rate of 5 to 9 mcg/kg/min should maintain continuous neuromuscular blockade in the range of 89% to 99% in most patients under balanced anesthesia.

In patients undergoing cardiopulmonary bypass with induced hypothermia, the rate of infusion required to maintain adequate surgical relaxation during hypothermia (25° to 28°C) is approximately half the rate required during normothermia.

Atracuraim Infusion Rates
Concentrations for 0.2 and 0.5 mg/ml

Drug delivery rate (mcg/kg/min)	Infusion delivery rate (ml/kg/min)	
	0.2 mg/ml[1]	0.5 mg/ml[2]
5	0.025	0.01
6	0.03	0.012
7	0.035	0.014
8	0.04	0.016
9	0.045	0.018
10	0.05	0.02

[1] 2 ml of 1% (10 mg/ml) added to 98 ml diluent.
[2] 5 ml of 1% (10 mg/ml) added to 95 ml diluent.

Admixture compatibility: Prepare infusion solutions by admixing atracurium with an appropriate diluent: 5% Dextrose Injection, 0.9% Sodium Chloride Injection or 5% Dextrose and 0.9% Sodium Chloride Injection. Do not use Lactated Ringer's Injection. The amount of infusion solution required per minute will depend upon the concentration and dose desired (see table). Use infusion solutions within 24 hours of preparation. Discard unused solutions.

Atracurium has an acid pH; do not mix with alkaline solutions (eg, barbiturates) in the same syringe or administer simultaneously during IV infusion through the same needle. The drug may be inactivated and precipitated.

Storage/Stability: Atracurium loses potency at the rate of 6% per year under refrigeration (5°C; 41°F). Rate of loss in potency increases to ≈ 5% per month at 25°C (77°F). Refrigerate at 2° to 8°C (36° to 46°F) to preserve potency. Do not freeze. Upon removal from refrigeration, use atracurium within 14 days even if refrigerated.

Store solutions containing 0.2 or 0.5 mg/ml either under refrigeration or at room temperature for 24 hours without significant loss of potency.

Rx	**Tracrium** (Glaxo-Wellcome)	**Injection:** 10 mg/ml[1]	In 5 ml single-use and 10 ml multi-dose vials.[2]

[1] With benzenesulfonic acid.
[2] With 0.9% benzyl alcohol.

Nondepolarizing Neuromuscular Blockers

VECURONIUM BROMIDE

Warning:
Do not administer unless facilities for intubation, artificial respiration, oxygen therapy and reversal agents are immediately available. Be prepared to assist or control respiration.

Actions:

Pharmacology: Vecuronium bromide, a nondepolarizing neuromuscular blocking agent of intermediate duration, possesses the pharmacologic actions of the curariform class. It competes for cholinergic receptors at the motor end-plate, and its effects are reversed by acetylcholinesterase inhibitors. Vecuronium is about ⅓ more potent than pancuronium, but its duration of activity is shorter at initially equipotent doses. The time to onset of paralysis decreases and the duration of maximum effect increases with increasing doses.

Pharmacokinetics:

Onset, peak and duration of action – The ED_{90} (dose required to produce 90% suppression of the muscle twitch response with balanced anesthesia) averages 0.057 mg/kg (0.049 to 0.062 mg/kg). Following an initial IV dose of 0.08 to 0.1 mg/kg, vecuronium produces the first depression of twitch in 1 minute, good intubation conditions within 2.5 to 3 minutes and maximum neuromuscular blockade within 3 to 5 minutes. Under balanced anesthesia, the recovery time to 25% of control is ≈ 25 to 40 minutes after injection; recovery is usually 95% complete in 45 to 65 minutes.

Repeated maintenance doses have little or no cumulative effect on duration of blockade. The first maintenance dose is generally required in 25 to 40 minutes, and subsequent doses are required at 12 to 15 minute intervals.

Recovery index (time from 25% to 75% recovery) is ≈ 15 to 25 minutes under balanced or halothane anesthesia, more rapid than recovery from pancuronium.

Absorption/Distribution – Following a single IV dose, the distribution half-life is ≈ 4 minutes. Plasma protein binding is 60% to 80%.

Metabolism/Excretion – Only unchanged vecuronium bromide has been detected in human plasma. One metabolite, 3-deacetyl vecuronium, has been identified in urine and in bile at concentrations of 10% and 25%, respectively, of the injected dose. Elimination half-life is 65 to 75 minutes in healthy surgical patients and in renal failure patients. A shortened half-life of ≈ 35 to 40 minutes has been reported in late pregnancy. The volume of distribution at steady state is ≈ 300 to 400 ml/kg; systemic rate of clearance is ≈ 3 to 4.5 ml/min/kg.

In patients with cirrhosis or cholestasis, recovery time may be doubled. Renal failure does not appear to significantly affect recovery times.

Urine recovery of vecuronium bromide varies from 3% to 35% in 24 hours. Approximately 25% to 50% may be excreted in bile within 42 hours.

Indications:
To use as an adjunct to general anesthesia, to facilitate endotracheal intubation and to provide skeletal muscle relaxation during surgery or mechanical ventilation.

Contraindications:
Hypersensitivity to vecuronium.

Warnings:

Myasthenia gravis: In patients who have myasthenia gravis or myasthenic (Eaton-Lambert) syndrome, small doses of vecuronium may have profound effects. In such patients, a peripheral nerve stimulator and use of a small test dose may be of value in monitoring the response to muscle relaxants.

Long-term use: Long-term IV infusion to support mechanical ventilation in ICU has not been studied sufficiently to support dosage recommendations.

Whenever the use of vecuronium or any neuromuscular blocking agent is contemplated in the ICU, it is recommended that neuromuscular transmission be monitored continuously during administration and recovery with the help of a nerve stimulator. Use of a peripheral nerve stimulator for adequate monitoring of neuromuscular blocking effect will preclude inadvertent excess dosing. Additional doses of vecuronium, or any other neuromuscular blocking agent, should not be given before there is a definite response to T_1 (first twitch). If no response is elicited, infusion administration should be discontinued until a response returns.

Renal/Hepatic function impairment: Vecuronium is well tolerated without significant prolongation of neuromuscular blocking effect in patients with renal failure who have been optimally prepared for surgery by dialysis. If anephric patients cannot be prepared for nonelective surgery, prolongation of neuromuscular blockade may occur; therefore, consider a lower initial dose of the drug.

Patients with cirrhosis or cholestasis have prolonged recovery times. Current data do not permit dosage recommendations in patients with impaired liver function.

Pregnancy: Category C. Safety for use during pregnancy has not been established. Use only when clearly needed and when the potential benefits outweigh the unknown potential hazards to the fetus.

Children: Infants < 1 year of age but > 7 weeks, also tested under halothane anesthesia, are moderately more sensitive to vecuronium on a mg/kg basis than adults and take ≈ 1½ times as long to recover. Available information does not permit recommendations for usage in neonates.

Precautions:

Altered circulation time: Conditions associated with slower circulation time (cardiovascular disease, old age and edematous states resulting in increased volume of distribution) may contribute to a delay in onset time; therefore, do not increase dosage.

Benzyl alcohol: Benzyl alcohol, contained in some of these products as a preservative, has been associated with a fatal "gasping syndrome" in premature infants.

Severe obesity or neuromuscular disease may pose airway or ventilatory problems requiring special care before, during and after the use of vecuronium.

Malignant hyperthermia (MH): Many drugs used in anesthetic practice are suspected of being capable of triggering MH. Data are insufficient to establish whether vecuronium is capable of triggering MH.

Electrolyte imbalance and diseases which lead to electrolyte imbalance, such as adrenal cortical insufficiency, have altered neuromuscular blockade. Depending on the nature of the imbalance, either enhancement or inhibition may be expected.

Drug Interactions:

Vecuronium Bromide Drug Interactions

Precipitant drug	Object drug*		Description
Antibiotics (eg, aminoglycosides, tetracyclines, bacitracin, polymyxin B, colistin and sodium colistimethate)	Vecuronium	↑	Parenteral/intraperitoneal administration of high doses of certain antibiotics may intensify or produce neuromuscular blockade on their own. If these or other newly introduced antibiotics are used with vecuronium during surgery, consider the possibility of unexpected prolongation of neuromuscular block.
Inhalational anesthetics (eg, enflurane, isoflurane and halothane)	Vecuronium	↑	Inhalational anesthetics given with vecuronium will enhance neuromuscular blockade. Potentiation is most prominent with use of enflurane and isoflurane. With the above agents, the initial dose of vecuronium may be the same as with balanced anesthesia unless the inhalational anesthetic has been administered for a sufficient time at a sufficient dose to have reached clinical equilibrium. If vecuronium is first administered > 5 minutes after the start of the inhalation of enflurane, isoflurane or halothane, or when steady state has been achieved, the intubating dose of vecuronium may be decreased by ≈ 15%.
Magnesium salts	Vecuronium	↑	Magnesium salts, administered for the management of toxemia of pregnancy, may enhance the neuromuscular blockade of vecuronium.
Quinidine	Vecuronium	↑	Recurrent paralysis may occur with injection of quinidine during recovery from use of other muscle relaxants. Consider this possibility with vecuronium.
Succinylcholine	Vecuronium	↑	Prior administration of succinylcholine may enhance vecuronium's neuromuscular blocking effect and its duration of action. If succinylcholine is used first, delay the administration of vecuronium until the succinylcholine effect shows signs of wearing off.

* ↑ = Object drug increased.

Nondepolarizing Neuromuscular Blockers

VECURONIUM BROMIDE

Adverse Reactions:

The most frequent adverse reaction to nondepolarizing blocking agents as a class is an extension of the drug's pharmacological action. This may vary from skeletal muscle weakness to profound and prolonged skeletal muscle paralysis resulting in respiratory insufficiency or apnea.

Vecuronium in doses up to 3 times those needed for clinical relaxation did not produce clinically significant changes in systolic, diastolic or mean arterial pressure.

Inadequate reversal of the neuromuscular blockade is possible. Manage these adverse reactions by manual or mechanical ventilation until recovery. Little or no increase in intensity of blockade or duration of action of vecuronium is noted from the use of thiobarbiturates, narcotic analgesics, nitrous oxide or droperidol. (See Overdosage.)

Hypersensitivity: Hypersensitivity reactions such as bronchospasm, flushing, redness, hypotension, tachycardia and other reactions commonly associated with histamine release are unlikely to occur.

Overdosage:

Excessive doses can produce enhanced pharmacological effects. This may be manifested by skeletal muscle weakness, decreased respiratory reserve, low tidal volume or apnea. Use a peripheral nerve stimulator to assess the degree of residual neuromuscular blockade and to differentiate residual neuromuscular blockade from other causes of decreased respiratory reserve.

Administration and Dosage:

For IV use only. Individualize dosage.

Vecuronium has no known effect on consciousness, pain threshold or cerebration. Administration must be accompanied by adequate anesthesia.

Initial adult dose: 0.08 to 0.1 mg/kg (1.4 to 1.75 times the ED_{90}) as an IV bolus injection to produce good or excellent nonemergency intubation conditions in 2.5 to 3 minutes. Under balanced anesthesia, clinically required neuromuscular blockade lasts ≈ 25 to 30 minutes, with recovery to 25% of control achieved in ≈ 25 to 40 minutes and recovery to 95% of control in 25 to 40 minutes. In the presence of potent inhalation anesthetics, vecuronium's neuromuscular blocking effect is enhanced. If vecuronium is first administered > 5 minutes after the start of inhalation agents or when steady state has been achieved, the initial dose may be reduced by ≈ 15%.

Prior administration of succinylcholine may enhance vecuronium's neuromuscular blocking effect and duration of action. If intubation is performed using succinylcholine, a reduction of initial dose of vecuronium to 0.04 to 0.06 mg/kg with inhalation anesthesia and 0.05 to 0.06 mg/kg with balanced anesthesia may be required.

Maintenance dosage: During prolonged surgical procedures, 0.01 to 0.015 mg/kg is recommended. The first maintenance dose is generally required within 25 to 40 minutes. Use clinical criteria to determine the need for maintenance doses. Because the drug lacks cumulative effects, subsequent maintenance doses may be administered at ≈ 12 to 15 minute intervals under balanced anesthesia, and slightly longer under inhalation agents. (If less frequent administration is desired, administer higher maintenance doses.)

If larger doses are necessary, initial doses ranging from 0.15 mg/kg up to 0.28 mg/kg have been given with proper ventilation during surgery under halothane without cardiovascular effects.

After an intubating dose of 0.08 to 0.1 mg/kg, a continuous infusion of 0.001 mg/kg/min can be initiated ≈ 20 to 40 minutes later. Infusion of vecuronium should be initiated only after early evidence of spontaneous recovery from the bolus dose.

Children (10 to 17 years): Administer adult dosage.

Nondepolarizing Neuromuscular Blockers

VECURONIUM BROMIDE

Admixture compatibility: 0.9% Sodium Chloride, 5% Dextrose in Saline or Water, Lactated Ringer's Solution and Sterile Water for Injection.

Storage/Stability: Store at 15° to 30°C (59° to 86°F). Protect from light. May be stored at room temperature or refrigerated. When reconstituted with supplied bacteriostatic water for injection, use within 5 days.

When reconstituted with sterile water for injection or other compatible IV solutions, refrigerate vial. Use within 24 hours. Single use only. Discard unused portion.

Rx	**Norcuron** (Organon)	**Powder for Injection:** 10 mg[1]	In 10 ml vials with and without diluent.[2]
		20 mg[1]	In 20 ml vials without diluent.

[1] With mannitol.

[2] Contains 0.9% benzyl alcohol.

PIPECURONIUM BROMIDE

Warning:
Administer pipecuronium in carefully adjusted dosage by or under the supervision of experienced clinicians familiar with the drug's actions and the possible complications of its use. Do not administer unless facilities for intubation, artificial respiration, oxygen therapy and an antagonist are within immediate reach. Clinicians administering long-acting neuromuscular blocking agents should employ a peripheral nerve stimulator to monitor drug response, need for additional relaxant and adequacy of spontaneous recovery or antagonism.

Actions:

Pharmacology: Pipecuronium bromide, a long-acting nondepolarizing neuromuscular blocker, possesses the characteristic pharmacological actions of this drug class (curariform). It competes for cholinergic receptors at the motor end-plate. This action is antagonized by acetylcholinesterase inhibitors, such as neostigmine.

Pharmacokinetics: The individual cumulative ED_{95} (dose required to produce 95% suppression of T_1 [first twitch] of the train-of-four or 95% suppression of single-twitch response) during balanced anesthesia has averaged 41 mcg/kg (range, 20 to 91 mcg/kg). Maximum blockade is achieved in ≈ 5 minutes following single doses of 70 to 85 mcg/kg. Under balanced anesthesia, following single doses of 70 mcg/kg, time to recovery to 25% of control (clinical duration) ranged from 30 to 175 minutes. Clinical duration following 80 to 85 mcg/kg single doses varied between 40 to 211 minutes. Pipecuronium has an onset time and clinical duration similar to those of pancuronium bromide at comparable doses.

No significant differences were observed in mean clinical duration of single 100 mcg/kg doses compared with doses of 80 to 85 mcg/kg. Doses >100 mcg/kg are not recommended because of the possibility of even longer duration of action.

The mean time for spontaneous recovery from 25% to 50% of control T_1 is ≈ 24 minutes (range, 8 to 131 minutes).

Pipecuronium can be administered following recovery from succinylcholine when the latter is used to facilitate endotracheal intubation. Preliminary data suggest that, if a single dose of 50 mcg/kg is administered under these conditions, prolongation in clinical duration may be noted (range, 23 to 95 minutes following succinylcholine vs 8 to 50 minutes without it). Initial doses of 70 to 85 mcg/kg used without succinylcholine have produced good to excellent intubation conditions within 2.5 to 3 minutes of injection, which is before maximum blockade.

Mean clinical duration of first maintenance doses of 10 to 15 mcg/kg given at 25% recovery of control T_1 is ≈ 50 minutes (range, 17 to 175 minutes).

Obesity – Clinical durations > 120 minutes for the dose of 70 mcg/kg or > 150 minutes for doses of ≥ 80 mcg/kg occurred in ≈ 8% of cases. In ≈ ⅓ of such cases, dosage was administered to obese patients (defined as ≥ 30% above ideal body weight for height) based on actual body weight. Prolonged clinical duration was ≈ 2 times more common in obese patients.

Renal function impairment – There is an inverse relationship between renal function and clinical duration; the mean clinical duration more than doubles when the calculated creatinine clearance decreases from 100 to 40 ml/min.

Preliminary Pharmacokinetic Parameters of Pipecuronium[1]

	Mean (range)[2]	
Parameter	Normal renal and hepatic function (n = 4)	Renal transplant (n = 7)
Clearance (L/hr/kg)	0.12 (0.1 - 0.14)	0.08 (0.02 - 0.12)
Volume of distribution at steady state (L/kg)	0.25 (0.12 - 0.37)	0.37 (0.28 - 0.51)
Half-life distribution (min)	6.22 (1.34 - 10.66)	4.33 (1.69 - 6.17)
Half-life elimination (hr)	1.7 (0.9 - 2.7)	4 (2 - 8.2)

[1] Due to the small number of subjects and the interpatient variation, this information is a general guide only. Definitive concentration-effect and pharmacokinetic relationships have not yet been established.

[2] Determined after rapid administration of a single bolus dose of 70 mcg/kg.

PIPECURONIUM BROMIDE

The 3–deacetyl metabolite has been detected in the urine of humans undergoing coronary artery bypass surgery. Fifty-six percent of the administered dose was recovered in the urine, of which 41% was unchanged drug, and the remaining 15% was the 3–deacetyl metabolite. No metabolites were found in the plasma.

Indications:

As an adjunct to general anesthesia; to provide skeletal muscle relaxation during surgery; to provide skeletal muscle relaxation for endotracheal intubation.

Pipecuronium is only recommended for procedures anticipated to last ≥ 90 minutes.

Warnings:

Antagonism of neuromuscular blockade: Antagonists (such as neostigmine) should not be administered prior to the demonstration of some spontaneous recovery from neuromuscular blockade. The use of a nerve stimulator to document recovery and antagonism of neuromuscular blockade is recommended.

Evaluate patients for adequate clinical evidence of antagonism (eg, 5–second head lift, adequate phonation, ventilation and upper airway maintenance). As with other neuromuscular blocking agents, physicians should be alert to the possibility that the action of the drugs used to antagonize neuromuscular blockade may wear off before plasma levels of pipecuronium have declined sufficiently.

Antagonism may be delayed in the presence of debilitation, carcinomatosis, and concomitant use of certain broad-spectrum antibiotics or anesthetic agents and other drugs that enhance neuromuscular blockade or separately cause respiratory depression. Management is same as that of prolonged neuromuscular blockade.

Edrophonium doses of 0.5 mg/kg are not as effective as neostigmine doses of 0.04 mg/kg in antagonizing pipecuronium-induced neuromuscular block and is often inadequate. Therefore, the use of edrophonium 0.5 mg/kg is not recommended to antagonize pipecuronium-induced neuromuscular blockade. The use of greater (1 mg/kg) doses of edrophonium or of pyridostigmine has not been investigated.

Hemodynamics: Clinically significant bradycardia, hypotension and hypertension have occurred. The most common observations, comparing vital signs immediately prior to initial dosage with pipecuronium and 2 minutes after injection, are a slight decrease in heart rate and systolic and diastolic blood pressure.

Myasthenia gravis or myasthenic (Eaton-Lambert) syndrome: Small doses of nondepolarizing neuromuscular blocking agents may have profound effects. Shorter acting muscle relaxants may be more suitable for these patients.

Long-term use: Pipecuronium is not recommended for use in patients requiring prolonged mechanical ventilation in the ICU or prior to or following other nondepolarizing neuromuscular blocking agents.

Renal function impairment: Because it is primarily excreted by the kidney, and because some shorter acting drugs (vecuronium and atracurium) have a more predictable duration of action in patients with renal dysfunction, use with extra caution in patients with renal failure (see Administration and Dosage; Actions).

Pregnancy: Category C. There are no adequate and well controlled studies in pregnant women. Use during pregnancy only if the potential benefit justifies the potential risk to the fetus.

Obstetrics (cesarean section) – There are insufficient data on placental transfer of pipecuronium and possible related effect(s) upon the neonate following cesarean section delivery. In addition, the duration of action of pipecuronium exceeds the duration of operative obstetrics (cesarean section). Therefore, pipecuronium is not recommended for use in patients undergoing cesarean section.

Children: Infants (3 months to 1 year) under balanced anesthesia or halothane anesthesia manifest similar dose response to pipecuronium as do adults on a mcg/kg basis. Children (1 to 14 years of age) under balanced anesthesia or halothane anesthesia, may be less sensitive than adults. Infants appear to be more sensitive to pipecuronium, but the duration of action is shorter in infants. There are no data on either onset time or clinical duration of larger doses in infants or children. There are no data on maintenance dosing in infants and children.

Precautions:

Bradycardia: Pipecuronium has little or no effect on the heart rate, and it will not counteract the bradycardia produced by many opioid anesthetics or vagal stimulation.

Increased volume of distribution: Conditions associated with an increased volume of distribution (eg, slower circulation time in cardiovascular disease, old age, edematous states) may be associated with a delay in onset time. Because higher doses may

PIPECURONIUM BROMIDE

produce a longer duration of action, the initial dosage should not usually be increased to enhance onset time.

Obesity: The most common patient condition associated with prolonged clinical duration is obesity, defined as ≥ 30% over ideal body weight. Base dose on ideal body weight for height in obese patients (see Administration and Dosage).

Malignant hyperthermia (MH): Human MH has not been reported with the administration of pipecuronium. Because pipecuronium is never used alone, and because the occurrence of MH during anesthesia is possible even in the absence of known triggering agents, clinicians should be familiar with early signs, confirmatory diagnosis and treatment of MH prior to the start of any anesthetic.

CNS: Pipecuronium has no known effect on consciousness, pain threshold or cerebration. Therefore administration must be accompanied by adequate anesthesia.

Fluid/Electrolyte imbalance: Experience with other drugs has suggested that acute (eg, diarrhea) or chronic (eg, adrenocortical insufficiency) electrolyte imbalance may alter neuromuscular blockade. Because electrolyte imbalance and acid-base imbalance are usually mixed, either enhancement or inhibition may occur.

Drug Interactions:

Pipecuronium Bromide Drug Interactions			
Precipitant drug	Object drug*		Description
Anesthetics, inhalational	Pipecuronium	⬆	Use of volatile inhalation anesthetics enhances the activity of other neuromuscular blocking agents on the order of enflurane > isoflurane > halothane. Minimal effects are generally observed on onset time and peak effect. In routine use of neuromuscular blocking agents, only clinical duration is generally affected (prolonged). Use of isoflurane has resulted in an increase in mean clinical duration of 12%. In 25 patients first anesthetized with enflurane for ≥ 5 minutes, the mean clinical duration was increased by 50%. Therefore, anticipate a prolonged clinical duration following initial or maintenance doses and prolonged recovery from the neuromuscular blocking effect of pipecuronium.
Antibiotics (eg, aminoglycosides; tetracyclines; bacitracin; polymyxin B; colistin; sodium colistimethate)	Pipecuronium	⬆	Parenteral/intraperitoneal administration of high doses of certain antibiotics may intensify or produce neuromuscular block on their own. If these antibiotics are used in conjunction with pipecuronium during surgery, consider prolongation of neuromuscular block a possibility.
Magnesium salts	Pipecuronium	⬆	Administration for the management of toxemia of pregnancy may enhance neuromuscular blockade.
Quinidine	Pipecuronium	⬆	Experience concerning injection of quinidine during recovery from use of other muscle relaxants suggests that recurrent paralysis may occur. This possibility must also be considered for pipecuronium.
Succinylcholine	Pipecuronium	⬆	Pipecuronium can be administered following recovery from succinylcholine when the latter is used to facilitate endotracheal intubation. The use of pipecuronium before succinylcholine, in order to attenuate some of the side effects of succinylcholine, is not recommended. (See Pharmacokinetics.)

* ⬆ = Object drug increased.

Adverse Reactions:

The most frequent side effect of nondepolarizing blocking agents is an extension of the drug's pharmacological action beyond the time period needed for surgery and anesthesia. Clinical signs may vary from skeletal muscle weakness to skeletal muscle paralysis resulting in respiratory insufficiency or apnea. This may be due to the drug's effect or inadequate antagonism.

Nondepolarizing Neuromuscular Blockers

PIPECURONIUM BROMIDE

Cardiovascular: Hypotension (2.5%); bradycardia (1.4%); hypertension, myocardial ischemia, cerebrovascular accident, thrombosis, atrial fibrillation, ventricular extrasystole (< 1%).

Metabolic/Nutritional: Hypoglycemia, hyperkalemia, increased creatinine (< 1%).

Musculoskeletal: Muscle atrophy, difficult intubation (< 1%).

Respiratory: Dyspnea, respiratory depression, laryngismus, atelectasis (< 1%).

Miscellaneous: Hypesthesia, CNS depression, anuria, rash, urticaria (< 1%).

Overdosage:

Treatment: Support ventilation by artificial means until no longer required. Intensified monitoring of vital organ function is required for the period of paralysis and during an extended period post-recovery.

Administration and Dosage:

For IV use only. Administer by or under the supervision of experienced clinicians familiar with the use of neuromuscular blocking agents. Individualize dosage.

The dosage information that follows serves as an initial guide to clinicians familiar with other neuromuscular block to acquire experience with pipecuronium. The monitoring of twitch response is recommended to evaluate recovery from pipecuronium and decrease the hazards of overdosage if additional doses are administered.

Clinicians administering long-acting neuromuscular blocking agents such as pipecuronium should employ a peripheral nerve stimulator to monitor drug response, need for additional relaxant and adequacy of spontaneous recovery or antagonism.

Individualize dosage: The table below is to assist those physicians who wish to adjust dosage based on ideal body weight and renal function.

For small patients with decreased renal function, the initial dose is < 70 to 85 mcg/kg, ie, < 2 times the average ED_{95} dose, which is generally the recommended intubating dose for neuromuscular blocking agents. Use extra care during intubation of any patient in whom, in order to decrease the possibility of prolonged clinical duration, < 70 mcg/kg is used for intubation. Dosing in accordance with the following table may reduce the variability in clinical duration to bring ≈ 20% more patients to within ± 30 minutes of the duration predicted by the dose adjusted by ideal body weight and calculated creatinine clearance.

Calculated Dose of Pipecuronium (mg)[1]							
Creatinine clearance (ml/min)[3]	Ideal body weight (kg)[2]						Dose in mcg/kg
	50	60	70	80	90	100	
≤ 40	2.5[4]	3[4]	3.5[4]	4[4]	4.5[4]	5[4]	50[4]
60	2.5[4]	3[4]	3.8	4.9	6.2	7.7	55
80	2.6	3.7	5	6.5	8.3	10[5]	70
≥ 100	3.2	4.6	6.3	8.2	9[5]	10[5]	85 to 100[5]

[1] Based on ideal body weight (IBW) in kg and estimated creatinine clearance; mg = ml if 10 mg vial is reconstituted with 10 ml.

[2] IBW (kg): Men = (106 + [6 lbs/inch in height > 5 ft])/2.2. Women = (100 + [5 lbs/inch in height > 5 ft])/2.2. Use actual body weight in the calculation if it is < IBW.

[3] Estimated Ccr = [{(140 − age in years) × IBW (kg)} ÷ {72 x serum creatinine (mg/dl)}] × 0.85 (for females only).

[4] Minimum calculated dose for intubation; anticipate prolonged clinical blockade.

[5] Maximum calculated dose for intubation; anticipate use of maintenance doses.

Endotracheal intubation: The recommended initial dose under balanced anesthesia, halothane, isoflurane or enflurane anesthesia in patients with normal renal function who are not obese is 0.07 to 0.085 mg/kg (70 to 85 mcg/kg). Good to excellent intubating conditions are generally provided within 2.5 to 3 minutes. Maximum blockade, usually > 95%, is achieved in ≈ 5 minutes. Doses in this range provide ≈1 to 2 hours of clinical relaxation under balanced anesthesia (range, 47 to 124 minutes). Under halothane, isoflurane and enflurane anesthesia, expect extension of the period of clinical relaxation.

For obese patients (≥ 30% above ideal body weight for height), it is particularly important to consider dosage adjustment according to ideal body weight.

Nondepolarizing Neuromuscular Blockers

PIPECURONIUM BROMIDE

Use following succinylcholine: If succinylcholine is used to facilitate endotracheal intubation, pipecuronium may be administered after recovery from succinylcholine paralysis. In patients with normal renal function who are not obese, starting doses of 0.05 mg/kg of pipecuronium are recommended and will provide ≈ 45 minutes of clinical relaxation. In nonobese patients with normal renal function, higher pipecuronium doses of 0.07 to 0.085 mg/kg, if administered after recovery from succinylcholine, are associated with approximately the same clinical duration as pipecuronium without prior succinylcholine administration.

Maintenance dosing: Maintenance doses of 0.01 to 0.015 mg/kg (10 to 15 mcg/kg) administered at 25% recovery of control T_1, provide ≈ 50 minutes (range, 17 to 175 minutes) clinical duration under balanced anesthesia. Consider a lower dose in patients receiving inhalation anesthetics. In all cases, guide dosing based on the clinical duration following initial dose or prior maintenance dose, and do not administer until signs of neuromuscular function are evident.

Children: Infants (3 months to 1 year) under balanced anesthesia or halothane anesthesia manifest similar dose response to pipecuronium as do adults on a mcg/kg basis. Children (1 to 14 years) under balanced anesthesia or halothane anesthesia may be less sensitive than adults. The clinical duration of doses averaging 0.04 mg/kg (40 mcg/kg) in infants and 0.057 mg/kg (57 mcg/kg) in children, ranged from 10 to 44 minutes and from 18 to 52 minutes, respectively. These doses were ≈ 1.2 times ED_{95}.

IV compatibility: 0.9% NaCl solution; 5% Dextrose in Saline; 5% Dextrose in Water; Lactated Ringer's; Sterile Water for Injection; Bacteriostatic Water for Injection.

Pipecuronium is not recommended for dilution into or administration from large volume IV solutions.

Storage/Stability: Store at 2° to 30°C (35° to 86°F). Protect from light.

When reconstituted with Bacteriostatic Water for Injection – Contains benzyl alcohol. Use within 5 days. May be stored at room temperature or refrigerated.

When reconstituted with compatible IV solutions – Refrigerate vial. Use within 24 hours. Single use only. Discard unused portion.

Rx	**Arduan** (Organon)	**Powder for Injection (lyophilized)**[1]: 10 mg	In 10 ml vials.

[1] Freeze-dried cake with 380 mg mannitol.

Nondepolarizing Neuromuscular Blockers

DOXACURIUM CHLORIDE

Warning:

Administer in carefully adjusted doses by or under the supervision of experienced clinicians who are familiar with the drug's actions and the possible complications of its use. Do not administer unless facilities for intubation, artificial respiration, oxygen therapy and an antagonist are immediately available. Employ a peripheral nerve stimulator to monitor drug response, need for additional relaxants and adequacy of spontaneous recovery or antagonism.

Doxacurium has no known effect on consciousness, pain threshold or cerebration; to avoid patient distress, do not induce neuromuscular blockade before unconsciousness.

Actions:

Pharmacology: Doxacurium chloride is a long-acting, nondepolarizing skeletal muscle relaxant for IV administration. It binds competitively to cholinergic receptors on the motor end-plate to antagonize the action of acetylcholine, resulting in a block of neuromuscular transmission. This action is antagonized by acetylcholinesterase inhibitors, such as neostigmine.

Doxacurium is ≈ 2.5 to 3 times more potent than pancuronium and 10 to 12 times more potent than metocurine. Doxacurium in doses of 1.5 to 2 x ED_{95} has a clinical duration of action similar to that of equipotent doses of pancuronium and metocurine. The average ED_{95} (dose required to produce 95% suppression of the adductor pollicis muscle twitch response to ulnar nerve stimulation) is 0.025 mg/kg (range, 0.02 to 0.033) in adults receiving balanced anesthesia.

The onset and clinically effective duration (time from injection to 25% recovery) of doxacurium administered alone or after succinylcholine during stable balanced anesthesia are shown in the following table:

Pharmacodynamic Dose Response to Doxacurium During Balanced Anesthesia[1]

Parameter	Initial doxacurium dose (mg/kg)		
	0.025[2] (n = 34)	0.05 (n = 27)	0.08 (n = 9)
Time to maximum block (min)	9.3 (5.4 - 16)	5.2 (2.5 - 13)	3.5 (2.4 - 5)
Clinical duration (min; time to 25% recovery)	55 (9 - 145)	100 (39 - 232)	160 (110 - 338)

[1] Values shown are means (range).
[2] Doxacurium administered after 10% to 100% recovery from an intubating dose of succinylcholine.

Initial doses of 0.05 mg/kg (2 x ED_{95}) and 0.08 mg/kg (3 x ED_{95}) given during thiopental-narcotic anesthesia induction produce good-to-excellent conditions for tracheal intubation in 5 and 4 minutes (which are before maximum block), respectively.

The mean time for spontaneous T_1 (first twitch) recovery from 25% to 50% of control following initial doses of doxacurium is ≈ 26 minutes (range, 7 to 104) during balanced anesthesia. The mean time for spontaneous T_1 recovery from 25% to 75% is 54 minutes (range, 14 to 184).

Most patients required pharmacologic reversal prior to full spontaneous recovery from neuromuscular block. As with other long-acting neuromuscular blocking agents, doxacurium may be associated with prolonged times to full spontaneous recovery. Following an initial dose of 0.025 mg/kg, some patients may require as long as 4 hours to exhibit full spontaneous recovery.

Cumulative neuromuscular blocking effects are not associated with repeated administration of maintenance doses of doxacurium at 25% T_1 recovery. As with initial doses, however, the duration of action following maintenance doses may vary considerably among patients.

The doxacurium ED_{95} for children 2 to 12 years of age receiving halothane anesthesia is ≈ 0.03 mg/kg. Children require higher doses on a mg/kg basis than adults to achieve comparable levels of block. The onset, time and duration of block are shorter in children than adults. During halothane anesthesia, doses of 0.03 and 0.05 mg/kg produce maximum block in ≈ 7 and 4 minutes, respectively. The duration of clinically effective block is ≈ 30 minutes after an initial dose of 0.03 mg/kg and ≈ 45 minutes after 0.05 mg/kg.

Nondepolarizing Neuromuscular Blockers

DOXACURIUM CHLORIDE

The neuromuscular block produced by doxacurium may be antagonized by anticholinesterase agents. The more profound the neuromuscular block at reversal, the longer the time and the greater the dose of anticholinesterase required for recovery of neuromuscular function.

Hemodynamics – In healthy adult patients, children (2 to 12 years of age) and patients with serious cardiovascular disease undergoing coronary artery bypass grafting, cardiac valvular repair or vascular repair, doxacurium produced no dose-related effects on mean arterial blood pressure or heart rate.

Doses of 0.03 to 0.08 mg/kg (1.2 to 3 x ED_{95}) were not associated with dose-dependent changes in mean plasma histamine concentration. Adverse experiences typically associated with histamine release (eg, bronchospasm, hypotension, tachycardia, cutaneous flushing, urticaria) are very rare.

Pharmacokinetics: The pharmacokinetics are linear. The pharmacokinetics are similar in healthy young adult and elderly patients. The time to maximum block is longer in elderly patients than in young adult patients (11.2 vs 7.7 minutes at 0.025 mg/kg). In addition, the clinically effective durations of block are more variable and tend to be longer in healthy elderly patients.

A longer half-life can be expected in patients with end-stage kidney disease; in addition, these patients may be more sensitive to the neuromuscular blocking effects of doxacurium. The time to maximum block was slightly longer and the clinically effective duration of block was prolonged in patients with end-stage kidney disease.

Sensitivity to the neuromuscular blocking effects of doxacurium was highly variable in patients undergoing liver transplantation. Three of seven patients developed ≤ 50% block, indicating that a reduced sensitivity to doxacurium may occur in such patients. In those patients who developed > 50% neuromuscular block, the time to maximum block and the clinically effective duration tended to be longer than in healthy young adult patients.

Pharmacokinetic and Pharmacodynamic Parameters of Doxacurium[1]

	Healthy young adult patients (22 to 49 years)				Kidney transplant patients	Liver transplant patients	Healthy elderly patients (67 to 72 yrs)
	Dose (mg/kg)				Dose (mg/kg)	Dose (mg/kg)	Dose (mg/kg)
Parameter	0.015 (n = 9)	0.025 (n = 8)	0.05 (n = 8)	0.08 (n = 8)	0.015 (n = 8)	0.015 (n = 7)	0.025 (n = 8)
Elimination half-life (min)	99 (48 - 193)	86 (25 - 171)	123 (61 - 163)	98 (47 - 163)	221 (84 - 592)	115 (69 - 148)	96 (50 - 114)
Volume of distribution at steady state (L/kg)	0.22 (0.11 - 0.43)	0.15 (0.1 - 0.21)	0.24 (0.13 - 0.3)	0.22 (0.16 - 0.33)	0.27 (0.17 - 0.55)	0.29 (0.17 - 0.35)	0.22 (0.14 - 0.4)
Plasma clearance (ml/min/kg)	2.66 (1.35 - 6.66)	2.22 (1.02 - 3.95)	2.62 (1.21 - 5.7)	2.53 (1.88 - 3.38)	1.23 (0.48 - 2.4)	2.3 (1.96 - 3.05)	2.47 (1.58 - 3.6)
Maximum block (%)	86 (59 - 100)	97 (88 - 100)	100	100	98 (95 - 100)	70 (0 - 100)	96 (90 - 100)
Clinically effective duration of block[2] (min)	36 (19 - 80)	68 (35 - 90)	91 (47 - 132)	177 (74 - 268)	80 (29 - 133)	52 (20 - 91)	97 (36 - 179)

[1] Values shown are means (range).

[2] Time from injection to 25% recovery of the control twitch height.

Consecutively administered maintenance doses of 0.005 mg/kg, each given at 25% T_1 recovery following the preceding dose, do not result in a progressive increase in the plasma concentration of doxacurium or a progressive increase in the depth or duration of block produced by each dose.

Doxacurium is not metabolized; the major elimination pathway is excretion of unchanged drug in urine and bile. In studies of healthy adult patients, 24% to 38% of an administered dose was recovered as parent drug in urine over 6 to 12 hours after dosing. High bile concentrations (relative to plasma) have been found 35 to 90 minutes after administration. The overall extent of biliary excretion is unknown.

Plasma protein binding is ≈ 30%.

Nondepolarizing Neuromuscular Blockers

DOXACURIUM CHLORIDE

Indications:

Adjunct to general anesthesia, to provide skeletal muscle relaxation during surgery; to provide skeletal muscle relaxation for endotracheal intubation or to facilitate mechanical ventilation.

Contraindications:

Hypersensitivity to the drug.

Warnings:

Antagonism of neuromuscular block: Antagonists (such as neostigmine) should not be administered prior to the demonstration of some spontaneous recovery from neuromuscular block. The time for recovery of neuromuscular function following administration of neostigmine is dependent upon the level of residual neuromuscular block at the time of attempted reversal; longer recovery times may be anticipated when neostigmine is administered at more profound levels of block (eg, at $< 25\%$ T_1 recovery).

Benzyl alcohol: Doxacurium injection contains benzyl alcohol. In newborn infants, benzyl alcohol has been associated with an increased incidence of neurological and other complications that are sometimes fatal.

Renal/Hepatic function impairment: Consider the possibility of prolonged neuromuscular block in patients undergoing renal transplantation and the possibility of a variable onset and duration of neuromuscular block in patients undergoing liver transplantation when doxacurium is used.

Elderly: In elderly patients, the onset of maximum block is slower and the duration of neuromuscular block is more variable and may be longer than in young patients.

Pregnancy: Category C. There are no adequate or well controlled studies in pregnant women. Use during pregnancy only if the potential benefit justifies the risk to the fetus.

Obstetrics (cesarean section) – Because the duration of action of doxacurium exceeds the usual duration of operative obstetrics (cesarean section), doxacurium is not recommended for use in patients undergoing cesarean section.

Lactation: It is not known whether doxacurium is excreted in breast milk. Exercise caution following administration to a nursing woman.

Children: Doxacurium has not been studied in children < 2 years of age. See Actions and Administration and Dosage for use in children 2 to 12 years of age.

Precautions:

Neuromuscular diseases: Neuromuscular blocking agents may have a profound effect in patients with neuromuscular diseases (eg, myasthenia gravis and the myasthenic syndrome). In these and other conditions in which prolonged neuromuscular block is a possibility (eg, carcinomatosis), use a peripheral nerve stimulator and a small test dose of doxacurium to assess the level of neuromuscular block and to monitor dosage requirements. Shorter acting muscle relaxants may be more suitable.

Burn victims: Resistance to nondepolarizing neuromuscular blocking agents may develop in patients with burns depending upon the time elapsed since the injury and the size of the burn.

Acid-base or serum electrolyte abnormalities may potentiate or antagonize the action of neuromuscular blocking agents. Their action may be enhanced by magnesium salts administered for the management of eclampsia or preeclampsia.

Obesity: Administration of doxacurium on the basis of actual body weight is associated with a prolonged duration of action in obese patients (see Actions). Base the dose upon ideal body weight in obese patients (see Administration and Dosage).

Malignant hyperthermia (MH): Doxacurium has not been studied in MH-susceptible patients. Because MH can develop in the absence of established triggering agents, be prepared to recognize and treat MH in any patient receiving general anesthesia.

Long-term use: Information on the use of doxacurium in the ICU is limited. No evidence of tachyphylaxis, accumulation or prolonged recovery has been observed.

When doxacurium is used in the ICU, monitor neuromuscular transmission continuously during administration with the help of a nerve stimulator. Do not give additional doses of doxacurium or any other neuromuscular blocking agent before there is a definite response to T_1 or to the first twitch. If no response is elicited, bolus administration should be delayed until a response returns.

Nondepolarizing Neuromuscular Blockers

DOXACURIUM CHLORIDE

Drug Interactions:

Doxacurium Chloride Drug Interactions			
Precipitant drug	Object drug*		Description
Antibiotics (eg, aminoglycosides, tetracyclines, bacitracin, polymyxins, lincomycin, clindamycin, colistin and sodium colistimethate)	Doxacurium	⬆	May enhance the neuromuscular blocking action of nondepolarizing agents.
Carbamazepine Phenytoin	Doxacurium	⬇	Carbamazepine and phenytoin lengthen the time of onset of neuromuscular block induced by doxacurium and shorten the duration of block.
Inhalational anesthetics	Doxacurium	⬆	Isoflurane, enflurane and halothane decrease the ED_{50} of doxacurium by 30% to 45% and may also prolong the duration of action by up to 25%.
Lithium Local anesthetics Magnesium salts Procainamide Quinidine	Doxacurium	⬆	May enhance the neuromuscular blocking action of nondepolarizing agents.

* ⬆ = Object drug increased. ⬇ = Object drug decreased.

Adverse Reactions:

The most frequent adverse effect of nondepolarizing blocking agents is an extension of the pharmacological action beyond the time needed for surgery and anesthesia. This effect may vary from skeletal muscle weakness to profound and prolonged skeletal muscle paralysis resulting in respiratory insufficiency and apnea that require manual or mechanical ventilation until recovery (see Overdosage). Inadequate reversal of neuromuscular block from doxacurium is possible.

Cardiovascular: Hypotension, flushing (0.3%); ventricular fibrillation, myocardial infarction (< 0.1%).

Dermatologic: Urticaria, injection site reaction (< 0.1%).

Respiratory: Bronchospasm, wheezing (< 0.1%).

Special senses: Diplopia (< 0.1%).

Miscellaneous: Difficult neuromuscular block reversal, prolonged drug effect, fever (< 0.1%).

Overdosage:

Overdosage with neuromuscular blocking agents may result in neuromuscular block beyond the time needed for surgery and anesthesia. The primary treatment is maintenance of a patent airway and controlled ventilation until recovery of normal neuromuscular function. Once evidence of recovery is observed, further recovery may be facilitated by administration of an anticholinesterase agent (eg, neostigmine, edrophonium) in conjunction with an appropriate anticholinergic agent.

Administration and Dosage:

Approved by the FDA in March 1991.

For IV use only.

Individualization of dosages:

Elderly/renal function impairment – The potential for a prolongation of block may be reduced by decreasing the initial dose and titrating the dose.

Obese patients (≥ 30% more than ideal body weight [IBW] for height) – Determine the dose using the patient's IBW, according to the following formulae:

Men: IBW (kg) = (106 + [6 × inches in height above 5 feet])/2.2

Women: IBW (kg) = (100 + [5 × inches in height above 5 feet])/2.2

Severe liver disease – Dosage requirements are variable; some patients may require a higher than normal initial dose to achieve clinically effective block. Once adequate block is established, the clinical duration of block may be prolonged in such patients relative to patients with normal liver function.

Nondepolarizing Neuromuscular Blockers

DOXACURIUM CHLORIDE

Other conditions – As with other nondepolarizing neuromuscular blocking agents, a reduction of doxacurium dose must be considered in cachetic or debilitated patients, in patients with neuromuscular diseases, severe electrolyte abnormalities, or carcinomatosis, and in other patients in whom potentiation of neuromuscular block or difficulty with reversal is anticipated. Increased doses of doxacurium may be required in burn patients (see Precautions).

Adults:

Initial doses – When administered as a component of a thiopental/narcotic induction-intubation paradigm as well as for production of long-duration neuromuscular block during surgery, 0.05 mg/kg (2 × ED_{95}) produces good-to-excellent conditions for tracheal intubation in 5 minutes in ≈ 90% of patients. Lower doses may result in a longer time for development of satisfactory intubation conditions. Clinically effective neuromuscular block may be expected to last ≈ 100 minutes on average (range, 39 to 232) following 0.05 mg/kg administered to patients receiving balanced anesthesia.

Reserve an initial dose of 0.08 mg/kg (3 × ED_{95}) for instances in which a need for very prolonged neuromuscular block is anticipated. In ≈ 90% of patients, good-to-excellent intubation conditions may be expected in 4 minutes after this dose; however, clinically effective block may be expected to persist ≥ 160 minutes (range, 110 to 338).

If doxacurium is administered during steady-state isoflurane, enflurane or halothane anesthesia, consider reduction of the dose by one-third.

When succinylcholine is administered to facilitate tracheal intubation in patients receiving balanced anesthesia, an initial dose of 0.025 mg/kg (ED_{95}) doxacurium provides ≈ 60 minutes (range, 9 to 145) of clinically effective neuromuscular block for surgery. For a longer duration of action, a larger initial dose may be administered.

Maintenance doses – Maintenance dosing will generally be required ≈ 60 minutes after an initial dose of 0.025 mg/kg or 100 minutes after an initial dose of 0.05 mg/kg during balanced anesthesia. Repeated maintenance doses administered at 25% T_1 recovery may be expected to be required at relatively regular intervals in each patient. The interval may vary considerably between patients. Maintenance doses of 0.005 and 0.01 mg/kg each provide an average 30 minutes (range, 9 to 57) and 45 minutes (range, 14 to 108), respectively, of additional clinically effective neuromuscular block. For shorter or longer desired durations, smaller or larger maintenance doses may be administered.

Children: When administering during halothane anesthesia, an initial dose of 0.03 mg/kg (ED_{95}) produces maximum neuromuscular block in ≈ 7 minutes (range, 5 to 11) and clinically effective block for an average of 30 minutes (range, 12 to 54). Under halothane anesthesia, 0.05 mg/kg produces maximum block in ≈ 4 minutes (range, 2 to 10) and clinically effective block for 45 minutes (range, 30 to 80). Maintenance doses are generally required more frequently in children than in adults. Because of the potentiating effect of halothane seen in adults, a higher dose of doxacurium may be required in children receiving balanced anesthesia than in children receiving halothane anesthesia to achieve a comparable onset and duration of neuromuscular block. Doxacurium has not been studied in children < 2 years of age.

Admixture incompatibility:

Y-site administration – Doxacurium injection may not be compatible with alkaline solutions with a pH > 8.5 (eg, barbiturate solutions).

Admixture compatibility: 5% Dextrose Injection; 0.9% Sodium Chloride Injection; 5% Dextrose and 0.9% Sodium Chloride Injection; Lactated Ringer's Injection; 5% Dextrose/Lactated Ringer's Injection; sufentanil citrate; alfentanil HCl; fentanyl citrate.

Storage/Stability: Store at room temperature of 15° to 25°C (59° to 77°F). Do not freeze.

Doxacurium diluted up to 1:10 in 5% Dextrose Injection or 0.9% Sodium Chloride Injection is physically and chemically stable when stored in polypropylene syringes at 5° to 25° C (41° to 77° F), for up to 24 hours. Immediate use of the diluted product is preferred; discard any unused portion of diluted doxacurium after 8 hours.

Rx	**Nuromax** (Glaxo Wellcome)	**Injection:** 1 mg/ml	In 5 ml multiple-dose vials.[1]

[1] With 0.9% benzyl alcohol.

Depolarizing Neuromuscular Blockers

SUCCINYLCHOLINE CHLORIDE

Warning:
Use succinylcholine only if skilled in the management of artificial respiration and when facilities are instantly available for tracheal intubation and for providing adequate ventilation of the patient, including the administration of oxygen under positive pressure and the elimination of carbon dioxide. The clinician must be prepared to assist or control respiration.

Actions:

Pharmacology: Succinylcholine is an ultrashort-acting depolarizing skeletal muscle relaxant. Like acetylcholine, it combines with cholinergic receptors of the motor endplate to produce depolarization observed as fasciculations. Neuromuscular transmission is then inhibited so long as an adequate concentration of succinylcholine remains at the receptor site; the neuromuscular block produces a flaccid paralysis.

Paralysis usually appears in the following muscles consecutively: Levator muscles of the eyelids, mastication muscles, limb muscles, abdominal muscles, glottis muscles, the intercostals, the diaphragm and all other skeletal muscles.

Succinylcholine has no effect on consciousness, pain threshold or cerebration; use only with adequate anesthesia. While it has no direct effect upon the myocardium, changes in rhythm may result from vagal stimulation, such as may result from surgical procedures (particularly in children) or from potassium-mediated alterations in electrical conductivity. These effects are enhanced by cyclopropane and halogenated anesthetics. Succinylcholine slightly increases intraocular pressure, which may persist after the onset of complete paralysis. Tachyphylaxis occurs with repeated doses. It has no direct effect on the uterus or other smooth muscles. Because the drug is highly ionized and has a low lipid solubility, it does not readily cross the placenta.

When succinylcholine is given over a prolonged period of time, the characteristic depolarizing neuromuscular block (Phase I block) may change to a block that superficially resembles a nondepolarizing block (Phase II block). This may be associated with prolonged respiratory depression or apnea in patients who manifest the transition to Phase II block. After confirmation by peripheral nerve stimulation, reverse with anticholinesterase drugs such as neostigmine (see Precautions).

Pharmacokinetics:

Onset and duration – Following IV injection, complete muscular relaxation occurs within 30 to 60 seconds and with single administration, lasts ≈ 4 to 6 minutes. Following IM injection, onset of action may vary from 2 to 3 minutes. Muscular relaxation of longer duration can be achieved by repeated injections at appropriate intervals or by continuous IV infusion.

Metabolism – The drug is rapidly hydrolyzed by plasma cholinesterase to succinylmonocholine (a nondepolarizing muscle relaxant), then more slowly to succinic acid and choline. Succinylmonocholine can accumulate and cause prolonged paralysis due to its slower rate of hydrolysis. Correlation has been found between pseudocholinesterase levels and duration of action. About 10% is excreted unchanged in the urine.

Indications:

Anesthesia: Adjunct to general anesthesia to facilitate endotracheal intubation, and to induce skeletal muscle relaxation during surgery or mechanical ventilation.

Contraindications:

Hypersensitivity to succinylcholine or any components of these products; patients with genetically determined disorders of plasma pseudocholinesterase; personal or familial history of malignant hyperthermia; myopathies associated with elevated creatine phosphokinase (CPK) values; acute narrow-angle glaucoma; penetrating eye injuries.

Warnings:

Malignant hyperthermia (MH): The abrupt onset of MH, a rare hypermetabolic process of skeletal muscle, may be triggered by succinylcholine. Early premonitory signs include: Muscle rigidity, particularly involving jaw muscles; tachycardia and tachypnea unresponsive to increased depth of anesthesia; evidence of increased oxygen requirement and carbon dioxide production (change in color of the CO_2 absorber); rising temperature; metabolic acidosis. Considerations important to the management of this problem are: Early recognition of premonitory signs; immediate discontinuation of anesthesia and succinylcholine (either agent may induce the syndrome); implementation of supportive measures including administration of oxygen and sodium bicarbonate, lowering body temperature, restoration of fluid and

SUCCINYLCHOLINE CHLORIDE

electrolyte balance, maintenance of adequate urinary output and administration of IV dantrolene (see the dantrolene monograph). Establish a standard protocol to implement when the syndrome becomes apparent.

Controlling respiration: Use succinylcholine only when facilities for endotracheal intubation, artificial respiration and oxygen administration are instantly available. Be prepared to assist or control respiration.

Myasthenia gravis patients have shown resistance to succinylcholine.

Myalgia: Succinylcholine may cause myalgia. Aspirin 600 mg 1 hour before anesthesia has been shown to reduce myalgia.

Pregnancy: Category C. Safety for use during pregnancy has not been established. It is not known whether the drug can cause fetal harm when administered to a pregnant woman or can affect reproduction capacity. Use in pregnant women only when clearly needed and when potential benefits outweigh potential hazards.

Pseudocholinesterase levels are decreased by ≈ 24% during pregnancy and for several days postpartum. Therefore, pregnant patients may be expected to show greater sensitivity (prolonged apnea) to succinylcholine than nonpregnant patients.

Labor and delivery – Succinylcholine is commonly used to provide muscle relaxation during cesarean section. While small amounts cross the placenta, the amount that enters fetal circulation after a single 1 mg/kg dose to the mother should not endanger the fetus. However, because the amount of drug that crosses the placenta depends on the concentration gradient between the maternal and fetal circulations, residual neuromuscular blockade (apnea and flaccidity) may occur in the neonate after repeated high doses to the mother or in the presence of atypical pseudocholinesterase in the mother.

Lactation: It is not known whether this drug is excreted in breast milk. Exercise caution when succinylcholine is administered to a nursing woman.

Children: There are rare reports of ventricular dysrhythmias and cardiac arrest secondary to acute rhabdomyolysis with hyperkalemia in healthy children. Many of these children were subsequently found to have a skeletal muscle myopathy, such as Duchenne's muscular dystrophy, which had clinical signs that were not obvious. The syndrome often presents as sudden cardiac arrest within minutes after the administration of succinylcholine. These children are usually, but not exclusively, males and most frequently ≤ 8 years of age. There have also been reports in adolescents. There may be no signs or symptoms to alert the practitioner to which patients are at risk. A careful history and physical may identify developmental delays suggestive of a myopathy. A preoperative creatine kinase could identify some but not all patients at risk. Because of the abrupt onset of this symptom, routine resuscitative measures are likely to be unsuccessful. Careful monitoring of the electrocardiogram may alert the practitioner to peaked T-waves (an early sign). Administration of IV calcium, bicarbonate and glucose with insulin, with hyperventilation have resulted in successful resuscitation in some of the reported cases. Extraordinary and prolonged resuscitative efforts have been effective in some cases. As in adults, the incidence of bradycardia in children is higher following the second succinylcholine dose.

Precautions:

Use with caution in cardiovascular, hepatic, pulmonary, metabolic or renal disorders. Administer with great caution to patients with severe burns, electrolyte imbalance, hyperkalemia, those receiving quinidine and those who are digitalized or recovering from severe trauma, as serious cardiac arrhythmias or cardiac arrest may result. Observe caution in patients with pre-existing hyperkalemia or those who are paraplegic, who have suffered spinal cord injury or have degenerative or dystrophic neuromuscular disease, because such patients tend to become severely hyperkalemic when succinylcholine is given.

Prolonged blockade may occur in patients with hypokalemia, hypocalcemia, hepatic disorders, cardiovascular and pulmonary disorders.

Low plasma pseudocholinesterase may be associated with a prolonged paralysis of respiration following succinylcholine. Low levels are often found in patients with severe liver disease or cirrhosis, anemia, burns, malnutrition, dehydration, cancer, collagen diseases, abnormal body temperatures, myxedema, pregnancy, exposure to neurotoxic insecticides; in those receiving antimalarial drugs, anticancer drugs, irradiation, MAO inhibitors, oral contraceptives, pancuronium, chlorpromazine, echothiophate iodide or neostigmine; or in those with a recessive hereditary trait. Administer minimal doses with extreme care to such patients. If low plasma pseudocholinesterase activity is suspected, administer a test dose of 5 to 10 mg or produce relaxation by the cautious administration of a 0.1% IV drip.

Depolarizing Neuromuscular Blockers

SUCCINYLCHOLINE CHLORIDE

Nondepolarizing blockade: During repeated or prolonged administration of succinylcholine, the characteristic Phase I block may convert to a Phase II block. Prolonged respiratory depression or apnea may be observed in patients manifesting this transition. The transition from Phase I to Phase II block was reported in seven of seven patients studied under halothane anesthesia after an accumulated dose of 2 to 4 mg/kg succinylcholine (administered in repeated, divided doses). The onset of Phase II block coincided with the onset of tachyphylaxis and prolongation of spontaneous recovery. In another study, using balanced anesthesia (N_2O/O_2/narcotic-thiopental) and succinylcholine infusion, the transition was less abrupt with great variability in the dose required to produce Phase II block. Of 32 patients studied, 24 developed Phase II block. Tachyphylaxis was not associated with the transition, and 50% of the patients who developed Phase II block experienced prolonged recovery.

When Phase II block is suspected, base the decision to reverse the block with an anticholinesterase drug upon a positive diagnosis using a peripheral nerve stimulator, because an anticholinesterase agent will potentiate a succinylcholine-induced Phase I block. Phase II block is indicated by fade of responses to successive stimuli (preferably "train of four"). Accompany anticholinesterase drugs to reverse Phase II block by appropriate doses of atropine to prevent cardiac arrhythmias. After adequate reversal of Phase II block with an anticholinesterase agent, observe the patient for at least 1 hour for signs of return of muscle relaxation. Do not attempt reversal unless: (1) A peripheral nerve stimulator is used to determine the presence of Phase II block, and (2) spontaneous recovery of muscle twitch has occurred for at least 20 minutes and has reached a plateau with further recovery proceeding slowly; this delay ensures complete hydrolysis of succinylcholine by pseudocholinesterase prior to administration of the anticholinesterase agent.

Concurrent use of a depolarizing and a nondepolarizing (competitive) muscle relaxant is not recommended because a prolonged mixed block may occur. In this instance, determine the dominant feature of the block by the use of a nerve stimulator and treat accordingly.

Ophthalmic: Succinylcholine causes a slight, transient increase in intraocular pressure immediately after its injection and during the fasciculation phase; slight increases may persist after onset of complete paralysis. Use with caution, if at all, during intraocular surgery and in patients with glaucoma.

Patients with fractures or muscle spasm require caution because the muscle fasciculations may cause additional trauma.

Reduce muscle fasciculations and hyperkalemia by administering a small dose of a nondepolarizing relaxant prior to succinylcholine. If other relaxants are to be used during the procedure, consider the possibility of a synergistic or antagonistic effect.

Intracranial pressure: Succinylcholine may cause a transient increase in intracranial pressure; however, adequate anesthetic induction prior to administration of succinylcholine will minimize this effect.

Intragastric pressure: Succinylcholine may increase intragastric pressure, which could result in regurgitation and possible aspiration of stomach contents.

Depolarizing Neuromuscular Blockers

SUCCINYLCHOLINE CHLORIDE

Drug Interactions:

Succinylcholine Drug Interactions			
Precipitant drug	Object drug*		Description
Amphotericin B and thiazide diuretics	Succinylcholine	↑	Amphotericin B and thiazide diuretics may increase effects of succinylcholine secondary to induced electrolyte imbalance. Patients with hypocalcemia and hypokalemia usually require reduced succinylcholine doses.
Cimetidine	Succinylcholine	↑	Cimetidine inhibits pseudocholinesterase.
Cyclophosphamide	Succinylcholine	↑	Cyclophosphamide decreases plasma pseudocholinesterase.
Diazepam	Succinylcholine	↓	Diazepam may reduce the duration of neuromuscular blockade produced by succinylcholine.
Inhalation anesthetics (eg, cyclopropane, diethyl ether, halothane and nitrous oxide)	Succinylcholine	↑	Coadministration with succinylcholine may increase incidence of bradycardia, arrhythmias, sinus arrest and apnea, as well as the occurrence of malignant hyperthermia in susceptible individuals.
IV procaine	Succinylcholine	↑	IV procaine competes for the enzyme and may prolong the effect of succinylcholine.
Narcotic analgesics	Succinylcholine	↑	Narcotic analgesics may increase the incidence of bradycardia and sinus arrest.
Nondepolarizing muscle relaxants	Succinylcholine	↑	Consider the possibility of a synergistic or antagonistic effect with succinylcholine.
Phenelzine, promazine, oxytocin, certain nonpenicillin antibiotics, quinidine, beta-adrenergic blocking agents, procainamide, lidocaine, trimethaphan, lithium carbonate, furosemide, magnesium sulfate, quinine, chloroquine and isoflurane	Succinylcholine	↑	All of these drugs may enhance the neuromuscular blocking action of succinylcholine.
Succinylcholine	Digitalis glycosides	↑	Succinylcholine may cause a sudden potassium extrusion from muscle cells, possibly causing arrhythmias or ventricular fibrillation in digitalized patients. Toxicity (cardiac arrhythmias) of both drugs may be increased.

* ↑ = Object drug increased. ↓ = Object drug decreased.

Adverse Reactions:

As with other neuromuscular blockers, the potential for releasing histamine is present following succinylcholine use. However, serious histamine-mediated flushing, hypotension and bronchoconstriction are uncommon in normal clinical usage.

Adverse reactions consist primarily of an extension of the drug's pharmacological actions. Profound and prolonged muscle relaxation may occur, resulting in respiratory depression to the point of apnea. Hypersensitivity and anaphylactic reactions have been reported rarely. The following reactions have been reported:

As with other neuromuscular blockers, the potential for releasing histamine is present following succinylcholine use. However, serious histamine-mediated flushing, hypotension and bronchoconstriction are uncommon in normal clinical usage.

Adverse reactions consist primarily of an extension of the drug's pharmacological actions. Profound and prolonged muscle relaxation may occur, resulting in respi-

Depolarizing Neuromuscular Blockers

SUCCINYLCHOLINE CHLORIDE

ratory depression to the point of apnea. Hypersensitivity and anaphylactic reactions have been reported rarely. The following reactions have been reported:

Cardiovascular: Bradycardia (frequently noted after a second IV injection of a 2% solution in children); tachycardia; hypertension; hypotension; cardiac arrest; arrhythmias.

Respiratory: Respiratory depression or apnea.

Miscellaneous: Malignant hyperthermia (see Warnings); increased intraocular pressure (see Precautions); muscle fasciculation; postoperative muscle pain; excessive salivation; hyperkalemia; rash; myoglobinemia; myoglobinuria; perioperative dreams (children); myalgia; jaw rigidity; rhabdomyolysis with possible myoglobinuric acute renal failure.

Overdosage:

Overdosage with succinylcholine may result in neuromuscular block beyond the time needed for surgery and anesthesia. This may be manifested by skeletal muscle weakness, decreased respiratory reserve, low tidal volume or apnea. The primary treatment is maintenance of a patent airway and respiratory support until recovery of normal respiration is assured. Depending on the dose and duration of succinylcholine administration, the characteristic depolarizing neuromuscular block (Phase I) may change to a block with characteristics superficially resembling a nondepolarizing block (Phase II).

Administration and Dosage:

Individualize dosage.

To avoid patient distress, administer after unconsciousness has been induced.

Short surgical procedures: The average dose required to induce muscle relaxation of short duration is 0.6 mg/kg IV. The optimum dose varies among individuals and may range from 0.3 to 1.1 mg/kg. Maximum paralysis may persist for ≈ 2 minutes. Recovery takes place within 4 to 6 minutes.

Following an injection of an effective dose of succinylcholine, relaxation sufficient for endotracheal intubation generally occurs in ≈ 1 minute. Administer more succinylcholine at appropriate intervals if relaxation is not complete.

Long surgical procedures: Dosage depends on duration of procedure and the need for muscle relaxation. Average rate for an adult ranges between 2.5 and 4.3 mg/min. Solutions containing 0.1% to 0.2% (1 to 2 mg/ml) are commonly used for continuous IV drip. The more dilute solution is probably preferable for ease of control of the administration rate of relaxation. Give this 1 mg/ml IV drip solution at 0.5 to 10 mg/minute to obtain required amount of relaxation. The 0.2% solution may be useful when it is desirable to avoid overburdening circulation with a large volume of fluid.

Prolonged muscular relaxation may be achieved with intermittent IV injections. Give an initial dose of 0.3 to 1.1 mg/kg then give 0.04 to 0.07 mg/kg at appropriate intervals to maintain the required degree of relaxation.

Children:

IV – For infants and small children, 2 mg/kg; for older children and adolescents, 1 mg/kg. IV bolus use may result in profound bradycardia or, rarely, asystole. As in adults, the incidence of bradycardia is higher after a second dose. Reduce occurrence of bradyarrhythmias by pretreatment with atropine.

IM – In the absence of a suitable vein for IV administration, a dose of 3 to 4 mg/kg (not exceeding a total dose of 150 mg) is suggested. The onset of effect is usually observed in ≈ 2 to 3 minutes.

Preparation of solution: Use only freshly prepared solutions. Succinylcholine is incompatible with alkaline solutions and will precipitate if mixed or administered simultaneously. Discard unused solutions within 24 hours. Inject separately; do not mix in the same syringe or administer simultaneously through the same needle with solutions of short-acting barbiturates, such as sodium thiopental or other drugs with an alkaline pH.

Storage/Stability: Refrigerate at 2° to 8°C (36° to 46°F). Multi-dose vials are stable for ≤ 14 days at room temperature without significant loss of potency.

Powder for infusion does not require refrigeration.

Depolarizing Neuromuscular Blockers

SUCCINYLCHOLINE CHLORIDE			
Rx	**Anectine** (Glaxo Wellcome)	**Injection:** 20 mg/ml	In 10 ml vials.[1]
Rx	**Quelicin** (Abbott)		In 5 ml *Abboject* (single-dose) syringe and 10 ml vials.[2]
Rx	**Succinylcholine Chloride** (Organon)		In 10 ml vials.[3]
Rx	**Quelicin** (Abbott)	**Injection:** 50 mg/ml	In 10 ml amps.
Rx	**Quelicin** (Abbott)	**Injection:** 100 mg/ml	In 5 ml and 10 ml vials.
Rx	**Anectine Flo-Pack** (Glaxo Wellcome)	**Powder for Infusion:** 500 mg	In vials.
		Powder for Infusion: 1 g	In vials.

[1] With methylparaben.
[2] With methyl- and propylparabens.
[3] With benzyl alcohol.

Centrally Acting

CARISOPRODOL

Actions:

Pharmacology: Carisoprodol is a congener of meprobamate. The mode of action of carisoprodol has not been clearly identified, but may be related to its sedative properties. Carisoprodol does not directly relax tense skeletal muscles in man. In animals, the drug produces muscle relaxation by blocking interneuronal activity in the descending reticular formation and spinal cord.

Pharmacokinetics: The onset of action is rapid (30 minutes) and the duration is 4 to 6 hours. It is metabolized in the liver and excreted in the urine.

Indications:

Musculoskeletal conditions: As an adjunct to rest, physical therapy and other measures for the relief of discomfort associated with acute, painful musculoskeletal conditions.

Contraindications:

Acute intermittent porphyria; allergic or idiosyncratic reactions to carisoprodol or related compounds such as meprobamate.

Warnings:

Idiosyncratic reactions may appear rarely within minutes or hours of the first dose of carisoprodol. Symptoms include: Extreme weakness, transient quadriplegia, dizziness, ataxia, temporary loss of vision, diplopia, mydriasis, dysarthria, agitation, euphoria, confusion and disorientation. Symptoms usually subside over the next several hours. Supportive and symptomatic therapy, including hospitalization, may be necessary.

Drug dependence: In one study, abrupt cessation of 100 mg/kg/day (about 5 times the recommended daily adult dosage) was followed in some patients by mild withdrawal symptoms such as abdominal cramps, insomnia, chills, headache and nausea. Delirium and convulsions did not occur. In clinical use, psychological dependence and abuse have been rare, and there have been no reports of significant abstinence signs. Nevertheless, use the drug with caution in addiction-prone individuals.

Renal/Hepatic function impairment: Exercise caution in administration to patients with compromised liver or kidney function.

Pregnancy: Safety for use during pregnancy has not been established. Use during pregnancy or in women of childbearing potential only when clearly needed and when the potential benefits outweigh the potential hazards to the fetus.

Lactation: Carisoprodol is excreted in breast milk at concentrations 2 to 4 times that of maternal plasma. Consider this factor when use of the drug is contemplated in lactating patients.

Children: Not recommended for use in children under 12 years of age.

Precautions:

Hazardous tasks: May impair the mental or physical abilities required for the performance of potentially hazardous tasks; patients should observe caution while driving or performing other tasks requiring alertness, coordination or physical dexterity.

Adverse Reactions:

CNS: Dizziness; drowsiness; vertigo; ataxia; tremor; agitation; irritability; headache; depressive reactions; syncope; insomnia.

Cardiovascular: Tachycardia; postural hypotension; facial flushing.

GI: Nausea; vomiting; hiccoughs; epigastric distress.

Miscellaneous:

Allergic or idiosyncratic (occasional) – Usually seen within the first to fourth doses in patients having had no previous contact with the drug. Skin rash, erythema multiforme, pruritus, eosinophilia and fixed drug eruption with cross-reaction to meprobamate have been reported. Severe reactions are manifested by asthmatic episodes, fever, weakness, dizziness, angioneurotic edema, smarting eyes, hypotension and anaphylactoid shock.

If such reactions occur, discontinue carisoprodol and initiate appropriate symptomatic therapy. Refer to Management of Acute Hypersensitivity Reactions.

Centrally Acting

CARISOPRODOL

Overdosage:

Symptoms: Stupor, coma, shock, respiratory depression and, very rarely, death. The effects of an overdosage of carisoprodol and alcohol or other CNS depressants or psychotropic agents can be additive even when one of the drugs has been taken in the usual recommended dosage.

Treatment: Includes usual supportive measures. Refer to General Management of Acute Overdosage.

Although carisoprodol overdosage experience is limited, the following treatments have been successful with the related drug, meprobamate: Diuresis, osmotic (mannitol) diuresis, peritoneal dialysis and hemodialysis (carisoprodol is dialyzable).

Monitor urine output and avoid overhydration. Observe for possible relapse due to incomplete gastric emptying and delayed absorption. Carisoprodol can be measured in biological fluids by gas chromatography.

Patient Information:

May take with food or meals if GI upset occurs.

May cause drowsiness or dizziness. Patients should observe caution while driving or performing other tasks requiring alertness, coordination or physical dexterity. Avoid alcohol and other CNS depressants.

If dizziness (postural hypotension) occurs, avoid sudden changes in posture; use caution when climbing stairs, etc.

Administration and Dosage:

Adults: 350 mg 3 or 4 times daily; take the last dose at bedtime.

Rx	**Carisoprodol** (Various, eg, Major, Mutual, Parmed, Schein)	**Tablets:** 350 mg	In 30s, 60s, 100s, 500s, 1000s and UD 100s.
Rx	**Soma** (Wallace)		(Soma/37 Wallace 2001). White. In 100s, 500s and UD 500s.

Centrally Acting

CHLORPHENESIN CARBAMATE

Actions:

Pharmacology: Chlorphenesin is chemically related to mephenesin. Its mode of action has not been identified, but may be related to its sedative properties. It has no direct action on striated muscle, the motor endplate or the nerve fiber. It does not directly relax tense skeletal muscles.

Pharmacokinetics: The drug is readily absorbed from the GI tract. Peak plasma concentrations of chlorphenesin are reached 1 or 3 hours after administration and half-life is approximately 3.5 hours.

Indications:

Musculoskeletal conditions: As an adjunct to rest, physical therapy and other measures for relief of discomfort associated with acute, painful musculoskeletal conditions.

Contraindications:

Hypersensitivity to chlorphenesin carbamate.

Warnings:

Hypersensitivity: Occasionally, anaphylactoid reactions and drug fever occur. Such reactions indicate discontinuing the drug. Refer to Management of Acute Hypersensitivity Reactions.

Hepatic function impairment: Use with caution in patients with preexisting liver disease or impaired hepatic function.

Pregnancy: Safety for use has not been established. Use during pregnancy and in women of childbearing potential only if clearly needed and when the potential benefits outweigh the potential hazards.

Lactation: Safety for use has not been established. Use in the nursing mother only when clearly needed and when the potential benefits outweigh the potential hazards.

Children: Safety and efficacy are not established. Use is not recommended.

Precautions:

Duration: Safe use for periods exceeding 8 weeks has not been established.

Hazardous tasks: May impair mental or physical abilities required for the performance of potentially hazardous tasks; patients should observe caution while driving or performing other tasks requiring alertness, coordination or physical dexterity.

Tartrazine sensitivity: This product contains tartrazine, which may cause allergic-type reactions (including bronchial asthma) in susceptible individuals. Although the incidence of tartrazine sensitivity in the general population is low, it is frequently seen in patients who also have aspirin hypersensitivity.

Adverse Reactions:

Hematologic: Leukopenia, thrombocytopenia, agranulocytosis, pancytopenia (rare).

Hypersensitivity: Anaphylactoid reactions and drug fever (see Warnings).

CNS: Drowsiness; dizziness; confusion; paradoxical stimulation; insomnia; increased nervousness; headache. Dose reduction will usually control these symptoms.

GI: Nausea; epigastric distress; GI bleeding (two cases, not established as drug-related).

Overdosage:

Symptoms: One patient who attempted suicide by ingesting 12 g was slightly nauseated and drowsy for about 6 hrs, but recovered with routine supportive therapy.

Treatment: Includes usual supportive measures. Refer to General Management of Acute Overdosage.

Patient Information:

May cause drowsiness or dizziness. Patients should observe caution while driving or performing other tasks requiring alertness, coordination or physical dexterity. Avoid alcohol and other CNS depressants.

Administration and Dosage:

Initial: 800 mg 3 times daily until the desired effect is obtained.

Maintenance: May reduce to 400 mg 4 times daily, or less, as required.

Safe use for periods exceeding 8 weeks has not been established.

Rx	**Maolate** (Upjohn)	**Tablets**: 400 mg	Tartrazine. (Maolate). Tan, scored. In 50s and 500s.

Centrally Acting

CHLORZOXAZONE

Actions:

Pharmacology: Mode of action is not identified, but may be related to its sedative properties. Acts primarily at the spinal cord level and subcortical areas of the brain, inhibiting multisynaptic reflex arcs involved in producing and maintaining skeletal muscle spasm of varied etiology. This results in reduced skeletal muscle spasm, relief of pain and increased mobility of involved muscles. It does not directly relax tense skeletal muscles.

Pharmacokinetics: Serum levels can be detected in the first 30 minutes after administration and peak in 1 to 2 hours. Onset of action is 1 hour; effects last 3 to 4 hours. The drug is rapidly metabolized and excreted in urine, primarily as a glucuronide conjugate. Half-life is ≈ 60 minutes; < 1% of a dose is excreted unchanged in urine in 24 hours.

Indications:

Musculoskeletal conditions: As an adjunct to rest, physical therapy and other measures for the relief of discomfort associated with acute, painful musculoskeletal conditions.

Contraindications:

Intolerance to chlorzoxazone.

Warnings:

Hypersensitivity: Use with caution in patients with known allergies or a history of allergic drug reactions. If a sensitivity reaction occurs such as urticaria, redness or itching, discontinue use. Refer to Management of Acute Hypersensitivity Reactions.

Pregnancy: Safety for use has not been established. Use only when clearly needed and when the potential benefits outweigh the potential hazards.

Precautions:

Hepatic effects: If signs or symptoms of liver dysfunction are observed, discontinue use.

Hazardous tasks: May produce drowsiness or dizziness; patients should observe caution while driving or performing other tasks requiring alertness, coordination or physical dexterity.

Adverse Reactions:

The drug is well tolerated and seldom produces undesirable adverse reactions.

GI: GI disturbances; GI bleeding (rare).

CNS: Drowsiness; dizziness; lightheadedness; malaise; overstimulation.

Dermatologic: Allergic-type skin rashes, petechiae, ecchymoses (rare).

Hypersensitivity: Angioneurotic edema, anaphylaxis (very rare). See Warnings.

Hepatic: Chlorzoxazone was suspected of causing liver damage in some patients. The clinical picture was compatible with either a viral or drug-induced hepatitis. In most cases the patients recovered when the drug was stopped.

Miscellaneous: Urine discoloration.

Overdosage:

Symptoms: Initially, nausea, vomiting or diarrhea together with drowsiness, dizziness, lightheadedness or headache may occur. Early in the course, there may be malaise or sluggishness followed by marked loss of muscle tone, making voluntary movement impossible. Deep tendon reflexes may be decreased or absent. The sensorium remains intact, and there is no peripheral loss of sensation. Respiratory depression may occur with rapid, irregular respiration and intercostal and substernal retraction. Blood pressure is lowered, but shock has not been observed.

Treatment: Treatment is supportive. Cholinergic drugs or analeptic drugs are of no value and should not be used. Refer to General Management of Acute Overdosage.

Centrally Acting

CHLORZOXAZONE

Patient Information:

Take with food or water if GI upset occurs. Notify physician of skin rash or itching.

May cause drowsiness, dizziness or lightheadedness. Observe caution while driving or performing other tasks requiring alertness, coordination or physical dexterity. Avoid alcohol and other CNS depressants.

Medication may discolor urine orange or purple-red.

Administration and Dosage:

Adults:

Usual dosage – 250 mg 3 or 4 times daily. Initial dosage for painful musculoskeletal conditions is 500 mg 3 or 4 times daily. If response is inadequate, increase to 750 mg 3 or 4 times daily. As improvement occurs, dosage can usually be reduced.

Rx	**Chlorzoxazone** (Various, eg, Goldline)	**Tablets:** 250 mg	In 100s and 1000s.
Rx	**Paraflex** (McNeil Pharm.)	**Caplets:** 250 mg	(Paraflex). Peach. In 100s.
Rx	**Remular-S** (Inter. Ethical)	**Tablets:** 250 mg	In 100s.
Rx	**Chlorzoxazone** (Various, eg, Goldline, IDE, Royce, Rugby, Schein)	**Tablets:** 500 mg	In 100s, 500s and 1000s.
Rx	**Parafon Forte DSC** (McNeil Pharm.)	**Caplets:** 500 mg	(McNeil Parafon Forte DSC). Lt. green, scored. In 100s, 500s and UD 100s.

Centrally Acting

CYCLOBENZAPRINE HCl

Actions:

Pharmacology: Cyclobenzaprine, structurally related to the tricyclic antidepressants (TCAs), relieves skeletal muscle spasm of local origin without interfering with muscle function. It is ineffective in muscle spasm due to CNS disease. In animals, the drug reduces or abolishes muscle hyperactivity, does not act at the neuromuscular junction or directly on skeletal muscle, and acts primarily within the CNS at the brain stem as opposed to spinal cord levels; however, its action on the latter may contribute to its overall skeletal muscle relaxant activity. The net effect is a reduction of tonic somatic motor activity, influencing both gamma and alpha motor systems.

Animal studies also show a similarity between the effects of cyclobenzaprine and TCAs, including reserpine antagonism, norepinephrine potentiation, potent peripheral and central anticholinergic effects and sedation. In animals, cyclobenzaprine causes a slight to moderate increase in heart rate.

Pharmacokinetics: Cyclobenzaprine is well absorbed after oral administration, but there is a large intersubject variation in plasma levels. Peak plasma levels are reached in 4 to 6 hours. The onset of action occurs in 1 hour with a duration of 12 to 24 hours. It is highly bound to plasma proteins, extensively metabolized primarily to glucuronide-like conjugates and excreted primarily via the kidneys. Elimination half-life is 1 to 3 days.

Clinical trials: Cyclobenzaprine significantly improves the signs and symptoms of skeletal muscle spasm as compared with placebo. Clinical responses include improvement in muscle spasm, local pain and tenderness, increased range of motion and less restriction in activities of daily living. Clinical improvement was observed as early as the first day of therapy. In controlled trials comparing cyclobenzaprine, diazepam and placebo, cyclobenzaprine demonstrated comparable or greater improvement in muscle spasm when compared with diazepam. Side effects were comparable.

Indications:

Musculoskeletal conditions: Adjunct to rest and physical therapy for relief of muscle spasm associated with acute painful musculoskeletal conditions.

Unlabeled uses: Cyclobenzaprine (10 to 40 mg/day) appears to be a useful adjunct in the management of the fibrositis syndrome.

Contraindications:

Hypersensitivity to cyclobenzaprine; concomitant use of monoamine oxidase (MAO) inhibitors or within 14 days after their discontinuation (see Drug Interactions); acute recovery phase of myocardial infarction (MI) and in patients with arrhythmias, heart block or conduction disturbances, or congestive heart failure (CHF); hyperthyroidism.

Warnings:

Spasticity: Cyclobenzaprine is not effective in the treatment of spasticity associated with cerebral or spinal cord disease, or in children with cerebral palsy.

Duration: Use only for short periods (up to 2 or 3 weeks); effectiveness for more prolonged use is not proven. Muscle spasm associated with acute, painful musculoskeletal conditions is generally of short duration; specific therapy for longer periods is seldom warranted.

Similarity to TCAs: Cyclobenzaprine is closely related to the TCAs. In short-term studies for indications other than muscle spasm associated with acute musculoskeletal conditions, and usually at doses greater than those recommended, some of the more serious CNS reactions noted with the TCAs have occurred. Because of pharmacologic similarities to tricyclic drugs, consider certain withdrawal symptoms with cyclobenzaprine, although they have not been reported. Abrupt cessation of treatment after prolonged administration may produce nausea, headache and malaise; these do not indicate addiction.

Pregnancy: Category B. Use only when clearly needed and when the potential benefits outweigh the unknown potential hazards to the fetus.

Lactation: It is not known whether cyclobenzaprine is excreted in breast milk. Some of the TCAs are excreted in breast milk. Exercise caution when administering cyclobenzaprine to a nursing woman.

Children: Safety and efficacy in children < 15 years of age have not been established.

CYCLOBENZAPRINE HCl

Precautions:

Anticholinergic effects: Because of its anticholinergic action, use with caution in patients with a history of urinary retention, angle-closure glaucoma and increased intraocular pressure.

Hazardous tasks: May impair mental or physical abilities required for performance of hazardous tasks; patients should observe caution while driving or performing other tasks requiring alertness, coordination and physical dexterity.

Drug Interactions:

Because of similarities to the TCAs, consider all interactions listed in the Tricyclic Antidepressants monograph.

MAO inhibitors: Hyperpyretic crisis, severe convulsions and death have occurred in patients receiving TCAs and MAO inhibitors. Cyclobenzaprine may interact similarly.

Adverse Reactions:

Because of the similarities to TCAs, consider all reactions listed in the Adverse Reaction section in the Tricyclic Antidepressants monograph.

Cardiovascular: Tachycardia, syncope, arrhythmias, vasodilation, palpitations, hypotension (< 1%); chest pain; edema; hypertension; myocardial infarction; heart block; stroke.

CNS: Drowsiness (39%); dizziness (11%); fatigue, tiredness, asthenia, blurred vision, headache, nervousness (1% to 3%); convulsions, ataxia, vertigo, dysarthria, paresthesia, tremors, hypertonia, malaise, tinnitus, diplopia (< 1%); decreased or increased libido; abnormal gait; delusions; peripheral neuropathy; Bell's palsy; alteration in EEG patterns; extrapyramidal symptoms.

Psychiatric: Confusion (1% to 3%); disorientation, insomnia, depressed mood, abnormal sensations, anxiety, agitation, abnormal thinking and dreaming, hallucinations, excitement (< 1%).

GI: Dry mouth (27%); nausea, constipation, dyspepsia, unpleasant taste (1% to 3%); vomiting, anorexia, diarrhea, GI pain, gastritis, thirst, flatulence, ageusia (< 1%); paralytic ileus; tongue discoloration; stomatitis; parotid swelling.

GU: Urinary frequency or retention (< 1%); impaired urination; dilation of urinary tract; impotence; testicular swelling; gynecomastia; breast enlargement; galactorrhea.

Hepatic: Abnormal liver function, hepatitis, jaundice, cholestasis (< 1%).

Dermatologic: Sweating, skin rash, urticaria, pruritus (< 1%); photosensitization; alopecia.

Musculoskeletal: Muscle twitching, local weakness (< 1%); myalgia.

Hematologic/Lymphatic: Purpura; bone marrow depression; leukopenia; eosinophilia; thrombocytopenia.

Metabolic/Nutritional: Elevation and lowering of blood sugar levels; weight gain or loss.

Miscellaneous: Edema of face and tongue (< 1%); inappropriate ADH syndrome; dyspnea.

Overdosage:

Symptoms: High doses may cause temporary confusion, disturbed concentration, transient visual hallucinations, agitation, hyperactive reflexes, muscle rigidity, vomiting or hyperpyrexia, in addition to the effects listed under adverse reactions. Overdosage may cause drowsiness, hypothermia, tachycardia and other cardiac arrhythmias such as bundle branch block, ECG evidence of impaired conduction and CHF, dilated pupils, convulsions, severe hypotension, stupor and coma. Paradoxical diaphoresis has been reported.

Treatment: Treatment includes usual supportive measures. Refer to General Management of Acute Overdosage. Obtain an ECG and closely monitor cardiac function if there is any evidence of dysrhythmia.

Physostigmine, 1 to 3 mg IV, has been used to reverse anticholinergic effects. However, profound bradycardia and asystole may occur as a result. The role of physostigmine is not clear; avoid its use if other therapeutic agents are successful in reversing cardiac dysrhythmias.

Dialysis is probably of no value because of low plasma concentrations of the drug.

Centrally Acting

CYCLOBENZAPRINE HCl

Patient Information:

May cause drowsiness, dizziness or blurred vision. Patients should observe caution while driving or performing other tasks requiring alertness, coordination or physical dexterity.

Avoid alcohol and other CNS depressants.

May cause dry mouth.

Administration and Dosage:

Give 10 mg 3 times daily (range, 20 to 40 mg daily in divided doses). Do not exceed 60 mg/day. Do not use longer than 2 or 3 weeks.

Rx	**Cyclobenzaprine HCl** (Various, eg, Goldline, Major, Moore, Parmed, Rugby, Schein)	**Tablets**: 10 mg	In 30s, 100s and 1000.
Rx	**Flexeril** (Merck)		(MSD 931). Yellow, film coated. In 100s and UD 100s.

METAXALONE

Actions:

Pharmacology: The mechanism of action of metaxalone has not been established, but it may be due to general CNS depression. The drug has no direct action on the contractile mechanism of striated muscle, the motor endplate or the nerve fiber. Metaxalone does not directly relax tense skeletal muscles.

Pharmacokinetics: Onset of action is 1 hour and duration of action is 4 to 6 hours. Peak plasma levels of approximately 300 mcg/ml occur 2 hours after administration of 800 mg metaxalone. The half-life is 2 to 3 hours; metabolites are excreted in the urine.

Indications:

Musculoskeletal conditions: As an adjunct to rest, physical therapy and other measures for the relief of discomfort associated with acute, painful musculoskeletal conditions.

Contraindications:

Hypersensitivity to metaxalone; known tendency to drug-induced hemolytic or other anemias; significantly impaired renal or hepatic function.

Warnings:

Hepatic function impairment: Administer with great care to patients with preexisting liver damage and perform serial liver function studies as required. Elevations in cephalin flocculation tests without concurrent changes in other liver function parameters have been noted.

Pregnancy: Human experience has not revealed evidence of fetal injury, but the possibility of infrequent or subtle damage to the human fetus cannot be excluded. Do not use during pregnancy, especially during early pregnancy, or in women who may become pregnant, unless the potential benefits outweigh the potential hazards to the fetus.

Lactation: It is not known whether this drug is excreted in breast milk. Safety for use in the nursing mother has not been established.

Children: Safety and efficacy for use in children ≤ 12 years of age have not been established.

Drug Interactions:

Drug/Lab test interactions: False-positive **Benedict's tests**, due to an unknown reducing substance, have been noted. A glucose-specific test will differentiate findings.

Adverse Reactions:

GI: Nausea; vomiting; GI upset.

CNS: Drowsiness; dizziness; headache; nervousness; irritability.

Miscellaneous: Hypersensitivity reaction (light rash with or without pruritus); leukopenia; hemolytic anemia; jaundice.

Overdosage:

Employ gastric lavage and supportive therapy as indicated. No documented case of major toxicity has been reported. to General Management of Acute Overdosage.

Patient Information:

May cause drowsiness or dizziness. Patients should observe caution while driving or performing other tasks requiring alertness, coordination and physical dexterity.

Avoid alcohol and other CNS depressants.

Notify physician if skin rash or yellowish discoloration of the skin or eyes occurs.

Administration and Dosage:

Adults and children (> 12 years): 800 mg 3 to 4 times daily.

Rx	**Skelaxin** (Carnrick)	**Tablets**: 400 mg	(C 8662). Pale rose, scored. In 100s and 500s.

Centrally Acting

METHOCARBAMOL

Actions:

Pharmacology: Mechanism of action has not been established, but may be due to general CNS depression. The drug has no direct action on the contractile mechanism of striated muscle, motor endplate or nerve fiber. It does not directly relax tense skeletal muscles.

Pharmacokinetics: Methocarbamol has an onset of action of 30 minutes. Peak plasma levels occur approximately 2 hours after administration of 2 g. The half-life is from 1 to 2 hours; inactive metabolites are excreted in the urine and small amounts in the feces.

Indications:

Musculoskeletal conditions: Adjunctive to rest, physical therapy, and other measures for the relief of discomfort associated with acute, painful musculoskeletal conditions.

Tetanus: May have a beneficial effect in the control of neuromuscular manifestations of tetanus.

Contraindications:

Hypersensitivity to methocarbamol or any ingredient of the product.

Parenteral: Due to the presence of polyethylene glycol 300 in the vehicle, do not administer parenteral methocarbamol to patients with known or suspected renal pathology.

Warnings:

Pregnancy: Safe use of methocarbamol has not been established with regard to possible adverse effects upon fetal development. Therefore, do not use the drug in women who are or may become pregnant, particularly during early pregnancy unless in the judgment of the physician, the potential benefits outweigh the possible hazards.

Lactation: It is not known whether methocarbamol is excreted in breast milk. Exercise caution when administering to a nursing woman. The American Academy of Pediatrics classifies methocarbamol as compatible with breastfeeding.

Children: Safety and efficacy in children < 12 years old are not established, except in tetanus. See directions for use in tetanus under Administration and Dosage.

Precautions:

Rate of injection should not exceed 3 ml/minute. Since solution is hypertonic, avoid vascular extravasation. A recumbent position reduces likelihood of adverse reactions.

Total parenteral dosage should not exceed 3 g per day for > 3 consecutive days, except in the treatment of tetanus.

Epilepsy: Use the injectable form cautiously in suspected or known epileptics.

Drug Interactions:

Drug/Lab test interactions: Methocarbamol may cause a color interference in certain screening tests for **5-hydroxyindoleacetic acid (5-HIAA)** and **vanilmandelic acid (VMA)**.

Adverse Reactions:

Parenteral: Certain reactions may have been due to an overly rapid rate of IV injection.

Cardiovascular – Syncope; hypotension; bradycardia. In most cases of syncope, there was spontaneous recovery. In others, epinephrine, injectable steroids or injectable antihistamines were employed to hasten recovery.

CNS – Dizziness; lightheadedness; vertigo; headache; drowsiness; fainting; mild muscular incoordination. Reports of convulsive seizures during IV use include instances in epileptics. Psychic trauma of the procedure may be a contributing factor. Several observers have reported success in terminating epileptiform seizures with methocarbamol, but its use in patients with epilepsy is not recommended.

Ophthalmic – Blurred vision; conjunctivitis with nasal congestion; nystagmus; diplopia.

Dermatologic – Urticaria; pruritus; rash; flushing.

Miscellaneous – GI upset; metallic taste; sloughing or pain at the injection site; thrombophlebitis; anaphylactic reaction; fever.

Oral: Lightheadedness; dizziness; drowsiness; nausea; urticaria; pruritus; rash; conjunctivitis with nasal congestion; blurred vision; headache; fever.

METHOCARBAMOL

Overdosage:

Symptoms: Overdose, often in conjunction with alcohol or other CNS depressants, is marked by coma and other signs of CNS depression.

Treatment: Supportive. Refer to General Management of Acute Overdosage.

Patient Information:

May cause drowsiness, dizziness or lightheadedness. Patients should observe caution while driving or performing other tasks requiring alertness, coordination or physical dexterity.

Avoid alcohol and other CNS depressants.

Urine may darken to brown, black or green.

Notify physician if skin rash, itching, fever or nasal congestion occurs.

Administration and Dosage:

Parenteral: For IV and IM use only. *Not recommended for SC administration.* Do not exceed total adult dosage of 3 g for > 3 consecutive days except in the treatment of tetanus. Repeat this course after a lapse of 48 hours if the condition persists. Base dosage and frequency of injection on severity of the condition and the therapeutic response.

For the relief of symptoms of moderate degree, 1 g may be adequate. Injection need not be repeated, as tablets will sustain the relief. For severe cases or in postoperative conditions in which oral administration is not feasible, 2 to 3 g may be required.

IV – Administer undiluted directly IV at a maximum rate of 3 ml/minute. May also be added to an IV drip of Sodium Chloride Injection or 5% Dextrose Injection; do not dilute one vial given as a single dose to > 250 ml for IV infusion. Avoid vascular extravasation which may result in thrombophlebitis. The patient should be recumbent during and for at least 10 to 15 minutes following injection.

IM – Do not inject > 5 ml into each gluteal region; repeat at 8 hour intervals, if needed. As symptoms are relieved, change to tablets.

Tetanus – Methocarbamol does not replace the usual procedure of debridement, tetanus antitoxin, penicillin, tracheotomy, attention to fluid balance and supportive care. Add methocarbomal injection to the regimen as soon as possible.

Adults: Inject 1 or 2 g directly into the IV tubing. An additional 1 or 2 g may be added to the infusion bottle so that a total of up to 3 g is given as the initial dose. Repeat procedure every 6 hours until conditions allow for the insertion of a nasogastric tube. Crushed methocarbamol tablets suspended in water or saline may then be given through the nasogastric tube. Total daily oral doses up to 24 g may be required.

Children: A minimum initial dose of 15 mg/kg is recommended. Give by injection into the tubing or by IV infusion with an appropriate quantity of fluid. Repeat every 6 hours as indicated.

Oral (Adults):

Initial – 1.5 g 4 times daily.

Maintenance – 1 g 4 times daily; 750 mg every 4 hours; or 1.5 g 3 times daily. For the first 48 to 72 hours, 6 g/day are recommended. (For severe conditions 8 g daily may be administered.) Thereafter, reduce to approximately 4 g daily.

Rx	**Methocarbamol** (Various, eg, IDE, Lederle, Major)	**Tablets**: 500 mg	In 100s and 500s.
Rx	**Robaxin** (Robins)		Saccharin. (Robaxin AHR). Light orange. Film coated. In 100s, 500s, UD 100s.
Rx	**Methocarbamol** (Various, eg, IDE, Lederle, Major)	**Tablets**: 750 mg	In 100s and 500s.
Rx	**Robaxin-750** (Robins)		Saccharin. (AHR Robaxin-750). Orange. Film coated. In 100s, 500s and Dis-co–Pak 100s.
Rx	**Methocarbamol** (Various)	**Injection**: 100 mg per ml	In 10 ml vials.
Rx	**Robaxin** (Robins)		In 10 ml vials.[1]

[1] In solution of polyethylene glycol 300. After mixing with IV infusion fluids, do not refrigerate.

ORPHENADRINE CITRATE

Actions:

Pharmacology: The mode of action of orphenadrine has not been identified, but may be related to its analgesic properties. It acts centrally at the brain stem; it does not directly relax tense skeletal muscles. It possesses anticholinergic actions.

Pharmacokinetics: Peak plasma levels occur 2 hours after administration of 100 mg orphenadrine; duration of action is 4 to 6 hours. The half-life is approximately 14 hours for the parent drug, and 2 to 25 hours for metabolites. Excretion is via urine and feces. Most of orphenadrine is degraded to eight known metabolites.

Indications:

Musculoskeletal conditions: As an adjunct to rest, physical therapy and other measures for relief of discomfort associated with acute, painful musculoskeletal conditions.

Unlabeled uses: Orphenadrine 100 mg at bedtime may be beneficial in the treatment of quinine-resistant leg cramps.

Contraindications:

Glaucoma; pyloric or duodenal obstruction; stenosing peptic ulcers; prostatic hypertrophy; obstruction of the bladder neck; cardiospasm (megaesophagus) and myasthenia gravis; hypersensitivity to orphenadrine.

Warnings:

Hypersensitivity reactions may occur. Refer to Management of Acute Hypersensitivity Reactions.

Pregnancy: Category C. It is not known whether orphenadrine can cause fetal harm or affect reproduction capacity. Use in pregnancy only when clearly needed.

Lactation: It is not known whether orphenadrine is excreted in breast milk.

Children: Safety and efficacy for use in children have not been established. Not recommended for use in the pediatric age group.

Precautions:

Cardiac disease: Use with caution in patients with cardiac decompensation, coronary insufficiency, cardiac arrhythmias or tachycardia.

Long-term therapy: Safety of continuous long-term therapy has not been established; periodically monitor blood, urine and liver function values.

Hazardous tasks: May cause transient episodes of lightheadedness, dizziness or syncope. Patients should observe caution while driving or performing other tasks requiring alertness, coordination or physical dexterity.

Sulfite sensitivity: Some of these products contain sulfites which may cause allergic-type reactions (eg, hives, itching, wheezing, anaphylaxis) in certain susceptible persons. Although the overall prevalence of sulfite sensitivity in the general population is probably low, it is seen more frequently in asthmatics or in atopic nonasthmatic persons. Specific products containing sulfites are identified in the product listings.

Drug Interactions:

Orphenadrine Drug Interactions

Precipitant drug	Object drug*		Description
Amantadine	Orphenadrine	↑	Anticholinergic effects may be increased.
Orphenadrine	Haloperidol	↔	Worsening of schizophrenic symptoms, decreased haloperidol levels and development of tardive dyskinesia may occur.
Orphenadrine	Phenothiazines	↓	Therapeutic effects of phenothiazines may be decreased.

* ↑ = Object drug increased. ↓ = Object drug decreased. ↔ = Undetermined effect.

Adverse Reactions:

Adverse effects are mainly due to the anticholinergic effects of orphenadrine and are usually associated with higher doses.

Dry mouth is the first side effect to appear. When daily dose is increased, possible effects include:

Cardiovascular: Tachycardia, palpitation, transient syncope.

CNS: Weakness, headache, dizziness, lightheadedness, confusion (in elderly patients), hallucinations, agitation, tremor, drowsiness.

GI: Vomiting, nausea, constipation, gastric irritation.

Centrally Acting

ORPHENADRINE CITRATE

GU: Urinary hesitancy and retention.

Ophthalmic: Blurred vision, pupil dilation, increased ocular tension.

Hematologic: Rarely, aplastic anemia; a causal relationship has not been established.

Hypersensitivity: Urticaria and other dermatoses (sometimes pruritic). Rarely, anaphylactic reaction following IM injection (rare). See Warnings.

Overdosage:

Symptoms: The lethal dose of orphenadrine in adults is 2 to 3 g. Intoxication is very rapid and death can occur within 3 to 5 hours preceded by deep coma, seizures and shock. Serious cardiac rhythm disturbances are common.

Treatment: Prevent further absorption by gastric lavage. Hemodialysis may not be helpful.

Patient Information:

May cause drowsiness, dizziness, blurred vision or fainting. Observe caution while driving or performing tasks requiring alertness, coordination or physical dexterity.

Avoid alcohol and other CNS depressants.

May cause dry mouth, difficult urination, constipation, headache and GI upset. Notify physician if these effects persist, or if skin rash or itching, rapid heart rate, palpitations or mental confusion occurs.

Administration and Dosage:

Oral: 100 mg each morning and evening. Do not crush or chew sustained release preparations.

Parenteral: 60 mg IV or IM. May repeat every 12 hours.

Rx	**Orphenadrine Citrate** (Various, eg, Major)	**Tablets:** 100 mg	In 30s, 100s, 500s and 1000s.
Rx	**Norflex** (3M Pharm)	**Tablets, sustained release:** 100 mg	(3M 221). White. In 100s and 500s.
Rx	**Orphenadrine Citrate** (Various, eg, Hyrex, Rugby, Schein)	**Injection:** 30 mg per ml	In 2 ml amps and 10 ml vials.
Rx	**Banflex** (Forest Pharm.)		In 10 ml vials.
Rx	**Flexoject** (Mayrand)		In 2 ml amps and 10 ml vials.
Rx	**Flexon** (Various, eg, Keene)		In 10 ml vials.
Rx	**Myolin** (Roberts Hauck)		In 10 ml vials.
Rx	**Norflex** (3M Pharm)		In 2 ml amps.[1]

[1] With sodium bisulfite.

Centrally Acting

DIAZEPAM

The following is an abbreviated monograph. For complete prescribing information, refer to the Benzodiazepines monograph in the Antianxiety Agents section.

Actions:

Pharmacology: In animals, diazepam acts on the thalamus and hypothalamus, inducing calming effects. Diazepam has no demonstrable peripheral autonomic blocking action, nor does it produce extrapyramidal side effects; however, animals treated with diazepam do have a transient ataxia at higher doses.

Major muscle relaxant actions occur in two proposed sites: At the spinal level resulting in enhancement of GABA-mediated presynaptic inhibition, and at supraspinal sites, probably in the brain stem reticular formation.

Indications:

An adjunct for the relief of skeletal muscle spasm due to reflex spasm to local pathology (such as inflammation of the muscles or joints, or secondary to trauma); spasticity caused by upper motor neuron disorders (eg, cerebral palsy and paraplegia); athetosis; stiff-man syndrome. Injectable diazepam may also be used as an adjunct in tetanus.

Also used as an antianxiety agent (see Benzodiazepines monograph in the Antianxiety Agents section) and an anticonvulsant (see the Diazepam monograph in the Anticonvulsants section).

Administration and Dosage:

Oral: Individualize dosage for maximum beneficial effect.

Adults – 2 to 10 mg 3 or 4 times daily.

Geriatric or debilitated patients – 2 to 2.5 mg 1 or 2 times daily initially, increasing as needed and tolerated.

Children – 1 to 2.5 mg 3 or 4 times daily initially, increasing as needed and tolerated (not for use in children > 6 months of age).

Intensol – Dosages are same as those listed above. Mix with liquid or semi-solid food such as water, juices, soda or soda-like beverages, applesauce and puddings. Stir in gently. Consume the entire mixture immediately. Do not store for future use.

Sustained release – 15 to 30 mg once daily.

Parenteral: Use lower doses (2 to 5 mg) and slow dosage increases for elderly or debilitated patients and when other sedatives are given. When acute symptoms are controlled with the injectable form, administer oral therapy if further treatment is required.

Neonates (≤ 30 days of age) – Safety and efficacy have not been established. Prolonged CNS depression has been observed in neonates, apparently due to inability to biotransform diazepam into inactive metabolites.

Children – Give slowly over 3 minutes in a dosage not to exceed 0.25 mg/kg. After a 15 to 30 minute interval, the initial dosage can be safely repeated. If relief is not obtained after a third administration, begin adjunctive therapy appropriate to the condition being treated.

IM: Inject deeply into the muscle.

IV: Inject slowly, taking at least 1 minute for each 5 mg (1 ml). Do not use small veins (ie, dorsum of hand or wrist). Avoid intra-arterial administration or extravasation. Do not mix or dilute with other solutions or drugs.

Adults – 5 to 10 mg, IM or IV initially, then 5 to 10 mg in 3 to 4 hours, if necessary. For tetanus, larger doses may be required.

Children – For tetanus in infants > 30 days of age, 1 to 2 mg IM or IV slowly; repeat every 3 to 4 hours as necessary. In children ≥ 5 years of age, 5 to 10 mg. Repeat every 3 to 4 hours if necessary to control tetanus spasms. Have respiratory assistance available.

Centrally Acting

DIAZEPAM

c-iv	**Diazepam** (Various, eg, Barr, Major, Mylan, Parmed, Rugby, Zenith)	**Tablets**: 2 mg	In 100s, 500s, 1000s and 5000s.
c-iv	**Valium** (Roche)		(2 Valium/ Roche). White, scored. In 100s, 500s and Tel-E-Dose 100s.
c-iv	**Diazepam** (Various,eg, Barr, Major, Mylan, Rugby, Zenith)	**Tablets**: 5 mg	In 100s, 500s, 1000s, 2500s and 5000s.
c-iv	**Valium** (Roche)		(5 Valium / Roche). Yellow, scored. In 100s, 500s and Tel-E-Dose 100s.
c-iv	**Diazepam** (Various, eg, Barr, Major, Mylan, Rugby, Zenith)	**Tablets**: 10 mg	In 100s, 500s, 1000s, 2500s and 5000s.
c-iv	**Valium** (Roche)		(10 Valium / Roche). Blue, scored. In 100s, 500s and Tel-E-Dose 100s.
c-iv	**Diazepam** (Roxane)	**Oral Solution**: 5 mg/5 ml	Wintergreen-spice flavor. In UD 5 and 10 ml.
c-iv	**Diazepam Intensol** (Roxane)	**Concentrated Oral Solution**: 5 mg/ml	In 30 ml with calibrated dropper.
c-iv	**Diazepam** (Various, eg, Elkins-Sinn, Lederle, LyphoMed, Winthrop)	**Injection**: 5 mg/ml	In 2 ml amps, 1, 2, 5 and 10 ml vials and 1 and 2 ml syringes.
c-iv	**Valium** (Roche)		In 2 ml amps,[1] 10 ml vials[1] and 2 ml Tel -E-Ject disp. syringes.[1]
c-iv	**Zetran** (Hauck)		In 10 ml vials[1]

[1] With 40% propylene glycol, 10% ethyl alcohol, 5% sodium benzoate and 1.5% benzyl alcohol.

Centrally Acting

BACLOFEN

Actions:

Pharmacology: The precise mechanism of action is unknown. Baclofen can inhibit both monosynaptic and polysynaptic reflexes at the spinal level, possibly by hyperpolarization of afferent terminals, although actions at supraspinal sites may also contribute to its clinical effect. It is a structural analog of the inhibitory neurotransmitter gamma-aminobutyric acid (GABA) and may exert its effects by stimulation of the $GABA_B$ receptor subtype. Baclofen has CNS depressant properties as indicated by production of sedation with tolerance, somnolence, ataxia and respiratory and cardiovascular depression.

When introduced directly into the intrathecal space, effective CSF concentrations are achieved with resultant plasma concentrations 100 times less than those occurring with oral administration.

Pharmacokinetics:

Oral – Baclofen is rapidly and extensively absorbed and eliminated. Absorption may be dose-dependent, being reduced with increasing doses. It is excreted primarily by the kidney in unchanged form with intersubject variation in absorption or elimination.

Intrathecal –

Bolus: The onset of action is generally 0.5 to 1 hour after an intrathecal bolus dose. Peak spasmolytic effect is seen at ≈ 4 hours after dosing and effects may last 4 to 8 hours. Onset, peak response and duration of action may vary with individual patients depending on the dose and severity of symptoms. After a bolus lumbar injection of 50 or 100 mcg in seven patients, the average CSF elimination half-life was 1.51 hours over the first 4 hours, and the average CSF clearance was ≈ 30 ml/hour.

Continuous infusion: The antispastic action is first seen at 6 to 8 hours after initiation of continuous infusion. Maximum activity is observed in 24 to 48 hours. The mean CSF clearance was ≈ 30 ml/hour in 10 patients on continuous intrathecal infusion.

The pharmacokinetics of CSF clearance of baclofen calculated from intrathecal bolus or continuous infusion studies approximates CSF turnover, suggesting elimination is by bulk-flow removal of CSF.

Concurrent plasma concentrations during intrathecal administration are expected to be low (0 to 5 ng/ml). Limited data suggest that a lumbar-cisternal concentration gradient of ≈ 4:1 is established along the neuroaxis during baclofen infusion.

Children: The onset, peak response and duration of action is similar to those seen in adult patients.

Indications:

Oral: For the alleviation of signs and symptoms of spasticity resulting from multiple sclerosis, particularly for the relief of flexor spasms, concomitant pain, clonus and muscular rigidity. Patients should have reversible spasticity so that treatment will aid in restoring residual function.

May be of some value in patients with spinal cord injuries and other spinal cord diseases.

Intrathecal: Management of severe spasticity of spinal cord origin in patients who are unresponsive to oral baclofen therapy or who experience intolerable CNS side effects at effective doses. Intended for use by the intrathecal route in single bolus test doses (via spinal catheter or lumbar puncture) and, for chronic use, only in implantable pumps approved by the FDA specifically for baclofen administration into the intrathecal space.

Intrathecal therapy may be considered an alternative to destructive neurosurgical procedures. Prior to implantation of a device for chronic intrathecal infusion, patients must show a response in a screening trial (see Administration and Dosage).

Unlabeled uses:

Oral – Treatment of trigeminal neuralgia (tic douloureux), (50 to 60 mg/day); tardive dyskinesia (40 mg/day) in combination with neuroleptics; intractable hiccoughs.

Intrathecal – 25, 50 or 100 mcg appears to be beneficial in children for reducing spasticity in cerebral palsy.

Contraindications:

Hypersensitivity to baclofen.

Oral: Treatment of skeletal muscle spasm resulting from rheumatic disorders; stroke, cerebral palsy and Parkinson's disease (because efficacy has not been established).

Intrathecal: IV, IM, SC or epidural administration.

Centrally Acting

BACLOFEN

Warnings:

Intrathecal administration: Because of the possibility of potentially life-threatening CNS depression, cardiovascular collapse or respiratory failure, physicians must be adequately trained and educated in chronic intrathecal infusion therapy.

Do not implant the pump system until the patient's response to bolus injection is adequately evaluated. Evaluation (consisting of a screening procedure; see Administration and Dosage) requires that baclofen be administered into the intrathecal space via catheter or lumbar puncture. Because of the risks associated with the screening procedure and dosage adjustment following pump implantation, conduct these phases in a medically supervised and adequately equipped environment following the instructions outlined in Administration and Dosage.

Fatalities: There were 16 deaths among the 576 patients treated with baclofen intrathecal in premarketing and postmarketing studies. Because these patients were treated in uncontrolled clinical settings, it is impossible to determine definitively what role, if any, baclofen played in their deaths.

Infection: Patients should be infection-free prior to the screening trial with baclofen injection because a systemic infection may interfere with an assessment of the patient's response.

Patients should be infection-free prior to pump implantation because an infection may increase the risk of surgical complications. Moreover, a systemic infection may complicate attempts to adjust the pump's dosing rate.

Abrupt drug withdrawal: Hallucinations and seizures have occurred on abrupt withdrawal. An isolated case of manic psychosis has been reported. Except in cases of serious adverse reactions, reduce dose slowly when drug is discontinued.

Stroke: Baclofen has not significantly benefited patients with stroke; they also have poor drug tolerance.

Renal function impairment: Because baclofen is primarily excreted unchanged through the kidneys, administer with caution to patients with impaired renal function. Dosage reduction may be necessary.

Pregnancy: Category C. Oral baclofen increases the incidence of omphaloceles (ventral hernias) in rat fetuses given ≈ 13 times the maximum oral dose recommended for human use; this dose also caused reductions in food intake and weight gain in dams. There are no studies in pregnant women. Use only when clearly needed and when potential benefits outweigh potential hazards to the fetus.

Lactation: In mothers treated with oral baclofen in therapeutic doses, the active substance passes into the breast milk. It is not known whether detectable levels of drug are present in the breast milk of nursing mothers receiving intrathecal baclofen. As a general rule, undertake nursing while a patient is receiving intrathecal baclofen only if the potential benefit justifies the potential risk to the infant.

Children:

Oral – Safety for use in children < 12 years of age has not been established. Oral baclofen is not recommended for use in children.

Intrathecal – Safety in children < 4 years of age has not been established.

Precautions:

Epilepsy: Monitor the clinical state and EEG at regular intervals, as deterioration in seizure control and EEG changes have occurred in patients taking this drug.

Need for spasticity: Use with caution where spasticity is utilized to sustain upright posture and balance in locomotion or whenever spasticity is utilized to obtain increased function.

Ovarian cysts have been found by palpation in ≈ 4% of multiple sclerosis patients treated with baclofen for ≤ 1 year. In most cases, these cysts disappeared spontaneously while patients continued to receive the drug. Ovarian cysts are estimated to occur spontaneously in ≈ 1% to 5% of the normal female population.

Psychotic disorders: Cautiously treat patients suffering from psychotic disorders, schizophrenia or confusional states and keep under careful surveillance, because exacerbations of these conditions have been observed with oral administration.

Autonomic dysreflexia: Use with caution in patients with a history of autonomic dysreflexia. The presence of nociceptive stimuli or abrupt withdrawl may cause an autonomic dysreflexic episode.

Hazardous tasks: Because of the possibility of sedation, patients should observe caution while driving or performing other tasks requiring alertness, coordination or physical dexterity.

Centrally Acting

BACLOFEN

Adverse Reactions:

Oral: Drowsiness (10% to 63%); hypotension (< 9%); weakness, dizziness/lightheadedness (5% to 15%); nausea/vomiting (4% to 12%); headache (4% to 8%); insomnia (2% to 7%); urinary frequecy, constipation (2% to 6%); lethargy/fatigue (2% to 4%); confusion (1% to 11%); slurred speech, blurred vision, seizures (rare).

Intrathecal: The most commonly observed adverse events that were not seen at an equivalent incidence among placebo-treated patients were: Drowsiness; dizziness; nausea; hypotension; headache; seizures; weakness.

Most frequent (≥ 1%) –

Spasticity of spinal origin: Hypotonia (25.3%); somnolence (20.9%); dizziness (7.9%); paresthesia (6.7%); nausea and vomiting (5.6%); headache, constipation (5.1%); convulsion, urinary retention, dry mouth, accidental injury, asthenia, confusion, death, pain, speech disorder, hypotension, amblyopia, diarrhea, hypoventilation, coma, impotence, peripheral edema, urinary incontinence, insomnia, anxiety, depression, dyspnea, fever, pneumonia, urinary frequency, urticaria, anorexia, diplopia, dysautonomia, hallucinations, hypertension (< 5%).

Spasticity of cerebral origin: Hypotonia (34.7%); somnolence (18.7%); headache (10.7%); convulsion (10%); urinary retention, dizziness (8%); nausea (7.3%); hypertonia (6%); nausea and vomiting, hypoventilation, paresthesia, hypotension, increased salivation, back pain, constipation, pain, pruritus, diarrhea, peripheral edema, abnormal thinking, agitation, asthenia, chills, coma, dry mouth, pneumonia, speech disorder, tremor, urinary incontinence, impaired urination (< 5%).

Fatalities – See Warnings.

In addition, the following adverse reactions (in decreasing order of frequency within each body system) were reported:

CNS – Respiratory depression; difficulty concentrating; decreased coordination; memory loss/forgetfulness; nystagmus; accommodation disorder; anxiety; hypothermia; burning buttocks/feet; cerebellar dysmetria; cerebrovascular accident; depression; disorientation; unsteady gait/balance alteration; hallucinations; moodiness; paranoia; head/neck pressure; delayed responsiveness; somnolence; difficulty swallowing; vertigo; dystonia.

GI – Dry mouth; diarrhea/bowel incontinence; decreased appetite; dehydration; ileus; decreased taste.

Cardiovascular – Bradycardia; deep vein thrombosis; skin flushing; diaphoresis; orthostatic hypotension; paleness; swelling of lower extremities.

Respiratory – Chest tightness; aspiration pneumonia.

GU – Urinary incontinence; sluggish bladder; bladder spasms; sexual dysfunction.

Dermatologic – Urticaria of face and hands; alopecia; face edema.

Miscellaneous – Septicemia; weight loss; subdural hemorrhage; suicide attempt; suicide ideation; double vision.

After discontinuation: Pump pocket infections; wound dehiscence; gynecological fibroids; pump overpressurization.

Oral: Additional adverse reactions are reported below:

CNS – Euphoria; excitement; depression; hallucinations; paresthesia; muscle pain; tinnitus; coordination disorder; tremor; rigidity; dystonia; ataxia; nystagmus; strabismus; miosis; mydriasis; diplopia; dysarthria (rare).

Cardiovascular – Dyspnea; palpitations; chest pain; syncope (rare).

GI – Dry mouth; anorexia; taste disorder; abdominal pain; diarrhea; positive test for occult blood in stool (rare).

GU – Enuresis; urinary retention; dysuria; impotence; inability to ejaculate; nocturia; hematuria (rare).

Miscellaneous – Rash; pruritus; ankle edema; excessive perspiration; weight gain; nasal congestion.

Lab test abnormalities – Increased AST; elevated alkaline phosphatase; elevation of blood sugar.

Overdosage:

Oral:

Symptoms – Vomiting; muscular hypotonia; muscle twitching; drowsiness; accommodation disorders; coma; respiratory depression; seizures.

Treatment – In the alert patient, empty the stomach promptly by induced emesis followed by lavage. In the obtunded patient, secure the airway with a cuffed endotracheal tube before beginning lavage (do not induce emesis). Maintain adequate respiratory exchange; do not use respiratory stimulants. Atropine has been used to improve ventilation, heart rate, blood pressure and core body temperature.

BACLOFEN

Intrathecal:

Symptoms – Pay special attention to recognizing the signs and symptoms of overdosage, especially during the initial screening and dose-titration phase of treatment, but also during re-introduction of intrathecal baclofen after a period of interruption in therapy. Symptoms may include: Drowsiness; lightheadedness; dizziness; somnolence; respiratory depression; seizures; rostral progression of hypotonia; loss of consciousness progressing to coma of up to 72 hour duration. In most cases reported, coma was reversible without sequelae after infusion was stopped. Symptoms of overdose were reported in a sensitive adult patient after receiving a 25 mcg intrathecal bolus.

Treatment – There is no specific antidote; however, the following steps should ordinarily be undertaken: (1) Remove residual solution from the pump as soon as possible; (2) intubate patients with respiratory depression, if necessary, until the drug is eliminated.

Anecdotal reports suggest that IV physostigmine may reverse central side effects, notably drowsiness and respiratory depression. Use caution in administering physostigmine IV, however, because its use has been associated with the induction of seizures, bradycardia and cardiac conduction disturbances. A dose of 1 to 2 mg physostigmine may be tried IV over 5 to 10 min. Monitor patients closely during this time. Repeat 1 mg doses at 30 to 60 minute intervals in an attempt to maintain adequate respiration and alertness if the patient shows a positive response. Physostigmine may not be effective in reversing large overdoses, and patients may need to be maintained with respiratory support.

If lumbar puncture is not contraindicated, consider withdrawing 30 to 40 ml of CSF to reduce CSF baclofen concentration.

Patient Information:

May cause drowsiness, dizziness and fatigue. Patients should observe caution while driving or performing other tasks requiring alertness, coordination or physical dexterity.

Avoid alcohol and other CNS depressants.

Do not discontinue therapy except on advice of physician. Abrupt withdrawal may result in hallucinations.

May cause frequent urge to urinate or painful urination, constipation, nausea, headache, insomnia or confusion. Notify physician if these effects persist.

Administration and Dosage:

Oral: Individualize dosage. Start at a low dosage and increase gradually until the optimum effect is achieved (usually 40 to 80 mg daily).

The following dosage schedule is suggested: 5 mg 3 times daily for 3 days; 10 mg 3 times daily for 3 days; 15 mg 3 times daily for 3 days; 20 mg 3 times daily for 3 days. Thereafter, additional increases may be necessary, but the total daily dose should not exceed 80 mg daily (20 mg 4 times daily).

The lowest effective dose is recommended. If benefits are not evident after a reasonable trial period, withdraw the drug slowly.

Intrathecal: Refer to the manufacturer's manual for the implantable intrathecal infusion pump for specific instructions and precautions for programming the pump or refilling the reservoir.

Screening phase – Prior to pump implantation and initiation of chronic infusion of baclofen, patients must demonstrate a positive clinical response to a bolus dose administered intrathecally in a screening trial. The screening trial employs baclofen, which must be diluted to a concentration of 50 mcg/ml. The screening procedure is as follows: Administer an initial bolus containing 50 mcg/ml into the intrathecal space by barbotage over a period of ≥ 1 minute. Observe the patient over the ensuing 4 to 8 hours. A positive response consists of a significant decrease in muscle tone or frequency or severity of spasm. If the initial response is less than desired, a second bolus injection may be administered 24 hours after the first. This second screening bolus dose consists of 75 mcg/1.5 ml. Again, observe the patient for an interval of 4 to 8 hours. If the response is still inadequate, a final bolus screening dose of 100 mcg/2 ml may be administered 24 hours later.

Do not consider patients who do not respond to a 100 mcg intrathecal bolus as candidates for an implanted pump for chronic infusion.

Children – The starting screening dose for pediatric patients is the same as in adult patients (eg, 50 mcg). However, for very small patients, a screening dose of 25 mcg may be tried first.

Post-implant dose titration period – To determine the initial total daily dose of baclofen following implant, double the screening dose that gave a positive effect,

BACLOFEN

and administer over a 24–hour period, unless the efficacy of the bolus dose was maintained for > 8 hours, in which case the starting daily dose should be the screening dose delivered over a 24–hour period. Do not increase the dose in the first 24 hours (eg, until the steady state is achieved).

Spasticity of spinal cord origin: After the first 24 hours, increase slowly by 10% to 30% increments and only once every 24 hours, until the desired clinical effect is achieved. If there is not a substantive clinical response to increases in the daily dose, check for proper pump function and catheter patency.

Monitor patients closely in a fully equipped and staffed environment during the screening phase and dose-titration period immediately following implant. Resuscitative equipment should be immediately available for use in case of life-threatening or intolerable side effects.

Spasticity of cerebral origin – After the first 24 hours, increase the daily dose slowly by 5% to 15% once every 24 hours until the desired clinical effect is achieved.

Children: After the first 24 hours, increase the daily dose slowly by 5% to 15% only once every 24 hours, until the desired effect is achieved.

Maintenance therapy – The clinical goal is to maintain muscle tone as close to normal as possible and to minimize the frequency and severity of spasms to the extent possible, without inducing intolerable side effects. Very often the maintenance dose needs to be adjusted during the first few months of therapy while patients adjust to changes in life-style because of the alleviation of spasticity. During periodic refills of the pump, the daily dose may be increased by 5% to 20% (10% to 40% for spasticity of spinal cord origin), but no more than 20% (40% for spasticity of spinal cord origin) to maintain adequate symptom control. The daily dose may be reduced by 10% to 20% if patients experience side effects. Most patients require gradual increases in dose over time to maintain optimal response during chronic therapy. A sudden large requirement for dose escalation suggests a catheter complication (eg, catheter kink or dislodgement).

Maintenance dosage for long-term continuous infusion has ranged from 12 to 2003 mcg/day, with most patients adequately maintained on 300 to 800 mcg/day. There is limited experience with daily doses > 1000 mcg/day. Determination of the optimal dose requires individual titration. Use the lowest dose with an optimal response.

Spasticity of cerebral origin: Maintenance dosage for long-term continuous infusion of baclofen has ranged from 22 mcg/day to 1400 mcg/day, with most patients adequately maintained on 90 to 703 mcg/day. In clinical trials, only 3 of 150 patients required daily doses > 1000 mcg/day.

Children: Use same dosing recommendations for patients with spasticity of cerebral origin. Pediatric patients under 12 years of age seemed to require a lower daily dose in clinical trials. Average daily dose for patients < 12 years of age was 274 mcg/day, with a range of 24 to 1199 mcg/day. Dosage requirement for pediatric patients > 12 years of age does not seem to be different from that of adult patients. Determination of the optimal baclofen dose requires individual titration. Use the lowest dose with an optimal response.

Potential need for dose adjustments in chronic use – During long-term treatment, ≈ 5% of patients become refractory to increasing doses. There is not sufficient experience to make firm recommendations for tolerance treatment; however, this "tolerance" has been treated on occasion in the hospital by a "drug holiday" consisting of the gradual reduction of baclofen intrathecal over a 2– to 4–week period and switching to alternative methods of spasticity management. After the "drug holiday," sensitivity to baclofen may return, and baclofen intrathecal may be restarted at the initial continuous infusion dose.

It may be important to maintain some degree of muscle tone and allow occasional spasms to help support circulatory function and possibly prevent the formation of deep vein thrombosis.

Except in overdose-related emergencies, the dose should ordinarily be reduced slowly if the drug is discontinued for any reason.

Attempt to discontinue concomitant oral antispasticity medication to avoid possible overdose or adverse drug interactions, preferably prior to initiation of baclofen infusion, with careful monitoring. Avoid abrupt reduction or discontinuation of concomitant antispastics, however, during chronic therapy.

Pump dose adjustment and titration – In most patients, it will be necessary to increase the dose gradually over time to maintain effectiveness; a sudden requirement for substantial dose escalation typically indicates a catheter complication.

Centrally Acting

BACLOFEN

Reservoir refilling must be performed by fully trained and qualified personnel following the directions provided by the pump manufacturer. Carefully calculate refill intervals to prevent depletion of the reservoir, as this would result in the return of severe spasticity.

Use extreme caution when filling an FDA-approved implantable pump equipped with an injection port that allows direct access to the intrathecal catheter. Direct injection into the catheter through the access port may cause a life-threatening overdose.

Dilution instructions – Dilute all strengths (10 mg/5 ml and 10 mg/20 ml) with sterile preservative-free Sodium Chloride for Injection to a 50 mcg/ml concentration for bolus injection into the subarachnoid space.

Delivery regimen – Baclofen intrathecal is most often administered in a continuous infusion mode immediately following implant. For those patients implanted with programmable pumps who have achieved relatively satisfactory control on continuous infusion, further benefit may be attained using more complex schedules of delivery. For example, patients who have increased spasms at night may require a 20% increase in their hourly infusion rate. Program changes in flow rate to start 2 hours before the time of desired clinical effect.

Baclofen oral liquid 5 mg/ml instructions for reconstitution: Grind 15 baclofen tablets in a glass mortar to create a fine powder. Add 10 ml of glycerin to wet the powder, triturating the powder to form a fine paste. Gradually add 15 ml of simple syrup to the paste and transfer the contents to the final container (amber glass bottle). Rinse the mortar with an additional 15 ml of simple syrup and transfer to the final container. Repeat this last step to bring the volume of the final container to 60 ml. Label the bottle "shake well before using" and "refrigerate." Assign an expiration date of 35 days to the completed product.

Storage/Stability:

Oral – Do not store above 30°C (86°F).

Intrathecal – Does not require refrigeration. Do not store above 30°C (86°F). Do not freeze. Do not heat sterilize.

Rx	**Baclofen** (Various, eg, Geneva, Major, Rugby, Schein, UDL, URL, Zenith)	**Tablets:** 10 mg	In 100s, 250s, 500s, 1000s and UD 100s.
Rx	**Lioresal** (Geigy)		(Lioresal 1010). White, scored. Oval. In 100s and UD 100s.
Rx	**Baclofen** (Various, eg, Geneva, Major, Rugby, Schein, UDL, URL, Zenith)	**Tablets:** 20 mg	In 100s, 250s, 500s, 1000s and UD 100s.
Rx	**Lioresal** (Geigy)		(Lioresal 2020). White, scored. Capsule shape. In 100s and UD 100s.
Rx	**Lioresal** (Medtronic)	**Intrathecal:** 10 mg/20 ml (500 mcg/ml)	Preservative-free. In single-use amps (1 amp refill kit).
		10 mg/5 ml (2000 mcg/ml)	Preservative-free. In single-use amps (2 or 4 amp refill kits).

Direct Acting

DANTROLENE SODIUM

Warning:

Dantrolene has a potential for hepatotoxicity. Do not use in conditions other than those recommended. The incidence of symptomatic hepatitis (fatal and nonfatal) reported in patients taking up to 400 mg/day is much lower than in those taking ≥ 800 mg/day. Even sporadic short courses of these higher dose levels within a treatment regimen markedly increased the risk of serious hepatic injury. Liver dysfunction, as evidenced by liver enzyme elevations, has been observed in patients exposed to the drug for varying periods of time. Overt hepatitis has been most frequently observed between the third and twelfth months of therapy. Risk of hepatic injury appears to be greater in females, in patients > 35 years of age and in patients taking other medications in addition to dantrolene.

Monitor hepatic function, including frequent determinations of AST or ALT. If no observable benefit is derived from therapy after 45 days, discontinue use.

Use the lowest possible effective dose for each patient.

Actions:

Pharmacology: In isolated nerve-muscle preparation, dantrolene produced relaxation by affecting contractile response of the skeletal muscle at a site beyond the myoneural junction and directly on the muscle itself. In skeletal muscle, the drug dissociates the excitation-contraction coupling, probably by interfering with the release of calcium from the sarcoplasmic reticulum. This effect appears more pronounced in fast muscle fibers than in slow ones, but generally affects both. A CNS effect occurs, with drowsiness, dizziness and generalized weakness occasionally present. Although dantrolene does not appear to directly affect the CNS, the extent of its indirect effect is unknown. The administration of IV dantrolene is also associated with loss of grip strength and weakness in the legs.

Malignant hyperthermia – In anesthetic-induced malignant hyperthermia syndrome, evidence points to an intrinsic abnormality of muscle tissue. In affected humans, "triggering agents" may induce a sudden rise in myoplasmic calcium by accelerating its release from sarcoplasmic reticulum. This rise in myoplasmic calcium activates acute catabolic processes common to the malignant hyperthermia crisis.

Dantrolene may prevent such changes within the muscle cell by interfering with calcium release from the sarcoplasmic reticulum to the myoplasm. Thus, physiologic, metabolic and biochemical changes associated with the crisis may be reversed or attenuated. Administration of IV dantrolene, combined with supportive measures, is effective in reversing the hypermetabolic process of malignant hyperthermia. Oral dantrolene will also attenuate or prevent the development of signs of malignant hyperthermia, provided that currently accepted practices in the management of such patients are adhered to; IV dantrolene should also be available for use should the signs of malignant hyperthermia appear.

Pharmacokinetics:

Absorption/Distribution – Absorption after oral administration is incomplete and slow but consistent, and dose-related blood levels are obtained.

Slightly greater amounts of dantrolene are associated with red blood cells than with the plasma fraction of blood. Significant amounts are reversibly bound to plasma proteins, mostly albumin; this binding is readily reversible. Its plasma protein binding is affected by some drugs (see Drug Interactions).

Metabolism – Metabolic patterns are similar in adults and children. Dantrolene is found in measurable amounts in blood and urine; the major metabolites noted are the 5-hydroxy analog and the acetamido analog. Mean half-life in adults is 9 hours after a 100 mg oral dose and 4 to 8 hours after IV administration. Since it is probably metabolized by hepatic microsomal enzymes, metabolism enhancement by other drugs is possible. However, neither phenobarbital nor diazepam appears to affect metabolism.

DANTROLENE SODIUM

Indications:

Spasticity:

Oral – For the control of clinical spasticity resulting from upper motor neuron disorders such as spinal cord injury, stroke, cerebral palsy or multiple sclerosis. It is of particular benefit to the patient whose functional rehabilitation has been retarded by the sequelae of spasticity. Such patients must have presumably reversible spasticity where relief of spasticity will aid in restoring residual function.

Malignant hyperthermia:

IV – Management of the fulminant hypermetabolism of skeletal muscle characteristic of malignant hyperthermia crisis, along with appropriate supportive measures.

Preoperatively, and sometimes postoperatively, to prevent or attenuate the development of clinical and laboratory signs of malignant hyperthermia in individuals judged to be susceptible to malignant hyperthermia.

Oral – Preoperatively to prevent or attenuate the development of signs of malignant hyperthermia in susceptible patients who require anesthesia or surgery. Currently accepted clinical practices in the management of such patients must still be adhered to (careful monitoring for early signs of malignant hyperthermia, minimizing exposure to triggering mechanisms and prompt use of IV dantrolene and indicated supportive measures if signs of malignant hyperthermia appear).

Following a malignant hyperthermia crisis to prevent recurrence of malignant hyperthermia.

Unlabeled uses: Exercise-induced muscle pain; neuroleptic malignant syndrome; heat stroke.

Contraindications:

Oral: Active hepatic disease, such as hepatitis and cirrhosis; where spasticity is utilized to sustain upright posture and balance in locomotion or to obtain or maintain increased function; treatment of skeletal muscle spasm resulting from rheumatic disorders.

Warnings:

Hepatic effects: Fatal and nonfatal liver disorders of an idiosyncratic or hypersensitivity type may occur. At the start of therapy, perform baseline liver function studies (AST, ALT, alkaline phosphatase, total bilirubin). If abnormalities exist, the potential for hepatotoxicity could be enhanced.

Perform liver function studies at appropriate intervals during therapy. If such studies reveal abnormal values, generally discontinue therapy. Consider reinitiation or continuation only when drug benefits have been of major importance. Some laboratory values may return to normal with continued therapy; others may not.

If symptoms of hepatitis accompanied by liver function test abnormalities or jaundice appear, discontinue therapy. If caused by dantrolene and detected early, abnormalities may revert to normal when the drug is discontinued.

Therapy has been reinstituted in a few patients who have developed clinical or laboratory evidence of hepatocellular injury. Attempt reinstitution only in patients who clearly need dantrolene, after previous symptoms and laboratory abnormalities have cleared. Hospitalize the patient and restart the drug in very small and gradually increasing doses. Monitor laboratory values frequently and withdraw the drug immediately if there is any indication of recurrent liver involvement. Some patients have reacted with liver abnormality upon administration of a challenge dose, while others have not.

Use with caution in females and in patients > 35 years of age; there is a greater likelihood of drug-induced, potentially fatal hepatocellular disease in these populations.

Long-term use: Safety and efficacy have not been established. Chronic studies in animals at dosages > 30 mg/kg/day showed growth or weight depression, signs of hepatopathy and possible occlusion nephropathy; all were reversible upon cessation of treatment.

Continued long-term administration is justified if use of the drug: Significantly reduces painful or disabling spasticity such as clonus; significantly reduces the intensity or degree of nursing care required; rids the patient of any annoying manifestation of spasticity considered important by the patient.

Brief withdrawal for 2 to 4 days will frequently demonstrate exacerbation of the manifestations of spasticity and may serve to confirm a clinical impression.

In view of the potential for liver damage in long-term use, discontinue therapy if benefits are not evident within 45 days.

Direct Acting

DANTROLENE SODIUM

Malignant hyperthermia (MH): IV use is not a substitute for previously known supportive measures. These measures include discontinuing the suspected triggering agents, attending to increased oxygen requirements, managing the metabolic acidosis, instituting cooling when necessary, attending to urinary output and monitoring electrolyte imbalance.

There have been occasional reports of death following malignant hyperthermia crisis even when treated with IV dantrolene; incidence figures are not available. Most of these deaths can be accounted for by late recognition, delayed treatment, inadequate dosage, lack of supportive therapy, intercurrent disease or the development of delayed complications such as renal failure or disseminated intravascular coagulopathy. In some cases, there are insufficient data to completely rule out therapeutic failure of dantrolene.

Rare reports of fatality in MH crisis, despite initial satisfactory response to IV dantrolene, involve patients who could not be weaned from dantrolene after initial treatment.

Hepatic function impairment: Use with caution in patients with a history of previous liver disease or dysfunction.

Carcinogenesis: An increased incidence of benign and malignant mammary tumors and hepatic lymphangiomas and hepatic angiosarcomas has occurred in animals. Carcinogenicity in humans cannot be fully excluded; weigh this possible risk of chronic administration against the benefits of the drug for the individual patient.

Pregnancy: Category C (parenteral). Dantrolene is embryocidal in the rabbit and decreases pup survival in the rat when given at doses seven times the human oral dose. There are no adequate and well controlled studies in pregnant women. Use only when clearly needed and when the potential benefits outweigh the potential hazards to the fetus.

Labor and delivery – In one uncontrolled study, 100 mg/day of prophylactic oral dantrolene was administered to term pregnant patients awaiting labor and delivery. Dantrolene readily crossed the placenta, with maternal and fetal whole blood levels approximately equal at delivery; neonatal levels then fell approximately 50% per day for 2 days before declining sharply. No neonatal respiratory and neuromuscular side effects were detected at low dose. More data, at higher doses, are needed before definitive conclusions can be made.

One patient developed postpartum uterine atony following dantrolene administration after a cesarean section.

Lactation: Do not use in nursing women.

Children: Safety for use in children < 5 years of age has not been established. Because of the possibility that adverse effects could become apparent only after many years, a benefit-risk consideration of long-term use is particularly important.

Precautions:

Special risk patients: Use with caution in patients with impaired pulmonary function, particularly those with obstructive pulmonary disease; severely impaired cardiac function due to myocardial disease.

Extravasation: Because of the high pH of the IV formulation, prevent extravasation into the surrounding tissues.

Hazardous tasks: Patients should use caution while driving or performing other tasks requiring alertness, coordination or physical dexterity.

Photosensitivity: Photosensitization may occur; therefore, caution patients to take protective measures (eg, sunscreens, protective clothing) against exposure to ultraviolet light or sunlight until tolerance is determined.

DANTROLENE SODIUM

Drug Interactions:

Dantrolene Drug Interactions			
Precipitant drug	Object drug*		Description
Clofibrate	Dantrolene	↓	Plasma protein binding of dantrolene may be reduced.
Dantrolene	Verapamil	↑	Hyperkalemia and myocardial depression occurred in one patient during concurrent use.
Estrogens	Dantrolene	↑	Although a definite drug interaction is not established, hepatotoxicity occurred more often in women > 35 years old receiving these agents concurrently.
Warfarin	Dantrolene	↓	Plasma protein binding of dantrolene may be reduced.

* ↑ = Object drug increased ↓ = Object drug decreased

Adverse Reactions:

Oral: Most frequent – Drowsiness; dizziness; weakness; general malaise; fatigue; diarrhea. These effects are generally transient, occur early in treatment and can often be obviated by beginning with a low dose and increasing gradually until an optimal regimen is established. Diarrhea may be severe and may necessitate temporary withdrawal of therapy. If diarrhea recurs upon readministration, discontinue use.

GI – Constipation; GI bleeding; anorexia; dysphagia; gastric irritation; abdominal cramps; hepatitis (see Warnings).

CNS – Speech disturbance; seizure; headache; lightheadedness; visual disturbance; diplopia; alteration of taste; insomnia; mental depression/confusion; increased nervousness.

Cardiovascular – Tachycardia; erratic blood pressure; phlebitis.

GU – Increased urinary frequency; hematuria; crystalluria; difficult erection; urinary incontinence; nocturia; dysuria; urinary retention.

Dermatologic – Abnormal hair growth; acne-like rash; pruritus; urticaria; eczematoid eruption; sweating.

Musculoskeletal – Myalgia; backache.

Miscellaneous – Chills; fever; feeling of suffocation; excessive tearing; pleural effusion with pericarditis.

Parenteral: The following adverse reactions are in approximate order of severity: Pulmonary edema developing during treatment of MH crisis (diluent volume and mannitol needed to deliver IV dantrolene possibly contributed); thrombophlebitis following IV dantrolene (actual incidence figures not available); urticaria and erythema (possibly associated with IV dantrolene); death (see Warnings).

None of the serious reactions occasionally reported with long-term oral dantrolene use, such as hepatitis, seizures, and pleural effusion with pericarditis, have been reasonably associated with short-term dantrolene IV therapy.

Overdosage:

There is no known antidote. Employ general supportive measures along with immediate gastric lavage. Administer IV fluids in fairly large quantities to avert the possibility of crystalluria. Maintain an adequate airway; have artificial resuscitation equipment available. Monitor ECG; observe patient carefully. No experience has been reported with dialysis.

Patient Information:

May cause drowsiness, dizziness or lightheadedness. Patients should exercise caution while driving or performing other tasks requiring alertness, coordination or physical dexterity.

Avoid alcohol and other CNS depressants.

Avoid prolonged exposure to sunlight; photosensitivity may occur.

May cause weakness, malaise, fatigue, nausea and diarrhea. Notify physician if these effects persist.

Notify physician if skin rash, itching, bloody or black tarry stools or yellowish discoloration of the skin or eyes occurs.

Dantrolene IV may decrease grip strength and increase weakness of leg muscles, especially walking down stairs.

Exercise caution at meals on the day of administration because difficulty swallowing and choking has been reported.

Direct Acting

DANTROLENE SODIUM

Administration and Dosage:

Chronic spasticity: Prior to administration, consider the potential response to treatment. Decreased spasticity sufficient to allow a daily function not otherwise attainable should be the therapeutic goal. Establish a therapeutic goal (regain and maintain a specific function such as therapeutic exercise program, utilization of braces, transfer maneuvers, etc) before beginning therapy. Increase dosage until the maximum performance compatible with the dysfunction due to underlying disease is achieved. No further increase in dosage is then indicated.

Titrate and individualize dosage. In view of the potential for liver damage in long-term use, discontinue therapy if benefits are not evident within 45 days.

Adults – Begin with 25 mg once daily; increase to 25 mg, 2 to 4 times daily; then by increments of 25 mg up to as high as 100 mg, 2 to 4 times daily if necessary. Most patients will respond to 400 mg/day or less; higher doses are rarely needed. (See Warning Box.) Maintain each dosage level for 4 to 7 days to determine response. Adjust dosage to achieve maximal benefit without adverse effects.

Children – Use a similar approach. Start with 0.5 mg/kg twice daily; increase to 0.5 mg/kg, 3 or 4 times daily; then by increments of 0.5 mg/kg, up to 3 mg/kg, 2 to 4 times daily if necessary. Do not exceed doses higher than 100 mg 4 times daily.

Malignant hyperthermia:

Preoperative prophylaxis – Dantrolene may be given orally or IV to patients judged susceptible to malignant hyperthermia as part of the overall patient management to prevent or attenuate development of clinical and laboratory signs of MH.

Oral – Give 4 to 8 mg/kg/day orally in 3 or 4 divided doses for 1 or 2 days prior to surgery, with last dose given ≈ 3 to 4 hours before scheduled surgery with a minimum of water. This dosage will usually be associated with skeletal muscle weakness and sedation (sleepiness or drowsiness) or excessive GI irritation (nausea or vomiting); adjust within the recommended dosage range to avoid incapacitation or excessive GI irritation.

IV – 2.5 mg/kg ≈ 1 hour before anesthesia and infused over ≈ 1 hour. Additional dantrolene IV may be indicated during anesthesia and surgery by malignant hyperthermia signs or prolonged surgery. Individualize additional doses.

Treatment – As soon as the malignant hyperthermia reaction is recognized, discontinue all anesthetic agents. Use of 100% oxygen is recommended. Administer dantrolene by continuous rapid IV push beginning at a minimum dose of 1 mg/kg, and continuing until symptoms subside or a maximum cumulative dose of 10 mg/kg has been reached. If the physiologic and metabolic abnormalities reappear, repeat the regimen. Note: Administration should be continuous until symptoms subside. The effective dose to reverse the crisis depends upon the degree of susceptibility to malignant hyperthermia, the amount and time of exposure to the triggering agent and the time elapsed between onset of the crisis and initiation of treatment.

Children – Dose is the same as for adults.

Post-crisis follow-up – Following a malignant hyperthermia crisis, give 4 to 8 mg/kg/day orally, in 4 divided doses for 1 to 3 days to prevent recurrence. IV dantrolene may be used when oral administration is not practical. The IV dose must be individualized, starting with 1 mg/kg or more as the clinical situation dictates.

Preparation of solution: Add 60 ml of Sterile Water for Injection, USP (without a bacteriostatic agent) to each vial, and shake until solution is clear. Protect from direct light and use within 6 hours. Store reconstituted solutions at controlled room temperature (15° to 30°C or 59° to 86°F). Avoid prolonged exposure to light.

Rx	**Dantrium** (Procter & Gamble Pharm.)	**Capsules**: 25 mg	Lactose. Orange and light brown. In 100s, 500s and UD 100s.
		50 mg	Lactose. Orange and dark brown. In 100s.
		100 mg	Lactose. Orange and light brown. In 100s and UD 100s.
Rx	**Dantrium Intravenous** (Procter & Gamble Pharm.)	**Powder for Injection**: 20 mg/vial. (≈ 0.32 mg/ml after reconstitution)	With 3 g mannitol per vial. In 70 ml vials.

SKELETAL MUSCLE RELAXANT COMBINATIONS

Uses: The methocarbamol and aspirin combinations and the carisoprodol and aspirin (with or without codeine) combinations are indicated as adjuncts to rest, physical therapy and other measures for relief of discomfort associated with acute, painful musculoskeletal conditions. The other combinations are classified as *"probably effective"* for this indication. Components of these combinations include:

MUSCLE RELAXANTS: Methocarbamol; Chlorzoxazone; Carisoprodol; Orphenadrine Citrate; (see individual monographs).

ANALGESICS: Acetaminophen; Aspirin; Codeine; (see individual monographs).

CAFFEINE (see individual monograph), used as a CNS stimulant, also has minor analgesic activity.

Rx	**Methocarbamol w/ASA** (Various, eg, Moore, Par)	**Tablets**: 400 mg methocarbamol and 325 mg aspirin *Dose: 2 tablets 4 times daily*	In 15s, 30s, 40s, 100s, 500s and 1000s.
Rx	**Robaxisal** (Robins)		Pink and white. In 100s, 500s and Dis-Co 100s.
Rx	**Carisoprodol Compound** (Various, eg, Moore, Rugby)	**Tablets**: 200 mg carisoprodol and 325 mg aspirin *Dose: 1 or 2 tablets 4 times daily*	In 15s, 30s, 40s, 100s, 500s and 1000s.
Rx	**Sodol Compound** (Major)		In 100s and 500s.
Rx	**Soma Compound** (Wallace)		(Soma CC Wallace-2103). White and orange. In 100s, 500s and UD 100s.
c-III	**Soma Compound w/Codeine** (Wallace)	**Tablets**: 200 mg carisoprodol, 325 mg aspirin and 16 mg codeine phosphate *Dose: 1 or 2 tablets 4 times daily*	(Soma CC Wallace-2403). White and yellow. In 100s.[1]
Rx	**Flexaphen** (Trimen)	**Capsules**: 250 mg chlorzoxazone and 300 mg acetaminophen *Dose: 2 capsules 4 times daily*	Tan. In 100s.
Rx	**Mus-Lax** (Jones Medical)		Red. In 100s.
Rx	**Lobac** (Seatrace)	**Capsules**: 200 mg salicylamide, 20 mg phenyltoloxamine and 300 mg acetaminophen *Dose: 2 capsules 4 times daily*	(Seatrace). Eggshell. In 24s and 100s.
Rx	**Norgesic** (3M Pharm)	**Tablets**: 25 mg orphenadrine citrate, 385 mg aspirin and 30 mg caffeine *Dose: 1 or 2 tablets 3 or 4 times daily*	(Norgesic 3M). Green, white and yellow. In 100s and 500s. Lactose
Rx	**Norgesic Forte** (3M Pharm)	**Tablets**: 50 mg orphenadrine citrate, 770 mg aspirin and 60 mg caffeine *Dose: or 1 tablet 3 or 4 times daily*	(Norgesic Forte 3M). Green, white and yellow, scored. In 100s and 500s. Lactose.

[1] With sodium metabisulfite.

ANTIPARKINSON AGENTS

Parkinsons's Disease: Parkinsonism is a neurological disease with a variety of origins characterized by tremor, rigidity, akinesia, and disorders of posture and equilibrium. The onset is slow and progressive with symptoms advancing over months to years.

Although the biochemical basis of parkinsonism is complex, the primary defect appears to be an imbalance of neurotransmitters (ie, a relative excess of acetylcholine and a deficiency/absence of dopamine in the basal ganglia). Other central neurotransmitters may have some modifying influence on these primary substances. This defect may be part of a more generalized, structural and enzymatic defect.

Currently, therapy for Parkinson's disease is palliative, as there is no cure for this disease. The goal of therapy is to provide maximum relief from the symptoms and to attempt to maintain the independence and mobility of the patient.

Drug therapy of Parkinson's disease is aimed at correcting or modifying these neurotransmitter defects by inhibiting the effects of acetylcholine or enhancing the effects of dopamine.

Anticholinergic agents: Centrally acting anticholinergics tend to diminish the characteristic tremor. Patients with minimal involvement who are functioning relatively well may not require medication. However, as the disease progresses, the anticholinergics may be considered.

Dopaminergic agents: Dopamine deficiency appears to be the central feature of the pathogenesis of parkinsonism. **Levodopa**, the immediate precursor of dopamine, directly increases dopamine content in the brain; it is currently the most effective treatment for parkinsonism. Other drugs are available that also affect the dopamine content of the brain: **Bromocriptine** and **pergolide** directly stimulate dopamine receptors. Pergolide is 10 to 1000 times more potent than bromocriptine on a milligram per milligram basis; **amantadine** may increase dopamine at the receptor either by releasing intact striatal dopamine stores or by blocking neuronal dopamine reuptake; **selegiline** increases dopaminergic activity through inhibition of monoamine oxidase type B, however, other mechanisms may exist such as interference of dopamine reuptake at the synapse.

Levodopa is used for symptomatic patients with moderate disabilities; therapy is usually initiated with a combination of levodopa and carbidopa (a dopa decarboxylase inhibitor that prevents peripheral metabolism of levodopa). Unfortunately, the response to levodopa gradually diminishes after 2 to 5 years in most patients, at which time the dopaminergic agonists, bromocriptine or pergolide, selegiline or amantadine may be added to the drug regimen. Amantadine may also be used in patients with minimal involvement when the patients cannot tolerate an anticholinergic drug.

The table below summarizes the drug therapy available for parkinsonism:

Drug Therapy for Parkinsonism

	Indications					
Drugs	Post-encephalitic	Arterio-sclerotic	Idiopathic	Drug/chemical induced	Adjunct to Levodopa/Carbidopa	Usual daily dose range (mg)
Anticholinergics						
Procyclidine	✔	✔	✔	✔		7.5-20
Trihexyphenidyl	✔	✔	✔	✔	✔	1-15
Benztropine	✔	✔	✔	✔		0.5-6.5
Biperiden	✔	✔	✔	✔		2-8
Ethopropazine	✔	✔	✔	✔		50-600
Diphenhydramine	✔	✔	✔	✔		10-400
Dopaminergic Agents						
Levodopa	✔	✔	✔	✔[1]		500-8000
Carbidopa/ levodopa	✔		✔	✔[1]		10/100-200/2000
Amantadine	✔	✔	✔	✔		200-400
Bromocriptine	✔		✔			12.5-100
Pergolide					✔	1-5
Selegiline					✔	10

[1] Not effective in drug-induced extrapyramidal symptoms.

Anticholinergics

ANTICHOLINERGIC AGENTS

Actions:

Pharmacology: The anticholinergic agents, although generally less effective than levodopa, are useful in the treatment of all forms of parkinsonism: Postencephalitic, arteriosclerotic, idiopathic and drug-induced extrapyramidal symptoms. They reduce the incidence and severity of akinesia, rigidity and tremor by about 20%; secondary symptoms such as drooling are also reduced. In addition to suppressing central cholinergic activity, these agents may also inhibit the reuptake and storage of dopamine at central dopamine receptors, thereby prolonging the action of dopamine.

The naturally occurring belladonna alkaloids (atropine, scopolamine, hyoscyamine) are active anticholinergic agents; however, they have largely been replaced by synthetic agents (eg, benztropine, trihexyphenidyl) with a more selective CNS activity. Peripheral anticholinergic side effects (eg, urinary retention, tachycardia, constipation) frequently limit the size of dosages utilized.

Antihistamines (eg, diphenhydramine) with central anticholinergic effects are also used; they may have a lower incidence of peripheral side effects than the belladonna alkaloids or synthetic derivatives. These agents are generally better tolerated by elderly patients. Some antihistamines provide mild antiparkinson effects, and are useful for initiating therapy in patients with minimal symptoms. Because of their sedative effects, the antihistamines may be useful in certain patients with insomnia.

Ethopropazine is a phenothiazine with prominent anticholinergic effects. It is less effective than the synthetic anticholinergic agents.

In spite of limited efficacy, anticholinergics are useful in mild cases of Parkinson's disease where risks and demands of levodopa therapy are not warranted.

Pharmacokinetics: Little pharmacokinetic data are available for these agents. The following table lists some of the available parameters.

Various Antiparkinson Anticholinergic Pharmacokinetic Parameters				
Anticholinergic	Time to peak concentration (hrs)	Peak concentration (mcg/L)	Half-life (hrs)	Oral bioavailability (%)
Benztropine[1]				
Biperiden	1-1.5	4-5	18.4-24.3	29
Diphenhydramine	2-4	65-90	4-15	50-72
Ethopropazine[1]				
Procyclidine	1.1-2	80	11.5-12.6	52-97
Trihexyphenidyl	1-1.3	87.2	5.6-10.2	≈100

[1] No data available.

Indications:

Adjunctive therapy in all forms of parkinsonism (postencephalitic, arteriosclerotic and idiopathic) and in the control of drug-induced extrapyramidal disorders. Refer to individual drug monographs for specific indications of individual agents.

Contraindications:

Hypersensitivity to any component; glaucoma, particularly angle-closure glaucoma (simple type glaucomas do not appear to be adversely affected); pyloric or duodenal obstruction; stenosing peptic ulcers; prostatic hypertrophy or bladder neck obstructions; achalasia (megaesophagus); myasthenia gravis; megacolon.

Benztropine: Children < 3 years of age; use with caution in older children.

Warnings:

Ophthalmic: Incipient narrow-angle glaucoma may be precipitated by these drugs. Performgonioscopy and closely monitor intraocular pressures at regular intervals.

Elderly: Geriatric patients, particularly > 60 years of age, frequently develop increased sensitivity to anticholinergic drugs and require strict dosage regulation. Occasionally, mental confusion and disorientation may occur; agitation, hallucinations and psychotic-like symptoms may develop.

Pregnancy: Category C. Safety for use during pregnancy has not been established. Use only when clearly needed and when the potential benefits outweigh the potential hazards to the fetus.

Lactation: Safety for use in the nursing mother has not been established. An inhibitory effect on lactation may occur. Although infants are particularly sensitive to anticholinergic agents, no adverse effects have been reported in nursing infants whose mothers were taking atropine.

Children: Safety and efficacy for use in children have not been established.

ANTICHOLINERGIC AGENTS

Precautions:

Concomitant conditions: Use caution in patients with tachycardia, cardiac arrhythmias, hypertension, hypotension, prostatic hypertrophy (particularly in the elderly), or any tendency toward urinary retention, liver or kidney disorders, and obstructive disease of the GI or GU tract.

CNS: When used to treat extrapyramidal reactions resulting from phenothiazines in psychiatric patients, antiparkinson agents may exacerbate mental symptoms and precipitate a toxic psychosis. The possibility of antiparkinson agents masking the development of persistent extrapyramidal symptoms with prolonged phenothiazine therapy has not been investigated. Whether to administer prophylactic anticholinergics to prevent drug-induced extrapyramidal effects is controversial.

In addition, 19% to 30% of patients given anticholinergics develop depression, confusion, delusions or hallucinations. Also, **benztropine** given in large doses or to susceptible patients may cause weakness and inability to move particular muscle groups. Dosage may have to be adjusted.

Tardive dyskinesia may appear in some patients on long-term therapy with phenothiazines and related agents, or may occur after therapy has been discontinued. Antiparkinson agents do not alleviate the symptoms of tardive dyskinesia and, in some instances, may aggravate such symptoms.

Heat illness: Give with caution during hot weather, especially when given concomitantly with other atropine-like drugs to the elderly, the chronically ill, alcoholics, those who have CNS disease and those who work in a hot environment. Anhidrosis may occur more readily when some disturbance of sweating already exists. Decrease dosage so that the ability to maintain body heat equilibrium by perspiration is not impaired. Severe anhidrosis and fatal hyperthermia have occurred.

Dry mouth: If dry mouth is so severe that there is difficulty in swallowing or speaking, or if loss of appetite and weight occurs, reduce dosage or discontinue the drug temporarily.

Abuse potential: Some patients may use these agents for mood elevations or psychedelic experiences. Cannabinoids, barbiturates, opiates and alcohol may have additive effects with anticholinergics. It is important to be aware of this potential abuse situation.

Hazardous tasks: May impair mental or physical abilities; patients should observe caution while driving or performing other tasks requiring alertness.

Drug Interactions:

Amantadine and anticholinergic coadministration may result in an increased incidence of anticholinergic side effects. These effects disappear when the anticholinergic dose is reduced.

Digoxin serum levels may be increased by anticholinergics when digoxin is administered as a slow dissolution oral tablet.

Haloperidol and anticholinergic coadministration may result in worsening of schizophrenic symptoms, decreased haloperidol serum concentrations and development of tardive dyskinesia.

Levodopa: Anticholinergics may decrease gastric motility resulting in increased gastric deactivation of levodopa and decreased intestinal absorption, possibly leading to a reduction in levodopa's efficacy. Other reports refute these findings.

Phenothiazines: The pharmacologic/therapeutic actions of phenothiazines may be reduced by concurrent anticholinergics. An increase in the incidence of anticholinergic side effects has occurred.

Adverse Reactions:

Hypersensitivity: Skin rash; urticaria; other dermatoses.

CNS: Disorientation; confusion; memory loss; hallucinations; psychoses; agitation; nervousness; delusions; delirium; paranoia; euphoria; excitement; lightheadedness; dizziness; headache; listlessness; depression; drowsiness; weakness; giddiness; paresthesia; heaviness of the limbs.

Cardiovascular: Tachycardia; palpitations; hypotension; postural hypotension; mild bradycardia.

GI: Dry mouth; acute suppurative parotitis; nausea; vomiting; epigastric distress; constipation; dilation of the colon; paralytic ileus; development of duodenal ulcer.

Ophthalmic: Blurred vision; mydriasis; diplopia; increased intraocular tension; angle-closure glaucoma; dilation of pupils.

Renal: Urinary retention; urinary hesitancy; dysuria.

Musculoskeletal: Muscular weakness; muscular cramping.

Miscellaneous: Elevated temperature; flushing; numbness of fingers; decreased sweating, hyperthermia, heat stroke (see Precautions); difficulty in achieving or maintaining an erection.

Because **ethopropazine** is a phenothiazine, the following side effects are theoretically possible: EEG slowing; seizures; ECG abnormalities (eg, tachycardia); rare hematologic reactions (agranulocytosis, pancytopenia, purpura); certain endocrine disturbances; jaundice; pigmentation of the cornea, lens, retina or skin; visual hallucinations.

Overdosage:

Symptoms: Characterized by the adverse reactions and may also include: Circulatory collapse; cardiac arrest; respiratory depression or arrest; CNS depression preceded or followed by stimulation; intensification of mental symptoms or toxic psychosis in mentally ill patients treated with neuroleptic drugs (eg, phenothiazines); shock; coma; stupor; seizures; convulsions; ataxia; anxiety; incoherence; hyperactivity; combativeness; anhidrosis; hyperpyrexia; fever; hot, dry, flushed skin; dry mucous membranes; dysphagia; foul-smelling breath; decreased bowel sounds; dilated and sluggish pupils.

Treatment: Immediately following acute ingestion, remove remaining drug from stomach by inducing emesis or by gastric lavage (contraindicated in precomatose, convulsive or psychotic states). Activated charcoal is an effective adsorbent.

Treatment of overdosage is symptomatic. To relieve the peripheral effects, 5 mg of pilocarpine may be given orally at repeated intervals.

Artificial respiration and oxygen therapy may be needed for respiratory depression. A short-acting barbiturate or diazepam may be used for CNS excitement or convulsions; use with caution to avoid subsequent depression; institute supportive care for depression. Urinary retention may require catheterization. Hyperpyrexia is best treated with alcohol sponges, ice bags or other cold applications. To counteract mydriasis and cycloplegia, a local miotic may be used. Darken room for photophobia. Treat circulatory collapse with fluids and vasopressors. The relapse intervals lengthen as the anticholinergic agent is metabolized; observe patient for 8 to 12 hours after last relapse.

Physostigmine salicylate reverses most cardiovascular and CNS effects of overdosage. In *adults,* 1 to 2mg IM or IV given slowly (no more than 1 mg/min) is effective. In *children,*start with 0.02mg/kg IM or by slow IV injection (no more than 0.5mg/min). If necessary, repeat at 5- to 10-minute intervals until a therapeutic effect or a maximum dose of 2mg is attained. Avoid rapid injection to reduce the possibility of physostigmine-induced convulsions. Give physostigmine cautiously. It can precipitate seizures, cholinergic crisis, bradyarrhythmias and asystole. Use in a setting where advanced life support is available.

Patient Information:

If GI upset occurs, may be taken with food.

May cause drowsiness, dizziness or blurred vision; observe caution while driving or performing other tasks requiring alertness until response to drug is known.

Avoid alcohol and other CNS depressants.

May cause dry mouth; sucking hard candy, adequate fluid intake or good oral hygiene may relieve this symptom. Difficult urination or constipation may occur; constipation may be relieved by use of stool softeners. Notify physician if effects persist.

Notify physician if rapid or pounding heartbeat, confusion, eye pain or rash occurs.

Use caution in hot weather. This medication may increase susceptibility to heat stroke.

Administration and Dosage:

Dosage depends upon the age of the patient, etiology of the disease and individual responsiveness. The dosage required for treatment of drug-induced extrapyramidal symptoms will depend on the severity of the side effects. Maintain flexible dosage to permit individualized dosing. In general, younger and postencephalitic patients require and tolerate somewhat higher doses than older patients and those with arteriosclerotic or idiopathic-type parkinsonism.

Give before or after meals, as determined by patient's reaction. Postencephalitic patients (more prone to excessive salivation) may prefer to take it after meals and may, in addition, require small amounts of atropine. If the mouth dries excessively, take before meals, unless it causes nausea. If taken after meals, thirst can be allayed by mint candies, chewing gum or water.

Anticholinergics

BELLADONNA ALKALOIDS

Complete prescribing information begins in the Antiparkinson Agents monograph.

Belladonna alkaloids may be used in symptomatic treatment of parkinsonism, in addition to their use as antispasmodics. For complete prescribing information on the belladonna alkaloids (atropine, scopolamine HBr, hyoscyamine sulfate and levorotatory alkaloids of belladonna) see Gastrointestinal Anticholinergics/Antispasmodics monograph.

PROCYCLIDINE

Complete prescribing information begins in the Antiparkinson Agents monograph.

Indications:

Parkinsonism: Treatment of parkinsonism, including the postencephalitic, arteriosclerotic and idiopathic types. Partial control of the parkinsonism symptoms is the usual therapeutic accomplishment. Procyclidine is usually more efficacious in the relief of rigidity than tremor; but tremor, fatigue, weakness and sluggishness are frequently improved. It can be substituted for all previous medications in mild and moderate cases. For the control of more severe cases, add other drugs to procyclidine therapy, as warranted.

Drug-induced extrapyramidal symptoms: Procyclidine relieves the symptoms of extrapyramidal dysfunction which accompany phenothiazine and rauwolfia therapy. It also controls sialorrhea resulting from neuroleptic medication.

Administration and Dosage:

Parkinsonism (for patients who have received no other therapy): Initially, 2.5 mg 3 times daily after meals. If well tolerated, gradually increase dose to 5 mg; administer 3 times daily, and occasionally before retiring, if necessary. In some cases, smaller doses may be effective.

Transferring patients from other therapy – Substitute 2.5 mg 3 times daily for all or part of the original drug. Procyclidine is then increased as required; the other drug is correspondingly omitted or decreased until complete replacement is achieved. Individualize dosage.

For drug-induced extrapyramidal symptoms: Begin with 2.5 mg 3 times daily; increase by 2.5 mg daily increments until the patient obtains relief of symptoms. Individualize dosage. In most cases, results will be obtained with 10 to 20 mg daily.

Rx	**Kemadrin** (Glaxo Wellcome)	**Tablets:** 5 mg	(Kemadrin S3A). White, scored. In 100s.

Anticholinergics

TRIHEXYPHENIDYL HCl

Complete prescribing information begins in the Antiparkinson Agents monograph.

Indications:

Adjunct in the treatment of all forms of parkinsonism (postencephalitic, arteriosclerotic and idiopathic); adjuvant therapy with levodopa; for the control of drug-induced extrapyramidal disorders. The sustained release dosage form is indicated for maintenance therapy after patients have been stabilized on tablets or elixir.

Administration and Dosage:

Parkinsonism: Initially, administer 1 to 2 mg the first day; increase by 2 mg increments at intervals of 3 to 5 days, until a total of 6 to 10 mg is given daily. Many patients derive maximum benefit from a total daily dose of 6 to 10 mg; however, postencephalitic patients may require a total daily dose of 12 to 15 mg. Trihexyphenidyl is tolerated best if divided into 3 doses and taken at mealtimes. High doses may be divided into 4 parts, administered at mealtimes and at bedtime.

Concomitant use with levodopa – The usual dose of each may need to be reduced. Conversely, trihexyphenidyl decreases the total bioavailability of levodopa. Careful adjustment is necessary, depending on side effects and degree of symptom control. Trihexyphenidyl 3 to 6 mg/day in divided doses is usually adequate.

Concomitant use with other anticholinergics: May be substituted, in whole or in part, for other anticholinergics. The usual procedure is partial substitution initially, with progressive reduction in the other medication as the dose of trihexyphenidyl is increased.

Drug-induced extrapyramidal disorders: Size and frequency of dose are determined empirically. Start with a single 1 mg dose. Daily dosage usually ranges between 5 to 15 mg, although reactions have been controlled on as little as 1 mg/day. If reactions are not controlled in a few hours, progressively increase subsequent doses until control is achieved. Control may be more rapidly achieved by temporarily reducing tranquilizer dose when instituting trihexyphenidyl; then adjust both drugs until desired ataractic effect is retained without onset of extrapyramidal reactions.

It is sometimes possible to maintain the patient on reduced dosage after the reactions have remained under control for several days. These reactions have remained in remission for long periods after discontinuing therapy.

Sustained release: Because of the relatively high dosage in sustained release capsules, do not use for initial therapy. Once patients are stabilized on conventional dosage forms, they may be switched to sustained release capsules on a milligram per milligram of total daily dose basis. Administer as a single dose after breakfast or in 2 divided doses 12 hours apart. Most patients will be adequately maintained on the sustained release form, but some may develop an exacerbation of parkinsonism and may require treatment with tablets or elixir.

Rx	**Trihexyphenidyl HCl** (Various, eg, Balan, Bioline, Bolar, Danbury, Goldline, Major, Moore, Raway, Schein, UDL)	**Tablets:** 2 mg	In 30s, 100s, 250s, 1000s and UD 100s.
Rx	**Artane** (Lederle)		(Artane 2 LL A11). White, scored. In 100s, 1000s and UD 100s.
Rx	**Trihexy-2** (Geneva)		White. In 100s and 1000s.
Rx	**Trihexyphenidyl HCl** (Various, eg, Balan, Bioline, Bolar, Danbury, Goldline, Lannett, Major, Moore, Schein, UDL)	**Tablets:** 5 mg	In 100s, 250s, 1000s and UD 100s.
Rx	**Artane** (Lederle)		(Artane 5 LL A12). White, scored. In 100s, UD 100s.
Rx	**Trihexy-5** (Geneva)		White. In 100s and 1000s.
Rx	**Artane Sequels** (Lederle)	**Capsules, sustained release:** 5 mg	(A9L). Blue, oval. In unit-of-issue 60s.
Rx	**Artane** (Lederle)	**Elixir:** 2 mg/5 ml	Alcohol, sorbitol. Lime-mint flavor. In 480 ml.

Anticholinergics

BENZTROPINE MESYLATE

Complete prescribing information begins in the Antiparkinson Agents monograph.

Indications:

For use as an adjunct in the therapy of all forms of parkinsonism. May also be used in the control of extrapyramidal disorders (except tardive dyskinesia) due to neuroleptic drugs (eg, phenothiazines).

Administration and Dosage:

Injection is useful for psychotic patients with acute dystonic reactions or other reactions which make oral medication difficult or impossible, or when a more rapid response is desired.

Since there is no significant difference in onset of action after IV or IM injection, there is usually no need to use the IV route. Improvement is sometimes noticeable a few minutes after injection. In emergency situations, when the condition of the patient is alarming, 1 to 2 ml will normally provide quick relief. If the parkinsonian effect begins to return, repeat the dose.

Dosage titration: Because of cumulative action, initiate therapy with a low dose, increase in increments of 0.5 mg gradually at 5 or 6 day intervals to the smallest amount necessary for optimal relief. Maximum daily dose is 6 mg.

Generally, older patients and thin patients cannot tolerate large doses.

Dosage intervals: Some patients experience greatest relief by taking the entire dose at bedtime; others react more favorably to divided doses, 2 to 4 times a day. The drug's long duration of action makes it particularly suitable for bedtime medication; its effects may last throughout the night, enabling patients to turn in bed during the night more easily, and to rise in the morning.

Parkinsonism: 1 to 2 mg/day, with a range of 0.5 to 6 mg/day, orally or parenterally.

Idiopathic parkinsonism – Start with 0.5 to 1 mg at bedtime; 4 to 6 mg per day may be required.

Postencephalitic parkinsonism – 2 mg per day in one or more doses. In highly sensitive patients, begin therapy with 0.5 mg at bedtime; increase as necessary.

Concomitant therapy: If other antiparkinson agents are to be reduced or discontinued, do so gradually. Many patients obtain greatest relief with combination therapy.

Drug-induced extrapyramidal disorders: Administer 1 to 4 mg once or twice daily.

Acute dystonic reactions – 1 to 2 ml IM or IV usually relieves the condition quickly. After that, 1 to 2 ml orally 2 times daily usually prevents recurrence.

Extrapyramidal disorders which develop soon after initiating treatment with neuroleptic drugs are likely to be transient. A dosage of 1 to 2 mg orally 2 or 3 times a day usually provides relief within 1 or 2 days. After 1 or 2 weeks, withdraw drug to determine its continued need. If such disorders recur, reinstitute benztropine.

Certain drug-induced extrapyramidal disorders which develop slowly may not respond to benztropine.

Rx	**Benztropine Mesylate** (Various, eg, Geneva, Harber, Moore, Par, Parmed, Rugby, Schein)	**Tablets:** 0.5 mg	In 100s and UD 100s.
Rx	**Cogentin** (MSD)		(MSD 21). White, scored. In 100s.
Rx	**Benztropine Mesylate** (Various, eg, Geneva, Goldline, Lederle, Moore, Purepac, Rugby, Schein, Vangard)	**Tablets:** 1 mg	In 100s, 1000s and UD 100s.
Rx	**Cogentin** (MSD)		(MSD 635). White, scored. Oval. In 100s, UD 100s.
Rx	**Benztropine Mesylate** (Various, eg, Geneva, Goldline, Lederle, Moore, Purepac, Rugby, Schein, Vangard)	**Tablets:** 2 mg	In 100s, 1000s and UD 100s.
Rx	**Cogentin** (MSD)		(MSD 60). White, scored. In 100s, 1000s, UD 100s.
Rx	**Cogentin** (MSD)	**Injection:** 1 mg/ml	In 2 ml amps.

Anticholinergics

BIPERIDEN

Complete prescribing information begins in the Antiparkinson Agents monograph.

Indications:

Adjunct in the therapy of all forms of parkinsonism (postencephalitic, arteriosclerotic and idiopathic). Useful in the control of extrapyramidal disorders secondary to neuroleptic drug therapy (eg, phenothiazines).

Administration and Dosage:

Parkinsonism: 2 mg 3 or 4 times daily, orally. Individualize dosage with dosing titrated to a maximum of 16 mg/24 hours.

Drug-induced extrapyramidal disorders: Oral: 2 mg 1 to 3 times daily.

Parenteral – 2 mg IM or IV. Repeat every half-hour until symptoms are resolved, but do not give more than 4 consecutive doses per 24 hours.

Rx	**Akineton** (Knoll)	**Tablets:** 2 mg (as HCl)	(11). White, scored. In 100s and 1000s.
		Injection: 5 mg/ml (as lactate)	In 1 ml amps.

ETHOPROPAZINE HCl

Complete prescribing information begins in the Antiparkinson Agents monograph.

A phenothiazine derivative.

Indications:

Effective as an adjunct in the therapy of all forms of parkinsonism (postencephalitic, idiopathic and arteriosclerotic). Although chemically a phenothiazine derivative, it is distinct from other drugs of its class. Ethopropazine is useful in the control of extrapyramidal disorders due to CNS drugs such as reserpine and phenothiazines.

Administration and Dosage:

Initially: 50 mg once or twice daily; increase gradually, if necessary.

Mild to moderate symptoms: 100 to 400 mg daily.

Severe cases: Gradually increase to 500 or 600 mg or more daily.

Rx	**Parsidol** (Parke-Davis)	**Tablets:** 10 mg	White. In 100s.
		50 mg	White, scored. In 100s.

DIPHENHYDRAMINE

For complete prescribing information and product availability, see Antihistamines group monograph. Also see the Antiparkinson Agents monograph.

Indications:

For parkinsonism and drug-induced extrapyramidal reactions in the elderly unable to tolerate more potent agents; mild cases of parkinsonism (including drug-induced) in other age groups; in other cases of parkinsonism (including drug-induced) in combination with centrally-acting anticholinergic agents.

Administration and Dosage:

Oral: Adults – 25 to 50 mg 3 to 4 times daily.

Children > 20 lbs (9 kg) – 12.5 to 25 mg 3 or 4 times daily or 5 mg/kg/day. Do not exceed 300 mg/day or 150 mg/m^2/day.

Parenteral: Administer IV or deeply IM.

Adults – 10 to 50 mg; 100 mg if required. Maximum daily dosage is 400 mg.

Children – 5 mg/kg/day or 150 mg/m^2/day, divided into 4 doses. Maximum daily dosage is 300 mg.

LEVODOPA

In order to reduce the high incidence of adverse reactions, individualize therapy and gradually increase dosage to the desired therapeutic level.

Actions:

Pharmacology: The symptoms of Parkinson's disease are related to depletion of striatal dopamine. Dopamine does not cross the blood-brain barrier; however, levodopa, the metabolic precursor of dopamine, does cross the blood-brain barrier. It is decarboxylated into dopamine in the basal ganglia and in the periphery. Hence, blood dopamine is markedly increased, accounting for many of levodopa's pharmacologic and adverse effects.

Pharmacokinetics:

Absorption/Distribution – Levodopa is absorbed from the small bowel; peak plasma levels occur in 0.5 to 2 hours, and may be delayed in the presence of food. The rate of absorption is dependent upon the rate of gastric emptying, pH of gastric juice, and the length of time the drug is exposed to degradative enzymes of gastric mucosa and intestinal flora.

Metabolism/Excretion – The drug is extensively metabolized (> 95%) in the periphery and by the liver; <1% of unchanged drug penetrates the CNS. Plasma half-life ranges from 1 to 3 hours. It is excreted primarily in the urine. The major urinary metabolites of levodopa appear to be dihydroxyphenylacetic acid (DOPAC) and homovanillic acid (HVA). In 24 hour urine samples, HVA accounts for 13% to 42% of the ingested dose of levodopa.

Indications:

Treatment of idiopathic, postencephalitic and symptomatic parkinsonism which may follow injury to the nervous system by carbon monoxide and manganese intoxication, and in elderly patients with parkinsonism associated with cerebral arteriosclerosis.

Concomitant therapy: Levodopa is often used in combination with carbidopa, which inhibits decarboxylation of levodopa and makes more levodopa available for transport to the brain (see Levodopa/Carbidopa monograph).

Selegiline and pergolide are each used as adjuncts in the management of parkinsonian patients being treated with levodopa/carbidopa; the dose of the levodopa/carbidopa may be decreased with concomitant therapy (see individual monographs).

Unlabeled uses: Levodopa has been used with some benefit to relieve herpes zoster (shingles) pain and restless legs syndrome.

Contraindications:

Hypersensitivity to the drug; narrow-angle glaucoma; patients on MAOI therapy (does not apply to MAOI-type B agents such as selegiline). Discontinue MAOIs 2 weeks prior to initiating levodopa therapy.

Because levodopa may activate a malignant melanoma, do not use in patients with suspicious, undiagnosed skin lesions or history of melanoma.

Warnings:

Concomitant conditions: Administer cautiously to patients with severe cardiovascular or pulmonary disease, bronchial asthma, occlusive cerebrovascular disease, renal, hepatic or endocrine disease, affective disorders, major psychoses and cardiac arrhythmias. Periodically evaluate hepatic, hematopoietic, cardiovascular and renal functions during extended therapy in all patients.

Myocardial infarction: Administer cautiously to patients with a history of myocardial infarction who have residual atrial, nodal or ventricular arrhythmias. Use in a facility with a coronary or intensive care unit.

Upper GI hemorrhage may occur in those patients with a history of peptic ulcer.

Psychiatric patients: Observe all patients for the development of depression with suicidal tendencies. Treat psychotic patients with caution.

Pregnancy: Safety for use during pregnancy has not been established. Use only when clearly needed and when potential benefits outweigh potential hazards to the fetus. At dosages in excess of 200mg/kg/day, levodopa has an adverse effect in rodents on fetal and postnatal growth and viability.

Lactation: Do not use in nursing mothers.

Children: Safety for use in children < 12 years has not been established.

Precautions:

Wide-angle glaucoma: Patients with chronic wide-angle glaucoma may be treated cautiously with levodopa, if the intraocular pressure is well controlled and the patient is carefully monitored for changes in intraocular pressure during therapy.

LEVODOPA

"On-off" phenomenon: Some patients who initially respond to levodopa therapy may develop the "on-off" phenomenon, a condition where patients suddenly oscillate between improved clinical status and loss of therapeutic effect (abrupt onset of akinesia). This effect may occur within minutes or hours and is associated with long-term levodopa treatment. Approximately 15% to 40% of patients develop this phenomenon after 2 to 3 years of treatment; this frequency increases after 5 years. In other patients, a deteriorating response to levodopa occurs ("wearing-off" effect).

Suggestions to alleviate these conditions include keeping the dose low, reserving the drug for severe cases, or the use of a "drug holiday" which includes complete withdrawal of levodopa for a period of time (5 to 14 days) followed by a slow reintroduction of the drug at a lower dose. A protein-restricted diet and adjunctive therapy (eg, pergolide, selegiline), allowing for a decreased levodopa dose, may also be beneficial. Further study is needed.

Tartrazine sensitivity: Some of these products contain tartrazine, which may cause allergic-type reactions (including bronchial asthma) in certain susceptible individuals. Although the overall incidence of tartrazine sensitivity is low, it is frequently seen in patients who also have aspirin hypersensitivity. Specific products containing tartrazine are identified in the product listings.

Drug Interactions:

Levodopa Drug Interactions

Precipitant drug	Object drug*		Description
Antacids	Levodopa	↑	Levodopa bioavailability may be increased, possibly increasing its efficacy.
Anticholinergics	Levodopa	↓	Increased gastric deactivation and decreased intestinal absorption of levodopa may occur.
Benzodiazepines	Levodopa	↓	Levodopa's therapeutic value may be attenuated.
Hydantoins	Levodopa	↓	Levodopa's effectiveness may be reduced.
Methionine	Levodopa	↓	Levodopa's effectiveness may be reduced.
Metoclopramide	Levodopa	↔	Levodopa's bioavailability may be increased; levodopa may decrease the effects of metoclopramide on gastric emptying and lower esophageal pressure.
MAO inhibitors	Levodopa	↑	Hypertensive reactions occur with levodopa and MAOI coadministration. Avoid concurrent use. The MAO-type B inhibitor selegiline is used with levodopa and is not associated with such a reaction.
Papaverine	Levodopa	↓	Levodopa's effectiveness may be reduced.
Pyridoxine	Levodopa	↓	Levodopa's effectiveness is reduced.
Tricyclic antidepressants	Levodopa	↓	Delayed absorption and decreased bioavailability of levodopa may occur. Hypertensive episodes have occurred.

* ↑ = Object drug increased ↓ = Object drug decreased ↔ = Undetermined effect

Drug/Lab test interactions: The **Coombs test** has occasionally become positive during extended therapy. Elevations of **uric acid** have occurred with the colorimetric method, but not with the uricase method.

Drug/Food interactions: In six of nine patients, meals reduced the peak plasma concentrations of levodopa by 29%; the peak was delayed by 34 minutes. A protein-restricted diet may also help minimize the "fluctuations" (decreased response to levodopa at the end of each day or at various times of day) that occur in some patients.

Adverse Reactions:

Elevations of BUN, AST, ALT, LDH, bilirubin, alkaline phosphatase, or protein-bound iodine have been reported; the significance of these findings is not known. Occasional reduction in WBC, hemoglobin and hematocrit have occurred.

Leukopenia has occurred; it required temporary cessation of levodopa therapy.

Frequent: Adventitious movements, such as choreiform or dystonic movements (10% to 90%); anorexia (50%); nausea and vomiting (80%) with or without abdominal pain and distress; dry mouth; dysphagia; dysgeusia (4.5% to 22%); sialorrhea; ataxia; increased hand tremor; headache; dizziness; numbness; weakness and faintness; bruxism; confusion; insomnia; nightmares; hallucinations and delusions; agitation and anxiety; malaise; fatigue; euphoria.

LEVODOPA

Less frequent: Cardiac irregularities or palpitations; orthostatic hypotension (symptomatic 5%); bradykinesia (the "on-off" phenomenon; see Precautions); mental changes, including paranoid ideation, psychotic episodes, depression with or without suicidal tendencies, and dementia; urinary retention; muscle twitching and blepharospasm (may be taken as an early sign of overdosage; consider dosage reduction); trismus; burning sensation of the tongue; bitter taste; diarrhea; constipation; flatulence; flushing; skin rash; increased sweating; bizarre breathing patterns; urinary incontinence; diplopia; blurred vision; dilated pupils; hot flashes; weight gain or loss; dark sweat or urine.

Rare: GI bleeding; duodenal ulcer; hypertension; phlebitis; hemolytic anemia; agranulocytosis; oculogyric crises; sense of stimulation; hiccoughs; edema; loss of hair; hoarseness; priapism; activation of latent Horner's syndrome.

Overdosage:

Treatment: For acute overdosage, employ general supportive measures, along with immediate gastric lavage. Administer IV fluids judiciously and maintain an adequate airway. Refer to General Management of Acute Overdosage.

Monitor ECG and carefully observe the patient for the possible development of arrhythmias; if required, give appropriate antiarrhythmic therapy. Consider the possibility of multiple drug ingestion.

Patient Information:

Effects may be delayed from several weeks to a few months.

May cause GI upset; take with food.

Avoid vitamin products containing vitamin B_6 (pyridoxine HCl). See Drug Interactions.

Observe caution while driving or performing other tasks requiring alertness.

If fainting, lightheadedness or dizziness (orthostatic hypotension) occurs, avoid sudden changes in posture; notify physician of this effect.

Medication may cause darkening of the urine or sweat. This effect is not harmful.

Diabetic patients: Medication may interfere with urine tests for sugar or ketones. Report any abnormal results to physician before adjusting dosage of antidiabetic medications.

Notify physician if any of the following occur: Uncontrollable movements of the face, eyelids, mouth, tongue, neck, arms, hands or legs; mood or mental changes; irregular heartbeats or palpitations; difficult urination; severe or persistent nausea and vomiting.

Administration and Dosage:

Determine the optimal daily dose for maximal improvement with tolerated side effects and titrate for each patient.

Initial: Administer 0.5 to 1g daily, divided into 2 or more doses; give with food.

Increase gradually in increments not exceeding 0.75g/day every 3 to 7 days, as tolerated. Do not exceed 8g/day, except for exceptional patients. A significant therapeutic response may not be obtained for 6 months.

In the event general anesthesia is required, therapy may be continued as long as the patient is able to take oral fluids and medication. If therapy is temporarily interrupted, the usual daily dosage may be administered as soon as the patient is able to take oral medication. Whenever therapy has been interrupted for longer periods, adjust dosage gradually; however, in many cases, the patient can be rapidly titrated to his previous therapeutic dosage.

Rx	**Larodopa** (Roche)	**Tablets:** 100 mg	Pink, scored. In 100s.
Rx	**Larodopa** (Roche)	**Tablets:** 250 mg	Pink, scored. In100s.
Rx	**Larodopa** (Roche)	**Tablets:** 500 mg	Pink, scored. In100s.
Rx	**Dopar** (Procter & Gamble)	**Capsules:** 100 mg	Tartrazine. (Eaton 013). Green. In 100s.
Rx	**Dopar** (Procter & Gamble)	**Capsules:** 250 mg	Tartrazine. (Eaton 014). Green and white. In 100s.
Rx	**Dopar** (Procter & Gamble)	**Capsules:** 500 mg	Tartrazine. (Eaton 015). Green. In 100s.

CARBIDOPA

Carbidopa is used only with levodopa. See levodopa monograph.

> **Warning:**
> When carbidopa is to be given to patients being treated with levodopa, give the two drugs at the same time, starting with no more than 20% to 25% of the previous daily dosage of levodopa. At least 8 hours should elapse between the last dose of levodopa and initiation of therapy with carbidopa and levodopa.

Actions:

Pharmacology: Carbidopa inhibits decarboxylation of peripheral levodopa. It does not cross blood-brain barrier and does not affect levodopa metabolism within the CNS.

Since its decarboxylase inhibiting activity is limited to extracerebral tissues, administration of carbidopa with levodopa makes more levodopa available for transport to the brain. Carbidopa does not have any overt pharmacodynamic actions in the recommended doses. Normally, pyridoxine HCl (vitamin B_6), in oral doses of 10 to 25 mg, may reverse the effects of levodopa by increasing the rate of aromatic amino acid decarboxylation. Carbidopa inhibits this action of pyridoxine HCl.

Since levodopa competes with certain amino acids, levodopa absorption may be impaired in some patients on a high protein diet.

Clinical trials: Carbidopa reduces the amount of levodopa required by about 70% to 75%. When administered with levodopa, carbidopa increases plasma levels and plasma half-life of levodopa, and decreases plasma and urinary dopamine and homovanillic acid. Coadministration produces greater urinary excretion of levodopa in proportion to excretion of dopamine than separate administration. Reduced formation of dopamine in extracerebral tissues, such as the heart, may protect against dopamine-induced cardiac arrhythmias.

Indications:

Carbidopa has no effect when given alone. It is indicated only for use with levodopa.

For use with levodopa in the treatment of the symptoms of idiopathic Parkinson's disease, postencephalitic parkinsonism and symptomatic parkinsonism which may follow injury to the nervous system by carbon monoxide intoxication and manganese intoxication.

Carbidopa permits administration of lower doses of levodopa, more rapid dosage titration and a somewhat smoother response. However, patients with markedly irregular ("on-off") response to levodopa do not benefit from the addition of carbidopa. Carbidopa is effective in patients who do not have adequate reduction in nausea and vomiting when the carbidopa/levodopa combination provides < 70 mg/day of carbidopa. Carbidopa is used with levodopa in the occasional patient whose dosage requirement of carbidopa and levodopa necessitates separate titration of each entity.

Unlabeled uses: Carbidopa is also used to reduce the peripheral metabolism of L-5-hydroxytryptophan (L-5HTP) when used to treat post-anoxic intention myoclonus (see the L-5HTP monograph in the Keeping Up section).

Contraindications:

Patients hypersensitive to carbidopa or levodopa.

Warnings:

Neuroleptic malignant-like syndrome including muscular rigidity, elevated body temperature, mental changes and increased serum creatine phosphokinase has been reported when antiparkinsonian agents were withdrawn abruptly. Therefore, carefully observe patients when the dosage of levodopa is reduced abruptly or discontinued, especially if the patient is receiving neuroleptics.

Discontinue levodopa at least 8 hours before concomitant therapy with carbidopa/levodopa is started. When combination therapy is initiated, reduce levodopa to 20% to 25% of the previous levodopa dosage (see Administration and Dosage).

Carbidopa does not decrease adverse reactions due to central effects of levodopa.

Dyskinesias: Carbidopa permits more levodopa to reach the brain and more dopamine to be formed. Dyskinesias may occur sooner and at lower dosages with coadministration than with levodopa alone, and may require dosage reduction.

Elderly patients may require less carbidopa/levodopa due to an age related decrease in peripheral dopa decarboxylase.

Pregnancy: Although effects in pregnancy are unknown, both levodopa and carbidopa/levodopa have caused visceral and skeletal malformations in rabbits. Use only when clearly needed and when potential benefits outweigh potential hazards to the fetus.

Lactation: Do not administer to the nursing mother.

Children: Safety for use in children < 18 years old is not established.

CARBIDOPA

Drug Interactions:

Tricyclic antidepressants: Concomitant use has, in rare reports, caused adverse reactions, including hypertension and dyskinesia.

Adverse Reactions:

Carbidopa has not been demonstrated to have any overt pharmacodynamic actions in the recommended doses. The only adverse reactions reported have been with concomitant use of carbidopa and levodopa. (See levodopa monograph.)

Levels of BUN, creatinine and uric acid are lower during concomitant administration of carbidopa and levodopa than with levodopa alone.

Administration and Dosage:

Carbidopa/levodopa combinations are the preferred method of administration (see Levodopa/Carbidopa monograph) but occasionally a patient may require individual titration of these drugs.

Determine optimal daily dosage by careful titration. Peripheral dopa decarboxylase is saturated by carbidopa at approximately 70 to 100 mg/day. Patients who require only low doses of levodopa (eg, < 700 mg when given as carbidopa/levodopa 1:10) will receive doses of carbidopa which theoretically do not saturate peripheral dopa decarboxylase.

Maximum daily dose: Do not exceed 200 mg. If the patient is taking carbidopa/levodopa, calculate the total amount of additional carbidopa to be administered each day.

Patients receiving carbidopa/levodopa who require additional carbidopa: Some patients may not have adequate reduction in nausea and vomiting when the dosage of carbidopa is < 70 mg a day, and the dosage of levodopa is < 700 mg a day. When these patients are taking 10 mg carbidopa/100 mg levodopa, 25 mg carbidopa may be given with the first dose each day. Additional doses of 12.5 mg or 25 mg may be given during the day with each dose. When patients are taking 25 mg carbidopa/250 mg levodopa, 25 mg carbidopa may be given with any dose, as required, for optimum therapeutic response.

Dosage adjustment: Add or omit to 1 tablet per day. Because therapeutic and adverse responses occur more rapidly with combined therapy than with levodopa alone, closely monitor patients. Dyskinesias may require dosage reduction. Blepharospasm may be a useful early sign of excess dosage.

Other standard antiparkinson agents may be continued while carbidopa and levodopa are administered; the dosage of such drugs may require adjustment.

If general anesthesia is required, continue therapy as long as patient is allowed to take oral fluids and medication. When therapy is temporarily interrupted, resume usual daily dosage as soon as patient is able to take oral medication.

Rx	**Lodosyn**[1] (Merck)	**Tablets:** 25 mg carbidopa	(MSD 129). Orange, scored. In 100s.

[1] Most patients may be maintained on carbidopa/levodopa combination products. *Lodosyn* is available to physicians for use in patients requiring individual titration of carbidopa and levodopa.

LEVODOPA AND CARBIDOPA

These agents are used in combination since carbidopa inhibits decarboxylation of levodopa and makes more levodopa available for transport to the brain. For complete information on each of the components refer to the individual monographs.

Actions:

Pharmacology: The sustained release formulation is designed to release the ingredients over a 4 to 6 hour period. There is less variation in plasma levodopa levels than with the conventional formulation. However, the sustained release form is less systemically bioavailable (70% to 75%) and may require increased daily doses to achieve the same level of symptomatic relief.

Pharmacokinetics: The half-life of levodopa may be prolonged following the sustained release form because of continuous absorption. In elderly subjects, the mean time to peak levodopa concentration was 2 hours for sustained release vs 0.5 hours for conventional. The maximum levodopa concentration of levodopa following the sustained release form was about 35% of the conventional form.

Clinical trials: In clinical trials, patients receiving the sustained release form did not experience quantitatively significant reductions in "off" time (motor fluctuations) compared to the conventional form; however, global ratings of improvement were better.

Indications:

Treatment of symptoms of idiopathic Parkinson's disease (paralysis agitans), postencephalitic parkinsonism and symptomatic parkinsonism which may follow injury to the nervous system by carbon monoxide and manganese intoxication.

Warnings:

CNS effects: Certain adverse CNS effects (eg, dyskinesias) will occur at lower dosages and sooner during therapy with the sustained release form.

Drug Interactions:

Drug/Food interactions: Administration of a single dose of the sustained release form with food increased the extent of levodopa availability by 50% and increased peak levodopa concentrations by 25%.

Adverse Reactions:

In clinical trials, the adverse reaction profile of the sustained release form did not differ substantially from that of the conventional form.

Administration and Dosage:

The optimum daily dose must be determined by careful titration in each patient.

Patients not receiving levodopa:

Sinemet – 1 tablet of 25 mg carbidopa/100 mg levodopa 3 times daily or 10 mg carbidopa/100 mg levodopa 3 or 4 times daily. Dosage may be increased by 1 tablet every day or every other day, as necessary, until a dosage of 8 tablets a day is reached.

Tablets of the two ratios (eg, 1:4, 25/100 or 1:10, 10/100 and 25/250) may be given separately or combined as needed to provide the optimum dosage.

Provide at least 70 to 100 mg carbidopa per day. When more carbidopa is required, substitute one 25/100 tablet for each 10/100 tablet. When more levodopa is required, substitute the 25/250 tablet for the 25/100 or 10/100 tablet.

Sinemet CR – 1 tablet twice daily at intervals of not less than 6 hours. Doses and dosing intervals may be increased or decreased based on response. Most patients have been adequately treated with 2 to 8 tablets per day (divided doses) at intervals of 4 to 8 hours while awake. Higher doses (≥ 12 tablets per day) and intervals < 4 hours have been used but are not usually recommended. If an interval of < 4 hours is used or if the divided doses are not equal, give the smaller doses at the end of the day. Allow at least a 3 day interval between dosage adjustments.

Sinemet CR may be administered as whole or half tablets which should not be crushed or chewed.

Patients currently treated with levodopa: Levodopa must be discontinued at least 8 hours before therapy with levodopa/carbidopa. Substitute the combination drug at a dosage that will provide approximately 25% of the previous levodopa dosage.

Sinemet – Suggested starting dosage is 1 tablet of 25 mg carbidopa/250 mg levodopa 3 or 4 times a day for patients taking > 1500 mg levodopa or 25 mg carbidopa/100 mg levodopa for patients taking < 1500 mg levodopa.

Sinemet CR – Usually 1 tablet twice daily.

LEVODOPA AND CARBIDOPA

Patients currently treated with conventional carbidopa/levodopa preparations: Substitute dosage with *Sinemet CR* at an amount that provides ≈ 10% more levodopa per day, although this may need to be increased to a dosage that provides up to 30% more levodopa per day. Use intervals of 4 to 8 hours while awake.

Guidelines for Initial Conversion from *Sinemet* to *Sinemet CR*

Sinemet Total daily levodopa dose (mg)	*Sinemet CR* Suggested dosage regimen
300 to 400	1 tablet twice daily
500 to 600	1½ tablets twice daily or 1 tablet 3 times daily
700 to 800	Total of 4 tablets in ≥ 3 divided doses (eg, 1½ tablets am, 1½ tablets early pm, 1 tablet later pm)
900 to 1000	Total of 5 tablets in ≥ 3 divided doses (eg, 2 tablets am, 2 tablets early pm, 1 tablet later pm)

Combination therapy: Other antiparkinson drugs can be given concurrently; dosage adjustment may be necessary.

Sinemet (25/100 or 10/100) can be added to the dosage regimen of *Sinemet CR* in selected patients with advanced disease who need additional levodopa.

Rx	**Carbidopa & Levodopa** (Lemmon)	**Tablets:** 10 mg carbidopa and 100 mg levodopa	(93 292). Blue, mottled, scored. In 100s and 1000s.
Rx	**Sinemet-10/100** (DuPont Pharm)		(647). Dark blue, scored. Oval. In 100s and UD 100s.
Rx	**Carbidopa & Levodopa** (Lemmon)	**Tablets:** 25 mg carbidopa and 100 mg levodopa	(93 293). Yellow, mottled, scored. In 100s and 1000s.
Rx	**Sinemet-25/100** (DuPont Pharm)		(650). Yellow, scored. Oval. In 100s and UD 100s.
Rx	**Carbidopa & Levodopa** (Lemmon)	**Tablets:** 25 mg carbidopa and 250 mg levodopa	(93 294). Blue, mottled, scored. In 100s and 1000s.
Rx	**Sinemet-25/250** (DuPont Pharm)		(654). Light blue, scored. Oval. In 100s and UD 100s.
Rx	**Sinemet CR** (DuPont Pharm)	**Tablets, sustained release:** 25 mg carbidopa, 100 mg levodopa	(601). Pink. Biconvex. Oval. In 100s and UD 100s.
		50 mg carbidopa and 200 mg levodopa	(521). Peach, scored. Oval, biconvex. In 100s and UD 100s.

AMANTADINE HCl

This is an abbreviated monograph. For full prescribing information, refer to the Antiviral Agents monograph.

Actions:

Pharmacology: The exact mechanism of action is unknown, but amantadine is thought to release dopamine from intact dopaminergic terminals that remain in the substantia nigra of parkinson patients. Dopamine release may also occur from other central sites.

Amantadine is less effective than levodopa in the treatment of Parkinson's disease, but slightly more effective than anticholinergic agents. Although anticholinergic-type side effects have been noted with amantadine when used in patients with drug-induced extrapyramidal reactions, there is a lower incidence of these side effects than with anticholinergic antiparkinson drugs.

Indications:

Parkinson's disease/syndrome and drug-induced extrapyramidal reactions: Idiopathic Parkinson's disease (paralysis agitans); postencephalitic parkinsonism; arteriosclerotic parkinsonism; drug-induced extrapyramidal reactions; symptomatic parkinsonism following injury to the nervous system by carbon monoxide intoxication.

Administration and Dosage:

Parkinson's disease: 100 mg twice/day when used alone. Onset of action is usually within 48 hrs. Initial dose is 100 mg/day for patients with serious associated medical illnesses or those receiving high doses of other antiparkinson drugs. After one to several weeks at 100 mg once/day, increase to 100 mg twice/day, if necessary. Patients whose responses are not optimal at 200 mg/day may occasionally benefit from an increase up to 400 mg/day in divided doses; supervise closely. Patients initially benefiting from amantadine often experience decreased efficacy after a few months. Benefit may be regained by increasing to 300 mg/day, or by temporary discontinuation for several weeks. Other antiparkinson drugs may be necessary.

Concomitant therapy – Some patients who do not respond to anticholinergic antiparkinson drugs may respond to amantadine. When each is used with marginal benefit, concomitant use may produce additional benefit.

When amantadine and levodopa are initiated concurrently, the patient can exhibit rapid therapeutic benefits. Maintain the dose at 100 mg/day or twice/day, while levodopa is gradually increased to optimal benefit. When amantadine is added to optimal, well tolerated doses of levodopa, additional benefit may result; this includes minimizing the fluctuations in improvement which sometimes occur on levodopa alone. Patients who require a reduction in their usual dose of levodopa because of side effects may regain lost benefit with addition of amantadine.

Renal function impairment: The following table is designed to yield steady-state plasma concentrations of 0.7 to 1 mcg/ml.

Suggested Dosage Guidelines for Amantadine in Impaired Renal Function

Creatinine clearance (ml/min/1.73 m^2)	Estimated half-life (hours)	Suggested maintenance regimen[1]
100	11	100 mg twice a day or 200 mg daily
80	14	100 mg twice a day
60	19	200 mg alternated with 100 mg daily
50	23	100 mg daily
40	29	100 mg daily
30	40	200 mg twice weekly
20	66	100 mg three times weekly
10	178	200 mg alternated with 100 mg every 7 days
Three times weekly chronic hemodialysis	199	200 mg alternated with 100 mg every 7 days

[1] Loading dose on first day of 200 mg.

Reproduced with permission from Horadam VW, Sharp JG, Smilack JD, et al. Pharmacokinetics of amantadine HCl in subjects with normal and impaired renal function. *Ann Intern Med* 1981;94 (Part 1):454-58.

AMANTADINE HCl

Drug-induced extrapyramidal reactions: 100 mg twice/day. Patients with suboptimal responses may benefit from 300 mg/day in divided doses.

Rx	**Amantadine HCl** (Various, eg, URL)	**Capsules:** 100 mg	In 100s.
Rx	**Symadine** (Solvay)		(RR 4140). Red. In 100s.
Rx	**Symmetrel** (DuPont)		Parabens. (Symmetrel/DuPont). Red. In 100s, 500s & UD 100s.
Rx	**Amantadine HCl** (Various, eg, Barre-National, Copley)	**Syrup:** 50 mg/5 ml	In pt.
Rx	**Symmetrel** (DuPont)		Parabens, sorbitol. In pt.

BROMOCRIPTINE MESYLATE

This is an abbreviated monograph. Bromocriptine is also used in the treatment of amenorrhea/galactorrhea, female infertility, acromegaly and prevention of physiological lactation. For full prescribing information, refer to the monograph in the Miscellaneous chapter.

Actions:

Pharmacology: Bromocriptine, a dopamine agonist, may relieve akinesia, rigidity and tremor in patients with Parkinson's disease. It produces its therapeutic effect by directly stimulating the dopamine receptors in the corpus striatum. Experiments in rodents suggest a direct action of bromocriptine on striatal dopamine receptors.

As adjunctive treatment to levodopa (alone or with a peripheral decarboxylase inhibitor), bromocriptine therapy may provide additional therapeutic benefits in those patients who are currently maintained on optimal dosages of levodopa, those who are beginning to develop tolerance to levodopa therapy, and those who are experiencing levodopa "end of dose failure." Bromocriptine may permit reducing the maintenance dose of levodopa and thus, may ameliorate the occurrence or severity of adverse reactions associated with long-term levodopa therapy such as abnormal involuntary movements (eg, dyskinesias) and the marked swings in motor function ("on-off" phenomenon). Continued efficacy of bromocriptine during treatment of > 2 years has not been established.

Data are insufficient to evaluate benefit from treating newly diagnosed Parkinson's disease with bromocriptine. Studies show more adverse reactions (notably nausea, hallucinations, confusion and hypotension) in bromocriptine-treated patients than in levodopa/carbidopa-treated patients. Patients unresponsive to levodopa are poor candidates for bromocriptine.

Indications:

Parkinson's disease: In the treatment of idiopathic or postencephalitic Parkinson's disease.

Administration and Dosage:

Parkinson's disease: Initiate treatment at a low dosage and individualize; increase the daily dosage slowly until a maximum therapeutic response is achieved. If possible, maintain the dosage of levodopa during this introductory period.

Initially, use 1.25 mg (one-half of a 2.5 mg tablet) twice daily with meals. Assess dosage titrations every 2 weeks to ensure that the lowest dosage producing an optimal therapeutic response is not exceeded. If necessary, increase the dosage every 2 to 4 weeks by 2.5 mg/day with meals. If it is necessary to reduce the dose because of adverse reactions, reduce dose gradually in 2.5 mg increments. Usual range is 10 to 40 mg/day.

The safety of bromocriptine has not been demonstrated in dosages exceeding 100 mg/day.

Rx	**Parlodel SnapTabs** (Sandoz)	**Tablets:** 2.5 mg (as mesylate)	(Parlodel 2½). White, scored. In 30s and 100s.
Rx	**Parlodel** (Sandoz)	**Capsules:** 5 mg (as mesylate)	(Parlodel 5 mg). Caramel/white. In 30s & 100s.

SELEGILINE HCl (L-Deprenyl)

Actions:

Pharmacology: Selegiline hydrochloride is a levorotatory acetylenic derivative of phenethylamine. The mechanism of action in the adjunctive treatment of Parkinson's disease is not fully understood. Inhibition of monoamine oxidase (MAO) type B activity is of primary importance; selegiline may act through other mechanisms to increase dopaminergic activity.

Selegiline is an irreversible inhibitor of MAO by acting as a 'suicide' substrate for the enzyme; ie, it is converted by MAO to an active moiety that combines irreversibly with the active site or the enzyme's essential FAD cofactor. Because selegiline has greater affinity for type B than for type A active sites, it can serve as a selective inhibitor of MAO type B at the recommended dose.

MAOs are widely distributed throughout the body; their concentration is especially high in liver, kidney, stomach, intestinal wall and brain. MAOs are currently subclassified into two types, A and B, which differ in their substrate specificity and tissue distribution in humans. Intestinal MAO is predominantly type A, while most of that in the brain is type B. In CNS neurons, MAO plays an important role in the catabolism of catecholamines (dopamine, norepinephrine and epinephrine) and serotonin. MAOs are also important in the catabolism of various exogenous amines found in a variety of food and drugs. MAO in the GI tract and liver (primarily type A) provides vital protection from exogenous amines (eg, tyramine) that have the capacity, if absorbed intact, to cause a hypertensive crisis.

Selegiline may have pharmacological effects unrelated to MAO type B inhibition. There is some evidence that it may increase dopaminergic activity by other mechanisms, including interfering with dopamine reuptake at the synapse. Effects resulting from selegiline administration may also be mediated through its metabolites. Two of its three principal metabolites, amphetamine and methamphetamine, have pharmacological actions of their own; they interfere with neuronal uptake and enhance release of several neurotransmitters (eg, norepinephrine, dopamine, serotonin). However, the extent to which these metabolites contribute to the effects of selegiline are unknown.

Pharmacokinetics:

Absorption/Distribution – Selegiline is rapidly absorbed; ≈ 73% of a dose is absorbed; maximum plasma concentration occurs 0.5 to 2 hours following administration. Following use of a single oral 10 mg dose in 12 healthy subjects, serum levels of intact selegiline were below the limit of detection (< 10 ng/ml).

Metabolism/Excretion – The drug is rapidly metabolized. Three metabolites, N-desmethyldeprenyl (the major metabolite; mean half-life 2 hours), amphetamine (mean half-life 17.7 hours), and methamphetamine (mean half-life 20.5 hours), were found in serum and urine. Over 48 hours, 45% of the dose appeared in the urine as these 3 metabolites. Unchanged selegiline is not detected in urine.

The rate of MAO-B regeneration following discontinuation of treatment has not been quantitated. It is this rate, dependent upon de novo protein synthesis, that seems likely to determine how fast normal MAO-B activity can be restored.

Clinical trials: Selegiline's benefit in Parkinson's disease has only been documented as an adjunct to levodopa/carbidopa. Its effectiveness as a sole treatment is unknown, but attempts to treat Parkinson's disease with nonselective MAO inhibitor monotherapy have been unsuccessful.

Indications:

Parkinson's disease: Adjunct in the management of Parkinsonian patients being treated with levodopa/carbidopa who exhibit deterioration in the quality of their response to this therapy.

Contraindications:

Hypersensitivity to the drug; use with meperidine (this contraindication is often extended to other opioids; see Drug Interactions).

Warnings:

Maximum dose: Do not use at daily doses exceeding those recommended (10 mg/day) because of the risks associated with nonselective inhibition of MAO.

The selectivity of selegiline for MAO-B may not be absolute even at the recommended daily dose of 10 mg/day and selectivity is further diminished with increasing daily doses. The precise dose at which selegiline becomes a nonselective inhibitor of all MAOs is unknown, but may be in the range of 30 to 40 mg/day.

Pregnancy: Category C. It is not known whether selegiline can cause fetal harm when administered to a pregnant woman or can affect reproduction capacity. Use during pregnancy only if clearly needed.

Lactation: It is not known whether selegiline is excreted in breast milk.

Children: The effects of selegiline in children have not been evaluated.

SELEGILINE HCl (L-Deprenyl)

Precautions:

Hypertensive crisis: In theory, because MAO-A of the gut is not inhibited, patients treated with selegiline at a dose of 10 mg/day can take medications containing pharmacologically active amines and consume tyramine-containing foods without risk of uncontrolled hypertension. Clinical experience appears to confirm this prediction. The pathophysiology of the tyramine reaction is complicated and, in addition to its ability to inhibit MAO-B selectively, selegiline's apparent freedom from this reaction has been attributed to an ability to prevent tyramine and other indirect acting sympathomimetics from displacing norepinephrine from adrenergic neurons.

It seems prudent to assume that selegiline can only be used safely without dietary restrictions at doses where it presumably selectively inhibits MAO-B (eg, 10 mg/day). Attention to the dose-dependent nature of selegiline's selectivity is critical if it is to be used without elaborate restrictions placed on diet and concomitant drug use.

Levodopa side effects: Some patients given selegiline may experience an exacerbation of levodopa-associated side effects, presumably due to the increased amounts of dopamine reacting with supersensitive post-synaptic receptors. These effects may be mitigated by reducing the dose of levodopa/carbidopa by ≈10% to 30%.

Drug Interactions:

Selegine Drug Interactions

Precipitant drug	Object drug *		Description
Selegiline	Fluoxetine	↑	Death has occurred following initiation of nonselective MAOIs shortly after discontinuation of fluoxetine. To date, this has not been reported with selegiline; however, in general, avoid this combination. At least 5 weeks should elapse between discontinuation of fluoxetine and initiation of an MAOI; at least 14 days between discontinuation of an MAOI and initation of fluoxetine.
Selegiline	Meperidine	↑	Because of reports of fatal interactions, MAOIs are ordinarily contraindicated for use with meperidine. This warning is often extended to other opioids. In general, avoid this combination. Stupor, muscular rigidity, severe agitation and elevated temperature have been reported in a man receiving selegiline and meperidine. This is typical of the interaction of meperidine and MAOIs. Other serious reactions (eg, severe agitation, hallucinations, death) have occurred.

* ↑ = Object drug increased

Adverse Reactions:

The following events led to discontinuation of treatment with selegiline (in decreasing order of frequency): Nausea; hallucinations; confusion; depression; loss of balance; insomnia; orthostatic hypotension; increased akinetic involuntary movements; agitation; arrhythmias; bradykinesia; chorea; delusions; hypertension; new or increased angina pectoris; syncope.

Selegiline Adverse Reactions (%)

Adverse reactions	Selegiline (n = 49)	Placebo (n = 50)	Adverse reactions	Selegiline (n = 49)	Placebo (n = 50)
Nausea	10	3	Ache, generalized	1	0
Dizziness/lightheaded/ fainting	7	1	Anxiety/tension	1	1
Abdominal pain	4	2	Diarrhea	1	0
Confusion	3	0	Insomnia	1	1
Hallucinations	3	1	Lethargy	1	0
Dry mouth	3	1	Leg pain	1	0
Vivid dreams	2	0	Low back pain	1	0
Dyskinesias	2	5	Palpitations	1	0
Headache	2	1	Urinary retention	1	0
			Weight loss	1	0

SELEGILINE HCl (L-Deprenyl)

The following adverse reactions were reported in prospectively monitored clinical trials (n = 920).

CNS:

Motor/Coordination/Extrapyramidal – Increased tremor; chorea; loss of balance; restlessness; blepharospasm; increased bradykinesia; facial grimace; falling down; heavy leg; stiff neck; tardive dyskinesia; dystonic symptoms; dyskinesia; involuntary movements; freezing; festination; increased apraxia; muscle cramps.

Mental status/behavioral/psychiatric – Hallucinations; dizziness; confusion; anxiety; depression; drowsiness; behavior/mood changes; dreams/nightmares; tiredness; delusions; disorientation; lightheadedness; lethargy; malaise; apathy; overstimulation; vertigo; personality change; sleep disturbance; restlessness; weakness; transient irritability.

Pain/Altered sensation – Headache; back/leg pain; tinnitus; migraine; supraorbital pain; throat burning; generalized ache; chills; numbness of fingers/toes; taste disturbance.

Cardiovascular: Orthostatic hypotension; hypertension; arrhythmia; palpitations; new/increased angina pectoris; hypotension; tachycardia; peripheral edema; sinus bradycardia; syncope.

GI: Nausea; vomiting; constipation; weight loss; anorexia; poor appetite; dysphagia; diarrhea; heartburn; rectal bleeding, GI bleeding (exacerbation of preexisting ulcer disease).

GU: Slow urination; transient nocturia; prostatic hypertrophy; urinary hesitancy/retention/frequency; sexual dysfunction.

Dermatologic: Increased sweating; diaphoresis; facial hair; hair loss; hematoma; rash; photosensitivity.

Miscellaneous: Asthma; diplopia; shortness of breath; speech affected; dry mouth; blurred vision.

Adverse reactions reported at doses > 10 mg/day include: Muscle twitch; myoclonic jerks; impaired memory; increased energy; transient euphoria; bruxism; transient anorgasmia; decreased penile sensation.

Overdosage:

Symptoms: Some individuals exposed to doses of 600 mg of dl-selegiline suffered hypotension and psychomotor agitation.

Since the selective inhibition of MAO-B is achieved only at doses in the range recommended for the treatment of Parkinson's disease (eg, 10 mg/day), overdoses are likely to cause significant inhibition of both MAO-A and B. Consequently, the signs and symptoms of overdose may resemble those observed with nonselective MAO inhibitors. Refer to the MAOI monograph in the Antidepressants section.

Treatment: The following is based on the assumption that selegiline overdose may be modeled by nonselective MAO inhibitor poisoning. Treat hypotension and vascular collapse with IV fluids and, if necessary, blood pressure titration with an IV infusion of a dilute pressor agent. Adrenergic agents may produce a markedly increased pressor response. Refer to General Management of Acute Overdosage.

Patient Information:

Advise patients of possible need to reduce levodopa dosage after therapy initiation.

Advise patients not to exceed the daily recommended dose of 10 mg. Explain the risk of using higher daily doses of selegiline, and provide a brief description of the tyramine reaction. It may be useful to inform patients (or their families) about the signs and symptoms associated with MAO inhibitor-induced hypertensive reactions. In particular, urge patients to immediately report any severe headache, other atypical or unusual symptoms not previously experienced.

Administration and Dosage:

Parkinsonian patients receiving levodopa/carbidopa therapy who demonstrate a deteriorating response to this treatment: 10 mg per day administered as divided doses of 5 mg each taken at breakfast and lunch. There is no evidence that additional benefit will be obtained from the administration of higher doses. In general, avoid higher doses because of the increased risk of side effects.

After 2 to 3 days of treatment, attempt to reduce the dose of levodopa/carbidopa. A reduction of 10% to 30% appears typical. Further reductions of levodopa/carbidopa may be possible during continued selegiline therapy.

Rx	**Carbex** (Du Pont Pharma)	**Tablets:** 5 mg	Lactose. (E620). White, oval. In 60s.
Rx	**Selegiline HCl** (Endo Labs)		In 60s and 500s.
Rx	**Eldepryl** (Somerset)	**Capsules:** 5 mg	Lactose. Aqua blue. In 60s and 300s.

PERGOLIDE MESYLATE

Actions:

Pharmacology: Pergolide mesylate is a potent dopamine receptor agonist at both D_1 and D_2 receptor sites. It is 10 to 1000 times more potent than bromocriptine on a mg per mg basis. Pergolide inhibits the secretion of prolactin; it causes a transient rise in serum concentrations of growth hormone and a decrease in serum concentrations of luteinizing hormone. In Parkinson's disease, pergolide is believed to exert its therapeutic effect by directly stimulating postsynaptic dopamine receptors in the nigrostriatal system.

Pharmacokinetics:

Absorption/Distribution – Following oral administration, ≈ 55% of the dose can be recovered from the urine and 5% from expired CO_2, suggesting that a significant fraction is absorbed. Pergolide is ≈ 90% bound to plasma proteins.

Metabolism/Excretion – At least 10 metabolites have been detected, including N–despropylpergolide, pergolide sulfoxide and pergolide sulfone. Pergolide sulfoxide and sulfone are dopamine agonists in animals. It is not known whether any other metabolites are active. The major route of excretion is via the kidney.

Clinical trials: In a study, of patients with mild to moderate Parkinson's disease who were intolerant to levodopa/carbidopa, pergolide use permitted a 5% to 30% reduction in daily levodopa dose. Patients on pergolide maintained an equivalent or better clinical status than they exhibited at baseline. These patients had been on levodopa/carbidopa for 3.9 years (range, 2 days to 16.8 years).

Indications:

Parkinson's disease: Adjunctive treatment to levodopa/carbidopa in the management of the signs and symptoms of Parkinson's disease.

Contraindications:

Hypersensitivity to pergolide or other ergot derivatives.

Warnings:

Symptomatic hypotension: In clinical trials, ≈ 10% of patients taking pergolide with levodopa vs 7% taking placebo with levodopa experienced symptomatic orthostatic or sustained hypotension, especially during initial treatment. With gradual dosage titration, tolerance to the hypotension usually develops. Warn patients of the risk, begin therapy with low doses, and increase the dosage in carefully adjusted increments over a period of 3 to 4 weeks (see Administration and Dosage).

Hallucinosis: In controlled trials, pergolide with levodopa caused hallucinosis in about 14% of patients as opposed to 3% taking placebo with levodopa. It caused discontinuation of treatment in about 3% of those enrolled; tolerance was not observed.

Fatalities: In one trial, 2 of 187 patients on placebo died vs 1 of 189 patients on pergolide. Of the 2299 patients on pergolide in premarketing studies, 143 died while on the drug or shortly after discontinuing it. The study patients were elderly, ill and at high risk for death. It seems unlikely that pergolide played any role in these deaths, but the possibility that pergolide shortens patient survival cannot be excluded.

Carcinogenesis/Fertility impairment: A 2 year carcinogenicity study was conducted in mice and rats; the highest doses tested were ≈ 340 and 12 times the maximum human oral dose. A low incidence of uterine neoplasms occurred in both rats and mice. Endometrial adenomas and carcinomas were observed in rats. Endometrial sarcomas were observed in mice. The occurrence of these neoplasms is probably attributable to the high estrogen/progesterone ratio which would occur in rodents as a result of the prolactin-inhibiting action of pergolide. The endocrine mechanisms believed to be involved in the rodents are not present in humans.

In male and female mice, fertility was maintained at 0.6 and 1.7 mg/kg/day, but decreased at 5.6 mg/kg/day. Prolactin may be involved in stimulating and maintaining progesterone levels required for implantation in mice and, therefore, the impaired fertility at high dose may occur because of depressed prolactin levels.

Pregnancy: Category B. There are no adequate and well controlled studies in pregnant women. Among women who received pergolide for endocrine disorders, there were 33 pregnancies that resulted in healthy babies and four pregnancies that resulted in congenital abnormalities (two major, two minor); a causal relationship has not been established. Use during pregnancy only if clearly needed.

Lactation: It is not known whether this drug is excreted in breast milk. Pergolide may interfere with lactation. Because of the potential for serious adverse reactions to nursing infants, decide whether to discontinue nursing or to discontinue the drug, taking into account the importance of the drug to the mother.

Children: Safety and efficacy for use in children have not been established.

PERGOLIDE MESYLATE

Precautions:

Cardiac dysrhythmias: Exercise caution in patients prone to cardiac dysrhythmias. In a study comparing pergolide and placebo, patients on pergolide had significantly more episodes of atrial premature contractions and sinus tachycardia.

The use of pergolide in patients on levodopa may cause or exacerbate preexisting states of confusion and hallucinations (see Warnings) or preexisting dyskinesia.

Drug Interactions:

Dopamine antagonists (eg, neuroleptics: Phenothiazines, butyrophenones, thioxanthines) or **metoclopramide** may diminish the effectiveness of pergolide, a dopamine agonist.

Because pergolide mesylate is ≈ 90% bound to plasma proteins, exercise caution if pergolide is coadministered with other drugs known to affect protein binding.

Adverse Reactions:

Pergolide Adverse Reactions (%)

Adverse Reaction	Pergolide (n = 189)	Placebo (n = 187)
Body as a Whole:		
Pain	7	2.1
Abdominal pain	5.8	2.1
Injury, accident	5.8	7
Headache	5.3	6.4
Asthenia	4.2	4.8
Chest pain	3.7	2.1
Flu syndrome	3.2	2.1
Neck pain	2.7	1.6
Back pain	1.6	2.1
Surgical procedure	1.6	< 1
Chills	1.1	0
Facial edema	1.1	0
Infection	1.1	0
Cardiovascular:		
Postural hypotension	9	7
Vasodilation	3.2	< 1
Palpitation	2.1	< 1
Hypotension	2.1	< 1
Syncope	2.1	1.1
Hypertension	1.6	1.1
Arrhythmia	1.1	< 1
Myocardial infarction	1.1	< 1
GI:		
Nausea	24.3	12.8
Constipation	10.6	5.9
Diarrhea	6.4	2.7
Dyspepsia	6.4	2.1
Anorexia	4.8	2.7
Dry mouth	3.7	< 1
Vomiting	2.7	1.6
Musculoskeletal:		
Arthralgia	1.6	2.1
Bursitis	1.6	< 1
Myalgia	1.1	< 1
Twitching	1.1	0
CNS:		
Dyskinesia	62.4	24.6
Dizziness	19.1	13.9
Hallucinations	13.8	3.2
Dystonia	11.6	8.
Confusion	11.1	9.6
Somnolence	10.1	3.7
Insomnia	7.9	3.2
Anxiety	6.4	4.3
Tremor	4.2	7.5
Depression	3.2	5.4
Abnormal dreams	2.7	4.3
Personality disorder	2.1	< 1
Psychosis	2.1	0
Abnormal gait	1.6	1.6
Akathisia	1.6	0
Extrapyramidal syndrome	1.6	1.1
Incoordination	1.6	< 1
Paresthesia	1.6	3.2
Akinesia	1.1	1.1
Hypertonia	1.1	0
Neuralgia	1.1	< 1
Speech disorder	1.1	1.6
Respiratory:		
Rhinitis	12.2	5.4
Dyspnea	4.8	1.1
Epistaxis	1.6	< 1
Hiccup	1.1	0
Dermatologic:		
Rash	3.2	2.1
Sweating	2.1	2.7
Special Senses:		
Abnormal vision	5.8	5.4
Diplopia	2.1	0
Taste perversion	1.6	0
Eye disorder	1.1	0
GU:		
Urinary frequency	2.7	6.4
Urinary tract infection	2.7	3.7
Hematuria	1.1	< 1
Miscellaneous:		
Peripheral edema	7.4	4.3
Edema	1.6	0
Weight gain	1.6	0
Anemia	1.1	< 1

PERGOLIDE MESYLATE

Most common:

CNS – Dyskinesia; hallucinations; somnolence; insomnia.

GI – Nausea; constipation; diarrhea; dyspepsia.

Respiratory – Rhinitis.

Discontinuation: Of approximately 1200 patients, 27% receiving pergolide discontinued treatment due to adverse events; most commonly related to the nervous system (15.5%), primarily hallucinations (7.8%) and confusion (1.8%).

Fatalities: See Warnings.

Additional adverse reactions that occurred in ≤ 1% of approximately 1800 patients:

Body as a whole – Fever (1%); enlarged abdomen, malaise, neoplasm, hernia, pelvic pain, sepsis, cellulitis, moniliasis, abscess, jaw pain, hypothermia (0.1% to 1%); acute abdominal syndrome, LE syndrome (< 0.1%).

Cardiovascular – Congestive heart failure (1%); tachycardia, heart arrest, abnormal ECG, angina pectoris, thrombophlebitis, bradycardia, ventricular extrasystoles, cerebrovascular accident, ventricular tachycardia, cerebral ischemia, atrial fibrillation, varicose vein, pulmonary embolus, AV block, shock (0.1% to 1%); vasculitis, pulmonary hypertension, pericarditis, migraine, heart block, cerebral hemorrhage (< 0.1%).

GI – Dysphagia (1%); flatulence, abnormal liver function tests, increased appetite, salivary gland enlargement, thirst, gastroenteritis, gastritis, periodontal abscess, intestinal obstruction, gingivitis, esophagitis, cholelithiasis, tooth caries, hepatitis, stomach ulcer, melena, hepatomegaly, hematemesis, eructation (0.1% to 1%); sialadenitis, peptic ulcer, pancreatitis, jaundice, glossitis, fecal incontinence, duodenitis, colitis, cholecystitis, aphthous stomatitis, esophageal ulcer (< 0.1%).

Endocrine – Hypothyroidism, adenoma, diabetes mellitus, inappropriate ADH (0.1% to 1%); endocrine disorder, thyroid adenoma (< 0.1%).

Hematologic/Lymphatic – Leukopenia, lymphadenopathy, leukocytosis, thrombocytopenia, petechia, megaloblastic anemia, cyanosis (0.1% to 1%); purpura, lymphocytosis, eosinophilia, thrombocythemia, acute lymphoblastic leukemia, polycythemia, splenomegaly (< 0.1%).

Metabolic/Nutritional – Weight loss (1%); dehydration, hypokalemia, hypoglycemia, iron deficiency anemia, hyperglycemia, gout, hypercholesterolemia (0.1% to 1%); electrolyte imbalance, cachexia, acidosis, hyperuricemia (< 0.1%).

Musculoskeletal – Bone pain, tenosynovitis, myositis, bone sarcoma, arthritis (0.1% to 1%); osteoporosis, muscle atrophy, osteomyelitis (< 0.1%).

CNS – Nervousness, choreoathetosis, amnesia, paranoid reaction, abnormal thinking (1%); neuropathy, delusion, convulsion, increased or decreased libido, euphoria, emotional lability, vertigo, myoclonus, coma, apathy, paralysis, neurosis, hyperkinesia, ataxia, acute brain syndrome, torticollis, meningitis, manic reaction, hypokinesia, hostility, agitation, hypotonia (0.1% to 1%); stupor, neuritis, intracranial hypertension, hemiplegia, facial paralysis, brain edema, myelitis (< 0.1%).

Respiratory – Pneumonia, pharyngitis, increased cough (1%); sinusitis, bronchitis, voice alteration, hemoptysis, asthma, lung edema, pleural effusion, laryngitis, emphysema, apnea, hyperventilation (0.1% to 1%); pneumothorax, lung fibrosis, larynx edema, hypoxia, hypoventilation, hemothorax, lung carcinoma (< 0.1%).

Dermatologic – Skin discoloration, pruritis, acne, skin ulcer, alopecia, dry skin, skin carcinoma, seborrhea, hirsutism, herpes simplex, eczema, fungal dermatitis, herpes zoster (0.1% to 1%); vesiculobullous rash, subcutaneous nodule, skin nodule, benign skin neoplasm, lichenoid dermatitis (< 0.1%).

Special Senses – Otitis media, conjunctivitis, tinnitus, deafness, ear or eye pain, glaucoma, eye hemorrhage, photophobia, visual field defect (0.1% to 1%); blindness, cataract, retinal detachment, retinal vascular disorder (< 0.1%).

GU – Urinary incontinence, dysmenorrhea (1%); dysuria, breast pain, menorrhagia, impotence, cystitis, urinary retention, abortion, vaginal hemorrhage, vaginitis, priapism, kidney calculus, fibrocystic breast, lactation, uterine hemorrhage, urolithiasis, salpingitis, pyuria, metrorrhagia, menopause, kidney failure, breast carcinoma, cervical carcinoma (0.1% to 1%); amenorrhea, bladder carcinoma, breast engorgement, epididymitis, hypogonadism, leukorrhea, nephrosis, pyelonephritis, urethral pain, uricaciduria, withdrawal bleeding (< 0.1%).

PERGOLIDE MESYLATE

Overdosage:

Symptoms: There is no clinical experience with massive overdosage. The largest overdose involved a young hospitalized adult patient who intentionally took 60 mg of pergolide. He experienced vomiting, hypotension and agitation. Another patient receiving a daily dosage of 7 mg of pergolide unintentionally took 19 mg/day for 3 days, after which his vital signs were normal but he experienced severe hallucinations. Within 36 hours of resumption of the prescribed dosage level, the hallucinations stopped. One patient unintentionally took 14 mg/day for 23 days instead of her prescribed 1.4 mg/day dosage. She experienced severe involuntary movements and tingling in her arms and legs. Another patient who inadvertently received 7 mg instead of the prescribed 0.7 mg experienced palpitations, hypotension and ventricular extrasystoles. The highest total daily dose (prescribed for several patients with refractory Parkinson's disease) has exceeded 30 mg.

Animal studies indicate that the manifestations of overdosage in man might include nausea, vomiting, convulsions, decreased blood pressure and CNS stimulation.

Treatment: Management of overdosage may require supportive measures to maintain arterial blood pressure. Monitor cardiac function; an antiarrhythmic agent may be necessary. If signs of CNS stimulation are present, a phenothiazine or other butyrophenone neuroleptic agent may be indicated; the efficacy of such drugs in reversing the effects of overdose has not been assessed.

Protect the patient's airway and support ventilation and perfusion. Meticulously monitor and maintain, within acceptable limits, the patient's vital signs, blood gases, serum electrolytes, etc. Absorption of drugs from the GI tract may be decreased by giving activated charcoal, which, in many cases, is more effective than emesis or lavage. Consider charcoal instead of or in addition to gastric emptying. Repeated doses of charcoal over time may hasten elimination of some drugs that have been absorbed. Safeguard the patient's airway when employing gastric emptying or charcoal.

There is no experience with dialysis or hemoperfusion, and these procedures are unlikely to be of benefit.

Patient Information:

Inform patients and their families of the common adverse consequences of the use of pergolide (see Adverse Reactions) and the risk of hypotension (see Warnings).

Administration and Dosage:

Initiate with a daily dose of 0.05 mg for the first 2 days. Gradually increase the dosage by 0.1 or 0.15 mg/day every third day over the next 12 days of therapy. The dosage may then be increased by 0.25 mg/day every third day until an optimal therapeutic dosage is achieved.

Pergolide is usually administered in divided doses 3 times per day. During dosage titration, the dosage of concurrent levodopa/carbidopa may be cautiously decreased.

In clinical studies, the mean therapeutic daily dosage of pergolide was 3 mg/day. The average concurrent daily dosage of levodopa/carbidopa (expressed as levodopa) was approximately 650 mg/day. The efficacy of pergolide at doses above 5 mg/day has not been systematically evaluated.

Rx	**Permax** (Athena Neurosciences)	**Tablets**: 0.05 mg	(4131). Ivory, scored. In 30s.
		0.25 mg	(4133). Green, scored. In 30s.
		1 mg	(4135). Pink, scored. In 100s.

chapter 7

gastrointestinal drugs

ANTACIDS

Actions:

Pharmacology: Antacids neutralize gastric acidity, resulting in an increase in the pH of the stomach and duodenal bulb. Additionally, by increasing the gastric pH above 4, they inhibit the proteolytic activity of pepsin. Antacids do not "coat" the mucosal lining, but may have a local astringent effect. Antacids also increase the lower esophageal sphincter tone. Aluminum ions inhibit smooth muscle contraction, thus inhibiting gastric emptying. Use aluminum-containing products with caution in patients with gastric outlet obstruction.

A *systemic* antacid (eg, sodium bicarbonate) is readily absorbed and capable of producing systemic electrolyte disturbances and alkalosis. A *nonsystemic* antacid forms compounds that are not absorbed to a significant extent and thus does not exert an appreciable systemic effect, unless use is chronic, high-dose or the patient has confounding pathology. However, nonsystemic antacids may alter urinary pH in some patients.

Acid neutralizing capacity (ANC) is a consideration in selecting an antacid. It varies for commercial antacid preparations and is expressed as mEq/ml. Milliequivalents of ANC is defined by the mEq of HCl required to keep an antacid suspension at pH 3.5 for 10 minutes in vitro. An antacid must neutralize at least 5 mEq/dose. Also, any ingredient must contribute at least 25% of the total ANC of a given product to be considered an antacid. Antacids with high ANC are usually more effective in vivo. Sodium bicarbonate and calcium carbonate have the greatest neutralizing capacity, but are not suitable for chronic therapy due to systemic effects. Suspensions have greater neutralizing capacity than powders or tablets. For maximum effectiveness, chew tablets thoroughly. If ingested in the fasting state, antacids reduce acidity for approximately 20 to 40 minutes because of rapid gastric emptying. If ingested 1 hour after meals, they reduce gastric acidity for at least 3 hours.

Alginic acid, an ingredient found with sodium bicarbonate in some antacid products, is not an antacid; however, in the presence of saliva, it reacts with sodium bicarbonate to form sodium alginate. Its protective effect is due to its foaming, viscous and floating properties.

Phosphate binding – Aluminum-containing antacids bind with phosphate ions in the intestine to form insoluble aluminum phosphate, which is excreted in the feces. This is of value in treating hyperphosphatemia of chronic renal failure. Calcium carbonate can also suppress phosphate concentrations. The aluminum salt with useful phosphate binding capacity is aluminum hydroxide.

Indications:

Hyperacidity: Symptomatic relief of upset stomach associated with hyperacidity (heartburn, gastroesophageal reflux, acid indigestion and sour stomach); hyperacidity associated with peptic ulcer and gastric hyperacidity.

Aluminum carbonate: Treatment, control or management of hyperphosphatemia or for use with a low phosphate diet to prevent formation of phosphate urinary stones.

Calcium carbonate: Treating calcium deficiency states (ie, postmenopausal/senile osteoporosis). See Calcium monograph in Minerals and Electrolytes, Oral section.

Magnesium oxide: Treatment of magnesium deficiencies or magnesium depletion from malnutrition, restricted diet, alcoholism or magnesium-depleting drugs.

Unlabeled uses: Antacids with aluminum and magnesium hydroxides or aluminum hydroxide alone effectively prevent significant stress ulcer bleeding. Antacids are also effective in treatment and maintenance of duodenal ulcer, and may be effective in treating gastric ulcer. Antacids are also recommended, initially, for gastroesophageal reflux disease.

Aluminum hydroxide has been used to reduce phosphate absorption in hyperphosphatemia in patients with chronic renal failure.

Calcium carbonate may also be used to bind phosphate.

ANTACIDS

Warnings:

Sodium content of antacids may be significant. Patients with hypertension, congestive heart failure, marked renal failure or those on restricted or low-sodium diets should use a low sodium preparation. The sodium content of most commercial antacid preparations is found in the product listings.

"Acid rebound": Antacids may cause dose-related rebound hyperacidity since they may increase gastric secretion or serum gastrin levels. Early data implicated calcium carbonate as the only agent that caused "acid rebound"; however, it is now clear that most antacids may result in this effect. In addition, the effect may not be clinically significant, since the "acid rebound" may be compensated for by buffers in the antacid.

Milk-alkali syndrome, an acute illness with symptoms of headache, nausea, irritability and weakness, or a chronic illness with alkalosis, hypercalcemia and possibly, renal impairment, has occurred following the concurrent use of high-dose calcium carbonate and sodium bicarbonate.

Hypophosphatemia: Prolonged use of aluminum-containing antacids may result in hypophosphatemia in normophosphatemic patients if phosphate intake is not adequate. In its more severe forms, hypophosphatemia can lead to anorexia, malaise, muscle weakness and osteomalacia.

Renal function impairment: Use magnesium-containing products with caution, particularly when > 50 mEq magnesium is given daily. Hypermagnesemia and toxicity may occur due to decreased clearance of the magnesium ion. Approximately 5% to 20% of orally administered magnesium salts can be systemically absorbed.

Prolonged use of aluminum-containing antacids in patients with renal failure may result in or worsen dialysis osteomalacia. Elevated tissue aluminum levels contribute to the development of the dialysis encephalopathy and osteomalacia syndromes. Small amounts of aluminum are absorbed form the GI tract and renal excretion of aluminum is impaired in renal failure. Aluminum is not well removed by dialysis because it is bound to albumin and transferrin, which do not cross dialysis membranes. As a result, aluminum is deposited in bone, and dialysis osteomalacia may develop when large amounts of aluminum are ingested orally by patients with impaired renal function.

Pregnancy: A pregnant woman should consult a physician before using an antacid.

Precautions:

GI hemorrhage: Use aluminum hydroxide with care in patients who have recently suffered massive upper GI hemorrhage.

Lipid effects: In one study, administration of an aluminum hydroxide-containing antacid reduced LDL cholesterol by 18.5% after 4 months in hypercholesterolemic patients. Although HDL was also reduced (to a lesser extent), the HDL/LDL ratio increased by 13%. Similar results were noted in a smaller pilot study. In another study, calcium carbonate reduced LDL by 4.4% and increased HDL by 4.1%. Further studies are needed to determine the role of antacids in hypercholesterolemia.

Buffered aspirin solutions: Caution against use of these antacid/analgesic combinations in chronic pain syndromes. Alkalinization of urine accelerates aspirin excretion, and systemic alkalosis and increased sodium load may occur.

Drug Interactions:

Antacid Drug Interactions

	Antacid[1]				
Drug	Aluminum salts	Calcium salts	Magnesium salts	Sodium bicarbonate	Magnesium - aluminum combinations
Allopurinol	↓				
Amphetamines				↑	
Benzodiazepines	↑		↓	↓	↓
Captopril					↓
Chloroquine	↓		↓		
Corticosteroids	↓		↓		↓
Dicumarol			↑		
Diflunisal	↓				
Digoxin	↓		↓		
Ethambutol	↓				

ANTACIDS

Antacid Drug Interactions

Drug	Antacid[1] Aluminum salts	Calcium salts	Magnesium salts	Sodium bicarbonate	Magnesium - aluminum combinations
Flecainide				↑	
Fluoroquinolones		↓			↓
Histamine H_2 antagonists	↓		↓		↓
Hydantoins		↓	↓		↓
Iron salts	↓	↓	↓	↓	↓
Isoniazid	↓				
Ketoconazole				↓	↓
Levodopa					↑
Lithium				↓	
Methenamine				↓	
Methotrexate				↓	
Nitrofurantoin			↓		
Penicillamine	↓		↓		↓
Phenothiazines	↓		↓		↓
Quinidine		↑	↑	↑	↑
Salicylates		↓		↓	↓
Sodium polystyrene sulfonate					‡[2]
Sulfonylureas			↑	↓	↑
Sympathomimetics				↑	
Tetracyclines	↓	↓	↓	↓	↓
Thyroid hormones	↓				
Ticlopidine	↓		↓		↓
Valproic acid					↑

[1] Pharmacologic effect increased (↑) or decreased (↓) by antacids.
[2] Concomitant use may cause metabolic alkalosis in patients with renal impairment.

Antacids may interfere with drugs by: 1. *Increasing the gastric pH* altering disintegration, dissolution, solubility, ionization and gastric emptying time. Absorption of weakly acidic drugs is decreased, possibly resulting in decreased drug effect (eg, digoxin, phenytoin, chlorpromazine, isoniazid). Weakly basic drug absorption is increased possibly resulting in toxicity or adverse reactions (eg, pseudoephedrine, levodopa).

2. *Adsorbing or binding* drugs to their surface resulting in decreased bioavailability (eg, tetracycline). Magnesium trisilicate and magnesium hydroxide have the greatest ability to adsorb drugs; calcium carbonate and aluminum hydroxide have an intermediate ability to adsorb drugs.

3. *Increasing urinary pH* affecting the rate of drug elimination. The effect is inhibition of the excretion of basic drugs (eg, quinidine, amphetamines) and enhanced excretion of acidic drugs (eg, salicylates). Sodium bicarbonate has the most pronounced effect on urinary pH.

Staggering the administration times of the interacting drug and the antacid by at least 2 hours will often help avoid undesirable drug interactions. Refer to individual product monographs for information.

Adverse Reactions:

Magnesium-containing antacids: Laxative effect as saline cathartic, may cause diarrhea; hypermagnesemia in renal failure patients (see Warnings).

ANTACIDS

Aluminum-containing antacids: Constipation (may lead to intestinal obstruction);aluminum-intoxication, osteomalacia and hypophosphatemia (see Precautions); accumulation of aluminum in serum, bone and the CNS (aluminum accumulation may be neurotoxic); encephalopathy.

Antacids: Dose-dependent rebound hyperacidity and milk-alkali syndrome (see Warnings).

Patient Information:

Chewable tablets: Thoroughly chew before swallowing. Follow with a glass of water.

Effervescent tablets: Allow to completely dissolve in water. Allow most of the bubbling to stop before drinking.

Drug interaction precaution: Antacids may interact with certain prescription drugs. If you are presently taking a prescription drug, do not take an antacid without checking with your physician or pharmacist.

Magnesium-containing products may act as a saline cathartic in larger doses and produce a laxative effect and may cause diarrhea; aluminum and calcium-containing products may cause constipation. Magnesium/aluminum antacid mixtures are used to avoid bowel function changes.

Notify physician if relief is not obtained or if there are any symptoms that suggest bleeding, such as black tarry stools or "coffee ground" vomitus.

Taking too much of these products can cause the stomach to secrete excess stomach acid. Consult your physician or pharmacist about the appropriate dose.Do not use the maximum dosage of antacids for > 2 weeks, except under the supervision of a physician.

Administration and Dosage:

Administration and dosage depends on the condition being treated and the agent being used. See individual products for specific information.

Liquid doseforms are usually preferred because of their rapid action and greater activity; however, tablets may be more acceptable and convenient, particularly when patients are away from home or where the liquid would be inconvenient to carry. Other doseforms are available but do not appear to offer any significant advantage.

MAGNESIA (Magnesium Hydroxide)

For complete prescribing information, refer to the Antacids group monograph.

Administration and Dosage:

Antacid dose, adults and children over 12:

Liquid – 5 to 15 ml up to 4 times daily with water.
Liquid, concentrated – 2.5 to 7.5 ml up to 4 times daily with water.
Tablets – 622 mg to 1244 mg up to 4 times daily.
Laxative dose – See product listing in Laxative monograph.

				Sodium[1] (mg)	ANC[1] (mEq)
otc	**Phillips' Chewable** (Sterling Health)	**Tablets, chewable:** 311 mg	Sucrose. (Phillips). Mint flavor. In 100s and 200s.		
otc	**Milk of Magnesia** (Various, eg, Geneva, Goldline, Rugby, Schein, UDL)	**Liquid:** 400 mg/5 ml	In 360 ml, pt and gal, UD 15 and 30 ml.		
otc	**Phillips' Milk of Magnesia** (Sterling Health)		Original, mint and cherry flavors. In 120 360 and 780 ml.		
otc	**Concentrated Phillips' Milk of Magnesia** (Sterling Health)	**Liquid:** 800 mg/5 ml	Sorbitol, sugar. Strawberry and orange vanilla creme flavors. In 240 ml.		

[1] Acid neutralizing capacity and sodium content per tablet or 5 ml.

ALUMINUM HYDROXIDE GEL

For complete prescribing information, refer to the Antacids group monograph.

Administration and Dosage:

Tablets/Capsules: 500 to 1500 mg 3 to 6 times daily, between meals and at bedtime.

Suspension: 5 to 30 ml as needed between meals and at bedtime or as directed.

				Sodium[1] (mg)	ANC[1] (mEq)
otc	**Amphojel** (Wyeth-Ayerst)	**Tablets:** 300 mg	In 100s.		
otc	**Alu-Tab** (3M Pharm)	**Tablets:** 500 mg	Green, film coated. In 250s.		10.6
otc	**Amphojel** (Wyeth-Ayerst)	**Tablets:** 600 mg	(Wyeth). Saccharin. In 100s.		
otc	**Alu-Cap** (3M Pharm)	**Capsules:** 400 mg	Red/green. In 100s.		8.5
otc	**Dialume** (RPR)	**Capsules:** 500 mg	In 500s.	≤ 1.2	
otc	**Aluminum Hydroxide Gel** (Various, eg, Goldline, Major, Pharm Assoc, Rugby, UDL)	**Suspension:** 320 mg per 5 ml	In 360 and 480 ml, UD 15 and 30 ml.		
otc	**Amphojel** (Wyeth-Ayerst)		Saccharin. In 355 ml.	< 2.3	10
otc	**Concentrated Aluminum Hydroxide Gel** (Roxane)	**Suspension:** 450 mg per 5 ml	Peppermint flavor. In 500 ml and UD 30 ml.	1-2	
		675 mg per 5 ml	Creamsicle flavor. In 180 and 500 ml, UD 20 and 30 ml.		
otc	**Concentrated Aluminum Hydroxide Gel** (Various, eg, Pharm Assoc, Roxane)	**Liquid:** 600 mg per 5 ml	In 30, 180 and 480 ml.		
otc	**AlternaGEL** (J & J-Merck)		In 150 and 360 ml.		

[1] Acid neutralizing capacity and sodium content per capsule, tablet or 5 ml.

ALUMINUM CARBONATE GEL, BASIC

For complete prescribing information, refer to the Antacids group monograph.

Indications:

In addition to its use as an antacid, it is also used for hyperphosphatemia.

Administration and Dosage:

Antacid: 2 capsules or tablets or 10 ml of regular suspension (in water or fruit juice) as often as every 2 hours, up to 12 times daily.

				Sodium[1] (mg)	ANC[1] (mEq)
otc	**Basaljel** (Wyeth-Ayerst)	**Tablets:** Equiv. to 608 mg dried aluminum hydroxide gel or 500 mg aluminum hydroxide	(Wyeth 473). Scored. In 100s.		
		Capsules: Equiv. to 608 mg dried aluminum hydroxide gel or 500 mg aluminum hydroxide	In 100s and 500s.		
		Suspension: Equiv. to 400 mg aluminum hydroxide per 5 ml	Menthol, saccharin, sorbitol. Peppermint flavor. In 355 ml.		

[1] Acid neutralizing capacity and sodium content per capsule, tablet or 5 ml.

CALCIUM CARBONATE

For complete prescribing information, refer to the Antacids group monograph.

Contains 40% calcium; 20 mEq calcium/g.

Administration and Dosage:

0.5 to 1.5 g, as needed.

				Sodium[1] (mg)	ANC[1] (mEq)
otc	**Amitone** (Menley & James)	**Tablets, chewable:** 350 mg	Sucrose. Peppermint flavor. In 100s.	<2	
otc *sf*	**Mallamint** (Roberts)	**Tablets, chewable:** 420 mg	Mint flavor. In 1000s, Sani-Pak 1000s and 4 dose boxes.	< 0.1	
otc	**Calcium Carbonate** (Various, eg, Medirex, Vangard)	**Tablets:** 500 mg	In 100s, 120s and UD 100s.		
otc	**Antacid Tablets** (Goldline)	**Tablets, chewable:** 500 mg	Sucrose. Assorted flavors. In 150s.	≤ 2	
otc	**Dicarbosil** (BIRA)		Peppermint flavor. White. In rolls of 12.	< 2	10
otc	**Equilet** (Mission)		In 150s.	< 0.35	
otc	**Tums** (SK-Beecham)		Sucrose. Peppermint, assort. flavors. In 36s, 75s, 150s and 400s.	≤ 2	
otc	**Chooz** (Schering-Plough)	**Gum tablets:** 500 mg	Sucrose, glucose. Mint flavor. In 16s.		
otc	**Calcium Carbonate** (Various, eg, Major, Moore)	**Tablets:** 600 mg	In 60s, 72s, 150s and UD 100s.		
otc	**Calcium Carbonate** (Various, eg, Lilly, Rugby)	**Tablets:** 650 mg	In 100s and 1000s.		
otc	**Extra Strength Alkets Antacid** (Roberts)	**Tablets, chewable:** 750 mg	Peppermint. In 96s.		
otc	**Extra Strength Antacid** (Various, eg, Goldline, Major)		In 96s.		
otc	**Extra Strength Tums E-X** (SK-Beecham)		Sucrose. Assorted flavors. In 24s, 48s and 96s.	≤ 2	
otc	**Alka-Mints** (Bayer)	**Tablets, chewable:** 850 mg	Sorbitol. (Alka-Mints). Spearmint. In 30s.	< 0.5	16
otc	**Maalox Antacid Caplets** (RPR)	**Tablets:** 1000 mg	(A-C). In 24s and 50s.	≤ 9.2	
otc	**Tums Ultra** (SK-Beecham)	**Tablets, chewable:** 1000 mg	Sucrose. Assorted fruit and mint flavors. In 36s and 72s.	≤ 4	
otc	**Calcium Carbonate** (Roxane)	**Tablets:** 1250 mg	In 100s and UD 100s.		
otc	**Calcium Carbonate** (Roxane)	**Suspension:** 1250 mg per 5 ml	Sorbitol. Mint flavor. In 500 ml, UD 5 ml.		
otc	**Mylanta** (J&J-Merck)	**Lozenges:** 600 mg	Corn syrup, sucrose. Cool mint creme and cherry creme flavors. In 18s and 50s.		11.4

[1] Acid-neutralizing capacity and sodium content per tablet, lozenge or 5 ml.

MAGNESIUM OXIDE

For complete prescribing information, refer to the Antacids group monograph.

Administration and Dosage:

Capsules: 140 mg 3 to 4 times daily.

Tablets: 400 to 800 mg/day.

				Sodium[1] (mg)	ANC[1] (mEq)
otc	**Mag-Ox 400** (Blaine)	**Tablets:** 400 mg	In 100s, 1000s and UD 100s.		
otc	**Maox 420** (Manne Co)	**Tablets:** 420 mg	Tartrazine. In 250s and 1000s.		21
otc	**Magnesium Oxide** (Various, eg, Major)	**Tablets** :500 mg	In 100s.		
otc	**Uro-Mag** (Blaine)	**Capsules:** 140 mg	In 100s and 1000s.		

[1] Acid neutralizing capacity and sodium content per capsule or tablet.

MAGALDRATE (Aluminum Magnesium Hydroxide Sulfate)

For complete prescribing information, refer to the Antacids group monograph.

Magaldrate is a chemical entity of aluminum and magnesium hydroxides (not a physical mixture). It contains the equivalent of 29% to 40% magnesium oxide and 18% to 26% aluminum oxide.

Administration and Dosage:

Suspension/Liquid: 5 to 10 ml between meals and at bedtime.

				Sodium[1] (mg)	ANC[1] (mEq)
otc	**Riopan** (Whitehall)	**Suspension:** 540 mg per 5 ml	Saccharin, sorbitol. Mint flavor. In 360 ml.		
otc	**Magaldrate** (Various, eg, Moore)	**Liquid:** 540 mg per 5 ml	In 355 ml.		
otc	**Iosopan** (Goldline)		In 355 ml.		

[1] Acid neutralizing capacity and sodium content per 5 ml.

SODIUM BICARBONATE

For complete prescribing information, refer to the Antacids group monograph.

Contains 27% sodium.

Administration and Dosage:

0.3 to 2 g 1 to 4 times daily.

				Sodium[1] (mg)	ANC[1] (mEq)
otc	**Sodium Bicarbonate** (Various, eg, Rugby)	**Tablets:** 325 mg	In 1000s.		
otc	**Bell/ans** (C.S. Dent)	**Tablets:** 520 mg	Ginger/Wintergreen flavor. In 30s and 60s.	144	
otc	**Sodium Bicarbonate** (Various, eg, Rugby)	**Tablets:** 650 mg	In 1000s.		

[1] Acid-neutralizing capacity and sodium content per tablet.

SODIUM CITRATE

For complete prescribing information, refer to the Antacids group monograph.

Administration and Dosage:

30 ml daily.

				Sodium[1] (mg)	ANC[1] (mEq)
otc	**Citra pH** (ValMed)	**Solution:** 450 mg	Sucrose. Clear. In 30 ml.	105.67	

[1] Acid neutralizing capacity and sodium content per 5 ml.

Capsules and Tablets

ANTACID COMBINATIONS

Refer to the general discussion of these products in the Antacids group monograph.

Content given in mg per tablet or gelcap. 23 mg sodium = 1 mEq.

	Product & distributor	Aluminum Hydroxide	Magnesium Hydroxide	Calcium Carbonate	Other Content	Sodium (mg)	How supplied
otc	**Maalox tablets** (Rhone-Poulenc Rorer)	200	200		Saccharin, sorbitol		chewable. Mint flavor. In 100s.
otc	**Mintox Tablets** (Major)				Saccharin		Chewable. Mint flavor. In 100s.
otc	**RuLox #1 Tablets** (Rugby)						Chewable. Mintflavor. In 100s and 1000s.
otc	**Extra Strength Maalox Tablets** (Rhone-Poulenc Rorer)	350	350		30 mg simethicone, sugar, dextrose, saccharin, sorbitol		chewable. Mint creme flavor. In 38s and 75s.
otc	**RuLox #2 Tablets** (Rugby)	400	400		Sorbitol		Chewable. Mint flavor. In 100s and 1000s.
otc	**Duracid Tablets** (Fielding)			325	175 mg aluminum hydroxide-magnesium carbonate		Chewable. In 100s.
otc *sf*	**Titralac Extra Strength Tablets** (3M Pharm.)			750	Saccharin	0.6	Chewable. Spearmint flavor. In 100s.
otc	**Marblen Tablets** (Fleming)			520	400 mg magnesium carbonate		Peach-apricot flavor. In 100s and 1000s.
otc	**Alkets Tablets** (Roberts Hauck)			500	Dextrose	≤ 2	Chewable. Peppermint flavor. In 36s, 96s and 150s.
otc	**Mi-Acid Gelcaps** (Major)			311	232 mg magnesum carbonate, parabens, EDTA		In 50s
otc	**Mylanta Gelcaps** (J & J Merck)				232 mg magnesium carbonate, parabens, EDTA		In 24s and 50s.
otc	**Mylagen Gelcaps** (Goldline)				232 mg magnesium carbonate		In 24s
otc	**Gas-Ban** (Roberts Med)			300	40 mg simethicone		In UD 8s and 1000s.

Capsules and Tablets

ANTACID COMBINATIONS

	Product & distributor	Aluminum Hydroxide	Magnesium Hydroxide	Calcium Carbonate	Other Content	Sodium (mg)	How supplied
otc *sf*	**Calglycine Antacid** (Rugby)			420	150 mg Glycine.		In 250s and 1000s.
otc *sf*	**Titralac Tablets** (3M Pharm.)				Saccharin	0.3	Chewable. Spearmint flavor. In 40s, 100s and 1000s.
otc	**Titralac Plus Tablets** (3M Pharm.)				21 mg simethicone, saccharin	1.1	Chewable. Spearmint flavor. In 100s.
otc	**Alenic Alka Tablets** (Rugby)	80			20 mg magnesium trisilicate, sodium bicarbonate, calcium stearate, sugar	18.4	Chewable. Butterscotch flavor. In 100s.
otc	**Foamicon Tablets** (Invamed				Alginic acid, sodium bicarbonate, 20 mg magnesium trisilicate, calcium stearate, sugar, sucrose	18.4	Chewable. White. In 100s.
otc	**Genaton Tablets** (Goldline)				Alginic acid, sodium bicarbonate, 20 mg magnesium trisilicate, sucrose, sugar	18.4	Chewable. In 100s.
otc	**Gaviscon Tablets** (SK-Beecham				Alginic acid, sodium bicarbonate, 20 mg magnesium trisilicate, sucrose, calcium stearate	18.4	Chewable. In 30s and 100s.

Capsules and Tablets

ANTACID COMBINATIONS

	Product & distributor	Aluminum Hydroxide	Magnesium Hydroxide	Calcium Carbonate	Other Content	Sodium (mg)	How supplied
otc	**Double Strenght Gaviscon-2 Tablets** (SK-Beecham)	160			Alginic acid, sodium bicarbonate, 40 mg magnesium trisilicate, sucrose	36.8	Chewable. In 48s.
otc	**Gaviscon Extra Strength Relief Formula Tablets** (SK-Beecham)				105 mg magnesium carbonate, alginic acid, sodium bicarbonate, sucrose, calcium stearate	29.9	Chewable. In 30s and 100s
otc	**Extra Strength Alenic Alka Tablets** (Rugby)				105 mg magnesium carbonate	29.9	Chewable. Butterscotch flavor. In 100s.
otc	**Extra Strength Genaton Tablets** (Goldline)				105 mg magnesium carbonate, alginic acid, sodium bicarbonate, sucrose, calcium stearate	29.9	Chewable. In 100s
otc	**Almacone Tablets** (Rugby)	200	200		20 mg simethicone		Chewable. Yellow/white. Peppermint flavor. In 100s and 1000s
otc	**Mylanta Tablets** (J & J-Merck)				20 mg simethicone, sorbitol	0.77	Chewable. (Stuart 620). Yellow and white, layered. In 12s, 40s, 48s, 100s and 180s.
otc	**RuLox Plus Tablets** (Rugby)				25 mg simethicone, sugar, saccharin, dextrose		Chewable. Lemon and cherry flavors. In 50s.
otc	**Magalox Plus** (Invamed				25 mg simethicone, sugar.		In 100s.
otc	**Gelusil Tablets** (Parke-Davis)	200	200		25 mg simetihicone, sorbitol, sugar	< 5	Chewable. Peppermint flavor. In 100s.
otc	**Maalox Plus Tablets** (Rhone-Poulenc Rorer)				25 mg simethicone, dextrose, saccharin, sorbitol, sugar		Chewable. Lemon creme and cherry creme flavors. In 50s, 100s and 144s.
otc	**Mintox Plus Tablets** (Major)	200	200		25 mg simethicone, saccharin, sucrose		Chewable. In 100s.
otc	**Extra Strength Maalox Plus Tablets** (Rhone-Poulenc Rorer)	350	350		30 mg simethicone, sugar, dextrose, saccharin, sorbitol		Chewable. Mint creme flavor. In 38s and 75s.

Capsules and Tablets

ANTACID COMBINATIONS

	Product & distributor	Aluminum Hydroxide	Magnesium Hydroxide	Calcium Carbonate	Other Content	Sodium (mg)	How supplied
otc	**Mylanta Double Strength Tablets** (J&J-Merck)	400	400		40 mg simethicone, saccharin, sorbitol		Chewable. Mint and cherry flavors. In 24s and 60s.
otc	**Tempo Tablets** (Thompson Medical)	133	81	414	20 mg simethicone, corn syrup, sorbitol	3	Chewable. In 10s, 30s and 60s.
otc	**Calcium Rich Rolaids Tablets** (Warner-Lambert)		80	412		0.4	Chewable. Original, cherry, spearmint and assorted fruit flavors. In 12s, 36s, 75s and 150s.
otc	**Advanced Formula Di-Gel Tablets** (Schering-Plough)		128	280	20 mg simethicone, sucrose		Chewable. Mint and lemon-orange flavors. In 30s, 60s and 90s.
otc	**Riopan Plus Tablets** (Whitehall)				480 mg magaldrate, 20 mg simethicone, sorbitol, sucrose		Chewable. Cool mint flavor. In 50s and 100s.
otc	**Riopan Plus Double Strength Tablets** (Whitehall)				1080 mg magaldrate, 20 mg simethicone, saccharin, sorbitol, sucrose		Chewable. Cool mint flavor. In 60s

sf - Sugar free.

Liquids

ANTACID COMBINATIONS

Refer to the general discussion of these products in the Antacids group monograph.

Content given in mg per 5 ml. 23 mg sodium = 1mEq.

	Product & Distributor	Aluminum Hydroxide	Magnesium Hydroxide	Calcium Carbonate	Other Content	Sodium (mg)	How Supplied
otc	**Nephrox Liquid** (Fleming)	320			10% mineral oil		Watermelon flavor. In pt.
otc	**Alamag Suspension** (Goldline)	225	200		Sorbitol, sucrose, parabens	< 1.25	Mint flavor. In 355 ml.
otc	**Maalox Suspension** (Rhone-Poulenc Rorer)				Saccharin, sorbitol, parabens		Mint creme and cherry creme flavors. In 148, 355 and 769 ml.
otc	**Magnox Suspension** (Lennod)						Mint flavor. In 360 ml.
otc	**Alamag Plus Suspension** (Goldline)				25 mg simethicone, parabens, saccharin, sorbitol		Lemon flavor. In 355 ml.
otc	**Magnalox Liquid** (Schein)						In 360 ml.
otc	**Antacid Suspension** (Geneva)						In 360 ml.
otc	**Mintox Suspension** (Major)				Parabens, saccharin, sorbitol	1.4	Mint flavor. In 355 and 780 ml.
otc	**RuLox Suspension** (Rugby)						Mint flavor. In 360 and 769 ml and gal.
otc	**Aludrox Suspension** (Wyeth-Ayerst)	307	103		Simethicone, saccharin, sorbitol, parabens		In 355 ml.
otc	**Extra Strength Maalox Suspension** (Rhone-Poulenc Rorer)	500	450		40 mg simethicone, parabens, saccharin, sorbitol		Cherry creme, lemon creme and mint creme flavors. In 148, 355 and 769 ml.
otc	**Maalox Therapeutic Concentrate Suspension** (Rhone-Poulenc Rorer)	600	300		Parabens, sorbitol		Mint flavor. In 355 ml.

Liquids

ANTACID COMBINATIONS

	Product & Distributor	Aluminum Hydroxide	Magnesium Hydroxide	Calcium Carbonate	Other Content	Sodium (mg)	How Supplied
otc	**Kudrox Double Strength Suspension** (Schwarz Pharma Kremers Urban)	500	450		40 mg simethicone, parabens, saccharin, sorbitol		Lemon Swiss creme flavor. In 355 ml.
otc	**Extra Strength Mintox Plus Liquid** (Major)				40 mg simethicone, parabens, saccharin, sorbitol		Lemon Swiss creme flavor. In 355 ml.
otc	**Simaal Gel 2 Liquid** (Schein)	500	400		40 mg simethicone		In 360 ml.
otc	**Gaviscon Extra Strength Relief Formula Liquid** (SK-Beecham)	254			237.5 mg magnesium carbonate, parabens, EDTA, saccharin, sorbitol, simethicone, sodium alginate		Cool mint flavor. In 355 ml.
otc	**Alenic Alka Liquid** (Rugby)	31.7			137.3 mg magnesium carbonate, sodium alginate, EDTA, saccharin, sorbitol, parabens	13	Spearmint flavor. In 355 ml.
otc	**Gaviscon Liquid** (SK-Beecham)				119.3 mg magnesium carbonate, sodium alginate, EDTA, saccharin, sorbitol, parabens	13	Cool mint flavor. In 177 and 355 ml.
otc	**Genaton Liquid** (Goldline)				137.3 mg magnesium carbonate, sodium alginate, EDTA, saccharin, sorbitol	13	Spearmint flavor. In 355 ml.
otc	**Marblen Liquid** (Fleming)			520	400 mg magnesium carbonate		Peach/Apricot flavor. In 473 ml.
otc *sf*	**Titralac Plus Liquid** (3M Personal Health Care)			500	20 mg simethicone, parabens, saccharin, sorbitol	0.15	Mint flavor. In 360 ml.

ANTACID COMBINATIONS

Liquids

	Product & Distributor	Aluminum Hydroxide	Magnesium Hydroxide	Calcium Carbonate	Other Content	Sodium (mg)	How Supplied
otc	**Almacone Liquid** (Rugby)	200	200		20 mg simethicone		In 360 ml and gal.
otc	**Di-Gel Liquid** (Schering-Plough)				20 mg simethicone, saccharin, sorbitol, parabens		Mint and lemon-orange flavors. In 180 and 360 ml.
otc	**Gelusil Liquid** (Parke-Davis)				25 mg simethicone, saccharin, sorbitol, menthol		Peppermint flavor. In 355 ml.
otc	**Mi-Acid Liquid** (Major)				20 mg simethicone, parabens, sorbitol		In 355 and 780 ml.
otc	**Mylagen Liquid** (Goldline)				20 mg simethicone, parabens, sorbitol, sucrose	< 1.25	In 355 ml.
otc	**Mygel Suspension** (Geneva)				20 mg simethicone		In 360 ml.
otc	**Mylanta Liquid** (J&J-Merck)				20 mg simethicone, sorbitol	0.68	In 150, 360, 720 ml and UD 30 ml.
otc	**Simaal Gel Liquid** (Schein)				20 mg simethicone		In 360 ml.
otc	**Alumina, Magnesia, and Simethicone Suspension** (Roxane)	213	200		20 mg simethicone, parabens, sorbitol		In UD 15 and 30 ml.

Liquids

ANTACID COMBINATIONS

	Product & Distributor	Aluminum Hydroxide	Magnesium Hydroxide	Calcium Carbonate	Other Content	Sodium (mg)	How Supplied
otc	**Gas Ban DS Liquid** (Roberts)	400	400		40 mg simehticone		In 150 ml.
otc	**Mygel II Suspension** (Geneva)				40 mg simethicone		In 360 ml.
otc	**Almacone II Double Strength Liquid** (Rugby)				40 mg simethicone, saccharin, sorbitol		In 360 ml and gal.
otc	**Mylagen II Liquid** (Goldline)				40 mg simethicone, parabens, sorbitol, sucrose	< 1.25	In 355 ml.
otc	**Mi-Acid II Liquid** (Major)				40 mg simethicone, parabens, sorbitol		In 355 ml.
otc	**Mylanta Double Strength Liquid** (J&J-Merck)				40 mg simethicone, sorbitol, parabens		Cherry and cool mint creme flavors. In 150 and 360 ml.
otc	**Extra Strength Maalox Plus Suspension** (Rhone-Poulenc Rorer)	500	450		40 mg simethicone, saccharin, sorbitol, parabens		Cherry creme, lemon creme and mint creme flavors. In 148, 355 and 769 ml.
otc	**RuLox Plus Suspension** (Rugby)						Lemon creme flavor. In 355 ml.

Liquids

ANTACID COMBINATIONS

	Product & Distributor	Aluminum Hydroxide	Magnesium Hydroxide	Calcium Carbonate	Other Content	Sodium (mg)	How Supplied
otc	**Maalox Heartburn Relief Liquid** (Rhone-Poulenc Rorer)				140 mg aluminum hydroxide-magnesium carbonate (codried gel), 175 mg magnesium carbonate, tartrazine, saccharin, magnesium alginate, parabens, sorbitol		Cool mint creme flavor. In 296 ml.
otc	**Iosopan Plus Liquid** (Goldline)				540 mg magaldrate, 40 mg simethicone		In 355 ml.
otc	**Lowsium Plus Suspension** (Rugby)				540 mg magaldrate, 40 mg simethicone		In 360 ml.
otc	**Magaldrate Plus Suspension** (Various, eg, Halsey, Moore)				540 mg magaldrate, 40 mg simethicone		In 360 ml.
otc	**Riopan Plus Suspension** (Whitehall)				540 mg magaldrate, 40 mg simethicone, saccharin, sorbitol		Mint flavor. In 360 ml.
otc	**Riopan Plus Double Strength Suspension** (Whitehall)				1080 mg magaldrate, 40 mg simethicone, saccharin, sorbitol		Mint or cherry creme flavors. In 360 ml.

Powders and Effervescent Tablets

ANTACID COMBINATIONS

Refer to the general discussion of these products in the Antacids group monograph.

Content given per dose or tablet.

	Product and Distributor	Sodium Bicarbonate (mg)	Other Content	Sodium (mg)	How Supplied
otc *sf*	**Citrocarbonate Effervescent Granules** (Roberts-Hauck)	780	1820 mg sodium citrate anhydrous	700.6	In 150 g.
otc	**Bromo Seltzer Effervescent Granules** (Warner-Lambert)	2781	325 mg acetaminophen, 2224 mg citric acid (when dissolved forms 2848 mg sodium citrate), sugar	761	In 127.5 g.
otc	**Sparkles Effervescent Granules** (Lafayette)	2000	1500 mg citric acid, simethicone		In UD 50s.
otc	**Gold Alka-Seltzer Effervescent Tablets** (Bayer)	958[1]	832 mg citric acid, 312 mg potassium bicarbonate	311	In 20s and 36s.
otc	**Original Alka-Seltzer Effervescent Tablets** (Bayer)	1700	325 mg aspirin, 1000 mg citric acid, 9 mg phenylalanine	506	Aspartame. Lemon-lime flavor. In 24s.
otc	**Original Alka-Seltzer Effervescent Tablets** (Bayer)	1916[1]	325 mg aspirin, 1000 mg citric acid	567	In 36s.
otc	**Extra Strength Alka-Seltzer Effervescent Tablets** (Bayer)	1985[1]	500 mg aspirin, 1000 mg citric acid	588	In 12s and 24s.

[1] Heat-treated.

SUCRALFATE

Actions:

Pharmacology: Sucralfate, a basic aluminum salt of sulfated sucrose, is a polysaccharide with antipeptic activity. In the acidic medium of gastric juice, the aluminum ion splits off, leaving a highly polar anion which is essentially nonabsorbable. It exerts a local rather than systemic action. Sucralfate forms an ulcer-adherent complex with proteinaceous exudate. The ulcer-adherent complex covers the ulcer site and protects it against acid, pepsin and bile salts. Sucralfate has minimal acid neutralizing capacity.

Sucralfate aids in ulcer healing by forming the protective layer at the ulcer site, providing a barrier to hydrogen ion diffusion, inhibiting pepsin's action 32% and adsorbing bile salts. The acid neutralizing effects do not contribute to antiulcer effects.

Pharmacokinetics: Sucralfate is minimally absorbed (3% to 5%) from the GI tract. Approximately 90% is excreted in the stool. The small amounts of the sulfated disaccharide absorbed are excreted primarily in the urine.

Clinical trials:

Tablets –

Acute duodenal ulcer: In two multicenter placebo controlled trials, endoscopic evaluation at 2 and 4 weeks demonstrated statistically significant sucralfate-placebo differences at 4 weeks but not at 2 weeks. At 4 weeks, the overall ulcer healing rate for sucralfate and placebo ranged from 75% to 92% and 58% to 64%, respectively.

Maintenance therapy: In two double-blind randomized placebo controlled trials, endoscopic evaluation at 4, 6 and 12 months revealed the following results:

Duodenal Ulcer Recurrence Rate with Sucralfate Tablets (%)

Drug	Months of therapy					
	1[1]	2[1]	3[1]	4[1]	6[2]	12[2]
Sucralfate	20	30	38	42	19	27
Placebo	33	46	55	63	54	65

[1] Sucralfate (n = 122); placebo (n = 117). "As needed" antacids not permitted.

[2] Sucralfate (n = 48); placebo (n = 46). "As needed" antacids permitted.

Suspension – In a multicenter, double-blind, placebo controlled study of sucralfate suspension, a dosage regimen of 1 g (10 ml) four times daily was demonstrated to be superior to placebo in ulcer healing.

Healing Rates for Acute Doudenal Ulcer: Sucralfate Suspension

Treatment	Healing Rates (%)		
	Week 1	Week 2	Week 3
Sucralfate (n =145)	16	46	66
Placebo (n =147)	7	27	39

Equivalence of sucralfate suspension to sucralfate tablets has not been demonstrated.

Indications:

Duodenal ulcer: Short-term treatment (up to 8 weeks) of active duodenal ulcer.

Tablets:

Maintenance therapy for duodenal ulcer patients at reduced dosage after healing of acute ulcers.

Unlabeled uses: Sucralfate has been used in the following conditions: Accelerating healing of gastric ulcers; long-term treatment of gastric ulcers; treatment of reflux and peptic esophagitis; treatment of NSAID- and aspirin-induced GI symptoms and mucosal damage; prevention of stress ulcers and GI bleeding in critically ill patients. Since increased gastric pH may be implicated in causing nosocomial infections in critically ill patients, sucralfate may offer an advantage over antacids and histamine H_2 antagonists in stress ulcer prophylaxis.

Sucralfate in suspension has also been used in treatment of oral and esophageal ulcers due to radiation, chemotherapy and sclerotherapy.

SUCRALFATE

Warnings:

Chronic renal failure/dialysis: During sucralfate administration, small amounts of aluminum are absorbed from the GI tract. Concomitant use with other aluminum-containing products (eg, antacids) may increase the total body burden of aluminum. Patients with normal renal function receiving these agents concomitantly adequately excrete aluminum in the urine. However, patients with chronic renal failure or receiving dialysis have impaired excretion of absorbed aluminum, and aluminum does not cross dialysis membranes. Aluminum accumulation and toxicity (eg, aluminum osteodystrophy, osteomalacia, encephalopathy) have occurred. Use with caution in these patients.

Pregnancy: Category B. There are no adequate and well controlled studies in pregnant women. Use this drug during pregnancy only if clearly needed.

Lactation: It is not known whether this drug is excreted in breast milk. Exercise caution when sucralfate is administered to a nursing mother.

Children: Safety and efficacy in children have not been established.

Precautions:

Ulcer recurrence: Duodenal ulcer is a chronic recurrent disease. While short-term treatment can completely heal the ulcer, do not expect a successful course to alter post-healing frequency or severity of duodenal ulceration.

Drug Interactions:

Sucralfate Drug Interactions

Precipitant drug	Object drug*		Description
Sucralfate	Antacids, aluminum-containing	⬆	The total body burden of aluminum may be increased with sucralfate coadministration. See Warnings.
Sucralfate	Anticoagulants	⬇	A decrease in the hypoprothrombinemic effect of warfarin may occur.
Sucralfate	Digoxin	⬇	Serum digoxin levels may be reduced, decreasing the therapeutic effects.
Sucralfate	Hydantoins	⬇	Phenytoin absorption may be decreased.
Sucralfate	Ketoconazole	⬇	Ketoconazole bioavailability may be decreased.
Sucralfate	Quinidine	⬇	Serum quinidine levels may be reduced, decreasing the therapeutic effects.
Sucralfate	Quinolones	⬇	Bioavailability of the quinolones may be decreased. Administering the quinolone ≥ 2 hours before sucralfate may eliminate the interaction.

* ⬆ = Object drug increased. ⬇ = Object drug decreased.

Adverse Reactions:

Adverse reactions in clinical trials were minor and rarely led to drug discontinuation.

Constipation was the most frequent complaint (2%). Other adverse effects include: Diarrhea, nausea, vomiting, gastric discomfort, indigestion, flatulence, dry mouth, rash, pruritus, back pain, headache, dizziness, sleepiness, vertigo (< 0.5%); laryngospasm; facial swelling; hypersensitivity reactions (including urticaria, angioedema, respiratory difficulty, rhinitis).

Overdosage:

Risks associated with overdosage appear minimal.

Patient Information:

Take on an empty stomach at least 1 hour before meals and at bedtime.

Do not take antacids ½ hour before or after taking sucralfate.

SUCRALFATE

Administration and Dosage:

Active duodenal ulcer:

Adults – 1 g 4 times a day on an empty stomach (1 hour before meals and at bedtime).

Take antacids as needed for pain relief, but not within ½ hour before or after sucralfate.

While healing with sucralfate may occur within the first 2 weeks, continue treatment for 4 to 8 weeks unless healing is demonstrated by x-ray or endoscopic examination.

Maintenance therapy (tablets only):

Adults – 1 g twice daily.

Rx	**Sucralfate** (Biocraft)	**Tablets:** 1 g	(Biocraft 105). White, scored. Capsule shape. In 30s, 100s and 500s.
Rx	**Carafate** (Hoechst Marion Roussel)	**Tablets:** 1 g	(Carafate 1712). Light pink, scored. In 100s, 120s, 500s and UD 100s.
		Suspension: 1 g per 10 ml	Sorbitol, methylparaben. In 420 ml.

GASTROINTESTINAL ANTICHOLINERGICS/ANTISPASMODICS

Anticholinergics are also known as antimuscarinic drugs. In addition to the Anticholinergics/Antispasmodics discussed below, related drugs include: Anticholinergic Antiparkinson Agents, Cycloplegic Mydriatics and Urinary Antispasmodics. See specific monographs.

GI anticholinergics are used primarily to decrease motility (smooth muscle tone) in GI, biliary and urinary tracts and for antisecretory effects. Antispasmodics, related compounds, decrease GI motility by acting on smooth muscle.

Gastrointestinal Anticholinergic/Antispasmodic Dosage

Drug	Adult Dosage	
	Oral	Parenteral
Anticholinergics		
Atropine	0.4-0.6 mg	0.4-0.6 mg
Scopolamine		0.32-0.65 mg
L-hyoscyamine	0.125-0.25 mg tid-qid (0.375 to 0.7 mg q 12 hrs – sustained release)	0.25-0.5 mg q 4 h
L-alkaloids of belladonna	0.25-0.5 mg tid	
Belladonna alkaloids	0.18-0.3 mg tid-qid	
Quaternary Anticholinergics		
Methscopolamine bromide	2.5 mg ac; 2.5-5 mg hs	
Anisotropine MBr	50 mg tid	
Clidinium bromide	2.5-5 mg tid-qid	
Glycopyrrolate	1-2 mg bid-tid	0.1-0.2 mg tid-qid
Hexocyclium	25 mg qid	
Isopropamide iodide	5-10 mg q 12 hrs	
Mepenzolate bromide	25-50 mg qid	
Methantheline bromide	50-100 mg q 4-6 hrs	
Propantheline bromide	7.5-15 mg tid; 30 mg hs	
Tridihexethyl chloride	25-50 mg tid-qid	
Antispasmodics		
Dicyclomine HCl	20-40 mg qid	20 mg qid
Oxyphencyclimine HCl	10 mg bid	

Actions:

Pharmacology: These agents inhibit the muscarinic actions of acetylcholine at postganglionic parasympathetic neuroeffector sites including smooth muscle, secretory glands and CNS sites. Large doses may block nicotinic receptors at the autonomic ganglia and at the neuromuscular junction.

Specific anticholinergic responses are dose-related. Small doses inhibit salivary and bronchial secretions and sweating; moderate doses dilate the pupil, inhibit accommodation and increase heart rate (vagolytic effect); larger doses decrease motility of GI and urinary tracts; very large doses inhibit gastric acid secretion.

Pharmacokinetics:

Absorption/Distribution –

Belladonna alkaloids are rapidly absorbed after oral use. They readily cross blood-brain barrier, and affect the CNS. The major difference between these agents is that atropine at usual therapeutic doses is a stimulant, whereas scopolamine is a CNS depressant. Undesirable peripheral and central effects occur at doses sufficient to control GI motility and gastric acid secretion.

Atropine has a half-life of about 2.5 hours; 94% of a dose is eliminated through the urine in 24 hours.

Quaternary anticholinergics: Synthetic or semisynthetic derivatives structurally related to the belladonna alkaloids, they are poorly and unreliably absorbed orally. Since they do not cross the blood-brain barrier, CNS effects are negligible. They are also less likely to affect the pupil or ciliary muscle of the eye. Duration of action is more prolonged than alkaloids. In addition, they may cause some degree of ganglionic blockade; neuromuscular blockade may occur at toxic doses.

Antispasmodics: The tertiary ammonium compounds have little or no antimuscarinic activity, and therefore, no significant effect on gastric acid secretion. They exhibit a nonspecific direct relaxant effect on smooth muscle.

GASTROINTESTINAL ANTICHOLINERGICS/ANTISPASMODICS

Indications:

The general uses for these agents are listed below. Refer to the individual product listings for specific indications.

Peptic ulcer: Adjunctive therapy for peptic ulcer. These agents suppress gastric acid secretion. There is no conclusive evidence they aid in the healing of a peptic ulcer, decrease the rate of recurrence or prevent complications. Anticholinergics are used much less frequently in modern ulcer management.

Other GI conditions: Functional GI disorders (diarrhea, pylorospasm, hypermotility, neurogenic colon), irritable bowel syndrome (spastic colon, mucous colitis), acute enterocolitis, ulcerative colitis, diverticulitis, mild dysenteries, pancreatitis, splenic flexure syndrome and infant colic.

Biliary tract: For spastic disorders of the biliary tract. Given in conjunction with a narcotic analgesic.

Urogenital tract: Uninhibited hypertonic neurogenic bladder.

Bradycardia: Atropine is used in the suppression of vagally-mediated bradycardias.

Preoperative medication: Atropine, scopolamine, hyoscyamine and glycopyrrolate are used as preanesthetic medication to control bronchial, nasal, pharyngeal and salivary secretions; and to block cardiac vagal inhibitory reflexes during induction of anesthesia and intubation. Scopolamine is used for preanesthetic sedation and for obstetric amnesia.

Antidotes for poisoning by cholinergic drugs: Atropine is used for poisoning by organophosphorous insecticides, chemical warfare nerve gases and as an antidote for mushroom poisoning due to muscarine in certain species such as Amanita muscaria (see Pralidoxime Chloride).

Miscellaneous uses: Calming delirium; motion sickness (scopolamine), see Antiemetic/Antivertigo Agents; parkinsonism, see Antiparkinson Agents.

Unlabeled uses:

Bronchial asthma – Atropine and related agents are effective in some patients with cholinergic-mediated bronchospasm. Use in chronic lung disease is not generally recommended; these agents reduce bronchial secretions resulting in decreased fluidity and thickening of residual secretion.

Glycopyrrolate may be effective in the treatment of bronchial asthma; doses of 1 mg (nebulization) and 1.3 mg (solution) have been used.

Contraindications:

Hypersensitivity to anticholinergic drugs. Patients hypersensitive to belladonna or to barbiturates may be hypersensitive to **scopolamine.**

Ocular: Narrow-angle glaucoma; adhesions (synechiae) between the iris and lens.

Cardiovascular: Tachycardia; unstable cardiovascular status in acute hemorrhage; myocardial ischemia.

GI: Obstructive disease (eg, achalasia, pyloroduodenal stenosis or pyloric obstruction, cardiospasm); paralytic ileus; intestinal atony of the elderly or debilitated; severe ulcerative colitis; toxic megacolon complicating ulcerative colitis; hepatic disease.

GU: Obstructive uropathy (eg, bladder neck obstruction due to prostatic hypertrophy); renal disease.

Musculoskeletal: Myasthenia gravis.

Atropine is contraindicated in asthma patients.

Dicyclomine: Infants < 6 months of age (see Warnings).

Warnings:

Heat prostration can occur with anticholinergic drug use (fever and heat stroke due to decreased sweating) in the presence of a high environmental temperature.

Diarrhea may be an early symptom of incomplete intestinal obstruction, especially in patients with ileostomy or colostomy. Treatment of diarrhea with these drugs is inappropriate and possibly harmful.

Parkinsonism: Vomiting, malaise, sweating and salivation may occur in patients with parkinsonism upon sudden withdrawal of large doses of **scopolamine.**

Anticholinergic psychosis has been reported in sensitive individuals given anticholinergic drugs. CNS signs and symptoms include confusion, disorientation, short-term memory loss, hallucinations, dysarthria, ataxia, coma, euphoria, decreased anxiety, fatigue, insomnia, agitation and mannerisms, and inappropriate affect. These CNS signs and symptoms usually resolve 12 to 24 hours after drug discontinuation.

Gastric ulcer may produce a delay in gastric emptying time and may complicate therapy (antral stasis).

GASTROINTESTINAL ANTICHOLINERGICS/ANTISPASMODICS

Elderly: Elderly patients may react with excitement, agitation, drowsiness and other untoward manifestations to even small doses of anticholinergic drugs.

Pregnancy: Category B (glycopyrrolate, parenteral); *Category C* (hyoscyamine, atropine, scopolamine, isopropamide, propantheline, methantheline). Hyoscyamine crosses the placenta; atropine and scopolamine cross the placenta rapidly after IV use. Effects on the fetus depend on maturity of its parasympathetic nervous system. In neonates, scopolamine may depress respiration and contribute to neonatal hemorrhage due to reduction in Vitamin K-dependent clotting factors.

Safety for use during pregnancy has not been established. Use only when clearly needed and when the potential benefits outweigh the potential hazards to the fetus.

Labor and delivery – Scopolamine does not affect uterine contractions during labor or increase duration of labor. It crosses the placenta but has not been reported to affect the fetus adversely.

Lactation: Hyoscyamine is excreted in breast milk; other anticholinergics (especially atropine) may be excreted in milk, causing infant toxicity, and may reduce milk production. Documentation is lacking or conflicting. Generally, do not use in nursing women.

Children: Safety and efficacy are not established. Hyoscyamine has been used in infant colic. **Isopropamide** is not recommended in children under 12. Safety and efficacy of **glycopyrrolate** in children under 12 are not established for peptic ulcer.

There are reports of infants in the first 3 months of life, administered **dicyclomine** syrup, who experienced respiratory distress, seizures, syncope, asphyxia, pulse rate fluctuations, muscular hypotonia and coma. These symptoms occurred within minutes of ingestion and lasted 20 to 30 minutes; this suggests that they were a consequence of local irritation or aspiration rather than a pharmacologic effect. A few deaths have been reported in infants ≤ 3 months of age. Two of these were associated with excessively high dicyclomine blood levels. Dicyclomine is contraindicated in infants < 6 months old.

Precautions:

Use with caution in:

Ocular – Glaucoma; light irides. If there is mydriasis and photophobia, wear dark glasses. Use caution in the elderly because of increased incidence of glaucoma.

GI – Hepatic disease; early evidence of ileus, as in peritonitis; ulcerative colitis (large doses may suppress intestinal motility and precipitate or aggravate toxic megacolon); hiatal hernia associated with reflux esophagitis (anticholinergics may aggravate it).

GU – Renal disease; prostatic hypertrophy. Patients with prostatism can have dysuria and may require catheterization.

Cardiovascular – Coronary heart disease; congestive heart failure; cardiac arrhythmias; tachycardia; hypertension.

Pulmonary – Debilitated patients with chronic lung disease; reduction in bronchial secretions can lead to inspissation and formation of bronchial plugs. Use cautiously in patients with asthma or allergies.

Miscellaneous: Autonomic neuropathy; hyperthyroidism.

In pain or severe anxiety, scopolamine is usually given with analgesics or sedatives to avoid behavioral disturbances. Risk of hyperpyrexia is increased in patients with fever. In elderly patients, confusional states are more common.

Special risk patients: Use cautiously in infants, small children, blondes, and persons with Down's syndrome, brain damage or spastic paralysis.

Hazardous tasks: May produce drowsiness, dizziness or blurred vision; observe caution while driving or performing other tasks requiring alertness.

Tartrazine sensitivity: Some of these products contain tartrazine, which may cause allergic-type reactions (including bronchial asthma) in certain susceptible persons. Although the overall incidence of tartrazine sensitivity in the general population is low, it is often seen in patients who have aspirin hypersensitivity. Specific products containing tartrazine are identified in the product listings.

Sulfite sensitivity: Some of these products contain sulfites that may cause allergic-type reactions including anaphylactic symptoms and life-threatening asthmatic episodes in certain susceptible persons. Although the overall prevalence of sulfite sensitivity in the general population is probably low, it is seen more frequently in asthmatic or atopic nonasthmatic persons.

Drug Interactions:

Amantadine: Coadministration of anticholinergics may result in an increase in anticholinergic side effects. Consider decreasing the anticholinergic dose.

Atenolol: The pharmacologic effects may be increased by concurrent anticholinergic administration. Metoprolol and propranolol were not affected in two studies.

Digoxin: Pharmacologic effects may be increased by anticholinergic coadministration. This may be product specific, ie, slow dissolving digoxin tablets interact whereas digoxin capsules and elixir are not affected. However, since USP standards require a minimum dissolution rate, tablets available in the US are not likely to be affected.

Phenothiazines: The antipsychotic effectiveness may be decreased by anticholinergic coadministration. Anticholinergic side effects may also be increased by concurrent therapy. Adjust the phenothiazine dose as necessary.

Tricyclic antidepressants: Anticholinergic coadministration may increase anticholinergic side effects (eg, dry mouth, constipation, urinary retention) due to an additive effect. A tricyclic antidepressant with less anticholinergic activity may be beneficial.

Drug/Lab test interactions: The iodine in **isopropamide iodide** may alter **thyroid function tests** and will suppress I^{131} uptake. Substitute a thyroid function test unaffected by exogenous iodides.

Adverse Reactions:

Cardiovascular: Palpitations; bradycardia (following low doses of atropine); tachycardia (after higher doses).

CNS: Headache; flushing; nervousness; drowsiness; weakness; dizziness; confusion; insomnia; fever (especially in children); mental confusion or excitement especially in elderly patients with even small doses. Large doses may produce CNS stimulation (restlessness, tremor). In the presence of pain, **scopolamine** may produce excitement, restlessness, hallucinations or delirium. Parenteral **dicyclomine** may cause temporary lightheadedness.

Dermatologic: Severe allergic reactions including anaphylaxis, urticaria and other dermal manifestations. Local irritation may occur with parenteral **dicyclomine.**

GI: Xerostomia; altered taste perception; nausea; vomiting; dysphagia; heartburn; constipation; bloated feeling; paralytic ileus.

GU: Urinary hesitancy and retention; impotence.

Ophthalmic: Blurred vision; mydriasis; photophobia; cycloplegia; increased intraocular pressure; dilated pupils.

Miscellaneous: Suppression of lactation; nasal congestion; decreased sweating.

Overdosage:

Symptoms:

GI – Dry mouth; thirst; vomiting; nausea; abdominal distention; difficulty swallowing.

CNS – Theoretically, a curare-like action may occur (ie, neuromuscular blockade leading to muscular weakness and paralysis); CNS stimulation; delirium; drowsiness; restlessness; anxiety; stupor; fever; disorientation; dizziness; headache; seizures; hallucinations; ataxia; convulsions; coma; psychotic behavior; other signs of an acute organic psychosis.

Cardiovascular – Circulatory failure; rapid pulse and respiration; vasodilation; tachycardia with weak pulse; hypertension; hypotension; respiratory depression; palpitations.

GU – Urinary urgency with difficulty in micturition.

Ocular – Blurred vision; photophobia; dilated pupils.

Miscellaneous – Leukocytosis; flushed hot dry skin; rash; respiratory failure.

Children, especially those with mongolism, spastic paralysis or brain damage, are more sensitive than adults to toxic effects.

Treatment: Induce emesis or perform gastric lavage, then administer activated charcoal slurry, and supportive and symptomatic therapy, as indicated. See also General Management of Acute Overdosage.

Physostigmine by slow IV injection of 0.2 to 4 mg has been used to reverse anticholinergic effects. Since physostigmine is rapidly metabolized, the patient may relapse into coma after 1 to 2 hours; repeat doses as necessary to a total of 6 mg (2 mg in children). However, profound bradycardia, asystole and seizures may occur (see Antidotes monograph). The role of physostigmine is not clear; avoid it if other therapeutic agents successfully reverse cardiac dysrhythmias.

Neostigmine methylsulfate 0.25 to 2.5 mg IV, repeated as needed, may be given.

Diazepam, short-acting barbiturates, IV sodium thiopental (2% solution) or chloral hydrate (100 to 200 ml of a 2% solution) by rectal infusion may control excitement. Hyoscyamine is dialyzable, but hemodialysis is ineffective for atropine poisoning. Treat hyperpyrexia with physical cooling measures.

If the curare-like effect progresses to paralysis of respiratory muscles, institute artificial respiration and maintain until effective respiratory action returns.

Patient Information:

Usually taken 30 to 60 minutes before a meal.

May cause drowsiness, dizziness or blurred vision; patients should observe caution while driving or performing other tasks requiring alertness.

Notify physician if skin rash, flushing or eye pain occurs.

May cause dry mouth, difficulty in urination, constipation or increased sensitivity to light; notify physician if these effects persist or become severe.

Belladonna Alkaloids

L-HYOSCYAMINE SULFATE

For complete prescribing information, refer to the Gastrointestinal Anticholinergics/Antispasmodics group monograph.

Indications:

GI: To aid in the control of gastric secretion, visceral spasm, hypermotility in spastic colitis, spastic bladder, pylorospasm and associated abdominal cramps. To relieve symptoms in functional intestinal disorders (eg, mild dysenteries and diverticulitis), infant colic, biliary and renal colic. As adjunctive therapy in peptic ulcer; irritable bowel syndrome (irritable colon, spastic colon, mucus colitis, acute enterocolitis, functional GI disorders); neurogenic bowel disturbances including splenic flexure syndrome and neurogenic colon; to reduce pain and hypersecretion in pancreatitis.

Respiratory tract: As a "drying agent" in the relief of symptoms of acute rhinitis.

CNS: In parkinsonism to reduce rigidity and tremors and to control associated sialorrhea and hyperhidrosis. May be used for poisoning by anticholinesterase agents.

GU: Cystitis; renal colic.

Cardiovascular: Certain cases of partial heart block associated with vagal activity.

Parenteral: Reduces duodenal motility to facilitate the diagnostic radiologic procedure, hypotonic duodenography. May also improve radiologic visibility of the kidneys.

Preoperative medication: Parenteral hyoscyamine is indicated as a pre-operative antimuscarinic to reduce salivary, tracheobronchial, and pharyngeal secretions; to reduce volume and acidity of gastric secretions; to block cardiac vagal inhibitory reflexes during induction of anesthesia and intubation. Hyoscyamine protects against peripheral muscarinic effects such as bradycardia and excessive secretions produced by halogenated hydrocarbons and cholinergic agents such as physostigmine, neostigmine, and pyridostigmine given to reverse actions of curariform agents.

Administration and Dosage:

Oral:

Adults – 0.125 to 0.25 mg, 3 or 4 times/day orally or sublingually; or 0.375 to 0.75 mg in sustained release form every 12 hours.

Children – Individualize dosage according to weight.

Parenteral: 0.25 to 0.5 mg SC, IM or IV, 2 to 4 times daily, as needed.

Rx	**Anaspaz** (Ascher)	**Tablets:** 0.125 mg	(225/295). In 100s, 500s.
Rx	**ED-SPAZ** (Edwards)		White, scored. In 100s.
Rx	**Donnamar** (Marnel)		In 100s.
Rx	**Gastrosed** (Roberts/Hauck)		In 100s.
Rx	**Levsin** (Schwarz Pharma Kremers Urban)		(K-U 531). White, scored. In 100s and 500s.
Rx	**Cystospaz** (Poly-Medica)	**Tablets:** 0.15 mg	(W 2225). Blue. In 100s.
Rx	**A-Spas S/L** (Hyrex)	**Tablets, sublingual:** 0.125 mg	White. In 100s.
Rx	**Levsin/SL** (Schwarz Pharma Kremers Urban)		(Schwarz 532). Blue-green, scored. Octagonal. Peppermint flavor. In 100s, 500s.
Rx	**Levbid** (Schwarz Pharma Kremers Urban)	**Tablets, extended release:** 0.375 mg	(SP538). Orange, scored. Capsule shape. In 100s.
Rx	**Cystospaz-M** (Poly-Medica)	**Capsules, timed release:** 0.375 mg	(W 2260). Blue. In 100s.
Rx	**Hyoscyamine Sulfate** (Ethex)		(Ethex /017). Clear. In 100s.
Rx	**Levsinex Timecaps** (Schwarz Pharma Kremers Urban)		(Kremers Urban 537). Brown/clear. In 100s & 500s.

Belladonna Alkaloids

L-HYOSCYAMINE SULFATE

Rx	**Hyoscyamine Sulfate** (Goldline)	**Solution:** 0.125 mg/ml	5% alcohol. In 15 ml w/dropper.
Rx	**Gastrosed** (Roberts/Hauck)		Alcohol free. In 5 ml.
Rx	**Levsin Drops** (Schwarz Pharma Kremers Urban)		5% alcohol. Sorbitol. Orange flavor. In 15 ml.
Rx	**Levsin** (Schwarz Pharma Kremers Urban)	**Elixir:** 0.125 mg/5 ml	20% alcohol. Sorbitol. Orange flavor. In pt.
Rx	**Levsin** (Schwarz Pharma Kremers Urban)	**Injection:** 0.5 mg/ml	In 1 ml amps and 10 ml[1] vials.

[1] With 1.5% benzyl alcohol and 0.1% sodium metabisulfite.

ATROPINE SULFATE

For complete prescribing information, refer to the Gastrointestinal Anticholinergics/Antispasmodics group monograph.

For information on atropine sulfate inhalation and ophthalmic preparations, refer to individual monographs.

Indications:

Antisialogogue for preanesthetic medication to prevent or reduce secretions of the respiratory tract.

Treatment of parkinsonism. Rigidity and tremor are relieved by the apparently selective depressant action.

Restore cardiac rate and arterial pressure during anesthesia when vagal stimulation produced by intra-abdominal surgical traction causes a sudden decrease in pulse rate and cardiac action.

Lessen the degree of atrioventricular heart block when increased vagal tone is a major factor in the conduction defect as in some cases due to digitalis.

Overcome severe bradycardia and syncope due to a hyperactive carotid sinus reflex.

Antidote (with external cardiac massage) for cardiovascular collapse from the injudicious use of a choline ester (cholinergic) drug, pilocarpine, physostigmine or isofluorophate.

Relieve pylorospasm, hypertonicity of small intestine and hypermotility of colon.

Relax the spasm of biliary and ureteral colic and bronchial spasm.

Relaxation of the upper GI tract and colon during hypertonic radiography.

Diminish the tone of the detrusor muscle of the urinary bladder in the treatment of urinary tract disorders.

Control the crying and laughing episodes in patients with brain lesions.

In cases of closed head injuries which cause acetylcholine to be released or to be present in cerebrospinal fluid, which in turn causes abnormal EEG patterns, stupor and neurological signs.

Relieve hypertonicity of the uterine muscle.

Management of peptic ulcer.

Control rhinorrhea of acute rhinitis or hay fever.

Poisoning: Treatment of anticholinesterase poisoning from organophosphorus insecticides; as an antidote for mushroom poisoning due to muscarine, in certain species such as *Amanita muscaria*.

Belladonna Alkaloids

ATROPINE SULFATE

Administration and Dosage:

Adults: 0.4 to 0.6 mg.

Children:

Atropine Dosage Recommendations in Children		
Weight		Dose
lb	kg	mg
7 to 16	3.2 to 7.3	0.1
16 to 24	7.3 to 10.9	0.15
24 to 40	10.9 to 18.1	0.2
40 to 65	18.1 to 29.5	0.3
65 to 90	29.5 to 40.8	0.4
> 90	40.8	0.4 to 0.6

Hypotonic radiography: 1 mg IM.

Surgery: Give SC, IM or IV. The average adult dose is 0.5 mg (range 0.4 to 0.6 mg). As an antisialogogue, it is usually injected IM prior to induction of anesthesia. In children, it has been suggested to use a dose of 0.01 mg/kg to a maximum of 0.4 mg, repeated every 4 to 6 hours as needed. A recommended infant dose is 0.04 mg/kg (infants < 5 kg) or 0.03 mg/kg (infants > 5 kg), repeated every 4 to 6 hours as needed. During surgery, the drug is given IV when reduction in pulse rate and cessation of cardiac action are due to increased vagal activity. However, if the anesthetic is cyclopropane, use doses less than 0.4 mg and give slowly to avoid production of ventricular arrhythmia. Usual doses reduce severe bradycardia and syncope associated with hyperactive carotid sinus reflex.

Bradyarrhythmias: The usual IV adult dosage ranges from 0.4 to 1 mg every 1 to 2 hours as needed; larger doses, up to a maximum of 2 mg, may be required. In children, IV dosage ranges from 0.01 to 0.03 mg/kg. Atropine is also a specific antidote for cardiovascular collapse resulting from injudicious administration of choline ester. When cardiac arrest has occurred, external cardiac massage or other method of resuscitation is required to distribute the drug after IV injection.

Poisoning: In anticholinesterase poisoning from exposure to insecticides, give large doses of at least 2 to 3 mg parenterally; repeat until signs of atropine intoxication appear. In "rapid" type of mushroom poisoning, give in doses sufficient to control parasympathomimetic signs before coma and cardiovascular collapse supervene.

Rx	**Atropine Sulfate** (Abbott)	**Injection:** 0.05 mg/ml	In 5 ml Abboject syringes.
Rx	**Atropine Sulfate** (Abbott)	**Injection:** 0.1 mg/ml	In 5 and 10 ml Abboject syringes.
Rx	**Atropine Sulfate** (Various, eg, American Regent, Burroughs Wellcome, Elkins-Sinn, Lilly, Loch, LyphoMed, Moore, Rugby, Schein, Vortech)	**Injection:** 0.3 mg/ml	In 1 and 30 ml vials.
		0.4 mg/ml	In 1 ml amps and 1, 20 and 30 ml vials.
		0.5 mg/ml	In 1 and 30 ml vials and 5 ml syringes.
		0.8 mg/ml	In 0.5 and 1 ml amps and 0.5 ml syringes.
		1 mg/ml	In 1 ml amps & vials and 10 ml syringes.
Rx	**Sal-Tropine** (Hope)	**Tablets:** 0.4 mg	In 100s.

Belladonna Alkaloids

SCOPOLAMINE HBr (Hyoscine HBr)

For complete prescribing information, refer to the Gastrointestinal Anticholinergics/Antispasmodics group monograph.

Indications:

Preanesthetic sedation and obstetric amnesia in conjunction with analgesics; also used for calming delirium.

Motion sickness (see Antiemetic/Antivertigo Agents monograph).

Administration and Dosage:

Give SC or IM; may give IV after dilution with Sterile Water for Injection.

Adults: 0.32 to 0.65 mg.

Children: 0.006 mg/kg (0.003 mg/lb). Maximum dosage, 0.3 mg.

Rx	**Scopolamine HBr** (Various, eg, Loch, LyphoMed)	**Injection:** 0.3 mg/ml	In 1 ml vials.
Rx	**Scopolamine HBr** (Various, eg, Burroughs Wellcome, LyphoMed)	**Injection:** 0.4 mg/ml	In 0.5 ml amps and 1 ml vials.
Rx	**Scopolamine HBr** (Burroughs Wellcome)	**Injection:** 0.86 mg/ml	In 0.5 ml amps.[1]
Rx	**Scopolamine HBr** (Various, eg, Loch, LyphoMed)	**Injection:** 1 mg/ml	In 1 ml vials.

[1] With alcohol and mannitol.

LEVOROTATORY ALKALOIDS OF BELLADONNA

For complete prescribing information, refer to the Gastrointestinal Anticholinergics/Antispasmodics group monograph.

Indications:

GI: Spasm; peptic ulcer; pylorospasm; spastic colitis; intestinal and biliary colic.

GU: Dysmenorrhea; renal colic; enuresis; nocturia.

Respiratory tract: Hypersecretion; bronchial asthama.

CNS: Vagal inhibition; parkinsonism (postencephalitic); motion sickness.

Administration and Dosage:

Oral:

Adults – 0.25 to 0.5 mg, 3 times daily.
Children (over 6 years) – 0.125 to 0.25 mg, 3 times daily.

Rx	**Bellafoline** (Sandoz)	**Tablets:** 0.25 mg	(Sandoz 78/30). White, scored. In 100s.

Belladonna Alkaloids

BELLADONNA

For complete prescribing information, refer to the Gastrointestinal Anticholinergics/Antispasmodics group monograph.

Belladonna, a crude botanical preparation, contains the anticholinergic alkaloids hyoscyamine (which racemizes to atropine on extraction), scopolamine (hyoscine) and other minor alkaloids. Belladonna leaf contains approximately 0.35% alkaloids. Pharmaceutical preparations of belladonna include *belladonna tincture,* which contains 27 to 33 mg alkaloids/100 ml.

Indications:

GI: As adjunctive therapy in the treatment of peptic ulcer, functional digestive disorders (including spastic, mucous and ulcerative colitis), diarrhea, diverticulitis, pancreatitis.

GU: Dysmenorrhea, nocturnal enuresis.

CNS: Parkinsonism (idiopathic and postencephalitic). Large doses may provide some symptomatic relief; tremor, rigidity, sialorrhea and oculogyric crises are reduced; posture, gait and speech are improved.

Other: Motion sickness; nausea and vomiting of pregnancy.

Administration and Dosage:

Belladonna Tincture: Adults - 0.6 to 1 ml, 3 to 4 times daily.

Children - 0.03 ml/kg (0.8 ml/m^2) 3 times daily.

Rx	**Belladonna Tincture** (Various, eg, Lannett, Life, Lilly, Rugby, Texas Drug)	**Liquid**: 27 to 33 mg belladonna alkaloids/ 100 ml	65% to 70% alcohol. In 120 ml, pt and gal.

Quaternary Anticholinergics

METHSCOPOLAMINE BROMIDE

For complete prescribing information, refer to the Gastrointestinal Anticholinergics/Antispasmodics group monograph.

Indications:

Adjunctive therapy in the treatment of peptic ulcer.

Administration and Dosage:

2.5 mg 30 minutes before meals and 2.5 to 5 mg at bedtime.

Rx	**Pamine** (Kenwood/ Bradley)	**Tablets**: 2.5 mg	White. In 100s and 500s.

ANISOTROPINE METHYLBROMIDE

For complete prescribing information, refer to the Gastrointestinal Anticholinergics/Antispasmodics group monograph.

Indications:

Adjunctive therapy in the treatment of peptic ulcer.

Administration and Dosage:

50 mg 3 times daily.

Rx	**Anisotropine Methylbromide** (Various, eg, Balan, Rugby)	**Tablets**: 50 mg	In 100s.

CLIDINIUM BROMIDE

For complete prescribing information, refer to the Gastrointestinal Anticholinergics/Antispasmodics group monograph.

Indications:

Adjunctive therapy in the treatment of peptic ulcer.

Administration and Dosage:

Adults: 2.5 to 5 mg, 3 or 4 times daily before meals and at bedtime.

Geriatric or debilitated patients: 2.5 mg, 3 times daily before meals.

Rx	**Quarzan** (Roche)	**Capsules**: 2.5 mg	(Quarzan 2.5 Roche). Green and red. In 100s.
		5 mg	(Quarzan 5.0 Roche). Green and gray. In 100s.

Quaternary Anticholinergics

GLYCOPYRROLATE

For complete prescribing information, refer to the Gastrointestinal Anticholinergics/Antispasmodics group monograph.

Indications:

Oral: Adjunctive therapy in the treatment of peptic ulcer.

Parenteral: Used preoperatively to reduce salivary, tracheobronchial and pharyngeal secretions; to reduce the volume and free acidity of gastric secretions; to block cardiac vagal inhibitory reflexes during induction of anesthesia and intubation. May be used intraoperatively to counteract drug-induced or vagal traction reflexes with the associated arrhythmias. Glycopyrrolate protects against the peripheral muscarinic effects (eg, bradycardia and excessive secretions) of cholinergic agents such as neostigmine and pyridostigmine given to reverse the neuromuscular blockade due to nondepolarizing muscle relaxants.

Administration and Dosage:

Not recommended for children under age 12 for the management of peptic ulcer.

Oral: 1 mg 3 times daily or 2 mg 2 to 3 times daily.

Maintenance – 1 mg 2 times daily.

Parenteral:

Peptic ulcer – 0.1 to 0.2 mg IM or IV 3 or 4 times daily.

Preanesthetic medication – 0.002 mg/lb (0.004 mg/kg) IM, 30 minutes to 1 hour prior to anesthesia. Children less than 2 years of age may require up to 0.004 mg/lb. Children under 12, give 0.002 to 0.004 mg/lb IM.

Intraoperative medication – Adults, 0.1 mg IV. Repeat as needed at 2 to 3 minute intervals. Children, give 0.002 mg/lb (0.004 mg/kg) IV, not to exceed 0.1 mg in a single dose; may be repeated at 2 to 3 minute intervals.

Reversal of neuromuscular blockade – Adults and children, 0.2 mg for each 1 mg neostigmine or 5 mg pyridostigmine. Administer IV simultaneously.

Rx	**Robinul** (Robins)	**Tablets:** 1 mg	(AHR 7824). White, scored. In 100s and 500s.
Rx	**Robinul Forte** (Robins)	**Tablets:** 2 mg	(AHR 2/7840). White, scored. In 100s.
Rx	**Glycopyrrolate** (Various, eg, American Regent, LyphoMed, Quad, Schein, Texas Drug, VHA)	**Injection:** 0.2 mg per ml	In 1, 2, 5 and 20 ml vials.
Rx	**Robinul** (Robins)		In 1, 2, 5 and 20 ml vials.[1]

[1] With 0.9% benzyl alcohol.

MEPENZOLATE BROMIDE

For complete prescribing information, refer to the Gastrointestinal Anticholinergics/Antispasmodics group monograph.

Indications:

Adjunctive therapy in the treatment of peptic ulcer.

Administration and Dosage:

Adults: 25 to 50 mg 4 times daily with meals and at bedtime.

Children: Safety and efficacy have not been established.

Rx	**Cantil** (Hoechst Marion Roussel)	**Tablets:** 25 mg	Tartrazine. (Merrell 37). Yellow. In 100s.

Quaternary Anticholinergics

METHANTHELINE BROMIDE

For complete prescribing information, refer to the Gastrointestinal Anticholinergics/Antispasmodics group monograph.

Indications:

Adjunctive therapy in the treatment of peptic ulcer.

Treatment of an uninhibited hypertonic neurogenic bladder.

Administration and Dosage:

Adults: 50 to 100 mg every 6 hours.

Pediatric:

Newborns – 12.5 mg 2 times daily, then 12.5 mg 3 times daily. *Infants* (1 to 12 months) –12.5 mg 4 times daily, increased to 25 mg 4 times daily. *Children* (over 1 year) – 12.5 to 50 mg 4 times daily.

Rx	**Banthine** (Schiapparelli Searle)	**Tablets:** 50 mg	(Searle 1501). Peach, scored. In 100s.

PROPANTHELINE BROMIDE

For complete prescribing information, refer to the Gastorintestinal anticholinergics/Antispasmodics group monograph.

Indications:

Adjunctive therapy in the treatment of peptic ulcer.

Unlabeled uses: Has been used for its antisecretory and antispasmodic effects.

Administration and Dosage:

Adults: 15 mg 30 minutes before meals and 30 mg at bedtime. For patients with mild manifestations, geriatric patients or those of small stature, take 7.5 mg, 3 times daily.

Children:

Peptic ulcer – Safety and efficacy have not been established.

Antisecretory – 1.5 mg/kg/day divided 3 to 4 times daily.

Antispasmodic – 2 to 3 mg/kg/day divided every 4 to 6 hours and at bedtime.

Rx	**Pro-Banthine** (Schiapparelli Searle)	**Tablets:** 7.5 mg	(Searle 611). White, sugar coated. In 100s.
	Propantheline Bromide (Various, eg, Balan, Goldline, Harber, Major, Moore, Par, Richlyn, Roxane, Rugby)	**Tablets:** 15 mg	In 100s, 500s, 1000s, and UD 100s.
	Pro-Banthine (Schiapparelli Searle)		(Searle 601) Peach, sugar coated. In 100s, 500s, and UD 100s.

TRIDIHEXETHYL CHLORIDE

For complete prescribing information, refer to the Gastrointestinal Anticholinergics/Antispasmodics group monograph.

Indications:

Adjunctive therapy in peptic ulcer treatment.

Administration and Dosage:

25 to 50 mg 3 or 4 times daily before meals and at bedtime. Bedtime dose: 50 mg.

Rx	**Pathilon** (Lederle)	**Tablets:** 25 mg	(LL/P4). Pink. Film coated. In 100s.

Antispasmodics

DICYCLOMINE HCl

For complete prescribing information, refer to the Gastrointestinal Anticholinergics/Antispasmodics group monograph.

Indications:

Treatment of functional bowel/irritable bowel syndrome (irritable colon, spastic colon, mucous colitis).

Administration and Dosage:

Oral: Adults- The only oral dose shown to be effective is 160 mg/day in 4 equally divided doses. However, because of side effects, begin with 80 mg/day (in 4 equally divided doses). Increase dose to 160 mg/day unless side effects limit dosage.

Parenteral: IM only. Not for IV use.

Adults – 80 mg/day in 4 divided doses.

Rx	**Dicyclomine HCl** (Various, eg, Bolar, Geneva, Goldline, Lederle, Major, Rugby, Schein)	**Capsules:** 10 mg	In 30s, 100s, 120s, 1000s, and UD 100s.
Rx	**Bentyl** (Hoechst Marion Roussel)		(Merrell 120/Bentyl or Bentyl 10). In 100s, 500s, and UD 100s.
Rx	**Byclomine** (Major)		In 100s, 250s, 1000s, and UD 100s.
Rx	**Di-Spaz** (Vortech)		In 1000s.
Rx	**Dicyclomine HCl** (Various, eg, Bolar, Geneva, Goldline, Lederle, Major, Rugby, Schein)	**Tablets:** 20 mg	In 15s, 20s, 30s, 100s, 120s, 250s, 1000s, and UD 100s.
Rx	**Bentyl** (Hoechst Marion Roussel)		(Merrell 123 or Bentyl 20) In 100s, 500s, 1000s, and UD 100s.
Rx	**Byclomine** (Major)		In 100s, 250s, 1000s, and UD 100s.
Rx	**Dicyclomine HCl** (Various, eg, Moore, Ritchie)	**Capsules:** 20 mg	In 100s, and 1000s.
Rx	**Dicyclomine HCl** (Various, eg, Gen-King, Goldline, Harber, Moore, Qualitest, Rugby, Schein)	**Syrup:** 10 mg/5 ml	In 118 ml, pt, and gal.
Rx	**Bentyl** (Hoechst Marion Roussel)		Saccharin in pt.
Rx	**Dicyclomine HCl** (Various, eg, Baxter, Goldline, Major, Moore, Ritchie, Rugby, Schein, Steris)	**Injection:** 10 mg/ml	In 2 and 10 ml vials.
Rx	**Antispas** (Keene)		In 10 ml vials.[1]
Rx	**Bentyl** (Hoechst Marion Roussel)		In 2 ml amps and 10 ml vials.[1]
Rx	**Dibent** (Hauck)		In 10 ml vials.[1]
Rx	**Dilomine** (Kay Drug)		In 10 ml vials.[1]
Rx	**Di-Spaz** (Vortech)		In 10 ml vials.[1]
Rx	**Or-Tyl** (Ortega)		In 10 ml vials.[1]

Antispasmodics

OXYPHENCYCLIMINE HCl

For complete prescribing information, refer to the Gastrointestinal Anticholinergics/Antispasmodics group monograph.

Indications:

Adjunctive therapy in the treatment of peptic ulcer.

Administration and Dosage:

Adults: 5 to 10 mg 2 or 3 times daily, preferably in the morning and at bedtime. Some respond to 5 mg 2 times day, while some may require higher dosage 3 times day.

Children: Not for use in children less than 12 years of age.

Rx	**Daricon** (Beecham Labs)	**Tablets:** 10 mg	White, scored. In 60s and 500s.	597

GASTROINTESTINAL ANTICHOLINERGIC COMBINATIONS

GASTROINTESTINAL ANTICHOLINERGIC COMBINATIONS

Refer to the general discussion of these products in the GI Anticholinergics/Antispasmodics group monograph.

Combination anticholinergic preparations may include the following components:

SEDATIVES and ANTIANXIETY AGENTS. See: Barbiturates, Prochlorperazine, Hydroxyzine, Meprobamate, Chlordiazepoxide.

ERGOTAMINE TARTRATE provides inhibition of the sympathetic nervous system.

GI ANTICHOLINERGIC COMBINATIONS, CAPSULES AND TABLETS

Refer to the general discussion of these products in the GI Anticholinergics/Antispasmodics group monograph.

Content given per tablet or capsule.

	Product and Distributor	Anticholinergic	Sedative, Antianxiety Agent or Other	Daily Dose (Tablets)	How Supplied
Rx	**Barbidonna No. 2 Tablets** (Wallace)	0.025 mg atropine sulfate 0.0074 mg scopolamine HBr 0.1286 mg hyoscyamine sulfate	32 mg phenobarbital	3	Lactose. (Wallace 311). Lt. brown, scored. In 100s.
Rx	**Barbidonna Tablets** (Wallace)	0.025 mg atropine sulfate 0.0074 mg scopolamine HBr 0.1286 mg hyoscyamine sulfate	16 mg phenobarbital	3 to 6	Lactose. (Wallace 301). White, scored. In 100s and 500s.
Rx	**Belladonna Alkaloids w/Phenobarbital Tablets** (Various, eg, Goldline, Major, Westward)	0.0194 mg atropine sulfate 0.0065 mg scopolamine HBr 0.1037 mg hyoscyamine HBr or sulfate	16.2 mg phenobarbital	3 to 8	In 50s, 100s, 1000s and UD 100s.
Rx	**Donnatal Capsules and Tablets** (Robins)				**Capsules**: Lactose, sucrose. (AHR 4207). Green and white. In 100s and 1000s. **Tablets**: Lactose, sucrose. (R). White, scored. In 100s, 1000s and Dis-Co pack 100s.
Rx	**Hyosophen Tablets** (Rugby)				(Rugby 3920). White, scored. In 100s and 1000s.
Rx	**Malatal Tablets** (Hauck)				In 1000s.
Rx	**Spasmolin Tablets** (Various, eg, Global)				In 100s and 1000s.
Rx	**Butibel Tablets** (Wallace)	15 mg belladonna extract	15 mg butabarbital sodium	4 to 8	(Butibel 37/046). Red. In 100s.
Rx	**Chardonna-2 Tablets** (Schwarz Pharma Kremers Urban)	15 mg belladonna extract	15 mg phenobarbital	3 to 8	(KU 202). Gray. In 100s.

GI ANTICHOLINERGIC COMBINATIONS, CAPSULES AND TABLETS

	Product and Distributor	Anticholinergic	Sedative, Antianxiety Agent or Other	Daily Dose (Tablets)	How Supplied
Rx	**Levsin w/Phenobarbital Tablets** (Schwarz Pharma Kremers Urban)	0.125 mg hyoscyamine sulfate	15 mg phenobarbital	3 to 8	(KU 534). Pink, scored. In 100s.
Rx	**Bellacane Tablets** (Treiner Co)				In 100s.
Rx	**Chlordiazepoxide w/Clidinium Bromide Capsules** (Various, eg, Eon, Goldline, Major, Moore, Schein)	2.5 mg clidinium	5 mg chlordiazepoxide HCl	3 to 8	In 100s, 500s, 1000s and UD 100s.
Rx	**Clindex Capsules** (Rugby)				Lactose. (Rugby 3490). White. In 100s, 250s, 500s and 1000s.
Rx	**Librax Capsules** (Roche)				Parabens, lactose. Green. In 100s, 500s and Tel-E-Dose 100s.
Rx	**Phenerbel-S Tablets** (Rugby)	0.2 mg l-alkaloids of belladonna	40 mg phenobarbital, 0.6 mg ergotamine tartrate	2	(Rugby/4234). In 100s.
Rx	**Bellergal-S Tablets** (Sandoz)				Lactose,sucrose, tartrazine. (78-31) Green, orange and yellow. In 100s.

GI ANTICHOLINERGIC COMBINATIONS, TABLETS, SUSTAINED RELEASE

Refer to the general discussion of these products in the GI Anticholinergics/Antispasmodics group monograph.

Content given per tablet.

	Product and Distributor	Anticholinergic	Sedative or Antianxiety Agent	Other Content	Daily Dose (Tablets)	How Supplied
Rx	**Donnatal Extentabs** (Robins)	0.0582 mg atropine sulfate, 0.0195 mg scopolamine HBr, 0.3111 mg hyoscyamine sulfate	48.6 mg phenobarbital	Sucrose	2 to 3	(AHR Donnatal Extentab). Green. In 100s, 500s and UD 100s.
Rx	**Bel-Phen-Ergot SR Tablets** (Goldline)	0.2 mg l-alkaloids of belladonna	40 mg phenobarbital, 0.6 mg ergotamine tartrate	Lactose	2	In 100s.
Rx	**Bellacane SR Tablets** (Treiner Co)					In 100s.

GI ANTICHOLINERGIC COMBINATIONS, LIQUIDS

Refer to the general discussion of these products at the beginning of the GI Anticholinergics/Antispasmodics group monograph.

Content given per 5 ml liquid and 1 ml drops.

	Product and Distributor	Anticholinergic	Sedative	Other Content	Daily Dose	How Supplied
Rx	**Donnatal Elixir** (Robins)	0.0194 mg atropine sulfate, 0.0065 mg scopolamine HBr, 0.1037 mg hyoscyamine HBr or sulfate	16.2 mg phenobarbital	23% alcohol, glucose, saccharin	15 to 40 ml *Children*: 4.5 kg to 45.4 kg - 0.5 to 5 ml q4h or 0.75 to 7.5 ml q6h, respectively	Green. Citrus flavor. In 120 ml, pt, gal and Dis-Co pack 5 ml (100s).
Rx	**Hyosophen Elixir** (Rugby)			23% alcohol, sugar, sorbitol		In 120 ml, pt and gal.
Rx	**Antispasmodic Elixir**[1] (Various, eg, Goldline, Halsey, Moore, Qualitest, RID, UDL)					In 120 ml, pt and gal.
Rx	**Susano Elixir** (Halsey)			23% alcohol, tartrazine		Green. Lime flavor. In pt and gal.
Rx	**Bellacane Elixir** (Treiner Co)					In pt and gal.

GASTROINTESTINAL ANTICHOLINERGIC COMBINATIONS

GI ANTICHOLINERGIC COMBINATIONS, LIQUIDS

	Product and Distributor	Anticholinergic	Sedative	Other Content	Daily Dose	How Supplied
Rx	**Butibel Elixir** (Wallace)	15 mg belladonna extract	15 mg butabarbital sodium	7% alcohol, sucrose, saccharin	20 to 40 ml. *Children* ≥ *6* - 10 ml; *Children* < *6* - 5 to 10 ml	Orange flavor. In pt.
Rx sf	**Antrocol Elixir** (ECR)	0.195 mg atropine sulfate	16 mg phenobarbital	20% alcohol	15 to 40 ml. *Children* - 0.5 ml per 15 lbs every 4 to 6 hours	In pt.
Rx	**Levsin PB Drops** (Schwarz Pharma KU)	0.125 mg hyoscyamine sulfate	15 mg phenobarbital	5% alcohol	6 to 12 ml. *Children 2 to 12* – 1 to 6 ml	Red. Cherry flavor. In 15 ml.

[1] May contain alcohol.

H. PYLORI AGENTS

Helicobacter pylori is found in ≈ 100% of chronic active antral gastritis cases, 90% to 95% of duodenal ulcer patients and 50% to 80% of gastric ulcer patients. The treatment of documented *H. pylori* infection in patients with confirmed peptic ulcer on first presentation or recurrence has been recommended by the National Institutes of Health in a 1994 Consensus Conference. Once *H. pylori* eradication has been achieved, reinfection rates are < 0.5% per year, and ulcer recurrence rates are dramatically reduced.

Numerous clinical trials have been done to determine the optimal regimen for *H. pylori* eradication, but there remains no golden standard of therapy to date. When selecting a regimen, take into account efficacy, tolerability, compliance and cost. Consideration of these factors will aid in selection of the most appropriate regimen. *H. pylori* is easily suppressed but, to ensure successful eradication, requires the use of two antimicrobial agents with either a bismuth compound, an antisecretory agent or both. These combinations have been shown to enhance *H. pylori* cure, shorten the duration of treatment and decrease treatment failure due to antimicrobial resistance.

The following is a brief description of the individual agents used in *H. pylori* eradication regimens and their role in eradication. Consult the individual drug monographs for complete prescribing information.

Amoxicillin: 500 mg 4 times daily.

This agent works by inhibiting the synthesis of bacterial cell walls. It demonstrates topical activity and is stable in an acid environment but is most active at a neutral pH. *H. pylori* is very sensitive to amoxicillin both in vitro and in vivo. Bacterial resistance to amoxicillin has not been reported. More common adverse effects include diarrhea, along with other GI effects, and hypersensitivity or allergic reactions. Take without regard to meals.

Tetracycline: 500 mg 4 times daily.

This agent works by inhibiting bacterial protein synthesis. It acts topically and is active at a low pH. *H. pylori* is very sensitive to tetracycline. Bacterial resistance to tetracycline has not been reported. Adverse effects include diarrhea, along with other GI effects, esophageal ulcers and photosensitivity reactions. Take on an empty stomach with plenty of water. Do not give simultaneously with dairy products (eg, milk, cheese), antacids, laxatives or iron-containing products. If these agents are used, take them at least 2 hours before or after tetracycline.

Metronidazole: 250 mg 4 times daily.

The exact mechanism of this agent is not well understood. It demonstrates selective toxicity to anaerobic or microaerophilic microorganisms and for anoxic or hypoxic cells. The drug diffuses into the cells and leads to the development of compounds that bind to DNA and inhibit synthesis, causing cell death. The activity of metronidazole is relatively independent of pH. Resistance is very high in areas of the world where it is used frequently for other indications because organisms with defective nitroreductase activity are readily resistant to metronidazole. Resistance develops less often when metronidazole is given with bismuth or a second antimicrobial agent, Adverse effects of metronidazole include peripheral neuropathy, metallic taste, nausea and a disulfiram-type reaction manifested by flushing, tachycardia, nausea, vomiting and other GI symptoms when used with alcohol. Metronidazole can be taken with food to minimize GI upset.

Clarithromycin: 500 mg 2 or 3 times daily.

Clarithromycin is a macrolide antibiotic that inhibits bacterial protein synthesis. It is more acid stable than erythromycin, better absorbed and more effective against *H. pylori*. Resistance can develop when clarithromycin is used alone. Adverse effects include diarrhea, abnormal taste and nausea. Clarithromycin may be taken without regard to meals.

Bismuth: 525 mg 4 times daily.

Bismuth compounds are topical compounds that disrupt the integrity of bacterial cell walls. The mechanism and role of bismuth in *H. pylori* eradication is multifactorial. Bismuth compounds are thought to lyse *H. pylori* near the gastric surface; prevent the adhesion of *H. pylori* to the gastric epithelium; inhibit its urease, phospholipase and proteolytic activity; and decrease resistance development when used with antimicrobial agents such as metronidazole. Adverse effects of bismuth compounds may include a temporary and harmless darkening of the tongue and stool, diarrhea and the potential for CNS toxicities when used in high doses. Take bismuth compounds without regard to meals.

Antisecretory agents (H_2 antagonists, Proton pump inhibitors): Provide rapid symptom relief and accelerated ulcer healing when used with antimicrobial agents for *H. pylori* eradication. Proton pump inhibitors may have a direct effect on inhibiting the growth of *H. pylori* and also appear to have a synergistic effect when combined with antimicrobial agents.

H. PYLORI AGENTS

Eradication of H. pylori:

Single antimicrobial agents: Monotherapy is not recommended because of the potential for the development of antimicrobial resistance.

Dual therapy:

Proton pump inhibitors plus amoxicillin – Significant variation exists among numerous studies that have been conducted to date with eradication rates ranging from 30% to 80%. Therefore, dual therapy with these two agents is not recommended.

Proton pump inhibitors plus clarithromycin – A number of studies have looked at the use of these agents in combination for *H. pylori* eradication, and the overall eradication appears to be ≈ 71%. Currently, the American College of Gastroenterology recommends adding a second antimicrobial agent to this regimen to enhance successful eradication.

Double antimicrobial therapy plus an antisecretory drug:

Regimens Used in the Eradication of *H. pylori* [1]

Regimen	Dosing	Duration	Eradication
Metronidazole Omeprazole Clarithromycin	500 mg twice daily with meals 20 mg twice daily with meals 500 mg twice daily with meals	1 week	87% to 91%
Amoxicillin Omeprazole Clarithromycin	1 g twice daily with meals 20 mg twice daily before meals 500 mg twice daily with meals	1 to 2 weeks	77% to 83%
Metronidazole Omeprazole Amoxicillin	500 mg twice daily with meals 20 mg twice daily before meals 1 g twice daily with meals	1 to 2 weeks	77% to 83%

[1] Extending therapy to 10 to 14 days in the above regimens may provide additional benefit. Histamine$_2$ blockers may be used with two antibiotics, but a longer treatment course (10 to14 days), higher antibiotic doses and 3 times daily administration are required.

Triple-therapy regimens: These regimens have proved to be very effective in eradicating *H. pylori.* The primary disadvantage of these regimens is compliance because of the variety and number of medications used. Likewise, adverse effects are more common in patients taking these regimens compared with alternatives.

Regimens Used in the Eradication of *H. Pylori* [1]

Regimen	Dosing	Duration	Eradication
Bismuth subsalicylate Metronidazole Tetracycline	525 mg 4 times daily with meals and at bedtime 250 mg 4 times daily with meals and at bedtime 500 mg 4 times daily	2 weeks 1 week	88% to 90% 86% to 90%
Bismuth subsalicylate Metronidazole Tetracycline Omeprazole	525 mg 4 times daily with meals and at bedtime 250 mg 4 times daily with meals and at bedtime 500 mg 4 times daily 20 mg 2 times daily before meals	1 week	94% to 98%
Bismuth subsalicylate Metronidazole Amoxicillin	525 mg 4 times daily with meals and at bedtime 250 mg 4 times daily with meals and at bedtime 500 mg 4 times daily with meals and at bedtime	2 weeks 1 week	80% to 86% 75% to 81%

[1] One week of 4 times daily therapy may be sufficient in the absence of antibiotic resistance. Adding a proton pump inhibitor facilitates shorter treatment periods. Until more data is available, the use of H_2 antagonists or proton pump inhibitors with the above regimens is appropriate to enhance ulcer healing and provide symptomatic relief.

Quadruple therapy regimens (two antibiotics, bismuth, antisecretory agent): Like triple therapy regimens these have proven to be effective in *H. pylori* eradication. The primary disadvantage of these regimens is compliance. In addition, because of the variety and number of medications used, adverse effects are more common in patients taking these regimens compared with alternatives.

H. PYLORI AGENTS

FDA Approved Regimens for the Eradication of *H. pylori*			
Regimen	Dosing	Eradication	Comments
Omeprazole Clarithromycin	40 mg once daily followed by a 2-week course of 20 mg once daily 500 mg 3 times daily for 2 weeks	64% to 74%	The American College of Gastroenterology recommends that either tetracycline or amoxicillin be added to this regimen.
Ranitidine bismuth citrate Clarithromycin	400 mg twice daily for 4 weeks 500 mg 3 times daily for 2 weeks	82%	The American College of Gastroenterology recommends that either tetracycline or amoxicillin be added to this regimen.
Metronidazole Tetracycline HCl Bismuth subsalicylate	250 mg 4 times daily at meals and bedtime 500 mg 4 times daily at meals and bedtime 525 mg 4 timesa day at meals and bedtime	82%	*Helidac* therapy combines bismuth subsalicylate, metronidazole and tetracycline in a consumer-tested, patient-friendly kit.

Practice Guidelines from the American College of Gastroenterology: In the 1996 Consensus Statement on Medical Treatment of Peptic Ulcer Disease, the American College of Gastroenterolog does not recommend single-antibiotic combinations of either clarithromycin or amoxicillin with proton pump inhibitors because efficacy is < 70% (cure), and a high-dose, 2–week treatment period is required. The Consensus Statement recommends a two-antibioic combination of clarithromycin, metronidazole or amoxicillin in regimens that do not employ a bismuth compound. In addition, the American College of Gastroenterology suggests adding either tetracycline or amoxicillin to the recently approved ranitidine-bismuth citrate-clarithromycin combination to enhance successful *H. pylori* eradication. Combining a proton pump inhibitor, either omeprazole or lansoprazole, with two antibiotics is thought to enhance effectiveness and allow for a shorter duration of treatment.

There are a number of factors that limit the effectiveness of regimens designed to eradicate *H. pylori*. The first, antibiotic resistance, is seen with metronidazole and clarithromycin but has not been reported with bismuth, amoxicillin or tetracycline. Because prior antibiotic exposure predicts drug resistance in individuals, take this factor into consideration when selecting a regimen. Although data are limited, studies have demonstrated that eradication of *H. pylori* is possible with metronidazole-containing regimens despite the presence of resistant organisms, but eradication rates are significantly lower. Alternatively, the American College of Gastroenterology suggests possible drug regimens to employ in cases of metronidazole resistance. These include, bismuth, clarithromycin and tetracycline or omeprazole, amoxicillin and clarithromycin. On the other hand, clarithromycin resistance is more bothersome because resistant organisms do not respond favorably to clarithromycin-containing regimens.

Second, mild adverse effects (eg, diarrhea, metallic taste, black stools) do occur in ≈ 30% to 50% of patients. Therefore, shorter treatment periods in this group of patients may be better tolerated.

Finally, patient compliance is often a problem because of cumbersome regimens and adverse effects.

Maintenance therapy with antisecretory agents: Limited data exist regarding the role of maintenance therapy in *H. pylori* eradication. Currently, it is advisable to continue maintenance until *H. pylori* cure has been confirmed in patients with a history of complications, frequent or troublesome recurrences or refractory ulcers.

Confirming successful eradication is important in patients with a history of complicated or refractory ulcers but is controversial in those with uncomplicated ulcers who remain asymptomatic after therapy.

Refractory ulcers in patients receiving antibiotic therapy for H. pylori eradication is often due to failure to successfully eradicate *H. pylori* infection. Resistance patterns, as well as noncompliance, and concurrent NSAID use may play a role in refractory cases.

RANITIDINE BISMUTH CITRATE

For complete pharmacology, refer to the Histamine H_2 Antagonists group monograph.

Actions:

Pharmacokinetics:

Absorption – Following ingestion, ranitidine bismuth citrate dissociates in intragastric fluid, giving rise to ranitidine and soluble and insoluble forms of bismuth.

Following a single oral 400 mg dose of ranitidine bismuth citrate to healthy volunteers, mean peak ranitidine plasma concentration of 455 ng/ml occurred at 0.5 to 5 hours. The rate and extent of absorption of ranitidine derived from ranitidine bismuth citrate increased proportionally with increasing doses up to 1600 mg. Ranitidine plasma concentrations showed no evidence of accumulation during a 28–day dosing period.

Oral absorption of bismuth is variable. A mean peak bismuth plasma concentration of 3.3 ng/ml occurs at 15 to 60 minutes after a 400 mg dose. The rate and extent of absorption of bismuth from ranitidine bismuth citrate do not increase with increasing doses up to 800 mg but increase more than proportionally with increasing doses above 800 mg. The rate of absorption of bismuth derived from an 800 mg dose of ranitidine bismuth citrate is decreased by 50%, and the extent of absorption is decreased by 25% when taken 30 minutes after a meal compared with 30 minutes before a meal. The absorption of bismuth from an 800 mg dose of ranitidine bismuth citrate increased when gastric pH exceeded 6. The increased pH resulted from the administration of an 800 mg dose of ranitidine bismuth citrate given 3 hours previously. Mucosal penetration and absorption of bismuth from ranitidine bismuth citrate is not affected by the degree of gastritis, the presence of *Helicobacter pylori* or an active ulcer. Small amounts of bismuth accumulate in plasma during twice-daily dosing with ranitidine bismuth citrate. In a 28–day study at 800 mg twice a day (twice the recommended daily dose), peak bismuth concentrations did not exceed 20 ng/ml at any time in any patient, with a median peak concentration of 6.3 ng/ml on day 28. Median peak and trough concentrations on day 28 were 105% and 68% of predicted steady-state peak and trough concentrations. In a study of 400 mg twice a day for 12 weeks (3 times the recommended duration), trough bismuth concentrations did not exceed predicted accumulation in any patient, and a median trough concentration of 2.8 ng/ml at week 12.

Distribution – The volume of distribution for ranitidine is 1.7 L/kg. Serum protein binding of ranitidine averages 15%. Bismuth is 98% bound to human plasma proteins, primarily albumin.

Metabolism – Ranitidine is metabolized to the N-oxide, S-oxide and N-desmethyl metabolites, accounting for ≈ 4%, 1% and 1% of the dose, respectively. It is not known whether bismuth undergoes any biotransformation.

Excretion – The elimination half-life of ranitidine derived from ranitidine bismuth citrate is 2.8 to 3.1 hours. The principal route of elimination for ranitidine is renal, accounting for 30% of the dose. Renal clearance averages 530 ml/min, indicating active tubular secretion. Total clearance is 760 ml/min. Elimination of bismuth is polyexponential, with a terminal elimination half-life of 11 to 28 days. Bismuth has an average renal clearance of 30 to 60 ml/min, indicating net tubular secretion. Less than 1% of bismuth derived from ranitidine bismuth citrate is recovered in urine after oral administration. Up to 28% of bismuth was recovered in the feces during a 6–day postdose period. Bismuth also undergoes minor excretion in the bile.

Renal impairment: The renal clearance of ranitidine and bismuth are correlated with renal function (eg, creatinine clearance). Ranitidine and bismuth concentrations may be elevated in renally impaired patients as a result of decreased renal elimination.

Clinical trials:

Eradication of H. pylori associated with active duodenal ulcer – Ranitidine bismuth citrate alone and in combination with clarithromycin was evaluated in two double-blind, randomized, multicenter, placebo controlled trials. oF 409 patients enrolled, 265 had *H. pylori* infection and active duodenal ulcer prior to the study. Ranitidine bismuth citrate 400 mg twice a day for 4 weeks plus clarithromycin 500 mg 3 times a day for the first 2 weeks was found to have a significantly higher *H. pylori* eradication rate when compared with clarithromycin 500 mg 3 times a day for 2 weeks, ranitidine bismuth citrate 400 mg twice a day for 4 weeks or placebo.

Indications:

Active duodenal ulcers: Ranitidine bismuth citrate in combination with clarithromycin is indicated for the treatment of patients with an active duodenal ulcer associated with *H. pylori* infection. The eradication of *H. pylori* has been demonstrated to reduce the risk of duodenal ulcer recurrence.

Do not prescribe ranitidine bismuth citrate alone for the treatment of active duodenal ulcer.

RANITIDINE BISMUTH CITRATE

Contraindications:

Hypersensitivity to ranitidine bismuth citrate or any of its ingredients; hangover.

Warnings:

Clarithromycin therapy: It is recommended that all patients not eradicated of *H. pylori* following ranitidine bismuth citrate plus clarithromycin treatment be considered to have *H. pylori* resistant to clarithromycin. Patients who fail to respond to therapy should not be re-treated with a regimen containing clarithromycin.

Elderly: Ulcer healing and relapse rates in elderly patients (≥ 65 years of age) were no different from those in younger age groups. The incidence rate for adverse events and laboratory abnormalities also were not different from those seen in other age groups. In a pharmacokinetic study, serum levels of ranitidine were increased in elderly patients, but serum bismuth levels were equivalent to those seen in the overall population.

Pregnancy: Category C.

Combination therapy with clarithromycin – There are no adequate and well controlled studies in pregnant women. Do not use clarithromycin in pregnant women except in clinical circumstances where no alternative therapy is appropriate. If pregnancy occurs while taking this drug, apprise the patient of the hazard to the fetus.

Teratology studies have been performed in pregnant rats at oral doses up to 1800 mg/kg/day (18 times the recommended human dose based on body surface area) and pregnant rabbits at oral doses up to 300 mg/kg/day (6 times the recommended human dose based on body surface area) and have revealed no evidence of harm to the fetus due to ranitidine bismuth citrate.

Five patients became pregnant while they were receiving ranitidine bismuth citrate alone at varied doses. Three of these patients had normal pregnancies and newborns, one had a voluntary abortion and one delivered a baby with postaxial polydactyly. This Caucasian woman had a history of unexplained spontaneous abortions. She had received ranitidine bismuth citrate for 7 days prior to conception and for 20 days after conception. The investigator considered the event unrelated to ranitidine bismuth citrate.

Because animal reproduction studies are not always predictive of human response, this drug should be used during pregnancy only if clearly needed.

Lactation: It is not known whether ranitidine bismuth citrate is excreted in breast milk. Exercise caution when ranitidine bismuth citrate is administered to a nursing woman. Both ranitidine and bismuth are excreted in rat milk.

Children: Safety and efficacy of ranitidine bismuth citrate plus clarithromycin in children have not been established.

Precautions:

Darkening of the tongue: The bismuth derived from ranitidine bismuth citrate may cause a temporary and harmless darkening of the tongue or stool. Stool darkening should not be confused with melena (blood in the stool).

Porphyria: Ranitidine bismuth citrate in combination with clarithromycin should not be used in patients with a history of acute porphyria.

Renal function impairment: This combination therapy is not recommended in patients with creatinine clearance < 25 ml/min. (See Administration and Dosage.)

Urine tests: False-positive tests for urine protein with *Multistix* may occur during ranitidine therapy; therefore, testing with sulfosalicylic acid is recommended.

RANITIDINE BISMUTH CITRATE

Drug Interactions:

Ranitidine Bismuth Citrate Drug Interactions			
Precipitant drug	Object drug*		Description
Antacid	Ranitidine bismuth citrate	⬇	Coadministration with a high dose of antacid (170 mEq) results in a 28% decrease in plasma concentrations of ranitidine and may decrease plasma concentrations of bismuth from ranitidine bismuth citrate.
Clarithromycin	Ranitidine bismuth citrate	⬆	Coadministration of ranitidine bismuth citrate with clarithromycin resulted in increased plasma ranitidine concentrations (57%), increased plasma bismuth trough concentrations (48%) and increased 14-hydroxy-clarithromycin plasma concentrations (31%).
Ranitidine bismuth citrate	Aspirin	⬇	Coadministration with aspirin results in a slightly decreased rate of salicylate absorption that is clinically unimportant.

* ⬆ = Object drug increased. ⬇ = Object drug decreased.

For information on drug interactions associated with ranitidine, refer to the Histamine H_2 Antagonists monograph.

Adverse Reactions:

Ranitidine Bismuth Citrate Adverse Reactions[1] (%)				
Adverse Reaction	Placebo (n = 469)	Ranitidine bismuth citrate tablets 800 mg (n = 903)	Clarithromycin 1500 mg (n = 120)	Ranitidine bismuth citrate tablets 800 mg + Clarithromycin 1500 mg (n = 120)
GI				
Diarrhea	1	2	5	8
Nausea and vomiting	1	< 1	2	3
Constipation	< 1	1	0	0
CNS				
Headache	< 1	1	<1	5
Dizziness	< 1	< 1	2	0
Dermatologic				
Pruritus	0	< 1	0	3
GU				
Gynecological problems	0	< 1	6	3
Miscellaneous				
Taste disturbance	< 1	< 1	11	10
Sleep disorder	< 1	< 1	< 1	2
Chest symptoms	< 1	0	0	2

[1] Total daily doses.

Adverse reactions occurring in < 1% of patients included:

CNS: Tremors (rare). The relationship of this reaction to ranitidine bismuth citrate has been unclear.

GI: Abdominal discomfort, gastric pain.

Hepatic: Transient changes in the liver enzymes.

Hypersensitivity: Rash, anaphylaxis (rare).

For information on adverse reactions associated with ranitidine, refer to the Histamine H_2 Antagonists monograph.

Overdosage:

There has been limited experience with overdosage. Adverse events related to overdosage with ranitidine are usually reversible, nonspecific and non-life threatening and result in no adverse sequelae. Although not seen in clinical trials with ranitidine bismuth citrate, bismuth intoxication from prolonged overdosage or deliberate self-poisoning can result in neurotoxicity and nephrotoxicity and possibly other symptoms seen with the use of soluble bismuth compounds. In the event of an overdose or suspected bismuth toxicity, measures should be employed to remove unab-

RANITIDINE BISMUTH CITRATE

sorbed material from the GI tract, and symptom monitoring and other supportive therapy should be employed, if indicated.

Administration and Dosage:

Approved by the FDA on August 8, 1996.

Eradication of H. pylori infection: The recommended dosage of ranitidine bismuth citrate is 400 mg twice a day for 4 weeks in conjunction with clarithromycin 500 mg 3 times a day for the first 2 weeks. Ranitidine bismuth citrate and clarithromycin can be taken with or without food.

Ranitidine Bismuth Citrate Dosing Regimen

Days 1 to 14	Days 15 to 28
Ranitidine bismuth citrate 400 mg twice a day + clarithromycin 500 mg 3 times a day	Ranitidine bismuth citrate 400 mg twice a day

Renal function impairment: Because the principal route of excretion is renal, exercise care when administering this combination therapy to renally impaired patients. This combination therapy is not recommended in patients with creatinine clearance < 25 ml/min.

Storage/Stability: Store between 2° and 30°C (36° and 86°F) in a dry place. Protect from light.

Rx	**Tritec** (Glaxo Wellcome)	**Tablet**: 400 mg	(Tritec) Blue. Film coated, elongated. Octagonal shape. In 100s and UD 100s.

BISMUTH SUBSALICYLATE, METRONIDAZOLE AND TETRACYCLINE HCl COMBINATION

For more information, refer to the *H. pylori* agents and individual monographs.

Actions:

Pharmacokinetics: There is no information about the gastric mucosal concentrations of bismuth, metronidazole and tetracycline after administration of these agents concomitantly or in combination with an acid suppressive agent. The systemic pharmacokinetic information presented below is based on studies in which each product was administered alone.

Bismuth subsalicylate – Upon oral administration, bismuth subsalicylate is almost completely hydrolyzed in the GI tract to bismuth and salicylic acid.

Less than 1% of bismuth from oral doses of bismuth subsalicylate is absorbed from the GI tract into systemic circulation. Absorbed bismuth is distributed throughout the body and is highly bound to plasma proteins (> 90%). Bismuth has multiple dispositon half-lives with an intermediate half-life of 5 to 11 days and a terminal half-life of 21 to 72 days. Elimination is primarily through urinary and biliary routes with a 50 ml/min renal clearance. The mean trough blood bismuth concentration after 2 weeks of 787 mg bismuth subsalicylate 4 times daily under fasting conditions was 5.1 ng/ml. In another study, the mean trough blood bismuth concentration after 2 weeks oral administration of 525 mg 4 times daily was 5 ng/ml with the highest value being 32 ng/ml.

More than 80% of the salicylic acid is absorbed from oral doses of bismuth subsalicylate chewable tablets. Salicylic acid is ≈ 90% plasma protein bound. The volume of distribution is ≈ 170 ml/kg. Salicylic acid is extensively metabolized, and ≈ 10% is excreted unchanged in the urine. The terminal half-life of salicylic acid following a single oral dose of 525 mg bismuth subsalicylate is between 2 and 5 hours; the mean peak plasma salicylic acid concentration was 13.1 mcg/ml under fasting conditions. The mean steady-state serum total salicylate concentration after 2 weeks oral administration of 525 mg bismuth subsalicylate 4 times daily was 24 mcg/ml with the highest value being 70 mcg/ml.

Metronidazole – Following oral administration, metronidazole is well absorbed with peak plasma concentrations occurring between 1 and 2 hours after administration. Plasma concentrations of metronidazole are proportional to the administered dose, with 250 mg producing a peak plasma concentration of 6 mcg/ml.

Metronidazole is the major component appearing in the plasma, with lesser quantities of the 2-hydroxymethyl metabolite also being present. Less than 20% is bound to plasma proteins. Metronidazole also appears in cerebrospinal fluid, saliva and breast milk in concentrations similar to those found in plasma. The average elimination half-life is 8 hours. The major elimination route of metronidazole and its metabolites is via the urine (60% to 80% of the dose), with fecal excretion accounting for 6% to 15% of the dose. The metabolites that appear in the urine result primarily from side-chain oxidation and glucuronide conjugation, with unchanged metronidazole accounting for ≈ 20% of the total. Renal clearance is ≈ 10 ml/min/1.73 m^2.

Decreased renal function does not alter the single-dose pharmacokinetics of metronidazole. In patients with decreased liver function, plasma clearance of metronidazole is decreased.

Tetracycline HCl – Tetracyclines are readily absorbed and are bound to plasma proteins in varying degrees. They are concentrated by the liver in the bile and excreted in the urine and feces at high concentrations in a biologically active form.

The relative contribution of systemic vs local antimicrobial activity against *H. pylori* for agents used in eradication therapy has not been established.

Microbiology: Bismuth subsalicylate, metronidazole and tetracycline individually have demonstrated in vitro activity against most susceptible strains of *H. pylori* isolated from patients with duodenal ulcers. (See *H. pylori* introduction.)

Metronidazole – Metronidazole resistance has been increasing in the US and mostly occurs in patients previously treated with metronidazole. Some *H. pylori* strains isolated from patients treated with bismuth, metronidazole and tetracycline demonstrate an increase in metronidazole minimum inhibitory concentrations, indicating decreasing susceptibility and increasing resistance.

It is recommended that all patients not eradicated of *H. pylori* following bismuth subsalicylate, metronidazole and tetracycline treatment be considered to have *H. pylori* resistance to metronidazole. Patients who fail therapy should not be retreated with a regimen containing metronidazole.

Clinical trials: A long-term study treated patients for active duodenal ulcer and frequently monitored them for ulcer recurrence for ≤ 1 year after therapy. This study compared patients who received bismuth subsalicylate (BSS), metronidazole (MTZ) and tetracycline (TCN) with ranitidine for 2 weeks with those who received ranitidine alone.

BISMUTH SUBSALICYLATE, METRONIDAZOLE AND TETRACYCLINE HCl COMBINATION

Duodenal Ulcer Recurrence Rates at 6 Months: Combination Therapy vs Ranitidine[1]		
Therapy	All patients	*H. pylori* negative patients post-treatment
BSS/MTZ/TCN + ranitidine	4% (1/25)	6% (1/18)
Ranitidine alone	85% (17/20)	100% (1/1)

[1] Includes all patients randomized to therapy who were *H. pylori* positive at baseline who had ulcer healing and 24 or 48 weeks of endoscopic follow-up data.

Duodenal Ulcer Recurrence Rates at 1 Year: Combination Therapy vs Ranitidine[1]		
Therapy	All patients	*H. pylori* negative patients post-treatment
BSS/MTZ/TCN + ranitidine	9% (2/22)	13% (2/16)
Ranitidine alone	95% (18/19)	100% (1/1)

[1] Includes all patients randomized to therapy who were *H. pylori* positive at baseline who had ulcer healing and 24 or 48 weeks of endoscopic follow-up data.

Indications:

Active duodenal ulcer: Bismuth subsalicylate, metronidazole and tetracycline, in combination with an H_2 antagonist, are indicated for the treatment of patients with an active duodenal ulcer associated with *H. pylori* infection. The eradication of *H. pylori* reduces the risk of duodenal ulcer recurrence.

Contraindications:

Pregnant or nursing women; pediatric patients; patients with renal or hepatic impairment; those hypersensitive to bismuth subsalicylate, metronidazole or other nitroimidazole derivatives or any of the tetracyclines; those allergic to aspirin or salicylates.

Warnings:

Bismuth subsalicylate:

Neurotoxicity – There have been rare reports of neurotoxicity associated with excessive doses of bismuth subsalicylate. Effects have been reversible with discontinuation of therapy.

Dark stools/tongue – Bismuth subsalicylate may cause a temporary and harmless darkening of the tongue and black stool. Do not confuse stool darkening with melena.

Children and teenagers who have or who are recovering from chicken pox or flu should not use this medicine to treat nausea or vomiting. If nausea or vomiting is present, patients are advised to consult a physician because this could be an early sign of Reye's syndrome.

Metronidazole:

CNS – Convulsive seizures and peripheral neuropathy, the latter characterized mainly by numbness or paresthesia of an extremity, have been reported. The prevalence and severity of the neuropathy are directly related to the cumulative dose and duration of therapy, being most prevalent in patients taking high doses for prolonged treatment periods. The appearance of abnormal neurologic signs demands the prompt discontinuation of metronidazole therapy. Administer metronidazole with caution to patients with CNS diseases.

Hematologic – Metronidazole is a nitroimidazole. Use with care in patients with evidence or history of blood dyscrasia. Mild leukopenia has been observed; however, no persistent hematologic abnormalities attributable to metronidazole have been observed.

Candidiasis – Known or previously unrecognized candidiasis may present more prominent symptoms during therapy with metronidazole and requires treatment with a candicidal agent.

Hepatic function impairment – Patients with severe hepatic disease metabolize metronidazole slowly with resultant accumulation of metronidazole and its metabolites in the plasma.

Carcinogenesis – Metronidazole has shown evidence of carcinogenic activity in a number of studies involving chronic oral administration in mice and rats.

Pregnancy – Category B. Metronidazole crosses the placenta and enters fetal circulation rapidly. There are no adequate and well controlled studies in pregnant women. Use during pregnancy only if clearly needed.

Tetracycline:

Blood urea nitrogen (BUN) – The antianabolic action of the tetracyclines may cause an increase in BUN. While this is not a problem in those with normal renal function, higher serum levels of tetracycline in patients with significantly impaired renal function may lead to azotemia, hyperphosphatemia and acidosis.

Superinfection – As with other antibiotics, tetracycline use may result in overgrowth of nonsusceptible organisms, including fungi. If superinfection occurs, discontinue tetracycline and institute appropriate therapy.

Pseudotumor cerebri (benign intracranial hypertension) in adults has been associated with tetracycline use. The usual clinical manifestations are headache and blurred vision. While this condition and related symptoms usually resolve soon after tetracycline discontinuation, the possibility for permanent sequelae exists.

Photosensitivity – Photosensitization may occur; therefore, caution patients to take protective measures (eg, sunscreens, protective clothing) against exposure to ultraviolet light or sunlight until tolerance is determined.

Pregnancy – Category D. Results of animal studies indicate that tetracyclines cross the placenta, are found in fetal tissues and can have toxic effects on the developing fetus (often related to retardation of skeletal development). Evidence of embryotoxicity has also been noted in animals treated early in pregnancy. If this drug is used during pregnancy or if the patient becomes pregnant while taking this drug, apprise of the potential hazard to the fetus.

Pregnant women with renal disease may be more prone to develop tetracycline-associated liver failure.

Children – The use of tetracycline during tooth development (last half of pregnancy, infancy and childhood to 8 years of age) may cause permanent tooth discoloration (yellow-gray-brown). This adverse reaction is more common during long-term drug use but has been observed following repeated short-term courses. Enamel hypoplasia has also been reported. Do not use tetracycline in this patient population.

Elderly: Elderly patients may suffer from asymptomatic renal and hepatic dysfunction. Use caution when administering this therapy to this patient population.

Lactation: Metronidazole and tetracycline are secreted in breast milk. Because of the potential for tumorigenicity shown for metronidazole in mice and rat studies and the potential for serious adverse reactions in nursing infants from tetracyclines, decide whether to discontinue nursing or to discontinue therapy, taking into account the importance of the therapy to the mother. Metronidazole is secreted in breast milk in concentrations similar to those found in plasma (see Contraindications).

Children: Safety and efficacy in children infected with *H. pylori* have not been established.

Drug Interactions:

For complete drug interaction data, refer to the individual monographs.

There is an anticipated reduction in **tetracycline** systemic absorption because of an interaction with **bismuth** or calcium carbonate, an excipient of **bismuth subsalicylate** tablets. The clinical significance of this is unknown as the relative contribution of systemic vs local antimicrobial activity against *H. pylori* for these agents has not been established.

Drug/Lab test interactions: Bismuth absorbs x-rays and may interfere with x-ray diagnostic procedures of the GI tract.

Metronidazole may interfere with certain types of determinations of serum chemistry values, such as aspartate aminotransferase (AST), alanine aminotransferase (ALT), lactate dehydrogenase (LDH), triglycerides and hexokinase glucose. Values of zero may be observed. All of the assays in which interference has been reported involve enzymatic coupling of the assay to oxidation-reduction of nicotine adenine dinucleotide ($NAD^+ \leftrightarrow NADH$). Interference is due to the similarity in absorbance peaks of NADH (340 nm) and metronidazole (322 nm) at pH 7.

Drug/Food interactions: Milk or dairy products impair tetracycline absorption.

Adverse Reactions:

The most common adverse reactions (≥ 1%) reported in clinical trials when all three components of the therapy were given concomitantly are listed in the table below. The majority of the adverse reactions were related to the GI tract, were reversible and infrequently led to discontinuation of therapy. For specific adverse reaction data relating to each agent, refer to individual monographs.

BISMUTH SUBSALICYLATE, METRONIDAZOLE AND TETRACYCLINE HCl COMBINATION

Bismuth Subsalicylate, Metronidazole and Tetracycline Combination Adverse Reactions (≥ 1%)

Adverse reaction	BSS/MTZ/TCN[1] n = 197	Adverse reaction	BSS/MTZ/TCN[1] n = 197
Nausea	10.2	Vomiting	1.5
Diarrhea	5.1	Asthenia	1
Abdominal Pain	3	Constipation	1
Melena	2.5	Insomnia	1
Anal discomfort	1.5	Pain	1
Anorexia	1.5	Upper Respiratory Infection	1
Dizziness	1.5		
Paresthesia	1.5		

[1] Most patients were on concomitant acid suppression therapy.

Overdosage:

If all three components of this therapy are involved in an overdose, acute treatment should focus on the salicylate intoxication. There is neither a pharmacologic basis nor data suggesting an increased toxicity of the combination compared with individual components.

Bismuth subsalicylate: The main concern of an acute bismuth subsalicylate overdose focuses on the salicylate burden and not on bismuth. Each 262.4 mg tablet of bismuth subsalicylate contains an amount of salicylate comparable with ≈ 130 mg aspirin. Acute ingestion of < 150 mg/kg of aspirin (eg, < 1 bismuth subsalicylate tablet per kg) is not expected to lead to toxicity. Mild to moderate toxicity may result from the ingestion of 150 to 300 mg/kg, while severe toxicity may occur from ingestions > 300 mg/kg.

Symptoms – Initial symptoms of salicylate toxicity include hyperpnea, nausea, vomiting, tinnitus, hyperpyrexia, lethargy, tachycardia and confusion. In severe cases, these symptoms may progress to severe hyperpnea, convulsions, pulmonary or cerebral edema, respiratory failure, cardiovascular collapse, coma and death.

Treatment – There is no specific antidote for salicylate poisoning. If there are no contraindications, induce vomiting as soon as possible with syrup of ipecac, or institute gastric lavage, provided that ≤ 1 hour has elapsed since ingestion. Activated charcoal and a cathartic may be administered as primary decontamination therapy in those cases where > 1 hour has elapsed since ingestion or to further decontaminate the GI tract in those who have already received ipecac or gastric lavage. Plasma salicylate levels may be useful; a common nomogram can be used to help predict the severity of intoxication. Provide supportive and symptomatic treatment with emphasis on correcting fluid, electrolyte, blood glucose and acid-base disturbances. Elimination may be enhanced by urinary alkalinization, hemodialysis or hemoperfusion. Because hemodialysis aids in correcting acid-base disturbances, this method may be preferred over hemoperfusion.

For overdose management information on metronidazole and tetracycline, refer to the individual monographs.

Patient Information:

Each dose includes four pills: two pink round chewable tablets (bismuth subsalicylate), one white tablet (metronidazole) and one pale orange and white capsule (tetracycline HCl). Take each dose 4 times/day with meals and at bedtime. Chew and swallow the bismuth subsalicylate tablets (pink tablets), and swallow the metronidazole tablet (white tablet) and the tetracycline capsule (pale orange and white capsule) whole with a full glass of water (8 ounces).

Drink adequate amounts of fluid, particularly with the bedtime tetracycline dose to reduce the risk of esophageal irritation and ulceration.

In case of a missed dose, continue the normal dosing schedule until the medication is gone. Do not take double doses. If more than four doses are missed, contact the physician.

This treatment regimen includes salicylates. If ringing in the ears occurs while taking with aspirin, consult the physician concerning discontinuation of the aspirin therapy until treatment is completed.

Concurrent use of tetracylines may render oral contraceptives less effective. Advise the patient to use a different or additional form of contraception. Breakthrough bleeding has been reported. Women who become pregnant while taking components of the therapy should notify their physician immediately.

Avoid alcoholic beverages while taking metronidazole and for ≥ 1 day afterward.

BISMUTH SUBSALICYLATE, METRONIDAZOLE AND TETRACYCLINE HCl COMBINATION

May cause photosensitivity. Avoid prolonged exposure to the sun and other ultraviolet light. Use sunscreens and wear protective clothing until tolerance is determined.

Bismuth subsalicylate may cause temporary and harmless darkening of the tongue and black stool. Do not confuse stool darkening with melena.

Administration and Dosage:

Adults: Take 525 mg bismuth subsalicylate, 250 mg metronidazole and 500 mg tetracycline plus an H_2 antagonist 4 times daily at meals and bedtimes for 14 days. Chew and swallow the bismuth subsalicylate tablets. Swallow the metronidazole tablet and tetracycline capsule whole with a full glass of water (8 ounces). Take concomitantly prescribed H_2 antagonist therapy as directed.

Ingestion of adequate amounts of fluid, particularly with the bedtime dose of tetracycline HCl, is recommended to reduce the risk of esophageal irritation and ulceration.

Missed doses can be made up by continuing the normal dosing schedule until the medication is gone. Do not take double doses. If more than four doses are missed, contact the physician.

Rx	**Helidac** (Procter & Gamble)	**Tablets:** 262.4 mg bismuth subsalicylate	(PG 11). Pink, chewable. In 8s.
		250 mg metronidazole	(PG 10). White. In 4s.
		Capsules: 500 mg tetracycline.	(PG 12). Pale orange and white. In 4s.

H. PYLORI AGENTS

The following agents are used in the treatment of *H. pylori*. For additional prescribing information, refer to the *H. pylori* introduction or the individual monographs.

OMEPRAZOLE

Indications:

Eradication of H. pylori: In combination with clarithromycin for treatment of patients with an active duodenal ulcer associated with *H. pylori* infection.

Administration and Dosage:

Omeprazole 40 mg once daily and clarithromycin 500 mg 3 times a day for days 1 to 14 and omeprazole 20 mg once daily for days 15 to 28.

CLARITHROMYCIN

Indications:

Eradication of H. pylori: Clarithromycin in combination with omeprazole for the treatment of patients with an active duodenal ulcer associated with *H. pylori* infection.

Administration and Dosage:

Omeprazole 40 mg once daily and clarithromycin 500 mg 3 times a day for days 1 to 14 and omeprazole 20 mg once daily for days 15 to 28.

BISMUTH

Indications:

Eradication of H. pylori: In combination with other products for the eradication of *H. pylori.*

Administration and Dosage:

525 mg 4 times a day in combination with other products.

TETRACYCLINE

Indications:

Eradication of H. pylori: In combination with other products for the eradication of *H. pylori.*

Administration and Dosage:

500 mg 4 times a day in combination with other products.

METRONIDAZOLE

Indications:

Eradication of H. pylori: In combination with other products for the eradication of *H. pylori.*

Administration and Dosage:

250 mg 4 times a day in combination with other products.

HISTAMINE H_2 ANTAGONISTS

Actions:

Pharmacology: Histamine H_2 antagonists are reversible competitive blockers of histamine at the H_2 receptors, particularly those in the gastric parietal cells. The H_2 antagonists are highly selective, do not affect the H_1 receptors, and are not anticholinergic agents. Potent inhibitors of all phases of gastric acid secretion, they inhibit secretions caused by histamine, muscarinic agonists and gastrin. They also inhibit fasting and nocturnal secretions, and secretions stimulated by food, insulin, caffeine, pentagastrin and betazole. In addition, the volume and the hydrogen ion concentration of gastric juice are reduced. Cimetidine, ranitidine and famotidine have no effect on gastric emptying, and cimetidine and famotidine have no effect on lower esophageal sphincter pressure. Ranitidine, nizatidine and famotidine have little or no effect on fasting or postprandial serum gastrin. Ranitidine is 5 to 12 times more potent and famotidine is 30 to 60 times more potent than cimetidine on a molar basis in controlling gastric acid hypersecretion, although there is no indication that the greater potency offers any advantage.

The histamine H_2 antagonists are effective in alleviating symptoms and in preventing complications of peptic ulcer disease. The drugs have similar adverse reaction profiles. Cimetidine appears to have the greatest degree of antiandrogenic (eg, gynecomastia, impotence) and CNS (eg, mental confusion) effects. Cimetidine inhibits the cytochrome P450 oxidase system that affects other drugs (eg, warfarin, theophylline). Ranitidine also affects the microsomal enzyme system, but its influence on elimination of other drugs is not significant. Famotidine and nizatidine do not affect the cytochrome P450 enzyme system.

Treatment failures have been documented with all of the H_2 antagonists. Since all of the drugs act to inhibit gastric acid secretion, it is doubtful that ulcers "resistant" to one drug will heal with another.

Cimetidine –

Antisecretory activity:

Nocturnal – Cimetidine 800 mg at bedtime reduces mean hourly hydrogen ion (H^+) activity by > 85% over 8 hours in duodenal ulcer patients, with no effect on daytime acid secretion. The 1600 mg bedtime dose produces 100% inhibition of mean hourly H^+ activity over an 8 hour period in ulcer patients, but also reduces H^+ activity by 35% for an additional 5 hours the next morning. Both the 400 mg twice daily and 300 mg 4 times daily doses decrease nocturnal acid secretion in a dose-related manner, 47% to 83% over 6 to 8 hours and 54% over 9 hours, respectively.

By the first hour after a standard meal, 300 mg inhibited gastric acid secretion in ulcer patients by at least 50% and during the next 2 hours by at least 75%. A 300 mg breakfast dose continued for at least 4 hours, with partial suppression of the rise in gastric acid secretion following lunch in duodenal ulcer patients.

Total pepsin output is also reduced as a result of the decrease in volume of gastric juice. Cimetidine 300 mg inhibited the rise in intrinsic factor concentration produced by betazole, but some intrinsic factor was secreted at all times.

Ranitidine – Basal, nocturnal and betazole-stimulated secretion are most sensitive to inhibition by ranitidine, responding almost completely to doses of 100 mg or less. Ranitidine does not affect pepsin secretion or pentagastrin-stimulated intrinsic factor secretion. Other pharmacological actions include an increase in gastric nitrate-reducing organisms; small, transient dose-related increases in serum prolactin after IV bolus injections of 100 mg or more and possible impairment of vasopressin release. No effect on prolactin levels has been noted with recommended oral or IV doses.

Famotidine – Both the acid concentration and volume of gastric secretion are suppressed while changes in pepsin secretion are proportional to volume output. Exocrine pancreatic function is not affected. After oral use, the onset of antisecretory effect occurred within 1 hour; the maximum effect was dose-dependent, occurring within 1 to 3 hours. Duration of secretion inhibition by doses of 20 and 40 mg was 10 and 12 hours, respectively.

After IV administration, the maximum effect was achieved within 30 minutes. Single IV doses of 10 and 20 mg inhibited nocturnal secretion for 10 and 12 hours, respectively.

There is no cumulative effect with repeated doses. The nocturnal intragastric pH was raised by evening doses of 20 and 40 mg to mean values of 5 and 6.4, respectively. When famotidine was given after breakfast, the basal daytime interdigestive pH at 3 and 8 hours after 20 or 40 mg was raised to about 5.

HISTAMINE H_2 ANTAGONISTS

Nizatidine's effect on gastric acid secretion is presented in the following table:

Effect of Oral Nizatidine on Gastric Acid Secretion						
		% Inhibition of gastric acid output by dose (mg)				
Method	Time after dose (hrs)	20-50	75	100	150	300
Basal	up to 8	45-57	–	72	–	–
Nocturnal	up to 10	57	–	73	–	90
Betazole	up to 3	–	93	–	100	99
Pentagastrin	up to 6	–	25	–	64	67
Meal	up to 4	41	64	–	98	97
Caffeine	up to 3	–	73	–	85	96

Total pepsin output was reduced in proportion to the reduced volume of gastric secretions. Oral administration of 75 to 300 mg nizatidine increased betazole-stimulated secretion of intrinsic factor. There was no effect on hormone levels, including androgens.

Pharmacokinetics:

Pharmacokinetic Properties of Histamine H_2 Antagonists									
							Elimination (%)		
							Urine, unchanged		
H_2 receptor antagonist	Bioavailability (%)	Time to peak plasma concentration (hrs)	Peak plasma concentration[1] (mcg/ml)	Half-life (hrs)	Protein binding (%)	Volume of distribution (L/kg)	Oral	IV	Metabolized
Cimetidine	60-70	0.75-1.5	0.7-3.2 (300 mg dose) (3.5-7.5 IV)	≈ 2[2]	13-25	0.8-1.2	48	75	30-40
Famotidine	40-45	1-3	0.076-0.1 (40 mg dose)	2.5-3.5[3]	15-20	1.1-1.4	25-30	65-70	30-35
Nizatidine	> 90	0.5-3	0.7-1.8/ 1.4-3.6 (150/300 mg dose)	1-2[3]	≈ 35	0.8-1.5	60	na[4]	< 18
Ranitidine	50-60 (90-100 IM)	1-3 (0.25 IM)	0.44-0.55 (0.58 IM)	2-3[3]	15	1.2-1.9	30-35	68-79	< 10

[1] Dose-dependent.
[2] Increased in renal and hepatic impairment and in the elderly.
[3] Increased in renal impairment.
[4] na = not applicable.

Additional pharmacokinetic data for these agents are discussed individually.

Cimetidine – Absorption may be decreased by antacids, but is unaffected by food. Both oral and parenteral administration provide comparable serum levels. Plasma concentrations of 0.5 to 1 mcg/ml are required to suppress basal or gastric acid secretion; however, plasma concentrations of cimetidine have not correlated with duodenal ulcer healing. Blood concentrations remain above those required to provide 80% inhibition of basal gastric acid secretion for 4 to 5 hours following a 300 mg dose. Cimetidine is widely distributed. Following oral administration, about 30% to 40% is metabolized in the liver, the sulfoxide being the major metabolite. Cimetidine is not significantly removed by hemodialysis or peritoneal dialysis.

Ranitidine – Absorption of oral ranitidine is not significantly impaired by the administration of food. Coadministration of antacids may reduce its absorption. Hepatic metabolism results in three metabolites. Maintenance of serum concentrations necessary to inhibit 50% of stimulated gastric acid secretion (36 to 94 ng/ml) is 12 hours orally and 6 to 8 hours IV. Blood levels, however, bear no consistent relationship to dose or degree of acid inhibition.

Famotidine – Plasma levels after multiple doses of famotidine are similar to those after single doses. Famotidine is eliminated by renal (65% to 70%) and metabolic (30% to 35%) routes. The only metabolite identified is the S-oxide.

HISTAMINE H_2 ANTAGONISTS

Nizatidine – A concentration of 1000 mcg/L is equivalent to 3 mcmol/L; a dose of 300 mg is equivalent to 905 micromoles. Plasma concentrations 12 hours after administration are < 10 mcg/L. Plasma clearance is 40 to 60 L/hour. Because of the short half-life and rapid clearance, drug accumulation would not be expected in individuals with normal renal function who take either 300 mg at bedtime or 150 mg bid. Nizatidine exhibits dose proportionality over recommended dose range.

Antacids consisting of aluminum and magnesium hydroxides with simethicone decrease nizatidine absorption by about 10%. With food, AUC and maximum concentration increase by ≈ 10%.

In humans, < 7% of an oral dose is metabolized as N2-monodesmethyl-nizatidine, an H_2-receptor antagonist. Other likely metabolites are the N2-oxide (less than 5% of the dose) and the S-oxide (< 6% of the dose). More than 90% of an oral dose of nizatidine is excreted in the urine within 12 hours. Renal clearance is about 500 ml/min, which indicates excretion by active tubular secretion. Less than 6% is eliminated in the feces.

Clinical trials:

Comparative studies –

Duodenal Ulcer Healing Rates – Comparison of H_2 Antagonists[1]

Drug	Dose (mg/day)	Healing rate 4 week	8 week
Cimetidine	1000	60% to 84%	82% to 95%
Famotidine	40	67% to 77%	
Nizatidine	300	73% to 81%	
Ranitidine	300	63% to 77%	

[1] Combined results. Studies did not compare all drugs simultaneously.

In the treatment of gastric ulcers, healing rates after 6 weeks of therapy with ranitidine 150 mg twice daily or cimetidine 300 mg 4 times daily were 65% to 70%; after 8 weeks of treatment, the rates increased to 75% to 85%.

Studies evaluating an evening meal or bedtime dose of ranitidine 150 mg or cimetidine 400 mg for duodenal ulcer maintenance therapy indicated the relapse rate was lower in ranitidine patients. However, these doses are not equipotent in reducing gastric acid secretion. A one year multicenter study indicated that nizatidine 150 mg at night is similar in efficacy to ranitidine in preventing ulcer recurrence.

Indications:

Duodenal ulcer:

Short-term treatment – Most patients heal within 4 weeks; there is rarely reason to use full dosage for > 6 to 8 weeks.

Maintenance therapy – Reduced dosages after healing of active ulcer. Patients have been maintained on continued cimetidine (400 mg at bedtime) for up to 5 years.

Gastric ulcer:

Treatment (benign, active) – Short-term treatment. Most patients heal in 6 wks.

Maintenance (ranitidine) – Reduced dosage after healing of acute ulcer.

Gastroesophageal reflux disease (GERD), including endoscopically diagnosed erosive esophagitis: Ranitidine and nizatidine are also indicated for symptomatic relief of associated heartburn.

Erosive esophagitis, maintenance (ranitidine).

Pathological hypersecretory conditions (cimetidine, famotidine, ranitidine): Eg, Zollinger-Ellison syndrome, systemic mastocytosis, multiple endocrine adenomas.

Upper GI bleeding (cimetidine): Prevention in critically ill patients.

Heartburn, acid indigestion and sour stomach:

Cimetidine (otc only) – Relief of these symptoms.

Famotidine (otc only) – Relief of these symptoms and prevention of these symptoms brought on by consuming food and beverages.

Unlabeled uses:

Histamine H_2 antagonists – As part of a multi-drug regimen to eradicate *Helicobacter pylori* in the treatment of peptic ulcer.

Cimetidine – Oral 400 to 600 mg or IV 300 mg, 60 to 90 minutes before anesthesia to prevent aspiration pneumonitis.

Doses of 1 g/day have been used with variable success to treat primary hyperparathyroidism and to control secondary hyperparathyroidism in chronic hemodialysis patients.

Treatment of chronic viral warts in children (25 to 40 mg/kg/day, divided doses).

HISTAMINE H_2 ANTAGONISTS

The combination of H_1 and H_2 antagonists may be useful in chronic idiopathic urticaria not responding to H_1 antagonists alone. It may also be useful for itching and flushing in anaphylaxis, pruritus, urticaria and contact dermatitis (IV).

Cimetidine IV may be useful in acetaminophen overdose by reducing formation of the toxic intermediate via the cytochrome P450 oxidase system, thereby protecting against hepatotoxicity.

Cimetidine has been used for dyspepsia (400 mg twice/day); however, other studies do not confirm its effectiveness.

Cimetidine may improve overall survival in patients with colorectal cancer.

Other potential uses include: Prophylaxis of stress-induced ulcers; tinea capitis; herpes virus infection; hirsute women.

Ranitidine – Ranitidine has shown some value in protection against aspiration of acid during anesthesia. In one study, oral ranitidine 2 to 3.5 mg/kg was effective in decreasing gastric acidity in children before anesthesia induction.

Ranitidine 150 mg twice daily may be effective in preventing gastroduodenal mucosal damage that may be associated with long-term NSAIDs, including aspirin.

Ranitidine controls acute upper GI bleeding (150 mg IV or 300 mg/day orally).

Effective in preventing stress ulcers IV (0.125 to 0.25 mg/kg/hr) or orally.

Famotidine – Famotidine may be effective in upper GI bleeding (20 mg twice daily).

Prevention of stress ulcers (40 mg/day).

During and before anesthesia to prevent pulmonary aspiration of gastric acid (40 mg IM or orally).

Histamine H_2 Antagonists: Summary of Indications

✓ – Labeled x – Unlabeled	Cimetidine	Famotidine	Nizatidine	Ranitidine
Duodenal ulcer				
Treatment	✓	✓	✓	✓
Maintenance	✓	✓	✓	✓
GERD (including erosive esophagitis)	✓	✓	✓	✓
Gastric ulcer				
Treatment	✓	✓	✓	✓
Maintenance				✓
Pathological hypersecretory conditions	✓	✓		✓
Heartburn/acid indigestion/sour stomach	✓[1,2]	✓[1,3]		
Erosive esophagitis, maintenance				✓
Prevent upper GI bleeding	✓	x		x
Peptic ulcer[4]	x	x	x	x
Prevent aspiration pneumonitis	x	x		x
Prophylaxis of stress ulcers	x	x		x
Prevent gastric NSAID damage				x
Hyperparathyroidism	x			
Secondary hyperparathyroidism in hemodialysis	x			
Tinea capitis	x			
Herpes virus infection	x			
Hirsute women	x			
Chronic idiopathic urticaria	x			
Anaphylaxis (dermatological)	x			
Acetaminophen overdose	x			
Dyspepsia	x			
Warts	x			
Colorectal cancer	x			

[1] *otc* use only.
[2] Relief of symptoms only.
[3] Relief and prevention of symptoms.
[4] As part of a multi-drug regimen to eradicate *Helicobacter pylori*.

HISTAMINE H_2 ANTAGONISTS

Contraindications:

Hypersensitivity to individual agents or to other H_2-receptor antagonists.

Warnings:

Benzyl alcohol, contained in some of these products as a preservative, has been associated with a fatal "gasping syndrome" in premature infants.

Hypersensitivity: Rare cases of anaphylaxis have occurred as well as rare episodes of hypersensitivity (eg, bronchospasm, laryngeal edema, rash, eosinophilia). Refer to Management of Acute Hypersensitivity Reactions.

Renal function impairment: Since these agents are excreted primarily via the kidneys, decreased clearance may occur; reduced dosage may be necessary (see Administration and Dosage).

Hepatic function impairment: Observe caution. Decreased clearance may occur; these agents are partly metabolized in the liver. In normal renal function with uncomplicated hepatic dysfunction, **nizatidine** disposition is similar to that in healthy individuals.

Elderly: Safety and efficacy appear similar to those of younger age; however, the elderly may have reduced renal function. Ulcer healing rates, adverse events and laboratory abnormalities in patients 65 to 82 years old on **ranitidine** were no different from younger patients. Decreased **cimetidine** clearance may be more common.

Pregnancy: (Category B – cimetidine, famotidine, ranitidine. Category C – nizatidine). Cimetidine crosses the placenta. There are no adequate and well controlled studies with these agents in pregnant women. Use only when clearly needed and when the potential benefits outweigh the potential hazards to the fetus.

Lactation:

Cimetidine is excreted in breast milk with milk:plasma ratios of approximately 5:1 to 12:1. Potential daily infant ingestion is approximately 6 mg. Do not nurse.

Ranitidine is excreted in breast milk with milk:plasma ratios of 1:1 to 6.7:1. Exercise caution when administering to a nursing mother.

Nizatidine is excreted in breast milk in a concentration of 0.1% of the oral dose in proportion to plasma concentrations. Decide whether to discontinue nursing or discontinue the drug, taking into account the importance of the drug to the mother.

Famotidine is excreted in the breast milk of rats. It is not known whether it is excreted in human breast milk. Decide whether to discontinue nursing or to discontinue the drug, taking into account the importance of the drug to the mother.

Children: Safety and efficacy are not established. **Cimetidine** is not recommended for children < 16 years old, unless anticipated benefits outweigh potential risks. In very limited experience, cimetidine 20 to 40 mg/kg/day has been used. OTC use is not recommended in children < 12 years of age.

Precautions:

Gastric malignancy: Symptomatic response to these agents does not preclude gastric malignancy. Transient healing of gastric ulcers (rare) has occurred with **cimetidine** despite subsequently documented malignancy. Follow gastric ulcer patients closely.

Reversible CNS effects (eg, mental confusion, agitation, psychosis, depression, anxiety, hallucinations, disorientation) have occurred with **cimetidine,** predominantly in severely ill patients. These confusional states usually develop within 2 to 3 days after initiation of therapy and clear within 3 to 4 days following discontinuation. Advancing age (≥ 50 years) and preexisting liver or renal disease appear to be contributing factors. In several cases, the mental confusion has been associated with elevated trough serum concentrations (> 1.25 mcg/ml).

Hepatocellular injury may occur with **nizatidine** as evidenced by elevated liver enzymes (AST, ALT or alkaline phosphatase). In some cases, there was a marked elevation of AST, ALT enzymes (> 500 IU/L) and, in a single instance, ALT was > 2000 IU/L. The overall occurrence of elevated liver enzymes and elevations to 3 times the upper limit of normal, however, did not significantly differ from placebo-treated patients. All abnormalities were reversible after discontinuation of nizatidine.

Occasionally, reversible hepatitis, hepatocellular or hepatocanalicular or mixed, with or without jaundice have occurred with oral **ranitidine.** ALT values have increased to at least twice pretreatment levels with IV ranitidine administered for ≥ 5 days.

Laboratory test monitoring for liver abnormalities is appropriate.

HISTAMINE H_2 ANTAGONISTS

Rapid IV administration of **cimetidine** has been followed by rare instances of cardiac arrhythmias and hypotension. Bradycardia, tachycardia and premature ventricular beats in association with rapid administration of IV **ranitidine** may occur rarely, usually in patients predisposed to cardiac rhythm disturbances.

Antiandrogenic effect: **Cimetidine** has a weak antiandrogenic effect in animals. Gynecomastia in patients treated for ≥ 1 month may occur. In patients with pathological hypersecretory states, this occurred in about 4% of cases; in all others, the incidence was about 0.3% to 1%. No evidence of endocrine dysfunction was found; the condition remained unchanged or returned to normal with continuing treatment.

Immunocompromised patients: Decreased gastric acidity, including that produced by acid-suppressing agents such as H_2 antagonists, may increase the possibility of strongyloidiasis.

Drug Interactions:

Cimetidine reduces the hepatic metabolism of drugs metabolized via the cytochrome P–450 pathway, delaying elimination and increasing serum levels. Drugs metabolized by hepatic microsomal enzymes, particularly those of low therapeutic ratio or in patients with renal or hepatic impairment, may require dosage adjustment. Concomitant cimetidine with any of the following drugs may result in their increased pharmacologic effects or toxicity.

Cimetidine Drug Interactions (Decreased Hepatic Metabolism)		
Benzodiazepines[1]	Metronidazole	Sulfonylureas
Caffeine	Moricizine	Tacrine
Calcium channel blockers	Pentoxifylline	Theophyllines[2]
Carbamazepine	Phenytoin	Triamterene
Chloroquine	Propafenone	Tricyclic antidepressants
Labetalol	Propranolol	Valproic acid
Lidocaine	Quinidine	Warfarin
Metoprolol	Quinine	

[1] Does not include agents metabolized by glucuronidation (lorazepam, oxazepam, temazepam).
[2] Does not include dyphylline.

Ranitidine (which weakly binds to cytochrome P450 in vitro), **famotidine** and **nizatidine** do not inhibit the cytochrome P450-linked oxygenase enzyme system in the liver. Drug interactions with these agents mediated by inhibition of hepatic metabolism are not expected. However, some interactions may occur with these agents (see table).

Following are additional interactions that may occur with cimetidine as well as potential interactions with the other H_2 antagonists:

Histamine H_2 Antagonist Drug Interactions			
Precipitant drug	Object drug*		Description
Cimetidine	Ferrous salts Indomethacin Ketoconazole Tetracyclines	⬇	Pharmacologic effects of these agents may be decreased by cimetidine due to decreased absorption.
Cimetidine	Carmustine	⬆	Bone marrow suppression (toxicity) of carmustine may be enhanced by cimetidine, possibly due to additive effect or inhibition of carmustine metabolism.
Cimetidine	Digoxin	⬇	Serum digoxin concentrations may decrease during coadministration.
Cimetidine	Flecainide	⬆	Pharmacologic effects of flecainide may be increased.
Cimetidine	Fluconazole	⬇	Fluconazole plasma levels may be reduced, possibly due to decreased absorption.
Cimetidine	Fluorouracil	⬆	Fluorouracil serum concentrations may be increased following chronic cimetidine use.
Cimetidine	Narcotic analgesics	⬆	Toxic effects (eg, respiratory depression) may be increased.

HISTAMINE H_2 ANTAGONISTS

Histamine H_2 Antagonist Drug Interactions			
Precipitant drug	Object drug*		Description
Cimetidine Ranitidine	Procainamide	⬆	Cimetidine may increase plasma levels of procainamide and its cardioactive metabolite n-acetylprocainamide (NAPA) by decreasing renal tubular secretion. Ranitidine may decrease the renal clearance and increase AUC of procainamide. One study reported no effect of ranitidine on procainamide or NAPA elimination.
Cimetidine	Succinylcholine	⬆	The neuromuscular blocking effects may be increased by cimetidine. Prolonged respiratory depression with extended periods of apnea may occur.
Cimetidine	Tocainide	⬇	Cimetidine may decrease the pharmacologic effects of tocainide.
Nizatidine	Salicylates	⬆	Increased serum salicylate levels occurred when nizatidine was administered to patients receiving very high doses of aspirin (3.9 g/day).
Ranitidine	Diazepam	⬇	Diazepam's pharmacologic effects may be decreased due to decreased GI absorption by ranitidine. Stagger-ing administration times may avoid this interaction.
Ranitidine	Sulfonylureas	⬆	Ranitidine may increase the hypoglycemic effect of glipizide; one glyburide patient developed severe hypoglycemia after ranitidine. This did not occur in two studies with glyburide or tolbutamide. Glipizide dosage adjustment may be needed.
Ranitidine	Theophyllines	⬌	Case reports indicate theophylline plasma levels may be increased by ranitidine, possibly increasing pharmacologic and toxic effects. However, controlled studies indicate an interaction does not occur. If this interaction occurs, it is rare.
Ranitidine	Warfarin	⬆	Ranitidine may interfere with warfarin clearance (data conflict; significance not established). Hypoprothrombinemic effects may increase; may need adjustment.
H_2 antagonists	Ethanol	⬆	Concurrent use may increase plasma ethanol levels and AUC. This interaction may have minimal clinical importance.
Antacids Anticholinergics Metoclopramide	H_2 antagonists	⬇	These agents may decrease the absorption of cimetidine. However, one study suggested cimetidine absorption is unaffected by concomitant multiple-dose antacid administration. Ranitidine absorption may be decreased by concurrent antacids; data conflict. Avoid simultaneous administration. Bioavailability of famotidine and nizatidine may be slightly decreased; no special precautions are necessary.
Cigarette smoking	Cimetidine	⬇	Cigarette smoking reverses cimetidine-induced inhibition of nocturnal gastric secretion, hindering ulcer healing. Cigarette use is closely related to ulcer recurrence.

* ⬆ = Object drug increased. ⬇ = Object drug decreased. ⬌ = Undetermined effect.

Drug/Lab test interactions: False-positive tests for urobilinogen may occur during **nizatidine** therapy. False-positive tests for urine protein with *Multistix* may occur during **ranitidine** therapy; testing with sulfosalicylic acid is recommended.

Drug/Food interactions: Food may increase bioavailability of **famotidine** and **nizatidine;** this is of no clinical consequence. **Cimetidine** and **ranitidine** are not affected.

HISTAMINE H_2 ANTAGONISTS

Adverse Reactions:

Histamine H_2 Antagonist Adverse Reactions

	Adverse reaction	Cimetidine	Famotidine	Nizatidine	Ranitidine
CNS	Headache	1%[1]	4.7%	†	†
	Somnolence/Fatigue	1%	†	2.4%	rare
	Dizziness	1%	1.3%	†	rare
	Confusional states[2]	1%	†	rare	rare
	Hallucinations	1%	†		rare
	Agitation/Anxiety		†		†
	Depression		†		rare
	Insomnia		†	†	rare
Dermatologic	Exfoliative dermatitis/ erythroderma	†		†	
	Alopecia	rare[2]	†		rare
	Rash	†	†	†	†
	Erythema multiforme	rare			rare
	Pruritus/Urticaria		†	0.5%	
GI	Nausea		†	†	†
	Vomiting		†	†	†
	Abdominal discomfort		†	†	†
	Diarrhea	1%	1.7%	†	†
	Constipation		1.2%	†	†
	Pancreatitis	rare[2]			rare
	Cholestatic/Hepatocellular effects	rare to 1%[2]		rare	†
Hematologic	Agranulocytosis	rare			rare
	Granulocytopenia	rare			†[2]
	Thrombocytopenia	rare	†	†	†[2]
	Autoimmune hemolytic/aplastic anemia	rare			rare
Other	Cardiac arrhythmias[3]/Arrest	rare		rare	rare
	Gynecomastia	0.3%-4%		rare	†
	Impotence	1%[2]	†	†	†
	Loss of libido		†	†	†
	Arthralgia	rare[2]	†		rare
	Bronchospasm	†	†		
	Hypersensitivity reactions	rare[2]			rare
	Transient pain at injection site	†[4]	†	na[5]	†

† Occurs, no incidence reported or not well established.
[1] May be severe.
[2] Reversible.
[3] With rapid IV administration.
[4] IM.
[5] na – Not applicable.

HISTAMINE H_2 ANTAGONISTS

In addition to the adverse effects listed in the table, the following have been reported:

Cimetidine: Reversible exacerbation of joint symptoms with preexisting arthritis, including gouty arthritis (1%); peripheral neuropathy; delirium; cutaneous vasculitis; phytobezoar formation; galactorrhea; neutropenia (including agranulocytosis) in patients with serious concomitant illnesses receiving drugs or treatment known to produce neutropenia.

Rare – Reversible interstitial nephritis and urinary retention; myalgia; polymyositis; epidermal necrolysis; strongyloidiasis hyperinfection in immunocompromised patients (extremely rare; see Precautions).

Impotence – Reversible impotence in patients with pathological hypersecretory disorders (eg, Zollinger-Ellison syndrome) receiving cimetidine, particularly in high doses, for 12 to 79 months (mean, 38 months). However, in large scale surveillance studies at regular dosages, the incidence has not exceeded that of the general population.

Ranitidine: Vertigo, reversible blurred vision (suggestive of a change in accommodation), malaise, reversible leukopenia, pancytopenia (sometimes with marrow hypoplasia), anaphylaxis, angioneurotic edema (rare). Transient local burning or itching may occur with IV administration.

Famotidine: Anorexia; dry mouth; musculoskeletal pain; paresthesias; grand mal seizure (one report); acne; dry skin; flushing; tinnitus; taste disorder; fever; asthenia; palpitations; orbital edema; conjunctival injection.

Nizatidine: Sweating (1%); asymptomatic ventricular tachycardia; hyperuricemia unassociated with gout or nephrolithiasis; eosinophilia; fever.

Lab test abnormalities: Small increases in serum creatinine and elevated ALT levels (at least twice pretreatment levels) occurred with **ranitidine.** Small possibly dose-related increases in plasma creatinine and serum transaminase occurred with **cimetidine**; these are not common and do not signify deteriorating renal function. Elevated AST, ALT and alkaline phosphatase levels occur with **nizatidine** (see Precautions).

Overdosage:

Symptoms: There is no experience with deliberate overdosage. Toxic doses in animals are associated with rapid respiration or respiratory failure, tachycardia, muscular tremors, vomiting, restlessness, pallor of mucous membranes or redness of mouth and ears, hypotension, collapse and cholinergic-type effects including lacrimation, salivation, emesis, miosis and diarrhea.

Reported ingestions of up to 20 g **cimetidine** have been associated with transient adverse effects similar to those encountered in normal clinical experience. Two deaths have occurred in adults who reportedly ingested > 40 g on a single occasion.

Famotidine doses of up to 640 mg/day have been given to patients with pathological hypersecretory conditions with no serious adverse effects.

Treatment: Symptomatic and supportive. Remove unabsorbed material from the GI tract, monitor the patient and employ supportive therapy. Refer to General Management of Acute Overdosage.

With **nizatidine**, renal dialysis for 4 to 6 hours increased plasma clearance by approximately 84%.

Physostigmine has been reported to arouse obtunded patients with evidence of **cimetidine**-induced CNS toxicity; data are insufficient to recommend this use.

Patient Information:

Inform physician or pharmacist of any concomitant drug therapy, especially when taking **cimetidine.**

Stagger doses of antacids and **cimetidine** or **ranitidine.**

These agents may be taken without regard to meals.

OTC: Do not take maximum daily dosage for > 2 weeks continuously except under the advice and supervision of a physician.

CIMETIDINE

For complete prescribing information, refer to the Histamine H_2 Antagonists group monograph.

Indications:

Duodenal ulcer: Short-term treatment and maintenance therapy.

Benign gastric ulcer: Short-term treatment.

Gastroesophageal reflux disease (GERD), erosive.

Pathological hypersecretory conditions.

GI bleeding: Prevention of upper GI bleeding in critically ill patients.

Heartburn, acid indigestion and sour stomach (otc only): Relief of these symptoms.

Administration and Dosage:

Approved by the FDA in 1977.

Oral:

Duodenal ulcer –

Short-term treatment of active duodenal ulcer: 800 mg at bedtime. Alternate regimens are 300 mg 4 times a day with meals and at bedtime, or 400 mg twice a day. Give antacids as needed for pain relief. While healing often occurs during the first few weeks, continue treatment for 4 to 6 weeks unless healing is demonstrated by endoscopy.

Maintenance therapy: 400 mg at bedtime.

Active benign gastric ulcer – For short-term treatment, 800 mg at bedtime or 300 mg 4 times a day with meals and at bedtime. The preferred regimen is 800 mg at bedtime based on convenience and lowered potential for drug interaction. There is no information concerning usefulness of treatment periods longer than 8 weeks.

Erosive gastroesophageal reflux disease (GERD) –

Adults: 1600 mg daily in divided doses (800 mg twice daily or 400 mg 4 times a day) for 12 weeks. Use beyond 12 weeks has not been established.

Pathological hypersecretory conditions – 300 mg 4 times a day with meals and at bedtime. If necessary, give 300 mg doses more often. Individualize dosage. Do not exceed 2400 mg/day; continue as long as clinically indicated.

Heartburn, acid indigestion and sour stomach (otc only) – 200 mg (2 tablets) with water as symptoms occur or as directed, up to twice daily (up to 4 tablets in 24 hrs). Do not take maximum dose for > 2 weeks contiuously unless otherwise directed by a physician.

Children: Do not give to children < 12 years of age unless otherwise directed.

Parenteral: For hospitalized patients with pathological hypersecretory conditions or intractable ulcers, or patients unable to take oral medication. The usual dose is 300 mg IM or IV every 6 to 8 hours. If it is necessary to increase dosage, do so by more frequent administration of a 300 mg dose, not to exceed 2400 mg/day.

Prevention of upper GI bleeding – Continuous IV infusion of 50 mg/hour. Patients with creatinine clearance < 30 ml/min should receive half the recommended dose. Treatment beyond 7 days has not been studied.

GERD – The doses and regimen for parenteral administration in patients with GERD have not been established.

IM – Administer undiluted.

IV – Dilute in 0.9% Sodium Chloride Injection or other compatible IV solution to a total volume of 20 ml; inject ≥ 2 minutes.

Intermittent IV infusion – Dilute 300 mg in at least 50 ml of 5% Dextrose Injection or other compatible IV solution; infuse over 15 to 20 minutes.

Continuous IV infusion – 37.5 mg/hour (900 mg/day). For patients requiring a more rapid elevation of gastric pH, continuous infusion may be preceded by a 150 mg loading dose administered by IV infusion as described above. Dilute 900 mg cimetidine injection in a compatible IV fluid (see Stability) for a constant rate infusion over a 24 hour period.

Note: Cimetidine may be diluted in 100 to 1000 ml; however, a volumetric pump is recommended if the volume for 24 hour infusion is < 250 ml.

Plastic containers – Do not add drugs to the solution in these containers or introduce any additives.

Stability – Stable for 48 hours at room temperature when added to commonly used IV solutions (eg, 0.9% Sodium Chloride Injection, 5% or 10% Dextrose Injection, Lactated Ringer's Solution, 5% Sodium Bicarbonate Injection) or when added to a total parenteral nutrition admixture containing amino acids, dextrose, fat emulsion, electrolytes and vitamins. When diluted to a concentration of 15 mg/ml in sterile water for injection and stored in glass vials, cimetidine was stable for 14 days at 22°C (71°F) and for 42 days at 4°C (39.2°F).

Premixed, single-dose: Avoid exposure of the premixed product to excessive heat. The product should be stored at controlled room temperature (15° to 30°C; 59° to 86°F). Brief exposure up to 40°C does not adversely affect premixed product.

CIMETIDINE

Admixture incompatibility – Incompatible with aminophylline and barbiturates in IV solutions. Incompatible in the same syringe with pentobarbital sodium and a pentobarbital sodium/atropine sulfate combination. In one study, cimetidine and aminophylline were chemically stable and physically compatible for 48 hours at room temperature when admixed in 5% Dextrose in Water.

Severely impaired renal function: Accumulation may occur. Use the lowest dose; 300 mg every 12 hours orally or IV has been recommended. According to the patient's condition, dosage frequency may be increased to every 8 hours or even further with caution. Whether hemodialysis reduces the level of circulating cimetidine is controversial. Give the dose at the end of hemodialysis. When liver impairment is also present, further dosage reductions may be necessary.

otc	**Tagamet HB** (SK-Beecham)	**Tablets**: 100 mg	In 16s, 32s and 64s.
Rx	**Cimetidine** (Various, eg, Endo, Goldline, Major, Mylan, Novopharm, Penn Labs, Schein)	**Tablets**: 200 mg	In 100s, 500s and 1000s.
Rx	**Tagamet** (SK-Beecham)		(Tagamet 200 SB). Light green. In 100s.
Rx	**Cimetidine** (Various, eg, Endo, Goldline, Major, Mylan, Novopharm, Penn Labs, Schein)	**Tablets**: 300 mg	In 100s, 500s and 1000s.
Rx	**Tagamet** (SK-Beecham)		(Tagamet 300 SB). Light green. In 100s & UD 100s.
Rx	**Cimetidine** (Various, eg, Endo, Goldline, Major, Mylan, Novopharm, Penn Labs, Schein)	**Tablets**: 400 mg	In 100s, 500s, and 1000s.
Rx	**Tagamet** (SK-Beecham)		(Tagamet 400 SB). Light green. Capsule shape. In 60s & UD 100s.
Rx	**Cimetidine** (Various, eg, Endo, Goldline, Major, Mylan, Novopharm, Penn Labs, Schein)	**Tablets**: 800 mg	In 100s, 500s and 1000s.
Rx	**Tagamet** (SK-Beecham)		(Tagamet 800 SB). Light green. Oval. In 30s & UD 100s.
Rx	**Cimetidine Oral Solution** (Barre-National)	**Liquid**: 300 mg (as HCl) per 5 ml	2.8% alcohol, parabens, saccharin, sorbitol. Mint-peach flavor. In 240 and 470 ml.
Rx	**Tagamet** (SK-Beecham)		2.8% alcohol, saccharin, parabens, sorbitol. Mint-peach flavor. In 240 ml and UD 5 ml (10s).
Rx	**Cimetidine** (Endo)	**Injection**: 150 mg (as HCl) per ml	5 mg phenol per ml. In 2 ml vials and 8 ml multi-dose vials.
Rx	**Tagamet** (SK-Beecham)	**Injection**: 300 mg (as HCl) per 2 ml	With phenol. In single-dose vials, disp. syringes and *ADD-Vantage* vials and 8 ml multiple-dose vials.
Rx	**Tagamet** (SK-Beecham)	**Injection, premixed:** 300 mg (as HCl) in 50 ml 0.9% sodium chloride	In single-dose containers.

RANITIDINE HCl

For complete prescribing information, refer to the Histamine H_2 Antagonists group monograph.

Indications:

Duodenal ulcer: Short-term treatment and maintenance therapy.

Gastric ulcer: Short-term treatment (benign, active) and maintenance therapy.

Pathological hypersecretory conditions.

Gastroesophageal reflux disease (GERD).

Erosive esophagitis:

Treatment of endoscopically diagnosed erosive esophagitis, and for symptomatic relief of associated heartburn.

Maintenance of healing erosive esophagitis.

Administration and Dosage:

Approved by the FDA in June 1983.

Oral:

Duodenal ulcer –

Short-term treatment of active duodenal ulcer: 150 mg orally twice daily. An alternate dosage of 300 mg once daily at bedtime can be used for patients in whom dosing convenience is important; 100 mg twice daily is as effective as the 150 mg dose. Smaller doses are equally effective in inhibiting gastric acid secretion.

Maintenance therapy – 150 mg at bedtime.

Pathological hypersecretory conditions – 150 mg orally twice a day. More frequent doses may be necessary. Individualize dosage and continue as long as indicated. Doses up to 6 g/day have been used.

Gastric ulcer (oral doseforms only) –

Benign, active: 150 mg twice daily.

Maintenance: 150 mg at bedtime.

GERD – 150 mg twice daily.

Erosive esophagitis –

Treatment: 150 mg 4 times daily.

Maintenance: 150 mg twice daily.

EFFERdose (tablets and granules) – Dissolve each dose in ≈ 6 to 8 oz of water before drinking.

Storage/Stability –

Syrup: Store between 4° and 25°C (39° and 77°F).

Parenteral: Do not exceed recommended rates of administration.

IM – 50 mg (2 ml) every 6 to 8 hours. (No dilution necessary.)

IV injection – 50 mg (2 ml) every 6 to 8 hours. Dilute 50 mg in 0.9% Sodium Chloride or other compatible IV solution to a total volume of 20 ml; inject over ≥ 5 min.

Intermittent IV infusion – 50 mg (2 ml) every 6 to 8 hours. Dilute 50 mg in 100 ml 5% Dextrose Injection or other compatible IV solution, or use 100 ml of 0.5 mg/ml premixed solution and infuse over 15 to 20 minutes; do not exceed 400 mg/day.

Premixed injection – Requires no dilution and should be infused over 15 to 20 minutes. Administer by slow IV drip infusion only. Do not introduce additives into the solution. If used with a primary IV fluid system, discontinue primary solution during premixed infusion.

Continuous IV infusion – Add ranitidine injection to 5% Dextrose Injection or other compatible IV solution (see Stability). Deliver at a rate of 6.25 mg/hr (eg, 150 mg [6 ml] ranitidine injection in 250 ml of 5% Dextrose Injection at 10.7 ml/hr).

For Zollinger-Ellison patients, dilute ranitidine injection in 5% Dextrose Injection or other compatible IV solution (see Stability) to a concentration ≤ 2.5 mg/ml. Start the infusion at a rate of 1 mg/kg/hr. If after 4 hours either the measured gastric acid output is > 10 mEq/hr or the patient becomes symptomatic, adjust the dose upwards in 0.5 mg/kg/hr increments and remeasure the acid output. Doses up to 2.5 mg/kg/hr and infusion rates as high as 220 mg/hr have been used.

Storage/Stability – Stable for 48 hours at room temperature when added to or diluted with most commonly used IV solutions (eg, 0.9% Sodium Chloride Injection, 5% or 10% Dextrose Injection, Lactated Ringer's Solution, 5% Sodium Bicarbonate Injection).

Studies have shown ranitidine is stable in minibags with 5% Dextrose or 0.9% NaCl when frozen (–30°C; –22°F) for 30 days in concentrations of 0.5, 1 and 2 mg/ml and for 100 days at a concentration of 2 mg/ml or refrigerated (4°C; 39°F) for 10 days in a concentration of 1 mg/ml. Concentrations of 83 to 250 mcg/ml in standard TPN solutions decreased by < 10% when stored at room temperature for < 48 hours. TPN solutions with 4.25% and 2.125% crystalline amino acids and 50 and 100 mcg/ml concentrations of ranitidine were stable 24 hours at room temperature.

RANITIDINE HCl

Renal impairment (Ccr < 50 ml/min): 150 mg orally every 24 hours or 50 mg parenterally every 18 to 24 hours. The frequency of dosing may be increased to every 12 hours or further with caution. Hemodialysis reduces the level of circulating ranitidine. Adjust dosage timing so that a scheduled dose coincides with the end of hemodialysis.

otc	**Zantac 75** (Glaxo Wellcome)	**Tablets:** 75 mg ranitidine.	Five-sided. In 4s, 10s and 20s.
Rx	**Zantac** (Glaxo Wellcome)	**Tablets:** 150 mg (as HCl)	(Zantac 150 Glaxo). Peach. Film coated. Five sided. In 60s, 500s and UD 100s.
Rx	**Zantac** (Glaxo Wellcome)	300 mg (as HCl)	(Zantac 300 Glaxo). Yellow. Film coated. Capsule shape. In 30s, 250s and UD 100s.
Rx	**Zantac EFFERdose** (Glaxo Wellcome)	**Tablets, effervescent:** 150 mg	Aspartame, 16.84 mg phenylalanine. (Zantac 150 427). White/pale yellow. In 30s and 60s.
Rx	**Zantac GELdose** (Glaxo Wellcome)	**Capsules:** 150 mg	Sorbitol. (Zantac 150 Glaxo). Beige. In 60s and UD 60s.
		300 mg	Sorbitol. (Zantac 300 Glaxo). Beige. In 30s and UD 30s.
Rx	**Ranitidine HCl** (UDL)	**Syrup:** 15 mg (as HCl) per ml	In UD 10 ml.
Rx	**Zantac** (Glaxo Wellcome)		7.5% alcohol, saccharin, sorbitol, parabens. Peppermint flavor. In 480 ml.
Rx	**Zantac EFFERdose** (Glaxo Wellcome)	**Granules, effervescent:** 150 mg	Aspartame, 16.84 mg phenylalanine. White/pale yellow. In 1.44 g packets (30s and 60s).
Rx	**Zantac** (Glaxo Wellcome)	**Injection:** 0.5 mg (as HCl) per ml	Preservative free. In 100 ml single-dose plastic containers.[1]
		25 mg (as HCl) per ml	In 2, 10 and 40 ml vials and 2 ml syringes.[2]

[1] Premixed in 0.45% sodium chloride.
[2] With phenol.

NIZATIDINE

For complete prescribing information, refer to the Histamine H_2 Antagonists group monograph.

Indications:

Duodenal ulcer: Short-term treatment and maintenance therapy.

Benign gastric ulcer (active): Short-term treatment.

Gastroesophageal reflux disease (GERD): For erosions, ulcerations and associated heartburn.

Administration and Dosage:

Approved by the FDA in April 1988.

Active duodenal ulcer: 300 mg once daily at bedtime. An alternative dosage regimen is 150 mg twice daily.

Maintenance of healed duodenal ulcer: 150 mg once daily at bedtime.

GERD: 150 mg twice daily.

Moderate to severe renal insufficiency:

Nizatidine Dosage in Renal Insufficiency

	Dosage	
Creatinine clearance	Active duodenal ulcer	Maintenance therapy
20 to 50 ml/min	150 mg/day	150 mg every other day
< 20 ml/min	150 mg every other day	150 mg every 3 days

Extemporaneous liquid preparation: When a typical 150 or 300 mg dose was mixed in various commercial juices (eg, *Gatorade,* apple juice, *Ocean Spray*), nizatidine solutions were stable for at least 48 hours under refrigeration and at room temperature (except in *V8* and *Cran-Grape* juices, which had 10% loss of nizatidine potency at room temperature).

otc	**Axid AR** (Whitehall-Robins)	**Tablets:** 75 mg	In 6s, 12s, 18s and 30s.
Rx	**Axid Pulvules** (Lilly)	**Capsules:** 150 mg	Yellow. In 60s.
		300 mg	Yellow/brown. In 30s.

FAMOTIDINE

For complete prescribing information, refer to the Histamine H_2 Antagonists group monograph.

Indications:

Duodenal ulcer: Short-term treatment and maintenance therapy.

Benign gastric ulcer: Short-term treatment.

Pathological hypersecretory conditions.

Gastroesophageal reflux disease (GERD): Short-term treatment. Also for esophagitis due to GERD, including erosive or ulcerative disease (short-term treatment).

Heartburn, acid indigestion and sour stomach (otc only): Relief of these symptoms. Also for prevention of these symptoms brought on by consuming food and beverages.

Administration and Dosage:

Approved by the FDA in October 1986.

Oral:

Duodenal ulcer –

Acute therapy: 40 mg/day at bedtime. Most heal in 4 weeks; there is rarely reason to use full dosage for > 6 to 8 weeks. 20 mg twice/day is also effective.

Maintenance therapy: 20 mg once a day at bedtime.

Benign gastric ulcer –

Acute therapy: 40 mg orally once a day at bedtime.

Pathological hypersecretory conditions – Individualize dosage. The adult starting dose is 20 mg every 6 hours; some patients may require a higher starting dose. Continue as long as clinically indicated. Doses up to 160 mg every 6 hours have been administered to some patients with severe Zollinger-Ellison syndrome.

GERD – 20 mg twice daily for up to 6 weeks. For esophagitis including erosions and ulcerations and accompanying symptoms due to GERD, 20 or 40 mg twice daily for up to 12 weeks.

Heartburn, acid indigestion and sour stomach (otc only) –

Relief: 10 mg (1 tablet) with water.

Prevention: 10 mg 1 hour before eating a meal that is expected to cause symptoms.

FAMOTIDINE

Can be used up to twice daily (up to 2 tablets in 24 hrs). Do not take maximum dose for > 2 weeks continuously unless otherwise directed by a physician.

Children: Do not give to children < 12 years of age unless otherwise directed.

Concomitant use of antacids – Antacids may be given concomitantly if needed.

Severe renal insufficiency (Ccr < 10 ml/min) – The elimination half-life may exceed 20 hours, reaching ≈ 24 hours in anuric patients. Although no relationship of adverse effects to high plasma levels has been established, to avoid excess accumulation of the drug, the dose may be reduced to 20 mg at bedtime or the dosing interval may be prolonged to 36 to 48 hours, as indicated.

Parenteral:

IV – In some hospitalized patients with pathological hypersecretory conditions or intractable ulcers, or in patients unable to take oral medication, give famotidine IV 20 mg every 12 hours. Doses and regimen for GERD are not established.

Preparation of IV solutions – Dilute 2 ml famotidine IV (solution containing 10 mg/ml) with 0.9% Sodium Chloride Injection or other compatible IV solution to a total volume of either 5 or 10 ml and inject over not less than 2 minutes.

Preparation of IV infusion solutions – Famotidine IV may also be administered as an infusion, 2 ml diluted with 100 ml of 5% Dextrose or other compatible solution, and infused over 15 to 30 minutes. A premixed solution is also available containing famotidine premixed with 0.9% sodium chloride.

Stability – Solution is stable for 48 hours at room temperature when added to or diluted with most commonly used IV solutions (eg, Water for Injection, 0.9% Sodium Chloride Injection, 5% or 10% Dextrose Injection, Lactated Ringer's Injection, 5% Sodium Bicarbonate Injection). Famotidine, 20 to 50 mg/L, is also stable with various total parenteral nutrition solutions: 24 hours at 4°C (39°F), then 24 hours at 20° to 22°C (68° to 72°F) in a mixture of dextrose, amino acids and fat emulsion; up to 72 hours at room temp in dextrose, amino acids, electrolytes, vitamins, minerals and fat emulsion; 35 days under refrigeration in dextrose, amino acids, electrolytes and trace elements.

Storage – Do not store powder at > 40°C (104°F). After reconstitution of powder, store oral suspension at < 30°C (86°F). Do not freeze. Discard unused suspension after 30 days. Store the premixed solutions at room temperature; avoid exposure to excessive heat (brief exposure to temperatures up to 35°C [95°F] does not adversely affect the product).

Store injection (non-premixed) at 2° to 8°C (36° to 46°F). When mixed with dextrose or sodium chloride in polyvinyl chloride minibags, famotidine is stable for 14 days at 4°C (39°F), or when frozen for 28 days and subsequently refrigerated for 14 days. Also, when stored at – 20°C (– 4°F) in polypropylene syringes, famotidine is stable for 3 weeks in dextrose and for 8 weeks in sodium chloride. One study showed stability of famotidine admixed in dextrose or saline in polyvinyl chloride minibags and polypropyline syringes for 15 days at room temperature.

otc	**Pepcid AC Acid Controller** (J & J Merck)	**Tablets:** 10 mg	In 12s.
Rx	**Pepcid** (Merck)	**Tablets:** 20 mg	(MSD 963). Beige. Film coated. In unit-of-use 30s, 90s, 100s, UD 100s.
		40 mg	(MSD 964). Lt. brownish-orange. Film coated. In unit-of-use 30s, 90s, 100s & UD 100s.
Rx	**Pepcid** (Merck)	**Powder for Oral Suspension:** 40 mg per 5 ml when reconstituted	Cherry-banana-mint flavor. In bottles of 400 mg.
Rx	**Pepcid** (Merck)	**Injection:** 10 mg per ml	Mannitol. In 2 ml single-dose vials[1] & 4 ml multi-dose vials.[2]
Rx	**Pepcid** (Merck)	**Injection, premixed:** 20 mg per 50 ml in 0.9% NaCl	In single-dose 50 ml *Galaxy* containers.

[1] Preservative free.

[2] With 0.9% benzyl alcohol.

MISOPROSTOL

Warning:

Misoprostol is contraindicated because of its abortifacient property in pregnant women. Advise patients of the abortifacient property and warn them not to give the drug to others. Do not use in women of childbearing potential unless the patient requires nonsteroidal anti-inflammatory drugs (NSAIDs) and is at high risk of complications from gastric ulcers associated with use of NSAIDs, or is at high risk of developing gastric ulceration. In such patients, misoprostol may be prescribed if the patient:

- Is capable of complying with effective contraceptive measures;
- Has received both oral and written warnings of the hazards of misoprostol, the risk of possible contraception failure and the danger to other women of childbearing potential should the drug be taken by mistake;
- Has had a negative *serum* pregnancy test within 2 weeks prior to beginning therapy;
- Will begin therapy only on second or third day of next normal menstrual period.

Actions:

Pharmacology: Misoprostol was approved by the FDA in 1988.

Misoprostol, a synthetic prostaglandin E_1 analog, has both antisecretory (inhibiting gastric acid secretion) and (in animals) mucosal protective properties. NSAIDs inhibit prostaglandin synthesis; a deficiency of prostaglandins within the gastric mucosa may lead to diminishing bicarbonate and mucous secretion and may contribute to the mucosal damage caused by these agents. Misoprostol can increase bicarbonate and mucus production.

Prostaglandin receptor binding is saturable, reversible and stereospecific. The sites have a high affinity for misoprostol, for its acid metabolite, and for other E type prostaglandins, but not for F or I prostaglandins and unrelated compounds, such as histamine or cimetidine. It is likely that these specific receptors allow misoprostol taken with food to be effective topically, despite the lower serum concentrations attained.

Misoprostol produces a moderate decrease in pepsin concentration during basal conditions, but not during histamine stimulation. It has no significant effect on fasting or postprandial gastrin nor on intrinsic factor output.

Effects on gastric acid secretion – Misoprostol over the range of 50 to 200 mcg inhibits basal and nocturnal gastric acid secretion, and acid secretion in response to a variety of stimuli, including meals, histamine, pentagastrin and coffee. Activity is apparent 30 minutes after oral administration and persists for at least 3 hours. Only the 200 mcg dose had substantial effects on nocturnal secretion or on histamine and meal-stimulated secretion.

Uterine effects – Misoprostol produces uterine contractions that may endanger pregnancy (see Warnings). In studies in women undergoing elective termination of pregnancy during the first trimester, misoprostol caused partial or complete expulsion of the uterine contents in 11% of the subjects and increased uterine bleeding in 41%.

Pharmacokinetics: Misoprostol is extensively absorbed, and undergoes rapid de-esterification to its free acid, which is responsible for its clinical activity and, unlike the parent compound, is detectable in plasma. In healthy volunteers, misoprostol is rapidly absorbed after oral administration with a time to reach peak concentration of misoprostol acid of 12 $\pm$ 3 minutes and a terminal half-life of 20 to 40 minutes.

Mean plasma levels after single doses show a linear relationship with doses over the range of 200 to 400 mcg. No accumulation was noted in multiple-dose studies; plasma steady state was achieved within 2 days. After oral administration of radiolabeled misoprostol, $\approx$ 80% of detected radioactivity appears in urine.

Misoprostol does not affect the hepatic mixed function oxidase (cytochrome P-450) enzyme system in animals. The serum protein binding of misoprostol acid is < 90% and is concentration-independent in the therapeutic range.

MISOPROSTOL

Clinical trials: A series of small short-term (about 1 week) placebo controlled studies in healthy human volunteers using misoprostol 200 mcg 4 times a day with tolmetin and naproxen or 100 and 200 mcg 4 times a day with ibuprofen showed reduction of the rate of significant endoscopic injury from about 70% to 75% on placebo to 10% to 30% on misoprostol. Doses of 25 to 200 mcg 4 times a day reduced aspirin-induced mucosal injury and bleeding.

Two 12 week randomized, double-blind trials in osteoarthritic patients who had GI symptoms but no ulcer on endoscopy while taking an NSAID compared the ability of 100 or 200 mcg of misoprostol or placebo to prevent gastric ulcer formation. Patients were equally divided between ibuprofen, piroxicam and naproxen and continued this treatment throughout the 12 weeks. The 200 mcg dose caused a marked, statistically significant reduction in gastric ulcers in both studies. The 100 mcg dose was somewhat less effective, with a significant result in only one of the studies.

In another clinical trial, 239 patients receiving aspirin 650 to 1300 mg 4 times a day for rheumatoid arthritis and who had endoscopic evidence of duodenal or gastric inflammation were randomized to misoprostol 200 mcg 4 times a day or placebo for 8 weeks while continuing to receive aspirin. Misoprostol did not interfere with the efficacy of aspirin in these patients with rheumatoid arthritis.

Indications:

Prevention of NSAID- (including aspirin) induced gastric ulcers in patients at high risk of complications from a gastric ulcer, eg, the elderly and patients with concomitant debilitating disease, as well as patients at high risk of developing gastric ulceration, such as patients with a history of ulcer. Take misoprostol for the duration of NSAID therapy.

Unlabeled uses: In doses of at least 400 mcg/day, misoprostol appears effective in treating duodenal ulcers, and may be useful in treating duodenal ulcers unresponsive to histamine H_2 antagonists; however, it does not prevent duodenal ulcers in patients on NSAIDs (see Warnings).

In one study, misoprostol 200 mcg 4 times daily for 12 weeks (concurrently with cyclosporine and prednisone) reduced the incidence of acute graft rejection in renal transplant recipients by improving renal function.

Contraindications:

History of allergy to prostaglandins; pregnancy (see Warnings).

Warnings:

Duodenal ulcers: Misoprostol does not prevent duodenal ulcers in patients on NSAIDs. It had no effect, compared to placebo, on GI pain or discomfort associated with NSAIDs.

Renal function impairment: Pharmacokinetic studies in patients with varying degrees of renal impairment showed an approximate doubling of half-life, maximum concentration and area under the curve (AUC), but no clear correlation between degree of impairment and AUC was shown. No routine dosage adjustment is recommended, but dosage may need to be reduced if usual dose is not tolerated.

Fertility impairment: Misoprostol, when administered to breeding male and female rats at doses 6.25 times to 625 times the maximum recommended human therapeutic dose, produced dose related pre- and post-implantation losses and a significant decrease in the number of live pups born at the highest dose. These findings suggest the possibility of a general adverse effect on fertility in males and females.

Elderly: In subjects > 64 years of age, the AUC for misoprostol acid is increased; however, no routine dosage adjustment is recommended. Reduce the dose if the usual dose is not tolerated.

Pregnancy: Category X. Misoprostol may cause miscarriage. Uterine contractions, uterine bleeding and expulsion of the products of conception occur. Miscarriages caused by misoprostol may be incomplete. In studies in women undergoing elective termination of pregnancy during the first trimester, misoprostol caused partial or complete expulsion of the products of conception in 11% of subjects and increased uterine bleeding in 41%. If a woman is or becomes pregnant while taking this drug, discontinue the drug and apprise the patient of potential hazards to the fetus.

Lactation: It is unlikely that misoprostol is excreted in breast milk, since it is rapidly metabolized. However, it is not known if the active metabolite (misoprostol acid) is excreted in breast milk. Therefore, do not administer to nursing mothers because the potential excretion of misoprostol acid could cause significant diarrhea in nursing infants.

Children: Safety and efficacy in children < 18 years of age have not been established.

MISOPROSTOL

Precautions:

Women of childbearing potential: Advise women of childbearing potential that they must not be pregnant when misoprostol therapy is initiated, and that they must use an effective contraception method while taking misoprostol. See Warnings.

Diarrhea (13% to 40%) is dose-related and usually develops early in the course of therapy (after 13 days), usually is self-limiting (often resolving after 8 days), but sometimes requires discontinuation of misoprostol (2% of the patients). The incidence of diarrhea can be minimized by administering after meals and at bedtime, and by avoiding coadministration of misoprostol with magnesium-containing antacids.

Drug Interactions:

Antacids reduce the total availability of misoprostol acid but this does not appear clinically important.

Drug/Food interactions: Maximum plasma concentrations of misoprostol acid are diminished when taken with food.

Adverse Reactions:

GI: Diarrhea (13% to 40%); abdominal pain (7% to 20%); nausea (3.2%); flatulence (2.9%); dyspepsia (2%); vomiting (1.3%); constipation (1.1%).

GU: Spotting (0.7%); cramps (0.6%); hypermenorrhea (0.5%); menstrual disorder (0.3%); dysmenorrhea (0.1%). Postmenopausal vaginal bleeding may be related to misoprostol administration. If it occurs, perform diagnostic workup to rule out gynecological pathology.

Miscellaneous: Headache (2.4%).

Overdosage:

Symptoms: The toxic dose in humans has not been determined. Cumulative total daily doses of 1600 mcg have been tolerated with only symptoms of GI discomfort. In animals, the acute toxic effects are diarrhea, GI lesions, focal cardiac, hepatic and renal tubular necrosis, testicular atrophy, respiratory difficulties and CNS depression. Clinical signs that may indicate an overdose are sedation, tremor, convulsions, dyspnea, abdominal pain, diarrhea, fever, palpitations, hypotension or bradycardia.

Treatment: Treat with supportive therapy; refer to Management of Acute Overdosage.

It is not known if misoprostol acid is dialyzable. However, because misoprostol is metabolized like a fatty acid, it is unlikely that dialysis would be appropriate treatment for overdosage.

Patient Information:

Misoprostol can cause miscarriage, often associated with potentially dangerous bleeding. This may result in hospitalization, surgery, infertility or death. Do not take misoprostol if pregnant and do not become pregnant while taking this medication. If pregnancy occurs during misoprostol therapy, discontinue the drug and contact physician immediately.

Take misoprostol only according to the directions given by the physician.

Do not give misoprostol to anyone else.

Administration and Dosage:

Adults: 200 mcg 4 times daily with food. If this dose cannot be tolerated, 100 mcg can be used. Take misoprostol for the duration of NSAID therapy as prescribed. Take with meals, the last dose of the day taken at bedtime.

Renal impairment: Dosage adjustment is not routinely needed, but dosage can be reduced if the 200 mcg dose is not tolerated.

Rx	**Cytotec** (Searle)	**Tablets:** 100 mcg	(Searle 1451). White. In UD 100s and unit-of-use 60s and 120s.
		200 mcg	(Searle 1461). White, scored. Hexagonal. In UD 100s and unit-of-use 60s and 100s.

OMEPRAZOLE

Actions:

Pharmacology: Omeprazole belongs to a class of antisecretory compounds, the substituted benzimidazoles, that do not exhibit anticholinergic or H_2 histamine antagonistic properties, but that suppress gastric acid secretion by specific inhibition of the H^+/K^+ ATPase enzyme system at the secretory surface of the gastric parietal cell. Because this enzyme system is the "acid (proton) pump" within the gastric mucosa, omeprazole has been characterized as a gastric acid pump inhibitor; it blocks the final step of acid production. This effect is dose-related and inhibits both basal and stimulated acid secretion regardless of the stimulus. In animals, after rapid disappearance from plasma, omeprazole is found within the gastric mucosa for ≥ 1 day.

Antisecretory activity – Onset after oral administration of omeprazole occurs within 1 hour and peaks within 2 hours. Inhibition of secretion is ≈ 50% of maximum at 24 hours, and the duration of inhibition lasts ≤ 72 hours. The antisecretory effect thus lasts far longer than would be expected from the very short (< 1 hour) plasma half-life, apparently due to prolonged binding to the parietal H^+/K^+ ATPase enzyme. When the drug is discontinued, secretory activity returns over 3 to 5 days. The inhibitory effect of omeprazole on acid secretion increases with repeated once-daily dosing, plateauing after 4 days.

Results from numerous studies on the antisecretory effect of multiple doses of 20 and 40 mg omeprazole in healthy volunteers and patients are shown below. The "max" value represents determinations at a time of maximum effect (2 to 6 hours after dosing), while "min" values are those 24 hours after the last omeprazole dose.

Mean Antisecretory Effects of Omeprazole After Multiple Daily Dosing (%)

Parameter	Omeprazole 20 mg		Omeprazole 40 mg	
	Max	Min	Max	Min
Decrease in basal acid output	78[1]	58 - 80	94[1]	80 - 93
Decrease in peak acid output	79[1]	50 - 59	88[1]	62 - 68
Decrease in 24 hr intragastric acidity	NA	80 - 97	NA	92 - 94

[1] Single-dose studies.

Single daily oral doses of omeprazole 10 to 40 mg have produced 100% inhibition of 24 hour intragastric acidity in some patients.

Serum gastrin effects – In studies involving > 200 patients, serum gastrin levels increased during the first 1 to 2 weeks of once-daily therapeutic omeprazole doses parallel with inhibition of acid secretion. No further increase in serum gastrin occurred with continued treatment. In comparison with histamine H_2-receptor antagonists, the median increases produced by 20 mg omeprazole were higher (1.3- to 3.6-fold vs 1.1- to 1.8-fold). Gastrin values usually returned to pretreatment levels within 1 to 2 weeks after discontinuation of therapy.

Other effects – No effect on gastric emptying was demonstrated after a single 90 mg dose. In healthy subjects, a single IV dose (0.35 mg/kg) had no effect on intrinsic factor secretion. No dose-dependent effect has been observed on basal or stimulated pepsin output. However, when intragastric pH is maintained at ≥ 4, basal pepsin output is low, and pepsin activity is decreased.

As seen with other agents that elevate intragastric pH, omeprazole administered for 14 days in healthy subjects produced a significant increase in the intragastric concentrations of viable bacteria. The pattern of the bacterial species was unchanged from that commonly found in saliva. All changes resolved within 3 days of stopping treatment.

Pharmacokinetics:

Absorption/Distribution – Omeprazole contains an enteric coated granule formulation (because omeprazole is acid-labile). Absorption is rapid, with peak plasma levels occurring within 0.5 to 3.5 hours. Peak plasma concentrations of omeprazole and AUC are approximately proportional to doses ≤ 40 mg, but because of a saturable first-pass effect, a greater than linear response in peak plasma concentration and AUC occurs with doses > 40 mg. Absolute bioavailability is ≈ 30% to 40% at doses of 20 to 40 mg, due to presystemic metabolism. Plasma half-life is 0.5 to 1 hour, and total body clearance is 500 to 600 ml/min. Protein binding is ≈ 95%. The bioavailability of omeprazole increases slightly upon repeated administration.

OMEPRAZOLE

Metabolism/Excretion – Little unchanged drug is excreted in urine. The majority of the dose (≈ 77%) is eliminated in urine as at least six metabolites. Two are hydroxyomeprazole and the corresponding carboxylic acid. The remainder of the dose was excreted in feces. This implies a significant biliary excretion of the metabolites of omeprazole. Three metabolites, the sulfide and sulfone derivatives and hydroxyomeprazole, have been identified in plasma. These metabolites have little or no antisecretory activity.

Hepatic function impairment: In patients with chronic hepatic disease, the bioavailability increased to ≈ 100%, reflecting decreased first-pass effect; plasma half-life increased to nearly 3 hours. Plasma clearance averaged 70 ml/min, compared with 500 to 600 ml/min in healthy subjects.

Renal function impairment: In patients with chronic renal impairment (creatinine clearance, 10 to 62 ml/min/1.73 m^2), the disposition of omeprazole was similar to that in healthy volunteers, but with a slight increase in bioavailability. Because urinary excretion is a primary route of excretion of omeprazole metabolites, their elimination slowed in proportion to the decreased creatinine clearance.

Elderly: The elimination rate of omeprazole was somewhat decreased, and bioavailability was increased. Omeprazole was 76% bioavailable with a 40 mg oral dose in elderly volunteers vs 58% in young volunteers. Nearly 70% of the dose was recovered in urine as metabolites; no unchanged drug was detected. The plasma clearance of omeprazole was 250 ml/min, and its plasma half-life averaged 1 hour.

Races: An increase in AUC of ≈ 4-fold was noted in Asian subjects compared with Caucasians. Consider dose adjustment for hepatically impaired and Asian subjects, particularly where maintenance of healing of erosive esophagitis is indicated.

Clinical trials:

Active duodenal ulcer – In a study of 293 patients with endoscopically documented duodenal ulcer, the percentage of patients healed (per protocol) at 4 weeks was significantly higher with omeprazole 20 mg once a day than with ranitidine 150 mg twice a day, and healing occurred significantly faster in patients treated with omeprazole.

Gastroesophageal reflux disease (GERD) –

Short-term treatment: In a study comparing 20 and 40 mg omeprazole in patients with symptomatic esophagitis and endoscopically diagnosed erosive esophagitis, the 40 mg dose was not superior to the 20 mg dose in the percentage healing rate. In comparison with histamine H_2-receptor antagonists in patients with erosive esophagitis, grade 2 or above, a 20 mg dose of omeprazole was significantly more effective than the active controls. Complete daytime and nighttime heartburn relief occurred significantly faster in patients treated with omeprazole than in those taking placebo or histamine H_2-receptor antagonists.

Maintenance treatment: In a study, omeprazole 10 and 20 mg daily were compared with ranitidine 150 mg twice daily in patients with endoscopically confirmed healed esophagitis. The percentages of patients in endoscopic remission at 12 months were as follows: Omeprazole 10 mg daily, 58%; omeprazole 20 mg daily, 77%; ranitidine, 46%. For maintenance after healing, in patients who initially had grades 3 or 4 erosive esophagitis, 20 mg/day omeprazole was effective, while 10 mg/day was not.

Pathological hypersecretory conditions – In studies of patients with pathological hypersecretory conditions, such as Zollinger-Ellison (ZE) syndrome with or without multiple endocrine adenomas, omeprazole significantly inhibited gastric acid secretion and controlled associated symptoms of diarrhea, anorexia and pain; 20 mg every other day to 360 mg/day maintained basal acid secretion < 10 mEq/hr was effective in patients without prior gastric surgery, and < 5 mEq/hr was effective in patients with prior gastric surgery.

Omeprazole was well tolerated for > 5 years in some patients. In most ZE patients, serum gastrin levels were not changed. However, serum gastrin increased in some patients. At least 11 patients with ZE syndrome on long-term treatment developed gastric carcinoids. This finding was believed to be a manifestation of the underlying condition, rather than the result of omeprazole administration.

Indications:

Gastric ulcer: Short-term treatment (4 to 8 weeks) of active benign gastric ulcer.

Active duodenal ulcer: Short-term treatment of active duodenal ulcer. Most patients heal within 4 weeks, although some may require an additional 4 weeks.

Gastroesophageal reflux disease (GERD):

Erosive esophagitis – Short-term treatment (4 to 8 weeks) of erosive esophagitis diagnosed by endoscopy.

Poorly responsive symptomatic GERD – Short-term treatment (4 to 8 weeks) of symptomatic GERD (esophagitis) poorly responsive to customary medical treatment, usually including histamine H_2-receptor antagonists.

Eradication of H. pylori – In combination with clarithromycin for treatment of patients with *H. pylori* infection and active duodenal ulcer.

Maintenance – To maintain healing of erosive esophagitis.

Pathological hypersecretory conditions (eg, Zollinger-Ellison syndrome, multiple endocrine adenomas and systemic mastocytosis): Long-term treatment.

Unlabeled uses: Omeprazole, in combination with amoxicillin, appears to be effective in the eradication of *H. pylori*.

Contraindications:

Hypersensitivity to any component of the formulation.

Warnings:

Maintenance therapy: Omeprazole should not be used as maintenance therapy for treatment of patients with duodenal ulcer disease.

Duration of therapy (GERD): The efficacy of omeprazole used for > 8 weeks has not been established. In the rare patient not responding to 8 weeks of treatment, an additional 4 weeks of treatment may help. If there is recurrence of erosive or symptomatic GERD poorly responsive to customary medical treatment, an additional 4 to 8 week course of omeprazole may be considered.

Atrophic gastritis has been noted occasionally in gastric corpus biopsies from patients treated long-term with omeprazole.

Carcinogenesis: In two 24 month carcinogenicity studies in rats, omeprazole at daily doses ≈ 4 to 352 times the human dose, produced gastric enterochromaffin-like (ECL) cell carcinoids in a dose-related manner in male and female rats; the incidence was markedly higher in female rats, which had higher blood levels of omeprazole. In addition, ECL cell hyperplasia was present in all treated groups of both sexes. In one study, female rats were treated with 35 times the human dose for 1 year, then taken off the drug and studied for an additional year. No carcinoids were seen in these rats. An increased incidence of treatment-related ECL cell hyperplasia was observed after 1 year (94% treated vs 10% controls). By the second year, the difference between treated and control rats was much smaller (46% vs 26%). An unusual primary malignant tumor in the stomach was seen in one rat (2%).

Elderly: Bioavailability may be increased (see Pharmacokinetics).

Pregnancy: Category C. In rabbits, doses 17 to 172 times the human dose produced dose-related increases in embryo lethality, fetal resorptions and pregnancy disruptions. In rats, dose-related embryo/fetal toxicity and postnatal developmental toxicity were observed in offspring of parents treated with 35 to 345 times the human dose. There are no adequate or well controlled studies in pregnant women. Use during pregnancy only if the potential benefit justifies the risk to the fetus.

Lactation: It is not known whether omeprazole is excreted in breast milk. In rats, omeprazole administration during late gestation and lactation at doses of 35 to 345 times the human dose resulted in decreased weight gain in pups. Decide whether to discontinue nursing or to discontinue the drug, taking into account the importance of the drug to the mother.

Children: Safety and efficacy in children have not been established.

Precautions:

Gastric malignancy: Symptomatic response to therapy with omeprazole does not preclude gastric malignancy.

OMEPRAZOLE

Drug Interactions:

There may be interactions with other drugs also metabolized via the cytochrome P450 system, although no interaction with theophylline or propranolol has been found in healthy subjects. Because of its profound and long lasting inhibition of gastric acid secretion, omeprazole may interfere with absorption of drugs where gastric pH is a determinant of their bioavailability (eg, ketoconazole, ampicillin esters, iron salts). In clinical trials, antacids were used concomitantly with omeprazole.

Omeprazole Drug Interactions

Precipitant drug	Object drug *		Description
Clarithromycin	Omeprazole	↑	Co-administration of omeprazole and clarithromycin may result in increases in plasma levels of omeprazole, clarithromycin and 14-hydroxy-clarithromycin.
Omeprazole	Clarithromycin		
Omeprazole	Diazepam	↑	Omeprazole produced a 130% increase in the half-life of diazepam, probably due to inhibition of oxidative metabolism. Plasma concentrations were also increased and total clearance of diazepam was decreased. Clinical significance was not determined.
Omeprazole	Phenytoin	↑	Omeprazole reduced the plasma clearance of phenytoin by 15% and increased its half-life by 27%, probably due to inhibition of oxidative metabolism. Clinical significance was not determined.
Omeprazole	Warfarin	↑	Omeprazole may prolong the elimination of warfarin via inhibition of oxidative metabolism.

* ↑ = Object drug increased.

Adverse Reactions:

Omeprazole is generally well tolerated. In clinical trials of 3096 patients (including duodenal ulcer, Zollinger-Ellison syndrome and resistant ulcer patients), the following adverse experiences occurred in ≥ 1% of patients:

Selected Omeprazole Adverse Reactions (%): Omeprazole vs Ranitidine

Adverse reaction	Omeprazole (n = 465)	Placebo (n = 64)	Ranitidine (n = 195)
CNS			
Headache	6.9	6.3	7.7
Dizziness	1.5	0	2.6
Asthenia	1.1	1.6	1.5
GI			
Diarrhea	3	3.1	2.1
Abdominal pain	2.4	3.1	2.1
Nausea	2.2	3.1	4.1
Vomiting	1.5	4.7	1.5
Constipation	1.1	0	0
Miscellaneous			
Upper-respiratory infection	1.9	1.6	2.6
Rash	1.5	0	0
Cough	1.1	0	1.5
Back pain	1.1	0	0.5

OMEPRAZOLE

Adverse reactions occurring in < 1% of patients (relationship to omeprazole unclear):

Body as a whole – Fever; pain; fatigue; malaise; abdominal swelling.

Cardiovascular – Chest pain/angina; tachycardia; bradycardia; palpitation; elevated blood pressure; peripheral edema.

CNS – Vertigo; insomnia; confusion; nervousness; tremors; apathy; somnolence; anxiety disorders; paresthesia; dream abnormalities; hemifacial dysesthesia; depression; agression; hallucinations.

Dermatologic – Rash; severe generalized skin reactions including toxic epidermal necrolysis (rare, some fatal); Stevens-Johnson syndrome; erythema multiforme (some severe); skin inflammation; urticaria; angioedema; pruritus; alopecia; dry skin; hyperhidrosis.

GI – Pancreatitis (some fatal); anorexia; irritable colon; fecal discoloration; esophageal candidiasis; mucosal atrophy of the tongue; dry mouth; flatulence; gastric fundic gland polyps (rare) that are benign and appear to be reversible with treatment discontinuation.

Gastro-duodenal carcinoids have been reported in patients with ZE syndrome on long-term treatment with omeprazole. This finding is believed to be a manifestation of the underlying condition, which is known to be associated with such tumors.

GU – Acute interstitial nephritis (some with positive rechallenge); urinary tract infection; microscopic pyuria; urinary frequency; elevated serum creatinine; proteinuria; hematuria; glycosuria; testicular pain; gynecomastia.

Hematologic – Pancytopenia; thrombocytopenia; neutropenia; anemia; hemolytic anemia; leukocytosis; gout; agranulocytosis (some fatal). Agranulocytosis occurred in a 65-year-old diabetic male on several drugs in addition to omeprazole; the relationship of the agranulocytosis to omeprazole is uncertain.

Hepatic – Elevated AST, ALT, γ-glutamyl transpeptidase, alkaline phosphatase and bilirubin (jaundice) (mild and rare); overt liver disease (rare), including hepatocellular, cholestatic or mixed hepatitis; liver necrosis (some fatal); hepatic failure (some fatal); hepatic encephalopathy.

Metabolic/Nutritional – Hyponatremia; hypoglycemia; weight gain.

Musculoskeletal – Muscle cramps; myalgia; muscle weakness; joint pain; leg pain.

Respiratory – Epistaxis; pharyngeal pain; bronchospasms.

Special Senses – Tinnitus; taste perversion.

Elderly: The incidence of clinical adverse experiences in patients > 65 years of age was similar to that in patients ≤ 65 years of age.

Combination therapy with clarithromycin: Adverse experiences observed in controlled clinical trials using combination therapy with omeprazole and clarithromycin that differed from those previously described for omeprazole alone were: Taste perversion (15%); tongue discoloration (2%); rhinitis (2%); pharyngitis (1%); flu syndrome (1%).

Overdosage:

Rare reports have been received of overdosage with omeprazole. Doses ranged from 320 to 900 mg (16 to 45 times the usual recommended dose).

Symptoms: Confusion; drowsiness; blurred vision; tachycardia; nausea; diaphoresis; flushing; headache; dry mouth. Symptoms were transient and no serious clinical outcome has been reported. No specific antidote for omeprazole overdosage is known.

Treatment: Omeprazole is extensively protein bound and is therefore not readily dialyzable. Treatment should be symptomatic and supportive. Refer to General Management of Acute Overdosage.

Patient Information:

Take before eating.

Swallow capsule whole; do not open, chew or crush.

OMEPRAZOLE

Administration and Dosage:

Active duodenal ulcer:

Adults – 20 mg daily for 4 to 8 weeks (see Indications).

GERD:

Erosive esophagitis or poorly responsive GERD –

Adults: 20 mg daily for 4 to 8 weeks (see Indications).

Maintenance of healing erosive esophagitis – 20 mg daily.

Reduction of risk of duodenal ulcer recurrence:

Omeprazole and Clarithromycin: Combination Therapy	
Days 1 - 14	Days 15 - 28
Omeprazole 40 mg qd (in the morning) plus clarithromycin 500 mg tid	Omeprazole 20 mg qd

For additional prescribing information for clarithromycin, refer to the clarithromycin monograph.

Gastric ulcer: The recommended adult oral dose is 40 mg once a day for 4 to 8 weeks.

Pathological hypersecretory conditions: Individualize dosage. Initial adult dose is 60 mg /day. Doses up to 120 mg 3 times/day have been administered. Administer daily dosages > 80 mg in divided doses. Some patients with Zollinger-Ellison syndrome have been treated continuously for > 5 years.

No dosage adjustment is necessary for patients with renal impairment, hepatic dysfunction or for the elderly.

Take before eating. Do not open, crush or chew the capsule; swallow whole. In the clinical trials, antacids were used concomitantly with omeprazole.

Storage/Stability: Store omeprazole delayed release capsules in a tight container. Protect from light and moisture. Store between 15° and 30°C (59° and 86°F).

Rx	**Prilosec** (Astra Merck)	**Capsules, delayed release:** 10 mg	Lactose. (606 Prilosec 10). Apricot and amethyst. In 30s, 100s and UD 100s.
		20 mg	Lactose. (742 Prilosec 20). Amethyst. In 30s, 1000s and UD 100s.

LANSOPRAZOLE

Actions:

Pharmacology: Lansoprazole belongs to a class of antisecretory compounds, the substituted benzimidazoles, that do not exhibit anticholinergic or histamine H_2-receptor antagonist properties, but that suppress gastric acid secretion by specific inhibition of the (H^+, K^+)-ATPase enzyme system at the secretory surface of the gastric parietal cell. Because this enzyme system is regarded as the acid (proton) pump within the parietal cell, lansoprazole has been characterized as a gastric acid-pump inhibitor because it blocks the final step of acid production. This effect is dose-related and leads to inhibition of both basal and stimulated gastric acid secretion regardless of the stimulus.

Antisecretory activity – Given orally, lansoprazole significantly decreases the basal acid output and significantly increases mean gastric pH and percent of time the gastric pH is > 3 and > 4. Lansoprazole also significantly reduces meal-stimulated gastric acid output and secretion volume, as well as pentagastrin-stimulated acid output. In patients with hypersecretion of acid, lansoprazole significantly reduces basal and pentagastrin-stimulated gastric acid secretion. Lansoprazole inhibits normal increases in secretion volume, acidity and acid output induced by insulin.

Because of the normal, physiologic effect caused by the inhibition of gastric acid secretion, blood flow in the antrum, pylorus and duodenal bulb decrease ≈ 17%. Lansoprazole increases serum pepsinogen levels and decreases pepsin activity under basal conditions in response to meal stimulation or insulin injection. As with other agents that elevate intragastric pH, increases in gastric pH are associated with increases in nitrate-reducing bacteria and elevation of nitrite concentration in gastric juice in patients with gastric ulcer.

Median fasting serum gastrin levels increase 50% to 100% from baseline but remain within normal range after treatment. These elevations reach a plateau within 2 months of therapy and return to pretreatment levels within 4 weeks after discontinuation of therapy.

Pharmacokinetics:

Absorption/Distribution – Absorption of lansoprazole begins only after the granules leave the stomach. Absorption is rapid with mean peak plasma levels occurring after ≈ 1.7 hours and is relatively complete with absolute bioavailability > 80%. Peak plasma concentrations (C_{max}) and the area under the plasma concentration curve (AUC) of lansoprazole are approximately proportional. Lansoprazole does not accumulate, and its pharmacokinetics are unaltered by multiple dosing. In healthy subjects, the mean plasma half-life was 1.5 hours. Both C_{max} and AUC are diminished by ≈ 50% if the drug is given 30 minutes after food as opposed to during fasting. There is no significant food effect if the drug is given before meals. Lansoprazole is 97% bound to plasma proteins.

Metabolism – Lansoprazole is extensively metabolized in the liver. Two metabolites have been identified in measurable quantities in plasma (the hydroxylated sulfinyl and sulfone derivatives). These metabolites have very little or no antisecretory activity. Lansoprazole is thought to be transformed into two active species that inhibit acid secretion by (H^+, K^+)-ATPase within the parietal cell canaliculus, but are not present in the systemic circulation. The plasma elimination half-life of lansoprazole does not reflect its duration of suppression of gastric acid secretion. Thus, the plasma elimination half-life is < 2 hours while the acid inhibitory effect lasts > 24 hours.

Excretion – Following single-dose oral administration, virtually no unchanged lansoprazole was excreted in the urine. After a single oral dose, ≈ 33% is excreted in the urine, and 66% was recovered in feces. This implies a significant biliary excretion of the metabolites.

Renal function impairment: Some pharmacokinetics are changed with renal and hepatic function impairment (see Warnings).

LANSOPRAZOLE

Clinical trials: In a crossover study comparing 15 and 30 mg lansoprazole with 20 mg omeprazole for 5 days, the following effects on intragastric pH were noted:

Mean Antisecretory Effects After Single and Multiple Daily Dosing: Lansoprazole vs Omeprazole

Parameter	Baseline value	Lansoprazole 15 mg Day 1	Lansoprazole 15 mg Day 5	Lansoprazole 30 mg Day 1	Lansoprazole 30 mg Day 5	Omeprazole 20 mg Day 1	Omeprazole 20 mg Day 5
Mean 24 hour pH	2.1	2.7	4	3.6	4.9	2.5	4.2
Mean nighttime pH	1.9	2.4	3	2.6	3.8	2.2	3
% time gastric pH > 3	18	33	59	51	72	30	61
% time gastric pH > 4	12	22	49	41	66	19	51

After the initial dose in this study, increased gastric pH was seen within 1 to 2 hours with lansoprazole 30 mg, within 2 to 3 hours with lansoprazole 15 mg and within 3 to 4 hours with omeprazole 20 mg. After multiple daily dosing, gastric pH increased within the first hour postdose with lansoprazole 30 mg and within 1 to 2 hours postdose with lansoprazole 15 mg and omeprazole 20 mg. Inhibition of gastric acid secretion (measured by intragastric pH) returns gradually to normal 2 to 4 days after multiple doses. There is no indication of rebound gastric acidity.

Duodenal ulcer – A comparative study of lansoprazole 15 and 30 mg/day with ranitidine 300 mg HS in 280 patients with endoscopically documented duodenal ulcer was conducted. The 15 mg dose of lansoprazole was superior to ranitidine at 4 weeks, but there was a lack of significant difference at 2 weeks; the absence of a difference between 30 mg of lansoprazole and ranitidine leaves the comparative effectiveness of the two agents undetermined.

Helicobacter pylori – Results from two US randomized, double-blind clinical studies showed that 30 mg lansoprazole plus 500 mg clarithromycin and 1 g amoxicillin given twice daily for 14 days eradicted *H. pylori* in 92% and 86% of patients.

Erosive esophagitis – In another study, 30 mg lansoprazole was compared with ranitidine 150 mg twice daily in 151 patients with erosive reflux esophagitis that were poorly responsive to a minimum of 12 weeks of treatment with either cimetidine 800 mg/day, ranitidine 300 mg/day, famotidine 40 mg/day or nizatidine 300 mg/day. Lansoprazole 30 mg was more effective than ranitidine 150 mg twice daily in healing reflux esophagitis. This study indicates that lansoprazole may be useful in patients failing on a histamine H_2-receptor antagonist.

Pathological hypersecretory conditions including Zollinger-Ellison syndrome – In open studies of 57 patients with pathological hypersecretory conditions, such as Zollinger-Ellison (ZE) syndrome with or without multiple endocrine adenomas, lansoprazole significantly inhibited gastric acid secretion and controlled associated symptoms of diarrhea, anorexia and pain.

Indications:

Duodenal ulcer:

Treatment – Short-term treatment (up to 4 weeks) for healing and symptomatic relief of active duodenal ulcer.

In combination with clarithromycin and amoxicillin as triple therapy for the eradication of *H. pylori* infection in patients with active or recurrent duodenal ulcers.

Maintenance – To maintain healing of duodenal ulcers. Controlled studies do not extend beyond 12 months.

Erosive esophagitis treatment:

Treatment – Short-term treatment (up to 8 weeks) for healing and symptomatic relief of all grades of erosive esophagitis. For patients who do not heal with lansoprazole for 8 weeks (5% to 10%) give an additional 8 weeks of treatment. If there is a recurrence of erosive esophagitis, consider an additional 8–week course of lansoprazole.

Maintenance – Lansoprazole is indicated to maintain healing of erosive esophagitis. Controlled studies do not extend beyond 12 months.

Pathological hypersecretory conditions including Zollinger-Ellison syndrome: Long-term treatment of pathological hypersecretory conditions, including Zollinger-Ellison syndrome.

Contraindications:

Hypersensitivity to any component of the formulation.

LANSOPRAZOLE

Warnings:

Renal function impairment: In severe renal insufficiency, plasma protein binding decreased by 1% to 1.5% after administration of 60 mg. Patients with renal insufficiency had a shortened elimination half-life and decreased total AUC (free and bound). However, AUC for free lansoprazole in plasma was not related to the degree of renal impairment, and C_{max} and T_{max} were not different from subjects with healthy kidneys.

Hepatic function impairment: In patients with various degrees of chronic hepatic disease, the mean plasma half-life of the drug was prolonged from 1.5 to 3.2 to 7.2 hours. An increase in mean AUC of up to 500% was observed at steady state in hepatically impaired patients compared with healthy subjects. Consider dose reduction in patients with severe hepatic disease. (See Administration and Dosage).

Carcinogenesis: Gastric biopsy specimens from the body of the stomach from ≈ 150 patients treated continuously with lansoprazole for ≥ 1 year have not shown evidence of gastric enterochromaffin-like (ECL) cell effects similar to those seen in rat studies. Longer term data are needed to rule out the possibility of an increased risk of the development of gastric tumors in patients receiving long-term therapy with lansoprazole.

Elderly: The clearance of lansoprazole is decreased in the elderly, with an increase of elimination half-life ≈ 50% to 100%. Because the mean half-life in the elderly remains between 1.9 to 2.9 hours, repeated once-daily dosing does not result in accumulation of lansoprazole. Peak plasma levels were not increased in the elderly.

Ulcer healing rates and rates of adverse events in elderly patients are similar to those in a younger age group. The initial dosing regimen need not be altered, but subsequent doses > 30 mg/day should not be administered unless additional gastric acid suppression is necessary.

Pregnancy: Category B. There are no adequate and well controlled studies in pregnant women. Use during pregnancy only if clearly needed.

Lactation: Lansoprazole or its metabolites are excreted in the milk of rats. It is not known whether lansoprazole is excreted in human breast milk. Because of the potential for serious adverse reactions in breast feeding infants from lansoprazole and because of the potential for tumorigenicity shown for lansoprazole in rat carcinogenicity studies, decide whether to discontinue nursing or to discontinue the drug, taking into account the importance of the drug to the mother.

Children: Safety and efficacy in children < 18 years of age have not been established.

Precautions:

Gastric malignancy: Symptomatic response to therapy with lansoprazole does not preclude the presence of gastric malignancy.

Drug Interactions:

Lansoprazole is metabolized through the cytochrome P450 system via the CYP3A and CYP2C19 isozymes; however, lansoprazole does not have clinically significant interactions with other drugs metabolized by the cytochrome P450 system.

Lansoprazole causes a profound and long lasting inhibition of gastric acid secretion; therefore, it is theoretically possible that lansoprazole may interfere with the absorption of drugs where gastric pH is an important determinant of bioavailability (eg, ketoconazole, ampicillin, iron salts, digoxin).

Lansoprazole Drug Interactions

Precipitant drug	Object drug*		Description
Lansoprazole	Ketoconazole	⬇	The effects of ketoconazole may be decreased.
Lansoprazole	Theophylline	⬇	When administered concomitantly, a minor increase (10%) in the clearance of theophylline was seen. Because of the small magnitude and the direction of the effect on theophylline clearance, this interaction is unlikely to be of clinical concern.
Sucralfate	Lansoprazole	⬇	Coadministration delayed absorption and reduced lansoprazole bioavailability by ≈ 17%. Therefore, take lansoprazole 30 minutes prior to sucralfate.

* ⬇ = Object drug decreased.

Drug/Food interactions: Both C_{max} and AUC are diminished by ≈ 50% if the drug is given 30 minutes after food as opposed to in the fasting condition. There is no significant food effect if the drug is given before meals.

LANSOPRAZOLE

Adverse Reactions:

In general, lansoprazole treatment has been well tolerated in both short-term and long-term trials. The following adverse events were reported in ≥ 1% of patients: Diarrhea (3.6%); abdominal pain (1.8%); nausea (1.4%). Headache was also seen at > 1% incidence but was more common with placebo. The incidence of diarrhea is similar between placebo and lansoprazole 15 and 30 mg patients (2.9%, 1.4% and 4.2%, respectively), but higher with lansoprazole 60 mg (7.4%). The most commonly reported adverse event during maintenance therapy was diarrhea. The most frequently reported adverse events for the triple therapy regimen were diarrhea (7%), headache (6%) and taste disturbance (5%).

Other adverse reactions are as follows (<1%):

Cardiovascular: Angina, cerebrovascular accident, hypertension/hypotension, myocardial infarction, palpitations, shock (circulatory failure), vasodilation.

CNS: Agitation, amnesia, anxiety, apathy, confusion, depression, dizziness/syncope, hallucinations, hemiplegia, aggravated hostility, decreased libido, nervousness, paresthesia, abnormal thinking.

Dermatologic: Acne, alopecia, pruritus, rash, urticaria.

Endocrine: Diabetes mellitus, goiter, hyperglycemia/hypoglycemia.

GI: Melena, anorexia, bezoar, cardiospasm, cholelithiasis, constipation, dry mouth/thirst, dyspepsia, dysphagia, eructation, esophageal stenosis, esophageal ulcer, esophagitis, fecal discoloration, flatulence, gastric nodules/fundic gland polyps, gastroenteritis, GI hemorrhage, hematemesis, increased appetite, increased salivation, rectal hemorrhage, stomatitis, tenesmus, ulcerative colitis.

GU: Abnormal menses, albuminuria, breast enlargement/gynecomastia, breast tenderness, glycosuria, hematuria, impotence, kidney calculus.

Hematologic: Anemia, hemolysis.

Metabolic/Nutritional: Gout, weight gain/loss.

Musculoskeletal: Arthritis/arthralgia, musculoskeletal pain, myalgia.

Respiratory: Asthma, bronchitis, increased cough, dyspnea, epistaxis, hemoptysis, hiccough, pneumonia, upper respiratory inflammation/infection.

Special senses: Amblyopia, deafness, eye pain, visual field defect, otitis media, taste perversion, tinnitus.

Miscellaneous: Asthenia, candidiasis, chest pain (not otherwise specified), edema, fever, flu syndrome, halitosis, infection (not otherwise specified), malaise.

Lab test abnormalities: Abnormal liver function tests; increased AST, ALT, creatinine, alkaline phosphatase, globulins, GGTP, glucocorticoids, LDH, gastrin levels; increased/decreased/abnormal WBC and platelets; abnormal AG ratio; abnormal RBC; bilirubinemia; eosinophilia; hyperlipemia; increased/decreased electrolytes; increased/decreased cholesterol.

In the placebo controlled studies, when ALT and AST were evaluated, 0.4% of placebo patients and 0.3% of lansoprazole patients had enzyme elevations > three times the upper limit of normal range at the final treatment visit. None of these patients reported jaundice at any time during the study.

Overdosage:

In one case of overdose, the patient consumed 600 mg of lansoprazole with no adverse reaction. Lansoprazole is not removed from the circulation by hemodialysis.

Patient Information:

Take before eating.

For patients who have difficulty swallowing capsules, lansoprazole can be opened, and the intact granules contained within can be sprinkled on one tablespoon of applesauce and swallowed immediately. Do not chew or crush the granules.

Antacids may be used while taking this medicine.

Administration and Dosage:

Approved by the FDA on May 10, 1995.

Take before eating.

Duodenal ulcer treatment: 15 mg once daily for 4 weeks.

Duodenal ulcer (healed) maintenance: 15 mg once daily.

Duodenal ulcers associated with H. pylori:

Triple therapy – 30 mg lansoprazole plus 500 mg clarithromycin and 1 g amoxicillin given twice daily for 14 days.

Double therapy – 30 mg lansoprazole plus 1 g amoxicillin 3 times daily for 14 days for patients intolerant or resistant to clarithromycin.

LANSOPRAZOLE

Erosive esophagitis treatment: 30 mg/day for up to 8 weeks. For patients who do not heal with lansoprazole for 8 weeks (5% to 10%) give an additional 8 weeks of treatment. If there is a recurrence of erosive esophagitis, consider an additional 8-week course of lansoprazole.

Eriosive esophagitis (healing) maintenance: 15 mg once daily.

Pathological hypersecretory conditions including Zollinger-Ellison syndrome: Individualize dosage. The recommended starting dose is 60 mg/day. Adjust doses to individual patient needs and continue for as long as clinically indicated. Dosages up to 90 mg twice daily have been administered. Administer daily dosages of > 120 mg in divided doses. Some patients with Zollinger-Ellison syndrome have been treated continuously with lansoprazole for > 4 years.

Hepatic function impairment: Consider dosage adjustment in patients with severe liver disease.

Elderly/Renal function impairment: No dosage adjustment is necessary.

Nasogastric (NG) tube: For patients who have an NG tube in place, lansoprazole can be opened and the intact granules mixed in 40 mg of apple juice and injected through the NG tube into the stomach. After administering the granules, flush the NG tube with addtional apple juice to clear the tube.

Difficulty swallowing: For patients who have difficulty swallowing capsules, lansoprazole can be opened, and the intact granules contained within can be sprinkled on one tablespoon of applesauce and swallowed immediately. Do not chew or crush the granules.

Storage/Stability: Store lansoprozole in a tight container. Protect from moisture.

Rx	**Prevacid** (TAP Pharm)	**Capsules, delayed release**: 15 mg	Sugar sphere, sucrose. Pink/green. In 100s, 1000s, unit-of-use 30s and UD 100s.
		30 mg	Sugar sphere, sucrose. Pink/black. In 100s, 1000s and UD 100s.

SIMETHICONE

Actions:

Pharmacology: The defoaming action relieves flatulence by dispersing and preventing the formation of mucus-surrounded gas pockets in the GI tract. It acts in the stomach and intestines to change the surface tension of gas bubbles, enabling them to coalesce; thus, gas is freed and eliminated more easily by belching or passing flatus.

Indications:

For relief of the painful symptoms of excess gas in the digestive tract. Used as an adjunct in the treatment of many conditions in which gas retention may be a problem, such as: Postoperative gaseous distention, air swallowing, functional dyspepsia, peptic ulcer, spastic or irritable colon, or diverticulosis.

Unlabeled uses: Simethicone has been used for treating the symptoms of infant colic. It is generally administered with meals.

Administration and Dosage:

Capsules: 125 mg, 4 times daily after each meal and at bedtime.

Tablets: 40 to 125 mg, 4 times daily after each meal and at bedtime. Chew thoroughly.

Drops: Take after meals and at bedtime. Shake well before using.

Children < 2 years of age – 20 mg 4 times daily up to 240 mg/day. For ease of administration, dosage can be mixed with 30 ml cool water, infant formula or other suitable liquids.

Children 2 to 12 years of age – 40 mg 4 times daily.

Adults – 40 to 80 mg 4 times daily up to 500 mg/day.

otc	**Simethicone** (Various, eg, Carolina Medical, Geneva)	**Drops**: 40 mg per 0.6 ml	In 30 ml w/calibrated oral syringe.
otc	**Flatulex** (Dayton)		In 30 ml w/calibrated dropper.
otc	**Gas Relief** (Rugby)		In 30 ml.
otc	**Mylicon** (J & J-Merck)		In 30 ml dropper bottle.
otc	**Phazyme** (Reed & Carnrick)		Saccharin. In 30 ml w/dropper.
otc	**Mylanta Gas** (J & J-Merck)	**Tablets, chewable**: 40 mg	(Stuart 450). White, scored. In 100s, 500s and UD 100s.
otc	**Degas** (Invamed)	**Tablets, chewable**: 80 mg	Sucrose. In 100s.
otc	**Simethicone** (Various, eg, Parmed, Schein)		In 100s.
otc	**Gas Relief** (Rugby)		Sugar, dextrose. In 100s.
otc	**Gax-X** (Sandoz)		(Gas-X). White, scored. In 12s, 30s.
otc	**Major-Con** (Major)		In 100s.
otc	**Maalox Anti-Gas** (R-P Rorer)		Sucrose. Lemon flavor. In 12s.
otc	**Mylanta Gas** (J & J-Merck)		(Stuart 858). Pink, scored. In 12s, 48s, 100s and UD 100s.
otc	**Extra Strength Gas-X** (Sandoz)	**Tablets, chewable**: 125 mg	(Gas-X). Yellow, scored. In 18s.
otc	**Gas Relief** (Rugby)		In 60s.
otc	**Maximum Strength Mylanta Gas** (J & J-Merck)		Sorbitol. White, scored. In 12s and 60s.
otc	**Phazyme** (Reed & Carnrick)	**Tablets**: 60 mg	Enteric coated inner core. In 50s, 100s and 1000s.
otc	**Phazyme 95** (Reed & Carnrick)	**Tablets**: 95 mg	Enteric coated inner core. In 50s, 100s, 500s and Consumer Pak 10s.
otc	**Maximum Strength Phazyme 125** (Reed & Carnrick)	**Capsules**: 125 mg	Red. In 50s.

SIMETHICONE

otc	**Gas-X Extra Strength** (Sandoz)	**Capsules, softgel:** 125 mg	Sorbitol. In 10s and 30s.

CHARCOAL

Actions:

Pharmacology: Charcoal is an adsorbent, detoxicant and soothing agent. It reduces the volume of intestinal gas and relieves related discomfort.

Indications:

For relief of intestinal gas, diarrhea and GI distress associated with indigestion and accompanying cramps or odor.

For the prevention of nonspecific pruritus associated with kidney dialysis treatment.

For use as an antidote in poisonings, see individual monograph in the Miscellaneous section.

Warnings:

Diarrhea: If diarrhea persists for > 2 days or is accompanied by fever, consult physician.

High dosage or prolonged use does not cause side effects or harm the patient's nutritional state.

Children: Do not use in children < 3 years of age.

Drug Interactions:

Activated charcoal can adsorb drugs while they are in the GI tract. Therefore, take charcoal 2 hours before or 1 hour after other medication.

Charcoal Drug Interactions

Precipitant drug	Object drug*			Description
Charcoal	Acetaminophen Barbiturates Carbamazepine Digitoxin Digoxin Furosemide Glutethimide Hydantoins Methotrexate Nizatidine Phenothiazines	Phenylbutazones Propoxyphene Salicylates Sulfones Sulfonylureas Tetracyclines Theophyllines Tricyclic antidepressants Valproic acid	⬇	Charcoal can reduce absorption of these drugs and actually remove them from the systemic circulation which may reduce the effectiveness of a given agent. Charcoal is also used as an antidote for drug overdoses (refer to the individual monograph in the Miscellaneous section).

* ⬇ = Object drug decreased.

Administration and Dosage:

Usual adult dosage is 520 mg after meals or at first sign of discomfort. Repeat as needed, up to 4.16 g daily.

otc	**Charcoal Plus** (Kramer)	**Tablets:** 250 mg	In 120s.
otc	**Charcoal** (Various, eg, Nature's Bounty, Rugby)	**Capsules:** 260 mg	In 50s and 100s.
otc	**CharcoCaps** (Requa)		In 8s, 36s and 100s.

CHARCOAL AND SIMETHICONE

Actions:

Pharmacology: Charcoal reduces the volume of gas. Simethicone disperses and prevents the formation of mucus-surrounded gas pockets, and allows for their elimination. For further information on simethicone, refer to the individual monograph.

Indications:

For the relief of gas pain and associated symptoms.

Administration and Dosage:

1 tablet 3 times daily and at bedtime (*Flatulex*) or 2 tablets 3 times daily after meals (*Charcoal Plus*).

otc	**Flatulex** (Dayton)	**Tablets:** 250 mg activated charcoal and 80 mg simethicone	Green. In 100s.

METOCLOPRAMIDE

Actions:

Pharmacology: Metoclopramide stimulates motility of the upper GI tract without stimulating gastric, biliary or pancreatic secretions. Its mode of action is unclear, but it appears to sensitize tissues to the action of acetylcholine. The effect on motility does not depend on intact vagal innervation, but it can be abolished by anticholinergic drugs.

Metoclopramide increases the tone and amplitude of gastric (especially antral) contractions, relaxes the pyloric sphincter and the duodenal bulb, and increases peristalsis of the duodenum and jejunum, resulting in accelerated gastric emptying and intestinal transit. It increases the resting tone of the lower esophageal sphincter. It has little, if any, effect on colon or gallbladder motility. In patients with gastroesophageal reflux and reduced lower esophageal sphincter pressure (LESP), single oral doses produce dose-related increases in LESP. Effects on LESP begin at about 5 mg and increase through 20 mg. The increase in LESP from a 5 mg dose lasts about 45 minutes and that of 20 mg lasts between 2 and 3 hours. Increased rate of stomach emptying has been observed with single oral doses of 10 mg.

Like the phenothiazines and related dopamine antagonists, metoclopramide produces sedation and, rarely, may produce extrapyramidal reactions. It also induces release of prolactin and transiently increases circulating aldosterone levels.

The antiemetic properties of metoclopramide appear to be a result of its antagonism of central and peripheral dopamine receptors. Dopamine produces nausea and vomiting by stimulation of the medullary chemoreceptor trigger zone (CTZ), and metoclopramide blocks stimulation of the CTZ by agents like levodopa or apomorphine which are known to increase dopamine levels or to possess dopamine-like effects. Metoclopramide also inhibits the central and peripheral effects of apomorphine and abolishes the slowing of gastric emptying caused by apomorphine.

In gastroesophageal reflux, the principal effect of metoclopramide is on symptoms of postprandial and daytime heartburn with less observed effect on nocturnal symptoms. If symptoms are confined to particular situations, such as following the evening meal, consider use of metoclopramide as single doses prior to the provocative situation, rather than using the drug throughout the day. In one study, patients with episodes of evening or nocturnal heartburn had significant improvement in the incidence and symptoms of heartburn following treatment with a single 10 mg dose either before or after the evening meal or at bedtime for 1 to 3 months. Healing of esophageal ulcers and erosions has been endoscopically demonstrated at the end of a 12 week trial using doses of 15 mg 4 times daily. As there is no documented correlation between symptoms and healing of esophageal lesions, endoscopically monitor patients with documented lesions.

Pharmacokinetics:

Absorption/Distribution – Metoclopramide is rapidly and well absorbed. Onset of action is 1 to 3 minutes following an IV dose, 10 to 15 minutes following IM administration, and 30 to 60 minutes following an oral dose. Effects persist for 1 to 2 hours.

Relative to an IV dose of 20 mg, the absolute oral bioavailability of metoclopramide is 80% ± 15.5%. Peak plasma concentrations occur at about 1 to 2 hours after a single oral dose. Similar time to peak is observed after individual doses at steady state. The area under the drug concentration-time curve increases linearly with doses from 20 to 100 mg; peak concentrations also increase linearly with dose. The whole body volume of distribution is high (about 3.5 L/kg) which suggests extensive distribution of drug to the tissues.

Metabolism/Excretion – Approximately 85% of an orally administered dose appears in the urine within 72 hours. Of the 85% eliminated in the urine, about one-half is present as free or conjugated metoclopramide. The average elimination half-life in individuals with normal renal function is 5 to 6 hours. The drug is not extensively bound to plasma proteins (about 30%).

Renal impairment affects the clearance of metoclopramide. In a study of patients with varying degrees of renal impairment, a reduction in creatinine clearance was correlated with a reduction in plasma clearance, renal clearance, non-renal clearance, and increase in elimination half-life. Decrease the dose in renal function impairment to avoid drug accumulation (see Administration and Dosage).

METOCLOPRAMIDE

Indications:

Diabetic gastroparesis: Relief of symptoms associated with acute and recurrent diabetic gastroparesis (diabetic gastric stasis). Usual manifestations of delayed gastric emptying (ie, nausea, vomiting, heartburn, persistent fullness after meals, anorexia) respond within different time intervals. Significant relief of nausea occurs early and improves over 3 weeks. Relief of vomiting and anorexia may precede the relief of abdominal fullness by ≥ 1 week.

Oral:

Symptomatic gastroesophageal reflux – Short-term (4 to 12 weeks) therapy for adults with symptomatic documented gastroesophageal reflux who fail to respond to conventional therapy.

Parenteral: For prevention of nausea and vomiting associated with emetogenic cancer chemotherapy.

Prophylaxis of postoperative nausea and vomiting when nasogastric suction is undesirable.

Single doses may facilitate small bowel intubation when the tube does not pass the pylorus with conventional maneuvers.

Stimulates gastric emptying and intestinal transit of barium in cases where delayed emptying interferes with radiological examination of the stomach or small intestine.

Unlabeled uses: Used to improve lactation. Doses of 30 to 45 mg/day have increased milk secretion, possibly by elevating serum prolactin levels. (See Warnings.)

Studies have indicated some potential value of metoclopramide in the following conditions: Nausea and vomiting of a variety of etiologies (uncontrolled studies report 80% to 90% efficacy), including emesis during pregnancy and labor (see Warnings); gastric ulcer; anorexia nervosa (due to GI stimulation); to improve patient response to ergotamine, analgesics and sedatives in migraine, perhaps by enhancing absorption of the other medications; treatment of postoperative gastric bezoars (10 mg 3 or 4 times daily); diabetic cystoparesis (atonic bladder); esophageal variceal bleeding.

Contraindications:

When stimulation of GI motility might be dangerous (eg, in the presence of GI hemorrhage, mechanical obstruction or perforation); pheochromocytoma (the drug may cause a hypertensive crisis, probably due to release of catecholamines from the tumor; control such crises with phentolamine); sensitivity or intolerance to metoclopramide; epileptics or patients receiving drugs likely to cause extrapyramidal reactions (the frequency and severity of seizures or extrapyramidal reactions may be increased).

Warnings:

Depression has occurred in patients with and without prior history of depression. Symptoms have ranged from mild to severe and have included suicidal ideation and suicide. Give metoclopramide to patients with a prior history of depression only if the expected benefits outweigh the potential risks.

Extrapyramidal symptoms, manifested primarily as acute dystonic reactions, occur in approximately 0.2% to 1% of patients treated with the usual adult dosages of 30 to 40 mg/day. These usually are seen during the first 24 to 48 hours of treatment, occur more frequently in children and young adults, and are even more frequent at the higher doses used in prophylaxis of vomiting due to cancer chemotherapy. These symptoms may include involuntary movements of limbs and facial grimacing, torticollis, oculogyric crisis, rhythmic protrusion of tongue, bulbar type of speech, trismus or dystonic reactions resembling tetanus. Rarely, dystonic reactions may present as stridor and dyspnea, possibly due to laryngospasm. If symptoms occur, they usually subside following 50 mg diphenhydramine IM. Benztropine 1 to 2 mg IM may also be used to reverse these reactions.

Parkinson-like symptoms have occurred, more commonly within the first 6 months after beginning treatment with metoclopramide, but occasionally after longer periods. These symptoms generally subside within 2 to 3 months following discontinuance of metoclopramide. Give metoclopramide cautiously, if at all, to patients with preexisting Parkinson's disease, since such patients may experience exacerbation of parkinsonian symptoms when taking metoclopramide.

METOCLOPRAMIDE

Tardive dyskinesia, a syndrome consisting of potentially irreversible, involuntary, dyskinetic movements, may develop in patients treated with metoclopramide. Although prevalence of the syndrome appears to be highest among the elderly, especially elderly women, it is impossible to predict which patients are likely to develop the syndrome. Both the risk of developing the syndrome and the likelihood that it will become irreversible are believed to increase with the duration of treatment and the total cumulative dose. Less commonly, the syndrome can develop after relatively brief treatment periods at low doses; in these cases, symptoms appear more likely to be reversible.

There is no known treatment for established cases of tardive dyskinesia although the syndrome may remit, partially or completely, within several weeks to months after metoclopramide is withdrawn. Metoclopramide itself, however, may suppress (or partially suppress) the signs of tardive dyskinesia, thereby masking the underlying disease process. The effect of this symptomatic suppression upon the long-term course of the syndrome is unknown. Therefore, the use of metoclopramide for the symptomatic control of tardive dyskinesia is not recommended.

Hypertension: In one study of hypertensive patients, IV metoclopramide released catecholamines. Use caution in hypertensive patients.

Anastomosis or closure of the gut: Giving a promotility drug such as metoclopramide could theoretically put increased pressure on suture lines following a gut anastomosis or closure. Although adverse events related to this possibility have not been reported to date, consider the possibility when deciding whether to use metoclopramide or nasogastric suction in the prevention of postoperative nausea and vomiting.

Carcinogenesis: Elevated prolactin levels persist during chronic administration. Approximately one-third of human breast cancers are prolactin-dependent in vitro; use caution if metoclopramide is contemplated in a patient with previously detected breast cancer. Although galactorrhea, amenorrhea, gynecomastia and impotence have occurred with prolactin-elevating drugs, the clinical significance of elevated serum prolactin levels is unknown. An increase in mammary neoplasms has been found in rodents after chronic administration of prolactin-stimulating neuroleptic drugs; however, studies have not shown an association and evidence is not conclusive.

Pregnancy: Category B. Metoclopramide crosses the placenta. However, there are no adequate and well controlled studies in pregnant women. In several case reports, no effects on the fetus occurred following the use of metoclopramide during pregnancy for nausea and vomiting and reflux esophagitis. Use only when clearly needed and when the potential benefits outweigh the potential hazards to the fetus.

Lactation: Metoclopramide is excreted into breast milk and may concentrate at about twice the plasma level at 2 hours postdose. In a mother receiving 30 mg/day, the amount to the infant would be < 45 mcg/kg/day, which is much less than the maximum daily recommended dose in infants. Therefore, there appears to be no risk to the nursing infant with maternal doses ≤ 45 mg/day. However, exercise caution when administering to a nursing mother.

Children: Infants and children (ages 21 days to 3.3 years) with symptomatic gastroesophageal reflux have been treated with metoclopramide at a dosage of 0.5 mg/kg/day; symptoms improved, the duration of the disease was shortened, and surgery was avoided. One infant with GI manifestations of congenital myotonic dystrophy was successfully treated with metoclopramide (0.3 mg/kg/day).

Methemoglobinemia has occurred in premature and full term neonates given metoclopramide orally, IV or IM, 1 to 4 mg/kg/day for 1 to ≥ 3 days; this did not occur at 0.5 mg/kg/day. Reverse methemoglobinemia by IV administration of methylene blue.

Precautions:

Hypoglycemia: Gastroparesis (gastric stasis) may be responsible for poor diabetic control. Exogenously administered insulins may act before food has left the stomach, leading to hypoglycemia.

Hazardous tasks: May cause drowsiness; observe caution while driving or performing other tasks requiring alertness, coordination or physical dexterity.

METOCLOPRAMIDE

Drug Interactions:

Metoclopramide Drug Interactions			
Precipitant drug	Object drug*		Description
Metoclopramide	Alcohol	↑	Metoclopramide increases the rate of absorption of alcohol by decreasing the time it takes alcohol to reach the small intestine where it is rapidly absorbed.
Metoclopramide	Cimetidine	↓	Bioavailability of cimetidine may be reduced due to decreased absorption as a result of faster gastric transit time.
Metoclopramide	Cyclosporine	↑	A faster gastric emptying time may allow for an increase in cyclosporine absorption, possibly increasing its immunosuppressive and toxic effects.
Metoclopramide	Digoxin	↓	Digoxin absorption, plasma levels and therapeutic effects may be decreased. The capsule, elixir and tablets with a high dissolution rate are least affected.
Metoclopramide	Levodopa	↑	These agents have opposite effects on dopamine receptors. The bioavailability of levodopa may be increased, and levodopa may decrease the effects of metoclopramide on gastric emptying and lower esophageal pressure. Metoclopramide is relatively contraindicated in Parkinson's disease patients.
Levodopa	Metoclopramide	↓	
Metoclopramide	MAO inhibitors	↑	Since metoclopramide releases catecholamines in patients with essential hypertension, use cautiously, if at all, in patients receiving MAO inhibitors.
Metoclopramide	Succinylcholine	↑	By inhibiting plasma cholinesterase, metoclopramide may increase the neuromuscular blocking effects of succinylcholine.
Anticholinergics Narcotic analgesics	Metoclopramide	↓	The effects of metoclopramide on GI motility are antagonized by these agents.

* ↑ = Object drug increased ↓ = Object drug decreased

Adverse Reactions:

Approximately 20% to 30% of patients experience side effects that are usually mild, transient and reversible upon drug withdrawal. Incidence also correlates with dose and duration of metoclopramide use. Doses of 2 mg/kg for control of cisplatin-induced vomiting have produced CNS and GI side effects with an incidence of 81% and 43%, respectively.

Extrapyramidal symptoms (EPS; 1% to 9%): Acute dystonic reactions, the most common type of EPS associated with metoclopramide, occur in approximately 0.2% of patients treated with 30 to 40 mg/day. In cancer chemotherapy patients receiving 1 to 2 mg/kg/dose, the incidence is 2% in patients ≥ 30 years of age and ≥ 25% in children and young adults who have not had prophylactic administration of diphenhydramine. Symptoms include involuntary movements of limbs, facial grimacing, torticollis, oculogyric crisis, rhythmic protrusion of tongue, bulbar type of speech, trismus, opisthotonus (tetanus-like reactions) and rarely, stridor and dyspnea possibly due to laryngospasm; ordinarily these symptoms are readily reversed by diphenhydramine (see Warnings).

Parkinson-like symptoms may include bradykinesia, tremor, cogwheel rigidity, mask-like facies (see Warnings).

Tardive dyskinesia most frequently is characterized by involuntary movements of the tongue, face, mouth or jaw, and sometimes by involuntary movements of the trunk or extremities; movements may be choreoathetotic in appearance (see Warnings).

Motor restlessness (akathisia) may consist of feelings of anxiety, agitation, jitteriness, and insomnia, as well as inability to sit still, pacing and foot-tapping. These symptoms may disappear spontaneously or respond to a reduction in dosage.

METOCLOPRAMIDE

Cardiovascular: Hypotension; hypertension (see Warnings); supraventricular tachycardia; bradycardia.

CNS: (12% to 24%) - Restlessness, drowsiness, fatigue, lassitude (≈ 10%); akathisia (1% to 8%); dizziness (3%; ≈ 70% in cancer chemotherapy patients treated with 1 to 22 mg/kg doses); anxiety; dystonia; insomnia; headache; myoclonus; confusion; mental depression with suicidal ideation (see Warnings); convulsive seizures; hallucinations.

Endocrine: Galactorrhea, amenorrhea, gynecomastia, impotence secondary to hyperprolactinemia (see Warnings); fluid retention secondary to transient elevation of aldosterone. Elevated serum prolactin levels may cause galactorrhea, reversible amenorrhea, nipple tenderness and gynecomastia in males.

GI: (2% to 9%) - Nausea and bowel disturbances, primarily diarrhea.

Hematologic: Neutropenia; leukopenia; agranulocytosis; methemoglobinemia (especially with overdosage in neonates). (See Overdosage.)

Hypersensitivity: A few cases of rash, urticaria or bronchospasm, especially in patients with a history of asthma. Rarely, angioneurotic edema, including glossal or laryngeal edema.

Miscellaneous: Urinary frequency; incontinence; visual disturbances; porphyria; neuroleptic malignant syndrome (NMS), potentially fatal, is comprised of the symptom complex of hyperthermia, altered consciousness, muscular rigidity and autonomic dysfunction; transient flushing of the face and upper body, without alterations in vital signs, following high IV doses; cases of hepatotoxicity, characterized by such findings as jaundice and altered liver function tests, when metoclopramide was administered with other drugs with known hepatotoxic potential.

Overdosage:

Symptoms: Drowsiness, disorientation and extrapyramidal reactions which are self-limiting and usually disappear within 24 hours. Muscle hypertonia, irritability and agitation are common.

Treatment: Anticholinergic or antiparkinson drugs or antihistamines with anticholinergic properties may help control extrapyramidal reactions. Hemodialysis appears ineffective in removing metoclopramide, probably because of the small amount of the drug in blood relative to tissues. Similarly, continuous ambulatory peritoneal dialysis does not remove significant amounts of drug. It is unlikely that dosage would need to be adjusted to compensate for losses through dialysis.

Methemoglobinemia has occurred in premature and full-term neonates who were given overdoses of metoclopramide (1 to 4 mg/kg/day orally, IM or IV for 1 to ≥ 3 days). Methemoglobinemia has not been reported in neonates treated with 0.5 mg/kg/day in divided doses. Methemoglobinemia can be reversed by the IV administration of methylene blue. Also see General Management of Acute Overdosage.

Patient Information:

May produce drowsiness and dizziness; observe caution while driving or performing other tasks requiring alertness, coordination or physical dexterity.

Notify physician if involuntary movement of eyes, face or limbs occurs.

Take medication 30 minutes before each meal.

Administration and Dosage:

Diabetic gastroparesis: 10 mg 30 minutes before each meal and at bedtime for 2 to 8 weeks.

Determine initial route of administration by the severity of symptoms. With only the earliest manifestations of diabetic gastric stasis, initiate oral administration. If symptoms are severe, begin with parenteral therapy. Administer 10 mg IV over 1 to 2 minutes. Parenteral administration up to 10 days may be required before symptoms subside, then oral administration may be instituted. Reinstitute therapy at the earliest manifestation.

Symptomatic gastroesophageal reflux: 10 to 15 mg orally up to 4 times daily 30 minutes before each meal and at bedtime. If symptoms occur only intermittently or at specific times of the day, single doses up to 20 mg prior to the provoking situation may be preferred rather than continuous treatment. Occasionally, patients who are more sensitive to the therapeutic or adverse effects of metoclopramide (eg, elderly) will require only 5 mg per dose. Guide therapy directed at esophageal lesions by endoscopy. Therapy > 12 weeks has not been evaluated and cannot be recommended.

Prevention of postoperative nausea and vomiting: Inject IM near the end of surgery. The usual adult dose is 10 mg; however, doses of 20 mg may be used.

METOCLOPRAMIDE

Prevention of chemotherapy-induced emesis: Infuse slowly IV over not less than 15 minutes, 30 minutes before beginning cancer chemotherapy; repeat every 2 hours for 2 doses, then every 3 hours for 3 doses.

The initial 2 doses should be 2 mg/kg if highly emetogenic drugs such as cisplatin or dacarbazine are used alone or in combination. For less emetogenic regimens, 1 mg/kg/dose may be adequate.

If extrapyramidal symptoms occur, administer 50 mg diphenhydramine IM.

IV admixture: When diluted in a parenteral solution, administer IV slowly over a period of not less than 15 minutes.

Preparation/Storage of solution – For doses > 10 mg, dilute injection in 50 ml of a parenteral solution. The preferred parenteral solution is Sodium Chloride Injection, which when combined with metoclopramide, can be stored frozen for up to 4 weeks. Metoclopramide is degraded when admixed and frozen with Dextrose 5% in Water. Metoclopramide diluted in Sodium Chloride Injection, Dextrose 5% in Water, Dextrose 5% in 0.45% Sodium Chloride, Ringer's Injection or Lactated Ringer's Injection may be stored up to 48 hours (without freezing) after preparation if protected from light. All dilutions may be stored unprotected from light under normal light conditions up to 24 hours after preparation.

Direct IV injection: Inject undiluted metoclopramide slowly IV allowing 1 to 2 minutes for 10 mg, since a transient but intense feeling of anxiety and restlessness, followed by drowsiness, may occur with rapid administration.

Facilitation of small bowel intubation – If the tube has not passed the pylorus with conventional maneuvers in 10 minutes, administer a single undiluted dose slowly IV over 1 to 2 minutes.

Recommended single dose –
Adults: 10 mg (2 ml).
Children (6 to 14 years): 2.5 to 5 mg (0.5 to 1 ml).
Children (< 6 years): 0.1 mg/kg.

Radiological examinations – In patients where delayed gastric emptying interferes with radiological examination of the stomach or small intestine, a single dose may be administered slowly IV over 1 to 2 minutes.

Rectal administration: For outpatient treatment when oral dosing is not possible, suppositories containing 25 mg metoclopramide have been extemporaneously compounded (5 pulverized oral tablets in polyethylene glycol). Administer 1 suppository 30 to 60 minutes before each meal and at bedtime.

Renal/Hepatic function impairment: Since metoclopramide is excreted principally through the kidneys, in those patients whose creatinine clearance is < 40 ml/min, initiate therapy at approximately one-half the recommended dosage. Depending on clinical efficacy and safety considerations, the dosage may be increased or decreased as appropriate.

See Overdosage section for information regarding dialysis.

Metoclopramide undergoes minimal hepatic metabolism, except for simple conjugation. Its safe use has been described in patients with advanced liver disease whose renal function was normal.

Admixture compatibilities/incompatibilities:

Physically and chemically compatible up to 48 hours – Cimetidine; mannitol; potassium acetate; potassium chloride; potassium phosphate.

Physically compatible up to 48 hours – Ascorbic acid; benztropine; cytarabine; dexamethasone sodium phosphate; diphenhydramine; doxorubicin; heparin sodium; hydrocortisone sodium phosphate; lidocaine; magnesium sulfate; multivitamin infusion (must be refrigerated) vitamin B complex with ascorbic acid.

Incompatible – Cephalothin; chloramphenicol; sodium bicarbonate.

METOCLOPRAMIDE

Rx	**Metoclopramide HCl** (Various, eg, Goldline, Invamed, Major)	**Tablets:** 5 mg metoclopramide HCl (as monohydrochloride monohydrate)	In 100s, 500s and 1000s.
Rx	**Reglan** (Robins)		Lactose. (Reglan 5 AHR). Green. Elliptical. In 100s and *Dis-Co* UD 100s.
Rx	**Metoclopramide HCl** (Various, eg, Geneva, Goldline, Invamed, Major, Martec, Parmed, Rugby, Schein, Warner-C)	**Tablets:** 10 mg (as monohydrochloride monohydrate)	In 100s, 500s, 1000s, 2500s and UD 100s.
Rx	**Maxolon** (SK-Beecham)		Lactose. (BMP 192). Blue, scored. In 100s.
Rx *sf*	**Reglan** (Robins)		(Reglan AHR 10). Pink, scored. Capsule shape. In 100s, 500s and *Dis-Co* UD 100s.
Rx	**Metoclopramide HCl** (Various, eg, Goldline, Major, Roxane, Rugby, Warner-C)	**Syrup:** 5 mg/5 ml (as monohydrochloride monohydrate)	In 480 ml and UD 10 ml.
Rx *sf*	**Reglan** (Robins)		Parabens, sorbitol. In 480 ml and *Dis–Co* UD 10 ml (100s).
Rx	**Metoclopramide Intensol** (Roxane)	**Concentrated solution:** 10 mg (as HCl) per ml	EDTA, sorbitol. In 10 and 30 ml with calibrated dropper.
Rx	**Metoclopramide HCl** (Various, eg, DuPont, Smith & Nephew SoloPak)	**Injection:** 5 mg/ml (as monohydrochloride monohydrate)	In 2, 10, 20 and 30 ml vials and 2 ml amps.
Rx	**Octamide PFS** (Adria)		Preservative free. In 2, 10 and 30 ml single-dose vials.
Rx	**Reglan** (Robins)		Preservative free. In 2 and 10 ml amps and 2, 10 and 30 ml vials.

sf - Sugar free.

DEXPANTHENOL (Dextro-Pantothenyl Alcohol)

Actions:

Pharmacology: Dexpanthenol is the alcohol analog of D-pantothenic acid. Pantothenic acid is a precursor of coenzyme A, which is a cofactor for enzyme-catalyzed reactions involving transfer of acetyl groups. The final step in acetylcholine synthesis is the choline acetylase transfer of an acetyl group from acetylcoenzyme A to choline. Acetylcholine, the neurohumoral transmitter in the parasympathetic system, maintains normal intestinal functions. Decreased acetylcholine content results in decreased peristalsis and in extreme cases, adynamic ileus. Dexpanthenol's mechanism of action is unknown.

Choline, in addition to being the precursor for acetylcholine, is essential for normal transport of fat, as a constituent of the phospholipid lecithin and as an intermediary methyl donor in intermediary metabolism. Choline has the same pharmacological actions as acetylcholine, but is less active; single oral 10 g doses produce no obvious pharmacodynamic response.

In one study, urinary concentrations of pantothenic acid increased 10- to 50-fold above baseline during a 4 hour period following 100 mg dexpanthenol. Within 24 hours, urinary levels were only slightly above baseline.

Indications:

Prophylactic use immediately after major abdominal surgery to minimize the possibility of paralytic ileus; intestinal atony causing abdominal distention; postoperative or postpartum retention of flatus; postoperative delay in resumption of intestinal motility; paralytic ileus.

Contraindications:

Hemophilia; ileus due to mechanical obstruction.

DEXPANTHENOL (Dextro-Pantothenyl Alcohol)

Warnings:

Hypersensitivity: If signs of a hypersensitivity reaction appear, discontinue drug. Refer to Management of Acute Hypersensitivity Reactions.

Pregnancy: Category C. It is not known whether dexpanthenol can cause fetal harm when administered to a pregnant woman or can affect reproduction capacity. Give to a pregnant woman only when clearly needed.

Lactation: It is not known whether this drug is excreted in breast milk. Exercise caution when administering the drug to a nursing woman.

Children: Safety and efficacy for use in children have not been established.

Precautions:

Mechanical obstruction: If ileus is secondary to mechanical obstruction, direct primary attention to the obstruction. Management of adynamic ileus includes: Correction of any fluid and electrolyte imbalance (especially hypokalemia), anemia and hypoproteinemia; treatment of infection; avoidance of drugs which decrease GI motility; GI tract decompression when considerably distended by nasogastric suction or by use of a long intestinal tube.

Drug Interactions:

Antibiotics, barbiturates or narcotics: Allergic reactions have occurred rarely during concomitant use of dexpanthenol.

Succinylcholine: Temporary respiratory difficulty occurred following dexpanthenol administration 5 minutes after succinylcholine was discontinued. Succinylcholine's effects appeared to have been prolonged. Do not administer within 1 hour of succinylcholine.

Adverse Reactions:

Itching; tingling; difficulty breathing; red patches of skin; generalized dermatitis; urticaria; slight drop in blood pressure; intestinal colic (30 minutes after administration); vomiting; diarrhea (10 days postsurgery); agitation in an elderly patient.

Administration and Dosage:

Prevention of postoperative adynamic ileus: 250 or 500 mg IM. Repeat in 2 hours, followed by doses every 6 hours until danger of adynamic ileus has passed.

Treatment of adynamic ileus: 500 mg IM. Repeat in 2 hours, followed by doses every 6 hours, as needed.

IV administration: Not for direct IV administration. The 500 mg dose has been mixed with IV bulk solutions such as glucose or Lactated Ringer's and infused slowly IV.

Rx	**Dexpanthenol** (Various, eg, Schein)	**Injection:** 250 mg per ml	In 10 ml and 2 ml vials.
Rx	**Ilopan** (Adria)		In 2 ml amps and UD *Stat-Pak* 2 ml disp. syringes.[1]

[1] Syringes contain no more than 0.5% chlorobutanol.

DEXPANTHENOL WITH CHOLINE BITARTRATE

For complete prescribing information, refer to the Dexpanthenol monograph.

Indications:

May help relieve gas retention associated with splenic flexure syndrome, cholecystitis, gastritis, gastric hyperacidity, irritable colon, regional ileitis, postantibiotic and postoperative gas retention or during laxative withdrawal.

Administration and Dosage:

Take 2 to 3 tablets 3 times daily.

Rx	**Ilopan-Choline** (Adria)	**Tablets:** 50 mg dexpanthenol and 25 mg choline bitartrate	(Adria 231). White. In 100s and 500s.

CISAPRIDE

Warning:
Serious cardiac arrhythmias including ventricular tachycardia, ventricular fibrillation, torsade de pointes and QT prolongation have been reported in patients taking cisapride with other drugs that inhibit cytochrome P450 IIIA4, such as ketoconazole, itraconazole, miconazole IV, troleandomycin, erythromycin, fluconazole and clarithromycin. Some of these events have been fatal.

Actions:

Pharmacology: Cisapride is an oral GI prokinetic agent. The mechanism of action appears to be primarily enhancement of release of acetylcholine at the myenteric plexus. Cisapride does not induce muscarinic or nicotinic receptor stimulation, nor does it inhibit acetylcholinesterase activity. It is less potent than metoclopramide in dopamine receptor-blocking effects in rats. It does not increase or decrease basal or pentagastrin-induced gastric acid secretion. In vitro cisapride is a serotonin-4 (5-HT_4) receptor agonist. This action may result in increased GI motility and cardiac rate.

Esophagus – Single doses of cisapride (4 to 10 mg IV) increased the lower esophageal sphincter pressure (LESP) and lower esophageal peristalsis compared to placebo or metoclopramide. In patients with gastroesophageal reflux disease (GERD) and an LESP of < 10 mm Hg, cisapride increased the strength of esophageal peristalsis and more than doubled LESP, raising it to normal values. The increase in LESP was partially reversed by atropine, suggesting that the effect is partly, but not exclusively, cholinergically mediated. A single 20 mg cisapride dose to healthy volunteers similarly increased LESP, starting 45 minutes after dosing, with a peak response at 75 minutes. Doses < 20 mg were ineffective. Oral cisapride (10 mg 3 times daily for several days) to patients with GERD resulted in a significant increase in LESP and an increased esophageal acid clearance.

Stomach – Cisapride (single 10 mg doses IV or 10 mg orally 3 times daily up to 6 weeks) significantly accelerated gastric emptying of both liquids and solids. Acceleration of gastric emptying, measured over 4 hours after a test meal lunch, was greatest when 10 mg was given both in the morning and again before the test meal, intermediate with 20 mg single dose in the morning and least when only 10 mg was given the morning of the test meal. The increases in gastric emptying were proportional to the plasma levels of cisapride measured over the same 4 hours that the gastric emptying test was conducted.

Pharmacokinetics: Cisapride is rapidly absorbed after oral administration; peak plasma concentrations are reached 1 to 1.5 hours after dosing. Onset of action is ≈ 30 to 60 minutes after oral use. Absolute bioavailability is 35% to 40%. When gastric acidity was reduced by a high-dose histamine H_2 receptor blocker and sodium bicarbonate in fasting subjects, there was a decrease in rate, and to a lesser degree extent, of cisapride tablet absorption (this has not been established for the suspension). Cisapride is ≈ 98% bound to plasma proteins, mainly albumin. Volume of distribution is ≈ 180 L, indicating extensive tissue distribution.

The plasma clearance is about 100 ml/min. The mean terminal half-life ranges from 6 to 12 hours; longer half-lives, up to 20 hours, have occurred following IV administration. The drug is extensively metabolized, mainly via the cytochrome P450 IIIA4 enzyme system; unchanged drug accounts for < 10% of urinary and fecal recovery following oral administration. Norcisapride, formed by N-dealkylation, is the principal metabolite in plasma, feces and urine.

After cessation of repeated dosing, elimination half-lives (8 to 10 hours) were in the same order as after single dosing. There is some evidence that degree of accumulation of cisapride or its metabolites may be somewhat higher in patients with hepatic or renal impairment and in elderly patients compared to young healthy volunteers, but differences are not consistent and do not require dosage adjustment.

Clinical trials: Two placebo controlled studies, one using a cisapride dose of 10 mg 4 times daily, the other both 10 and 20 mg 4 times daily, showed effects on nighttime heartburn, although the 10 mg dose in the second study was only marginally effective. There were no consistent effects on daytime heartburn, symptoms of regurgitation or histopathology of the esophagus. Use of antacids was only infrequently affected and slightly decreased. In a third controlled trial, neither 10 nor 20 mg taken 4 times was superior to placebo.

CISAPRIDE

Indications:

Heartburn: Symptomatic treatment of patients with nocturnal heartburn due to gastroesophageal reflux disease.

Contraindications:

Patients in whom an increase in GI motility could be harmful (eg, in the presence of GI hemorrhage, mechanical obstruction, perforation); hypersensitivity or intolerance to the drug; concomitant administration of ketoconazole, itraconazole, miconazole IV, fluconazole, erythromycin, clarithromycin or troleandomycin (see Warnings and Drug Interactions).

Warnings:

Cardiac effects: Rare cases of serious cardiac arrhythmias, including ventricular arrhythmias and torsade de pointes associated with QT prolongation, have been observed in patients taking cisapride with ketoconazole, itraconazole, miconazole IV, erythromycin, clarithromycin or fluconazole. Some of these patients did not have known cardiac histories; however, most had been receiving multiple other medications and had pre-exisiting cardiac disease or risk factors for arrhythmias. Some of these cases have been fatal (see warning box).

Concomitant use with ketoconazole is contraindicated because it has resulted in markedly elevated cisapride plasma concentrations. Due to potent in vitro inhibition of the hepatic enzyme system mainly responsible for the metabolism of cisapride (cytochrome P450 IIIA4), itraconazole, miconazole IV, clarithromycin, erythromycin, fluconazole and troleandomycin can lead to elevated cisapride plasma concentrations. Therefore, concomitant use with cisapride is also contraindicated.

Fertility impairment: In female rats, cisapride at oral doses of ≥ 40 mg/kg/day prolonged the breeding interval required for impregnation. Similar effects were also observed at maturity in the female offspring of the female rats treated with oral doses of cisapride at ≥ 10 mg/kg/day. Cisapride at an oral dose of 160 mg/kg/day also exerted contragestational/pregnancy disrupting effects in female rats.

Elderly: Steady-state plasma levels are generally higher in older than in younger patients due to a moderate prolongation of the elimination half-life. Therapeutic doses, however, are similar to those used in younger adults. The rate of adverse experiences in patients > 65 years of age was similar to that in younger adults.

Pregnancy: Category C. Cisapride was embryotoxic and fetotoxic in rats at a dose of 160 mg/kg/day (100 times the maximum recommended human dose) and in rabbits at a dose ≥ of 20 mg/kg/day (≈ 12 times the maximum recommended human dose) or higher. It also produced reduced birth weights of pups in rats at 40 and 160 mg/kg/day and adversely affected the pup survival. There are no adequate and well controlled studies in pregnant women. Use during pregnancy only if the potential benefit justifies the potential risk to the fetus.

Lactation: Cisapride is excreted in breast milk at concentrations ≈ 1/20 of those observed in plasma. Particular care must be taken if the nursing infant or mother is taking a drug that might alter cisapride's metabolism. Exercise caution when administering to a nursing woman.

Children: Safety and efficacy in children have not been established.

Precautions:

QT prolongation: Weigh potential benefits against risks prior to administration in patients with conditions associated with QT prolongation, such as congenital prolonged QT syndrome, uncorrected electrolyte disturbances or in patients who are taking other medications known to prolong QT interval.

CISAPRIDE

Drug Interactions:

Acceleration of gastric emptying by cisapride could affect the rate of absorption of other drugs. Closely follow patients receiving narrow therapeutic ratio drugs or other drugs that require careful titration; reassess plasma levels if they are being monitored.

Cisapride Drug Interactions

Precipitant drug	Object drug*		Description
Anticholinergics	Cisapride	↓	Concurrent use would be expected to compromise the beneficial effects of cisapride.
Azole antifungals Ketoconazole Itraconazole Miconazole IV Fluconazole	Cisapride	↑	Ketoconazole potently inhibits the metabolism of cisapride, resulting in a mean eightfold increase in cisapride's AUC; prolongation of the QT interval on the ECG may occur. In vitro data indicate that itraconazole, miconazole IV and fluconazole, also markedly inhibit cytochrome P450 IIIA4, mainly responsible for metabolism of cisapride. Concurrent use is contraindicated (see Warnings).
Macrolides Clarithromycin Erythromycin Troleandomycin	Cisapride	↑	In vitro data indicate that troleandomycin, erythromycin and clarithromycin markedly inhibit cytochrome P450 IIIA4, mainly responsible for metabolism of cisapride. Concurrent use is contraindicated (see Warnings).
H_2 antagonists Cimetidine	Cisapride	↑	Increased peak plasma level and AUC of cisapride may occur; ranitidine has no effect on cisapride absorption. GI absorption of cimetidine and ranitidine is accelerated by cisapride.
Cisapride	H_2 antagonists Cimetidine Ranitidine	↑	
Cisapride	Anticoagulants	↑	Since coagulation times may be increased, it is advisable to check them 1 week after the start and discontinuation of cisapride therapy. Adjust the anticoagulant dose if necessary.

* ↑ = Object drug increased. ↓ = Object drug decreased.

Adverse Reactions:

Cisapride Adverse Reactions (%)

Adverse reaction	Cisapride (n = 1042)	Placebo (n = 686)	Adverse reaction	Cisapride (n = 1042)	Placebo (n = 686)
GI			*Body as a whole*		
Diarrhea	14.2[1]	10.3	Pain	3.4	2.3
Abdominal pain	10.2[1]	7.7	Fever	2.2	1.5
Nausea	7.6	7.6	*CNS*		
Constipation	6.7[1]	3.4	Headache	19.3	17.1
Flatulence	3.5[1]	3.1	Insomnia	1.9	1.3
Dyspepsia	2.7	1	Anxiety	1.4	1
Respiratory			Nervousness	1.4	0.7
Rhinitis	7.3[1]	5.7	*Dermatologic*		
Sinusitis	3.6	3.5	Rash	1.6	1.6
Upper respiratory tract infection	3.1	2.8	Pruritus	1.2	1
			Miscellaneous		
Coughing	1.5	1.2	Viral infection	3.6	3.2
GU			Arthralgia	1.4	1.2
Urinary tract infection	2.4	1.9	Abnormal vision	1.4	0.3
Micturition frequency	1.2	0.6	Vaginitis	1.2	0.9

[1] Incidence was more frequent with doses of 20 mg than 10 mg cisapride.

CISAPRIDE

The following adverse events reported in > 1% of patients were more frequently reported with placebo: Dizziness; vomiting; pharyngitis; chest pain; fatigue; back pain; depression; dehydration; myalgia.

Miscellaneous: Dry mouth, somnolence, palpitation, migraine, tremor, edema (≤ 1%); seizures, extrapyramidal effects, tachycardia, elevated liver enzymes, hepatitis, thrombocytopenia, leukopenia, aplastic anemia, pancytopenia, sinus tachycardia, granulocytopenia (rare).

Overdosage:

Symptoms: Reports of overdosage include an adult who took 540 mg and for 2 hours experienced retching, borborygmi, flatulence, stool and urinary frequency. Single oral doses of 160 to 4000 mg/kg were lethal in animals. Symptoms of acute toxicity were ptosis, tremors, convulsions, dyspnea, loss of righting reflex, catalepsy, catatonia, hypotonia and diarrhea.

Treatment: Treatment should include gastric lavage or activated charcoal, close observation and general supportive measures. Refer to General Management of Acute Overdosage.

Patient Information:

Although cisapride does not affect psychomotor function nor induce sedation or drowsiness when used alone, advise patients that the sedative effects of benzodiazepines and of alcohol may be accelerated.

Counsel patients against concomitant use of oral ketoconazole, itraconazole, miconazole IV, erythromycin, clarithromycin, fluconazole or troleandomycin.

Administration and Dosage:

Approved by the FDA on July 29, 1993.

Adults: Initiate therapy with 10 mg (one 10 mg tablet or 10 ml of the suspension) 4 times daily at least 15 minutes before meals and at bedtime. In some patients the dosage will need to be increased to 20 mg or 20 ml, given as above, to obtain a satisfactory result.

Elderly: Steady-state plasma levels are generally higher due to a moderate prolongation of the elimination half-life. Therapeutic doses, however, are similar to those used in younger adults.

Storage/Stability: Store at room temperature 15° to 30° C (59° to 86° F). Protect tablets from moisture. The 20 mg tablets should be protected from light.

Rx	**Propulsid** (Janssen)	**Tablets:** 10 mg	Lactose. (Janssen P/10). White, scored. In 100s and 500s.
		20 mg	Lactose. (Janssen P/20). Blue. In 100s.
		Suspension: 1 mg/ml	Parabens, sorbitol. Cherry cream flavor. In 450 ml.

DIGESTIVE ENZYMES

Actions:

Pharmacology: Pancreatin and pancrelipase hydrolyze fats to glycerol and fatty acids, change protein into proteoses and derived substances, and convert starch into dextrins and sugars. Administration reduces the fat and nitrogen content in the stool. These agents exert their primary effects in the duodenum and upper jejunum. Pancreatic enzymes are normally secreted in great excess. There is a tenfold reserve for exocrine pancreatic enzyme secretion. Generally, steatorrhea and malabsorption occur only after a ≥ 90% reduction in secretion of lipase and proteolytic enzymes. It has been estimated that ≈ 8000 units of lipase per hour should be delivered into the duodenum postprandially. Even if all the enzymes taken orally reached the proximal intestine in active form, ingestion of 24,000 units of lipase (8000 units per hour) for 3 postprandial hours would be required. If one could deliver sufficient pancreatic enzymes to the small intestine, malabsorption could be corrected. It is rarely possible to achieve complete relief of steatorrhea although major improvement in fat absorption can be achieved in most patients.

There are many factors which may influence the ability to deliver pancreatic enzymes to the duodenum including asynchrony of gastric emptying of food and enzyme, sensitivity of pancreatic enzymes to permanent inactivation by gastric acid and pepsin secreted in response to the meal, and acidic precipitation of bile acids.

Pancreatic lipase is irreversibly inactivated at pH ≤ 4. An enteric coating may prevent destruction or inactivation by gastric pepsin and acid pH, but may inhibit enzyme delivery to the duodenum. Cimetidine or antacids may increase the amount of pancreatin in the duodenum by decreasing its destruction by the gastric acid.

Pancreatic Extract Activity

Enzyme concentrate	Source	Minimal USP standards (USP units/mg)		
		Lipase	Protease	Amylase
Pancrelipase	Porcine	24	100	100
Pancreatin	Bovine, porcine or vegetable	2	25	25

Indications:

Enzyme replacement therapy in patients with deficient exocrine pancreatic secretions, cystic fibrosis, chronic pancreatitis, postpancreatectomy, ductal obstructions caused by cancer of the pancreas or common bile duct, pancreatic insufficiency and for steatorrhea of malabsorption syndrome and postgastrectomy (Billroth II and Total) or, post-GI surgery (eg, Billroth II gastroenterostomy).

Presumptive test for pancreatic function, especially in pancreatic insufficiency due to chronic pancreatitis.

Contraindications:

Hypersensitivity to pork protein or enzymes; acute pancreatitis; acute exacerbations of chronic pancreatic diseases.

Warnings:

Replacement therapy: Pancreatic exocrine replacement therapy should not delay or supplant treatment of the primary disorder.

Pregnancy: Category C. It is not known whether the drug can cause fetal harm when administered to a pregnant woman or can affect reproduction capacity. Give to a pregnant woman only if clearly needed. The enteric coating component, diethyl phthalate, has been teratogenic in rats with high intraperitoneal dosing.

Lactation: It is not known whether pancreatin is excreted in breast milk. Exercise caution when administering to a nursing mother.

Precautions:

Excessive doses may cause nausea, abdominal cramps or diarrhea. Extremely high doses have been associated with hyperuricosuria and hyperuricemia.

Pork sensitivity: Use pork products with caution in patients sensitive to pork. Discontinue use if symptoms of sensitivity appear and initiate symptomatic and supportive treatment if necessary. Individuals previously sensitized to trypsin, pancreatin or pancrelipase may have allergic reactions.

Irritation of skin/mucous membranes: Do not spill powder on hands since it may irritate skin. The dust of finely powdered concentrates irritates the nasal mucosa and the respiratory tract. Inhalation of airborne powder can precipitate an asthma attack. Asthma can also occur in patients sensitized to pancreatic enzyme concentrates.

DIGESTIVE ENZYMES

Drug Interactions:

Antacids: Calcium carbonate or magnesium hydroxide may negate the beneficial effect of the enzymes.

Iron: The serum iron response to oral iron may be decreased by concomitant pancreatic extracts.

Adverse Reactions:

The most frequently reported adverse reactions are GI in nature. Less frequently, allergic-type reactions have also been observed. Perianal irritation may occur with pancreatin and rarely, inflammation with large doses.

Overdosage:

Overdosage may cause diarrhea or transient intestinal upset.

Patient Information:

Take before or with meals.

Do not inhale powder dosage form or powder from capsules since it may irritate skin or mucous membranes.

To protect enteric coating, do not crush or chew the microspheres/tablets in the enteric coated capsule formulations. Microsphere contact with foods having a pH > 5.5 can dissolve the enteric shell.

Do not change brands without consulting with the physician or pharmacist.

Administration and Dosage:

Microspheres/Microtablets: To protect enteric coating, do not crush or chew the microspheres or microtablets. Where swallowing of capsules is difficult, they may be opened and shaken onto a small quantity of soft non-hot food (eg, applesauce, gelatin), which does not require chewing. Swallow immediately without chewing as the proteolytic action may cause irritation of the mucosa. Follow with a glass of juice or water to ensure complete swallowing of the microspheres/microtablets. Contact of the microspheres/microtablets with foods having a pH > 5.5 can dissolve the protective enteric shell. Use any mixture of food or liquid with the microspheres/ microtablets immediately; do not store.

Brand interchange: These products are not bioequivalent. Therefore, do not substitute one brand for another without first consulting the physician.

PANCRELIPASE

For complete prescribing information, refer to the Digestive Enzymes group monograph.

Administration and Dosage:

Adjust dosage according to the severity of the exocrine pancreatic enzyme deficiency. Estimate dosage by assessing which dose minimizes steatorrhea and maintains good nutritional status. The assessment of the end points in children is aided by charting growth curves.

Capsules and tablets:

Children –

< 6 months old, dosage not established.

6 months to 1 year, 2000 units lipase per meal.

1 to 6 years, 4000 to 8000 units lipase with each meal and 4000 units with snacks.

7 to 12 years, 4000 to 12,000 units lipase (or more if necessary) with each meal and with snacks.

Adults – 4000 to 48,000 units lipase with each meal and with snacks.

In patients with pancreatectomy or obstruction of pancreatic ducts, administer 8000 to 16,000 units lipase at 2 hour intervals or as directed by physician (Viokase). In severe deficiencies, the dose may be increased to 64,000 to 88,000 units lipase with meals or the frequency of administration may increase to hourly intervals if nausea, cramps or diarrhea do not occur.

Powder (in cystic fibrosis): 0.7 g with meals.

PANCRELIPASE

Content given per capsule, tablet or 0.7 g powder.

	Product and Distributor	Lipase (units)	Protease (units)	Amylase (units)	Other Content	How Supplied
Rx	**Pancrease MT 4 Capsules** (McNeil)	4,500	12,000	12,000		(McNeil Pancrease MT 4). Yellow/clear. In 100s.
Rx	**Pancrease Capsules** (McNeil)	4,500	25,000	20,000	Sugar	Dye free. Enteric coated microspheres. (McNeil Pancrease). White. In 100s and 250s.
Rx	**Pancrelipase Capsules** (Geneva)	4,000	25,000	20,000		Enteric coated pellets. White. In 100s and 250s.
Rx	**Protilase Capsules** (Rugby)					Enteric coated spheres. In 100s and 500s.
Rx	**Cotazym-S Capsules** (Organon)	5,000	20,000	20,000		Enteric coated spheres. (Organon 388). Clear. In 100s and 500s.
Rx	**Cotazym Capsules** (Organon)	8,000	30,000	30,000	25 mg calcium carbonate	(Organon 381). In 100s and 500s.
Rx	**Ku-Zyme HP Capsules** (Schwarz Pharma Kremers-Urban)	8,000	30,000	30,000	Lactose	(Kremers Urban 525). White. In 100s.
Rx	**Viokase Tablets** (Robins)					(Viokase/AHR 9111). Tan. In 100s and 500s.
Rx	**Pancrease MT 10 Capsules** (McNeil)	10,000	30,000	30,000	Parabens	Enteric coated microtablets. (McNeil Pancrease MT 10). Pink/clear. In 100s.
Rx	**Creon 10 Capsules, Delayed Release** (Solvay)	10,000	37,500	33,200		Delayed release. (Solvay 1210). Brown/transparent. In 100s and 250s.
Rx	**Ilozyme Tablets** (Adria)	11,000	≥ 30,000	≥ 30,000		(200). Buff. In 250s.
Rx	**Zymase Capsules** (Organon)	12,000	24,000	24,000		Enteric coated spheres. In 100s.
Rx	**Ultrase MT 12 Capsules** (Scandipharm)	12,000	39,000	39,000		(Ultrase MT12). White/yellow. In 100s.
Rx	**Pancrease MT 16 Capsules** (McNeil)	16,000	48,000	48,000	Parabens	Enteric coated microtablets. (McNeil Pancrease MT 16). Salmon/clear. In 100s.
Rx	**Viokase Powder** (Robins)	16,800	70,000	70,000	Lactose	In 113.5 and 227 g.
Rx	**Ultrase MT 20 Capsules** (Scandipharm)	20,000	65,000	65,000		(Ultrase MT20). Gray/yellow. In 100s.
Rx	**Creon 20 Capsules, Delayed Release** (Solvay)	20,000	75,000	66,400		Delayed release. (Solvay 1220). Brown/transparent. In 100s an 250s.
Rx	**Pancrease MT 20 Capsules** (McNeil)	20,000	44,000	56,000	Parabens	(McNeil/Pancrease MT 20). White w/yellow bands. In 100s.

PANCREATIN

For complete prescribing information, refer to the Digestive Enzymes group monograph.

Administration and Dosage:

Take 1 to 2 with meals or snacks. Adjust according to individual requirements for control of steatorrhea.

Content given per tablet or capsule.

	Product and Distributor	Pancreatin (mg)	Lipase (units)	Protease (units)	Amylase (units)	How Supplied
Rx	**Donnazyme Tablets** (Robins)	500	1,000	12,500	12,500	Parabens, sucrose. Green. In 100s.
otc sf	**Pancrezyme 4X Tablets** (Vitaline)	2,400	12,000	60,000	60,000	In 90s
otc sf	**4X Pancreatin 600 mg Tablets** (Vitaline)					In 90s.
otc sf	**Hi-Vegi-Lip Tablets** (Freeda)	2,400	4,800	60,000	60,000	In 100s and 250s.
otc sf	**8X Pancreatin 900 mg Tablets** (Vitaline)	7,200	22,500	180,000	180,000	In 60s.
Rx	**Creon Capsules** (Solvay)	300	8,000	13,000	30,000	Enteric coated microspheres. (Solvay 1200). Brown/yellow. In 100s and 250s.
Rx	**Creon 10** (Solvay)		10,000	37,500	33,200	(Solvay 1210). Brown/transparent. In 100s and 250s.
Rx	**Creon 20** (Solvay)		20,000	75,000	66,400	(Solvay 1220). Bron/transparent. In 100s and 250s.
Rx	**Digepepsin Tablets** (Kenwood/Bradley)	300				250 mg pepsin, 150 mg bile salts. Brown. Dual coated. In 60s.

GASTRIC ACIDIFIERS

Actions:

Pharmacology: Gastric acidifiers counterbalance a deficiency of hydrochloric acid in the gastric juice and destroy or inhibit growth of putrefactive microorganisms in ingested food. A deficiency of hydrochloric acid is often associated with pernicious anemia, allergies, gastric carcinoma and congenital achlorhydria.

Contraindications:

Gastric hyperacidity or peptic ulcer.

GLUTAMIC ACID HCl

For complete prescribing information, refer to the Gastric Acidifiers group monograph.

Administration and Dosage:

1 to 3 capsules 3 times daily before meals.

340 mg contains approximately 1.8 mEq hydrochloric acid.

otc	**Glutamic Acid HCl** (Various)	**Capsules:** 340 mg	In 100s.

DEHYDROCHOLIC ACID

Actions:

Pharmacology: Dehydrocholic acid is an oxidation product of cholic acid (a natural bile acid). At recommended dosage levels, dehydrocholic acid exerts laxative and hydrocholeretic (increased volume and water content of bile) actions. The mechanisms of action are unknown. Unlike the natural bile acids and their conjugates, dehydrocholic acid does not readily form micelles (small aggregates of bile acids, fats and phospholipids necessary for normal fat absorption).

Indications:

Temporary relief of constipation.

Adjunctive therapy of biliary stasis, without complete mechanical obstruction of the common or hepatic bile ducts, where hydrocholeresis is desired.

Contraindications:

Significant cholelithiasis; presence of jaundice; marked hepatic insufficiency; complete obstruction of the common or hepatic bile ducts or of the GI or GU tracts; hypersensitivity to bile acids or their conjugates; use as a diuretic or adjunct.

Warnings:

Rectal bleeding or failure to have a bowel movement after use as a laxative may indicate a serious condition. Discontinue use and consult a physician.

Duration: Do not use as a laxative for > 1 week unless directed otherwise.

GI effects: Do not use as a laxative if abdominal pain, nausea or vomiting are present unless directed otherwise.

Elderly: Use with caution. If promotion of true bile flow is desired, use a cholagogue.

Children: No data supporting a recommended pediatric dose are available. Therefore, do not use in children < 12 years of age.

Adverse Reactions:

Hypersensitivity (pruritus, dermatitis).

Administration and Dosage:

250 to 500 mg 3 times daily after meals. Thereafter, titrate dosage to individual patient's needs. Do not exceed 1.5 g in 24 hours.

When used as a laxative, a bowel movement is generally produced in 6 to 12 hours.

Rx	**Dehydrocholic Acid** (Various, eg, Goldline)	**Tablets:** 250 mg	In 100s.
otc	**Cholan-HMB** (Ciba Consumer)		Lactose. Dye free. (Cholan HMB). In 100s.
otc	**Decholin** (Miles Pharm.)		Lactose. In 100s.

MISCELLANEOUS DIGESTIVE PRODUCTS

These products are used in the symptomatic treatment of various digestive dysfunctions, to supplement deficiencies of natural digestive enzymes and for a variety of vague GI disorders. Treat specific deficiency states with the deficient substance rather than with a mixture of components.

Components of these combinations include:

DIGESTIVE ENZYMES: Pepsin and papain aid in protein digestion.

Pancreatic enzymes (see individual monograph) aid in the intestinal digestion of starch, fat and protein.

Cellulase aids in dietary cellulose digestion.

DEHYDROCHOLIC ACID (see individual monograph) and *DESOXYCHOLIC ACID* increase secretion of bile and aid in digestion of fats.

ANTICHOLINERGICS relieve spasm and reduce hypermotility (see GI Anticholinergic/Antispasmodic monograph).

BARBITURATES (see individual monograph) and *PHENYLTOLOXAMINE CITRATE*, an antihistamine, are used for their sedative effects.

Administration and Dosage:

Capsules and tablets: Take 1 to 3 with or after meals (see individual dosing instructions).

Rx	**Arco-Lase Plus** (Arco)	**Tablets**: 30 mg amylase, 6 mg protease, 25 mg lipase, 2 mg cellulase, 0.1 mg hyoscyamine sulfate, 0.02 mg atropine sulfate, 7.5 mg phenobarbital	In 50s.
Rx	**Digepepsin** (Kenwood/Bradley)	**Tablets**: 250 mg pepcin, 300 mg pancreatin, 150 mg bile salts	In 60s.
Rx	**Digestozyme** (Various, eg, Major)	**Tablets**: 300 mg pancreatin, 250 mg pepsin, 25 mg dehydrocholic acid	In 50s, 100s and 1000s.
otc	**Gustase** (Geriatric Pharm.)	**Tablets**: 30 mg amylase, 6 mg protease, 2 mg cellulase	In 42s, 100s and 500s.
Rx	**Gustase Plus** (Geriatric Pharm.)	**Tablets**: 30 mg amylase, 6 mg protease, 2 mg cellulase, 2.5 mg homatropine MBr, 8 mg phenobarbital	In 42s, 100s and 500s.
Rx	**Kutrase** (Schwarz Pharma Kremers Urban)	**Capsules**: 30 mg amylase, 6 mg protease,75 mg lipase, 2 mg cellulase, 0.0625 mg hyoscyamine sulfate, 15 mg phenyltoloxamine citrate	Lactose. (Kremers Urban 475). Green and white. In 100s.
Rx	**Ku-Zyme** (Schwarz Pharma Kremers Urban)	**Capsules**: 30 mg amylase, 6 mg protease, 75 mg lipase, 2 mg cellulase	Lactose. (Kremers Urban 522). Yellow and white. In 100s.
otc	**Arco-Lase** (Arco)	**Tablets, chewable**: 30 mg amylase, 6 mg protease, 25 mg lipase, 2 mg cellulase	Mint flavor. In 50s.
otc	**Enzyme** (Nature's Bounty)	**Tablets, chewable**: 30 mg amylase, 6 mg protease, 2 mg cellulase, 25 mg lipase	In 100s.
otc	**Papaya Enzyme** (Nature's Bounty)	**Tablets, chewable**: 60 mg papain (from papaya leaves) and 60 mg amylase	In 100s.

URSODIOL (Ursodeoxycholic acid)

Warning:

Gallbladder stone dissolution with ursodiol treatment requires months of therapy. Complete dissolution does not occur in all patients and recurrence of stones within 5 years has been observed in up to 50% of patients who do dissolve their stones on bile acid therapy. Carefully select patients for therapy with ursodiol, and consider alternative therapies.

Actions:

Pharmacology: Ursodiol, intended for dissolution of radiolucent gallstones, is a naturally occurring bile acid found in small quantities in normal human bile and in larger quantities in the biles of certain species of bears. Ursodiol suppresses hepatic synthesis and cholesterol secretion, and also inhibits intestinal absorption of cholesterol. It has little inhibitory effect on synthesis and secretion into bile of endogenous bile acids, and does not appear to affect phospholipid secretion into bile.

With repeated dosing, bile ursodeoxycholic acid concentrations reach steady state in about 3 weeks. Although insoluble in aqueous media, cholesterol can be solubilized in at least two ways in the presence of dihydroxy bile acids. In addition to solubilizing cholesterol in micelles, ursodiol acts by an apparently unique mechanism to cause dispersion of cholesterol as liquid crystals in aqueous media. Thus, even though administration of high doses (eg, 15 to 18 mg/kg/day) does not result in a concentration of ursodiol higher than 60% of the total bile acid pool, ursodiol-rich bile solubilizes cholesterol. The overall effect of ursodiol is to increase the concentration level at which saturation of cholesterol occurs. The various actions of ursodiol combine to change the bile of patients with gallstones from cholesterol-precipitating to cholesterol-solubilizing.

After ursodiol dosing is stopped, its concentration in bile falls exponentially, declining to about 5% to 10% of its steady-state level in about 1 week.

Pharmacokinetics: About 90% of a therapeutic dose of ursodiol is absorbed in the small bowel after oral administration. After absorption, ursodiol enters the portal vein and undergoes extraction from portal blood by the liver (ie, "first-pass" effect) where it is conjugated with either glycine or taurine and is then secreted into the hepatic bile ducts. Ursodiol in bile is concentrated in the gallbladder and expelled into the duodenum in gallbladder bile via the cystic and common ducts by gallbladder contractions provoked by physiologic responses to eating.

Small quantities of ursodiol appear in the systemic circulation and very small amounts are excreted into urine. A small portion of orally administered drug undergoes bacterial degradation with each cycle of enterohepatic circulation. Ursodiol can be both oxidized and reduced, yielding either 7-keto-lithocholic acid or lithocholic acid, respectively. Free ursodiol, 7-keto-lithocholic acid and lithocholic acid are relatively insoluble in aqueous media and larger proportions of these compounds are excreted via the feces. Reabsorbed free ursodiol is reconjugated by the liver. Eighty percent of lithocholic acid formed in the small bowel is excreted in the feces, but the 20% that is absorbed is sulfated in the liver to relatively insoluble lithocholyl conjugates which are excreted into bile and lost in feces. Absorbed 7-keto-lithocholic acid is stereospecifically reduced in the liver to chenodiol.

Clinical trials: Based on clinical trials in 868 patients with radiolucent gallstones treated for 6 to 78 months with ursodiol doses ranging from about 5 to 20 mg/kg/day, a dose of about 8 to 10 mg/kg/day appeared to be best. Complete stone dissolution occurs in about 30% of unselected patients with uncalcified gallstones < 20 mm in maximal diameter treated for up to 2 years. Patients with calcified gallstones prior to treatment, or patients who develop stone calcification or gallbladder nonvisualization on treatment, and patients with stones larger than 20 mm in maximal diameter rarely dissolve their stones. The chance of gallstone dissolution is increased up to 50% in patients with floating or floatable stones (ie, those with high cholesterol content), and is inversely related to stone size for those < 20 mm in maximal diameter. Complete dissolution was observed in 81% of patients with stones up to 5 mm in diameter. Age, sex, weight, degree of obesity and serum cholesterol level are not related to the chance of stone dissolution with ursodiol.

Partial stone dissolution occurring within 6 months of beginning therapy with ursodiol appears to be associated with a > 70% chance of eventual complete stone dissolution with further treatment; partial dissolution observed within 1 year of starting therapy indicates a 40% probability of complete dissolution.

URSODIOL (Ursodeoxycholic acid)

Stone recurrence after dissolution with ursodiol therapy was seen within 2 years in 30% of patients. Stone recurrence occurs in up to 50% of patients within 5 years of complete stone dissolution with ursodiol therapy. Obtain serial ultrasonographic examinations to monitor for recurrence of stones; establish radiolucency of the stones before instituting another course of ursodiol. A prophylactic dose of ursodiol has not been established.

Alternative therapies – Watchful waiting has the advantage that no therapy may ever be required. For patients with silent or minimally symptomatic stones, the rate of development of moderate to severe symptoms or gallstone complications is between 2% and 6% per year; 7% to 27% in 5 years. Presumably the rate is higher for patients already having symptoms.

Surgery (cholecystectomy) offers the advantage of immediate and permanent stone removal, but carries a high risk in some patients. About 5% of cholecystectomized patients have residual symptoms of retained common duct stones. The spectrum of surgical risk varies as a function of age and the presence of disease other than cholelithiasis.

Indications:

Gallstone disolution: Dissolution of gallstones in patients with radiolucent, noncalcified, gallbladder stones < 20 mm in greatest diameter in whom elective cholecystectomy would be undertaken except for the presence of increased surgical risk due to systemic disease, advanced age, idiosyncratic reaction to general anesthesia, or for those patients who refuse surgery.

Contraindications:

Presence of calcified cholesterol stones, radiopaque stones or radiolucent bile pigment stones (ursodiol will not dissolve these stones, hence, patients with such stones are not candidates for ursodiol); patients with compelling reasons for cholecystectomy including unremitting acute cholecystitis, cholangitis, biliary obstruction, gallstone pancreatitis or biliary-gastrointestinal fistula; allergy to bile acids; chronic liver disease.

Warnings:

Length of therapy: Safety of use of ursodiol beyond 24 months is not established.

Gallbladder nonvisualization: Nonvisualizing gallbladder by oral cholecystogram prior to the initiation of therapy is not a contraindication to ursodiol therapy. However, gallbladder nonvisualization developing during ursodiol treatment predicts failure of complete stone dissolution and therapy should be discontinued.

Carcinogenesis: Bile acids might be involved in the pathogenesis of human colon cancer in patients who have undergone a cholecystectomy; direct evidence is lacking.

Pregnancy: Category B. There have been no adequate and well controlled studies in pregnant women, but inadvertent exposure of four women to therapeutic doses of the drug in the first trimester of pregnancy during the ursodiol trials led to no evidence of effects on the fetus or newborn baby. The possibility that ursodiol can cause fetal harm cannot be ruled out; hence, do not use the drug during pregnancy.

Lactation: It is not known whether ursodiol is excreted in breast milk. Exercise caution when ursodiol is administered to a nursing mother.

Children: Safety and efficacy for use in children have not been established.

Precautions:

Hepatic effects: Ursodiol therapy has not been associated with liver damage. Lithocholic acid, a naturally occurring bile acid and metabolite of ursodiol, is known to be a liver-toxic metabolite. This bile acid is formed in the gut from ursodiol less efficiently and in smaller amounts than that seen from chenodiol. Lithocholic acid is detoxified in the liver by sulfation and although man appears to be an efficient sulfater, it is possible that some patients may have a congenital or acquired deficiency in sulfation, thereby predisposing them to lithocholate-induced liver damage. Therefore, measure AST and ALT at the initiation of therapy, after 1 and 3 months of therapy, and every 6 months thereafter.

Patients with significant abnormalities in liver tests at any point should be monitored frequently; evaluate carefully for worsening gallstone disease which, in the controlled clinical trials, has been the only identified cause of significant liver test abnormality. Discontinue therapy with ursodiol if increased levels persist.

URSODIOL (Ursodeoxycholic acid)

Drug Interactions:

Ursodiol Drug Interactions			
Precipitant drug	Object drug*		Description
Antacids	Ursodiol	⬇	Aluminum-based antacids adsorb bile acids in vitro and interfere with the action of ursodiol by reducing its absorption.
Bile acid sequestrants	Ursodiol	⬇	Cholestyramine and colestipol may interfere with the action of ursodiol by reducing its absorption.
Clofibrate Estrogens Oral Contraceptives	Ursodiol	⬇	These agents (and perhaps other lipid-lowering drugs) increase hepatic cholesterol secretion, and encourage cholesterol gallstone formation and hence may counteract the effectiveness of ursodiol.

* ⬇ = Object drug decreased.

Adverse Reactions:

Dermatologic: Pruritus; rash; urticaria; dry skin; sweating; hair thinning. One patient with preexisting psoriasis apparently developed exacerbation of itching which remitted on withdrawal of the drug.

GI: Nausea; vomiting; dyspepsia; metallic taste; abdominal pain; biliary pain; cholecystitis; constipation; stomatitis; flatulence. Doses of 8 to 10 mg/kg/day rarely cause diarrhea (< 1%); in one study, incidence of mild, transient diarrhea was 6%.

Miscellaneous: Headache; fatigue; anxiety; depression; sleep disorder; arthralgia; myalgia; back pain; cough; rhinitis.

Overdosage:

The most likely manifestation of severe overdose with ursodiol would probably be diarrhea; treat symptomatically. Treatment includes usual supportive measures. Refer to General Management of Acute Overdosage.

Administration and Dosage:

Radiolucent gallbladder stones: 8 to 10 mg/kg/day given in 2 or 3 divided doses.

Obtain ultrasound images of the gallbladder at 6 month intervals for the first year of therapy to monitor gallstone response. If gallstones appear to have dissolved, continue therapy and confirm dissolution on a repeat ultrasound within 1 to 3 months. Most patients who eventually achieve complete stone dissolution will show partial or complete dissolution at the first on-treatment reevaluation. If partial stone dissolution is not seen by 12 months, likelihood of success is greatly reduced.

Storage: Do not store above 86°F (30°C).

Rx	**Actigall** (Ciba)	**Capsules:** 300 mg	White and pink. In 100s.

MONOCTANOIN

Actions:

Pharmacology: Monoctanoin is a semisynthetic esterified glycerol intended for cholesterol stone dissolution via perfusion of the common bile duct. The mixed mono-diglyceride has the following approximate composition: Glyceryl-l-mono-octanoate (80% to 85%); glyceryl-l-mono-decanoate and glyceryl-l-2-di-octanoate (10% to 15%); and free glycerol (maximum 2.5%).

Monoctanoin is readily hydrolyzed by pancreatic and other digestive lipases. The liberated fatty acids are excreted or absorbed and metabolized in a normal fashion.

Treatment results in complete stone dissolution about 33% of the time and in reduction in stone size in approximately 33% of patients. When reduced in size, these stones may pass spontaneously or may be more susceptible to simple physical extraction. Complete dissolution is much more likely when there is a single stone (almost 50%) than when there are multiple stones (about 20%). Complete dissolution is lower in diabetic patients (about 10%).

Indications:

Gallstone dissolution: A solubilizing agent for cholesterol (radiolucent) gallstones retained in the biliary tract following cholecystectomy, via perfusion of the common bile duct, when other means of removing cholesterol stones retained in the common bile duct have failed or cannot be undertaken.

Contraindications:

Impaired hepatic function; significant biliary tract infection; history of recent duodenal ulcer or jejunitis; porto-systemic shunting (such that there is saturation of the hepatic uptake and metabolism of material absorbed from the gut lumen); acute pancreatitis, or any active life-threatening problems that would be complicated by perfusion into the biliary tract.

Warnings:

Rate of administration: Intended for biliary tract perfusion only; not for parenteral use. Monoctanoin is irritating to GI and biliary tracts. The irritation seems closely related to biliary tract pressure and rate of perfusion; monitor both closely. Such irritation is reversible and disappears 2 to 7 days after therapy. (See Adverse Reactions.)

Ascending cholangitis has occurred, possibly related to obstruction in the common bile duct. If fever, anorexia, chills, leukocytosis, severe right upper quadrant abdominal pain or increasing jaundice occurs, discontinue treatment.

GI effects: Biopsies from the gastric antrum, duodenum and bile ducts have shown diffuse erythema in the antral and duodenal mucosa. Duodenal erosion and inflammatory cell infiltration have occurred. Multiple duodenal ulcerations adjacent to the infusion catheter were observed in one patient. No mucosal abnormalities were seen 1 month after therapy was discontinued.

Pregnancy: Category C. It is not known whether monoctanoin can cause fetal harm when administered to a pregnant woman or if it can affect reproduction capacity. Use during pregnancy only when clearly needed and when potential benefits outweigh potential hazards to the fetus.

Lactation: It is not known whether monoctanoin is excreted in breast milk. Exercise caution when administering to a nursing woman.

Children: Safety and efficacy for use in children have not been established.

Precautions:

Hepatic function: Monitor liver function tests in all patients. Use caution in patients with obstructive jaundice due to stones.

MONOCTANOIN

Adverse Reactions:

The incidences of adverse reactions are based on 326 patients. Overall, most adverse reactions were mild GI symptoms related to perfusion rate and biliary pressure. Some were tolerated; some abated with reduced perfusion rate and discontinuation during meals.

GI: Abdominal pain/discomfort (50.3%); nausea (32%); vomiting (20%); diarrhea (19%); anorexia (3%); loose stool (1.5%); indigestion (1.2%); increased serum amylase, burning epigastrium, increased fistula drainage, bile shock (< 1%).

Miscellaneous: Fever (6.3%); leukopenia, pruritus, fatigue/lethargy, intolerance, chills, depression, diaphoresis, headache, hypokalemia, allergic reaction (< 1%). One patient developed lupus erythematosus, which abated when the drug was discontinued. Five deaths have been attributed to cholangitis, gallbladder perforation and biliary peritonitis, pulmonary embolism, preexisting jaundice and pancreatitis and sepsis, CHF and renal failure, respectively.

Administration and Dosage:

Determine the value of monoctanoin therapy. Gallstones must be radiolucent and readily accessible to the perfusate. If recently removed stones are available, analyze them for composition or incubate in monoctanoin at body temperature with stirring. If analysis shows the stone to be other than cholesterol or if no dissolution is observed after 72 hours of incubation, do not institute or discontinue therapy.

Do not administer IV or IM. Perfuse into the biliary tract either directly via catheter inserted through the T-tube or a catheter inserted through the mature sinus tract through a nasobiliary tube placed endoscopically. The gravity feed method is recommended if a positive pressure infusion pump is not available. The tip of the catheter must be placed as close to the stone(s) as possible (preferably within 1 cm) to ensure stone contact and complete bathing. Monoctanoin is effective only when in direct contact with the stone.

Add 13 ml of Sterile Water for Injection to each 120 ml vial to reduce the viscosity and enhance the bathing of the stone(s). This dilution reduces the viscosity by nearly 50%. The drug should enter the body at 37°C (98.6°F) and be maintained at this temperature during administration.

Continuously perfuse on a 24 hour basis at a rate of 3 to 5 ml/hr. Continuous perfusion usually requires 2 to 10 days for elimination or size reduction of stones. If, after 10 days, cholangiography shows neither elimination nor reduction in size or density of stones, perform endoscopy to determine advisability of additional perfusion based on friability, softness or reduction of stone density.

If abdominal pain, nausea, diarrhea or emesis occurs and is not tolerated, stop perfusion for 1 hour, aspirate duct, then restart; if symptoms persist, stop perfusion for 1 hour, aspirate duct, then restart at a reduced rate of 3 ml/hr; if symptoms still persist, temporarily discontinue perfusion during meals.

Storage/Stability: When stored at temperatures below 15°C (59°F), the drug may form a semisolid. To reliquify, heat to 21° to 27°C (70° to 80°F). Store at room temperature 15° to 30°C (59° to 86°F).

Rx	**Moctanin** (Ethitek)	**Infusion:** Glyceryl-l-mono-octanoate (80-85%), glyceryl-l-mono-decanoate (10-15%), glyceryl-l-2-di-octanoate (10-15%), free glycerol (2.5% maximum)	In 120 ml ready-for-use bottles with disposable bottle hangers.

LAXATIVES

Laxatives promote bowel evacuation. Nonprescription laxatives are frequently misused due to lack of understanding of normal bowel function. Restrict self-medication to short-term therapy of constipation; chronic use of laxatives (particularly stimulants) may lead to dependence. Prior to institution of laxative use, consider living habits affecting bowel function including disease state and drug history. Rational therapy and prevention of constipation includes: Adequate fluid intake (4 to 6 glasses [8 oz] of water daily), proper dietary habits including sufficient bulk or roughage, responding to the urge to defecate and daily exercise.

Actions:

Pharmacology:

Pharmacologic Actions of Laxatives

	Laxatives	Onset of action (hrs)	Site of action	Mechanism of action	Comments
Saline	Magnesium sulfate Magnesium hydroxide Magnesium citrate Sodium phosphate	0.5-3	Small & large intestine	Attract/retain water in intestinal lumen increasing intraluminal pressure; cholecystokinin release	May alter fluid and electrolyte balance. Sulfate salts are considered the most potent.
	Sod. phosphate/ biphosphate enema	0.03-0.25	Colon		
Irritant/Stimulant	Cascara Senna Phenolphthalein Bisacodyl Tablets Casanthranol	6-10	Colon	Direct action on intestinal mucosa; stimulate myenteric plexus; alters water and electrolyte secretion	Bile must be present for phenolphthalein to produce its effects. May prefer castor oil when more complete evacuation is required.
	Bisacodyl suppository	0.25-1			
	Castor oil	2-6	Small intestine		Castor oil is converted to ricinoleic acid (active component) in the gut.
Bulk-Producing	Methylcellulose Psyllium Polycarbophil	12-24 (up to 72)	Small & large intestine	Holds water in stool; mechanical distention; malt soup extract reduces fecal pH	Safest and most physiological.
Lubricant	Mineral oil	6-8	Colon	Retards colonic absorption of fecal water; softens stool	May decrease absorption of fat soluble vitamins.
Surfactants	Docusate	24-72	Small & large intestine	Detergent activity; facilitates admixture of fat & water to soften stool	Beneficial when feces are hard or dry, or in anorectal conditions where passage of a firm stool is painful.
Miscellaneous	Glycerin suppository	0.25-0.5	Colon	Local irritation; hyperosmotic action	Sodium stearate in preparation causes the local irritation.
	Lactulose	24-48	Colon	Delivers osmotically active molecules to colon	Also indicated in portal-systemic encephalopathy.

Indications:

Short-term treatment of constipation; certain stimulant, lubricant and saline laxatives are used to evacuate the colon for rectal and bowel examinations. Lubricant laxatives or fecal softeners are useful prophylactically in patients who should not strain during defecation (ie, following anorectal surgery, myocardial infarction). Psyllium is also useful in patients with irritable bowel syndrome, diverticular disease, spastic colon and hemorrhoids. Polycarbophil is indicated for constipation or diarrhea associated with conditions such as irritable bowel syndrome and diverticulosis; it is also for acute non-specific diarrhea. Mineral oil enema is indicated for relief of fecal impaction.

LAXATIVES

Unlabeled uses: Psyllium appears to be useful in the reduction of cholesterol levels as an adjunct to a dietary program. In two studies of 101 patients with mild to moderate hypercholesterolemia, 3.4 g psyllium 3 times a day for 8 weeks resulted in a mean reduction in cholesterol of approximately 5% to 15% and an 8% to 20% reduction in LDL.

Contraindications:

Hypersensitivity to any ingredient; nausea, vomiting or other symptoms of appendicitis; acute surgical abdomen; fecal impaction (except mineral oil enema); intestinal obstruction; undiagnosed abdominal pain.

Do not use **bisacodyl tannex** in patients with ulcerative lesions of the colon or in children < 10 years old.

Do not give **docusate sodium** if mineral oil is being given.

Warnings:

Fluid and electrolyte balance: Excessive laxative use may lead to significant fluid and electrolyte imbalance. Monitor patients periodically.

Preparations containing sodium should not be used by individuals on a sodium restricted diet or in the presence of edema, congestive heart failure or hypertension.

Megacolon, imperforate anus or CHF – Do not use sodium phosphate and sodium biphosphate in these patients; hypernatremic dehydration may occur.

Abuse/Dependency – Chronic use of laxatives, particularly stimulants, may lead to laxative dependency, which in turn may result in fluid and electrolyte imbalances, steatorrhea, osteomalacia and vitamin and mineral deficiencies. Also known as laxative abuse syndrome (LAS), it is difficult to diagnose. It is often seen in women with depression, personality disorders or anorexia nervosa. Many agents can be detected in urine or stool samples; however, it is important to follow up negative test results if LAS is suspected since patients may be intermittent abusers or change laxative products frequently.

Cathartic colon, a poorly functioning colon, results from the chronic abuse of stimulant cathartics. Pathologic presentation resembles ulcerative colitis.

Melanosis coli is a darkened pigmentation of the colonic mucosa resulting from chronic use of anthraquinone derivatives. It resolves within 5 to 11 months of drug discontinuation.

Bisacodyl tannex: Use with caution when multiple enemas are administered. Tannic acid is hepatotoxic if absorbed in sufficient quantity. Deaths have occurred from hepatic damage due to tannic acid used in barium enema examination.

Lipid pneumonitis may result from oral ingestion and aspiration of mineral oil, especially when patient reclines. The young, elderly, debilitated and dysphagic are at greatest risk.

Renal function impairment: Up to 20% of the magnesium in magnesium salts may be absorbed. Do not use products containing phosphate, sodium, magnesium or potassium salts in the presence of renal dysfunction. Use sodium phosphate and sodium biphosphate with caution in these patients; hyperphosphatemia, hypernatremia, acidosis and hypocalcemia may occur.

Pregnancy: Category C. Docusate sodium, cascara sagrada, mineral oil, senna) Do not use castor oil during pregnancy; its irritant effect may induce premature labor. Mineral oil may decrease absorption of fat-soluble vitamins. Improper use of saline cathartics can lead to dangerous electrolyte imbalance. If needed, limit use to bulk forming or surfactant laxatives.

Lactation: Cascara sagrada is excreted in breast milk. There may be an increased incidence of diarrhea in the nursing infant. It is not known whether docusate sodium or lactulose are excreted in breast milk.

Children: Physical manipulation of a glycerin suppository in infants often initiates defecation; hence, adverse effects are minimal. Do not administer enemas to children < 2 years of age. Do not use bisacodyl tannex in children < 10 years of age.

An 11-month-old infant died following an overdose of a sodium phosphate enema. A 6-week-old infant developed magnesium poisoning following 16 doses of ≈ 1.7 ml over 48 hrs of a magnesium hydroxide mixture (550 mg/10 ml) for constipation.

LAXATIVES

Precautions:

Rectal bleeding or failure to respond to therapy may indicate a serious condition which may require further medical attention.

Phenolphthalein may cause a skin hypersensitivity characterized by a fixed drug eruption. Discontinue the drug if this occurs.

Discoloration of acid urine to yellow-brown may occur with cascara sagrada or senna. Pink-red, red-violet or red-brown discoloration of alkaline urine may occur with phenolphthalein, cascara sagrada or senna.

Impaction or obstruction may be caused by bulk-forming agents if temporarily arrested in their passage through the alimentary canal (eg, patients with esophageal strictures). Use in patients with intestinal ulcerations, stenosis or disabling adhesions may be hazardous.

Tartrazine sensitivity: Some of these products contain tartrazine, which may cause allergic-type reactions (including bronchial asthma) in susceptible individuals. Although the incidence of tartrazine sensitivity in the general population is low, it is frequently seen in patients who also have aspirin hypersensitivity. Specific products containing tartrazine are identified in the product listings.

Drug Interactions:

Mineral oil: Surfactants (ie, docusate) may facilitate absorption, thus increasing the toxicity of mineral oil.

Milk or antacids: Concomitant administration of **bisacodyl** tablets may cause the enteric coating to dissolve, resulting in gastric lining irritation or dyspepsia.

Lipid soluble vitamins (vitamins A, D, E and K): Absorption may decrease during prolonged administration with **mineral oil.**

Tetracycline: Laxatives containing aluminum, calcium or magnesium (ie, polycarbophil) impair absorption of tetracycline, due to release of free calcium.

Adverse Reactions:

Excessive bowel activity (griping, diarrhea, nausea, vomiting); perianal irritation; weakness; dizziness; fainting; palpitations; sweating; bloating; flatulence.

Abdominal cramps have occurred.

Esophageal, gastric, small intestinal and rectal obstruction due to the accumulation of mucilaginous components of bulk laxatives have occurred.

Large doses of mineral oil may cause anal seepage, resulting in itching (pruritis ani), irritation, hemorrhoids and perianal discomfort.

Bisacodyl suppositories may cause proctitis and inflammation. Not recommended for long-term use.

Patient Information:

Direct attention to proper dietary fiber intake, adequate fluids and regular exercise.

Do not use in the presence of abdominal pain, nausea or vomiting.

Laxative use is only a temporary measure; do not use longer than 1 week. When regularity returns, discontinue use. Prolonged, frequent or excessive use may result in dependence or electrolyte imbalance.

Notify physician if unrelieved constipation, rectal bleeding or symptoms of electrolyte imbalance (eg, muscle cramps or pain, weakness, dizziness) occurs.

Pink-red, red-violet or red-brown discoloration of alkaline urine may occur with cascara sagrada, phenolphthalein or senna.

Yellow-brown discoloration of acid urine may occur with cascara sagrada or senna.

Refrigerate magnesium citrate solutions to retain potency and palatability.

Take with a full glass of water or juice.

Mineral oil: Preferably administered on an empty stomach.

Bisacodyl tablets: Swallow whole; do not take within 1 hour of antacids or milk.

SALINE LAXATIVES

For complete prescribing information, refer to the Laxatives group monograph.

otc	**Epsom Salt** (Various, eg, Dixon-Shane, Humco, Purepac)	**Granules**: Magnesium sulfate. 40mEq magnesium/5g *Dose:* Adults – 10 to 15 g in glass of water. Children – 5 to 10 g in glass of water.	In 150 and 240 g and 1 and 4 lb.
otc	**Milk of Magnesia – Concentrated** (Various, eg, Roxane, Vangard)	**Liquid**: Magnesium hydroxide *Dose:* 10 to 20 ml.	Lemon flavor. In 100, 400 and 480 ml and UD 10, 15 and 20 ml.
otc	**Phillips' Milk of Magnesia, Concentrated** (Glenbrook)	**Liquid**: Magnesium hydroxide. *Dose:* 15 to 30 ml.	Sorbitol, sugar. Strawberry and orange vanilla creme flavors. In 240 ml.
otc	**Milk of Magnesia** (Various, eg, Apothecon, Geneva, Goldline, Major, Moore, Purepac, Roxane, Rugby, Schein, URL)	**Liquid**: Magnesium hydroxide. 7% to 8.5% aqueous suspension; 80 mEq magnesium per 30 ml *Dose:* Adults – 30 to 60 ml/day, taken with liquid. Children ≥ 2 years – 5 to 30ml, depending on age.	In 180, 360, 480, 720 and 960 ml, and UD 15 and 30 ml.
otc	**Phillips' Milk of Magnesia** (Glenbrook)		Mint and regular flavors. In120, 360 and 780 ml.
otc	**Citrate of Magnesia** (Dixon-Shane)	**Solution**: Magnesium citrate *Dose:* Adults – 1 glassful (approx. 240 ml) as needed. Children – ½ the adult dose; repeat if necessary.	In 300 ml.
otc *sf*	**Fleet Phospho-soda** (Fleet)	**Solution**: 18 g sodium phosphate and 48 g sodium biphosphate per 100 ml (96.4mEq sodium per 20 ml) *Dose:* Adults – 20 to 30 ml mixed with ½ glass cool water. Children – 5 to 15 ml.	Regular and ginger-lemon flavors. In 45, 90 and 237 ml.
otc *sf*	**Sodium Phosphates** (Roxane)		Lemon flavor. In UD 30 ml.

Irritant or Stimulant Laxatives

CASCARA SAGRADA

For complete prescribing information, refer to the Laxative group monograph.

otc	**Cascara Sagrada** (Various, eg, Dixon-Shane, Rugby)	**Tablets:** 325 mg *Dose:* 1 tablet at bedtime.	In 100s and 1000s.
otc	**Cascara Sagrada Aromatic Fluid Extract** (Various, eg, Major, Purepac, Rugby)	**Liquid:** ≈ 18% alcohol *Dose:* 5 ml.	In 120 ml and pt.

CALCIUM SALTS OF SENNOSIDES A & B (The laxative principle of senna)

For complete prescribing information, refer to the Laxatives group monograph.

otc	**Ex-Lax Gentle Nature** (Sandoz)	**Tablets:** 20 mg *Dose:* Adults – 1 to 2 tablets with water at bedtime. Children (≥ 6 years) – 1 tablet/day	In 16s.

Irritant or Stimulant Laxatives

PHENOLPHTHALEIN

Complete prescribing information for these products begins in the Laxatives group monograph.

Yellow phenolphthalein is 2 to 3 times more potent than white phenolphthalein.

Dose: 60 to 194 mg, preferably at bedtime.

otc	**Alophen Pills** (Warner Lambert)	**Tablets**: 60 mg phenolphthalein	Sucrose, sugar. In 100s.
otc	**Ex-Lax Unflavored** (Sandoz Consumer)	**Tablets**: 90 mg yellow phenolphthalein	Sucrose. In 8s, 30s and 60s.
otc	**Lax Pills** (G & W)		In 30s and 60s.
otc	**Laxative Pills** (Rugby)		Sugar coated. In 30s.
otc	**Espotabs** (Combe)	**Tablets**: 97.2 mg yellow phenolphthalein	Lactose, sucrose. In 12s,30s and 60s.
otc	**Feen-a-mint** (Schering-Plough)		In 20s.
otc	**Modane** (Adria)	**Tablets**: 130 mg phenolphthalein	Lactose, sucrose. (A 513).Red. Sugar coated. In 10s, 30s and 100s.
otc	**Prulet** (Mission)	**Tablets**: 60 mg white phenolphthalein	Green, scored. Lemon-lime flavor. In 12s and 40s.
otc	**Ex-Lax Maximum Relief** (Sandoz)	**Tablets**: 135 mg yellow phenolphthalein	Sucrose. (Ex-Lax). In 24s.
otc	**Feen-a-mint Chocolated** (Schering-Plough)	**Tablets, chewable**: 65 mg yellow phenolphthalein	Sugar. Chocolate mint flavor. In 4s, 18s and 36s.
otc	**Ex-Lax Chocolated** (Sandoz Consumer)	**Tablets, chewable**: 90 mg yellow phenolphthalein	Sugar. In 6s, 18s, 48s and 72s.
otc	**Evac-U-Gen** (Walker)	**Tablets, chewable**: 97.2 mg yellow phenolphthalein	Corn syrup, lactose, saccharin, sugar. In 35s and 100s.
otc	**Feen-a-mint** (Schering-Plough)		Sugar, methylsalicylate. Scored. Square shape. Mint flavor. In 20s.
otc	**Medilax** (Mission)	**Tablets, chewable**: 120 mg phenolphthalein	Aspartame, 1.5 mg phenylalanine. Citrus flavor. In 24s.
otc	**Phenolax** (Upjohn)	**Wafers**: 64.8 mg phenolphthalein	Tartrazine, glucose, sucrose. (Phenolax). In 100s.
otc	**Evac-U-Lax Tablets** (Hauck)	**Wafers, chewable**: 80 mg phenolphthalein	In 1000s.
otc	**Feen-a-mint** (Schering-Plough)	**Gum**: 97.2 mg yellow phenolphthalein	Sugar. Peppermint flavor. In 5s, 16s and 40s.

SENNA

For complete prescribing information, refer to the Laxatives group monograph.

otc	**Senexon** (Rugby)	**Tablets**: Standard senna concentrate equivalent to 5.6 mg of senosides A and B. *Dose:* Adults – 2 tablets at bedtime (up to 8/day). Children > 60 lbs (27 kg) – 1 tablet at bedtime (up to 4/day).	Sucrose. In 100s and 1000s.
otc	**Senolax** (Schein)	**Tablets**: 187 mg senna concentrate *Dose:* Adults – 2 tablets (up to 8/day) Children (6 to 12 years) – 1 tablet (up to 4/day)	In 100s and 1000s.

Irritant or Stimulant Laxatives

SENNA			
otc	**Senokot** (Purdue Frederick)	**Tablets:** 187 mg standardized senna concentrate	Lactose. In 20s, 50s, 100s, 1000s and UD 100s.
		Granules: 326 mg standardized senna concentrate per tsp	Sucrose. In 60, 170 & 340 g.
		Suppositories: 652 mg standardized senna concentrate *Dose:* Adults – 2 tablets (up to 8/day), 1 tsp granules (up to 4 tsp/day) or 1 suppository at bedtime (repeat in 2 hrs if necessary). Children (6 to < 12 years) – 1 tablet (up to 4/day), > 60 lbs (27 kg) – ½ tsp granules (up to 2 tsp/day) or ½ suppository at bedtime.	In 6s.
		Syrup: 218 mg/5 ml standardized senna extract *Dose:* Adults – 10 to 15 ml at bedtime (up to 30 ml/day). Children (5 to 15 years) – 5 to 10 ml at bedtime (up to 20 ml/day). Children (1 to 5 years) – 2.5 to 5 ml at bedtime (up to 10 ml/day). Children (1 month to 1 year) – 1.25 to 2.5 ml at bedtime (up to 5 ml/day).	7% alcohol. In 60 and 240 ml.
otc	**Senna-Gen** (Goldline)	**Tablets:** 8.6 mg sennocides. *Dose:* Adults – 2 tablets at bedtime (up to 8/day). Children > 60 lbs (27 kg) – 1 tablet at bedtime (up to 4/day).	Lactose. In 1000s.
otc	**Senokotxtra** (Purdue Fredrick)	**Tablets:** 374 mg senna concentrate *Dose:* Adults – 1 tablet at bedtime (up to 4/day)	In 12s.
otc	**Black-Draught** (Chattem)	**Tablets:** 600 mg senna equivalent	Sucrose. In 30s.
		Granules: 1.65 g senna equivalent per ½ tsp *Dose:* Adults – 2 tablets at bedtime (up to 3/day) or ¼ to ½ level tsp granules with water.	Tartrazine, sucrose. In 22.5 g.
otc	**Gentlax** (Blair)	**Granules:** 326 mg standardized senna concentrate per tsp *Dose:* Adults – 1 tsp once/day (up to 4 tsp/day). Children 6 to < 12 years – ½ tsp once/day (up to 2 tsp/day).	Malt extract, sucrose. In 180 g.
otc	**Dr. Caldwell Senna Laxative** (Gebauer)	**Liquid:** 33.3 mg/ml senna concentrate *Dose:* Adults – 15 to 30 ml with or after meals or at bedtime. Children (6 to 15 years) – 10 to 15 ml at bedtime. Children (2 to 5 years) – 5 to 10 ml at bedtime.	4.9% alcohol, salicylic acid, sucrose. In 150 and 360 ml.
otc	**Fletcher's Castoria** (Mentholatum)	**Liquid:** 33.3 mg/ml senna concentrate *Dose:* Children (6 to 15 years) – 10 to 15 ml. Children (2 to 5 years) – 5 to 10 ml.	3.5% alcohol, sucrose. In 75 and 150 ml.
otc	**Dosalax** (Richwood)	**Syrup:** Extract of senna fruit	7% alcohol, parabens, sucrose. In 237 ml.

Irritant or Stimulant Laxatives

CASTOR OIL

For complete prescribing information, refer to the Laxatives group monograph.

otc	**Castor Oil** (Various, eg, Apothecon, Dixon-Shane, Paddock, Purepac)	**Liquid:** *Dose:* Adults – 15 to 60 ml. Children (2 to 12 years) – 5 to 15 ml.	In 60 and 120 ml and pt.
otc	**Fleet Flavored Castor Oil** (Fleet)	**Emulsion**: 67% castor oil with emulsifying agents. *Dose:* Adults – 45 ml. Children (2 to 12 years) – 15 ml.	In 90 ml.
otc	**Purge** (Fleming)	**Liquid**: 95% castor oil. Lemon flavor. *Dose:* Adults – 30 to 60 ml. Children - Adjust between infant and adult dosage. Infants - 2.5 to 7.5 ml.	In 30 and 60 ml.
otc *sf*	**Emulsoil** (Paddock)	**Emulsion:** 95% castor oil with emulsifying agents. *Dose:* Adults – 15 to 60 ml mixed with ½ to 1 glass liquid. Children – 5 to 10 ml mixed with ½ to 1 glass liquid.	In 60 ml.
otc *sf*	**Neoloid** (Kenwood/Bradley)	**Oil**: 36.4% castor oil with 0.1% sodium benzoate, 0.2% potassium sorbate. *Dose:* Adults – 30 to 60 ml. Children –Adjust between infant and adult dosage. Infants – 2.5 to 7.5 ml.	Mint flavor. In 118 ml.

sf - Sugar free.

BISACODYL

For complete prescribing information, refer to the Laxatives group monograph.

Administration and Dosage:

Tablets: Swallow whole; do not chew. Do not take within 1 hour of antacids or milk.

Adults – 10 to 15 mg (usually 10) in a single dose once daily. Up to 30 mg has been used for preparation of lower GI tract for special procedures.

Children (6 to < 12 years) – 5(0.3 mg/kg) once daily.

Suppositories:

Adults – 10 mg once daily to induce bowel movement.

Children (6 to < 12 years) – 5 mg once daily.

otc	**Bisacodyl** (Various, eg, Major, Moore, Parmed, Upsher-Smith, URL)	**Tablets, enteric coated:** 5 mg	In 25s, 100s, 1000s and UD 100s.
otc	**Dulcagen** (Goldline)		Yellow. In 100s.
otc	**Dulcolax** (CIBA Cons.)		Lactose, sucrose, parabens. In 10s, 25s, 50s, 100s, 1000s.
otc	**Fleet Laxative** (Fleet)		In 24s.
otc	**Bisacodyl** (Various, eg, Major, Moore, Parmed, URL)	**Suppositories:** 10 mg	In 8s, 12s and 100s.
otc	**Bisacodyl Uniserts** (Upsher-Smith)		In UD 12s.
otc	**Bisco-Lax** (Raway)		In UD 12s, 50s, 100s, 500s and 1000s.
otc	**Dulcagen** (Goldline)		In 12s and 100s.
otc	**Dulcolax** (CIBA Cons.)		In 2s, 4s, 8s, 16s and 50s.
otc	**Fleet Laxative** (Fleet)		In 4s.

Bulk-Producing Laxatives

MISCELLANEOUS

For complete prescribing information, refer to the Laxatives group monograph.

Administration and Dosage:

Take with a full glass of water; encourage additional fluid intake.

Citrucel:

Adults and children ≥ 12 years – 1 heaping tbsp (19 g) in 8 oz cold water, 1 to 3 times daily.

Children (6 to < 12 years) – ½ the adult dose in 4 oz cold water, 1 to 3 times daily.

Unifiber is classified as a dietary fiber supplement. It is not FDA approved as a bulk-producing laxative. Dose is 1 to 2 tbsp in liquid once or twice daily.

Maltsupex:

Tablets – Adults, 12 to 64 g/day. Initially, 4 tabs 4 times daily (meals and bedtime).

Powder – Adults, up to 32 g twice daily for 3 or 4 days, then 16 to 32 g at bedtime. Children 6 to 12 years, up to 16 g twice daily for 3 or 4 days; 2 to 6 years, 8 g twice daily for 3 or 4 days. Infants, > 1 month (bottlefed), 8 to 16 g daily in formula for 3 or 4 days, then 4 to 8 g daily in formula; > 1 month (breastfed), 4 g in 2 to 4 oz water or fruit juice twice daily for 3 or 4 days.

Liquid – Adults, 2 tbsp twice daily for 3 or 4 days, then 1 to 2 tbsp at bedtime. Children 6 to 12 years, 1 to 2 tbsp once or twice daily for 3 or 4 days; 2 to 6 years, ½ tbsp once or twice daily for 3 or 4 days. Infants, > 1 month (bottlefed), ½ to 2 tbsp daily in formula for 3 or 4 days, then 1 to 2 tsp daily in formula; > 1 month (breastfed), 1 to 2 tsp in 2 to 4 oz water or fruit juice once or twice daily for 3 or 4 days.

otc	**Citrucel** (SK-Beecham)	**Powder**: 2 g methylcellulose per heaping tbsp	Sucrose. Orange flavor. In 19 g (20s), 480, 720 and 900 g.
otc sf	**Citrucel Sugar Free** (SK-Beecham)	**Powder**: 2 g methylcellulose, 52 mg phenylalanine per heaping tbsp	Aspartame. In 258 and 507 g.
otc	**Unifiber** (Dow B. Hickam)	**Powder**: Powdered cellulose	In 150, 270 and 480 g.
otc	**Maltsupex** (Wallace)	**Tablets**: 750 mg adiastatic barley malt extract	In 100s.
		Powder: 8 g adiastatic barley malt extract per tbsp	In 240 and 480 g.
		Liquid: 16 g adiastatic barley malt extract per tbsp	In 240 and 480 ml.

POLYCARBOPHIL

For complete prescribing information, refer to the Laxatives group monograph.

Actions:

Pharmacology: Calcium polycarbophil is a hydrophilic agent. As a *bulk laxative,* it retains free water within the intestinal lumen, and indirectly opposes dehydrating forces of the bowel, promoting well-formed stools. In *diarrhea,* when the intestinal mucosa is incapable of absorbing water at normal rates, it absorbs free fecal water, forming a gel and producing formed stools. Thus, in both diarrhea and constipation, it works by restoring a more normal moisture level and providing bulk.

Indications:

Treatment of constipation or diarrhea associated with conditions such as irritable bowel syndrome and diverticulosis; acute nonspecific diarrhea.

Administration and Dosage:

Adults: 1 g 1 to 4 times daily or as needed. Do not exceed 6 g in 24 hours.

Children: 500 mg 1 to 3 times daily or as needed. Do not exceed 3 g/day.

(3 to < 6 years) – 500 mg 1 to 2 times daily or as needed. Do not exceed 1.5 g/day.

For severe diarrhea, repeat dose every 30 min; do not exceed maximum daily dose.

When using as a laxative, drink 8 oz water or other liquid with each dose.

Bulk-Producing Laxatives

POLYCARBOPHIL

otc	**FiberCon** (Lederle)	**Tablets**: 500 mg (as calcium). Sodium free	(LL F66). Film coated. In 36s, 60s and 90s.
otc	**Equalactin** (Numark)	**Tablets, chewable**: 500 mg (as calcium)	Sorbitol. In 16s and 36s.
otc	**Mitrolan** (Robins)	**Tablets, chewable**: 500 mg (as calcium) < 0.02 mEq (0.46 mg) sodium/tablet	Sucrose. In 36s and 100s.
otc	**FiberNorm** (G & W)	**Tablets**: 625 mg calcium polycarbophil	In 60s.
otc	**Konsyl Fiber** (Konsyl)		In 90s.
otc	**Fiber-Lax** (Rugby)	**Tablets**: 625 mg calcium polycarbophil (equivalent to 500 mg polycarbophil)	In 60s.
otc	**Fiberall** (Ciba Consumer)	**Tablets, chewable**: 1250 mg calcium carbophil (= 1 g polycarbophil)	Dextrose. Scored. Lemon flavor. In 18s.

PSYLLIUM

For complete prescribing information, refer to the Laxatives group monograph.

otc	**Fiberall Natural Flavor** (Ciba Consumer)	**Powder**: 3.4 g psyllium hydrophilic mucilloid, wheat bran, < 10 mg sodium, < 60 mg potassium and < 6 cal/ dose *Dose:* 1 rounded tsp (5 to 5.9 g) in 8 oz cool water or juice, 1 to 3 x day.	In 284 and 426 g.
otc	**Fiberall Orange Flavor** (Ciba Consumer)		Saccharin. In 284 and 426 g.
otc	**Hydrocil Instant** (Solvay Pharm.)	**Powder**: 3.5 g psyllium hydrophilic mucilloid / dose *Dose:* 1 packet or level scoopful (3.7 g) in liquid, morning & evening	In 250 g and UD 3.7 g packets (30s & 500s).
otc	**Konsyl** (Konsyl Pharm.)	**Powder**: 100% psyllium. *Dose:* 1 packet or rounded tsp (6 g) in liquid, 1 to 3 times daily.	In 300 and 450 g and UD 6 g packets (25s).
otc	**Konsyl-Orange** (Konsyl Pharm.)	**Powder**: 3.4 g psyllium fiber per tbsp.	Sucrose. Orange flavor. In 12 and 538 g.
otc	**Maalox Daily Fiber Therapy** (R-P Rorer)	**Powder**: ≈ 3.4 g psyllium hydrophilic mucilloid/dose, 35 calories per 12 g.	Sucrose. Orange and citrus flavors. In 369 g.
otc	**Maalox Daily Fiber Therapy Sugar Free** (R-P Rorer)	**Powder**: ≈ 3.4 g psyllium hydrophilic mucilloid/dose, 21 mg/tsp phenylalanine, 9 calories per 5.8 g.	Aspartame. In 283 and 369 g.
otc	**Metamucil** (Procter & Gamble)	**Powder**: ≈ 3.4 g psyllium hydrophilic mucilloid, 3.5 g carbohydrates, < 10 mg sodium, 31 mg potassium & 14 calories per dose *Dose:* 1 rounded tsp (7 g) in liquid, 1 to 3 times a day.	Dextrose. In 210, 420, 630 and 960 g and 30 and 100 UD single-dose packs (100s).
otc	**Metamucil, Orange Flavor** (Procter & Gamble)	**Powder**: ≈ 3.4 g psyllium hydrophilic mucilloid, 7.1 g carbohydrate, < 10 mg sodium, 31 mg potassium and 30 calories / dose *Dose:* 1 rounded tbsp (11 g) in liquid, 1 to 3 times a day.	In 210, 420, 630 and 960 g and UD 30s.
otc	**Metamucil, Sugar Free** (Procter & Gamble)	**Powder**: ≈ 3.4 g psyllium hydrophilic mucilloid, 0.3 g carbohydrates, < 10 mg sodium, 31 mg potassium and 1 calorie per dose *Dose:* 1 rounded tsp (3.7 g) in liquid, 1 to 3 times a day.	Aspartame, 6 mg phenylalanine. In 111, 222, 333 and 507 g and UD single-dose packs (100s).

Bulk-Producing Laxatives

PSYLLIUM

otc	**Metamucil** (Procter & Gamble)	**Wafers:** ≈ 1.7 g psyllium mucilloid, 18 g carbohydrate, 18 mg sodium, 4.5 g fat, 96 calories per dose	Sugar, fructose, molasses, sucrose. In 24s.
otc	**Metamucil, Sugar Free, Orange Flavor** (Procter & Gamble)	**Powder:** ≈ 3.4 mg psyllium hydrophilic mucilloid, 1.4 mg carbohydrate, < 10 mg sodium, 31 mg potassium and 5 calories per dose. *Dose:* 1 rounded tsp (5.2 g) in liquid 1 to 3 times a day.	Aspartame, 30 mg phenylalanine per dose. In 141, 261, 387 and 621 g.
otc	**Mylanta Natural Fiber Supplement** (J & J Merck)	**Powder:** 3.4 mg psyllium hydrophilic mucilloid fiber/dose *Dose:* 1 rounded tsp in 8 oz. liquid, up to 3 times a day.	Sucrose. Orange flavor. In 390 g.
otc	**Natural Vegetable** (Various, eg, Dixon-Shane, Geneva Marsam, Moore, Schein)	**Powder:** 3.4 g psyllium hydrophilic mucilloid with dextrose, < 10 mg sodium and 14 calories per dose *Dose:* 1 rounded tsp (7 g) in liquid, 1 to 3 times daily.	In 210, 420 and 630 g.
otc	**Reguloid, Orange** (Rugby)	**Powder:** 3.4 g psyllium mucilloid & 70% sucrose/rounded tbsp *Dose:* Adults – 1 rounded tbsp, 2 to 3 times daily. Children – ½ adult dose	Orange flavor. In 420 and 630 g.
otc	**Reguloid, Sugar Free Orange** (Rugby)	**Powder:** ≈ 3.4 g psyllium hydrophilic mucilloid, < 0.01 g sodium and ≈ 5 calories per rounded tsp *Dose:* Adults – 1 rounded tsp (5.2 g) in 8 oz liquid 1 to 3 times/day. Children (6 to 12) – ½ adult dose in 8 oz liquid 1 to 3 times/day.	Aspartame, 30 mg phenylalanine per dose. In 246 and 387 g.
otc	**Reguloid, Sugar Free Regular** (Rugby)	**Powder:** ≈ 3.4 g psyllium hydrophilic mucilloid, < 0.01 g sodium and ≈ 1 calorie per 3.7 g dose *Dose:* Adults – 1 rounded tsp (3.7 g) in 8 oz liquid, 1 to 3 times/day. Children (6 to 12) – ½ adult dose in 8 oz liquid 1 to 3 times a day.	Aspartame, 6 mg phenylalanine per dose. In 222 and 333 g.
otc	**Restore** (InAgra)	**Powder:** 3.4 g hydrophilic mucilloid fiber per 12 g	Saccharin, sucrose. Orange flavor. In 390 and 538 g.
otc sf	**Restore Sugar Free** (InAgra)		Aspartame, 30 mg phenylalanine per tsp, saccharin. Orange flavor. In 300 and 425 g.
otc	**Serutan** (Menley & James)	**Powder:** 3.4 g psyllium (< 0.1 g sodium) per heaping tsp *Dose:* 1 heaping tsp in 240 ml water, 1 to 3 times daily, preferably with meals.	Dextrose (regular flavor). In regular and fruit flavors. In 210, 420 and 630 g.
otc	**Syllact** (Wallace)	**Powder:** 3.3 g psyllium seed husks and ≈ 14 calories per rounded tsp *Dose:* 1 rounded tsp in 8 oz liquid, 1 to 3 times daily. Children ≥ 6 – ½ adult dose in 8 oz liquid	Dextrose, saccharin. Fruit flavor. In 300 g.
otc	**Konsyl-D** (Konsyl Pharm)	**Powder:** 3.4 g psyllium hydrophilic mucilloid, 14 calories per rounded tsp *Dose:* Adults – 1 tsp (6.5 g) in 8 oz liquid 1 to 3 times per day. Children – ½ adult dose	Dextrose. In 325 & 500 g & UD 6.5 g (25s).

Bulk-Producing Laxatives

PSYLLIUM

otc	**Modane Bulk** (Adria)	**Powder:** 50% psyllium hydrophilic mucilloid and 50% dextrose per dose *Dose:* Adults – 1 rounded tsp in 8 oz liquid, 1 to 3 times a day. Children (6-13) – ½ adult dose in 8 oz liquid	2 mg sodium, 37 mg potassium and 14 calories per tsp. In 396 g.
otc	**Reguloid, Natural** (Rugby)		14 calories per tsp. Sodium free. In 420 and 630 g.
otc	**V-Lax** (Century)		In 120 and 480 g.
otc	**Alramucil** (Alra)	**Effervescent Powder:** 3.6 g psyllium hydrophilic mucilloid, potassium and sodium bicarbonate, < 0.01 g sodium and 4 calories per packet *Dose:* 1 packet in 8 oz water, 1 to 3 times a day.	Sucrose, saccharin. Regular and orange flavors. In 30s.
otc	**Metamucil Lemon-Lime Flavor** (Procter & Gamble)	**Effervescent Powder:** ≈ 3.4 g psyllium hydrophilic mucilloid, sodium and potassium bicarbonate, < 10 mg sodium, calcium carbonate, 290 mg potassium and 1 calorie per dose *Dose:* 1 packet in 8 oz water 1 to 3 times daily.	Aspartame, 30 mg phenylalanine per dose. In single dose packets (30s and 100s).
otc	**Metamucil Orange Flavor** (Procter & Gamble)	**Effervescent Powder:** ≈ 3.4 g psyllium hydrophilic mucilloid, sodium and potassium bicarbonate, 310 mg potassium, < 10 mg sodium and 1 calorie per dose *Dose:* 1 packet in 8 oz water, 1 to 3 times a day.	Aspartame, 30 mg phenylalanine per dose. In single dose packets (30s).
otc	**Perdiem Fiber** (Rhone-Poulenc Rorer)	**Granules:** 4.03 g psyllium, 1.8 mg sodium, 36.1 mg potassium and 4 calories/rounded tsp (6 g) *Dose:* Adults – 1 to 2 rounded tsp with 8 oz liquid, once or twice daily. Do not chew. Children (7 to 11) – 1 rounded tsp with 8 oz liquid once or twice daily	Sucrose. Dye free. Mint flavor. In 100 and 250 g.
otc	**Serutan** (Menley & James)	**Granules:** 2.5 g psyllium and < 0.03 g sodium per heaping tsp *Dose:* Adults – 1 to 3 heaping tsp on cereal or other food, 1 to 3 times daily. Children (6 to 12) – ½ adult dose with 8 oz liquid.	Saccharin, sugar. In 180 and 540 g.
otc	**Siblin** (Warner-Lambert Consumer)	**Granules:** 2.5 g blond psyllium seed coatings per rounded tsp *Dose:* Adults – 1 rounded tsp up to 12 times daily in liquid. Children (6 to 12) – ½ rounded tsp up to 12 times daily.	Sugar. In 480 g.
otc	**Fiberall** (Ciba Consumer)	**Wafers:** 3.4 g psyllium hydrophilic mucilloid, 0.03 g sodium and 78 calories per wafer. With wheat bran and oats. *Dose:* Adults – 1 or 2 wafers with 8 oz liquid, 1 to 3 times a day. Children (6 to 12) – ½ adult dosage.	Corn syrup, molasses, sugar. Oatmeal raisin and fruit & nut flavors. In 14s.

Emolient Laxatives

MINERAL OIL

For complete prescribing information, refer to the Laxatives group monograph.

Administration and Dosage:

Dose:

Adults – 5 to 45 ml.

Children – 5 to 20 ml. Although usual directions are to give at bedtime, caution is advised because of lipid pneumonitis (see Laxative group monograph).

otc	**Mineral Oil** (Various, eg, Apothecon, Barre, Century, Lannett, Paddock, Pharm Assoc., Purepac, Roxane, UDL)	**Liquid:** Heavy mineral oil	In 30 and 180 ml, pt, qt and gal.
otc	**Neo-Cultol** (Fisons)	**Jelly:** Refined mineral oil	Sugar. Chocolate flavor. In 180 ml.
otc	**Milkinol** (Schwarz Pharma Kremers-Urban)	**Emulsion:** Mineral oil with an emulsifier	In 355 ml.
otc sf	**Agoral Plain** (Warner-Lambert)	**Emulsion:** 1.4 g mineral oil/5 ml w/agar, tragacanth, egg albumin, acacia, glycerin	In 480 ml.
otc sf	**Kondremul Plain** (Fisons)	**Emulsion:** Mineral oil	Irish moss, acacia, glycerin. Maple walnut flavor. In 480 ml.

Fecal Softeners

DOCUSATE SODIUM (Dioctyl Sodium Sulfosuccinate; DSS)

For complete prescribing information, refer to the Laxatives group monograph.

Administration and Dosage:

Increase the daily fluid intake by drinking a glass of water with each dose.

Adults and older children: 50 to 500 mg.

Children (6 to 12): 40 to 120 mg.

Children (3 to 6): 20 to 60 mg.

Children (< 3): 10 to 40 mg.

Give higher doses for initial therapy; individualize dosage.

Liquid: Give in milk, fruit juice or infant formula to mask taste. In enemas, add 50 to 100 mg (5 to 10 ml liquid) to a retention or flushing enema.

otc	**Dialose** (J & J-Merck)	**Tablets:** 100 mg	Lactose, sugar. In 36s.
otc	**Regutol** (Schering-Plough)		Lactose, sugar. In UD 30s, 60s, 90s.
otc	**Docusate Sodium** (Roxane)	**Capsules:** 50 mg	In 100s, UD 100s.
otc	**Colace** (Mead Johnson)		In 30s, 60s, 250s, 1000s and UD 100s.
otc	**Docusate Sodium** (Various, eg, Geneva, Lederle, Major, Purepac, Rugby, Schein, URL)	**Capsules:** 100 mg	In 100s, 1000s and UD 100s.
otc	**Colace** (Mead Johnson)		In 30s, 60s, 250s, 1000s and UD 100s.
otc	**Disonate** (Lannett)		Amber. In 100s, 500s, 1000s.
otc	**DOK** (Major)		In 1000s.
otc	**DOS Softgel** (Goldline)		Red-orange. Oval. In 60s, 100s, 1000s.
otc	**D-S-S** (Warner Chilcott)		(WC 247). In 100s, 1000s and UD 100s.
otc	**Modane Soft** (Adria)		Sorbitol. In UD 30s.
otc	**Regulax SS** (Republic)		In 100s.
otc	**Disonate** (Lannett)	**Capsules:** 240 mg	Amber. In 100s, 500s and 1000s.
otc	**Docusate Sodium** (Various, eg, Geneva, Goldline, Major, Purepac, Rugby, Schein, URL, Vitarine)	**Capsules:** 250 mg	In 100s and 1000s.
otc	**Dioeze** (Century)		In 100s and 1000s.
otc	**DOK** (Major)		In 100s and 1000s.
otc	**DOS Softgels** (Goldline)		Red-orange. In 30s, 100s and 500s.
otc	**Regulax SS** (Republic)		In 100s.
otc	**Correctol Extra Gentle** (Schering-Plough)	**Capsules, soft gel:** 100 mg	Rose. In 30s.
otc	**Silace** (Silarx)	**Syrup:** 20 mg per 5 ml.	≤ 1% alcohol. In 473 ml.
otc	**Docusate Sodium** (Roxane)	**Syrup:** 50 mg per 15 ml	Saccharin, sucrose. In UD 15 and 30 ml (100s).

Fecal Softeners

DOCUSATE SODIUM (Dioctyl Sodium Sulfosuccinate; DSS)

otc	**Docusate Sodium** (Various, eg, Geneva, Lederle, Major, PBI, Schein)	**Syrup:** 60 mg per 15 ml	In pt and gal.
otc	**Diocto** Goldline, Moore, PBI, Rugby, URL)		In pt and gal.
otc	**Colace** (Mead Johnson)		≤ 1% alcohol, menthol, sucrose. In 240 & 480 ml.
otc	**Disonate** (Lannett)		In 240 ml, pt and gal.
otc	**DOK** (Major)		In pt and gal.
otc	**Diocto** (Various, eg, Goldline, Moore, Rugby)	**Liquid:** 150 mg per 15 ml	In pt and gal.
otc	**Colace** (Mead Johnson)		With calibrated dropper. In 30 and 480 ml.
otc	**Disonate** (Lannett)		In pt.
otc	**DOK** (Major)		In pt.
otc	**Doxinate** (Hoechst-Marion Roussel)	**Solution:** 50 mg per ml	5% alcohol. In 60 ml and gal.

DOCUSATE CALCIUM (Dioctyl Calcium Sulfosuccinate)

For complete prescribing information, refer to the Laxatives group monograph.

Administration and Dosage:

Adults: 240 mg daily until bowel movements are normal.

Children (≥ 6 years): 50 to 150 mg daily.

otc	**Surfak Liquigels** (Upjohn)	**Capsules:** 50 mg	≤ 1.3% alcohol, sorbitol. Orange. In 30s and 100s.
otc	**Docusate Calcium** (Various, eg, Dixon-Shane, Geneva Marsam, Major, Parmed, Rugby, Schein)	**Capsules:** 240 mg	In 100s, 250s, 500s, 1000s and UD 100s.
otc	**DC Softgels** (Goldline)		Red, oblong. In 100s and 500s.
otc	**Pro-Cal-Sof** (Vangard)		In 1000s, UD 100s, Metripak 640s.
otc	**Sulfalax Calcium** (Major)		In 500s.
otc	**Surfak Liquigels** (Upjohn)		≤ 3% alcohol, sorbitol. Red. In 7s, 30s, 100s, 500s and UD 100s.

DOCUSATE POTASSIUM (Dioctyl Potassium Sulfosuccinate)

For complete prescribing information, refer to the Laxatives group monograph.

Administration and Dosage:

Adults: 100 to 300 mg daily until bowel movements are normal.

Children (≥ 6 years): 100 mg at bedtime.

otc	**Dialose** (J & J-Merck)	**Tablets:** 100 mg	Lactose, sugar. In 36s.
otc	**Diocto-K** (Rugby)	**Tablets:** 100 mg	Pink. In 100s.
otc	**Kasof** (J & J-Merck)	**Capsules:** 240 mg	Sorbitol. Brown. In 30s and 60s.

Hyperosmolar Agents

GLYCERIN

For complete prescribing information, refer to the Laxatives group monograph.

Administration and Dosage:

Suppositories: Insert one suppository high in the rectum and retain 15 minutes; it need not melt to produce laxative action.

Rectal liquid: With gentle, steady pressure, insert stem with tip pointing towards navel. Squeeze unit until nearly all the liquid is expelled, then remove. A small amount of liquid will remain in unit.

otc	**Glycerin, USP** (Various, eg, Dixon-Shane, Goldline, Major, Moore, Purepac, Rugby, Schein, URL)	**Suppositories:** Glycerin and sodium stearate	**Adults:** In 10s, 12s, 25s, 50s and 100s.
			Pediatric: In 10s, 12s and 25s.
otc	**Sani-Supp** (G & W Labs)		**Adults:** In 10s, 25s and 50s.
			Pediatric: In 10s and 25s.
otc	**Fleet Babylax** (Fleet)	**Liquid:** 4 ml per applicator	In 6 applicators.

Enemas

MISCELLANEOUS ENEMAS

For complete prescribing information, refer to the Laxatives group monograph.

otc	**Fleet** (Fleet)	**Disposable Enema:** 7 g sodium phosphate and 19 g sodium biphosphate per 118 ml delivered dose (4.4 g sodium per dose) *Dose:* Adults – 118 ml. Children (≥ 2 years) – ½ the adult dose.	In squeeze bottles. **Pediatric:** In 67.5 ml. **Adult:** In 133 ml.
otc	**Fleet Bisacodyl** (Fleet)	**Disposable Enema:** 10 mg bisacodyl per 30 ml delivered dose *Dose:* Adults – 30 ml.	In 37 ml squeeze bottles.
otc	**Fleet Bisacodyl Prep** (Fleet)	**Enema:** 10 mg bisacodyl in 10 ml aqueous suspension per packet *Dose:* Cleansing enema – 1 packet in 1.5 L water. Barium enema – 1 packet into barium suspension.	In 36 packets.
otc	**Fleet Mineral Oil** (Fleet)	**Disposable Enema:** Mineral oil *Dose:* Adults – 118 ml. Children (> 2 years) – ½ adult dose.	In 133 ml plastic squeeze bottles.
otc	**Therevac-SB** (Jones Medical)	**Disposable Enema:** 283 mg docusate sodium in a base of soft soap, PEG 400 and glycerin per 3.9 g capsule *Dose:* 3.9 g.	In 30 disposable capsules per bottle.
otc	**Therevac-Plus** (Jones Medical)	**Disposable Enema:** 283 mg docusate sodium and 20 mg benzocaine in a base of soft soap, PEG 400 and glycerin per 3.9 g capsule *Dose:* 3.9 g.	In 50 disposable capsules per bottle.

BISACODYL TANNEX

For complete prescribing information, refer to the Laxatives group monograph.

Administration and Dosage:

Cleansing enema: 2.5 g (1 packet) in 1 L warm water.

Barium enema: 2.5 or 5 g in 1 L barium suspension.

Total dosage for one colonic examination should not exceed 7.5 g. Do not give > 10 g within a 72 hour period.

Do not administer to children < 10 years of age.

Rx	**Clysodrast** (Rhone-Poulenc Rorer)	**Powder:** 1.5 mg bisacodyl and 2.5 g tannic acid per packet	In 25s and 50s.

CO_2 RELEASING SUPPOSITORIES

For complete prescribing information, refer to the Laxatives group monograph.

otc	**Ceo-Two** (Beutlich)	**Suppositories:** Sodium bicarbonate and potassium bitartrate in a water soluble polyethylene glycol base Before inserting, moisten suppository with warm water.	In 10s.

Bowel Evacuants

POLYETHYLENE GLYCOL-ELECTROLYTE SOLUTION (PEG-ES)

For complete prescribing information, refer to the Laxatives group monograph.

Actions:

Pharmacology: Oral solution induces diarrhea (onset 30 to 60 min) which rapidly cleanses the bowel, usually within 4 hours. Polyethylene glycol 3350 (PEG 3350), a nonabsorbable solution, acts as an osmotic agent. By using sodium sulfate as the major sodium source, active sodium absorption is markedly reduced. The electrolyte concentration results in virtually no net absorption or secretion of ions. Large volumes may be given without significant changes in water or electrolyte balance.

Indications:

For bowel cleansing prior to GI examination.

Unlabeled uses: PEG electrolyte solutions are useful in the management of acute iron overdose in children. In children < 3 years old, 0.5 L/hour was successful.

Contraindications:

GI obstruction; gastric retention; bowel perforation; toxic colitis, megacolon or ileus.

Warnings:

Do not add flavorings or additional ingredients to solution before use.

Pregnancy: Category C. Safety not established. Use only when clearly needed and when the benefits outweigh the potential hazards to the fetus.

Children: Safety and efficacy for use in children have not been established.

Several studies in infants and children ranging in age from 3 weeks to 18 years showed that the use of PEG-electrolyte solutions are safe and effective in bowel evacuation. In healthy children, bowel preparation for surgery using these solutions generally required less time and volume (25 to 40 ml/kg/hour for 4 to 10 hours).

Precautions:

Barium enema: Patient prep may be less satisfactory with this solution; it may interfere with barium coating of colonic mucosa using double-contrast technique.

Regurgitation/Aspiration: Observe unconscious or semiconscious patients with impaired gag reflex and those who are otherwise prone to regurgitation or aspiration during use, especially if given via a nasogastric tube. If GI obstruction or perforation is suspected, rule out these contraindications before administration.

If a patient experiences severe bloating, distention or abdominal pain, slow or temporarily discontinue administration until symptoms abate.

Severe ulcerative colitis: Use with caution.

Drug Interactions:

Oral medication given within 1 hour of start of therapy may be flushed from the GI tract and not absorbed.

Adverse Reactions:

Nausea, abdominal fulness and bloating are the most common adverse reactions (occurring in up to 50% of patients). Abdominal cramps, vomiting and anal irritation occur less frequently. These adverse reactions are transient and subside rapidly. Isolated cases of urticaria, rhinorrhea and dermatitis have been reported which may represent allergic reactions.

Administration and Dosage:

The patient should fast approximately 3 to 4 hours prior to ingestion of the solution; solid foods should never be given < 2 hours before solution is administered.

One method is to schedule patients for midmorning exam, allowing 3 hours for drinking and 1 hour to complete bowel evacuation. Another method is to give the solution the evening before the exam, particularly if the patient is to have a barium enema. No foods except clear liquids are permitted after solution administration.

Adult dosage is 4 L orally of solution prior to GI exam. May be given via a nasogastric tube to patients unwilling or unable to drink the preparation. Drink 240 ml every 10 minutes until 4 L are consumed or until the rectal effluent is clear. Rapid drinking of each portion is preferred to drinking small amounts continuously. Nasogastric tube administration is at the rate of 20 to 30 ml/minutes (1.2 to 1.8 L/hour). The first bowel movement should occur in ≈ 1 hour.

Preparation of solution: Tap water may be used to reconstitute the solution. Shake container vigorously several times to ensure that the powder is completely dissolved.

After reconstitution to 4 L volume with water, the solution contains PEG 3350 17.6 mmol/L, sodium 125 mmol/L, sulfate 40 mmol/L (*Colyte* 80 mmol/L), chloride 35 mmol/L, bicarbonate 20 mmol/L and potassium 10 mmol/L (mmol/L = mEq/L).

Bowel Evacuants

POLYETHYLENE GLYCOL-ELECTROLYTE SOLUTION (PEG-ES)

Storage: Refrigerate reconstituted solution (chilling before administration improves palatability); use within 48 hours.

Rx	**Co-Lav** (Copley)	**Powder for solution:** 60 g PEG 3350, 1.46 g NaCl, 0.745 g KCl, 1.68 g sodium bicarb and 5.68 g sodium sulfate per L	In 4 L jug.
Rx	**Colovage** (Dynapharm)	**Powder for Oral Solution:** 146 mg NaCl, 168 mg sodium bicarb, 568 mg sodium sulfate anhydrous, 74.5 mg KCl, 6 g PEG 3350/100 ml.	Makes one gallon when reconstituted
Rx	**CoLyte** (Schwarz Pharma)	**Powder for Oral Solution: 1 gal:** 227.1 g PEG 3350, 21.5 g sodium sulfate, 6.36 g sodium bicarb, 5.53 g NaCl, 2.82 g KCl.	
		4 L: 240 g PEG 3350, 22.72 g sodium sulfate, 6.72 g sodium bicarb, 5.84 g NaCl, 2.98 g KCl.	
Rx	**Go-Evac** (Copley)	**Powder for solution:**59 g PEG 3350, 5.685 g sodium sulfate, 1.685 g sodium bicarb, 1.465 g sodium chloride and 0.743 g potassium chloride per L	In 4 L jug.
Rx	**GoLYTELY** (Braintree Labs)	**Powder for Oral Solution:** 236 g PEG 3350, 22.74 g sodium sulfate, 6.74 g sodium bicarb, 5.86 g NaCl, 2.97 g KCl.	In disposable container.
Rx	**NuLytely** (Braintree)	**Powder for Reconstitution:** 420 g PEG 3350, 5.72 g sodium bicarb, 11.2 g NaCl, 1.48 g KCl.	In 4 L disposable jugs.
Rx	**OCL** (Abbott)	**Oral Solution:** 146 mg NaCl, 168 mg sodium bicarb, 1.29 g sodium sulfate decahydrate, 75 mg KCl, 6 g PEG 3350, 30 mg polysorbate-80/100 ml.	In 1500 ml (3 pack).

MISCELLANEOUS BOWEL EVACUANTS

For complete prescribing information, refer to the Laxatives group monograph.

otc	**X-Prep Liquid** (Gray)	Senna extract, 7% alcohol, 50 g sugar. In 74 ml.
otc	**Dulcolax Bowel Prep Kit** (B-I)	4 Bisacodyl tablets (5 mg each). Yellow. Enteric coated.[1] 1 Bisacodyl suppository (10 mg).
otc	**Tridrate Bowel Evacuant Kit** (Lafayette)	300 ml magnesium citrate solution. 3 Bisacodyl tablets (5 mg each). 1 Bisacodyl suppository (10 mg).
otc sf	**Evac-Q-Kit** (Adria)	300 ml *Evac-Q-Mag*: Mg and K citrate, citric acid. Saccharin. Cherry flavor. Carbonated. 2 *Evac-Q-Tabs*: 130 mg phenolphthalein per tablet.[1] 2 *Evac-Q-Sert* suppositories: Sodium bicarbonate and potassium bitartrate in polyethylene glycol base.
otc sf	**Evac-Q-Kwik** (Adria)	300 ml *Evac-Q-Mag*: Mg and K citrate, citric acid. Saccharin. Cherry flavor. Carbonated. 2 *Evac-Q-Tabs*: 130 mg phenolphthalein per tablet.[1] 1 *Evac-Q-Kwik* suppository: 10 mg bisacodyl.
otc	**X-Prep Bowel Evacuant Kit-1** (Gray)	74 ml *X-Prep* liquid: Senna fruit, 50 g sugar, 7% alcohol. 2 *Senokot-S* tablets: Standardized senna concentrate and 50 mg docusate sodium per tablet, lactose. 1 *Rectolax* suppository: 10 mg bisacodyl.
otc	**X-Prep Bowel Evacuant Kit-2** (Gray)	74 ml *X-Prep* liquid: Senna fruit, 50 g sugar, 7% alcohol. 30 g *Citralax* granules: Effervescent Mg citrate/sulfate. 1 *Rectolax* suppository: 10 mg bisacodyl.
otc	**Fleet Prep Kit 1** (Fleet)	45 ml *Phospho-soda* (2.4 g sodium biphosphate and 0.9 g sodium phosphate per 5 ml). 4 Bisacodyl tablets (5 mg each). Enteric coated. 1 Bisacodyl suppository (10 mg).

Bowel Evacuants

MISCELLANEOUS BOWEL EVACUANTS

otc	**Fleet Prep Kit 2** (Fleet)	45 ml *Phospho-soda* (2.4 g sodium biphosphate and 0.9 g sodium phosphate per 5 ml). 4 Bisacodyl tablets (5 mg each). Enteric coated. 1 Bagenema: Enema unit w/9 ml liquid castile soap.
otc	**Fleet Prep Kit 3** (Fleet)	45 ml *Phospho-soda* (2.4 g sodium biphosphate and 0.9 g sodium phosphate per 5 ml). 4 Bisacodyl tablets (5 mg each). Enteric coated. 30 ml Bisacodyl enema (10 mg).
otc	**Fleet Prep Kit 4** (Fleet)	45 ml flavored castor oil emulsion. 4 Bisacodyl tablets (5 mg each). Enteric coated. 1 Bisacodyl suppository (10 mg).
otc	**Fleet Prep Kit 5** (Fleet)	45 ml flavored castor oil emulsion. 4 Bisacodyl tablets (5 mg each). Enteric coated. 1 Bagenema: Enema unit with 9 ml liquid castile soap.
otc	**Fleet Prep Kit 6** (Fleet)	45 ml flavored castor oil emulsion. 4 Bisacodyl tablets (5 mg each). Enteric coated. 30 ml Bisacodyl enema (10 mg).

[1] Contains lactose and sucrose. *sf* - Sugar free.

LACTULOSE

Actions:

Pharmacology: Lactulose, a synthetic disaccharide analog of lactose containing galactose and fructose, decreases blood ammonia concentrations and reduces the degree of portal-systemic encephalopathy.

The human GI tissue does not have an enzyme capable of hydrolysis of this disaccharide; as a result, oral doses pass to the colon virtually unchanged. After reaching the colon, lactulose is metabolized by bacteria (*Lactobacillus, Bacteroides, Escherichia coli* and *Streptococcus faecalis*) resulting in the formation of low molecular weight acids (lactic acid, formic acid, acetic acid) and carbon dioxide. These products produce an increased osmotic pressure and slightly acidify the colonic contents, resulting in an increase in stool water content and stool softening. Since the colonic contents are more acidic than the blood, ammonia can migrate from the blood into the colon. The acid colonic contents convert NH_3 to the ammonium ion $[NH_4]^+$, trapping it and preventing its absorption. The laxative action of the lactulose metabolites then expels the trapped ammonium ion from the colon.

Lactulose may also interfere with glutamine-dependent non-bacterial ammonia production in the intestinal wall.

Pharmacokinetics: Lactulose is poorly absorbed. When given orally, only small amounts reach the blood. Urinary excretion is ≤ 3% and is essentially complete within 24 hours. Lactulose does not exert its effect until it reaches the colon. Transit time through the colon may be slow; therefore, 24 to 48 hours may be required to produce a normal bowel movement.

Indications:

Chronulac, Constilac, Duphalac: Treatment of constipation.

Cephulac, Cholac, Enulose: Prevention and treatment of portal-systemic encephalopathy, including hepatic pre-coma and coma. Lactulose reduces blood ammonia levels by 25% to 50%; this generally parallels improved mental state and EEG patterns.

Clinical response has been observed in about 75% of patients. An increase in protein tolerance is also frequent. In chronic portal-systemic encephalopathy, lactulose has been given for > 2 years in controlled studies.

Contraindications:

Patients who require a low galactose diet.

Warnings:

Electrocautery procedures: A theoretical hazard may exist for patients being treated with lactulose who may undergo electrocautery procedures during proctoscopy or colonoscopy. Accumulation of H_2 gas in significant concentration in the presence of an electrical spark may result in an explosion. Although this complication has not been reported with lactulose, patients should have a thorough bowel cleansing with a nonfermentable solution. Insufflation of CO_2 as an additional safeguard may be pursued, but is considered a redundant measure.

Pregnancy: Category B. Safety of lactulose during pregnancy and its effect on fetus or mother have not been evaluated in humans. Use only when clearly needed and when potential benefits outweigh potential hazards to the mother and fetus.

Lactation: It is not known whether lactulose is excreted in breast milk. Exercise caution when administering lactulose to a nursing mother.

Children: Safety and efficacy for use in children have not been established. Infants receiving lactulose may develop hyponatremia and dehydration.

Precautions:

Monitoring: In the overall management of portal-systemic encephalopathy, there is serious underlying liver disease with complications such as electrolyte disturbance (eg, hypokalemia and hypernatremia) which may require other specific therapy. Elderly, debilitated patients who receive lactulose for > 6 months should have serum electrolytes (potassium, chloride) and carbon dioxide measured periodically.

Diabetics: Lactulose syrup contains galactose (< 2.2 g/15 ml) and lactose (< 1.2 g/15 ml). Use with caution in these individuals.

Concomitant laxative use: Do not use other laxatives, especially during the initial phase of therapy for portal-systemic encephalopathy; the resulting loose stools may falsely suggest adequate lactulose dosage.

Drug Interactions:

Neomycin and other anti-infectives: Reports conflict about concomitant use of lactulose syrup. The elimination of certain colonic bacteria may interfere with the desired degradation of lactulose and prevent the acidification of colonic contents. Monitor the patient if concomitant oral anti-infectives are given.

LACTULOSE

Antacids: Nonabsorbable antacids given concurrently with lactulose may inhibit the desired lactulose-induced drop in colonic pH.

Adverse Reactions:

Gaseous distention with flatulence, belching, abdominal discomfort such as cramping (20%). Excessive dosage can lead to diarrhea. Nausea and vomiting have occurred.

Overdosage:

There have been no reports of accidental overdose. It is expected that diarrhea and abdominal cramps would be the major symptoms. Discontinue the medication.

Patient Information:

May be mixed with fruit juice, water or milk to increase palatability.

May cause belching, flatulence or abdominal cramps; notify physician if these effects become bothersome or if diarrhea occurs.

Do not take other laxatives while on lactulose therapy.

In the event that an unusual diarrheal condition occurs, contact your physician.

Administration and Dosage:

Chronulac, Constilac, Duphalac:

Treatment of constipation – 15 to 30 ml (10 to 20 g lactulose) daily, increased to 60 ml/day, if necessary.

Cephulac, Cholac, Enulose: Prevent and treat portal-systemic encephalopathy:

Oral –

Adults: 30 to 45 ml, tid or qid. Adjust dosage every day or two to produce 2 or 3 soft stools daily. Hourly doses of 30 to 45 ml may be used to induce rapid laxation in the initial phase of therapy. When the laxative effect has been achieved, reduce dosage to recommended daily dose. Improvement may occur within 24 hours, but may not begin before 48 hours or later. Continuous long-term therapy is indicated to lessen severity and prevent recurrence of portal-systemic encephalopathy.

LACTULOSE

Children: There is little information on use in children and adolescents. The goal is to produce 2 or 3 soft stools daily. Recommended initial daily oral dose in infants is 2.5 to 10 ml in divided doses. For older children and adolescents, the total daily dose is 40 to 90 ml. If the initial dose causes diarrhea, reduce immediately. If diarrhea persists, discontinue use.

Rectal – Administer to adults during impending coma or coma stage of portal-systemic encephalopathy when the danger of aspiration exists or when endoscopic or intubation procedures interfere with oral administration. The goal of treatment is reversal of the coma stage so the patient can take oral medication. Reversal of coma may occur within 2 hours of the first enema. Start recommended oral doses before enema is stopped entirely.

Lactulose may be given as a retention enema via a rectal balloon catheter. Do not use cleansing enemas containing soap suds or other alkaline agents.

Mix 300 ml lactulose with 700 ml water or physiologic saline and retain for 30 to 60 minutes. The enema may be repeated every 4 to 6 hours. If the enema is inadvertently evacuated too promptly, it may be repeated immediately.

May be more palatable when mixed with fruit juice, water or milk.

Storage: Store below 86°F (30°C); do not freeze.

Rx	**Cephulac** (Hoechst Marion Roussel)	**Syrup**: 10 g lactulose per 15 ml. (< 2.2 g galactose, < 1.2 g lactose and ≤ 1.2 g of other sugars).	In 480 ml, 1.9 L, UD 30 ml.
Rx	**Cholac** (Alra)		In 240, 480 and 960 ml, 1.9 L, gal and UD 30 ml.
Rx	**Chronulac** (Hoechst Marion Roussel)		In 240, 960 ml, UD 30 ml.
Rx	**Constilac** (Alra)		In 240, 480 and 960 ml, 1.9 L, gal and UD 30 ml.
Rx	**Constulose** (Barre-National)		In 237, 473 and 946 ml and 1.89 L.
Rx	**Duphalac** (Solvay Pharm.)		In 240, 480 and 960 ml and UD 30 ml.
Rx	**Enulose** (Barre-National)		In pt and 1.89 L.
Rx	**Lactulose** (Various, eg, Moore, Schiapparelli Searle)		In 240 and 960 ml and UD 30 ml.
Rx	**Evalose** (Copley)	**Syrup**: 10 g lactulose/15 ml (< 1.6 g galactose, < 1.2 g lactose and ≤ 1.2 g other sugars).	Cola flavor. In 240, 960 ml.
Rx	**Heptalac** (Copley)		Cola flavor. In 473, 1920 ml.

LAXATIVE COMBINATIONS, CAPSULES AND TABLETS

Refer to the general discussion of these products beginning in the Laxatives group monograph.

Ingredients:

In addition to the laxatives listed on the previous pages, these combinations include:

DEHYDROCHOLIC ACID, used as a choleretic (see individual monograph).

CASANTHRANOL is a stimulant laxative.

Administration and Dosage:

1 or 2 at bedtime with a full glass of water.

		Docusate (mg)	Senna Concentrate (mg)	Phenolphthalein (mg)	Casanthranol (mg)	Cascara Sagrada (mg)	Sodium Carboxymethylcellulose (mg)	Other Content and How Supplied
otc	**Gentlax S Tablets** (Blair)	50[1]	8.6[2]					Lactose. In 60s.
otc	**Senokot-S Tablets** (Purdue Frederick)	50[1]	187					Lactose. In 30s, 60s, 1000s and UD 100s.
otc	**Doxidan Capsules** (Upjohn)	60[3]		65				Sorbitol. Maroon. In 10s, 30s, 100s, 1000s and UD 100s.
otc	**Docucal-P Softgels (Capsules)** (Parmed)							In 100s and 1000s.
otc	**Ex-Lax, Extra Gentle Pills (Tablets)** (Sandoz Consumer)	75[1]		65				Sucose. Pink. In 24s.
otc	**Phillips' Laxative Gelcaps (Capsules)** (Sterling Health)	83[1]		90				Sorbitol. (Phillips). In 30s.
otc	**Colax Tablets** (Rugby)	100[1]		65				In 30s.
otc	**Correctol Tablets** (Schering-Plough)							Sugar. In 15s, 30s, 60s and 90s.
otc	**Dialose Plus Tablets** (J & J-Merck)							Sugar. In 100s.
otc	**Dialose Plus Capsules** (J & J-Merck)							In 36s, 100s and 500s.
otc	**Disolan Capsules** (Lannett)							Blue and yellow. In 100s, 500s and 1000s.
otc	**Feen-a-mint Pills (Tablets)** (Schering-Plough)							Sugar. In 15s, 30s and 60s.
otc	**Femilax Tablets** (G & W Labs)							In 30s, 60s and 90s.
otc	**Modane Plus Tablets** (Adria)							Sucrose. In 10s, 30s and 100s.
otc	**Unilax Capsules** (B.F. Ascher)	230[1]		130				Sorbitol. In 15s and 60s.

LAXATIVE COMBINATIONS, CAPSULES AND TABLETS

		Docusate (mg)	Senna Concentrate (mg)	Phenolphthalein (mg)	Casanthranol (mg)	Cascara Sagrada (mg)	Sodium Carboxymethylcellulose (mg)	Other Content and How Supplied
otc	**Docusate w/ Casanthranol Caps** (Various, eg, Geneva, Major, Schein)	100[1]			30			In 100s, 1000s and UD 100s.
otc	**Disanthrol Capsules** (Lannett)							In 100s and 1000s.
otc	**D-S-S plus Capsules** (Warner-Chilcott)							Maroon. In 100s, 1000s and UD 100s.
otc	**Genasoft Plus Softgels (Capsules)** (Goldline)							Maroon. In 60s.
otc	**Peri-Colace Capsules** (Mead Johnson)							Maroon. In 30s, 60s, 250s, 1000s and UD 100s.
otc	**Peri-Dos Softgels (Capsules)** (Goldline)							Maroon. In 100s and 1000s.
otc	**Pro-Sof Plus Capsules** (Vangard)							In 100s, 1000s and UD 32s and 100s.
otc	**Regulace Capsules** (Republic)							In 100s.
otc	**Docusate Potassium w/Casanthranol Capsules** (Various, eg, UDL, URL)	100[4]			30			In 100s, 1000s and UD 100s.
otc	**Diocto-K Plus Capsules** (Rugby)							Sorbitol. Yellow. In 100s and 1000s.
otc	**Dioctolose Plus Capsules** (Goldline)							Yellow. In 100s and 1000s.
otc	**DSMC Plus Capsules** (Geneva)							Yellow. In 100s.
otc	**Disoplex Capsules** (Lannett)	100[1]					400	Pink. In 100s, 500s and 1000s.
otc	**Disolan Forte Capsules** (Lannett)	100[1]			30		400	Yellow. In 100s, 500s and 1000s.
otc *sf*	**Herbal Laxative Tablets** (Nature's Bounty)		125[5]			20[6]		5 mg buckthorn bark PDR. In 100s.
otc	**Veracolate Tablets** (Numark)			32.4		75[7]		0.05 min oleoresin capsicum. In 100s.
otc	**Nature's Remedy Tablets** (SK Beecham Consumer)					150		100 mg aloe, lactose. In 12s, 30s and 60s.

[1] As sodium.
[2] As sennosides.
[3] As calcium.
[4] As potassium.
[5] As senna leaves.
[6] As cascara sagrada bark.
[7] As extract.

LAXATIVE COMBINATIONS, LIQUIDS

Refer to the general discussion of these products beginning in the Laxatives group monograph.

Dose: Usual adult dose is 5 to 45 ml with a full glass of water at bedtime.

otc	**Diocto C** (Various, eg, Barre National, Moore, Rugby, URL)	**Syrup:** 60 mg docusate sodium and 30 mg casanthranol per 15 ml	In 240 ml, pt and gal.
otc	**Docusate Sodium w/Casanthranol** (Various, eg, Geneva, Major, Schein)		In pt and gal.
otc	**Peri-Colace** (Mead Johnson)		10% alcohol. Sorbitol, sucrose. In 240 and 480 ml.
otc sf	**Liqui-Doss** (Ferndale)	**Emulsion:** Mineral oil in an emulsifying base	Alcohol free. In pt.
otc sf	**Kondremul w/Phenolphthalein** (Fisons)	**Emulsion:** 55% mineral oil, 150 mg phenolphthalein per 15 ml w/Irish Moss	In pt.
otc sf	**Agoral** (Warner-Lambert)	**Emulsion:** 4.2 g mineral oil and 0.2 g phenolphthalein per 15 ml with agar, tragacanth, egg albumin, acacia, glycerin and saccharin	Plain, marshmallow and raspberry flavors. In 480 ml.
otc	**Haley's M-O** (Sterling Health)	**Liquid:** 900 mg magnesium hydroxide and 3.75 ml mineral oil per 15 ml	Saccharin. Regular or flavored. In 120, 360 and 780 ml.
otc	**Black-Draught** (Chattem)	**Syrup:** 90 mg per 15 ml casanthranol with senna extract, fluid rhubarb aromatic, methyl salicylate and menthol	5% alcohol. Tartrazine, sugar. In 150 ml.
otc	**Silace-C** (Silarx)	**Syrup:** 30 mg casanthranol, 60 mg docusate sodium per 15 ml	10% alcohol. In 473 ml.

sf - Sugar free.

LAXATIVE COMBINATIONS, POWDERS AND GRANULES

Refer to the general discussion of these products beginning in the Laxatives group monograph.

Dose: Usual adult dose is 1 or 2 rounded tsp, 1 to 3 times daily, with a full glass of water.

otc	**Syllamalt** (Wallace)	**Powder:** 4 g malt soup extract, 3 g psyllium seed husks and 13 calories/rounded tsp	In 300 g.
otc	**Perdiem** (Rhone-Poulenc Rorer)	**Granules:** 3.25 g psyllium, 0.74 g senna, 1.8 mg sodium, 35.5 mg potassium and 4 calories per rounded teaspoonful (6 g)	Dye free. Sucrose. In 100 and 250 g.

DIFENOXIN HCl WITH ATROPINE SULFATE

Actions:

Pharmacology: Difenoxin is an antidiarrheal agent chemically related to meperidine. Atropine sulfate is present to discourage deliberate overdosage.

Animal studies have shown that difenoxin manifests its antidiarrheal effect by slowing intestinal motility. The mechanism of action is by a local effect on the gastrointestinal wall.

Difenoxin is the principal active metabolite of diphenoxylate and is effective at one-fifth the dosage of diphenoxylate.

Pharmacokinetics: Difenoxin is rapidly and extensively absorbed orally. Mean peak plasma levels of 160 ng/ml occur within 40 to 60 minutes in most patients following a 2 mg dose. Plasma levels decline to less than 10% of their peak values within 24 hours and to less than 1% of their peak values within 72 hours. This decline parallels the appearance of difenoxin and its metabolites in the urine. Difenoxin is metabolized to an inactive hydroxylated metabolite. Both the drug and its metabolites are excreted, mainly as conjugates, in urine and feces.

Indications:

Adjunctive therapy in management of acute nonspecific diarrhea and acute exacerbations of chronic functional diarrhea.

Contraindications:

Diarrhea associated with organisms that penetrate the intestinal mucosa (eg, toxigenic *E coli, Salmonella* sp, *Shigella*;) and pseudomembranous colitis associated with broad-spectrum antibiotics. Antiperistaltic agents may prolong or worsen diarrhea.

Children under 2 years of age because of the decreased margin of safety of drugs in this class in younger age groups.

Hypersensitivity to difenoxin, atropine or any of the inactive ingredients; jaundice.

Warnings:

Difenoxin HCl with atropine sulfate is not innocuous; strictly adhere to dosage recommendations. It is not recommended for children under 2 years of age. Overdosage may result in severe respiratory depression and coma, possibly leading to permanent brain damage or death (see Overdosage).

Fluid and electrolyte balance: The use of this drug does not preclude the administration of appropriate fluid and electrolyte therapy. Dehydration, particularly in children, may further influence the variability of response and may predispose to delayed difenoxin intoxication. Drug-induced inhibition of peristalsis may result in fluid retention in the colon, and this may further aggravate dehydration and electrolyte imbalance. If severe dehydration or electrolyte imbalance is manifested, withhold the drug until appropriate corrective therapy has been initiated.

Ulcerative colitis: Agents which inhibit intestinal motility or delay intestinal transit time have induced toxic megacolon. Consequently, carefully observe patients with acute ulcerative colitis. Discontinue promptly if abdominal distention occurs or if other untoward symptoms develop.

Liver and kidney disease: Use with extreme caution in patients with advanced hepatorenal disease and in all patients with abnormal liver function tests since hepatic coma may be precipitated.

Atropine: A subtherapeutic dose of atropine has been added to difenoxin to discourage deliberate overdosage. A recommended dose is not likely to cause prominent anticholinergic side effects, but avoid in patients in whom anticholinergic drugs are contraindicated. Observe the warnings and precautions for use of anticholinergic agents. In children, signs of atropinism may occur even with recommended doses, particularly in patients with Down's Syndrome.

Pregnancy: Category C. Reproduction studies in rats and rabbits with doses up to 75 times the human therapeutic dose demonstrated no evidence of teratogenesis. Pregnant rats receiving oral doses 20 times the maximum human dose had an increase in delivery time as well as a significant increase in the percent of stillbirths. Neonatal survival in rats was also reduced with most deaths occurring within 4 days of delivery. There are no well controlled studies in pregnant women. Use during pregnancy only if the potential benefit justifies the potential risk to the fetus.

Lactation: Because of the potential for serious adverse reactions in nursing infants, decide whether to discontinue nursing or to discontinue the drug, taking into account the importance of the drug to the mother.

Children: Contraindicated in children under 2 years of age. Safety and efficacy in children below the age of 12 have not been established. See Overdosage section for information on hazards from accidental poisoning in children.

DIFENOXIN HCl WITH ATROPINE SULFATE

Precautions:

Drug abuse and dependence: Addiction to (dependence on) difenoxin is theoretically possible at high dosage. Therefore, do not exceed recommended dosage. Because of the structural and pharmacological similarities of difenoxin to drugs with definite addiction potential, administer with caution to patients receiving addicting drugs, to addiction-prone individuals, or to those whose histories suggest they may increase the dosage on their own initiative.

Drug Interactions:

Monoamine oxidase (MAO) inhibitors: Since the chemical structure of difenoxin is similar to meperidine, concurrent use with MAO inhibitors may, in theory, precipitate a hypertensive crisis.

Barbiturates, tranquilizers, narcotics and alcohol may be potentiated by coadministration of difenoxin. Closely monitor patients.

Adverse Reactions:

Anticholinergic: In view of the small amount of atropine present (0.025 mg/tablet), effects such as dryness of the skin and mucous membranes, flushing, hyperthermia, tachycardia and urinary retention are very unlikely to occur, except perhaps in children.

Many adverse effects reported during clinical investigation are difficult to distinguish from symptoms of diarrheal syndrome. However, the following events have occurred:

CNS: Dizziness, lightheadedness (5%); drowsiness (4%); headache (2.5%); tiredness, nervousness, insomnia, confusion (< 1%).

GI: Nausea (7%), vomiting, dry mouth (3%); epigastric distress, constipation (≤ 1%).

Ophthalmic: Burning eyes, blurred vision (infrequent).

Overdosage:

Symptoms: Initial signs may include dryness of the skin and mucous membranes, flushing, hyperthermia and tachycardia followed by lethargy or coma, hypotonic reflexes, nystagmus, pinpoint pupils and respiratory depression.

Treatment: Gastric lavage, establishment of a patent airway and, possibly, mechanically assisted respiration are advised. Refer to General Management of Acute Overdosage.

Naloxone may be used in the treatment of respiratory depression. When administered IV, the onset is generally apparent within 2 minutes. Naloxone may also be administered SC or IM providing a slightly less rapid onset but a more prolonged effect.

Since the duration of action of difenoxin is longer than that of naloxone, improvement of respiration following administration may be followed by recurrent respiratory depression. Continuous observation is necessary until the effect of difenoxin on respiration (which may persist for many hours) has passed. Supplemental IM naloxone doses may be used to produce a longer lasting effect. Treat all possible overdosages as serious; observe for at least 48 hours, preferably under continuous hospital care.

Although signs of overdosage and respiratory depression may not be evident soon after ingestion of difenoxin, respiratory depression may occur 12 to 30 hours later.

Patient Information:

Adhere strictly to recommended dosage schedules. Keep out of reach of children since accidental overdosage may result in severe, even fatal, respiratory depression.

Drowsiness or dizziness may occur. Exercise caution in activities requiring mental alertness, coordination or physical dexterity, eg, driving or operating dangerous machinery.

Administration and Dosage:

Adults: Recommended starting dose: 2 tablets, then 1 tablet after each loose stool; 1 tablet every 3 to 4 hours as needed. The total dosage during any 24 hour treatment period should not exceed 8 tablets. For diarrhea in which clinical improvement is not observed in 48 hours, continued administration is not recommended. For acute diarrhea and acute exacerbations of functional diarrhea, treatment beyond 48 hours is usually not necessary.

Children: Studies in children < 12 years old are inadequate to evaluate safety and efficacy. Contraindicated in children < 2 years old.

C-IV	**Motofen** (Carnrick)	**Tablets:** 1 mg difenoxin (as HCl) and 0.025 mg atropine sulfate	Dye free. (C 8674). White, scored. Five-sided. In 50s, 100s.

DIPHENOXYLATE HCl WITH ATROPINE SULFATE

Actions:

Pharmacology: Diphenoxylate, a constipating meperidine congener, lacks analgesic activity. High doses (40 to 60 mg) cause opioid activity, (eg, euphoria, suppression of morphine abstinence syndrome, physical dependence after chronic use).

Pharmacokinetics: Bioavailability of tablet vs liquid is ≈ 90%. Diphenoxylate is rapidly, extensively metabolized to diphenoxylic acid (difenoxine), the active major metabolite. Elimination half-life is ≈ 12 to 14 hrs. An average of 14% of drug and metabolites are excreted over 4 days in urine, 49% in feces. Urinary excretion of unmetabolized drug is < 1%; difenoxine plus its glucuronide conjugate constitutes ≈ 6%.

Indications:

Adjunctive therapy in the management of diarrhea.

Contraindications:

Children < 2 years old due to greater variability of response; hypersensitivity to diphenoxylate or atropine; obstructive jaundice; diarrhea associated with pseudomembranous enterocolitis or enterotoxin-producing bacteria (see Warnings).

Warnings:

Diarrhea: Diphenoxylate may prolong or aggravate diarrhea associated with organisms that penetrate intestinal mucosa (ie, toxigenic *Escherichia coli, Salmonella, Shigella*) or in pseudomembranous enterocolitis associated with broad-spectrum antibiotics. Do not use diphenoxylate in these conditions. In some patients with acute ulcerative colitis, diphenoxylate may induce toxic megacolon. Discontinue therapy if abdominal distention or other untoward symptoms develop.

Fluid/electrolyte balance: Dehydration, particularly in younger children, may influence variability of response and may predispose to delayed diphenoxylate intoxication. Inhibition of peristalsis may result in fluid retention in the intestine, which may further aggravate dehydration and electrolyte imbalance. If severe dehydration or electrolyte imbalance occurs, withhold the drug until initiating corrective therapy.

Hepatic function impairment: Use with extreme caution in patients with advanced hepatorenal disease or abnormal liver function; hepatic coma may be precipitated.

Pregnancy: Category C. There are no adequate and well controlled studies in pregnant women. Use in women of childbearing potential only when clearly needed and when the potential benefits outweigh the potential hazards to the fetus.

Lactation: Exercise caution when administering to a nursing mother. Diphenoxylic acid may be excreted in breast milk and atropine is excreted in breast milk.

Children: Use with caution; signs of atropinism may occur with recommended doses, particularly in Down's syndrome patients. Use with caution in young children due to variable response. Not recommended in children < 2 years old.

Precautions:

Drug abuse and dependence: In recommended doses, diphenoxylate has not produced addiction and is devoid of morphine-like subjective effects. At high doses, it exhibits codeine-like subjective effects; therefore, addiction to diphenoxylate is possible. A subtherapeutic dose of atropine may discourage deliberate abuse.

Hazardous tasks: May cause drowsiness or dizziness; observe caution while driving or performing other tasks requiring alertness, coordination or physical dexterity.

Drug Interactions:

Monoamine oxidase inhibitors: Since the chemical structure of diphenoxylate is similar to meperidine, concurrent use may precipitate hypertensive crises.

Barbiturates, tranquilizers and alcohol: Diphenoxylate may potentiate the depressant action. Closely observe the patient when these medications are used concomitantly.

Adverse Reactions:

Atropine effects: Dry skin and mucous membranes, flushing, hyperthermia, tachycardia, urinary retention, especially in children.

CNS: Dizziness; drowsiness; sedation; headache; malaise; lethargy; restlessness; euphoria; depression; numbness of extremities; confusion.

GI: Anorexia; nausea; vomiting; abdominal discomfort; paralytic ileus; toxic megacolon; pancreatitis.

Hypersensitivity: Pruritus; gum swelling; angioneurotic edema; urticaria; anaphylaxis.

Overdosage:

Symptoms: Initial signs include dry skin and mucous membranes, mydriasis, restlessness, flushing, hyperthermia and tachycardia followed by lethargy or coma, hypotonic reflexes, nystagmus and pinpoint pupils. Severe, even fatal, respiratory depression may result. Signs of overdosage and respiratory depression may not be evident soon after ingestion; respiratory depression may occur 12 to 30 hours later.

DIPHENOXYLATE HCl WITH ATROPINE SULFATE

Treatment: includes usual supportive measures. Refer to General Management of Acute Overdosage. Gastric lavage, induction of emesis, establishment of a patent airway, and, possibly, mechanically assisted respiration are advised. Use naloxone for respiratory depression (see individual monograph). Diphenoxylate's duration of action is longer than that of naloxone; improved respiration after administration may be followed by recurrent respiratory depression. Consequently, continuous observation for at least 48 hours is necessary until diphenoxylate's effect on respiration has passed. Activated charcoal may significantly decrease bioavailability of diphenoxylate. In non-comatose patients, 100 g activated charcoal slurry can be given immediately after induction of vomiting or gastric lavage.

Patient Information:

Do not exceed prescribed dosage. Avoid alcohol and other CNS depressants.

May cause drowsiness or dizziness; use caution while driving or performing other tasks requiring alertness, coordination or physical dexterity.

May cause dry mouth.

Notify physician if diarrhea persists or if fever, palpitations or abnormal distention occur.

Administration and Dosage:

Adults: Individualize dosage. Initial dose is 5 mg 4 times a day.

Children: See Warnings. In children 2 to 12 years of age, use liquid form only. The recommended initial dosage is 0.3 to 0.4 mg/kg daily, in 4 divided doses.

Diphenoxylate w/Atropine Pediatric Dosage

Age (years)	Approximate weight kg	Approximate weight lb	Dosage (ml) (4 times daily)
2	11-14	24-31	1.5-3
3	12-16	26-35	2-3
4	14-20	31-44	2-4
5	16-23	35-51	2.5-4.5
6-8	17-32	38-71	2.5-5
9-12	23-55	51-121	3.5-5

This pediatric schedule is the best approximation of an average dose recommendation which may be adjusted downwards according to the overall nutritional status and degree of dehydration encountered in the sick child.

Reduce dosage as soon as initial control of symptoms is achieved. Maintenance dosage may be as low as ¼ of the initial daily dosage. Do not exceed recommended dosage. Clinical improvement of acute diarrhea is usually observed within 48 hours. If clinical improvement of chronic diarrhea is not seen within 10 days after a maximum daily dose of 20 mg, symptoms are unlikely to be controlled by further use.

c-v	**Diphenoxylate HCl w/Atropine Sulfate** (Various, eg, Halsey, Major, Mylan, Purepac, Rugby, Schein)	**Tablets:** 2.5 mg diphenoxylate HCl and 0.025 mg atropine sulfate	In 100s, 500s, 1000s, 2500s and UD 100s.
c-v	**Logen** (Goldline)		White. In 100s, 500s & 1000s.
c-v	**Lomotil** (Searle)		Sorbitol, sucrose. (Searle 61). White. In 100s, 500s, 1000s, 2500s, UD 100s.
c-v	**Lonox** (Geneva)		White. In 100s, 500s, 1000s & UD 100s.
c-v	**Diphenoxylate HCl w/ Atropine Sulfate** (Various, eg, Goldline, Major, Roxane, Rugby)	**Liquid:** 2.5 mg diphenoxylate HCl and 0.025 mg atropine sulfate per 5 ml	In 60 ml, UD 4 and 10 ml.
c-v	**Lomanate** (Various, eg, Barre-National, CMC)		In 60 ml.
c-v	**Lomotil** (Searle)		15% alcohol. Sorbitol. Cherry flavor. In 60 ml w/dropper.

LOPERAMIDE HCl

Actions:

Pharmacology: Loperamide slows intestinal motility and affects water and electrolyte movement through the bowel. It inhibits peristalsis by a direct effect on the circular and longitudinal muscles of the intestinal wall. It reduces daily fecal volume, increases viscosity and bulk density and diminishes the loss of fluid and electrolytes. Tolerance to the antidiarrheal effect has not been observed.

In morphine-dependent monkeys, loperamide at higher than recommended doses prevented signs of morphine withdrawal. However, in humans, opiate-like effects have not been demonstrated after > 2 years of therapeutic use of loperamide.

Pharmacokinetics:

Absorption/Distribution – Loperamide is 40% absorbed after oral administration and does not penetrate well into the brain. Peak plasma levels occur approximately 5 hours after capsule administration, 2.5 hours after liquid administration and are similar for both formulations.

Metabolism/Excretion – The apparent elimination half-life is 10.8 hrs (range, 9.1 to 14.4 hrs). Of a 4 mg oral dose, 25% is excreted unchanged in the feces, and 1.3% is excreted in the urine as free drug and glucuronic acid conjugate within 3 days.

Indications:

Rx: Control and symptomatic relief of acute nonspecific diarrhea and of chronic diarrhea associated with inflammatory bowel disease.

For reducing the volume of discharge from ileostomies.

OTC: Control of symptoms of diarrhea, including Traveler's Diarrhea.

Unlabeled uses: In one study, the combination of loperamide (4 mg loading dose, 2 mg after each loose stool) plus trimethoprim-sulfamethoxazole for 3 days resulted in more rapid relief from traveler's diarrhea than either agent alone.

Contraindications:

Hypersensitivity to the drug and in patients who must avoid constipation.

OTC use: Bloody diarrhea; body temperature > 101°F.

Warnings:

Diarrhea: Do not use loperamide in acute diarrhea associated with organisms that penetrate the intestinal mucosa (enteroinvasive *Escherichia coli*, Salmonella and *Shigella*) or in pseudomembranous colitis associated with broad-spectrum antibiotics.

Acute ulcerative colitis: In some patients with acute ulcerative colitis, agents which inhibit intestinal motility or delay intestinal transit time may induce toxic megacolon. Discontinue therapy promptly if abdominal distention occurs or if other untoward symptoms develop in patients with acute ulcerative colitis.

Fluid/electrolyte depletion may occur in patients who have diarrhea. Loperamide use does not preclude administration of appropriate fluid and electrolyte therapy.

Pregnancy: Category B. There are no adequate and well controlled studies in pregnant women. Safety for use during pregnancy is not established. Use only when clearly needed and when potential benefits outweigh potential hazards to fetus.

Lactation: It is not known whether loperamide is excreted in breast milk. Safety for use in the nursing mother has not been established.

Children: Not recommended for use in children < 2 years old. Use special caution in young children because of the greater variability of response in this age group. Dehydration may further influence variability of response. Dosage has not been established for children in treatment of chronic diarrhea.

Precautions:

Acute diarrhea: If clinical improvement is not observed in 48 hours, discontinue use.

Hepatic dysfunction: Monitor patients with hepatic dysfunction closely for signs of CNS toxicity because of the apparent large first-pass biotransformation.

Drug abuse and dependence: Physical dependence in humans has not been observed.

Adverse Reactions:

Adverse experiences are generally minor and self-limiting; they are more commonly observed during the treatment of chronic diarrhea: Abdominal pain, distention or discomfort; constipation; dry mouth; nausea; vomiting; tiredness; drowsiness or dizziness; hypersensitivity reactions (including skin rash).

Overdosage:

Symptoms: Constipation, CNS depression and GI irritation. In clinical trials, nausea and vomiting occurred in an adult who took 60 mg within 24 hours. Ingestion of up to 60 mg loperamide in a single dose caused no significant adverse effects in healthy subjects. A 15-month-old, 8 kg child developed opioid toxicity (eg, pale skin, increased pulse rate, respiratory depression) following a 1 g dose of loperamide.

LOPERAMIDE HCl

Treatment: Activated charcoal administered promptly after loperamide ingestion can reduce the amount of drug absorbed into systemic circulation by up to ninefold.

Monitor for CNS depression for at least 24 hrs; if it occurs, give naloxone. Children may be more sensitive to CNS effects. If responsive to naloxone, monitor vital signs for symptom recurrence for at least 24 hrs after last naloxone dose. In view of loperamide's prolonged action and naloxone's short duration (1 to 3 hrs) (see individual monograph), monitor closely; repeat naloxone as indicated.

Patient Information:

May cause drowsiness or dizziness; patients should observe caution while driving or performing other tasks requiring alertness, coordination or physical dexterity.

May cause dry mouth. Drink plenty of clear fluids to help prevent dehydration, which may accompany diarrhea.

Notify physician if diarrhea does not stop after a few days or if abdominal pain or distention or fever occurs. Do not exceed prescribed dosage.

Administration and Dosage:

Rx: Acute diarrhea: Adults: 4 mg followed by 2 mg after each unformed stool. Do not exceed 16 mg/day. Clinical improvement is usually observed within 48 hours.

Children: First day dosage schedule

Loperamide Pediatric Dosage (First Day Schedule)

Age (years)	Weight (kg)	Doseform	Amount
2-5	13-20	liquid	1 mg tid
6-8	20-30	liquid or capsule	2 mg bid
8-12	> 30	liquid or capsule	2 mg tid

This dosage may be adjusted downwards according to the overall nutritional status and degree of dehydration encountered in the sick child.

Subsequent doses – Administer 1 mg/10 kg only after a loose stool. Total daily dosage should not exceed recommended dosages for the first day.

Chronic diarrhea:

Adults – 4 mg followed by 2 mg after each unformed stool until diarrhea is controlled; then, individualize dosage. When optimal daily dosage (average, 4 to 8 mg) has been established, administer as a single dose or in divided doses.

If clinical improvement is not observed after treatment with 16 mg/day for at least 10 days, symptoms are unlikely to be controlled by further use. Continue administration if diarrhea cannot be adequately controlled with diet or specific treatment.

Children: Dose has not been established.

LOPERAMIDE HCl

OTC: Acute diarrhea, including Traveler's Diarrhea:

Adults – 4 mg after first loose bowel movement followed by 2 mg after each subsequent loose bowel movement but no more than 8 mg/day for no more than 2 days.

Children – *9 to 11 years old (60 to 95 lbs),* 2 mg after first loose bowel movement followed by 1 mg after each subsequent loose bowel movement but no more than 6 mg/day for no more than 2 days; *6 to 8 years old (48 to 59 lbs),* 1 mg after first loose bowel movement followed by 1 mg after each subsequent loose bowel movement but no more than 4mg/day for no more than 2 days; *< 6 years old (up to 47 lbs),* consult physician (not for use in children < 6).

otc	**Imodium A-D Caplets** (McNeil-CPC)	**Tablets:** 2 mg	Lactose. In 6s and 12s.
otc	**Kaopectate II Caplets** (Upjohn)		Lactose. In 6s and 12s.
otc	**Maalox Anti-Diarrheal Caplets** (R-P Rorer)		Lactose. In 12s.
Rx	**Loperamide** (Various, eg, Mylan, Novopharm)	**Capsules:** 2 mg	In 100s, 500s and 1000s.
Rx	**Imodium** (Janssen)		Lactose. Two-tone green. In 100s, 500s, UD 100s.
otc	**Neo-Diaral** (Roberts)		In UD 8s and 250s.
otc	**Loperamide** (Various, eg, Barre-National, Roxane)	**Liquid:** 1 mg/5 ml	In 60 and 118 ml.
otc	**Imodium A-D** (McNeil-CPC)		5.25% alcohol. Cherry/licorice flavor. In 60, 90 and 120 ml.
otc	**Pepto Diarrhea Control** (Procter & Gamble)	**Liquid:** 1 mg/ml	5.25% alcohol, parabens. Cherry flavor. In 60 and 120 ml.

BISMUTH SUBSALICYLATE (BSS)

Actions:

Pharmacology: Bismuth subsalicylate (BSS) appears to have antisecretory and antimicrobial effects in vitro and may have some anti-inflammatory effects. The salicylate moiety provides the antisecretory effect, while the bismuth moiety may exert direct antimicrobial effects against bacterial and viral enteropathogens.

Pharmacokinetics: BSS undergoes chemical dissociation in the GI tract. Two BSS tablets yield 204 mg salicylate. Following ingestion, salicylate is absorbed, with > 90% recovered in the urine; plasma levels are similar to levels achieved after a comparable dose of aspirin. Absorption of bismuth is negligible.

Indications:

For indigestion without causing constipation; nausea; control of diarrhea, including Traveler's Diarrhea, within 24 hours. Also relieves abdominal cramps.

Unlabeled uses: Bismuth subsalicylate has been used to prevent Traveler's Diarrhea (enterotoxigenic *Escherichia coli*), in doses of 2.1 g/day (2 tablets qid before meals and at bedtime) for up to 3 weeks during brief periods of high risk. The suspension has also been used (4.2 g/day). BSS has been effective in up to 65% of patients.

BSS has also been used for chronic infantile diarrhea (2.5 ml every 4 hours for children 2 to 24 months old; 5 ml for those 24 to 48 months old; 10 ml for those 48 to 70 months old) and for symptoms of Norwalk virus-induced gastroenteritis.

Precautions:

Impaction may occur in infants and debilitated patients.

Radiologic examinations: May interfere with radiologic examinations of GI tract. Bismuth is radiopaque.

Drug Interactions:

Bismuth Subsalicylate (BSS) Drug Interactions

Precipitant drug	Object drug*		Description
BSS	Aspirin	⬆	BSS contains salicylate. If taken with aspirin and ringing of the ears occurs, discontinue use.
BSS	Tetracyclines	⬇	Bismuth may decrease GI absorption and bioavailability of tetracyclines, reducing their efficacy.

* ⬆ = Object drug increased ⬇ = Object drug decreased

Patient Information:

Shake liquid well before using. Chew tablets or allow to dissolve in mouth.

Stool may temporarily appear gray-black.

If diarrhea is accompanied by high fever or continues for > 2 days, consult physician.

Administration and Dosage:

Adults: 2 tablets or 30 ml.

Children: 9 to 12 years – 1 tablet or 15 ml.
6 to 9 years – ⅔ tablet or 10 ml.
3 to 6 years – ⅓ tablet or 5 ml.
< 3 years – Consult physician.

Repeat dosage every 30 min to 1 hour, as needed, up to 8 doses in 24 hrs.

otc	**Bismatrol** (Major)	**Tablets, chewable:** 262 mg	Saccharin. In 240 ml.
otc sf	**Pepto-Bismol** (Procter & Gamble)		< 2 mg sodium/tablet. Saccharin, mannitol. (Pepto-Bismol). Pink. Original and cherry flavors. In 30s, 42s (cherry). In 24s, 42s (original).
otc sf	**Pepto-Bismol** (Procter & Gamble)	**Caplets:** 262 mg (99 mg salicylate)	< 2 mg sodium. In 24s and 40s.
otc	**Pink Bismuth** (Various, eg, Goldline)	**Liquid:** 262 mg/15 ml	In 240 ml.
otc sf	**Pepto-Bismol** (Procter & Gamble)		5 mg sodium/15 ml. Saccharin. In 120, 240, 360 & 480 ml.
otc	**Bismatrol Extra Strength** (Major)	**Liquid:** 524 mg/15 ml	In 240 ml.
otc sf	**Pepto-Bismol Max Strength** (P & G)		< 5 mg sodium/15 ml. Saccharin. In 120, 240 and 360 ml.

ANTIDIARRHEAL COMBINATION PRODUCTS

Indications:

For the symptomatic treatment of diarrhea by reducing intestinal motility or adsorbing fluid.

Warnings:

Diarrhea from other causes: Do not use antiperistaltic agents for diarrhea associated with pseudomembranous enterocolitis or in diarrhea caused by toxigenic bacteria.

Salicylate absorption may occur from bismuth subsalicylate; therefore, observe caution in patients with bleeding disorders or salicylate sensitivity and in children.

Ingredients: The use of the ingredients in combination in the following products as nonspecific antidiarrheal agents has, to a large extent, been empiric. Adequate controlled clinical studies demonstrating the efficacy of these antidiarrheal combinations are lacking. The FDA has determined that the following ingredients are not generally recognized as safe and effective and are misbranded when present in otc antidiarrheal preparations: Aluminum hydroxide, atropine sulfate, calcium carbonate, carboxymethylcellulose, glycine, homatropine methylbromide, hyoscyamine sulfate, *Lactobacillus acidophilus* and *bulgaricus*, opium (powdered and tincture), paregoric, phenyl salicylate, scopolamine hydrobromide and zinc phenolsulfonate.

In 1986, in the tentative final monograph for these agents, the FDA considered attapulgite a Category I agent (safe and effective) and placed kaolin and pectin in Category III (insufficient data to permit classification). Recently, however, an FDA advisory committee recommended that the FDA reverse the classifications, making attapulgite Category III and kaolin and pectin Category I. Further studies are pending. A final monograph is expected in late 1994.

ACTIVATED ATTAPULGITE, KAOLIN and *PECTIN* are used for their adsorbent and protectant actions.

BISMUTH SALTS have antacid and adsorbent properties.

otc	**Kao-Spen** (Century)	**Suspension:** 5.2 g kaolin, 260 mg pectin/30 ml *Dose:* 60 to 120 ml after each bowel movement	Peppermint flavor. In 120 ml, pt and gal.
otc	**Kaolin w/Pectin** (Various, eg, Roxane, Wyeth-Ayerst)	**Suspension:** 90 g kaolin, 2 g pectin/30 ml *Dose:* After each bowel movement *Adults* - 60 to 120 ml/dose *Children - 6 to 12 years:* 30 to 60 ml/dose *3 to 6 years:* 15 to 30 ml/dose	In 180 ml, pt and UD 30 ml.
otc	**Kapectolin** (Various, eg, Goldline, Major)		In 360 ml.
otc	**Kaopectate Advanced Formula** (Upjohn)	**Liquid:** 750 mg attapulgite per 15 ml.	Alcohol free. Methylparaben, sucrose. In regular and peppermint flavors. In 354 ml.
otc	**Parepectolin** (Rhone-Poulenc Rorer)	**Concentrated liquid:** 600 mg attapulgite/15 ml *Dose:* After each bowel movement up to 7 doses/day *Adults* – 30 ml/dose *Children - 6 to 12 years:* 15 ml/dose *3 to < 6 years:* 7.5 ml/dose	Sucrose. In 240 ml.
otc	**K-Pek** (Rugby)	**Suspension:** 600 mg attapulgite/15 ml *Dose:* After each bowel movement up to 7 doses/day *Adults* – 30 ml *Children - 6 to < 12 years:* 15 ml/dose *3 to < 6 years:* 7.5 ml/dose	Sucrose. Regular flavor in 237 ml, pt and gal. Peppermint flavor in 237 ml.
otc	**K-C** (Century)	**Suspension:** 5.2 g kaolin, 260 mg pectin, 260 mg bismuth subcarbonate/30 ml *Dose:* 10 to 20 ml every 6 hours	Peppermint flavor. In 120 ml, pt and gal.

ANTIDIARRHEAL COMBINATION PRODUCTS

otc	**Kaodene Non-Narcotic** (Pfeiffer)	**Liquid:** 3.9 g kaolin, 194.4 mg pectin/30 ml, bismuth subsalicylate *Dose:* 1 to 3 doses/day or after each loose stool *Adults* – 45 ml/dose *Children - 6 to 12 years:* 22.5 ml/dose *3 to 6 years:* 15 ml/dose	Alcohol free. Sucrose. In 120 ml.
otc	**Children's Kaopectate** (Upjohn)	**Liquid:** 600 mg attapulgite/15 ml *Dose:* After each bowel movement up to 7 doses/day *Adults* – 30 ml/dose *Children – 6 to < 12 years:* 15 ml/dose *3 to < 6 years:* 7.5 ml/dose	Alcohol free. Sucrose. Cherry flavor. In 180 ml.
otc	**Donnagel** (Wyeth-Ayerst)	**Tablets, chewable:** 600 mg attapulgite *Dose:* After each bowel movement up to 7 doses/day *Adults* – 2/dose *Children - 6 to 11 years:* 1/dose *3 to 5 years:* ½ tab/dose	Saccharin, sorbitol. (AHR Donnagel). Green with darker green specks. Beveled. In 18s.
		Liquid: 600 mg attapulgite/15 ml *Dose:* After each bowel movement up to 7 doses/day *Adults* - 30 ml/dose *Children – 6 to 11 years:* 15 ml/dose *3 to 5 years:* 7.5 ml/dose	1.4% alcohol, saccharin, sorbitol. In 120 and 240 ml.
otc	**Rheaban Maximum Strength** (Pfizer)	**Caplets:** 750 mg activated attapulgite *Dose:* After each bowel movement up to 6 doses/day *Adults* – 2/dose *Children – 6 to 12 years* – 1/dose	Sucrose. White. In 12s.
otc	**Diasorb** (Columbia)	**Tablets:** 750 mg activated attapulgite *Dose:* After each bowel movement up to 3 doses/day *Adults* – 4/dose *Children – 6 to 12 years:* 2/dose *3 to 6 years:* 1/dose	Sorbitol. In 24s.
		Liquid: 750 mg activated attapulgite/5 ml *Dose:* After each bowel movement up to 3 doses/day *Adults* – 20 ml/dose *Children – 6 to 12 years:* 10 ml/dose *3 to 6 years:* 5 ml/dose	Sugar free. Sorbitol, saccharin. Cola flavor. In 120 ml.
otc	**Kaopectate Maximum Strength** (Upjohn)	**Caplets:** 750 mg attapulgite *Dose:* After each bowel movement up to 6 doses/day *Adults* - 2/dose *Children - 6 to 12 years:* 1/dose	Sucrose. In 12s and 20s.

MESALAMINE (5-aminosalicylic acid, 5–ASA)

Actions:

Pharmacology: Sulfasalazine is split by bacterial action in the colon into sulfapyridine (SP) and mesalamine (5–ASA). It is thought that the mesalamine component is therapeutically active in ulcerative colitis. The usual oral dose of sulfasalazine for active ulcerative colitis in adults is 3 to 4 g per day in divided doses, which provides 1.6 g free mesalamine to the colon. Each suspension enema delivers up to 4 g mesalamine to the left side of the colon; each suppository delivers 500 mg to the rectum.

The mechanism of action of mesalamine (and sulfasalazine) is unknown, but appears to be topical rather than systemic. Mucosal production of arachidonic acid (AA) metabolites, both through cyclooxygenase pathways (ie, prostanoids) and through lipoxygenase pathways (ie, leukotrienes [LTs] and hydroxyeicosatetraenoic acids [HETEs]) is increased in patients with chronic inflammatory bowel disease, and it is possible that mesalamine diminishes inflammation by blocking cyclooxygenase and inhibiting prostaglandin (PG) production in the colon.

Pharmacokinetics:

Absorption/Distribution –

Rectal: Mesalamine administered rectally as a suspension enema is poorly absorbed from the colon and is excreted principally in the feces during subsequent bowel movements. The extent of absorption is dependent upon the retention time of the drug product, and there is considerable individual variation. At steady state, approximately 10% to 30% of the daily 4 g dose can be recovered in cumulative 24 hour urine collections. Other than the kidneys, the organ distribution and other bioavailability characteristics of absorbed mesalamine are not known. The compound undergoes acetylation, but whether this process takes place at colonic or systemic sites has not been elucidated.

Oral:

Tablets – Mesalamine tablets are coated with an acrylic-based resin that delays release of mesalamine until it reaches the terminal ileum and beyond. Approximately 28% is absorbed after oral ingestion, leaving the remainder available for topical action and excretion in the feces. Absorption is similar with or without food. Mesalamine from oral mesalamine tablets appears to be more extensively absorbed than that released from sulfasalazine. Maximum plasma levels of mesalamine and N-acetyl-5-ASA following multiple doses are about 1.5 to 2 times higher than those following an equivalent dose of sulfasalazine; combined parent drug and metabolite areas under the concentration-time curve and urine drug dose recoveries are also about 1.3 to 1.5 times higher. The time to reach maximum plasma concentration for mesalamine and its metabolite is usually delayed (due to the delayed release formulation) and ranges from 4 to 12 hours.

Capsules – Mesalamine capsules are ethylcellulose-coated, controlled release formulations designed to release therapeutic quantities of the drug throughout the GI tract; 20% to 30% of mesalamine is absorbed. In contrast, when mesalamine is administered orally as an unformulated 1 g aqueous suspension, mesalamine is approximately 80% absorbed. Plasma mesalamine concentration peaked at approximately 1 mcg/ml 3 hours after administration of a 1 g dose and declined in a biphasic manner. Mean terminal half-life was 42 minutes after IV administration. N-acetyl-5–ASA peaked at approximately 3 hours at 1.8 mcg/ml, and its concentration followed a biphasic decline.

Metabolism/Excretion –

Rectal: Whatever the metabolic site, most absorbed mesalamine is excreted in urine as the N-acetyl–5–ASA metabolite. Patients demonstrated plasma levels of 2 mcg/ml 10 to 12 hours after administration; about 66% of this was the N-acetyl metabolite. While the elimination half-life of mesalamine is short (0.5 to 1.5 hr), the acetylated metabolite exhibits a half-life of 5 to 10 hours. In addition, steady-state plasma levels demonstrated a lack of accumulation of either free or metabolized drug during repeated daily administrations.

Oral:

Tablets – Following oral administration, the absorbed mesalamine is rapidly acetylated in the gut mucosal wall and by the liver. It is excreted mainly by the kidneys as N-acetyl-5-ASA. The half-lives of elimination for mesalamine and the metabolite are usually about 12 hours, but are variable ranging from 2 to 15 hours. There is large intersubject variability in plasma concentrations of mesalamine and N-acetyl-5-ASA and in their elimination half-lives following use of the tablets.

Capsules – Elimination of free mesalamine and salicylates in feces increased proportionately with the dose. N-acetyl-5–ASA was the primary compound excreted in the urine (19% to 30%).

MESALAMINE (5-aminosalicylic acid, 5–ASA)

Indications:

Chronic inflammatory bowel disease:

Oral – Remission and treatment of mildly to moderately active ulcerative colitis.

Rectal – Treatment of active mild to moderate distal ulcerative colitis, proctosigmoiditis or proctitis.

Contraindications:

Hypersensitivity to mesalamine, salicylates or any component of the formulation.

Warnings:

Intolerance/Colitis exacerbation: Mesalamine has been implicated in the production of an acute intolerance syndrome or exacerbation of colitis (≈ 3% of patients) characterized by cramping, acute abdominal pain and bloody diarrhea, and occasionally fever, headache, malaise, pruritus, conjunctivitis and rash. Symptoms usually abate when mesalamine is discontinued. Re-evaluate the patient's history of sulfasalazine intolerance, if any. If a rechallenge is performed to validate the hypersensitivity, do it under close supervision and only if clearly needed, giving consideration to reduced dosage. One patient previously sensitive to sulfasalazine was rechallenged with 400 mg oral mesalamine; within 8 hours she experienced headache, fever, intensive abdominal colic and profuse diarrhea and was readmitted as an emergency. She responded poorly to steroids; 2 weeks later, a pancolectomy was required.

Pancolitis: While using mesalamine some patients have developed pancolitis. However, extension of upper disease boundary or flare-ups occurred less often in mesalamine patients than in placebo patients.

Hypersensitivity: In a clinical trial, most patients who were hypersensitive to sulfasalazine were able to take mesalamine enemas without evidence of any allergic reaction. Nevertheless, exercise caution when mesalamine is initially used in patients known to be allergic to sulfasalazine. Instruct these patients to discontinue therapy if signs of rash or fever become apparent.

Renal function impairment: Renal impairment, including minimal change nephropathy, and acute and chronic interstitial nephritis, has occurred. In animals, the kidney is the principal target organ for toxicity; at doses ≈ 15 to 20 times the recommended human dose, mesalamine causes renal papillary necrosis. Exercise caution when using mesalamine in patients with renal dysfunction or a history of renal disease. Evaluate renal function of all patients prior to therapy and periodically during therapy.

The possibility of increased absorption of mesalamine and concomitant renal tubular damage as noted in preclinical studies must be kept in mind. Carefully monitor patients who receive concurrent oral products which liberate mesalamine and those with preexisting renal disease with urinalysis, BUN and creatinine studies.

Pregnancy: Category B. There are no adequate and well controlled studies in pregnant women for either sulfasalazine or 5–ASA. Use during pregnancy only if clearly needed. Mesalamine is known to cross the placental barrier.

Lactation: Low concentrations of mesalamine and higher concentrations of N-acetyl-5-ASA have been detected in breast milk. Clinical significance has not been determined. However, exercise caution when administering to a nursing woman.

Children: Safety and efficacy for use in children have not been established.

Precautions:

Pericarditis has occurred rarely with mesalamine-containing products including sulfasalazine. Cases of pericarditis have also occurred as manifestations of inflammatory bowel disease. In cases reported with mesalamine rectal suspension, there have been positive rechallenges. In one of these cases, however, a second rechallenge with sulfasalazine was negative throughout a 2 month follow-up. Investigate chest pain or dyspnea in mesalamine-treated patients with this in mind. Discontinuation of the drug may be warranted in some patients, but rechallenge can be performed under careful clinical observation.

Sulfite sensitivity: Some of these products contain sulfites that may cause allergic-type reactions (including anaphylactic symptoms and life-threatening or less severe asthmatic episodes) in certain susceptible people. The overall prevalence of sulfite sensitivity in the general population is unknown and probably low. It is seen more frequently in asthmatic or atopic nonasthmatic people. Specific products containing sulfites are identified in the product listings.

Epinephrine is the preferred treatment for serious allergic or emergency situations even though epinephrine injection contains sodium or potassium metabisulfite. The alternatives to using epinephrine in a life-threatening situation may not be satisfactory. The presence of a sulfite(s) in epinephrine injection should not deter the administration of the drug for treatment of serious allergic or other emergency situations.

MESALAMINE (5-aminosalicylic acid, 5–ASA)

Adverse Reactions:

Mesalamine is usually well tolerated. Most adverse effects have been mild and transient.

Mesalamine Adverse Reactions (%)[1]

Adverse reaction	Oral		Rectal	
	Tablets (n = 152)	Capsules (n = 451)	Suppository (n = 168)	Suspension (n = 815)
GI				
Abdominal pain/cramps/discomfort	18	1.1	3	8.1
Bloating	—	—	—	1.5
Colitis exacerbation	3	0.4	1.2	
Constipation	5	< 1	—	< 1
Diarrhea	7	3.5	3	2.1
Dyspepsia	6	—	—	—
Eructation	16	< 1	—	—
Flatulence/Gas	3	—	3.6	6.1
Hemorrhoids	—	—	—	1.4
Nausea	13	3.1	1.2	5.8
Pain on insertion of enema	—	—	—	1.4
Rectal pain/soreness/burning	—	—	1.8	1.2
Vomiting	5	1.1	—	—
CNS				
Asthenia	7	—	1.2	< 1
Chills	3	—	—	—
Dizziness	8	< 1	3	1.8
Fever	7	0.9	1.2	3.2
Headache	35	2.2	6.5	6.5
Insomnia	✓[2]	< 1	—	< 1
Malaise/Fatigue/Weakness	1-2	< 1	—	3.4
Sweating	3	< 1	—	—
Respiratory				
Cold/Sore throat	—	—	1.8	2.3
Cough increased	1-2	—	—	—
Pharyngitis	11	—	—	—
Rhinitis	5	—	—	—
Dermatologic				
Acne	1-2	0.2	1.2	—
Itching	—	—	—	1.2
Pruritus	3	< 1	—	—
Rash/Spots	6	1.3	1.2	2.8
Musculoskeletal				
Arthralgia	5	< 1	—	—
Arthritis	1-2	—	—	—
Back pain	7	—	—	1.3
Hypertonia	5	—	—	—
Leg/Joint pain	✓[2]	< 1	—	2.1
Myalgia	3	< 1	—	—
Miscellaneous				
Chest pain	3	—	—	—
Conjunctivitis	1-2	< 1	—	—
Dysmenorrhea	3	—	—	—
Edema	3	< 1	1.2	< 1
Flu syndrome	3	—	—	5.3
Hair loss[3]	✓[2]	< 1	—	< 1
Pain	14	—	—	—
UTI/Urinary burning	✓[2]	—	—	< 1

[1] Data are pooled from separate studies and are not necessarily comparable.

[2] ✓ = *Occurred, no incidence reported.*

[3] Mild hair loss characterized by "more hair in the comb." There are at least six additional cases in the literature of mild hair loss with mesalamine or sulfasalazine. Retreatment is not always associated with repeated hair loss.

MESALAMINE (5-aminosalicylic acid, 5–ASA)

Other adverse reactions reported with oral mesalamine include the following:

Cardiovascular: Pericarditis (see Precautions); myocarditis; vasodilation; migraine; palpitations; pericarditis; fatal myocarditis; chest pain; T-wave abnormalities.

CNS: Anxiety; depression; somnolence; emotional lability; hyperesthesia; vertigo; nervousness; confusion; paresthesia; tremor; peripheral neuropathy; transverse myelitis; Guillain-Barre syndrome.

Dermatologic: Psoriasis; pyoderma gangrenosum; dry skin; erythema nodosum; urticaria; eczema; nail disorder; photosensitivity; lichen planus.

GI: Anorexia; pancreatitis (also for rectal); gastroenteritis; gastritis; increased appetite; cholecystitis; dry mouth; oral ulcers; perforated peptic ulcer; bloody diarrhea; tenesmus; duodenal ulcer, dysphagia; esophageal ulcer; fecal incontinence; GI bleeding; oral moniliasis; rectal bleeding; stool abnormalities (color/texture change).

GU: Interstitial nephritis, nephropathy (see Warnings); dysuria; urinary urgency; hematuria; epididymitis; menorrhagia; amenorrhea; metrorrhagia; hypomenorrhea; nephrotic syndrome; urinary frequency; albuminuria; nephrotoxicity.

Hematologic: Agranulocytosis; thrombocytopenia; eosinophilia; leukopenia; anemia; lymphadenopathy; ecchymosis; thrombocythemia.

Respiratory: Sinusitis; interstitial pneumonitis; asthma exacerbation; pulmonary infiltrates; fibrosing alveolitis.

Special senses: Ear/Eye pain; taste perversion; blurred vision; tinnitus.

Miscellaneous: Neck pain; abdominal enlargement; facial edema; gout; hypersensitivity pneumonitis; asthenia; breast pain; Kawasaki-like syndrome.

Lab test abnormalities: Elevated AST, ALT, alkaline phosphatase, serum creatinine, BUN, amylase, lipase, GGTP and LDH. Hepatitis occurs rarely. More commonly, asymptomatic elevations of liver enzymes have occurred which usually resolve during continued use or with discontinuation of the drug.

Overdosage:

Symptoms: Mesalamine is an aminosalicylate, and symptoms of salicylate toxicity may be possible, such as tinnitus, vertigo, headache, confusion, drowsiness, sweating, hyperventilation, vomiting and diarrhea. Severe intoxication with salicylates can lead to disruption of electrolyte balance and blood pH, hyperthermia and dehydration.

One case of overdosage has been reported. A 3-year-old male ingested 2 g of mesalamine tablets. He was treated with ipecac and charcoal, and no adverse events occurred. Oral doses in mice and rats of $\approx$ 5000 mg/kg cause significant lethality.

Treatment: Conventional therapy for salicylate toxicity may be beneficial in the event of acute overdosage. This includes prevention of further GI tract absorption by emesis and, if necessary, by gastric lavage. Correct fluid and electrolyte imbalance by the administration of appropriate IV therapy. Maintain adequate renal function.

Patient Information:

Tablets: Swallow tablets whole; do not break the outer coating, which is designed to remain intact to protect the active ingredient. In 2% to 3% of patients, intact or partially intact tablets are found in the stool. If this occurs repeatedly, notify the physician.

Suppository: Remove the foil wrapper. Avoid excessive handling of the suppository which is designed to melt at body temperature. Insert completely into rectum with gentle pressure, pointed end first.

Suspension: Patient instructions are included with the product. Shake well. Remove protective sheath from applicator tip; gently insert applicator tip into the rectum.

MESALAMINE (5-aminosalicylic acid, 5–ASA)

Administration and Dosage:

Oral:

Tablets – 800 mg 3 times daily for a total dose of 2.4 g/day for 6 weeks.

Capsules – 1 g 4 times daily for a total dose of 4 g for up to 8 weeks.

Suppository: One suppository (500 mg) 2 times daily. Retain the suppository in the rectum for 1 to 3 hours or more if possible to achieve maximum benefit. While the effect may be seen within 3 to 21 days, the usual course of therapy is 3 to 6 weeks depending on symptoms and sigmoidoscopic findings. Studies have not assessed whether the suppositories will modify relapse rates after the 6 week short-term treatment.

Suspension: The usual dosage of mesalamine suspension enema in 60 ml units is one rectal instillation (4 g) once a day, preferably at bedtime, and retained for ≈ 8 hours. While the effect may be seen within 3 to 21 days, the usual course of therapy is 3 to 6 weeks depending on symptoms and sigmoidoscopic findings. Studies have not assessed whether the suspension enema will modify relapse rates after the 6 week short-term treatment.

Shake the bottle well to make sure the suspension is homogenous. Remove the protective sheath from the applicator tip. Holding the bottle at the neck will not cause any of the medication to be discharged. The position most often used is to lie on the left side (to facilitate migration into the sigmoid colon), with the lower leg extended and the upper right leg flexed forward for balance. An alternative is the knee-chest position. Gently insert the applicator tip in the rectum pointing toward the umbilicus. A steady squeezing of the bottle will discharge most of the preparation. Patient instructions are included with every 7 units.

Rx	**Asacol** (Procter & Gamble)	**Tablets, delayed release**: 400 mg	Lactose. (Asacol NE). Red-brown. Capsule shape. In 100s.
Rx	**Pentasa** (Hoechst-Marion Roussel)	**Capsules, controlled release**: 250 mg	Sugar. (2010 Pentasa 250 mg). Green/ blue. In 240s and UD 80s.
Rx	**Rowasa** (Solvay)	**Suppositories**: 500 mg	Light tan. In 12s and 24s.
		Rectal Suspension: 4 g per 60 ml	Potassium metabisulfite. In units of 7 disposable bottles.

OLSALAZINE SODIUM

Actions:

Pharmacology: Olsalazine sodium is a sodium salt of a salicylate compound that is effectively bioconverted to 5–aminosalicylic acid (mesalamine; 5–ASA), which has anti-inflammatory activity in ulcerative colitis. Approximately 98% to 99% of an oral dose will reach the colon where each molecule is rapidly converted into two molecules of 5-ASA by colonic bacteria and the low prevailing redox potential found in this environment. More than 0.9 g mesalamine would usually be made available in the colon from 1 g olsalazine. The liberated 5-ASA is absorbed slowly, resulting in very high local concentrations in the colon.

Mechanism of mesalamine is unknown, but appears topical rather than systemic. It possibly diminishes colonic inflammation by blocking cyclooxygenase and inhibiting colon prostaglandin production in bowel mucosa.

In rats the kidney is the major target organ of olsalazine toxicity. At an oral daily dose of ≥ 400 mg/kg, olsalazine treatment produced nephritis and tubular necrosis in a 4 week study, interstitial nephritis and tubular calcinosis in a 6 month study and renal fibrosis, mineralization and transitional cell hyperplasia in a 1 year study.

Pharmacokinetics: Approximately 2.4% of a single 1 g oral dose is absorbed. Maximum serum concentrations appear after approximately 1 hour, and are low (eg, 1.6 to 6.2 mcmol/L) even after a 1 g single dose. Olsalazine has a very short serum half-life of ≈ 0.9 hours and is > 99% bound to plasma proteins. Urinary recovery is < 1%. Total oral olsalazine recovery ranges from 90% to 97%.

About 0.1% of an oral dose is metabolized in liver to olsalazine-O-sulfate (olsalazine-S), which has a half-life of 7 days and accumulates to steady state in 2 to 3 weeks. Patients on daily 1 g doses for 2 to 4 yrs show a stable plasma concentration of olsalazine-S (3.3 to 12.4 mcmol/L). Olsalazine-S is > 99% plasma protein bound. Its long half-life is mainly due to slow dissociation from the protein binding site. Less than 1% of olsalazine and olsalazine-S appears undissociated in plasma.

Serum concentrations of 5-ASA are detected after 4 to 8 hours. The peak levels of 5–ASA after an oral dose of 1 g olsalazine are low (0 to 4.3 mcmol/L). Of the total urinary 5-ASA, > 90% is in the form of N-acetyl-5-ASA (Ac-5-ASA).

Ac-5-ASA is acetylated (deactivated) in at least two sites, colonic epithelium and liver. Ac-5-ASA is found in serum, with peak values of 1.7 to 8.7 mcmol/L after a single 1 g dose. In urine, ≈ 20% of total 5-ASA is found almost exclusively as Ac-5-ASA. Remaining 5-ASA is partially acetylated and excreted in feces. After dosing, the concentration of 5-ASA in the colon has been calculated to be 18 to 49 mmol/L. No accumulation of 5-ASA or Ac-5-ASA in plasma has been detected. 5–ASA and Ac-5-ASA are 74% and 81% bound to plasma proteins, respectively.

Clinical trials: In one controlled study, ulcerative colitis patients in remission were randomized to olsalazine 500 mg tid or placebo; relapse rates at 6 months were compared. For the 52 olsalazine patients, 12 relapses occurred; for the 49 placebo patients, 22 relapses occurred. This difference in relapse rates was significant.

In a second controlled study, 164 ulcerative colitis patients in remission were randomized to olsalazine 500 mg twice a day or sulfasalazine 1 g twice a day and relapse rates were compared after 6 months. The relapse rate for olsalazine was 19.5% while that for sulfasalazine was 12.2%; the difference was not significant.

Indications:

Maintenance of remission of ulcerative colitis in patients intolerant of sulfasalazine.

Contraindications:

Hypersensitivity to salicylates.

Warnings:

Carcinogenesis: In animals, olsalazine was tested at daily doses of 200 to 2000 mg/kg/day (approximately 10 to 100 times the human maintenance dose). Urinary bladder transitional cell carcinomas were found in three male rats (6%); liver hemangiosarcomata were found in two male mice (4%).

Pregnancy: Category C. Olsalazine produces fetal developmental toxicity ie, reduced fetal weights, retarded ossifications and immaturity of visceral organs when given during organogenesis to pregnant rats in doses 5 to 20 times the human dose (100 to 400 mg/kg). There are no adequate and well controlled studies in pregnant women. Use during pregnancy only if potential benefit justifies potential risk to the fetus.

Lactation: Oral olsalazine given to lactating rats in doses 5 to 20 times the human dose produced growth retardation in their pups. It is not known whether this drug is excreted in human milk. Exercise caution when administering to a nursing woman.

Children: Safety and efficacy in children have not been established.

Precautions:

Diarrhea: About 17%, resulting in drug withdrawal in 6%; appears dose-related, but may be difficult to distinguish from underlying disease symptoms.

OLSALAZINE SODIUM

Exacerbation of the symptoms of colitis thought to have been caused by mesalamine or sulfasalazine has been noted.

Renal abnormalities were not reported in clinical trials with olsalazine; however, the possibility of renal tubular damage due to absorbed mesalamine or its n-acetylated metabolite must be kept in mind, particularly for patients with pre-existing renal disease. In these patients, monitor urinalysis, BUN and creatinine determination.

Adverse Reactions:

Overall, 10.4% of patients discontinued olsalazine because of an adverse experience compared with 6.7% of placebo patients.

Olsalazine Adverse Reactions

Adverse Reactions	Olsalazine (n = 441)	Placebo (n = 208)	Adverse Reactions	Olsalazine (n = 441)	Placebo (n = 208)
CNS			*Miscellaneous*		
Headache	5%	4.8%	Arthralgia	4%	2.9%
Fatigue/Drowsiness/Lethargy	1.8%	2.9%	Upper Respiratory Infection	1.5%	—
Depression	1.5%	—	*Withdrawal from therapy* (No. Patients)		
Vertigo/Dizziness	1%				
Insomnia	—	2.4%			
GI			Diarrhea	26	10
Diarrhea	11.1%	6.7%	Nausea	3	2
Pain/Cramps	10.1%	7.2%	Abdominal Pain	5	0
Nausea	5%	3.9%	Rash/Itching	5	0
Dyspepsia	4%	4.3%	Headache	3	0
Bloating	1.5%	1.4%	Heartburn	2	0
Anorexia	1.3%	1.9%	Rectal Bleeding	1	0
Vomiting	1%	—	Insomnia	1	0
Stomatitis	1%		Dizziness	1	0
Blood in Stool	—	3.4%	Anorexia	1	0
Dermatologic			Lightheadedness	1	0
Rash	2.3%	1.4%	Depression	1	0
Itching	1.3%		Miscellaneous	4	3

A causal relationship to the drug has not been demonstrated for the following.

Cardiovascular/Pulmonary: Pericarditis; second degree heart block; hypertension; orthostatic hypotension; peripheral edema; chest pains; tachycardia; palpitations; bronchospasm; shortness of breath.

Neurologic: Paresthesia; tremors; mood swings; irritability; fever; chills.

Dermatologic: Erythema nodosum; photosensitivity; erythema; hot flashes; alopecia.

GI: Pancreatitis; rectal bleeding; flare in symptoms; rectal discomfort; epigastric discomfort; flatulence; granulomatous hepatitis and nonspecific, reactive hepatitis. A patient developed mild cholestatic hepatitis with sulfasalazine and when changed to olsalazine 2 weeks later. Withdrawal of olsalazine led to complete recovery.

GU: Urinary frequency; dysuria; hematuria; proteinuria; impotence; menorrhagia.

Hematologic: Leukopenia; neutropenia; lymphopenia; eosinophilia; thrombocytopenia; anemia; reticulocytosis.

Musculoskeletal: Muscle cramps.

Lab test abnormalities: Elevated ALT or AST.

Special senses: Dry mouth; dry eyes; watery eyes; blurred vision.

Overdosage:

Symptoms of acute toxicity were decreased motor activity and diarrhea in all species tested and, in addition, vomiting in dogs.

Patient Information:

Take with food. Take in evenly divided doses.

Contact your physician if diarrhea occurs (reported in ≈ 17% in clinical trials.

Administration and Dosage:

1 g per day in 2 divided doses.

Rx	**Dipentum** (Pharmacia)	**Capsules:** 250 mg	(Dipentum 250 mg). Beige. In 100s and 500s.

chapter 8

anti-infectives

PENICILLINS

Actions:

Pharmacology: Penicillins are bactericidal antibiotics that include natural and semisynthetic derivatives. These agents contain the 6-β-aminopenicillanic acid nucleus and have a similar mechanism of action. All penicillins share cross-allergenicity. Significant differences among agents include: Resistance to gastric acid inactivation; resistance to inactivation by penicillinase; spectrum of antimicrobial activity. In addition to the prototype penicillin G, this class includes an acid stable penicillin G derivative (penicillin V), penicillinase-resistant penicillins, the aminopenicillins and the extended spectrum derivatives. Bacampicillin is hydrolyzed in vivo to ampicillin; amoxicillin is closely related to ampicillin. Several of these penicillins are also available in combination with agents that inactivate β–lactamase enzymes (eg, clavulanic acid, sulbactam), thereby extending the antibiotic spectrum to include many bacteria normally resistant to it and to other β-lactam antibiotics (see Pharmacokinetics). The available combinations include ampicillin/sulbactam; amoxicillin/potassium clavulanate; ticarcillin/potassium clavulanate and piperacillin/tazobactam sodium.

Penicillins

	Routes of administration	Penicillinase-resistant	Acid stable	% Protein bound	May be taken with meals
Natural					
Penicillin G	IM-IV	no	no	60	†[1]
Penicillin V	Oral	no	yes	80	yes
Penicillinase-Resistant					
Cloxacillin	Oral	yes	yes	95	no
Dicloxacillin	Oral	yes	yes	98	no
Methicillin	IM-IV	yes	†[1]	40	†[1]
Nafcillin	IM-IV-Oral	yes	yes	87 to 90	no
Oxacillin	IM-IV-Oral	yes	yes	94	no
Aminopenicillins					
Amoxicillin	Oral	no	yes	20	yes
Amoxicillin/potassium clavulanate	Oral	yes	yes	20/30	yes
Ampicillin	IM-IV-Oral	no	yes	20	no
Ampicillin/sulbactam	IM-IV	yes	†[1]	28/38	†[1]
Bacampicillin	Oral	no	yes	20	yes[2]
Extended Spectrum					
Carbenicillin	Oral	no	yes	50	no
Mezlocillin	IM-IV	no	†[1]	16 to 42	†[1]
Piperacillin	IM-IV	no	†[1]	16	†[1]
Piperacillin/tazobactam sodium	IV	yes	†[1]	30/30	†[1]
Ticarcillin	IM-IV	no	†[1]	45	†[1]
Ticarcillin/potassium clavulanate	IV	yes	†[1]	45/9	†[1]

[1] Available only for IM or IV use.
[2] Tablets only; not the suspension.

Mechanism – Penicillins inhibit the biosynthesis of cell wall mucopeptide. They are bactericidal against sensitive organisms when adequate concentrations are reached, and they are most effective during the stage of active multiplication. Inadequate concentrations may produce only bacteriostatic effects.

Pharmacokinetics:

Absorption – Oral preparations of penicillin G are slightly affected by normal gastric acidity (pH 2 to 3.5); however, a pH < 2 may partially or totally inactivate it. Oral penicillin G is absorbed (about 30%) chiefly in the duodenum. Since gastric acidity, stomach emptying time and other factors affecting absorption may vary considerably, serum levels may be reduced to nontherapeutic levels in certain individuals. Penicillin V is preferred for oral therapy since it achieves blood levels 2 to 5 times higher than the same dose of penicillin G and shows less individual variation. Methicillin is the only acid labile penicillinase-resistant penicillin, and is only used parenterally. Nafcillin's oral absorption is inferior to oxacillin, cloxacillin and dicloxacillin. Ampicillin and carbenicillin indanyl have good GI absorption, but amoxicillin and bacampicillin are more completely absorbed.

Absorption of most penicillins is affected by food; these medications are best taken on an empty stomach, 1 hour before or 2 hours after meals. Penicillin V may be given with meals; however blood levels may be slightly higher when given on an empty stomach. Amoxicillin, bacampicillin tablets and amoxicillin/potassium clavulanate may be given without regard to meals.

Peak serum levels occur approximately 1 hour after oral use. After a 500 mg oral dose, peak serum concentrations for oxacillin, cloxacillin and dicloxacillin range from 5 to 7, 7.5 to 14.4 and 10 to 17 mcg/ml, respectively. One hour after a 1 g oral nafcillin dose, average serum concentration was 1.19 mcg/ml (range, 0 to 3.12). IM injections of 1 g nafcillin, 560 mg oxacillin and 1 g methicillin produced peak serum levels in 0.5 to 1 hour of 7.61, 15 and 17 mcg/ml, respectively.

Parenteral penicillin G (sodium and potassium) gives rapid and high but transient blood levels; derivatives provide prolonged penicillin blood levels with IM use. Procaine penicillin G, an equimolecular suspension of procaine and penicillin G, must be given IM; it dissolves slowly at the injection site and plateaus in about 4 hours; levels decline gradually over 15 to 20 hours. Benzathine penicillin G IM is absorbed very slowly from the injection site and is hydrolyzed to penicillin G; hence, serum levels are much lower but more prolonged, sustaining serum levels for up to 4 weeks.

Distribution – Penicillins are bound to plasma proteins, primarily albumin, in varying degrees (see table in Pharmacology section). They diffuse readily into most body tissues and fluids, including kidneys, liver, lungs, heart, skin, synovial fluid, intestines, bile, peritoneal fluid, bronchial and wound secretions, bone, prostate, pericardial and ascitic fluids, spleen and other tissues. Penetration into cerebrospinal fluid (CSF), the brain and the eye occurs only with inflammation. CSF levels usually do not exceed 5% of penicillin G's peak serum concentration. Penicillins cross the placenta and appear in amniotic fluid and cord serum.

Excretion – Penicillins are excreted largely unchanged in the urine by glomerular filtration and active tubular secretion. Nonrenal elimination includes hepatic inactivation and excretion in bile; this is only a minor route for all penicillins except nafcillin and oxacillin. Excretion by renal tubular secretion can be delayed by coadministration of probenecid. Excretion is delayed in neonates and infants. Elimination half-life of most penicillins is short (≤ 1.5 hr). Impaired renal function prolongs the serum half-life of penicillins eliminated primarily by renal excretion. The half-life is not greatly affected for nafcillin, oxacillin, cloxacillin and dicloxacillin due to increased biotransformation and biliary excretion. Because piperacillin is excreted by biliary and renal routes, it can be used safely in appropriate dosage in patients with severe renal impairment and in the treatment of hepato-biliary infections.

β-lactamase inhibitors (clavulanic acid and sulbactam) have weak antimicrobial activity, but irreversibly inactivate bacterial β-lactamase enzymes. Used with β-lactam antibiotics, they protect antibiotics from inactivation by β-lactamase-producing organisms.

Clavulanic acid, used in combination with amoxicillin and ticarcillin, inhibits plasmid-mediated β-lactamases (eg, *Haemophilus influenzae, Neisseria gonorrheae, E coli,* salmonella, shigella, staphylococci) and chromosomal-mediated β-lactamases (eg, *Klebsiella, Bacteroides fragilis* and *Legionella*). It does not inhibit β-lactamases produced by *Enterobacter, Serratia, Morganella, Citrobacter, Pseudomonas* or *Acinetobacter* species.

Clavulanic acid is well absorbed orally and widely distributed to many body tissues. Half-life is approximately 1 hour; 35% to 45% is excreted unchanged in the urine during the first 6 hours after administration. Probenecid does not alter renal excretion of clavulanic acid.

Sulbactam, another β-lactamase inhibitor, extends the bacterial spectrum of ampicillin to include such β-lactamase-producing organisms as *S aureus, H influenzae, B fragilis* and most strains of *E coli.*

PENICILLINS

Microbiology: The following table indicates the organisms that are generally susceptible to the penicillins in vitro:

Organisms Generally Susceptible to Penicillins

	Organisms	Natural penicillins		Penicillinase-resistant					Aminopenicillins					Extended spectrum				
	✓ = generally susceptible	Penicillin G	Penicillin V	Cloxacillin	Dicloxacillin	Methicillin	Nafcillin	Oxacillin	Amoxicillin	Ampicillin	Bacampicillin	Amoxicillin/potassium clavulanate	Ampicillin/ sulbactam	Carbenicillin	Mezlocillin	Piperacillin	Ticarcillin	Ticarcillin/potassium clavulanate
Gram-positive	Staphylococci	✓[1]	✓[1]	✓	✓	✓	✓	✓	✓[1]	✓[1]	✓[1]	✓	✓	✓[1]		✓[1]	✓[1]	✓
	Staphylococcus aureus	✓[1]	✓[1]	✓	✓	✓	✓	✓				✓	✓	✓[1]	✓[1]	✓[1]	✓[1]	✓
	Streptococci	✓	✓			✓				✓			✓					
	Streptococcus pneumoniae	✓	✓	✓	✓	✓	✓	✓	✓	✓	✓	✓	✓	✓	✓	✓	✓	✓
	Beta-hemolytic streptococci	✓	✓				✓		✓	✓	✓	✓	✓	✓	✓	✓	✓	✓
	Streptococcus faecalis	✓	✓						✓	✓	✓	✓	✓	✓	✓	✓	✓	✓
	Streptococcus viridans	✓	✓				✓		✓			✓	✓			✓		✓
	Corynebacterium diphtheriae	✓	✓															
	Bacillus anthracis	✓	✓							✓			✓					
	Listeria monocytogenes	✓	✓							✓			✓					
Gram-negative	Escherichia coli	✓							✓	✓	✓	✓	✓	✓	✓	✓	✓	✓
	Hemophilus influenzae								✓	✓	✓	✓	✓	✓	✓	✓[2]	✓	✓
	Klebsiella sp											✓	✓		✓	✓		✓
	Neisseria gonorrhoeae	✓[1]	✓						✓	✓	✓	✓	✓	✓	✓	✓	✓	✓
	Neisseria meningitidis	✓								✓		✓	✓			✓	✓	✓
	Proteus mirabilis	✓							✓	✓	✓	✓	✓	✓	✓	✓	✓	✓
	Salmonella sp	✓								✓			✓	✓	✓	✓	✓	✓
	Shigella sp	✓								✓			✓		✓	✓		
	Morganella morganii												✓	✓	✓	✓	✓	✓
	Proteus vulgaris												✓	✓	✓	✓	✓	✓
	Providencia sp																	
	Providencia rettgeri												✓	✓	✓	✓	✓	✓
	Providencia stuartii												✓		✓			✓
	Enterobacter sp	✓										✓	✓	✓	✓	✓	✓	✓
	Citrobacter sp													✓	✓	✓	✓	✓
	Pseudomonas aeruginosa													✓	✓	✓	✓	✓
	Serratia sp													✓	✓	✓	✓	✓
	Acinetobacter sp												✓		✓	✓		✓
	Streptobacillus moniliformis	✓	✓															
	Moraxella (Branhamella) catarrhalis											✓	✓			✓		✓
Anaerobic	Clostridium sp	✓	✓						✓	✓		✓	✓	✓	✓	✓	✓	✓
	Peptococcus sp	✓	✓						✓	✓		✓	✓	✓	✓	✓	✓	✓
	Peptostreptococcus sp	✓	✓						✓			✓	✓	✓	✓	✓	✓	✓
	Bacteroides sp	✓[3]											✓	✓	✓	✓	✓	✓
	Fusobacterium sp	✓											✓	✓	✓	✓	✓	✓
	Eubacterium sp	✓													✓	✓	✓	✓
	Treponema pallidum	✓	✓															
	Actinomyces bovis	✓	✓													✓		
	Veillonella sp														✓	✓		✓

[1] Non-penicillinase-producing.
[2] Non-beta-lactamase-producing.
[3] B fragilis is resistant.

PENICILLINS

Indications:

Oral: Penicillins are generally indicated in the treatment of r infections due to penicillin-sensitive microorganisms.

Penicillin V is preferred over penicillin G for oral use c

Penicillinase-resistant penicillins: The percentage of staph to penicillin G outside the hospital is increasing, appro age found in the hospital. Therefore, use a penicillinase-r therapy for any suspected staphylococcal infection until culture and results are known.

When treatment is initiated before definitive culture and sensitivity results are known, consider that these agents are only effective in the treatment of infections caused by pneumococci, group A beta-hemolytic streptococci and penicillin G-resistant and penicillin G–sensitive staphylococci.

Parenteral: In patients with severe infection, or when there is nausea, vomiting, gastric dilatation, cardiospasm or intestinal hypermotility. Parenteral aqueous penicillin G (eg, potassium, sodium) is the dosage form of choice in severe infections caused by penicillin-sensitive microorganisms when rapid and high penicillin serum levels are required.

For specific labeled indications, refer to individual drug monographs.

Contraindications:

History of hypersensitivity to penicillins, cephalosporins or imipenem.

Do not treat severe pneumonia, empyema, bacteremia, pericarditis, meningitis and purulent or septic arthritis with an oral penicillin during the acute stage.

Warnings:

Hypersensitivity: Serious and occasionally fatal immediate hypersensitivity reactions have occurred. The incidence of anaphylactic shock is between 0.015% and 0.04%. Anaphylactic shock resulting in death has occurred in approximately 0.002% of the patients treated. Although anaphylaxis is more frequent following parenteral therapy, it may occur with oral use. Accelerated reactions (including urticaria and laryngeal edema) and delayed reactions (serum sickness-like reactions) may also occur. These reactions are likely to be immediate and severe in penicillin-sensitive individuals with a history of atopic conditions (see Adverse Reactions).

Hypersensitivity myocarditis is not dose-dependent and may occur at any time during treatment. The initial reaction involves rash, fever and eosinophilia. The second stage reflects cardiac involvement: Sinus tachycardia, ST-T changes, slight increase in cardiac enzymes (creatine phosphokinase) and cardiomegaly.

A urticarial rash, not representing a true penicillin allergy, occasionally occurs with **ampicillin** (9%). This reaction is more frequent in patients on allopurinol (14% to 22.4%), patients with lymphatic leukemia (90%) and in those with infectious mononucleosis (43% to 100%). Typically, the rash appears 7 to 10 days after the start of oral ampicillin therapy and remains for a few days to a week after drug discontinuance. In most cases, the rash is maculopapular, pruritic and generalized.

Before therapy, inquire about previous hypersensitivity reactions to penicillins, cephalosporins and other allergens. Skin testing with benzylpenicilloyl-polylysine may be used to evaluate penicillin hypersensitivity (see individual monograph in In Vivo Diagnostic Aids section).

Desensitization: Patients with a positive skin test to one of the penicillin determinants can be desensitized, which is a relatively safe procedure. This is recommended in instances when penicillin must be given (eg, neurosyphilis, congenital syphilis, syphilis in pregnancy) where no proven alternatives exist. This can be done orally, IV or SC; however, oral is thought to be safest and easiest. Various protocols are described, but each protocol utilizes the same principles, which involve gradually increasing doses of penicillin, increasing each dose every 15 to 20 minutes. For example, one oral protocol using penicillin V uses 14 total doses, each dose given 15 minutes apart. The units per dose are doubled at each interval (eg, 100, 200, 400, 800) for a total cumulative dose of 1.3 million units over 4 hours. After desensitization, maintain patients on penicillin for the duration of therapy.

Cross-allergenicity with cephalosporins: Individuals with a history of penicillin hypersensitivity have experienced severe reactions when treated with a cephalosporin. The incidence of cross-allergenicity between penicillins and cephalosporins is estimated to range from 5% to 16%; however, it is possible the incidence is much lower, possibly 3% to 7%.

Urticaria, other skin rashes and serum sickness-like reactions may be controlled by antihistamines and, if necessary, corticosteroids. Discontinue use unless the condition being treated is life-threatening and amenable only to penicillin therapy. Serious anaphylactoid reactions require emergency measures. See Management of Acute Hypersensitivity Reactions.

ng abnormalities: **Ticarcillin, mezlocillin or piperacillin** may induce hemorrhagic anifestations associated with abnormalities of coagulation tests (eg, bleeding time, prothrombin time, platelet aggregation). Upon withdrawal of the drug, bleeding should cease and coagulation abnormalities revert to normal. Observe patients with renal impairment, in whom excretion of these drugs is delayed, for prolonged bleeding manifestations.

Cystic fibrosis patients have a higher incidence of side effects (eg, fever, rash) when treated with extended spectrum penicillins (eg, piperacillin, carbenicillin). This may be due to the higher IgE, IgG and eosinophil levels in this population.

Pregnancy: Category B. There are no adequate or well controlled studies in pregnant women. Penicillins cross the placenta. Use during pregnancy only if clearly needed.

Labor and delivery – Oral aminopenicillins are poorly absorbed during labor. It is not known whether use has immediate or delayed adverse effects on the fetus, or alters normal labor.

Lactation: Penicillins are excreted in breast milk in low concentrations; use may cause diarrhea, candidiasis or allergic response in the nursing infant.

Children: Safety and efficacy of carbenicillin, piperacillin and the β-lactamase inhibitor/penicillin combinations have not been established in infants and children < 12 years old. Penicillins are excreted largely unchanged by the kidney. Because of incompletely developed renal function in infants, the rate of elimination will be slow. Penicillinase-resistant penicillins (especially methicillin) may not be completely excreted, with abnormally high blood levels resulting. Oral aminopenicillins are not absorbed as well in neonates as in adults. Use caution in administering to newborns and evaluate organ system function frequently. Frequent blood levels are advisable, with dosage adjustments when necessary. Monitor all newborns closely for clinical and laboratory evidence of toxic or adverse effects.

Precautions:

Monitoring: Perform bacteriologic studies to determine causative organisms and their susceptibility so that appropriate therapy is administered.

Obtain blood cultures, white blood cell and differential cell counts prior to initiation of therapy and at least weekly during therapy with penicillinase-resistant penicillins. Measure AST and ALT during therapy to monitor for liver function abnormalities.

Perform periodic urinalysis, BUN and creatinine determinations during therapy with penicillinase-resistant penicillins, and consider dosage alterations if these values become elevated. If renal impairment is known or suspected, reduce the total dosage and monitor blood levels to avoid possible neurotoxic reactions.

Monitoring is particularly important in newborns and other infants, and when high dosages are used.

Streptococcal infections: Therapy must be sufficient to eliminate the organism (a minimum of 10 days); otherwise, sequelae (eg, endocarditis, rheumatic fever) may occur. Take cultures after treatment to confirm that streptococci have been eradicated.

Sexually transmitted diseases: When treating gonococcal infections in which primary and secondary syphilis are suspected, perform proper diagnostic procedures, including darkfield examinations and monthly serological tests for at least 4 months. All cases of penicillin-treated syphilis should receive clinical and serological examinations every 6 months for 2 to 3 years.

Renal function impairment: Since carbenicillin is primarily excreted by the kidney, patients with severe renal impairment (creatinine clearance, < 10 ml/min) will not achieve the therapeutic urine levels of carbenecillin.

In patients with creatinine clearance 10 to 20 ml/min, it may be necessary to adjust dosage to prevent accumulation of the drug.

Resistance: The number of strains of staphylococci resistant to penicillinase-resistant penicillins has been increasing; widespread use of penicillinase-resistant penicillins may result in an increasing number of resistant staphylococcal strains. Interpret resistance to any penicillinase-resistant penicillin as evidence of clinical resistance to all. Cross-resistance with cephalosporin derivatives also occurs frequently.

Pseudomembranous colitis has occurred with the use of broad spectrum antibiotics due to overgrowth of clostridia; therefore, it is important to consider its diagnosis in patients who develop diarrhea in association with antibiotic use. Mild cases may respond to drug discontinuation alone. Manage moderate-to-severe cases with fluid, electrolyte and protein supplementation. If it is not relieved by drug withdrawal or when it is severe, oral vancomycin is the treatment of choice.

PENICILLINS

Procaine sensitivity: If sensitivity to the procaine in **penicillin G procaine** is suspected, inject 0.1 ml of a 1% to 2% procaine solution intradermally. Development of erythema, wheal, flare or eruption indicates procaine sensitivity; treat by the usual methods. Do not use procaine penicillin preparations.

Parenteral administration: Inadvertent intravascular administration, including direct intra-arterial injection or injection immediately adjacent to arteries, has resulted in severe neurovascular damage, including transverse myelitis with permanent paralysis, gangrene requiring amputation of digits and more proximal portions of extremities, and necrosis and sloughing at and surrounding the injection site. Such severe effects have occurred following injections into the buttock, thigh and deltoid areas. Other serious complications include immediate pallor, mottling or cyanosis of the extremity, both distal and proximal to the injection site, followed by bleb formation; severe edema requiring anterior or posterior compartment fasciotomy in the lower extremity. These severe effects have most often occurred in infants and small children. Promptly consult specialist if any evidence of compromise of the blood supply occurs at, proximal to or distal to the site of injection.

Quadriceps femoris fibrosis and atrophy have occurred following repeated IM injections of penicillin preparations into the anterolateral thigh.

Take particular care with IV administration because of the possibility of thrombophlebitis. Higher than recommended IV doses of most of the penicillins may cause neuromuscular excitability or convulsions.

Avoid SC and fat layer injections; pain and induration may occur. If these occur, apply an ice pack.

Electrolyte imbalance: Administer **aqueous penicillin G** IV in high doses (> 10 million units) slowly because of electrolyte imbalance from either the potassium or sodium content. When sodium restriction is necessary (eg, cardiac patients), make periodic electrolyte determinations and monitor cardiac status.

Patients given continuous IV therapy with **potassium penicillin G** in high dosage (> 10 million units daily) may suffer severe or even fatal potassium poisoning, particularly if renal insufficiency is present. Hyperreflexia, convulsions, coma, cardiac arrhythmias and cardiac arrest may be indicative of this syndrome. High dosage of **sodium salts of penicillins** may result in or aggravate CHF due to high sodium intake. Individuals with liver disease or those receiving cytotoxic therapy or diuretics rarely demonstrated a decrease in serum potassium concentrations with high doses of **piperacillin.**

Sodium penicillin G contains 2 mEq sodium per million units, **potassium penicillin G** contains 1.7 mEq potassium and 0.3 mEq sodium per million units. The sodium content of other IV penicillin derivatives is listed below:

Sodium Content of IV Penicillins

Penicillin	Maximum daily dose (g)	Sodium content (mEq/g)[1]	Sodium (mEq/day)[1,2]
Ampicillin sodium	12	2.9	34.8
Methicillin sodium	12	3	36
Mezlocillin sodium	24	1.85	44.4
Nafcillin sodium	9	2.9	26
Oxacillin sodium	12	2.5	30
Piperacillin sodium	24	1.85	44.4
Ticarcillin disodium	24	4.7 to 5	112.8 to 120

[1] 1 mEq sodium equals 23 mg.
[2] Based on maximum daily dose.

Hypokalemia has occurred in a few patients receiving **mezlocillin, ticarcillin** and **piperacillin.** It may also occur in patients with low potassium reserves and in patients receiving cytotoxic therapy or diuretics. Monitor serum potassium and supplement when necessary.

Superinfection: Use of antibiotics (especially prolonged or repeated therapy) may result in bacterial or fungal overgrowth of nonsusceptible organisms. Such overgrowth may lead to a secondary infection. Take appropriate measures if this occurs.

Indwelling IV catheters encourage superinfections.

Tartrazine sensitivity: Some of these products contain tartrazine, which may cause allergic-type reactions (including bronchial asthma) in susceptible individuals. Although the incidence of tartrazine sensitivity in the general population is low, it is frequently seen in patients who also have aspirin hypersensitivity. Specific products containing tartrazine are identified in the product listings.

PENICILLINS

Sulfite sensitivity: Some of these products contain sodium formaldehyde sulfoxylate, a sulfite that may cause allergic-type reactions including anaphylactic symptoms and life-threatening or less severe asthmatic episodes in certain susceptible people. The overall prevalence of sulfite sensitivity in the general population is unknown and probably low. Sulfite sensitivity is seen more frequently in asthmatic than in non-asthmatic people.

Drug Interactions:

Penicillin Drug Interactions			
Precipitant drug	Object drug*		Description
Penicillins, parenteral	Aminoglycosides, parenteral	↔	Although these agents are often used together to achieve a synergistic action, certain penicillins may inactivate certain aminoglycosides in vitro. Do not mix in the same IV solution. Also, oral neomycin may reduce the serum concentrations of oral penicillin.
Penicillins, parenteral	Anticoagulants	↑	Large IV doses of penicillins can increase bleeding risks of anticoagulants by prolonging bleeding time. Conversely, nafcillin has been associated with warfarin resistance.
Penicillins, oral	Beta blockers	↔	Ampicillin may reduce the bioavailability of atenolol. Case reports indicated that beta blockers may potentiate anaphylactic reactions of penicillin.
Penicillins	Contraceptives, oral	↓	The efficacy of oral contraceptives may be reduced. Although infrequently reported, the use of an additional form of contraception during penicillin therapy is advisable.
Penicillins, parenteral	Heparin	↑	An increased risk of bleeding may occur, possibly due to additive effects.
Allopurinol	Ampicillin	↑	The rate of ampicillin-induced skin rash appears much higher when coadministered with allopurinol than with either drug by itself (see Warnings).
Chloramphenicol	Penicillins	↔	Synergistic effects may develop, but antagonism has been reported in animal studies.
Erythromycin	Penicillins	↔	In vitro tests and clinical studies have demonstrated both antagonism and synergism with coadministration.
Tetracyclines	Penicillins	↓	The bacteriostatic action of tetracycline derivatives may impair the bactericidal effects of penicillins.

* ↑ = Object drug increased ↓ = Object drug decreased ↔ = Undetermined effect

Drug/Lab test interactions: False-positive **urine glucose** reactions may occur with penicillin therapy if Clinitest, Benedict's Solution or Fehling's Solution are used. It is recommended that enzymatic glucose oxidase tests (such as *Clinistix* or *Tes-Tape*) be used. Positive **Coombs' tests** have occurred. Positive direct antiglobulin tests (DAT) have been reported after large IV doses of **piperacillin; clavulanic acid** has also been reported to cause a positive DAT. High urine concentrations of some penicillins may produce false-positive protein reactions (pseudoproteinuria) with the following methods: Sulfosalicylic acid and boiling test, acetic acid test, biuret reaction and nitric acid test. The bromphenol blue (*Multi-Stix*) reagent strip test has been reported to be reliable.

Drug/Food interactions: Absorption of most penicillins is affected by food; these medications are best taken on an empty stomach, 1 hour before or 2 hours after meals. Penicillin V may be given with meals; however, blood levels may be slightly higher when taken on an empty stomach. Amoxicillin, amoxicillin/potassium clavulanate and bacampicillin tablets may be given without regard to meals; absorption of bacampicillin suspension is affected by food.

PENICILLINS

Adverse Reactions:

Hypersensitivity: Adverse reactions (estimated incidence, 1% to 10%) are more likely to occur in individuals with previously demonstrated hypersensitivity. In penicillin-sensitive individuals with a history of allergy, asthma or hay fever, the reactions may be immediate and severe. (See Warnings).

Allergic symptoms include urticaria, angioneurotic edema, laryngospasm, bronchospasm, hypotension, vascular collapse; death; maculopapular to exfoliative dermatitis; vesicular eruptions; erythema multiforme (rarely, Stevens-Johnson syndrome); reactions resembling serum sickness (chills, fever, edema, arthralgia, arthritis, malaise); laryngeal edema; skin rashes; prostration.

GI: Glossitis; stomatitis; gastritis; sore mouth or tongue; dry mouth; furry tongue; black "hairy" tongue; abnormal taste sensation; nausea; vomiting; abdominal pain or cramp; epigastric distress; diarrhea or bloody diarrhea; rectal bleeding; flatulence; enterocolitis; pseudomembranous colitis (see Precautions). Incidence of symptoms, particularly diarrhea, is less with amoxicillin and bacampicillin than with ampicillin.

Hematologic/Lymphatic: Anemia; hemolytic anemia; thrombocytopenia; thrombocytopenic purpura; eosinophilia; leukopenia; granulocytopenia; neutropenia; bone marrow depression; agranulocytosis; a reduction of hemoglobin or hematocrit; prolongation of bleeding and prothrombin time; decrease in WBC and lymphocyte counts; increase in lymphocytes, monocytes, basophils and platelets. These reactions are usually reversible on discontinuation of therapy, and are believed to be hypersensitivity phenomena. A slight thrombocytosis occurred in < 1% of patients treated with amoxicillin and clavulanate potassium.

Bleeding abnormalities: Hemorrhagic manifestations associated with abnormalities of coagulation tests such as clotting and prothrombin time have occurred (see Warnings).

Renal: Interstitial nephritis (eg, oliguria, proteinuria, hematuria, hyaline casts, pyuria) and nephropathy are infrequent and usually associated with high doses of parenteral penicillins (most frequently **methicillin**); this has also occurred with all of the penicillins. Such reactions are hypersensitivity responses and are usually associated with fever, skin rash and eosinophilia. Methicillin-induced nephropathy does not appear to be dose-related and is generally reversible upon prompt discontinuation of the drug. Elevations of creatinine or BUN may occur.

CNS: Penicillins have caused neurotoxicity (manifested as lethargy, neuromuscular irritability, hallucinations, convulsions and seizures) when given in large IV doses especially in patients with renal failure. Mental disturbances including anxiety, confusion, agitation, depression, hallucinations, weakness, seizures, combativeness and expressed "fear of impending death" have been reported in individuals following single dose therapy for gonorrhea with **penicillin G procaine**, which may have been a reaction to procaine. Reactions have been transient, lasting from 15 to 30 minutes. Dizziness, fatigue, insomnia, reversible hyperactivity and prolonged muscle relaxation have occurred.

Local: Pain (accompanied by induration) at the site of injection; ecchymosis; deep vein thrombosis; hematomas. Vein irritation and phlebitis can occur, particularly when undiluted solution is injected directly into the vein. Tissue necrosis due to extravasated **nafcillin** has been successfully modified with hyaluronidase.

Miscellaneous: Vaginitis; anorexia; hyperthermia, itchy eyes, transient hepatitis and cholestatic jaundice (rare); sciatic neuritis caused by IM injection of penicillin. The Jarisch-Herxheimer reaction has been reported in the treatment of syphilis.

Lab test abnormalities: Elevations of AST, ALT, bilirubin and LDH have been noted in patients receiving semisynthetic penicillins (particularly **oxacillin** and **cloxacillin**); such reactions are more common in infants. Elevations of serum alkaline phosphatase and hypernatremia, and reduction in serum potassium, albumin, total proteins and uric acid may occur. Evidence indicates glutamic oxaloacetic transaminase (GOT) is released at the site of IM injection of **ampicillin**. Increased amounts of this enzyme in the blood do not necessarily indicate liver involvement.

PENICILLINS

Overdosage:

Penicillin overdosage can result in neuromuscular hyperexcitability or convulsive seizures. Dose-related toxicity may arise with the use of massive doses of IV penicillins (40 to 100 million units/day), particularly in patients with severe renal impairment. Manifestations may include agitation, confusion, asterixis, hallucinations, stupor, coma, multifocal myoclonus, seizures and encephalopathy. Hyperkalemia is also possible.

In case of overdosage, discontinue penicillin, treat symptomatically and institute supportive measures as required. Refer to General Management of Acute Overdosage. If necessary, hemodialysis may be used to reduce blood levels of penicillin, although the degree of effectiveness of this procedure is questionable. The metabolic by-products of carbenicillin indanyl sodium, indanyl sulfate and glucuronide, as well as free carbenicillin, are dialyzable. In renal function impairment, aminopenicillins can be removed by hemodialysis, but not peritoneal dialysis. The molecular weight, degree of protein binding and pharmacokinetic profile of sulbactam and clavulanic acid suggest these compounds may also be removed by hemodialysis.

Patient Information:

Complete full course of therapy.

Take on an empty stomach 1 hour before or 2 hours after meals. Absorption of penicillin V, amoxicillin, bacampicillin tablets and amoxicillin/potassium clavulanate is not significantly affected by food.

Take each oral dose with a full glass of water, not fruit juice or carbonated beverage (cloxacillin, penicillin G).

Take at even intervals, preferably around the clock.

Notify physician if skin rash, itching, hives, severe diarrhea, shortness of breath, wheezing, black tongue, sore thoat, nausea, vomiting, fever, swollen joints or any unusual bleeding or bruising occurs.

Discard any liquid forms of penicillin after 7 days if stored at room temperature or after 14 days if refrigerated.

Administration and Dosage:

Therapy may be initiated prior to obtaining results of bacteriologic studies when there is reason to believe the causative organisms may be susceptible. Once results are known, adjust therapy.

Dosage for any individual patient must take into consideration the severity of infection, the susceptibility of the organisms causing the infection and the status of the patient's host defense mechanism. Duration of therapy depends on the severity of the infection.

Continue treatment of all infections for a minimum of 48 to 72 hours beyond the time that the patient becomes asymptomatic or evidence of bacterial eradication has been obtained, unless single dose therapy is employed. A minimum of 10 days treatment is recommended for any infection caused by group A beta-hemolytic streptococci to prevent the occurrence of acute rheumatic fever or acute glomerulonephritis.

Patients with a history of rheumatic fever and receiving continuous prophylaxis may harbor increased numbers of penicillin-resistant organisms.

Natural Penicillins

PENICILLIN G (AQUEOUS), PARENTERAL

For complete prescribing information, refer to the Penicillins group monograph.

Administration and Dosage:

Children: 100,000 to 250,000 units/kg/day in divided doses every 4 hours.

Infants:

Over 7 days and > 2000 g – 100,000 units/kg/day in divided doses every 6 hours (meningitis – 200,000 units).

Over 7 days and < 2000 g – 75,000 units/kg/day in divided doses every 8 hours (meningitis – 150,000 units).

Under 7 days and > 2000 g – 50,000 units/kg/day in divided doses every 8 hours (meningitis – 150,000 units).

Under 7 days and < 2000 g – 50,000 units/kg/day in divided doses every 12 hours (meningitis – 100,000 units).

Streptococci in groups A, C, G, H, L and M are very sensitive to penicillin G. Some group D organisms are sensitive to the high serum levels obtained with aqueous penicillin G.

Parenteral Penicillin G Use and Dosages

Organisms/Infections	Dosage
Labeled uses:	
Meningococcal meningitis	1 to 2 million units IM every 2 hours; or 20 to 30 million units/day continuous IV drip for 14 days or until afebrile for 7 days; or 200,000 to 300,000 units/kg/day every 2 to 4 hours divided doses for a total of 24 doses.
Actinomycosis For cervicofacial cases	1 to 6 million units/day
For thoracic and abdominal disease	12 to 20 million units/day IV for 6 weeks. May be followed by oral penicillin V, 500 mg 4 times daily for 2 to 3 months
Clostridial infections	20 million units/day as adjunct to antitoxin
Fusospirochetal infections: Severe infections of oropharynx, lower respiratory tract and genital area	5 to 10 million units/day
Rat-bite fever (Spirillum minus, Streptobacillus moniliformis), Haverhill fever	12 to 20 million units/day for 3 to 4 weeks
Listeria infections (Listeria monocytogenes):	
Meningitis (adults)	15 to 20 million units/day for 2 weeks
Endocarditis (adults)	15 to 20 million units/day for 4 weeks
Pasteurella infections (Pasteurella multocida): Bacteremia and meningitis	4 to 6 million units/day for 2 weeks
Erysipeloid (Erysipelothrix rhusiopathiae): Endocarditis	12 to 20 million units/day for 4 to 6 weeks
Gram-negative bacillary bacteremia (Escherichia coli, Enterobacter aerogenes, Alcaligenes faecalis, Salmonella, Shigella, Proteus mirabilis)	≥ 20 million units/day
Diphtheria: Adjunct to antitoxin to prevent carrier state	2 to 3 million units/day in divided doses for 10 to 12 days
Anthrax: (B anthracis is often resistant)	Minimum 5 million units/day; 12 to 20 million units/day have been used
Pneumococcal infections (S pneumoniae):	
Empyema	5 to 24 million units/day in divided doses every 4 to 6 hours
Meningitis	20 to 24 million units/day for 14 days
Suppurative arthritis, osteomyelitis, mastoiditis, endocarditis, peritonitis, pericarditis	12 to 20 million units/day for ≥ 2 to 4 weeks

Natural Penicillins

PENICILLIN G (AQUEOUS), PARENTERAL

Parenteral Penicillin G Use and Dosages	
Organisms/Infections	Dosage
Syphilis:[1]	
Neurosyphilis	12 to 24 million units/day IV (2 to 4 million units every 4 hours) for 10 to 14 days. Many recommend benzathine penicillin G 2.4 million units IM weekly for 3 weeks following the completion of this regimen.
Congenital syphilis: Symptomatic or asymptomatic infants	*Newborns:* 50,000 units/kg/day IV every 8 to 12 hours for 10 to 14 days. If > 1 day of therapy is missed, restart the entire course. *Infants (after newborn period):* 50,000 units/kg every 4 to 6 hours for 10 to 14 days.
Gonococcal infections:[1] Infants with disseminated gonococcal infection or gonococcal ophthalmia (hospitalization recommended)	If the gonococcal isolate is proven to be susceptible to penicillin: 100,000 units/kg/day in 2 equal doses (4 equal doses per day for infants > 1 week old). Increase the dose to 150,000 units/kg/day for meningitis.
Unlabeled uses:	
Lyme disease (Borrelia burgdorferi):	
Erythema chronicum migrans	Use oral penicillin V
Neurologic complications (eg, meningitis, encephalitis)	200,000 to 300,000 units/kg/day (up to 20 million units) IV for 10 to 14 days
Carditis	200,000 to 300,000 units/kg/day (up to 20 million units) IV for 10 days with cardiac monitoring and a temporary pacemaker for complete heart block
Arthritis	200,000 to 300,000 units/kg/day (up to 20 million units) IV for 10 to 20 days

[1] CDC 1989 Sexually Transmitted Diseases Treatment Guidelines. *Morbidity and Mortality Weekly Report* 1989 Sep 1;38 (No. S-8):1-43.

Since alpha-hemolytic streptococci resistant to penicillin may be found when patients are receiving continuous oral penicillin for secondary prevention of rheumatic fever, prophylactic agents other than penicillin may be prescribed in addition to their continuous rheumatic fever prophylactic regimen.

Natural Penicillins

PENICILLIN G (AQUEOUS), PARENTERAL

Penicillin G potassium contains 1.7 mEq potassium and 0.3 mEq sodium per million units; Penicillin G sodium contains 2 mEq sodium per million units.

Give recommended daily dosage IM or by continuous IV infusion.

Administer 10 or 20 million units by IV infusion only.

IM: Keep total volume of injection small. The IM route is the preferred route of administration. Solutions containing up to 100,000 units/ml may be used with a minimum of discomfort. Use greater concentrations as required.

Continuous IV infusion: When larger doses are required, administer aqueous solutions by means of continuous IV infusion. Determine volume and rate of fluid administration required by the patient in a 24 hour period. Add appropriate daily dosage to this fluid.

Intrapleural or other local infusion: If fluid is aspirated, give infusion in a volume equal to ¼ or ½ the amount of fluid aspirated; otherwise, prepare as for the IM injection.

Intrathecal use: Must be highly individualized. Use only with full consideration of the possible irritating effects of penicillin when used by this route. The preferred route of therapy in bacterial meningitis is IV, supplemented by IM injection. It has been suggested that intrathecal use has no place in therapy.

Preparation of solutions: Depending on the route of administration, use Sterile Water for Injection, Isotonic Sodium Chloride Injection or Dextrose Injection. Penicillins are rapidly inactivated in the presence of carbohydrate solutions at alkaline pH.

Stability/Storage: The dry powder is stable and does not require refrigeration. Sterile solutions may be kept in the refrigerator for 1 week without loss of potency. Solutions prepared for IV infusion are stable at room temperature for at least 24 hours.

Premixed, frozen solution – Thaw frozen container at room temperature (25°C; 77°F) or in a refrigerator (5°C; 41°F). Do not force thaw by immersion in water baths or by microwave irradiation.

The thawed solution is stable for 24 hours at room temperature or for 14 days under refrigeration. Do not refreeze thawed antibiotics.

R	**Penicillin G Potassium** (Baxter)	**Injection, premixed, frozen:** 1,000,000 units	In 50 ml.
		2,000,000 units	In 50 ml.
		3,000,000 units	In 50 ml.
Rx	**Penicillin G Potassium** (Apothecon)	**Powder for Injection:** 1,000,000 units	In vials.
Rx	**Pfizerpen** (Roerig)		In vials.
Rx	**Penicillin G Potassium** (Apothecon)	**Powder for Injection:** 5,000,000 units	In vials.
Rx	**Pfizerpen** (Roerig)		In vials.
Rx	**Penicillin G Potassium** (Apothecon)	**Powder for Injection:** 10,000,000 units	In vials.
Rx	**Penicillin G Potassium** (Apothecon)	**Powder for Injection:** 20,000,000 units per vial	In vials.
Rx	**Pfizerpen** (Roerig)		In vials.
Rx	**Penicillin G Sodium** (Apothecon)	**Powder for Injection:** 5,000,000 units per vial	In vials.

Natural Penicillins

PENICILLIN G POTASSIUM, ORAL

For complete prescribing information, refer to the Penicillins group monograph.

Administration and Dosage:

250 mg = 400,000 units.

Administer at least 1 hour before or 2 hours after meals.

Streptococci in groups A, C, G, H, L and M are very sensitive to penicillin G. Other groups, including group D (enterococci), are resistant.

Penicillin V is the preferred agent for oral therapy.

Children (< 12 years): 25,000 to 90,000 units/kg/day in 3 to 6 divided doses. 40,000 to 80,000 units/kg/day divided every 6 hours has been suggested.

Oral Penicillin G Uses and Dosages

Organisms/Infections	Dosage
Streptococcal infections of the upper respiratory tract (ie, otitis media, scarlet fever and mild erysipelas):	
Mild infections	200,000 to 250,000 units every 6 to 8 hours for 10 days.
Moderately severe infections	400,000 to 500,000 units every 8 hours for 10 days or 800,000 units every 12 hours.
Pneumococcal infections: Mild to moderately severe infections of the respiratory tract (eg, otitis media)	400,000 to 500,000 units every 6 hours until afebrile for at least 2 days.
Staphylococcal infections: Mild infections of skin and skin structures	200,000 to 500,000 units every 6 to 8 hours until infection is cured.
Fusospirochetosis (Vincent's gingivitis and pharyngitis) of the oropharynx: Mild to moderately severe infections	400,000 to 500,000 units every 6 to 8 hours. Obtain necessary dental care in infections involving the gum tissue.
Prevention of recurrent rheumatic fever and/or chorea	200,000 to 250,000 units twice daily on a continuing basis.

Rx	**Penicillin G Potassium** (Various, eg, Purepac, Rugby, URL)	**Tablets:** 200,000 units	In 100s and 1000s.
Rx	**Penicillin G Potassium** (Various, eg, Dixon-Shane, Geneva Marsam, Goldline, Major, Rugby, URL)	**Tablets:** 250,000 units	In 100s and 1000s.
Rx	**Penicillin G Potassium** (Various, eg, Dixon-Shane, Geneva Marsam, Goldline, Major, Moore, Mylan, Rugby, Schein, URL, Warner Chilcott)	**Tablets:** 400,000 units	In 100s and 1000s.
Rx	**Pentids '400'** (Apothecon)		Lactose. (165). White, scored. Oval. In 100s.
Rx	**Penicillin G Potassium** (Rugby)	**Tablets:** 500,000 units	In 100s.
Rx	**Pentids '800'** (Apothecon)	**Tablets:** 800,000 units	Tartrazine, lactose. (168). Yellow, scored. Oval. In 100s.
Rx	**Pentids '400' for Syrup** (Apothecon)	**Powder for Oral Solution:** 400,000 units per 5 ml when reconstituted	Tartrazine, saccharin. Fruit flavor. In 100 and 200 ml.

Natural Penicillins

PENICILLIN G PROCAINE, AQUEOUS (APPG)

For complete prescribing information, refer to the Penicillins group monograph.

Indications:

A long-acting parenteral penicillin indicated in the treatment of moderately severe infections due to penicillin G-sensitive microorganisms sensitive to low and persistent serum levels achievable with this dosage form. When high sustained serum levels are required, use aqueous penicillin G, either IM or IV.

Administration and Dosage:

Administer by deep IM injection into the upper, outer quadrant of the buttock. In infants and small children, the midlateral aspect of the thigh may be preferable. When doses are repeated, rotate the injection site.

Streptococci in groups A, C, G, H, L and M are very sensitive to penicillin G. Other groups, including group D (enterococci), are resistant. Use aqueous penicillin for streptococcal infections with bacteremia.

An increasing number of strains of staphylococci are resistant to penicillin G, emphasizing the need for culture and sensitivity studies.

Gonorrhea: Some isolates of *Neisseria gonorrhoeae* have decreased susceptibility to penicillin, but penicillin in large doses remains the drug of choice for these strains. Strains producing penicillinase, however, are resistant to penicillin G and another drug should be used.

Retreatment – The CDC recommends follow-up cultures 3 to 7 days after treatment is completed. In the male, a gram-stained smear is adequate if positive; otherwise, obtain a culture specimen from the anterior urethra. In the female, obtain culture specimens from both the endocervical and anal canal sites. Retreatment in the male is indicated if urethral discharge persists for ≥ 3 days following initial therapy and the smear or culture remains positive. If gonorrhea persists after a non-spectinomycin treatment regimen, treat with **spectinomycin** 2 g IM or **ceftriaxone** 250 mg IM.*

Perform a serologic test for syphilis at the time of diagnosis. If patients with gonorrhea have concurrent syphilis, give additional treatment appropriate to the stage of syphilis.

Adults and children: 600,000 to 1.2 million units/day IM in one or two doses (up to a maximum of 4.8 million units/day) for 10 days to 2 weeks.

Newborns: 50,000 units/kg IM once daily. Avoid use in these patients since sterile abscesses and procaine toxicity are of much greater concern than in older children.

Severe pneumonia, empyema, bacteremia, pericarditis, meningitis, peritonitis and purulent or septic arthritis of pneumococcal etiology are better treated with aqueous penicillin G during the acute stage.

Penicillin G Procaine Uses and Dosages

Organisms/Infections	Dosage
Pneumococcal infections: Moderately severe uncomplicated pneumonia and middle ear and paranasal sinus infections	600,000 to 1.2 million units/day
Streptococcal infections (group A): Moderately severe to severe tonsillitis, erysipelas, scarlet fever, upper respiratory tract (ie, otitis media) and skin and skin structure infections	600,000 to 1.2 million units/day for a minimum of 10 days
Bacterial endocarditis – Only in extremely sensitive infections *(S viridans, S bovis)*	1.2 million units 4 times daily for 2 to 4 weeks plus streptomycin 500 mg twice daily for the first 2 weeks
Staphylococcal infections: Moderately severe to severe infections of the skin and skin structure	600,000 to 1.2 million units/day
Diphtheria: Adjunctive therapy with antitoxin	300,000 to 600,000 units/day
Carrier state	300,000 units/day for 10 days
Anthrax: Cutaneous	600,000 to 1.2 million units/day

* CDC 1989 Sexually Transmitted Diseases Treatment Guidelines. *Morbidity and Mortality Weekly Report* 1989 Sept 1;38 (No. S-8):1-43.

Natural Penicillins

PENICILLIN G PROCAINE, AQUEOUS (APPG)

Penicillin G Procaine Uses and Dosages	
Organisms/Infections	Dosage
Vincent's gingivitis and pharyngitis (fusospirochetosis):	600,000 to 1.2 million units/day. Obtain necessary dental care in infections involving gum tissue.
Erysipeloid:	600,000 to 1.2 million units/day
Rat-bite fever (Streptobacillus moniliformis and Spirillum minus):	600,000 to 1.2 million units/day
Gonorrheal infections (uncomplicated):	4.8 million units divided into at least two doses at one visit; 1 g oral probenecid is given 30 minutes before the injections. Obtain follow-up cultures from the original site(s) of infection 7 to 14 days after therapy. In women, it is also desirable to obtain culture test-of-cure from both the endocervical and anal canals. Note: Treat gonorrheal endocarditis intensively with aqueous penicillin G
Syphilis: Primary, secondary and latent with a negative spinal fluid (adults and children > 12 years of age):	600,000 units daily for 8 days; total 4.8 million units
Neurosyphilis[1] (as an alternative to the recommended regimen of penicillin G aqueous)	2 to 4 million units/day plus probenecid 500 mg orally 4 times daily, both for 10 to 14 days; many recommend benzathine penicillin G 2.4 million units weekly for 3 doses following the completion of this regimen.
Congenital syphilis:[1] Symptomatic and asymptomatic infants	50,000 units/kg/day (administered once IM) for 10 to 14 days
Yaws, Bejel and Pinta:	Treat same as syphilis in corresponding stage of disease

Storage: Refrigerate (stable for 24 months); avoid freezing.

Rx	**Crysticillin 300 A.S.** (Apothecon)	**Injection:** 300,000 units per ml	In 10 ml vials.[2]
Rx	**Pfizerpen-AS** (Roerig)		In 10 ml vials.[3]
Rx	**Crysticillin 600 A.S.** (Apothecon)	**Injection:** 500,000 units per ml (600,000 units/1.2 ml)	In 12 ml vials.[4]
Rx	**Wycillin** (Wyeth-Ayerst)	**Injection:** 600,000 units per unit dose	In 1 ml Tubex.[5]
Rx	**Wycillin** (Wyeth-Ayerst)	**Injection:** 1,200,000 units per unit dose	In 2 ml Tubex.[5]
Rx	**Wycillin** (Wyeth-Ayerst)	**Injection:** 2,400,000 units per unit dose	In 4 ml disp. syringe.[5]

[1] CDC 1989 Sexually Transmitted Diseases Treatment Guidelines. *Morbidity and Mortality Weekly Report* 1989 Sept 1;38 (No. S-8):1–43.
[2] With parabens, lecithin, povidone and sodium formaldehyde sulfoxylate.
[3] With parabens, sorbitol, polyvinylpyrrolidone and lecithin.
[4] With parabens, phenol, povidone, lecithin and sodium formaldehyde sulfoxylate.
[5] With parabens, lecithin and povidone.

Natural Penicillins

PENICILLIN G BENZATHINE, PARENTERAL

For complete prescribing information, refer to the Penicillins group monograph.

Administration and Dosage:

Administer by deep IM injection in the upper outer quadrant of the buttock. In infants and small children, the midlateral aspect of the thigh may be preferable. Do not inject benzathine penicillin into the gluteal region of children < 2 years of age. When doses are repeated, rotate the injection site.

Adults: 1.2 million units in one dose.

Children (> 27 kg): 900,000 to 1.2 million units in one dose.

Children and infants (< 27 kg): 300,000 to 600,000 units in one dose.

Neonates: 50,000 units/kg in one dose.

Parenteral Penicillin G Benzathine Uses and Dosages

Organisms/Infections	Dosage
Streptococcal (group A): Prevention of recurrent rheumatic fever.	1.2 million units every 4 weeks
Syphilis:[1] *Early syphilis* - Primary, secondary or latent syphilis of < 1 year's duration.	2.4 million units IM in single dose
Syphilis of > 1 year's duration, gummas and cardiovascular syphilis - Latent, cardiovascular or late benign syphilis.	2.4 million units once weekly for three weeks
Neurosyphilis	Aqueous penicillin G, 12 to 24 million units/day IV (2 to 4 million units every 4 hours) for 10 to 14 days. Many recommend benzanthine penicillin G, 2.4 million IM units weekly for 3 doses following completion of this regimen. or Aqueous procaine penicillin G, 2.4 million units/day IM *plus* probenecid 500 mg orally 4 times daily, both for 10 to 14 days. Many recommend benzathine penicillin G, 2.4 million units IM weekly for 3 doses following completion of this regimen.
Syphilis in pregnancy	Dosage schedule appropriate for stage of syphilis recommended for nonpregnant patients.
Congenital syphilis - Older children with definite acquired syphilis and a normal neurologic examination.	50,000 units/kg IM, up to the adult dose of 2.4 million units.
Yaws, bejel and pinta	1.2 million units in a single dose
Erysipeloid (Erysipelothrix rhusiopathiae): Uncomplicated infection.	1.2 million units in a single dose

[1] CDC 1989 Sexually Transmitted Diseases Treatment Guidelines. *Morbidity and Mortality Weekly Report* 1989 Sep 1;38(No. S-8):1-43.

Storage: Refrigerate (stable for 24 months); avoid freezing.

Rx	**Bicillin L-A** (Wyeth-Ayerst)	**Injection:** 300,000 units per ml	In 10 ml vials.[2]
		600,000 units/dose	In 1 ml Tubex.[2]
		1,200,000 units/dose	In 2 ml Tubex.[2]
		2,400,000 units/dose	In 4 ml syringe.[2]
Rx	**Permapen** (Roerig)	**Injection:** 1,200,000 units per dose	In 2 ml Isoject.[3]

[2] With lecithin, povidone, methyl and propyl parabens.

[3] With lecithin, methyl and propyl parabens.

PENICILLIN G BENZATHINE AND PROCAINE COMBINED

For complete prescribing information, refer to the Penicillins group monograph.

Indications:

Treatment of moderately severe infections due to microorganisms that are susceptible to the serum levels of penicillin G achievable with this dosage form. Guide therapy by bacteriological studies and clinical response. When high, sustained serum levels are required, use IV or IM aqueous penicillin G (potassium or sodium). This drug should not be used in the treatment of venereal diseases, including syphilis and gonorrhea, or yaws, bejel and pinta. The following infections will usually respond to adequate doses of this drug:

Streptococcal infections: Moderately severe to severe infections of the upper respiratory tract, skin and soft tissue infections, scarlet fever and erysipelas.

Pneumococcal infections: Moderately severe pneumonia and otitis media.

Administration and Dosage:

Administer by deep IM injection in the upper outer quadrant of the buttock. In infants and small children, the midlateral aspect of the thigh may be preferable. When doses are repeated, rotate the injection site.

Streptococcal infections: Streptococci in groups A, C, G, H, L and M are very sensitive to penicillin G. Other groups, including group D (enterococci), are resistant. Penicillin G sodium or potassium is recommended for streptococcal infections with bacteremia.

Treatment with the recommended dosage is usually given in a single session using multiple IM sites when indicated. An alternative dosage schedule may be used, giving half the total dose on day 1 and half on day 3. This will also ensure adequate serum levels over a 10 day period; however, use only when the patient's cooperation can be assured.

Adults and children (> 60 lbs; 27 kg) – 2.4 million units.
Children (30 to 60 lbs; 14 to 27 kg) – 900,000 to 1.2 million units.
Infants and children (< 30 lbs; 14 kg) – 600,000 units.

Pneumococcal infections (except pneumococcal meningitis):

Children – 600,000 units.

Adults – 1.2 million units. Repeat every 2 or 3 days until the patient has been afebrile for 48 hours. Severe pneumonia, empyema, bacteremia, pericarditis, meningitis, peritonitis and arthritis of pneumococcal etiology are better treated with aqueous penicillin G during the acute stage.

Storage: Refrigerate.

Rx	**Bicillin C-R** (Wyeth-Ayerst)	**Injection:** 300,000 units/ml (150,000 units each penicillin G benzathine and penicillin G procaine)	In 10 ml vials.[1]
		600,000 units/dose (300,000 units each penicillin G benzathine and penicillin G procaine)	In 1 ml Tubex.[1]
		1,200,000 units/dose	In 2 ml Tubex.[1]
		2,400,000 units/dose	In 4 ml syringe.[1]
Rx	**Bicillin C-R 900/300** (Wyeth-Ayerst)	**Injection:** 900,000 units penicillin G benzathine and 300,000 units penicillin G procaine per dose	In 2 ml Tubex.[1]

[1] With parabens, lecithin and povidone.

Natural Penicillins

PENICILLIN V (Phenoxymethyl Penicillin)

For complete prescribing information, refer to the Penicillins group monograph.

Administration and Dosage:

250 mg = 400,000 units.

Each g of penicillin V potassium contains 2.6 mmol (2.6 mEq) potassium.

Severe pneumonia, empyema, bacteremia, pericarditis, meningitis and arthritis should not be treated with oral penicillin V during the acute stage.

Streptococci in groups A, C, G, H, L and M are very sensitive to penicillin. Other groups, including group D (enterococci), are resistant.

An increasing number of strains of staphylococci are resistant to penicillin G (and V), emphasizing the need for culture and susceptibility studies.

Adults: 125 to 500 mg 4 times a day; in renal impairment (creatinine clearance, ≤ 10 ml/min) – Do not exceed 250 mg every 6 hours.

Children: 25 to 50 mg/kg/day in divided doses every 6 to 8 hours.

Penicilliln V Uses and Dosages

Organisms/Infections	Dosage
Labeled uses:	
Streptococcal infections: Infections of the upper respiratory tract, including scarlet fever and mild erysipelas	125 to 250 mg every 6 to 8 hours for 10 days for mild to moderately severe infections
Pharyngitis in children	250 mg 2 times daily for 10 days
Otitis media and sinusitis	250 to 500 mg every 6 hours for 2 weeks
Prevention of bacterial endocarditis[1]: As an alternative regimen to amoxicillin for patients undergoing dental, oral, esophageal or respiratory tract procedures	(see ampicillin monograph for alternate regimen) Alternate regimen - see ampicillin Penicillin allergy - see clindamycin, cephalexin, cefadroxil, azithromycin or clarithromycin
Pneumococcal infections: Mild to moderately severe respiratory tract infections including otitis media	250 to 500 mg every 6 hours until afebrile at least 2 days
Staphylococcal infections: Mild infections of skin and soft tissue	250 to 500 mg every 6 to 8 hours
Fusospirochetosis (Vincent's infection) of the oropharynx: Mild to moderately severe infections	250 to 500 mg every 6 to 8 hours
Unlabeled uses:	
Prophylactic treatment of children with sickle cell anemia (to reduce the incidence of *S pneumoniae* septicemia)	125 mg 2 times daily
Anaerobic infections: Mild to moderate infections	250 mg 4 times daily
Lyme disease (Borrelia burgdorferi):	
Erythema chronicum migrans:	
Pregnant or lactating women, tetracycline treatment failures	250 to 500 mg 4 times a day for 10 to 20 days
Children < 2 years of age	50 mg/kg/day (up to 2 g/day) in 4 divided doses for 10 to 20 days
Neurologic complications (eg, meningitis, encephalitis), carditis, arthritis	Use penicillin G IV

[1] American Heart Association Statement. *JAMA* 1997;277:1794-1801.

Storage/Stability: Reconstituted oral suspension is stable for 24 to 48 hours at room temperature (not exceeding 25°C; 77°F.)

Natural Penicillins

PENICILLIN V (Phenoxymethyl Penicillin)

Rx	**V-Cillin K** (Lilly)	**Tablets:** 125 mg	Lactose. In 100s.
Rx	**Penicillin VK** (Various, eg, Dixon-Shane, Major, Mylan, Parmed, Rugby, URL, Warner Chilcott)	**Tablets:** 250 mg	In 100s and 1000s.
Rx	**Beepen-VK** (SK-Beecham)		Lactose. In 1000s.
Rx	**Betapen-VK** (Apothecon)		Lactose. Film coated. In 100s and 1000s.
Rx	**Ledercillin VK** (Lederle)		Lactose. (L10 LL). White, scored. In 100s, 1000s and unit-of-issue 480s.
Rx	**Pen-V** (Goldline)		White. Oval or round. In 100s and 1000s.
Rx	**Pen•Vee K** (Wyeth-Ayerst)		Lactose. (Wyeth 59). White, scored. In 100s, 500s and UD 100s.
Rx	**Robicillin VK** (Robins)		In 100s and 1000s.
Rx	**V-Cillin K** (Lilly)		Lactose. In 100s and 500s.
Rx	**Veetids '250'** (Apothecon)		Lactose. Film coated. In 100s and 1000s.
Rx	**Penicillin VK** (Various, eg, Dixon-Shane, Geneva Marsam, Major, Mylan, Parmed, Rugby, URL, Warner Chilcott)	**Tablets:** 500 mg	In 100s, 500s, 1000s and UD 100s.
Rx	**Beepen-VK** (SK-Beecham)		Lactose. In 500s.
Rx	**Betapen-VK** (Apothecon)		Lactose. Film coated. In 100s and 500s.
Rx	**Ledercillin VK** (Lederle)		(L9 LL). White, scored. In 100s and 500s.
Rx	**Pen-V** (Goldline)		White. Oval or round. In 100s and 1000s.
Rx	**Pen•Vee K** (Wyeth-Ayerst)		(Wyeth 390). White, scored. In 100s, 500s and UD 100s.
Rx	**V-Cillin K** (Lilly)		Lactose. In 100s and 500s.
Rx	**Veetids '500'** (Apothecon)		Lactose. Film coated. In 100s and 1000s.
Rx	**Penicillin VK** (Various, eg, Major, Rugby, URL, Warner Chilcott)	**Powder for Oral Solution:** 125 mg per 5 ml when reconstituted	In 100 and 200 ml.
Rx	**Beepen-VK** (SK-Beecham)		Saccharin, sucrose. In 100 and 200 ml.
Rx	**Betapen-VK** (Apothecon)		DL-menthol, saccharin, sucrose. In 100 and 200 ml.
Rx	**Pen•Vee K** (Wyeth-Ayerst)		Saccharin, sucrose. In 100 and 200 ml.
Rx	**V-Cillin K** (Lilly)		Saccharin, sucrose. In 100, 150 and 200 ml.
Rx	**Veetids '125'** (Apothecon)		DL-menthol, saccharin, sucrose. In 100 and 200 ml.

Natural Penicillins

PENICILLIN V (Phenoxymethyl Penicillin)

Rx	**Penicillin VK** (Various, eg, Rugby, URL, Warner Chilcott)	**Powder for Oral Solution:** 250 mg per 5 ml when reconstituted	In 100 and 200 ml.
Rx	**Beepen-VK** (SK-Beecham)		Saccharin, sucrose. In 100 and 200 ml.
Rx	**Betapen-VK** (Apothecon)		DL-menthol, saccharin, sucrose. In 100 and 200 ml.
Rx	**Ledercillin VK** (Lederle)		Saccharin, sugar. Cherry flavor. In 100, 150 and 200 ml.
Rx	**Pen•Vee K** (Wyeth-Ayerst)		Saccharin, sucrose. In 100, 150 and 200 ml.
Rx	**V-Cillin K** (Lilly)		Saccharin, sucrose. In 100, 150 and 200 ml.
Rx	**Veetids '250'** (Apothecon)		DL-menthol, saccharin, sucrose. In 100 and 200 ml.

Penicillinase-Resistant Penicillins

METHICILLIN SODIUM

Complete prescribing information for these products begins in the Penicillins group monograph.

Indications:

Treatment of infections due to penicillinase-producing staphylococci. May be used to initiate therapy when a staphylococcal infection is suspected. (See Indications in the group monograph concerning use of penicillinase-resistant penicillins.)

Oral penicillinase-resistant penicillins should not be used as initial therapy. Oral therapy may be used as follow-up therapy as soon as the clinical condition warrants.

Administration and Dosage:

IM: Take care to avoid sciatic nerve injury.

IV: Take care due to possibility of thrombophlebitis, especially in the elderly.

Treatment of osteomyelitis and endocarditis may require a longer term of intensive therapy.

Adults: 4 to 12 g/day in divided doses every 4 to 6 hours; in severe renal impairment (creatinine clearance ≤ 10 ml/min) do not exceed 2 g every 12 hours.

Children: 100 to 300 mg/kg/day in divided doses every 4 to 6 hours.

Infants:

Over 7 days and > 2000 g – 100 mg/kg/day in divided doses every 6 hours; for meningitis – 200 mg/kg/day.

Over 7 days and < 2000 g – 75 mg/kg/day in divided doses every 8 hours; for meningitis – 150 mg/kg/day.

Under 7 days and > 2000 g – 75 mg/kg/day in divided doses every 8 hours; for meningitis – 150 mg/kg/day.

Under 7 days and < 2000 g – 50 mg/kg/day in divided doses every 12 hours; for meningitis – 100 mg/kg/day.

Preparation of solutions: Reconstitute with Sterile Water for Injection or Sodium Chloride Injection. If another agent is used in conjunction with methicillin therapy, do not physically mix with methicillin, but administer separately.

IM – Dilute as indicated in the table below. Each reconstituted ml contains approximately 500 mg methicillin.

Methicillin IM Administration Dilution	
Vial size	Minimum amount of diluent
1 g	1.5 ml
4 g	5.7 ml
6 g	8.6 ml

IV administration – Dilute each ml of reconstituted solution with 25 ml Sodium Chloride Injection.

Reconstitute piggyback units according to manufacturer's product label.

Compatible IV solutions: The drug will lose < 10% activity at room temperature (21°C; 70°F) during an 8 hour period when given in the solutions listed below. Dilute methicillin for IV infusion only in these solutions: 5% Dextrose in Normal Saline; 10% D-Fructose in Water or in Normal Saline; Lactated Potassic Saline Injection; 5% Plasma Hydrolysate in Water; 10% Invert Sugar in Normal Saline‡; 10% Invert Sugar plus 0.3% Potassium Chloride in Water; *Travert* 10% Electrolyte #1, #2 or #3.

Rx	**Staphcillin** (Apothecon)	**Powder for Injection:** (Contains 3 mEq sodium/g) 1 g	In vials and piggyback vials.
		4 g	In vials.
		6 g	In vials.
		10 g	In bulk vials.

‡ At a concentration of 2 mg/ml, methicillin is stable for only 4 hours. Concentrations between 10 and 30 mg/ml are stable for 8 hours.

Penicillinase-Resistant Penicillins

NAFCILLIN SODIUM

Complete prescribing information for these products begins in the Penicillins group monograph.

Indications:

The treatment of infections due to penicillinase-producing staphylococci. They may be used to initiate therapy in any patient in whom a staphylococcal infection is suspected. (See Indications in the group monograph for use of penicillinase-resistant penicillins.)

Administration and Dosage:

Use parenteral therapy initially in severe infections. Very severe infections may require very high doses. Change to oral therapy as condition warrants.

Parenteral: IV: 3 to 6 g per 24 hours. Use this route for short-term therapy (24 to 48 hours) because of occasional occurrence of thrombophlebitis, particularly in the elderly.

IM – Adults – 500 mg every 4 to 6 hours.

Infants and children – 25 mg/kg twice daily.

Neonates – 10 mg/kg twice daily. Other suggested doses include: Weight < 2000 g – 50 mg/kg/day divided every 12 hours (age < 7 days) or 75 mg/kg/day divided every 8 hours (age > 7 days).

Weight > 2000 g – 50 mg/kg/day divided every 8 hours (age < 7 days) or 75 mg/kg/day divided every 6 hours (age > 7 days).

Oral: Serum levels of nafcillin after oral administration are low and unpredictable.

Adults – 250 to 500 mg every 4 to 6 hours for mild to moderate infections. In severe infections – 1 g every 4 to 6 hours.

Children –

Staph infections: 50 mg/kg/day in 4 divided doses. For neonates, 10 mg/kg 3 to 4 times daily. If inadequate, change to parenteral nafcillin sodium.

Scarlet fever and pneumonia: 25 mg/kg/day in 4 divided doses.

Streptococcal pharyngitis: 250 mg, 3 times daily for 10 days. (Penicillin V is the drug of choice for streptococcal infections.)

Preparation of solutions: IV – Dilute in 15 to 30 ml Sterile Water for Injection or Sodium Chloride for Injection; inject over 5 to 10 min. or longer. Stability studies show that nafcillin sodium at concentrations of 2 to 40 mg/ml loses < 10% activity at 21°C (70°F) for 24 hours or at 4°C (40°F) for 96 hours in the following IV solutions: Isotonic sodium chloride; Sterile Water for Injection; 5% Dextrose in Water; 5% Dextrose in 0.4% Sodium Chloride Solution; Ringer's Solution; M/6 Sodium Lactate Solution. Discard unused portions of IV solution after time period stated. Use only those solutions listed above for IV infusion. Concentration of the antibiotic should be within the range of 2 to 40 mg/ml.

IM – Reconstitute with Sterile Water for Injection or Sodium Chloride Injection. Administer clear solution immediately by deep intragluteal injection. After reconstitution, refrigerate (2° to 8°C; 36° to 46°F) and use within 7 days or keep at room temperature (25°C; 77°F) and use within 3 days or keep frozen (– 20°C; – 4°F) for up to 3 months.

Penicillinase-Resistant Penicillins

NAFCILLIN SODIUM

Rx	**Unipen** (Wyeth-Ayerst)	**Tablets:** 500 mg	(Wyeth 464). White, scored. Film coated. Capsule shape. In 50s.
Rx	**Unipen** (Wyeth-Ayerst)	**Capsules:** 250 mg	(Wyeth 57). Green and yellow. In 100s.
Rx	**Nafcillin Sodium** (Geneva Marsam)	**Powder for Injection:** 500 mg[1]	In vials.
Rx	**Nafcil** (Apothecon)		In vials.
Rx	**Nallpen** (SK-Beecham)		In vials.
Rx	**Unipen** (Wyeth-Ayerst)		In vials.
Rx	**Nafcillin Sodium** (Geneva Marsam)	**Powder for Injection:** 1 g[1]	In vials, piggyback and *ADD-Vantage vials.*
Rx	**Nafcil** (Apothecon)		In vials, piggyback vials and *ADD-Vantage vials.*
Rx	**Nallpen** (SK-Beecham)		In vials, piggyback and *ADD-Vantage vials.*
Rx	**Unipen** (Wyeth-Ayerst)		In vials, piggyback and *ADD-Vantage vials.*
Rx	**Nafcillin Sodium** (Geneva Marsam)	**Powder for Injection:** 2 g[1]	In vials, piggyback and *ADD-Vantage vials.*
Rx	**Nafcil** (Apothecon)		In vials, piggyback and *ADD-Vantage vials.*
Rx	**Nallpen** (SK-Beecham)		In vials, piggyback and *ADD-Vantage vials.*
Rx	**Unipen** (Wyeth-Ayerst)		In vials, piggyback and *ADD-Vantage vials.*
Rx	**Nafcillin Sodium** (Geneva Marsam)	**Powder for Injection:** 10 g[1]	In bulk package.
Rx	**Nafcil** (Apothecon)		In bulk package.
Rx	**Nallpen** (SK-Beecham)		In bulk package.
Rx	**Unipen** (Wyeth-Ayerst)		In bulk package.

[1] Contains 2.9 mEq sodium/gram.

Penicillinase-Resistant Penicillins

OXACILLIN SODIUM

For complete prescribing information, refer to the Penicillins group monograph.

Indications:

Treatment of infections due to penicillinase-producing staphylococci. May be used to initiate therapy when a staphylococcal infection is suspected. (See Indications in the group monograph concerning use of penicillinase-resistant penicillins.)

Administration and Dosage:

Oral:

Mild to moderate infections of skin, soft tissue or upper respiratory tract –

Adults and children (> 20 kg): 500 mg every 4 to 6 hrs for at least 5 days.

Children (< 20 kg): 50 mg/kg/day in divided doses every 6 hrs for at least 5 days.

In serious or life-threatening infections, such as staphylococcal septicemia or other deep-seated severe infection – Following initial parenteral treatment, oral oxacillin may be given for follow-up therapy. Continue therapy 1 to 2 weeks after the patient is afebrile and cultures are sterile. Treatment of osteomyelitis may require several months of intensive therapy.

Adults: 1 g every 4 to 6 hours.

Children: ≥ 100 mg/kg/day in equally divided doses every 4 to 6 hours.

Parenteral: Consider for patients who are unable to take oral form. Oral use is most appropriate as prolonged follow-up therapy after successful initial parenteral use.

Mild to moderate upper respiratory or localized skin or soft tissue infections –

Adults and children (≥ 40 kg): 250 to 500 mg every 4 to 6 hours.

Children (< 40 kg): 50 mg/kg/day in equally divided doses every 6 hours.

Absorption and excretion data indicate that 25 mg/kg/day in prematures and neonates provided adequate therapeutic levels.

Severe infections (lower respiratory tract or disseminated infections) –

Adults and children (≥ 40 kg): ≥ 1 g every 4 to 6 hours.

Children (< 40 kg): ≥ 100 mg/kg/day in equally divided doses every 4 to 6 hrs.

Very severe infections may require very high doses and prolonged therapy. Maximum daily dose for adults is 12 g/day and for children 100 to 300 mg/kg/day.

Other suggested doses for children and neonates include –

Children: 50 to 100 mg/kg/day divided every 6 hours.

Neonates: Weight < 2000 g – 50 mg/kg/day divided every 12 hours (age < 7 days) or 100 mg/kg/day divided every 8 hours (age > 7 days).

Weight > 2000 g: 75 mg/kg/day divided every 8 hours (age < 7 days) or 150 mg/kg/day divided every 6 hours (age > 7 days).

Preparation of solutions: Reconstitute vials only with Sterile Water for Injection or Sodium Chloride (normal saline) Injection in the appropriate volume.

IM – Reconstitute to a dilution of 250 mg/1.5 ml. Discard unused solution after 3 days at room temperature (21°C; 70°F) or 7 days under refrigeration (4°C; 40°F).

Direct IV – Reconstitute with Sterile Water for Injection or Sodium Chloride Injection. Administer slowly over approximately 10 minutes to avoid vein irritation.

Continuous IV – Prior to diluting with IV solution, reconstitute as directed.

IV solutions: Use only the solutions listed below for IV infusions. At concentrations from 0.5 to 40 mg/ml, these dilutions are stable at least 6 hours at room temperature: 5% Dextrose in Normal Saline; 10% D-Fructose in Water or Normal Saline; Lactated Potassic Saline Injections; 10% Invert Sugar in Normal Saline; 10% Invert Sugar plus 0.3% Potassium Chloride in Water; *Travert* 10% Electrolyte #1, #2 or #3.

Rx	**Oxacillin Sodium** (Various, eg, Geneva, Major, Marsam, Rugby, Schein)	**Capsules:** 250 mg	In 100s.
Rx	**Bactocill** (SK-Beecham)		Lactose. (BMP 143). In 100s.
Rx	**Prostaphlin** (Apothecon)		In 48s, 100s and UD 100s.
Rx	**Oxacillin Sodium** (Various, eg, Geneva, Major, Rugby, Schein)	**Capsules:** 500 mg	In 100s.
Rx	**Bactocill** (SK-Beecham)		Lactose. (BMP 144). In 100s.
Rx	**Prostaphlin** (Apothecon)		In 48s, 100s and UD 100s.
Rx	**Prostaphlin** (Apothecon)	**Powder for Oral Solution:** 250 mg/5 ml when reconstituted	Saccharin, sucrose. In 100 ml.

Penicillinase-Resistant Penicillins

OXACILLIN SODIUM

Rx	**Oxacillin Sodium**[1](Apothecon)	**Powder for Injection:** 250 mg	In vials.
Rx	**Bactocill**[2] (SK-Beecham)		In vials.
Rx	**Oxacillin Sodium**[1] (Apothecon)	**Powder for Injection:** 500 mg	In vials.
Rx	**Bactocill**[2](SK-Beecham)		In vials.
Rx	**Prostaphlin** (Apothecon)		In vials.
Rx	**Oxacillin Sodium**[1] (Apothecon)	**Powder for Injection:** 1 g	In vials and piggyback vials.
Rx	**Bactocill**[2] (SK-Beecham)		In vials, piggyback and *Add-Vantage* vials.
Rx	**Prostaphlin** (Apothecon)		In vials and piggyback vials.
Rx	**Oxacillin Sodium**[1] (Apothecon)	**Powder for Injection:** 2 g	In vials and piggyback vials.
Rx	**Bactocill**[2] (SK-Beecham)		In vials, piggyback and *Add-Vantage* vials.
Rx	**Prostaphlin** (Apothecon)		In vials and piggyback vials.
Rx	**Oxacillin Sodium**[1] (Apothecon)	**Powder for Injection:** 4 g	In vials.
Rx	**Bactocill**[2] (SK-Beecham)		In bulk vials.
Rx	**Prostaphlin** (Apothecon)		In vials.
Rx	**Oxacillin Sodium**[1] (Apothecon)	**Powder for Injection:** 10 g	In bulk vials.
Rx	**Bactocill**[2](SK-Beecham)		In bulk vials.
Rx	**Prostaphlin** (Apothecon)		In bulk vials.

[1] Contains 2.5 mEq sodium/g.
[2] Contains 3.1 mEq sodium/g.

DICLOXACILLIN SODIUM

For complete prescribing information, refer to the Penicillins group monograph.

Indications:

Treatment of infections due to penicillinase-producing staphylococci. May be used to initiate therapy when a staphylococcal infection is suspected. (See Indications in the group monograph concerning use of penicillinase-resistant penicillins.)

Administration and Dosage:

For mild to moderate upper respiratory and localized skin and soft tissue infections:

Adults and children (> 40 kg) – 125 mg every 6 hours.

Children (< 40 kg) – 12.5 mg/kg/day in equal doses every 6 hours.

For more severe infections, such as lower respiratory tract or disseminated infections:

Adults and children (> 40 kg) – 250 mg every 6 hours.

Children (< 40 kg) – 25 mg/kg/day in equally divided doses every 6 hours.

Another suggested dosage for children is 12 to 25 mg/kg/day divided every 6 hours.

Use in the newborn is not recommended.

Storage/Stability: When the reconstituted oral solution is stored in polypropylene oral syringes for unit dose purposes, it is stable for 7 days (ambient conditions), 10 days (refrigerated) and 21 days (frozen). The manufacturer states a 14 day stability when reconstituted and refrigerated in its original container.

Penicillinase-Resistant Penicillins

DICLOXACILLIN SODIUM

Rx	**Dynapen** (Apothecon)	**Capsules:** 125 mg	Lactose. In 24s and 100s.
Rx	**Dicloxacillin Sodium** (Various, eg, Apothecon, Geneva, Lederle, Goldline, Major, Moore, Rugby, URL, Warner-Chilcott)	**Capsules:** 250 mg	In 100s.
Rx	**Dycill** (SK-Beecham)		Lactose. In 100s.
Rx	**Dynapen** (Apothecon)		Lactose. In 24s, 100s and UD 100s.
Rx	**Pathocil** (Wyeth-Ayerst)		Lactose. Purple and white. (Wyeth 360). In 100s.
Rx	**Dicloxacillin Sodium** (Various, eg, Apothecon, Geneva, Goldline, Lederle, Major, Moore, Rugby, URL, Warner-Chilcott)	**Capsules:** 500 mg	In 40s and 100s.
Rx	**Dycill** (SK-Beecham)		In 100s.
Rx	**Dynapen** (Apothecon)		Lactose. In 50s.
Rx	**Pathocil** (Wyeth-Ayerst)		Lactose. Purple and white. (Wyeth 593). In 50s.
Rx	**Dynapen** (Apothecon)	**Powder for Oral Suspension:** 62.5 mg/5 ml reconstituted[1]	In 80, 100 and 200 ml.
Rx	**Pathocil** (Wyeth-Ayerst)		In 100 ml.

[1] With saccharin and sucrose.

CLOXACILLIN SODIUM

For complete prescribing information, refer to the Penicillins group monograph.

Indications:

Treatment of infections due to penicillinase-producing staphylococci. May be used to initiate therapy when a staphylococcal infection is suspected. (See Indications in the group monograph concerning use of penicillinase-resistant penicillins.)

Administration and Dosage:

Mild to moderate upper respiratory and localized skin and soft tissue infections:
Adults and children (> 20 kg) – 250 mg every 6 hours.
Children (< 20 kg) – 50 mg/kg/day in equally divided doses every 6 hours.

Severe infections (lower respiratory tract or disseminated infections):
Adults and children (> 20 kg) – ≥ 500 mg every 6 hours.
Children (< 20 kg) – ≥ 100 mg/kg/day in equal doses every 6 hours.

Another suggested dosage for infants and children is 50 to 100 mg/kg/day, up to a maximum of 4 g/day, divided every 6 hours.

Rx	**Cloxacillin Sodium** (Various, eg, Biocraft, Geneva, Major, Rugby, Schein, Warner-Chilcott)	**Capsules:** 250 mg	In 100s.
Rx	**Cloxapen** (SK-Beecham)		In 100s.
Rx	**Tegopen** (Apothecon)		In 100s.
Rx	**Cloxacillin Sodium** (Various, eg, Biocraft, Geneva, Major, Rugby, Schein, Warner-C)	**Capsules:** 500 mg	In 100s.
Rx	**Cloxapen** (SK-Beecham)		In 100s.
Rx	**Tegopen** (Apothecon)		In 100s.
Rx	**Cloxacillin Sodium** (Various, eg, Biocraft, Major, Rugby, Warner-Chilcott)	**Powder for Oral Solution:** 125 mg per 5 ml when reconstituted	In 100 and 200 ml.
Rx	**Tegopen** (Apothecon)		In 100 and 200 ml.[1]

[1] With saccharin and sucrose.

Aminopenicillins

AMPICILLIN

For complete prescribing information for these products begins in the Penicillins group monograph.

Indications:

Treatment of infections caused by susceptible strains of *Shigella, Salmonella* (including *S typhosa*), *Escherichia coli, Hemophilus influenzae, Proteus mirabilis, Neisseria gonorrhoeae* and enterococci. It is also effective in the treatment of meningitis due to *N meningitidis* and in infections caused by susceptible gram-positive organisms: Penicillin G-sensitive staphylococci, streptococci and pneumococci.

Ampicillin Uses and Dosages	
Organisms/Infections	Dosage
Labeled uses: *Respiratory tract and soft tissue infections:*	Parenteral: Patients ≥ 40 kg – 250 to 500 mg every 6 hours; < 40 kg – 25 to 50 mg/kg/day in divided doses at 6 to 8 hour intervals. Oral: Patients ≥ 20 kg – 250 mg every 6 hours; < 20 kg – 50 mg/kg/day in divided doses at 6 to 8 hour intervals.
Bacterial meningitis: H influenzae, S pneumoniae or *N meningitidis*	8 to 14 g/day (100 to 200 mg/kg/day for children) in divided doses every 3 to 4 hours. Initial treatment is usually by IV drip, followed by frequent (every 3 to 4 hour) IM injections.
Septicemia:	Parenteral: 150 to 200 mg/kg/day. Give IV at least 3 days; continue IM every 3 to 4 hrs.
Gonococcal infections:[1] Disseminated gonococcal infection (hospitalization recommended)	When the infecting organism is proven to be penicillin-sensitive, parenteral treatment may be switched to ampicillin 1 g every 6 hours (or equivalent).
Rape victims (prophylaxis of infection): Alternative regimen for pregnant women or when tetracycline is contraindicated.	3.5 g orally with 1 g probenecid.
Prevention of bacterial endocarditis:[2]: As an alternative to amoxicillin, or for patients unable to take oral medications undergoing dental, oral, esophageal or respiratory tract procedures.	2 g (50 mg/kg for children) IM or IV within 30 minutes before procedure.
As an alternative to amoxicillin or in combination with gentamicin B or high-risk patients undergoing genitourinary or nonesophageal gastrointestinal procedures	*Moderate risk*: 2 g (50 mg/kg for children) IM or IV within 30 minutes of starting the procedure. *High-risk*: 2 g (50 mg/kg not to exceed 2 g in children) IM or IV plus gentamicin 1.5 mg/kg (not to exceed 120 mg in adults) within 30 minutes of starting procedure; 6 hours later, ampicillin 1 g (25 mg/kg for children) IM or IV or amoxicillin 1 g (25 mg/kg for children) orally.
Unlabeled use: Prophylaxis in cesarean section in certain high risk patients	Single IV dose, administered immediately after cord clamping.

[1] CDC 1989 Sexually Transmitted Diseases Treatment Guidelines. *Morbidity and Mortality Weekly Report* 1989 Sept. 1;38(No.S-8):1-43

[2] American Heart Association Statement. *JAMA* 1997;277:1794-1801

Administration and Dosage:

Reserve parenteral form (IM or IV) for moderately severe and severe infections and for patients unable to take oral medication. Change to oral therapy as soon as appropriate.

Renal impairment: Increase dosing interval to 12 hours in severe renal impairment (creatinine clearance ≤ 10 ml/min).

In the treatment of chronic urinary tract and intestinal infections, frequent bacteriologic and clinical appraisal is necessary. Higher doses should be used for persistent or severe infections. In persistent infections, therapy may be required for several

Aminopenicillins

AMPICILLIN

weeks. It may be necessary to continue clinical or bacteriologic follow-up for several months after cessation of therapy.

In the treatment of complications of gonorrheal urethritis, such as prostatitis and epididymitis, prolonged and intensive therapy is recommended. Cases of gonorrhea with a suspected primary lesion of syphilis should have dark-field examinations before receiving treatment. In all other cases where concomitant syphilis is suspected, perform monthly serologic tests for a minimum of 4 months.

Adults: 1 to 12 g daily in divided doses every 4 to 6 hours.

Children: 50 to 200 mg/kg/day in divided doses every 4 to 6 hours.

Infants (over 7 days and > 2000 g) – 100 mg/kg/day in divided doses every 6 hours (meningitis 200 mg/kg/day).

Over 7 days and < 2000 g – 75 mg/kg/day in divided doses every 8 hours (meningitis 150 mg/kg/day).

Under 7 days and > 2000 g – 75 mg/kg/day in divided doses every 8 hours (meningitis 150 mg/kg/day).

Under 7 days and < 2000 g – 50 mg/kg/day in divided doses every 12 hours (meningitis 100 mg/kg/day).

Preparation of solutions: Use only freshly prepared solutions. Administer IM and IV injections within 1 hour after preparation since the potency may decrease significantly after this period. Reconstitute with Sterile or Bacteriostatic Water for Injection (piggyback vials may be reconstituted with Sodium Chloride Injection).

Direct IV administration – Administer slowly over at least 10 to 15 minutes.

Caution: More rapid administration may result in convulsive seizures.

IV drip (standard vials) – Dilute as above for direct IV use prior to further dilution with compatible IV solutions.

IV drip (piggyback vials) – After reconstitution, administer alone or further dilute with suitable IV solutions. To assure compatibility and stability of ampicillin solutions for IV use, use only the solutions specified below:

IV Solutions Compatible with Ampicillin

IV solution	Concentrations up to (mg/ml)	Stability (hours)
0.9% Sodium Chloride	30	8
5% Dextrose in Water	2	4
5% Dextrose in Water	10-20	2
5% Dextrose in 0.45% Sodium Chloride Solution	2	4
10% Invert Sugar in Water	2	4
M/6 Sodium Lactate Solution	30	8
Lactated Ringer's Solution	30	8
Sterile Water for Injection	30	8

Stability studies on ampicillin sodium in various IV solutions indicate that the drug will lose < 10% activity at room temperature (21°C; 70°F) for the time periods and concentrations stated.

Oral: Reconstituted oral solution is stable for 7 days at room temperature (not exceeding 25°C; 77°F).

AMPICILLIN WITH PROBENECID

For complete prescribing information, refer to the Penicillins group monograph.

Indications:

Treatment of uncomplicated infections (urethral, endocervical or rectal) caused by *Neisseria gonorrhoeae* in adults.

Administration and Dosage:

Administer 3.5 g ampicillin and 1 g probenecid as a single dose.

Rx	**Polycillin-PRB** (Apothecon)	**Powder For Oral Suspension:** 3.5 g ampicillin (as trihydrate) & 1 g probenecid per bottle	In single-dose bottles.
Rx	**Probampacin** (Various, eg, Goldline, Schein)		In single-dose bottles.

Aminopenicillins

AMPICILLIN SODIUM, PARENTERAL

For complete prescribing information, refer to the Penicillins group monograph.
(Contains 3 mEq sodium/g.)

Rx	**Ampicillin Sodium** (Various, eg, Apothecon, Elkins-Sinn, Geneva Marsam)	**Powder for Injection:** 125 mg	In vials.
Rx	**Omnipen-N** (Wyeth-Ayerst)		In vials and *ADD-Vantage* vials.
Rx	**Polycillin-N** (Apothecon)		In vials.
Rx	**Ampicillin Sodium** (Various, eg, Apothecon, Elkins-Sinn, Geneva Marsam)	**Powder for Injection:** 250 mg	In vials.
Rx	**Omnipen-N** (Wyeth-Ayerst)		In vials and *ADD-Vantage* vials.
Rx	**Polycillin-N** (Apothecon)		In vials.
Rx	**Totacillin-N** (SK-Beecham)		In vials.
Rx	**Ampicillin Sodium** (Various, eg, Apothecon, Elkins-Sinn, Geneva Marsam, Lilly)	**Powder for Injection:** 500 mg	In vials and piggyback vials.
Rx	**Omnipen-N** (Wyeth-Ayerst)		In vials, piggyback and *ADD-Vantage* vials.
Rx	**Polycillin-N** (Apothecon)		In vials
Rx	**Totacillin-N** (SK-Beecham)		In vials and piggyback vials.
Rx	**Ampicillin Sodium** (Various, eg, Apothecon, Elkins-Sinn, Geneva Marsam)	**Powder for Injection:** 1 g	In vials and piggyback vials.
Rx	**Omnipen-N** (Wyeth-Ayerst)		In vials, piggyback and *ADD-Vantage* vials.
Rx	**Polycillin-N** (Apothecon)		In vials and piggyback vials.
Rx	**Totacillin-N** (SK-Beecham)		In vials, piggyback and *ADD-Vantage* vials.
Rx	**Ampicillin Sodium** (Various, eg, Apothecon, Elkins-Sinn, Geneva Marsam)	**Powder for Injection:** 2 g	In vials and piggyback vials.
Rx	**Omnipen-N** (Wyeth-Ayerst)		In vials, piggyback and *ADD-Vantage* vials.
Rx	**Polycillin-N** (Apothecon)		In vials and piggyback vials.
Rx	**Totacillin-N** (SK-Beecham)		In vials, piggyback and *ADD-Vantage* vials.
Rx	**Ampicillin Sodium** (Various, eg, Apothecon, Elkins-Sinn, Geneva Marsam)	**Powder for Injection:** 10 g bulk	In vials.
Rx	**Omnipen-N** (Wyeth-Ayerst)		In vials.
Rx	**Polycillin-N** (Apothecon)		In vials.
Rx	**Totacillin-N** (SK-Beecham)		In vials.

Aminopenicillins

AMPICILLIN, ORAL

For complete prescribing information, refer to the Penicillins group monograph.

Rx	**Ampicillin** (Various, eg, Dixon-Shane)	**Capsules:** 250 mg (as trihydrate)	In 28s, 40s, 100s, 500s, 1000s and UD 100s.
Rx	**Polycillin** (Apothecon)		In 100s, 500s, 1000s and UD 100s.
Rx	**Principen** (Apothecon)		(Squibb 971). Red/gray. In 100s, 500s and UD 100s.
Rx	**Totacillin** (SK-Beecham)		In 500s.
Rx	**Omnipen** (Wyeth-Ayerst)	**Capsules:** 250 mg (anhydrous)	Lactose. (Wyeth 53). Violet and pink. In 500s.
Rx	**Ampicillin** (Various, eg, Biocraft, Dixon-Shane, Geneva, Mylan, Parmed)	**Capsules:** 500 mg (as trihydrate)	In 21s, 28s, 40s, 100s, 500s, 1000s and UD 100s.
Rx	**D-Amp** (Dunhall)		In 100s.
Rx	**Marcillin** (Marnel)		In 100s.
Rx	**Polycillin** (Apothecon)		In 100s, 500s, UD 100s.
Rx	**Principen** (Apothecon)		(Squibb 974). Red/gray. In 100s, 500s and UD 100s.
Rx	**Totacillin** (SK-Beecham)		In 500s.
Rx	**Omnipen** (Wyeth-Ayerst)	**Capsules:** 500 mg (anhydrous)	Lactose. (Wyeth 309). Violet and pink. In 100s, 500s.
Rx	**Polycillin Pediatric Drops** (Apothecon)	**Powder for Oral Suspension:** 100 mg per ml (as trihydrate) when reconstituted	Sucrose. In 20 ml.
Rx	**Ampicillin** (Various, eg, Biocraft, Dixon-Shane, Mylan, Schein, URL, Warner-C)	**Powder for Oral Suspension:** 125 mg per 5 ml (as trihydrate) when reconstituted	In 80, 100, 150 and 200 ml.
Rx	**Omnipen** (Wyeth-Ayerst)		Sucrose. In 100, 150 and 200 ml.
Rx	**Polycillin** (Apothecon)		Sucrose. In 100, 150 and 200 ml and UD 5 ml (25s).
Rx	**Principen** (Apothecon)		Sucrose. In 100, 150 and 200 ml and UD 5 ml.
Rx	**Totacillin** (SK-Beecham)		Sucrose. In 100, 200 ml.
Rx	**Ampicillin** (Various, eg, Biocraft, Dixon-Shane, Major, Mylan, Rugby, Schein, URL, Warner Chilcott)	**Powder for Oral Suspension:** 250 mg per 5 ml (as trihydrate) when reconstituted	Sucrose. In 80, 100, 150 and 200 ml.
Rx	**Omnipen** (Wyeth-Ayerst)		Sucrose. In 100, 150 and 200 ml.
Rx	**Polycillin** (Apothecon)		Sucrose. In 100, 150 and 200 ml and UD 5 ml (25s).
Rx	**Principen** (Apothecon)		Sucrose. In 100, 150 and 200 ml and UD 5 ml.
Rx	**Totacillin** (SK-Beecham)		Sucrose. In 100, 200 ml.
Rx	**Polycillin** (Apothecon)	**Powder for Oral Suspension:** 500 mg per 5 ml (as trihydrate) when reconstituted	Sucrose. In 100 ml and UD 5 ml (25s).

Aminopenicillins

AMPICILLIN SODIUM AND SULBACTAM SODIUM

For complete prescribing information, refer to the Penicillins group monograph.

Actions:

Pharmacokinetics: Peak serum concentrations of ampicillin and sulbactam are attained immediately following a 15 minute IV infusion. Ampicillin serum levels are similar to those produced by the administration of equivalent amounts of ampicillin alone. Peak ampicillin serum levels ranging from 109 to 150 mcg/ml are attained after administration of 2000 mg ampicillin plus 1000 mg sulbactam and 40 to 71 mcg/ml after administration of 1000 mg ampicillin plus 500 mg sulbactam. The corresponding mean peak serum levels for sulbactam range from 48 to 88 mcg/ml and 21 to 40 mcg/ml, respectively. After an IM injection of 1000 mg ampicillin plus 500 mg sulbactam, peak ampicillin serum levels ranging from 8 to 37 mcg/ml and peak sulbactam serum levels ranging from 6 to 24 mcg/ml are attained. The mean serum half-life of both drugs is ≈ 1 hour in healthy volunteers.

Approximately 75% to 85% of both ampicillin and sulbactam is excreted unchanged in the urine during the first 8 hours after administration to individuals with normal renal function. Higher and more prolonged serum levels can be achieved with the coadministration of probenecid. Ampicillin is ≈ 28% reversibly bound to human serum protein and sulbactam is ≈ 38% reversibly bound.

Microbiology: A wide range of β-lactamases found in microorganisms resistant to penicillins and cephalosporins are irreversibly inhibited by sulbactam. Although sulbactam alone possesses little useful antibacterial activity except against Neisseriaceae, sulbactam restores ampicillin activity against β-lactamase producing strains. Sulbactam has good inhibitory activity against clinically important plasmid mediated β-lactamases most often responsible for transferred drug resistance. Sulbactam has no effect on the activity of ampicillin against ampicillin-susceptible strains.

The presence of sulbactam in the formulation effectively extends the antibiotic spectrum of ampicillin to include many bacteria normally resistant to it and to other β-lactam antibiotics. Thus, this combination possesses the properties of a broad-spectrum antibiotic and a β-lactamase inhibitor.

Indications:

For the treatment of infections due to susceptible strains of the microorganisms in the conditions listed below.

Skin and skin structure infections caused by β-lactamase producing strains of *Staphylococcus aureus, Escherichia coli,** *Klebsiella* sp* (includ. *K pneumoniae**), *Proteus mirabilis,** *Bacteroides fragilis,** *Enterobacter* sp* and *Acinetobacter calcoaceticus.**

Intra-abdominal infections caused by β-lactamase producing strains of *E coli, Klebsiella* sp (includ. *K pneumoniae**), *Bacteroides* (including *B fragilis*), *Enterobacter* sp.*

Gynecological infections caused by β-lactamase producing strains of *E coli** and *Bacteroides* sp* (including *B fragilis**).

While this combination is indicated only for the conditions listed above, infections caused by ampicillin-susceptible organisms are also amenable to treatment due to the ampicillin content. Therefore, mixed infections caused by ampicillin-susceptible organisms and β-lactamase producing organisms susceptible to this combination should not require the addition of another antibiotic.

Adverse Reactions:

Lab test abnormalities: Increased AST, ALT, alkaline phosphatase and LDH. Decreased hemoglobin, hematocrit, RBC, WBC, neutrophils, lymphocytes, platelets and increased lymphocytes, monocytes, basophils, eosinophils and platelets; decreased serum albumin and total proteins; increased BUN and creatinine; presence of RBCs and hyaline casts in urine.

Local: Pain at IM injection site (16%); pain at IV injection site, thrombophlebitis (3%).

Systemic:

Most frequent – Diarrhea (3%); rash (< 2%). In < 1% of patients: Itching; nausea; vomiting; candidiasis; fatigue; malaise; headache; chest pain; flatulence; abdominal distension; glossitis; urine retention; dysuria; edema; facial swelling; erythema; chills; tightness in throat; substernal pain; epistaxis; mucosal bleeding.

Overdosage:

Neurological adverse reactions, including convulsions, may occur with the attainment of high CSF levels of β-lactams. Ampicillin may be removed from circulation by

* Efficacy for this organism in this organ system was studied in fewer than 10 infections.

hemodialysis. The molecular weight, degree of protein binding and pharmacokinetic profile of sulbactam suggest that this compound may also be removed by hemodialysis.

Administration and Dosage:

Give IV or IM. Adult dosage is 1.5 g (1 g ampicillin + 0.5 g sulbactam) to 3 g (2 g ampicillin + 1 g sulbactam) every 6 hrs. Do not exceed 4 g/day sulbactam.

Renal function impairment: The elimination kinetics of ampicillin and sulbactam are similarly affected; hence, the ratio of one to the other will remain constant whatever the renal function. In patients with renal impairment, give as follows:

Ampicillin/Sulbactam Dosage Guide For Patients With Renal Impairment

Ccr (ml/min/1.73m^2)	Half-life (hours)	Recommended dosage
≥ 30	1	1.5-3 g q 6-8 h
15-29	5	1.5-3 g q 12 h
5-14	9	1.5-3 g q 24 h

Children: Safety and efficacy in children < 12 years old have not been established.

Dissolution: Reconstitute powder for IV and IM use with any of the compatible diluents described below. Allow solutions to stand after dissolution so that any foaming will dissipate. This permits visual inspection for complete solubilization.

Preparation for IV use: 1.5 and 3 g bottles -Reconstitute to desired concentrations with any of the following diluents. Discard unused solutions after indicated times:

Preparation of Ampicillin/Sulbactam for IV Use

Diluent	Maximum concentration (mg/ml)	Stability
Sterile Water for Injection	45 (30/15)	8 hrs @ 25°C
	45 (30/15)	48 hrs @ 4°C
	30 (20/10)	72 hrs @ 4°C
0.9% Sodium Chloride Injection	45 (30/15)	8 hrs @ 25°C
	45 (30/15)	48 hrs @ 4°C
	30 (20/10)	72 hrs @ 4°C
5% Dextrose Injection	30 (20/10)	2 hrs @ 25°C
	30 (20/10)	4 hrs @ 4°C
	3 (2/1)	4 hrs @ 25°C
Lactated Ringer's Injection	45 (30/15)	8 hrs @ 25°C
	45 (30/15)	24 hrs @ 4°C
M/6 Sodium Lactate Injection	45 (30/15)	8 hrs @ 25°C
	45 (30/15)	8 hrs @ 4°C
5% Dextrose in 0.45% Saline	3 (2/1)	4 hrs @ 25°C
	15 (10/5)	4 hrs @ 4°C
10% Invert Sugar	3 (2/1)	4 hrs @ 25°C
	30 (20/10)	3 hrs @ 4°C

Aminopenicillins

AMPICILLIN SODIUM AND SULBACTAM SODIUM

If piggyback bottles are unavailable, use standard vials of sterile powder. Initially, reconstitute with Sterile Water for Injection to yield 375 mg/ml (250 mg ampicillin/125 mg sulbactam). Then immediately dilute to yield 3 to 45 mg/ml (2 to 30 mg ampicillin/1 to 15 mg sulbactam/ml). Injection slowly over at least 10 to 15 min or infuse in greater dilutions with 50 to 100 ml diluent over 15 to 30 min.

Preparation for IM injection: Reconstitute with Sterile Water for Injection or 0.5% or 2% Lidocaine HCl Injection. Consult the following table for recommended volumes needed to obtain 375 mg/ml solutions (250 mg ampicillin/125 mg sulbactam/ml). *Use only freshly prepared solutions; give within 1 hour after preparation.*

Preparation of Ampicillin/Sulbactam for IM Use

Vial size	Diluent to be added	Withdrawal volume
1.5 g	3.2 ml	4 ml
3 g	6.4 ml	8 ml

Stability and storage: Store at ≤ 30°C (86°F) prior to reconstitution. When concomitant aminoglycosides are indicated, reconstitute and administer this product and aminoglycosides separately; aminopenicillins inactivate aminoglycosides in vitro.

Rx	**Unasyn** (Roerig)	**Powder for Injection**: 1.5 g (1 g ampicillin sodium/0.5 g sulbactam sodium)	In vials, bottles and *Add-Vantage* vials.
		3 g (2 g ampicillin sodium/1 g sulbactam sodium)	In vials and bottles.

Aminopenicillins

BACAMPICILLIN HCl

For complete prescribing information, refer to the Penicillins group monograph.

Bacampicillin is hydrolyzed to ampicillin during absorption from the GI tract. Because bacampicillin is more completely absorbed than ampicillin, it is administered in lower total daily dosages, and sustains effective serum levels when given every 12 hours.

Indications:

Upper and lower respiratory tract infections (including acute exacerbations of chronic bronchitis) due to streptococci (β-hemolytic streptococci, *S pyogenes*), pneumococci (*S pneumoniae*), nonpenicillinase-producing staphylococci and *Hemophilus influenzae.*

Urinary tract infections due to *Escherichia coli, Proteus mirabilis* and *S faecalis* (enterococci).

Skin and skin structure infections due to streptococci and susceptible staphylococci.

Gonorrhea (acute uncomplicated urogenital infections) due to *Neisseria gonorrhoeae.*

Administration and Dosage:

Tablets may be given without regard to meals; administer suspension to fasting patients.

Upper respiratory tract infections (including otitis media) due to streptococci, pneumococci, nonpenicillinase-producing staphylococci and H influenzae; urinary tract infections due to *E coli, P mirabilis* and *S faecalis; skin and skin structure* infections due to streptococci and susceptible staphylococci:

Adults (≥ 25 kg) – 400 mg every 12 hours.
Children – 25 mg/kg/day in equally divided doses at 12 hour intervals.

Severe infections or those caused by less susceptible organisms:

Adults (≥ 25 kg) – 800 mg every 12 hours.
Children – 50 mg/kg/day in equally divided doses at 12 hour intervals.

Lower respiratory tract infections due to streptococci, pneumococci, nonpenicillinase-producing staphylococci and *H influenzae:*

Adults (≥ 25 kg) – 800 mg every 12 hours.
Children – 50 mg/kg/day in equally divided doses at 12 hour intervals.

Gonorrhea: The usual adult dosage (males and females) is 1.6 g bacampicillin plus 1 g probenecid as a single oral dose. No pediatric dosage has been established.

Larger doses may be needed for persistent or severe infections.

Rx	**Spectrobid** (Roerig)	**Tablets**: 400 mg (chemically equivalent to 280 mg ampicillin)	Lactose. White. Film coated. Oblong. In 100s.
		Powder for Oral Suspension: 125 mg per 5 ml reconstituted suspension (chemically equivalent to 87.5 mg ampicillin)	Saccharin, sugar. In 70 ml.

Aminopenicillins

AMOXICILLIN

Complete prescribing information for these products begins in the Penicillins group monograph.

The spectrum of amoxicillin is essentially identical to ampicillin, except that ampicillin is more effective against *Shigella* sp. Amoxicillin has the advantage of more complete absorption than ampicillin, a 3 times a day regimen for most infections and less diarrhea than ampicillin.

Indications:

Infections due to susceptible strains of the following organisms: Gram-negative – *Hemophilus influenzae, E coli, P mirabilis* and *N gonorrhoeae*. Gram-positive – Streptococci (including *S faecalis*), *S pneumoniae* and nonpenicillinase-producing staphylococci.

Administration and Dosage:

Larger doses may be required for persistent or severe infections.

The children's dose is intended for individuals whose weight will not cause the calculated dosage to be greater than that recommended for adults; the children's dose should not exceed the maximum adult dose.

Amoxicillin Uses and Dosages

Organisms/Infections	Dosage
Infections of the ear, nose and throat due to streptococci, pneumococci, nonpenicillinase-producing staphylococci and *H influenzae* *Infections of the GU tract due to E coli, P mirabilis and S faecalis* *Infections of the skin and soft tissues* due to streptococci, susceptible staphylococci and *E coli*	*Adults and children (> 20 kg)* – 250 to 500 mg every 8 hours. *Children* – 20 to 40 mg/kg/day in divided doses every 8 hours.
Infections of the lower respiratory tract due to streptococci, pneumococci, nonpenicillinase-producing staphylococci and *H influenzae*	*Adults and children (> 20 kg)* – 500 mg q 8 h. *Children* – 40 mg/kg/day in divided doses q 8 h.
Gonococcal infections: Uncomplicated urethral, endocervical or rectal infection (alternative regimen)[1]	*Adults* – If infection was acquired from a source proven not to have penicillin-resistant gonorrhea, a penicillin such as amoxicillin 3g plus 1g probenecid *followed by* doxycycline may be used.
Prevention of bacterial endocarditis:[2] For patients undergoing dental, oral, esophageal or respiratory tract procedures.	2 g (50 mg/kg for children) orally 1 hour before procedure.
For moderate-risk patients undergoing GU or nonesophageal GI procedures	2 g (50 mg/kg for children) orally 1 hour before procedure
Unlabeled use: *Chlamydia trachomatis* in pregnancy	As an alternative to erythromycin; 500 mg 3 times a day for 7 days.

[1] CDC 1989 Sexually Transmitted Diseases Treatment Guidelines. *Morbidity and Mortality Weekly Report* 1989 Sept 1;38 (No S-8):1-43.

[2] American Heart Association Statement. *JAMA* 1997;277:1794-1801.

Storage/Stability: Reconstituted oral suspension stable for 7 days at room temperature (not exceeding 25°C; 77°F).

Aminopenicillins

AMOXICILLIN

Rx	**Amoxil** (SK Beecham)	**Tablets, chewable:** 125 mg (as trihydrate)	Saccharin, sucrose. In 60s.
Rx	**Amoxicillin** (Various, eg, Biocraft, Geneva, Goldline, Major, Moore, Qualitest, Rugby, Schein)	**Tablets, chewable**: 250 mg (as trihydrate)	In 100s and 500s.
Rx	**Amoxil** (SK Beecham)		Saccharin, sucrose. In 100s.
Rx	**Amoxicillin** (Various, eg, Geneva Marsam, Goldline, Lemmon, Major, Mylan, Parmed, Rugby, Schein, URL, Warner Chilcott)	**Capsules**: 250 mg (as trihydrate)	In 50s, 100s, 500s and UD 1000s.
Rx	**Amoxil** (SK Beecham)		In 100s, 500s and UD 100s.
Rx	**Biomox** (Inter. Ethical Labs[1])		In 100s.
Rx	**Polymox** (Apothecon)		In 100s, 500s and UD 100s.
Rx	**Trimox 250** (Apothecon)		In 100s, 500s and UD 100s.
Rx	**Wymox** (Wyeth-Ayerst)		(Wyeth 559). Gray and green. In 100s & 500s.
Rx	**Amoxicillin** (Various, eg, Dixon-Shane, Geneva Marsam, Goldline, Lemmon, Major, Mylan, Parmed, Rugby, URL, Warner-C)	**Capsules**: 500 mg (as trihydrate)	In 50s, 100s, 500s and UD 100s.
Rx	**Amoxil** (SK Beecham)		In 100s, 500s and UD 100s.
Rx	**Biomox** (Inter. Ethical Labs[1]1)		In 100s.
Rx	**Polymox** (Apothecon)		In 50s, 100s, 500s, UD 100s.
Rx	**Trimox 500** (Apothecon)		In 50s, 500s and UD 100s.
Rx	**Wymox** (Wyeth-Ayerst)		(Wyeth 560). Gray and green. In 50s & 500s.
Rx	**Amoxil Pediatric Drops** (SK Beecham)	**Powder for Oral Suspension**: 50 mg per ml (as trihydrate) when reconstituted	Sucrose. In 15 and 30 ml.
Rx	**Polymox Drops** (Apothecon)		Sucrose. In 15 ml.
Rx	**Amoxicillin** (Various, eg, Dixon-Shane, Geneva Marsam, Major, Mylan, Parmed, Rugby, URL, Warner Chilcott)	**Powder for Oral Suspension**: 125 mg per 5 ml (as trihydrate) when reconstituted	In 80, 100, 150 and 200 ml.
Rx	**Amoxil** (SK Beecham)		Sucrose. In 80, 100 & 150 ml and UD 5 ml.
Rx	**Polymox** (Apothecon)		Sucrose. In 80, 100 & 150 ml and UD 5 ml.
Rx	**Trimox 125** (Apothecon)		Sucrose. In 80, 100, 150 ml and UD 5 ml.
Rx	**Wymox** (Wyeth-Ayerst)		Sucrose. In 100 and 150 ml.

Aminopenicillins

AMOXICILLIN

Rx	**Amoxicillin** (Various, eg, Dixon-Shane, Geneva-Marsam, Major, Mylan, Parmed, Rugby, Schein, URL, Warner Chilcott)	**Powder for Oral Suspension:** 250 mg per 5 ml (as trihydrate) when reconstituted	In 80, 100, 150 and 200 ml.
Rx	**Amoxil** (SK Beecham)		Sucrose. In 80, 100 & 150 ml and UD 5 ml.
Rx	**Biomox** (Inter. Ethical Labs[1])		In 100 and 150 ml.
Rx	**Polymox** (Apothecon)		Sucrose. In 80, 100 & 150 ml and UD 5 ml.
Rx	**Trimox 250** (Apothecon)		Sucrose. In 80, 100, 150 ml and UD 5 ml.
Rx	**Wymox** (Wyeth-Ayerst)		Sucrose. In 80, 100 & 150 ml.

[1] International Ethical Laboratories, Rio Piedras, Puerto Rico 00921 (809) 765-3510.

AMOXICILLIN AND POTASSIUM CLAVULANATE (Co-amoxiclav)

For complete prescribing information, refer to the Penicillins group monograph.

Actions:

Pharmacology: Amoxicillin has a spectrum of bacterial activity essentially identical to ampicillin, except that ampicillin is more effective against *Shigella* sp. Amoxicillin is more completely absorbed from the GI tract than ampicillin. Clavulanic acid, a β-lactam structurally related to the penicillins, inactivates β-lactamase enzymes commonly found in microorganisms resistant to penicillin. The combination of amoxicillin/clavulanic acid extends the antibiotic spectrum of amoxicillin to include bacteria normally resistant to amoxicillin and other β-lactam antibiotics (see Microbiology table in the group monograph).

Indications:

Lower respiratory infections caused by β-lactamase-producing strains of *Haemophilus influenzae* and *Moraxella (Branhamella) catarrhalis.*

Otitis media and sinusitis caused by β-lactamase-producing strains of *H. influenzae* and *M. catarrhalis.*

Skin and skin structure infections caused by β-lactamase-producing strains of *Staphylococcus aureus, Escherichia coli* and *Klebsiella* sp.

Urinary tract infections caused by β-lactamase-producing strains of *E. coli, Klebsiella* sp and *Enterobacter* sp.

While amoxicillin/potassium clavulanate is indicated only for the conditions listed above, infections caused by ampicillin-susceptible organisms are also amenable to this drug due to its amoxicillin content. Therefore, mixed infections caused by ampicillin-susceptible organisms and β-lactamase-producing organisms susceptible to amoxicillin/potassium clavulanate should not require an additional antibiotic. Therapy may be instituted prior to obtaining the results from bacteriologic studies when there is reason to believe the infection may involve any of the β-lactamase-producing organisms listed above. Once the results are known, adjust therapy.

Administration and Dosage:

May be administered without regard to meals; however, absorption of clavulanate potassium is enhanced when taken at the start of a meal. To minimize the potential for GI intolerance, give the drug at the start of a meal.

Tablet interchangeability: Because both the 250 and 500 mg tablets contain the same amount of clavulanic acid (125 mg as potassium salt), two 250 mg tablets are NOT equivalent to one 500 mg tablet. The 875 mg tablet also contains 125 mg potassium clavulanate. In addition, the 250 mg tablet and 250 mg chewable tablet do NOT contain the same amount of potassium clavulanate and should not be substituted for each other, as they are not interchangeable.

Usual dose:

Adults – One 500 mg tablet every 12 hours or one 250 mg tablet every 8 hours.

Suspension: Adults who have difficulty swallowing may be given the 125 mg/5 ml or 250 mg/5 ml suspension in place of the 500 mg tablet or give 200 mg/5 ml or 400 mg/5 ml suspension in place of the 875 mg tablet.

Severe infections and respiratory tract infections: One 875 mg tablet every 12 hours or one 500 mg tablet every 8 hours.

AMOXICILLIN AND POTASSIUM CLAVULANATE (Co-amoxiclav)

Chancroid (Haemophilus ducreyi infection):* One 500 mg tablet 3 times daily for 7 days as an alternative to erythromycin, azithromycin or ceftriaxone (not evaluated in the US).

Renal function impairment does not generally require a dose reduction unless impairment is severe. Severely impaired patients with a glomerular filtration rate (GFR) of < 30 ml/min should not receive the 875 mg tablet. Give patients with a GFR of 10 to 30 ml/min 500 or 250 mg every 12 hours, depending on the severity of infection. Give patients with a GFR < 10 ml/min 500 or 250 mg every 24 hours, depending on the severity of infection. Give hemodialysis patients 500 or 250 mg every 24 hours. They should receive an additional dose both during and at the end of dialysis.

Hepatic function impairment: Dose with caution and monitor hepatic function.

Children –

≥ 40 kg: Dose according to adult recommendations.

< 3 months old: 30 mg/kg/day divided every 12 hours, based on the amoxicillin component. Use of the 125 mg/5 ml oral suspension is recommended.

≥ 3 months old: Children's dose is based on amoxicillin content. Refer to the following table. Because of the different amoxicillin to clavulanic acid ratios in the 250 mg tablets (250/125) vs the 250 mg chewable tablets (250/62.5), do not use the 250 mg tablet until the child weighs ≥ 40 kg.

Amoxicillin/Potassium Clavulanate Dosing in Children ≥ 3 Months of Age		
	Dosing regimen	
Infections	200 mg/5ml or 400 mg/5 ml (q12hr)[1,2]	125 mg/5 ml or 250 mg/5 ml (q8hr)[2]
Otitis media,[3] sinusitus, lower respiratory tract infections, severe infections	45 mg/kg/day	40 mg/kg/day
Less severe infections	25 mg/kg/day	20 mg/kg/day

[1] The every-12-hour regimen is associated with significantly less diarrhea; however, the 200 and 400 mg formulations (suspension and chewable tablets) contain aspartame and should not be used by phenylketonurics.
[2] Each strength of the suspension is available as a chewable tablet for use by older children.
[3] Recommended duration is 10 days.

Storage/Stability: Refrigerate reconstituted suspension and discard after 10 days. Shake well before using.

* CDC 1993 Sexually Transmitted Diseases Treatment Guidelines. *Morbidity and Mortality Weekly Report* 1993 Sept 24;42(No.RR-14):i-102.

Aminopenicillins

AMOXICILLIN AND POTASSIUM CLAVULANATE (Co-amoxiclav)

Rx	**Augmentin** (SK-Beecham)	**Tablets**: 250 mg amoxicillin (as trihydrate) and 125 mg clavulanic acid[1]	0.63 mEq potassium. (Augmentin 250/125). White. Oval. In 30s and UD 100s.
		500 mg amoxicillin (as trihydrate) and 125 mg clavulanic acid[1]	0.63 mEq potassium. (Augmentin 500/125). White. Oval. In 20s, 30s and UD 100s.
		875 mg amoxicillin (as trihydrate) and 125 mg clavulanic acid[1]	0.63 mEq potassium. (Augmentin 875 SB). White, scored. Capsule shape. In 20s and UD 100s.
		Tablets, chewable: 125 mg amoxicillin (as trihydrate) and 31.25 mg clavulanic acid[1]	0.16 mEq potassium. Saccharin. (BMP 189). Yellow, mottled. In 30s.
		200 mg amoxicillin (as trihydrate) and 28.5 mg clavulanic acid[1]	0.14 mEq potassium. Saccharin, aspartame.[2] Pink, mottled. In 20s.
		250 mg amoxicillin (as trihydrate) and 62.5 mg clavulanic acid[1]	0.32 mEq potassium. Saccharin. (BMP 190). Yellow, mottled. In 30s.
		400 mg amoxicillin (as trihydrate) and 57 mg clavulanic acid[1]	0.29 mEq potassium. Saccharin, aspartame.[3] Pink, mottled. In 20s.
		Powder for Oral Suspension: 125 mg amoxicillin and 31.25 mg clavulanic acid[1] per 5 ml	0.16 mEq potassium/5 ml. Saccharin. Banana flavor. In 75, 100 and 150 ml.
		200 mg amoxicillin and 28.5 mg clavulanic acid[1] per 5 ml	0.14 mEq potassium/5 ml. Saccharin, aspartame.[4] Orange-raspberry flavor. In 50, 75 and 100 ml.
		250 mg amoxicillin and 62.5 mg clavulanic acid[1] per 5 ml	0.32 mEq potassium/5 ml. Saccharin. Orange flavor. In 75, 100 and 150 ml.
		400 mg amoxicillin and 57 mg clavulanic acid[1] per 5 ml	0.29 mEq potassium/5 ml. Saccharin, aspartame.[4] Orange-raspberry flavor. In 50, 75 and 100 ml.

[1] As the potassium salt.
[2] Contains 2.1 mg phenylalanine.
[3] Contains 4.2 mg phenylalanine.
[4] Contains 7 mg phenylalanine.

Extended Spectrum Penicillins

TICARCILLIN DISODIUM

Complete prescribing information begins in the Penicillins group monograph.

Indications:

For treatment of the following: Bacterial septicemia, skin/soft tissue infections, acute and chronic respiratory tract infections caused by susceptible strains of *Pseudomonas aeruginosa, Proteus* sp (both indole-positive and indole-negative), and *Escherichia coli.* Although clinical improvement has been shown, bacteriological cures cannot be expected in patients with chronic respiratory disease or cystic fibrosis.

Genitourinary tract infections (complicated and uncomplicated) due to susceptible strains of *P aeruginosa, Proteus* species (both indole-positive and indole-negative), *E coli, Enterobacter* and *Streptococcus faecalis* (enterococcus).

Infections due to susceptible anaerobic bacteria: Bacterial septicemia; lower respiratory tract infections such as empyema, anaerobic pneumonitis and lung abscess; intra-abdominal infections such as peritonitis and intra-abdominal abscess (typically resulting from anaerobic organisms resident in the normal GI tract); infections of the female pelvis and genital tract such as endometritis, pelvic inflammatory disease, pelvic abscess and salpingitis; skin and soft tissue infections.

Although ticarcillin is primarily indicated in gram-negative infections, consider its in vitro activity against gram-positive organisms in infections caused by both gram-negative and gram-positive organisms.

Based on the in vitro synergism between ticarcillin and gentamicin or tobramycin against certain strains of *P aeruginosa*, combined therapy has been successful using full therapeutic dosages.

Administration and Dosage:

Use IV therapy in higher doses in serious urinary tract and systemic infections. Intramuscular injections should not exceed 2 g/injection.

Seriously ill patients should receive higher doses. Ticarcillin is useful in infections in which protective mechanisms are impaired, such as acute leukemia, and during therapy with immunosuppressive or oncolytic drugs.

Ticarcillin Uses and Dosages

Organisms/Infections	Dosage
Bacterial septicemia, respiratory tract infections, skin and soft tissue infections, intra-abdominal infections and infections of the female pelvis and genital tract	*Adults:* 200 to 300 mg/kg/day by IV infusion in divided doses every 3, 4 or 6 hours (3 g every 3, 4 or 6 hours), depending on weight of patient and severity of infection. *Children (< 40 kg):* 200 to 300 mg/kg/day by IV infusion in divided doses every 4 or 6 h.[1]
Urinary tract infections: Complicated infections.	150 to 200 mg/kg/day IV infusion in divided doses every 4 or 6 hours. Usual dose for average adult (70 kg) is 3 g 4 times daily.
Uncomplicated infections.	*Adults:* 1 g IM or direct IV every 6 hours. *Children (< 40 kg)*: 50 to 100 mg/kg/day IM or direct IV in divided doses every 6 or 8 hours.
Neonates: Severe infections (sepsis) due to susceptible strains of *Pseudomonas* species, *Proteus* species and *E coli.*	Give IM or by 10 to 20 minute IV infusions.
< 2 kg –	*< 7 days* – 75 mg/kg/12 hr (150 mg/kg/day). *> 7 days* – 75 mg/kg/8 hr (225 mg/kg/day).
> 2 kg –	*< 7 days* – 75 mg/kg/8 hr (225 mg/kg/day). *> 7 days* – 100 mg/kg/8 hr (300 mg/kg/day).
Dosage in renal insufficiency:[2]	Initial loading dose of 3 g IV, then base IV doses on Ccr and type of dialysis.
Creatinine clearance (ml/min) –	
> 60	3 g every 4 hours.
30 to 60	2 g every 4 hours.
10 to 30	2 g every 8 hours.
< 10	2 g every 12 hours or 1 g IM every 6 hours.
< 10 with hepatic dysfunction	2 g every 24 hours or 1 g IM every 12 hours.
Patients on peritoneal dialysis	3 g every 12 hours.
Patients on hemodialysis	2 g every 12 hrs and 3 g after each dialysis.

[1] Daily dose for children should not exceed adult dosage.

[2] Half-life in patients with renal failure is approximately 13 hours.

Extended Spectrum Penicillins

TICARCILLIN DISODIUM

Use the following to calculate creatinine clearance from serum creatinine value:

$$\text{Males: } \frac{\text{Weight (kg)} \times (140 - \text{age})}{72 \times \text{serum creatinine (mg/dl)}} = \text{Ccr}$$

Females: 0.85 × above value

Children weighing > 40 kg should receive adult dose. In children under 40 kg, data are insufficient to recommend an optimum dose.

IM: Reconstitute each g ticarcillin with 2 ml Sterile Water for Injection, Sodium Chloride Injection or 1% lidocaine HCl solution (without epinephrine) to obtain 1 g ticarcillin per 2.6 ml solution and use promptly.

Inject well into a relatively large muscle, using usual techniques and precautions.

IV: Reconstitute each g of ticarcillin with 4 ml of desired IV solution. Each 1ml of the resulting solution will have an approximate average concentration of 200 mg. When dissolved, dilute further to desired volume. When injecting solution directly, administer as slowly as possible to avoid vein irritation.

For IV infusions, administer by continuous or intermittent IV drip. Administer intermittent infusion over a 30 minute to 2 hour period in 6 equally divided doses.

Reconstitute 3 g piggyback vials with a minimum of 30 ml of desired IV solution. A dilution of ≈ 1 g/20 ml or more will reduce the incidence of vein irritation.

Stability and Storage of Ticarcillin IV Solutions

Concentration	Compatible diluents	Stability (loss of potency < 10%) Controlled room temperature	Refrigeration
10 mg/ml & 50 mg/ml	Sodium Chloride Injection[1]	72 hours	14 days
	Dextrose Injection 5%[1]	72 hours	14 days
	Lactated Ringer's Injection[1]	48 hours	14 days

IV infusion: Use a 50 ml or 100 ml *ADD-Vantage* container of either Sodium Chloride Injection or 5% Dextrose in Water. The resulting concentration of the 3 g dose reconstituted in 50 ml diluent is ≈ 60 mg/ml. The resulting concentration of the 3 g dose reconstituted in 100 ml diluent is ≈ 30 mg/ml. Administer by continuous or intermittent IV drip. Give intermittent infusion over 30 minutes to 2 hours in equally divided doses. To avoid vein irritation, administer as slowly as possible.

The IV solutions, Sodium Chloride Injection and 5% Dextrose in Water, in concentrations of ≈ 30 or ≈ 60 mg/ml are stable for 72 hours when stored at room temperature (21° to 24°C; 70° to 75°F).

Incompatibilities: Do NOT mix ticarcillin together with gentamicin, amikacin or tobramycin in the same IV solution, due to the gradual inactivation of gentamicin, amikacin or tobramycin under these circumstances. The therapeutic effect of these drugs remains unimpaired when administered separately.

Rx	**Ticar** (SK-Beecham)	**Powder for Injection:** (Contains 5.2mEq sodium/g)	
		1 g (as disodium)	In vials.
		3 g (as disodium)	In vials, piggyback and *ADD-Vantage vials.*
		6 g (as disodium)	In vials.
		20 g (as disodium)	In bulk vials.
		30 g (as disodium)	In bulk vials.

[1] These solutions remain stable up to 100 mg/ml concentration. After reconstitution, they can be frozen (approximately -18° C; 0° F) and stored for up to 30 days without loss of potency. The stabilities of the thawed solutions are identical to the unfrozen ones listed above.

Extended Spectrum Penicillins

TICARCILLIN AND CLAVULANATE POTASSIUM

For complete prescribing information, refer to the Penicillins group monograph.

Actions:

Pharmacology: The formulation of ticarcillin with clavulanic acid protects ticarcillin from degradation by β-lactamase enzymes (see group monograph).

Indications:

Treatment of infections caused by susceptible strains of these designated organisms:

Septicemia including bacteremia, caused by β-lactamase-producing strains of *Klebsiella** sp, *Escherichia coli**, *Staphylococcus aureus** and *Pseudomonas aeruginosa** (and other *Pseudomonas* species*).

Lower respiratory infections caused by β-lactamase-producing strains of *S aureus, Hemophilus influenzae** and *Klebsiella* sp.*

Bone and joint infections caused by β-lactamase-producing strains of *S aureus.*

Skin and skin structure infections caused by β-lactamase-producing strains of *S aureus, Klebsiella* sp* and *E coli.**

Urinary tract infections (complicated and uncomplicated) caused by β-lactamase-producing strains of *E coli, Klebsiella* sp, *P aeruginosa**(and other *Pseudomonas* species*), *Citrobacter* sp*, *Enterobacter cloacae*, Serratia marcescens*, S aureus.**

Gynecologic infections: Endometritis caused by β-lactamase producing strains of *B melaninogenicus*, Enterobacter* sp (including *E cloacae**), *E coli, Klebsiella pneumoniae*, S aureus* and *Staphylococcus epidermidis.*

While this combination is indicated only for the conditions listed above, infections caused by ticarcillin-susceptible organisms are also amenable to this combination treatment due to its ticarcillin content.

Treatment of mixed infections and for presumptive therapy prior to the identification of the causative organisms.

Based on the in vitro synergism between this drug and aminoglycosides against certain strains of *P aeruginosa,* combined therapy has been successful, especially in patients with impaired host defenses. Use drugs in full therapeutic doses. When results of culture and susceptibility tests become available, adjust antimicrobial therapy.

Administration and Dosage:

Administer by IV infusion over 30 minutes.

Generally, continue treatment for at least 2 days after signs and symptoms of infection have disappeared. The usual duration is 10 to 14 days; however, in difficult and complicated infections, more prolonged therapy may be required.

Frequent bacteriologic and clinical appraisal is necessary during therapy of chronic urinary tract infections and may be required for several months after therapy has been completed; persistent infections may require treatment for several weeks; do not use doses smaller than those indicated.

In certain infections involving abscess formation, perform appropriate surgical drainage in conjunction with antimicrobial therapy.

When administering in combination with another antimicrobial (eg, an aminoglycoside), administer each drug separately.

Ticarcillin/Clavulanate Potassium Uses and Dosages

Infection	Dosage
Systemic and urinary tract infections:	
Adults (≥ 60 kg)	3.1 g[1] every 4 to 6 hours
(≤ 60 kg)[2]	200 to 300 mg/kg/day (based on ticarcillin content) in divided doses every 4 to 6 hrs
Gynecologic infections:	
Adults (≥ 60 kg)	
moderate infections	200 mg/kg/day in divided doses every 6 hours
severe infections	300 mg/kg/day in divided doses every 4 hours

* Efficacy for this organism in this organ system was studied in < 10 infections.
[1] 3 g ticarcillin plus 100 mg clavulanic acid.
[2] Dosage in children < 12 years of age is not established.

* Efficacy for this organism in this organ system was studied in < 10 infections.

Extended Spectrum Penicillins

TICARCILLIN AND CLAVULANATE POTASSIUM

Dosage of Ticarcillin/Clavulanate Potassium in Renal Insufficiency[1]	
Initial loading dose is 3.1g[2]. Follow with doses based on creatinine clearance and type of dialysis.	
Creatinine clearance (ml/min)	*Dosage*
> 60	3.1 g[2] every 4 hours
30 to 60	2 g every 4 hours
10 to 30	2 g every 8 hours
< 10	2 g every 12 hours
< 10 with hepatic dysfunction	2 g every 24 hours
Patients on peritoneal dialysis	3.1 g[2] every 12 hours
Patients on hemodialysis	2 g every 12 hours supplemented with 3.1 g[2] after each dialysis

[1] Half-life of ticarcillin in patients with renal failure is ≈ 13 hours.
[2] 3 g ticarcillin plus 100 mg clavulanic acid.

Use the following formula to calculate creatinine clearance from serum creatinine values:

$$\text{Males: } \frac{\text{Weight (kg)} \times (140 - \text{age})}{72 \times \text{serum creatinine (mg/dl)}} = \text{Ccr}$$

$$\text{Females: } 0.85 \times \text{above value}$$

IV: Reconstitute by shaking with ≈ 13 ml of Sterile Water for Injection or NaCl Injection. The resulting ticarcillin concentration is ≈ 200 mg/ml and 6.7 mg/ml clavulanic acid for the 3.1 g dose. Conversely, each 5 ml of the 3.1 g dose reconstituted with ≈ 13 ml of diluent will contain ≈ 1 g ticarcillin and 33 mg clavulanic acid.

Further dilute the solution with Sodium Chloride Injection, 5% Dextrose Injection or Lactated Ringer's Injection to a concentration between 10 to 100 mg/ml. Administer over 30 minutes by direct infusion or through a Y–type IV infusion set already in place. If this method or the "piggyback" method is used, temporarily discontinue administering any other solutions during the infusion of ticarcillin and clavulanate potassium.

The concentrated stock solution (200 mg/ml) is stable for up to 6 hours at room temperature (21° to 23°C; 70° to 75°F) or up to 72 hours under refrigeration (4°C; 40°F); if further diluted to a concentration between 10 mg/ml and 100 mg/ml with any of the recommended diluents, the following stability periods apply:

Stability and Storage for IV Solution of Ticarcillin/Clavulanate Potassium				
		Stability		
Concentration	Compatible diluents	Controlled room temp.	Refrigeration	Frozen
10 mg/ml to 100 mg/ml	Sodium Chloride Injection	24 hours	7 days	30 days
	5% Dextrose Injection	24 hours	3 days	7 days
	Lactated Ringer's Injection	24 hours	7 days	30 days

Unused solutions must be discarded after the time period stated above. Use all thawed solutions within 8 hours. Do not refreeze thawed solutions.

Premixed, frozen solutions: Store at ≤ –20°C (– 4°F). Thaw at room temperature 22°C (72°F) or in a refrigerator 4°C (40°F). Do not force thaw by immersion in water baths or by microwave irradiation. Thawed solution is stable for 7 days if stored under refrigeration or for 24 hours at room temperature. Do not refreeze.

Incompatibility: Incompatible with sodium bicarbonate.

Rx	**Timentin** (SK-Beecham Labs)	**Powder for Injection**: Contains 4.75 mEq sodium/g. 3 g ticarcillin (as disodium) and 0.1 g clavulanic acid	In 3.1 g vials, piggyback bottles, *ADD-Vantage* vials and 31 g pharmacy bulk packages.[1]
		Solution: Contains 18.7 mEq sodium/100 ml 3 g ticarcillin (as disodium) and 0.1 g clavulanic acid.	In 100 ml premixed, frozen vials.

[1] Pharmacy bulk package contains 30 g ticarcillin (as disodium) and 1 g clavulanic acid.

MEZLOCILLIN SODIUM

Complete prescribing information for these products begins in the Penicillins group monograph.

Indications:

Lower respiratory tract infections: Including pneumonia and lung abscess caused by *Hemophilus influenzae, Klebsiella* sp including *K pneumoniae, Proteus mirabilis, Pseudomonas* sp including *P aeruginosa, E coli*and *Bacteroides* sp including *B fragilis.*

Intra-abdominal infections: Including acute cholecystitis, cholangitis, peritonitis, hepatic abscess and intra-abdominal abscess caused by susceptible *E coli, P mirabilis, Klebsiella* sp, *Pseudomonas* sp, *Streptococcus faecalis* (enterococcus), *Bacteroides* sp, *Peptococcus* sp and *Peptostreptococcus* sp.

Urinary tract infections: Caused by susceptible *E coli; P mirabilis;* the indole-positive *Proteus* sp, *Morganella morganii; Klebsiella* sp; *Enterobacter* sp; *Serratia* sp; *Pseudomonas* sp; *S faecalis* (enterococcus).

Uncomplicated gonorrhea due to susceptible *Neisseria gonorrhoeae.*

Gynecological infections: Including endometritis, pelvic cellulitis and pelvic inflammatory disease associated with susceptible *N gonorrhoeae, Peptococcus* sp, *Peptostreptococcus* sp, *Bacteroides* sp, *E coli, P mirabilis, Klebsiella* sp and *Enterobacter* sp.

Skin and skin structure infections: Caused by susceptible *S faecalis* (enterococcus); *E coli; P mirabilis;* the indole-positive *Proteus* sp, *P vulgaris* and *Providencia rettgeri; Klebsiella* sp; *Enterobacter* sp; *Pseudomonas* sp; *Peptococcus* sp; *Bacteroides* sp.

Septicemia: Including bacteremia caused by susceptible *E coli, Klebsiella* sp, *Enterobacter* sp, *Pseudomonas* sp, *Bacteroides* sp and *Peptococcus* sp.

Streptococcal infections: Caused by *Streptococcus* sp including group A beta-hemolytic *Streptococcus* and *S pneumoniae;* however, such infections are ordinarily treated with more narrow spectrum penicillins. Mezlocillin's broad spectrum of activity makes it useful for treating mixed infections caused by susceptible strains of both gram-negative and gram-positive aerobic or anaerobic bacteria. It is not effective, however, against infections caused by penicillinase-producing *Staphylococcus aureus.*

Severe infections: In certain severe infections when the causative organisms are unknown, administer in conjunction with an aminoglycoside or a cephalosporin antibiotic as initial therapy. When results of culture and susceptibility tests become available, adjust antimicrobial therapy if indicated.

Pseudomonas infections: Mezlocillin is effective in combination with an aminoglycoside for the treatment of life-threatening infections caused by *P aeruginosa.* For the treatment of febrile episodes in immunosuppressed patients with granulocytopenia, combine with an aminoglycoside or a cephalosporin.

Prophylaxis: Perioperative administration may reduce the incidence of infection in patients undergoing surgical procedures that are classified as contaminated or potentially contaminated (eg, vaginal hysterectomy, colorectal surgery). Effective use depends on time of administration. To achieve effective tissue levels, give ½ to 1½ hours before surgery.

In patients undergoing Caesarean section, intraoperative (after clamping the umbilical cord) and postoperative use may reduce the incidence of postoperative infections.

For patients undergoing colorectal surgery, preoperative bowel preparation by mechanical cleansing as well as with a non-absorbable antibiotic (eg, neomycin) is recommended.

Administration and Dosage:

Administer IV for serious infections. IM doses should not exceed 2 g/injection. Individualize dosage.

Adults: The recommended adult dosage for serious infections is 200 to 300 mg/kg/day given in 4 to 6 divided doses. The usual dose is 3 g given every 4 hours (18 g/day) or 4 g given every 6 hours (16 g/day).

Extended Spectrum Penicillins

MEZLOCILLIN SODIUM

Infants and children: Limited data are available on the safety and effectiveness in the treatment of infants and children with serious infection.

Mezlocillin Dosage Guidelines for Neonates		
Body weight (g)	Age	
	≤ 7 Days	> 7 Days
≤ 2000	75 mg/kg every 12 hours (150 mg/kg/day)	75 mg/kg every 8 hours (225 mg/kg/day)
> 2000	75 mg/kg every 12 hours (150 mg/kg/day)	75 mg/kg every 6 hours (300 mg/kg/day)

For infants > 1 month of age and children < 12 years, administer 50 mg/kg every 4 hours (300 mg/kg/day); infuse IV over 30 minutes or administer by IM injection.

Renal function impairment: The rate of elimination of mezlocillin is dose-dependent and related to the degree of renal function impairment. After an IV dose of 3 g, the serum half-life is approximately 1 hour in patients with creatinine clearances > 60 ml/min, 1.3 hours in those with clearances of 30 to 59 ml/min, 1.6 hours in those with clearances of 10 to 29 ml/min, and approximately 3.6 hours in patients with clearances of < 10 ml/min. Dosage adjustments are not required in patients with mild impairment of renal function.

Renal failure and hepatic insufficiency – Measuring serum levels will provide additional guidance for adjusting dosage, but may not be practical.

Mezlocillin Uses and Dosages	
Organisms/Infections	Dosage
Urinary infection: Uncomplicated with normal renal function (creatinine clearance ≥ 30 ml/min).	100 to 125 mg/kg/day (6 to 8 g/day); 1.5 to 2 g every 6 hours IV or IM.
Uncomplicated with renal impairment	1.5 g every 8 hours
Complicated with normal renal function	150 to 200 mg/kg/day (12 g/day); 3 g every 6 hours IV.
Complicated with renal impairment – Creatinine clearance	
10 to 30 ml/min	1.5 g every 6 hours.
<10 ml/min	1.5 g every 8 hours.
Lower respiratory tract infection, intra-abdominal infection, gynecological infection, skin and skin structure infections, septicemia:	225 to 300 mg/kg/day (16 to 18 g/day); 4 g every 6 hours or 3 g every 4 hours IV.
Serious systemic infection with renal impairment – Creatinine clearance	
10 to 30 ml/min	3 g every 8 hours.
<10 ml/min	2 g every 8 hours.
Serious systemic infection undergoing hemodialysis for renal failure	3 to 4 g after each dialysis; then every 12 hours.
peritoneal dialysis	3 g every 2 hours
Life-threatening infections:	Up to 350 mg/kg/day; 4 g every 4 hours (24 g/day maximum).
In patients with renal impairment – Creatinine clearance	
10 to 30 ml/min	3 g every 6 hours.
<10 ml/min	2 g every 6 hours.
Acute, uncomplicated gonococcal urethritis:	1 to 2 g IV or IM; plus 1 g probenecid at time of dosing or up to ½ hour before.
Prophylaxis:	
To prevent postoperative infection in contaminated or potentially contaminated surgery	4 g IV, ½ to 1½ hr prior to start of surgery; 4 g IV, 6 and 12 hours later.
Caesarean section patients –	First dose: 4 g IV when umbilical cord is clamped; Second dose: 4 g IV, 4 hrs after first dose; Third dose: 4 g IV, 8 hrs after first dose.

Extended Spectrum Penicillins

MEZLOCILLIN SODIUM

IV administration: Administer IV by intermittent infusion or by direct IV injection. In combination with another antimicrobial, such as an aminoglycoside, give each drug separately in accordance with the recommended dosage and routes of administration for each drug.

Infusion – Reconstitute each g of mezlocillin by vigorous shaking with at least 9 to 10 ml of Sterile Water for Injection, 5% Dextrose Injection or 0.9% Sodium Chloride Injection. Further dilute to desired volume (50 to 100 ml) with an appropriate IV solution. The solution may then be administered over a period of 30 minutes by direct infusion or through a Y-type IV infusion set. If this method or the piggyback method of administration is used, temporarily discontinue the administration of any other solutions during the infusion.

Injection – May inject reconstituted solution directly into a vein or into IV tubing; when so administered, give slowly over a period of 3 to 5 minutes. To minimize venous irritation, the concentration of drug should not exceed 10%.

IM administration: Reconstitute each g of mezlocillin by vigorous shaking with 3 to 4 ml of Sterile Water for Injection or with 3 to 4 ml of 0.5% or 1% lidocaine HCl solution (without epinephrine). Do not exceed 2 g/injection.

Inject well within the body of a relatively large muscle, such as the upper outer quadrant of the buttock; aspirate to avoid unintentional injection into blood vessel. Slow injection (12 to 15 seconds) will minimize discomfort of IM administration.

Stability and Storage of Mezlocillin IV Solutions

Concentration	Compatible diluents	Stability (loss of potency < 10%) Controlled room temperature	Refrigeration
10 mg/ml & 100 mg/ml	Sterile Water for Injection[1]	48 hours	7 days
	0.9% Sodium Chloride Injection[1]	48 hours	7 days
	5% Dextrose Injection[1]	48 hours	7 days
	5% Dextrose in 0.225% Sodium Chloride Injection	72 hours	7 days
	Lactated Ringer's Injection	24 hours	7 days
	5% Dextrose in Electrolyte #75 Injection	72 hours	7 days
	5% Dextrose in 0.45% Sodium Chloride Injection[2]	48 hours	48 hours
	Ringer's Injection	24 hours	24 hours
	10% Dextrose Injection	24 hours	24 hours
	5% Fructose Injection	24 hours	24 hours
Up to 250 mg/ml	Sterile Water for Injection	24 hours	
	0.9% Sodium Chloride Injection	24 hours	
	0.5% and 1% Lidocaine HCl Solution (without epinephrine)	24 hours	

[1] These solutions are stable for up to 28 days when frozen at −12°C (10°F).
[2] This solution is stable from 10 mg/ml to 50 mg/ml refrigerated.

If precipitation occurs under refrigeration, warm product to 37°C (98.6°F) for 20 minutes in a water bath and shake well.

Store vials and infusion bottles at or below 30°C (86°F). Product may darken slightly depending on storage conditions, but potency is not affected.

Rx	**Mezlin** (Miles Pharm.)	**Powder for Injection:** Contains 1.85 mEq sodium/g 1 g mezlocillin (as sodium)	In vials.
		2 g mezlocillin (as sodium)	In vials and infusion bottles.
		3 g mezlocillin (as sodium)	In vials and infusion bottles and *ADD-Vantage* vials.
		4 g mezlocillin (as sodium)	In vials, infusion bottles and *ADD-Vantage* vials.
		20 g mezlocillin (as sodium)	In pharmacy bulk packages.

Extended Spectrum Penicillins

PIPERACILLIN SODIUM

For complete prescribing information, refer to the Penicillins group monograph.

Indications:

Treatment of mixed infections and presumptive therapy prior to the identification of the causative organisms. Also, it may be used as single drug therapy in some situations where two antibiotics are normally used.

Intra-abdominal infections (including hepatobiliary and surgical infections): Caused by *Escherichia coli; Pseudomonas aeruginosa;* enterococci; *Clostridium* sp; anaerobic cocci; *Bacteroides* sp, including *B fragilis.*

Urinary tract infections (UTIs): Caused by *E coli, Klebsiella* sp, *P aeruginosa, Proteus* sp, including *P mirabilis* and enterococci.

Gynecologic infections (including endometritis, pelvic inflammatory disease, pelvic cellulitis): Caused by *Bacteroides* sp, including *B fragilis;* anaerobic cocci; *Neisseria gonorrhoeae;* enterococci (*Streptococcus faecalis*).

Septicemia (including bacteremia): Caused by *E coli, Klebsiella* sp, *Enterobacter* sp, *Serratia* sp, *P mirabilis, S pneumoniae,* enterococci, *P aeruginosa, Bacteroides* sp and anaerobic cocci.

Lower respiratory tract infections: Caused by *E coli, Klebsiella* sp, *Enterobacter* sp, *P aeruginosa, Serratia* sp, *Hemophilus influenzae, Bacteroides* sp and anaerobic cocci. Although improvement has been noted in cystic fibrosis patients, long-term bacterial eradication may not be achieved.

Skin and skin structure infections: Caused by *E coli; Klebsiella* sp; *Serratia* sp; *Acinetobacter* sp; *Enterobacter* sp; *P aeruginosa;* indole-positive *Proteus* sp; *P mirabilis; Bacteroides* sp, including *B fragilis;* anaerobic cocci; enterococci.

Bone and joint infections: Caused by *P aeruginosa,* enterococci, *Bacteroides* sp and anaerobic cocci.

Gonococcal infections: Treatment of uncomplicated gonococcal urethritis.

Streptococcal infections: Infections caused by streptococcus species including group A β-hemolytic *Streptococcus* and *S pneumoniae;* however, these infections are ordinarily treated with more narrow spectrum penicillins.

Prophylaxis: For prophylactic use in surgery including intra-abdominal (GI and biliary) procedures, vaginal and abdominal hysterectomy and cesarean section. Effective prophylaxis depends on the time of administration; give ½ to 1 hour before the operation so that effective levels can be achieved in the wound prior to the procedure.

Stop the prophylactic use of piperacillin within 24 hours. Continuing administration of any antibiotic increases the possibility of adverse reactions, but in the majority of surgical procedures does not reduce the incidence of subsequent infections. If there are signs of infection, obtain specimens for culture so that appropriate therapy can begin.

Administration and Dosage:

Administer IM or IV. For serious infections, give 3 to 4 g every 4 to 6 hours as a 20 to 30 minute IV infusion. Maximum daily dose is 24 g/day, although higher doses have been used. Limit IM injections to 2 g/site.

Hemodialysis: Maximum dose is 6 g/day (2 g every 8 hours). Hemodialysis removes 30% to 50% of piperacillin in 4 hours; administer an additional 1 g after each dialysis.

Renal failure and hepatic insufficiency: Measure serum levels to provide additional guidance for adjusting dosage; however, this may not be practical.

Infants and children < 12 years of age: Dosages have not been established; however, the following dosages have been suggested:

Neonates – 100 mg/kg/dose every 12 hours.

Children – Cystic fibrosis, 350 to 500 mg/kg/day divided every 4 to 6 hours. Other conditions, 200 to 300 mg/kg/day, up to a maximum of 24 g/day divided every 4 to 6 hours.

Concomitant therapy with aminoglycosides has been used successfully, especially in patients with impaired host defenses. Use both drugs in full therapeutic doses.

Extended Spectrum Penicillins

PIPERACILLIN SODIUM

Piperacillin Uses and Dosages	
Organisms/Infections	Dosage
Serious infections (septicemia, nosocomial pneumonia, intra-abdominal infections, aerobic and anaerobic gynecologic infections and skin and soft tissue infections):	12 to 18 g/day IV (200 to 300 mg/kg/day) in divided doses every 4 to 6 hours.
Renal impairment –	
Creatinine clearance 20 to 40 ml/min	12 g/day; 4 g every 8 hours.
< 20 ml/min	8 g/day; 4 g every 12 hours.
Urinary tract infections: Complicated (normal renal function)	8 to 16 g/day IV (125 to 200 mg/kg/day) in divided doses every 6 to 8 hours.
Renal impairment	
Creatinine clearance 20 to 40 ml/min	9 g/day; 3 g every 8 hours.
< 20 ml/min	6 g/day; 3 g every 12 hours.
Uncomplicated UTI and most community-acquired pneumonia (normal renal function)	6 to 8 g/day IM or IV (100 to 125 mg/kg/d) in divided doses every 6 to 12 hours.
Uncomplicated UTI with renal impairment– Creatinine clearance < 20 ml/min	6 g/day; 3 g every 12 hours.
Uncomplicated gonorrhea infections:	2 g IM in a single dose with 1 g probenecid ½ hour prior to injection.
Prophylaxis: Intra-abdominal surgery	2 g IV just prior to surgery; 2 g during surgery; 2 g every 6 hours post-op for no more than 24 hours.
Vaginal hysterectomy	2 g IV just prior to surgery; 2 g 6 hrs after initial dose; 2 g 12 hrs after first dose.
Cesarean section	2 g IV after cord is clamped; 2 g 4 hours after initial dose; 2 g 8 hours after first dose.
Abdominal hysterectomy	2 g IV just prior to surgery; 2 g on return to recovery room; 2 g after 6 hours.

Diluents for Reconstitution of Piperacillin	
Sterile Water for Injection	Bacteriostatic* Sodium Chloride Injection
Bacteriostatic Water*for Injection	Dextrose 5% in Water
Sodium Chloride Injection	Dextrose 5% and 0.9% Sodium Chloride**
	Lidocaine HCl 0.5% to 1% (w/o epinephrine)

* Either parabens or benzyl alcohol.

** For IM use only. Lidocaine is contraindicated in patients with a known history of hypersensitivity to local anesthetics of the amide type.

Piperacillin Solutions		
IV Solutions	IV Admixtures	ADD-Vantage vials
Dextrose 5% in Water	Normal Saline [+ KCl 40 mEq]	Dextrose 5% in Water
0.9% Sodium Chloride	5% Dextrose in Water [+ KCl 40 mEq]	0.9% Sodium Chloride
Dextrose 5% and 0.9% Sodium Chloride	5% Dextrose/Normal Saline [+ KCl 40 mEq]	
Lactated Ringer's Injection	Ringer's Injection [+ KCl 40 mEq]	
Dextran 6% in 0.9% Sodium Chloride	Lactated Ringer's Injection [+ KCl 40 mEq]	

IV administration:

Reconstitution directions – Reconstitute each g piperacillin with at least 5 ml of a suitable diluent (except Lidocaine HCl 0.5% to 1% without epinephrine) listed above. Shake well until dissolved. Reconstituted solution may be further diluted to the desired volume (eg, 50 or 100 ml) in the above listed IV solutions and admixtures.

Reconstitution directions for bulk vial – Reconstitute the 40 g vial with 172 ml of a suitable diluent (except Lidocaine HCl 0.5% to 1% without epinephrine) listed above to achieve a concentration of 1 g per 5 ml.

Extended Spectrum Penicillins

PIPERACILLIN SODIUM

Directions for administration:

Intermittent IV infusion – Infuse diluted solution over a period of about 30 minutes. During infusion it is desirable to discontinue the primary IV solution.

IV injection (bolus) – Reconstituted solution should be injected slowly over a 3 to 5 minute period to help avoid vein irritation.

IM administration:

Reconstitution directions – Reconstitute each g of piperacillin with 2 ml of a suitable diluent listed in the previous table to achieve a concentration of 1 g per 2.5 ml. Shake well until dissolved.

Directions for administration – When indicated by clinical and bacteriological findings, IM administration of 6 to 8 g daily, in divided doses, may be used for initiation of therapy. In addition, consider IM administration of the drug for maintenance therapy after clinical and bacteriologic improvement has been obtained with IV piperacillin sodium treatment. Administration IM should not exceed 2 g per injection at any one site. The preferred site is the upper outer quadrant of the buttock (ie, gluteus maximus). Use the deltoid area only if well developed, and then only with caution to avoid radial nerve injury. Injections IM should not be made into the lower or mid-third of the upper arm.

Stability following reconstitution: Stable in both glass and plastic containers when reconstituted with recommended diluents and when diluted with the IV solutions and IV admixtures indicated above.

Extensive stability studies have demonstrated chemical stability (potency, pH and clarity) through 24 hours at room temperature, up to 1 week refrigerated, and up to 1 month frozen (–10° to –20°C;14 to –4°F). (*Note:* The 40 g bulk vial should not be frozen after reconstitution.) Appropriate consideration of aseptic technique and individual hospital policy, however, may recommend discarding unused portions after storage for 48 hours under refrigeration and recommend discarding after 24 hours storage at room temperature.

Rx	**Pipracil** (Lederle)	**Powder for injection:** Contains 1.85 mEq (42.5 mg) sodium/g 2 g	In vials, infusion bottles and *ADD-Vantage* vials.
		3 g	In vials, infusion bottles and *ADD-Vantage* vials.
		4 g	In vials, infusion bottles and *ADD-Vantage* vials.
		40 g	In pharmacy bulk vials.

CARBENICILLIN INDANYL SODIUM

Complete prescribing information for these products begins in the Penicillins group monograph.

Indications:

Treatment of acute and chronic infections of the upper and lower urinary tract and in asymptomatic bacteriuria due to susceptible strains of: *Escherichia coli, Proteus mirabilis, Morganella morganii, Providencia rettgeri, P vulgaris, Pseudomonas, Enterobacter* and enterococci. Also indicated in the treatment of prostatitis due to susceptible strains of: *E coli,* enterococcus *(S faecalis), P mirabilis* and *Enterobacter* species.

Administration and Dosage:

Urinary tract infections:

E coli, Proteus species and Enterobacter – 382 to 764 mg 4 times daily.

Pseudomonas and enterococci – 764 mg 4 times daily.

Prostatitis due to E coli, P mirabilis, Enterobacter and enterococcus (S faecalis): 764 mg 4 times daily.

Rx	**Geocillin** (Roerig)	**Tablets, film coated:** 382 mg carbenicillin (118 mg indanyl sodium ester)	Yellow. Capsule shape. In 100s and UD 100s.

Extended Spectrum Penicillins

PIPERACILLIN SODIUM AND TAZOBACTAM SODIUM

For complete prescribing information, refer to the Penicillins group monograph.

Actions:

Pharmacology: Piperacillin/tazobactam is an injectable antibacterial combination product consisting of the semisynthetic antibiotic piperacillin sodium and the beta-lactamase inhibitor tazobactam sodium.

Pharmacokinetics:

Absorption/Distribution – Piperacillin plasma concentrations, following a 30 minute infusion, were similar to those attained when equivalent doses of piperacillin were administered alone, with mean peak plasma levels of ≈ 134, 242 and 298 mcg/ml for the 2.25, 3.375 and 4.5 g piperacillin/tazobactam doses, respectively. The corresponding mean peak plasma concentrations of tazobactam were 15, 24 and 34 mcg/ml, respectively. Following a 30 minute IV infusion, steady-state plasma concentrations of piperacillin and tazobactam were similar to those attained after the first dose.

Metabolism/Excretion – The plasma half-life of piperacillin and tazobactam ranged from 0.7 to 1.2 hours in healthy subjects. Piperacillin is metabolized to a minor microbiologically active desethyl metabolite. Tazobactam is metabolized to a single metabolite that lacks pharmacological and antibacterial activities. Both piperacillin and tazobactam are eliminated via the kidney by glomerular filtration and tubular secretion. Piperacillin is excreted rapidly as unchanged drug with 68% of the administered dose excreted in the urine. Tazobactam and its metabolite are eliminated primarily by renal excretion with 80% of the administered dose excreted as unchanged drug and the remainder as the single metabolite. Piperacillin, tazobactam and desethyl piperacillin are also secreted into the bile. Both piperacillin and tazobactam are ≈ 30% bound to plasma proteins.

After administration to subjects with renal impairment (Ccr < 20 ml/min), the half-life of piperacillin and tazobactam increases 2- to 4-fold with decreasing creatinine clearance (Ccr). The half-life of piperacillin and of tazobactam increases by ≈ 25% and 18%, respectively, in patients with hepatic cirrhosis. However, this difference does not warrant dosage adjustment.

Indications:

For the treatment of patients with moderate to severe infections caused by piperacillin-resistant, piperacillin/tazobactam susceptible, β-lactamase producing strains of the microorganisms in the conditions listed below.

Appendicitis (complicated by rupture or abscess) and peritonitis caused by piperacillin-resistant, β-lactamase producing strains of *E. coli* or these members of the *Bacteroides fragilis* group: *B. fragilis, B. ovatus, B. thetaiotaomicron* or *B. vulgatus.*

Uncomplicated and complicated skin and skin structure infections, including cellulitis, cutaneous abscesses and ischemic/diabetic foot infections caused by piperacillin-resistant, β-lactamase producing strains of *S. aureus.*

Postpartum endometritis or pelvic inflammatory disease caused by piperacillin-resistant, β-lactamase producing strains of *E. coli.*

Community-acquired pneumonia (moderate severity only) caused by piperacillin-resistant, β-lactamase producing strains of *H. influenzae.*

Nosocomial pneumonia (moderate to severe) caused by piperacillin-resistant, β-lactamase producing strains of *S. aureus.*

Piperacillin/tazobactam is indicated only for the specified conditions listed above. Infections caused by piperacillin-susceptible organisms for which piperacillin is effective are also amenable to piperacillin/tazobactam treatment due to its piperacillin content. The treatment of mixed infections caused by piperacillin-susceptible organisms and piperacillin-resistant, β-lactamase producing organisms susceptible to piperacillin/tazobactam should not require adding another antibiotic.

Adverse Reactions:

Diarrhea (11.3%); headache, constipation (7.7%); nausea (6.9%); insomnia (6.6%); rash (including maculopapular, bullous, urticarial and eczematoid; 4.2%); vomiting, dyspepsia (3.3%); pruritus (3.1%); stool changes, fever (2.4%); agitation (2.1%); pain (1.7%); moniliasis, hypertension (1.6%); dizziness (1.4%); abdominal pain, chest pain (1.3%); edema, anxiety, rhinitis (1.2%); dyspnea (1.1%).

Nosocomial lower respiratory tract infections: Diarrhea (20%); constipation (8.4%); agitation (7.1%); nausea (5.8%); headache, insomnia (4.5%); oral thrush, erythematous rash (3.9%); anxiety, fever, pain, pruritus (3.2%); hiccough, vomiting (2.6%); dyspepsia, edema, fluid overload, stool changes (1.9%); anorexia, cardiac arrest, confusion, diaphoresis, duodenal ulcer, flatulence, hypertension, hypotension, injection site inflammation, pleural effusion, pneumothorax, rash, supraventricular tachycardia, thrombophlebitis, urinary incontinence (1.3%).

Lab test abnormalities: Decreases in hemoglobin and hematocrit, thrombocytopenia, increases in platelet count, eosinophilia, leukopenia, neutropenia (the leukopenia/neutropenia appears to be reversible and most frequently associated with prolonged administration [eg, ≥ 21 days of therapy]), positive direct Coombs' test, prolonged prothrombin time, prolonged partial thromboplastin time, transient elevations of AST, ALT, alkaline phosphatase and bilirubin, increases in serum creatinine and blood urea nitrogen, proteinuria, hematuria, pyuria, abnormalities in electrolytes (eg, increases and decreases in sodium, potassium, and calcium), hyperglycemia, decreases in total protein or albumin.

Administration and Dosage:

Approved by the FDA on October 22, 1993.

Administer by IV infusion over 30 minutes. The usual total daily dose for adults is 12 g/1.5 g for 7 to 10 days, given as 3.375 g every 6 hours.

Nosocomial pneumonia: Start with 3.375 g every 4 hours plus an aminoglycoside. Continue the aminoglycoside in patients from whom *P. aeruginosa* is isolated. If it is not isolated, the aminoglycoside may be discontinued at the discretion of the treating physician as guided by the severity of the infection and the patient's clinical and bacteriological progress.

Renal function impairment: In patients with renal insufficiency (Ccr < 40 ml/min), adjust the IV dose to the degree of actual renal function impairment. In patients with nosocomial pneumonia receiving concomitant aminoglycoside therapy, adjust the aminoglycoside dosage according to the manufacturer's recommendations.

Piperacillin Sodium and Tazobactam Sodium Dosage Recommendations	
Creatinine Clearance (ml/min)	Recommended Dosage Regimen
20-40	8 g/1 g/day in divided doses of 2.25 g every 6 hours
< 20	6 g/0.75 g/day in divided doses of 2.25 g every 8 hours

Hemodialysis: The maximum dose is 2.25 g every 8 hours. In addition, because hemodialysis removes 30% to 40% of a dose in 4 hours, give one additional 0.75 g dose following each dialysis period.

Compatible IV diluents include 0.9% Sodium Chloride for Injection, Sterile Water for Injection, Dextran 6% in Saline, Dextrose 5%, Bacteriostatic Saline/Parabens, Bacteriostatic Water/Parabens, Bacteriostatic Saline/Benzyl Alcohol, Bacteriostatic Water/Benzyl Alcohol. Lactated Ringer's solution is not compatible. Dilute to at least 50 ml.

Intermittent IV infusion: During the infusion it is desirable to discontinue the primary infusion solution. When concomitant therapy with aminoglycosides is indicated, reconstitute piperacillin/tazobactam and the aminoglycoside and administer separately (due to the in vitro inactivation of the aminoglycoside by the penicillin).

Storage/Stability: Use single dose vials immediately after reconstitution. Discard any unused portion after 24 hours if stored at room temperature or after 48 hours if stored at refrigerated temperature (2° to 8°C [36° to 46°F]). Stability in the IV bags has been demonstrated for up to 24 hours at room temperature and up to 1 week at refrigerated temperature. Stability in an ambulatory IV infusion pump has been demonstrated for a period of 12 hours at room temperature.

Rx	**Zosyn** (Wyeth-Ayerst)	**Powder for Injection:** 2 g piperacillin/ 0.25 g tazobactam	4.69 mEq sodium. In 2.25 g vials.
		3 g piperacillin/ 0.375 g tazobactam	7.04 mEq sodium. In 3.375 g vials.
		4 g piperacillin/ 0.5 g tazobactam	9.39 mEq sodium. In 4.5 g and piggyback infusion vials.

CEPHALOSPORINS AND RELATED ANTIBIOTICS

Actions:

Pharmacology: Structurally and pharmacologically related to penicillins. Cefoxitin and cefotetan (cephamycins) and loracarbef (a carbacephem) are included due to their similarity.

Most cephalosporins and related compounds are divided into first, second and third generation agents (see table). Within each group, differentiation is primarily by pharmacokinetics; groups are divided by antibacterial spectrum. In general, progression from first to third generation reveals broadening gram-negative spectrum, loss of efficacy against gram-positive organisms, greater efficacy against resistant organisms and increased cost. However, this classification scheme is becoming less clearly defined as newer agents enter the market. The decision to use a specific agent in the clinical setting should be primarily based on bacterial spectrum, route of administration, side effect profile and indications.

Mechanism – Cephalosporins inhibit mucopeptide synthesis in the bacterial cell wall, making it defective and osmotically unstable. The drugs are usually bactericidal, depending on organism susceptibility, dose, tissue concentrations and the rate at which organisms are multiplying. They are more effective against rapidly growing organisms forming cell walls.

Pharmacokinetics:

Pharmacokinetic Parameters of Cephalosporins

			Half-Life						
	Drug	Routes	Normal renal function (minutes)	ESRD[1] (hours)	Hemodialysis (hours)	Protein bound (%)	Recovered unchanged in urine (%)	Peak serum level 1 g IV dose (mcg/ml)	Sodium (mEq/g)
First	Cephalexin	Oral	50-80	19-22	4-6	10	> 90	—	—
	Cefadroxil	Oral	78-96	20-25	3-4	20	> 90	—	—
	Cephradine	Oral/IM-IV	48-80	8-15	—	8-17	> 90	86	6[2]
	Cephalothin	IM-IV	30-50	3-15	3	70	68-70	30	2.8
	Cephapirin	IM-IV	24-36	1.8-4	1.8	54	68-70	73	2.4
	Cefazolin	IM-IV	90-120	3-7	9-14	80-86	80-96	185-189	2-2.1
Second	Cefaclor	Oral	35-54	2-3	1.6-2.1	25	60-85	—	—
	Cefamandole	IM-IV	30-60	8-11	7	70	65-85	139	3.3
	Cefoxitin	IM-IV	40-60	20	4	73	85-99	64-110	2.3
	Cefuroxime	Oral/IM-IV	80	16-22[3]	3.5	33-50	66-100	100[4]	2.4[3]
	Cefonicid	IM-IV	270	11	—	98	95-99	221.3	3.7
	Cefmetazole	IV	72	—	—	65	85	—	2
	Cefotetan	IM-IV	180-276	13-35	5	88-90	51-81	158	3.5
	Cefprozil	Oral	78	5.2-5.9	decreased	36	60	—	—
	Loracarbef	Oral	60	32	4	25	> 90	—	—
Third	Cefixime	Oral	180-240	11.5	—	65	50	—	—
	Cefpodoxime[5]	Oral	120-180	9.8	—	21-29	29-33	—	—
	Cefoperazone	IM-IV	102-156	1.3-2.9	2	82-93	20-30	73-153	1.5
	Cefotaxime	IM-IV	60	3-11	2.5	30-40	20-36	42-102	2.2
	Ceftizoxime	IM-IV	84-114	25-30	6	30	80	60-87	2.6
	Ceftriaxone	IM-IV	348-522	15.7	14.7	85-95	33-67	151	3.6
	Ceftazidime	IM-IV	114-120	14-30	—	< 10-17	80-90	69-90	2.3
	Ceftibuten	Oral	144	13.4-22.3	2-4	65	56	—	—
	Cefepime	IM-IV	102-138	17-21	11-16	20	85	79	—

[1] ESRD = End stage renal disease (Ccr < 10 ml/min/1.73 m^2).
[2] Also available in sodium free form.
[3] Injection only.
[4] Following 1.5 g IV dose.
[5] Extended spectrum agent.

CEPHALOSPORINS AND RELATED ANTIBIOTICS

Organisms Generally Susceptible to Cephalosporins

✓ = generally susceptible
‡ = demonstrated in vitro activity

	Organisms	First Generation						Second Generation				
		Cephalexin	Cefadroxil	Cephradine	Cephalothin	Cephapirin	Cefazolin	Cefaclor	Cefamandole	Cefoxitin	Cefuroxime	Cefonicid
Gram-positive	*Staphylococci*[1]	✓[2]	✓	✓	✓	✓	✓	✓[2]	✓	✓	✓	✓[2]
	Streptococci, beta-hemolytic	✓	✓	✓	✓	✓	✓	✓	✓	✓	✓	✓
	Streptococcus pneumoniae	✓	✓	✓	✓	✓	✓	✓	✓	✓	✓	✓
	Streptococcus pyogenes											
Gram-negative	*Acinetobacter* sp											
	Citrobacter sp										✓[2]	‡
	Enterobacter sp						✓[2]		✓		✓[2]	‡
	Escherichia coli	✓	✓	✓	✓	✓	✓	✓	✓	✓	✓	✓
	Haemophilus influenzae	✓		✓	✓	✓	✓	✓[3]	✓[3]	✓[3]	✓[3]	✓[3]
	Haemophilus parainfluenzae										‡	
	Hafnia alvei											
	Klebsiella sp	✓	✓	✓	✓	✓	✓	✓	✓	✓	✓	✓
	Moraxella (Branhamella) catarrhalis	‡						✓			‡	
	Morganella (Proteus) morganii								✓	✓	✓[2]	✓
	Neisseria gonorrhoeae							‡		✓	✓	‡
	Neisseria meningitidis										✓	
	Proteus mirabilis	✓	✓	✓	✓	✓	✓	✓	✓	✓	✓	✓
	Proteus vulgaris								✓[2]	✓		✓
	Providencia sp									✓	✓	
	Providencia rettgeri								✓	✓	✓	✓
	Pseudomonas aeruginosa											
	Salmonella sp				✓						✓	
	Salmonella typhi											
	Serratia sp											
	Shigella sp				✓						✓	
Anaerobes	*Bacteroides* sp							✓	✓	✓	✓	
	Bacteroides fragilis									✓		
	Clostridium sp								✓	✓	✓	‡
	Clostridium difficile											
	Eubacterium sp											
	Fusobacterium sp								✓		✓	‡
	Peptococcus sp							‡	✓	✓	✓	‡
	Peptostreptococcus sp							‡	✓	✓	✓	‡

[1] Coagulase-positive, coagulase-negative and penicillinase-producing.
[2] Some strains are resistant.
[3] Including some β-lactamase-producing strains.

CEPHALOSPORINS AND RELATED ANTIBIOTICS

Organisms Generally Susceptible to Cephalosporins

Second Generation (Cont.)				Third Generation									Organisms	
Cefmetazole	Cefotetan	Cefprozil	Loracarbef	Cefixime	Cefpodoxime[4]	Cefoperazone	Cefotaxime	Ceftizoxime	Ceftriaxone	Ceftazidime	Ceftibuten	Cefepime[8]	✓= generally susceptible ‡= demonstrated in vitro activity	
✓	✓	✓	✓		✓[2]	✓	✓[3]	✓	✓	✓		✓[5]	*Staphylococci*[1]	Gram-positive
✓	✓	✓	✓	✓	✓	✓	✓	✓	✓	✓		‡	*Streptococci*, beta-hemolytic	Gram-positive
✓	✓	✓	✓	✓	✓	✓	✓	✓	✓	✓	✓[6]	✓	*Streptococcus pneumoniae*	Gram-positive
											✓	✓[7]	*Streptococcus pyogenes*	Gram-positive
						✓[2]	✓	✓	‡	‡		‡	*Acinetobacter* sp	Gram-negative
‡	‡	‡	‡	‡	‡	✓	✓	‡	‡	✓		‡	*Citrobacter* sp	Gram-negative
‡	✓					✓	✓	✓	✓	✓		✓	*Enterobacter* sp	Gram-negative
✓	✓	‡	✓	✓	✓	✓	✓	✓	✓	✓		✓	*Escherichia coli*	Gram-negative
✓[3]	✓[3]	✓[3]	✓[3]	✓[3]	✓[3]	✓[3]	✓[3]	✓[3]	✓[3]	✓[3]	✓[3]	‡[3]	*Haemophilus influenzae*	Gram-negative
			‡	‡[3]	‡		✓		✓	‡			*Haemophilus parainfluenzae*	Gram-negative
												‡	*Hafnia alvei*	Gram-negative
✓	✓	‡	‡	‡	✓	✓	✓	✓	✓	✓		✓	*Klebsiella* sp	Gram-negative
‡		✓	✓[3]	✓[3]	✓			‡		✓	✓[3]	‡[3]	*Moraxella (Branhamella) catarrhalis*	Gram-negative
✓	✓					✓	✓	✓	✓	‡		‡	*Morganella (Proteus) morganii*	Gram-negative
‡	✓	‡	‡[1]	‡	✓[2]	✓[3]	✓	✓	✓	‡			*Neisseria gonorrhoeae*	Gram-negative
	‡					‡	✓	‡	✓	✓			*Neisseria meningitidis*	Gram-negative
✓	✓	‡	‡	✓	✓	✓	✓	✓	✓	✓		✓	*Proteus mirabilis*	Gram-negative
✓	✓			‡	‡	✓	✓	✓	✓	✓		‡	*Proteus vulgaris*	Gram-negative
✓	✓			‡			‡	‡	‡	‡		‡	*Providencia* sp	Gram-negative
‡	✓			‡	‡	✓	✓	✓	‡	‡		‡	*Providencia rettgeri*	Gram-negative
						✓	✓[2]	✓[2]	✓[2]	✓		✓	*Pseudomonas aeruginosa*	Gram-negative
‡	‡	‡	‡	‡		‡	‡	‡	‡	‡			*Salmonella* sp	Gram-negative
	‡						‡	‡	‡				*Salmonella typhi*	Gram-negative
	‡			‡		✓	✓	✓	✓	✓		‡	*Serratia* sp	Gram-negative
‡	‡	‡	‡	‡		‡	‡	‡	‡	‡			*Shigella* sp	Gram-negative
✓	✓[2]	‡				✓	✓	‡	✓				*Bacteroides* sp	Anaerobes
✓	✓					✓	✓	✓	‡				*Bacteroides fragilis*	Anaerobes
✓	✓	‡	‡			✓	✓	‡	‡	‡			*Clostridium* sp	Anaerobes
		‡				‡							*Clostridium difficile*	Anaerobes
						‡			‡				*Eubacterium* sp	Anaerobes
✓	✓	‡	‡			‡	✓	‡	‡				*Fusobacterium* sp	Anaerobes
‡	✓		‡			✓	✓	✓	‡	‡			*Peptococcus* sp	Anaerobes
‡	✓	‡	‡		‡	✓	✓	✓	‡	‡			*Peptostreptococcus* sp	Anaerobes

[1] Coagulase-positive, coagulase-negative and penicillinase-producing.
[2] Some strains are resistant.
[3] Including some β-lactamase-producing strains.
[4] Extended spectrum agent.
[5] Methicillin-susceptible strains only.
[6] Penicillin-susceptible strains only.
[7] Lancefield's Group A streptococci.
[8] Some other references consider this fourth generation.

CEPHALOSPORINS AND RELATED ANTIBIOTICS

Absorption – Cephalexin, cephradine, cefaclor, cefixime, cefprozil, cefadroxil, ceftibuten and loracarbef are well absorbed from the GI tract; absorption of these agents (except cefadroxil and cefprozil) may be delayed by food, but the amount absorbed is not affected. Peak plasma levels of loracarbef (capsules) are decreased by food and occur later. The absorption of oral cefuroxime and cefpodoxime is increased when given with food.

Distribution – Cephalosporins are widely distributed to most tissues and fluids. First and second generation agents do not readily enter cerebrospinal fluid (CSF), except cefuroxime, even when meninges are inflamed. Third generation compounds (little data for cefixime) and cefuroxime readily diffuse into the CSF of patients with inflamed meninges. However, CSF levels of cefoperazone are relatively low. Therapeutic levels are reached in bone after usual doses of most agents. Cefazolin penetrates acutely inflamed bone at higher concentrations than in normal bone.

High concentrations of ceftriaxone, cefamandole and cefoperazone are attained in bile. Therapeutic levels of ceftizoxime, cefuroxime, cefotetan, ceftazidime, cefoxitin and cefonicid are attained in bile. Bile levels of cefazolin can reach or exceed serum levels by up to 5 times in patients without obstructive biliary disease.

Metabolism/Excretion – Cefuroxime axetil is metabolized to free cefuroxime plus acetaldehyde and acetic acid. Cephalothin and cephapirin are metabolized to less active compounds; however, desacetylcephapirin contributes to the drug's antibacterial activity. Desacetylcefotaxime, a major metabolite of cefotaxime, contributes to the bactericidal activity and increases the spectrum to include anaerobes, specifically *Bacteroides* sp; the synergy with the parent drug appears to extend the dosing interval to 8 to 12 hours due to the prolonged metabolite half-life. Cefpodoxime proxetil is a prodrug that is de-esterified to its active metabolite, cefpodoxime. Most cephalosporins and metabolites are primarily excreted renally. Cefoperazone is excreted mainly in the bile; peak serum levels and serum half-lives are unchanged, even in patients with severe renal insufficiency. In hepatic dysfunction, serum half-life and urinary excretion are increased.

Microbiology: Refer to the previous tables for organisms generally susceptible to cephalosporins.

β-lactamase resistance – First generation cephalosporins are generally inactivated by β-lactamase-producing organisms. Newer agents are distinguished by an increasing resistance to β-lactamase inactivation. Cefonicid and cefixime have a high degree of stability to some β–lactamases. Cefoxitin, cefuroxime, ceftriaxone, cefotaxime, ceftizoxime and cefotetan have a high degree of stability in the presence of both penicillinases and cephalosporinases produced by gram-negative and gram-positive bacteria. Cefoperazone and ceftazidime are also highly stable in the presence of β–lactamases produced by most gram-negative pathogens, and are active against organisms that are resistant to other β–lactam antibiotics because of β-lactamase production. Cefepime has a broad spectrum of activity against gram-positive and gram-negative bacteria but has a low affinity for chromosomally-encoded beta-lactamases.

Indications:

For specific approved indications, refer to individual drug monographs.

Surgery: Some of these agents are indicated for preoperative, intraoperative and postoperative prophylaxis to reduce infection in patients undergoing surgical procedures classified as contaminated or potentially contaminated (eg, GI surgery, cesarean section, vaginal hysterectomy or cholecystectomy in high-risk patients).

Contraindications:

Hypersensitivity to cephalosporins or related antibiotics (see Warnings).

Warnings:

Cross-allergenicity with penicillin: Administer cautiously to penicillin-sensitive patients. There is evidence of partial cross-allergenicity; cephalosporins cannot be assumed to be an absolutely safe alternative to penicillin in the penicillin-allergic patient. The estimated incidence of cross-sensitivity is 5% to 16%; however, it is possibly as low as 3% to 7%.

Serum sickness-like reactions (erythema multiforme or skin rashes accompanied by polyarthritis, arthralgia and, frequently, fever) have been reported; these reactions usually occurred following a second course of therapy. Signs and symptoms occur after a few days of therapy and resolve a few days after drug discontinuation with no serious sequelae. Antihistamines and corticosteroids may be of benefit in managing symptoms.

Seizures: Several cephalosporins have been implicated in triggering seizures, particularly in patients with renal impairment when the dosage was not reduced. If seizures associated with drug therapy occur, discontinue the drug. Anticonvulsant therapy can be given if clinically indicated.

CEPHALOSPORINS AND RELATED ANTIBIOTICS

Coagulation abnormalities: **Moxalactam** (with which most experience is reported), **cefamandole** and **cefoperazone** can interfere with hemostasis through three different mechanisms: Hypoprothrombinemia with or without bleeding (due to destruction of vitamin K-producing intestinal bacteria; a molecular attachment common to these three drugs, a methyltetrazolethiol side chain that prevents activation of prothrombin); platelet dysfunction; very rarely, immune-mediated thrombocytopenia. A total of 2.5% of clinical trial patients treated for ≥ 4 days with moxalactam experienced bleeding which was usually serious. At least 13 deaths occurred. Alterations in prothrombin times (PT) occur rarely in patients treated with **ceftriaxone. Cefotetan** also contains the methyltetrazolethiol side chain, but bleeding has not yet been a problem. However, several case reports have noted hypoprothrombinemia.

Bleeding associated with *hypoprothrombinemia* can be prevented with vitamin K. Give moxalactam patients 10 mg vitamin K/week prophylactically. Inhibition of *platelet function,* which may be accompanied by prolonged bleeding time, is dose-dependent and can generally be avoided by limiting dosage to 4 g/day. Monitor bleeding time in patients with normal renal function who receive > 4 g moxalactam/day for > 3 days. Reduce dosage in all patients with significantly impaired renal function. If bleeding time becomes unduly prolonged, discontinue these agents.

If bleeding occurs and PT is prolonged, give vitamin K. Fresh frozen plasma, packed red cells and platelet concentrates may be indicated. Discontinue moxalactam if bleeding is due to platelet dysfunction; use cefamandole, cefoperazone, ceftriaxone and cefotetan with caution. Bleeding may also be related to complications of underlying diseases (eg, sepsis, malignancy, renal and hepatic dysfunction) or may result from combined effects of underlying diseases and drug therapy. When bleeding occurs, rule out disseminated intravascular coagulation (DIC) since DIC is more likely to occur in patients with sepsis, malignancy or hepatic disease.

Predisposing factors to cephalosporin bleeding abnormalities include hepatic and renal dysfunction, thrombocytopenia and the concomitant use of "high dose" heparin (> 20,000 units/day), oral anticoagulants or other drugs that affect hemostasis (eg, aspirin). Elderly, malnourished or debilitated patients are more likely to experience bleeding abnormalities than other patients.

Pseudomembranous colitis occurs with cephalosporins (and other broad spectrum antibiotics); consider its diagnosis in patients who develop diarrhea with antibiotic use. Colitis may range in severity from mild to life-threatening. Treatment alters normal flora of the colon and may permit overgrowth of *Clostridia* species. A toxin produced by *C. difficile* is a primary cause of antibiotic-associated colitis. Cholestyramine and colestipol resins bind the toxin in vitro.

Mild cases of colitis may respond to drug discontinuation alone. Manage moderate to severe cases by sigmoidoscopy, bacteriologic studies and with fluid, electrolyte and protein supplementation, as indicated. When the colitis is not relieved by drug discontinuation, or when it is severe, oral vancomycin or metronidazole (see individual monographs) is treatment of choice. Rule out other causes of colitis.

Prescribe broad spectrum antibiotics with caution in individuals with a history of GI disease, especially colitis.

Renal function impairment: Cephalosporins may be nephrotoxic; use with caution in the presence of markedly impaired renal function (creatinine clearance [Ccr] rate of < 50 ml/min/1.73 m^2). In the elderly and in patients with known or suspected renal impairment, monitor carefully prior to and during therapy.

Reduce total daily antibiotic dosage in patients with transient or persistent reduction of urinary output due to renal insufficiency; high and prolonged serum concentrations can occur in such patients from usual doses. See individual product monographs for information on dosage adjustments in impaired renal function.

Hepatic function impairment: **Cefoperazone** is extensively excreted in bile. Serum half-life increases twofold to fourfold in patients with hepatic disease or biliary obstruction. If higher dosages are used (> 4 g), monitor serum concentrations.

Pregnancy: Category B; (Category C - Moxalactam). Safety for use during pregnancy is not established. Use only when potential benefits outweigh potential hazards to the fetus. Cephalosporins appear safe for pregnant patients, but relatively few controlled studies exist. Few case reports are available for the newer agents.

These agents cross the placenta; peak umbilical cord concentrations for the various agents range from 3 to 29 mcg/ml following doses of 0.5 to 2 g. These data yielded a maternal:fetal serum ratio range of 0.16 to 1. Drug levels in cord blood after administration of **cefazolin** are approximately ¼ to ⅓ maternal drug levels. **Cefotetan** reaches therapeutic levels in cord blood.

In addition, the pharmacokinetic parameters of these drugs appear to change in the pregnant woman; tendencies are toward shorter half-lives, lower serum levels, larger volumes of distribution and increased clearance.

Lactation: Most of these agents are excreted in breast milk in small quantities. Levels range from 0.16 to 4 mcg/ml, or a breast milk:maternal serum ratio of 0.01 to 0.5 following 0.5 to 2 g doses. However, consider these problems for the nursing infant: Modification/alteration of bowel flora; pharmacological effects; interference with interpretation of culture results if a fever/infection workup is needed.

Children: When using cephalosporins in infants, consider the relative benefit to risk. In neonates, accumulation of cephalosporin antibiotics (with resulting prolongation of drug half-life) has occurred.

In children ≥ 3 months of age, higher doses of **cefoxitin** have been associated with an increased incidence of eosinophilia and elevated AST.

In children ≥ 6 months of age, **ceftizoxime** has been associated with transient elevated levels of eosinophils, AST, ALT and CPK.

Safety and efficacy in children < 1 month (**cefaclor, cefamandole, cefazolin** and **parenteral cephradine**), < 3 months (**cefuroxime**), < 6 months (**cefixime, cefpodoxime**), < 9 months (**oral cephradine**) and < 1 year (**ceforanide**) have not been established.

Safety and efficacy of **cefoperazone** and **cefotetan** in children not established.

Precautions:

Parenteral use: Inject IM preparations deep into musculature; properly dilute IV preparations and administer over an appropriate time interval. See individual product monographs. Prolonged or high dosage IV use may be associated with thrombophlebitis; use small IV needles, larger veins and alternate infusion sites.

Gonorrhea: In the treatment of gonorrhea, all patients should have a serologic test for syphilis. Patients with incubating syphilis (seronegative without clinical signs of syphilis) are likely to be cured by the regimens used for gonorrhea.

Superinfection: Use of antibiotics (especially prolonged or repeated therapy) may result in bacterial or fungal overgrowth of nonsusceptible organisms. Such overgrowth may lead to a secondary infection. Take appropriate measures if this occurs.

Drug Interactions:

Cephalosporin Drug Interactions

Precipitant drug	Object drug*		Description
Cephalosporins	Ethanol	⬆	Alcoholic beverages consumed concurrently with or up to 72 hours after cefamandole, cefoperazone, moxalactam or cefotetan may produce acute alcohol intolerance (disulfiram-like reaction). These four antibiotics possess a methyltetrazolethiol side chain that may inhibit aldehyde dehydrogenase. The reaction begins within 30 minutes after alcohol ingestion and may subside 30 minutes to several hours afterwards; the reaction may occur up to 3 days after the last dose of the antibiotic.
Cephalosporins	Aminoglycosides	⬆	Aminoglycoside nephrotoxicity may be potentiated by concurrent use of some cephalosporins, specifically cephalothin. Monitor renal function closely.
Cephalosporins	Anticoagulants	⬆	Hypoprothrombinemic effects of anticoagulants may be increased by cephalosporins with the methyltetrazolethiol side chain (cefamandole, cefoperazone, cefotetan, moxalactam). Bleeding complications may occur (see Warnings). Bleeding disorders have occurred with some of the other cephalosporins; therefore, the risk might be increased in anticoagulated patients. The concurrent use of heparin may also theoretically increase the risk of bleeding.
Cephalosporins	Polypeptide antibiotics	⬆	The nephrotoxic effects of colistimethate may be increased by cephalothin. Monitor renal function.
Probenecid	Cephalosporins	⬆	Probenecid may increase and prolong cephalosporin plasma levels by competitively inhibiting renal tubular secretion. This is most significant for cephalosporins eliminated primarily by tubular secretion.

* ⬆ = Object drug increased

Drug/Lab test interactions: A false-positive reaction for **urine glucose** may occur with Benedict's solution, Fehling's solution or with *Clinitest* tablets, but not with enzyme-based tests such as *Clinistix* and *Tes-Tape*. **Moxalactam** does not interfere with

CEPHALOSPORINS AND RELATED ANTIBIOTICS

Clinitest. There may be a false-positive test for *proteinuria* with acid and denaturization-precipitation tests.

Cephradine may cause false-positive reactions in urinary protein tests that use sulfosalicylic acid.

Cefuroxime may cause a false-negative reaction in the ferricyanide test for **blood glucose**.

A false-positive direct **Coombs' test** has occurred in some patients receiving cephalosporins, particularly those with azotemia, in hematologic studies, in transfusion cross-matching procedures when **antiglobulin tests** are performed on the minor side or in Coombs' testing of newborns of mothers receiving cephalosporins before parturition. This reaction is nonimmunological.

Cephalosporins may falsely elevate **urinary 17-ketosteroid** values.

High concentrations of **cephalothin** or **cefoxitin** (> 100 mcg/ml) may interfere with measurement of *creatinine levels* by the Jaffe reaction and produce false results. Serum samples from patients on cefoxitin should not be analyzed for creatinine if obtained within 2 hrs of drug use. **Cefotetan** may affect these measurements.

Drug/Food interactions: Food increases absorption of cefpodoxime and oral cefuroxime.

Adverse Reactions:

Most common: GI disturbances and hypersensitivity phenomena. The latter are more likely to occur in individuals who have previously demonstrated hypersensitivity and in those with a history of allergy, asthma, hay fever or urticaria.

Miscellaneous: Hypotension; fever; dyspnea; interstitial pneumonitis; candidal overgrowth consisting of oral candidiasis, vaginitis, genital moniliasis, vaginal discharge and genito-anal pruritus; elevated CPK (after IM **ceforanide**); reversible hyperactivity; nervousness; insomnia; confusion; hypertonia; dizziness; somnolence.

Hypersensitivity: (See Warnings.) Allergic reactions may include: Stevens-Johnson syndrome; erythema multiforme; toxic epidermal necrolysis; renal dysfunction; toxic nephropathy; hepatic dysfunction including cholestasis, aplastic anemia, hemolytic anemia, hemorrhage.

Serum sickness-like reactions – See Warnings.

GI: Nausea; vomiting; diarrhea; anorexia; dysgeusia; glossitis; abdominal pain; flatulence; heartburn; stomach cramps; gallbladder sludge; cholestasis; dyspepsia. Colitis, including pseudomembranous colitis, can appear during or after treatment (see Warnings). Adverse GI effects after parenteral use of some cephalosporins.

Hematologic: Eosinophilia; transient neutropenia; lymphocytosis; leukocytosis; leukopenia; thrombocythemia; thrombocytopenia; agranulocytosis; granulocytopenia; hemolytic anemia; bone marrow depression; pancytopenia; decreased platelet function; bleeding in association with hypoprothrombinemia; anemia; aplastic anemia; hemorrhage; transient thrombocytosis. Lymphocytosis, lymphopenia, monocytosis, basophilia, jaundice, glycosuria, bronchospasm, palpitations and epistaxis (**ceftriaxone**, rare). Neutropenia due to an immunologic reaction and characterized by rapid destruction of peripheral neutrophils may require drug discontinuation. Transient fluctuations in leukocyte count, predominantly lymphocytosis, in infants and young children (**cefaclor**). Slight decreases in neutrophil count, decreased hemoglobin or hematocrit, disturbances in vitamin K-dependent clotting function (increased PT), increased platelets and increased bleeding have occurred (see Warnings).

Hepatic: Elevated AST, ALT, GGTP, total bilirubin, alkaline phosphatase, LDH; hepatomegaly; hepatitis; significantly elevated liver enzymes with clinical signs and symptoms of hepatitis (**cefoperazone**, one case). Values tend to return to normal after the end of therapy. Cholestatic jaundice has occurred (**cefaclor, cephalexin** and **cefamandole**).

Renal: Transitory elevations in BUN with and without elevated serum creatinine (frequency increases in patients > 50 years old and in children < 3); pyuria; dysuria; reversible interstitial nephritis; hematuria; toxic nephropathy; acute renal failure (rare); decreased creatinine clearance in patients with prior renal impairment (**cefamandole**); casts in the urine (**ceftriaxone**).

CNS: Headache; dizziness; lethargy; fatigue; paresthesia; confusion; diaphoresis; flushing; generalized tonic-clonic seizures, mild hemiparesis and extreme confusion following large doses in renal failure (**cefazolin**).

Local: IM administration commonly results in pain, induration, temperature elevation and tenderness. Sterile abscesses have occurred following accidental SC injection. Administration IV or IM has produced local swelling, inflammation, burning, cellulitis, paresthesia, phlebitis and thrombophlebitis.

CEPHALOSPORINS AND RELATED ANTIBIOTICS

Overdosage:

Parenteral cephalosporins: Inappropriately large doses may cause seizures, particularly in renal impairment. Reduce dosage when renal function is impaired. If seizures occur, promptly discontinue drug; administer anticonvulsants if clinically indicated; consider hemodialysis in cases of overwhelming overdosage.

Patient Information:

For oral preparations: Complete full course of therapy.

May cause GI upset; may take with food or milk. Take cefpodoxime and cefuroxime with food to increase absorption.

A false-positive reaction for urine glucose may occur with the nonspecific urine tests. Use an enzyme-based test.

Cephradine: Diabetics-Notify physician before changing diet or dosage of medication.

Administration and Dosage:

Duration of therapy: Continue administration for a minimum of 48 to 72 hours after fever abates or after evidence of bacterial eradication has been obtained. A minimum of 10 days treatment is recommended for group A β-hemolytic streptococci infections to guard against the risk of rheumatic fever or glomerulonephritis.

Perioperative prophylaxis: Discontinue prophylactic use within 24 hours after the surgical procedure. In surgery where infection may be particularly devastating (eg, open heart surgery, prosthetic arthroplasty), may continue prophylactic use for 3 to 5 days following surgery completion. If there are signs of infection, obtain cultures and perform sensitivity tests so appropriate therapy may be instituted.

CEFPODOXIME PROXETIL

For complete prescribing information, refer to the Cephalosporins group monograph.

Indications:

Lower respiratory tract:

Acute, community-acquired pneumonia caused by *Streptococcus pneumoniae* or *Haemophilus influenzae* (non-beta-lactamase-producing strains only).

Chronic bronchitis – Acute bacterial exacerbation caused by *S. pneumoniae, H. influenzae* (non-beta-lactamase-producing strains only) or *M. catarrhalis.*

Data are insufficient to establish efficacy in pneumonia or acute bacterial exacerbations of chronic bronchitis caused by β-lactamase-producing *H. influenzae.*

Upper respiratory tract:

Acute otitis media caused by *S. pneumoniae, H. influenzae* (including β-lactamase-producing strains), or *Moraxella (Branhamella) catarrhalis.*

Pharyngitis/tonsillitis caused by *S. pyogenes.*

Only IM penicillin is effective in prophylaxis of rheumatic fever. Cefpodoxime is generally effective in eradication of streptococci from the oropharynx. However, efficacy for prophylaxis of subsequent rheumatic fever is not established.

Sexually transmitted diseases:

Acute, uncomplicated urethral and cervical gonorrhea caused by *Neisseria gonorrhoeae* (including penicillinase-producing strains).

Acute, uncomplicated ano-rectal infections in women due to *N. gonorrhoeae* (including penicillinase-producing strains).

Efficacy of cefpodoxime in males with rectal infections caused by *N. gonorrhoeae* is not established. Data do not support use of cefpodoxime in treatment of pharyngeal infections due to *N. gonorrhoeae* in men or women.

Skin and skin structures:

Uncomplicated infections caused by *Staphylococcus aureus* (including penicillinase-producing strains) or *S. pyogenes.* Surgically drain abscesses as clinically indicated.

In clinical trials, successful treatment of uncomplicated skin and skin structure infections was dose-related. The effective therapeutic dose for skin infections was higher than those used in other recommended indications.

Urinary tract:

Uncomplicated infections (cystitis) caused by *Escherichia coli, Klebsiella pneumoniae, Proteus mirabilis* or *S. saprophyticus.*

In considering the use of cefpodoxime in the treatment of cystitis, weigh cefpodoxime's lower bacterial eradication rates against the increased eradication rates and different safety profiles of some other classes of approved agents.

Administration and Dosage:

Approved by the FDA on August 7, 1992.

Administer with food to enhance absorption.

CEFPODOXIME PROXETIL

Dosage/Duration of Cefpodoxime			
Type of infection	Total daily dose	Dose frequency	Duration
Adults ≥ 13 years of age			
Acute community-acquired pneumonia	400 mg	200 mg every 12 hrs	14 days
Acute bacterial exacerbations of chronic bronchitis	400 mg	200 mg every 12 hrs	10 days
Uncomplicated gonorrhea (men and women) and rectal gonococcal infections (women)	200 mg	single dose	
Skin and skin structure	800 mg	400 mg every 12 hrs	7 to 14 days
Pharyngitis/tonsillitis	200 mg	100 mg every 12 hrs	5 to 10 days
Uncomplicated urinary tract infection	200 mg	100 mg every 12 hrs	7 days
Children (age 5 months through 12 years):			
Acute otitis media	10 mg/kg/day (max 400 mg/day)	10 mg/kg every 24 hrs (max 400 mg/dose) or 5 mg/kg every 12 hrs (max 200 mg/dose)	10 days
Pharyngitis/tonsillitis	10 mg/kg/day (max 200 mg/day)	5 mg/kg every 12 hours (max 100 mg/dose)	5 to 10 days

Renal function impairment: For patients with severe renal impairment (creatinine clearance [Ccr] < 30 ml/min), increase the dosing intervals to every 24 hours. Hemodialysis patients use a dose frequency of 3 times/week after hemodialysis.

When only the serum creatinine level is available, the calculation given in the front matter (based on sex, weight and age of the patient) may be used to estimate Ccr (ml/min). For this estimate to be valid, the serum creatinine level should represent a steady state of renal function.

Cirrhosis: Cefpodoxime pharmacokinetics in cirrhotic patients (with or without ascites) are similar to those in healthy subjects. Dose adjustment is not necessary.

Storage/Stability: Store the suspension in a refrigerator at 2° to 8°C (36°C to 46°F). Discard unused portion after 14 days.

Rx	**Vantin** (Upjohn)	**Tablets:** 100 mg	Lactose. (U3617). Orange. Film coated. In 20s, 100s and UD 100s.
		200 mg	Lactose. (U3618). Coral red. Film coated. In 20s, 100s and UD 100s.
		Granules for suspension: 50 mg/5 ml	Lactose, sucrose. Lemon creme flavor. In 100 ml.
		100 mg/5 ml	Lactose, sucrose. Lemon creme flavor. In 100 ml.

CEFACLOR

For complete prescribing information, refer to the Cephalosporins group monograph.

Indications:

Lower respiratory tract infections, including pneumonia caused by *Streptococcus pneumoniae, H. influenzae* and *S. pyogenes* (group A β-hemolytic streptococci).

Upper respiratory tract infections, including pharyngitis and tonsillitis caused by *S. pyogenes* (group A β-hemolytic streptococci).

Otitis media caused by *S. pneumoniae, H. influenzae,* staphylococci and *S. pyogenes* (group A β-hemolytic streptococci).

Skin and skin structure infections caused by *Staphylococcus aureus* and *S. pyogenes* (group A β-hemolytic streptococci).

Urinary tract infections including pyelonephritis and cystitis caused by *Escherichia coli, Proteus mirabilis, Klebsiella* sp and coagulase-negative staphylococci.

Tablets, extended release:

Acute bacterial exacerbations of chronic bronchitis due to *H. influenzae* (non-β-lactamase-producing strains only), *M. catarrhalis* (including β-lactamase-producing strains) or *S. pneumoniae.*

CEFACLOR

Secondary bacterial infections of acute bronchitis due to *H. influenzae* (non-β-lactamase-producing strains only), *M. catarrhalis* (including β-lactamase-producing strains) or *S. pneumoniae.*

Pharyngitis and tonsillitis due to *S. pyogenes.*

Uncomplicated skin/skin structure infections due to *S. aureus* (methicillin-susceptible).

Unlabeled uses: A single 2 g dose may be effective for acute uncomplicated UTI in select populations.

Administration and Dosage:

Adults: Usual dosage is 250 mg every 8 hours. In severe infections or those caused by less susceptible organisms, dosage may be doubled.

Tablets, extended release – Administer with food to enhance absorption. Do not cut, crush or chew.

Acute bacterial exacerbations of chronic bronchitis: 500 mg/12 hours for 7 days.
Secondary bacterial infection of acute bronchitis: 500 mg/12 hours for 7 days.
Pharyngitis or tonsillitis: 375 mg/12 hours for 10 days.
Uncomplicated skin and skin structure infections: 375 mg/12 hours for 7 to 10 days.

Children: Give 20 mg/kg/day in divided doses every 8 hours. In more serious infections, otitis media and infections caused by less susceptible organisms, administer 40 mg/kg/day, with a maximum dosage of 1 g/day.

Twice daily treatment option – For otitis media and pharyngitis, the total daily dosage may be divided and administered every 12 hours.

Storage/Stability: Refrigerate suspension after reconstitution; discard after 14 days.

Rx	**Cefaclor** (Various, eg, Apothecon, Mylan, Rugby, UDL, URL)	**Capsules:** 250 mg	In 15s, 100s, 500s and 1000s.
Rx	**Ceclor Pulvules** (Lilly)		(3061). White and purple. In 15s, 100s and UD 100s.
Rx	**Cefaclor** (Various, eg, Apothecon, Mylan, Rugby, UDL, URL)	**Capsules:** 500 mg	In 15s, 100s and 500s.
Rx	**Ceclor Pulvules** (Lilly)		(3062). Gray and purple. In 15s, 100s and UD 100s.
Rx	**Ceclor CD** (Lilly)	**Tablets, extended release:** 375 mg	(4220). Blue. In 60s.
		500 mg	(4221). Blue. In 60s.
Rx	**Cefaclor** (Various, eg, Apothecon, Mylan, Rugby, URL)	**Powder for oral suspension:** 125 mg/5 ml	In 75 and 150 ml.
		187 mg/5 ml	In 50 and 100 ml.
		250 mg/5 ml	In 75 and 150 ml.
		375 mg/5 ml	In 50 and 100 ml.
Rx	**Ceclor** (Lilly)	**Powder for oral suspension:** 125 mg/5 ml	Sucrose. Strawberry flavor. In 75 and 150 ml.
		187 mg/5 ml	Sucrose. Strawberry flavor. In 50 and 100 ml.
		250 mg/5 ml	Sucrose. Strawberry flavor. In 75 and 150 ml.
		375 mg/5 ml	Sucrose. Strawberry flavor. In 50 and 100 ml.

CEPHALEXIN

Complete prescribing information for these products begins in the Cephalosporins group monograph.

Indications:

Respiratory tract infections due to *Streptococcus pneumoniae* and *S pyogenes.*

Otitis media caused by *S pneumoniae, H influenzae,* staphylococci, streptococci and *M catarrhalis* (monohydrate only).

Skin and skin structure infections caused by staphylococci or streptococci.

Bone infections caused by staphylococci or *Proteus mirabilis.*

GU infections, including acute prostatitis, caused by *E coli, P mirabilis* and *K pneumoniae*

CEPHALEXIN

Unlabeled uses: Prevention of bacterial endocarditis in penicillin-allergic patients undergoing dental, oral, esophageal or respiratory tract procedures who have not exhibited an immediate-type hypersensitivity reaction to penicillins.

Administration and Dosage:

Adults: 1 to 4 g/day in divided doses. Usual dose – 250 mg every 6 hours. Streptococcal pharyngitis, skin and skin structure infections, uncomplicated cystitis in patients > 15 years – 500 mg every 12 hours. May need larger doses for more severe infections or less susceptible organisms. If dose is > 4 g/day, use parenteral drugs.

Children:

Monohydrate – 25 to 50 mg/kg/day in divided doses. For streptococcal pharyngitis in patients > 1 year and for skin and skin structure infections, divide total daily dose and give every 12 hours. In severe infections, double the dose.

Otitis media: 75 to 100 mg/kg/day in 4 divided doses.

β-hemolytic streptococcal infections: Continue treatment for at least 10 days.

HCl monohydrate – Safety and efficacy not established for use in children.

Bacterial endocarditis prophylaxis – 2 g orally 1 hour before procedure (50 mg/kg for children).

CEPHALEXIN MONOHYDRATE

Rx	**Cephalexin** (Various, eg, Apothecon, Geneva, Goldline, Lederle, Major, Moore, Rugby)	**Capsules**: 250 mg	In 100s, 500s, and UD 100s.
Rx	**Keflex** (Dista)		(402). White/dark green. In 20s, 100s, UD 100s.
Rx	**Cephalexin** (Various, eg, Apothecon, Geneva, Goldline, Lederle, Major, Moore, Rugby)	**Capsules**: 500 mg	In 40s, 100s, 250s, 500s and UD 100s.
Rx	**Biocef** (Inter. Ethical Labs)		In 100s.
Rx	**Keflex** (Dista)		(403). Two-tone green. In 20s, 100s and UD 100s.
Rx	**Cephalexin** (Various, eg, Goldline, Lederle, Major, Moore)	**Tablets**: 250 mg	In 100s.
Rx	**Cephalexin** (Various, eg, Goldline, Lederle, Major, Moore, Schein, Zenith)	**Tablets**: 500 mg	In 100s and 500s.
Rx	**Cephalexin** (Major)	**Tablets**: 1 g	In 24s.
Rx	**Cephalexin** (Various, eg, Apothecon, Geneva, Goldline, Lederle, Major, Moore, Rugby)	**Oral Suspension**:[1] 125 mg/5 ml	In 100 and 200 ml.
Rx	**Keflex** (Dista)		In 100 and 200 ml.
Rx	**Cephalexin** (Various, eg, Apothecon, Geneva, Goldline, Lederle, Major, Moore, Rugby)	**Oral Suspension**:[1] 250 mg/5 ml	In 100 and 200 ml.
Rx	**Keflex** (Dista)		In 100, 200 and UD 5 ml.
Rx	**Biocef** (Inter. Ethical Labs)	**Powder for oral suspension**: 125 mg/5 ml (reconstituted)	In 100 ml.
		250 mg/5 ml (reconstituted)	In 100 ml.

[1] Refrigerate reconstituted suspension; discard after 14 days.

CEPHALEXIN HCl MONOHYDRATE

Cephalexin HCl monohydrate does not require conversion in the stomach before absorption.

Rx	**Keftab** (Dista)	**Tablets:** 500 mg	(4143). Dark green. In 100s.

CEFADROXIL

For complete prescribing information, refer to the Cephalosporins group monograph.

Indications:

Urinary tract infections caused by *Escherichia coli, Proteus mirabilis* and *Klebsiella* sp.

Skin and skin structure infections caused by staphylococci or streptococci.

Pharyngitis and tonsillitis caused by group A β-hemolytic streptococci.

Unlabeled uses: Prevention of bacterial endocarditis in penicillin-allergic patients undergoing dental, oral, esophageal or respiratory tract procedures who have not exhibited an immediate-type hypersensitivity reaction to penicillins.

Administration and Dosage:

Can be given without regard to meals. Shake suspension well before using.

Urinary tract infections: For uncomplicated lower urinary tract infection (ie, cystitis), the usual dosage is 1 or 2 g/day in single or 2 divided doses. For all other urinary tract infections, the usual dosage is 2 g/day in 2 divided doses.

Skin and skin structure infections: 1 g/day in single or 2 divided doses.

Pharyngitis and tonsillitis:

Group A β-hemolytic streptococci – 1 g/day in single or 2 divided doses for 10 days.

Children:

Urinary tract infections, skin and skin structure infections – 30 mg/kg/day in divided doses every 12 hours.

Pharyngitis, tonsillitis – 30 mg/kg/day in single or 2 divided doses. For β–hemolytic streptococcal infections, continue treatment for at least 10 days.

Bacterial endocarditis prophylaxis: 2 g orally 1 hour before the procedure (50 mg/kg for children).

Renal impairment: Adjust dosage according to creatinine clearance rates to prevent drug accumulation.

Initial adult dose – 1 g; the maintenance dose (based on creatinine clearance rate, ml/min/1.73 m^2) is 500 mg at the intervals below:

Cefadroxil Dosage in Renal Impairment	
Creatinine Clearance (ml/min)	Dosage Interval (hours)
0-10	36
10-25	24
25-50	12
> 50	No adjustment

Rx	**Cefadroxil** (Various, eg, Major)	**Capsules:** 500 mg[1]	In 100s.
Rx	**Duricef** (Mead Johnson)		In 50s, 100s and UD 100s.
Rx	**Cefadroxil** (Various, eg, Major)	**Tablets:** 1 g[1]	In 24s.
Rx	**Duricef** (Mead Johnson)		In 50s, 100s and UD 100s.
Rx	**Cefadroxil** (Various, eg, Major)	**Oral Suspension:**[2] 125 mg/5 ml	In 50 and 100 ml.
Rx	**Duricef** (Mead Johnson)		Orange-pineapple flavor. In 50 and 100 ml.
Rx	**Cefadroxil** (Various, eg, Major)	**Oral Suspension:**[2] 250 mg/5 ml	In 50 and 100 ml.
Rx	**Duricef** (Mead Johnson)		Orange-pineapple flavor. In 50 and 100 ml.
Rx	**Cefadroxil** (Various, eg, Major)	**Oral Suspension:**[2] 500 mg/5 ml	In 100 ml.
Rx	**Duricef** (Mead Johnson)		Orange-pineapple flavor. In 50, 75 and 100 ml.

[1] As monohydrate.

[2] Refrigerate reconstituted suspension; discard after 14 days.

CEPHRADINE

Complete prescribing information for these products begins in the Cephalosporins group monograph.

Indications:

Oral:

Respiratory tract infections (eg, tonsillitis, pharyngitis and lobar pneumonia) caused by group A β-hemolytic streptococci and Streptococcus pneumoniae.

Otitis media caused by group A β-hemolytic streptococci, *S pneumoniae, Haemophilus influenzae* and staphylococci.

Skin and skin structure infections caused by staphylococci (penicillinase/nonpenicillinase-producing) and β-hemolytic streptococci.

Urinary tract infections, including prostatitis, caused by Escherichia coli, Proteus mirabilis and *Klebsiella* species.

Cephradine may be used in the treatment of some enterococcal (*S faecalis*) infections confined to the urinary tract. The high concentrations of cephradine achieved in the urinary tract will be effective against many strains of enterococci for which disc susceptibility studies indicate relative resistance. Ampicillin is the drug of choice for enterococcal urinary tract (*S faecalis*) infections.

Parenteral:

Respiratory tract infections due to *S pneumoniae, Klebsiella* sp, *H influenzae, S aureus* (penicillinase/nonpenicillinase-producing) and group A β-hemolytic streptococci.

Urinary tract infections due to *E coli, P mirabilis* and *Klebsiella* sp.

Skin and skin structure infections due to *S aureus* (penicillinase/nonpenicillinase-producing) and group A β-hemolytic streptococci.

Bone infections due to *S aureus* (penicillinase/nonpenicillinase-producing).

Septicemia due to *S pneumoniae, S aureus* (penicillinase/nonpenicillinase producing), *P mirabilis* and *E coli.*

Perioperative prophylaxis administration (preoperatively, intraoperatively and postoperatively) may reduce the incidence of certain postoperative infections in patients undergoing surgical procedures (eg, vaginal hysterectomy) that are classified as contaminated or potentially contaminated.

In cesarean section, intraoperative (after clamping the umbilical cord) and postoperative use may reduce the incidence of certain postoperative infections.

Effective perioperative use depends on time of administration. Give 30 to 90 minutes before surgery, which is sufficient time to achieve effective tissue levels.

Administration and Dosage:

Oral: May be given without regard to meals.

Adults –

Skin, skin structures and respiratory tract infections(other than lobar pneumonia): Usual dose is 250 mg every 6 hours or 500 mg every 12 hours.

For lobar pneumonia: 500 mg every 6 hours or 1 g every 12 hours.

For uncomplicated urinary tract infections: The usual dose is 500 mg every 12 hours. In more serious infections and prostatitis, 500 mg every 6 hours or 1 g every 12 hours. Severe or chronic infections may require larger doses (up to 1 g every 6 hours).

Children – No adequate information is available on the efficacy of twice a day regimens in children less than 9 months of age. For children over 9 months, the usual dose is 25 to 50 mg/kg/day, in equally divided doses every 6 or 12 hours. For otitis media due to H influenzae, 75 to 100 mg/kg/day in equally divided doses every 6 or 12 hours is recommended; do not exceed 4 g/day.

All patients, regardless of age and weight – Larger doses (up to 1 g 4 times/day) may be given for severe or chronic infections.

Parenteral: Parenteral therapy may be followed by oral. To minimize pain and induration, inject IM deep into a large muscle mass.

Adults – Daily dose is 2 to 4 g in equally divided doses 4 times/day, IM or IV. In bone infections, the usual dosage is 1 g IV, 4 times/day. A dose of 500 mg, 4 times/day is adequate in uncomplicated pneumonia, skin and skin structure infections and most urinary tract infections. In severe infections, dose may be increased by giving every 4 hours or by increasing dose up to a maximum of 8 g/day.

Perioperative prophylaxis: Recommended doses are 1 g IV or IM administered 30 to 90 minutes prior to start of surgery, followed by 1 g every 4 to 6 hours after the first dose for 1 or 2 doses, or for up to 24 hours postoperatively.

Cesarean section: Give 1 g IV as soon as the umbilical cord is clamped. Give the second and third doses as 1 g IM or IV at 6 and 12 hours after the first dose.

Infants and children: 50 to 100 mg/kg/day in 4 equally divided doses; determine by age, weight and infection severity. Weigh benefits of use in infants < 1 yr against risks. In neonates, accumulation of other cephalosporins (with resultant half-life prolongation) may occur. Do not exceed adult dose.

Pediatric Dosage of Cephradine

Weight		50 mg/kg/day		100 mg/kg/day	
lbs	kg	Approx. single dose (mg q 6 h)	Volume needed @ 208 mg/ml	Approx. single dose (mg q 6 h)	Volume needed @ 227 mg/ml
10	4.5	56	0.27 ml	112	0.5 ml
20	9.1	114	0.55 ml	227	1 ml
30	13.6	170	0.82 ml	340	1.5 ml
40	18.2	227	1.1 ml	455	2 ml
50	22.7	284	1.4 ml	567	2.5 ml

Renal impairment dosage:

Patients not on dialysis – Use the following initial dosage schedule as a guideline based on creatinine clearance. Further modification in the dosage schedule may be required because of individual variations in absorption.

Cephradine Dosage in Renal Impairment

Ccr (ml/min)	Dose (mg)	Time Interval (hours)
> 20	500	6
5 to 20	250	6
<5	250	12

Patients on chronic, intermittent hemodialysis – 250 mg initially; repeat at 12 hours and after 36 to 48 hours. Children may require dosage modification proportional to their weight and severity of infection.

IM: Add Sterile Water for Injection or Bacteriostatic Water for Injection.

IV: A 3 mcg/ml serum concentration can be maintained for each mg of cephradine/kg of body weight per hour of infusion.

Direct IV – Add 5 ml of diluent to the 250 or 500 mg vials, 10 ml to the 1 g vial or 20 ml to the 2 g bottle. Inject slowly over 3 to 5 minutes or give through tubing.

Diluents for direct IV injection are: Sterile Water for Injection; 5% Dextrose Injection; Sodium Chloride Injection.

Continuous or intermittent IV infusion – Add 10 or 20 ml of Sterile Water for Injection or a suitable infusion fluid to the 1 g vial or 2 g bottles, respectively, to prepare solution. Withdraw entire contents; transfer to an IV infusion container.

2 g IV bottle: Reconstitute with 40 ml; infuse directly.

Infusion solutions include: 5% and 10% Dextrose Injection; Sodium Chloride Injection; M/6 Sodium Lactate; Dextrose and Sodium Chloride Injection; 10% Invert Sugar in Water; *Normosol-R; Ionosol B* with 5% Dextrose. Use Sterile Water for Injection at a concentration of 30 to 50 mg/ml.

Stability and Storage: Use IM or direct IV solutions within 2 hours at room temperature. Solutions refrigerated at 5°C (41°F) retain potency for 24 hours. The IV infusion solutions retain potency for 10 hours at room temperature or 48 hours at 5°C (41°F); infusion solutions in Sterile Water for Injection, frozen immediately after reconstitution, are stable for 6 weeks at –20°C (–4°F). For prolonged infusions, replace the infusion every 10 hours with fresh solution. Protect from concentrated light or direct sunlight.

Oral suspension – Do not store above 86°F prior to reconstitution. After reconsitution, suspensions retain their potency for 7 days at room temperature and 14 days if refrigerated.

Admixture incompatibility: Do not mix cephradine with other antibiotics. Do not use with Lactated Ringer's Injection.

CEPHRADINE

Rx	**Cephradine** (Various, eg, Baxter, Biocraft, Geneva, Lederle, Lemmon, Major, Parmed, Rugby, Schein, Zenith)	**Capsules:** 250 mg	In 24s, 100s, 500s and UD 100s.
Rx	**Velosef** (Apothecon)		(Squibb 113). In 24s, 100s, UD 100s.
Rx	**Cephradine** (Various, eg, Baxter, Biocraft, Geneva, Lederle, Lemmon, Major, Parmed, Rugby, Schein, Zenith)	**Capsules:** 500 mg	In 24s, 100s, 500s and UD 100s.
Rx	**Velosef** (Apothecon)		(Squibb 114). In 24s, 100s, UD 100s.
Rx	**Cephradine** (Various, eg, Barr, Biocraft, Geneva, Major, Parmed, Schein	**Oral Suspension:** 125 mg/5 ml when reconstituted	In 100 ml.
Rx	**Velosef** (Apothecon)		Fruit flavor. In 100, 200 and UD 5 ml.
Rx	**Cephradine** (Various, eg, Barr, Biocraft, Geneva, Major, Parmed, Schein	**Oral Suspension:** 250 mg/5 ml when reconstituted	In 100 ml.
Rx	**Velosef** (Apothecon)		Fruit flavor. In 100, 200 and UD 5 ml.
Rx	**Velosef** (Apothecon)	**Powder for Injection:**[1] 250 mg	In vials.
		500 mg	In vials.
		1 g	In vials.
		2 g	In 100 ml infusion bottles.

[1] Contains 6 mEq (136 mg) sodium per g.

LORACARBEF

Complete prescribing information for these products begins in the Cephalosporins group monograph.

Indications:

Lower respiratory tract:

Secondary bacterial infection of acute bronchitis and acute bacterial exacerbations of chronic bronchitis caused by *S pneumoniae,* or *H influenzae* or *M catarrhalis* (both including β-lactamase-producing strains).

Pneumonia caused by *S pneumoniae* or *H influenzae* (non-β-lactamase-producing strains only).

Upper respiratory tract:

Otitis media caused by *S pneumoniae, H influenzae* (including β-lactamase-producing strains), *M catarrhalis* (including β-lactamase-producing strains), *S pyogenes.*

Acute maxillary sinusitis caused by *S pneumoniae, H influenzae* (non-β-lactamase-producing strains only) or *M catarrhalis* (including β-lactamase-producing strains).

In a patient population with significant numbers of β-lactamase-producing organisms, loracarbef's clinical cure and bacteriological eradication rates were somewhat less than those observed with a product containing a β-lactamase inhibitor. Take into account loracarbef's decreased potential for toxicity vs products containing β-lactamase inhibitors along with susceptibility patterns of common microbes.

Pharyngitis and tonsillitis caused by *S pyogenes.* Usual drug of choice in treatment and prevention of streptococcal infections, including prophylaxis of rheumatic fever, is IM penicillin. Loracarbef is generally effective in eradicating *S pyogenes* from the nasopharynx; however, data establishing efficacy of loracarbef in subsequent prevention of rheumatic fever are not available at present.

Skin and skin structure:

Uncomplicated skin and skin structure infections caused by *S aureus* (including penicillinase-producing) or *S pyogenes.* Surgically drain abscesses as indicated.

Urinary tract:

Uncomplicated UTIs (cystitis) caused by *E coli* or *S saprophyticus.**

* Efficacy for this organism in this organ system was studied in fewer than 10 infections.

LORACARBEF

In considering the use of loracarbef in the treatment of cystitis, weigh its lower bacterial eradication rates and lower potential for toxicity against the increased eradication rates and increased potential for toxicity demonstrated by some other classes.

Uncomplicated pyelonephritis caused by *E coli.*

Administration and Dosage:

Approved by the FDA on December 31, 1991.

Administer at least 1 hour before or 2 hours after a meal.

Dosage/Duration of Loracarbef

Population/Infection	Dosage (mg)	Duration (days)
Adults ≥ 13 years of age		
Lower respiratory tract		
Secondary bacterial infection of acute bronchitis	200 - 400 q 12 h	7
Acute bacterial exacerbation of chronic bronchitis	400 q 12 h	7
Pneumonia	400 q 12 h	14
Upper respiratory tract		
Pharyngitis/Tonsillitis	200 q 12 h	10[1]
Sinusitis	400 q 12 h	10
Skin and skin structure		
Uncomplicated	200 q 12 h	7
Urinary tract		
Uncomplicated cystitis	200 q 24 h	7
Uncomplicated pyelonephritis	400 q 12 h	14
Infants and children (6 months to 12 years)		
Upper respiratory tract		
Acute otitis media[2]	30 mg/kg/day in divided doses q 12 h	10
Pharyngitis/Tonsillitis	15 mg/kg/day in divided doses q 12 h	10[1]
Skin and skin structure		
Impetigo	15 mg/kg/day in divided doses q 12 h	7

[1] In treatment of infections due to *S pyogenes*, administer for at least 10 days.

[2] Use suspension; it is more rapidly absorbed than capsules, resulting in higher peak plasma concentrations when given at the same dose.

Loracarbef Pediatric Suspension Dosage

Weight		Daily dose 15 mg/kg/day				Daily dose 30 mg/kg/day			
		100 mg/5 ml twice daily		200 mg/5 ml twice daily		100 mg/5 ml twice daily		200 mg/5 ml twice daily	
lb	kg	ml	tsp	ml	tsp	ml	tsp	ml	tsp
15	7	2.6	0.5	—	—	5.2	1	2.6	0.5
29	13	4.9	1	2.5	0.5	9.8	2	4.9	1
44	20	7.5	1.5	3.8	0.75	—	—	7.5	1.5
57	26	9.8	2	4.9	1	—	—	9.8	2

LORACARBEF

Renal function impairment: Use usual dose and schedule in patients with creatinine clearance (Ccr) levels ≥ 50 ml/min. Patients with Ccr between 10 and 49 ml/min may be given half the recommended dose at the usual dosage interval. Patients with Ccr levels < 10 ml/min may receive recommended dose given every 3 to 5 days; patients on hemodialysis should receive another dose following dialysis.

When only serum creatinine is available, the following formula may be used to convert this value into Ccr. The equation assumes the patient's renal function is stable.

$$\text{Males: } \frac{\text{Weight (kg)} \times (140 - \text{age})}{72 \times \text{serum creatinine (mg/dl)}} = \text{Ccr}$$

Females: 0.85 × above value

Reconstitution of oral suspension – Add 30 or 60 ml water in 2 portions to the dry mixture in the 50 or 100 ml bottle, respectively.

Storage/Stability: After mixing, the suspension may be kept at room temperature, 15° to 30°C (59° to 86°F), for 14 days without significant loss of potency. Keep tightly closed. Discard unused portion after 14 days.

Rx	Lorabid (Lilly)	**Pulvules (capsules)**: 200 mg	(3170). Blue/gray. In 30s.
		400 mg	(3171). Blue/pink. In 30s.
		Capsules: 500 mg cephalexin monohydrate.	Red. In 100s.
		Oral suspension: 100 mg/5 ml	Parabens, sucrose. Strawberry bubble gum flavor. In 50 and 100 ml.
		200 mg/5 ml	Parabens, sucrose. Strawberry bubble gum flavor. In 50 and 100 ml.
		Powder for suspension: 100 mg/5 ml	Parabens, sucrose. Strawberry bubble gum flavor. In 100 ml.
		200 mg/5 ml	Parabens, sucrose. Strawberry bubble gum flavor. In 50 and 100 ml.

CEFPROZIL

For complete prescribing information, refer to the Cephalosporins group monograph.

Indications:

Pharyngitis/tonsillitis caused by *Streptococcus pyogenes.*

Note: Usual drug of choice in treatment and prevention of streptococcal infections, including rheumatic fever prophylaxis, is IM penicillin. Cefprozil is generally effective in eradicating *S pyogenes* from nasopharynx; however, substantial data establishing efficacy in subsequent prevention of rheumatic fever are not available.

Otitis media caused by *S pneumoniae, Haemophilus influenzae* and *Moraxella catarrhalis.*

Note: In the treatment of otitis media due to beta-lactamase producing organisms, cefprozil had bacteriologic eradication rates somewhat lower than those observed with a product containing a specific beta-lactamase inhibitor. In considering the use of cefprozil, balance lower overall eradication rates against the susceptibility patterns of the common microbes in a given geographic area and the increased potential for toxicity with products containing beta-lactamase inhibitors.

Secondary bacterial infection of acute bronchitis and acute bacterial exacerbation of chronic bronchitis caused by *S pneumoniae, H influenzae* (beta-lactamase positive and negative strains) and *Moraxella catarrhalis.*

Uncomplicated skin and skin structure infections caused by *Staphylococcus aureus* (including penicillinase-producing strains) and *S pyogenes.*

Administration and Dosage:

Approved by the FDA in December 1991.

Cefprozil Dosage and Duration

Population/Infection	Dosage (mg)	Duration (days)
Adults (≥ 13 years of age)		
Pharyngitis/Tonsillitis	500 q 24 h	10[1]
Secondary bacterial infection of acute bronchitis and acute bacterial exacerbation of chronic bronchitis	500 q 12 h	10
Uncomplicated skin and skin structure infections	250 q 12 h, 500 q 24 h or 500 q 12 h	10
Children (2 to 12 years)		
Pharyngitis/Tonsillitis	7.5 mg/kg q 12 h	10[1]
Uncomplicated skin and skin structure infections	20 mg/kg q 24 h	10
Infants and children (6 months to 12 years)		
Otitis media	15 mg/kg q 12 h	10

[1] For infections due to *S pyogenes,* administer for ≥ 10 days.

Renal function impairment: For creatinine clearance (Ccr) of 30 to 120 ml/min, use standard dosage and dosing interval. For Ccr < 30 ml/min, use a dosage 50% of standard at the standard dosing interval.

Cefprozil is in part removed by hemodialysis; therefore, administer after the completion of hemodialysis.

Storage/Stability:

Suspension – Refrigerate after reconstitution; discard after 14 days.

Rx	**Cefzil** (Bristol Labs)	**Tablets:** 250 mg (as anhydrous)	(BMS 7720 250). Light orange. Film coated. In 100s and UD 100s.
		500 mg (as anhydrous)	(BMS 7721 500). White. Film coated. In 50s, 100s and UD 100s.
Rx	**Cefzil** (Bristol Labs)	**Powder for suspension:** 125 mg/5 ml (as anhydrous)	Sucrose, aspartame, 28 mg/5 ml phenylalanine. Bubble gum flavor. In 50, 75 and 100 ml.
		250 mg/5 ml (as anhydrous)	Sucrose, aspartame, 28 mg/5 ml phenylalanine. Bubble gum flavor. In 50, 75 and 100 ml.

CEFTIBUTEN

For complete prescribing information, refer to the Cephalosporins group monograph.

Indications:

Acute bacterial exacerbations of chronic brochitis due to *Haemophilus influenzae* (including β-lactamase-produing strains), *Moraxella catarrhalis* (including β-lactamase-producing strains) and *Streptococcus pneumoniae* (penicillin-susceptible strains only).

In acute bacterial exacerbations of chronic bronchitis clinical trials where *Moraxella catarrhalis* was isolated from infected sputum at baseline, ceftibuten clinical efficacy was 22% less than control.

Acute bacterial otitis media due to *H influenzae* (including β-lactamase-producing strains), *M catarrhalis* (including β-lactamase-producing strains) or *S pyogenes.*

Although ceftibuten used empirically was equivalent to comparators in the treatment of clinically or microbiologically documented acute otitis media, the efficacy against *S pneumoniae* was 23% less than control. Therefore, give ceftibuten empirically only when adequate antimicrobial coverage against *S pneumoniae* has been previously administered.

Pharyngitis and tonsillitis due to *S pyogenes.*

Only penicillin by the IM route has been shown to be effective in the prophylaxis of rheumatic. Ceftibuten is generally effective in the eradication of *S pyogenes* from the oropharynx; however, data establishing efficacy for prophylaxis of subsequent rheumatic fever are not available.

Administration and Dosage:

Approved by the FDA on December 20, 1995.

Ceftibuten suspension must be administered at least 2 hours before or 1 hour after a meal.

Ceftibutin Dosage and Duration			
Type of infection	Daily maximum dose	Dose and frequency	Duration
Adults ≥ 12 years of age Acute bacterial exacerbations of chronic bronchitis due to *H influenzae, M catarrhalis* or *Streptococcus pneumoniae* Pharyngitis and tonsillitis due to S pyogenes Acute bacterial otitis media due to *H influenzae, M catarrhalis* or *S pyogenes*	400 mg	400 mg qd	10 days
Children Pharyngitis and tonsillitis due to *S pyogenes* Acute bacterial otitis media due to *H influenzae, M catarrhalis* or *S pyogenes*	400 mg	9 mg/kg qd	10 days

Ceftibuten Oral Suspension Pediatric Dosage Chart[1]

Weight			
kg	lb	90 mg/5 ml	180 mg/5 ml
10	22	5 ml (1 tsp) qd	2.5 ml (½ tsp) qd
20	44	10 ml (2 tsp) qd	5 ml (1 tsp) qd
40	88	20 ml (4 tsp) qd	10 ml (2 tsp)qd

[1] Children > 45 kg should receive the maximum daily dose of 400 mg

Renal function impairment: Ceftibuten may be administered at normal doses in the presence of impaired renal function with creatinine clearance of ≥ 50 ml/min. The recommendations for dosing in patient with varying degrees of renal insufficiency are presented in the following table.

CEFTIBUTEN

Ceftibuten Dosage in Renal Impairment	
Creatinine clearance (ml/min)	Recommended dosing schedule
> 50	9 mg/kg or 400 mg q 24 h (normal dosing schedule)
30 - 49	4.5 mg/kg or 200 mg q 24 h
5 - 29	2.25 mg/kg or 100 mg q 24 h

Hemodialysis patients: In patients undergoing hemodialysis two or three times weekly, a single 400 mg dose of ceftibuten capsules or a single dose of 9 mg/kg (maximum of 400 mg) oral suspension may be administered at the end of each hemodialysis session.

Directions for Mixing Ceftibuten Suspensin			
Final concentration	Bottle size	Amount of Water	Directions
90 mg per 5 ml	30 ml	Suspend in 28 ml of water	First, tap bottle to loosen powder. Then, add water in two portions, shaking well after each aliquot.
	60 ml	Suspend in 53 ml of water	
	120 ml	Suspend in 103 ml of water	
180 mg per 5 ml	30 ml	Suspend in 28 ml of water	
	60 ml	Suspend in 53 ml of water	
	120 ml	Suspend in 103 ml of water	

Storage/Stability:

Suspension – After mixing, the suspension may be kept for 14 days and must be stored in the refrigerator. Keep tightly closed. Shake well before each use. Discard any unused portion after 14 days.

Rx	**Cedax** (Schering)	**Capsules:** 400 mg	Parabens. (Cedax 400). White. In 20s, 100s and UD 40s.
		Suspension, oral: 90 mg/5 ml	Sucrose. Cherry flavor. In 30, 60 and 120 ml.
		180 mg/5 ml	Sucrose. Cherry flavor. In 30, 60 and 120 ml.

CEPHALOTHIN SODIUM

Complete prescribing information for these products begins in the Cephalosporins group monograph.

Indications:

Respiratory tract infections caused by *Streptococcus pneumoniae*, staphylococci (penicillinase/nonpenicillinase-producing), group A β-hemolytic streptococci, *Klebsiella* species and *Haemophilus influenzae.*

Skin and soft tissue infections, including peritonitis, caused by staphylococci (penicillinase/nonpenicillinase-producing), group A β-hemolytic streptococci, *Escherichia coli, Proteus mirabilis* and *Klebsiella* species.

Genitourinary tract infections caused by *E coli, P mirabilis* and *Klebsiella* species.

Septicemia, including endocarditis, caused by *S pneumoniae,* staphylococci (penicillinase/nonpenicillinase-producing), group A β-hemolytic streptococci, *S viridans, E coli, P mirabilis* and *Klebsiella* species.

Gastrointestinal infections caused by *Salmonella* and *Shigella* species.

Meningitis caused by *S pneumoniae,* group A β-hemolytic streptococci and staphylococci (penicillinase/nonpenicillinase-producing).

Because only low drug levels are found in the cerebrospinal fluid, the drug is not reliable in treatment of meningitis and cannot be recommended for that purpose. However, the drug has been effective in a number of cases of meningitis and may be considered for unusual circumstances in which other, more reliable, antibiotics cannot be used.

CEPHALOTHIN SODIUM

Bone and joint infections caused by staphylococci (penicillinase/nonpenicillinase-producing).

Perioperative prophylaxis to reduce the incidence of certain postoperative infections in patients undergoing contaminated or potentially contaminated surgical procedures (eg, vaginal hysterectomy). Perioperative use also may be effective in surgical patients in whom infection at the operative site would present a serious risk (eg, open heart surgery, prosthetic arthroplasty).

Administration and Dosage:

Adults: 500 mg to 1 g every 4 to 6 hours.

Uncomplicated pneumonia, furunculosis with cellulitis, most urinary tract infections – 500 mg every 6 hours.

Severe infections – Increase the dose to 1 g or administer 500 mg every 4 hours.

Life-threatening infections – Up to 2 g every 4 hours.

Normal renal function (bacteremia, septicemia or other severe or life-threatening infections): The IV dosage is 4 to 12 g daily. In conditions such as septicemia, 6 to 8 g per day may be administered IV for several days at the beginning of therapy; reduce the dosage gradually.

Infants and children: The dosage is proportionately less according to age, weight and severity of infection. Daily administration of 100 mg/kg (80 to 160 mg/kg or 40 to 80 mg/lb) in divided doses is effective for most infections susceptible to cephalothin.

Perioperative prophylaxis:

Preoperative – 1 to 2 g administered IV ½ to 1 hour prior to initial incision.

Intraoperative – 1 to 2 g during surgery, administered according to the duration of surgery.

Postoperative – 1 to 2 g every 6 hours; discontinue within 24 hours after surgery. If there are signs of infection, obtain specimens for culture and sensitivity testing and institute appropriate therapy.

Children – 20 to 30 mg/kg given at the times designated above.

Renal function impairment: Give an IV loading dose of 1 to 2 g. Determine the continued dosage schedule by degree of renal impairment, severity of infection and susceptibility of the causative organism. Base maximum doses on the following recommendations:

Cephalothin Dosage in Renal Impairment		
Renal function	Creatinine clearance (ml/min)	Maximum adult dosage (maintenance)
Mild impairment	50 - 80	2 g every 6 hours
Moderate impairment	25 - 50	1.5 g every 6 hours
Severe impairment	10 - 25	1 g every 6 hours
Marked impairment	2 - 10	0.5 g every 6 hours
Essentially no function	< 2	0.5 g every 8 hours

CEPHALOTHIN SODIUM

Administer IV or by deep IM injection. The IV route may be preferable in bacteremia, septicemia or other severe or life-threatening infections.

IM: Administer deeply IM into a large muscle mass (eg, the gluteus or lateral aspect of the thigh) to minimize pain and induration.

Intermittent IV administration: Slowly inject a solution of 1 g in 10 ml diluent directly into the vein over 3 to 5 minutes, or give through IV tubing.

Intermittent infusion with Y-type administration set: Can be accomplished while bulk IV solutions are infused. However, during infusion, discontinue the other solutions.

Continuous IV infusion: 1 or 2 g of cephalothin, diluted and mixed with at least 10 ml of Sterile Water for Injection, may be added to an IV container of one of the following IV solutions: Acetated Ringer's Injection; 5% Dextrose Injection; 5% Dextrose in Lactated Ringer's Injection; Ionosol B in D5-W; *Isolyte M* with 5% Dextrose; Lactated Ringer's Injection; *Normosol-M* in D5-W; *Plasma-Lyte Injection; Plasma-Lyte-M* in 5% Dextrose; Ringer's Injection; 0.9% Sodium Chloride Injection.

Intraperitoneal: Cephalothin has been added to peritoneal dialysis fluid in concentrations up to 6 mg/100 ml and instilled into the peritoneal cavity throughout an entire dialysis (16 to 30 hours); 44% was absorbed. Serum levels of 10 mcg/ml were reported; accumulation and untoward local or systemic reactions were not evident.
Intraperitoneal administration of 0.1% to 4% cephalothin solutions in saline has been used to treat peritonitis or contaminated peritoneal cavities. (The total daily dosage should take into account the amount given by the intraperitoneal route.)

Preparation of solution: For IM use, reconstitute each gram with 4 ml Sterile Water for Injection. If the vial contents do not completely dissolve, add an additional small amount of diluent (0.2 to 0.4 ml) and warm the contents slightly.

Storage/Stability: Concentrated solutions will darken, especially at room temperature; slight discoloration is permissible.

Room temperature – Give solutions for IM injection within 12 hours after reconstitution. Start IV infusions within 12 hours and complete within 24 hours. For prolonged infusion, replace with a freshly prepared solution at least every 24 hours.

Refrigeration – The solution is stable for 96 hours after reconstitution. Redissolve solutions which precipitate by warming to room temperature and constantly agitating.

Freezing – Solutions in Sterile Water for Injection, 5% Dextrose Injection or 0.9% Sodium Chloride Injection frozen immediately after reconstitution in the original container are stable for 12 weeks when stored at –20°C (-4°F); do not refreeze.

Rx	**Cephalothin Sodium** (Baxter)	**Injection:**[1] 1 g in 5% Dextrose	Premixed, frozen. In 50 ml single dose *Viaflex Plus* containers.
		2 g in 5% Dextrose	Premixed, frozen. In 50 ml single dose *Viaflex Plus* containers.
Rx	**Cephalothin Sodium** (Various, eg, Pasadena)	**Powder for Injection:**[2] 1 g	In 10 ml vials and 100 ml piggyback vials.
Rx	**Keflin, Neutral** (Lilly)		In 10 and 100 ml vials and Faspak.
Rx	**Keflin, Neutral** (Lilly)	**Powder for Injection:**[2] 2 g	In 100 ml vials and Faspak.

[1] Contains 2.4 mEq sodium/g.
[2] Contains 2.8 mEq sodium/g.

CEPHAPIRIN SODIUM

Complete prescribing information for these products begins in the Cephalosporins group monograph.

Indications:

Respiratory tract infections caused by *Streptococcus pneumoniae, Staphylococcus aureus* (penicillinase/nonpenicillinase-producing), *Klebsiella* sp, *Hemophilus influenzae* and group A β-hemolytic streptococci.

Skin and skin structure infections caused by *S aureus* (penicillinase/nonpenicillinase-producing), *S epidermidis* (methicillin-susceptible strains), *Escherichia coli, Proteus mirabilis, Klebsiella* sp and group A β-hemolytic streptococci.

Urinary tract infections caused by *S aureus*(penicillinase/nonpenicillinase-producing), *E coli, P mirabilis* and *Klebsiella* species.

Septicemia caused by *S aureus* (penicillinase/nonpenicillinase-producing), *S viridans, E coli, Klebsiella* sp and group A β-hemolytic streptococci.

Endocarditis caused by *S viridans* and *S aureus* (penicillinase/nonpenicillinase-producing).

Osteomyelitis caused by *S aureus* (penicillinase/nonpenicillinase-producing), *Klebsiella* sp, *P mirabilis* and group A β-hemolytic streptococci.

Perioperative prophylaxis: Preoperative and postoperative administration may reduce the incidence of certain postoperative infections in patients undergoing contaminated or potentially contaminated surgical procedures (eg, vaginal hysterectomy).

Perioperative use may also be effective in surgical patients in whom infection at the operative site would present a serious risk (eg, open heart surgery and prosthetic arthroplasty).

Administration and Dosage:

Adults: 500 mg to 1 g every 4 to 6 hours IM or IV. The lower dose is adequate for certain infections, such as skin and skin structure and most urinary tract infections; the higher dose is recommended for more serious infections.

Serious or life-threatening infections: Up to 12 g daily. Use the IV route when high doses are indicated.

Renal function impairment – Depending upon the causative organism and the severity of infection, patients with reduced renal function (moderately severe oliguria or serum creatinine > 5 mg/100 ml) may be treated adequately with a lower dose, 7.5 to 15 mg/kg every 12 hours. Patients who are to be dialyzed should receive the same dose just prior to dialysis and every 12 hours thereafter.

Perioperative prophylaxis – 1 to 2 g IM or IV administered ½ to 1 hour prior to start of surgery; 1 to 2 g during surgery (administration modified depending on duration of operation); 1 to 2 g IV or IM every 6 hours for 24 hours postoperatively.

Give the preoperative dose just prior to surgery (½ to 1 hour) so that adequate antibiotic levels are present in the serum and tissues at initial surgical incision. Administer cephapirin, if necessary, at appropriate intervals during surgery to provide sufficient levels of the antibiotic at the anticipated moments of greatest exposure to infective organisms.

In surgery in which the occurrence of infection may be particularly devastating (eg, open heart surgery and prosthetic arthroplasty), prophylactic administration may be continued for 3 to 5 days following surgery.

Children: Dosage is in accordance with age, weight and severity of infection. Recommended total daily dose is 40 to 80 mg/kg (20 to 40 mg/lb) administered in 4 equally divided doses.

Infants: Cephapirin has not been extensively studied in infants; therefore, in the treatment of children < 3 months of age, consider the relative benefit to risk.

IM: Reconstitute the 500 mg and 1 g vials with 1 or 2 ml of Sterile Water for Injection or Bacteriostatic Water for Injection, respectively. Each 1.2 ml contains 500 mg of cephapirin. Inject deep in the muscle mass.

IV: Patients with bacteremia, septicemia or other severe or life-threatening infections may be poor risks because of resistance-lowering conditions such as malnutrition, trauma, surgery, diabetes, heart failure and malignancy. The IV route may be preferable in these patients particularly if shock is present or impending.

Intermittent IV injection – Dilute the 500 mg or 1 or 2 g vial with 10 ml or more diluent and give slowly over 3 to 5 minutes, or administer with IV infusions.

Piggyback vials contain labeled quantities of cephapirin for IV use. Diluent and volume are specified on the label.

Intermittent IV infusion with Y-tube – Can be accomplished while bulk IV solutions are being infused. However, during infusion, discontinue the other solution. When Y–tube arrangement is used, dilute 4 g vial with 40 ml Bacteriostatic Water for Injection, Dextrose Injection or Sodium Chloride Injection.

CEPHAPIRIN SODIUM

Pharmacy bulk package – Add 67 ml of Sodium Chloride Injection or Dextrose Injection. The resulting solution contains 250 mg cephapirin activity per ml. Reconstituted solutions are stable for 24 hours at room temperature or 10 days under refrigeration.

Stability:

Stability of Cephapirin in Various Diluents			
Diluent	Approximate Concentration (mg/ml)	Stability Time 25°C	Stability Time 4°C
Water for Injection	50 to 400	12 hrs	10 days
Bacteriostatic Water for Injection	250 to 400	48 hrs	10 days
Normal Saline	20 to 100	24 hrs	10 days
5% Dextrose in Water	20 to 100	24 hrs	10 days

Solutions can be frozen immediately after reconstitution and stored at −15°C (5°F) for 60 days before use. After thawing at room temperature (25°C; 77°F), solutions are stable for at least 12 hours at room temperature or 10 days under refrigeration (4°C; 39°F).

Compatibility with infusion solutions: Stable and compatible for 24 hours at room temperature at concentrations between 2 and 30 mg/ml in the following solutions: Sodium Chloride Injection; 5% Sodium Chloride in Water; 5%, 10% and 20% Dextrose in Water; Sodium Lactate Injection; 10% Invert Sugar in Normal Saline or Water; 5% Dextrose = 0.2% or 0.45% Sodium Chloride Injection; 5% Dextrose in Normal Saline; Lactated Ringer's Injection; Lactated Ringer's with 5% Dextrose; Ringer's Injection; Sterile Water for Injection; 5% Dextrose in Ringer's Injection; *Normosol R; Normosol R* in 5% Dextrose Injection; *Ionosol D-CM; Ionosol G* in 10% Dextrose Injection.

Cephapirin 4 mg/ml is stable and compatible for 10 days under refrigeration (4°C; 39°F) or 14 days in the frozen state (−15°C; 5°F) followed by 24 hours at room temperature (25°C; 77°F) in all solutions listed above.

Rx	**Cephapirin Sodium** (Lyphomed)	**Powder for Injection:**[1] 500 mg	In 10 ml vials.
Rx	**Cefadyl** (Apothecon)		In vials.
Rx	**Cephapirin Sodium** (Lyphomed)	**Powder for Injection:**[1] 1 g	In 10 and 100 ml vials.
Rx	**Cefadyl** (Apothecon)		In vials and piggyback vials.
Rx	**Cephapirin Sodium** (Various, eg, Lyphomed, VHA Supply)	**Powder for Injection:**[1] 2 g	In 20 and 100 ml vials.
Rx	**Cefadyl** (Apothecon)		In vials and piggyback vials.
Rx	**Cephapirin Sodium** (Lyphomed)	**Powder for Injection:**[1] 4 g	In 100 ml vials.
Rx	**Cefadyl** (Apothecon)		In piggyback vials.
Rx	**Cephapirin Sodium** (Lyphomed)	**Powder for Injection:**[1] 20 g	In 100 ml vials.
Rx	**Cefadyl** (Apothecon)		In bulk packages.

[1] Contains 2.36 mEq sodium per g.

CEFAZOLIN SODIUM

Complete prescribing information for these products begins in the Cephalosporins group monograph.

Indications:

Respiratory tract infections due to *Streptococcus pneumoniae, Klebsiella species, Haemophilus influenzae, Staphylococcus aureus* (penicillinase/non-penicillinase-producing) and group A β-hemolytic streptococci.

Genitourinary tract infections due to *Escherichia coli, Proteus mirabilis, Klebsiella* species and some strains of *Enterobacter* and enterococci.

Skin and skin structure infections due to *S aureus* (penicillinase/nonpenicillinase-producing) and group A β-hemolytic streptococci and other strains of streptococci.

Biliary tract infections due to *E coli*, various strains of streptococci, *P mirabilis, Klebsiella* species and *S aureus.*

Bone and joint infections due to *S aureus.*

Septicemia due to *S pneumoniae, S aureus* (penicillinase/nonpenicillinase-producing), *P mirabilis, E coli* and *Klebsiella* species.

Endocarditis due to *S aureus*(penicillinase/nonpenicillinase-producing) and group A β-hemolytic streptococci. Recommended by the American Heart Association for penicillin-allergic patients unable to take oral medications and undergoing dental, oral, esophageal or respiratory tract procedures who have not exhibited an immediate-type hypersensitivity reaction to penicillins.

Perioperative prophylaxis may reduce the incidence of certain postoperative infections in patients undergoing contaminated or potentially contaminated surgical procedures (eg, vaginal hysterectomy and cholecystectomy in high risk patients such as those over 70 years of age, with acute cholecystitis, obstructive jaundice or common duct bile stones).

May also be effective in surgical patients in whom infection at the operative site would present a serious risk (eg, open heart surgery and prosthetic arthroplasty).

Administration and Dosage:

Total daily dosages are the same for IV and IM administration.

Mild infections caused by susceptible gram-positive cocci: 250 to 500 mg every 8 hours.

Moderate to severe infections: 500 mg to 1 g every 6 to 8 hours.

Pneumococcal pneumonia: 500 mg every 12 hours.

Severe, life-threatening infections (eg, endocarditis, septicemia): 1 to 1.5 g every 6 hours. Rarely, 12 g per day have been used.

Acute uncomplicated urinary tract infections: 1 g every 12 hours.

Perioperative prophylaxis:

Preoperative – 1 g IV or IM, ½ to 1 hour prior to surgery.

Intraoperative (2 hours or more) – 0.5 to 1 g IV or IM during surgery at appropriate intervals.

Postoperative – 0.5 to 1 g IV or IM every 6 to 8 hours for 24 hours after surgery. Prophylactic administration may be continued for 3 to 5 days, especially where the occurrence of infection may be particularly devastating (eg, open heart surgery, prosthetic arthroplasty).

Renal function impairment: All reduced dosage recommendations apply after an initial loading dose appropriate to the severity of the infection.

Cefazolin Dosage in Renal Impairment

Serum Creatinine (mg %)	Ccr (ml/min)	Dose: Mild to Moderate Infection (mg)	Dose: Moderate to Severe Infection (mg)	Dosage Interval (hrs)
≤ 1.5	≥ 55	250 to 500	500 to 1000	6-8
1.6-3	35-54	250 to 500	500 to 1000	≥ 8
3.1-4.5	11-34	125 to 250	250 to 500	12
≥ 4.6	≤10	125 to 250	250 to 500	18-24

Children:

Mild to moderately severe infections – A total daily dosage of 25 to 50 mg/kg (approximately 10 to 20 mg/lb) in 3 or 4 equal doses.

Severe infections – Total daily dosage may be increased to 100 mg/kg (45 mg/lb).

CEFAZOLIN SODIUM

Pediatric Dosage of Cefazolin[1]

Weight		25 mg/kg/day				50 mg/kg/day			
		Approx. single dose		Volume needed @ 125 mg/ml		Approx. single dose		Volume needed @ 225 mg/ml	
lbs	kg	mg q 8 h	mg q 6 h	mg q 8 h	mg q 6 h	mg q 8 h	mg q 6 h	mg q 8 h	mg q 6 h
10	4.5	40	30	0.35 ml	0.25 ml	75	55	0.35 ml	0.25 ml
20	9.1	75	55	0.6 ml	0.45 ml	150	110	0.7 ml	0.5 ml
30	13.6	115	85	0.9 ml	0.7 ml	225	170	1 ml	0.75 ml
40	18.2	150	115	1.2 ml	0.9 ml	300	225	1.35 ml	1 ml
50	22.7	190	140	1.5 ml	1.1 ml	375	285	1.7 ml	1.25 ml

[1] Infants (premature and < 1 month): Safety not established; use is not recommended.

Renal function impairment – Recommendations apply after an initial loading dose. Ccr 40 to 70 ml/min, 60% of normal daily dose every 12 hrs; Ccr 20 to 40 ml/min, 25% of normal daily dose every 12 hrs; Ccr 5 to 20 ml/min, 10% of normal daily dose every 24 hrs.

Prevention of bacterial endocarditis – 1 g (25 mg/kg for children) IM or IV within 30 minutes before procedure.

IM administration: Inject into a large muscle mass. Pain on injection is infrequent.

Intermittent IV infusion: Administer in a volume control set or in a separate, secondary IV container. Reconstituted 500 mg or 1 g may be diluted in 50 to 100 ml of: 0.9% NaCl Injection; 5% or 10% Dextrose Injection; 5% Dextrose in Lactated Ringer's Injection; 5% Dextrose and 0.2%, 0.45% or 0.9% NaCl; Lactated Ringer's Injection; 5% or 10% Invert Sugar in Sterile Water for Injection; 5% Sodium Bicarbonate (*Ancef*); Ringer's Injection; *Normosol-M* in D5-W; *Ionosol B* w/Dextrose 5%; *Plasma-Lyte* with 5% Dextrose.

Direct IV injection: Dilute reconstituted 500 mg or 1 g in minimum of 10 ml Sterile Water for Injection. Inject slowly into vein or through IV tubing over 3 to 5 min.

Preparation of solution: IM: Reconstitute with Sterile Water, Bacteriostatic Water or 0.9% Sodium Chloride Injections. Shake well until dissolved.

IV: Dilute as required.

Stability and storage: Reconstituted cefazolin is stable for 24 hours at room temperature, 96 hours refrigerated (5°C; 41°F). Solutions in Sterile Water for Injection, 5% Dextrose Injection or 0.9% Sodium Chloride Injection frozen immediately after reconstitution in original container are stable up to 12 weeks when stored at –20°C (–4°F). If warmed, avoid heating after thawing is complete; do not refreeze. Thaw premixed frozen solution at room temperature. Do not introduce additives. After thawing, stable 48 hours at room temperature and 10 days refrigerated. Do not refreeze.

Rx	**Cefazolin Sodium** (Apothecon)	**Powder for Injection:** 250 mg	In vials.
Rx	**Ancef** (SKF)		In vials[1].
Rx	**Cefazolin Sodium** (Apothecon)	**Powder for Injection:** 500 mg	In vials and piggyback vials.
Rx	**Ancef** (SKF)		In vials and piggyback vials[1].
Rx	**Cefazolin Sodium** (Apothecon)	**Powder for Injection:** 1 g	In vials and piggyback vials.
Rx	**Ancef** (SKF)		In vials and piggyback vials[1].
Rx	**Kefzol** (Lilly)		In vials[1].
Rx	**Cefazolin Sodium** (Apothecon)	**Powder for Injection:** 5 g	In pharmacy bulk packages.
Rx	**Ancef** (SKF)		In bulk vials[1].

CEFAZOLIN SODIUM

Rx	**Cefazolin Sodium** (Apothecon)	**Powder for Injection**: 10 g	In pharmacy bulk packages.
Rx	**Ancef** (SKF)		In bulk vials[1].
Rx	**Kefzol** (Lilly)		In 100 ml bulk vials[1].
Rx	**Cefazolin Sodium** (Apothecon)	**Powder for Injection**: 20 g	In pharmacy bulk packages.
Rx	**Ancef** (SKF)	**Injection:**[1]500 mg in 5% Dextrose in Water	Premixed, frozen. In 50 ml plastic containers.
		1 g in 5% Dextrose in Water	Premixed, frozen. In 50 ml plastic containers.
Rx	**Kefzol** (Lilly)	**Injection:**1 g	In 10 ml Redi-vials, Faspacks and *ADD-Vantage* vials.
Rx	**Zolicef** (Apothecon)	**Powder for Injection:**[1]500 mg	In 10 ml vials.
		1 g	In 10 ml vials.

[1] Contains 2.1 mEq sodium/g.

CEFMETAZOLE SODIUM

Complete prescribing information for these products begins in the Cephalosporins.

Indications:

Urinary tract infections (complicated or uncomplicated) caused by E coli.

Lower respiratory tract infections: Pneumonia and bronchitis caused by *S pneumoniae, S aureus* (penicillinase-and non-penicillinase-producing strains), *E coli, H influenzae* (non-penicillinase-producing strains).

Skin and structure infections: S aureus (penicillinase- and non-penicillinase-producing strains), *S epidermidis, S pyogenes, S agalactiae, E coli, P mirabilis, P vulgaris**, *M morganii**, *P stuartii**, *K pneumoniae, K oxytoca**, *B fragilis, B melaninogenicus.**

*Intra-abdominal infections: E coli, K pneumoniae**, *K oxytoca**, *B fragilis, C perfringens.**

Prophylaxis: Preoperative administration may reduce the incidence of certain postoperative infections in patients who undergo cesarean section, abdominal or vaginal hysterectomy, cholecystectomy (high-risk patients) and colorectal surgery.

* Efficacy of this organism in this organ system was studied in fewer than 10 infections.

CEFMETAZOLE SODIUM

Administration and Dosage:

Adults: General guidelines - 2 g IV every 6 to 12 hours for 5 to 14 days.

Prophylaxis:

Cefmetazole Dosing Regimen for Prophylaxis	
Surgery	Dosing Regimen
Vaginal hysterectomy	2 g single dose 30 to 90 min before surgery or 1 g doses 30 to 90 minbefore surgery and repeated 8 and 16 hours later
Abdominal hysterectomy	1 g doses 30 to 90 min before surgery and repeated 8 and 16 hours later
Cesarean section	2 g single dose after clamping cord or 1 g doses after clamping cord; repeated at 8 and 16 hours
Colorectal surgery	2 g single dose 30 to 90 minutes before surgery or 2 g doses 30 to 90 minutes before surgery and repeated 8 and 16 hours later
Cholecystectomy (high risk)	1 g doses 30 to 90 minutes before surgery and repeated 8 and 16 hours later

Renal function impairment:

Cefmetazole Dosage Guidelines in Renal Function Impairment			
Renal Function	Creatinine Clearance (ml/min/1.73 m^2)	Dose (g)	Frequency (hrs)
Mild impairment	50-90	1 to 2	q 12
Moderate impairment	30-49	1 to 2	q 16
Severe impairment	10-29	1 to 2	q 24
Essentially no function	< 10	1 to 2	q 48[1]

[1] Administered after hemodialysis.

Reconstitution: Reconstitute with Sterile Water for Injection, Bacteriostatic Water for Injection or 0.9% Sodium Chloride Injection.

Stability and storage: Following reconstitution, cefmetazole maintains satisfactory potency for 24 hours at room temperature (25°C; 77°F) , for 7 days under refrigeration (8°C; 46°F) and for 6 weeks in the frozen state (≤ -20°C; -4°F).

Primary solutions may be further diluted to concentrations of 1 to 20 mg/ml in 0.9% Sodium Chloride Injection, 5% Dextrose Injection or Lactated Ringer's Injection and maintain potency for 24 hours at room temperature (25°C; 77°F), for 7 days under refrigeration (8°C; 46°F) and for 6 weeks in the frozen state (≤-20°C; -4°F).

Do not refreeze thawed solutions. Discard unused solutions or frozen material.

Rx	**Zefazone** (Upjohn)	**Powder for Injection:** 1 g	In vials.
		2 g	In vials.

CEFAMANDOLE NAFATE

Complete prescribing information for these products begins in the Cephalosporins group monograph.

Indications:

Lower respiratory infections, including pneumonia caused by *Streptococcus pneumoniae, Haemophilus influenzae, Klebsiella* sp, *Staphylococcus aureus* (penicillinase/nonpenicillinase-producing), β-hemolytic streptococci and *Proteus mirabilis.*

Urinary tract infections caused by *Escherichia coli, Proteus* sp (both indole-negative and positive), *Enterobacter* sp, *Klebsiella* sp, group D streptococci (*Note:* Most enterococci, eg, *S faecalis* are resistant) and *S epidermidis.*

Peritonitis caused by *E coli* and *Enterobacter* species.

Septicemia caused by *E coli, S aureus* (penicillinase/nonpenicillinase-producing), *S pneumoniae, S pyogenes* (group A β-hemolytic streptococci), *H influenzae, Klebsiella* sp.

Skin and skin structure infections caused by *S aureus* (penicillinase/nonpenicillinase-producing), *S pyogenes* (group A β-hemolytic streptococci), *H influenzae, E coli, Enterobacter* sp and *P mirabilis.*

Bone, joint infections caused by *S aureus* (penicillinase/nonpenicillinase-producing).

Mixed infections: Nongonococcal pelvic inflammatory disease in females, lower respiratory and skin infections. Cefamandole has been successful in infections in which several organisms were isolated. Most *Bacteroides fragilis* strains are resistant in vitro; however, infections caused by susceptible strains have been treated successfully.

Concomitant aminoglycoside therapy: In confirmed or suspected gram-positive or gram-negative sepsis or in patients with other serious infections in which causative organism is not identified, cefamandole may be used concomitantly with an aminoglycoside. Monitor renal function carefully, especially with higher dosages.

Perioperative prophylaxis may reduce the incidence of certain postoperative infections in patients undergoing surgical procedures that are classified as contaminated or potentially contaminated (eg, GI surgery, cesarean section, vaginal hysterectomy or cholecystectomy in high risk patients such as those with acute cholecystitis, obstructive jaundice or common bile duct stones).

In major surgery in which the risk of postoperative infection is low but serious (cardiovascular surgery, neurosurgery or prosthetic arthroplasty), cefamandole may effectively prevent such infections.

Discontinue use after 24 hours; however, in prosthetic arthroplasty, continue for 72 hours. If signs of infection occur, obtain culture specimens for identification of the causative organism so that appropriate antibiotic therapy may be instituted.

Administration and Dosage:

Administer IV or by deep IM injection into a large muscle mass to minimize pain.

Adults: Usual dosage range is 500 mg to 1 g every 4 to 8 hours; 500 mg every 6 hours is adequate in uncomplicated pneumonia and skin structure infections. In uncomplicated urinary tract infections, 500 mg every 8 hours; in more serious urinary tract infections, the dose may be increased to 1 g every 8 hours. In severe infections, administer 1 g at 4 to 6 hour intervals. In life-threatening infections or infections due to less susceptible organisms, up to 2 g every 4 hours may be needed.

Infants and children: 50 to 100 mg/kg/day in equally divided doses every 4 to 8 hours is effective for most infections susceptible to cefamandole. This may be increased to 150 mg/kg/day (not to exceed the maximum adult dose) for severe infections.

Perioperative prophylaxis:

Adults – 1 or 2 g IM or IV, ½ to 1 hour prior to the surgical incision, followed by 1 or 2 g every 6 hours for 24 to 48 hours.

Children (3 months of age and older) – 50 to 100 mg/kg/day in equally divided doses by the routes and schedule designated above.

In patients undergoing prosthetic arthroplasty, administer up to 72 hours.

In patients undergoing cesarean section, administer the initial dose just prior to surgery or immediately after the cord has been clamped.

Renal function impairment: Reduce dosages and monitor the serum levels. After an initial dose of 1 to 2 g (depending on the severity of infection), follow maintenance dosage in table. Determine further dosage by degree of renal impairment, severity of infection and susceptibility of the causative organism.

When only serum creatinine is available, use the following formula to obtain creatinine clearance. The serum creatinine should represent steady-state renal function.

$$\text{Males:} \quad \frac{\text{Weight (kg)} \times (140 - \text{age})}{72 \times \text{serum creatinine (mg/dl)}} = \text{Ccr}$$

Females: 0.85 × above value

CEFAMANDOLE NAFATE

Maintenance Cefamandole Dosage Guide for Patients with Renal Impairment

Renal Function	Creatinine Clearance (ml/min/1.73 m²)	Life-threatening Infections (Maximum Dosage)	Less Severe Infections
Normal Impairment	> 80	2 g q 4 h	1-2 g q 6 h
Mild Impairment	50-80	1.5 g q 4 h or 2 g q 6 h	0.75-1.5 g q 6 h
Moderate Impairment	25-50	1.5 g q 6 h or 2 g q 8 h	0.75-1.5 g q 8 h
Severe Impairment	10-25	1 g q 6 h or 1.25 g q 8 h	0.5-1 g q 8 h
Marked Impairment	2-10	0.67 g q 8 h or 1 g q 12 h	0.5-0.75 g q 12 h
None	< 2	0.5 g q 8 h or 0.75 g q 12 h	0.25-0.5 g q 12 h

IM: Dilute each gram with 3 ml of one of the following diluents: Sterile Water for Injection; Bacteriostatic Water for Injection; 0.9% Sodium Chloride Injection; Bacteriostatic Sodium Chloride Injection. Shake well until dissolved.

IV: The IV route may be preferable for bacterial septicemia, localized parenchymal abscesses (ie, intra-abdominal abscess), peritonitis or other severe or life-threatening infections when patients may be poor risks because of lowered resistance. In patients with normal renal function, the IV dosage is 3 to 12 g daily. In conditions such as bacterial septicemia, give 6 to 12 g/day IV initially for several days, and gradually reduce.

Concomitant aminoglycoside therapy – If combination therapy with cefamandole and an aminoglycoside is indicated, administer in different sites. Do not mix an aminoglycoside with cefamandole in the same IV fluid container.

Intermittent IV – Reconstitute each gram with 10 ml of Sterile Water for Injection, 5% Dextrose Injection or 0.9% Sodium Chloride Injection. Slowly inject into the vein over 3 to 5 minutes, or through IV fluid containing: 0.9% Sodium Chloride Injection; 5% Dextrose Injection; 5% or 10% Dextrose and 0.2%, 0.45% or 0.9% Sodium Chloride Injection; Sodium Lactate Injection (M/6).

Intermittent IV infusion with a Y-type administration set or volume control set can also be accomplished while any of the mentioned IV fluids are being infused. However, during infusion, discontinue the other solution. When a Y-tube arrangement is used, add 100 ml of the appropriate diluent to the 1 or 2 g piggyback (100 ml) vial. If Sterile Water for Injection is used as the diluent, reconstitute with approximately 20 ml/g to avoid a hypotonic solution.

Continuous IV infusion – Dilute each gram with 10 ml of Sterile Water for Injection. An appropriate quantity of the resulting solution may be added to an IV container of one of the fluids listed under *Intermittent IV* administration.

Stability:

Room temperature – Reconstituted cefamandole is stable for 24 hours at room temperature (25°C; 77°F). During storage, carbon dioxide develops inside the vial after reconstitution. This pressure may be dissipated prior to withdrawal of the vial contents, or it may be used to aid withdrawal if the vial is inverted over the syringe needle and the contents are allowed to flow into the syringe.

Refrigeration – The solution is stable for 96 hours when refrigerated (5°C; 41°F).

Freezing – Solutions in Sterile Water for Injection, 5% Dextrose Injection or 0.9% Sodium Chloride Injection frozen immediately after reconstitution in the original container are stable for 6 months when stored at -20°C (-4°F). If the product is warmed (to a maximum of 37°C; 99°F), avoid heating after thawing is complete; do not refreeze.

Rx	**Mandol** (Lilly)	**Powder for Injection:**[1] 1 g	In 10 and 100 ml vials, *ADD-Vantage* vials and Faspacks.
		2 g	In 20 and 100 ml vials, *ADD-Vantage* vials and Faspacks.
		10 g	In 100 ml vials.

[1] Contains 3.3 mEq sodium/g.

CEFOXITIN SODIUM

For complete prescribing information, refer to the Cephalosporins group monograph.

Indications:

Cefoxitin and cephalothin were comparable for management of infections caused by susceptible gram-positive cocci and gram-negative rods. Many infections caused by gram-negative bacteria resistant to some cephalosporins and penicillins respond to cefoxitin.

Lower respiratory tract infections (pneumonia and lung abscess) caused by *Streptococcus pneumoniae*, other streptococci (excluding enterococci, eg, *S faecalis*), *Staphylococcus aureus* (penicillinase/nonpenicillinase-producing), *Escherichia coli, Klebsiella* species, *Haemophilus influenzae* and *Bacteroides* species.

Urinary tract infections caused by *E coli, Klebsiella* species, *Proteus mirabilis*, indole-positive *Proteus* (ie, *Morganella morganii* and *P vulgaris*) and *Providencia* species (including *P rettgeri*). Uncomplicated gonorrhea due to *Neisseria gonorrhoeae* (penicillinase/nonpenicillinase-producing).

Intra-abdominal infections (peritonitis and intra-abdominal abscess), caused by *E coli, Klebsiella* species, *Bacteroides* species including *B fragilis* and *Clostridium* species.

Gynecological infections (endometritis, pelvic cellulitis and pelvic inflammatory disease) caused by *E coli, N gonorrhoeae* (penicillinase/nonpenicillinase-producing), *Bacteroides* species including the *B fragilis* group, *Clostridium* species, *Peptococcus* species, *Peptostreptococcus* species and group B streptococci.

Septicemia caused by *S pneumoniae, S aureus* (penicillinase/nonpenicillinase-producing), *E coli, Klebsiella* species and *Bacteroides* species including *B fragilis*.

Bone/joint infections caused by *S aureus* (penicillinase/nonpenicillinase-producing).

Skin and skin structure infections caused by *S aureus* (penicillinase/nonpenicillinase-producing), *S epidermidis*, streptococci (excluding enterococci, eg, *S faecalis*), *E coli, P mirabilis, Klebsiella* species, *Bacteroides* species including the *B fragilis* group, *Clostridium* species, *Peptococcus* species and *Peptostreptococcus* species.

Perioperative prophylaxis may reduce incidence of certain postoperative infections following surgical procedures (eg, vaginal hysterectomy, GI surgery, transurethral prostatectomy) classified as contaminated or potentially contaminated and in those in whom operative site infection would present serious risk (eg, prosthetic arthroplasty). In cesarean section, intraoperative (after clamping umbilical cord) and postoperative use may reduce incidence of postoperative infections.

Give cefoxitin 30 to 60 minutes before the operation, to achieve effective levels in the wound during the procedure. Prophylactic administration should usually be stopped within 24 hours.

Administration and Dosage:

Adult dosage range is 1 to 2 g every 6 to 8 hours. Determine dosage and route of administration by susceptibility of the causative organisms, severity of infection and the patient's condition (see table for dosage guidelines). Maintain antibiotic therapy for group A β-hemolytic streptococcal infections for at least 10 days to guard against the risk of rheumatic fever or glomerulonephritis.

Cefoxitin Dosage Guidelines

Type of Infection	Daily Dosage	Frequency and Route
Uncomplicated (pneumonia, urinary tract, cutaneous)[1]	3 to 4 g	1 g every 6 to 8 hours IV or IM
Moderately severe or severe	6 to 8 g	1 g every 4 hours or 2 g every 6 to 8 hours IV
Infections commonly requiring higher dosage (eg, gas gangrene)	12 g	2 g every 4 hours or 3 g every 6 hours IV

[1] Including patients in whom bacteremia is absent or unlikely.

Uncomplicated gonorrhea: 2 g IM with 1 g oral probenecid given concurrently or up to 30 minutes before cefoxitin.

Prophylactic use, surgery: Administer 2 g IV or IM 30 to 60 minutes prior to surgery followed by 2 g every 6 hours after the first dose for no more than 24 hours (continued for 72 hours after prosthetic arthroplasty).

Prophylactic use, cesarean section: Administer 2 g IV as soon as the umbilical cord is clamped. If a three dose regimen is used, give the second and third 2 g dose IV, 4 and 8 hours after the first dose.

Prophylactic use, transurethral prostatectomy: Administer 1 g prior to surgery; 1 g every 8 hours for up to 5 days.

CEFOXITIN SODIUM

Renal function impairment:

Adults – Initial loading dose is 1 to 2 g. Maintenance doses:

Maintenance Cefoxitin Dosage in Renal Impairment			
Renal Function	Ccr (ml/min/1.73 m^2)	Dose (g)	Frequency (hrs)
Mild impairment	30-50	1-2	8-12
Moderate impairment	10-29	1-2	12-24
Severe impairment	5-9	0.5-1	12-24
Essentially no function	< 5	0.5-1	24-48

When only serum creatinine level is available, use the following to obtain creatinine clearance. Serum creatinine should represent steady-state renal function.

$$\text{Males: } \frac{\text{Weight (kg)} \times (140 - \text{age})}{72 \times \text{serum creatinine (mg/dl)}} = \text{Ccr}$$

Females: 0.85 × above value

Hemodialysis: Administer a loading dose of 1 to 2 g after each hemodialysis. Give the maintenance dose as indicated in the table above.

Infants and Children ≥3 months – 80 to 160 mg/kg/day divided every 4 to 6 hours. Use higher dosages for more severe or serious infections. Do not exceed 12 g/day.

Prophylactic use (≥ 3 months): 30 to 40 mg/kg/dose every 6 hours.

Renal function impairment: Modify consistent with recommendations for adults.

CDC recommended treatment schedules for gonorrhea and acute pelvic inflammatory disease (PID)†:

Disseminated gonococcal infection – 1 g cefoxitin IV, 4 times/day for at least 7 days for disseminated infections caused by PPNG.

Gonococcal ophthalmia in adults – For PPNG, use 1 g cefoxitin IV, 4 times/day.

Acute PID – For hospitalized patients, give 100 mg doxycycline, IV, twice/day plus 2 g cefoxitin, IV, 4 times/day. Continue drugs IV for at least 4 days and at least 48 hours after patient improves. Continue 100 mg oral doxycycline, twice/day after discharge to complete 10 to 14 days of therapy. For outpatients, give 2 g cefoxitin IM with 1 g oral probenecid, then 100 mg oral doxycycline, twice/day for 10 to 14 days.

Preparation of solution:

Preparation of Cefoxitin Solution			
Package Size	Diluent to Add (ml)	≈ Withdrawable Volume (ml)	≈ Concentration (mg/ml)
1 g vial (IM)	2	2.5	400
2 g vial (IM)	4	5	400
1 g vial (IV)	10	10.5	95
2 g vial (IV)	10 or 20	11.1 or 21	180 or 95
1 g infusion bottle (IV)	50 or 100	50 or 100	20 or 10
2 g infusion bottle (IV)	50 or 100	50 or 100	40 or 20
10 g bulk (IV)	43 or 93	49 or 98.5	200 or 100

IV use – Reconstitute 1 g with at least 10 ml of Sterile Water for Injection, and 2 g with 10 to 20 ml. May reconstitute 10 g vial with 43 or 93 ml Sterile Water for Injection or any solutions listed under IV Compatibility and Stability. Benzyl alcohol as a preservative has caused toxicity in neonates. This has not occurred in infants > 3 months of age, but they may also be at risk. Do not use benzyl alcohol in infants.

IM use – Reconstitute each g with 2 ml Sterile Water for Injection or 2 ml 0.5% lidocaine HCl (without epinephrine) to minimize IM injection discomfort.

Administration of solution:

IV administration is preferable for patients with bacteremia, bacterial septicemia or other severe or life-threatening infections, or for patients who are poor risks because of lowered resistance from debilitating conditions (malnutrition, trauma, surgery, diabetes, heart failure, malignancy), particularly if shock is present or impending.

Intermittent IV administration – 1 or 2 g in 10 ml of Sterile Water for Injection over 3 to 5 minutes; may also give over longer periods through an existing system. Temporarily discontinue administration of any other solutions at the same site.

† *Morbidity and Mortality Weekly Report* 1985 (Oct 18); 34 (Suppl 4S);75S-108S and *Morbidity and Mortality Weekly Report* 1987 (Sep 11); 36 (Suppl 5S);1S-18S.

CEFOXITIN SODIUM

Continuous IV infusion – For higher doses, add solution to an IV container of 5% Dextrose Injection, 0.9% Sodium Chloride Injection, 5% Dextrose and 0.9% Sodium Chloride Injection or 5% Dextrose Injection w/0.02% Sodium Bicarbonate Solution.

Storage/Stability: Store dry powder below 30°C (86°F). Avoid exposure to temperatures above 50°C (122°F). The dry material, as well as solutions, darkens depending on storage conditions; product potency, however, is not adversely affected.

Premixed frozen – Maintains satisfactory potency after thawing for 24 hours at room temperature and 21 days if stored under refrigeration (2° to 8°C; 36° to 46°F). Discard any unused thawed solutions. Do not refreeze.

Admixture incompatibility – Do not add solutions of cefoxitin to aminoglycoside solutions because of potential interaction; administer separately to the same patient. After time periods listed in the table, discard unused solution.

Stability/Storage for Diluents of Cefoxitin

Diluent	24 hrs at room temp.	Refrigeration		Freezer	
		48 hours	1 week	26 weeks	30 weeks
Sterile Water for Injection	✓[1,2,3,4]	✓[2,4]	✓[1,3]		✓[1,3]
Bacteriostatic Water for Injection	✓[1,3]		✓[1,3]		✓[1,3]
0.9% Sodium Chloride Injection	✓[1,4,5,6]	✓[4,5,6]	✓[1]	✓[5,6]	✓[1]
5% Dextrose Injection	✓[1,4,6]	✓[4,6]	✓[1]	✓[6]	✓[1]
10% Dextrose Injection	✓[4]	✓[4]			
Lactated Ringer's	✓[4,6]	✓[4,6]		✓[6]	
5% Dextrose in Lactated Ringer's	✓[4]	✓[4]			
Neut (Sodium Bicarbonate)	✓[4]	✓[4]			
Normosol-M in D5-W	✓[4]	✓[4]			
Ionosol B with 5% Dextrose	✓[4]	✓[4]			
10% Mannitol	✓[4]	✓[4]			
5% Dextrose and 0.9% NaCl	✓[4]	✓[4]			
5% Dextrose with 0.02% Sodium Bicarbonate Solution	✓[4]	✓[4]			
5% Dextrose w/ 0.2% or 0.45% NaCl	✓[4]	✓[4]			
Ringer's Injection	✓[4]	✓[4]			
5% or 10% Invert Sugar in Water	✓[4]	✓[4]			
10% Invert Sugar in Saline	✓[4]	✓[4]			
5% Sodium Bicarbonate Injection	✓[4]	✓[4]			
M/6 Sodium Lactate Solution	✓[4]	✓[4]			
Polyonic M56 in 5% Dextrose	✓[4]	✓[4]			
2.5% and 5% Mannitol	✓[4]	✓[4]			
Isolyte E	✓[4]	✓[4]			
Isolyte E with 5% Dextrose	✓[4]	✓[4]			
0.5% or 1% Lidocaine without Epinephrine	✓[3]		✓[3]		✓[3]

[1] When reconstituted to 1 g/10 ml.
[2] After reconstitution and subsequent storage in plastic syringes.
[3] After reconstitution for IM use.
[4] After reconstitution and further dilution in 50 to 1000 ml.
[5] After storage in IV bags, plastic tubing, drip chambers, volume control devices.
[6] After storage in IV bags.

CEFOXITIN SODIUM

Rx	**Mefoxin** (Merck)	**Powder for Injection:**[1] 1 g	In vials, infusion bottles and *ADD-Vantage* vials.
		2 g	In vials, infusion bottles and *ADD-Vantage* vials.
		10 g	In bulk bottles.
		Injection: 1 g in 5% Dextrose in Water	Premixed, frozen. In 50 ml plastic containers.
		2 g in 5% Dextrose in Water	Premixed, frozen. In 50 ml plastic containers.

[1] Contains 2.3 mEq sodium/g.

CEFEPIME HCl

For complete prescribing information, refer to the Cephalosporins group monograph.

Indications:

Uncomplicated and complicated urinary tract infections (including pyelonephritis) caused by *Escherichia coli* or *Klebsiella pneumoniae*, when the infection is severe or caused by *E. coli, K. pneumoniae*, or *Proteus mirabilis*, when the infection is mild to moderate, including cases associated with concurrent bacteremia with these microorganisms.

Uncomplicated skin and skin structure infections caused by *Staphylococcus aureus* (methicillin-susceptible strains only) or *Streptococcus pyogenes*.

Pneumonia (moderate to severe) caused by *S. pneumoniae*, including cases associated with concurrent bacteremia, *Pseudomonas aeruginosa, K. pneumoniae* or *Enterobacter* sp.

Administration and Dosage:

Approved by the FDA on January 18, 1996.

Recommended Dosage Schedule for Cefepime			
Site and type of infection	Dose	Frequency	Duration (days)
Mild to moderate uncomplicated or complicated urinary tract infections, including pyelonephritis, due to *E. coli, K. pneumoniae* or *P. mirabilis*.[1]	0.5 to 1 g IV/IM[2]	q12h	7 to 10
Severe uncomplicated or complicated urinary tract infections, including pyelonephritis, due to *E. coli* or *K. pneumoniae*.	2 g IV	q12h	10
Moderate to severe pneumonia due to *S. pneumoniae, Pseudomonas aeruginosa, Klebsiella pneumoniae* or *Enterobacter* sp.	1 to 2 g IV	q12h	10
Moderate to severe uncomplicated skin and skin structure infections due to *S. aureus* or *S. pyogenes*.	2 g IV	q12h	10

[1] Including cases associated with concurrent bacteremia.

[2] IM route of administration is indicated only for mild to moderate, uncomplicated or complicated UTIs due to *E. coli* when the IM route is a more appropriate route of drug administration.

Renal function impairment: In patients with impaired renal function (creatinine clearance < 60 ml/min), adjust the dose of cefepime to compensate for the slower rate of renal elimination. The recommended initial dose should be the same as in patients with normal renal function.

In patients undergoing hemodialysis, ≈ 68% of the total amount of cefepime present in the body at the start of dialysis will be removed during a 3–hour dialysis period. A repeat dose, equivalent to the initial dose, should be given at the completion of each dialysis session.

In elderly patients, adjust dosage and administration in the presence of renal insufficiency.

In patients undergoing continuous ambulatory peritonial dialysis, administer cefepime at normal recommended doses at a dosage interval of every 48 hours.

Recommended Cefepime Maintenance Schedule in Patients with Renal Impairment			
Creatinine clearance (ml/min)	Recommended maintenance schedule		
> 60	500 mg q 12h[1]	1 g q 12h	2 g q 12h
30 to 60	500 mg q 24h	1 g q 24h	2 g q 24h
11 to 29		500 mg q 24h	1 g q 24h
≤ 10	250 mg q 24h	250 mg q 24h	500 mg q 24h

[1] Normal recommended dosing schedule.

IV administration: Administer over ≈ 30 minutes. Dilute with 50 to 100 ml of a compatible IV fluid. Cefepime is compatible at concentrations of 1 to 40 mg/ml with 0.9% Sodium Chloride Injection, 5% and 10% Dextrose Injection, M/6 Sodium Lactate Injection, 5% Dextrose and 0.9% Sodium Chloride Injection, Lactated Ringers and 5% Dextrose Injection, *Normosol-R* or *Normosol-M* in 5% Dextrose injection.

CEFEPIME HCl

Cefepime Admixture Stability				
Cefepime concentration (mg/ml)	Admixture and concentration	IV Infusion solutions	Stability time for RT/L[1] (20° to 25°C) (hours)	Stability time for refrigeration (2° to 8°C)
40	Amikacin 6 mg/ml	NS[2] or D5W[3]	24	7 days
40	Ampicillin 1 mg/ml	D5W[3]	8	8 hours
40	Ampicillin 10 mg/ml	D5W[3]	2	8 hours
40	Ampicillin 1 mg/ml	NS[2]	24	48 hours
40	Ampicillin 10 mg/ml	NS[2]	8	48 hours
4	Ampicillin 40 mg/ml	NS[2]	8	8 hours
4 to 40	Clindamycin Phosphate 0.25 to 6 mg/ml	NS[2] or D5W[3]	24	7 days
4	Heparin 10 to 50 units/ml	NS[2] or D5W[3]	24	7 days
4	Potassium chloride 10 to 40 mEq/L	NS[2] or D5W[3]	24	7 days
4	Theophylline 0.8 mg/ml	D5W[3]	24	7 days
1 to 4	na	*Aminosyn II* 4.25% with electrolytes and calcium	8	3 days
0.125 to 0.25	na	*Inpersol* with 4.25% dextrose	24	7 days

[1] Ambient room temperature and light.
[2] 0.9% sodium chloride injection.
[3] 5% dextrose injection.

Admixture compatibility/incompatibility – Intermittent IV infusion with a Y-type administration set can be accomplished with compatible solutions; however, during infusion of a solution containing cefepime, it is desirable to discontinue the other solution.

Solutions of cefepime, like those of most β-lactam antibiotics, should not be added to solutions of ampicillin at a concentration > 40 mg/ml, and should not be added to metronidazole, vancomycin, gentamicin, tobramycin, netilmicin sulfate or aminophylline because of potential interaction. However, if concurrent therapy with cefepime is indicated, each of these antibiotics can be administered separately.

IM administration: Reconstitute cefepime with the following diluents: 0.9% sodium chloride, 5% dextrose injection, 0.5% or 1% lidocaine HCl or bacteriostatic water for injection with parabens or benzyl alcohol.

Storage/Stability: Store at controlled room temperature 20° to 25°C (68° to 77°F) for 24 hours or store in the refrigerator at 2° to 8°C (36° to 46°F) for 7 days. Protect from light.

Rx	**Maxipime** (Bristol-Myers Squibb)	**Powder for Injection:** 500 mg	In 15 ml vial.
		1g	In 15 ml and *ADD-Vantage* vials, piggyback bottle.
		2 g	In 20 ml vials and piggyback bottle.

CEFUROXIME

For complete prescribing information, refer to the Cephalosporins group monograph.

Indications:

Oral:

Tablets –

Pharyngitis and tonsillitis caused by *S. pyogenes* (group A β-hemolytic streptococci).

Otitis media (acute bacterial) caused by *S. pneumoniae, H. influenzae* (including beta lactamase-producing strains), *M. catarrhalis* and *S. pyogenes.*

Acute bacterial exacerbations of chronic bronchitis and secondary bacterial infections of acute bronchitis caused by *S. pneumoniae, H. influenzae* (including beta lactamase-negative strains) or *H. parainfluenzae* (including beta lactamase-negative strains).

Urinary tract infections (uncomplicated) caused by *E. coli* or *K. pneumoniae.*

Skin and skin structure infections (uncomplicated) caused by *S. aureus* (including beta lactamase-producing strains) and *S. pyogenes.*

Uncomplicated gonorrhea (urethral and endocervical) caused by nonpenicillinase-producing strains of *N. gonorrhoeae.*

Suspension – Treatment of children 3 months to 12 years of age.

Pharyngitis/Tonsillitis caused by *S. pyogenes.*

Otitis media (acute bacterial) caused by *S. pneumoniae, H. influenzae* (including beta lactamase-producing strains), *M. catarrhalis* (including beta lactamase-producing strains) or *S. pyogenes.*

Impetigo caused by *S. aureus* (including beta lactamase-producing strains) or *S. pyogenes.*

Penicillin IM is the usual drug of choice in treatment and prevention of streptococcal infections, including prophylaxis of rheumatic fever. Cefuroxime axetil generally eradicates streptococci from the nasopharynx; however, substantial data establishing efficacy in subsequent prevention of rheumatic fever are not available.

Parenteral:

Lower respiratory infections, including pneumonia caused by *S. pneumoniae, H. influenzae* (including ampicillin-resistant), *Klebsiella* sp, *S. aureus* (penicillinase/nonpenicillinase-producing), *S. pyogenes, E. coli.*

Urinary tract infections caused by *E. coli* and *Klebsiella* sp.

Skin and skin structure infections caused by *S. aureus* (penicillinase/ nonpenicillinase-producing), *S. pyogenes, E. coli, Klebsiella* sp and *Enterobacter* sp.

Septicemia caused by *S. aureus* (penicillinase/nonpenicillinase-producing), *S. pneumoniae, E. coli, H. influenzae* (including ampicillin-resistant strains) and *Klebsiella* sp.

Meningitis caused by *S. pneumoniae, H. influenzae* (including ampicillin-resistant strains), *N. meningitidis* and *S. aureus* (penicillinase/nonpenicillinase-producing).

Gonorrhea – Uncomplicated and disseminated gonococcal infections due to *N. gonorrhoeae* (penicillinase/nonpenicillinase-producing) in both males and females.

Bone/joint infections caused by *S. aureus* (penicillinase/nonpenicillinase-producing).

Mixed infections – Clinical microbiological studies in skin and skin structure infections frequently reveal the growth of susceptible strains of both aerobic and anaerobic organisms. Cefuroxime has been used successfully in these mixed infections in which several organisms have been isolated. In certain cases of confirmed or suspected gram-positive or gram-negative sepsis, or in patients with other serious infections in which the causative organism has not been identified, the drug may be used concomitantly with an aminoglycoside. The recommended doses of both antibiotics may be given, depending on the severity of the infection and on the patient's condition.

Preoperative prophylaxis may reduce incidence of certain postoperative infections in patients undergoing surgical procedures (eg, vaginal hysterectomy) classified as clean-contaminated or potentially contaminated. Stop prophylaxis within 24 hours. Preoperative use is effective during open heart surgery when operative site infections present a serious risk. For these patients, continue therapy at least 48 hours after procedure ends. If infection is present, obtain culture specimens; institute appropriate therapy.

Patient Information:

The tablet should be swallowed whole, not crushed, since the crushed tablet has a strong, persistent, bitter taste. Children who cannot swallow the tablet whole should receive the oral suspension. Discontinuation of therapy due to taste or problems of administering this drug occurred in 1.4% of children given the oral suspension. Complaints about taste (which may impair compliance) occurred in 5% of children.

CEFUROXIME

Administration and Dosage:

Oral: Tablets and suspension are NOT bioequivalent and are NOT substitutable on a mg/mg basis.

Tablets – The tablets may be given without regard to meals.

Dosage for Cefuroxime Axetil Tablets

Population/Infection	Dosage	Duration (days)
Adults (≥ 13 years)		
Pharyngitis/tonsillitis	250 mg bid	10
Acute bacterial exacerbations of chronic bronchitis and secondary bacterial infections of acute bronchitis	250 or 500 mg bid	10
Uncomplicated skin and skin structure infections	250 or 500 mg bid	10
Uncomplicated urinary tract infections	125 or 250 mg bid	7 to 10
Uncomplicated gonorrhea	1000 mg once	single dose
Children who can swallow tablets whole		
Pharyngitis/tonsillitis	125 mg bid	10
Acute otitis media	250 mg bid	10

Suspension – Must be administered with food. Shake well each time before using. The suspension may be administered to children ranging in age from 3 months to 12 years, according to dosages in the following table:

Dosage for Cefuroxime Axetil Suspension

Population/infection (*infants and children, 3 months to 12 years*)	Dosage	Daily maximum dose	Duration (days)
Pharyngitis/tonsillitis	20 mg/kg/day divided bid	500 mg	10
Acute otitis media	30 mg/kg/day divided bid	1000 mg	10
Impetigo	30 mg/kg/day divided bid	1000 mg	10

Renal failure: Since cefuroxime is renally eliminated, its half-life will be prolonged in patients with renal failure.

Reconstitution of suspension: Shake the bottle to loosen the powder. Add the total amount of water for reconstitution (see table below). Invert the bottle and vigorously rock the bottle from side to side so that water rises through the powder. Once the sound of the powder against the bottle disappears, turn the bottle upright and vigorously shake it in a diagonal direction.

Amount of Water for Reconstitution of Cefuroxime Suspension

Bottle size	Water required for reconstitution
50 ml	18 ml
100 ml	33 ml
200 ml	66 ml

Each teaspoonful (5 ml) contains the equivalent of 125 mg cefuroxime axetil.

CEFUROXIME

Parenteral:

Dosage –

Adults: 750 mg to 1.5 g IM or IV every 8 hours, usually for 5 to 10 days.

Cefuroxime Dosage Guidelines		
Type of Infection	Daily Dosage (g)	Frequency
Uncomplicated urinary tract, skin and skin structure, disseminated gonococcal, uncomplicated pneumonia	2.25	750 mg every 8 hours
Severe or complicated	4.5	1.5 g every 8 hours
Bone and joint	4.5	1.5 g every 8 hours
Life-threatening or due to less susceptible organisms	6	1.5 g every 6 hours
Bacterial meningitis	9	≤ 3 g every 8 hours
Uncomplicated gonococcal	1.5 g IM[1]	Single dose

[1] Administered at 2 different sites together with 1 g oral probenecid.

Preoperative prophylaxis – For clean-contaminated or potentially contaminated surgical procedures, administer 1.5 g IV prior to surgery (≈ ½ to 1 hour before). Thereafter, give 750 mg IV or IM every 8 hours when the procedure is prolonged.

For preventive use during open heart surgery, give 1.5 g IV at the induction of anesthesia and every 12 hours thereafter for a total of 6 g.

Renal function impairment – Reduce dosage.

Parenteral Cefuroxime Dosage in Renal Impairment (Adults)	
Creatinine clearance (ml/min)	Dose and frequency
> 20	750 mg to 1.5 g every 8 hours
10 to 20	750 mg every 12 hours
< 10	750 mg every 24 hours[1]

[1] Since cefuroxime is dialyzable, give patients on hemodialysis a further dose at the end of the dialysis.

When only serum creatinine is available, refer to the following formula:

$$\text{Males: } \frac{\text{Weight (kg)} \times (140 - \text{age})}{72 \times \text{serum creatinine (mg/dl)}} = \text{Ccr}$$

Females: 0.85 × above value

Infants and children (> 3 months): 50 to 100 mg/kg/day in equally divided doses every 6 to 8 hours. Use 100 mg/kg/day (not to exceed the maximum adult dose) for more severe or serious infections.

Bone and joint infections – 150 mg/kg/day (not to exceed maximum adult dose) in equally divided doses every 8 hours.

Bacterial meningitis – Initially, 200 to 240 mg/kg/day IV in divided doses every 6 to 8 hours.

In renal insufficiency, modify dosage frequency per adult guidelines.

Administration:

IV – May be preferable for patients with bacterial septicemia or other severe or life-threatening infections, or for patients who may be poor risks because of lowered resistance, particularly if shock is present or impending.

Direct intermittent IV: Slowly inject solution into a vein over 3 to 5 minutes or give it through the tubing by which the patient receives other IV solutions.

Intermittent IV infusion with a Y-type administration set: Dose through the tubing by which the patient is receiving other IV solutions. However, during infusion, temporarily discontinue administration of other solutions at the same site.

Continuous IV infusion: A solution may be added to an IV bottle containing one of the following fluids: 0.9% Sodium Chloride Injection; 5% or 10% Dextrose Injection; 5% Dextrose and 0.45% or 0.9% Sodium Chloride Injection; M/6 Sodium Lactate Injection.

IM – Give by deep IM injection into a large muscle mass. Prior to IM injection, aspiration is necessary to avoid injection into a blood vessel.

CEFUROXIME

Preparation of Cefuroxime Solution

	Kefurox			*Zinacef*		
Strength	Diluent to add (ml)	Volume to be withdrawn (ml)	Approximate concentration (mg/ml)	Diluent to add (ml)	Volume to be withdrawn	Approximate concentration (mg/ml)
750 mg vial	3.6 (IM)	3.6[1]	220	3 (IM)	Total[1]	220
750 mg vial	9 (IV)	8	100	8 (IV)	Total	90
1.5 g vial	14 (IV)	Total	100	16 (IV)	Total	90
750 mg infusion pack	50 (IV)	—	15	100 (IV)		7.5
750 mg infusion pack	100 (IV)	—	7.5			
1.5 g infusion pack	50 (IV)	—	30	100 (IV)	—	15
1.5 g infusion pack	100 (IV)	—	15			
750 mg bottle	50 (IV)	—	15			
750 mg bottle	100 (IV)	—	7.5			
1.5 g bottle	50 (IV)	—	30			
1.5 g bottle	100 (IV)	—	15			
750 mg *ADD-Vantage*	50 (IV)	—	15			
750 mg *ADD-Vantage*	100 (IV)	—	7.5			
1.5 g *ADD-Vantage*	50 (IV)	—	30			
1.5 g *ADD-Vantage*	100 (IV)	—	15			
7.5 g pharmacy bulk package				77 (IV)	Amount needed[2]	95

[1] Cefuroxime sodium is a suspension at IM concentrations.

[2] 8 ml of solution contains 750 mg cefuroxime; 16 ml of solution contains 1.5 g cefuroxime.

Use Sterile Water for Injection, 5% Dextrose in Water, 0.9% Sodium Chloride or any solution listed in the Compatibility/Stability IV section. If Sterile Water for Injection is used, reconstitute with ≈ 20 ml/g to avoid a hypotonic solution.

Admixture compatibility/stability: Discard unused solutions after specified time periods.

IV – When the 750 mg, 1.5 g and 7.5 g pharmacy bulk vials are reconstituted as directed with Sterile Water for Injection, the solutions for IV administration maintain potency for 24 hours at room temperature and for 48 hours (750 mg and 1.5 g vials) and for 7 days (pharmacy bulk vial) when refrigerated at 5° C (41° F). More dilute solutions such as 750 mg or 1.5 g plus 50 to 100 ml Sterile Water for Injection, 5% Dextrose Injection or 0.9% Sodium Chloride Injection maintain potency for 24 hours at room temperature and for 7 days refrigerated.

These solutions may be further diluted to concentrations between 1 and 30 mg/ml in the following solutions, and will lose ≤ 10% activity for 24 hours at room temperature or for at least 7 days under refrigeration: 0.9% Sodium Chloride Injection; M/6 Sodium Lactate Injection; Ringer's Injection; Lactated Ringer's Injection; 5% Dextrose and 0.225%, 0.45% or 0.9% Sodium Chloride Injection; 5% or 10% Dextrose Injection; 10% Invert Sugar in Water for Injection.

The following are compatible for 24 hours at room temperature when admixed in IV infusion: Heparin (10 and 50 units/ml) in 0.9% Sodium Chloride Injection and Potassium Chloride (10 and 40 mEq/L) in 0.9% Sodium Chloride Injection.

Sodium bicarbonate injection is not recommended for dilution.

Premixed, frozen solution: Thaw at room temperature or under refrigeration. Do not force thaw by immersion in water bath or by microwave irradiation. Components of the solution may precipitate in the frozen state and will dissolve upon reaching room temperature with little or no agitation. Potency is not affected. Mix after solution has reached room temperature. Do not add supplementary medication. The thawed solution is stable for 28 days under refrigeration (5° C; 41° F) or for 24 hours at room temperature (25° C; 77° F). Do not refreeze.

IM – When reconstituted with Sterile Water for Injection, suspensions for IM injection maintain satisfactory potency for 24 hours at room temperature and for 48 hours when refrigerated at 5° C (41° F).

CEFUROXIME

Frozen, reconstituted –

Zinacef: Reconstitute 750 mg or 1.5 or 7.5 g vial as directed for IV administration. Immediately withdraw total contents of 750 mg or 1.5 g vial or 8 or 16 ml from the 7.5 g bulk vial and add to a *Viaflex Mini-bag* containing 50 or 100 ml of 0.9% Sodium Chloride Injection or 5% Dextrose Injection and freeze. Frozen solutions are stable for 6 months when stored at –20°C (–4°F). Thaw frozen solutions at room temperature. Do not refreeze. Do not force thaw by immersion in water bath, or by microwave irradiation. Thawed solutions may be stored for 24 hours at room temperature or 7 days in refrigerator.

Incompatibility: Do not add cefuroxime to aminoglycoside solutions. However, each may be administered separately to the same patient.

Storage/Stability:

Parenteral – Store cefuroxime in the dry state between 15° and 30° C (59° and 86° F) and protect from light. Powder, solutions and suspensions tend to darken, depending on storage conditions, without adversely affecting the product's potency.

Premixed, frozen – Do not store above –20°C (–4°F).

Suspension – Shake the oral suspension well before each use. Store reconstituted suspension between 2° and 25°C (36° and 77°F), either in the refrigerator or at room temperature. Discard after 10 days.

Tablets – Store between 15° and 30°C (59° and 86°F). Protect from excessive moisture.

Rx	**Ceftin** (Glaxo Wellcome)	**Tablets:** (as axetil) 125 mg	(Glaxo 395). White. Capsule shape. Film coated. In 20s, 60s and UD 100s.
		250 mg	(Glaxo 387). Light blue. Capsule shape. Film coated. In 20s, 60s and UD 100s.
		500 mg	(Glaxo 394). Dark blue. Capsule shape. Film coated. In 20s, 60s and UD 50s.
		Suspension: 125 mg/5 ml (as axetil) when reconstituted	Sucrose. Tutti-frutti flavor. In 50, 100 and 200 ml bottles.
Rx	**Cefuroxime Sodium** (Various,eg, Marsam)	**Powder for Injection:**[1] 750 mg (as sodium).	In 10 ml vials and 100 ml piggyback vials.
Rx	**Kefurox** (Lilly)		In 10 and 100 ml vials, Faspak and *ADD-Vantage* vials.
Rx	**Zinacef** (Glaxo Wellcome)		In vials, infusion pack and *ADD-Vantage* vials.
Rx	**Cefuroxime Sodium** (Various, eg, Marsam)	**Powder for Injection:**[1] 1.5 g (as sodium)	In 20 ml vials and 100 ml piggyback vials.
Rx	**Kefurox** (Lilly)		In 20 and 100 ml vials, Faspak and *ADD-Vantage* vials.
Rx	**Zinacef** (Glaxo)		In vials and infusion pack.
Rx	**Cefuroxime Sodium** (Various, eg, Marsam)	**Powder for Injection:**[1] 7.5 g (as sodium) per vial	In pharmacy bulk package.
Rx	**Zinacef** (Glaxo)		In pharmacy bulk package.
Rx	**Kefurox** (Lilly)		In pharmacy bulk package.
Rx	**Zinacef** (Glaxo)	**Injection:**[1] 750 mg (as sodium)	Premixed, frozen. In 50 ml.
		1.5 g (as sodium)	Premixed, frozen. In 50 ml.

[1] Contains 2.4 mEq sodium/g.

CEFONICID SODIUM

For complete prescribing information, refer to the Cephalosporins group monograph.

Indications:

Lower respiratory tract infections due to *Streptococcus pneumoniae; Klebsiella pneumoniae; Escherichia coli; Haemophilus influenzae* (ampicillin-resistant and ampicillin-sensitive).

Urinary tract infections due to *E coli; Proteus* sp (which may include the organisms now called *Proteus vulgaris, Providencia rettgeri* and *Morganella morganii*); and *K pneumoniae*.

Skin and skin structure infections due to *Staphylococcus aureus* and *S epidermidis; S pyogenes* (group A *Streptococcus*) and *S agalactiae* (group B *Streptococcus*).

Septicemia due to *S pneumoniae* and *E coli*.

Bone and joint infections due to *S aureus*.

Preoperative prophylaxis: A single 1 g dose administered before surgery may reduce the incidence of postoperative infections in patients undergoing surgical procedures classified as contaminated or potentially contaminated (eg, colorectal surgery, vaginal hysterectomy or cholecystectomy in high risk patients), or in patients in whom infection at the operative site would present a serious risk (eg, prosthetic arthroplasty, open heart surgery). Although cefonicid is as effective as cefazolin in preventing infection following coronary artery bypass surgery, no placebo controlled trials have evaluated any cephalosporin antibiotic in preventing infections following coronary artery bypass surgery or prosthetic heart valve replacement.

In cesarean section, the use of cefonicid (after the umbilical cord has been clamped) may reduce the incidence of certain postoperative infections.

Administration and Dosage:

Adults: Usual dose is 1 g/24 hours, IV or by deep IM injection. Doses > 1 g/day are rarely necessary; however, up to 2 g/day have been well tolerated.

General Cefonicid Dosage Guidelines (IM or IV)

Type of infection	Daily dosage (g)	Frequency
Uncomplicated urinary tract	0.5	once every 24 hrs
Mild to moderate	1	once every 24 hrs
Severe or life-threatening	2[1]	once every 24 hrs
Surgical prophylaxis	1	1 hr preoperatively

[1] When administering 2 g IM doses once daily, divide dose in half and give each half in a different large muscle mass.

Preoperative prophylaxis: Administer 1 g 1 hour prior to appropriate surgical procedures, to provide protection from most infections due to susceptible organisms for approximately 24 hours after administration. Intraoperative and postoperative administration are not necessary. Daily doses may be administered for 2 additional days in patients undergoing prosthetic arthroplasty or open heart surgery.

In cesarean section, administer only after the umbilical cord has been clamped.

Renal function impairment requires modification of dosage. Following an initial loading dosage of 7.5 mg/kg, IM or IV, follow the maintenance schedule below. Individualize further dosing. It is not necessary to administer additional dosage following dialysis.

Cefonicid Dosage in Adults with Reduced Renal Function

Creatinine clearance (ml/min/1.73 m^2)	Mild to moderate infections	Severe infections
60-79	10 mg/kg q 24 hr	25 mg/kg q 24 hr
40-59	8 mg/kg q 24 hr	20 mg/kg q 24 hr
20-39	4 mg/kg q 24 hr	15 mg/kg q 24 hr
10-19	4 mg/kg q 48 hr	15 mg/kg q 48 hr
5-9	4 mg/kg q 3 to 5 days	15 mg/kg q 3 to 5 days
< 5	3 mg/kg q 3 to 5 days	4 mg/kg q 3 to 5 days

IM injection: Inject well within the body of a relatively large muscle and aspirate. When administering 2 g IM doses once daily, divide the dose in half and give in different large muscle masses.

CEFONICID SODIUM

IV administration:

Direct (bolus) injection – Administer reconstituted solution slowly over 3 to 5 minutes, directly or through tubing for patients receiving parenteral fluids.

Infusion – Dilute reconstituted cefonicid in 50 to 100 ml of one of the following solutions: 0.9% Sodium Chloride Injection; 5% or 10% Dextrose Injection; 5% Dextrose and 0.2%, 0.45% or 0.9% Sodium Chloride Injection; Ringer's Injection; Lactated Ringer's Injection; 5% Dextrose and Lactated Ringer's Injection; 10% Invert Sugar in Sterile Water for Injection; 5% Dextrose and 0.15% Potassium Chloride Injection; Sodium Lactate Injection.

Preparation of solution:

Single dose vials – Reconstitute with Sterile Water for Injection according to the following table. Shake well.

Pharmacy bulk vials – Reconstitute with Sterile Water for Injection, Bacteriostatic Water for Injection or Sodium Chloride Injection according to the following table:

Preparation of Cefonicid Solution

Vial size	Diluent to add (ml)	≈ Available volume (ml)	≈ Average concentration
500 mg	2	2.2	220 mg/ml
1 g	2.5	3.1	325 mg/ml
10 g	25	31	333 mg/ml
	45	51	200 mg/ml

For IV infusion, dilute reconstituted solution in 50 to 100 ml of the parenteral fluids listed under IV administration.

Piggyback vials – Reconstitute with 50 to 100 ml Sodium Chloride Injection or other IV solution listed under IV administration. Give with primary IV fluids as a single dose.

Storage/Stability: After reconstitution or dilution, all of these solutions are stable for 24 hours at room temperature or for 72 hours if refrigerated (5°C; 41°F).

A solution of 1 g cefonicid in 18 ml Sterile Water for Injection is isotonic.

Rx	**Monocid** (SmithKline Beecham)	**Powder for Injection:**[1] 500 mg	In vials.
		1 g	In vials and piggyback vials.
		10 g	In pharmacy bulk vials.

[1] Contains 3.7 mEq sodium/g.

CEFTRIAXONE SODIUM

For complete prescribing information, refer to the Cephalosporins group monograph.

Indications:

Lower respiratory tract infections caused by *Streptococcus pneumoniae, Staphylococcus aureus, Haemophilus influenzae, H parainfluenzae, Klebsiella pneumoniae, Serratia marcescens, Escherichia coli, E aerogenes, Proteus mirabilis.*

Skin and skin structure infections caused by *S aureus, S epidermidis, Streptococcus pyogenes,* Viridans group streptococci, *E coli, Enterobacter cloacae, K oxytoca, K pneumoniae, P mirabilis, Pseudomonas aeruginosa, Morganella morganii, S marcescens, Acinetobacter calcoaceticus, Bacteroides fragilis, Peptostreptococcus* sp.

Urinary tract infections (complicated and uncomplicated) caused by *E coli, P mirabilis, P vulgaris, Morganella morganii* and *Klebsiella* sp (including *K pneumoniae*).

Uncomplicated gonorrhea (cervical/urethral and rectal) caused by *Neisseria gonorrhoeae,* including both penicillinase/nonpenicillinase-producing strains (considered treatment of choice) and pharyngeal gonorrhea caused by nonpenicillinase-producing strains of *N gonorrhoeae.*

Pelvic inflammatory disease caused by *N gonorrhoeae.*

Bacterial septicemia caused by *S aureus, S pneumoniae, E coli, H influenzae* and *K pneumoniae.*

Bone and joint infections caused by *S aureus, S pneumoniae, Streptococcus* sp (excluding enterococci), *E coli, P mirabilis, K pneumoniae, S pneumoniae, Streptococcus, S pneumoniae, Streptococcus* and *Enterobacter* sp.

Intra-abdominal infections caused by *E coli, K pneumoniae, B fragilis, Clostridium* sp (most strains of *C difficile* are resistant), *Peptostreptococcus* sp.

Meningitis caused by *H influenzae, N meningitidis* and *S pneumoniae.* Has been used successfully in a limited number of cases of meningitis and shunt infections caused by *S epidermidis* and *E coli.*

CEFTRIAXONE SODIUM

Prophylaxis: The use of a single preoperative dose may reduce the incidence of postoperative infections in patients undergoing surgical procedures classified as contaminated or potentially contaminated (eg, vaginal or abdominal hysterectomy) and in surgical patients for whom infection at the operative site would present serious risk (eg, coronary artery bypass surgery). Ceftriaxone is as effective as cefazolin in preventing infection following coronary artery bypass surgery.

Unlabeled uses: Ceftriaxone 2 to 4 g daily IV for 10 to 14 days is effective in treating neurologic complications, arthritis and carditis associated with Lyme disease in patients refractory to penicillin G.

Administration and Dosage:

Administer IV or IM. Continue for at least 2 days after signs and symptoms of infection have disappeared. Usual duration is 4 to 14 days; in complicated infections, longer therapy may be required. For *S pyogenes,* continue for at least 10 days.

Adults: Usual daily dose is 1 to 2 g once a day (or in equally divided doses twice a day) depending on type and severity of infection. Do not exceed total daily dose of 4 g.

Uncomplicated gonococcal infections – Give a single IM dose of 250 mg.

Surgical prophylaxis – Give a single 1 g dose ½ to 2 hours before surgery.

Children: To treat serious infections other than meningitis, administer 50 to 75 mg/kg/day (not to exceed 2 g) in divided doses every 12 hours.

Meningitis – 100 mg/kg/day (not to exceed 4 g). Thereafter, a total daily dose of 100 mg/kg/day (not to exceed 4 g/day) is recommended. May give daily dose once per day or in equally divided doses every 12 hours. Usual duration is 7 to 14 days.

Skin and skin structure infections – Give 50 to 75 mg/kg once daily (or in equally divided doses twice daily), not to exceed 2 g.

No dosage adjustment is necessary; however, monitor blood levels.

CDC recommended treatment schedules for chancroid, gonorrhea and acute pelvic inflammatory disease (PID)†:

Chancroid (Haemophilus ducreyi infection) – 250 mg IM as a single dose.

Gonococcal infections –

Uncomplicated: 125 mg IM once plus doxycycline.

Conjunctivitis: 1 g IM single dose.

Disseminated: 1 g IM or IV every 24 hours.

Meningitis/Endocarditis: 1 to 2 g IV every 12 hours for 10 to 14 days (meningitis) or for at least 4 weeks (endocarditis).

Children (< 45 kg): With bacteremia or arthritis, use 50 mg/kg (maximum, 1 g) IM or IV in a single dose for 7 days. For meningitis, increase duration to 10 to 14 days and maximum dose to 2 g.

Infants: 25 to 50 mg/kg/day IV or IM in a single daily dose, not to exceed 125 mg. For disseminated infection, continue for 7 days, with a duration of 7 to 14 days with documented meningitis.

Acute PID (ambulatory) – 250 mg IM plus doxycycline.

Reconstitution of Ceftriaxone

	Vial/Bottle dosage size	Amount of diluent to add (ml)	Resultant concentration (mg/ml)
IM[1]	250 mg	0.9	250
	500 mg	1.8	250
	1 g	3.6	250
	2 g	7.2	250
IV[2]	250 mg	2.4	100
	500 mg	4.8	100
	1 g	9.6	100
	2 g	19.2	100
Piggyback[3]	1 g	10	
	2 g	20	

[1] If required, use more dilute solutions. Inject well within the body of a large muscle.
[2] Administer by intermittent infusion. Concentrations between 10 and 40 mg/ml are recommended; however, lower concentrations may be used.
[3] After reconstitution, further dilute to 50 or 100 ml with appropriate IV diluent.

10 g bulk container: This dosage size is not for direct administration. Reconstitute with 95 ml of an appropriate IV diluent. Before parenteral administration, withdraw the required amount, then further dilute to the desired concentration.

† CDC 1993 Sexually Transmitted Diseases Treatment Guidelines. *Morbidity and Mortality Weekly Report* 1993 Sep 24; 42 (No. RR-14):1-102.

CEFTRIAXONE SODIUM

Admixture compatibility: Do not physically mix with other antimicrobial drugs because of possible incompatibility.

Storage/Stability: Protect from light. After reconstitution, protection from normal light is not necessary.

IM – Solutions remain stable (loss of potency < 10%) for these time periods:

Stability/Storage of Ceftriaxone (IM)

Diluent	Concentration (mg/ml)	Storage	
		Room temp (25° C)	Refrigerated (4° C)
Sterile Water for Injection	100	3 days	10 days
	250	24 hours	3 days
0.9% Sodium Chloride Solution	100	3 days	10 days
	250	24 hours	3 days
5% Dextrose Solution	100	3 days	10 days
	250	24 hours	3 days
Bacteriostatic Water and 0.9% Benzyl Alcohol	100	24 hours	10 days
	250	24 hours	3 days
1% Lidocaine Solution (without epinephrine)	100	24 hours	10 days
	250	24 hours	3 days

IV – At concentrations of 10, 20 and 40 mg/ml, solutions stored in glass or PVC containers and IV solutions at concentrations of 100 mg/ml in the IV piggyback glass containers remain stable (loss of potency < 10%) for the following time periods:

Stability/Storage of Ceftriaxone (IV)

Diluent	Storage	
	Room temp (25° C)	Refrigerated (4° C)
Sterile Water	3 days	10 days
0.9% Sodium Chloride Solution	3 days	10 days
5% or 10% Dextrose Solution	3 days	10 days
5% Dextrose and 0.9% Sodium Chloride Solution[1]	3 days	Incompatible
5% Dextrose and 0.45% Sodium Chloride Solution	3 days	Incompatible

[1] Data available for 10 to 40 mg/ml concentrations in this diluent in PVC containers only.

The following IV solutions are stable at room temperature (25°C; 77°F) for 24 hours at concentrations between 10 and 40 mg/ml: Sodium Lactate (PVC container), 10% Invert Sugar (glass container), 5% Sodium Bicarbonate (glass container), *Freamine* III (glass container), *Normosol-M* in 5% Dextrose (glass and PVC containers), *Ionosol-B* in 5% Dextrose (glass container), 5% or 10% Mannitol (glass container).

Solutions reconstituted with 5% Dextrose or 0.9% Sodium Chloride solution at concentrations between 10 mg/ml and 40 mg/ml, and then frozen (–20°C; –4°F) in PVC or polyolefin containers, remain stable for 26 weeks. Thaw frozen solutions at room temperature before use. After thawing, discard unused portions. Do not refreeze.

Rx	**Rocephin** (Roche)	**Powder for Injection:**[1] 250 mg	In vials.
		500 mg	In vials.
		1 g	In vials, piggyback vials and *ADD-Vantage* vials.
		2 g	In vials, piggyback vials and *ADD-Vantage* vials.
		10 g	In bulk containers.
		Injection:[1] 1 g	Premixed, frozen. In 50 ml plastic containers.
		2 g	Premixed, frozen. In 50 ml plastic containers.

[1] Contains 3.6 mEq sodium/g.

CEFIXIME

Complete prescribing information for these products begins in the Cephalosporins group monograph.

Indications:

Uncomplicated urinary tract infections caused by *E coli* and *P mirabilis.*

Otitis media caused by *H influenzae* (beta-lactamase positive and negative strains), *Moraxella catarrhalis* and *S pyogenes.*

Pharyngitis and tonsillitis caused by *S pyogenes.*

Acute bronchitis and acute exacerbations of chronic bronchitis caused by *S pneumoniae* and *H influenzae* (beta-lactamase positive and negative strains.

Uncomplicated gonorrhea (cervical/urethral) caused by *N gonorrhoeae* (penicillinase- and non-penicillinase-producing strains).

Administration and Dosage:

Adults: 400 mg/day as a single 400 mg tablet (recommended for gonococcal infections) or as 200 mg every 12 hours.

Children: 8 mg/kg/day suspension as a single daily dose or as 4 mg/kg every 12 hours. Treat children > 50 kg or > 12 years of age with the recommended adult dose.

Pediatric Dosage of Cefixime

Weight		Dose/Day		
lb	kg	mg	tsp of suspension	ml
13	6	46	0.5	2.4
27.5	12.5	100	1	5
42	19	152	1.5	7.6
55	25	200	2	10
77	35	280	3	14

Treat otitis media with the suspension. In clinical studies, the suspension resulted in higher peak blood levels than the tablet administered at the same dosage.

For *S pyogenes* infections, administer cefixime for at least 10 days.

Renal function impairment:

Cefixime Dosage in Renal Impairment

Creatinine clearance (ml/min)	Dosage
> 60	Standard
21-60 or renal hemodialysis	75% of standard
≤ 20 or continuous ambulatory peritonial dialysis	50% of standard

Rx	**Suprax** (Lederle)	**Tablets:** 200 mg	(Suprax 200 LL). White, scored. Fllm coated. In 100s.
		400 mg	(Suprax 400 LL). White, scored. Film coated. In 50s. and 100s.
		Powder for Oral Suspension: 100 mg/5 ml	Strawberry flavor. In 50 and 100 ml.

CEFOPERAZONE SODIUM

Complete prescribing information for these products begins in the Cephalosporins group monograph.

Indications:

Respiratory tract infections caused by Streptococcus pneumoniae, *Haemophilus influenzae, Staphylococcus aureus* (penicillinase/nonpenicillinase-producing), *S pyogenes** (group A β-hemolytic streptococci), *Pseudomonas aeruginosa, Klebsiella pneumoniae, Escherichia coli, Proteus mirabilis* and *Enterobacter* sp.

Peritonitis and other intra-abdominal infections caused by *E coli, P aeruginosa**, enterococci, anaerobic gram-negative bacilli (including *Bacteroides fragilis*).

Bacterial septicemia caused by *S pneumoniae, S agalactiae*, S aureus,* enterococci, *P aeruginosa*, E coli, Klebsiella* sp*, *Proteus* sp* (indole-positive and indole-negative), *Clostridium* sp* and anaerobic gram-positive cocci.*

Skin and skin structure infections caused by *S aureus* (penicillinase/nonpenicillinase-producing), *S pyogenes,** and *P aeruginosa* and enterococci.

Pelvic inflammatory disease, endometritis and other female genital tract infections caused by *N gonorrhoeae, S epidermidis*, S agalactiae, E coli, Clostridium* sp*, enterococci, *Bacteroides* sp (including *B fragilis*), anaerobic gram-positive cocci.

Urinary tract infections caused by enterococci*, *E coli* and *P aeruginosa.*

Administration and Dosage:

Administer IM or IV.

Usual adult dose is 2 to 4 g/day administered in equally divided doses every 12 hours.

In severe infections or infections caused by less sensitive organisms, the total daily dose or frequency may be increased. Patients have been successfully treated with a total daily dosage of 6 to 12 g divided into 2, 3 or 4 administrations ranging from 1.5 to 4 g/dose. A total daily dose of 16 g by constant infusion has been given without complications. Steady-state serum concentrations were ≈ 150 mcg/ml.

Hepatic disease or biliary obstruction: Cefoperazone is extensively excreted in bile. The serum half-life is increased twofold to fourfold in patients with hepatic disease or biliary obstruction. In general, total daily dosage above 4 g should not be necessary. If higher dosages are used, monitor serum concentrations.

Renal function impairment: Because renal excretion is not the main route of elimination, patients with renal failure require no adjustment in dosage when usual doses are administered. When high doses are used, monitor serum drug concentrations.

Hemodialysis – The half-life is reduced slightly during hemodialysis. Thus, schedule dosing to follow a dialysis period. In patients with both hepatic dysfunction and significant renal disease, do not exceed 1 to 2 g daily without monitoring serum concentration.

IV administration:

Vials – In general, concentrations of between 2 and 50 mg/ml are recommended. Vials of sterile powder may be initially reconstituted with a minimum of 2.8 ml diluent per g of cefoperazone. Use any compatible diluent listed appropriate for IV administration. Reconstitute, using 5 ml of compatible diluent per g of cefoperazone. Withdraw the entire quantity for further dilution and administer via an IV administration system using one of the following methods:

Piggyback units:

Intermittent infusion – Further dilute reconstituted cefoperazone in 20 to 40 ml of diluent per g and administer over 15 to 30 minutes.

Continuous infusion – After dilution to a final concentration of between 2 and 25 mg per ml, use cefoperazone for continuous infusion.

IM administration: Any suitable diluent listed may be used to prepare solutions for IM injection. Where concentrations ≥ 250 mg/ml are to be administered, prepare solutions using 0.5% Lidocaine HCl Injection.

After reconstitution, the following volumes and concentrations will be obtained:

Volume and Concentration Following Reconstitution of Cefoperazone

Package size	Concentration (mg/ml)	Diluent to add (ml)	Withdrawable volume (ml)
1 g vial	333	2.6	3
	250	3.8	4
2 g vial	333	5	6
	250	7.2	8

* Efficacy of this organism in this organ system was studied in fewer than 10 infections.

CEFOPERAZONE SODIUM

Preparation of solution: Reconstitute powder for IV or IM use with any compatible solution for infusion mentioned below. After reconstitution, allow any foaming to dissipate to permit visual inspection for complete solubilization. Vigorous prolonged agitation may be needed to solubilize cefoperazone in higher concentrations (> 333 mg/ml). Maximum solubility of cefoperazone is ≈ 475 mg/ml compatible diluent.

IV use – Reconstitute with 5% Dextrose Injection; 5% Dextrose and Lactated Ringer's Injection; 5% Dextrose and 0.2% or 0.9% Sodium Chloride Injection; 10% Dextrose Injection; Lactated Ringer's Injection; 0.9% Sodium Chloride Injection; *Normosol M* and 5% Dextrose Injection; *Normosol R.*

IM use – Reconstitute with Bacteriostatic Water for Injection (benzyl alcohol or parabens); 0.5% Lidocaine HCl Injection; Sterile Water for Injection.

Do not use preparations containing benzyl alcohol in neonates.

Storage/Stability: The following parenteral diluents and approximate concentrations of cefoperazone provide stable solutions under the following conditions for the indicated time periods. (After indicated time periods, discard unused portions.)

Compatibility, Stability and Storage of Cefoperazone

Diluent	24 hours room temperature (15° to 25°C)	5 days refrigeration (2° to 8°C)	Freezer: 3 weeks (-20° to -10°C)	Freezer: 5 weeks (-20° to -10°C)	Approximate concentration (mg/ml)
Bacteriostatic Water for Injection (benzyl alcohol or parabens)	✓	✓			300
5% Dextrose Injection	✓	✓	✓[1]		2-50
5% Dextrose & Lactated Ringer's Inj.	✓				2-50
5% Dextrose & 0.2% or 0.9% Sodium Chloride Injection	✓	✓	✓[2]		2-50
10% Dextrose Injection	✓				2-50
Lactated Ringer's Injection	✓	✓			2
0.5% Lidocaine HCl Injection	✓	✓			300
0.9% Sodium Chloride Injection	✓	✓		✓[3]	2-300
Normosol M & 5% Dextrose Injection	✓	✓			2-50
Normosol R	✓	✓			2-50
Sterile Water for Injection	✓	✓		✓	300

[1] The 50 mg/ml injection only.
[2] The 2 mg/ml injection only.
[3] The 300 mg/ml injection only.

Thaw frozen samples at room temperature before use. After thawing, discard unused portions. Do not refreeze.

Sterile powder – Prior to reconstitution, protect sterile powder from light and store at or below 25°C (77°F). After reconstitution, protection from light is not necessary.

Frozen solution – Do not store above 20°C (–4°F). After thawing, solution is stable for 10 days at 5°C (4°F) and for 48 hours at room temperature. Do not refreeze.

Admixture incompatibility – Do not mix cefoperazone directly with an aminoglycoside. If concomitant therapy is necessary, use sequential intermittent IV infusion provided that separate secondary IV tubing is used and the primary IV tubing is irrigated between doses. Administer cefoperazone prior to the aminoglycoside.

Rx	**Cefobid** (Roerig)	**Powder for Injection:**[1] 1 g	In vials and Piggyback units.
		2 g	In vials and Piggyback units.
		Injection:[1] 1 g	Premixed, frozen. In 50 ml plastic containers.[2]
		2 g	Premixed, frozen. In 50 ml plastic containers.[3]

[1] Contains 1.5 mEq sodium/g.
[2] With 2.3 g dextrose hydrous.
[3] With 1.8 g dextrose hydrous.

CEFOTAXIME SODIUM

Complete prescribing information for these products begins in the Cephalosporins group monograph.

Indications:

Lower respiratory tract infections, including pneumonia, caused by *Streptococcus pneumoniae, S pyogenes** (group A streptococci) and other streptococci (excluding enterococci, eg, *S faecalis*), *Staphylococcus aureus* (penicillinase/nonpenicillinase-producing), *Escherichia coli, Klebsiella* sp, *Haemophilus influenzae* (including ampicillin-resistant strains), *H parainfluenzae, Proteus mirabilis, Serratia marcescens** and *Enterobacter* sp, indole-positive *Proteus* and *Pseudomonas* sp.

Urinary tract infections caused by *Enterococcus* sp, *S epidermidis, S aureus** (penicillinase/nonpenicillinase-producing), *Citrobacter* species, *Enterobacter* species, *E coli, Klebsiella* species, *P mirabilis, P vulgaris*, P inconstans* group B, *Morganella morganii*, Providencia rettgeri*, S marcescens* and *Pseudomonas* sp. Also, uncomplicated gonorrhea caused by *Neisseria gonorrhoeae,* including penicillinase-producing strains.

Gynecological infections, including pelvic inflammatory disease, endometritis and pelvic cellulitis caused by *S epidermidis,* streptococci, *Enterococcus, Enterobacter* sp*, *Klebsiella* sp*, *E coli, P mirabilis, Bacteroides* species (including *B fragilis*)*, *Clostridium* species and anaerobic cocci (including *Peptostreptococcus, Peptococcus*).

Bacteremia/Septicemia caused by *E coli, Klebsiella* sp, *S marcescens, S aureus* and streptococci.

Skin and skin structure infections caused by *S aureus* (penicillinase/nonpenicillinase-producing), *S epidermidis, S pyogenes* (group A streptococci) and other streptococci, *Enterococcus, Acinetobacter* sp*, *Citrobacter* sp, *E coli, Enterobacter, Klebsiella* sp, *P mirabilis, M morganii, P rettgeri*, P vulgaris*, Pseudomonas* sp, *S marcescens, Bacteroides* sp and anaerobic cocci (including *Peptostreptococcus*, Peptococcus*).

Intra-abdominal infections including peritonitis caused by streptococci*, *E coli, Klebsiella* sp, *Bacteroides* sp and anaerobic cocci (including *Peptostreptococcus** and *Peptococcus*, P mirabilis** and *Clostridium* sp).

Bone or joint infections caused by *S aureus* (penicillinase/nonpenicillinase-producing strains), streptococci, *Pseudomonas* sp and *P mirabilis.**

CNS infections (eg, meningitis and ventriculitis) caused by *N meningitidis, H influenzae, S pneumoniae, K pneumoniae** and *E coli.**

Although many strains of enterococci (eg, *S faecalis*) and *Pseudomonas* species are resistant to cefotaxime in vitro, it has been used successfully in treating patients with infections caused by susceptible organisms.

Perioperative prophylaxis may reduce the incidence of certain postoperative infections in patients undergoing surgical procedures (eg, abdominal or vaginal hysterectomy, GI and GU surgery) that are classified as contaminated or potentially contaminated. Effective perioperative use depends on the time of administration. For patients undergoing GI surgery, preoperative bowel preparation by mechanical cleansing as well as with a nonabsorbable antibiotic (eg, neomycin) is recommended.

Cesarean section – Intraoperative (after clamping the umbilical cord) and postoperative use may reduce the incidence of certain postoperative infections.

If there are signs of infection, obtain specimens for identification of the causative organism so that appropriate therapy may be instituted.

Concomitant aminoglycoside therapy – In certain cases of confirmed or suspected gram-positive or gram-negative sepsis, or other serious infections in which the causative organism has not been identified, cefotaxime may be used concomitantly with an aminoglycoside. The dosage recommended for both antibiotics may be given, and dosage depends on the severity of the infection and the patient's condition. Monitor renal function, especially if higher dosages of the aminoglycosides are used or if therapy is prolonged, because of the potential nephrotoxicity and ototoxicity of aminoglycoside antibiotics. Some β-lactam antibiotics also have a certain degree of nephrotoxicity. Although not noted when cefotaxime was given alone, nephrotoxicity may be potentiated if it is used concomitantly with an aminoglycoside.

* Efficacy for this organism in this organ system has been studied in fewer than 10 infections.

CEFOTAXIME SODIUM

Administration and Dosage:

Adults: Administer IV or IM. The maximum daily dosage should not exceed 12 g. Determine dosage and route of administration by susceptibility of the causative organisms, severity of the infection and the patient's condition (see table for dosage guidelines).

Cefotaxime Dosage Guidelines for Adults

Type of Infection	Daily Dosage (g)	Frequency and Route
Gonorrhea	1	1 g IM (single dose)
Uncomplicated infections	2	1 g every 12 hours IM or IV
Moderate to severe	3 to 6	1 to 2 g every 8 hours IM or IV
Infections commonly needing higher dosage (eg, septicemia)	6 to 8	2 g every 6 to 8 hours IV
Life-threatening infections	up to 12	2 g every 4 hours IV

Perioperative prophylaxis – 1 g IV or IM, 30 to 90 minutes prior to surgery.

Cesarean section – Administer the first 1 g dose IV as soon as the umbilical cord is clamped. Administer the second and third doses as 1 g IV or IM at 6 and 12 hour intervals after the first dose.

Pediatric – It is not necessary to differentiate between premature and normal gestational age infants. The following dosage recommendations may serve as a guide:

Cefotaxime Dosage Guidelines in Pediatrics

Age	Weight (kg)	Dosage Schedule	Route
0 to 1 week	—	50 mg/kg every 12 hours	IV
1 to 4 weeks	—	50 mg/kg every 8 hours	IV
1 month to 12 years	< 50[1]	50 to 180 mg/kg/day in 4 to 6 divided doses[2]	IV or IM

[1] For children ≥ 50 kg, use adult dosage.

[2] Use higher doses for more severe or serious infections including meningitis.

Renal function impairment: Determine dosage by degree of renal impairment, severity of infection and susceptibility of the causative organism. In patients with estimated creatinine clearances of less than 20 ml/min/1.73m^2, reduce dosage by one-half.

When only serum creatinine is available, the following formula may be used to convert this value into creatinine clearance. The serum creatinine should represent steady-state renal function.

$$\text{Males: } \frac{\text{Weight (kg)} \times (140 - \text{age})}{72 \times \text{serum creatinine (mg/dl)}} = \text{Ccr}$$

$$\text{Females: } 0.85 \times \text{above value}$$

CDC recommended treatment schedules for gonorrhea:*

Disseminated gonococcal infection – Give 500 mg cefotaxime IV 4 times per day for at least 7 days.

Gonococcal ophthalmia in adults – For penicillinase-producing *Neisseria gonorrhoeae* (PPNG), give 500 mg, IV, 4 times per day.

IV administration: The IV route is preferable for patients with bacteremia, bacterial septicemia, peritonitis, meningitis, or other severe or life-threatening infections, or for patients who may be poor risks because of lowered resistance resulting from such debilitating conditions as malnutrition, trauma, surgery, diabetes, heart failure or malignancy, particularly if shock is present or impending.

Intermittent IV – 1 or 2 g in 10 ml of Sterile Water for Injection over 3 to 5 minutes; may also be given over a longer period of time through the tubing system by which the patient may be receiving other IV solutions. However, temporarily discontinue administration of other solutions at the same site.

Continuous IV infusion – May add to IV bottles containing solutions discussed below.

IM administration: Inject well within the body of a relatively large muscle (ie, gluteus maximus). Divide doses of 2 g and administer in different IM sites.

* *Morbidity and Mortality Weekly Report* 1985 (Oct 18); 34 (Supp 4S):76S-108S.

CEFOTAXIME SODIUM

Preparation of solution: Use the following table as a guide for reconstitution:

Volume and Concentration Following Reconstitution of Cefotaxime			
Package Size	Diluent to Add (ml)	≈ Withdrawable Volume (ml)	≈ Concentration (mg/ml)
1 g vial	3 (IM)	3.4	300
2 g vial	5 (IM)	6	330
1 g vial	10 (IV)	10.4	95
2 g vial	10 (IV)	11	180
1 g infusion	50-100	50-100	10-20
2 g infusion	50-100	50-100	20-40
10 g bottle	47	52	200
10 g bottle	97	102	100

Shake to dissolve. Solutions range in color from light yellow to amber, depending on concentration, diluent used, and length and condition of storage. A solution of 1 g cefotaxime in 14 ml of Sterile Water for Injection is isotonic.

IV – Reconstitute with at least 10 ml of Sterile Water for Injection. Infusion bottles may be reconstituted with 50 or 100 ml of 0.9% Sodium Chloride Injection or 5% Dextrose Injection.

IM – Reconstitute with Sterile Water or Bacteriostatic Water for Injection.

Compatibility, Stability and Storage: Solutions reconstituted as described above maintain potency for 24 hours at room temperature (≤ 22°C; 72°F), for 10 days under refrigeration (≤ 5°C; 4°F) and for at least 13 weeks frozen. After reconstitution and subsequent storage in disposable glass or plastic syringes, cefotaxime is stable for 24 hours at room temperature, 5 days under refrigeration and 13 weeks frozen.

Reconstituted solutions may be further diluted up to 50 to 1000 ml with the following solutions and will maintain potency for 24 hours at room temperature and at least 5 days under refrigeration: 0.9% Sodium Chloride; 5% or 10% Dextrose; 5% Dextrose and 0.2%, 0.45% or 0.9% Sodium Chloride; Lactated Ringer's Solution; Sodium Lactate Injection (M/6); 10% Invert Sugar.

IV bags: Solutions of cefotaxime in 0.9% Sodium Chloride Injection and 5% Dextrose Injection in IV bags are stable for 24 hours at room temperature, 5 days under refrigeration and 13 weeks frozen.

Thaw frozen samples at room temperature before use; do not heat. After the periods mentioned above, discard any unused solutions or frozen material. Do not refreeze.

Cefotaxime solutions exhibit maximum stability in the pH 5 to 7 range. Do not use with diluents having a pH above 7.5 (eg, Sodium Bicarbonate Injection).

Admixtures: Do not admix with aminoglycoside solutions. If cefotaxime and aminoglycosides are to be administered to the same patient, administer separately.

Storage:

Powder – Store cefotaxime in the dry state below 30°C (86°F). The dry material, as well as the solutions, tends to darken depending on storage conditions; protect from elevated temperatures and excessive light.

Frozen solutions – Thawed solutions are stable for 24 hours at room temperature (≤ 22°C; 72°F) or for 10 days under refrigeration (≤ 5°C; 4°F).

Rx	**Claforan** (Hoechst Marion Roussel)	**Powder for Injection:**[1] 500 mg	In vials. In 10s.
		1 g	In vials, packages of 10s, 25s, 50s. Infusion bottles in 10s. *ADD-Vantage* system vials in 25s.
		2 g	In vials, packages of 10s, 25s, 50s. Infusion bottles in 10s. *ADD-Vantage* system vials in 25s.
		10 g	In bulk vials.
		Injection:[1] 1 g	Premixed, frozen. In 50 ml, package of 24s.
		2 g	Premixed, frozen. In 50 ml, package of 24s.

[1] Contains 2.2 mEq sodium/g.

CEFTIZOXIME SODIUM

For complete prescribing information, refer to the Cephalosporins group monograph.

Indications:

Lower respiratory tract infections caused by *Streptococcus* sp (including *S pneumoniae,* but excluding enterococci), *Klebsiella* sp, *Proteus mirabilis, Escherichia coli, Haemophilus influenzae* (including ampicillin-resistant strains), *Staphylococcus aureus* (penicillinase/ nonpenicillinase-producing), *Serratia* sp, *Enterobacter* sp and *Bacteroides* sp.

Urinary tract infections caused by *S aureus* (penicillinase/nonpenicillinase-producing), *E coli, Pseudomonas* sp including *P aeruginosa, Proteus mirabilis, P vulgaris, Providencia rettgeri, Morganella morganii, Klebsiella* sp, *Serratia* sp including *S marcescens* and *Enterobacter* sp.

Gonorrhea: Uncomplicated cervical and urethral gonorrhea caused by *N gonorrhoeae.*

Pelvic inflammatory disease (PID) caused by *N gonorrhoeae, E coli* or *S agalactiae.*

Intra-abdominal infections caused by *E coli, S epidermidis, Streptococcus* sp (excluding enterococci), *Enterobacter* sp, *Klebsiella* sp, *Bacteroides* sp including *B fragilis* and anaerobic cocci, including *Peptococcus* sp and *Peptostreptococcus* sp.

Septicemia caused by *Streptococcus* sp including *S pneumoniae,* but excluding enterococci, *Staphylococcus aureus* (penicillinase/nonpenicillinase-producing), *E coli, Bacteroides* sp including *B fragilis, Klebsiella* sp and *Serratia* sp.

Skin and skin structure infections caused by *S aureus* (penicillinase/nonpenicillinase-producing), *S epidermidis, E coli, Klebsiella* sp, *Streptococcus* sp including *S pyogenes* (group A β-hemolytic, but excluding enterococci), *P mirabilis, Serratia* sp, *Enterobacter* sp, *Bacteroides* sp including *B fragilis* and anaerobic cocci, including *Peptococcus* sp and *Peptostreptococcus* sp.

Bone and joint infections caused by *S aureus* (penicillinase/nonpenicillinase-producing), *Streptococcus* sp (excluding enterococci), *P mirabilis, Bacteroides* sp and anaerobic cocci, including *Peptococcus* sp and *Peptostreptococcus* sp.

Meningitis caused by *H influenzae.* Used to treat limited cases of meningitis caused by *S pneumoniae.*

Administration and Dosage:

Adults: Usual dosage is 1 or 2 g every 8 to 12 hours. Individualize dosage.

Ceftizoxime Dosage Guidelines in Adults		
Type of infection	Daily dose (g)	Frequency and route
Uncomplicated urinary tract	1	500 mg every 12 hours IM or IV
PID[1]	6	2 g every 8 hours IV
Other sites	2-3	1 g every 8 to 12 hours IM or IV
Severe or refractory	3-6	1 g every 8 hours IM or IV 2 g every 8 to 12 hours IM[1] or IV
Life-threatening [2]	9-12	3 to 4 g every 8 hours IV

[1] Dosages up to 2 g every 4 hours have been given.
[2] Divide 2 g IM doses and give in different large muscle masses.

Urinary tract infections: Because of the serious nature of urinary tract infections due to *P aeruginosa* and because many strains of *Pseudomonas* species are only moderately susceptible to ceftizoxime, higher dosage is recommended. Institute other therapy if the response is not prompt.

Gonorrhea, uncomplicated: A single 1 g IM injection is the usual dose.

Life-threatening infections: The IV route may be preferable for patients with bacterial septicemia, localized parenchymal abscesses (such as intra-abdominal abscess), peritonitis or other severe or life-threatening infections.

In those patients with normal renal function, the IV dosage is 2 to 12 g daily. In conditions such as bacterial septicemia, 6 to 12 g/day IV may be given initially for several days, and the dosage gradually reduced according to clinical response and laboratory findings.

Pediatric:

Children (≥ 6 months) – 50 mg/kg every 6 to 8 hours. Dosage may be increased to 200 mg/kg/day. Do not exceed the maximum adult dose for serious infection.

Renal function impairment requires modification of dosage. Following an initial loading dose of 500 mg to 1 g IM or IV, use the maintenance dosing schedule in the following table. Determine further dosing by therapeutic monitoring, severity of the infection and susceptibility of the causative organisms.

CEFTIZOXIME SODIUM

When only serum creatinine is available, calculate creatinine clearance from the formula below. The serum creatinine should represent steady-state renal function.

Males: $$\frac{\text{Weight (kg)} \times (140 - \text{age})}{72 \times \text{serum creatinine (mg/dl)}} = \text{Ccr}$$

Females: 0.85 × above value

Hemodialysis – No additional supplemental dosing is required following hemodialysis; give the dose (according to the table below) at the end of dialysis.

Ceftizoxime Dosage in Adults with Renal Impairment

Renal function	Creatinine clearance (ml/min)	Less severe infections	Life-threatening infections
Mild impairment	50-79	500 mg q 8 h	750 mg to 1.5 g q 8 h
Moderate to severe impairment	5-49	250 to 500 mg q 12 h	500 mg to 1 g q 12 h
Dialysis patients	0-4	500 mg q 48 h or 250 mg q 24 h	500 mg to 1 g q 48 h or 500 mg q 24 h

IV administration: Direct (bolus) injection, slowly over 3 to 5 minutes, directly or through tubing for patients receiving parenteral fluids (see list below). For intermittent or continuous infusion, dilute reconstituted ceftizoxime in 50 to 100 ml of one of the following: NaCl Injection; 5% or 10% Dextrose Injection; 5% Dextrose and 0.9%, 0.45% or 0.2% NaCl Injection; Ringer's Injection; Lactated Ringer's Injection; 5% Sodium Bicarbonate in Sterile Water for Injection; 5% Dextrose in Lactated Ringer's Injection (only when reconstituted with 4% Sodium Bicarbonate Inj.).

Preparation of solution: Reconstitute with Sterile Water for Injection. Shake well.

Volume and Concentration Following Reconstitution of Ceftizoxime

Package size	Diluent to add (ml)	≈ Available volume (ml)	≈ Concentration (mg/ml)
1 g vial	3 (IM)	3.7	270
2 g vial[1]	6 (IM)	7.4	270
1 g vial	10 (IV)	10.7	95
2 g vial	20 (IV)	21.4	95
10 g vial	30 (bulk vial)	37	1 g/3.5 ml
	45 (bulk vial)	51	1 g/5 ml

[1] Divide 2 g IM doses and give in different large muscle masses.

Piggyback vials – Reconstitute with 50 to 100 ml of any IV solution listed above. Shake well. Administer as a single dose with primary IV fluids.

A solution of 1 g ceftizoxime in 13 ml Sterile Water for Injection is isotonic.

Frozen injection – Thaw container at room temperature. Do not introduce additives into the solution.

Storage: After reconstitution or dilution in the IV fluids above, these solutions are stable for 24 hours at room temperature and for 96 hours if refrigerated (5°C; 41°F).

After thawing the frozen injection, the solution is stable for 24 hours at room temperature or for 10 days if refrigerated. Do not refreeze.

Rx	**Cefizox** (Fujisawa)	**Powder for Injection:**[1] 500 mg (as sodium)	In 10 ml single dose fliptop vials.
		1 g (as sodium)	In 20 ml single dose fliptop vials and 100 ml piggyback vials.
		2 g (as sodium)	In 20 ml single dose fliptop vials and 100 ml piggyback vials.
		10 g (as sodium)	In pharmacy bulk package.
		Injection: In 5% Dextrose in Water[1] 1 g (as sodium)	Frozen, premixed. In 50 ml single dose plastic containers.
		2 g (as sodium)	Frozen, premixed. In 50 ml single dose plastic containers.

[1] Contains 2.6 mEq sodium/g.

CEFOTETAN DISODIUM

For complete prescribing information, refer to the Cephalosporins group monograph.

Indications:

Urinary tract infections caused by *Escherichia coli, Klebsiella* sp (including *K pneumoniae*) and *Proteus* sp (including *P vulgaris, P mirabilis, Providencia rettgeri* and *Morganella morganii*).

Lower respiratory tract infections caused by *Streptococcus pneumoniae, Staphylococcus aureus* (penicillinase/nonpenicillinase-producing), *H influenzae* (including ampicillin-resistant strains), *Klebsiella* sp (including *K pneumoniae*), *E coli.*

Skin/Skin structure infections caused by *S aureus* (penicillinase/nonpenicillinase-producing), *S epidermidis, S pyogenes, Streptococcus* sp (excluding enterococci) and *E coli.*

Gynecologic infections caused by *S aureus** (including penicillinase/nonpenicillinase-producing), *S epidermidis, Streptococcus* sp (excluding enterococci), *E coli, P mirabilis, Neisseria gonorrhoeae, Bacteroides* sp (excluding *B distasonis, B ovatus, B thetaiotaomicron*), *Fusobacterium* sp and gram-positive anaerobic cocci (including *Peptococcus* and *Peptostreptococcus* sp*).

Intra-abdominal infections caused by *E coli, Klebsiella* sp (including *K pneumoniae**), *Streptococcus* sp (excluding enterococci) and *Bacteroides* sp (excluding *B distasonis, B ovatus, B thetaiotaomicron*).

Bone and joint infections caused by *S aureus.**

Concomitant antibiotic therapy: If cefotetan and an aminoglycoside are used concomitantly, carefully monitor renal function, especially if higher dosages of the aminoglycoside are to be administered or if therapy is prolonged, because of the potential nephrotoxicity and ototoxicity of aminoglycosides. Although to date, nephrotoxicity has not been noted when cefotetan was given alone, it is possible that nephrotoxicity may be potentiated if used concomitantly with an aminoglycoside.

Perioperative prophylaxis: Preoperative administration may reduce incidence of certain postoperative infections in patients undergoing surgical procedures classified as clean contaminated or potentially contaminated (eg, cesarean section, abdominal or vaginal hysterectomy, transurethral surgery, GI and biliary tract surgery).

If there are signs and symptoms of infection, obtain specimens for identification of causative organism so that appropriate therapeutic measures may be initiated.

Administration and Dosage:

Adults: The usual dosage is 1 or 2 g IV or IM every 12 hours for 5 to 10 days. Determine proper dosage and route of administration by the condition of the patient, severity of the infection and susceptibility of the causative organism.

General Cefotetan Dosage Guidelines		
Type of Infection	Daily Dose	Frequency and Route
Urinary Tract	1 to 4 g	500 mg every 12 hours IV or IM
		1 or 2 g every 24 hours IV or IM
		1 or 2 g every 12 hours IV or IM
Other Sites	2 to 4 g	1 or 2 g every 12 hours IV or IM
Severe	4 g	2 g every 12 hours IV
Life-threatening	6 g[1]	3 g every 12 hours IV

[1] Maximum daily dosage should not exceed 6 g.

Prophylaxis: To prevent postoperative infection in clean contaminated or potentially contaminated surgery in adults, give a single 1 or 2 g IV dose 30 to 60 minutes prior to surgery. In patients undergoing cesarean section, give the dose as soon as the umbilical cord is clamped.

Renal function impairment: Reduce the dosage schedule using these guidelines:

Cefotetan Dosage in Renal Impairment		
Ccr (ml/min)	Dose	Frequency
> 30	Usual Recommended Dose[2]	Every 12 hours
10-30	Usual Recommended Dose[2]	Every 24 hours
< 10	Usual Recommended Dose[2]	Every 48 hours

[2] Determined by type/severity of infection, susceptibility of causative organism.

* Efficacy for this organism in this organ system was studied in fewer than ten infections.

CEFOTETAN DISODIUM

Alternatively, the dosing interval may remain constant at 12 hour intervals, but reduce dose by one-half for patients with a creatinine clearance of 10 to 30 ml/min, and by one-quarter for patients with a creatinine clearance of less than 10 ml/min.

When only serum creatinine is available, use the following formula to estimate creatinine clearance. Serum creatinine level should represent steady-state renal function.

$$\text{Males: } \frac{\text{Weight (kg)} \times (140 - \text{age})}{72 \times \text{serum creatinine (mg/dl)}} = \text{Ccr}$$

Females: 0.85 × above value

Dialysis – Cefotetan is dialyzable; for patients undergoing intermittent hemodialysis, give one-quarter of the usual recommended dose every 24 hours on days between dialysis and one-half the usual recommended dose on the day of dialysis.

IV: The IV route is preferable for patients with bacteremia, bacterial septicemia or other severe or life-threatening infections, or for patients who may be poor risks because of lowered resistance resulting from such debilitating conditions as malnutrition, trauma, surgery, diabetes, heart failure or malignancy, particularly if shock is present or impending.

Intermittent IV administration – Inject a solution containing 1 or 2 g in Sterile Water for Injection over 3 to 5 minutes. Using an infusion system, the solution may be given over a longer period through the tubing system by which the patient may be receiving other IV solutions. Butterfly or scalp vein-type needles are preferred. However, during infusion of cefotetan, temporarily discontinue the administration of other solutions at the same site.

IM: As with all IM preparations, inject well within the body of a relatively large muscle such as the upper outer quadrant of the buttock (ie, gluteus maximus).

Preparation of Solution:

For IV use – Reconstitute with Sterile Water for Injection.

For IM use – Reconstitute with Sterile Water for Injection, Bacteriostatic Water for Injection, Normal Saline USP or 0.5% or 1% Lidocaine HCl.

Volume and Concentration Following Reconstitution of Cefotetan

Vial Size (g)	Amount of Diluent to Add (ml)	≈ Withdrawable Volume (ml)	≈ Average Concentration (mg/ml)
IV			
1	10	10.5	95
2	10-20	11-21	182-195
IM			
1	2	2.5	400
2	3	4	500

Infusion bottles (100 ml) may be reconstituted with 50 to 100 ml of 5% Dextrose Solution or 0.9% Sodium Chloride Solution.

Compatibility and stability: Reconstituted as described above, cefotetan maintains potency for 24 hours at room temperature (25°C; 77°F), for 96 hours refrigerated (5°C; 40°F) and for at least 1 week frozen. After reconstitution and subsequent storage in disposable glass or plastic syringes, cefotetan is stable for 24 hours at room temperature and 96 hours refrigerated.

Thaw frozen samples at room temperature before use. After the periods mentioned above, discard any unused solutions or frozen materials. Do not refreeze.

Admixtures – Do not admix with solutions containing aminoglycosides. If cefotetan and aminoglycosides are to be administered to the same patient, they must be administered separately and not as a mixed injection.

Storage – Do not store vials above 22°C (72°F); protect from light.

CEFOTETAN DISODIUM

Rx	**Cefotan** (Zeneca)	**Powder for Injection**: Contains 3.5 mEq sodium/g	
		1 g	In 10 and 100 ml vials.
		2 g	In 20 and 100 ml vials.
		10 g	In 100ml vials
		Injection: 1 g/50 ml	Dextrose. Frozen, iso-osmotic, premixed. In 50 ml single-dose *Galaxy* containers.
		2 g/50 ml	Dextrose. Frozen, iso-osmotic, premixed. In 50 ml single-dose *Galaxy* containers.

CEFTAZIDIME

Complete prescribing information for these products begins in the Cephalosporins group monograph.

Indications:

Lower respiratory tract infections, including pneumonia, caused by *Pseudomonas aeruginosa* and other *Pseudomonas* species; *Haemophilus influenzae,* including ampicillin-resistant strains; *Klebsiella* species; *Enterobacter* species; *Proteus mirabilis; Escherichia coli; Serratia* species; *Citrobacter* species; *Staphylococcus pneumoniae; S aureus* (methicillin-susceptible strains).

Skin and skin structure infections, caused by *P aeruginosa; Klebsiella* species; *E coli; Proteus* species, including *P mirabilis*and indole-positive *Proteus; Enterobacter* species; *Serratia* species; *S aureus* (methicillin-susceptible strains); *S pyogenes* (group A β–hemolytic streptococci).

Urinary tract infections, both complicated and uncomplicated, caused by *P aeruginosa; Enterobacter* species; *Proteus* species, including *P mirabilis* and indole-positive *Proteus; Klebsiella* species; *E coli.*

Bacterial septicemia caused by *P aeruginosa; Klebsiella* species; *H influenzae; E coli; Serratia* species; *S pneumoniae; S aureus* (methicillin-susceptible strains).

Bone and joint infections, caused by *P aeruginosa; Klebsiella* species; *Enterobacter* species; *S aureus* (methicillin-susceptible strains).

Gynecological infections, including endometritis, pelvic cellulitis and other infections of the female genital tract, caused by *E coli.*

Intra-abdominal infections, including peritonitis caused by *E coli; Klebsiella* species; *S aureus* (methicillin-susceptible strains); polymicrobial infections caused by aerobic and anaerobic organisms and *Bacteroides* species (many strains of *B fragilis* are resistant).

CNS infections, including meningitis caused by *H influenzae* and *Neisseria meningitidis.* Ceftazidime has also been used successfully in a limited number of cases of meningitis due to *P aeruginosa* and *S pneumoniae.*

Concomitant antibiotic therapy: Ceftazidime may be used concomitantly with other antibiotics (eg, aminoglycosides, vancomycin and clindamycin) in severe and life-threatening infections and in the immunocompromised patient. Dose depends on the severity of the infection and the patient's condition.

Administration and Dosage:

Determine dosage and route by the susceptibility of the causative organisms, severity of infection and patient's condition and renal function.

Ceftazidime Dosage Guidelines		
Patient/Infection site	Dose	Frequency
Adults Usual recommended dose	1 g IV or IM	q 8-12 h
Uncomplicated urinary tract infections	250 mg IV or IM	q 12 h
Complicated urinary tract infections	500 mg IV or IM	q 8-12 h
Uncomplicated pneumonia; mild skin and skin structure infections	500 mg to 1 g IV or IM	q 8 h
Bone and joint infections	2 g IV	q 12 h
Serious gynecological and Intra-abdominal infections	2 g IV	q 8 h
Meningitis		
Very severe life-threatening infections, especially in immunocompromised patients		
Pseudomonal lung infections in cystic fibrosis patients w/normal renal function[1]	30 to 50 mg/kg IV to a max 6 g/day	q 8 h
Neonates (0 to 4 weeks)	30 mg/kg IV	q 12 h
Infants and children (1 month to 12 years)	30 to 50 mg/kg IV to g/day[2]	q 8 h

[1] Although clinical improvement has been shown, bacteriological cures cannot be expected in patients with chronic respiratory disease and cystic fibrosis.

[2] Reserve the higher dose for immunocompromised children or children with cystic fibrosis or meningitis.

Hepatic function impairment: No dosage adjustment is required.

CEFTAZIDIME

Renal function impairment: Ceftazidime is excreted by the kidneys, almost exclusively by glomerular filtration. In patients with impaired renal function (GFR < 50 ml/min), reduce dosage to compensate for slower excretion. In patients with suspected renal insufficiency, give an initial loading dose of 1 g. Estimate GFR to determine the appropriate maintenance dose.

Ceftazidime Dosage in Renal Impairment		
Creatinine clearance (ml/min)	Recommended unit dose of ceftazidime	Frequency of dosing
31-50	1 g	q 12 h
16-30	1 g	q 24 h
6-15	500 mg	q 24 h
≤ 5	500 mg	q 48 h

When only serum creatinine is available, use the following formula to estimate creatinine clearance. Serum creatinine should represent steady-state renal function.

$$\text{Males: } \frac{\text{Weight (kg)} \times (140 - \text{age})}{72 \times \text{serum creatinine (mg/dl)}} = \text{Ccr}$$

Females: $0.85 \times$ above value

In patients with severe infections who would normally receive 6 g ceftazidime daily were it not for renal insufficiency, the unit dose given in the table above may be increased by 50% or the dosing frequency increased appropriately. Determine further dosing by therapeutic monitoring, severity of the infection and susceptibility of the causative organism.

In children, as for adults, adjust creatinine clearance for body surface area or lean body mass and reduce the dosing frequency in cases of renal insufficiency.

Dialysis – Give a 1 g loading dose, followed by 1 g after each hemodialysis period.

Ceftazidime can also be used in patients undergoing intraperitoneal dialysis (IPD) and continuous ambulatory peritoneal dialysis (CAPD). Give a loading dose of 1 g, followed by 500 mg every 24 hours. In addition to IV use, ceftazidime can be incorporated in the dialysis fluid at a concentration of 250 mg per 2 L of dialysis fluid.

Preparation of Ceftazidime Solutions			
Package size	Diluent to add (ml)	≈ Available volume (ml)	≈ Ceftazidime concentration (mg/ml)
IM			
500 mg vial	1.5	1.8	280
1 g vial	3	3.6	280
IV			
500 mg vial	5	5.3	100
1 g vial	5 or 10	5.6 or 10.6	180 or 100
2 g vial	10	2-11.5	170-180
Infusion pack			
1 g vial	50 or 100[1]	50 or 100	20 or 10
2 g vial	50 or 100[1]	50 or 100	40 or 20
Bulk package			
6 g vial	26	30	200

[1] *Note:* Addition should be in two stages (see *IV infusion*).

Inject IV or deeply IM into a large muscle mass such as the upper outer quadrant of the gluteus maximus or lateral part of the thigh.

IM: Reconstitute with one of the following diluents: Sterile or Bacteriostatic Water for Injection or 0.5% or 1% Lidocaine HCl Injection. Refer to the Preparation of Ceftazidime Solutions table.

IV: This route is preferable for patients with bacterial septicemia, bacterial meningitis, peritonitis or other severe or life-threatening infections, or for patients who may be poor risks because of lowered resistance resulting from malnutrition, trauma, surgery, diabetes, heart failure or malignancy, particularly if shock is present or impending.

Direct intermittent IV administration – Reconstitute ceftazidime as directed in the table with Sterile Water for Injection. Slowly inject directly into the vein over a period of 3 to 5 minutes or give through the tubing of an administration set while the patient is also receiving one of the compatible IV fluids.

CEFTAZIDIME

IV infusion – Reconstitute the 1 or 2 g infusion pack with 100 ml Sterile Water for Injection or one of the compatible IV fluids. Alternatively, reconstitute the 500 mg, 1 or 2 g vial and add an appropriate quantity of the resulting solution to an IV container with one of the compatible IV fluids.

Intermittent IV infusion (Y–type) can be accomplished with compatible solutions. However, during infusion of ceftazidime solution, discontinue other solution.

Compatibility and stability:

IM – When reconstituted as directed with Sterile or Bacteriostatic Water for Injection or 0.5% or 1% Lidocaine HCl Injection, the solution maintains potency for 18 to 24 hours at room temperature or for 7 to 10 days if refrigerated. Solutions in Sterile Water for Injection, frozen immediately after reconstitution in the original container, are stable for 3 months at –20°C (–4°F). Once thawed, do not refreeze. Thawed solutions may be stored for 8 to 24 hours at room temperature or 4 days in a refrigerator.

IV – When reconstituted as directed with Sterile Water for Injection, the solution maintains potency for 18 to 24 hours at room temperature or for 7 to 10 days under refrigeration. Solutions in Sterile Water for Injection in the original container or in 0.9% Sodium Chloride or 5% Dextrose Injection in PVC small volume containers, frozen immediately after reconstitution, are stable for 3 months at –20°C (–4°F). For larger volumes, when it is necessary to warm the frozen product (to a maximum of 40°C; 104°F), avoid heating after thawing is complete. Once thawed, do not refreeze. Store thawed solutions for 8 to 24 hrs at room temp. or for 4 days in a refrigerator.

Ceftazidime is compatible with the more common IV infusion fluids. Solutions at concentrations between 1 mg/ml and 40 mg/ml in the following infusion fluids may be stored for up to 18 to 24 hours at room temperature or 7 to 10 days if refrigerated: 0.9% Sodium Chloride; M/6 Sodium Lactate; Ringer's; Lactated Ringer's; 5% or 10% Dextrose; 5% Dextrose and 0.225%, 0.45% or 0.9% Sodium Chloride; 10% Invert Sugar in Water; *Normosol M* in 5% Dextrose.

Ceftazidime is less stable in Sodium Bicarbonate Injection than in other IV fluids. It is not recommended as a diluent. Solutions in 5% Dextrose and 0.9% Sodium Chloride Injection are stable for at least 6 hours at room temperature in plastic tubing, drip chambers and volume control devices of common IV infusion sets.

Ceftazidime at a concentration of 4 mg/ml is compatible for 18 to 24 hours at room temperature or 7 to 10 days under refrigeration in 0.9% Sodium Chloride Injection or 5% Dextrose Injection when admixed with: Cefuroxime 3 mg/ml; heparin 10 or 50 units/ml; or potassium chloride 10 or 40 mEq/L.

Admixtures – Do not add aminoglycoside antibiotics to ceftazidime. Give separately.

CEFTAZIDIME

Rx	**Ceptaz** (Glaxo Wellcome)	**Powder for Injection:**[1] 349 mg/g	In 500 mg, 1 g and 2 g vials, 1 and 2 g infusions and 10 g.
Rx	**Fortaz** (Glaxo Wellcome)	**Powder for Injection:**[2] 500 mg	In vials.
Rx	**Tazidime** (Lilly)		In 10 ml vials.
Rx	**Fortaz** (Glaxo Wellcome)	**Powder for Injection:**[2] 1 g	In vials and infusion packs.
Rx	**Tazicef** (SK-Beecham)		In vials and Piggyback vials.
Rx	**Pentacef** (SK-Beecham)		In vials and piggyback vials.
Rx	**Tazidime** (Lilly)		In 20 and 100 ml vials.
Rx	**Fortaz** (Glaxo Wellcome)	**Powder for Injection**[2]: 2 g	In vials and infusion packs.
Rx	**Pentacef** (SK-Beecham)		In vials and Piggyback vials
Rx	**Tazicef** (SK-Beecham)		In vials and Piggyback vials.
Rx	**Tazidime** (Lilly)		In 50 and 100 ml vials.
Rx	**Fortaz** (Glaxo Wellcome)	**Powder for Injection:**[2] 6 g	In bulk package.[2]
Rx	**Pentacef** (SK-Beecham)		In pharmacy bulk vials.
Rx	**Tazicef** (SK-Beecham)		In bulk package.
Rx	**Tazidime** (Lilly)		In 100 ml vial.
Rx	**Ceptaz** (Glaxo Wellcome)	**Powder for Injection:** 500 mg	In 1 and 2 g vials, 1 and 2 g infusions and 10 g bulk packages.
Rx	**Fortaz** (Glaxo Wellcome)	**Injection:** 1 g	Premixed, frozen. In 50 ml.[3]
		2 g	Premixed, frozen. In 50 ml.[4]

[1] As pentahydrate with L-arginine.
[2] Contains 2.3 mEq sodium/g.
[3] With 2.2 g dextrose hydrous.
[4] With 1.6 g dextrose hydrous.

MEROPENEM

Actions:

Pharmacology: Meropenem is a broad-spectrum carbapenem antibiotic. The bactericidal activity of meropenem results from the inhibition of cell-wall synthesis. Meropenem readily penetrates the cell wall of most gram-positive and gram-negative bacteria to reach penicillin-binding-protein (PBP) targets.

Pharmacokinetics: Meropenem has dose-dependent kinetics. At the end of a 30-minute IV infusion of a single dose of meropenem in normal volunteers, mean peak plasma concentrations are ≈ 23 mcg/ml (range: 14 to 26 mcg/ml) for the 500 mg dose and 49 mcg/ml (range: 39 to 68 mcg/ml) for the 1 g dose. A 5-minute IV bolus injection of meropenem in normal volunteers results in mean peak plasma concentrations of ≈ 45 mcg/ml (range: 18 to 65 mcg/ml) for the 500 mg dose and 112 mcg/ml (range: 83 to 140 mcg/ml) for the 1 g dose.

Following IV doses of 500 mg, mean plasma concentrations of meropenem usually decline to ≈ 1 mcg/ml at 6 hours after administration.

In subjects with normal renal function, the elimination half-life of meropenem is ≈ 1 hour. Meropenem is excreted by the kidney with a half-life of 0.8 to 1.24 hours; 65% to 83% of the dose is recovered in the urine as meropenem and 20% to 28% as the inactive open β-lactam metabolite. Urinary concentrations of meropenem > 10 mcg/ml are maintained for ≤ 5 hours after a 500 mg dose. No meropenem accumulation in plasma or urine was observed with regimens using 500 mg administered every 8 hours or 1 g administered every 6 hours in volunteers with normal renal function.

Plasma protein binding of meropenem is ≈ 2%. There is one metabolite that is microbiologically inactive. The volume of meropenem distribution is 15.7 to 26.68 L. Meropenem penetrates well into most body fluids and tissues, including cerebrospinal fluid, achieving concentrations matching or exceeding those required to inhibit most susceptible bacteria. After a single IV dose of meropenem, the highest mean meropenem concentrations were found in tissues and fluids at 1 hour (0.5 to 1.5 hours) after the start of infusion, except where indicated in the tissues and fluids listed in the table below.

Meropenem Concentrations in Selected Tissues (Highest Concentrations Reported)

Tissue	IV dose (g)	Mean [mcg/ml or mcg/g][1]	Range [mcg/ml or mcg/g]
Endometrium	0.5	4.2	1.7-10.2
Myometrium	0.5	3.8	0.4-8.1
Ovary	0.5	2.8	0.8-4.8
Cervix	0.5	7	5.4-8.5
Fallopian tube	0.5	1.7	0.3-3.4
Skin	0.5, 1	3.3, 5.3	0.5-12.6, 1.3-16.7
Colon	1	2.6	2.5-2.7
Bile	1	14.6 (3 h)	4-25.7
Gall bladder	1	-	3.9
Interstitial fluid	1	26.3	20.9-37.4
Peritoneal fluid	1	30.2	7.4-54.6
Lung	1	4.8 (2 h)	1.4-8.2
Bronchial mucosa	1	4.5	1.3-11.1
Muscle	1	6.1 (2 h)	5.3-6.9
Fascia	1	8.8	1.5-20
Heart valves	1	9.7	6.4-12.1
Myocardium	1	15.5	5.2-25.5
CSF (inflamed)	20 mg/kg[2]	1.1 (2 h)	0.2-2.8
	40 mg/kg[3]	3.3 (3 h)	0.9-6.5
CSF (uninflamed)	1	0.2 (2 h)	0.1-0.3

[1] At 1 hour unless otherwise noted.
[2] In pediatric patients 5 months to 8 years of age.
[3] In pediatric patients 1 month to 15 years of age.

The pharmacokinetics of meropenem in pediatric patients ≥ 2 years of age are essentially similar to those in adults. In children 6 months to 12 years of age, meropenem 10 mg/kg IV produced a mean peak concentration of 28.7 mg/L, and 20 mg/kg IV produced a mean peak concentration of 60.2 mg/L. The half-life was 1 to 1.11 hours and volume of distribution was 0.4 to 0.5 L/kg. Urinary recovery of meropenem averaged 65% of the administered dose. Compared with adults, volume of distribution and clearance were increased, while half-life and amount eliminated unchanged in the urine were similar. In infants and children ages 2 months to

12 years administered meropenem 10 to 40 mg/kg in a pharmacokinetic study, no age- or dose-dependent effects on pharmacokinetic parameters were observed. Mean half-life was 1.13 hours, mean volume of distribution at steady-state was 0.43 L/kg, mean residence time was 1.57 hours, clearance was 5.63 ml/min/kg and renal clearance was 2.53 ml/min/kg. Approximately 55% of the administered dose was recovered in the urine unchanged 12 hours after administration. The elimination half-life is slightly prolonged (1.5 hours) in pediatric patients 3 months to 2 years of age.

Pharmacokinetic studies with meropenem in patients with renal insufficiency have shown that the plasma clearance of meropenem correlates with creatinine clearance. In patients with moderate renal dysfunction (Ccr 30 to 80 ml/min), mean half-life has been prolonged to 1.93 to 3.36 hours. In patients with greater dysfunction (Ccr 2 to 30 mg/min), mean half-life has been further prolonged to 3.82 to 5.73 hours. Patients undergoing hemodialysis (patients with end-stage renal disease) had mean predialysis half-lives of 7 to 10 hours. Hemodialysis shortened elimination half-life to 1.4 to 2.9 hours during the dialysis period. Dosage adjustments are necessary in subjects with renal impairment (see Adminstration and Dosage). A pharmacokinetic study with meropenem in elderly patients with renal insufficiency has shown a reduction in plasma clearance of meropenem that correlates with age-associated reduction in creatinine clearance. The mean terminal half-life is prolonged slightly to 1.27 hours. A pharmacokinetic study with meropenem in patients with hepatic impairment has shown that there are no effects of liver disease on the pharmacokinetics of meropenem.

Microbiology: Its strongest affinities are toward PBP 2, 3 and 4 of *Escherichia coli* and *Pseudomonas aeruginosa*; and PBPs 1, 2 and 4 of *Staphylococcus aureus*. Bactericidal concentrations (defined as a 3 $\log_{10}$ reduction in cell counts within 12 to 24 hours) are typically 1 to 2 times the bacteriostatic concentrations of meropenem, with the exception of *Listeria monocytogenes*, against which lethal activity is not observed.

Meropenem has significant stability to hydrolysis by β-lactamases of most categories, both penicillinases and cephalosporinases produced by gram-positive and gram-negative bacteria, with the exception of matallo-β-lactamases. Do not use to treat methicillin-resistant staphylococci. Cross resistance is sometimes observed with strains resistant to other carbapenems. In vitro tests show meropenem to act synergistically with aminoglycoside antibiotics against some isolates of *P. aeruginosa*.

Meropenem has been shown to be active against most strains of the following microorganisms, both in vitro and in clinical infections as described in the Indications section.

Gram-positive aerobes – Streptococcus pneumoniae (excluding penicillin-resistant strains); Viridans group streptococci. Note: Penicillin-resistant strains had meropenem MIC_{90} values of 1 or 2 mcg/ml; this value is above the 0.12 mcg/ml susceptible breakpoint for this species.

Gram-negative aerobes – E. coli; Haemophilus influenzae (β-lactamase and non-β-lactamase-producing); *Klebsiella pneumoniae; Neisseria meningitidis; P. aeruginosa.*

Anaerobes – Bacteroides fragilis; B. thetaiotaomicron; Peptostreptococcus sp.

The following in vitro data are available, but their clinical significance is unknown.

Meropenem exhibits in vitro minimum inhibitory concentrations (MICs) of 0.12 mcg/ml against most (≥ 90%) strains of *S. pneumoniae*, ≤ 0.5 mcg/ml against most (≥ 90%) strains of *H. influenzae* and ≤ 4 mcg/ml against most (≥ 90%) strains of the other microorganisms in the following list; however, the safety and effectiveness of meropenem in treating clinical infections due to these microorganisms have not been established in adequate and well controlled clinical trials.

Gram-positive aerobes – S. aureus (β-lactamase and non-β-lactamase producing); *S. epidermidis* (β-lactamase and non-β-lactamase producing). Note: Staphylococci that are resistant to methicillin/oxacillin must be considered resistant to meropenem.

Gram-negative aerobes – Acinetobacter sp; *Aeromonas hydrophila; Campylobacter jejuni; Citrobacter diversus; Citrobacter freundii; Enterobacter cloacae; H. influenzae* (ampicillin-restant, non-β-lactamase producing strains [BLNAR strains]); *Hafnia alvei; K. oxytoca; Moraxella catarrhalis* (β-lactamase and non-β-lactamase producing strains); *Morganella morganii; Pasteurelia multocida; Proteus mirabilis; P. vulgaris; Salmonella* sp; *Serratia marcescens; Shigella* sp; *Yersinia enterocolitica*

Anaerobes – Bacteroides distasonis; B. ovatus; B. uniformis; B. ureolyticus; B. vulgatus; Clostridium difficile; C. perfringens; Eubacterium lentum; Fusobacterium sp; *Prevotella bivia; Prevotella intermedia; Prevotella melaninogenica; Prophyromonas asaccharolytica; Propionibacterium acnes.*

Clinical trials:

Intra-abdominal infection – Meropenem was compared with imipenem/cilastatin in the treatment of intra-abdominal infection requiring surgery. Patients with diffuse or local peritonitis of moderate severity, complicated in most cases by gangrenous appendicitis, stomach perforation or gallbladder disease, were treated with either meropenem or imipenem/cilastatin. Both agents were administered IV at a dosage of 1 g every 8 hours. Therapy was continued for a mean of 7.7 days in the meropenem group and 8.6 days in the imipenem/cilastatin group. Surgical excision and drainage was performed on the first day of therapy or before the start of this antibiotic regimen. Therapy was judged successful in all patients evaluated in both groups. No cases of post-operative wound infection or superinfection at other sites were observed.

Meningitis – Meropenem 40 mg/kg every 8 hours was compared with cefotaxime 75 to 100 mg/kg every 8 hours in 190 children aged 3 months to 14 years with bacterial meningitis. Concurrent dexamethasone was administered to 185 patients. Among patients with no preexisting neurological abnormalities prior to antimicrobial therapy, cure without audiological or neurological sequelae occurred in 79% of meropenem-treated patients and 83% of cefotaxime-treated patients. Among patients with preexisting neurological abnormalities, cure without audiological or neurological sequelae occurred in 47% of the meropenem-treated patients and 60% of the cefotaxime-treated patients. At the end of therapy, among patients without middle ear effusion, hearing impairment was evident in 33% of meropenem-treated patients and 28% of cefotaxime-treated patients. The severity of impairment was similar in the two groups. Bacterial eradication among patients with culture proven meningitis was 100% in both groups.

Indications:

For the treatment of the following infections when caused by susceptible strains of the designated microorganisms:

Intra-abdominal infections: Complicated appendicitis and peritonitis caused by viridans group streptococci, *E. coli, K. pneumoniae, P. aeruginosa, B. fragilis, B. thetaiotaomicron* and *Peptostreptococcus* sp.

Bacterial meningitis (pediatric patients ≥ 3 months only): Bacterial meningitis caused by *S. pneumoniae, H. influenzae* (β- lactamase and non-β-lactamase-producing strains) and *N. meningitidis.*

Contraindications:

Hypersensitivity to any component of this product or to other drugs in the same class or in patients who have demonstrated anaphylactic reactions to β-lactams.

Warnings:

Pseudomembranous colitis has been reported with nearly all antibacterial agents, including meropenem and may range in severity from mild to life-threatening. Therefore, it is important to consider this diagnosis in patients who develop diarrhea subsequent to the administration of antibacterial agents.

After the diagnosis of pseudomembranous colitis has been established, initiate appropriate therapeutic measures. Mild cases of pseudomembranous colitis usually respond to drug discontinuation alone. In moderate-to-severe cases, give consideration to management with fluids and electrolytes, protein supplementation and treatment with an antibacterial drug clinically effective against *C. difficile* colitis.

Hypersensitivity: Serious and occasionally fatal hypersensitivity (anaphylactic) reactions have been reported in patients receiving therapy with β-lactams. These reactions are more likely to occur in individuals with a history of sensitivity to multiple allergens.

There have been reports of individuals with a history of penicillin hypersensitivity who have experienced severe hypersensitivity reactions when treated with other β-lactams. If an allergic reaction to meropenem occurs, discontinue the drug immediately. Serious anaphylactic reactions require immediate emergency treatment with epinephrine, oxygen, intravenous steroids and airway management, including intubation. Other therapy may also be administered as indicated. Refer to Management of Acute Hypersensitivity Reactions.

Renal function impairment: In patients with renal dysfunction, thrombocytopenia has been observed but no clinical bleeding was reported. (See Administration and Dosage.)

Pregnancy: Category B. Reproductive studies have been performed with meropenem in rats at doses of ≤ 1000 mg/kg/day, and cynomolgus monkeys at doses of ≤ 360 mg/kg/day. These studies revealed no evidence of impaired fertility or harm to the fetus because of meropenem, although there were slight changes in body weight. However, there are no adequate and well controlled studies in pregnant women. Because animal reproduction studies are not always predictive of human response, use this drug during pregnancy only if clearly needed.

Lactation: It is not known whether this drug is excreted in breast milk. Because many drugs are excreted in breast milk, use caution when administering to a nursing woman.

Children: The safety and efficacy of meropenem have not been established for children < 3 months of age (see Administration and Dosage).

Precautions:

Monitoring: While meropenem possesses the characteristic low toxicity of the β-lactam group of antibiotics, periodic assessment of organ system functions, including renal, hepatic and hematopoietic is advisable during prolonged therapy.

Seizures and other CNS adverse experiences have been reported during treatment with meropenem. These adverse experiences have occurred most commonly in patients with CNS disorders (eg, brain lesions or history of seizures) or with bacterial meningitis or compromised renal function.

Superinfection: As with other broad-spectrum antibiotics, prolonged use of meropenem may result in overgrowth of nonsusceptible organisms. Repeated evaluation of the patient is essential. If superinfection does occur during therapy, take appropriate measures.

Drug Interactions:

Probenicid competes with meropenem for active tubular secretion and thus inhibits the renal excretion of meropenem. This led to statistically significant increases in the elimination half-life (38%) and in the extent of systemic exposure (56%). Therefore, the coadministration of probenecid with meropenem is not recommended.

Adverse Reactions:

Local: Inflammation at the injection site (3%); phlebitis/thrombophlebitis (1.2%); injection site reaction (1.1%); pain at the injection site (0.4%); edema at the injection site (0.2%).

Systemic: Diarrhea (5%); nausea, vomiting (3.9%); headache (2.8%); rash (1.7%); pruritus (1.6%); apnea (1.2%); constipation (1.2%); bleeding events (GI hemorrhage, melena, epistaxis, hemoperitoneum) (0.7%).

Body as a whole: Pain, abdominal pain, chest pain, sepsis, shock, fever, abdominal enlargement, back pain, hepatic failure (< 1%).

Cardiovascular: Heart failure, heart arrest, tachycardia, hypertension, myocardial infarction, pulmonary embolus, bradycardia, hypotension, syncope (< 1%).

CNS: Insomnia, agitation/delirium, confusion, dizziness, nervousness, paresthesia, hallucinations, somnolence, anxiety, depression (< 1%); seizures (0.5%).

Dermatologic: Urticaria, sweating (< 1%).

GI: Oral moniliasis, anorexia, cholestatic jaundice/jaundice, flatulence, ileus (<1%).

GU: Dysuria, kidney failure, presence of urine red blood cells (< 1%).

Hematologic: Increased platelets, increased eosinophils, prolonged prothrombin time, prolonged partial thromboplastin time, decreased platelets, positive direct or indirect Coombs test, decreased hemoglobin, decreased hematocrit, decreased WBC, shortened prothrombin time, shortened partial thromboplastin time, anemia (< 1%).

Hepatic: Increased ALT, AST, alkaline phosphatase, LDH and bilirubin (< 1%).

Metabolic/Nutritional: Peripheral edema, hypoxia (< 1%).

Renal: Increased creatinine and BUN (< 1%).

Respiratory: Respiratory disorder, dyspnea (< 1%).

Children:

Bacterial infection – Diarrhea (4.3%); rash (1.4%); vomiting (1%).

Meningitis – Rash (mostly diaper area moniliasis), diarrhea (3.5%); oral moniliasis (2%); glossitis (1%).

Laboratory abnormalities seen in pediatric-aged patients are similar to those reported in adult patients.

Overdosage:

Overdosing might occur if large doses are given to patients with reduced renal function. The largest dose of meropenem administered in clinical trials has been 2 g given IV every 8 hours. At this dosage, no adverse pharmacological effects or increased safety risks have been observed. In the event of an overdose, discontinue meropenem and give general supportive treatment until renal elimination takes place. Meropenem and its metabolite are readily dialyzable and effectively removed by hemodialysis.

Administration and Dosage:

Approved June 2, 1996.

Adults: 1 g by IV administration every 8 hours. Give over ≈ 15 to 30 minutes or as an IV bolus injection (5 to 20 ml) over ≈ 3 to 5 minutes.

MEROPENEM

Renal function impairment: Reduce dosage in patients with creatinine clearance < 50 ml/min.

Recommended Meropenem IV Dosage Schedule for Adults with Impaired Renal Function		
Creatinine clearance (ml/min)	Dose (dependent on type of infection)	Dosing interval
26 to 50	recommended dose (1000 mg)	every 12 hours
10 to 25	one-half recommended dose	every 12 hours
< 10	one-half recommended dose	every 24 hours

When only serum creatinine is available, the following formula (Cockcroft and Gault equation) may be used to estimate creatinine clearance.

$$\text{Males: } \frac{\text{Weight (kg)} \times (140 - \text{age})}{72 \times \text{serum creatinine (mg/dl)}} = \text{Ccr}$$

$$\text{Females: } 0.85 \times \text{above value}$$

Use in pediatric patients: For pediatric patients from ≥ 3 months of age, the meropenem dose is 20 or 40 mg/kg every 8 hours (maximum dose is 2 g every 8 hours), depending on the type of infection (intra-abdominal or meningitis). Administer pediatric patients weighing > 50 kg 1 g every 8 hours for intra-abdominal infections and 2 g every 8 hours for meningitis. Give over ≈ 15 to 30 minutes or as an IV bolus injection (5 to 20 ml) over ≈ 3 to 5 minutes.

Recommended Meropenem IV Dosage Schedule for Pediatrics with Normal Renal Function		
Type of infection	Dose (mg/kg)	Dosing interval
Intra-abdominal	20	every 8 hours
Meningitis	40	every 8 hours

Admixture compatibility/stability: Do not mix with solutions containing other drugs.

Stability of Solutions of Meropenem for Infusion		
Solution	Number of hours stable at controlled room temperature 15° to 25°C (59° to 77°F)	Number of hours stable at 4°C (39°F)
0.9% Sodium Chloride Injection	4	24
5% Dextrose Injection	1	4
10% Dextrose Injection	1	2
5% Dextrose and 0.9% Sodium Chloride Injection	1	2
5% Dextrose and 0.2% Sodium Chloride Injection	1	4
0.15% Potassium Chloride in 5% Dextrose Injection	1	6
0.02% Sodium Bicarbonate in 5% Dextrose Injection	1	6
5% Dextrose Injection in *Normosol-M*	1	8
5% Dextrose Injection in Ringers Lactate Injection	1	4
2.5% Dextrose and 0.45% Sodium Chloride Injection	3	12
2.5% Mannitol Injection	2	16
Ringers Injection	4	24
Ringers Lactate Injection	4	12
Sodium Lactate Injection 1/6 N	2	24
5% Sodium Bicarbonate Injection	1	4
Sterile Water for Injection	2	12

Storage: Store at controlled room temperature 20° to 25°C (68° to 77°F).

Rx	**Merrem IV** (Zeneca)	**Powder for Injection:** 500 mg	In 20 and 100 ml vials and 15 ml *ADD-Vantage* vials.
		1 g	In 30 and 100 ml vials and 15 ml *ADD-Vantage* vials.

IMIPENEM-CILASTATIN

Actions:

Pharmacology: This product is a formulation of imipenem, a thienamycin antibiotic, and cilastatin sodium, the inhibitor of the renal dipeptidase, dehydropeptidase 1, which is responsible for the extensive metabolism of imipenem when it is administered alone. Cilastatin, by inhibiting this dipeptidase, prevents the metabolism of imipenem, thereby increasing urinary recovery and decreasing possible renal toxicity. The bactericidal activity of imipenem results from the inhibition of cell wall synthesis, related to binding to penicillin binding proteins (PBP) 1A, 1B, 2, 4, 5 and 6 of *Escherichia coli* and 1A, 1B, 2, 4 and 5 of *Pseudomonas aeruginosa*. The lethal effect is related to binding to PBP 2 and PBP 1B.

Pharmacokinetics:

Absorption/Distribution –

IV infusion over 20 minutes results in peak plasma levels of imipenem antimicrobial activity that range from 14 to 24 mcg/ml for the 250 mg dose, from 21 to 58 mcg/ml for the 500 mg dose and from 41 to 83 mcg/ml for the 1 g dose. Plasma levels declined to ≤ 1 mcg/ml in 4 to 6 hours. Peak plasma levels of cilastatin following a 20 minute IV infusion range from 15 to 25 mcg/ml for the 250 mg dose, from 31 to 49 mcg/ml for the 500 mg dose and from 56 to 88 mcg/ml for the 1 g dose.

The plasma half-life of each component is ≈ 1 hour. Urine imipenem concentrations > 10 mcg/ml can be maintained for up to 8 hours at the 500 mg dose.

After a 1 g dose, the following average levels (mcg/ml or mcg/g) of imipenem were measured (usually 1 hour post-dose except where indicated) in the following tissues and fluids: Peritoneal 23.9 (2 hours); pleural 22; interstitial 16.4; fallopian tubes 13.6; endometrium 11.1; lung 5.6; bile 5.3 (2.25 hours); myometrium 5; skin 4.4; fascia 4.4; vitreous humor 3.4 (3.5 hours); aqueous humor 2.99 (2 hours); CSF (inflamed) 2.6 (2 hours); bone 2.6; sputum 2.1; CSF (uninflamed) 1 (4 hours).

IM: Following IM administration of 500 or 750 mg doses, peak plasma levels of imipenem antimicrobial activity occur within 2 hours and average 10 and 12 mcg/ml, respectively. For cilastatin, peak plasma levels average 24 and 33 mcg/ml, respectively, and occur within 1 hour. When compared to IV administration, imipenem is ≈ 75% bioavailable following IM administration while cilastatin is ≈ 95% bioavailable. The absorption of imipenem from the IM injection site continues for 6 to 8 hours while that for cilastatin is essentially complete within 4 hours. This prolonged absorption of imipenem following IM use results in an effective plasma half-life of ≈ 2 to 3 hours and plasma levels which remain above 2 mcg/ml for at least 6 or 8 hours following a 500 or 750 mg dose, respectively. This plasma profile for imipenem permits IM administration every 12 hours with no accumulation of cilastatin and only slight accumulation of imipenem.

Plasma Concentrations of Imipenem, IV vs IM (mcg/ml)

	500 mg dose		750 mg dose	
Time	IV	IM	IV	IM
25 min	45.1	6	57	6.7
1 hr	21.6	9.4	28.1	10
2 hr	10	9.9	12	11.4
4 hr	2.6	5.6	3.4	7.3
6 hr	0.6	2.5	1.1	3.8
12 hr	nd[1]	0.5	nd[1]	0.8

[1] nd = Not detectable (< 0.3 mcg/ml).

Imipenem urine levels remain above 10 mcg/ml for the 12 hour dosing interval following IM administration of 500 or 750 mg doses. Total urinary excretion of imipenem and cilastatin averages 50% and 75%, respectively, following either dose.

Metabolism/Excretion – Imipenem, when administered alone, is metabolized in the kidneys by dehydropeptidase 1 resulting in relatively low levels in urine. Cilastatin, an inhibitor of this enzyme, prevents renal metabolism of imipenem. The protein binding of imipenem and cilastatin is ≈ 20% and 40%, respectively. Within 10 hours of administration, ≈ 70% of imipenem and cilastatin is recovered in urine.

Microbiology: Imipenem has in vitro activity against a wide range of gram-positive and gram-negative organisms. It has a high degree of stability in the presence of β–lactamases, including penicillinases and cephalosporinases produced by gram-negative and gram-positive bacteria. It is a potent inhibitor of β–lactamases from certain gram-negative bacteria resistant to many β–lactam antibiotics (eg, *Pseudomonas aeruginosa, Serratia* sp, *Enterobacter* sp).

In vitro, imipenem is active against most strains of clinical isolates in the following microorganisms: Gram-positive aerobes; streptococcus; gram-negative aerobes; gram-positive anaerobes; gram-negative anaerobes.

In vitro tests show imipenem to act synergistically with aminoglycoside antibiotics against some isolates of *Pseudomonas aeruginosa.*

Indications:

IV: Treatment of serious infections caused by susceptible strains of the designated microorganisms in the diseases listed below:

Lower respiratory tract infections – Staphylococcus aureus (penicillinase-producing), *Escherichia coli, Klebsiella* sp, *Enterobacter* sp, *Haemophilus influenzae, Haemophilus parainfluenzae, Acinetobacter* sp, *Serratia marcescens.*

Urinary tract infections (complicated and uncomplicated) – Enterococus faecalis, S. aureus (penicillinase-producing), *E. coli, Klebsiella* sp, *Enterobacter* sp, *Proteus vulgaris, Providencia rettgeri, M. morganii, P. aeruginosa.*

Intra-abdominal infections – E. faecalis, S. aureus (penicillinase-producing), *Staphylococcus epidermidis, E. coli, Klebsiella* sp, *Enterobacter* sp, *Proteus* sp (indole-positive and indole-negative), *Morganella morganii, P. aeruginosa, Citrobacter* sp, *Clostridium* sp, *Bacteroides* sp including *B. fragilis, Fusobacterium* sp; gram-positive anaerobes including *Peptococcus* sp, *Peptostreptococcus* sp, *Eubacterium* sp, *Propionibacterium* sp, *Bifidobacterium* sp.

Gynecologic infections – E. faecalis; S. aureus (penicillinase-producing), *S. epidermidis, Streptococcus agalactiae* (group B streptococcus), *E. coli, Klebsiella* sp, *Proteus* sp (indole-positive and indole-negative), *Enterobacter* sp, *Bifidobacterium* sp, *Bacteroides* sp including *B. fragilis, Gardnerella vaginalis*; gram-positive anaerobes including *Peptococcus* sp, *Peptostreptococcus* sp, *Propionibacterium* sp.

Bacterial septicemia – E. faecalis, S. aureus (penicillinase-producing), *E. coli, Klebsiella* sp, *P. aeruginosa, Serratia* sp, *Enterobacter* sp, *Bacteroides* sp including *B. fragilis.*

Bone and joint infections – E. faecalis; S. aureus (penicillinase-producing), *S. epidermidis, Enterobacter* sp, *P. aeruginosa.*

Skin and skin structure infections – E. faecalis, S. aureus (penicillinase-producing), *S. epidermidis, E. coli, Klebsiella* sp, *Enterobacter* sp, *P. vulgaris, P. rettgeri, M. morganii, P. aeruginosa, Serratia* sp, *Citrobacter* sp, *Acinetobacter* sp, *Bacteroides* sp including *B. fragilis, Fusobacterium* sp; gram-positive anaerobes including *Peptococcus* sp and *Peptostreptococcus* sp.

Endocarditis – S. aureus (penicillinase-producing).

Polymicrobic infections, including those in which *S. pneumoniae* (pneumonia, septicemia), group A β–hemolytic streptococcus (skin and skin structure) or nonpenicillinase-producing *S. aureus* is one of the causative organisms. However, these monobacterial infections are usually treated with narrower spectrum antibiotics (eg, penicillin). Although clinical improvement has been observed in patients with cystic fibrosis, chronic pulmonary disease and lower respiratory tract infections caused by *P. aeruginosa,* bacterial eradication may not be achieved.

IM: Treatment of serious infections of mild to moderate severity where IM therapy is appropriate. Not intended for severe or life-threatening infections, including bacterial sepsis or endocarditis, or in instances of major physiological impairments (eg, shock).

Lower respiratory tract infections, including pneumonia and bronchitis as an exacerbation of COPD, caused by *S. pneumoniae* and *H. influenzae.*

Intra-abdominal infections, including acute gangrenous or perforated appendicitis and appendicitis with peritonitis, caused by group D streptococcus including *E. faecalis; Streptococcus viridans* group; *E. coli; Klebsiella pneumoniae; P. aeruginosa; Bacteroides* sp including *B. fragilis, B. distasonis, B. intermedius* and *B. thetaiotaomicron; Fusobacterium* sp; *Peptostreptococcus* sp.

Skin and skin structure infections, including abscesses, cellulitis, infected skin ulcers and wound infections caused by *S. aureus* (including penicillinase-producing strains); *Streptococcus pyogenes;* group D streptococcus including *E. faecalis; Acinetobacter* sp including *A. calcoaceticus; Citrobacter* sp; *E. coli; Enterobacter cloacae; K. pneumoniae; P. aeruginosa; Bacteroides* sp including *B. fragilis.*

Gynecologic infections, including postpartum endomyometritis, caused by group D streptococcus including *E. faecalis; E. coli; K. pneumoniae; B. intermedius; Peptostreptococcus* sp.

As with other β–lactam antibiotics, some strains of *P. aeruginosa* may develop resistance fairly rapidly; periodically perform appropriate susceptibility testing.

Infections resistant to other antibiotics (eg, cephalosporins, penicillins, aminoglycosides) have responded to treatment with imipenem.

Contraindications:

Hypersensitivity to any component of this product.

IM: Hypersensitivity to local anesthetics of the amide type and in patients with severe shock or heart block due to the use of lidocaine HCl diluent.

IMIPENEM-CILASTATIN

Warnings:

Resistance: As with other β-lactam antibiotics, some strains of *Pseudomonas aeruginosa* may develop resistance fairly rapidly during treatment with imipenem-cilastatin. During therapy of *P. aeruginosa* infections, perform periodic susceptibility testing when clinically appropriate.

Pseudomembranous colitis has occurred with virtually all antibiotics. Consider its diagnosis in patients developing diarrhea while on antibiotics. Severity ranges from mild to life-threatening. Mild cases may respond to drug discontinuation. More severe cases may require sigmoidoscopy, appropriate bacteriological studies, fluid, electrolyte and protein supplementation and a drug such as oral vancomycin, as indicated. Isolating the patient may be advisable. Consider other causes of colitis.

Hypersensitivity: Serious and occasionally fatal hypersensitivity (anaphylactic) reactions have occurred in patients receiving therapy with β-lactams. They are more apt to occur in persons with a history of sensitivity to multiple allergens. Patients with a history of penicillin hypersensitivity have experienced severe reactions when treated with another β-lactam. If a reaction occurs, discontinue the drug. Serious reactions require immediate emergency measures. See Management of Acute Hypersensitivity Reactions.

Renal function impairment: Do not give imipenem-cilastatin IV to patients with creatinine clearance (Ccr) of $\leq$ 5 ml/min/1.73 m^2, unless hemodialysis is instituted within 48 hours. For patients on hemodialysis, imipenem-cilastatin IV is recommended only when the benefit outweighs the potential risk of seizures.

Pregnancy: Category C. There are no adequate and well controlled studies in pregnant women. Use only when potential benefits outweigh potential hazards.

Lactation: It is not known whether this drug is excreted in breast milk. Exercise caution when administering to a nursing woman.

Children: Safety and efficacy in children < 12 years old have not been established.

Precautions:

Monitoring: While imipenem has the characteristic low toxicity of the β-lactam group of antibiotics, periodically assess organ system functions, including renal, hepatic and hematopoietic, during prolonged therapy.

CNS adverse experiences (eg, myoclonic activity, confusional states, seizures) have occurred with the IV formulation, especially when recommended dosages were exceeded. They are most common in patients with CNS disorders (eg, brain lesions, history of seizures) who also have compromised renal function and are rare when no underlying CNS disorder exists. Closely adhere to recommended dosage schedules, especially in patients with known factors that predispose to convulsive activity. Continue anticonvulsants in patients with a known seizure disorder. If focal tremors, myoclonus or seizures occur, neurologically evaluate patient and institute anticonvulsants. Re-examine the dosage and determine whether to decrease dosage or discontinue the drug. If these effects occur with the IM formulation, discontinue the drug.

Cross-allergenicity: Individuals with a history of penicillin sensitivity may experience cross-sensitivity to imipenem-cilastatin. Use caution when administering to patients with a history of penicillin allergy.

Superinfection: Use of antibiotics (especially prolonged or repeated therapy) may result in bacterial or fungal overgrowth of nonsusceptible organisms. Such overgrowth may lead to secondary infection. Take appropriate measures if superinfection occurs.

Drug Interactions:

Ganciclovir: Generalized seizures have occurred in patients receiving concomitant imipenem-cilastatin IV and ganciclovir. Do not use concomitantly.

Probenecid: Probenecid and concurrent imipenem-cilastatin results in only minimal increases in imipenem plasma levels and half-life; therefore, it is not recommended that probenecid be given concurrently.

Adverse Reactions:

IV:

Lab test abnormalities –

Hepatic: Increased AST, ALT, alkaline phosphatase, bilirubin and LDH.

Hemic: Increased eosinophils, monocytes, lymphocytes, basophils; decreased neutrophils (including agranulocytosis), hemoglobin, hematocrit; increased/decreased WBCs and platelets; positive Coombs' test; abnormal prothrombin time.

Electrolytes: Decreased serum sodium; increased potassium and chloride.

Renal: Increased BUN and creatinine.

Urinalysis: Presence of protein, RBCs, WBCs, casts, bilirubin or urobilinogen in the urine.

Local – Phlebitis/thrombophlebitis (3.1%); pain at the injection site (0.7%); erythema at the injection site (0.4%); vein induration (0.2%); infused vein infection (0.1%).

Cardiovascular – Hypotension (0.4%); palpitations, tachycardia (< 0.2%).

CNS – Fever (0.5%); seizures (0.4%); dizziness (0.3%); somnolence (0.2%); encephalopathy, tremor, confusion, myoclonus, paresthesia, vertigo, headache, psychic disturbances including hallucinations (< 0.2%).

Dermatologic – Rash (0.9%); pruritus (0.3%); urticaria (0.2%); erythema multiforme, Stevens-Johnson syndrome, angioneurotic edema, toxic epidermal necrolysis, facial edema, flushing, cyanosis, skin texture changes, candidiasis, hyperhidrosis, pruritus vulvae (< 0.2%).

GI – Nausea (2%); diarrhea (1.8%); vomiting (1.5%); pseudomembranous colitis, hemorrhagic colitis, hepatitis, jaundice, staining of the teeth, gastroenteritis, abdominal pain, glossitis, tongue papillar hypertrophy, heartburn, pharyngeal pain, increased salivation (< 0.2%).

Hematologic – Pancytopenia, bone marrow depression, thrombocytopenia, neutropenia, leukopenia, hemolytic anemia (< 0.2%).

Respiratory – Chest discomfort, dyspnea, hyperventilation, thoracic spine pain (< 0.2%).

Miscellaneous – Transient hearing loss, tinnitus, polyarthralgia, taste perversion, asthenia/weakness, oliguria/anuria, polyuria, acute renal failure, urine discoloration (< 0.2%).

IM:

Lab test abnormalities

Hemic: Decreased hemoglobin and hematocrit; eosinophilia; increased/decreased WBCs and platelets; decreased erythrocytes; increased prothrombin time.

Hepatic: Increased AST, ALT, alkaline phosphatase and bilirubin.

Renal: Increased BUN and creatinine.

Urinalysis: Presence of RBCs, WBCs, casts and bacteria in the urine.

Local – Pain at the injection site (1.2%).

Systemic – Nausea, diarrhea (0.6%); vomiting (0.3%); rash (0.4%).

Overdosage:

In the case of overdosage, discontinue the drug. Treat symptomatically and institute supportive measures as required. Refer to General Management of Acute Overdosage. Imipenem-cilastatin is hemodialyzable; however, usefulness of this procedure in the overdosage setting is questionable.

Administration and Dosage:

Dosage recommendations represent the quantity of imipenem to be administered. An equivalent amount of cilastatin is also present in the solution.

Base the initial dosage on the type or severity of infection and administer in equally divided doses. Base subsequent dosing on severity of illness, degree of susceptibility of the pathogen(s), weight and creatinine clearance.

Renal function impairment: Patients with creatinine clearance (Ccr) of < 20 ml/min/1.73 m^2 for IM and ≤ 70 ml/min/1.73 m^2 for IV require dosage adjustment (see table). Base doses on 70 kg body weight.

Serum creatinine alone may not be a sufficiently accurate measure of renal function. Ccr may be estimated from the following equation:

$$\text{Males: } \frac{\text{Weight (kg)} \times (140 - \text{age})}{72 \times \text{serum creatinine (mg/dl)}} = \text{Ccr}$$

Females: 0.85 × above value

Imipenem-Cilastatin IV Dosage in Renal Impairment			
Ccr (ml/min/1.73 m^2)	Renal function impairment	Fully susceptible organisms including gram-positive and gram-negative aerobes and anaerobes	Moderately susceptible organisms, primarily some strains of *P. aeruginosa*
31-70	Mild	500 mg q 8 h	500 mg q 6 h
21-30	Moderate	500 mg q 12 h	500 mg q 8 h
6-20	Severe to marked	250 mg q 12 h	500 mg q 12 h
0-5[1]	None, but on hemodialysis		

[1] Do not administer imipenem-cilastatin unless hemodialysis is instituted within 48 hours.

IV: Give a 125, 250 or 500 mg dose by IV infusion over 20 to 30 min. Infuse a 750 or 1 g dose over 40 to 60 min. In patients who develop nausea, slow the infusion rate.

Because of high antimicrobial activity, do not exceed 50 mg/kg/day or 4 g/day, whichever is lower. There is no evidence that higher doses provide greater efficacy.

IMIPENEM-CILASTATIN

Imipenem-Cilastatin IV Dosing Schedule for Adults with Normal Renal Function

Type or severity of infection	Fully susceptible organisms including gram-positive and gram-negative aerobes and anaerobes	Moderately susceptible organisms, primarily some strains of *P. aeruginosa*
Mild	250 mg q 6 h	500 mg q 6 h
Moderate	500 mg q 8 h or 500 mg q 6 h	500 mg q 6 h or 1 g q 8 h
Severe, life-threatening	500 mg q 6 h	1 g q 8 h or 1 g q 6 h
Uncomplicated UTI	250 mg q 6 h	250 mg q 6 h
Complicated UTI	500 mg q 6 h	500 mg q 6 h

IM: Total daily IM dosages > 1500 mg/day are not recommended.

Duration of therapy depends on the type and severity of the infection. Generally, continue for at least 2 days after signs and symptoms of infection have resolved. Safety and efficacy of treatment beyond 14 days have not been established.

Administer by deep IM injection into a large muscle mass (such as the gluteal muscles or lateral part of the thigh) with a 21 gauge 2″ needle. Aspiration is necessary to avoid inadvertent injection into a blood vessel.

Imipenem-Cilastatin IM Dosage Guidelines

Type/Location of infection	Severity	Dosage regimen
Lower respiratory tract Skin and skin structure Gynecologic	Mild/Moderate	500 or 750 mg q 12 h depending on the severity of infection
Intra-abdominal	Mild/Moderate	750 mg q 12 h

Children – 25 mg/kg/dose every sixth hour to children aged 3 months to 3 years with a maximal daily dose of 2 g. In children ≥ 3 years, the recommended dose is 15 mg/kg/dose every sixth hour.

Hemodialysis – Imipenem-cilastatin is cleared by hemodialysis. Administer after hemodialysis and at 12 hour intervals timed from the end of that dialysis session. For patients on hemodialysis, imipenem-cilastatin is recommended only when the benefits outweigh the potential risk of seizures. There is inadequate information to recommend usage for patients undergoing peritoneal dialysis. Carefully monitor dialysis patients, especially those with CNS diseases.

Preparation of solution:

IV – Restore contents of infusion bottles with 100 ml diluent (see *Compatibility*).

IM – Prepare with 1% lidocaine HCl solution (without epinephrine). Prepare the 500 mg vial with 2 ml and the 750 mg vial with 3 ml lidocaine HCl.

Compatibility:

Diluents – Imipenem-cilastatin in infusion bottles and vials, reconstituted as directed with the following diluents, maintains satisfactory potency for 4 hours at room temperature and for 24 hours when refrigerated (5°C; 41°F): 0.9% Sodium Chloride Injection; 5% or 10% Dextrose Injection; 5% Dextrose and 0.9% Sodium Chloride Injection; 5% Dextrose Injection with 0.225% or 0.45% saline solution; 5% Dextrose Injection with 0.15% potassium chloride solution; Mannitol 2.5%, 5% and 10%. Do not freeze solutions.

Storage:

IV – Store dry powder at < 25°C (77°F).

IM – Store dry powder at < 30°C (86°F).

Rx	**Primaxin I.V.** (Merck)	**Powder for Injection:** 250 mg imipenem equivalent and 250 mg cilastatin equivalent. Contains 0.8 mEq sodium.	In vials, infusion bottles and *ADD-Vantage* vials.
		500 mg imipenem equivalent and 500 mg cilastatin equivalent. Contains 1.6 mEq sodium.	In vials, infusion bottles and *ADD-Vantage* vials.
Rx	**Primaxin I.M.** (Merck)	**Powder for Injection:** 500 mg imipenem equivalent and 500 mg cilastatin equivalent. Contains 1.4 mEq sodium.	In vials.
		750 mg imipenem equivalent and 750 mg cilastatin equivalent. Contains 2.1 mEq sodium.	In vials.

AZTREONAM

Actions:

Pharmacology: Aztreonam, a synthetic bactericidal antibiotic, is the first of a new class of antibiotics identified as monobactams. The monobactams have a monocyclic β-lactam nucleus and are structurally different from other β-lactams (eg, penicillins, cephalosporins, cephamycins). Aztreonam has a wide spectrum of activity against gram-negative aerobic pathogens. The bactericidal action results from the inhibition of bacterial cell-wall synthesis due to the high affinity of aztreonam for penicillin-binding protein (PBP) 3.

Pharmacokinetics:

Absorption/Distribution – Single 30 minute IV infusions of 500 mg, 1 and 2 g doses in healthy subjects produced peak serum levels of 54, 90 and 204 mcg/ml, respectively, immediately after administration; at 8 hours, serum levels were 1, 3 and 6 mcg/ml, respectively.

Following single IM injections of 500 mg and 1 g, maximum serum concentrations occur at ≈ 1 hour.

The serum half-life averaged 1.7 hours (range, 1.5 to 2) in subjects with normal renal function, independent of the dose and route. In healthy subjects, based on a 70 kg person, the serum clearance is 91 ml/min, and renal clearance is 56 ml/min. The apparent mean volume of distribution at steady state averaged 12.6 L.

Elderly: The average elimination half-life appears slightly longer in healthy elderly males.

Renal/hepatic impairment: In patients with impaired renal function, the serum half-life is prolonged. Serum half-life is slightly prolonged in patients with hepatic impairment because the liver is a minor pathway of excretion.

Lactation: The concentration in breast milk at 2 hours after a single 1 g IV dose (six patients) was 0.2 mcg/ml; in amniotic fluid at 6 to 8 hours after a single 1 g IV dose (five patients), it was 2 mcg/ml. The concentration in peritoneal fluid obtained 1 to 6 hours after multiple 2 g IV doses ranged between 12 and 90 mcg/ml in seven of eight patients studied.

Metabolism/Excretion – After IM injection of single 500 mg and 1 g doses, urinary levels were ≈ 500 and 1200 mcg/ml, respectively, within the first 2 hours, declining to 180 and 470 mcg/ml in the 6- to 8-hour specimens. Aztreonam is excreted in the urine equally by active tubular secretion and glomerular filtration. In an IV or IM dose, ≈ 60% to 70% was recovered in the urine by 8 hours; recovery was complete by 12 hours. About 12% of a single IV dose was recovered in the feces.

Administration IV or IM of a single 500 mg or 1 g dose every 8 hours for 7 days to healthy subjects produced no apparent accumulation; serum protein binding averaged 56% and was independent of dose.

Microbiology: Aztreonam exhibits potent and specific activity in vitro against a wide spectrum of gram-negative aerobic pathogens including *Pseudomonas aeruginosa.* Aztreonam does not induce β-lactamase activity, and its molecular structure confers a high degree of resistance to hydrolysis by β-lactamases; therefore, it is usually active against gram-negative aerobic organisms. Aztreonam maintains its antimicrobial activity over a pH of 6 to 8. Aztreonam is effective in clinical infections against most strains of the following organisms: *Escherichia coli; Enterobacter* sp; *Klebsiella pneumoniae* and *K. oxytoca; Proteus mirabilis; P. aeruginosa; Serratia marcescens; Haemophilus influenzae,* including ampicillin-resistant and other penicillinase-producing strains; *Citrobacter* sp.

While in vitro studies have demonstrated susceptibility to aztreonam in most of these strains, clinical efficacy for infections other than those included in the indications section has not been documented, such as: *Neisseria gonorrhoeae* (including penicillinase-producing strains); *P. vulgaris; Morganella morganii* (formerly *Proteus morganii*); *Providencia* species, including *P. stuartii* and *P. rettgeri; Pseudomonas* sp; *Shigella* sp; *Pasteurella multocida; Yersinia enterocolitica; Aeromonas hydrophila; N. meningitidis.*

Aztreonam and aminoglycosides are synergistic in vitro against most strains of *P. aeruginosa,* many strains of Enterobacteriaceae and other gram-negative aerobic bacilli.

Aztreonam has little effect on the anaerobic intestinal microflora in in vitro studies. *Clostridium difficile* and its cytotoxin were not found in animal models following administration of aztreonam.

Indications:

Treatment of the following infections caused by susceptible gram-negative microorganisms:

Urinary tract infections (complicated and uncomplicated), including pyelonephritis and cystitis (initial and recurrent) caused by *E. coli, K. pneumoniae, P. mirabilis, P. aeruginosa, E. cloacae, K. oxytoca, Citrobacter* sp and *S. marcescens.*

AZTREONAM

Lower respiratory tract infections, including pneumonia and bronchitis, caused by *E. coli, K. pneumoniae, P. aeruginosa, H. influenzae, P. mirabilis, Enterobacter* sp and *S. marcescens.*

Septicemia caused by *E. coli, K. pneumoniae, P. aeruginosa, P. mirabilis, S. marcescens* and *Enterobacter* sp.

Skin and skin structure infections, including those associated with postoperative wounds, ulcers and burns, caused by *E. coli, P. mirabilis, S. marcescens, Enterobacter* sp, *P. aeruginosa, K. pneumoniae* and *Citrobacter* sp.

Intra-abdominal infections, including peritonitis caused by *E. coli, Klebsiella* sp including *K. pneumoniae, Enterobacter* sp including *E. cloacae, P. aeruginosa, Citrobacter* sp including *C. freundii* and *Serratia* sp including *S. marcescens.*

Gynecologic infections, including endometritis and pelvic cellulitis, caused by *E. coli, K. pneumoniae, Enterobacter* sp including *E. cloacae* and *P. mirabilis.*

Surgery: For adjunctive therapy to surgery to manage infections caused by susceptible organisms.

Concurrent initial therapy with other antimicrobials and aztreonam is recommended before the causative organism(s) is known in seriously ill patients who are also at risk of having an infection due to gram-positive aerobic pathogens. If anaerobic organisms are also suspected, initiate therapy concurrently with aztreonam.

Unlabeled uses: 1 g IM may be beneficial for acute uncomplicated gonorrhea in patients with penicillin-resistant gonococci, as an alternative to spectinomycin.

Contraindications:

Hypersensitivity to aztreonam or any other component in the formulation.

Warnings:

Pseudomembranous colitis has been reported with nearly all antibacterial agents, including aztreonam, and may range in severity from mild to life-threatening. Therefore, it is important to consider this diagnosis in patients who develop diarrhea subsequent to the administration of antibacterial agents.

After the diagnosis of pseudomembranous colitis has been established, initiate therapeutic measures. Mild cases usually respond to drug discontinuation alone. In moderate to severe cases, consider management with fluids and electrolytes, protein supplementation and treatment with an antibacterial drug clinically effective against *C. difficile* colitis.

Epidermal necrolysis: Rare cases of toxic epidermal necrolysis have been reported in association with aztreonam in patients undergoing bone marrow transplant with multiple risk factors including graft vs host disease, sepsis, radiation therapy and other concomitantly administered drugs associated with toxic epidermal necrolysis.

Hypersensitivity: Make careful inquiry for a history of hypersensitivity reactions. Monitor patients who have had immediate hypersensitivity reactions (eg, anaphylactic or urticarial) to penicillins or cephalosporins. If an allergic reaction to aztreonam occurs, discontinue the drug and institute supportive treatment. Refer to Management of Acute Hypersensitivity Reactions. It has been suggested that aztreonam does not exhibit cross-sensitivity with penicillins or other β-lactams.

Renal/Hepatic function impairment: Appropriate monitoring is recommended.

Pregnancy: Category B. Aztreonam crosses the placenta and enters fetal circulation. There are no adequate and well controlled studies in pregnant women. Use during pregnancy only if clearly needed.

Lactation: Aztreonam is excreted in breast milk in concentrations that are < 1% of maternal serum (see Actions). Consider temporary discontinuation of nursing.

Children: Safety and efficacy for use in infants and children have not been established. However, aztreonam has been used in children in clinical trials (see Administration and Dosage).

Precautions:

Superinfection: Use of antibiotics (especially prolonged or repeated therapy) may result in bacterial (including gram-positive *S. aureus* and *S. faecalis*) or fungal overgrowth of nonsusceptible organisms. Such overgrowth may lead to a secondary infection. Take appropriate measures if superinfection occurs.

Drug Interactions:

Probenecid or furosemide: Concomitant administration causes clinically insignificant increases in aztreonam serum levels.

Antibiotics (eg, cefoxitin, imipenem) may induce high levels of β-lactamase in vitro in some gram-negative aerobes such as *Enterobacter* and *Pseudomonas* sp, resulting in antagonism to many β-lactam antibiotics including aztreonam. Do not use β-lactamase-inducing antibiotics concurrently with aztreonam.

Aminoglycosides: If an aminoglycoside is used concurrently with aztreonam, especially if high dosages of the former are used or if therapy is prolonged, monitor renal function because of potential nephrotoxicity and ototoxicity of aminoglycoside antibiotics.

Adverse Reactions:

Local: Phlebitis/thrombophlebitis following IV administration (1.9%); discomfort/swelling at the injection site following IM administration (2.4%).

Cardiovascular: Transient ECG changes (ventricular bigeminy and PVC), hypotension, flushing (< 1%).

CNS: Seizure, confusion, headache, vertigo, paresthesia, insomnia, dizziness (< 1%).

Dermatologic: Rash (1% to 1.3%); toxic epidermal necrolysis, purpura, erythema multiforme, urticaria, exfoliative dermatitis, petechiae, pruritus, diaphoresis (< 1%).

GI: Diarrhea, nausea, vomiting (1% to 1.3%); abdominal cramps, *C. difficile*-associated diarrhea (including pseudomembranous colitis; symptoms may occur during or after antibiotic treament), GI bleeding (< 1%).

Hematologic: Pancytopenia, neutropenia, thrombocytopenia, anemia, eosinophilia, leukocytosis, thrombocytosis (< 1%).

Hypersensitivity: Anaphylaxis, angioedema, bronchospasm (< 1%).

Special senses: Tinnitus, diplopia, mouth ulcer, altered taste, numb tongue, sneezing, nasal congestion, halitosis (< 1%).

Miscellaneous: Vaginal candidiasis, vaginitis, breast tenderness, weakness, muscular aches, fever, malaise, chest pain, dyspnea, wheezing, hepatitis, jaundice (< 1%).

Lab test abnormalities: Elevations of AST, ALT and alkaline phosphatase, increases in prothrombin and partial thromboplastin times, positive Coombs test and increases in serum creatinine (< 1%).

Overdosage:

If necessary, clear aztreonam from the serum by hemodialysis or peritoneal dialysis.

Administration and Dosage:

Give IM or IV. Individualize dosage.

Aztreonam Dosage Guide (Adults)

Type of infection	Dose[1]	Frequency (hours)
Urinary tract infection	500 mg or 1 g	8 or 12
Moderately severe systemic infections	1 or 2 g	8 or 12
Severe systemic or life-threatening infections	2 g	6 or 8

[1] Maximum recommended dose is 8 g/day.

IV route is recommended for patients requiring single doses > 1 g or those with bacterial septicemia, localized parenchymal abscess (eg, intra-abdominal abscess), peritonitis or other severe systemic or life-threatening infections. For infections due to *P. aeruginosa*, a dosage of 2 g every 6 or 8 hours is recommended, at least upon therapy initiation.

Duration of therapy depends on the severity of infection. Generally, continue aztreonam for at least 48 hours after the patient becomes asymptomatic or evidence of bacterial eradication has been obtained. Persistent infections may require treatment for several weeks. Do not use doses smaller than those indicated.

Children: 30 mg/kg every 6 to 8 hours has been used in children for various infections; 50 mg/kg every 4 to 6 hours has been used for *P. aeruginosa* infections.

Renal function impairment: Prolonged aztreonam serum levels may occur in patients with transient or persistent renal insufficiency. Therefore, reduce dosage by 50% in patients with estimated creatinine clearances (Ccr) between 10 and 30 ml/min/1.73 m^2 after an initial loading dose of 1 or 2 g.

When only the serum creatinine concentration is available, the following formula may be used to approximate creatinine clearance. The serum creatinine should represent steady-state renal function.

$$\text{Males: } \frac{\text{Weight (kg)} \times (140 - \text{age})}{72 \times \text{serum creatinine (mg/dl)}} = \text{Ccr}$$

$$\text{Females: } 0.85 \times \text{above value}$$

In patients with severe renal failure (creatinine clearance < 10 ml/min/1.73 m^2), such as those supported by hemodialysis, give 500 mg, 1 or 2 g initially. The maintenance dose should be 25% of the usual initial dose given at the usual fixed interval of 6, 8 or 12 hours. For serious or life-threatening infections, in addition to the maintenance doses, give 12.5% of the initial dose after each hemodialysis session.

AZTREONAM

Elderly: Renal status is a major determinant of dosage in the elderly. Serum creatinine may not be an accurate determinant of renal status. Therefore, obtain estimates of Ccr and make appropriate dosage modifications.

IV: Bolus injection may be used to initiate therapy. Slowly inject directly into a vein or into the tubing of a suitable administration set, over 3 to 5 minutes.

Infusion – With any intermittent infusion of aztreonam and another drug not pharmaceutically compatible, flush the common delivery tube before and after delivery of aztreonam with an infusion solution compatible with both drug solutions. Do not deliver the drugs simultaneously. Complete the infusion within 20 to 60 minutes. With a Y-type administration set, give careful attention to the calculated volume of aztreonam solution required so that the entire dose will be infused. If a volume control administration set is used to deliver an initial dilution of aztreonam during use, the final aztreonam dilution should provide a concentration ≤ 2% w/v.

IM: Inject deeply into a large muscle mass (eg, upper outer quadrant of gluteus maximus or lateral thigh). Aztreonam is well tolerated; do not admix with local anesthetics.

Preparation of solutions: Constituted aztreonam yields a colorless to light straw yellow solution that may develop a slight pink tint on standing (potency is not affected).

IV solutions – For bolus injection: Constitute the contents of the 15 or 30 ml vial with 6 to 10 ml Sterile Water for Injection.

For infusion – Constitute the contents of the 100 ml bottle to a final concentration ≤ 2% w/v (at least 50 ml of any infusion solution listed below per g of aztreonam). Most solutions may be frozen in the original container immediately after constitution.

Further dilute with one of the following IV infusion solutions: Sodium Chloride Injection, 0.9%; Ringer's or Lactated Ringer's Injection; Dextrose Injection, 5% or 10%; Dextrose and Sodium Chloride Injection, 5%:0.9%, 5%:0.45% or 5%:0.2%; Sodium Lactate Injection (M/6 Sodium Lactate); *Ionosol B* and 5% Dextrose; *Isolyte E* or *Isolyte E* with 5% Dextrose; *Isolyte M* with 5% Dextrose; *Normosol R*; *Normosol R* and 5% Dextrose; *Normosol M* and 5% Dextrose; Mannitol Injection, 5% or 10%; Lactated Ringer's and 5% Dextrose Injection; *Plasma-Lyte M* and 5% Dextrose; *10% Travert* Injection; *10% Travert and Electrolyte No. 1, 2 or 3* Injection.

IM solutions – The following diluents may be used: Sterile Water for Injection; Bacteriostatic Water for Injection (with benzyl alcohol or methyl- and propylparabens); Sodium Chloride Injection, 0.9%; Bacteriostatic Sodium Chloride Injection (with benzyl alcohol or parabens).

Admixture compatibilities: IV infusion solutions of aztreonam prepared with NaCl Injection 0.9% or Dextrose Injection 5%, to which clindamycin, gentamicin, tobramycin or cefazolin have been added, are stable for ≤ 48 hours at room temperature or 7 days refrigerated. Ampicillin admixtures with aztreonam in NaCl Injection 0.9% are stable for 24 hours at room temperature and 48 hours under refrigeration; stability in Dextrose Injection 5% is 2 hours at room temperature and 8 hours refrigerated. Aztreonam-cloxacillin and aztreonam-vancomycin admixtures are stable in *Dianeal 137* (peritoneal dialysis solution) with 4.25% Dextrose for ≤ 24 hours at room temperature.

Storage/Stability: Use solutions for IV infusion at concentrations ≤ 2% w/v within 48 hours following constitution if kept at controlled room temperature (15° to 30°C; 59° to 86°F) or within 7 days if refrigerated (2° to 8°C; 36° to 46°F). Frozen infusion solutions, except for solutions prepared with Mannitol Injection 10% or Lactated Ringer's and 5% Dextrose Injection that have not been tested, may be stored for up to 3 months at –20°C (–4°F). Use frozen solutions that have been thawed and maintained at controlled room temperature or by overnight refrigeration within 24 or 72 hours, respectively, after removal from the freezer. Do not refreeze solutions. After preparation, promptly use solutions at concentrations exceeding 2% w/v, except those prepared with Sterile Water for Injection or NaCl Injection; use the two excepted solutions within 48 hours if stored at controlled room temperature or within 7 days if refrigerated.

Rx	**Azactam** (Squibb)	**Powder for Injection (lyophylized cake):** 500 mg[1]	In single-dose 15 ml vials and single-dose 100 ml infusion bottles.
		1 g[1]	In single-dose 15 ml vials and single-dose 100 ml infusion bottles.
		2 g[1]	In 30 ml single-dose vials and single-dose 100 ml infusion bottles.

[1] With ≈ 780 mg L-arginine per g aztreonam.

CHLORAMPHENICOL

Warning:

Serious and fatal blood dyscrasias (aplastic anemia, hypoplastic anemia, thrombocytopenia and granulocytopenia) occur after chloramphenicol administration. Aplastic anemia, which later terminated in leukemia, has been reported. Blood dyscrasias have occurred after both short-term and prolonged therapy. Chloramphenicol must not be used when less potentially dangerous agents are effective. *It must not be used to treat trivial infections (ie, influenza, colds, throat infections), infections other than indicated, or as prophylaxis for bacterial infections.*

It is essential that adequate blood studies be performed during treatment. While blood studies may detect early peripheral blood changes, such as leukopenia, reticulocytopenia or granulocytopenia before they become irreversible, such studies cannot be relied upon to detect bone marrow depression prior to development of aplastic anemia. To facilitate appropriate studies and observation, patients should be hospitalized.

Actions:

Pharmacology: Chloramphenicol binds to 50 S ribosomal subunits of bacteria and interferes with or inhibits protein synthesis. In vitro, chloramphenicol exerts mainly a bacteriostatic effect on a wide range of gram-negative and gram-positive bacteria.

Pharmacokinetics:

Absorption – Chloramphenicol base is absorbed rapidly from the intestinal tract and is 75% to 90% bioavailable. In adults, at doses of 1 g every 6 hours for 8 doses, the average peak serum level was 11.2 mcg/ml 1 hour after the first dose, and 18.4 mcg/ml after the fifth 1 g dose. Mean serum levels ranged from 8 to 14 mcg/ml over the 48 hour period.

The inactive prodrug, chloramphenicol palmitate, is rapidly hydrolyzed to active chloramphenicol base. Bioavailability is approximately 80% for the palmitate ester. The bioavailability of the IV succinate is approximately 70%. Hydrolysis of the succinate is probably by esterases of the liver, kidney and lungs. Approximately 30% is eliminated in the urine as unhydrolyzed ester.

Distribution – The therapeutic range for total serum chloramphenicol concentration is: Peak, 10 to 20 mcg/ml; trough, 5 to 10 mcg/ml. The drug is approximately 60% bound to plasma proteins. Because of the significantly greater concentration of free drug in the serum of premature infants, the therapeutic range for total serum concentration of chloramphenicol may be lower.

Chloramphenicol diffuses rapidly, but its distribution is not uniform. Highest concentrations are found in liver and kidney, and lowest concentrations are found in brain and cerebrospinal fluid (CSF). However, chloramphenicol enters the CSF, even in the absence of meningeal inflammation, appearing in concentrations 45% to 99% of those found in the blood. Measurable levels are also detected in pleural and ascitic fluids, saliva, milk and in the aqueous and vitreous humors. Transport across the placental barrier occurs with somewhat lower concentrations in the cord blood of newborns than in maternal blood.

Metabolism/Excretion – Total urinary excretion of chloramphenicol ranges from 68% to 99% over 3 days. From 5% to 15% is excreted as free chloramphenicol; the remainder consists of inactive metabolites via the liver, principally the glucuronide. Since the glucuronide is excreted rapidly, most chloramphenicol detected in the blood is in the active free form. Small amounts of active drug are found in bile and feces.

The elimination half-life of chloramphenicol is approximately 4 hours, and correlates well with serum bilirubin concentration. Protein binding and clearance are decreased in patients with severe liver dysfunction, leading to potentially toxic serum concentrations of free drug.

Microbiology: Chloramphenicol is effective against a wide range of gram-positive and -negative bacteria, and is active in vitro against rickettsiae, the lymphogranuloma-psittacosis group and *Vibrio cholerae*. It is particularly active against *Salmonella typhi* and *Haemophilus influenzae*.

Indications:

Serious infections for which less potentially dangerous drugs are ineffective or contraindicated caused by susceptible strains of *Salmonella* species; *H influenzae*, specifically, meningeal infections; rickettsiae; lymphogranuloma-psittacosis group; various gram-negative bacteria causing bacteremia, meningitis or other serious gram-negative infections; infections involving anaerobic organisms, when *Bacteroides fragilis* is suspected; other susceptible organisms which have been demonstrated to be resistant to all other appropriate antimicrobial agents.

CHLORAMPHENICOL

If presumptive therapy is initiated, perform in vitro sensitivity tests concurrently, so that the drug may be discontinued if less potentially dangerous agents are indicated.

Acute infections caused by *S typhi*. Chloramphenicol is a drug of choice. In treatment of typhoid fever, some authorities recommend that chloramphenicol be used at therapeutic levels for 8 to 10 days after the patient becomes afebrile, to lessen the possibility of relapse. It is not recommended for the routine treatment of the typhoid "carrier state".

Cystic fibrosis regimens.

Contraindications:

History of hypersensitivity to, or toxicity from, chloramphenicol.

Chloramphenicol must not be used to treat trivial infections (ie, colds, influenza, throat infections), infections other than indicated, or as prophylaxis for bacterial infections.

Warnings:

Blood dyscrasias: See Warning Box. Serious and fatal blood dyscrasias (aplastic anemia, hypoplastic anemia, thrombocytopenia and granulocytopenia) occur. An irreversible type of marrow depression leading to aplastic anemia with a high rate of mortality is characterized by appearance of bone marrow aplasia or hypoplasia weeks or months after therapy. Peripherally, pancytopenia is most often observed, but only one or two of the three major cell types (erythrocytes, leukocytes and platelets) may be depressed. This complication appears unrelated to administration route. One estimate based on 149 cases stated that the route was oral in 83%, parenteral in 14% and rectal in 3%. Several cases of aplastic anemia have been associated with chloramphenicol ophthalmic ointment.

A dose-related reversible type of bone marrow depression may occur and is associated with sustained serum levels at peak ≥ 25 mcg/ml, trough ≥ 10 mcg/ml. This type of marrow depression is characterized by vacuolization of the erythroid cells, a decrease in red cell iron uptake, an increase in circulating serum iron with saturation of iron-binding globulin (usually within 6 to 10 days) and reduction of reticulocytes (usually within 5 to 7 days) and leukopenia; it responds promptly to withdrawal of the drug.

Renal/Hepatic function impairment: Excessive blood levels may result from the use of the recommended dose in patients with impaired liver or kidney function, including that due to immature metabolic processes in the infant. Adjust dosage accordingly or, preferably, determine the blood concentration at appropriate intervals.

Pregnancy: There are no studies to establish the safety of this drug in pregnancy. Since it readily crosses the placental barrier, cautious use is particularly important during pregnancy at term or during labor because of potential toxic effects on the fetus (gray syndrome).

Lactation: Chloramphenicol appears in breast milk with a milk:plasma ratio of 0.5. Use with caution, if at all, during lactation, because of the possibility of toxic effects on the nursing infant.

Children: Use with caution and in reduced dosages in premature and full-term infants to avoid gray syndrome toxicity. (See Adverse Reactions.) Monitor drug serum levels carefully during therapy of the newborn.

Precautions:

Hematology: Evaluate baseline and periodic blood studies approximately every 2 days during therapy. Discontinue the drug upon appearance of reticulocytopenia, leukopenia, thrombocytopenia, anemia or any other findings attributable to chloramphenicol. Such studies do not exclude the possible later appearance of the irreversible type of bone marrow depression. Avoid concurrent therapy with other drugs that may cause bone marrow depression.

Avoid repeated courses if at all possible. Do not continue treatment longer than required to produce a cure.

Acute intermittent porphyria or glucose-6-phosphate dehydrogenase deficiency: Use with caution in patients with these conditions.

Superinfection: Use of antibiotics (especially prolonged or repeated therapy) may result in bacterial or fungal overgrowth of nonsusceptible organisms. Such overgrowth may lead to a secondary infection. Take appropriate measures if superinfection occurs.

CHLORAMPHENICOL

Drug Interactions:

Chloramphenicol Drug Interactions			
Precipitant drug	Object drug*		Description
Barbiturates	Chloramphenicol	⬇	Decreased chloramphenicol serum levels may occur, and barbiturate clearance may be decreased, resulting in increased levels or toxicity.
Chloramphenicol	Barbiturates	⬆	
Rifampin	Chloramphenicol	⬇	Concomitant administration may reduce serum chloramphenicol levels, presumably through hepatic enzyme induction.
Chloramphenicol	Anticoagulants	⬆	Anticoagulant action may be enhanced.
Chloramphenicol	Cyclophosphamide	⬇	Decreased or delayed activation of cyclophosphamide may occur, although it is unclear if a significant decrease in its effect would occur.
Chloramphenicol	Hydantoins	⬆	Serum hydantoin levels may be increased, possibly resulting in toxicity. In addition, chloramphenicol levels may be increased or decreased.
Hydantoins	Chloramphenicol	⬌	
Chloramphenicol	Iron salts	⬆	Serum iron levels may be increased.
Chloramphenicol	Penicillins	⬌	Synergistic effects may develop in the treatment of certain microorganisms, but antagonism may also occur.
Chloramphenicol	Sulfonylureas	⬆	Clinical manifestations of hypoglycemia may occur with concurrent use.
Chloramphenicol	Vitamin B_{12}	⬇	Hematologic effects of vitamin B_{12} may be decreased in patients with pernicious anemia by concurrent chloramphenicol.

* ⬆ = Object drug increased. ⬇ = Object drug decreased. ⬌ = Undetermined effect.

Adverse Reactions:

Hematologic: (see Warnings).

Blood dyscrasias – The most serious adverse effect is bone marrow depression.

Aplastic anemia is estimated to occur in 1:40,000 cases (range 1:19,000 to 1:200,000). There have been reports of aplastic anemia attributed to the drug which later terminated in leukemia.

Hemoglobinuria – Paroxysmal nocturnal hemoglobinuria has been reported.

GI: Nausea; vomiting; glossitis; stomatitis; diarrhea; enterocolitis (low incidence).

CNS: Headache; mild depression; mental confusion; delirium. Optic and peripheral neuritis have been reported, usually following long-term therapy; if this occurs, promptly withdraw the drug.

Hypersensitivity: Fever; macular and vesicular rashes; angioedema; urticaria; anaphylaxis. Herxheimer reactions have occurred during therapy for typhoid fever.

Miscellaneous:

Gray syndrome – Toxic reactions including fatalities (approximately 40%) have occurred in the premature infant and newborn; the signs and symptoms associated with these reactions have been referred to as the "gray syndrome". The following summarizes the clinical and laboratory studies:

- In most cases, therapy was instituted within the first 48 hours of life.
- Symptoms first appeared after 3 to 4 days of treatment with high doses.
- Symptoms appeared in the following order: Abdominal distension with or without emesis; progressive pallid cyanosis; vasomotor collapse, frequently accompanied by irregular respiration; death within a few hours of onset. Other initial symptoms may include refusal to suck, loose green stools, flaccidity, ashen color, decrease in temperature and refractory lactic acidosis. Death occurs in approximately 40% of the patients within 2 days of initial symptoms.
- Progression of symptoms was accelerated with higher doses.
- Serum level studies revealed unusually high drug concentrations (≥ 40 mcg/ml after repeated doses) with doses in excess of 25 mg/kg/day in newborns.
- Termination of therapy upon early evidence of associated symptoms frequently reversed the process with complete recovery.
- Preexisting liver dysfunction may be a significant risk factor.

CHLORAMPHENICOL

Patient Information:

Preferably taken on an empty stomach at least 1 hour before or 2 hours after meals. Take with food if GI upset occurs.

Take at evenly spaced intervals (every 6 hours) around the clock.

Notify physician if fever, sore throat, tiredness or unusual bleeding or bruising occurs.

Administration and Dosage:

Therapeutic concentrations generally should be maintained as follows: Peak 10 to 20 mcg/ml; trough 5 to 10 mcg/ml.

Monitoring serum levels is important because of the variability of chloramphenicol's pharmacokinetics. Monitor serum concentrations weekly; monitor more often in patients with hepatic dysfunction, in therapy > 2 weeks or with potentially interacting drugs (see Drug Interactions).

Adults: 50 mg/kg/day in divided doses every 6 hours for typhoid fever and rickettsial infections. Exceptional infections (ie, meningitis, brain abscess) due to moderately resistant organisms may require dosage up to 100 mg/kg/day to achieve blood levels inhibiting the pathogen; decrease high doses as soon as possible.

Renal/hepatic function impairment reduces the ability to metabolize and excrete the drug. Impaired metabolic processes require that doses be adjusted based on drug concentration in the blood. An initial loading dose of 1 g followed by 500 mg every 6 hours has been recommended in impaired hepatic function.

Children: 50 to 75 mg/kg/day in divided doses every 6 hours has been recommended for most indications. For meningitis, 50 to 100 mg/kg/day in divided doses every 6 hours has been recommended.

Newborns (See Gray syndrome under Adverse Reactions.) 25 mg/kg/day in 4 doses every 6 hours usually produces and maintains adequate concentrations in blood and tissues. Give increased dosage demanded by severe infections only to maintain the blood concentration within an effective range. After the first 2 weeks of life, full-term infants ordinarily may receive up to 50 mg/kg/day in 4 doses every 6 hours.

Neonates (< 2 kg) – 25 mg/kg once daily.

Neonates from birth to 7 days (> 2 kg) – 25 mg/kg once daily.

Neonates over 7 days (> 2 kg) – 50 mg/kg/day in divided doses every 12 hours.

These dosage recommendations are extremely important because blood concentration in all premature and full-term infants < 2 weeks of age differs from that of other infants due to variations in the maturity of the metabolic functions of the liver and kidneys. When these functions are immature (or seriously impaired in adults), the drug is found in high concentrations which tend to increase with succeeding doses.

Infants and children with immature metabolic processes: 25 mg/kg/day usually produces therapeutic concentrations. In this group particularly, carefully monitor the concentration of drug in the blood.

IV administration: Chloramphenicol sodium succinate is intended for IV use only; it is ineffective when given IM. It must be hydrolyzed to its active form, and there is a lag in achieving adequate blood levels following infusion. Administer IV as a 10% solution injected over at least 1 minute. Prepare by adding 10 ml of an aqueous diluent (eg, Water for Injection or 5% Dextrose Injection). Substitute oral dosage as soon as feasible.

Rx	**Chloramphenicol** (Various, eg, Qualitest)	**Capsules**: 250 mg	In 100s.
Rx	**Chloromycetin Kapseals** (Parke-Davis)		Lactose. (P-D 379). In 100s.
Rx	**Chloramphenicol Sodium Succinate** (Various, eg, Lyphomed)	**Powder for Injection:** 100 mg/ml (as sodium succinate) when reconstituted	1 g in 15 ml vials.
Rx	**Chloromycetin Sodium Succinate** (Parke-Davis)		2.25 mEq sodium per g. In 1 g vials.

FLUOROQUINOLONES

Actions:

Pharmacology: The fluoroquinolones are synthetic, broad-spectrum antibacterial agents related to the other quinolones, nalidixic acid and cinoxacin. These agents contain a 6-fluoro and 7-piperazine substituent which greatly enhances their antimicrobial efficacy when compared to nalidixic acid. The fluorine molecule provides increased potency against gram-negative organisms and broadens the spectrum to include gram-positive organisms; the piperazine moiety is responsible for antipseudomonal activity. These agents are bactericidal; they interfere with the enzyme DNA gyrase needed for the synthesis of bacterial DNA.

Pharmacokinetics:

Pharmacokinetics of Fluoroquinolones

Fluoroquinolone	Bioavailability (%)	Max urine concentration (mcg/ml) (dose)	Mean peak plasma concentration (mcg/ml) (dose)	Area under curve (AUC) (mcg • hr/ml) (dose)	Protein binding (%)	t½ (hr)	Urine recovery unchanged (%)
Ciprofloxacin Oral	70-80	160-700 (500 mg)	1.2 (250 mg) 2.4 (500 mg) 4.3 (750 mg) 5.4 (1000 mg)	4.8 (250 mg) 11.6 (500 mg) 20.2 (750 mg) 30.8 (1000 mg)	20-40	4	40-50
IV		> 200 (200 mg) > 400 (400 mg)	4.3 (400 mg)	4.8 (200 mg) 11.6 (400 mg)	20-40	5-6	50-70
Enoxacin	90	nd	0.83 (200 mg) 2 (400 mg)	16 (400 mg)	40	3-6	> 40
Lomefloxacin	95-98	> 300 (400 mg)	4.2 (400 mg)	5.6 (100 mg) 10.9 (200 mg) 26.1 (400 mg)	10	8	65
Norfloxacin	30-40	200-500 (400 mg)	0.8 (200 mg) 1.5 (400 mg)	5.4 (400 mg)	10-15	3-4.5	26-32
Ofloxacin Oral	≈ 98	220 (200 mg)	1.5 (200 mg) 2.4 (300 mg) 2.9 (400 mg)	14.1 (200 mg) 21.2 (300 mg) 31.4 (400 mg)	32	5-7	70-80
IV		nd[1]	2.7 (200 mg) 4 (400 mg)	43.5 (400 mg)	32	5-10	nd[1]

[1] nd = no data.

Norfloxacin: Absorption/Distribution – Absorption is rapid. Food may decrease absorption. Steady-state norfloxacin levels will be attained within 2 days of dosing. Urinary concentrations of ≥ 200 mcg/ml are attained 2 to 3 hours after a single 400 mg dose. Mean urinary concentrations of norfloxacin remain above 30 mcg/ml for at least 12 hours following a 400 mg dose. Norfloxacin is least soluble at urinary pH of 7.5; greater solubility occurs at pHs above and below this value.

Metabolism/Excretion: Norfloxacin is eliminated through metabolism, biliary excretion and renal excretion. Renal excretion occurs by both glomerular filtration and tubular secretion, as evidenced by the high rate of renal clearance (≈ 275 ml/min). Within 24 hours of administration, 5% to 8% of the dose is recovered in the urine as six less active metabolites. Fecal recovery accounts for another 30%. In healthy elderly volunteers (65 to 75 years of age), norfloxacin is eliminated more slowly because of decreased renal function. Drug absorption appears unaffected. Disposition of norfloxacin in patients with creatinine clearance (Ccr) rates > 30 ml/min/1.73 m^2 is similar to that in healthy volunteers. In patients with Ccr rates ≤30 ml/min/1.73 m^2, the renal elimination decreases so that the effective serum half-life is 6.5 hours; dosage alteration is necessary. See Administration and Dosage.

Enoxacin: Absorption/Distribution – Peak plasma levels are achieved in 1 to 3 hours. Effect of food on absorption has not been studied. In elderly, mean peak plasma concentrations are 50% higher than in young adults. Enoxacin diffuses into cervix, fallopian tube and myometrium at levels ≈ 1 to 2 times those in plasma, and into kidney and prostate at levels ≈ 2 to 4 times plasma levels.

Metabolism/Excretion: Five metabolites have been identified in the urine and account for 15% to 20% of a dose. Some isozymes of the cytochrome P-450 hepatic microsomal enzyme system are inhibited by enoxacin, resulting in significant drug interactions with some agents (see Drug Interactions). Clearance is reduced in renal impairment; dosage adjustment is necessary (see Administration and Dosage).

FLUOROQUINOLONES

Ciprofloxacin: Absorption/Distribution – Ciprofloxacin is rapidly and well absorbed from the GI tract after oral administration with no substantial loss by first-pass metabolism. When given concomitantly with food, there is a delay in the absorption of the drug, resulting in peak concentrations that are closer to 2 hours after dosing rather than 1 hour. The overall absorption, however, is not substantially affected. Maximum serum concentrations are attained 1 to 2 hours after oral dosing. Mean concentrations 12 hours after dosing with 250, 500 or 750 mg are 0.1, 0.2 and 0.4 mcg/ml, respectively. Following 60 minute IV infusions of 200 and 400 mg, mean maximum serum concentrations achieved were 2.1 and 4.6 mcg/ml, respectively; concentrations at 12 hours were 0.1 and 0.2 mcg/ml, respectively. Ciprofloxacin is widely distributed throughout the body. Tissue concentrations often exceed serum concentrations in both men and women, particularly in genital tissue. The drug diffuses into the cerebrospinal fluid (CSF); however, CSF concentrations are generally only about 10% of peak serum concentrations.

Metabolism/Excretion: Four metabolites have been identified in urine which, together, account for approximately 15% of an oral dose. The metabolites have antimicrobial activity, but are less active than unchanged ciprofloxacin. After IV administration, three metabolites have been identified in urine which account for ≈ 10% of the IV dose. After a 250 mg oral dose, urine concentrations usually exceed 200 mcg/ml during the first 2 hours and are ≈ 30 mcg/ml at 8 to 12 hours after dosing. Following a 200 or 400 mg IV dose, urine concentrations usually exceed 200 and 400 mcg/ml, respectively, during the first 2 hours and are generally > 15 and > 30 mcg/ml, respectively, at 8 to 12 hours after dosing. Urinary ciprofloxacin excretion is virtually complete within 24 hours after dosing. Renal clearance is ≈ 300 ml/min; active tubular secretion plays a significant role. Although bile concentrations are several fold higher than serum after oral dosing, only a small amount is recovered from the bile. Approximately 20% to 35% of an oral dose is recovered from feces within 5 days after dosing. In patients with reduced renal function, the half-life is slightly prolonged; dosage adjustments may be required. See Administration and Dosage.

Ofloxacin: Absorption/Distribution – Maximum serum concentrations are achieved 1 to 2 hours after an oral dose. The amount absorbed increases proportionately with the dose. The effect of food on absorption has not been studied. Elimination is biphasic; half-lives are approximately 4 to 5 hours and 20 to 25 hours, although accumulation at steady state can be estimated using a half-life of 9 hours. Steady-state concentrations are achieved after four doses and are ≈ 50% higher than concentrations after single doses. Ofloxacin is widely distributed to body tissues and fluids.

Metabolism/Excretion: Ofloxacin has a pyridobenzoxazine ring that appears to decrease the extent of parent compound metabolism; < 5% of a dose is recovered in the urine as the desmethyl or N-oxide metabolites. Elimination is mainly by renal excretion; 4% to 8% is excreted in the feces. In healthy elderly volunteers with normal renal function, the apparent half-life is 6 to 8 hours (compared to ≈ 5 hours in younger adults); however, absorption is unaffected by age. Clearance is reduced in patients with renal function impairment (Ccr ≤ 50 ml/min); dosage adjustment is necessary. See Administration and Dosage.

Lomefloxacin: Absorption/Distribution – Absorption is rapid. Following coadministration with food, rate of absorption is delayed (time to reach maximum plasma concentration delayed by 41%, maximum concentration decreased by 18%) and the extent of absorption (AUC) is decreased by 12%. At 24 hours post-dose, single doses of 200 or 400 mg result in mean plasma levels of 0.1 and 0.24 mcg/ml, respectively. Steady-state concentrations are achieved within 48 hours of initiating once-daily dosing. The mean urine concentration exceeds 35 mcg/ml for at least 24 hours after dosing. Urine pH appears to affect the solubility of lomefloxacin, with solubilities ranging from 3.03 to 7.8 mg/ml at pH of 8.12 to 5.2, respectively.

Metabolism/Excretion: Mean renal clearance is 145 ml/min in subjects with normal renal function, which may indicate tubular secretion. Approximately 9% of a dose is recovered in the urine as the glucuronide metabolite; four other metabolites have been identified and account for < 0.5% of the dose. Approximately 10% of a dose is recovered unchanged in the feces. In healthy elderly volunteers, plasma clearance was reduced by ≈ 25% and the AUC was increased by ≈ 33%, which may be due to decreased renal function in this population. In patients with Ccr between 10 and 40 ml/min/1.73 m^2, the mean AUC after a single dose increased 335% over the AUC in patients with Ccr > 80 ml/min/1.73 m^2, and mean half-life increased to 21 hours. In patients with Ccr < 10 ml/min/1.73 m^2, AUC increased 700% and half-life increased to 45 hours. Adjustment of dosage is necessary. See Administration and Dosage.

FLUOROQUINOLONES

Microbiology:

Table I: Organisms Generally Susceptible to Fluoroquinolones In Vitro

	Organism	Ciprofloxacin	Enoxacin	Lomefloxacin	Norfloxacin	Ofloxacin
Gram-negative	Acinetobacter sp	✓			✓	✓
	Aeromonas sp	✓	✓[1]	✓[1]	✓[1]	✓
	Alcaligenes sp				✓	
	Brucella melitensis	✓				
	Campylobacter sp	✓			✓	✓[1]
	Citrobacter sp	✓	✓[1]	✓[1]	✓[1]	✓[1]
	Edwardsiella tarda	✓			✓	
	Enterobacter sp	✓	✓[1]	✓	✓[1]	✓[1]
	Escherichia coli	✓	✓	✓	✓	✓
	Flavobacterium sp				✓	
	Hafnia alvei			✓	✓	
	Haemophilus ducreyi	✓	✓			
	Haemophilus influenzae	✓		✓	✓	✓
	Haemophilus parainfluenzae	✓		✓	✓	✓
	Klebsiella pneumoniae	✓	✓[1]	✓	✓[1]	✓[1]
	Klebsiella sp	✓	✓	✓	✓	✓
	Legionella sp	✓		✓	✓	✓
	Listeria monocytogenes	✓				
	Moraxella (Branhamella) catarrhalis	✓		✓	✓	✓
	Morganella morganii	✓	✓	✓	✓	✓
	Neisseria gonorrhoeae	✓	✓		✓	✓
	Neisseria meningitidis	✓			✓	✓
	Pasteurella multocida	✓				
	Plesiomonas shigelloides					✓
	Proteus mirabilis	✓	✓	✓	✓	✓
	Proteus vulgaris	✓	✓	✓	✓	✓
	Providencia alcalifaciens		✓	✓	✓	
	Providencia rettgeri	✓		✓	✓	✓
	Providencia stuartii	✓	✓		✓	✓
	Pseudomonas aeruginosa	✓	✓	✓	✓	✓
	Pseudomonas fluorescens					✓
	Salmonella sp	✓			✓	✓
	Serratia sp	✓	✓[1]	✓	✓[1]	✓[1]
	Shigella sp	✓			✓	✓
	Vibrio sp	✓			✓[1]	✓[1]
	Xanthomonas (Pseudomonas) maltophilia					✓
	Yersinia enterocolitica	✓			✓	✓

FLUOROQUINOLONES

Table I: Organisms Generally Susceptible to Fluoroquinolones In Vitro

	Organism	Ciprofloxacin	Enoxacin	Lomefloxacin	Norfloxacin	Ofloxacin
Gram-positive	Staphylococcus aureus	✓[2]		✓[2]	✓[2]	✓[2]
	coagulase-negative sp	✓				
	epidermidis	✓	✓	✓[2]	✓	✓[2]
	hemolyticus	✓			✓	
	saprophyticus	✓	✓	✓	✓	✓
	Streptococci group D				✓	
	agalactiae				✓	✓
	faecalis	✓			✓	✓
	pneumoniae	✓				✓
	pyogenes	✓				✓
	Bacillus cereus				✓	

[1] May be species-dependent.
[2] Including methicillin-susceptible and methicillin-resistant strains.

These agents have in vitro activity against a wide range of gram-negative and gram-positive organisms. Ciprofloxacin, lomefloxacin and norfloxacin are generally inactive against anaerobic bacteria. Refer to Table I for a listing of organisms generally susceptible to fluoroquinolones in vitro.

Ciprofloxacin – Most strains of streptococci are only moderately susceptible as are *Mycobacterium tuberculosis, M fortuitum* and *Chlamydia trachomatis. Mycoplasma pneumoniae, M hominis* and *Ureaplasma urealyticum* are susceptible in vitro. Some strains of *Pseudomonas aeruginosa* may develop resistance fairly rapidly.

Ciprofloxacin does not cross-react with other antimicrobial agents such as beta-lactams or aminoglycosides; however, additive activity may result when it is combined with beta-lactams, aminoglycosides, clindamycin or metronidazole.

Norfloxacin – U urealyticum is susceptible in vitro. Resistance to norfloxacin due to spontaneous mutation in vitro is rare (< 1%). Development of resistance is greatest in the following: *Pseudomonas aeruginosa*; *Klebsiella pneumoniae*; *Acinetobacter* sp; enterococci. Norfloxacin is not generally active against obligate anaerobes.

Ofloxacin – The following organisms are susceptible in vitro:

Anaerobes: Bacteroides fragilis; *Clostridium perfringens* and *B intermedius* and *C welchii*; *Gardnerella vaginalis*; *Peptococcus niger*; *Peptostreptococcus* sp.

Other: Chlamydia pneumoniae;*C trachomatis* (also active in vivo); *M tuberculosis*; *Mycoplasma pneumoniae*; *U urealyticum*.

Many strains of other streptococcal sp, enterococcus sp and anaerobes are resistant. It is not active against *Treponema pallidum*. Although cross-resistance has been observed between ofloxacin and other fluoroquinolones, some organisms resistant to other quinolones may be susceptible to ofloxacin.

Lomefloxacin – Most group A, B, D and G streptococci, *S pneumoniae, Pseudomonas cepacia, U urealyticum, Mycoplasma hominis* and anaerobic bacteria are resistant.

Cross-resistance has occurred between lomefloxacin and other quinolone-class antimicrobial agents, but not between lomefloxacin and other antimicrobials, such as aminoglycosides, penicillins, tetracyclines, cephalosporins or sulfonamides. Lomefloxacin is active in vitro against some strains of cephalosporin- and aminoglycoside-resistant gram-negative bacteria.

Indications:

For specific approved indications, refer to individual drug monographs.

Unlabeled uses:

Ciprofloxacin 750 mg twice daily appears effective in patients with cystic fibrosis who have pulmonary exacerbations associated with susceptible microorganisms. However, restrict use to patients > 14 years of age. Also, long-term therapy is inadvisable due to emergence of resistant organisms. It may also be useful in the treatment of malignant external otitis (750 mg twice daily) and for tuberculosis in combination with rifampin and other antituberculosis agents. It has been used as part of a multi-drug regimen (1500 mg/day divided every 12 hours) for the treatment of *Mycobacterium avium* complex infection, a common infection in AIDS patients.

FLUOROQUINOLONES

Fluoroquinolones may also be useful in the following conditions (some agents are specifically indicated for these conditions; refer to drug monographs): Bronchitis; pneumonia (including Legionella and Mycoplasma); prostatitis; osteomyelitis (selected types); prophylaxis in urological surgery; traveler's diarrhea; gonorrheal cervicitis or urethritis; pelvic inflammatory disease; sinusitis; otitis media; septic arthritis; bacterial meningitis; bacteremia (pseudomonal or staphylococcal); endocarditis. Further study is needed.

Contraindications:

Hypersensitivity to fluoroquinolones or the quinolone group of antibacterial agents (cinoxacin and nalidixic acid).

Warnings:

Photosensitivity: Moderate to severe phototoxic reactions have occurred in patients exposed to direct or indirect sunlight or to artificial ultraviolet light (eg, sunlamps) during or following treatment with **lomefloxacin**. These reactions have also occurred in patients exposed to shaded or diffuse light, including exposure through glass. Advise patients to discontinue lomefloxacin therapy at the first signs or symptoms of a phototoxicity reaction such as a sensation of skin burning, redness, swelling, blisters, rash, itching or dermatitis.

These reactions have occurred with and without the use of sunscreens or sunblocks and with single doses of lomefloxacin. In a few cases, recovery was prolonged for several weeks. As with some other types of phototoxicity, there is the potential for exacerbation of the reaction on re-exposure to sunlight or artificial ultraviolet light prior to complete recovery from the reaction. In rare cases, reactions have recurred up to several weeks after stopping therapy.

Avoid direct exposure to direct or indirect sunlight (even when using sunscreens or sunblocks) while taking lomefloxacin and other fluoroquinolones for several days following therapy. Discontinue therapy at first signs or symptoms of phototoxicity.

Convulsions, increased intracranial pressure and toxic psychosis have occurred. CNS stimulation may also occur, which may lead to tremor, restlessness, lightheadedness, confusion and hallucinations. Use with caution in patients with known or suspected CNS disorders, (eg, severe cerebral arteriosclerosis, epilepsy) or other factors which predispose to seizures. If these reactions occur, stop the drug and institute appropriate measures.

Syphilis: **Ofloxacin** and **enoxacin** are not effective for syphilis. High doses of antimicrobial agents for short periods of time to treat gonorrhea may mask or delay symptoms of incubating syphilis. All patients should have a serologic test for syphilis at the time of gonorrhea diagnosis. Patients treated with ofloxacin and enoxacin should have a follow-up serologic test after 3 months.

Chronic bronchitis due to S pneumoniae: **Lomefloxacin** is not indicated for the empiric treatment of acute bacterial exacerbation of chronic bronchitis when it is probable that *S pneumoniae* is a causative pathogen since it exhibits in vitro resistance to lomefloxacin. Use only if sputum gram stain demonstrates an adequate quality of specimen and there is a predominance of gram-negative and not gram-positive organisms.

Hypersensitivity reactions, serious and occasionally fatal, have occurred in patients receiving quinolone therapy, some following the first dose. Some reactions were accompanied by cardiovascular collapse, loss of consciousness, tingling, pharyngeal or facial edema, dyspnea, urticaria and itching. If an allergic reaction occurs, discontinue the drug. Refer to Management of Acute Hypersensitivity Reactions.

Pseudomembranous colitis has been reported with nearly all antibacterial agents, including fluoroquinolones, and may range from mild to life-threatening in severity. Therefore, it is important to consider this diagnosis in patients who present with diarrhea subsequent to the administration of antibacterial agents. After the diagnosis of pseudomembranous colitis has been established, initiate therapeutic measures. Mild cases of pseudomembranous colitis usually respond to discontinuation of drug alone. In moderate to severe cases, consider management with fluid and electrolytes, protein supplementation, and treatment with an antibacterial drug clinically effective against *C difficile* colitis.

Renal function impairment: Alteration in dosage regimen is necessary. See Administration and Dosage.

Carcinogenesis: Mice exposed to UVA light while receiving **lomefloxacin** developed a phototoxic response. Time to development of skin tumors was 16 weeks; with other quinolones and UVA light, times to skin tumor development ranged from 28 to 52 weeks. Well-differentiated squamous cell carcinomas developed in 92% of mice, which were non-metastatic and endophytic. Lomefloxacin alone did not result in skin or systemic tumors.

FLUOROQUINOLONES

Fertility impairment: Decreased spermatogenesis and subsequent decreased fertility occurred in animals given **enoxacin** doses that produced plasma levels 3 times higher than those in humans at the recommended therapeutic dosage.

Elderly: Norfloxacin is eliminated more slowly because of decreased renal function; absorption appears unaffected. The apparent half-life of **ofloxacin** is 6 to 8 hours, compared to ≈ 5 hours in younger adults; absorption is unaffected. **Lomefloxacin** plasma clearance was reduced by ≈ 25% and the AUC was increased by ≈ 33% in the elderly, which may be due to decreased renal function in this population. **Enoxacin** plasma concentrations are 50% higher in the elderly than in young adults.

Pregnancy: Category C. Do not use in pregnant women. There are no adequate and well controlled studies in pregnant women. Use during pregnancy only if the potential benefit justifies the potential risk to the fetus.

Norfloxacin produces embryonic loss in monkeys when given in doses 10 times the maximum human dose.

Ciprofloxacin and **norfloxacin** caused lameness in immature dogs due to permanent cartilage lesions, and caused arthropathy in immature animals.

Ofloxacin in doses equivalent to 10 to 50 times the maximum therapeutic dose were fetotoxic (ie, decreased fetal body weight, increased fetal mortality) in rats and rabbits, and minor skeletal variations occurred in rats; it also caused arthropathy in immature animals.

Lomefloxacin increased the incidence of fetal loss in monkeys at approximately 3 to 6 times the recommended human dose. In rabbits, maternal toxicity and associated fetotoxicity, decreased placental weight and variations of the coccygeal vertebrae occurred at doses 2 times the recommended human dose.

Enoxacin caused dose-related maternal toxicity (eg, venous irritation, weight loss) and fetal toxicity (increased post-implantation loss and stunted fetuses) following IV doses of 10 to 50 mg/kg. At 50 mg/kg, the incidence of fetal malformations was significantly increased in the presence of overt maternal and fetal toxicity.

Lactation: **Norfloxacin** was not detected in breast milk following the administration of 20 mg to nursing mothers; however, this was a low dose. **Ciprofloxacin** is excreted in breast milk; however, the amount ingested by the infant appears to be low. **Ofloxacin** as a single 200 mg dose resulted in breast milk concentrations in nursing females that were similar to those found in plasma. It is not known whether **lomefloxacin** or **enoxacin** are excreted in breast milk. Because of the potential for serious adverse reactions in nursing infants, decide whether to discontinue nursing or to discontinue the drug, taking into account the importance of the drug to the mother.

Children: Do not use in children. Safety and efficacy of **lomefloxacin, enoxacin** and **ofloxacin** in children < 18 years of age have not been established. **Ciprofloxacin, enoxacin, lomefloxacin** and **ofloxacin** cause arthropathy and osteochondrosis in immature animals. Administration of **norfloxacin** and **ciprofloxacin** caused lameness in immature dogs due to permanent cartilage lesions.

Precautions:

Monitoring: Periodic assessment of organ system functions, including renal, hepatic and hematopoietic is advisable during prolonged therapy.

Ophthalmologic abnormalities, including cataracts and multiple punctate lenticular opacities, have occurred during therapy with some quinolones. With multiple-dose therapy, ophthalmic tissue levels of the quinolones were significantly higher than plasma levels. A causal relationship has not been established.

Crystalluria: Needle-shaped crystals were found in the urine of some volunteers who received either placebo or 800 or 1600 mg norfloxacin. While crystalluria is not expected to occur under usual conditions with 400 mg twice daily, do not exceed the daily recommended dosage. Crystalluria related to ciprofloxacin has occurred only rarely in man because human urine is usually acidic. The patient should drink sufficient fluids to ensure proper hydration and adequate urinary output. Avoid alkalinity of the urine and do not exceed the recommended daily dose.

Phototoxicity reactions, moderate to severe, have occurred in patients who are exposed to direct sunlight while receiving some drugs in this class. See Warnings.

Superinfection: Use of antibiotics (especially prolonged or repeated therapy) may result in bacterial or fungal overgrowth of nonsusceptible organisms. Such overgrowth may lead to a secondary infection. Take appropriate measures if superinfection occurs.

FLUOROQUINOLONES

Drug Interactions:

Fluoroquinolone Drug Interactions			
Precipitant drug	Object drug*		Description
Antacids Didanosine Iron salts Sucralfate Zinc salts	Fluoroquinolones	⬇	Interference of GI absorption of the fluoroquinolones, resulting in decreased serum levels. Avoid simultaneous use; administer antacids 2 to 4 hours before or after the fluoroquinolone.
Antineoplastic agents	Fluoroquinolones	⬇	Fluoroquinolone serum levels may be decreased.
Azlocillin	Ciprofloxacin	⬆	The clearance of ciprofloxacin is decreased, possibly increasing its pharmacologic effects. This combination may be beneficial for some serious gram-negative infections, although it is not known if toxicity also increases.
Bismuth subsalicylate	Enoxacin	⬇	Enoxacin bioavailability is decreased when bismuth subsalicylate is given with or 60 minutes after enoxacin. Avoid concurrent use.
Cimetidine	Fluoroquinolones	⬆	Cimetidine may interfere with the elimination of the fluoroquinolones.
Nitrofurantoin	Norfloxacin	⬇	Antibacterial effect of norfloxacin in the urinary tract may be antagonized.
Probenecid	Fluoroquinolones	⬆	Ciprofloxacin renal clearance is reduced 50%, and its serum concentration is increased 50%; diminished norfloxacin and lomefloxacin urinary excretion has also occurred.
Ciprofloxacin Enoxacin Norfloxacin	Caffeine	⬆	Total body clearance of caffeine is reduced, possibly resulting in increased pharmacologic effects. Ofloxacin and lomefloxacin do not appear to affect caffeine. Enoxacin trough plasma levels were also 20% higher.
Ciprofloxacin Norfloxacin	Cyclosporine	⬆	The nephrotoxic effect of cyclosporine may be increased.
Enoxacin	Digoxin	⬆	Digoxin serum levels may be increased. Monitor digoxin levels.
Ciprofloxacin	Hydantoins	⬇	Phenytoin serum levels may be reduced, producing a decrease in therapeutic effects.
Fluoroquinolones	Anticoagulants	⬆	The effects of the anticoagulant may be increased. Monitor prothrombin time.
Fluoroquinolones	Cyclosporine	⬆	Nephrotoxic effects may be increased. Closely monitor renal function. Conflicting data exist.
Fluoroquinolones	Theophylline	⬆	Decreased clearance and increased plasma levels and toxicity of theophylline has occurred with concurrent ciprofloxacin and enoxacin. Data conflict with norfloxacin and ofloxacin; some studies report no interaction, others suggest increased theophylline levels. Lomefloxacin does not appear to alter theophylline levels. Monitor theophylline levels.

* ⬆ = Object drug increased. ⬇ = Object drug decreased.

Drug/Food interactions: Food may decrease the absorption of **norfloxacin**. Food delays the absorption of **ciprofloxacin**, resulting in peak concentrations that are closer to 2 hours after dosing rather than 1 hour; however, overall absorption is not substantially affected. Dairy products such as milk and yogurt reduce the absorption of ciprofloxacin; avoid concurrent use. The bioavailability of ciprofloxacin may also be decreased by enteral feedings. Food delays the rate of absorption of **lomefloxacin** (time to reach maximum plasma concentration delayed by 41%, maximum concentration decreased by 18%) and decreases the extent of absorption (AUC) by 12%.

FLUOROQUINOLONES

Adverse Reactions:

Fluoroquinolone Adverse Reactions (%)						
	Adverse reactions	Ciprofloxacin[1]	Enoxacin	Lomefloxacin	Norfloxacin	Ofloxacin[1]
GI	Nausea	5.2	2-9	3.7	2.8	3-10
	Abdominal pain/ discomfort	1.7	≤ 2	< 1	0.3-1	1-3
	Diarrhea	2.3	1-2	1.4	✓[2]	1-4
	Vomiting	2	6-9	< 1	✓[2]	1-3
	Dry/painful mouth	< 1	< 1	< 1	✓[2]	1-3
	Dyspepsia/Heartburn	✓[2]	1	< 1	0.3-1	< 1
	Constipation	✓[2]	< 1	< 1	0.3-1	< 1
	Flatulence	✓[2]	< 1	< 1	0.3-1	1-3
	Pseudomembranous colitis[3]	✓[2]	✓[2]	✓[2]	✓[2]	✓[2]
CNS	Headache	1.2	≤ 2	3.2	2.7	1-9
	Dizziness	< 1	≤ 3	2.3	1.8	1-5
	Fatigue/Lethargy/ Malaise	< 1	< 1	< 1	0.3-1	1-3
	Somnolence/ Drowsiness	< 1	< 1	< 1	0.3-1	1-3
	Depression	< 1	< 1	< 1	0.3-1	< 1
	Insomnia	< 1	1	< 1	0.3-1	3-7
	Seizures/Convulsions[3]	< 1	< 1	< 1	rare	✓[2]
	Confusion	✓[2]	< 1	< 1	✓[2]	
	Psychotic reactions	< 1			✓[2]	
	Paresthesia	< 1	< 1	< 1	✓[2]	< 1
	Hallucinations	< 1				< 1
Dermatologic	Photosensitivity[3]	< 1	< 1	2.4	✓[2]	✓[2]
	Rash	1.1	≤ 1	< 1	0.3-1	1-3
	Pruritus		1	< 1	✓[2]	1-3
	Toxic epidermal necrolysis	✓[2]	< 1		✓[2]	
	Stevens-Johnson syn- drome	✓[2]	< 1		✓[2]	
	Exfoliative dermatitis	✓[2]			✓[2]	
	Hypersensitivity[3]	< 1		✓[2]	✓[2]	✓[2]
Other	Visual disturbances	< 1	< 1	< 1	✓[2]	1-3
	Hearing loss	< 1			✓[2]	< 1
	Vaginitis	< 1	< 1	< 1		1-3
	Hypertension	< 1		< 1		<1
	Palpitations	< 1	< 1			<1
	Syncope	< 1	< 1	< 1		< 1
	Chills	< 1	< 1	< 1		<1
	Edema	< 1	< 1	< 1		< 1
	Fever		< 1		✓[2]	1-3

FLUOROQUINOLONES

	Adverse reactions	Ciprofloxacin[1]	Enoxacin	Lomefloxacin	Norfloxacin	Ofloxacin[1]
Abnormal laboratory values	↑ALT/↑ AST	1.9/1.7	< 1	≤ 0.4	1.8/1.8	≥ 1/0
	↑ Alkaline phosphatase	0.8	< 1	0.1	1.4	
	↑ LDH	0.4			✓[2]	
	↑ Bilirubin	0.3	< 1	0.1		
	Eosinophilia	0.6	< 1	≤ 0.1	1.8	≥ 1
	Leukopenia	0.4	< 1	≤ 0.1	1.2	
	↑ or ↓ Platelets	0.1	< 1	≤ 1	✓[2]	
	Pancytopenia	0.1				
	↑ ESR/ Lymphocytopenia			0.1		≥ 1
	Neutropenia				1.2	
	↑ Serum creatinine	1.1			✓[2]	
	↑ BUN	0.9		0.1	✓[2]	
	Crystalluria/ Cylinduria/ Candiduria	✓[2]			✓[2]	
	Hematuria	✓[2]				≥ 1
	Glucosuria/Pyuria					≥ 1
	Proteinuria/ Albuminuria	✓[2]	< 1	≤ 0.1		≥ 1
	↑ γ-glutamyltransferase	< 0.1		≤ 0.1		
	↑ Serum amylase	< 0.1				
	↑ Uric acid	< 0.1				
	↑ or ↓ Blood glucose	< 0.1		≤ 0.1		≥ 1
	↓ Hemoglobin/ hematocrit	< 0.1	< 1	≤ 0.1	✓[2]	
	↑ or ↓ Potassium	< 0.1	< 1	0.1		
	Anemia	< 0.1		≤ 0.1		
	Bleeding/↑ PT	< 0.1		≤ 0.1		
	↑ Monocytes	< 0.1		0.3		
	Leukocytosis	< 0.1	< 1			≥ 1
	↑ Triglycerides/ cholesterol	✓[2]				

Table title: Fluoroquinolone Adverse Reactions (%)

[1] Includes data for oral and IV formulations.
[2] ✓ = Adverse reaction observed, incidence not reported.
[3] See Warnings or Precautions.

Other adverse reactions listed only for the individual agents:

Ciprofloxacin:

GU – Acidosis, interstitial nephritis, nephritis, renal failure, polyuria, urinary retention, urethral bleeding (< 1%); vaginal candidiasis; renal calculi.

Cardiovascular – Angina pectoris, atrial flutter, cardiopulmonary arrest, cerebral thrombosis, myocardial infarction, ventricular ectopy (< 1%); postural hypotension.

Respiratory – Bronchospasm, dyspnea, epistaxis, hemoptysis, hiccoughs, laryngeal/pulmonary edema, pulmonary embolism (<1%).

Special Senses – Bad taste in mouth, eye pain, tinnitus (< 1%); nystagmus.

Miscellaneous – Restlessness (1.1%); oral/cutaneous candidiasis, intestinal perforation, GI bleeding, nightmares, irritability, tremor, ataxia, anorexia, urticaria, flushing, hyperpigmentation, erythema nodosum (< 1%); hepatic necrosis; exacerbation of myasthenia gravis; dysphasia; agranulocytosis; cholestatic jaundice.

Norfloxacin:

Miscellaneous – Erythema; myoclonus (rare); erythema multiforme; hepatitis; pancreatitis; stomatitis; arthralgia.

FLUOROQUINOLONES

Ofloxacin:

GU – Vaginal discharge, genital pruritus (1% to 3%); burning/irritation/pain of female genitalia, dysmenorrhea, menorrhagia, metrorrhagia, urinary frequency/pain (< 1%).

Cardiovascular – Chest pain (1% to 3%); vasodilation (< 1%).

Respiratory – Cough, rhinorrhea (< 1%).

Special Senses – Dysgeusia (1% to 3%); photophobia (< 1%).

CNS – Sleep disorders, nervousness (1% to 3%); anxiety, cognitive change, dream abnormality, euphoria, vertigo (< 1%).

Miscellaneous – Decreased appetite (1% to 3%); arthralgia, asthenia, diaphoresis, myalgia, thirst, vasculitis, weight loss (< 1%).

Lomefloxacin:

GU – Dysuria, hematuria, strangury, micturition disorder, anuria, leukorrhea, intermenstrual bleeding, perineal pain, vaginal moniliasis, orchitis, epididymitis (< 1%).

Cardiovascular – Hypotension, tachycardia, bradycardia, arrhythmia, extrasystoles, cyanosis, cardiac failure, angina pectoris, myocardial infarction, pulmonary embolism, cerebrovascular disorder, cardiomyopathy, phlebitis (< 1%).

Respiratory – Dyspnea, respiratory infection, epistaxis, respiratory disorder, bronchospasm, cough, increased sputum, stridor (< 1%).

CNS – Coma, hyperkinesia, tremor, vertigo, nervousness, anorexia, anxiety, agitation, increased appetite, depersonalization, paroniria (< 1%).

GI – GI inflammation/bleeding, dysphagia, tongue discoloration, bad taste (< 1%).

Special Senses – Earache, tinnitus, conjunctivitis, eye pain (< 1%).

Dermatologic – Urticaria, eczema, skin exfoliation, skin disorder (< 1%).

Miscellaneous – Flushing, increased sweating, back/chest pain, asthenia, facial edema, influenza-like symptoms, decreased heat tolerance, purpura, lymphadenopathy, increased fibrinolysis, thirst, gout, hypoglycemia, leg cramps, arthralgia, myalgia (< 1%); abnormalities of urine specific gravity or serum electrolytes (≤ 0.1%).

Enoxacin:

GI – Anorexia, bloody stools, gastritis, stomatitis (< 1%).

CNS – Nervousness, anxiety, tremor, agitation, myoclonus, depersonalization, hypertonia (< 1%).

Dermatologic – Urticaria, hyperhidrosis, mycotic infection, erythema multiforme (< 1%).

Special Senses – Vertigo (3%); unusual taste (1%); tinnitus, conjunctivitis (< 1%).

Respiratory – Dyspnea, cough, epistaxis (< 1%).

GU – Vaginal moniliasis, urinary incontinence, renal failure (< 1%).

Miscellaneous – Asthenia, back/chest pain, myalgia, arthralgia, tachycardia, vasodilation, purpura (< 1%).

Overdosage:

Symptoms: One patient developed oliguric acute renal failure following ingestion of 21 g of ciprofloxacin (serum concentration, 12 mcg/ml). The patient responded to prednisone therapy.

Treatment: Empty the stomach by inducing vomiting or by gastric lavage. Observe patient carefully and give symptomatic and supportive treatment. Maintain adequate hydration. Refer to General Management of Acute Overdosage.

Hemodialysis or peritoneal dialysis may aid in the removal of **ciprofloxacin**, particularly if renal function is compromised. **Ofloxacin, enoxacin, norfloxacin** and **lomefloxacin** are not efficiently removed by dialysis.

Patient Information:

Drink fluids liberally.

Do not take antacids containing magnesium or aluminum or products containing iron or zinc simultaneously or within 4 hours before or 2 hours after dosing.

May cause dizziness or lightheadedness; observe caution while driving or performing other tasks requiring alertness, coordination or physical dexterity. CNS stimulation may occur (eg, tremor, restlessness, confusion); use with caution in patients predisposed to seizures or with other CNS disorders.

Take **norfloxacin** and **enoxacin** 1 hour before or 2 hours after meals. Do not take **ofloxacin** with food. **Ciprofloxacin** and **lomefloxacin** can be taken without regard to meals; however, the preferred time of ciprofloxacin dosing is 2 hours after a meal.

Hypersensitivity reactions may occur, even following the first dose; discontinue the drug at the first sign of skin rash or other allergic reaction.

Avoid excessive sunlight/artificial ultraviolet light; discontinue drug if phototoxicity occurs. Avoid re-exposure to ultraviolet light. Reactions may recur up to several weeks after stopping therapy. See Warnings.

CIPROFLOXACIN

Complete prescribing information for these products begins in the Fluoroquinolones group monograph.

Indications:

For the treatment of infections caused by susceptible strains of the designated microorganisms in the conditions listed below:

Lower respiratory infections caused by *Escherichia coli, Klebsiella pneumoniae, Enterobacter cloacae, Proteus mirabilis, Pseudomonas aeruginosa, Haemophilus influenzae, Haemophilus parainfluenzae* and *Streptococcus pneumoniae.*

Skin and skin structure infections caused by *E coli, K pneumoniae, E cloacae, P mirabilis, Proteus vulgaris, Providencia stuartii, Morganella morganii, Citrobacter freundii, Streptococcus pyogenes, P aeruginosa* and *Staphylococcus aureus* (penicillinase- and nonpenicillinase-producing strains) and *Staphylococcus epidermidis.*

Bone/joint infections caused by *E cloacae, Serratia marcescens* and *P aeruginosa.*

Urinary tract infections caused by *E coli, K pneumoniae, E cloacae, Serratia marcescens, P mirabilis, Providencia rettgeri, M morganii, Citrobacter diversus, C freundii, P aeruginosa, S epidermidis* and *Enterococcus faecalis.*

Infectious diarrhea caused by *E coli* (enterotoxigenic strains), *Campylobacter jejuni, Shigella flexneri* and *Shigella sonnei* when antibacterial therapy is indicated.

Typhoid fever (enteric fever) caused by *Salmonella typhi.* Efficacy in the eradication of the chronic typhoid carrier state has not been demonstrated.

Sexually transmitted diseases: Uncomplicated cervical and urethral gonorrhea due to *Neisseria gonorrhoeae.*

Administration and Dosage:

Approved by the FDA in 1987.

Ciprofloxacin Dosage Guidelines

Location of infection	Type or severity	Unit dose	Frequency	Daily dose
Urinary tract	mild/moderate	250 mg (200 mg IV)	q 12 h	500 mg (400 mg IV)
	severe/complicated	500 mg (400 mg IV)	q 12 h	1000 mg (800 mg IV)
Lower respiratory tract Bone and joint Skin & skin structure	mild/moderate	500 mg (400 mg IV)	q 12 h	1000 mg (800 mg IV)
	severe/complicated	750 mg	q 12 h	1500 mg
Infectious diarrhea	mild/moderate/severe	500 mg	q 12 h	1000 mg
Typhoid fever	mild/moderate	500 mg	q 12 h	1000 mg
Urethral/Cervical gonococcal infections	uncomplicated	250 mg	single dose	-

The duration of treatment depends upon the severity of infection. Generally, continue ciprofloxacin for at least 2 days after the signs and symptoms of infection have disappeared. The usual duration is 7 to 14 days; however, for severe and complicated infections, more prolonged therapy may be required. Bone and joint infections may require treatment for 4 to 6 weeks or longer. Infectious diarrhea may be treated for 5 to 7 days. Typhoid fever should be treated for 10 days.

Renal function impairment: The following table provides dosage guidelines; however, monitoring of serum drug levels provides the most reliable basis for dosage adjustment:

Ciprofloxacin Dosage in Impaired Renal Function

Creatinine clearance (ml/min)	Dose
> 50 (oral); ≥ 30 (IV)	See usual dosage
30-50	250-500 mg q 12 h
5-29	250-500 mg q 18 h (oral); 200-400 mg q 18-24 h (IV)
Hemodialysis or peritoneal dialysis	250-500 mg q 24 h (after dialysis)

When only the serum creatinine concentration is known, this formula may be used to estimate Ccr. Serum creatinine should represent a steady state of renal function.

$$\text{Males: } \frac{\text{Weight (kg)} \times (140 - \text{age})}{72 \times \text{serum creatinine (mg/dl)}} = \text{Ccr}$$

Females: 0.85 × above value

CIPROFLOXACIN

In patients with severe infections and severe renal impairment, a unit dose of 750 mg may be administered orally at the intervals noted in the table; however, carefully monitor patients and measure serum ciprofloxacin concentration periodically. Peak concentrations (1 to 2 hours after dosing) should generally range from 2 to 4 mcg/ml. For patients with changing renal function or with renal impairment and hepatic insufficiency, measurement of serum levels will provide additional guidance for adjusting dosage.

CDC recommended treatment schedules for chancroid and gonorrhea†:

Chancroid (H ducreyi infection) – 500 mg orally 2 times a day for 3 days (alternative regimen).

Gonococcal infections –

Disseminated: 500 mg orally 2 times a day to complete a full week of therapy after treatment with initial regimen (ceftriaxone 1 g IM or IV every 24 hours) for 24 to 48 hours after improvement begins.

Uncomplicated: 500 mg orally in a single dose plus doxycycline.

IV: Administer by IV infusion over 60 minutes. Slow infusion of a dilute solution into a large vein will minimize patient discomfort and reduce the risk of venous irritation.

Vials – Prepare the IV dose by aseptically withdrawing the appropriate volume of concentrate from the vials. Dilute before use with a suitable IV solution to a final concentration of 1 to 2 mg/ml (see Compatibility/Stability).

Admixture compatibility/stability – Stable up to 14 days at refrigerated or room temperature (5° to 25°C; 41° to 77°F) when diluted with 0.9% NaCl Injection, USP or 5% Dextrose Injection, USP. Protect from light and freezing. If a Y-type IV infusion set or a piggyback method is used, temporarily discontinue the administration of any other solutions during the ciprofloxacin infusion.

Admixture incompatibility: Ciprofloxacin is incompatible with the following agents: Aminophylline; amoxicillin sodium (alone and with potassium clavulanate); clindamycin; mezlocillin.

Rx	**Cipro** (Bayer)	**Tablets:** 100 mg	(Cipro 100). Yellow. Film-coated. In *Cipro Cystitis Packs* 6s.
		250 mg	(Cipro 250). Yellowish. Film coated. In 100s and UD 100s.
		500 mg	(Cipro 500). Yellowish. Film coated. Capsule shape. In 100s and UD 100s.
		750 mg	(Cipro 750). Yellowish. Film coated. Capsule shape. In 50s and UD 100s.
Rx	**Cipro I.V.** (Bayer)	**Injection:** 200 mg	Lactic acid. In 20 ml vials (1%) and 100 ml in 5% dextrose flexible containers (0.2%).
		400 mg	Lactic acid. In 40 ml vials (1%) and 200 ml in 5% dextrose flexible containers (0.2%).

NORFLOXACIN

For complete prescribing information, refer to the Fluoroquinolones group monograph.

Indications:

For the treatment of adults with the following infections caused by susceptible strains of the designated microorganisms in the conditions listed below:

Urinary tract infections: Uncomplicated infections (including cystitis) caused by *Enterococcus faecalis, E coli, K pneumoniae, P mirabilis, P aeruginosa, S epidermidis, S saprophyticus, C freundii, Enterobacter aerogenes, Enterobacter cloacae, P vulgaris, S aureus* or *S agalactiae;* complicated infections caused by *Enterococcus faecalis, E coli, K pneumoniae, P mirabilis, P aeruginosa* or *Serratia marcescens.*

Sexually transmitted diseases: Uncomplicated urethral and cervical gonorrhea caused by *N gonorrhoeae.*

Prostatitis due to *E coli.*

Administration and Dosage:

Approved by the FDA in 1986.

Take 1 hour before or 2 hours after meals with glass of water. Patients should be well hydrated.

† CDC 1993 Sexually Transmitted Diseases Treatment Guidelines. *Morbidity and Mortality Weekly Report* 1993 Sep 24; 42 (No. RR-14): 1–102.

NORFLOXACIN

Recommended Norfloxacin Dosage					
Infection	Description	Dose	Frequency	Duration	Daily dose
Urinary tract infections (UTI)	Uncomplicated (cystitis) due to *E coli, K pneumoniae* or *P mirabilis*	400 mg	q 12 h	3 days	800 mg
	Uncomplicated due to other organisms	400 mg	q 12 h	7-10 days	800 mg
	Complicated	400 mg	q 12 h	10-21 days	800 mg
Sexually transmitted diseases	Uncomplicated gonorrhea	800 mg	single dose	1 day	800 mg
Prostatitis	Acute or chronic	400 mg	q 12 h	28 days	800 mg

Renal function impairment: In patients with a Ccr rate ≤ 30 ml/min/1.73 m^2, administer 400 mg once daily for the duration given above.

When only the serum creatinine is known, the following formula may be used to estimate Ccr. The serum creatinine should represent a steady state of renal function.

$$\text{Males: } \frac{\text{Weight (kg)} \times (140 - \text{age})}{72 \times \text{serum creatinine (mg/dl)}} = \text{Ccr}$$

Females: 0.85 × above value

Elderly: Dose based on normal or impaired renal function.

CDC recommended treatment schedules for gonorrhea:†

Gonococcal infections, uncomplicated – 800 mg as a single dose (alternative regimen to ciprofloxacin or ofloxacin).

Rx	**Noroxin** (Roberts)	**Tablets:** 400 mg	(MSD 705 Noroxin). Dark pink. Film coated. In 100s and UD 20s and 100s.

† CDC 1993 Sexually Transmitted Diseases Treatment Guidelines. *Morbidity and Mortality Weekly Report* 1993 Sept 24; 42 (No. RR-14): 1–102.

OFLOXACIN

For complete prescribing information, refer to the Fluoroquinolones group monograph.

Indications:

For the treatment of adults with the following infections caused by susceptible strains of the designated microorganisms. Use IV administration when this route is advantageous to the patient (eg, patient cannot tolerate an oral dosage form).

In the absence of vomiting or other factors interfering with the absorption of orally administered drug, patients receive essentially the same systemic antimicrobial therapy after equivalent doses of ofloxacin administered by either the oral or the IV route. Therefore, the IV formulation does not provide a higher degree of efficacy or more potent antimicrobial activity than an equivalent dose of the oral formulation.

Lower respiratory tract infections: Acute bacterial exacerbations of chronic bronchitis or community-acquired pneumonia due to *H influenzae* or *S pneumoniae.*

Sexually transmitted diseases: See Warnings. Acute, uncomplicated urethral and cervical gonorrhea due to *N gonorrhoeae;* nongonococcal urethritis and cervicitis due to *Chlamydia trachomatis;* mixed infections of urethra and cervix due to both organisms.

Skin and skin structure infections (uncomplicated) due to *S aureus, S pyogenes* or *P mirabilis.*

Urinary tract infections: Uncomplicated cystitis due to *Citrobacter diversus, Enterobacter aerogenes, E coli, K pneumoniae, P mirabilis* or *P aeruginosa;* complicated UTIs due to *E coli, K pneumoniae, P mirabilis, Citrobacter diversus* or *P aeruginosa.*

Prostatitis due to *E coli.*

Administration and Dosage:

Approved by the FDA in 1990.

Usual daily dose is 200 to 400 mg every 12 hours as described in the following table:

Ofloxacin Dosage Guidelines (Oral and IV)

Infection	Description	Unit dose	Frequency	Duration	Daily dose
Lower respiratory tract	Exacerbation of chronic bronchitis	400 mg	q 12 h	10 days	800 mg
	Pneumonia	400 mg	q 12 h	10 days	800 mg
Sexually transmitted diseases	Acute, uncomplicated gonorrhea	400 mg	single dose	1 day	400 mg
	Cervicitis/urethritis due to *C trachomatis*	300 mg	q 12 h	7 days	600 mg
	Cervicitis/urethritis due to *C trachomatis and N gonorrhoeae*	300 mg	q 12 h	7 days	600 mg
Skin and skin structure	Mild to moderate	400 mg	q 12 h	10 days	800 mg
Urinary tract	Cystitis due to *E coli or K pneumoniae*	200 mg	q 12 h	3 days	400 mg
	Cystitis due to other organisms	200 mg	q 12 h	7 days	400 mg
	Complicated UTIs	200 mg	q 12 h	10 days	400 mg
Prostatitis		300 mg	q 12 h	6 weeks[1]	600 mg

[1] Because there are no safety data presently available to support the use of the IV formulation for > 10 days, switch to oral therapy or other appropriate therapy after 10 days.

Renal function impairment: Adjust dosage in patients with a Ccr value of ≤ 50 ml/min. After a normal initial dose, adjust the dosing interval as follows: Ccr 10-50 ml/min, use a 24 hour interval and do not adjust dosage; Ccr < 10 ml/min, use a 24 hour interval and one-half the recommended dosage.

When only the serum creatinine is known, the following formula may be used to estimate Ccr. Serum creatinine should represent a steady state of renal function.

$$\text{Males: } \frac{\text{Weight (kg)} \times (140 - \text{age})}{72 \times \text{serum creatinine (mg/dl)}} = \text{Ccr}$$

Females: 0.85 × above value

OFLOXACIN

CDC recommended treatment schedules for chlamydia, epididymitis, pelvic inflammatory disease (PID) and gonorrhea†:

Chlamydia – 300 mg orally 2 times a day for 7 days (alternative regimen).

Epididymitis – 300 mg orally 2 times a day for 10 days (alternative regimen).

PID, outpatient – 400 mg orally 2 times a day for 14 days plus clindamycin or metronidazole.

Gonococcal infections, uncomplicated – 400 mg orally in a single dose plus doxycycline.

IV: Administer by IV infusion only. Do not give IM, intrathecally, intraperitoneally or SC. Avoid rapid or bolus IV infusion; administer slowly over a period of not less than 60 min.

Single-use vials – Must be diluted prior to use (see Compatible IV solutions). The resulting concentration is 4 mg/ml. Prepare the desired dosage as follows:

Preparation of Ofloxacin Dosage From Single-Use Vials

Desired strength (mg)	Volume to withdraw (ml)		Volume of diluent	Infusion time (min)
	From 10 ml vial	From 20 ml vial		
200	5	10	qs 50 ml	60
300	7.5	15	qs 75 ml	60
400	10	20	qs 100 ml	60

Compatible IV solutions – 0.9% Sodium Chloride; 5% Dextrose; 5% Dextrose/0.9% Sodium Chloride; 5% Dextrose in Lactated Ringer's; 5% Sodium Bicarbonate; *Plasma-Lyte* 56 in 5% Dextrose; 5% Dextrose, 0.45% Sodium Chloride and 0.15% Potassium Chloride; Sodium Lactate (M/6); Water for Injection.† Efficacy for this organism in this organ system was studied in fewer than 10 infections.

Premixed bottles/flexible containers – No further dilution is necessary; already premixed in 5% Dextrose.

Storage/Stability – Preservative free; discard unused portions. Store premixed flexible containers at ≤ 25° C (77° F). Brief exposure up to 40° C (104° F) does not adversely affect the product. Avoid excessive heat and protect from freezing and light.

Rx	**Floxin** (Ortho)	**Tablets:** 200 mg	(Floxin 200). Pale gold. Film coated. In 50s and UD 100s.
		300 mg	(Floxin 300). Pale gold. Film coated. In 50s and UD 100s.
		400 mg	(Floxin 400). Pale gold. Film coated. In 50s and UD 100s.
		Injection: 200 mg[1]	In 50 ml single-use premixed flexible containers in 5% dextrose.
		400 mg[1]	In 10 and 20 ml single-use vials in Water for Injection, and 100 ml single-use premixed bottles or flexible containers in 5% dextrose.

[1] Preservative free.

† CDC 1993 Sexually Transmitted Diseases Treatment Guidelines. *Morbidity and Mortality Weekly Report* 1993 Sept 24; 42 (No. RR-14): 1–102.

ENOXACIN

Complete prescribing information for these products begins in the Fluoroquinolones group monograph.

Indications:

For the treatment of adults (≥ 18 years of age) with infections caused by susceptible strains of the designated microorganisms in the conditions listed below:

Sexually transmitted diseases: Uncomplicated urethral or cervical gonorrhea due to *Neisseria gonorrhoeae.*

Urinary tract infections: Uncomplicated (cystitis) due to *Escherichia coli, Staphylococcus epidermidis* or *S saprophyticus;* complicated due to *E coli, Klebsiella pneumoniae, Proteus mirabilis, Pseudomonas aeruginosa, S epidermidis* or *Enterobacter cloacae.*

Administration and Dosage:

Approved by the FDA on December 31, 1991.

Take at least 1 hour before or 2 hours after a meal.

Enoxacin Dosage Guidelines

Infection	Description	Dose	Frequency	Duration	Daily dose
Urinary tract infections	Uncomplicated (cystitis)	200 mg	q 12 h	7 days	400 mg
	Complicated	400 mg	q 12 h	14 days	800 mg
Sexually transmitted diseases	Uncomplicated gonorrhea	400 mg	single dose	1 day	400 mg

Renal function impairment: Adjust dosage in patients with a creatinine clearance (Ccr) ≤ 30 ml/min/1.73 m^2. After a normal initial dose, use a 12 hour interval and one-half the recommended dose.

When only the serum creatinine is known, the following formula may be used to estimate Ccr. Serum creatinine should represent a steady state of renal function.

$$\text{Males: } \frac{\text{Weight (kg)} \times (140 - \text{age})}{72 \times \text{serum creatinine (mg/dl)}} = \text{Ccr}$$

Females: 0.85 × above value

Elderly: Dosage adjustment is not necessary with normal renal function; however, adjust according to previous guidelines in patients with compromised renal function.

CDC recommended treatment schedules for gonorrhea:†

Gonococcal infections, uncomplicated – 400 mg as a single dose (alternative regimen to ciprofloxacin or ofloxacin).

Rx	**Penetrex** (Rhone-Poulenc Rorer)	**Tablets:** 200 mg	(5100). Light blue. Film coated. In 50s.
		400 mg	(5140). Dark blue. Film coated. In 50s.

† CDC 1993 Sexually Transmitted Diseases Treatment Guidelines. *Morbidity and Mortality Weekly Report* 1993 Sept 24; 42 (RR-14): 1–102.

LOMEFLOXACIN HCl

Complete prescribing information for these products begins in the Fluoroquinolones group monograph.

Indications:

For the treatment of adults with mild to moderate infections caused by susceptible strains of the designated microorganisms in the conditions listed below:

Lower respiratory tract infections:

Acute bacterial exacerbation of chronic bronchitis caused by *Haemophilus influenzae* or *Moraxella (Branhamella) catarrhalis. Note:* Lomefloxacin is not indicated for the empiric treatment of acute bacterial exacerbation of chronic bronchitis when it is probable that *Streptococcus pneumoniae* is a causative pathogen (see Warnings).

Urinary tract infections:

Uncomplicated (cystitis) caused by *Escherichia coli, Klebsiella pneumoniae, Proteus mirabilis* or *Staphylococcus saprophyticus.*

Complicated caused by *E. coli, K. pneumoniae, P. mirabilis, Pseudomonas aeruginosa, Citrobacter diversus* or *Enterobacter cloacae.*

Prophylaxis: Preoperatively to reduce the incidence of urinary tract infections in the early postoperative period (3 to 5 days postsurgery) in patients undergoing transurethral procedures. Efficacy in decreasing the incidence of other infections in the early postoperative period has not been established. Do not use in minor urologic procedures for which prophylaxis is not indicated (eg, simple cystoscopy, retrograde pyelography).

Administration and Dosage:

Approved by the FDA on February 21, 1992.

Lomefloxacin may be taken without regard to meals (see Actions).

Recommended Daily Dose of Lomefloxacin					
Body system	Infection	Dose	Frequency	Duration	Daily dose
Lower respiratory tract	Acute bacterial exacerbation of chronic bronchitis	400 mg	once daily	10 days	400 mg
Urinary tract	Cystitis	400 mg	once daily	10 days	400 mg
	Complicated urinary tract infections	400 mg	once daily	14 days	400 mg

Elderly: No dosage adjustment is needed for elderly patients with normal renal function (Ccr ≥ 40 ml/min/1.73 m^2).

Renal function impairment: Lomefloxacin is primarily eliminated by renal excretion. Modification of dosage is recommended in patients with renal dysfunction. In patients with a Ccr > 10 but < 40 ml/min/1.73 m^2, the recommended dosage is an initial loading dose of 400 mg followed by daily maintenance doses of 200 mg once daily for the duration of treatment. It is suggested that serial determinations of lomefloxacin levels be performed to determine any necessary alteration in the appropriate next dosing interval. If only the serum creatinine is known, the following formula may be used to estimate Ccr:

$$\text{Males: } \frac{\text{Weight (kg)} \times (140 - \text{age})}{72 \times \text{serum creatinine (mg/dl)}} = \text{Ccr}$$

Females: 0.85 × above value

Dialysis patients: Hemodialysis removes only a negligible amount of lomefloxacin (3% in 4 hours). Hemodialysis patients should receive an initial loading dose of 400 mg followed by maintenance doses of 200 mg once daily for duration of treatment.

Cirrhosis: Cirrhosis does not reduce the non-renal clearance of lomefloxacin. Base the need for a dosage reduction in this population on the degree of renal function and plasma concentrations.

Prophylaxis: A single 400 mg dose 2 to 6 hrs prior to surgery when oral pre-operative prophylaxis for transurethral surgical procedures is considered appropriate.

CDC recommended treatment schedules for gonorrhea:†

Gonococcal infections, uncomplicated – 400 mg as a single dose (alternative regimen to ciprofloxacin or ofloxacin).

Rx	**Maxaquin** (Searle)	**Tablets:** 400 mg	(Maxaquin 400). White, scored. Film coated. Oval. In 20s & UD 100s.

† CDC 1993 Sexually Transmitted Diseases Treatment Guidelines. *Morbidity and Mortality Weekly Report* 1993 Sept 24;42(RR-14):59.

SPARFLOXACIN

Complete prescribing information for these products begins in the Fluoroquinolones group monograph.

Indications:

For the treatment of adults (≥ 18 years of age) with the following infections caused by susceptible strains of the designated microorganisms in the conditions listed below:

Community-acquired pneumonia caused by *Chlamydia pneumoniae, Haemophilus influenzae, Haemophilus parainfluenzae, Moraxella catarrhalis, Mycoplasma pneumoniae* or *Streptococcus pneumoniae.*

Acute bacterial exacerbations of chronic bronchitis caused by *C. pneumoniae, Enterobacter cloacae, H. influenzae, H. parainfluenzae, Klebsiella pneumoniae, M. catarrhalis, Staphylococcus aureus* or *S. pneumoniae.*

Administration and Dosage:

Approved by the FDA on December 20, 1996.

Sparfloxacin can be taken with or without food.

The recommended daily dose of sparfloxacin in patients with normal renal function is two 200 mg tablets taken on the first day as a loading dose. Thereafter, take one 200 mg tablet every 24 hours for a total of 10 days of therapy (11 tablets).

Renal function impairment: The recommended daily dose of sparfloxacin in patients with renal impairment (creatinine clearance < 50 ml/min) is two 200 mg tablets taken on the first day as a loading dose. Thereafter, take one 200 mg tablet every 48 hours for a total of 9 days of therapy (6 tablets).

Rx	**Zagam** (Rhone-Poulenc Rorer)	**Tablets:** 200 mg	(RPR 201). White. Round. Film coated. In 55s and Blister Pack 11s.

LEVOFLOXACIN

Complete prescribing information for these products begins in the Fluoroquinolones group monograph.

Indications:

Acute maxiliary sinusitis due to *Streptococcus pneumoniae, Haemophilus influenzae* or *Moraxella catarrhalis.*

Acute bacterial exacerbation of chronic bronchitis due to *Staphylococcus aureus, S. pneumoniae, H. influenzae, H. parainfluenzae* or *M. catarrhalis.*

Community acquired pneumonia due to *S. aureus, S. pneumoniae, H. influenzae, H. parainfluenzae, Klebsiella pneumoniae, M. catarrhalis, Chlamydia pneumoniae, Legionella pneumophila* or *Mycoplasma pneumoniae.*

Uncomplicated skin and skin structure infections (mild to moderate) including abscesses, cellulitis, furuncles, impetigo, pyoderma, wound infections due to *S. aureus* or *Streptococcus pyogenes.*

Complicated urinary tract infections (mild to moderate) due to *Enterococcus faecalis, Enterobacter cloacae, Escherichia coli, Klebsiella pneumoniae, Proteus mirabilis* or *Pseudomonas aeruginosa.*

Acute pyelonephritis (mild to moderate) caused by *E. coli.*

Administration and Dosage:

Tablets: The usual dose is 500 mg orally every 24 hours as described in the following dosing chart. These recommendations apply to patients with normal renal function. Administer oral doses at least 2 hours before or 2 hours after antacids containing magnesium or aluminum, as well as sucralfate, metal cations such as iron and multivitamin preparations with zinc.

Levofloxacin Dosing				
Infection*	Unit dose	Frequency	Duration	Daily dose
Acute bacterial exacerbation of chronic bronchitis	500 mg	every 24 hours	7 days	500 mg
Community acquired pneumonia	500 mg	every 24 hours	7-14 days	500 mg
Acute maxillary sinusitis	500 mg	every 24 hours	10-14 days	500 mg
Uncomplicated SSSI	500 mg	every 24 hours	7-10 days	500 mg
Complicated UTI	250 mg	every 24 hours	10 days	250 mg
Acute pyelonephritis	250 mg	every 24 hours	10 days	250 mg

* Due to the designated pathogens (see Indications).

Levofloxacin Dosing with Renal Function Impairment		
Renal status	Initial dose	Subsequent dose
Acute bacterial exacerbation of chronic bronchitis/Community acquired pneumonia/Acute maxillary sinusitis/Uncomplicated SSSI		
Ccr[1] from 50 to 80 ml/min	No dosage adustment required	
Ccr[1] from 20 to 49 ml/min	500 mg	250 mg every 24 hours
Ccr[1] from 10 to 19 ml/min	500 mg	250 mg every 48 hours
Hemodialysis	500 mg	250 mg every 48 hours
CAPD[2]	500 mg	250 mg every 48 hours
Complicated UTI/Acute pyelonephritis		
Ccr[1] ≥ 20 ml/min	No dosage adjustment required	
Ccr[1] from 10 to 19 ml/min	250 mg	250 mg every 48 hours

[1] Ccr = creatinine clearance.
[2] CAPD = chronic ambulatory peritoneal dialysis.

Injection: Administer by IV only, slowly over a period of not less than 60 minutes.

Admixture compatibilities:

- 0.9% Sodium Chloride Injection
- 5% Dextrose Injection
- 5% Dextrose/0.9% Sodium Chloride Injection
- 5% Dextrose in Lactated Ringers
- *Plasma-Lyte* 56/5% Dextrose Injection
- 5% Dextrose, 0.45% Sodium Chloride
- 0.15% Potassium Chloride Injection
- Sodium Lactate Injection (M/6)

LEVOFLOXACIN

Storage/Stability:

Lovefloxacin tablets should be stored at 15° to 30°C (59° to 85°F) in well-closed containers.

Lovefloxacin injection, when diluted in a compatible intravenous fluid to a concentration of 5 mg/ml is stable for 72 hours when stored ≤ 25°C (77°F) and for 14 days when stored under refrigeration at 5°C (41°F) in plastic IV containers. Solutions that are diluted in a compatible intravenous solution and frozen in glass bottles or plastic IV containers are stable for 6 months when stored at –20°C (–4°F). Thaw frozen solutions at room temperature 25°C (77°F) or in a refrigerator 8°C (46°F). Do not force thaw by microwave irradiation or by bath immersion. Do not refreeze after initial thawing.

Rx	**Levaquin** (McNeil Pharmaceutical)	**Tablets:** 250 mg	(McNeil 1520 250.) Terra cotta pink. Film coated. Rectangular. In 50s and UD 100s.
		500 mg	(McNeil 1525 500.) Peach. Film coated. Rectangular. In 50s and UD 100s.
		Injection: 500 mg	In single-use 20 ml vials.
		Injection (premix): 250 mg	In 50 ml flexible containers with 5% Dextrose solution.
		500 mg	In 100 ml flexible containers with 5% Dextrose solution.

TETRACYCLINES

Actions:

Pharmacokinetics:

Absorption/Distribution – Tetracyclines are adequately but incompletely absorbed in children and adults in the fasting state. The percentage of an oral dose absorbed is highest for doxycycline and minocycline, and intermediate for oxytetracycline, methacycline, demeclocycline and tetracycline. Achlorhydria has no effect on absorption. Food decreases absorption of tetracyclines, except doxycycline and minocycline; take these two agents with food.

Doxycycline and minocycline are highly lipid soluble, and readily penetrate into the cerebrospinal fluid (CSF), brain, eye and prostate. In addition, minocycline displays good penetration of saliva, making it useful in eliminating meningococci from asymptomatic carriers. Tetracycline and demeclocycline are intermediate in terms of lipid solubility, whereas oxytetracycline is the least lipid soluble. Oxytetracycline diffuses readily through the placenta into fetal circulation, into pleural fluid and under some circumstances into the CSF.

Metabolism/Excretion – Hemodialysis removes 20% to 30% of tetracycline, but has little effect on doxycycline or minocycline. Peritoneal dialysis has no effect on any of the tetracyclines.

The tetracyclines are concentrated by the liver in the bile and excreted in the urine and feces, largely unchanged; therefore, make appropriate dosage adjustments in patients with impaired renal function. Conventional tetracyclines are contraindicated in anuria. Doxycycline and minocycline are excreted largely by nonrenal routes; their serum half-lives do not significantly increase in renal impairment. Doxycycline is secreted in an inactive form into the intestinal lumen and eliminated with feces; hence, its half-life is largely independent of renal or hepatic function. Minocycline is metabolized, and its half-life is prolonged in oliguria.

Tetracycline Pharmacokinetic Variables and Dosage Regimens

Tetracyclines	Serum Protein Binding (%)	Normal Serum Half-Life (hrs)	% Excreted Unchanged in Urine	Usual Oral Adult Maintenance Dosage	Lipid Solubility
Tetracycline	65	16 to 12	60	250 mg q 6 h or 500 mg q 6 to 12 h	Intermediate
Demeclocycline	65 to 91	12 to 16	39	150 mg q 6 h or 300 mg q 12 h	Intermediate
Doxycycline	80 to 95	15 to 25	30 to 42	150 mg q 12 h or 100 mg q 24 h	High
Methacycline	80 to 90	14 to 16	50 to 60	150 mg q 6 h or 300 mg q 12 h	
Minocycline	70 to 80	11 to 18	16 to 12	100 mg q 12 h	High
Oxytetracycline	20 to 40	16 to 12	70	250 to 500 mg q 6 h	Low

Microbiology: The tetracyclines are bacteriostatic. They exert their antimicrobial effect by inhibition of protein synthesis. Tetracyclines are active against a wide range of gram-negative and gram-positive organisms (see Indications). The tetracyclines have similar antimicrobial spectra, and cross-resistance is common.

Indications:

Infections caused by the following microorganisms: Rickettsiae (Rocky Mountain spotted fever, typhus fever and the typhus group, Q fever, rickettsialpox and tick fevers); Mycoplasma pneumoniae (PPLO, Eaton agent); agents of psittacosis and ornithosis; agents of lymphogranuloma venereum and granuloma inguinale; the spirochetal agent of relapsing fever *(Borrelia recurrentis)*.

Infections caused by the following gram-negative microorganisms: *Hemophilus ducreyi* (chancroid); *Yersinia pestis* and *Francisella tularensis* (formerly *Pasteurella pestis* and *P tularensis*); *Bartonella bacilliformis; Bacteroides* sp; *Campylobacter fetus* (formerly *Vibrio fetus*); *V cholerae* (formerly *V comma*); *Brucella* sp (in conjunction with streptomycin).

Infections caused by the following microorganisms, when bacteriologic testing indicates appropriate susceptibility to the drug:

Gram-negative – Escherichia coli; Enterobacter aerogenes (formerly *Aerobacter aerogenes*); *Shigella* sp; *Acinetobacter calcoaceticus* (formerly *Mima* and *Herellea* sp); *H influenzae* (respiratory infections); *Klebsiella* sp (respiratory and urinary infections).

Gram-positive – Streptococcus sp including *S pneumoniae.* Up to 44% of strains of *S pyogenes* and 74% of *S faecalis* are resistant to tetracyclines. Therefore, do not use tetracyclines unless the organism has been demonstrated to be sensitive.

TETRACYCLINES

For upper respiratory infections due to group A β-hemolytic streptococci, including prophylaxis of rheumatic fever, penicillin is the usual drug of choice.

Staphylococcus aureus, skin and soft tissue infections. Tetracyclines are not the drugs of choice in the treatment of any type of staphylococcal infection.

Treatment of trachoma, although the infectious agent is not always eliminated, as judged by immunofluorescence.

When penicillin is contraindicated, tetracyclines are alternatives for treatment of infections due to: *Neisseria gonorrhoeae; Treponema pallidum* and *T pertenue* (syphilis and yaws); *Listeria monocytogenes; Clostridium* sp; *Bacillus anthracis; Fusobacterium fusiforme* (Vincent's infection); *Actinomyces* sp; *N meningitidis* (IV only).

Acute intestinal amebiasis: Tetracyclines may be a useful adjunct to amebicides.

Oral tetracyclines:

Adults – Treatment of uncomplicated urethral, endocervical or rectal infections caused by *Chlamydia trachomatis.*

Severe acne (where it may be useful as adjunctive therapy).

Inclusion conjunctivitis (which may be treated with oral tetracyclines or with a combination of oral and topical agents).

Doxycycline, oral – Treatment of uncomplicated gonococcal infections in adults (except for anorectal infections in men); gonococcal arthritis-dermatitis syndrome; acute epididymo-orchitis caused by *N gonorrhoeae* and *C trachomatis;* nongonococcal urethritis caused by *C trachomatis* and *Ureaplasma urealyticum.*

Minocycline, oral – Treatment of asymptomatic carriers of *N meningitidis* to eliminate meningococci from the nasopharynx. In order to preserve the usefulness of minocycline in this indication, perform diagnostic laboratory procedures, including serotyping and susceptibility testing, to establish the carrier state and the correct treatment. Reserve the drug for situations in which the risk of meningococcal meningitis is high. *Not* indicated for the treatment of meningococcal infection.

Oral minocycline has been successful in *Mycobacterium marinum* infections.

Minocycline is also indicated for the treatment of uncomplicated urethral, endocervical or rectal infections in adults caused by *U urealyticum;* uncomplicated gonococcal urethritis in men due to *N gonorrhoeae.*

Methacycline – Mycoplasma pneumonia; nongonococcal urethritis caused by *C trachomatis;* early Lyme disease.

Unlabeled uses: **Demeclocycline** has been used successfully in the treatment of chronic hyponatremia associated with the syndrome of inappropriate antidiuretic hormone (SIADH) secretion. Experience with this therapy is limited.

Doxycycline has been used to prevent "Traveler's Diarrhea" commonly caused by enterotoxigenic *E coli.*

Minocycline has been used as an alternative to sulfonamides in nocardiosis.

Tetracycline instilled through a chest tube is employed as a pleural sclerosing agent in malignant pleural effusions. Tetracycline plus gentamicin is recommended for *V vulnificus* infections caused by wound infection after trauma or by ingestion of contaminated seafood.

Tetracycline suspension has been used as a mouthwash in the treatment of nonspecific mouth ulcerations, aphthous ulcers and canker sores. Dosages have ranged from 5 to 10 ml of 125 mg/ml 3 times/day for 5 to 7 days.

Lyme disease (the etiologic agent is a spirochete, *Borrelia burgdorferi*): Oral **tetracycline** 250 mg daily for 10 days is the drug of choice for stage I disease (skin rash: erythema chronicum migrans) in adults; **doxycycline** has also been recommended for early disease. Both agents have been recommended for stage II disease (mild cardiac and neurologic illness), and they are being evaluated for treatment of stage III disease (arthritis). However, the efficacy of tetracycline at the recommended dose for early Lyme disease has been questioned.

Refer to individual product listings for CDC recommendations for treatment of sexually transmitted diseases.

Contraindications:

Hypersensitivity to any of the tetracyclines.

Warnings:

Photosensitivity: Photosensitivity manifested by an exaggerated sunburn reaction has been observed in some individuals taking tetracyclines. Advise patients who are apt to be exposed to direct sunlight or ultraviolet light that this reaction can occur with tetracycline drugs, and discontinue treatment at the first evidence of skin erythema.

In patients taking **demeclocycline**, exaggerated sunburn reactions are characterized by severe burns of exposed surfaces, resulting from direct exposure to sunlight during therapy with moderate or large doses. Phototoxic reactions are most frequent with demeclocycline, and occur less frequently with the other tetracyclines; minocycline is least likely to cause phototoxic reactions.

TETRACYCLINES

Parenteral therapy: Reserve for situations in which oral therapy is not indicated. Institute oral therapy as soon as possible. If given IV over prolonged periods, thrombophlebitis may result. IM use produces lower blood levels than recommended oral dosages. If high blood levels are needed rapidly, administer IV.

Nephrogenic diabetes insipidus: Administration of **demeclocycline** has resulted in appearance of the diabetes insipidus syndrome (polyuria, polydipsia and weakness) in some patients on long-term therapy. The syndrome has been shown to be nephrogenic, dose-dependent and reversible on discontinuation of therapy.

Hazardous tasks: Lightheadedness, dizziness or vertigo may occur with **minocycline.** Patients should observe caution while driving or performing other tasks requiring alertness. These symptoms may disappear during therapy and always disappear rapidly when the drug is discontinued.

Renal function impairment: If renal impairment exists, even usual doses may lead to excessive systemic accumulation of the tetracyclines (with the exception of doxycycline and minocycline) and possible liver toxicity. Use lower than usual doses; if therapy is prolonged, drug serum level determinations may be advisable.

The hazard of liver toxicity is of particular importance in parenteral administration to pregnant or postpartum patients with pyelonephritis.

The antianabolic action of tetracyclines may cause an increase in BUN. In significantly impaired renal function, higher serum tetracycline levels may lead to azotemia, hyperphosphatemia and acidosis. This does not occur with doxycycline.

Hepatic function impairment: Doses > 2 g/day IV can be extremely dangerous. In the presence of renal dysfunction, and particularly in pregnancy, IV tetracycline > 2 g/day has been associated with death secondary to liver failure. When need for intensive treatment outweighs its potential dangers (especially during pregnancy or in known or suspected renal and liver impairment), monitor renal and liver function tests. Serum tetracycline concentrations should not exceed 15 mcg/ml. Do not prescribe other potentially hepatotoxic drugs concomitantly.

Pregnancy: Category D (doxycycline; methacycline). (See Warnings about use during tooth development.) Tetracyclines should not be used during pregnancy. They readily cross the placenta; concentrations of oxytetracycline in cord blood are ≈ 50% of those of the mother. Tetracyclines are found in fetal tissues and can have toxic effects on the developing fetus (retardation of skeletal development). Evidence of embryotoxicity has also been noted in animals treated early in pregnancy.

Lactation: Tetracyclines are excreted in breast milk. A dosage of 2 g/day for 3 days has achieved a milk:plasma ratio of 0.6 to 0.8. Because of the potential for serious adverse reactions decide whether to discontinue nursing or discontinue the drug.

Children: Tetracyclines should not generally be used in children under 8 years of age, unless other drugs are not likely to be effective, or are contraindicated.

Teeth – The use of tetracyclines during the period of tooth development (from the last half of pregnancy through the eighth year of life) may cause permanent discoloration (yellow-gray-brown) of deciduous and permanent teeth. This adverse reaction is more common during long-term use of the drugs, but has been observed following repeated short-term courses. Enamel hypoplasia has also been reported. Doxycycline and oxytetracycline may be less likely to affect teeth.

Bone – Tetracycline forms a stable calcium complex in any bone-forming tissue. Decreased fibula growth rate occurred in premature infants given 25 mg/kg oral tetracycline every 6 hrs. This was reversible when drug was discontinued.

Precautions:

Pseudotumor cerebri (benign intracranial hypertension) in adults has been associated with tetracycline use. Usual clinical manifestations are headache and blurred vision. Bulging fontanels have been associated with tetracycline use in infants. While both conditions and related symptoms usually resolve soon after tetracycline discontinuation, the possibility for permanent sequelae exists.

Outdated products: Under no circumstances should outdated tetracyclines be administered; the degradation products of tetracyclines are highly nephrotoxic and have, on occasion, produced a Fanconi-like syndrome.

Laboratory tests: In sexually transmitted diseases when coexistent syphilis is suspected, perform darkfield examination before treatment is started and repeat the blood serology monthly for at least 4 months.

In long-term therapy, perform periodic laboratory evaluation of organ systems, including hematopoietic, renal and hepatic studies.

Superinfection: Use of antibiotics (especially prolonged or repeated therapy) may result in bacterial or fungal overgrowth of nonsusceptible organisms. Such overgrowth may lead to a secondary infection. Take appropriate measures if superinfection occurs. Superinfection of the bowel by staphylococci may be life-threatening.

TETRACYCLINES

Sulfite sensitivity: Some of these products contain sulfites that may cause allergic-type reactions (including anaphylactic symptoms and life-threatening or less severe asthmatic episodes) in certain susceptible people. The overall prevalence of sulfite sensitivity in the general population is unknown and probably low. It is seen more frequently in asthmatic or atopic nonasthmatic people. Specific products containing sulfites are identified in the product listings.

Drug Interactions:

Antacids containing **aluminum, calcium, zinc or magnesium** and **bismuth salts** and other **divalent** and **trivalent cations** impair absorption of tetracyclines due to formation of a poorly soluble chelate, possibly decreasing the antimicrobial efficacy. Administer tetracyclines at least 2 hours before or after these agents.

Anticoagulants, oral: Tetracyclines may alter normal hemostasis; therefore these agents may increase the hypoprothrombinemic effects of concurrent anticoagulants. Monitor prothrombin activity.

Barbiturates, carbamazepine and **hydantoins** may increase the rate of metabolism, and therefore, decrease the half-life and serum levels of doxycycline. Antimicrobial effectiveness may be decreased.

Cimetidine may decrease the GI absorption of tetracyclines due to a pH-dependent inhibition of dissolution; antimicrobial effectiveness may be decreased.

Digoxin: Tetracyclines may increase the serum levels of **digoxin** in a small portion (< 10%) of patients; this could lead to digoxin toxicity. These effects may last for months after tetracycline administration is discontinued.

Insulin: Tetracyclines may reduce insulin requirements. Controlled studies are needed. Monitor blood glucose.

Iron salts, oral may decrease the GI absorption of tetracyclines due to formation of poorly soluble chelate; antimicrobial effectiveness may be decreased. Give iron salts in non-enteric coated, non-sustained release form at least 3 hours before or 2 hours after tetracyclines.

Lithium: Tetracycline may increase or decrease lithium levels. Monitor serum lithium.

Methoxyflurane and tetracycline coadministration may increase the nephrotoxic effects of both drugs. Avoid this combination.

Oral contraceptives: Coadministration of tetracyclines may decrease the pharmacologic effects of oral contraceptives; breakthrough bleeding or pregnancy may occur.

Penicillins: Bacteriostatic drugs (eg, tetracycline) may interfere with the bactericidal action of penicillins; avoid concomitant administration.

Sodium bicarbonate may impair the GI absorption of tetracyclines; this may depend on differences in tetracycline product formulations. Alkalinization of the urine may also alter urinary tetracycline excretion.

Drug/Lab test interactions: Following a course of therapy, persistence for several days in both urine and blood of bacteriosuppressive levels of **demeclocycline** may interfere with culture studies. These levels should not be considered therapeutic.

Drug/Food interactions: Food and some dairy products interfere with absorption of tetracyclines. Administer oral tetracycline 1 hour before or 2 hours after meals. Doxycycline has a low affinity for calcium binding. Gastrointestinal absorption of minocycline and doxycycline is not significantly affected by food or dairy products.

Adverse Reactions:

GI:

Oral and parenteral – Anorexia; nausea; vomiting; diarrhea; epigastric distress; bulky loose stools; stomatitis; sore throat; glossitis; hoarseness; black hairy tongue; dysphagia; enterocolitis; inflammatory lesions (with monilial overgrowth) in the anogenital region, including proctitis and pruritis ani.

Oral – Esophageal ulcers, most commonly in patients with an esophageal obstructive element or hiatal hernia. Having the patient remain standing for at least 90 seconds after medication ingestion and taking the medication with a full glass of water at least 1 hour before going to bed may minimize this problem.

Dermatologic: Maculopapular and erythematous rashes; exfoliative dermatitis (uncommon). Photosensitivity (See Warnings). Onycholysis and discoloration of the nails (rare). Onycholysis has been reported to occur in up to 25% of patients experiencing phototoxic reactions to tetracyclines. This may also occur without phototoxicity. Blue-gray pigmentation of the skin and mucous membranes has been reported, primarily with **minocycline.**

Stevens-Johnson syndrome (rare) has occurred with **minocycline.**

Renal: Rise in BUN (dose-related). (See Warnings).

TETRACYCLINES

Hepatic: Fatty liver; hepatotoxicity, hepatitis (rare); increases in liver enzymes. Hepatic cholestasis (rare) is usually associated with high dosage levels. (See Warnings).

CNS: Lightheadedness, dizziness or vertigo has been reported with **minocycline**; (see Warnings). Transient myopathy has been reported.

Hypersensitivity: Urticaria; angioneurotic edema; anaphylaxis; anaphylactoid purpura; pericarditis; exacerbated systemic lupus erythematosus; polyarthralgia; serum sickness-like reactions, (eg, fever, rash, arthralgia); pulmonary infiltrates with eosinophilia.

Hematologic: Hemolytic anemia; thrombocytopenia; thrombocytopenic purpura; neutropenia; eosinophilia.

Miscellaneous: Pseudotumor cerebri (adults); bulging fontanels (infants). (See Warnings.) Nephrogenic diabetes insipidus has been reported with **demeclocycline**. (See Warnings.) When given over prolonged periods, tetracyclines reportedly produce brown-black microscopic discoloration of thyroid glands. No abnormal thyroid function studies are known to occur. Drug deposition in the eye may produce abnormal pigmentation of conjunctiva. Tooth discoloration in adults is rare.

Local: Irritation may occur with IM administration.

Patient Information:

Take on empty stomach, at least 1 hour before or 2 hours after meals (**doxycycline** and **minocycline** may be taken with food or milk). Take with full glass of water (240 ml).

Avoid simultaneous dairy products (milk, cheese), antacids, laxatives or iron-containing products. If an antacid must be taken, take at least 2 hrs before or after tetracycline.

Avoid prolonged exposure to sunlight or sunlamps; may cause photosensitivity (especially **demeclocycline**).

Administration and Dosage:

Avoid rapid IV administration. Thrombophlebitis may result from prolonged IV therapy.

Continue therapy at least 24 to 48 hours after symptoms and fever subside. Treat all infections due to group A β-hemolytic streptococci for at least 10 days.

TETRACYCLINE HCl

Complete prescribing information for these products begins in the Tetracyclines group monograph.

Administration and Dosage:

Oral:

Adults – Usual dose: 1 to 2 g/day in 2 or 4 equal doses.

Mild to moderate infections: 500 mg, 2 times/day or 250 mg, 4 times/day.

Severe infections: 500 mg, 4 times/day.

Children (over 8 years of age) – Daily dose is 10 to 20 mg/lb (25 to 50 mg/kg) in 4 equal doses.

Brucellosis – 500 mg 4 times/day for 3 weeks, accompanied by 1 g streptomycin IM twice/day the first week, and once daily the second week.

Syphilis – 30 to 40 g in equally divided doses over 10 to 15 days. Perform close follow-up and laboratory tests.

Gonorrhea – 1.5 g initially, then 500 mg every 6 hours, to a total of 9 g.

Gonorrhea in patients sensitive to penicillin – Initially, 1.5 g; follow with 500 mg every 6 hours for 4 days to a total of 9 g.

Uncomplicated urethral, endocervical or rectal infections caused by Chlamydia trachomatis – 500 mg 4 times/day for at least 7 days.

Severe acne (long-term therapy) – Initially, 1 g/day in divided doses. For maintenance, give 125 to 500 mg/day.

CDC recommended treatment schedules for sexually transmitted diseases†:

Chlamydia trachomatis—Uncomplicated urethral, endocervical or rectal infections in adults – 500mg 4 times/day for 7 days.

Gonococcal infections - Uncomplicated urethral, endocervical or rectal infections in adults – 3 g amoxicillin, 3.5 g oral ampicillin, 4.8 million units IM aqueous procaine penicillin G or 250 mg IM ceftriaxone. Each (except ceftriaxone) should be accompanied by 1 g oral probenecid. Follow with 500 mg tetracycline, 4 times/day for 7 days.

In adults allergic to penicillins, cephalosporins or probenecid: 500 mg 4 times/day for 7 days.

In PPNG-endemic and –hyperendemic areas – 250 mg IM ceftriaxone plus 100 mg oral doxycycline twice daily for 7 days or 500 mg oral tetracycline 4 times a day for 7 days. If tetracyclines are contraindicated or not tolerated, follow the single-dose regimen with erythromycin.

† *MMWR* 1985 (Oct 18); 34 (Suppl 4S):75S-108S and 1987 (Sep 11); 36 (Suppl 5S):1S-18S.

TETRACYCLINE HCl

Penicillinase-producing Neisseria gonorrhoeae – 2 g IM spectinomycin or 250 mg IM ceftriaxone. Follow with 500 mg tetracycline, 4 times/day for 7 days.

Children (> 8 years) allergic to penicillins or cephalosporins: 40 mg/kg/day in 4 divided doses for 5 days.

Disseminated gonococcal infections in patients allergic to penicillins or cephalosporins – 500 mg 4 times/day for at least 7 days.

Lymphogranuloma venereum - Genital, inguinal or anorectal – 500 mg 4 times/day for at least 2 weeks.

Nongonococcal urethritis – 500 mg,4 times/day for 7 days.

Acute pelvic inflammatory disease - Ambulatory treatment – 2 g IM cefoxitin, 3 g amoxicillin, 3.5 g oral ampicillin, 4.8 million units IM aqueous procaine penicillin G at 2 sites or 250 mg IM ceftriaxone. Each (except for ceftriaxone) should be accompanied by 1 g oral probenecid. Follow with 500 mg tetracycline, 4 times/day. (However, doxycycline is preferred.)

Children over 7 years of age: 150 mg/kg/day IV cefuroxime or 100 mg/kg/day IV ceftriaxone followed by 30 mg/kg/day IV tetracycline in 3 doses, continued for at least 4 days. Thereafter, continue tetracycline orally to complete at least 14 days of therapy.

Syphilis (penicillin-allergic patients) - Early – 500 mg 4 times/day for 15 days. *More than 1 year's duration:* 500 mg 4 times/day for 30 days.

Sexually transmitted epididymo-orchitis – 3 g oral amoxicillin, 3.5 g oral ampicillin, 4.8 million units IM aqueous procaine penicillin G at 2 sites (each with 1 g oral probenecid), 2 g IM spectinomycin or 250 mg IM ceftriaxone followed by 500 mg tetracycline, 4 times/day for 10 days.

Urethral syndrome in women – 500 mg 4 times/day for 7 days.

Rape victims - Prophylaxis – 500 mg 4 times/day for 7 days.

Rx	**Tetracycline HCl Syrup** (Various, eg, Gen-King, Goldline, Harber, Major, Rugby)	**Oral Suspension:** 125 mg/5 ml	In 60 and 480 ml.
Rx	**Achromycin V** (Lederle)		Cherry flavor. In 473 ml.
Rx	**Sumycin Syrup** (Apothecon)		Fruit flavor. In 473 ml.
Rx	**Tetralan Syrup** (Lannett)		Cherry flavor. In 480 ml.
Rx	**Tetracycline HCl** (Richlyn)	**Capsules:** 100 mg	In 1000s.
Rx	**Tetracycline** (Various, eg, Geneva, Goldline, Major, Moore, Rugby)	**Capsules:** 250 mg	In 20s, 28s, 30s, 40s, 60s, 100s, 500s, 1000s and UD 32s and 100s.
Rx	**Achromycin V** (Lederle)		(Lederle A3 250 mg). Blue/yellow. In 100s, 1000s, UD 100s, unit-of-issue 120s, 240s, 336s, 480s, 1200s.
Rx	**Panmycin** (Upjohn)		Tartrazine. Grey and yellow. In 100s and 1000s.
Rx	**Robitet Robicaps** (Robins)		Pink/brown. In 100s, 1000s.
Rx	**Sumycin '250'**(Apothecon)		In 100s, 1000s and UD 100s.
Rx	**Teline** (Hauck)		In 100s and 1000s.
Rx	**Tetracap** (Circle)		In 100s.
Rx	**Tetracyn** (Pfizer)		Black/white. In 100s, 1000s.
Rx	**Tetralan "250"** (Lannett)		White/orange. In 100s, 1000s.
Rx	**Tetracycline** (Dr.'s Pharm.)	**Tablets:** 250 mg	In 30s and 60s.
Rx	**Sumycin '250'** (Apothecon)		In 100s and 1000s.

TETRACYCLINE HCl

Rx	**Tetracycline HCl** (Various, eg, Bioline, Geneva)	**Capsules:** 500 mg	In 20s, 28s, 40s, 50s, 100s, 500s, 1000s and UD 100s.
Rx	**Achromycin V** (Lederle)		(Lederle A5 500 mg). Blue/yellow. In 100s, 1000s, UD 100s, unit-of-issue 240s.
Rx	**Robitet Robicaps** (Robins)		Cream/brown. In 100s, 500s.
Rx	**Sumycin '500'** (Apothecon)		In 100s, 500s and UD 100s.
Rx	**Teline-500** (Hauck)		In 100s.
Rx	**Tetracyn 500** (Pfizer)		Black/blue. In 100s.
Rx	**Tetralan-500** (Lannett)		Black/yellow. In 100s, 1000s.
Rx	**Tetracycline** (Dr.'s Pharm.)	**Tablets:** 500 mg	In 30s and 60s.
Rx	**Sumycin '500'** (Apothecon)		In 100s and 500s.

DEMECLOCYCLINE HCl

Complete prescribing information for these products begins in the Fluoroquinolones group monograph.

Caution: May cause photosensitivity (see group monograph).

Administration and Dosage:

Adults:

Daily dose – 4 divided doses of 150 mg each or 2 divided doses of 300 mg each.

Children (over 8 years of age):

Usual daily dose – 3 to 6 mg/lb (6 to 12 mg/kg), depending upon the severity of the disease, divided into 2 or 4 doses.

Gonorrhea patients sensitive to penicillin: Initially, 600 mg; follow with 300 mg every 12 hours for 4 days to a total of 3 g.

Rx	**Declomycin** (Lederle)	**Capsules:** 150 mg	(LL D9). In 100s.
		Tablets: 150 mg	(LL D11). In 100s.
		300 mg	(LL D12). In 48s.

[1] With 40 mg procaine HCl per vial.

DOXYCYCLINE

Complete prescribing information for these products begins in the Tetracyclines group monograph.

Administration and Dosage:

Oral: The therapeutic antibacterial serum activity will usually persist for 24 hours.

Adults –

Usual dose: 200 mg on the first day of treatment (100 mg every 12 hours); follow with a maintenance dose of 100 mg/day. The maintenance dose may be administered as a single dose or as 50 mg every 12 hours.

More severe infections (particularly chronic urinary tract infections): 100 mg every 12 hours.

Children (over 8 years of age) –

100 pounds or less (<45 kg): 2 mg/lb (4.4 mg/kg) divided into 2 doses on the first day of treatment; follow with 1 mg/lb (2.2 mg/kg) given as a single daily dose or divided into 2 doses on subsequent days.

More severe infections: Up to 2 mg/lb (4.4 mg/kg) may be used. For children over 100 pounds (45 kg), use the usual adult dose.

Acute gonococcal infection – 200 mg immediately, then 100 mg at bedtime on the first day. Follow by 100 mg 2 times/day for 3 days.

Single visit dose: Immediately give 300 mg; follow with 300 mg in 1 hour, which may be administered with food, milk or carbonated beverage.

Primary and secondary syphilis – 300 mg/day in divided doses for at least 10 days.

Uncomplicated urethral, endocervical or rectal infections in adults caused by Chlamydia trachomatis – 100 mg twice daily for at least 7 days.

Unlabeled Use – Doxycycline has been used to prevent "Traveler's Diarrhea" commonly caused by enterotoxigenic *Escherichica coli.* In limited trials, this prophylactic (100 mg/day) therapy appears to be superior to placebo.

Endometritis, salpingitis, parametritis or peritonitis – Give 100 mg doxycycline IV, twice daily and 2 g cefoxitin IV, 4 times/day. Continue IV administration for at least 4 days and for at least 48 hours after patient improves. Then continue oral doxycycline (100 mg), twice daily to complete 10 to 14 days total therapy.

Parenteral: Do not inject IM or SC. The duration of IV infusion may vary with the dose (100 to 200 mg per day), but is usually 1 to 4 hours. A recommended minimum infusion time for 100 mg of a 0.5 mg/ml solution is 1 hour. Continue therapy for at least 24 to 48 hours after symptoms and fever have subsided. Therapeutic antibacterial serum activity usually persists for 24 hours following recommended dosage.

Renal impairment – Doxycycline at recommended doses does not lead to excessive accumulation in patients with renal impairment.

Adults – The usual dosage is 200 mg IV on the first day of treatment, administered in 1 or 2 infusions. Subsequent daily dosage is 100 to 200 mg, depending upon the severity of infection, with 200 mg administered in 1 or 2 infusions.

Primary and secondary syphilis: 300 mg daily for at least 10 days.

Children (over 8 years) – ≤ 100 pounds (45 kg), give 2 mg/lb (4.4 mg/kg) on the first day of treatment, in 1 or 2 infusions. Subsequent daily dosage is 1 to 2 mg/lb (2.2 to 4.4 mg/ kg) given as 1 or 2 infusions, depending on the severity of the infection. For children > 100 pounds (45 kg), use the usual adult dose.

Children (< 8 years) – Safety of IV use has not been established (see Warnings, p. 341b).

Preparation of solution: To prepare a solution containing 10 mg/ml, reconstitute the contents of the vial with 10 ml (for the 100 mg/vial) or 20 ml (for the 200 mg/vial) of Sterile Water for Injection or any of the IV infusion solutions listed below. Dilute the 100 mg vial further with 100 to 1000 ml (or 200 to 2000 ml for the 200 mg vial) of the following IV solutions: Sodium Chloride Injection; 5% Dextrose Injection; Ringer's Injection; 10% Invert Sugar in Water; Lactated Ringer's Injection; 5% Dextrose in Lactated Ringer's; *Normosol-M* in D5–W; *Normosol-M* in D5–W; *Plasma-Lyte 56* in 5% Dextrose; *Plasma-Lyte 148* in 5% Dextrose. This will result in the recommended concentrations of 0.1 to 1 mg/ml.

Storage: When diluted with Lactated Ringer's Injection or 5% Dextrose in Lactated Ringer's, complete infusion of the solution (0.1 to 1 mg/ml) within 6 hours after reconstitution to assure stability. Use solutions within this time period or discard.

When diluted with the remaining solutions listed above, doxycycline may be stored up to 72 hours prior to infusion, if refrigerated and protected from light. Complete infusion within 12 hours to ensure stability; discard remaining solution.

Stability: Solutions at concentrations of 10 mg/ml in Sterile Water for Injection, when frozen immediately after reconstitution, are stable for 8 weeks when stored at –20°C. If product is warmed, avoid heating after thawing is complete. Do not refreeze.

DOXYCYCLINE

CDC recommended treatment schedules for sexually transmitted diseases†:

Chlamydia trachomatis –

Uncomplicated urethral, endocervical or rectal infections in adults: 100 mg, 2 times/day for 7 days.

Gonococcal infections –

Uncomplicated urethral, endocervical or rectal infections in adults: 3 g oral amoxicillin, 3.5 g oral ampicillin, 4.8 million units IM aqueous procaine penicillin G or 250 mg IM ceftriaxone. Each (except for ceftriaxone) should be accompanied by 1 g oral probenecid. Follow with 100 mg doxycycline, twice daily for 7 days.

In adults allergic to penicillins, cephalosporins or probenecid: 100 mg, twice daily for 7 days.

In PPNG-endemic and –hyperendemic areas: 250 mg IM ceftriaxone plus 100 mg oral doxycycline twice daily for 7 days or 500 mg oral tetracycline 4 times a day for 7 days. If tetracyclines are contraindicated or not tolerated, follow the single-dose regimen with erythromycin.

Penicillinase-producing Neisseria gonorrhoeae: 2 g IM spectinomycin or 250 mg IM ceftriaxone. Follow with 100 mg doxycycline, twice daily for 7 days.

Disseminated gonococcal infections in patients allergic to penicillins or cephalosporins: 100 mg, twice daily for a least 7 days.

Lymphogranuloma venereum:

Genital, inguinal or anorectal – 100 mg, twice daily for at least 2 weeks.

Nongonococcal urethritis – 100 mg, twice daily for 7 days.

Acute pelvic inflammatory disease:

Ambulatory treatment – 250 mg single IM dose of ceftriaxone plus 100 mg oral doxycycline twice daily for 10 to 14 days. Other effective third generation cephalosporins may be substituted in the appropriate doses for ceftriaxone.

Inpatient treatment – 100 mg IV doxycycline twice daily, plus 2 g IV cefoxitin 4 times a day. Continue drugs IV for at least 4 days and at least 48 hours after patient improves. Then continue doxycycline 100 mg orally twice daily to complete 10 to 14 days of total therapy.

Sexually transmitted epididymo-orchitis: 3 g oral amoxicillin, 3.5 g oral ampicillin, 4.8 million units IM aqueous procaine penicillin G at 2 sites (each with 1 g oral probenecid), 2 g IM spectinomycin or 250 mg IM ceftriaxone followed by 100 mg doxycycline, twice daily for 10 days.

Urethral syndrome in women: 100 mg, twice daily for 7 days.

Rape victims:

Prophylaxis – 100 mg, twice daily for 7 days.

† Morbidity and Mortality Weekly Report 1985 (Oct 18); 34 (Suppl 4S):75S-108S and 1987 (Sep 11); 36 (Suppl 5S):1S-18S.

Rx	**Doxycycline** (Various, eg, Geneva, Goldline, Lederle, Lemmon, Squibb-Mark, Warner-Chilcott, Zenith)	**Capsules**: 50 mg (as hyclate)	In 50s, 60s, 100s, 500s and UD 50s and 100s.
Rx	**Doxychel** Hyclate (Rachelle)		In 50s and 500s.
Rx	**Vibramycin** (Pfizer)		(094). In 50s and UD 100s.
Rx	**Monodox** (Oclassen)	**Capsules**: 50 mg (as monohydrate)	In 100s.
Rx	**Doxychel Hyclate** (Rachelle)	**Tablets**: 50 mg (as hyclate)	In 50s and 500s.
Rx	**Doxycycline** (Various, eg, Geneva, Goldline, Lederle, Lemmon, Squibb-Mark, Warner-Chilcott, Zenith)	**Capsules**: 100 mg (as hyclate)	In 10s, 11s, 14s, 20s, 40s, 50s, 100s, 200s, 500s and UD 100s.
Rx	**Doxy Caps** (Edwards)		In 50s.
Rx	**Doxychel Hyclate** (Rachelle)		In 50s, 500s and UD 100s.
Rx	**Vibramycin** (Pfizer)		(095). In 50s, 500s and UD 100s.
Rx	**Monodox** (Oclassen)	**Capsules**: 100 mg (as monohydrate)	(Monodox 100 M 259). Yellow/brown. In 50s and 250s.
Rx	**Doryx** (Parke-Davis)	**Capsules, coated pellets**: 100 mg (as hyclate)	(Doryx). Yellow and blue. In 50s.

DOXYCYCLINE

Rx	**Doxycycline** (Various, eg, Geneva, Goldline, Lederle, Lemmon, Major, Purepac, Rugby, Squibb-Mark, Warner-Chilcott, Zenith)	**Tablets:** 100 mg (as hyclate)	In 20s, 28s, 30s, 32s, 50s, 200s, 500s and UD 100s.
Rx	**Bio-Tab** (Inter. Ethical Labs)		Film coated. In 50s, 100s and 500s.
Rx	**Doxychel Hyclate** (Rachelle)		In 50s and 500s
Rx	**Vibra-Tabs** (Pfizer)		(099). Film coated. In 50s, 500s and UD 100s.
Rx	**Vibramycin** (Pfizer)	**Powder for Oral Suspension:** 25 mg (as monohydrate) per 5 ml when reconstituted	Raspberry flavor. In 60 ml.
Rx	**Vibramycin** (Pfizer)	**Syrup:** 50 mg (as calcium) per 5 ml	Raspberry flavor. In 60 ml.
Rx	**Doxycycline** (Various, eg, Dupont Crit Care, Elkins-Sinn, Loch, Lyphomed)	**Powder for Injection:** 100 mg (as hyclate)	In vials.
Rx	**Doxy 100** (Lyphomed)		In vials.
Rx	**Doxychel Hyclate** (Rachelle)		In vials.
Rx	**Vibramycin IV** (Pfizer)		In vials.
Rx	**Doxycycline** (Various, eg, DuPont Crit Care, Elkins-Sinn, Loch, Lyphomed)	**Powder for Injection:** 200 mg (as hyclate)	In vials.
Rx	**Doxy 200** (Lyphomed)		In vials.
Rx	**Doxychel Hyclate** (Rachelle)		In vials.
Rx	**Vibramycin IV** (Roerig)		In vials.

MINOCYCLINE

Complete prescribing information for these products begins in the Tetracyclines group monograph.

Administration and Dosage:

Oral:

Usual dosage –

Adults: 200 mg initially, followed by 100 mg every 12 hours. If more frequent doses are preferred, give 100 or 200 mg initially; follow with 50 mg, 4 times/day.

Children (over 8 years of age): Initially, 4 mg/kg; follow with 2 mg/kg every 12 hours.

Syphilis – Administer usual dose over a period of 10 to 15 days. Close follow-up, including laboratory tests, is recommended.

Uncomplicated urethral, endocervical or rectal infections in adults caused by Chlamydia trachomatis or Ureaplasma urealyticum – 100 mg, 2 times/day for at least 7 days.

Uncomplicated gonococcal urethritis in men – 100 mg, 2 times/day for 5 days.

Gonorrhea patients sensitive to penicillin – 200 mg initially, followed by 100 mg every 12 hours for a minimum of 4 days, with post-therapy cultures within 2 to 3 days.

Meningococcal carrier state – 100 mg every 12 hours for 5 days.

Mycobacterium marinum infections – Although optimal doses are not established, 100 mg twice daily for 6 to 8 weeks has been successful in a limited number of cases.

Parenteral:

Adults – 200 mg followed by 100 mg every 12 hours; do not exceed 400 mg in 24 hours.

Children (over 8 years of age) – Usual pediatric dose is 4 mg/kg, followed by 2 mg/kg every 12 hours.

Preparation of solution: Initially dissolve the drug and then further dilute to 500 to 1000 ml with either Sodium Chloride Injection, Dextrose Injection, Dextrose and Sodium Chloride Injection, Ringer's Injection or Lactated Ringer's Injection, but not in other solutions containing calcium (a precipitate may form).

MINOCYCLINE

Storage: The prepared solution is stable at room temperature for 24 hours without significant loss of potency. Discard unused portions after that period. Administer the final dilution immediately.

Rx	**Dynacin** (Medicis Dermatologics)	**Capsules:** 50 mg (as HCl)	Yellow. In 100s.
Rx	**Minocycline HCL** (Various, eg, Warner Chilcott)		(WC 815). Olive/brown. In 100s.
Rx	**Dynacin** (Medicis Dermatologics)	**Capsules:** 100 mg (as HCl)	Dark gray/yellow. In 50s.
Rx	**Minocycline HCL** (Various, eg, Warner Chilcott)		(WC 816). White/olive. In 50s.
Rx	**Minocin** (Lederle)	**Capsules, pellet filled:** 50 mg (as HCl)	(Lederle M45 50 mg). Yellow and green. In 100s.
		100 mg (as HCl)	(Lederle M46 100 mg). Green. In 50s.
		Oral Suspension: 50 mg (as HCl) per 5 ml	5% alcohol. Custard flavor. In 60 ml.
Rx	**Minocin IV** (Lederle)	**Powder for Injection:** 100 mg	In vials.

OXYTETRACYCLINE

Complete prescribing information for these products begins the Tetracyclines group monograph.

Administration and Dosage:

Oral: See Tetracycline HCl.

Parenteral:

Adults – The usual daily dose is 250 mg administered once every 24 hours or 300 mg given in divided doses at 8 to 12 hour intervals.

Children (over 8 years of age) – 15 to 25 mg/kg, up to a maximum of 250 mg per single daily injection. Dosage may be divided and given at 8 to 12 hour intervals.

Rx	**Oxytetracycline HCl** (Various, eg, Balan, Dixon-Shane, Major, Parmed, Rugby)	**Capsules:** 250 mg (as HCl)	In 100s and 1000s.
Rx	**Terramycin** (Pfizer)		(Terramycin Pfizer 073). Yellow. In 100s and 500s.
Rx	**Uri-Tet** (American Urologicals)		In 100s.
Rx	**Terramycin IM** (Various, eg, Roerig, Texas Drug)	**Injection:** 50 mg per ml with 2% lidocaine	In 2 ml amps and 10 ml vials.
Rx	**Terramycin IM** (Roerig)	**Injection:** 125 mg per ml with 2% lidocaine	In 2 ml amps.

MACROLIDES

For complete prescribing information, refer to individual monographs.

Actions:

Pharmacology: Macrolide antibiotics, which include azithromycin, clarithromycin, dirithromycin, erythromycin and troleandomycin, reversibly bind to the P site of the 50S ribosomal subunit of susceptible organisms and inhibit RNA-dependent protein synthesis by stimulating the dissociation of peptidyl t-RNA from ribosomes. They may be bacteriostatic or bactericidal, depending on such factors as drug concentration.

Rearrangement of erythromycin's 9-oxime derivative, followed by reduction and N-methylation, yields the ring-expanded derivative azithromycin, an azalide. Alkylation of the hydroxyl group at C-6 yields clarithromycin. The classical erythromycins A, B, C and D and oleandomycin are 14-membered macrolides; azithromycin is a 15-membered-ring macrolide.

Despite differing structures, macrolides have similar antibacterial spectrum, mechanisms of action and resistance, but relatively different pharmacokinetics (see table).

Macrolides are weak bases; their activity increases in alkaline pH. Macrolides enter pleural fluid, ascitic fluid, middle-ear exudates and sputum. When meninges are inflamed, macrolides may enter the CSF.

Erythromycin base, the active form, is marketed in acid-resistant enteric-coated form to retard gastric inactivation. Converting the base to its acid-stable salt (stearate), ester (ethyl succinate and propionate) or salt of an ester (estolate) also improves oral bioavailability. For IV injection, a relatively water-soluble salt, lactobionate, is available.

Dirithromycin is a pro-drug. Available as an enteric-coated tablet, it is converted non-enzymatically during intestinal absorption into the microbiologically active moiety erythromycylamine.

Macrolides are used for respiratory, genital, GI tract and skin and soft tissue infections, especially when beta-lactam antibiotics or tetracyclines are contraindicated.

Pharmacokinetics:

Various Pharmacokinetic Parameters of Macrolides

Macrolide	Protein binding (%)	Metabolism	Elimination	Bioavailability (%)	Effect of food	C_{max}* (mcg/ml)	T_{max}* (hr)	Half-life (hr)
Azithromycin	50 (0.02 mg/L) 7 (1 mg/L)		4.5% excreted unchanged in urine; primarily excreted unchanged in bile	≈ 40	Food decreases absorption, C_{max} and AUC by ≈ 50%; take on empty stomach	0.4	2-3	68[1]
Clarithromycin		Metabolized to active metabolite (14-OH clarithromycin)	Primarily renal; rate approximates normal GFR	≈ 50	Food delays onset of absorption and formation of metabolite; does not affect extent of bioavailability. Take without regard to meals	1-3	1.7	3-7
Dirithromycin	15-30[2]	Non-enzymatic conversion to erythromycylamine	81%-97% fecal/hepatic[2]	≈ 10	Take with food or within an hour of having eaten	0.3 - 0.4[2]	3.9 - 4.1[2]	2-36
Erythromycin	70-74	Hepatic; demethylation	< 5% (oral) and 12% to 15% (IV) excreted unchanged in urine; significant quantity excreted in bile		Base or stearate: Take on an empty stomach. Estolate, ethylsuccinate, delayed release base: Take without regard to meals			1.4
Troleandomycin			20% excreted in urine; significant quantity excreted in bile		Take on an empty stomach	2	2	

* C_{max} = Maximum concentration; T_{max} = Time to reach maximum concentration.

[1] Average terminal half-life.

[2] Value listed for erythromycylamine, the active moiety.

MACROLIDES

Azithromycin has an extended half-life and high tissue penetration. Without a loading dose, minimum plasma concentrations take 5 to 7 days to reach steady state. It is rapidly absorbed and widely distributed throughout the body. It is also rapidly distributed into tissues and reaches high concentrations within cells; therefore, significantly higher concentrations are achieved in tissues compared to plasma or serum. The prolonged half-life appears to be due to uptake and subsequent release of drug from tissues.

Clarithromycin is rapidly absorbed, reaching peak concentrations in serum 2 hours after dosing, regardless of dose size.

Microbiology:

Organisms Generally Susceptible to Macrolides In Vitro

	Organisms (✓ = generally susceptible)	Azithromycin	Clarithromycin	Dirithromycin	Erythromycin	Troleandomycin[1]
Gram-positive aerobes	*Staphylococcus aureus*	✓	✓	✓	✓	
	Streptococcus pyogenes	✓	✓	✓	✓	✓
	Streptococcus pneumoniae	✓	✓	✓	✓	✓
	Streptococcus agalactiae	✓	✓	✓	✓	
	Streptococcus sp	✓	✓	✓		
	Streptococcus viridans	✓	✓	✓	✓	
	Listeria monocytogenes		✓	✓	✓	
	Corynebacterium diphtheriae				✓	
	Corynebacterium minutissimum				✓	
Gram-negative aerobes	*Haemophilus influenzae*	✓	✓		†[2]	
	Haemophilus ducreyi	✓				
	Moraxella catarrhalis	✓	✓	✓	✓	
	Bordetella pertussis	✓	✓	✓	✓	
	Legionella pneumophila	✓	✓	✓	✓	
	Campylobacter jejuni	✓	✓			
	Neisseria gonorrhoeae		✓		✓	
	Pasteurella multocida		✓			
Anaerobes	*Bacteroides bivius*	✓				
	Bacteroides melaninogenicus		✓			
	Clostridium perfringens	✓	✓			
	Propionibacterium acnes		✓	✓		
	Peptococcus niger		✓			
	Peptostreptococcus sp	✓				
Other	*Borrelia burgdorferi*	✓				
	Chlamydia trachomatis	✓	✓		✓	
	Mycobacterium kansasii		✓			
	Mycoplasma pneumoniae	✓	✓	✓	✓	
	Treponema pallidum	✓			✓	
	Ureaplasma urealyticum	✓			✓	
	Entamoeba histolytica				✓	

[1] Data is limited for troleandomycin.

[2] Many strains resistant to erythromycin alone; may be susceptible to erythromycin plus a sulfonamide.

The in vitro spectrum of erythromycin covers primarily gram-positive microorganisms and gram-negative cocci.

Azithromycin is less active than erythromycin against most *Staphylococcus* and *Streptococcus* sp, but it is more potent against other organisms, including many gram-negative bacteria considered resistant to erythromycin. Azithromycin may expand the therapeutic range traditionally assigned to macrolides.

Clarithromycin exhibits the same spectrum of in vitro activity as erythromycin, but appears to have significantly increased potency against those organisms.

Troleandomycin, an acetylated ester of oleandomycin, is less active than erythromycin and offers no advantage. It can also cause hepatotoxicity.

CLARITHROMYCIN

Actions:

Pharmacology: Clarithromycin is a semi-synthetic macrolide antibiotic. It exerts its antibacterial action by binding to the 50S ribosomal subunit of susceptible organisms and inhibiting protein synthesis.

Pharmacokinetics: Clarithromycin is rapidly absorbed from the GI tract after oral administration. The absolute bioavailability of 250 mg tablets is ≈ 50%. Food slightly delays onset of absorption and the formation of the antimicrobially active metabolite, 14–OH clarithromycin. In adults given the suspension (250 mg), food appeared to decrease mean peak plasma clarithromycin levels by 17% and the extent of absorption by 10% (food increased mean peak plasma levels by 27% and 42%, respectively, in children given 7.5 mg/kg).

In fasting healthy subjects, peak serum concentrations were attained within 2 hours (tablet) and around 3 hours (suspension) after oral dosing. The elimination half-life was ≈ 3 to 4 hours with 250 mg every 12 hours (tablet or suspension) and increased to 5 to 7 hours with the 500 mg tablet every 8 to 12 hours. With a 250 mg tablet every 12 hours 14–OH clarithromycin attains a peak steady-state concentration of ≈ 0.6 mcg/ml (0.7 mcg/ml with suspension) and has an elimination half-life of 5 to 6 hours (5 to 7 hours with suspension). The steady-state concentration of 14–OH clarithromycin is generally attained within 2 to 3 days.

After a 250 mg tablet every 12 hours, ≈ 20% of the dose is excreted in the urine as the unchanged parent drug. After a 500 mg tablet every 12 hours, the urinary excretion of clarithromycin is ≈ 30%. The renal clearance of clarithromycin is, however, relatively independent of the dose and approximates the normal glomerular filtration rate. The major metabolite found in urine is 14–OH clarithromycin which accounts for an additional 10% to 15% of the dose.

Steady-state concentrations of clarithromycin and 14–OH clarithromycin following 500 mg doses every 12 hours in adult patients with HIV infection were similar to those in healthy volunteers. In adult HIV-infected patients, steady-state clarithromycin C_{max} values ranged from 2 to 4 mcg/ml and 5 to 10 mcg/ml, respectively. In children with HIV taking 15 mg/kg every 12 hours, parent drug peak levels were generally 6 to 15 mcg/ml.

Clarithromycin is metabolized in the liver by hydroxylation and N-methylation. The steady-state concentrations of clarithromycin in subjects with impaired hepatic function did not differ from those in healthy subjects; however, the 14–OH clarithromycin concentrations were lower in the hepatically impaired subjects. The decreased formation of 14–OH clarithromycin was at least partially offset by an increase in renal clearance of clarithromycin in subjects with impaired hepatic function when compared to healthy subjects. The pharmacokinetics of clarithromycin were also altered in subjects with impaired renal function (see Warnings).

Clarithromycin and the 14–OH clarithromycin metabolite distribute readily into body tissues and fluids. No data are available on CSF penetration.

The plasma levels of clarithromycin and 14–OH clarithromycin were increased by the concomitant administration of omeprazole. For clarithromycin, the mean C_{max} was 10% greater, the mean C_{min} was 27% greater and the mean AUC was 15% greater when clarithromycin was administered with omeprazole than when clarithromycin was administered alone. Similar results were seen for 14–OH clarithromycin, the mean C_{max} was 45% greater, the mean C_{min} was 57% greater and the mean AUC was 45% greater. Clarithromycin concentrations in the gastric tissue and mucus were also increased by concomitant administration of omeprazole.

Microbiology: The 14–OH clarithromycin metabolite has clinically significant antimicrobial activity. Against *Haemophilus influenzae*, 14–OH clarithromycin is twice as active as the parent compound. However, for *Mycobacterium avium* complex (MAC) isolates, the 14–OH metabolite is 4 to 7 times less active than clarithromycin.

Beta-lactamase production should have no effect on clarithromycin activity.

Indications:

For the treatment of mild to moderate infections caused by susceptible strains of the designated microorganisms in the following conditions.

Adults:

Pharyngitis/Tonsillitis due to *Streptococcus pyogenes.*

Acute maxillary sinusitis due to *Haemophilus influenzae, Moraxella catarrhalis* or *S. pneumoniae.*

Acute bacterial exacerbation of chronic bronchitis due to *H. influenzae, M. catarrhalis* or *S. pneumoniae.*

Pneumonia due to *Mycoplasma pneumoniae* or *S. pneumoniae.*

Uncomplicated skin and skin structure infections due to *Staphylococcus aureus* or *S. pyogenes.* Abscesses usually require surgical drainage.

Disseminated mycobacterial infections due to *Mycobacterium avium* and *M. intracellulare.*

CLARITHROMYCIN

Prevention of disseminated Mycobacterium avium complex disease in patients with advanced HIV infection.

Helicobacter pylori – Clarithromycin in combination with omeprazole is indicated for the treatment of patients with an active duodenal ulcer associated with *H. pylori* infection. The eradication of *H. pylori* has been demonstrated to reduce the risk of duodenal ulcer recurrence.

Children:

Pharyngitis/Tonsillitis due to *S. pyogenes.*

Acute maxillary sinusitis due to *H. influenzae, M. catarrhalis* or *S. pneumoniae.*

Acute otitis media due to *H. influenzae, M. catarrhalis* or *S. pneumoniae.*

Uncomplicated skin and skin structure infections due to *S. aureus* or *S. pyogenes.* Abscesses usually require surgical drainage.

Disseminated mycobacterial infections due to *M. avium* and *M. intracellulare.*

Prevention of disseminated Mycobacterium avium complex disease in patients with advanced HIV infection.

Unlabeled uses: Prevention of bacterial endocarditis in penicillin-allergic patients undergoing dental, oral, esophageal or respiratory tract procedures.

Contraindications:

Hypersensitivity to clarithromycin, erythromycin or any of the macrolide antibiotics; patients receiving terfenadine or astemizole who have preexisting cardiac abnormalities (eg, arrhythmias, bradycardia, QT interval prolongation, ischemic heart disease, CHF) or electrolyte disturbances.

Warnings:

Pseudomembranous colitis has occurred with nearly all antibacterial agents, including macrolides, and may range in severity from mild to life-threatening. Therefore, it is important to consider this diagnosis in patients who present with diarrhea subsequent to the administration of antibacterial agents.

Treatment with antibacterial agents alters the normal flora of the colon and may permit overgrowth of clostridia. Studies indicate that a toxin produced by *Clostridium difficile* is a primary cause of "antibiotic-associated colitis."

After the diagnosis of pseudomembranous colitis has been established, initiate therapeutic measures. Mild cases of pseudomembranous colitis usually respond to discontinuation of the drug alone. In moderate to severe cases, give consideration to management with fluids and electrolytes, protein supplementation and treatment with an antibacterial drug effective against *C. difficile* colitis.

Renal/Hepatic function impairment: Clarithromycin is principally excreted via the liver and kidney and may be administered without dosage adjustment to patients with hepatic impairment and normal renal function. However, in the presence of severe renal impairment (creatinine < 30 ml/min) with or without coexisting hepatic impairment, decreased dosage or prolonged dosing intervals may be appropriate.

Elderly: Maximum concentrations and AUC of clarithromycin and 14–OH clarithromycin are increased. These changes in pharmacokinetics parallel known age-related decreases in renal function. In clinical trials, elderly patients did not have an increased incidence of adverse events when compared to younger patients. Consider dosage adjustment in elderly patients with severe renal impairment.

Pregnancy: Category C. Clarithromycin has adverse effects on pregnancy outcome or embryo-fetal development in monkeys, rats, mice and rabbits. There are no adequate and well controlled studies in pregnant women. Do not use clarithromycin in pregnant women except in clinical circumstances where no alternative therapy is appropriate. If pregnancy occurs while taking this drug, apprise the patient of the hazard to the fetus.

Lactation: Clarithromycin is excreted in the milk of animals; other drugs of this class are excreted in human breast milk. It is not known whether clarithromycin is excreted in human breast milk. Exercise caution when administering to a nursing woman.

Children: Safety and efficacy in children < 6 months of age have not been established.

Drug Interactions:

Like erythromycin, concurrent use of clarithromycin with drugs metabolized by the cytochrome P450 system may be associated with elevated serum levels of these drugs. Some of these interactions are described in the following table. Other drugs include, but are not limited to, alfentanil, bromocriptine, disopyramide, hexobarbital, lovastatin, phenytoin, pimozide and valproate. Also consider all drug interactions with erythromycin (see individual monograph).

Clarithromycin Drug Interactions			
Precipitant drug	Object drug*		Description
Clarithromycin	Anticoagulants, oral	↑	Oral anticoagulant effects may be potentiated. Carefully monitor PT.
Clarithromycin	Antihistamines, nonsedating Terfenadine Astemizole	↑	Following coadministration, plasma levels of the active acid metabolite of terfenadine were 3-fold higher on average. Do not use concurrently in patients who have preexisting cardiac abnormalities or electrolyte disturbances (see Contraindications).
Clarithromycin	Carbamazepine	↑	Increased concentrations of carbamazepine may occur. Consider monitoring carbamazepine levels.
Clarithromycin	Cisapride	↑	Serious cardiac arrhythmias (some fatal) including ventricular tachycardia, ventricular fibrillation, torsade de pointes and QT prolongation have been reported in patients taking cisapride with other drugs that inhibit cytochrome P450 IIIA4.
Clarithromycin	Cyclosporine	↑	Elevated cyclosporine with increased risk of toxicity (nephrotoxicity, neurotoxicity) may occur.
Clarithromycin	Digoxin	↑	Serum digoxin levels may be elevated because of clarithromycin's inhibitory effect on gut flora that metabolize digoxin. Serum digoxin levels should be carefully monitored while patients are receiving digoxin and clarithromycin simultaneously.
Clarithromycin	Ergot alkaloids	↑	Acute ergot toxicity characterized by severe peripheral vasopasm and dysesthesia has occurred.
Clarithromycin	Tacrolimus	↑	Plasma tacrolimus (FK506) levels may be increased, increasing the risk of toxicity.
Clarithromycin	Theophyllines	↑	Concurrent use may be associated with increased serum theophylline. Consider monitoring theophylline levels in patients receiving high doses of theophylline or with baseline concentrations in the upper therapeutic range. In two studies, theophylline steady-state levels of C_{max}, C_{min} and AUC increased ≈ 20%.
Clarithromycin	Triazolam	↑	CNS effects (eg, somnolence, confusion) have occurred.
Clarithromycin	Zidovudine	↔	Simultaneous use in HIV-infected patients resulted in decreased steady-state zidovudine levels; however, peak serum zidovudine concentrations may be increased or decreased.
Fluconazole	Clarithromycin	↑	Concomitant fluconazole 200 mg daily and clarithromycin 500 mg twice daily to 21 healthy volunteers led to increases in the mean steady-state clarithromycin C_{min} and AUC of 33% and 18%, respectively. Steady-state concentrations of the antimicrobially active metabolite 14-OH clarithromycin were not significantly affected by concomitant fluconazole.

* ↑ = Object drug increased. ↔ = Undetermined effect.

Drug/Food interactions: Following tablet administration, food delays both the onset of clarithromycin absorption and the formation of 14–OH clarithromycin (the active metabolite), but does not affect the extent of bioavailability. Following the suspension, food decreases mean peak clarithromycin levels and extent of absorption. However, clarithromycin may be given without regard to meals.

Adverse Reactions:

The majority of side effects observed in clinical trials were of a mild and transient nature. Fewer than 3% of adult patients without mycobacterial infections and fewer than 2% of children without mycobacterial infections discontinued therapy because of drug-related side effects.

The most frequently reported adverse events in adult patients were: Diarrhea, nausea, abnormal taste (3%); dyspepsia, abdominal pain/discomfort, headache (2%). In children, the most frequently reported events were: Diarrhea, vomiting (6%); abdominal pain, rash (3%); headache (2%).

CLARITHROMYCIN

Post-Marketing experience: Allergic reactions ranging from urticaria and mild skin eruptions to rare cases of anaphylaxis and Stevens-Johnson syndrome; glossitis; stomatitis; oral moniliasis; vomiting; dizziness; isolated reports of hearing loss, which is usually reversible, occurring chiefly in elderly women; alterations of the sense of smell, usually in conjunction with taste perversion; transient CNS events including behavioral changes, confusional states, depersonalization, disorientation, hallucinations, insomnia, nightmares, tinnitus and vertigo; hepatic dysfunction, including increased liver enzymes and hepatocellular cholestatic hepatitis, with or without jaundice (infrequently). Hepatic dysfunction may be severe and is usually reversible. In very rare instances, hepatic failure with fatal outcome has been reported and generally has been associated with serious underlying diseases or concomitant medications.

Rarely, erythromycin and clarithromycin have been associated with ventricular arrhythmias, including ventricular tachycardia and torsade de pointes, in individuals with prolonged QT_c intervals.

Lab test abnormalities:

Hepatic – Elevated ALT, AST, GGT, alkaline phosphatase, LDH, total bilirubin (< 1%).
Hematologic – Decreased WBC (< 1%); elevated prothrombin time (1%).
Renal – Elevated BUN (4%); elevated serum creatinine (< 1%).

Patient Information:

Clarithromycin may be given without regard to meals and can be taken with milk.

Suspension: Shake well before each use. Do not refrigerate.

Administration and Dosage:

Approved by the FDA in October 1991.

Clarithromycin Dosage Regimen for Active Duodenal Ulcer Associated with H. pylori Infection (28-Day Therapy)	
Days 1 - 14	Days 15 - 28
500 mg tablet three times daily plus omeprazole 2 x 20 mg every morning	Omeprazole 20 mg every morning

Adults:

Clarithromycin Dosage Guidelines		
Infection	Dosage (every 12 hr)	Normal duration (days)
Pharyngitis/Tonsillitis	250 mg	10
Acute maxillary sinusitis	500 mg	14
Acute exacerbation of chronic bronchitis due to:		
S. pneumoniae	250 mg	7 to 14
M. catarrhalis	250 mg	7 to 14
H. influenzae	500 mg	7 to 14
Pneumonia due to:		
S. pneumoniae	250 mg	7 to 14
M. pneumoniae	250 mg	7 to 14
Uncomplicated skin and skin structure	250 mg	7 to 14

Children: Usual recommended daily dosage is 15 mg/kg/day divided every 12 hours for 10 days.

Pediatric Dosage Guidelines (Based on Body Weight)				
Dosing calculated on 7.5 mg/kg q 12 h				
Weight		Dose	125 mg/5 ml	250 mg/5 ml
kg	lbs	(q 12 h)	(q 12 h)	(q 12 h)
9	20	62.5 mg	2.5 ml	1.25 ml
17	37	125 mg	5 ml	2.5 ml
25	55	187.5 mg	7.5 ml	3.75 ml
33	73	250 mg	10 ml	5 ml

Mycobacterial infections: Recommended as the primary agent for the treatment of disseminated *Mycobacterium avium* complex (MAC). Use in combination with other antimycobacterial drugs that have shown in vitro activity against MAC (eg, ethambutol, clofazimine, rifampin). The US Public Health Service Task Force has provided recommendations for the treatment of MAC. Continue therapy for life if clinical and mycobacterial improvements are observed.

CLARITHROMYCIN

Dosage (treatment and prevention) –

Adults: 500 mg twice daily.

Children: 7.5 mg/kg twice daily up to 500 mg twice daily. Refer to the Pediatric Dosage table for dosing recommendations.

Bacterial endocarditis prophylaxis – 500 mg (15 mg/kg for children) orally 1 hour before procedure.

Renal/Hepatic function impairment: May be administered without dosage adjustment in the presence of hepatic impairment if there is normal renal function. However, in the presence of severe renal impairment (Ccr < 30 ml/min) with or without coexisting hepatic impairment, halved doses or prolongation of dosing intervals may be needed.

Storage/Stability:

Tablets and granules for oral suspension – Store at controlled room temperature 15° to 30°C (59° to 86°F) in a well closed container. Protect from light.

Reconstituted suspension – Shake well before each use. Do not refrigerate. After mixing, store at 15° to 30°C (59° to 86°F), and use within 14 days.

Rx	**Biaxin** (Abbott)	**Tablets:** 250 mg	(KT). Yellow. Film coated. Oval. In 60s and UD 100s.
		500 mg	(KL). Yellow. Film coated. Oval. In 60s and UD 100s.
		Granules for Oral Suspension (after reconstitution): 125 mg/5 ml	Sucrose. Fruit punch flavor. In 50 and 100 ml.
		250 mg/5 ml	Sucrose. Fruit punch flavor. In 50 and 100 ml.

AZITHROMYCIN

Actions:

Pharmacology: Azithromycin is an azalide antibiotic, a subclass of the macrolides. Azithromycin is derived from erythromycin; however, it differs chemically from erythromycin in that a methyl-substituted nitrogen atom is incorporated into the lactone ring. Azithromycin acts by binding to the 50S ribosomal subunit of susceptible organisms and thus interfering with microbial protein synthesis. Nucleic acid synthesis is not affected.

Pharmacokinetics:

Adults – Following oral administration, azithromycin is rapidly absorbed and widely distributed throughout the body. Rapid distribution into tissues and high concentration within cells result in significantly higher azithromycin concentrations in tissues than in plasma or serum.

The pharmacokinetic parameters of azithromycin capsules in plasma after a 500 mg loading dose on day 1 followed by 250 mg every day on days 2 through 5 in healthy young adults (ages 18 to 40 years old) are listed in the following table.

Azithromycin Pharmacokinetics (n = 12)

Parameter (mean)	Day 1	Day 5
C_{max} (mcg/ml)	0.41	0.24
T_{max} (hr)	2.5	3.2
AUC 0-24 (mcg•hr/ml)	2.6	2.1
C_{min} (mcg/ml)	0.05	0.05
Urinary excretion (% dose)	4.5	6.5

Plasma azithromycin concentrations declined in a polyphasic pattern resulting in an average terminal half-life of 68 hours. On the recommended dosing regimen, C_{min} and C_{max} remained essentially unchanged from day 2 through day 5. However, without a loading dose, C_{min} levels required 5 to 7 days to reach steady state.

The pharmacokinetic parameters in elderly men were similar to those in young adults; however, in elderly women, although higher peak concentrations (increased by 30% to 50%) were observed, no significant accumulation occurred.

The high values in adults for apparent steady-state volume of distribution (31.1 L/kg) and plasma clearance (630 ml/min) suggest that the prolonged half-life is due to extensive uptake and subsequent release of drug from tissues. Selected tissue (or fluid) to plasma/serum concentration ratios are shown in the following table:

AZITHROMYCIN

Azithromycin Levels After Recommended Clinical Dosage Regimen (Adults)				
Tissue or fluid	Time after dose (hr)	Tissue or fluid concentration (mcg/g or mcg/ml)[1]	Plasma or serum level (mcg/ml)	Tissue (fluid): Plasma (serum) ratio[1]
Skin	72-96	0.4	0.012	35
Lung	72-96	4	0.012	> 100
Sputum	2-4	1	0.64	2
Sputum	10-12	2.9	0.1	30
Tonsil	9-18	4.5	0.03	> 100
Tonsil	180	0.9	0.006	> 100
Cervix	19	2.8	0.04	70

[1] High tissue concentrations should not be interpreted to be quantitatively related to clinical efficacy. The antimicrobial activity of azithromycin is pH-related. Azithromycin is concentrated in cell lysosomes which have a low intraorganelle pH, at which the drug's activity is reduced. However, the extensive distribution of drug to tissues may be relevant to clinical activity.

Only very low concentrations were noted in CSF (< 0.01 mcg/ml) in the presence of non-inflamed meninges.

The serum protein binding of azithromycin is variable, decreasing from 51% at 0.02 mcg/ml to 7% at 2 mcg/ml.

Biliary excretion of azithromycin, predominantly as unchanged drug, is a major route of elimination. Over the course of a week, approximately 6% of the administered dose appears as unchanged drug in urine. Food decreases the absorption of azithromycin capsules, reducing the C_{max} by 52% and the AUC by 43%. When azithromycin suspension was administered with food to 28 healthy adult males, the rate of absorption (C_{max}) was increased by 56% while the extent of absorption (AUC) was unchanged. Azithromycin concentrates in phagocytes and fibroblasts; concentration in phagocytes may contribute to drug distribution to inflamed tissues.

Children – In two clinical studies, azithromycin for oral suspension was dosed at 10 mg/kg on day 1, followed by 5 mg/kg on days 2 through 5 to two groups of children (ages 1 to 5 years and 5 to 15 years, respectively). The mean pharmacokinetic parameters at day 5 were C_{max} = 0.216 mcg/ml, T_{max} = 1.9 hours and AUC_{0-24} = 1.822 mcg•hr/ml for the 1 to 5 year-old group. Mean pharmacokinetic parameters at day 5 for the 5 to 15 year olds were C_{max} = 0.383 mcg/ml, T_{max} = 2.4 hours and AUC_{0-24} = 3.109 mcg•hr/ml.

There are no pharmacokinetic data on azithromycin suspension when administered at a dose of 12 mg/kg/day in the presence or absence of food. (For the pediatric pharyngitis/tonsillitis dose, see Administration and Dosage).

Microbiology: Azithromycin is active against a variety of organisms. Refer to the table in the Macrolides introduction.

Indications:

For the treatment of patients with mild to moderate infections caused by susceptible strains of the designated microorganisms in the specific conditions listed below:

Adults:

Acute bacterial exacerbations of chronic obstructive pulmonary disease due to *Haemophilus influenzae, Moraxella catarrhalis* or *Streptococcus pneumoniae.*

Community-acquired pneumonia of mild severity due to *S pneumoniae* or *H influenzae* in patients appropriate for outpatient oral therapy (see Warnings).

Pharyngitis/Tonsillitis caused by *S pyogenes* in individuals who cannot use first-line therapy.

Note: Penicillin IM is the usual drug of choice in the treatment of *S pyogenes* infections and the prophylaxis of rheumatic fever. Azithromycin is often effective in the eradication of susceptible strains of *S pyogenes* from the nasopharynx. Because some strains are resistant to azithromycin, perform susceptibility tests when patients are treated with azithromycin.

Skin/Skin structure infections, uncomplicated due to *Staphylococcus aureus, S pyogenes* or *S agalactiae.* Abscesses usually require surgical drainage.

Sexually transmitted diseases – Non-gonococcal urethritis and cervicitis due to *Chlamydia trachomatis.*

Children:

Acute otitis media caused by *H influenzae, M catarrhalis* or *S pneumoniae.*

Pharyngitis/Tonsillitis caused by *S pyogenes* in individuals who cannot use first-line therapy.

AZITHROMYCIN

Note: Penicillin IM is the usual drug of choice in the treatment of *S pyogenes* infections and the prophylaxis of rheumatic fever. Azithromycin is often effective in the eradication of susceptible strains of *S pyogenes* from the nasopharynx. Because some strains are resistant to azithromycin, perform susceptibility tests when patients are treated with azithromycin.

Unlabeled uses: Prevention of bacterial endocarditis in penicillin-allergic patients undergoing dental, oral, esophageal or respiratory tract procedures.

Contraindications:

Hypersensitivity to azithromycin, erythromycin or any macrolide antibiotic.

Warnings:

Pneumonia: Azithromycin is only safe and effective in the treatment of community-acquired pneumonia of mild severity due to *S pneumoniae* and *H influenzae* in patients appropriate for outpatient oral therapy. Do not use in patients with pneumonia who are judged to be inappropriate for outpatient oral therapy because of moderate to severe illness or risk factors such as any of the following: Nosocomially acquired infections; known or suspected bacteremia; conditions requiring hospitalization; significant underlying health problems that may compromise the patient's ability to respond to their illness (including immunodeficiency or functional asplenia); elderly or debilitated patients.

Gonorrhea or syphilis: Azithromycin at the recommended dose should not be relied upon to treat gonorrhea or syphilis. Antimicrobial agents used in high doses for short periods of time to treat non-gonococcal urethritis may mask or delay the symptoms of incubating gonorrhea or syphilis. All patients with sexually transmitted urethritis or cervicitis should have a serologic test for syphilis and appropriate cultures for gonorrhea performed at the time of diagnosis. Initiate appropriate antimicrobial therapy and follow-up tests for these diseases if infection is confirmed.

Pseudomembranous colitis has been reported with nearly all antibacterial agents and may range in severity from mild to life-threatening. Therefore, it is important to consider this diagnosis in patients who present with diarrhea subsequent to the administration of antibacterial agents.

Treatment with antibacterial agents alters the normal flora of the colon and may permit overgrowth of clostridia. Studies indicate that a toxin produced by *Clostridium difficile* is a primary cause of "antibiotic-associated colitis."

After the diagnosis of pseudomembranous colitis has been established, initiate therapeutic measures. Mild cases of pseudomembranous colitis usually respond to discontinuation of the drug alone. In moderate to severe cases, give consideration to management with fluids and electrolytes, protein supplementation and treatment with an antibacterial drug effective against *C difficile* colitis.

Cardiac effects: During post-marketing, one patient with a history of arrhythmias experienced torsade de pointes and subsequent MI following a course of azithromycin therapy. Ventricular arrhythmias, including ventricular tachycardia and torsade de pointes, in individuals with prolonged QT intervals have not been reported in clinical trials with azithromycin; however, it has occurred with macrolide products.

Hypersensitivity: Rare serious allergic reactions, including angioedema and anaphylaxis, have been reported in patients on azithromycin therapy. Despite initially successful symptomatic treatment of the allergic symptoms, when symptomatic therapy was discontinued, the allergic symptoms recurred soon thereafter in some patients without further azithromycin exposure. These patients required prolonged periods of observation and symptomatic treatment. The relationship of these episodes to the long tissue half-life of azithromycin and subsequent prolonged exposure to antigen is unknown at present.

If an allergic reaction occurs, discontinue and institute appropriate therapy. Physicians should be aware that reappearance of the allergic symptoms may occur when symptomatic therapy is discontinued.

AZITHROMYCIN

Renal/Hepatic function impairment: Because azithromycin is principally eliminated via the liver, exercise caution when azithromycin is administered to patients with impaired hepatic function. There are no data regarding azithromycin usage in patients with renal impairment; thus, exercise caution when prescribing azithromycin in these patients.

Elderly: Pharmacokinetic parameters in older volunteers (65 to 85 years old) were similar to those in younger volunteers (18 to 40 years old) for the 5 day therapeutic regimen. Dosage adjustment does not appear to be necessary for older patients with normal renal and hepatic function receiving treatment with this dosage regimen.

Pregnancy: Category B. There are no adequate and well controlled studies in pregnant women. Use during pregnancy only if clearly needed.

Lactation: It is not known whether azithromycin is excreted in breast milk. Exercise caution when administering to a nursing woman.

Children:

Acute otitis media – Safety and effectiveness in children < 6 months of age have not been established.

Pharyngitis/Tonsillitis – Safety and effectiveness in children < 2 years of age have not been established.

Precautions:

Use of antibiotics (especially prolonged or repeated therapy) may result in bacterial or fungal overgrowth of nonsusceptible organisms. Such overgrowth may lead to a secondary infection. Take appropriate measures if superinfection occurs.

Photosensitization (photoallergy or phototoxicity) may occur; therefore, caution patients to take protective measures against exposure to ultraviolet or sunlight (ie, sunscreens, protective clothing) until tolerance is determined.

Drug Interactions:

Azithromycin Drug Interactions

Precipitant drug	Object drug*		Description
Antacids	Azithromycin	↓	Aluminum- and magnesium-containing antacids reduce the peak serum levels but not the extent of azithromycin absorption.
Azithromycin	Tacrolimus	↑	Azithromycin may increase the plasma levels of tacrolimus, increasing the risk of toxicity.
Azithromycin	Theophylline	↔	Azithromycin did not affect the plasma levels or pharmacokinetics of theophylline administered as a single IV dose. The effect of azithromycin on multiple doses is not known. However, concurrent use of macrolides and theophylline has been associated with increases in serum concentrations of theophylline. Therefore, until further data are available, carefully monitor theophylline levels in patients receiving azithromycin and theophylline concomitantly.
Azithromycin	Warfarin	↔	Azithromycin did not affect the prothrombin time (PT) response to a single dose of warfarin. However, concurrent use of macrolides and warfarin has been associated with increased anticoagulant effects. Carefully monitor PT in all patients treated with azithromycin and warfarin concomitantly.

* ↑ = Object drug increased. ↓ = Object drug decreased. ↔ = Undetermined effect.

Also consider all drug interactions listed with erythromycin (see individual monograph).

Drug/Food interactions: Food decreases absorption of azithromycin capsules, reducing maximum concentration by 52% and bioavailability by 43%. When azithromycin suspension was administered with food to 28 healthy adult males, the rate of absorption (C_{max}) was increased by 56% while the extent of absorption (AUC) was unchanged. Take 1 hour before or 2 hours after a meal. Do not take with food.

Adverse Reactions:

Rare serious allergic reactions, including angioedema and anaphylaxis, have been reported in patients on azithromycin therapy. Despite initially successful symptomatic treatment of the allergic symptoms, when symptomatic therapy was discontinued, the allergic symptoms recurred soon thereafter in some patients without further azithromycin exposure. These patients required prolonged periods of observation and symptomatic treatment. The relationship of these episodes to the long tissue half-life of azithromycin and subsequent prolonged exposure to antigen is unknown at present (see Warnings).

Most side effects are mild to moderate in severity and are reversible upon discontinuation of the drug. Approximately 0.7% of the patients (adults and children) from the multiple-dose clinical trials discontinued therapy because of treatment-related side effects. Most of the side effects leading to discontinuation were related to the GI tract (eg, nausea, vomiting, diarrhea, abdominal pain). Rare, but potentially serious side effects, were angioedema (1 case), cholestatic jaundice (1 case) and torsade de pointes with subsequent myocardial infarction (see Warnings).

Adults:

Single 1 g dose regimen – The most common side effects were related to the GI system and were more frequently reported in the multiple-dose regimen. Side effects that occurred with a frequency of ≥ 1% included: Diarrhea/loose stools (7%); nausea, abdominal pain (5%); vomiting (2%); dyspepsia, vaginitis (1%).

Multiple-dose regimen – Overall, the most common side effects in patients receiving the multiple-dose regimen were related to the GI system with diarrhea/loose stools (5%), nausea and abdominal pain (3%) being the most frequently reported. The following adverse reactions occurred in ≤ 1% of patients:

Cardiovascular – Palpitations; chest pain.
GI – Dyspepsia; flatulence; vomiting; melena; cholestatic jaundice.
GU – Monilia; vaginitis; nephritis.
CNS – Dizziness; headache; vertigo; somnolence; fatigue.
Hypersensitivity – Rash; photosensitivity; angioedema (see Warnings).

AZITHROMYCIN

Children: The types of side effects in children were comparable to those seen in adults, with different incidence rates for the two dosage regimens recommended in children.

Acute otitis media – For the recommended dosage regimen of 10 mg/kg on day 1 followed by 5 mg/kg on days 2 to 5, the most frequent side effects were diarrhea/loose stools (2%), abdominal pain (2%), vomiting (1%) and nausea (1%).

Pharyngitis/tonsillitis – For the recommended dosage regimen of 12 mg/kg on days 1 to 5, the most frequent side effects were diarrhea/loose stools (6%), vomiting (5%), abdominal pain (3%), nausea (2%) and headache (1%). The following adverse reactions occurred with a frequency of 1% or less:

Cardiovascular – Chest pain.

GI – Dyspepsia; constipation; anorexia; flatulence; gastritis.

CNS – Headache; hyperkinesia; dizziness; agitation; nervousness; insomnia; fatigue; fever; malaise.

Hypersensitivity – Rash.

Special senses – Conjunctivitis.

Lab test abnormalities:

Adults – Elevated serum creatine phosphokinase, potassium, ALT, GGT and AST (1% to 2%); leukopenia, neutropenia, decreased platelet count and elevated serum alkaline phosphatase, bilirubin, BUN, creatinine, blood glucose, LDH and phosphate (≤ 1%). When follow-up was provided, changes in laboratory tests appeared to be reversible. In multiple-dose clinical trials involving > 3000 patients, three patients discontinued therapy because of treatment-related liver enzyme abnormalities and one because of a renal function abnormality.

Children – Significant abnormalities (irrespective of drug relationship) occurring during clinical trials were all reported at a frequency of less than 1%, but were similar in type to the adult pattern.

In multiple-dose clinical trials involving almost 3000 pediatric patients, no patients discontinued therapy because of treatment-related abnormalities.

Patient Information:

Caution patients to take azithromycin at least 1 hour prior to a meal or at least 2 hours after a meal. Azithromycin should not be mixed or taken with food.

Caution patients not to take aluminum- and magnesium-containing antacids and azithromycin simultaneously.

Patients should discontinue azithromycin immediately and contact a physician if any signs of an allergic reaction oocur.

Administration and Dosage:

Approved by the FDA in November 1991.

Adults: Administer at least 1 hour before or 2 hours after a meal. Do not administer with food.

Mild to moderate acute bacterial exacerbations of chronic obstructive pulmonary disease, community-acquired pneumonia of mild severity, pharyngitis/tonsillitis (as second-line therapy), and uncomplicated skin and skin structure infections 500 mg as a single dose on the first day followed by 250 mg once daily on days 2 through 5.

Non-gonococcal urethritis and cervicitis – Give a single 1 g dose.

CDC recommended treatment schedules for chancroid and chlamydia† – 1 g as a single dose.

Bacterial endocarditis prophylaxis: 500 mg (15 mg/kg for children) orally 1 hour before procedure.

Children:

Acute otitis media – The recommended dose of azithromycin for oral suspension for the treatment of children with acute otitis media is 10 mg/kg as a single dose on the first day (not to exceed 500 mg/day, followed by 5 mg/kg on days 2 through 5 (not to exceed 250 mg/day). See the following table.

† CDC 1993 Sexually Transmitted Diseases Treatment Guidelines. *Morbidity and Mortality Weekly Report* 1993 Sept 24;42 (No. RR-14):1–102.

Pediatric Dosage Guidelines for Otitis Media (≥ 6 months of age)						
Dosing calculated on 10 mg/kg on day 1 dose, followed by 5 mg/kg on days 2 to 5						
Weight		Amount of 100 mg/5 ml Suspension		Amount of 200 mg/5 ml Suspension		Total ml per treatment course
kg	lbs	Day 1	Days 2 to 5	Day 1	Days 2 to 5	
10	22	5 ml	2.5 ml			15 ml
20	44			5 ml	2.5 ml	15 ml
30	66			7.5 ml	3.75 ml	22.5 ml
40	88			10 ml	5 ml	30 ml

Pharyngitis/tonsillitis – The recommended dose for children with Pharyngitis/tonsillitis is 12 mg/kg qd for 5 days (not to exceed 500 mg/day). See the following.

Pediatric Dosage Guidelines for Pharyngitis/Tonsillitis (≥ 2 years of age)			
Dosing calculated on 12 mg/kg once daily days 1 through 5			
Weight		Amount of 200 mg/5 ml suspension	
kg	lbs	Days 1 to 5	Total ml per treatment course
8	18	2.5 ml	12.5 ml
17	37	5 ml	25 ml
25	55	7.5 ml	37.5 ml
33	73	10 ml	50 ml
40	88	12.5	62.5 ml

Preparation of oral solution:

Preparation of Azithromycin Oral Solution			
Azithromycin/Bottle	Water to add	Total volume after constitution	Resulting azithromycin concentration
300 mg	9 ml	15 ml	100 mg/5 ml
600 mg	9 ml	15 ml	200 mg/5 ml
900 mg	12 ml	22.5 ml	200 mg/5ml

Storage/Stability: Store capsules below 30° C (86° F).
Store reconstituted solution between 5° and 30° C (41° and 86° F).

Rx	**Zithromax** (Pfizer)	**Capsules**: 250 mg azithromycin (as dihydrate)	Lactose. (Pfizer 305). Red. In 50s, UD 50s and Z-Pak 6s (3).
		Suspension: 100 mg/5 ml azithromycin (as dihydrate) after reconstitution	Sucrose. In bottles containing 300 mg powder.
		Suspension: 200 mg/5 ml azithromycin (as dihydrate) after reconstitution	Sucrose. In bottles containing 600 or 900 mg powder.

DIRITHROMYCIN

Actions:

Pharmacology: Dirithromycin, a semi-synthetic macrolide antibiotic, is a pro-drug converted non-enzymatically during intestinal absorption into the microbiologically active moiety erythromycylamine. Erythromycylamine, the microbiologically active product of dirithromycin hydrolysis, exerts its activity by binding to the 50S ribosomal subunits of susceptible microorganisms resulting in inhibition of protein synthesis.

Pharmacokinetics:

Absorption – Dirithromycin is rapidly absorbed and converted by nonenzymatic hydrolysis to the microbiologically active compound erythromycylamine. The absolute bioavailability of the oral formulation is ≈ 10%. The pharmacokinetic parameters of erythromycylamine in plasma after single-and multiple-dose oral administration of 500 mg dirithromycin once daily for 10 days in 10 fasting healthy subjects (19 to 50 years of age) were as follows:

Erythromycylamine Pharmacokinetics		
	Mean	
Parameter (n=10)	Day 1	Day 10
C_{max} (mcg/ml)	0.3	0.4
T_{max} (hr)	3.9	4.1
AUC_{0-24}(mcg•hr/ml)	0.9	1.8

Distribution – The protein binding of erythromycylamine ranges from 15% to 30%. Erythromycylamine is widely distributed throughout the body with a mean apparent volume of distribution of 800 L.

Rapid distribution of erythromycylamine into tissues and high levels within cells result in significantly higher levels in tissues than in plasma or serum.

Steady-State Tissue Concentrations of Erythromycylamine after 500 mg Dirithromycin Once/Day				
Tissue	Time after last last dose (hr)	Mean tissue concentration (mcg/g or mcg/10^7 cells)	Corresponding mean plasma or serum concentration (mcg/ml)	Tissue/plasma (serum) ratio[1]
Tonsil	14	3.47	0.17	20.4
Healthy lung	12	3.79	0.13	29.2
Pathologic/infected lung	12	3.85	0.13	29.6
Infected bronchial mucosa	12	1.7	0.13	13.1
Alveolar macrophages	5	0.37	0.35	1.1

[1] High tissue concentrations should not be interpreted to be qualitatively related to clinical efficacy. Erythromycylamine is concentrated in cell lysosomes, which have a low organelle pH at which drug activity is reduced.

Metabolism/Excretion – Erythromycylamine is primarily eliminated in the bile and undergoes little or no hepatic metabolism. Thus, the primary route of elimination is fecal/hepatic with 81% to 97% of the dose eliminated in this manner. Approximately 2% of the administered dose is eliminated through the kidney, mainly within the first 36 hours following drug administration.

The mean plasma half-life of erythromycylamine was estimated to be about 8 hr (range, 2 to 36 hr), while a mean urinary terminal elimination half-life of about 44 hr (range, 16 to 65 hr) and a mean apparent total body clearance of approximately 23 L/hr (20 to 32 L/hr) were observed in patients with normal renal function.

Microbiology: Dirithromycin/Erythromycylamine are active against a variety of organisms. Refer to the table in the Macrolides introduction.

Indications:

For the treatment of individuals ≥ 12 years of age with mild to moderate infections caused by susceptible strains of the designated microorganisms in the specific conditions listed below.

Acute bacterial exacerbations of chronic bronchitis due to *Moraxella catarrhalis* or *Streptococcus pneumoniae.* See Warnings.

Secondary bacterial infection of acute bronchitis due to *M catarrhalis* or *S pneumoniae.*

Community-acquired pneumonia due to *Legionella pneumophila, Mycoplasma pneumoniae* or *S pneumoniae.*

Pharyngitis/Tonsillitis due to *S pyogenes.*

The usual drug of choice in the treatment and prevention of streptococcal infections and the prophylaxis of rheumatic fever is penicillin. Dirithromycin generally is effective in the eradication of *S pyogenes* from the nasopharynx; however, data establishing the efficacy of dirithromycin in the subsequent prevention of rheumatic fever are not available at present.

Uncomplicated skin and skin structure infections due to *Staphylococcus aureus* (methicillin-susceptible strains). Abscesses usually require surgical drainage. See Warnings.

Contraindications:

Hypersensitivity to dirithromycin, erythromycin or any other macrolide antibiotic.

Warnings:

Terfenadine drug interaction: In a study of six healthy males, dirithromycin did not affect terfenadine metabolism. The subjects received terfenadine alone (60 mg bid) for 8 days, then terfenadine with dirithromycin (500 mg qd) for 10 days (both drugs were thus dosed to steady state). The pharmacokinetics of terfenadine and its acid metabolite and the electrocardiographic QT_c interval were measured in both periods (with terfenadine alone, and with terfenadine plus dirithromycin). In five men, terfenadine was undetectable (< 5 ng/ml) throughout the study; in one man, the terfenadine C_{max} was 8.1 ng/ml with terfenadine alone and 7.2 ng/ml with terfenadine plus dirithromycin. The mean C_{max}, T_{max} and AUC of the acid metabolite of terfenadine were not significantly changed. The mean QT_c interval was 369 msec with terfenadine alone and 367 with terfenadine plus dirithromycin.

Serious cardiac dysrhythmias, some resulting in death, have occurred in patients receiving terfenadine concomitantly with other macrolide antibiotics. In addition, most macrolides are contraindicated in patients receiving terfenadine therapy who have preexisting cardiac abnormalities (eg, arrhythmia, bradycardia, QT_c interval prolongation, ischemic heart disease, congestive heart failure) or electrolyte disturbances. Until further use data are available, it is prudent to monitor the terfenadine levels when dirithromycin and terfenadine are coadministered.

DIRITHROMYCIN

Bacteremias: Dirithromycin should not be used in patients with known, suspected or potential bacteremias as serum levels are inadequate to provide antibacterial coverage of the blood stream.

Respiratory infections: Because the safety and efficacy of dirithromycin in the treatment of respiratory disease secondary to *H influenzae* have not been demonstrated, dirithromycin is NOT indicated for the empiric treatment of acute bacterial exacerbations of chronic or secondary bacterial infecton of acute bronchitis. Infections known, suspected or considered potentially to be caused by *Haemophilus* species should be treated by an antibacterial agent indicated for such treatment.

Skin/Skin structure infections: Because the safety and efficacy of dirithromycin in the treatment of uncomplicated skin and skin structure infections due to *S pyogenes* have not been demonstrated, dirithromycin is NOT indicated for the empiric treatment of uncomplicated skin and skin structure infections. Infections known, suspected or potentially caused by *S pyogenes* should be treated with an antibacterial agent indicated for such treatment.

Pseudomembranous colitis has been reported with nearly all antibacterial agents, including dirithromycin, and may range in severity from mild to life-threatening. Therefore, it is important to consider this diagnosis in patients who present with diarrhea subsequent to the administration of antibacterial agents. Treatment with antibacterial agents alters the normal flora of the colon and may permit overgrowth of clostridia. Studies indicate that a toxin produced by *Clostridium difficile* is a primary cause of "antibiotic-associated colitis."

After the diagnosis of pseudomembranous colitis has been established, initiate therapeutic measures. Mild cases of pseudomembranous colitis usually respond to discontinuation of the drug alone. In moderate-to-severe cases, consider management with fluids and electrolytes, protein supplementation and treatment with an antibacterial drug clinically effective against *C difficile* colitis.

Renal function impairment: The mean peak plasma concentration (C_{max}) and AUC tended to increase as creatinine clearance decreased; however, based on data available to date, no dosage adjustment should be necessary inpatients with impaired renal function, including dialysis patients.

Hepatic function impairment: In patients with mild (Child's Grade A) hepatic impairment, mean peak serum concentration, AUC and volume of distribution increased somewhat with multiple-dose administration; however, based on the magnitude of these changes, no dosage adjustment should be necessary in patients with mildly impaired hepatic function. The pharmacokinetics of dirithromycin in patients with moderate or severe hepatic function impairment (Child's Grade B or greater) have not been studied.

Elderly: In a multiple-dose study in which 19 healthy elderly subjects (65 to 83 years of age) were given 500 mg dirithromycin every day for 10 days, C_{max} and AUC tended to increase with age; however, neither C_{max} nor AUC was statistically or clinically significantly altered with age. Therefore, based on these pharmacokinetic results, no dosage adjustment should be necessary in elderly patients.

Pregnancy: Category C. A study in mice demonstrated that fetal weight was significantly depressed at the 1000 mg/kg dose (8 times the maximum recommended human dose), and there was an increased occurrence of incomplete ossification among these fetuses (a manifestation of retarded development). This decrease in ossification was also seen in rats given 1000 mg/kg/day for 2 weeks prior to mating, throughout the mating period and throughout gestation.

There are no adequate and well controlled studies in pregnant women. Use during pregnancy only if the potential benefit justifies the potential risk to the fetus.

DIRITHROMYCIN

Lactation: It is not known whether either dirithromycin or erythromycylamine is excreted in breast milk. Dirithromycin is excreted in milk of rodents; other drugs of this class are excreted in human milk. Use caution when administering to a nursing woman.

Children: Safety and efficacy in children < 12 years of age have not been established.

Precautions:

Superinfection: Use of antibiotics (especially prolonged or repeated therapy) may result in bacterial or fungal overgrowth of nonsusceptible organisms. Such overgrowth may lead to a secondary infection. Take appropriate measures if this occurs.

Drug Interactions:

Dirithromycin Drug Interactions			
Precipitant drug	Object drug*		Description
Dirithromycin	Antihistamines, nonsedating Terfenadine	↔	An interaction does not appear to occur. However, it is prudent to monitor terfenadine levels during concurrent use. See Warnings.
Dirithromycin	Theophyllines	↔	Most patients treated with dirithromycin receiving theophylline may not require empiric adjustment of the theophylline dosage or monitoring of theophylline plasma concentrations. However, monitor theophylline plasma levels, with dosage adjustment as appropriate, when pulmonary disease requires maintaining a given theophylline plasma level for optimal pulmonary function or when theophylline levels are at the higher end of the therapeutic range.
Antacids	Dirithromycin	⬆	When given immediately antacids, the absorption of dirithromycin is slightly enhanced.
H_2 antagonists	Dirithromycin	⬆	When given immediately after H_2-antagonists, dirithromycin absorption is slightly enhanced.

* ⬆ = Object drug increased. ↔ = Undetermined effect.

Also consider all drug interactions with erythromycin (see individual monograph.)

Drug/Food interactions: Dirithromycin should be administered with food or within an hour of having eaten. The effect of food on bioavailability was evaluated after administration of two 250 mg tablets 1 or 4 hours before food and immediately after a standard breakfast. Results indicated an increase in absorption of erythromycylamine when dirithromycin was administered after food, while a significant decrease in C_{max} (33%) and AUC (31%) occurred when administered 1 hour before food. Dietary fat had little or no effect on the bioavailability of dirthromycin.

Adverse Reactions:

Dirithromycin Adverse Reactions (%): Dirithromycin vs Erythromycin		
Adverse reaction	Dirithromycin	Erythromycin
Abdominal pain	9.7	7.5
Headache	8.6	8.2
Nausea	8.3	7.5
Diarrhea	7.7	7.3
Platelet count increased	3.8	4.8
Vomiting	3	2.8
Dyspepsia	2.6	2.1
Potassium increased	2.6	0
Dizziness/Vertigo	2.3	2.3
Pain (non-specific)	2.2	1.6
Asthenia	2	1.9
GI disorder	1.6	1.4
Increased cough	1.5	2.6
Flatulence	1.5	1.5
Rash	1.4	2.6
Bicarbonate decreased	1.4	2
CPK increased	1.2	0.9
Eosinophils increased	1.2	0.6

DIRITHROMYCIN

Dirithromycin Adverse Reactions (%): Dirithromycin vs Erythromycin		
Adverse reaction	Dirithromycin	Erythromycin
Seg neutrophils increased	1.2	1.3
Dyspnea	1.2	1.2
Pruritus/Urticaria	1.2	1
Insomnia	1	0.7

Other adverse reactions occuring during the clinical trials with dirithromycin included the following (> 0.1% to < 1%).

Abnormal stools, allergic reaction (not further defined), amblyopia, anorexia, anxiety, constipation, dehydration, depression, dry mouth, dysmenorrhea, edema, epistaxis, eye disorder (not further defined), fever, flu syndrome, gastritis, gastroenteritis, hemoptysis, hyperventilation, malaise, mouth ulceration, myalgia, neck pain, nervousness, palpitaion, paresthesia, peripheral edema, somnolence, sweating, syncope, taste perversion, thirst, tinnitus, tremor, urinary frequency, vaginal moniliasis, vaginitis, vasodilation.

Other adverse laboratory reactions occurring during the clinical trials with dirithromycin included the following (> 0.1% to <1%).

Decreased: Albumin, chloride, hematocrit, hemoglobin, seg neutrophils, phosphorus, platelet count and total protein.

Increased: Alkaline phosphatase, ALT, AST, bands, basophils, total bilirubin, creatinine, GGT, leukocyte count, lymphocytes, monocytes, phosphorous and uric acid.

Overdosage:

Symptoms: The toxic symptoms following an overdose of a macrolide antibiotic may include nausea, vomiting, epigastric distress and diarrhea.

Treatment: Forced diuresis, peritoneal dialysis, hemodialysis or hemoperfusion have not been established as beneficial for an overdose of dirithromycin. Hemodialysis has been shown to be ineffective in hastening the elimination erythromycylamine from plasma in patients with chronic renal failure.

Patient Information:

Take dirithromycin with food or within 1 hour of having eaten.

Do not cut, chew or crush the tablets.

Administration and Dosage:

Approved by the FDA in June 1995.

Administer with food or within 1 hour of having eaten. Do not cut, crush or chew the tablets.

Recommended Dosage Schedule for Dirithromycin (≥ 12 years of age)			
Infection (Mild to Moderate Severity)	Dose	Frequency	Duration (days)
Acute bacterial exacerbations of chronic bronchitis due to *Moraxella catarrhalis* or *Streptococcus pneumoniae*. Not for empiric therapy (see Warnings).	500 mg	once a day	7
Secondary bacterial infection of acute bronchitis due to *M catarrhalis* or *S pneumoniae*. Not for empiric therapy (see Warnings).	500 mg	once a day	7
Community-acquired pnemonia due to *Legionella pneumophila, Mycoplasma pneumoniae* or *S pneumoniae*	500 mg	once a day	14
Pharyngitis/Tonsillitis due to *Streptococcus pyogenes*	500 mg	once a day	10
Uncomplicated skin and skin structure infections due to *Staphylococcus aureus* (methicillin-susceptible). Not for empiric therapy (see Warnings).	500 mg	once a day	7

Rx	**Dynabac** (Bock)	**Tablets, enteric coated:** 250 mg	(UC5364). White. Elliptical shape. In 60s.

ERYTHROMYCIN

Actions:

Pharmacology: Erythromycin is a macrolide antibiotic which may be bactericidal or bacteriostatic. Erythromycin binds to the 50 S ribosomal subunits of susceptible bacteria and suppresses protein synthesis without affecting nucleic acid synthesis.

The strength of erythromycin products is expressed as erythromycin base equivalents. Because of differences in absorption and biotransformation, varying quantities of each erythromycin salt form are required to produce the same free erythromycin serum levels. For example, expressed in base equivalents, 400 mg erythromycin ethylsuccinate produces the same free erythromycin serum levels as 250 mg of erythromycin base, stearate or estolate.

Pharmacokinetics:

Absorption – Erythromycin base is acid labile and is usually formulated in enteric coated or film coated forms for oral administration. Acid stable salts and esters (estolate, ethylsuccinate, stearate) are well absorbed. Generally, administer the base and stearate preparations in the fasting state or immediately before meals. Absorption of the estolate and ethylsuccinate preparations and the base in a delayed release dosage form is unaffected or enhanced by food.

Distribution – Erythromycin is approximately 70% bound to plasma proteins. It diffuses into most body fluids, including prostatic fluid, where it reaches concentrations approximately 40% of those in plasma. Low concentrations are normally achieved in the spinal fluid, but passage of the drug across the blood-brain barrier increases in meningitis. Erythromycin crosses the placenta and is excreted in breast milk.

Metabolism/Excretion – In normal hepatic function, the drug is concentrated in the liver and excreted via the bile. Erythromycin's plasma half-life is approximately 1.4 hours in patients with normal renal function; it is prolonged to 4.8 to 5.8 hours in anuria. From 12% to 15% of IV erythromycin is excreted in active form in the urine. After oral use, < 5% is recovered in urine. Erythromycin is not dialyzable.

Urine alkalinization (pH 8.5) increases erythromycin's gram-negative antibacterial activity; several investigators suggest coadministration of urinary alkalinizers (eg, sodium bicarbonate) and erythromycin for urinary tract infections.

Microbiology: Erythromycin is usually active against the following organisms in vitro:

Gram positive – Staphylococcus aureus (resistant organisms may emerge during treatment); *Streptococcus pyogenes* (group A beta-hemolytic streptococci); alpha-hemolytic streptococci (viridans group); *S pneumonia; Corynebacterium diphtheriae; C minutissimum.*

Gram-negative – Moraxella catarrhalis; Neisseria gonorrhoeae; Legionella pneumophila; Bordetella pertussis.

Mycoplasma – Mycoplasma pneumoniae; Ureaplasma urealyticum

Other – Chlamydia trachomatis; Entamoeba histolytica; Treponema pallidum; Listeria monocytogenes.

Haemophilus influenzae – Many strains are resistant to erythromycin alone but are susceptible to erythromycin and sulfonamides together.

Indications:

Indicated for treatment of infections caused by susceptible strains of the designated microorganisms in the diseases listed below:

Upper respiratory tract infections of mild to moderate severity caused by: *Streptococcus pyogenes* (group A beta-hemolytic streptococci); *S pneumoniae; H influenzae* (with concomitant sulfonamides).

Lower respiratory tract infections of mild to moderate severity caused by: *S pyogenes* (group A beta-hemolytic streptococci); *S pneumoniae.*

Respiratory tract infections due to *Mycoplasma pneumoniae*

Skin/skin structure infections of mild to moderate severity caused by: *S pyogenes; Staphylococcus aureus* (resistant staphylococci may emerge during treatment).

Pertussis (whooping cough) caused by *Bordetella pertussis.* Effective in eliminating the organism from the nasopharynx of infected patients. May be helpful in the prophylaxis of pertussis in exposed susceptible individuals.

Diphtheria: Adjunct to antitoxin in infections due to *Corynebacterium diphtheriae,* to prevent establishment of carriers and to eradicate the organism in carriers.

Erythrasma: Treatment of infections due to *C minutissimum.*

Intestinal amebiasis caused by *Entamoeba histolytica* (oral erythromycin only). Extraenteric amebiasis requires treatment with other agents.

Pelvic inflammatory disease (PID), acute caused by *Neisseria gonorrhoeae:* Erythromycin lactobionate IV followed by oral erythromycin as an alternative to penicillin in patients with a history of penicillin sensitivity.

Conjunctivitis of the newborn, pneumonia of infancy, urogenital infections during pregnancy caused by *Chlamydia trachomatis.*

ERYTHROMYCIN

Uncomplicated urethral, endocervical or rectal infections in adults due to *C trachomatis* when tetracyclines are contraindicated or not tolerated.

Nongonococcal urethritis caused by *Ureaplasma urealyticum* when tetracyclines are contraindicated or not tolerated.

Primary syphilis caused by *Treponema pallidum:* Erythromycin (oral only) as an alternative to penicillin in penicillin-allergic patients.

Legionnaire's disease caused by *Legionella pneumophila.* Although no controlled clinical efficacy studies have been conducted, in vitro and limited preliminary clinical data suggest effectiveness.

Rheumatic fever: Prevention of initial or recurrent attacks as an alternative in patients who are allergic to penicillins or sulfonamides

Bacterial endocarditis (due to alpha-hemolytic streptococci, Viridans group): Prevention as an alternative in patients allergic to penicillins.

Listeria monocytogenes infections.

Unlabeled uses:

Neisseria gonorrhoeae – Uncomplicated urethral, endocervical or rectal infection and in penicillinase-producing *N gonorrhoeae* (PPNG); in pregnancy.

Treponema pallidum – Early syphilis (primary, secondary or early latent syphilis of < 1 year duration).

Campylobacter jejuni – Erythromycin has been used successfully in prolonged diarrhea associated with campylobacter enteritis.

Lymphogranuloma venereum – Genital, inguinal or anorectal.

Hemophilus ducreyi (chancroid) – Treat until ulcers or lymph nodes are healed.

Prior to elective colorectal surgery, to reduce wound complications, erythromycin base with oral neomycin is a popular preoperative combination.

Other uses, as alternative to penicillins, include: Anthrax; Vincent's gingivitis; erysipeloid; tetanus; actinomycosis; *Nocardia* infections (with a sulfonamide); *Eikenella corrodens* infections; *Borrelia* infections (including early Lyme disease).

Contraindications:

Hypersensitivity to erythromycin.

Erythromycin estolate: Preexisting liver disease.

Warnings:

Pseudomembranous colitis has occurred with virtually all broad-spectrum antibiotics (including macrolides, semi-synthetic penicillins and cephalosporins). Therefore, consider its diagnosis in patients who develop diarrhea in association with antibiotic use. Broad-spectrum antibiotics alter the normal flora of the colon; this may permit overgrowth of Clostridia. A toxin produced by *Clostridium difficile* is a primary cause of antibiotic-associated colitis. Such colitis may range in severity from mild to life-threatening.

Mild cases usually respond to discontinuation. Management of moderate to severe cases should include sigmoidoscopy, bacteriologic studies and fluid, electrolyte and protein supplementation. When colitis does not improve after discontinuation, or when it is severe, oral vancomycin or metronidazole is the drug of choice; rule out other causes.

Hepatotoxicity: Erythromycin administration has been associated with the infrequent occurrence of cholestatic hepatitis. This effect is most common with erythromycin estolate; however, it has also occurred with other erythromycin salts. Laboratory findings include abnormal hepatic function, peripheral eosinophilia and leukocytosis. Symptoms may include malaise, nausea, vomiting, abdominal cramps and fever. Jaundice may or may not be present. In some instances, severe abdominal pain may simulate the pain of biliary colic, pancreatitis, perforated ulcer or an acute abdominal surgical problem. In other instances, clinical symptoms and results of liver function tests have resembled findings in extrahepatic obstructive jaundice. Although initial symptoms have developed after a few days of treatment, they generally have followed 1 or 2 weeks of continuous therapy. Symptoms reappear promptly, usually within 48 hours after the drug is readministered to sensitive patients. The syndrome seems to result from a form of sensitization, occurs chiefly in adults, and is reversible when medication is discontinued.

Hypersensitivity: Serious allergic reactions, including anaphylaxis, have occurred. Refer to Management of Acute Hypersensitivity Reactions.

Hepatic function impairment: Erythromycin is principally excreted by the liver. Exercise caution in administering to patients with impaired hepatic function. There have been reports of hepatic dysfunction with or without jaundice.

ERYTHROMYCIN

Pregnancy: Category B. Safety for use during pregnancy has not been established. Erythromycin crosses the placental barrier but fetal levels are low (5% to 20% of maternal concentrations). There are no adequate and well controlled studies in pregnant women. Use only when clearly needed. **Erythromycin estolate** abnormally elevated liver function tests in 10% of pregnant patients.

Lactation: Erythromycin is excreted in breast milk, and may concentrate (observed milk: plasma ratio of 0.5 to 3). Although no infant adverse effects are reported, potential problems for the nursing infant include modification of bowel flora, pharmacologic effects and interference with fever work-ups. Erythromycin is considered compatible with breastfeeding by the American Academy of Pediatrics.

Precautions:

Superinfection: Use of antibiotics (especially prolonged or repeated therapy) may result in bacterial or fungal overgrowth of nonsusceptible organisms. Take appropriate measures if superinfection occurs.

Drug Interactions:

Erythromycin Drug Interactions

Precipitant drug	Object drug*		Description
Erythromycin	Alfentanil	↑	The alfentanil clearance may be decreased and its elimination half-life increased.
Erythromycin	Anticoagulants	↑	The anticoagulant effect is increased; hemorrhage has occurred.
Erythromycin	Antihistamines – Astemizole Terfenadine	↑	Astemizole and terfenadine plasma levels (including metabolite levels) may be increased, which may lead to serious cardiovascular adverse events.
Erythromycin	Bromocriptine	↑	Serum bromocriptine levels may be increased, resulting in an increase in pharmacologic and toxic effects.
Erythromycin	Carbamazepine	↑	Carbamazepine toxicity sufficient to require hospitalization or resuscitative measures may result.
Erythromycin	Cyclosporine	↑	Increased cyclosporine concentrations with renal toxicity may occur.
Erythromycin	Digoxin	↑	Increased serum digoxin levels may occur in a small population of patients (≈ 10%); toxic effects may occur.
Erythromycin	Disopyramide	↑	Increased disopyramide plasma levels may occur. Arrhythmias and increased QTc intervals have occurred.
Erythromycin	Ergot alkaloids	↑	Acute ergotism manifested as peripheral ischemia has occurred.
Erythromycin	Lincosamides	↓	Under some conditions, coadministration may be antagonistic.
Erythromycin	Methylprednisolone	↑	Methylprednisolone clearance may be decreased.
Erythromycin	Penicillins	↔	Both antagonism and synergism have occurred with coadministration.
Erythromycin	Theophyllines	↔	Increased theophylline serum levels with toxicity are possible. Decreased erythromycin levels may also occur.
Erythromycin	Triazolam	↑	Triazolam bioavailability may be increased, resulting in increased CNS depression.

* ↑ = Object drug increased, ↓ = Object drug decreased, ↔ = Undetermined effect

Drug/Food interactions: Antimicrobial effectiveness of erythromycin stearate and certain formulations of erythromycin base may be reduced. Take at least 2 hours before or after a meal. Erythromycin estolate and ethylsuccinate and the base in a delayed release form may be administered without regard to meals.

ERYTHROMYCIN

Adverse Reactions:

Local: Venous irritation and phlebitis have occurred with parenteral administration, but the risk of such reactions may be reduced if the infusion is given slowly, in dilute solution, by continuous IV infusion or intermittent infusion over 20 to 60 minutes.

Special senses: There have been isolated reports of reversible hearing loss occurring chiefly in patients with renal or hepatic insufficiency, in the elderly (> 50 years old) and in those receiving high doses (> 4 g/day). In rare instances involving IV use, the ototoxic effect has been irreversible.

Hypersensitivity: Serious allergic reactions, including anaphylaxis, have occurred. Mild allergic reactions include rashes with or without pruritus, urticaria, bullous fixed eruptions and eczema. See Warnings.

GI: The most frequent dose-related side effects following oral use include abdominal cramping and discomfort, anorexia, nausea, vomiting and diarrhea. Pseudomembranous colitis associated with erythromycin therapy has occurred (see Warnings). Several cases of nausea and vomiting following IV erythromycin lactobionate have occurred.

Hepatic: Hepatotoxicity is most commonly associated with **erythromycin estolate** (see Warnings).

Cardiovascular: Rarely, production of ventricular arrhythmias, including ventricular tachycardia and torsade de pointes in individuals with prolonged QT intervals.

Overdosage:

Symptoms: Symptoms may include nausea, vomiting, epigastric distress and diarrhea. The severity of the epigastric distress and diarrhea are dose-related. Reversible mild acute pancreatitis has occurred. Hearing loss, with or without tinnitus and vertigo, may occur, especially in patients with renal or hepatic insufficiency.

Treatment: Treatment includes usual supportive measures. Refer to General Management of Acute Overdosage. Induce prompt elimination of unabsorbed drug. However, unless 5 times the normal single dose has been ingested, GI decontamination should not be necessary. An accidental ingestion of erythromycin should not be predicted to have minimal toxicity unless there is a good approximation of how much was ingested and unless only a single medication was involved. Control allergic reactions with conventional therapy as indicated. Hemodialysis and peritoneal dialysis are not particularly effective.

Patient Information:

Preferably taken on an empty stomach (at least 1 hour before or 2 hours after meals); if GI upset occurs, may be taken with food. Erythromycin estolate, ethylsuccinate and certain brands of erythromycin base enteric coated tablets may be taken without regard to meals; consult the current package literature.

Complete full course of therapy; take until finished.

Take each dose with an adequate amount of water (180 to 240 ml).

Take at evenly spaced intervals during the day, preferably around the clock.

Notify physician if nausea, vomiting, diarrhea or stomach cramps, severe abdominal pain, yellow discoloration of the skin or eyes, darkened urine, pale stools or unusual tiredness occurs.

ERYTHROMYCIN, IV

Complete prescribing information for these products begins in the Erythromycin group monograph.

Administration and Dosage:

Erythromycin IV is indicated when oral use is impossible, or when severity of the infection requires immediate high serum levels. Replace IV therapy with oral as soon as possible.

Continuous infusion is preferable, but intermittent infusion in 20 to 60 minute periods at intervals of ≤ 6 hours is also effective. Due to irritative properties of erythromycin, IV push is unacceptable.

Severe infections: 15 to 20 mg/kg/day. Up to 4 g/day in very severe infections.

Preparation of solution:

Vials – Prepare the initial solution by adding 10 ml Sterile Water for Injection, USP to the 500 mg vial or 20 ml Sterile Water for Injection, USP to the 1 g vial. Use only Sterile Water for Injection, USP as other diluents may cause precipitation during reconstitution. Do not use diluents containing preservatives or inorganic salts. Note: When the product is reconstituted as directed above, the resulting solution contains an effective microbial preservative. After reconstitution, each ml contains 50 mg erythromycin activity.

Add the initial dilution to one of the following diluents before administration to give a concentration of 1 g/L (1 mg/ml) erythromycin activity for continuous infusion or 1 to 5 mg/ml for intermittent infusion: 0.9% Sodium Chloride Injection, USP; Lactated Ringer's Injection, USP; *Normosol-R*.

The following solutions may also be used providing they are first buffered with 4% sodium bicarbonate or *Neut* by adding 1 ml of the 4% Sodium Bicarbonate Injection or *Neut* per 100 ml of solution: 5% Dextrose Injection, USP; 5% Dextrose and Lactated Ringer's Injection; 5% Dextrose and 0.9% Sodium Chloride Injection.

Piggyback vial – Add 100 ml 0.9% Sodium Chloride Injection, USP or Lactated Ringer's Injection, USP or *Normosol-R* to the dispensing vial. Immediately after adding diluent, shake the product to aid dissolution. Lack of immediate agitation will greatly increase time required for complete dissolution. May also be reconstituted using 100 ml of the following solutions to which 1 ml of 4% Sodium Bicarbonate Injection or *Neut* has first been added: 5% Dextrose Injection, USP; 5% Dextrose and Lactated Ringer's Injection; 5% Dextrose and 0.9% Sodium Chloride Injection, USP; *Normosol-M* and 5% Dextrose Injection; *Normosol-R* and 5% Dextrose Injection.

The 4% sodium bicarbonate injection or *Neut* must be added to these solutions so that their pH is in the optimum range for erythromycin lactobionate stability. Acidic solutions of erythromycin lactobionate are unstable and lose their potency rapidly. A pH of at least 5.5 is desirable for the final diluted solution of erythromycin lactobionate.

Storage/Stability: The *initial* solution is stable for 2 weeks if refrigerated or for 24 hours at room temperature. Completely administer the final diluted solution within 8 hours in order to assure proper potency since it is not suitable for storage.

Use the solution in the piggyback vial within 8 hours if stored at room temperature and 24 hours if stored in the refrigerator. If the solution is to be frozen, freeze at −10° to −20°C (14° to −4°F) within 4 hours of preparation. Frozen solution may be stored for 30 days. Thaw the frozen solution in the refrigerator and use within 8 hours after thawing is completed. Thawed solution must not be refrozen.

Rx	**Erythromycin Lactobionate** (Various, eg, Abbott, Elkins-Sinn, Lederle, Lyphomed)	**Powder for Injection:** 500 mg (as lactobionate)	In vials and piggyback vials.
		1 g (as lactobionate)	In vials.
Rx	**Ilotycin Gluceptate** (Dista)	**Injection**: 1 g erythromycin (as gluceptate) per vial	In 30 ml vials.

ERYTHROMYCIN, ORAL

Complete prescribing information for these products begins in the Erythromycin group monograph.

Administration and Dosage:

Dosages and product strengths are expressed as erythromycin base equivalents. Because of differences in absorption and biotransformation, varying quantities of each salt form are required to produce the same free erythromycin serum levels. For example, expressed in base equivalents, 400 mg erythromycin ethylsuccinate produces the same free erythromycin serum levels as 250 mg of erythromycin base, stearate or estolate.

Optimal serum levels of erythromycin are reached when erythromycin base or stearate is taken in the fasting state or immediately before meals. Erythromycin ethylsuccinate, estolate and enteric coated erythromycin may be administered without regard to meals.

Usual dosage: Adults – 250 mg (or 400 mg ethylsuccinate) every 6 hours, or 500 mg every 12 hours, or 333 mg every 8 hours. May increase up to ≥ 4 g/day, according to severity of infection. If twice-a-day dosage is desired, the recommended dose is 500 mg every 12 hours. Twice-a-day dosing is not recommended when doses > 1 g daily are administered.

Children – 30 to 50 mg/kg/day (15 to 25 mg/lb/day) in divided doses. Proper dosage is determined by age, weight and severity of infection. For more severe infections, dosage may be doubled.

Erythromycin Uses and Dosages

Indication (Organism)	Dosage (Stated as erythromycin base)
Labeled uses:	
Upper respiratory tract infections of mild to moderate severity	
Streptococcus pyogens (Group A beta-hemolytic streptococcus)	250 to 500 mg 4 times a day or 20 to 50 mg/kg/day in divided doses for 10 days.
S pneumoniae	250 to 500 mg every 6 hours
Haemophilus influenzae (used concomitantly with a sulfonamide)	Erythromycin ethylsuccinate: 50 mg/kg/day. Sulfisoxazole: 150 mg/kg/day. Combination given for 10 days.
Lower respiratory tract infections of mild to moderate severity	
S pyogenes	250 to 500 mg 4 times a day or 20 to 50 mg/kg/day in divided doses for 10 days.
S pneumoniae	250 to 500 mg every 6 hours.
Respiratory tract infections	
Mycoplasma pneumoniae (Eaton agent, PPLO)	500 mg every 6 hours for 5 to 10 days. Treat severe infections for up to 3 weeks.
Skin and skin structure infections of mild to moderate severity	
S pyogenes	250 to 500 mg 4 times a day or 20 to 50 mg/kg/day in divided doses for 10 days.
Staphylococcus aureus (resistant organisms may emerge)	250 mg every 6 hours or 500 mg every 12 hours, maximum 4 g/day.
Pertussis (whooping cough)	
Bordetella pertussis: Effective in eliminating the organism from the nasopharynx of infected patients. May be helpful in prophylaxis of pertussis in exposed individuals.	40 to 50 mg/kg/day in divided doses for 5 to 14 days, or 500 mg 4 times a day for 10 days.
Diphtheria	
Corynebacterium diphtheriae: Adjunct to antitoxin to prevent establishment of carriers and to eradicate organism in carriers.	500 mg every 6 hours for 10 days.
Erythrasma	
C minutissiumum	250 mg 3 times daily for 21 days.
Intestinal amebiasis	
Entamoeba histolyticia: Oral erythromycin only.	*Adults:* 250 mg 4 times daily for 10 to 14 days. *Children:* 30 to 50 mg/kg/day in divided doses for 10 to 14 days.

ERYTHROMYCIN, ORAL

Erythromycin Uses and Dosages	
Indication (Organism)	Dosage (Stated as erythromycin base)
Pelvic inflammatory disease (PID), acute *Neisseria gonorrhoeae:* Erythromycinlactobionate IV followed by oral erythromycin.[1]	500 mg IV every 6 hours for 3 days, then 250 mg orally every 6 hours for 7 days. An alternative regimen for ambulatory management of PID is 500 mg orally 4 times a day for 10 to 14 days.[2]
Conjunctivitis of the newborn, pneumonia of infancy, urogenital infections during pregnancy *Chlamydia trachomatis*	50 mg/kg/day in 4 divided doses for 14 days (conjunctivitis) or 21 days (pneumonia); 500 mg 4 times daily for 7 days or 250 mg 4 times daily for 14 days (urogenital infections).
Urethral, endocervical or rectal infections, uncomplicated *C trachomatis*[1]	500 mg 4 times daily for 7 days or 250 mg 4 times daily for 14 days.[2]
Nongonococcal urethritis *Ureaplasma urealyticum*[1]	500 mg 4 times daily for at least 7 days.
Primary syphilis *Treponema pallidum:* (Oral only)[1]	20 g in divided doses over 10 days.
Legionnaire's disease *Legionella pneumophila:* No controlled clinical efficacy studies have been conducted, but data suggest effectiveness	1 to 4 g daily in divided doses or 500 mg to 1 g 4 times daily for 21 days.
Rheumatic fever *S pyogenes* (group A beta-hemolytic streptococci): Prevention of initial or recurrent attacks.[1]	250 mg 2 times daily.
Listeria monocytogenes	*Adults:* 250 mg every 6 hours or 500 mg every 12 hours, maximum 4 g/day.
Unlabeled uses: *Campylobacter jejuni:* Has been successful in severe or prolonged diarrhea associated with *Campylobacter enteritis* or enterocolitis.[2]	500 mg 4 times a day for 7 days.
Lymphogranuloma venereum: Genital, inguinal or anorectal.[2]	500 mg 4 times a day for 21 days.
Hemophilus ducreyi (chancroid): Treat until ulcers or lymph nodes are healed.[2]	500 mg 4 times a day for 7 days.
Neisseria gonorrhoeae: Uncomplicated urethral, endocervical or rectal infections and in penicillinase-producing *N gonorrhoeae* (PPNG)[2] In pregnancy[2]	500 mg 4 times a day for 7 days or spectinomycin 2 g IM followed by erythromycin regimen. 500 mg 4 times a day for 7 days.
Treponema pallidum: Early syphilis (primary, secondary or latent syphilis of < 1 year duration)	500 mg 4 times a day for 14 days.
Prior to elective colorectal surgery, to reduce wound complications	Combination of erythromycin base and neomycin is a popular preoperative preparation.
Clostridium tetani: Tetanus[1]	500 mg every 6 hours for 10 days.

[1] Use as alternative drug in penicillin or tetracycline hypersensitivity or when penicillin or tetracycline are contraindicated or not tolerated.
[2] CDC 1989 Sexually Transmitted Diseases Treatment Guidelines. *Morbidity and Mortality Weekly Report* 1989 Sept 1;38(No. S-8):1-43.

ERYTHROMYCIN BASE

Complete prescribing information begins in the Erythromycin group monograph.

Rx	**E-Mycin** (Boots)	**Tablets, enteric coated:** 250 mg	Orange. In 40s, 100s, 500s and UD 100s.
Rx	**Ery-Tab** (Abbott)		Delayed release. Pink. In 30s, 40s, 100s, 500s and UD 100s.
Rx	**Robimycin Robitabs** (Robins)		Lactose. Green. In 100s and 500s.
Rx	**E-Base Caplets and Tablets** (Barr)	**Tablets, enteric coated:** 333 mg	Delayed release. (E-Base/333 barr). White. In 100s, 500s and 1000s.
Rx	**E-Mycin** (Boots)		White. In 30s, 100s, 500s and UD 100s.
Rx	**Ery-Tab** (Abbott)		Delayed release. White. In 30s, 100s, 500s and UD 100s.
Rx	**Erythromycin** (Various, eg, Boots, Parmed)	**Tablets, delayed release:** 333 mg	In 100s.
Rx	**E-Base** (Barr)	**Tablets, enteric coated:** 500 mg	(E-Base/500 mg barr). White. Capsule shape. In 100s, 500s.
Rx	**Ery-Tab** (Abbott)		Delayed release. Pink. In 100s and UD 100s.
Rx	**PCE Dispertab** (Abbott)	**Tablets with polymer coated particles:** 500 mg	(EK). White. Oval. In 100s.
Rx	**Erythromycin Filmtabs** (Abbott)	**Tablets, film coated:** 250 mg	Pink. In 100s, 500s and UD 100s.
Rx	**Erythromycin Filmtabs** (Abbott)	**Tablets, film coated:** 500 mg	Pink. In 100s.
Rx	**Eryc** (Parke-Davis)	**Capsules, delayed release, enteric coated pellets:** 250 mg	(P-D 696). Clear and orange. In 40s, 100s, 500s and UD 100s.
Rx	**Erythromycin Base** (Various, eg, Abbott, Parmed)	**Capsules, delayed release:** 250 mg	In 100s and 500s.

ERYTHROMYCIN ESTOLATE

Complete prescribing information begins in the Erythromycin group monograph.

Rx	**Ilosone** (Dista)	**Tablets:** 500 mg (as estolate)	White, scored. Capsule shape. In 50s.
Rx	**Erythromycin Estolate** (Various, eg, Barr, Geneva, Major, Parmed, Rugby, Schein, URL)	**Capsules:** 250 mg (as estolate)	In 100s.
Rx	**Ilosone Pulvules** (Dista)		Ivory and red. In 100s and UD 100s.
Rx	**Erythromycin Estolate** (Various, eg, Dixon-Shane)	**Suspension:** 125 mg (as estolate) per 5 ml	In 480 ml.
Rx	**Ilosone** (Dista)		Sucrose. Orange flavor. In 480 ml.
Rx	**Erythromycin Estolate** (Various, eg, Dixon-Shane)	**Suspension:** 250 mg (as estolate) per 5 ml	In 480 ml.
Rx	**Ilosone** (Dista)		Sucrose. Cherry flavor. In 100 & 480 ml.

ERYTHROMYCIN STEARATE

Complete prescribing information begins in the Erythromycin group monograph.

Rx	**Erythromycin Stearate** (Various, eg, Barr, Geneva, Major, Mylan, Rugby, Schein, Warner Chilcott, Zenith)	**Tablets, film coated:** 250 mg (as stearate)	In 100s, 500s and 1000s.
Rx	**Eramycin** (Wesley)		In 100s and 500s.
Rx	**Erythromycin Stearate** (Various, eg, Geneva, Lederle, Major, Moore, Mylan, Purepac, Rugby, URL, Warner-C, Zenith)	**Tablets, film coated:** 500 mg (as stearate)	In 100s, 500s and UD 100s.

ERYTHROMYCIN ETHYLSUCCINATE

Complete prescribing information begins in the Erythromycin group monograph.

Expressed in base equivalents, 400 mg erythromycin ethylsuccinate produces the same free erythromycin serum levels as 250 mg of erythromycin base, stearate or estolate.

Rx	**EryPed** (Abbott)	**Tablets, chewable:** 200 mg (as ethylsuccinate)	Sugar. Fruit flavor. Scored. In 40s.
Rx	**Erythromycin Ethylsuccinate** (Various, eg, Abbott, Barr, Geneva, Lederle, Major, Moore, Parmed, Rugby, Schein)	**Tablets:** 400 mg (as ethylsuccinate)	In 100s and 500s.
Rx	**E.E.S. 400** (Various, eg, Abbott, Dixon-Shane)		Film coated. In 100s, 500s and UD 100s.
Rx	**Erythromycin Ethylsuccinate** (Various, eg, Barr, Lederle, Major, Purepac, Rugby, Schein, URL, Warner Chilcott)	**Suspension:** 200 mg (as ethylsuccinate) per 5 ml	In 100, 200 and 480 ml.
Rx	**E.E.S. 200** (Various, eg, Abbott, Dixon-Shane)		In 100 and 480 ml.
Rx	**EryPed 200** (Abbott)		Sucrose. Fruit flavor. In 100, 200 ml, UD 5 ml.
Rx	**Erythromycin Ethylsuccinate** (Various, eg, Lederle, Major, Schein, Warner Chilcott)	**Suspension:** 400 mg (as ethylsuccinate) per 5 ml	In 480 ml.
Rx	**E.E.S. 400** (Various, eg, Abbott, Dixon-Shane)		In 100 and 480 ml.
Rx	**EryPed 400** (Abbott)		Sucrose. Banana flavor. In 60, 100, 200 and UD 5 ml (100s).
Rx	**EryPed Drops** (Abbott)	**Suspension:** 100 mg (as ethylsuccinate)/2.5 ml	Sucrose. Fruit flavor. In 50 ml.
Rx	**E.E.S. Granules** (Abbott)	**Powder for Oral Suspension:** 200 mg (as ethylsuccinate)/5 ml when reconstituted	Sucrose. Cherry flavor. In 100 and 200 ml.
Rx	**EryPed** (Abbott)	**Granules for Oral Suspension:** 400 mg (as ethylsuccinate)/5 ml when reconstituted	In 60, 100 and 200 ml.

TROLEANDOMYCIN (Triacetyloleandomycin)

Actions:

Pharmacology: Synthetically derived acetylated ester of the macrolide oleandomycin.

Pharmacokinetics: Peak serum levels of 2 mcg/ml are attained 2 hours following a 500 mg dose. Serum levels are still detected 12 hours later; 20% of the drug is recovered in the urine. Significant quantities are also excreted in bile.

Indications:

Streptococcus pneumoniae: Pneumococcal pneumonia due to susceptible strains.

Streptococcus pyogenes: Group A β-hemolytic streptococcal infections of the upper respiratory tract. Troleandomycin is generally effective in the eradication of streptococci from the nasopharynx. However, substantial data establishing efficacy in the subsequent prevention of rheumatic fever are not available.

Contraindications:

Hypersensitivity to troleandomycin.

Warnings:

Hepatic effects: Troleandomycin has been associated with an allergic cholestatic hepatitis. Some patients receiving troleandomycin for > 2 weeks or in repeated courses have developed jaundice accompanied by right upper quadrant pain, fever, nausea, vomiting, eosinophilia and leukocytosis. These have reversed on drug discontinuance. Readministration reproduces hepatotoxicity, often within 24 to 48 hours. Monitor liver function tests and discontinue drug if abnormalities develop.

Hepatic function impairment: Troleandomycin is principally excreted by the liver. Exercise caution in administering to patients with impaired hepatic function.

Pregnancy: Safety for use during pregnancy has not been established.

Precautions:

Superinfection: Use of antibiotics (especially prolonged or repeated therapy) may result in bacterial or fungal overgrowth of nonsusceptible organisms. Such overgrowth may lead to a secondary infection. Take appropriate measures if this occurs.

Drug Interactions:

Troleandomycin Drug Interactions

Precipitant drug	Object drug *		Description
Troleandomycin	Carbamazepine	⬆	Carbamazepine toxicity sufficient to require resuscitative measures may result.
Troleandomycin	Contraceptives, oral	⬆	Concurrent use may result in an increased risk of intrahepatic cholestasis due to decreased metabolism and accumulation of the contraceptive.
Troleandomycin	Ergot alkaloids	⬆	Acute ergotism manifested as peripheral ischemia has occurred.
Troleandomycin	Methylprednisolone	⬆	The clearance of methylprednisolone is greatly reduced. This has been used as a therapeutic advantage to reduce the dose.
Troleandomycin	Theophyllines	⬆	Increased theophylline serum levels with toxicity may occur.
Troleandomycin	Triazolam	⬆	Triazolam bioavailability may be increased, resulting in increased CNS depression.

* ⬆ = Object drug increased

Adverse Reactions:

Most frequent: Abdominal cramping and discomfort (dose-related).

Infrequent: Nausea; vomiting; diarrhea.

Hypersensitivity: Anaphylaxis; urticaria and other skin rashes.

Patient Information:

Take at evenly spaced intervals during the day, preferably around the clock. Complete full course of therapy; take until gone.

Administration and Dosage:

Continue therapy for 10 days when used for streptococcal infection.

Adults: 250 to 500 mg, 4 times a day.

Children: 125 to 250 mg (6.6 to 11 mg/kg) every 6 hours.

Rx	**Tao** (Roerig)	**Capsules:** 250 mg oleandomycin (as troleandomycin)	Lactose. (Roerig 159). In 100s.

SPECTINOMYCIN

Actions:

Pharmacology: Spectinomycin, structurally different from related aminoglycosides, inhibits protein synthesis in bacterial cell. Site of action is 30S ribosomal subunit.

Pharmacokinetics: Rapidly absorbed after IM injection. A 2 g injection produces average peak serum concentrations of 100 mcg/ml at 1 hour; a 4 g injection, 160 mcg/ml at 2 hours. Eight hours after a 2 or 4 g injection, plasma concentrations are 15 and 31 mcg/ml, respectively. The majority is excreted in urine in biologically active form.

Microbiology: Active in vitro against most strains of Neisseria gonorrhoeae, studies show no cross-resistance between spectinomycin and penicillin.

Indications:

Acute gonorrheal urethritis and proctitis in the male and acute gonorrheal cervicitis and proctitis in the female due to susceptible strains of N gonorrhoeae. Treat men and women with known recent exposure to gonorrhea as those with gonorrhea.

Contraindications:

Hypersensitivity to spectinomycin.

Warnings:

Syphilis: Not effective for syphilis. Antibiotics used to treat gonorrhea may mask or delay symptoms of incubating syphilis. All patients with gonorrhea should have a serologic test for syphilis at time of diagnosis and a follow-up test after 3 months.

Pharyngeal infections: Not effective in pharyngeal infections due to *N gonorrhoeae.*

Pregnancy: Safety for use during pregnancy has not been established.

Children: Safety for use has not been established.

Precautions:

Monitoring: Monitor clinical effectiveness to detect resistance by *N gonorrhoeae.*

The diluent provided with this product contains benzyl alcohol which has been associated with a fatal gasping syndrome in infants.

Hypersensitivity: A few cases of anaphylaxis or anaphylactoid reactions have been reported. Have epinephrine immediately available. Refer to Management of Acute Hypersensitivity Reactions.

Adverse Reactions:

In single and multiple dose studies in healthy volunteers, a reduction in urine output was noted; however, renal toxicity has not been demonstrated.

Single dose: Sore injection site; urticaria; dizziness; nausea; chills; fever; insomnia.

Multiple dose: Decrease in hemoglobin, hematocrit and creatinine clearance; elevation of alkaline phosphatase, BUN and ALT.

Administration and Dosage:

For IM use only. Shake vials vigorously immediately after adding diluent and before withdrawing dose. Inject 5 ml (2 g) IM deep into upper outer quadrant of gluteus. Also recommended for treatment after failure of previous antibiotic therapy. In geographic areas where antibiotic resistance is prevalent, initial treatment with 4 g (10 ml) IM is preferred, and may be divided between 2 gluteal injection sites.

CDC recommended treatment schedules for gonorrhea†:

Uncomplicated urethral, endocervical or rectal gonococcal infections, alternative regimen – For patients who cannot take ceftriaxone, the preferred alternative is spectinomycin 2 g IM as a single dose followed by doxycycline.

Children ≥ 45 kg (100 lbs) should receive adult regimens. Children < 45 kg (100 lbs) with uncomplicated vulvovaginitis, cervicitis, urethritis, pharyngitis or proctitis and who cannot tolerate ceftriaxone may receive 40 mg/kg IM once.

Gonococcal infections in pregnancy – Treat pregnant women allergic to β-lactams with 2 g IM followed by erythromycin.

Disseminated gonococcal infection – Treat patients allergic to β-lactams with 2 g IM every 12 hours.

Stability: Use reconstituted suspension within 24 hours.

Rx	**Trobicin** (Upjohn)	**Powder for Injection:** 400 mg (as HCl) per ml when reconstituted	In 2 g vial w/3.2 ml diluent.[1]
			In 4 g vial w/6.2 ml diluent.[1]

[1] Bacteriostatic water for injection with 0.9% benzyl alcohol.

† CDC 1989 Sexually Transmitted Diseases Treatment Guidelines. *Morbidity and Mortality Weekly Report* 1989 Sept 1;38 (No. S-8):1-43.

VANCOMYCIN

Actions:

Pharmacology: Vancomycin is a tricyclic glycopeptide antibiotic which inhibits cell-wall biosynthesis. It also alters bacterial-cell-membrane permeability and RNA synthesis.

Pharmacokinetics:

Absorption/Distribution – Systemic absorption of oral vancomycin is generally poor, although clinically significant serum concentrations have occurred in patients with active C difficile-induced colitis. With doses of 2 g daily, very high concentrations of drug can be found in the feces (> 3100 mg/kg) and very low concentrations (< 1 mcg/ml) can be found in the serum of patients with normal renal function who have pseudomembranous colitis.

Parenteral: In subjects with normal kidney function, multiple IV dosing of 1 g (15 mg/kg) infused over 60 minutes produces mean plasma concentrations of ≈ 63 mcg/ml immediately after the completion of infusion, ≈ 23 mcg/ml 2 hours after infusion, and ≈ 8 mcg/ml 11 hours after the end of the infusion. Multiple dosing of 500 mg infused over 30 minutes produces mean plasma concentrations of ≈ 49 mcg/ml at the completion of infusion, ≈ 19 mcg/ml 2 hours after infusion, and ≈ 10 mcg/ml 6 hours after infusion. The plasma concentrations during multiple dosing are similar to those after a single dose. Vancomycin IV penetrates inflamed meninges at levels about 15% of those found in serum (mean, 2.5 mcg/ml in adults, 3.1 mcg/ml in infants). In the presence of inflammation, it also penetrates into pleural, pericardial, ascitic and synovial fluids, urine, peritoneal dialysis fluid, atrial appendage tissue and bile (≈ 15%). It is ≈ 55% protein bound.

Metabolism/Excretion – In the first 24 hours, about 75% of a dose is excreted in urine by glomerular filtration. Urine concentrations of 90 to 300 mcg/ml are achieved 1 hour after a 500 mg IV dose. Creatinine clearance is linearly associated with vancomycin clearance. Elimination half-life is 4 to 6 hours in adults and 2 to 3 hours in children. Accumulation occurs in renal failure. Serum half-life in anephric patients is approximately 7.5 days. About 60% of an intraperitoneal dose administered during peritoneal dialysis is absorbed systemically in 6 hours. Serum concentrations of about 10 mcg/ml are achieved by intraperitoneal injection of 30 mg/kg. In anephric patients, the drug is slowly eliminated by unknown routes and mechanisms. Vancomycin is not significantly removed by hemodialysis or continuous ambulatory peritoneal dialysis, although there have been reports of increased clearance with hemoperfusion and hemofiltration.

Microbiology: At clinically achievable concentrations, vancomycin is active only against gram-positive bacteria. In vitro, at concentrations of 0.5 to 5 mcg/ml, it is active against many strains of streptococci, staphylococci, *Clostridium difficile, Corynebacterium, Listeria monocytogenes, Lactobacillus* sp, *Actinomyces* sp, *Clostridium* sp and *Bacillus* sp. It is bacteriostatic against enterococci.

No cross-resistance between vancomycin and any other antibiotic has been reported.

The combination of vancomycin and an aminoglycoside acts synergistically in vitro against many strains of *S aureus,* nonenterococcal group D streptococci, enterococci and *Streptococcus* sp (viridans group).

Indications:

Parenteral: Serious or severe infections not treatable with other antimicrobials, including the penicillins and cephalosporins.

Severe staphylococcal infections (including methicillin-resistant staphylococci) in patients who cannot receive or who have failed to respond to penicillins and cephalosporins, or who have infections with resistant staphylococci. Infections may include endocarditis, bone infections, lower respiratory tract infections, septicemia and skin and skin structure infections.

Endocarditis –

Staphylococcal: Vancomycin is effective alone.

Streptococcal: Vancomycin is effective alone or in combination with an aminoglycoside for endocarditis caused by Streptococcus viridans or *S bovis.* It is only effective in combination with an aminoglycoside for endocarditis caused by enterococci (eg, *S faecalis*).

Diphtheroid: Vancomycin is effective for diphtheroid endocarditis, and has been used successfully with rifampin, an aminoglycoside or both in early onset prosthetic valve endocarditis caused by *S epidermidis* or diphtheroids.

Prophylactic: Although no controlled clinical efficacy studies have been conducted, IV vancomycin has been suggested for prophylaxis against bacterial endocarditis in penicillin-allergic patients who have congenital heart disease or rheumatic or other acquired or valvular heart disease when these patients undergo dental procedures or surgical procedures of the upper respiratory tract.

Pseudomembranous colitis/staphylococcal enterocolitis caused by C difficile – The parenteral form may be administered orally; parenteral use alone is unproven. The oral use of parenteral vancomycin is not effective for other infections.

Oral: Staphylococcal enterocolitis and antibiotic-associated pseudomembranous colitis produced by *C difficile*. The parenteral product may also be given orally for these infections. Oral vancomycin is *not* effective for other types of infection.

Contraindications:

Hypersensitivity to vancomycin.

Warnings:

Ototoxicity has occurred in patients receiving vancomycin. It may be transient or permanent. It has occurred mostly in patients who have been given excessive doses, who have an underlying hearing loss, or who are receiving concomitant therapy with another ototoxic agent, such as an aminoglycoside. Serial tests of auditory function may be helpful in order to minimize the risk of ototoxicity.

Hypotension: Rapid bolus administration (eg, over several minutes) may be associated with exaggerated hypotension, including shock, and, rarely, cardiac arrest. To avoid hypotension, administer in a dilute solution over not less than 60 minutes. Stopping the infusion usually results in prompt cessation of these reactions. Frequently monitor blood pressure and heart rate.

Pseudomembranous colitis: In rare instances, pseudomembranous colitis has occurred due to C difficile developing in patients who received IV vancomycin.

Reversible neutropenia has occurred in patients receiving vancomycin. Periodically monitor the leukocyte count of patients on prolonged therapy or those receiving concomitant drugs that may cause neutropenia.

Tissue irritation: Vancomycin is irritating to tissue and must be given by a secure IV route of administration. Pain, tenderness and necrosis occur with IM injection or inadvertent extravasation. Thrombophlebitis may occur, the frequency and severity of which can be minimized by administering the drug slowly as a dilute solution (2.5 to 5 g/L) and by rotating the sites of infusion. The safety and efficacy of vancomycin administration by the intrathecal (intralumbar or intraventricular) routes have not been assessed.

Renal function impairment: Because of its nephrotoxicity, use carefully in renal insufficiency. The risk of toxicity may be appreciably increased by high serum concentrations or prolonged therapy. Factors that may increase the risk of nephrotoxicity include use in elderly and neonatal patients and concomitant use with other nephrotoxic drugs.

Elderly: Total systemic and renal clearance of vancomycin may be reduced in the elderly. The natural decrement of glomerular filtration with increasing age may lead to elevated vancomycin serum concentrations if dosage is not adjusted. Adjust dosage schedules in elderly patients.

Pregnancy: Category C. In a controlled clinical study, the potential ototoxic and nephrotoxic effects of vancomycin on infants were evaluated when the drug was administered to pregnant women for serious staphylococcal infections complicating IV drug abuse. Vancomycin was found in cord blood. No sensorineural hearing loss or nephrotoxicity attributable to the drug was noted. One infant whose mother received vancomycin in the third trimester experienced conductive hearing loss that was not attributable to administration of the drug. Because the number of patients treated in this study was limited, and the drug was administered only in the second and third trimesters, it is not known whether vancomycin can cause fetal harm. Give to a pregnant woman only if clearly needed.

Lactation: Vancomycin is excreted in breast milk. Exercise caution when adminstering the drug to a nursing woman. Because of the potential for adverse events, decide whether to discontinue nursing or to discontinue the drug, taking into account the importance of the drug to the mother.

Children: In premature and full-term neonates it may be appropriate to confirm desired vancomycin serum concentrations. Concomitant administration of vancomycin and anesthetic agents has been associated with erythema and histamine-like flushing (see Drug Interactions).

Precautions:

Monitoring: Perform serial tests of auditory function and monitor serum levels. When monitoring vancomycin serum levels, draw a serum sample 1.5 to 2.5 hours after the completion of a 1 hour infusion. Peak levels are generally expected to be in the 30 to 40 ng/ml range. The relationship between vancomycin levels and ototoxicity and nephrotoxicity is not well established.

VANCOMYCIN

Systemic absorption: Clinically significant serum concentrations may occur in some patients who have taken multiple oral doses for active C difficile-induced pseudomembranous colitis or who have inflammatory disorders of the intestinal mucosa; the risk is greater with the presence of renal impairment.

Route of administration: For IV use only.

Red Man (or Redneck) syndrome is characterized by a sudden and profound fall in blood pressure with or without a maculopapular rash over the face, neck, upper chest and extremities. The reaction appears to be at least partially mediated through a histaminergic response.

The reaction is usually stimulated by a too rapid IV infusion (dose given over a few minutes), but it has been reported rarely when given as recommended (up to a 2 hour administration) and following oral or intraperitoneal administration. This is not an allergic-type reaction. The onset may occur anytime within a few minutes of starting an IV infusion, to a short time after infusion completion. The rash generally resolves several hours after termination of administration.

Monitor blood pressure throughout the infusion; if treatment is necessary, fluids, antihistamines or corticosteroids may be beneficial. Pretreatment with either H_1 blockers, H_2 blockers or both may protect against the hypotension that may occur. Also, desensitization may be useful in managing certain refractory hypersensitivity cases by using sequential increments of vancomycin over several days, allowing for adminstration of therapeutic doses.

Superinfection: Use of antibiotics (especially prolonged therapy) may result in overgrowth of non-susceptible organisms. Such overgrowth may lead to a secondary infection. Take appropriate measures if superinfection occurs.

Drug Interactions:

Vancomycin Drug Interactions			
Precipitant drug	Object drug*		Description
Vancomycin	Aminoglycosides	↑	The risk of nephrotoxicity may be increased above that associated with aminoglycoside use alone.
Vancomycin	Anesthetics	↑	Concomitant use has been associated with erythema and histamine-like flushing in children.
Vancomycin	Neurotoxic/ Nephrotoxic agents	↑	Concurrent or sequential systemic or topical use requires careful monitoring.
Vancomycin	Nondepolarizing muscle relaxants	↑	Neuromuscular blockade may be enhanced.

* ↑ = Object drug increased

Adverse Reactions:

Renal: Renal failure (rare), principally manifested by increased serum creatinine or BUN concentrations especially in patients given large doses. Interstitial nephritis (rare), mostly in patients who were given aminoglycosides concomitantly or who had preexisting kidney dysfunction; when vancomycin was discontinued, azotemia resolved in most patients.

Special senses: Hearing loss (most patients had kidney dysfunction or a preexisting hearing loss or were receiving concomitant treatment with an ototoxic drug); vertigo, dizziness, tinnitus (rare).

Hematologic: Neutropenia (appears to be promptly reversible when the drug is discontinued), usually starting ≥ 1 week after onset of therapy or after a total dosage of > 25 g; thrombocytopenia (rare).

Miscellaneous: Anaphylaxis, drug fever, nausea, chills, eosinophilia, rashes (including exfoliative dermatitis), Stevens-Johnson syndrome (infrequent); vasculitis (rare).

Parenteral: Hypotension; wheezing; dyspnea; urticaria; pruritus; inflammation at the site of injection; Redneck or Red Man syndrome (see Precautions).

Overdosage:

Supportive care is advised, with maintenance of glomerular filtration. Vancomycin is poorly removed by dialysis. Hemofiltration and hemoperfusion with polysulfone resin have increased vancomycin clearance.

Patient Information:

Complete full course of therapy; do not discontinue therapy without notifying physician.

VANCOMYCIN

Administration and Dosage:

Oral:

Adults – 500 mg to 2 g/day given in 3 or 4 divided doses for 7 to 10 days.

Alternatively, dosages of 125 mg 3 or 4 times daily for C difficile colitis may be as effective as the 500 mg dose regimen.

Children – 40 mg/kg/day in 3 or 4 divided doses for 7 to 10 days. Do not exceed 2 g/day.

Neonates – (See Warnings.) 10 mg/kg/day in divided doses.

Preparation of solution – Add 115 ml distilled or deionized water to the 10 g container. Each 6 ml of solution provides ≈ 500 mg vancomycin.

The contents of the 1 g vial may be mixed with distilled or deionized water (20 ml). When reconstituted, each 5 ml contains ≈ 250 mg vancomycin. Mix thoroughly to dissolve.

The appropriate oral solution dose may be diluted in 1 oz of water and given to the patient to drink. Common flavoring syrups may be added to the solution to improve the taste for oral administration. The diluted material may be administered via nasogastric tube.

Parenteral: Administer each dose over at least 60 minutes. Intermittent infusion is the preferred administration method.

Adults – 500 mg IV every 6 hours or 1 g every 12 hours.

Children – 10 mg/kg per dose given every 6 hours.

Infants and neonates – Initial dose of 15 mg/kg, followed by 10 mg/kg every 12 hours for neonates in the first week of life and every 8 hours thereafter up to the age of 1 month.

Preparation of solution – Reconstitute by adding 10 ml Sterile Water for Injection to the 500 mg vial or 20 ml to the 1 g vial. Further dilution is required.

Dilute reconstituted solutions containing 500 mg or 1 g vancomycin with at least 100 or 200 ml, respectively, of diluent.

Compatible diluents – 5% Dextrose Injection, 5% Dextrose Injection and 0.9% NaCl, Lactated Ringer's Injection, Lactated Ringer's and 5% Dextrose Injection, *Normosol-M* and 5% Dextrose, 0.9% NaCl Injection, *Isolyte E,* Acetated Ringer's Injection.

Prevention of bacterial endocarditis in penicillin-allergic patients undergoing GU or nonesaphageal GI procedures:

Moderate-risk – 1 g (20 mg/kg for children) IV over 1 to 2 hours; complete infusion within 30 minutes of starting the procedure.

High-risk – 1 g (20 mg/kg for children) over 1 to 2 hours plus gentamicin 1.5 mg (not to exceed 120 mg in adults) IV or IM; complete infusion/injection within 30 minutes of starting the procedure.

GU/GI procedures (penicillin allergic patients) – 1 g IV over 1 hour (children, 20 mg/kg) plus 1.5 mg/kg (children, 2 mg/kg) gentamicin IV or IM (not to exceed 80 mg) 1 hour before procedure; may repeat once 8 hours after initial dose.

Renal function impairment: Adjust dosage; check serum levels regularly. In premature infants and the elderly, dosage reduction may be necessary due to decreasing renal function.

For most patients, if creatinine clearance (Ccr) can be measured or estimated accurately, the dosage may be calculated by using the following table.

Vancomycin Dosage in Impaired Renal Function

Ccr (ml/min)	Dose (mg/24 hr)
100	1545
90	1390
80	1235
70	1080
60	925
50	770
40	620
30	465
20	310
10	155

The table is not valid for functionally anephric patients on dialysis. For such patients, give a loading dose of 15 mg/kg to achieve therapeutic serum levels promptly and a maintenance dose of 1.9 mg/kg/24 hr. In patients with marked renal impairment, it may be more convenient to give maintenance doses of 250 to 1000 mg once every several days rather than administering the drug on a daily basis. In anuria a dose of 1000 mg every 7 to 10 days has been recommended.

VANCOMYCIN

When only serum creatinine is available, use the formula below to calculate estimated Ccr. Serum creatinine should represent a steady state of renal function.

$$\text{Males: } \frac{\text{Weight (kg)} \times (140 - \text{age})}{72 \times \text{serum creatinine (mg/dl)}} = \text{Ccr}$$

Females: 0.85 × above value

Stability/Storage: Oral and parenteral solutions are stable for 14 days if refrigerated after initial reconstitution. After further dilution, the parenteral solution is stable for 24 hours at room temperature and for 2 months under refrigeration (< 6% loss of potency) after dilution with Dextrose 5% or Sodium Chloride 0.9%.

Rx	**Vancocin** (Lilly)	**Pulvules:** 125 mg	Blue and brown. In Identi-Dose 20s.
		250 mg	Blue and lavender. In *Identi-Dose* 20s.
		Powder for Oral Solution: 1 g	In bottles.
		10 g	In bottles.
Rx	**Vancomycin HCl** (ESI Lederle)	**Powder for Oral Solution:** 1 g	In bottles.
Rx	**Vancomycin HCl** (Various, eg, Elkins-Sinn, Schein)	**Powder for Injection:** 500 mg	In vials.
Rx	**Lyphocin** (Lyphomed)		In 10 ml vials.
Rx	**Vancocin** (Lilly)		In 10 ml vials and 500 mg ADD-Vantage vials.
Rx	**Vancoled** (Lederle)		In vials.
Rx	**Vancomycin HCl** (Various, eg, Elkins-Sinn, Schein)	**Powder for Injection:** 1 g	In vials.
Rx	**Lyphocin** (Lyphomed)		In 10 ml vials.
Rx	**Vancocin** (Lilly)		In 10 ml vials and 500 mg ADD-Vantage vials.
Rx	**Vancoled** (Lederle)		In vials.
Rx	**Lyphocin** (Lyphomed)	**Powder for Injection:** 5 g	In 100 ml vials.
Rx	**Vancoled** (Lederle)		In pharmacy bulk package.
Rx	**Vancocin** (Lilly)	**Powder for Injection:** 10 g	In 100 ml vials.

LINCOSAMIDES

Warning:

These agents can cause severe and possibly fatal colitis, characterized by severe persistent diarrhea, severe abdominal cramps and possibly, the passage of blood and mucus. Endoscopic examination may reveal pseudomembranous colitis. A toxin(s) produced by *Clostridia* is a primary cause of antibiotic-associated colitis.

When significant diarrhea occurs, discontinue the drug or, if necessary, continue only with close observation of the patient. Large bowel endoscopy is recommended.

Mild colitis may respond to stopping drug. Promptly manage moderate to severe cases with fluid, electrolyte and protein supplements as indicated. Systemic corticosteroids and corticosteroid retention enemas may help relieve the colitis. Also consider other causes such as previous sensitivities to drugs or other allergens.

Antiperistaltic agents such as opiates and diphenoxylate with atropine may prolong or aggravate the condition. Diarrhea, colitis and pseudomembranous colitis can begin up to several weeks following cessation of therapy.

Vancomycin is effective in antibiotic-associated pseudomembranous colitis produced by *C difficile*.(See individual monograph for complete information.)

Reserve for serious infections where less toxic antimicrobial agents are inappropriate (see Indications). Do not use in patients with nonbacterial infections (ie, most upper respiratory tract infections).

Actions:

Pharmacology: Lincomycin and clindamycin (7–deoxy, 7–chloro derivative of lincomycin), known collectively as lincosamides, bind exclusively to the 50 S subunit of bacterial ribosomes and suppress protein synthesis.

Since bacterial resistance to these agents has been demonstrated, perform susceptibility testing. Cross-resistance has been demonstrated between these two agents.

Clindamycin is preferred because it is better absorbed and more potent.

Pharmacokinetics: Administration with food markedly impairs lincomycin (but not clindamycin) oral absorption. Both agents achieve significant tissue penetration; lincomycin may reach cerebrospinal fluid (CSF) concentration 40% of serum levels with inflamed meninges, but neither crosses well if meninges are normal.

Lincomycin levels above the MIC for most gram-positive organisms are maintained with oral doses of 500 mg for 6 to 8 hours and for 14 hours after a 600 mg IV infusion. Following a 600 mg IM dose, detectable levels persist for 24 hours.

Clindamycin serum levels exceed MIC for most indicated organisms at least 6 hrs after recommended doses. Maintain levels above in vitro MIC for most indicated organisms by giving clindamycin phosphate every 8 to 12 hrs to adults, every 6 to 8 hrs to children or by continuous IV infusion. Equilibrium is reached by dose 3.

Dialysis – Hemo- and peritoneal dialysis do not remove either agent from blood.

Select Pharmacokinetic Parameters of Lincosamides

Lincosamides	Bioavailability (%)	Mean peak serum level[1] (mcg/ml)	Time to peak serum level (hours)	Protein binding (%)	Half-Life (hours): Normal	Half-Life (hours): Anephric	Half-Life (hours): Liver disease	Elimination (%): Hepatic	Elimination (%): Unchanged in urine (range)	Elimination (%): Feces
Clindamycin[2]										
Oral	23-38	4	1-2							
IM		4.9	1-3	≈ 90	2.4-3	3.5-5	7-14	85	10-15	3.6
IV		14.7	0[3]							
Lincomycin										
Oral	30	2.6	2-4						4 (1-31)	
IM		9.5	0.5	70-72	4.4-6.4	10	11.8	50-70	17.3 (2-25)	40
IV		19	0						13.8 (5-30)	

[1] Clindamycin 300 mg; lincomycin, oral 500 mg, IM/IV 600 mg.
[2] Clindamycin palmitate and phosphate are rapidly hydrolyzed to the base.
[3] By end of infusion, peak levels are reached.

LINCOSAMIDES

Microbiology:

Organisms Generally Susceptible to Lincosamides

✓ = generally susceptible		Lincosamides	
	Microorganism	Lincomycin	Clindamycin
Gram-positive	Staphylococcus aureus	✓	✓
	S epidermidis[1]	✓	✓
	Streptococcus pneumoniae	✓	✓
	S pyogenes	✓	✓
	β-hemolytic streptococci	✓	✓
	S viridans	✓	✓
	Pneumococci		✓
	Corynebacterium diphtheriae	✓	✓
	Nocardia asteroides	✓	✓
Anaerobes	Bacteroides sp	✓	✓[2]
	Fusobacterium		✓
	Propionibacterium (same as C acnes)	✓	✓
	Eubacterium	✓	✓
	Actinomyces sp	✓	✓
	Peptococcus	✓	✓
	Peptostreptococcus	✓	✓
	Microaerophilic streptococci		✓
	Clostridium perfringens	✓	✓
	C tetani	✓	✓
	Veillonella		✓

[1] Penicillinase and nonpenicillinase.
[2] Including B fragilis and B melaninogenicus.

Indications:

For the treatment of serious infections due to susceptible strains of streptococci, pneumococci and staphylococci. Reserve use for penicillin-allergic patients or when penicillin is inappropriate. Because of the risk of colitis (see Warning Box), consider the nature of the infection and the suitability of less toxic alternatives (eg, erythromycin).

Refer to individual monographs for complete information.

Contraindications:

Hypersensitivity to lincosamides; treatment of minor bacterial or viral infections.

Warnings:

Meningitis: **Clindamycin** does not diffuse adequately into CSF; not for meningitis.

Hypersensitivity: Use with caution in patients with a history of asthma or significant allergies. If hypersensitivity occurs, discontinue the drug and institute emergency treatment. Refer to Management of Acute Hypersensitivity Reactions.

Renal function impairment: Cautiously give **clindamycin** to patients with severe renal or hepatic disease accompanied by severe metabolic aberrations; monitor serum clindamycin levels during high-dose therapy. Use of **lincomycin** in preexisting liver disease is not recommended unless special clinical circumstances so indicate.

Elderly: Older patients with associated severe illness may not tolerate diarrhea well; carefully monitor these patients for changes in bowel frequency.

Pregnancy: Safety has not been established. Clindamycin and lincomycin cross the placenta in amounts ≈ 50% and 25% of maternal serum levels, respectively.

Lactation: **Clindamycin** appears in breast milk in ranges of 0.7 to 3.8 mcg/ml following doses of 300 mg orally to 600 mg IV every 6 hours. **Lincomycin** appears in breast milk in ranges of 0.5 to 2.4 mcg/ml. Breastfeeding is probably best discontinued when taking these agents to avoid potential problems in the infant. However, the American Academy of Pediatrics considers clindamycin to be compatible with breastfeeding.

Children: **Lincomycin** is not indicated for use in the newborn. When **clindamycin** is administered to newborns and infants, monitor organ system functions. Each ml of clindamycin and lincomycin contains 9.45 mg benzyl alcohol.

LINCOSAMIDES

Precautions:

Monitoring: Prolonged therapy — Perform liver/kidney function tests, blood counts.

IV infusion: Do NOT inject IV undiluted as a bolus; infuse over at least 10 to 60 minutes as directed in Administration and Dosage.

GI disease: Use cautiously in patients with GI disease, particularly colitis.

Benzyl alcohol: Some of these products contain benzyl alcohol which has been associated with fatal "gasping syndrome" in premature infants.

Superinfection: Use of antibiotics may result in bacterial or fungal overgrowth of nonsusceptible organisms, particularly yeasts. Such overgrowth may lead to a secondary infection. Take appropriate measures if superinfection occurs.

Tartrazine sensitivity: Some products contain tartrazine, which may cause allergic-type reactions (including bronchial asthma) in susceptible individuals. Although incidence of tartrazine sensitivity in the general population is low, it is frequently seen in patients who also have aspirin hypersensitivity. Refer to product listings.

Drug Interactions:

Lincosamide Drug Interactions

Precipitant drug	Object drug*		Description
Erythromycin	Lincosamides	⬇	Antagonism has occurred in vitro between clindamycin and erythromycin.
Kaolin-Pectin	Lincosamides	⬇	GI absorption is decreased for lincomycin and delayed for clindamycin when they are administered with kaolin-pectin antidiarrheals.
Lincosamides	Neuromuscular blockers (nondepolarizing)	⬆	The actions of the neuromuscular blockers may be enhanced, possibly contributing to profound and severe respiratory depression.

* ⬆ = Object drug increased ⬇ = Object drug decreased

Drug/Food interactions: Food impairs the absorption of lincomycin; do not take anything by mouth (except water) for 1 to 2 hours before and after lincomycin. Clindamycin absorption is not affected by food.

Adverse Reactions:

GI: Nausea; vomiting; diarrhea (clindamycin 3.4% to 30%); pseudomembranous colitis (clindamycin 0.01% to 10%; 3 to 4 times more frequent with oral administration).

Hematologic: Neutropenia; leukopenia; agranulocytosis; thrombocytopenic purpura.

Hypersensitivity: Skin rashes, urticaria, erythema multiforme, some cases resembling Stevens-Johnson syndrome (rare); anaphylaxis.

Hepatic: Jaundice; liver function test abnormalities (serum transaminase elevations).

Renal: Dysfunction has been characterized by azotemia, oliguria and proteinuria (rare).

Cardiovascular: Hypotension & cardiopulmonary arrest after too rapid IV use (rare).

Local: Pain following injection. Induration and sterile abscess have occurred after IM injection and thrombophlebitis after IV infusion with clindamycin; give deep IM injections and avoid prolonged use of IV catheters.

Clindamycin:

GI – Abdominal pain; esophagitis; anorexia; unpleasant or metallic taste (following higher doses of IV clindamycin).

Hypersensitivity – Maculopapular rash; generalized morbilliform-like rash.

Body as a whole – Transient eosinophilia; polyarthritis (rare).

Lincomycin:

GI – Glossitis; stomatitis; pruritus ani.

Hematologic – Aplastic anemia, pancytopenia (rare).

Hypersensitivity – Angioneurotic edema; serum sickness.

Special Senses – Tinnitus; vertigo.

Body as a whole – Vaginitis; exfoliative, vesiculobullous dermatitis (rare).

Patient Information:

May cause diarrhea; notify physician if this occurs.

Take each dose with a full glass of water. Complete full course of therapy.

Do not take anything by mouth (except water) for 1 to 2 hours before and after lincomycin. Clindamycin may be taken without regard to meals.

LINCOMYCIN

For complete prescribing information, refer to the Lincosamides group monograph.

Indications:

Treatment of serious infections due to susceptible strains of streptococci, pneumococci and staphylococci resistant to other antibiotics. Administer concomitantly with other antimicrobial agents when indicated.

Administration and Dosage:

Oral: Take at least 1 to 2 hours before or after eating to ensure optimum absorption.

Adults –

Serious infections: 500 mg every 8 hours.

More severe infections: ≥ 500 mg every 6 hours. With β-hemolytic streptococcal infections, continue treatment for at least 10 days to diminish the likelihood of subsequent rheumatic fever or glomerulonephritis.

Children > 1 month of age –

Serious infections: 30 mg/kg/day (15 mg/lb/day) divided into 3 or 4 equal doses.

More severe infections: 60 mg/kg/day (30 mg/lb/day) divided into 3 or 4 equal doses.

IM: IM administration is well tolerated.

Adults –

Serious infections: 600 mg every 24 hours.

More severe infections: 600 mg every 12 hours or more often.

Children > 1 month of age –

Serious infections: 10 mg/kg (5 mg/lb) every 24 hours.

More severe infections: 10 mg/kg (5 mg/lb) every 12 hours or more often.

IV: Dilute to 1 g/100 ml (minimum) and infuse over 1 hour. Severe cardiopulmonary reactions have occurred when given at greater than the recommended concentration and rate. IV administration in 250 to 500 ml of 5% Dextrose in Water or normal saline produces no local irritation or phlebitis.

Adults – Determine dose by the severity of the infection.

Serious infections: 600 mg to 1 g every 8 to 12 hours.

Severe to life-threatening situations: Doses of 8 g/day have been given.

Maximum recommended dose: 8 g/day.

Children > 1 month of age – Infuse 10 to 20 mg/kg/day (5 to 10 mg/lb/day), depending on severity of infection, in divided doses as described above for adults.

Subconjunctival injection: 75 mg/0.25 ml injected subconjunctivally results in ocular fluid levels of antibiotic (lasting for at least 5 hours) with MICs sufficient for most susceptible pathogens.

Renal function impairment: When required, an appropriate dose is 25% to 30% of that recommended for patients with normal renal function.

Admixture compatibilities/incompatibilities: Compatible and incompatible determinations are physical observations only, not chemical determinations. Adequate clinical evaluation of safety and efficacy of these combinations has not been performed.

Lincomycin Admixtures: Compatible for 24 Hours at Room Temperature Unless Otherwise Indicated

Infusion solutions:	*Antibiotics in infusion solutions:*
5% and 10% Dextrose in Water	Penicillin G Sodium (satisfactory for 4 hours)
5% and 10% Dextrose in Saline	Cephalothin
Ringer's Solution	Cephaloridine
Sodium Lactate ⅙ Molar	Colistimethate (satisfactory for 4 hours)
Travert 10% – Electrolyte No. 1	Ampicillin
Dextran in 6% Saline	Methicillin
Vitamins in infusion solutions:	Chloramphenicol
B-Complex	Polymyxin B Sulfate
B-Complex with Ascorbic Acid	

Incompatibilities – Lincomycin is incompatible with novobiocin, kanamycin and phenytoin sodium.

Rx	**Lincocin** (Upjohn)	**Capsules:** 500 mg (as HCl)	Lactose. Powder blue and dark blue. In 24s and 100s.
		Capsules, pediatric: 250 mg (as HCl)	Lactose. Blue. In 24s.
Rx	**Lincocin** (Upjohn)	**Injection:** 300 mg (as HCl)/ml	In 2 and 10 ml vials.[1]
Rx	**Lincorex** (Hyrex)		In 10 ml vials.

[1] With 0.9% benzyl alcohol.

CLINDAMYCIN

For complete prescribing information, refer to the Lincosamides group monograph.

Indications:

Parenteral and oral:

Anaerobes – Serious respiratory tract infections such as empyema, anaerobic pneumonitis and lung abscess; serious skin and soft tissue infections; septicemia, intra-abdominal infections such as peritonitis and intra-abdominal abscess (typically resulting from anaerobic organisms resident in the normal GI tract); infections of the female pelvis and genital tract such as endometritis, nongonococcal tubo-ovarian abscess, pelvic cellulitis and postsurgical vaginal cuff infection.

Streptococci and staphylococci – Serious respiratory tract infections; serious skin and soft tissue infections.

Pneumococci – Serious respiratory tract infections.

Parenteral:

Streptococci – Septicemia.

Staphylococci – Septicemia; acute hematogenous osteomyelitis.

Adjunctive therapy – In the surgical treatment of chronic bone and joint infections due to susceptible organisms.

Unlabeled uses: Clindamycin (1200 to 2400 mg/day) may be beneficial as an alternative to sulfonamides in combination with pyrimethamine in the acute treatment of CNS toxoplasmosis in AIDS patients.

Clindamycin (600 mg 4 times/day IV or 300 to 450 mg orally 4 times/day) with primaquine may be beneficial in *Pneumocystis carinii* pneumonia.

Clindamycin is effective in the treatment of *Chlamydia trachomatis* infections in women. See CDC recommendations for acute PID in the Dosage section.

Clindamycin 300 mg twice daily for 7 days is effective in bacterial vaginosis due to *Gardnerella* vaginalis and may be an alternative to metronidazole.

Prevention of bacterial endocarditis – For penicillin-allergic patients undergoing dental, oral, esophageal or respiratory tract procedures.

Parenterally for penicillin-allergic patients unable to take oral medications.

Administration and Dosage:

Anaerobic infections: Use parenteral form initially. May be followed by oral therapy.

β-hemolytic streptococcal infections: Continue treatment for at least 10 days.

Oral: Take with a full glass of water or with food to avoid esophageal irritation. Clindamycin absorption is not affected by food.

Adults –

Serious infections: 150 to 300 mg every 6 hours.

More severe infections: 300 to 450 mg every 6 hours.

Children –

Clindamycin HCl:

Serious infections – 8 to 16 mg/kg/day divided into 3 or 4 equal doses.

More severe infections – 16 to 20 mg/kg/day divided into 3 or 4 equal doses.

Clindamycin palmitate HCl:

Serious infections – 8 to 12 mg/kg/day divided into 3 or 4 equal doses.

Severe infections – 13 to 25 mg/kg/day divided into 3 or 4 equal doses. In children weighing ≤ 10 kg, administer 37.5 mg 3 times daily as the minimum dose.

Parenteral:

Adults –

Serious infections due to aerobic gram-positive cocci and the more sensitive anaerobes: 600 to 1200 mg/day in 2 to 4 equal doses.

More severe infections, particularly those due to *B fragilis, Peptococcus* sp or *Clostridium* sp other than *C perfringens:* 1.2 to 2.7 g/day in 2 to 4 equal doses. For more serious infections, these doses may have to be increased.

In life-threatening situations due to aerobes or anaerobes, doses of 4.8 g/day have been given IV to adults. Single IM injections > 600 mg are not recommended.

Children (> 1 month of age) – 20 to 40 mg/kg/day in 3 or 4 equal doses, depending on the severity of infection.

Alternatively, children may be dosed based on body surface area:
Serious infections: 350 mg/m²/day;
more serious infections: 450 mg/m²/day.

Neonates (< 1 month of age) – 15 to 20 mg/kg/day in 3 to 4 equal doses.

CDC recommendation for acute pelvic inflammatory disease†*:* 900 mg IV every 8 hours plus gentamicin loading dose 2 mg/kg IV or IM, followed by 1.5 mg/kg every 8 hours. Continue for at least 48 hours after patient improves.

† CDC 1989 Sexually Transmitted Diseases Treatment Guidelines. *Morbidity and Mortality Weekly Report* 1989; Sept 1;38(No. S-8):1-43.

CLINDAMYCIN

After discharge from hospital, continue with oral doxycycline 100 mg 2 times a day for 10 to 14 days total. Alternatively, continue with oral clindamycin 450 mg 5 times daily for 10 to 14 days.

Bacterial endocarditis prophylaxis:

Oral – 600 mg (20 mg/kg for children) 1 hour before procedure.

Parenteral – 600 mg (20 mg/kg for children) IV within 30 minutes before procedure.

Dilution and infusion rates: Dilute clindamycin phosphate prior to IV administration to a concentration of not more than 18 mg/ml.

Clindamycin Infusion Rates		
Dose (mg)	Diluent (ml)	Time (min)
300	50	10
600	50	20
900	50-100	30
1200	100	40

Do not administer > 1200 mg in a single 1 hour infusion.

Compatibility in IV solutions:

Clindamycin Compatibility in IV Solution		
Compatible at room temperature for 24 hours		Incompatible
IV solutions containing: sodium chloride dextrose calcium potassium	vitamin B complex cephalothin kanamycin gentamicin penicillin carbenicillin	ampicillin phenytoin sodium barbiturates aminophylline magnesium sulfate calcium gluconate

Reconstitution – Add 75 ml water to 100 ml bottle of palmitate in 2 portions; shake.

Storage/Stability – Store unreconstituted palmitate product at room temperature 15° to 30°C (59° to 86°F). Do NOT refrigerate the reconstituted solution; it may thicken and be difficult to pour when chilled. The solution is stable for 2 weeks at room temperature.

Clindamycin phosphate is stable in 0.9% Sodium Chloride Injection, 5% Dextrose in Water Injection and Lactated Ringer's Solution, in both glass and polyvinyl chloride containers, at concentrations of 6, 9, 12 and 18 mg/ml for 8 weeks frozen (–10°C), 32 days refrigerated (4°C) and 16 days at room temperature (25°C).

Rx	**Clindamycin HCl** (Various, eg, URL)	**Capsules:** 75 mg (as HCl)	In 100s.
Rx	**Cleocin** (Upjohn)		Tartrazine, lactose. Lavender. In 100s.
Rx	**Clindamycin HCl** (Various, eg, Biocraft, Geneva, Major, Moore, URL)	**Capsules:** 150 mg (as HCl)	In 100s.
Rx	**Cleocin** (Upjohn)		Tartrazine, lactose. Lavender and maroon. In 16s, 100s and UD 100s.
Rx	**Cleocin** (Upjohn)	**Capsules:** 300 mg (as HCl)	Lactose. Maroon. In 16s, 100s and UD 100s.
Rx	**Cleocin Pediatric** (Upjohn)	**Granules for Oral Solution:** 75 mg/5 ml (as palmitate)	Sucrose, parabens. In 100 ml.

CLINDAMYCIN

Rx	**Clindamycin Phosphate** (Various, eg, Abbott, Astra, Elkins-Sinn, Geneva, Lederle, Lyphomed, Smith & Nephew SoloPak)	**Injection:** 150 mg (as phosphate) per ml	In 2, 4, 6 and 60 ml vials.
Rx	**Cleocin Phosphate** (Upjohn)		In 2, 4 and 6 ml vials[1] and 4 and 6 ml *ADD-Vantage* vials[1], 50 ml Galaxy plastic containers and 60 ml pharmacy bulk package.

[1] With benzyl alcohol and EDTA.

AMINOGLYCOSIDES, PARENTERAL

Actions:

Pharmacology: Aminoglycosides are bactericidal antibiotics used primarily in the treatment of gram-negative infections. They irreversibly bind to the 30S subunit of bacterial ribosomes, misreading of the genetic code. The ribosomes separate from messenger RNA; cell death ensues.

Pharmacokinetics:

Absorption – Absorption from the GI tract is poor. Aminoglycosides are occasionally used orally for enteric infections (see Aminoglycosides, Oral monograph). Absorption from IM injection is rapid, with peak blood levels achieved within 1 hour.

Distribution – Aminoglycosides are widely distributed in extracellular fluids; peak serum concentrations may be lower than usual in patients whose extracellular fluid volume is expanded (eg, patients with edema or ascites). These drugs cross the placental barrier. Concentrations are found in bile, tissues, sputum, bronchial secretions and synovial, interstitial, peritoneal, abscess and pleural fluids. Concentrations in renal cortex are several times higher than usual serum levels. Aminoglycosides exhibit low protein binding, except for streptomycin. They do not achieve significant cerebrospinal fluid (CSF) levels in healthy patients. Although penetration is enhanced in the presence of inflamed meninges, only low levels are achieved. When intrathecal gentamicin is given with systemic gentamicin, CSF levels are substantially increased, depending on location of injection. Peak CSF concentrations following intralumbar administration generally occur 1 to 6 hours after injection.

Newborn infants, postpartum females and patients with ascites, spinal cord injury and cystic fibrosis may have an enlarged apparent volume of distribution. Obesity will artificially contract the apparent volume of distribution because adipose tissue contains less water than lean body mass of equal weight.

Excretion is by glomerular filtration, largely as unchanged drug; thus, high urine levels are attained. Probenecid does not affect renal tubular transport. The serum half-lives of all the agents are between 2 to 3 hours in patients with normal renal function. Approximately 53% to 98% of a single IV dose is excreted in the urine in 24 hours. However, when renal function is impaired, significant accumulation and subsequent toxicity may occur rapidly if dosage is not adjusted. The serum half-life is longer in young infants, as the immature renal system is unable to excrete these drugs rapidly; during the first days of life, the half-life may exceed 5 to 6 hours. Prolonged half-life may also be noted in the elderly. In severely burned patients, the half-life may be significantly decreased and result in serum concentrations lower than anticipated. Febrile and anemic states may be associated with a shorter serum half-life; dosage adjustment is usually not necessary. Aminoglycosides are removed by hemodialysis (4 to 6 hours removes approximately 50%) and peritoneal dialysis (range, removal of 23% in 8 hours to only 4% in 22 hours).

Serum levels: Because of the narrow range between therapeutic and toxic serum levels, careful attention to dosage calculations is essential, especially in patients with renal impairment, geriatric and female patients, those requiring high peak serum levels, patients on prolonged (> 10 days) therapy, patients with unstable renal function or those undergoing dialysis, those with abnormal extracellular fluid volume, or with prior exposure to ototoxic or nephrotoxic drugs. Age markedly affects peak concentration in children; it is generally lower in young children and infants. Monitor drug serum levels. Peak levels indicate therapeutic levels. Trough serum level determinations (just before next dose) best indicate drug accumulation. Obtain serum levels within 48 hours of start of therapy and every 3 to 4 days assuming stable renal function; also, levels are indicated when dose is changed or in changing renal function. Generally, to measure peak levels, draw a serum sample about 30 minutes after IV infusion or 1 hour after an IM dose. For trough levels, obtain serum samples at 8 hours or just prior to the next dose.

Various Pharmacokinetic Parameters of the Aminoglycosides

Aminoglycoside	Half-life (hrs) Normal	Half-life (hrs) ESRD	Therapeutic serum levels (peak) (mcg/ml)	Toxic serum levels (mcg/ml) Peak[1]	Toxic serum levels (mcg/ml) Trough[2]	Dose (mg/kg/day) (normal Ccr)
Amikacin	2-3	24-60	16-32	> 35	> 10	15
Gentamicin	2	24-60	4-8	> 12	> 2	3-5
Kanamycin	2-3	24-60	15-40	> 35	> 10	15
Netilmicin	2-2.7	40	6-10	> 16	> 4	3-6.5
Streptomycin	2.5	100	20-30	> 50	—	15
Tobramycin	2-2.5	24-60	4-8	> 12	> 2	3-5

[1] Measured 1 hour after IM administration.
[2] Measured immediately prior to next dose.

AMINOGLYCOSIDES, PARENTERAL

Microbiology: The bactericidal activity of aminoglycosides is through inhibition of bacterial protein synthesis. One-way cross resistance is frequently noted. Three mechanisms for the development of bacterial resistance to aminoglycosides have been identified: Alteration of the drug target site (the bacterial ribosome); reduction or elimination of transport of the drug into the bacterial cell; inactivation of the drug by enzymatic modification (aminoglycoside inactivating enzymes; most significant).

Perform culture and sensitivity testing. Treat susceptible organisms with less toxic agents, especially if renal function is compromised. Resistance develops slowly, except with streptomycin. Development of streptomycin resistance may be a single step process and may occur rapidly. Most streptococci species (particularly group D), including *S pneumoniae*, anaerobic organisms (including *Bacteroides* sp and *Clostridia* sp) and anaerobic cocci are resistant to aminoglycosides.

Organisms Generally Susceptible to Aminoglycosides

	Organisms	Amikacin	Gentamicin	Kanamycin	Netimicin	Streptomycin	Tobramycin
Gram-positive	Mycobacterium tuberculosis	✓[1]				✓[2]	
	Staphylococci	✓[3]	✓[3]		✓[3]		✓
	S aureus	✓	✓	✓[3]	✓[3]		✓
	S epidermidis	✓		✓	✓		
	Streptococci					✓[2]	
	S faecalis		✓[2]		✓[2]	✓[2]	✓[2]
Gram-negative	Acinetobacter sp	✓		✓	✓		
	Brucella sp					✓	
	Citrobacter sp	✓	✓	✓	✓	✓	✓
	Enterobacter sp	✓	✓	✓	✓	✓	✓
	Escherichia coli	✓	✓	✓	✓	✓	✓
	Hemophilus influenzae	✓		✓		✓[2]	
	Hemophilus ducreyi					✓	
	Klebsiella sp	✓	✓	✓	✓	✓[2]	✓
	Morganella morganii						✓
	Neisseria sp	✓		✓	✓	✓	
	Proteus sp	✓[4]	✓[4]	✓[4]	✓	✓	✓[4]
	Providencia sp	✓	✓	✓	✓	✓	✓
	Pseudomonas sp	✓			✓		
	P aeruginosa	✓	✓[2]		✓	✓	✓
	Salmonella sp	✓	✓	✓	✓	✓	✓
	Serratia sp	✓	✓	✓	✓	✓	✓
	Shigella sp	✓	✓	✓	✓	✓	✓
	Yersinia (Pasteurella) pestis	✓	✓	✓	✓	✓	✓

[1] ✓ = generally susceptible
[2] Usually used concomitantly with other anti-infectives.
[3] Penicillinase-producing and nonpenicillinase-producing.
[4] Indole-positive and indole-negative.

Indications:

The indications for specific agents are listed in individual drug monographs on the following pages. Reserve these drugs for treatment of infections caused by organisms not sensitive to less toxic agents. Safety for treatment periods > 14 days has not been established.

Unlabeled uses: In cystic fibrosis patients, the use of inhaled aminoglycosides may be beneficial in certain populations (eg, younger patients). Clinical outcome is not improved but deterioration of pulmonary function tests may be slowed or prevented.

AMINOGLYCOSIDES, PARENTERAL

Contraindications:

Previous reactions to these agents. With the exception of the use of streptomycin in tuberculosis, these agents are generally not indicated in long-term therapy because of the ototoxic and nephrotoxic hazards of extended administration.

Warnings:

Toxicity: Aminoglycosides are associated with significant nephrotoxicity or ototoxicity. These agents are excreted primarily by glomerular filtration; thus, the serum half-life will be prolonged and significant accumulation will occur in patients with impaired renal function. Toxicity may develop even with conventional doses, particularly in patients with prerenal azotemia or impaired renal function.

Ototoxicity – Neurotoxicity, manifested as both auditory (cochlear) and vestibular ototoxicity, can occur with any of these agents. Auditory changes are irreversible, usually bilateral and may be partial or total. Risk of hearing loss increases with the degree of exposure to either high peak or high trough serum concentrations and continues to progress after drug withdrawal. The risk is greater in patients with renal impairment and with preexisting hearing loss. High frequency deafness usually occurs first and can be detected by audiometric testing. When feasible, obtain serial audiograms. There may be no clinical symptoms to warn of developing cochlear damage. Tinnitus or vertigo may occur, and are evidence of vestibular injury. Other manifestations of neurotoxicity may include numbness, skin tingling, muscle twitching and convulsions. Total or partial irreversible bilateral deafness may occur after drug discontinuation. Aminoglycoside-induced ototoxicity is usually irreversible. Vestibular toxicity is more predominant with gentamicin and streptomycin; auditory toxicity is more common with kanamycin, amikacin and netilmicin. Tobramycin affects both functions equally. Relative ototoxicity is: Streptomycin = Kanamycin > Amikacin = Gentamicin = Tobramycin > Netilmicin. Kanamycin, amikacin and streptomycin appear in this relative comparison based on high dose (kanamycin, amikacin) and antituberculosis (streptomycin) therapy.

Renal toxicity may be characterized by decreased creatinine clearance, cells or casts in the urine, decreased urine specific gravity, oliguria, proteinuria or evidence of nitrogen retention (increasing BUN, nonprotein nitrogen [NPN] or serum creatinine). Renal damage is usually reversible. The relative nephrotoxicity of these agents is estimated to be: Kanamycin = Amikacin = Gentamicin = Netilmicin > Tobramycin > Streptomycin.

Monitoring – Closely observe all patients treated with aminoglycosides. Monitoring renal and eighth cranial nerve function at onset of therapy is essential for patients with known or suspected renal impairment and also in those whose renal function is initially normal, but who develop signs of renal dysfunction. Evidence of renal impairment or ototoxicity requires drug discontinuation or appropriate dosage adjustments. When feasible, monitor drug serum concentrations. Avoid concomitant use with other ototoxic, neurotoxic or nephrotoxic drugs. Other factors which may increase risk of toxicity are dehydration and advanced age.

Burn patients: In patients with extensive burns, altered pharmacokinetics may result in reduced serum concentrations of aminoglycosides. In such patients, measurement of serum concentration is especially important for dosage determination.

Hypomagnesemia may occur in more than ⅓ of patients whose oral diet is restricted or who are eating poorly.

Neuromuscular blockade: Neurotoxicity can occur after intrapleural and interperitoneal installation of large doses of an aminoglycoside; however, the reaction has followed IV, IM and oral administration. Aminoglycosides may aggravate muscle weakness because of a potential curare-like effect on the neuromuscular junction. Use with caution in patients with neuromuscular disorders (eg, myasthenia gravis, parkinsonism, infant botulism).

Neuromuscular blockade resulting in respiratory paralysis has occurred with aminoglycosides, especially if given with or soon after anesthesia or muscle relaxants (see Drug Interactions).

During or following gentamicin and netilmicin therapies, paresthesias, tetany, positive Chvostek and Trousseau signs, and mental confusion have been described in patients with hypomagnesemia, hypocalcemia and hypokalemia. When this occurred in infants, tetany and muscle weakness occurred. Both adults and infants required appropriate corrective electrolyte therapy.

Some patients who have had previous neurotoxic reactions to aminoglycosides have been treated with **netilmicin** without further neurotoxicity.

Use caution in newborns of mothers on magnesium sulfate; these hypermagnesemic infants may experience respiratory arrest after receiving aminoglycosides.

AMINOGLYCOSIDES, PARENTERAL

Nephrotoxicity may occur. Risk factors include the elderly, patients with a history of renal impairment who are treated for longer periods or with higher doses than those recommended, a recent course of aminoglycosides (within 6 weeks), concurrent use of other nephrotoxic agents, frequent dosing, potassium depletion and decreased intravascular volume. Adverse renal effects can occur in patients with initially normal renal function. Of patients receiving an aminoglycoside for several days or more, approximately 8% to 26% will develop mild renal impairment which is generally reversible.

Since renal function may alter appreciably during therapy, test renal function daily or more frequently. Examine urine for increased excretion of protein and for presence of cells and casts, keeping in mind the effects of the primary illness on these tests. Obtain one or more of the following laboratory measurements at the onset of therapy, frequently during therapy and at, or shortly after, the end of therapy: Creatinine clearance (Ccr) rate (either carefully measured or estimated from published nomograms or equations based on patient's age, sex, body weight and serial creatinine concentrations; preferred over BUN); serum creatinine concentration (preferred over BUN); BUN. More frequent testing is desirable if renal function is changing. If signs of renal irritation appear such as casts, white or red cells and albumin, increase hydration; a dosage reduction may be desirable (see Administration and Dosage for individual agents). These signs usually disappear when treatment is completed. However, if azotemia or a progressive decrease of urine output occurs, stop treatment. Reduce dosage if other evidence of renal dysfunction occurs (decreased Ccr or urine specific gravity, or increased BUN, creatinine or oliguria).

The risk of toxic reactions is low in well hydrated patients with normal renal function who do not receive **netilmicin, gentamicin** or **kanamycin** injections at higher doses or for longer periods of time than recommended.

Hydration – These drugs reach high concentrations in the renal system; keep patients well hydrated to minimize chemical irritation of tubules. Well hydrated patients with normal renal function have low risk of nephrotoxic reactions if recommended dosage is not exceeded.

Streptomycin, given to patients with preexisting renal insufficiency, calls for extreme caution. In severely uremic patients, a single dose may produce high blood levels for several days and the cumulative effect may produce ototoxic sequelae. Alkalinize the urine to minimize or prevent renal irritation.

Elderly patients may have reduced renal function that is not evident in the results of routine screening tests, such as BUN or serum creatinine. A Ccr determination may be more useful. Monitoring of renal function and drug levels during treatment is particularly important in such patients.

Pregnancy: Category D (amikacin, gentamicin, kanamycin, netilmicin, tobramycin). Aminoglycosides can cause fetal harm when given to pregnant women. These agents cross the placenta. Fetal serum levels may reach 16% to 50% of maternal levels. There are reports of total irreversible bilateral congenital deafness in children whose mothers received **streptomycin** during pregnancy. Prolonged use of **gentamicin** during pregnancy may result in otological damage to the fetus. Serious side effects to the mother, fetus or newborn have not been reported with other aminoglycosides, but the potential for harm exists. Although there is no clearly defined risk, such experience cannot exclude the possibility of infrequent or subtle damage to the fetus. If these drugs are used during pregnancy, or if the patient becomes pregnant while taking these drugs, apprise her of the potential hazards to the fetus.

Lactation: Small amounts of **streptomycin, kanamycin** and **netilmicin** are excreted in breast milk. Decide whether to discontinue nursing or discontinue the drug, taking into account the importance of the drug to the mother.

Children: Use with caution in premature infants and neonates because of their renal immaturity and the resulting prolongation of serum half-life of these drugs.

A syndrome of apparent CNS depression, characterized by stupor and flaccidity to coma and deep respiratory depression, has been reported in very young infants given **streptomycin**in doses greater than those recommended. Do not exceed recommended doses in infants.

Precautions:

Intrathecal gentamicin: A patient with multiple sclerosis for 7 years was given intralumbar gentamicin; disseminated microscopic brainstem lesions were found at autopsy. Tissue rarefaction and marked swelling of axis cylinders with occasional calcification, loss of oligodendroglia and astroglia and poor inflammatory response were seen. Use of excessive (40 to 160 mg) doses of intrathecal gentamicin has produced neuromuscular disturbances (eg, ataxia, paresis, incontinence).

Cross-allergenicity among the aminoglycosides has been demonstrated and depends largely on inactivation by bacterial enzymes.

AMINOGLYCOSIDES, PARENTERAL

Monitoring: Collect urine specimens for examination during therapy (see Nephrotoxicity). Monitor peak and trough serum concentrations periodically to assure adequate levels and to avoid potentially toxic levels. Also monitor serum calcium, magnesium and sodium (see Adverse Reactions).

Eighth cranial nerve function testing – Serial audiometric tests are suggested, particularly when renal function is impaired or prolonged aminoglycoside therapy is required; also repeat such tests periodically after treatment if there is evidence of a hearing deficit or vestibular abnormality before or during therapy, or when consecutive or concomitant use of other potentially ototoxic drugs is unavoidable. Discontinue therapy if tinnitus or subjective hearing loss develops, or if follow-up audiograms show loss of high frequency perception. Aminoglycoside-induced ototoxicity is usually irreversible.

Factors that may increase risk of aminoglycoside-induced ototoxicity include renal impairment (especially if dialysis is required), excessive dosage, dehydration, concomitant administration of ethacrynic acid or furosemide, or previous use of other ototoxic drugs.

Cochlear damage is usually manifested initially by small changes in audiometric test results at the high frequencies and may not be associated with subjective hearing loss; vestibular dysfunction is usually manifested by nystagmus, vertigo, nausea, vomiting or acute Meniere's syndrome.

Syphilis: In the treatment of sexually transmitted disease, if concomitant syphilis is suspected, perform a darkfield examination before treatment is started. Perform monthly serologic tests for at least 4 months.

Topical use: Aminoglycosides are quickly and almost totally absorbed when applied topically in association with surgical procedures, except to the urinary bladder. Irreversible deafness, renal failure, and death due to neuromuscular blockade have occurred following irrigation of both small and large surgical fields with an aminoglycoside preparation. Consider potential toxicity.

Benzyl alcohol, contained in some of these products as a preservative, has been associated with a fatal "gasping syndrome" in premature infants.

Superinfection: Use of antibiotics (especially prolonged or repeated therapy) may result in bacterial or fungal overgrowth of nonsusceptible organisms. Such overgrowth may lead to a secondary infection. Take appropriate measures if this occurs.

Sulfite sensitivity: Some products contain sulfites that may cause allergic-type reactions including anaphylactic symptoms and life-threatening/less severe asthmatic episodes in susceptible persons. Overall prevalence in general population is unknown and probably low. It is more frequent in asthmatics or atopic nonasthmatics.

Drug Interactions:

Aminoglycoside Drug Interactions			
Precipitant drug	Object drug*		Description
Cephalosporins Enflurane Methoxyflurane Vancomycin	Aminoglycosides	↑	Risk of nephrotoxicity may increase above that with aminoglycoside alone. Monitor patients. With cephalosporins, bactericidal activity against certain pathogens may be enhanced (see Administration).
Indomethacin IV	Aminoglycosides	↑	In preterm infants, the use of indomethacin for closure of patent ductus arteriosus resulted in aminoglycoside accumulation in one study.
Loop diuretics	Aminoglycosides	↑	Auditory toxicity appears to increase during concomitant use. Hearing loss of varying degrees may occur; it may be irreversible. Monitor patients.
Penicillins	Aminoglycosides	↑	Synergism of these agents is well documented; however, certain penicillins may inactivate certain aminoglycosides. The problem may be greatest in vitro (see Administration).
Aminoglycosides	Neuromuscular blockers, depolarizing and nondepolarizing	↑	The neuromuscular blocking effects are enhanced by aminoglycosides. Prolonged respiratory depression may occur.
Aminoglycosides	Polypeptide antibiotics	↑	Concurrent use of thes agents may increase the risk of respiratory paralysis and renal dysfunction.

* ↑ = Object drug increased

AMINOGLYCOSIDES, PARENTERAL

Adverse Reactions:

Aminoglycoside Adverse Reactions (%)

	Adverse Reaction	Amikacin	Gentamicin	Kanamycin	Netimicin	Streptomycin	Tobramycin
Central/Peripheral nervous system	Headache	rare	✓[1]	rare	< 0.1		✓
	Encephalopathy		✓		✓		
	Confusion		✓				✓
	Fever		✓		0.1	✓	✓
	Lethargy		✓				✓
	Disorientation				< 0.1		✓
	Neuromuscular blockade[2]	✓		✓	✓	✓	
	Paresthesia	rare		rare	< 0.1		
	Convulsions		✓		✓		
	Muscle twitching		✓		✓		
	Myasthenia gravis-like syndrome		✓		✓		
	Numbness		✓		✓		
	Peripheral neuropathy		✓		✓		
	Skin tingling		✓		✓		
GI	Vomiting	rare	✓	rare	< 0.1	✓	✓
	Nausea	rare	✓	rare		✓	✓
	Diarrhea			rare	< 0.1		✓
Hematologic	Anemia	rare	✓		< 0.1		✓
	Eosinophilia	rare	✓		0.4	✓	✓
	Leukopenia		✓		< 0.1	✓	✓
	Thrombocytopenia		✓		< 0.1	✓	✓
	Granulocytopenia		✓				✓
Hyper-sensitivity	Rash	rare	✓	rare	≤ 0.5	✓	✓
	Urticaria		✓			✓	✓
	Itching		✓		≤ 0.5		✓
	Anaphylaxis/Anaphylactoid reaction		✓			✓	
Special senses	Dizziness		✓		✓		✓
	Tinnitus		✓		✓		✓
	Vertigo		✓		✓	✓	✓
	Roaring in ears		✓				✓
	Hearing loss/deafness	✓	✓	✓[3]		✓	✓
	Loss of balance	✓		✓[3]			
	Visual disturbances/blurred vision		✓		< 0.1		
Renal[1]	Oliguria	✓	✓	✓	✓		✓
	Proteinuria	✓	✓	✓	✓		✓
	Rising serum creatinine[2]	✓	✓	✓	✓		✓
	Casts	✓	✓		✓		
	Rising BUN[2]		✓	✓	✓		✓
	Red and white cells in urine	✓		✓	✓		
	Azotemia	✓		✓		✓	
	Rising NPN[2]		✓				✓
	Decreasing Ccr			✓	✓		
Lab test abnormalities	Increased AST/ALT		✓		1.5		✓
	Increased bilirubin		✓		1.5		✓
	Increased serum LDH		✓				✓
Other	Apnea	✓	✓	✓	✓	✓	✓
	Drug fever	rare		rare			
	Pain/Irritation at injection site		✓	✓	≈ 0.4		✓
	Hypotension	rare	✓		< 0.1		
	Acute muscular paralysis	✓		✓			
	Decreased serum Ca, Na, K, Mg[2]		✓				✓

[1] ✓ = Reported; no incidence given
[2] See Warnings
[3] Partially reversible to irreversible bilateral hearing loss.

AMINOGLYCOSIDES, PARENTERAL

Renal:

Renal function changes are usually reversible upon discontinuation. See Warnings.

Other adverse reactions listed only for the individual agents:

Amikacin: Arthralgia, tremor (rare).

Gentamicin:

CNS – Acute organic brain syndrome; depression; pseudotumor cerebri; respiratory depression.

GI – Decreased appetite; hypersalivation; stomatitis; weight loss.

Hematologic – Increased and decreased reticulocyte count; transient agranulocytosis.

Hypersensitivity – Generalized burning; laryngeal edema; purpura.

Miscellaneous – Alopecia; hypertension; joint pain; pulmonary fibrosis; splenomegaly; subcutaneous atrophy or fat necrosis (rare); transient hepatomegaly; leg cramps; increased CSF protein; arachnoiditis or burning at injection site after intrathecal administration (see Warnings); a Fanconi-like syndrome, with aminoaciduria and metabolic acidosis.

Kanamycin: Granular casts; "malabsorption syndrome" characterized by an increase in fecal fat, decrease in serum carotene and fall in xylose absorption (prolonged therapy).

Netilmicin: Increased alkaline phosphatase (1.5%); severe pain, induration and hematomas following injection (≈ 0.4%); thrombocytosis (0.2%); prolonged PT (0.1%); hyperkalemia, palpitations, immature circulating WBCs, leukemoid reaction (< 0.1%); nystagmus; a Fanconi-like syndrome, with aminoaciduria and metabolic acidosis.

Streptomycin:

Hypersensitivity – Angioneurotic edema; exfoliative dermatitis.

Neurotoxic: Facial, circumoral or peripheral paresthesia; muscular weakness.

Miscellaneous – Amblyopia; hemolytic anemia; hepatic necrosis; myocarditis; pancytopenia; serum sickness; toxic epidermal necrolysis.

Tobramycin: Cylindruria; delirium; leukocytosis.

Overdosage:

Symptoms: The severity of the signs and symptoms following overdose are dependent on the dose administered, patient's renal function, state of hydration and age, and whether or not other medications with similar toxicities are being administered concurrently. Toxicity may occur in patients treated > 10 days or in patients with reduced renal function where dose has not been appropriately adjusted.

Nephrotoxicity following the parenteral administration of an aminoglycoside is most closely related to the area under the curve. Nephrotoxicity is more likely if trough concentrations fail to fall below the intended concentration. Patients who are elderly, have abnormal renal function, are receiving other nephrotoxic drugs or are volume depleted are at greater risk for developing acute tubular necrosis. Auditory and vestibular toxicities have been associated with aminoglycoside overdose. These toxicities occur in patients treated > 10 days, in patients with abnormal renal function, in dehydrated patients, or in patients receiving medications with additive auditory toxicities. These patients may not have signs or symptoms or may experience dizziness, tinnitus, vertigo and a loss of high-tone acuity as ototoxicity progresses. Ototoxic signs and symptoms may not begin to occur until long after the drug has been discontinued.

AMINOGLYCOSIDES, PARENTERAL

Neuromuscular blockade or respiratory paralysis may occur following aminoglycoside administration. Neuromuscular blockade, respiratory failure and prolonged respiratory paralysis may occur more commonly in patients with myasthenia gravis or Parkinson's disease. Prolonged respiratory paralysis may also occur in patients receiving neuromuscular blockers. If neuromuscular blockade occurs, it may be reversed by the administration of calcium salts but mechanical assistance may be necessary.

If an aminoglycoside were ingested, toxicity would be less likely because they are poorly absorbed from an intact GI tract.

Treatment: The initial intervention is to establish an airway and ensure oxygenation and ventilation. Initiate resuscitative measures promptly if respiratory paralysis occurs. Adequately hydrate patients, and carefully monitor fluid balance, Ccr and plasma levels.

Peritoneal dialysis or hemodialysis will aid in removal from the blood. This is especially important if renal function is, or becomes, compromised. Hemodialysis is preferable because it is more efficient in reducing serum levels. Complexation with ticarcillin or carbenicillin (12 to 30 g/day) appears as effective as hemodialysis in lowering excessive aminoglycoside serum concentrations. In newborns, consider exchange transfusions.

Range of Aminoglycoside Half-Lives (Hours) During Dialysis[1]

Aminoglycosides	Interdialysis	Hemodialysis	Peritoneal dialysis
Kanamycin	40-96	5	12
Gentamicin	21-59	6-11	5-29
Tobramycin	27-70	3-10	10-37
Amikacin	28-87	4-7	18-29
Netilmicin	24-52	5	—

[1] Patient renal function creatinine clearance ≤ 5 ml/min.

Administration and Dosage:

Synergism: In vitro studies indicate that aminoglycosides combined with penicillins or cephalosporins act synergistically against some strains of gram-negative organisms and enterococci (Streptococcus faecalis). Aminoglycosides may exhibit a synergistic effect when combined with carbenicillin or ticarcillin for *Pseudomonas* infections. Tests for antibiotic synergy are necessary. See also Admixture Incompatibility and Drug Interactions.

Admixture incompatibility: Beta-lactam antibiotics (eg, penicillins, cephalosporins) may inactivate aminoglycosides when admixed. Ticarcillin and carbenicillin are the worst β-lactam offenders; tobramycin and gentamicin are more susceptible than netilmicin or amikacin. This is most likely to occur: When the agents are mixed in the same container; during the aminoglycoside assay procedure; and in poor renal function. Concomitant cephalosporins may also falsely elevate creatinine determinations.

Ticarcillin and carbenicillin may also decrease aminoglycoside serum levels (see Overdosage).

Inactivation of tobramycin has not occurred in patients with normal renal function if they are given the drugs by separate routes. Kanamycin and methicillin inactivate each other in vitro, but this has not been seen in patients who receive them by different routes.

Guard against in vitro inactivation of aminoglycosides by β-lactam antibiotics in patients on combination therapy: 1) Place sample on ice immediately after drawing the specimen; test immediately. If testing is delayed, freeze serum as soon as possible; 2) draw the aminoglycoside level when the β-lactam antibiotic is at its trough level; 3) inactivation can still occur when the specimen is frozen (eg, kanamycin and ampicillin). If samples are to be frozen for a long period of time, inactivate the penicillin with penicillinase prior to freezing.

Dosing interval: Although further studies are needed, preliminary evidence indicates that aminoglycosides may be administered on a once daily basis without compromising efficacy and without increasing the potential for nephrotoxicity and ototoxicity. It is possible that the incidence of nephrotoxicity may even be decreased.

STREPTOMYCIN SULFATE

For complete prescribing informatin, refer to the Aminoglycosides group monograph.

SPECIAL NOTE: See WARNING BOX in the group monograph concerning toxicity.

Indications:

Mycobacterium tuberculosis: The Advisory Council for Elimination of TB, the American Thoracic Society and CDC recommend that either streptomycin or ethambutol be added as a fourth drug in a regimen containing isoniazid, rifampin and pyrazinamide for initial TB treatment unless the likelihood of INH or rifampin resistance is very low. Reasses need for a fourth drug when susceptibility testing results are known.

Streptomycin is also indicated for therapy of TB when one or more of the above drugs is contraindicated because of toxicity or intolerance. The management of TB has become more complex as a consequence of increasing rates of drug resistance and concomitant HIV infection. Additional consultation from experts may be desirable in those settings. Refer also to the introduciton in the Antituberculous Drugs group monograph.

Nontuberculous infections: Use only in infections caused by organisms shown to be susceptible, and when less potentially hazardous therapeutic agents are ineffective or contraindicated. Organisms usually sensitive include: *Pasteurella pestis* (plague); *Francistularensis* (tularemia); *Brucella,* Calymmatobacterium granulomatis (donovanosis, granuloma inguinale); *Haemophilus ducreyi* (chancroid); *H influenzae* (in respiratory, endocardial and meningeal infections with another agent); *Klebsiella pneumoniae* pneumonia (with another agent); *E coli, Proteus* sp, *A aerogenes, K pneumoniae* and *Entercoccus faecalis* in UTIs; *S viridans* and *E faecalis* (in endocardial infections with penicillin); gram-negative bacilli (in bacteremia, with another agent).

Unlabeled uses: Streptomycin 11 to 13 mg/kg/24 hrs IV or 15 mg/kg/day IM may be used as part of a multiple-drug regimen (generally three to five agents) for *Mycobacterium avium* complex, a common infection in AIDS patients.

Administration and Dosage:

Administer by the IM route.

Tuberculosis: The standard regimen for the treatment of drug-susceptible TB has been 2 months of INH, rifampin and pyrazinamide followed by 4 months of INH and rifampin (patients with concomitant TB and HIV infection may require treatment for a longer period). When streptomycin is added to this regimen because of suspected or proven drug resistance, the recommended dosing for streptomycin is as follows:

Streptomycin Dosing for TB			
	Daily	Twice weekly	Thrice weekly
Children	20-40 mg/kg max 1 g	25-30 mg/kg max 1.5 g	25-30 mg/kg max 1.5 g
Adults	15 mg/kg max 1 g	25-30 mg/kg max 1.5 g	25-30 mg/kg max 1.5 g

STREPTOMYCIN SULFATE

Streptomycin is usually administered daily as a single IM injection. Give a total dose of < 120 g over the course of therapy unless there are no other therapeutic options. In patients > 60 years of age, use a reduced dosage. Therapy with streptomycin may be terminated when toxic symptoms have appeared, when impending toxicity is feared, when organisms become resistant, or when full treatment effect has been obtained. The total period of drug treatment of TB is a minimum of 1 year.

Tularemia: 1 to 2 g/day in divided doses for 7 to 14 days, or until the patient is afebrile for 5 to 7 days.

Plague: 2 g daily in two divided doses for minimum of 10 days.

Bacterial endocarditis:

Streptococcal – In penicillin-sensitive alpha and non-hemolytic streptococci (sensitive to ≤ 0.1 mcg/ml penicillin), use streptomycin for 2 weeks with penicillin: 1 g twice daily for 1 week, 0.5 g twice daily for the second week. If patient is > 60 years of age, give 0.5 g twice daily for the entire 2 week period.

Enterococcal – 1 g b.i.d. for 2 weeks and 0.5 g b.i.d. for 4 weeks in combination with penicillin.

Concomitant agents: For use with other agents to which infecting organism is also sensitive, streptomycin is a secondary choice. Gram-negative bacillary bacteremia, meningitis and pneumonia; brucellosis; granuloma inguinale; chancroid; UTI.

Adults: 1 to 2 g in divided doses every 6 to 12 hours for moderate to severe infections. Doses should generally not exceed 2 g per day.

Children: 20 to 40 mg/kg/day (8 to 20 mg/lb/day) in divided doses every 6 to 12 hours. (Take particular care to avoid excessive dosage in children.)

Storage/Stability: Store under refrigeration at 2° to 8°C (36° to 46°F).

Rx	**Streptomycin Sulfate** (Pfizer)	**Injection:** 400 mg/ml	In 2.5 ml amps.

KANAMYCIN SULFATE

For complete prescribing information, refer to the Aminoglycosides, Parenteral group monograph.

SPECIAL NOTE: See WARNING BOX in the group monograph concerning toxicity.

Warning:

Carefully observe elderly patients, patients with preexisting tinnitus or vertigo or known subclinical deafness, those having received prior ototoxic drugs, and patients receiving a total dose of > 15 g kanamycin sulfate for signs of eighth nerve damage. Loss of hearing may occur, even with normal renal function.

Indications:

Consider initial therapy for one or more of the following: *Escherichia coli, Proteus* sp (both indole-positive and indole-negative), *Enterobacter aerogenes, Klebsiella pneumoniae, Serratia marcescens* and *Acinetobacter* sp. May be used as initial therapy with a penicillin or cephalosporin before obtaining results of susceptibility testing. Not the drug of choice for staphylococcal infections; may be indicated for inital therapy of severe infections where the strain is thought to be susceptible in patients allergic to other antibiotics, or in mixed staphylococcal/gram-negative infections.

Not indicated in oong-term therapy (eg, tuberculosis) because of the toxic hazard associated with extended administration.

Unlabeled uses: Kanamycin 11 to 13 mg/kg/24 hours IV or 15 mg/kg/day IM may be used as part of a multiple-drug regimen (generally three to five agents) for *Mycobacterium avium* complex, a common infection in AIDS patients.

Administration and Dosage:

Do not exceed a total of 1.5 g/day by any route.

IM: Inject deeply into upper outer quadrant of gluteal muscle. For adults or children, 7.5 mg/kg every 12 hours (15 mg/kg/day). If continuously high blood levels are desired, give daily dose of 15 mg/kg in equally divided doses every 6 or 8 hours. Usual treatment duration is 7 to 10 days. Doses of 7.5 mg/kg give mean peak levels of 22 mcg/ml. At 8 hours after a 7.5 mg/kg dose, mean serum levels are 3.2 mcg/ml.

Uncomplicated infections should respond in 24 to 48 hours. If a clinical response does not occur within 3 to 5 days, stop therapy and reevaluate. Failure may be due to resistance of organism or presence of septic foci requiring surgical drainage.

IV: Do not admix with other antibacterial agents; administer separately.

Adults – Do not exceed 15 mg/kg/day. Give slowly. Prepare by adding contents of 500 mg vial to 100 to 200 ml sterile diluent (Normal Saline or 5% Dextrose in Water) or the contents of a 1 g vial to 200 to 400 ml of sterile diluent. Give over 30 to 60 minutes. Divide daily dose itno 2 to 3 equal doses.

Children – Use sufficient diluent to infuse the drug over 30 to 60 minutes.

KANAMYCIN SULFATE

Renal failure: Follow therapy by appropriate serum assays. If not feasible, reduce frequency of administration. Calculate the dosage interval with the following formula: Serum creatinine (mg/dl) × 9 = dosage interval (in hours).

Intraperitoneal (following exploration for peritonitis or after peritoneal contamination due to fecal spill during surgery): 500 mg in 20 ml sterile distilled water instilled through a polyethylene catheter into the wound. If possible, postpone instillation until patient has recovered from anesthesia and muscle relaxants. Absorption after intraperitoneal instillation is similar to IM use. After a single instillation of 250 or 500 mg, peak serum levels of 13.5 and 24 mcg/ml, respectively, occurred in one study.

Aerosol treatment: 250 mg 2 to 4 times a day. Withdraw 250 mg (1 ml) from 500 mg vial, dilute with 3 ml Normal Saline and nebulize.

Other routes: Concentrations of 0.25% have been used as irrigating solutions in abscess cavities, pleural space, peritoneal and ventricular cavities.

Stability: Darkening of vials during shelf life does not indicate loss of potency.

Rx	**Kanamycin Sulfate** (Various, eg, Lyphomed, S & N SoloPak)	**Injection:** 500 mg	In 2 ml vials.[1]
Rx	**Kantrex** (Apothecon)		In 2 ml vials.[2]
Rx	**Kanamycin Sulfate** (Various, eg, Lyphomed, S & N SoloPak)	**Injection:** 1 g	In 3 ml vials.[1]
Rx	**Kantrex** (Apothecon)		In 3 ml vials.[2]
Rx	**Kanamycin Sulfate** (Various, eg, Lyphomed, S & N SoloPak)	**Pediatric Injection:** 75 mg	In 2 ml vials.[1]
Rx	**Kantrex** (Apothecon)		In 2 ml vials.[2]

[1] May contain sulfites.
[2] With sodium bisulfite.

GENTAMICIN

For complete prescribing information, refer to the Aminoglycosides, Parenteral group monograph.

Indications:

Treatment of serious infections caused by susceptible strains of *Pseudomonas aeruginosa, Proteus* sp (indole-positive and indole-negative), *Escherichia coli, Klebsiella* sp, *Enterobacter* sp, *Serratia* sp, *Citrobacter* sp and *Staphylococcus* sp (coagulase-positive and coagulase-negative).

Effective in bacterial neonatal sepsis; bacterial septicemia; serious bacterial infections of the CNS (meningitis), urinary tract, respiratory tract, GI tract (including peritonitis), skin, bone and soft tissue (including burns).

Not indicated in uncomplicated initial episodes of urinary tract infections, unless causative organisms are susceptible to these antibiotics and are not susceptible to antibiotics with less potential for toxicity. Perform bacterial cultures.

Gram-negative infections: Consider as initial therapy in suspected or confirmed gram-negative infections; therapy may be started before obtaining results of susceptibility testing, but continue therapy based on susceptibility test results, infection severity and the concepts in the Warning Box (see Warnings).

Unknown causative organisms: In serious infections, administer gentamicin as initial therapy in conjunction with a penicillin or cephalosporin before obtaining results of susceptibility tests. Following identification of the organism and its susceptibility, continue appropriate antibiotic therapy.

Combination therapy: Effective in combination with carbenicillin for the treatment of life-threatening infections caused by *P aeruginosa.* Also effective when combined with a penicillin for treatment of endocarditis caused by group D streptococci. In the neonate with suspected bacterial sepsis or staphylococcal pneumonia, penicillin is usually indicated concomitantly with gentamicin.

Staphylococcal infections: While not the antibiotic of first choice, consider gentamicin when penicillins or other less toxic drugs are contraindicated, when bacterial susceptibility tests and clinical judgment indicate its use and in mixed infections caused by susceptible strains of staphylococci and gram-negative organisms.

Intrathecal administration is indicated as adjunctive therapy to systemic gentamicin sulfate in the treatment of serious CNS infections (meningitis, ventriculitis) caused by susceptible *Pseudomonas* sp. Perform bacteriologic tests to determine that the causative organisms are susceptible to gentamicin.

Unlabeled uses: An alternative regimen for pelvic inflammatory disease is gentamicin 2 mg/kg IV followed by 1.5 mg/kg 3 times daily (normal renal function) plus clindamycin 600 mg IV 4 times daily. Continue for at least 4 days and at least 48 hours after patient improves; then continue clindamycin 450 mg orally 4 times daily for 10 to 14 days total therapy.

Administration and Dosage:

Monitoring: Because of the potential for toxicity, serum level monitoring is recommended when the drug is used in patients with impaired renal function, when doses in excess of 3 mg/kg/day are used, or when the drug is used in any patient in whom altered pharmacokinetics are suspected (ie, patients with extensive burns).

Generally, the peak concentration (at 30 to 60 minutes after IM injection or immediately after a slow IV infusion) is expected to be in the range of 4 to 6 mcg/ml. When monitoring peak concentrations, avoid prolonged levels > 12 mcg/ml. When monitoring trough concentrations (just prior to the next dose), avoid levels > 2 mcg/ml. When determining the adequacy of a serum level for a particular patient, consider susceptibility of the causative organism, infection severity and the status of the patient's host-defense mechanisms.

Dosage: May be given IM or IV. For patients with serious infections and normal renal function, give 3 mg/kg/day in 3 equal doses every 8 hours. For patients with life-threatening infections, administer up to 5 mg/kg/day in 3 or 4 equal doses. Reduce dosage to 3 mg/kg/day as soon as clinically indicated.

Obese patients – Base dosage on an estimate of lean body mass.

Children – 6 to 7.5 mg/kg/day (2 to 2.5 mg/kg every 8 hours).

Infants and neonates – 7.5 mg/kg/day (2.5 mg/kg every 8 hours).

Premature or full term neonates (≤ 1 week of age) – 5 mg/kg/day (2.5 mg/kg every 12 hours). A regimen of either 2.5 mg/kg every 18 hours or 3 mg/kg every 24 hours may also provide satisfactory peak and trough levels in preterm infants < 32 weeks gestational age.

Duration of therapy is usually 7 to 10 days. In difficult and complicated infections, a longer course of therapy may be necessary. In such cases, monitor renal, auditory and vestibular function, since toxicity is more apt to occur with treatment extended beyond 10 days. Reduce dosage if clinically indicated.

GENTAMICIN

Prevention of bacterial endocarditis: In high risk patients undergoing GU or nonesophageal GI procedures.

High-risk – 2 g (50 mg/kg not to exceed 2 g in children) IM or IV plus gentamicin 1.5 mg/kg (not to exceed 120 mg in adults) within 30 minutes of starting procedure; 6 hours later, ampicillin 1 g (25 mg/kg for children) IM or IV or amoxicillin 1 g (25 mg/kg for children) orally.

High-risk penicillin-allergic – 1 g (20 mg/kg for children) IV over 1 to 2 hours plus gentamicin 1.5 mg/kg (not to exceed 120 mg in adults) IV or IM; complete infusion/injection within 30 minutes of starting the procedure.

GU or GI procedures (standard regimen) – 2 g (50 mg/kg for children) ampicillin plus 1.5 mg/kg (2 mg/kg for children) gentamicin not to exceed 80 mg, both IM or IV one-half hour prior to procedure followed by 1.5 mg (25 mg/kg for children) amoxicillin.

Renal function impairment: Adjust dosage; whenever possible, monitor serum concentrations of gentamicin. One method of dosage adjustment is to increase the interval between the doses administered.

Rule of eights – The serum creatinine concentration roughly correlates with the serum half-life of gentamicin. Creatinine clearance is better, but still roughly correlates with serum aminoglycoside levels. Approximate the interval between doses (in hours) by multiplying the serum creatinine level (mg/dl) by 8. For example, a patient weighing 60 kg with a serum creatinine level of 2 mg/dl could be given 60 mg (1 mg/kg) every 16 hours (2 x 8).

In patients with serious systemic infections and renal impairment, administer the antibiotic more frequently, but in reduced dosage. Measure serum concentrations of gentamicin so that appropriate levels result. Peak and trough concentrations, measured intermittently during therapy, will provide optimal guidance for adjusting dosage.

After the usual initial dose, a rough guide for determining reduced dosage at 8 hour intervals is to divide the normally recommended dose by the serum creatinine level. For example, after an initial dose of 60 mg (1 mg/kg), a patient weighing 60 kg with a serum creatinine level of 2 mg/dl could be given 30 mg every 8 hours (60 ÷ 2).

The status of renal function may change over the course of the infectious process. Deteriorating renal function may require a greater reduction in dosage than that specified in the above guidelines for patients with stable renal impairment. The above dosage schedules are not rigid recommendations, but are provided as rough guides to dosage when the measurement of gentamicin serum levels is not feasible.

Several predictive methods and published nomograms have been compared, none of which performed as well as individualized pharmacokinetic dosing with serum levels.

Hemodialysis – The amount of gentamicin removed from the blood may vary depending on several factors, including the dialysis method used. An 8 hour hemodialysis may reduce serum concentrations of gentamicin by approximately 50%. The recommended dosage at the end of each dialysis period is 1 to 1.7 mg/kg, depending on the severity of infection. In children, administer a dose of 2 to 2.5 mg/kg.

IV: The dose for IV and IM administration is identical; IV administration is useful for treating patients with bacterial septicemia or those in shock. It may also be the preferred route for some patients with CHF, hematologic disorders, severe burns or reduced muscle mass. A 1 to 2 mg/kg loading dose may be used, followed by a maintenance dose.

For intermittent IV administration in adults, dilute a single dose in 50 to 200 ml sterile isotonic saline or in a sterile solution of 5% Dextrose in Water. In infants and children, the volume of diluent should be less. Infuse over a period of ½ to 2 hours.

Admixture incompatibility – Do not physically premix gentamicin with other drugs; administer separately in accordance with route and dosage schedule.

GENTAMICIN

Intrathecal: Administer only the 2 mg/ml intrathecal preparation without preservatives.

Dosage will vary depending upon factors such as age and weight of the patient, site of injection, degree of obstruction to CSF flow and the amount of CSF estimated to be present. In general, the recommended dose for infants and children ≥ 3 months of age is 1 to 2 mg once a day. For adults, administer 4 to 8 mg once a day.

Continue administration as long as sensitive organisms are demonstrated in the CSF. Since the intralumbar or intraventricular dose is administered immediately after specimens are taken for laboratory study, continue treatment for at least 1 day after negative results have been obtained from CSF cultures or stained smears.

The suggested method for administering the intrathecal injection into the lumbar area is as follows: Perform the lumbar puncture and remove a specimen of the spinal fluid for laboratory tests, then insert syringe containing injection into the hub of the spinal needle. Allow a quantity of CSF (approximately 10% of the estimated total CSF volume) to flow into the syringe and mix with the gentamicin. Inject the resultant solution over a period of 3 to 5 minutes with the bevel of the needle directed upward.

If the CSF is grossly purulent, or if it is unobtainable, dilute gentamicin with sterile normal saline before injection.

May also be administered directly into the subdural space or directly into the ventricles, including administration by use of an implanted reservoir.

Rx	**Gentamicin Sulfate** (Various, eg, Elkins-Sinn, Lyphomed, Major, Moore, Pasadena, Schein)	**Injection:** 40 mg per ml (as sulfate)	In 2 and 20 ml vials and 1.5 and 2 ml cartridge-needle units.
Rx	**Garamycin** (Schering)		In 2 and 20 ml vials[1] and 1.5 and 2 ml disp. syringes.[1]
Rx	**Jenamicin** (Hauck)		In 20 ml vials.[1]
Rx	**Pediatric Gentamicin Sulfate** (Elkins-Sinn)	**Injection:** 10 mg per ml (as sulfate)	In 2 ml vials.
Rx	**Garamycin Pediatric** (Schering)		In 2 ml vials.[1]
Rx	**Garamycin Intrathecal** (Schering)	**Injection:** 2 mg per ml (as sulfate)	Preservative free. In 2 ml amps.

[1] With parabens, EDTA and sodium bisulfite.

TOBRAMYCIN SULFATE

Information beginning in the Aminoglycoside group monograph must be considered when using these products.

SPECIAL NOTE: See WARNING BOX concerning aminoglycoside toxicity.

Indications:

Treatment of serious infections caused by susceptible strains of *Pseudomonas aeruginosa, Escherichia coli, Proteus* sp (indole-positive and indole-negative) including *P mirabilis, Morganella morganii* and *P vulgaris, Providencia* sp including *P rettgeri, Klebsiella-Enterobacter-Serratia* group, *Citrobacter* sp and staphylococci, including *S aureus* (coagulase-positive and coagulase-negative).

Septicemia (neonates, children, adults) caused by *P aeruginosa, E coli, Klebsiella* sp.

Lower respiratory tract infections caused by *P aeruginosa, Klebsiella* sp, *Enterobacter* sp, *Serratia* sp, *E coli, S aureus* (penicillinase- and nonpenicillinase-producing).

Serious CNS infections (meningitis) caused by susceptible organisms.

Intra-abdominal infections, including peritonitis, caused by *E coli, Klebsiella* sp and *Enterobacter* sp.

Skin, bone and skin structure infections caused by *P aeruginosa, Proteus* sp, *E coli, Klebsiella* sp, *Enterobacter* sp and *S aureus.*

Complicated and recurrent urinary tract infections (UTIs) caused by *P aeruginosa, Proteus* sp (indole-positive and indole-negative), *E coli, Klebsiella* sp, *Enterobacter* sp, *Serratia* sp, *S aureus, Providencia* sp, *Citrobacter* sp. Not for uncomplicated initial episodes of UTIs unless the organisms are not susceptible to less toxic antibiotics.

Tobramycin may be considered in serious staphylococcal infections when penicillin or other potentially less toxic drugs are contraindicated and when bacterial susceptibility testing and clinical judgment indicate its use.

In patients in whom serious life-threatening gram-negative infection is suspected, including those in whom concurrent therapy with a penicillin or cephalosporin and an aminoglycoside may be indicated, initiate tobramycin before susceptibility study results are obtained. Base decision to continue therapy on these results, infection severity and concepts discussed in Warning Box (see Warnings).

Administration and Dosage:

Dosage: Use the patient's ideal body weight for dosage calculation. For obese patients, calculate appropriate dosage by using patient's estimated lean body weight plus 40% of the excess as the basic weight on which to figure mg/kg. Following 1 mg/kg IM, maximum serum concentrations reach about 4 mcg/ml, and measurable levels persist for as long as 8 hours. Therapeutic serum levels range from 4 to 6 mcg/ml. Serum concentrations of the drug given by IV infusion over 1 hour are similar to those obtained by IM use.

Duration: Usual duration of treatment is 7 to 10 days. A longer course may be necessary in difficult and complicated infections. In such cases, monitor renal, auditory and vestibular functions; toxicity can occur when treatment extends > 10 days.

Monitor serum concentrations, both peak and trough, to ensure adequate levels and avoid toxicity; avoid prolonged concentrations > 12 mcg/ml. Examine urine for decreased specific gravity and for increased excretion of protein, cells and casts.

Adults with serious infections: Administer 3 mg/kg/day in 3 equal doses every 8 hours.

Life-threatening infections – Administer up to 5 mg/kg/day in 3 or 4 equal doses. Reduce dosage to 3 mg/kg/day as soon as clinically indicated. To prevent increased toxicity due to excessive blood levels, do not exceed 5 mg/kg/day, unless serum levels are monitored.

Children: Administer 6 to 7.5 mg/kg/day in 3 or 4 equally divided doses (2 to 2.5 mg/kg every 8 hours or 1.5 to 1.9 mg/kg every 6 hours).

Premature or full-term neonates (≤ 1 week of age): Administer up to 4 mg/kg/day in 2 equal doses every 12 hours. Preliminary data suggest that 2.5 mg/kg every 18 hours or 3 mg/kg every 24 hours may achieve safe and effective peak and trough serum concentrations in newborn infants weighing < 1 kg at birth.

Renal function impairment: Whenever possible, determine serum concentrations. Following a loading dose of 1 mg/kg, adjust subsequent dosage, either with reduced doses administered at 8 hour intervals or with normal doses given at prolonged intervals. Both of these methods are suggested as guides when serum levels of tobramycin cannot be measured directly. They are based on either creatinine clearance (Ccr; preferred) or serum creatinine, because these values correlate with the half-life of tobramycin. Use the dosage schedules derived from either method with careful clinical and laboratory observations of the patient; modify as necessary. These calculation methods may be misleading in patients who have undergone severe wasting and in the elderly. Do not use either method when dialysis is performed.

TOBRAMYCIN SULFATE

Reduced dosage at 8 hour intervals – When the Ccr is ≤ 70 ml/min, or when serum creatinine is known, determine the amount of the reduced dose by multiplying the normal dose by the percent of normal dose from the accompanying nomogram.

REDUCED DOSAGE NOMOGRAM†

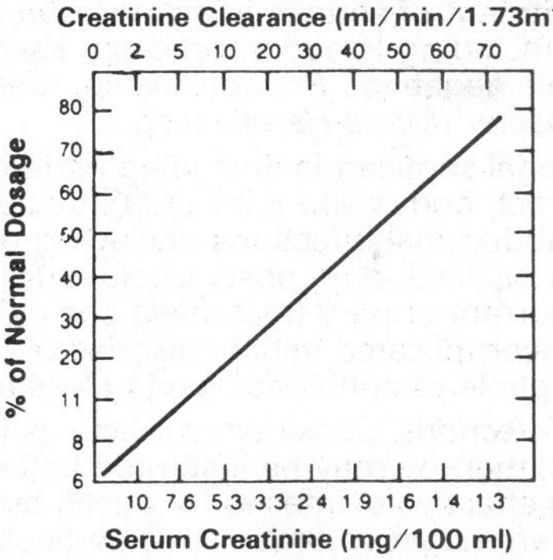

†Scales have been adjusted to facilitate dosage calculations.

An alternate guide for determining reduced dosage at 8 hour intervals (for patients whose steady-state serum creatinine values are known) is to divide the normally recommended dose by the patient's serum creatinine.

Normal dosage at prolonged intervals – If the Ccr is not available and the patient's condition is stable, determine a dosage frequency (in hours) for the normal dosage by multiplying the patient's serum creatinine by 6.

Several predictive methods and published nomograms have been compared for gentamicin, none of which performed as well as individualized pharmacokinetic dosing with serum levels. This would probably also be true for tobramycin.

Hemodialysis removes approximately 50% of a dose in 6 hours. In anephric patients maintained by regular dialysis, the usual dose of 1.5 to 2 mg/kg given after every dialysis usually maintains therapeutic, nontoxic serum levels. In patients receiving intermittent peritoneal dialysis, patients dialyzed twice weekly should receive a 1.5 to 2 mg/kg loading dose followed by 1 mg/kg every 3 days. Where dialysis occurs every 2 days, a 1.5 mg/kg loading dose is given after the first dialysis and 0.75 mg/kg after each subsequent dialysis.

IV administration: The IV dose is the same as the IM dose. The usual volume of diluent (0.9% Sodium Chloride Injection or 5% Dextrose Injection) for adult doses is 50 to 100 ml. For children, the volume of diluent should be proportionately less than for adults. Infuse the diluted solution over a period of 20 to 60 minutes. Infusion periods of < 20 minutes are not recommended, because peak serum levels may exceed 12 mcg/ml.

Admixture incompatibility – Do not physically premix with other drugs. Administer separately according to the recommended dose and route.

Rx	**Nebcin** (Lilly)	**Injection:** 10 mg/ml after reconstitution	In 6 and 8 ml *ADD-Vantage* vials w/diluent.[1]
Rx	**Tobramycin Sulfate** (Various, eg, Abbott, Apothecon, Geneva, Lederle)	**Injection:** 40 mg/ml	In 1.5 and 2 ml syringes and 2 and 30 ml vials.
Rx	**Nebcin** (Lilly)		In 1.5 and 2 ml *Hyporets*[1] and 2 and 30 ml vials.[1]
Rx	**Tobramycin Sulfate** (Various, eg, Abbott, Apothecon, Geneva, Lederle)	**Pediatric Injection:** 10 mg/ml	In 2 ml vials.
Rx	**Nebcin** (Lilly)		In 2 ml vials.[1]
Rx	**Nebcin** (Lilly)	**Powder for injection:** 30 mg/ml after reconstitution	In 1.2 g vials.

[1] With phenol, EDTA, sodium bisulfite. May also contain sulfuric acids.

AMIKACIN SULFATE

Information beginning in the Aminoglycosides group monograph must be considered when using these products.

SPECIAL NOTE: See WARNING BOX concerning aminoglycoside toxicity.

Indications:

Organisms: Short-term treatment of serious infections due to susceptible strains of gram-negative bacteria, including Pseudomonas sp, *Escherichia coli, Proteus* sp (indole-positive and indole-negative), *Providencia* sp, *Klebsiella* sp, *Enterobacter* sp, *Serratia* sp and *Acinetobacter (Mima-Herellea)* sp.

Infections: Effective in bacterial septicemia (including neonatal sepsis); in serious infections of the respiratory tract, bones and joints, CNS (including meningitis) and skin and soft tissue; in intra-abdominal infections (including peritonitis); and in burns and postoperative infections (including postvascular surgery). Also effective in serious complicated and recurrent urinary tract infections (UTIs) due to these organisms. Not indicated in uncomplicated initial episodes of UTIs unless the causative organisms are not susceptible to antibiotics having less toxicity.

Suspected gram-negative infections: Consider amikacin as initial therapy in suspected gram-negative infections; therapy may be instituted before obtaining the results of susceptibility testing. It is effective in infections caused by gentamicin or tobramycin resistant strains of gram-negative organisms, particularly *P rettgeri, P stuartii, S marcescens*and *P aeruginosa.*Continue therapy based on susceptibility test results, infection severity, patient response and the concepts discussed in the Warning Box (see Warnings).

Staphylococcal infections: Consider as initial therapy under certain conditions in the treatment of known or suspected staphylococcal disease, such as: Severe infections where the causative organism may be either a gram-negative bacterium or a staphylococcus; infections due to susceptible strains of staphylococci in patients allergic to other antibiotics; and in mixed staphylococcal/gram-negative infections.

Neonatal sepsis: In severe infections, concomitant therapy with a penicillin-type drug may be indicated because of the possibility of infections due to gram-positive organisms, such as streptococci or pneumococci.

Unlabeled uses: Intrathecal/intraventricular administration has been suggested at 8 mg/24 hours.

Amikacin 15 mg/kg/day IV in divided doses every 8 to 12 hours may be used as part of a multiple-drug regimen (generally three to five agents) for *Mycobacterium avium* complex, a common infection in AIDS patients.

Administration and Dosage:

Monitor the patient's renal status. Evidence of impairment in renal, vestibular or auditory function requires drug discontinuation or dosage adjustment. Examine urine for increased protein excretion, the presence of cells and casts and decreased specific gravity. Monitor serum concentrations and avoid prolonged peak concentrations > 35 mcg/ml. In healthy adult volunteers, average peak serum concentrations of about 12, 16 and 21 mcg/ml are obtained 1 hour after IM administration of 250 mg (3.7 mg/ kg), 375 mg (5 mg/kg) and 500 mg (7.5 mg/kg) single doses, respectively. At 10 hours, serum levels are about 0.3, 1.2 and 2.1 mcg/ml, respectively.

Adults, children and older infants: Use the patient's ideal body weight for dosage calculation. Administer IM or IV. Administer 15 mg/kg/day divided into 2 or 3 equal doses at equally divided intervals. Treatment of heavier patients should not exceed 1.5 g/day. In uncomplicated UTIs, use 250 mg twice daily.

Neonates – A loading dose of 10 mg/kg is recommended, followed by 7.5 mg/kg every 12 hours. Preliminary IM studies in newborns of different weights (<1.5 kg, 1.5 to 2 kg, >2 kg) at a dose of 7.5 mg/kg revealed that, like other aminoglycosides, serum half-life values were correlated inversely with postnatal age and renal clearances of amikacin. Lower dosages may be safer during the first 2 weeks of life.

Duration: The usual duration of treatment is 7 to 10 days. Do not exceed 15 mg/kg/day. If treatment beyond 10 days is considered, monitor amikacin serum levels, renal, auditory and vestibular functions daily. Uncomplicated infections due to sensitive organisms should respond in 24 to 48 hours. If definite clinical response does not occur within 3 to 5 days, stop therapy and reevaluate. Failure of the infection to respond may be due to resistance of the organism or to the presence of septic foci requiring surgical drainage.

AMIKACIN SULFATE

Renal function impairment: Whenever possible, monitor serum concentrations. Adjust doses in patients with impaired renal function by administering normal doses at prolonged intervals or by administering reduced doses at a fixed interval. Both methods are based on the patient's creatinine clearance (Ccr; preferred) or serum creatinine values, since these have been found to correlate with aminoglycoside half-lives. Use these dosage schedules in conjunction with clinical and laboratory observations of the patient, and modify as necessary. These methods of dosage calculation may be misleading in patients who have undergone severe wasting and in the elderly. Neither method should be used when dialysis is being performed.

Normal dosage at prolonged intervals – If the Ccr is not available and the patient's condition is stable, calculate a dosage interval (in hours) for the normal dose by multiplying the patient's serum creatinine by 9.

Reduced dosage at fixed time intervals – Measure serum concentrations to assure accurate administration and to avoid concentrations > 35 mcg/ml. Initiate therapy by administering a normal dose, 7.5 mg/kg, as a loading dose.

To determine maintenance doses administered every 12 hours, reduce the loading dose in proportion to the reduction in the patient's Ccr:

$$\text{Maintenance dose every 12 hours} = \frac{\text{observed Ccr (ml/min)}}{\text{normal Ccr (ml/min)}} \times \text{calculated loading dose (mg)}$$

An alternate rough guide for determining reduced dosage at 12 hour intervals (for patients whose steady-state serum creatinine values are known) is to divide the normally recommended dose by the patient's serum creatinine.

Several predictive methods and published nomograms have been compared for gentamicin, none of which performed as well as individualized pharmacokinetic dosing with serum levels. This would probably also be true for amikacin.

Dialysis – Approximately half the normal mg/kg dose can be given after hemodialysis; in peritoneal dialysis, a parenteral dose of 7.5 mg/kg is given, and then amikacin is instilled in peritoneal dialysate at a concentration desired in serum.

IV administration: Dose is identical to IM dose.

Adults – Single doses of 500 mg (7.5 mg/kg), administered as an infusion over a period of 30 minutes, produced a mean peak serum concentration of 38 mcg/ml at the end of the infusion, and levels of 24, 18 and 0.75 mcg/ml at 30 minutes, 1 hour and 10 hours postinfusion, respectively. Repeated infusions of 7.5 mg/kg every 12 hours were well tolerated and caused no drug accumulation.

Preparation of solution – Prepare the solution for IV use by adding the contents of a 500 mg vial to 100 or 200 ml of sterile diluent. Administer the solution to adults over 30 to 60 minutes. Do not exceed 15 mg/kg/day, and divide into either 2 or 3 equal doses at equal intervals.

Infants – In pediatric patients, the amount of fluid used will depend on the amount ordered for the patient. It should be a sufficient amount to infuse the amikacin over 30 to 60 minutes. Infants should receive a 1 to 2 hour infusion.

Admixture compatibility: Amikacin is stable for 24 hours at room temperature at concentrations of 0.25 and 5 mg/ml in the following solutions: 5% Dextrose Injection; 5% Dextrose and 0.2% Sodium Chloride Injection; 5% Dextrose and 0.45% Sodium Chloride Injection; 0.9% Sodium Chloride Injection; Lactated Ringer's Injection; *Normosol M* in 5% Dextrose Injection (or *Plasma-Lyte 56* Injection in 5% Dextrose in Water); *Normosol R* in 5% Dextrose Injection (or *Plasma-Lyte 148* Injection in 5% Dextrose in Water).

Admixture incompatibility: Do not physically premix amikacin with other drugs; administer separately.

Rx	**Amikacin** (Various, eg, Bedford Labs, Elkins-Sinn)	**Injection:** 250 mg/ml	In 2 and 4 ml vials[1].
Rx	**Amikin** (Apothecon)		In 2 and 4 ml vials[2] and 2 ml disp syringes.[2]
	Amikacin (Various, eg, Gensia)	**Pediatric Injection:** 50 mg/ml	0.13% sodium metabisulfite, 0.5% sodium citrate dihydrate. In 2 and 4 ml vials.
Rx	**Amikin** (Apothecon)		In 2 ml vials.[2]

[1] May contain sodium metabisulfite, sodium citrate dihydrate or sulfuric acid.
[2] With sodium bisulfite and sulfuric acid.

NETILMICIN SULFATE

Information beginning in the Aminoglycoside group monograph must be considered when using these products.

SPECIAL NOTE: See WARNING BOX concerning aminoglycoside toxicity.

Indications:

For the short-term treatment of patients with serious or life-threatening bacterial infections caused by susceptible strains of the following organisms:

Complicated urinary tract infections caused by *Escherichia coli, Klebsiella pneumoniae, Pseudomonas aeruginosa, Enterobacter* sp, *Proteus mirabilis, Proteus* sp (indole-positive), *Serratia* and *Citrobacter* sp and *Staphylococcus aureus.*

Septicemia caused by *E coli, K pneumoniae, P aeruginosa, Enterobacter* sp, *Serratia* sp and *P mirabilis.*

Skin and skin structure infections caused by *E coli, K pneumoniae, P aeruginosa, Enterobacter* sp, *Serratia* sp, *P mirabilis, Proteus* sp (indole-positive) and *S aureus* (penicillinase and nonpenicillinase-producing strains).

Intraabdominal infections including peritonitis and intraabdominal abscess caused by *E coli, K pneumoniae, P aeruginosa, Enterobacter* sp, *P mirabilis, Proteus* sp (indole-positive), and *S aureus* (penicillinase and nonpenicillinase-producing strains).

Lower respiratory tract infections caused by *E coli, K pneumoniae, P aeruginosa, Enterobacter* sp, *Serratia* sp, *P mirabilis, Proteus* sp (indole-positive) and *S aureus* (penicillinase and nonpenicillinase-producing strains).

Consider netilmicin as initial therapy in suspected or confirmed gram-negative infections; therapy may be instituted before obtaining results of susceptibility testing. Continue therapy based on the susceptibility test results, infection severity and the concepts contained in the Warning Box (see Warnings).

While not the antibiotic class of first choice, consider netilmicin for the treatment of serious staphylococcal infections when penicillins or other less potentially toxic drugs are contraindicated and when bacterial susceptibility tests and clinical judgment indicate their use. It may also be considered in mixed infections caused by susceptible strains of staphylococci and gram-negative organisms.

Netilmicin is indicated for those infections for which potentially less toxic antimicrobial agents are ineffective or contraindicated. It is not indicated in the treatment of uncomplicated initial episodes of urinary tract infection unless the causative organisms are resistant to antimicrobial agents having less potential toxicity.

In serious infections when the causative organisms are unknown, netilmicin may be administered as initial therapy in conjunction with a penicillin- or cephalosporin-type drug before obtaining results of susceptibility testing. In neonates with suspected sepsis, a penicillin-type drug is also usually indicated as concomitant therapy with netilmicin. If anaerobic organisms are suspected, also give other suitable antimicrobial therapy. Following identification of the organism and its susceptibility, continue appropriate antibiotic therapy.

Netilmicin has been used effectively in combination with carbenicillin or ticarcillin for the treatment of life-threatening infections caused by *P aeruginosa*. It also has been effective in the treatment of serious infections caused by some organisms resistant to other aminoglycosides.

Administration and Dosage:

Dosage: Administer IM or IV. The recommended dosage for both methods is identical. The following dosage recommendations are intended as guides for initial therapy, or for when the measurement of netilmicin serum levels during therapy is not feasible.

Obtain patient's pretreatment body weight for calculation of correct dosage. Base the dosage in obese patients on an estimate of the lean body mass.

Patients with normal renal function:

Adults –

Complicated UTIs: 1.5 to 2 mg/kg every 12 hours (3 to 4 mg/kg/day).

Serious systemic infections: 1.3 to 2.2 mg/kg every 8 hours or 2 to 3.25 mg/kg every 12 hours (4 to 6.5 mg/kg/day).

Infants and children (6 weeks through 12 years of age) – Administer 1.8 to 2.7 mg/kg every 8 hours or 2.7 to 4 mg/kg every 12 hours (5.5 to 8 mg/kg/day).

Neonates (< 6 weeks of age) Administer 2 to 3.25 mg/kg every 12 hours (4 to 6.5 mg/kg/day).

NETILMICIN SULFATE

Duration: Limit the duration of treatment to short-term whenever feasible. The usual duration of treatment is 7 to 14 days. In complicated infections, a longer course of therapy may be necessary. Although prolonged courses of netilmicin therapy have been well tolerated, it is particularly important to monitor patients carefully for changes in renal, auditory and vestibular functions. Adjust dosage if clinically indicated.

Measure serum concentrations (both peak and trough) periodically during therapy to determine the safety and efficacy of the administered dosage.

Peak serum concentrations range from 4 to 12 mcg/ml. Adjust dosage to attain the desired peak and trough concentrations and to avoid prolonged peak serum concentrations > 16 mcg/ml. When monitoring trough concentrations (just prior to the next dose), adjust dosage to avoid levels > 4 mcg/ml. Generally, desirable peak and trough concentrations range from 6 to 10 and 0.5 to 2 mcg/ml, respectively.

To determine the adequacy of a serum level, consider the susceptibility of the causative organism, the severity of the infection and the status of the patient's host-defense mechanisms.

Renal function impairment: Individualize dosage. Dosage adjustment based on serum drug concentrations during treatment is the most accurate.

If netilmicin serum concentrations are not available and renal function is stable, serum creatinine and creatinine clearance (Ccr) values are the most reliable, readily available indicators of the degree of renal impairment to guide dosage adjustment. The BUN level is much less reliable for this purpose. Periodically reassess renal function during therapy.

Deteriorating renal function may require a greater reduction in dosage than that specified in the guidelines given below for patients with stable renal impairment.

The initial or loading dose is the same as that for a patient with normal renal function. Three suggested methods to adjust the total daily dosage for the degree of renal impairment are:

1) Divide the suggested dosage value for patients with normal renal function by the serum creatinine level to obtain the adjusted size of each dose.

2) Determine the adjusted daily dose of netilmicin by multiplying the dose for patients with normal renal function by:

$$\frac{\text{Patient's Ccr}}{\text{Normal Ccr}}$$

3) Alternatively, use the following graph to obtain the percentage of the dose selected; administer at 8 hour intervals:

REDUCED DOSAGE NOMOGRAM

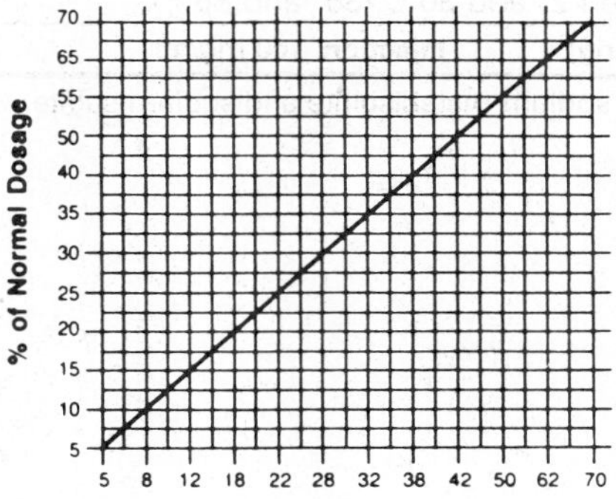

Creatinine Clearance (ml/min/1.73 m²)

NETILMICIN SULFATE

Ccr can be estimated from serum creatinine levels by the following formula:

$$\text{Males: } \frac{\text{Weight (kg)} \times (140 - \text{age})}{72 \times \text{serum creatinine (mg/dl)}} = \text{Ccr}$$

Females: 0.85 × above value

The adjusted total daily dose may be administered as one dose at 24 hour intervals, or as 2 or 3 equally divided doses at 12 hour or 8 hour intervals, respectively. Generally, each individual dose should not exceed 3.25 mg/kg.

Hemodialysis – In adults with renal failure who are undergoing hemodialysis, the amount of netilmicin removed from the blood may vary, depending upon the dialysis equipment and methods used. In adults, a dose of 2 mg/kg at the end of each dialysis period is recommended until the results of tests measuring serum levels become available. Adjust dosage appropriately based on these tests.

Burn patients: In patients with extensive body surface burns, altered pharmacokinetics may result in reduced serum concentrations. Measurement of netilmicin serum concentrations is particularly important as a basis for dosage adjustment.

Alternate dosing method (normal or impaired renal function): An alternate method of determining dosage regimen (dose and dosing interval) applicable to all ages and all states of renal function is to employ pharmacokinetic parameters derived from measurements of serum concentrations. This is probably the most reliable and accurate method.

IV administration: In adults, a single dose may be diluted in 50 to 200 ml of one of the parenteral solutions listed below. In infants and children, the volume of diluent should be less, according to the fluid requirements of the patient. The solution may be infused over a period of ½ to 2 hours.

Admixture compatibility: Tested at concentrations of 2.1 to 3 mg/ml, netilmicin is stable in the following large volume parenteral solutions for up to 72 hours when stored in glass containers, both when refrigerated and at room temperature. Do not use after this time period. Sterile Water for Injection; 0.9% Sodium Chloride Injection alone or with 5% Dextrose; 5% or 10% Dextrose Injection in Water or 5% Dextrose with Electrolyte #48 or #75; Ringer's and Lactated Ringer's, and Lactated Ringer's with 5% Dextrose Injection; *10% Travert with Electrolyte #2* or *#3 Injection*; *Isolyte E, M or P* with 5% Dextrose Injection; 10% Dextran 40 or 6% Dextran 75 in 5% Dextrose Injection; *Plasma-Lyte 56 or 148* Injection with 5% Dextrose; *Plasma-Lyte M* Injection with 5% Dextrose; *Ionosol B* in D5-W; *Normosol-R*; *Plasma-Lyte 148* Injection (approx. pH 7.4); 10% Fructose Injection; Electrolyte #3 with 10% Invert Sugar Injection; *Normosol-M or R* in D5-W; *Isolyte H or S* with 5% Dextrose; *Isolyte S*; *Plasma-Lyte 148* Injection in Water; *Normosol-R* pH 7.4.

Storage: Store between 2° and 30°C (36° and 86°F).

Rx	**Netromycin** (Schering)	**Injection:** 100 mg/ml	In 1.5 ml vials.[1]

[1] With benzyl alcohol, EDTA, sodium metabisulfite and sodium sulfite.

AMINOGLYCOSIDES, ORAL

For more complete information on aminoglycosides, refer to the Aminoglycosides, Parenteral group monograph.

SPECIAL NOTE: See WARNING BOX in Aminoglycosides, Parenteral group monograph concerning toxicity.

Actions:

Pharmacokinetics: Oral aminoglycosides are poorly absorbed; therefore use only for suppression of GI bacterial flora. The small absorbed fraction is rapidly excreted with normal kidney function. The unabsorbed drug is eliminated unchanged in the feces. Most intestinal bacteria are rapidly eliminated with bacterial suppression persisting for 48 to 72 hours. Nonpathogenic yeasts and occasionally resistant strains of *Enterobacter aerogenes* replace the intestinal bacteria.

Indications:

Suppression of intestinal bacteria.

Hepatic coma.

See individual monographs for specific information.

Contraindications:

Presence of intestinal obstruction; hypersensitivity to aminoglycosides.

Warnings:

Increased absorption: Although negligible amounts are absorbed through intact mucosa, consider the possibility of increased absorption from ulcerated or denuded areas.

Nephrotoxicity/Ototoxicity: Because of reported cases of deafness and potential nephrotoxic effects, closely observe patients. Perform urine and blood examinations and audiometric tests prior to and during extended therapy, especially in those with hepatic or renal disease. If renal insufficiency develops, reduce dosage or discontinue the drug. Refer to the Warning Box in the Aminoglycosides, Parenteral monograph concerning aminoglycoside toxicity.

Pregnancy: Safety for use during pregnancy has not been established. Use only when clearly needed and when the potential benefits outweigh the potential hazards.

Neomycin – Category D. Aminoglycosides can cause fetal harm when administered to a pregnant woman. Aminoglycosides cross the placenta. Although serious side effects to fetus or newborn have not been reported in the treatment of pregnant women, the potential for harm exists. If neomycin is used during pregnancy, or if the patient becomes pregnant while taking this drug, apprise the patient of the potential hazard to the fetus.

Lactation: Neomycin is excreted in cow milk following a single IM injection. It is not known whether neomycin is excreted in human breast milk. Other aminoglycosides are excreted in human breast milk. Because of the potential for serious adverse reactions from the aminoglycosides in nursing infants, decide whether to discontinue nursing or to discontinue the drug, taking into account the importance of the drug to the mother.

Children: The safety and efficacy of oral neomycin in patients < 18 years of age have not been established. If treatment is necessary, use with caution; do not exceed a treatment period of 3 weeks because of absorption from the GI tract.

Precautions:

Muscular disorders: Use with caution in patients with muscular disorders such as myasthenia gravis or parkinsonism; these drugs may aggravate muscle weakness because of their potential curare-like effect on neuromuscular junction.

GI effects:

Neomycin – Orally administered neomycin increases fecal bile acid excretion and reduces intestinal lactase activity.

Paromomycin – Use with caution in individuals with ulcerative lesions of the bowel to avoid renal toxicity through inadvertent absorption.

Superinfection: Use of antibiotics (especially prolonged or repeated therapy) may result in bacterial or fungal overgrowth of nonsusceptible organisms. Such overgrowth may lead to a secondary infection. Take appropriate measures if superinfection occurs.

AMINOGLYCOSIDES, ORAL

Drug Interactions:

Oral Aminoglycoside Drug Interactions			
Precipitant drug	Object drug*		Description
Aminoglycosides	Anticoagulants	↑	A small rise in warfarin-induced hypoprothrombinemia may occur, possibly due to interference in absorption of dietary vitamin K by aminoglycosides.
Aminoglycosides	Digoxin	↓	Rate and extent of digoxin absorption may be reduced; however, in a small number of patients (< 10%), this may be offset by a reduction in digoxin's metabolism.
Aminoglycosides	Methotrexate	↓	Methotrexate's absorption and bioavailability may be decreased.
Aminoglycosides	Neuromuscular blockers — Depolarizing and nondepolarizing	↑	The actions of the neuromuscular blockers may be enhanced; prolonged respiratory depression may occur.
Aminoglycosides	Polypeptide antibiotics	↑	Concurrent use may increase the risk of respiratory paralysis and renal dysfunction.
Aminoglycosides	Vitamin A	↓	Serum retinol and plasma carotene levels may be decreased.

* ↑ = Object drug increased ↓ = Object drug decreased

Adverse Reactions:

Nausea, vomiting and diarrhea are most common. The "malabsorption syndrome" characterized by increased fecal fat, decreased serum carotene and fall in xylose absorption has occurred with prolonged therapy. *Clostridium difficile* associated colitis has occurred following neomycin therapy. Nephrotoxicity and ototoxicity have occurred following prolonged and high dosage therapy in hepatic coma.

Overdosage:

Because of low absorption, it is unlikely that acute overdosage would occur with oral neomycin sulfate. However, prolonged administration could result in sufficient systemic drug levels to produce neurotoxicity, ototoxicity or nephrotoxicity. Hemodialysis will remove neomycin sulfate from the blood.

Patient Information:

Complete full course of therapy; take until gone. May cause nausea, vomiting or diarrhea.

Notify physician if ringing in the ears, hearing impairment or rash, problems urinating or dizziness occurs.

Drink plenty of fluids.

Neomycin: Before administering the drug, inform patients or members of their families of possible toxic effects on the eighth cranial nerve. The possibility of acute toxicity increases in premature infants and neonates.

KANAMYCIN SULFATE

For complete prescribing information, refer to the Aminoglycosides, Oral group monograph.

Indications:

Suppression of intestinal bacteria: For short-term adjunctive therapy.

Hepatic coma: Prolonged administration is effective adjunctive therapy by reduction of the ammonia-forming bacteria in the intestinal tract. The subsequent reduction in blood ammonia has resulted in neurologic improvement.

Administration and Dosage:

Suppression of intestinal bacteria: As an adjunct to mechanical cleansing of the large bowel in short-term therapy – 1 g every hour for 4 hours, followed by 1 g every 6 hours for 36 to 72 hours.

Hepatic coma: 8 to 12 g/day in divided doses.

Rx	**Kantrex** (Apothecon)	**Capsules:** 500 mg (as sulfate)	Lactose. In 20s & 100s.

NEOMYCIN SULFATE

Refer to the general discussion of these products in the Aminoglycosides, Oral group monograph.

Indications:

Suppression of intestinal bacteria of the bowel (eg, preoperative preparation of the bowel). It is given concurrently with enteric coated erythromycin.

Hepatic coma: Administration has been effective adjunctive therapy in hepatic coma by reduction of the ammonia-forming bacteria in the intestinal tract. The subsequent reduction in blood ammonia has resulted in neurologic improvement.

Unlabeled uses: Many studies have documented lipid-lowering efficacy of neomycin. Alone, it reduced LDL cholesterol levels by 24%. Combined with niacin, it reduced LDL cholesterol level to below the 90th percentile in 92% of patients.

Administration and Dosage:

Preoperative prophylaxis for elective colorectal surgery:

Recommended Bowel Preparation Regimen (Proposed Surgery Time 8 am)[1]			
Therapy	Day 3 before surgery	Day 2 before surgery	Day 1 before surgery
Diet	Minimum residue or clear liquid	Minimum residue or clear liquid	Clear liquid
Bisacodyl, 1 oral cap	6 pm (–62 hrs)		
Magnesium sulfate, 30 ml of a 50% solution orally		10 am (–46 hrs). Repeat at 2 pm (–42 hrs) and 6 pm (–38 hrs).	10 am (–22 hrs). Repeat at 2 pm (–18 hrs).
Enema		7 pm (–37 hrs) & 8 pm (–36 hrs). Repeat hourly until no solid feces return with last enema.	None
Supplemental IV fluids			As needed
Neomycin and erythromycin tablets, 1 g each, orally			1 pm (–19 hrs). Repeat at 2 pm (–18 hrs) and 11 pm (–9 hrs).

[1] On day of surgery, patient should evacuate rectum at 6:30 am (–1½ hrs) for 8 am procedure.

Hepatic coma (as adjunct): The following regimen has been used: Withdraw protein from diet; avoid diuretics; supportive therapy, including transfusions, as needed.

Adults – 4 to 12 g/day in divided doses.

Children – 50 to 100 mg/kg/day in divided doses. Continue treatment over a period of 5 to 6 days; during this time, return protein to the diet incrementally. Chronic hepatic insufficiency may require up to 4 g/day over an indefinite period.

Rx	**Neomycin Sulfate** (Various, eg, Eon, Geneva, Goldline, Rugby, Schein)	**Tablets:** 500 mg	In 100s.
Rx	**Neo-Tabs** (Pharma-Tek)		In 100s.
Rx	**Mycifradin** (Upjohn)	**Oral Solution:** 125 mg per 5 ml	Parabens. In 480 ml.
Rx	**Neo-fradin** (Pharma-Tek)		Parabens. In 480 ml.

PAROMOMYCIN SULFATE

Refer to the general discussionof these products in the Aminoglycosides, Oral group monograph.

Indications:

Intestinal amebiasis (acute and chronic): Note: Paromomycin is not effective in extraintestinal amebiasis. (See monograph in Amebicides section.)

Hepatic coma: As adjunctive therapy.

Unlabeled uses: Has been recommended for other parasitic infections — *Dientamoeba fragilis* (25 to 30 mg/kg/day in 3 doses for 7 days); *Diphyllobothrium latum, Taenia saginata, T solium, Dipylidium caninum* (adults: 1 g every 15 min for 4 doses; pediatric: 11 mg/kg every 15 min for 4 doses); *Hymenolepis nana* (45 mg/kg/day for 5 to 7 days).

Administration and Dosage:

Intestinal amebiasis: Adults and children - Usual dose is 25 to 35 mg/kg/day, in 3 doses with meals for 5 to 10 days.

Management of hepatic coma:

Adults – Usual dose: 4 g/day in divided doses at regular intervals for 5 to 6 days.

Rx	**Humatin** (Parke-Davis)	**Capsules:** 250 mg	In 16s.

COLISTIN SULFATE

Actions:

Pharmacokinetics: Colistin sulfate is not significantly absorbed into the systemic circulation.

Microbiology: Colistin has in vitro bactericidal activity against most gram-negative enteric pathogens, especially enteropathogenic *Escherichia coli* and *Shigella* sp, but not *Proteus* sp. In infants and children, it has effectively controlled acute infections of the intestinal tract due to these pathogens. Susceptible strains of *E coli* and *Shigella* sp in vitro or in vivo rarely develop resistance. Cross-resistance to polymyxin B sulfate does exist, but cross-resistance to broad spectrum antibiotics has not been encountered.

Indications:

Diarrhea in infants and children, caused by susceptible strains of enteropathogenic *E coli.*

Gastroenteritis due to *Shigella* organisms. Clinical response may vary due to the absence of tissue levels in the bowel wall.

Contraindications:

Hypersensitivity to colistin sulfate.

Warnings:

Superinfection: Use of antibiotics (especially prolonged or repeated therapy) may result in bacterial or fungal overgrowth of nonsusceptible organisms (ie, *Proteus*). Such overgrowth may lead to secondary infection. Take appropriate measures if superinfection occurs.

Renal function impairment: Although colistin sulfate is not absorbed systemically in measurable amounts, it is assumed that slight absorption may occur. Therefore, a potential for renal toxicity exists in the presence of azotemia or if dosages above those recommended are used.

Precautions:

Monitoring: Assess renal function prior to initiation of therapy.

Administration and Dosage:

Usual dose is 5 to 15 mg/kg/day given in 3 divided doses. Higher doses may be necessary.

Preparation: Reconstitute with 37 ml distilled water. Slowly add one-half of the diluent, replace the cap and shake well. Add remaining diluent and repeat shaking.

Storage/Stability: When reconstituted, it is stable for 2 weeks when kept below 15°C (59°F).

Rx	**Coly-Mycin S** (Parke-Davis)	**Powder for Oral Suspension:** 25 mg colistin (as sulfate) per 5 ml when reconstituted	Menthol, parabens, saccharin, sorbitol, sucrose. Chocolate flavor. In 60 ml bottles.

COLISTIMETHATE SODIUM

Actions:

Pharmacokinetics: Higher initial blood levels are obtained following IV administration. Blood levels peak at between 5 and 10 mcg/ml between 2 and 3 hours after IM administration. Serum half-life is 2 to 3 hours.

Average urinary levels range from about 270 mcg/ml at 2 hours to about 15 mcg/ml at 8 hours after IV administration and from about 200 to 25 mcg/ml during a similar period following IM administration.

Microbiology: Colistimethate has bactericidal activity against the following gram-negative bacilli: Enterobacter aerogenes, Escherichia coli, Klebsiella pneumoniae and *Pseudomonas aeruginosa.*

Indications:

Treatment of acute or chronic infections due to sensitive strains of certain gram-negative bacilli. Particularly indicated when the infection is caused by sensitive strains of *P aeruginosa.* Clinically effective in treatment of infections due to the following gram-negative organisms: *E aerogenes, E coli, K pneumoniae* and *P aeruginosa.* Pending results of bacteriologic cultures and sensitivity tests, colistimethate may be used to initiate therapy in serious infections that are suspected to be due to gram-negative organisms.

Contraindications:

Hypersensitivity to colistimethate sodium; infections due to *Proteus* or *Neisseria* species.

Warnings:

Maximum dosage: Do not exceed 5 mg/kg/day in patients with normal renal function.

Neurologic effects may occur transiently. These include circumoral paresthesias or numbness, tingling or formication of the extremities, generalized pruritus, vertigo, dizziness and slurring of speech. Warn patients not to drive vehicles or use hazardous machinery while on therapy. Dosage reduction may alleviate symptoms. Therapy need not be discontinued, but observe such patients carefully. Overdosage can result in renal insufficiency, muscle weakness and apnea.

Renal function impairment: Since colistimethate is eliminated mainly by renal excretion, use with caution when the possibility of impaired renal function exists. Consider the decline in renal function with advanced age.

When actual renal impairment is present, use colistimethate with extreme caution; reduce the dosage in proportion to the extent of the impairment. Administration of amounts in excess of renal excretory capacity will lead to high serum levels. This can result in further impairment of renal function, initiating a cycle which, if not recognized, can lead to acute renal insufficiency, renal shutdown and further concentration of the antibiotic to toxic levels in the body. Interference with nerve transmission at neuromuscular junctions may occur and result in muscle weakness and apnea.

Signs indicating the development of impaired renal function are diminishing urine output and rising BUN or serum creatinine. If present, discontinue therapy immediately. If a life-threatening situation exists, reinstate therapy at a lower dosage after blood levels have fallen.

Pregnancy: Colistimethate sodium is transferred across the placental barrier, and blood levels of about 1 mcg/ml are obtained in the fetus following IV administration to the mother. Safety for use during pregnancy has not been established. Use only when clearly needed and when the potential benefits outweigh the potential hazards.

Precautions:

Respiratory effects: Respiratory arrest has occurred following IM administration. Impaired renal function increases the possibility of apnea and neuromuscular blockade, generally because of failure to follow recommended guidelines, overdosage, failure to reduce dose commensurate with degree of renal impairment or concomitant use of other antibiotics or drugs with neuromuscular blocking potential. If apnea occurs, treat with assisted respiration, oxygen and calcium chloride injections.

Nephrotoxicity: A decrease in urine output or increase in BUN or serum creatinine can be signs of nephrotoxicity, which is probably a dose-dependent effect. These manifestations are reversible following discontinuation. Increases of BUN have occurred at dose levels of 1.6 to 5 mg/kg/day. Values returned to normal following cessation.

COLISTIMETHATE SODIUM

Drug Interactions:

Colistimethate Drug Interactions			
Precipitant drug	Object drug*		Description
Aminoglycosides	Colistimethate	↑	Concurrent use may increase the risk of respiratory paralysis and renal dysfunction.
Cephalothin	Colistimethate	↑	Concurrent use may increase the risk of renal dysfunction.
Colistimethate	Nondepolarizing muscle relaxants	↑	Neuromuscular blockade may be enhanced.

* ↑ = Object drug increased.

Adverse Reactions:

Respiratory arrest (see Precautions); decreased urine output or increased BUN or serum creatinine (see Precautions); paresthesia; tingling of the extremities or the tongue; generalized itching or urticaria; drug fever; GI upset; vertigo; slurring of speech. The subjective symptoms reported by the adult may not be manifest in infants or young children, thus requiring close attention to renal function.

Administration and Dosage:

For IM or IV use.

Adults and children: 2.5 to 5 mg/kg/day in 2 to 4 divided doses for patients with normal renal function, depending upon the severity of the infection. Reduce the daily dose in the presence of any renal impairment.

Suggested Modification of Colistimethate Dosage Schedules for Adults with Impaired Renal Function						
Renal function			Dosage			
Degree of impairment	Plasma creatinine (mg/dl)	Urea clearance % (of normal)	Dose[1] (mg)	Frequency (times per day)	Total daily dose (mg)	Approx. daily dose (mg/kg)
Normal	0.7 - 1.2	80 - 100	100 - 150	4 to 2	300	5
Mild	1.3 - 1.5	40 - 70	75 - 115	2	150 - 230	2.5 - 3.8
Moderate	1.6 - 2.5	25 - 40	66 - 150	2 or 1	133 - 150	2.5
Severe	2.6 - 4	10 - 25	100 - 150	q 36 h	100	1.5

[1] Suggested unit dose is 2.5 to 5 mg/kg; increase time interval between injections in presence of impaired renal function.

IV administration:

Direct intermittent administration – Inject one-half the total daily dose over a period of 3 to 5 minutes every 12 hours.

Continuous infusion – Slowly inject one-half the daily dose over 3 to 5 minutes. Add the remaining half of the total daily dose of colistimethate to one of the following: 0.9% Sodium Chloride; 5% Dextrose in Water; 5% Dextrose with 0.9% Sodium Chloride; 5% Dextrose with 0.45% Sodium Chloride; 5% Dextrose with 0.225% Sodium Chloride; Lactated Ringer's solution. Swirl gently to avoid frothing.

Administer by slow IV infusion starting 1 to 2 hours after the initial dose over the next 22 to 23 hours in the presence of normal renal function. In the presence of impaired renal function, reduce infusion rate. Choice of IV solution and volume to be employed are dictated by requirements of fluid and electrolyte management.

Stability – Freshly prepare any infusion solution containing colistimethate and use for no longer than 24 hours.

Rx	**Coly-Mycin M** (Parke-Davis)	**Injection (lyophilized cake):** 150 mg colistin (as colistimethate sodium) for reconstitution	In vials.

POLYMYXIN B SULFATE

Warning:

When this drug is given intramuscularly or intrathecally, administer only to hospitalized patients to provide constant physician supervision.

Carefully determine renal function; reduce dosage in patients with renal damage and nitrogen retention. Patients with nephrotoxicity due to polymyxin B sulfate usually show albuminuria, cellular casts and azotemia. Diminishing urine output and a rising BUN are indications to discontinue therapy.

Neurotoxic reactions may be manifested by irritability, weakness, drowsiness, ataxia, perioral paresthesia, numbness of the extremities and blurring of vision. These are usually associated with high serum levels found in patients with impaired renal function or nephrotoxicity. Avoid concurrent use of other nephrotoxic and neurotoxic drugs, particularly kanamycin, streptomycin, paromomycin, colistin, tobramycin, neomycin and gentamicin.

The drug's neurotoxicity can result in respiratory paralysis from neuromuscular blockade, especially when the drug is given soon after anesthesia or muscle relaxants.

Actions:

Pharmacology: Polymyxin is bactericidal against almost all gram-negative bacilli except the *Proteus* group; it increases the permeability of bacterial cell membranes.

Pharmacokinetics: Polymyxin B sulfate is not absorbed from the normal GI tract. Since the drug loses 50% of its activity in the presence of serum, active blood levels are low. Repeated injections may give a cumulative effect. Levels tend to be higher in infants and children. Tissue diffusion is poor; the drug does not pass blood-brain barrier into cerebrospinal fluid (CSF). Drug is excreted slowly by kidneys. In therapeutic dosage, it causes some nephrotoxicity with slight tubule damage.

Microbiology: All gram-positive bacteria, fungi and gram-negative cocci, *Neisseria gonorrhoeae* and *N meningitidis,* are resistant.

Indications:

Acute infections caused by susceptible strains of *Pseudomonas* aeruginosa. It may be used topically and subconjunctively in the treatment of infections of the eye caused by susceptible strains of *P aeruginosa.*

It may be indicated (when less toxic drugs are ineffective or contraindicated) in serious infections caused by susceptible strains of the following organisms: *Hemophilus influenzae* (meningeal infections); *Escherichia coli* (urinary tract infections); *Enterobacter aerogenes* (bacteremia); *Klebsiella pneumoniae* (bacteremia).

Note: In meningeal infections, administer polymyxin B sulfate only intrathecally.

Contraindications:

Hypersensitivity to the polymyxins.

Warnings:

Pregnancy: Safety for use during pregnancy has not been established.

Precautions:

Monitoring: Determine baseline renal function prior to therapy. Frequently monitor renal function and drug levels during therapy. The use of doses higher than those recommended is dangerous and potentially fatal. In doses of 3 mg/kg/day (30,000 units), polymyxin B may cause nephrotoxicity in patients with normal renal function, but lower doses may cause renal damage in patients with preexisting renal impairment.

Superinfection: Use of antibiotics (especially prolonged or repeated therapy) may result in bacterial or fungal overgrowth of nonsusceptible organisms. Such overgrowth may lead to a secondary infection. Take appropriate measures if this occurs.

Drug Interactions:

Polymyxin B Drug Interactions

Precipitant drug	Object drug*		Description
Aminoglycosides	Polymyxin B	⬆	Concurrent use may increase the risk of respiratory paralysis and renal dysfunction.
Polymyxin B	Nondepolarizing muscle relaxants	⬆	Neuromuscular blockade may be enhanced.

* ⬆ = Object drug increased

POLYMYXIN B SULFATE

Adverse Reactions:

Nephrotoxic: Albuminuria; cylindruria; azotemia; rising blood levels without increase in dosage.

Neurotoxic: Facial flushing; dizziness progressing to ataxia; drowsiness; peripheral paresthesias (circumoral and stocking-glove); apnea due to concurrent use of curariform muscle relaxants, other neurotoxic drugs or inadvertent overdosage.

Meningeal irritation with intrathecal administration (eg, fever, headache, stiff neck and increased cell count and protein in CSF).

Miscellaneous: Drug fever; urticarial rash; severe pain or thrombophlebitis at injection sites.

Administration and Dosage:

IV: Dissolve 500,000 units polymyxin B sulfate in 300 to 500 ml of 5% Dextrose in Water for continuous IV drip.

Adults and children – 15,000 to 25,000 units/kg/day in individuals with normal renal function. Reduce this amount from 15,000 units/kg downward for individuals with renal impairment. Infusions may be given every 12 hours; however, the total daily dose must not exceed 25,000 units/kg/day.

Infants with normal renal function may receive up to 40,000 units/kg/day.

IM: Not recommended routinely because of severe pain at injection sites, particularly in infants and children. Dissolve 500,000 units in 2 ml sterile distilled water (Water for Injection, USP) or sterile physiologic saline (Sodium Chloride Injection) or 1% procaine HCl solution.

Adults and children – 25,000 to 30,000 units/kg/day. Reduce dosage in the presence of renal impairment. Dosage may be divided and given at either 4 or 6 hour intervals.

Infants with normal renal function may receive up to 40,000 units/kg/day.

Note: Doses as high as 45,000 units/kg/day have been used in limited clinical studies in treating premature and newborn infants for sepsis caused by *Pseudomonas aeruginosa*.

Intrathecal: A treatment of choice for *P aeruginosa* meningitis. Dissolve 500,000 units in 10 ml sterile physiologic saline for a concentration of 50,000 units/ml.

Adults and children (> 2 years of age) – 50,000 units once daily intrathecally for 3 to 4 days, then 50,000 units once every other day for at least 2 weeks after cultures of the CSF are negative and glucose content has returned to normal.

Children (< 2 years of age) – 20,000 units once daily, intrathecally for 3 to 4 days or 25,000 units once every other day. Continue with a dose of 25,000 units once every other day for at least 2 weeks after cultures of the CSF are negative and glucose content has returned to normal.

Storage of solution: Refrigerate and discard any unused portion after 72 hours.

Rx	**Polymyxin B Sulfate** (Roerig)	**Injection:** 500,000 units	In vials.
Rx	**Aerosporin** (Glaxo Wellcome)	**Powder for Injection:** 500,000 units	In vials.

BACITRACIN

Warning:

Nephrotoxicity: Parenteral (IM) bacitracin may cause renal failure due to tubular and glomerular necrosis. Restrict use to infants with staphylococcal pneumonia and empyema when due to organisms shown to be susceptible. Use only where laboratory facilities are adequate and constant supervision is possible.

Carefully determine renal function prior to therapy, and daily during therapy. Do not exceed the recommended daily dose, and maintain fluid intake and urinary output at proper levels to avoid renal toxicity. If renal toxicity occurs, discontinue the drug. Avoid the concurrent use of other nephrotoxic drugs, particularly streptomycin, kanamycin, polymyxin B, colistin and neomycin.

Actions:

Pharmacology: Bacitracin exerts pronounced antibacterial action in vitro against a variety of gram-positive and a few gram-negative organisms. However, among systemic diseases, only staphylococcal infections qualify for consideration of bacitracin therapy. Bacitracin is assayed against a standard, and its activity is expressed in units, with 1 mg having a potency of not less than 50 units.

Pharmacokinetics: Absorption after IM injection is rapid and complete. A dose of 200 or 300 units/kg every 6 hrs gives serum levels of 0.2 to 2 mcg/ml in individuals with normal renal function. It is widely distributed in all body organs and is demonstrable in ascitic and pleural fluids. It is excreted slowly by glomerular filtration.

Indications:

Limit use of IM bacitracin to the treatment of infants with pneumonia and empyema caused by staphylococci shown to be sensitive to the drug (see Warning Box).

Unlabeled uses: Oral use in antibiotic-associated colitis has been successful.

Contraindications:

Hypersensitivity or toxic reaction to bacitracin.

Precautions:

Fluid intake: Maintain adequate fluid intake orally, or if necessary, parenterally.

Superinfection: Use of antibiotics (especially prolonged or repeated therapy) may result in bacterial or fungal overgrowth of nonsusceptible organisms. Such overgrowth may lead to a secondary infection. Take appropriate measures if this occurs.

Drug Interactions:

Bacitracin Drug Interactions

Precipitant drug	Object drug*		Description
Aminoglycosides	Bacitracin	↑	Concurrent use may increase risk of respiratory paralysis and renal dysfunction.
Bacitracin	Nondepolarizing muscle relaxants	↑	Neuromuscular blockade may be enhanced.

* ↑ = Object drug increased

Adverse Reactions:

Albuminuria; cylindruria; azotemia; rising blood levels without increase in dosage; nausea and vomiting; pain at injection site; skin rashes.

Administration and Dosage:

IM use only. Give in upper outer quadrant of buttocks, alternating sides and avoiding multiple injections in the same region because of transient pain following injection.

Infants < 2.5 kg: 900 units/kg/24 hours, in 2 or 3 divided doses.

Infants > 2.5 kg: 1000 units/kg/24 hours, in 2 or 3 divided doses.

Preparation of solutions: Dissolve in Sodium Chloride Injection containing 2% procaine HCl. Antibiotic concentration in solution should not be < 5000 units/ml nor > 10,000 units/ml. Do not use diluents containing parabens; cloudy solutions and precipitate formation have occurred. Reconstitution of the 50,000 unit vial with 9.8 ml of diluent will result in a concentration of 5000 units/ml.

Storage/Stability: Refrigerate the unreconstituted product at 2° to 8°C (36° to 46°F). Solutions are stable for 1 week when refrigerated at 2° to 8°C (36° to 46°F).

Rx	**Bacitracin USP** (*Various, eg, Schein, Upjohn*)	**Powder for Injection:** 50,000 units	In vials.
Rx	**Baci-IM** (Pharma-Tek)		In vials.

NOVOBIOCIN

> **Warning:**
> Use only for serious infections where less toxic drugs are ineffective or contraindicated because of: (1) High frequency of adverse reactions, principally urticaria and maculopapular dermatitis. Hepatic dysfunction and blood dyscrasias are less frequent. (2) Rapid and frequent emergence of resistant strains, especially staphylococci.

Actions:

Pharmacology: Novobiocin, primarily bacteriostatic, interferes with bacterial cell wall synthesis.

Pharmacokinetics: Novobiocin is well absorbed from the GI tract. Peak serum levels, which occur in 2 to 3 hours, are higher when taken in the fasting state. The drug is highly bound to serum proteins (> 90%) and diffusion into body fluids is poor. Small amounts may penetrate into the cerebrospinal fluid if the meninges are inflamed. Excretion is primarily via the bile; 3% is excreted in the urine.

Microbiology: In vitro, it is active against Staphylococcus aureus and some *Proteus vulgaris* strains. In vitro, *S aureus* rapidly develops resistance.

Indications:

Serious infections due to susceptible *S aureus* when other effective antibiotics are contraindicated. May be useful in the few urinary tract infections caused by *Proteus* sp sensitive to novobiocin but resistant to other therapy.

Contraindications:

Hypersensitivity to novobiocin.

Warnings:

Hypersensitivity: Novobiocin possesses a high index of sensitization. If allergic reactions develop during treatment and are not readily controlled by the usual measures, discontinue use. Refer to Management of Acute Hypersensitivity Reactions.

Pregnancy: Category C. It is not known whether novobiocin causes fetal harm when administered to a pregnant woman or can affect reproduction capacity. Use only when clearly needed.

Lactation: Safety and efficacy for use in the nursing mother have not been established. Novobiocin reaches low levels in breast milk (0.34 to 0.54 mg/dl); kernicterus may develop in the neonate. Effects on the neonate may include modification of bowel flora, direct effects and interference of cultures for fever evaluation.

Children: Novobiocin affects bilirubin metabolism apparently by inhibiting glycuronyl transferase; avoid use in newborns and premature infants.

Precautions:

Monitoring: Routinely perform hepatic and hematologic studies. Discontinue use if liver dysfunction develops and if hematologic studies show evidence of leukopenia or blood dyscrasias.

Superinfection: Use of antibiotics (especially prolonged or repeated therapy) may result in bacterial or fungal overgrowth of nonsusceptible organisms. Such overgrowth may lead to a secondary infection. Take appropriate measures if superinfection occurs.

Drug Interactions:

Drug/Lab test interactions: Novobiocin may cause "pseudojaundice" (yellow skin and plasma). This may interfere with **serum bilirubin** and **icterus index determinations.**
The drug may interfere with the hepatic uptake or biliary excretion of **sulfobromophthalein** in the bromsulphalein test.

Adverse Reactions:

Hematologic: Blood dyscrasias including leukopenia, eosinophilia, hemolytic anemia, pancytopenia, agranulocytosis and thrombocytopenia.

Hypersensitivity: Reactions consist of skin eruptions, including urticarial, erythematous, maculopapular or scarlatiniform rash (10% to 15% of patients receiving therapy for ≥ 1 week develop a rash). See Warnings. Erythema multiforme (Stevens-Johnson syndrome) has occurred, but is rare.

Hepatic: Jaundice; elevation of unconjugated bilirubin; impaired bromsulphalein excretion; yellow discoloration of plasma, skin and sclerae due to lipochrome pigment metabolite.

Miscellaneous: Nausea; vomiting; loose stools and diarrhea (fairly common but usually does not necessitate discontinuing therapy); intestinal hemorrhage; alopecia.

NOVOBIOCIN

Patient Information:

Complete full course of therapy.

Notify physician of skin rash or hives; yellowish discoloration of skin or eyes; fever; sore throat; or unusual bleeding or bruising.

Administration and Dosage:

Adults: 250 mg every 6 hours or 500 mg every 12 hours. Continue for at least 48 hours after temperature has returned to normal and evidence of infection has disappeared. In severe or unusually resistant infections, give 0.5 g every 6 hours or 1 g every 12 hours.

Children: 15 mg/kg/day for moderate acute infections; up to 30 to 45 mg/kg/day for severe infections. Give in divided doses.

Rx	**Albamycin** (Upjohn)	**Capsules:** 250 mg novobiocin (as sodium)	White and maroon. In 100s.

METRONIDAZOLE

Metronidazole is also available for topical and intravaginal use. For further information refer to the individual monographs in the Topicals chapter. It is also used orally as an amebicide; refer to the individual monograph in the Amebicides section.

> **Warning:**
> Metronidazole is carcinogenic in rodents. Avoid unnecessary use.

Actions:

Pharmacology: Metronidazole, a nitroimidazole, is active against various anaerobic bacteria and protozoa. Its mode of action is not well understood. It appears to enter the cells of microorganisms that contain nitroreductase, where its nitro group is reduced. Unstable intermediate compounds are formed which bind to DNA and inhibit synthesis, causing cell death.

Pharmacokinetics:

Absorption – Metronidazole is well absorbed after oral administration (similar to IV values). Peak serum levels occur at about 1 to 2 hours. Oral bioavailability is not affected by food, but peak serum levels will be delayed up to 2 hours.

Distribution – Metronidazole has a large apparent volume of distribution. It diffuses well into all tissues, achieving therapeutic levels in bone, pelvic tissues, bile, saliva, seminal fluid, breast milk, placenta, abscesses (including hepatic abscesses), empyema fluid, middle ear fluid and cerebrospinal fluid (approximately 50% of serum cncentration in patients with normal meninges, approximates serum concentration in patients with inflamed meninges). Less than 20% of the circulating drug is bound to plasma proteins. Plasma concentrations are proportional (linear) to the administered dose, both IV and oral. A dosage regimen of 15 mg/kg loading dose, followed by 7.5 mg/kg every 6 hours, produces peak steady-state plasma concentrations averaging 25 mcg/ml, with trough concentrations averaging 18 mcg/ml. Multiple dosing results in some drug accumulation.

Metabolism – Metronidazole is the major component appearing in the plasma, along with lesser quantities of the 2–hydroxymethyl metabolite and an acidic metabolite. The metabolites that appear in the urine result primarily from side-chain oxidation and glucuronide conjugation, with unchanged metronidazole accounting for approximately 20% of the total. Both the parent compound and the 2–hydroxymethyl metabolite possess in vitro bactericidal activity against most strains of anaerobic bacteria and in vitro trichomonacidal activity.

Excretion – The major route of elimination of metronidazole and its metabolites is via the urine (60% to 80% of the dose); fecal excretion accounts for 6% to 15% of the dose. Renal clearance is approximately 10 ml/min/1.73 m^2.

Metronidazole has an average elimination half-life in healthy subjects of 8 hours. The hydroxy-metabolite has a half-life of ≈ 15 hours. In patients with creatinine clearances (Ccr) > 10 ml/min, the accumulation of metronidazole or its metabolites is unlikely to produce toxicity. Patients with Ccr < 10 ml/min (not receiving dialysis) will accumulate both metabolites. Metronidazole and its two major metabolites are removed by hemodialysis. Mean dialysis clearance values for parent compound and metabolites range from 60 to 125 ml/min, depending on the membrane used. Metronidazole is also removed by peritoneal dialysis. Plasma clearance is decreased in patients with decreased liver function.

Pharmacokinetic parameters are not significantly altered in patients with serious anaerobic infections or during pregnancy. However, neonates have a slower elimination of metronidazole; half-life may be as high as 22 hours. Dosage adjustment may be necessary.

Microbiology: Metronidazole is active in vitro against most obligate anaerobes, but does not appear to possess activity against facultative anaerobes or obligate aerobes. It is generally bactericidal against susceptible organisms, at concentrations equal to or slightly higher than the minimal inhibitory concentrations (MICs). Metronidazole is active against anaerobic gram-negative bacilli, including *Bacteroides* sp (eg, *B fragilis, B distasonis, B ovatus, B thetaiotaomicron, B vulgatus*); *Fusobacterium* sp; anaerobic gram-positive bacilli, including *Clostiridium* sp and susceptible strains of *Eubacterium;* anaerobic gram-positive cocci, including *Peptococcus* sp and *Peptostreptococcus* sp; anaerobic protozoa, including *Trichomonas vaginalis, Entamoeba histolytica, Giardia lamblia* and *Balantidium coli.*

Perform bacteriologic studies to determine the causative organisms and their susceptibility; however, therapy may be started while awaiting these results.

Indications:

Anaerobic infections: Treatment of serious infections caused by susceptible anaerobic bacteria. Effective in *B fragilis* infections resistant to clindamycin, chloramphenicol and penicillin.

METRONIDAZOLE

Intra-abdominal infections (peritonitis, intra-abdominal abscess and liver abscess) caused by *Bacteroides* sp (*B fragilis, B distasonis, B ovatus, B thetaiotaomicron, B vulgatus*), *Clostridium* sp, *Eubacterium* sp, *Peptostreptococcus* sp and *Peptococcus* sp.

Skin and skin structure infections, caused by *Bacteroides* sp including the *B fragilis* group, *Clostridium* sp, *Peptococcus* sp, *Peptostreptococcus* sp and *Fusobacterium* sp.

Gynecologic infections (endometritis, endomyometritis, tubo-ovarian abscess and postsurgical vaginal cuff infection), caused by *Bacteroides* sp including the *B fragilis* group, *Clostridium* sp, *Pepotococcus* sp and *Peptostreptococcus* sp.

Bacterial septicemia caused by *Bacteroides* sp including the *B fragilis* group and *Clostridium* sp.

Bone and joint infections caused by *Bacteroides* sp including the *B fragilis* group, as adjunctive therapy.

CNS infections (meningitis and brain abscess), caused by *Bacteroides* sp including the *B fragilis* group.

Lower respiratory tract infections (pneumonia, empyema and lung abscess) caused by *Bacteroides* sp including the *B fragilis* group.

Endocarditis caused by *Bacteroides* sp including the *B fragilis* group.

Prophylaxis: Preoperative, intraoperative and postoperative IV metronidazole may reduce the incidence of postoperative infection in patients undergoing elective colorectal surgery which is classified as contaminated or potentially contaminated.

Discontinue within 12 hours after surgery. If there are signs of infection, obtain specimens for cultures to identify the causative organisms.

Metronidazole is also indicated for amebiasis and trichomoniasis, intravaginally for bacterial vaginosis and topically for acne rosacea (see individual monographs).

Unlabeled uses: Metronidazole has shown efficacy, alone and in combination, as prophylaxis in reducing infection rates in gynecologic and abdominal surgery.

Hepatic encephalopathy – Metronidazole has compared favorably to neomycin.

Crohn's disease – Metronidazole (500 mg/day) has been successful, with particular improvement of perianal manifestations (up to 20 mg/kg) (see Precautions).

Antibiotic-associated pseudomembranous colitis – Metronidazole is as effective as vancomycin (1 to 2 g/day for 7 to 10 days).

Helicobacter pylori – A combination of metronidazole (250 mg 3 times a day) and bismuth for 4 weeks appears to be effective in the eradication of *H pylori* for up to 12 months. The addition of tetracycline may increase the length of remission.

The CDC has recommended the use of oral metronidazole for bacterial vaginosis (500 mg twice daily for 7 days)* and for giardiasis (alternative to quinacrine; 250 mg 3 times daily for 7 days).†Single-dose therapy for bacterial vaginosis (2 g) also appears to be as effective as multiple-dose therapy.

Contraindications:

Hypersensitivity to metronidazole or other nitroimidazole derivatives; pregnancy (first trimester in patients with trichomoniasis; see Warnings).

Warnings:

Neurologic effects: Seizures (associated with high cumulative doses) and peripheral neuropathy (characterized by numbness or paresthesia of an extremity) have occurred. Peripheral neuropathy occurs rarely when metronidazole is used in low doses for short durations. Carefully monitor patients receiving high doses for long periods (eg, Crohn's disease). In some cases, neuropathy is not reversible. Appearance of abnormal neurologic signs demands prompt discontinuation of therapy. Administer metronidazole with caution to patients with CNS diseases.

Hepatic function impairment: Patients with severe hepatic disease metabolize metronidazole slowly. Accumulation of the drug and its metabolites may occur. Cautiously administer doses below those usually recommended.

Carcinogenesis: Metronidazole has shown evidence of carcinogenic activity with chronic oral administration in rodents. In several long-term studies in rats, there was an increase in the incidence of neoplasms, particularly mammary and hepatic tumors, among female rats. Also, metronidazole has shown mutagenic activity in a number of in vitro assay systems.

Elderly: Since the pharmacokinetics of metronidazole may be altered in the elderly, monitoring of serum levels may be necssary to adjust the dosage accordingly.

* CDC 1989 Sexually Transmitted Diseases Treatment Guidelines. *Morbidity and Mortality Weekly Report* 1989 Sept 1;38 (No.2–8):1–43.

† CDC 1985 STD Treatment Guidelines. *Morbidity and Mortality Weekly Report* 1985 Oct 18;34 (No. 4s):75S-108S.

METRONIDAZOLE

Pregnancy: Category B. Metronidazole crosses the placenta and enters fetal circulation rapidly. There are no adequate and well controlled studies in pregnant women. Use during pregnancy only if clearly needed.

Restrict metronidazole for trichomoniasis in the second and third trimesters to those in whom local palliative treatment has been inadequate to control symptoms.

Lactation: Safety for use in the nursing mother has not been established. Metronidazole is secreted in breast milk in concentrations similar to those found in plasma. Its half-life in breast milk is about 9 to 10 hours. A nursing mother should express and discard any breast milk produced while on the drug and resume nursing 24 to 48 hours after the drug is discontinued.

Children: Safety and efficacy in children have not been established, except for the treatment of amebiasis. Newborns demonstrate a diminished capacity to eliminate metronidazole. The elimination half-life is inversely related to gestational age. In infants whose gestational ages were between 28 and 40 weeks, the corresponding elimination half-lives ranged from 109 to 22.5 hours.

Precautions:

Crohn's disease patients are known to have an increased incidence of GI and certain extraintestinal cancers. There have been some reports in the medical literature of breast and colon cancer in Crohn's disease patients who have been treated with metronidazole at high doses for extended periods of time. A cause and effect relatinship has not been established. (See Unlabeled uses.)

Candidiasis, known or previously unrecognized, may present more prominent symptoms during therapy and requires treatment with a candicidal agent.

Hematologic effects: Metronidazole is a nitroimidazole; use with care in patients with evidence or history of blood dyscrasia. Mild leukopenia has been seen during administration; however, no persistent hematologic abnormalities attributable to the drug have been observed. Perform total and differential leukocyte counts before and after therapy.

Amebic liver abscess: Metronidazole does not obviate the need for aspiration of pus.

Drug Interactions:

Metronidazole Drug Interactions

Precipitant drug	Object drug*		Description
Barbiturates	Metronidazole	⬇	Therapeutic failure of metronidazole may occur.
Cimetidine	Metronidazole	⬆	Decreased metronidazole clearance and increased serum levels may occur; however, data conflict.
Metronidazole	Anticoagulants	⬆	The anticoagulant effect of warfarin may be enhanced.
Metronidazole	Disulfiram	⬆	Concurrent use may result in an acute psychosis or confusional state.
Metronidazole	Ethanol	⬆	A disulfiram-like reaction including symptoms of flushing, palpitations, tachycardia, nausea, vomiting, etc, may occur with concurrent use. Although the risk for most patients may be slight, caution is advised.
Metronidazole	Hydantoins	⬆	The total clearance of phenytoin may be decreased and its eliminatin half-life prolonged.
Metronidazole	Lithium	⬆	In patients stabilized on relatively high lithium doses, short-term metronidazole has been associated with increased lithium levels and toxicity in some cases.

* ⬆ = Object drug increased. ⬇ = Object drug decreased.

Drug/Lab test interactions: The drug may interfere with chemical analyses for AST, ALT, LDH, triglycerides and hexokinase glucose. Zero values may occur.

Adverse Reactions:

CNS: Seizures and peripheral neuropathy, the latter characterized mainly by numbness or paresthesia of an extremity; dizziness; vertigo; incoordination; ataxia; confusion; irritability; depression; weakness; insomnia; headache; syncope.

GI: Nausea, sometimes accompanied by headache, anorexia and occasionally, vomiting; diarrhea; epigastric distress; abdominal cramping; constipation; proctitis; sharp, unpleasant metallic taste; a modification of the taste of alcoholic beverages; furry tongue, glossitis, stomatitis (these may be associated with a sudden overgrowth of *Candida*). Paradoxically, metronidazole has been implicated in causing pseudomembranous colitis.

Hematologic: Reversible neutropenia (leukopenia); reversible thrombocytopenia (rare).

Renal/GU: Dysuria; cystitis; polyuria; incontinence; sense of pelvic pressure; proliferation of *Candida* in the vagina; dyspareunia; decreased libido. Darkened urine (deep red-brown color) has been reported. The pigment appears to be a metabolite of metronidazole and it seems to have no clinical significance.

Cardiovascular: Flattening of the T-wave may be seen in ECG tracings.

Hypersensitivity: Urticaria; erythematous rash; flushing; nasal congestion; dryness of the mouth (or vagina or vulva); fever.

Local: Thrombophlebitis after IV infusion can be minimized or eliminated by avoiding prolonged use of indwelling IV catheters.

Miscellaneous: Fleeting joint pains, sometimes resembling "serum sickness." One case of metronidazole-induced pancreatitis, confirmed with rechallenge, has been reported.

Overdosage:

Symptoms: Nausea, vomiting and ataxia. Neurotoxic effects (seizures and peripheral neuropathy) have been reported after 5 to 7 days of 6 to 10.4 g every other day. Single oral doses, up to 15 g, have been reported in suicide attempts and accidental overdoses. Use of doses higher than those recommended (27 mg/kg 3 times a day for 20 days and a 75 mg/kg loading dose followed by 7.5 mg/kg maintenance doses) have been used with no adverse effects.

Treatment: No specific antidote for metronidazole overdose exists. Treatment consists of usual supportive measures. Refer to General Management of Acute Overdosage.

Patient Information:

May cause GI upset; take with food. Avoid alcoholic beverages.

Complete full course of therapy; take until gone. May cause darkening of urine

An unpleasant metallic taste may be noticeable.

Administration and Dosage:

Anaerobic bacterial infections: In the treatment of most serious anaerobic infections, metronidazole is usually administered IV initially.

Loading dose – 15 mg/kg infused over 1 hour (≈ 1 g for a 70 kg adult).

Maintenance dose – 7.5 mg/kg infused over 1 hour every 6 hours (≈ 500 mg for a 70 kg adult). Administer the first maintenance dose 6 hours following the initiation of loading dose. Do not exceed a maximum of 4 g in 24 hours.

The usual duration of therapy is 7 to 10 days; however, infections of the bone and joints, lower respiratory tract and endocardium may require longer treatment.

Administer by slow IV, continuous or intermittent drip infusion only. Do not use equipment containing aluminum (eg, needles, hubs). If used with a primary IV fluid system, discontinue the primary solution during infusion. Do not give by direct IV bolus injection because of the low pH (0.5 to 2) of the reconstituted product. The drug must be further diluted and neutralized for infusion. Do not introduce additives into the solution.

Oral – Following IV therapy, use oral metronidazole when conditions warrant. The usual adult oral dosage is 7.5 mg/kg every 6 hours. Do not exceed a maximum of 4 g in 24 hours.

Prophylaxis: To prevent postoperative infection in contaminated or potentially contaminated colorectal surgery, the recommended adult dosage is 15 mg/kg infused over 30 to 60 minutes and completed ≈ 1 hour before surgery, followed by 7.5 mg/kg infused over 30 to 60 minutes at 6 and 12 hours after the initial dose.

Complete administration of the initial preoperative dose ≈ 1 hour before surgery so that adequate drug levels are present in the serum and tissues at the time of initial incision, and administer, if necessary, at 6 hour intervals to maintain effective drug levels. Limit prophylactic use to the day of surgery only, following the above guidelines.

It has also been suggested that a dose of 1500 mg infused at the beginning of surgery achieves significantly higher concentrations against *B fragilis* than the 500 mg infusion and may be beneficial in ensuring adequate metronidazole levels.

Hepatic disease patients metabolize metronidazole slowly; accumulation of metronidazole and its metabolites occurs. Therefore, reduce doses below those usually recommended. Monitor plasma metronidazole levels and observe for toxicity.

Renal disease: Do not specifically reduce the dose in anuric patients, since accumulated metabolites may be rapidly removed by dialysis.

METRONIDAZOLE

Elderly: Dosage adjustment may be necessary; monitor serum levels.

Preparation of parenteral solution: NOTE: Order of mixing is important. (1) Reconstitution; (2) Dilution in IV solution; (3) pH neutralization with sodium bicarbonate injection.

Do not use aluminum-containing equipment with metronidazole IV. The solution will interact, turning an orange/rust color, although drug potency is not affected.

Reconstitution – Add 4.4 ml of one of the following diluents to the vial and mix thoroughly: Sterile Water for Injection; Bacteriostatic Water for Injection; 0.9% Sodium Chloride Injection; Bacteriostatic 0.9% Sodium Chloride Injection. The resultant volume is 5 ml with an approximate concentration of 100 mg/ml.

The pH of the reconstituted product will be between 0.5 to 2; the solution is clear, and pale yellow to yellow-green in color. Do not use if cloudy or precipitated.

Dilution in IV solutions – Add the properly reconstituted product to a glass or plastic IV container. Do not exceed a concentration of 8 mg/ml. Use any of the following: 0.9% Sodium Chloride Injection; 5% Dextrose Injection; Lactated Ringer's Injection.

Neutralization for IV infusion – Prior to administration, neutralize the IV solution containing metronidazole with approximately 5 mEq sodium bicarbonate injection for each 500 mg used. Mix thoroughly. The pH of the neutralized IV solution will be ≈ 6 to 7. Carbon dioxide gas will be generated with neutralization. It may be necessary to relieve gas pressure within the container.

When the contents of one vial (500 mg) are diluted and neutralized to 100 ml, the resultant concentration is 5 mg/ml. Do not exceed an 8 mg/ml concentration in the neutralized IV solution; neutralization will decrease aqueous solubility and precipitation may occur. *Do not refrigerate neutralized solutions;* precipitation may occur.

Ready-to-use: Do not use plastic containers in series connections; it could result in air embolism due to residual air (≈ 15 ml) being drawn from the primary container before administration of the fluid from the secondary container is complete.

Storage/Stability: Reconstituted *Flagyl IV* is stable for 96 hours when stored below 30°C (86°F) in room light. Use diluted and neutralized IV solutions within 24 hours. Store ready-to-use solution at 15° to 30°C (59° to 86°F); protect from light.

METRONIDAZOLE

Rx	**Metronidazole** (Various, eg, Eon, Geneva, Goldline, Lemmon, Major, Parmed, Rugby, Schein, Zenith)	**Tablets**: 250 mg	In 100s, 250s, 280s, 500s, 1000s and UD 100s.
Rx	**Flagyl** (Searle)		(Searle 1831 Flagyl 250). Blue. Film coated. In 50s, 100s, 250s, 2500s and UD 100s.
Rx	**Protostat** (Ortho)		(Ortho 1570). White, scored. Capsule shaped. In 100s.
Rx	**Metronidazole** (Various, eg, Eon, Geneva, Goldline, Lemmon, Major, Moore, Parmed, Rugby, Schein, Zenith)	**Tablets**: 500 mg	In 50s, 100s, 200s, 500s and UD 100s.
Rx	**Flagyl** (Searle)		(Flagyl 500). Blue. Film coated. Oblong. In 50s, 100s, 500s and UD 100s.
Rx	**Protostat** (Ortho)		(Ortho 1571). White, scored. Capsule shape. In 50s.
Rx	**Flagyl 375** (Searle)	**Capsules**: 375 mg	(375 Flagyl). Gray/light green. In 50s, 100s and UD 100s.
Rx	**Flagyl IV** (Searle)	**Powder for Injection, lyophilized**: 500 mg (as HCl)	In vials.[1]
Rx	**Metronidazole** (Abbott)	**Injection, ready-to-use**: 500 mg per 100 ml	In 100 ml vials.
Rx	**Metronidazole Redi-Infusion** (Elkins-Sinn)		Preservative free. In 100 ml vials.[2]
Rx	**Flagyl IV RTU** (Searle)		In 100 ml plastic containers.[2]
Rx	**Metro I.V.** (McGaw)		In 100 ml plastic containers.[3]

[1] With 415 mg mannitol.
[2] 14 mEq sodium per vial.
[3] 13.5 mEq sodium per vial.

FLUCYTOSINE (5–FC; 5–Fluorocytosine)

> **Warning:**
> Use with extreme caution in patients with renal impairment. Close monitoring of hematologic, renal and hepatic status of all patients is essential.

Actions:

Pharmacology: Flucytosine has in vitro and in vivo activity against *Candida* and *Cryptococcus*, but the exact mode is not known. It is rarely used alone; generally it is used in combination with amphotericin B (see Drug Interactions).

Pharmacokinetics:

Absorption/Distribution – Well absorbed after oral use with peak serum levels in 2 hrs. Well distributed into aqueous humor, joints, peritoneal fluid and other body fluids and tissues; CSF concentrations are about 65% to 90% of serum levels. Plasma protein binding is minimal. Toxicity occurs at blood levels > 100 mcg/ml.

Metabolism/Excretion – ≈ 80% to 90% of a dose is excreted unchanged in urine by glomerular filtration; < 10% is found unchanged in the feces. Serum half-life is 2 to 5 hours in patients with normal renal function; half-life increases significantly in renal failure. The drug is easily removed by hemodialysis or peritoneal dialysis.

Indications:

Serious infections caused by susceptible strains of *Candida* or *Cryptococcus*.

Candida: Septicemia, endocarditis and urinary tract infections have been effectively treated. Trials in pulmonary infections have been limited.

Cryptococcus: Meningitis and pulmonary infections. Good responses in septicemias and urinary tract infections have occurred.

Unlabeled uses: Flucytosine has been used for the treatment of chromomycosis.

Contraindications:

Hypersensitivity to flucytosine.

Warnings:

Bone marrow depression: Give with extreme caution to patients with bone marrow depression. Patients may be more prone to bone marrow depression if they have a hematologic disease, are being treated with radiation or marrow-suppressant drugs, or have a history of treatment with such drugs or radiation. Frequently monitor hepatic function and the hematopoietic system during therapy.

Renal function impairment: Give with extreme caution; drug accumulation may occur. Monitor blood levels to determine the adequacy of renal excretion in such patients. Adjust dosage or dosing interval to maintain blood levels at < 100 mcg/ml.

Pregnancy: Category C. Teratogenic in rat and mouse at 40 mg/kg/day; teratogenicity appears species-related. There are no adequate and well controlled studies in pregnant women. Use only if potential benefit justifies potential risk to fetus.

Lactation: It is not known whether this drug is excreted in breast milk. Because of potential serious adverse reactions in nursing infants, discontinue nursing or the drug, taking into account importance of drug to mother.

Children: Safety and efficacy in children have not been established.

Precautions:

Before therapy is instituted, determine hematologic, renal status and electrolytes. Monitor hepatic function at frequent intervals during therapy.

Drug Interactions:

Amphotericin B may increase the therapeutic action and toxicity of flucytosine.

Cytosine may inactivate the antifungal activity of flucytosine.

Drug/Lab test interactions: Flucytosine interferes with creatinine value determinations with the dry-slide enzymatic method (Kodak Ektachem analyzer). Use Jaffe method.

Adverse Reactions:

Respiratory: Respiratory arrest; chest pain; dyspnea.

Dermatologic: Rash; pruritus; urticaria; photosensitivity.

GI: Nausea; emesis; abdominal pain; diarrhea; anorexia; dry mouth; duodenal ulcer; GI hemorrhage; hepatic dysfunction; jaundice; ulcerative colitis; bilirubin elevation; elevation of hepatic enzymes.

GU: Azotemia; creatinine and BUN elevation; crystalluria; renal failure.

Hematologic: Anemia; agranulocytosis; aplastic anemia; eosinophilia; leukopenia; pancytopenia; thrombocytopenia.

CNS: Ataxia; hearing loss; headache; paresthesia; parkinsonism; peripheral neuropathy; pyrexia; vertigo; sedation; confusion; hallucinations; psychosis.

FLUCYTOSINE (5–FC; 5–Fluorocytosine)

Miscellaneous: Cardiac arrest; fatigue; hypoglycemia; hypokalemia; weakness.

Overdosage:

Symptoms: There is no experience with intentional overdosage. It is reasonable to expect pronounced manifestations of the known clinical adverse reactions. Prolonged serum concentration > 100 mcg/ml may be associated with an increased incidence of toxicity, especially GI (diarrhea, nausea, vomiting), hematologic (leukopenia, thrombocytopenia) and hepatic (hepatitis).

Treatment: Prompt gastric lavage or emetic use is recommended. Maintain adequate fluid intake by IV route if necessary; flucytosine is excreted unchanged via renal tract. Monitor hematologic parameters frequently; monitor liver and kidney function carefully. Should any abnormalities appear in any of these parameters, institute appropriate therapeutic measures. Refer to General Management of Acute Overdosage. Since hemodialysis rapidly reduced serum concentrations in anuric patients, consider this method in overdosage management.

Patient Information:

May cause GI upset (nausea, vomiting). Reduce or avoid by taking capsules a few at a time over a 15 minute period. Notify physician if effects become intolerable.

Administration and Dosage:

The usual dosage is 50 to 150 mg/kg/day in divided doses at 6 hour intervals. To reduce or avoid nausea or vomiting, take capsules a few at a time over 15 minutes. If BUN or serum creatinine is elevated, or if there are other signs of renal impairment, the initial dose should be at the lower level (see Warnings).

Rx	**Ancobon** (Roche)	**Capsules:** 250 mg	(Ancobon Roche 250). Green and gray. In 100s.
		500 mg	(Ancobon Roche 500). White and gray. In 100s.

NYSTATIN, ORAL

Actions:

Pharmacology: A polyene antibiotic with antifungal activity. Nystatin probably acts by binding to sterols in the cell membrane of the fungus, with a resultant change in membrane permeability allowing leakage of intracellular components.

Pharmacokinetics: Sparingly absorbed after oral use, with no detectable blood levels at recommended doses. Most unabsorbed drug is passed unchanged in stool. Exhibits no appreciable activity against bacteria or trichomonads.

Indications:

Treatment of intestinal candidiasis.

For information on nystatin oral suspension and troches for the treatment of oral candidiasis, refer to the monograph in the Mouth and Throat Products section.

Contraindications:

Hypersensitivity to nystatin.

Warnings:

Pregnancy: No adverse effects or complications have been attributed to nystatin in infants born to women treated with nystatin.

Adverse Reactions:

Nystatin is virtually nontoxic and nonsensitizing and is well tolerated by all age groups including debilitated infants, even on prolonged administration. Large oral doses have occasionally produced diarrhea, GI distress, nausea and vomiting.

Patient Information:

Continue therapy for at least 2 days after symptoms have disappeared.

Administration and Dosage:

500,000 to 1,000,000 units 3 times daily. Continue treatment for at least 48 hours after clinical cure to prevent relapse.

Rx	**Nystatin** (Various, eg, Major, Rugby)	**Tablets:** 500,000 units	In 15s, 30s, 100s, 500s, 1000s.
Rx	**Mycostatin** (Apothecon)		Lactose. (580). Film coated. In 100s, Unimatic 100s.
Rx	**Nilstat** (Lederle)		(LL N5). Pink. Convex. Film coated. In 100s, UD 100s.

MICONAZOLE

For information on vaginal and topical miconazole antifungal, refer to individual monographs.

Actions:

Pharmacology: Miconazole, an imidazole derivative, exerts a fungicidal effect by altering the permeability of the fungal cell membrane. Its mechanism of action may also involve an alteration of RNA and DNA metabolism or an intracellular accumulation of peroxides toxic to the fungal cell.

Pharmacokinetics:

Absorption/Distribution – Recommended doses of miconazole produce serum concentrations which exceed in vitro minimum inhibitory concentration (MIC) values for the fungal species noted in the microbiology section. Doses > 9 mg/kg produce peak blood levels > 1 mcg/ml in most cases. Intrathecal administration of a 20 mg dose produces CSF concentrations > 1 mcg/ml for 24 hours; CSF levels following IV administration are undetectable. Penetration of the drug into inflamed joints, the vitreous body of the eye and the peritoneal cavity is good; penetration into sputum and saliva is poor. Greater than 90% is bound to serum protein.

Metabolism/Excretion – Miconazole is rapidly metabolized in the liver. About 14% to 22% of the administered dose is excreted in the urine, mainly as inactive metabolites. The terminal elimination half-life is 20 to 25 hours. The pharmacokinetic profile is unaltered in patients with renal insufficiency, including those on hemodialysis.

Microbiology: The in vitro antifungal activity is broad. Clinical efficacy has been demonstrated against the following: *Coccidioides immitis; Candida albicans; Cryptococcus neoformans; Pseudoallescheria boydii* (*Petriellidium boydii, Allescheria boydii*); *Paracoccidioides brasiliensis.*

Indications:

Treatment of the following severe systemic fungal infections: Coccidioidomycosis, candidiasis, cryptococcosis, pseudoallescheriosis (petriellidiosis, allescheriosis), paracoccidioidomycosis and for the treatment of chronic mucocutaneous candidiasis.

In the treatment of fungal meningitis or *Candida* urinary bladder infections, IV infusion alone is inadequate. It must be supplemented with intrathecal administration or bladder irrigation. Follow appropriate diagnostic procedures and determine MICs.

Use only to treat severe systemic fungal disease.

Contraindications:

Hypersensitivity to miconazole.

Warnings:

Cardiac effects: Cardiorespiratory arrest or anaphylaxis has occurred, possibly due to excessively rapid administration in some cases. Rapid injection of undiluted miconazole may produce transient tachycardia or arrhythmia.

Pregnancy: Category C. There are no adequate and well controlled studies in pregnant women. Give to a pregnant woman only if clearly needed.

Children: Safety for use in children < 1 year of age has not been extensively studied. There are reports of 21 neonates who received 3 to 50 mg/kg/day with no unanticipated adverse reactions. Seven of 11 evaluable children recovered or improved.

Precautions:

Give by IV infusion. Start treatment under stringent conditions of hospitalization. Subsequently, it may be given to suitable patients under ambulatory conditions with close clinical monitoring. Give initial 200 mg dose with the physician in attendance. Monitor hemoglobin, hematocrit, electrolytes and lipids. Since *Pseudoallescheria* is difficult to distinguish histologically from species of *Aspergillus,* grow cultures.

Systemic fungal mycoses may be complications of chronic underlying conditions which, in themselves, may require appropriate measures.

Drugs containing cremophor-type vehicles (eg, PEG 40, castor oil) cause electrophoretic abnormalities of the lipoprotein. These effects are reversible upon discontinuation of treatment, but are usually not an indication to discontinue treatment.

Drug Interactions:

Amphotericin B: Limited data indicate that miconazole and amphotericin B are antagonistic both in vitro and in vivo. The antifungal activity of the two drugs when used in combination is less than that of either drug used alone.

Anticoagulants, oral: An enhanced anticoagulant effect has occurred; carefully monitor the anticoagulant effect; reductions of anticoagulant doses may be indicated.

Phenytoin levels were increased in one patient on miconazole; toxicity resulted.

Due to structural similarity with ketoconazole, consider the possibility of similar drug interactions occurring with miconazole (see ketoconazole monograph).

MICONAZOLE

Adverse Reactions:

Dermatologic: Phlebitis at infusion site (29%); pruritus (21%); rash (9%). If pruritus and skin rashes are severe, discontinuation of treatment may be necessary.

GI: Nausea (18%); vomiting (7%); diarrhea; anorexia. Nausea and vomiting can be lessened with antihistaminic or antiemetic drugs given prior to infusion, or by reducing the dose, slowing the rate of infusion or avoiding administration at mealtime.

Hematologic: Transient decreases in hematocrit have been observed following infusion. Thrombocytopenia, aggregation of erythrocytes or rouleau formation on blood smears has occurred.

Body as a whole: Fever and chills (10%), drowsiness, flushes, transient decreases in serum sodium, anaphylaxis. Hyperlipemia has occurred and is reported to be due to the vehicle, *Cremophor EL* (PEG 40, castor oil).

Administration and Dosage:

Adults: The following daily doses are recommended:

Recommended Miconazole Daily Doses

Organism	Total daily dosage range[1] (mg)	Duration of therapy (weeks)
Coccidioidomycosis	1800 to 3600	3 to > 20
Cryptococcosis	1200 to 2400	3 to > 12
Pseudoallescheriosis	600 to 3000	5 to > 20
Candidiasis	600 to 1800	1 to > 20
Paracoccidioidomycosis	200 to 1200	2 to > 16

[1] May be divided over 3 infusions.

Repeated courses may be necessitated by relapse or reinfection.

Children:

< 1 year old – 15 to 30 mg/kg/day.

1 to 12 years old – 20 to 40 mg/kg/day. Do not exceed 15 mg/kg/dose.

IV: For doses ≤ 2400 mg/day, dilute in at least 200 ml of fluid per amp. The diluent of choice is 0.9% Sodium Chloride Injection or, alternatively, 5% Dextrose Injection. Infuse at a rate of approximately 2 hours/amp. For doses > 2400 mg/day, adjust infusion rate and diluent according to patient tolerability.

Continue treatment until clinical and laboratory tests no longer indicate presence of active fungal infection. Inadequate treatment periods may yield poor response and lead to early recurrence of clinical symptoms. Dosing intervals, sites and duration of treatment vary and depend on the causative organism.

Intrathecal: Administer undiluted solution by various intrathecal routes (20 mg per dose) as an adjunct to IV treatment in fungal meningitis. Succeeding intrathecal injections may be alternated between lumbar, cervical and cisternal punctures every 3 to 7 days.

Bladder instillation: 200 mg diluted solution for *Candida* of the urinary bladder.

Rx	**Monistat i.v.** (Janssen)	**Injection:** 10 mg per ml	In 20 ml amps.[2]

[2] With PEG 40, castor oil and parabens.

KETOCONAZOLE

For information on topical ketoconazole, refer to the individual monograph in the Topical Anti-infectives section.

> **Warning:**
> Ketoconazole has been associated with hepatic toxicity, including some fatalities. Closely monitor patients and inform them of the risk. See Warnings.

Actions:

Pharmacology: Ketoconazole, an imidazole broad-spectrum antifungal agent, impairs the synthesis of ergosterol, the main sterol of fungal cell membranes, allowing increased permeability and leakage of cellular components.

Pharmacokinetics:

Absorption/Distribution – Bioavailability depends on an acidic pH for dissolution and absorption (see Precautions). Peak plasma levels of 1.6 to 6.9 mcg/ml occur 1 to 2 hours after a 200 mg oral dose taken with a meal. Administration with food may decrease absorption. In vitro, plasma protein binding is about 95% to 99%, mainly to albumin. At recommended doses, cerebrospinal fluid penetration is negligible. Detectable concentrations are achieved in urine, saliva, sebum and cerumen.

Metabolism/Excretion – The drug undergoes extensive hepatic metabolism to inactive metabolites. Plasma elimination is biphasic; half-life is 2 hours during the first 10 hours, 8 hours thereafter. The major excretory route is enterohepatic. From 85% to 90% is excreted in bile and feces, 10% to 15% in urine, 2% to 4% unchanged.

Renal failure does not alter ketoconazole dosing requirements; the drug does not appear to be dialyzable.

Microbiology: Active against clinical infections with Blastomyces dermatitidis, Candida sp, *Coccidioides immitis, Histoplasma capsulatum, Paracoccidioides brasiliensis, Phialophora* sp, *Trichophyton* sp, *Epidermophyton* sp and *Microsporum* sp. In animals, activity has been demonstrated against *Malassezia furfur* and *Cryptococcus neoformans.*

Indications:

Treatment of the following systemic fungal infections: Candidiasis, chronic mucocutaneous candidiasis, oral thrush, candiduria, blastomycosis, coccidioidomycosis, histoplasmosis, chromomycosis and paracoccidioidomycosis.

Treatment of severe recalcitrant cutaneous dermatophyte infections not responding to topical therapy or oral griseofulvin or in patients unable to take griseofulvin.

Unlabeled uses: Ketoconazole has been used successfully in the treatment of onychomycosis (caused by *Trichophyton* and *Candida* sp); pityriasis versicolor (Tinea versicolor); tinea pedis, corporis and cruris (200 to 400 mg/day); tinea capitis (3.3 to 6.6 mg/kg/day); and vaginal candidiasis.

High-dose (800 to 1200 mg/day) ketoconazole has shown some success in treating CNS fungal infections.

Ketoconazole in doses of 400 mg every 8 hours has been used in the treatment of advanced prostate cancer (see Warnings).

Ketoconazole 800 to 1200 mg/day has been used to effectively treat Cushing's syndrome due to its ability to inhibit adrenal steroidogenesis.

Contraindications:

Hypersensitivity to ketoconazole. Do not use for the treatment of fungal meningitis because it penetrates poorly into the CSF (see Unlabeled uses).

Warnings:

Hepatotoxicity, primarily of the hepatocellular type, has been associated with ketoconazole including rare fatalities. The incidence has been about 1:10,000 exposed patients, but this probably represents under-reporting. The median duration of therapy in patients who developed symptomatic hepatotoxicity was about 28 days, although the range extended to as low as 3 days. The hepatic injury is usually reversible upon discontinuation of treatment. Several cases of hepatitis have occurred in children.

Prompt recognition of liver injury is essential. Measure liver function (eg, AST, ALT, alkaline phosphatase, bilirubin) before starting treatment and frequently during treatment. Monitor patients receiving ketoconazole concurrently with other potentially hepatotoxic drugs, particularly those patients requiring prolonged therapy or those with a history of liver disease.

Transient minor elevations in liver enzymes have occurred. Discontinue drug if these persist or worsen, or are accompanied by symptoms of possible liver injury.

Prostatic cancer: In clinical trials involving 350 patients with metastatic prostatic cancer, 11 deaths were reported within 2 weeks of starting high-dose ketoconazole (1200 mg/day). It is not known whether death was related to therapy. High ketoconazole doses are known to suppress adrenal corticosteroid secretion.

KETOCONAZOLE

Hypersensitivity: Anaphylaxis occurs rarely after the first dose. Hypersensitivity reactions, including urticaria, have been reported. Have epinephrine 1:1000 immediately available. Refer to Management of Acute Hypersensitivity Reactions.

Pregnancy: Category C. Teratogenic effects (syndactylia and oligodactylia), embryotoxic effects and dystocia have been seen in animals at doses in excess of the maximum human dose. There are no adequate and well controlled studies in pregnant women. Use only if the potential benefit justifies the potential risk to the fetus.

Lactation: Ketoconazole is probably excreted in breast milk; mothers who are under treatment should not nurse.

Children: Safety for use in children < 2 years of age has not been established. Do not use in pediatric patients unless the potential benefits outweigh the risks.

Precautions:

Hormone levels: Ketoconazole lowers serum testosterone. Testosterone levels are impaired with doses of 800 mg/day and abolished by 1600 mg/day. Once therapy has been discontinued, levels return to baseline values. It also decreases ACTH-induced corticosteroid serum levels at similar high doses. Closely follow the recommended dose of 200 to 400 mg/day.

Gastric acidity: Ketoconazole requires acidity for dissolution and absorption. If antacids, anticholinergics or H_2 blockers are needed, give at least 2 hours after administration. In achlorhydria, dissolve each tablet in 4 ml aqueous solution of 0.2 N HCl. Use a glass or plastic straw to avoid contact with teeth. Follow with a glass of water.

Drug Interactions:

Ketoconazole Drug Interactions

Precipitant Drug	Object Drug*		Description
Antacids	Ketoconazole	⬇	Increased gastric pH may inhibit ketoconazole absorption. Consider giving antacids ≥ 2 hrs after ketoconazole.
Histamine H_2 antagonists	Ketoconazole	⬇	Increased gastric pH may inhibit ketoconazole absorption.
Isoniazid	Ketoconazole	⬇	Bioavailability of ketoconazole may be decreased.
Rifampin	Ketoconazole	⬇	Decreased serum levels of either drug may occur. Avoid concurrent use if possible.
Ketoconazole	Anticoagulants, oral	⬆	The anticoagulant response may be enhanced.
Ketoconazole	Antihistamines – Astemizole Terfenidine	⬆	Astemizole and terfenadine plasma levels (including metabolite levels) may be increased, which may lead to serious cardiovascular adverse events.
Ketoconazole	Corticosteroids	⬆	Corticosteroid bioavailability may be increased and clearance may be decreased, possibly resulting in toxicity.
Ketoconazole	Cyclosporine	⬆	Increased cyclosporine concentrations may occur, possibly resulting in toxicity. Since the effect on cyclosporine levels is consistent and predictable, this interaction has been used beneficially to decrease cyclosporine dosage in some patients.
Ketoconazole	Theophyllines	⬇	Theophylline serum levels may be decreased.

* ⬆ = Object drug increased ⬇ = Object drug decreased

KETOCONAZOLE

Adverse Reactions:

Most reactions are mild, transient and rarely require discontinuation. The rare occurrences of hepatic dysfunction require special attention.

GI: Nausea/vomiting (3% to 10%); abdominal pain (1.2%); diarrhea (< 1%); hepatotoxicity.

CNS: Headache, dizziness, somnolence, photophobia (< 1%).

Psychiatric: Suicidal tendencies, severe depression (rare).

Miscellaneous: Pruritus (1.5%); fever, chills, impotence, gynecomastia, thrombocytopenia, leukopenia, hemolytic anemia, bulging fontanelles (< 1%). Hypersensitivity including urticaria (see Warnings). Oligospermia has occurred at dosages above those approved but not at dosages up to 400 mg/day; sperm counts were obtained infrequently at these dosages.

Overdosage:

Institute supportive measures, including gastric lavage with sodium bicarbonate. Refer to General Management of Acute Overdosage.

Patient Information:

Do not take with antacids; if antacids are required, delay administration by 2 hours.

Take with food to alleviate GI disturbance.

May produce headache, dizziness and drowsiness; observe caution while driving or performing other tasks requiring alertness, coordination or physical dexterity.

Notify physician of any signs or symptoms suggesting liver dysfunction (eg, unusual fatigue, anorexia, nausea, vomiting, jaundice, dark urine, pale stools), or if abdominal pain, fever or diarrhea become pronounced.

Administration and Dosage:

Prior to starting therapy, determine laboratory and clinical documentation of infection. Continue therapy until tests indicate that active fungal infection has subsided.

Adults: Initially, 200 mg once daily. In very serious infections, or if clinical response is insufficient, increase dose to 400 mg once daily.

Children:

(> 2 years) – 3.3 to 6.6 mg/kg/day as a single daily dose.

(< 2 years) – Daily dosage has not been established.

Inadequate treatment periods may yield poor response and lead to early recurrence of clinical symptoms. Minimum treatment for candidiasis is 1 or 2 weeks and for the other indicated systemic mycoses, 6 months. Chronic mucocutaneous candidiasis usually requires maintenance therapy.

Minimum treatment of recalcitrant dermatophyte infections is 4 weeks in cases involving glabrous skin. Palmar and plantar infections may respond more slowly. Apparent cures may subsequently recur after discontinuation of therapy in some cases.

Rx	**Nizoral** (Janssen)	**Tablets:** 200 mg	(Janssen/Nizoral). White, scored. In 100s and UD 100s.

AMPHOTERICIN B

For topical amphotericin B, refer to the monograph in the Topical Anti-infectives section.

Warning:

Use primarily for treatment of patients with progressive and potentially fatal fungal infections. Do not use to treat the common clinically inapparent forms of fungal disease that show only positive skin or serologic tests. Do not use to treat noninvasive forms of fungal disease such as oral thrush, vaginal candidiasis and esophageal candidiasis in patients with normal neutrophil counts.

Actions:

Pharmacology: Amphotericin B is a polyene antibiotic produced by a strain of streptomyces nodosus that is fungistatic or fungicidal, depending on the concentration obtained in body fluids and on the susceptibility of the fungus. It acts by binding to sterols (primarily ergosterol) in the fungal cell membrane with a resultant change in membrane permeability, allowing leakage of a variety of intracellular components. Mammalian cell membranes also contain sterols, and the damage to human cells (toxicity) and fungal cells (antibiotic effect) may share common mechanisms.

Liposomal encapsulation or incorporation in a lipid complex can substantially affect a drug's functional properties relative to those of the unencapsulated or nonlipid-associated drug. In addition, different liposomal or lipid-complexed products with a common active ingredient may vary from one another in the chemical composition and physical form of the lipid component. Such differences may affect functional properties of these drug products.

Pharmacokinetics:

Absorption/Distribution –

Amphotericin B deoxycholate: An initial IV infusion of 1 to 5 mg/day, gradually increased to 0.4 to 0.6 mg/kg/day, produces peak plasma concentrations of ≈ 0.5 to 2 mcg/ml. Amphotericin B is highly protein bound (> 90%) and is poorly dialyzable. Approximately two-thirds of concurrent plasma concentrations have been detected in fluids from inflamed pleura, peritoneum, synovium and aqueous humor; concentrations in the cerebrospinal fluid seldom exceed 2.5% of those in the plasma; little amphotericin B penetrates into vitreous humor or normal amniotic fluid. Complete details of tissue distribution are not known.

Amphotericin B cholesteryl: The pharmacokinetics of amphotericin B cholesteryl were nonlinear. Steady-state volume of distribution (Vss) and total plasma clearance (CLt) increased with escalating doses, resulting in less than proportional increases in plasma concentration over a dose range of 0.5 to 8.0 mg/kg/day. After doses of 3 to 6 mg/kg/day, the Vss ranged from 3.8 to 4.5 L/kg, the distribution half-life from 3.5 to 3.4 minutes, the maximum plasma concentration achieved at the end of an infusion was 2.6 to 3.4 mcg/ml and the area under the plasma concentration time curve at steady-state was 29 to 50 mcg/ml. The increased volume of distribution probably reflected uptake by tissues. The covariates of body weight and dose level accounted for a substantial portion of the variability of the pharmacokinetic estimates between patients. The unexplained variability in clearance was 26%.

Metabolism/Excretion – Metabolic pathways of amphotericin B are not known. It has a relatively short initial serum half-life of 24 hours, followed by a second elimination phase with a half-life of ≈ 15 days. Liposomal amphotericin B has a mean terminal elimination half-life of 173.4 hours. The drug is slowly excreted by the kidneys with 2% to 5% as the biologically active form. After treatment is discontinued, amphotericin B can be detected in the urine for at least 7 weeks. The cumulative urinary output over 7 days amounts to ≈ 40% of the drug infused.

Following a 1 mg/kg/hour infusion, 25% of the total amphotericin B concentration measured in plasma was in the amphotericin B cholesteryl complex, dropping to 9.3% at 1 hour and 7.5% at 24 hours after the end of the infusion. At doses ranging from 3 to 6 mg/kg/day, the CLt was 0.105 to 0.121 L/hr/kg and the elimination half-life was 27.5 to 28.8 hours.

Children: Based on studies in a small number of premature infants and children, amphotericin B pharmacokinetics differ from those seen in adults and vary with the age of the child. Therefore, consider these differences when determining a dosing regimen and individualize doses based on therapeutic drug monitoring.

Microbiology:

Amphotericin B deoxycholate, a polyene antibiotic, is active in vitro against many species of fungi. *Histoplasma capsulatum, Coccidioides immitis, Candida* sp, *Blastomyces dermatitidis, Rhodotorula* sp, *Cryptococcus neoformans, Sporothrix schenckii, Mucor mucedo* and *Aspergillus fumigatus* are inhibited by concentrations ranging from 0.03 to 1 mcg/ml in vitro. It has no effect on bacteria, rickettsiae and viruses.

Liposomal amphotericin B is active in animal models against *Aspergillus fumigatus, Candida albicans, C. guillermondi, C. stellatoideae* and *C. tropicalis, Cryptococcus* sp, *Coccidioidomyces* sp, *Histoplasma* sp and *Blastomyces* sp in which endpoints were clearance of microorganisms from target organ(s) or prolonged survival of infected animals.

Amphotericin B cholesteryl is active in vitro against *Aspergillus* and *Candida* sp.

Clinical trials: In a randomized, double-blind study of amphotericin B cholesteryl (4 mg/kg/day) and amphotericin B deoxycholate (0.8 mg/kg/day) as empiric treatment in febrile neutropenic patients, it was demonstrated that in patients with normal baseline renal function the incidence of nephrotoxicity was significantly lower with amphotericin B cholesteryl than with amphotericin B deoxycholate.

Indications:

Amphotericin B deoxycholate: Administer amphotericin B for injection primarily to those patients with progressive potentially life-threatening fungal infections.

Fungal infection – Specifically intended to treat cryptococcosis (torulosis); North American blastomycosis; systemic candidiasis; the disseminated forms of moniliasis, coccidioidomycosis and histoplasmosis; zygomycosis including mucormycosis (phycomycosis) caused by species of the genera *Mucor, Rhizopus, Absidia, Entomophthora* and *Basidiobolus;* sporotrichosis *(S. schenckii);* aspergillosis *(A. fumigatus).*

May be helpful in the treatment of American mucocutaneous leishmaniasis, but it is not the drug of choice in primary therapy.

Liposomal amphotericin B is indicated for the treatment of invasive fungal infections in patients refractory to or intolerant of conventional amphotericin B therapy.

Amphotericin B cholesteryl: For the treatment of invasive aspergillosis in patients where renal impairment or unacceptable toxicity precludes the use of amphotericin B deoxycholate in effective doses and in patients with invasive aspergillosis where prior amphotericin B deoxycholate therapy has failed.

Unlabeled uses: Prophylactic use to prevent fungal infection in patients with bone marrow transplantation (0.1 mg/kg/day).

Contraindications:

Hypersensitivity to amphotericin B, unless the condition requiring treatment is life-threatening and amenable only to amphotericin B therapy.

Warnings:

Fatal fungal diseases: Amphotericin B is frequently the only effective treatment for potentially fatal fungal diseases. Balance its possible lifesaving effect against its dangerous side effects.

Nephrotoxicity: Renal damage, the most important toxic effect, is a limiting factor for the use of amphotericin B. Renal dysfunction usually improves upon interruption of therapy, dose reduction or increased dosing interval; however, some permanent impairment often occurs, especially in patients receiving large doses (> 5 g). Decreased glomerular filtration rate and renal blood flow, increased serum creatinine and renal tubular dysfunction are prominent. Sodium loading may be effective in reducing nephrotoxicity of amphotericin B in sodium-depleted patients, but this may be a problem in patients with cardiac or hepatic disease.

In some patients, hydration and sodium repletion prior to amphotericin B administration may reduce the risk of developing nephrotoxicity. Supplemental alkali medication may decrease renal tubular acidosis complications.

Acute reactions including fever, shaking chills, hypotension, anorexia, vomiting, nausea, headache and tachypnea are common 1 to 3 hours after starting an IV infusion. These reactions are usually more severe with the first few doses of amphotericin B and usually diminish with subsequent doses. Acute infusion-related reactions can be managed by pretreatment with antihistamines and corticosteroids or by reducing the rate of infusion and by prompt administration of antihistamines and corticosteroids.

Nephrocalcinosis is also commonly observed and usually improves upon interruption of therapy; however, some permanent impairment often occurs, especially in those patients receiving large amounts (> 5 g) of amphotericin B deoxycholate. Supplemental alkali medication may decrease renal tubular acidosis complications.

Rapid infusion: Avoid rapid infusion because it has been associated with hypotension, hypokalemia, arrhythmias and shock.

Leukoencephalopathy has been reported following use of amphotericin B. The literature has suggested that total body irradiation may be a predisposition.

Rhinocerebral phycomycosis, a fulminating disease, generally occurs in association with diabetic ketoacidosis. Diabetic control must be instituted before successful treatment with amphotericin B can be accomplished. Pulmonary phycomycosis, which is more common in association with hematologic malignancies, is often an incidental finding at autopsy. A cumulative dose of at least 3 g amphotericin B is recommended. Although a total dose of 3 to 4 g will infrequently cause lasting renal impairment, it is a reasonable minimum where there is clinical evidence of deep tissue invasion. Rhinocerebral phycomycosis usually follows a rapidly fatal course; therapy must be more aggressive than that for more indolent mycoses.

Hypersensitivity: Anaphylaxis has been reported with amphotericin B. If severe respiratory distress occurs, discontinue the infusion immediately. Do not give further infusions. Have cardiopulmonary resuscitation facilities available during administration.

Renal function impairment: Use with care in patients with reduced renal function; frequent monitoring is recommended (see Precautions).

Elderly: Sixty-one patients ≥ 65 years of age were treated with amphotericin B cholesteryl. Forty-nine elderly patients ≥ 65 years of age were treated with 5 mg/kg/day liposomal amphotericin B. No unexpected adverse events have been reported.

Pregnancy: Category B. Systemic fungal infections have been successfully treated in pregnant women with amphotericin B without obvious effects to the fetus, but the number of cases reported has been small. Adequate and well controlled studies have not been conducted; therefore, use during pregnancy only if clearly needed.

Lactation: It is not known whether amphotericin B is excreted in breast milk. However, consider discontinuing nursing or eliminating IV amphotericin B.

Children: Safety and efficacy in children have not been established. Systemic fungal infections have been successfully treated in children without reports of unusual side effects. Limit administration to the least amount compatible with an effective therapeutic regimen.

Precautions:

Monitoring: Perform BUN and serum creatinine or endogenous creatinine clearance tests at least weekly during therapy. If BUN exceeds 40 mg/dl or if serum creatinine exceeds 3 mg/dl, discontinue the drug or reduce dosage until renal function improves. Weekly hemograms, serum potassium and magnesium determinations are also advisable. Low serum magnesium levels have been noted during treatment. Discontinue therapy if liver function test results are abnormal (elevated bromsulphalein, alkaline phosphatase and bilirubin).

Monitor renal function frequently during amphotericin B therapy. It is also advisable to monitor liver function, serum electrolytes (particularly magnesium and potassium), blood counts and hemoglobin concentrations on a regular basis. Use laboratory test results as a guide to subsequent dose adjustments. Monitor complete blood count and prothrombin time as medically indicated.

Record the patient's temperature, pulse, respiration and blood pressure every 30 minutes for 2 to 4 hours after administration.

Prevention of adverse reactions: Most patients will exhibit some intolerance, often at less than full therapeutic dosage. Severe reactions may be lessened by giving aspirin, antipyretics (eg, acetaminophen), antihistamines and antiemetics before the infusion and by maintaining sodium balance. Administration on alternate days may decrease anorexia and phlebitis. Small doses of IV adrenal corticosteroids given prior to or during the infusion may decrease febrile reactions. Keep the dosage and duration of such corticosteroid therapy to a minimum (see Drug Interactions). In three patients, dantrolene was a successful adjunctive agent for the prophylaxis (50 mg oral) and treatment (50 mg IV) of amphotericin B-induced rigors. Adding a small amount of heparin to the infusion (500 to 2000 units), rapid infusion rate, removal of needle after infusion, rotation of infusion sites, administration through a large central vein and using a pediatric scalp-vein needle may lessen the incidence of thrombophlebitis. Extravasation may cause chemical irritation. Meperidine (25 to 50 mg IV) has been shown in some patients to decrease the duration of shaking chills and fever that may accompany infusion of amphotericin B.

Resistance: Variants with reduced susceptibility to amphotericin B have been isolated from several fungal species after serial passage in cell culture media containing the drug and from some patients receiving prolonged therapy with amphotericin B. The relevance of drug resistance to clinical outcome has not been established.

Prolonged therapy is usually necessary. Unpleasant reactions are common, and some are potentially dangerous. Use only in hospitalized patients or in those under close medical observation. Reserve use for those patients in whom a diagnosis of the progressive, potentially fatal forms of susceptible mycotic infections has been firmly established, preferably by positive culture or histologic study.

AMPHOTERICIN B

Therapy interruption: Whenever medication is interrupted for > 7 days, resume therapy with the lowest dosage level; increase gradually.

Pulmonary reactions characterized by acute dyspnea, hypoxemia and interstitial infiltrates have been observed in neutropenic patients receiving amphotericin B and leukocyte transfusions. Although pulmonary toxicity has occurred in association with either agent used alone, it was more frequent when amphotericin B was given after or during initiation of leukocyte transfusions. Administer amphotericin B cautiously in patients receiving leukocyte transfusions and separate the infusion as far as possible from the time of a leukocyte transfusion.

Laboratory test abnormalities:

Serum electrolyte abnormalities – Hypomagnesemia, hyperkalemia, hypocalcemia; hypercalcemia; hypokalemia.

Liver function test abnormalities – Increased AST, ALT, GGT, bilirubin, alkaline phosphatase and LDH.

Renal function test abnormalities – Increased BUN and serum creatinine.

Other test abnormalities – Acidosis, hypermylasemia, hypoglycemia, hyperglycemia, hyperuricemia, hypophosphatemia.

Drug Interactions:

Amphotericin B Drug Interactions			
Precipitant drug	Object drug*		Description
Antineoplastic agents	Amphotericin B	↑	Concurrent administration may enhance the potential for renal toxicity, bronchospasm and hypotension.
Corticosteroids and corticotropin	Amphotericin B	↑	Concurrent administration may potentiate hypokalemia and predispose the patient to cardiac dysfunction. Do not give unless necessary to control adverse reactions.
Zidovudine	Amphotericin B lipid complex	↑	Concurrent administration increases myelotoxicity and nephrotoxicity. If used concomitantly, closely monitor renal and hematologic function.
Amphotericin B	Cyclosporine/ Tacrolimus	↑	Coadministration of cyclosporine or tacrolimus causes an increase in serum creatinine levels.
Amphotericin B	Digitalis glycosides	↑	Concurrent administration may induce hypokalemia and may potentiate digitalis toxicity.
Amphotericin B	Flucytosine	↑	A synergistic relationship with amphotericin B has been reported. Flucytosine toxicity may be increased by increasing its cellular uptake or impairing renal excretion.
Amphotericin B	Imidazoles	↔	Antagonism between amphotericin B and imidazole derivatives such as miconazole and ketoconazole that inhibit ergosterol synthesis, has been reported in both in vitro and in vivo animal studies. The clinical significance of these findings has not been determined.
Amphotericin B	Nephrotoxic agents	↑	Nephrotoxic effects of cyclosporine appear to be increased. Take extra care when administering amphotericin B with other nephrotoxic agents.
Amphotericin B	Neuromuscular blocking agents	↑	Amphotericin B-induced hypokalemia may enhance the curariform affect of skeletal muscle relaxants.
Amphotericin B	Thiazides	↑	Electrolyte depletion may be intensified, particularly hypokalemia. Monitor potassium levels.

* ↑ = Object drug increased. ↔ = Undetermined effect.

Adverse Reactions:

Most frequent:

General toxic reactions – Fever (sometimes with shaking chills usually occurring within 15 to 20 minutes after initiation of treatment); headache; anorexia; malaise; generalized pain, including muscle and joint pains.

Cardiovascular – Hypotension; hypertension; tachycardia; tachypnea.

CNS – Confusion; headache; depression; thinking abnormal.

AMPHOTERICIN B

Dermatologic – Rash; pruritis; maculopapular rash.

GI – Nausea; vomiting; dyspepsia; diarrhea; cramping; epigastric pain; abdominal pain; melena; stomatitis; anorexia.

GU – Hematuria.

Hematologic – Normochromic, normocytic anemia; prothrombin time increased; anemia; coagulation disorder.

Metabolic/Nutritional – Bilirubinemia; increased serum creatinine; acidosis.

Renal – Decreased renal function abnormalities including: Azotemia, hypokalemia, hyposthenuria, renal tubular acidosis, and nephrocalcinosis (see Warnings); permanent damage is often related to a large total dose (> 5 g).

Respiratory – Respiratory failure; respiratory disorder; pneumonia; dyspnea; hypoxia; epistaxis; cough increased; lung disorder; hemoptysis; hyperventilation; apnea.

Local – Venous pain at the injection site with phlebitis and thrombophlebitis.

Miscellaneous – Weight loss; multiple organ failure; infection; rash; sweating; pain; chest pain; back pain; sepsis; face edema; mucous membrane disorder; asthenia; arrhythmias; peripheral edema; edema; eye hemorrhage.

Less frequent (or rare):

Cardiovascular – Arrhythmias; ventricular fibrillation; cardiac arrest; hypertension; hypotension; cardiac failure; pulmonary edema; shock; myocardial infarction; atrial fibrillation; bradycardia; congestive heart failure; heart arrest; hemorrhage; phlebitis; syncope; ventricular extrasystoles; postural hypotension; supraventricular tachycardia; hemoptysis; pulmonary embolus; cardiomyopathy; hypersensitivity pneumonitis; dyspnea; thrombophlebitis; pleural effusion.

CNS – Peripheral neuropathy; convulsions; encephalopathy; extrapyrimidal syndrome; dizziness; somnolence; agitation; stupor; tremor; anxiety; paresthesia; hallucinations; neuropathy; peripheral neuropathy; hypertonia; cerebral vascular accident; other neurologic symptoms.

Dermatologic – Maculopapular rash; pruritus (without rash); exfoliative dermatitis; erythema multiforme; skin disorder.

GI – Melena or hemorrhagic gastroenteritis; GI disorder; GI hemorrhage; hematemesis; dyspepsia; cramping; epigastric pain; diarrhea; hepatomegaly; cholangitis; cholecystitis.

Hematologic – Coagulation defects; thrombocytopenia; leukopenia; agranulocytosis; eosinophilia; leukocytosis; hypochromic anemia; leukocytosis; blood dyscrasias.

Hepatic – Acute liver failure; hepatitis; jaundice; veno-occlusive liver disease; hepatic failure.

Hypersensitivity – Anaphylactoid and other allergic reactions; bronchospasm; wheezing; asthma (see Warnings).

Renal – Acute renal failure; anuria; oliguria; kidney function abnormal.

Special Senses – Hearing loss; tinnitus; transient vertigo; blurred vision; diplopia; visual impairment.

Miscellaneous – Anaphylactoid reactions (see Warnings); flushing; dyspnea; impotence; myasthenia; arthralgia; myalgia; malaise; anuria; renal tubular acidosis; dysuria; abdomen enlarged; face edema; infection; injection site pain; injection site reaction.

Overdosage:

Amphotericin B overdose has been reported to cause cardio-respiratory arrest. Out of 15 patients reported to have received one or more doses of liposomal amphotericin B between 7 and 13 mg/kg, none had a serious acute reaction. If overdose is suspected, discontinue therapy, monitor clinical status and administer supportive therapy. Refer to General Management of Acute Overdosage. Amphotericin B is not hemodialyzable.

Administration and Dosage:

Amphotericin B deoxycholate:

Test dose – An initial test dose of 1 mg in 20 ml of dextrose injection 5% administered IV over 20 to 30 minutes may be preferred.

Administer by slow IV infusion over 6 hours at a concentration of 0.1 mg/ml.

Individualize dosage. Therapy is usually instituted with a daily dose of 0.25 mg/kg and gradually increased as tolerance permits. Data are insufficient to define total dosage requirements and duration of treatment necessary for eradication of mycoses such as phycomycosis. Optimal dose is unknown. Do not exceed a total daily dose of 1.5 mg/kg. Total daily dosage may range up to 1 mg/kg; alternate daily dosages range up to 1.5 mg/kg. Several months of therapy are usually necessary; a shorter period of therapy may be inadequate and lead to relapse.

Severe and rapidly progressive fungal infection – Therapy may be initiated with a daily dose of 0.3 mg/kg IV over 2 to 6 hours.

AMPHOTERICIN B

Impaired cardio-renal function or a severe reaction to the test dose – Initiate therapy with smaller daily doses (eg, 5 to 10 mg). Depending on the patient's cardio-renal status, doses may gradually be increased by 5 to 10 mg/day to a final daily dosage of 0.5 to 0.7 mg/kg.

Sporotrichosis – Usual dose per injection is 20 mg. Therapy has ranged up to 9 months.

Aspergillosis has been treated for ≤ 11 months with a total dose of ≤ 3.6 g/day.

Rhinocerebral phycomycosis – A cumulative dose of at least 3 g per day amphotericin B is recommended (see Warnings).

Unlabeled administration – Because of amphotericin's poor CNS penetration, fungal meningitis may require intrathecal or intraventricular administration. Doses range from 0.1 mg initially, increased gradually up to 0.5 mg every 48 to 72 hours.

Bladder irrigations have been used for the treatment of candidal cystitis with minimal toxicity. It has been administered in concentrations ranging from 5 to 15 mg/dl, instilled periodically or continuously for 5 to 10 days.

IV infusion of 45 minutes to 2 hours has been successful without resulting in hypotension and other local side effects.

Liposomal amphotericin B: The recommended daily dosage for adults and children is 5 mg/kg given as a single infusion. Administer IV at a rate of 2.5 mg/kg/hr. If the infusion time exceeds 2 hours, mix the contents by shaking the infusion bag every 2 hours.

Renal toxicity has been shown to be dose-dependent. Make decisions about dose adjustments only after taking into account the overall clinical condition of the patient.

Amphotericin B cholesteryl: For adults and children, therapy may begin at a daily dose of 3 to 4 mg/kg as required. The dose may be increased to 6 mg/kg/day if there is not improvement or if there is evidence of progression of the fungal infection.

Administer diluted in 5% Dextrose for Injection by IV infusion at a rate of 1 mg/kg/hr. A test dose immediately preceding the first dose is advisable when commencing all new courses of treatment. Infuse a small amount of drug (eg, 10 ml of the final preparation containing between 1.6 to 8.3 mg) over 15 to 30 minutes, and observe the patient carefully for the next 30 minutes.

The infusion time may be shortened to a minimum of 2 hours for patients who show no evidence of intolerance or infusion-related reactions. If the patient experiences acute reactions or cannot tolerate the infusion volume, the infusion time may be extended.

Preparation of solutions:

Amphotericin B deoxycholate – For initial concentration of 5 mg/ml, rapidly inject 10 ml Sterile Water for Injection without a bacteriostatic agent directly into the lyophilized cake, using a sterile needle (minimum diameter: 20 gauge). Shake the vial immediately until the colloidal solution is clear. The infusion solution, providing 0.1 mg/ml, is then obtained by further dilution (1:50) with 5% Dextrose Injection of pH above 4.2.

Ascertain the pH of each container of Dextrose Injection before use. Commercial Dextrose Injection usually has a pH above 4.2; however, if it is below 4.2, then add 1 or 2 ml of buffer to the Dextrose Injection before it is used to dilute the concentrated solution of amphotericin B. The recommended buffer has the following composition: Dibasic sodium phosphate (anhydrous) 1.59 g; monobasic sodium phosphate (anhydrous) 0.96 g; Water for Injection, dilute to 100 ml.

Sterilize the buffer before adding to the Dextrose Injection, either by filtration through a bacterial retentive stone, mat or membrane, or by autoclaving for 30 minutes at 15 lb pressure (121°C).

Caution: Do not reconstitute with saline solutions. Use of any other diluent or presence of a bacteriostatic agent in the diluent may cause precipitation.

An in-line membrane filter may be used for IV infusion. To assure passage of the antibiotic colloidal dispersion, the filter's mean pore diameter should be ≥ 1 micron.

Liposomal amphotericin B – Shake the vial gently until there is no yellow sediment at the bottom. Withdraw the appropriate dose of liposomal amphotericin B from the required number of vials into one or more sterile 20 ml syringes using an 18–gauge needle. Remove the needle from each syringe filled with liposomal amphotericin B, and replace with a 5–micron filter needle. Each filter needle may be used to filter the content of ≤ 4 vials. Insert the filter needle of the syringe into an IV bag containing 5% Dextrose Injection, and empty the contents of the syringe into the bag. The infusion concentration should be 1 mg/ml. For pediatric patients and patients with cardiovascular disease the drug may be diluted with 5% Dextrose Injection to a final infusion concentration of 2 mg/ml.

AMPHOTERICIN B

Amphotericin B cholesteryl must be reconstituted by addition of Sterile Water for Injection. Using sterile syringe and a 20–gauge needle, rapidly add the following volumes to the vial to provide a liquid containing 5 mg/ml. Shake gently by hand, rotating the vial until all solids have dissolved. Note that the fluid may be opalescent or clear.

- 50 mg/vial add 10 ml Sterile Water for Injection
- 100 mg/vial add 20 ml Sterile Water for InjectionFor infusion, further dilute the reconstituted liquid to a final concentration of $\approx$ 0.6 mg/ml.

Do not reconstitute the lyophilized powder with saline or dextrose solutions or admix the reconstituted liquid with saline or electrolytes.

Admixture incompatibility:

Liposomal amphotericin B – Do not dilute with saline solutions or mix with other drugs or electrolytes as the compatibility of liposomal amphotericin B with these materials has not been established. Flush an existing IV line with 5% Dextrose Injection before infusion of liposomal amphotericin B, or use a separate infusion line.

Do not use an in-line filter.

Amphotericin B cholesteryl – Do not filter or use an in-line filter with amphotericin B cholesteryl.

Storage/Stability: The manufacturer recommends that the solution be protected from light during administration. Although solutions of amphotericin B are light sensitive, loss of drug activity is reported to be negligible when solutions are exposed to light for 8 hours. Therefore, it is probably not necessary to cover infusion containers if administered within 8 hours of reconstitution.

Amphotericin B deoxycholate – Refrigerate vials; protect against exposure to light. The concentrate (after reconstitution) may be stored in the dark at room temperature for 24 hours or under refrigeration for 1 week with minimal loss of potency and clarity. Discard any unused material. Use solutions prepared for IV infusions promptly.

Liposomal amphotericin B – Prior to admixture, store liposomal amphotericin B at 2° to 8°C (36° to 46°F). Protect from exposure to light. Do not freeze. Retain liposomal amphotericin B in the carton until time of use. The admixed liposomal amphotericin B and 5% Dextrose Injection may be stored for $\leq$ 48 hours at 2° to 8°C (36° to 46°F) and an additional 6 hours at room temperature. Discard any unused material.

Amphotericin B cholesteryl – Store unopened vials at 15° to 30°C (59° to 86°F). After reconstitution, refrigerate the drug at 2° to 8°C (36° to 46°F), and use within 24 hours. Do not freeze. After further dilution with 5% Dextrose for Injection, store in a refrigerator (2° to 8°C; 36° to 46°F), and use within 24 hours.

Rx	**Amphotericin B** (Pharma-Tek)	**Injection (lyophylized cake)**: 50 mg (as deoxycholate)	In vials.[1]
Rx	**Fungizone Intravenous** (Bristol-Myers Squibb)		In vials.[1]
Rx	**Abelcet** (Liposome Co.)	**Suspension for Injection**: 100 mg/20 ml (as liposomal complex)	In single-use vials with 5-micron filter needles.
Rx	**Amphotec** (Sequus Pharmaceuticals)	**Powder for Injection, lyophilized**: 50 mg (as cholesteryl)	In 20 ml vials.[2]
		100 mg (as cholesteryl)	In 50 ml vials.[2]
🍁	**Fungizone** (Squibb)	**Powder for Injection, lyophilized**: 50 mg	In 20 ml vials.[2]

[1] With 41 mg sodium desoxycholate.

[2] With 52.8 mg sodium cholesteryl sulfate.

GRISEOFULVIN

Actions:

Pharmacology: Griseofulvin, an antibiotic derived from a species of *Penicillium*, is deposited in the keratin precursor cells, which are gradually exfoliated and replaced by noninfected tissue; it has a greater affinity for diseased tissue. The drug is tightly bound to the new keratin, which becomes highly resistant to fungal invasions.

Pharmacokinetics: The peak serum level found in fasting adults given 0.5 g griseofulvin microsize occurs at about 4 hours and ranges between 0.5 to 2 mcg/ml. Some individuals are consistently "poor absorbers" and tend to attain lower blood levels at all times. The serum level may be increased by giving the drug with a meal with a high fat content. GI absorption varies considerably among individuals, due to insolubility of the drug in aqueous media of the upper GI tract. The efficiency of GI absorption of the ultramicrocrystalline formulation is ≈ 1.5 times that of conventional microsized griseofulvin. This factor permits the oral intake of ⅔ as much ultramicrocrystalline griseofulvin as the microsized form; but there is no evidence that this confers any significant clinical differences in regard to safety and efficacy.

Microbiology: Fungistatic with in vitro activity against species of *Microsporum, Epidermophyton* and *Trichophyton*. It has no effect on bacteria or other fungi.

Indications:

Ringworm infections: Treatment of ringworm infections of the skin, hair and nails, namely: Tinea corporis, tinea pedis, tinea cruris, tinea barbae, tinea capitis, tinea unguium (onychomycosis) when caused by one or more of the following genera of fungi: *Trichophyton rubrum; T. tonsurans; T. mentagrophytes; T. interdigitalis; T. verrucosum; T. megnini; T. gallinae; T. crateriform; T. sulphureum; T. schoenleini; Microsporum audouini; M. canis; M. gypseum; Epidermophyton floccosum.*

Note: Prior to therapy, identify the types of fungi responsible for the infection. Use of this drug is not justified in minor or trivial infections which will respond to topical agents alone.

Griseofulvin is NOT effective in bacterial infections; candidiasis (moniliasis); histoplasmosis; actinomycosis; sporotrichosis; chromoblastomycosis; coccidioidomycosis; North American blastomycosis; cryptococcosis (torulosis); tinea versicolor; nocardiosis.

Contraindications:

Hypersensitivity to griseofulvin; porphyria; hepatocellular failure.

Warnings:

Prophylaxis: Safety and efficacy for prophylaxis of fungal infections have not been established.

Hypersensitivity reactions (eg, skin rashes, urticaria, angioneurotic edema) may occur and necessitate withdrawal of therapy. Institute appropriate counter measures; refer to Management of Acute Hypersensitivity Reactions.

Carcinogenesis: Chronic feeding of griseofulvin to mice, at levels ranging from 0.5% to 2.5% of the diet, resulted in the development of liver tumors. Smaller particle sizes resulted in an enhanced effect. Thyroid tumors developed in male rats receiving griseofulvin at levels of 2%, 1% and 0.2% of the diet.

In subacute toxicity studies, griseofulvin produced hepatocellular necrosis in mice, but not in other species. Griseofulvin produced disturbances in porphyrin metabolism, a colchicine-like effect on mitosis and cocarcinogenicity with methylcholanthrene in cutaneous tumor induction in laboratory animals.

Pregnancy: Category C. Griseofulvin was embryotoxic and teratogenic in rats. Rare cases of conjoined twins have been reported in patients taking griseofulvin during the first trimester of pregnancy. Do not give to pregnant women or women contemplating pregnancy.

Precautions:

Prolonged therapy: Closely observe patients on prolonged therapy. Periodically monitor renal, hepatic and hematopoietic function.

Penicillin cross-sensitivity is possible because griseofulvin is derived from species of *Penicillium*; however, known penicillin-sensitive patients have been treated without difficulty.

Lupus erythematosus, lupus-like syndromes or exacerbation of lupus erythematosus have occurred in patients receiving griseofulvin.

Photosensitivity may occur; caution patients to take protective measures (eg, sunscreens, protective clothing) against exposure to ultraviolet light or sunlight.

Photosensitivity reactions may aggravate lupus erythematosus.

GRISEOFULVIN

Drug Interactions:

Griseofulvin Drug Interactions			
Precipitant drug	Object drug*		Description
Griseofulvin	Anticoagulants	⬇	Griseofulvin may decrease the hypoprothrombinemic activity of warfarin; patients may require anticoagulant dosage adjustment.
Griseofulvin	Contraceptives, oral	⬇	Loss of contraceptive effectiveness may occur, possibly leading to breakthrough bleeding, amenorrhea or unintended pregnancy.
Griseofulvin	Cyclosporine	⬇	Cyclosporine levels may be reduced, resulting in a decrease in pharmacologic effects.
Griseofulvin	Salicylates	⬇	Serum salicylate concentrations may be decreased.
Barbiturates	Griseofulvin	⬇	Serum griseofulvin levels may be decreased.

* ⬇ = Object drug decreased.

Adverse Reactions:

Most common: Hypersensitivity reactions, such as skin rashes, urticaria, and rarely, angioneurotic edema may occur. See Warnings.

Occasional: Oral thrush; nausea; vomiting; epigastric distress; diarrhea; headache; fatigue; dizziness; insomnia; mental confusion; impairment of performance of routine activities.

Rare: Griseofulvin interferes with porphyrin metabolism. Proteinuria; leukopenia; hepatic toxicity; GI bleeding; menstrual irregularities; paresthesias of the hands and feet after extended therapy. Discontinue administration if granulocytopenia occurs. When rare, serious reactions occur with griseofulvin, they are usually associated with high dosages, long periods of therapy or both.

Patient Information:

Beneficial effects may not be noticeable for some time; continue taking medication for entire course of therapy.

Photosensitivity reactions may occur; avoid prolonged exposure to sunlight or sunlamps.

Notify physician if fever, sore throat or skin rash occurs.

Oral suspension: Store at room temperature in a light resistant container.

Administration and Dosage:

Accurate diagnosis of the infecting organism is essential.

Duration of therapy: Continue medication until the infecting organism is completely eradicated, as indicated by appropriate clinical or laboratory examination. Representative treatment periods are: Tinea capitis, 4 to 6 weeks; tinea corporis, 2 to 4 weeks; tinea pedis, 4 to 8 weeks; tinea unguium (depending on rate of growth) – fingernails, at least 4 months, toenails, at least 6 months.

Hygiene: Observe good hygiene to control sources of infection or reinfection. Concomitant use of appropriate topical agents is usually required, particularly in treatment of tinea pedis. In some forms of athlete's foot, yeasts and bacteria may be involved, as well as fungi. Griseofulvin will not eradicate the bacterial or monilial infection.

Adults: Tinea corporis, tinea cruris, tinea capitis - A single or divided daily dose of 500 mg microsize (330 to 375 mg ultramicrosize) will give a satisfactory response in most patients.

Tinea pedis, tinea unguium – 0.75 to 1 g microsize (660 to 750 mg ultramicrosize) per day in divided doses.

Children: Approximately 11 mg microsize/kg/day (5 mg/lb/day) or 7.3 mg ultramicrosize/kg/day (3.3 mg/lb/day) is an effective dose for most children. The following dosage schedule is suggested:

Griseofulvin Dosage for Children Based on Weight			
Weight		Daily dose (mg)	
lb	kg	microsize	ultramicrosize
30 to 50	13.6 to 23	125 to 250	82.5 to 165
> 50	> 23	250 to 500	165 to 330

Clinical experience indicates that a single daily dose is effective in children with tinea capitis.

Children (≤ 2 years of age) – Dosage not established.

GRISEOFULVIN MICROSIZE

Complete prescribing information begins in the Griseofulvin group monograph.

Rx	**Fulvicin U/F** (Schering)	**Tablets:** 250 mg	(Schering AUF or 948). White, scored. In 60s and 250s.
Rx	**Grifulvin V** (Ortho Derm)		(Ortho 211). White, scored. In 100s.
Rx	**Fulvicin U/F** (Schering)	**Tablets:** 500 mg	(Schering AUG or 496). White, scored. In 60s and 250s.
Rx	**Grifulvin V** (Ortho Derm)		(Ortho 214). White, scored. In 100s and 500s.
Rx	**Grisactin 500** (Wyeth-Ayerst)		(Grisactin 500444). Scored. In 60s.
Rx	**Grisactin 250** (Wyeth-Ayerst)	**Capsules:** 250 mg	(Grisactin 250443). In 100s and 500s.
Rx	**Grifulvin V** (Ortho Derm)	**Oral Suspension:** 125 mg/5 ml	0.2% alcohol, saccharin, sucrose. In 120 ml.

GRISEOFULVIN ULTRAMICROSIZE

Complete prescribing information begins in the Griseofulvin group monograph.

The efficiency of GI absorption of griseofulvin ultramicrosize is approximately 1.5 times that of conventional microsized griseofulvin. This factor permits the oral intake of two-thirds as much ultramicrosize as the microsize form, but there is no evidence that this confers any significant clinical difference in regard to safety and efficacy.

Rx	**Fulvicin P/G** (Schering)	**Tablets:** 125 mg	(Schering 228). White, scored. In 100s.
Rx	**Grisactin Ultra** (Wyeth-Ayerst)		(Grisactin Ultra 125). White. Square. In 100s.
Rx	**Gris-PEG** (Allergan Herbert)		(Gris-PEG 125). White, scored. Elliptical. Film coated. In 100s.
Rx	**Fulvicin P/G** (Schering)	**Tablets:** 165 mg	(Fulvicin P/G 654). Off-white, scored. Oval. In 100s.
Rx	**Ultramicrosize Griseofulvin** (Various, eg, Sidmak)		In 100s.
Rx	**Fulvicin P/G** (Schering)	**Tablets:** 250 mg	(Schering 507). White, scored. In 100s.
Rx	**Grisactin Ultra** (Wyeth-Ayerst)		(Grisactin Ultra 250). White. Square. In 100s.
Rx	**Gris-PEG** (Allergan Herbert)		(Gris-PEG 250). White, scored. Capsule shape. Film coated. In 100s and 500s.
Rx	**Fulvicin P/G** (Schering)	**Tablets:** 330 mg	(Fulvicin P/G 352). Off-white, scored. Oval. In 100s.
Rx	**Grisactin Ultra** (Wyeth-Ayerst)		(Grisactin Ultra 330). White, scored. Oval. In 100s.
Rx	**Ultramicrosize Griseofulvin** (Various, eg, Sidmak)		In 100s.

FLUCONAZOLE

Actions:

Pharmacology: Fluconazole, a synthetic broad spectrum bis-triazole antifungal agent, is a highly selective inhibitor of fungal cytochrome P-450 and sterol C-14 alpha-demethylation. Mammalian cell demethylation is much less sensitive to fluconazole inhibition. The subsequent loss of normal sterols correlates with the accumulation of 14 alpha-methyl sterols in fungi and may be responsible for the fungistatic activity of fluconazole.

In healthy volunteers, fluconazole administration (doses ranging from 200 to 400 mg once daily for up to 14 days) was associated with small and inconsistent effects on testosterone concentrations, endogenous corticosteroid concentrations and the ACTH-stimulated cortisol response.

Pharmacokinetics:

Absorption/Distribution – The pharmacokinetic properties of fluconazole are similar following administration by the IV or oral routes. In healthy volunteers, the bioavailability of oral fluconazole is > 90% compared with IV administration. Bioequivalence was established between the 100 mg tablet and both suspension strengths when administered as a single 200 mg dose.

Peak plasma concentrations (C_{max}) in fasted healthy volunteers occur between 1 and 2 hours with a terminal plasma elimination half-life of ≈ 30 hrs (range, 20 to 50) after oral administration. A single oral 400 mg dose leads to a mean C_{max} of 6.72 mcg/ml (range, 4.12 to 8.08); after single oral doses of 50 to 400 mg, plasma concentrations and AUC are dose-proportional. A single 150 mg oral dose to 10 lactating women resulted in a mean C_{max} of 2.61 mcg/ml (range, 1.57 to 3.65).

Steady-state concentrations are reached within 5 to 10 days following oral doses of 50 to 400 mg given once daily. Administration of a loading dose (day 1) of twice the usual daily dose results in plasma concentrations close to steady state by day 2. The apparent volume of distribution approximates that of total body water. Plasma protein binding is low (11% to 12%). Following either single or multiple oral doses for up to 14 days, fluconazole penetrates into all body fluids studied (see table).

Tissue/Fluid Concentration of Fluconazole

Tissue or fluid	Concentration[1] (tissue/plasma ratio)
Cerebrospinal fluid[2]	0.5-0.9
Saliva	1
Sputum	1
Blister fluid	1
Urine	10
Normal skin	10
Nails	1
Blister skin	2
Vaginal tissue	1
Vaginal fluid	0.4-0.7

[1] Relative to plasma concentrations in subjects with normal renal function.
[2] Independent of degree of meningeal inflammation.

Metabolism/Excretion – In healthy volunteers, fluconazole is cleared primarily by renal excretion, with ≈ 80% of the dose appearing in the urine unchanged, ≈ 11% as metabolites. The pharmacokinetics of fluconazole are markedly affected by reduction in renal function. There is an inverse relationship between the elimination half-life and creatinine clearance. The dose may need to be reduced in patients with impaired renal function (see Administration and Dosage). A 3 hour hemodialysis session decreases plasma concentrations by ≈ 50%.

Doses of 200 to 400 mg once daily for up to 2 weeks in healthy volunteers were associated with small, inconsistent effects on testosterone and endogenous corticosteroid concentrations and the ACTH-stimulated cortisol response.

Microbiology: Fluconazole exhibits in vitro activity against *Cryptococcus neoformans* and *Candida* sp. Fungistatic activity has also been demonstrated in normal and immunocompromised animal models for systemic and intracranial fungal infections due to *C neoformans* and for systemic infections due to *C albicans.* Development of resistance to fluconazole has not been studied; however, there have been reports of cases of superinfection with *Candida* species other than *C albicans,* which are often inherently nonsusceptible to fluconazole (eg, *C krusei*). Such cases may require alternative antifungal therapy.

FLUCONAZOLE

In common with other azole antifungal agents, most fungi show a higher apparent sensitivity to fluconazole in vivo than in vitro. Activity has been demonstrated against fungal infections caused by *Aspergillus flavus* and *A fumigatus* in mice. Fluconazole is active in animal models of endemic mycoses, including one model of *Blastomyces dermatitidis* pulmonary infections, one model of *Coccidioides immitis* intracranial infections and several models of *Histoplasma capsulatum* pulmonary infection.

Coadministration of fluconazole and amphotericin B in infected normal and immunosuppressed mice showed a small additive antifungal effect in systemic infection with *C albicans,* no interaction in intracranial infection with *C neoformans,* and antagonism of the two drugs in systemic infection with *A fumigatus.*

Clinical trials:

Cryptococcal meningitis – Fluconazole (200 mg/day) was compared to amphotericin B (0.3 mg/kg/day) for cryptococcal meningitis in AIDS patients. Mortality among high-risk patients was 33% and 40% for amphotericin B and fluconazole, respectively, with overall deaths 14% and 18%, respectively.

Vaginal candidiasis – In two studies of patients with vaginal candidiasis, the results of the 150 mg single-dose fluconazole regimen were comparable to the control regimen (clotrimazole or miconazole intravaginally for 7 days) at the 1 month post-treatment evaluation. The therapeutic cure rate (complete resolution of signs and symptoms [clinical cure] along with a negative KOH examination and negative culture for *Candida* [microbiologic eradication]) was 55% for both groups. Approximately 75% of patients had acute vaginitis and achieved 80% clinical cure, 67% mycologic eradication and 59% therapeutic cure with fluconazole, which was comparable to controls. The remaining 25% of patients had recurrent vaginitis and achieved 57% clinical cure, 47% mycologic eradication and 40% therapeutic cure; the numbers are too small to make a meaningful comparison with controls.

Indications:

Candidiasis:

Treatment – Oropharyngeal and esophageal candidiasis.

Candidal urinary tract infections, peritonitis and systemic candidal infections including candidemia, disseminated candidiasis and pneumonia.

Vaginal candidiasis (vaginal yeast infections due to *Candida*).

Prophylaxis – To decrease the incidence of candidiasis in patients undergoing bone marrow transplantation who receive cytotoxic chemotherapy or radiation therapy.

Cryptococcal meningitis: Treatment of cryptococcal meningitis.

Contraindications:

Hypersensitivity to fluconazole or to any excipients in the product. There is no information regarding cross hypersensitivity between fluconazole and other azole antifungal agents; use with caution in patients with hypersensitivity to other azoles.

Warnings:

Causative organisms: Obtain specimens for fungal culture and other relevant laboratory studies (serology, histopathology) prior to therapy to isolate and identify causative organisms. Therapy may be instituted before the results are known; however, once these results become available, adjust anti-infective therapy accordingly.

Hepatic injury: Fluconazole has been associated with rare cases of serious hepatic toxicity. The spectrum has ranged from mild transient elevations in transaminases to clinical hepatitis, cholestasis and fulminant hepatic failure, including fatalities. Instances of fatal hepatic reactions occurred primarily in patients with serious underlying medical conditions (predominantly AIDS or malignancy) and often while taking multiple concomitant medications. In cases of fluconazole-associated hepatotoxicity, no obvious relationship to total daily dose, duration of therapy, sex or age of the patient has been observed. Fluconazole hepatotoxicity has usually, but not always, been reversible on discontinuation of therapy. Patients who develop abnormal liver function tests during fluconazole therapy should be monitored for the development of more severe hepatic injury. Fluconazole should be discontinued if clinical signs and symptoms consistent with liver disease develop that may be attributable to fluconazole. Transient hepatic reactions, including hepatitis and jaundice have occurred among patients with no other identifiable risk factors. In each of these cases, liver function returned to baseline on discontinuation of fluconazole.

Anaphylaxis: In rare cases, anaphylaxis has occurred.

Dermatologic changes: Patients have rarely developed exfoliative skin disorders during treatment with fluconazole. In patients with serious underlying diseases (predominantly AIDS and malignancy), these have rarely resulted in a fatal outcome. Patients who develop rashes during treatment with fluconazole should be monitored closely and the drug discontinued if lesions progress.

FLUCONAZOLE

Carcinogenesis/Fertility impairment: Male rats treated with 5 and 10 mg/kg/day had an increased incidence of hepatocellular adenomas.

Onset of parturition was slightly delayed in rats at 20 mg/kg orally. With doses of 5, 20 and 40 mg/kg, dystocia and prolongation of parturition were observed in a few dams at 20 mg/kg (approximately 5 to 15 times the recommended human dose) and 40 mg/kg, but not at 5 mg/kg. The effects on parturition in rats are consistent with the species-specific, estrogen-lowering property produced by high doses of fluconazole. Such a hormone change has not been observed in women treated with fluconazole. (See Pharmacology.)

Pregnancy: Category C. Fluconazole was administered orally to pregnant rabbits during organogenesis in two studies at 5, 10 and 20 mg/kg and at 5, 25 and 75 mg/kg, respectively. Maternal weight gain was impaired at all dose levels and abortions occurred at 75 mg/kg (approximately 20 to 60 times the recommended human dose); no adverse fetal effects were detected. In several studies in which pregnant rats were treated orally with fluconazole during organogenesis, maternal weight gain was impaired and placental weights were increased at 25 mg/kg. There were no fetal effects at 5 or 10 mg/kg; increases in fetal anatomical variants (eg, supernumerary ribs, renal pelvis dilation) and delays in ossification were observed at 25 and 50 mg/kg and higher doses. At doses ranging from 80 mg/kg (approximately 20 to 60 times the recommended human dose) to 320 mg/kg, embryolethality in rats was increased and fetal abnormalities included wavy ribs, cleft palate and abnormal cranio-facial ossification. These effects are consistent with the inhibition of estrogen synthesis in rats and may be a result of known effects of lowered estrogen on pregnancy, organogenesis and parturition.

There are no adequate and well controlled studies in pregnant women. Use in pregnancy only if the potential benefit justifies the possible risk to the fetus.

Lactation: Fluconazole is excreted in breast milk at concentrations similar to plasma. Therefore, the use of fluconazole in nursing mothers is not recommended.

Children: Efficacy has not been established in children. A small number of patients from age 3 to 13 years have been treated safely with fluconazole using doses of 3 to 6 mg/kg daily. Safety and efficacy of the single-dose regimen for vaginal candidiasis in patients < 18 years of age have not been established.

Precautions:

Single-dose use: Weigh the convenience and efficacy of the single dose regimen for treatment of vaginal yeast infections against the acceptability of a higher incidence of adverse reactions with fluconazole (26%) vs intravaginal agents (16%).

Drug Interactions:

Fluconazole Drug Interactions			
Precipitant drug	Object drug*		Description
Cimetidine	Fluconazole	↓	Cimetidine resulted in a reduction in fluconazole AUC and C_{max}.
Hydrochlorothiazide	Fluconazole	↑	Concomitant use resulted in a significant increase in fluconazole C_{max} and AUC, which can be attributed to reduced renal clearance.
Rifampin	Fluconazole	↓	A single oral fluconazole dose after chronic rifampin resulted in a decrease in AUC and a shorter half-life of fluconazole.
Fluconazole	Antihistamines, nonsedating	↑	Although terfenadine levels were not affected by fluconazole, terfenadine metabolite AUC increased.
Fluconazole	Contraceptives, oral	↔	Concurrent use with an OC containing ethinyl estradiol/levonorgestrel produced an overall mean increase in the levels of the OC components; however, in some cases there were decreases up to 47% and 33% of ethinyl estradiol and levonorgestrel levels, respectively.
Fluconazole	Cyclosporine	↑	Significant increases in cyclosporine C_{max}, C_{min} and AUC values occurred following fluconazole use.
Fluconazole	Phenytoin	↑	Coadministration resulted in an increase of phenytoin AUC values.
Fluconazole	Theophylline	↑	Theophylline AUC, C_{max} and half-life were significantly increased and clearance was decreased.

Fluconazole Drug Interactions			
Precipitant drug	Object drug*		Description
Fluconazole	Sulfonylureas	⬆	Fluconazole resulted in significant increases in C_{max} and AUC of tolbutamide, glyburide and glipizide. Several subjects experienced symptoms consistent with hypoglycemia; some required oral glucose treatment.
Fluconazole	Warfarin	⬆	A single warfarin dose after 14 days of fluconazole resulted in an increase in the PT response (area under the prothrombin time-time curve). Of 13 subjects, 1 experienced a twofold increase in PT response.
Fluconazole	Zidovudine	⬆	There was a significant increase in zidovudine AUC following fluconazole administration.

* ⬆ = Object drug increased. ⬇ = Object drug decreased. ⟷ = Undetermined effect.

Adverse Reactions:

Patients receiving single doses: In 448 patients with vaginal candidiasis receiving single 150 mg doses, the overall incidence of adverse reactions was 26%. In 422 patients receiving active comparative agents, the incidence was 16%. Effects reported with fluconazole were: Headache (13%); nausea (7%); abdominal pain (6%); diarrhea (3%); dyspepsia, dizziness, taste perversion (1%); angioedema, anaphylactic reaction (rare). Most reactions were mild to moderate in severity.

Patients receiving multiple doses: In > 4000 patients treated with fluconazole in clinical trials ≥ 7 days, 16% experienced adverse events. Treatment was discontinued in 1.5% of patients due to adverse clinical events and in 1.3% of patients due to laboratory test abnormalities. Clinical adverse events were reported more frequently in HIV-infected patients (21%) than in non-HIV infected patients (13%); however, the patterns in both patients were similar. The proportions of patients discontinuing therapy due to clinical adverse events were similar in the two groups (1.5%).

The following adverse events have occurred: Nausea (3.7%); headache (1.9%); skin rash (1.8%); vomiting (1.7%), abdominal pain (1.7%); diarrhea (1.5%); seizures; exfoliative skin disorders (including Stevens-Johnson syndrome and toxic epidermal necrolysis) (see Warnings); alopecia; leukopenia; thrombocytopenia; hypercholesterolemia, hypertriglyceridemia; hypokalemia; serious hepatic reactions (see Warnings).

Lab test abnormalities: In two comparative trials a statistically significant increase was observed in median AST levels from a baseline value of 30 to 41 IU/L in one trial and 34 to 66 IU/L in the other. The overall rate of serum transaminase elevations of more than 8 times the upper limit of normal was approximately 1% in fluconazole-treated patients in clinical trials. These elevations occurred in patients with severe underlying disease, predominantly AIDS or malignancies, most of whom were receiving multiple concomitant medications, including many known to be hepatotoxic. The incidence of abnormally elevated serum transaminases was greater in patients taking fluconazole concomitantly with one or more of the following medications: Rifampin, phenytoin, isoniazid, valproic acid or oral sulfonylurea hypoglycemic agents.

Overdosage:

Symptoms: There has been one reported case of overdosage; a 42-year-old patient infected with HIV developed hallucinations and exhibited paranoid behavior after reportedly ingesting 8.2 g of fluconazole. The patient's condition improved within 48 hours. In mice and rats receiving very high doses of fluconazole, clinical effects included decreased motility and respiration, ptosis, lacrimation, salivation, urinary incontinence, loss of righting reflex and cyanosis; death was sometimes preceded by clonic convulsions.

Treatment: In the event of overdose, institute symptomatic treatment (with supportive measures and gastric lavage if clinically indicated). Refer to General Management of Acute Overdosage.

Fluconazole is largely excreted in urine. A 3 hour hemodialysis session decreases plasma levels by approximately 50%.

FLUCONAZOLE

Administration and Dosage:

Single dose:

Vaginal candidiasis – 150 mg as a single oral dose.

Multiple dose: Individualize dosage. Since oral absorption is rapid and almost complete, the daily dose of fluconazole is the same for oral and IV administration. In general, a loading dose of twice the daily dose is recommended on the first day of therapy to result in plasma levels close to steady state by the second day of therapy.

For infections other than vaginal candidiasis, base the daily dose on the infecting organism and patient response to therapy. Continue treatment until clinical parameters or lab tests indicate that active fungal infection has subsided. An inadequate treatment period may lead to recurrence of active infection. Patients with AIDS and cryptococcal meningitis or recurrent oropharyngeal candidiasis usually require maintenance therapy to prevent relapse.

Oropharyngeal candidiasis – 200 mg on first day, followed by 100 mg once daily. Clinical evidence of oropharyngeal candidiasis generally resolves within several days, but continue treatment for 2 weeks to decrease likelihood of relapse.

Esophageal candidiasis – 200 mg on the first day, followed by 100 mg once daily. Doses up to 400 mg/day may be used, based on the patient's response. Treat patients with esophageal candidiasis for a minimum of 3 weeks and for at least 2 weeks following resolution of symptoms.

Candidiasis, other – For candidal UTIs and peritonitis, 50 to 200 mg/day has been used. For systemic candidal infections (including candidemia, disseminated candidiasis and pneumonia), optimal dosage and duration have not been determined, although doses up to 400 mg/day have been used.

Prevention of candidiasis in bone marrow transplant – 400 mg once daily. In patients who are anticipated to have severe granulocytopenia (< 500 neutrophils/mm^3), start fluconazole prophylaxis several days before anticipated onset of neutropenia, and continue 7 days after neutrophil count rises above 1000 cells/mm^3.

Cryptococcal meningitis – 400 mg on the first day, followed by 200 mg once daily. A dosage of 400 mg once daily may be used, based on the patient's response to therapy. The duration of treatment for initial therapy of cryptococcal meningitis is 10 to 12 weeks after the cerebrospinal fluid becomes culture negative. The dosage of fluconazole for suppression of relapse of cryptococcal meningitis in patients with AIDS is 200 mg once daily.

Children:

Fluconazole Dosage in Children

Pediatric Patients	Adults
3 mg/kg	100 mg
6 mg/kg	200 mg
12 mg/kg[1]	400 mg

[1] Some older children may have clearances similar to that of adults. Absolute doses exceeding 600 mg/day are not recommended.

Experience in neonates is limited to pharmacokinetic studies in premature newborns. Based on the prolonged half-life seen in premature newborns (gestational age 26 to 29 weeks), these children, in the first 2 weeks of life, should receive the same dosage (mg/kg) as in older children, but administered every 72 hours. After the first 2 weeks, dose these children once daily.

Oropharyngeal candidiasis – The recommended dosage is 6 mg/kg on the first day, followed by 3 mg/kg once daily. Administer treatment for at least 2 weeks to decrease the likelihood of relapse.

Esophageal candidiasis – The recommended dosage is 6 mg/kg on the first day followed by 3 mg/kg once daily. Doses up to 12 mg/kg/day may be used based on medical judgment of the patient's response to therapy. Treat patients with esophageal candidiasis for a minimum of 3 weeks and for at least 2 weeks following the resolution of symptoms.

Systemic Candida infections – For the treatment of candidemia and disseminated Candida infections, daily doses of 6 to 12 mg/kg/day have been used in an open, noncomparative study of a small number of children.

Cryptococcal meningitis – The recommended dosage is 12 mg/kg on the first day, followed by 6 mg/kg once daily. A dosage of 12 mg/kg once daily may be used, based on medical judgment of the patient's response to therapy. The recommended duration of treatment for initial therapy of cryptococcal meningitis is 10 to 12 weeks after the CSF becomes culture negative. For supression of relapse of cryptococcal meningitis in children with AIDS, the recommended dose is 6 mg/kg once daily.

FLUCONAZOLE

Renal function impairment: Fluconazole is cleared primarily by renal excretion as unchanged drug. There is no need to adjust single dose therapy for vaginal candidiasis in patients with impaired renal function. In patients with impaired renal function who will receive multiple doses, give an initial loading dose of 50 to 400 mg. After the loading dose, base the daily dose on the following table:

Fluconazole Dose in Impaired Renal Function	
Creatinine clearance (ml/min)	Percentage of recommended dose
> 50	100%
11-50	50%
Patients receiving regular hemodialysis	One recommended dose after each dialysis

These are suggested dose adjustments based on pharmacokinetics following administration of multiple doses. Further adjustment may be needed depending upon clinical condition.

When serum creatinine is the only measure of renal function available, use the following formula to estimate the creatinine clearance.

$$\text{Males:} \quad \frac{\text{Weight (kg)} \times (140 - \text{age})}{72 \times \text{serum creatinine (mg/dl)}} = \text{Ccr}$$

Females: 0.85 × above value

Children – Although the pharmacokinetics of fluconazole has not been studied in children with renal insufficiency, dosage reduction in children with renal insufficiency should parallel that recommended for adults. The following formula may be used to estimate Ccr in children:

$$K \times \frac{\text{linear length or height (cm)}}{\text{serum creatinine (mg/100 ml)}}$$

(Where K = 0.55 for children > 1 year of age and 0.45 for infants).

Directions for mixing oral suspension: To reconstitute, add 24 ml distilled water or purified water to fluconazole bottle and shake vigorously to suspend powder. Each bottle will deliver 35 ml of suspension. The concentrations of the reconstituted suspensions are 10 mg/ml (350 mg bottle) and 40 mg/ml (1400 mg bottle).

Injection: Fluconazole injection has been used safely for up to 14 days of IV therapy. Administer the IV infusion of fluconazole at a maximum rate of ≈ 200 mg/hr, given as a continuous infusion. Fluconazole injections are intended only for IV administration. Do not use if the solution is cloudy or contains a precipitate or if the seal is not intact.

Directions for IV use – Do not remove unit from overwrap until ready for use. The overwrap is a moisture barrier. The inner bag maintains the sterility of the product. Do not use plastic containers in series connections; such use could result in air embolism due to residual air being drawn from the primary container before administration of the fluid from the secondary container is completed.

Tear overwrap down side at slit and remove solution container. Some opacity of the plastic due to moisture absorption during the sterilization process may be observed. This is normal and does not affect the solution quality or safety. The opacity will diminish gradually. After removing overwrap, check for minute leaks by squeezing inner bag firmly. If leaks are found, discard solution as sterility may be impaired.

Admixture incompatibility – Do not add supplementary medication.

Storage/Stability: Shake oral suspension well before using. Store reconstituted suspension between 5° and 30°C (4° and 86°F). Discard unused portion after 2 weeks. Protect from freezing.

FLUCONAZOLE

Rx	**Diflucan** (Roerig)	**Tablets:** 50 mg	(Diflucan 50 Roerig). Pink. Trapezoid shape. In 30s.
		100 mg	(Diflucan 100 Roerig). Pink. Trapezoid shape. In 30s and UD 100s.
		150 mg	(Diflucan 150 mg Roerig). Pink. Oval. In 1s.
		200 mg	(Diflucan 200 Roerig). Pink. Trapezoid shape. In 30s and UD 100s.
Rx	**Diflucan** (Roerig)	**Powder for oral suspension:** 10 mg/ml when reconstituted	Sucrose. Orange flavor. In 350 mg.
		40 mg/ml when reconstituted	Sucrose. Orange flavor. In 1400 mg.
Rx	**Diflucan** (Roerig)	**Injection:** 2 mg/ml	In 100 or 200 ml bottles or *Viaflex Plus* (available with sodium chloride[1] or dextrose diluents[2]).

[1] Contains 9 mg/ml sodium chloride.
[2] Contains 56 mg/ml dextrose, hydrous.

ITRACONAZOLE

Warning:

Coadministration of terfenadine with itraconazole is contraindicated. Serious cardiovascular adverse events, including death, ventricular tachycardia and torsade de pointes have occurred due to increased terfenadine concentrations induced by itraconazole.

Another oral azole antifungal, ketoconazole, inhibits the metabolism of astemizole, resulting in elevated plasma concentrations of astemizole and its active metabolite desmethylastemizole, which may prolong QT intervals. Based on results of an in vitro study and the chemical resemblance of itraconazole and ketoconazole, coadministration of astemizole and itraconazole is contraindicated.

Coadministration of cisapride with itraconazole is contraindicated. Serious cardiovascular adverse events including death, ventricular tachycardia and torsades de pointes have occurred in patients taking itraconazole concomitantly with cisapride.

Actions:

Pharmacology: Itraconazole is a synthetic triazole antifungal agent. In vitro, itraconazole inhibits the cytochrome P-450-dependent synthesis of ergosterol, which is a vital component of fungal cell membranes.

Pharmacokinetics: Plasma concentrations reported were measured by high performance liquid chromatography (HPLC) specific for itraconazole. When itraconazole in plasma is measured by a bioassay, values reported are ≈ 3.3 times higher than those obtained by HPLC due to the bioactive metabolite, hydroxyitraconazole.

In six healthy volunteers, the total plasma clearance averaged 381 ml/min and the apparent volume of distribution averaged 796 L. The observed absolute oral bioavailability was 55%. Itraconazole may undergo saturation metabolism with multiple dosing. Doubling the dose results in approximately a threefold increase in the itraconazole plasma concentrations.

Itraconazole Pharmacokinetics (Single-Dose)

	Itraconazole (n = 6)				Itraconazole[1] (n = 27)		Hydroxy-itraconazole	
Parameter	50 mg (fed)	100 mg (fed)	100 mg (fasted)	200 mg (fed)	Fed	Fasted	Fed	Fasted
C_{max} (ng/ml)	45	132	38	289	239	140	397	286
T_{max} (hrs)	3.2	4	3.3	4.7	4.5	3.9	5.1	4.5
AUC (ng•hr/ml)	567	1899	722	5211	3423	2094	7978	5191
Half-life (hrs)	—	—	—	—	21	21	12	12

[1] 200 mg single dose.

Itraconazole Pharmacokinetics (Steady-State)		
Parameter	Itraconazole[1] (n = 27)	Hydroxyitraconazole
C_{max} (ng/ml)	2282	3488
C_{min} (ng/ml)	1855	3349
T_{max} (hrs)	4.6	3.4
AUC (ng•hr/ml)	22,569	38,572
Half-life (hrs)	64	56

[1] 200 mg twice daily for 15 days with food.

Itraconazole is extensively metabolized by the liver into a large number of metabolites including hydroxyitraconazole, the major metabolite. Fecal excretion of the parent drug varies between 3% and 18% of the dose. Renal excretion of the parent drug is < 0.03% of the dose. About 40% of the dose is excreted as inactive metabolites in the urine. No excreted single metabolite represents > 5% of a dose.

Plasma concentrations of itraconazole in subjects with renal insufficiency were comparable to those obtained in healthy subjects. The effect of hepatic impairment on the plasma concentration is unknown. Carefully monitor plasma concentrations in patients with hepatic impairment.

The plasma protein binding of itraconazole is 99.8% and that of hydroxyitraconazole is 99.5%. Itraconazole is not removed by hemodialysis.

In animal studies, itraconazole is extensively distributed into lipophilic tissues. Concentrations of itraconazole in fatty tissues, omentum, liver, kidney and skin tissues are 2 to 20 times the corresponding plasma concentrations. Aqueous fluids such as cerebrospinal fluid and saliva contain negligible amounts of the drug.

Microbiology: Itraconazole exhibits in vitro activity against *Blastomyces dermatitidis, Histoplasma capsulatum* and *duboisii, Aspergillus flavus* and *fumigatus* and *Cryptococcus neoformans.* Itraconazole also exhibits varying in vitro activity against *Sporothrix schenckii, Trichophyton* sp, *Candida albicans* and *Candida* sp. The bioactive metabolite hydroxyitraconazole has not been evaluated against *Histoplasma capsulatum* and *Blastomyces dermatitidis.*

Clinical trials:

Onychomycosis – Patients with onychomycosis of the toenails received 200 mg once daily for 12 consecutive weeks. Results demonstrated mycological cure in 54% of patients, defined as simultaneous occurrence of negative KOH plus negative culture. Thirty-five percent of patients were considered an overall success (mycological cure plus clear nail or minimal nail involvement with significantly decreased signs); 14% of patients demonstrated mycological cure plus clinical cure (clearance of all signs with or without residual nail deformity). The mean time to overall success was ≈ 10 months. In the overall success group, 21% had a relapse.

Indications:

Antifungal: Treatment of the following fungal infections in immunocompromised and non-immunocompromised patients:

Blastomycosis (pulmonary and extrapulmonary).

Histoplasmosis (including chronic cavitary pulmonary disease and disseminated, non-meningeal histoplasmosis).

Aspergillosis (pulmonary and extrapulmonary) in patients who are intolerant of or refractory to amphotericin B therapy.

Onychomycosis due to dermatophytes (tinea unguium) of the toenail with or without fingernail involvement.

Unlabeled uses: Itraconazole appears to be beneficial in the treatment of the following conditions: Dosage is generally 50 to 400 mg/day; duration of therapy varies from 1 day to ≥ 6 months depending on the condition and mycological response.

Itraconazole Unlabeled Uses		
Superficial mycoses	Systemic mycoses	Miscellaneous
Dermatophytoses	Candidiasis	Subcutaneous mycoses
Tinea capitis	Cryptococcal infections	Sporotrichosis
Tinea corporis	Meningitis	Chromomycosis
Tinea cruris	Disseminated	Leishmaniasis, cutaneous
Tinea pedis	Dimorphic infections	Fungal keratitis
Tinea manuum	Paracoccidioidomycosis	Alternariosis
Pityriasis versicolor	Coccidioidomycosis	Zygomycosis
Sebopsoriasis		
Candidiasis		
Vaginal		
Chronic mucocutaneous		

Contraindications:

Coadministration of terfenadine, astemizole, cisapride, triazolam or oral midazolam (see Warning Box and Drug Interactions); hypersensitivity to the drug or its excipients (there is no information regarding cross hypersensitivity between itraconazole and other azole antifungal agents; use caution in prescribing to patients with hypersensitivity to other azoles).

Do not administer for treatment of onychomycosis to pregnant women or to women contemplating pregnancy.

Warnings:

Cultures: Obtain specimens for fungal cultures and other relevant laboratory studies (wet mount, histopathology, serology) prior to therapy to isolate and identify causative organisms. Therapy may be instituted before the results of the cultures and other laboratory studies are known; however, once these results become available, adjust anti-infective therapy accordingly.

Hepatitis: Three cases of reversible idiosyncratic hepatitis occurred among > 2500 patients taking itraconazole. One other patient developed fulminant hepatitis and died during administration. Since this patient was on multiple medications, the causal association with itraconazole is uncertain. If clinical signs and symptoms consistent with liver disease develop that may be attributable to itraconazole, discontinue the drug.

HIV-infected patients: The response rate of histoplasmosis in HIV-infected patients appears to be similar to non-HIV-infected patients. The clinical course of histoplasmosis in HIV-infected patients is more severe and usually requires maintenance therapy to prevent relapse. Studies to investigate the efficacy and safety of itraconazole, including optimal dosage and duration in HIV-infected patients, are ongoing. Because hypochlorhydria has occurred in HIV-infected individuals, the absorption of itraconazole in these patients may be decreased.

Carcinogenesis: Male rats treated with 25 mg/kg/day (3.1 times the maximum recommended human dose) had a slightly increased incidence of soft tissue sarcoma. These sarcomas may have been a consequence of hypercholesterolemia, which is a response of rats to chronic itraconazole administration. Female rats treated with 50 mg/kg/day (6.25 times the maximum recommended human dose) had an increased incidence of squamous cell carcinoma of the lung.

Pregnancy: Category C. Itraconazole caused a dose-related increase in maternal toxicity, embryotoxicity and teratogenicity in rats and mice at dosage levels of approximately 40 to 160 mg/kg/day (5 to 20 times the maximum recommended human dose). In rats, the teratogenicity consisted of major skeletal defects; in mice, it consisted of encephaloceles or macroglossia. Use in pregnancy for systemic fungal infections only if the benefit outweighs the potential risk.

Do not administer itraconazole for the treatment of onychomycosis to pregnant women or to women contemplating pregnancy. Do not administer itraconazole to women of childbearing potential for the treatment of onychomycosis unless they are taking effective measures to prevent pregnancy and the patient begins therapy on the second or third day of the next normal menstrual period. Effective contraception should be continued throughout itraconazole therapy and for 2 months following treatment.

Lactation: Itraconazole is excreted in breast milk; therefore, do not administer to a nursing woman.

Children: Safety and efficacy have not been established. A small number of patients from 3 to 16 years of age have been treated with 100 mg/day for systemic fungal infections and no serious adverse effects have been reported.

ITRACONAZOLE

Itraconazole, when administered to rats, can produce bone defects. While no such toxicity has been reported in adult patients, the long-term effect of itraconazole in children is unknown.

Precautions:

Monitoring: Monitor hepatic enzyme test values in patients with pre-existing hepatic function abnormalities. Monitor hepatic enzyme test values periodically in all patients receiving continuous treatment for > 1 month or at any time a patient develops signs or symptoms suggestive of liver dysfunction.

Decreased gastric acidity: Under fasted conditions, itraconazole absorption was decreased in the presence of decreased gastric acidity. The absorption of itraconazole may be decreased with the concomitant administration of antacids or gastric acid secretion suppressors. Studies conducted under fasted conditions demonstrated that administration with 240 ml (8 oz) of a cola beverage resulted in increased absorption of itraconazole in AIDS patients with relative or absolute achlorhydria (see Drug/Food interactions). This increase relative to the effects of a full meal is unknown.

Drug Interactions:

Both itraconazole and its major metabolite, hydroxyitraconazole, are inhibitors of the cytochrome P450 3A4 enzyme system. Coadministration of itraconazole and drugs primarily metabolized by the cytochrome P450 3A4 enzyme system may result in increased plasma concentrations of the drugs that could increase or prolong both therapeutic and adverse effects. Therefore, unless otherwise specified, appropriate dosage adjustments may be necessary.

Itraconazole Drug Interactions

Precipitant drug	Object drug*		Description
Itraconazole	Antihistamines, nonsedating Astemizole Terfenadine	↑	Increased terfenadine plasma levels have occurred, resulting in rare instances of life-threatening cardiac dysrhythmias and death. Coadministration with astemizole may result in the same effect. Avoid concurrent use. See Warning box.
Itraconazole	Calcium blockers	↑	Edema has occurred with concomitant use of itraconazole and dihydropyridine (eg, amlodipine, nifedipine) calcium blockers.
Itraconazole	Cyclosporine plus HMG-CoA reductase inhibitors	↑	There have been rare reports of rhabdomyolysis involving renal transplant patients receiving the combination of itraconazole, cyclosporine and the HMG-CoA reductase inhibitors lovastatin or simvastatin. Rhabdomyolysis has been observed in patients receiving HMG-CoA reductase inhibitors alone or concomitantly with cyclosporine. Increased cyclosporine levels may occur. Reduce the cyclosporine dose by 50% when using itraconazole doses > 100 mg/day. Monitor cyclosporine levels.
Itraconazole	Digoxin	↑	Increased digoxin levels may occur. Monitor digoxin levels initially and then frequently thereafter.
Itraconazole	Midazolam (oral) Triazolam	↑	Coadministration has resulted in elevated plasma concentrations of oral midazolam or triazolam. This may potentiate and prolong hypnotic and sedative effects. These agents should not be used concurrently. If midazolam is administered parenterally, the sedative effect may be prolonged.
Itraconazole	Quinidine	↑	Tinnitus and decreased hearing have occurred.
Itraconazole	Sulfonylureas	↑	Hypoglycemia may occur. Monitor blood glucose.
Itraconazole	Tacrolimus	↑	Coadministration has led to increased tacrolimus plasma concentrations.
Itraconazole	Warfarin	↑	The anticoagulant effect of warfarin may be enhanced. Monitor prothrombin time or INR.

Itraconazole Drug Interactions			
Precipitant drug	Object drug*		Description
Itraconazole	Cisapride	↑	Concomitant administration of ketoconazole with cisapride has resulted in markedly elevated cisapride plasma concentrations, prolonged QT intervals, and has rarely been associated with ventricular arrhythmias and torsades de pointes. Due to potent in vitro inhibition of the hepatic enzyme system mainly responsible for the metabolism of cisapride (cytochrome P450 3A4), itraconazole is also expected to markedly raise cisapride plasma concentrations; therefore, concomitant use is contraindicated.
H_2 antagonists	Itraconazole	↓	Reduced plasma itraconazole levels may occur.
Phenytoin	Itraconazole	↓	Reduced plasma itraconazole levels may occur. Also, phenytoin metabolism may be altered.
Itraconazole	Phenytoin	↑	
Rifampin	Itraconazole	↓	Reduced plasma itraconazole levels may occur.

* ↑ = Object drug increased ↓ = Object drug decreased

Drug/Food interactions: Absorption of itraconazole under fasted conditions in individuals with relative or absolute achlorhydria, such as patients with AIDS or volunteers taking gastric acid secretion suppressors (eg, H_2 antagonists), was increased when itraconazole was administered with a cola beverage. Eighteen males with AIDS received single 200 mg doses of itraconazole under fasted conditions with 240 ml of water or a cola beverage in a crossover design. The absorption of itraconazole was increased when itraconazole was coadministered with a cola beverage with AUC and C_{max} increasing 75% and 95%, respectively.

Adverse Reactions:

Adverse Reactions During Use of Itraconazole in Systemic Fungal Infections vs Onychomycosis (%)		
	Incidence	
Adverse reaction	Systemic fungal infections (n = 602)	Onychomycosis (n = 112)
GI		
Nausea	10.6	—
Vomiting	5.1	—
Elevated liver enzymes (> 2 times normal range)	—	4
GI disorders, general	—	4
Diarrhea	3.3	—
Abdominal pain	1.5	—
Anorexia	1.2	—
Body as a whole		
Edema	3.5	—
Fatigue	2.8	—
Fever	2.5	—
Malaise	1.2	1
Myalgia	—	1
Cardiovascular		
Hypertension	3.2	2
Orthostatic hypotension	—	1
Vasculitis	—	1
Dermatologic		
Rash	8.6[1]	3
Pruritus	2.5	—
CNS		
Headache	3.8	1
Dizziness/Vertigo	1.7	1
Libido decreased	1.2	—
Somnolence	1.2	—

Adverse Reactions During Use of Itraconazole in Systemic Fungal Infections vs Onychomycosis (%)		
	Incidence	
Adverse reaction	Systemic fungal infections (n = 602)	Onychomycosis (n = 112)
Miscellaneous		
Hepatic function abnormal	2.7	—
Hypokalemia	2	—
Albuminuria	1.2	—
Impotence	1.2	—

[1] Tends to occur more frequently in immunocompromised patients receiving immunosuppressant medications.

Adverse events infrequently reported in all studies included constipation, gastritis, depression, insomnia, tinnitus, menstrual disorder, adrenal insufficiency, gynecomastia and male breast pain.

In postmarketing experience with itraconazole, allergic reactions including rash, pruritus, urticaria, angioedema and in rare instances, anaphylaxis and Stevens-Johnson syndrome, have been reported. In addition, there have been reports of elevated liver enzymes, hepatitis (rare), hypertriglyceridemia (rare) and neuropathy (isolated cases).

Overdosage:

Itraconazole is not removed by dialysis. In the event of accidental overdosage, employ supportive measures, including gastric lavage with sodium bicarbonate. Refer to General Management of Acute Overdosage.

Patient Information:

Take itraconazole after a full meal.

Patients should report any signs and symptoms that may suggest liver dysfunction so that the appropriate laboratory testing can be done. Such signs and symptoms may include unusual fatigue, anorexia, nausea, vomiting, jaundice, dark urine or pale stool.

Administration and Dosage:

Approved by the FDA on September 11, 1992.

Take with a full meal to ensure maximal absorption.

Blastomycosis/Histoplasmosis: The recommended dose is 200 mg once daily. If there is no obvious improvement or there is evidence of progressive fungal disease, increase the dose in 100 mg increments to a maximum of 400 mg daily. Give doses > 200 mg/day in two divided doses.

Aspergillosis: Recommended daily dose is 200 to 400 mg.

Life-threatening situations: Although studies did not provide for a loading dose, it is recommended that a loading dose of 200 mg 3 times a day (600 mg/day) be given for the first 3 days.

Continue treatment for a minimum of 3 months and until clinical parameters and laboratory tests indicate that the active fungal infection has subsided. An inadequate period of treatment may lead to recurrence of active infection.

Onychomycosis: Recommended dose is 200 mg once daily for 12 consecutive weeks.

Rx	**Sporanox** (Janssen)	**Capsules:** 100 mg	Sucrose, sugar. (Janssen Sporanox 100). Blue/pink. In 30s and UD 30s.

TERBINAFINE HCl

Actions:

Pharmacology: Terbinafine HCl is a synthetic allylamine derivative, which exerts its antifungal effect by inhibiting squalene epoxidase, a key enzyme in sterol biosynthesis in fungi. This action results in a deficiency in ergosterol and a corresponding accumulation of squalene within the fungal cell and causes fungal cell death.

Pharmacokinetics: Terbinafine is well absorbed (> 70%). First-pass metabolism is ≈ 40%. Peak plasma concentrations of 1 mcg/ml appear ≤ 2 hours after a single 250 mg dose, the area under the plasma concentration-time curve (AUC) is ≈ 4.56 mcg•hr/ml. An increase in the AUC of terbinafine of < 20% is observed when terbinafine is taken with food.

In patients with renal impairment (creatinine clearance ≤ 50 ml/min) or hepatic cirrhosis, the clearance of terbinafine is decreased by ≈ 50%. In plasma, terbinafine is > 99% bound to plasma proteins, and there are no specific binding sites. At steady-state, in comparison to a single dose, the peak concentration of terbinafine is 25% higher and plasma AUC increases by a factor of 2.5; the increase in plasma AUC is consistent with an effective half-life of ≈ 36 hours. Terbinafine is distributed to the sebum and skin. A terminal half-life of 200 to 400 hours may represent the slow elimination of terbinafine from tissues such as skin and adipose.

Prior to excretion, terbinafine is extensively metabolized. No metabolites have been identified that have antifungal activity similar to terbinafine. Approximately 70% of the administered dose is eliminated in the urine.

Microbiology: Terbinafine is active against most strains of the following organisms both in vitro and in clinical infections: *Trichophyton mentagrophytes; Trichophyton rubrum.* Terbinafine exceeds in vitro MICs against most strains of the following organisms which can infect the nail; however, safety and efficacy of terbinafine in treating nail infections due to these organisms have not been established: *Microsporum gypseum and nanum; Trichophyton verrucosum; Epidermophyton floccosum; Candida albicans; Scopulariopsis brevicaulis.*

Clinical trials: The efficacy of terbinafine tablets in the treatment of onychomycosis is illustrated by the response of patients with toenail or fingernail infections who participated in placebo controlled clinical trials. Results of the toenail study were assessed at week 48. Fifty-nine percent experienced effective treatment, and 38% demonstrated mycological cure plus clinical cure. Results of the fingernail study, as assessed at week 24, demonstrated mycological cure in 79% of patients, effective treatment in 75% of patients and mycological cure plus clinical cure in 59% of patients.

Indications:

Onychomycosis: Treatment of onychomycosis of the toenail or fingernail due to dermatophytes.

Contraindications:

Hypersensitivity to terbinafine or any component of the product; pre-existing liver disease or renal impairment (creatinine clearance ≤ 50 ml/min).

Warnings:

Ophthalmic: Changes in the ocular lens and retina have been reported following the use of terbinafine.

Neutropenia: Isolated cases of severe neutropenia have been reported but were reversible with discontinuation of treatment with or without supportive therapy. If clinical signs and symptoms suggest a secondary infection, obtain a complete blood count (CBC). If the neutrophil count is ≤ 1000 cells/mm^3, discontinue treatment and start supportive management.

Dermatologic: There have been isolated reports of serious skin reactions (eg, Stevens-Johnson syndrome and toxic epidermal necrolysis). If progressive skin rash occurs, discontinue treatment.

Pregnancy: Category B. There are no adequate and well controlled studies in pregnant women. Because treatment of onychomycosis can be postponed until after pregnancy is completed, it is recommended that terbinafine tablets not be initiated during pregnancy.

Lactation: After oral administration, terbinafine is present in the breast milk of nursing mothers. The ratio of terbinafine in milk to plasma is 7:1. Treatment with terbinafine tablets is not recommended in nursing mothers.

Children: Safety and efficacy in children have not been established.

Precautions:

Monitoring:

Immunodeficiency – Monitor CBC in patients receiving treatment for > 6 weeks.

TERBINAFINE HCl

Hepatic – Monitor hepatic function (hepatic enzyme) test in patients administered terbinafine for > 6 weeks.

Symptomatic hepatobiliary dysfunction: If hepatobiliary dysfunction or cholestatic hepatitis develops, discontinue treatment.

Drug Interactions:

Terbinafine Drug Interactions			
Precipitant drug	Object drug*		Description
Cimetidine	Terbinafine	↑	Terbinafine clearance is decreased 33% by cimetidine.
Rifampin	Terbinafine	↓	Terbinafine clearance is increased 100% by rifampin.
Terfenadine	Terbinafine	↑	Terbinafine clearance is decreased 16% by terfenadine.
Terbinafine	Caffeine	↑	Terbinafine decreases the clearance of IV caffeine by 19%.
Terbinafine	Cyclosporine	↓	Terbinafine increases the clearance of cyclosporine by 15%.

* ↑ = Object drug increased. ↓ = Object drug decreased. ↔ = Undetermined effect.

Adverse Reactions:

Oral:

Adverse Events Reported With Oral Terbinafine		
Adverse Event	Oral terbinafine (%) (n = 465)	Placebo (%) (n = 137)
GI		
Diarrhea	5.6	2.9
Dyspepsia	4.3	2.9
Abdominal pain	2.4	1.5
Nausea	2.6	2.9
Flatulence	2.2	2.2
Dermatologic		
Rash	5.6	2.2
Pruritus	2.8	1.5
Urticaria	1.1	0
Miscellaneous		
Liver enzyme abnormalities	3.3	1.4
Headache	12.9	9.5
Taste disturbance	2.8	0.7
Visual disturbance	1.1	1.5

Other (rare): Symptomatic idiosyncratic hepatobiliary dysfunction (including cholestatic hepatitis); serious skin reactions; severe neutropenia; allergic reactions (including anaphylaxis); taste disturbance (including taste loss, which is usually recovered within several weeks after discontinuation of the drug).

Lab test abnormalities: Decreases in absolute lymphocyte counts (ALC).

Overdosage:

There is no information on human overdosage with oral terbinafine. Single oral doses in rats and mice up to 400 times the therapeutic dose produce sedation, drowsiness, ataxia, dyspnea, exophthalmus and piloerection. Animal mortality was < 50% at this dose level.

Patient Information:

Use the medication for the recommended treatment time.

Administration and Dosage:

Onychomycosis:

Fingernail – 250 mg/day for 6 weeks.

Toenail – 250 mg/day for 12 weeks.

The optimal clinical effect is seen some months after mycological cure and cessation of treatment. This is related to the period required for outgrowth of healthy nail.

Storage: Store tablets below 25°C (77°F). Protect from light.

Rx	**Lamisil** (Sandoz)	**Tablet:** 250 mg	(Lamisil 250). White to yellow-tinged white. Biconvex. In 30s and 100s.

SULFONAMIDES

In addition to the sulfonamides listed on the following pages, other preparations that contain sulfonamides include: Ophthalmic; vaginal; burn preparations (eg, mafenide, silver sulfadiazine). See individual monographs or sections.

Actions:

Pharmacology: Sulfonamides exert their bacteriostatic action by competitive antagonism of para-aminobenzoic acid (PABA), an essential component in folic acid synthesis. Microorganisms that require exogenous folic acid and do not synthesize folic acid are not susceptible to the action of sulfonamides.

Pharmacokinetics:

Absorption/Distribution – The oral sulfonamides are readily absorbed from the GI tract. Approximately 70% to 100% of an oral dose is absorbed. These agents are distributed throughout all body tissues and readily enter the cerebrospinal fluid, pleura, synovial fluids, the eye, the placenta and the fetus. Sulfonamides are bound to plasma proteins in varying degrees. Wide interpatient variation in serum levels may result from identical doses. "Free" sulfonamide serum levels of 5 to 15 mg/dl may be therapeutically effective for most infections. Avoid levels > 20 mg/dl.

Metabolism – The duration of antibacterial activity depends on the rate of metabolism and renal excretion. Metabolism occurs in the liver by conjugation, acetylation and other metabolic pathways to inactive metabolites. Sulfonamide acetylation requires a coenzyme which is a pantothenic acid derivative; individuals who are pantothenic acid deficient or are slow acetylators have an increased risk of toxicity from sulfonamide accumulation.

Excretion – Renal excretion is mainly by glomerular filtration; tubular reabsorption occurs in varying degrees. Urinary solubility of these compounds is pH dependent. Some of the acetylated metabolites are less soluble and may contribute to crystalluria and renal complications. To prevent the possibility of crystalluria, alkalinization of the urine and adequate fluid intake are recommended when using the less soluble sulfonamides (eg, sulfadiazine, sulfamerazine). Small amounts are eliminated in the feces, and in bile, breast milk and other secretions.

Microbiology: Sulfonamides have a broad antibacterial spectrum which includes both gram-positive and gram-negative organisms.

Resistance develops in organisms which produce excessive amounts of PABA; resistance may also be due to destruction of the sulfonamide molecule. The increasing frequency of resistant organisms is a limitation to the usefulness of the sulfonamides alone, especially in the treatment of chronic and recurrent urinary tract infections. Cross-resistance between sulfonamides is common, once resistance develops. Minimize resistance by initiating treatment promptly with adequate doses and continue for a sufficient period. In vitro sensitivity tests are not always reliable; carefully coordinate the test with bacteriologic and clinical response.

SULFONAMIDES

Indications:

Sulfonamide Indications							
Indications ✓ – Labeled × – Unlabeled	Multiple Sulfas	Sulfacytine	Sulfadiazine	Sulfamethizole	Sulfamethoxazole	Sulfasalazine	Sulfisoxazole
Chancroid	✓		✓		✓		✓
Colitis, ulcerative						✓	
Inclusion conjunctivitis	✓		✓		✓		✓
Malaria[1]	✓		✓		✓		✓
Meningitis, *H influenzae*[2]	✓		✓				✓
Meningitis, meningococcal[3]	✓		✓		✓		✓
Nocardiosis	✓		✓		✓		✓
Otitis media, acute[4]	✓		✓		✓		✓
Rheumatic fever			✓				
Toxoplasmosis[5]	✓		✓		✓		✓
Trachoma	✓		✓		✓		✓
Urinary tract infections[6] (pyelonephritis, cystitis)	✓	✓	✓	✓	✓		✓
Ankylosing spondylitis						×	
Colitis, collagenous						×	
Crohn's disease						×	
Otitis media, recurrent							×
Rheumatoid arthritis						×	

[1] As adjunctive therapy due to chloroquine-resistant strains of *P falciparum*.
[2] As adjunctive therapy with parenteral streptomycin.
[3] When the organism is susceptible and for prophylaxis when sulfonamide-sensitive group A strains prevail.
[4] Due to *H influenzae* when used with penicillin or erythromycin.
[5] As adjunctive therapy with pyrimethamine.
[6] In the absence of obstructive uropathy or foreign bodies, when caused by *E coli, Klebsiella-Enterobacter, S aureus, P mirabilis* and *P vulgaris*.

Contraindications:

Hypersensitivity to sulfonamides or chemically related drugs (eg, sulfonylureas, thiazide and loop diuretics, carbonic anhydrase inhibitors, sunscreens with PABA, local anesthetics); pregnancy at term, lactation (see Warnings); infants < 2 months old (except in congenital toxoplasmosis as adjunct with pyrimethamine); porphyria (see Warnings); salicylate hypersensitivity; intestinal/urinary obstruction (**sulfasalazine**).

Warnings:

Group A beta-hemolytic streptococcal infections: Do not use for treatment of these infections. In an established infection, they will not eradicate the streptococcus and will not prevent sequelae, such as rheumatic fever and glomerulonephritis.

Severe reactions including deaths due to sulfonamides have been associated with hypersensitivity reactions, agranulocytosis, aplastic anemia, other blood dyscrasias and renal and hepatic damage. Irreversible neuromuscular and CNS changes and fibrosing alveolitis may occur. Sore throat, fever, pallor, purpura or jaundice may be early indications of serious blood disorders. Perform complete blood counts.

Porphyria: In patients with porphyria, these drugs have precipitated an acute attack.

Photosensitivity: Photosensitization (photoallergy or phototoxicity) may occur; therefore, caution patients to take protective measures (ie, sunscreens, protective clothing) against exposure to ultraviolet light or sunlight until tolerance is determined.

Renal/Hepatic function impairment: Use with caution. The frequency of renal complications is considerably lower in patients receiving the more soluble sulfonamides (sulfisoxazole and sulfamethizole). Obtain urinalysis with microscopic examinations and perform liver and kidney function tests during long-term treatment. Maintain adequate fluid intake to prevent crystalluria and stone formation.

Fertility impairment: Oligospermia and infertility have been described in men treated with **sulfasalazine**. Withdrawal of the drug appears to reverse these effects.

Pregnancy: Safety for use during pregnancy is not established. Sulfonamides cross the placenta; fetal levels average 70% to 90% of maternal serum levels. Significant levels may persist in the neonate if these drugs are given near term; jaundice, hemolytic anemia and kernicterus may occur. Most reports do not demonstrate congenital malformations, but teratogenicity (eg, cleft palate, other bony abnormalities) has occurred in some animal species. Do not use at term.

Lactation: Sulfonamides are excreted in breast milk in low concentrations. Milk:plasma ratios for sulfonamides are as low as 0.06 (sulfisoxazole). According to the American Academy of Pediatrics, breast feeding and sulfonamide use are compatible since sulfonamide excretion into breast milk does not pose a significant risk to the healthy full-term neonate. However, do not nurse premature infants or those with hyperbilirubinemia or G–6–PD deficiency.

Children: Do not use in infants < 2 months old (except for congenital toxoplasmosis as adjunctive therapy with pyrimethamine). **Sulfacytine** is not recommended for children < 14 years. There are insufficient clinical data on prolonged or recurrent therapy with **sulfamethoxazole** in chronic renal diseases of children < 6 years.

Precautions:

Allergy or asthma: Give with caution to patients with severe allergy or bronchial asthma. If toxicity or hypersensitivity reactions occur, discontinue immediately.

Hemolytic anemia, frequently dose-related, may occur in G-6-PD deficient individuals.

Drug Interactions:

Sulfonamide Drug Interactions

Precipitant Drug	Object Drug*		Description
Sulfonamides	Anticoagulants, oral	↑	Warfarin's anticoagulation action may be enhanced. Hemorrhage could occur
Sulfisoxazole	Barbiturate anesthetics	↑	The anesthetic effects of thiopental may be enhanced
Sulfonamides	Cyclosporine	↔	Cyclosporine concentrations are decreased, and the risk of nephrotoxicity may be increased
Sulfasalazine	Digoxin	↓	Digoxin's bioavailability may be decreased, possibly resulting in a reduced therapeutic effect
Sulfasalazine	Folic acid	↓	Signs of folate deficiency have occurred (eg, low serum folate, megaloblastic anemia, macrocytosis, reticulocytosis), but specific symptoms related to the deficiency have not been reported
Sulfonamides	Hydantoins	↑	Serum hydantoin levels may be increased
Sulfonamides	Methotrexate	↑	The risk of methotrexate-induced bone marrow suppression may be enhanced
Sulfonamides	Sulfonylureas	↑	Increased sulfonylurea half-lives and hypoglycemia

* ↑ = Object drug increased ↓ = Object drug decreased ↔ = Undetermined effect.

Drug/Lab test interactions: Sulfonamides may produce false-positive **urinary glucose tests** when performed by Benedict's method. Sulfisoxazole may interfere with the **Urobilistix test** and may produce false-positive results with sulfosalicylic acid tests for urinary protein.

Adverse Reactions:

Hematologic: Agranulocytosis; aplastic anemia; thrombocytopenia; leukopenia; hemolytic anemia; purpura; hypoprothrombinemia; cyanosis; methemoglobinemia; megaloblastic (macrocytic) anemia; Heinz body anemia.

Hypersensitivity: Stevens-Johnson type erythema multiforme; parapsoriasis varioliformis acuta (Mucha-Habermann syndrome); generalized skin eruptions; allergic myocarditis; epidermal necrolysis, with or without corneal damage; urticaria; serum sickness; pruritus; exfoliative dermatitis; anaphylactoid reactions; periorbital edema; conjunctival, scleral injection; photosensitization; arthralgia; allergic myocarditis; transient pulmonary changes with eosinophilia and decreased pulmonary function.

GI: Nausea; emesis; abdominal pains; diarrhea; bloody diarrhea; anorexia; pancreatitis; stomatitis; impaired folic acid absorption; hepatitis; hepatocellular necrosis; pseudomembranous enterocolitis; glossitis.

SULFONAMIDES

CNS: Headache; peripheral neuropathy; mental depression; convulsions; ataxia; hallucinations; tinnitus; vertigo; insomnia; hearing loss; drowsiness; transient lesions of posterior spinal column; transverse myelitis; apathy.

Renal: Crystalluria; hematuria; proteinuria; elevated creatinine; nephrotic syndrome; toxic nephrosis with oliguria and anuria.

Miscellaneous: Drug fever; chills; pyrexia; alopecia; arthralgia; myalgia; pulmonary infiltrates; periarteritis nodosum; L.E. phenomenon.

The sulfonamides bear chemical similarities to some goitrogens, diuretics (acetazolamide and the thiazides) and oral hypoglycemic agents. Goiter production, diuresis and hypoglycemia have occurred rarely in patients receiving sulfonamides. Cross-sensitivity may exist with these agents (see Contraindications).

Sulfasalazine produces an orange-yellow color urine when the urine is alkaline. Similar discoloration of the skin has also occurred.

Overdosage:

Therapeutic doses of 2 to 5 g/day may produce toxicity or fatalities. The aniline radical is largely responsible for the effects on the blood or hematopoietic system.

Symptoms:

GI – Anorexia; colic; nausea; vomiting.

CNS – Dizziness; headache; drowsiness; unconsciousness.

Toxic fever – Precedes serious manifestations and may develop ≥ 1 day after the fever due to infection has subsided.

Serious manifestations – Acidosis; acute hemolytic anemia; agranulocytosis; sensitivity reactions; dermatitis (maculopapular); toxic neuritis; hepatic jaundice; death (occurring several days after first dose).

Treatment: Discontinue the drug immediately. Within 1 or 2 days after discontinuation, the less serious symptoms disappear; grave symptoms require 1 to 3 weeks for remission. Empty the stomach if large doses have been ingested. Alkalinize the urine to enhance solubility and excretion. Force fluids if kidney function is normal, up to 4 L/day, to increase excretion. If anuria is present, treat for renal failure. Catheterization of the ureters may be indicated for complete renal blockage by crystals. For agranulocytosis, give antibiotic therapy to combat infection, and blood or platelet transfusions for severe anemia or thrombocytopenia.

Patient Information:

Complete full course of therapy.

Take on an empty stomach with a full glass of water.

Avoid prolonged exposure to sunlight; photosensitivity may occur. If outside, wear protective clothing and apply sunscreen to exposed areas.

Notify physician if any of the following occurs: Blood in urine, rash, ringing in ears, difficulty in breathing, fever, sore throat or chills.

Sulfasalazine: Take with food if GI irritation occurs. May cause an orange-yellow discoloration of the urine or skin. May permanently stain soft contact lenses yellow.

Oral suspension: Shake well; refrigerate after opening. Discard unused portion after 14 days.

Administration and Dosage:

See individual products for specific guidelines based on indication.

CDC recommended treatment schedules for sexually transmitted diseases†:

Lymphogranuloma venereum – As an alternative regimen to doxycycline, sulfisoxazole 500 mg 4 times a day for 21 days or equivalent sulfonamide course.

Treatment of uncomplicated urethral, endocervical or rectal Chlamydia trachomatic infections – As an alternative regimen to doxycycline or tetracycline (or if erythromycin is not tolerated), sulfisoxazole 500 mg 4 times a day for 10 days or equivalent sulfonamide course.

† *Morbidity and Mortality Weekly Report* 1989 (Sept 1);38 (No. S-8):1-43.

SULFADIAZINE

Complete prescribing information begins in the Sulfonamides group monograph.

Administration and Dosage:

Adults: Loading dose - 2 to 4 g. *Maintenance dose* - 4 to 8 g/day in 4 to 6 divided doses.

Children (> 2 months): Loading dose - 75 mg/kg (or 2 g/m^2). *Maintenance dose* - 120 to 150 mg/kg/day (4 g/m^2/day) in 4 to 6 divided doses. *Maximum dose* - 6 g/day.

Infants (< 2 months): Contraindicated, except as adjunctive therapy with pyrimethamine in the treatment of congenital toxoplasmosis. *Loading dose* - 75 to 100 mg/kg. *Maintenance dose* - 100 to 150 mg/kg/day in 4 divided doses.

Other recommended doses for toxoplasmosis (for 3 to 4 weeks) include: Infants (< 2 months) - 25 mg/kg/dose 4 times daily. *Children (> 2 months)* - 25 to 50 mg/kg/dose 4 times daily.

Prevention of recurrent attacks of rheumatic fever (not for initial treatment of streptococcal infections): Patients > 30 kg (> 66 lbs) – 1 g/day; < 30 kg (< 66 lbs) – 0.5 g/day.

Rx	**Sulfadiazine** (Various, eg, Lannett)	**Tablets:** 500 mg	In 100s and 1000s.
Rx	**Sulfadiazine** (Eon)		In 100s and 1000s.

SULFACYTINE

Complete prescribing information begins in the Sulfonamides group monograph.

Administration and Dosage:

Loading dose: 500 mg. *Maintenance dose* - 250 mg 4 times daily for 10 days.

Not recommended in children < 14 years of age.

Rx	**Renoquid** (Glenwood)	**Tablets:** 250 mg	In 100s.

SULFISOXAZOLE

For complete prescribing information, refer to the Sulfonamides group monograph.

Administration and Dosage:

Loading dose: 2 to 4 g. *Maintenance dose* - 4 to 8 g/day in 4 to 6 divided doses. Although recommended, a loading dose is unnecessary because sulfisoxazole is rapidly absorbed and appears in high concentrations in the urine.

Children and infants (> 2 months): Initial dose - 75 mg/kg. *Maintenance dose* -120 to 150 mg/kg/day (4 g/m^2/day) in 4 to 6 divided doses (max, 6 g/day).

Rx	**Sulfisoxazole** (Various, eg, Geneva, Goldline, Major, Moore, Parmed, Rugby, Schein, URL, Zenith)	**Tablets:** 500 mg	In 100s, 1000s and UD 100s.

SULFAMETHOXAZOLE

Complete prescribing information begins in the Sulfonamides group monograph.

Administration and Dosage:

Adults: Mild to moderate infections - 2 g initially; maintenance dose is 1 g morning and evening thereafter. *Severe infections* - 2 g initially, then 1 g 3 times daily.

Children and infants (> 2 months): Initially, 50 to 60 mg/kg; maintenance dose is 25 to 30 mg/kg morning and evening. Do not exceed 75 mg/kg/day.

Another recommended dose is 50 to 60 mg/kg/day divided every 12 hours, not to exceed 3 g/24 hours.

Rx	**Sulfamethoxazole** (Various, eg, Bolar, Geneva, Parmed, Rugby, URL)	**Tablets:** 500 mg	In 100s and 1000s.
Rx	**Gantanol** (Roche)		(Roche Gantanol). Green, scored. In 100s and Tel-E-Dose 100s.
Rx	**Urobak** (Shionogi)		Scored. In 100s, 1000s.
Rx	**Gantanol** (Roche)	**Oral Suspension:** 500 mg per 5 ml	Saccharin, sorbitol, sucrose, EDTA. Cherry flavor. In pt.

SULFAMETHIZOLE

Complete prescribing information begins in the Sulfonamides group mongraph.

Administration and Dosage:

Adults: 0.5 to 1 g 3 or 4 times daily.

Children and infants (> 2 months): 30 to 45 mg/kg/day in 4 divided doses.

Rx	**Thiosulfil Forte** (W-A)	**Tablets:** 500 mg	White, scored. Oval. In 100s.

SULFASALAZINE

For complete prescribing information, refer to the Sulfonamides group monograph.

About one-third of an oral dose of sulfasalazine is absorbed from the small intestine. The remaining two-thirds passes to the colon where it is split into 5–aminosalicylic acid (5–ASA) and sulfapyridine. Most of the sulfapyridine thus liberated is absorbed, whereas only about one-third of the 5-ASA is absorbed, the remainder being excreted in the feces.

Administration and Dosage:

Individualize dosage. Administer in evenly divided doses over each 24 hour period; intervals between nighttime doses should not exceed 8 hours. Administer after meals. Doses of ≥ 4 g/day tend to increase adverse reactions.

GI intolerance (eg, anorexia, nausea, vomiting) after the first few doses is probably due to mucosal irritation and may be alleviated by distributing the total daily dose more evenly or by giving enteric coated tablets. If such symptoms occur after the first few days of treatment, they are probably due to increased serum levels of total sulfapyridine and may be alleviated by halving the dose and subsequently increasing it gradually over several days. If symptoms continue, stop the drug for 5 to 7 days, then reinstitute at a lower daily dose.

It is often necessary to continue medication, even when clinical symptoms, including diarrhea, have been controlled. When endoscopic examination confirms satisfactory improvement, reduce dosage to maintenance level. If diarrhea recurs, increase dosage to previously effective levels.

Desensitization regimens: Upon reinstituting sulfasalazine, various regimens comprise a total daily dose of 50 to 250 mg which is doubled every 4 to 7 days until desired therapeutic level is achieved. Small doses are best achieved with oral suspension. If sensitivity symptoms recur, discontinue drug. Do not attempt desensitization in patients with a history of agranulocytosis or anaphylactoid reaction to the drug.

Initial therapy: Adults - 3 to 4 g/day in evenly divided doses; however, initial doses of 1 to 2 g/day may lessen adverse GI effects. Doses of ≥ 4 g/day increase the risk of toxicity. *Children (≥ 2 years old)* - 40 to 60 mg/kg/24 hours in 4 to 6 divided doses.

Maintenance therapy: Adults - 2 g/day (500 mg 4 times daily). *Children* - 20 to 30 mg/kg/day, in 4 divided doses, maximum 2 g/day.

Rx	**Sulfasalazine** (Various, eg, Geneva, Goldline, Lederle, Major, Parmed, Rugby, Schein, URL)	**Tablets:** 500 mg	In 100s, 250s, 500s, 1000s and UD 100s.
Rx	**Azulfidine** (Pharmacia)		(101). Gold, scored. In 100s, 500s, UD 100s, 1000s.
Rx	**Sulfasalazine** (Various, eg, Bolar, Genetco, Major, Moore, Parmed, Qualitest, Rugby, URL)	**Tablets, enteric coated:** 500 mg	In 100s, 500s and 1000s.
Rx	**Azulfidine EN-tabs** (Pharmacia)		(102). Gold, elliptical. In 100s and 500s.

QUININE SULFATE

Actions:

Pharmacology: Quinine, a cinchona alkaloid, acts primarily as a blood schizonticide. Its antimalarial action is unclear. It was once believed to be due to the intercalation of the quinoline moiety into the DNA of the parasite, thereby reducing the effectiveness of DNA to act as a template, as well as depression of the oxygen uptake and carbohydrate metabolism of plasmodia. More recently it is thought that pH elevation in intracellular organelles of the parasites by quinine plays a role in the mechanism.

Quinine has a skeletal muscle relaxant effect, increasing the refractory period by direct action on the muscle fiber, decreasing the excitability of the motor end-plate by a curariform action, and affecting the distribution of calcium within the muscle fiber. It also has oxytocic effects. It is an optical isomer of quinidine, and has cardiovascular effects similar to quinidine.

Pharmacokinetics:

Absorption – Quinine is readily absorbed orally, mainly from the upper small intestine. Absorption is almost complete, even in patients with marked diarrhea. Peak plasma concentrations occur within 1 to 3 hours after a single oral dose. Chronic administration of 1 g/day produces an average plasma concentration of 7 mcg/ml.

Tinnitus and hearing impairment rarely occur at plasma concentrations of < 10 mcg/ml. However, an occasional patient may have some evidence of cinchonism such as tinnitus (see Warnings).

Distribution – Quinine is ≈ 70% to 85% protein bound. The concentration of the alkaloid in cerebrospinal fluid is only 2% to 7% of that in the plasma. However, it can cross the placenta and readily reach fetal tissues.

Metabolism/Excretion – The cinchona alkaloids are primarily metabolized in the liver; < 5% is excreted unaltered in the urine. There is no accumulation in the body upon continued administration. Half-life is 4 to 5 hours. After termination of therapy, the plasma level falls rapidly and only a negligible concentration is detectable after 24 hours.

The metabolites are excreted in the urine, many as hydroxy derivatives; small amounts also appear in the feces, gastric juice, bile and saliva. Renal excretion of quinine is twice as rapid when the urine is acidic as when it is alkaline; greater tubular reabsorption of the alkaloidal base occurs in an alkaline medium.

The pharmacokinetics of quinine are affected by malarial infection, with volume of distribution and systemic clearance decreasing. Also, protein binding increases to > 90% in patients with cerebral malaria, in pregnant patients and in children.

Indications:

Chloroquine-resistant falciparum malaria: Either alone, with pyrimethamine and a sulfonamide or with a tetracycline. It is also considered alternative therapy for chloroquine-sensitive strains of *P. falciparum, P. malariae, P. ovale* and *P. vivax*. Mefloquine and clindamycin may also be used with quinine depending on where the malaria was acquired (eg, Southeast Asia, Bangladesh, East Africa).

Unlabeled uses: Nocturnal recumbency leg cramps, prevention and treatment.
Dose: 260 to 300 mg at bedtime.

Contraindications:

Hypersensitivity to quinine; glucose-6-phosphate dehydrogenase (G–6–PD) deficiency; optic neuritis; tinnitus; history of blackwater fever and thrombocytopenic purpura (associated with previous quinine ingestion); pregnancy (see Warnings).

Warnings:

Cinchonism: Repeated doses or overdosage of quinine may precipitate cinchonism. The mildest symptoms include tinnitus, headache, nausea and slightly disturbed vision, which usually subside rapidly upon discontinuation of the drug. When quinine is continued or after large single doses, symptoms also involve the GI tract, the nervous and cardiovascular systems and the skin.

Tinnitus and impaired hearing may occur at plasma quinine concentrations > 10 mcg/ml, a level not normally attained with quinine 260 to 520 mg/day. In a hypersensitive patient, as little as 300 mg may produce tinnitus.

Glucose-6–phosphate dehydrogenase (G–6–PD) deficiency: In patients with G–6–PD deficiency, primaquine should only be administered if essential and under close supervision. A weekly, as opposed to daily, regimen is recommended to reduce the risk of hemolysis.

Hemolysis (with the potential for hemolytic anemia) has been associated with a G-6-PD deficiency in patients taking quinine. Stop therapy immediately if hemolysis appears.

QUININE SULFATE

Cardiac disease: Use with caution in patients with cardiac arrhythmias; quinine has quinidine-like activity. In patients with atrial fibrillation, quinine use requires the same precautions as those for quinidine. May cause cardiotoxicity.

Hypersensitivity: Discontinue quinine if there is any evidence of hypersensitivity. Cutaneous flushing, pruritus, skin rashes, fever, gastric distress, dyspnea, ringing in the ears and visual impairment may occur, particularly with only small doses of quinine. Extreme flushing of the skin accompanied by intense, generalized pruritus is most common. Hemoglobinuria and asthma are idiosyncratic. Refer to Management of Acute Hypersensitivity Reactions.

Pregnancy: Category X. Quinine has an oxytocic action that appears to occur only with doses that are higher than those recommended. It also crosses the placenta. Congenital malformations have occurred primarily with large doses (30 g) for attempted abortion. In about 50%, the malformation was deafness related to auditory nerve hypoplasia. Other abnormalities were limb anomalies, visceral defects and visual changes.

Lactation: Quinine is excreted in breast milk in small amounts. Although no adverse effects have been reported in the nursing infant, rule out patients at risk for G–6-PD deficiency before breastfeeding.

Drug Interactions:

Quinine Drug Interactions			
Precipitant drug	Object drug *		Description
Antacids, aluminum-containing	Quinine	⬇	Aluminum-containing antacids may delay or decrease absorption of concurrent quinine.
Cimetidine	Quinine	⬆	Cimetidine may reduce quinine's oral clearance and increase its elimination half-life.
Mefloquine	Quinine	⬆	Do not use concurrently with quinine. If these agents are to be used in the initial treatment of severe malaria, delay mefloquine administration at least 12 hours after the last dose of quinine. ECG abnormalities or cardiac arrest may occur. The risk of convulsions may also be increased with coadministration.
Rifamycins (rifabutin, rifampin)	Quinine	⬇	Rifamycins, potent inducers of hepatic microsomal enzymes, increased the hepatic clearance of quinine. Enzyme induction can persist for several days following discontinuation of the rifamycin.
Urinary alkalinizers (eg, acetazolamide, sodium bicarbonate)	Quinine	⬆	Urinary alkalinizers administered concurrently with quinine may increase quinine blood levels with potential for toxicity.
Quinine	Anticoagulants, oral	⬆	Quinine may depress the hepatic enzyme system that synthesizes the vitamin K dependent clotting factors and thus may enhance the action of warfarin and other oral anticoagulants.
Quinine	Digoxin	⬆	Digoxin serum concentrations may be increased by concurrent quinine. Monitor digoxin levels periodically.
Quinine	Neuromuscular blocking agents (depolarizing and nondepolarizing)	⬆	The neuromuscular blockade of these agents may be potentiated by quinine, and may result in respiratory difficulties.
Quinine	Succinylcholine	⬆	Quinidine may produce a decrease in plasma cholinesterase activity, resulting in a slowed metabolic rate for succinylcholine.

* ⬆ = Object drug increased. ⬇ = Object drug decreased.

Drug/Lab test interactions: Elevated values for urinary 17-ketogenic steroids may occur with the Zimmerman method.

QUININE SULFATE

Adverse Reactions:

Body as a whole: Cinchonism (see Warnings).

Hematologic: Acute hemolysis; hemolytic anemia; thrombocytopenic purpura; agranulocytosis; hypoprothrombinemia.

Ophthalmic: Visual disturbances, including disturbed color vision and perception; photophobia; blurred vision with scotomata; night blindness; amblyopia; diplopia; diminished visual fields; mydriasis; optic atrophy.

CNS: Tinnitus (see Warnings); deafness; vertigo; headache; fever; apprehension; restlessness; confusion; syncope; excitement; delirium; hypothermia; convulsions; dizziness.

GI: Nausea; vomiting; epigastric pain; hepatitis; gastrointestinal disturbance.

Hypersensitivity: Cutaneous rashes (urticarial, papular, scarlatinal); pruritus; flushing; sweating; facial edema; asthmatic symptoms. See Warnings.

Cardiovascular: Anginal symptoms.

Miscellaneous: Vasculitis; hypoglycemia; lichenoid photosensitivity.

Overdosage:

Symptoms: The more common signs and symptoms are tinnitus, dizziness, skin rash and GI disturbance (intestinal cramping). With higher doses, cardiovascular and CNS effects may occur, including headache, fever, vomiting, apprehension, confusion and convulsions. Other effects are listed in Adverse Reactions.

Fatalities with quinine have occurred from single oral doses of 2 to 8 g; a single fatality reported with a dose of 1.5 g may reflect an idiosyncratic effect. Several cases of blindness following large overdoses of quinine, with partial recovery of vision in each instance, have been reported.

Treatment: Employ gastric lavage or induce emesis. Support blood pressure and maintain renal function; provide mechanical ventilation if needed. Use sedatives, oxygen and other supportive measures as necessary. Maintain fluid and electrolyte balance with IV fluids. Refer also to General Management of Acute Overdosage.

Urinary acidification will promote renal excretion of quinine. In the presence of hemoglobinuria, however, acidification of the urine may augment renal blockade. Quinine is readily dialyzable by hemodialysis or hemoperfusion.

Angioedema or asthma may require epinephrine, corticosteroids or antihistamines.

In the acute phase of toxic amaurosis caused by quinine, IV vasodilators may have a salutory effect. Stellate block has also been used effectively for quinine-associated blindness. Residual visual impairment occasionally yields to vasodilators.

Patient Information:

Take with food or after meals to minimize GI irritation.

Medication may cause diarrhea, nausea, stomach cramps or pain, vomiting or ringing in the ears; notify physician if these become pronounced.

May produce blurred vision, vertigo, restlessness, confusion or dizziness; patients should observe caution while driving or performing other tasks requiring alertness.

Stop the drug if there is any evidence of allergy such as flushing, itching, rash, fever, stomach pain, difficult breathing, ringing in the ears and vision problems.

Administration and Dosage:

Adults: 260 to 650 mg 3 times a day for 6 to 12 days.

Children: 10 mg/kg every 8 hours for 5 to 7 days.

Storage/Stability: Dispense in a tight, light-resistant container as defined in the USP. Use child-resistant closure. Store at controlled room temperature 15° to 30°C (59° to 86°F). Protect from light.

Rx	**Quinine Sulfate** (Various, eg, Moore, Zenith)	**Capsules:** 200 mg	In 100s, 500s, 1000s.
		260 mg	In 100s, 500s, 1000s.
		325 mg	In 100s, 500s, 1000s.
Rx	**Quinine Sulfate** (Various, eg, Moore, Zenith)	**Tablets:** 260 mg	In 100s, 500s, 1000s.

MEFLOQUINE HCl

Actions:

Pharmacology: Mefloquine is an antimalarial agent which acts as a blood schizonticide. Its exact mechanism of action is unknown, but it may act by raising intravesicular pH in parasite acid vesicles. It is a structural analog of quinine.

Pharmacokinetics: Studies of healthy males showed a significant lagtime after administration; terminal elimination half-life varied widely (13 to 24 days) with a mean of ≈ 3 weeks. Mefloquine is a mixture of enantiomeric molecules whose rates of release, absorption, transport, action, degradation and elimination may differ.

Additional studies showed slightly greater drug concentrations for longer periods. Absorption half-life was 0.36 to 2 hours; terminal elimination half-life was 15 to 33 days. Concentrations of the primary metabolite surpassed the concentrations of mefloquine. In multiple-dose studies, mean metabolite to mefloquine ratio at steady state ranged between 2.3 and 8.6.

Total drug clearance, which is essentially all hepatic, is ≈ 30 ml/min. Volume of distribution, ≈ 20 L/kg, indicates extensive distribution. The drug is highly bound (98%) to plasma proteins and concentrated in blood erythrocytes, the target cells in malaria, at a relatively constant erythrocyte-to-plasma concentration ratio of ≈ 2.

The pharmacokinetics of mefloquine in patients with compromised renal function and compromised hepatic function have not been studied.

Strains of *Plasmodium falciparum* resistant to mefloquine have been reported.

Indications:

Treatment of acute malaria infections: Mild to moderate acute malaria caused by mefloquine-susceptible strains of *P. falciparum* (both chloroquine-susceptible and resistant strains) or *P. vivax.* There are insufficient clinical data to document mefloquine's effect in malaria caused by *P. ovale* or *P. malariae.*

Prevention of malaria: Prophylaxis of *P. falciparum* and *P. vivax* malarial infections, including prophylaxis of chloroquine-resistant strains of *P. falciparum.* The use of mefloquine alone is recommended by the CDC for travel to areas of risk where chloroquine-resistant *P. falciparum* exists.

Contraindications:

Hypersensitivity to mefloquine or related compounds.

Warnings:

Acute P. vivax malaria: Patients with acute *P. vivax* malaria treated with mefloquine are at high risk of relapse because mefloquine does not eliminate exoerythrocytic (hepatic phase) parasites. To avoid relapse, after initial treatment of the acute infection with mefloquine, patients should subsequently be treated with an 8–aminoquinoline (eg, primaquine).

Infection due to P. falciparum: In case of life-threatening, serious or overwhelming malarial infections due to *P. falciparum,* treat patients with an IV antimalarial drug. Following completion of IV treatment, mefloquine may be given orally to complete the course of therapy.

Pregnancy: Category C. Mefloquine is teratogenic in rats and mice at a dose of 100 mg/kg/day. In rabbits, 160 mg/kg/day was embryotoxic and teratogenic and 80 mg/kg/day was teratogenic but not embryotoxic. There are no adequate and well controlled studies in pregnant women. Use during pregnancy only if potential benefit justifies potential risk to the fetus. Warn women of childbearing potential traveling to areas where malaria is endemic against becoming pregnant and to practice reliable contraceptive measures during prophylaxis and for 2 months after the last dose.

Lactation: Mefloquine is excreted in breast milk. Based on a study in a few subjects, low concentrations (3% to 4%) of mefloquine were excreted in breast milk following a dose equivalent to 250 mg of the free base. Because of the potential for serious adverse reactions in nursing infants from mefloquine, decide whether to discontinue the drug, taking into account the importance of the drug to the mother.

Children: Safety and efficacy have not been established. Two studies of mefloquine in children living in endemic areas for *P. falciparum* were conducted. All these children had at least a low level of parasitemia and 18% to 40% had significant parasitemia with or without mild malaria symptoms. When given a single 20 to 30 mg/kg dose, all children with fever became afebrile, and 92% with significant parasitemia had a satisfactory response. Nausea and vomiting occurred in ≈ 10% and 20%, respectively, and dizziness was seen in ≈ 40% of children.

Precautions:

Monitoring: This drug has not been administered for periods > 1 year. If it is to be given for a prolonged period, perform periodic evaluations including liver function tests.

Perform periodic hepatic function evaluation during prolonged prophylaxis.

MEFLOQUINE HCl

Cardiac disease: Parenteral animal studies show that mefloquine, a myocardial depressant, possesses 20% of the antifibrillatory action of quinidine and produces 50% of the increase in the PR interval reported with quinine. Mefloquine's effect on the compromised cardiovascular system has not been evaluated. However, transitory and clinically silent ECG alterations have been reported during mefloquine use. Alterations include sinus bradycardia, sinus arrhythmia, first-degree AV block, prolongation of the QT_c interval and abnormal T waves. Weigh the benefits of therapy against possible adverse effects in cardiac disease patients.

Ocular lesions were observed in rats fed mefloquine daily for 2 years. All surviving rats given 30 mg/kg/day had ocular lesions in both eyes characterized by retinal degeneration, opacity of the lens and retinal edema. Similar but less severe lesions were observed in 80% of female and 22% of male rats fed 12.5 mg/kg/day for 2 years. At doses of 5 mg/kg/day, only corneal lesions were observed (9% of rats studied). Periodic ophthalmic examinations are recommended.

Psychiatric disturbances: Exercise caution in patients with psychiatric disturbances because mefloquine has been associated with emotional disturbances.

Hazardous tasks: Exercise caution while driving or operating hazardous machinery, as dizziness, a disturbed sense of balance, neurological and psychiatric reactions have occurred during and following the use of mefloquine. These effects may occur after therapy is discontinued due to the drug's long half-life. During prophylactic use, if signs of unexplained anxiety, depression, restlessness or confusion are noticed, these may be considered prodromal to a more serious event. In these cases, discontinue the drug.

Drug Interactions:

Mefloquine Drug Interactions			
Precipitant drug	Object drug*		Description
Beta-adrenergic blockers	Mefloquine	⬆	ECG abnormalities or cardiac arrest may occur with concurrent mefloquine. There is one report of cardiopulmonary arrest with full recovery in a patient taking propranolol.
Chloroquine	Mefloquine	⬆	The risk of convulsions may be increased with concomitant mefloquine.
Halofantrine	Mefloquine	⬆	Do not use concurrently because of the danger of a potentially fatal prolongation of the QT_c interval.
Mefloquine	Quinine or Quinidine	⬆	Do not use concurrently with mefloquine. If these agents are to be used in the initial treatment of severe malaria, delay mefloquine administration at least 12 hours after the last dose of quinine or quinidine. ECG abnormalities or cardiac arrest may occur. Although no cardiovascular action of mefloquine, a myocardial depressant, has been observed during clinical trials, parenteral studies in animals show that it possesses 20% of the antifibrillatory action of quinidine and produces 50% of the increase in the PR interval reported with quinine. The risk of convulsions may also be increased with concurrent mefloquine and quinine.
Mefloquine	Valproic acid	⬇	Valproic acid and concurrent mefloquine resulted in loss of seizure control and lower than expected valproic acid blood levels. Therefore, monitor valproic acid blood levels and adjust the dosage as necessary.

* ⬆ = Object drug increased. ⬇ = Object drug decreased.

Adverse Reactions:

At doses used for acute malaria, symptoms possibly attributable to the drug cannot be distinguished from symptoms usually attributable to the disease itself.

Prophylaxis of malaria: Vomiting (3%); dizziness, syncope, extrasystoles (< 1%).

Treatment of malaria: The most frequently observed adverse reactions included: Dizziness; myalgia; nausea; fever; headache; vomiting; chills; diarrhea; skin rash; abdominal pain; fatigue; loss of appetite; tinnitus. Side effects occurring in < 1% included: Bradycardia; hair loss; emotional problems; pruritus; asthenia; transient emotional disturbances; telogen effluvium (loss of resting hair); seizures.

Postmarketing: Vertigo; visual disturbances; CNS disturbances (eg, psychotic manifestations, hallucinations, confusion, anxiety, depression, convulsions); insomnia; abnormal dreams; forgetfulness; motor and sensory neuropathy; hypertension;

MEFLOQUINE HCl

hypotension; flushing; tachycardia; palpitations; urticaria; Stevens-Johnson syndrome and erythema multiforme.

Post-marketing surveillance indicates that the same adverse experiences are reported during prophylaxis, as well as acute treatment.

Lab test abnormalities: Decreased hematocrit; transient elevation of transaminases; leukopenia; thrombocytopenia. These alterations were observed in patients with acute malaria who received treatment doses of the drug and were attributed to the disease itself. During prophylactic mefloquine to indigenous populations in malaria-endemic areas, the following occasional alterations in lab values were observed: Transient elevation of transaminases; leukocytosis; thrombocytopenia.

Overdosage:

Induce vomiting or perform gastric lavage, as appropriate. Monitor cardiac function and neurologic and psychiatric status for at least 24 hours. Provide symptomatic and intensive supportive treatment as required, particularly for cardiovascular disturbances. See a physician immediately because of the potential cardiotoxic effect. Treat vomiting or diarrhea with standard fluid therapy. Refer to General Management of Acute Overdosage.

Patient Information:

Hazardous tasks: May produce dizziness; patients should observe caution while driving or performing other tasks requiring alertness and physical dexterity.

Administration and Dosage:

Treatment of mild to moderate malaria in adults caused by P. vivax or mefloquine-susceptible strains of P. falciparum: 5 tablets (1250 mg) as a single dose. Do not take on an empty stomach. Give with at least 240 ml (8 oz) water.

Patients given mefloquine for acute *P. vivax* malaria are at high risk of relapse; mefloquine does not eliminate exoerythrocytic (hepatic phase) parasites. To avoid such relapse, subsequently treat with 8-aminoquinolone (eg, primaquine).

Malaria prophylaxis: Adult - 250 mg once weekly for 4 weeks, then 250 mg every other week. The CDC recommends a single dose taken weekly starting 1 week before travel, continued weekly during travel and for 4 weeks after leaving such areas.†

Children – CDC recommends these pediatric doses weekly, starting 1 week before travel, continued weekly during travel and for 4 weeks after leaving such areas: 15 to 19 kg, ¼ tab; 20 to 30 kg, ½ tab; 31 to 45 kg, ¾ tab; > 45 kg, 1 tab.†

Initiate prophylactic drug use 1 week prior to departure to an endemic area. It is suggested the same day of the week be used for each dose. To avoid development of malaria after return from an endemic area, continue prophylaxis for 4 additional weeks. Do not take on an empty stomach. Administer with at least 240 ml (8 oz) water.

Storage/Stability: Store at 15° to 30°C (59° to 86°F).

Rx	**Lariam** (Roche)	**Tablets**: 250 mg	(Lariam 250 Roche). White, scored. In *Tel-E-Dose* 25s.

DOXYCYCLINE

Indications:

Malaria prophylaxis: Prophylaxis of malaria due to *Plasmodium falciparum* in short-term travelers (< 4 months) to areas with chloroquine or pyrimethamine-sulfadoxine resistant strains.

Administration and Dosage:

Begin doxycycline prophylaxis 1 to 2 days before travel to malarious areas and continue daily during travel in the malarious area and for 4 weeks after the traveler leaves the area.

Adults: 100 mg once daily.

Children: 2 mg/kg/day up to adult dose of 100 mg/day.

For complete listing of available products, see the Doxycycline monograph in the Tetracyclines section.

† *Morbidity and Mortality Weekly Report* 1990 (Mar 9);39 (RR-3):1-10 and 1990 (Sep 14);39:630.

4–AMINOQUINOLINE COMPOUNDS

Actions:

Pharmacology: Chloroquine's exact mechanism of action is not known, but several mechanisms have been suggested. It concentrates in parasite acid vesicles and raises internal pH. The "non-weak base effect" inhibits parasite growth at extracellular drug concentrations; this may occur due to active chloroquine-concentrating mechanism in parasite acid vesicles. Another mechanism may involve ferriprotoporphyrin IX aggregates, which are released by parasitized erythrocytes during hemoglobin degradation and serve as chloroquine receptors, causing membrane damage with lysis of parasites or erythrocytes. Chloroquine may also influence hemoglobin digestion or interfere with parasite/nucleoprotein synthesis.

Pharmacokinetics: Absorbed readily from GI tract, peak plasma levels are reached in 1 to 6 hours. Plasma protein binding is 55%. Drug concentrates in liver, spleen, kidney and brain and is strongly bound in melanin-containing cells such as in eyes and skin. Chloroquine is eliminated very slowly and may persist in tissues for a prolonged period. Up to 70% of a dose may be excreted unchanged in urine and up to 25% as a metabolite. Renal excretion is enhanced by urinary acidification.

Microbiology: Active against the erythrocytic forms of *Plasmodium vivax* and *malariae* and most strains of *P. falciparum* (but not the gametocytes of *P. falciparum*).

These drugs do not prevent relapses or infection of *P. vivax* or *malariae* malaria; not effective against exoerythrocytic parasite forms. Highly effective in suppressing *P. vivax* or *malariae* malaria, terminating acute attacks and significantly lengthening interval between treatment and relapse. In *P. falciparum* malaria, they abolish acute attack and completely cure infection unless due to resistant strain. Hydroxychloroquine is not effective against chloroquine-resistant *P. falciparum* strains.

Indications:

Malaria: Prophylaxis and treatment of acute attacks of malaria due to *P. vivax, P. malariae, P. ovale* and susceptible strains of *P. falciparum.* Chloroquine phosphate is the drug of choice in this situation. Chloroquine HCl is used when oral therapy is not feasible. For radical cure of *P. vivax* and *P. malariae* malaria, concomitant primaquine therapy is required.

Unlabeled uses: Chloroquine has been used to suppress rheumatoid arthritis and in the treatment of systemic and discoid lupus erythematosus, scleroderma, pemphigus, lichen planus, polymyositis, sarcoidosis and porphyria cutanea tarda.

For other uses, refer to individual product monographs.

Contraindications:

Retinal or visual field changes; hypersensitivity; long-term therapy in children (hydroxychloroquine). Consider an exception in acute malarial attacks caused by *Plasmodia* strains susceptible only to 4–aminoquinolines.

Warnings:

Resistance: Certain strains of *P. falciparum* are resistant to 4-aminoquinoline compounds; normally adequate doses fail to prevent or cure malaria or parasitemia.

Retinopathy: Irreversible retinal damage has occurred with long-term or high dosages. Retinopathy may be dose-related. During prolonged therapy, perform baseline and periodic ophthalmologic exams. If there is any indication of abnormality in visual acuity/field or retinal macular areas or any visual symptoms not explainable by difficulties of accommodation or corneal opacities, stop drug immediately; observe for possible progression. Retinal changes/visual disturbances may progress after therapy cessation.

Glucose-6-phosphate dehydrogenase (G-6-PD) deficiency: Use with caution in patients with G-6–PD deficiencies.

Muscular weakness: Periodically question and examine patients who are on long-term therapy; test knee and ankle reflexes to detect muscular weakness. If weakness occurs, discontinue therapy.

Psoriasis or porphyria: Use of these drugs may exacerbate these conditions. Do not use in these conditions unless the benefit outweighs the possible hazard.

Hepatic function impairment: These drugs concentrate in liver; use with caution in hepatic disease or alcoholism, or in conjunction with hepatotoxic drugs.

Pregnancy: Use only when clearly needed and when potential benefits outweigh potential hazards to the fetus.

Lactation: Safety for use has not been established; these agents are excreted in breast milk. A nursing infant may consume ≈ 0.55% of a 300 mg maternal dose over 24 hours. One study determined the milk:blood ratio of the nursing mother to be 0.358.

4–AMINOQUINOLINE COMPOUNDS

Children: Children are especially sensitive to the 4-aminoquinoline compounds. Fatalities following accidental ingestion of relatively small doses and sudden deaths from parenteral chloroquine have been recorded. Do not exceed a single dose of 5 mg base/kg of chloroquine HCl in infants or children.

Precautions:

Monitoring: Perform periodic CBCs during prolonged therapy. If any severe blood disorder not attributable to the disease appears, consider discontinuing therapy. Measure glucose-6-phosphate dehydrogenase (G-6-PD) in susceptible individuals prior to initiating therapy. Although probably safe when given in normal therapeutic doses, these compounds may induce hemolysis in G-6-PD deficient individuals in the presence of infection or stressful conditions. An acute drop in hematocrit, hemoglobin and red blood cell count may occur.

Drug Interactions:

4-Aminoquinoline Drug Interactions

Precipitant drug	Object drug *		Description
Cimetidine	Chloroquine	⬆	Cimetidine may reduce the oral clearance rate and metabolism of chloroquine
Chloroquine	Kaolin or magnesium trisilicate	⬇	GI absorption of chloroquine may be decreased by concomitant administration of these agents.

* ⬆ = Object drug increased. ⬇ = Object drug decreased.

Adverse Reactions:

Cardiovascular: Hypotension; ECG changes (particularly inversion or depression of the T wave, widening of QRS complex); cardiomyopathy (rare).

CNS: Mild, transient headache; psychic stimulation; psychotic episodes, convulsions (rare).

GI: Anorexia; nausea; vomiting; diarrhea; abdominal cramps.

Ophthalmic: Irreversible retinal damage (see Warnings); visual disturbances (blurred vision, difficulty of focusing or accommodation); nyctalopia; scotomatous vision with field defects of paracentral, pericentral ring types and typically temporal scotomas, eg, difficulty reading with words tending to disappear, seeing half an object, misty vision, fog before eyes.

Miscellaneous: Agranulocytosis; hair loss; pruritus; neuromyopathy, blood dyscrasias, lichen planus-like eruptions, skin/mucosal pigment changes, pleomorphic skin eruptions. A few cases of a nerve-type deafness have occurred after prolonged high doses.

Overdosage:

Symptoms: Symptoms may occur within 30 minutes in overdosage (or rarely with lower doses in hypersensitive patients) and consist of headache, drowsiness, visual disturbances, nausea, vomiting, cardiovascular collapse and convulsions followed by sudden and early respiratory and cardiac arrest. Respiratory depression, cardiovascular collapse, shock, convulsions and death have occurred with overdose of parenteral chloroquine HCl, especially in infants and children. The ECG may reveal atrial standstill, nodal rhythm, prolonged intraventricular conduction and bradycardia progressing to ventricular fibrillation or arrest. In a retrospective study, it was determined that ingestion of > 5 g of chloroquine was an accurate predictor of fatal outcome in adults.

Treatment: Treatment is symptomatic; the stomach must be immediately evacuated by emesis or gastric lavage until the stomach is completely emptied. After lavage, activated charcoal (a dose not less than five times estimated dose ingested) may inhibit further absorption if given within 30 minutes of ingestion.

Control convulsions before attempting gastric lavage. If due to cerebral stimulation, cautious administration of a short-acting barbiturate may be tried. Treat anoxia-induced convulsions by oxygen, mechanical ventilation or, in shock with hypotension, by vasopressor therapy. Tracheal intubation or tracheostomy may be necessary. Peritoneal dialysis and exchange transfusions have been suggested.

For at least 6 hours, closely observe an asymptomatic patient who survives the acute phase. Force fluids and acidify the urine with 8 g ammonium chloride in divided doses (for adults) to help promote excretion.

4–AMINOQUINOLINE COMPOUNDS

In one study, 10 of 11 patients who ingested > 5 g of chloroquine survived after treatment with diazepam and epinephrine for several days along with mechanical ventilation. The use of diazepam has also been successful in other reports.

Patient Information:

May cause GI upset; take with food. Complete full course of therapy.

Report visual disturbances or difficulty in hearing or ringing in ears to physician.

Keep out of reach of children; overdosage is especially dangerous in children.

Medication may cause diarrhea, loss of appetite, nausea, stomach pain or vomiting, muscle weakness or rash. Notify physician if pronounced or bothersome.

CHLOROQUINE PHOSPHATE

Chloroquine phosphate 500 mg is equivalent to 300 mg chloroquine base and 400 mg hydroxychloroquine sulfate.

Indications:

Malaria: Prophylaxis and treatment of acute attacks of malaria due to *P. vivax*, *P. malariae*, *P. ovale* and susceptible strains of *P. falciparum*.

Amebiasis: Also used for treatment of extraintestinal amebiasis (see Amebicides section).

Administration and Dosage:

Children's doses, expressed in mg/kg, should not exceed the recommended adult dose.

Suppression:

Adults – 300 mg (base) weekly, on the same day each week. Begin 1 to 2 weeks prior to exposure; continue for 4 weeks after leaving endemic area.

If suppressive therapy is not begun prior to exposure, double the initial loading dose (adults - 600 mg base; children - 10 mg base/kg) and give in 2 divided doses, 6 hours apart.

Children – Administer 5 mg base/kg weekly, up to a maximum adult dose of 300 mg base.[1]

Children's Chloroquine Dose Based on Age

Age (years)	Chloroquine base equivalent
< 1	37.5 mg
1 to 3	75 mg
4 to 6	100 mg
7 to 10	150 mg
11 to 16	225 mg

CDC recommended schedule for chloroquine as an alternative to mefloquine[1]: Travelers to areas of risk where chloroquine-resistant *P. falciparum* is endemic and for whom mefloquine is contraindicated may elect to use an alternative regimen. Chloroquine alone taken weekly is recommended for travelers who cannot use mefloquine or doxycycline, especially pregnant women and children < 15 kg. In addition, give these travelers a single treatment dose of sulfadoxine/pyrimethamine to keep during travel and to take promptly in the event of a febrile illness during their travel when professional medical care is not readily available. Continue weekly chloroquine prophylaxis after presumptive treatment with sulfadoxine/pyrimethamine.

4–Aminoquinoline Compounds

CHLOROQUINE PHOSPHATE

Acute attack:

Chloroquine Phosphate Dose in Acute Malarial Attack			
		Dosage (in mg of base)	
Dose	Time	Adults	Children
Initial dose	Day 1	600 mg	10 mg/kg
2nd dose	6 hours later	300 mg	5 mg/kg
3rd dose	Day 2	300 mg	5 mg/kg
4th dose	Day 3	300 mg	5 mg/kg

Rx	**Chloroquine Phosphate** (Various, eg, CMC, Gallipot)	**Tablets:** 250 mg (equiv. to 150 mg base)	In 100s and 1000s.
Rx	**Aralen Phosphate** (Sanofi Winthrop)	**Tablets:** 500 mg (equiv. to 300 mg base)	Pink. Film coated. In 25s.
Rx	**Aralen Phosphate** (Sanofi Winthrop)	**Injection:** 5 mg (equiv. to 200 mg base)	In 5 amps.

[1] *Morbidity and Mortality Weekly Report* 1990 (Mar 9);39 (RR-3):1–10.

4–Aminoquinoline Compounds

CHLOROQUINE HCl

Chloroquine HCl 50 mg is equivalent to 40 mg chloroquine base.

Indications:

Malaria: Treatment of malaria when oral therapy is not feasible.

Amebiasis: Also used for treatment of extraintestinal amebiasis (see Amebicides section).

Administration and Dosage:

Adults: 160 to 200 mg base (4 to 5 ml) IM initially; repeat in 6 hours if necessary. Do not exceed 800 mg (base) total dose in the first 24 hours. Begin oral dosage as soon as possible and continue for 3 days until ≈ 1.5 g base has been administered.

Other suggested dosages include 2.5 mg base/kg every 4 hours or 3.5 mg/kg every 6 hours; repeat if necessary, maximum 25 mg/kg/day.

Children: Infants and children are extremely susceptible to overdosage. Severe reactions and deaths have occurred. The recommended single dose is 5 mg base/kg; repeat in 6 hours. Do not exceed 10 mg/kg/24 hours.

Rx	**Aralen HCl** (Sanofi Winthrop)	**Injection:** 50 mg (equiv. to 40 mg base)/ml	In 5 ml amps.

HYDROXYCHLOROQUINE SULFATE

Hydroxychloroquine sulfate 200 mg is equivalent to 155 mg hydroxychloroquine base and 250 mg chloroquine phosphate.

Indications:

Malaria: Prophylaxis and treatment of acute attacks of malaria due to *P. vivax, P. malariae, P. ovale* and susceptible strains of *P. falciparum.*

Lupus erythematosus and rheumatoid arthritis: Also used for the treatment of discoid and systemic lupus erythematosus and rheumatoid arthritis (see monograph in Antirheumatic Agents section).

Administration and Dosage:

Children's doses, expressed in mg/kg, should not exceed the recommended adult dose.

Suppression: Adults - 310 mg base weekly on the same day each week. Begin 1 to 2 weeks prior to exposure; continue for 4 weeks after leaving endemic area.

If suppressive therapy is not begun prior to exposure, double the initial loading dose (adults – 620 mg base; children – 10 mg base/kg) and give in 2 doses, 6 hours apart.

Children – Administer 5 mg base/kg weekly, up to a maximum adult dose.

Children's Hydroxychloroquine Dose Based on Age

Age (years)	Hydroxychloroquine base equivalent
< 1	37.5 mg
1 to 3	75 mg
4 to 6	100 mg
7 to 10	150 mg
11 to 16	225 mg

Acute attack:

Hydroxychloroquine Dose in Acute Malarial Attack

Dose	Time	Dosage (mg of base) Adults	Dosage (mg of base) Children
Initial dose	Day 1	620 mg	10 mg/kg
2nd dose	6 hours later	310 mg	5 mg/kg
3rd dose	Day 2	310 mg	5 mg/kg
4th dose	Day 3	310 mg	5 mg/kg

An alternative method, using a single dose of 620 mg base, has also been proven effective.

Rx	**Hydroxychloroquine Sulfate** (Various, eg, Copley, Geneva, Moore, Zenith)	**Tablets:** 200 mg (equiv. to 155 mg base)	White. In 100s, 500s and 1000s.
Rx	**Plaquenil Sulfate** (Sanofi Winthrop)		In 100s and 500s.

8–Aminoquinoline Compound

PRIMAQUINE PHOSPHATE

Actions:

Pharmacology: An 8-aminoquinoline, primaquine is structurally similar to the 4-aminoquinolines but possesses markedly different antimalarial activities.

Primaquine may disrupt the parasite's mitochondria and bind to native DNA. The resulting structural changes create a major disruption in the metabolic process. The gametocyte and exoerythrocyte forms are inhibited. Some gametocytes are destroyed while others are rendered incapable of undergoing maturation division in the mosquito gut. By eliminating tissue (exoerythrocyte) infection, primaquine prevents development of blood (erythrocytic) forms responsible for relapses in *P. vivax* malaria.

Pharmacokinetics: After oral administration, peak plasma concentrations of primaquine are reached in 1 to 3 hours. Primaquine, as compared to other antimalarials, is found in relatively low concentrations in the tissues. Highest concentrations are in the liver, lungs, brain, heart and skeletal muscle.

Primaquine is rapidly metabolized to a carboxylic acid derivative and then to further metabolites which have varying degrees of activity. Approximately 1% is excreted unchanged in the urine.

Microbiology: Active against *Plasmodium vivax, P. ovale* and the gametocytial forms of *P. falciparum.*

Indications:

P. Vivax malaria: Recommended only for the radical cure of *P. vivax* malaria, the prevention of relapse in *P. vivax* malaria or following the termination of chloroquine phosphate suppressive therapy in an area where *P. vivax* malaria is endemic.

Contraindications:

Concomitant administration of quinacrine and primaquine (see Drug Interactions); the acutely ill suffering from systemic disease manifested by tendency to granulocytopenia (eg, rheumatoid arthritis and lupus erythematosus); concurrent administration of other potentially hemolytic drugs or bone marrow depressants.

Warnings:

Hemolytic reactions (moderate to severe) may occur in the following groups of people while receiving primaquine: Glucose-6-phosphate dehydrogenase (G-6-PD) deficient patients; individuals with idiosyncratic reactions (manifested by hemolytic anemia, methemoglobinemia or leukopenia); individuals with nicotinamide adenine dinucleotide (NADH) methemoglobin reductase deficiency; or individuals with a family or personal history of favism. Discontinue if marked darkening of the urine or sudden decrease in hemoglobin concentration or leukocyte count occurs.

Pregnancy: Safety for use during pregnancy has not been established. Use only when clearly needed and when potential benefits outweigh potential hazards to the fetus.

Precautions:

Monitoring: Anemia, methemoglobinemia and leukopenia have occurred following large doses; do not exceed recommended dose. Perform routine blood examinations (particularly blood cell counts and hemoglobin determinations) during therapy.

Drug Interactions:

Quinacrine may potentiate the toxicity of antimalarial compounds which are structurally related to primaquine. Do not administer primaquine to patients who have recently received quinacrine.

Adverse Reactions:

GI: Nausea; vomiting; epigastric distress; abdominal cramps.

Hematologic: Leukopenia; hemolytic anemia in G-6-PD deficient individuals; methemoglobinemia in NADH methemoglobin reductase deficient individuals.

Overdosage:

Symptoms: Abdominal cramps; vomiting; burning, epigastric distress; CNS and cardiovascular disturbances; cyanosis; methemoglobinemia; moderate leukocytosis or leukopenia; anemia. The most striking symptoms are granulocytopenia and acute hemolytic anemia in sensitive persons. Acute hemolysis occurs, but patients recover completely if the dosage is discontinued.

Treatment is symptomatic.

8–Aminoquinoline Compound

PRIMAQUINE PHOSPHATE

Patient Information:

Complete full course of therapy.

If GI upset occurs, may be taken with food. If stomach upset (nausea, vomiting or stomach pain) continues, notify physician.

Notify physician if a darkening of the urine occurs.

Administration and Dosage:

Primaquine phosphate 26.3 mg is equivalent to 15 mg primaquine base.

Patients suffering from an attack of *P. vivax* malaria or having parasitized red blood cells should receive a course of chloroquine phosphate which quickly destroys the erythrocytic parasites and terminates the paroxysm. Administer primaquine concurrently to eradicate the exoerythrocytic parasites in a dosage of 15 mg (base) daily for 14 days.

CDC recommended treatment schedule:* Begin therapy during the last 2 weeks of, or following a course of, suppression with chloroquine or a comparable drug.
Adults – 26.3 mg (15 mg base) daily for 14 days.
Children – 0.5 mg/kg/day (0.3 mg base/kg/day; for 14 days.

Rx	**Primaquine Phosphate** (Various, eg, Quality Care, Sanofi Winthrop)	**Tablets:** 26.3 mg (equivalent to 15 mg base)	Lactose. In 20s, 100s.
Rx	**Primaquine Phosphate** (Various, eg, Medisca, Palisades)	**Powder**	5, 25, 100, 500 g

* *Morbidity and Mortality Weekly Report* 1990 (Mar 9);39(No. RR-3):1-10.

Folic Acid Antagonists

PYRIMETHAMINE

Actions:

Pharmacology: Pyrimethamine is a folic acid antagonist; its therapeutic action is based on differential requirement between host and parasite for nucleic acid precursors involved in growth as it selectively inhibits plasmodial dihydrofolate reductase. Pyrimethamine inhibits the enzyme dihydrofolate reductase, which catalyzes the reduction of dihydrofolate to tetrahydrofolate. This activity is highly selective against plasmodia and *Toxoplasma gondii.* It does not destroy gametocytes but arrests sporogony in the mosquito. Pyrimethamine possesses blood schizonticidal and some tissue schizonticidal activity against malaria parasites of humans.

Pharmacokinetics: Pyrimethamine is well absorbed after oral use. Peak plasma concentrations occur in 2 to 6 hrs. Plasma half-life is ≈ 4 days; suppressive concentrations are maintained for ≈ 2 weeks. It is ≈ 87% plasma protein-bound. It is hepatically metabolized. Several metabolites appear in the urine.

Indications:

Chemoprophylaxis of malaria due to susceptible strains of plasmodia. Fast-acting schizonticides (chloroquine or quinine) are preferable for acute attacks. However, concurrent pyrimethamine will initiate transmission control and suppressive cure for susceptible strains of plasmodia.

Toxoplasmosis: Use with a sulfonamide; synergism exists with this combination.

Contraindications:

Hypersensitivity; documented megaloblastic anemia due to folate deficiency.

Warnings:

Hypersensitivity reactions, occasionally severe, can occur at any dose, particularly if given with a sulfonamide. See Management of Acute Hypersensitivity Reactions.

Folic acid deficiency: If signs of folate deficiency develop, reduce dosage or discontinue drug according to patient response. Folinic acid (leucovorin) may be given in a dosage of 5 to 15 mg/day (oral, IM or IV) until normal hematopoiesis is restored. Use with caution in possible folate deficiency (eg, malabsorption syndrome, alcoholism, pregnancy, phenytoin usage).

Renal/Hepatic function impairment: Use with caution.

Pregnancy: Category C. There are no adequate and well controlled studies in pregnant women. Use pyrimethamine during pregnancy only if the potential benefit justifies the potential risk to the fetus. Concurrent administration of folinic acid is strongly recommended when used to treat toxoplasmosis during pregnancy.

Lactation: Pyrimethamine is excreted in breast milk. Milk samples from lactating mothers after pyrimethamine use had measurable drug concentrations with peak concentration at 6 hours postadministration. It is estimated that after a single 75 mg oral pyrimethamine dose, ≈ 3 to 4 mg of drug would be passed on to the feeding child over 48 hours. Because of the potential for serious adverse reactions in nursing infants from pyrimethamine, decide whether to discontinue nursing or discontinue the drug, taking into account the importance of the drug to the mother.

Precautions:

Monitoring: For toxoplasmosis, perform semiweekly blood counts, including platelet counts.

G-6-PD: May precipitate hemolytic anemia in patients with glucose-6–phosphate dehydrogenase deficiency, generally in the presence of other stressful events.

Drug Interactions:

Pyrimethamine Drug Interactions

Precipitant drug	Object drug*		Description
Antifolic drugs (eg, methotrexate, sulfonamides, TMP-SMZ)	Pyrimethamine	↑	Concurrent use of antifolic acids and pyrimethamine may increase the risk of bone marrow suppression. Discontinue pyrimethamine if signs of folate deficiency develop (see Warnings).
Pyrimethamine	Lorazepam	↑	Mild hepatotoxicity has been reported when lorazepam and pyrimethamine were administered concomitantly.

* ↑ = Object drug increased.

Folic Acid Antagonists

PYRIMETHAMINE

Adverse Reactions:

GI: Anorexia, vomiting (large doses); atrophic glossitis. Vomiting may be minimized by giving with meals; it usually disappears promptly upon reduction of dosage.

Hematologic: Megaloblastic anemia, leukopenia, thrombocytopenia, pancytopenia, hematuria (large doses).

Cardiac: Rhythm disorders (large doses).

Rare: Insomnia; diarrhea; headache; lightheadedness; dryness of the mouth or throat; fever; malaise; dermatitis; abnormal skin pigmentation; depression; seizures; pulmonary eosinophilia; hyperphenylalaninemia.

Overdosage:

Symptoms: Acute intoxication involves GI symptoms or CNS stimulation. Initial symptoms are GI and include abdominal pain, nausea and severe and repeated vomiting possibly including hematemesis. CNS toxicity is manifested by initial excitability, generalized and prolonged convulsions which may be followed by respiratory depression, circulatory collapse and death within a few hours. Neurological symptoms appear rapidly (30 min to 2 hours after drug ingestion), suggesting that in gross overdosage, pyrimethamine has a direct toxic effect on the CNS.

The fatal dose is variable; the smallest reported fatal single dose is 250 to 300 mg. There are reports of children who have recovered after taking 375 to 625 mg.

Treatment: There is no specific antidote for pyrimethamine. Gastric lavage is effective. A parenteral barbiturate may control convulsions. Administer folinic acid (leucovorin) to counteract effects on the hematopoietic system. Treatment includes the usual supportive measures. Refer to General Management of Acute Overdosage.

Patient Information:

May cause anorexia or vomiting; take with food or meals.

At first appearance of a skin rash, discontinue the drug and seek medical attention.

Administration and Dosage:

Chemoprophylaxis of malaria:

Adults and children (> 10 years old) – 25 mg once weekly.
Children (4 to 10 years old) – 12.5 mg once weekly.
Infants and children (< 4 years old) – 6.25 mg once weekly.

Extend regimens to include suppressive cure through any characteristic periods of early recrudescence and late relapse for at least 6 to 10 weeks in each case.

Treatment of acute attacks: Recommended in areas where only susceptible plasmodia exist. Not recommended for use alone to treat acute attacks of malaria in nonimmune persons. Fast-acting schizonticides (chloroquine or quinine) are indicated for treatment of acute attacks. However, concomitant pyrimethamine, 25 mg daily for 2 days, will initiate transmission control and suppressive cure.

If pyrimethamine must be used alone in semi-immune persons for acute attack:

Adults and children (> 10 years old) : 50 mg daily for 2 days.
Children (4 to 10 years old): 25 mg daily for 2 days.

Follow clinical cure by the chemoprophylaxis regimen described above.

Toxoplasmosis: At the high dosage, there is marked variation in tolerance. Young patients may tolerate higher doses than older patients.

Adults – Initially, 50 to 75 mg daily with 1 to 4 g of a sulfonamide of the sulfapyrimidine type. Continue for 1 to 3 weeks, depending on response and tolerance. Dosage for each drug may then be reduced by one-half and continued for an additional 4 or 5 weeks.

Pediatric dosage is 1 mg/kg/day divided into 2 equal daily doses; after 2 to 4 days, reduce to one-half and continue for ≈ 1 month. The usual pediatric sulfonamide dosage is used in conjunction with pyrimethamine.

Another recommended dosage is a loading dose of 2 mg/kg/day for 3 days, then a maintenance dose of 1 mg/kg/day or divided twice daily for 4 weeks; maximum dose of 25 mg/day.

Convulsive disorders: Use lower initial dose to avoid potential CNS toxicity.

Storage/Stability: Store at 15° to 25°C (59° to 77°F) in a dry place and protect from light.

Rx	**Daraprim** (Glaxo Wellcome)	**Tablets**: 25 mg	(Daraprim A3A). White, scored. In 100s.

ANTITUBERCULOUS DRUGS

Antituberculous drugs are categorized as primary and retreatment agents, indicating their approximate place and usefulness in treatment of tuberculosis. The foundation of treatment should include the primary agents, most of which are bactericidal (ie, destructive to mycobacteria) and are necessary for sterilization of the tuberculous lesions.

The retreatment agents are generally less effective or more toxic than the primary group. A number of these agents are bacteriostatic (ie, inhibit the growth or multiplication of mycobacteria). They are indicated for use in combination with the primary drugs for partial or complete drug-resistant organisms or to treat extrapulmonary tuberculosis.

Antituberculosis Drugs

Drugs	Activity	Route	Pediatric Daily Dose (mg/kg)	Adult Daily Dose (mg/kg/day)	Usual Adult Daily Dose	Max. Daily Dose (Children &Adults)	Toxicity
Primary Agents							
Isoniazid[1]	Bactericidal	oral	10-20 (20-40 twice weekly)	5-10 once daily (15 mg/kg twice weekly)	300 mg	300 mg (900 mg twice wkly)	Hepatic Neurologic
Rifampin	Bactericidal	oral	10-20 (10-20 twice weekly)	10 once daily (10 mg/kg twice weekly)	600 mg	600 mg	Hepatic Hematologic
Ethambutol[2]	Bacteriostatic	oral	15-25 (50 twice weekly)	15-25 once daily (50 twice weekly)	800-1600 mg	2.5 g	Optic neuritis
Pyrazinamide[2]	Bactericidal	oral	15-30 (50-70 twice weekly)	15-30 once daily (50-70 twice weekly)	1-2 g	2 g	Hepatic Hyperuricemia
Streptomycin[2]	Bactericidal	IM	20-40 (25-30 twice weekly)	7-15 once daily (25-30 twice weekly)	0.75-1 g	1 g (750 mg > 60 yrs)	Eighth nerve Renal
Retreatment Agents							
P-amino-salicylic acid	Bacteriostatic	oral	150-200	200, 4 equal doses 6–hourly	12-16 g	12 g	GI intolerance
Ethionamide	Bacteriostatic	oral	15-20	7-15, 4 equal doses 6–hourly	0.75-1 g	1 g	GI intolerance Hepatic
Cycloserine	Bacteriostatic	oral	10-20	10-15, 4 equal doses 6–hourly	0.75-1 g	1 g	Psychoses Seizures
Capreomycin	Bactericidal	IM	15	15 once daily	1 g	1 g	Eighth nerve Renal
Kanamycin	Bactericidal	IM	7.5-15	15 once daily	0.5-1 g	1 g	Eighth nerve Renal

* Adapted from Hoeprich PD, et al. *Infectious Diseases,*ed. 4. Philadelphia: J.B. Lippincott Co., 1989.

1 Always include in retreatment regimen if susceptibility remains.

2 May use as primary or retreatment.

The most generally effective and widely used regimen for pulmonary tuberculosis is the combination of the primary agents, isoniazid 300 mg and rifampin 600 mg, both given in single daily doses. Sputum conversion (ie, failure of growth of *M tuberculosis* in cultures) occurs within 1 month in the majority of patients and within 3 months in > 95% of previously untreated cases with drug susceptible organisms. The major disadvantage of the combination is that as many as 20% to 30% of patients develop laboratory evidence of impaired hepatic function; most will have no symptoms and liver function returns to normal despite drug continuation. It is estimated that < 5% of patients develop symptoms (anorexia, nausea, vomiting), jaundice and progressive deterioration of liver function; if symptoms occur, discontinue isoniazid/rifampin immediately and substitute another regimen temporarily or permanently.

Treatment regimens of isoniazid-streptomycin-ethambutol (initial therapy) followed by isoniazid-ethambutol have typically been continued for 18 to 24 months. Regimens of isoniazid-rifampin for 12 months, or isoniazid-rifampin for 20 weeks, followed by isoniazid-ethambutol for 12 months following sputum conversion, have proven to be highly effective.

Other regimens recommended include: (a) Isoniazid (5 mg/kg/day, up to 500 mg in adults or 10 to 20 mg/kg/day, up to 300 mg in children) and ethambutol, 15 mg/kg/day for 18 to 24 months – a third drug may be used for the initial 2 to 3 months; (b) after sputum conversion an 18 month, twice weekly regimen of isoniazid, 15 mg/kg/dose and streptomycin, 25 mg/kg/dose *or* isoniazid and ethambutol, 50 mg/kg/dose.

ANTITUBERCULOUS DRUGS

Short-course regimen: The American Thoracic Society and the Tuberculosis Control Division of the Centers for Disease Control have recommended a 9 month regimen of isoniazid-rifampin as an acceptable alternative for adults with previously untreated, drug susceptible, uncomplicated pulmonary tuberculosis. In some circumstances after 2 weeks to 2 months of daily therapy, treatment may be continued with twice weekly supervised doses of isoniazid (15 mg/kg) and rifampin (600 mg). Add ethambutol if isoniazid resistance is suspected. Patients with extrapulmonary tuberculosis, those who have received previous therapy for tuberculosis and those following irregular or inconsistent regimens because of toxicity are not candidates for short-course chemotherapy.

A more recent regimen is isoniazid, rifampin and pyrazinamide daily for 2 months followed by isoniazid-rifampin daily (or twice weekly with increased isoniazid dose) for 4 months. If isoniazid resistance is suspected, add ethambutol during the initial phase. Continuing pyrazinamide > 2 months does not appear to improve outcome. Substituting ethambutol or streptomycin for pyrazinamide appears to decrease efficacy.

Although good results with regimens < 6 months have been reported, relapse rates are unacceptably high. Rifampin and isoniazid are essential components of any regimen < 9 or 12 months for at least the first 2 months.

In Southeast Asia and Central and South America, primary drug resistance is common. Therefore, patients should be given ethambutol in addition to isoniazid-rifampin until susceptibility tests are completed.

Retreatment regimens generally consist of two or three agents that were not previously used. Always include isoniazid in the retreatment regimen if susceptibility remains; occasionally isoniazid is recommended when in vitro resistance is determined since the degree of resistance may vary. Treat patients resistant to isoniazid with rifampin 600 mg/day combined with ethambutol and streptomycin; pyrazinamide may also be used in place of ethambutol. If the patient is resistant to streptomycin, capreomycin (preferred) or kanamycin are recommended. Ethionamide, p–aminosalicylic acid and cycloserine are rarely required. Continuous therapy for 18 to 24 months is generally required; delete the most toxic agents during treatment if possible.

HIV: If patients with HIV develop tuberculosis, use standard antituberculous regimen. The recommended regimen is short-course 9 month (see above). However, treatment period may need to be longer. Preventive therapy with isoniazid may also be considered (see Chemoprophylaxis). Again, may need to extend treatment period.

Pregnancy: Tuberculosis in pregnancy should be treated, but presents a therapeutic dilemma. The best therapeutic choices with the least danger to the fetus appear to be combinations of isoniazid, ethambutol and rifampin.

Resistance to these drugs is not uncommon, but is relatively low in North American- and European-born patients. In the US, ≈ 7% are resistant to one or more drugs; 3% to 5% are resistant to isoniazid. Primary resistance to rifampin is low.

ANTITUBERCULOUS DRUGS

Chemoprophylaxis: Isoniazid for 1 year in a single daily dose of 300 mg for adults and 10 to 14 mg/kg (not > 300 mg/day) for children prevents active pulmonary tuberculosis. Isoniazid diminishes mycobacterial population of roentgenographically detectable, quiescent pulmonary lesions or of pulmonary foci which are radiologically inapparent. The US Public Health Service has demonstrated significant reduction of morbidity in treated subjects. Chemoprophylaxis reduces risk of active disease in those treated, and also prevents spread of disease to uninfected persons. Evidence suggests 6 month therapy may be comparable. Therapy for < 6 months is of little value and therapy for > 1 year provides no additional benefit. Additionally, one study revealed that patients (n= 27,000) taking prophylactic isoniazid for 24 to 52 weeks had a reduction in tuberculosis development of 65% to 93% with minimal side effects.

However, wide-spread prophylactic treatment is questioned because of isoniazid-induced hepatitis risk. The following priorities are recommended and widely accepted in identifying candidates for chemoprophylaxis. (1) Household members and other close associates of persons with recently diagnosed tuberculosis. (2) Tuberculin reactors with chest roentgenograms demonstrating nonprogressive, healed or quiescent lesions, and in whom there are neither positive bacteriologic findings nor a history of adequate chemotherapy. (3) Persons whose tuberculin reaction has become positive within the last 2 years. (4) Tuberculin reactors at increased risk of developing tuberculous disease (ie, prolonged adrenocorticosteroid therapy, immunosuppressive therapy, diabetes mellitus, silicosis, leukemia, Hodgkin's disease, post-gastrectomy). (5) Regardless of age, persons with AIDS, ARC or HIV-seropositivity who are skin test positive, or have a negative skin test but a history of prior significant reaction to PPD. (6) Any positive tuberculin reactor > 35 years and particularly children < 7 years.

Isoniazid prophylaxis is indicated during pregnancy by some for recent tuberculin converters and in any tuberculin reactor with inactive disease. Therapy for most other pregnant candidates should probably be withheld until the postpartum period.

ISONIAZID (Isonicotinic acid hydrazide; INH)

Refer to the general discussion inf the Antituberculous Drugs monograph.

> **Warning:**
>
> Severe and sometimes fatal hepatitis associated with isoniazid therapy may occur or develop even after many months of treatment. The risk of developing hepatitis is age-related. Approximate case rates by age are 0 per 1000 for persons < 20 years of age, 3 per 1000 for persons 20 to 34, 12 per 1000 for persons 35 to 49, 23 per 1000 for persons 50 to 64, and 8 per 1000 for persons > 65 years of age.
>
> Risk of hepatitis increases with daily alcohol consumption. Precise fatality rate for isoniazid-related hepatitis is not available; however, in 13,838 persons taking isoniazid, there were eight deaths among 174 cases of hepatitis.
>
> Carefully monitor and interview patients at monthly intervals. Serum transaminase concentration becomes elevated in about 10% to 20% of patients, usually during the first few months of therapy but can occur at any time. Enzyme levels generally return to normal despite continuance of the drug, but in some cases, progressive liver dysfunction occurs. Instruct patients to report immediately any of the prodromal symptoms of hepatitis, such as fatigue, weakness, malaise, anorexia, nausea or vomiting. If these symptoms appear, or if signs suggestive of hepatic damage are detected, discontinue isoniazid promptly since continued use of the drug in such cases may cause a more severe form of liver damage.
>
> Reinstitute isoniazid after symptoms and laboratory abnormalities have become normal. Restart the drug in very small doses; gradually increase doses and withdraw immediately if there is any indication of recurrent liver involvement.
>
> Defer preventive treatment in persons with acute hepatic diseases.

Actions:

Pharmacology: Isoniazid (INH) acts against actively growing tubercle bacilli. It is bactericidal and interferes with lipid and nucleic acid biosynthesis in growing organisms.

Pyridoxine (vitamin B_6) deficiency is sometimes observed in adults taking high doses of INH, and is probably due to the drug's competition with pyridoxal phosphate for the enzyme apotryptophanase.

Pharmacokinetics:

Absorption – INH is rapidly and completely absorbed orally and parenterally and produces peak blood levels within 1 to 2 hours; these decline to ≤ 50% within 6 hours. However, the rate and extent of absorption is decreased by food.

Distribution – INH readily diffuses into all body fluids including cerebrospinal (90% serum concentrations), pleural and ascitic, tissues, organs, and excreta (saliva, sputum, feces). It also passes through the placental barrier and into breast milk in concentrations comparable to those in plasma.

Metabolism – The half-life of INH is widely variable and dependent on acetylator status. Isoniazid is primarily acetylated by the liver; this process is genetically controlled. Liver disease can prolong the clearance of isoniazid. Fast acetylators metabolize the drug about 5 to 6 times faster than slow acetylators. Several minor metabolites have been identified, one or more of which may be "reactive" (monoacetylhydrazine is suspected), and responsible for liver damage. Approximately 50% of Blacks and Caucasians are "slow acetylators" and the rest are "rapid acetylators"; the majority of Eskimos and Orientals are "rapid acetylators". The rate of acetylation does not significantly alter the effectiveness of INH. However, slow acetylation may lead to higher blood levels of the drug, and thus to an increase in toxic reactions. Rapid acetylators may be more likely to develop hepatitis, since hepatotoxicity is caused by the acetylated metabolite of INH; however, this remains controversial.

Excretion – Approximately 50% to 70% of a dose of isoniazid is excreted as unchanged drug and metabolites by the kidneys in 24 hours. Elimination is largely independent of renal function.

Indications:

Used for all forms of tuberculosis in which organisms are susceptible.

Also recommended as preventive therapy (chemoprophylaxis) for specific situations (see the Antituberculous Drugs Introduction).

IM administration is intended for use whenever oral administration is not possible.

Unlabeled uses: Isoniazid (300 to 400 mg/day, increased over 2 weeks to 20 mg/kg/day) may improve severe tremor in patients with multiple sclerosis.

Contraindications:

Patients with previous isoniazid-associated hepatic injury or other severe adverse reactions, (eg, drug fever, chills, arthritis; acute liver disease of any etiology).

ISONIAZID (Isonicotinic acid hydrazide; INH)

Warnings:

Hypersensitivity: Stop all drugs and evaluate at the first sign of a hypersensitivity reaction. If isoniazid must be reinstituted, give only after symptoms have cleared. Restart the drug in very small and gradually increasing doses and withdraw immediately if there is any indication of recurrent hypersensitivity reaction. Refer to Management of Acute Hypersensitivity Reactions.

Renal/Hepatic function impairment: Monitor patients with active chronic liver disease or severe renal dysfunction.

Carcinogenesis: Isoniazid induces pulmonary tumors in a number of strains of mice.

Pregnancy: Isoniazid exerts an embryocidal effect in both rats and rabbits, but no isoniazid-related congenital anomalies have been found in reproduction studies in mammalian species (mice, rats and rabbits). Prescribe during pregnancy only when therapeutically necessary. Weigh the benefit of preventive therapy against a possible risk to the fetus. Start preventive treatment generally after delivery because of the increased risk of tuberculosis for new mothers.

Refer to the Antituberculous Drugs Introduction for treatment regimens suggested during pregnancy.

Lactation: Since isoniazid appears in breast milk, observe breastfed infants of isoniazid-treated mothers for any evidence of adverse effects.

Precautions:

Periodic ophthalmologic examinations during isoniazid therapy are recommended even when visual symptoms do not occur.

Pyridoxine administration is recommended in individuals likely to develop peripheral neuropathies secondary to INH therapy (see Adverse Reactions). Prophylactic doses of 6 to 50 mg of pyridoxine daily have been recommended.

Drug Interactions:

Alcohol ingestion on a daily basis may be associated with a higher incidence of isoniazid-related hepatitis.

Aluminum salts may reduce the oral absorption of isoniazid, thereby decreasing its serum levels. Administer isoniazid 1 to 2 hours before aluminum salts.

Anticoagulants, oral: Anticoagulant activity may be enhanced by concurrent isoniazid.

Benzodiazepines: Isoniazid may inhibit the metabolic clearance of benzodiazepines that undergo oxidative metabolism (eg, diazepam, triazolam), possibly increasing the activity of the benzodiazepine.

Carbamazepine toxicity or isoniazid hepatotoxicity may result from concurrent use. Monitor carbamazepine concentrations and liver function.

Cycloserine in combination with isoniazid may result in increased cycloserine CNS side effects, most notably dizziness.

Disulfiram and isoniazid coadministration may result in acute behavioral and coordination changes.

Enflurane: In rapid acetylators of isoniazid, high output renal failure may occur due to nephrotoxic concentrations of inorganic fluoride. Isoniazid may produce high concentrations of hydrazine which then facilitates defluorination of enflurane. Monitor renal function in patients receiving these agents concurrently.

Halothane: Hepatotoxicity and hepatic encephalopathy have occurred when rifampin and isoniazid were given after halothane anesthesia.

Hydantoins: Serum hydantoin levels may be increased by isoniazid due to inhibition of hepatic microsomal enzymes. An increase in the pharmacologic or toxic effects of the hydantoins may occur. This may be most significant in slow acetylators of isoniazid.

Ketoconazole serum concentrations may be decreased by isoniazid, possibly resulting in antifungal treatment resistance.

Meperidine coadministration may result in a hypotensive episode or CNS depression.

Rifampin and isoniazid coadministration may result in a higher rate of hepatotoxicity than with either agent alone. If alterations in liver function tests occur, consider discontinuation of one or both agents.

Drug/Food interactions: Since isoniazid has some monoamine oxidase inhibitor activity, an interaction may occur with tyramine-containing foods (see Monoamine Oxidase Inhibitors group monograph). Diamine oxidase may also be inhibited, causing exaggerated responses (eg, headache, palpitations, sweating, hypotension, flushing, diarrhea, itching) to foods containing histamine (eg, tuna, sauerkraut juice, yeast extract).

ISONIAZID (Isonicotinic acid hydrazide; INH)

Adverse Reactions:

Toxic effects are usually encountered with higher doses of isoniazid; the most frequent are those affecting the nervous system and the liver.

Metabolic/Endocrine: Pyridoxine deficiency; pellagra; hyperglycemia; metabolic acidosis; gynecomastia. Isoniazid may cause hypocalcemia and hypophosphatemia due to alterations of vitamin D metabolism.

CNS: Peripheral neuropathy, the most common toxic effect, is characterized by symmetrical numbness and tingling of the extremities. The incidence correlates closely with the dose of isoniazid, ie, ≈ 2%, 10% to 20% and 44% of patients may develop pyridoxine deficiency-induced peripheral neuropathy while taking 3 to 5 mg/kg/day, 10 mg/kg/day and 16 to 24 mg/kg/day, respectively. Patients predisposed to this condition include the malnourished, slow isoniazid acetylators, pregnant women, elderly, diabetics and patients with chronic liver disease, including alcoholics. Some advocate pyridoxine (B_6) prophylaxis for all patients, others advocate prophylaxis only for those predisposed. Recommended prophylactic doses range from 6 to 50 mg daily, but the lower doses of 6 to 25 mg appear more common. Treatment of established neuropathy requires 50 to 200 mg pyridoxine daily.

Other neurotoxic effects uncommon with conventional doses: Convulsions; toxic encephalopathy; optic neuritis and atrophy; memory impairment; toxic psychosis.

GI: Nausea; vomiting; epigastric distress.

Hepatic: Elevated serum transaminase levels (AST, ALT); bilirubinemia; bilirubinuria; jaundice; occasionally, severe and sometimes fatal hepatitis. The common prodromal symptoms are anorexia, nausea, vomiting, fatigue, malaise and weakness. Mild and transient elevation of serum transaminase levels occurs in 10% to 20% of patients taking isoniazid. This abnormality usually appears in the first 4 to 6 months of treatment, but can develop at any time during therapy. Enzyme levels return to normal in most instances, and there is no need to discontinue medication. Occasionally, progressive liver damage with accompanying symptoms may occur. In such cases, discontinue the drug immediately. The frequency of progressive liver damage increases with age. It is rare in individuals < 20 years, but is seen in as many as 2.3% of those patients > 50 years old.

Concurrent ethanol use may increase the risk of hepatitis. In addition, it is more commonly believed that rapid acetylators are at greater risk; however, the same has been shown for slow acetylators.

Hematologic: Agranulocytosis; hemolytic, sideroblastic or aplastic anemia; thrombocytopenia; eosinophilia.

Hypersensitivity: Fever; skin eruptions (morbilliform, maculopapular, purpuric or exfoliative); lymphadenopathy; vasculitis (see Warnings).

Miscellaneous: Rheumatic syndrome and systemic lupus erythematosus-like syndrome. Local irritation has been observed at the site of IM injection.

Overdosage:

Symptoms: Occur within 30 minutes to 3 hours. Nausea, vomiting, dizziness, slurring of speech, blurring of vision and visual hallucinations (including bright colors and strange designs) are among the early manifestations. With marked overdosage, respiratory distress and CNS depression, progressing rapidly from stupor to profound coma, are to be expected along with severe, intractable seizures. Ingestion of 80 to 150 mg/kg usually results in severe seizures and a high likelihood of fatality. Severe metabolic acidosis, acetonuria and hyperglycemia are typical laboratory findings.

Treatment: INH overdosage can be fatal, but good response has been reported in most patients adequately treated within the first few hours after drug ingestion.

Secure the airway and establish adequate respiratory exchange. Gastric lavage is advised within the first 2 to 3 hours, but not until convulsions are under control. To control convulsions, administer a short-acting IV barbiturate or diazepam, followed by pyridoxine IV (usually 1 mg per 1 mg of isoniazid ingested). Pyridoxine can be toxic, but doses of 70 to 357 mg/kg have been administered without incident.

Obtain blood samples for immediate determination of gases, electrolytes, BUN, glucose, etc; type and crossmatch blood in preparation for possible hemodialysis.

Rapid control of metabolic acidosis is fundamental to management. Give sodium bicarbonate IV immediately and repeat as needed, adjusting subsequent dosage on the basis of laboratory findings (ie, serum sodium, pH).

Start forced osmotic diuresis early and continue for some hours after clinical improvement has been noted to hasten renal clearance of the drug and help prevent relapse. Monitor fluid intake and output.

Hemodialysis is advised for severe cases. If this is not available, peritoneal dialysis can be used concomitantly with forced diuresis. In addition, protect against hypoxia, hypotension, aspiration pneumonitis, etc.

ISONIAZID (Isonicotinic acid hydrazide; INH)

Patient Information:

Take on an empty stomach, at least 1 hour before or 2 hours after meals; it may be taken with food to decrease GI upset.

Take as directed. Do not discontinue except on advice of physician.

Minimize daily alcohol consumption while on INH due to increased hepatitis risk.

Avoid certain foods (ie, fish-skipjack, tuna, and perhaps tyramine-containing products) (see Monoamine Oxidase Inhibitor group monograph).

Notify physician of weakness, fatigue, loss of appetite, nausea and vomiting, yellowing of skin or eyes, darkening of urine, or numbness or tingling in hands and feet.

Administration and Dosage:

Treatment of tuberculosis: Use in conjunction with other effective antituberculosis agents. If the bacilli become resistant, therapy must be changed to agents to which the bacilli are susceptible.

Adults – 5 mg/kg/day (up to 300 mg total) in a single dose.

Infants and children – 10 to 20 mg/kg/day (300 mg total) in a single dose, depending on the severity of infection.

Preventive treatment: Adults - 300 mg/day in a single dose.

Infants and children – 10 mg/kg/day (up to 300 mg total) in a single dose.

Continuous administration of isoniazid for a sufficient period is an essential part of the regimen, because relapse rates are higher if chemotherapy is stopped prematurely. In the treatment of tuberculosis, resistant organisms may multiply and the emergence of resistant organisms may necessitate a change in the regimen.

Concomitant administration of 6 to 50 mg/day pyridoxine is recommended in the malnourished and in those predisposed to neuropathy (eg, alcoholics and diabetics). See Adverse Reactions.

Rx	**Isoniazid** (Various, eg, Schein)	**Tablets:** 50 mg	In 100s, 500s and 1000s.
Rx	**Laniazid** (Lannett)		Scored. In 100s and 500s.
Rx	**Isoniazid** (Various, eg, Barr, Baxter, Geneva, Halsey, Major, Moore, Qualitest, Rugby, Schein)	**Tablets:** 100 mg	In 100s, 1000s and UD 100s.
Rx	**Laniazid** (Lannett)		Scored. In 100s, 500s, 1000s.
Rx	**Isoniazid** (Various, eg, Barr, Baxter, Geneva, Halsey, Major, Moore, Rugby, Schein)	**Tablets:** 300 mg	In 30s, 100s, 1000s & UD 100s.
Rx	**Laniazid C.T.** (Lannett)		White, scored. Convex. In 100s and 1000s.
Rx	**Isoniazid** (Carolina Medical)	**Syrup:** 50 mg per 5 ml	Sorbitol. Orange flavor. In pt.
Rx	**Laniazid** (Lannett)		Sorbitol. Raspberry flavor. In 480 ml.
Rx	**Nydrazid** (Apothecon)	**Injection:** 100 mg per ml	In 10 ml vials.[1]

[1] With 0.25% chlorobutanol.

ISONIAZID COMBINATIONS

ISONIAZID acts against actively growing tubercle bacilli. See individual monograph.

PYRIDOXINE is included as a supplement due to the increased need for pyridoxine induced by isoniazid treatment. See individual monograph.

RIFAMPIN is used as an adjunct to isoniazid in the treatment of tuberculosis. See individual monograph.

Rx	**Rifater** (Hoechst Marion Roussel)	**Tablets:** 120 mg rifampin, 50 mg isoniazid, 300 mg pyrazinamide	In 60s and UD 100s.
Rx	**Rifamate** (Hoechst Marion Roussel)	**Capsules:** 150 mg isoniazid and 300 mg rifampin	Red. In 60s.
Rx	**Rimactane/INH Dual Pack** (Ciba)	**Pack:** Thirty 300 mg isoniazid tab, sixty 300 mg rifampin caps	In 30 day supplies.

RIFAMPIN

Refer to the general discussion in the Antituberculous Drugs monograph.

Actions:

Pharmacology: Rifampin inhibits DNA-dependent RNA polymerase activity in susceptible cells. Specifically, it interacts with bacterial RNA polymerase, but does not inhibit the mammalian enzyme. Cross-resistance has only been shown with other rifamycins.

Pharmacokinetics:

Oral –

Absorption/Distribution: Rifampin, 600 mg administered orally, is almost completely absorbed and achieves mean peak plasma levels within 1 to 4 hours. The peak level averages 7 mcg/ml but may vary from 4 to 32 mcg/ml. In children, mean peak serum levels range from 3.5 to 15 mcg/ml. Food interferes with absorption. It is 80% protein bound but very lipid soluble; it penetrates and concentrates in many body tissues, including the cerebrospinal fluid, which is increased with meningitis (12% to 25% of serum concentrations).

Metabolism: Rifampin is metabolized in the liver by deacetylation; the metabolite is still active against *Mycobacterium tuberculosis*. About 40% is excreted in bile and undergoes enterohepatic circulation; however, the deacetylated metabolite is poorly absorbed. The half-life is approximately 3 hours after a 600 mg oral dose, up to 5.1 hours after a 900 mg oral dose. With repeated administration, the half-life decreases and averages approximately 2 to 3 hours. In children, the half-life is 2.9 hours following a dose of 10 mg/kg.

Excretion: 6% to 30% of rifampin is excreted in the urine; 30% to 60% in the deacetylated form, approximately 50% unchanged. Dosage adjustment is not necessary in renal failure, but is with hepatic dysfunction. Neither peritoneal dialysis nor hemodialysis removes significant amounts of rifampin from the plasma.

IV – Following administration of a 300 or 600 mg IV dose in 12 volunteers, mean peak plasma concentrations were 9 and 17 mcg/ml, respectively. The average plasma concentrations remained detectable for 8 and 12 hours, respectively. The elimination of the larger dose was not as rapid. After repeated once daily infusions of 600 mg in five patients for 7 days, concentrations decreased from 5.8 mcg/ml 8 hours after the infusion on day 1 to 2.6 mcg/ml 8 hours after the infusion on day 7.

In children, the mean peak serum concentration was 26 mcg/ml following a 300 mg/m^2 infusion, 11.7 to 41.5 mcg/ml 1 to 4 days after initiation of therapy, and 13.6 to 37.4 mcg/ml 5 to 14 days after initiation of therapy. The half-life was 1.17 to 3.24 hours.

Microbiology: Rifampin has initial in vitro activity against the following organisms; however, clinical efficacy has not been established: *M leprae*; *Haemophilus influenzae*; *Staphylococcus aureus*; *S epidermidis*. Both penicillinase- and non-penicillinase- producing strains and β-lactam resistant staphylococci (MRSA) are initially susceptible in vitro.

Indications:

Tuberculosis:

Oral – Treatment of all forms of tuberculosis in conjunction with at least one other antituberculous drug. Frequently used regimens include: Isoniazid and rifampin; ethambutol and rifampin; isoniazid, ethambutol and rifampin; isoniazid, pyrazinamide and rifampin.

IV – Initial treatment and retreatment of tuberculosis when the drug cannot be taken by mouth.

Neisseria meningitidis carriers: Treatment of asymptomatic carriers of N meningitidis to eliminate meningococci from the nasopharynx. Not indicated for treatment of meningococcal infection.

To avoid indiscriminate use, perform diagnostic laboratory procedures, including serotyping and susceptibility testing. Reserve the drug for situations in which the risk of meningococcal meningitis is high. Since rapid emergence of resistance can occur, perform culture and susceptibility tests in the event of persistent positive cultures.

Unlabeled uses: Rifampin has a broad antibacterial spectrum. Some uses showing promise with a reasonable amount of human data include: Infections caused by *Staphylococcus aureus* and *S epidermidis* (eg, endocarditis, osteomyelitis, prostatitis), usually in combination with other effective drugs; gram-negative bacteremia in infancy; Legionella (*Legionella pneumophilia*) when not responsive to erythromycin; leprosy (in combination with dapsone); prophylaxis of meningitis due to *Haemophilus influenzae*.

Contraindications:

Hypersensitivity to any rifamycin.

RIFAMPIN

Warnings:

Hepatotoxicity: There have been fatalities associated with jaundice in patients with liver disease or patients receiving rifampin concomitantly with other hepatotoxic agents. Since an increased risk may exist for individuals with liver disease, weigh benefits against risk of further liver damage. Carefully monitor liver function, especially AST and ALT, prior to therapy and then every 2 to 4 weeks during therapy. Withdraw rifampin if signs of hepatocellular damage occur.

Hyperbilirubinemia, resulting from competition between rifampin and bilirubin for excretory pathways of the liver at the cell level, can occur in the early days of treatment. An isolated report showing a moderate rise in bilirubin or transaminase level is not in itself an indication to interrupt treatment. Make the decision based on repeat tests and the patient's clinical condition.

Porphyria: Isolated reports have associated porphyria exacerbation with rifampin administration.

Meningococci resistance: The possibility of rapid emergence of resistant meningococci restricts use to short-term treatment of asymptomatic carrier state. Not for treatment of meningococcal disease.

Hypersensitivity reactions have occurred during intermittent therapy or when treatment was resumed following accidental or intentional interruption and were reversible with rifampin discontinuation and appropriate therapy. Refer to General Management of Acute Hypersensitivity Reactions. See Adverse Reactions.

Hepatic function impairment: Dosage adjustment is necessary.

Carcinogenesis: A few cases of accelerated growth of lung carcinoma have occurred in man, but a causal relationship has not been established. An increase in the incidence of hepatomas in female mice (of a strain known to be particularly susceptible to the spontaneous development of hepatomas) was observed when rifampin was administered in doses 2 to 10 times the average daily human dose for 60 weeks. Rifampin possesses immunosuppressive potential in animals and humans. Antitumor activity in vitro has also occurred.

Pregnancy: Category C. The effect of rifampin (alone or in combination with other antituberculous drugs) on the human fetus is not known. Rifampin crosses the placental barrier and appears in cord blood. It is teratogenic in rodents given oral doses of 15 to 25 times the human dose. An increase in congenital malformations, primarily spina bifida and cleft palate, has occurred in the offspring of rodents given oral doses of 150 to 250 mg/kg/day. Imperfect osteogenesis and embryotoxicity occurred in rabbits given doses up to 20 times the usual human daily dose. When administered during the last few weeks of pregnancy, rifampin can cause postnatal hemorrhages in the mother and infant for which treatment with vitamin K may be indicated. Carefully weigh possible teratogenic potential in women capable of bearing children against benefits of therapy (see also Antituberculous Drugs introduction).

Carefully observe neonates of rifampin-treated mothers for any adverse effects.

Lactation: Rifampin is excreted in breast milk with a milk/plasma ratio of 0.2 to 0.6. Decide whether to discontinue nursing or discontinue the drug, taking into account the importance of the drug to the mother.

Precautions:

Monitoring: Obtain a complete blood count prior to instituting therapy and periodically throughout the course of therapy. Because of a possible transient rise in transaminase and bilirubin values, obtain blood for baseline clinical chemistries before rifampin dosing.

Intermittent therapy may be used if the patient cannot or will not self-administer drugs on a daily basis. Closely monitor patients on intermittent therapy for compliance, and caution against intentional or accidental interruption of prescribed therapy because of increased risk of serious adverse reactions.

Urine, feces, saliva, sputum, sweat and tears may be colored red-orange. Soft contact lenses may be permanently stained. Advise patients of these possibilities. Rifampin may impart a yellow color to cerebrospinal fluid.

IV: For IV infusion only. Must not be administered by IM or SC route. Avoid extravasation during injection; local irritation and inflammation due to extravascular infiltration of the infusion have been observed. If these occur, discontinue and restart at another site.

Thrombocytopenia has occurred, primarily with high dose intermittent therapy, but has also been noted after resumption of interrupted treatment. It rarely occurs during well supervised daily therapy. This effect is reversible if the drug is discontinued as soon as purpura occurs. Cerebral hemorrhage and fatalities have occurred when rifampin administration has continued or resumed after appearance of purpura.

RIFAMPIN

Drug Interactions:

Rifampin is known to induce the hepatic microsomal enzymes that metabolize various drugs listed in the table below. The therapeutic effects of these drugs may be decreased.

Rifampin Drug Interactions Due to Hepatic Microsomal Enzyme Induction		
Acetaminophen	Corticosteroids	Mexiletine
Anticoagulants, oral	Cyclosporine	Quinidine
Barbiturates	Digitoxin	Sulfones
Benzodiazepines[1]	Disopyramide	Sulfonylureas
Beta-blockers	Estrogens	Theophyllines[2]
Chloramphenicol	Hydantoins	Tocainide
Clofibrate	Methadone	Verapamil
Contraceptives, oral		

[1] Benzodiazepines metabolized by oxidation.
[2] Dyphylline probably does not interact.

Digoxin serum concentrations may be decreased by rifampin.

Enalapril: A significant increase in blood pressure occurred in a patient receiving enalapril and rifampin concurrently.

Halothane: Hepatotoxicity and hepatic encephalopathy have occurred when rifampin and isoniazid were given after halothane anesthesia.

Isoniazid and rifampin coadministration may result in a higher rate of hepatotoxicity than with either agent alone. If alterations in liver function tests occur, consider discontinuation of one or both agents.

Ketoconazole: Treatment failure of either ketoconazole or rifampin may occur.

Drug/Lab test interactions: Therapeutic levels of rifampin inhibit standard assays for serum **folate** and **vitamin B_{12}**. Consider alternative methods when determining folate and vitamin B_{12} concentrations in the presence of rifampin.

Transient abnormalities in liver function tests (eg, elevation in serum bilirubin, abnormal bromsulphalein [BSP] excretion, alkaline phosphatase and serum transaminases), and reduced biliary excretion of contrast media used for visualization of the gallbladder have also been observed. Therefore, perform these tests before the morning dose of rifampin.

Drug/Food interactions: Food interferes with the absorption of rifampin, possibly resulting in decreased peak plasma concentrations. Take on an empty stomach.

Adverse Reactions:

High doses of rifampin (> 600 mg) given once or twice weekly have resulted in a high incidence of adverse reactions including: The "flu-like" syndrome (eg, fever, chills, malaise); hematopoietic reactions (eg, leukopenia, thrombocytopenia, acute hemolytic anemia); cutaneous, GI and hepatic reactions; shortness of breath; shock; renal failure. Recent studies indicate that regimens using twice-weekly doses of rifampin 600 mg plus isoniazid 15 mg/kg are much better tolerated.

GI: (1% to 2%) — Heartburn; epigastric distress; anorexia; nausea; vomiting; gas; cramps; diarrhea; sore mouth and tongue; pseudomembranous colitis; pancreatitis.

Hepatic: Asymptomatic elevations of liver enzymes (up to 14%) and hepatitis (< 1%). Hepatitis or shock-like syndrome with hepatic involvement (rare); abnormal liver function tests; transient abnormalities in liver function tests (elevations in serum bilirubin, BSP, alkaline phosphatase, serum transaminases). Perform BSP test prior to the morning dose of rifampin to avoid false-positive results.

Dermatologic: Rash (1% to 5%); pruritus; urticaria; pemphigoid reaction; flushing.

CNS: Headache; drowsiness; fatigue; dizziness; inability to concentrate; mental confusion; generalized numbness; behavioral changes; myopathy (rare).

Hematologic: Eosinophilia; transient leukopenia; hemolytic anemia; decreased hemoglobin; hemolysis; thrombocytopenia (see Precautions).

Musculoskeletal: Ataxia; muscular weakness; pain in extremities; osteomalacia; myopathy.

Ophthalmic: Visual disturbances; exudative conjunctivitis.

Renal: Hemoglobinuria; hematuria; renal insufficiency; acute renal failure. These are considered hypersensitivity reactions (see Warnings).

Miscellaneous: Menstrual disturbances; fever; elevations in BUN and elevated serum uric acid; possible immunosuppression; isolated reports of abnormal growth of lung tumors; reduced 25-hydroxycholecalciferol levels; edema of face and extremities; shortness of breath; wheezing; decrease in blood pressure; shock.

RIFAMPIN

Overdosage:

Symptoms: Nausea, vomiting and increasing lethargy will probably occur shortly after ingestion; unconsciousness may occur with severe hepatic involvement. Brownish-red or orange discoloration of skin, urine, sweat, saliva, tears and feces is proportional to amount ingested. Liver enlargement, possibly with tenderness, can develop within a few hours after severe overdosage, and jaundice may develop rapidly. Hepatic involvement may be more marked in patients with prior impairment of hepatic function. Other physical findings remain essentially normal.

Direct and total bilirubin levels may increase rapidly with severe overdosage; hepatic enzyme levels may be affected, especially with prior impairment of hepatic function. A direct effect on the hematopoietic system, electrolyte levels or acid-base balance is unlikely.

Non-fatal overdoses with as high as 12 g of rifampin have been reported. One case of fatal overdose occurred in a 26-year-old man after self-administering 60 g.

Treatment: Nausea and vomiting are likely to be present. Gastric lavage is probably preferable to inducing emesis. Instill activated charcoal slurry into stomach after evacuation of gastric contents to help absorb any remaining drug in GI tract. Antiemetic medication may be required to control severe nausea or vomiting.

Forced diuresis (with measured intake and output) will promote excretion of the drug. Bile drainage may be indicated in the presence of serious impairment of hepatic function lasting more than 24 to 48 hours; extracorporeal hemodialysis may be required. In patients with previously adequate hepatic function, reversal of liver enlargement and impaired hepatic excretory function probably will be noted within 72 hours, with rapid return toward normal thereafter.

Patient Information:

Take on an empty stomach, at least 1 hour before or 2 hours after meals.

Take medication on a regular basis; avoid missing doses. Do not discontinue therapy except on advice of physician.

Medication may cause a reddish-orange discoloration of urine, stools, saliva, tears, sweat and sputum. This is to be expected and is not harmful. May also permanently discolor soft contact lenses.

Notify physician of flu-like symptoms (fever, chills, muscle and bone pain, headache), excessive tiredness or weakness, anorexia, nausea, vomiting, sore throat, unusual bleeding or bruising, yellowish discoloration of skin or eyes, skin rash or itching.

Administration and Dosage:

Oral: Administer once daily, either 1 hour before or 2 hours after meals.

Data is not available to determine dosage for children < 5 years of age. For pediatric and adult patients in whom capsule swallowing is difficult or when lower doses are needed, a rifampin suspension can be prepared (see Preparation of Extemporaneous Oral Suspension).

Oral and IV:

Tuberculosis: Adults – 600 mg once daily.

Children – 10 to 20 mg/kg, not to exceed 600 mg/day.

Use with at least one other antituberculous agent. In general, continue therapy until bacterial conversion and maximal improvement have occurred.

In general, continue therapy for tuberculosis for 6 to 9 months or until at least 6 months have elapsed from conversion of sputum to culture negativity. In patients who cannot be relied upon for compliance, intermittent therapy with 600 mg/day 2 or 3 times per week under close supervision may be prescribed and substituted for the daily regimen after 1 to 2 months of an initial daily phase of therapy.

The 6 month regimen ordinarily consists of an initial 2 month phase of rifampin, isoniazid and pyrazinamide and, if clinically indicated, streptomycin or ethambutol, followed by 4 months of rifampin and isoniazid.

The 9 month regimen ordinarily consists of rifampin and isoniazid, usually supplemented during the initial phase by pyrazinamide, streptomycin or ethambutol.

Either of the above regimens is recommended as standard therapy.

Meningococcal carriers: Once daily for 4 consecutive days in the following doses:
Adults – 600 mg.
Children – 10 to 20 mg/kg, not to exceed 600 mg/day.
The following dosage has also been recommended –
Adults: 600 mg every 12 hours for 2 days; *children (≥ 1 month of age)* – 10 mg/kg every 12 hours for 2 days; *children (< 1 month of age)* – 5 mg/kg every 12 hours for 2 days.

Preparation/Stability of solution for IV infusion: Reconstitute the lyophilized powder by transferring 10 ml of Sterile Water for Injection to a vial containing 600 mg of rifampin for injection. Swirl vial gently to completely dissolve the antibiotic. The resultant solution contains rifampin 60 mg/ml and is stable at room temperature for 24 hours. Withdraw a volume equivalent to the amount of rifampin calculated to be administered and add to 500 ml of infusion medium. Mix well and infuse at a rate allowing for complete infusion in 3 hours. In some cases, the amount of rifampin calculated to be administered may be added to 100 ml of infusion medium and infused in 30 minutes. The 500 and 100 ml dilutions should be prepared and used within a total 4 hour period. Precipitation of rifampin from the infusion solution may occur beyond this time.

Dextrose 5% for injection is the recommended infusion medium. Sterile Saline may be used when dextrose is contraindicated, but the stability of rifampin is slightly reduced. Other solutions are not recommended.

Preparation of extemporaneous oral suspension (according to Merrell Dow Pharmaceuticals): Preparation of suspension (to contain rifampin 10 mg/ml) – 1) Empty the contents of four rifampin 300 mg (or eight rifampin 150 mg) capsules into a 4 oz amber glass bottle. 2) Add 20 ml of simple syrup (Syrup, NF). Shake vigorously. 3) Add 100 ml of simple syrup. Shake again.

Storage – The suspension is stable for 4 weeks when stored at room temperature (25° ± 3°C) or in refrigerator (2° to 8°C; 36° to 46°F).

Rx	**Rifadin** (Hoechst Marion Roussel)	**Capsules**: 150 mg	(Rifadin 150). Maroon and scarlet. In 30s.
Rx	**Rifadin** (Hoechst Marion Roussel)	**Capsules**: 300 mg	(Rifadin 300). Maroon and scarlet. In 30s, 60s, 100s.
Rx	**Rimactane** (Ciba)		(Ciba 154). Scarlet and caramel. In 30s, 60s, 100s.
Rx	**Rifadin** (Hoechst Marion Roussel)	**Powder for Injection**: 600 mg	In vials.

RIFABUTIN

Actions:

Pharmacology: Rifabutin, an antimycobacterial agent, is a semisynthetic ansamycin antibiotic derived from rifamycin S. Rifabutin inhibits DNA-dependent RNA polymerase in susceptible strains of Escherichia coli and *Bacillus subtilis* but not in mammalian cells. In resistant strains of *E coli,* rifabutin, like rifampin, did not inhibit this enzyme. It is not known whether rifabutin inhibits DNA-dependent RNA polymerase in *Mycobacterium avium* or in *M intracellulare* which comprise *M avium* complex (MAC).

Pharmacokinetics: Following a single oral dose of 300 mg to healthy adult volunteers, rifabutin was readily absorbed from the GI tract with mean peak plasma levels (Cmax) of 375 ng/ml (range, 141 to 1033 ng/ml) attained in 3.3 hours (tmax range, 2 to 4 hours). Plasma concentrations post-Cmax declined in an apparent biphasic manner. Kinetic dose-proportionality has been established over the 300 to 600 mg dose range in healthy adult volunteers and in early symptomatic human immunodeficiency virus (HIV)-positive patients over a 300 to 900 mg dose range. Rifabutin was slowly eliminated from plasma in healthy adult volunteers, presumably because of distribution-limited elimination, with a mean terminal half-life of 45 hours (range, 16 to 69 hours). Although the systemic levels of rifabutin following multiple dosing decreased by 38%, its terminal half-life remained unchanged. Rifabutin, due to its high lipophilicity, demonstrates a high propensity for distribution and intracellular tissue uptake. Estimates of apparent steady-state distribution volume (9.3 L/kg) in HIV-positive patients, following IV dosing, exceed total body water by approximately 15 fold. Substantially higher intracellular tissue levels than those seen in plasma have been observed. The lung to plasma concentration ratio, obtained at 12 hours, was ≈ 6.5 in four surgical patients. Mean rifabutin steady-state trough levels (24 hours post-dose) ranged from 50 to 65 ng/ml in HIV-positive patients and in healthy adult volunteers. About 85% of the drug is bound in a concentration-independent manner to plasma proteins over a concentration range of 0.05 to 1 mcg/ml.

Mean systemic clearance in healthy adult volunteers following a single oral dose was 0.69 L/hr/kg (range, 0.46 to 1.34 L/hr/kg); renal and biliary clearance of unchanged drug each contribute approximately 5%. About 30% of the dose is excreted in the feces; 53% of the oral dose is excreted in the urine, primarily as metabolites. Of the five metabolites that have been identified, 25-O-desacetyl and 31-hydroxy are the most predominant, and show a plasma metabolite:parent area under the curve ratio of 0.1 and 0.07, respectively. The 25-O-desacetyl metabolite has an activity equal to the parent drug and contributes up to 10% to the total antimicrobial activity.

Absolute bioavailability assessed in HIV-positive patients averaged 20%. At least 53% of the orally administered dose is absorbed from the GI tract. The bioavailability from the capsule dosage form, relative to a solution, was 85% in healthy adult volunteers. High-fat meals slow the rate without influencing the extent of absorption. The overall pharmacokinetics are modified only slightly by alterations in hepatic function or age. Compared to healthy volunteers, steady-state kinetics are more variable in elderly patients (> 70 years of age) and in symptomatic HIV-positive patients. Somewhat reduced drug distribution and faster drug elimination in compromised renal function may result in decreased drug concentrations.

Microbiology: Rifabutin has demonstrated in vitro activity against MAC organisms isolated from both HIV-positive and HIV-negative people. The vast majority of isolates from MAC-infected, HIV-positive people are *M avium,* whereas in HIV-negative people, about 40% of the MAC isolates are *M intracellulare.* Rifabutin has in vitro activity against many strains of *M tuberculosis.*

Cross-resistance between rifampin and rifabutin is commonly observed with *M tuberculosis* and *M avium* complex isolates. Isolates of *M tuberculosis* resistant to rifampin are likely to be resistant to rifabutin.

Susceptibility of M Avium Complex Strains to Rifampin and Rifabutin

		% of strains susceptible/resistant to different concentrations of rifabutin (mcg/ml)			
Susceptibility to rifampin (mcg/ml)	Number of strains	Susceptible to 0.5	Resistant to 0.5 only	Resistant to 1	Resistant to 2
Susceptible to 1	30	100	0	0	0
Resistant to 1 only	163	88.3	11.7	0	0
Resistant to 5	105	38	57.1	2.9	2
Resistant to 10	225	20	50.2	19.6	10.2
Total	523	49.5	36.7	9	4.8

RIFABUTIN

Clinical trials: Two randomized, double-blind clinical trials compared rifabutin (300 mg/day) to placebo in patients with CDC-defined AIDS and CD4 counts ≤ 200 cells/mcl; median CD4 cell count at study entry was 40 to 42 cells/mcl. Endpoints included the following: (1) MAC bacteremia, defined as at least one blood culture positive for *M avium* complex bacteria; (2) clinically significant disseminated MAC disease, defined as MAC bacteremia accompanied by signs or symptoms of serious MAC infection, including one or more of the following: Fever, night sweats, rigors, weight loss, worsening anemia, elevations in alkaline phosphatase; and (3) survival.

MAC bacteremia – Participants who received rifabutin were one-third to one-half as likely to develop MAC bacteremia as were participants who received placebo.

In one study, the 1 year cumulative incidence of MAC bacteremia was 9% for patients randomized to rifabutin and 22% for placebo. In another study, these rates were 13% and 28% for rifabutin-treated and placebo-treated patients, respectively.

Most cases of MAC bacteremia (approximately 90% in these studies) occurred among participants whose CD4 count at study entry was ≤ 100 cells/mcl. The median and mean CD4 counts at onset of MAC bacteremia were 13 cells/mcl and 24 cells/mcl, respectively. These studies did not investigate the optimal time to begin MAC prophylaxis.

Clinically significant disseminated MAC disease – In association with the decreased incidence of bacteremia, patients on rifabutin showed reductions in the signs and symptoms of disseminated MAC disease, including fever, night sweats, weight loss, fatigue, abdominal pain, anemia and hepatic dysfunction.

Survival – The 1 year survival rates in one study were 77% for rifabutin and 77% for placebo. In the other study, the 1 year survival rates were 77% for rifabutin and 70% for placebo.

Indications:

Prevention of disseminated Mycobacterium avium complex (MAC) disease in patients with advanced HIV infection.

Contraindications:

Hypersensitivity to this drug or to any other rifamycins.

Warnings:

Active tuberculosis: Rifabutin prophylaxis must not be administered to patients with active tuberculosis. Tuberculosis in HIV-positive patients is common and may present with atypical or extrapulmonary findings. Patients are likely to have a nonreactive purified protein derivative (PPD) despite active disease. In addition to chest X-ray and sputum culture, the following studies may be useful in the diagnosis of tuberculosis in the HIV-positive patient: Blood culture, urine culture or biopsy of a suspicious lymph node.

Immediately evaluate patients who develop complaints consistent with active tuberculosis while on rifabutin prophylaxis, so that those with active disease may be given an effective combination regimen of antituberculosis medications. Administration of single-agent rifabutin to patients with active tuberculosis is likely to lead to the development of tuberculosis that is resistant both to rifabutin and to rifampin.

There is no evidence that rifabutin is effective prophylaxis against *M tuberculosis*. Patients requiring prophylaxis against both *M tuberculosis* and *M avium* complex may be given isoniazid and rifabutin concurrently.

Fertility impairment: Fertility was impaired in male rats given 160 mg/kg (32 times the recommended human daily dose).

Pregnancy: Category B. In rats given 200 mg/kg/day (40 times the recommended human daily dose) there was a decrease in fetal viability. In rats, 40 mg/kg/day caused an increase in fetal skeletal variants. In rabbits, 80 mg/kg/day caused maternotoxicity and an increase in fetal skeletal anomalies. There are no adequate and well controlled studies in pregnant women. Use in pregnant women only if the potential benefit justifies the potential risk to the fetus.

Lactation: It is not known whether rifabutin is excreted in breast milk. Because of the potential for serious adverse reactions in nursing infants, decide whether to discontinue nursing or discontinue the drug, taking into account the importance of the drug to the mother.

Children: Safety and efficacy in children have not been established. Limited safety data are available from treatment use in 22 HIV-positive children with MAC who received rifabutin in combination with at least two other antimycobacterials for periods from 1 to 183 weeks. Mean doses (mg/kg) for these children were: 18.5 (range, 15 to 25) for infants 1 year of age; 8.6 (range, 4.4 to 18.8) for children 2 to 10 years of age; and 4 (range, 2.8 to 5.4) for adolescents 14 to 16 years of age. There is no evidence that doses > 5 mg/kg/day are useful. Adverse experiences were similar to those observed in the adult population, and included leukopenia, neutropenia and rash. Doses of rifabutin may be administered mixed with foods such as applesauce.

RIFABUTIN

Precautions:

Monitoring: Because rifabutin may be associated with neutropenia, and more rarely thrombocytopenia, consider obtaining hematologic studies periodically in patients receiving prophylaxis.

Drug Interactions:

Rifabutin Drug Interactions

Precipitant drug	Object drug*		Description
Rifabutin	Zidovudine	⬇	In 10 healthy adults and 8 HIV-positive patients, steady-state zidovudine plasma levels were decreased after repeated rifabutin dosing; mean decrease in C_{max} and AUC was 48% and 32%, respectively. Rifabutin does not affect inhibition of HIV by zidovudine.
Rifabutin	Didanosine	⟷	Rate and extent of systemic availability of didanosine were not altered after repeated rifabutin dosing.

* ⬇ = Object drug decreased. ⟷ = Undetermined or no effect.

Rifabutin has liver enzyme-inducing properties. The related drug rifampin is known to reduce the activity of a number of other drugs. Because of the structural similarity of rifabutin and rifampin, rifabutin may be expected to have similar interactions. However, unlike rifampin, rifabutin appears not to affect the acetylation of isoniazid. Rifabutin appears to be a less potent enzyme inducer than rifampin. The significance of this finding for clinical drug interactions is not known. Dosage adjustment of other drugs may be necessary if they are given concurrently with rifabutin. For further information, refer to the Rifampin monograph.

Drug/Food interactions: High-fat meals slow the rate of absorption without influencing the extent. Rifabutin doses may be mixed with foods such as applesauce.

Adverse Reactions:

Rifabutin is generally well tolerated. Discontinuation of therapy due to an adverse event was required in 16% of patients receiving rifabutin vs 8% with placebo. Primary reasons for discontinuation were rash (4%), GI intolerance (3%) and neutropenia (2%).

Rifabutin Adverse Reactions (%)

Adverse reaction	Rifabutin (n = 566)	Placebo (n = 580)	Adverse reaction	Rifabutin (n = 566)	Placebo (n = 580)
Lab test abnormalities			Chest pain	1	1
Increased alkaline phosphatase (> 450 U/L)	< 1	3	Fever	2	1
			Headache	3	5
			Pain	1	2
Increased AST (> 150 U/L)	7	12	*GI*		
			Anorexia	2	2
Increased ALT (> 150 U/L)	9	11	Diarrhea	3	3
Anemia (Hgb <8 g/dl)	6	7	Dyspepsia	3	1
			Eructation	3	1
Eosinophilia	1	1	Flatulence	2	1
Leukopenia (WBC <1500/mm³)	17	16	Nausea	6	5
			Nausea/vomiting	3	2
Neutropenia (ANC <750/mm³)	25	20	Vomiting	1	1
			Other		
Thrombocytopenia (platelets < 50,000/ mm³)	5	4	Myalgia	2	1
			Insomnia	1	1
			Rash	11	8
Body as a whole			Taste perversion	3	1
Abdominal pain	4	3	Discolored urine	30	6
Asthenia	1	1			

Other adverse reactions include: Flu-like syndrome, hepatitis, hemolysis, arthralgia, myositis, chest pressure or pain with dyspnea, skin discoloration (< 1%); seizure; parathesia; aphasia; confusion; non-specific T wave changes on ECG.

When rifabutin was administered at doses from 1050 to 2400 mg/day, generalized arthralgia and uveitis occurred. These adverse experiences abated when rifabutin was discontinued.

The incidence of neutropenia in patients treated with rifabutin was significantly greater than in patients treated with placebo. Although thrombocytopenia was not significantly more common among rifabutin-treated patients, it has been clearly linked to thrombocytopenia in rare cases. One patient developed thrombotic thrombocytopenic purpura, which was attributed to rifabutin.

Overdosage:

Treatment: While there is no experience in the treatment of overdose with rifabutin, clinical experience with rifamycins suggest that gastric lavage to evacuate gastric contents (within a few hours of overdose), followed by instillation of an activated charcoal slurry into the stomach, may help absorb any remaining drug from the GI tract.

Rifabutin is 85% protein bound and distributed extensively into tissues. It is not primarily excreted via the urinary route (< 10% as unchanged drug); therefore, neither hemodialysis nor forced diuresis is expected to enhance the systemic elimination of unchanged rifabutin from the body in a patient with rifabutin overdose.

Patient Information:

Advise patients of the signs and symptoms of both MAC and tuberculosis, and instruct them to consult their physicians if they develop new complaints consistent with either of these diseases. In addition, since rifabutin may rarely be associated with myositis and uveitis, advise patients to notify their physicians if they develop signs or symptoms suggesting either of these disorders.

Urine, feces, saliva, sputum, perspiration, tears and skin may be colored brown-orange with rifabutin and some of its metabolites. Soft contact lenses may be permanently stained. Make patients aware of these possibilities.

Patients using oral contraceptives should consider changing to nonhormonal methods of birth control since rifabutin, like rifampin, may decrease their efficacy.

Administration and Dosage:

Approved by the FDA on December 23, 1992.

Usual dose: 300 mg once daily. For those patients with propensity to nausea, vomiting or other GI upset, administration of rifabutin at doses of 150 mg twice daily taken with food may be useful.

Rx	**Mycobutin** (Adria)	**Capsules:** 150 mg	(Adria/Mycobutin). Opaque red/brown. In 100s.

ETHAMBUTOL HCl

Refer to the general discussion in the Antituberculous Drugs monograph.

Actions:

Pharmacology: Ethambutol diffuses into actively growing mycobacterium cells such as tubercle bacilli. It inhibits the synthesis of one or more metabolites, thus causing impairment of cell metabolism, arrest of multiplication, and cell death. No cross-resistance with other agents has been demonstrated.

Pharmacokinetics:

Absorption/Distribution – Ethambutol absorption is not influenced by food. Following a single oral dose of 15 to 25 mg/kg, ethambutol attains a peak of 2 to 5 mcg/ml in serum 2 to 4 hours after administration. Serum levels are similar after prolonged dosing. The serum level is undetectable 24 hours after the last dose except in some patients with abnormal renal function. Cerebrospinal fluid concentrations may attain 10% to 50% of simultaneous serum concentrations in the presence of meningeal inflammation.

Metabolism – During the 24 hours following oral administration, about 20% of ethambutol is metabolized by the liver.

Excretion – Approximately 50% of unchanged drug is excreted in the urine, 8% to 15% as metabolites and 20% to 25% unchanged in the feces. Marked accumulation may occur with renal insufficiency.

Microbiology: Ethambutol is effective against strains of *Mycobacterium tuberculosis,* but does not seem to be active against fungi, viruses or other bacteria. *M tuberculosis* strains previously unexposed to ethambutol have been uniformly sensitive to concentrations of ≤ 8 mcg/ml, depending on the nature of the culture media. When used alone for treatment of tuberculosis, tubercle bacilli from these patients have developed resistance by in vitro susceptibility tests; the development of resistance has been unpredictable and appears to occur in a stepwise manner. Ethambutol has reduced incidence of mycobacterial resistance to isoniazid when used concurrently.

Indications:

Pulmonary tuberculosis: Use in conjunction with at least one other antituberculous drug.

In patients who have received previous therapy, mycobacterial resistance to other drugs used in initial therapy is frequent. In retreatment patients, combine ethambutol with at least one of the second-line drugs not previously administered to the patient, and to which bacterial susceptibility has been indicated.

Contraindications:

Hypersensitivity to ethambutol; known optic neuritis, unless clinical judgment determines that it may be used.

Warnings:

Renal function impairment: Patients with decreased renal function require reduced dosage (as determined by serum levels) since this drug is excreted by the kidneys.

Pregnancy: The effects of combinations of ethambutol with other antituberculous drugs on the fetus are not known. Administration to pregnant patients has produced no detectable effect upon the fetus; use only when clearly needed and when the potential benefits outweigh the potential hazards to the fetus.

In fetuses born of mice treated with high doses of ethambutol during pregnancy, a low incidence of cleft palate, exencephaly and abnormality of the vertebral column were observed. Minor abnormalities of the cervical vertebra were seen in the newborn of rats treated with high doses of ethambutol during pregnancy. Rabbits receiving high doses during pregnancy gave birth to two fetuses with monophthalmia, one with a shortened right forearm accompanied by bilateral wrist-joint contracture and one with hare lip and cleft palate.

Children: Not recommended for use in children < 13 years.

Precautions:

Monitoring: Perform periodic assessment of renal, hepatic and hematopoietic systems during long-term therapy.

Visual effects: This drug may have adverse effects on vision. The effects are generally reversible when the drug is discontinued promptly. In rare cases, recovery may be delayed for up to 1 year or more, and the effect may possibly be irreversible. Patients have then received the drug again without recurrence of loss of visual acuity. Acuity changes may be unilateral or bilateral; therefore, each eye must be tested separately and both eyes tested together. Perform testing before beginning therapy and periodically during drug administration (monthly when a patient is receiving > 15 mg/kg/day). Use Snellen eye charts for testing of visual acuity. Physical examination should include ophthalmoscopy, finger perimetry and testing of color discrimination.

ETHAMBUTOL HCl

In patients with visual defects such as cataracts, recurrent inflammatory conditions of the eye, optic neuritis, and diabetic retinopathy, the evaluation of changes in visual acuity is more difficult; the variations in vision may be due to the underlying disease conditions. In such patients, consider the relationship between benefits expected and possible visual deterioration, since evaluation of visual changes is difficult.

Advise patients to report promptly any change in visual acuity. Changes in color perception are probably the first signs of toxicity. These changes can be detected with the use of hue charts. If evaluation confirms visual change and fails to reveal other causes, discontinue drug and reevaluate patient at frequent intervals. Consider progressive decreases in visual acuity during therapy to be due to the drug.

Patients developing visual abnormality during treatment may show subjective visual symptoms before, or simultaneously with, the demonstration of decreases in visual acuity; periodically question all patients receiving ethambutol about blurred vision and other subjective eye symptoms.

Drug Interactions:

Aluminum salts may delay and reduce the absorption of ethambutol. Separate their administration by several hours.

Adverse Reactions:

Hypersensitivity: Anaphylactoid reactions; dermatitis; pruritus.

Ophthalmic: May produce decreases in visual acuity, which appear to be due to optic neuritis and to be related to dose and duration of treatment. See Precautions.

GI: Anorexia; nausea; vomiting; GI upset; abdominal pain.

CNS: Fever; malaise; headache; dizziness; mental confusion; disorientation; possible hallucinations. Numbness and tingling of the extremities due to peripheral neuritis have occurred infrequently.

Metabolic: Elevated serum uric acid levels; precipitation of acute gout; transient impairment of liver function as indicated by abnormal liver function.

Miscellaneous: Toxic epidermal necrolysis; thrombocytopenia; joint pain.

Patient Information:

May cause stomach upset; take with food.

Notify physician if changes in vision (eg, blurring, red-green color blindness) or skin rash occurs.

Administration and Dosage:

Do not use ethambutol alone. Administer once every 24 hours only. Absorption is not significantly altered by administration with food. Continue therapy until bacteriological conversion has become permanent and maximal clinical improvement has occurred.

Initial treatment: In patients who have not received previous antituberculous therapy, administer 15 mg/kg (7 mg/lb) as a single oral dose once every 24 hours. Isoniazid has been administered concurrently in a single, daily oral dose.

Retreatment: In patients who have received previous antituberculous therapy, administer 25 mg/kg (11 mg/lb) as a single oral dose once every 24 hours. Concurrently administer at least one other antituberculous drug to which the organisms have been demonstrated to be susceptible by in vitro tests. Suitable drugs usually include those not previously used in the treatment of the patient. After 60 days of administration, decrease the dose to 15 mg/kg and administer as a single oral dose once every 24 hours.

During the period when a patient is receiving a daily dose of 25 mg/kg, monthly eye examinations are advised (see Precautions).

Children: Not recommended for use in children < 13 years old.

Rx	**Myambutol** (Lederle)	**Tablets:** 100 mg	(LL M6). White, coated. Convex. In 100s.
		400 mg	(LL M7). White, scored. Film coated. In 1000s, UD 100s, unit-of-use 100s.

PYRAZINAMIDE

Refer to the general discussion in the Antituberculous Drugs monograph.

Actions:

Pharmacology: Pyrazinamide, the pyrazine analog of nicotinamide, is an antituberculous agent. Pyrazinamide may be bacteriostatic or bactericidal against *Mycobacterium tuberculosis* depending on the concentration of the drug attained at the site of infection. The mechanism of action is unknown.

Pharmacokinetics:

Absorption/Distribution – Pyrazinamide is well absorbed from the GI tract and attains peak plasma concentrations within 2 hours. Plasma concentrations generally range from 30 to 50 mcg/ml with doses of 20 to 25 mg/kg. It is widely distributed in body tissues and fluids including the liver, lungs and cerebrospinal fluid.

Metabolism/Excretion – The half-life is 9 to 10 hours; it may be prolonged in patients with impaired renal or hepatic function. Pyrazinamide is hydrolyzed in the liver to its major active metabolite, pyrazinoic acid. Pyrazinoic acid is hydroxylated to the main excretory product, 5-hydroxypyrazinoic acid.

Approximately 70% of an oral dose is excreted in urine, mainly by glomerular filtration, within 24 hours.

Indications:

Initial treatment of active tuberculosis in adults and children when combined with other antituberculous agents.

The current recommendation of the CDC for drug-susceptible disease is to use a 6 month regimen for initial treatment of active tuberculosis, consisting of isoniazid, rifampin and pyrazinamide given for 2 months, followed by isoniazid and rifampin for 4 months.

After treatment failure with other primary drugs in any form of active tuberculosis.

Contraindications:

Severe hepatic damage; hypersensitivity; acute gout.

Warnings:

Combination therapy: Use only in conjunction with other effective antituberculous agents. Treat patients with drug-resistant disease with regimens individualized to their situation. Pyrazinamide frequently will be an important component of such therapy.

Hyperuricemia: Pyrazinamide inhibits renal excretion of urates, frequently resulting in hyperuricemia which is usually asymptomatic. Patients started on pyrazinamide should have baseline serum uric acid determinations. Discontinue the drug and do not resume if signs of hyperuricemia accompanied by acute gouty arthritis appear.

Renal function impairment: It does not appear that patients with impaired renal function require a reduction in dose. It may be prudent to select doses at the low end of the dosing range, however.

Hepatic function impairment: Patients started on pyrazinamide should have baseline liver function determinations. Closely follow those patients with preexisting liver disease or those at increased risk for drug-related hepatitis (eg, alcohol abusers). Discontinue pyrazinamide and do not resume if signs of hepatocellular damage appear.

Elderly: Clinical studies of pyrazinamide did not include sufficient numbers of patients ≥ 65 years of age to determine whether they respond differently from younger patients. Other reported clinical experience has not identified differences in responses between the elderly and younger patients. In general, dose selection for an elderly patient should be cautious, usually starting at the low end of the dosing range, reflecting the greater frequency of decreased hepatic or renal function, and of concomitant disease or other drug therapy.

Pregnancy: Category C. It is not known whether pyrazinamide can cause fetal harm when administered to a pregnant woman or can affect reproduction capacity. Give to a pregnant woman only if clearly needed.

Lactation: Pyrazinamide has been found in small amounts in breast milk. Therefore, it is advised that pyrazinamide be used with caution in nursing mothers, taking into account the risk-benefit of this therapy.

Children: Pyrazinamide regimens employed in adults are probably equally effective in children. Pyrazinamide appears to be well tolerated in children.

PYRAZINAMIDE

Precautions:

Monitoring: Determine baseline liver function studies (especially ALT and AST) and uric acid levels prior to therapy. Perform appropriate laboratory testing at periodic intervals and if any clinical signs or symptoms occur during therapy.

HIV infection: In patients with concomitant HIV infection, be aware of current recommendations of CDC. It is possible these patients may require a longer course of treatment.

Diabetes mellitus: Use with caution in patients with a history of diabetes mellitus, as management may be more difficult.

Primary resistance of M tuberculosis to pyrazinamide is uncommon. In cases with known or suspected drug resistance, perform in vitro susceptibility tests with recent cultures of *M tuberculosis* against pyrazinamide and the usual primary drugs. There are few reliable in vitro tests for pyrazinamide resistance. A reference laboratory capable of performing these studies must be employed.

Drug Interactions:

Drug/Lab test interactions: Pyrazinamide has been reported to interfere with Acetest and *Ketostix* urine tests to produce a pink-brown color.

Adverse Reactions:

Fever, porphyria, dysuria (rare); gout (see Warnings).

Hepatic: The principal adverse effect is a hepatic reaction (see Warnings). Hepatotoxicity appears to be dose-related, and may appear at any time during therapy.

GI: Nausea; vomiting; anorexia.

Hematologic/Lymphatic: Thrombocytopenia and sideroblastic anemia with erythroid hyperplasia, vacuolation of erythrocytes, increased serum iron concentration and adverse effects on blood clotting mechanisms (rare).

Miscellaneous: Mild arthralgia and myalgia (frequent); hypersensitivity reactions including rashes, urticaria, pruritus; fever, acne, photosensitivity, porphyria, dysuria, interstitial nephritis (rare).

Overdosage:

Overdosage experience is limited. In one case report of overdose, abnormal liver function tests developed. These spontaneously reverted to normal when the drug was stopped. Employ clinical monitoring and supportive therapy. Refer to General Management of Acute Overdosage. Pyrazinamide is dialyzable.

Patient Information:

Instruct patients to notify their physicians promptly if they experience any of the following: Fever, loss of appetite, malaise, nausea and vomiting, darkened urine, yellowish discoloration of the skin and eyes, pain or swelling of the joints.

Compliance with the full course of therapy must be emphasized; stress the importance of not missing any doses.

Administration and Dosage:

Administer pyrazinamide with other effective antituberculous drugs. It is administered for the initial 2 months of a 6 month or longer treatment regimen for drug susceptible patients. Treat patients who are known or suspected to have drug-resistant disease with regimens individualized to their situation. Pyrazinamide frequently will be an important component of such therapy.

HIV infection: Patients with concomitant HIV infection may require longer courses of therapy. Be alert to any revised recommendations from CDC for this group of patients.

Usual dose: 15 to 30 mg/kg once daily. Older regimens employed 3 to 4 divided doses daily, but the most current recommendations are once a day. Do not exceed 3 g/day. The CDC recommendations do not exceed 2 g/day when given as a daily regimen.

Alternative dosing: Alternatively, a twice weekly dosing regimen (50 to 70 mg/kg twice weekly based on lean body weight) has been developed to promote patient compliance on an outpatient basis. In studies evaluating the twice weekly regimen, doses of pyrazinamide in excess of 3 g twice weekly have been administered. This exceeds the recommended maximum 3 g/daily dose. However, an increased incidence of adverse reactions has not been reported.

Rx	**Pyrazinamide** (Lederle)	**Tablets:** 500 mg	(P36 LL). White, scored. In 100s and 500s.

AMINOSALICYLATE SODIUM (Para–Aminosalicylate Sodium)

Aminosalicylate sodium is the sodium salt of para-aminosalicylic acid (PAS). It contains 73% aminosalicylic acid equivalent and 10.9% sodium (54.5 mg sodium/500 mg tab).

Actions:

Pharmacology: Aminosalicylate sodium is bacteriostatic against Mycobacterium tuberculosis. It inhibits the onset of bacterial resistance to streptomycin and isoniazid.

Pharmacokinetics:

Absorption/Distribution – PAS is readily absorbed from GI tract; the sodium salt is absorbed more rapidly than free acid. It is widely distributed, concentrates in pleural and caseous tissue, but achieves low cerebrospinal fluid concentration.

Metabolism – The half-life of PAS is about 1 hour. It is metabolized in the liver; > 50% is acetylated.

Excretion – Over 80% is excreted through the kidneys as metabolites and free acid. Excretion is retarded in the presence of renal dysfunction.

Indications:

Treatment of tuberculosis in combination with other antituberculous drugs when due to susceptible strains of tubercle bacilli.

Unlabeled uses: PAS has been shown to have serum lipid-lowering activity.

Contraindications:

Severe hypersensitivity to aminosalicylate sodium and its congeners.

Warnings:

Hypersensitivity: Stop all medication if symptoms of hypersensitivity develop. Refer to General Management of Acute Hypersensitivity Reactions.After the symptoms have abated, restart medications one at a time, in very small but gradually increasing doses, to determine if the symptoms were drug-induced and, if so, which medication was responsible. Oral hyposensitization can only occasionally be accomplished. See Adverse Reactions.

Renal/Hepatic function impairment: Use with caution.

Precautions:

Gastric ulcer: Use cautiously in patients with gastric ulcer.

Crystalluria may be prevented by maintaining the urine at a neutral or alkaline pH.

Tablet deterioration: Aminosalicylate sodium deteriorates rapidly in contact with water, heat and sunlight. A brownish or purplish color of powder or tablets, especially of a solution made with them, is indicative of such deterioration. If deterioration is evident, discard the drug.

Use with caution in patients with known or impending congestive heart failure and in other situations in which excess sodium is potentially harmful.

Drug Interactions:

Digoxin: Oral absorption of digoxin may be reduced with a subsequent reduction in serum levels by PAS. Digoxin doses need to be increased.

Vitamin B_{12} (oral) deficiency may be induced due to PAS interference of its GI absorption; parenteral vitamin B_{12} may be required.

Adverse Reactions:

Most common:

GI – Nausea; vomiting; diarrhea; abdominal pain.

Less common:

Hypersensitivity – Fever; various skin eruptions; infectious mononucleosis-like syndrome; leukopenia; agranulocytosis; thrombocytopenia; hemolytic anemia; jaundice; hepatitis; encephalopathy; Loffler's syndrome; vasculitis. See Warnings.

Endocrine – Goiter with or without myxedema.

Patient Information:

Take as directed. Do not stop taking before consulting your doctor.

May cause stomach upset. Take with food or meals.

Do not use products that are brown or purple in color. Aminosalicylate will not work if it becomes wet or is left in extreme heat or direct sunlight. Therefore, do not store in the kitchen or bathroom cabinet.

Notify your doctor if fever, sore throat, unusual bleeding or bruising, or skin rash occurs.

AMINOSALICYLATE SODIUM (Para–Aminosalicylate Sodium)

Administration and Dosage:

Administer aminosalicylate sodium with other antituberculous drugs.

Adults: 14 to 16 g/day in 2 to 3 divided doses.

Children: 275 to 420 mg/kg/day in 3 to 4 divided doses daily.

Rx	**Sodium P.A.S.** (Lannett)	**Tablets:** 0.5 g	In 100s, 500s and 1000s.
Rx	**Paser** (Jacobus)	**Granules:** 4 g	In 30s.

ETHIONAMIDE

Refer to the general discussion in the Antituberculous Drugs monograph.

Actions:

Pharmacology: Bacteriostatic against Mycobacterium tuberculosis.

Pharmacokinetics: Oral administration of ethionamide yields peak plasma concentrations in 3 hours. It is widely and rapidly distributed, including into the cerebrospinal fluid. The drug is metabolized in the liver and < 1% is excreted in the urine unchanged.

Indications:

Recommended for any form of active tuberculosis when treatment with first-line drugs (isoniazid, rifampin) has failed. Use only with other effective antituberculous agents.

Contraindications:

Severe hypersensitivity to ethionamide; severe hepatic damage.

Warnings:

Pregnancy: Teratogenic effects have been demonstrated in small animals receiving doses in excess of those recommended in humans. Use during pregnancy only when clearly needed and when the potential benefits outweigh the potential hazards to the fetus.

Children: Optimum dosage for children has not been established. This does not preclude use of the drug when crucial to therapy.

Precautions:

Monitoring: Make determinations of serum transaminase (AST, ALT) prior to and every 2 to 4 weeks during therapy.

Pretreatment examinations should include in vitro susceptibility tests of recent cultures of *M tuberculosis* from the patient as measured against ethionamide and the usual first-line antituberculous drugs.

Diabetes mellitus: Management of the diabetes may be more difficult and hepatitis occurs more frequently.

Adverse Reactions:

CNS: Depression, drowsiness and asthenia (common); convulsions; peripheral neuritis and neuropathy; olfactory disturbances; blurred vision; diplopia; optic neuritis; dizziness; headache; restlessness; tremors; psychosis.

GI: Anorexia, nausea and vomiting are most common (50% unable to tolerate doses > 500 mg); diarrhea; metallic taste; hepatitis (5%); jaundice; stomatitis.

Miscellaneous: Postural hypotension; skin rash; acne; alopecia; thrombocytopenia; pellagra-like syndrome; gynecomastia; impotence; menorrhagia; increased difficulty managing diabetes mellitus.

Patient Information:

May cause stomach upset, loss of appetite, metallic taste or salivation. Notify physician if these effects persist or are severe. Taking with food may help reduce GI upset.

Administration and Dosage:

Administer with at least 1 other effective antituberculous drug.

Average adult dose: 0.5 to 1 g/day in divided doses.

Children: A dose of 15 to 20 mg/kg/day (maximum 1 g) has been recommended.

Concomitant administration of pyridoxine is recommended.

Rx	**Trecator-SC** (Wyeth-Ayerst)	**Tablets:** 250 mg	(Wyeth 4130). Orange. Sugar coated. In 100s.

CYCLOSERINE

Refer to the general discussion in the Antituberculous Drugs monograph.

Actions:

Pharmacology: Inhibits cell wall synthesis in susceptible strains of gram-positive and gram-negative bacteria and in *Mycobacterium tuberculosis.* This structural analogue of D-alanine antagonizes D-alanine's role in bacterial cell wall synthesis.

Pharmacokinetics:

Absorption/Distribution – When given orally, cycloserine is rapidly absorbed, reaching peak plasma concentrations in 3 to 8 hours. It is widely distributed throughout body fluids and tissues; cerebrospinal fluid levels are similar to plasma.

Metabolism/Excretion – Approximately 35% of the drug is metabolized; 50% of a parenteral dose is excreted unchanged in the urine in the first 12 hours. About 65% of the drug is recoverable in 72 hours. Renal insufficiency will lead to toxic accumulation; it may be removed by dialysis.

Indications:

Treatment of active pulmonary and extrapulmonary tuberculosis (including renal disease) when organisms are susceptible, after failure of adequate treatment with the primary medications. Use in conjunction with other effective chemotherapy.

May be effective in the treatment of acute urinary tract infections caused by susceptible strains of gram-positive and gram-negative bacteria, especially Enterobacter sp and *Escherichia coli.* It is usually less effective than other antimicrobial agents in the treatment of urinary tract infections caused by bacteria other than mycobacteria. Consider using only when the more conventional therapy has failed and when the organism has demonstrated sensitivity.

Contraindications:

Hypersensitivity to cycloserine; epilepsy; depression, severe anxiety or psychosis; severe renal insufficiency; excessive concurrent use of alcohol.

Warnings:

CNS toxicity: Discontinue the drug or reduce dosage if patient develops allergic dermatitis or symptoms of CNS toxicity, such as convulsions, psychosis, somnolence, depression, confusion, hyperreflexia, headache, tremor, vertigo, paresis or dysarthria. The risk of convulsions is increased in chronic alcoholics.

Toxicity is closely related to excessive blood levels (> 30 mcg/ml), which are due to high dosage or inadequate renal clearance. The therapeutic index in tuberculosis is small.

Monitor patients by hematologic, renal excretion, blood level and liver function studies.

Renal function impairment: Patients will accumulate cycloserine and may develop toxicity if the dosage regimen is not modified. Patients with severe impairment should not receive the drug.

Pregnancy: Category C. It is not known whether this drug can cause fetal harm when administered to a pregnant woman or can affect reproduction capacity. Use only if clearly needed.

Lactation: Because of the potential for serious adverse reactions in nursing infants, decide whether to discontinue nursing or to discontinue the drug, taking into account the importance of the drug to the mother.

Children: Safety and dosage not established for pediatric use.

Precautions:

Obtain cultures and determine susceptibility before treatment.

Determine blood levels weekly for patients having reduced renal function, for individuals receiving > 500 mg/day, and for those with symptoms of toxicity. Adjust dosage to maintain blood level < 30 mcg/ml.

Anticonvulsant drugs or sedatives may be effective in controlling symptoms of CNS toxicity, such as convulsions, anxiety and tremor. Closely observe patients receiving > 500 mg/day for such symptoms. Pyridoxine may prevent CNS toxicity, but its efficacy has not been proven.

Anemia: Administration has been associated in a few cases with vitamin B_{12} or folic acid deficiency, megaloblastic anemia and sideroblastic anemia. If evidence of anemia develops, institute appropriate studies and therapy.

Drug Interactions:

Alcohol and cycloserine are incompatible; alcohol increases the possibility and risk of epileptic episodes.

Isoniazid in combination with cycloserine may result in increased cycloserine CNS side effects, most notably dizziness.

CYCLOSERINE

Adverse Reactions:

CNS: (related to dosages > 500 mg/day): Convulsions; drowsiness and somnolence; headache; tremor; dysarthria; vertigo; confusion and disorientation with loss of memory; psychoses, possibly with suicidal tendencies, character changes, hyperirritability, aggression; paresis; hyperreflexia; paresthesias; major and minor (localized) clonic seizures; coma.

Cardiovascular: Sudden development of congestive heart failure has been reported.

Hypersensitivity: (not related to dosage): Skin rash.

Miscellaneous: Elevated transaminase, especially in patients with liver disease.

Overdosage:

Symptoms: Acute toxicity can occur if > 1 g is ingested; chronic toxicity is dose-related and can occur if > 500 mg/day is administered. Toxic effects may include CNS depression with accompanying drowsiness, mental confusion, headache, vertigo, hyperirritability, paresthesias, dysarthrias and psychosis. Paresis, convulsions and coma may occur after larger doses.

Treatment: Management includes supportive therapy. Charcoal may be more effective than emesis or lavage; consider charcoal instead of or in addition to gastric emptying. Hemodialysis removes the drug from the bloodstream; reserve for patients with life-threatening toxicity. Pyridoxine 200 to 300 mg/day may treat the neurotoxic effects. Refer also to General Managment of Acute Overdosage.

Patient Information:

May cause drowsiness. Observe caution when driving or performing other tasks requiring alertness. Avoid excessive alcohol consumption.

Notify physician if skin rash, mental confusion, dizziness, headache or tremors occur.

Administration and Dosage:

Administer 500 mg to 1 g daily in divided doses monitored by blood levels. The usual initial dosage is 250 mg twice daily at 12 hour intervals for the first 2 weeks. Do not exceed 1 g/day.

Pyridoxine 200 to 300 mg/day may prevent the neurotoxic effects.

Children: A dose of 10 to 20 mg/kg/day (maximum 0.75 to 1 g) has been recommended.

Rx	**Seromycin Pulvules** (Dura)	**Capsules:** 250 mg	In 40s.

STREPTOMYCIN SULFATE

The following is an abbreviated monograph for streptomycin sulfate. For complete prescribing information, see individual monograph in Aminoglycosides, Parenteral section.

Indications:

Recommended in the treatment of all forms of *Mycobacterium tuberculosis* when the infecting organisms are susceptible. Use only in combination with other antituberculous drugs.

For nontuberculous infection indications, see individual monograph in Aminoglycosides, Parenteral section.

Administration and Dosage:

Administer by the IM route only.

Combined therapy for adults: 1g streptomycin and an appropriate dosage of additional antitubercular drugs (usually isoniazid, ethambutol or rifampin). Elderly patients should have a smaller daily dose of streptomycin in accordance with age, renal function and eighth nerve function.

Discontinue the streptomycin or reduce dosage to 1 g 2 to 3 times weekly. Therapy with streptomycin may be terminated when toxic symptoms appear, impending toxicity is feared, organisms have become resistant, or full therapeutic effect has been obtained. The total period of treatment for tuberculosis is a minimum of 1 year; however, indications for terminating streptomycin therapy may occur at any time.

Children: A dose of 20 to 40 mg/kg/day (maximum 0.75 to 1g) has been recommended.

As with other aminoglycosides, reduce dosage in patients with impaired renal function.

For a complete listing of streptomycin sulfate products, refer to individual monograph in Aminoglycosides, Parenteral section.

CAPREOMYCIN

Refer to the general discussion in the Antituberculous Drugs monograph.

Warning:

The use of capreomycin in patients with renal insufficiency or preexisting auditory impairment must be undertaken with great caution, and weigh the risk of additional eighth nerve impairment or renal injury against benefits to be derived from therapy.

Since other parenteral antituberculous agents (eg, streptomycin) also have similar and sometimes irreversible toxic effects, particularly on eighth cranial nerve and renal function, simultaneous administration of these agents with capreomycin is not recommended. Use concurrent nonantituberculous drugs (eg, aminoglycoside antibiotics) having ototoxic or nephrotoxic potential only with great caution.

Actions:

Pharmacology: A polypeptide antibiotic isolated from *Streptomyces capreolus.*

Pharmacokinetics:

Distribution – Capreomycin sulfate is not absorbed in significant quantities from the GI tract and must be administered parenterally. Peak serum concentrations following IM administration of 1g are achieved in 1 to 2 hours. Low serum concentrations are present at 24 hours. Doses of 1 g daily for ≥ 30 days produce no significant accumulation in subjects with normal renal function.

Excretion – Capreomycin is excreted essentially unaltered; 52% is excreted in the urine within 12 hours. Urine concentrations average 1680 mcg/ml during the 6 hours following a 1 g dose.

Microbiology: Active against human strains of *Mycobacterium tuberculosis.*

Cross-resistance – Varying degrees of cross-resistance between capreomycin and kanamycin and neomycin have occurred. No cross-resistance has been observed between capreomycin and isoniazid, aminosalicylate sodium, cycloserine, streptomycin, ethionamide or ethambutol.

Indications:

Intended for use concomitantly with other antituberculous agents in pulmonary infections caused by capreomycin-susceptible strains of *M tuberculosis,* when the primary agents (eg, isoniazid, rifampin) have been ineffective or cannot be used because of toxicity or the presence of resistant tubercle bacilli.

Perform susceptibility studies to determine the presence of a capreomycin-susceptible strain of *M tuberculosis.*

Contraindications:

Hypersensitivity to capreomycin.

Warnings:

Hypersensitivity: Has occurred when capreomycin and other antituberculous drugs were given concomitantly. Refer to General Management of Acute Hypersensitivity Reactions.

Renal function impairment: Dosage reduction is necessary. See Administration and Dosage.

Pregnancy: Category C. Well controlled studies have not been performed in pregnant women. Use only if clearly needed and when potential benefits justify potential risks to the fetus. Safety for use during pregnancy has not been established.

Lactation: It is not known whether this drug is excreted in breast milk. Therefore, exercise caution when administering capreomycin to nursing mothers.

Children: Safety for use in infants and children has not been established.

Precautions:

Ototoxicity: Perform audiometric measurements and assessment of vestibular function prior to initiation of therapy and at regular intervals during treatment.

Nephrotoxicity: Perform regular tests of renal function throughout treatment, and reduce dose in patients with renal impairment. Renal injury with tubular necrosis, elevation of BUN or serum creatinine and abnormal sediment has been noted. Monitor renal function both before therapy is started and on a weekly basis during treatment. Slight elevation of the BUN or serum creatinine has been observed in a significant number of patients receiving prolonged therapy. The appearance of casts, red cells and white cells in the urine has been noted in a high percentage of these cases.

CAPREOMYCIN

Elevation of the BUN > 30 mg/dl or any other evidence of decreasing renal function with or without a rise in BUN level should indicate careful evaluation of the patient; reduce the dosage or withdraw the drug. The clinical significance of abnormal urine sediment and slight elevation in the BUN (or serum creatinine) during long-term therapy has not been established.

Hypokalemia may occur during therapy; therefore, determine serum potassium levels frequently.

Drug Interactions:

Aminoglycosides and capreomycin coadministration may increase the risk of respiratory paralysis and renal dysfunction.

Nondepolarizing neuromuscular blocking agents: Neuromuscular blockade may be enhanced by concurrent capreomycin due to a synergistic effect on myoneural function.

Adverse Reactions:

Nephrotoxicity: In 36% of 722 patients treated with capreomycin, elevation of the BUN >20 mg/dl has been observed. In many instances, there was also depression of PSP excretion and abnormal urine sediment. In 10% of this series, the BUN elevation exceeded 30 mg/dl.

Toxic nephritis was reported in one patient with tuberculosis and portal cirrhosis who was treated with capreomycin (1 g) and aminosalicylate sodium daily for 1 month. This patient developed renal insufficiency and oliguria and died. Autopsy showed subsiding acute tubular necrosis.

Electrolyte disturbances resembling Bartter's syndrome occurred in one patient.

Ototoxicity: Subclinical auditory loss was noted in approximately 11% of patients. This has been a 5 to 10 decibel loss in the 4,000 to 8,000 CPS range. Clinically apparent hearing loss occurred in 3% of 722 subjects. Some audiometric changes were reversible. Other cases with permanent loss were not progressive following withdrawal of capreomycin.

Tinnitus and vertigo have also occurred.

Other: Pain and induration and excessive bleeding at the injection sites; sterile abscesses.

Hematologic: Leukocytosis and leukopenia have been observed. The majority of patients treated have had eosinophilia exceeding 5% while receiving daily injections of capreomycin. This subsided with reduction of the capreomycin dosage to 2 or 3 g weekly.

Rare cases of thrombocytopenia have occurred.

Hepatic: Serial tests of liver function have demonstrated a decrease in BSP excretion without change in AST or ALT in the presence of preexisting liver disease. Abnormal results in liver function tests have occurred in many persons receiving capreomycin in combination with other antituberculous agents which are also known to cause changes in hepatic function. The role of capreomycin is not clear; however, periodic determinations of liver function are recommended.

Hypersensitivity: Urticaria and maculopapular skin rashes, associated in some cases with febrile reactions. See Warnings.

Overdosage:

Adverse reactions listed above may be seen in capreomycin overdose. Management includes supportive therapy. Refer to General Management of Acute Overdosage.

Hemodialysis may be useful in patients with significant renal disease.

Administration and Dosage:

Give by deep IM injection into a large muscle mass; superficial injections may be associated with increased pain and sterile abscesses. Always administer in combination with at least one other antituberculous agent to which the patient's strain of tubercle bacilli is susceptible.

Usual dose: 1 g daily (not to exceed 20 mg/kg/day) given IM for 60 to 120 days, followed by 1 g IM 2 or 3 times weekly.

Note: Maintain therapy for tuberculosis for 12 to 24 months. If facilities for administering injectable medication are not available, a change to oral therapy is indicated upon the patient's release from the hospital.

Children: A dose of 15mg/kg/day (maximum 1 g) has been recommended.

CAPREOMYCIN

Renal function impairment: Reduce the dosage based on creatinine clearance (Ccr) using the guidelines in the table. These dosages are designed to achieve a mean steady-state capreomycin level of 10 mg/L.

Capreomycin Dosage in Renal Function Impairment

Ccr (ml/min)	Capreomycin clearance (L/kg/h × 10^{-2})	Half-life (hours)	Dose[1] (mg/kg) for the following dosing intervals: 24 hr	48 hr	72 hr
0	0.54	55.5	1.29	2.58	3.87
10	1.01	29.4	2.43	4.87	7.31
20	1.49	20.0	3.58	7.16	10.7
30	1.97	15.1	4.72	9.45	14.2
40	2.45	12.2	5.87	11.7	
50	2.92	10.2	7.01	14	
60	3.40	8.8	8.16		
80	4.35	6.8	10.4		
100	5.31	5.6	12.7		
110	5.78	5.2	13.9		

[1] Initial maintenance dose estimates are given for optional dosing intervals; longer dosing intervals are expected to provide greater peak and lower trough serum capreomycin levels than shorter dosing intervals.

Preparation of solution: Dissolve in 2 ml of 0.9% Sodium Chloride Injection or Sterile Water for Injection. Allow 2 to 3 minutes for complete dissolution. For administration of a 1 g dose, give the entire contents of the vial. For dosages < 1 g, the following dilution table may be used.

Preparation of Capreomycin Solution

Concentration[1] (Approx.)	Diluent added to 1 g vial	Volume of solution
350 mg/ml	2.15 ml	2.85 ml
300 mg/ml	2.63 ml	3.33 ml
250 mg/ml	3.3 ml	4 ml
200 mg/ml	4.3 ml	5 ml

[1] Stated in terms of mg of capreomycin activity.

Storage/Stability: The solution may acquire a pale straw color and darken with time, but this is not associated with loss of potency or the development of toxicity. After reconstitution, solutions may be stored for 48 hours at room temperature and up to 14 days under refrigeration.

Rx	**Capastat Sulfate** (Dura)	**Powder for Injection:** 1 g (as sulfate) per 10 ml vial.

AMEBICIDES

The agents listed in this group are recommended for the following disorders (see individual monographs):

Intestinal amebiasis:	*Extraintestinal amebiasis:*
Paromomycin	Metronidazole
Iodoquinol	Emetine HCl
Metronidazole	Chloroquine
Emetine HCl	

PAROMOMYCIN

Actions:

Pharmacology: Paromomycin is an amebicidal and antibacterial aminoglycoside obtained from a strain of *Streptomyces rimosus,* and is active in intestinal amebiasis. Its in vitro and in vivo antibacterial activity closely parallels that of neomycin; complete cross-resistance exists between promomycin, kanamycin and neomycin. Effective against enteric bacteria *Salmonella* and *Shigella.*

Gastrointestinal absorption of paromomycin is poor; almost 100% of the drug is recovered in the stool.

Indications:

Acute and chronic intestinal amebiasis.

Adjunctive therapy in the management of hepatic coma.

Not indicated in extraintestinal amebiasis because it is not absorbed.

Unlabeled uses: Has been recommended for other parasitic infections — *Dientamoeba fragilis* (25 to 30 mg/kg/day in 3 doses for 7 days); *Diphyllobothrium latum, Taenia saginata, T solium, Dipylidium caninum* (adults: 1 g every 15 min for 4 doses; pediatric: 11 mg/kg every 15 min for 4 doses); *Hymenolepsis nana* (45 mg/kg/day for 5 to 7 days).

Contraindications:

Hypersensitivity reactions to paromomycin; intestinal obstruction.

Precautions:

Ototoxicity and renal damage: Inadvertent absorption through ulcerative bowel lesions may result in eighth cranial nerve damage and renal damage.

Superinfection: Use of antibiotics (especially prolonged or repeated therapy) may result in bacterial or fungal overgrowth of nonsusceptible organisms. Such overgrowth may lead to secondary infections. Take appropriate measures if superinfection occurs.

Drug Interactions:

Since paromomycin is an aminoglycoside, consider the interactions that may occur with the other oral aminoglycosides as potentially occurring with paromomycin as well (see Aminoglycosides, Oral section).

Adverse Reactions:

GI: Doses > 3 g daily have reportedly produced nausea, abdominal cramps and diarrhea.

Patient Information:

Complete full course of therapy.

May cause nausea, vomiting or diarrhea.

Notify physician if ringing in the ears, hearing impairment or dizziness occurs.

Administration and Dosage:

Intestinal amebiasis:

Adults and children – 25 to 35 mg/kg/day in 3 divided doses with meals for 5 to 10 days.

Management of hepatic coma:

Adults – 4 g daily in divided doses administered at regular intervals for 5 to 6 days.

Rx	**Humatin** (Parke-Davis)	**Capsules:** 250 mg (as sulfate)	In 16s.

IODOQUINOL (Diiodohydroxyquin)

Actions:

Pharmacology: Iodoquinol is effective against the trophozoites and cysts of Entamoeba histolytica located in the large intestine. Because it is poorly absorbed in the GI tract, the drug can reach high concentrations in the intestinal lumen, and produce its potent amebicidal effect precisely at the site of infection, without significant systemic absorption (approximately 8%). This is useful for the prevention of extraintestinal (liver, lung) complications of amebic dysentery. The drug is not effective in amebic hepatitis and amebic abscess of the liver.

Indications:

Treatment of intestinal amebiasis.

Not indicated for treatment of chronic diarrhea, particularly in children, because of potential association with optic atrophy and permanent loss of vision.

Contraindications:

Hypersensitivity to any 8-hydroxyquinoline (eg, iodoquinol, iodochlorhydroxyquin) or iodine-containing preparations; hepatic damage.

Warnings:

Optic neuritis, optic atrophy and peripheral neuropathy have occurred following prolonged high dosage therapy; avoid long-term therapy.

Pregnancy: Safety for use during pregnancy and in the nursing mother has not been established.

Precautions:

Use with caution in patients with thyroid disease.

Drug Interactions:

Protein bound iodine levels may be increased during treatment and interfere with the results of certain **thyroid** function tests. These effects may persist for as long as 6 months after discontinuance of therapy.

Adverse Reactions:

Dermatologic: Various forms of skin eruptions (acneiform, papular, pustular, bullae, vegetating or tuberous iododerma); urticaria; pruritus.

GI: Nausea; vomiting; abdominal cramps; diarrhea; pruritus ani.

Miscellaneous: Fever; chills; headache; vertigo; enlargement of thyroid. Optic neuritis, optic atrophy and peripheral neuropathy have occurred in association with prolonged high dosage 8-hydroxyquinoline therapy.

Patient Information:

Complete full course of therapy.

May cause nausea, vomiting, diarrhea or GI upset.

Administration and Dosage:

Adults: 650 mg 3 times daily after meals for 20 days.

Children: 40 mg/kg daily (maximum 650 mg/dose) in 3 divided doses for 20 days. Do not exceed 1.95 g in 24 hours for 20 days.

Rx	**Yodoxin** (Glenwood)	**Tablets**: 210 mg	In 100s and 1000s.
		650 mg	In 100s and 1000s.
		Powder	In 25 g.

METRONIDAZOLE

The following is an abbreviated monograph for metronidazole. Complete prescribing information begins in the full monograph in the Antibiotics section of the Anti-Infectives chapter.

> **Warning:**
> Metronidazole has been shown to be carcinogenic in rodents. Avoid unnecessary use.

Actions:

Microbiology: Metronidazole is a nitroimidazole that possesses direct trichomonacidal and amebicidal activity against *Trichomonas vaginalis*and *Entamoeba histolytica.*The in vitro minimal inhibitory concentration (MIC) for most strains of these organisms is ≤ 1 mcg/ml. Metronidazole's mechanism of antiprotozoal action is unknown.

Indications:

Amebiasis: Treatment of acute intestinal amebiasis (amebic dysentery) and amebic liver abscess. In amebic liver abscess, therapy does not obviate the need for aspiration or drainage of pus.

Trichomoniasis, symptomatic: Treatment in females and males when the presence of the trichomonad has been confirmed by appropriate laboratory procedures (wet smears or cultures).

Trichomoniasis, asymptomatic: Treatment of asymptomatic females with endocervicitis, cervicitis or cervical erosion. Since there is evidence that presence of the trichomonad can interfere with accurate assessment of abnormal cytological smears, perform additional smears after eradication of the parasite.

Treatment of asymptomatic partners: T vaginalis infection is a sexually transmitted disease. Therefore, in order to prevent reinfection, simultaneously treat asymptomatic sexual partners of treated patients if the organism has been found to be present. Since there can be difficulty in isolating the organism from the asymptomatic male carrier, negative smears and cultures cannot be relied upon. Women may become reinfected if the male partner is not treated. Therefore, it may be advisable to treat an asymptomatic male partner with a negative culture or when no culture has been attempted.

Anaerobic bacterial infections: Refer to the use of metronidazole as an antibiotic in the Anti-Infectives chapter.

Unlabeled uses: The CDC has recommended the use of oral metronidazole for *Gardnerella vaginalis* (500 mg twice daily for 7 days) and for giardiasis (alternative to quinacrine; 250 mg 3 times daily for 7 days).

Patient Information:

May cause GI upset; take with food.

Complete full course of therapy; take until gone.

Avoid alcoholic beverages.

May cause darkening of urine.

An unpleasant metallic taste may be noticeable.

During treatment for trichomoniasis, it is recommended that the patient refrain from sexual intercourse or the male partner wear a condom to avoid reinfection.

METRONIDAZOLE

Administration and Dosage:

Amebiasis:

Acute intestinal amebiasis (acute amebic dysentery) – 750 mg 3 times daily for 5 to 10 days.

Amebic liver abscess – 500 or 750 mg 3 times daily for 5 to 10 days.

Children – 35 to 50 mg/kg/24 hours (maximum 750 mg/dose) in 3 divided doses for 10 days.

Trichomoniasis:

1 day treatment – 2 g given either as a single dose or in 2 divided doses of 1 g each given in the same day.

7 day course of treatment –

Adults: 250 mg 3 times daily for 7 consecutive days;

Children: 5 mg/kg/dose 3 times daily for 7 days.

Cure rates, as determined by vaginal smears, signs and symptoms, may be higher after a 7 day course of treatment than after the 1 day treatment regimen. Individualize dosage. Single dose treatment can assure compliance, especially if administered under supervision, in those patients who cannot be relied upon to continue the 7 day regimen. A 7 day course of treatment may minimize reinfection of the female long enough to treat sexual contacts. Further, some patients may tolerate one course of therapy better than the other.

Do not treat pregnant patients during the first trimester. If treated during the second or third trimester in those whom local palliative treatment has been inadequate to control symptoms, do not use the 1 day course of therapy as it results in higher serum levels which reach the fetal circulation.

When repeat courses of drug are required, 4 to 6 weeks should elapse between courses and reconfirm presence of trichomonad by appropriate laboratory measures. Perform total and differential leukocyte counts before and after retreatment.

Patients with severe hepatic disease metabolize metronidazole slowly, with resultant accumulation of metronidazole and its metabolites in the plasma. Accordingly, cautiously administer doses below those usually recommended. Monitor plasma metronidazole levels and toxicity.

Do not specifically reduce the dose of metronidazole in anuric patients since accumulated metabolites may be rapidly removed by dialysis.

Rx	**Metronidazole** (Various, eg, Baxter, Geneva, Goldline, Lederle, Lemmon, Moore, Rugby, Schein)	**Tablets**: 250 mg	In 100s, 250s, 500s, 1000s and UD 32s and 100s.
Rx	**Flagyl** (Searle)		(Searle 1831 Flagyl 250). Blue. Film coated. In 50s, 100s, 250s, 1000s, 2500s and UD 100s.
Rx	**Metric 21** (Fielding)		In 100s.
Rx	**Protostat** (Ortho)		(Ortho 1570). White, scored. Capsule shape. In 100s.
Rx	**Metronidazole** (Various, eg, Baxter, Geneva, Goldline, Lederle, Lemmon, Moore, Rugby, Schein)	**Tablets**: 500 mg	In 100s, 200s, 250s, 500s and UD 32s and 100s.
Rx	**Flagyl** (Searle)		(Flagyl 500). Blue. Film coated. Oblong. In 50s, 100s, 500s and UD 100s.
Rx	**Protostat** (Ortho)		(Ortho 1571). White, scored. Capsule shape. In 50s.
Rx	**Flagyl 375** (Searle)	**Capsules**: 375 mg	(375 Flagyl). Gray/light green. In 50s, 100s and UD 100s.

CHLOROQUINE PHOSPHATE

The following is an abbreviated monograph for chloroquine phosphate. For complete prescribing information, see 4–Aminoquinoline Compounds in the Antimalarial Preparations section.

Indications:

Treatment of extraintestinal amebiasis.

Administration and Dosage:

Adults: 1 g (600 mg base) daily for 2 days, followed by 500 mg (300 mg base) daily for at least 2 to 3 weeks. Treatment is usually combined with an effective intestinal amebicide.

Rx	**Chloroquine Phosphate** (Various)	**Tablets:** 250 mg (equiv. to 150 mg base)	In 40s, 100s and 1000s.
Rx	**Aralen Phosphate** (Sanofi Winthrop)	**Tablets:** 500 mg (equiv. to 300 mg base)	Pink. Film coated. In 25s.

CHLOROQUINE HCl

For complete prescribing information, refer to the 4–Aminoquinoline Compounds in the Antimalarial Preparations section.

Indications:

Treatment of extraintestinal amebiasis when oral therapy is not feasible.

Administration and Dosage:

Adults: 4 to 5 ml (200 to 250 mg; 160 to 200 mg base) IM daily for 10 to 12 days. Substitute or resume oral administration as soon as possible.

Rx	**Aralen HCl** (Sanofi Winthrop)	**Injection:** 50 mg (equiv. to 40 mg base) per ml	In 5 ml amps.

CIDOFOVIR

Warning:

Renal impairment is the major toxicity of cidofovir. To minimize possible nephrotoxicity, IV prehydration with Normal Saline and administration of probenecid must be used with each cidofovir infusion. Monitor renal function (serum creatinine and urine protein) prior to each dose of cidofovir and modify the dose for changes in renal function as appropriate.

Granulocytopenia has been observed in association with cidofovir treatment. Monitor neutrophil counts during cidofovir therapy.

Actions:

Pharmacology: Cidofovir is a nucleotide analog. Cidofovir suppresses cytomegalovirus (CMV) replication by selective inhibition of viral DNA synthesis. Biochemical data support selective inhibition of CMV DNA polymerase by cidofovir diphosphate, the active intracellular metabolite of cidofovir. Cidofovir diphosphate inhibits herpes virus polymerases at concentrations that are 8- to 600-fold lower than those needed to inhibit human cellular DNA polymerases alpha, beta and gamma. Incorporation of cidofovir into the growing viral DNA chain results in reductions in the rate of viral DNA synthesis.

Resistance – CMV isolates with reduced susceptibility to cidofovir have been selected in vitro in the presence of high concentration of cidofovir. IC_{50} values for selected resistant isolates ranged from 7 to 15 μM.

Cross resistance – Cidofovir-resistant isolates selected in vitro following exposure to increasing concentrations of cidofovir were assessed for susceptibility to ganciclovir and foscarnet. All were cross-resistant to ganciclovir, but remained susceptible to foscarnet. Ganciclovir or ganciclovir/foscarnet-resistant isolates that are cross resistant to cidofovir have been obtained from drug-naive patients and from patients following ganciclovir or ganciclovir/foscarnet therapy. To date, the majority of ganciclovir-resistant isolates are UL97 gene product (phosphokinase) mutants and remain susceptible to cidofovir. However, reduced susceptibility to cidofovir has been reported for DNA polymerase mutants of CMV that are resistant to ganciclovir. To date, all clinical isolates that exhibit high level resistance to ganciclovir, because of mutations in the DNA polymerase gene, have been shown to be cross-resistant to cidofovir. Cidofovir is active against some, but not all, CMV isolates that are resistant to foscarnet. The incidence of foscarnet-resistant isolates that are resistant to cidofovir is not known.

A few triple-drug resistant isolates have been described. Genotypic analysis of two of these triple-resistant isolates revealed several point mutations in the CMV DNA polymerase gene.

Pharmacokinetics: Cidofovir must be administered with probenecid. Renal tubular secretion contributes to the elimination of cidofovir.

Cidofovir Pharmacokinetic Parameters Following 3 and 5 mg/kg Infusions With and Without Probenecid

Parameters	Cidofovir Administered Without Probenicid		Cidofovir Administered With Probenecid	
	3 mg/kg	5 mg/kg	3 mg/kg	5 mg/kg
AUC (mcg•hr/ml)	20.0	28.3	25.7	40.8
C_{max} (end of infusion) (mcg/ml)	7.3	11.5	9.8	19.6
Vdss (ml/kg)	537		410	
Clearance (ml/min/1.73 m²)	179		148	
Renal Clearance (ml/min/1.73 m²)	150		98.6	

In vitro, cidofovir was < 6% bound to plasma or serum proteins over the cidofovir concentration range 0.25 to 25 mcg/ml. CSF concentrations of cidofovir following IV infusion of cidofovir 5 mg/kg with concomitant probenecid and IV hydration were undetectable (< 0.1 mcg/ml, assay detection threshold) at 15 minutes after the end of a 1-hour infusion in one patient whose corresponding serum concentration was 8.7 mcg/ml.

CIDOFOVIR

Clinical trials:

Delayed vs immediate therapy – In an open-label trial, previously untreated patients with peripheral CMV retinitis were randomized to either immediate treatment with cidofovir (5 mg/kg once a week for 2 weeks, then 5 mg/kg every other week), or delayed cidofovir treatment until progression of CMV retinitis occurred. Of 25 and 23 patients in the immediate and delayed groups respectively, 23 and 21 were evaluable for retinitis progression as determined by retinal photography. Based on masked readings of retinal photographs, the median (95% confidence internal [CI]) times to retinitis progression were 120 days (40, 134) and 22 days (10, 27) for the immediate and delayed therapy groups, respectively. This difference was statistically significant. Median (95% CI) times to the alternative endpoint of retinitis progression or study drug discontinuation (including adverse events, withdrawn consent and systemic CMV disease) were 52 days (37, 85) and 22 days (13, 27) for the immediate and delayed therapy groups, respectively. This difference was statistically significant.

Indications:

CMV retinitis: For the treatment of CMV retinitis in patients with acquired immunodefiency syndrome (AIDS).

The safety and efficacy of cidofovir have not been established for treatment of other CMV infections (such as pneumonitis or gastroenteritis), congenital or neonatal CMV disease, or CMV disease in non-HIV-infected individuals.

Contraindications:

Hypersensitivity to cidofovir; a history of clinically severe hypersensitivity to probenecid or other sulfa-containing medications; direct intraocular injection.

Warnings:

Direct intraocular injection may be associated with significant decreases in intraocular pressure and impairment of vision.

Nephrotoxicity: Dose-dependent nephrotoxicity is the major dose-limiting toxicity related to cidofovir administration. Dose adjustment or discontinuation is required for changes in renal function while on therapy. Proteinuria may be an early indicator of cidofovir-related nephrotoxicity. Continued administration of cidofovir may lead to additional proximal tubular cell injury that may result in glycosuria; decreases in serum phosphate, uric acid and bicarbonate; and elevations in serum creatinine. Patients with these adverse events occurring concurrently and meeting a criteria of Fanconi's syndrome have been reported. Renal function may not return to baseline after drug discontinuation.

Hematological toxicity: Neutropenia may occur during cidofovir therapy. Monitor neutrophil count while receiving cidofovir therapy.

Metabolic acidosis: Fanconi's syndrome and decreases in serum bicarbonate associated with evidence of renal tubular damage have been reported. Serious metabolic acidosis, in association with liver failure, pancreatitis, mucormycosis, aspergillus, disseminated mycobacterial infection and progression to death occurred in one patient.

Ocular hypotony: Among the subset of patients monitored for intraocular pressure changes, ocular hypotony (≥ 50% change from baseline) was reported in five patients. Hypotony was reported in one patient with concomitant diabetes mellitus. Risk of ocular hypotony may be increased in patients with preexisting diabetes.

Renal function impairment: It is recommended that cidofovir not be initiated in patients with baseline serum creatinine > 1.5 mg/dL or creatinine clearances ≤ 55 ml/min. In these patients, use cidofovir when the potential benefits exceed the potential risks.

Carcinogenesis/Fertility impairment: Mammary adenocarcinomas have occurred in rats and mice, and Zymbal's gland carcinomas have occurred in rats. Studies showed inhibition of spermatogenesis in rats and monkeys. However, no adverse effects on fertility or reproduction were seen following once weekly IV injections of cidovovir in male rats for 13 consecutive weeks.

Elderly: No studies of the safety and efficacy of cidofovir in patients > 60 years of age have been conducted. Because elderly individuals frequently have reduced glomerular filtration, pay particular attention to assessing renal function before and during cidofovir administration.

Pregnancy: Category C. Cidofovir was embryotoxic (reduced fetal body weights) in rats and in rabbits. An increased incidence of fetal external, soft tissue and skeletal anomalies (meningocele, short snout and short maxillary bones) occurred in rabbits. There are no adequate and well controlled studies in pregnant women. Use cidofovir during pregnancy only if the potential benefit justifies the potential risk to the fetus.

CIDOFOVIR

Lactation: It is not known whether cidofovir is excreted in breast milk. Since many drugs are excreted in breast milk and because of the potential for adverse reactions as well as the potential for tumorigenicity shown for cidofovir in animal studies, do not administer cidofovir to nursing women. The US Public Health Service Centers for Disease Control and Prevention advises HIV-infected women not to breastfeed and to avoid postnatal transmission of HIV to a child who may not yet be infected.

Children: Safety and effectiveness in children have not been studied. The use of cidofovir in children with AIDS warrants extreme caution due to the risk of long-term carcinogenicity and reproductive toxicity. Administer cidofovir to children only after careful evaluation and only if the potential benefits of treatment outweigh the risks.

Precautions:

Monitoring: Monitor serum creatinine, urine protein and white blood cell counts with differential prior to each dose. In patients with proteinuria, administer IV hydration and repeat the test. Periodically monitor intraocular pressure, visual acuity and ocular symptoms.

Drug Interactions:

Nephrotoxic agents: Avoid concomitant administration of cidofovir and agents with nephrotoxic potential (eg, amphotericin B, aminoglycosides, foscarnet and IV pentamidine).

Adverse Reactions:

Renal: Renal toxicity (53%); proteinuria (80%); serum creatinine elevations (29%) (see Warnings).

Body as a whole: Allergic reaction; face edema; malaise; back pain; chest pain; neck pain; sarcoma; sepsis.

Cardiovascular: Hypotension; postural hypotension; pallor; syncope; tachycardia.

GI: Nausea, vomiting (65%); diarrhea (27%); anorexia (22%); abdominal pain (17%); colitis; constipation; tongue discoloration; dyspepsia; dysphagia; flatulence; gastritis; hepatomegaly; abnormal liver function tests; melena; oral candidiasis; rectal disorder; stomatitis; aphthous stomatitis; mouth ulceration; dry mouth.

Hematologic/Lymphatic: Thrombocytopenia; neutropenia (< 750/mm^3; 31%); anemia (20%).

Metabolic/Nutritional: Edema; dehydration; hyperglycemia; hyperlipemia; hypocalcemia; hypokalemia; increased alkaline phosphatase; increased SGOT; increased SGPT; weight loss.

Musculoskeletal: Arthralgia; myasthenia; myalgia.

CNS: Headache (27%); asthenia (46%); amnesia; anxiety; confusion; convulsion; depression; dizziness; abnormal gait; hallucinations; insomnia; neuropathy; paresthesia; somnolence; vasodilation.

Respiratory: Asthma; bronchitis; coughing; dyspnea (22%); hiccup; increased sputum; lung disorder; pharyngitis; pneumonia (9%); rhinitis; sinusitis.

Dermatologic: Alopecia (25%); rash (30%); acne; skin discoloration; dry skin; herpes simplex; pruritus; rash; sweating; urticaria.

Special senses: Amblyopia; conjunctivitis; eye disorder; hypotony (12%) (see Warnings); iritis; retinal detachment; taste perversion; uveitis; abnormal vision.

GU: Decreased creatinine clearance; glycosuria; hematuria; urinary incontinence; urinary tract infection.

Miscellaneous: Fever (57%); infections (24%); chills (24%).

Overdosage:

Overdosage with cidofovir has not been reported; however, hemodialysis and hydration may reduce drug plasma concentrations in patients who receive an overdosage of cidofovir. Probenecid may reduce the potential for nephrotoxicity in patients who receive an overdose of cidofovir through reduction of active tubular secretion.

Patient Information:

Advise patients that cidofovir is not a cure for CMV retinitis, and that they may continue to experience progression of retinitis during and following treatment. Advise patients receiving cidofovir to have regular follow-up ophthalmologic examinations. Patients may also experience other manifestations of CMV disease despite cidofovir therapy.

HIV-infected patients may continue taking antiretroviral therapy. However, because probenecid reduces metabolic clearance of zidovudine, advise those taking zidovudine to temporarily discontinue zidovudine administration or decrease their zidovudine dose by 50% on days of cidofovir administration only.

CIDOFOVIR

Inform patients of the major toxicity of cidofovir, namely renal impairment, and that dose modification, including reduction, interruption and possibly discontinuation, may be required. Emphasize close monitoring of renal function (routine urinalysis and serum creatinine) while on therapy.

Emphasize the importance of completing a full course of probenecid with each cidofovir dose. Warn patients of potential adverse events caused by probenecid (eg, headache, nausea, vomiting and hypersensitivity reactions). Hypersensitivity/allergic reactions may include rash, fever, chills and anaphylaxis. Administration of probenecid after a meal or use of antiemetics may decrease the nausea. Prophylactic or therapeutic antihistamines or acetaminophen may be used to ameliorate hypersensitivity reactions.

Cidofovir caused reduced testes weight and hypospermia in animals. Such changes may occur in humans and cause infertility. Advise women of childbearing potential that cidofovir is embryotoxic in animals and not to use the drug during pregnancy. Women of childbearing potential should use effective contraception during and for 1 month following treatment. Men should practice barrier contraceptive methods during and for 3 months following treatment.

Administration and Dosage:

Approved by the FDA on June 26, 1996.

Do not administer by intraocular injection.

Dosage: The recommended dosage, frequency or infusion rate must not be exceeded. Cidofovir must be diluted in 100 ml 0.9% Saline Solution prior to administration. To minimize potential nephrotoxicity, probenecid and IV saline prehydration must be administered with each cidofovir infusion.

Induction treatment: The recommended dose of cidofovir is 5 mg/kg body weight (given as an IV infusion at a constant rate over 1 hour) administered once weekly for 2 consecutive weeks.

Maintenance treatment: The recommended maintenance dose of cidofovir is 5 mg/kg body weight (given as an IV infusion at a constant rate over 1 hour) administered once every 2 weeks.

Probenecid: Probenecid must be administered orally with each cidofovir dose. Two grams must be administered 3 hours prior to the cidofovir dose, and 1 g administered at 2 and again at 8 hours after completion of the 1-hour cidofovir infusion (for a total of 4 g).

Ingestion of food prior to each dose of probenecid may reduce drug-related nausea and vomiting. Administration of an antiemetic may reduce the potential for nausea associated with probenecid ingestion. In patients who develop allergic or hypersensitivity symptoms to probenecid, consider the use of an appropriate prophylactic or therapeutic antihistamine or acetaminophen.

Hydration: Patients should receive a total of 1 L of 0.9% Saline Solution IV with each infusion of cidofovir. Infuse the saline solution over a 1- to 2-hour period immediately before the cidofovir infusion. Patients who can tolerate the additional fluid load should receive a second liter. If administered, the second liter of saline should be initiated either at the start of the cidofovir infusion or immediately afterwards, and should be infused over a 1- to 3-hour period.

Nephrotoxicity: For increases in serum creatinine (0.3 to 0.4 mg/dL), reduce the cidofovir dose from 5 mg/kg to 3 mg/kg. Discontinue cidofovir therapy for an increase in serum creatinine of ≥ 0.5 mg/dL or development of ≥ 3+ proteinuria.

Renal function impairment:

Dosing of Cidofovir with Renal Function Impairment		
Creatinine Clearance	Induction	Maintenance
(ml/min)	(once weekly for 2 weeks)	(once every 2 weeks)
41 - 55	2.0 mg/kg	2.0 mg/kg
30 - 40	1.5 mg/kg	1.5 mg/kg
20 - 29	1.0 mg/kg	1.0 mg/kg
≤ 19	0.5 mg/kg	0.5 mg/kg

Storage/Stability: Store at controlled room temperature 20° to 25°C (68° to 77°F).

Admixtures may be stored under refrigeration (2° to 8°C; 36° to 46°F) for no more than 24 hours. Allow refrigerated admixtures to equilibrate to room temperature prior to use.

Rx	**Vistide** (Gilead Sciences)	**Injection:** 75 mg/ml	5 ml amp

FAMCICLOVIR

Actions:

Pharmacology: Famciclovir undergoes rapid biotransformation to the active antiviral compound penciclovir, which has inhibitory activity against herpes simplex virus types 1 (HSV-1) and 2 (HSV-2) and varicella zoster virus (VZV). In cells infected with HSV-1, HSV-2 or VZV, viral thymidine kinase phosphorylates penciclovir to a monophosphate form that, in turn, is converted to penciclovir triphosphate by cellular kinases. In vitro studies demonstrate that penciclovir triphosphate inhibits HSV-2 polymerase competitively with deoxyguanosine triphosphate. Consequently, herpes viral DNA synthesis and, therefore, replication are selectively inhibited.

Pharmacokinetics:

Absorption/Distribution – The absolute bioavailability of famciclovir is 77%. The area under the plasma concentration-time curve (AUC) is 8.6 mcg•hr/ml. The maximum concentration (C_{max}) is 3.3 mcg/ml and the time to C_{max} (T_{max}) is 0.9 hours.

After a 1-hour intravenous infusion of penciclovir at doses of 5 to 20 mg/kg, the volume of distribution (Vd_b) of penciclovir was 83.1 L and 125 L, respectively. Penciclovir is < 20% bound to plasma proteins over the concentration range of 0.1 to 20 mcg/ml. The blood/plasma ratio of penciclovir is ≈ 1.

Penciclovir C_{max} decreased ≈ 50% and T_{max} was delayed by 1.5 hours when a capsule formulation of famciclovir was administered with food (nutritional content was ≈ 910 Kcal and 26% fat). There was no effect on the extent of availability (AUC) of penciclovir. There was an 18% decrease in C_{max} and a delay in T_{max} of about 1 hour when famciclovir was given 2 hours after a meal as compared to its administration 2 hours before a meal because there was no effect on the extent of systemic availability of penciclovir, it appears that famciclovir can be taken without regard to meals.

Metabolism – Following oral administration, famciclovir is deacetylated and oxidized to form penciclovir. Metabolites that are inactive include 6-deoxy penciclovir, monoacetylated penciclovir and 6-deoxy monoacetylated penciclovir. Little or no famciclovir is detected in plasma or urine. The conversion of 6-deoxy penciclovir to penciclovir is catalyzed by aldehyde oxidase.

Excretion – Following the oral administration of a single 500 mg dose of radiolabeled famciclovir, 73% and 27% of administered radioactivity were recovered in urine and feces over 72 hours, respectively. Penciclovir accounted for 82% and 6–deoxy penciclovir accounted for 7% of the radioactivity excreted in the urine. Approximately 60% of administered radiolabeled dose was collected in urine in the first 6 hours.

After IV administration of penciclovir the mean total plasma clearance of penciclovir was 36.6 L/hr. Penciclovir renal clearance accounted for 74.5% of total plasma clearance.

Renal clearance of penciclovir following the oral administration of a single 500 mg dose of famciclovir was 27.7 L/hr.

The plasma elimination half-life of penciclovir was 2 hours after IV administration of penciclovir and 2.3 hours after oral administration of 500 mg famciclovir. The half-life in seven patients with herpes zoster was 3 hours.

Renal insufficiency: Apparent plasma clearance, renal clearance and the plasma-elimination rate constant of penciclovir decreased linearly with reductions in renal function. After the administration of a single 500 mg famciclovir oral dose to healthy volunteers and to volunteers with varying degrees of renal insufficiency, the following results were obtained.

Pharmacokinetics of Famciclovir in Patients with Renal Function Impairment

Parameter (mean)	CL_{CR}[1] ≥ 60 (ml/min; n = 15)	CL_{CR} 40-59 (ml/min; n = 5)	CL_{CR} 20-39 (ml/min; n = 4)	CL_{CR} < 20 (ml/min; n = 3)
CL_{CR} (ml/min)	88.1	49.3	26.5	12.7
CL_R (L/hr)	30.1	13[2]	4.2	1.6
CL/F[3] (L/hr)	66.9	27.3	12.8	5.8
Half-life (hr)	2.3	3.4	6.2	13.4

[1] CL_{CR} is measured creatinine clearance.
[2] n = 4.
[3] CL/F consists of bioavailability factor and famciclovir to penciclovir conversion factor.

A dosage adjustment is recommended for patients with renal insufficiency (see Administration and Dosage).

Hepatic insufficiency: Well compensated chronic liver disease (chronic hepatitis, chronic ethanol abuse or primary biliary cirrhosis) had no effect on the extent of availability (AUC) of penciclovir following a single dose of 500 mg famciclovir. However, there was a 44% decrease in penciclovir mean maximum plasma concentration and the time to maximum plasma concentration was increased by 0.75 hours in patients with hepatic insufficiency compared to normal volunteers. No dosage adjustment is recommended for patients with well compensated hepatic impairment. The pharmacokinetics of penciclovir have not been evaluated in patients with severe uncompensated hepatic impairment.

Elderly subjects: Based on cross-study comparisons, mean penciclovir AUC was 40% larger and penciclovir renal clearance was 22% lower after the oral administration of famciclovir in elderly volunteers (ages 65 to 79 years) compared to younger volunteers. Some of this difference may be due to differences in renal function between the two groups.

Microbiology: In cell culture studies, penciclovir has antiviral activity against the herpes viruses HSV-1, HSV-2 and VZV. Penciclovir-resistant mutants of HSV and VZV can result from qualitative changes in viral thymidine kinase or DNA polymerase. The most commonly encountered acyclovir-resistant mutants that are deficient in viral thymidine kinase are also resistant to penciclovir. The possibility of viral resistance to penciclovir should be considered in patients who show poor clinical response during therapy.

Clinical trials:

Herpes zoster – Famciclovir was studied in a placebo controlled, double-blind trial of 419 otherwise healthy patients with uncomplicated herpes zoster who were treated with famciclovir 500 mg three times daily, famciclovir 750 mg three times daily or placebo. Treatment was begun within 72 hours of initial lesion appearance and therapy was continued for 7 days. The times to full crusting, loss of vesicles, loss of ulcers and loss of crusts were shorter for famciclovir (500 mg) treated patients than for placebo treated patients in the overall study population. The median time to full crusting in famciclovir (500 mg) treated patients was 5 days compared with 7 days in placebo treated patients. No additional efficacy was demonstrated with the higher dose of famciclovir (750 mg three times daily), when compared with famciclovir 500 mg three times daily. In the total population, 65.2% of patients had a positive viral culture at some time during their acute infection. Patients treated with famciclovir 500 mg had a shorter median duration of viral shedding (time to last positive viral culture) than did placebo treated patients (1 day and 2 days, respectively).

There were no overall differences in the duration of acute pain (eg, pain before rash healing) between famciclovir and placebo treated groups. In addition, there was no difference in the incidence of postherpetic neuralgia (eg, pain after rash healing) between the treatment groups. In the 186 patients (44.4% of total study population) who did develop postherpetic neuralgia, the median duration of postherpetic neuralgia was shorter in patients treated with famciclovir 500 mg than in those treated with placebo (63 days and 119 days, respectively).

A second double-blind controlled trial in 545 otherwise healthy patients with uncomplicated herpes zoster treated within 72 hours of initial lesion appearance compared famciclovir 250 mg three times daily, famciclovir 500 mg three times daily, famciclovir 750 mg three times daily and acyclovir 800 mg five times daily for 7 days. Patients treated with famciclovir and acyclovir had comparable times to full lesion crusting and times to loss of acute pain. There were no statistically significant differences in the time to loss of postherpetic neuralgia between famciclovir and acyclovir treated groups.

Genital herpes infections – In two placebo controlled trials, 626 otherwise healthy patients with a recurrence of genital herpes were treated with famciclovir 125 mg twice daily, famciclovir 250 mg twice daily, famciclovir 500 mg twice daily or placebo for 5 days. In the two studies combined, the median time to healing in famciclovir 125 mg treated patients was 4 days compared with 5 days in placebo treated patients and the median time to cessation of viral shedding was 1.8 vs 3.4 days in famciclovir 125 mg and placebo recipients, respectively. The median time to loss of all symptoms was 3.2 days in famciclovir (125 mg) treated patients vs 3.8 days in placebo treated patients. When used to treat acute recurrent genital herpes, no additional efficacy was demonstrated with higher doses of famciclovir when compared with famciclovir 125 mg twice daily.

FAMCICLOVIR

Indications:

Acute herpes zoster: Management of acute herpes zoster (shingles).

Genital herpes: Treatment of recurrent episodes of genital herpes.

Contraindications:

Hypersensitivity to famciclovir.

Warnings:

Renal function impairment: Dosage adjustment is recommended when administering famciclovir to patients with creatinine clearance values < 60 ml/min. (see Administration and Dosage).

Carcinogenesis/Mutagenesis/Fertility impairment: A significant increase in the incidence of mammary adenocarcinoma was seen in female rats receiving 600 mg/kg/day. Marginal increases in the incidence of subcutaneous tissue fibrosarcomas or squamous cell carcinomas of the skin were seen in female rats (dosed at 600 mg/kg/day) and male mice (dosed at 600 mg/kg/day). No increases in tumor incidence were reported for male rats treated at doses up to 240 mg/kg/day or in female mice at doses up to 600 mg/kg/day.

Famciclovir induced increases in polyploidy in human lymphocytes in vitro in the absence of chromosomal damage (1200 mcg/ml). Penciclovir was positive in the L5178Y mouse lymphoma assay for gene mutation/chromosomal aberrations. In human lymphocytes, penciclovir caused chromosomal aberrations in the absence of metabolic activation (250 mcg/ml). Penciclovir caused an increased incidence of micronuclei in mouse bone marrow in vivo when administered IV at doses highly toxic to bone marrow (500 mg/kg), but not when administered orally.

Testicular toxicity was observed in rats, mice and dogs following repeated administration of famciclovir or penciclovir. Famciclovir had no effect on general reproductive performance or fertility in female rats at doses up to 1000 mg/kg/day.

Elderly: The effect on rash resolution was more pronounced in patients ≥ 50 years of age.

Pregnancy: Category B. There are no adequate and well controlled studies in pregnant women. Use during pregnancy only if the benefit to the patient clearly exceeds the potential risk to the fetus.

Lactation: It is not known whether famciclovir is excreted in breast milk. Because of the potential for tumorigenicity shown for famciclovir in rats, decide whether to discontinue nursing or to discontinue the drug, taking into account the importance of the drug to the mother.

Children: Safety and efficacy in children < 18 years of age have not been established.

FAMCICLOVIR

Drug Interactions:

The conversion of 6–deoxy penciclovir to penciclovir is catalyzed by aldehyde oxidase. Interactions with other drugs metabolized by this enzyme could potentially occur.

Drug Interactions			
Precipitant drug	Object drug*		Description
Cimetidine	Famciclovir	↑	Penciclovir AUC and urinary recovery increased 18% and 12%, respectively, in 12 healthy volunteers following the administration of a single 500 mg famciclovir dose after pretreatment with cimetidine 400 mg twice daily for 7 days. The magnitude of this effect is considered to be of no clinical importance.
Probenecid	Famciclovir	↑	Concurrent use with probenecid or other drugs significantly eliminated by active renal tubular secretion may result in increased plasma concentrations of penciclovir.
Theophylline	Famciclovir	↑	Penciclovir AUC and C_{max} increased 22% and 26%, respectively, following a single oral dose of 500 mg famciclovir in 12 healthy volunteers who were pretreated with theophylline 300 mg twice daily for 7 days. Renal clearance of penciclovir decreased by 12%. The magnitude of this effect is considered to be of no clinical importance.
Famciclovir	Digoxin	↑	After single-dose administration of digoxin and famciclovir in 12 healthy male volunteers, the C_{max} of digoxin increased 19% as compared with digoxin administered alone.

* ↑ = Object drug increased.

Drug/Food interactions: When famciclovir was administered with food, penciclovir C_{max} decreased ≈ 50%. Because the systemic availability of penciclovir (AUC) was not altered, it appears that famciclovir may be taken without regard to meals.

Adverse Reactions:

The most frequent adverse events associated with famciclovir were headache and nausea.

Famciclovir Adverse Reactions (%)				
	Herpes zoster		Genital herpes	
Adverse reaction	Famciclovir (n = 273)	Placebo (n = 146)	Famciclovir (n = 640)	Placebo (n = 225)
CNS				
Headache	22.7	17.8	23.6	16.4
Dizziness	3.3	4.1	5.5	4.9
Insomnia	1.5	1.4	2.5	2.2
Somnolence	2.6	2.7	1.6	0.4
Paresthesia	2.6	0	1.3	0
GI				
Nausea	12.5	11.6	10	8
Diarrhea	7.7	4.8	4.5	7.6
Abdominal pain	1.1	3.4	3.9	5.8
Dyspepsia	1.1	1.4	3.4	2.2
Flatulence	1.5	0.7	1.9	2.2
Constipation	4.4	4.8	1.4	0.9
Vomiting	4.8	3.4	1.3	0.9
Anorexia	2.6	4.1	1.1	0.9

Famciclovir Adverse Reactions (%)				
	Herpes zoster		Genital herpes	
Adverse reaction	Famciclovir (n = 273)	Placebo (n = 146)	Famciclovir (n = 640)	Placebo (n = 225)
Body as a whole				
Fatigue	4.4	3.4	6.3	4.4
Pain	2.6	2.7	2	1.8
Injury	2.6	0	0.8	1.3
Fever	3.3	4.1	0.8	0.4
Rigors	1.5	2.7	0.5	0.4
Respiratory				
URI	0.7	0.7	3.3	2.7
Pharyngitis	2.6	4.8	2.7	2.2
Sinusitis	2.6	1.4	1.3	1.3
Musculoskeletal				
Back pain	1.5	2.7	1.9	2.2
Arthralgia	1.5	2.1	1.3	0
Dermatologic				
Pruritus	3.7	2.7	0.9	0
Zoster/Genital herpes-related signs/symptoms/complications	2.9	3.4	1.7	2.2

Confusion (including delirium, disorientation, confusional state) has been reported very rarely. Most of these spontaneous reports have occurred in the elderly.

Overdosage:

No acute overdosage has been reported. Give appropriate symptomatic and supportive therapy. Penciclovir is removed by hemodialysis.

Patient Information:

May be taken without regard to meals.

Herpes zoster: Begin medication as soon as herpes zoster is diagnosed.

Genital herpes: Inform patients that famciclovir is not a cure for genital herpes. There are no data evaluating whether famciclovir will prevent transmission of infection to others. As genital herpes is a sexually transmitted disease, patients should avoid contact with lesions or avoid intercourse when lesions or symptoms are present to avoid infecting partners. Genital herpes can also be transmitted in the absence of symptoms through asymptomatic viral shedding.

Begin medication at the first sign or symptom (eg, pain, tenderness, burning, itching, tingling, vesicles, ulcers or crusts) if medical management of genital herpes recurrence is indicated. The effectiveness of famciclovir has not been established when treatment is started more than 6 hours after onset of symptoms or lesions.

FAMCICLOVIR

Administration and Dosage:

Approved by the FDA on June 29, 1994 (1S classification).

Herpes zoster: The recommended dosage is 500 mg every 8 hours for 7 days. Therapy should be initiated promptly as soon as herpes zoster is diagnosed.

Genital herpes (recurrent episodes): The recommended dosage is 125 mg twice daily for 5 days. Initiate therapy at the first sign or symptom if medical management of a genital herpes recurrence is indicated.

Famciclovir Dosage in Renal Function Impairment

Creatinine clearance (ml/min)	Dose regimen
Herpes zoster	
≥ 60	500 mg every 8 hours
40 to 59	500 mg every 12 hours
20 to 39	500 mg every 24 hours
< 20	250 mg every 48 hours
Recurrent genital herpes	
≥40	125 mg every 12 hours
20 to 39	125 mg every 24 hours
< 20	125 mg every 48 hours

Hemodialysis patients: The recommended dose of famciclovir is 250 mg (herpes zoster) or 125 mg (genital herpes) administered following each dialysis treatment.

Rx	**Famvir** (SmithKline Beecham)	**Tablets:** 125 mg	Lactose. (Famvir 125). White. Film coated. In 30s and UD 100s.
		250 mg	Lactose. (Famvir 250). White. Film coated. In 30s.
		500 mg	Lactose. (Famvir 500). White. Oval. Film coated. In 30s and UD 50s.

STAVUDINE (d4T)

> **Warning:**
>
> Stavudine is indicated for the treatment of adults with advanced HIV infection who are intolerant of approved therapies with proven clinical benefit or who have experienced significant clinical or immunologic deterioration while receiving these therapies or for whom such therapies are contraindicated. At present, there are no results from controlled trials evaluating the effect of stavudine therapy on the clinical progression of HIV infection, such as the incidence of opportunistic infections or survival. Because therapy with zidovudine prolongs survival in patients with advanced HIV disease, consider zidovudine initial therapy for the treatment of HIV infection.
>
> The major clinical toxicity of stavudine is peripheral neuropathy. This occurred in 15% to 21% of patients in the controlled trials.
>
> Patients receiving stavudine or any other antiretroviral therapy may continue to develop opportunistic infections and other complications of HIV infection and, therefore, should remain under close clinical observation by physicians experienced in the treatment of patients with HIV-associated diseases.

Actions:

Pharmacology: Stavudine is a synthetic thymidine nucleoside analog active against the human immunodeficiency virus (HIV). It inhibits the replication of HIV in human cells in vitro. Stavudine is phosphorylated by cellular kinases to stavudine triphosphate which exerts antiviral activity. Stavudine triphosphate has an intracellular half-life of 3.5 hours in CEM and peripheral blood mononuclear cells. Stavudine triphosphate inhibits HIV replication by two known mechanisms: 1) It inhibits HIV reverse transcriptase by competing with the natural substrate deoxythymidine triphosphate; and 2) it inhibits viral DNA synthesis by causing DNA chain termination because stavudine lacks the 3′-hydroxyl group necessary for DNA elongation. Stavudine triphosphate also inhibits cellular DNA polymerase beta and gamma, and markedly reduces mitochondrial DNA synthesis.

Pharmacokinetics:

Adults –

Absorption: Following oral administration to HIV-infected patients, stavudine is rapidly absorbed with a mean absolute bioavailability of 86.4%. Peak plasma concentrations (C_{max}) increased in a dose-related manner for doses ranging from 0.03 to 4 mg/kg and occurred ≤ 1 hour after dosing. Area under the plasma concentration-time curve (AUC) increased in proportion to dose after both single and multiple doses. There was no significant accumulation with repeated administration every 6, 8 or 12 hours. When stavudine (70 mg) was administered to 16 asymptomatic HIV-infected patients under fasting conditions, 1 hour before a standardized high-fat meal (773 Kcal, 53% fat) or immediately after the meal, systemic exposure (AUC) was similar. Mean C_{max} of stavudine was reduced from 1.44 mcg/ml in the fasting state to 0.75 mcg/ml after the meal, and the median time to reach C_{max} was prolonged from 0.6 to 1.5 hours.

Distribution: Following 1 hour IV infusions of 0.0625 to 1 mg/kg, mean volume of distribution (Vd) was 58 L, suggesting that stavudine distributes into extravascular spaces. Mean apparent Vd following single oral doses ranging from 0.03 to 4 mg/kg was 66 L. In three patients who received oral doses of 1.3, 3 or 4 mg/kg, stavudine was measured in CSF samples at concentrations of 0.08, 0.2 and 0.48 mcg/ml at 0.5, 1.75 and 5 hours post-dose, respectively. Binding to serum proteins was negligible. Stavudine distributes equally between red blood cells and plasma.

Metabolism: After incubation of [^{14}C]-stavudine for 6 hours with human liver slices, 87% of radioactivity was accounted for by parent drug, 2% was metabolized to thymine and 7% was associated with unidentified polar compounds.

Excretion: Plasma clearance and terminal elimination half-life were independent of dose over an IV dosing range of 0.0625 to 1 mg/kg and an oral dosing range of 0.03 to 4 mg/kg. Following 1 hour infusions, plasma concentrations declined in a biphasic manner with a mean terminal elimination half-life of 1.15 hours. After single oral doses, the mean terminal elimination half-life was 1.44 hours. Mean total body clearance, after IV infusion, was 594 ml/min and was independent of dose and body weight. Following single-dose oral administration, mean apparent oral clearance was independent of dose, having a value of 559 ml/min. Renal elimination accounted for about 40% of the overall clearance regardless of the route of administration; there is active tubular secretion in addition to glomerular filtration. Mean cumulative urinary excretion of unchanged drug over 6 to 24 hours after administration of an oral dose was 39% of the dose.

STAVUDINE (d4T)

Children –

Absorption: Stavudine was rapidly absorbed following oral administration to HIV-infected children with a mean absolute bioavailability of 78.5% and 69.2% for capsules and solution, respectively. First-dose and multiple-dose (after 152 weeks of treatment) pharmacokinetic profiles were similar, indicating no accumulation.

Distribution: Following IV infusions of 0.125 to 2 mg/kg, mean Vd was 13.2 L, suggesting that stavudine distributes into extravascular spaces. After 12 weeks of treatment, the stavudine concentration in CSF samples from 7 patients ranged from 0.01 to 0.12 mcg/ml at times ranging from 2 to 3 hours post-dose. CSF concentrations corresponded to 16% to 97% of the level in simultaneous plasma samples.

Elimination: Plasma concentrations declined with a mean terminal elimination half-life of 1.09 hours following the end of a 1-hour infusion. After a single oral dose, mean terminal half-life was 0.91 hours. Mean total body clearance after IV infusion was 181.13 ml/min. Mean apparent oral clearance after administration of solution (n = 10; age < 6 years) and capsule (n = 8; age > 6 years) formulations was 16.45 and 11.01 ml/min/kg, respectively.

Renal insufficiency – The apparent oral clearance of stavudine decreased as creatinine clearance (Ccr) decreased. The terminal elimination half-life was prolonged up to 8 hours. C_{max} and T_{max} were not significantly affected by reduced renal function. Based on these preliminary observations, it is recommended that stavudine dosage be modified in patients with reduced Ccr (see Administration and Dosage).

Microbiology: The relationship between in vitro susceptibility of HIV to stavudine and the inhibition of HIV replication in humans or clinical response to therapy has not been established.

The development of resistance to stavudine was studied using HIV-1 isolates obtained from 13 patients treated with stavudine for 18 to 22 months. Ten of the 13 patients had been treated with zidovudine before stavudine and 3 patients were reported to be zidovudine-naive. Drug sensitivity testing indicated that 3 of the 11 post-treatment isolates displayed 4- to 12-fold decreases in their sensitivity to stavudine; five became resistant to zidovudine and three were resistant to didanosine. A stavudine-resistant HIV-1 isolate from one patient was cross-resistant to both zidovudine and didanosine. Of the other two isolates, one was cross-resistant to zidovudine, and the other to didanosine.

Analysis of clinical isolates identified multiple mutations in the reverse transcriptase gene. Mutations that confer resistance to zidovudine were observed in 7 of the 13 isolates from patients after stavudine treatment, and correlated with the observed zidovudine-resistant phenotype.

Clinical trials: In a multi-center, randomized, double-blind trial of stavudine (40 mg twice daily for patients weighing ≥ 60 kg, and 30 mg twice daily for those weighing < 60 kg) vs continued zidovudine (200 mg 3 times/day) in HIV-infected adults who had received at least 24 weeks of prior zidovudine treatment, the mean change from baseline in CD4 cell counts at 12 weeks was +22 cells/mm^3 (range, -185 to +375 cells/mm^3) in patients taking stavudine. At 12 weeks, the mean change in CD4 cell counts from baseline among patients who were continued on zidovudine was -22 cells/mm^3 (range, -215 to +430 cells/mm^3).

Indications:

HIV infection: Treatment of adults with advanced HIV infection who are intolerant of approved therapies with proven clinical benefit or who have experienced significant clinical or immunologic deterioration while receiving these therapies or for whom such therapies are contraindicated.

Contraindications:

Hypersensitivity to stavudine or to any components of the formulation.

Warnings:

Progression of HIV: At present, there are no results from controlled trials evaluating the effect of stavudine therapy on the clinical progression of HIV infection, such as the incidence of opportunistic infections or survival.

Initial therapy for HIV: Because therapy with zidovudine prolongs survival in patients with advanced HIV disease, consider zidovudine initial therapy for treating HIV.

Peripheral neuropathy: The major clinical toxicity of stavudine is peripheral neuropathy. This occurred in 15% to 21% of patients in controlled trials. Monitor patients for development of neuropathy, usually characterized by numbness, tingling or pain in feet or hands. Stavudine-related peripheral neuropathy may resolve if therapy is withdrawn promptly. Symptoms may worsen temporarily following therapy discontinuation. If symptoms resolve completely, resumption of treatment may be considered at a reduced dose (see Administration and Dosage). Patients with a history of peripheral neuropathy are at increased risk for developing neuropathy. If stavudine must be given in this clinical setting, careful monitoring is essential.

STAVUDINE (d4T)

Pancreatitis was reported in 1% of patients enrolled in controlled clinical trials and was associated with 14 deaths, five of which were attributed to drug toxicity.

Mutagenesis: Stavudine produced positive results in the in vitro human lymphocyte clastogenesis and mouse fibroblast assays, and in the in vivo mouse micronucleus test. In the in vitro assays, stavudine elevated the frequency of chromosome aberrations in human lymphocytes and increased the frequency of transformed foci in mouse fibroblast cells. In the in vivo micronucleus assay, stavudine was clastogenic in bone marrow cells following oral stavudine administration to mice at dosages of 600 to 2000 mg/kg/day for 3 days.

Pregnancy: Category C. In rat fetuses, the incidence of a common skeletal variation, unossified or incomplete ossification of sternebra, was increased at 399 times human exposure. A slight post-implantation loss was noted at 216 times the human exposure. An increase in early rat neonatal mortality (birth to 4 days of age) occurred at 399 times the human exposure. A study in rats showed that stavudine is transferred to the fetus through the placenta. The concentration in fetal tissue was approximately one-half that in maternal plasma. There are no adequate and well controlled studies in pregnant women. Use during pregnancy only if clearly needed.

Lactation: Studies in which lactating rats were administered a single dose (5 or 100 mg/kg) of stavudine demonstrated that the drug is readily excreted into breast milk. It is not known whether stavudine is excreted in human breast milk. Because of the potential for adverse reactions from stavudine in nursing infants, instruct mothers to discontinue nursing if they are receiving stavudine.

Children: Safety and efficacy of stavudine for treatment of HIV in children have not been established. Limited data are available from 37 children aged 5 months to 15 years who received stavudine in doses ranging from 0.125 to 4 mg/kg/day for a median duration of 37 weeks (range, 8 to 75 weeks). Serious adverse events that have been observed include AST and ALT elevations and one case of neuropathy.

Precautions:

Laboratory tests: Mild to moderate increases in AST and ALT occurred commonly in clinical trials, and tended to resolve following interruption of therapy (see Administration and Dosage).

Drug Interactions:

Drug/Food interactions: C_{max} of stavudine was decreased by ≈ 45% when administered with food; however, systemic availability (AUC) was unchanged.

Adverse Reactions:

The major clinical toxicity is peripheral neuropathy, which is dose-related (see Warnings). This toxicity In Phase I trials, peripheral neuropathy occurred in 29%, 19%, 53%, 70%, 67% and 64% of patients at doses of 0.5, 1, 2, 4, 8 and 12 mg/kg/day, respectively. Modest elevation of hepatic transaminases was commonly seen in controlled trials.

Adverse events that occurred in > 1% of adult patients receiving stavudine in the Phase III controlled comparative trial and in the Parallel Track Program are provided in the following table.

Stavudine Adverse Reactions (%)

Adverse reaction	Phase III		Parallel Track Program	
	Stavudine (40 mg bid) (n = 172)	Zidovudine (200 mg tid) (n = 185)	Stavudine (40 mg bid) (n = 4623)	Stavudine (20 mg bid) (n = 4603)
Body as a whole				
Headache	55	52	3	3
Chills/Fever	38	49	5	6
Asthenia	28	36	2	2
Abdominal pain	26	27	4	5
Back pain	20	17	< 1	< 1
Pain	18	21	3	2
Malaise	17	17	1	2
Weight loss	10	11	< 1	< 1
Allergic reaction	9	7	< 1	< 1
Flu syndrome	9	6	<1	< 1
Lymphadenopathy	5	4	< 1	< 1
Pelvic pain	2	2	0	< 1
Neoplasms	2	1	4	4
Death	< 1	0	5	5

Stavudine Adverse Reactions (%)

Adverse reaction	Phase III Stavudine (40 mg bid) (n = 172)	Phase III Zidovudine (200 mg tid) (n = 185)	Parallel Track Program Stavudine (40 mg bid) (n = 4623)	Parallel Track Program Stavudine (20 mg bid) (n = 4603)
Cardiovascular				
Chest pain	8	11	< 1	< 1
Vasodilation	3	1	< 1	< 1
Hypertension	2	3	< 1	< 1
Peripheral vascular disorder	2	< 1	< 1	< 1
Syncope	1	< 1	< 1	< 1
GI				
Diarrhea	50	47	4	5
Nausea/vomiting	35	46	6	6
Anorexia	10	21	< 1	< 1
Dyspepsia	9	15	< 1	< 1
Constipation	7	4	<1	< 1
Ulcerative stomatitis	3	6	< 1	< 1
Aphthous stomatitis	1	2	< 1	< 1
Pancreatitis	1	< 1	1	1
Musculoskeletal				
Myalgia	35	36	2	1
Arthralgia	19	19	< 1	< 1
CNS				
Other peripheral neurologic symptoms	40	36	5	6
Insomnia	26	34	1	1
Anxiety	22	17	< 1	< 1
Neuropathy	15	6	21	15
Depression	14	21	< 1	< 1
Nervousness	10	11	< 1	< 1
Dizziness	9	8	< 1	< 1
Confusion	3	2	< 1	< 1
Migraine	3	< 1	< 1	0
Somnolence	2	< 1	< 1	< 1
Tremor	2	0	< 1	< 1
Neuralgia	1	0	< 1	< 1
Dementia	0	0	1	2
Respiratory				
Dyspnea	13	10	< 1	1
Pneumonia	3	2	4	5
Asthma	2	1	< 1	< 1
Dermatologic				
Rash	33	32	3	3
Sweating	19	18	< 1	< 1
Pruritus	12	11	< 1	1
Maculopapular rash	6	6	< 1	< 1
Skin benign neoplasm	4	5	< 1	< 1
Urticaria	3	3	< 1	< 1
Exfoliative dermatitis	1	< 1	0	< 1
Special senses				
Conjunctivitis	5	2	< 1	< 1
Abnormal vision	3	8	< 1	< 1

Stavudine Adverse Reactions (%)				
	Phase III		Parallel Track Program	
Adverse reaction	Stavudine (40 mg bid) (n = 172)	Zidovudine (200 mg tid) (n = 185)	Stavudine (40 mg bid) (n = 4623)	Stavudine (20 mg bid) (n = 4603)
GU				
Dysuria	3	1	< 1	< 1
Genital pain	2	1	0	0
Dysmenorrhea	2	0	0	0
Vaginitis	2	0	0	0
Urinary frequency	1	2	< 1	< 1
Hematuria	1	< 1	< 1	< 1
Impotence	1	< 1	< 1	< 1
Neoplasm urogenital	1	< 1	0	0

Stavudine Lab Test Abnormalities				
	Phase III Study		Parallel Track Program	
Lab tests	Stavudine (40 mg bid) (n = 172)	Zidovudine (200 mg tid) (n = 185)	Stavudine (40 mg bid) (n = 4623)	Stavudine (40 mg bid) (n = 4603)
AST (> 5 × ULN[1])	8	13	5	5
ALT (> 5 × ULN)	12	13	10	9
Alkaline phosphatase (> 5 × ULN)	1	0	4	4
Bilirubin (> 2.5 × ULN)	1	3	na[2]	na[2]
Anemia (< 8 g/dl)	0	2	3	3
Leukopenia (WBC < 1000/mm^3)	0	0	1	1
Neutropenia (neutrophils < 750/mm^3)	3	8	11	12
Thrombocytopenia (platelets < 50,000/mm^3)	1	2	4	4
Amylase (> 1.4 × ULN)	9	10	na[2]	na[2]

[1] ULN = upper limit of normal.
[2] na = Not applicable.

Overdosage:

Experience with adults treated with 12 to 24 times the recommended daily dosage revealed no acute toxicity. Complications of chronic overdosage include peripheral neuropathy and hepatic toxicity. It is not known whether stavudine is eliminated by peritoneal dialysis or hemodialysis.

Patient Information:

Inform patients that stavudine is not a cure for HIV infection, and that they may continue to acquire illnesses associated with AIDS or ARC, including opportunistic infections. Stavudine has not been shown to reduce the incidence or frequency of such illnesses; advise patients to remain under a physician's care when using stavudine.

Inform patients that the most common toxicity of stavudine is peripheral neuropathy. Symptoms include tingling, burning, pain or numbness in the hands or feet. Counsel patients that this toxicity occurs with greater frequency in patients with a history of peripheral neuropathy. Advise them to report these symptoms to their physician and that dose changes may be necessary. They should also be cautioned about the use of other medications that may exacerbate peripheral neuropathy.

Tell patients that the long-term effects of stavudine are unknown at this time. Advise them that stavudine therapy has not been shown to reduce the risk of transmission of HIV to others through sexual contact or blood contamination.

STAVUDINE (d4T)

Administration and Dosage:

Approved by the FDA on June 24, 1994.

Adults: The interval between oral doses should be 12 hours. C_{max} was decreased by ≈ 45% when stavudine was administered with food; however, the systemic availability (AUC) was unchanged. Thus, it appears that stavudine may be taken without regard to meals. The recommended starting dose based on body weight is as follows:

Patients ≥ 60 kg – 40 mg twice daily.
Patients < 60 kg – 30 mg twice daily.

Dosage adjustment: Monitor patients for the development of peripheral neuropathy which is usually characterized by numbness, tingling or pain in the feet or hands. If these symptoms develop, interrupt stavudine therapy. Symptoms may resolve if therapy is withdrawn promptly. In some cases, symptoms may worsen temporarily following discontinuation of therapy. If symptoms resolve completely, resumption of treatment may be considered using the following dosage schedule:

Patients ≥ 60 kg – 20 mg twice daily.
Patients < 60 kg – 15 mg twice daily.

Manage clinically significant elevations of hepatic transaminases in the same way.

Renal function impairment – Stavudine may be administered to adult patients with impaired renal function. The following schedule is recommended:

Stavudine Dosage in Renal Function Impairment

Creatinine clearance (ml/min)	Recommended stavudine dose by patient weight	
	≥ 60 kg	< 60 kg
> 50	40 mg every 12 hours	30 mg every 12 hours
26 - 50	20 mg every 12 hours	15 mg every 12 hours
10 - 25	20 mg every 24 hours	15 mg every 24 hours

There are insufficient data to recommend a dose for patients with Ccr < 10 ml/min or for patients undergoing dialysis.

Rx	**Zerit** (B-M Squibb)	**Capsules:** 15 mg	Lactose. (BMS 1964 15). Lt. yellow/dark red. In 60s.
		20 mg	Lactose. (BMS 1965 20). Lt. brown. In 60s.
		30 mg	Lactose. (BMS 1966 30). Lt. orange/dark orange. In 60s.
		40 mg	Lactose. (BMS 1967 40). Dark orange. In 60s.
Rx	**Zerit** (B-M Squibb)	**Powder for oral solution:** 1 mg/ml	Sucrose, parabens. Dye-free. Fruit flavored. In 200s.

VALACYCLOVIR HCl

Actions:

Pharmacology: Valacyclovir is the hydrochloride salt of L-valyl ester of the antiviral drug acyclovir. Valacyclovir is rapidly converted to acyclovir, which has in vitro and in vivo inhibitory activity against herpes simplex virus types I (HSV-1) and II (HSV-2) and varicella-zoster virus (VZV). In cell culture, acyclovir has the highest antiviral activity against HSV-1, followed by (in decreasing order of potency) HSV-2 and VZV.

The inhibitory activity of acyclovir is highly selective due to its affinity for the enzyme thymidine kinase (TK). This viral enzyme converts acyclovir into acyclovir monophosphate, a nucleotide analog. The monophosphate is further converted into diphosphate by cellular guanylate kinase and into triphosphate by a number of cellular enzymes. In vitro, acyclovir triphosphate stops replication of herpes viral DNA in three ways: 1) Competitive inhibition of viral DNA polymerase, 2) incorporation and termination of the growing viral DNA chain and 3) inactivation of the viral DNA polymerase. The greater antiviral activity of acyclovir against HSV compared with VZV is due to its more efficient phosphorylation by the viral TK.

Pharmacokinetics:

Absorption/Distribution – After oral administration, valacyclovir is rapidly absorbed from the GI tract and is rapidly and nearly completely converted to acyclovir and L-valine by first-pass intestinal or hepatic metabolism.

Absolute bioavailability of acyclovir after valacyclovir administration is 54.5%. Acyclovir bioavailability from valacyclovir administration is not altered by administration with food (30 minutes after an 873 Kcal breakfast, including 51 g of fat).

VALACYCLOVIR HCl

There was a lack of dose proportionality in acyclovir maximum concentration (C_{max}) and area under the acyclovir concentration-time curve (AUC) after single-dose administration of 100, 250, 500, 750 and 1000 mg valacyclovir to eight healthy volunteers. The mean C_{max} was 0.83, 2.15, 3.28, 4.17 and 5.65 mcg/ml, respectively, and the mean AUC was 2.28, 5.76, 11.59, 14.11 and 19.52 hr•mcg/ml, respectively. There was also a lack of dose proportionality in acyclovir C_{max} and AUC after the multiple-dose administration of 250, 500 and 1000 mg of valacyclovir 4 times daily for 11 days in parallel groups of eight healthy volunteers. The mean C_{max} was 2.11, 3.69 and 4.96 mcg/ml, respectively, and the mean AUC was 5.66, 9.88 and 15.7 hr•mcg/ml, respectively.

The binding of valacyclovir to human plasma proteins ranged from 13.5% to 17.9%.

Metabolism – Valacyclovir is rapidly and nearly completely converted to acyclovir and L-valine by first-pass intestinal metabolism, hepatic metabolism or both. Acyclovir is converted to a small extent to inactive metabolites by aldehyde oxidase and by alcohol and aldehyde dehydrogenase. Neither valacyclovir nor acyclovir metabolism is associated with liver microsomal enzymes. Plasma concentrations of unconverted valacyclovir are low and transient, generally becoming non-quantifiable by 3 hours after administration. Peak plasma valacyclovir concentrations are generally < 0.5 mcg/ml at all doses. After single-dose administration of 1 g, average plasma valacyclovir concentrations were 0.5, 0.4 and 0.8 mcg/ml in patients with hepatic dysfunction, renal insufficiency and in healthy volunteers who received concomitant cimetidine and probenecid, respectively.

Excretion – The pharmacokinetic disposition of acyclovir from valacyclovir is consistent with previous experience from IV and oral acyclovir. Following the oral administration of a single 1 g valacyclovir dose to four healthy subjects, 45.6% and 47.12% was recovered in urine and feces over 96 hours, respectively. Acyclovir accounted for 88.6% excreted in the urine. Renal clearance of acyclovir following the administration of a single 1 g valacyclovir dose to 12 healthy volunteers was ≈ 255 ml/min, which represents 41.9% of total acyclovir apparent plasma clearance.

The plasma elimination half-life of acyclovir typically averaged 2.5 to 3.3 hours in volunteers with normal renal function.

End-stage renal disease (ESRD): Following administration of valacyclovir to volunteers with ESRD, the average acyclovir half-life is ≈ 14 hours. During hemodialysis, the acyclovir half-life is ≈ 4 hours. Approximately 33% of acyclovir is removed by dialysis during a 4 hour hemodialysis session. Apparent plasma clearance of acyclovir in dialysis patients and healthy volunteers was 86.3 ml/min/1.73 m^2 and 679.16 ml/min/1.73 m^2, respectively. A dosage reduction is recommended in patients with estimated creatinine clearances < 50 ml/min (see Administration and Dosage).

Elderly: After single-dose administration of 1 g valacyclovir in healthy geriatric volunteers (mean age, 74 years), the half-life of acyclovir was 3.11 hours compared with 2.91 hours in healthy volunteers (mean age, 41.2 years). Dosage modification may be necessary in geriatric patients with reduced renal function (see Administration and Dosage).

Hepatic function impairment: Administration of valacyclovir to patients with moderate (biopsy-proven cirrhosis) or severe (with and without ascites and biopsy-proven cirrhosis) liver disease indicated that the rate but not the extent of conversion of valacyclovir to acyclovir was reduced, and the acyclovir half-life was not affected. Dosage modification is not recommended for patients with cirrhosis.

HIV infection: In nine patients with advanced HIV infection (CD4 cell counts < 50 cells/mm^3) who received valacyclovir at a dosage of 1 g 4 times daily for 30 days, the pharmacokinetics of valacyclovir and acyclovir were not different from that observed in healthy volunteers.

Clinical trials:

Herpes zoster – Two randomized double-blind clinical trials in immunocompetent patients with localized herpes zoster were conducted. Valacyclovir was compared with placebo in patients < 50 years of age, and with acyclovir in patients > 50 years of age. All patients were treated within 72 hours of appearance of zoster rash. In patients < 50 years of age, the median time to cessation of new lesion formation was 2 days for those treated with valacyclovir vs 3 days with placebo. In patients > 50 years of age, the median time to cessation of new lesions was 3 days in patients treated with either valacyclovir or acyclovir. In patients < 50 years of age, no difference was found in the duration of pain after rash healing (post-herpetic neuralgia) between the recipients of valacyclovir and placebo. In patients > 50 years of age who reported pain after rash healing (post-herpetic neuralgia), there was a nonsignificant trend toward a shorter median duration of pain after healing in patients treated with valacyclovir for 7 or 14 days (40 or 43 days) compared with patients treated with acyclovir for 7 days (59 days).

VALACYCLOVIR HCl

Recurrent genital herpes – Two double-blind placebo controlled trials in immunocompetent patients with recurrent genital herpes were conducted. Patients self-initiated therapy within 24 hours of the first sign or symptom of a recurrent genital herpes episode. In one study, patients were randomized to receive 5 days of treatment with either 500 mg valacyclovir twice a day (n = 360) or placebo (n = 259). The median time to healing was 4 days in the valacyclovir group vs 6 days in the placebo group, and the median time to cessation of viral shedding in patients with at least 1 positive culture (42% of the overall study population) was 2 days in the valacyclovir group vs 4 days in the placebo group. The median time to cessation of pain was 3 days in the valacyclovir group vs 4 days in the placebo group.

Indications:

Herpes zoster: Treatment of herpes zoster (shingles) in immunocompetent adults.

Recurrent genital herpes: Episodic treatment of recurrent genital herpes in immunocompetent adults.

Contraindications:

Hypersensitivity or intolerance to valacyclovir, acyclovir or any component of the formulation.

Warnings:

Thrombotic thrombocytopenic purpura/hemolytic uremic syndrome (TTP/HUS), in some cases resulting in death, has been reported in patients with advanced HIV infection and in bone marrow and renal transplant recipients. Valacyclovir is not indicated for the treatment of immunocompromised patients. TTP/HUS has not been seen in immunocompetent patients receiving valacyclovir in clinical trials.

Renal function impairment: Exercise caution when giving valacyclovir to patients with renal impairment or those receiving potentially nephrotoxic agents as this may increase the risk of renal dysfunction or the risk of reversible CNS symptoms such as those that occur infrequently in patients treated with IV acyclovir. A dosage reduction may be recommended (see Administration and Dosage).

Elderly: The pharmacokinetics of acyclovir following single- and multiple-dose oral administration of valacyclovir in geriatric volunteers varied with renal function. Dosage reduction may be required in geriatric patients, depending on the underlying renal status of the patient (see Administration and Dosage).

Pregnancy: Category B. There are no adequate and well controlled studies of valacyclovir or acyclovir in pregnant women. As of December 1994, outcomes of live births have been documented in 380 women exposed to systemic acyclovir during the first trimester of pregnancy. The occurrence rate of birth defects approximates that found in the general population. However, the small size of the registry is insufficient to evaluate the risk for less common defects or to permit reliable and definitive conclusions regarding the safety of acyclovir in pregnant women and their developing fetuses. Use valacyclovir during pregnancy only if the potential benefit justifies the potential risk to the fetus.

Pregnancy exposure registry – To monitor maternal-fetal outcomes of pregnant women exposed to valacyclovir, Glaxo Wellcome maintains a Valacyclovir in Pregnancy Registry. Physicians are encouraged to register their patients by calling (800) 722-9292, ext. 58465.

Lactation: There is no experience with valacyclovir. However, acyclovir concentrations have been documented in breast milk in two women following oral administration of acyclovir and ranged from 0.6 to 4.1 times corresponding plasma levels. These concentrations would potentially expose the nursing infant to a dose of acyclovir as high as 0.3 mg/kg/day. Administer valacyclovir to a nursing mother with caution and only when indicated. Give consideration to temporary discontinuation of nursing, as the safety of valacyclovir has not been established in infants.

Children: Safety and efficacy have not been established.

Drug Interactions:

Cimetidine/Probenecid: Administration of these agents, separately or together, reduced the rate, but not the extent, of conversion of valacyclovir to acyclovir. The renal clearance of acyclovir was reduced. An additive increase in acyclovir AUC and C_{max} was observed when valacyclovir was administered to healthy volunteers who were taking cimetidine, probenecid or a combination of both.

VALACYCLOVIR HCl

Adverse Reactions:

Adverse Reactions: Valacyclovir vs Acyclovir or Placebo (%)						
	Herpes zoster				Genital herpes	
	≥ 50 Years of age		18 to 50 Years of age		18 to 79 Years of age	
Adverse reaction	Valacyclovir 1 g 3 x daily (n = 765)	Acyclovir 800 mg 5 x daily (n = 376)	Valacyclovir 1 g 3 x daily (n = 202)	Placebo (n = 195)	Valacyclovir 1 g 2 x daily (n = 1235)	Placebo (n = 439)
Nausea	16	19	10	8	8	8
Headache	13	13	17	12	17	14
Vomiting	7	8	4	3	< 1	< 1
Diarrhea	5	7	4	6	4	6
Constipation	5	5	1	3	< 1	< 1
Asthenia	4	5	3	4	2	4
Dizziness	4	6	2	2	3	3
Abdominal pain	3	3	2	2	2	3
Anorexia	3	3	< 1	2	< 1	< 1

Overdosage:

There have been no reports of overdosage with valacyclovir. However, it is known that precipitation of acyclovir in renal tubules may occur when the solubility (2.5 mg/ml) is exceeded in the intratubular fluid. In the event of acute renal failure and anuria, the patient may benefit from hemodialysis until renal function is restored.

Patient Information:

Herpes zoster: Advise patients to initiate treatment as soon as possible after a diagnosis of herpes zoster. There are no data on treatment initiated > 72 hours after onset.

Recurrent genital herpes: Tell patients to avoid contact with lesions and to avoid intercourse when lesions or symptoms are present to avoid infecting others. If medical management of herpes recurrence is indicated, advise patients to initiate therapy at the first sign or symptom of an episode.

Administration and Dosage:

Approved by the FDA on June 23, 1995 (1S classification).

Valacyclovir may be given without regard to meals.

Herpes zoster: The recommended dosage is 1 g 3 times daily for 7 days. Initiate therapy at the earliest sign or symptom of herpes zoster; it is most effective when started within 48 hours of the onset of zoster rash. No data are available on efficacy of treatment started > 72 hours after rash onset.

Recurrent genital herpes: The recommended dosage is 500 mg twice daily for 5 days. If medical management of a genital herpes recurrence is indicated, advise patients to initiate therapy at the first sign or symptom of an episode. There are no data on the efficacy of treatment started > 24 hours after the onset of signs or symptoms.

Acute or chronic renal impairment:

Valacyclovir Dosage Adjustments for Renal Impairment				
Creatinine clearance (ml/min)	Herpes zoster		Genital herpes	
	Dose	Frequency	Dose	Frequency
≥ 50	1 g	every 8 hours	500 mg	every 12 hours
30 to 49	1 g	every 12 hours	500 mg	every 12 hours
10 to 29	1 g	every 24 hours	500 mg	every 24 hours
< 10	500 mg	every 24 hours	500 mg	every 24 hours

Hemodialysis: During hemodialysis, the half-life of acyclovir after administration of valacyclovir is ≈ 4 hours. About 33% of acyclovir in the body is removed by dialysis during a 4 hour hemodialysis session. Patients requiring hemodialysis should receive the recommended dose of valacyclovir after hemodialysis.

Peritoneal dialysis: Supplemental doses of valacyclovir should not be required following chronic ambulatory peritoneal dialysis (CAPD) or continuous arteriovenous hemofiltration/hemodialysis (CAVHD).

Storage/Stability: Store at 15° to 25°C (59° to 77°F).

Rx	**Valtrex** (Glaxo Wellcome)	**Tablets:** 500 mg	Caplets. (Valtrex 500 mg). Blue. Film coated. In 42s and UD 100s.

RITONAVIR

> **Warning:**
> Coadministraiton of ritonavir with certain nonsedating antihistamines, sedative hypnotics or antiarrhythmics may result in potentially serious or life-threatening adverse events due to possible effects of ritonavir on the hepatic metabolism of certain drugs (see Contraindications and Drug Interactions).

Actions:

Pharmacology: Ritonavir is an inhibitor of HIV protease with activity against the human immunodeficiency virus (HIV). Ritonavir is a petidomimetic inhibitor of both the HIV-1 and HIV-2 proteases. Inhibition of HIV protease renders the enzyme incapable of processing the *gag-pol* polyprotein precursor which leads to production of noninfectious immature HIV particles.

The potential for HIV cross-resistance between protease inhibitors has not been fully explored. Therefore, it is unknown what effect ritonavir therapy will have on the activity of concomitantly or subsequently administered protease inhibitors. Serial HIV isolates obtained from six patients during ritonavir therapy showed a decrease in ritonavir susceptibility in vitro, but did not demonstrate a concordant decrease in susceptibility to saquinavir in vitro when compared with matched baseline isolates. However, isolates form two of these patients demonstrated decreased susceptibility to indinavir in vitro (8–fold). Cross-resistance between ritonavir and reverse transcriptase inhibitors is unlikely because of the different enzyme targets involved.

Pharmacokinetics: After a 600 mg dose of oral solution, peak concentrations of ritonavir were achieved ≈ 2 hours and 4 hours after dosing under fasting and nonfasting (514 KCal; 9% fat, 12% protein and 79% carbohydrate) conditions, respectively. When the oral solution was given under non-fasting conditions, Peak ritonavir concentrations decreased 23% and the extent of absorption decreased 7% relative to fasting conditions. Dilution of the oral solution, within 1 hour of administration, with 240 ml of chocolate milk, *Advera* or *Ensure* did not significantly affect the extent and rate of ritonavir absorption. After a single 600 mg dose under non-fasting conditions, in two separate studies, the capsule and oral soltuion formulations yielded mean areas uder the plasma concentration-time curve (AUCs) of 129.5 and 129 mcg•hr/ml, respectively. Relative to fasting conditions, the extent of absorption of ritonavir from the capsule formulation was 15% higher when administered with a meal (771 KCal; 46% fat, 18% protein and 37% carbohydrate).

Nearly all of the plasma radioactivity after a single oral 600 mg dose of ^{14}C-ritonavir oral solution was attributed to unchanged ritonavir. Five ritonavir metabolites have been identified in urine and feces. The isopropylthiazole oxidation metabolite (M-2) is the major metabolite and has antiviral activity similar to that of the parent drug; however, the concentrations of this metabolite in plasma are low. Studies utilizing human liver microsomes have demonstrated that cytochrome P450 3A (CYP3A) is a major isoform involved in ritonavir metabolism, although CYP2D6 also contributes to the formation of M-2.

In a study of five subjects receiving a 600 mg dose of oral solution, 11.3% of the dose was excreted into the urine; 3.5% of the dose excreted was unchanged parent drug. In that study, 86.4% of the dose was excreted in the feces with 33.8% of the dose excreted as unchanged parent drug.

Ritonavir Pharmacokinetic Characteristics

Parameter	Values (mean)	Parameter	Values (mean)
C_{max} SS[1]	11.2 mcg/ml	CL/F[2]	4.6 L/h
C_{trough} SS[1]	3.7 mcg/ml	CL_R	< 0.1 L/h
V_β/F[2]	0.41 L/kg	RBC/Plasma ratio	0.14
CL/F[2]	8.8 L/h	Percent bound[3]	98% to 99%

[1] SS = Steady state; ritonavir doses of 600 mg q 12 h.
[2] Single ritonavir 600 mg dose.
[3] Primarily bound to human serum albumin and alpha-1 acid glycoprotein over the ritonavir concentration range of 0.01 to 30 μg/ml.

Clinical trials:

Advanced patients with prior antiviral therapy – A study of 1090 patients was a randomized, double-blind trial conducted in HIV-infected patients with at least 9 months of prior antiretroviral therapy and baseline CD_4 cell counts ≤ 100 cells/mm^3. Ritonavir 600 mg twice a day or placebo was added to each patient's baseline antiretroviral terapy regimen. The 6–month cumulative incidence of clinical disease progression or death was 17% for patients randomized to ritonavir compared with

34% for patients randomized to placebo. The 6–month cumulative mortality was 5.8% for patients randomized to ritonavir and 10.1% for patients randomized to placebo.

Patients without prior antiretroviral therapy – In an ongoing study, 356 antiretroviral-naive HIV-infected patients (mean baseline CD_4 = 364 cells/mm^3) were randomized to receive either ritonavir 600 mg twice a day, zidovudine 200 mg twice a day or a combination of these drugs. In analyses of average CD_4 cell count changes from baseline over the first 16 weeks of the study, both ritonavir therapy and combination therapy produced greater mean increases in CD_4 cell counts than did zidovudine monotherapy. The CD_4 cell count increases for ritonavir monotherapy were larger than the increases for the combination therapy.

Indications:

HIV infection: Combination with nucleoside analogs or as monotherapy for the treatment of HIV infection when therapy is warranted.

Contraindications:

Hypersensitivity to the drug or any of its ingredients.

Ritonavir is expected to produce large increases in the plasma concentrations of the following drugs: Amiodarone, astemizole, bepridil, bupropion, cisapride, clozapine, encainiede, flecainide, meperidine, piroxicam, propafenone, propoxyphene, quinidine, rifabutin and terfenadine. These agents have recognized risks of arrhythmias, hematologic abnormalities, seizures or other potentially serious adverse effects. Do not administer these drugs concomitantly with ritonavir.

Coadministration is likely to produce large increases in these highly metabolized sedatives and hypnotics: Alprazolam, clorazepate, diazepam, estazolam, flurazepam, midazolam, triazolam and zolpidem. Due to the potential for extreme sedation and respiratory depression from these agents, do not administer with ritonavir.

Warnings:

Hepatic function impairment: Ritonavir is principally metabolized by the liver. Exercise caution when administering this drug to patients with impaired hepatic function.

Pregnancy: Category B. Developmental toxicity observed in rats (early resorptions, decreased fetal body weight and ossification delays and developmental variations) occurred at a maternally toxic dosage at an exposure equivalent to ≈ 30% of that achieved with the proposed therapeutic dose. A slight increase in the rate of cryptorchidism was also noted in rats at an exposure ≈ 20% of that achieved with the proposed therapeutic dose. Developmental toxicity observed in rabbits (resorptions, decreased litter size and decreased fetal weights) also occurred at a maternally toxic dosage equivalent to 1.8 times the proposed therapeutic dose.

There are no adequate and well controlled studies in pregnant women. Use during pregnancy only if clearly needed.

Lactation: It is not known whether this drug is excreted in breast milk. Exercise caution when administering to a nursing woman. The US Public Health Service Centers for Disease Control and Prevention advises HIV-infected women not to breastfeed to avoid postnatal transmission of HIV to a child who may not be infected.

Children: Safety and efficacy in children < 12 years of age have not been established.

Precautions:

Laboratory tests: Ritonavir has been associated with alterations in triglycerides, AST, ALT, GGT, CPK and uric acid. Perform appropriate laboratory testing prior to initiating ritonavir therapy and at periodic intervals or if any clinical signs and symptoms occur during therapy.

Percentage of Patients with Marked Chemistry and Hematology Laboratory Value Abnormalities with Ritonavir Therapy

		Naive patients			Advanced patients	
Variable	Limit	Ritonavir + AZT	Ritonavir	AZT	Ritonavir	Placebo
Chemistry values	high					
Glucose	(> 250 mg/dl)	2	-	0.9	0.4	1.1
Uric acid	(> 12 mg/dl)	-	-	-	3.6	0.2
Creatinine	(> 3.6 mg/dl)	-	-	-	0.2	0.2
Potassium	(> 6 mEq/L)	-	-	-	0.4	0.2
Chloride	(> 122 mEq/L)	-	0.9	-	-	-
Total bilirubin	(> 3.6 mg/dl)	-	-	-	1.2	0.2
Alkaline phosphatase	(> 550 IU/L)	-	0.9	-	1.4	1.7
AST	(> 180 IU/L)	2.9	6.5	1.7	3.8	4.3

Percentage of Patients with Marked Chemistry and Hematology Laboratory Value Abnormalities with Ritonavir Therapy						
		Naive patients			Advanced patients	
Variable	Limit	Ritonavir + AZT	Ritonavir	AZT	Ritonavir	Placebo
ALT	(> 215 IU/L)	3.9	3.6	2.6	6.1	2.6
GGT	(> 300 IU/L)	2	2.8	0.9	14.7	6.7
LDH	(> 1170 IU/L)	-	-	-	1	0.2
Triglycerides	(> 1500 mg/dl)	1	2.8	-	10.1	0.2
Triglycerides fasting	(>1500 mg/dl)	2.1	1.4	-	7.9	0.4
CPK	(> 1000 IU/L)	7	7.5	7.1	8.6	4.5
Amylase	(> 2 × ULN[1])	-	0.9	-	0.2	-
Chemistry values	low					
Albumin	(< 2 g/dl)	-	-	-	0.2	0.6
Sodium	(< 123 mEq/L)	-	-	-	0.2	-
Potassium	(< 3 mEq/L)	-	0.9	-	2	1.1
Chloride	(< 84 mEq/L)	-	0.9	-	-	0.4
Magnesium	(< 1 mEz/L)	-	-	-	0.4	0.4
Calcium	(< 6.9 mEz/L)	-	-	-	1.2	0.9
Hematology values	low					
Hemoglobin	(< 8 g/dL)	-	-	-	2.8	2.4
Hematocrit	(< 30%)	2	-	-	11.7	16
RBC	(< 3 × 10^{12}/L)	1	-	1.7	14.9	19.7
WBC	(< 2.5 × 10^9/L)	-	-	3.5	25.1	51.4
Platelet count	(< 20 × 10^9/L)	-	-	-	0.4	0.6
Neutrophils	(≤ 0.5 × 10^9/L)	-	-	-	4	6.9
Hematology values	high					
WBC	(> 25 × 10^9/L)	-	-	-	1.6	0.7
Neutrophils	(> 20 × 10^9/L)	-	-	-	1.8	0.9
Eosinophils	(> 1 × 10^9/L)	-	1.9	0.9	1.8	2.6
Prothrombin time	(> 1.5 × ULN[1])	1	-	-	1	1.3

[1] ULN = upper limit of the normal range.

- Indicates no events reported.

Drug Interactions:

Ritonavir Drug Interactions			
Precipitant drug	Object drug*		Description
Clarithromycin	Ritonavir	↑	Coadministration for 4 days increased the ritonavir AUC by 12% and C_{max} by 15%, and the clarithromycin AUC increased by 77% and C_{max} by 31%.
Ritonavir	Clarithromycin	↑	
Didanosine	Ritonavir	↔	Coadministration for 4 days decreased the didanosine AUC by 13% and the C_{max} by 16%.
Ritonavir	Didanosine	↓	
Fluconazole	Ritonavir	↑	Coadministration for 4 days increased the ritonavir AUC by 12% and the C_{max} by 15%.
Fluoxetine	Ritonavir	↑	Concurrent use increased the ritonavir AUC by 19%.
Rifampin	Ritonavir	↓	Coadministration decreased the ritonavir AUC by 35% and the C_{max} by 25%.
Ritonavir	Desipramine	↑	Concurrent use increased the 2-0H desipramine metabolite AUC by 145% and the C_{max} by 23%.
Ritonavir	Disulfiram Metronidazole	↑	Ritonavir formulations contain alcohol, which can produce reactions when co-administered with disulfiram or other drugs that produce disulfiram-like reactions.
Ritonavir	Ethinyl estradiol	↓	Coadministration decreased the ethinyl estradiol AUC by 40% and the C_{max} by 32%.

RITONAVIR

Ritonavir Drug Interactions			
Precipitant drug	Object drug*		Description
Ritonavir	Narcotic analgesics	⟷	AUC of the narcotics may be increased or decreased.
Ritonavir	Rifabutin	⬆	Coadministration increased the 25-O-desacetyl metabolite AUC 4-fold and the C_{max} 25-fold.
Ritonavir	Saquinavir	⬆	Ritonavir extensively inhibits the metabolism of saquinavir resulting in increased saquinavir plasma concentrations.
Ritonavir	Sulfamethoxazole	⬇	The AUC of sulfamethoxazole was decreased by 20%.
Ritonavir	Theophylline	⬇	Coadministration decreased the theophylline AUC by 43% and the C_{max} by 27%.
Ritonavir	Trimethoprim	⬆	The AUC of trimethoprim was increased by 20%.
Ritonavir	Zidovudine	⬇	Coadministration for 4 days decreased the zidovudine AUC by 12% and the C_{max} by 27%.

* ⬆ = Object drug increased. ⬇ = Object drug decreased. ⟷ = Undetermined effect.

Agents Whose AUCs May Be Increased by Ritonavir		
Alpha blockers	Antimalarials	Erythromycin
Antiarrhythmatics	Antineoplastics	Immunosuppressants
Antidepressants	Beta blockers	Methyllphenidiate
Antiemetics	Calcium blockers	Pentoxifylline
Antifungals	Cimetidine	Phenothiazines
Antihyperlipidemics	Corticosteroids	Warfarin

Agents Whose AUCs May Be Decreased by Ritonavir	
Atovaquone	Diphenoxylate
Clofibrate	Metoclopramide
Daunorubicin	Sedatives/Hypnotics

Drug/Food interactions: When the oral solution was given under non-fasting conditions, peak ritonavir concentrations decreased 23% and extent of absorption decreased 7% relative to fasting conditions. Extent of absorption of ritonavir from the capsule was 15% higher when given with a meal relative to fasting conditions. The manufacturer recommends taking ritonavir with meals, if possible.

Adverse Reactions:

The most frequent clinical adverse events, other than asthenia, among patients receiving ritonavir were GI and neurological disturbances including nausea, diarrhea, vomiting, anorexia, abdominal pain, taste perversion and circumoral and peripheral paresthesias.

Body as a whole: Abdomen enlarged, accidental injury, allergic reaction, back pain, cachexia, chest pain, chill, facial edema, diabetes mellitus, facial pain, flu syndrome, hormone level altered, hypothermia, kidney pain, neck pain, neck rigidity, pain (unspecified), substernal chest pain, photosensitivity reaction (< 2%).

Cardiovascular: Hemorrhage, hypotension, migraine, palpitation, peripheral vascular disorder, postural hypotension, syncope, tachycardia (< 2%).

GI: Abnormal stools, bloody diarrhea, cheilitis, cholangitis, colitis, dry mouth, dysphagia, eructation, esophagitis, gastritis, gastroenteritis, GI disorder, GI hemorrhage, gingivitis, hepatitis, hepatomegaly, ileitis, liver damage, liver function tests abnormal, mouth ulcer, oral moniliasis, pancreatitis, periodontal abscess, rectal disorder, tenesmus, thirst (< 2%).

Hematologic/Lymphatic: Anemia, ecchymosis, leukopenia, lymphadenopathy, lymphocytosis, thrombocytopenia (< 2%).

Metabolic/Nutritional: Avitaminosis, dehydration, edema, glycosuria, gout, hypercholesterolemia, peripheral edema, weight loss (< 2%).

Musculoskeletal: Arthralgia, arthrosis, joint disorder, muscle cramps, muscle weakness, myositis, twitching (< 2%).

CNS: Abnormal dreams, abnormal gait, agitation, amnesia, anxiety, aphasia, ataxia, confusion, convulsions, depression, diplopia, emotional lability, euphoria, grand mal convulsions, hallucinations, hyperesthesia, incoordination, libido decreased, ner-

RITONAVIR

vousness, neuralgia, neuropathy, paralysis, peripheral neuropathy, peripheral sensory neuropathy, personality disorder, tremor, vertigo (< 2%).

Respiratory: Asthma, dyspnea, epistaxis, hiccough, hypooventilation, increased cough, interstitial pneumonia, lung disorder, rhinitis (< 2%).

Dermatologic: Acne, contact dermatitis, dry skin, eczema, folliculitis, maculopapular rash, molluscum contagiosum, pruritus, psoriasis, seborrhea, urticaria, vesiculobullous rash (< 2%).

Special senses: Abnormal electro-oculogram, abnormal electroretinogram, abonromal vision, amblyopia/blurred vision, blepharitis, ear pain, eye pain, hearing impairment, increased cerumen, iritis, parosmia, photophobia, taste loss, tinnitus, uveitis, visual field defect (< 2%).

GU: Dysuria, hematuria, impotence,k kidney calculus, kidney failure, nocturia, penis disorder, polyuria, pyelonephritis, urethritis, urinary frequency (< 2%).

Overdosage:

Symptoms: One patient in clinical trials took ritonavir 1500 mg/day for 2 days. The patient reported paresthesias which resolved after the dose was decreased.

The approximate lethal dose was found to be > 20 times the related human dose in rats and 10 times the related human dose in mice.

Treatment: Consists of general supportive measures including monitoring of vital signs and observation of the clinical status of the patient. If indicated, eliminate unabsorbed drug by emesis or gastric lavage; observe usual precautions to maintain the airway. Administration of activated charcoal may also be used to aid in the removal of unabsorbed drug. Ritonavir is extensively metabolized by the liver and is highly protein bound. Dialysis is unlikely to aid in removal of the drug.

Patient Information:

Ritonavir is not a cure for HIV infection. Patients may continue to acquire illnesses associated with advanced HIV infection, including opportunistic infections.

Long-term effects are unknown at this time. Ritonavir has not been shown to reduce the risk of transmitting HIV through sexual contact or blood contamination.

Take ritonavir every day as prescribed. Do not alter the dose or discontinue ritonavir without consulting a doctor. If a dose is missed, take the next dose as soon as possible. However, if a dose is skipped, do not double the next dose.

Ritonavir interacts with some drugs when taken together. Report the use of any other medications, including prescription and nonprescription drugs, to a physician (see Drug Interactions).

The taste of ritonavir oral solution may be improved by mixing with chocolate milk, *Ensure* or *Advera* within 1 hour of dosing. If possible, take ritonavir with food.

Administration and Dosage:

Approved by the FDA on March 6, 1996.

The recommended dosage is 600 mg twice daily. If possible, take with food. Some patients experience nausea upon initiation of 600 mg twice daily dosing; dose escalation may provide some relief: 300 mg twice daily for 1 day, 400 mg twice daily for 2 days, 500 mg twice daily for 1 day and then 600 mg twice daily thereafter. In addition, patients initiating combination regimens with ritonavir and nucleosides may improve GI tolerance by initiating ritonavir alone and subsequently adding nucleosides before completing 2 weeks of ritonavir monotherapy.

Storage/Stability: Store capsules in a refrigerator between 36° to 46°F (2° to 8°C). Protect from light.

Store ritonavir solution in a refrigerator between 36° to 46°F (2° to 8°C).

Refrigeration of ritonavir oral solution by the patient is recommended, but not required if used within 30 days and stored below 25°C (77°F). Store product in the original container. Avoid exposure to excessive heat. Keep cap tightly closed.

Rx	**Norvir** (Abbott)	**Capsules:** 100 mg	(100 mg PI). White. In 84s.
		Oral Solution: 80 mg/ml	Saccharin. Peppermint or caramel flavored. In 240 ml.

INDINAVIR SULFATE

Warning:
Indinavir is indicated for the treatment of HIV infection in adults when antiretroviral therapy is warranted. This indication is based on analyses of surrogate endpoints in studies of up to 24 weeks in duration. At present, there are no results from controlled clinical trials evaluating the effect of therapy with indinavir on clinical progression of HIV infection, such as survival or the incidence of opportunistic infections.

Actions:

Pharmacology: Indinavir is an inhibitor of the human immunodeficiency virus (HIV) protease. HIV protease is an enzyme required for the proteolytic cleavage of the viral polyprotein precursors into the individual functional proteins found in infectious HIV. Indinavir binds to the protease active site and inhibits the activity of the enzyme. This inhibition prevents cleavage of the viral polyproteins resulting in the formation of immature noninfectious viral particles. The relationship between in vitro susceptibility of HIV to indinavir and inhibition of HIV replication in humans has not been established.

Drug resistance – Isolates of HIV with reduced susceptibility to the drug have been recovered from some patients treated withindinavir. Viral resistance was correlated with the accumulation of mutations that resulted in the expression of amino acid substitutions in the viral protease. Eleven amino acid residue positions, at which substitutions are associated with resistance, have been identified. Resistance was mediated by the co-expression of multiple and variable substitutions at these positions. In general, higher levels of resistance were associated with the co-expression of greater numbers of substitutions.

Cross-resistance between indinavir and HIV reverse transcriptase inhibitors is unlikely because the enzyme targets involved are different. Cross-resistance was noted between indinavir and the protease inhibitor ritonavir. Varying degrees of cross-resistance have been observed between indinavir and other HIV-protease inhibitors.

Pharmacokinetics:

Absorption – Indinavir was rapidly absorbed in the fasted state with a time to peak plasma concentration (T_{max}) of 0.8 hours. A greater than dose-proportional increase in indinavir plasma concentrations was observed over the 200 to 1000 mg dose range. At a dosing regimen of 800 mg every 8 hours, steady-state area under the plasma concentration-time curve (AUC) was 30,691 nM•hour, peak plasma concentration (C_{max}) was 12,617 nM and plasma concentration 8 hours post-dose (trough) was 251 nM. High calorie, fat and protein meals decrease the AUC and C_{max} (see Drug Interactions).

Distribution – Indinavir was ≈ 60% bound to human plasma proteins over a concentration range of 81 to 16,300 nM.

Metabolism – Following a 400 mg dose of ^{14}C-indinavir, 83% and 19% of the total radioactivity was recovered in feces and urine, respectively; radioactivity due to parent drug in feces and urine was 19.1% and 9.4%, respectively. Seven metabolites have been identified, one glucuronide conjugate and six oxidative metabolites. In vitro studies indicate that cytochrome P450 3A4 (CYP344) is the major enzyme responsible for formation of the oxidative metabolites.

Excretion – Less than 20% of indinavir is excreted unchanged in the urine. Mean urinary excretion of unchanged drug was 10.4% and 12% following a single 700 and 1000 mg dose, respectively. Indinavir was rapidly eliminated with a half-life of 1.8 hours. Significant accumulation was not observed after multiple dosing at 800 mg every 8 hours.

Clinical trials: In ongoing, multicenter, double-blind, randomized clinical endpoint trials in patients with no prior antiretroviral therapy, the effects of indinavir on CD4 cell counts and serum viral RNA were evaluated in HIV-1 seropositive adults over a 24 week period. At baseline, patients were randomized to one of three treatment groups: Indinavir alone, zidovudine alone and indinavir plus zidovudine. The mean baseline CD4 cell count over all patients was 145 to 254.4 cells/mm^3 and the serum viral RNA was 4.28 to 4.4 log_{10} copies/ml (19,210 to 25,330 copies/ml).

At 24 weks of therapy, 37% of patients receiving indinavir alone, 36% to 56% of patients receiving indinavir in combination with zidovudine, and 2% to 7% of patients receiving zidovudine alone had serum viral RNA levels ≤ 500 copies/ml, the limit of detection of the assay; the clinical significance of this finding is unknown.

In an ongoing multicenter, double-blind, randomized trial in HIV-1 seropositive patients with prior zidovudine experience (median time of zidovudine therapy, 30.9 months), patients were randomized to 1 of 3 treatment groups: Indinavir, zidovudine plus lamivudine or indinavir plus zidovudine plus lamivudine. At 24 weeks of therapy, 35% of patients receiving indinavir alone, 91% of patients receiving indinavir in combination with zidovudine and lamivudine and 0% of patients receiving zidovudine plus lamivudine had serum viral RNA levels ≤ 500 copies/ml, the limit of detection of the assay; the clinical significance of this finding is unknown.

In an open-label study, zidovudine– and didanosine-naive HIV-infected patients were randomized to 1 of 3 treatment groups: Indinavir 600 mg every 6 hours, zidovudine plus didanosine, and indinavir plus zidovudine plus didanosine. At 24 weeks of therapy, all three groups had a significant increase in CD4 cell counts and decrease in serum viral RNA compared to baseline; however, there were no differences in mean CD4 cell count changes between treatment arms. Patients treated with indinavir plus zidovudine plus didanosine had a greater mean decline in serum viral RNA than those treated with indinavir alone or zidovudine plus didanosine.

A randomized trial studied 70 HIV-seropositive patients receiving indinavir at one of three doses (800 mg every 8 hours, 1000 mg every 8 hours and 800 mg every 6 hours). At 24 weeks, changes in CD4 cell counts and serum viral RNA were similar in all three treatment groups.

Indications:

HIV infection: Treatment of HIV infection in adults when antiretroviral therapy is warranted.

Contraindications:

Hypersensitivity to any component of the product.

Warnings:

Concomitant agents: Do not administer indinavir concurrently with terfenadine, astemizole, cisapride, triazolam and midazolam because competition for CYP344 by indinavir could result in inhibition of the metabolism of these drugs and create the potential for serious or life-threatening events (eg, cardiac arrhythmias, prolonged sedation).

Renal function impairment: Nephrolithiasis, including flank pain with or without hematuria (including microscopic hematuria), has been reported in ≈ 4% of patients. In general, these events were not associated with renal dysfunction and resolved with hydration and temporary interruption of therapy (eg, 1 to 3 days). Following the acute episode, 9.2% of patients discontinued therapy.

To ensure adequate hydration, it is recommended that the patient drink at least 1.5 liters (≈ 48 ounces) of liquids during the course of 24 hours.

Hepatic function impairment: Patients with mild to moderate hepatic insufficiency and clinical evidence of cirrhosis had evidence of decreased metabolism of indinavir resulting in ≈ 60% higher mean AUC following a single 400 mg dose. The half-life increased to 2.8 hours.

Pregnancy: Category C. Treatment-related increases over controls in the incidence of supernumerary ribs (at doses at or below those in humans) and of cervical ribs (at doses comparable to or slghtly greater than those in humans) were seen in rats.

There are no adequate and well controlled studies in pregnant women. Use during pregnancy only if the potential benefit justifies the potential risk to the fetus.

Lactation: Studies in lactating rats have demonstrated that indinavir is excreted in milk. Although it is not known whether indinavir is excreted in breast milk, there exists the potential for adverse effects from indinavir in nursing infants. Instruct mothers to discontinue nursing if they are receiving indinavir. This is consistent with the recommendation by the US Public Health Service Centers for Disease Control and Prevention that HIV-infected mothers not breastfeed their infants to avoid risking postnatal transmission of HIV.

Children: Safety and efficacy have not been established.

Precautions:

Hyperbilirubinemia: Asymptomatic hyperbilirubinemia (total bilirubin ≥ 2.5 mg/dl), reported predominantly as elevated indirect bilirubin, has occurred in ≈ 10% of patients. In < 1%, this was associated with elevations in ALT or AST.

Drug Interactions:

Indinavir Drug Interactions

Precipitant drug	Object drug*		Description
Indinavir	Astemizole Cisapride Midazolam Terfenadine Triazolam	⬆	Because competition for CYP344 by indinavir could result in inhibition of the metabolism of these drugs and create the potential for serious or life-threatening events (eg, cardiac arrhythmias, prolonged sedation), indinavir should not be administered concurrently with any of these agents (see Warnings).

INDINAVIR SULFATE

Indinavir Drug Interactions			
Precipitant drug	Object drug*		Description
Clarithromycin	Indinavir	↑	Coadministration for 1 week resulted in a 29% increase in indinavir AUC and a 53% increase in clarithromycin AUC.
Indinavir	Clarithromycin	↑	
Didanosine	Indinavir	↓	If indinavir and didanosine are administered concomitantly, administer at least 1 hour apart on an empty stomach; a normal (acidic) gastric pH may be necessary for optimum absorption of indinavir, whereas acid rapidly degrades didanosine which is formulated with buffering agents to increase pH.
Fluconazole	Indinavir	↓	Concurrent use for 1 week resulted in a 19% decrease in indinavir AUC.
Ketoconazole	Indinavir	↑	Coadministration resulted in a 68% ± 48% increase in indinavir AUC.
Quinidine	Indinavir	↑	Concurrent use resulted in a 10% increase in indinavir AUC.
Rifampin	Indinavir	↓	Because rifampin is a potent inducer of P450, which could markedly diminish plasma concentrations of indinavir, coadministration is not recommended.
Indinavir	Isoniazid	↑	Coadministration for 1 week resulted in a 13% increase in isoniazid AUC.
Indinavir	Lamivudine	↓	Coadministration of indinavir with zidovudine and lamivudine for 1 week resulted in a 36% increase in zidovudine AUC and a 6% decrease in lamivudine AUC.
Indinavir	Oral contraceptives	↑	Coadministration of indinavir for 1 week resulted in a 24% increase in ethinyl estradiol AUC and a 26% increase n norethindrone AUC.
Indinavir	Rifabutin	↑	Coadministration for 10 days resulted in a 32% ± 19% decrease in indinavir AUC and a 204% ± 142% increase in rifabutin AUC.
Rifabutin	Indinavir	↓	
Indinavir	Stavudine	↑	Coadministration for 1 week resulted in a 25% increase in stavudine AUC.
Indinavir	Trimethoprim/Sulfamethoxazole	↑	Coadministration for 1 week resulted in a 19% increase in trimethoprim AUC, and no change in sulfamethoxazole AUC.
Indinavir	Zidovudine	↑	Coadministration for 1 week resulted in a 13% ± 48% increase in indinavir AUC and a 17% ± 23% increase in zidovudine AUC.
Zidovudine	Indinavir	↑	

Drug/Food interactions: Administration of indinavir with a meal high in calories, fat and protein (784 kcal, 48.6 g fat, 31.3 g protein) resulted in a 77% reduction in AUC and an 84% reduction in C_{max}. Administration with lighter meals (eg, a meal of dry toast with jelly, apple juice and coffee with skim milk and sugar or a meal of corn flakes, skim milk and sugar) resulted in little or no change in AUC, C_{max} or trough concentration. Administration of a single 400 mg dose of indinavir with 8 oz of grapefruit juice resulted in a decrease in indinavir AUC (26%).

Adverse Reactions:

Adverse Reactions: Indinavir vs Zidovudine (≥ 2%)			
Adverse reaction	Indinavir (n = 196)	Indinavir + zidovudine (n = 196)	Zidovudine (n = 195)
Body as a whole			
Abdominal pain	8.7	8.2	5.1
Asthenia/fatigue	3.6	9.2	7.7
Flank pain	2.6	1	0
Malaise	0.5	2	1.5
GI			
Nausea	11.7	32.1	14.4
Diarrhea	4.6	4.1	2.1

Adverse Reactions: Indinavir vs Zidovudine (≥ 2%)			
Adverse reaction	Indinavir (n = 196)	Indinavir + zidovudine (n = 196)	Zidovudine (n = 195)
Vomiting	4.1	12.2	4.6
Acid regurgitation	2	2	0.5
Anorexia	0.5	2	3.1
Dry mouth	0.5	0	2.1
CNS			
Headache	5.6	11.7	5.1
Insomnia	3.1	1.5	0
Dizziness	1	3.6	0.5
Somnolence	1	1.5	3.6
Miscellaneous			
Taste perversion	2.6	3.6	2.1
Back pain	2	1	1.5

Indinavir vs Zidovudine: Selected Lab Test Abnormalities (%)			
Lab test abnormalities	Indinavir (n = 196)	Indinavir + zidovudine (n = 196)	Zidovudine (n = 195)
Hematology			
Decreased hemoglobin <8 g/dl	0.5	1.1	0.5
Decreased platelet count <50 THS/mm³	0.5	0.5	0
Decreased neutrophil < 0.75 THS/mm³	1.1	1.6	3.8
Blood chemistry			
Increased ALT > 500% ULN[1]	3.1	3.2	2.1
Increased AST > 500% ULN	2.1	2.1	1.1
Total serum bilirubin > 2.5 mg/dl	7.8	7.4	0.5
Increased serum amylase > 200% ULN	1	2.1	0.5

[1] Upper limit of the normal range.

Adverse reactions occurring in < 2% of patients in all Phase II/Phase III studies and considered at least possibly related to or of unknown relationship to treatment and of at least moderate intensity are listed below by body system.

Body as a whole: Abdominal distention; chest pain; chills; fever; flank pain; flu-like illness; fungal infection; malaise; pain; syncope.

Cardiovascular: Cardiovascular disorder; palpitation.

CNS: Agitation; anxiety; anxiety disorder; bruxism; decreased mental acuity; depression; dizziness; dream abnormality; dysesthesia; excitement; fasciculation; hypesthesia; nervousness; neuralgia; neurotic disorder; paresthesia; peripheral neuropathy; sleep disorder; somnolence; tremor; vertigo.

Dermatologic: Body odor; contact dermatitis; dermatitis; dry skin; flushing; folliculitis; herpes simplex; herpes zoster; night sweats; pruritus; seborrhea; skin disorder; skin infection; sweating; urticaria.

GI: Acid regurgitation; anorexia; aphthous stomatitis; cheilitis; cholecystitis; cholestasis; constipation; dry mouth; dyspepsia; eructation; flatulence; gastritis; gingivitis; glossodynia; gingival hemorrhage; increased appetite; infectious gastroenteritis; jaundice; liver cirrhosis.

GU: Dysuria; hematuria; hydronephrosis; nocturia; prmenstrual syndrome; proteinuria; renal colic; urinary frequency; urinary tract infection; urine abnormality; urine sediment abnormality; urolithiasis.

Hematologic/Lymphatic: Anemia; lymphadenopathy; spleen disorder.

Musculoskeletal: Arthralgia; back pain; leg pain; myalgia; muscle cramps; muscle weakness; musculoskeletal pain; shoulder pain; stiffness.

INDINAVIR SULFATE

Respiratory: Cough; dyspnea; halitosis; pharyngeal hyperemia; pharyngitis; pneumonia; rales/rhonchi; respiratory failure; sinus disorder; sinusitis; upper respiratory infection.

Special senses: Accommodation disorder; blurred vision; eye pain; eye swelling; orbital edema; taste disorder.

Miscellaneous: Rash; food allergy; hyperbilirubinemia and nephrolithiasis occurred more frequently at doses > 2.4 g/day compared with doses < 2.4 g/day (see Warnings).

Overdosage:

It is not known whether indinavir is dialyzable by peritoneal or hemodialysis.

Patient Information:

Indinavir is not a cure for HIV and patients may continue to develop opportunistic infections and other complications associated with HIV disease. Indinavir has not been shown to reduce the incidence or frequency of such illnesses. The long-term effects of indinavir are unknown. Indinavir has not been shown to reduce the risk of transmission of HIV to others through sexual contact or blood contamination.

Advise patients to remain under the care of a physician when using indinavir and not to modify or discontinue treatment without first consulting the physician. Therefore, if a dose is missed, patients should take the next dose at the regularly scheduled time and should not double this dose.

For optimal absorption, administer indinavir without food but with water 1 hour before or 2 hours after a meal. Alternatively, administer with other liquids such as skim milk, juice, coffee or tea, or with a light meal (eg, dry toast with jelly, juice and coffee with skim milk and sugar; or corn flakes, skim milk and sugar). Ingestion of indinavir with a meal high in calories, fat and protein reduces the absorption of indinavir.

Indinavir capsules are sensitive to moisture. Instruct patients to store indinavir in the original container and to keep the desiccant in the bottle.

Administration and Dosage:

Approved by the FDA on March 13, 1995.

The recommended dosage is 800 mg (two 400 mg capsules) orally every 8 hours. The dosage is the same whether indinavir is used alone or in combination with other antiretroviral agents. The antiretroviral activity of indinavir may be increased when used in combination with approved reverse transcriptase inhibitors.

Administer at intervals of 8 hours. For optimal absorption, administer without food but with water 1 hour before or 2 hours after a meal or administer with other liquids such as skim milk, juice, coffe or tea, or with a light meal (eg, dry toast with jelly, juice and coffee with skim milk and sugar; or corn flakes, skim milk and sugar).

If indinavir and didanosine are administered concomitantly, they should be administered at least 1 hour apart on an empty stomach.

In addition to adequate hydration, medical management in patients who experience nephrolithiasis may include temporary interruption of therapy (eg, 1 to 3 days) during the acute episode of nephrolithiasis or discontinuation of therapy.

Cirrhosis: Reduce the dosage of indinavir to 600 mg every 8 hours in patients with mild-to-moderate hepatic insufficiency due to cirrhosis.

Storage/Stability: Store in a tighlty closed container at room temperature, 15° to 30°C (59° to 86°F). Protect from moisture. Indinavir capsules are sensitive to moisture. Dispense and store in the original container. Keep the desiccant in the original bottle.

Rx	**Crixivan** (Merck)	**Capsules:** 200 Mg	Lactose. (Crixivan 200 mg). Blue. In 270s and 360s.
		400 mg	Lactose. (Crixivan 400 mg). Green. In 180s.

ZIDOVUDINE (Azidothymidine; AZT; Compound S)

Warning:

Zidovudine may be associated with hematologic toxicity including granulocytopenia and severe anemia particularly in patients with advanced human immunodeficiency (HIV) disease (see Warnings). Prolonged use of zidovudine has been associated with symptomatic myopathy similar to that produced by HIV.

Rare occurrences of lactic acidosis in the absence of hypoxemia, and severe hepatomegaly with steatosis have occurred with antiretroviral nucleoside analogs, including zidovudine and zalcitabine, and are potentially fatal (see Warnings).

Actions:

Pharmacology: Zidovudine is a thymidine analog and an inhibitor of the in vitro replication of some retroviruses, including HIV. Cellular thymidine kinase converts zidovudine into zidovudine monophosphate and finally to the triphosphate derivative by other cellular enzymes. Zidovudine triphosphate interferes with the HIV viral RNA-dependent DNA polymerase (reverse transcriptase) and thus, inhibits viral replication. It also inhibits cellular α-DNA polymerase, but at concentrations 100-fold higher than those required to inhibit reverse transcriptase. In vitro, zidovudine triphosphate is incorporated into growing chains of DNA by viral reverse transcriptase, and the DNA chain is terminated.

Pharmacokinetics:

Absorption/Distribution – The following pharmacokinetic data was obtained in adults. Overall, the pharmacokinetics in pediatric patients > 3 months of age are similar to that in adults. After oral dosing, zidovudine is rapidly absorbed from the GI tract with peak serum concentrations occurring within 0.5 to 1.5 hours. The rate of absorption of the syrup is greater than that of the capsules. Dose-dependent kinetics were observed over the range of 2 mg/kg every 8 hours to 10 mg/kg every 4 hours. Zidovudine plasma protein binding is 34% to 38%. Mean steady-state predose and 1.5 hours post-dose concentrations were 0.16 mcg/ml (range, 0 to 0.84 mcg/ml) and 0.62 mcg/ml (range, 0.05 to 1.46 mcg/ml), respectively, following chronic oral use of 250 mg every 4 hours (n=21; 3 to 5.4 mg/kg).

Metabolism/Excretion – Zidovudine is rapidly metabolized in the liver to the inactive 3′-azido-3′-deoxy-5′-O-β-D-glucopyranuronosylthymidine (GAZT) which has an apparent elimination half-life of 1 hr (range, 0.61 to 1.73). The mean zidovudine half-life was ≈ 1 hr (range, 0.78 to 1.93). Urinary recovery of zidovudine and GAZT was 14% and 74% of an oral dose, respectively, and the total urinary recovery averaged 90% (range, 63% to 95%). However, as a result of first-pass metabolism, the average oral capsule bioavailability is 65% (range, 52% to 75%).

Following IV dosing (1 to 5 mg/kg) total body clearance averaged 1900 ml/min/70 kg and the apparent volume of distribution was 1.6 L/kg. Renal clearance is ≈ 400 ml/min/70 kg, indicating glomerular filtration and active tubular secretion by the kidneys. The zidovudine CSF/plasma concentration ratios measured at 2 to 4 hours following IV dosing of 2.5 and 5 mg/kg were 0.2 and 0.64, respectively.

Microbiology: Zidovudine acts additively or synergistically with a number of anti-HIV agents, including zalcitabine, didanosine and interferon alfa, in inhibiting the replication of HIV in cell culture.

The emergence of resistance is a function of both duration of zidovudine therapy and stage of disease. Asymptomatic patients developed resistance at significantly slower rates than patients with advanced disease. Combination therapy with zalcitabine does not appear to prevent the emergence of zidovudine-resistant isolates.

Zidovudine has antiviral activity against some mammalian retroviruses in addition to HIV. Inhibitory activity was exhibited against the Epstein-Barr virus (clinical significance not known). Many Enterobacteriaceae, including strains of *Shigella, Salmonella, Klebsiella, Enterobacter, Citrobacter* and *Escherichia coli* are inhibited in vitro by low concentrations of zidovudine (0.005 to 0.5 mcg/ml). Clinical significance is not known. Synergy of zidovudine with trimethoprim has been observed against some of these bacteria. Limited data suggest that bacterial resistance to zidovudine develops rapidly. Although *Giardia lamblia* is inhibited by 1.9 mcg/ml of zidovudine, no activity was observed against other protozoal pathogens.

ZIDOVUDINE (Azidothymidine; AZT; Compound S)

Indications:

Oral:

Monotherapy –

Adults: Initial treatment of HIV-infected adults with CD4 cell count ≤ 500/mm³. Monotherapy with zidovudine was found to be clinically superior to didanosine or zalcitabine monotherapy for the initial management of HIV-infected patients who have not received previous antiretroviral treatment. However, for some patients with advanced disease on prolonged zidovudine therapy, modifying the antiviral regimen may be more effective in delaying disease progression than remaining on zidovudine monotherapy.

Children: For HIV-infected children > 3 months of age who have HIV-related symptoms or who are asymptomatic with abnormal laboratory values indicating significant HIV-related immunosuppression.

Maternal-Fetal HIV transmission: Prevention of maternal-fetal HIV transmission as part of a regimen that includes oral zidovudine beginning between 14 and 34 weeks of gestation, IV zidovudine during labor, and zidovudine syrup to the newborn after birth. However, transmission to infants may still occur in some cases despite the use of this regimen.

Combination therapy with zalcitabine – Treatment of selected patients with advanced HIV disease (CD4 cell count ≤ 300 cells/mm³). In patients without prior exposure to zidovudine, this indication is based on greater increases in CD4 cell counts that were maintained longer for patients treated with combination therapy vs monotherapy with zidovudine.

IV: For the management of certain adult patients with symptomatic HIV infection (AIDS and advanced ARC) who have a history of cytologically confirmed *Pneumocystis carinii* pneumonia (PCP) or an absolute CD4 (T4 helper/inducer) lymphocyte count of < 200/mm³ in the peripheral blood before therapy is begun.

Contraindications:

Life-threatening allergic reactions to any of the components of the product.

Warnings:

Safety/Efficacy: The full safety and efficacy profile of zidovudine is not completely defined, especially with prolonged use and in HIV-infected individuals who have less advanced disease. Several serious adverse events have been reported with the use of zidovudine in clinical practice. Reports of pancreatitis, sensitization reactions (including anaphylaxis in one patient; see Hypersensitivity), vasculitis and seizures have been rare. These events, except for sensitization, have also been associated with HIV disease. Changes in skin and nail pigmentation have been associated with zidovudine.

Hematologic effects: Use with extreme caution in patients who have bone marrow compromise evidenced by granulocyte count < 1000/mm³ or hemoglobin < 9.5 g/dl. Anemia and granulocytopenia are the most significant adverse events observed. There have been reports of reversible pancytopenia.

Significant anemia most commonly occurred after 4 to 6 weeks of therapy and in many cases required dose adjustment, discontinuation of drug or blood transfusions. Frequent blood counts are strongly recommended for advanced HIV disease patients, less frequent for asymptomatic and early HIV disease depending on overall status. If anemia or granulocytopenia develops, dosage adjustments may be necessary.

Myopathy and myositis with pathological changes, similar to that produced by HIV disease, have been associated with prolonged use of zidovudine.

Lactic acidosis/severe hepatomegaly with steatosis: Rare occurrences of lactic acidosis in the absence of hypoxemia, and severe hepatomegaly with steatosis have been reported with the use of antiretroviral nucleoside analogs, including zidovudine and zalcitabine, and are potentially fatal; it is not known whether these events are causally related to the drugs. Consider lactic acidosis whenever a patient receiving zidovudine develops unexplained tachypnea, dyspnea or fall in serum bicarbonate level. Under these circumstances, suspend zidovudine therapy until the diagnosis of lactic acidosis has been excluded. Exercise caution when administering zidovudine to any patient, particularly obese women, with hepatomegaly, hepatitis or other known risk factors for liver disease. Follow these patients closely while on therapy. Suspend treatment in the setting of rapidly elevating aminotransferase levels, progressive hepatomegaly or metabolic/lactic acidosis of unknown etiology.

Combination therapy: No benefit from combination therapy with zalcitabine has been observed in a study of patients with extensive prior exposure to zidovudine (median 18 months) and CD4 cell counts < 150 cells/mm³; combination therapy is therefore not recommended for these patients.

ZIDOVUDINE (Azidothymidine; AZT; Compound S)

Hypersensitivity: Sensitization reactions, including anaphylaxis in one patient, have occurred with zidovudine therapy. Patients experiencing a rash should undergo medical evaluation. Refer to Management of Acute Hypersensitivity Reactions.

Renal/Hepatic function impairment: Zidovudine is eliminated from the body primarily by renal excretion following metabolism in the liver (glucuronidation). In patients with severely impaired renal function, dosage reduction is recommended (see Administration and Dosage). Although very little data are available, patients with severely impaired hepatic function may be at greater risk of toxicity.

Carcinogenesis/Mutagenesis: In mice, seven late-appearing (after 19 months) vaginal neoplasms (five non-metastasizing squamous cell carcinomas, one squamous cell papilloma, one squamous polyp) occurred in animals given the highest dose of zidovudine; one squamous cell papilloma occurred with the middle dose. In rats, two late-appearing (after 20 months) non-metastasizing vaginal squamous cell carcinomas occurred in animals given the highest dose.

Zidovudine was weakly mutagenic in the absence of metabolic activation only at the highest concentrations tested (4000 and 5000 mcg/ml) in mouse lymphoma cells. In the presence of metabolic activation the drug was weakly mutagenic at concentrations of ≥ 1000 mcg/ml. In cultured human lymphocytes, zidovudine caused dose-related structural chromosomal abnormalities at concentrations ≥ 3 mcg/ml.

Pregnancy: Category C. In rats and rabbits, there was embryo/fetal toxicity as evidenced by an increase in the incidence of fetal resorptions (150 to 500 mg/kg/day). In rats, a dose of 3000 mg/kg/day caused marked maternal toxicity and an increase in the incidence of fetal malformations.

A randomized, double-blind, placebo controlled trial was conducted in HIV-infected pregnant women to determine the utility of zidovudine for the prevention of maternal-fetal HIV-transmission. Congenital abnormalities occurred with similar frequency between infants born to mothers who received zidovudine and infants born to mothers who received placebo.

To monitor maternal-fetal outcomes of pregnant women exposed to zidovudine, an Antiretroviral Pregnancy registry has been established. Physicians are encouraged to register patients by calling (800) 722–9292, ext. 58465.

Lactation: The US Public Health Centers for Disease Control and Prevention advises HIV-infected women not to breastfeed to avoid postnatal transmission of HIV to a child who may not yet be infected.

It is not known whether zidovudine is excreted in breast milk or whether zidovudine reduces the potential for transmission of HIV in breast milk. Lactating mice given zidovudine were found to have milk concentrations of zidovudine 5 times the corresponding serum concentration. Milk concentrations of zidovudine declined at a slower rate than serum levels.

Children: A positive test for HIV-antibody in children < 15 months of age may represent passively acquired maternal antibodies, rather than an active antibody response to infection in the infant. Thus, the presence of HIV-antibody in a child < 15 months of age must be interpreted with caution, especially in the asymptomatic infant. Pursue confirmatory tests such as serum P_{24} antigen or viral culture in such children.

Drug Interactions:

Zidovudine Drug Interactions

Precipitant drug	Object drug*		Description
Acetaminophen	Zidovudine	⬇	Acetaminophen may decrease the AUC of zidovudine.
Bone marrow suppressive/ cytotoxic agents (eg, adriamycin, dapsone, flucytosine, vincristine, vinblastine)	Zidovudine	⬆	Coadministration of zidovudine with drugs that are nephrotoxic, cytotoxic or interfere with RBC/WBC number or function may increase the risk of hematologic toxicity.
Fluconazole	Zidovudine	⬆	Concurrent use may increase the zidovudine AUC and half-life at steady state.
Ganciclovir	Zidovudine	⬆	Concurrent use increases the risk of hematologic toxicities in some patients with advanced HIV disease. If combination use is necessary, dose reduction or interruption of one or both agents may be necessary. Monitor hematologic parameters frequently.

ZIDOVUDINE (Azidothymidine; AZT; Compound S)

Zidovudine Drug Interactions			
Precipitant drug	Object drug*		Description
Interferon alfa	Zidovudine	⬆	Hematologic toxicities have been seen with concomitant use. If combination use is necessary, dose reduction or interruption of one or both agents may be necessary. Monitor hematologic parameters frequently.
Interferon beta-1b	Zidovudine	⬆	Zidovudine serum levels may be elevated.
Nucleoside analogs	Zidovudine	⬆	Experimental nucleoside analogs which are being evaluated in AIDS and ARC patients may affect RBC/WBC number or function and may increase the potential for hematologic toxicity of zidovudine. Some analogs affecting DNA replication antagonize the in vitro antiviral activity of zidovudine against HIV; avoid concomitant use.
Probenecid	Zidovudine	⬆	Probenecid may increase zidovudine levels by inhibiting glucuronidation or reducing renal excretion. Some patients have developed flu-like symptoms consisting of myalgia, malaise or fever and maculopapular rash.
Rifamycins	Zidovudine	⬇	The AUC of zidovudine may be decreased.
Trimethoprim	Zidovudine	⬆	Serum levels of zidovudine and its metabolite may be increased.
Zidovudine	Acyclovir	⬆	Severe drowsiness and lethargy may occur with concurrent use.
Zidovudine	Phenytoin	⟷	Phenytoin levels have been reported to increase, decrease or not change with concurrent use. In addition, zidovudine clearance was decreased by phenytoin.
Phenytoin	Zidovudine	⬆	

* ⬆ = Object drug increased. ⬇ = Object drug decreased. ⟷ = Undetermined effect.

Drug/Food interactions: Administration of capsules with food decreased peak plasma concentrations by > 50%; however, bioavailability as determined by AUC may not be affected.

Adverse Reactions:

The most frequent adverse events and abnormal laboratory values reported in the placebo controlled clinical trial of oral zidovudine were granulocytopenia and anemia. The occurrence of hematologic toxicities was inversely related to CD4 (T4) lymphocyte number, hemoglobin and granulocyte count at study entry, and directly related to dose and duration of therapy. The anemia appeared to be the result of impaired erythrocyte maturation as evidenced by increasing macrocytosis (MCV) while on drug. Similar results occurred in children.

Zidovudine Adverse Reactions (≥ 5% Advanced Adult HIV Patients) (%)					
Adverse Reaction	Zidovudine (n = 144)	Placebo (n = 137)	Adverse Reaction	Zidovudine (n = 144)	Placebo (n = 137)
Body as a whole			*GI*		
Asthenia	19	18	Anorexia	11	8
Diaphoresis	5	4	Diarrhea	12	18
Fever	16	12	Dyspepsia	5	4
Headache	42	37	GI pain	20	19
Malaise	8	7	Nausea	46	18
CNS			Vomiting	6	3
Dizziness	6	4	*Other*		
Insomnia	5	1	Dyspnea	5	3
Paresthesia	6	3	Myalgia	8	2
Somnolence	8	9	Rash	17	15
			Taste perversion	5	8

ZIDOVUDINE (Azidothymidine; AZT; Compound S)

Several serious adverse reactions have been reported in clinical practice. Myopathy and myositis with pathological changes, similar to that produced by HIV disease, have been associated with prolonged use. Reports of hepatomegaly with steatosis, hepatitis, pancreatitis, lactic acidosis, sensitization reactions (including anaphylaxis in one patient; see Warnings), hyperbilirubinemia, vasculitis and seizures have been rare. A single case of macular edema has been reported. Other reactions include:

Body as a whole: Body odor; chills; edema of the lip; flu syndrome; hyperalgesia; abdominal/back/chest pain; lymphadenopathy.

Dermatologic: Acne; pruritus; urticaria; skin/nail pigmentation changes; rash; sweating.

Cardiovascular: Vasodilation; syncope.

GI: Constipation; dysphagia; edema of the tongue; eructation; flatulence; bleeding gums; rectal hemorrhage; mouth ulcer; diarrhea.

Musculoskeletal: Arthralgia; muscle spasm; tremor; twitch.

CNS: Anxiety; confusion; depression; emotional lability; nervousness; syncope; loss of mental acuity; vertigo; dizziness; paresthesia; somnolence.

Respiratory: Cough; epistaxis; pharyngitis; rhinitis; sinusitis; hoarseness; dyspnea.

Special senses: Amblyopia; hearing loss; photophobia; taste perversion.

GU: Dysuria; polyuria; urinary frequency; urinary hesitancy.

Zidovudine Adverse Reactions (Early Symptomatic and Asymptomatic Adult HIV Patients) (%)

	Early Symptomatic HIV Disease		Asymptomatic HIV Infection		
Adverse reaction	Zidovudine (n = 361)	Placebo (n = 352)	Zidovudine 500 mg (n = 453)	Zidovudine 1500 mg[1] (n = 457)	Placebo (n = 428)
Body as a whole					
Asthenia	69	62	8.6	10.1	5.8
Headache	—	—	62.5	58	52.6
Malaise	—	—	53.2	55.6	44.9
Dizziness	—	—	17.9	20.8	15.2
GI					
Anorexia	—	—	20.1	19.3	10.5
Constipation	—	—	6.4	8.1	3.5
Dyspepsia	6	1	—	—	—
Nausea	61	41	51.4	57.3	29.9
Vomiting	25	13	17.2	16.4	9.8

[1] Three times the currently recommended dose in asymptomatic patients.

Children (the adverse effects reported in adults may also occur in children):

Body as a whole – Granulocytopenia (39%; advanced HIV disease); anemia (23%; advanced HIV disease); fever (3.2%); phlebitis/bacteremia, headache (1.6%).

GI – Vomiting (4.8%); abdominal pain (3.2%); nausea, diarrhea, weight loss (0.8%).

CNS – Decreased reflexes (5.6%); insomnia (2.4%); nervousness/irritability (1.6%); seizure (0.8%).

Cardiovascular – ECG abnormality (2.4%); left ventricular dilation, cardiomyopathy, S_3 gallop, CHF, generalized edema (0.8%).

GU – Hematuria/viral cystitis (0.8%).

Maternal-Fetal transmission of HIV prevention:

Hematologic – The most commonly reported adverse reactions were anemia (22% of infants) and neutropenia (21% of infants).

Overdosage:

Cases of acute overdoses in both children and adults have occurred with doses up to 50 g; none were fatal. The only consistent finding was spontaneous or induced nausea and vomiting. Hematologic changes were transient and not severe. Some patients experienced nonspecific CNS symptoms such as headache, dizziness, drowsiness, lethargy and confusion. One patient had a grand mal seizure possibly related to zidovudine 3 hours after ingesting 36 g. All patients recovered without permanent sequelae. Hemodialysis and peritoneal dialysis appear to have a negligible effect on zidovudine while elimination of its primary metabolite, GAZT, is enhanced.

ZIDOVUDINE (Azidothymidine; AZT; Compound S)

Patient Information:

Zidovudine is not a cure for HIV infections, and patients may continue to acquire illnesses associated with AIDS or ARC, including opportunistic infections. Patients should seek medical care for any significant change in their health status.

The major toxicities of zidovudine are granulocytopenia or anemia that may require transfusions or dose modifications including possible discontinuation. Frequency and severity of these toxicities are greater in patients with more advanced disease and in those who initiate therapy later in the course of their infection. It is extremely important to have blood counts followed closely while on therapy, especially patients with advanced symptomatic HIV disease.

Warn patients about the use of other medications (eg, ganciclovir, interferon) that may exacerbate the toxicity of zidovudine (see Drug Interactions).

Advise patients to contact their physician if they experience shortness of breath, muscle weakness, symptoms of hepatitis or pancreatitis, or any other unexpected adverse reaction. Inform patients that nausea and vomiting may also occur.

Long-term effects of zidovudine are unknown at this time.

Zidovudine therapy has not been shown to reduce the risk of transmission of HIV to others through sexual contact or blood contamination.

Advise pregnant women considering use of the drug to prevent maternal-fetal transmission of HIV that transmission may still occur in some cases despite therapy. Long-term consequences of in utero and infant exposure are unknown. HIV-infected women should not breastfeed.

Oral: Take exactly as prescribed. Do not share medication and do not exceed the recommended dose.

Administration and Dosage:

Oral:

Monotherapy –

Adults:

Symptomatic HIV infection (including AIDS) – 100 mg (one 100 mg capsule or 2 teaspoonfuls [10 ml] syrup) every 4 hours (600 mg daily dose). The effectiveness of this dose compared to higher dosing regimens in improving neurologic dysfunction associated with HIV disease is unknown. A small study found a greater effect of higher doses on improvement of neurological symptoms in patients with preexisting neurological disease.

Asymptomatic HIV infection – 100 mg every 4 hours while awake (500 mg/day).

Children (3 months to 12 years): The recommended starting dose is 180 mg/m^2 every 6 hours (720 mg/m^2/day), not to exceed 200 mg every 6 hours.

Maternal-Fetal HIV transmission:

Maternal dosing (> 14 weeks of pregnancy) – 100 mg orally 5 times per day until the start of labor. During labor and delivery, administer IV zidovudine at 2 mg/kg over 1 hour followed by a continuous IV infusion of 1 mg/kg/hr until clamping of the umbilical cord.

Infant dosing – 2 mg/kg orally every 6 hours starting within 12 hours after birth and continuing through 6 weeks of age. Infants unable to receive oral dosing may be given zidovudine IV at 1.5 mg/kg, infused over 30 minutes, every 6 hours.

Combination therapy with zalcitabine – Zidovudine 200 mg orally with zalcitabine 0.75 mg every 8 hours.

Monitor hematologic indices every 2 weeks to detect serious anemia or granulocytopenia. In patients with hematologic toxicity, reduction in hemoglobin may occur as early as 2 to 4 weeks, and granulocytopenia usually occurs after 6 to 8 weeks. Hematologic toxicities appear to be related to pretreatment bone marrow reserve and to dose and duration of therapy.

ZIDOVUDINE (Azidothymidine; AZT; Compound S)

Dose adjustment – Significant anemia (hemoglobin of < 7.5 g/dl or reduction of > 25% from baseline) or significant granulocytopenia (granulocyte count of < 750/mm^3 or reduction of > 50% from baseline) may require a dose interruption until evidence of marrow recovery is observed. For less severe anemia or granulocytopenia, dose reduction may be adequate. In patients who develop significant anemia, dose modification does not necessarily eliminate the need for transfusion. If marrow recovery occurs following dose modification, gradual increases in dose may be appropriate depending on hematologic indices and patient tolerance.

Renal function impairment: In end-stage renal disease patients maintained on hemodialysis or peritoneal dialysis, recommended dosing is 100 mg every 6 to 8 hours.

Storage/stability:

Capsules/Syrup – Protect from light.

IV: 1 to 2 mg/kg infused over 1 hour at a constant rate; administer every 4 hours, around the clock. Avoid rapid infusion or bolus injection. Do not give IM. Patients should receive the IV infusion only until oral therapy can be administered. The IV dosing regimen equivalent to the oral administration of 100 mg every 4 hours is approximately 1 mg/kg IV every 4 hours.

Preparation – Dilute prior to administration. Remove the calculated dose from the vial; add to 5% Dextrose Injection to achieve a concentration of ≤ 4 mg/ml.

IV admixture incompatibility – Admixture in biologic or colloidal fluids (eg, blood products, protein solutions) is not recommended.

Storage/stability – After dilution, the solution is physically and chemically stable for 24 hours at room temperature and 48 hours if refrigerated at 2° to 8°C (36° to 46°F). As an additional precaution, administer the diluted solution within 8 hours if stored at 25°C (77°F) or 24 hours if refrigerated at 2° to 8°C to minimize the potential administration of a microbially contaminated solution. Store undiluted vials at 15° to 25°C (59° to 77°F) and protect from light.

Rx	**Retrovir** (Glaxo Wellcome)	**Capsules:** 100 mg	(Wellcome Y9C 100). White with blue band. In 100s.
		Syrup: 50 mg/5 ml	Strawberry flavor. In 240 ml.
		Injection: 10 mg/ml	In 20 ml single use vial.
		Tablets: 300 mg	(GXCW3 300). White. Round, biconvex. Film-coated. In 60s.

LAMIVUDINE (3TC)

Warning:

Lamivudine is indicated for use in combination with zidovudine (AZT) for the treatment of human immunodeficiency virus (HIV) infection when antiretroviral therapy is warranted based on clinical or immunological evidence of disease progression. This indication is based on analyses of surrogate endpoints. At present, there are no results from controlled clinical trials evaluating the effect of therapy with lamivudine plus zidovudine on the clinical progression of HIV infection, such as the incidence of opportunistic infections or survival.

Patients receiving lamivudine plus AZT may continue to develop opportunistic infections and other complications of HIV infection, and should remain under close observation by physicians experienced in treating HIV-associated diseases.

Actions:

Pharmacology: Lamivudine (formerly known as 3TC) is synthetic nucleoside analog with activity against HIV. In vitro, lamivudine is phosphororylated to its active 5'-triphosphate metabolite (L-TP), which has an intracellular half-life of 10.5 to 15.5 hours. The principal mode of action of L-TP is inhibition of HIV reverse transcription via viral DNA chain termination. L-TP also inhibits the RNA- and DNA-dependent DNA polymerase activities of reverse transcriptase.

Pharmacokinetics:

Absorption/Distribution – Lamivudine was rapidly absorbed after oral administration in HIV-infcted patients. Absolute bioavailability in 12 adult patients was 86% for the tablet and 87% for the oral solution. After oral administration of 2 mg/kg twice a day to nine adults with HIV, the peak serum lamivudine concentration (C_{max}) was 1.5 mcg/ml. The area under the plasma concentration vs time curve (AUC) and C_{max} increased in proportion to oral dose over the range from 0.25 to 10 mg/kg. Absorption of lamivudine was slower and C_{max} was lower in the fed state vs the fasted state, but there was no significant difference in AUC (see Drug Interactions)

The apparent volume of distribution after IV administration to 20 patients was 1.3 L/kg, suggesting that lamivudine distributes into extravascular spaces. Volume of distribution was independent of dose and did not correlate with body weight. Binding of lamivudine to human plasma proeins is low (< 36%). In vitro, over the concentration range of 0.1 to 100 pg/ml, the amount of lamivudine associated with erythrocytes ranged rom 53% to 57% and was independent of concentration.

Children: Lamivudine pharmacokinetics after monotherapy were assessed after 1, 2, 4, 8, 12 and 20 mg/kg/day. In the nine infants and children receiving 8 mg/kg/day (the usual recommended pediatric dose), absolute bioavailability was 66%, which is less than the 86% observed in adolescents and adults. The mechanism for this diminished absolute bioavailabiltiy in infants and children is unknown. Systemic clearance decreased with increasing age in pediatric patients.

After oral administration of 8 mg/kg/day to 11 pediatric patients ranging from 4 months to 14 years of age, C_{max} was 1.1 mcg/ml and half-life was 2 hours (in adults with similar blood sampling, the half-life was 3.7 hours). Total exposure to lamivudine, as reflected by mean AUC values, was comparable between pediatric patients receiving an 8 mg/kg/day dose and adults receiving a 4 mg/kg/day dose.

Metabolism – Metabolism of lamivudine is a minor route of elimination. The only known metabolite of lamivudine is the trans-sulfoxide metabolite. Within 12 hours after a single oral dose of lamivudine in six HIV-infected adults, 5.2% of the dose was excreted as the trans-sulfoxide metabolite in the urine. Serum concentrations of this metabolite have not been determined.

Excretion – The majority is eliminated unchanged in urine. In 20 patients given a single IV dose, renal clearance was 0.22 L/hr•kg, representing 71% of total clearance. In most single dose studies, the observed mean elimination half-life ranged from 5 to 7 hours. Total clearance was 0.37 L/hr•kg. Oral clearance and elimination half-life were independent of dose and body weight from 0.25 to 10 mg/kg.

Renal function impairment:

Lamivudine Pharmacokinetis in Renal Function Impairment (Single 300 mg Oral Dose)			
	Creatinine clearance criterion		
Parameter	> 60 ml/min (n = 6)	10 to 30 ml/min (n = 4)	< 10 ml/min (n = 6)
Creatinine clearance (ml/min)	111	28	6
C_{max} (mcg/ml)	2.6	3.6	5.8
AUC (mcg•h/ml)	11	48	157
Cl/F (ml/min)	464	114	36

LAMIVUDINE (3TC)

Exposure (AUC), C_{max} and half-life increased with diminishing renal function (as expressed by Ccr). Apparent total oral clearance (Cl/F) of lamivudine decreased as Ccr decreased. T_{max} was not significantly affected by renal function. Based on these observations, it is recommended that the dosage of lamivudine be modified in patients with renal impairment (see Administration and Dosage). The effects of renal impairment on lamivudine pharmacokinetics inpediatric patients are not known.

Microbiology: Susceptibility of clinical isolates to lamivudine and zidovudine was monitored in controlled clinical trials. In patients receiving lamivudine monotherapy or combination therapy with lamivudine plus zidovudine, HIV-1 isolates from most patients became phenotypically and genotypically resistant to lamivudine within 12 weeks. In some patients harboring zidovudine-resistant virus, phenotypic sensitivity to zidovudine was restored by 12 weeks of treatment. Combination therapy with lamivudine plus zidovudine delayed the emergence of mutations conferring resistance to zidovudine.

The relationship between in vitro susceptibility of HIV to lamivudine and the inhibition of HIV replication in humans has not been established. In HIV-1–infected MT-4 cells, lamivudine in combination with zidovudine had synergistic antiretroviral activity.

Indications:

HIV infection: Lamivudine in combination with zidovudine is indicated for the treatment of HIV infection when therapy is warranted based on clinical or immunological evidence of disease progression. At present, there are no results from controlled trials evaluating the effect of lamivudine plus zidovudine on clinical progression of HIV infection, such as the incidence of opportunistic infections or survival.

Contraindications:

Hypersensitivity to any of the components of the products.

Warnings:

Zidovudine prescribing information: The complete prescribing information for zidovudine should be consulted before combination therapy with lamivudine and zidovudine is initiated.

Renal function impairment: Reduction of the dosage of lamivudine is recommended for patients with impaired renal function (see Administration and Dosage).

Pregnancy: Category C. Some evidence of early embryolethality was seen in the rabbit at doses similar to those produced by the usual adult dose and higher, but there was no indication of this effect in the rat at orally administered doses up to 130 times the usual adult dose. Studies in pregnant rats and rabbits showed that lamivudine is transferred to the fetus through the placenta. There are no adequate and well controlled studies in pregant women. Use during pregnancy only if the potential benefits outweigh the risks.

Antiretroviral pregnancy registry – To monitor maternal-fetal outcomes of pregnant women exposed to lamivudine, an Antiretroviral Pregnancy Registry has been established. Physicians are encouraged to register patients by calling (800)722–9292, ext 58465.

Lactation: A study in which lactating rats were administered 45 mg/kg of lamivudine showed that lamivudine concentrations in milk were slightly greater than those in plasma. Although it is not known if lamivudine is excreted in human breast milk, there is the potential for adverse effects from lamivudine in nursing infants. Instruct mothers to discontinue nursing if they are receiving lamivudine. This instruction is consistent with the CDC recommendation that HIV-infected mothers not breastfeed their infants to avoid risking postnatal transmission of HIV infection.

Children: Following lamivudine monotherapy, AUC and half-life are lower in infants and children compared with adolescents and adults (see Pharmacokinetics). There are no data on the use of lamivudine in combination with zidovudine in pediatric patients.

Pancreatitis – In children with a history of pancreatitis or other significant risk factors for development of pancreatitis, use the combination of lamivudine and zidovudine with extreme caution and only if there is no satisfactory alternative therapy. Stop treatment with lamivudine immediately if clinical signs, symptoms or laboratory abnormalities suggestive of pancreatitis occur (see Adverse Reactions).

LAMIVUDINE (3TC)

Drug Interactions:

Lamivudine Drug Interactions			
Precipitant drug	Object drug*		Description
Lamivudine	Zidovudine	↑	Coadministration of lamivudine with zidovudine resulted in an increase of 39% of zidovudine C_{max}.
Trimethoprim-Sulfamethoxazole	Lamivudine	↑	Coadministration resulted in an increase of 44% in lamivudine AUC, a decrease of 29% in oral clearance and a decrease of 30% in renal clearance. The pharmacokinetic properties of TMP and SMZ were not altered by coadministration.

* ↑ = Object drug increased.

Drug/Food interactions: An investigational 25 mg dosage form of lamivudine was given orally to 12 asymptomatic HIV-infected patients on two occasions, once in the fasted state and once with food (1099 kcal; 75 g fat, 34 g protein, 72 g carbohydrate). Absorption was slower in the fed state (T_{max}, 3.2 hours) compared with the fasted state (T_{max}, 0.9 hours); C_{max} in the fed state was 40% lower than in the fasted state. There was no significant difference in systemic exposure (AUC) in the fed and fasted states; therefore, lamivudine may be administered with or without food.

Adverse Reactions:

Adults:

Selected Adverse Reactions (≥ 5% Frequency) in Adults in Four Controlled Clinical Trials (%)		
Adverse Event	Lamivudine 150 mg bid plus zidovudine (n = 251)	Zidovudine (n = 230)
Body as a whole		
Headache	35	27
Malaise and fatigue	27	23
Fever or chills	10	12
Skin rashes	9	6
GI		
Nausea	33	29
Diarrhea	18	22
Nausea and vomiting	13	12
Anorexia or decreased appetite	10	7
Abdominal pain	9	11
Abdominal cramps	6	3
Dyspepsia	5	5
CNS		
Neuropathy	12	10
Insomnia and other sleep disorders	11	7
Dizziness	10	4
Depressive disorders	9	4
Respiratory		
Nasal signs and symptoms	20	11
Cough	18	13
Musculoskeletal		
Musculoskeletal pain	12	10
Myalgia	8	6
Arthralgia	5	5
Lab test abnormalities		
Neutropenia (ANC[1] < 750/mm^3)	7.2	5.4
Amylase (> 2 ULN)	4.2	1.5
ALT (> 5 × ULN[2])	3.7	3.6
Anemia (Hgb < 8 g/dl)	2.9	1.8
AST (> 5 × ULN)	1.7	1.8
Bilirubin (> 2.5 ULN)	0.8	0.4
Thrombocytopenia (platelets < 50,000/mm^3)	0.4	1.3

[1] ANC = Absolute neutrophil count

[2] ULN = Upper limit of normal

LAMIVUDINE (3TC)

Pancreatitis was observed in 3 of the 656 adult patients (< 0.5%) who received lamivudine in controlled clinical trials.

Children: Limited information on the incidence of adverse events in children receiving monotherapy is available from one open-label uncontrolled sudy. Of 97 patients, 14% developed pancreatitis while receiving monotherapy. In a second ongoing study in 47 pediatric patients (age range, 3 months to 18 years) enrolled in an open-label evaluation of lamivudine/didanosine, lamivudine/zidovudine and lamivudine/zidovudine/didanosine, 15% developed pancreatitis (see Warnings).

Paresthesias and peripheral neuropathies were reported in 13 patients (13%) and resulted in treatment discontinuation in 3 patients.

Selected Laboratory Abnormalities in Pediatric Patients (%; n = 97)		
Test (abnormal level)	Patients with normal baselines	Patients with abnormal baselines
Neutropenia (ANC < 750/mm^3)	22	45
Anemia (Hgb < 8 g/dl)	2	24
Thrombocytopenia (platelets < 40,000/mm^3)	0	25
ALT (> 5 × ULN)	4	29
AST (> 5 × ULN)	0	19
Amylase (> 2 ULN)	3	23

Overdosage:

One case of an adult ingesting 6 g of lamivudine was reported; there were no clinical signs or symptoms noted and hematologic tests remained normal. It is not known whether lamivudine can be removed by peritoneal dialysis or hemodialysis. There is no known antidote for lamivudine.

Patient Information:

Lamivudine is not a cure for HIV infection and patients may continue to experience illnesses associated with HIV infection, including opportunistic infections. Treatment with lamivudine has not been shown to reduce the frequency of such illnesses and patients should remain undr the care of a physician when using lamivudine.

Advise patients that the use of lamivudine has not been shown to reduce the risk of transmission of HIV to others through sexual contact or blood contamination.

Advise patients that the long-term effects of lamivudine are unknown at this time.

Advise patients of the importance of taking lamivudine exactly as it is prescribed.

Advise parents to monitor pediatric patients for symptoms of pancreatitis.

Administration and Dosage:

Approved by the FDA on November 17, 1995.

Adults and adolescents (12 to 16 years of age): The recommended dose is 150 mg twice daily in combination with zidovudine. Consult the complete prescribing information for zidovudine for information on its dosage and administration.

For adults withlow body weights (< 50 kg; < 110 lbs), the recommended dose is 2 mg/kg twice daily in combination with zidovudine. No data are available to support a dosage recommendation for adolescents with low body weight (< 50 kg).

Children (3 months to 12 years of age): The recommended dose is 4 mg/kg twice daily (up to a maximum of 150 mg twice a day) administered with zidovudine.

Renal function impairment: It is recommended that doses of lamivudine be adjusted in accordance with renal function in patients > 16 years of age.

Adjustment of Lamivudine Dosage in Patients with Renal Function Impairment	
Creatinine clearance (ml/min)	Recommended lamivudine dosage
≤ 50	150 mg twice daily
30 - 49	150 mg once daily
15 - 29	150 mg first dose, then 100 mg once daily
5 - 14	150 mg first dose, then 50 mg once daily
< 5	50 mg first dose, then 25 mg once daily

Insufficient data are available to recommend a dosage of lamivudine in dialysis.

Storage: Store solution at 2° to 25°C (36° to 77°F) tightly closed.

Rx	**Epivir** (Glaxo Wellcome)	**Tablets:** 150 mg	(150 GXCJ7). White. Diamond shaped. Film coated. In 60s.
		Oral Solution: 10 mg/ml	Sucrose. Strawberry-banana flavor. In 240 ml.

SAQUINAVIR MESYLATE

Warning:
The indication for saquinavir for the treatment of HIV infection is based on changes in surrogate markers. At present, there are no results from controlled clinical trials evaluating the effect of regimens containing saquinavir on patient survival or the clinical progression HIV infection, such as the occurrence of opportunistic infections or malignancies.

Actions:

Pharmacology: Saquinavir is an inhibitor of the human immunodeficiency virus (HIV) protease. HIV protease cleaves viral polyprotein precursors to generate functional proteins in HIV-infected cells. The cleavage of viral polyprotein precursors is essential for maturation of infectious virus. Saquinavir is a synthetic peptide-like substrate analog that inhibits the activity of HIV protease and prevents the cleavage of viral polyproteins.

Pharmacokinetics:

Absorption – Following multiple dosing (600 mg 3 times daily) in HIV-infected patients, the steady-state area under the plasma concentration-time curve (AUC) was 2.5 times higher than that observed after a single dose. HIV-infected patients administered saquinavir 600 mg 3 times daily, after a meal or substantial snack, had AUC and maximum plasma concentration (C_{max}) values which were about twice those observed in healthy volunteers receiving the same treatment regimen.

Absolute bioavailability averaged 4% in 8 healthy volunteers who received a single 600 mg dose following a high fat breakfast (48 g protein, 60 g carbohydrate, 57 g fat, 1006 kcal). The low bioavailability is thought to be due to a combination of incomplete absorption and extensive first-pass metabolism.

Distribution – The mean steady-state voume of distributin following IV administration of a 12 mg dose was 700 L, suggesting saquinavir partitions into tissues. Saquinavir was ≈ 98% bound to plasma proteins over a concentration range of 15 to 700 ng/ml. In two patients receiving saquinavir 600 mg 3 times daily, CSF concentrations were negligible.

Metabolism/Excretion – In vitro, the metabolism of saquinavir is cytochrome P450 mediated with specific isoenzyme, CYP3A4, responsible for > 90% of the hepatic metabolism. In vitro, saquinavir is rapidly metabolized to a range of mono- and di-hydroxylated inactive compounds; 88% and 1% of the orally administered dose was recovered in feces and urine, respectively, within 48 hours of dosing; 81% and 3% of an IV dose was recovered in feces and urine, respectively, within 48 hours of dosing. In mass balance studies, 13% of circulating radioactivity in plasma was attributed to unchanged drug after oral administration and the remainder attributed to saquinavir metabolites. Following IV administration, 66% of circulating radioactivity was attributed to unchanged drug and the remainder attributed to saquinavir metabolites, suggesting that saquinavir undergoes extensive first-pass metabolism.

Systemic clearance of saquinavir was rapid, 1.14 L/hr/kg after IV doses of 6, 36 and 72 mg. The mean residence time of saquinavir was 7 hours.

Microbiology:

Anitviral activity in vitro – In cell culture, saquinavir demonstrated additive to synergistic effects against HIV in double and triple combination regimens with reverse transcriptase inhibitors zidovudine (AZT), zalcitabine (ddC) and didanosine (ddI), without enhanced cytotoxicity.

Cross-resistance to other antiretrovirals – The potential for HIV cross-resistance between protease inhibitors has not been fully explored. Therefore, it is unknown what effect saquinavir therapy will have on the activity of subsequent protease inhibitors. Cross-resistance between saquinavir and reverse transcriptase inhibitors is unlikely because of the different enzyme targets involved. AZT-resistant HIV isolates have been shown to be sensitive to saquinavir in vitro.

Clinical trials:

Advanced patients without prior AZT therapy – A study compared saquinavir doses of 75, 200 and 600 mg 3 times daily in combination with AZT 200 mg 3 times daily to saquinavir 600 mg 2 times daily alone and AZT alone. In analyses of average CD4 changes over 16 weeks, treatment with the combination of saquinavir 600 mg 3 times daily plus AZT produced greater CD4 cell increases than AZT monotherapy. The CD4 changes of AZT in combination with doses of saquinavir < 600 mg 3 times daily were no greater than that of AZT alone.

Advanced patients with prior AZT therapy – Patients (mean baseline CD4 = 165) with prolonged AZT treatment (median, 713 days) were randomized to receive either saquinavir 600 mg 3 times daily plus ddC plus AZT (triple combination), saquinavir 600 mg 3 times daily plus AZT or ddC plus AZT. In analyses of average CD4 changes over 24 weeks, the triple combination produced greater increases in CD4 cell counts compared with that of ddC plus AZT. There were no significant differences in CD4 changes among patients receiving saquinavir plus AZT and ddC plus AZT.

An ongoing study is comparing saquinavir 600 mg plus ddC to ddC monotherapy and saquinavir monotherapy in patients with advanced HIV infection and at least 16 weeks of prior AZT treatment. The study remains blinded with respect to clinical endpoints of disease progression; however, analyses of CD4 changes over 16 weeks were conducted for a cohort of 423 patients. These analyses showed that the combination of saquinavir plus ddC was associated with greater CD4 increases than either ddC or saquinavir as monotherapy.

Comparisons of data across studies suggest that when saquinavir was added to a regimen of prolonged prior zidovudine, there was little activity contributed by continuing AZT.

Indications:

HIV infection: In combination with nucleoside analogs for the treatment of advanced HIV infection in selected patients. This indication is based on changes in surrogate markers in patients who initiated saquinavir concomitantly with either AZT (in previously untreated patients) or ddC (in patients previously treated with prolonged zidovudine therapy). At present, no resuts are available from trials evaluating the activity of saquinavir in combination with nucleoside analogs other than AZT or ddC. There are no results available from clinical trials confirming the clinical benefit of combination therapy with saquinavir on HIV disease progression or survival.

Contraindications:

Clinically significant hypersensitivity to saquinavir or to any of the components in the capsule.

Photosensitization (photoallergy or phototoxicity) may occur; therefore, caution patients to take protective measures against exposure to ultraviolet or sunlight (ie, sunscreens, protective clothing) until tolerance is determined.

Warnings:

Hepatic function impairment: Exercise caution when administering saquinavir to patients with hepatic insufficiency because patients with baseline liver function tests > 5 times the normal upper limit were not included in clinical studies.

Pregnancy: Category B. Use during pregnancy after taking into account the importance of the drug to the mother.

Lactation: It is not known whether saquinavir is excreted in breast milk. Because of the potential for serious adverse reactions in nursing infants from saquinavir, decide whether to discontinue nursing or discontinue the drug, taking into account the importance of saquinavir to the mother.

Children: Safety and efficacy in HIV-infected children or adolescents < 16 years of age have not been established.

Precautions:

Toxicity: If a serious or severe toxicity occurs during treatment with saquinavir, interrupt therapy until the etiology of the event is identified or the toxicity resolves. At that time, resumption of treatment with full dose saquinavir may be considered.

Monitoring: Perform clinical chemistry tests prior to initiating saquinavir therapy and at appropriate intervals thereafter.

Drug Interactions:

Saquinavir Drug Interactions			
Precipitant drug	Object drug*		Description
Ketoconazole	Saquinavir	⬆	Concomitant administration resulted in steady-state saquinavir AUC and C_{max} values that were three times those seen with saquinavir alone. No dose adjustment is required.
Rifamycins	Saquinavir	⬇	Coadministration of rifampin decreased the steady-state AUC and C_{max} of saquinavir by ≈ 80%. Steady-state AUC of saquinavir was decreased by 40% when saquinavir was coadministered with rifabutin.

* ⬆ = Object drug increased. ⬇ = Object drug decreased.

Other drugs that induce CYP3A4 (eg, phenobarbital, phenytoin, dexamethasone, carbamazepine) may reduce saquinavir plasma conentrations. If therapy with such drugs is warranted, consider using alternatives when a patient is taking saquinavir.

Coadministration of terfenadine or astemizole with drugs that are known to be potent inhibitors of the cytochrome P4503A pathway (eg, ketoconazole, itraconazole) may lead to elevated plasma concentrations of terfenadine or astemizole, which may in turn prolong QT intervals leading to rare cases of serious cardiovascular adverse events. Although saquinavir is not a strong inhibitor of cytochrome P4503A, use alternatives to terfenadine or astemizole when a patient taking saquinavir requires antihistamines. Other compunds that are substrates of CYP3A4 (eg, calcium channel blockers, clindamycin, dapsone, quinidine, triazolam) may have elevated plasma concentrations when coadministered with saquinavir; therefore, monitor patients for toxicities associated with such drugs.

Drug/Food interactions: Absolute bioavailability averaged 4% in eight healthy volunteers who received a single 600 mg dose following a high fat breakfast (48 g protein, 60 g carbohydrate, 57 g fat, 1006 kcal). The low bioavailability may be due to a combination of incomplete absorption and extensive first-pass metabolism. The mean 24 hour AUC after a single 600 mg oral dose in healthy volunteers was increased from 24 (under fasting conditions to 161 ng•hr/ml when saquinavir was given following a high fat breakfast. Saquinavir 24 hour AUC and C_{max} following the administration of a higher calorie meal (943 kcal, 54 g fat) were on average two times higher than after a lower calorie, lower fat meal (355 kcal, 8 g fat). The effect of food persists for up to 2 hours.

Adverse Reactions:

The majority of adverse events were of mild intensity. The most frequently reported adverse events among patients receiving saquinavir were diarrhea, abdominal discomfort and nausea. Rare occurrences of the following serious adverse experiences have been reported during clinical trials of saquinavir: Confusion, ataxia and weakness; acute myeloblastic leukemia; hemolytic anemia; attempted suicide; Stevens-Johnson syndrome; seizures; severe cutaneous reaction associated with increased liver funciton tests; isolated elevation of transaminases, thrombophlebitis, headache and thrombocytopenia; exacerbation of chronic liver disease with Grade 4 elevated liver function tests, jaundice, ascites and right and left upper quadrant abdominal pain.

Saquinavir Adverse Reactions (%)

	Study 1			Study 2		
Adverse reaction	SAQ + AZT (n = 99)	SAQ + ddC + AZT (n = 98)	ddC + AZT (n = 100)	ddC (n = 145)	SAQ (n = 159)	SAQ + ddC (n = 147)
GI						
Diarrhea	3	1	=	1.4	3.8	3.4
Abdominal discomfort	2	3.1	4	1.4	1.3	0.7
Nausea		3.1	3	0.7	1.9	0.7
Dyspepsia	1	1	2	2.1		0.7
Abdominal pain	2	1	2	0.7	1.9	0.7
Mucosa damage	=	=	4	1.4	=	0.7
Buccal mucosa ulceration	=	2	2	9	2.5	4.1
Neurologic						
Headache	2	2	2	4.1	0.6	0.7
Paresthesia	2	3.1	4	0.7	1	1
Extremity numbness	2	1	4	=	=	0.7
Dizziness	=	2	1	=	=	=
Peripheral neuropathy	=	1	2	5.5	=	4.8
Body as a whole						
Asthenia	6.1	9.2	10	0.7	1.3	0.7
Appetite disturbances	=	1	2	=	=	=
Dermatologic						
Rash	=	=	3	0.7	1.3	1.4
Pruritus	=	=	2	=	=	=
Musculoskeletal						
Musculoskeletal pain	2	2	4	=	0.6	0.7

Saquinavir Adverse Reactions (%)						
	Study 1			Study 2		
Adverse reaction	SAQ + AZT (n = 99)	SAQ + ddC + AZT (n = 98)	ddC + AZT (n = 100)	ddC (n = 145)	SAQ (n = 159)	SAQ + ddC (n = 147)
Myalgia	1	=	3	1.4	=	=
Lab test abnormalities						
Calcium (high)	1	0	0	< 1	0	0
Creatine phosphokinase	10	12	7	6	4	7
Glucose (low)	0	0	0	4	5	4
Glucose (high)	0	0	0	0	< 1	< 1
Phosphorus	2	1	0	0	0	0
Potassium (high)	0	0	0	1	< 1	< 1
Potassium (low)	0	0	0	0	< 1	0
Serum amylase	2	1	1	< 1	< 1	2
AST	2	2	0	3	< 1	< 1
ALT	0	3	1	3	< 1	< 1
Total bilirubin	1	0	0	0	< 1	0
Uric acid	0	0	1	NA	NA	NA
Neutrophils (low)	2	2	8	0	0	0
Hemoglobin (low)	0	0	1	0	< 1	0
Platelets (low)	0	0	2	0	0	< 1

= Indicates no events reported. NA - Not assessed.

Other clinical adverse experiences of any intensity are listed below by body system.

Body as a whole: Allergic reaction; chest pain; edema; fever; intoxication; parasites external; retrosternal pain; shivering; wasting syndrome; weight decrese; abscess; angina tonsillaris; candidiasis; hepatitis; herpes simples; herpes zoster; infection (bacterial/mycotic/staphylococcal); influenza; lymphadenopathy; tumor.

Cardiovascular: Cyanosis; heart murmur; heart valve disorder; hypertension; hypotension; syncope; vein distended.

Metabolic: Dehydration; dry eye syndrome; hyperglycemia; weight increase; xerophothalmia.

GI: Cheilitis; constipation; dysphagia; eructation; bloodstained/discolored feces; gastralgia; gastritis; GI inflammation; gingivitis; glossitis; rectal hemorrhage; hemorrhoids; hepatomegaly; hepatosplenomegaly; melena; pain; painful defecation; pancreatitis; parotid disorder; pelvic salivary glands disorder; stomatitis; tooth disorder; vomiting.

Hematologic: Anemia; microhemorrhages; pancytopenia; splenomegly; thrombocytopenia.

Musculoskeletal: Arthralgia; arthritis; back pain; muscle cramps; musculoskeletal disorders; stiffness; tissue changes; trauma.

CNS: Ataxia; frequent bowel movements; confusion; convusions; dysarthria; dysesthesia; heart rate disorder; hyperesthesia; hyperreflexia; hyporeflexia; dry mouth; face numbness; facial pain; paresis; poliomyelitis; progressive multifocal leukoencephalopathy; spasms; tremor.

Psychiatric: Agitation; amnesia; anxiety; depession; dreaming excessive; euphoria; hallucination; insomnia; reduced intellectual ability; irritability; lethargy; libido disorder; overdose effect; psychic disorder; somnolence; speech disorder.

GU: Prostate enlarged; vaginal discharge; micturiton disorder; urinary tract infection.

Respiratory: Bronchitis; cough; dyspnea; epistaxis; hemoptysis; laryngitis; pharyngitis; pneumonia; respiratory disorder rhinitis; sinusitis; upper respiratory tract infection.

Dermatologic: Acne; dermatitis; seborrheic dermatitis; eczema; erythema; folliculitis; furunculosis; hair changes; hot flushes; photosensitivity reaction; skin pigment

SAQUINAVIR MESYLATE

changes; maculopapular rash; skin disorder/nodule/ulceration; sweating increased; urticaria; verruca; xeroderma.

Special senses: Blepharitis; earache; ear pressure; eye irritation; hearing decreased; otitis; taste alteration; tinnitus; visual disturbance.

Overdosage:

No acute toxicities or sequelae were noted in one patient who ingested 8 g saquinavir as a single dose. The patient was treated with induction of emesis within 2 to 4 hours after ingestion. In an exploratory Phase II study with saquinavir at 7200 mg/day, no serious toxicities were reported through the first 25 weeks of treatment.

Patient Information:

Inform patients that saquinavir is not acure for HIV infection and that they may continue to acquire illnesses associated with advanced HIV infection, including opportunistic infections. Saquinavir has not been shown to reduce the incidence or frequency of such illnesses; advise patients to remain under the care of a physician while using saquinavir.

Tell patients that the long-term effects of saquinavir are unknown at this time. Inform them that saquinavir therapy has not been shown to reduce the risk of transmitting HIV to others through sexual conduct or blood contamination.

Advise patients that saquinavir should be taken within 2 hours after a full meal. When saquinavir is taken without food, concentrations of saquinavir in the blood are substantially reduced and may result in no antiviral activity.

Photosensitization (photoallergy or phototoxicity) may occur; therefore, caution patients to take protective measures against exposure to ultraviolet or sunlight (ie, sunscreens, protective clothing) until tolerance is determined.

Administration and Dosage:

Approved by the FDA on December 6, 1995.

The recommended dose for saquinavir in combination with a nucleoside analog is three 200 mg capsules 3 times daily taken within 2 hours after a full meal. The recommended doses of ddC or AZT as part of combination therapy are: ddC 0.75 mg 3 times daily, or AZT 200 mg 3 times daily as appropriate.

Dose adjustment for combination therapy with saquinavir: For toxicities that may be associated with saquinavir, interrupt the drug. Saquinavir at doses < 600 mg 3 times daily are not recommended since lower doses have not shown antiviral activity. For recipients of combination therapy with saquinavir and nucleoside analogs, dose adjustment of the nucleoside analog should be based on the known toxicity profile of the individual drug.

Rx	**Invirase** (Roche)	**Capsules:** 200 mg	Lactose. (Roche 0245). Lt. brown/green. In 270s.

NEVIRAPINE

Warning:

The duration of benefit from antiretroviral therapy may be limited. Consider alteration of antiretroviral therapies if disease progression occurs while patients are receiving nevirapine.

Resistant HIV virus emerges rapidly and uniformly when nevirapine is administered as monotherapy. Therefore, always administer nevirapine in combination with at least one additional antiretroviral agent.

Nevirapine has been associated with severe rash, which in some cases, has been life-threatening. When severe rash occurs, discontinue nevirapine.

Actions:

Pharmacology: Nevirapine is a non-nucleoside reverse transcriptase inhibitor (NNRTI) with activity against human immunodeficiency virus type 1 (HIV-1). Nevirapine is structurally a member of the dipyridodiazepinone chemical class of compounds.

Nevirapine binds directly to reverse transcriptase (RT) and blocks the RNA-dependent and DNA-dependent DNA polymerase activities by causing a disruption of the enzyme's catalytic site. The activity of nevirapine does not compete with template or nucleoside triphosphates. HIV-2 RT and eukaryotic DNA polymerases (such as human DNA polymerases α, β, γ or δ) are not inhibited by nevirapine.

In vitro HIV susceptibility – The relationship between in vitro susceptibility of HIV-1 to nevirapine and the inhibition of HIV-1 replication in humans has not been established. The in vitro antiviral activity of nevirapine was measured in peripheral blood mononuclear cells, monocyte derived macrophages and lymphoblastoid cell lines. IC_{50} values (50% inhibitory concentration) ranged from 10 to 100 nM against laboratory and clinical isolates of HIV-1. In cell culture, nevirapine demonstrated additive to synergistic activity against HIV in drug combination regimens with zidovudine (AZT), didanosine (ddI), stavudine (d4t), lamivudine (3TC) and saquinavir.

Resistance – HIV isolates with reduced susceptibility (100- to 250-fold) to nevirapine emerge in vitro. Genotypic analysis showed mutations in the HIV RT gene at amino acid positions 181 or 106, depending upon the virus strain and cell line employed. Time to emergence of nevirapine resistance in vitro was not altered when selection included nevirapine in combination with several other NNRTIs.

Cross-resistance – Rapid emergence of HIV strains which are cross-resistant to NNRTIs has been observed in vitro. Data on cross-resistance between the NNRTI nevirapine and nucleoside analog RT inhibitors are limited. Cross-resistance between nevirapine and HIV protease inhibitors is unlikely because the enzyme targets involved are different.

Pharmacokinetics:

Absorption and bioavailability – Nevirapine is readily absorbed (> 90%) after oral administration in healthy volunteers and in adults with HIV-1 infection. Absolute bioavailability was 93% for a 50 mg tablet and 91% for an oral solution. Peak plasma nevirapine concentrations of 2 mcg/ml (7.5 μM) were attained within 4 hours following a single 200 mg dose. Following multiple doses, nevirapine peak concentrations appear to increase linearly in the dose range of 200 to 400 mg/day. Steady-state trough nevirapine concentrations of 4.5 mcg/ml were attained at 400 mg/day.

Food – When nevirapine 200 mg was administered to 24 healthy adults (12 female, 12 male) with either a high fat breakfast (857 kcal, 50 g fat, 53% of calories from fat) or antacid, the extent of nevirapine absorption (AUC) was comparable to that observed under fasting conditions. In a separate study in HIV-1–infected patients (n = 6), nevirapine steady-state systemic exposure was not significantly altered by didanosine, which is formulated with an alkaline buffering agent. Administer nevirapine with or without food, antacids or didanosine.

Distribution – Nevirapine is highly lipophilic and is essentially nonionized at physiologic pH. Following IV administration to healthy adults, the volume of distribution of nevirapine was 1.21 L/kg, suggesting that nevirapine is widely distributed in humans. Nevirapine readily crosses the placenta and is found in breast milk. Nevirapine is ≈ 60% bound to plasma proteins in the plasma concentration range of 1 to 10 mcg/ml. Nevirapine concentrations in human cerebrospinal fluid were 45% of concentrations in plasma; this ratio is approximately equal to the fraction not bound to plasma protein.

Metabolism/Elimination – In vivo studies in humans and in vitro studies with human liver microsomes have shown that nevirapine is extensively biotransformed via cytochrome P450 (oxidative) metabolism to several hydroxylated metabolites. In vitro studies with human liver microsomes suggest that oxidative metabolism of nevirapine is mediated primarily by cytochrome P450 isozymes from the CYP3A family, although other isozymes may have a secondary role. In a mass balance/excretion study in eight healthy male volunteers dosed to steady-state with nevirapine 200 mg given twice daily followed by a single 50 mg dose of ^{14}C-nevirapine, ≈ 91.4% of the dose was recovered, with urine (81.3%) representing the primary route of excretion compared to feces (10.1%). Greater than 80% of the radioactivity in urine was made up of glucuronide conjugates of hydroxylated metabolites. Thus cytochrome P450 metabolism, glucuronide conjugation and urinary excretion of glucuronidated metabolites represent the primary route of nevirapine biotransformation and elimination in humans. Only a small fraction (< 5%) of the radioactivity in urine (representing < 3% of the total dose) was made up of parent compound; therefore, renal excretion plays a minor role in elimination of the parent compound.

Nevirapine has been shown to be an inducer of hepatic cytochrome P450 metabolic enzymes. The pharmacokinetics of autoinduction are characterized by an ≈ 1.5– to 2–fold increase in the apparent oral clearance of nevirapine as treatment continues from a single dose to 2 to 4 weeks of dosing with 200 to 400 mg/day. Autoinduction also results in a corresponding decrease in the terminal phase half-life of nevirapine in plasma from ≈ 45 hours (single dose) to ≈ 25 to 30 hours following multiple dosing with 200 to 400 mg/day.

Race – An evaluation of nevirapine plasma concentrations (pooled data from several clinical trials) from HIV-1–infected patients (27 African-American, 24 Hispanic, 189 Caucasian) revealed no marked difference in nevirapine steady-state trough concentrations (median $Cmin_{ss}$ = 4.7 mcg/ml African-American, 3.8 mcg/ml Hispanic, 4.3 mcg/ml Caucasian) with long-term nevirapine treatment at 400 mg/day. However, the pharmacokinetics of nevirapine have not been evaluated specifically in the effects of ethnicity.

Clinical trials:

Resistance – Phenotypic and genotypic changes in HIV-1 isolates from patients treated with either nevirapine (n = 24) or nevirapine and AZT (n = 14) were monitored in Phase I/II trials over 1 to ≥ 12 weeks. After 1 week of nevirapine monotherapy, isolates from three of three patients had decreased susceptibility to nevirapine in vitro; one or more of the RT mutations at amino acid positions 103, 106, 108, 181, 188 and 190 were detected in some patients as early as 2 weeks after therapy initiation. By week eight of nevirapine monotherapy, 100% of the patients tested (n = 24) had HIV isolates with a > 100–fold decrease in susceptibility to nevirapine in vitro compared with baseline and had one or more of the nevirapine-associated RT resistance mutations; 19 of 24 patients (80%) had isolates with a position 181 mutation regardless of dose. Nevirapine + AZT combination therapy did not alter the emergence rate of nevirapine-resistant virus or the magnitude of nevirapine resistance in vitro; however, a different RT mutation pattern, predominantly distributed amongst amino acid positions 103, 106, 188 and 190 was observed. In patients (6 of 14) whose baseline isolates possessed a wild type RT gene, nevirapine + AZT combination therapy did not appear to delay emergence of AZT-resistant RT mutations. The clinical relevance of phenotypic and genotypic changes associated with nevirapine therapy has not been established.

No history of prior antiretroviral therapy – One study compared treatment with nevirapine + AZT + ddI vs nevirapine + AZT vs AZT + ddI in 151 HIV-1–infected patients (median age 36 years, 94% Caucasian, 93% male) with CD4+ cell counts of 200 to 600 cells/mm^3 (mean, 376 cells/mm^3) and a mean baseline plasma HIV-1 RNA concentration of 4.41 $\log_{10}$ copies/ml (25,704 copies/ml). Treatment doses were 200 mg daily nevirapine for 2 weeks, followed by 200 mg twice daily or placebo; AZT, 200 mg 3 times daily; ddI, 125 or 200 mg twice daily. Changes in CD4+ cell counts at 24 weeks: Mean levels of CD4+ cell counts in those randomized to nevirapine + AZT + ddI and AZT + ddI remained significantly above baseline; however, there was no significant difference between these arms. Changes in HIV-1 viral RNA at 24 weeks: There was no significant difference as measured by mean changes in plasma viral RNA between those randomized to nevirapine + AZT + ddI and AZT + ddI. However, the proportion of patients whose HIV-1 RNA decreased below the limit of detection (400 copies/ml) was significantly greater for the nevirapine + AZT + ddI group (27/36 or 75%), when compared to the AZT + ddI group (18/39 or 46%) or the nevirapine + AZT group (0/28 or 0%); the clinical significance of this finding is unknown.

Indications:

HIV-1 infection: In combination with nucleoside analogs for the treatment of HIV-1 infected adults who have experienced clinical and immunologic deterioration.

Contraindications:

Hypersensitivity to any of the components contained in the product.

Warnings:

Skin reactions: Severe and life-threatening skin reactions have occurred in patients treated with nevirapine including Stevens-Johnson syndrome (SJS). Discontinue nevirapine in patients developing a severe rash accompanied by constitutional symptoms such as fever, blistering, oral lesions, conjunctivitis, swelling, muscle or joint aches or general malaise.

The majority of rashes associated with nevirapine occur within the first 6 weeks of initiation of therapy. Therefore, monitor patients carefully for the appearance of rash during this period. Instruct patients not to increase the 200 mg/day dosage if any rash occurs during the 2-week lead-in dosing period until the rash resolves.

Rashes are usually mild to moderate, maculopapular, erythematous cutaneous eruptions with or without pruritus, located on the trunk, face and extremities.

Alteration of antiretroviral therapy: The duration of benefit from antiretroviral therapy may be limited. Alteration of antiretroviral therapy should be considered if disease progression occurs while patients are receiving nevirapine.

Resistant virus emerges rapidly and uniformly when nevirapine is administered as monotherapy. Therefore, always administer nevirapine in combination with at least one additional antiretroviral agent.

Renal/Hepatic function impairment: The pharmacokinetics of nevirapine have not been evaluated in patients with either hepatic or renal dysfunction. Therefore, use with caution in these patient populations.

Hepatotoxicity – Abnormal liver function tests have been reported with nevirapine, some in the first few weeks of therapy, including cases of hepatitis. Interrupt administration in patients experiencing moderate or severe liver function test abnormalities until liver function tests return to baseline values. Discontinue treatment permanently if liver function abnormalities recur on readministration.

NEVIRAPINE

Pregnancy: Category C. No teratogenicity was observed in reproductive studies performed in pregnant rats and rabbits. There are no adequate and well controlled studies in pregnant women. Administer nevirapine during pregnancy only if the potential benefit justifies the risk to the fetus.

Lactation: Preliminary results from an ongoing pharmacokinetic study (ACTG 250) of 10 HIV-1 infected pregnant women who were administered a single oral dose of 100 or 200 mg nevirapine at a median of 5.8 hours before delivery indicate that nevirapine readily crosses the placenta and is found in breast milk. Instruct patients receiving nevirapine to discontinue nursing.

Children: Safety and efficacy has not been established. Nevirapine is metabolized more rapidly in pediatric patients than in adults.

Precautions:

Monitoring: Perform clinical chemistry tests, which include liver function tests, prior to initiating nevirapine therapy and at appropriate intervals during therapy.

Drug Interactions:

Nevirapine Drug Interactions			
Precipitant drug	Object drug*		Description
Rifampin Rifabutin	Nevirapine	⬇	Steady-state nevirapine trough concentrations were reduced in patients who received rifabutin and rifampin, known inducers of CYP3A. Nevirapine is an inducer of CYP3A, with maximal induction occurring within 2 to 4 weeks of initiating multiple-dose therapy. There are insufficient data to assess whether dose adjustments are necessary when nevirapine and rifampin or rifabutin are coadministered. Therefore, these drugs should only be used in combination if clearly indicated and with careful monitoring.
Nevirapine	Protease inhibitors	⬇	Nevirapine may decrease plasma concentrations of protease inhibitors. These drugs should not be administered concomitantly with nevirapine.
Nevirapine	Oral contraceptives	⬇	Nevirapine may decrease plasma concentrations of oral contraceptives (also other hormonal contraceptives); therefore, these drugs should not be administered concomitantly with nevirapine.

* ⬇ = Object drug decreased.

Adverse Reactions:

The most frequent adverse events related to nevirapine therapy are rash, fever, nausea, headache and abnormal liver function tests. Other frequent reactions include:

Comparative Incidence of Selected Nevirapine (NVP) Drug-Related Events				
Adverse reaction	NVP + ZDV + ddI (n = 197)	ZDV + ddI (n = 201)	NVP + ZDV (n = 55)	ZDV (n = 30)
Rash	8	2	20	3
Fever	3	3	11	3
Nausea	5	4	9	3
Headache	3	3	11	0
Diarrhea	2	2	0	0
Abdominal pain	1	2	2	0
Ulcerative stomatitis	0	0	4	0
Peripheral neuropathy	0	2	0	0
Paresthesia	1	0	2	0
Myalgia	1	0	2	7
Hepatitis	1	0	4	0

Patients with Marked Laboratory Abnormalities After Nevirapine Administration (%)[1]		
Abnormality parameters	Nevirapine (n = 252)	Control (n = 255)
Hematology		
Decreased Hg (< 8 g/dl)	1.2	2
Decreased platelets (< 50,000/mm^3)	0.8	0.8
Decreased neutrophils (< 750/mm^3)	11.1	10.2
Blood chemistry		
Increased ALT (> 250 U/L)	3.4	3.5
Increased AST (> 250 U/L)	2.0	2.4
Increased GGT (> 450 U/L)	2.4	1.2
Increased total bilirubin (> 2.5 mg/dl)	0.4	1.2

[1] Data combined for controlled trials.

Overdosage:

There is no known antidote for nevirapine overdosage. No acute toxicities or sequelae were reported for one patient who ingested 800 mg of nevirapine in one day.

Administration and Dosage:

Initial therapy: 200 mg tablet daily for 14 days.

Maintenance: 200 mg tablet twice daily in combination with nucleoside analog antiretroviral agents. For concomitantly administered nucleoside therapy, the manufacturer's recommended dosage and monitoring should be followed.

Missed doses: Patients who interrupt nevirapine dosing for more than 7 days should restart the recommended dosing, using one 200 mg tablet daily for the first 14 days (lead-in), followed by one 200 mg twice daily.

Storage/Stability: Store at 15° to 30°C (59° to 86°F). Keep bottle tightly closed.

Rx	**Viramune** (Roxane)	**Tablets:** 200 mg	Lactose. (54 193). White, scored. Oval, biconvex. In 100s and UD 100s.

NELFINAVIR MESYLATE

Warning:
Nelfinavir is indicated for the treatment of human immunodeficiency virus (HIV) infection when antiretroviral therapy is warranted. This indication is based on surrogate marker changes in patients who received nelfinavir in combination with nucleoside analogues or alone for ≤ 24 weeks. At present, there are no results from controlled trials evaluating the effect of therapy with nelfinavir on clinical progression of HIV infection, such as survival or the incidence of opportunistic infections.

Actions:

Pharmacology: Nelfinavir is an inhibitor of the HIV-1 protease. Inhibition of the viral protease prevents cleavage of the gagpol polyprotein resulting in the production of immature, non-infectious virus.

The antiviral activity of nelfinavir in vitro has been demonstrated in both acute and chronic HIV infections in lymphoblastoid cell lines, peripheral blood lymphocytes and monocytes/macrophages. Nelfinavir was found to be active against several laboratory strains of HIV-1 and several clinical isolates of HIV-1 and the HIV-2 strain ROD. The EC_{95} (95% effective concentration) of nelfinavir ranges from 7 to 196 nM. In combination with reverse transcriptase inhibitors, nelfinavir demonstrated additive (didanosine or stavudine) to synergistic (zidovudine, lamivudine or zalcitabine) antiviral activity in vitro without enhanced cytotoxicity. Drug combination studies with protease inhibitors (ritonavir, saquinavir or indinavir) showed variable results ranging from antagonistic to synergistic.

Drug resistance – One or more virus protease mutations at amino acid positions 30, 35, 36, 46, 71, 77 and 88 were detected in > 10% of patients with evaluable isolates.

Cross-resistance – HIV isolates from five patients during nelfinavir therapy showed a 5- to 93-fold decrease in nelfinavir susceptibility in vitro when compared with matched baseline isolates but did not demonstrate a concordant decrease in susceptibility to indinavir, ritonavir, saquinavir or 141W94, in vitro. Cross-resistance between nelfinavir and reverse transcriptase inhibitors is unlikely because different enzyme targets are involved.

Pharmacokinetics:

Absorption – After single and multiple oral doses of 500 to 750 mg with food, peak nelfinavir plasma concentrations were typically achieved in 2 to 4 hours. After multiple dosing with 750 mg 3 times daily for 28 days (steady-state), peak plasma concentrations (C_{max}) averaged 3 to 4 mcg/ml and plasma concentrations prior to the morning dose (trough) were 1 to 3 mcg/ml (trough sample collection times averaged 11 hours after the previous evening dose). A greater than dose-proportional increase in nelfinavir plasma concentrations was observed after single doses; however, this was not observed after multiple dosing.

Effect of food: Maximum plasma concentrations and area under the plasma concentration-time curve (AUC) were 2- to 3-fold higher under fed conditions compared with fasting.

Distribution – The apparent volume of distribution following oral administration of nelfinavir was 2 to 7 L/kg. Nelfinavir in serum is extensively protein-bound (> 98%).

Metabolism – Unchanged nelfinavir comprised 82% to 86% of the total plasma. In vitro multiple cytochrome P450 isoforms including CYP3A are responsible for metabolism of nelfinavir. One major and several minor oxidative metabolites were found in plasma. The major oxidative metabolite has in vitro antiviral activity comparable to the parent drug.

Excretion – The terminal half-life in plasma was typically 3.5 to 5 hours. The majority (87%) of an oral 750 mg dose was recovered in the feces; fecal radioactivity consisted of numerous oxidative metabolites (78%) and unchanged nelfinavir (22%). Only 1% to 2% of the dose was recovered in the urine, of which unchanged nelfinavir was the major component.

Hepatic/Renal function impairment: The pharmacokinetics of nelfinavir have not been studied in patients with hepatic or renal insufficiency; however, < 2% of nelfinavir is excreted in the urine, so the impact of renal impairment on nelfinavir elimination should be minimal.

Indications:

HIV: For the treatment of HIV infection when antiretroviral therapy is warranted. This indication is based on surrogate marker changes in patients who received nelfinavir in combination with nucleoside analogues or alone for ≤ 24 weeks.

NELFINAVIR MESYLATE

Contraindications:

Hypersensitivity to any components of the product; concurrent administration with terfenadine, astemizole, cisapride, rifampin, triazolam or midazolam (see Drug Interactions).

Warnings:

Hepatic function impairment: Nelfinavir is principally metabolized by the liver. Exercise caution when administering this drug to patients with hepatic impairment.

Pregnancy: Category B. There are no adequate and well-controlled studies in pregnant women. Use during pregnancy only if clearly needed.

Lactation: The US Public Health Service Centers for Disease Control and Prevention advises HIV-infected women not to breastfeed to avoid postnatal transmission of HIV to a child who may not yet be infected. Studies in lactating rats have demonstrated that nelfinavir is excreted in milk. It is not known whether nelfinavir is excreted in breast milk.

Children: A similar adverse event profile was seen during the pediatric clinical trial as in adult patients. The evaluation of the antiviral activity of nelfinavir in pediatric patients is ongoing.

The safety, effectiveness and pharmacokinetics of nelfinavir have not been evaluated in pediatric patients < 2 years old (see Administration and Dosage).

Precautions:

Resistance/Cross-resistance: It is unknown what effect nelfinavir therapy will have on the activity of subsequently administered protease inhibitors.

Hemophilia: There have been reports of increased bleeding, including spontaneous skin hematomas and hemarthrosis, in patients with hemophilia type A and B treated with protease inhibitors. In some patients, additional factor VIII was given. In more than half of the reported cases, treatment with protease inhibitors was continued or reintroduced. A causal relationship has not been established.

Drug Interactions:

Nelfinavir is an inhibitor of CYP3A (cytochrome P450 3A). Coadministration of nelfinavir and drugs primarily metabolized by CYP3A may result in increased plasma concentrations of the other drug which could increase or prolong both its therapeutic and adverse effects. Nelfinavir is metabolized in part by CYP3A. Coadministration of nelfinavir and drugs that induce CYP3A may decrease nelfinavir plasma concentrations and reduce its therapeutic effect. Coadministration of nelfinavir and drugs that inhibit CYP3A may increase nelfinavir plasma concentrations (see Contraindications). Drug interactions are not expected between nelfinavir and dapsone, trimethoprim/sulfamethoxazole, clarithromycin, azithromycin, erythromycin, itraconazole and fluconazole.

Nelfinavir Drug Interactions

Precipitant drug	Object drug*		Description
Anticonvulsants (eg, carbamazepine, phenobarbital, phenytoin)	Nelfinavir	↓	Concurrent use may decrease nelfinavir plasma concentrations.
Indinavir	Nelfinavir	↑	Coadministration of indinavir with nelfinavir resulted in an 83% increase in nelfinavir plasma AUC and a 51% increase in indinavir plasma AUC. The safety of this combination has not been established.
Nelfinavir	Indinavir		
Ketoconazole	Nelfinavir	↑	Coadministration of ketoconazole with nelfinavir resulted in a 35% increase in nelfinavir plasma AUC. This change was not considered clinically significant and no dose adjustment is needed.
Rifabutin	Nelfinavir	↓	Coadministration of rifabutin with nelfinavir resulted in a 32% decrease in nelfinavir plasma AUC and a 207% increase in rifabutin plasma AUC. It is recommended that the dose of rifabutin be reduced to one-half the usual dose when administered with nelfinavir.
Nelfinavir	Rifabutin	↑	
Rifampin	Nelfinavir	↓	Coadministration of rifampin with nelfinavir resulted in an 82% decrease in nelfinavir plasma AUC. Do not coadminister nelfinavir and rifampin.

NELFINAVIR MESYLATE

Nelfinavir Drug Interactions			
Precipitant drug	Object drug*		Description
Ritonavir	Nelfinavir	⬆	Coadministration of ritonavir with nelfinavir resulted in a 152% increase in nelfinavir plasma AUC and very little change in ritonavir plasma AUC. The safety of this combination has not been established.
Saquinavir	Nelfinavir	⬆	Coadministration of saquinavir with nelfinavir resulted in an 18% increase in nelfinavir plasma AUC and a 392% increase in saquinavir plasma AUC. If used in combination, no dose adjustments are needed.
Nelfinavir	Saquinavir		
Nelfinavir	Antihistamines, nonsedating, Astemizole Terfenadine	⬆	Administration of terfenadine with nelfinavir resulted in the appearance of unchanged terfenadine in plasma; therefore, do not administer nelfinavir concurrently with terfenadine because of the potential for serious and life-threatening cardiac arrhythmias. Because a similar interaction is likely, do not administer concurrently with astemizole.
Nelfinavir	Didanosine	⬌	It is recommended that didanosine be administered on an empty stomach; therefore, administer nelfinavir (with food) 1 hour after or > 2 hours before didanosine.
Nelfinavir	Oral contraceptives	⬇	Coadministration of nelfinavir with oral contraceptives resulted in a 47% decrease in ethinyl estradiol and an 18% decrease in norethindrone plasma concentrations. Use alternate or additional contraceptive measures during therapy with nelfinavir.
Nelfinavir	Zidovudine Lamivudine	⬇	Coadministration of zidovudine and lamivudine with nelfinavir resulted in a 35% decrease in zidovudine plasma AUC. A dose adjustment is not needed when zidovudine is administered with nelfinavir.

* ⬆ = Object drug increased. ⬇ = Object drug decreased. ⬌ = Undetermined effect.

NELFINAVIR MESYLATE

Adverse Reactions:

Percentage of Patients with Treatment-Emergent[1] Adverse Reactions of Moderate or Severe Intensity						
	Naive patients			Experienced patients		
Adverse events	Placebo + AZT/3TC (n = 101)	500 mg TID nelfinavir + AZT/3TC (n = 97)	750 mg TID nelfinavir + AZT/3TC (n = 100)	Placebo + d4T (n = 109)	500 mg TID nelfinavir + d4T (n = 98)	750 mg TID nelfinavir + d4T (n = 101)
GI						
Abdominal pain	1%	0	0	3%	2%	4%
Diarrhea	3%	14%	20%	10%	28%	32%
Nausea	4%	3%	7%	1%	3%	2%
Flatulence	0	5%	2%	4%	8%	3%
Hematology abnormalities						
Hemoglobin	6%	3%	2%	0	0	0
Neutrophils	4%	3%	5%	1%	1%	4%
Lymphocytes	1%	6%	1%	1%	1%	0
Laboratory abnormalities						
ALT	6%	1%	1%	1%	3%	2%
AST	4%	1%	0	0	3%	3%
Creatine kinase	7%	2%	2%	4%	5%	6%
Miscellaneous						
Asthenia	2%	1%	1%	4%	3%	1%
Rash	1%	1%	3%	0	4%	3%

[1] Includes those adverse events at least possibly related to study drug or of unknown relationship and excludes concurrent HIV conditions.

Body as a whole: Accidental injury; allergic reaction; back pain; fever; headache; malaise; pain.

GI: Anorexia; dyspepsia; epigastric pain; GI bleeding; hepatitis; mouth ulceration; pancreatitis; vomiting.

Hematologic/Lymphatic: Anemia; leukopenia; thrombocytopenia.

Metabolic: Increases in alkaline phosphatase, amylase, creatine phosphokinase, lactic dehydrogenase, AST, ALT, gamma glutamyl transpeptidase; hyperlipemia; hyperuricemia; hypoglycemia; dehydration; liver function tests abnormal.

Musculoskeletal: Arthralgia; arthritis; cramps; myalgia; myasthenia; myopathy.

CNS: Anxiety; depression; dizziness; emotional lability; hyperkinesia; insomnia; migraine; paresthesia; seizures; sleep disorder; somnolence; suicide ideation.

Respiratory: Dyspnea; pharyngitis; rhinitis; sinusitis.

Dermatologic: Dermatitis; folliculitis; fungal dermatitis; maculopapular rash; pruritus; sweating; urticaria.

GU: Kidney calculus; sexual dysfunction; urine abnormality.

Special senses: Acute iritis; eye disorder.

Lab test abnormalities: Few patients experienced significant laboratory abnormalities.

Overdosage:

There is no specific antidote for overdose with nelfinavir. If indicated, eliminate unabsorbed drug by emesis or gastric lavage, or administer activated charcoal. Because nelfinavir is highly protein bound, dialysis is unlikely to be of benefit.

Patient Information:

For optimal absorption, advise patients to take nelfinavir with food.

The most frequent adverse event associated with nelfinavir is diarrhea, which can usually be controlled with non-prescription drugs such as loperamide.

Instruct patients taking oral contraceptives to use alternate or additional contraceptive measures.

Administration and Dosage:

Approved by the FDA on March 14, 1997.

Take with a meal or light snack.

NELFINAVIR MESYLATE

Adults: The recommended dose is 750 mg (three 250 mg tablets) 3 times a day in combination with nucleoside analogues (antiviral activity is enhanced).

Pediatric patients (2 to 13 years): 20 to 30 mg/kg/dose, 3 times daily.

Pediatric Dose of Nelfinavir to be Administered Three Times Daily				
Body weight		Number of level 1 g scoops	Number of level teaspoons	Number of tablets
kg	lbs			
7 to < 8.5	15.5 to < 18.5	4	1	-
8.5 to < 10.5	18.5 to < 23	5	1¼	-
10.5 to < 12	23 to < 26.5	6	1½	-
12 to < 14	26.5 to < 31	7	1¾	-
14 to < 16	31 to < 35	8	2	-
16 to < 18	35 to < 39.5	9	2¼	-
18 to < 23	39.5 to < 50.5	10	2½	2
≥ 23	≥ 50.5	15	3¾	3

Oral powder – The oral powder may be mixed with a small amount of water, milk, formula, soy formula, soy milk or dietary supplement; once mixed, the entire contents must be consumed in order to obtain the full dose. Acidic food or juice (eg, orange juice, apple juice or apple sauce) are not recommended because of bitter taste. Do not reconstitute with water in its original container.

Storage/Stability: Store tablets and powder at 15° to 30°C (59° to 86°F). Once mixed, store the oral powder for ≤ 6 hours.

Rx	**Viracept** (Agouron)	**Tablets:** 250 mg	(Viracept/250 mg). Capsule shape. Lt. blue. In 270s.
		Powder: 50 mg/g	Aspartame, sucrose[1]. In multiple dose bottles containing 144 g powder w/1 g scoop.

[1] 11.2 mg/g phenylalanine

RIBAVIRIN

Warning:

In patients requiring mechanical ventilator assistance, pay strict attention to procedures that have been shown to minimize the accumulation of drug precipitate that can result in mechanical ventilator dysfunction and associated increased pulmonary pressures.

Deterioration of respiratory function has been associated with ribavirin use in adults with chronic obstructive lung disease or asthma and in infants (see Warnings).

Actions:

Pharmacology:

Antiviral effects – Ribavirin has antiviral inhibitory activity in vitro against respiratory syncytial virus (RSV), influenza virus and herpes simplex virus. The mechanism of action is unknown. Reversal of the in vitro antiviral activity by guanosine or xanthosine suggests ribavirin may act as an analog of these cellular metabolites.

Immunologic effects – Neutralizing antibody responses to RSV were decreased in aerosolized ribavirin-treated infants compared with placebo-treated infants. In rats, ribavirin resulted in lymphoid atrophy of thymus, spleen and lymph nodes. Humoral immunity was reduced in guinea pigs and ferrets. Cellular immunity was also mildly depressed in animal studies. Clinical significance of these observations is unknown.

Pharmacokinetics:

Absorption – Ribavirin administered by aerosol is absorbed systemically. Four pediatric patients inhaling ribavirin aerosol by face mask for 2.5 hours each day for 3 days had plasma concentrations ranging from 0.44 to 1.55 μM (mean, 0.76 μM). The plasma half-life was 9.5 hours. Three pediatric patients inhaling ribavirin aerosol by face mask or mist tent for 20 hours/day for 5 days had plasma concentrations ranging from 1.5 to 14.3 μM (mean, 6.8 μM).

Distribution – Bioavailability of the aerosol is unknown and may depend on mode of delivery. After aerosol use, peak plasma concentrations are less than the concentration that reduced RSV plaque formation in tissue culture by 85% to 98%. Respiratory tract secretions are likely to contain ribavirin in concentrations many times higher than those required to reduce plaque formation. However, RSV is an intracellular virus and it is unknown whether plasma concentrations or respiratory secretion concentrations of the drug better reflect intracellular concentrations in the respiratory tract.

Accumulation of drug or metabolites in red blood cells occurs, plateauing in red cells in ≈ 4 days. Accumulation gradually declines with an apparent half-life of 40 days. Accumulation following inhalation is not well defined.

Indications:

Severe lower respiratory tract infections: Treatment of carefully selected hospitalized infants and young children with severe lower respiratory tract infections due to RSV.

The presence of underlying conditions such as prematurity, immunosuppression or cardiopulmonary disease may increase the severity of the infection and its risk to the patient. High risk infants and young children with such conditions may benefit from treatment.

Unlabeled uses: Aerosol ribavirin has shown some success against influenza A and B. *Oral* ribavirin (600 mg to 1800 mg/day for 10 to 14 days) has been variously effective against other viral diseases including acute and chronic hepatitis, herpes genitalis, measles and Lassa fever.

Contraindications:

Hypersensitivity to the drug or its components.

Pregnancy or the potential for pregnancy during exposure to the drug. Although there are no pertinent human data, ribavirin is teratogenic (malformation of skull, palate, eye, jaw, limbs, skeleton and GI tract) or embryolethal in most species in which it has been tested.

Warnings:

Assisted ventilation: Some subjects requiring assisted ventilation have experienced serious difficulties because of inadequate ventilation and gas exchange. Drug precipitation within the ventilatory apparatus, including the endotracheal tube, has resulted in increased positive aend expiratory pressure and increased positive inspiratory pressure. Accumulation of fluid in tubing ("rain out") has also been noted.

Pulmonary function significantly deteriorated during ribavirin aerosol treatment in six of six adults with chronic obstructive lung disease and in four of six asthmatic adults. Dyspnea and chest soreness also occurred in the latter group. Minor abnormalities in pulmonary function were also seen in healthy adult volunteers.

Respiratory function: Carefully monitor respiratory function during treatment. If ribavirin aerosol treatment produces sudden deterioration of respiratory function, stop treatment and reinstitute only with extreme caution, continuous monitoring and consideration of concomitant administration of bronchodilators.

Deaths: Deaths during or shortly after treatment with aerosolized ribavirin have been reported in 20 cases of patients treated with ribavirin (12 of these patients were being treated for RSV infections). Sevral cases have been characterized as "possibly related" to ribavirin by the treating physician; these were in infants who experienced worsening respiratory status related to bronchospasm while being treated with the drug. Several other cases have been attributed to mechanical ventilator malfunction in which ribavirin precipitation within the ventilator apparatus lead to excessively high pulmonary pressures and diminished oxygenation.

Anemia: Although anemia has not been reported with aerosol use, it occurs frequently with oral and IV ribavirin, and most infants treated with the aerosol have not been evaluated 1 to 2 weeks posttreatment when anemia is likely.

Carcinogenesis: Ribavirin induces cell transformation in an in vitro mammalian system. However, in vivo carcinogenicity studies are incomplete. Results thus far suggest that chronic feeding of ribavirin to rats at doses of 16 to 60 mg/kg can induce benign mammary, pancreatic, pituitary and adrenal tumors.

Pregnancy: Category X. Ribavirin has demonstrated significant teratogenic or embryocidal potential in all animal species in which adequate studies have been conducted. The incidence and severity of teratogenic effects increased with escalation of the drug dose. Although clinical studies have not been performed, ribavirin may cause fetal harm in humans. See Contraindications.

Lactation: Ribavirin aerosol use in nursing mothers is not indicated because RSV infection is self-limited in this population. Ribavirin is toxic to lactating animals and their offspring. It is not known whether the drug is excreted in breast milk.

Adverse Reactions:

Body as a whole: Rash; conjunctivitis.

Cardiovascular: Cardiac arrest; hypotension; bradycardia; digitalis toxicity; bigeminy; tachycardia.

Hematologic: Reticulocytosis.

Pulmonary: Worsening of respiratory status; bronchospasm; pulmonary edema; hypoventilation; cyanosis; dyspnea; bacterial pneumonia; pneumothorax; apnea; atelectasis; ventilator dependence (see Warnings).

Health care workers: Headache (51%); conjunctivitis (32%); rhinitis, nausea, rash, dizziness, pharyngitis, lacrimation (10 to 20%). Several cases of bronchospasm and chest pain were also reported, usually in individuals with known underlying reactive airway disease. There are several case reports of damage to contact lenses after prolonged close exposure to aerosolized ribavirin. Most signs and symptoms reported as having occurred in exposed health care workers resolved within minutes to hours of discontinuing close exposure to aerosolized ribavirin.

Administration and Dosage:

For aerosol administration only.

Mechanically ventilated infants: The recommended dose and administration schedule for infants who require mechanical ventilation is the same as for those who do not. Either a pressure or volume cycle ventilator may be used in conjunction with the SPAG-2. In either case, suction endotracheal tubes every 1 to 2 hours and monitor pulmonary pressures frequently (every 2 to 4 hours). For both pressure and volume ventilators, heated wire connective tubing and bacteria filters in series in the expiratory limb of the system (which must be changed frequently, eg, every 4 hours) must be used to minimize the risk of ribavirin precipitation in the system and the subsequent risk of ventilator dysfunction. Use water column pressure release valves in the ventilator circuit for pressure cycled ventilators. They may also be utilized with volume cycled ventilators.

Treatment is carried for 12 to 18 hours per day for 3 to 7 days. The aerosol is delivered to an infant oxygen hood fromt the SPAG-2 aerosol generator. Administration by face mask or oxygen tent may be necessary if a hood cannot be used. However, the volume and condensation area are larger in a tent and this may alter the drug's delivery dynamics. Ribavirin aerosol is not to be administered with any other aerosol generating device or together with other aerosolized medications.

Reconstitute drug with a minimum of 75 ml of sterile water for injection or inhalation in the original 100 ml vial. Shake well. Transfer to the clean, sterilized 500 ml wide-mouth Erlenmeyer flask (SPAG-2 Reservoir) and further dilute to a final volume of 300 ml with sterile water for injection or inhalation. The final concentration should be 20 mg/ml. *Important* — This water does not have any antimicrobial agent or other substance added. Discard solutions placed in the SPAG-2 unit at least every 24 hours and when the liquid level is low before adding newly reconstituted solution. Using the recommended drug concentration of 20 mg/ml ribavirin as the starting solution in the SPAG unit's drug reservoir, the average aerosol concentration for a 12–hour period is 190 mcg/L of air.

Storage/Stability: Store lyophilized drug powder at 15° to 25°C (59° to 78°F) in a dry place. May store reconstituted solutions at room temperature (20° to 30°C, 68° to 86°F) for ≤ 24 hours.

Rx	**Virazole** (ICN)	**Lyophilized pwder for aerosol reconstitution:** 6 g ribavirin/100 ml vial. Contains 20 mg per ml when reconstituted with 300 ml sterile water.	In vials.

AMANTADINE HCl

Amantadine is also used as an antiparkinson agent. For information regarding this use, refer to amantadine in the Antiparkinson Agents section.

Actions:

Pharmacology: Amantadine's antiviral activity against influenza A virus is not completely understood. Its mode of action appears to be the prevention of the release of infectious viral nucleic acid into the host cell. It may also interfere with viral penetration into cells. The reaction appears to be virus specific (for influenza A) but not host specific. Amantadine does not appear to interfere with the immunogenicity of inactivated influenza A virus vaccine.

Amantadine is not effective against type B influenza. When administered within 24 to 48 hours after onset of illness, amantadine reduces the duration of fever and other systemic symptoms with a more rapid return to routine daily activities and improvement in peripheral airway function.

Pharmacokinetics:

Absorption/Distribution – After oral administration of a single dose of 100 mg, maximum blood levels are reached in ≈ 4 hours, based on the mean time of the peak urinary excretion rate; the peak excretion rate is ≈ 5 mg/hr; the mean half-life of the excretion rate is ≈ 15 hours.

Compared with otherwise healthy adults, clearance of amantadine is significantly reduced in adults with renal insufficiency. Elimination half-life increases 2- to 3-fold when creatinine clearance is < 40 ml/min/1.73 m^2 and averages 8 days in patients on chronic maintenance hemodialysis.

The renal clearance of amantadine is reduced and plasma levels are increased in otherwise healthy elderly patients age 65 years and older. The drug plasma levels in elderly patients receiving 100 mg daily have been reported to approximate those determined in younger adults taking 200 mg daily. Whether these changes are due to the normal decline in renal function or other age related factors is not known.

Metabolism/Excretion – Amantadine is readily absorbed, is not metabolized, and is excreted in the urine.

Indications:

Influenza A virus respiratory tract illness: Prevention or chemoprophylaxis of and treatment of respiratory tract illness caused by influenza A virus strains. Indicated especially for high risk patients because of underlying disease (eg, cardiovascular, pulmonary, metabolic, neuromuscular or immunodeficiency disease), close household or hospital ward contacts of index cases, immunocompromised patients and health care and community services personnel. Early immunization is the prophylaxis method of choice. When early immunization is contraindicated, not feasible or not available, amantadine can be used for chemoprophylaxis.

Amantadine prophylaxis recommendations:

1.) Short-term prophylaxis during the course of a presumed influenza A outbreak (eg, in institutions for persons at high risk), particularly when the vaccine may be relatively ineffective.
2.) Adjunct to late immunization of high risk individuals. It is not too late to immunize even when influenza A is known to be in the community. Since the development of a protective response following vaccination takes about 2 weeks, use amantadine in the interim.
3.) To reduce disruption of medical care and to reduce spread of virus to high risk persons when influenza A virus outbreaks occur. Prophylaxis is desirable for those physicians, nurses and other personnel who have extensive contact with high risk patients but who failed to receive the recommended annual influenza vaccination before the onset of influenza A activity.
4.) To supplement vaccination protection in those with impaired immune responses. Consider chemoprophylaxis for high risk patients who may have a poor response to influenza vaccine, eg, those with severe immunodeficiency.
5.) As chemoprophylaxis throughout the influenza season for those few high risk individuals for whom influenza vaccine is contraindicated because of anaphylactic hypersensitivity to egg protein or prior severe reactions associated with influenza vaccination.

Parkinson's disease and drug-induced extrapyramidal reactions: See amantadine in the Antiparkinson Agents section.

Contraindications:

Hypersensitivity to amantadine.

Warnings:

Seizures: Closely observe patients with a history of epilepsy or other seizures for increased seizure activity. Dosage reduction is recommended (see Administration and Dosage).

AMANTADINE HCl

Exercise care in patients with liver disease, history of recurrent eczematoid rash, or psychosis or severe psychoneurosis not controlled by chemotherapeutic agents.

Congestive heart failure (CHF): CHF or peripheral edema requires careful observation and dosage titration; patients have developed CHF while receiving amantadine.

Renal function impairment: Reduce the dose in renal impairment. Amantadine is not metabolized and is mainly excreted in the urine; therefore, it accumulates in plasma and the body when renal function declines. See Administration and Dosage.

Elderly: Reduce dose in individuals 65 years of age and older.

Pregnancy: Category C. Amantadine in high doses is embryotoxic and teratogenic in animals. Cardiovascular malformation was reported in an infant exposed to amantadine during the first trimester. There are no adequate and well controlled studies of amantadine in pregnant women. Use only when clearly needed and when the potential benefits outweigh the potential hazards to the fetus.

Lactation: Amantadine is excreted in breast milk. Exercise caution when administering to a nursing woman.

Children: Safety and efficacy for use in neonates and infants < 1 year of age have not been established.

Precautions:

May cause CNS effects or blurred vision; observe caution while driving or performing other tasks requiring alertness.

Do not discontinue abruptly; a few patients with Parkinson's disease experienced a parkinsonian crisis (ie, a sudden marked clinical deterioration) when this medication was stopped suddenly.

Drug Interactions:

Anticholinergic drugs: Reduce the dose of anticholinergic drugs or of amantadine if atropine-like effects appear when these drugs are used concurrently.

Hydrochlorothiazide plus triamterene: Decreased urinary excretion of amantadine with subsequent increased plasma concentrations occurred when hydrochlorothiazide plus triamterene was administered concurrently with amantadine.

Adverse Reactions:

Most frequent (5% to 10%): Nausea; dizziness; lightheadedness; insomnia.

Less frequent (1% to 5%): Depression; anxiety; irritability; hallucinations; confusion; anorexia; dry mouth; constipation; ataxia; livedo reticularis; peripheral edema; orthostatic hypotension; headache.

Infrequent (0.1% to 1%): CHF; psychosis; urinary retention; dyspnea; fatigue; skin rash; vomiting; weakness; slurred speech; visual disturbance.

Rare (< 0.1%): Convulsions; leukopenia; neutropenia; eczematoid dermatitis; oculogyric episodes.

Overdosage:

Symptoms: Nausea, vomiting, anorexia and CNS effects (including hyperexcitability, tremors, ataxia, blurred vision, lethargy, depression, slurred speech and convulsions). Ventricular arrhythmias manifested by torsade de pointes and ventricular fibrillation were observed in a patient who ingested 2.5 g amantadine. Death has occurred from a major overdose.

Treatment:

There is no specific antidote. CNS toxicity – IV physostigmine, 1 to 2 mg slowly administered every 1 to 2 hours in adults or 0.5 mg at 5 to 10 minute intervals up to a maximum of 2 mg/hour in children.

Acute overdosing – Employ general supportive measures along with immediate gastric lavage or induction of emesis. Refer to General Management of Acute Overdosage. Force fluids; administer IV if necessary. Urinary acidification may increase elimination from the body. Monitor blood pressure, pulse, respiration, temperature, electrolytes, urine pH and urinary output. Observe the patient for hyperactivity and convulsions; administer sedatives and anticonvulsants if required. Give appropriate antiarrhythmic and vasopressor therapy when warranted.

Hemodialysis does not remove significant amounts of amantadine.

Patient Information:

May cause blurred vision; observe caution while driving or performing other tasks requiring alertness.

If dizziness or lightheadedness occurs, avoid sudden changes in posture; notify physician of this effect.

Notify physician if mood or mental changes, swelling of the extremities, difficult urination or shortness of breath occurs.

AMANTADINE HCl

Administration and Dosage:

Influenza A virus illness:

Prophylaxis – Start in anticipation of contact or as soon as possible after exposure. Continue daily for at least 10 days following a known exposure. The infectious period extends from shortly before onset of symptoms to up to 1 week after. When vaccine is unavailable or contraindicated, administer for up to 90 days in case of possible repeated and unknown exposures. Because amantadine does not appear to suppress antibody response, it can be used in conjunction with inactivated influenza A virus vaccine until protective antibody responses develop; administer for 2 to 3 weeks after vaccine has been given.

Symptomatic management – Start as soon as possible after onset of symptoms and continue for 24 to 48 hours after symptoms disappear.

Adults – 200 mg daily as a single dose or 100 mg twice a day. Splitting the dose may reduce the frequency of CNS side effects.

Children (9 to 12 years) – 100 mg twice a day.

Children (1 to 9 years) – 2 to 4 mg/lb/day (4.4 to 8.8 mg/kg/day) given once daily or divided twice daily; not to exceed 150 mg per day.

The following table may serve as a guideline for dosage:

Amantadine Dosage by Patient Age and Renal Function

Renal function	Dosage[1]
No recognized renal disease	
1 to 9 yrs[2]	4.4 to 8.8 mg/kg/day once daily or divided twice daily, not to exceed 150 mg/day
10 to 64 yrs[3]	200 mg once daily or divided twice daily
≥ 65 yrs	100 mg once daily[4]
Renal function impairment Creatinine clearance: ($ml/min/1.73m^2$)	
30 to 50	200 mg 1st day; 100 mg daily thereafter
15 to 29	200 mg 1st day; then 100 mg on alternate days
< 15	200 mg every 7 days
Hemodialysis patients	200 mg every 7 days

[1] For prophylaxis, take amantadine each day for the duration of influenza A activity in the community (generally 6 to 12 weeks). For therapy, institute amantadine as soon as possible after onset of symptoms and continue for 24 to 48 hours after symptoms disappear (generally 5 to 7 days).

[2] Use in children < 1 year old is not evaluated adequately. In one study, a dose of 6.6 mg/kg/day was well tolerated by children > 2 years old.

[3] Reduce dosage to 100 mg/day for persons with an active seizure disorder, because they may be at increased risk of seizure frequency when given 200 mg/day.

[4] Recommended to minimize risk of toxicity; renal function normally declines with age, and side effects are more frequent in the elderly.

Rx	**Amantadine HCl** (Various, eg, Geneva, Goldline, Major, Parmed, PBI, Rugby, Schein, URL, Warner-Chilcott)	**Capsules:** 100 mg	In 100s, 250s, 500s and UD 100s.
Rx	**Symadine** (Solvay)		(RR 4140). Red. In 100s.
Rx	**Symmetrel** (DuPont)		Lecithin. (DuPont Symmetrel). Red. In 100s, 500s and UD 100s.
Rx	**Symmetrel** (DuPont)	**Syrup:** 50 mg per 5 ml	Sorbitol. Raspberry flavor. In 480 ml.

FOSCARNET SODIUM (Phosphonoformic acid; PFA)

Warning:

Renal impairment is the major toxicity of foscarnet. Continual assessment of a patient's risk, frequent monitoring of serum creatinine with dose adjustment for changes in renal function and adequate hydration with administration are imperative (see Administration and Dosage).

Seizures, related to alterations in plasma minerals and electrolytes, have been associated with foscarnet treatment. Therefore, patients must be carefully monitored for such changes and their potential sequelae. Mineral and electrolyte supplementation may be required.

Foscarnet is indicated for use only in immunocompromised patients with CMV retinitis and mucocutaneous acyclovir-resistant HSV infections (see Indications).

Actions:

Pharmacology: Foscarnet is an organic analog of inorganic pyrophosphate that inhibits replication of known herpes viruses in vitro including cytomegalovirus (CMV) and herpes simplex virus types 1 and 2 (HSV-1, HSV-2).

Foscarnet exerts its antiviral activity by a selective inhibition at the pyrophosphate binding site on virus-specific DNA polymerases at concentrations that do not affect cellular DNA polymerases. Foscarnet does not require activation (phosphorylation) by thymidine kinase or other kinases, and therefore is active in vitro against HSV mutants deficient in thymidine kinase and CMV UL97 mutants. HSV strains resistant to acyclovir or CMV strains resistant to ganciclovir may be sensitive to foscarnet. However, acyclovir or ganciclovir resistant mutants with alterations in the viral DNA polymerase may be resistant to foscarnet and may not respond to therapy with foscarnet. The combination of foscarnet and ganciclovir has enhanced activity in vitro.

The quantitative relationship between the in vitro susceptibility of human CMV or herpes simplex virus 1 and 2 to foscarnet and clinical response to therapy has not been established and virus sensitivity testing has not been standardized.

Resistance – All foscarnet resistant mutants are known to be generated through mutation in the viral DNA polymerase gene. CMV strains with double mutations conferring resistance to both foscarnet and ganciclovir have been isolated from patients with AIDS. Consider the possibility of viral resistance in patients who show poor clinical response or experience persistent viral excretion during therapy.

Pharmacokinetics: Foscarnet is 14% to 17% bound to plasma protein at plasma drug concentrations of 1 to 1000 mcM.

The foscarnet terminal half-life determined by urinary excretion was 87.5 ± 41.8 hours, possibly because of release of foscarnet from bone. Postmortem data on several patients in European clinical trials provide evidence that foscarnet does accumulate in bone in humans; however, the extent to which this occurs has not been determined. In animal studies (mice), 40% of an IV dose of foscarnet was deposited in bone in young animals and 7% was deposited in adult animals.

Foscarnet Pharmacokinetic Characteristics

Parameter	60 mg/kg q 8 h	90 mg/kg q 12 h
C_{max} at steady-state (mcM)	589	623
C_{trough} at steady-state (mcM)	114	63
Volume of distribution (L/kg)	0.41	0.52
Plasma half-life (hr)	4	3.3
Systemic clearance (L/hr)	6.2	7.1
Renal clearance (L/hr)	5.6	6.4
CSF: plasma ratio	0.69[1]	0.68[2]

[1] 50 mg/kg q 8 h for 28 days, samples taken 3 hrs after end of 1 hr infusion.

[2] 90 mg/kg q 12 h for 28 days, samples taken 1 hr after end of 2 hr infusion.

Approximately 80% to 90% of IV foscarnet is excreted unchanged in the urine of patients with normal renal function. Both tubular secretion and glomerular filtration account for urinary elimination of foscarnet.

FOSCARNET SODIUM (Phosphonoformic acid; PFA)

Renal function impairment –

Pharmacokinetic Parameters After a Single 60 mg/kg Dose of Foscarnet in Four Groups of Adults with Varying Degrees of Renal Function				
Parameter	Group 1 (n=6)	Group 2 (n=6)	Group 3 (n=6)	Group 4 (n=4)
Creatinine clearance (ml/min)	108	68	34	70
Foscarnet CL (ml/min/kg)	2.13	1.33	0.45	0.43
Foscarnet half-life (hr)	1.93	3.35	13	25.3

Group 1 patients had normal renal function, defined as a creatinine clearance (Ccr) of > 80 ml/min, Group 2 Ccr was 50 to 80 ml/min, Group 3 Ccr was 25 to 49 ml/min and Group 4 Ccr was 10 to 24 ml/min.

Total systemic clearance (CL) of foscarnet decreased and half-life increased with diminishing renal function (as expressed by creatinine clearance). Based on these observations, it is necessary to modify the dosage of foscarnet in patients with renal impairment.

Clinical trials:

CMV retinitis – A prospective, randomized, controlled clinical trial was conducted in 24 patients with AIDS and CMV retinitis. Patients received induction treatment of 60 mg/kg every 8 hours for 3 weeks, followed by maintenance treatment with 90 mg/kg/day until retinitis progression (appearance of a new lesion or advancement of the border of a posterior lesion > 750 microns in diameter). The 13 patients randomized to treatment with foscarnet had a significant delay in progression of CMV retinitis compared with untreated controls. Median times to retinitis progression from study entry were 93 days (range, 21 to > 364) and 22 days (range, 7 to 42), respectively.

In another prospective clinical trial of CMV retinitis in AIDS patients, 33 were treated with 2 to 3 weeks of foscarnet induction (60 mg/kg 3 times daily) and then randomized to two maintenance dose groups, 90 and 120 mg/kg/day. Median times from study entry to retinitis progression were 96 days (range, 14 to > 176) and 140 days (range, 16 to > 233), respectively. This was not statistically significant.

In another study, 107 patients with newly diagnosed CMV retinitis were randomized to treatment with foscarnet (induction 60 mg/kg twice a day for 2 weeks, maintenance 90 mg/kg once daily) and 127 were randomized to treatment with ganciclovir (induction 5 mg/kg twice a day, maintenance 5 mg/kg once daily). The median time to progression on the two drugs was similar (foscarnet 59 days and ganciclovir 56 days).

Relapsed CMV retinitis – A randomized, open-label comparison of foscarnet or ganciclovir monotherapy to the combination of both drugs for the treatment of persistently active or relapsed CMV retinitis in patients with AIDS was conducted. Subjects were randomized to one of three treatments: Foscarnet 90 mg/kg twice a day induction followed by 120 mg/kg once daily maintenance (Fos), ganciclovir 5 mg/kg twice a day induction followed by 10 mg/kg once daily maintenance (Gcv) or the combination of the two drugs, consisting of continuation of the subject's current therapy and induction dosing of the other drug followed by maintenance with foscarnet 90 mg/kg once daily plus ganciclovir 5 mg/kg once daily. Assessment of retinitis progression was performed by masked evaluation of retinal photographs. The median times to retinitis progression or death were 39 days for the foscarnet group, 61 days for the ganciclovir group and 105 days for the combination group. For the alternative endpoint of retinitis progression (censoring on death) the median times were 39 days for the foscarnet group, 61 days for the ganciclovir group and 132 days for the combination group. Because of censoring on death, the latter analysis may overestimate the treatment effect. Treatment modifications caused by toxicity were more common in the combination group than in the foscarnet or ganciclovir monotherapy groups.

HSV infections – A prospective, comparative trial was conducted in 25 AIDS patients with mucocutaneous, acyclovir-resistant HSV infections. Fourteen patients were randomized to either foscarnet (n = 8) at a dose of 40 mg/kg 3 times daily or vidarabine (n = 6) at a dose of 15 mg/kg/day; eleven patients received foscarnet without being randomized. Lesions in the eight patients randomized to foscarnet healed after 11 to 25 days; seven of the eleven nonrandomized patients treated with foscarnet had healed lesions in 10 to 30 days. Vidarabine was discontinued because of intolerance or poor therapeutic response. Five of these patients were subsequently treated with foscarnet and two had healed lesions in 15 and 24 days. In a second prospective, randomized trial, 40 AIDS patients and three bone marrow transplant recipients with mucocutaneous, acyclovir-resistant HSV infections were randomized to receive foscarnet at a dose of either 40 mg/kg twice daily or three times daily.

FOSCARNET SODIUM (Phosphonoformic acid; PFA)

Fifteen of the 43 patients had healing of their lesions in 11 to 72 days with no difference in response between the two treatment groups.

Indications:

CMV retinitis: Treatment of CMV retinitis in patients with AIDS.

Combination: Combination therapy with ganciclovir for patients who have relapsed after monotherapy with either drug.

HSV infections: Treatment of acyclovir-resistant mucocutaneous HSV infections in immunocompromised patients.

Contraindications:

Hypersensitivity to foscarnet.

Warnings:

Mineral and electrolyte imbalances: Foscarnet has been associated with changes in serum electrolytes including hypocalcemia (15%), hypophosphatemia (8%), hyperphosphatemia (6%), hypomagnesemia (15%) and hypokalemia (16%). Foscarnet is associated with a dose-related decrease in ionized serum calcium, which may not be reflected in total serum calcium. This effect is most likely related to foscarnet's chelation of divalent metal ions such as calcium. Therefore, advise patients to report symptoms of low ionized calcium such as perioral tingling, numbness in the extremities and paresthesias. Be prepared to treat these as well as severe manifestations of electrolyte abnormalities, such as tetany, cardiac disturbances and seizures. The rate of infusion may affect the decrease in ionized calcium; slowing the rate may decrease or prevent symptoms.

Particular caution and careful management of serum electrolytes is advised in patients with altered calcium or other electrolyte levels before treatment and especially in those with neurologic or cardiac abnormalities and those receiving other drugs known to influence minerals and electrolytes.

Accidental exposure: Accidental skin and eye contact with foscarnet sodium solution may cause local irritation and burning sensation. If accidental contact occurs, flush the exposed area with water.

Seizures: Foscarnet was associated with seizures in 18/189 (10%) of AIDS patients in five controlled studies. Several cases were associated with death. Three cases were associated with overdoses of foscarnet (see Overdosage). Risk factors associated with seizures include impaired baseline renal function, low total serum calcium and underlying CNS conditions.

Other CMV infections: Safety and efficacy have not been established for the treatment of other CMV infections (eg, pneumonitis, gastroenteritis); congenital or neonatal CMV disease; non-immunocompromised individuals.

Other HSV infections: Safety and efficacy have not been established for treatment of other HSV infections (eg, retinitis, encephalitis); congenital or neonatal HSV disease; or HSV in non-immunocompromised individuals.

Nephrotoxicity: The major toxicity of foscarnet is renal impairment, which occurs to some degree in most patients. Approximately 33% of patients with AIDS and CMV retinitis who received IV foscarnet without adequate hydration in clinical studies developed significant impairment of renal function, manifested by a rise in serum creatinine concentration to ≥ 2 mg/dl. Therefore, use foscarnet with caution in all patients, especially those with a history of renal function impairment. Patients vary in their sensitivity to foscarnet-induced nephrotoxicity, and initial renal function may not be predictive of the potential for drug-induced renal impairment.

Renal impairment is most likely to become clinically evident during the second week of induction therapy but may occur at any time during treatment; therefore, monitor renal function carefully (see Monitoring).

Elevations in serum creatinine are usually reversible following discontinuation or dose adjustment. Because of foscarnet's potential to cause renal impairment, dose adjustment based on serum creatinine is necessary. Hydration may reduce the risk of nephrotoxicity. It is recommended that 750 to 1000 ml of normal saline or 5% dextrose solution be given prior to the first infusion of foscarnet to establish diuresis. With subsequent infusions, 750 to 1000 ml of hydration fluid should be given with 90 to 120 mg/kg of foscarnet, and 500 ml with 40 to 60 mg/kg of foscarnet. Hydration fluid may need to be decreased if clinically warranted. After the first dose, administer the hydration fluid concurrently with each infusion of foscarnet.

Mutagenesis: Foscarnet showed genotoxic effects in the BALB/3T3 in vitro transformation assay at concentrations > 0.5 mcg/ml and an increased frequency of chromosome aberrations in the sister chromatid exchange assay at 1000 mcg/ml. A high dose of foscarnet (350 mg/kg) caused an increase in micronucleated polychromatic erythrocytes in vivo in mice at doses that produced exposures (AUC) comparable to that anticipated clinically.

FOSCARNET SODIUM (Phosphonoformic acid; PFA)

Elderly: No studies of the efficacy or safety of foscarnet in people > 65 years of age have been conducted. Because these individuals frequently have reduced glomerular filtration, pay particular attention to assessing renal function before and during administration.

Pregnancy: Category C. Daily SC doses up to 75 mg/kg administered to rabbits and 150 mg/kg administered to rats during gestation caused an increase in the frequency of skeletal anomalies/variations. On the basis of estimated drug exposure (as measured by AUC), the 150 mg/kg dose in rats and 75 mg/kg dose in rabbits were ≈ 1/8 (rat) and 1/3 (rabbit) the estimated maximal daily human exposure. These studies are inadequate to define the potential teratogenicity at levels to which women will be exposed. There are no adequate and well controlled studies in pregnant women. Use during pregnancy only if clearly needed.

Lactation: In lactating rats administered 75 mg/kg, foscarnet was excreted in maternal milk at concentrations three times higher than peak maternal blood concentrations. It is not known whether foscarnet is excreted in breast milk. Exercise caution if foscarnet is administered to a nursing woman.

Children: The safety and efficacy of foscarnet in children have not been studied. Foscarnet is deposited in teeth and bone, and deposition is greater in young and growing animals. Foscarnet adversely affects development of tooth enamel in mice and rats. The effects of this deposition on skeletal development have not been studied. Because deposition in human bone also occurs, it is likely that it does so to a greater degree in developing bone in children. Administer to children only after careful evaluation and only if the potential benefits for treatment outweigh the risks.

Precautions:

Monitoring:

Renal – The majority of patients will experience some decrease in renal function due to foscarnet administration. Therefore, it is recommended that Ccr, either measured or estimated using the modified Cockcroft and Gault equation based on serum creatinine, be determined at baseline, 2 to 3 times/week during induction therapy and at least once every 1 to 2 weeks during maintenance therapy, with foscarnet dose adjusted accordingly (see Administration and Dosage). More frequent monitoring may be required for some patients. It is also recommended that a 24 hour Ccr be determined at baseline and periodically thereafter to ensure correct dosing. Discontinue foscarnet if Ccr drops to < 0.4 ml/min/kg.

Electrolytes – Because of foscarnet's propensity to chelate divalent metal ions and alter levels of serum electrolytes, closely monitor patients for such changes. It is recommended that a schedule similar to that recommended for serum creatinine (see above) be used to monitor serum calcium, magnesium, potassium and phosphorus. Particular caution is advised in patients with decreased total serum calcium or other electrolyte levels before treatment, as well as in patients with neurologic or cardiac abnormalities, and in patients receiving other drugs known to influence serum calcium levels. Correct any clinically significant metabolic changes. Patients who experience mild (eg, perioral numbness or paresthesias) or severe symptoms (eg, seizures) of electrolyte abnormalities should have serum electrolyte and mineral levels assessed as close in time to the event as possible. Carefully monitor electrolytes, including calcium and magnesium (see Monitoring).

Careful monitoring and appropriate management of electrolytes, calcium, magnesium and creatinine are of particular importance in patients with conditions that may predispose them to seizures (see Warnings).

Toxicity/local irritation: Infuse solutions containing foscarnet only into veins with adequate blood flow to permit rapid dilution and distribution and avoid local irritation (see Administration and Dosage). Local irritation and ulcerations of penile epithelium have occurred in male patients receiving foscarnet, possibly related to the presence of the drug in urine. One case of vulvovaginal ulceration has occurred. Adequate hydration with close attention to personal hygiene may minimize the occurrence of such events.

Granulocytopenia has been reported in 17% of patients receiving foscarnet in controlled studies; however, only 1% (2/189) were terminated from these studies because of neutropenia.

Anemia occurred in 33% of patients.

FOSCARNET SODIUM (Phosphonoformic acid; PFA)

Drug Interactions:

Foscarnet Drug Interactions

Precipitant drug	Object drug*		Description
Nephrotoxic drugs (eg, aminoglycosides, amphotericin B, IV pentamidine)	Foscarnet	⬆	Because of foscarnet's tendency to cause renal impairment, avoid the use of foscarnet in combination with potentially nephrotoxic drugs unless the potential benefits outweigh the risks to the patient.
Foscarnet	Ganciclovir	⬌	The pharmacokinetics of foscarnet and ganciclovir were not altered in 13 patients receiving either concomitant therapy or daily alternating therapy for maintenance of CMV disease.
Foscarnet	Pentamidine	⬆	Concomitant treatment of four patients with foscarnet and IV pentamidine may have caused hypocalcemia; one patient died with severe hypocalcemia. Toxicity associated with concomitant use of aerosolized pentamidine has not been reported.

* ⬆ = Object drug increased. ⬌ = Undetermined effect.

Calcium: Foscarnet decreases serum levels of ionized calcium. Exercise particular caution when other drugs known to influence serum calcium levels are used concurrently.

Adverse Reactions:

The most frequently reported events were: Fever (65%); nausea (47%); anemia (33%); diarrhea (30%); abnormal renal function, decreased Ccr (27%); vomiting, headache (26%); seizure (10%) (see Warnings and Precautions).

Adverse events categorized as "severe" were: Death (14%); abnormal renal function (14%); marrow suppression (10%); anemia (9%); seizures (7%). Although death was specifically attributed to foscarnet in only one case, other complications of foscarnet (eg, renal impairment, electrolyte abnormalities, seizures) may have contributed to patient deaths (see Warnings and Precautions).

Injection site: Injection site pain or inflammation (1% to 5%).

Body as a whole: Fever, fatigue, rigors, asthenia, malaise, pain, infection, sepsis, death (≥ 5%); back/chest pain, edema, influenza-like symptoms, bacterial/fungal infections, facial edema, moniliasis, abscess (1% to 5%).

Cardiovascular: Hypertension, palpitations, ECG abnormalities including sinus tachycardia, first degree AV block and non-specific ST-T segment changes, hypotension, flushing, cerebrovascular disorder (1% to 5%); cardiac arrest, arrhythmias (< 1%).

CNS: Headache, paresthesia, dizziness, involuntary muscle contractions, hypoesthesia, neuropathy, seizures (including grand mal; see Warnings) (≥ 5%); tremor, ataxia, dementia, stupor, generalized spasms, sensory disturbances, meningitis, aphasia, abnormal coordination, leg cramps, EEG abnormalities (1% to 5%); coma (< 1%).

Dermatologic: Rash, increased sweating (≥ 5%); pruritus, skin ulceration, seborrhea, erythematous rash, maculopapular rash, skin discoloration (1% to 5%).

Endocrine: Antidiuretic hormone disorders (< 1%).

GI: Anorexia, nausea, diarrhea, vomiting, abdominal pain (≥ 5%); constipation, dysphagia, dyspepsia, rectal hemorrhage, dry mouth, melena, flatulence, ulcerative stomatitis, pancreatitis (1% to 5%); increased amylase (< 1%).

GU: Alterations in renal function, including increased serum creatinine, decreased Ccr and abnormal renal function (see Warnings) (≥ 5%); albuminuria, dysuria, polyuria, urethral disorder, urinary retention, urinary tract infections, acute renal failure, nocturia (1% to 5%); hematuria (< 1%).

Hematologic: Anemia, granulocytopenia, leukopenia (≥ 5%); thrombocytopenia, platelet abnormalities, thrombosis, WBC abnormalities, lymphadenopathy (1% to 5%); pancytopenia (< 1%).

Hepatic: Abnormal A-G ratio, abnormal hepatic function, increased AST and ALT (1% to 5%).

Metabolic/Nutritional: Mineral/electrolyte imbalances (see Warnings), including hypokalemia, hypocalcemia, hypomagnesemia, hypo- or hyperphosphatemia (≥ 5%); hyponatremia, decreased weight, increased alkaline phosphatase, increased LDH, increased BUN, acidosis, cachexia, thirst (1% to 5%); dehydration, increased creatine phosphokinase, hypoproteinemia (< 1%).

Musculoskeletal: Arthralgia, myalgia (1% to 5%).

FOSCARNET SODIUM (Phosphonoformic acid; PFA)

Neoplasms: Lymphoma-like disorder, sarcoma (1% to 5%).

Psychiatric: Depression, confusion, anxiety (≥ 5%); insomnia, somnolence, nervousness, amnesia, agitation, aggressive reaction, hallucination (1% to 5%).

Respiratory: Coughing, dyspnea (≥ 5%); pneumonia, sinusitis, pharyngitis, rhinitis, respiratory disorders or insufficiency, pulmonary infiltration, stridor, pneumothorax, hemoptysis, bronchospasm (1% to 5%).

Special senses: Vision abnormalities (≥ 5%); taste perversions, eye abnormalities, eye pain, conjunctivitis (1% to 5%).

Overdosage:

Symptoms: In controlled clinical trials, overdosage was reported in 10 patients. All 10 patients experienced adverse events, and all except one made a complete recovery. One patient died after receiving a total daily dose of 12.5 g for 3 days instead of the intended 10.9 g. The patient suffered a grand mal seizure, became comatose and died three days later. The cause of death was listed as respiratory/cardiac arrest. The other nine patients received doses ranging from 1.14 times to 8 times their recommended doses with an average of 4 times their recommended doses. Overall, three patients had seizures, three had renal function impairment, four had paresthesias, either in limbs or periorally, and five had documented electrolyte disturbances primarily involving calcium and phosphate.

Treatment: There is no specific antidote. Hemodialysis and hydration may be of benefit in reducing drug plasma levels in patients who receive an overdosage, but these have not been evaluated in a clinical trial setting. Observe the patient for signs and symptoms of renal impairment and electrolyte imbalance. Institute medical treatment if clinically warranted. Refer to General Management of Acute Overdosage.

Patient Information:

CMV retinitis: Foscarnet is not a cure for CMV retinitis; patients may continue to experience progression of retinitis during or following treatment. Regular ophthalmologic examinations are necessary.

HSV infections: Foscarnet is not a cure for HSV infections. While complete healing may occur, relapse occurs in most patients. Because relapse may be due to acyclovir-sensitive HSV, sensitivity testing of the viral isolate is advised. Repeated treatment with foscarnet has led to development of resistance associated with poorer response. In this case, sensitivity testing of the viral isolate also is advised.

The major toxicities of foscarnet are renal impairment, electrolyte disturbances and seizures; dose modifications and possibly discontinuation may be required.

Close monitoring while on therapy is essential. Advise patients of the importance of perioral tingling, numbness in the extremities or paresthesias during or after infusion as possible symptoms of electrolyte abnormalities. Should such symptoms occur, stop the infusion, obtain appropriate laboratory samples for assessment of electrolyte concentrations and consult a physician before resuming treatment. The rate of infusion must be ≤ 1 mg/kg/min.

The potential for renal impairment may be minimized by accompanying administration with hydration adequate to establish and maintain diuresis during dosing.

Administration and Dosage:

Caution: Do not administer by rapid or bolus IV injection. Toxicity may be increased as a result of excessive plasma levels. Take care to avoid unintentional overdose; carefully control the rate of infusion by using an infusion pump. In spite of the use of an infusion pump, overdoses have occurred.

Hydration may reduce the risk of nephrotoxicity. It is recommended that 750 to 1000 ml of normal saline or 5% dextrose solution should be given prior to the first infusion of foscarnet to establish diuresis. With subsequent infusions, 750 to 1000 ml of hydration fluid should be given with 90 to 120 mg/kg of foscarnet and 500 ml with 40 to 60 mg/kg of foscarnet. Hydration fluid may need to be decreased if clinically warranted. After the first dose, the hydration fluid should be administered concurrently with each infusion of foscarnet.

Administer by controlled IV infusion, either by using a central venous line or a peripheral vein. The standard 24 mg/ml solution may be used without dilution when using a central venous catheter for infusion. When a peripheral vein catheter is used, dilute the 24 mg/ml solution to 12 mg/ml with 5% Dextrose in Water or with a Normal Saline Solution prior to administration to avoid local irritation of peripheral veins. Because the dose is calculated on the basis of body weight, it may be desirable to remove and discard any unneeded quantity from the bottle before starting with the infusion to avoid overdosage.

FOSCARNET SODIUM (Phosphonoformic acid; PFA)

Induction treatment:

CMV retinitis – The recommended initial dose for patients with normal renal function is either 90 mg/kg (1.5- to 2-hour infusion) every 12 hours or 60 mg/kg over a minimum of 1 hour every 8 hours for 2 to 3 weeks depending on clinical response.

HSV infections – The recommended initial dose for acyclovir-resistant HSV patients with normal renal function is 40 mg/kg (minimum 1 hour infusion) either every 8 or 12 hours for 2 to 3 weeks or until healed.

An infusion pump must be used to control the rate of infusion. Adequate hydration is recommended to establish diuresis, both prior to and during treatment to minimize renal toxicity (see Warnings), provided there are no clinical contraindications.

Maintenance treatment: 90 to 120 mg/kg/day (individualized for renal function) given as an IV infusion over 2 hours. Because the superiority of the 120 mg/kg/day has not been established in controlled trials and given the likely relationship of higher plasma foscarnet levels to toxicity, it is recommended that most patients be started on maintenance treatment with a dose of 90 mg/kg/day. Escalation to 120 mg/kg/day may be considered should early reinduction be required because of retinitis progression. Some patients who show excellent tolerance to foscarnet may benefit from initiation of maintenance treatment at 120 mg/kg/day earlier in their treatment. An infusion pump must be used to control the rate of infusion with all doses. Again, hydration to establish diuresis both prior to and during treatment is recommended to minimize renal toxicity.

Patients who experience progression of retinitis while receiving maintenance therapy may be retreated with the induction and maintenance regimens given above.

Renal function impairment: Use with caution in patients with abnormal renal function because reduced plasma clearance of foscarnet will result in elevated plasma levels. In addition, foscarnet has the potential to further impair renal function (see Warnings). Safety and efficacy data for patients with baseline serum creatinine levels > 2.8 mg/dL or measured 24–hour creatinine clearances < 50 ml/min are limited. Carefully monitor renal function at baseline and during induction and maintenance therapy with appropriate dose adjustments. If Ccr falls below the limits of the dosing nomograms (0.4 ml/min/kg) during therapy, discontinue foscarnet and monitor the patient daily until resolution of renal impairment is ensured.

Dose adjustment – Individualize foscarnet dosing according to the patient's renal function status. Refer to the table below for recommended doses and adjust the dose as indicated.

To use this dosing guide, actual 24 hour Ccr (ml/min) must be divided by body weight (kg) or the estimated Ccr in ml/min/kg can be calculated from serum creatinine (mg/dl) using the following formula (modified Cockcroft and Gault equation):

$$\text{Males: } \frac{\text{Weight (kg)} \times (140 - \text{age})}{72 \times \text{serum creatinine (mg/dl)}} = \text{Ccr}$$

Females: 0.85 × above value

Foscarnet Dosing Guide Based on Ccr for Induction				
	HSV: Equivalent to		CMV: Equivalent to	
Ccr (ml/min/kg)	40 mg/kg q 12 hr	40 mg/kg q 8 hr	60 mg/kg q 8 hr	90 mg/kg q 12 hr
> 1.4	40 q 12 hr	40 q 8 hr	60 q 8 hr	90 q 12 hr
> 1 to 1.4	30 q 12 hr	30 q 8 hr	45 q 8 hr	70 q 12 hr
> 0.8 to 1	20 q 12 hr	35 q 12 hr	50 q 12 hr	50 q 12 hr
> 0.6 to 0.8	35 q 24 hr	25 q 12 hr	40 q 12 hr	80 q 24 hr
> 0.5 to 0.6	25 q 24 hr	40 q 24 hr	60 q 24 hr	60 q 24 hr
≥ 0.4 to 0.5	20 q 24 hr	35 q 24 hr	50 q 24 hr	50 q 24 hr
< 0.4	Not recommended	Not recommended	Not recommended	Not recommended

Foscarnet Dosing Guide Based on Ccr for Maintenance		
	CMV: Equivalent to	
Ccr (ml/min/kg)	90 mg/kg/day	120 mg/kg/day
> 1.4	90 q 24 hr	120 q 24 hr
> 1 to 1.4	70 q 24 hr	90 q 24 hr
> 0.8 to 1	50 q 24 hr	65 q 24 hr
> 0.6 to 0.8	80 q 48 hr	105 q 48 hr
> 0.5 to 0.6	60 q 48 hr	80 q 48 hr
≥ 0.4 to 0.5	50 q 48 hr	65 q 48 hr
< 0.4	Not recommended	Not recommended

FOSCARNET SODIUM (Phosphonoformic acid; PFA)

Admixture incompatibility: Other drugs and supplements can be administered to a patient receiving foscarnet. However, take care to ensure that foscarnet is only administered with Normal Saline or 5% Dextrose Solution and that no other drug or supplement is administered concurrently via the same catheter. Foscarnet is chemically incompatible with 30% Dextrose Solution, amphotericin B and solutions containing calcium such as Ringer's Lactate and TPN. Physical incompatibility with other IV drugs includes: Acyclovir sodium, diphenhydramine, dobutamine, droperidol, ganciclovir, gentamicin, haloperidol, isethionate, morphine sulfate, trimetrexate, pentamidine, vancomycin, trimethoprim/sulfamethoxazole, diazepam, midazolam, digoxin, phenytoin, leucovorin and prochlorperazine. Because of foscarnet's chelating properties, a precipitate can potentially occur when divalent cations are administered concurrently in the same catheter.

Storage/Stability: Store at room temperature 15° to 30°C (59° to 86°F) and do not freeze. At a concentration of 12 mg/ml in Normal Saline Solution, foscarnet is stable for 30 days at 5°C (41°F).

Rx	**Foscavir** (Astra)	**Injection:** 24 mg/ml	In 250 and 500 ml bottles.

DIDANOSINE (ddI; dideoxyinosine)

Warning:

Pancreatitis, which has been fatal in some cases, is the major clinical toxicity associated with didanosine therapy. Consider pancreatitis whenever a patient receiving didanosine develops abdominal pain and nausea, vomiting or elevated biochemical markers. Under these circumstances, suspend use until the diagnosis of pancreatitis is excluded (see Warnings).

Patients receiving didanosine or any antiretroviral therapy may continue to develop opportunistic infections and other complications of HIV infection, and should remain under close clinical observation by physicians experienced in the treatment of patients with HIV-associated diseases.

Actions:

Pharmacology: Didanosine is a synthetic purine nucleoside analog of deoxyadenosine, active against the human immunodeficiency virus (HIV). The chemical name for didanosine is 2′,3′-dideoxyinosine; it is also called ddI. It inhibits in vitro replication of HIV (also known as HTLV III or LAV) in human primary cell cultures and in established cell lines. After didanosine enters the cell, it is converted by cellular enzymes to the active antiviral metabolite, dideoxyadenosine triphosphate (ddATP). The intracellular half-life of ddATP varies from 8 to 24 hours.

A common feature of dideoxynucleosides (the class of compounds to which didanosine belongs) is the lack of a free 3′-hydroxyl group. In nucleic acid replication, the 3′-hydroxyl of a naturally occurring nucleoside is the acceptor for covalent attachment of subsequent nucleoside 5′-monophosphates; its presence is therefore requisite for continued DNA chain extension. Because ddATP lacks a 3′-hydroxyl group, incorporation of ddATP into viral DNA leads to chain termination and, thus, inhibition of viral replication. In addition, ddATP further contributes to inhibition of viral replication through interference with the HIV-RNA dependent DNA polymerase (reverse transcriptase) by competing with the natural nucleoside triphosphate, dATP, for binding to the active site of the enzyme.

Pharmacokinetics: Didanosine is rapidly degraded at acidic pH. Therefore, all oral formulations contain buffering agents designed to increase gastric pH. When the tablets are administered, each adult and pediatric dose must consist of 2 tablets to achieve adequate acid-neutralizing capacity for maximal absorption. For pediatric patients < 1 year of age, only 1 tablet is necessary.

Bioequivalence of dosage formulations – A study of 18 asymptomatic, HIV-seropositive patients comparing a 375 mg dose of powder for oral solution and buffered tablets indicated that didanosine is 20% to 25% more bioavailable from the tablet than the solution. A 375 mg dose of the buffered powder for oral solution produced similar plasma concentrations to a 300 mg (2 x 150 mg tablets) dose of the tablets. Mean peak plasma concentrations (C_{max}) were 1.6 mcg/ml (range, 0.4 to 2.9) for the buffered solution and 1.6 mcg/ml (range, 0.5 to 2.6) for the tablet. Mean area under the plasma concentration vs time curve (AUC) values were 3 mcg • hr/ml (range, 1.6 to 5.1) for the buffered solution and 2.6 mcg • hr/ml (range, 1.1 to 3.9) for the chewable tablet.

DIDANOSINE (ddI; dideoxyinosine)

Effect of food on oral absorption – Administer all didanosine formulations on an empty stomach. The administration of didanosine tablets within 5 minutes of a meal results in a 50% decrease in mean C_{max} and AUC values.

Adults – The pharmacokinetics of didanosine were evaluated in 69 adult patients with AIDS or severe AIDS-Related Complex (ARC) after single and multiple IV and oral doses. Patients received a 60 minute IV infusion once or twice a day for 2 weeks, at total daily doses ranging from 0.8 to 33 mg/kg. Oral doses equivalent to twice the IV dose were administered for an additional 4 weeks. Plasma concentrations were obtained on the first day of dosing and at steady state after IV and oral dosing.

Absorption: Although there was significant variability between patients, the C_{max} and AUC values increased in proportion to dose over the range of doses administered. At doses of ≤ 7 mg/kg, the average absolute bioavailability was 33% after a single dose and 37% after 4 weeks of dosing. Pharmacokinetic parameters at steady state were not significantly different from values obtained after the initial IV or oral dose.

Distribution: The steady-state volume of distribution after IV administration averaged 54 L (range, 22 to 103). In a study of five adults, the concentration in the CSF 1 hour after infusion averaged 21% of the simultaneous plasma concentration.

Elimination: After oral administration, average elimination half-life was 1.6 hours (range, 0.52 to 4.64). Total body clearance averaged 800 ml/min (range, 412 to 1505). Renal clearance represented ≈ 50% of total body clearance (average, 400 ml/min; range, 95 to 860) when didanosine was given either IV or orally. This indicates that active tubular secretion, in addition to glomerular filtration, is responsible for the renal elimination. Urinary recovery after a single dose was ≈ 55% (range, 27% to 98%), and 20% (range, 3% to 31%) of the dose after IV and oral administration, respectively. There was no evidence of accumulation after either IV or oral dosing.

Children – The pharmacokinetics of didanosine have been evaluated in two pediatric studies. In one study, 16 children and 4 adolescents received a single IV dose ranging from 40 to 90 mg/m^2 and multiple, twice-daily oral doses of 80 to 180 mg/m^2 of didanosine. In another study, 48 pediatric patients received a single IV dose and then multiple, 3 times daily oral doses ranging from 20 to 180 mg/m^2.

Absorption: Although there was significant variability between patients, the C_{max} and AUC values increased in proportion to dose in both studies. These findings were similar to those in adult patients. The absolute bioavailability varied between patients in one study and averaged 32% (range, 13% to 53%) and 42% (range, 21% to 78%), after the first oral dose and at steady state, respectively. The other study also demonstrated significant variability in the oral absorption of didanosine with an average absolute bioavailability of 19% (range, 2% to 89%). In one study, the average steady-state AUC was 1.4, 1.6 and 2.3 mcg•hr/ml after the administration of oral doses of 80, 120 and 180 mg/m^2, respectively. The average corresponding steady-state C_{max} values were 0.8, 1.4 and 1.7 mcg/ml, respectively.

Distribution: In one study, the volume of distribution after IV administration averaged 35.6 L/m^2 (range, 18.4 to 60.7). In this study, the concentration of didanosine ranged from 0.04 to 0.12 mcg/ml in CSF samples collected from seven patients at times ranging from 1.5 to 3.5 hours after a single IV or oral dose. These CSF concentrations corresponded to 12% to 85% (mean, 46%) of the concentration in a simultaneous plasma sample.

Elimination: In one study, the elimination half-life following oral administration averaged 0.8 hours (range, 0.51 to 1.2). Total body clearance following IV administration averaged 532 ml/min/m^2 (range, 294 to 920). Mean renal clearance ranged from 190 to 319 ml/min/m^2 after the first oral dose and from 231 to 265 ml/min/m^2 at steady state. Urinary recovery averaged 17% (range, 5.4% to 30.4%) at steady state. There was no evidence of accumulation of didanosine after the administration of oral doses for an average of 26 days.

Metabolism: The metabolism of didanosine has not been evaluated in humans. When didanosine was administered to dogs as a single IV or oral dose, extensive metabolism occurred. The major metabolite identified in the urine, allantoin, represented ≈ 61% after oral administration. Three putative metabolites tentatively identified in the urine were hypoxanthine, xanthine and uric acid. Based on data from animal studies, it is presumed that the metabolism of didanosine in humans will occur by the same pathways responsible for elimination of endogenous purines.

The intracellular half-life of ddATP, the metabolite presumed to be responsible for the antiretroviral activity of didanosine, is 8 to 24 hours in vitro.

In vitro human plasma protein binding is < 5%.

DIDANOSINE (ddI; dideoxyinosine)

Microbiology: The relationship between in vitro susceptibility of HIV to didanosine and the inhibition of HIV replication in man or clinical response to therapy is not established.

Didanosine has in vitro antiviral activity in a variety of HIV-infected T cell and monocyte/macrophage cell cultures. The concentration of drug necessary to inhibit viral replication 50% ranges from 2.5 to 10 mcM (1mcM = 0.2 mcg/ml) in T cells and from 0.01 to 0.1 mcM in monocyte/macrophage cell cultures.

The development of clinically significant didanosine resistance in patients with HIV infection receiving didanosine therapy has not been studied adequately and the frequency of didanosine-resistant isolates in the general population remains unknown.

Didanosine inhibits human hepatitis B virus replication in vitro; the clinical significance is unknown.

Clinical trials:

Controlled clinical trials, results – A randomized, double-blind, controlled clinical trial compared two doses of didanosine (250 to 375 mg twice daily) to zidovudine in patients (n = 913) who had tolerated ≥ 4 months of prior zidovudine therapy.

Median duration of prior zidovudine was 13.7 months. The median entry CD4 cell count was 95 cells/mcl; 60% of patients had ARC, 30% had AIDS and 10% had asymptomatic HIV disease. Median treatment duration during the study was 11.4 months.

Overall, participants randomized to didanosine at the recommended dose had a statistically significant delay in time to first new AIDS-defining event or death compared to those randomized to zidovudine. There was no statistically significant difference between the high-dose didanosine and zidovudine arms in time to first new AIDS-defining event or death.

At 1 year the proportion of patients who developed a new AIDS-defining event or death was 40% with zidovudine, vs 28% and 34% for didianosine at the recommended dose and high dose, respectively. There were no survival differences observed among the treatment arms.

The mean change in CD4 cell counts by week 12 was + 13 and + 11 for high dose and recommended dose didanosine, respectively, vs –9 for zidovudine. At week 24, the mean change was –9, –7 and –27, respectively. The 50:50 response (see Phase I trials) was 10% for high-dose didanosine, 9% for didanosine at the recommended dose, and 3% for zidovudine. The 10:10 response was 37%, 34% and 17%, respectively.

Phase I trials –

Adults: Median CD4 count at entry was 62 cells/mcl. Dosages ranged from 0.8 to 66 mg/kg/day for a median duration of 38 weeks (range, 0 to 99). The median average daily dose was 10.3 mg/kg. Analyses included the following:

a) Presence of a "response," where response was defined as i) the greater of a 50 cell or 50% increase over baseline CD4 cell count maintained for a minimum of any consecutive 4 weeks during therapy (50:50); ii) the greater of a 10 cell or 10% increase over baseline CD4 cell count maintained for a minimum of any consecutive 4 weeks during therapy (10:10).

b) Percent change from baseline in CD4 cell count at various time points on therapy.

c) Longitudinal changes during study weeks 0 to 12: Time weighted average of serial CD4 cell counts corrected for (normalized by) baseline CD4 cell count (NAUC). NAUCs that exceed a value of 1 indicate that the average CD4 level during therapy is increased over the baseline CD4 cell count.

Results:

a) Response – i) 22% of patients receiving didanosine had a 50:50 response in CD4 counts vs 2% to 12% of the historical control patients; ii) 50% of patients receiving didanosine had a 10:10 response in CD4 counts vs 17% to 31% of the historical control patients.

b) Percent change from baseline – In patients receiving didanosine the increase from baseline CD4 cell counts was 29% at 4 weeks, 27% at 8 weeks and 14% at 12 weeks. In comparison, historical control groups had progressive declines in CD4 cell counts.

c) Longitudinal changes during study weeks 0 to 12 – Seventy percent of patients receiving didanosine had NAUC values exceeding 1, vs 34% to 46% of the historical control patients. The mean NAUC in patients receiving didanosine was 1.38 vs 0.99 to 1.04 in historical control groups.

DIDANOSINE (ddI; dideoxyinosine)

Children: Patients received doses from 60 to 540 mg/m²/day. Based on an increased incidence of pancreatitis observed at the higher doses administered, all patients treated at doses > 360 mg/m²/day were dose-reduced to this level or lower. Due to multiple-dose adjustments, 77% of patients received average daily doses ≤ 300 mg/m²/day. Results were obtained from open-label studies without controls.

Activity of didanosine was based on the criteria previously described for the adult patients. Weight gain in children was also analyzed as either a 10% increase in weight (for smaller children) or a 2.5 kg increase (for children > 25 kg), also occurring at any time during therapy and maintained for at least 4 weeks.

The effect of didanosine on survival and the incidence of opportunistic infections in children could not be assessed in these studies, and data evaluating the impact of didanosine therapy on clinical parameters of HIV infection in children are not currently available. Therefore, consider zidovudine as initial therapy for the treatment of advanced HIV infection, unless contraindicated.

Thirty-seven percent of patients had a 10:10 response in CD4 counts, and 23% had a 50:50 response. The percent increase from baseline CD4 counts was 27% at 8 weeks. A weight response occurred in 39% of patients.

In general, hematologic parameters were stable during treatment with didanosine. In addition, improvement in platelet counts was seen in 3 of 6 patients with idiopathic thrombocytopenic purpura who entered the pediatric studies with this diagnosis. Some children exhibited improvements in detailed neuropsychometric tests. An increment in an individual's IQ score of 10% and a minimum of 8 points relative to baseline was considered a response. Improvement was seen in 12 of 43 evaluable patients with a baseline IQ < 115. In the absence of a control group, the contribution of drug to this increase is uncertain.

Indications:

For the treatment of adult patients with advanced HIV infection who have received prolonged prior zidovudine therapy.

For the treatment of adult and pediatric patients (> 6 months of age) with advanced HIV infection who have demonstrated intolerance or significant clinical or immunologic deterioration during zidovudine therapy.

Because zidovudine prolongs survival and decreases the incidence of opportunistic infections in patients with advanced HIV disease, consider zidovudine as initial therapy for the treatment of advanced HIV infection, unless contraindicated.

Contraindications:

Hypersensitivity to any of the components of the formulations.

Warnings:

Peripheral neuropathy occurs in patients treated with didanosine; the frequency appears to be dose-related. Monitor patients for the development of a neuropathy that is usually characterized by distal numbness, tingling, or pain in the feet or hands. In the controlled trial comparing two doses of didanosine to zidovudine, the 1 year rates of grades 2, 3 or 4 peripheral neuropathy were 14%, 13% and 14% for high-dose didanosine at the recommended dose, and zidovudine, respectively.

Incidence of Neuropathy with Didanosine

Parameter	All phase I (n = 170)	≤ 12.5 mg/kg/day (n = 91)	Phase I > 12.5 mg/kg/day (n = 79)
Neuropathy	42%	34%	51%
Neuropathy requiring dose modification	22%	12%	34%

Among the 91 adult Phase I patients who received an average oral daily dose approximately ≤ 750 mg/day, 12% had neuropathy severe enough to require dose modification; 34% of patients in these studies treated with ≤ 12.5 mg/kg/day developed neuropathy.

Neuropathy occurred more frequently in patients with a history of neuropathy or neurotoxic drug therapy. These patients may be at increased risk of neuropathy during didanosine therapy.

Neuropathy has occurred rarely in children treated with didanosine. However, because signs and symptoms of neuropathy are difficult to assess in children, alert physicians of this possibility.

DIDANOSINE (ddI; dideoxyinosine)

Pancreatitis which has been fatal in some cases is the major clinical toxicity associated with didanosine therapy (see Warning Box). Pancreatitis must be considered whenever a patient receiving didanosine develops abdominal pain, nausea, vomiting or elevated biochemical markers. Under these circumstances, suspend use of didanosine until the diagnosis of pancreatitis is excluded. When treatment with other drugs known to cause pancreatic toxicity is required (eg, IV pentamidine), consider suspension of didanosine.

Incidence of Pancreatitis with Didanosine			
Controlled Study			
	Didanosine		
Parameter	High dose (n = 311)	Recommended dose (n = 298)	Zidovudine (n = 304)
Pancreatitis	3.2%	2%	0.66%
Abdominal pain/nausea and elevated amylase	< 0.1%	0.2%	0.3%
Elevated amylase	4.5%	3.4%	< 1%
Abdominal pain/nausea	0.3%	0.7%	1.3%
Phase I Studies			
Parameter	All phase I (n = 170)	≤ 12.5 mg/kg/day (n = 91)	> 12.5 mg/kg/day (n = 79)
Pancreatitis	17%	9%	27%
Abdominal pain	8%	10%	6%
Increased amylase	16%	18%	15%
Abdominal pain and increased amylase	6%	7%	6%

In the Expanded Access Program for didanosine, 30% of patients treated with didanosine who had a history of pancreatitis, developed pancreatitis. Use only with extreme caution in this population.

Closely follow patients with a heightened risk of pancreatitis, such as those with a history of pancreatitis, alcohol consumption, elevated triglycerides or evidence of advanced HIV infection. Patients with renal impairment may be at greater risk for pancreatitis if treated without dose adjustment.

In pediatric studies, pancreatitis occurred in 3% of patients treated at entry doses < 300 mg/m²/day and in 13% treated at higher doses. In pediatric patients with symptoms similar to those described above, suspend didanosine until the diagnosis of pancreatitis is excluded.

Hepatic failure: In the controlled clinical trial comparing two doses of didanosine to zidovudine, the 1 year rates of grade 3 to 4 liver function test alteration was 21% for high-dose didanosine, 13% for didanosine at the recommended dose and 14% for zidovudine. Fatal liver failure of unknown etiology occurred during didanosine therapy in 1/170 patients in the Phase I studies and 14/7806 in the Expanded Access Program.

Retinal depigmentation: Four pediatric patients demonstrated retinal depigmentation at doses > 300 mg/m²/day. Two of the patients, treated at doses of 540 mg/m²/day, had progression of disease when treated with lower doses. One patient treated at lower doses has continued therapy without progression of disease. Children receiving didanosine should undergo dilated retinal examination every 6 months or if a change in vision occurs.

Myopathy: Evidence of a dose-limiting skeletal muscle toxicity has been observed in mice and rats (but not in dogs) following long-term (> 90 days) dosing with didanosine at doses that were approximately 1.2 to 12 times the estimated human exposure. Human myopathy has been associated with administration of other nucleoside analogs.

Renal function impairment: Patients with renal impairment (serum creatinine > 1.5 mg/dl or creatinine clearance < 60 ml/min) may be at greater risk of toxicity from didanosine due to decreased drug clearance; consider a dose reduction. The magnesium hydroxide content of each tablet (15.7 mEq) may present an excessive magnesium load to patients with significant renal impairment, particularly after prolonged dosing.

Hepatic function impairment: Patients with hepatic impairment may be at greater risk for toxicity due to altered metabolism; a dose reduction may be necessary.

DIDANOSINE (ddI; dideoxyinosine)

Mutagenesis: In an in vitro cytogenic study, high concentrations of didanosine (≥ 500 mcg/ml) elevated the frequency of cells bearing chromosome aberrations. Another in vitro study revealed that didanosine produces chromosome aberrations at ≥ 500 mcg/ml after 48 hours of exposure. Similar chromosomal aberration effects were induced by the natural nucleoside of didanosine (2′-deoxyinosine), suggesting that these effects of didanosine were not due to a direct genotoxic interaction.

At significantly elevated doses in vitro, the genotoxic effects of didanosine are similar in magnitude to those seen with natural DNA nucleosides.

Pregnancy: Category B. At approximately 12 times the estimated human exposure, didanosine was slightly toxic to female rats and their pups during mid and late lactation. These rats showed reduced food intake and body weight gains but the physical and functional development of the offspring was not impaired and there were no major changes in the F2 generation. There are no adequate and well controlled studies in pregnant women. Use during pregnancy only if clearly needed.

Lactation: It is not known whether didanosine is excreted in breast milk. Because of the potential for serious adverse reactions from didanosine in nursing infants, instruct mothers to discontinue nursing when taking didanosine.

Children: See Indications, Warnings and Administration and Dosage.

Precautions:

Opportunistic infections: Patients receiving didanosine or any other antiretroviral therapy may continue to develop opportunistic infections and other complications of HIV infection and, therefore, should remain under close clinical observation by physicians experienced in the treatment of patients with associated HIV diseases.

Progression of HIV infection: At present there are no results from controlled studies regarding the effect of didanosine therapy on the clinical progression of HIV infection, such as incidence of opportunistic infections and survival.

Phenylketonuria: Didanosine tablets contain 22.5 mg phenylalanine (33.7 mg in the 150 mg tablet).

Sodium-restricted diets: Each buffered tablet contains 264.5 mg sodium. Each single-dose packet of buffered powder for oral solution contains 1380 mg sodium.

Hyperuricemia: Didanosine has been associated with asymptomatic hyperuricemia; consider suspending treatment if clinical measures aimed at reducing uric acid levels fail.

Diarrhea: Didanosine buffered powder for oral solution was associated with diarrhea in 34% of patients in the Phase I adult studies. No data are available to demonstrate whether other formulations are associated with lower rates of diarrhea. However, if diarrhea develops in a patient receiving buffered powder for oral solution, consider a trial of chewable/dispersible buffered tablets.

Drug Interactions:

Didanosine Drug Interactions

Precipitant drug	Object drug *		Description
Didanosine	Fluoroquinolones	⬇	Plasma concentrations of some quinolone antibiotics are decreased when administered with antacids containing magnesium or aluminum. Therefore, do not administer quinolone antibiotics within 2 hours of taking didanosine tablets or pediatric powder for oral solution.
Didanosine	Tetracyclines	⬇	As with other products containing magnesium or aluminum antacid components, do not simultaneously administer didanosine tablets or pediatric powder for oral solution with tetracycline.

* ⬇ = Object drug decreased

Administer drugs whose absorption can be affected by the level of acidity in the stomach (eg, ketoconazole, dapsone) at least 2 hours prior to dosing with didanosine.

Coadministration of didanosine with drugs that are known to cause peripheral neuropathy or pancreatitis may increase the risk of these toxicities. Closely observe patients who receive these drugs.

Drug/Food interactions: Ingestion of didanosine with food reduces the absorption of didanosine by as much as 50%. Therefore, administer on an empty stomach.

DIDANOSINE (ddI; dideoxyinosine)

Adverse Reactions:

The major toxicities are pancreatitis and peripheral neuropathy (see Warnings).

Didanosine Adverse Reactions (Adults) (%)			
	Didanosine		
Adverse reaction	Recommended dose (n = 298)	High dose (n = 311)	Zidovudine (n = 304)
Diarrhea	28	20	21
Neuropathy (all grades)	20	17	17
Chills/Fever	12	9	11
Rash/Pruritus	9	7	5
Abdominal pain	7	10	8
Asthenia	7	5	9
Headache	7	10	7
Pain	7	7	3
Nausea/Vomiting	7	6	6
Infection	6	5	5
Pancreatitis	6	10	2
Pneumonia	5	6	5
Sarcoma	3	3	4
Myopathy	3	2	6
Anorexia	2	1	2
Dry mouth	2	3	0
Convulsion	2	2	2
Thinking abnormally	2	1	1
Dyspnea	2	3	3
Allergic reaction	1	2	1
Anxiety/Nervousness/Twitching	1	2	2
Confusion	1	2	0
Depression	1	2	3
Lab test abnormalities			
Leukopenia (< 2000/mcl)	16	13	22
Amylase (≥ 5 x ULN*)	15	22	5
Granulocytopenia (< 750/mcl)	8	8	15
Thrombocytopenia (< 50,000/mcl)	2	2	3
ALT (> 5 x ULN*)	6	8	6
AST (> 5 x ULN*)	7	8	6
Alkaline phosphatase (> 5 x ULN*)	1	4	1
Hemoglobin (< 8 g/dl)	3	2	5
Bilirubin (> 5 x ULN*)	1	2	1
Uric acid (> 5 x ULN*)	2	1	1

* ULN = Upper limit of normal

Children: In pediatric studies, pancreatitis occurred in 3% of patients treated at entry doses < 300 mg/m^2/day and in 13% of patients treated at higher doses.

Body as a whole: Abscess, cellulitis, cyst, dehydration, flu syndrome, hernia, neck rigidity, numbness of hands/feet (≤ 1%).

Cardiovascular: Chest pain, hypotension, hypertension, migraine, palpitation, peripheral vascular disorder, syncope (≤ 1%).

GI: Colitis, constipation, eructation, flatulence, gastroenteritis, GI hemorrhage, moniliasis (oral), sialadenitis, stomach ulcer hemorrhage (≤ 1%).

CNS: Acute brain syndrome, amnesia, aphasia, ataxia, convulsion (grand mal), dizziness, hyperesthesia, hypertonia, ileus, incoordination, intracranial hemorrhage, malaise, paralysis, paranoid reaction, psychosis, sleep disorder, speech disorder, tremor (≤ 1%).

Metabolic/Nutritional: Anomaly, arthralgia, arthritis, edema (peripheral), hemiparesis, hypokalemia, joint disorder, leg cramp (≤ 1%).

DIDANOSINE (ddI; dideoxyinosine)

Respiratory: Asthma, bronchitis, cough increased, epistaxis, laryngitis, lung function decreased, pharyngitis, pneumonia (interstitial), respiratory disorder (≤ 1%).

Special senses: Blurred vision, conjunctivitis, diplopia, dry eye, ear disorder, glaucoma, otitis (externa and media), retinitis (≤ 1%).

GU: Impotence, kidney calculus/failure/abnormal function, nocturia, urinary frequency, vaginal hemorrhage (≤ 1%).

Dermatologic: Herpes simplex, pruritus, skin disorder, sweating (≤ 1%).

Hematologic/Lymphatic: Hemorrhage, lymphoma-like reaction, microcytic anemia (≤ 1%).

Didanosine Adverse Reactions (Children)

Adverse reaction	< 300 mg/m^2/day (n = 60)	All patients (n = 98)
Body as whole		
Chills/Fever	82%	82%
Anorexia	52%	51%
Asthenia	42%	41%
Pain	27%	31%
Malaise	38%	29%
Failure to thrive	13%	9%
Weight loss	10%	8%
Flu syndrome	7%	7%
Change in appetite	10%	6%
Alopecia	7%	5%
Dehydration	7%	5%
Increased appetite	5%	0%
GI		
Diarrhea	82%	81%
Nausea/Vomiting	57%	58%
Liver abnormalities	32%	38%
Abdominal pain	32%	35%
Stomatitis/Mouth sores	17%	16%
Pancreatitis	3%	13%
Constipation	10%	12%
Oral thrush	13%	9%
Melena	7%	7%
Dry mouth	7%	4%
Lympho-Hematologic		
Ecchymosis	15%	15%
Hemorrhage	10%	10%
Petechiae	3%	7%
Musculoskeletal		
Arthritis	12%	11%
Myalgia	12%	9%
Muscle atrophy	12%	8%
Decreased strength	3%	6%
Cardiovascular		
Vasodilation	22%	22%
Arrhythmia	10%	6%
CNS		
Headache	58%	55%
Nervousness	33%	27%
Insomnia	10%	8%
Dizziness	5%	7%
Poor coordination	8%	6%
Lethargy	7%	4%
Neurologic	2%	< 1%
Seizure	1%	< 1%
Respiratory		
Cough	87%	85%
Rhinitis	48%	48%
Dyspnea	27%	23%
Asthma	28%	21%
Rhinorrhea	20%	21%
Epistaxis	13%	14%
Pharyngitis	17%	14%
Hypoventilation	10%	8%
Sinusitis	8%	7%
Rhonchi/Rales	8%	6%
Congestion	5%	3%
Pneumonia	1%	< 1%
Skin and appendages		
Rash/Pruritus	72%	70%
Skin disorder	12%	13%
Eczema	13%	12%
Sweating	8%	7%
Impetigo	5%	6%
Excoriation	7%	4%
Erythema	5%	4%
Special senses		
Ear pain/Otitis	13%	11%
Photophobia	8%	5%
Strabismus	8%	5%
Visual impairment	5%	5%
Other		
Urinary frequency	5%	4%
Diabetes mellitus	1%	< 1%
Diabetes insipidus	1%	< 1%

DIDANOSINE (ddI; dideoxyinosine)

Laboratory Test Abnormalities with Didanosine				
Laboratory test (seriously abnormal level)	Children		Adults	
	Normal baseline	Abnormal baseline	Normal baseline	Abnormal baseline
Leukopenia (< 2000/mcl)	3%	36%	5%	37%
Granulocytopenia (< 1000/mcl)	24%	62%	3%	56%
Thrombocytopenia (< 50,000/mcl)	2%	67%	1%	25%
Anemia (Hgb < 8 g/dl)	4%	27%	5%	0
ALT (> 5 x ULN*)	3%	25%	10%	12%
AST (> 5 x ULN*)	0	36%	10%	12%
Alkaline phosphatase (> 5 x ULN*)	0	0	4%	17%
Bilirubin (> 5 x ULN*)	2%	0	3%	0
Uric acid (> 1.25 x ULN*)	0	0	6%	50%
Amylase (≥ 5 x ULN*)	0	0	3%	0

* ULN = Upper limit of normal

Overdosage:

There is no known antidote for overdosage. Experience in the Phase I studies in which didanosine was initially administered at doses 10 times the currently recommended dose indicates that the complications of chronic overdosage would include pancreatitis, peripheral neuropathy, diarrhea, hyperuricemia or, possibly, hepatic dysfunction. It is not known whether didanosine is dialyzable by peritoneal or hemodialysis.

Administration and Dosage:

Approved by the FDA in October 1991.

Dosage: Use a 12 hour dosing interval. Administer all formulations on an empty stomach.

Adults: Take 2 tablets at each dose so that adequate buffering is provided to prevent gastric acid degradation of didanosine. The recommended starting dose in adults is dependent on weight as outlined in the table below:

Adult Didanosine Dosing		
Patient weight (kg)	Tablets	Buffered powder
≥ 60	200 mg bid	250 mg bid
< 60	125 mg bid	167 mg bid

Children: To prevent gastric acid degradation, children > 1 year of age should receive a 2 tablet dose; children < 1 year old should receive a 1 tablet dose. The recommended dose in children is dependent on body surface area as outlined in the table below. Doses equivalent to 100 to 300 mg/m^2/day of the pediatric powder are being further evaluated in controlled clinical trials. The optimal dose has not been established; some investigators recommend doses of up to 300 mg/m^2/day divided into 3 daily doses.

Pediatric Didanosine Dosing (based on 200 mg/m^2/day average recommended dose)[1]			
Body surface area (m^2)	Tablets	Pediatric powder (m^2)	
		Dose	Vol/10 mg/ml admixture
1.1-1.4	100 mg bid	125 mg bid	12.5 ml bid
0.8-1	75 mg bid	94 mg bid	9.5 ml bid
0.5-0.7	50 mg bid	62 mg bid	6 ml bid
< 0.4	25 mg bid	31 mg bid	3 ml bid

[1] Based on didanosine pediatric powder.

Dose adjustment: If clinical signs suggest pancreatitis, suspend dose and carefully evaluate the possibility of pancreatitis. Resume dosing only after pancreatitis has been ruled out.

Many patients who have presented with symptoms of neuropathy will tolerate a reduced dose after resolution of these symptoms following drug discontinuation.

There are insufficient data to recommend dose adjustment in patients with impaired renal or hepatic function. Consider a dose reduction in patients with renal insufficiency or hepatic impairment.

DIDANOSINE (ddI; dideoxyinosine)

Method of preparation:

Adults –

Chewable/dispersible buffered tablets: Thoroughly chew tablets or manually crush or disperse 2 tablets in at least 1 ounce of water prior to consumption. To disperse tablets, add 2 tablets to at least 1 ounce of water. Stir until a uniform dispersion forms, and drink entire dispersion immediately.

Buffered powder for oral solution:

1. Open packet carefully and pour contents into approximately 4 ounces of water. Do not mix with fruit juice or other acid-containing liquid.
2. Stir until the powder completely dissolves (approximately 2 to 3 minutes).
3. Drink the entire solution immediately.

Children –

Chewable/dispersible buffered tablets: Chew tablets or manually crush or disperse 1 or 2 tablets in water prior to consumption, as described for adults.

Pediatric powder for oral solution: Prior to dispensing, the pharmacist must constitute dry powder with Purified Water, USP, to an initial concentration of 20 mg/ml and immediately mix the resulting solution with antacid to a final concentration of 10 mg/ml as follows:

20 mg/ml initial solution – Reconstitute the product to 20 mg/ml by adding 100 or 200 ml Purified Water, USP, to the 2 or 4 g of powder, respectively, in the product bottle. Prepare final admixture as described below.

10 mg/ml final admixture – 1. Immediately mix one part of the 20 mg/ml initial solution with one part of either *Mylanta Double Strength Liquid* or *Maalox TC Suspension* for a final dispensing concentration of 10 mg/ml. For patient home use, dispense the admixture in flint-glass bottles with child-resistant closures. This admixture is stable for 30 days under refrigeration at 2° to 8°C (36° to 46°F).

2. Instruct the patient to shake the admixture thoroughly prior to use and to store the tightly closed container in the refrigerator at 2° to 8°C (36° to 46°F), up to 30 days.

Spill, leak and disposal procedure: Avoid generating dust during clean-up of powdered products; use wet mop or damp sponge. Clean surface with soap and water as necessary. Contain larger spills.

Rx	**Videx** (Bristol-Myers Squibb)	**Tablets, buffered, chewable/dispersible:**[1] 25 mg	(Videx BL 25). White. Mint flavor. In 60s.
		50 mg	(Videx BL 50). White. Mint flavor. In 60s.
		100 mg	(Videx BL 100). White. Mint flavor. In 60s.
		150 mg	(Videx BL 150). White. Mint flavor. In 60s.
		Powder for Oral Solution, buffered:[2] 100 mg	In single-dose packets.
		167 mg	In single-dose packets.
		250 mg	In single-dose packets.
		375 mg	In single-dose packets.
		Powder for Oral Solution, pediatric: 2 g	In bottles.
		4 g	In bottles.

[1] Buffered with dihydroaluminum sodium carbonate, magnesium hydroxide and sodium citrate. With aspartame and sugar.

[2] Buffered with dibasic sodium phosphate, sodium citrate and citric acid. With sucrose.

ACYCLOVIR (Acycloguanosine)

Actions:

Pharmacology: A synthetic acyclic purine nucleoside analog, acyclovir has in vitro inhibitory activity against Herpes simplex virus types 1 and 2 (HSV–1 and HSV–2), varicella zoster, Epstein-Barr and cytomegalovirus. Acyclovir is preferentially taken up and selectively converted to the active triphosphate form by HSV-infected cells. Acyclovir triphosphate interferes with HSV DNA polymerase and inhibits viral DNA replication. In vitro, acyclovir triphosphate can be incorporated into growing chains of DNA by viral DNA polymerase and, to a much smaller extent, by cellular DNA polymerase. When incorporation occurs, the DNA chain is terminated.

The relationship between in vitro susceptibility of HSV to antiviral drugs and clinical response has not been established.

Pharmacokinetics:

Absorption/Distribution – Proportionality between dose and plasma levels is seen after single doses or at steady-state after multiple dosing. When acyclovir was administered to adults at 5 mg/kg (≈ 250 mg/m^2) by 1 hour infusions every 8 hours, mean steady-state peak and trough concentrations were 9.8 mcg/ml (5.5 to 13.8 mcg/ml) and 0.7 mcg/ml (0.2 to 1 mcg/ml), respectively. Similar concentrations are achieved in children > 1 year old when doses of 250 mg/m^2 are given every 8 hours. Oral acyclovir is slowly and incompletely absorbed from the GI tract. Peak concentrations are reached in 1.5 to 2 hours; absorption is unaffected by food. Bioavailability is between 15% and 30% and decreases with increasing doses. Concentrations achieved in CSF are ≈ 50% of plasma values. Plasma protein binding is 9% to 33%. Acyclovir is widely distributed in tissues and body fluids, including brain, kidney, lung, liver, muscle, spleen, uterus, vaginal mucosa, vaginal secretions, CSF and herpetic vesicular fluid.

Metabolism/Excretion – Renal excretion of unchanged drug by glomerular filtration and tubular secretion following IV use accounts for 62% to 91% of the dose. Mean renal excretion of unchanged drug following oral use is 14.4% (8.6% to 19.8%). The only major urinary metabolite is 9–carboxymethoxymethylguanine; this may account for up to 14% of the dose in patients with normal renal function. An insignificant amount is recovered in feces and expired CO_2; there is no evidence of tissue retention.

Half-life and total body clearance depend on renal function:

Acyclovir Half-Life and Total Body Clearance Based on Renal Function		
Creatinine clearance (ml/min/1.73 m^2)	Half-life (h)	Total body clearance (ml/min/1.73 m^2)
> 80	2.5	327
50-80	3	248
15-50	3.5	190
0 (Anuric)	19.5	29

The half-life and total body clearance of acyclovir in pediatric patients > 1 year of age are similar to those in adults with normal renal function.

Clinical trials:

Genital herpes (oral therapy) –

Initial episodes: Oral acyclovir reduced the duration of acute infection and lesion healing. Duration of pain and new lesion formation were decreased in some patients. The promptness of initiation of therapy or the patient's prior exposure to HSV may influence the degree of benefit from therapy.

Recurrent episodes: In patients with frequent recurrences (≥ 6 episodes per year), oral acyclovir given for 4 months to 3 years prevented or reduced the frequency or severity of recurrences in > 95% of patients. In a study of 283 patients who received 400 mg twice daily for 3 years, 45%, 52% and 63% of patients remained free of recurrences in the first, second and third years, respectively. Serial analysis of the 3 month recurrence rates for the 283 patients showed that 71% to 87% were recurrence-free in each quarter, indicating that the effects are consistent over time.

In general, do not use for suppression of recurrent disease in mildly affected patients. Immunocompromised patients with recurrent HSV can be treated with either intermittent or chronic suppressive therapy. Clinically significant resistance, although rare, is more likely to be seen with prolonged or repeated therapy in severely immunocompromised patients with active lesions.

Herpes zoster – In two studies of 270 patients with localized cutaneous zoster infection, acyclovir 800 mg 5 times daily for 7 to 10 days shortened the times to lesion scabbing, healing and complete cessation of pain, and reduced the duration of viral shedding, the duration of new lesion formation and the prevalence of localized zoster-associated neurologic symptoms (paresthesia, dysesthesia, hyperesthesia).

ACYCLOVIR (Acycloguanosine)

Chickenpox – In 110 patients (5 to 16 years of age) who presented within 24 hours of the onset of a typical chickenpox rash, acyclovir 4 times daily for 5 to 7 days at oral doses of 10, 15 or 20 mg/kg depending on age reduced the maximum number of lesions (336 vs > 500; lesions beyond 500 were not counted). Acyclovir also shortened the mean time to 50% healing (7.1 vs 8.7 days), reduced the number of vesicular lesions by the second day of treatment (49 vs 113) and decreased the proportion of patients with fever (temperature > 38°C [100°F]) by the second day (19% vs 57%).

In two studies, 883 patients (2 to 18 years of age) were enrolled within 24 hours of the onset of a typical chickenpox rash. In the larger study (n = 815, 2 to 12 years of age), acyclovir 20 mg/kg orally up to 800 mg 4 times daily for 5 days reduced the median maximum number of lesions (277 vs 386), the median number of vesicular lesions by the second day of treatment (26 vs 40) and the proportion of patients with moderate to severe itching by the third day of treatment (15% vs 34%). In addition, in both studies acyclovir also decreased the proportion of patients with fever (> 38°C [100°F]), anorexia and lethargy by the second day of treatment and decreased the mean number of residual lesions on day 28.

Indications:

Parenteral: Treatment of initial and recurrent mucosal and cutaneous HSV-1 and HSV-2 and varicella-zoster (shingles) infections in immunocompromised patients.

Herpes simplex encephalitis in patients > 6 months of age.

Severe initial clinical episodes of genital herpes in patients who are not immunocompromised.

Oral: Treatment of initial episodes and management of recurrent episodes of genital herpes in certain patients. Severity of the disease (and hence, patient selection) depends upon the immune status of the patient, frequency and duration of episodes and degree of cutaneous or systemic involvement.

Acute treatment of herpes zoster (shingles) and chickenpox (varicella).

Unlabeled uses: Other potential uses of oral or parenteral acyclovir include:

Unlabeled Uses of Acyclovir

Cytomegalovirus and HSV infection following bone marrow or renal transplantation	Herpes simplex ocular infections
	Herpes simplex proctitis
Disseminated primary eczema herpeticum	Herpes simplex whitlow
Herpes simplex-associated erythema multiforme	Herpes zoster encephalitis
	Infectious mononucleosis
Herpes simplex labialis	Varicella pneumonia

Contraindications:

Hypersensitivity to acyclovir or any component of the formulation.

Warnings:

Testicular atrophy occurred in rats administered acyclovir intraperitoneally at 320 or 80 mg/kg/day for 1 and 6 months, respectively. Some recovery of sperm production was evident 30 days post-dose.

Pregnancy: Category C. In a non-standard test in rats given 3 SC doses of 100 mg/kg (plasma levels of 63 and 125 times human levels), there was maternal toxicity and fetal abnormalities such as head and tail anomalies. There are no adequate and well controlled studies in pregnant women. Use during pregnancy only if the potential benefit outweighs the potential risk to the fetus. Potential uses in pregnancy would be for life-threatening infections such as disseminated maternal HSV infection and varicella pneumonia.

Lactation: Acyclovir concentrations in breast milk in women following oral administration have ranged from 0.6 to 4.1 times corresponding plasma levels. These concentrations would potentially expose the nursing infant to a dose of acyclovir up to 0.3 mg/kg/day. Exercise caution when administering to a nursing woman.

Children: Safety and efficacy of oral acyclovir in children < 2 years of age have not been established.

Precautions:

Diagnosis: Proof of HSV infection rests on viral isolation and identification in tissue culture. Although the cutaneous vesicular lesions associated with HSV are often characteristic, other etiologic agents can cause similar lesions.

Genital herpes: Avoid sexual intercourse when visible lesions are present because of the risk of infecting intimate partners.

ACYCLOVIR (Acycloguanosine)

Herpes zoster infections: Adults ≥ 50 years of age tend to have more severe shingles, and acyclovir treatment showed more significant benefit for older patients. Treatment was begun within 72 hours of rash onset in these studies, and was more useful if started within the first 48 hours.

Chickenpox: Although chickenpox in otherwise healthy children is usually a self-limited disease of mild to moderate severity, adolescents and adults tend to have more severe disease. Treatment was initiated within 24 hours of the typical chickenpox rash in the controlled studies, and there is no information regarding the effects of treatment begun later in the disease course. It is unknown whether the treatment of chickenpox in childhood has any effect on long term immunity. However, there is no evidence to indicate that acyclovir treatment of chickenpox would have any effect on either decreasing or increasing the incidence or severity of subsequent recurrences of herpes zoster (shingles) later in life. IV acyclovir is indicated for the treatment of varicella-zoster infections in immunocompromised patients.

Do not exceed the recommended dosage, frequency or length of treatment. Base dosage adjustments on estimated creatinine clearance.

Renal effects: Precipitation of acyclovir crystals in renal tubules can occur if the maximum solubility of free acyclovir (2.5 mg/ml at 37°C in water) is exceeded or if the drug is administered by bolus injection. Serum creatinine and blood urea nitrogen (BUN) rise and creatinine clearance decreases.

Bolus administration of the drug leads to a 10% incidence of renal dysfunction, while infusion of 5 mg/kg (250 mg/m^2) over one hour was associated with a lower frequency (4.6%). Concomitant use of other nephrotoxic drugs, pre-existing renal disease and dehydration make further renal impairment with acyclovir more likely. In most instances, alterations of renal function were transient and resolved spontaneously or with improvement of water and electrolyte balance, with drug dosage adjustments or with drug discontinuation. However, these changes may progress to acute renal failure.

Hydration: Accompany IV infusion by adequate hydration. Since maximum urine concentration occurs within the first 2 hours following infusion, establish sufficient urine flow during that period to prevent precipitation in renal tubules.

Encephalopathic changes: Approximately 1% of patients receiving acyclovir IV have manifested encephalopathic changes characterized by either lethargy, obtundation, tremors, confusion, hallucinations, agitation, seizures or coma. Use with caution in those patients who have underlying neurologic abnormalities; those with serious renal, hepatic or electrolyte abnormalities or significant hypoxia and those who have manifested prior neurologic reactions to cytotoxic drugs.

Resistance: Exposure of HSV isolates to acyclovir in vitro can lead to the emergence of less sensitive viruses. In severely immunocompromised patients, prolonged or repeated courses of acyclovir may result in resistant viruses which may not fully respond to continued acyclovir therapy.

Drug Interactions:

Acyclovir Drug Interactions			
Precipitant drug	Object drug*		Description
Probenecid	Acyclovir	⬆	Acyclovir bioavailability and terminal plasma half-life may be increased, and renal clearance may be decreased.
Zidovudine	Acyclovir	⬆	Severe drowsiness and lethargy may occur.

* ⬆ = Object drug increased.

Adverse Reactions:

Parenteral:

Frequency ≥ 1% – Inflammation or phlebitis at injection site (≈ 9%); transient elevations of serum creatinine or BUN (5% to 10%, the higher incidence usually occurring following rapid [< 10 minutes] IV infusion); nausea or vomiting (≈ 7%); itching, rash, hives (≈ 2%); elevation of transaminases (1% to 2%); encephalopathic changes characterized by either lethargy, obtundation, tremors, confusion, hallucinations, agitation, seizures or coma (≈ 1%; see Precautions).

Frequency < 1% - Anemia; anuria; hematuria; hypotension; edema; anorexia; lightheadedness; thirst; headache; diaphoresis; fever; neutropenia; thrombocytopenia; abnormal urinalysis (characterized by an increase in formed elements in urine sediment); painful urination; pulmonary edema with cardiac tamponade; abdominal pain; chest pain; thrombocytosis; leukocytosis; neutrophilia; ischemia of digits; hypokalemia; purpura fulminans; pressure on urination; hemoglobinemia; rigors.

ACYCLOVIR (Acycloguanosine)

Oral:

Oral Acyclovir Adverse Reactions (Treatment of Herpes Simplex)			
Body system	Short-term administration	Long-term administration	Intermittent administration
GI	Nausea/vomiting (2.7%); diarrhea (0.3%)	Nausea (4.8%); diarrhea (2.4%)	Diarrhea (2.7%); nausea (2.4%)
CNS	Headache (0.6%); dizziness, fatigue (0.3%)	Headache (0.9% to 1.9%)	Headache (2.2%)
Dermatologic	Skin rash (0.3%)	Skin rash (1.3% to 1.7%)	Skin rash (1.5%)
Other	Anorexia, edema, inguinal adenopathy, leg pain, medication taste, sore throat (0.3%)	Asthenia (1.2%); paresthesia (0.8% to 1.2%)	

Oral Acyclovir Adverse Reactions (Treatment of Herpes Zoster and Chickenpox)				
	Herpes zoster		Chickenpox	
Adverse Reaction	Acyclovir	Placebo	Acyclovir	Placebo
Malaise	11.5%	11.1%	—	—
Nausea	8%	11.5%	—	—
Headache	5.9%	11.1%	—	—
Vomiting	2.5%	2.5%	0.6%	—
Diarrhea	1.5%	0.3%	3.2%	2.2%
Constipation	0.9%	2.4%	—	—
Abdominal pain	—	—	0.6%	—
Rash	—	—	0.6%	—
Flatulence	—	—	0.4%	0.8%

Overdosage:

Symptoms: Precipitation of acyclovir in renal tubules may occur when the solubility (2.5 mg/ml) in the intratubular fluid is exceeded.

Parenteral – Overdosage has occurred with bolus injections, or inappropriately high doses, and in patients whose fluid and electrolyte balance was not properly monitored. Elevations in BUN, serum creatinine and subsequent renal failure resulted.

Oral – Doses as high as 800 mg 6 times daily for 5 days have been administered without acute untoward effects. This should not be construed as a recommended dosage for patients with more severe herpes.

Treatment: Acyclovir is dialyzable. A 6 hour hemodialysis results in a 60% decrease in plasma acyclovir concentration. Peritoneal dialysis appears less efficient in removing acyclovir from the blood. In the event of acute renal failure and anuria, the patient may benefit from hemodialysis until renal function is restored.

Patient Information:

Avoid sexual intercourse when visible herpes lesions are present.

Oral acyclovir does not eliminate latent HSV virus and is not a cure.

Do not exceed recommended dosage; do not share medication with others.

Notify physician if frequency and severity of recurrences do not improve.

ACYCLOVIR (Acycloguanosine)

Administration and Dosage:

Approved by the FDA in 1984.

Parenteral: Avoid rapid or bolus IV, IM or SC injection. Initiate therapy as soon as possible following onset of signs and symptoms. For IV infusion only. Administer over at least 1 hour to prevent renal tubular damage.

IV Acyclovir Dosage/Management Guidelines		
	Dosage	
Indication	Adults	Children (< 12 years)
Mucosal and cutaneous HSV infections in immunocompromised patients	5 mg/kg infused at a constant rate over 1 hour every 8 hours (15 mg/kg/day) for 7 days[1]	250 mg/m^2 infused at a constant rate over 1 hour every 8 hours (750 mg/m^2/day) for 7 days[1]
Varicella-zoster infections (shingles) in immunocompromised patients[2]	10 mg/kg infused at a constant rate over 1 hour every 8 hours for 7 days[3]	500 mg/m^2 infused at a constant rate over at least 1 hour every 8 hours for 7 days[3]
Herpes simplex encephalitis	10 mg/kg infused at a constant rate over at least 1 hour every 8 hours for 10 days	500 mg/m^2 infused at a constant rate over at least 1 hour every 8 hours for 10 days[4]

[1] For severe initial clinical episodes of herpes genitalis, use the same dose for 5 days.
[2] Base dosage for obese patients on ideal body weight (10 mg/kg).
[3] Do not exceed 500 mg/m^2 every 8 hours.
[4] Children > 6 months of age.

Renal function impairment, acute or chronic – Adjust the dosing interval as indicated below:

Parenteral Acyclovir Dosage in Renal Function Impairment		
Creatinine clearance (ml/min/1.73 m^2)	Percent of recommended dose	Dosing interval (hours)
> 50	100%	8
25 - 50	100%	12
10 - 25	100%	24
0 - 10	50%	24

Hemodialysis – The mean plasma half-life of acyclovir during hemodialysis is approximately 5 hours; a 60% decrease in plasma concentrations follows a 6 hour dialysis period. Therefore, administer a dose after each dialysis.

Preparation of IV solution – Dissolve the contents of the 500 or 1000 mg vial in 10 or 20 ml Sterile Water for Injection, respectively, to yield a final concentration of 50 mg/ml acyclovir (pH ≈ 11). Do not use bacteriostatic water containing benzyl alcohol or parabens; it is incompatible and may cause precipitation.

Add the calculated dose to an appropriate IV solution at a volume selected for administration during each 1 hour infusion. Infusion concentrations of approximately 7 mg/ml or lower are recommended. In clinical studies, the average 70 kg adult received approximately 60 ml of fluid per dose. Higher concentrations (eg, 10 mg/ml) may produce phlebitis or inflammation at the injection site upon inadvertent extravasation. The addition of acyclovir to biologic or colloidal fluids (eg, blood products, protein solutions) is not recommended.

ACYCLOVIR (Acycloguanosine)

Oral:

Herpes simplex –

Initial genital herpes: 200 mg every 4 hours, 5 times daily for 10 days. In patients with extremely severe episodes in which prostration, CNS involvement, urinary retention or inability to take oral medication requires hospitalization and more aggressive management, initiate therapy with IV acyclovir (see above).

Chronic suppressive therapy for recurrent disease: 400 mg 2 times daily for up to 12 months, followed by reevaluation. Reevaluate the frequency and severity of the patient's HSV after 1 year of therapy to assess the need for continuation of therapy; frequency and severity of episodes of untreated genital herpes may change over time. Reevaluation usually requires a trial off acyclovir to assess the need for reinstitution of suppressive therapy. Some patients, such as those with very frequent or severe episodes before treatment, may warrant uninterrupted suppression for > 1 year.

Alternative regimens have included doses ranging from 200 mg 3 times daily to 200 mg 5 times daily.

Intermittent therapy: 200 mg every 4 hours, 5 times daily for 5 days. Initiate therapy at the earliest sign or symptom (prodrome) of recurrence.

Herpes zoster, acute treatment – 800 mg every 4 hours, 5 times daily for 7 to 10 days.

Chickenpox – 20 mg/kg (not to exceed 800 mg) 4 times daily for 5 days. Initiate at earliest sign or symptom.

Renal impairment, acute or chronic –

Oral Acyclovir Dosage in Renal Function Impairment

Normal dosage regimen (5x daily)	Creatinine clearance (ml/min/1.73 m²)	Adjusted dosage regimen	
		Dose (mg)	Dosing interval
200 mg every 4 hours	> 10	200	Every 4 hours, 5x daily
	0 - 10	200	Every 12 hours
400 mg every 12 hours	> 10	400	Every 12 hours
	0 - 10	200	Every 12 hours
800 mg every 4 hours	> 25	800	Every 4 hours, 5x daily
	10 - 25	800	Every 8 hours
	0 - 10	800	Every 12 hours

Hemodialysis – For patients that require hemodialysis, adjust dosing schedule so that a dose is administered after each dialysis. No supplemental dose is necessary after peritoneal dialysis.

Stability/Storage: Use reconstituted solution within 12 hours. Once diluted for administration, use each dose within 24 hours. Refrigeration of reconstituted solutions may result in formation of a precipitate which redissolves at room temperature.

ACYCLOVIR (Acycloguanosine)

Rx	**Acyclovir** (Various, eg, Teva, Zenith-Goldline)	**Tablets:** 400 mg	In 100s, 500s and 1000s.
Rx	**Zovirax** (Glaxo Wellcome)		(Zovirax). White. Shield shaped. In 100s.
Rx	**Acyclovir** (Various, eg, Teva, Zenith-Goldline)	**Tablets:** 800 mg	In 100s and 500s.
Rx	**Zovirax** (Glaxo Wellcome)		(Zovirax 800 mg). Blue. Oval. In 100s, UD 100s and Shingles Relief Pak 35s.
Rx	**Acyclovir** (Various, eg, Teva, Zenith-Goldline)	**Capsules:** 200 mg	In 100s.
Rx	**Zovirax** (Glaxo Wellcome)		(Wellcome Zovirax 200). Blue. In 100s and UD 100s.
Rx	**Zovirax** (Glaxo Wellcome)	**Suspension:** 200 mg/5 ml	Banana flavor. In 473 ml.[1]
		Powder for Injection: 500 mg/vial (as sodium)	In 10 ml vials.
		1000 mg/vial (as sodium)	In 20 ml vials.

[1] With 0.1% methylparaben, 0.02% propylparaben and sorbitol.

Warning:

The clinical toxicity of ganciclovir includes granulocytopenia, anemia and thrombocytopenia. In animal studies, ganciclovir was carcinogenic, teratogenic and caused aspermatogenesis.

Ganciclovir IV is indicated for use only in the treatment of cytomegalovirus (CMV) retinitis in immunocompromised patients and for the prevention of CMV disease in transplant patients at risk for CMV disease.

Ganciclovir capsules are indicated only for prevention of CMV disease in patients with advanced HIV infection at risk for CMV disease and for maintenance treatment of CMV retinitis in immunocompromised patients.

Because oral ganciclovir is associated with a risk of more rapid rate of CMV retinitis progression, use only in those patients for whom this risk is balanced by the benefit associated with avoiding daily IV infusions.

Actions:

Pharmacology: Ganciclovir, a synthetic guanine derivative active against cytomegalovirus (CMV), is an acyclic nucleoside analog of 2'-deoxyguanosine that inhibits replication of herpes viruses both in vitro and in vivo. Sensitive human viruses include CMV, herpes simplex virus-1 and -2, herpes virus type 6, Epstein-Barr virus, varicella zoster virus and hepatitis B virus.

Ganciclovir must be converted to the corresponding triphosphate in order to exert its antiviral activity. In herpes simplex virus-infected cells, the initial conversion to the monophosphate is catalyzed by a viral thymidine kinase. In contrast, in CMV-infected cells, a protein kinase homologue may be responsible for the initial phosphorylation of ganciclovir. Cellular kinases, in CMV-infected cells, subsequently phosphorylate ganciclovir monophosphate to the diphosphate and active triphosphate moieties. Levels of ganciclovir-triphosphate are as much as 100-fold greater in CMV-infected cells than in uninfected cells, indicating a preferential phosphorylation of ganciclovir in virus-infected cells. Ganciclovir triphosphate, once formed, appears quite stable and persists for days in the CMV-infected cell. The antiviral activity of ganciclovir-triphosphate is believed to be the result of inhibition of viral DNA synthesis by two known modes: (1) Competitive inhibition of viral DNA polymerases; and (2) direct incorporation into viral DNA, resulting in eventual termination of viral DNA elongation. The cellular DNA polymerase alpha is also inhibited, but at a higher concentration than required for inhibition of viral DNA polymerase.

The median concentration of ganciclovir that effectively inhibits the replication of either laboratory strains or clinical isolates of CMV (ED_{50}) has ranged from 0.02 to 3.48 mcg/ml. The relationship of in vitro sensitivity of CMV to ganciclovir and clinical response has not been established. Ganciclovir inhibits mammalian cell proliferation in vitro at higher concentrations; IC_{50} values range from 30 to 725 mcg/ml, with the exception of bone marrow-derived colony-forming cells that are more sensitive with IC_{50} values ranging from 0.028 to 0.7 mcg/ml.

Pharmacokinetics:

Absorption – The absolute bioavailability of oral ganciclovir under fasting conditions was ≈ 5% and following food it was 6% to 9%. When given with a meal containing 602 calories and 46.5% fat, the steady-state area under serum concentration vs time curve (AUC) increased and there was a significant prolongation of time to peak serum concentrations (see Drug Interactions).

At the end of a 1-hour IV infusion of 5 mg/kg, total AUC ranged between 22.1 and 26.8 mcg•hr/ml and C_{max} ranged between 8.27 and 9 mcg/ml.

Distribution – The steady-state volume of distribution after IV administration was 0.74 L/kg. Cerebrospinal fluid concentrations obtained 0.25 and 5.67 hours post-dose in three patients who received 2.5 mg/kg ganciclovir IV every 8 or 12 hours ranged from 0.31 to 0.68 mcg/ml, representing 24% to 70% of the respective plasma concentrations. Binding to plasma proteins was 1% to 2% over ganciclovir concentrations of 0.5 and 51 mcg/ml.

For ganciclovir capsules, no correlation was observed between AUC and reciprocal weight (range: 55 to 128 kg); oral dosing according to weight is not required.

Metabolism – Following oral administration of a single 1000 mg dose, 86% of the administered dose was recovered in the feces, and 5% was recovered in the urine. No metabolite accounted for 1% to 2% recovered in urine or feces.

Excretion – When administered IV, ganciclovir exhibits linear pharmacokinetics over the range of 1.6 to 5 mg/kg. When administered orally, it exhibits linear kinetics up to a total daily dose of 4 g/day. Renal excretion of unchanged drug by glomerular filtration and active tubular secretion is the major route of elimination. In patients with normal renal function, 91.3% of IV ganciclovir was recovered unmetabolized in the urine. Systemic clearance of IV ganciclovir was 3.52 ml/min/kg while renal clearance was 3.2 ml/min/kg, accounting for 91% of the systemic clearance. After oral administration, steady state is achieved within 24 hours. Renal clearance following oral administration was 3.1 ml/min/kg. Half-life was 3.5 hours following IV administration and 4.8 hours following oral use.

Renal function impairment: Because the major elimination pathway for ganciclovir is renal, dosage must be reduced according to creatinine clearance (Ccr; see Administration and Dosage). The pharmacokinetics following IV administration were evaluated in 10 immunocompromised patients with renal impairment who received doses ranging from 1.25 to 5 mg/kg.

IV Ganciclovir Pharmacokinetics in Patients with Renal Impairment

Ccr (ml/min)	Dose (mg/kg)	Clearance (ml/min)	Half-life (hours)
50 - 79 (n = 4)	3.2 - 5	128	4.6
25 - 49 (n = 3)	3 - 5	57	4.4
< 25 (n = 3)	1.25 - 5	30	10.7

The pharmacokinetics following oral administration were evaluated in 8 solid organ transplant recipients; dose was modified according to estimated Ccr.

Oral Ganciclovir in Patients with Renal Impairment

Ccr (ml/min)	Dose (mg/kg)	AUC_{0-24} (mcg•hr/ml)	Half-life (hours)
50 - 69 (n = 4)	1000 mg q 8 hr	49.1 ± 12.2	NC[2]
25 - 49 (n = 1)	1000 mg q day	27.4	18.2
10 - 24 (n = 1)	500 mg q day	10.7	15.7
< 10 (n = 2)	500 mg 3 times weekly[1]	25.6 ± 5.9	NC[2]

[1] After hemodialysis.
[2] NC = Not calculated; half-life exceeded sampling interval.

Hemodialysis reduces plasma concentrations of ganciclovir by about 50% after both IV and oral administration.

Race – The effects of race were studied in subjects receiving a dose regimen of 1000 mg every 8 hours. Although the numbers of African Americans (16%) and Hispanics (20%) were small, there appeared to be a trend towards a lower steady-state C_{max} and AUC_{0-8} in these subpopulations as compared to Caucasians.

Children – At an IV dose of 4 or 6 mg/kg in 27 neonates (ages 2 to 49 days), the pharmacokinetic parameters were, respectively, C_{max} of 5.5 and 7 mcg/ml, systemic clearance of 3.14 and 3.56 ml/min/kg and half-life of 2.4 hours for both.

Clinical trials:

IV –

Immunocompromised patients: Of 314 immunocompromised patients enrolled in an open label study of the treatment of life- or sight-threatening CMV disease, 121 patients had a positive culture for CMV within 7 days prior to treatment.

Virologic Response to IV Ganciclovir Treatment

Culture source	No. patients cultured	No. (%) patients responding	Median days to response
Urine	107	93 (87%)	8
Blood	41	34 (83%)	8
Throat	21	19 (90%)	7
Semen	6	6 (100%)	15

Transplant recipients: In 149 CMV seropositive heart allograft recipients and 72 CMV culture positive allogeneic bone marrow transplant recipients, ganciclovir prevented recrudescence of CMV shedding in the heart allograft patients and suppressed CMV shedding in the bone marrow allograft patients.

Patients with Positive CMV Cultures Following IV Ganciclovir				
	Heart allograft		Bone marrow allograft	
Time	Ganciclovir	Placebo	Ganciclovir	Placebo
Pre-Treatment	2%	8%	100%	100%
Week 2	3%	16%	6%	68%
Week 4	5%	43%	0%	80%

Oral – The antiviral activity of ganciclovir capsules was confirmed in two randomized, controlled trials comparing IV vs oral ganciclovir for the maintenance treatment of CMV retinitis in patients with acquired immunodeficiency syndrome (AIDS). Only a small proportion of patients remained culture-positive during maintenance therapy with either IV or oral ganciclovir. There were no statistically significant differences in the rates of positive cultures between the treatment groups. The antiviral effect of oral ganciclovir in the patients in the two studies is summarized in the following table:

Patients with Positive CMV Following Oral Ganciclovir				
	Patients with newly diagnosed CMV retinitis[1]		Patients with stable, previously treated CMV retinitis[2]	
	IV	Oral	IV	Oral[3]
At start of maintenance	13.5%	24.3%	3%	3.6%
Anytime during maintenance	6.3%	9.1%	2.2%	7.1%

[1] 3 weeks of treatment with IV ganciclovir before start of maintenance.
[2] 4 weeks to 4 months treatment with IV ganciclovir before start of maintenance.
[3] Data from 6 times daily and 3 times daily regimens pooled.

Viral resistance – CMV resistance to ganciclovir in individuals with AIDS and CMV retinitis who have not previously been treated with ganciclovir does occur but appears to be infrequent. Viral resistance has been observed in patients receiving prolonged treatment with ganciclovir IV. However, because of the limited number of viral isolates tested, it is difficult to estimate the overall frequency of reduced sensitivity in patients receiving ganciclovir. Nonetheless, consider the possibility of viral resistance in patients who show poor clinical response or experience persistent viral excretion during therapy. The principal mechanism of resistance to ganciclovir in CMV is the decreased ability to form the active triphosphate moiety. Mutations in the viral DNA polymerase have also been reported to confer viral resistance to ganciclovir. In two randomized controlled trials, the incidence of reduced sensitivity appeared to be no more common during treatment with oral ganciclovir than during IV treatment.

Indications:

IV:

CMV retinitis – Treatment of CMV retinitis in immunocompromised patients, including patients with AIDS.

CMV disease – Prevention of CMV disease in transplant recipients at risk for CMV disease.

Oral:

CMV retinitis – Alternative to the IV formulation for maintenance treatment of CMV retinitis in immunocompromised patients, including patients with AIDS, in whom retinitis is stable following appropriate induction therapy and for whom the risk of more rapid progression is balanced by the benefit associated with avoiding daily IV infusions.

CMV disease – Prevention of CMV disease in individuals with advanced HIV infection at risk for developing CMV disease.

Unlabeled uses: Ganciclovir may also be beneficial in some immunocompromised patients in the treatment of other CMV infections (eg, pneumonitis, gastroenteritis, hepatitis [see Warnings]).

Contraindications:

Hypersensitivity to ganciclovir or acyclovir.

Warnings:

CMV disease: Safety and efficacy have not been established for congenital or neonatal CMV disease, treatment of established CMV disease other than retinitis or use in non-immunocompromised individuals. The safety and efficacy of oral ganciclovir have not been established for treating any manifestation of CMV disease other than maintenance treatment of CMV retinitis.

Diagnosis of CMV retinitis is ophthalmologic and should be made by indirect ophthalmoscopy. Other conditions in the differential diagnosis of CMV retinitis include candidiasis, toxoplasmosis, histoplasmosis, retinal scars and cotton wool spots, any of which may produce a retinal appearance similar to CMV. The diagnosis may be supported by a culture of CMV from urine, blood, throat, etc, but a negative CMV culture does not rule out CMV retinitis.

Retinal detachment has been observed in subjects with CMV retinitis both before and after initiation of therapy with ganciclovir. Its relationship to therapy is unknown. Retinal detachment occurred in 11% of patients treated with IV ganciclovir and in 8% of patients treated with oral ganciclovir. Patients with CMV retinitis should have frequent ophthalmologic evaluations to monitor the status of their retinitis and to detect any other retinal pathology.

Hematologic: Do not administer if the absolute neutrophil count is < 500/mm^3 or the platelet count is < 25,000/mm^3. Granulocytopenia (neutropenia), anemia and thrombocytopenia have been observed in patients treated with ganciclovir. The frequency and severity of these events vary widely in different patient populations (see Adverse Reactions). Therefore, use with caution in patients with pre-existing cytopenias or with a history of cytopenic reactions to other drugs, chemicals or irradiation. Granulocytopenia usually occurs during the first or second week of treatment, but may occur at any time during treatment. Cell counts usually begin to recover within 3 to 7 days after discontinuing drug. Colony-stimulating factors have increased neutrophil and WBC counts in patients receiving IV ganciclovir for CMV retinitis.

Renal function impairment: Use ganciclovir with caution because the half-life and plasma/serum concentrations of ganciclovir will be increased because of reduced renal clearance (see Administration and Dosage).

Hemodialysis reduces plasma levels of ganciclovir by approximately 50%.

Carcinogenesis/Mutagenesis/Fertility impairment: In mice, daily oral doses of 1000 mg/kg may have caused an increased incidence of tumors in the preputial gland of males, nonglandular mucosa of the stomach of males and females, and reproductive tissues (ovaries, uterus, mammary glands, clitoral gland and vagina) and liver in females. A slightly increased incidence of tumors occurred in the preputial gland (males) and nonglandular mucosa (males and females) of the stomach in mice given 20 mg/kg/day. Consider ganciclovir a potential carcinogen in humans.

Ganciclovir caused point mutations and chromosomal damage in mammalian cells in vitro and in vivo. Because of the mutagenic and teratogenic potential of ganciclovir, advise women of childbearing potential to use effective contraception during treatment. Similarly, advise men to practice barrier contraception during and for at least 90 days following treatment with ganciclovir.

Ganciclovir increased mutations in mouse lymphoma cells and DNA damage in human lymphocytes in vitro.

Animal data indicate that ganciclovir causes inhibition of spermatogenesis and subsequent infertility. These effects were reversible at lower doses and irreversible at higher doses. Although data in humans have not been obtained regarding this effect, it is considered probable that ganciclovir, at the recommended doses, causes temporary or permanent inhibition of spermatogenesis. Animal data also indicate that suppression of fertility in females may occur.

Elderly: The pharmacokinetic profile in elderly patients has not been established. Because elderly individuals frequently have a reduced glomerular filtration rate, pay particular attention to assessing renal function before and during administration of ganciclovir (see Administration and Dosage).

Pregnancy: Catagory C. Ganciclovir is embryotoxic in rabbits and mice following IV administration and teratogenic in rabbits. Fetal resorptions were present in at least 85% of rabbits and mice administered 2 times the human exposure. Effects observed in rabbits included: Fetal growth retardation, embryolethality, teratogenicity and maternal toxicity. Teratogenic changes included cleft palate, anophthalmia/microphthalmia, aplastic organs (kidney and pancreas), hydrocephaly and brachygnathia. In mice, effects observed were maternal/fetal toxicity and embryolethality.

Daily IV doses administered to female mice prior to mating, during gestation and during lactation caused hypoplasia of the testes and seminal vesicles in the month-old male offspring, as well as pathologic changes in the nonglandular region of the stomach.

Ganciclovir may be teratogenic or embryotoxic at dose levels recommended for human use. There are no adequate and well controlled studies in pregnant women. Use during pregnancy only if the potential benefits justify the potential risk to the fetus.

Lactation: It is not known whether ganciclovir is excreted in breast milk. However, because carcinogenic and teratogenic effects occurred in animals treated with ganciclovir, the possibility of serious adverse reactions from ganciclovir in nursing infants is considered likely. Instruct mothers to discontinue nursing if they are receiving ganciclovir. The minimum interval before nursing can safely be resumed after the last dose of ganciclovir is unknown.

Children: Safety and efficacy in children have not been established. The use of ganciclovir in children warrants extreme caution regarding the probability of long-term carcinogenicity and reproductive toxicity. Administer to children only after careful evaluation and only if the potential benefits of treatment outweigh the risks. Oral ganciclovir has not been studied in children < 13 years of age.

There has been very limited clinical experience using IV ganciclovir for the treatment of CMV retinitis in patients < 12 years of age. Two children (9 and 5 years of age) showed improvement or stabilization of retinitis for 23 and 9 months, respectively. These children received induction treatment with 2.5 mg/kg 3 times daily followed by maintenance therapy with 6 to 6.5 mg/kg once a day, 5 to 7 days per week. When retinitis progressed during once-daily maintenance therapy, both children were treated with the 5 mg/kg twice-daily regimen. Two other children (2.5 and 4 years of age) who received similar induction regimens showed only partial or no response to treatment. Another child, a 6-year-old with T-cell dysfunction, showed stabilization of retinitis for 3 months while receiving continuous infusions of IV ganciclovir at doses of 2 to 5 mg/kg/day. Continuous infusion treatment was discontinued due to granulocytopenia.

Eleven of the 72 patients in the placebo controlled trial in bone marrow transplant recipients were children, ranging from 3 to 10 years of age (5 treated with IV ganciclovir and 6 with placebo). Five of the pediatric patients treated with ganciclovir received 5 mg/kg IV twice daily for up to 7 days; 4 patients went on to receive 5 mg/kg once daily up to day 100 post-transplant. Results were similar to those observed in adult transplant recipients treated with IV ganciclovir. Two of the 6 placebo-treated pediatric patients developed CMV pneumonia vs none of the 5 treated with ganciclovir. The spectrum of adverse events in the pediatric group was similar to that observed in the adult patients.

The spectrum of adverse reactions reported in 120 immunocompromised pediatric clinical trial participants with serious CMV infections receiving IV ganciclovir were similar to those reported in adults. Granulocytopenia (17%) and thrombocytopenia (10%) were the most common adverse events reported.

Precautions:

Monitoring: Because of the frequency of neutropenia, anemia and thrombocytopenia in patients receiving ganciclovir, it is recommended that complete blood counts and platelet counts be performed frequently, especially in patients in whom ganciclovir or other nucleoside analogs have previously resulted in leukopenia, or in whom neutrophil counts are < 1000/mm^3 at the beginning of treatment. Because dosing with ganciclovir must be modified in patients with renal impairment, and because of the incidence of increased serum creatinine levels that have been observed in transplant recipients treated with IV ganciclovir, patients should have serum creatinine or creatinine clearance values followed carefully.

Large doses/rapid infusion: The maximum single dose administered was 6 mg/kg by IV infusion over 1 hour. Larger doses have resulted in increased toxicity. It is likely that more rapid infusions would also result in increased toxicity (see Overdosage).

Phlebitis/Pain at injection site: Initially, reconstituted solutions of IV ganciclovir have a high pH (pH 11). Despite further dilution in IV fluids, phlebitis or pain may occur at the site of IV infusion. Take care to infuse solutions containing ganciclovir only into veins with adequate blood flow to permit rapid dilution and distribution.

Hydration: Since ganciclovir is excreted by the kidneys and normal clearance depends on adequate renal function, administration of ganciclovir should be accompanied by adequate hydration.

Photosensitivity: Photosensitization (photoallergy or phototoxicity) may occur; therefore, caution patients to take protective measures against exposure to ultraviolet or sunlight (eg, sunscreens, protective clothing) until tolerance is determined.

GANCICLOVIR (DHPG)

Drug Interactions:

Ganciclovir Drug Interactions

Precipitant drug	Object drug*		Description
Ganciclovir	Cytotoxic drugs	⬆	Cytotoxic drugs that inhibit replication of rapidly dividing cell populations such as bone marrow, spermatogonia and germinal layers of skin and GI mucosa may have additive toxicity when administered concomitantly with ganciclovir. Therefore, consider the concomitant use of drugs such as dapsone, pentamidine, flucytosine, vincristine, vinblastine, adriamycin, amphotericin B, trimethoprim/sulfamethoxazole combinations or other nucleoside analogs only if potential benefits outweigh the risks.
Imipenem-cilastatin	Ganciclovir	⬆	Generalized seizures occurred in patients who received ganciclovir and imipenem-cilastatin. Do not use these drugs concomitantly unless the potential benefits outweigh the risks.
Nephrotoxic drugs	Ganciclovir	⬆	Increases in serum creatinine were observed following concurrent use of ganciclovir and either cyclosporine or amphotericin B.
Probenecid	Ganciclovir	⬆	Ganciclovir AUC increased 53% (range, -14% to 299%) in the presence of probenecid. Renal clearance of ganciclovir decreased 22% (range, -54% to -4%), which is consistent with an interaction involving competition for renal tubular secretion.
Ganciclovir	Didanosine	⬆	Steady-state didanosine AUC increased 111% (range, 10% to 493%) when didanosine was administered either 2 hours prior to or simultaneously with ganciclovir. A decrease in steady-state ganciclovir AUC of 21% (range, -44% to 5%) was observed when didanosine was administered 2 hours prior to administration of ganciclovir, but ganciclovir AUC was not affected by the presence of didanosine when the two drugs were administered simultaneously.
Didanosine	Ganciclovir	⬇	
Ganciclovir	Zidovudine	⬆	Mean steady-state ganciclovir AUC decreased 17% (range, -52% to 23%) in the presence of zidovudine. Steady-state zidovudine AUC increased 19% (range, -11% to 74%) in the presence of ganciclovir. Because both drugs can cause granulocytopenia and anemia, many patients will not tolerate combination therapy at full dosage.
Zidovudine	Ganciclovir	⬇	

* ⬆ = Object drug increased. ⬇ = Object drug decreased.

Drug/Food interactions: When ganciclovir was administered orally with food at a total daily dose of 3 g/day (either 500 mg every 3 hours 6 times daily or 1000 mg 3 times daily), the steady-state absorption as measured by AUC and C_{max} were similar following both regimens. When ganciclovir capsules were given with a meal containing 602 calories and 46.5% fat at a dose of 1000 mg every 8 hours to 20 HIV-positive subjects, the steady-state AUC increased by 22% (range, 6% to 68%) and there was a significant prolongation of time to peak serum concentrations (T_{max}) from 1.8 to 3 hours and a higher C_{max} (0.85 vs 0.96 mcg/ml).

Adverse Reactions:

AIDS patients: Three controlled, randomized, phase III trials comparing ganciclovir IV with ganciclovir capsules for maintenance treatment of CMV retinitis have been completed. During these trials, ganciclovir (both doseforms) was prematurely discontinued in 9% of subjects because of adverse events, new or worsening intercurrent illnesses or laboratory abnormalities. In a placebo controlled, randomized, phase III trial of ganciclovir capsules for prevention of CMV disease in patients with AIDS, treatment was prematurely discontinued because of adverse events, new or worsening intercurrent illnesses or laboratory abnormalities in 19.5% of subjects treated with ganciclovir capsules and 16% of the subjects receiving placebo.

Selected Adverse Reactions Oral vs IV Ganciclovir Maintenance Treatment (%)		
Adverse reaction	Oral (3000 mg/day) (n = 326)	IV (5 mg/kg/day) (n = 179)
Body as a whole		
Fever	38	48
Abdominal pain	17	19
Infection	9	13
Chills	7	10
Sepsis	4	15
GI		
Diarrhea	41	44
Nausea	26	25
Anorexia	15	14
Vomiting	13	13
Flatulence	6	3
Hemic/ Lymphatic		
Leukopenia	29	41
Anemia	19	25
Thrombocytopenia	6	6
CNS		
Neuropathy	8	9
Paresthesia	6	10
Other		
Rash	15	10
Sweating	11	12
Pruritus	6	5
Vitreous disorder	6	4
Pneumonia	6	8
Catheter-related		
Total catheter events	6	22
Catheter infection	4	9
Catheter sepsis	1	8
Neutropenia (ANC/mm^3)	(n = 320)	(n = 175)
< 500	5.6	14.3
500 to < 750	5.3	8
750 to < 1000	6	15
Total ANC ≤ 1000	17	38
Anemia hemoglobin (g/dl)	(n = 320)	(n = 175)
< 6.5	0.6	3
6.5 < 8	3	9
8 < 9.5	7.8	9
Total Hb < 9.5	12	26

Overall, subjects treated with IV ganciclovir experienced lower minimum ANCs and hemoglobin levels, consistent with more neutropenia and anemia, compared with those who received oral ganciclovir.

For the majority of subjects, maximum serum creatinine levels were < 1.5 mg/dl and no difference was noted between IV and oral ganciclovir for the occurrence of renal impairment. Serum creatinine elevations > 2.5 mg/dl occurred in < 2% of all subjects, and no significant differences were noted in the time from the start of maintenance to the occurrence of elevations in serum creatinine values.

Transplant recipients:

Granulocytopenia/Thrombocytopenia with IV Ganciclovir (%)				
	Heart allograft[1]		Bone marrow allograft[2]	
Hematologic Effect	Ganciclovir (n = 76)	Placebo (n = 73)	Ganciclovir IV (n = 57)	Control (n = 55)
Neutropenia				
Minimum ANC < $500/mm^3$	4	3	12	6
Minimum ANC 500 - $1000/mm^3$	3	8	29	17
Total ANC ≤ $1000/mm^3$	7	11	41	23

GANCICLOVIR (DHPG)

Granulocytopenia/Thrombocytopenia with IV Ganciclovir (%)				
	Heart allograft[1]		Bone marrow allograft[2]	
Hematologic Effect	Ganciclovir (n = 76)	Placebo (n = 73)	Ganciclovir IV (n = 57)	Control (n = 55)
Thrombocytopenia				
Platelet count < 25,000/mm^3	3	1	32	28
Platelet count 25,000 - 50,000/mm^3	5	3	25	37
Total Platelet 50,000/mm^3	8	4	57	65

[1] Mean duration of treatment = 28 days.
[2] Mean duration of treatment = 45 days.

Elevated Serum Creatinine with IV Ganciclovir (%)						
	Heart allograft		Bone marrow allograft			
Maximum serum creatinine levels	Ganciclovir IV (n = 76)	Placebo (n = 73)	Ganciclovir IV (n = 20)	Control (n = 20)	Ganciclovir IV (n = 37)	Placebo (n = 35)
Serum creatinine ≥ 2.5 mg/dl	18	4	20	0	0	0
Serum creatinine ≥ 1.5 - < 2.5 mg/dl	58	69	50	35	43	44

Other adverse reactions:

Body as a whole: Asthenia (6%); headache (4%); injection site inflammation, pain (2%); abdomen enlarged, abscess, back pain, cellulitis, chest pain, chills, fever, drug level increased (ganciclovir), edema, face edema, injection site abscess/edema/hemorrhage/pain/phlebitis, lab test abnormality, malaise, photosensitivity reaction, neck pain/rigidity (≤ 1%).

GI: Aphthous stomatitis (4%); abnormal liver function test, dyspepsia, esophagitis; nausea, vomiting (2%); constipation, dysphagia, eructation, fecal incontinence, hemorrhage, hepatitis, melena, mouth ulceration, tongue disorder (≤ 1%).

Hematologic: Eosinophilia, hypochromic anemia, marrow depression, pancytopenia, splenomegaly (≤ 1%).

Respiratory: Cough increased, dyspnea, pharyngitis (≤ 1%).

CNS: Abnormal dreams, abnormal gait, abnormal thinking, agitation, amnesia, anxiety, ataxia, coma, confusion, depression, dizziness, dry mouth, emotional lability, euphoria, hypertonia, hypesthesia, insomnia, libido decreased, manic reaction, myoclonus, nervousness, psychosis, seizures, somnolence, tremor, trismus (≈ 5%).

Dermatologic: Acne, alopecia, dry skin, fixed eruption, herpes simplex, maculopapular rash, skin discoloration, urticaria, vesiculobullous rash (≤ 1%).

Special senses: Abnormal vision, amblyopia, blindness, conjunctivitis, deafness, eye pain, glaucoma, retinitis, photophobia, taste perversion, tinnitus (≤ 1%).

Metabolic/Nutritional: Increased alkaline phosphatase, creatinine, creatine phosphokinase, lactic dehydrogenase, AST, ALT, hypokalemia, pancreatitis, decreased blood sugar, weight loss (≤ 1%).

Cardiovascular: Phlebitis (2%); arrhythmia, deep thrombophlebitis, hypertension, hypotension, migraine, vasodilatation (≤ 1%).

GU: Breast pain, creatinine clearance decreased/increased, hematuria, increased BUN, kidney failure, kidney function abnormal, urinary frequency, urinary tract infection.

Musculoskeletal: Arthralgia, bone pain, leg cramps, myalgia, myasthenia (≤ 1%).

Miscellaneous: The following adverse reactions may be fatal: Pancreatitis, sepsis and multiple organ failure.

Adverse reactions reported in post-marketing surveillance:

Reported on two or more occasions – Acidosis, anaphylactic reaction, bronchospasm, cardiac arrest, cardiac conduction abnormality, cataracts, cholestasis, cholangitis, congenital anomaly, encephalopathy, extrapyramidal reaction, hallucinations, hemolytic anemia, hepatic failure, hepatitis, hyponatremia, impotence, infertility, intestinal ulceration, intracranial hypertension, leukemia, lymphoma, myocardial infarction, pericarditis, Stevens-Johnson syndrome, stroke, torsades de pointes, transverse myelitis, unexplained death, vasculitis, ventricular tachycardia.

Reported once – Allograft rejection, arthritis, asthma, bleeding disorder, cachexia, corneal erosion, cyanosis, diplopia, dry eyes, dysethesia, ear infection, elevated triglyceride levels, endocarditis, exfoliative dermatitis, exacerbation of psoriasis, facial palsy, gangrene, gingival hypertrophy, Guillain-Barre syndrome, hemolytic-uremic syndrome, hypernatremia, hypomagnesemia, icterus, inappropriate serum ADH, increased sweating, irritability, loss of memory, loss of sense of smell, multiple organ failure, myelopathy, myocarditis, nephritis, ophthalmoplegia, parathyroid disorder, Parkinsonism-like reaction, pneumothorax, peripheral ischemia, perforated intestine, pneumonia, proteinuria, pseudotumor cerebri, pulmonary fibrosis, pulmonary embolism, respiratory distress syndrome, rhabdomyolysis, sperm production abnormal, testicular hypotrophy, thyroid disorder, Wolff-Parkinson-White syndrome.

Overdosage:

IV: Overdosage with IV ganciclovir has been reported in 17 patients (13 adults and 4 children < 2 years of age). Five patients experienced no adverse events following overdosage at the following doses: 7 doses of 11 mg/kg over a 3-day period (adult), single dose of 3500 mg (adult), single dose of 500 mg (72.5 mg/kg) followed by 48 hours of peritoneal dialysis (4 month-old), single dose of approximately 60 mg/kg followed by exchange transfusion (18 month-old), 2 doses of 500 mg instead of 31 mg (21 month-old).

Irreversible pancytopenia developed in one adult with AIDS and CMV colitis after receiving 3000 mg IV ganciclovir on each of two consecutive days. He experienced worsening GI symptoms and acute renal failure that required short-term dialysis. Pancytopenia persisted until his death from a malignancy several months later. Other adverse events reported following overdosage include: Persistent bone marrow suppression (one adult with neutropenia and thrombocytopenia after a single dose of 6000 mg), reversible neutropenia or granulocytopenia (four adults, overdoses ranging from 8 mg/kg daily for 4 days to a single dose of 25 mg/kg), hepatitis (one adult receiving 10 mg/kg daily and one 2 kg infant after a single 40 mg dose), renal toxicity (one adult with transient worsening of hematuria after a single 500 mg dose and one adult with elevated creatinine [5.2 mg/dl] after a single 5000 to 7000 mg dose) and seizure (one adult with known seizure disorder after 3 days of 9 mg/kg). In addition, one adult received 0.4 ml (instead of 0.1 ml) by intravitreal injection and experienced temporary loss of vision and central retinal artery occlusion secondary to increased intraocular pressure related to the injected fluid volume.

Oral: There have been no reports of overdosage with oral ganciclovir. Doses as high as 6000 mg/day did not result in overt toxicity other than transient neutropenia.

Treatment: Dialysis may be useful in reducing serum concentrations. Adequate hydration should be maintained. Consider the use of hematopoietic growth factors.

Patient Information:

Ganciclovir is not a cure for CMV retinitis, and immunocompromised patients may continue to experience progression of retinitis during or following treatment. Advise patients to have regular ophthalmologic examinations at a minimum of every 6 weeks while being treated. Some patients will require more frequent follow-up.

The major toxicities of ganciclovir are granulocytopenia and thrombocytopenia. Dose modifications may be required, including possible discontinuation. Emphasize the importance of close monitoring of blood counts while on therapy. Inform patients that ganciclovir has been associated with increases in serum creatinine.

Advise patients to take oral ganciclovir with food to maximize bioavailability.

Patients with AIDS may be receiving zidovudine. Treatment with zidovudine and ganciclovir will not be tolerated by many patients and may result in severe granulocytopenia. Patients with AIDS may be receiving didanosine. Counsel patients that concurrent treatment with both ganciclovir and didanosine can significantly increase didanosine serum concentrations.

Advise patients that ganciclovir may cause infertility. Advise women of childbearing potential that ganciclovir should not be used during pregnancy; use effective contraception during ganciclovir treatment. Similarly, advise men to practice barrier contraception during and for at least 90 days following ganciclovir treatment.

Although there is no information, consider ganciclovir a potential carcinogen.

Transplant recipients: Counsel transplant recipients regarding the high frequency of impaired renal function, particularly in patients receiving concomitant administration of nephrotoxic agents such as cyclosporine and amphotericin B.

Administration and Dosage:

Approved by the FDA in 1989.

IV: Do not administer by rapid or bolus IV injection. The toxicity may be increased as a result of excessive plasma levels. Do not exceed the recommended infusion rate. IM or SC injection of reconstituted ganciclovir may result in severe tissue irritation because of high pH.

GANCICLOVIR (DHPG)

CMV retinitis (normal renal function):

Induction – The recommended initial dose is 5 mg/kg (given IV at a constant rate over 1 hour) every 12 hours for 14 to 21 days. Do not use oral ganciclovir for induction treatment.

Maintenance –

IV: Following induction treatment, the recommended maintenance dose is 5 mg/kg given as a constant rate IV infusion over 1 hour once daily 7 days per week, or 6 mg/kg once daily 5 days per week.

Oral: Following induction treatment, the recommended maintenance dose of oral ganciclovir is 1000 mg 3 times daily with food. Alternatively, the dosing regimen of 500 mg 6 times daily every 3 hours with food, during waking hours, may be used.

For patients who experience progression of CMV retinitis while receiving maintenance treatment with either formulation of ganciclovir, reinduction treatment is recommended.

Prevention of CMV disease in transplant recipients: The recommended initial dose of IV ganciclovir for patients with normal renal function is 5 mg/kg (given IV at a constant rate over 1 hour) every 12 hours for 7 to 14 days, followed by 5 mg/kg once daily 7 days per week or 6 mg/kg once daily 5 days per week.

The duration of treatment with IV ganciclovir in transplant recipients is dependent on the duration and degree of immunosuppression. In controlled clinical trials in bone marrow allograft recipients, treatment was continued until day 100 to 120 post-transplantation. CMV disease occurred in several patients who discontinued treatment with ganciclovir prematurely. In heart allograft recipients, the onset of newly diagnosed CMV disease occurred after treatment with ganciclovir was stopped at day 28 post-transplant, suggesting that continued dosing may be necessary to prevent late occurrence of CMV disease in this patient population.

Prevention of CMV disease in patients with advanced HIV infection and normal renal function: The recommended dose of ganciclovir capsules is 1000 mg three times daily with food.

Renal impairment:

IV – Refer to the following table for recommended doses and adjust the dosing interval as indicated.

IV Ganciclovir Dose in Renal Impairment				
Creatinine clearance (ml/min)	Ganciclovir induction dose (mg/kg)	Dosing interval (hours)	Ganciclovir maintenance dose (mg/kg)	Dosing interval (hours)
≥ 70	5	12	5	24
50 to 69	2.5	12	2.5	24
25 to 49	2.5	24	1.25	24
10 to 24	1.25	24	0.625	24
< 10	1.25	3 times per week following hemodialysis	0.625	3 times per week following hemodialysis

Hemodialysis: Dosing for patients undergoing hemodialysis should not exceed 1.25 mg/kg 3 times per week, following each hemodialysis session. Give shortly after completion of the hemodialysis session, because hemodialysis reduces plasma levels by approximately 50%.

Oral – In patients with renal impairment, modify the dose of oral ganciclovir as follows:

Oral Ganciclovir Dose in Renal Impairment	
Creatinine clearance (ml/min)	Ganciclovir doses
≥ 70	1000 mg TID or 500 mg q 3h, 6x/day
50 to 69	1500 mg QD or 500 mg TID
25 to 49	1000 mg QD or 500 mg BID
10 to 24	500 mg QD
< 10	500 mg three times per week, following hemodialysis

Ccr can be related to serum creatinine by the following formula:

$$\text{Males:} \quad \frac{\text{Weight (kg)} \times (140 - \text{age})}{72 \times \text{serum creatinine (mg/dl)}} = \text{Ccr}$$

Females: 0.85 × above value

GANCICLOVIR (DHPG)

Patient monitoring: Because of the frequency of granulocytopenia and thrombocytopenia, it is recommended that neutrophil counts and platelet counts be performed frequently, especially in patients in whom ganciclovir or other nucleoside analogs have previously resulted in leukopenia, or in whom neutrophil counts are < 1000/mm^3 at the beginning of treatment. Because dosing with ganciclovir must be modified in patients with renal impairment, and because of the incidence of increased serum creatinine levels that have been observed in transplant recipients treated with IV ganciclovir, patients should have serum creatinine or Ccr values followed carefully.

Reduction of dose: Dose reductions are required for patients with renal impairment and for those with neutropenia or thrombocytopenia. Therefore, perform frequent white blood cell counts. Severe neutropenia (ANC < 500/mm^3) or severe thrombocytopenia (platelets < 25,000/mm^3) require a dose interruption until evidence of marrow recovery is observed (ANC > 750/mm^3).

Preparation of IV solution: Each 10 ml clear glass vial contains ganciclovir sodium equivalent to 500 mg of the free base form of ganciclovir and 46 mg of sodium. Prepare the contents of the vial for administration in the following manner:

Reconstituted solution –

1. Reconstitute lyophilized ganciclovir by injecting 10 ml of Sterile Water for Injection, USP, into the vial. Do not use bacteriostatic water for injection containing parabens; it is incompatible with ganciclovir and may cause precipitation.
2. Shake the vial to dissolve the drug.
3. Visually inspect the reconstituted solution for particulate matter and discoloration prior to proceeding with infusion solution. Discard the vial if particulate matter or discoloration is observed.
4. Reconstituted solution in the vial is stable at room temperature for 12 hours. Do not refrigerate.

Infusion solution – Based on patient weight, remove the appropriate volume of the reconstituted solution (ganciclovir concentration 50 mg/ml) from the vial and add to an acceptable (see below) infusion fluid (typically 100 ml) for delivery over the course of 1 hour. Infusion concentrations > 10 mg/ml are not recommended. The following infusion fluids have been determined to be chemically and physically compatible with ganciclovir IV solution: 0.9% Sodium Chloride, 5% Dextrose, Ringer's Injection and Lactated Ringer's Injection, USP.

Handling and disposal: Exercise caution in the handling and preparation of ganciclovir. Solutions of IV ganciclovir are alkaline (pH 11). Avoid direct contact with the skin or mucous membranes of the powder contained in ganciclovir capsules or of ganciclovir IV solutions. If such contact occurs, wash thoroughly with soap and water; rinse eyes thoroughly with plain water. Do not open or crush ganciclovir capsules.

Because ganciclovir shares some of the properties of antitumor agents (eg, carcinogenicity and mutagenicity), give consideration to handling and disposal according to guidelines issued for antineoplastic drugs.

Storage/Stability: Reconstituted solution in the vial is stable at room temperature for 12 hours. Do not refrigerate. Because nonbacteriostatic infusion fluid must be used with ganciclovir IV solution, the infusion solution must be used within 24 hours of dilution to reduce the risk of bacterial contamination. Refrigerate the infusion solution. Freezing is not recommended.

Rx	**Cytovene** (Roche)	**Capsules:** 250 mg	(Roche CY250). Green. In 180s.
		Powder for injection, lyophilized: 500 mg/vial ganciclovir (as sodium)	In 10 ml vials.

ZALCITABINE (Dideoxycytidine; ddC)

Warning:

The use of zalcitabine has been associated with significant clinical adverse reactions, some of which are potentially fatal. Zalcitabine can cause severe peripheral neuropathy; therefore use with extreme caution in patients with preexisting neuropathy. Zalcitabine may also rarely cause pancreatitis, and patients who develop any symptoms suggestive of pancreatitis while using zalcitabine should have therapy suspended immediately until this diagnosis is excluded.

Rare occurrences of lactic acidosis in the absence of hypoxemia and severe hepatomegaly with steatosis have been reported with the use of nucleoside analogs, including zidovudine and zalcitabine, and are potentially fatal. In addition, rare cases of hepatic failure and death, considered possibly related to underlying hepatitis B and zalcitabine monotherapy, have been reported (see Warnings).

Because of clinical uncertainty regarding the most appropriate use of nucleoside analogs, it is recommended that the decisions regarding the use of zalcitabine therapy be made in consultation with a physician experienced in the treatment of HIV infections.

Actions:

Pharmacology: Zalcitabine, active against the human immunodeficiency virus (HIV), is a synthetic pyrimidine nucleoside analog of the naturally occurring nucleoside 2′-deoxycytidine in which the 3′-hydroxyl group is replaced by hydrogen. Within cells, zalcitabine is converted to the active metabolite, dideoxycytidine 5′-triphosphate (ddCTP), by cellular enzymes. This metabolite serves as an alternative substrate to deoxycytidine triphosphate (dCTP) for HIV-reverse transcriptase and inhibits the in vitro replication of HIV-1 by inhibition of viral DNA synthesis. Because ddCTP lacks the 3-hydroxyl group required for DNA chain elongation, its incorporation into a growing DNA chain leads to premature chain termination. The metabolite serves as a competitive inhibitor of the natural substrate dCTP for the active site of the viral reverse transcriptase and thus further inhibits viral DNA synthesis. The active metabolite, ddCTP, also has a high affinity for cellular mitochondrial DNA polymerase gamma and appears to be incorporated into the DNA of cells in culture. Furthermore, the cellular DNA polymerase beta is able to utilize ddCTP causing chain termination. The half-life of ddCTP in established cell lines and in human peripheral blood mononuclear cells in culture is in the range of 2.6 to 10 hours.

Pharmacokinetics:

Adults –

Absorption/Distribution: Following oral administration to HIV-infected patients, the mean absolute bioavailability of zalcitabine was > 80%. The absorption rate of a 1.5 mg oral dose was reduced when administered with food. This resulted in a 39% decrease in mean maximum plasma concentrations (C_{max}) from 25.2 to 15.5 ng/ml, and a twofold increase in time to achieve C_{max} from a mean of 0.8 hours under fasting conditions to 1.6 hours when the drug was given with food. The extent of absorption was decreased by 14% (from 72 to 62 ng•hr/ml).

The steady-state volume of distribution following IV administration of a 1.5 mg dose averaged 0.534 L/kg. Cerebrospinal fluid obtained from 9 patients at 2 to 3.5 hours following 0.06 or 0.09 mg/kg IV infusion showed measurable concentrations of zalcitabine. The CSF:plasma concentration ratio ranged from 9% to 37% (mean, 20%), demonstrating drug penetration through the blood-brain barrier.

Metabolism/Excretion: Zalcitabine is phosphorylated intracellularly to zalcitabine triphosphate, the active substrate for HIV-reverse transcriptase. Concentrations of zalcitabine triphosphate are too low for quantitation. Metabolism has not been fully evaluated. Zalcitabine does not appear to undergo a significant degree of metabolism by the liver. Renal excretion appears to be the primary route of elimination, and it accounted for approximately 70% of an orally administered dose within 24 hours after dosing. The mean elimination half-life is 2 hours and generally ranges from 1 to 3 hours. Total body clearance following an IV dose averages 285 ml/min. Less than 10% of a dose appears in the feces.

In patients with impaired kidney function, prolonged elimination of zalcitabine may be expected. Results from 7 patients with renal impairment (estimated Ccr < 55 ml/min) indicate that the half-life was prolonged (up to 8.5 hours) in these patients compared with those with normal renal function. C_{max} was higher in some patients after a single dose. In patients with normal renal function, the pharmacokinetics of zalcitabine were not altered during 3 times daily multiple dosing. Accumulation of drug in plasma during this regimen was negligible. The drug was < 4% bound to plasma proteins, indicating that drug interactions involving binding-site displacement are unlikely (see Drug Interactions).

ZALCITABINE (Dideoxycytidine; ddC)

Children – Limited pharmacokinetic data have been reported for five HIV-positive children using doses of 0.03 and 0.04 mg/kg administered orally every 6 hours. The mean bioavailability of zalcitabine in this study was 54% and mean apparent systemic clearance was 150 ml/min/m^2.

Microbiology: The emergence of HIV variants with reduced susceptibility (resistance) to zalcitabine has been demonstrated in a small number of patients who received monotherapy for > 1 year. Combination therapy of zalcitabine plus zidovudine does not appear to prevent the emergence of zidovudine-resistant isolates. However, studies with zidovudine-resistant virus isolates indicate that zidovudine-resistant strains remain sensitive to zalcitabine.

Clinical trials:

Monotherapy – Zalcitabine was compared to didanosine for treatment of advanced HIV infection (mean CD4 cell count, 37 cells/mm^3) in patients who were intolerant to zidovudine or had disease progression while receiving zidovudine. Zalcitabine was at least as effective as didanosine in terms of time to an AIDS-defining event or death, while for survival alone the results favored zalcitabine.

Combination therapy –

Zidovudine-naive patients: Zidovudine-naive patients receiving zalcitabine with zidovudine had a greater rise in CD4 cell counts, which was maintained longer with combination therapy vs zidovudine monotherapy.

Zidovudine-exposed patients: Patients who had previously received zidovudine received zalcitabine alone, zalcitabine in combination with zidovudine or zidovudine alone. Patients had an entry CD4 cell count of ≤ 300 cells/mm^3. Overall there were no significant treatment differences in disease progression or death for the three groups. All treatment arms eventually showed decline in CD4 cell count.

Indications:

Monotherapy: Treatment of HIV infection in adults with advanced HIV disease who either are intolerant to zidovudine or who have disease progression while receiving zidovudine.

Combination therapy with zidovudine: For the treatment of selected patients with advanced HIV infection (CD4 cell count ≤ 300/mm^3).

Contraindications:

Hypersensitivity to zalcitabine or any components of the product.

Warnings:

Peripheral neuropathy: The major clinical toxicity is peripheral neuropathy (22% to 35%) of subjects. By comparison, neuropathy occurred in ≤ 14% of zidovudine-treated patients. Rates were similar among patients treated with zalcitabine monotherapy and in combination with zidovudine.

Zalcitabine-related peripheral neuropathy is a sensorimotor neuropathy characterized initially by numbness and burning dysesthesia involving the distal extremities. These symptoms may be followed by sharp shooting pains or severe continuous burning pain if the drug is not withdrawn. The neuropathy may progress to severe pain requiring narcotic analgesics and is potentially irreversible, especially if zalcitabine is not stopped promptly. In some patients, symptoms of neuropathy may initially progress despite discontinuation of zalcitabine. With prompt discontinuation, the neuropathy is usually slowly reversible.

There are no data regarding the use of zalcitabine in patients with preexisting peripheral neuropathy since these patients were excluded from clinical trials; therefore, use with extreme caution in these patients. Avoid zalcitabine in individuals with moderate or severe peripheral neuropathy, as evidenced by symptoms accompanied by objective findings.

Pancreatitis: Documented fatal pancreatitis has occurred with zalcitabine alone or in combination with zidovudine. Pancreatitis is an uncommon complication of zalcitabine monotherapy, occurring in 1.1% of patients. The occurrence of asymptomatic elevated serum amylase of any etiology while on zalcitabine monotherapy was 1.6%.

Closely follow patients with a history of pancreatitis or known risk factors for the development of pancreatitis while on zalcitabine. In 528 patients with history of pancreatitis or increased amylase, 5.3% developed pancreatitis and an additional 4.4% developed asymptomatic elevated serum amylase.

Stop treatment immediately if clinical signs or symptoms (eg, nausea, vomiting, abdominal pain) or if abnormalities in lab values (eg, hyperamylasemia associated with dysglycemia, rising triglyceride level, decreasing serum calcium) suggestive of pancreatitis occur. If clinical pancreatitis develops, it is recommended that zalcitabine be permanently discontinued. Interrupt treatment if therapy with another drug known to cause pancreatitis is required (see Drug Interactions).

ZALCITABINE (Dideoxycytidine; ddC)

Hepatic toxicity: Lactic acidosis in the absence of hypoxemia and severe hepatomegaly with steatosis has been reported rarely with nucleoside analogs, including zidovudine and zalcitabine, and are potentially fatal. In addition, rare cases of hepatic failure (one which coincided with renal failure) and death possibly related to underlying hepatitis B and zalcitabine monotherapy have occurred. Approach treatment with zalcitabine with caution in patients with preexisting liver disease, liver enzyme abnormalities, a history of ethanol abuse or hepatitis. Interrupt or discontinue therapy in the setting of deterioration of liver function tests, hepatic steatosis, progressive hepatomegaly or unexplained lactic acidosis. In clinical trials, drug interruption was recommended if liver function tests exceeded > 5 times the upper limit of normal.

Oral ulcers: Severe oral ulcers occurred in ≈ 3% of patients in two trials. Less severe oral ulcerations occurred at higher frequencies in other clinical trials.

Esophageal ulcers: Infrequent cases of esophageal ulcers have been attributed to zalcitabine therapy. Consider interruption of therapy in patients who develop esophageal ulcers that do not respond to specific treatment for opportunistic pathogens in order to assess a possible relationship to zalcitabine.

Cardiomyopathy/Congestive heart failure (CHF) have occurred with the use of nucleoside antiretroviral agents in AIDS patients; infrequent cases have occurred in patients receiving zalcitabine. Approach treatment with caution in patients with baseline cardiomyopathy or history of CHF.

Anaphylactoid reaction: There has been one report of an anaphylactoid reaction occurring in a patient receiving both zalcitabine and zidovudine. In addition, there have been several reports of urticaria without other signs of anaphylaxis.

Combination therapy: In vitro combination studies have demonstrated that zalcitabine and zidovudine have an additive or synergistic antiviral effect, depending on the cell line used, without increased cytotoxicity over that observed for either agent alone. Because severe adverse effects may be attributable to either the zalcitabine or the zidovudine components of combination therapy, or to their combination, consult complete product information for zidovudine before initiating combination therapy or reinstituting zidovudine monotherapy following an adverse reaction.

No benefit from combination therapy has been observed from studies of zidovudine-exposed patients with CD4 cell counts < 150 cells/mm^3. Combination therapy is not recommended in these patients.

Renal function impairment: Patients with renal impairment (estimated Ccr < 55 ml/min) may be at a greater risk of toxicity due to decreased drug clearance. Dosage reduction is recommended (see Administration and Dosage).

Mutagenesis: Human peripheral blood lymphocytes were exposed to zalcitabine, and at ≥ 1.5 mcg/ml, dose-related increases in chromosomal aberrations were seen. Oral doses of zalcitabine at 2500 and 4500 mg/kg were clastogenic in the mouse micronucleus assay.

Pregnancy: Category C. Zalcitabine is teratogenic in mice and rats. Increased embryolethality was observed and average fetal body weight was significantly decreased in mice and rats. There are no adequate and well controlled studies in pregnant women. Use during pregnancy only if the potential benefit justifies the potential risk to the fetus. Fertile women should not receive zalcitabine unless they are using an effective contraceptive during therapy.

Lactation: It is not known whether zalcitabine is excreted in breast milk. Decide whether to discontinue nursing or the drug, taking into account the importance of the drug to the mother. It is currently recommended in the US that HIV-infected women do not breastfeed infants regardless of the use of antiretroviral agents.

Children: Safety and efficacy of zalcitabine in combination with zidovudine or as monotherapy in HIV-infected children < 13 years of age have not been established.

ZALCITABINE (Dideoxycytidine; ddC)

Precautions:

Monitoring: Perform periodic complete blood counts and clinical chemistry tests. Monitor serum amylase levels in those individuals who have a history of elevated amylase, pancreatitis, ethanol abuse, who are on parenteral nutrition or who are otherwise at high risk of pancreatitis. Carefully monitor for signs or symptoms suggestive of peripheral neuropathy, particularly in individuals with a low CD4 cell count or who are at a greater risk of developing peripheral neuropathy while on therapy. (See Warnings.)

Lymphoma: High doses of zalcitabine for 3 months in mice (resulting in plasma concentrations > 1000 times those seen in patients taking the recommended dose) induced an increased incidence of thymic lymphoma. A predisposition to chemically induced thymic lymphoma and high rates of spontaneous lymphoreticular neoplasms have previously been noted in this strain of mice.

HIV infection complications: Patients receiving zalcitabine or any other antiretroviral therapy may continue to develop opportunistic infections and other complications of HIV infection, and should remain under close clinical observation by healthcare personnel experienced in the treatment of patients with HIV.

Drug Interactions:

Zalcitabine Drug Interactions

Precipitant drug	Object drug*		Description
Antacids	Zalcitabine	⬇	Zalcitabine absorption is moderately reduced (≈ 25%) when coadministered with magnesium/aluminum-containing antacids. Do not ingest simultaneously.
Chloramphenicol Cisplatin Dapsone Didanosine Disulfiram Ethionamide Glutethimide Gold Hydralazine Iodoquinol Isoniazid Metronidazole Nitrofurantoin Phenytoin Ribavirin Vincristine	Zalcitabine	⬆	These drugs have been associated with peripheral neuropathy. Avoid concomitant use when possible. Concomitant use of zalcitabine with didanosine is not recommended. In addition, drugs such as amphotericin, foscarnet and aminoglycosides may increase the risk of developing peripheral neuropathy or other zalcitabine-associated toxicities by interfering with the renal clearance of zalcitabine (and thereby raising systemic exposure). Patients who require the use of one of these drugs with zalcitabine should have frequent clinical and laboratory monitoring with dosage adjustment for any significant change in renal function.
Cimetidine	Zalcitabine	⬆	Concomitant use decreases zalcitabine elimination, most likely by inhibition of renal tubular secretion.
Metoclopramide	Zalcitabine	⬇	Zalcitabine bioavailability is mildly reduced (≈ 10%).
Pentamidine (and other agents that have potential to cause pancreatitis)	Zalcitabine	⬆	Interrupt treatment when the use of a drug that has the potential to cause pancreatitis is required. Death due to fulminant pancreatitis possibly related to zalcitabine and IV pentamidine was reported. If IV pentamidine is required to treat *Pneumocystis carinii* pneumonia, interrupt treatment with zalcitabine.
Probenecid	Zalcitabine	⬆	Concomitant use decreases zalcitabine elimination, most likely by inhibition of renal tubular secretion.

* ⬆ = Object drug increased. ⬇ = Object drug decreased.

Drug/Food interactions: The absorption rate of a 1.5 mg dose is reduced when administered with food resulting in a 39% decrease in mean Cmax and a twofold increase in time to achieve Cmax. The extent of absorption is decreased by 14%.

ZALCITABINE (Dideoxycytidine; ddC)

Adverse Reactions:

Zidovudine Adverse Reactions (%): Zalcitabine vs Didanosine		
Adverse reaction	Zalcitabine 0.75 mg q 8 h (n = 237)	Didanosine 250 mg q 12 h (n = 230)
CNS		
Fatigue	3.8	2.6
Headache	2.1	1.3
Fever	1.7	0.4
GI		
Abdominal pain	3	7
Oral lesions/Stomatitis	3	0
Vomiting/Nausea	3.4	7
Diarrhea	2.5	17
Neurological		
Convulsions	1.3	2.2
Peripheral neuropathy	28.3	13
Metabolic and Nutritional		
Elevated amylase	3.4	5.2
Pancreatitis	0	1.7
Miscellaneous		
Abnormal hepatic function	8.9	7
Rash/Pruritus/Urticaria	3.4	3.9

Zalcitabine Adverse Reactions (%): Monotherapy or Combination Therapy (with Zidovudine)			
Adverse reaction	Zalcitabine (n = 287)	Zidovudine (n = 286)	Zalcitabine + Zidovudine (n = 428)
GI			
Constipation	0.4	0.4 - 1.1	0.2 - 1.4
Melena	1.1	0.4	0.2
Flatulence/Gas	0.7	1.4	0.7
Diarrhea	0.4 9.5	1.4 10.6	1.2 - 10.6
Acute pharyngitis	1.8	1.1	2.4
Oral ulcers	3.2 - 7	2.8	0.9 - 5.6
Nausea	0.7 - 3.5	1.1 - 7	0.5 - 8.2
Dysphagia	0.4 - 4.2	1.1	0.7 - 3.5
Vomiting	1.1 3.5	1.4 - 4.6	0.7 - 6.6
Swallowing, painful	0.4 - 2.1	1.1	0.5 - 2.1
Mouth lesion	1.1 - 3.2	0.7 - 1.4	0.2 - 2.6
Abdominal pain	1.4 - 8.1	1.4 - 7.7	1.9 - 7.1
Metabolic/Nutritional			
Hypoglycemia	1.8 - 6.3	1.1 - 6.3	1.4 - 7.8
Triglyceride abnormal	0.7	0.7 - 1.4	0.2
Hypophosphatemia	0.7 - 2.1	0.4 - 1.8	0.5 - 1.2
Hypernatremia	0.4	1.1	0.5 - 1.4
Hyponatremia	3.5	0.4 - 1.4	1.2
Bilirubin increased	2.1 - 4.9	2.8 - 5.3	2.6 - 5.4
Appetite, loss of	3.9	6.7	0.9 - 7.3
Abnormal weight loss	0.7 - 4.9	1.1 - 6.3	0.5 - 9.4
Hypomagnesemia	0.4 - 1.1	0.7	0.2 - 0.5
Hypocalcium	1.1 - 2.1	0.7 - 1.8	0.7 - 2.1
Creatinine	0.4 - 1.1	0.4	0.7 - 1.4
Amylase increased	8.1	1.4 - 2.8	2.1 - 4.2
Hyperglycemia	1.1 - 5.6	2.1 - 3.9	1.6 - 4.5

ZALCITABINE (Dideoxycytidine; ddC)

Zalcitabine Adverse Reactions (%): Monotherapy or Combination Therapy (with Zidovudine)			
Adverse reaction	Zalcitabine (n = 287)	Zidovudine (n = 286)	Zalcitabine + Zidovudine (n = 428)
Musculoskeletal			
Joint pain	1.1	0.4	1.9
Weakness in leg muscle	2.1	1.8	4.2
Myalgia	0.4 - 6	1.8 - 10.2	0.5 - 8
Muscle weakness, upper	0.7	2.1	1.4
CPR elevated	0.4 - 0.7	1.1 - 1.4	1.2
Weakness, gen. muscle	0.4	1.4	0.5 - 1.9
CNS			
Dizziness	1.1	1.4	1.4
Confusion	0.4 - 1.8	0.7	0.5
Loss of memory	1.8	0	0.2 - 0.5
Concentration, decreased	1.1	0.7	0.5
Anxiety state	0.7	0.4 - 1.4	1.2
Depression	0.4 - 2.1	0.4 - 3.9	0.7 - 4
Headache	1.4 - 12.3	1.8 - 16.2	2.6 - 15.3
Insomnia	0.7	0.4 - 2.8	0.2 - 4.2
Renal			
Dysurea	0.7	1.1	1.2
Urination (frequency)	0.4	0.4 - 1.8	1.2
Respiratory			
Nasal discharge	3.5	6	0.2 - 6.4
Cough	6.3	7.7	0.2 - 8.2
Rales/Rhonchi	1.1	0.7	0
Dyspnea/Respiratory distress	0.7 - 2.8	5.6	2.8
Dermatologic			
Pruritic disorder	1.1 - 4.9	0.4 - 4.2	0.5 - 4
Rash	2.1 - 11.2	1.4 - 8.8	0.7 - 9.4
Night sweats	0.7 - 2.8	2.5	0.5 - 3.8
Lip blister, lesions	0.4 - 1.1	0	0.2
Special senses			
Ear problem, pain	0	1.1	0.5
Smell dysfunction	0.4 - 1.1	0	0
Miscellaneous			
Fever	4.9 - 16.8	9.2 - 17.6	3.8 - 16.2
Malaise/Fatigue	1.8 - 13.3	2.8 - 17.3	3.5 - 18.1
Chest pain, unspec.	0.4 - 1.4	0.4 - 3.9	0.2 - 2.8
General debilitation	1.1	0.4 - 1.8	0.2
Chills	0.7 - 1.4	1.1	0.5 - 2.1
LDH, abnormal lab results	0.7	0.4 - 1.4	0.7
GGT abnormal	2.8	3.2 - 3.5	0.7 - 0.9
Lymphadenopathy	0.4 - 1.4	1.1	0.5
Vaginal discharge	0	1.1	0

Body as a whole: Asthenia, cachexia, chest tightness or pain, chills, cutaneous/allergic reaction, debilitation, difficulty moving, dry eyes/mouth, edema, facial pain or swelling, fatigue, fever, flank pain, flushing, increased sweating, lymphadenopathy, malaise, night sweats, pain, pelvic/groin pain, rigors, weight decrease (< 3%).

Cardiovascular: Abnormal cardiac movement, arrhythmia, atrial fibrillation, cardiac failure, cardiac dysrhythmias, cardiomyopathy, heart racing, hypertension, palpitation, subarachnoid hemorrhage, syncope, tachycardia, ventricular ectopy (< 3%).

ZALCITABINE (Dideoxycytidine; ddC)

CNS: Abnormal coordination, aphasia, ataxia, Bell's palsy, confusion, convulsion, decreased concentration, decreased neurological function, disequilibrium, dizziness, dysphonia, facial nerve palsy, focal motor seizures, grand mal seizure, hyperkinesia, hypertonia, hypokinesia, memory loss, migraine, neuralgia, neuritis, paralysis, seizures, speech disorder, status epilepticus, stupor, tremor, twitch, vertigo (< 3%).

Dermatologic: Acne, alopecia, bullous eruptions, carbuncle/furuncle, cellulitis, cold sore, dermatitis, dry skin, dry rash desquamation, erythematous rash, exfoliative dermatitis, finger inflammation, follicular rash, impetigo, infection, itchy rash, lip blisters/lesions, macular/papular rash, maculopapular rash, moniliasis, mucocutaneous/skin disorder, nail disorder, photosensitivity reaction, pruritus, skin lesions, skin fissure, skin ulcer, urticaria (< 3%).

Endocrine: Abnormal triglycerides, abnormal lipase, altered serum glucose, diabetes mellitus, glycosuria, gout, hot flushes, hyperglycemia, hyperkalemia, hyperlipidemia, hypernatremia, hyperuricemia, hypocalcemia, hypokalemia, hypomagnesemia, increased nonprotein nitrogen, polydipsia (< 3%).

GI: Abdominal bloating or cramps, acute pancreatitis, anal/rectal pain, anorexia, bleeding gums, colitis, constipation, dental abscess, dry mouth, dyspepsia, dysphagia, enlarged abdomen, epigastric pain, eructation, esophageal pain, esophageal ulcers, esophagitis, flatulence, gagging with pills, gastritis, GI hemorrhage, gingivitis, glossitis, gum disorder, heartburn, hemorrhagic pancreatitis, hemorrhoids, increased saliva, left quadrant pain, melena, nausea, vomiting, odynophagia, painful sore gums, pancreatitis, rectal hemorrhage, rectal mass, rectal ulcers, salivary gland enlargement, sore tongue, sore throat, tongue disorder, tongue ulcer, toothache, unformed/loose stools, vomiting (< 3%).

GU: Abnormal renal function, acute renal failure, albuminuria, bladder pain, dysuria, genital lesion/ulcer, increased blood urea nitrogen, micturition frequency, nocturia, painful penis sore, penile edema, polyuria, renal cyst, renal calculus, testicular swelling, toxic nephropathy, urinary retention, vaginal itch, vaginal ulcer, vaginal pain, vaginal/cervix disorder (< 3%).

Hematologic: Absolute neutrophil count alteration, anemia, epistaxis, decreased hematocrit, granulocytosis, hemoglobinemia, leukopenia, neutrophilia, platelet alteration, purpura, thrombocytopenia, thrombus, unspecified hematologic toxicity, white blood cell alteration (< 3%).

Hepatic: Abnormal gamma-glutamyl transferase and lactate dehydrogenase, bilirubinemia, cholecystitis, decreased alkaline phosphatase, hepatitis, hepatocellular damage, hepatomegaly, increased alkaline phosphatase/AST/ALT (< 3%).

Musculoskeletal: Arthralgia, arthritis, arthropathy, arthrosis, back pain, backache, bone pains/aches, bursitis, cold extremities, extremity pain, increased creatine phosphokinase, joint pain, joint inflammation, joint swelling, leg cramps, muscle weakness, muscle disorder, muscle stiffness, muscle cramps, myalgia, myopathy, myositis, neck pain, rib pain, stiff neck (< 3%).

Psychiatric: Acute psychotic disorder, acute stress reaction, agitation, amnesia, anxiety, confusion, decreased motivation, decreased sexual desire, depersonalization, depression, emotional lability, euphoria, hallucination, impaired concentration, insomnia, manic reaction, mood swings, nervousness, paranoid state, somnolence, suicide attempt (< 3%).

Respiratory: Acute nasopharyngitis, chest congestion, coughing, cyanosis, dry nasal mucosa, dyspnea, flu-like symptoms, hemoptysis, pharyngitis, sinus congestion, sinus pain, sinusitis, wheezing (< 3%).

Special senses: Abnormal/blurred/decreased vision, burning eyes, decreased taste, ear pain/problem/blockage, eye abnormality/inflammation/itching/pain/irritation/redness/hemorrhage, fluid in ears, hearing loss, increased tears, loss of taste, mucopurulent conjunctivitis, parosmia, photophobia, taste perversion, tinnitus, unequal-sized pupils, xerophthalmia, yellow sclera (< 3%).

ZALCITABINE (Dideoxycytidine; ddC)

Lab test abnormalities:

Zalcitabine Laboratory Test Abnormalities (%)					
Lab test abnormality	Zalcitabine (n = 285)	Zidovudine (n = 283)	Zalcitabine + Zidovudine (n = 423)	Zalcitabine 0.75 mg q 8 h (n = 237)	Didanosine 250 mg q 12 h (n = 230)
Anemia (< 7.5 g/dl)	6	4.2	5.7	8.4	7.4
Leukopenia (< 1500/mm^3)	9.1	12.7	13.9	13.1	9.6
Neutropenia (< 750/mm^3)	15.1	18.7	22.7	16.9	11.7
Eosinophilia (> 1000 or 25%)	6.3	4.6	5	2.5	1.7
Thrombocytopenia (< 50,000/mm^3)	2.8	2.1	3.1	1.3	4.8
ALT (> 250 U/L)	3.2	3.9	3.1	—	—
AST (> 250 U/L)	3.2	4.2	3.5	—	—
AST (> 5 × ULN)	—	—	—	7.6	5.7
Alkaline phosphatase (> 625 U/L)	1.4	1.1	1.2	—	—

Overdosage:

Acute: Inadvertent pediatric overdoses have occurred with doses up to 1.5 mg/kg. The children had prompt gastric lavage and treatment with activated charcoal and had no sequelae. Mixed overdoses including zalcitabine and other drugs have led to drowsiness and vomiting or increased GGT or creatine phosphokinase. There is no experience with acute overdosage at higher doses and sequelae are unknown. There is no known antidote. It is not known whether zalcitabine is dialyzable by peritoneal dialysis or hemodialysis.

Chronic: In a study in which zalcitabine was administered at doses 25 times (0.25 mg/kg every 8 hours) the currently recommended dose, one patient discontinued zalcitabine after 1.5 weeks of treatment subsequent to the development of a rash and fever.

In early Phase 1 studies, all patients receiving zalcitabine at ≈ 6 times the current total daily recommended dose experienced peripheral neuropathy by week 10; 80% who received ≈ 2 times the current total daily recommended dose experienced peripheral neuropathy by week 12.

Patient Information:

Zalcitabine is not a cure for HIV infection; patients may continue to develop illnesses associated with advanced HIV infection including opportunistic infections. Since it is frequently difficult to determine whether symptoms are due to drug effect or underlying disease, encourage patients to report all changes in their condition to their physician. Use of zalcitabine or other antiretroviral drugs does not preclude the ongoing need to maintain practices designed to prevent transmission of HIV.

Instruct patients that the major toxicity of zalcitabine is peripheral neuropathy. Pancreatitis and hepatic toxicity are other serious and potentially life-threatening toxicities. Advise patients of the early symptoms of these conditions and instruct them to promptly report these symptoms to their physician. Since development of peripheral neuropathy appears dose-related, advise patients to follow prescribed dose.

Women of childbearing age should use effective contraception while on zalcitabine.

Administration and Dosage:

Approved by the FDA on June 19, 1992.

Monotherapy: 0.75 mg every 8 hours (2.25 mg total daily dose).

Combination therapy with zidovudine: 0.75 mg administered concomitantly with 200 mg zidovudine every 8 hours (2.25 mg zalcitabine total daily dose and 600 mg zidovudine total daily dose).

Renal function impairment: Dosage reduction is recommended: Ccr 10 to 40 ml/min, 0.75 mg every 12 hours; Ccr < 10 ml/min, 0.75 mg every 24 hours.

ZALCITABINE (Dideoxycytidine; ddC)

Dose adjustment:

Monotherapy and combination therapy – For toxicities likely to be associated with zalcitabine (see Warnings and Precautions), interrupt or reduce dose. For severe toxicities or those persisting after dose reduction, interrupt zalcitabine therapy. For recipients of combination therapy with zalcitabine and zidovudine, base dose adjustments for either drug on the known toxicity profile of the individual drugs. For toxicities that are associated with either zidovudine or zalcitabine (eg, hepatic toxicity), interrupt or reduce dose of both drugs. For any interruption of zalcitabine (especially if zalcitabine is permanently discontinued), adjust zidovudine dosage schedule from 200 mg every 8 hours to 100 mg every 4 hours. For severe toxicities or toxicities in which the causative drug is unclear or which persist after dose interruption or reduction of one drug, interrupt or reduce dose of the other drug.

Peripheral neuropathy – Patients developing moderate discomfort with signs or symptoms of peripheral neuropathy should stop zalcitabine. Zalcitabine-associated peripheral neuropathy may continue to worsen despite interruption of therapy. Reintroduce the drug at 50% dose (0.375 mg every 8 hours) only if all findings related to peripheral neuropathy have improved to mild symptoms. Permanently discontinue the drug when patients experience severe discomfort related to peripheral neuropathy or moderate discomfort progresses. If other moderate to severe clinical adverse reactions or lab abnormalities (eg, increased liver function tests) occur, then interrupt zalcitabine (or both zalcitabine and zidovudine in combination therapy) until the adverse reaction abates. Carefully reintroduce therapy at lower doses if appropriate. If adverse reactions recur, discontinue therapy.

Hematologic toxicities – In patients with poor bone marrow reserve, particularly those patients with advanced symptomatic HIV disease, frequent monitoring of hematologic indices is recommended to detect serious anemia or granulocytopenia (see Warnings). Significant toxicities, such as anemia (hemoglobin < 7.5 g/dl or reduction > 25% of baseline) or granulocytopenia (granulocyte count < 750/mm^3 or reduction of > 50% from baseline), may require a treatment interruption of zalcitabine and zidovudine until evidence of marrow recovery is observed. For less severe anemia or granulocytopenia, a reduction in the zidovudine daily dose may be adequate. In patients who experience hematologic toxicity, reduction in hemoglobin may occur as early as 2 to 4 weeks after initiation of therapy and granulocytopenia usually occurs after 6 to 8 weeks of therapy. In patients who develop significant anemia, dose modification does not necessarily eliminate the need for transfusion. If marrow recovery occurs following dose modification, gradual increases in dose may be appropriate depending on hematologic indices and patient intolerance.

Rx	**Hivid** (Roche)	**Tablets**: 0.375 mg	Lactose. (Hivid 0.375 Roche). Beige, oval. Film coated. In 100s.
		0.75 mg	Lactose. (Hivid 0.750 Roche). Gray, oval. Film coated. In 100s.

RIMANTADINE HCl

Actions:

Pharmacology: Rimantadine is a synthetic antiviral agent. The mechanism of action is not fully understood. It appears to exert its inhibitory effect early in the viral replicative cycle, possibly inhibiting the uncoating of the virus. Genetic studies suggest that a virus protein specified by the virion M_2 gene plays an important role in the susceptibility of influenza A virus to inhibition by rimantadine.

Rimantadine is safe and effective in preventing signs and symptoms of infection caused by various strains of influenza A virus. Early vaccination on an annual basis as recommended by the CDC's Immunization Practices Advisory Committee is the method of choice in the prophylaxis of influenza unless vaccination is contraindicated, not available or not feasible. Since rimantadine does not completely prevent the host immune response to influenza A infection, individuals who take this drug may still develop immune responses to natural disease or vaccination and may be protected when later exposed to antigenically related viruses. Following vaccination during an influenza outbreak, consider rimantadine prophylaxis for the 2 to 4 week time period required to develop an antibody response. However, the safety and effectiveness of prophylaxis have not been demonstrated for > 6 weeks.

Consider rimantadine therapy for adults who develop an influenza-like illness during known or suspected influenza A infection in the community. When administered within 48 hours after onset of signs and symptoms of infection caused by influenza A virus strains, rimantadine reduces the duration of fever and systematic symptoms.

Pharmacokinetics: There are no data establishing a correlation between plasma concentration and antiviral effect. The tablet and syrup formulations of rimantadine are equally absorbed after oral administration. The mean peak plasma concentration after a single 100 mg dose was 74 ng/ml (range, 45 to 138 ng/ml). The time to peak concentration was 6 hours in healthy adults (age, 20 to 44 years). The single dose elimination half-life in this population was 25.4 hours (range, 13 to 65 hours). The single-dose elimination half-life in a group of healthy 71- to 79-year-old subjects was 32 hours (range, 20 to 65 hours). Plasma protein binding is about 40%.

After the administration of 100 mg twice daily to healthy volunteers (age, 18 to 70 years) for 10 days, area under the curve (AUC) values were ≈ 30% greater than predicted from a single dose. Plasma trough levels at steady state ranged between 118 and 468 ng/ml. In a comparison of three groups of healthy older subjects (age, 50 to 60, 61 to 70 and 71 to 79 years), the 71- to 79-year-old group had average AUC values, peak concentrations and elimination half-life values at steady state that were 20% to 30% higher than the other two groups. Steady-state concentrations in elderly nursing home patients (age, 68 to 102 years) were two- to fourfold higher than those seen in healthy young and elderly adults.

In a group (n = 10) of children 4 to 8 years old who were given a single dose (6.6 mg/kg) of syrup, plasma concentrations ranged from 446 to 988 ng/ml at 5 to 6 hours and from 170 to 424 ng/ml at 24 hours. In some children, the drug was detected in plasma 72 hours after the last dose. Following oral administration, rimantadine is extensively metabolized in the liver with < 25% of the dose excreted in the urine as unchanged drug. Three hydroxylated metabolites have been found in plasma. These metabolites, an additional conjugated metabolite and parent drug account for 74% of a single 200 mg dose excreted in urine over 72 hours.

In a group of patients with chronic liver disease, the majority of whom were stabilized cirrhotics, the pharmacokinetics of rimantadine were not appreciably altered following a single 200 mg oral dose compared to six healthy subjects. After administration of a single 200 mg dose to patients with severe hepatic dysfunction, AUC was approximately threefold larger, elimination half-life was approximately twofold longer and apparent clearance was about 50% lower when compared to historic data from healthy subjects.

Studies of the effects of renal insufficiency on the pharmacokinetics of rimantadine have given inconsistent results. Following administration of a single 200 mg oral dose to eight patients with a creatinine clearance (Ccr) of 31 to 50 ml/min and six patients with Ccr of 11 to 30 ml/min, the apparent clearance was 37% and 16% lower, respectively, and plasma metabolite concentrations were higher when compared to healthy subjects (n = 9, Ccr > 50 ml/min). After a single 200 mg oral dose was given to eight hemodialysis patients (Ccr 0 to 10 ml/min), there was a 1.6-fold increase in the elimination half-life and a 40% decrease in apparent clearance compared to healthy subjects. Hemodialysis did not contribute to the clearance of rimantadine.

RIMANTADINE HCl

Microbiology: Rimantadine is inhibitory to the in vitro replication of influenza A virus isolates from each of the three antigenic subtypes (H1N1, H2N2 and H3N2) that have been isolated from man. Rimantadine has little or no activity against influenza B virus. Rimantadine does not appear to interfere with the immunogenicity of inactivated influenza A vaccine. A quantitative relationship between the in vitro susceptibility of influenza A virus to rimantadine and clinical response to therapy has not been established. Rimantadine-resistant strains of influenza A virus have emerged among freshly isolated epidemic strains in closed settings where rimantadine has been used. Resistant viruses have been shown to be transmissible and to cause typical influenza illness.

Indications:

Adults: Prophylaxis and treatment of illness caused by various strains of influenza A virus.

Children: Prophylaxis against influenza A virus.

Contraindications:

Hypersensitivity to drugs of the adamantine class, including rimantadine and amantadine.

Warnings:

Renal/Hepatic function impairment: The safety and pharmacokinetics of rimantadine in renal and hepatic insufficiency have only been evaluated after single dose administration. In a single dose study of patients with anuric renal failure, the apparent clearance was ≈ 40% lower and the elimination half-life was 1.6-fold greater than that in healthy controls. In a study of 14 persons with chronic liver disease (mostly stabilized cirrhotics), no alterations in the pharmacokinetics were observed after a single dose of rimantadine. However, the apparent clearance of rimantadine following a single dose to 10 patients with severe liver dysfunction was 50% lower than that reported for healthy subjects. Because of the potential for accumulation of rimantadine and its metabolites in plasma, exercise caution when patients with renal or hepatic insufficiency are treated with rimantadine.

Pregnancy: Category C. There are no adequate and well controlled studies in pregnant women. Rimantadine crosses the placenta in mice. Rimantadine is embryotoxic in rats when given at a dose of 200 mg/kg/day (11 times the recommended human dose) which consisted of increased fetal resorption; this dose also produced a variety of maternal effects including ataxia, tremors, convulsions and significantly reduced weight gain. In rabbits, there was evidence of a developmental abnormality in the form of a change in the ratio of fetuses with 12 or 13 ribs. This ratio is normally about 50:50 in a litter but was 80:20 after rimantadine treatment. In pregnant rats using doses of 30, 60 and 120 mg/kg/day (1.7, 3.4 and 6.8 times the recommended human dose), maternal toxicity drug gestation was noted at the two higher doses of rimantadine, and at the highest dose there was an increase in pup mortality during the first 2 to 4 days postpartum. Decreased fertility of the F1 generation was also noted for the two higher doses. For these reasons, use during pregnancy only if the potential benefit justifies the risk to the fetus.

Lactation: Rimantadine should not be administered to nursing mothers because of the adverse affects noted in offspring of rats treated with rimantadine during the nursing period. Rimantadine is concentrated in rat milk in a dose-related manner: 2 to 3 hours following administration of rimantadine, rat breast milk levels were approximately twice those observed in serum.

Children: In children, rimantadine is recommended for the prophylaxis of influenza A. Safety and efficacy of rimantadine in the treatment of symptomatic influenza infection in children have not been established. Prophylaxis studies with rimantadine have not been performed in children < 1 year of age.

Precautions:

Seizures: An increased incidence of seizures has been reported in patients with a history of epilepsy who received the related drug amantadine. In clinical trials, the occurrence of seizure-like activity was observed in a small number of patients with a history of seizures who were not receiving anticonvulsant medication while taking rimantadine. If seizures develop, discontinue the drug.

Resistance: Consider transmission of rimantadine-resistant virus when treating patients whose contacts are at high risk for influenza A illness. Influenza A virus strains resistant to rimantadine can emerge during treatment and may be transmissible and cause typical influenza illness. Of patients with initially sensitive virus upon treatment with rimantadine, 10% to 30% shed rimantadine-resistant virus. Clinical response, although slower in those patients, was not significantly different from those who did not shed resistant virus.

Drug Interactions:

Rimantadine Drug Interactions			
Precipitant drug	Object drug*		Description
Acetaminophen	Rimantadine	⬇	Coadministration with acetaminophen reduced the peak concentration and AUC values for rimantadine by ≈ 11%.
Aspirin	Rimantadine	⬇	Peak plasma and AUC of rimantadine were reduced ≈ 10% by aspirin.
Cimetidine	Rimantadine	⬆	When a single 100 mg dose of rimantadine was administered 1 hour after cimetidine (300 mg 4 times a day) in healthy adults, the apparent total rimantadine clearance was reduced by 16%.

* ⬆ = Object drug increased. ⬇ = Object drug decreased.

Adverse Reactions:

The most frequently reported adverse events involved the GI and CNS. Rates increased significantly using higher than recommended doses. In most cases, symptoms resolved rapidly with discontinuation of treatment.

Adverse Reactions: Rimantadine vs Placebo		
Adverse reaction	Rimantadine (n = 1027)	Placebo (n = 986)
CNS		
Insomnia	2.1%	0.9%
Dizziness	1.9%	1.1%
Headache	1.4%	1.3%
Nervousness	1.3%	0.6%
Fatigue	1%	0.9%
Asthenia	1.4%	0.5%
GI		
Nausea	2.8%	1.6%
Vomiting	1.7%	0.6%
Anorexia	1.6%	0.8%
Dry mouth	1.5%	0.6%
Abdominal pain	1.4%	0.8%

Adverse Reactions: Rimantadine vs Amantadine			
Adverse reaction	Rimantadine (n =145)	Placebo (n = 143)	Amantadine (n =148)
Insomnia	3.4%	0.7%	7%
Nervousness	2.1%	0.7%	2.8%
Impaired concentration	2.1%	1.4%	2.1%
Dizziness	0.7%	0	2.1%
Depression	0.7%	0.7%	3.5%
Total % with adverse reactions	6.9%	4.1%	14.7%
Total % withdrawn due to adverse reactions	6.9%	3.4%	14%

GI: Diarrhea, dyspepsia (0.3% to 1%); constipation, dysphagia, stomatitis.

CNS: Impairment of concentration, ataxia, somnolence, agitation, depression (0.3% to 1%); gait abnormality, euphoria, hyperkinesia, tremor, hallucination, confusion, convulsions (< 0.3%); agitation, diaphoresis, hypesthesia.

Special senses: Tinnitus (0.3% to 1%); taste loss/change, parosmia (< 0.3%); eye pain.

Respiratory: Dyspnea (0.3% to 1%); bronchospasm, cough (< 0.3%).

Cardiovascular: Pallor, palpitation, hypertension, cerebrovascular disorder, cardiac failure, pedal edema, heart block, tachycardia, syncope (< 0.3%).

RIMANTADINE HCl

Miscellaneous: Rash (0.3% to 1%); non-puerperal lactation (< 0.3%); increased lacrimation, increased micturition frequency, fever, rigors.

Elderly – In general, the incidence of adverse events in the elderly was higher; 10.6% of those treated with rimantadine compared with 8.3% in the placebo group experienced events related to the CNS. The profile of these events was similar to that for the most frequent adverse events reported in other controlled trials. Pooled data from controlled studies of prophylaxis and treatment of influenza with rimantadine in persons > 65 years of age showed an increase in adverse clinical events associated with the recommended dose of rimantadine (100 mg twice a day) compared to controls as follows: Central and peripheral nervous systems (12.5% vs 8.7%); GI (17% vs 11.3%).

Overdosage:

As with any overdose, administer supportive therapy as indicated. Overdoses of a related drug, amantadine, have been reported with reactions consisting of agitation, hallucinations, cardiac arrhythmia and death. The administration of IV physostigmine (a cholinergic agent) at doses of 1 to 2 mg in adults and 0.5 mg in children repeated as needed as long as the dose did not exceed 2 mg/hr has been reported anecdotally to be beneficial in patients with CNS effects from overdoses of amantadine. Refer to General Management of Acute Overdosage.

Administration and Dosage:

Approved by the FDA on September 17, 1993.

Prophylaxis:

Adults – The recommended dose of rimantadine is 100 mg twice a day. In patients with severe hepatic dysfunction, renal failure (Ccr ≤ 10 ml/min) and elderly nursing home patients, a dose reduction to 100 mg daily is recommended.

Children (< 10 years of age) – Administer once a day at a dose of 5 mg/kg, not exceeding 150 mg. For children ≥ 10 years of age, use the adult dose.

Treatment:

Adults – The recommended dose is 100 mg twice a day. In patients with severe hepatic dysfunction, renal failure (Ccr ≤ 10 ml/min) and elderly nursing home patients, a dose reduction to 100 mg daily is recommended. Initiate therapy as soon as possible, preferably within 48 hours after onset of signs and symptoms of influenza A infection. Continue therapy for ≈ 7 days from the initial onset of symptoms.

Renal/Hepatic function impairment: Because of the potential for accumulation of rimantadine metabolites during multiple dosing, monitor patients with any degree of renal insufficiency for adverse effects, with dosage adjustments being made as necessary.

Rx	**Flumadine** (Forest)	**Tablets:** 100 mg	(Flumadine 100 Forest). Orange. Oval. Film coated. In 20s, 100s, 500s and 1000s.
		Syrup: 50 mg per 5 ml	Saccharin, sorbitol, parabens. Raspberry flavor. In 60, 240 and 480 ml.

TRIMETHOPRIM (TMP)

Actions:

Pharmacology: Trimethoprim blocks production of tetrahydrofolic acid from dihydrofolic acid by binding to and reversibly inhibiting the enzyme dihydrofolate reductase. This binding is much stronger for the bacterial enzyme than for the corresponding mammalian enzyme. Bacterial biosynthesis of nucleic acids and proteins is blocked by trimethoprim's interference with the normal bacterial metabolism of folinic acid.

Pharmacokinetics:

Absorption/Distribution – Oral trimethoprim is rapidly absorbed. Mean peak serum levels of approximately 1 mcg/ml occur 1 to 4 hours after a single 100 mg dose. Approximately 44% is serum protein bound. Urine concentrations are considerably higher than blood concentrations. After a single oral dose of 100 mg, urine levels ranged from 30 to 160 mcg/ml during the 0 to 4 hour period and declined to approximately 18 to 91 mcg/ml during the 8 to 24 hour period.

Metabolism/Excretion – Trimethoprim is metabolized less than 20%. The half-life is 8 to 10 hours. Elimination is delayed in patients with renal function impairment and half-life is prolonged. Excretion is chiefly by the kidneys through glomerular filtration and tubular secretion. After oral administration, 50% to 60% is excreted in the urine within 24 hours; ≈ 80% is unmetabolized, and ≈ 4% is detectable in feces.

Microbiology: In vitro, the spectrum of antibacterial activity includes common urinary tract pathogens except Pseudomonas aeruginosa.

Using the dilution method for determining the minimum inhibitory concentrations (MIC), the MIC for susceptible organisms is ≤ 8 mcg/ml. Resistant species have an MIC of ≥ 16 mcg/ml.

Representative Trimethoprim MICs For Susceptible Organisms

Bacteria	Trimethoprim MIC (mcg/ml)
Escherichia coli	0.05-1.5
Proteus mirabilis	0.5-1.5
Klebsiella pneumoniae	0.5-5
Enterobacter species	0.5-5
Staphylococcus species (coagulase-negative)	0.15-5

Normal vaginal and fecal flora are the source of most pathogens causing urinary tract infections (UTIs). Concentrations in vaginal secretions are consistently greater (1.6 fold) than those in serum. Sufficient trimethoprim is excreted in the feces to markedly reduce or eliminate susceptible organisms. Dominant fecal organisms (non-*Enterobacteriaceae, Bacteroides* and *Lactobacillus* species), are generally not susceptible.

Trimethoprim acts synergistically with sulfonamides, blocking sequential steps in the biosynthesis of folic acid. See trimethoprim-sulfamethoxazole monograph.

Indications:

For the treatment of initial uncomplicated UTIs due to susceptible strains including: *E coli, P mirabilis, K pneumoniae, Enterobacter* species, and coagulase-negative *Staphylococcus* species, including *S saprophyticus.*

Perform culture and susceptibility tests. May initiate therapy prior to obtaining test results.

Contraindications:

Hypersensitivity to trimethoprim; megaloblastic anemia due to folate deficiency.

Warnings:

Hematologic effects: Trimethoprim rarely interferes with hematopoiesis, especially in large doses or for prolonged periods. Sore throat, fever, pallor, or purpura may be early indications of serious blood disorders; obtain complete blood counts. Discontinue drug if the count of any formed blood element is significantly reduced.

Renal/Hepatic function impairment: Use with caution.

Pregnancy: Category C. Teratogenic in small animals at 40 times the human dose; increased fetal loss occurred with 6 times the human therapeutic dose.

Trimethoprim crosses the placenta, producing similar levels in fetal and maternal serum and in amniotic fluid. In a report of 186 pregnancies in which the mother received either placebo or trimethoprim/sulfamethoxazole, the incidence of congenital abnormalities was 4.5% (3 of 66) for placebo and 3.3% (4 of 120) for the drug combination. There were no abnormalities in 10 children exposed during the first trimester or in 35 children exposed to trimethoprim/sulfamethoxazole at conception or shortly after.

TRIMETHOPRIM (TMP)

Trimethoprim may interfere with folic acid metabolism; use only when potential benefits outweigh potential hazards to the fetus.

Lactation: Following 160 mg twice daily for 5 days, milk concentrations ranged from 1.2 to 2.4 mcg/ml; observed milk:plasma ratios were 1.25. Because it may interfere with folic acid metabolism, use caution when administering to nursing women.

Children: Safety for use in infants < 2 months has not been established. The efficacy for use in children < 12 has not been established.

Precautions:

Folate deficiency: Use with caution. Folates may be administered concomitantly without interfering with antibacterial action.

Drug Interactions:

Phenytoin's pharmacologic effects may be increased by coadministration of trimethoprim, apparently due to inhibition of hepatic metabolism.

Adverse Reactions:

Dermatologic: Rash (3% to 7%); pruritus; exfoliative dermatitis. In high-dose studies, an increased incidence of mild to moderate maculopapular, morbilliform and pruritic rashes occurred 7 to 14 days after therapy began.

GI: Epigastric distress; nausea; vomiting; glossitis.

Hematologic: Thrombocytopenia; leukopenia; neutropenia; megaloblastic anemia; methemoglobinemia.

Miscellaneous: Fever; elevation of serum transaminase and bilirubin; increased BUN and serum creatinine levels.

Overdosage:

Acute:

Symptoms – After ingestion of ≥ 1 g, nausea, vomiting, dizziness, headaches, mental depression, confusion, and bone marrow depression may occur (see Chronic Overdosage).

Treatment – Gastric lavage and general supportive measures. Urine acidification increases renal elimination. Peritoneal dialysis is not effective and hemodialysis is only moderately effective.

Chronic:

Symptoms – Use at high doses or for extended periods may cause bone marrow depression manifested as thrombocytopenia, leukopenia or megaloblastic anemia.

Treatment – Discontinue use and give leucovorin, 3 to 6 mg IM daily for 3 days, or as required to restore normal hematopoiesis. Alternatively, 5 to 15 mg daily of oral leucovorin has been recommended.

Patient Information:

Take for full course of therapy until medication is gone.

Administration and Dosage:

Adults: 100 mg every 12 hours or 200 mg every 24 hours for 10 days.

Renal impairment: If creatinine clearance is 15 to 30 ml/min, give 50 mg every 12 hours. If it is < 15 ml/min, use is not recommended.

Children: Effectiveness has not been established.

Storage: Protect the 200 mg tablet from light.

Rx	**Trimethoprim** (Various, eg, Biocraft, Major, Moore, Parmed, Rugby, Schein)	**Tablets:** 100 mg	In 14s, 30s, 100s and UD 100s.
Rx	**Proloprim** (Glaxo Wellcome)		(Proloprim 09A). White, scored. In 100s.
Rx	**Trimpex** (Roche)		(Trimpex 100 Roche). White, scored. In 100s and Tel–E–Dose 100s.
Rx	**Trimethoprim** (Various, eg, Biocraft, Moore, Rugby,)	**Tablets:** 200 mg	In 100s.
Rx	**Proloprim** (Glaxo Wellcome)		(Proloprim 200). Yellow, scored. In 100s.

TRIMETHOPRIM AND SULFAMETHOXAZOLE (Co-Trimoxazole; TMP-SMZ)

See also individual monographs for trimethoprim and sulfonamides.

Actions:

Pharmacology: Sulfamethoxazole (SMZ) inhibits bacterial synthesis of dihydrofolic acid by competing with para-aminobenzoic acid. Trimethoprim (TMP) blocks the production of tetrahydrofolic acid by inhibiting the enzyme dihydrofolate reductase. Thus, this combination blocks two consecutive steps in the bacterial biosynthesis of essential nucleic acids and proteins. In vitro, bacterial resistance develops more slowly with this combination than with either drug alone.

Pharmacokinetics:

Absorption/Distribution – TMP-SMZ is rapidly and completely absorbed following oral administration. Peak plasma levels occur in 1 to 4 hours following oral administration and 1 to 1.5 hours after IV infusion. The 1:5 ratio of TMP to SMZ achieves an approximate 1:20 ratio of peak serum concentrations. Detectable amounts of TMP–SMZ are present in the blood 24 hours after administration. During 3 days of administration of 160 mg TMP/800 mg SMZ twice daily, the mean steady-state plasma TMP concentration was 1.72 mcg/ml. The steady-state mean plasma levels of free and total SMZ were 57.4 mcg/ml and 68 mcg/ml, respectively. Approximately 44% of TMP and 70% of SMZ are protein bound. Both distribute to sputum, vaginal fluid and middle ear fluid, pass the placental barrier, and are excreted in breast milk; TMP also distributes to bronchial secretion. Two to three times the serum concentration of TMP is achieved in prostatic fluid. Therapeutic concentrations are achieved in vaginal secretions, cerebrospinal fluid, pulmonary tissue, pleural effusion, bile, sputa and aqueous humor. It is also detectable in breast milk, amniotic fluid and fetal serum. Following oral administration, the half-lives of TMP (8 to 11 hours) and SMZ (10 to 12 hours) are similar. Following IV administration, the mean plasma half-life was 11.3 $\pm$ 0.7 hours for TMP and 12.8 $\pm$ 1.8 hours for SMZ. Patients with severely impaired renal function exhibit an increase in the half-lives of both components, requiring dosage regimen adjustment.

Metabolism/Excretion – TMP is metabolized to a relatively small extent; SMZ undergoes biotransformation to inactive compounds. The metabolism of SMZ occurs predominantly by N_4-acetylation, although the glucuronide conjugate has been identified. The principal metabolites of TMP are the 1- and 3-oxides and the 3′- and 4′-hydroxy derivatives. The free forms are the therapeutically active forms.

Excretion is chiefly by the kidneys through both glomerular filtration and tubular secretion. Urine concentrations are considerably higher than serum concentrations. Concurrent administration does not affect the excretion pattern of either drug. The average percentage of the dose recovered in urine from 0 to 72 hours after a single oral dose is 84.5% for total sulfonamide and 66.8% for free TMP. Of the total sulfonamide, 30% is excreted as free SMZ, with the remaining as N_4-acetylated metabolite.

Microbiology: The antibacterial activity of TMP–SMZ includes the common urinary tract pathogens except *Pseudomonas aeruginosa*. The following are usually susceptible: *Escherichia coli, Klebsiella* and *Enterobacter* sp, *Morganella morganii, Proteus mirabilis* and indole-positive *Proteus* sp including *P vulgaris*. The following pathogens isolated from middle ear exudate and bronchial secretions are usually susceptible: *Haemophilus influenzae* (including ampicillin-resistant strains), *Streptococcus pneumoniae, Shigella flexneri* and *S sonnei*.

Indications:

Oral and parenteral:

Urinary tract infections (UTIs) due to susceptible strains of E coli, Klebsiella and Enterobacter species, M morganii, P mirabilis and P vulgaris – Treat initial uncomplicated UTIs with a single antibacterial agent.

Parenteral therapy is indicated in severe or complicated infections when oral therapy is not feasible.

Shigellosis enteritis caused by susceptible strains of *S flexneri* and *S sonnei* in children and adults.

Pneumocystis carinii pneumonia (PCP) – Treatment of PCP in children and adults.

Oral:

Pneumocystis carinii pneumonia – Prophylaxis against PCP in individuals who are immunosuppressed and considered to be at increased risk.

Acute otitis media in children due to susceptible strains of *H influenzae* or *S pneumoniae*. There are limited data on the safety of repeated use in children < 2 years of age. Not indicated for prophylactic use or prolonged administration.

Acute exacerbations of chronic bronchitis in adults due to susceptible strains of *H influenzae* and *S pneumoniae*.

Travelers' diarrhea in adults due to susceptible strains of enterotoxigenic *E coli*.

TRIMETHOPRIM AND SULFAMETHOXAZOLE (Co-Trimoxazole; TMP-SMZ)

Unlabeled uses: Treatment of cholera and salmonella-type infections and nocardiosis.

TMP 40 mg and SMZ 200 mg daily at bedtime, a minimum of 3 times weekly or postcoitally has been used to prevent recurrent UTIs in females.

Low-dose TMP–SMZ has been studied in the prophylaxis of neutropenic patients with *P carinii* infections or leukemia patients to reduce the incidence of gram-negative rod bacteremia.

Prophylaxis with TMP-SMZ (320/1600 mg/day) appears beneficial in reducing the incidence of bacterial infection (especially of the urinary tract and blood) following renal transplantation, and may provide protection against *P carinii* pneumonia.

Treatment of acute and chronic prostatitis – 160 mg TMP/800 mg SMZ twice daily has been used for chronic bacterial prostatitis for up to 12 weeks.

Contraindications:

Hypersensitivity to trimethoprim or sulfonamides; megaloblastic anemia due to folate deficiency; pregnancy at term and lactation (see Warnings); infants < 2 months old.

The sulfonamides are chemically similar to some goitrogens, diuretics (acetazolamide and the thiazides) and oral hypoglycemic agents. Goiter production, diuresis and hypoglycemia occur rarely in patients receiving sulfonamides. Cross-sensitivity may exist with these agents.

Warnings:

Streptococcal pharyngitis: Do not use to treat streptococcal pharyngitis. Patients with group A β-hemolytic streptococcal tonsillopharyngitis have a greater incidence of bacteriologic failure with this combination than with penicillin.

Hematologic effects: Sulfonamide-associated deaths, although rare, have occurred from hypersensitivity of the respiratory tract, Stevens-Johnson syndrome, toxic epidermal necrolysis, fulminant hepatic necrosis, agranulocytosis, aplastic anemia and other blood dyscrasias. Both TMP and SMZ can interfere with hematopoiesis. In elderly patients receiving diuretics (primarily thiazides), an increased incidence of thrombocytopenia with purpura occurred. Discontinue the drug at the first appearance of skin rash or any sign of adverse reaction. Rash, sore throat, fever, arthralgia, cough, shortness of breath, pallor, purpura or jaundice may be early indications of serious reactions. Obtain complete blood counts frequently. If significant reduction in the count of any formed blood element is noted, discontinue therapy.

IV use at high doses or for extended periods of time may cause bone marrow depression manifested as thrombocytopenia, leukopenia or megaloblastic anemia. If signs of bone marrow depression occur, give leucovorin as needed to restore normal hematopoiesis. Oral leucovorin, 5 to 15 mg/day has been recommended.

Pneumocystis carinii pneumonitis in patients with Acquired Immunodeficiency Syndrome (AIDS): Because of their unique immune dysfunction, AIDS patients may not tolerate or respond to TMP–SMZ. The incidence of side effects, particularly rash, fever, leukopenia, elevated aminotransferase values, hyperkalemia and hyponatremia in these patients is greatly increased compared with non-AIDS patients.

Adverse effects are generally less severe in patients receiving TMP-SMZ for prophylaxis. A history of mild intolerance to TMP-SMZ in AIDS patients does not appear to predict intolerance of subsequent secondary prophylaxis. However, if a patient develops skin rash or any sign of adverse reaction, re-evaluate therapy.

Renal/Hepatic function impairment: Use with caution. Maintain adequate fluid intake to prevent crystalluria and stone formation. Perform urinalyses and renal function tests during therapy, particularly in impaired renal function.

Elderly: There may be an increased risk of severe adverse reactions, particularly when complicating conditions exist (eg, impaired kidney or liver function, concomitant use of other drugs). Severe skin reactions, generalized bone marrow suppression or a decrease in platelets (with or without purpura) are the most frequently reported severe adverse reactions. In those concurrently receiving certain diuretics, primarily thiazides, an increased incidence of thrombocytopenia with purpura has occurred. Make appropriate dosage adjustments for impaired kidney function.

Pregnancy: Category C. Do not use at term. Sulfonamides readily cross the placenta. Fetal levels average 70% to 90% of maternal levels. Toxicities observed in the neonate include jaundice, hemolytic anemia and kernicterus. Trimethoprim crosses the placenta, producing similar levels in fetal and maternal serum. There are no large, well controlled studies; however, in one study of 186 pregnancies where the mother received either placebo or oral TMP–SMZ, the incidence of congenital abnormalities was 4.5% (3 of 66) in those who received placebo and 3.3% (4 of 120) in those receiving TMP–SMZ. There were no abnormalities in 10 children whose mothers received the drug during the first trimester or in 35 children whose mothers had taken the drug at conception or shortly thereafter.

Because TMP-SMZ may interfere with folic acid metabolism, use during pregnancy only if the potential benefits outweigh the potential hazards to the fetus.

Lactation: TMP–SMZ is not recommended in the nursing period because sulfonamides are excreted in breast milk and may cause kernicterus. Premature infants and infants with hyperbilirubinemia or G–6–PD deficiency are also at risk for adverse effects.

Children: Not recommended for infants < 2 months old. See Indications.

Precautions:

Special risk patients: Use with caution in patients with possible folate deficiency (eg, elderly patients, chronic alcoholics, anticonvulsant therapy, malabsorption syndrome, patients in malnutrition states), severe allergy or bronchial asthma. In G-6-PD deficient individuals, hemolysis may occur; it is frequently dose-related.

Extravascular infiltration: If local irritation and inflammation due to extravascular infiltration of the infusion occurs, discontinue the infusion and restart at another site.

Benzyl alcohol, contained in some of these products as a preservative, has been associated with a fatal "gasping syndrome" in premature infants.

Superinfection: Use of antibiotics (especially prolonged or repeated therapy) may result in bacterial or fungal overgrowth of nonsusceptible organisms. Such overgrowth may lead to a secondary infection. Take appropriate measures if this occurs.

Sulfite sensitivity: Sulfites may cause allergic-type reactions (eg, hives, itching, wheezing, anaphylaxis) in susceptible persons. Although the prevalence of sulfite sensitivity in the general population is probably low, it is more frequent in asthmatics or atopic nonasthmatic persons. Products containing sulfites are identified in the product listings.

Drug Interactions:

TMP-SMZ Drug Interactions

Precipitant drug	Object drug*		Description
TMP-SMZ	Anticoagulants	↑	The prothrombin time of warfarin may be prolonged. Monitor coagulation tests and adjust dosage as required.
TMP-SMZ	Cyclosporine	↓	A decrease in the therapeutic effect of cyclosporine and an increased risk of nephrotoxicity have occurred.
TMP-SMZ	Dapsone	↑	Increased serum levels of both dapsone and TMP may occur.
Dapsone	TMP-SMZ	↑	
TMP-SMZ	Diuretics	↑	In elderly patients, concomitant use has increased incidence of thrombocytopenia with purpura.
TMP-SMZ	Hydantoins	↑	Phenytoin's hepatic clearance may be decreased and the half-life prolonged.
TMP-SMZ	Methotrexate	↑	Sulfonamides can displace methotrexate (MTX) from plasma protein binding sites, thus increasing free MTX concentrations; bone marrow depressant effects may be potentiated.
TMP-SMZ	Sulfonylureas	↑	The hypoglycemic response may be increased.
TMP-SMZ	Zidovudine	↑	The serum levels of zidovudine may be increased due to a decreased renal clearance.

* ↑ = Object drug increased. ↓ = Object drug decreased.

Drug/Lab test interactions: Trimethoprim can interfere with a serum methotrexate assay as determined by the competitive binding protein technique (CBPA) when a bacterial dihydrofolate reductase is used as the binding protein. No interference occurs if methotrexate is measured by a radioimmunoassay.

TMP-SMZ may interfere with the Jaffe alkaline picrate reaction assay for creatinine, resulting in overestimations of about 10% in the range of normal values.

Adverse Reactions:

Parenteral therapy: Local reaction, pain and slight irritation on IV administration (infrequent); thrombophlebitis (rare).

Most common: GI disturbances (nausea, vomiting, anorexia); allergic skin reactions (eg, rash, urticaria).

Hematologic: Agranulocytosis; aplastic, hemolytic or megaloblastic anemia; thrombocytopenia; leukopenia; neutropenia; hypoprothrombinemia; eosinophilia; methemoglobinemia; hyperkalemia; hyponatremia.

TRIMETHOPRIM AND SULFAMETHOXAZOLE (Co-Trimoxazole; TMP-SMZ)

Hypersensitivity: Erythema multiforme; Stevens-Johnson syndrome; generalized skin eruptions; rash; toxic epidermal necrolysis; urticaria; serum sickness-like syndrome; pruritus; exfoliative dermatitis; anaphylactoid reactions; conjunctival and scleral injection; photosensitization; allergic myocarditis; angioedema; drug fever; chills; Henoch-Schoenlein purpura; systemic lupus erythematosus; generalized allergic reactions; periarteritis nodosa.

GI: Glossitis; anorexia; stomatitis; nausea; emesis; abdominal pain; diarrhea; pseudomembranous enterocolitis; hepatitis (including cholestatic jaundice and hepatic necrosis); pancreatitis; elevation of serum transaminase and bilirubin.

CNS: Headache; mental depression; convulsions; ataxia; hallucinations; tinnitus; vertigo; insomnia; apathy; fatigue; weakness; nervousness; aseptic meningitis; peripheral neuritis.

GU: Renal failure; interstitial nephritis; BUN and serum creatinine elevation; toxic nephrosis with oliguria and anuria; crystalluria.

Musculoskeletal: Arthralgia; myalgia.

Respiratory: Pulmonary infiltrates.

Overdosage:

Symptoms:

Acute – Signs and symptoms observed with either TMP or SMZ alone include: Anorexia; colic; nausea; vomiting; dizziness; headache; drowsiness; unconsciousness; pyrexia; hematuria; crystalluria; depression; confusion; blood dyscrasias and jaundice (late manifestations).

Chronic – High doses or use for extended periods may cause bone marrow depression manifested as thrombocytopenia, leukopenia or megaloblastic anemia. Give leucovorin; 5 to 15 mg/day has been recommended.

Treatment: Treatment includes usual supportive measures. Refer to General Management of Acute Overdosage. Perform gastric lavage or emesis, force oral fluids and administer IV fluids if urine output is low and renal function is normal. Acidifying urine will increase renal elimination of TMP. Monitor patient with blood counts and appropriate blood chemistries, including electrolytes. If significant blood dyscrasia or jaundice occurs, institute specific therapy for these complications. Peritoneal dialysis is not effective and hemodialysis is only moderately effective in eliminating TMP and SMZ.

Patient Information:

Complete full course of therapy. Take each oral dose with a full glass of water.

Maintain adequate fluid intake.

Notify physician immediately if sore throat, fever, chills, pale skin, yellowing of skin or eyes, rash or unusual bleeding or bruising occurs.

Administration and Dosage:

Administration and Dosage of TMP-SMZ

Organisms/Infections	Dosage	
Urinary tract infections, shigellosis and acute otitis media:		
Adults:	160 mg TMP/800 mg SMZ every 12 hours for 10 to 14 days (5 days for shigellosis).	
Children (≥ 2 months of age):	8 mg/kg TMP/40 mg/kg SMZ per day given in 2 divided doses every 12 hours for 10 days (5 days for shigellosis).	
Guideline for proper dosage:	Dose every 12 hours:	
Weight (kg)	Teaspoonfuls	Tablets
10	1 (5 ml)	-
20	2 (10 ml)	1
30	3 (15 ml)	1½
40	4 (20 ml)	2 (or 1 double strength tablet)

TRIMETHOPRIM AND SULFAMETHOXAZOLE (Co-Trimoxazole; TMP-SMZ)

Administration and Dosage of TMP-SMZ

Organisms/Infections	Dosage	
Patients with impaired renal function	Recommended dosage regimen:	
Ccr (ml/min):		
> 30	Usual regimen	
15-30	½ usual regimen	
< 15	Not recommended	
IV: Adults and children > 2 months with normal renal function for severe UTIs and shigellosis.	8 to 10 mg/kg/day (based on TMP) in 2 to 4 divided doses every 6, 8 or 12 hours for up to 14 days for severe UTIs and 5 days for shigellosis.	
Travelers' diarrhea in adults:	160 mg TMP/800 mg SMZ every 12 hrs for 5 days.	
Acute exacerbations of chronic bronchitis in adults:	160 mg TMP/800 mg SMZ every 12 hrs for 14 days.	
Pneumocystis carinii pneumonia:		
Treatment:	15 to 20 mg/kg TMP/100 mg/kg SMZ per day in divided doses every 6 hours for 14 to 21 days.	
Guideline for proper dosage in children	Dose every 6 hours:	
Weight (kg)	Teaspoonfuls	Tablets
8	1 (5 ml)	-
16	2 (10 ml)	1
24	3 (15 ml)	1½
32	4 (20 ml)	2 (or 1 double strength tablet)
IV for adults and children > 2 months:	15 to 20 mg/kg/day (based on TMP) in 3 or 4 divided doses every 6 to 8 hours for up to 14 days.	
Prophylaxis:		
Adults:	160 mg TMP/800 mg SMZ given orally every 24 hours.	
Children:	150 mg/m² TMP/ 750 mg/m² SMZ per day given orally in equally divided doses twice a day, on 3 consecutive days per week. The total daily dose should not exceed 320 mg TMP/1600 mg SMZ.	
Guideline for proper dosage in children	Dose every 12 hours	
Body surface area (m²)	Teaspoonfuls	Tablets
0.26	½ (2.5 ml)	-
0.53	1 (5 ml)	½
1.06	2 (10 ml)	1

[1] Also recommended by the Public Service Task Force on Antipneumocystis Prophylaxis. CDC 1993 Sexually Transmitted Diseases Treatment Guidelines. *Morbidity and Mortality Weekly Report* 1993 Sep 24;42 (No. RR-14):1–102.

Parenteral:

IV – Administer over 60 to 90 minutes. Avoid rapid infusion or bolus injection. Do not give IM. When administered by an infusion device, thoroughly flush all lines used to remove any residual TMP-SMZ. The following infusion systems have been tested and found satisfactory: Unit-dose glass containers; unit-dose polyvinyl chloride; polyolefin containers.

Preparation of solution – Infusion must be diluted; add the contents of each 5 ml amp to 125 ml of 5% Dextrose in Water. Do not mix with other drugs or solutions. Do not refrigerate and use within 6 hours. If a dilution of 5 ml per 100 ml D5W is desired, use within 4 hours. When fluid restriction is desirable, add each 5 ml amp

TRIMETHOPRIM AND SULFAMETHOXAZOLE (Co-Trimoxazole; TMP-SMZ)

to 75 ml of D5W. Mix solution just prior to use and administer within 2 hours. If solution is cloudy or precipitates after mixing, discard and prepare fresh solution.

Storage/Stability – Store infusion at room temperature (15° to 30°C; 59° to 86°F). Do not refrigerate. Protect from light. After initial entry into the multi-dose vials, use the remaining contents within 48 hours.

Rx	**Trimethoprim and Sulfamethoxazole** (Various, eg, Geneva, Goldline, Lederle, Lemmon, Moore, Rugby, Schein, URL)	**Tablets:** 80 mg trimethoprim and 400 mg sulfamethoxazole	In 100s and 500s.
Rx	**Bactrim** (Roche)		(Bactrim-Roche). Lt. green, scored. Capsule shape. In 100s.
Rx	**Cotrim** (Lemmon)		(Cotrim 93). White, scored. In 100s and 500s.
Rx	**Septra** (Glaxo Wellcome)		(Septra Y2B). Pink, scored. In 100s.
Rx	**Trimethoprim and Sulfamethoxazole DS** (Various, eg, Goldline, Geneva, Lederle, Lemmon, Moore, Rugby, Schein, URL)	**Tablets, Double Strength:** 160 mg trimethoprim and 800 mg sulfamethoxazole	In 100s and 500s.
Rx	**Bactrim DS** (Roche)		(Bactrim-DS 01 Roche). White. Capsule shape. In 100s, 250s and 500s.
Rx	**Cotrim D.S.** (Lemmon)		(Cotrim DS). White, scored. Oval. In 100s and 500s.
Rx	**Septra DS** (Glaxo Wellcome)		(Septra DS O2C). Pink, scored. Oval. In 100s, 250s and UD 100s.
Rx	**Trimethoprim and Sulfamethoxazole** (Various, eg, Geneva, Goldline, Lemmon, Moore, Rugby, Schein)	**Oral Suspension:** 40 mg trimethoprim and 200 mg sulfamethoxazole per 5 ml	In 150, 200 and 480 ml.
Rx	**Bactrim Pediatric** (Roche)		Cherry flavor. In 480 ml.[1]
Rx	**Cotrim Pediatric** (Lemmon)		Cherry flavor. In 473 ml.[2]
Rx	**Septra** (Glaxo Wellcome)		Cherry flavor in 20, 100, 150, 200 and 473 ml.[3] Grape flavor in 473 ml.[3]
Rx	**Sulfatrim** (Various, eg, URL)		In 473 ml.
Rx	**Trimethoprim and Sulfamethoxazole** (Various, eg, Sanofi)	**Injection:** 80 mg trimethoprim and 400 mg sulfamethoxazole per 5 ml	In 5 ml *Carpuject*.
Rx	**Bactrim IV** (Roche)		In 10 and 30 ml multiple-dose vials.[4]
Rx	**Septra IV** (Glaxo Wellcome)		In 5 ml vials and 10 and 20 ml multiple-dose vials.[4]

[1] With 0.3% alcohol, saccharin, sorbitol, sucrose, parabens, EDTA.
[2] With ≤ 0.5% alcohol, saccharin, sorbitol.
[3] With 0.26% alcohol, 0.1% methylparaben, 0.1% sodium benzoate, saccharin, sorbitol.
[4] With 40% propylene glycol, 10% ethyl alcohol, 0.3% diethanolamine, 0.1% sodium metabisulfite and 1% benzyl alcohol.

ERYTHROMYCIN ETHYLSUCCINATE AND SULFISOXAZOLE

Indications:

Children: Acute otitis media caused by susceptible strains of *Hemophilus influenzae.*

Administration and Dosage:

Do not administer to infants < 2 months old; systemic sulfonamides are contraindicated in this age group.

Acute otitis media: 50 mg/kg/day erythromycin and 150 mg/kg/day (to a maximum of 6 g/day), sulfisoxazole. Give in equally divided doses 4 times daily for 10 days. Administer without regard to meals. The following dosage schedule is recommended:

Erythromycin/Sulfisoxazole Dosage Based on Weight

Weight		
kg	lb	Dose (every 6 hours)
< 8	< 18	Adjust dosage by body weight
8	18	2.5 ml
16	35	5 ml
24	53	7.5 ml
> 45	> 100	10 ml

Rx	**Erythromycin and Sulfisoxasole** (Various, eg, Barr, Geneva Marsam, Goldline, Harber, Lederle, Major, Moore, Rugby, Schein, URL)	**Granules for Oral Suspension:** Erythromycin ethylsuccinate (equivalent to 200 mg erythromycin activity) and sulfisoxazole acetyl (equivalent to 600 mg sulfisoxazole) per 5 ml when reconstituted	In 100, 150 and 200 ml.
Rx	**Eryzole** (Alra)		Sucrose. Strawberry flavor. In 100, 150 and 200 ml.
Rx	**Pediazole** (Ross)		Sucrose. Strawberry-banana flavor. In 100, 150, 200 and 250 ml.

FURAZOLIDONE

Actions:

Pharmacology: Furazolidone exerts bactericidal activity via interference with several bacterial enzyme systems, minimizing the development of resistant organisms. It neither significantly alters the normal bowel flora nor results in fungal overgrowth.

Pharmacokinetics: There are limited data in humans. Previously it was thought that very little drug was absorbed following oral administration. However, recent data indicate significant absorption. It is rapidly and extensively metabolized, possibly in the intestine. Colored metabolites are excreted in the urine.

Microbiology: Its broad antibacterial spectrum covers the majority of GI tract pathogens, including *Escherichia coli*, staphylococci, *Salmonella*, *Shigella* and *Proteus* species, *Aerobacter aerogenes*, *Vibrio cholerae* and *Giardia lamblia*.

Indications:

Specific and symptomatic treatment of bacterial or protozoal diarrhea and enteritis caused by susceptible organisms.

Unlabeled uses: Furazolidone 7.5 mg/kg plus oral rehydration therapy for 5 days was more effective than oral rehydration therapy alone in the treatment of acute infantile diarrhea (when fecal leukocytes were present) in children 3 to 73 months of age.

Furazolidone appears effective in the treatment of typhoid fever in adults (800 mg/day for 14 days) and for the treatment of giardiasis in children (67 to 266 mg/day for 10 days).

Furazolidone may also be useful in treating traveler's diarrhea, cholera and bacteremic salmonellosis.

Contraindications:

Do not administer to infants < 1 month of age.

Prior sensitivity to furazolidone.

Warnings:

Pregnancy: Category C. Safety for use during pregnancy has not been established. Use only when clearly needed and when the potential benefits outweigh the potential hazards to the fetus. Theoretically, furazolidone could produce hemolytic anemia in a glucose-6-phosphate dehydrogenase (G-6-PD) deficient neonate if given at term.

Lactation: Safety for use in the nursing mother has not been established. Drug concentration in breast milk has not been determined.

Precautions:

Orthostatic hypotension and hypoglycemia may occur.

Hemolysis may occur in G-6-PD deficient individuals.

Hypertensive crisis: When considering the administration of larger than recommended doses, or for > 5 days, consider the possibility of hypertensive crises.

Monoamine oxidase (MAO) inhibition: Furazolidone inhibits the enzyme MAO. Doses of 400 mg/day for 5 days increased tyramine and amphetamine sensitivity two- to threefold. See Drug Interactions. Use caution if administering with other MAOIs.

FURAZOLIDONE

Drug Interactions:

Furazolidone Drug Interactions			
Precipitant Drug	Object Drug*		Description
Furazolidone	Alcohol	↑	A disulfiram-like reaction (eg, facial flushing, light-headedness, weakness, lacrimation) has occurred. See Adverse Reactions.
Furazolidone	Anorexiants	↑	Increased sensitivity to the pressor response of the anorexiants due to MAO inhibition.
Furazolidone	Levodopa	↑	Both the efficacy and adverse effects of levodopa may be increased, specifically hypertensive crisis. This may occur for several weeks after stopping furazolidone.
Furazolidone	Meperidine	↑	Effects are difficult to characterize, but may include agitation, seizures, diaphoresis, fever and progress to coma and apnea.
Furazolidone	Sympathomimetics (indirect and mixed)	↑	Increased pressor sensitivity to the indirect- and mixed-acting sympathomimetics due to MAO inhibition. Direct-acting agents are not affected.
Furazolidone	Tricyclic antidepessants	↑	Variable effects, including hypertension, hyperpyrexia, seizures, tachycardia; acute psychosis has occurred.

* ↑ = Object drug increased.

Drug/Food interactions: Patients taking furazolidone may experience marked elevation of blood pressure, hypertensive crisis or hemorrhagic strokes if foods high in amine content are consumed concurrently or after therapy. For a list of foods, see the MAOI group monograph.

Adverse Reactions:

Hypersensitivity: Hypotension; urticaria; fever; arthralgia; vesicular morbilliform rash. These reactions subsided following withdrawal of the drug.

GI: Colitis; proctitis; anal pruritus; staphylococcic enteritis. Nausea or emesis occurs occasionally and may be minimized or eliminated by reducing or withdrawing the drug.

CNS: Headache; malaise.

Miscellaneous:

Disulfiram-like reaction – Rarely, individuals have exhibited a disulfiram-like reaction to alcohol characterized by flushing, fever, dyspnea, and in some instances, chest tightness. All symptoms disappeared within 24 hours with no lasting ill effects. During 9 years of clinical use, 43 cases have been reported (14 under experimental conditions with doses in excess of those recommended). Three experienced hypotension necessitating active therapy. Norepinephrine may be used for hypotensive episodes, since it is not potentiated by furazolidone. Avoid indirectly acting pressor agents. Avoid ingestion of alcohol in any form during therapy and for 4 days thereafter.

Other – Renal or hepatic toxicity have not been significant with furazolidone.

Hematologic: May cause mild reversible intravascular hemolysis in G6–PD deficient patients. Observe patients closely; discontinue the drug if there is any indication of hemolysis.

Do not administer to infants < 1 month of age because of possible hemolytic anemia due to immature enzyme systems (glutathione instability).

FURAZOLIDONE

Patient Information:

Avoid ingestion of alcohol during and within 4 days after furazolidone therapy (a disulfiram-like reaction may occur; see Adverse Reactions).

Avoid foods containing tyramine, especially if therapy extends beyond 5 days (see Drug Interactions).

Avoid over-the-counter or prescription medications containing sympathomimetic drugs (eg, cold and hay fever remedies, anorexiants).

Medication may color the urine brown.

May cause nausea, vomiting or headache. Notify physician if these symptoms become severe.

Administration and Dosage:

Dosage is based on an average dose of 5 mg/kg/day given in 4 equally divided doses. Do not exceed 8.8 mg/kg/day due to the possibility of nausea and emesis. If these are severe, reduce dosage.

Adults: 100 mg 4 times daily.

Children:

(≥ 5 years of age) – 25 to 50 mg 4 times daily (tablet or liquid).
(1 to 4 years) – 17 to 25 mg 4 times daily (liquid).
(1 month to 1 year) – 8 to 17 mg 4 times daily (liquid).

If satisfactory clinical response is not obtained within 7 days, the pathogen is refractory to furazolidone; discontinue the drug. Adjunctive therapy with other antibacterial agents or bismuth salts is not contraindicated.

Rx	**Furoxone** (Procter & Gamble Pharm.)	**Tablets:** 100 mg	Sucrose. (Eaton 072). Green, scored. In 20s and 100s.
		Liquid: 50 mg per 15 ml	Saccharin. In 60 and 473 ml.

PENTAMIDINE ISETHIONATE

Actions:

Pharmacology: Pentamidine isethionate, an aromatic diamidine antiprotozoal agent, has activity against *Pneumocystis carinii*.The mode of action is not fully understood. In vitro studies indicate that the drug interferes with nuclear metabolism and inhibits the synthesis of DNA, RNA, phospholipids and protein synthesis.

Pharmacokinetics:

Absorption/Distribution – s well absorbed after IM administration. It is detectable in the blood briefly, due to extensive tissue binding.

The mean concentrations of pentamidine determined 18 to 24 hours after inhalation therapy were 23.2 ng/ml in bronchoalveolar lavage fluid and 705 ng/ml in sediment after administration of a 300 mg single dose via the Respirgard;® II nebulizer. The mean concentrations of pentamidine determined 18 to 24 hours after a 4 mg/kg IV dose were 2.6 ng/ml in bronchoalveolar lavage fluid and 9.3 ng/ml in sediment. In the patients who received aerosolized pentamidine, the peak plasma levels of pentamidine were at or below the lower limit of detection of the assay (2.3 ng/ml).

Metabolism/Excretion – Approximately of the dose is excreted unchanged by the kidneys in the first 6 hours; however, small amounts are found in the urine up to 6 to 8 weeks following administration. Pentamidine may accumulate in renal failure. Following a single 2 hour IV infusion of 4 mg/kg of pentamidine the mean maximum plasma concentration, half-life and clearance were 612 ± 371 ng/ml, 6.4 ± 1.3 hr and 248 ± 91 L/hr respectively.

Plasma concentrations after aerosol administration are substantially lower than those observed after a comparable IV dose. The extent of pentamidine accumulation and distribution following chronic inhalation therapy are not known.

Indications:

Injection: Treatment of *Pneumocystis carinii* pneumonia (PCP).

Inhalation: Prevention of PCP in high-risk, HIV-infected patients defined by one or both of the following criteria:

1) a history of one or more episodes of PCP
2) a peripheral CD4+ (T4 helper/inducer) lymphocyte count ≤ 200 cu mm.

Unlabeled uses: Pentamidine has been used in the treatment of trypanosomiasis and visceral leishmaniasis.

Contraindications:

Injection: Once the diagnosis of PCP has been established, there are no absolute contraindications to the use of pentamidine.

Inhalation: Patients with a history of an anaphylactic reaction to inhaled or parenteral pentamidine isethionate.

Warnings:

Development of acute PCP still exists in patients receiving pentamidine prophylaxis. Therefore, any patient with symptoms suggestive of the presence of a pulmonary infection, including but not limited to dyspnea, fever or cough, should receive a thorough medical evaluation and appropriate diagnostic tests for possible acute PCP and for other opportunistic and non-opportunistic pathogens. The use of pentamidine may alter the clinical and radiographic features of PCP and could result in an atypical presentation, including but not limited to mild diseases or focal infection.

Prior to initiating pentamidine prophylaxis, evaluate symptomatic patients to exclude the presence of PCP. The recommended dose of pentamidine for the prevention of PCP is insufficient to treat acute PCP.

Fatalities due to severe hypotension, hypoglycemia and cardiac arrhythmias have been reported, both by the IM and IV routes. Severe hypotension may result after a single dose. Limit administration of the drug to patients in whom *P carinii* has been demonstrated. Closely monitor patients for serious adverse reactions.

Pregnancy: Category C. Safety and efficacy for use during pregnancy have not been established. Use only when clearly needed and when the potential benefits outweigh the unknown potential hazards to the fetus.

Lactation: It is not known whether pentamidine is excreted in breast milk. Because of the potential for serious adverse reactions in nursing infants decide whether to discontinue nursing or to discontinue the drug, taking into account the importance of the drug to the mother.

Children: Safety and efficacy of inhalation solution have not been established.

Precautions:

Use with caution in patients with hypertension, hypotension, hypoglycemia, hyperglycemia, hypocalcemia, leukopenia, thrombocytopenia, anemia, hepatic or renal dysfunction, ventricular tachycardia, pancreatitis, Stevens-Johnson syndrome.

PENTAMIDINE ISETHIONATE

Hypotension: Patients may develop sudden, severe hypotension after a single dose, whether given IV or IM. Therefore, patients receiving the drug should be supine; monitor blood pressure closely during drug administration and several times thereafter until the blood pressure is stable. Have equipment for emergency resuscitation readily available. If pentamidine is administered IV, infuse over 60 minutes.

Hypoglycemia: Pentamidine-induced hypoglycemia has been associated with pancreatic islet cell necrosis and inappropriately high plasma insulin concentrations. Hyperglycemia and diabetes mellitus, with or without preceding hypoglycemia, have also occurred, sometimes several months after therapy. Therefore, monitor blood glucose levels daily during therapy and several times thereafter.

Pulmonary: Inhalation of pentamidine isethionate may induce bronchospasm or cough particularly in patients who have a history of smoking or asthma. In clinical trials, cough and bronchospasm were the most frequently reported adverse experiences associated with pentamidine administration (38% and 15%, respectively of patients receiving the 300 mg dose); however less than 1% of the doses were interrupted or terminated due to these effects. For the majority of patients, cough and bronchospasm were controlled by administration of an aerosolized bronchodilator (only 1% of patients withdrew from the study due to treatment-associated cough or bronchospasm). In patients who experience bronchospasm or cough, administration of an inhaled bronchodilator prior to giving each pentamidine dose may minimize recurrence of the symptoms.

Extrapulmonary infection with P carinii has been reported infrequently with inhalation use. Most have been reported in patients who have a history of PCP. Consider the presence of extrapulmonary pneumocystosis when evaluating patients with unexplained signs and symptoms.

Laboratory tests to perform before, during and after therapy:

1. Daily BUN, serum creatinine and blood glucose.
2. Complete blood count and platelet counts.
3. Liver function test, including bilirubin, alkaline phosphatase, AST and ALT.
4. Serum calcium.
5. ECG at regular intervals.

Adverse Reactions:

Injection: 244 of 424 (57.5%) patients treated with pentamidine injection developed some adverse reaction. Most of the patients had acquired immunodeficiency syndrome (AIDS). In the following, "severe" refers to life-threatening reactions or reactions that required immediate corrective measures and led to discontinuation of pentamidine.

Severe – Leukopenia (< 1000/cu mm) 2.8%; hypoglycemia (< 25 mg/dl) 2.4%; thrombocytopenia (< 20,000/cu mm) 1.7%; hypotension (< 60 mm Hg systolic) 0.9%; acute renal failure (serum creatinine > 6 mg/dl) 0.5%; hypocalcemia (0.2%); Stevens-Johnson syndrome and ventricular tachycardia (0.2%); fatalities due to severe hypotension, hypoglycemia and cardiac arrhythmias.

Moderate – Elevated serum creatinine (2.4 to 6 mg/dl) 23.1%; sterile abscess, pain or induration at the IM injection site (11.1%); elevated liver function tests (8.7%); leukopenia (7.5%); nausea, anorexia (5.9%); hypotension (4%); fever, hypoglycemia (3.5%); rash (3.3%); bad taste in mouth, confusion/hallucinations (1.7%); anemia (1.2%); neuralgia, thrombocytopenia (0.9%); hyperkalemia, phlebitis (0.7%); dizziness without hypotension (0.5%).

Each of the following was reported in one patient: Abnormal ST segment of ECG, bronchospasm, diarrhea, hypocalcemia and hyperglycemia.

Aerosol:

Most Frequent – Fatigue, metallic taste, shortness of breath, decreased appetite (53% to 72%); dizziness, rash, cough (31% to 47%); nausea, pharyngitis, chest pain/congestion, night sweats, chills, vomiting, bronchospasm (10% to 23%).

Less frequent – Pneumothorax, diarrhea, headache, anemia (generally associated with zidovudine use), myalgia, abdominal pain, edema (1% to 5%).

Causal relationship unknown (≤ 1%):

Cardiovascular – Tachycardia; hypotension; hypertension; palpitations; syncope; cerebrovascular accident; vasodilation; vasculitis.

Metabolic – Hypoglycemia; hyperglycemia; hypocalcemia.

GI – Gingivitis; dyspepsia; oral ulcer/abscess; gastritis; gastric ulcer; hypersalivation; dry mouth; splenomegaly; melena; hematochezia; esophagitis; colitis; pancreatitis.

Hematologic – Pancytopenia; neutropenia; eosinophilia; thrombocytopenia.

Hepatic – Hepatitis; hepatomegaly; hepatic dysfunction.

Renal – Renal failure; flank pain; nephritis.

PENTAMIDINE ISETHIONATE

CNS – Tremors; confusion; anxiety; memory loss; seizure; neuropathy; paresthesia; insomnia; hypesthesia; drowsiness; emotional lability; vertigo; paranoia; neuralgia; hallucination; depression; unsteady gait.

Respiratory – Rhinitis; laryngitis; laryngospasm; hyperventilation; hemoptysis; gagging; eosinophilic or interstitial pneumonitis; pleuritis; cyanosis; tachypnea; rales.

Dermatologic – Pruritis; erythema; dry skin; desquamation; urticaria.

Special Senses – Eye discomfort; conjunctivitis; blurred vision; blepharitis; loss of taste and smell.

Miscellaneous – Incontinence; miscarriage; arthralgia; allergic reactions; extrapulmonary pneumocystosis.

Administration and Dosage:

Injection:

Adults and children – 4 mg/kg once a day for 14 days administered deep IM or IV only. The benefits and risks of therapy for more than 14 days are not well defined. Dosage in renal failure should be patient-specific. If necessary, reduce dosage, use a longer infusion time or extend the dosing interval.

Preparation of solution:

IM – Dissolve the contents of 1 vial in 3 ml of Sterile Water for Injection.

IV – Dissolve the contents of 1 vial in 3 to 5 ml of Sterile Water for Injection or 5% Dextrose Injection. Further dilute the calculated dose in 50 to 250 ml of 5% Dextrose solution.

Infuse the diluted IV solution over 60 minutes.

Aerosol:

Prevention of PCP – 300 mg once every 4 weeks administered via the *Respirgard* II nebulizer by Marquest.

Deliver the dose until the nebulizer chamber is empty (approximately 30 to 45 minutes). The flow rate should be 5 to 7 L/min from a 40 to 50 pounds per square inch (PSI) air or oxygen source. Alternatively, a 40 to 50 PSI air compressor can be used with flow limited by setting the flowmeter at 5 to 7 L/min or by setting the pressure at 22 to 25 PSI. Do not use low pressure (less than 20 PSI) compressors.

Reconstitution – The contents of one vial must be dissolved in 6 ml Sterile Water for Injection, USP. It is important to use *only* sterile water; saline solution will cause the drug to precipitate. Place the entire reconstituted contents of the vial into the Respirgard® II nebulizer reservoir for administration. Do not mix the pentamidine solution with any other drugs.

Stability and storage:

Injection – IV solutions of 1 and 2.5 mg/ml prepared in 5% Dextrose Injection are stable at room temperature for up to 48 hours. Store dry product between 15° to 30°C (59° to 86°F). Protect from light. Discard unused portion.

Aerosol – Use freshly prepared solutions. After reconstitution with sterile water, the solution is stable for 48 hours in the original vial at room temperature if protected from light. Store dry product at controlled room temperature 15° to 30°C (59° to 86°F).

Rx	**Pentam 300** (Lyphomed)	**Injection**: 300 mg	In single-dose vials.
Rx	**Pentacarinat** (Armour)		In single-dose vials.
Rx	**Pentamidine Isethionate** (Abbott)	**Powder for Injection, lyophilized**: 300 mg	In single-dose flip-top vials.
Rx	**NebuPent** (Lyphomed)	**Aerosol**: 300 mg	In single dose vials.

EFLORNITHINE HCl (DFMO)

Actions:

Pharmacology: Eflornithine is an antiprotozoal agent for IV injection. Its activity has been attributed to inhibition of the enzyme ornithine decarboxylase. Eflornithine differs from other currently available antiprotozoal drugs in both structure and mode of action. It is a specific, enzyme-activated, irreversible inhibitor of ornithine decarboxylase. In all mammalian and many non-mammalian cells, decarboxylation of ornithine by ornithine decarboxylase is an obligatory step in the biosynthesis of polyamines such as putrescine, spermidine and spermine, which are ubiquitous in living cells and thought to play important roles in cell division and differentiation.

Pharmacokinetics: Following IV administration to humans, approximately 80% of the administered dose is excreted unchanged in the urine within 24 hours, and the terminal plasma elimination half-life is approximately 3 hours. Eflornithine's excretion through the kidney approximates that of creatinine clearance. Therefore, in patients with impaired renal function, dose adjustments are necessary to compensate for the slower excretion of the drug.

Eflornithine does not bind significantly to human plasma proteins. It crosses the blood-brain barrier and produces cerebrospinal fluid:blood ratios between 0.13 and 0.51 (studies in 5 patients).

Microbiology: In tissue culture, eflornithine inhibits growth of *Trypanosoma brucei brucei*. This effect is reversed by the addition of polyamine putrescine to the culture medium.

Eflornithine is active in treatment of African trypanosomal infections in various animal models, including *Trypanosoma brucei gambiense* infection in a monkey model.

Indications:

Treatment of meningoencephalitic stage of *Trypanosoma brucei gambiense* infection (sleeping sickness). Extended follow-up of patients is required to assure adequate further therapy should relapse occur (see Precautions).

Warnings:

Concentrate: Must be diluted before use.

Hematologic effects:

Myelosuppression – The safe and effective use of eflornithine demands thorough knowledge of the natural history of trypanosomiasis due to *T brucei gambiense* and of the condition of the patient. The most frequent, serious, toxic effect of eflornithine is myelosuppression, which may be unavoidable if successful treatment is to be completed. Base decisions to modify dosage or to interrupt or cease treatment upon the response to treatment, the severity of the observed adverse event(s) and the availability of support facilities.

Anemia (hemoglobin < 10 g/dl, a decrease of ≥ 2 g/dl hemoglobin during treatment of hematocrit < 35%, or a decrease of > 5% in hematocrit during treatment) occurred in about 55% of monitored patients, but was generally found to be reversible upon stopping treatment. Many of these patients were chronically anemic prior to the start of therapy.

Leukopenia (≤ 4,000 WBC/mm^3) occurred in about 37% of the patients monitored. The minimum value usually occurred within 8 days of the start of therapy, and the condition usually resolved after discontinuation of therapy.

Thrombocytopenia (< 100,000 platelets/mm^3) developed in approximately 14% of the patients in clinical trials. In these patients, thrombocytopenia was reversible with interruption of or after completion of eflornithine therapy.

Seizures: Eflornithine has been temporally associated with seizures, an adverse event that can also be caused by the underlying disease. Seizures occurred in approximately 8% of patients treated with IV eflornithine in clinical trials. The etiology of the seizures (intrinsic meningoencephalitis or drug or combination) has not been determined. Be aware of the potential for seizure activity.

Occasional hearing impairment has occurred. When feasible, it is recommended that serial audiograms be obtained.

Relapse: Due to limited data on the risk of relapse after eflornithine therapy for Stage II *gambiense trypanosomiasis*, physicians are advised to follow their patients for at least 24 months to assure further therapy should relapses occur.

Renal function impairment: Since approximately 80% of the IV dose is eliminated unchanged in the urine, exercise caution in patients with renal impairment.

Fertility impairment: Decreased spermatogenetic effects in rats and rabbits were observed at doses equivalent to one-half the recommended human dose and in mice at approximately twice the human dose.

Antiprotozoals

EFLORNITHINE HCl (DFMO)

Pregnancy: Category C. Eflornithine is contragestational in rats, rabbits and mice when given, respectively, in doses 0.5, 0.5 and 2 times the human dose. There are no adequate and well controlled studies in pregnant women. Use during pregnancy only if the potential benefit justifies the potential risk to the fetus. In postnatal studies, retarded development occurred in rat pups on doses slightly higher than the human dose.

Lactation: It is not known whether this drug is excreted in breast milk. Because of the potential for serious adverse reactions in nursing infants from eflornithine, decide whether to discontinue nursing or to discontinue the drug, taking into account the importance of the drug to the mother.

Children: Safety and efficacy in children have not been established.

Precautions:

Monitoring: Perform complete blood counts, including platelet counts, before treatment, twice weekly during therapy, and weekly after completion of therapy until hematologic values return to baseline levels.

Adverse Reactions:

Most frequent: Anemia (55%), leukopenia (37%), thrombocytopenia (14%), see Warnings; diarrhea (9%); seizures (8%), see Warnings; hearing impairment (5%), see Warnings; vomiting (5%); alopecia (3%); abdominal pain, anorexia, headache, asthenia, facial edema, eosinophilia (2%); dizziness (1%).

Four percent of patients died during therapy or shortly after completion of treatment. It could not be established whether these deaths were caused by underlying disease or the use of eflornithine.

Overdosage:

In mice and rats given intraperitoneal doses of 3 g/kg, moderate CNS depression was observed after 2 to 4 hours. Convulsions were observed in 3 out of 10 rats, and 2 of them died within 3 hours following receipt of the drug.

Administration and Dosage:

Trypanosoma brucei gambiense(sleeping sickness) 100 mg/kg/dose (46 mg/lb/dose) administered every 6 hours by IV infusion for 14 days. Administer infusion over a minimum of 45 consecutive minutes. Other drugs should not be administered intravenously during the infusion of eflornithine.

Renal function impairment: In patients with impaired renal function, dose adjustments are necessary to compensate for the slower excretion of the drug. When only serum creatinine is available, the following formula (Cockcroft's equation) may be used to estimate creatinine clearance. The serum creatinine should represent a steady state of renal function:

$$\text{Males: } \frac{\text{Weight (kg)} \times (140 - \text{age})}{72 \times \text{serum creatinine (mg/dl)}} = \text{Ccr}$$

$$\text{Females: } 0.85 \times \text{above value}$$

Preparation for IV administration: Eflornithine concentrate is hypertonic and must be diluted with Sterile Water for Injection, USP, before infusion.

Solutions within 10% of plasma tonicity can be produced using 1 part eflornithine concentrate to 4 parts Sterile Water for Injection, USP, by volume as described below.

Using strict aseptic technique, withdraw the entire contents of each 100 ml vial. Inject 25 ml into each of four IV diluent bags, each of which contains 100 ml of Sterile Water, USP. The eflornithine concentration following dilution will be 40 mg/ml (5000 mg of eflornithine in 125 ml total volume).

Storage/Stability: The diluted drug must be used within 24 hours of preparation. Store bags containing diluted eflornithine at 4°C (39°F) to minimize the risk of microbial proliferation. Store undiluted vial at room temperature, preferably below 30°C (86°F). Protect from freezing and light.

Rx	**Ornidyl** (Hoechst Marion Roussel)	**Injection Concentrate**: 200 mg/ ml (as monohydrate)	In 100 ml vials.

Antiprotozoals

ATOVAQUONE

Actions:

Pharmacology: Atovaquone, an analog of ubiquinone, is an antiprotozoal with anti-pneumocystis activity. The mechanism of action against *Pneumocystis carinii* has not been fully elucidated. In *Plasmodium* species, the site of action appears to be the cytochrome bc_1 complex (Complex III). Several metabolic enzymes are linked to the mitochondrial electron transport chain via ubiquinone. Inhibition of electron transport by atovaquone will result in indirect inhibition of these enzymes. The ultimate metabolic effects of such blockade may include inhibition of nucleic acid and ATP synthesis.

Pharmacokinetics:

Absorption – Atovaquone is a highly lipophilic compound with a low aqueous solubility. Bioavailability is highly dependent on formulation and diet. The suspension provides an approximately twofold increase in bioavailability in the fasting or fed state compared to the previously marketed tablet formulation. Absolute bioavailability of a 750 mg dose given under fed conditions in nine HIV-infected volunteers was 47% (vs 23% with the tablet). Absorption is enhanced approximately twofold when given with food (see Drug Interactions). Plasma concentrations do not increase proportionally with dose; when given with food at doses of 500, 750 and 1000 mg once daily, average steady-state concentrations were 11.7, 12.5 and 13.5 mcg/ml, respectively, and C_{max} concentrations were 15.1, 15.3 and 16.8 mcg/ml.

Distribution – Following IV administration, volume of distribution at steady state was 0.6 L/kg. Atovaquone is extensively bound to plasma proteins (> 99.9%). CSF concentrations are < 1% of plasma concentrations.

Metabolism/Excretion – Plasma clearance following IV administration in HIV-infected volunteers was 10.4 ml/min. Half-life was 62.5 hours following IV use and ranged from 67 to 77.6 hours following the suspension. The long half-life is due to presumed enterohepatic cycling and eventual fecal elimination. In healthy volunteers, > 94% of the dose was recovered unchanged in the feces over 21 days; there was little or no excretion in the urine (< 0.6%). There is indirect evidence that atovaquone may undergo limited metabolism; however, a specific metabolite has not been identified.

Children: Preliminary analysis indicates that atovaquone pharmacokinetics are age-dependent. Children between 2 and 13 years of age had steady-state plasma concentrations of 16.8 and 37.1 mcg/ml when given doses of 10 and 30 mg/kg, respectively. Children between 3 and 24 months had concentrations of 5.7 and 8.9 mcg/ml, respectively.

Clinical trials:

Trimethoprim-sulfamethoxazole (TMP-SMZ) comparative study – One study compared the safety and efficacy of atovaquone to that of TMP-SMZ for the treatment of AIDS patients with histologically confirmed *Pneumocystis carinii* pneumonia (PCP). Only patients with mild to moderate PCP were eligible for enrollment; 160 received atovaquone (750 mg) and 162 received TMP-SMZ (320/1600 mg), both 3 times daily for 21 days. Therapy success was defined as improved clinical and respiratory measures persisting at least 4 weeks after therapy cessation. Failures included lack of response, drug discontinuation due to an adverse experience and unevaluable patients.

There was significant difference in mortality rates between the treatment groups: 8% of patients treated with atovaquone and 2.5% receiving TMP-SMZ died during the 21 day treatment course or 8 week follow-up period. Of the 13 patients treated with atovaquone who died, four died of PCP and five died with a combination of bacterial infections and PCP; bacterial infections did not appear to be a factor in any of the four deaths among TMP-SMZ-treated patients.

A correlation between plasma atovaquone concentrations and death was demonstrated; in general, patients with lower plasma concentrations were more likely to die. Of those patients for whom day 4 atovaquone plasma concentration data are available, 63% of the patients with concentrations < 5 mcg/ml died during participation in the study. However, only 2% with day 4 plasma concentrations ≥ 5 mcg/ml died. Failure rate due to lack of response was significantly larger with atovaquone while failure rate due to adverse experiences was significantly larger with TMP-SMZ.

Antiprotozoals

ATOVAQUONE

Outcome of Treatment for PCP-Positive Patients: Atovaquone vs TMP-SMZ (%)		
Outcome of therapy	Atovaquone (n = 160)	TMP-SMZ (n = 162)
Therapy success	62	64
Therapy failure		
Lack of response	17	6
Adverse experience	7	20
Unevaluable	14	10
Required alternate PCP therapy during study	34	34

Pentamidine comparative study – One study compared the safety and efficacy of atovaquone to that of pentamidine for the treatment of histologically confirmed mild or moderate PCP in AIDS patients. Approximately 80% of the patients had a history of intolerance to trimethoprim or sulfonamides (the primary therapy group) or were experiencing intolerance to TMP-SMZ with treatment of an episode of PCP at the time of enrollment in the study (the salvage treatment group). Patients received either atovaquone 750 mg 3 times daily for 21 days or pentamidine isethionate 3 to 4 mg/kg single IV infusion daily for 21 days.

There was no difference in mortality rates between the treatment groups. Among the 135 patients with confirmed PCP, 14% receiving atovaquone and 14% receiving pentamidine died during the 21 day treatment course or 8 week follow-up period. Of those patients for whom day 4 atovaquone plasma concentrations are available, 60% with concentrations < 5 mcg/ml died during participation in the study. However, only 9% with day 4 plasma concentrations ≥ 5 mcg/ml died.

Outcome of Treatment for PCP-Positive Patients: Atovaquone vs Pentamidine (%)				
	Primary treatment		Salvage treatment	
Outcome of therapy	Atovaquone (n = 56)	Pentamidine (n = 53)	Atovaquone (n = 14)	Pentamidine (n = 11)
Therapy success	57	40	93	64
Therapy failure				
Lack of response	29	17		
Adverse experience	3.6	36		27
Unevaluable	11	8	7	9
Required alternate PCP therapy during study	34	55		36

Chronic use – Atovaquone has not been systematically evaluated as a chronic suppressive agent to prevent the development of PCP in patients at high risk for PCP. In a pilot dosing study of atovaquone in AIDS patients, five of 31 patients had PCP breakthroughs: One patient at 750 mg once daily (after 20 days), three patients at 750 mg twice daily (after 14, 70 and 97 days), and one patient at 1500 mg twice daily (after 74 days).

Indications:

Pneumocystis carinii pneumonia: Acute oral treatment of mild to moderate PCP in patients who are intolerant to trimethoprim-sulfamethoxazole (TMP-SMZ).

Contraindications:

Development or history of potentially life-threatening allergic reactions to any of the components of the formulation.

Warnings:

Severe PCP/prophylaxis: Clinical experience has been limited to patients with mild to moderate PCP. Treatment of more severe episodes of PCP has not been systematically studied. Atavaquone has not been evaluated as an agent for PCP prophylaxis.

Elderly: Atovaquone has not been systematically evaluated in patients > 65 years of age. Exercise caution when treating elderly patients reflecting the greater frequency of decreased hepatic, renal and cardiac function in this population.

ATOVAQUONE

Pregnancy: Category C. Atovaquone caused maternal toxicity in rabbits at plasma concentrations that were approximately equal to the estimated human exposure. Mean fetal body lengths and weights were decreased and there were higher numbers of early resorption and post-implantation loss per diem. It is not clear whether these effects were caused by atovaquone or were secondary to maternal toxicity. Concentrations of atovaquone in rabbit fetuses averaged 30% of the concurrent maternal plasma concentrations. In a separate study in rats, concentrations in rat fetuses were 18% (middle gestation) and 60% (late gestation) of concurrent maternal plasma concentrations. There are no adequate and well controlled studies in pregnant women. Use during pregnancy only if the potential benefit justifies the potential risk to the fetus.

Lactation: It is not known whether atovaquone is excreted in breast milk. Exercise caution when administering atovaquone to a nursing woman. In a rat study, atovaquone concentrations in the milk were 30% of the concurrent atovaquone concentrations in the maternal plasma.

Children: Safety and efficacy have not been established. Clinical experience is limited to a study in children who were at risk of developing PCP. Preliminary analysis suggests that the pharmacokinetics are age-dependent. No treatment-limiting adverse events were observed.

Precautions:

Absorption of orally administered atovaquone is limited but can be significantly increased when the drug is taken with food. Plasma concentrations correlate with the likelihood of successful treatment and survival. Therefore, consider parenteral therapy with other agents for patients who have difficulty taking atovaquone with food (see Drug Interactions). GI disorders may limit absorption of orally administered drugs. Patients with these disorders also may not achieve plasma concentrations of atovaquone associated with response to therapy in controlled trials.

Concurrent pulmonary conditions: Based on the spectrum of in vitro antimicrobial activity, atovaquone is not effective therapy for concurrent pulmonary conditions such as bacterial, viral or fungal pneumonia or mycobacterial diseases. Clinical deterioration in patients may be due to infections with other pathogens, as well as progressive PCP. Carefully evaluate all patients with acute PCP for other possible causes of pulmonary disease and treat with additional agents as appropriate.

Drug Interactions:

Atovaquone is highly bound to plasma protein (> 99.9%). Therefore, use caution when administering atovaquone concurrently with other highly plasma protein bound drugs with narrow therapeutic indices as competition for binding sites may occur. However, the extent of plasma protein binding of atovaquone in human plasma is not affected by the presence of therapeutic concentrations of phenytoin (15 mcg/ml), nor is the binding of phenytoin affected by the presence of atovaquone.

Atovaquone Drug Interactions

Precipitant drug	Object drug*		Description
Rifamycins	Atovaquone	⬇	Concurrent use with rifampin results in a significant decrease in average steady-state plasma concentrations. Rifabutin may interact similarly.
Atovaquone	TMP-SMZ	⬇	Coadministration resulted in a 17% and 8% decrease in average steady-state concentrations of TMP and SMZ in plasma, respectively. However, this effect is minor and would not be expected to produce any clinically significant events.
Atovaquone	Zidovudine	⬆	In one study, concurrent use resulted in a 24% decrease in zidovudine apparent oral clearance, leading to a 35% increase in AUC. The glucuronide metabolite:parent ratio decreased from a mean of 4.5 (zidovudine alone) to 3.1. However, this effect is minor and would not be expected to produce any clinically significant events.

* ⬆ = Object drug increased. ⬇ = Object drug decreased.

Antiprotozoals

ATOVAQUONE

Drug/Food interactions: Administering atovaquone with food enhances its absorption by approximately twofold. In one study, 16 healthy volunteers received a single dose of 750 mg after an overnight fast and following a breakfast (23 g fat: 642 kCal). The mean AUC values were 324 and 801 hr•mcg/ml under fasting and fed conditions, respectively. In a multi-dose study in 19 HIV-infected volunteers receiving atovaquone 500 mg daily, AUC values were 169 and 280 hr•mcg/ml under fasting and fed conditions, respectively; C_{max} was 8.8 and 15.1 mcg/ml, respectively.

Adverse Reactions:

Because many patients who participated in clinical trials had complications of advanced HIV disease, it was often difficult to distinguish adverse events caused by atovaquone from those caused by underlying medical conditions. There were no life-threatening or fatal adverse experiences caused by atovaquone.

Adverse Reactions: Atovaquone vs TMP-SMZ (%)

Adverse reactions	Atovaquone (n = 203)	TMP-SMZ (n = 205)
Rash (including maculopapular)	23	34
Nausea	21	44
Diarrhea	19	7
Headache	16	22
Vomiting	14	35
Fever	14	25
Insomnia	10	9
Asthenia	8	8
Pruritus	5	9
Monilia, oral	5	10
Abdominal pain	4	7
Constipation	3	17
Dizziness	3	8
Patients discontinuing therapy due to an adverse experience	9	24
Patients reporting at least one adverse experience	63	65
Laboratory test abnormality		
Anemia (Hgb < 8 g/dl)	6	7
Neutropenia (ANC < 750 cells/mm^3)	3	9
Elevated ALT (> 5 × ULN[1])	6	16
Elevated AST (> 5 × ULN)	4	14
Elevated alkaline phosphatase (> 2.5 × ULN)	8	6
Elevated amylase (> 1.5 × ULN)	7	12
Hyponatremia (< 0.96 × LLN[2])	7	26

[1] ULN = upper limit of normal range
[2] LLN = lower limit of normal range

Of patients receiving atovaquone, 4% discontinued therapy due to development of rash. The majority of cases of rash among patients were mild and did not require the discontinuation of dosing. The only other clinical adverse experience that led to premature discontinuation by more than one patient was the development of vomiting (< 1%). The most common adverse experience requiring discontinuation in the TMP-SMZ group was rash (8%). Therapy was prematurely discontinued due to elevations in ALT/AST in 2% of atovaquone patients and 7% with TMP-SMZ.

ATOVAQUONE

Adverse Reactions: Atovaquone vs Pentamidine (%)		
Adverse reactions	Atovaquone (n = 73)	Pentamidine (n = 71)
Fever	40	25
Nausea	22	37
Rash	22	13
Diarrhea	21	31
Insomnia	19	14
Headache	18	28
Vomiting	14	17
Cough	14	1
Abdominal pain	10	11
Pain	10	10
Sweating	10	3
Monilia, oral	10	3
Asthenia	8	14
Dizziness	8	14
Anxiety	7	10
Anorexia	7	10
Sinusitis	7	6
Dyspepsia	5	10
Rhinitis	5	7
Taste perversion	3	13
Hypoglycemia	1	15
Hypotension	1	10
Patients discontinuing therapy due to an adverse experience	7	41
Patients reporting at least one adverse experience	63	72
Laboratory test abnormality		
Anemia (Hgb < 8 g/dl)	4	9
Neutropenia (ANC < 750 cells/mm^3)	5	9
Hyponatremia (< 0.96 × LLN[1])	10	10
Hyperkalemia (> 1.18 × ULN[2])	0	5
Alkaline phosphatase (> 2.5 × ULN)	5	2
Hyperglycemia (> 1.8 × ULN)	9	13
Elevated AST (> 5 × ULN)	0	5
Elevated amylase (> 1.5 × ULN)	8	4
Elevated creatinine (> 1.5 × ULN)	0	7

[1] LLN = lower limit of normal range
[2] ULN = upper limit of normal range

Only 7% of patients discontinued treatment with atovaquone due to adverse events while 41% of patients who received pentamidine discontinued treatment for this reason. Of the five patients who discontinued therapy with atovaquone, three reported rash (4%). Rash was not severe in any patient. No other reason for discontinuation of atovaquone was cited more than once. The most frequently cited reasons for discontinuation of pentamidine therapy were hypoglycemia (11%) and vomiting (9%).

Laboratory abnormality was the reason for discontinuation of treatment in two of 73 patients who received atovaquone. One patient (1%) had elevated creatinine and BUN levels and one patient (1%) had elevated amylase levels. Laboratory abnormalities were the sole or contributing factor in 14 patients who prematurely discontinued pentamidine therapy. In the 71 patients who received pentamidine, laboratory parameters most frequently reported as reasons for discontinuation were hypoglycemia (11%), elevated creatinine levels (6%) and leukopenia (4%).

Antiprotozoals

ATOVAQUONE

Patient Information:

Stress the importance of taking the prescribed dose. Instruct patients to take their daily doses with meals as the presence of food will significantly improve the absorption of the drug.

Administration and Dosage:

Approved by the FDA on November 25, 1992.

Adults: 750 mg administered with food twice daily for 21 days (total daily dose 1500 mg). Failure to administer atovaquone with food may result in lower atovaquone plasma concentrations and may limit response to therapy (see Precautions and Drug Interactions).

Storage/Stability: Do not freeze.

Rx	**Mepron** (Glaxo Wellcome)	**Suspension**[1]: 750 mg/5 ml	Benzyl alcohol. Saccharin. Citrus flavor. In 210 ml.

[1] The tablet form is being phased out over time; atovaquone will be available only as a suspension.

Folate Antagonists

TRIMETREXATE GLUCURONATE

Warning:
Trimetrexate must be used with concurrent leucovorin (leucovorin protection) to avoid potentially serious or life-threatening toxicities (see Precautions and Administration and Dosage).

Actions:

Pharmacology: Trimetrexate, a 2,4-diaminoquinazoline, non-classical folate antagonist, is a synthetic inhibitor of the enzyme dihydrofolate reductase (DHFR). In vitro, trimetrexate is a competitive inhibitor of DHFR from bacterial, protozoan and mammalian sources. DHFR catalyzes the reduction of intracellular dihydrofolate to the active coenzyme, leading directly to interference with thymidylate biosynthesis, as well as inhibition of folate-dependent formyltransferases, and indirectly to inhibition of purine biosynthesis. The end result is disruption of DNA, RNA and protein synthesis, with consequent cell death. Leucovorin (folinic acid) is readily transported into mammalian cells by an active, carrier-mediated process and can be assimilated into cellular folate pools following its metabolism. In vitro, leucovorin provides a source of reduced folates necessary for normal cellular biosynthetic processes. Because the *Pneumocystis carinii* organism lacks the reduced folate carrier-mediated transport system, leucovorin is prevented from entering the organism. Therefore, at concentrations achieved with therapeutic doses of trimetrexate plus leucovorin, the selective transport of trimetrexate, but not leucovorin, into the *P carinii* organism allows the concurrent administration of leucovorin to protect normal host cells from the cytotoxicity of trimetrexate without inhibiting the antifolate's inhibition of *P carinii*. It is not known if considerably higher doses of leucovorin would affect trimetrexate's effect on *P carinii*.

Pharmacokinetics: Trimetrexate pharmacokinetics were assessed in six patients with acquired immunodeficiency syndrome (AIDS) who had *P carinii* pneumonia (PCP; n = 4) or toxoplasmosis (n = 2). Trimetrexate was administered IV as a bolus injection at a dose of 30 mg/m^2/day every 6 hours for 21 days. Clearance was 38 ± 15 ml/min/m^2 and volume of distribution at steady state (Vd_{ss}) was 20 ± 8 L/m^2. The plasma concentration time profile declined in a biphasic manner over 24 hours with a terminal half-life of 11 ± 4 hours.

The pharmacokinetics of trimetrexate without the concomitant administration of leucovorin have been evaluated in cancer patients with advanced solid tumors using various dosage regimens. Following the single-dose administration of 10 to 130 mg/m^2 to 37 patients, plasma concentrations were obtained for 72 hours. The alpha phase half-life was 57 ± 28 minutes, followed by a terminal phase with a half-life of 16 ± 3 hours. The plasma concentrations in the remaining patients exhibited a triphasic decline with half-lives of 8.6 ± 6.5 minutes, 2.4 ± 1.3 hours and 17.8 ± 8.2 hours.

Trimetrexate clearance in cancer patients has been reported as 53 ± 41 ml/min (n = 14) and 32 ± 18 ml/min/m^2 (n = 23) following single-dose administration. After a 5 day infusion to 16 patients, plasma clearance was 30 ± 8 ml/min/m^2.

Renal clearance in cancer patients has varied from about 4 ± 2 to 10 ± 6 ml/min/m^2 and 10% to 30% is excreted unchanged in the urine. Considering the free fraction of trimetrexate, active tubular secretion may possibly contribute to the renal clearance. Renal clearance has been associated with urine flow, suggesting the possibility of tubular reabsorption as well.

The Vd_{ss} of trimetrexate in cancer patients after single-dose administration and for whom plasma concentrations were obtained for 72 hours was 36.9 ± 17.6 L/m^2 (n = 23) and 0.62 ± 0.24 L/kg (n = 14). Following a constant infusion for 5 days, Vd_{ss} was 32.8 ± 16.6 L/m^2.

There have been inconsistencies in the reporting of trimetrexate protein binding. The in vitro plasma protein binding of trimetrexate using ultrafiltration is approximately 95% over the concentration range of 18.75 to 1000 ng/ml. There is a suggestion of capacity-limited binding (saturable binding) at concentrations > 1000 ng/ml, with free fraction progressively increasing to about 9.3% as concentration is increased to 15 mcg/ml. Other reports have declared trimetrexate to be > 98% bound at concentrations of 0.1 to 10 mcg/ml; however, specific free fractions were not stated. The free fraction of trimetrexate also has been reported to be about 15% to 16% at a concentration of 60 ng/ml, increasing to about 20% at a concentration of 6 mcg/ml.

Folate Antagonists

TRIMETREXATE GLUCURONATE

Trimetrexate metabolism in man has not been characterized. Preclinical data strongly suggest that the major metabolic pathway is oxidative O-demethylation, followed by conjugation to either glucuronide or the sulfate. N-demethylation and oxidation is a related minor pathway. Preliminary findings in humans indicate the presence of a glucuronide conjugate with DHFR inhibition and a demethylated metabolite in urine. Data suggest the presence of one or more metabolites with DHFR inhibition activity.

Fecal recovery of trimetrexate over 48 hours after IV administration ranged from 0.09% to 7.6% of the dose as determined by DHFR inhibition and 0.02% to 5.2% of the dose as determined by HPLC.

The pharmacokinetics of trimetrexate have not been determined in patients with renal insufficiency or hepatic dysfunction.

Microbiology: Trimetrexate inhibits, in a dose-related manner, in vitro growth of the trophozoite stage of rat *P carinii* cultured on human embryonic lung fibrolast cells. Leucovorin alone did not alter either the growth of the trophozoites or the anti-pneumocystis activity of trimetrexate. Resistance to trimetrexate's antimicrobial activity against *P carinii* has not been studied.

Clinical trials:

Trimetrexate vs trimethoprim-sulfamethoxazole (TMP-SMZ) – This double-blind, randomized trial was designed to compare the safety and efficacy of trimetrexate/leucovorin (TMTX/LV) to that of TMP-SMZ for the treatment of histologically confirmed, moderate-to-severe PCP in patients with AIDS. Of the 220 patients with histologically confirmed PCP, 109 were randomized to receive TMTX/LV (45 mg/m^2 of TMTX daily for 21 days plus 20 mg/m^2 of LV every 6 hours for 24 days), and 111 to TMP-SMZ (5 mg/kg TMP plus 25 mg/kg SMZ 4 times daily for 21 days). Response to therapy, defined as alive and off ventilatory support at completion of therapy, without a requirement for a change in anti-pneumocystis therapy, or addition of supraphysiologic doses of steroids, occurred in 50% of patients in each treatment group. The observed mortality in the TMTX/LV treatment group was approximately twice that in the TMP-SMZ treatment group. Thirty of 109 (27%) patients treated with TMTX/LV and 18 of 111 (16%) patients receiving TMP-SMZ died during the 21 day treatment course or 4 week follow-up period. Twenty-seven of 30 deaths in the TMTX/LV arm were attributed to PCP; all 18 deaths in the TMP-SMZ arm were attributed to PCP. A significantly smaller proportion of patients who received TMTX/LV compared to TMP-SMZ failed therapy due to toxicity (10% vs 25%), and a significantly greater proportion of patients failed due to lack of efficacy (40% vs 24%). Six patients (12%) who responded to TMTX/LV relapsed during the 1 month follow-up period; no patient responding to TMP-SMZ relapsed during this period.

Treatment IND – The FDA granted a Treatment IND for trimetrexate with leucovorin protection in February 1988 to make trimetrexate therapy available to HIV-infected patients with histologically confirmed PCP who had disease refractory to, or who were intolerant of TMP-SMZ or IV pentamidine. Of the 577 evaluable patients, 227 patients were intolerant of both TMP-SMZ and pentamidine (IST; patients intolerant of both standard therapies), 146 were intolerant of one therapy and refractory to the other (RIST; patients refractory to one therapy and intolerant of the other) and 204 were refractory to both therapies (RST; refractory to both standard therapies). This was a very ill patient population; 38% required ventilatory support at entry. These studies did not have concurrent control groups. The overall survival rate 1 month after completion of TMTX/LV as salvage therapy was 48%. Patients who had not responded to treatment with both TMP-SMZ and pentamidine, of whom 63% required mechanical ventilation at entry, achieved a survival rate of 25% following treatment with TMTX/LV. Survival was 67% in patients who were intolerant to both TMP-SMZ and pentamidine. In the Treatment IND, 12% of patients discontinued TMTX/LV for toxicity.

Indications:

As an alternative therapy with concurrent leucovorin administration (leucovorin protection) for the treatment of moderate-to-severe *Pneumocystis carinii* pneumonia (PCP) in immunocompromised patients, including patients with acquired immunodeficiency syndrome (AIDS), who are intolerant of, or are refractory to trimethoprim-sulfamethoxazole therapy or for whom TMP/SMZ is contraindicated.

Unlabeled uses: Trimetrexate is being investigated for treatment of non-small cell lung, prostate and colorectal cancer.

TRIMETREXATE GLUCURONATE

Contraindications:

Clinically significant sensitivity to trimetrexate, leucovorin or methotrexate.

Warnings:

Concurrent leucovorin: Trimetrexate must be used with concurrent leucovorin to avoid potentially serious or life-threatening complications including bone marrow suppression, oral and GI mucosal ulceration, and renal and hepatic dysfunction. Leucovorin therapy must extend for 72 hours past the last dose of trimetrexate. Inform patients that failure to take the recommended dose and duration of leucovorin can lead to fatal toxicity. Closely monitor patients for the development of serious hematologic adverse reactions (see Precautions and Administration and Dosage).

Hypersensitivity: An anaphylactoid reaction has occurred in a cancer patient receiving trimetrexate as a bolus injection.

Fertility impairment: No studies have been conducted to evaluate the potential of trimetrexate to impair fertility. However, during standard toxicity studies conducted in mice and rats, degeneration of the testes and spermatocytes, including the arrest of spermatogenesis, was observed.

Pregnancy: Category D. Trimetrexate can cause fetal harm when administered to a pregnant woman. Trimetrexate is fetotoxic and teratogenic in rats and rabbits. Rats administered 1.5 and 2.5 mg/kg/day IV on gestational days 6 to 15 showed substantial postimplantation loss and severe inhibition of maternal weight gain; 0.5 and 1 mg/kg/day on gestational days 6 to 15 retarded normal fetal development and was teratogenic. Rabbits given daily doses of 2.5 and 5 mg/kg/day on gestational days 6 to 18 resulted in significant maternal and fetotoxicity; 0.1 mg/kg/day was teratogenic in the absence of significant maternal toxicity. These effects were observed using doses 1/20 to 1/2 the equivalent human therapeutic dose based on a mg/m^2 basis. Teratogenic effects included skeletal, visceral, ocular and cardiovascular abnormalities. If trimetrexate is used during pregnancy, or if the patient becomes pregnant while taking this drug, apprise the patient of the potential hazard to the fetus. Advise women of childbearing potential to avoid becoming pregnant.

Lactation: It is not known if trimetrexate is excreted in breast milk. Because of the potential for serious adverse reactions in nursing infants, it is recommended that breastfeeding be discontinued if the mother is treated with trimetrexate.

Children: Safety and efficacy of trimetrexate for the treatment of histologically confirmed PCP has not been established for patients < 18 years of age. Under the Compassionate Use Protocol, two children (9 and 15 months of age) were treated with trimetrexate and leucovorin using a dose of 45 mg/m^2/day of trimetrexate for 21 days and 20 mg/m^2/day of leucovorin for 24 days. There were no serious or unexpected adverse effects.

Precautions:

Monitoring: Mild elevations in transaminase and alkaline phosphatase have been observed and are usually not cause for modifications of therapy (see Administration and Dosage). Patients receiving trimetrexate with leucovorin protection should be seen frequently by a physician. Perform blood tests at least twice a week during therapy to assess the following parameters: Hematology (absolute neutrophil counts [ANC], platelets); renal function (serum creatinine, BUN); hepatic function (AST, ALT, alkaline phosphatase).

Special risk patients: Patients receiving trimetrexate may experience hematologic, hepatic, renal and GI toxicities. Use caution in treating patients with impaired hematologic, renal or hepatic function. Treat and carefully monitor patients who require concomitant therapy with nephrotoxic, myelosuppressive or hepatotoxic drugs with trimetrexate at the discretion of the physician. To allow for full therapeutic doses of trimetrexate, discontinue treatment with zidovudine during trimetrexate therapy. Trimetrexate-associated myelosuppression, stomatitis and GI toxicities can generally be ameliorated by adjusting the dose of leucovorin.

Seizures have been reported rarely (<1%) in AIDS patients receiving trimetrexate; however, a causal relationship has not been established.

TRIMETREXATE GLUCURONATE

Pulmonary conditions: Trimetrexate has not been evaluated clinically for the treatment of concurrent pulmonary conditions such as bacterial, viral or fungal pneumonia or mycobacterial diseases. In vitro activity has been observed against *Toxoplasma gondii, Mycobacterium avium* complex, gram-positive cocci and gram-negative rods. If clinical deterioration is observed in patients, carefully evaluate them for other possible causes of pulmonary disease and treat with additional agents as appropriate.

Drug Interactions:

Since trimetrexate is metabolized by a P–450 enzyme system, drugs that induce or inhibit this drug metabolizing enzyme system may elicit important drug interactions that may alter trimetrexate plasma concentrations. Agents that might be coadministered with trimetrexate in AIDS patients for other indications that could elicit this activity include erythromycin, rifampin, rifabutin, ketoconazole and fluconazole. In vitro, cimetidine caused a significant reduction in trimetrexate metabolism and acetaminophen altered the relative concentration of trimetrexate metabolites, possibly by competing for sulfate metabolites. In vitro, nitrogen substituted imidazole drugs (eg, clotrimazole, ketoconazole, miconazole) were potent, non-competitive inhibitors of trimetrexate metabolism. Carefully monitor patients being treated with these drugs and receiving concurrent trimetrexate.

Adverse Reactions:

Because many patients who participated in clinical trials had complications of advanced HIV disease, it is difficult to distinguish adverse events caused by trimetrexate from those resulting from underlying medical conditions. Laboratory toxicities were generally manageable with dose modification of trimetrexate/leucovorin (see Administration and Dosage). Of the patients receiving TMP-SMZ, 29% discontinued therapy due to adverse events vs 10% of patients treated with TMTX/LV. Hematologic toxicity was the principal dose-limiting side effect. An anaphylactoid reaction occurred in a cancer patient receiving trimetrexate as a bolus injection.

Trimetrexate Adverse Reactions (%)

Adverse reaction	TMTX/LV (n = 109)	TMP-SMZ (n = 111)
Non-laboratory:		
Fever	8.3	12.6
Rash/Pruritus	5.5	12.6
Nausea/Vomiting	4.6	13.5
Confusion	2.8	2.7
Fatigue	1.8	0
Hematologic toxicity:		
Neutropenia (≤ 1000/mm^3)	30.3	33.3
Thrombocytopenia (≤ 75,000/mm^3)	10.1	15.3
Anemia (Hgb < 8 g/dl)	7.3	9
Hepatotoxicity:		
Increased AST (> 5 x ULN)	13.8	9
Increased ALT (> 5 x ULN)	11	11.7
Increased alkaline phosphatase (> 5 x ULN)	4.6	2.7
Increased bilirubin (2.5 x ULN)	1.8	0.9
Renal:		
Increased serum creatinine (> 3 x ULN)	0.9	1.8
Electrolyte imbalance:		
Hyponatremia	4.6	9
Hypocalcemia	1.8	0
Number of patients with ≥ 1 adverse event	53.2	54.1

TRIMETREXATE GLUCURONATE

Overdosage:

Symptoms: Trimetrexate administered without concurrent leucovorin can cause lethal complications. There has been no extensive experience in humans receiving single IV doses of trimetrexate > 90 mg/m²/day with concurrent leucovorin. The toxicities seen at this dose were primarily hematologic.

Treatment: In the event of overdose, stop trimetrexate and administer leucovorin at a dose of 40 mg/m² every 6 hours for 3 days.

Administration and Dosage:

Approved by the FDA on December 17, 1993.

Trimetrexate must be given with concurrent leucovorin (leucovorin protection) to avoid potentially serious or life-threatening toxicities. Leucovorin must be given daily during trimetrexate treatment and for 72 hours past the last trimetrexate dose.

Trimetrexate is administered at a dose of 45 mg/m² once daily by IV infusion over 60 to 90 minutes. Leucovorin may be administered IV at a dose of 20 mg/m² over 5 to 10 minutes every 6 hours for a total daily dose of 80 mg/m², or orally as 4 doses of 20 mg/m² spaced equally throughout the day. Round up the oral dose to the next higher 25 mg increment. The recommended course of therapy is 21 days of trimetrexate and 24 days of leucovorin.

Dosage modifications:

Hematologic toxicity – Modify trimetrexate and leucovorin doses based on the worst hematologic toxicity according to the following table. If leucovorin is given orally, round up doses to the next higher 25 mg increment.

Dose Modifications for Hematologic Toxicity

Toxicity Grade	Neutrophils per mm³	Platelets per mm³	Trimetrexate	Leucovorin
1	> 1,000	> 75,000	45 mg/m² once daily	20 mg/m² every 6 hours
2	750-1,000	50,000-75,000	45 mg/m² once daily	40 mg/m² every 6 hours
3	500-749	25,000-49,999	22 mg/m² once daily	40 mg/m² every 6 hours
4	< 500	< 25,000	Day 1-9 discontinue Day 10-21 interrupt up to 96 hours[1]	40 mg/m² every 6 hours

[1] If Grade 4 hematologic toxicity occurs prior to day 10, discontinue trimetrexate. Administer leucovorin (40 mg/m² every 6 hours) for an additional 72 hours. If Grade 4 hematologic toxicity occurs at day 10 or later, trimetrexate may be held up to 96 hours to allow counts to recover. If counts recover to Grade 3 within 96 hours, administer trimetrexate at a dose of 22 mg/m² and maintain leucovorin at 40 mg/m² every 6 hours. When counts recover to Grade 2 toxicity, trimetrexate dose may be increased to 45 mg/m², but the leucovorin dose should be maintained at 40 mg/m² for the duration of treatment. If counts do not improve to ≤ Grade 3 toxicity within 96 hours, discontinue trimetrexate. Administer leucovorin at a dose of 40 mg/m² every 6 hours for 72 hours following the last dose of trimetrexate.

Hepatic toxicity – Transient elevations of transaminases and alkaline phosphatase have occurred in trimetrexate patients. Treatment interruption is advisable if transaminase levels or alkaline phosphatase levels increase to > 5 times the upper limit of normal range.

Renal toxicity – Interruption of trimetrexate is advisable if serum creatinine levels increase to > 2.5 mg/dl and the elevation is considered secondary to trimetrexate.

Other toxicities – Interruption of treatment is advisable in patients with severe mucosal toxicity that interferes with oral intake. Discontinue treatment for fever (oral temperature ≥ 40.5°C [105°F]) that cannot be controlled with antipyretics. Leucovorin therapy must extend for 72 hours past the last dose of trimetrexate.

Folate Antagonists

TRIMETREXATE GLUCURONATE

Reconstitution and dilution: Reconstitute with 2 ml of 5% Dextrose Injection or Sterile Water for Injection to yield a concentration of 12.5 mg/ml (complete dissolution should occur within 30 seconds). The reconstituted product will appear as a pale greenish-yellow solution and must be inspected visually for particulate matter prior to dilution. Do not use if cloudiness or precipitate is observed. Filter this solution (0.22 mcM) prior to dilution. Do not reconstitute with solutions containing either chloride ion or leucovorin, since precipitation occurs instantly.

Further dilute reconstituted solution with 5% Dextrose Injection to yield a final concentration of 0.25 to 2 mg/ml. Administer the diluted solution by IV infusion over 60 minutes. The IV line must be flushed thoroughly with at least 10 ml of 5% Dextrose Injection before and after administering trimetrexate.

Trimetrexate and leucovorin solutions must be administered separately. Leucovorin protection may be administered prior to or following trimetrexate. In either case the IV line must be flushed thoroughly with at least 10 ml of 5% Dextrose Injection between infusions. Dilute leucovorin according to the manufacturer's instructions and administer over 5 to 10 minutes every 6 hours.

Handling and disposal: If trimetrexate contacts the skin or mucosa, immediately and thoroughly wash with soap and water. Procedures for proper disposal of cytotoxic drugs should be considered.

Storage/Stability: Store vials at controlled room temperature and protect from exposure to light. After reconstitution, the solution is stable under refrigeration or at room temperature for up to 24 hours. Do not freeze reconstituted solution. Discard the unused portions after 24 hours.

Rx	**Neutrexin** (US Bioscience)	**Powder for injection, lyophilized:** 25 mg trimetrexate	In 5 ml vials with or without 50 mg leucovorin.

DAPSONE (DDS)

Actions:

Pharmacology: Dapsone (4,4-diaminodiphenylsulphone; DDS), a sulfone, is bactericidal as well as bacteriostatic against *Mycobacterium leprae.* The mechanism of action in dermatitis herpetiformis has not been established.

Pharmacokinetics:

Absorption/Distribution – Dapsone is rapidly and nearly completely absorbed from the GI tract; peak plasma concentrations are reached in 4 to 8 hours. Daily administration of 200 mg for at least 8 days is necessary to achieve a plateau level of 0.1 to 7 mcg/ml (average 2.3). Approximately 70% to 90% of dapsone is plasma protein bound. Its main metabolite is monoacetyl dapsone (MADDS) which is nearly 100% protein bound. Enterohepatic circulation accounts for appreciable tissue levels of dapsone 3 weeks after therapy is discontinued.

Metabolism/Excretion – Dapsone is acetylated in the liver, and the degree of acetylation is genetically determined. The plasma half-life ranges from 10 to 50 hours (average 28 hours). Repeat tests in the same individual show the clearance rate to be constant. Daily administration (50 to 100 mg) in leprosy patients will provide blood levels in excess of the usual minimum inhibitory concentration even for patients with a short dapsone half-life.

About 70% to 85% is excreted in urine as conjugates and unidentified water-soluble metabolites. Excretion of the drug is slow and a constant blood level can be maintained with the usual dosage.

Indications:

Dermatitis herpetiformis.

Leprosy: All forms of leprosy (Hansen's disease) except for cases of proven dapsone resistance.

Unlabeled uses: Treatment of relapsing polychondritis; prophylaxis of malaria; inflammatory bowel disorders; Leishmaniasis; *Pneumocystis carinii* pneumonia; rheumatic/connective tissue disorders (eg, rheumatoid arthritis, lupus erythematosus); brown recluse spider bites. Doses used generally range from 50 to 200 mg/day.

Contraindications:

Hypersensitivity to dapsone or its derivatives.

Warnings:

Hematologic effects: Deaths associated with dapsone administration have been reported from agranulocytosis, aplastic anemia and other blood dyscrasias. Sore throat, fever, pallor, purpura or jaundice may occur.

Severe anemia – Treat prior to initiation of therapy and monitor hemoglobin. Hemolysis and methemoglobin may be poorly tolerated by patients with severe cardiopulmonary disease.

Hypersensitivity: Cutaneous reactions (especially bullous), include exfoliative dermatitis, toxic erythema, erythema multiforme, toxic epidermal necrolysis, morbilliform and scarlatiniform reactions, urticaria and erythema nodosum. These are some of the most serious and rare complications of dapsone therapy. They are directly due to drug sensitization. If new or toxic dermatologic reactions occur, promptly discontinue sulfone therapy and institute appropriate therapy.

Sulfone syndrome is an unusual and potentially fatal hypersensitivity reaction. It consists of fever, malaise, jaundice with hepatic necrosis, exfoliative dermatitis, lymphadenopathy, methemoglobinemia and hemolytic anemia.

Leprosy reactional states, including cutaneous, are not hypersensitivity reactions to dapsone and do not require discontinuation (see Precautions).

Carcinogenesis: Dapsone is carcinogenic (sarcomagenic) in small animals.

Pregnancy: Category C. Extensive but uncontrolled experience and two published surveys in pregnant women have not shown that dapsone increases the risk of fetal abnormalities if administered during all trimesters. Because of the lack of controlled studies, use during pregnancy only if necessary.

In general, for leprosy, the United States Public Health Service (USPHS) recommends maintenance of dapsone. Dapsone has been important for the management of some pregnant dermatitis herpetiformis patients. It is generally not considered to have an effect on the later growth, development and functional maturation of the child.

Lactation: Dapsone is excreted in breast milk in substantial amounts. Hemolytic reactions can occur in neonates. Because of the potential for tumorigenicity shown in animal studies, discontinue nursing or discontinue the drug.

DAPSONE (DDS)

Precautions:

Monitoring: Perform blood counts weekly for the first month, monthly for 6 months and semi-annually thereafter. If a significant reduction in leukocytes, platelets or hematopoiesis occurs, discontinue dapsone; follow the patient intensively.

Hemolysis and Heinz body formation may be exaggerated in individuals with glucose-6-phosphate dehydrogenase (G-6-PD) deficiency, methemoglobin reductase deficiency or hemoglobin M. This reaction is frequently dose-related. Give dapsone with caution to these patients or patients exposed to other agents or conditions such as infection or diabetic ketosis capable of producing hemolysis.

Hepatic effects: Toxic hepatitis and cholestatic jaundice have been reported early in therapy. Hyperbilirubinemia may occur more often in G-6-PD deficient patients. When feasible, baseline and subsequent monitoring of liver function is recommended. If abnormal, discontinue dapsone until the source of the abnormality is established.

Peripheral neuropathy is an unusual complication in nonleprosy patients. Motor loss is predominant. If muscle weakness appears, withdraw dapsone. Recovery on withdrawal is usually substantially complete. The mechanism of recovery is reportedly by axonal regeneration. In leprosy, this complication may be difficult to distinguish from a leprosy reactional state.

Phototosensitivity: Phototoxicity may occur; caution patients to take protective measures (ie, sunscreens, protective clothing) against exposure to ultraviolet light or sunlight until tolerance is determined.

Leprosy reactional states are abrupt changes in clinical activity occurring in leprosy with any effective treatment and are classified into two groups.

Type 1 (reversal reaction; downgrading) may occur in borderline or tuberculoid leprosy patients soon after chemotherapy is started, and is presumed to result from a reduction in the antigenic load. The patient has an enhanced delayed hypersensitivity response to residual infection leading to swelling ("reversal") of existing skin and nerve lesions. If severe, or if neuritis is present, use large doses of steroids and hospitalize the patient. In general, continue antileprosy treatment and therapy to suppress the reaction, using measures such as analgesics, steroids or surgical decompression of swollen nerve trunks. Contact USPHS* for advice in management.

Type 2 (erythema nodosum leprosum; ENL; lepromatous reaction) occurs mainly in lepromatous patients and small numbers of borderline patients. Approximately 50% of treated patients show this reaction in the first year. The principal clinical features are fever and tender erythematous skin nodules sometimes associated with malaise, neuritis, orchitis, albuminuria, joint swelling, iritis, epistaxis or depression. Skin lesions can become pustular or ulcerate. Histologically, there is a vasculitis with an intense polymorphonuclear infiltrate. Elevated circulating immune complexes are considered the mechanism of the reaction. If severe, hospitalize patients. In general, antileprosy treatment is continued. Analgesics, steroids and other agents (eg, thalidomide, clofazimine) available from USPHS* are used to suppress the reaction.

DAPSONE (DDS)

Drug Interactions:

Dapsone Drug Interactions			
Precipitant drug	Object drug*		Description
Charcoal, activated	Dapsone	⬇	Activated charcoal may decrease dapsone's GI absorption and enterohepatic recycling.
Didanosine	Dapsone	⬇	Possible therapeutic failure of dapsone, leading to an increase in infection.
Folic acid antagonists	Dapsone	⬆	Folic acid antagonists such as pyrimethamine may increase the likelihood of hematologic reactions. Weekly concomitant use has caused agranulocytosis during the second and third months of therapy.
Para-aminobenzoic acid	Dapsone	⬇	Para-aminobenzoic acid may antagonize the effect of dapsone by interfering with the primary mechanism of action.
Probenecid	Dapsone	⬆	Probenecid reduces urinary excretion of dapsone metabolites, increasing plasma concentrations.
Rifampin	Dapsone	⬇	Rifampin lowers dapsone levels seven to tenfold by accelerating plasma clearance.
Trimethoprim	Dapsone	⬆	Increased serum levels of both drugs may occur, possibly increasing the pharmologic and toxic effects of each drug.
Dapsone	Trimethoprim	⬆	

* ⬆ = Object drug increased. ⬇ = Object drug decreased.

Adverse Reactions:

Hematologic: Dose-related hemolysis is the most common adverse effect, including hemolytic anemia (in patients with or without G-6-PD deficiency). Hemolysis develops in almost every individual treated with 200 to 300 mg dapsone per day. Doses of ≤ 100 mg in healthy individuals and ≤ 50 mg in individuals with G-6-PD deficiency do not cause hemolysis. Almost all patients demonstrate the interrelated changes of a loss of 1 to 2 g hemoglobin, an increase in the reticulocytes (2% to 12%), a shortened red cell life span and a rise in methemoglobin. G-6-PD deficient patients have greater responses.

Hypoalbuminemia without proteinuria has occurred.

Dermatologic: Drug-induced lupus erythematosus; phototoxicity.

CNS: Peripheral neuropathy (see Precautions); headache; psychosis; insomnia; vertigo; paresthesia.

GI: Nausea; vomiting; abdominal pain; anorexia.

Renal: Albuminuria; the nephrotic syndrome; renal papillary necrosis.

Miscellaneous: Blurred vision; tinnitus; fever; male infertility; tachycardia; an infectious mononucleosis-like syndrome; pancreatitis; pulmonary eosinophilia.

Overdosage:

Symptoms: Nausea, vomiting and hyperexcitability can appear a few minutes and up to 24 hours after ingestion of an overdose. Methemoglobin-induced depression, convulsions and severe cyanosis require prompt treatment.

Treatment: Empty the stomach by lavage. In normal and methemoglobin reductase deficient patients, methylene blue, 1 to 2 mg/kg, given slowly IV is the treatment of choice. The effect is complete in 30 minutes, but may have to be repeated if methemoglobin reaccumulates. For nonemergencies, if treatment is needed, methylene blue may be given orally in doses of 3 to 5 mg/kg every 4 to 6 hours. Methylene blue reduction depends on G-6-PD; do not give to fully expressed G-6-PD deficient patients. Hemolysis may be treated by blood transfusions to replace damaged cells. Other supportive measures include oxygen and IV fluids.

Use of activated charcoal in intoxicated patients increased the rate of elimination by 3 to 5 times. The half-life of dapsone and MADDS was reduced by 50%.

Patient Information:

May cause photosensitivity; avoid prolonged exposure to sunlight or sunlamps.

DAPSONE (DDS)

Administration and Dosage:

Dermatitis herpetiformis: Individualize dosage. Start with 50 mg daily in adults and correspondingly smaller doses in children. If full control is not achieved within the range of 50 to 300 mg daily, higher doses may be tried. Reduce dosage to a minimum maintenance level as soon as possible. In responsive patients, there is a prompt reduction in pruritus followed by clearance of skin lesions. There is no effect on the GI component of the disease.

Dapsone levels are influenced by acetylation rates. Patients with high acetylation rates or who are receiving treatment affecting acetylation may require a dosage adjustment.

Maintenance dosage may be reduced or eliminated on a strict gluten free diet; the average time for dosage reduction is 8 months with a range of 4 months to 2½ years and for dosage elimination 29 months with a range of 6 months to 9 years.

Leprosy: To reduce a secondary dapsone resistance, the WHO Expert Committee on Leprosy and the USPHS* recommend therapy be commenced and maintained at full dosage (100 mg/day) without interruption in combination with one or more anti-leprosy drugs.

Recommended dosage – The schedule amounts to 50 to 100 mg daily in adults, with correspondingly smaller doses for children.

Bacteriologically negative tuberculoid and indeterminate disease – An adult dosage of 100 mg daily with 6 months of rifampin 600 mg/day is recommended. Under WHO, daily rifampin may be replaced by 600 mg rifampin monthly if supervised. After all signs of clinical activity are controlled (usually after an additional 6 months), continue dapsone therapy a minimum of 3 years for tuberculoid and indeterminate patients.

Lepromatous and borderline patients – Administer dapsone (100 mg/day) for 2 years with rifampin 600 mg daily. Under WHO daily rifampin may be replaced by 600 mg rifampin monthly, if supervised. One may elect the concurrent administration of a third anti-leprosy drug, usually either clofazimine 50–100 mg daily or ethionamide 250–500 mg daily. Dapsone 100 mg daily is continued 3–10 years until all signs of clinical activity are controlled with skin scrapings and biopsies negative for one year. Dapsone should then be continued for an additional 10 years for borderline patients and for life for lepromatous patients.

Suspect secondary dapsone resistance whenever a lepromatous or borderline lepromatous patient receiving dapsone treatment relapses clinically and bacteriologically. If such cases show no response to regular and supervised dapsone therapy within 3 to 6 months, consider dapsone resistance confirmed clinically. Determination of drug sensitivity after prior arrangement is available without charge from USPHS.* Treat patients with proven dapsone resistance with other drugs.

Children: The recommended dosage is 1 to 2 mg/kg/day for a minimum of 3 years; maximum is usual adult dosage of 100 mg/day.

Rx	**Dapsone** (Jacobus)	**Tablets:** 25 mg	(Jacobus 25 102). White, scored. In 100s.
		100 mg	(Jacobus 100 101). White, scored. In 100s.

* Gillis W. Long National Hansen's Disease Center; Carville, LA 70721: (800) 642-7771.

CLOFAZIMINE

Actions:

Pharmacology: Clofazimine exerts a slow bactericidal effect on *Mycobacterium leprae* (Hansen's bacillus). It inhibits mycobacterial growth and binds preferentially to mycobacterial DNA. The drug also exerts anti-inflammatory properties in controlling erythema nodosum leprosum reactions. Precise mechanism of action is unknown.

Pharmacokinetics:

Absorption/Distribution – Absorption rate ranges from 45% to 62% after oral administration. Average serum concentrations in patients treated with 100 and 300 mg daily were 0.7 and 1 mcg per ml, respectively.

Clofazimine is highly lipophilic and is deposited predominantly in fatty tissue and in the reticuloendothelial system. It is taken up by macrophages.

Metabolism/Excretion – After ingestion of a single 300 mg dose, elimination of unchanged drug and its metabolites in urine in 24 hours was negligible. Clofazimine is retained in the human body for a long time. Half-life after repeated doses is estimated to be at least 70 days. Part of the drug recovered from feces may represent excretion via bile. A small amount is eliminated in sputum, sebum and sweat.

Microbiology: Measurement of the minimum inhibitory concentration (MIC) of clofazimine against leprosy bacilli in vitro is not yet feasible. Although bacterial killing may begin shortly after starting the drug, it cannot be measured in patient biopsy tissues until approximately 50 days after therapy starts.

Clofazimine does not show cross-resistance with dapsone or rifampin. Rarely are microorganisms other than mycobacteria inhibited by the drug.

Indications:

Leprosy: Treatment of lepromatous leprosy, including dapsone-resistant lepromatous leprosy and lepromatous leprosy complicated by erythema nodosum leprosum.

Combination drug therapy has been recommended for initial treatment of multibacillary leprosy to prevent the development of drug resistance.

Warnings:

GI effects: Severe abdominal symptoms have necessitated exploratory laparotomies in patients receiving clofazimine. Rare reports have included splenic infarction, bowel obstruction and GI bleeding. Death has been reported following severe abdominal symptoms. Autopsies have revealed crystalline deposits of clofazimine in the intestinal mucosa, liver, gallbladder, bile, spleen, adrenals, subcutaneous fat, mesenteric lymph nodes, muscles, bone and skin.

Use with caution in patients who have GI problems such as abdominal pain and diarrhea. Give dosages of > 100 mg daily for as short a period as possible and only under close medical supervision. If a patient complains of colicky or burning pain in the abdomen, nausea, vomiting or diarrhea, reduce the dose and, if necessary, increase the interval between doses or discontinue the drug.

Pregnancy: Category C. Clofazimine crosses the human placenta. The infant skin was deeply pigmented at birth. No evidence of teratogenicity was found in these infants. There are no adequate and well controlled studies in pregnant women. Use during pregnancy only if clearly needed and when the potential benefits outweigh the potential hazards to the fetus.

There was evidence of fetotoxicity in the mouse at 12 to 25 times the human dose. Skin and fatty tissue of offspring became discolored ≈ 3 days after birth; this was attributed to the presence of the drug in maternal milk.

Lactation: Clofazimine is excreted in breast milk. Do not administer to a nursing woman unless clearly indicated.

Children: Safety and efficacy in children have not been established. Several cases of children treated with clofazimine have been reported in the literature.

Precautions:

Skin discoloration due to the drug may result in depression. Two suicides have been reported in patients receiving clofazimine. For skin dryness and ichthyosis, apply oil to the skin.

Drug Interactions:

Dapsone: Preliminary data which suggest that dapsone may inhibit the anti-inflammatory activity of clofazimine have not been confirmed. If leprosy-associated inflammatory reactions develop in patients being treated with dapsone and clofazimine, it is still advisable to continue treatment with both drugs.

CLOFAZIMINE

Adverse Reactions:

In general, clofazimine is well tolerated when administered in dosages no greater than 100 mg daily. The most consistent adverse reactions are usually dose-related and reversible when the drug is discontinued.

Dermatologic: Pigmentation (pink to brownish black) in 75% to 100% of patients within a few weeks of treatment; ichthyosis, dryness (8% to 28%); rash, pruritus (1% to 5%); phototoxicity, erythroderma, acneiform eruptions, monilial cheilosis (< 1%).

CNS: Dizziness, drowsiness, fatigue, headache, giddiness, neuralgia, taste disorder (< 1%).

Psychiatric: Depression secondary to skin discoloration; two suicides have occurred (< 1%).

Lab test abnormalities: Elevated albumin, serum bilirubin and AST, eosinophilia, hypokalemia (< 1%).

GI: Abdominal/epigastric pain, diarrhea, nausea, vomiting, GI intolerance (40% to 50%); bowel obstruction and GI bleeding (see Warnings), anorexia, constipation, weight loss, hepatitis, jaundice, eosinophilic enteritis, enlarged liver (< 1%).

Ophthalmic: Conjunctival and corneal pigmentation due to clofazimine crystal deposits; dryness; burning; itching; irritation.

Miscellaneous: Splenic infarction (see Warnings), thromboembolism, anemia, cystitis, bone pain, edema, fever, lymphadenopathy, vascular pain, diminished vision (< 1%); discolored urine, feces, sputum or sweat; elevated blood sugar or ESR.

Overdosage:

No specific data are available. In case of overdose, empty the stomach by inducing vomiting or by gastric lavage. Treatment includes usual supportive measures. Refer to General Management of Acute Overdosage.

Patient Information:

Take with meals.

Warn patients that clofazimine may discolor the skin from red to brownish black, as well as discoloring the conjunctivae, lacrimal fluid, sweat, sputum, urine and feces. Skin discoloration, although reversible, may take several months or years to disappear after the conclusion of therapy.

Administration and Dosage:

Take with meals.

Clofazimine should be used preferably in combination with one or more other antileprosy agents to prevent the emergence of drug resistance.*

Dapsone-resistant leprosy: Give 100 mg clofazimine/day in combination with one or more other antileprosy drugs for 3 years, followed by monotherapy with 100 mg clofazimine/day. Clinical improvement usually can be detected between the first and third months of treatment and is usually clearly evident by the sixth month.

Dapsone-sensitive multibacillary leprosy: Combination therapy with two other antileprosy drugs is recommended. Give the triple-drug regimen for at least 2 years and continue, if possible, until negative skin smears are obtained. At this time, monotherapy with an appropriate antileprosy drug can be instituted.

Erythema nodosum leprosum: Treatment depends on the severity of symptoms. In general, continue basic antileprosy treatment; if nerve injury or skin ulceration is threatened, give corticosteroids. Where prolonged corticosteroid therapy becomes necessary, clofazimine 100 to 200 mg daily for up to 3 months may be useful in eliminating or reducing corticosteroid requirements. Dosages > 200 mg daily are not recommended; taper dosage to 100 mg daily as quickly as possible after the reactive episode is controlled. Keep patient under medical surveillance.

Storage: Store below 86°F; protect from moisture.

Rx	**Lamprene** (Geigy)	**Capsules:** 50 mg	Brown. In 100s.

* For information about combination drug regimens, contact the Gillis W. Long Hansen's Disease Center, Carville, LA 70721: (800) 642-2477.

ANTHELMINTICS

The following table lists the major parasitic infections, causative organisms and drugs of choice for treatment. For investigational antiparasitic agents available from the Centers for Disease Control, refer to the CDC Anti-Infective Agents monograph.

Major Parasite Infections			
	Infection (common name)	Organism	Drug(s) of Choice
Intestinal Nematodes	Ascariasis[1] (Roundworm)	*Ascaris lumbricoides*	Mebendazole, Pyrantel pamoate or Diethylcarbamazine
	Uncinariasis (Hookworm)	*Ancylostoma duodenale* *Necator americanus*	Mebendazole or Pyrantel pamoate[2]
	Strongyloidiasis (Threadworm)	*Strongyloides stercoralis*	Thiabendazole
	Trichuriasis (Whipworm)	*Trichuris trichiura*	Mebendazole
	Enterobiasis[3] (Pinworm)	*Enterobius vermicularis*	Mebendazole, Pyrantel pamoate or Albendazole
	Capillariasis	*Capillaria philippinensis*	Mebendazole, Thiabendazole or Albendazole
Tissue Nematodes	Trichinosis	*Trichinella spiralis*	Steroids for severe symptoms plus Thiabendazole, Albendazole, Flubendazole[6] or Mebendazole[2]
	Cutaneous larva migrans (Creeping eruption)	*Ancylostoma braziliense* and others	Thiabendazole, Albendazole or Ivermectin[4]
	Onchocerciasis (River blindness)	*Onchocerca volvulus*	Suramin[5], Diethylcarbamazine or Ivermectin[4]
	Dracontiasis (Guinea worm)	*Dracunculus medinensis*	Thiabendazole or Mebendazole
	Angiostrongyliasis (Rat lungworm)	*Angiostrongylus cantonensis*	Thiabendazole or Mebendazole
	Loiasis	*Loa loa*	Diethylcarbamazine
Cestodes	Taeniasis		
	(Beef tapeworm)	*Taenia saginata*	Praziquantel[2] or Niclosamide[6]
	(Pork tapeworm)	*Taenia solium*	Praziquantel[2], Niclosamide[6] or Albendazole
	Diphyllobothriasis (Fish tapeworm)	*Diphyllobothrium latum*	Praziquantel[2] or Niclosamide[6]
	Dog tapeworm	*Dipylidium caninum*	Praziquantel[2]
	Hymenolepiasis (Dwarf tapeworm)	*Hymenolepis nana*	Praziquantel[2] or Niclosamide[6]
	Hydatid cysts	*Echinococcus granulosus*	Albendazole or Praziquantel
Trematodes	Schistosomiasis	*Schistosoma mansoni*	Praziquantel or Oxamniquine
		Schistosoma japonicum	Praziquantel
		Schistosoma haematobium	Praziquantel
		Schistosoma mekongi	Praziquantel
	Hermaphroditic Flukes		
	Fasciolopsiasis (Intestinal fluke)	*Fasciolopsis buski*	Praziquantel
		Heterophyes heterophyes *Metagonimus yokogawai*	Praziquantel
	Clonorchiasis (Chinese liver fluke)	*Clonorchis sinensis*	Praziquantel
	Fascioliasis (Sheep liver fluke)	*Fasciola hepatica*	Praziquantel or Bithionol[4]
	Opisthorchiasis (Liver fluke)	*Opisthorchis viverrini*	Praziquantel
	Paragonimiasis (Lung fluke)	*Paragonimus westermani*	Praziquantel or Bithionol[4] (alternate)

[1] The following drugs are also indicated in Ascariasis: Piperazine citrate (if intestinal or biliary obstruction) and thiabendazole.

[2] Unlabeled use.

[3] The following drugs are also indicated in Enterobiasis: Piperazine and thiabendazole.

[4] Available from the CDC.

[5] Available from the CDC, although generally not recommended.

[6] Not available in the US.

MEBENDAZOLE

Refer to the general discussion of these products in the Anthelmintics introduction.

Actions:

Pharmacology: Mebendazole inhibits the formation of the worms' microtubules and irreversibly blocks glucose uptake by the susceptible helminths, thereby depleting endogenous glycogen stored within the parasite that is required for survival and reproduction of the helminth. Mebendazole does not affect blood glucose concentrations in the host.

Pharmacokinetics: Mebendazole is poorly absorbed (5% to 10%) after oral administration. Peak plasma levels are reached in 2 to 4 hours. Following administration of 100 mg of mebendazole twice daily for 3 consecutive days, plasma levels of mebendazole and its primary metabolite did not exceed 0.03 mcg/ml and 0.09 mcg/ml, respectively. Approximately 2% of the drug is excreted in the urine during the first 24 to 48 hours. Most of the dose is excreted in the feces as unchanged drug or primary metabolites.

Microbiology: Active against *Trichuris trichiura* (whipworm), *Enterobius vermicularis* (pinworm), *Ascaris lumbricoides* (roundworm), *Ancylostoma duodenale* (common hookworm) and *Necator americanus* (American hookworm). Parasite immobilization and death are slow, and complete clearance from the GI tract may take up to 3 days after treatment. Efficacy varies as a function of such factors as preexisting diarrhea and GI transit time, degree of infection and helminth strains.

Indications:

Helminths: Treatment of *Trichuris trichiura* (whipworm), *Enterobius vermicularis* (pinworm), *Ascaris lumbricoides* (roundworm), *Ancylostoma duodenale* (common hookworm) or *Necator americanus* (American hookworm), in single or mixed infections.

Contraindications:

Hypersensitivity to mebendazole.

Warnings:

Hydatid disease: There is no evidence that mebendazole is effective for hydatid disease.

Pregnancy: Category C. Mebendazole was embryotoxic and teratogenic in pregnant rats at single oral doses as low as 10 mg/kg. This drug is not recommended for use in pregnant women. Based on a limited number of women, the incidence of spontaneous abortion, malformation and teratogenesis did not exceed that in the general population. During pregnancy, especially during the first trimester, use mebendazole only if the potential benefit justifies the potential risk to the fetus.

Lactation: It is not known whether mebendazole is excreted in breast milk. Because many drugs are excreted in breast milk, excercise caution when mebendazole is administered to a nursing woman.

Children: Safety and efficacy for use in children < 2 years of age have not been established; consider the relative benefit vs risk.

Drug Interactions:

Carbamazepine and **hydantoins** may reduce the plasma levels of concomitant mebendazole, possibly decreasing its therapeutic effect.

Adverse Reactions:

GI: Transient abdominal pain and diarrhea have occurred in cases of massive infection and expulsion of worms.

Hematologic: Two patients receiving high doses of mebendazole for echinococcosis developed a severe but reversible neutropenia apparently because of marrow suppression.

Miscellaneous: Fever, a possible response to drug-induced tissue necrosis, has occurred.

MEBENDAZOLE

Overdosage:

GI complaints lasting up to a few hours may occur. Induce vomiting and purging. Refer to General Management of Acute Overdosage.

Patient Information:

Chew or crush tablet and mix with food.

Parasite death may be slow. Removal from digestive tract may take up to 3 days after treatment. Effectiveness depends on factors such as degree of infection or resistance of parasite to treatment, presence of diarrhea and how quickly things pass through the digestive system. Laxative therapy and fasting are not necessary.

If not cured in 3 weeks, a second treatment is recommended.

Pinworm infections are easily spread to others. If one family member has a pinworm infection, treat all family members in close contact with the patient. This decreases the chance of spreading the infection.

Strict hygiene is essential to prevent reinfection. Disinfect toilet facilities daily. Change and launder undergarments, bed linens, towels and nightclothes daily.

Administration and Dosage:

The same dosage schedule applies to children and adults.

Tablets may be chewed, swallowed or crushed and mixed with food. No special procedures, such as fasting or purging, are required.

If the patient is not cured 3 weeks after treatment, a second treatment course is advised.

Trichuriasis, ascariasis and hookworm infection: One tablet morning and evening on 3 consecutive days. In one study, treatment with a single 500 mg dose was effective against *A. lumbricoides.*

Enterobiasis: A single tablet given once.

Rx	**Vermox** (Janssen)	**Tablets, chewable:** 100 mg	In 12s.
Rx	**Mebendazole** (Copley)		In 12s.

DIETHYLCARBAMAZINE CITRATE

Refer to the general discussion of these products in the Anthelmintics introduction.

Actions:

Pharmacology: Diethylcarbamazine does not resemble other antiparasitic compounds. It is a synthetic organic compound which is highly specific for several common parasites and does not contain any toxic metallic elements.

The drug is effective against the following organisms: *Wuchereria bancrofti, Onchocerca volvulus, Loa loa* and *Ascaris lumbricoides.*

Diethylcarbamazine has demonstrated a low order of toxicity in animals.

Indications:

Treatment of Bancroftian filariasis, onchocerciasis, ascariasis, tropical eosinophilia, loiasis.

Precautions:

Administer carefully to avoid or to control allergic or other untoward reactions.

Adverse Reactions:

Wuchereria bancrofti: Mild reactions are transient but fairly frequent. Headache, lassitude, weakness or general malaise are most common. Nausea, vomiting and skin rash occasionally occur. These effects are not considered serious and do not usually require discontinuation of therapy. However, it may be necessary to stop therapy when severe allergic phenomena appear in conjunction with skin rash. It has not yet been determined what proportion or type of reactions result from the death of the parasites rather than from the influence of the drug.

Onchocerciasis: Facial edema and pruritus, especially of the eyes, are often encountered. Severe reactions may develop after a single dose when intense infestations are treated. In such cases, only 1 dose should be given on the first day, 2 doses the second day and 3 daily thereafter for 30 days. If very severe reactions occur, discontinue the drug and start antihistamine therapy. After 1 or 2 days, therapy may be resumed, but if severe allergic phenomena again supervene, use the drug only with extreme caution.

Ascariasis: Giddiness, nausea, vomiting and malaise may occur more frequently following treatment of ascariasis in children who are malnourished or who suffer from various debilitating diseases.

Administration and Dosage:

Bancroft's filariasis, onchocerciasis and loiasis: Usual dose is 2 mg/kg 3 times a day immediately following meals. When the disease is in the acute stage, continue treatment for 3 to 4 weeks. Recurrences have been more frequent with smaller doses. When, as a public health measure, it is desirable to treat large numbers of patients known to harbor microfilariae, use the same dosage schedule for 3 to 5 days. Laboratory tests in randomly selected patients are helpful in assessing efficacy of therapy.

Ascariasis:

Outpatients – 13 mg/kg, given once a day for 7 days, should reduce the number of worms by 85% to 100%. No pretreatment fasting or post-treatment purging is required. Expulsion of ascarids usually begins 1 or 2 days after therapy initiation.

Children – Give 6 to 10 mg/kg 3 times daily for 7 to 10 days. In particularly obstinate cases, an additional course consisting of 10 mg/kg 3 times daily is indicated.

Tropical eosinophilia: 13 mg/kg/day for 4 to 7 days.

Rx	**Hetrazan**[1] (Wyeth-Ayerst)	**Tablets:** 50 mg	In 100s.

[1] Hetrazan is available from Wyeth-Ayerst Labs without charge for compassionate use only. For more information, physicians should contact: Wyeth-Ayerst Labs, P.O. Box 8299, Philadelphia, PA 19101, (610) 688–4400.

PYRANTEL

Refer to the general discussion of these products in the Anthelmintics introduction.

Actions:

Pharmacology: Pyrantel is a depolarizing neuromuscular blocking agent, resulting in spastic paralysis of the worm. It also inhibits cholinesterases. It is active against *Enterobius vermicularis* (pinworm) and *Ascaris lumbricoides* (roundworm); it is also effective against *Ancylostoma duodenale* (hookworm).

Pharmacokinetics: Pyrantel is poorly absorbed from the GI tract. Plasma levels of unchanged drug are low. Greater than 50% is excreted in feces as unchanged drug; ≤ 7% of the dose is found in the urine as parent drug and metabolites.

Indications:

Helminths: Treatment of ascariasis (roundworm infection) and enterobiasis (pinworm infection).

Contraindications:

Hepatic disease; pregnancy (see Warnings); hypersensitivity to pyrantel.

Warnings:

Pregnancy: Do not use during pregnancy unless otherwise directed by a physician.

Children: Safety and efficacy for use in children < 2 years have not been established.

Drug Interactions:

Piperazine: In ascariasis, pyrantel and piperazine are mutually antagonistic; therefore, concomitant use is unwise.

Theophylline serum levels increased in a pediatric patient following pyrantel pamoate administration. Further study is needed.

Adverse Reactions:

GI: Anorexia; nausea; vomiting; abdominal cramps; diarrhea.

CNS: Headache; dizziness; drowsiness; insomnia.

Dermatologic: Rash.

Patient Information:

A single dose is required. The dose is based on body weight.

May be taken with food, milk, juice or on an empty stomach anytime during the day. Be certain to take the entire dose.

Using a laxative after taking the drug to facilitate removal of the parasites is not necessary.

Pinworm infections are easily spread to others. If one family member has a pinworm infection, treat all family members in close contact with the patient. This decreases the chance of spreading the infection.

Strict hygiene is essential to prevent reinfection. Disinfect toilet facilities daily. Change and launder undergarments, bed linens, towels and nightclothes daily.

A package insert is available for patients containing the following information: Symptoms of pinworm infestations; how to find and identify the pinworm; pinworm life cycle; how it is spread from person to person.

Administration and Dosage:

A single dose of 11 mg/kg (5 mg/lb). Maximum total dose is 1 g.

May be administered without regard to ingestion of food or time of day. Purging is not necessary. May be taken with milk or fruit juices.

otc	**Pin-Rid** (Apothecary)	**Capsules, soft gel:** 180 mg pyrantel pamoate (equiv. to 62.5 mg pyrantel base)	In 24s.
otc	**Reese's Pinworm** (Reese)		In 24s.
otc	**Antiminth** (Pfizer Labs)	**Oral Suspension:** 50 mg pyrantel (as pamoate) per ml	Sorbitol. Caramel-currant flavor. In 60 ml.
otc	**Pin-Rid** (Apothecary)	**Liquid:** 50 mg pyrantel (as pamoate) per ml	Sucrose, saccharin, parabens. Cherry flavor. In 30 ml.
otc	**Pin-X** (Effcon)		Sorbitol, parabens. Caramel flavor. In 30 ml.
otc	**Reese's Pinworm** (Reese)		In 30 ml.

THIABENDAZOLE

Refer to the general discussion of these products in the Anthelmintics introduction.

Actions:

Pharmacokinetics: Thiabendazole is rapidly absorbed and peak plasma concentrations occur within 1 to 2 hours. It is metabolized almost completely and appears in the urine as conjugates. In 48 hours, ≈ 5% of the administered dose is recovered from feces and ≈ 90% from urine. Most is excreted within the first 24 hours.

Microbiology: Thiabendazole is vermicidal or vermifugal against *Enterobius vermicularis* (pinworm); *Ascaris lumbricoides* (roundworm); *Strongyloides stercoralis* (threadworm); *Necator americanus* and *Ancylostoma duodenale* (hookworm); *Trichuris trichiura* (whipworm); *Ancylostoma braziliense* (dog and cat hookworm); and *Toxocara canis* and *Toxocara cati* (ascarids).

Thiabendazole's effect on larvae of *Trichinella spiralis* that have migrated to muscle is questionable. It suppresses egg or larval production and may inhibit the subsequent development of those eggs or larvae which are passed in the feces. While the exact mechanism is unknown, the drug inhibits the helminth-specific enzyme fumarate reductase. The anthelmintic activity against *Trichuris trichiura* (whipworm) is least predictable.

Indications:

Helminths: Treatment of strongyloidiasis (threadworm infection), cutaneous larva migrans (creeping eruption) and visceral larva migrans.

Although not indicated as primary therapy, when enterobiasis (pinworm) occurs with any of the conditions listed above, additional therapy is not required for most patients. Use thiabendazole only in the following infestations when more specific therapy is not available or cannot be used or when further therapy with a second agent is desirable: Uncinariasis (hookworm: *Necator americanus* and *Ancylostoma duodenale*); Trichuriasis (whipworm); Ascariasis (large roundworm).

Also indicated for alleviating symptoms of trichinosis during the invasive phase.

Contraindications:

Hypersensitivity to thiabendazole.

Warnings:

CNS effects: Because CNS side effects may occur, avoid activities requiring mental alertness.

Hypersensitivity: If hypersensitivity reactions occur, discontinue the drug immediately. Erythema multiforme has been associated with therapy; in severe cases (eg, Stevens-Johnson syndrome), fatalities have occurred. Refer to Management of Acute Hypersensitivity Reactions.

Pregnancy: Category C. There are no adequate and well controlled studies in pregnant women. Use during pregnancy only if the potential benefit outweighs the risk to the fetus.

Lactation: It is not known whether this drug is excreted in breast milk. Because of the potential for serious adverse reactions in nursing infants, decide whether to discontinue nursing or drug taking into account importance of drug to mother.

Children: Safety and efficacy for the treatment of Strongyloidiasis, Ascariasis, Uncinariasis, Trichuriasis and Trichinosis in children weighing < 13.6 kg (30 lbs) has been limited.

Precautions:

Monitoring: Monitor patients with hepatic or renal dysfunction carefully.

Supportive therapy is indicated for anemic, dehydrated or malnourished patients prior to initiation of therapy.

Metabolite: Some patients may excrete a metabolite that imparts an odor to urine similar to that occurring after ingestion of asparagus.

Thiabendazole is not suitable for the treatment of mixed infections with ascaris because it may cause these worms to migrate. Use only in patients in whom susceptible worm infestation has been diagnosed; do not use prophylactically.

Laboratory tests: Rarely, a transient rise in cephalin flocculation and AST has occurred in patients receiving thiabendazole.

Drug Interactions:

Xanthines: Thiabendazole may compete with these agents for sites of metabolism in the liver, thus elevating the serum levels of the xanthine to potentially toxic levels. Monitor xanthine serum levels and reduce the dose if necessary.

THIABENDAZOLE

Adverse Reactions:

CNS: Dizziness; weariness; drowsiness; giddiness; headache; numbness; hyperirritability; convulsions; collapse; psychic disturbances.

GI: Anorexia; nausea; vomiting; diarrhea; epigastric distress; jaundice; cholestasis; parenchymal liver damage.

GU: Hematuria; enuresis; malodor of the urine; crystalluria.

Hypersensitivity: Pruritus; fever; facial flush; chills; conjunctival injection ("red eye"); angioedema; anaphylaxis; skin rashes (including perianal); erythema multiforme (including Stevens-Johnson syndrome); lymphadenopathy. See Warnings.

Special senses: Tinnitus; abnormal sensation in eyes; xanthopsia (objects appear yellow); blurring of vision; drying of mucous membranes (eg, mouth, eyes).

Body as a whole: Appearance of live Ascaris in the mouth and nose; hypotension; transient leukopenia; hyperglycemia.

Overdosage:

Symptoms: Possible transient disturbances of vision and psychic alterations.

Treatment: There is no specific antidote. Use symptomatic and supportive measures. Induce emesis or carefully perform gastric lavage. Refer to General Management of Acute Overdosage.

Patient Information:

May cause stomach upset. Take with food.

Chewable tablets: Chew thoroughly before swallowing.

Cleansing enemas are not needed after drug therapy.

Duration of therapy varies from 2 or more days depending upon the condition being treated.

Pinworm infections are easily spread to others. If one family member has a pinworm infection, treat all family members in close contact with the patient. This decreases the chance of spreading the infection.

Repeat therapy in 7 days to prevent reinfection.

Strict hygiene is essential to prevent reinfection. Disinfect toilet facilities daily. Change and launder undergarments, bed linens, towels and nightclothes daily.

May produce drowsiness or dizziness. Use caution when driving or performing other tasks requiring alertness.

Administration and Dosage:

< 150 lbs (68 kg): 10 mg/lb/dose (22 mg/kg/dose).

≥ 150 lbs: 1.5 g/dose.

The usual dosage schedule for all conditions is 2 doses per day. Maximum daily dose is 3 g after meals if possible.

Dietary restriction, complementary medications and cleansing enemas are not needed.

Thiabendazole Dosage Regimen for Each Indication

Indication	Regimen	Comments
Strongyloidiasis[1] Ascariasis[1] Uncinariasis[1] Trichuriasis[1]	2 doses/day for 2 successive days	May also use single dose of 20 mg/lb (44 mg/kg) but with higher incidence of side effects.
Cutaneous larva migrans (creeping eruption)	2 doses/day for 2 successive days	If active lesions are still present 2 days after end of therapy, a second course is recommended.
Trichinosis[1]	2 doses/day for 2 to 4 successive days. Individualize dosage	Optimal dosage has not been established.
Visceral larva migrans	2 doses/day for 7 successive days	Safety and efficacy data on the 7 day treatment are limited.

[1] Clinical experience with thiabendazole in children weighing < 13.6 kg (30 lbs) is limited.

Rx	**Mintezol** (Merck)	**Tablets, chewable:** 500 mg	Lactose, saccharin. (MSD 907). White, scored. Orange flavor. In 36s.
		Oral Suspension: 500 mg/5 ml	Sorbic acid, sorbitol. In 120 ml.

OXAMNIQUINE

Refer to the general discussion of these products in the Anthelmintics introduction.

Actions:

Pharmacokinetics: Oxamniquine is well absorbed; plasma concentrations reach a peak at 1 to 1.5 hours after oral administration of therapeutic doses, with a plasma half-life of 1 to 2.5 hours. It is extensively metabolized to inactive acidic metabolites which are largely excreted in the urine.

Microbiology: Male schistosomes are more susceptible than female; however, after treatment with oxamniquine, the residual female schistosomes cease to lay eggs, thus losing the parasitological aspect of their pathological significance.

Indications:

All stages of *Schistosoma mansoni* infection, including acute and chronic phase with hepatosplenic involvement.

Unlabeled uses: Concurrent low dose administration of oxamniquine plus praziquantel has been used successfully as a single-dose treatment of schistosomiasis.

Warnings:

Convulsions: Epileptiform convulsions have occurred rarely within the first few hours after ingestion, most often in patients with a previous seizure history. Use with care in such individuals and keep them under medical supervision with facilities available to treat a convulsion. EEG abnormalities have also developed in patients with normal pretreatment recordings.

Pregnancy: Category C. Oxamniquine was embryocidal in rabbits and mice when given in doses 10 times the human dose. There are no adequate and well controlled studies in pregnant women. Use only when clearly needed and when the potential benefits outweigh the potential hazards to the fetus.

Lactation: It is not known whether this drug is excreted in breast milk. Exercise caution when administering to a nursing mother.

Adverse Reactions:

CNS: Transitory dizziness/drowsiness (33%); headache; epileptiform convulsions (rare, see Warnings); EEG abnormalities.

GI: Nausea; vomiting; abdominal pain; anorexia.

Dermatologic: Urticaria.

Minor and transient abnormalities were observed after treatment (not drug-related and of no clinical significance). They included rare instances of mild to moderate liver enzyme elevations, but no evidence of hepatotoxicity, even in patients with severe hepatosplenic involvement.

Patient Information:

Take after food to improve tolerance.

Administration and Dosage:

Generally well tolerated. Tolerance improves when doses are given after food.

Adults: 12 to 15 mg/kg as a single oral dose in patients with Western Hemisphere strains of *S. mansoni.* Recommended dosage according to weight is as follows:

Recommended Oxamniquine Adult Dosage	
Weight (kg)	Dose (mg)
30 to 40	500
41 to 60	750
61 to 80	1000
81 to 100	1250

Children (< 30 kg): 20 mg/kg given in 2 divided doses of 10 mg/kg in one day with 2 to 8 hours between doses.

Rx	**Vansil** (Pfizer Labs)	**Capsules:** 250 mg	Lactose. Green and yellow. In 24s.

PRAZIQUANTEL

Refer to the general discussion of these products in the Anthelmintics introduction.

Actions:

Pharmacology: Praziquantel increases cell membrane permeability in susceptible worms, resulting in a loss of intracellular calcium, massive contractions and paralysis of their musculature. The drug further results in vacuolization and disintegration of the schistosome tegument. This effect is followed by attachment of phagocytes to the parasite and death.

Pharmacokinetics: Praziquantel is rapidly absorbed (80%), reaching maximal serum concentration in 1 to 3 hours. Cerebrospinal fluid levels are ≈ 14% to 20% the total amount of drug in plasma. It undergoes significant first-pass biotransformation; elimination half-life of parent drug is 0.8 to 1.5 hrs; 4 hrs for metabolites. Metabolites are excreted primarily in urine and have little or no activity.

Indications:

For infections due to: *Schistosoma mekongi, S. japonicum, S. mansoni* and *S. hematobium*; liver flukes, *Clonorchis sinensis/Opisthorchis viverrini* (approval of this indication was based on studies in which the two species were not differentiated).

Unlabeled uses: Praziquantel demonstrates promise for the treatment of neurocysticercosis. Further study is needed. It may also be beneficial in the treatment of other tissue flukes (eg, *Opisthorchis felineus, Paragonimus westermani* and other species, *Fasciola hepatica*), intestinal flukes (eg, *Heterophyes heterophyes, Fasciolopsis buski*) and intestinal cestodes (eg, *Diphyllobothrium latum, Taenia saginata* and *solium, Dipylidium caninum, Hymenolepis nana*).

Concurrent low dose administration of oxamniquine plus praziquantel has been used successfully as a single-dose treatment of schistosomiasis.

Contraindications:

Previous hypersensitivity to praziquantel; ocular cysticercosis.

Warnings:

Ocular cysticercosis: Because parasite destruction within the eyes may cause irreparable lesions, do not treat ocular cysticercosis with praziquantel.

Pregnancy: Category B. An increase in the abortion rate was found in rats at three times the single human therapeutic dose. There are no adequate and well controlled studies in pregnant women. Use this drug during pregnancy only if clearly needed.

Lactation: Praziquantel appeared in breast milk at a concentration of ≈ 25% that of maternal serum. Do not nurse during treatment or the subsequent 72 hrs.

Children: Safety in children < 4 years of age has not been established.

Precautions:

Hazardous tasks: May produce drowsiness; observe caution while driving or performing other tasks requiring alertness on the day of and following treatment.

Minimal increases in liver enzymes have occurred in some patients.

When schistosomiasis or fluke infection is found to be associated with cerebral cysticercosis, hospitalize the patient for the duration of treatment.

Drug Interactions:

Hydantoins: Serum praziquantel concentrations may be reduced, possibly leading to treatment failures.

Adverse Reactions:

Well tolerated. Side effects are usually mild and transient and do not need treatment but may be more frequent or serious in patients with a heavy worm burden.

In order of severity: Malaise; headache; dizziness; abdominal discomfort (with or without nausea); rising temperature; urticaria (rare). Such symptoms can, however, also result from the infection itself. In patients with liver impairment caused by the infection, no adverse effects occurred that necessitated restriction in use.

PRAZIQUANTEL

Overdosage:

In the event of overdose, give a fast-acting laxative.

Patient Information:

Take with liquids during meals. Do not chew tablets.

May cause dizziness or drowsiness; observe caution while driving or performing other tasks requiring alertness.

Administration and Dosage:

Schistosomiasis: 3 doses of 20 mg/kg as a 1 day treatment.

Clonorchiasis and opisthorchiasis: 3 doses of 25 mg/kg as a 1 day treatment.

The interval between the doses should be not < 4 and not > 6 hours.

Swallow the tablets unchewed with some liquid during meals. Keeping the tablets in the mouth may reveal a bitter taste which can produce gagging or vomiting.

Rx	**Biltricide** (Bayer)	**Tablets:** 600 mg	White, tri-scored. Film coated. In 6s.

ALBENDAZOLE

Refer to the general discussion of these products in the Anthelmintics introduction.

Actions:

Pharmacology: Albendazole's principal mode of action is its inhibitory effect on tubulin polymerization, which results in the loss of cytoplasmic microtubules.

Pharmacokinetics:

Absorption – Albendazole is poorly absorbed from the GI tract because of its low aqueous solubility. Albendazole concentrations are negligible or undetectable in plasma as it is rapidly converted to the sulfoxide metabolite prior to reaching the systemic circulation. The systemic anthelmintic activity has been attributed to the primary metabolite, albendazole sulfoxide. Oral bioavailability appears to be enhanced when albendazole is coadministered with a fatty meal (estimated fat content 40 g) as evidenced by higher (up to 5–fold on average) plasma concentrations of albendazole sulfoxide as compared with the fasted state.

Maximal plasma concentrations of albendazole sulfoxide are typically achieved 2 to 5 hours after dosing and are on average 1.31 mcg/ml (0.46 to 1.58 mcg/ml) following oral doses of albendazole (400 mg) when administered with a fatty meal. Plasma concentrations of albendazole sulfoxide increase in a dose-proportional manner over the therapeutic dose range following ingestion of a fatty meal (fat content 43.1 g). The mean apparent terminal elimination half-life of albendazole sulfoxide typically ranged from 8 to 12 hours in 25 healthy subjects, as well as in 14 hydatid and 8 neurocysticercosis patients.

Following 4 weeks of treatment with albendazole (200 mg three times daily), 12 patients' plasma concentrations of albendazole sulfoxide were ≈ 20% lower than those observed during the first half of the treatment period, suggesting that albendazole may induce its own metabolism.

Distribution – Albendazole sulfoxide is 70% bound to plasma protein and is widely distributed throughout the body; it has been detected in urine, bile, liver, cyst wall, cyst fluid and cerebral spinal fluid (CSF). Concentrations in plasma were 3– to 10–fold and 2– to 4–fold higher than those simultaneously determined in cyst fluid and CSF, respectively. Limited in vitro and clinical data suggest that albendazole sulfoxide may be eliminated from cysts at a slower rate than observed in plasma.

Metabolism/Excretion – Albendazole is rapidly converted in the liver to the primary metabolite, albendazole sulfoxide, which is further metabolized to albendazole sulfone and other primary oxidative metabolites that have been identified in human urine. Following oral administration, albendazole has not been detected in human urine. Urinary excretion of albendazole sulfoxide is a minor elimination pathway with < 1% of the dose recovered in the urine. Biliary elimination presumably accounts for a portion of the elimination as evidenced by biliary concentrations of albendazole sulfoxide similar to those achieved in plasma.

Special populations:

Renal function impairment – The pharmacokinetics of albendazole in patients with impaired renal function have not been studied. However, because renal elimination of albendazole and its primary metabolite, albendazole sulfoxide, is negligible, it is unlikely that clearance of these compounds would be altered in these patients.

Hepatic function impairment – In patients with evidence of extrahepatic obstruction, the systemic availability of albendazole sulfoxide is increased, as indicated by a 2–fold increase in maximum serum concentration and a 7–fold increase in area under the curve (AUC). The rate of absorption/conversion and elimination of albendazole sulfoxide appeared to be prolonged with mean T_{max} and serum elimination half-life values of 10 hours and 31.7 hours, respectively. Plasma concentrations of parent albendazole were measurable in only one of five patients.

Children – Albendazole sulfoxide pharmacokinetics were similar to those observed in fed adults.

Elderly – Although no studies have investigated the effect of age on albendazole sulfoxide pharmacokinetics, data in 26 hydatid cyst patients (up to 79 years) suggest pharmacokinetics similar to those in young healthy subjects.

Microbiology: Albendazole is active against the larval forms of *Echinococcus granulosus* and *Taenia solium*.

ALBENDAZOLE

Indications:

Neurocysticercosis: For the treatment of parenchymal neurocysticercosis due to active lesions caused by larval forms of the pork tapeworm, *T. solium*.

Hydatid disease: For the treatment of cystic hydatid disease of the liver, lung and peritoneum caused by the larval form of the dog tapeworm, *E. granulosus*.

When medically feasible, surgery is considered the treatment of choice for hydatid disease. When administering albendazole in the pre- or post-surgical setting, optimal killing of cyst contents is achieved when three courses of therapy have been given.

Contraindications:

Hypersensitivity to the benzimidazole class of compound or any components of albendazole.

Warnings:

Hepatic function impairment: Albendazole has been associated with mild to moderate elevations of hepatic enzymes in ≈ 16% of patients. These have returned to normal upon discontinuation of therapy. Perform liver function tests (transaminases) before the start of each treatment. If enzymes are significantly increased, discontinue albendazole therapy. Therapy can be reinstituted when liver enzymes have returned to pretreatment levels, but perform laboratory tests frequently during repeated therapy.

Fertility impairment: Patients should not become pregnant for at least 1 month following cessation of albendazole therapy.

Elderly: Experience in patients ≥ 65 years of age is limited. No problems associated with an older population have been observed.

Pregnancy: Category C. Albendazole has been shown to be teratogenic in animals. There are no adequate and well controlled studies of albendazole administration in pregnant women. Do not use albendazole in pregnant women except in clinical circumstances where no alternative management is appropriate. If a patient becomes pregnant while taking this drug, discontinue albendazole immediately.

Lactation: It is not known whether albendazole is excreted in breast milk. Because many drugs are excreted in breast milk, use caution when administering to a nursing woman.

Children: Experience in children < 6 years of age is limited. In hydatid disease, infection in infants and young children is uncommon, but no problems have been encountered in those who have been treated. In neurocysticercosis, infection is more frequently encountered. In studies involving pediatric patients as young as 1 year of age, no significant problems were encountered, and the efficacy appeared similar to the adult population.

Precautions:

Monitoring:

White blood cell count – Albendazole has been shown to cause occasional (< 1% of treated patients) reversible reductions in total white blood cell count. Rarely, more significant reductions may be enountered including granulocytopenia, agranulocytosis or pancytopenia. Perform blood counts at the start of each 28–day treatment cycle and every 2 weeks during each 28–day cycle. Albendazole may be continued if the total white blood cell count decrease appears modest and does not progress.

Coadministration: Patients being treated for neurocysticercosis should receive appropriate steroid and anticonvulsant therapy as required. Consider oral or IV corticosteroids to prevent cerebral hypertensive episodes during the first week of anticysticeral therapy.

Cysticercosis may, in rare cases, involve the retina. Before initiating therapy for neurocysticercosis, examine the patient for the presence of retinal lesions. If such lesions are visualized, weigh the need for anticysticeral therapy against the possibility of retinal damage caused by albendazole-induced changes to the retinal lesion.

ALBENDAZOLE

Drug Interactions:

Albendazole Drug Interactions			
Precipitant drug	Object drug*		Description
Dexamethasone	Albendazole	↑	Steady-state trough concentrations of albendazole sulfoxide were ≈ 56% higher when 8 mg dexamethasone was coadministered with each dose of albendazole (15 mg/kg/day) in eight neurocysticercosis patients.
Praziquantel	Albendazole	↑	Praziquantel (40 mg/kg) increased mean maximum plasma concentration and AUC of albendazole sulfoxide by ≈ 50% in healthy subjects.
Cimetidine	Albendazole	↑	Albendazole sulfoxide concentrations in bile and cystic fluid were increased (≈ 2-fold) in hydatid cyst patients treated with cimetidine.

* ↑ = Object drug increased.

Adverse Reactions:

Adverse Reaction Incidence in Hydatid Disease and Neurocysticercosis (%)		
Adverse reaction	Hydatid disease	Neurocysticercosis
Abnormal liver function tests	15.6	< 1
Abdominal pain	6	0
Nausea/Vomiting	3.7	6.2
Headache	1.3	11
Dizziness/Vertigo	1.2	< 1
Raised intracranial pressure	0	1.5
Meningeal signs	0	1
Reversible alopecia	1.6	< 1
Fever	1	0

The following adverse reactions were observed at an incidence of < 1%.

Hematologic: Leukopenia (0.7%); granulocytopenia, pancytopenia, agranulocytosis, thrombocytopenia (rare).

Dermatologic: Rash; urticaria.

Hypersensitivity: Allergic reactions.

Renal: Acute renal failure.

Overdosage:

One case of overdosage has been reported with albendazole in a patient who took at least 16 g over 12 hours. No untoward effects were reported. In case of overdosage, symptomatic therapy (eg, gastric lavage and activated charcoal) and general supportive measures are recommended. Refer to General Management of Acute Overdosage.

ALBENDAZOLE

Patient Information:

Albendazole may cause fetal harm; therefore, begin treatment after a negative pregnancy test in women of childbearing age.

Caution women of childbearing age against becoming pregnant while on albendazole or within 1 month of completing treatment.

Take with food.

Administration and Dosage:

Dosing of Albendazole According to the Parasitic Infection			
Indication	Weight	Dose	Duration
Hydatid disease	≥ 60 kg	400 mg twice a day with meals	28-day cycle followed by a 14-day albendazole-free interval, for a total of three cycles[1]
	< 60 kg	15 mg/kg/day given in divided doses twice a day with meals (maximum total daily dose 800 mg)	
Neurocysticercosis	≥ 60 kg	400 mg twice a day with meals	8 to 30 days
	< 60 kg	15 mg/kg/day given in divided doses twice a day with meals (maximum total daily dose 800 mg)	

[1] When administering albendazole in the pre- or post-surgical setting, optimal killing of cyst contents is achieved when three courses of therapy have been given.

Patients being treated for neurocysticercosis should receive appropriate steroid and anticonvulsant therapy as required. Consider oral or IV corticosteroids to prevent cerebral hypertensive episodes during the first week of treatment.

Storage/Stability: Store between 20° and 25°C (68° and 77°F).

Rx	**Albenza** (SmithKline Beecham)	**Tablets:** 200 mg	Lactose, saccharin. Biconvex. In film-coated *Tiltab*. In 112s.

IVERMECTIN

Actions:

Pharmacology: Ivermectin is a semisynthetic anthelmintic agent. It is derived from the avermectins, a class of highly active broad-spectrum anti-parasitic agents isolated from the fermentation products of *Streptomyces avermitilis.*

Compounds of the avermectin class bind selectively and with high affinity to glutamate-gated chloride ion channels that occur in invertebrate nerve and muscle cells. This leads to an increase in the permeability of the cell membrane to chloride ions with hyperpolarization of the nerve or muscle cell, resulting in paralysis and death of the parasite. Compounds of this class may also interact with other ligand-gated chloride channels, such as those gated by the neurotransmitter gamma-aminobutyric acid (GABA).

The selective activity of compounds of this class is attributable to the fact that some mammals do not have glutamate-gated chloride channels and that the avermectins have a low affinity for mammalian ligand-gated chloride channels.

Pharmacokinetics:

Absorption/Distribution – Following oral administration, plasma concentrations are approximately proportional to the dose. In two studies, after single 12 mg doses in fasting, healthy volunteers (representing a mean dose of 165 mcg/kg), the mean peak plasma concentrations of the major component (H_2B_{1a}) were 46.6 ng/ml (range: 16.4 to 101.1) and 30.6 ng/ml (range: 13.9 to 68.4), respectively, at ≈ 4 hours after dosing. The apparent plasma half-life of ivermectin is ≈ 16 hours following oral administration. Ivermectin does not readily cross the blood-brain barrier.

Metabolism/Excretion – Ivermectin is metabolized in the liver, and ivermectin or its metabolites are excreted almost exclusively in the feces over an estimated 12 days, with < 1% of the administered dose excreted in the urine.

Microbiology: Ivermectin is active against various life-cycle stages of many but not all nematodes. It is active against the tissue microfilariae of *Onchocerca volvulus* but not against the adult form. Its activity against *Strongyloides stercoralis* is limited to the intestinal stages.

Clinical trials:

Strongyloidiasis – Two studies showed the efficacy was significantly greater for ivermectin (a single dose of 170 to 200 mcg/kg) than for albendazole (200 mg twice daily for 3 days). Another study showed ivermectin administered as a single dose of 200 mcg/kg for 1 day was as efficacious as thiabendazole administered at 25 mg/kg twice daily for 3 days.

Onchocerciasis – In a double-blind, placebo controlled study involving adult patients with moderate to severe onchocercal infection, patients who received a single dose of 150 mcg/kg ivermectin experienced an 83.2% and 99.5% decrease in skin microfilariae (geometric mean) 3 days and 3 months after the dose, respectively. A marked reduction of > 90% was maintained for up to 12 months after the single dose. As with other microfilaricidal drugs, there was an increase in the microfilariae count in the anterior chamber of the eye at day 3 after treatment in some patients. At 3 and 6 months after the dose, a significantly greater percentage of patients treated with ivermectin had decreases in microfilariae count in the anterior chamber than patients treated with placebo.

Children: In a separate open study involving pediatric patients 6 to 13 years of age (n=103; weight range: 17 to 41 kg), similar decreases in skin microfilariae counts were observed for up to 12 months after dosing.

Indications:

Strongyloidiasis: Treatment of intestinal (eg, nondisseminated) strongyloidiasis caused by the nematode parasite *Strongyloides stercoralis.*

Onchocerciasis: Treatment of onchocerciasis caused by the nematode parasite *Onchocerca volvulus.*

Contraindications:

Hypersensitivity to any component of this product.

Warnings:

Mazzotti reaction: Historical data have shown that microfilaricidal drugs, such as diethylcarbamazine citrate (DEC-C), may cause cutaneous or systemic reactions of varying severity (the Mazzotti reaction) and ophthalmological reactions in patients with onchocerciasis. These reactions are probably caused by allergic and inflammatory responses to the death of microfilariae. Patients treated with ivermectin for onchocerciasis may experience these reactions in addition to clinical adverse reactions possibly, probably or definitely related to the drug itself.

The Mazzotti-type and ophthalmologic reactions associated with the treatment of onchocerciasis or the disease itself would not be expected to occur in strongyloidiasis patients treated with ivermectin.

Oral hydration, recumbency, IV normal saline or parenteral corticosteroids have been used to treat postural hypotension. Antihistamines or aspirin have been used for most mild to moderate Mazzotti reactions.

Ophthalmological conditions were examined in 963 adult patients before treatment, at day 3 and at months 3 and 6 after treatment with 100 to 200 mcg/kg ivermectin. Changes observed were primarily deterioration from baseline 3 days posttreatment. Most changes either returned to baseline condition or improved over baseline severity at the 3– and 6–month visits.

Pregnancy: Category C. Ivermectin was teratogenic in mice, rats and rabbits when given in repeated doses of 0.2, 8.1 and 4.5 times the maximum recommended human dose, respectively (on a mg/m^2/day basis). Teratogenicity was characterized in the three species tested by cleft palate; clubbed forepaws were additionally observed in rabbits. There are no adequate and well controlled studies in pregnant women. Do not use ivermectin during pregnancy because safety in pregnancy has not been established.

Lactation: Ivermectin is excreted in breast milk in low concentrations. Treat mothers who intend to breastfeed only when the risk of delayed treatment to the mother outweighs the possible risk to the newborn.

Children: Safety and efficacy in pediatric patients weighing < 15 kg (33 lbs) have not been established.

Precautions:

Hyperreactive onchodermatitis: After treatment with microfilaricidal drugs, patients with hyperreactive onchodermatitis (sowdah) may be more likely than others to experience severe adverse reactions, especially edema and aggravation of onchodermatitis.

Immunocompromised hosts: In immunocompromised (including HIV-infected) patients being treated for intestinal strongyloidiasis, repeated courses of therapy may be required. Adequate and well controlled clinical studies have not been conducted in such patients to determine the optimal dosing regimen. Several treatments (eg, at 2–week intervals) may be required, and cure may not be achievable. Control of extra-intestinal strongyloidiasis in these patients is difficult, and suppressive therapy (eg, once per month) may be helpful.

Adverse Reactions:

In comparative trials, patients treated with ivermectin experienced more abdominal distention and chest discomfort than patients treated with albendazole. Ivermectin was better tolerated than thiabendazole in comparative studies involving 37 patients treated with thiabendazole.

Strongyloidiasis:

Body as a whole – Asthenia/fatigue, abdominal pain (0.9%).
CNS – Dizziness (2.8%); somnolence, tremor, vertigo (0.9%).
Dermatologic – Pruritus (2.8%); rash, urticaria (0.9%).
GI – Diarrhea, nausea (1.8%); anorexia, constipation, vomiting (0.9%).

Onchocerciasis:

Mazzotti reaction – Pruritus (27.5%); skin involvement including edema, papular and pustular or frank urticarial rash (22.7%); fever (22.6%); inguinal lymph node enlargement and tenderness (12.6% and 13.9%, respectively); axillary lymph node enlargement and tenderness (11% and 4.4%, respectively); arthralgia/synovitis (9.3%); cervical lymph node enlargement and tenderness (5.3% and 1.2%, respectively); other lymph node enlargement and tenderness (3% and 1.9%, respectively). (see Warnings).

Ophthalmologic – Limbitis (4.6%); punctate opacity (1.6%) (see Warnings).

The following ophthalmological side effects occur because of the disease itself but have also been reported after treatment with ivermectin: Abnormal sensation in the eyes; anterior uveitis; chorioretinitis or choroiditis; conjunctivitis; eyelid edema; keratitis; limbitis. These have rarely been severe or associated with loss of vision and have generally resolved without corticosteroid treatment.

Miscellaneous – Tachycardia (3.5%); peripheral edema (3.2%); facial edema (1.2%); orthostatic hypotension (1.1%); headache, myalgia (< 1%); hypotension (mainly orthostatic hypotension); worsening of bronchial asthma.

A similar safety profile was observed in an open study in pediatric patients 6 to 13 years of age.

Lab test abnormalities: Eosinophilia, decrease in leukocyte count (3%); elevation in ALT or AST (2%); hemoglobin increase (1%); leukopenia, anemia (one patient).

Overdosage:

Symptoms: Significant lethality was observed in mice and rats after single oral doses of 25 to 50 mg/kg and 40 to 50 mg/kg, respectively. At these doses, treatment-related signs observed in these animals included ataxia, bradypnea, decreased activity, emesis, mydriasis, ptosis and tremors.

In accidental intoxication with or significant exposure to unknown quantities of veterinary formulations of ivermectin in humans by ingestion, inhalation, injection or exposure to body surfaces, the following adverse effects have been reported most frequently: Asthenia, diarrhea, dizziness, edema, headache, nausea, rash and vomiting. Other adverse effects that have been reported include: Abdominal pain, ataxia, dyspnea, paresthesia, seizure and urticaria.

Treatment: In case of accidental poisoning, supportive therapy, if indicated, should include parenteral fluids and electrolytes, respiratory support (oxygen and mechanical ventilation if necessary) and pressor agents if clinically significant hypotension is present. Induce emesis or gastric lavage as soon as possible, followed by purgatives and other routine anti-poison measures if needed to prevent absorption of ingested material.

Patient Information:

Take ivermectin with water.

Strongyloidiasis: Remind the patient of the need for repeated stool examinations to document clearance of infection.

Onchocerciasis: Remind the patient that treatment with ivermectin does not kill the adult *Onchocerca* parasites; therefore, repeated follow-up and re-treatment is usually required.

Administration and Dosage:

Approved by the FDA in November 1996.

Strongyloidiasis: A single oral dose designed to provide ≈ 200 mcg/kg. Take tablets with water. In general, additional doses are not necessary. However, perform follow-up stool examinations to verify eradication of infection.

Dosage Guidelines for Ivermectin for Strongyloidiasis

Body weight (kg)	Single oral dose (# of tablets)
15-24	0.5
25-35	1
36-50	1.5
51-65	2
66-79	2.5
≥ 80	200 mcg/kg

Onchocerciasis: A single oral dose designed to provide ≈ 150 mcg/kg. Take tablets with water. The most commonly used dose interval is 12 months. For the treatment of individual patients, consider re-treatment at intervals as short as 3 months.

Dosage Guidelines for Ivermectin for Onchocerciasis

Body weight (kg)	Single oral dose (# of tablets)
15-25	0.5
26-44	1
45-64	1.5
65-84	2
≥ 85	150 mcg/kg

Rx	**Stromectol** (Merck)	**Tablets:** 6 mg	(MSD 139). White, scored. Round, flat. In UD 10s.

URINARY ANTI-INFECTIVES

Urinary tract antiseptics and anti-infectives are effective in inhibiting bacterial proliferation in the urinary tract. Concentrated in the renal tubules, these drugs may be used to treat urinary tract infections. They do not generally achieve significant serum or tissue concentrations and are therefore not useful in systemic or localized infections in other tissues. The urinary tract antiseptics have been commonly used for treatment and prevention of urinary tract infections.

Other anti-infective agents with more general utility are considered primary agents for the treatment of acute urinary tract infections (UTIs). These include:

- Aminoglycosides, parenteral
- Cephalosporins
- Fluoroquinolones
- Penicillins
- Sulfonamides
- Tetracyclines
- Trimethoprim
- Trimethoprim/Sulfamethoxazole

See individual monographs for complete prescribing information.

METHYLENE BLUE

Actions:

Pharmacology: Methylene blue is a dye that is a weak germicide and is used as a mild genitourinary antiseptic. However, its use in these conditions is now obsolete; it has largely been replaced by other agents. It is primarily bacteriostatic; bactericidal properties are very mild.

This compound has an oxidation-reduction action and a tissue staining property. In high concentrations, methylene blue converts the ferrous iron of reduced hemoglobin to the ferric form; as a result, methemoglobin is produced. This action is the basis for the antidotal action of methylene blue in cyanide poisoning (see monograph in the Miscellaneous chapter). In contrast, low concentrations of methylene blue are capable of hastening the conversion of methemoglobin to hemoglobin. Oral absorption is reported to be 53% to 97% (74% average).

Indications:

GU antiseptic: A mild genitourinary antiseptic for cystitis and urethritis. However, other agents have replaced methylene blue for this purpose.

Diagnostic: Used as a diagnostic agent and indicator dye.

Methemoglobinemia: For treatment of idiopathic and drug-induced methemoglobinemia

Antidote: Antidote for cyanide poisoning (see individual monograph in the Miscellaneous chapter).

Unlabeled uses: May be useful in the management of patients with oxalate and phosphate urinary tract calculi.

Contraindications:

Renal insufficiency; patients allergic to methylene blue; glucose–6–phosphate dehydrogenase (G-6-PD) deficient patients (methylene blue may induce hemolysis).

Adverse Reactions:

Turns the urine and sometimes the stool and skin blue-green. May cause bladder irritation, and in some cases, nausea, vomiting and diarrhea. Large doses may cause fever.

Patient Information:

Take after meals with a glass of water.

May discolor the urine, skin or stool blue-green.

Administration and Dosage:

Take 65 to 130 mg 3 times daily after meals with a full glass of water.

Rx	**Methblue 65** (Manne Co)	**Tablets:** 65 mg	In 100s and 1000s.
Rx	**Urolene Blue** (Star)		In 100s and 1000s.

NALIDIXIC ACID

Actions:

Pharmacology: Nalidixic acid, a bactericidal agent, appears to interfere with DNA polymerization.

Pharmacokinetics:

Absorption/Distribution – Nalidixic acid is well absorbed; peak serum levels of 20 to 40 mcg/ml are attained 1 to 2 hours after an oral 1 g dose. The drug concentrates in renal tissue and seminal fluid; it does not penetrate prostatic tissue.

Metabolism/Excretion – Hepatic metabolism to hydroxynalidixic acid (activity similar to nalidixic acid) and inactive conjugates is followed by rapid renal excretion. Protein binding is ≈ 93% to 97% for nalidixic acid and 63% for hydroxynalidixic acid. Approximately 2% to 3% of nalidixic acid and 13% of hydroxynalidixic acid appear in the urine. Plasma half-life in normal renal function is 1.5 hours; half-life in urine is about 6 hours. Renal failure significantly affects renal clearance of nalidixic acid, increasing serum concentrations and decreasing urine levels of parent and metabolites. Approximately 4% of nalidixic acid is excreted in the feces.

Microbiology: Nalidixic acid is bactericidal and has marked antibacterial activity over the urinary pH against gram-negative bacteria (eg, *Proteus mirabilis, P morganii, P vulgaris, Providencia rettgeri, Escherichia coli, Enterobacter* and *Klebsiella* species). *Pseudomonas* strains are generally resistant. Conventional chromosomal resistance to full dosage emerges in ≈ 2% to 14% of patients during treatment.

Indications:

Urinary tract infections caused by susceptible gram-negative microorganisms, including the majority of *Proteus* strains, *Klebsiella* and *Enterobacter* species and *E coli.*

Contraindications:

Hypersensitivity to nalidixic acid; history of convulsive disorders.

Warnings:

CNS: Brief convulsions, increased intracranial pressure and toxic psychosis (rare) usually occur from overdosage or with predisposing factors, such as epilepsy, cerebral vascular insufficiency, parkinsonism, mental instability or cerebral arteriosclerosis. They usually rapidly disappear upon drug discontinuation. If these reactions occur, discontinue use and institute therapeutic measures. If CNS symptoms do not disappear within 48 hours, perform diagnostic procedures even if risky to the patient. In infants and children receiving therapeutic doses, intracranial hypertension, increased intracranial pressure with bulging anterior fontanelle, papilledema and headache have occasionally occurred. A few cases of sixth cranial nerve palsy were reported. Signs and symptoms usually disappear rapidly upon discontinuation.

Hematologic: Nalidixic acid has caused hemolytic anemia in patients with or without glucose–6–phosphate dehydrogenase deficiency (G-6-PD).

Renal function impairment: Therapeutic concentrations in the urine, without increased toxicity due to drug accumulation in the blood, have occurred in patients on full dosage with creatinine clearances as low as 2 to 8 ml/min. However, exercise caution.

Pregnancy: Category B. Safe use during the first trimester has not been established. The drug has been used during the last two trimesters without apparent ill effects on mother or child. No drug-linked congenital defects have been reported.

Labor and delivery – Use caution when giving nalidixic acid in the days prior to delivery because of the theoretical risk that exposure in utero may lead to significant blood levels in the neonate immediately after birth. Advise patients using nalidixic acid during pregnancy to discontinue use at the first sign of labor.

Lactation: Data are scant; reported milk:plasma ratios are 0.08 to 0.13. Milk levels of 4 mcg/ml have been noted. Although the amounts are small, hemolytic anemia has been reported in one infant whose mother received 1 g nalidixic acid, 4 times/day.

Children: Nalidixic acid and related drugs can produce erosions of the cartilage in weight-bearing joints and other signs of arthropathy in animals. No joint lesions have been reported in humans; however, use care in prepubertal children.

Precautions:

Monitoring: Perform periodic blood counts and renal and liver function tests if treatment is continued for > 2 weeks.

Special risk patients: Use with caution in liver disease, epilepsy or severe cerebral arteriosclerosis patients.

Resistance: If bacterial resistance emerges, it is usually within 48 hours, permitting rapid change to another drug. If clinical response is unsatisfactory or if relapse occurs, repeat cultures and sensitivity tests. Underdosage (< 4 g/day for adults) may predispose to resistance. Cross-resistance with cinoxacin has occurred.

NALIDIXIC ACID

Photosensitivity: Photosensitization (photoallergy or phototoxicity) may occur; therefore, caution patients to take protective measures against exposure to ultraviolet or sunlight (ie, sunscreens, protective clothing) until tolerance is determined.

Drug Interactions:

Anticoagulants: Nalidixic acid may enhance the anticoagulant effects by displacing significant amounts of these drugs from serum albumin binding sites.

Drug/Lab test interactions: Urinary metabolites of nalidixic acid liberate glucuronic acid and produce false-positive **urinary glucose** results when Benedict's or Fehling's solutions or Clinitest reagent tablets are used. Avoid this problem by using Clinistix or Tes-Tape. **Urinary 17–keto and ketogenic steroids** may be falsely elevated due to an interaction between nalidixic acid and the m–dinitrobenzene used in the assay. In such cases, use the Porter-Silber method.

Adverse Reactions:

CNS: Drowsiness; weakness; headache; dizziness; vertigo; toxic psychosis, brief convulsions (rare); intracranial hypertension; increased intracranial pressure with bulging anterior fontanel, papilledema and headache; sixth cranial nerve palsy in children and infants (see Warnings).

Ophthalmic: Reversible subjective visual disturbances occur infrequently (generally with each dose during the first few days) and include overbrightness of lights, change in color perception, focusing difficulty, decrease in visual acuity and double vision. They usually disappear promptly with reduced dosage or discontinuation.

GI: Abdominal pain; nausea; vomiting; diarrhea.

Hypersensitivity: Rash; pruritus; urticaria; angioedema; eosinophilia; arthralgia with joint stiffness and swelling; anaphylactoid reaction (rare).

Hematologic: Thrombocytopenia, leukopenia or hemolytic anemia, sometimes associated with G-6-PD deficiency (rare).

Miscellaneous: Cholestatic jaundice, cholestasis, paresthesia, metabolic acidosis (rare).

Photosensitivity reactions (eg, erythema and painful bullae on exposed skin surfaces) usually resolve completely in 2 weeks to 2 months after discontinuing the drug. However, bullae may continue to appear with successive exposures to sunlight or with mild skin trauma for up to 3 months after discontinuation.

Overdosage:

Symptoms: Toxic psychosis, convulsions, increased intracranial pressure, metabolic acidosis, vomiting, nausea and lethargy may occur in patients taking more than the recommended dosage.

Treatment: Reactions are short lived (2 to 3 hours) because the drug is rapidly excreted. If overdosage is noted early, gastric lavage is indicated. If absorption has occurred, increase fluid administration and have supportive measures available. Anticonvulsants may be indicated in severe cases.

Patient Information:

May cause GI upset; take with food.

May produce drowsiness, dizziness or blurred vision; observe caution while driving or performing other tasks requiring alertness, coordination or physical dexterity.

Avoid prolonged exposure to sunlight; photosensitivity may occur.

If seizures, psychotic behavior (eg, hallucinations, incoherent speech, confusion) or severe headaches occur while on nalidixic acid, contact the physician immediately.

Administration and Dosage:

Underdosage (< 4 g/day) during initial treatment may predispose to emergence of bacterial resistance.

Adults:

Initial therapy – 1 g 4 times/day (total dose 4 g/day) for 1 or 2 weeks.

Prolonged therapy – May be reduced to 2 g/day after the initial treatment period.

Children (3 months to ≤ 12 years of age):

Initial therapy – 55 mg/kg/day (25 mg/lb/day) in 4 equally divided doses.

Prolonged therapy – May be reduced to 33 mg/kg/day (15 mg/lb/day).

Do not administer to infants < 3 months of age.

Rx	**NegGram** (Sanofi Winthrop)	**Caplets:** 250 mg	Scored. In 56s.
		500 mg	Scored. In 56s and 500s.
		1 g	Scored. In 100s.
		Suspension: 250 mg per 5 ml	Saccharin, sorbitol. Raspberry flavor. In 480 ml.

CINOXACIN

Actions:

Pharmacology: Cinoxacin, a synthetic organic acid chemically related to nalidixic acid, inhibits DNA replication. The drug is active within the range of urinary pH.

Pharmacokinetics:

Absorption/Distribution – Cinoxacin is rapidly absorbed after oral administration. Mean peak plasma concentrations of 15 mcg/ml occur ≈ 2 hours after a single 500 mg dose and detectable levels persist 10 to 12 hours. Food decreases peak serum concentrations by about 30%, although the total extent of absorption is not altered. It is > 60% protein bound.

Metabolism/Excretion – Average urine concentrations of 300 mcg/ml occur within 4 hours; urine concentrations usually exceed the MIC (ie, 10 to 30 mcg/ml). The mean serum half-life is 1 to 1.5 hours with normal renal function; renal failure increases half-life. Oral cinoxacin is 97% excreted in the urine within 24 hours. Approximately 60% of cinoxacin is excreted unchanged, 40% as inactive metabolites.

Microbiology: Cinoxacin has in vitro activity against a wide variety of aerobic gram-negative bacilli, particularly strains of *Enterobacteriaceae.* It is active against most strains of the following organisms: *Escherichia coli, Klebsiella* sp, *Enterobacter* sp *Proteus mirabilis* and *P vulgaris.*

Cinoxacin is NOT active against Pseudomonas, enterococci or staphylococci. Cross-resistance with nalidixic acid has been demonstrated. Conventional chromosomal resistance to cinoxacin has been reported in ≈ 4% of patients treated with recommended doses; bacterial resistance to cinoxacin has not been shown to be transferable via R-factor (plasmids).

Indications:

Urinary tract infections: Treatment of initial and recurrent urinary tract infections in adults caused by the following susceptible microorganisms: *E coli, P mirabilis, P vulgaris, Klebsiella* sp (including *K pneumoniae*) and *Enterobacter* sp.

Effective in preventing urinary tract infections for up to 5 months in women with a history of recurrent urinary tract infections.

Contraindications:

Hypersensitivity to cinoxacin or other quinolones.

Warnings:

Convulsions and abnormal EEGs have been reported in a few patients receiving quinolone class antimicrobials. Convulsions, increased intracranial pressure and toxic psychoses have also occurred in patients receiving other drugs in this class.

Quinolones may also cause CNS stimulation with tremors, restlessness, lightheadedness, confusion or hallucinations. If these reactions occur in patients receiving cinoxacin, discontinue the drug and institute appropriate measures. As with all quinolones, use with caution in patients with known or suspected CNS disorders (eg, severe cerebral arteriosclerosis, epilepsy) that predispose to seizures.

Hypersensitivity: Serious and occasionally fatal hypersensitivity (anaphylactic) reactions, some following the first dose, have occurred in patients receiving quinolone class antimicrobials. Some reactions were accompanied by cardiovascular collapse, loss of consciousness, tingling, pharyngeal or facial edema, dyspnea, urticaria and itching. Only a few patients had a history of previous hypersensitivity reactions. If an allergic reaction to cinoxacin occurs, discontinue the drug. Refer to Management of Acute Hypersensitivity Reactions.

Renal function impairment: Since cinoxacin is primarily eliminated by the kidney, decrease dosage in patients with reduced renal function. Administration is not recommended for anuric patients.

Pregnancy: Category B. There are no adequate and well controlled studies in pregnant women. Since cinoxacin causes arthropathy in immature animals (see Children), its use during pregnancy is not recommended.

Lactation: It is not known whether cinoxacin is excreted in breast milk. Because other drugs in this class are excreted in breast milk and because of the potential for serious adverse reactions in nursing infants, discontinue nursing or discontinue the drug, taking into account the importance of the drug to the mother.

Children: Safety and efficacy of use in adolescents and children < 18 years of age have not been established. Cinoxacin and other quinolones have produced erosions of the cartilage in weight-bearing joints and other signs of arthropathy in immature animals of various species.

Precautions:

Monitoring: As with any potent drug, periodic assessment of organ system function, including renal, hepatic and hematopoietic function is advisable during prolonged therapy.

CINOXACIN

Crystalluria: Although not expected to occur with usual cinoxacin doses, patients should be well hydrated; avoid alkalinization of urine.

Hazardous tasks: Patients should use caution while driving or performing other tasks requiring alertness, coordination or physical dexterity.

Photosensitivity: Photosensitization (photoallergy or phototoxicity) may occur; therefore, caution patients to take protective measures against exposure to ultraviolet or sunlight (ie, sunscreens, protective clothing) until tolerance is determined.

Drug Interactions:

Probenecid pretreatment will block tubule secretion of cinoxacin, and thus, will reduce the elimination rate, increase half-life, decrease urine concentrations by 20% and double serum concentrations.

Also consider drug interactions listed with the Fluoroquinolones (see monograph in Anti-Infectives chapter).

Drug/Food interactions: Food decreases peak serum cinoxacin by ≈ 30%, although total extent of absorption is not altered.

Adverse Reactions:

The overall incidence of adverse reactions is approximately 4%.

GI: Nausea (< 3%); anorexia, vomiting, abdominal cramps/pain, diarrhea, perineal burning, distorted taste sensation (1%).

CNS: Headache, dizziness (1%); insomnia, drowsiness, tingling sensation, photophobia, tinnitus (< 1%).

Hypersensitivity: Rash, urticaria, pruritus, edema, angioedema, eosinophilia (< 3%); anaphylactoid reactions (rare); toxic epidermal necrolysis (very rare); erythema multiforme; Stevens-Johnson syndrome.

Hematologic: Thrombocytopenia (rare).

Lab test abnormalities: Laboratory values reported to be abnormally elevated were, in order of frequency – BUN, AST, ALT, serum creatinine, alkaline phosphatase and reduction in hematocrit/hemoglobin (each ≤ 1%).

Overdosage:

Symptoms: Anorexia, nausea, vomiting epigastric distress and diarrhea may follow an overdose of cinoxacin. The severity of epigastric distress and the diarrhea are dose-related. Headache, dizziness, insomnia, photophobia, tinnitus and a tingling sensation have occurred in some patients. If other symptoms are present, they are probably secondary to an underlying disease state, an allergic reaction or the ingestion of a second medication with toxicity.

Treatment: Patients who have ingested an overdose of cinoxacin shoud be kept well hydrated to prevent crystalluria. Protect the patient's airway and support ventilation and perfusion. Meticulously monitor and maintain, within acceptable limits, the patient's vital signs, blood gases, serum electrolytes, etc. Absorption of drugs from the GI tract may be decreased by giving activated charcoal, which, in many cases, is more effective than emesis or lavage. Forced diuresis, peritoneal dialysis, hemodialysis or charcoal hemoperfusion have not been established as beneficial for a cinoxacin overdose. Refer to General Management of Acute Overdosage.

CINOXACIN

Patient Information:

May be taken without regard to meals, but drink fluids liberally.

May cause dizziness; observe caution while driving or performing other tasks requiring alertness, coordination or physical dexterity.

Avoid excessive sunlight during therapy. If phototoxicity occurs, discontinue therapy.

Administration and Dosage:

The usual adult dosage is 1 g/day, in 2 or 4 divided doses for 7 to 14 days. Although susceptible organisms may be eradicated within a few days after therapy has begun, the full treatment course is recommended.

Renal function impairment: A reduced dosage must be employed. After an initial dose of 500 mg, use the following maintenance dosage schedule:

Cinoxacin Maintenance Dosage Guide for Renal Impairment

Creatinine clearance (ml/min/1.73 m^2)	Renal Function	Dosage
> 80	Normal	500 mg bid
80-50	Mild impairment	250 mg tid
50-20	Moderate impairment	250 mg bid
< 20	Marked impairment	250 mg daily

Administration of cinoxacin to anuric patients is not recommended.

When only serum creatinine is available, use the following formula to convert this value into creatinine clearance. The serum creatinine should represent a steady-state of renal function.

$$\text{Males: } \frac{\text{Weight (kg)} \times (140 - \text{age})}{72 \times \text{serum creatinine (mg/dl)}} = \text{Ccr}$$

$$\text{Females: } 0.85 \times \text{above value}$$

Preventive therapy: A single dose of 250 mg at bedtime for up to 5 months has been shown to be effective in women with a history of recurrent urinary tract infections.

Rx	**Cinobac** (Oclassen)	**Capsules:** 250 mg	Orange and green. In 40s.
Rx	**Cinoxacin** (Biocraft)		(Biocraft 163). Blue/yellow. In 40s and 100s.
Rx	**Cinoxacin** (Various, eg, Biocraft, Goldline, Moore, Rugby)	**Capsules:** 500 mg	In 50s and 100s.
Rx	**Cinobac** (Oclassen)		Orange and green. In 50s.

FOSFOMYCIN TROMETHAMINE

Actions:

Pharmacology: Fosfomycin is a synthetic, broad-spectrum bactericidal antibiotic for oral administration.

Fosfomycin has in vitro activity against a broad range of gram-positive and gram-negative aerobic microorganisms which are associated with uncomplicated urinary tract infections. Fosfomycin is bactericidal in urine at therapeutic doses. The bactericidal action of fosfomycin is because of its inactivation of the enzyme enolpyruvyl transferase, thereby irreversibly blocking the condensation of uridine diphosphate-N-acetylglucosamine with p-enolpyruvate, one of the first steps in bacterial cell wall synthesis. It also reduces adherence of bacteria to uroepithelial cells.

Pharmacokinetics:

Absorption – Fosfomycin is rapidly absorbed following oral administration and converted to the free acid fosfomycin. Absolute oral bioavailability under fasting conditions is 37%. After a single 3 g dose, the mean maximum serum concentration (C_{max}) achieved was 26.1 mcg/ml within 2 hours. The oral bioavailability is reduced to 30% under fed conditions. Following a single 3 g oral dose with a high-fat meal, the mean C_{max} achieved was 17.6 mcg/ml within 4 hours.

Distribution – The mean apparent steady-state volume of distribution is 136.1 L following oral administration. It is not bound to plasma proteins.

Fosfomycin is distributed to the kidneys, bladder wall, prostate and seminal vesicles. Following a 50 mg/kg dose to patients undergoing urological surgery for bladder carcinoma, the mean concentration in the bladder, taken at a distance from the neoplastic site, was 18 mcg/g of tissue at 3 hours after dosing. Fosfomycin crosses the placental barrier.

Excretion – Fosfomycin is excreted unchanged in both urine and feces. Following oral administration, the mean total body clearance and mean renal clearance were 16.8 and 6.3 L/hr, respectively. Approximately 38% of a 3 g dose is recovered from urine and 18% is recovered from feces. Following IV administration, the mean total body clearance and mean renal clearance of fosfomycin were 6.1 L/hr and 5.5 L/hr, respectively.

A mean urine fosfomycin concentration of 706 mcg/ml was attained within 2 to 4 hours after a single oral 3 g dose under fasting conditions. The mean urinary concentration was 10 mcg/ml in samples collected 72 to 84 hours following a single oral dose.

Following a 3 g dose administered with a high fat meal, a mean urine concentration of 537 mcg/ml was attained within 6 to 8 hours. Although the rate of urinary excretion was reduced under fed conditions, the cumulative amount of fosfomycin excreted in the urine was the same, 1118 mg (fed) vs 1140 mg (fasting). Further, urinary concentrations ≥ 100 mcg/ml were maintained for the same duration, 26 hours, indicating that fosfomycin can be taken without regard to food. Following oral administration, the mean half-life for elimination ($t_{1/2}$) is 5.7 hours.

Renal function impairment: In five patients undergoing hemodialysis, the $t_{1/2}$ of fosfomycin during hemodialysis was 40 hours. In patients with varying degrees of renal impairment (creatinine clearances varying from 54 to 7 ml/min), the $t_{1/2}$ increased from 11 hours to 50 hours. The percent of fosfomycin recovered in urine decreased from 32% to 11% indicating that renal impairment significantly decreases the excretion of fosfomycin.

Microbiology: There is generally no cross-resistance between fosfomycin and other classes of antibacterial agents such as beta-lactams and aminoglycosides.

Fosfomycin has been shown to be active against most strains of the following microorganisms, both in vitro and in clinical infections:

Aerobic gram-positive microorganisms – Enterococcus faecalis.

Aerobic gram-negative microorganisms – Escherichia coli.

Fosfomycin exhibits in vitro minimum inhibitory concentrations of ≤ 64 mcg/ml against most (≥ 90%) strains of the following microorganisms; however, the safety and effectiveness of fosfomycin in treating clinical infections caused by these microorganisms has not been established in adequate and well controlled clinical trials:

Aerobic gram-positive microorganisms – Enterococcus faecium.

Aerobic gram-negative microorganisms – Citrobacter diversus; Citrobacter freundii; Enterobacter aerogenes; Klebsiella oxytoca; Klebsiella pneumoniae; Proteus mirabilis; Proteus vulgaris; Serratia marcescens.

Clinical trials: In controlled studies of acute cystitis, a single dose of fosfomycin was compared with three other oral antibiotics. Based on differences in microbiologic eradication rates at 5 to 11 days post-therapy, fosfomycin was inferior to ciprofloxacin and trimethoprim/sulfamethoxazole and equivalent to nitrofurantoin.

Indications:

Uncomplicated urinary tract infections: Treatment of uncomplicated urinary tract infections (acute cystitis) in women caused by susceptible strains of *E. coli* and *E. faecalis.* Fosfomycin is not indicated for the treatment of pyelonephritis or perinephric abscess.

Contraindications:

Known hypersensitivity to the drug.

Warnings:

Elderly: Based on limited data regarding 24–hour urinary drug concentrations, no differences in urinary excretion of fosfomycin have been observed in elderly subjects. No dosage adjustment is necessary in the elderly. There were no clinically significant differences in the bacteriological effectiveness or safety profiles of fosfomycin for women > 65 years of age.

Pregnancy: Category B. When administered IM as the sodium salt at a dose of 1 g to pregnant women, fosfomycin crosses the placental barrier. However, there are no adequate and well controlled studies in pregnant women. Use this drug during pregnancy only if clearly needed.

Lactation: It is not known whether fosfomycin is excreted in breast milk. Decide whether to discontinue nursing or to discontinue the drug, taking into account the importance of the drug to the mother.

Children: Safety and efficacy in children ≤ 12 years of age have not been established.

Precautions:

Acute cystitis: Do not use more than one single dose of fosfomycin to treat a single episode of acute cystitis. Repeated daily doses of fosfomycin did not improve the clinical success or microbiological eradication rates compared with single dose therapy, but did increase the incidence of adverse events.

Drug Interactions:

Metoclopramide: When coadministered with fosfomycin, metoclopramide lowers the serum concentration and urinary excretion of fosfomycin. Other drugs that increase GI motility may produce similar effects.

Adverse Reactions:

Adverse Reactions in Fosfomycin and Comparator Populations (%)

Adverse reaction	Fosfomycin (n = 1233)	Nitrofurantoin (n = 374)	Trimethoprim/ Sulfamethoxazole (n = 428)	Ciprofloxacin (n = 445)
Diarrhea	9	6.4	2.3	3.1
Vaginitis	5.5	5.3	4.7	6.3
Rhinitis	4.5	-	-	-
Nausea	4.1	7.2	8.6	3.4
Headache	3.9	5	5.4	3.4
Back pain	3	-	-	-
Dysmenorrhea	2.6	-	-	-
Pharyngitis	2.5	-	-	-
Abdominal pain	2.2	+	+	1.7
Rash	1.4	+	+	1.1
Dizziness	1.3	1.8	2.3	2.2
Dyspepsia	1.1	2.1	0.7	1.1
Asthenia	1.1	0.3	0.5	0

+ Occurs, but significance is unknown.

The following adverse events occurred in clinical trials at a rate of < 1%: Abnormal stools, anorexia, constipation, dry mouth, dysuria, ear disorder, fever, flatulence, flu syndrome, hematuria, infection, insomnia, lymphadenopathy, menstrual disorder, migraine, myalgia, nervousness, paresthesia, pruritus, ALT increased, skin disorder, somnolence, vomiting, unilateral optic neuritis (one patient).

FOSFOMYCIN TROMETHAMINE

Post-marketing experience: Angioedema, aplastic anemia, asthma (exacerbation), cholestatic jaundice, hepatic necrosis, toxic megacolon (all rare).

Lab test abnormalities: Increased eosinophil count, increased or decreased WBC count, increased bilirubin, increased ALT, increased AST, increased alkaline phosphatase, decreased hematocrit, decreased hemoglobin, increased and decreased platelet count. The changes were generally transient and were not clinically significant.

Overdosage:

In acute toxicology studies, oral administration of high doses of fosfomycin up to 5 g/kg were well-tolerated in mice and rats, produced transient and minor incidences of watery stool in rabbits, and produced diarrhea with anorexia in dogs 2 to 3 days after single-dose administration. These doses represent 50 to 125 times the human therapeutic dose.

There have been no reported cases of overdosage. In the event of overdosage, treatment should be symptomatic and supportive. Refer to General Management of Acute Overdosage.

Patient Information:

Fosfomycin can be taken with or without food.

Symptoms should improve in 2 to 3 days after taking fosfomycin; if not improved, the patient should contact their health care provider.

Do not take in its dry form. Always mix fosfomycin with water before ingesting.

Administration and Dosage:

Approved by the FDA on December 19, 1996.

The recommended dosage for women ≥ 18 years of age for uncomplicated urinary tract infection (acute cystitis) is one packet of fosfomycin. Fosfomycin may be taken with or without food.

Do not take in its dry form. Always mix fosfomycin with water before ingesting.

Pour the entire contents of a single-dose packet of fosfomycin into 90 to 120 ml (3 to 4 ounces) of water and stir to dissolve. Do not use hot water. Take immediately after dissolving in water.

Rx	**Monurol** (Forest)	**Granules:** 3 g	In single-dose packets.

NITROFURANTOIN

Actions:

Pharmacology: Nitrofurantoin is a synthetic nitrofuran that is bacteriostatic in low concentrations (5 to 10 mcg/ml) and bactericidal in higher concentrations. Nitrofurantoin may inhibit acetylcoenzyme A, interfering with bacterial carbohydrate metabolism. It may also disrupt bacterial cell wall formation.

Pharmacokinetics:

Absorption/Distribution – Well absorbed from the GI tract after oral administration. The macrocrystalline form is absorbed more slowly due to slower dissolution and causes less GI distress. Bioavailability of micro- and macrocrystalline forms is enhanced by concomitant ingestion of food. Therapeutic serum and tissue concentrations are not achieved after usual oral doses, except in the urinary tract. Protein binding is about 60%.

Metabolism/Excretion – Approximately 50% to 70% of the drug is rapidly metabolized by body tissues. The plasma half-life is about 20 minutes in healthy individuals and increases to 60 minutes in the anephric patient. In patients with impaired renal function, nitrofurantoin accumulates in the serum. Renal excretion is via glomerular filtration and tubular secretion. About 30% to 50% of a dose is excreted unchanged in the urine. Usual doses produce urinary levels of 50 to 250 mcg/ml in patients with normal renal function. If creatinine clearance is < 40 ml/min, antibacterial concentrations attained in the urine are inadequate, and the subsequent elevated blood levels increase the danger of toxicity. Antibacterial activity is greater in an acidic urine. Acid urine enhances tubular reabsorption of nitrofurantoin, enhancing antibacterial activity in the renal tissues and lowering urinary concentrations. However, do not alkalinize urine to increase urinary concentration of nitrofurantoin, because the antimicrobial activity is decreased at a higher pH.

Microbiology: The MIC in urine for most susceptible organisms is ≤ 32 mcg/ml. Resistant species generally have an MIC of ≥ 100 mcg/ml. Most gram-negative bacilli and gram-positive cocci associated with urinary tract infections are susceptible, including: *Escherichia coli, Klebsiella* and *Enterobacter* sp, enterococci (eg, *Enterococcus faecalis*), *Staphylococcus aureus* and *S saprophyticus.* Some strains of *Enterobacter* and *Klebsiella* sp are resistant. Most strains of *Proteus* and *Serratia* species are resistant. It has no activity against *Pseudomonas* sp. Susceptible bacteria do not readily develop resistance to nitrofurantoin during therapy. However, plasmid-mediated, transferable resistance has been demonstrated. Although in vitro susceptibility of *Salmonella, Shegella, Neisseria, Streptococcus pyogenes, S pneumoniae, Corynebacterium* and many anaerobes has been demonstrated, nitrofurantoin is of little clinical importance for infections caused by these organisms.

Indications:

Urinary tract infections: Treatment of urinary tract infections due to susceptible strains of *E coli*, enterococci, *S aureus* (not for treatment of pyelonephritis or perinephric abscesses) and certain strains of *Klebsiella* and *Enterobacter* species.

Contraindications:

Renal function impairment (creatinine clearance < 60 ml/min), anuria or oliguria (treatment is much less effective and carries an increased risk of toxicity because of impaired excretion of the drug); hypersensitivity to nitrofurantoin.

Pregnant patients at term, during labor and delivery, or when the onset of labor is imminent, and in infants under 1 month of age (possibility of hemolytic anemia due to immature enzyme systems [glutathione instability]).

Warnings:

Pulmonary reactions:

Acute – Manifested by sudden onset of dyspnea, chest pain, cough, fever and chills, pulmonary infiltration with consolidation or pleural effusion on x-ray; elevated sedimentation rate and eosinophilia are also present. Resolution of clinical and radiological abnormalities occurs within 24 to 48 hours after discontinuation. Rechallenge is dangerous and will produce similar symptoms.

Subacute/chronic – Associated with prolonged therapy. These reactions are characterized by insidious development of dyspnea, nonproductive cough and malaise after 1 to 6 months or more of therapy. Pulmonary function tests demonstrate a restrictive pattern. Radiographs show an interstitial pneumonitis. Usually, symptoms regress with discontinuation of the drug over weeks to months. Pulmonary function may be permanently impaired, even after cessation of nitrofurantoin. Death has been reported.

Hemolysis: Hemolytic anemia of the primaquine sensitivity type has been induced by nitrofurantoin. The hemolysis appears to be linked to a glucose-6-phosphate dehydrogenase (G-6-PD) deficiency in the red blood cells of affected patients. At any sign of hemolysis, discontinue the drug. Hemolysis ceases when the drug is withdrawn.

Hepatic reactions including hepatitis, cholestatic jaundice, chronic active hepatitis, and hepatic necrosis, occur rarely. Fatalities have been reported. The onset of chronic active hepatitis may be insidious. Periodically monitor patients receiving long-term therapy for changes in liver function. If hepatitis occurs, withdraw the drug and take appropriate measures.

Pregnancy: Category B. In mice, at doses of 19 and 68 times the human dose, induction of papillary adenomas, growth retardation and a low incidence of minor and common malformations occurred. Safety for use during pregnancy has not been established. Use in women of childbearing potential only when clearly needed and when the potential benefits outweigh the potential hazards to the fetus. Do not give to pregnant patients with G–6–PD deficiency because of the risk of hemolysis in the mother and fetus, although fetal hemolysis has not been documented. Contraindicated in pregnant women at term.

Labor and delivery – Nitrofurantoin use is contraindicated during labor and delivery. See Contraindications.

Lactation: Nitrofurantoin is excreted into breast milk in very low concentrations. Concentrations of 0.3 to 0.5 mcg/ml were reported in two women who received 100 mg nitrofurantoin every 6 hours for 1 day followed by either 100 or 200 mg the next morning. However, infants with G–6–PD deficiency may be adversely affected. Safety for use in the nursing mother has not been established.

Children: Contraindicated in infants < 1 month of age. See Contraindications.

Precautions:

Monitoring: Obtain specimens for culture and susceptibility testing prior to and during drug administration.

Peripheral neuropathy may occur and may become severe or irreversible. Fatalities have been reported. Predisposing conditions such as renal impairment, anemia, diabetes, electrolyte imbalance, vitamin B deficiency and debilitating disease may enhance such occurrences.

Superinfection: Use of antibiotics (especially prolonged or repeated therapy) may result in bacterial or fungal overgrowth of nonsusceptible organisms. Such overgrowth may lead to a secondary infection. Take appropriate measures if superinfection occurs.

Drug Interactions:

Nitrofurantoin Drug Interactions			
Precipitant drug	Object drug*		Description
Anticholinergics	Nitrofurantoin	⬇	Anticholinergic drugs increase nitrofurantoin bioavailability by delaying gastric emptying and increasing absorption.
Magnesium salts	Nitrofurantoin	⬇	Magnesium salts may delay or decrease the absorption of nitrofurantoin.
Uricosurics	Nitrofurantoin	⬇	Administration of high doses of probenecid with nitrofurantoin decreases renal clearance and increases serum levels of nitrofurantoin. The result could be increased toxic effects.

* ⬆ = Object drug increased.

Drug/Lab test interactions: A false-positive reaction for glucose in the urine may occur. This has been observed with Benedict's and Fehling's solutions but not with the glucose enzymatic test.

Drug/Food interactions: Bioavailability of nitrofurantoin is increased by food.

Adverse Reactions:

GI: Anorexia, nausea, emesis (most frequent); abdominal pain, diarrhea parotitis, pancreatitis (less frequent).

Hepatic: Hepatic reactions, including hepatitis, cholestatic jaundice, chronic active hepatitis and hepatic necrosis (rare).

Pulmonary: Sensitivity reactions (acute, subacute or chronic) are documented with outcomes ranging from complete resolution to death. See Warnings.

Dermatologic: Exfoliative dermatitis and erythema multiforme (including Stevens-Johnson syndrome) have been reported rarely; maculopapular, erythematous or eczematous eruption; pruritus; urticaria; angioedema.

Hypersensitivity: Anaphylaxis; asthmatic attack in patients with history of asthma; drug fever; arthralgia; myalgia; chills; sialadenitis.

NITROFURANTOIN

Hematologic: Glucose-6–phosphate dehydrogenase deficiency anemia (see Warnings); granulocytopenia; agranulocytosis; leukopenia; thrombocytopenia; eosinophilia; megaloblastic anemia; hemolytic anemia. In most cases, these hematologic abnormalities resolved following cessation of therapy. Aplastic anemia (rare).

CNS: Peripheral neuropathy (see Precautions); headache; dizziness; nystagmus; drowsiness; asthenia; vertigo; confusion; depression; euphoria, psychotic reactions (rare).

Miscellaneous: Transient alopecia; superinfections in GU tract by resistant organisms; benign sintracranial hypertension; changes in ECG; collapse; cyanosis; a lupus-like syndrome associated with pulmonary reactions; muscular aches.

Lab test abnormalities: Increased AST, increased ALT, decreased hemoglobin, increased serum phosphorus.

Overdosage:

Symptoms: Occasional incidents of acute overdosage of nitrofurantoin have not resulted in any specific symptoms other than vomiting.

Treatment: Induction of emesis is recommended. There is no specific antidote, but a high fluid intake should be maintained to promote urinary excretion of the drug. It is dialyzable.

Patient Information:

Complete full course of therapy; do not discontinue without notifying physician.

May cause GI upset; take with food or milk.

May cause brown discoloration of the urine.

Notify physician if fever, chills, cough, chest pain, difficult breathing, skin rash, numbness or tingling of the fingers or toes, or intolerable GI upset occurs.

Administration and Dosage:

Give with food or milk to improve drug absorption and, in some patients, tolerance. Continue for at least 1 week, or for at least 3 days after sterile urine is obtained. Continued infection indicates need for reevaluation.

Adults: 50 to 100 mg 4 times/day with meals and at bedtime. For long-term suppressive therapy, reduce dosage (50 to 100 mg at bedtime).

Children: 5 to 7 mg/kg/24 hrs given in 4 divided doses. For long-term suppressive therapy, doses as low as 1 mg/kg/24 hrs, given in single or in 2 divided doses, may be adequate. Contraindicated in children less than 1 month of age.

The following table is based on an average weight in each range receiving 5 to 6 mg/kg of body weight per 24 hours, given in four divided doses. It can be used to calculate an average dose of oral suspension (5 mg/ml).

Nitrofurantoin Dosage in Children Based on Body Weight

Body weight		No. of teaspoonsful
lbs	kg	4 times a day
15 to 26	7 to 11	½ (2.5 ml)
27 to 46	12 to 21	1 (5 ml)
47 to 68	22 to 30	1½ (7.5 ml)
69 to 91	31 to 41	2 (10 ml)

Rx	**Furadantin** (Dura)	**Oral Suspension:** 25 mg per 5 ml	Saccharin, sorbitol. In 60 and 470 ml.

NITROFURANTOIN MACROCRYSTALS

The large crystal size improves GI tolerance.

Rx	**Macrodantin** (Procter & Gamble Pharm)	**Capsules:** 25 mg	(Macrodantin 25 mg 0149–0007). White. In 100s.
Rx	**Nitrofurantoin** (Various, eg, Goldline, Major, Moore, Rugby, URL, Warner Chilcott, Zenith)	**Capsules:** 50 mg	In 100s, 500s and 1000s.
Rx	**Macrodantin** (Procter & Gamble Pharm.)		(Macrodantin 50 mg 0149–0008). Yellow/white. In 100s, 500s, 1000s and UD 100s.
Rx	**Nitrofurantoin** (Various, eg, Goldline, Major, Moore, Rugby, URL, Warner Chilcott, Zenith)	**Capsules:** 100 mg	In 100s, 500s and 1000s.
Rx	**Macrodantin** (Procter & Gamble Pharm)		(Macrodantin 100 mg 0149–0009). Yellow. In 100s, 500s, 1000s and UD 100s.
Rx	**Macrobid** (Procter & Gamble Pharm)	**Capsules:** 100 mg (as 25 mg macrocrystals, 75 mg monohydrate)	(Macrobid). Sugar, lactose. Black and yellow. In 100s.

Methenamine and Methenamine Salts

METHENAMINE

Actions:

Pharmacology: In acid urine, methenamine is hydrolyzed to ammonia and formaldehyde, which is bactericidal. Methenamine does not liberate formaldehyde in the serum. The acid salts (mandelate and hippurate) help maintain a low urine pH.

Pharmacokinetics:

Absorption – Methenamine is readily absorbed following oral administration; 10% to 30% of the drug will be hydrolyzed by the gastric juices unless it is protected by an enteric coating.

Metabolism/Excretion – Approximately 10% to 25% of methenamine is metabolized in the liver and has a half-life of 3 to 6 hours. Generation of formaldehyde depends upon urinary pH, the concentration of methenamine and the duration that the urine is retained in the bladder. Peak concentrations of formaldehyde occur at a urine pH of ≤ 5.5 and are seen approximately 2 hours after a dose of methenamine hippurate and 3 to 8 hours after a dose of methenamine mandelate. A urinary formaldehyde concentration of > 25 mcg/ml is necessary for antimicrobial activity. Steady-state urinary formaldehyde concentrations are achieved in 2 to 3 days. Formaldehyde levels range from 1 to 85 mcg/ml, and decrease with increasing pH, urinary volume or flow rate.

In some instances, supplementary urine acidification may be desirable, especially in infections caused by urea-splitting organisms (which raise the urine pH). Ingestion of acidifying agents (eg, mandelic acid, hippuric acid, ammonium chloride, monobasic sodium phosphate) or acid-producing foods (eg, cranberries, plums, prunes) aid in maintaining an acid urine; however, effects may be negligible. Ammonium chloride 8 to 12 g/day, methionine 8 to 15 g/day and cranberry juice 1200 to 4000 ml/day, have all been recommended, but with marginal results. There is no reliable oral urinary acidifier at present. Monitor urine pH.

Excretion occurs via glomerular filtration and tubular secretion. Approximately 90% of the methenamine moiety is excreted in the urine within 24 hours. The influence of renal dysfunction on the pharmacology of methenamine is unknown.

Microbiology: The nonspecific antibacterial action of formaldehyde is effective against gram-positive and gram-negative organisms and fungi. *Escherichia coli,* enterococci and staphylococci are usually susceptible. *Enterobacter aerogenes* and *Proteus vulgaris* are generally resistant. Urea-splitting organisms (eg, *Proteus, Pseudomonas*) may be resistant since they raise the pH of the urine inhibiting the release of formaldehyde. An effective urine concentration of formaldehyde must persist for a minimum of 2 hours.

Methenamine is effective clinically against most common urinary tract pathogens since most bacteria are sensitive to free formaldehyde concentrations of 20 mcg/ml.

Methenamine is particularly suited for therapy of chronic infections, since bacteria and fungi do not develop resistance to formaldehyde.

Indications:

Urinary tract infections: Prophylaxis or suppression/elimination of frequently recurring urinary tract infections when long-term therapy is considered necessary. Use only after eradication of the infection by other appropriate antimicrobial agents.

Contraindications:

Renal insufficiency; severe dehydration; severe hepatic insufficiency (because it facilitates ammonia production in the intestine); use alone for acute infections with parenchymal involvement causing systemic symptoms; hypersensitivity to the drug; concurrent sulfonamides since an insoluble precipitate may form with formaldehyde in the urine.

Warnings:

Pregnancy: Category C. Safe use of methenamine in early pregnancy has not been established. Safety in the last trimester is suggested, but not proven. Methenamine passes into the fetus, but there is no evidence that methenamine salts cause fetal abnormalities. It is not known whether the drug can cause fetal harm when administered to a pregnant woman or can affect reproduction capacity. Give to pregnant women only if clearly needed.

Lactation: Methenamine passes into breast milk; levels are about equivalent to maternal serum and peak in 1 hour. One estimate revealed that an infant would receive about 0.15 to 0.4 mg methenamine/feeding. No adverse effects on the nursing infant have been reported.

Methenamine and Methenamine Salts

METHENAMINE

Precautions:

Large doses (8 g daily for 3 to 4 weeks) have caused bladder irritation, painful and frequent micturition, proteinuria and gross hematuria.

Acid urine pH should be maintained, especially when treating infections due to urea-splitting organisms such as *Proteus* and strains of *Pseudomonas.* When acidification is contraindicated or unattainable (as with some urea-splitting bacteria) the drug is not recommended.

Serum transaminases have elevated mildly during treatment in a few instances and returned to normal while patients were still receiving methenamine hippurate. Perform liver function studies periodically on patients receiving methenamine hippurate, especially those with liver dysfunction.

Gout: Methenamine salts may cause precipitation of urate crystals in the urine.

Tartrazine sensitivity: Some of these products contain tartrazine, which may cause allergic-type reactions (including bronchial asthma) in certain susceptible individuals. Although the overall incidence of tartrazine sensitivity in the general population is low, it is frequently seen in patients who also have aspirin hypersensitivity. Specific products containing tartrazine are identified in the product listings.

Drug Interactions:

Methenamine Drug Interactions

Precipitant drug	Object drug*		Description
Sulfonamides	Methenamine	⬇	An insoluble precipitate between the sulfonamide and formaldehyde may form in the urine.
Urinary alkalinizers	Methenamine	⬇	Alkalinizing agents may decrease the efficacy of methenamine by inhibiting its conversion to formaldehyde.

* ⬇ = Object drug decreased.

Drug/Lab test interactions: Methenamine may interfere with laboratory urine determinations of **17-hydroxycorticosteroids, catecholamines** and **vanillylmandelic acid** (false increases); and **5-hydroxyindoleacetic acid** (false decrease).

Methenamine taken during pregnancy can interfere with laboratory tests of **urine estriol** (resulting in unmeasurably low values) when an acid hydrolysis procedure is used. This is due to the presence in the urine of methenamine or formaldehyde. Use enzymatic hydrolysis in place of acid hydrolysis.

Adverse Reactions:

Overall incidence: Approximately 1% to 7%.

GI: Nausea; vomiting; cramps; stomatitis; anorexia.

GU: Bladder irritation, dysuria, proteinuria, hematuria, urinary frequency/urgency, crystalluria (large doses).

Dermatologic: Pruritus (rare); urticaria; erythematous eruptions; rash.

Miscellaneous: Headache, dyspnea, lipoid pneumonitis, generalized edema (rare).

Overdosage:

Treatment: Immediately after ingestion of an overdose, further absorption of the drug may be minimized by inducing vomiting or by gastric lavage, followed by administration of activated charcoal. Force fluids, either oral or parenteral, to tolerance.

Patient Information:

It may be necessary to attempt to acidify the urine (eg, ascorbic acid, cranberry juice).

Take with food to minimize GI upset.

Drink sufficient fluids to ensure adequate urine flow.

Avoid excessive intake of alkalinizing foods (milk products) or medication (bicarbonate, acetazolamide).

Complete full course of therapy; take until gone.

Notify physician if skin rash, painful urination or intolerable GI upset occurs.

Methenamine and Methenamine Salts

METHENAMINE HIPPURATE

Complete prescribing information for these products begins in the Methenamine monograph.

Administration and Dosage:

Adults and children > 12 years of age: 1 g twice daily.

Children (6 to 12 years of age): 0.5 to 1 g twice daily.

Rx	**Hiprex** (Hoechst Marion Roussel)	**Tablets:** 1 g	Tartrazine, saccharin. (Merrell 277). Yellow, scored. In 100s.
Rx	**Urex** (3M Pharmaceuticals)		Saccharin. (3M Urex). White, scored. In 100s.

METHENAMINE MANDELATE

Complete prescribing information for these products begins in the Methenamine monograph.

Administration and Dosage:

Adults: 1 g 4 times daily, after meals and at bedtime.

Children (6 to 12 years of age): 0.5 g, 4 times daily.

Children (< 6 years of age): 0.25 g/30 lb (14 kg), 4 times daily.

Rx	**Methenamine Mandelate** (Various, Major, Rugby)	**Tablets, enteric coated:** 0.5 g	In 100s and 1000s.
Rx	**Mandelamine** (Parke-Davis)		(166). Brown. Film coated. In 100s.
Rx	**Methenamine Mandelate** (Various, eg, Rugby)	**Tablets, enteric coated:** 1 g	In 100s and 1000s.
Rx	**Mandelamine** (Parke-Davis)		(167). Purple. Film coated. In 100s.
Rx	**Methenamine Mandelate** (Various, eg, Barre-National, Schein)	**Suspension:** 0.5 g/5 ml	In 480 ml.

URINARY ANTI-INFECTIVE COMBINATIONS

Ingredients:

The following anti-infective agents are used in these combinations:

OXYTETRACYCLINE
SULFONAMIDES
METHENAMINE
METHYLENE BLUE

Additional ingredients include:

PHENAZOPYRIDINE HCL, used as a urinary analgesic.
SODIUM SALICYLATE and *PHENYL SALICYLATE*, used as analgesics.
BELLADONNA ALKALOIDS, used as urinary antispasmodics.
SODIUM BIPHOSPHATE (SODIUM ACID PHOSPHATE) and *BENZOIC ACID*, used to acidify the urine.

Administration and Dosage:

Usual adult doses are listed, unless otherwise specified. Take doses with a full glass of water.

SULFONAMIDE COMBINATIONS

Rx	**Urobiotic-250** (Pfizer)	**Capsules:** 250 mg oxytetracycline (as HCl), 250 mg sulfamethizole, 50 mg phenazopyridine HCl *Dose:* 1 capsule 4 times daily	In 50s.
Rx	**Azo-Sulfisoxazole** (Various, eg, Major)	**Tablets:** 500 mg sulfisoxazole, 50 mg phenazopyridine HCl *Dose:* 4 tablets initially, then 2 tablets 4 times daily, up to 2 days. Continue treatment beyond 2 days with sulfisoxazole only	In 100s and 1000s.

METHENAMINE COMBINATIONS

Rx	**Trac Tabs 2X** (Hyrex)	**Tablets:** 120 mg methenamine, 30 mg phenyl salicylate, 0.06 mg atropine sulfate, 0.03 mg hyoscyamine sulfate, 7.5 mg benzoic acid, 6 mg methylene blue *Dose:* 1 or 2 tablets 4 times daily	In 100s and 1000s.
Rx	**Prosed/DS** (Star)	**Tablets:** 81.6 mg methenamine, 36.2 mg phenyl salicylate, 10.8 mg methylene blue, 9 mg benzoic acid, 0.06 mg atropine sulfate, 0.06 mg hyoscyamine sulfate *Dose:* 1 tablet 4 times daily	Parabens, sugar. (Prosed/DS). Dark blue. Sugar coated. In 100s and 1000s.
Rx	**Urogesic Blue** (Edwards)	**Tablets:** 81.6 mg methenamine, 40.8 mg sodium biphosphate, 36.2 mg phenyl salicylate, 10.8 mg methylene blue, 0.12 mg hyoscyamine sulfate *Dose:* 1 tablet 4 times daily	Sucrose, parabens. (MD-20). Purple. Oval. Sugar coated. In 100s.
Rx	**Urimar-T** (Marnel)	**Tablets:** 81.6 mg methenamine, 40.8 mg sodium biphosphate, 36.2 mg phenyl salicylate, 10.8 mg methylene blue, 0.12 mg hyoscyamine sulfate *Dose:* 1 tablet 4 times daily	In 100s.
Rx	**Uro-Phosphate** (ECR Pharm)	**Tablets:** 300 mg methenamine, 434.78 mg sodium biphosphate *Dose:* 1 or 2 tablets at 4 to 6 hour intervals	(9531). White. Film coated. In 100s.
Rx	**Uroquid-Acid No. 2** (Beach)	**Tablets:** 500 mg methenamine mandelate, 500 mg sodium acid phosphate monohydrate *Dose:* Initial - 2 tablets 4 times daily Maintenance - 2 to 4 tablets daily in divided doses	(Beach 1114). Yellow. Film coated. Capsule shape. In 100s.

METHENAMINE COMBINATIONS

Rx	**Urisedamine** (PolyMedica)	**Tablets**: 500 mg methenamine mandelate, 0.15 mg hyoscyamine *Dose:* 2 tablets 4 times daily Children (≥ 6 years) – Reduce dosage in proportion to age and weight	Sucrose. (W2210). Light blue. Capsule shape. In 100s.
Rx	**Atrosept** (Geneva)	**Tablets**: 40.8 mg methenamine, 18.1 mg phenyl salicylate, 0.03 mg atropine sulfate, 0.03 mg hyoscyamine (as sulfate), 4.5 mg benzoic acid, 5.4 mg methylene blue *Dose:* Adults – 2 tablets 4 times daily Children (≥ 6 years) – Reduce dosage in proportion to age and weight	(220). Deep blue. Sugar coated. In 100s and 1000s.
Rx	**Dolsed** (American Urologicals)		(Dolsed). Deep blue. Sugar coated. In 100s and 1000s.
Rx	**UAA** (Econo Med)		(UAA). Blue. Sugar coated. In 100s and 1000s.
Rx	**Uridon Modified** (Rugby)		Blue. Sugar coated. In 100s and 1000s.
Rx	**Urinary Antiseptic No. 2** (Various, eg, Eon)		In 100s and 1000s.
Rx	**Urised** (PolyMedica)		(W 2183). Purple. Sugar coated. In 100s and 500s.
Rx	**Uritin** (Various, eg, Goldline)		In 1000s.
otc	**Cystex** (Numark)	**Tablets**: 162 mg methenamine, 162.5 mg sodium salicylate, 32 mg benzoic acid *Dose:* Adults and children > 16 years old – 2 tablets 4 times daily with meals and at bedtime	In 40s and 100s.

NEOMYCIN AND POLYMYXIN B IRRIGANT

Actions:

Pharmacology: Polymyxin B sulfate is bactericidal to most gram-negative bacilli, particularly against Pseudomonas infections. Neomycin sulfate is bactericidal against a wide range of gram-negative organisms including *Proteus vulgaris* and gram-positive organisms. When used topically, these drugs are rarely irritating.

Indications:

Urinary bladder irrigant: Continuous irrigant or rinse for short-term use (up to 10 days) in the urinary bladder of abacteriuric patients to help prevent bacteriuria and gram-negative rod bacter- emia associated with the use of indwelling catheters.

Contraindications:

Hypersensitivity to any component.

Precautions:

Recent UT surgery: Safety and efficacy have not been established for use in patients with recent lower urinary tract surgery.

Neomycin toxicity: Neomycin is nephrotoxic and ototoxic, particularly when given parenterally in higher than recommended doses. Cases of nephrotoxicity or ototoxicity have been reported following its topical use for extensive burns and wound irrigation. Although the possibility of these reactions is remote with use of the minimal amount in bladder irrigations, such reactions may occur if irrigations are continued beyond the recommended maximum of 10 days; observe caution.

Superinfection: Use of antibiotics (especially prolonged or repeated therapy) may result in bacterial or fungal overgrowth of nonsusceptible organisms. Such overgrowth may lead to a secondary infection. Take appropriate measures if superinfection occurs.

Adverse Reactions:

The prevalence of neomycin hypersensitivity has increased; however, topical application to mucous membranes rarely results in local or systemic reactions.

Administration and Dosage:

Not for injection.

For use with catheter systems permitting continuous irrigation of the urinary bladder: Add 1 ml irrigant to 1 L isotonic saline solution. Connect the container to the inflow lumen of the three-way catheter. Connect the outflow lumen via a sterile disposable plastic tube to a disposable plastic collection bag.

Adjust flow rate to 1 L/24 hours. If the patient's urine output exceeds 2 L/day, increase flow rate to 2 L/24 hours.

The rinse of the bladder must be continuous. Do not interrupt the inflow or rinse solution for more than a few minutes.

Rx	**Neosporin G.U. Irrigant** (Glaxo Wellcome)	**Solution:** 40 mg neomycin (as sulfate) and 200,000 units polymyxin B sulfate per ml	In 1 ml amps (10s and 50s) and 20 ml multi-dose vials.[1]

[1] With methylparaben.

CITRIC ACID, GLUCONO-DELTA-LACTONE AND MAGNESIUM CARBONATE IRRIGANT (Hemiacidrin)

Actions:

Pharmacology: The action of hemiacidrin on susceptible apatite calculi results from an exchange of magnesium from the irrigating solution for the insoluble calcium contained in the stone matrix or calcification. The magnesium salts thereby formed are soluble in the gluconocitrate irrigating solution resulting in the dissolution of the calculus. Struvite calculi are composed mainly of magnesium ammonium phosphates which are solubilized by hemiacidrin due to its acidic pH.

Hemiacidrin is not effective for dissolution of calcium oxalate, uric acid or cysteine stones.

Indications:

Solution: Local irrigation for dissolution of renal calculi composed of apatite (a calcium carbonate-phosphate compound) or struvite (magnesium ammonium phosphates) in patients who are not candidates for surgical removal of the calculi.

As adjunctive therapy to dissolve residual apatite or struvite calculi and fragments after surgery or to achieve partial dissolution of renal calculi to facilitate surgical removal.

For dissolution of bladder calculi of the struvite or apatite variety by local intermittent irrigation through a urethral catheter or cystostomy catheter as an alternative or adjunct to surgical procedures.

For use as an intermittent irrigating solution to prevent or minimize encrustations of indwelling urinary tract catheters.

Powder for solution: For use in preparing solutions for irrigating indwelling urethral catheters and the urinary bladder, to dissolve or prevent formation of calcifications.

Unlabeled uses: Hemiacidrin has been used as a renal pelvis irrigation, with meticulous attention to intrapelvic pressure and urosepsis.

Contraindications:

Solution: Urinary tract infections (see Warnings); presence of demonstrable urinary tract extravasation.

Powder for solution: Biliary calculi; therapy or preventive therapy above the ureteral-vesical junction, therefore contraindicated for use with ureteral catheters, nephrostomy or pyelostomy tubes or renal lavage for dissolving calculi.

Warnings:

Urinary tract infection: Stop the drug immediately if patient develops fever, urinary tract infection, signs and symptoms consistent with urinary tract infection, persistent flank pain, or if hypermagnesemia or elevated serum creatinine develops.

Urea-splitting bacteria reside within struvite and apatite stones which therefore serve as a source of infection. Dissolution therapy with hemiacidrin in the presence of an infected urinary tract may lead to sepsis and death. Obtain urine specimens for culture prior to initiating chemolytic therapy of the renal pelvis. Institute appropriate antibiotic therapy to treat any infection detected. A sterile urine must be present prior to initiating therapy. An infected stone can serve as a continual source for infection; therefore, continue antibiotic therapy throughout the course of dissolution therapy.

Severe hypermagnesemia has occurred. Use caution when irrigating the renal pelvis of patients with impaired renal function. Observe patients for early signs and symptoms of hypermagnesemia including nausea, lethargy, confusion and hypotension. Severe hypermagnesemia may result in hyporeflexia, dyspnea, apnea, coma, cardiac arrest and subsequent death. Monitor serum magnesium levels and evaluate deep tendon reflexes. Treatment of hypermagnesemia should include discontinuation of hemiacidrin followed by therapy with IV calcium gluconate, fluids and diuresis in severe cases.

Not indicated for dissolution of calcium oxalate, uric acid or cysteine calculi.

Pregnancy: Category C. It is not known whether hemiacidrin can cause fetal harm when administered to a pregnant woman or can affect reproduction capacity. Give to a pregnant woman only if clearly needed.

Lactation: Magnesium is known to be excreted into breast milk. However, it is not known whether hemiacidrin is excreted in breast milk. Exercise caution when hemiacidrin is administered to a nursing woman.

Precautions:

Vesicoureteral reflux frequently occurs in patients with indwelling urethral or cystostomy catheters. Cystogram prior to initiation of hemiacidrin is essential for such patients. If reflux is demonstrated, all precautions recommended for renal pelvis irrigation must be taken.

CITRIC ACID, GLUCONO-DELTA-LACTONE AND MAGNESIUM CARBONATE IRRIGANT (Hemiacidrin)

Catheter care: Hospitalization is prolonged for days to weeks when chemolytic therapy is used in lieu of, or following, surgery. Reserve this therapy for selected patients. Care must be taken during chemolysis of renal calculi with hemiacidrin to maintain the patency of the irrigating catheter. Calculus fragments and debris may obstruct the outflow catheter. Continued irrigation under those circumstances leads to increased intrapelvic pressure with a danger of tissue damage or absorption of the irrigating solution. Catheter outflow blockage may be prevented by flushing the catheter with saline and repositioning of the catheter. Frequent monitoring of the system should be performed by a nurse, an aide or any person with sufficient skills to be able to detect any problems with the patency of the catheter. At the first sign of obstruction, discontinue the irrigation and disconnect the system.

Intrapelvic pressures must be maintained at or below 25 cm of water. The preferred method of pressure control is the insertion of an open Y connection pop-off valve into the infusion line allowing immediate decompression if pressure exceeds 25 cm of water. An alternative method has been proposed to direct or stop the flow of the irrigating solution to prevent increased intrapelvic pressure: Placement of a pinch clamp on the inflow line which can be used by the patient or nurse to stop the irrigation at the first sign of flank pain. However, extreme caution must be taken when relying on cooperation of the patient. Patients may not be sufficiently alert to detect signs and symptoms of outflow obstruction. This is especially true in elderly patients, sedated patients or those with severe neurological dysfunction with varying degrees of sensory loss or motor paralysis.

Monitoring: Throughout the course of therapy, monitor patients to ensure safety. Obtain serum creatinine phosphate and magnesium every few days. Collect urine specimens for culture and antibacterial sensitivity every 3 days or less and at the first sign of fever. Stop the irrigation if any culture exhibits growth and initiate appropriate antibacterial therapy. The irrigation may be started again after a course of antibacterial therapy upon demonstration of a sterile urine. Struvite calculi frequently contain bacteria within the stone; therefore, continue antibacterial therapy throughout the course of dissolution therapy. Hypermagnesemia or an elevated serum creatinine level are indications to halt the irrigation until they return to pre-irrigation levels. Evidence of severe urothelial edema on X-ray is also an indication for temporarily halting the irrigation until the complication resolves.

Drug Interactions:

Magnesium-containing medications: Concurrent use may contribute to production of hypermagnesemia and is not recommended.

Adverse Reactions:

Solution: The most common adverse reaction in selected case series is transient flank pain which occurs in most patients. Additional reactions include: Urothelial ulceration or edema (13%); fever (20% but up to 40% in some case series); urinary tract infection, back pain, dysuria, transient hematuria, nausea, hypermagnesemia, hyperphosphatemia, elevated serum creatinine, candidiasis, bladder irritability (1% to 10%); septicemia, ileus, vomiting, thrombophlebitis (< 1%). Death from sepsis has occurred.

Powder for solution: Occasional temporary pain or burning sensation from this procedure; discontinue use if this occurs.

Administration and Dosage:

Solution:

Renal calculi – It is essential that patients be free from urinary tract infections prior to initiating chemolytic therapy. A nephrostomy tube is placed at surgery or percutaneously to permit lavage of the calculi. A single catheter may be sufficient if the calculus is not obstructing the ureter or ureteropelvic junction. In patients with an obstructed ureter, a retrograde catheter can be placed through the ureter to the renal pelvis via a cystoscope. This second catheter is used to irrigate the calculus while the percutaneous nephrostomy tube is used for drainage. Pressure measurements are made under fluoroscopy to assure that 2 to 3 ml/min can be infused without causing pain, pyelovenous or pyelotubular backflow or manometric evidence of elevated pressure within the collecting system.

For postoperative patients, irrigation should not be started before the fourth or fifth postoperative day. Irrigation of the renal pelvis is begun with sterile saline only after a sterile urine has been demonstrated. The saline is infused at a rate of 60 ml/hr initially, and the rate is increased until pain or an elevated pressure (25 cm H_2O) appears, or until a maximum flow rate of 120 ml/hr is achieved. Inspect the site of insertion for leakage. If leakage occurs, the irrigation is discontinued temporarily to allow for complete healing around the nephrostomy tube.

CITRIC ACID, GLUCONO-DELTA-LACTONE AND MAGNESIUM CARBONATE IRRIGANT (Hemiacidrin)

If no leakage or flank pain occurs, start irrigation with hemiacidrin with a flow rate equal to maximum rate achieved with the saline solution. Place a clamp on the inflow tube and instruct patients and nursing personnel to stop the irrigating solution whenever pain develops. Nursing personnel who are responsible for performing the irrigation must be instructed concerning location of the nephrostomy tube(s) and direction of flow of irrigating solution to ensure against misconnection of inflowing and egress tubes. Perform nephrostomograms periodically to assure proper placement of catheter tip and to assess efficacy. If stones fail to change size after several days of adequate irrigation, discontinue the procedure.

Upon demonstration of complete dissolution of the calculus, the inflow tube is clamped and left in place for a few days to ensure that no obstruction exists, after which time the nephrostomy tube is removed.

Bladder calculi – Chemolysis of bladder calculi is used as an alternative to cystoscopic or surgical removal of the stones in patients who refuse surgery or cystoscopic removal or in whom these procedures constitute an unwarranted risk. Following appropriate studies to evaluate possible vesicoureteral reflux, 30 ml of hemiacidrin is instilled through a urinary catheter into the bladder and the catheter is clamped for 30 to 60 minutes. The clamp is then released and the bladder is drained. This is repeated 4 to 6 times a day. A continuous drip through a 3 way Foley catheter is an alternative means of dissolving bladder stones. In the presence of bladder spasm and associated high pressure reflux, all precautions required for irrigation of the renal pelvis must be observed.

Indwelling urinary tract catheter encrustation – Periodic instillation of hemiacidrin is indicated to minimize or prevent encrustation of indwelling catheters which frequently results in plugging of the catheter and discomfort to the patient. This is accomplished by instilling 30 ml of the solution through the catheter and then clamping the catheter for 10 minutes, after which the clamp is removed to allow drainage of the bladder. This process is repeated 3 times a day.

Powder for solution: Irrigating indwelling catheters – Administer as a 10% solution (sterile) in distilled water. Irrigation is carried out with 30 to 60 ml 2 to 3 times daily by means of a rubber syringe.

Preparation of the solution: Always add powder to the water; do not add water to the powder when preparing solutions.

Dissolve the contents of one 300 g bottle in 3000 ml of sterile distilled water, or any smaller quantity of powder in the proportionately smaller amount of water. Since powder may be reactive upon addition to water, add slowly to the water, with constant agitation, in a container larger than that which the amount of solution actually requires. Do not stopper or cap the container during preparation. Thoroughly mix the solution for as long as possible (up to 15 to 20 minutes). This can be achieved through the use of a mechanical mixer where available. Solutions often vary in color from almost colorless to a definite clear yellow solution.

After thorough mixing, filter the solution through a coarse filter to remove any undissolved matter. Alternatively, if desired, allow the solution to stand and decant. (A 10% solution was filtered after 24 hours and the residue dried at 105°C for 8 hours, then weighed. The weight of the residue equalled 0.008% of the solution.)

The residue which may be noted on a filter consists primarily of the insolubles present in the original magnesium hydroxycarbonate, which has about 0.03% to 0.05% acid insolubles in the form of a small amount of silica (or calcium, as the silicate) and iron oxides which remain undissolved when the solution is prepared. It may be yellow or even brown or black in color.

Storage (solution): Minimize exposure of hemiacidrin to heat or cold. Store at controlled room temperature (15° to 30°C; 59° to 86°F). Avoid excessive heat or cold (keep from freezing). Brief exposure to temperatures up to 40°C (104°F) or temperatures down to 5°C (41°F) does not adversely affect the product.

Rx	**Renacidin** (Guardian)	**Powder for Solution:** 156 to 171 g citric acid (anhydrous), 21 to 30 g d-gluconic acid (as lactone) w/75 to 87 g purified Mg hydroxycarbonate, 9 to 15 g Mg acid citrate, 2 to 6 g Ca (as carbonate) and 17 to 21 g water (combined & free) per 300 g bottle	In 150 or 300 g.
		Solution: 6.602 g citric acid (anhydrous), 0.198 g glucono-delta-lactone, 3.177 g magnesium carbonate and 0.023 g benzoic acid per 100 ml	In 500 ml.

HEXITOL IRRIGANTS

Actions:

Pharmacology: Hexitol irrigants are nonelectrolytic and nonhemolytic urologic irrigation solutions. The amount of solution absorbed intravascularly during transurethral prostatic surgery is variable and depends primarily on the extent and duration of the surgery. Mannitol is confined to the extracellular space, only slightly metabolized, rapidly excreted in the urine and is, therefore, an effective osmotic diuretic. The sorbitol-containing products will be metabolized to carbon dioxide (70%) and dextrose (30%) or excreted by the kidneys.

Indications:

In transurethral prostatic resection or other transurethral surgical procedures.

Contraindications:

Anuria; injection.

Warnings:

Use caution in significant cardiopulmonary or renal dysfunction (see Precautions).

Systemic effects: Irrigating fluids used during transurethral prostatectomy may enter the systemic circulation in relatively large volumes. Therefore, the irrigation solution must be considered as a systemic drug. The osmotic diuresis it may produce can significantly alter cardiopulmonary and renal dynamics.

Diabetes mellitus: Hyperglycemia from metabolism of sorbitol may occur in patients with diabetes mellitus.

Sorbitol solution: Use with caution in patients unable to metabolize sorbitol rapidly enough to avoid the development of hyperosmolar states.

Precautions:

Cardiovascular effects: Carefully evaluate cardiovascular status of the patient, particularly one with cardiac disease, before and during transurethral prostatic resection when mannitol irrigant is used. The quantity of fluid absorbed into systemic circulation may cause expansion of extracellular fluid, leading to fulminating CHF.

Fluid and electrolyte balance: Systemic absorption of the solutions may cause a shift of sodium free intracellular fluid into the extracellular compartment, lowering serum sodium concentration and aggravating any preexisting hyponatremia.

A significant diuresis resulting from the irrigating solution may obscure and intensify inadequate hydration or hypovolemia. Excessive loss of water and electrolytes may lead to hypernatremia.

Adverse Reactions:

Since significant systemic absorption occurs, the potential for systemic effects must be considered. The following effects have been noted from *intravenous infusion:*

Cardiovascular/pulmonary disorders: Pulmonary congestion; hypotension; tachycardia; angina-like pains; thrombophlebitis.

Electrolyte Disturbance: Acidosis; electrolyte loss; marked diuresis; urinary retention; edema; dry mouth; thirst; dehydration.

Miscellaneous: Blurred vision; convulsions; nausea; vomiting; rhinitis; chills; vertigo; backache; urticaria; diarrhea.

Additional reactions associated with sorbitol solution include slight increases in postoperative serum glucose and inhibition of intestinal absorption of vitamin B_{12}.

Administration and Dosage:

Do not use unless solution is clear and seal unbroken. Use as required for irrigation.

Storage: Promptly use the contents of opened containers; discard unused portions of the solution. Do not warm above 66°C (150°F). Protect from freezing and avoid storage above 40°C (104°F).

MANNITOL

For complete prescribing information, refer to the Hexitol Irrigants group monograph.

Rx	**Resectisol** (Kendall McGaw)	**Solution**: 5 g per 100 ml in distilled water (275 mOsm/L)	In 2000 ml.

SORBITOL

For complete prescribing information, refer to the Hexitol Irrigants group monograph.

Rx	**Sorbitol** (McGaw)	**Solution**: 3.3% (183 mOsm/L)	In 2000 ml.
Rx	**Sorbitol** (Travenol)	**Solution**: 3% (165 mOsm/L)	In 1500 and 3000 ml.

MANNITOL AND SORBITOL

For complete prescribing information, refer to the Hexitol Irrigants group monograph.

Rx	**Sorbitol-Mannitol** (Abbott)	**Solution**: 0.54 g mannitol and 2.7 g sorbitol per 100 ml (178 mOsm/L)	In 1500 and 3000 ml.

SUBY'S SOLUTION G

Indications:

To dissolve phosphatic calculi or incrustations in the bladder and urethra; to irrigate the bladder and urethra with an acidic solution.

Contraindications:

Do not use in presence of fulminating bladder infections, bleeding, ulcerations or other open wounds.

Not for injection into body tissue.

Not for irrigation during transurethral surgical procedures.

These solutions are conductive; do not use in the presence of electrical instrumentation.

Warnings:

For use in irrigation of the lower urinary tract only.

Not recommended for dissolving phosphate calculi in the renal pelvis because of the risk of creating back pressure that may reactivate an existing pyelonephritis.

Do not use solution to replace other indicated measures including correction of underlying metabolic disorders, surgical intervention and treatment of infection.

Pregnancy: Category C. It is not known whether this irrigation solution can cause fetal harm when given to a pregnant woman or can affect reproduction capacity. Administer to a pregnant woman only if clearly needed.

Precautions:

Avoid reflux of the solution up the ureters into the renal pelvis. Repeated or continuous use may cause bleeding. Solution is irritating to urethra; after each treatment, irrigate with sterile saline or water.

Four cases of sudden death were reported during lavage therapy with a similarly acting solution. The autopsy indicated that calcium phosphate sludge resulting from dissolving stone is a severe irritant to the renal pelvis and is probably absorbed to some degree as evidenced by a terminal serum phosphorus of three times the normal level in one case. Disintegration of calculi into phosphate sludge by acids might form a variety of toxic compounds in small quantities. Since pyelonephritis accompanies renal calculus disease in many cases, pyelorenal backflow of chemicals may aggravate the infectious process causing progression to a severe toxemia.

Adverse Reactions:

Discomfort or pain due to bladder irritation during irrigation. In the presence of undetected mucosal lesions, irrigation may initiate bleeding from the bladder.

Administration and Dosage:

Not for IV, SC or IM injection.

Administer 1 to 3 liters daily by intermittent irrigation or by tidal instillation and drainage to allow continuous irrigation of the bladder for periods of several hours. Intermittent irrigation of the bladder (after the manner of intermittent peritoneal dialysis) may be preferred to promote more prolonged contact of the irrigation with bladder stones; tidal (continuous in and out flow) irrigation may be less efficient and require larger amounts of irrigation fluid.

Use contents of opened container promptly to minimize the possibility of bacterial growth or pyrogen formation. Do not use solution unless clear and seal is intact. Discard unused portion.

Rx	**Suby's Solution G** (Various, eg, Abbott, Travenol)	**Solution:** 3.24 g citric acid (monohydrate), 0.43 g sodium carbonate (anhydrous) and 0.38 g magnesium oxide (anhydrous) per 100 ml	In 1000 ml.

ACETIC ACID FOR IRRIGATION

Indications:

For bladder irrigation.

Rx	**Acetic Acid for Irrigation** (Various, eg, Abbott, Baxter, Kendall McGaw)	**Solution:** 0.25%	In 250, 500 and 1000 ml.

GLYCINE (AMINOACETIC ACID) FOR IRRIGATION

Indications:

For urological irrigation.

Rx	**Glycine for Irrigation** (Various, eg, Abbott, Baxter, Kendall McGaw)	**Solution:** 1.5%	In 1500, 2000, 3000, 4000 and 5000 ml.

SODIUM CHLORIDE FOR IRRIGATION

Indications:

For use as an irrigating solution.

Rx	**Sodium Chloride for Irrigation** (Various, eg, Abbott, Baxter, Kendall McGaw)	**Solution (Isotonic):** 0.9%	In 150, 250, 500, 1000, 1500, 2000 and 4000 ml.
Rx	**Sodium Chloride for Irrigation** (Various, eg, Abbott, Baxter)	**Solution (Hypotonic):** 0.45%	In 500, 1000 and 1500 ml.

STERILE WATER FOR IRRIGATION

Indications:

For use as an irrigating solution.

Rx	**Sterile Water for Irrigation** (Various, eg, Abbott, Baxter, Kendall McGaw)		In 250, 500, 1000, 2000 and 4000 ml.

CDC ANTI-INFECTIVE AGENTS

In addition to the commercially available anti-infective agents, the Centers for Disease Control and Prevention (CDC) can supply several investigational agents upon request. These agents may be requested from the Drug Service, Division of Host Factors, Center for Infectious Disease, by calling 404-639-3670, 8:00 am to 4:30 pm EST Monday through Friday; for emergencies (evenings, weekends or holidays), call 404-639-2888.

Available CDC Anti-Infective Agents

Generic name	Trade name	Disease/Infestation	Organism
Bithionol	**Lorothidol** **(Bitin)**	Paragonimiasis Fascioliasis	*Paragonimus westermani* *Fasciola hepatica*
Dehydroemetine	**Mebadin**	Amebiasis Amebic dysentery	*Entamoeba histolytica*
Diloxanide furoate	**Furamide**	Amebiasis, asymptomatic cyst passers	*Entamoeba histolytica*
Melarsoprol (Mel B)	**Arsobal**	Trypanosomiasis (African sleeping sickness)	*Trypanosoma gambiense* *Trypanosoma rhodesiense*
Nifurtimox	**Lampit** **(Bayer 2502)**	Chagas' disease (megaesophagus, megacolon)	*Trypanosoma cruzi*
Sodium antimony gluconate or sodium stibogluconate	**Pentostam**	Leishmaniasis (kala azar, espundia ulcer, oriental sore)	*Leishmania brasiliensis* *Leishmania mexicana* *Leishmania donovani* *Leishmania tropica*
Suramin	**Fourneau 309** **Bayer 205**	Trypanosomiasis	*Trypanosoma gambiense* *Trypanosoma rhodesiense*
	Germanin **Moranyl** **Belganyl** **Naphuride** **Antrypol** **Naganol**	Onchocerciasis	*Onchocerca volvulus*

chapter 9

biologicals

IMMUNE SERUMS

The following general information applies to all immune sera. For specific information on individual agents, refer to specific monographs:

- Immune Globulin, IV
- Cytomegalovirus Immune Globulin, IV
- Immune Globulin, IM
- Hepatitis B Immune Globulin
- Tetanus Immune Globulin
- Varicella-Zoster Immune Globulin
- Rho (D) Immune Globulin
- Lymphocyte Immune Globulin

Actions:

Pharmacology: Standard immune globulins contain approximately 16.5% gamma globulin. Immune globulin IV contains 5% immune globulins. These products are obtained, purified and standardized from human serum or plasma. They are obtained from pooled plasma either of donors from the general population or of hyperimmunized donors (for immune globulins for specific diseases).

Indications:

To provide passive immunization to one or more infectious diseases. Protection derived will be of rapid onset, but of short duration (1 to 3 months). See individual monographs for specific indications.

Contraindications:

Allergic response to gamma globulin or anti-immunoglobulin A (IgA) antibodies.

Allergic response to thimerosal.

Persons with isolated immunoglobulin A (IgA) deficiency. Such persons have the potential for developing antibodies to IgA and could have anaphylactic reactions to subsequent administration of blood products that contain IgA.

Immune globulin, intramuscular: Patients who have severe thrombocytopenia or any coagulation disorder that would contraindicate IM use.

Warnings:

Route of administration: Do not give these products IV (except immune globulin IV and cytomegalovirus immune glovulin IV). IV injections can cause a precipitous fall in blood pressure and a picture similar to anaphylaxis. Administer IM.

Anaphylactic reactions (rare) may occur following injection of human immune globulin preparations. Anaphylaxis is more likely if immune globulin is given IV; therefore, except for immune globulin IV, these products must only be given IM. In highly allergic individuals, repeated injections may lead to anaphylactic shock.

Hypersensitivity: Give with caution to patients with prior systemic allergic reactions following use of human immunoglobulin preparations. Hypersensitivity reactions are rare; the incidence may be increased by use of large IM doses or repeated injections of immune globulin. Have epinephrine available for treatment of acute allergic symptoms. Refer to Management of Acute Hypersensitivity Reactions.

Pregnancy: Category C. No studies have been conducted in pregnant patients. Clinical experience suggests no adverse effects on the fetus per se; however, it is not known whether these agents can cause fetal harm.

Lactation: Safety for use in the nursing mother has not been established. It is not known whether immune globulin is excreted in breast milk.

Precautions:

Skin testing should not be performed. Intradermal injection of concentrated gamma globulin causes a localized area of inflammation which can be misinterpreted as a positive allergic reaction. It is actually localized chemical tissue irritation. Misinterpretation can cause necessary medication to be withheld from a patient not actually allergic to this material. True allergic responses to human gamma globulin given in the prescribed IM manner are extremely rare.

Admixture incompatibilities: Do not admix with other medications.

Drug Interactions:

Virus vaccines, live: Do not administer within 3 months of immune globulin administration because antibodies in the globulin preparation may interfere with the immune response to the vaccination. It may be necessary to revaccinate persons who received immune globulin shortly after live virus vaccination.

Adverse Reactions:

Local: Tenderness, pain, muscle stiffness at injection site; may persist several hours.

Systemic: Urticaria; angioedema. Less frequently reported reactions include: Emesis; chills; fever; myalgia; lethargy; chest tightness; nausea. Isolated cases of angioneurotic edema and nephrotic syndrome have occurred.

IMMUNE GLOBULIN INTRAVENOUS (IGIV)

For additional information, refer to the Immune Serums Introduction.

Actions:

Pharmacokinetics: IGIV provides immediate antibody levels, whereas IM administration involves a 2- to 5-day delay before adequate serum levels are attained. Half-life is ≈ 3 weeks.

Indications:

Immunodeficiency syndrome: For the maintenance treatment of patients who are unable to produce sufficient amounts of IgG antibodies. IGIV may be preferred to IM immunoglobulin, especially in patients who require an immediate and substantial increase in IV immunoglobulin levels, in patients with a small muscle mass and in patients with bleeding tendencies in whom IM injections are contraindicated. It may be used in disease states such as congenital agammaglobulinemia (eg, x-linked agammaglobulinemia), common variable hypogammaglobulinemia, x-linked immunodeficiency with or without hyper IgM, Wiskott-Aldrich syndrome and combined immunodeficiency.

Idiopathic thrombocytopenic purpura (ITP) (Gamimune N, Gammagard S/D, Polygam S/D, Sandoglobulin, Venoglobulin-I and Venoglubulin-S only): Some children and adults with ITP have shown a temporary increase in platelet counts upon administration of IGIV. Therefore, consider administration in situations that require a rapid, temporary rise in platelet count (eg, prior to surgery, to control excessive bleeding or as a measure to defer splenectomy). Not all patients will respond. Even in those patients who do respond, do not consider this treatment curative.

B-cell chronic lymphocytic leukemia (CLL) (Gammagard S/D, Polygam S/D): Prevention of bacterial infections in patients with hypogammaglobulinemia or recurrent bacterial infections associated with B-cell CLL. In one study, bacterial infections were significantly reduced in 41 patients receiving IGIV compared with 40 patients receiving placebo. The placebo group had twice as many bacterial infections.

Kawasaki syndrome (Iveegam only): Administration in conjunction with aspirin within 10 days of onset of disease resulted in a 65% to 78% decrease in the incidence of coronary artery abnormalities compared with treatment with aspirin alone.

Bone marrow transplantation (BMT) (Gamimune N only): Prevention of systemic and local infections, interstitial pneumonia of infectious and idiopathic etiologies and acute graft-vs-host disease in patients ≥ 20 years of age in the first 100 days post-transplant.

Pediatric HIV infection (Gamimune N only): To decrease the frequency of serious and minor bacterial infections and the frequency of hospitalization and to increase the time free of serious bacterial infections in children with clinical or immunologic evidence of HIV disease. The effect of IGIV in preventing serious bacterial infections was especially apparent in preventing severe bacteremia (including *Streptococcus pneumoniae* bacteremia) and acute pneumonia.

Unlabeled uses: IGIVs may also be useful in chronic fatigue syndrome; quinidine-induced thrombocytopenia (400 mg/kg/day for 2 to 5 days).

Warnings:

Aseptic meningitis syndrome (AMS) has been reported to occur infrequently in association with IGIV treatment. The syndrome occurs more frequently in association with high dose (2 g/kg) and usually begins within several hours to within 2 days of treatment. It is characterized by symptoms and signs including severe headache, nuchal rigidity, drowsiness, fever, photophobia, painful eye movements, nausea and vomiting.

Hypersensitivity: IGIV can cause a precipitous fall in blood pressure and the clinical picture of anaphylaxis, even when the patient is not known to be sensitive to immune globulin preparations. These reactions appear related to infusion rate. Closely follow infusion rates given under Administration and Dosage. Monitor vital signs continuously and observe for any symptoms throughout the infusion. Have epinephrine available. Refer to Management of Acute Hypersensitivity Reactions.

Administration and Dosage:

Administer IV only.

IGIV is well tolerated and less likely to produce side effects if infused at indicated rates.

Sandoglobulin: Administer only if the solution is approximately room temperature.

Immunodeficiency syndrome – 200 mg/kg/month by IV infusion. If clinical response or the IgG level achieved is insufficient (minimum serum level, 200 mg/dl), increase to 300 mg/kg or repeat the infusion more frequently. After the first bottle of 3% solution is infused and the patient shows good tolerance, subsequent infusions may be administered at a higher rate or concentration. Such increases should be made gradually, allowing 15 to 30 minutes before each increment.

IMMUNE GLOBULIN INTRAVENOUS (IGIV)

Rate of administration – Give the first infusion to previously untreated agammaglobulinemic or hypogammaglobulinemic patients as a 3% immunoglobulin solution. Start with a flow rate of 0.5 to 1 ml/min. After 15 to 30 minutes, further increase to 1.5 to 2.5 ml/min.

If high doses must be administered repeatedly after the first dose, a 6% solution may be used; the initial infusion rate should be 1 to 1.5 ml/min, increased after 15 to 30 minutes to a maximum of 2.5 ml/min.

Idiopathic thrombocytopenic purpura – 400 mg/kg for 2 to 5 consecutive days.

Reconstitution –

3% solution: Invert bottle so that solvent flows into the bottle.

Proceed only if solution is clear and at approximately room temperature.

Gammagard S/D:

Immunodeficiency syndrome – 200 to 400 mg/kg. Monthly doses of ≥ 100 mg/kg are recommended.

B-Cell CLL – 400 mg/kg every 3 to 4 weeks.

Idiopathic thrombocytopenic purpura – 1000 mg/kg. Need for additional doses can be determined by clinical response and platelet count. Give up to 3 doses on alternate days if required.

Rate of administration – Initially 0.5 ml/kg/hr. If rate causes the patient no distress, it may be gradually increased, not to exceed 4 ml/kg/hr.

Gammar-P I.V.:

Immunodeficiency syndrome – 200 to 400 mg/kg every 3 to 4 weeks. An initial loading dose of ≥ 200 mg/kg at more frequent intervals, 200 to 600 mg/kg at 3 week intervals once a therapeutic plasma level has been established can be used. Individualize treatment.

Rate of administration – 0.01 ml/kg/min, increasing to 0.02 ml/kg/min after 15 to 30 minutes. Most patients tolerate a gradual increase to 0.03 to 0.06 ml/kg/min. If adverse reactions develop, slowing the infusion rate will usually eliminate the reaction.

Venoglobulin-I:

Immunodeficiency syndrome – 200 mg/kg, administered monthly. If clinical response or the level of IgG achieved is insufficient, increase to 300 to 400 mg/kg/month or repeat infusion more frequently than once a month.

Rate of administration – Infuse at a rate of 0.01 to 0.02 ml/kg/min for the first 30 minutes. If rate causes the patient no distress, it may be increased to 0.04 ml/kg/min. If tolerated, subsequent infusions to the same patient may be at the higher rate. If adverse effects occur, the rate should be reduced or the infusion interrupted until the symptoms subside.

The drug can be administered sequentially into a primary IV line containing Normal Saline or flushed with Normal Saline without causing precipitation or turbidity. Not physically compatible with 5% Dextrose Solution.

Idiopathic thrombocytopenic purpura –

Induction: Up to 2000 mg/kg/day over 2 to 7 consecutive days.

Acute: Patients who respond to induction therapy by manifesting a platelet count of 30,000 to 50,000/mm^3 may be discontinued after 2 to 7 daily doses.

Maintenance: If platelet count falls to < 30,000/mm^3 or clinically significant bleeding occurs, give up to a single 2000 mg/kg infusion every 2 weeks or less as needed to maintain platelet count > 30,000/mm^3 in children or 20,000/mm^3 in adults.

Gamimune N:

Immunodeficiency syndrome – 100 to 200 mg/kg/month (2 to 4 ml/kg/month). The dosage may be given more frequently or increased as high as 400 mg/kg (8 ml/kg) if the clinical response is inadequate or the level of IgG is insufficient.

Idiopathic thrombocytopenic purpura – 400 mg/kg for 5 consecutive days or 1000 mg/kg/day for 1 day or 2 consecutive days.

Maintenance: If platelet count falls to < 30,000/mm^3 or if the patient manifests clinically significant bleeding, 400 mg/kg may be given as a single infusion. If an adequate response does not result, the dose can be increased to 800 to 1000 mg/kg given as a single infusion. Maintenance infusions may be administered intermittently as clinically indicated to maintain a platelet count > 30,000/mm^3.

BMT – 500 mg/kg (10 ml/kg) beginning on days 7 and 2 pre-transplant or at the time conditioning therapy for transplantation is begun, then weekly through the 90-day post-transplant period.

Pediatric HIV infection – 400 mg/kg (8 ml/kg) every 28 days.

Rate of administration – 0.01 to 0.02 ml/kg/min for 30 minutes by itself. If the patient does not experience any discomfort, the rate may be increased to a maximum of 0.08 ml/kg/min. If side effects occur, reduce the rate or interrupt the infusion until symptoms subside; resume at a rate tolerable by the patient.

IMMUNE GLOBULIN INTRAVENOUS (IGIV)

Iveegam:

Immunodeficiency syndrome – 200 mg/kg/month. If desired clinical results are not obtained, the dosage may be increased up to 4–fold or intervals shortened. Doses ≤ 800 mg/kg/month have been tolerated.

Kawasaki syndrome – 400 mg/kg/day for 4 consecutive days or a single dose of 2000 mg/kg given over a 10–hour period. Initiate treatment within 10 days of onset of the disease. Treatment regimen should include aspirin, 100 mg/kg each day through the 14th day of illness, then 3 to 5 mg/kg/day thereafter for 5 weeks.

Rate of administration – 1 ml/min to a maximum of 2 ml/min for 5% solution. May be further diluted with 5% Dextrose or saline; with gradually increasing dosage levels and protein concentrations (≤ 5% protein), adverse reactions were not observed.

Polygam S/D:

Immunodeficiency syndrome – 100 mg/kg/month. An initial dose of 200 to 400 mg/kg may be administered. Individualize treatment.

B-Cell CLL – 400 mg/kg every 3 to 4 weeks.

Idiopathic thrombocytopenic purpura – 1 g/kg. A need for additional doses can be determined by clinical response and platelet count. Give up to three separate doses on alternate days if required.

Rate of administration – Initially 0.5 ml/kg/hr. If rate causes the patient no distress, it may be gradually increased, not to exceed 4 ml/kg/hr. Patients who tolerate the 5% solution at 4 ml/kg/hr can receive the 10% concentration starting at 0.5 ml/kg/hr.

If rate causes the patient no distress, it may be increased, not to exceed 8 ml/kg/hr.

Venoglobulin-S:

Immunodeficiency syndrome – 200 mg/kg/month. If clinical response is inadequate or the level of serum IgG achieved is felt to be insufficient, the dose may be increased to 300 to 400 mg/kg/month or the infusion may be repeated more frequently than once per month.

Idiopathic thrombocytopenic purpura – 2000 mg/kg over ≤ 5 days for induction therapy.

Maintenance therapy – 1000 mg/kg may be administered as needed to maintain platelet counts of 30,000/mm^3 in children and 20,000/mm^3 in adults or to prevent bleeding episodes in the interval between infusions.

Rate of administration – Initially 0.01 to 0.02 ml/kg/min or 0.6 to 1.2 ml/kg/hr for the first 30 minutes. If the patient does not experience any discomfort, the rate for the 5% solution may be increased to 0.04 ml/kg/min or 2.4 ml/kg/hr and the rate for the 10% solution may be increased to 0.05 ml/kg/min or 3 ml/kg/hr. In studies where IGIV was used to treat ITP, rates of 0.8 ml/kg/min or 4.8 ml/kg/hr were tolerated.

Storage/Stability:

Sandoglobulin – Store at room temperature ≤ 30°C (86°F). Discard partially used vials.

Gamimune N and Iveegam – Store at 2° to 8°C (36° to 46°F). Do not freeze. Discard partially used vials.

Venoglobulin-I – Store at a temperature < 30°C (86°F).

Gammar-P I.V., Polygam S/D, Venoglobulin-S, Gammagard S/D – Store at ≤ 25°C (77°F). Avoid freezing. Administration of *Gammagard S/D* and *Polygam S/D* should begin ≤ 2 hours after reconstitution. Discard unused solution.

Rx	**Gamimune N** (Bayer)	**Injection**: 5%[1]	Preservative free. In 10, 50, 100 and 250 ml vials.
		Injection: 10%[2]	Preservative free. In 10, 50, 100 and 200 ml vials.
Rx	**Gammagard S/D** (Baxter)	**Powder for Injection (freeze-dried, solvent/detergent treated)**: 50 mg/ml	In 2.5, 5 or 10 g single-use bottles with Sterile Water for Injection, transfer device and administration set.
Rx	**Polygam S/D** (American Red Cross)	**Powder for Injection (freeze-dried, solvent/detergent treated)**: 50 mg/ml; 90% gammaglobulin	Preservative free. In 2.5, 5 and 10 g single-use bottles with diluent, transfer device and administration set.[3]
Rx	**Sandoglobulin** (Sandoz)	**Powder for Injection (lyophilized)**[4]: 1 g, 3 g, 6 g, 12 g	Preservative free. In vials or kits with 0.9% NaCl or bulk packs without diluent.

IMMUNE GLOBULIN INTRAVENOUS (IGIV)

Rx	**Venoglobulin-I** (Alpha Therapeutic)	**Powder for Injection (lyophilized):**[5] 50 mg/ml IgG	Preservative free. In 0.5 g with reconstitution kit, 2.5 or 5 g vial with or without reconstitution kit w/ Sterile Water for Injection and 10 g with reconstitution kit and administration set.
Rx	**Venoglobulin-S** (Alpha Therapeutic)	**Solution for Injection (solvent/ detergent treated):** 5% immune globulin IV (human)[6]	Preservative free. In 50, 100 and 200 ml with sterile IV administration set.
		10% immune globulin IV (human)[7]	Preservative free. In 50, 100 and 200 ml with sterile IV administration set.
Rx	**Gammar-P I.V.** (Centeon)	**Powder for Injection (lyophilized):** 5% IgG, 3% human albumin	Preservative free. With 5% sucrose, 0.5% NaCl. In 1, 2.5 and 5 g single-dose vials with diluent and 10 g with administration set and diluent. With vented transfer spike.
Rx	**Iveegam** (Immuno)	**Powder for Injection (freeze-dried):** 50 mg/ml IgG	Preservative free. In 1000 mg with diluent, double-ended spike and filter needle and 2500 and 5000 mg with diluent, double-ended spike and infusion set with filter.[8]
Rx	**Polygam** (American Red Cross)	**Powder for Injection (freeze-dried):** 50 mg/ml; 90% gammaglobulin.	In 0.5, 2.5, 5 and 10 g single-use bottles.[9]

[1] In 9% to 11% maltose.
[2] In 0.16 to 0.24 M glycine.
[3] With 20 mg glucose, 2 mg polyethylene glycol, 22.5 mg glycine, 1 mcg tri-n–butyl phosphate, 1 mcg octoxynol 9, 100 mcg polysorbate 80, 3 mg albumin (human) per ml.
[4] With ≈ 1.67 g sucrose per g.
[5] With 20 mg d-mannitol, < 6 mg polyethylene glycol, 10 mg/ml albumin (human) and 5 mg/ml NaCl.
[6] With 50 mg d-sorbitol, ≤ 1.3 mg albumin (human), ≤ 100 mcg polyethylene glycol, ≤ 100 mcg polysorbate 80 and ≤ 10 mcg tri-n-butyl phosphate per ml.
[7] With 50 mg d-sorbitol, ≤ 2.6 mg albumin (human), ≤ 200 mcg polyethylene glycol, ≤ 200 mcg polysorbate 80 and ≤ 20 mcg tri-n-butyl phosphate per ml.
[8] Final solution contains 50 mg/ml glucose.
[9] With ≈ 0.15 M sodium chloride, 20 mg glucose, 2 mg polyethylene glycol, 0.3 M glycine, 3 mg/ml albumin (human).

CYTOMEGALOVIRUS IMMUNE GLOBULIN INTRAVENOUS, HUMAN (CMV-IGIV)

For additional information, refer to the Immune Serums introduction.

Actions:

Pharmacology: This product contains IgG antibodies representative of the large number of healthy persons who contributed to the plasma pools from which the product was derived. The globulin contains a relatively high concentration of antibodies directed against cytomegalovirus (CMV). In persons who may be exposed to CMV, this product can raise the relevant antibodies to levels sufficient to attenuate or reduce the incidence of serious CMV disease. In two separate clinical trials, CMV-IGIV provided effective prophylaxis in renal transplant recipients at risk for primary CMV disease. In the first randomized trial, the incidence of virologically confirmed CMV-associated syndromes was reduced from 60% in controls (n = 35) to 21% in recipients of CMV immune globulin (n = 24); marked leukopenia was reduced from 37% in controls to 4% in globulin recipients. Fungal or parasitic superinfections were not seen in globulin recipients, but occurred in 20% of controls. Serious CMV disease was reduced from 46% to 13%. There was a concomitant, but not statistically significant reduction in the incidence of CMV pneumonia (17% of controls as compared with 4% of globulin recipients). There was no effect on rates of viral isolation or seroconversion although the rate of viremia was less in CMV-IGIV recipients. In a subsequent non-randomized trial in renal transplant recipients (n = 36), the incidence of virologically confirmed CMV-associated syndrome was reduced to 36% in the globulin recipients. The rates of CMV-associated pneumonia, CMV-associated hepatitis and concomitant fungal and parasitic superinfection were similar to those in the first trial.

Indications:

Cytomegalovirus (CMV): For the attenuation of primary CMV disease associated with kidney transplantation. Specifically, the product is indicated for kidney transplant recipients who are seronegative for CMV and who receive a kidney from a CMV seropositive donor. In a population of seronegative recipients of seropositive kidneys, ≈ 75% of the untreated recipients would be expected to develop CMV disease. Clinical studies have shown a 50% reduction in primary CMV disease in renal transplant patients given CMV-IGIV.

Administration and Dosage:

The maximum recommended total dosage per infusion is 150 mg/kg, administered according to the following schedule:

Dosage Schedule for CMV-IGIV

Time of infusion	Dosage (mg/kg)
Within 72 hours of transplant	150
2 weeks post-transplant	100
4 weeks post-transplant	100
6 weeks post-transplant	100
8 weeks post-transplant	100
12 weeks post-transplant	50
16 weeks post-transplant	50

Initial dose: Administer IV at 15 mg/kg/hr. If no untoward reactions occur after 30 minutes, the rate may be increased to 30 mg/kg/hr; if no untoward reactions occur after a subsequent 30 minutes, the infusion may be increased to 60 mg/kg/hr (volume not to exceed 75 ml/hour). Do not exceed this rate of administration. Monitor the patient closely during and after each rate change.

Subsequent doses: Administer at 15 mg/kg/hr for 15 minutes. If no untoward reactions occur, increase to 30 mg/kg/hr for 15 minutes and then increase to a maximum rate of 60 mg/kg/hr (volume not to exceed 75 ml/hr). Do not exceed this rate of administration. Monitor the patient closely during each rate change.

Potential adverse reactions are: Flushing; chills; muscle cramps; back pain; fever; nausea; vomiting; wheezing; drop in blood pressure. Minor adverse reactions have been infusion-rate related. If the patient develops a minor side effect (eg, nausea, back pain, flushing), slow the rate or temporarily interrupt the infusion. If anaphylaxis or drop in blood pressure occurs, discontinue infusion and use an antidote such as diphenhydramine and epinephrine. Refer to Management of Acute Hypersensitivity Reactions.

CYTOMEGALOVIRUS IMMUNE GLOBULIN INTRAVENOUS, HUMAN (CMV-IGIV)

Infusion: Begin infusion within 6 hours after entering the vial and complete within 12 hours of entering the vial. Monitor vital signs pre-infusion, mid-way and post-infusion as well as before any rate increase. Administer through an IV line using a constant infusion pump. Pre-dilution of CMV-IGIV before infusion is not recommended. Administer through a separate IV line. If this is not possible, it may be "piggybacked" into a pre-existing line if that line contains either Sodium Chloride Injection or one of the following dextrose solutions (with or without NaCl added): 2.5%, 5%, 10% or 20% Dextrose in Water. If a pre-existing line must be used, do not dilute the CMV-IGIV more than 1:2 with any of the above solutions. Admixtures of CMV-IGIV with any other solutions have not been evaluated. Filters are not necessary for the administration of CMV-IGIV, but an in-line filter may be used for the infusion.

Storage: Store between 2° to 8°C (36° to 46°F). Use within 6 hours after entering the vial.

Rx	**CytoGam** (Massachusetts Public Health Biologic Labs)	**Solution for injection:** 50 ± 10 mg/ml[1]	Solvent detergent treated. In 50 ml vials.

[1] With 50 mg sucrose and 10 mg albumin (human)/ml.

IMMUNE GLOBULIN INTRAMUSCULAR (IG; Gamma Globulin; ISG)

For additional information, refer to the Immune Serums introduction.

Indications:

Hepatitis A: The prophylactic value of IG is greatest when given before or soon after exposure to hepatitis A. Not indicated in persons with clinical manifestations of hepatitis A or in those exposed more than 2 weeks previously.

Measles (Rubeola): For the prevention or modification of measles in susceptible contacts (one who has not been vaccinated and has not had measles previously) exposed less than 6 days previously. May be especially indicated for susceptible household contacts of measles patients, particularly those under 1 year of age, for whom the risk of complications is highest. Do not give with measles vaccine. If a child older than 12 months has received IG, give measles vaccine about 3 months later, when the measles antibody titer will have disappeared.

If a susceptible child exposed to measles is immunocompromised, administer IG immediately. Children who are immunocompromised should not receive measles vaccine or any other live viral vaccine.

Immunoglobulin deficiency: IG therapy may prevent serious infection if circulating IgG levels of ≈ 200 mg/dl plasma are maintained. However, it may not prevent chronic infections of external secretory tissues such as the respiratory and GI tracts.

Prophylactic therapy, especially against infections due to encapsulated bacteria, is often effective in Bruton-type, sex-linked congenital agammaglobulinemia, agammaglobulinemia associated with thymoma and acquired agammaglobulinemia.

Varicella: Passive immunization against varicella in immunosuppressed patients is best accomplished with varicella zoster immune globulin. If unavailable, IG may be used.

Rubella: The routine use of IG for rubella prophylaxis in early pregnancy is of dubious value and cannot be justified. Some studies suggest that the use of IG in exposed susceptible women can lessen the likelihood of infection and fetal damage. See Administration and Dosage below.

Administration and Dosage:

For IM injection only.

Hepatitis A: A dose of 0.02 ml/kg (0.01 ml/lb) is recommended for household and institutional hepatitis A case contacts. The following doses are recommended for persons who plan to travel in areas where hepatitis A is common:

IG Dose for Common Hepatitis A Areas	
Length of Stay	Dose (ml/kg)
< 3 months	0.02
Prolonged (> 3 months)	0.06 (repeat every 4 to 6 months)

Measles (Rubeola): To prevent or modify measles in a susceptible person exposed less than 6 days previously, give 0.11 ml/lb (0.25 ml/kg). If a susceptible child who is also immunocompromised is exposed to measles, give 0.5 ml/kg (15 ml maximum) immediately.

Immunoglobulin deficiency: The usual dosage consists of an initial dose of 1.3 ml/kg followed in 3 or 4 weeks by 0.66 ml/kg (at least 100 mg/kg) to be given every 3 to 4 weeks. Some patients may require more frequent injections.

Varicella: Give 0.6 to 1.2 ml/kg promptly, if zoster immune globulin is unavailable.

Rubella: Some studies suggest that the use of IG in exposed susceptible women can lessen the likelihood of infection and fetal damage; therefore, a dose of 0.55 ml/kg within 72 hours of exposure has been recommended and may benefit those women who do not consider a therapeutic abortion.

Storage: Store between 2° to 8°C (35° to 46°F). Do not freeze.

Rx	**Gamastan** (Cutter Biological)	In 2 and 10 ml vials.[1]
Rx	**Gammar** (Armour)	In 2 and 10 ml vials.[1]

[1] Dissolved in 0.3 M glycine with thimerosal.

HEPATITIS B IMMUNE GLOBULIN (HBIG)

For additional information, refer to the Immune Serums introduction.

A sterile solution of immunoglobulin (10% to 18% protein) containing a high titer of antibody to hepatitis B surface antigen (HBsAg).

Indications:

Postexposure prophylaxis following either parenteral exposure (eg, accidental "needlestick"), direct mucous membrane contact (eg, accidental splash) or oral ingestion (eg, pipetting accident) involving HB_sAg-positive materials such as blood, plasma or serum.

Prophylaxis of infants born to HB_sAg-positive mothers: Such infants are at risk of being infected with hepatitis B virus and becoming chronic carriers. The risk is especially great if the mother is HB_eAg-positive. The carrier state can be prevented in about 75% of such infections in newborns given HBIG immediately after birth and in the early months of life; 98% are prevented when HBIG is given at birth and again at 3 months of age, then active immunization with hepatitis B vaccine is begun.

Individuals at increased risk of infection with hepatitis B virus may be candidates for active vaccination with hepatitis B vaccine. Administration of HBIG either preceding or concomitant with the commencement of active immunization with hepatitis B vaccine does not interfere with the active immune response to the vaccine, and provides for more rapid achievement of protective levels of hepatitis B antibody than when the vaccine alone is administered. Rapid achievement of protective levels of antibody to hepatitis B virus may be desirable in certain clinical situations as in cases of accidental inoculations with contaminated medical instruments.

Administration and Dosage:

Give injections IM, preferably in the gluteal or deltoid region.

Postexposure prophylaxis: The recommended dose is 0.06 ml/kg; the usual adult dose is 3 to 5 ml. Administer the appropriate dose as soon after exposure as possible (preferably within 7 days) and repeat 28 to 30 days after exposure.

Prophylaxis of infants born to HB_sAG-positive mothers: The recommended dose for at-risk newborns is 0.5 ml IM into the anterolateral thigh, as soon after birth as possible, preferably within 12 hours.

Prevention of carrier state: A similar or higher rate of prevention of the carrier state may be achieved in at-risk infants by administering HBIG 0.5 ml IM as soon after birth as possible, preferably no later than 24 hours and repeated at 3 months of age. At this time, an active vaccination program with hepatitis B vaccine is begun.

Individuals at increased risk: HBIG may be administered at the same time (but at a different site), or up to 1 month preceding hepatitis B vaccination without impairing the active immune response from hepatitis B vaccination.

Storage: Store at 2° to 8°C (35° to 46°F). Do not freeze.

Hepatitis B Virus Postexposure Recommendations*

	Hepatitis B Immune Globulin		Vaccine	
Exposure	Dose (IM)	Recommended Timing	Dose (IM)	Recommended Timing
Perinatal	0.5 ml	Within 12 hrs of birth	0.5 ml	Within 12 hrs of birth;[1] repeat at 1 and 6 months
Percutaneous[2]	0.06 ml/kg	Single dose within 24 hours	1 ml[3]	Within 7 days; repeat at 1 and 6 months
Sexual	0.06 ml/kg	Single dose within 14 days of sexual contact[4]	1 ml[5]	Within 7 days; repeat at 1 and 6 months

* Morbidity and Mortality Weekly Report 1985;34:313-35 and 1988;37:341-46.

Rx	**H-BIG** (Abbott)	In 4 and 5 ml vials.[6]
Rx	**Hep-B-Gammagee** (MSD)	In 5 ml vials.[6]
Rx	**HyperHep** (Cutter Biological)	In 1 and 5 ml vials[7] and 0.5 ml prefilled syringe.

[1] First dose can be given the same time as the HBIG dose, but at a different site.
[2] Needlestick, ocular or mucosal exposure.
[3] < 10 years old, give 0.5 ml.
[4] In heterosexuals, if vaccine is not given, give a second dose of HBIG and a course of the vaccine if the index patient remains HB_sAg-positive for 3 months after detection.
[5] Vaccine recommended for homosexual men and for regular sexual contacts of HBV carriers. Vaccine optional in initial treatment of heterosexual contacts of persons with acute HBV.
[6] Dissolved in 0.3 M glycine with 1:10,000 thimerosal.
[7] Dissolved in 0.21 to 0.32 M glycine with 80 to 120 mcg/ml thimerosal.

TETANUS IMMUNE GLOBULIN

For additional information, refer to the Immune Serums introduction.

Indications:

For passive immunization against tetanus. Passive immunization is indicated for any person with a wound that might be contaminated with tetanus spores (ie, a wound other than a clean, minor wound), when the following conditions exist: The history of active immunization with tetanus toxoid is unknown or uncertain. A history of having received "tetanus shots" is not sufficient unless it can be confirmed that prior "shots" were tetanus toxoid and not tetanus antitoxin or TIG; or that the person has received either less than two prior doses of tetanus toxoid or two prior doses of tetanus toxoid, but a delay of 24 hours or more has occurred between the time of injury and initiation of tetanus prophylaxis.

If given at the time of injury, it will not interfere with the primary immune response to tetanus toxoid given at the same time at a different site, should it be necessary to begin a series of active immunization.

Tetanus antibodies of homologous origin have a half-life of 3.5 to 4.5 weeks.

Administration and Dosage:

Good medical care is essential in the prevention of tetanus in fresh wounds. Thorough cleansing and removal of all foreign and necrotic material from the injury is important.

Administer IM. Do NOT inject IV.

Prophylaxis:

Adults – 250 units.

Children – In small children, the dose may be calculated by the body weight (4 units/kg). However, it may be advisable to administer the entire contents of the vial or syringe (250 units) regardless of the child's size, since theoretically the same amount of toxin will be produced in his body by the infecting tetanus organisms as in an adult.

Therapy: Several studies suggest the value of human tetanus antitoxin in the actual treatment of active tetanus using single doses of 3000 to 6000 units in combination with other accepted clinical procedures.

The table below is a guide to active and passive tetanus immunization at the time of wound cleansing or debridement. It presumes a reliable knowledge of the patient's immunization history.

Guide to Tetanus Prophylaxis in Wound Management

History of Tetanus Immunization (Doses)	Clean, Minor Wounds		All Other Wounds	
	Tetanus Toxoid	Tetanus Immune Globulin	Tetanus Toxoid	Tetanus Immune Globulin
Uncertain	Yes	No	Yes	Yes
0 to 1	Yes	No	Yes	Yes
2	Yes	No	Yes	No[1]
3 or more	No[2]	No	No[3]	No

Storage: Store between 2° and 8°C (35° and 46°F). Do not freeze.

Rx	**Hyper-Tet** (Cutter Biological)	In 250 unit vial[4] and 250 unit disp. syringe.[4]

[1] Unless wound is more than 24 hours old.
[2] Unless more than 10 years since last dose.
[3] Unless more than 5 years since last dose.
[4] Dissolved in 0.21 to 0.32 M glycine with 80 to 120 mcg thimerosal.

VARICELLA-ZOSTER IMMUNE GLOBULIN (HUMAN) (VZIG)

For additional information, refer to the Immune Serums introduction.

Actions:

Pharmacology: VZIG (Human) is the globulin fraction of human plasma, primarily immunoglobulin G (IgG) found in routine screening of normal volunteer blood donors. When absorbed into the circulation, the antibodies persist for ≥ 1 month and are sufficient to mitigate or prevent varicella infection. It significantly reduces mortality and morbidity from varicella among immunodeficient children.

Indications:

Passive immunization of susceptible immunodeficient individuals after significant exposure to varicella (see criteria below). Most effective if begun within 96 hrs of exposure. There is no evidence it modifies established Varicella-Zoster infections.

VZIG supplies are limited; restrict use to those meeting the following criteria:

1.) One of the following underlying illnesses or conditions:
   - a.) Neoplastic disease (eg, leukemia or lymphoma)
   - b.) Congenital or acquired immunodeficiency
   - c.) Immunosuppressive therapy with steroids, antimetabolites or other immunosuppressive treatment regimens.
   - d.) Newborn of mother who had onset of chickenpox within 5 days before delivery or within 48 hours after delivery
   - e.) Premature (≥ 28 weeks' gestation) if mother has no history of chickenpox
   - f.) Premature (< 28 weeks' gestation or ≤ 1000 g VZIG) regardless of maternal history

2.) One of the following types of exposure to chickenpox or zoster patient(s):
   - a.) Continuous household contact
   - b.) Playmate contact (>1 hour play indoors)
   - c.) Hospital contact (in same 2 to 4 bed room or adjacent beds in a large ward or prolonged face-to-face contact with an infectious staff member or patient)

3.) Susceptible to varicella zoster.

4.) Age of < 15 years; administer to immunocompromised adolescents and adults and to other older patients on an *individual basis.*

5.) If VZIG can be administered within 96 hours after exposure, but preferably sooner.

Not for prophylactic use in immunodeficient patients with history of varicella, unless patient's immunosuppression is associated with bone marrow transplantation.

Not recommended for nonimmunodeficient patients, including pregnant women, because the severity of chickenpox is much less than in immunosuppressed patients.

Administration and Dosage:

Administer as soon as possible after presumed exposure, as late as 96 hours after exposure. High risk susceptible patients who are exposed again more than 3 weeks after a prior dose of VZIG should receive another full dose.

Do not inject IV. Administer by deep IM injection in the gluteal or other large muscle mass. Inject 125 units per 10 kg (22 lbs), up to a maximum dose of 625 units (5 vials). The minimum dose is 125 units; do not give fractional doses. Administer entire contents of each vial. For patients ≤ 10 kg, administer 1.25 ml at a single site. For patients > 10 kg, give no more than 2.5 ml at a single site.

VZIG Dose Based on Weight

Weight of Patient		Dose	
Kilograms	Pounds	Units	Number of Vials
0 to 10	0 to 22	125	1
10.1 to 20	22.1 to 44	250	2
20.1 to 30	44.1 to 66	375	3
30.1 to 40	66.1 to 88	500	4
> 40	> 88	625	5

The regimen effectively modifies severity of chickenpox, and reduces frequency of death, pneumonia and encephalitis to < 25% expected without treatment.

Storage: Store at 2° to 8°C (35° to 46°F).

Rx	**Varicella-Zoster Immune Globulin (Human)** (American Red Cross, Northeast Region)[1]	**Injection:** A sterile 10% to 18% solution of the globulin fraction of human plasma, primarily IgG.	In single dose vials[2] containing 125 units of varicella-zoster virus antibody in 2.5 ml or less.

[1] Within Mass., VZIG is distributed by the Mass. Public Health Biologic Laboratories. Outside Mass., distribution is arranged by the American Red Cross Blood Services – Northeast Region through other regional distribution centers. VZIG is distributed free of charge to Mass. residents.

[2] In 0.3 M glycine as a stabilizer and 1:10,000 thimerosal.

RH_O (D) IMMUNE GLOBULIN

For additional information, refer to the Immune Serums introduction.

Actions:

Pharmacology: Effectively suppresses the immune response of nonsensitized Rh_O (D) negative individuals who receive Rh_O (D) positive blood as the result of a fetomaternal hemorrhage, abdominal trauma, amniocentesis, abortion, full-term delivery or transfusion accident.

Each vial of Rh_O (D) completely suppresses immunity to 15 ml of Rh-positive packed red blood cells (RBCs) (≈ 30 ml whole blood). One vial contains approximately
300 mcg immunoglobulin.

Indications:

Full term delivery: To prevent sensitization to the Rh_O (D) factor and to prevent hemolytic disease of the newborn (Erythroblastosis fetalis) in a subsequent pregnancy. It effectively suppresses the immune response of nonsensitized Rh-negative mothers after delivery of an Rh-positive infant.

Criteria for an Rh-incompatible pregnancy requiring administration are:

1.) The mother must be Rh_O (D)—negative.
2.) The mother has not been previously sensitized to Rh_O (D) factor.
3.) The infant must be Rh_O (D)-positive and direct antiglobulin negative.
4.) If the father can be determined to be Rh_O (D) antigen-negative, Rh_O (D) IG need not be given. Do not perform Rh_O (D) cross-match prior to administration.

Incomplete pregnancy: Administer to all nonsensitized Rh-negative women after spontaneous or induced abortions, ruptured tubal pregnancies, amniocentesis and other abdominal trauma, chorionic villus sampling, percutaneous umbilical-cord blood sampling, fetal surgery or manipulation or any occurrence of transplacental hemorrhage, unless the blood type of the fetus or the father has been determined to be Rh_O (D)-negative. Sensitization occurs more frequently in women undergoing induced abortions than in those aborting spontaneously.

For antepartum prophylaxis:

Note – In a case of abortion or ectopic pregnancy when Rh typing of the fetus is not possible, assume the fetus to be Rh_O (D)-positive and consider the patient a candidate for administration of Rh_O (D) immune globulin. If the father can be determined to be Rh_O (D)-negative, Rh_O (D) immune globulin need not be given.

Transfusions: To prevent Rh_O (D) sensitization in Rh_O (D)-negative patients accidentally transfused with Rh_O (D)-positive blood, which may include massive platelet transfusion.

Unlabeled uses: Although controversial, some physicians advocate administration prior to *external version* attempts for breech presentations (due to induced fetomaternal hemorrhage) and following *tubal ligation* after delivery of a Rh_O (D)-positive infant (to prevent problems should the sterilization fail or subsequent tubal reanastomoses occur).

Administration and Dosage:

Do not give IV.

Do not give Rh_O (D) immune globulin to: The postpartum infant; to a Rh_O (D)-positive individual; or to a Rh_O (D)-negative individual previously sensitized to the Rh_O (D) antigen.

Note: Although there is no need to administer Rh_O (D) immune globulin to a woman who is already sensitized to the Rh factor, there is no more risk than when it is given to a woman who is not sensitized. When in doubt, administer Rh_O (D) immune globulin.

Administer within 72 hours after Rh incompatible delivery, miscarriage, abortion or transfusion.

Preadministration laboratory procedure: Immediately postpartum, determine the infant's blood type (ABO, Rh_O [D]) and perform a direct antiglobulin test using umbilical cord, venous or capillary blood.

Confirm that the mother is RH_O (D)-negative.

Obstetrical usage: One vial prevents maternal sensitization to the Rh factor if the fetal packed RBC volume that entered the mother's blood due to fetomaternal hemorrhage is less than 15 ml (30 ml of whole blood). When the fetomaternal hemorrhage exceeds this, administer more than one vial.

Postpartum prophylaxis – Administer one vial IM, preferably within 72 hours of delivery. If an unusually large fetomaternal hemorrhage is suspected, determine the number of vials required as described below.

Antepartum prophylaxis – Inject one vial (approximately 300 mcg) IM at 26 to 28 weeks gestation and one vial within 72 hours after an Rh-incompatible delivery to prevent Rh isoimmunization during pregnancy.

RH_O (D) IMMUNE GLOBULIN

To determine number of vials required, determine volume of packed fetal RBCs by approved laboratory assay. The volume of fetomaternal hemorrhage divided by 2 gives the volume of packed fetal RBCs in maternal blood. Determine number of vials to be administered by dividing volume (ml) of packed RBCs by 15.

Following amniocentesis, miscarriage, abortion or ectopic pregnancy at or beyond 13 weeks' gestation – One vial IM.

Transfusion accidents: The number of vials to be administered depends on the volume of packed RBCs or whole blood transfused. Multiply the volume (in ml) of Rh-positive whole blood administered by the hematocrit of the donor unit. This value equals the volume of packed red blood cells transfused. Divide the volume (in ml) of packed RBCs by 15 to obtain the number of vials to be administered. If the dosage calculation results in a fraction, administer the next whole number of vials.

One vial dose: Withdraw the entire contents of the vial and inject IM.

Two or more vial dose: The contents of the total number of vials may be injected as a divided dose at different injection sites at the same time, or the total dosage may be divided and injected at intervals if the total dosage is injected within 72 hours postpartum or after a transfusion accident.

Storage: Store at 2° to 8°C (35° to 46°F). Do not freeze.

Rx	**Gamulin Rh** (Armour)	Each package contains one single dose vial of Rh_O (D) Immune Globulin[1], patient ID card, directions for use, lab control form and patient information brochure.
Rx	**HypRho-D** (Miles)	Each package contains one prefilled syringe of Rh_O (D) Immune Globulin[2], and directions for use.
Rx	**RhoGAM** (Ortho Diagnostics)	Each package contains one single dose vial or prefilled syringe of Rh_O (D) Immune Globulin[3], package insert, control form and patient ID card.

[1] Dissolved in 0.3 M glycine with 0.01% thimerosal.
[2] Dissolved in 0.21 to 0.32 M glycine with 80 to 120 mcg thimerosal.
[3] Dissolved in glycine 15 mg/ml with 0.003% thimerosal, 2.9 mg sodium chloride and 0.01% polysorbate 80.

RH_O (D) IMMUNE GLOBULIN MICRO-DOSE

For additional information, refer to the Immune Serums introduction.

One vial will suppress the immune response to 2.5 ml of Rh_O (D)-positive packed red blood cells. One vial contains approximately 50 mcg immunoglobulin.

This dose is indicated for the prevention of isoimmunization in Rh-negative women following spontaneous or induced abortion or termination of ectopic pregnancy up to and including 12 weeks gestation, unless the father is Rh-negative. At or beyond 13 weeks gestation, administer a full dose (300 mcg) RH_O (D) Immune Globulin.

Give one vial IM as soon as possible after termination of pregnancy.

Storage: Store at 2° to 8°C (35° to 46°F). Do not freeze.

Rx	**HypRho-D Mini-Dose** (Miles)	Each package contains one single dose syringe of Rh_O (D) Immune Globulin micro-dose[1], package insert.
Rx	**MICRhoGAM** (Ortho Diagnostics)	Each package contains one single dose prefilled syringe of Rh_O (D) Immune Globulin micro-dose[2], package insert, injection control form and patient ID card.
Rx	**Mini-Gamulin Rh** (Armour)	Each package contains one single dose vial of Rh_O (D) Immune Globulin micro-dose[3], package insert, injection control form and patient ID card.

[1] Dissolved in 0.21 to 0.32 M glycine with 80 to 120 mcg thimerosal.
[2] Dissolved in 15 mg glycine per ml with 0.003% thimerosal.
[3] Dissolved in 0.3 M glycine with 0.01% thimerosal, 2.9 mg sodium chloride and 0.01% polysorbate 80.

RH_o (D) IMMUNE GLOBULIN IV (HUMAN)

Actions:

Pharmacology: Rh_o (D) immune globulin IV (Rh_o [D] IGIV) is a sterile, freeze-dried gamma globulin (IgG) fraction containing antibodies to Rh_o (D). For use in the suppression of Rh isoimmunization, Rh_o (D) IGIV may be administered either IM or IV. For use in the treatment of immune thrombocytopenic purpura (ITP), the drug must be administered IV. The manufacturing process includes a solvent-detergent treatment step that is effective in inactivating lipid-enveloped viruses such as hepatitis B, hepatitis C and HIV. This process is designed to increase product safety by reducing the risk of virus transmission. This product contains ≈ 2 mcg IgA per 1500 International Units (300 mcg). In the past, a full dose of Rh_o (D) immune globulin has traditionally been referred to as a "300 mcg" dose. Potency and dosing recommendations are now expressed in IU by comparison to the WHO Anti-D standard. The conversion of "mcg" to "IU" is 1 mcg = 5 IU. Rh_o (D) immune globulin is prepared from human plasma by an anion-exchange column chromatography method. A 1500 IU (300 mcg) vial contains sufficient anti-Rh_o(D) to effectively suppress the immunizing potential of ≈ 17 ml of Rh_o (D) antigen-positive red blood cells.

Rh_o (D) IGIV is used to suppress the immune response of non-sensitized Rh_o (D) antigen-negative individuals following Rh_o (D) antigen-positive red blood cell exposure by fetomaternal hemorrhage during delivery of an Rh_o (D) antigen-positive infant, abortion (spontaneous or induced), amniocentesis, abdominal trauma or mismatched transfusion. The mechanism of action is not completely understood.

Rh_o (D) immune globulin, when administered within 72 hours of a full-term delivery of an Rh_o (D) antigen-positive infant by an Rh_o (D) antigen-negative mother, will reduce the incidence of Rh isoimmunization from between 12% and 13% to between 1% and 2%. The 1% to 2% range is due, for the most part, to isoimmunization during the last trimester of pregnancy. When treatment is given both antenatally at 28 weeks gestation and postpartum, the Rh immunization rate drops to ≈ 0.1%.

When 600 IU (120 mcg) of Rh_o (D) IGIV is given to pregnant women, passive anti-Rh_o (D) antibodies are not detectable in the circulation for > 6 weeks, and therefore, a dose of 1500 IU (300 mcg) should be used for antenatal administration.

In a clinical study with Rh_o (D) antigen-negative volunteers (9 males and 1 female), Rh_o (D) antigen-positive red cells were completely cleared from the circulation within 8 hours of IV administration. There was no indication of Rh isoimmunization of these subjects at 6 months after the clearance of the Rh_o (D) antigen-positive red cells (RBCs).

Rh_o (D) IGIV increases platelets in ITP patients. Platelet counts usually rise within 1 to 2 days and peak within 7 to 14 days after initiation of therapy. The duration of response is variable; however, the average duration is ≈ 30 days. The mechanism of action is not completely understood.

Pharmacokinetics:

IM vs IV administration – In a clinical study involving Rh_o (D) antigen-negative volunteers, two subjects were given 600 IU (120 mcg) IM and two subjects were given this dose IV. Peak levels (36 to 48 ng/ml) were reached within 2 hours of IV administration; for IM, peak levels (18 to 19 ng/ml) were reached at 5 to 10 days. The calculated areas under the curve were the same for both routes of administration. The half-life was about 24 and 30 days following IV and IM administration, respectively.

Clinical trials:

Childhood chronic ITP – In one study, 24 children with ITP > 6 months duration were treated initially with 250 IU/kg (50 mcg) Rh_o (D) IGIV (125 IU/kg on days 1 and 2), with subsequent doses ranging from 125 to 275 IU/kg. Response was defined as a platelet increase to at least 50,000/mm^3 and a doubling of the baseline value. Nineteen of 24 patients responded for an overall response rate of 79%, an overall mean peak platelet count of 229,400/mm^3 (range, 43,300 to 456,000) and a mean duration of response of 36.5 days (range, 6 to 84).

Childhood acute ITP – A trial comparing Rh_o (D) IGIV to high- and low-dose IGIV and prednisone was conducted in 146 children with acute ITP and platelet counts < 20,000/mm^3. Of 38 patients receiving Rh_o (D) IGIV (125 IU/kg on days 1 and 2), 32 patients (84%) responded (platelet count ≥ 50,000/mm^3) with a mean peak platelet count of 319,500/mm^3 (range, 61,000 to 892,000), with no statistically significant differences compared to other treatment arms. The mean times to achieving ≥ 20,000/mm^3 or ≥ 50,000/mm^3 platelets for patients receiving Rh_o (D) IGIV were 1.9 and 2.6 days, respectively.

Adult chronic ITP – Adults (n = 24) with ITP of > 6 months duration and platelet counts < 30,000/mm^3 or requiring therapy were treated with 100 to 375 IU/kg Rh_o (D) IGIV (mean dose, 231 IU/kg). Twenty-one of 24 patients responded (increase ≥ 20,000/mm^3) during the first two courses of therapy for an overall response rate of 88% and a mean peak platelet count of 92,300/mm^3 (range, 8,000 to 229,000).

RH_o (D) IMMUNE GLOBULIN IV (HUMAN)

ITP secondary to HIV infection – Children (n = 11) and adults (n = 52) with all Walter Reed classes of HIV infection and ITP, and with initial platelet counts of ≤ 30,000/mm^3 or otherwise requiring therapy, were treated with 100 to 375 IU/kg Rh_o (D) IGIV, administered for an average of 7.3 courses (range, 1 to 57) over a mean period of 407 days (range, 6 to 1952). Of 63 patients, 57 responded (increase ≥ 20,000/mm^3) during the first 6 courses of therapy for an overall response rate of 90%. The overall mean change in platelet count for 6 courses was 60,900/mm^3 (range, -2,000 to 565,000) and the mean peak platelet count was 81,700/mm^3 (range, 16,000 to 593,000).

Indications:

Pregnancy/Other obstetric conditions: Suppression of Rh isoimmunization in non-sensitized Rh_o (D) antigen-negative women within 72 hours after spontaneous or induced abortions, amniocentesis, chorionic vilus sampling, ruptured tubal pregnancy, abdominal trauma, transplacental hemorrhage or in the normal course of pregnancy unless the blood type of the fetus or father is known to be Rh_o (D) antigen-negative. In the case of maternal bleeding due to threatened abortion, administer Rh_o (D) immune globulin as soon as possible. Suppression of Rh isoimmunization reduces the likelihood of hemolytic disease in an Rh_o (D) antigen-positive fetus in present and future pregnancies.

Transfusion: Suppression of Rh isoimmunization in Rh_o (D) antigen-negative female children and female adults in their childbearing years transfused with Rh_o (D) antigen-positive RBCs or blood components containing Rh_o (D) antigen-positive RBCs. Initiate treatment within 72 hours of exposure. Give treatment (without preceding exchange transfusion) only if the transfused Rh_o (D) antigen-positive blood represents < 20% of the total circulating red cells. A 1500 IU (300 mcg) dose will suppress the immunizing potential of ≈ 17 ml of Rh_o (D) antigen-positive RBCs.

Immune thrombocytopenic purpura (ITP): Treatment of non-splenectomized Rh_o (D) antigen-positive children with chronic or acute ITP, adults with chronic ITP or children and adults with ITP secondary to HIV infection in clinical situations requiring an increase in platelet count to prevent excessive hemorrhage.

Contraindications:

Individuals known to have had an anaphylactic or severe systemic reaction to human globulin. Rh_o (D) immune globulin contains trace amounts of IgA (≈ 2 mcg per 1500 IU [300 mcg] vial). Individuals who are deficient in IgA may have the potential for developing IgA antibodies and have anaphylactic reactions. Weigh the potential benefit of treatment with Rh_o (D) immune globulin against the potential for hypersensitivity reactions.

Warnings:

Criteria for Rh_o (D) IGIV administration: The criteria for an Rh-incompatible pregnancy requiring administration of Rh_o (D) immune globulin at 28 weeks gestation and within 72 hours after delivery are: The mother must be Rh_o (D) antigen-negative; the mother is carrying a child whose father is either Rh_o (D) antigen-positive or Rh_o (D) unknown; the infant is either Rh_o (D) antigen-positive or Rh_o (D) unknown; and the mother must not be previously sensitized to the Rh_o (D) antigen (and thus possessing anti-Rh_o [D] antibodies).

Route of administration (ITP): Rh_o (D) IGIV must be administered IV for the treatment of ITP. Efficacy of the IM or SC routes has not been established.

Rh_o (D) antigen-negative or splenectomized patients: Do not administer to Rh_o (D) antigen-negative or splenectomized individuals as its efficacy in these patients has not been demonstrated.

Pregnancy: Category C. It is not known whether Rh_o (D) immune globulin can cause fetal harm when administered to a pregnant woman or can affect reproductive capacity. Give to a pregnant woman only if clearly needed.

Children: For the suppression of Rh isoimmunization in the mother. Do not administer to the infant.

Precautions:

Suppression of Rh isoimmunization: Rh_o (D) IGIV should not be administered to Rh_o (D) antigen-negative individuals who are Rh immunized [Rh antibody-positive], as evidenced by standard manual Rh antibody screening tests.

Fetomaternal hemorrhage – A large fetomaternal hemorrhage late in pregnancy or following delivery may cause a weak mixed field positive D^u test result. Assess such an individual for a large fetomaternal hemorrhage and adjust the dose of Rh_o (D) immune globulin accordingly. Administer Rh_o (D) immune globulin if there is any doubt about the mother's blood type.

RH_o (D) IMMUNE GLOBULIN IV (HUMAN)

Hemoglobin: If a patient has a lower than normal hemoglobin level (< 10 g/dl), give a reduced dose of 125 to 200 IU/kg to minimize the risk of increasing the severity of anemia in the patient. Rh_o (D) IGIV must be used with extreme caution in patients with a hemoglobin level that is < 8 g/dl due to the risk of increasing the severity of the anemia.

Laboratory tests: The presence of passively administered anti-Rh_o (D) antibodies in maternal or fetal blood can lead to a false-positive direct antiglobulin test. If there is an uncertainty about mother's Rh group or immune status, administer Rh_o (D) immune globulin to the mother.

Adverse Reactions:

Rh isoimmunization suppression: Adverse reactions to Rh_o (D) immune globulin are infrequent in Rh_o (D) antigen-negative individuals. In the clinical trial of 1186 Rh_o (D) antigen-negative pregnant women, no adverse events were attributed to the drug. Discomfort and slight swelling at the injection site and slight elevation in temperature have been reported in a small number of cases. As is the case with all drugs of this nature, there is a remote chance of an anaphylactic reaction in individuals with hypersensitivity to blood products. There was one report of an Rh_o (D) antigen-negative patient who had received one unit of Rh_o (D) antigen-positive blood and experienced chills, shaking, nausea, myalgia, vomiting, drowsiness, disorientation and lethargy after receiving 6000 IU.

ITP: Side effects related to the destruction of Rh_o (D) antigen-positive red cells, such as decreased hemoglobin, can be expected. At the recommended initial IV dose of 250 IU/kg, the mean maximum decrease in hemoglobin was 1.7 g/dl (range, +0.4 to -6.1 g/dl). At a reduced dose, ranging from 125 to 200 IU/kg, the mean maximum decrease in hemoglobin was 0.61 g/dl (range, +0.65 to -1.9 g/dl). Only 5 of the 137 (3.7%) patients had a maximum decrease in hemoglobin of > 4 g/dl.

In trials in subjects (n = 161) with childhood acute ITP, adults and children with chronic ITP and adults and children with ITP secondary to HIV, 60 of 846 (7%) infusions were associated with at least one adverse event that was considered to be related to the study medication. The most common adverse events were headache (19 infusions; 2%), chills (14 infusions; < 2%), and fever (9 infusions; 1%). All are expected adverse events associated with infusions of immunoglobulins.

One child with chronic ITP who received an initial dose of 250 IU/kg Rh_o (D) IGIV followed by 175 IU/kg on day 15 had a drop in hemoglobin from 12.4 to 7.6 g/dl after the second course of treatment. Rh_o(D) IGIV was subsequently withheld.

Overdosage:

In clinical studies with nonpregnant Rh_o (D) antigen-positive patients with ITP (n = 141) treated with 600 to 32,500 IU of Rh_o (D) IGIV, there were no signs or symptoms that warranted medical intervention. However, these same doses were associated with a mild, transient hemolytic anemia.

Administration and Dosage:

Approved by the FDA on March 24, 1995.

Rh_o (D) IGIV may be given IV or IM for the suppression of Rh isoimmunization.

Rh_o (D) IGIV must be given IV for the treatment of ITP.

Pregnancy: Administer IM or IV.

Administer 1500 IU (300 mcg) at 28 weeks gestation. If Rh_o (D) immune globulin is administered early in the pregnancy, it is recommended that it be given at 12 week intervals in order to maintain an adequate level of passively acquired anti-Rh (antibodies).

Administer a 600 IU (120 mcg) dose as soon as possible after delivery of a confirmed Rh_o (D) antigen-positive baby and within 72 hours after delivery. In the event that the Rh status of the baby is not known at 72 hours, administer Rh_o (D) immune globulin to the mother at 72 hours after delivery. If > 72 hours have elapsed, do not withhold Rh_o (D) immune globulin, but administer as soon as possible, up to 28 days after delivery.

Other obstetric conditions: Administer IM or IV.

Administer 600 IU (120 mcg) immediately after abortion, amniocentesis (after 34 weeks gestation) or any other manipulation late in pregnancy (after 34 weeks gestation) associated with increased risk of Rh isoimmunization. Administration should take place within 72 hours after the event.

Administer a 1500 IU (300 mcg) dose immediately after amniocentesis before 34 weeks gestation or after chorionic vilus sampling. Repeat this dose every 12 weeks during the pregnancy. In the case of threatened abortion, administer as soon as possible.

RH_o (D) IMMUNE GLOBULIN IV (HUMAN)

Transfusion: Administer within 72 hours after exposure for treatment of incompatible blood transfusions or massive fetal hemorrhage, as outlined in the following table.

Rh$_o$ (D) IGIV Dosage			
Route	Dose & Frequency	Rh+ blood/ml blood	Rh+ red cells/ml cells
IV	3000 IU (600 mcg) every 8 hours until the total dose is administered	45 IU (9 mcg)	90 IU (18 mcg)
IM	6000 IU (1200 mcg) every 12 hours until the total dose is administered.	60 IU (12 mcg)	120 IU (24 mcg)

ITP: An initial dose of 250 IU (50 mcg) per kg is recommended. If the patient has a hemoglobin level < 10 g/dl, give a reduced dose of 125 to 200 IU (25 to 40 mcg) per kg to minimize the risk of increasing the severity of the patient's anemia. The initial dose may be administered as a single dose or in two divided doses given on separate days. Monitor all patients to determine clinical response by assessing platelet counts, red cell counts, hemoglobin and reticulocyte levels. If subsequent therapy is required to elevate platelet counts, an IV dose of 125 to 300 IU (25 to 60 mcg) per kg is recommended. Determine the frequency and dose used in maintenance therapy by the patient's clinical response when assessing platelet counts, red cell counts, hemoglobin and reticulocyte levels.

Reconstitution:

IV administration – Aseptically reconstitute the product shortly before use with 2.5 ml of 0.9% sodium chloride injection (see following table). Inject the diluent slowly onto the inside wall of the vial and wet the pellet by gently swirling until dissolved. Do not shake. Infuse into a suitable vein over 3 to 5 minutes.

IM administration – Aseptically reconstitute the product shortly before use with 1.25 ml of 0.9% sodium chloride injection (see following table). Inject the diluent slowly onto the inside wall of the vial and wet the pellet by gently swirling until dissolved. Do not shake. Administer into the deltoid muscle of the upper arm or the anterolateral aspects of the upper thigh. Due to the risk of sciatic nerve injury, the gluteal region should not be used as a routine injection site. If the gluteal region is used, use only the upper, outer quadrant.

Reconstitution of Rh$_o$ (D) IGIV			
Vial size	Volume of diluent to be added to vial	Approximate available volume	Nominal concentration/ml
IV injection			
600 IU (120 mcg)	2.5 ml	2.4 ml	240 IU (48 mcg)
1500 IU (300 mcg)	2.5 ml	2.4 ml	600 IU (120 mcg)
IM injection			
600 IU (120 mcg)	1.25 ml	1.2 ml	480 IU (96 mcg)
1500 IU (300 mcg)	1.25 ml	1.2 ml	1200 IU (240 mcg)

Admixture compatibility/incompatibility: Reconstitute only with 0.9% sodium chloride injection. Do not administer with other products.

Storage/Stability: Store at 2° to 8°C (35° to 46°F). Do not freeze. If the reconstituted product is not used immediately, store it at room temperature for no longer than 4 hours. Do not freeze the reconstituted product. Use the product within 4 hours of reconstitution. Discard any unused portion.

Rx	**WinRho SD** (Univax)	**Injection**: 600 IU (120 mcg)	With 2.5 ml diluent. In 10s.
		Injection: 1500 IU (300 mcg)	With 2.5 ml diluent. In 10s.

LYMPHOCYTE IMMUNE GLOBULIN, ANTI-THYMOCYTE GLOBULIN (EQUINE) (LIG, ATG)

Warning:

Only physicians experienced in immunosuppressive therapy and management of renal transplant patients should use this product.

Patients receiving this drug should be managed in facilities equipped and staffed with adequate laboratory and supportive medical resources.

Actions:

Pharmacology: Lymphocyte immune globulin, anti-thymocyte globulin (equine), is a lymphocyte-selective immunosuppressant. It reduces the number of circulating, thymus-dependent lymphocytes that form rosettes with sheep erythrocytes. This antilymphocytic effect is believed to reflect an alteration of the function of the T-lymphocytes, which are responsible, in part, for cell-mediated immunity and are involved in humoral immunity. It also contains low concentrations of antibodies against other formed elements of the blood. In rhesus and cynomolgus monkeys, this drug reduces lymphocytes in the thymus-dependent areas of the spleen and lymph nodes. It also decreases the circulating sheep-erythrocyte-rosetting lymphocytes that can be detected, but ordinarily does not cause severe lymphopenia.

In general, when administered with other immunosuppressive therapy, such as antimetabolites and corticosteroids, the patient's own antibody response to horse gamma globulin is minimal.

Precise methods of determining potency have not been established; thus activity may potentially vary from lot to lot.

In general, ATG enables a 1 year graft survival rate of ≥ 80%. Graft and patient survival are dependent on whether the transplanted organ is harvested from a living or deceased host, the degree of antigenic matching, the combination of immunosuppressive drugs delivered and other factors.

Pharmacokinetics: Onset is rapid. Peak plasma level of equine IgG occurs after 5 days of infusion at 10 mg/kg/day. Peak values vary depending on recipient's ability to catabolize equine IgG. In a small study, mean peak plasma value was 727 ± 310 mcg/ml. Rosette-forming cells decrease immediately after beginning therapy. Recovery to normal values after therapy cessation is dependent on recipient's catabolic rate and, in some cases, upon length of therapy. Mean half-life is 5.7 days (range, 1.5 to 13 days). About 1% of equine IgG is excreted in urine, mostly intact.

Indications:

Renal transplantation: Management of allograft rejection in renal transplant patients. When administered with conventional therapy at the time of rejection, it increases the frequency of resolution of the acute rejection episode.

Also used as an adjunct to other immunosuppressives to delay onset of first rejection episode. Data have not consistently demonstrated improvement in functional graft survival associated with therapy to delay onset of first rejection episode.

Aplastic anemia: Treatment of moderate to severe aplastic anemia in patients unsuited for bone marrow transplantation. When administered with a regimen of supportive care, ATG may include partial or complete hematologic remission.

Unlabeled uses: As an immunosuppressant in the course of liver, bone-marrow, heart and other organ transplants; treatment of multiple sclerosis, myasthenia gravis, pure red-cell aplasia and scleroderma, although efficacy is not definitively established.

Contraindications:

Severe systemic reaction during prior administration of the drug or any other equine gamma globulin preparation.

Warnings:

Hematologic effects: Discontinue treatment if severe and unremitting thrombocytopenia or leukopenia occur.

Hemolysis – Clinically significant hemolysis is rare. Treatment may include transfusion of erythrocytes; if necessary, administer IV mannitol, furosemide, sodium bicarbonate and fluids. Severe and unremitting hemolysis may require discontinuation of therapy.

Thrombocytopenia is usually transient; platelet counts generally return to adequate levels without discontinuing therapy and without transfusions.

Hypersensitivity: Uncommon but serious, anaphylaxis may occur at any time during therapy. Stop infusion immediately; administer 0.3 ml aqueous epinephrine 1:1000 IM. Administer steroids, assist respiration and provide other resuscitative measures. Do not resume therapy. Respiratory distress or hypotension may indicate anaphylaxis. Pain in chest, flank or back may indicate anaphylaxis or hemolysis. Stop infusion; treat appropriately.

Pregnancy: Category C. Safety for use during pregnancy has not been established. Use only when clearly needed and when the potential benefits outweigh the potential hazards to the fetus.

Lactation: It is not known if ATG antibodies are excreted into breast milk.

Children: Experience with children has been limited. The drug has been administered safely to a small number of pediatric renal allograft recipients at dosage levels comparable to those used in adults on a mg per kg basis.

Precautions:

Infection: Because this agent is ordinarily given with corticosteroids and antimetabolites, monitor patients carefully for concurrent infection. If infection occurs, institute adjunctive therapy promptly. On the basis of the clinical circumstances, decide whether therapy will continue.

Concomitant immunosuppressive therapy: Safety and efficacy have not been demonstrated in renal transplant patients receiving concomitant immunosuppressive therapy.

When the dose of corticosteroids and other immunosuppressants is being reduced, some previously masked reactions to the drug may appear; observe patients carefully during therapy.

Chills and fever occur frequently. ATG may release endogenous leukocyte pyrogens. Prophylactic or therapeutic administration of antihistamines or corticosteroids generally controls this reaction.

Chemical phlebitis can be caused by infusion through peripheral veins. Avoid by administering the solution into a high-flow vein.

Itching and erythema probably result from the drug's effect on blood elements. Antihistamines control the symptoms.

Adverse Reactions:

Renal transplantation: Fever (33%); chills, leukopenia (14%); dermatological reactions (eg, rash, pruritus, urticaria, wheal, flare 13%); thrombocytopenia (11%); arthralgia, chest/back pain, clotted A/V fistula, diarrhea, dyspnea, headache, hypotension, nausea, vomiting, night sweats, pain at the infusion site, peripheral thrombophlebitis, stomatitis (1% to 5%); anaphylaxis, dizziness, weakness, faintness, edema, herpes simplex reactivation, hiccoughs, epigastric pain, hyperglycemia, hypertension, iliac vein obstruction, laryngospasm, localized infection, lymphadenopathy, malaise, myalgia, paresthesia, possible serum sickness, pulmonary edema, renal artery thrombosis, seizures, systemic infection, tachycardia, toxic epidermal necrosis, wound dehiscence (< 1%).

Aplastic anemia: Chills, arthralgia (50%); headache (17%); myalgia (10%); nausea, chest pain (7%); phlebitis (5%); diaphoresis, joint stiffness, periorbital edema, aches, edema, muscle ache, vomiting, agitation/lethargy, listlessness, lightheadedness, seizures, diarrhea, bradycardia, myocarditis, cardiac irregularity, hepatosplenomegaly, encephalitis or postviral encephalopathy, hypotension, CHF, hypertension, burning soles/palms, foot sole pain, lymphadenopathy, postcervical lymphadenopathy, tender lymph nodes, bilateral pleural effusion, respiratory distress, anaphylaxis, proteinuria (< 5%); abnormal tests of liver function (eg, AST, ALT, alkaline phosphatase) and renal function (eg, serum creatinine). In some trials, clinical and laboratory findings of serum sickness were seen in a majority of patients.

Post-marketing experience: Fever (51%); thrombocytopenia (30%); rashes (27%); chills (16%); leukopenia (14%); systemic infection (13%); abnormal renal function tests, serum sickness-like symptoms, dyspnea or apnea, arthralgia, chest/back/flank pain, diarrhea, nausea, vomiting (5% to 10%); hypertension, herpes simplex infection, pain, swelling or redness at the infusion site, eosinophilia, headache, myalgia, leg pains, hypotension, anaphylaxis, tachycardia, edema, localized infection, malaise, seizures, GI bleeding/ perforation, deep vein thrombosis, sour mouth/throat, hyperglycemia, acute renal failure, abnormal liver function tests, confusion, disorientation, cough, neutropenia, granulocytopenia, anemia, thrombophlebitis, dizziness, epigastric/stomach pain, lymphadenopathy, pulmonary edema, CHF, abdominal pain, nosebleed, vasculitis, aplasia, pancytopenia, abnormal involuntary movement, tremor, rigidity, sweating, laryngospasm, edema, hemolysis/hemolytic anemia, viral hepatitis, faintness, enlarged/ruptured kidney, paresthesias, renal artery thrombosis (< 5%).

LYMPHOCYTE IMMUNE GLOBULIN, ANTI-THYMOCYTE GLOBULIN (EQUINE) (LIG, ATG)

Administration and Dosage:

Skin testing: Test patients with an intradermal injection of 0.1 ml of a 1:1000 dilution (5 mcg horse IgG) in normal saline and a saline control. If this causes a wheal or erythema > 10 mm or both with or without pseudopod formation and itching or a marked local swelling, be particularly cautious during infusion. A systemic reaction such as a generalized rash, tachycardia, dyspnea, hypotension or anaphylaxis precludes any additional administration of the drug. The predictive value of this test is not proven; allergic reactions can occur in patients whose skin test is negative.

Renal allograft recipients:

Adults – 10 to 30 mg/kg/day.

Children – 5 to 25 mg/kg/day.

The drug has been used to delay the onset of the first rejection episode and at the time of the first rejection episode. Most patients who received it for the treatment of acute rejection had not received it at the time of transplantation. Usually, it is used concomitantly with azathioprine and corticosteroids. Exercise caution during repeat courses of therapy; carefully observe patients for signs of allergic reactions.

Delaying the onset of renal allograft rejection – Give a fixed dose of 15 mg/kg/day for 14 days, then every other day for 14 days, for a total of 21 doses in 28 days. Administer the first dose within 24 hours before or after the transplant.

Treatment of allograft rejection – The first dose can be delayed until the diagnosis of the first rejection episode. The recommended dose is 10 to 15 mg/kg/day for 14 days. Additional alternate day therapy up to a total of 21 doses can be given.

Aplastic anemia: 10 to 20 mg/kg daily for 8 to 14 days. Additional alternate-day therapy up to a total of 21 doses can be given. Because thrombocytopenia can be associated with ATG administration, patients receiving it may need prophylactic platelet transfusions to maintain platelets at clinically acceptable levels.

Infusion instructions: Dilute in saline solution before IV infusion. Invert the IV saline bottle so undiluted drug does not contact the air inside. Add the total daily dose to a sterile 0.45% or 0.9% saline solution. Ideally, concentration should not exceed 1 mg/ml.

Adding the drug to dextrose solutions is not recommended, as low-salt concentrations can cause precipitation. Highly acidic infusion solutions can also contribute to physical instability over time.

During clinical trials, most investigators infused into a vascular shunt, arterial venous fistula or a high-flow central vein through an in-line filter with a pore size of 0.2 to 1 micron to prevent inadvertent administration of any insoluble material that may develop in the product during storage. Using high-flow veins will minimize the occurrence of phlebitis and thrombosis.

Do not infuse a dose in < 4 hours.

Always keep a tray containing epinephrine, antihistamines, corticosteroids, syringes and an airway at the patient's bedside while this agent is being administered. Observe the patient continuously for possible allergic reactions throughout the infusion.

Admixture compatibility: Diluted ATG is physically and chemically stable for up to 24 hours in concentrations of up to 4 mg/ml in 0.9% sodium chloride, 5% dextrose with 0.225% sodium chloride and 5% dextrose with 0.45% sodium chloride.

Storage/Stability: Refrigerate at 2° to 8°C (36° to 46°F). Do not freeze; discard if frozen. Do not keep in diluted form for > 12 hours (including actual infusion time). Refrigerate diluted solution if prepared prior to time of infusion. Even if refrigerated, total time in dilution should not exceed 24 hours, including infusion time.

Rx	**Atgam** (Upjohn)	**Injection:** 50 mg per ml.	With 0.3 M glycine and 0.01% thimerosal. In 5 ml amps.

RESPIRATORY SYNCYTIAL VIRUS IMMUNE GLOBULIN INTRAVENOUS (HUMAN) (RSV-IGIV)

For additional information, refer to the Immune Serums introduction.

Actions:

Pharmacology: RSV-IGIV is a sterile liquid immunoglobulin G (IgG) containing neutralizing antibody to respiratory syncytial virus (RSV). The immunoglobulin is purified from pooled adult human plasma selected for high titers of neutralizing antibody against RSV. A widely utilized solvent-detergent viral inactivation process is used to decrease the possibility of transmission of bloodborne pathogens. Each milliliter contains 50 mg immunoglobulin, primarily IgG, and trace amounts of IgA and IgM.

Clinical trials: In randomized, controlled studies of RSV disease prophylaxis, monthly doses of 750 mg/kg RSV-IGIV were effective in reducing the incidence of RSV hospitalization in high-risk children. Children with bronchopulmonary dysplasia (BPD) may be at high risk for serious RSV disease up to 60 months of age. Children born prematurely may be at high risk for serious RSV disease during the first year of life.

PREVENT trial – RSV-IGIV reduced the incidence of RSV hospitalization by 41%, total days of RSV hospitalization by 53%, total RSV hospital days with increased supplemental oxygen requirement by 60% and total RSV hospital days with a moderate or severe lower respiratory tract infection by 54%. A trend in reduction in total ICU days (44%) was observed, although it was not statistically significant.

The incidence of any hospitalization due to respiratory illness was compared between placebo control and children receiving RSV-IGIV. The incidence in placebo controls was 26.5% vs 16.4% in the RSV-IGIV recipients. This represents a 38% reduction in the incidence of respiratory hospitalization for RSV-IGIV recipients. The total days of hospitalization for respiratory illness per 100 randomized children were compared between placebo controls and RSV-IGIV recipients. There were 317 days per 100 control children and 170 days per 100 RSV-IGIV children. This represents a 46% reduction in the total days of hospitalization for respiratory illness per 100 randomized children for RSV-IGIV recipients.

NIAID trial – The NIAID study was a study of the safety and efficacy of RSV-IGIV in the prophylaxis of RSV in 274 infants and children at high risk of RSV disease due to chronic pulmonary disease (principally BPD), congenital heart disease (CHD) or premature birth (< 35 weeks gestation). Compared with control children (n = 90), children randomized to receive 750 mg/kg RSV-IGIV showed a 57% reduction in the incidence of RSV hospitalization, a 59% reduction in total days of RSV hospitalization per 100 children, a 97% reduction in RSV ICU days per 100 children and 100% reduction in mechanical ventilation per 100 children.

Cardiac trial – The cardiac trial was conducted to further assess the safety and efficacy of RSV-IGIV in 429 children with CHD of < 48 months of age at enrollment. The mean age was 9 months and ranged from 0 to 47 months. Although trends toward RSV-IGIV efficacy were observed, the data were not statistically significant. The efficacy and safety of RSV-IGIV have not been established in children with CHD (see Warnings).

Open label trial – An additional supportive clinical trial was conducted to determine the safety and pharmacokinetics of monthly 750 mg/kg doses of RSV-IGIV in 68 children with BPD or prematurity. During the study, 7 children (10.3%) were hospitalized for RSV. RSV hospital days were 54/100 children, and ICU days were 15/100 children. RSV-IGIV has not been demonstrated to be effective for the treatment of RSV infection.

Indications:

Respiratory syncytial virus (RSV): Prevention of serious lower respiratory tract infection caused by RSV in children < 24 months of age with bronchopulmonary dysplasia (BPD) or a history of premature birth (≤ 35 weeks gestation). RSV-IGIV is safe and effective in reducing the incidence and duration of RSV hospitalization and the severity of RSV illness in these high-risk infants.

Contraindications:

History of a severe prior reaction associated with the administration of RSV-IGIV or other human immunoglobulin preparations. Patients with selective IgA deficiency have the potential for developing antibodies to IgA and could have anaphylactic or allergic reactions to blood products that contain IgA, including RSV-IGIV.

RESPIRATORY SYNCYTIAL VIRUS IMMUNE GLOBULIN INTRAVENOUS (HUMAN) (RSV-IGIV)

Warnings:

Fluid overload: Infants with underlying pulmonary disease may be sensitive to extra fluid volume. Infusion of RSV-IGIV, particularly in children with BPD, may precipitate symptoms of fluid overload. Overall, 8.4% of participants (1% premature and 13% BPD) received new or extra diuretics during the period 24 hours before through 48 hours after at least one of their infusions in the PREVENT trial. RSV-IGIV-related fluid overload was reported in 3 patients (1.2%) and RSV-IGIV-related respiratory distress was reported in 4 patients (1.6%); all had underlying BPD. These children were managed with diuretics or modification of the infusion rate and went on to receive subsequent infusions.

Complications related to fluid volume were recorded as a reason for incomplete or prolonged infusion in 2% of children receiving RSV-IGIV (2.5% BPD and 1.1% premature) and in 1.5% of children receiving placebo. Children with clinically apparent fluid overload should not be infused with RSV-IGIV.

Hypersensitivity: Severe reactions, such as anaphylaxis or angioneurotic edema, have been reported in association with IV immunoglobulins, even in patients not known to be sensitive to human immunoglobulins or blood products. Serious allergic reaction was noted in two patients in the PREVENT trial. These reactions were manifest as an acute episode of cyanosis, mottling and fever in one patient and respiratory distress in the other. The rate of allergic reaction appears to be low and consistent with rates observed for other IGIV products. If hypotension, anaphylaxis or severe allergic reaction occurs, discontinue infusion and administer epinephrine (1:1000) as required. Refer to Management of Acute Hypersensivity Reactions.

Pregnancy: Category C. It is not known whether RSV-IGIV can cause fetal harm when administered to a pregnant woman or affect reproduction capacity. Give to a pregnant woman only if clearly indicated.

Children: RSV-IGIV is indicated for use in children < 24 months of age. However, the safety and efficacy of RSV-IGIV in children with CHD have not been established. Although equivalent proportions of children in the RSV-IGIV and control groups in the CARDIAC trial had adverse events, a larger number of RSV-IGIV recipients had severe or life-threatening adverse events. These events were most frequently observed in infants with CHD with right to left shunts who underwent cardiac surgery.

Precautions:

Monitoring: Administer RSV-IGIV cautiously. During administration, monitor the patient's vital signs frequently for increases in heart rate, respiratory rate, retractions and rales. A loop diuretic such as furosemide or bumetanide should be available for management of fluid overload.

Rate of administration: Except for hypersensitivity reactions, adverse reactions to IGIVs may be related to the rate of administration. Careful adherence to the infusion rate outlined under Administration and Dosage is therefore important. Have loop diuretics available for the management of patients who are at risk for fluid overload. Although systemic allergic reactions are rare (see Adverse Reactions), have epinephrine and diphenhydramine available for treatment of acute allergic symptoms.

Aseptic meningitis syndrome (AMS): Rare occurrences of AMS have been reported in association with IGIV treatment. AMS usually begins within several hours to 2 days following IGIV treatment and is characterized by symptoms including severe headache, drowsiness, fever, photophobia, painful eye movements, muscle rigidity, nausea and vomiting. Cerebrospinal fluid studies generally demonstrate pleocytosis, predominantly granulocytic, and elevated protein levels. Thoroughly evaluate patients exhibiting such symptoms and signs to rule out other causes of meningitis. AMS may occur more frequently in association with high dose (2 g/kg) IGIV treatment. Discontinuation of IGIV treatment has resulted in remission of AMS within several days without sequelae.

Bloodborne viral transmission: RSV-IGIV is made from human plasma and, like other plasma products, carries the possibility for transmission of bloodborne pathogenic agents. The risk of transmission of recognized bloodborne viruses is considered to be low because of screening of plasma donors, an added viral inactivation step and removal properties in the Cohn-Oncley cold ethanol precipitation procedure used for purification of immune globulin products. Until 1993, cold ethanol manufactured immune globulins licensed in the US had not been documented to transmit any viral agent. However, during a brief period in late 1993 to early 1994, IGIV made by one US manufacturer was associated with transmission of hepatitis C virus.

RESPIRATORY SYNCYTIAL VIRUS IMMUNE GLOBULIN INTRAVENOUS (HUMAN) (RSV-IGIV)

To further guard against possible transmission of bloodborne viruses, RSV-IGIV is treated with a solvent-detergent viral inactivation procedure known to inactivate a wide spectrum of lipid enveloped viruses, including HIV-1, HIV-2, hepatitis B virus and hepatitis C virus. However, because new bloodborne agents may yet emerge, some of which may not be inactivated or eliminated by the manufacturing process or by solvent-detergent treatment, RSV-IGIV, like any other blood product, should be given only if a benefit is expected.

Discard after use: RSV-IGIV does not contain a preservative. Enter the single-use vial only once for administration purposes and begin the infusion within 6 hours. Closely adhere to the infusion schedule (see Administration and Dosage). Do not use if the solution is turbid.

Drug Interactions:

Live virus vaccines: Antibodies present in immune globulin preparations may interfere with the immune response to live virus vaccines, such as mumps, rubella and, particularly, measles. If such vaccines are given during or within 10 months after RSV-IGIV infusion, reimmunization is recommended, if appropriate. Studies have suggested that responses to non-live childhood vaccines (eg, DPT) are not substantially influenced by administration of IGIVs. Limited information available from infants who received RSV-IGIV concurrently with one or more doses of their primary immunization series indicates that antibody responses to diphtheria, tetanus, pertussis and *Haemophilus influenzae* b may be lower in RSV-IGIV recipients than in controls. It is not known whether antibody responses to trivalent oral polio vaccine might be affected by concurrent RSV-IGIV. Consider giving a booster dose of these vaccines 3 or 4 months after the last dose of RSV-IGIV in order to ensure immunity to DPT, *H influenza* b and OPV (oral poliovirus).

Adverse Reactions:

RSV-IGIV is generally well tolerated. In the PREVENT trial of RSV-IGIV in children with BPD or prematurity, there was no difference in the proportion of children in the RSV-IGIV and placebo groups who report adverse events.

RSV-IGIV Adverse Reactions (%)

Adverse Reaction	RSV-IGIV (n = 250)	Placebo (n = 260)	Adverse Reaction	RSV-IGIV (n = 250)	Placebo (n = 260)
Fever/pyrexia	6	2	Rash	1	2
Respiratory distress	2	< 1	Hypertension	1	0
Vomiting/emesis	2	1	Hypoxia/hypoxemia	1	1
Wheezing	2	2	Tachypnea	1	<1
Diarrhea	1	<1	Gastroenteritis	1	< 1
Rales	1	0	Injection site inflammation	1	1
Fluid overload	1	0	Overdose effect	1	< 1
Tachycardia/increased pulse rate	1	0			

Infrequent adverse reactions included: Edema; pallor; hypotension; heart murmur; gagging; cyanosis; sleepiness; cough; rhinorrhea; eczema; cold and clammy skin; conjunctival hemorrhage.

Reactions similar to those reported with other IGIVs may occur with RSV-IGIV. These include: Dizziness; flushing; blood pressure changes; anxiety; palpitations; chest tightness; dyspnea; abdominal cramps; pruritis; myalgia; arthralgia. Such reactions are often related to the rate of infusion. Immediate allergic, anaphylactic or hypersensitivity reactions may be observed (see Warnings). Rarely, aseptic meningitis syndrome (AMS) has been reported in association with IGIV treatment, particularly at high dosage (2 g/kg; see Precautions).

In the PREVENT trial, 3 children developed aseptic meningitis of unknown etiology. In the single blind, controlled NIAID trial in children with BPD, CHD or prematurity, adverse reactions were reported in 3% of all RSV-IGIV infusions. Five of 160 children were considered to have had mild fluid overload associated with infusion. The remaining adverse reactions consisted of mild decreases in oxygen saturation (n = 8) and fever (n = 5). In the open-label study in children with BPD or prematurity (n = 6), infusion-associated adverse reactions were noted in 14 of 294 (4.8%) infusions. Six adverse events were considered related to infusion, including 4 mild and 2 moderate events. In the CARDIAC study, children with CHD with right to left shunts appeared to have an increased frequency of cardiac surgery and had a greater frequency of severe and life-threatening adverse events associated with cardiac surgery (see Warnings).

RESPIRATORY SYNCYTIAL VIRUS IMMUNE GLOBULIN INTRAVENOUS (HUMAN) (RSV-IGIV)

Overdosage:

Although few data are available, clinical experience with other immune globulin preparations suggests that the major manifestations would be those related to fluid volume overload.

Administration and Dosage:

Approved by the FDA on January 18, 1996.

The maximum recommended total dosage per monthly infusion is 750 mg/kg, administered according to the following schedule:

RSV-IGIV Infusion Schedule

Time after start of infusion	Rate of infusion (ml/kg of body mass per hour)
0 to 15 minutes	1.5 ml/kg/hr
15 to 30 minutes	3 ml/kg/hr
30 minutes to end of infusion	6 ml/kg/hr

Administer RSV-IGIV intravenously at 1.5 ml/kg/hr for 15 minutes. If the clinical condition does not contraindicate a higher rate, increase the rate to 3 ml/kg/hr for 15 minutes and, finally, increase to a maximum rate of 6 ml/kg/hr. *Do not exceed this rate of administration.* Monitor the patient closely during and after each rate change. In especially ill children with BPD, slower rates of infusion may be indicated.

Consider factors such as other clinical illness, how well the child has grown and the risk of exposure from siblings or daycare when determining whether to use RSV-IGIV. Administer the first dose prior to commencement of the RSV season and subsequent doses monthly throughout the RSV season in order to maintain protection. In the Northern Hemisphere, the RSV season typically commences in November and runs through April. Infuse children from early November through April, unless RSV activity begins earlier or persists later in a community. It is recommended that RSV-IGIV be administered separately from other drugs or medications that the patient may be receiving. It is recommended that children infected with RSV continue to receive monthly doses for the duration of the RSV season.

Infusion: Begin infusion within 6 hours and complete within 12 hours after the single-use vial is entered. Assess the patient's vital signs and cardiopulmonary status prior to infusion, before each rate increase, and thereafter, at 30 minute intervals until 30 minutes following completion of the infusion. Administer RSV-IGIV through an IV line using a constant infusion pump (ie, *IVAC* pump or equivalent). Predilution of RSV-IGIV before infusion is not recommended. If possible, administer RSV-IGIV through a separate IV line, although it may be "piggy-backed" into a pre-existing line if that line contains one of the following dextrose solutions (with or without sodium chloride): 2.5%, 5%, 10% or 20% dextrose in water. If a preexisting line must be used, the RSV-IGIV should not be diluted more than 1:2 with any of the above-named solutions. While filters are not necessary, an in-line filter with a pore size > 15 micrometers may be used for the infusion of RSV-IGIV.

Admixture incompatibility: It is recommended that RSV-IGIV be administered separately from other drugs or medications that the patient may be receiving.

Storage/Stability: Store between 2° and 8°C (35.6° and 46.4°F). Do not freeze. Do not shake vial; avoid foaming. Discard after use.

Rx	**RespiGam** (MedImmune)	**Injection:** 2500 mg RSV immunoglobulin	Preservative free. Contains 5% sucrose, 1% albumin (human) and 1 to 1.5 mEq sodium per 50 ml. In single-use 50 ml vials.

ANTITOXINS AND ANTIVENINS

Antitoxins and antivenins are used for passive immunization. Antitoxins are antibodies which combine with the toxins and neutralize them. Most antitoxins for human use are derived from horse serum (eg, antivenins, diphtheria). However, there is a tetanus immune globulin of human origin. The following general information applies to antitoxins and antivenins. For specific indications and dosage guidelines, refer to individual product listings.

Warnings:

Hypersensitivity: In the parenteral administration of any biological product, observe every precaution to prevent or arrest allergic or other untoward reactions. A careful history should review possible sensitivity to the type of protein being injected. Administer animal serums with caution even in individuals with a negative sensitivity test.

Have epinephrine injection (1:1000) available while performing sensitivity tests or administering antitoxin. Refer to Management of Acute Hypersensitivity Reactions.

Precautions:

History and sensitivity testing: Before administration of any product prepared from animal serum, make a complete record of previous injections of "serum" of any type and any previous allergic manifestations of the patient. Test for sensitivity to animal serum. Do the scratch test or "eye" sensitivity test before proceeding to the intradermal tests. These tests should be performed by skilled personnel familiar with management of acute anaphylaxis. Fatalities have resulted from intradermal testing. Positive tests indicate probable sensitivity. A negative skin or conjunctival sensitivity test is usually reliable, but does not completely rule out systemic sensitivity. The following is a general procedure for sensitivity testing. Manufacturers' recommendations may vary. Consult package literature prior to use of a product.

Scratch test – Make a ¼" skin scratch through a drop of 1:100 dilution in normal saline. To serve as a control, make a similar scratch through a drop of normal saline on a different but comparable skin site. After 20 minutes, compare the sites. A positive sensitivity test consists of an urticarial wheal, with or without pseudopods, surrounded by a halo of erythema. A negative or minimal reaction, with no wheal or pseudopods, occurs at the control site.

Conjunctival test ("eye" test) – Instill into the conjunctival sac one drop of a 1:10 saline dilution. A drop of normal saline placed in the opposite conjunctival sac provides a control. A positive reaction consists of itching, burning, redness and lacrimation appearing within 10 to 30 minutes; these symptoms can be relieved by instilling a drop of epinephrine solution. The control eye should remain normal. If both eyes remain normal, the conjunctival test is negative.

Intradermal test – In patients with a negative allergy history and negative scratch or eye test, inject with 0.02 to 0.1 ml of 1:100 saline diluted serum; refer to manufacturers' recommendations for specific instructions. In patients with a history or allergy, especially to animal serums, inject with 1:1000 saline diluted serum. Inject a separate but comparable skin site intracutaneously with normal saline to serve as a control. After 10 to 30 minutes, compare the injection sites. A positive sensitivity test consists of an urticarial wheal, with or without pseudopods, surrounded by a halo of erythema. A negative or minimal reaction, with no wheal or pseudopods, occurs at the control site.

Desensitization: In the event of a positive sensitivity test or a doubtful reaction, perform careful desensitization of the patient. Serial injections of diluted antitoxin or antivenin may be made at 15 minute intervals, provided no reaction occurs. If a reaction occurs after an injection, wait an hour and then repeat the last dose which failed to cause a reaction.

Antihistamines: Concomitant use may interfere with sensitivity tests.

Adverse Reactions:

Systemic: Acute anaphylaxis is characterized by sudden onset of urticaria, respiratory distress and vascular collapse, and serum sickness (usually appearing 7 to 12 days after administration). Symptoms of lymphadenopathy, polyarthritis, arthralgias, skin rash and fever may develop. Anaphylaxis is largely related to the amount of serum administered, patient hypersensitivity and history of previous serum injection. The incidence of serum sickness with modern enzyme-treated serum is about 5% to 10%. This occurs more frequently after the largest dose.

Local: Pain or erythema and urticaria without constitutional disturbance may occur 7 to 10 days after administration and may last for about 2 days.

DIPHTHERIA ANTITOXIN

For additional information refer to the Antitoxins and Antivenins introduction.

Actions:

Pharmacology: A sterile solution of purified antitoxic substances obtained from the blood of horses immunized against diphtheria toxin. The efficacy of diptheria antitoxin decreases as the duration of pharyngeal diphtheria increases. The risk-benefit ratio appears to be better for diptheria antitoxin use in pharyngeal disease, compared to cuntaneous diptheria. IV effect is rapid; concentrations peak several hours after IM injection. Mean half-life is < 15 days.

Indications:

Diphtheria: For passive, transient protection against or treatment of diphtheria infections.

Warnings:

Pregnancy: Catagory C. Use only if clearly needed. Intact IgG crosses the placenta from the maternal circulation increasingly after 30 weeks gestation.

Lactation: It is not known if antitoxin antibodies are excreted into breast milk. Problems in humans have not been documented.

Children: Give children the same antitoxin dose as adults. At the same time, but in a different extremity and with a separate syringe, continue or complete the child's basic immunizing series with DTP or DT, as appropriate.

Administration and Dosage:

Administer IM or by slow IV infusion. Warm antitoxin to 32° to 34°C (90° to 95°F).

Therapeutic regimen: Any person with clinical symptoms of diphtheria should receive diphtheria antitoxin immediately without waiting for bacteriologic confirmation. Continue treatment until all local and general symptoms are controlled, or until some other etiologic agent has been identified.

1.) Perform sensitivity tests.
2.) Immediately give all of the required antitoxin IM or IV. Each hour's delay increases dosage requirement and decreases beneficial effects.
3.) Suggested ranges: Pharyngeal or laryngeal disease of 48 hours duration - 20,000 to 40,000 units; nasopharyngeal lesions - 40,000 to 60,000 units; extensive disease of ≥ 3 days duration or any patient with brawny swelling of the neck - 80,000 to 120,000 units.
4.) Give children the same dose as adults.
5.) Start appropriate antimicrobial agents in full therapeutic dosage.

Storage/Stability: Store between 2° to 8°C (35° to 46°F).

Rx	**Diphtheria Antitoxin** (Connaught)[1]	**Injection:** ≥ 500 units/ml	With 0.4% tricresol. In 20,000 units per vial.

[1] Distributed by the Centers for Disease Control and Prevention.

ANTIVENIN (CROTALIDAE) POLYVALENT

For additional information refer to the Antitoxins and Antivenins introduction.

Actions:

Pharmacology: Concentrated serum globulins from horses immunized with the following venoms: *Crotalus adamanteus* (eastern diamond rattlesnake), *C atrox* (western diamond rattlesnake), *C durissus terrificus* (tropical rattlesnake, Cascabel) and *Bothrops atrox* (Fer-de-lance). IV effect is rapid; concentration peaks in ≥ 8 hours after IM injection. Mean half-life is < 15 days.

The location of antivenins for rare species and names and telephone numbers of experts on venomous bites can be obtained at any hour from the Arizona Poison Control Center (602-626-6016).

Indications:

To neutralize the toxic effects of venoms of crotalids (pit vipers) native to North, Central and South America, including rattlesnakes (*Crotalus, Sistrurus*); copperhead and cottonmouth moccasins (*Agkistrodon*), including *A halys* of Korea and Japan; the Fer-de-lance and other species of *Bothrops*; the tropical rattler (*C durissus* and similar species); the Cantil (*A bilineatus*); and bushmaster (*Lachesis mutus*) of South and Central America.

ANTIVENIN (CROTALIDAE) POLYVALENT

Warnings:

Pit viper bites and envenomation: Symptoms, signs and severity of snake venom poisoning depend on many factors, including species, age and size of the snake; number and location of bite(s); depth of venom deposit; condition of the snake's fangs and venom glands; length of time the snake "hangs on"; age, general health and size of the victim; timing, type and efficacy of first aid treatment rendered to remove venom. In any snake bite, the actual amount of venom introduced is unknown. The type of clothing or leg-footwear through which the snake's fangs pass may affect the amount of venom delivered. Although most North American pit vipers tend to bite and introduce venom superficially, their fangs may get hung up in subcutaneous tissues during the biting act and penetrate deeper tissues during the attempt to release the bitten part. In some bites, fangs may penetrate into muscle. In such cases, the usual local superficial manifestations of envenomation may not appear early in the course of poisoning. In bites by some species, systemic evidence of envenomation may be present in the absence of significant local manifestations. It may be difficult to determine the severity of envenomation during the first several hours after a pit viper bite; estimates of severity may need to be revised as poisoning progresses. Not all pit viper bites result in envenomation. In approximately 20% of rattlesnake bites, the snake may not inject any venom. Local and systemic signs and symptoms of envenomation include the following:

Local (fang punctures) –

Swelling: Edema, usually seen around the bite area within 5 minutes, may progress rapidly and involve the entire extremity within an hour.

Ecchymosis and skin discoloration often appear in the bite area within a few hours. Vesicles may form in a few hours and are usually present at 24 hours. Hemorrhagic blebs and petechiae are common. Necrosis may develop, necessitating amputation.

Pain frequently begins shortly after a bite by most pit vipers. Pain may be absent after bites by Mojave rattlers.

Systemic – Weakness; faintness; nausea; sweating; numbness or tingling around the mouth, tongue, scalp, fingers, toes, bite area; muscle fasciculations; hypotension; prolonged bleeding and clotting times; hemoconcentration followed by decrease in erythrocytes; thrombocytopenia; hematuria; proteinuria; vomiting, including hematemesis; melena; hemoptysis; epistaxis.

In fatal poisoning, cause of death is frequently associated with destruction of erythrocytes and changes in capillary permeability, especially of the pulmonary vascular system, leading to pulmonary edema; hemoconcentration usually occurs early, probably as a result of plasma loss secondary to vascular permeability; hemoglobin may fall, and bleeding may occur throughout the body as early as 6 hours after the bite. Renal involvement is uncommon. Mojave rattler venom may cause neuromuscular changes leading to respiratory failure.

Supportive care – Treat suspected envenomation as a medical emergency. Until careful observation provides clear evidence that envenomation has not occurred or is minimal, follow these procedures: Monitor vital signs frequently. Draw blood as soon as possible for baseline lab studies, including type and cross-match, CBC, hematocrit, platelet count, prothrombin time, clot retraction, bleeding and coagulation times, BUN, electrolytes and bilirubin. During the first 4 or 5 days after a severe envenomation, perform hemoglobin, hematocrit and platelet counts several times a day. Obtain urine samples at frequent intervals, with special attention to microscopic examination for presence of erythrocytes. Chart fluid intake and urine output. To monitor progression of edema, measure the circumference of the bitten extremity every 15 to 30 minutes, just proximal to the bite and at one or more additional points, each several inches closer to the trunk.

Have available for immediate use: Oxygen and resuscitation equipment including airway, tourniquet, epinephrine, parenteral antihistamines and corticosteroids.

Start IV infusions: Use one line for supportive therapy, if needed, and the other line for administration of the antivenin and electrolytes.

Treat shock following envenomation like shock from hypovolemia of any cause, including administration of blood products or plasma expanders, as indicated.

Pregnancy: Catagory C. Use only if clearly needed, with appropriate consideration of the risk-benefit ratio. It is not known if antivenom antibodies cross the placenta. Intact IgG crosses the placenta from the maternal circulation increasingly after 30 weeks gestation.

Lactation: It is not known if antivenom antibodies are excreted into breast milk. Problems in humans have not been documented.

Children: Children may require larger doses than adults, because of a child's relatively small volume of body fluid in which to dilute the venom. Do not adjust pediatric doses by the weight of the patient.

ANTIVENIN (CROTALIDAE) POLYVALENT

Administration and Dosage:

Test for sensitivity to horse serum whenever a product containing hourse serum is administered (see introduction to this section). There is a possibility of a severe immediate reaction. Constant observation for untoward reactions is mandatory. Should any systemic reaction occur, discontinue use and initiate appropriate treatment. See also Management of Acute Hypersensitivity Reactions.

IV route is preferred; if shock is present, IV use is mandatory. Administer within 4 hours of bite; it is less effective when given after 8 hours, and may be of questionable value after 12 hours. However, in severe poisonings, administer antivenin even if 24 hours have elapsed since time of bite. Maximum blood levels of antivenin may not be obtained for ≥ 8 hours following IM administration.

Reconstituting dried antivenin: Withdraw diluent and inject into the vial of antivenin. Gentle agitation will hasten complete dissolution of the lyophilized drug.

For IV infusion, prepare a 1:1 to 1:10 dilution of reconstituted drug in Sodium Chloride Injection or 5% Dextrose Injection. Gently swirl to avoid foaming. Infuse initial 5 to 10 ml over 3 to 5 minutes, while observing patient; if no immediate systemic reactions appear, continue infusion with delivery at the maximum safe rate for IV fluid administration. To determine dilution, type of electrolyte solution and delivery rate, consider the patient's age, weight and cardiac status; severity of envenomation; estimated total amount of parenteral fluids needed and interval between bite and therapy initiation.

Give entire initial dose as soon as possible based on the best estimate of the severity of envenomation. The following doses are recommended:

No envenomation – No local or systemic manifestations. No dose given.

Minimal envenomation – Local swelling and other local changes; no systemic manifestations; normal laboratory findings. 20 to 40 ml (2 to 4 vials).

Moderate envenomation – Swelling progresses beyond the site of bite; one or more systemic manifestations; abnormal laboratory findings (eg, fall in hematocrit or platelets). 50 to 90 ml (5 to 9 vials).

Severe envenomation – Marked local response, severe systemic manifestations, significant alteration in laboratory findings. 100 to 150 ml or more (≥ 10 to 15 vials).

Base the need for additional antivenin on clinical response to initial dose and continuing assessment of severity of poisoning. If swelling progresses, if systemic symptoms increase in severity or if new manifestations appear, administer an additional 10 to 50 ml (1 to 5 vials) IV.

Children: Envenomation by large snakes in children or small adults requires larger doses of antivenin. The amount administered to a child is *not* based on weight (see Warnings).

IM: Administer into large muscle mass, preferably the gluteal area, taking care to avoid nerve trunks. Never inject into a finger or toe.

Storage/Stability: Store at room temperature, not exceeding 37°C (99°F). Do not freeze. Use reconstituted solution within 48 hours and dilutions within 12 hours. To avoid foaming and protein degradation, mix by gently swirling rather than shaking. The product self life expires within 60 months.

Rx	**Antivenin (Crotalidae) Polyvalent** (Wyeth-Ayerst)	**Injection**	**Combination Package** – 1 vial lyophilized serum[1], 1 vial 10 ml Bacteriostatic Water for Injection, USP[2] and one 1 ml vial normal horse serum[3] (diluted 1:10) as sensitivity testing material.

[1] With 0.25% phenol and 0.005% thimerosal.
[2] With 0.001% phenylmercuric nitrate.
[3] With 0.35% phenol and 0.005% thimerosal.

ANTIVENIN (MICRURUS FULVIUS) (North American Coral Snake Antivenin)

For additional information refer to the Antitoxins and Antivenins introduction.

Actions:

Pharmacology: Refined, concentrated, lyophilized preparation of serum globulins from healthy horses immunized with eastern coral snake *(Micrurus fulvius fulvius)* venom.

Two genera of coral snakes inhabit the US: *Micrurus* (including the eastern and Texas varieties), and *Micruroids* (the Arizonan or Sonoran variety). *Micrurus fulvius fulvious* inhabits an area from North Carolina south to Florida and west to the Mississippi River. *Micrurus fulvius tenere* inhabits an area including Louisiana, Arkansas, central Texas and northern Mexico. Several other species of coral snake inhabit much of Central and South America, including three genera, *Leptomicrurus, Micrurus* and *Micruoides.*

IV effect is rapid; IM absorption may not peak until the second day. Mean half-life is < 15 days.

Indications:

For passive, transient protection from the toxic effects of venoms of *Micrurus fulvius fulvius* (Eastern coral snake). Also neutralizes the venom of *fulvius tenere* (Texas coral snake). If indicated, the best effect results if antivenin administration begins within 4 hours of envenomation.

This antivenin partially neutralizes the venom of *dumerilii carinicauda* and minimally neutralizes the venom of *spixii.* It may also provide some protection against the venom of *nigrocinctus.*

Warnings:

Not effective against the venom of *euryxanthus* (Arizonan or Sonoran coral snake), found only in southeastern Arizona, southwestern New Mexico and portions of Mexico. Not effective in other snakes not described above.

Envenomation: Coral snake venom is chiefly paralytic (neurotoxic) and usually causes only minimal to moderate tissue reaction and pain at the bite area. Coral snakebites, like bites by crotalids, are not always followed by envenomation. However, severe and even fatal envenomation from a coral snakebite may be present without significant local tissue reaction.

Symptoms of envenomation usually begin 1 to 7 hours after the bite, but may be delayed for as long as 18 hours. If envenomation occurs, symptoms and signs may progress rapidly and precipitously. Paralysis has been observed 2.5 hours postbite and appears to be of a bulbar type, involving cranial motor nerves. Death from respiratory paralysis has occurred within 4 hours of the bite.

Systemic signs and symptoms may include euphoria, lethargy, weakness, nausea, vomiting, excessive salivation, ptosis of eyelids, dyspnea, abnormal reflexes, seizures and motor weakness or paralysis, including complete respiratory paralysis.

Local signs and symptoms may include scratch marks or fang puncture wounds, no edema to moderate edema, erythema, pain at the bite area and paresthesia in the bitten extremity.

Supportive therapy – Appropriate tetanus prophylaxis is indicated. Morphine or other narcotics that depress respiration are contraindicated. Use sedatives with extreme caution.

Pregnancy: Catagory C. Use only if clearly needed, with appropriate consideration of the risk-benefit ratio. It is not known if antivenom antibodies cross the placenta. Intact IgG crosses the placenta from the maternal circulation increasingly after 30 weeks gestation.

Lactation: It is not known if antivenom antibodies are excreted into breast milk. Problems in humans have not been documented.

Children: The pediatric dose is equivalent to the adult dose. Pediatric doses are not adjusted by the weight of the patient.

Administration and Dosage:

Test for sensitivity to horse serum (see introduction to this section). Whenever a product containing horse serum is administered, there is a possibility of a severe immediate reaction. Have appropriate therapeutic agents available (not corticosteroids). See also Management of Acute Hypersensitivity Reactions.

If practical, immobilize victim immediately and completely. If complete immobilization is not practical, splint bitten extremity to limit spread of venom.

If symptoms or signs of envenomation occur or are already present at the time the patient is first seen, give antivenin promptly IV. With vigorous treatment and careful observation, patients with complete respiratory paralysis have recovered.

Hemoglobinuria has occurred in animals. Therefore, continuous bladder drainage with careful attention to urinary output and blood electrolyte balance is recommended.

ANTIVENIN (MICRURUS FULVIUS) (North American Coral Snake Antivenin)

Reconstituting dried antivenin: Withdraw diluent and inject into the vial of antivenin. Gentle agitation will hasten complete dissolution of lyophilized drug. Do not shake.

Antivenin therapy: Depending on the nature and severity of the signs and symptoms of envenomation, administer the contents of 3 to 5 vials as the initial dose. Observe the patient carefully and administer additional antivenin as required. Some envenomed patients may need the contents of > 10 vials.

Administer therapeutic doses by slow IV injection or by IV infusion. In either case, give the first 1 to 2 ml of the antivenin dilution over 3 to 5 minutes and watch the patient carefully for evidence of an allergic reaction. If no signs or symptoms of anaphylaxis appear, continue the injection or infusion.

Adjust the rate of delivery by the severity of signs and symptoms of envenomation and tolerance of antivenin. Nonetheless, until the contents of 3 to 5 vials of antivenin have been given, administer at the maximum safe rate for IV fluids, based on body weight and general condition of the patient. For example, 250 to 500 ml over 30 minutes may be appropriate in a healthy adult, while small children may receive the first 100 ml rapidly, followed by a rate not to exceed 4 ml/min. Response to treatment may be rapid and dramatic.

Observe the patient carefully and administer additional antivenin as required. Some envonomed patients may need the contents of 10 to > 15 vials.

Storage/Stability: Store at 2° to 8°C (36° to 46°F). Do not expose to temperatures > 40°C (104°F). Do not freeze diluent. Product can tolerate 10 days in solution at room temperature. Use reconstituted solutions within 48 hours and dilutions within 12 hours. To avoid foaming and protein degradation, mix by gently swirling rather than shaking. Product shelf life expires within 60 months.

Rx	**Antivenin (Micrurus fulvius)** (Wyeth-Ayerst)	**Injection**	**Combination Package** – One vial antivenin[1] and one vial diluent (10 ml Bacteriostatic Water for Injection)[2].

[1] With 0.25% phenol and 0.005% thimerosal.
[2] With 1:100,000 phenylmercuric nitrate.

BLACK WIDOW SPIDER SPECIES ANTIVENIN (Latrodectus Mactans)

For additional information, refer to the Antitoxins and Antivenins introduction.

Actions:

Pharmacology: Prepared from blood serum of horses immunized against black widow spider venom. Moderately effective in pain relief. Can be life-saving. IV effect is rapid; concentration peaks 2 to 3 days after IM injection. Mean half-life is < 15 days.

Indications:

For passive, transient protection from toxic effects of bites by the black widow (*Lactrodecus mactans*) and similar spiders. Emphasize early use of this antivenin for prompt relief. The best effect occurs with antivenin administration within 4 hours after envenomation.

Warnings:

Envenomation:

Symptoms – Local muscular cramps begin from 15 minutes to several hours after bite, usually producing sharp pain similar to that caused by needle puncture. The exact sequence of symptoms depends on location of the bite. Venom acts on the myoneural junctions or nerve endings, causing ascending motor paralysis or destruction of peripheral nerve endings. Muscles most frequently affected first are thigh, shoulder and back. Later, pain becomes more severe, spreading to the abdomen, and weakness and tremor usually develop. Abdominal muscles assume a board-like rigidity, but tenderness is slight. Respiration is thoracic; patient is restless and anxious. Feeble pulse, cold, clammy skin, labored breathing and speech, light stupor and delirium may occur. Convulsions may also occur, particularly in small children. Temperature may be normal or slightly elevated. Urinary retention, shock, cyanosis, nausea, vomiting, insomnia and cold sweats have been reported. The syndrome following the bite of the black widow spider may be confused with any medical or surgical condition with acute abdominal symptoms.

The symptoms of black widow spider bite increase in severity for several hours, perhaps a day, and then very slowly become less severe, gradually passing off in 2 or 3 days, except in fatal cases. Residual symptoms such as general weakness, tingling, nervousness and transient muscle spasm may persist for weeks or months after recovery from the acute stage.

BLACK WIDOW SPIDER SPECIES ANTIVENIN (Latrodectus Mactans)

Supportive therapy is indicated by the condition of the patient. If possible, hospitalize patient. Additional treatment consists of prolonged warm baths and IV injection of 10 ml of calcium gluconate 10%, repeated as necessary to control muscle pain. Morphine may be required to control pain. Barbiturates may be used for extreme restlessness. However, because venom can cause respiratory paralysis, consider this when using morphine or a barbiturate. Corticosteroids have been used with varying degrees of success. Local treatment of the bite is of no value; nothing is gained by applying a tourniquet or attempting to remove venom by incision and suction.

In otherwise healthy individuals between the ages of 16 and 60, the use of antivenin may be deferred and treatment with muscle relaxants may be considered.

Pregnancy: Category C. It is not known whether the antivenin can cause fetal harm when administered to a pregnant woman or can affect reproduction capacity. Give to a pregnant woman only if clearly needed and when potential benefits outweigh potential hazards to the fetus.

Envenomation has produced spontaneous abortion.

Lactation: It is not known whether this drug is excreted in breast milk. Use caution when administering to a nursing woman.

Children: Controlled studies have not been conducted. However, there have been virtually no adverse effects in children receiving this product.

Administration and Dosage:

Test for sensitivity to horse serum (see introduction to this section).

Adults and children: Inject one vial (2.5 ml) of antivenin IM, preferably in the region of the anterolateral thigh so that a tourniquet may be applied in the event of a systemic reaction. Symptoms usually subside in 1 to 3 hours. Although one dose is usually adequate, a second dose may be necessary.

May also be given IV in 10 to 50 ml of saline over 15 minutes. This is the preferred route in severe cases, when the patient is < 12 years of age, or in shock. One vial is usually adequate.

Storage/Stability: Refrigerate at 2° to 8°C (36° to 46°F). Discard if frozen. Do not expose to excessive heat. After reconstitution, refrigerate and discard within 6 hours.

Rx	**Antivenin (Latrodectus mactans)** (Merck)	**Powder for Injection:** 6000 antivenin units per vial[1]	Supplied with a 2.5 ml vial of Sterile Water for Injection and a 1 ml vial of normal horse serum[1] (1:10 dilution) for sensitivity testing.

[1] With 1:10,000 thimerosal.

RABIES PROPHYLAXIS PRODUCTS

Although rabies rarely affects humans in the US, every year approximately 25,000 persons receive rabies prophylaxis. Appropriate management depends on the interpretation of the risk of infection and the efficacy and risk of prophylactic treatment. There are two types of immunizing products: Vaccines and globulins. Use both types of products concurrently for rabies postexposure prophylaxis.

Vaccines induce an active immune response that requires about 7 to 10 days to develop, but persists for as long as a year or more.

Human Diploid Cell Rabies Vaccine (HDCV) – An inactivated virus vaccine prepared from fixed rabies virus grown in human diploid cell culture.

Rabies Vaccine, Adsorbed (RVA) – A cell culture-derived vaccine prepared from the Kissling strain of rabies virus adapted to a diploid cell line of the fetal rhesus lung.

RVA differs from HDCV in several aspects: A different virus strain, cell line and concentration process are used in making RVA, and it is liquid rather than lyophilized. Also, approximately 6% of patients receiving HDCV develop an "immune complex-like" reaction, apparently due to the presence of a small amount of human serum albumin. Since this is not a component of the medium used to grow the rabies virus for RVA, this reaction should be less likely to occur. However, an allergic reaction to RVA has occurred in < 1% of patients. Other adverse reactions to RVA appear similar to HDCV. RVA should be used IM and should not be given intradermally. Administration and dosage is the same as for HDCV.

Globulins provide rapid passive immune protection that persists for a short time (half-life of about 21 days).

Rabies Immune Globulin, Human (RIG) – Antirabies gamma globulin, concentrated from plasma of hyperimmunized human donors.

Rationale of treatment: Individually evaluate each possible rabies exposure. Consult local or state public health officials if questions arise about the need for prophylaxis. Consider the following factors before specific treatment is initiated:

Species of biting animal – Carnivorous animals (especially skunks, foxes, coyotes, raccoons, dogs and cats) and bats are more likely to be infective than other animals. Unless the animal is tested and shown not rabid, initiate post-exposure prophylaxis upon bite or non-bite exposure to these animals. If treatment has been initiated and subsequent testing shows the exposing animal is not rabid, treatment can be discontinued.

Since the likelihood that a domestic dog or cat is infected with rabies varies from region to region, the need for post-exposure prophylaxis also varies. Bites of rabbits, hares, squirrels, chipmunks, rats, mice, hamsters, guinea pigs, gerbils and other rodents are rarely found to be infected with rabies and have not been known to cause human rabies in the US. In these cases, consult state or local health departments before a decision is made to initiate post-exposure antirabies prophylaxis.

Circumstances of biting incident – An unprovoked attack is more likely to mean that the animal is rabid. Bites inflicted during attempts to feed or handle an apparently healthy animal should generally be regarded as provoked.

Type of exposure – Rabies is transmitted by introducing the virus into open cuts or wounds in skin via mucous membranes. The likelihood of rabies infection varies with the nature and extent of the exposure.

Bite: Any penetration of the skin by teeth.

Nonbite: Scratches, abrasions, open wounds or mucous membranes contaminated with saliva or other potentially infectious material, such as brain tissue from a rabid animal. There have been two instances of airborne rabies acquired in laboratories and two probable airborne rabies cases acquired in one bat-infested cave.

Casual contact with a rabid animal, such as petting it (without a bite or nonbite exposure), is not an indication for prophylaxis.

The only documented cases of rabies due to human-to-human transmission occurred in four patients who received corneal transplants from persons who died of rabies undiagnosed at the time of death.

Pre-exposure prophylaxis: Pre-exposure immunization does not eliminate the need for prompt post-exposure prophylaxis following an exposure; it only reduces the post-exposure regimen.

RABIES PROPHYLAXIS PRODUCTS

Consider pre-exposure immunization for persons in high risk groups: Veterinarians, animal handlers, certain laboratory workers and persons, especially children, spending time (eg, ≥ 1 month) in foreign countries where rabies is a constant threat. Also consider others whose vocational or avocational pursuits bring them into contact with potentially rabid dogs, cats, foxes, skunks or bats. Pre-exposure immunization of immunosuppressed persons is not recommended.

Pre-exposure prophylaxis is given for several reasons. First, it may provide protection to persons with inapparent exposure to rabies. Secondly, it may protect persons whose post-exposure therapy might be expected to be delayed. Finally, although it does not eliminate the need for additional therapy after a rabies exposure, it simplifies therapy by eliminating the need for globulin and decreasing the number of doses of vaccine needed. This is of particular importance for persons at high risk of being exposed in countries where the available rabies immunizing products may carry a higher risk of adverse reactions.

Pre-exposure immunization consists of 3 doses of HDCV or RVA, 1 ml/dose, IM (ie, deltoid area), one each on days 0, 7 and 21 or 28. The intradermal dose is 0.1 ml in the deltoid area of either arm on days 0, 7 and 28. Administration of routine booster doses of vaccine depends on exposure risk category as noted below.

Criteria for Pre-Exposure Immunization

Risk category	Nature of risk	Typical populations	Pre-exposure regimen
Continuous	Virus present continuously, often in high concentrations. Aerosol, mucous membrane, bite or nonbite exposure possible. Specific exposures may go unrecognized.	Rabies research lab workers,[1] rabies biologics production workers.	Primary pre-exposure immunization course. Serology every 6 months. Booster immunization when antibody titer falls below acceptable level.[2]
Frequent	Exposure usually episodic, with source recognized or unrecognized. Aerosol, mucous membrane, bite or nonbite exposure.	Rabies diagnostic lab workers,[1] spelunkers, veterinarians and animal control and wildlife workers in rabies epizootic areas.	Primary pre-exposure immunization course. Booster immunization or serology every 2 years.[2]
Infrequent (greater than population-at-large)	Exposure nearly always episodic with source recognized. Mucous membrane, bite or nonbite exposure.	Veterinarians and animal control wildlife workers in areas of low rabies endemicity. Travelers to foreign rabies epizootic areas. Veterinary students.	Primary pre-exposure immunization course. No routine booster immunization or serology.
Rare (population-at-large)	Exposure always episodic, mucous membrane or bite with source recognized.	US population-at-large, including individuals in rabies epizootic areas.	No pre-exposure immunization.

[1] Judgment of relative risk and extra monitoring of immunization status of laboratory workers is the responsibility of the laboratory supervisor (see US Department of Health and Human Services' *Biosafety in Microbiological and Biomedical Laboratories*,1984).

[2] Preexposure booster immunization consists of one dose of HDCV, 1 ml/dose, IM or 0.1 ml ID. Acceptable antibody level is 1:5 titer (complete inhibition in RFFIT at 1:5 dilution). Boost if titer falls below 1:5.

Post-exposure prophylaxis:

Local wound treatment – Immediate and thorough washing of all bite wounds and scratches with soap and water is perhaps the most effective means of preventing rabies. Give tetanus prophylaxis and control bacterial infection as indicated.

Immunization – Post-exposure antirabies immunization should always include both passive immunization (preferably RIG) and vaccine, with one exception: Persons previously immunized with HDCV in recommended pre-exposure or post-exposure regimens or with other types of vaccines and who have a documented adequate rabies antibody titer should receive only vaccine. The globulin/vaccine combination is recommended for both bite and nonbite exposures, regardless of the interval between exposure and treatment.

Treatment – Use the following recommendations as a guide in conjunction with knowledge of the circumstances of the situation. Consult public health officials with questions about the need for rabies prophylaxis.

RABIES PROPHYLAXIS PRODUCTS

Treatment Recommendations for Post-Exposure Rabies

Animal species	Condition of animal at time of attack	Treatment of exposed person[1]
Domestic: Dog and cat	Healthy & available for 10 days of observation	None, unless animal develops rabies[2]
	Rabid/suspected rabid	RIG and vaccine[3]
	Unknown (escaped)	Consult public health officials. If treatment is indicated, give RIG and vaccine[3]
Wild: Skunk, bat, fox, coyote, raccoon, bobcat & other carnivores	Regard as rabid unless proven negative by laboratory test[4]	RIG and vaccine[3]
Other: Livestock, rodents, rabbits and hares	Consider individually: Bites of squirrels, hamsters, guinea pigs, gerbils, chipmunks, rats, mice, other rodents, rabbits and hares almost never call for antirabies prophylaxis.	

[1] If treatment is indicated, administer both RIG and vaccine as soon as possible, regardless of the interval from exposure.
[2] Begin treatment with RIG and vaccine at first sign of rabies in biting domestic animals during the usual holding period of 10 days. Kill and test the symptomatic animal immediately.
[3] Discontinue vaccine if fluorescent antibody tests of animal are negative.
[4] Kill and test animal as soon as possible. Holding for observation is not recommended.

Treatment Schedule for Post-Exposure Rabies Prophylaxis

Vaccination status	Treatment[1]
Not previously vaccinated	*Local wound cleansing:* All post-exposure treatment should begin with immediate, thorough cleansing of each wound with soap and water. *Rabies immune globulin:* Give 20 IU/kg. If anatomically feasible, infiltrate up to one-half the dose around the wound(s) and inject the balance IM in the gluteal area. Do not give RIG through the same syringe or into the same anatomical site as rabies vaccine. Because RIG may partially suppress active induction of antirabies antibody, give no more than the recommended dose. *Rabies vaccine:* Give 1 ml IM in the deltoid area on days 0, 3, 7, 14 and 28.
Previously vaccinated[2]	*Local wound cleansing:* All post-exposure treatments begin with immediate, thorough cleansing of each wound with soap and water. Do not administer RIG. *Rabies vaccine:* Give 1 ml IM in the deltoid area on days 0 and 3.

[1] These regimens apply to all age groups, including children.
[2] Any person with a history of pre- or post-exposure vaccination with HDCV or RVA; or with both a history of prior vaccination with any other type of rabies vaccine and a documented history of antibody response to that vaccination.

Recommendations for Post-Exposure Immunization
2 doses of HDVC, 1 ml/dose, IM, one each on days 0 and 3.
RIG, 20 IU/kg, one-half infiltrated at bite site (if possible), remainder IM; 5 doses of HDCV, 1 ml/dose, IM, one each on days 0, 3, 7, 14 and 28.

RABIES PROPHYLAXIS PRODUCTS

Passive immunization: Administer RIG once at the beginning of antirabies therapy. If not given when vaccination was begun, RIG can be given up to the eighth day after the first dose of vaccine. After that, RIG is not indicated, since an antibody response is presumed to have occurred. The recommended RIG dose is 20 IU/kg (≈ 9 IU/lb). Thoroughly infiltrate ≤ half the dose of RIG around the wound and administer the rest IM. Because RIG may partially suppress active production of antibody, do not exceed the recommended dose.

Active immunization: Administer the vaccine in conjunction with RIG on day 0. Give five 1 ml doses of the vaccine IM. Administer the first dose as soon as possible after the exposure; give an additional dose on each of days 3, 7, 14 and 28 after the first dose (day 0). WHO recommends a sixth dose at 90 days after the first dose. In unusual instances (eg, an immunosuppressed patient), serologic testing is indicated.

Previously immunized persons: When an immunized person who was vaccinated by the recommended regimen with HDCV or RVA or who had previously demonstrated rabies antibody is exposed to rabies, that person should receive two doses of HDCV or RVA 1 ml/dose, IM, one immediately and one 3 days later. If the person's immune status is not known, post-exposure antirabies treatment may be necessary. If antibody can be demonstrated in a serum sample collected before vaccine is given, treatment can be discontinued after at least two doses of HDCV.

RABIES VACCINE

Refer to the general discussion in the Rabies Prophylaxis Products introduction.

Actions:

Pharmacology: Rabies vaccine is available as a human diploid-cell vaccine (HDCV) and an adsorbed vaccine (RVA).

Pre-exposure immunization – High titer antibody responses of HDCV have been demonstrated. Seroconversion was often obtained with only one dose. With two doses 1 month apart, 100% of recipients developed specific antibody.

Post-exposure immunization efficacy was proven in conjunction with antirabies serum. Persons severely bitten by rabid dogs and wolves received the vaccine within hours of, and up to 14 days after, the bites. All individuals were fully protected against rabies.

Indications:

Pre-exposure immunization: Vaccinate persons with greater than usual risk of exposure to rabies virus by reason of occupation or avocation, including veterinarians, certain laboratory workers, animal handlers, forest rangers, spelunkers and persons staying > 1 month in countries (eg, India) where rabies is a constant threat.

Post-exposure prophylaxis: If a bite from a carrier animal is unprovoked, the animal is not apprehended and rabies is present in that species in the area, administer RIG and vaccine as indicated. Consider vaccine recipients adequately immunized if they previously completed pre- or post-exposure prophylaxis with any current rabies vaccine or have a documented adequate antibody response to duck-embryo rabies vaccine (DEV).

Contraindications:

Theoretically, rabies vaccine may be contraindicated in persons who have had life-threatening allergic reactions to rabies vaccine or any of its components, but carefully consider a patient's risk of developing rabies before deciding to discontinue vaccination.

Warnings:

Serious reactions: Report any serious reactions immediately to the State Health Department or the manufacturer/distributor of the vaccine.

Guillain-Barré syndrome: Two cases of acute polyradiculoneuropathy (Guillain-Barré syndrome) that resolved within 12 weeks, and a focal subacute CNS disorder temporally associated with HDCV have been reported.

Immune complex-like reactions: Recently, a significant increase has been noted in "immune complex-like" reactions (6%) in persons receiving booster doses of HDCV. The illness, characterized by onset at 2 to 21 days postbooster, presents with a generalized urticaria and may also include arthralgia, arthritis, angioedema, nausea, vomiting, fever and malaise. In no case were the illnesses life-threatening. This reaction occurred much less frequently in persons receiving primary immunization.

Hypersensitivity: May give antihistamines. Have epinephrine available to counteract anaphylactic reactions. Refer to Management of Acute Hypersensitivity Reactions.

While the concentration of antibiotics in each dose of vaccine is extremely small, persons with known hypersensitivity to any of these agents could manifest an allergic reaction.

RABIES VACCINE

Pregnancy: Category C. Give rabies vaccine to a pregnant woman only if clearly needed. Pregnancy is not a contraindication to post-exposure therapy. There have been no fetal abnormalities associated with rabies vaccination. If there is substantial risk of rabies exposure, pre-exposure prophylaxis may also be indicated during pregnancy.

Lactation: It is not known if rabies vaccine or corresponding antibodies are excreted in breast milk. Problems in humans have not been documented.

Children: Pediatric and adult doses are the same. Safety and efficacy are established in children. Safe and effective use of the Michigan/SKB vaccine is established for persons ≥ 6 years of age.

Precautions:

Route of administration:

Imovax Rabies Vaccine and Rabies Vaccine Adsorbed – Inject IM only in the deltoid area; possible vaccine failure may occur if injected in the gluteal area. Do not inject ID.

Imovax Rabies ID Vaccine – Inject ID only; do not inject IM.

Drug Interactions:

Rabies Vaccine Drug Interactions			
Precipitant drug	Object drug*		Description
Chloroquine	Rabies vaccine, ID	⬇	Long-term therapy with chloroquine may suppress the immune response to low-dose HDCV administered ID. Complete pre-exposure rabies vaccination 1 to 2 months before chloroquine administration begins. If this is not feasible, perform serologic tests several weeks after vaccination to determine the magnitude of the recipient's antibody response.
Immunosuppressants	Rabies vaccine	⬇	Like all inactivated vaccines, administration of rabies vaccine to persons receiving immunosuppressants, including high-dose corticosteroids, or radiation therapy, may result in an insufficient response to immunization. They may remain susceptible despite immunization. Do not give immunosuppressives during post-exposure therapy unless essential. It may be helpful to test steroid-treated patients for development of antirabies antibodies.
Rabies immune globulin	Rabies vaccine	⬇	Simultaneous administration may slightly delay the antibody response to rabies vaccine. Because of this possibility, follow CDC recommendations exactly and give no more than the recommended dose of RIG.

* ⬇ = Object drug decreased.

Adverse Reactions:

HDCV: Transient pain, erythema, swelling or itching at the injection site (25%). Treat such reactions with simple analgesics.

Mild systemic reactions (20%) – Headache, nausea, abdominal pain, muscle aches and dizziness. In general, ID administration results in fewer adverse reactions, except for a slight increase in transient local reactions. Serum-sickness-like reactions occur in 6% of those receiving ID booster doses 2 to 21 days after injection. These reactions may be due to albumin in the vaccine formula rendered allergenic by beta-propiolactone during the manufacturing process.

RVA: Transient pain, redness and swelling at the injection site (65% to 70%). In a few cases, these effects persist 48 hours and may be successfully treated with simple analgesics. Mild, transient constitutional reactions (8% to 10%); headache, nausea, slight fever or fatigue. Serum-sickness-like reaction (< 1%), between 7 and 14 days after booster vaccination, perhaps due to lack of albumin in the vaccine formula.

RABIES VACCINE

Administration and Dosage:

Dosage:

Pre-exposure prophylaxis – Vaccine doses on days 0, 7 and 21 to 28, and then every 2 to 5 years based on antibody titers. Give 1 ml IM (either *Imovax Rabies Vaccine* or *Rabies Vaccine Adsorbed*) or 0.1 ml ID (*Imovax Rabies ID Vaccine* only).

Post-exposure prophylaxis – Do not inject post-exposure vaccine intradermally. Give rabies immune globulin (20 IU/kg) as soon after exposure as possible, followed by IM vaccine doses (either manufacturer) on days 0, 3, 7, 14 and 28.

For patients who have previously received pre-exposure prophylaxis, give 1 ml of either vaccine IM only on days 0 and 3. Do not give RIG.

Route and site: The deltoid area is the only acceptable site for post-exposure vaccination of adults and older children. For younger children, use the outer aspect of the thigh. Never administer rabies vaccine in the gluteal area.

Travelers to endemic areas may receive vaccine by the ID route if the 3–dose series can be completed ≥ 30 days before departure; otherwise give the vaccine IM.

HDCV – IM in deltoid muscle or ID. Use only the IM route for post-exposure prophylaxis. ID injections given in the lateral aspect of the upper arm are less likely to result in adverse reactions, compared with ID injection in the forearm.

RVA – IM only, in deltoid muscle. Do not inject ID. Vaccinate children in the anterolateral aspect of the thigh muscle.

Booster dose: For occupational or other continuing risk, every 2 to 5 years based on antibody titers, in a single 1 ml IM or 0.1 ml ID injection.

Pre-exposure booster immunization – Test persons who work with live rabies virus in research laboratories or in vaccine production or with diagnostic tests for serum rabies antibody titer every 6 months. Give booster vaccine doses as needed to maintain an adequate titer. Give workers (eg, veterinarians, animal control and wildlife officers in areas where animal rabies is epizootic) booster doses every 2 years or have their serum rabies antibody titer determined every 2 years. If the titer is insufficient, give a booster dose. Veterinarians and similar workers in areas of low rabies endemicity do not require routine booster doses of rabies vaccine after completion of primary pre-exposure immunization or post-exposure prophylaxis.

Missed doses:

Pre-exposure prophylaxis – Prolonging the interval between doses does not interfere with immunity achieved after the concluding dose of the basic series.

Post-exposure prophylaxis – Prolonging the interval between doses may seriously delay achieving protective antibody titers, with potentially fatal consequences.

Stability: Refrigerate dried vaccine at 2° to 8°C (36° to 46°F). Do not freeze. HDCV can presumably tolerate 30 days at room temperature.

Rx	**Imovax Rabies Vaccine (Human Diploid Cell)** (Connaught)	**Powder for Injection:** Freeze-dried suspension of Wistar rabies virus strain PM-1503-3M grown in human diploid cell cultures (inactivated whole virus). Contains ≥ 2.5 IU rabies antigen per ml	In single dose vial[1] with disposable needle and syringe containing diluent and disposable needle for administration.
Rx	**Imovax Rabies I.D. Vaccine (Human Diploid Cell)**[2] (Connaught)	**Powder for Injection:** Freeze-dried suspension of Wistar rabies virus strain PM-1503-3M grown in human diploid cell cultures. Contains 0.25 IU rabies antigen per 0.1 ml intradermal dose	In single-dose syringe with 1 vial diluent.[3]
Rx	**Rabies Vaccine (Adsorbed)** (Various, eg, Michigan Department of Public Health, SK Beecham)	**Injection:** Challenge Virus Standard (CVS) Kissling/MDPH strain	In single-dose 1 ml vial.[4]

[1] With < 100 mg human albumin, < 150 mcg neomycin sulfate and 20 mcg phenol red indicator.
[2] This product is for pre-exposure use only by the intradermal route.
[3] With < 15 mg human albumin, < 22 mcg neomycin sulfate and 3 mcg phenol red indicator/dose.
[4] With ≤ 2 mg/ml aluminum phosphate and 0.01% thimerosal.

RABIES IMMUNE GLOBULIN, HUMAN (RIG)

Refer to the general discussion in the Rabies Prophylaxis Products introduction.

Actions:

Pharmacology: Provides passive protection when given immediately to individuals exposed to rabies virus. Studies of RIG with the first of five doses of human diploid cell vaccine (HDCV) confirmed that passive immunization with RIG provides maximum circulating antibody with minimum interference of active immunization by HDCV. After initiation of the vaccine series, it takes approximately 1 week to develop immunity to rabies; therefore, the value of immediate passive immunization with rabies antibody cannot be overemphasized.

Indications:

Rabies propohylaxis: For passive, transient post-exposure prevention of rabies infection. Administer as soon as possible after exposure, up to 8 days after first vaccine dose. Give RIG to all persons suspected of exposure to rabies with one exception: Persons who have been completely immunized with rabies vaccine and are known to have an adequate antibody titer should receive post-exposure vaccine booster doses only, not RIG.

Contraindications:

Do not administer in repeated doses once vaccine treatment has been initiated. Repeating the dose may interfere with maximum active immunity expected from the vaccine.

Warnings:

Hypersensitivity: There have been a few isolated occurrences of angioedema, urticara nephrotic syndrome and anaphylactic shock after injection. See also Management of Acute Hypersensitivity Reactions.

Pregnancy: Category C. Safety for use during pregnancy has not been established. Use only when clearly needed and when the potential benefits outweigh the potential hazards to the fetus. Intact IgG crosses the placenta from the maternal circulation increasingly after 30 weeks gestation.

Lactation: It is not known if antirabies antibodies are excreted in breast milk. Problems in humans have not been documented.

Children: RIG is generally safe and effective in children.

Precautions:

Allergic response: Use caution in individuals who are allergic to human immunoglobulin or thimerosal.

Drug Interactions:

Rabies immune Globulin Drug Interactions			
Precipitant drug	Object drug*		Description
RIG	Measles/ Mumps/ Rubella vaccine	⬇	RIG may diminish the antibody response through antigen-antibody antagonism. As a general rule, administer live virus vaccines 14 to 30 days before or 6 to 12 weeks after immune globulin administration. Alternately, administer live virus vaccines during this interval if corresponding antibody titers are measusred 3 months after RIG administration.
RIG	Rabies vaccine	⬇	Simultaneous administration may slightly delay the antibody response to rabies vaccine. Because of this possibility, follow CDC recommendations exactly and give no more than the recommended dose of RIG.

* ⬇ = Object drug decreased.

Adverse Reactions:

Local tenderness; muscle soreness or stiffness at the injection site; low grade fever; sensitization to repeated injections of human globulin in immunoglobulin-deficient patients; hypersensitivity (see Warnings).

RABIES IMMUNE GLOBULIN, HUMAN (RIG)

Administration and Dosage:

For IM administration only, preferably in gluteal muscle (upper, outer quadrant only) or deltoid muscle; do not administer IV. Immediate and thorough washing of all bite wounds and scratches with soap and water is perhaps the most effective measure for preventing rabies. Give RIG 20 IU/kg (0.133 ml/kg) as soon as possible after exposure, preferably with the first dose of vaccine. Use up to half the dose to infiltrate the wound site, if the nature and location of the wound site permits. Administer the balance of the dose IM at a different site and in a different extremity from the vaccine.

Storage: Refrigerate between 2° to 8°C (35° to 46°F). Do not freeze. *Imogam* can tolerate 4 days at room temperature; *Hyperab* can tolerate 30 days at 30°C (86°F).

Rx	**Hyperab** (Cutter)	**Injection:** 150 IU per ml	With 0.21 to 0.32 M glycine, 0.008% to 0.012% thimerosal. In 2 and 10 ml single-dose vials.
Rx	**Imogam** (Connaught)		With 0.3 M glycine, 0.008% to 0.012% thimerosal. In 2 and 10 ml single-dose vials.

AGENTS FOR ACTIVE IMMUNIZATION

In contrast to the immune serums and antitoxins, which contain exogenous antibodies to provide passive immunity, the Agents for Active Immunization include specific antigens which induce the endogenous production of antibodies. Agents that induce active immunity include vaccines and toxoids.

Vaccines contain whole (killed or attenuated live) microorganisms capable of inducing antibody formation, but which are not pathogenic. Toxoids are detoxified by-products derived from organisms which induce disease primarily through the elaboration of exotoxins. Although toxoids are not toxic, they are antigenic, and therefore stimulate specific antibody production. Active immunization induced through inoculation with vaccines and toxoids provides prolonged immunity, whereas passive immunization with immune sera or antitoxins is of short duration.

The table below indicates the recommended immunization schedule for infants and children. This schedule has been approved by the Advisory Committee on Immunization Practices (ACIP), The American Academy of Pediatrics (AAP) and the American Academy of Family Physicians (AAFP).

Recommended Immunization Schedules[1]

Vaccine	Birth	2 months	4 months	6 months	12 months	15 months	18 months	4-6 years	11-12 years	14-16 years
Hepatitis B	HB-1									
		HB-2		HB-3						
Diphtheria, tetanus, pertussis		DTP	DTP	DTP	DTP or DTaP at 15 months			DTP or DTaP	Td	
H influenzae type b		Hib	Hib	Hib	Hib					
Poliovirus		OPV	OPV	OPV				OPV		
Measles, mumps, rubella					MMR			MMR[2]		

[1] Recommended childhood immunization schedule-United States, January 1995. *MMWR* 1995 Jan 6;43:959–60.

[2] The second dose of measles-mumps-rubella vaccine should be administered either at 4 to 6 years or at 11 to 12 years.

Concomitant vaccination: Several routine pediatric vaccines may safely and effectively be administered simultaneously at separate injection sites. National authorities recommend simultaneous immunization at separate sites as indicated by age or health risk if return of a vaccine recipient for a subsequent visit is doubtful.

Immunization for other diseases is recommended for persons with a risk of exposure. Specific immunization requirements and recommendations for international travel can be obtained from the Superintendent of Documents, US Government Printing Office, Washington, DC 20402, in the publication "Health Information for International Travel." These can also be found in the following publication: Grabenstein JD. *ImmunoFacts: Vaccines & Immunologic Drugs.* St. Louis: Facts and Comparisons, 1995.

Hypersensitivity to vaccine components: Vaccine antigens produced in systems containing allergenic substances (ie, embryonated chicken eggs) may cause hypersensitivity reactions, including anaphylaxis. Such vaccines should not be given to persons with known hypersensitivity to these components. In contrast, influenza vaccine antigens (whole or split), although prepared in embryonated eggs, are highly purified and only rarely are associated with hypersensitivity reactions.

Live virus vaccines prepared by growing viruses in cell cultures are essentially devoid of allergenic substances. On very rare occasions, hypersensitivity reactions to measles vaccine have been reported in persons with anaphylactic hypersensitivity to eggs. Measles vaccine, however, can be given safely to egg-allergic individuals provided the allergies are not manifested by anaphylactic symptoms. The same precautions apply to mumps vaccine.

Some vaccines contain preservatives (eg, thimerosal) or trace amounts of antibiotics (eg, neomycin) to which patients may be hypersensitive.

AGENTS FOR ACTIVE IMMUNIZATION

Altered immunocompetence: Virus replication after administration of live, attenuated virus vaccines may be enhanced in persons with immune deficiency diseases and in those with suppressed capability for immune response (eg, leukemia, lymphoma, generalized malignancy or therapy with corticosteroids, alkylating agents, antimetabolites or radiation). Do not give live, attenuated virus vaccines to such patients. Do not give live, attenuated virus vaccines to a member of a household in which there is a family history of congenital or hereditary immunodeficiency until the immune competence of the recipient is known.

HIV infection: Special immunization recommendations are appropriate for persons infected with HIV.

Live bacterial or viral vaccines – Persons infected with HIV and persons who have developed AIDS are theoretically at risk of disseminated infection following immunization with a live, albeit attenuated, bacterial or viral vaccine.

Innactivated vaccines or toxoids – In general, immunization with an inactivated vaccine or toxoid poses no additional risk to persons infected with HIV and persons who have developed AIDS. But these persons may be less likely to develop an adequate immune response to vaccination and may remain susceptible to the disease at issue. While HIV-infected persons and AIDS patients may develop less than optimal immunity, compared with uninfected persons, immunization is often still recommended to confer at least partial protection. Optimally, complete the immunization of HIV-infected persons before they meet the criteria for AIDS.

Immunization of HIV-infected persons – In vitro studies demonstrate that proliferating CD4 cells are more susceptible to infection with HIV than nonproliferating cells, raising the possibility that immunization may be a cofactor in exacerbating the progression of HIV infection to AIDS. Nonetheless, no clinical data have substantiated the concern about antigenic stimulation causing deterioration of clinical status. CDC and WHO continue to recommend immunization of HIV-infected persons when the benefits of immunization outweigh the risks of infection.

Summary Recommendations for Routine Immunization of HIV-infected Persons in the US

Drug	Known asymptomatic	Symptomatic
DTP/Td	yes	yes
OPV	no	no
e-IPV[1]	yes	yes
MMR	yes	yes[2]
Hib[3]	yes	yes
Pneumococcal	yes	yes
Influenza	yes[2]	yes

[1] For adults ≥ 18 years of age, use only if indicated.
[2] Consider risk and benefit.
[3] Consider for HIV-infected adults also.

Severe febrile illnesses: Immunization of persons with severe febrile illnesses should generally be deferred until they have recovered.

Vaccination during pregnancy: On the grounds of a theoretical risk to the developing fetus, live, attenuated virus vaccines are not generally given to pregnant women or to those likely to become pregnant within 3 months after receiving vaccine(s). With some of these vaccines, particularly rubella, measles and mumps, pregnancy is a contraindication. When vaccine is to be given during pregnancy, waiting until the second or third trimester to minimize any concern over teratogenicity is a reasonable precaution. However, there has been no evidence of congenital rubella syndrome in infants born to susceptible mothers who received rubella vaccine during pregnancy.

Measles, mumps, rubella or oral polio vaccines may be safely administered to children of pregnant women. Experience to date has not revealed any risks of polio vaccine virus to the fetus.

There is no convincing evidence of risk to the fetus from immunization of pregnant women using inactivated virus vaccines, bacterial vaccines or toxoids. Tetanus and diphtheria toxoid (Td) should be given to inadequately immunized pregnant women because it affords protection against neonatal tetanus.

Adverse events following immunization: Modern vaccines are extremely safe and effective, but not completely so. Adverse events following immunization have been reported with all vaccines. These range from frequent, minor, local reactions to extremely rare, severe, systemic illness such as paralysis associated with oral polio vaccine.

BCG VACCINE

Actions:

Pharmacology: BCG vaccine for intravesical or percutaneous use is an attenuated, live culture preparation of the Bacillus of Calmette and Guerin (BCG) strain of Mycobacterium bovis. The Tice strain was developed at the University of Illinois from a strain originated at the Pasteur Institute.

Immunization with BCG vaccine lowers the risk of serious complications of primary tuberculosis in children. Estimates of efficacy from observational studies in areas where vaccination is performed at birth show that the incidence of tuberculous meningitis and miliary tuberculosis is 52% to 100% lower and that the incidence of pulmonary tuberculosis is 2% to 80% lower in vaccinated children < 15 years of age than in unvaccinated controls. However, estimates of vaccine efficacy may be distorted because of the following: Vaccination was not allocated randomly in observational studies; there were differences in BCG strains, methods and routes of administration; there were differences in the characteristics of the populations and environments in which the vaccines have been studied.

Indications:

Exposed tuberculin skin test-negative infants and children: BCG vaccination is recommended for infants and children with risk of intimate and prolonged exposure to persistently untreated or ineffectively treated patients with infectious pulmonary tuberculosis and who cannot be removed from the source of exposure and cannot be placed on long-term preventive therapy, or who are continuously exposed to persons with tuberculosis who have bacilli resistant to isoniazid and rifampin.

Groups with an excessive rate of new infections: BCG vaccination is also recommended for tuberculin-negative infants and children in groups in which the rate of new infections exceeds 1% per year and for whom the usual surveillance and treatment programs have been attempted but are not operationally feasible. These groups include persons without regular access to health care, those for whom usual health care is culturally or socially unacceptable, or groups who have demonstrated an inability to effectively use existing accessible care.

The US Immunization Practices Advisory Committee (ACIP) no longer recommends BCG vaccination for healthcare workers at risk of repeated exposure to tuberculosis but recommends that these individuals be under tuberculin skin testing surveillance and receive isoniazid prophylaxis in case of tuberculin skin test conversion.

For international travelers, the CDC recommends that BCG vaccination be considered only for travelers with insignificant reaction to tuberculin skin test who will be in a high-risk environment for prolonged periods of time without access to tuberculin skin test surveillance.

Tice BCG vaccine is also indicated for carcinoma in situ of the bladder. See individual monograph in the Antineoplastics section.

Contraindications:

Persons with impaired immune responses, whether congenital, disease-produced, drug- or therapy-induced (ie, cytotoxic drugs and radiation used in cancer therapy). Concurrent steroid use requires caution because of possibility of the vaccine establishing systemic infection; if necessary, treat infection with antituberculous drugs.

Warnings:

Route of administration: Do not inject IV, SC or intradermally. Use percutaneous administration with the multiple puncture disc (see Administration and Dosage).

Immune deficiency syndromes: Do not use in infants, children or adults with severe immune deficiency syndromes. Administer with caution to persons in groups at high risk for HIV infection. Children with a family history of immune deficiency disease should not be vaccinated. If they are, consult an infectious disease specialist and administer antituberculous therapy if clinically indicated.

Pregnancy: Category C. It is not known whether BCG vaccine can cause fetal harm when administered to a pregnant woman or can affect reproduction capacity. Give to a pregnant woman only if clearly needed.

Lactation: It is not known whether BCG vaccine is excreted in breast milk. Because of the potential for serious adverse reactions in nursing infants from BCG vaccine, decide whether to discontinue nursing or not to vaccinate, taking into account the importance of tuberculosis vaccination to the mother.

Children: Take precautions with respect to infants vaccinated with BCG and exposed to persons with active tuberculosis. See Administration and Dosage.

Precautions:

Aseptic technique: Tice BCG contains live bacteria; use with aseptic technique. Handle and dispose of all equipment, supplies, and receptacles in contact with BCG vaccine as biohazardous.

BCG VACCINE

Allergic reactions: Assess the possibility of allergic reactions.

Normal reaction: The intensity and duration of the local reaction depends on the depth of penetration of the multiple-puncture disc and individual variations in patients' tissue reactions. The initial skin lesions usually appear within 10 to 14 days and consist of small red papules at the site. The papules reach maximum diameter (about 3 mm) after 4 to 6 weeks, after which they may scale and then slowly subside.

Six months later, there is usually no visible sign of the vaccination, but on occasion a faintly discernible pattern of the disc points may be visible. On people whose skin tends to keloid formation, there may be slightly more visible evidence.

Vaccination is recommended only for those who are tuberculin negative to a recent skin test with 5 tuberculin units (5TU). Otherwise, vaccination of persons highly sensitive to mycobacterial antigens can result in hypersensitivity reactions including fever, anorexia, myalgia and neuralgia, which last a few days.

After vaccination, it is usually not possible to clearly distinguish between a tuberculin reaction caused by persistent postvaccination sensitivity and one caused by a virulent suprainfection. Caution is advised in attributing a positive skin test to BCG vaccination. Further investigate a sharp rise in the tuberculin reaction since the latest test (except in the immediate postvaccination period).

Lymphadenopathy: Occasionally, lymphadenopathy of the regional lymph node, which spontaneously resolves itself, is seen in young children. Only rarely does the node create a fistula followed by a short period of drainage. The usual treatment is to maintain cleanliness of the drainage site and allow the lesion to heal spontaneously without medical intervention.

Drug Interactions:

Antimicrobial or immunosuppressive agents may interfere with the development of the immune response; use only under medical supervision.

Adverse Reactions:

Lymphadenopathy (see Precautions); osteomyelitis (≈ 1 per 1,000,000 vaccinees); lupoid reactions; disseminated BCG infection and death (very rare; ≈ 1 per 5,000,000 vaccinees) occur almost exclusively in children with impaired immune responses.

Overdosage:

Accidental overdosages, if treated immediately with antituberculous drugs, have not led to complications. If vaccination response is allowed to progress it can still be treated successfully with antituberculous drugs but complications can include regional adenitis, lupus vulgaris, subcutaneous cold abscesses, ocular lesions, etc.

Patient Information:

Keep the vaccination site clean until the local reaction has disappeared.

Administration and Dosage:

Preparation: Add 1 ml Sterile Water for Injection, USP, to one amp of vaccine. Draw the mixture into a syringe and expel it back into the ampule three times to ensure thorough mixing.

Treatment and schedule: The vaccine is administered after fully explaining the risks and benefits to the vaccinee, parent or guardian. After the vaccine is prepared, the immunizing dose of 0.2 to 0.3 ml is dropped on the cleansed surface of the skin, and the vaccine is administered percutaneously utilizing a sterile multiple-puncture disc. After vaccination, the vaccine should flow into the wounds and dry. No dressing is required; however, it is recommended that the site be kept dry for 24 hours. Advise the patient that the vaccine contains live organisms. Although the vaccine will not survive in a dry state, infection of others is possible.

Repeat vaccination for those who remain tuberculin-negative to 5TU of tuberculin after 2 to 3 months.

Children: In infants < 1 month old, reduce the dosage of vaccine by one half by using 2 ml of Sterile Water when reconstituting. If a vaccinated infant remains tuberculin negative to 5TU on skin testing, and if indications for vaccination persist, the infant should receive a full dose after 1 year of age.

Storage/Stability: Refrigerate the intact amp at 2° to 8°C (36° to 46°F). Protect from light. Do not use after the expiration date printed on the label.

Keep reconstituted vaccine refrigerated, protect from light, use within 2 hours.

Rx	**TICE BCG** (Organon)	**Powder for Injection, lyophilized:** Tice strain[1] (1 to 8 x 10^8 CFU equivalent to approximately 50 mg)	In 2 ml amps.[2]

[1] Developed at the University of Illinois.
[2] Preservative free.

MIXED RESPIRATORY VACCINE

Actions:

Pharmacology: Mixed respiratory vaccine (MRV) is prepared from many strains of bacterial organisms commonly found in respiratory tract infections. Many of these strains are isolated in the preparation of autogenous vaccines for patients subject to respiratory infections.

These organisms consist of two general classes of streptococci (a variety of *viridans* and non-hemolytic types). Staphylococci is a mixture of several *aureus* strains. Four types of pneumococci are in this product. The other organisms in the vaccine are *Moraxella (Branhamella) catarrhalis, Klebsiella pneumoniae* (Friedlanders bacillus) and *Hemophilus influenzae.*

The mechanism of MRV is not known. Antigens injected into the skin are processed locally or in satellite lymph nodes by macrophages or lymphocytes. Subsequently this may lead to production of blocking antibody to specific antigens or activation of suppressor cells or helper cells that alter the immunologic status of the patient.

The antigens are metabolized in the macrophages of the immune system. It is not known how much of the antigenic material in bacterial vaccines passes through the immune barriers to be excreted or detoxified by other organs.

Clinical trials: Very few controlled studies have evaluated the effectiveness of MRV or delineated the kinds of illness likely to respond to MRV. Infectious asthma, chronic bronchitis, rhino-bronchitis and secretory otitis were conditions treated, but exact criteria for these diagnoses were generally vague. Criteria for judging severity of symptoms were generally subjective, but the same criteria were applied to both treated and control patients.

To various degrees, these studies indicated that patients given bacterial vaccines did better over the period of study and in some cases did less well later, after vaccines were discontinued. Many reports on the effectiveness of MRV have come from pediatric practices. The youngest patient reported is 3 years old.

Many diseases such as rhinitis, infectious asthma, chronic sinusitis, nasal polyposis and chronic, serous otitis are of unknown etiology. Bacterial or viral infections play a prominent role in these disorders. These disorders may respond transiently or incompletely to appropriate antibiotic, surgical, antihistamine and anti-inflammatory treatment. Bacterial vaccines have been used in the hopes of favorably altering the course of the chronic inflammatory process. There are numerous uncontrolled testimonial reports that indicate the benefits of mixed respiratory vaccines for a variety of common chronic disorders, including those listed above.

Indications:

Based on a review by the Panel on the safety, effectiveness and labeling of bacterial vaccines and bacterial antigens that have "No U.S. Standard of Potency" and other information, the Food and Drug Administration has directed that further investigation be conducted before this product is determined to be fully effective for the labeled indications.

Contraindications:

Rheumatoid arthritis; lupus erythematosus; other connective tissue disease; hypersensitivity to any component of the product (see Warnings). Occasionally a patient will develop excessively large, delayed local reactions after injection, and rarely, vague malaise or myalgia. Drastically reduce subsequent doses or discontinue.

Warnings:

Hypersensitivity: Systemic reactions are very rare. If any do occur, treat like other allergenic reactions using epinephrine and antihistamines. Delayed hypersensitivity to bacterial products is common, and if severe, may limit the dose that can be administered. If delayed skin reactions are accompanied by any systemic symptoms, stop administration. Refer also to Management of Acute Hypersensitivity Reactions.

Pregnancy: Category C. It is not known whether MRV can cause fetal harm when administered to a pregnant woman or can affect reproduction capacity. Give to a pregnant woman only if clearly needed.

Lactation: It is not known whether bacterial products appear in breast milk.

Adverse Reactions:

Immediate systemic reactions are rare. When suspicion has arisen, other antigens were given that were known to be associated with immediate hypersensitivity. Delayed, local reactions are frequent but are no cause for alarm unless accompanied by fever, malaise or myalgia.

Administration and Dosage:

Inject SC. Do not inject IV. Always agitate the suspension to ensure uniform distribution while withdrawing the dose from the vial.

MIXED RESPIRATORY VACCINE

Initial dose: An initial prophylactic dose of 0.05 ml SC is recommended. Increase doses by 0.05 to 0.1 ml at 4 to 7 day intervals until a maximum dose of 0.5 to 1 ml has been reached. In acute conditions, give an initial dose of 0.02 ml and administer increments of 0.02 to 0.05 ml at 3 to 5 day intervals. Patient sensitivity varies and for some, doses may be increased faster; for others, more slowly. Do not administer another dose until all local reactions resulting from the previous dose have disappeared.

Dosage increments: When doses are being advanced, the time interval can be every 3 to 4 days with the lower concentration and 5 to 7 days with the more concentrated vaccine. Local reaction and generalized symptoms determine the final maintenance dose.

Maintenance dose: Generally, give 0.5 ml at weekly or alternate week intervals. The hyposensitizing dose for children is the same as for adults. The maximum volume of antigen tolerated without undue pain and swelling may be less for the smaller patient.

Increasingly large delayed reactions may occur after administering maintenance doses for many months. Further administration of vaccine, even at smaller doses, may continue to increase the reaction. Stop vaccine immediately. A rest period of 2 to 6 months may allow the delayed hypersensitivity to subside, and injections may be resumed at a lower dose if still needed. Individualize dosage. Smaller increments in doses may be necessary for extremely sensitive patients.

General reactions such as fatigue, drowsiness or a definite aggravation of allergic symptoms require a reduction in the size of the subsequent doses or further dilution of the vaccine. Severe systemic reactions mandate a decrease of at least 50% in the next dose, followed by cautious increases.

Storage: Store at 2° to 8°C (36° to 46°F).

Rx	**MRV** (Hollister-Stier, Miles)	**Injection:** 2000 million organisms per ml from: *Staphylococcus aureus* 1200 million; *Streptococcus (viridans and non-hemolytic)* 200 million; *Streptococcus pneumoniae* 150 million; *Moraxella (Branhamella) catarrhalis* 150 million; *Klebsiella pneumoniae* 150 million; *Hemophilus influenzae* 150 million	In 20 ml vials with 0.4% phenol and dextrose.

STAPHAGE LYSATE (SPL)

Actions:

Pharmacology: Bacterial antigen made from *Staphylococcus,* staphage lysate (SPL) is a bacteriologically sterile staphylococcal vaccine containing components of *S aureus,* bacteriophage and culture medium ingredients.

In experimental conditions, *S aureus* or its cellular components may induce cell-mediated immunity. In uncontrolled studies in humans, favorable results have been reported using SPL for a variety of staphylococcal diseases, as well as for herpesvirus and aphthous ulcers (essentially treatment failures with other therapeutic modalities).

In vitro, SPL has stimulated lymphoproliferative responses in both T- and B-cell subpopulations present in peripheral and cord blood of healthy human subjects.

These findings appear to support the interpretation that SPL in staphylococcal-hypersensitive subjects acts as an immunopotentiator of nonspecific cell-mediated immunity.

Indications:

Treatment of either staphylococcal infections or polymicrobial infections with a staphylococcal component.

Based on a review by the Panel on Bacterial Vaccines and Bacterial Antigens with no US Standard of Potency and other information, the Food and Drug Administration has directed that further investigation be conducted before this product is determined fully effective for the labeled indication(s).

Contraindications:

Intranasal use during an acute asthmatic episode.

Warnings:

Allergies: Exercise caution when administering SPL intranasally to patients with known allergies (see Administration and Dosage).

STAPHAGE LYSATE (SPL)

Hypersensitivity: In common with all antigens employed to stimulate the production of antibodies that are protective in the event of subsequent disease, SPL presents the remote potential of host sensitization to staphylococcal or bovine protein. Anaphylaxis has never been observed in > 10 million doses, but consider this possibility and be prepared with emergency resuscitation equipment and medications. Refer to Management of Acute Hypersensitivity Reactions.

Pregnancy: Category B. There are no adequate and well controlled studies in pregnant women. Use during pregnancy only if clearly needed and if the potential benefits outweigh the potential hazards to the fetus.

Lactation: It is not known whether SPL is excreted in breast milk. Exercise caution when administering to a nursing mother.

Children: Safety and effectiveness in children have not been established.

Precautions:

Preservative free: SPL does not contain a preservative; it must be handled aseptically. Do not use if it becomes cloudy or turbid.

Amps: Use 1 ml amps for SC injection and intranasal aerosol inhalation only. When a parenteral dose of SPL is withdrawn from the amp, use the remainder immediately or discard.

Vials: Use the 10 ml vial for intranasal (aerosol or drop instillation), oral or topical administration only; do not use for SC injection.

Adverse Reactions:

SPL may cause general vaccine-type reactions (eg, malaise, fever, chills). Excessive reactions may be lessened by dose reduction.

Reactions at the site of injection (redness, itching or swelling) may occur in 2 to 3 hours and may last up to 3 days, steadily decreasing. These reactions indicate a normal response to SPL and, if excessive, may be lessened by dose reduction.

Patient Information:

SPL may cause vaccine-type or injection site reactions and, if excessive, these reactions may be lessened by dose reduction.

Administration and Dosage:

Routes of administration: SPL is administered by several routes including: SC injection; intranasal aerosol inhalation or nasal drop instillation; oral; topical; irrigation; combinations of these routes. The severity of the infection and the response of the patient are the guiding factors in determining the proper dosage regimen.

Skin testing: It is highly recommended that all new patients first be skin-tested with 0.025 to 0.05 ml intracutaneously to assess their relative sensitivity to SPL. Based on relative sensitivity to skin test, the initial dose of SPL is small, followed by incremental increases at prescribed intervals (according to urgency and tolerance), to a maximum dose. The dose is continued until improvement is certain, then the interval may be lengthened gradually to the longest interval that maintains adequate clinical control.

Tolerance: The limit of tolerance is the maximum quantity that can be given to a patient without producing signs of a general vaccine-type reaction (see Adverse Reactions).

Chronic, recurrent, refractory or deep-seated infections: Cautiously increase the frequency or the dose to achieve the desired therapeutic response.

Children usually should receive about one-half the adult dose. Infants are best treated with nasal drop instillation, sprays or topical application.

Acute infections:

Initial dose – 0.05 to 0.2 ml, followed by incremental increases (according to urgency and tolerance) of 0.1 to 0.2 ml at 1 to 2 day intervals, to a maximum dose of up to 0.5 ml.

Subacute and chronic infections:

Initial dose – 0.05 to 0.1 ml, followed by incremental increases (according to urgency and tolerance) of 0.1 to 0.2 ml at 2 to 4 day intervals, to a maximum dose of 0.2 to 0.5 ml.

SC administration: Administer in the deltoid region. Following the initial injection, subsequent injections are given in alternate arms, avoiding a previous site.

If an undue amount of local redness, itching or swelling ensues, await a partial subsidence of the reactions, proceed with one-half the previous dose and make incremental increases at longer intervals.

Following an SC injection, the unused contents of the 1 ml amp may be given orally, topically or intranasally to reinforce the SC dose.

STAPHAGE LYSATE (SPL)

Intranasal aerosol inhalation: SPL is rapidly absorbed through the anterior nares, the main reservoir of pathogenic staphylococci. The importance of intranasal aerosol inhalation is stressed because of the high absorptive characteristics of the nasal mucosa. When using this route, some patients may experience transient general vaccine-type reactions. If excessive, reactions may be lessened by dose reduction.

Intranasal aerosol inhalation allows direct access to the sinuses, throat and bronchi; when this route is combined with SC injection, better clinical results may be obtained.

A nebulizer with nasal tips is used, attached by rubber tubing having a hand-controlled air valve to an air supply (a DeVilbiss Air Compressor). Clean the nebulizer after each use according to the manufacturer's directions.

A measured dose of SPL is placed in nebulizer, adding sufficient sterile preservative free water or isotonic saline to a total volume of 1 ml for efficient atomization. Nebulization is achieved by closing air valve during inspiration, holding the breath a few seconds, and exhaling through the mouth, avoiding hyperventilation.

Patients without allergies –

Initial dose: 0.1 ml, followed by incremental increases (according to urgency and tolerance) of up to 0.2 ml at 1 to 3 days, to a maximum dose of 0.5 to 1 ml.

Patients with known allergies – Exercise caution when administering SPL by this route to patients with allergies such as bronchial asthma, pulmonary fibrosis, emphysema, bronchiectasis, hay fever and multiple allergies.

It is highly recommended that these patients first be skin-tested with 0.025 to 0.05 ml intracutaneously to assess their relative sensitivity to SPL. Based on relative sensitivity to the skin test, the initial dose varies from 0.05 to 0.1 ml, followed by incremental increases (according to urgency and tolerance) of 0.05 to 0.1 ml at weekly intervals, to a maximum dose of 0.25 to 0.5 ml. These doses can be increased cautiously at shorter intervals if the patient tolerates SPL well.

For faster immunologic response, SPL may be given concomitantly by SC injection or orally without aftereffects.

Nasal drop instillation: If intranasal aerosol inhalation equipment is not available, administer SPL by nasal drop instillation, particularly to patients with upper respiratory symptoms. Administer by this route either alone or concomitantly with other routes.

Before using SPL by nasal drop instillation, review all information under *Intranasal aerosol inhalation.*

When using this route, withdraw appropriate dose with sterile tuberculin syringe and needle, remove the needle, and use the syringe as a dropper. Divide the dose equally between each nostril and keep in contact with the nasal mucosa for a minimum of 2 minutes to achieve adequate absorption.

Oral: The specific therapy of staphylococcal enterocolitis should include an oral dose of 1 to 2 ml, in water, 1 to 3 times a day as long as necessary to maintain adequate clinical control.

For systemic action, SPL by SC injection or intranasally will reinforce the oral dose.

Topical application: Concomitantly with other routes of administration, SPL in the form of sprays, drops, packs or irrigations may be used to treat accessible lesions of the skin and mucous membranes, including eye and ear infections, burns, sinus tracts and ulcers. The usual dose varies from 0.25 to 2 ml, as often as indicated to maintain adequate clinical control.

Storage/Stability: Store at 2° to 8°C (35° to 46°F). Do not freeze. Do not use if cloudy or turbid. Preservative free; handle aseptically.

Rx	**SPL-Serologic Types I and III** (Delmont Labs)	**Solution:** per ml 120 to 180 million *Staphylococcus aureus colony forming units* and 100 to 1000 million *Staphylococcus bacteriophage plaque forming units*	In 1 ml amps[1] and 10 ml vials.[2]

[1] Preservative free. For SC injection and intranasal aerosol inhalation only.

[2] Preservative free. For intranasal aerosol inhalation or nose drops, oral administration or topical application only.

MENINGOCOCCAL POLYSACCHARIDE VACCINE

Actions:

Pharmacology: Meningitis can be caused by a variety of microorganisms including several sero-groups of meningococci. This vaccine will not stimulate protection against infections caused by organisms other than *Neisseria meningitidis* Groups A, C, Y and W-135. The presence of human serum bactericidal antibodies to meningococcal antigens is strongly correlated with immunity to meningococcal disease; meningococcal polysaccharides induce the formation of such antibodies in humans.

Clinical trials: In one study, group A polysaccharide vaccine was 100% effective in preventing systemic disease caused by group A organisms occurring ≥ 2 weeks after immunization. Another study using group C polysaccharide vaccine was at least 87% effective in preventing disease caused by group C organisms. With A and C combined, there was at least a fourfold increase in bactericidal antibodies in 95% of subjects in a separate study. Another study using groups A, C, Y and W-135 showed at least a fourfold increase in antibodies in > 90% of subjects. In children (ages 2 to 12), the following seroconversion rates were obtained following the vaccine: Group A – 72% to 99%; Group C – 58% to 99%; Group Y – 90% to 97%; Group W-135 – 82% to 89%.

Indications:

Persons ≥ 2 years of age at risk in epidemic or highly endemic areas.

Consider vaccination for:

Household or institutional contacts of meningococcal disease as an adjunct to appropriate antibiotic chemoprophylaxis.

Medical and laboratory personnel at risk of exposure to meningococcal disease.

Travelers planning to visit countries having epidemic meningococcal disease.

Terminal complement component deficiency patients.

Anatomic or functional asplenia patients.

Routine vaccination is not recommended in the US for the following reasons: (1) Meningococcal disease is infrequent (≈ 3000 cases per year); (2) no vaccine exists for serogroup B, which accounts for ≈ 50% of cases in the US; and (3) vaccine is not efficacious against group C disease in children < 2 years of age, which account for 28% of the group C cases in the US.

Contraindications:

Acute illness; pregnancy (see Warnings).

Warnings:

Immunosuppressive therapy: The expected immune response may not be obtained if the vaccine is used in persons receiving immunosuppressive therapy.

Hypersensitivity: Have epinephrine 1:1000 available to control anaphylactic reactions. Refer to Management of Acute Hypersensitivity Reactions.

Pregnancy: Category C. Effects on the human fetus and on reproduction capacity are unknown. Do not administer to a pregnant woman unless clearly required.

Children: Not recommended in children < 2 years of age.

Adverse Reactions:

Systemic: Headache (1.2% to 4.1%); malaise (≤ 2.6%); fever (0.4% to 3.1%); chills (≤ 1.7%).

Local: Tenderness (24.2% to 29.1%); pain (17.5% to 25.1%); erythema (0.8% to 31.7%); induration (4.8% to 8.3%).

Administration and Dosage:

Inject SC. Avoid injecting intradermally or IV since clinical studies have not established safety and efficacy. The immunizing dose is one SC injection of 0.5 ml.

Preparation of solution: Reconstitute the vaccine using the diluent supplied. Shake until dissolved.

Storage/Stability: Store freeze-dried vaccine and reconstituted vaccine between 2° to 8°C (35° to 46°F). Discard remainder of vaccine within 5 days after reconstitution.

Rx	**Menomune-A/C/Y/W-135** (Connaught Labs)	**Powder for Injection:** When reconstituted, each 0.5 ml contains 50 mcg "isolated product" from each of groups A, C, Y and W–135.	Freeze-dried. In single dose vials with diluent.[1]

[1] With lactose (2.5 to 5 mg per dose) and 1:10,000 thimerosal.

CHOLERA VACCINE

Actions:

Pharmacology: Cholera vaccine is a sterile suspension of equal parts of phenol-inactivated Ogawa and Inaba serotypes of killed *Vibrio cholerae (V comma)* in buffered sodium chloride injection. The vaccine contains 8 units of each serotype antigen (Ogawa and Inaba) per ml.

Cholera vaccine is used for active immunization against cholera. In field studies carried out in endemic cholera areas, cholera vaccines were approximately 50% effective in reducing incidence of disease and for only 3 to 6 months. Use of cholera vaccine does not prevent transmission of infection.

Indications:

Active immunization against cholera is indicated only for individuals traveling to or residing in countries where cholera is endemic or epidemic.

The risk of cholera to most US travelers is so low that vaccination is of dubious benefit. The World Health Organization no longer recommends cholera vaccination for travel to or from cholera-infected areas; however, some countries affected or threatened by cholera may require evidence of vaccination as a condition of entry. The traveler's best protection against cholera is to avoid food and water that might be contaminated.

Contraindications:

Presence of any acute illness; history of severe systemic reaction or allergic response following a prior dose of cholera vaccine.

Warnings:

Route of administration: Do not inject IV. Inject IM, SC or intradermally. Do not administer IM to persons with thrombocytopenia or any coagulation disorder that would contraindicate IM injection.

Hypersensitivity: Before the injection of any biological, take all precautions known for prevention of allergic or other side effects, including a review of the patient's history regarding possible sensitivity, and a knowledge of the recent literature pertaining to the use of the biological concerned. Have epinephrine 1:1000 available for immediate use when this product is injected. Refer to Management of Acute Hypersensitivity Reactions.

Pregnancy: Category C. It is not known whether cholera vaccine can cause fetal harm when administered to a pregnant woman or can affect reproductive capacity. However, as with other inactivated bacterial vaccines, its use is not contraindicated during pregnancy unless the intended recipient has manifested significant systemic or allergic reaction following administration of prior doses. Individualize use of cholera vaccine during pregnancy to reflect actual need.

Precautions:

Hepatitis B: Use a separate, sterilized syringe and needle for each patient to prevent transmission of hepatitis B virus and other infectious agents from one person to another.

Aspirate: Before delivering the dose IM or SC, aspirate to help avoid inadvertent injection into a blood vessel.

Drug Interactions:

Yellow fever vaccine: Some data suggest that administration of cholera and yellow fever vaccines within 3 weeks of each other may result in decreased levels of antibody response to both vaccines as compared with administration at longer intervals. However, there is no evidence that protection to either disease is diminished following simultaneous administration. When feasible, administer cholera and yellow fever vaccines at a minimal interval of 3 weeks, unless time constraints preclude this. If the vaccines cannot be administered at least 3 weeks apart, give simultaneously.

Adverse Reactions:

Local reactions manifested by erythema, induration, pain and tenderness at the site of injection occur in most recipients, and such local reactions may persist for a few days.

Recipients frequently develop malaise, headache and mild-to-moderate temperature elevations which may persist for 1 to 2 days.

CHOLERA VACCINE

Patient Information:

The traveler's best protection against cholera is to avoid food and water that may be contaminated.

Administration and Dosage:

Administer intradermally, SC or IM. The intracutaneous (intradermal) route is satisfactory for persons ≥ 5 years of age, but higher levels of antibody may be achieved in children < 5 years old by the SC and IM routes.

The primary immunizing course consists of 2 doses, 1 week to 1 month or more apart. The primary immunizing series does not need to be repeated for booster doses to be effective.

Primary and Booster Immunizations for Cholera Vaccine

	Route and Age			
	Intradermal[1]	SC or IM		
Dose number	≥ 5 years	6 mos-4 years	5-10 years	> 10 years
1 & 2[2]	0.2 ml	0.2 ml	0.3 ml	0.5 ml
Boosters[3]	0.2 ml	0.2 ml	0.3 ml	0.5 ml

[1] Higher levels of antibody may be achieved in children < 5 years old by the SC or IM routes.
[2] Primary immunization requires 2 doses given at intervals of 1 week to 1 month (or more).
[3] Give booster every 6 months where cholera is epidemic or endemic.

Storage: Refrigerate between 2° to 8°C (35° to 46°F). Do not freeze.

Rx	**Cholera Vaccine** (Wyeth-Ayerst)	**Injection:** Suspension of killed *Vibrio cholerae* (Inaba and Ogawa types), 8 units of each serotype per ml	In 1.5 and 20 ml vials.[4]

[4] With 0.5% phenol.

PLAGUE VACCINE

Actions:

Pharmacology: Yersinia pestis, the etiologic bacterial agent of plague, is infectious for animals and humans. Although *Y. pestis* infection of humans can assume various clinical forms, the most common clinical form is acute regional lymphadenitis, called bubonic plague. Less common clinical forms include septicemic, pneumonic and meningeal plague. Secondary pneumonia (pneumonic plague) is a severe complication of bubonic plague in which the infection reaches the lungs by the hematogenous spread of bacteria from the bubo. Plague is highly contagious by airborne transmission. Primary inhalation pneumonia is rare but is a potential threat after exposure to a patient with plague who has a cough or to moribund or dead animals. Less common complications of plague infection are meningitis, pharyngitis that may resemble acute tonsillitis and prominent GI symptoms of nausea, vomiting, diarrhea and abdominal pain. These symptoms may precede the bubo or, in septicemic plague, occur without a bubo. Mortality is high in untreated cases and the fulminant clinical course can produce death as quickly as 2 to 4 days after the onset of symptoms. Antibiotics (tetracyclines, chloramphenicol, streptomycin or sulfamethoxazole-trimethoprim) administered early in the course of the disease markedly reduce fatalities. After primary plague infection, humans develop acquired immunity which probably confers long-term protection from future plague infections. Secondary infections are likely to be milder and result in fewer fatalities. Although patients with uncomplicated infections who are promptly treated with antibiotics should not present a health hazard to other persons, those with cough or other signs of pneumonia pose a small but definite risk for person-to-person transmission of the plague bacillus through airborne droplets.

Humans play no role in the maintenance of plague in nature, but they are accidental hosts in the natural cycle of plague either after direct exposure, through the bite of an infective flea or handling of contaminated animal carcasses or tissues of rodents or other mammals. In sylvatic enzootic foci of plague, which occurs in the US, the important reservoirs are the ground squirrel, rock squirrel, prairie dog and pack rat. Infection from domestic cats has been increasing in the US with 15 human cases from 1977 to 1994, four of which were pneumonic plague. From 1944 to 1993, 362 cases of human plague were reported in the US, ≈ 90% occurring in New Mexico, Arizona, California and Colorado. Approximately 16% of the cases were fatal.

Clinical trials: Twenty-nine human subjects were immunized with 1 ml plague vaccine, then 0.2 ml at 3 months and 0.2 ml 6 months later. Thirty days after the initial dose of vaccine, 86% of the vaccinees had detectable passive hemagglutination (PHA) antibody titers against *Y. pestis* F1 antigen on sensitized sheep red blood cells. Subsequent booster doses of vaccine stimulated increased titers of PHA anti-F1 antibodies. After the second and third doses, 90% and 93% of the subjects, respectively, had detectable PHA titers. Two individuals (7%) did not develop detectable antibodies after three doses.

Military experience obtained in South Vietnam between 1961 and 1971 has provided indirect epidemiological evidence indicating that vaccination with plague vaccine reduces the incidence and severity of disease resulting from the bite of infected rodent fleas. The low incidence (approximately one case of plague per 1,000,000 man-years of exposure) of clinical plague in vaccinated Americans as compared to 333 cases per 1,000,000 man-years of exposure in Vietnamese civilians during a 10 year period strongly suggests that the plague vaccine is effective.

Indications:

Yersinia pestis: Active immunization of adults against infection with *Yersinia pestis.*

Contraindications:

Hypersensitivity to any component of this vaccine, including beef protein, soy, casein, sulfite, phenol and formaldehyde.

Patients with history of serious adverse reactions (eg, anaphylaxis or seizures) to plague vaccine injections should not be revaccinated.

Defer immunization during the course of any febrile illness.

Warnings:

Immunization against plague is recommended only for those persons at high risk of exposure. Vaccination may be considered for (1) laboratory personnel regularly working with *Y. pestis* or plague-infected rodents, particularly those engaged in *Y. pestis* aerosol experiments or working with *Y. pestis* organisms resistant to antimicrobics, (2) persons engaged in field operations or workers who reside in rural areas with enzootic or epidemic plague where avoidance of rodents and fleas is impossible and (3) persons whose vocation brings them into regular contact with wild rodents or infected animals in areas with enzootic plague.

PLAGUE VACCINE

Vaccination is not recommended for persons living in or traveling to areas of the US with enzootic plague or most travelers in countries reporting cases, particularly if their travel is limited to urban areas with modern accommodations.

Plague vaccination is not required for international travel. It may be considered for persons traveling to or residing in endemic and epizootic areas following natural disasters and when regular sanitary practices are interrupted such that plague can extend from its usual areas of endemicity into urban centers.

Plague disease: Plague vaccine is not indicated for treatment of active plague disease.

Exposure: Give persons either exposed to *Y. pestis* aerosols or to plague patients with pneumonia adequate doses of a suitable antibiotic over a 7 to 10 day period regardless of vaccination history.

Blood disorders: As with any IM injection, give with caution to individuals with thrombocytopenia or any coagulation disorder that would contraindicate IM injection (see Drug Interactions).

Immunocompromised patients: If plague vaccine is administered to immunosuppressed persons or persons receiving immunosuppressive therapy, the expected immune response may not be obtained. This includes patients with asymptomatic or symptomatic human immunodeficiency virus (HIV) infection, severe combined immunodeficiency, hypogammaglobulinemia or agammaglobulinemia, altered immune states due to diseases such as leukemia, lymphoma, or generalized malignancy, or an immune system compromised by treatment with corticosteroids, alkylating drugs, antimetabolites or radiation.

Hypersensitivity: Epinephrine injection 1:1000 must be immediately available following immunization should anaphylaxis or other allergic reactions occur due to any component of the vaccine. Refer to the Management of Acute Hypersensitivity Reactions.

Pregnancy: Category C. Whether plague vaccine can cause fetal harm when administered to a pregnant woman or can affect reproduction capacity is not known. Use during pregnancy only if the potential benefit justifies the risk to the fetus.

Lactation: It is not known if plague vaccine is excreted in breast milk.

Children: Plague vaccine is not indicated for pediatric use. Safety and efficacy have not been established. Although the Immunization Practices Advisory Committee has provided a dose and schedule table for the immunization of children, there are no safety and efficacy studies of plague vaccine in children to support the use of this vaccine in persons < 18 years of age.

Drug Interactions:

Anticoagulants: As with other IM injections, plague vaccine should be given with caution to individuals on anticoagulant therapy.

Cholera/Typhoid vaccine: When practical, plague vaccine should not be given on the same occasion as cholera vaccine or AKD or H-P typhoid vaccines to avoid the possibility of accentuated side effects.

Adverse Reactions:

Adverse reactions to plague vaccine have been mild following primary immunization and may result in general malaise; headache; fever; mild lymphadenopathy; erythema and induration at the injection site; sterile abscesses, urticarial and asthmatic phenomena (infrequent). These local reactions such as injection pain, erythema and induration are usually resolved within 48 hours of vaccination. However, severe reactions to plague vaccine, although infrequent, may occur.

PLAGUE VACCINE

Local or Systemic Adverse Reactions Seen Within 24 Hours After Immunization with Plague Vaccine (%)

Adverse reaction	Dose 1 (n = 67)	Dose 2 (n = 59)
Local:		
Tenderness	71.6	18.6
Arm motion	11.9	1.7
Erythema	4.5	0
Warmth	3	1.7
Edema	1.5	0
Systemic:		
Headache	19.4	6.8
Nausea	13.4	3.4
Malaise	10.4	5.1
Dizziness	6	0
Chills	4.5	3.4
Joint ache	4.5	0
Muscle ache	4.5	0
Anorexia	1.5	0
Diarrhea	1.5	0
Vomiting	1.5	0

Patient Information:

Fully inform patients of the benefits and risks of immunization with plague vaccine and instruct them to report any serious adverse reactions to the health care provider and to seek emergency medical help if wheezing or shortness of breath occurs.

Prior to administration of plague vaccine, instruct patients to wait in the physician's office for at least 20 minutes after inoculation in the event anaphylaxis develops.

Plague vaccine may be considered for persons traveling to endemic or epidemic plague areas. Consult current CDC advisories with regard to specific plague locales.

Advise travelers to endemic and epidemic plague areas to take all necessary precautions to avoid contact with *Y. pestis* (plague) infected wild rodents or their fleas and to other infected wild animals and domestic animals (see Warnings).

Inform the patient of the importance of completing the immunization schedule.

Persons expecting repeated or continuous exposure to *Y. pestis* should consult with a physician about booster immunization.

Administration and Dosage:

Plague vaccine is for IM injection, preferably into the deltoid muscle. A jet injector gun may be used to administer the vaccine. Do not inject IV.

Shake well before use to assure suspension uniformity prior to withdrawing the dose from the vial.

Primary immunization consists of a series of three injections. The first injection is 1 ml of plague vaccine, followed after 1 to 3 months by a 0.2 ml injection and the third injection of 0.2 ml 5 to 6 months after the second injection. The serum levels of anti-plague antibodies are generally increased by successive injections of plague vaccine. Some individuals not responding to the first two injections may produce an adequate response following the third injection, and others may not respond with the production of detectable anti-plague antibodies.

The duration of antibody following administration of the primary series of plague vaccine is brief (eg, 6 to 12 months) and booster doses of 0.2 ml at approximately 6 month intervals may be required for continued protection for individuals remaining in a known plague area. Booster doses at intervals of 1 to 2 years may be appropriate for persons who have received ≥ 3 booster doses at 6 month intervals. Where available, the determination of hemagglutination titers may be helpful in determining the need for a booster immunization.

Storage: Store at 2° to 8°C (35° to 46°F). Do not freeze.

Rx	**Plague Vaccine** (Greer)	**Injection:** 1.8 to 2.2 x 10^9 killed plague bacilli per ml	0.9% sodium chloride, 0.019% formaldehyde, 0.5% phenol, sodium sulfite. In 20 ml vials.

TYPHOID VACCINE

Actions:

Pharmacology: Typhoid vaccine is estimated to be > 70% effective in preventing typhoid fever, depending partly on the degree of exposure.

Oral – Typhoid vaccine live oral Ty21a is a live attenuated vaccine for oral administration. The vaccine contains the attenuated strain *Salmonella typhi* Ty21a. The vaccine strain is grown under controlled conditions and lyophilized. The lyophilized bacteria are filled into gelatin capsules coated with an organic solution to render them resistant to dissolution in stomach acid.

Parenteral – For purposes of clarity in this monograph, the parenteral doseforms will be abbreviated AKD (acetone-killed and dried), H-P (heat- and phenol-inactivated) and Vi (typhoid Vi capsular polysaccharide vaccine).

The Vi polysaccharide is extracted from *S. typhi* Ty2 strain. The organism is grown in a semi-synthetic medium without animal proteins. Each single dose of 0.5 ml is formulated to contain 25 mcg of purified Vi polysaccharide in a colorless isotonic phosphate buffered saline (pH 7 ± 0.3).

Typhoid vaccine for SC or intradermal use is a saline suspension containing ≤ 1000 million *S. typhi* (Ty2 strain) organisms per ml. The vaccine strain is grown on veal infusion agar, the bacteria are washed off the medium, suspended in buffered sodium chloride injection and killed by a combination of phenol and heat or by treatment with acetone.

There are 400 to 600 cases of typhoid fever (also called *typhus abdominalis*) per year diagnosed in the US. In 62% of these patients (statistics from 1977 to 1979), the disease was acquired outside of the US, while in 38%, the disease was acquired within the US. Of the cases acquired in the US, 23% were associated with typhoid carriers, 24% were due to food outbreaks, 23% were associated with the ingestion of contaminated food or water, 6% were due to household contact with an infected person and 4% were acquired following exposure to *S. typhi* in a laboratory setting.

Virulent strains of *S. typhi*, upon ingestion, are able to pass through the stomach acid barrier, colonize the intestinal tract, penetrate the lumen and enter the lymphatic system and blood stream, thereby causing disease.

The ability of *S. typhi* to cause disease and to induce a protective immune response is dependent upon the bacteria possessing a complete lipopolysaccharide. The *S. typhi* Ty21a vaccine strain is restricted in its ability to produce a complete lipopolysaccharide. However, a sufficient quantity of complete lipopolysaccharide is synthesized to evoke a protective immune response.

Efficacy –

Oral: Vaccination reduces disease incidence by 60% to 70%.

Parenteral:

AKD & H-P – Efficacy is 75% to 94% and 71% to 77% in the AKD and H-P vaccines, respectively, in preventing typhoid fever, depending on degree of exposure. Food and water discipline are the most important measures to avoid disease, even for vaccine recipients.

Vi – A 25 mcg dose produced a 4–fold rise in antibody titers in 88% to 96% of healthy American adults. The Vi polysaccharide vaccine reduced disease incidence by 49% to 87% in a trial among adults and children in Nepal. In a pediatric study in South Africa, blood culture-confirmed cases of typhoid fever were reduced 61%, 52% and 50% in the first, second and third years, respectively, after a single dose of Vi polysaccharide vaccine.

Typhoid fever, an acute, febrile enteric disease, is caused by *S. typhi.* Efficacy of protective immunity seems to depend on the size of the bacterial inoculum consumed. Counsel travelers to take standard food and water precautions to avoid typhoid fever. Select appropriate antibiotics to treat active infections (eg, chloramphenicol, ampicillin). Consider cholecystectomy or ciprofloxacin therapy for chronic carriers. No evidence indicates that typhoid vaccine is useful in controlling common-source outbreaks. Typhoid vaccine will not prevent infection or disease caused by other species of *Salmonella* or other bacteria that cause enteric disease.

Onset –

Oral: Finish the fourth capsule at least 1 week before travel.

Parenteral:

AKD & H-P – Protective antibody titers presumably develop within 1 to 2 weeks after the second dose.

Vi – Protective antibody titers develop within 2 weeks after a single dose.

Duration –

Oral: ≈ 5 years.

Parenteral:

AKD & H-P – > 2 years.

Vi – ≈ 2 years.

TYPHOID VACCINE

Indications:

Oral: For immunization of adults and children > 6 years of age against disease caused by *S. typhi.* Complete the vaccine regimen 1 week before potential exposure to typhoid bacteria.

Parenteral: For active immunity against typhoid fever. Complete the vaccine regimen 1 week before potential exposure to typhoid bacteria.

Routine immunization against typhoid fever is not recommended in the US. Selective immunization against typhoid fever is recommended under the following circumstances: 1) Expected intimate exposure to a household contact with typhoid fever or a known carrier, 2) travelers to typhoid-endemic areas (especially Africa, Asia and South and Central America), especially if prolonged exposure to potentially contaminated food and water is likely and travelers to areas of the world with a risk of exposure to typhoid fever, and 3) workers in microbiology laboratories with expected frequent contact with *S. typhi.*

Contraindications:

A person with typhoid fever or a chronic typhoid carrier.

Oral: Hypersensitivity to any component of the vaccine or the capsule. Do not administer the capsules during acute febrile illness or during an acute GI illness (eg, persistent diarrhea or vomiting).

Parenteral: A previous severe systemic or allergic reaction. In the presence of acute respiratory or other active infection, or intensive physical activity (particularly when environmental temperatures are high).

Warnings:

Hypersensitivity: Two hours after the IM injection of typhoid vaccine, a 20-year-old man presented with fever, shaking chills, myalgias, mild shortness of breath, headache, rapid pulse, elevated temperature, a blood pressure of 92/60 mmHg and elevated liver function tests. On the second day of hospitalization, he became hypotensive, developed facial and periorbital edema and showed interstitial edema with bilateral pleural effusions. Refer to the Management of Acute Hypersensitivity Reactions.

Immunodeficiency: If administered to immunosuppressed persons or persons receiving immunosuppressive therapy, the expected immune response may not be obtained. This includes patients with asymptomatic or symptomatic HIV infection, severe combined immunodeficiency, hypogammaglobulinemia or agammaglobulinemia, altered immune states due to diseases such as leukemia, lymphoma or generalized malignancy; or an immune system compromised by treatment with corticosteroids, alkylating drugs, antimetabolites or radiation.

Oral – Do not give typhoid vaccine capsules to immunocompromised persons, including persons with congenital or acquired immune deficiencies, whether due to genetics, disease or drug or radiation therapy, regardless of possible benefits from vaccination. This product contains live bacteria. Avoid use in HIV-positive persons. Use a parenteral, inactivated typhoid vaccine instead.

Pregnancy: Category C. It is not known whether typhoid vaccine can cause fetal harm when administered to pregnant women or can affect reproduction capacity. Give to a pregnant woman only if clearly needed.

Oral – Consider using parenteral inactivated typhoid vaccine in pregnant women at risk of typhoid fever.

Parenteral – Give to a pregnant woman only if clearly needed (if disease risk exceeds vaccination risks). It is not known if typhoid vaccine or corresponding antibodies cross the placenta. Generally, most IgG passage across the placenta occurs during the third trimester.

Lactation: There are no data to warrant the use of the product in nursing mothers. It is not known if the vaccine is excreted in breast milk.

Children:

Oral – Safety and efficacy have not been established for the oral vaccine in children < 6 years of age and is therefore not recommended for use in this age group.

Parenteral –

AKD and H-P: Reduce dosage volume to 0.25 ml for children < 10 years old. These vaccines are known to be effective in children as young as 6 months of age.

Vi: Vaccine is not recommended for children < 2 years old because no safety or efficacy data are available for that age group.

Precautions:

Protection: Not all recipients of typhoid vaccine will be fully protected against typhoid fever. Travelers should take all necessary precautions to avoid contact with or ingestion of potentially contaminated food or water sources.

TYPHOID VACCINE

Oral typhoid vaccine will not afford protection against enteric microorganisms other than *S. typhi*. An optimal booster dose has not yet been established. However, it is recommended that a booster dose consisting of 4 vaccine capsules taken on alternate days be given every 5 years under conditions of repeated or continued exposure to typhoid fever (see Administration and Dosage).

Drug Interactions:

Typhoid Vaccine Drug Interactions			
Precipitant drug	Object drug*		Description
Typhoid vaccine (Vi)	Anticoagulants	⬆	As with other drugs administered by IM injection, give Vi polysaccharide vaccine with caution to persons receiving anticoagulant therapy.
Typhoid vaccine	Plague vaccine	⬆	When practical, plague vaccine should not be given on the same occasion as AKD and H-P typhoid vaccines to avoid the possibility of accentuated side effects.
Plague vaccine	Typhoid vaccine		
Immunosuppressants	Typhoid vaccine	⬇	Like all inactivated and live vaccines, administration of typhoid vaccine to persons receiving immunosuppressant drugs, including high-dose corticosteroids or radiation therapy may result in an insufficient response to immunization. They may remain susceptible despite immunization.
Phenytoin	Typhoid vaccine	⬇	Concomitant phenytoin therapy may decrease antibody response to SC typhoid vaccination. Anticipate the possibility of suboptimal antibody response and consider risk/benefit ratios for each drug. Counsel these persons especially to observe good food and water discipline.
Sulfonamides	Typhoid vaccine (oral)	⬇	The vaccine should not be administered to individuals receiving sulfonamides and antibiotics since these agents may be active against the vaccine strain and prevent a sufficient degree of multiplication to occur in order to induce a protective immune response.

* ⬆ = Object drug increased ⬇ = Object drug decreased

Adverse Reactions:

Oral: Objectively monitored side effects did not occur at a statistically higher frequency in the vaccinated group than in the placebo group. Post-marketing surveillance outside of the US has found that side effects are infrequent, transient and resolve of their own accord. Reported adverse reactions include: Nausea, abdominal cramps, vomiting, skin rash or urticaria on the trunk or extremities.

Parenteral:

AKD and H-P – Most recipients of typhoid vaccine experience some degree of local and systemic response, usually beginning within 24 hours of administration and persisting for 1 or 2 days. Local reactions are usually manifested by erythema, induration and tenderness and should be expected in those injected intracutaneously.

Systemic manifestations may include: Malaise; headache; myalgia; elevated temperature; anaphylaxis (see Warnings).

Local and systemic reactions may follow typhoid vaccination, usually beginning within 6 to 24 hours of administration and persisting 1 or 2 days. Local reactions, occurring in 50% to 80% of recipients, include erythema, induration and tenderness (6% to 40%). Expect these reactions when the vaccine is injected intradermally. Systemic manifestations may include: Malaise, headache (9% to 30%); myalgia and elevated temperature (14% to 29%); hypotension (rare). Reactogenicity does not differ significantly for typhoid vaccines prepared using the AKD or H-P methods. Local reaction rates increase if vaccine is administered by jet injector.

Vi – Most adverse reactions to Vi polysaccharide are minor and transient local reactions. Local reactions may include erythema (4% to 11%): induration (5% to 18%); pain (26% to 56%); or tenderness (> 93%). These almost always resolve within 48 hours. Systemic effects may include: Fever ≥ 37.8°C (≥ 100°F; ≤ 2%); malaise (4% to 37%); myalgia (2% to 7%); nausea (2% to 8%); headache (11% to 27%); lymphadenopathy, cervical pain, vomiting, diarrhea, abdominal pain, tremor, hypotension, loss of consciousness, allergic reactions including urticaria and other events have been reported (rare). Because Vi vaccine contains negligible amounts of bacterial lipopolysaccharide, it produces reactions less than half as frequently as H-P or

TYPHOID VACCINE

AKD vaccines. No statistically significant difference in reaction rates were seen between first and subsequent doses of Vi polysaccharide.

Overdosage:

Oral: Five to eight doses of oral vaccine were administered to 155 healthy adult males. This dosage was, at a minimum, 5–fold higher than the currently recommended dose. No significant reactions (eg, vomiting, acute abdominal distress, fever) were observed. At the recommended dosage, the *S. typhi* Ty21a vaccine strain is not excreted in the feces; however, overdosing can increase the possibility of shedding the *S. typhi* Ty21a vaccine strain in the feces.

Patient Information:

Advise vaccine recipients to take standard food and water precautions to avoid typhoid fever. Vaccine protection can be overwhelmed by swallowing a large dose of typhoid bacteria.

Oral: It is essential that all 4 doses of vaccine be taken at the prescribed alternate day interval to obtain a maximal protective immune response.

Vaccine potency is dependent upon storage under refrigeration (2° to 8°C; 36° to 46°F). Store the vaccine under refrigeration at all times. It is essential to replace unused vaccine in the refrigerator between doses.

Swallow the vaccine capsule approximately 1 hour before a meal with a cold or lukewarm drink, not to exceed body temperature (37°C; 98.6°F). Do not chew the vaccine capsule; swallow as soon as possible.

Administration and Dosage:

Oral:

Primary immunization – One capsule on alternate days (eg, days 1, 3, 5 and 7), swallowed whole 1 hour before a meal with cold or lukewarm water, not to exceed body temperature (37°C; 98.6°F). The vaccine capsule should not be chewed; swallow as soon as possible after placing in the mouth. A complete immunization schedule is the ingestion of 4 vaccine capsules as described above. Unless a complete immunization schedule is followed, an optimum immune response may not be achieved. Not all recipients will be fully protected against typhoid fever. Travelers should take all necessary precautions to avoid contact or ingestion of potentially contaminated food or water.

Booster dose – The optimum booster schedule has not been determined. Efficacy persists for at least 5 years. Further, there is no experience with oral vaccine as a booster in persons previously immunized with parenteral typhoid vaccine. Despite these limitations, it is recommended that a booster dose consisting of 4 vaccine capsules taken on alternate days be given every 5 years under conditions of repeated or continued exposure to typhoid fever.

Parenteral: Shake vial well before withdrawing each dose.

Primary immunization –

AKD and H-P:

Adults and children (> 10 years old) – Two doses of 0.5 ml each, administered SC at an interval of ≥ 4 weeks.

Children (< 10 years old) – Two doses of 0.25 ml each, administered SC at an interval of ≥ 4 weeks.

In urgent situations, 3 doses of the appropriate volume may be given at weekly intervals, although efficacy may be reduced. Administer these vaccines subcutaneously. Only the H-P vaccine may be given intradermally and only for booster doses. Do not administer AKD vaccine intradermally because of a high frequency of local reactions. The AKD vaccine can be given by jet injection. Vials of H-P vaccine are not compatible with jet injectors.

Vi: For IM use only. Do not inject intravenously. Indicated only for persons ≥ 2 years old. Give a single 0.5 ml (25 mcg) IM dose. Inject adults in the deltoid muscle. Inject children in either the deltoid or vastus lateralis. Do not inject in the gluteal area or where there may be a nerve trunk. There are no published data on safety and efficacy with administration by jet injector.

Booster doses –

AKD and H-P:

Adults and children (> 10 years old) – 0.5 ml SC or 0.1 ml of the H-P product intracutaneously (intradermally).

Children (6 months to 10 years old) – 0.25 ml SC or 0.1 ml of the H-P product intracutaneously (intradermally).

Under conditions of continued or repeated exposure, give a booster dose every 3 years. In instances where an interval of > 3 years has elapsed since primary immunization or the last booster dose, a single booster dose is considered sufficient; it is not necessary to repeat the primary immunizing series.

TYPHOID VACCINE

Vi: Give a single 25 mcg dose every 2 years under conditions of repeated or continued exposure. Booster doses do not elicit higher antibody levels than primary immunization with the polysaccharide antigen.

Mefloquine may be given at least 24 hours before or after typhoid vaccine and chloroquine, pyrimethamine-sulfadoxine, immune globulins and other live vaccines may be given simultaneously.

Storage/Stability –

Oral: The oral vaccine is not stable when exposed to ambient temperatures. Ship and store between 2° and 8°C (36° to 46°F). If frozen, thaw capsules before use. Product can tolerate 48 hours at 25°C (77°F). Each package of vaccine shows an expiration date. This expiration date is valid only if the product has been maintained at these temperatures.

AKD and H-P: Store at 2° to 8°C (35° to 46°F). Do not freeze. Both AKD and H-P vaccine can tolerate 14 days at room temperature or 10 days at 46°C (114°F). Contact the manufacturer regarding exposure to freezing temperatures. Discard AKD vaccine 30 days after reconstitution.

Vi – Store at 2° to 8°C (35° to 46°F). Discard frozen vaccine.

Rx	**Vivotif Berna Vaccine** (Berna)	**Capsules, enteric coated:** 2 to 6 x 10^9 colony-forming units of viable *S. typhi* Ty21a and 5 to 50 x 10^9 bacterial cells of nonviable *S. typhi* Ty21a[1]	In a single foil blister containing 4 doses in a single package.
Rx	**Typhoid Vaccine (H-P)** (Wyeth-Ayerst)	**Injection suspension:** Heat- and phenol-inactivated. Killed Ty-2 strain of *S. typhi* organisms. Provides 8 units/ml, ≤ 1 billion/ml and ≤ 35 mcg nitrogen/ml	In 5 and 10 ml vials.[2]
Rx	**Typhoid Vaccine (AKD)**[3] (Wyeth-Ayerst)	**Powder for suspension:** Acetone inactivated, dried. Killed Ty-2 strain of *S. typhi* organisms. Provides 8 units/ml, ≤1 billion/ml[4]	In 50 dose vial with 20 ml diluent/dose.
Rx	**Typhim Vi** (Connaught)	**Injection:** 25 mcg purified Vi capsular polysaccharide/0.5 ml[5]	In 0.5 ml syringes and 20 and 50 dose vials.

[1] With 26 to 130 mg sucrose, 1 to 5 mg ascorbic acid, 1.4 to 7 mg amino acid mixture, 100 to 180 mg lactose and 3.6 to 4.4 mg magnesium stearate.
[2] With 0.5% phenol.
[3] Available for military use only.
[4] With 0.02 molar sodium phosphate, 0.5% sodium chloride, 0.5% phenol.
[5] With 4.15 mg NaCl, 0.065 mg disodium phosphate, 0.023 mg monosodium phosphate, 0.5 ml sterile water for injection.

PNEUMOCOCCAL VACCINE, POLYVALENT

Actions:

Pharmacology: The 23-valent vaccine affords protection against the 23 most prevalent or invasive pneumococcal types, accounting for at least 90% of pneumococcal blood isolates and at least 85% of all pneumococcal isolates from generally sterile sites.

Because the polysaccharide capsules are immunogenic, they stimulate antipneumococcal antibody production and prevent pneumococcal disease. The vaccine will protect only against the capsular types of pneumococci contained in the vaccine.

Indications:

For immunization against pneumococcal pneumonia and bacteremia caused by the types of pneumococci included in the vaccine.

Adults:* Immunocompetent adults at increased risk of pneumococcal disease or its complications because of chronic illnesses (eg, cardiovascular or pulmonary disease, diabetes mellitus, alcoholism, cirrhosis or CSF leaks) or adults ≥ 65 years old.

Immunocompromised adults at increased risk of pneumococcal disease or its complications (eg, persons with splenic dysfunction or anatomic asplenia, Hodgkin's disease, lymphoma, multiple myeloma, chronic renal failure, nephrotic syndrome or conditions such as organ transplantation associated with immunosuppression).

Asymptomatic or symptomatic HIV infection.

Children:* Children ≥ 2 years old with chronic illnesses specifically associated with increased risk of pneumococcal disease or its complications (eg, anatomic or functional asplenia [including sickle cell disease], nephrotic syndrome, CSF leaks and conditions associated with immunosuppression).

Children ≥ 2 years old with asymptomatic or symptomatic HIV infection.

Prevention of pneumococcal otitis media in children ≥ 2 years old who are at risk of developing middle ear infections.

Note – The CDC states that recurrent upper respiratory diseases, including otitis media and sinusitis, are *not* considered indications for vaccine use in children.

Special groups: Persons living in special environments or social settings with an identified increased risk of pneumococcal disease or its complications (eg, certain native American populations).* Persons > 2 years old, as follows: (1) Closed groups (eg, residential schools, nursing homes, other institutions); (2) groups epidemiologically at risk in the community when there is a generalized outbreak due to a single pneumococcal type included in the vaccine; (3) patients at high risk of influenza complications, particularly pneumonia.

Contraindications:

Hypersensitivity to any component of the vaccine; previous immunization with any polyvalent pneumococcal vaccine (see Adverse Reactions).

Immunosuppressive therapy: Do not attempt immunization of patients < 10 days prior to or during treatment with immunosuppressive drugs or irradiation.

Hodgkin's disease patients immunized < 7 to 10 days prior to immunosuppressive therapy have postimmunization antibody levels below preimmunization levels.

Patients who have received extensive chemotherapy or nodal irradiation have impaired antibody response to 12-valent vaccine. In some intensively treated patients, use of that vaccine depressed preexisting levels of antibody to some pneumococcal types; 23-valent vaccine is not recommended for these patients.

Infections: Defer administration in the presence of acute respiratory or other active infections, except when withholding the agent entails even greater risk.

Warnings:

Limited effectiveness: The vaccine may not be effective in preventing infection resulting from basilar skull fracture or from external communication with CSF, or in patients with altered humoral immune responses due to agammaglobulinemia, multiple myeloma, lymphoproliferative diseases or immunosuppressive drugs. The vaccine may be less effective in splenectomized patients.

When elective splenectomy is considered, give pneumococcal vaccine at least 2 weeks before the operation, if possible. Similarly, when immunosuppressive therapy is planned, as in candidates for organ transplants, the interval between vaccination and initiation of immunosuppressive therapy should be as long as possible.

Although vaccine failures have occurred in some of these groups, especially those who are immunocompromised, vaccination is still recommended for such persons because they are at high risk of developing severe disease.

Hypersensitivity: Epinephrine 1:1000 must be available to control immediate allergic reactions. Refer to Management of Acute Hypersensitivity Reactions.

* *Morbidity and Mortality Weekly Report* 1989 (February 10);38(5):64-76.

PNEUMOCOCCAL VACCINE, POLYVALENT

Pregnancy: Category C. Safety for use during pregnancy has not been established. Use only when clearly needed and when the potential benefits outweigh the potential hazards to the fetus. Ideally, vaccinate women at high risk before pregnancy.

Lactation: It is not known whether this drug is excreted in breast milk. Exercise caution when administering to a nursing woman.

Children: Not recommended for children < 2 years of age since they do not respond satisfactorily to the capsular types of the vaccine that are most often the cause of pneumococcal disease in this age group.

Certain groups at very high risk for pneumococcal disease (eg, sickle cell disease, nephrotic syndrome) may have lower peak levels of antibody response or more rapid rates of decline in antibody levels than do healthy adults. Insufficient data are available to permit formulation of guidelines for reimmunization of high risk children.

Precautions:

History of pneumococcal pneumonia or other pneumococcal infection: Patients may have high levels of pre-existing pneumococcal antibodies which may result in increased reactions to this vaccine. These reactions are mostly local, but are occasionally systemic. Exercise caution if such patients are considered for vaccination.

Cardiac/pulmonary disease: Exercise caution in those with severely compromised cardiac or pulmonary function; a systemic reaction could pose a significant risk.

Revaccination: Do not give a repeat (booster) injection to previously vaccinated subjects. Arthus and systemic reactions have been common among adults given second doses. Revaccination may result in more frequent and severe local reactions, especially in persons who have retained high antibody titers. Such reactions have occurred with booster doses given after long intervals from the initial vaccination. There is also evidence that booster doses do not increase antibody titers.

Without more information, do not routinely revaccinate persons who received 14-valent pneumococcal vaccine with 23-valent vaccine, as increased coverage is modest and duration of protection not well defined. However, strongly consider revaccination with 23-valent vaccine for persons who received 14-valent vaccine if they are at highest risk of fatal pneumococcal infection (eg, asplenic). Also consider revaccination for adults at highest risk who received 23-valent vaccine ≥ 6 years before and for those shown to have rapid decline in pneumococcal antibody levels (eg, patients with nephrotic syndrome, renal failure, or transplant recipients). Consider revaccination after 3 to 5 years for children with nephrotic syndrome, asplenia, or sickle cell anemia who would be ≤ 10 years old at revaccination.

Antibiotic prophylaxis: In patients who require antibiotic prophylaxis against pneumococcal infection, do not discontinue prophylaxis after vaccination.

Concomitant use of influenza virus vaccine with this vaccine gives satisfactory antibody response without an increase in adverse reactions.

Adverse Reactions:

Local: Erythema, induration and soreness at the injection site (≈ 72%), usually of < 48 hours duration, occur within 2 to 3 days after vaccination.

Systemic: Low grade fever (< 37.7 °C; 100 °F) and mild myalgia occur occasionally, usually within 24 hours following vaccination. However, acute febrile reactions (> 38.8 °C; 102 °F), rash and arthralgia have occurred rarely.

Patients with otherwise stabilized idiopathic thrombocytopenic purpura have experienced a relapse, occurring 2 to 14 days after vaccination, and lasting up to 2 weeks.

Reactions of greater severity, duration or extent are unusual.

Neurological disorders such as paresthesias and acute radiculoneuropathy, including Guillain-Barré syndrome, occur rarely in temporal association with use of pneumococcal vaccine. No cause and effect relationship has been established.

Anaphylactoid reactions have been rare (about 5 cases per million doses).

Administration and Dosage:

Give one 0.5 ml dose. Do not inject IV. Avoid intradermal administration. Administer SC or IM (preferably in the deltoid muscle or lateral mid-thigh).

Preparation and storage: Refrigerate at 2° to 8°C (36° to 46°F). Use the vaccine directly as supplied. No dilution or reconstitution is necessary. At room temperature, *Pnu-Imune 23* is stable for several days (temperature not exceeding 25°C; 77°F) and *Pneumovax 23* is stable for 1 month (temperature 15°C to 30°C; 59°F to 86°F).

Rx	**Pneumovax 23** (MSD)	**Injection:** 25 mcg each of 23 polysaccharide isolates per 0.5 ml dose	In 1 and 5 dose vials.[1]
Rx	**Pnu-Imune 23** (Lederle)		In 5 dose vials[2] and Lederject disp. syringes.[2]

[1] With 0.25% phenol.

[2] With 0.01% thimerosal.

HEMOPHILUS b CONJUGATE VACCINE

Hemophilus influenzae type b (Hemophilus b; Hib) is a leading cause of serious systemic bacterial disease in the US. Most cases of *H influenzae* meningitis among children are caused by capsular strains of type b. In addition to bacterial meningitis, Hemophilus b is responsible for other invasive diseases, including epiglottitis, sepsis, septic arthritis, osteomyelitis, pericarditis and pneumonia.

Actions:

Pharmacology: The principal virulence factor is the capsular polysaccharide purified from Hemophilus influenzae type b, strain Eag, and is a polymer of ribose, ribitol and phosphate.

Diphtheria toxoid-conjugate and protein-conjugate are prepared from the purified capsular polysaccharide covalently bound to diphtheria toxoid (D) and diphtheria CRM_{197} protein, respectively. The meningococcal protein conjugate is prepared from the purified capsular polysaccharide covalently bound to an outer membrane complex (OMPC) of the B11 strain of *Neisseria meningitidis* serogroup B.

An antibody concentration of ≥ 0.15 mcg/ml is correlated with protection; in 3 week post-vaccination serum, antibody levels ≥ 1 mcg/ml were correlated with long-term protection.

The development of stable humoral immunity requires recognition of foreign material by at least two separate sets of lymphocytes: The B-lymphocytes, which are precursors of antibody-forming cells, and the T–lymphocytes, which can modulate B-cell function. Some antigens (ie, polysaccharides) stimulate B-cells directly to produce antibody (T–independent). Responses to many other antigens are augmented by helper T-lymphocytes (T-dependent). Hib conjugate vaccines use a new technology, covalent bonding of the capsular polysaccharide of *Hemophilus influenzae* type b to either diphtheria toxoid, diphtheria CRM_{197} protein or to an OMPC of *Neisseria meningitidis*, to produce an antigen which is postulated to convert the T-independent antigen into a T–dependent antigen. The protein carries both its own antigenic determinants and those of the covalently bound polysaccharide. Therefore, the polysaccharide is postulated to be presented as a T-dependent antigen resulting in both an enhanced antibody response and an immunologic memory.

Immunogenicity Studies of Conjugate Vaccines by Age

	HibTITER			*PedvaxHIB*				*ProHIBiT*	
Parameter	1-6 mos.[1] (n = 423)	7-14 mos.[2] (n = 432)	15-23 mos. (n = 377)	2-14 mos.[2] (n = 365)	15-17 mos. (n = 59)	18-23 mos. (n = 59)	24-71 mos. (n = 52)	15-17 mos. (n = 43)	18-23 mos. (n = 180)
% subjects responding with ≥ 1 mcg/ml	99.2	≈100	97.6	88-92	83	97	92	53	73
Geometric mean titer of PRP antibody (mcg/ml)	22.4	27.9-32.7	11.4	4.6-6	3.1	7.4	10.6	1.2	3.1

[1] Following 3 doses.
[2] Following 2 doses.

Following immunization of 16- to 24-month-old children with a single dose of conjugate, 89% (109/123) had antibody levels ≥ 0.15 mcg/ml 12 months post-immunization, compared to 93% 1 month post-vaccination.

Indications:

For the routine immunization of children 2 months to 5 years of age (*HibTITER*), 2 to 71 months of age (*PedvaxHIB*) and 18 months to 5 years of age (*ProHIBiT*) against invasive diseases caused by *H influenzae* type b. The duration of protection and need for booster doses have not yet been determined.

Administration may be considered for children as young as 15 months of age (*ProHIBiT*) when it is expected that the child will not return at 18 months for Hemophilus b immunization. However, the percentage of children at 15 months of age responding with > 1 mcg/ml may not be as high as in children ≥ 18 months of age (see table).

The Immunization Practices Advisory Committee (ACIP) recommends that all children receive one of the conjugate vaccines licensed for infant use beginning routinely at 2 months of age. The vaccine series may be initiated as early as age 6 weeks.

Children < 24 months of age who have had invasive Hib disease should still receive the vaccine, since many children of that age fail to develop adequate immunity following natural disease. The vaccine can be initiated (or continued) at the time of hospital discharge.

HEMOPHILUS b CONJUGATE VACCINE

Chemoprophylaxis of household or daycare classroom contacts of children with Hib disease should be directed at both vaccinated and unvaccinated contacts because immune individuals may asymptomatically carry and transmit the organism.

Conjugate vaccines may be given simultaneously with diphtheria and tetanus toxoids and pertussis vaccine adsorbed (DPT); combined measles, mumps and rubella vaccine (MMR); oral poliovirus vaccine (OPV); or inactivated poliovirus vaccine (IPV).

Hemophilus b conjugate vaccines will not protect children against *H influenzae* other than type b or other microorganisms that cause meningitis or septic disease.

Contraindications:

Hypersensitivity to diphtheria toxoid or any component of the vaccine, including thimerosal.

Warnings:

The expected immune response may not be attained in persons deficient in producing antibody, whether due to genetic defect or to immunosuppressive therapy.

Any febrile illness or active infection is reason for delaying vaccine.

Hypersensitivity: Have epinephrine 1:1000 available for immediate use if an anaphylactoid reaction occurs. Refer to Management of Acute Hypersensitivity Reactions.

Hemophilus b disease may occur in the week after vaccination, prior to the onset of the protective effects of the vaccine.

Although some immune response to the diphtheria toxoid component of the conjugate vaccine may occur, it does not substitute for routine diphtheria immunization.

Pregnancy: Category C. It is not known whether these vaccines can cause fetal harm or affect reproduction capacity; they are NOT recommended for use in pregnant patients.

Children: ProHIBiT is not recommended for use in children < 15 months of age. *HibTITER* and *PedvaxHIB* are not recommended in children < 2 months of age; however, the ACIP states that the vaccine series may be initiated as early as age 6 weeks.

Drug Interactions:

Drug/Lab test interactions: Sensitive tests (eg, Latex Agglutination Kits) may detect PRP derived from the vaccine in urine of some vaccinees for up to 7 days following vaccination with PedvaxHIB.

Adverse Reactions:

Hemophilus b Vaccines Adverse Reactions		
Adverse reaction	< 24 hrs	> 24 hrs
Fever (> 38.3°C or 101°F)	1.1% to 3.8%[1]	1.5% to 2.1%
Erythema	1% to 3.3%	0.4% to 2.5%
Induration	1.5%	1% to 1.9%
Tenderness	3.7%	4.6%
Diarrhea/Vomiting	nd[2]	< 1.2%
Crying	nd[2]	< 1.2%

[1] Higher in older children.
[2] nd = no data reported.

Miscellaneous:

Other (causal relationship not established): Rash; hives; convulsions; early onset Hemophilus b disease; Guillain-Barré syndrome; irritability; sleepiness, respiratory infection/symptoms; ear infection/otitis media; thrombocytopenia (one case).

Administration and Dosage:

Administer IM doses in the outer aspect area of the vastus lateralis (mid-thigh) or deltoid. Do not inject IV.

Data are not available regarding interchangeability of hemophilus b conjugate vaccines with regard to safety, immunogenicity or efficacy. Ideally, use the same conjugate vaccine throughout entire vaccination series. Situations will arise in which the vaccine provider does not know which vaccine was previously used. It is prudent for vaccine providers to ensure that, at a minimum, an infant 2 to 6 months of age receives a primary series of three doses of conjugate vaccine.

HibTITER: 2 to 6 months old - Three separate IM injections of 0.5 ml given at approximately 2 month intervals.

7 to 11 months old (previously unvaccinated) – Two separate IM injections of 0.5 ml given approximately 2 months apart.

HEMOPHILUS b CONJUGATE VACCINE

12 to 14 months old (previously unvaccinated) – One IM injection.

All vaccinated children receive single booster dose at ≥ 15 months of age, not < 2 months after the previous dose. Previously unvaccinated children 15 to 60 months of age receive a single 0.5 ml IM injection in mid-thigh or deltoid muscle.

PedvaxHIB: 2 to 14 months old - Two separate IM injections of 0.5 ml given at 2 months of age and 2 months later (or as soon as possible thereafter). When the primary two dose regimen is completed before 12 months of age, a 0.5 ml booster dose is required at 12 months of age but not earlier than 2 months after the second dose.

≥ 15 months old (previously unvaccinated) – Give a single 0.5 ml IM injection.

Reconstitution – Use only the aluminum hydroxide diluent supplied.

ProHIBiT: 15 months to 5 years old - Administer a single 0.5 ml IM injection.

Vaccination Schedule for Hemophilus b Conjugate Vaccines

	HibTITER		*PedvaxHIB*		*ProHIBiT*	
Age at first dose (mos)	Primary series	Booster	Primary series	Booster	Primary series	Booster
2-6	3 doses, 2 months apart	15 mos.[1]	2 doses, 2 months apart	12 mos.[1]		
7-11	2 doses, 2 months apart	15 mos.[1]	2 doses, 2 months apart	15 mos.[1]		
12-14	1 dose	15 mos.[1]	1 dose	15 mos.[1]		
15-59	1 dose	—	1 dose	—	1 dose	—

[1] At least 2 months after previous dose.

Storage: HibTITER and *ProHIBiT* - Store at 2° to 8°C (36° to 46°F). Do not freeze.

PedvaxHIB – Before reconstitution, store at 2° to 8°C (36° to 46°F); store reconstituted vaccine at the same temperature and discard if not used within 24 hours. Do not freeze the reconstituted vaccine or the aluminum hydroxide diluent.

Rx	**Comvax** (Merck)	**Powder for Injection**: 7.5 mcg purified capsular polysaccharide, 125 mcg *Neisseria meningitidis* OMPC and 5 mg hepatitis B surface antigen/0.5 ml.	In 0.5 ml single dose vials.
Rx	**HibTITER** (Lederle/Praxis Biologicals)	**Injection**: 10 mcg capsular oligosaccharide ≈ 25 mcg diphtheria CRM_{197} protein/0.5 ml dose.	In 1, 5 and 10 dose vials.[1]
Rx	**ActHIB** (Connaught)	**Powder for Injection, lyophilized**: 10 mcg purified capsular polysaccharide, 24 mcg tetanus toxoid/0.5 ml	8.5% sucrose. In vials with 7.5 ml vials of diphtheria and tetanus toxoids and pertussis vaccine as diluents.[2]
Rx	**OmniHIB** (SK-Beecham)		In vials with prefilled 0.6 ml syringes of diluent.[2]
Rx	**PedvaxHIB** (MSD)	**Powder for Injection**: 15 mcg purified capsular polysaccharide, 250 mcg *Neisseria meningitidis* OMPC/dose when reconstituted[3]	In single-dose vials with vial of aluminum hydroxide diluent.
Rx	**ProHIBiT** (Connaught)	**Injection**: 25 mcg purified capsular polysaccharide, 18 mcg conjugated diphtheria toxoid protein/0.5 ml dose[4]	In 1, 5 and 10 dose vials.

[1] Multidose vials contain thimerosal 1:10,000.
[2] With 8.5% sucrose.
[3] In 0.9% sodium chloride with 2 mg lactose and thimerosal 1:20,000.
[4] Dissolved in sodium phosphate buffered isotonic sodium chloride solution.

MEASLES (RUBEOLA) VIRUS VACCINE, LIVE, ATTENUATED

For information on recommended immunization schedules, refer to Agents for Active Immunization.

> **Warning:**
> Trivalent measles-mumps-rubella (MMR) vaccine is the preferred immunizing agent for most children and many adults.

Actions:

Pharmacology: A more attenuated line of measles virus derived from Enders' attenuated Edmonston strain grown in cell cultures of chick embryo. It produces a modified measles infection in susceptible individuals. The vaccine is highly immunogenic and generally well tolerated. A single injection induces measles hemagglutination-inhibiting antibodies in ≥ 97% of susceptible persons. Vaccine-induced antibody levels persist for ≥ 13 years without substantial decline.

Indications:

Selective induction of active immunity against measles. Trivalent measles-mumps-rubella (MMR) vaccine is the preferred immunizing agent for most children and many adults. Almost all children and some adults need > 1 dose of MMR.

Prior to international travel, give individuals known to be susceptible to measles, mumps or rubella either a single-antigen vaccine or a polyvalent vaccine, as appropriate. Trivalent MMR vaccine is preferred for persons likely to be susceptible to mumps and rubella. If single-antigen vaccines are not readily available, give travelers trivalent MMR regardless of their immune status to mumps or rubella.

Contraindications:

Pregnancy (see Warnings); hypersensitivity reaction to this vaccine or any of its components (eg, eggs); patients receiving immunosuppressive therapy; blood dyscrasia, leukemia, lymphoma of any type, or other malignant neoplasms affecting the bone marrow or lymphatic systems; primary or acquired immunodeficiency; active untreated tuberculosis; family history of congenital or hereditary immunodeficiency, until the immune competence of the potential vaccine recipient is demonstrated.

Do not vaccinate persons who are immunosuppressed in association with AIDS or other clinical manifestations of infection with HIV, cellular immune deficiencies and hypogammaglobulinemic and dysgammaglobulinemic states. Nonetheless, ACIP and AAP recommend that asymptomatic children with HIV infection be vaccinated.

Defer immunization during the course of any acute illness.

Warnings:

Hypersensitivity: Have epinephrine 1:1000 available to control immediate allergic reactions. See also Management of Acute Hypersensitivity Reactions.

Hypersensitivity to eggs – Live measles vaccine is produced in chick embryo cell culture. Persons with a history of anaphylactic, anaphylactoid or other immediate reactions (eg, hives, swelling of mouth and throat, difficulty breathing, hypotension, shock) subsequent to egg ingestion should not be vaccinated. Evidence indicates that persons are not at increased risk if they have egg allergies that are not anaphylactic or anaphylactoid in nature. Such persons should be vaccinated in the usual manner. There is no evidence to indicate that persons with allergies to chicken or feathers are at increased risk of reaction to the vaccine.

Elderly: Most persons born in 1956 or earlier are likely to have been infected naturally and generally are considered not susceptible.

Pregnancy: Category C. It is not known whether the drug can cause fetal harm or can affect reproduction capacity. Therefore, do not give to pregnant women. Avoid pregnancy for 3 months following vaccination.

Contracting natural measles during pregnancy enhances fetal risk. Increased rates of spontaneous abortion, stillbirth, congenital defects and prematurity have occurred. There are no adequate studies of measles virus vaccine in pregnancy. However, it is assumed that the vaccine strain of virus is also capable of inducing adverse fetal effects for up to 3 months following vaccination.

Advisory committees recommend vaccination of postpubertal females presumed to be susceptible to measles and not known to be pregnant. If measles exposure occurs during pregnancy, consider providing temporary passive immunity with immune globulin (human).

Lactation: It is not known whether measles vaccine virus is secreted in breast milk. Exercise caution when administering to a nursing woman.

MEASLES (RUBEOLA) VIRUS VACCINE, LIVE, ATTENUATED

Children: Attenuated measles vaccine is safe and effective in persons ≥ 12 months of age. Younger persons may fail to respond due to circulating residual measles antibodies passively transferred from the child's mother. Revaccinate infants vaccinated when < 12 months of age after they reach 15 months of age. There is evidence to suggest that infants immunized when < 1 year old may not develop sustained antibody levels when later reimmunized. Weigh the advantage of early protection against the chance for failure to respond adequately on reimmunization. Trivalent MMR vaccine is the preferred agent for children and many adults.

Children and young adults known to be infected with human immunodeficiency viruses but without overt clinical mainfestations of immunosuppression may be vaccinated. However, monitor closely for vaccine-preventable diseases because immunization may be less effective than for uninfected persons.

Precautions:

Tuberculosis: Children under treatment for tuberculosis have not experienced exacerbation of the disease when immunized with measles vaccine.

Drug Interactions:

Measles Virus Vaccine Drug Interactions			
Precipitant drug	Object drug*		Description
Immunosuppressants	Measles vaccine	⬇	Administration of measles vaccine to patients receiving immunosuppressants, including corticosteroids or radiation therapy, may result in insufficient response to immunization. They may remain susceptible despite immunization.
Immune globulins	Measles vaccine	⬇	To avoid inactivation of the attenuated virus, administer the vaccine at least 14 to 30 days before or 6 to 8 weeks after the immune globulin. Alternately, check antibody titers or repeat the vaccine dose 3 months after IgG.
Interferon	Measles vaccine	⬇	Concurrent use may inhibit antibody response to the vaccine.
Measles vaccine	Meningococcal vaccine	⬇	Reduced seroconversion rate to meningococci may occur with concurrent immunization.
Measles vaccine	Tuberculin skin test	⬇	Measles vaccine may temporarily depress tuberculin skin sensitivity. Administer the test before or simultaneously with the vaccine.
Measles vaccine	Virus vaccines, other	⬇	To avoid the hypothetical concern over antigenic competition, give measles vaccine after or ≥ 1 month before other virus vaccines. However, several vaccines may be given simultaneously at separate injection sites (eg, DTP, OPV, MMR, Hib, hepatitis B).

* ⬇ = Object drug decreased

Drug/Lab test interactions: Methacholine inhalation challenge may be falsely positive for a few days after influenza, measles or other immunization. This effect appears to mimic the bronchospastic effect associated with acute respiratory infections. The effect has been observed in 44% to 90% of asthmatic patients, but apparently not among healthy subjects.

Live virus vaccines may cause delayed-hypersensitivity skin tests (eg, tuberculin, histoplasmin) to appear falsely negative. Evaluate such tests knowingly. The effect may persist for several weeks after vaccination. ACIP and AAP recommend that tuberculin tests be given prior to live-virus vaccination, simultaneously or ≥ 6 weeks after vaccination.

Adverse Reactions:

Anaphylaxis and anaphylactoid reactions have occurred.

Occasional: Moderate fever of 38.3° to 39.4°C (101° to 103°F) may occur during the month after vaccination. Generally, fever, rash, or both appear between the 5th and 12th days. Rash is usually minimal but rarely may be generalized. Cough and rhinitis have occurred.

Less common: High fever (> 39.4°C; 103°F); mild lymphadenopathy.

Rare: Diarrhea; vasculitis; erythema multiforme.

MEASLES (RUBEOLA) VIRUS VACCINE, LIVE, ATTENUATED

Killed measles: Marked swelling, redness and vesiculation at the injection site and systemic reactions including atypical measles have occurred in persons previously vaccinated with killed measles. Rarely, more severe reactions that require hospitalization, including prolonged high fevers, panniculitis and extensive local reactions, have been reported.

CNS: Children developing fever may rarely exhibit febrile convulsions. Afebrile convulsions or seizures have occurred rarely following vaccination with live attenuated measles vaccine. Syncope, particularly at the time of mass vaccination, has occurred.

Significant CNS reactions (eg, encephalitis, encephalopathy) occurring within 30 days after vaccination have been temporally associated with measles vaccine very rarely. In no case has it been shown that reactions were actually caused by vaccine. The risk following measles vaccine administration remains far less than that for encephalitis and encephalopathy with natural measles (1 per 2000 reported cases).

Rarely, ocular palsies, Guillain-Barre syndrome or ataxia have occurred after immunization with vaccines containing live attenuated measles virus. The ocular palsies occurred approximately 3 to 24 days following vaccination. A causal relationship has not been established.

Subacute sclerosing panencephalitis (SSPE) has occurred in children who did not have a history of natural measles but received measles vaccine. The association of SSPE cases to measles vaccination is about one case per million doses, far less than that associated with natural measles, 6 to 22 cases per million.

Local: Burning or stinging of short duration at injection site. Rare allergic reactions such as wheal and flare at the injection site or urticaria have occurred.

Hematologic: Thrombocytopenia, purpura (extremely rare).

Administration and Dosage:

Federal law requires that (1) the manufacturer and lot number of this vaccine (2) the date of its administration, and (3) the name, address and title of the person administering the vaccine be documented in the recipient's permanent medical record or in a permanent office log. Certain adverse events must be reported to the VAERS system, 1-800-822-7967.

Trivalent MMR vaccine is the preferred product for most vaccinations.

Inject the total volume of the single-dose vial or 0.5 ml of the multiple-dose vial of reconstituted vaccine SC, preferably at 15 months of age and into the outer aspect of the upper arm. Do not inject IV. The dosage is the same for all patients.

Use a sterile syringe free of preservatives, antiseptics and detergents for each injection, as these substances may inactivate the live virus vaccine. A 25-gauge, ⅝" needle is recommended. The 10 dose vial may be used with either syringe or jet injector; use the 50 dose vial by jet injection only.

Storage/Stability: Before reconstitution, store at 2° to 8°C (36° to 46°F). Freezing does not harm the vaccine. Protect from light at all times; such exposure may inactivate the virus. Use only the diluent supplied and use as soon as possible after reconstitution. Store reconstituted vaccine in a dark place at 2° to 8°C. Discard if not used within 8 hours. Vaccine powder can tolerate 7 days at room temperature.

Rx	**Attenuvax** (Merck)	**Powder for injection, lyophilized:** ≥ 1000 $TCID_{50}$ (tissue culture infectious doses) per 0.5 ml dose.	With 25 mcg neomycin and sorbitol. Preservative free. In single-dose vials with diluent, 10 dose vials with 7 ml diluent, and 50 dose vials with 30 ml diluent.

RUBELLA VIRUS VACCINE, LIVE

For information on recommended immunization schedules, refer to Agents for Active Immunization.

> **Warning:**
> Trivalent measles-mumps-rubella (MMR) vaccine is the preferred immunizing agent for most children and many adults.

Actions:

Pharmacology: Attenuated rubella vaccine induces a modified, noncommunicable rubella infection in susceptible persons. RA 27/3 strain elicits higher immediate postvaccination hemagglutination-inhibiting (HI), complement-fixing and neutralizing antibody levels than other strains of rubella vaccine and induces a broader profile of circulating antibodies, including anti-theta and anti-iota precipitating antibodies. RA 27/3 strain immunologically simulates natural infection more closely than other rubella virus strains. The increased levels and broader profile of antibodies produced by RA 27/3 strain appear to correlate with greater resistance to subclinical reinfection by the wild virus.

Onset of rubella vaccine is 2 to 6 weeks. It induces HI antibodies in at least 97% of susceptible children. Seroconversion is somewhat less in adults. Disease incidence is typically reduced by 95% in family and classroom cohorts. Antibody levels persist ≥ 10 years in most recipients. Specific rubella HI antibody titer of ≥ 1:8 is considered immune.

Indications:

Selective active immunization against rubella. The national rubella immunization program is intended to reduce the occurrence of congenital rubella syndrome (CRS) among offspring of women who contract rubella during pregnancy.

Children: Vaccination is routinely recommended for persons from 12 months of age to puberty. Give previously unimmunized children of susceptible pregnant women attenuated rubella (or preferably MMR) vaccine, since an immunized child is less likely to acquire natural rubella and introduce it into the household.

Adolescent or adult males: Vaccination is a useful procedure in preventing or controlling outbreaks of rubella in circumscribed populations.

Nonpregnant adolescent and adult females: Immunization of susceptible nonpregnant adolescent and adult females of childbearing potential is indicated, if precautions to avoid pregnancy are observed. When vaccinating postpubertal females, counsel these women to avoid pregnancy for 3 months following vaccination. Vaccinating susceptible postpubertal females confers individual protection against subsequently acquiring rubella infection during pregnancy, which in turn prevents infection of the fetus and CRS. It may be convenient to vaccinate rubella-susceptible women in the immediate postpartum period.

International travel: Prior to international travel, give individuals known to be susceptible to measles, mumps or rubella either a single-antigen vaccine or a polyvalent vaccine, as appropriate. Trivalent MMR vaccine is preferred for persons likely to be susceptible to mumps and rubella. Almost all children and some adults need > 1 dose of MMR vaccine. If single-antigen vaccines are not readily available, give travelers trivalent MMR regardless of their immune status to mumps or rubella.

Unlabeled uses: Intranasal administration may boost antibody titers, although this route is not confirmed as safe and effective by the FDA and is not commonly employed.

Contraindications:

Pregnancy (see Warnings); history of a hypersensitivity reaction to this vaccine or any of its components; patients receiving immunosuppressive therapy; blood dyscrasia, leukemia, lymphoma of any type, or other malignant neoplasms affecting the bone marrow or lymphatic systems; primary or acquired immunodeficiency; active untreated tuberculosis; family history of congenital or hereditary immunodeficiency, until the immune competence of the potential vaccine recipient is demonstrated.

Do not vaccinate persons who are immunosuppressed in association with AIDS or other clinical manifestations of infection with HIV, cellular immune deficiencies, and hypogammaglobulinemic and dysgammaglobulinemic states. Nonetheless, vaccinate asymptomatic children with HIV infection.

Defer immunization during the course of any acute illness.

RUBELLA VIRUS VACCINE, LIVE

Warnings:

Immunodeficiency: Do not use in immunodeficient persons, including persons with congenital or acquired immune deficiencies, whether due to genetics, disease, or drug or radiation therapy. Contains live viruses. Nonetheless, routine immunization of symptomatic and asymptomatic HIV-infected persons with MMR is recommended.

Hypersensitivity: Have epinephrine 1:1000 available to control immediate allergic reactions. See also Management of Acute Hypersensitivity Reactions.

Elderly: Most persons born in 1956 or earlier are likely to have been infected naturally and generally are considered not susceptible.

Pregnancy: Category C. Natural rubella infection of the fetus may result in congenital rubella syndrome. There is evidence suggesting transmission of attenuated rubella virus to the fetus, although the vaccine is not known to cause fetal harm when administered to pregnant women. Nonetheless, do not intentionally give attenuated rubella vaccine to pregnant females. If postpubertal females are vaccinated, counsel these women to avoid pregnancy for 3 months following vaccination. It may be convenient to vaccinate rubella-susceptible women in the immediate postpartum period.

In counseling women who are inadvertently vaccinated when pregnant or who become pregnant within 3 months of vaccination, the following information may be useful. In a 10 year survey of > 700 pregnant women who received rubella vaccine within 3 months before or after conception (of whom 189 received the current RA 27/3 strain), none of the newborns had abnormalities compatible with congenital rubella syndrome.

Generally, most IgG passage across the placenta occurs during third trimester.

Lactation: Vaccine-strain virus is secreted in breast milk and may be transmitted to infants in this manner. In the infants with serologic evidence of rubella infection, none exhibited severe disease. However, one exhibited mild clinical illness typical of acquired rubella.

Children: Safe and effective for children ≥ 12 months of age. Vaccination is not recommended for children < 12 months of age, since remaining maternal rubella neutralizing antibody may interfere with the immune response. Trivalent MMR vaccine is the preferred agent for children and many adults.

Drug Interactions:

Rubella Virus Vaccine Drug Interactions			
Precipitant drug	Object drug		Description
Immunosuppressants	Rubella vaccine	⬇	Administration of rubella vaccine to patients receiving immunosuppressants, including corticosteroids or radiation therapy, may result in insufficient response to immunization. They may remain susceptible despite immunization.
Immune globulins	Rubella vaccine	⬇	To avoid inactivation of the attenuated virus, administer the vaccine at least 14 to 30 days before or 6 to 8 weeks after the immune globulin. Alternately, check antibody titers or repeat the vaccine dose 3 months after IgG.
Interferon	Rubella vaccine	⬇	Concurrent use may inhibit antibody response to the vaccine.
Rubella vaccine	Meningococcal vaccine	⬇	Reduced seroconversion rate to meningococci may occur with concurrent immunization.
Rubella vaccine	Virus vaccines, other	⬇	To avoid the hypothetical concern over antigenic competition, give rubella vaccine after or ≥ 1 month before other virus vaccines. However, several vaccines may be given simultaneously at separate injection sites (eg, DTP, OPV, MMR, Hib, hepatitis B).

* ⬇ = Object drug decreased.

RUBELLA VIRUS VACCINE, LIVE

Adverse Reactions:

Reactions are usually mild and transient. Because the vaccine is slightly acidic, patients may experience burning or stinging of short duration at the injection site. Symptoms similar to those seen following natural rubella may occur and include: Regional lymphadenopathy; urticaria; rash; malaise; sore throat; fever; headache; polyneuritis; temporary arthralgia (infrequently associated with inflammation). Local pain, induration and erythema may occur at the injection site. Moderate fever (38° to 39.4° C; 101° to 102.9° F) occurs occasionally, high fever (> 39.4° C or 103° F) less commonly.

Encephalitis and other CNS reactions, erythema multiforme, optic neuritis and polyneuropathy (including Guillain-Barre syndrome) may occur. Because of decreases in platelet counts, thrombocytopenic purpura is a theoretical hazard.

Arthritis/Arthralgia: Chronic arthritis has been associated with natural rubella infection. Only rarely have vaccine recipients developed chronic joint symptoms. Following vaccination in children, reactions in joints are uncommon (≤ 3%) and generally of brief duration. In adult women, incidence rates for arthritis and arthralgia are generally higher (12% to 20%) and the reactions tend to be more marked and of longer duration. Symptoms may persist for months or, on rare occasions, for years. In adolescent girls, the reactions appear to be intermediate in incidence between those seen in children and in adult women. Even in older women (35 to 45 years of age), these reactions are generally well tolerated and rarely interfere with normal activities. Myalgia and paresthesia have been reported rarely. Advise postpubertal females of the frequent occurrence of generally self-limited arthralgia or arthritis beginning 2 to 4 weeks after vaccination.

Administration and Dosage:

Federal law requires that (1) the manufacturer and lot number of this vaccine, (2) the date of its administration, and (3) the name, address and title of the person administering the vaccine be documented in the recipient's permanent medical record or in a permanent office log. Certain adverse events must be reported to the VAERS system, 1–800-822-7967.

Inject total volume of reconstituted vaccine SC, into the outer aspect of the upper arm. Do not inject IV or administer intranasally.

Storage/Stability: Prior to and after reconstitution, store at 2° to 8°C (36° to 46°F) and protect from light. To reconstitute, use only the diluent supplied. Use as soon as possible after reconstitution. Discard reconstituted vaccine if not used within 8 hours. Ship vaccine at ≤ 10°C (50°F); it may be shipped on dry ice.

Rx	**Meruvax II** (Merck)	**Powder for Injection**: ≥1000 $TCID_{50}$ (tissue culture infectious doses) of rubella per 0.5 ml dose.	With 25 mcg neomycin. In single dose vials.

MUMPS VIRUS VACCINE, LIVE

For recommended immunization schedules, refer to Agents for Active Immunization.

> **Warning:**
> Trivalent measles-mumps-rubella (MMR) vaccine is the preferred immunizing agent for most children and many adults.

Actions:

Pharmacology: Prepared from the Jeryl Lynn (B level) strain grown in cell cultures of chick embryo. Attenuated mumps vaccine produces a modified, noncommunicable mumps infection in susceptible persons. Antibodies induced by this infection protect against subsequent infection. A single dose induced an effective antibody response in ≈ 97% of susceptible children and 93% of susceptible adults.

Mumps vaccine reduced disease incidence 95% in family and classroom cohorts for at least 20 months. Onset occurs in 2 to 3 weeks. Antibody levels persist ≥ 15 years in most recipients, with a rate of decline comparable to natural infection.

The vaccine will not offer protection when given after exposure to natural mumps.

Indications:

Selective active immunization against mumps. Prior to international travel, give individuals known to be susceptible to measles, mumps or rubella either a single-antigen vaccine or a polyvalent vaccine, as appropriate. Trivalent MMR vaccine is preferred for persons likely to be susceptible to mumps and rubella.

Almost all children and some adults need > 1 dose of MMR vaccine. If single-antigen vaccines are not readily available, give travelers trivalent MMR regardless of their immune status to mumps or rubella.

Contraindications:

Pregnancy (see Warnings); history of a hypersensitivity reaction to this vaccine or any of its components (eg, eggs); concomitant immunosuppressive therapy; patients with a blood dyscrasia, leukemia, lymphoma of any type, or other malignant neoplasms affecting the bone marrow or lymphatic systems; primary or acquired immunodeficiency; active untreated tuberculosis; family history of congenital or hereditary immunodeficiency, until the immune competence of the potential vaccine recipient is demonstrated.

Do not vaccinate persons who are immunosuppressed in association with AIDS or other clinical manifestations of infection with HIV, cellular immune deficiencies, and hypogammaglobulinemic and dysgammaglobulinemic states. Nonetheless, vaccinate asymptomatic children with HIV infection.

Do not vaccinate persons with a history of anaphylactoid or other immediate reactions (eg, hives, swelling of the mouth and throat, difficulty breathing, hypotension, shock) subsequent to egg ingestion since the vaccine is propagated in cell cultures of chick embryo. Skin-test persons suspected of being hypersensitive to egg protein, using a dilution of the vaccine as the antigen. Do not vaccinate persons with adverse reactions to such testing. Persons are apparently not at risk if they have egg allergies that are not anaphylactoid in nature; vaccinate such persons in the usual manner. There is no evidence that persons with allergies to chickens or feathers are at increased risk of reaction to the vaccine. Defer immunization during the course of any acute illness.

Warnings:

Allergy skin testing: Do not use for delayed hypersensitivity (anergy) skin testing. Use mumps skin test antigen, a killed viral product (see individual monograph).

Hypersensitivity: Have epinephrine 1:1000 available to control immediate allergic reactions. See also Management of Acute Hypersensitivity Reactions.

Immunodeficiency – Do not use in immunodeficient persons, including persons with congenital or acquired immune deficiencies, whether due to genetics, disease, or drug or radiation therapy. Contains live viruses. Nonetheless, routine immunization of symptomatic and asymptomatic HIV-infected persons with MMR is recommended.

Elderly: Persons born prior to 1957 are generally considered immune and need not be vaccinated.

Pregnancy: Category C. Although mumps virus can infect the placenta and fetus, there is no good evidence that it causes congenital malformations in humans. Attenuated mumps vaccine virus can infect the placenta, but virus has not been isolated from fetal tissues of susceptible women who were vaccinated and underwent elective abortions. Nonetheless, do not intentionally give attenuated mumps vaccine to pregnant females. If postpubertal females are vaccinated, counsel these women to avoid pregnancy for 3 months following vaccination. Generally most IgG passage across the placenta occurs during the third trimester.

MUMPS VIRUS VACCINE, LIVE

Lactation: It is not known if attenuated mumps virus or corresponding antibodies are excreted in breast milk.

Children: Mumps vaccine is safe and effective for children ≥ 12 months of age. Vaccination is not recommended for children < 12 months of age since remaining maternal virus neutralizing antibody may interfere with the immune response. Trivalent MMR vaccine is the preferred agent for children and many adults.

Drug Interactions:

Mumps Virus Vaccine Drug Interactions			
Precipitant drug	Object drug*		Description
Immunosuppressants	Mumps vaccine	⬇	Administration of mumps vaccine to patients receiving immunosuppressants, including corticosteroids or radiation therapy, may result in insufficient response to immunization. They may remain susceptible despite immunization.
Immune globulins	Mumps vaccine	⬇	To avoid inactivating attenuated virus, give the vaccine at least 14 to 30 days before or 6 to 8 weeks after immune globulin. Alternately, check antibody titers or repeat the vaccine 3 months after IgG.
Interferon	Mumps vaccine	⬇	Concurrent use may inhibit antibody response to the vaccine.
Mumps vaccine	Virus vaccines, other	⬇	To avoid the hypothetical concern over antigenic competition, give mumps vaccine after or ≥ 1 month before other virus vaccines. However, several vaccines may be given simultaneously at separate injection sites (eg, DTP, OPV, MMR, Hib, hepatitis B).

* ⬇ = Object drug decreased

Drug/Lab test interactions: Live virus vaccines may cause delayed-hypersensitivity skin tests (eg, tuberculin, histoplasmin) to appear falsely negative. Evaluate such tests knowingly. The effect may persist for several weeks after vaccination. ACIP and AAP recommend that tuberculin tests be given prior to live-virus vaccination, simultaneously, or 6 or more weeks after vaccination.

Adverse Reactions:

Burning or stinging of short duration at the injection site have occurred. Occasional reactions include mild fever, mild lymphadenopathy or diarrhea. Fever > 39.4°C (> 103°F) is uncommon. Rarely, parotitis and orchitis may occur. In most of these cases, prior exposure to natural mumps was established. Infrequently, optic neuritis may follow vaccination. Allergic reactions at the injection site or erythema multiforme occurred rarely. Very rarely, encephalitis, febrile seizures, nerve deafness and other nervous system reactions have occurred.

Administration and Dosage:

Federal law requires that (1) the manufacturer and lot number of this vaccine, (2) the date of its administration, and (3) the name, address and title of the person administering the vaccine be documented in the recipient's permanent medical record or in a permanent office log. Certain adverse events must be reported to the VAERS system, 1–800-822-7967.

Vaccination: 0.5 ml, for both children at 15 months of age and adults. Trivalent MMR vaccine is the preferred product for most vaccinations. Inject total volume of reconstituted vaccine SC, into the outer aspect of the upper arm. Do not inject IV. Use a sterile syringe free of preservatives, antiseptics and detergents. A 25-gauge⅝" needle is recommended.

Booster dose: If concern exists about mumps immune status, consider revaccination with appropriate monovalent or polyvalent vaccines. Routine MMR is recommended by ACIP as children enter kindergarten or first grade. AAP recommends a routine second vaccination as children enter middle or junior high school.

Storage/Stability: Prior to and after reconstitution, store at 2° to 8°C (36° to 46°F). Powder can tolerate 5 days room temperature. Protect from light. Reconstitute, only with diluent supplied and use as soon as possible. Discard within 8 hours.

Rx	**Mumpsvax** (Merck)	**Powder for Injection:** ≥ 20,000 TCID50 (tissue culture infectious doses) per 0.5 ml dose.	With 25 mcg neomycin. In single-dose vials with vials of diluent.

RUBELLA AND MUMPS VIRUS VACCINE, LIVE

For information on recommended immunization schedules, refer to Agents for Active Immunization.

Consider the prescribing information for rubella virus vaccine and for mumps virus vaccine when using this product (see individual monographs).

Indications:

Children (≥ 12 months of age): Simultaneous immunization against rubella and mumps.

Infants (< 12 months of age): Not recommended. Infants may retain maternal rubella and mumps neutralizing antibodies which may interfere with the immune response.

Revaccination: If concern exists about immune status, consider revaccination with appropriate monovalent or polyvalent vaccines. Routine revaccination with trivalent MMR vaccine is recommended by ACIP as children enter into kindergarten or first grade. AAP recommends a routine second vaccination as children enter into middle school or junior high school. Unnecessary doses of a vaccine are best avoided by ensuring that written documentation of vaccination is preserved and a copy given to each vaccinee or the vaccinee's agent.

Administration and Dosage:

Vaccination: 0.5 ml for children (preferably at 15 months of age) and adults. Trivalent MMR vaccine is the preferred product for most vaccinations. Inject the total volume of reconstituted vaccine SC, preferably into the outer aspect of the upper arm, with a 25-gauge ⅝" needle. Do not inject IV.

Storage/Stability: Prior to and after reconstitution, store at 2° to 8°C (36° to 46°F) and protect from light. To reconstitute, use only the diluent supplied. Use as soon as possible after reconstitution. Discard within 8 hours.

Rx	**Biavax II** (Merck)	**Powder for Injection:** Mixture of 2 viruses: ≥ 20,000 mumps $TCID_{50}$ (tissue culture infectious doses) and ≥ 1000 rubella $TCID_{50}$ per 0.5 ml dose	With 25 mcg neomycin. In single-dose vials with diluent.

MEASLES (RUBEOLA) AND RUBELLA VIRUS VACCINE, LIVE

For information on recommended immunization schedules, refer to Agents for Active Immunization.

Consider the prescribing information for measles (rubeola) virus vaccine and for rubella virus vaccine when using this product (see individual monographs).

Indications:

Children (≥ 15 months of age) and adults: Simultaneous immunization against measles and rubella.

Infants (< 15 months of age) may fail to respond to one or both components of the vaccine due to residual measles or rubella antibody of maternal origin in the circulation; the younger the infant, the lower the likelihood of seroconversion.

In geographically isolated or other relatively inaccessible populations for whom immunization programs are logistically difficult, and in population groups in which natural measles infection may occur in a significant proportion of infants before 15 months of age, it may be desirable to give the vaccine to infants at an earlier age. Weigh the advantage of early protection against the chance for failure of response; revaccinate these infants after they reach 15 months of age.

Revaccination: If prevention of sporadic measles outbreaks is the sole objective, consider revaccination with a monovalent measles vaccine. If concern also exists about immune status to mumps or rubella, consider revaccination with appropriate monovalent or polyvalent vaccines. Routine revaccination with trivalent MMR vaccine is recommended by ACIP as children enter into kindergarten or first grade. AAP recommends a routine second vaccination as children enter into middle school or junior high school.

Administration and Dosage:

Vaccination: 0.5 ml for children (preferably at 15 months of age) and adults. Trivalent MMR vaccine is the preferred product for most vaccinations. Inject the total volume of reconstituted vaccine SC, preferably into the outer aspect of the upper arm. Do not inject IV.

Storage/Stability: Prior to and after reconstitution, store at 2° to 8°C (36° to 46°F). Protect from light. To reconstitute, use only the diluent supplied and use as soon as possible after reconstitution. Discard if not used within 8 hours.

Rx	**M-R-Vax II** (Merck)	**Powder for Injection:** Mixture of 2 viruses: ≥ 1000 measles $TCID_{50}$ (tissue culture infectious doses) and ≥ 1000 rubella $TCID_{50}$ per 0.5 ml dose.	With 25 mcg neomycin. In single-dose vials with vial of diluent.

MEASLES, MUMPS AND RUBELLA VIRUS VACCINES, LIVE

For information on recommended immunization schedules, refer to Agents for Active Immunization.

Consider the prescribing information for measles virus vaccine, mumps virus vaccine and rubella virus vaccine when using this product (see individual monographs).

Indications:

Children (≥ 15 months of age) or adults: Simultaneous immunization against measles, mumps and rubella.

Infants (< 15 months of age): May fail to respond to one or all three components of the vaccine due to presence in the circulation of residual measles, mumps or rubella antibody of maternal origin; the younger the infant, the lower the likelihood of seroconversion.

In geographically isolated or other relatively inaccessible populations for whom immunization programs are logistically difficult, and in population groups in which natural measles infection may occur in a significant proportion of infants before 15 months of age, it may be desirable to give the vaccine to infants at an earlier age. Weigh the advantage of early protection against the chance for failure of response; revaccinate these infants after they reach 15 months of age.

Revaccination: Almost all children and some adults should receive a booster dose of MMR vaccine, in addition to a primary dose given after the age of 12 months. Routine revaccination with trivalent MMR vaccine is recommended by ACIP as children enter into kindergarten or first grade, since this procedure is easier to implement in public health clinics. AAP recommends a routine second vaccination as children enter into middle school or junior high school, a procedure that has epidemiologic advantages.

If concern also exists about immune status to mumps or rubella, consider revaccination with appropriate monovalent or polyvalent vaccines.

Administration and Dosage:

Vaccination: 0.5 ml for children (preferably at 15 months of age) and adults. Inject the total volume of reconstituted vaccine SC into the outer aspect of the upper arm with a 25-gauge ⅝" needle. Do not inject IV.

Storage/Stability: Prior to and after reconstitution, store at 2° to 8°C (36° to 46°F) and protect from light. To reconstitute, use only the diluent supplied. Use as soon as possible after reconstitution. Discard within 8 hours.

Rx	**M-M-R** II (Merck)	**Powder for Injection:** Mixture of 3 viruses: ≥ 1000 measles TCID50 (tissue culture infectious doses), ≥ 20,000 mumps $TCID_{50}$ and ≥ 1000 rubella $TCID_{50}$ per 0.5 ml dose.	With 25 mcg neomycin. In single dose vials with diluent.

POLIOVIRUS VACCINE, LIVE, ORAL, TRIVALENT (OPV; TOPV; Sabin)

For recommended immunization schedules, refer to Agents for Active Immunization.

Actions:

Pharmacology: Attenuated, live virus vaccine produces active immunity by simulating natural infection without producing symptoms of the disease. To accomplish this with live poliovirus vaccine, the virus must multiply in the intestinal tract. A primary series of this vaccine is designed to produce an antibody response to poliovirus types 1, 2 and 3 comparable to the immunity induced by the natural disease.

Antibodies develop within 1 to 2 weeks after several doses. Greater than 95% of children studied 5 years after immunization had protective antibodies against all three types of poliovirus. Type-specific neutralizing antibodies will be induced in at least 90% of susceptible persons.

OPV is preferred over IPV for routine immunization of children by the ACIP, AAP and the Institute of Medicine of the National Academy of Sciences, because OPV induces intestinal immunity, is simple to administer, is well accepted by patients, results in immunization of some contacts of vaccinated persons, and has a record of having essentially eliminated disease associated with wild poliovirus in the US.

Indications:

Prevention of poliomyelitis caused by poliovirus types 1, 2 and 3.

Children (infants from 6 to 12 weeks of age, all unimmunized children and adolescents through age 18): For routine prophylaxis.

Trivalent oral poliovirus vaccine (OPV) and inactivated poliovirus vaccine (IPV) both prevent poliomyelitis. OPV is the vaccine of choice for primary immunization of children in the US because: It induces intestinal immunity; is simple to administer; is well accepted by patients; results in immunization of some contacts of vaccinated persons; has essentially eliminated disease associated with wild poliovirus in this country. OPV is also recommended for control of epidemic poliomyelitis.

History of clinical poliomyelitis or prior vaccination with IPV in otherwise healthy individuals does not preclude the administration of OPV when otherwise indicated.

Adults: Routine poliomyelitis immunization for adults residing in the continental US is not necessary because of extreme unlikelihood of exposure. However, primary immunization with IPV is recommended whenever feasible for unimmunized adults with increased risk of exposure, as by travel to or contact with epidemic or endemic areas, and for those employed in hospitals, medical laboratories, clinics or sanitation facilities. If < 4 weeks are available before protection is needed, a single dose of OPV is recommended, with IPV given later if the person remains at increased risk. Immunization with IPV may be indicated for unimmunized parents and those in other special situations where protection may be needed. In a household with an immunocompromised member or among other close contacts, or in a household with an unimmunized adult, use only IPV for all those requiring poliovirus immunization.

Contraindications:

Defer immunization in the presence of any acute illness, persistent vomiting or diarrhea and in patients with any advanced debilitated condition.

Any person with immunosuppression, or any household member of an immunodeficient person. This includes those with combined immunodeficiency, hypogammaglobulinemia, agammaglobulinemia, thymic abnormalities, leukemia, lymphoma, generalized malignancy, lowered resistance to infection from therapy with corticosteroids, alkylating drugs, antimetabolites or radiation. Advise vaccine recipients to avoid such persons for at least 6 to 8 weeks.

To preclude vaccine-associated disease, do not give OPV to a member of a household in which there is a family history of immunodeficiency until the immune status of the intended recipient and other children in the family is determined to be normal. IPV is preferred for immunizing all persons in the circumstances described above. Give adults in such households 3 doses of IPV a month apart before the children receive OPV; the children may receive their first dose at the same time the adults receive their third dose of IPV.

Warnings:

Poliomyelitis: OPV is not effective in modifying or preventing cases of existing or incubating poliomyelitis.

Immunodeficiency: Do not use in immunodeficient persons, including persons with congenital or acquired immune deficiencies, whether due to genetics, disease, or drug or radiation therapy. Contains live viruses. Avoid use in HIV-positive persons, regardless of whether symptomatic or asymptomatic. Poliovirus is shed for 6 to 8 weeks in vaccinees' stools and by the pharyngeal route.

Pregnancy: Category C. Use only if clearly needed. Use OPV in pregnancy if exposure is imminent and immediate protection is needed.

POLIOVIRUS VACCINE, LIVE, ORAL, TRIVALENT (OPV; TOPV; Sabin)

Lactation: Breastfeeding does not generally interfere with successful immunization of infants, despite IgA antibody secretion in breast milk. In certain tropical epidemic areas where vaccination may be recommended for the infant at birth, the manufacturer suggests that immunization be withheld until the child is 3 days old. Advise women to abstain from breastfeeding for 2 to 3 hours before and after vaccination of their infants, to permit establishment of viruses in the gut. Because successful immunization is likely in newborn infants, complete the OPV series following the neonatal dose when the infant reaches 2 months of age.

Children: Administer 2, 4 and 15 or 18 months of age, and at 4 to 6 years of age. An additional dose at 6 months of age is optional.

Drug Interactions:

Oral Poliovirus Vaccine Drug Interactions

Precipitant drug	Object drug*		Description
Immunosuppressants	OPV	⬇	Administration of OPV to patients receiving immunosuppressants, including corticosteroids or radiation therapy, may result in insufficient response to OPV. They may remain susceptible despite immunization.
Vaccines, other	OPV	⬇	Cholera vaccine reduced the seroconversion rate to OPV Type 1 vaccine in one study. Separate by 1 month if possible. Several routine vaccines may be given simultaneously at separate injection sites (eg, DTP, MMR, Hib, hepatitis B).

* ⬇ = Object drug decreased

Adverse Reactions:

Vaccine-associated paralysis occurs with a frequency of 1 case per 2.6 million OPV doses. Of 105 cases of paralytic poliomyelitis from 1973 through 1984 (when 274.1 million OPV doses were distributed), 35 occurred in vaccine recipients. First doses are more likely to result in a case of paralysis than subsequent doses (1 case per 520,000 vs 1 case per 12.3 million). Since 1980, all reported domestic cases of paralytic polio have apparently been caused by OPV. Of 85 paralytic cases from 1980 to 1989, 80 involved vaccine-associated disease.

Administration and Dosage:

Federal law requires that (1) manufacturer and lot number of vaccine, (2) date of its administration, and (3) name, address and title of person administering vaccine be documented in recipient's permanent medical record or in a permanent office log. Certain adverse events must be reported to the VAERS system, 1-800-822-7967.

Administer orally; not for injection. Administer directly or mix with distilled water, chlorinated tap water, simple syrup, milk or on bread, sugar cube or cake.

Primary immunizing series: Three 0.5 ml doses, optimally starting at 6 to 12 weeks of age. Give the second dose not < 6 and preferably 8 weeks later, commonly at 4 months of age. Give the third dose 8 to 12 months after the second dose, commonly at 18 months of age. An optional additional dose of OPV may be given at 6 months of age in areas where poliomyelitis disease or risk is endemic.

Give older children (up to 18 years of age) 2 OPV doses, not < 6 and preferably 8 weeks apart, followed by a third dose, 6 to 12 months after the second dose.

On entering elementary school, give all children who have completed the primary series a single follow-up dose of OPV. All other should complete the primary series. This fourth dose is not required in those who received the third primary dose on or after their fourth birthday.

The multiple doses of OPV in the primary series are not administered as boosters, but to ensure that immunity to all 3 types of virus has been achieved.

Booster dose: The need for routine additional doses has not been determined. If persons need additional vaccine after 18 years of age, IPV is generally preferred because they are slightly more likely to develop OPV-induced poliomyelitis than children.

Storage/Stability: Store in a freezer. After thawing, use within 30 days. Not stable at room temperature. Do not expose to > 10 freeze-thaw cycles, with none exceeding 8°C (46°F). If the cumulative period of thaw is > 24 hours, store at 2° to 8°C (36° to 46°F) and use within 30 days. OPV is colorless or yellow or red tinge; color changes have no significance as long as product remains clear.

Rx	**Orimune** (Lederle Praxis)	**Oral Suspension:** Mixture of 3 viruses (Types 1, 2 and 3) propagated in monkey kidney tissue culture	In 0.5 ml single dose Dispettes.[1]

[1] With sorbitol and < 25 mcg each streptomycin and neomycin.

POLIOVIRUS VACCINE, INACTIVATED (IPV)

Actions:

Pharmacology: Poliovirus vaccine, inactivated (IPV) is a sterile suspension of three types of poliovirus: Type 1 (Mahoney), Type 2 (MEF-1), and Type 3 (Saukett). The viruses are grown in cultures of VERO cells, a continuous line of monkey kidney cells (IPOL) or in human diploid cell cultures *(Poliovax),* both by the microcarrier technique. This culture technique and improvements in purification, concentration and standardization of poliovirus antigen have resulted in a more potent and more consistently immunogenic vaccine than the poliovirus vaccine inactivated which was available in the US prior to 1988. These new methods allow for the production of vaccine that induces antibody responses in most children after administering fewer doses than with vaccine available prior to 1988. Studies in developed and developing countries with similar inactivated poliovirus vaccine produced by the same technology have shown that a direct relationship exists between the antigenic content of the vaccine, the frequency of seroconversion, and resulting antibody titer. Since the *Poliovax* vaccine will be available mainly as a backup to *IPOL,* this monograph will refer to prescribing information for *IPOL;* however, the prescribing information for *Poliovax* closely follows that of *IPOL.*

Clinical trials: Of 120 infants who received two doses of IPV at 2 and 4 months of age, detectable serum neutralizing antibody was induced after two doses of vaccine in 98.3% (Type 1), 100% (Type 2) and 97.5% (Type 3) of the children. In 83 children receiving three doses at 2, 4 and 12 months of age, detectable serum neutralizing antibodies were detected in 97.6% (Type 1) and 100% (Types 2 and 3) of the children. Paralytic polio has not been reported in association with administration of IPV.

Indications:

For active immunization of infants, children and adults for preventing poliomyelitis. Recommendations on the use of live and inactivated poliovirus vaccines are described in the ACIP Recommendations and the 1988 American Academy of Pediatrics Red Book.

Infants, children and adolescents:

General recommendations – It is recommended that all infants, unimmunized children and adolescents not previously immunized be vaccinated routinely against paralytic poliomyelitis. IPV should be offered to individuals who have refused poliovirus vaccine live oral trivalent (OPV) or in whom OPV is contraindicated. Adequately inform parents of the risks and benefits of both inactivated and oral polio vaccines so that they can make an informed choice.

OPV should not be used in households with immunodeficient individuals because OPV is excreted in the stool by healthy vaccinees and can infect an immunocompromised household member, which may result in paralytic disease. In a household with an immunocompromised member, use only IPV for all those requiring poliovirus immunization.

Children incompletely immunized – Children of all ages should have their immunization status reviewed and be considered for supplemental immunization as follows for adults. Time intervals between doses longer than those recommended for routine primary immunization do not necessitate additional doses as long as a final total of four doses is reached (see Administration and Dosage).

Previous clinical poliomyelitis (usually due to only a single poliovirus type) or incomplete immunization with OPV are not contraindications to completing the primary series of immunization with IPV.

Adults:

General recommendations – Routine primary poliovirus vaccination of adults (generally those ≥ 18 years of age) residing in the US is not recommended. Adults who have increased risk of exposure to either vaccine or wild poliovirus and have not been adequately immunized should receive polio vaccination in accordance with the schedule given in the Administration and Dosage section.

The following categories of adults run an increased risk of exposure to wild polioviruses:

1. Travelers to regions or countries where poliomyelitis is endemic or epidemic;
2. Health care workers in close contact with patients who may be excreting polioviruses;
3. Laboratory workers handling specimens that may contain polioviruses;
4. Members of communities or specific population groups with disease caused by wild polioviruses;
5. Incompletely vaccinated or unvaccinated adults in a household with (or other close contacts of) children given OPV provided that immunization of the child can be assured and not unduly delayed. Inform adult of the small OPV related risk to the contact.

POLIOVIRUS VACCINE, INACTIVATED (IPV)

Immunodeficiency and altered immune status: Patients with recognized immunodeficiency are at a greater risk of developing paralysis when exposed to live poliovirus than persons with a normal immune system. Under no circumstances should OPV be used in such patients or introduced into a household where such a patient resides.

Use IPV in all patients with immunodeficiency diseases and members of such patients' households when vaccination of such persons is indicated. This includes patients with asymptomatic HIV infection, AIDS or AIDS-related complex, severe combined immunodeficiency, hypogammaglobulinemia or aggammaglobulinemia; altered immune states due to diseases such as leukemia, lymphoma or generalized malignancy; or an immune system compromised by treatment with corticosteroids, alkylating drugs, antimetabolites or radiation. Patients with an altered immune state may develop a protective response against paralytic poliomyelitis after IPV administration.

Contraindications:

Hypersensitivity to any component of the vaccine, including neomycin, streptomycin and polymyxin B (see Warnings).

Defer vaccination of persons with any acute, febrile illness until after recovery; however, minor illnesses such as mild upper respiratory infection, are not in themselves reasons for postponing vaccine administration.

Warnings:

Hypersensitivity: Neomycin, streptomycin, and polymyxin B are used in producing this vaccine. Although purification procedures eliminate measurable amounts of these substances, traces may be present and allergic reactions may occur in persons sensitive to these substances. If anaphylaxis or anaphylactic shock occurs within 24 hours of administration of a dose, no further doses should be given. Epinephrine HCl (1:1000) and other appropriate agents should be available to control immediate allergic reactions. Refer to Management of Acute Hypersensitivity Reactions.

Pregnancy: Category C. It is not known whether IPV can cause fetal harm when administered to a pregnant woman or can affect reproduction capacity. Give to a pregnant woman only if clearly needed.

Children: Safety and efficacy of IPV have been shown in children > 6 weeks of age (see Administration and Dosage).

Precautions:

Patient review: Before injection of the vaccine, the physician should carefully review the recommendations for product use and the patient's medical history including possible hypersensitivities and side effects that may have occurred following previous doses of the vaccine.

HIV infection: Concerns have been raised that stimulation of the immune system of a patient with HIV infection by immunization with inactivated vaccines might cause deterioration in immunologic function. However, such effects have not been noted thus far among children with AIDS or among immunosuppressed individuals after immunizations with inactivated vaccines. The potential benefits of immunization of these children outweigh the undocumented risk of such adverse events.

Adverse Reactions:

In earlier studies with the vaccine grown in primary monkey kidney cells, transient local reactions at the site of injection have been observed. Erythema, induration and pain occurred in 3.2%, 1% and 13%, respectively, of vaccinees within 48 hours post-vaccination. Temperatures ≥ 39°C (≥ 102°F) were reported in up to 38% of vaccinees. Other symptoms noted included sleepiness, fussiness, crying, decreased appetite and spitting up of feedings. Because IPV was given in a different site but concurrently with Diphtheria and Tetanus Toxoids and Pertussis Vaccine Adsorbed (DTP), systemic reactions could not be attributed to a specific vaccine. However, these systemic reactions were comparable in frequency and severity to that reported for DTP given without IPV.

In another study using IPV in the US, there were no significant local or systemic reactions following injection of the vaccine. There were 7% (6/86), 12% (8/65) and 4% (2/45) of children with temperatures > 100.6°F, following the first, second and third doses, respectively. Most of the children received DTP at the same time as IPV and therefore it was not possible to attribute reactions to a particular vaccine; however, such reactions were not significantly different than when DTP is given alone.

Although no causal relationship between IPV and Guillain-Barré Syndrome (GBS) has been established, GBS has been temporally related to administration of another IPV.

POLIOVIRUS VACCINE, INACTIVATED (IPV)

Note: The National Childhood Vaccine Injury Act of 1986 requires the keeping of certain records and the reporting of certain events occurring after the administration of vaccine, including the occurrence of any contraindicating reaction. Poliovirus vaccines are listed vaccines covered by this Act and health care providers should ensure that they comply with the terms thereof.

Administration and Dosage:

Administer SC; do not administer IV. In infants and small children, the mid-lateral aspect of the thigh is the preferred site. In adults, administer the vaccine in the deltoid area.

Take care to avoid administering the injection into or near blood vessels and nerves. After aspiration, if blood or any suspicious discoloration appears in the syringe, do not inject; discard contents and repeat procedures using a new dose of vaccine administered at a different site.

Children:

Primary immunization – A primary series of IPV consists of three 0.5 ml doses administered SC. The interval between the first two doses should be at least 4 weeks, but preferably 8 weeks. The first two doses are usually administered with DTP immunization and are given at 2 and 4 months of age. The third dose should follow at least 6 months but preferably 12 months after the second dose. It may be desirable to administer this dose with MMR and other vaccines, but at a different site, in children 15 to 18 months of age. Give all children who received a primary series of IPV, or a combination of IPV and OPV, a booster dose of OPV or IPV before entering school, unless the first dose of the primary series was administered on or after the fourth birthday. The need to routinely administer additional doses is unknown at this time.

A final total of four doses is necessary to complete a series of primary and booster doses. Children and adolescents with a previously incomplete series of IPV should receive sufficient additional doses to reach this number.

Adults:

Unvaccinated adults – For unvaccinated adults at increased risk of exposure to poliovirus, a primary series of IPV is recommended. While the responses of adults to primary series have not been studied, the recommended schedule for adults is two doses given at a 1 to 2 month interval and a third dose given 6 to 12 months later. If < 3 months but > 2 months are available before protection is needed, give 3 doses at least 1 month apart. Likewise, if only 1 or 2 months are available, give 2 doses of IPV at least 1 month apart. If < 1 month is available, a single dose of either OPV or IPV is recommended.

Incompletely vaccinated adults – Adults who are at an increased risk of exposure to poliovirus and who have had at least one dose of OPV, < 3 doses of conventional IPV or a combination of conventional IPV or OPV totalling < 3 doses should receive at least 1 dose of OPV or IPV. Give additional doses to complete a primary series if time permits.

Completely vaccinated adults – Adults who are at an increased risk of exposure to poliovirus and who have previously completed a primary series with one or a combination of polio vaccines can be given a dose of either OPV or IPV.

Storage: The vaccine is stable if stored in the refrigerator between 2° and 8°C (35° and 46°F). The vaccine must not be frozen.

Rx	**IPOL** (Connaught)	**Injection:** Suspension of 3 types of poliovirus (Types 1, 2 and 3) grown in monkey kidney cell cultures	In 0.5 ml single-dose syringe with integrated needle.[1]

[1] Each dose contains 0.5% 2-phenoxyethanol, a maximum of 0.02% formaldehyde and not more than 200 ng streptomycin, 25 ng polymyxin B and 5 ng neomycin.

INFLUENZA VIRUS VACCINE

Actions:

Pharmacology: Inoculation of antigens prepared from inactivated influenza virus stimulates the production of specific antibodies. Protection is afforded only against those strains or closely related strains from which the vaccine is prepared.

An updated type A (H1N1) antigen will be a component of the influenza virus vaccines that will be used during the 1997-1998 influenza season, as well as the same A (H3N2) and B components that were used in the 1996-1997 vaccine. The antigens recommended by the FDA Vaccine Advisory Panel include A/Johannesburg/82/96 (H1N1) (A/Bayern/07/95-like), A/Nanchang/933/95 (H3N2) (A/Wuhan/359-95-like) and B/Harbin/07/94 (B/Beijing/184/93-like). Therefore, these strains will be included in the influenza virus vaccine for use during the 1997-1998 season. Remaining 1996-1997 vaccines should not be used for the 1997-1998 season. The vaccine is available as a "whole-virus", "split-virus" (subvirion) or "purified surface antigen" preparation. Having received a vaccination for the 1996-1997 flu season does not preclude the need to be revaccinated for the 1997-1998 season to provide optimal protection.

Indications:

For the production of immunity to influenza virus-containing antigens related to those in the vaccine. Influenza vaccine is strongly recommended for any person ≥ 6 months of age who, because of age or underlying medical condition, is at increased risk for complications of influenza. Healthcare workers and others (including household members) in close contact with high-risk people should also be vaccinated. In addition, influenza vaccine may be given to any person who wishes to reduce the chance of becoming infected with influenza. Guidelines for use of the vaccine in specific groups follow.

Groups at increased risk of influenza-related complications: 1. People ≥ 65 years of age.

2. Residents of nursing homes and other chronic-care facilities housing people of any age with chronic medical conditions.

3. Adults and children with chronic disorders of the pulmonary or cardiovascular systems, including children with asthma.

4. Adults and children who have required regular medical follow-up or hospitalization during the preceding year because of chronic metabolic diseases (including diabetes mellitus), renal dysfunction, hemoglobinopathies or immunosuppression (including immunosuppression caused by medications).

5. Children and teenagers (6 months to 18 years of age) who are receiving long-term aspirin therapy and, therefore, may be at risk of developing Reye's syndrome after influenza.

6. Women who will be in the second or third trimester of pregnancy during the influenza season.

Groups that can transmit influenza to high-risk people: People who are clinically or subclinically infected and who attend or live with high-risk people can transmit the influenza virus to them. Some high-risk people (eg, elderly, transplant recipients, people with AIDS) can have low antibody responses to influenza vaccine. Efforts to protect these high-risk people against influenza may be improved by reducing the chances of exposure to influenza from their care providers. Therefore, the following groups should be vaccinated:

1. Physicians, nurses and other personnel in both hospital and outpatient-care settings who have contact with high-risk people in all age groups, including infants.
2. Employees of nursing homes and chronic-care facilities who have contact with patients or residents.
3. Providers of home care to high-risk people (eg, visiting nurses, volunteer workers).
4. Household members (including children) of high-risk people.

General population: Any individual wishing to reduce the chance of acquiring an influenza infection. people who provide essential community service (eg, police, fire department employees) and students or other people in institutional settings may be considered for vaccination programs to minimize potential disruption of routine activities during outbreaks or epidemics, respectively.

People infected with human immunodeficiency virus (HIV): Little information exists regarding the frequency and severity of influenza illness in HIV-infected people, but reports suggest that symptoms may be prolonged and the risk of complications increased for some patients in this group. Because influenza may result in serious illness and complications, vaccination is a prudent precaution and will result in protective antibody levels in many recipients. However, the antibody response to vaccine may be low in people with advanced HIV disease and low CD4 + T-lymphocyte cell counts; a booster dose of vaccine has not improved the immune response for these individuals.

INFLUENZA VIRUS VACCINE

Foreign travelers: The risk of exposure to influenza during foreign travel varies, depending on season and destination. In the tropics, influenza can occur throughout the year; in the southern hemisphere, the season of greatest activity is April through September. Because of the short incubation period for influenza, exposure to the virus during travel can result in clinical illness that also begins while traveling, an inconvenience or potential danger, especially for people at increased risk for complications. People preparing to travel to the tropics at any time of year or to the southern hemisphere during April through September should review their influenza vaccination histories. If they were not vaccinated the previous fall/winter, they should consider influenza vaccination before travel. People in the high-risk categories should be especially encouraged to receive the most currently available vaccine. High-risk people given the previous season's vaccine before travel should be revaccinated in the fall/winter with the current vaccine.

Pregnancy: See Warnings.

Contraindications:

The use of products prepared from the embryonic fluid of chicken eggs is contraindicated in people with a history of allergy to eggs or egg products. The vaccine is also contraindicated in individuals hypersensitive to any component of the vaccine.

In people suspected of having an allergic condition, precede immunization procedures by a scratch test or an intradermal injection (0.05 to 0.1 ml) of vaccine diluted 1:100 in sterile saline to determine possible sensitivity to the minute residual egg protein that may be present in the vaccine. A positive skin reaction contraindicates immunization with the vaccine (see Warnings).

Defer immunization in the presence of acute respiratory disease or other active infection or acute febrile illness (see Precautions).

Warnings:

Impaired immune response: Patients with impaired immune responsiveness, whether caused by the use of immunosuppressive therapy (including irradiation, corticosteroids, antimetabolites, alkylating agents and cytotoxic agents), a genetic defect, HIV infection or other causes, may have a reduced antibody response in active immunization procedures.

Hypersensitivity: Have epinephrine 1:1000 immediately available. Refer to Management of Acute Hypersensitivity Reactions.

Immunosuppressed patients may experience a lower than expected antigenic response, although in one study, appropriate antibody responses occurred in patients with HIV who received trivalent influenza vaccine. Amantadine may be given to supplement the protection afforded by vaccination in high-risk patients.

Pregnancy: Category C. Pregnancy has not been demonstrated to be a risk factor for severe influenza infection, except in the largest pandemics of 1918–1919 and 1957–1958. However, vaccinate pregnant women with medical conditions that increase the risk of complications from influenza because influenza vaccine is considered safe for pregnant women without a specific severe egg allergy. To minimize any concern over the theoretical possibility of teratogenicity, give vaccine after the first trimester. However, it may be undesirable to delay vaccinating a pregnant woman who has a high-risk condition and will still be in the first trimester of pregnancy when influenza activity usually begins.

Lactation: Influenza vaccine does not affect the safety of breastfeeding for mothers or infants. Breastfeeding does not adversely affect immune response and is not a contraindication for vaccination.

Children: Safety and efficacy of *Fluvirin* in children 6 months to 4 years of age have not been established; do not administer unless potential benefits clearly outweigh the risks. Do not administer *Fluvirin* to children < 6 months. Safety and efficacy of other available products in children < 6 months have not been established.

Precautions:

Concurrent vaccination: Because children are accessible when pediatric vaccines are administered, it may be desirable to administer influenza vaccine simultaneously with routine pediatric vaccine but in a different site. Studies have not been done, but no diminution of immunogenicity or enhancement of adverse reactions is expected.

Pneumococcal vaccine and influenza vaccine can be given at the same time at different sites without increasing side effects. Note: Influenza vaccine is given annually; pneumococcal vaccine should be given only once.

High-risk children may receive influenza vaccine at the same time as measles-mumps-rubella, *Haemophilus b*, pneumococcal and oral polio vaccines, at different sites. Physicians may prefer to not give influenza vaccine within 3 days of vaccination with pertussis vaccine; however, the AAP recommends that influenza vaccine can be administered simultaneously (but at a different site and with a different syringe) with other routine vaccinations in children, including pertussis vaccine (DTP or DTaP). DTaP may be preferable in children ≥ 15 months because of fever risk with influenza vaccine.

Other neurologic disorders, including encephalopathies, have been temporally associated with influenza vaccination.

Febrile reaction: Because of the possibility of a febrile reaction following immunization, weigh the value of immunizing patients with a history of febrile convulsions. Do not vaccinate people with acute febrile illnesses until their temporary symptoms have abated. The likelihood of febrile convulsions is greater in children 6 months through 35 months of age. Minor illnesses with or without fever should not contraindicate the use of influenza vaccine, particularly among children with a mild upper respiratory tract infection or allergic rhinitis.

Seroconversion: Vaccination may not result in sero-conversion in all individuals.

Guillain-Barre syndrome (GBS), characterized by ascending paralysis, is usually self-limited and reversible. Although most people recover without residual weakness, ≈ 5% of cases are fatal. Before 1976, no association of GBS with influenza vaccination was recognized. However, that year, GBS appeared among people who had received A/New Jersey/76 swine influenza vaccine. No significant excess risk of GBS was found for recipients of influenza vaccine during the influenza seasons 1978–1979 to 1980–1981. Subsequent vaccines have not been associated with an increased frequency of GBS. Nonetheless, advise people who receive influenza vaccine of the possible risk as compared with the risk of influenza and its complications.

Sulfite sensitivity: Sulfites may cause allergic-type reactions (eg, hives, itching, wheezing, anaphylaxis) in certain susceptible people. Although the overall prevalence of sulfite sensitivity in the general population is probably low, it is seen more frequently in asthmatics or in atopic nonasthmatic people. Although not detectable in the final product by current assay procedures, the manufacturing process for some formulations utilizes sodium bisulfite.

Drug Interactions:

Influenza Virus Vaccine Drug Interactions

Precipitant drug	Object drug*		Description
Influenza virus vaccine	Phenytoin	↔	Although influenza vaccination reportedly inhibits the clearance of these agents, further studies have consistently failed to show any adverse effects of influenza vaccination among patients taking these drugs.
	Theophylline	↑	
	Warfarin	↑	

* ↑ = Object drug increased. ↔ = Undetermined effect.

Adverse Reactions:

Side effects of influenza vaccine are generally inconsequential in adults and occur at low frequency. Severe reactions are uncommon in adults and disabling effects are exceedingly rare.

Local: Soreness at injection site for up to 1 or 2 days (< 33%; most frequent).

Systemic: Two types: (1) Fever, malaise, myalgia and other symptoms of toxicity, although infrequent, occur more often in children and others who have had no exposure to the influenza virus antigen. These reactions, which begin 6 to 12 hours after vaccination and persist 1 to 2 days, are attributed to the influenza antigens (even though they are inactivated) and constitute most of the systemic side effects. (2) Immediate, presumably allergic, responses such as flare and wheal or various respiratory symptoms (extremely rare), probably resulting from sensitivity to some vaccine component, most likely residual egg protein (see Contraindications).

Administration and Dosage:

Do not inject IV. Give injections IM, preferably in the deltoid muscle for adults and older children; for infants and young children, the preferred site is the anterolateral aspect of the thigh.

Vaccination schedules: Organized vaccination campaigns where high-risk people are routinely accessible, such as in chronic-care facilities or worksites, may be optimally undertaken in November. Vaccination is desirable in September or October (1) if warranted by regional experience of earlier than normal epidemic activity (eg, in Alaska); or (2) for other people recommended for vaccination who receive medical check-ups or treatment during September or October and who may not be seen again until after November. In addition, make arrangements to assure vaccination of hospitalized high-risk adults and children who are discharged between September and the time influenza activity begins to decline in their community; give vaccine as part of the discharge procedure.

INFLUENZA VIRUS VACCINE

Children < 9 years of age who have not been previously vaccinated require two doses of vaccine with at least 1 month between doses. Schedule programs for childhood influenza vaccination so the second dose can be given before December. Vaccine can be given to both children and adults up to and even after influenza virus activity is documented in a region, although temporary chemoprophylaxis may be indicated when influenza outbreaks are occurring.

Influenza Vaccine Dosage Recommendations by Age Group

Age	Product type[1]	Dosage (ml)	Number of doses
> 12 years	whole-virus, split-virus or purified surface antigen	0.5	1
9-12 years	split-virus or purified surface antigen	0.5	1
3-8 years	split-virus or purified surface antigen	0.5	1 or 2[2]
6-35 months	split-virus or purified surface antigen	0.25	1 or 2[2]

[1] Because of the lower potential for causing febrile reactions, use only split (subvirion) or purified surface antigen vaccine in children. Immunogenicity and side effects of split, whole and purified surface antigen virus vaccine are similar in adults when used as recommended.

[2] ≥ 4 weeks between doses; both doses are recommended for maximum protection. However, if the individual received at least 1 dose of the 1978-1979 or later influenza vaccine, 1 dose is sufficient.

The only drugs currently available for the specific prophylaxis and therapy of influenza virus infections are amantadine HCl and rimantadine HCl (in children, only for prophylaxis). People who take the drugs may still develop immune responses that will protect them when exposed to antigenically-related viruses.

While amantadine and rimantadine chemoprophylaxis is effective against influenza A, it confers no protection against influenza B, and patient compliance could be a problem for continuous administration throughout epidemic periods, which generally last 6 to 12 weeks. *Under most circumstances do not use in lieu of vaccination.*

Consider amantadine and rimantadine for therapeutic use, particularly for people in the high-risk groups if they develop an illness compatible with influenza during a period of known or suspected influenza A activity in the community.

Storage/Stability: Store between 2° to 8°C (35° to 46°F). Freezing destroys potency.

Rx	**Fluzone** (Connaught)	**Injection (Split-Virus):** 15 mcg A/Johannesburg/F2/96 (H1N1) (A/Bayern/07/95-like), 15 mcg A/Nanchang/933/95 (H3N2) (A/Wuhan/359-95-like) and 15 mcg B/Harbin/7/94 (B/Beijing/184/93-like) hemagglutinin antigens per 0.5 ml	In 5 and 25 ml vials[1] and 0.5 ml syringes.[1]
Rx	**FluShield** (Wyeth-Ayerst)	**Injection (Purified Split-Virus):** 15 mcg A/Johannesburg/F2/96 (H1N1) (A/Bayern/07/95-like), 15 mcg A/Nanchang/933/95 (H3N2) (A/Wuhan/359-95-like) and 15 mcg of B/Harbin/7/94 (B/Beijing/184/93-like) hemagglutinin antigens per 0.5 ml	In 5 ml vial and 0.5 ml Tubex.
Rx	**Fluzone** (Connaught)	**Injection (Whole-Virus):** 15 mcg A/Johannesburg/F2/96 (H1N1) (A/Bayern/07/95-like), 15 mcg A/Nanchang/933/95 (H3N2) (A/Wuhan/359-95-like) and 15 mcg B/Harbin/7/94 (B/Beijing/184/93-like) hemagglutinin antigens per 0.5 ml	In 5 ml vials and syringes.[1]
Rx	**Fluvirin** (Adams)	**Injection (Purified Surface Antigen):** 15 mcg A/Johannesburg/F2/96 (H1N1) (A/Bayern/07/95-like), 15 mcg A/Nanchang/933/95 (H3N2) (A/Wuhan/359-95-like) and 15 mcg B/Harbin/7/94 (B/Beijing/184/93-like) hemagglutinin antigens per 0.5 ml[1]	In 5 ml vials and 0.5 ml pre-filled syringes.

[1] With 0.01% thimerosal.

JAPANESE ENCEPHALITIS VIRUS VACCINE

Actions:

Pharmacology: Japanese encephalitis (JE) virus vaccine is a sterile, lyophilized vaccine for SC use, prepared by inoculating mice intracerebrally with JE virus ("Nakayama-NIH" strain). JE, a mosquito-borne arboviral Flavivirus infection, is the leading cause of viral encephalitis in Asia. Infection leads to overt encephalitis in 1 of 20 to 1000 cases. Encephalitis usually is severe, resulting in a fatal outcome in 25% of cases and residual neuropsychiatric sequelae in 50% of cases. JE acquired during the first or second trimesters of pregnancy may cause intrauterine infection and miscarriage. Infections that occur during the third trimester of pregnancy have not been associated with adverse outcomes in newborns. The virus is transmitted in an enzootic cycle among mosquitoes and vertebrate amplifying hosts, chiefly domestic pigs and, in some areas, wild Ardeid (wading) birds. Viral infection rates in mosquitoes range from < 1% to 3%. JE virus is transmitted seasonally in most areas of Asia. The periods of greatest risk for JE viral transmission may vary regionally and within countries, and from year to year.

In areas where JE is endemic, annual incidence ranges from 1 to 10 per 10,000 people. Cases occur primarily in children < 10 years of age. Seroprevalence studies in these endemic areas indicate nearly universal exposure by adulthood. In addition to children < 10 years, an increase in JE incidence has been observed in the elderly.

Clinical trials: The efficacy of JE vaccine was demonstrated in a placebo-controlled, randomized clinical trial in Thai children. In this trial, children between 1 and 14 years of age received a monovalent or a bivalent vaccine or tetanus toxoid as a placebo. Immunization consisted of two SC 1 ml doses of vaccine, except in children < 3 years of age who received two 0.5 ml doses. One case (5 cases/100,000) of JE occurred in the monovalent vaccine group, one case (5 cases/100,000) in the bivalent vaccine group and 11 cases (51 cases/100,000) in the placebo group. The observed efficacy of both monovalent and bivalent vaccines was 91% (95% confidence interval, 54% to 98%). Side effects of vaccination, including headache, sore arm, rash, and swelling were reported at rates similar to those in the placebo group, usually < 1%. Symptoms did not increase after the second dose. A schedule of two doses, separated by 7 days, may be appropriate for use in residents of endemic or epidemic areas, where pre-existing exposure to Flaviviruses may contribute to the immune response.

A three-dose vaccination schedule is recommended for US travelers and military personnel, based on the CDC experience and on a controlled immunogenicity trial performed in US military personnel. The CDC experience demonstrated that neutralizing antibody was produced in < 80% of vaccinees following two doses of vaccine in US travelers, and antibody levels declined substantially in most vaccinees within 6 months. In 538 volunteers, two three-dose regimens were evaluated (day 0, 7 and 14 or day 0, 7 and 30). All vaccine recipients demonstrated neutralizing antibodies at 2 and 6 months after initiation of vaccination. The schedule of day 0, 7 and 30 produced higher antibody responses. Of the original study participants, 273 were tested at 12 months post-vaccination and there was no longer a statistical difference in antibody titers between the two vaccination regimens.

The full duration of protection is unknown. Of volunteers completing a three-dose regimen, 252 agreed to receive a booster dose of vaccine 1 year after the primary series. All participants still had antibody 12 months after the booster. Protective levels of neutralizing antibody persisted for 24 months in all 21 persons who had not received a booster. Definitive recommendations cannot be given on the timing of booster doses at this time.

Indications:

For active immunization against JE for persons > 1 year of age.

Consider JE vaccine in persons who plan to reside in or travel to areas where JE is endemic or epidemic during a transmission season. It is not recommended for all persons traveling to or residing in Asia. Consider the incidence of JE in the location of intended stay, the conditions of housing, nature of activities, duration of stay and the possibility of unexpected travel to high-risk areas in the decision to administer vaccine. In general, consider vaccinating persons spending ≥ 1 month in epidemic or endemic areas during the transmission season, especially if travel will include rural areas. Depending on the epidemic circumstances, consider for persons spending < 30 days whose activities, such as extensive outdoor activities in rural areas, place them at particularly high risk for exposure.

In all instances, travelers are advised to take personal precautions to reduce exposure to mosquito bites. (See Patient Information.)

Consult current CDC advisories with regard to JE epidemicity in specific locales.

JAPANESE ENCEPHALITIS VIRUS VACCINE

Contraindications:

Adverse reactions to a prior dose of JE vaccine manifesting as generalized urticaria and angioedema (report patients who develop allergic or unusual adverse events after vaccination through the Vaccine Adverse Event Reporting System [VAERS] at 1-800-822-7967); hypersensitivity to proteins of rodent or neural origin (JE vaccine is produced in mouse brains) or thimerosal.

Warnings:

Hypersensitivity: Adverse reactions to JE vaccine manifesting as generalized urticaria or angioedema may occur within minutes following vaccination. A possibly related reaction has occurred as late as 17 days after vaccination. Most reactions occur within 10 days with the majority occurring within 48 hours. (See Adverse Reactions.) Observe vaccinees for 30 minutes after vaccination and warn about the possibility of delayed generalized urticaria, often in a generalized distribution or angioedema of the extremities, face and oropharynx, especially of the lips. Advise vaccinees to remain in areas where they have ready access to medical care for 10 days after receiving JE vaccine, and instruct them to seek medical attention immediately upon onset of any reaction.

Persons should not embark on international travel within 10 days of JE vaccine immunization because of the possibility of delayed allergic reactions.

Persons with a history of urticaria after *Hymenoptera* envenomation, drugs, physical or other provocations or of idiopathic cause appear to have a greater risk of developing reactions to JE vaccine. Consider this history when weighing risks and benefits of the vaccine for an individual patient. When patients with such a history are offered JE vaccine, alert them to their increased risk for reaction and monitor appropriately. There are no data supporting the efficacy of prophylactic antihistamines or steroids in preventing JE vaccine-related allergic reactions.

Have epinephrine and other medications and equipment to treat anaphylaxis. Refer to Management of Acute Hypersensitivity Reactions.

Elderly: Advanced age may be a risk factor for developing symptomatic illness after infection. Consider this when advising elderly persons who plan to visit JE-endemic areas.

Pregnancy: Category C. It is not known whether JE vaccine can cause fetal harm when administered to a pregnant woman. Immunize pregnant women who must travel to an area where risk of JE is high when the theoretical risks of immunization are outweighed by the risk of infection to the mother and developing fetus; JE acquired during the first or second trimesters of pregnancy may cause intrauterine infection and miscarriage. Give to a pregnant woman only if clearly needed.

Lactation: It is not known whether JE vaccine is excreted in breast milk. Exercise caution when administering to a nursing woman.

Children: Safety and efficacy in infants < 1 year of age have not been established. Whenever possible defer immunization of infants until they are ≥ 1 year of age.

Precautions:

Patient history: Prior to injection of any vaccine, take all known precautions to prevent adverse reactions. This includes a review of the patient's history with respect to possible sensitivity to this vaccine, a similar vaccine or allergic disorders in general.

Transmission of infectious agents: Use a separate sterile syringe and needle or a disposable unit for each patient to prevent transmission of infectious agents from person to person. Do not recap needles; dispose of properly.

Antibody level: Although substantial neutralizing antibody titers are elicited by JE vaccine, in > 90% of US travelers without history of prior JE immunization or of prior exposure to JE, the precise relationship between antibody level and efficacy has not been established even though these titers persisted for at least 2 years after immunization.

Risks: The decision to administer JE vaccine should balance the risks for exposure to the virus and for developing illness, the availability and acceptability of repellents and other alternative protective measures, and the side effects of vaccination.

Research laboratory workers: Laboratory acquired JE has been reported in 22 cases. JE virus may be transmitted in a laboratory setting through needle sticks and other accidental exposures. Vaccine-derived immunity presumably protects against exposure through these percutaneous routes. Exposure to aerosolized JE virus, and particularly to high concentrations of virus (eg, during viral purification), potentially could lead to infection through mucous membranes and possibly directly into the CNS through the olfactory mucosa. It is unknown whether vaccine-derived immunity protects against such exposures, but immunization is recommended for all laboratory workers with a potential for exposure to infectious JE virus.

JAPANESE ENCEPHALITIS VIRUS VACCINE

As with any vaccine, vaccination with JE vaccine may not result in protection in all individuals. Long-term protection, as demonstrated by persistence of neutralizing antibody for > 2 years, has not yet been shown.

Adverse Reactions:

In clinical trials, side effects including headache, sore arm, rash and swelling occurred at rates similar to those in placebo groups, usually < 1%. Overall, 20% of vaccine recipients experience mild to moderate local side effects: Tenderness, redness, swelling (range, < 1% to 31%). Systemic effects include: Fever, headache, malaise, rash, chills, dizziness, muscle pain, nausea, vomiting, abdominal pain (5% to 10%); hives (0.2%); facial swelling (0.1%). Report adverse events to the VAERS system at 1-800-822-7967.

Some adverse reactions to JE vaccine occur within minutes, most within 48 hours, and nearly all within 10 days, although one reaction occurred 17 days after vaccination. Median time to reaction after a first dose of vaccine was 12 hours; 88% of reactions occurred within 3 days. The interval between a second dose and onset of symptoms was longer (median, 3 days; outer limit, 2 weeks). Symptoms did not increase in frequency or severity with increasing numbers of doses. Reactions occurred after a second or third dose when preceding doses had not evoked a reaction.

Since 1989, an apparently new pattern of adverse reactions has been reported among vaccinees in Europe, North America and Australia. The pattern is characterized by urticaria, often in a generalized distribution, or angioedema of the extremities or face, especially of the lips and oropharynx; three vaccinees developed respiratory distress. Distress or collapse due to hypotension or other causes led to hospitalization in several cases. Most reactions were treated successfully with antihistamines or oral corticosteroids; some patients were hospitalized for IV steroid therapy. Three patients developed erythema multiforme or nodosum and some patients had joint swelling. Some vaccinees complained of generalized itching without objective evidence of rash. Rates of serious allergic reactions (eg, generalized urticaria, angioedema) are ≈ 1 to 104 per 10,000 doses. Persons with certain allergic histories (eg, urticaria after *Hymenoptera* envenomation, drugs, physical or other provocations, idiopathic cause) appear to be 9.1 times more likely to experience an adverse reaction after vaccination. Due to the possibility of delayed allergic reactions, advise recipients to remain in areas where they have ready access to medical care for 10 days after receiving a dose (see Warnings).

Other serious adverse events reported after vaccination include: (1) A case of Guillain-Barre syndrome although this patient also was diagnosed as having mononucleosis 3 weeks before the onset of weakness; (2) a case of urticaria, hepatitis, eosinophilia and respiratory failure with effusion and infiltrate on chest radiograph 1 week after the second JE dose; (3) a case of respiratory and renal failure, with infiltrate on chest radiograph and AFB in sputum; and (4) a case of newly diagnosed hypertension in a young adult presenting with a headache several hours after receiving a first dose. The etiology of these adverse events is unconfirmed. Sudden death occurred 60 hours after receiving the first dose in a 21-year-old with a history of recurrent hypersensitivity and a prior episode of possible anaphylaxis. This person received a third dose of plague vaccine 12 to 15 hours prior to death. There was no evidence of urticaria or angioedema.

Patient Information:

JE vaccine is given to provide immunization against Japanese encephalitis virus. Complete a three-dose immunizing series, except in unusual circumstances. (see Contraindications and Administration and Dosage).

Give to a pregnant woman only if, in the opinion of a physician, withholding the vaccine entails even greater risk.

Report adverse events following JE vaccine through the Vaccine Adverse Event Reporting System (VAERS) at 1-800-822-7967 after immediately contacting the physician.

If the patient has a history of urticaria (hives) following *Hymenoptera* envenomation, drugs, physical or other provocation, or of idiopathic origin, adverse effects are more likely.

Adverse events consisting of arm soreness and local redness can occur shortly after vaccination. Adverse events consisting of headache, rash, edema and generalized urticaria or angioedema may occur shortly after vaccination or up to 17 days (usually within 10 days) following vaccination.

International travel should not be initiated within 10 days of JE vaccination because of the possibility of delayed adverse reactions. Instruct patients to seek medical attention immediately upon onset of any adverse reaction.

JAPANESE ENCEPHALITIS VIRUS VACCINE

Take personal precautions to avoid exposure to mosquito bites by the use of insect repellents and protective clothing. Avoiding outdoor activity, especially during twilight periods and in the evening, will reduce risk even further.

Administration and Dosage:

Approved by the FDA on December 10, 1992. Previously available in the US from 1983 through 1987 on an investigational basis through the CDC.

Primary immunization schedule:

Adults and children > 3 years of age – The recommended primary immunization series is three SC doses of 1 ml each given on days 0, 7 and 30.

Children 1 to 3 years of age – Give a series of three SC doses of 0.5 ml each on days 0, 7 and 30.

An abbreviated schedule of days 0, 7 and 14 can be used when the longer schedule is impractical because of time constraints. When it is impossible to follow one of the above recommended schedules, two doses given a week apart will induce antibodies in approximately 80% of vaccinees; however, this two-dose regimen should not be used except under unusual circumstances. Give the last dose at least 10 days before the commencement of international travel to ensure an adequate immune response and access to medical care in the event of delayed adverse reactions.

Infants < 1 year of age – There are no data on the safety and efficacy of JE vaccine. Whenever possible, defer immunization of infants until they are ≥ 1 year of age.

Booster dose: A booster dose of 1 ml (0.5 ml for children from 1 to 3 years of age) may be given after 2 years. In the absence of firm data on the persistence of antibody after primary immunization, a definite recommendation cannot be made on the spacing of boosters beyond 2 years.

Clean and disinfect the skin at the site of injection first. Shake vial thoroughly before each use. Cleanse top of rubber stopper of the vial with a suitable antiseptic and wipe away all excess before withdrawing vaccine. Inspect visually for extraneous particulate matter or discoloration prior to administration. If either of these conditions exist, do not administer the vaccine.

Concomitant vaccines: When JE vaccine and any other vaccines are given concurrently, use separate syringes and separate sites.

Reconstitution: Remove plastic tab of flip-off cap. Do not remove rubber stopper. Cleanse stopper with a suitable disinfectant. Reconstitute only with the supplied 1.3 ml (single-dose vial) or 11 ml (10 dose vial) of diluent (sterile water for injection). Shake vial thoroughly.

Storage/Stability: Store the vaccine between 2° to 8°C (35° to 46°F). Do not freeze. After reconstitution, store the vaccine between 2° to 8°C and use within 8 hours. Do not freeze reconstituted vaccine.

Rx	**JE-VAX** (Connaught)	**Powder for injection (lyophilized)**[1,2]	In single-dose vial with 1.3 ml diluent (sterile water for injection) and 10 dose vial with 11 ml diluent (sterile water for injection).

[1] Potency is determined by immunizing mice with either the test vaccine or the JE Reference Vaccine. Neutralizing antibodies are measured in a plaque-neutralization assay performed on sera from the immunized mice. The potency of the test vaccine must be no less than that of the reference vaccine.

[2] With thimerosal 0.007%. Each 1 ml dose contains ≈ 500 mcg gelatin, < 100 mcg formaldehyde and < 50 ng mouse serum protein.

YELLOW FEVER VACCINE

This vaccine is a live, attenuated virus preparation prepared by culturing the 17D strain virus in living chick embryo. Onset of immunity is 7 to 10 days; duration is ≥ 10 years.

Indications:

Induction of active immunity against yellow fever virus, primarily among travenlers to yellow fever endemic areas.

The World Health Organization (WHO) requires revaccination every 10 years to maintain travelers' vaccination certificates. US vaccination certificates are valid for 10 years, beginning 10 days after initial vaccination or revaccination.

Contraindications:

Hypersensitivity to the vaccine or to egg or chick embryo protein; pregnant women; children < 6 months (except in high risk areas); any form of immunodeficiency.

Warnings:

Immunodeficiency: Do not use in immunodeficient persons, including persons with congenital or acquired immune deficiencies, whether due to genetics, disease, or or radiation therapy. Contains live viruses. Avoid use in HIV-positive persons.

Hypersensitivity: Yellow fever vaccine is produced in chick embryos; do not administer to individuals hypersensitive to egg or chicken protein. Perform intradermal skin tests with the vaccine and sterile normal saline as a control on all such individuals. Inject 0.02 to 0.03 ml into the volar surface of the forearm. This should raise a noticeable intradermal wheal at each test site.

A positive sensitivity test consists of an urticarial wheal, with or without pseudopods, surrounded by an area of erythema and no response to the control. A positive reaction contraindicates vaccine administration. Have epinephrine 1:1000 and a tourniquet available while performing the sensitivity test.

An intradermal dose of 0.02 ml administered for hypersensitivity testing may induce immunity. However, in such individuals, the presence of specific protective antibodies must be confirmed through evaluation of serum obtained ≈ 4 weeks after skin testing. Contact the state or public health laboratory for assistance.

Immediate hypersensitivity reactions characterized by rash, urticaria or asthma are very rare (< 1 per 1,000,000) and occur principally in persons with histories of egg allergy. Have epinephrine 1:1000 available. Refer to Management of Acute Hypersensitivity Reactions.

Pregnancy: Category C. Avoid use unless travel to high-risk area is unavoidable. Generally, most IgG passage across the placenta occurs during the third trimester. Yellow fever vaccine virus crossed the placenta to one newborn among 41 mothers unknowingly vaccinated during pregnancy. The child appeared unaffected by infection, but yellow fever virus is known to be neurotropic. Avoid vaccination during pregnancy if at all possible.

Lactation: It is not known if yellow fever virus or corresponding antibodies are excreted in breast milk. Problems in humans have not been documented.

Children: The same dose is used for children as for adults. Do not administer to infants < 6 months of age, unless travel to high-risk area is unavoidable, to avoid a risk of encephalitis. Vaccinate pregnant women and infants 6 to 9 months of age only if they must travel and they cannot avoid mosquito bites. Vaccinate infants 4 to 6 months of age only if the risk of infection is high. Use the same dose for children and adults. Do not vaccinate infants < 4 months of age. They are especially vulnerable to swelling of the brain after vaccination.

Precautions:

Blood/Plasma transfusion: Defer vaccination with yellow fever vaccine for 8 weeks following blood or plasma transfusion.

Drug Interactions:

Yellow Fever Vaccine Drug Interactions			
Precipitant drug	Object drug*		Description
Cholera vaccine	Yellow fever vaccine	⬇	Concurrent cholera and yellow fever vaccinations impair the immune response to each vaccine. Separate these vaccinations by ≥ 3 weeks, if possible; may be administered on the same day if separation is not feasible.
Hepatitis B vaccine	Yellow fever vaccine	⬇	Concurrent vaccination against hepatitis B and yellow fever viruses in one study reduced the antibody titer expected from yellow fever vaccine. Separate these vaccinations by 1 month if possible.

YELLOW FEVER VACCINE

Yellow Fever Vaccine Drug Interactions

Precipitant drug	Object drug*		Description
Immune globulins	Yellow fever vaccine	⟷	Yellow fever vaccine does not interact with American-produced immune globulins, although it may be prudent to maintain an interval of several weeks between these drugs if time permits.
Preservatives	Yellow fever vaccine	⬇	Since yellow fever vaccine consists of live viruses, reconstitute it with a diluent that does not contain preservatives. Preservatives may inactivate constituent viruses and render the vaccine ineffective.
Yellow fever vaccine	Immunosuppressants	⬇	Like all live viral vaccines, administration to patients receiving immunosuppressant drugs, including steroids, or radiation may predispose patients to disseminated infections or insufficient response to immunization. They may remain susceptible despite immunization.

* ⬇ = Object drug decreased. ⟷ = Undetermined effect.

Adverse Reactions:

Frequent: Fever or malaise, usually appearing 7 to 14 days after administration (10%; treatment is symptomatic); myalgia and headache (2% to 5%). Fewer than 0.2% curtail regular activities.

Rare: Encephalitis has developed in very young infants; only two cases have been reported in the US. One death has been reported.

Anaphylaxis may occur, even in individuals with no history of hypersensitivity to any vaccine component (see Warnings).

Patient Information:

Advise vaccinated persons to take personal precautions to reduce exposure to mosquito bites. Travelers should stay in screened or air conditioned rooms, use insecticidal space sprays as necessary, and use mosquito repellents and protective clothing to avoid mosquito bites.

Administration and Dosage:

Adults and children: Administer a single immunizing dose of 0.5 ml SC.

Preparation: Reconstitute the vaccine using only the diluent supplied. The vaccine is slightly opalescent and light orange after reconstitution. Draw the volume of the diluent, shown on the diluent label, into a suitable size syringe and inject into the vial containing the vaccine. Slowly add diluent to vaccine, let set for 1 to 2 minutes and then carefully swirl mixture until suspension is uniform. Avoid vigorous shaking as it tends to cause foaming of the suspension. Use vaccine within 60 minutes of reconstitution.

Storage/Stability: Yellow fever vaccine is shipped in a container with dry ice; do not use vaccine unless shipping case contains some dry ice on arrival. Maintain vaccine continuously at a temperature between –30° to 5°C (–22° to 41°F). Elevated temperatures reduce half-life. Sterilize and discard all unused rehydrated vaccine and containers after 1 hour. Shelf life is 12 months.

Rx	**YF-Vax**[1] (Connaught)	**Powder for Injection**: Not less than 5.04 Log_{10} Plaque Forming Units (PFU) per 0.5 ml dose when reconstituted[2]	In single-dose vials with 1 ml diluent, and 5 and 20 dose vials.

[1] Supplied only to designated Yellow Fever Vaccination Centers authorized to issue certificates of Yellow Fever Vaccination.

[2] With gelatin and sorbitol.

HEPATITIS B VACCINE

Actions:

Pharmacology: The recombinant hepatitis vaccines are derived from HBsAg produced in yeast cells.

Hepatitis B vaccine induces protective anti-HBs in most individuals receiving the recommended three-dose regimen. Responsiveness is age-dependent; children respond more vigorously than adults. Immunocompromised and immunosuppressed persons do not respond as well as healthy individuals. Antibody titers ≥ 10 mIU/ml against HBsAg are recognized as conferring protection against hepatitis B. Seroconversion is defined as antibody titers ≥ 1 mIU/ml. Duration of protective effect is unknown. Anti-HBs levels may fall below 10 sample ratio units (protective level) over 3 to 4 years. Periodically determine anti-HBs level.

Hepatitis B vaccine was 80% to 95% effective in preventing acute hepatitis B, asymptomatic infection and antigenemia. Immunity (defined by predetermined serum titers of antibody which prevented hepatitis B infection) was obtained in 87% of vaccinated subjects after two doses; however, a third dose was needed in 96% of the population.

Follow-up data from clinical trials provide no evidence to suggest transmission of AIDS by this vaccine. The vaccines are prepared from recombinant yeast cultures and are free of association with human blood or blood products.

The vaccines, injected into the deltoid, induced protective antibody levels in 93% to 99% of healthy adults, adolescents, children and neonates who received the recommended regimen; in adults ≥ 40 years of age, the protective level is lower (88% to 89%).

Revaccination (booster doses) –

Adults and children with normal immune status: The antibody response to properly administered vaccine is excellent, and protection lasts for at least 5 years. Booster doses are not routinely recommended, nor is routine serologic testing to assess antibody levels in vaccine recipients necessary during this period.

Hemodialysis patients: The vaccine-induced protection is less complete and may persist only as long as antibody levels remain above 10 mIU/ml. Assess the need for booster doses by semiannual antibody testing; give booster doses when antibody levels are < 10 mIU/ml.

Vaccinated persons who experience percutaneous or needle exposure to HBsAg-positive blood: Serologic testing to assess immune status is recommended unless testing within the previous 12 months has indicated adequate antibody levels. If inadequate levels exist, treatment with HBIG or a booster dose of vaccine is indicated.

Nonresponders: Revaccination of persons who do not respond to the primary series produces adequate antibody in only one-third when the primary vaccination has been given in the deltoid. Therefore, revaccination of nonresponders to deltoid injection is not recommended. For persons who did not respond to a primary vaccine series given in the buttock, two small studies suggest that revaccination in the arm induces adequate antibody in over 75%. Strongly consider revaccination for such persons.

Postexposure prophylaxis – Hepatitis B Immune Globulin (HBIG), administered with hepatitis B vaccine at separate sites, does not interfere with induction of protective antibodies against hepatitis B virus.

Interchangeability with hepatitis B vaccines – It is possible to interchange the use of vaccines for completion of a series or for booster doses since studies indicate the antibody produced in response to each type of vaccine is comparable. However, the quantity of antigen or the dosage volume will vary. (Also see Contraindications.)

Indications:

For immunization against infection caused by all known subtypes of hepatitis B virus. Since hepatitis D virus (caused by the delta virus) can only infect and cause illness in persons infected with hepatitis B, immunity to hepatitis B also protects against hepatitis D.

Vaccination is recommended in persons of all ages, especially in those at increased risk of infection with hepatitis B virus.

Healthcare personnel: Dentists; oral surgeons, physicians; surgeons; nurses; paramedical personnel and custodial staff who may be exposed via blood or patient specimens; dental hygienists and nurses; blood bank and plasma fractionation workers; laboratory personnel handling blood, its products and patient specimens; dental, medical and nursing students.

HEPATITIS B VACCINE

Selected patients and patient contacts: Patients and staff in hemodialysis units and hematology/oncology units; patients requiring frequent or large volume blood transfusions or clotting factor concentrates (eg, persons with hemophilia, thalassemia); residents and staff of institutions for the mentally handicapped; classroom contacts of deinstitutionalized mentally handicapped persons who have persistent hepatitis B antigenemia and who show aggressive behavior; household and other intimate contacts of persons with persistent hepatitis B antigenemia.

Adolescents: Because a vaccination strategy limited to high-risk individuals has failed to substantially lower the overall incidence of hepatitis B infection, both the Immunization Practices Advisory Committee (ACIP) and the Committee on Infectious Diseases of the American Academy of Pediatrics (AAP) have endorsed universal infant immunization as part of a comprehensive strategy for the control of hepatitis B infection. These advisory groups further recommend broad-based vaccination of adolescents. The ACIP encourages universal hepatitis B vaccination of adolescents in communities where use of illicit injectable drugs, pregnancy among teenagers, or sexually transmitted diseases are common. Similarly, the AAP recommends that universal immunization of all adolescents should be implemented when resources permit with emphasis on those individuals in high-risk settings. (See Indications.)

Infants, including those born to HBsAg-positive mothers whether HBeAg-positive or -negative: CDC, ACIP and AAP recommend routine vaccination of all infants against hepatitis B.

Populations with high incidence of the disease: Alaskan Eskimos; Pacific islanders, Indochinese refugees; Haitian refugees; refugees from other HBV endemic areas; all infants of women born in areas where the infection is highly endemic.

Persons at increased risk due to their sexual practices: Persons who have heterosexual activity with multiple partners (eg, > 1 partner in a 6 month period), persons who repeatedly contract sexually transmitted diseases, homosexually active males and female prostitutes.

Others at increased risk: Certain military personnel; morticians and embalmers; prisoners; users of illicit injectable drugs; police and fire department personnel who render first aid or medical assistance; blood bank and plasma-fractionation workers; adoptees from countries of high HBV endemicity.

Unlabeled uses: Hepatitis B vaccination is appropriate for persons expected to receive human alpha–1 proteinase inhibitor, which is produced from heat-treated, pooled human plasma that may contain the causative agents of hepatitis and other viral diseases.

Contraindications:

Hypersensitivity to yeast or any component of the vaccines.

Warnings:

Hypersensitivity: Have epinephrine 1:1000 immediately available. Refer to Management of Acute Hypersensitivity Reactions.

Immunosuppressed patients may require larger vaccine doses and may not respond as well as healthy individuals. Refer to Administration and Dosage.

Unrecognized hepatitis B infection may be present at the time the vaccine is given, and the vaccine may not prevent hepatitis B in such patients because of the long incubation period.

Limitations: No hepatitis B vaccine will protect against hepatitis A, C and E viruses or other viruses known to infect the liver.

Elderly: Immunogenicity of hepatitis B vaccine is somewhat reduced in persons > 40 years of age.

Pregnancy: Category C. Safety for use during pregnancy has not been established. Use only when clearly needed and when the potential benefits outweigh potential hazards to the fetus.

Lactation: Safety for use in the nursing mother has not been established.

Children: Hepatitis B vaccine is well tolerated and highly immunogenic in infants and children of all ages. Newborns also respond well; maternally transferred antibodies do not interfere with the active immune response to the vaccine.

Precautions:

Infection: Serious active infection is reason to delay use of hepatitis B vaccine, except when withholding the vaccine entails a greater risk.

Special risk patients: Cautiously administer to individuals with severely compromised cardiopulmonary status or when a febrile or systemic reaction could be a significant risk.

HEPATITIS B VACCINE

Drug Interactions:

Other vaccines: ACIP states that, in general, simultaneous administration of certain live and inactivated pediatric vaccines has not resulted in impaired antibody responses or increased rates of adverse reactions. Use separate sites and syringes for simultaneous administration of injectable vaccines.

Hepatitis B Vaccine (HBV) Drug Interactions			
Precipitant drug	Object drug*		Description
Immunosuppressants	HBV	⬇	Administration of HBV to persons receiving immunosuppressant drugs, including high-dose corticosteroids or radiation therapy, may result in an insufficient response to immunization. They may remain susceptible despite immunization.
HBV	Yellow fever vaccine	⬇	In one study, concurrent vaccination against hepatitis B and yellow fever viruses reduced the antibody titer otherwise expected from yellow fever vaccine. Separate these vaccines by a month, if possible.
HBV	Anticoagulants	⬆	As with other drugs administered by IM injection, give hepatitis B vaccine with caution to persons receiving anticoagulant therapy.
Interleukin-2	HBV	⟷	Natural interleukin-2 may boost systemic immune response to HBsAg in immunodeficient nonresponders to hepatitis B vaccination, but a recombinant interleukin-2 did not augment response to hepatitis B vaccine in healthy adults in one study.

* ⬆ = Object drug increased. ⬇ = Object drug decreased. ⟷ = Undetermined effect.

Adverse Reactions:

Body as a whole: Fatigue/weakness; fever (≥ 100°F); malaise; sweating; achiness; sensation of warmth; chills; flushing; irritability; tingling.

CNS: Headache; lightheadedness; vertigo; dizziness; paresthesia; insomnia; disturbed sleep; somnolence; irritability; agitation; migraine; syncope; paresis; neuropathy including hypoesthesia, Guillain-Barre syndrome, Bell's palsy; transverse myelitis.

Dermatologic: Pruritus; rash (nonspecified); angioedema; urticaria; petechiae; erythema; eczema; purpura; herpes zoster.

GI: Nausea; vomiting; abdominal pain/cramps; dyspepsia; diminished appetite; anorexia; diarrhea; abnormal liver function tests.

Local: Injection site soreness (17% to 22%); erythema; swelling; warmth; induration; pain; tenderness; pruritus; ecchymosis; nodule formation.

Musculoskeletal: Arthralgia; myalgia; back, neck and shoulder pain; neck stiffness.

Respiratory: Pharyngitis; upper respiratory infection; rhinitis; influenza-like symptoms; cough; bronchospasm.

Miscellaneous: Lymphadenopathy; earache; hypotension; dysuria; tachycardia/palpitations; thrombocytopenia; conjunctivitis; keratitis; visual disturbances.

Administration and Dosage:

Route and site: For IM use. Never inject IV. The deltoid muscle is the preferred site in adults. Injections given in the buttocks frequently are given into fatty tissue instead of into muscle and have resulted in a lower seroconversion rate than expected. The anterolateral thigh is the recommended site in infants and young children. May be given SC to persons at risk of hemorrhage following IM injection (eg, hemophiliacs). The immune responses and clinical reactions following IM and SC use are comparable. However, the SC route may produce a less than optimal response, and an increased incidence of local reactions, including subcutaneous nodules, may occur.

HEPATITIS B VACCINE

Immunization Regimen of Hepatitis B Vaccine Doses				
	Initial		1 and 6 months	
Age group	Recombivax HB	Engerix-B	Recombivax HB	Engerix-B
Birth[1] to 10 years	2.5 mcg/0.25 ml or 2.5 mcg/0.5 ml	10 mcg/ 0.5 ml	2.5 mcg/0.25 ml or 2.5 mcg/0.5 ml	10 mcg/ 0.5 ml
11 to 19 years	5 mcg/0.5 ml	20 mcg/ml	5 mcg/0.5 ml	20 mcg/ml
≥ 20 years[2]	10 mcg/ml	20 mcg/ml	10 mcg/ml	20 mcg/ml
Dialysis/ immuno-compromised	40 mcg/ml	40 mcg/ 2 ml[3]	40 mcg/ml	40 mcg/ 2 ml[4]

[1] Infants born of HBsAg negative mothers. If the infant is born of an HBsAg-positive mother, give 0.5 ml of HBIG at birth, then give an appropriate dose of the vaccine (depending on brand) within 7 days of birth and 1 and 6 months later or 1, 2 and 12 months later; use 5 mcg of *Recombivax HB* or 10 mcg of *Engerix-B*.
[2] *Engerix-B* dose for 11–19 years age group is the same.
[3] Two 1 ml doses given at different sites.
[4] Two 1 ml doses given at different sites, plus an additional dose at 2 months.

Post-exposure prophylaxis: See also the HBIG monograph. In response to known or presumed exposure to hepatitis B surface antigen (eg, needle-stick, ocular or mucous-membrane exposure; human bites that penetrate the skin; sexual contact; infants born of HBsAg-positive mothers), give previously unvaccinated persons post-exposure prophylaxis. This consists of 0.06 ml/kg HBIG as soon as possible or within 24 hours after exposure, if possible (within 14 days in the case of sexual contact). Give the appropriate volume of either hepatitis B vaccine based on age within 7 days of exposure, and additional vaccine doses either 1 and 6 months after the first dose or 1, 2 and 12 months later.

Alternate schedule –

Engerix-B: Designed for certain populations (eg, neonates born of hepatitis B-infected mothers, others who have or might have been recently exposed to the virus, certain travelers to high-risk areas).

Alternate Dosing Schedule for Engerix-B				
Age group	Initial	1 month	2 months	12 months
Birth to 10 yrs	10 mcg/0.5 ml	10 mcg/0.5 ml	10 mcg/0.5 ml	10 mcg/0.5 ml[1]
Children > 10 yrs and adults	20 mcg/ml	20 mcg/ml	20 mcg/ml	20 mcg/ml[1]

[1] Recommended for infants born of infected mothers and for others for whom prolonged maintenance of protective titers is desired.

Recombivax HB: An alternate schedule has been recommended. Give doses at 0, 1 and 2 months to provide rapid induction of immunity. On this alternate schedule, give an additional dose 12 months after the first dose if prolonged protection is needed.

Routine infant immunization:

Recombivax HB – From birth through 10 years of age, each dose consists of 2.5 mcg/0.25 ml or 2.5 mcg/0.5 ml.

Engerix-B – From birth through 10 years of age, each dose consists of 10 mcg/0.5 ml.

Nonresponders: Give additional doses of vaccine to persons who do not develop protective levels of anti-HBs antibodies after an initial 3-dose series. Various approaches have been published, involving 1 to 3 extra doses, typically at 1 to 5 month intervals. Roughly 30% to 75% of this group will respond to the second vaccination series.

Revaccination (booster): See Pharmacology.

Engerix-B – Children ≤ 10 years of age – 10 mcg. *Adults and children > 10 years of age* – 20 mcg.

Hemodialysis patients – Assess need by semiannual antibody testing. Give 40 mcg (two 20 mcg doses) when antibody levels decline below 10 mIU/ml.

HEPATITIS B VACCINE

Prophylaxis of perinatal hepatitis B:

Recommended Schedule for Prophylaxis of Perinatal Hepatitis B in Infants Born to Mothers Known to be HBsAg-Positive		
Age of infant	Vaccine dose	HBIG dose
Birth (within 12 hrs)	First	First
1 month	Second	
6 months[1]	Third	

[1] If the 4–dose schedule for *Engerix-B* is used, give the third dose at 2 months of age and the fourth dose at 12 to 18 months.

Recommended Schedule for Prophylaxis of Perinatal Hepatitis B in Infants Born of Mothers Not Screened or Known to be HBsAg-Negative		
Age of infant	Vaccine dose[1]	HBIG dose
Birth (within 12 hours)	First	See footnote[2]
1 to 2 months[3]	Second	
6 months	Third	

[1] If mother was not screened, use appropriate dose for an infant of an HBsAg-positive mother. If the mother is later found to be HBsAg-positive, continue that dose. If the mother is later found to be HBsAg-negative, decrease *Recombivax HB* vaccine dose to appropriate level.

[2] If mother is later found to be HBsAg-positive, administer HBIG to infants as soon as possible, not later than 1 week after birth.

[3] Vaccinate infants of women who are HBsAg-negative beginning at birth or at 2 months of age.

Recombivax HB dialysis formulation is intended only for adult predialysis/dialysis patients.

Dosage – Recommended vaccination schedule is as follows: 1 ml initially, then 1 ml at 1 and 6 months.

Revaccination – A booster dose may be considered if the anti-HBs level is < 10 mIU/ml 1 to 2 months after the third dose.

Preparation: After thorough agitation, the vaccine is a slightly opaque, white suspension. Use as supplied; no dilution or reconstitution is necessary.

Storage/Stability: Store unopened and opened vials at 2° to 8°C (35° to 46°F). Do not freeze; freezing destroys potency. *Recombivax HB* can tolerate 7 days at room temperature without significant loss of potency when prefilled into syringes.

Rx	**Recombivax HB** (Merck)	**Injection (adult formulation)**: 10 mcg/ml hepatitis B surface antigen[1]	In 1 ml single-dose and 3 ml multi-dose vials.
		Injection (pediatric formulation): 2.5 mcg/0.5 ml hepatitis B surface antigen[1]	In 0.5 ml single-dose and 3 ml multi-dose vials.
		Injection (adolescent/high-risk infant formulation): 5 mcg/0.5 ml hepatitis B surface antigen[1]	In 0.5 ml single-dose vials.
		Injection (dialysis formulation): 40 mcg/ml hepatitis B surface antigen[1]	In 1 ml single-dose vials.
Rx	**Engerix-B** (SK-Beecham)	**Injection (adult formulation)**: 20 mcg/ml hepatitis B surface antigen[1]	In 1 ml single-dose and 10 ml multi-dose vials and 1 ml single-dose syringes (23 gauge, 1-inch needle).
		Injection (pediatric formulation): 10 mcg/0.5 ml hepatitis B surface antigen[1]	In 0.5 ml single-dose vials and 0.5 ml single-dose syringes (23 gauge, 1-inch needle).

[1] With 0.005% thimerosal.

HEPATITIS A VACCINE, INACTIVATED

Actions:

Pharmacology: The hepatitis A virus (HAV) belongs to the picornavirus family. Only one serotype of HAV has been described. The virus (strain HM 175) is propagated in MRC human diploid cells.

Hepatitis A is highly contagious, and the predominant mode of transmission is person-to-person via the fecal-oral route. Infection has been shown to be spread (1) by contaminated water or food; (2) by infected food handlers; (3) after breakdown in usual sanitary conditions or after floods or natural disasters; (4) by ingestion of raw or undercooked shellfish (oysters, clams, mussels) from contaminated waters; (5) during travel to areas of the world with poor hygienic conditions; (6) among institutionalized people; (7) in daycare centers where children have not been toilet trained; (8) by parenteral transmission, either blood transfusions or sharing needles with infected people.

The level of economic development influences the prevalence of hepatitis A and the age at which it is most likely to occur. In developing countries with poor hygiene and sanitation, about 90% of children are infected by age 5. As conditions improve, the prevalence decreases and the age at which infection occurs increases. Hence it is more likely to occur in adulthood, when disease is generally more severe and more likely to be fatal. In the US, attack rates for hepatitis A infection are cyclical and vary by population. The rates have increased gradually from 9.2 per 100,000 in 1983 to 14.6 per 100,000 in 1989.

The incubation period for hepatitis A averages 28 days (range, 15 to 50 days). The course of hepatitis A infection is extremely variable, ranging from asymptomatic infection to icteric hepatitis. However, most infected adults (76% to 97%) become symptomatic. Symptoms range from mild and transient to severe and prolonged and may include fever, nausea, vomiting and diarrhea in the prodromal phase, followed by jaundice in up to 88% of adults, as well as hepatomegaly and biochemical evidence of hepatocellular damage. Recovery is generally complete and followed by protection against HAV infection. However, illness may be prolonged, and relapse of clinical illness and viral shedding have been described.

Hepatitis A infection is often asymptomatic in children < 2 years of age, who nonetheless excrete the virus in their stool and thereby serve as a source of infection. In older patients and persons with underlying liver disease, it is generally much more severe. This is reflected in mortality rates. While an overall case fatality rate of 0.6% has been reported, a case fatality rate of 2.7% has been reported in patients ≥ 49 years of age. While 67% of cases occur in children, > 70% of deaths occur in those > 49 years of age.

There is no chronic carrier state. The virus replicates in the liver and is excreted in bile. The highest concentrations of HAV are found in stools of infected persons during the 2-week period immediately before the onset of jaundice and decline after jaundice appears. Children and infants may shed HAV for longer periods than adults, possibly lasting as long as several weeks after the onset of clinical illness. Chronic shedding of HAV in feces has not been demonstrated, but relapses of hepatitis A can occur in as many as 20% of patients; fecal shedding of HAV may recur at this time.

Clinical trials:

Immunogenicity in adults – In three clinical studies involving > 400 healthy adult volunteers given a single 1440 EL.U. dose of the hepatitis A vaccine, specific humoral antibodies against HAV were elicited in > 96% of subjects when measured 1 month after vaccination. By day 15, 80% to 98% of vaccinees had already seroconverted.

In two clinical trials in which a booster dose of 1440 EL.U. was given 6 months following the initial dose, 100% of vaccinees (n = 269) were seropositive 1 month after the booster dose. The titers obtained from this additional dose approximate those observed several years after natural infection.

Immunogenicity in children – In six studies involving children (n = 762; age 1 to 18 years), 99% seroconverted following two doses. When a booster (third) dose was given 6 months following the initial doses, all subjects were seropositive 1 month following the booster dose. The duration of protection afforded by hepatitis A vaccine has not been established; it is unknown if the protection provided to immunized children will last until adulthood.

Protective efficacy – Protective efficacy with hepatitis A vaccine has been demonstrated in children (age 1 to 16 years) in Thailand who were at high risk of HAV infection. There were 32 cases of clinical hepatitis A in the control group; in the hepatitis A vaccine group, only two cases were identified (mild both in terms of biochemical and clinical indices of hepatitis A disease). The calculated efficacy rate for prevention of clinical hepatitis A was 94%. Up to three additional cases of very mild clinical illness may have occurred in vaccinees. By including these as cases, the calculated efficacy rate for prevention of clinical hepatitis A would be 84%.

HEPATITIS A VACCINE, INACTIVATED

Indications:

Hepatitis A virus (HAV): For active immunization of persons ≥ 2 years of age against disease caused by HAV.

Primary immunization should be completed at least 2 weeks prior to expected exposure to HAV. Immunization with hepatitis A vaccine is indicated for those people desiring protection against hepatitis A who are, or will be, at increased risk of infection by HAV:

Travelers – Persons traveling to areas of higher endemicity for hepatitis A. These areas include, but are not limited to, Africa, Asia (except Japan), the Mediterranean basin, Eastern Europe, the Middle East, Central and South America, Mexico and parts of the Caribbean. Consult current CDC advisories with regard to specific locales.

Populations with high incidence of the disease – Native peoples of Alaska and the Americas.

Persons at increased risk due to their employment – Certain institutional workers (eg, caretakers for the developmentally challenged); employees of child day-care centers; laboratory workers who handle live hepatitis A virus; handlers of primate animals that may be harboring HAV.

Others – Persons engaging in high-risk sexual activity (such as homosexually active males); users of illicit injectable drugs; residents of a community experiencing an outbreak of hepatitis A; military personnel; people living in, or relocating to areas of high endemicity.

Contraindications:

Hypersensitivity to any component of the vaccine.

Warnings:

Hepatitis: Hepatitis A vaccine will not prevent hepatitis caused by other agents such as hepatitis B, C or E virus or other pathogens known to infect the liver.

Hypersensitivity: Epinephrine should be available for use in case of anaphylaxis or anaphylactoid reaction.

Pregnancy: Category C. Safety for use during pregnancy has not been established. Use only when clearly needed and when the potential benefits outweigh potential hazards to the fetus.

Lactation: It is not known whether the vaccine is excreted in breast milk. Exercise caution when administering to a nursing woman.

Children: Hepatitis A vaccine is well tolerated and highly immunogenic and effective in children ≥ 2 years of age.

Precautions:

Febrile illness is reason to delay use of hepatitis A vaccine, except when withholding the vaccine entails a greater risk.

Bleeding disorders: Administer cautiously to people with thrombocytopenia or a bleeding disorder as bleeding may occur following IM use.

Immunosuppressed persons or persons receiving immunosuppressive therapy may not obtain the expected immune response.

Transmission: A separate sterile syringe and needle (for single-dose vial) or a sterile disposable unit (prefilled syringe) must be used for each patient to prevent the transmission of infectious agents from person to person. Needles should not be recapped and should be disposed of properly.

Injection site: Do not inject into a blood vessel.

Drug Interactions:

Concomitant administration of a wide variety of other vaccines is unlikely to interfere with the immune response to hepatitis A vaccine. When concomitant administration is required, they should be given with different syringes and at different injection sites.

Adverse Reactions:

The US Department of Health and Human Services has established the Vaccine Adverse Events Reporting System (VAERS) to accept reports of suspected adverse events after the administration of any vaccine, including, but not limited to, the reporting of events required by the National Childhood Vaccine Injury Act of 1986. The toll-free number for VAERS forms and information is 1–800–822–7967.

The most frequently reported reaction was injection-site soreness (56% adults, 15% children); however, < 0.5% of soreness was reported as severe. Other reactions include the following:

Body as a whole: Fatigue, fever [> 37.5°C; 99.5°F], malaise (1% to 10%); anaphylaxis/anaphylactoid reactions, somnolence (rare).

HEPATITIS A VACCINE, INACTIVATED

CNS: Headache (14% adults, < 0.5% children); hypertonic episode, insomnia, photophobia, vertigo (< 1%); convulsions, encephalopathy, dizziness, neuropathy, myelitis, paresthesia, Guillain-Barre syndrome, multiple sclerosis (rare).

Dermatologic: Pruritus, rash, urticaria (< 1%); erythema multiforme, hyperhydrosis, angioedema (rare).

GI: Anorexia, nausea (1% to 10%); abdominal pain; diarrhea; dysgeusia; vomiting.

Local: Injection site soreness (56% adults, 15% children); injection site pain (9.5%); tenderness (8.1%); induration, redness, swelling (1% to 10%); hematoma (< 1%); localized edema (rare).

Musculoskeletal: Arthralgia, elevation of creatine phosphokinase, myalgia (< 1%).

Respiratory: Pharyngitis, other upper respiratory tract infections (< 1%); dyspnea (rare).

Miscellaneous: Lymphadenopathy (< 1%); congenital abnormality, jaundice, hepatitis, syncope (rare).

Patient Information:

For persons traveling to endemic or epidemic areas, consult current CDC advisories with regard to specific locales.

Travelers should take all necessary precautions to avoid contact with or ingestion of contaminated food or water.

The duration of immunity following a complete schedule of immunization with hepatitis A vaccine has not been established.

Administration and Dosage:

Approved by the FDA on February 22, 1995.

Route and site: For IM use. Do not inject IV, ID or SC. In adults, give the injection in the deltoid region. Do not administer in the gluteal region; may result in suboptimal response.

Concomitant agents: May be administered concomitantly with IG, although the ultimate antibody titer obtained may be lower than when the vaccine is given alone. Hepatitis A vaccine has been administered simultaneously with hepatitis B vaccine without interference with their respective immune responses. When concomitant administration of other vaccines or IG is required, they should be given with different syringes and at different injection sites.

Primary immunization regimen:

Adults – A single dose of 1440 EL.U.

Children (2 to 18 years of age) – Two doses, each containing 360 EL.U. given 1 month apart.

Booster dose – A booster dose is recommended anytime between 6 and 12 months after the initiation of the primary course in order to ensure the highest antibody titers.

In those with an impaired immune system, adequate anti-HAV response may not be obtained after the primary immunization course. Such patients may require administration of additional doses of vaccine.

Preparation: Shake vial/syringe well before withdrawal and use. With thorough agitation, the vaccine is an opaque white suspension. Discard if it appears otherwise.

No dilution or reconstitution is necessary. Use the full recommended dose of the vaccine.

Storage/Stability: Store between 2° and 8°C (36° and 47°F). Do not freeze.

Rx	**Havrix** (SmithKline Beecham)	**Injection (pediatric formulation)**: 360 EL.U./0.5 ml of viral antigen[1]	In single-dose vials.[2, 3]
		Injection (pediatric formulation): 720 EL.U./0.5 ml of viral antigen[1]	In single-dose vials and prefilled syringe.[2, 3]
		Injection (adult formulation): 1440 EL.U./1 ml of viral antigen[1]	In single-dose vials and prefilled syringe.[2, 3]

[1] EL.U. = ELISA (enzyme linked immunosorbent assay).

[2] Absorbed on 0.5 mg (pediatric) or 0.25 mg (adult) aluminum (as hydroxide).

[3] With 0.5% 2–phenoxyethanol, 0.3% amino acid supplement, 0.05 mg/ml polysorbate, < 5 mcg residual MRC cellular proteins (adult dose) and < 0.1 mg/ml formalin.

VARICELLA VIRUS VACCINE

Actions:

Pharmacology: Varicella virus vaccine is a preparation of the Oka/Merck strain of live, attenuated varicella virus. The virus was initially obtained from a child with natural

VARICELLA VIRUS VACCINE

varicella, then introduced into human embryonic lung cell cultures, adapted to and propagated in embryonic guinea pig cell cultures and finally propagated in human diploid cell cultures.

Varicella is a highly communicable disease in children, adolescents and adults caused by the varicella-zoster virus. The disease usually consists of 300 to 500 maculopapular or vesicular lesions accompanied by a fever (oral temperature > 37.8°C or > 100°F) in up to 70% of individuals. Approximately 3.5 million cases of varicella occurred annually from 1980 to 1994 in the US with the peak incidence occurring in children 5 to 9 years of age. The incidence rate of chickenpox is 8.3% to 9.1% per year in children 1 to 9 years of age. The attack rate of natural varicella following household exposure among healthy susceptible children was shown to be 87%. Although it is generally a benign, self-limiting disease, varicella may be associated with serious complications (eg, bacterial superinfection, pneumonia, encephalitis, Reye's Syndrome) or death.

Clinical trials:

Children – The majority of subjects who received varicella vaccine and were exposed to wild-type virus were either completely protected from chickenpox or developed a milder form of the disease.

In clinical trials with the current vaccine, it was observed that 0.2% to 1% of vaccinees per year reported breakthrough chickenpox for up to 3 years post single-dose vaccination. This represents an approximate 93% decrease from the total number of cases expected based on attack rates in children aged 1 to 9 over this same period (8.3% to 9.1%). In those who developed breakthrough chickenpox post-vaccination, the majority experienced mild disease.

Among a subset of vaccinees who were actively followed, 259 were exposed to an individual with chickenpox in a household setting. There were no reports of breakthrough chickenpox in 80% of exposed children; 20% reported a mild form of chickenpox. This represents a 77% reduction in the expected number of cases when compared with the historical attack rate of 87% in unvaccinated individuals following household exposure to chickenpox.

In one trial, a single dose of varicella vaccine protected 96% to 100% of children against chickenpox over a 2-year period. The study enrolled healthy individuals 1 to 14 years of age (vaccine, n = 491; placebo, n = 465). In the first year, 8.5% of placebo recipients contracted chickenpox, while no vaccine recipient did, for a calculated protection rate of 100% during the first varicella season. In the second year, when only a subset of individuals agreed to remain in the blinded study (vaccine, n = 163; placebo, n = 161), 96% protective efficacy was calculated for the vaccine group as compared with placebo.

Adults/Adolescents – In up to 2 years of active follow-up, 17 of 64 (27%) vaccinees reported breakthrough chickenpox following household exposure; of the 17 cases, 12 (71%) reported < 50 lesions, 5 reported 50 to 300 lesions and none reported > 300 lesions with an oral temperature > 100°F. In combined clinical studies of adolescents and adults (n = 1019) who received two doses of varicella vaccine and later developed breakthrough chickenpox (42 of 1019), 60% reported < 50 lesions, 38% reported 50 to 300 lesions and 2% reported > 300 lesions and an oral temperature > 100°F.

When compared with the previously reported attack rate of natural varicella of 87% following household exposure among unvaccinated children, this represents ≈ a 70% reduction in the expected number of cases in the household setting.

Immunogenicity – Seroconversion as defined by the acquisition of any detectable varicella antibodies was observed in 97% of vaccinees at ≈ 4 to 6 weeks post-vaccination in 6889 susceptible children 12 months to 12 years of age. Rates of breakthrough disease were significantly lower among children having varicella antibody titers > 5 compared with children having titers < 5. Titers > 5 were induced in ≈ 76% of children vaccinated with a single dose of vaccine. In a multicenter study involving susceptible adolescents and adults 13 years of age and older, two doses of varicella vaccine administered 4 to 8 weeks apart induced a seroconversion rate of ≈ 75% in 539 individuals 4 weeks after the first dose and of 99% in 479 individuals 4 weeks after the second dose. The average antibody response in vaccinees who received the second dose 8 weeks after the first dose was higher than that in those who received the second dose 4 weeks after the first dose. In another multicenter study involving adolescents and adults, two doses of varicella vaccine administered 8 weeks apart induced a seroconversion rate of 94% in 142 individuals 6 weeks after the first dose, 99% in 142 individuals six weeks after the first dose and 99% in 122 individuals six weeks after the second dose.

VARICELLA VIRUS VACCINE

Persistence of immune response – Studies in vaccinees examining chickenpox breakthrough rates over 5 years showed the lowest rates (0.2% to 2.9%) in the first 2 years post-vaccination, with somewhat higher but stable rates in years 3 through 5. The severity of reported breakthrough chickenpox, as measured by number of lesions and maximum temperature, appeared not to increase with time.

In clinical studies involving healthy children who received 1 dose of vaccine, detectable varicella antibodies were present in 98.8% at 1 year, 98.9% at 2 years, 97.5% at 3 years and 99.5% at 4 years post-vaccination. Antibody levels were present at least 1 year in 97.2% of healthy adolescents and adults who received two doses of live varicella vaccine separated by 4 to 8 weeks.

Herpes Zoster – Eight cases of herpes zoster have been reported in children during 44,994 person years of follow-up in clinical trials, resulting in a calculated incidence of at least 18 cases per 100,000 person years. One case of herpes zoster has been reported in the adolescent and adult age group during 7826 person years of follow-up in clinical trials resulting in a calculated incidence of 12.8 cases per 100,000 person years. All nine cases were mild and without sequelae.

Indications:

Varicella: Vaccination against varicella in individuals ≥ 12 months of age.

Contraindications:

Hypersensitivity to any component of the vaccine, including gelatin; history of anaphylactoid reaction to neomycin (each dose of reconstituted vaccine contains trace quantities of neomycin); individuals with blood dyscrasia, leukemia, lymphomas of any type, or other malignant neoplasms affecting the bone marrow or lymphatic systems; concomitant immunosuppressive therapy (see Drug Interactions); individuals with primary and acquired immunodeficiency states, including those who are immunosuppressed in association with AIDS or other clinical manifestations of infection with human immunodeficiency virus, cellular immune deficiencies, and hypogammaglobulinemic and dysgammaglobulinemic states; family history of congenital or hereditary immunodeficiency, unless the immune competence of the potential vaccine recipient is demonstrated; active untreated tuberculosis; any febrile respiratory illness or other active febrile infection; pregnancy (see Warnings).

Warnings:

Booster doses: The duration of protection of varicella vaccine is unknown at present and the need for booster doses is not defined. However, a boost in antibody levels has been observed in vaccinees following exposure to natural varicella as well as following a booster dose of varicella vaccine administered 4 to 6 years post-vaccination.

In a highly vaccinated population, immunity for some individuals may wane due to lack of exposure to natural varicella as a result of shifting epidemiology. Postmarketing surveillance studies are ongoing to evaluate the need and timing for booster vaccination.

Protection/Prevention: Vaccination with varicella vaccine may not result in protection of all healthy, susceptible children, adolescents and adults. It is not known whether varicella vaccine given immediately after exposure to natural varicella virus will prevent illness.

Acute lymphoblastic leukemia (ALL): Children and adolescents with ALL in remission can receive the vaccine under an investigational protocol. More information is available by contacting the varicella vaccine coordinating center: Bio-Pharm Clinical Services, Inc., 4 Valley Square, Blue Bell, PA 19422, (215) 283-0897.

Hypersensitivity: Have adequate treatment provisions, including epinephrine injection (1:1000), available for immediate use should an anaphylactoid reaction occur. Refer to Management of Acute Hypersensitivity Reactions.

Pregnancy: Category C. It is not known whether varicella vaccine can cause fetal harm or affect reproduction capacity when administered to a pregnant woman . However, natural varicella is known to sometimes cause fetal harm. Therefore, varicella vaccine should not be administered to pregnant females; furthermore, pregnancy should be avoided for 3 months following vaccination.

Lactation: It is not known whether varicella vaccine virus is secreted in breast milk. Therefore, because some viruses are secreted in breast milk, exercise caution if varicella vaccine is administered to a nursing woman.

Children: No clinical data are available on safety or efficacy of varicella vaccine in children < 1 year of age; administration to infants < 1 year of age is not recommended.

VARICELLA VIRUS VACCINE

Precautions:

Reye's syndrome: Vaccine recipients should avoid use of salicylates for 6 weeks after vaccination with varicella vaccine as Reye's syndrome has been reported following the use of salicylates during natural varicella infections.

Transmission: Individuals vaccinated with varicella vaccine may potentially be capable of transmitting the vaccine virus to close contacts. Therefore, vaccine recipients should avoid close association with susceptible high-risk individuals (eg, newborns, pregnant women, immunocompromised persons). Weigh the potential risk of transmission of vaccine virus against the risk of transmission of natural varicella virus in such circumstances.

Use a separate sterile needle and syringe for administration of each dose of varicella vaccine to prevent transfer of infectious diseases. Properly dispose of needles and do not recap.

Immunodeficiency: The safety and efficacy of varicella vaccine have not been established in children and young adults who are known to be infected with human immunodeficiency viruses with and without evidence of immunosuppression. Vaccination should be deferred in patients with a family history of congenital or hereditary immunodeficiency until the patient's own immune system has been evaluated.

Injection site: Do not inject into a blood vessel.

Drug Interactions:

Varicella Vaccine Drug Interactions

Precipitant drug	Object drug*		Description
Immune globulins	Varicella vaccine	↔	Vaccination should be deferred for at least 5 months following blood or plasma transfusions, or administration of immune globulin or varicella-zoster immune globulin (VZIG). Following administration of varicella vaccine, any immune globulin, including VZIG, should not be given for 2 months thereafter unless its use outweighs the benefits of vaccination.
Immunosuppressants	Varicella vaccine	⬇	Individuals who are on immunosuppressant drugs are more susceptible to infections than healthy individuals. Vaccination with live attenuated varicella vaccine can result in a more extensive vaccine-associated rash or disseminated disease in individuals on immunosuppressant doses of corticosteroids.
Salicylates	Varicella vaccine	⬆	Avoid use of salicylates for 6 weeks after varicella vaccine; Reye's syndrome has been reported following salicylate use during natural varicella infections.

* ⬆ = Object drug increased. ⬇ = Object drug decreased. ↔ = Undetermined effect.

Concomitant vaccines: Results from clinical studies indicate that varicella vaccine can be administered concomitantly with MMR II.

Limited data from an experimental product containing varicella vaccine suggest that varicella vaccine can be administered concomitantly with DTaP and *PedvaxHIB* (haemophilus b conjugate vaccine) using separate sites and syringes. However, there are no data relating to simultaneous administration of varicella vaccine with DTP or OPV.

Adverse Reactions:

The US Department of Health and Human Services has established a Vaccine Adverse Event Reporting System (VAERS) to accept all reports of suspected adverse events after the administration of any vaccine, including, but not limited to, the reporting of events required by the National Childhood Vaccine Injury Act of 1986. The toll-free number for VAERS forms and information is 1-800-822-7967.

In clinical trials, varicella vaccine was administered to 11,102 healthy children, adolescents and adults; the vaccine was generally well tolerated. In a study of 914 healthy children and adolescents, the only adverse reactions that occurred at a significantly greater rate in vaccine recipients than in placebo recipients were pain and redness at the injection site.

Children (1 to 12 years of age): In clinical trials involving healthy children monitored for up to 42 days after a single dose of varicella vaccine, the frequency of fever, injection-site complaints or rashes were reported as follows: Fever (≥ 39°C [102°F], 14.7%); injection site complaints (pain/soreness, swelling, erythema, rash, pruritus, hematoma, induration, stiffness; 19.3%); varicella-like rash (injection site, 3.4%; generalized, 3.8%).

VARICELLA VIRUS VACCINE

In addition, the most frequently (> 1%) reported adverse experiences, listed in decreasing order of frequency, include: Upper respiratory illness; cough; irritability; nervousness; fatigue; disturbed sleep; diarrhea; loss of appetite; vomiting; otitis; diaper rash/contact rash; headache; teething; malaise; abdominal pain; other rash; nausea; eye complaints; chills; lymphadenopathy; myalgia; lower respiratory illness; allergic reactions (including allergic rash, hives); stiff neck; heat rash/prickly heat; arthralgia; eczema/dry skin/dermatitis; constipation; itching; pneumonitis, febrile seizures (< 1%).

Adults and adolescents (≥ 13 years of age): In clinical trials involving healthy adolescents, the majority of whom received two doses of varicella vaccine and were monitored for up to 42 days after any dose, the frequency of fever, injection-site complaints or rashes were reported as follows: Fever (≥ 39°C [102°F], 9.5% to 10.2%); injection site complaints (soreness, erythema, swelling, rash, pruritus, pyrexia, hematoma, induration, numbness; 24.4% to 32.5%); varicella-like rash (injection site, 1% to 3%; generalized, 0.9% to 5.5%).

In addition, the most frequently (> 1%) reported adverse experiences, listed in decreasing order of frequency, include: Upper respiratory illness; headache; fatigue; cough; myalgia; disturbed sleep; nausea; malaise; diarrhea; stiff neck; irritability; nervousness; lymphadenopathy; chills; eye complaints; abdominal pain; loss of appetite; arthralgia; otitis; itching; vomiting; other rashes; constipation; lower respiratory illness; allergic reactions (including allergic rash, hives); contact rash; cold/canker sore.

Patient Information:

Inform the patient, parent or guardian of the benefits and risks of varicella vaccine, and instruct them to report any adverse reactions to their health-care provider.

Avoid pregnancy for 3 months following vaccination.

Administration and Dosage:

For SC administration; the outer aspect of the upper arm (deltoid) is the preferred site of injection. Do not inject intravenously. During clinical trials, some children received varicella vaccine intramuscularly resulting in seroconversion rates similar to those in children who received the vaccine by the SC route. Persistence of antibody and efficacy in those receiving IM injections have not been defined.

Children (1 to 12 years of age): A single 0.5 ml dose administered subcutaneously.

Adults and adolescents (≥ 13 years of age): A 0.5 ml dose administered subcutaneously at elected date and a second 0.5 ml dose 4 to 8 weeks later.

Reconstitution of vaccine: To reconstitute the vaccine, first withdraw 0.7 ml of diluent into the syringe to be used for reconstitution. Inject all the diluent in the syringe into the vial of lyophilized vaccine and gently agitate to mix thoroughly. Withdraw the entire contents into a syringe, change the needle and inject the total volume (about 0.5 ml) of reconstituted vaccine. It is recommended that the vaccine be administered immediately after reconstitution to minimize loss of potency. Discard if reconstituted vaccine is not used within 30 minutes. Caution: Use a sterile syringe free of preservatives, antiseptics and detergents for each injection or reconstitution of varicella vaccine because these substances may inactivate the vaccine virus. It is important to use a separate sterile syringe and needle for each patient to prevent transmission of infectious agents from one individual to another. To reconstitute the vaccine, use only the diluent supplied, as it is free of preservatives or other antiviral substances that might inactivate the vaccine virus. Do not freeze reconstituted vaccine. Do not give immune globulin (including VZIG) concurrently. When reconstituted, varicella vaccine is a clear, colorless to pale yellow liquid.

Storage/Stability: Varicella vaccine retains a potency level of ≥ 1500 PFU per dose for at least 18 months in a frost-free freezer with an average temperature of -15°C (+5°F) or colder. Varicella vaccine has a minimum potency level of ≈ 1350 PFU 30 minutes after reconstitution at room temperature (20 to 25°C; 68 to 77°F). For information regarding stability at temperatures other than those recommended for storage, call 1-800-9–VARIVAX. During shipment, to ensure that there is no loss of potency, the vaccine must be maintained at a temperature of -20°C (-4°F) or colder. Before reconstitution, store the lyophilized vaccine in a freezer at an average temperature of -15°C (+5°F) or colder. Storage in a frost-free freezer with an average temperature of -15°C (+5°F) or colder is acceptable. Before reconstitution, protect from light. Store the diluent separately at room temperature or in the refrigerator.

Rx	**Varivax** (Merck)	**Powder for Injection:** 1350 PFU of Oka/Merck varicella virus (live)	Sucrose. In single-dose vials: 1s and 10s.

TETANUS TOXOID

Warning:
Trivalent DTP is the preferred immunizing agent for most children up to their seventh birthday. Tetanus and diphtheria toxoids (Td) for adult use is the preferred immunizing agent for most adults and older children. For information about tetanus therapy, refer to the monograph on tetanus immune globulin. The only rational use of fluid tetanus toxoid is in assessing cell-mediated immunity.

Actions:

Pharmacology: Adsorbed tetanus toxoid induces specific protective antibodies against the exotoxin excreted by *Clostridium tetani*. The aluminum salt, a mineral adjuvant, prolongs and enhances the antigenic properties of tetanus toxoid by retarding the rate of absorption. Its duration is ≈ 10 years.

While the rate of seroconversion and promptness of antibody response are essentially equivalent for both the fluid and adsorbed forms of tetanus toxoid, adsorbed toxoids induce higher antitoxin titers and, hence, more persistent antitoxin levels. Therefore, adsorbed tetanus toxoid is strongly recommended for both primary and booster immunizations. Use fluid tetanus toxoid to immunize the rare patient who is hypersensitive to the aluminum adjuvant. The only other rational use remaining for fluid tetanus toxoid is in compounding dilutions of a reagent for delayed-hypersensitivity skin-testing.

Indications:

Adsorbed tetanus toxoid: Selective induction of active immunity against tetanus in selected patients. Tetanus and diphtheria toxoids for adult use (Td) is the preferred immunizing agent for most adults and children after their seventh birthday. All persons should maintain tetanus immunity by means of booster doses throughout life since tetanus spores are ubiquitous. Tetanus immunity is especially important for military personnel, farm and utility workers, those working with horses, firemen and all individuals whose occupation or vocation renders them liable to even minor lacerations and abrasions. Advise travelers to developing nations to maintain active tetanus immunity to obviate any need for therapy with equine tetanus antitoxin and thus avoid associated complications.

Fluid tetanus toxoid: For detection of delayed hypersensitivity and assessment of cell-mediated immunity. May be used for active immunization against tetanus, but a product containing adsorbed tetanus toxoid is preferred. Use fluid tetanus toxoid to immunize the rare patient who is hypersensitive to the aluminum adjuvant. For primary immunization of adults and children, four 0.5 ml doses of tetanus toxoid fluid must be given.

Contraindications:

Adsorbed tetanus toxoid: History of any type of neurological symptoms or signs following administration of this product. Use fluid tetanus toxoid to immunize the rare patient who is hypersensitive to the aluminum adjuvant.

An acute infection is reason for deferring administration of routine primary immunizing or routine recall doses, but not emergency recall doses.

The FDA recommends that elective tetanus immunization be deferred during any outbreak of poliomyelitis since injections are an important cause of provocative poliomyelitis.

Fluid tetanus toxoid: Hypersensitivity to tetanus toxoid or any product components.

Warnings:

Tetanus infection: Under no circumstances should tetanus toxoid be used to treat actual tetanus infections, nor should it be used for immediate prophylaxis of unimmunized individuals. Employ tetanus antitoxin, preferably tetanus immune globulin (human), in all such cases.

Immunodeficiency: Persons receiving immunosuppressive therapy or with other immunodeficiencies may have a diminished antibody response to active immunization. This is a reason for deferring primary diphtheria immunization until treatment is discontinued or for injecting an additional dose ≥ 1 month after treatment has ceased. Nonetheless, routine immunization of symptomatic and asymptomatic HIV-infected persons is recommended.

Hypersensitivity: Take every precaution to prevent and arrest allergic and other untoward reactions. A careful history should review possible sensitivity to the type of protein to be injected. Epinephrine 1:1000 and other appropriate agents should be readily available to combat unexpected allergic reactions. Refer to Management of Acute Hypersensitivity Reactions.

TETANUS TOXOID

Elderly: The elderly develop lower to normal antitoxin levels following tetanus immunization than younger persons. Skin test responsiveness may be delayed or reduced in magnitude in older persons.

Pregnancy: Category C. Use only if clearly needed, although Td is preferred. Based on extensive human experience, there is no evidence that tetanus toxoid is teratogenic. Give a previously unimmunized pregnant woman who may deliver her child under nonhygienic conditions 2 properly spaced doses of a product containing tetanus toxoid adsorbed (eg, Td), preferably during the last 2 trimesters. Incompletely immunized pregnant women should complete their 3 dose primary series. Give those immunized > 10 years previously a booster dose. It is not known if tetanus toxoid or corresponding antibodies cross the placenta. It is unlikely that intradermal tetanus toxoid crosses the placenta. Generally, most IgG passage across the placenta occurs during the third trimester.

Lactation: It is not known if tetanus toxoid or corresponding antibodies are excreted in breast milk. It is unlikely that intradermal tetanus toxoid is excreted in breast milk.

Children: Safety and efficacy of tetanus toxoid are known for children as young as 2 months. Nonetheless, trivalent DTwP or DTaP is the preferred immunizing agent for most children until their seventh birthday. Safety and efficacy as a delayed-hypersensitivity skin-test reagent have not been established.

Drug Interactions:

Tetanus Toxoid Drug Interactions

Precipitant drug	Object drug*		Description
Immunosuppressants	Tetanus toxoid, adsorbed	⬇	Administration of tetanus toxoid, adsorbed, to patients receiving immunosuppressants including corticosteroids or radiation therapy, may result in insufficient response to immunization. They may remain susceptible despite immunization.
Cimetidine	Tetanus toxoid, fluid	⬆	Cimetidine may enhance or augment delayed-hypersensitivity responses to skin-test antigens.
Chloramphenicol	Tetanus toxoid, adsorbed	⬇	Systemic chloramphenicol may impair amnestic response to tetanus toxoid. Avoid concurrent use.
Tetanus immune globulin	Tetanus toxoid, adsorbed	⬇	Concurrent use may delay development of active immunity by several days; however, this interaction is not clinically significant and does not preclude concurrent use.

* ⬆ = Object drug increased ⬇ = Object drug decreased

Adverse Reactions:

Adsorbed tetanus toxoid: A small amount of erythema and induration surrounding the injection site, persisting for a few days, is not unusual. A nodule may be palpable at the injection site for a few weeks. Allow such nodules to recede spontaneously and do not incise. Sterile abscesses (incidence, < 6 to 10 cases per million doses) and SC atrophy may also occur. Adverse reactions often associated with multiple prior booster doses may be manifested 2 to > 12 hours after administration by erythema, boggy edema, pruritus, lymphadenopathy and induration surrounding the site of injection. Pain and tenderness are usually not the primary complaints.

Low-grade fever; chills; malaise; generalized aches and pains; headaches; flushing; generalized urticaria or pruritus; tachycardia; anaphylaxis; hypotension; neurological complications.

Although the cause is unknown, hypersensitivity to the exotoxin or bacillary protein of the tetanus organism itself is assumed to be possible. In other persons, interaction between the injected antigen and high levels of preexisting tetanus antibody from prior booster doses seems to be the most likely cause of these Arthus-like responses. Do not give these persons even emergency doses of tetanus toxoid more frequently than every 10 years.

Fluid tetanus toxoid: Markedly hypersensitive persons may develop a local reaction at the injection site. Mild exaggeration of the patient's allergic symptoms, hives, anaphylactic reactions, shock and death from anaphylaxis may occur.

TETANUS TOXOID

Administration and Dosage:

Federal law requires that (1) the manufacturer and lot number of this vaccine, (2) the date of its administration, and (3) the name, address and title of the person administering the vaccine be documented in the recipient's permanent medical record or in a permanent office log. Certain adverse events must be reported to the VAERS system, 1-800-822-7967.

Tetanus toxoid, adsorbed: Administer IM, preferably into the deltoid or midlateral thigh muscles. In infants, the vastus lateralis (mid-thigh laterally) is the preferred site.

Tetanus toxoid, fluid: As a diluted skin-test reagent, administer intradermally typically to the volar surface of the forearm. For immunization, inject IM or SC.

Primary immunization for adults and children:

Primary Immunization of Tetanus Toxoid[1]		
	Tetanus toxoid	
Administration	Adsorbed	Fluid
Dose (route)	0.5 ml (IM)	0.5 ml (IM or SC)[2]
Number of injections	2	3
Interval (weeks)	4 to 8	4 to 8
Additional dose	Give a third dose of 0.5 ml approximately 6 to 12 months after second injection	Give a fourth dose of 0.5 ml approximately 6 to 12 months after third injection
Booster dose	0.5 ml every 10 years	0.5 ml every 10 years

[1] Adults and children beginning at 6 to 8 weeks of age.

[2] For use as a skin test cell-mediated immunity reagent, use 0.1 ml of 1:100 v/v or 0.02 ml of 1:10 v/v.

Concomitant vaccines: Several routine vaccines may safely and effectively be administered simultaneously at separate injection sites (eg, DTP or Td, MMR, OPV or IPV, Hib, hepatitis B). National authorities recommend simultaneous immunization at separate sites as indicated by age or health risk, if return of a vaccine recipient for a subsequent visit is doubtful.

Tetanus prophylaxis in wound management: Tetanus and diphtheria toxoids adsorbed for adults (Td) is the preferred preparation for active tetanus immunization in wound management of patients ≥ 7 years of age. This is to enhance diphtheria protection, since a large proportion of adults are susceptible. Tetanus immune globulin is the product of choice for passive immunization. Refer to individual monographs.

Storage/Stability: Store at 2° to 8°C (36° to 46°F). Do not freeze. Discard frozen toxoid.

TETANUS TOXOID, FLUID

For complete prescribing information, refer to the Tetanus Toxoid group monograph.

Rx	**Tetanus Toxoid, Fluid** (Connaught)	**Injection:** 4 Lf units tetanus per 0.5 ml dose	In 7.5 ml vials. Thimerosal.
Rx	**Tetanus Toxoid, Fluid** (Wyeth-Ayerst)	**Injection:** 5 Lf units tetanus per 0.5 ml dose	In 0.5 ml *Tubex* and 7.5 ml vials. Thimerosal.

TETANUS TOXOID, ADSORBED

For complete prescribing information, refer to the Tetanus Toxoid group monograph.

Rx	**Tetanus Toxoid, Adsorbed** (Biocine Sclavo)	**Injection:** 10 Lf units tetanus per 0.5 ml dose	Aluminum hydroxide and thimerosal. In 0.5 and 5 ml vials.
Rx	**Tetanus Toxoid, Adsorbed** (Connaught)	**Injection:** 5 Lf units tetanus per 0.5 ml dose	Aluminum potassium and thimerosal. In 5 ml vials.
Rx	**Tetanus Toxoid, Adsorbed** (Lederle-Praxis)	**Injection:** 5 Lf units tetanus per 0.5 ml dose	Aluminum phosphate and thimerosal. In 0.5 ml disp. syringes and 5 ml vials.

TETANUS TOXOID, ADSORBED

Rx	**Tetanus Toxoid, Adsorbed** (Wyeth-Ayerst)	**Injection:** 5 Lf units tetanus per 0.5 ml dose	Aluminum phosphate and thimerosal. In 0.5 ml *Tubex* and 5 ml vials.

DIPHTHERIA AND TETANUS TOXOIDS, COMBINED (DT; Td)

Refer to general discussion of Agents for Active Immunization.

Warning:

Trivalent DTP is the preferred immunizing agent for most children. Use whole-cell DTP (DTwP) for the first three doses; either DTwP or acellular DTP (DTaP) may be used for the fourth and fifth doses. Tetanus and diphtheria toxoids for adult use (Td) is the preferred immunizing agent for most adults and older children.

Specific information about the individual components of this drug appear in the individual monographs on diphtheria toxoid and tetanus toxoid.

Actions:

Pharmacology: These preparations combine diphtheria and tetanus toxins (detoxified by formaldehyde). Adequate immunization with diphtheria toxoid is thought to confer protection for at least 10 years. It significantly reduces both the risk of developing diphtheria and the severity of clinical illness. It does not, however, eliminate carriage of *Corynebacterium diphtheriae* in the pharynx or on the skin. A serum level ≥ 0.01 toxin neutralization units/ml is generally protective.

Tetanus toxoid is highly effective, with a failure rate in fully immunized persons of < 4 per 100 million. Protective levels of serum antitoxin (≥ 0.01 toxin neutralization units/ml) are achieved which persist for at least 10 years after full immunization.

Indications:

Pediatric (DT): Selective induction of active immunity against tetanus and diphtheria in infants and children from age 2 months to the seventh birthday. Maintain tetanus immunity by means of booster doses throughout life since tetanus spores are ubiquitous. Trivalent DTP is the preferred immunizing agent for most children up to their seventh birthday. Use diphtheria and tetanus toxoids for pediatric use (DT) only for children for whom pertussis vaccination alone is contraindicated.

Adult (Td): Induction of active immunity against tetanus and diphtheria. Tetanus and diphtheria toxoids for adult use (Td) is the preferred immunizing agent for most adults and children after their seventh birthday. All persons should maintain tetanus immunity by means of booster doses throughout life since tetanus spores are ubiquitous. Tetanus immunity is especially important for military personnel, farm and utility workers, those working with horses, firemen and all individuals whose occupation or vocation renders them susceptible to even minor lacerations and abrasions. Advise travelers to developing nations to maintain active tetanus immunity to obviate any need for therapy with equine tetanus antitoxin and thus avoid associated complications.

Contraindications:

Patients > 7 years of age (DT); history of serious adverse reaction to constituents of this drug.

An acute infection is reason for deferring administration of routine primary immunizing or recall booster doses, but not emergency recall booster doses.

Warnings:

Infections: Do not use for treatment of actual tetanus or diphtheria infections.

Immunodeficiency: Persons receiving immunosuppressive therapy or with other immunodeficiencies may have diminished antibody response to active immunization. This is a reason for deferring primary diphtheria immunization until discontinuing treatment or for injecting an additional dose ≥ 1 month after discontinuing treatment. Nonetheless, routine immunization of symptomatic and asymptomatic HIV-infected persons is recommended.

Hypersensitivity: Have epinephrine 1:1000 immediately available. Refer to Management of Acute Hypersensitivity Reactions.

Elderly: Use of DT is contraindicated after the seventh birthday. Tetanus and diphtheria toxoids for adult use (Td) is the preferred immunizing agent for most adults and older children. The elderly develop lower to normal antitoxin levels following tetanus immunization than younger persons.

Pregnancy: Category C. Use Td only if clearly needed. There is no evidence that tetanus toxoid is teratogenic. Give a previously unimmunized pregnant woman who may deliver her child under nonhygienic conditions two properly spaced doses of a product containing tetanus toxoid (eg, Td), preferably during the last two trimesters. Incompletely immunized pregnant women should complete the 3 dose series. Give those immunized > 10 years previously a booster dose. Generally, most IgG passage across the placenta occurs during the third trimester.

Lactation: It is not known if DT or Td antigens or corresponding antibodies are excreted in breast milk.

DIPHTHERIA AND TETANUS TOXOIDS, COMBINED (DT; Td)

Children: DT is indicated for children > 6 weeks and < 7 years of age in whom pertussis vaccination is contraindicated. Trivalent DTwP or DTaP is the preferred immunizing agent for most children up to their seventh birthday. Td is the preferred immunizing agent for most adults and children > 7 years of age.

Drug Interactions:

DT/Td Drug Interactions			
Precipitant drug	Object drug*		Description
DT/Td	Immunosuppressants	⬇	Like all inactivated vaccines, administration of DT/Td vaccine to persons receiving immunosuppressant drugs, including high-dose corticosteroids or radiation, may result in an insufficient response to immunization. They may remain susceptible despite immunization.
DT/Td	Anticoagulants	⬆	As with other drugs administered by IM injection, give with caution to persons receiving anticoagulants.

* ⬆ = Object drug increased. ⬇ = Object drug decreased.

Adverse Reactions:

Systemic: Transient low-grade fever, chills, malaise, generalized aches and pains, headaches, flushing, generalized urticaria or pruritus, tachycardia, anaphylaxis, hypotension, neurological complications. Although the cause is unknown, hypersensitivity to the toxin or bacillary protein of the tetanus organism itself is assumed to be possible. In other persons, interaction between the injected antigen and high levels of preexisting tetanus antibody from prior booster doses seems to be the most likely cause of the Arthus-like response. Do not give these persons even emergency doses of tetanus more frequently than every 10 years.

Local: Mild to moderate pain, tenderness, swelling and redness (8% to 10%); edema; erythema; induration surrounding the injection site for a few days. Persistent nodules and sterile abscesses may occur. A nodule may be palpable at injection site for a few weeks.

Severe local reactions (generally starting 2 to 8 hours after an injection) have been reported from tetanus toxoids prepared by different manufacturers. Hypersensitivity to the toxin or bacillary protein is a possible cause. Interreaction between the injected antigen and high levels of preexisting tetanus antibody (antitoxin) from prior booster doses seems the most likely cause of the Arthus-type response.

The National Childhood Vaccine Injury Act requires the healthcare provider to report to the Secretary of the Department of Health and Human Services through the Vaccine Adverse Event Reporting System (VAERS) the occurrence following immunization of any event set forth in the Vaccine Injury Table, including: Anaphylaxis or anaphylactic shock within 24 hours; encephalopathy or encephalitis within 7 days; shock-collapse or hypotonic-hyporesponsive collapse within 7 days; residual seizure disorder; any acute complication of sequelae (including death) of above events, or any event that would contraindicate further doses of vaccine.

The US Department of Health and Human Services has established VAERS to accept all reports of suspected adverse events after the administration of any vaccine, including but not limited to the reporting of events required by the National Childhood Vaccine Injury Act of 1986. The VAERS toll-free number for forms and information is 800-822-7967.

DIPHTHERIA AND TETANUS TOXOIDS, COMBINED (DT; Td)

Administration and Dosage:

The National Childhood Vaccine Injury Act requires that the manufacturer and lot number of the vaccine administered be recorded by the healthcare provider in the vaccine recipient's permanent medical record (or in a permanent office log or file), along with the date of administration of the vaccine and the name, address and title of the person administering the vaccine.

Interruption of the recommended schedule with a delay between doses does not interfere with the final immunity achieved, nor does it necessitate starting the series over again, regardless of the length of time elapsed between doses.

Shake vial well before withdrawing each dose.

Do not inject intracutaneously or SC. Ensure that injection does not enter a blood vessel. For adults, give IM in the vastus lateralis (mid-thigh laterally), gluteus or deltoid. For infants, the vastus lateralis is preferred. Avoid injection in the deltoid area in infants; also avoid the gluteus maximus due to the potential for sciatic nerve damage. During primary immunization, do not inject the same site more than once.

Children:

Primary immunizing series – Beginning at 6 to 8 weeks of age, two 0.5 ml doses, at an interval of 4 to 8 weeks, followed by a third reinforcing 0.5 ml dose 6 to 12 months later. The third dose is an integral part of the primary series. Do not consider basic immunization complete until the third dose has been given.

When immunization with DT begins in the first year of life (rather than immunization with DTwP), the primary series consists of three 0.5 ml doses, 4 to 8 weeks apart, followed by a fourth reinforcing 0.5 ml dose 6 to 12 months after the third dose.

Immunization of infants normally starts at 6 weeks to 2 months of age; always start immunization at once if diphtheria is present in the community. Give unimmunized children ≤ 1 year of age in whom pertussis immunization is contraindicated two 0.5 ml DT doses 4 to 8 weeks apart, followed by a third 0.5 ml dose 6 to 12 months after the second dose, to complete the primary series.

Adults and children (≥ 7 years of age): 2 primary doses of 0.5 ml each, given at an interval of 4 to 8 weeks, followed by a third (reinforcing) 0.5 ml dose 6 to 12 months later; basic immunization is not complete until the third dose is given.

Booster dose – Give routine recall (booster) 0.5 ml doses of tetanus and diphtheria toxoids for adult use (Td) at 10 year intervals throughout life to maintain immunity. Upon intimate exposure to diphtheria, an emergency recall booster dose of 0.5 ml (based on age) may be indicated. If emergency tetanus prophylaxis is indicated during the period between the third primary dose and the reinforcing dose, give a 0.5 ml dose of monovalent tetanus toxoid adsorbed. If given before 6 months have elapsed, count this dose as the primary dose. If given after 6 months, regard it as a reinforcing dose.

Wound management: For tetanus prophylaxis in wound management, refer to the Tetanus Toxoid monograph.

Storage: Store between 2° to 8°C (36° to 46°F). Do not freeze.

DIPHTHERIA AND TETANUS TOXOIDS, ADSORBED (FOR PEDIATRIC USE)

For complete prescribing information, refer to the Diphtheria and Tetanus Toxoids, Combined group monograph.

For use only in patients ≤ 6 years of age.

Rx	**Diphtheria & Tetanus Toxoids, Pediatric** (Connaught)	**Injection:** 6.6 Lf units diphtheria and 5 Lf units tetanus per 0.5 ml dose	In 5 ml multidose vials.[2]
Rx	**Diphtheria & Tetanus Toxoids, Pediatric** (Lederle-Praxis)	**Injection:** 12.5 Lf units diphtheria and 5 Lf units tetanus per 0.5 ml dose	In 5 ml multidose vials.[3]
Rx	**Diphtheria & Tetanus Toxoids, Pediatric** (Massachusetts Public Health Biologic Labs)	**Injection:** 7.5 Lf units diphtheria and 7.5 Lf units tetanus per 0.5 ml dose	In multidose vials.[1]
Rx	**Diphtheria & Tetanus Toxoids, Pediatric** (Wyeth-Ayerst)	**Injection:** 10 Lf units diphtheria and 5 Lf units tetanus per 0.5 ml dose	In 0.5 ml *Tubex*.[4] and 5 ml multidose vials.[4]

[1] With aluminum hydroxide, thimerosal.
[2] In saline with aluminum potassium sulfate, thimerosal.
[3] With aluminum phosphate, glycine, thimerosal.
[4] With aluminum phosphate, thimerosal.

DIPHTHERIA AND TETANUS TOXOIDS, ADSORBED (FOR ADULT USE)

For complete prescribing information, refer to the Diphtheria and Tetanus Toxoids, Combined group monograph.

Contains ≤ 2 Lf units of diphtheria toxoid per 0.5 ml.

Rx	**Diphtheria & Tetanus Toxoids, Adult** (Connaught)	**Injection:** 2 Lf units diphtheria and 5 Lf units tetanus per 0.5 ml dose	In 5 and 30 ml multidose vials.[2]
Rx	**Diphtheria & Tetanus Toxoids, Adult** (Lederle-Praxis)	**Injection:** 2 Lf units diphtheria and 5 Lf units tetanus per 0.5 ml dose	In 0.5 ml disp. syringes[3] and 5 ml multidose vials.[3]
Rx	**Diphtheria & Tetanus Toxoids, Adult** (Massachusetts Public Health Biologic Labs)	**Injection:** 2 Lf units diphtheria and 2 Lf units tetanus per 0.5 ml dose	In multidose vials.[4]
Rx	**Diphtheria & Tetanus Toxoids, Adult** (Wyeth-Ayerst)	**Injection:** 2 Lf units diphtheria and 5 Lf units tetanus per 0.5 ml dose	In 0.5 ml *Tubex*[4] and 5 ml multidose vials[4].

[1] With aluminum hydroxide, thimerosal.
[2] In saline with aluminum potassium sulfate, thimerosal.
[3] In saline with aluminum phosphate, glycine, thimerosal.
[4] With aluminum phosphate, thimerosal.

DIPHTHERIA AND TETANUS TOXOIDS AND WHOLE-CELL PERTUSSIS VACCINE, ADSORBED (DTwP)

Refer to general discussion of Agents for Active Immunization.

> **Warning:**
> *Note:* Trivalent DTP is the preferred immunizing agent for most children. Use whole-cell DTP (DTwP) for the first three doses; either DTwP or acellular DTP (DTaP) may be used for the fourth and fifth doses. Tetanus and diphtheria toxoids for adult use (Td) is the preferred immunizing agent for adults and older children.

Actions:

Pharmacology: These preparations combine diphtheria and tetanus toxins (detoxified by formaldehyde) with pertussis vaccine. Adequate immunization with diphtheria toxoid is thought to confer protection for at least 10 years. It significantly reduces both the risk of developing diphtheria and the severity of clinical illness. It does not, however, eliminate carriage of *Corynebacterium diphtheriae* in the pharynx or on the skin. A serum level ≥ 0.01 toxin neutralization units/ml is generally protective.

Tetanus toxoid is highly effective, with a failure rate in fully immunized persons of < 4 per 100 million. Protective levels of serum antitoxin (≥ 0.01 toxin neutralization units/ml) are achieved which persist for at least 10 years after full immunization.

A protective level of antipertussis antibodies has not been determined.

Indications:

For active immunization of infants and children through 6 years of age (between 6 weeks and the 7th birthday) against diphtheria, tetanus and pertussis. Recommended for both primary immunization and routine recall. Start immunization at once if whooping cough or diphtheria is present in the community.

Contraindications:

Not recommended for use in adults, in children ≥ 7 years of age or in children < 6 weeks of age; further doses of a vaccine containing pertussis antigens to children who have recovered from culture-confirmed pertussis; history of serious adverse reactions to a previous dose of a pertussis-containing vaccine; hypersensitivity to any component of the vaccine, including thimerosal; immediate anaphylactic reaction or encephalopathy occurring within 7 days following DTP vaccination (such encephalopathies may include major alterations in consciousness, unresponsiveness, generalized or focal seizures that persist more than a few hours and failure to recover within 24 hours or other generalized or focal neurological signs); during the course of any febrile illness or acute infection (a minor respiratory illness such as a mild upper respiratory infection is not usually reason to defer immunization).

If a contraindication to the pertussis vaccine component occurs, substitute diphtheria and tetanus toxoids for pediatric use (DT) for each of the remaining doses.

The occurrence of any type of neurological symptoms or signs, including one or more convulsions, following DTwP administration is generally a contraindication to further use. The presence of any evolving or changing disorder affecting the CNS contraindicates administration of pertussis vaccine regardless of whether the suspected neurological disorder is associated with occurrence of seizure activity of any type.

Warnings:

Infections: Do not use DTwP for treatment of actual tetanus, diphtheria or whooping cough infections.

Convulsions: The Immunization Practices Advisory Committee (ACIP) and the American Academy of Pediatrics (AAP) have reviewed the risks and benefits of pertussis vaccine for infants and children with a family history of convulsions. Based on this review, the ACIP and AAP believe that a family history of convulsions should not be a contraindication to DTP vaccination. Also, the ACIP believes that antipyretic use with DTwP vaccination may be reasonable in children with personal or family histories of convulsions.

There are no data on whether prophylactic use of antipyretic drugs (eg, acetaminophen) can decrease the risk of febrile convulsions. Data do suggest that acetaminophen will reduce the incidence of post-vaccination fever. ACIP and AAP suggest administering an appropriate dose of acetaminophen based on age at the time of vaccination and every 4 to 6 hours to children at higher risk for seizures than the general population (ie, children with a personal or family history of seizures.)

Hypersensitivity: Review the patient's history regarding possible sensitivity. Have epinephrine 1:1000 immediately available. Refer to Management of Acute Hypersensitivity Reactions.

DIPHTHERIA AND TETANUS TOXOIDS AND WHOLE-CELL PERTUSSIS VACCINE, ADSORBED (DTwP)

Pregnancy: Category C. DTP is generally contraindicated after the 7th birthday. It is not known if DTP antigens or corresponding antibodies cross the placenta. Generally, most IgG passage across the placenta occurs during the third trimester.

Lactation: It is not known if DTP antigens or corresponding antibodies are excreted into breast milk.

Children: Do not reduce or divide the DTP dose for preterm infants or any other children. DTP is contraindicated in children < 6 weeks of age, since the product may not be immunogenic. DTP is also contraindicated in children > 7 years of age because of their decreased risk of pertussis and increased likelihood of adverse effects. DTwP or DTaP is the preferred immunizing agent for most children up to their 7th birthday. Tetanus diphtheria toxoids for adult use (Td) is the preferred immunizing agent for adults and older children.

Precautions:

Adverse events: When an infant or child returns for the next dose in the series, question the parent concerning occurrence of any symptoms or signs of adverse reactions after the previous dose. If such are reported, further doses of DTwP are contraindicated; complete active immunization against diphtheria and tetanus with diphtheria and tetanus toxoids, adsorbed (pediatric) (see individual monograph).

Several events were previously listed as contraindications, but are now listed simply as precautions, warranting careful consideration: Temperature 40.5° C (105° F) within 48 hours after DTwP administration not due to another identifiable cause; collapse or shock-like state (hypotonic-hyporesponsive episode) within 48 hours; persistent inconsolable crying lasting ≥ 3 hours within 48 hours; or convulsions with or without fever within 3 days. There may be circumstances, such as a high local incidence of pertussis, in which the potential benefits outweigh possible risks, particularly because these events are not associated with permanent sequelae.

Immunodeficiency: Persons receiving immunosuppressive therapy or with other immunodeficiencies may have a diminished antibody response to active immunization. Defer vaccination in persons receiving immunosuppressive therapy. Nonetheless, routine immunization of symptomatic and asymptomatic HIV-infected persons is recommended.

Drug Interactions:

DTwP Drug Interactions			
Precipitant drug	Object drug*		Description
DTwP	Immunosuppressants	⬇	Like all inactivated vaccines, administration of DTwP vaccine to persons receiving immunosuppressant drugs, including high-dose corticosteroids or radiation therapy, may result in an insufficient response to immunization. They may remain susceptible despite immunization.
DTwP	Anticoagulants	⬆	As with other drugs administered by IM injection, give with caution to persons receiving anticoagulant therapy.

* ⬆ = Object drug increased. ⬇ = Object drug decreased.

Adverse Reactions:

The National Childhood Vaccine Injury Act requires the healthcare provider to report to the Secretary of the Department of Health and Human Services through the Vaccine Adverse Event Reporting System (VAERS) the occurrence following immunization of any event set forth in the Vaccine Injury Table, including: Anaphylaxis or anaphylactic shock within 24 hours; encephalopathy or encephalitis within 7 days; shock-collapse or hypotonic-hyporesponsive collapse within 7 days; residual seizure disorder; any acute complication of sequelae (including death) of above events, or any event that would contraindicate further doses of vaccine.

The US Department of Health and Human Services established VAERS to accept all reports of suspected adverse events after administration of any vaccine, including but not limited to the reporting of events required by the National Childhood Vaccine Injury Act of 1986. The VAERS toll-free number for forms and information is 800-822-7967.

DIPHTHERIA AND TETANUS TOXOIDS AND WHOLE-CELL PERTUSSIS VACCINE, ADSORBED (DTwP)

Local: Mild local and constitutional reactions (40% to 60%): Pain, induration and redness at the injection site, usually beginning within 72 hours after vaccination. Occasionally a nodule is induced at the injection site that can persist for several weeks. These reactions are self-limiting and usually require no treatment. Rarely, an abscess develops at the injection site. Mild constitutional reactions consist chiefly of febrile reactions (38.2° to 40.4°C; 101° to 104.7°F). Constitutional reactions usually begin within 12 hours after vaccination, persist for 1 to 7 days, and may be accompanied by irritability, malaise, sleepiness or vomiting.

Systemic: Reactions that constitute absolute contraindications to further vaccination with the pertussis component include: Convulsions; encephalopathy; focal neurological disease; collapse; shock; altered consciousness. Reactions such as thrombocytopenic purpura and demonstrable hypersensitivity reactions such as anaphylaxis, generalized urticarial eruptions, or Arthus-type reactions after administration of either pertussis or DTwP vaccines also constitute an absolute contraindication to additional immunization with these vaccines. Other reactions include excessive somnolence, excessive screaming (persistent crying or screaming for ≥ 3 hours), temperature > 40.5°C (105°F). Peripheral neuropathy can follow DTwP vaccination, possibly due in some cases to injection of vaccine too close to a peripheral nerve.

An expert panel assembled by the Institute of Medicine has concluded that no causal association exists between pertussis vaccination and SIDS.

Administration and Dosage:

The National Childhood Vaccine Injury Act requires that the manufacturer and lot number of the vaccine administered be recorded by the healthcare provider in the vaccine recipient's permanent medical record (or in a permanent office log or file), along with the date of administration of the vaccine and the name, address and title of the person administering the vaccine.

Interruption of the recommended schedule with a delay between doses does not interfere with the final immunity achieved, nor does it necessitate starting the series over again, regardless of the length of time elapsed between doses.

Inject IM. The midlateral muscle of the thigh is preferred for infants. Do not inject the same muscle site more than once during the course of basic immunization.

Primary immunization: For children 6 weeks through 6 years of age, administer 0.5 ml IM on 3 occasions beginning at 6 weeks of age, then at 4 to 8 week intervals with a reinforcing dose administered 1 year after the 3rd injection. Give preterm infants a full 0.5 ml dose at the normal chronologic age after birth.

Booster doses: Administer 0.5 ml IM when the child is 4 to 6 years of age (preferably prior to entering kindergarten or elementary school). However, if the 4th dose of the basic immunization series was administered after the 4th birthday, a recall (booster) of DTP prior to school entry is not necessary.

For booster doses thereafter, use the recommended dose of diphtheria and tetanus toxoids, adsorbed (adult) every 10 years. Do not immunize persons ≥ 7 years of age with pertussis vaccine.

Storage: Store between 2° to 8°C (36° to 46°F). Do not freeze.

Rx	**Diphtheria & Tetanus Toxoids & Pertussis Vaccine** (Connaught)	**Injection**: 6.5 Lf units diphtheria, 5 Lf units tetanus and 4 units pertussis per 0.5 ml dose	In 2.5, 5 and 7.5 ml multidose vials.[1]
Rx	**Diphtheria & Tetanus Toxoids & Pertussis Vaccine** (Massachusetts Public Health Biologic Labs)	**Injection:** 10 Lf units diphtheria, 5.5 Lf units tetanus and 4 units pertussis per 0.5 ml dose	In 5 ml multidose vials.[2]
Rx	**DTwP** (Michigan Dept. of Public Health/SKB)		In 5 ml multidose vials.[3]
Rx	**Tri-Immunol** (Lederle-Praxis)	**Injection:** 12.5 Lf units diphtheria, 5 Lf units tetanus and 4 units pertussis per 0.5 ml dose	In 7.5 ml multidose vials.[3]

[1] In saline solution with aluminum potassium sulfate, thimerosal.
[2] In saline solution with aluminum phosphate, thimerosal.
[3] In saline solution with aluminum, thimerosal.

DIPHTHERIA AND TETANUS TOXOIDS AND ACELLULAR PERTUSSIS VACCINE (DTaP)

Refer to general discussion of Agents for Active Immunization.

Warning:

Note: Trivalent DTP is the preferred immunizing agent for most children. Use whole-cell DTP for the first three doses; either DTwP or acellular DTP (DTaP) may be used for the fourth and fifth doses. Tetanus and diphtheria toxoids for adult use (Td) is the preferred immunizing agent for adults and older children.

Whole-cell and acellular DTP (DTwP and DTaP) products are not generically equivalent due to differences in composition and side effect incidence. Restrict acellular DTP vaccines to fourth and fifth doses of a primary immunizing series.

Actions:

Pharmacology: These preparations combine diphtheria and tetanus toxoids with acellular pertussis bacterial vaccine. The acellular pertussis component consists of pertussis toxin (PT) and filamentous hemagglutinin (FHA), treated with formaldehyde to inactivate the toxin into a toxoid. Adequate immunization with diphtheria toxoid is thought to confer protection for at least 10 years. It significantly reduces both the risk of developing diphtheria and the severity of clinical illness. It does not, however, eliminate carriage of *Corynebacterium diphtheriae* in the pharynx or on the skin. A serum level ≥ 0.01 toxin neutralization units/ml is generally protective.

Tetanus toxoid is highly effective, with a failure rate in fully immunized persons of < 4 per 100 million. Protective levels of serum antitoxin (≥ 0.01 toxin neutralization units/ml) are achieved which persist for at least 10 years after full immunization.

A protective level of antipertussis antibodies has not been determined.

Indications:

Induction of active immunity against diphtheria, tetanus and pertussis as the fourth or fifth dose in children, from age 15 months (*Tripedia*) or 17 months *(Acel-Imune)* through the 7th birthday. Recipients must have been previously immunized with 3 or 4 doses of whole-cell DTP (DTwP). Consider DTaP for administration to a child as young as 15 months if the child is not expected to return at 18 months of age for the fourth dose in the primary immunization series.

Unlabeled uses: DTaP is being investigated for immunizing adults against pertussis.

Contraindications:

Not recommended for use in adults or in children > 7 years of age or in children < 15 months of age; further doses of a vaccine containing pertussis antigens to children who have recovered from culture-confirmed pertussis; history of serious adverse reactions to a previous dose of a pertussis-containing vaccine; hypersensitivity to any component of the vaccine, including thimerosal; immediate anaphylactic reaction or encephalopathy occurring within 7 days following DTP vaccination (such encephalopathies may include major alterations in consciousness, unresponsiveness, generalized or focal seizures that persist more than a few hours and failure to recover within 24 hours or other generalized or focal neurological signs); defer immunization during any febrile illness or acute infection (a minor respiratory illness such as a mild upper respiratory infection is not usually reason to defer immunization).

If a contraindication to the pertussis vaccine component occurs, substitute diphtheria and tetanus toxoids for pediatric use (DT) for each of the remaining doses.

The occurrence of any type of neurological symptoms or signs, including one or more convulsions, following DTaP administration is generally a contraindication to further use. The presence of any evolving or changing disorder affecting the CNS contraindicates administration of pertussis vaccine regardless of whether the suspected neurological disorder is associated with occurrence of seizure activity of any type.

Warnings:

Convulsions: The Immunization Practices Advisory Committee (ACIP) and the American Academy of Pediatrics (AAP) recognize cases when children with stable CNS disorders, including well controlled seizures or satisfactorily explained single seizures, may receive pertussis vaccine. ACIP and AAP do not consider a family history of seizures to be a contraindication to pertussis vaccine. Studies suggesting that infants and children with a history of convulsions in first-degree family members (ie, siblings and parents) have an increased risk for neurologic events, compared to those without such histories may be flawed by selection bias or genetic confounding.

There are no data on whether prophylactic use of antipyretic drugs (eg, acetaminophen) can decrease the risk of febrile convulsions. Data do suggest that acetaminophen will reduce the incidence of post-vaccination fever. ACIP and AAP suggest administering an appropriate dose of acetaminophen based on age at the time of vaccination and every 4 to 6 hours to children at higher risk for seizures than the general population (ie, children with a personal or family history of seizures).

DIPHTHERIA AND TETANUS TOXOIDS AND ACELLULAR PERTUSSIS VACCINE (DTaP)

Pregnancy: Category C. DTP is generally contraindicated after the 7th birthday. It is not known if DTaP antigens or corresponding antibodies cross the placenta. Most IgG passage across the placenta occurs during the third trimester.

Lactation: It is not known if DTaP antigens or corresponding antibodies are excreted into breast milk.

Children: For use from age 15 or 17 months until a child's 7th birthday. Recipients must have been previously immunized with 3 or 4 doses of whole-cell DTP. Consider DTaP for administration to a child as young as 15 months if the child is not expected to return at 18 months of age for the fourth dose in the primary immunization series. DTaP is not yet currently recommended for children < 15 months old; studies in this age group are not complete. Do not reduce or divide the DTaP dose for preterm infants or any other children.

Children who have recovered from culture-confirmed pertussis do not need further doses of a pertussis-containing vaccine. Tetanus and diphtheria toxoids for adult use (Td) is the preferred immunizing agent for adults and older children.

Precautions:

Immunization history: Ascertain previous immunization history to confirm that at least 3 doses of DTwP have been given.

Adverse events: When an infant or child returns for the next dose in the series, question the parent concerning occurrence of any symptoms or signs of adverse reactions after the previous dose. If such are reported, further doses of DTaP are contraindicated; complete active immunization against diphtheria and tetanus with diphtheria and tetanus toxoids, adsorbed (pediatric) (see individual monograph).

Several events were previously listed as contraindications, but are now listed simply as precautions, warranting careful consideration: Temperature > 40.5°C (105°F) within 48 hours after DTP administration not due to another identifiable cause; collapse or shock-like state (hypotonic-hyporesponsive episode) within 48 hours; persistent inconsolable crying lasting ≥ 3 hours within 48 hours; or convulsions with or without fever within 3 days. There may be circumstances, such as a high local incidence of pertussis, in which the potential benefits outweigh possible risks, particularly because these events are not associated with permanent sequelae.

Immunodeficiency: Persons receiving immunosuppressive therapy or with other immunodeficiencies may have a diminished antibody response to active immunization. Consider deferral of vaccine administration. Nonetheless, routine immunization of symptomatic and asymptomatic HIV-infected persons is recommended.

Drug Interactions:

DTaP Drug Interactions			
Precipitant drug	Object drug*		Description
DTaP	Immunosuppressants	⬇	Like all inactivated vaccines, administration of DTaP vaccine to persons receiving immunosuppressant drugs, including high-dose corticosteroids or radiation, may result in an insufficient response to immunization. They may remain susceptible despite immunization.
DTaP	Anticoagulants	⬆	As with other drugs administered by IM injection, give with caution to persons receiving anticoagulants.

* ⬆ = Object drug increased. ⬇ = Object drug decreased.

Adverse Reactions:

The National Childhood Vaccine Injury Act requires the healthcare provider to report to the Secretary of the Department of Health and Human Services through the Vaccine Adverse Event Reporting System (VAERS) the occurrence following immunization of any event set forth in the Vaccine Injury Table, including: Anaphylaxis or anaphylactic shock within 24 hours; encephalopathy or encephalitis within 7 days; shock-collapse or hypotonic-hyporesponsive collapse within 7 days; residual seizure disorder; any acute complication of sequelae (including death) of above events, or any event that would contraindicate further doses of vaccine.

The US Department of Health and Human Services has established VAERS to accept all reports of suspected adverse events after the administration of any vaccine, including but not limited to the reporting of events required by the National Childhood Vaccine Injury Act of 1986. The VAERS toll-free number for forms and information is 800-822-7967.

DIPHTHERIA AND TETANUS TOXOIDS AND ACELLULAR PERTUSSIS VACCINE (DTaP)

DTaP vs DTwP: Some adverse reactions following DTaP occur less frequently than in recipients of DTwP, especially less pain and tenderness, erythema, induration, swelling and warmth at the injection site. Less drowsiness, fretfulness or irritability and fever also followed DTaP use, compared with DTwP. *Tripedia* cites less frequent vomiting, anorexia and high-pitched unusual cry, and *Acel-Imune* cites less frequent antipyretic drug use, compared to DTwP.

Fever of ≥ 38°C (100.4°F) occurred within 72 hours of DTaP administration (7% to 19%); fever > 39°C (102.2°F) occurred in 1.5%. Other occasional reactions that occurred included upper respiratory infection or rhinitis (6%), diarrhea or loose stools (3.5%), vomiting (2%) or rash (1.2%). As with other aluminum-containing vaccines, a nodule may occasionally be palpable at the injection site for several weeks. Sterile abscess formation or SC atrophy at the injection site may also occur.

Reactions not noted with DTaP in clinical trials, but noted with broader use of other drugs containing diphtheria, tetanus or pertussis antigens included urticaria, erythema multiforme, other rashes, arthralgias, or more rarely a severe anaphylactic reaction (eg, urticaria with swelling of the mouth, difficulty breathing, hypotension, shock). Other possible reactions: Neurological complications such as convulsions; encephalopathy; various mono- or polyneuropathies, including Guillan-Barré syndrome. Permanent neurological disability and death occurred rarely in temporal association to immunization with a pertussis antigen.

An expert panel assembled by the Institute of Medicine concluded that no causal association exists between pertussis vaccination and SIDS.

Administration and Dosage:

The National Childhood Vaccine Injury Act requires that the manufacturer and lot number of the vaccine administered be recorded by the healthcare provider in the vaccine recipient's permanent medical record (or in a permanent office log or file), along with the date of administration of the vaccine and the name, address and title of the person administering the vaccine.

Interrupting the recommended schedule or delaying subsequent doses does not require restarting the series. Use Td, rather than DTP, for any doses needed after a child's 7th birthday.

Administer IM; use no other route. The anterolateral aspect of the thigh or the deltoid muscle of the upper arm is preferred. Do not inject DTaP in the gluteal area or other areas where there may be a major nerve trunk.

Before administration, check the patient's immunization history to ensure that at least 3 doses of whole-cell DTP vaccine have previously been given. Shake vial well to obtain a uniform suspension before withdrawing each dose. Give the fourth dose of 0.5 ml at approximately 18 months of age, at least 6 months after the third DTwP dose. Give a fifth 0.5 ml dose at 4 to 6 years of age, preferably prior to entrance into kindergarten or elementary school.

Booster dose: If a 4th dose of the primary immunizing series was administered after a child's 4th birthday, a booster prior to school entry is not necessary. No doses of DTaP are needed after a child's 7th birthday. Tetanus and diphtheria toxoids for adult use (Td) is the preferred immunizing agent for adults and older children.

Storage/Stability: Store at 2° to 8°C (36° to 46°F). Do not freeze. Discard frozen vaccine.

Rx	**Acel-Imune** (Lederle-Praxis)	**Injection**: 5 Lf units diphtheria, 5 Lf units tetanus and 300 hemagglutinatin (HA) units of acellular pertussis vaccine per 0.5 ml	In 5 ml vials.[1]
Rx	**Tripedia** (Connaught)	**Injection**: 6.7 Lf units diphtheria, 5 Lf units tetanus and 46.8 mcg pertussis antigens (23.4 mg each of pertussis toxin and filamentous hemagglutinin) per 0.5 ml	In 7.5 ml vials.[2]
Rx	**Infanrix** (SmithKline Beecham)	**Injection**: 25 Lf units diphtheria, 10 Lf units tetanus and 25 mcg pertussis, 25 mcg FHA, 8 mcg pertactin per 0.5 ml	In 0.5 ml vials.

[1] With aluminum hydroxide and phosphate, thimerosal, gelatin, glycine, polysorbate 80.
[2] With aluminum potassium sulfate (alum), thimerosal, gelatin, polysorbate 80.

DIPHTHERIA AND TETANUS TOXOIDS AND WHOLE-CELL PERTUSSIS AND HAEMOPHILUS INFLUENZAE TYPE B CONJUGATE VACCINES (DTwP-HIB)

Refer to general discussion of Agents for Active Immunization.

Warning:

Note: Products containing diphtheria, tetanus and pertussis antigens are the preferred immunizing agents for most children. Tetanus and diphtheria toxoids for adult use (Td) is the preferred immunizing agent for adults and older children.

Specific information about the individual components appears in individual monographs on diphtheria toxoid, tetanus toxoid, pertussis vaccine and Hib vaccine.

Actions:

Pharmacology: This drug is a simple mixture of DTwP (Tri-Immunol) and Hib vaccine *(HibTITER)*. See specific monographs for details.

DTwP-Hib has been given to 6793 children as part of a series of studies to test the safety and immunogenicity of this combined product when compared to separate administration of DTwP and Hib. The vaccines were given at 2, 4 and 6 months of age or at 15 to 18 months of age. The antibody response to each of the components was measured (n = 189) and compared to separate administration of the vaccines (n = 189). After three doses, the antibody response to DTwP-Hib was equal to or higher for all four components. In addition, responses to specific pertussis antigens were found to be as high or higher in the DTwP-Hib product compared to separate administration of DTwP. Therefore, the immunogenicity of the combined vaccine is at least as good as the two vaccines given separately.

Adequate immunization against diphtheria and tetanus generally persists for 10 years. Protection against pertussis persists about 4 to 6 years. Hib antibody titers > 1 mcg/ml correlate with prolonged protection from disease, generally implying several years of protection.

Antidiphtheria and antitetanus antitoxin levels > 0.01 antitoxin units each per ml are considered protective. A protective level of antipertussis antibodies are not determined. Hib antibody titers > 0.15 mcg/ml correlate with clinical protection from disease.

Indications:

For the active immunization of children 2 months to 5 years of age for protection against diphtheria, tetanus, pertussis and *Haemophilus* b disease when indications for immunization with DTP vaccine and *Haemophilus* b conjugate vaccine coincide. Typically, this is at 2, 4, 6 and 15 months of age.

Children who have recovered from culture-confirmed pertussis need not receive further doses of a vaccine containing pertussis. However, these children should receive additional doses of diphtheria and tetanus toxoids, adsorbed, for pediatric use (DT) as well as *Haemophilus* b conjugate vaccine as appropriate to complete the series.

The American Academy of Pediatrics (AAP) has recommended that children who have experienced invasive *Haemophilus* b disease when < 24 months of age should continue immunization against *Haemophilus* b, but that children whose disease occurred at ≥ 24 months need not receive further doses of *Haemophilus* b conjugate vaccine. However, these children should receive additional doses of DTP (or if pertussis is contraindicated, DT should be used) as appropriate to complete the series.

Contraindications:

Further doses of a vaccine containing pertussis antigens to children who have recovered from culture-confirmed pertussis; history of serious adverse reactions to a previous dose of a pertussis-containing vaccine; hypersensitivity to any component of the vaccine, including thimerosal.

Contraindications to whole-cell pertussis vaccine administration adopted by ACIP and AAP include an immediate anaphylactic reaction or encephalopathy occurring within 7 days following DTP vaccination. Such encephalopathies may include major alteration in consciousness, unresponsiveness, generalized or focal seizures that persist more than a few hours and failure to recover within 24 hours or other generalized or focal neurological signs.

Any febrile illness or acute infection is reason for delaying immunization with this vaccine (mild afebrile illness such as a mild upper respiratory infection is not usually reason to defer immunization).

The occurrence of any type of neurological symptoms or signs, including one or more convulsions, following DTwP administration is generally a contraindication to further use. The presence of any evolving or changing disorder affecting the CNS contraindicates administration of pertussis vaccine regardless of whether the suspected neurological disorder is associated with occurrence of seizure activity of any type.

DIPHTHERIA AND TETANUS TOXOIDS AND WHOLE-CELL PERTUSSIS AND HAEMOPHILUS INFLUENZAE TYPE B CONJUGATE VACCINES (DTwP-HIB)

If a contraindication to the pertussis-vaccine component occurs, substitute diphtheria and tetanus toxoids for pediatric use (DT) and a monovalent Hib vaccine for each of the remaining doses.

Warnings:

Convulsions: The Immunization Practices Advisory Committee (ACIP) and the American Academy of Pediatrics (AAP) recognize certain circumstances in which children with stable CNS disorders, including well controlled seizures or satisfactorily explained single seizures, may receive pertussis vaccine. ACIP and AAP do not consider a family history of seizures to be a contraindication to pertussis vaccine. Studies suggesting that infants and children with a history of convulsions in first-degree family members (ie, siblings and parents) have an increased risk for neurologic events, compared to those without such histories may be flawed by selection bias or genetic confounding.

There are no data on whether prophylactic use of antipyretic drugs (eg, acetaminophen) can decrease the risk of febrile convulsions. Data do suggest that acetaminophen will reduce the incidence of post-vaccination fever. ACIP and AAP suggest administering an appropriate dose of acetaminophen based on age at the time of vaccination and every 4 to 6 hours to children at higher risk for seizures than the general population (ie, children with a personal or family history of seizures).

Pregnancy: Category C. Products containing DTP are generally contraindicated after the 7th birthday. It is not known if DTP or Hib antigens or corresponding antibodies cross the placenta. Generally, most IgG passage across the placenta occurs during the third trimester.

Lactation: It is not known if DTP or Hib antigens or corresponding antibodies are excreted in breast milk. Problems in humans have not been documented.

Children: Safety and efficacy in children < 6 weeks of age have not been established. Routine immunization of all infants beginning at 2 months of age is recommended in the US. Do not reduce or divide the dose for preterm infants or any other children. Children who have recovered from culture-confirmed pertussis do not need further doses of a pertussis-containing vaccine. DTP is contraindicated in children < 6 weeks of age, since the product may not be immunogenic. DTP is also contraindicated in children > 7 years of age, because of their decreased risk of pertussis and increased likelihood of adverse effects. Trivalent DTwP or DTaP is the preferred immunizing agent for most children up to their 7th birthday. Tetanus & diphtheria toxoids for adult use (Td) is the preferred agent for adults and older children.

Precautions:

Adverse events: Several events were previously listed as contraindications, but are now listed simply as precautions, warranting careful consideration: Temperature > 40.5°C (105°F) within 48 hours after DTP administration not due to another identifiable cause; collapse or shock-like state (hypotonic-hyporesponsive episode) within 48 hours; persistent inconsolable crying lasting ≥ 3 hours occurring within 48 hours; or convulsions with or without fever within 3 days. There may be circumstances, such as a high local incidence of pertussis, in which the potential benefits outweigh possible risks, particularly because these events are not associated with permanent sequelae.

Immunodeficiency: If this vaccine is used in persons deficient in producing antibody, whether due to genetic defect, illness or immunosuppressive therapy, the expected immune response may not result. ACIP recommends DTP and Hib immunization of symptomatic and asymptomatic children who are immunosuppressed in association with AIDS or any other immunodeficiency disease.

Drug Interactions:

DTwP-Hib Drug Interactions

Precipitant drug	Object drug*		Description
DTwP-Hib	Anticoagulants	⬆	As with other drugs administered by IM injection, give with caution to persons receiving anticoagulant therapy.
DTwP-Hib	Immunosuppressants	⬇	Like all inactivated vaccines, administration of DTwP-Hib vaccine to persons receiving immunosuppressant drugs, including high-dose corticosteroids, or radiation therapy may result in an insufficient response to immunization. They may remain susceptible despite immunization.

* ⬆ = Object drug increased ⬇ = Object drug decreased

DIPHTHERIA AND TETANUS TOXOIDS AND WHOLE-CELL PERTUSSIS AND HAEMOPHILUS INFLUENZAE TYPE B CONJUGATE VACCINES (DTwP-HIB)

Adverse Reactions:

The National Childhood Vaccine Injury Act further requires the healthcare provider to report to the Secretary of the Department of Health and Human Services through the Vaccine Adverse Event Reporting System (VAERS) the occurrence following immunization of any event set forth in the Vaccine Injury Table including: Anaphylaxis or anaphylactic shock within 24 hours; encephalopathy or encephalitis within 7 days; shock-collapse or hypotonic-hyporesponsive collapse within 7 days; residual seizure disorder; any acute complication or sequelae (including death) of above events, or any event that would contraindicate further doses of vaccine. The US Department of Health and Human Services established VAERS to accept all reports of suspected adverse events after vaccine administration, including but not limited to the reporting of events required by the National Childhood Vaccine Injury Act of 1986. The VAERS number for information is 800-822-7967.

DTwP-Hib was evaluated in 6793 children at 2, 4 and 6 months of age or at 15 to 18 months of age in three separate sites. The percent of doses administered associated with injection site reactions within 72 hours, or common systemic symptoms within 4 days, is summarized below:

Percentage of DTwP-Hib Doses Associated with Adverse Reactions (%)

Adverse reaction	Infants (542 doses)	Infants (7269 doses)	Toddlers (107 doses)
Local[1]			
Erythema	34	19	40
Pain/Tenderness	21	30	65
Swelling	20	20	43
Warmth	16	–	35
Systemic[2]			
Fever ≥ 38°C	24	40	33
Irritability	42	54	49
Drowsiness	26	–	9
Restless sleep	–	28	–
Loss of appetite	–	4	–
Vomiting	5	2	1
Diarrhea	9	1	10
Rash	3	–	0

[1] Within 72 hours of immunization.
[2] Within 4 days of immunization.

Consider adverse reactions that may occur when using DTwP or Hib vaccines separately (see specific monographs).

In patients who received DTwP-Hib, the most common response for seeking care included trauma, viral illness and respiratory illness (eg, upper respiratory infection, otitis media, bronchitis/bronchiolitis, pneumonia). One child became transiently pale and tremulous without loss of responsiveness 4 hours after immunization and was hospitalized with a diagnosis of seizure. No other hospital visits for seizure or hypotonic, hyporesponsive episodes were reported within 72 hours of immunization. These results were not different from those observed in infants who received DTP and Hib at separate injection sites.

As with other aluminum-containing vaccines, a nodule may be palpable at the injection site for several weeks. Although not seen in studies with DTwP-Hib, sterile abscess formation or subcutaneous atrophy at the injection site may also occur.

The occurrence of sudden infant death syndrome (SIDS) has been reported following administration of DTP. However, a large case-control study in the US revealed no causal relationship between receipt of DTP vaccine and SIDS. A recent study of 6497 infants found no increase in the rate of SIDS among DTwP-Hib recipients.

DIPHTHERIA AND TETANUS TOXOIDS AND WHOLE-CELL PERTUSSIS AND HAEMOPHILUS INFLUENZAE TYPE B CONJUGATE VACCINES (DTwP-HIB)

Administration and Dosage:

The National Childhood Vaccine Injury Act requires that the manufacturer and lot number be recorded by the healthcare provider in the vaccine recipient's permanent medical record (or in a permanent office log or file), along with the date of vaccine administration and the name, address and title of person administering the vaccine.

Interruption of the recommended schedules with a delay between doses does not interfere with the final immunity achieved; nor does it necessitate starting the series over again, regardless of the length of time elapsed between doses.

For IM use only. The preferred sites are the anterolateral aspect of the thigh or the deltoid muscle of the upper arm. The vaccine should not be injected in the gluteal area or areas where there may be a major nerve trunk.

For infants beginning at 2 months of age, the immunization series for DTwP-Hib consists of three doses of 0.5 ml each at approximately 2 month intervals, followed by a fourth dose of 0.5 ml at approximately 15 months of age.

DTwP-Hib may be substituted for DTP and Hib given separately, when recommended schedules for use of these coincide (see DTP and Hib recommended dosage schedules in the Agents for Active Immunization group monograph). There are no published data to support interchangeability of *Haemophilus* b conjugate vaccine in *Tetramune* and *HibTITER* with other *Haemophilus* b conjugate vaccines for primary series. The same conjugate vaccine should be used throughout primary series, consistent with data on vaccine licensure.

Previously unvaccinated younger children:

Recommended Immunization Schedules for DTwP-Hib (Previously Unvaccinated Younger Children)

Dose	Age	Immunization
1	2 months	DTwP-Hib
2	4 months	DTwP-Hib
3	6 months	DTwP-Hib
4	15-18 months	DTwP-Hib[1]
5	4-6 years	DTP or DTaP

[1] Children 15 to 18 months may receive DTaP plus *Haemophilus* B conjugate vaccine as separate injections.

Previously unvaccinated older children: Consider immunization schedules on an individual basis for children not vaccinated according to the recommended schedule. Three doses of a product containing DTP, given at ≈ 2 month intervals, are required followed by a fourth dose of a product containing DTP or DTaP ≈ 12 months later and a fifth dose of a product containing DTP or DTaP at 4 to 6 years of age. If the fourth dose of a pertussis-containing vaccine is not given until after the fourth birthday, no further doses of a pertussis-containing vaccine are necessary.

The number of doses of an Hib-containing product indicated depends on the age that immunization is begun. A child 7 to 11 months of age should receive 3 doses of a product containing Hib. A child 12 to 14 months of age should receive 2 doses of a product containing Hib. A child 15 to 59 months of age should receive 1 dose of a product containing Hib.

Vaccinate preterm infants with DTwP-Hib according to their chronological age of birth.

If a contraindication to the pertussis vaccine component occurs, substitute diphtheria and tetanus toxoids adsorbed, for pediatric use (DT) and *Haemophilus* b conjugate vaccine, as separate injections, for each of the remaining doses.

For passive immunization against tetanus and diphtheria, human tetanus immune globulin or diphtheria antitoxin are recommended. Use separate syringe and injection site.

DIPHTHERIA AND TETANUS TOXOIDS AND WHOLE-CELL PERTUSSIS AND HAEMOPHILUS INFLUENZAE TYPE B CONJUGATE VACCINES (DTwP-HIB)

Concomitant use: Several routine pediatric vaccines may safely and effectively be administered simultaneously at separate injection sites (eg, DTP, MMR, OPV or e-IPV, Hib, hepatitis B). National authorities recommend simultaneous immunization of separate sites as indicated by age or health risk, if return of a vaccine recipient for a subsequent visit is doubtful. Delay diphtheria toxoid administration until 3 to 4 weeks after diphtheria antitoxin use, to avoid the hypothetical possibility of antitoxin-toxoid interference. In order to attribute causality of adverse reactions, do not give influenza vaccine within 3 days of pertussis vaccination.

Hib, meningococcal and pneumococcal vaccines may safely and effectively be administered simultaneously at separate injection sites.

Storage/Stability: Store at 2° to 8°C (35° to 46°F). Do not freeze.

Rx	**Tetramune** (Lederle-Praxis)	**Injection:** 5 Lf units tetanus toxoid, 12.5 Lf units diphtheria toxoid, 4 units pertussis and 10 mcg *H influenzae* type b oligosaccharide per 0.5 ml.	In 5 ml vials.[1]
Rx	**TriHIBit** (Pasteur Merieux)	**Injection:** 5 Lf units tetanus toxoid, 6.7 Lf units diphtheria toxoid, 46.8 mcg pertussis antigens and 10 mcg *H influenzae* type b purefied capsular polysaccharide per 0.5 ml.	Sucrose, thimerosal. Kit containing 1 dose vial of lyophilized tetanus toxoid conjugate and one 7.5 ml vial or five single-dose vials of diphtheria and tetanus toxoids and acellular pertussis vaccine adsorbed.

[1] With 25 mcg CRM_{197} protein, > 0.85 mg aluminum, glycine, thimerosal.

ALLERGENIC EXTRACTS

Actions:

Pharmacology: Allergenic extracts are derived individually from various biological sources containing antigens which possess immunologic activity. They are categorized based standardization and doseform. Standardization systems include: 1) Standardized by biological activity (in allergenic units, AU), 2) weight-to-volume (w/v) standardized, and 3) protein nitrogen unit (PNU) standardized. Doseforms include: 1) aqueous, 2) glycerinated and 3) alum-precipitated.

The mechanism of action is not completely defined. Specific immunoglobulin G (IgG) appears in the serum following injection of allergenic extracts. IgG competes with specific IgE for a specific antigen. Bound to receptors on mast cell membranes, IgE produces an allergenic reaction by releasing histamine and other agents upon coupling with an antigen. Serum IgE levels decrease over time. Decreased leukocyte sensitivity to allergens and increased numbers of T–suppressor cells for IgE-producing plasma cells are also noted. The histamine release response of circulating basophils to a specific allergen may be reduced in some patients by hyposensitization.

Onset/Duration – Relief of symptoms is dose-related. It is rarely achieved before maintenance dosage levels are reached, which often takes 4 to 6 months, sometimes 12 months. Serum IgG levels remain elevated for weeks to months following injection and vary markedly between individuals.

Indications:

Diagnosis of specific allergies, when properly diluted.

Relief of allergic symptoms (eg, hay fever, rhinitis, allergic asthma, insect-sting anaphylaxis) due to specifically identified materials by means of a graduated schedule of doses.

Contraindications:

As initial therapy when an allergen can be environmentally avoided.

Frequent large local reactions or systemic reactions are relative contraindications for continued immunotherapy.

Foodstuff allergen extracts are diagnostic tools; efficacy for hyposensitization immunotherapy has not been demonstrated.

Warnings:

Cross-sensitivity: Cross-immunoreactivity has been documented within botanical genus groups, especially among grasses. Exercise caution in prescribing since the additive effects could precipitate an allergic reaction. Markedly increased exposure to allergens in the environment may have an additive effect when coupled with an allergen extract injection. Dosage reduction may be necessary.

Hypersensitivity: Anaphylactic reactions may occur with an overdose or in extremely sensitive individuals. Administer allergen extracts only where emergency facilities are immediately available. Refer to Management of Acute Hypersensitivity Reactions.

Pregnancy: Category C. Controlled studies of hyposensitization with allergen extracts thoughout pregnancy failed to demonstrate any fetal or maternal risk. Because histamine can produce uterine contraction, avoid any reaction which releases significant amounts of histamine, whether from natural allergen exposure or from hyposensitization overdose. IgG crosses the placenta, especially in the third trimester. Administer during pregnancy only if clearly needed and with caution. Although pregnancy is not an indication to stop allergen extract therapy in women receiving maintenance doses without side effects, some allergists empirically decrease the maintenance dose by 50% throughout gestation.

Lactation: Minimal amounts of IgG are excreted in breast milk. No problems in humans have been documented. Various nutritional, immunologic and other advantages of breastfeeding have been described, especially in children of atopic mothers.

Children: Dosage for children is generally the same as for adults. The larger dosage volumes may produce relatively greater discomfort. To achieve the total dose required, the volume of the dose may be distributed among several injection sites.

Precautions:

Mixed allergens are not to be used for skin testing. In the case of a negative reaction, a mixture fails to indicate whether one of the individual components at the full labeled concentration is capable of evoking a positive reaction. If the patient responds positively, there is no indication which component of the mixture produced the antigenic response. Treatment with nonreactive allergens can lead to sensitization and induction of IgE production.

Combining allergens: Do not combine allergens to which the patient is extremely sensitive with allergens for which only a nominal sensitivity is shown. Administer separately to individualize and better control dosage.

ALLERGENIC EXTRACTS

Seasonal exposure: Delay the start of immunotherapy until after any period of symptoms from seasonal environmental exposure. Typical allergic symptoms may follow shortly after an injection, particularly when the sum of the antigen load from the environment and from the injection exceeds the patient's antigen tolerance.

Routine immunizations: While routine immunizations may theoretically exacerbate autoimmune diseases, studies have failed to demonstrate this. Give hyposensitization cautiously to patients with autoimmune diseases and only if the risk from exposure exceeds the risk of exacerbating the underlying condition.

Drug Interactions:

Drug/Lab test interactions: **H_1 histamine antagonists** and **tricyclic antidepressants** may produce a false-negative reaction to cutaneous diagnostic testing with allergen extracts, unless a 72 hour period of antihistamine abstinence is observed. Long-acting antihistamines may interfere for weeks. **H_2 antagonists** do not decrease skin-test responsiveness alone, but may enhance suppression synergistically with H_1 antihistamines. **Topical corticosteroids** suppress dermal reactivity to allergan extracts locally.

Adverse Reactions:

Most serious reactions begin within 30 minutes of an injection. Observe patients for at least 30 minutes after every injection, even once they have achieved maintenance therapy.

Local: Erythema and swelling at the injection site are common, but not significant unless they persist > 24 hours or exceed the diameter of a nickel (about 2 cm).

Systemic: Anaphylaxis, including fainting, pallor, bradycardia, hypotension, angioedema, wheezing, cough, conjunctivitis, rhinitis, generalized urticaria (see Warnings).

Patient Information:

Comply with full course of therapy. To achieve efficacy, take regularly and in the proper dosage. Medication will not cure allergies, but will help control them.

Notify physician of increased environmental exposure to natural allergens; a dosage reduction may be required.

Missed dose: Depending on the amount of time elapsed, dosage reduction may be required. Do *not* double the dose to make up for the missed dose. More frequent injections may be necessary to return to maintenance doses.

Notify physician if erythema, swelling or generalized urticaria persists.

Notify physician immediately if fainting, wheezing, hypotension or bradycardia occurs.

Administration and Dosage:

Begin immunotherapy with very small doses; increase progressively until maintenance levels are reached. Dosages vary depending on the type of standardization used. Individualize dosage.

Do not inject IV. SC injection is preferable because it is less painful, allows better delineation of reaction size and slows the absorption rate, thus lowering the likelihood of an anaphylactic reaction. Although IM administration is acceptable, it is more painful and more difficult to assess the local reaction.

Combining allergens: Do not combine allergens to which the patient is extremely sensitive with allergens for which only a nominal sensitivity is shown. Distinct treatment schedules for each formula are frequently employed. (See Precautions.)

Children: Dosage is the same as for adults; divide large volume doses among several injection sites.

Diagnostic testing: Perform puncture (prick) or intradermal testing with appropriate dilutions, employing positive and negative controls. Consult manufacturer's literature for each allergen. Do not conduct test with alum-precipitated allergen extracts.

Therapeutic dosing: Typical doses are given SC every 3 to 14 days (or 7 to 14 days with alum-precipitated allergen extracts). Progress to the maximum tolerated dose or a weekly maintenance dose. Consult manufacturer's literature for each allergen.

Admixtures: Limit combinations of allergens so that each allergen will be present at a therapeutic concentration. Do not combine allergens of different standardization types. Stability varies with diluent, storage condition and concentration. Stability will be shortest in the low concentration ranges.

Storage: Store between 2° and 8°C (36° to 46°F).

ALLERGENIC EXTRACTS AQUEOUS AND GLYCERINATED ALLERGENIC EXTRACTS

For complete prescribing information, refer to the Allergenic Extracts group monograph.

Rx	**Allergenic Extracts, Aqueous and Glycerinated** (Various, eg, ALK, Allergy Laboratories, Allermed, ALO, Antigen Laboratories, Center, Greer, Iatric, Meridian, Miles, Nelco)	**Injection:** Over 900 distinct allergens available in these categories: Animal products, foods, grass pollens, insect products, molds, tree pollens, weed pollens and other inhalants	Extracts supplied in various aqueous diluents or with varying concentrations of glycerin. In multidose vials of 2, 5, 10, 20, 30 and 50 ml.

ALUM-PRECIPITATED ALLERGENIC EXTRACTS

For complete prescribing information, refer to the Allergenic Extracts group monograph.

Rx	**Allpyral** (Miles)	**Injection:** Alum-precipitated extracts, prepared by pyridine extraction	In multidose vials of 10 and 30 ml at 5000, 10,000 and 20,000 PNU/ml.
Rx	**Center-Al** (Center)	**Injection:** Alum-precipitated extracts	In multidose vials of 10 and 30 ml at 10,000 and 20,000 PNU/ml.

HYMENOPTERA VENOM/VENOM PROTEIN

For complete prescribing information, refer to the Allergenic Extracts group monograph.

Rx	**Albay, Venomil** (Miles)	**Injection:** Purified venoms of honey bee, wasp, white faced hornet, yellow hornet, yellow jacket and mixed vespids (both hornets and yellow jacket)	In vials of 12, 120 and 550 mcg.
Rx	**Pharmalgen** (ALK)		In vials of 120 and 1100 mcg.

TUBERCULIN TESTS

Actions:

Pharmacology: The various PPD solutions are generically equivalent, but differ from PPD multipuncture devices and from old tuberculin products. Intradermal PPD is more sensitive and more specific than any tuberculin delivered by multipuncture device.

Tuberculin testing products contain soluble growth products derived from the tubercle bacillus. When administered intradermally, a hypersensitivity reaction, manifesting as induration and erythema, appears in sensitive individuals. A positive reaction indicates that the patient has had, at some time, a tuberculous infection, but may indicate previous BCG vaccination. A positive test does not indicate an active infection, but indicates that further evaluation is needed.

Two agents are used for tuberculin testing: Old tuberculin (OT) is a culture filtrate standardized to a uniform potency; Purified Protein Derivative (PPD) is a more refined preparation, and is recommended by the American Thoracic Society.

Both OT and PPD are used in multiple puncture-type devices as screening tools. PPD is also used in the intradermal (Mantoux) test to confirm a positive reaction with the puncture test.

PPD tests are 95% (multi-puncture, 93.8%) sensitive, implying that 5% (multi-puncture, 6.2%) of infected test recipients will test falsely negative. PPD tests are 98% (multi-puncture, 89%) specific, implying that 2% (multi-puncture, 10.9%) of uninfected test recipients will test falsely positive. A tuberculin Tine-Test is 92% sensitive and *Mono-Vacc* is 98.8% sensitive (compared to a Mantoux test), implying 8% or 1.2%, respectively, of infected test recipients will test falsely negative. Old tuberculin tests are 96% specific, implying that 4% of uninfected test recipients will test falsely positive. Skin reactions may occur in individuals infected by nontuberculous mycobacteria (eg, *Mycobacterium avium, Mycobacterium intracellulare*). Specificity is highest among people living in Arctic areas or at high elevations and lowest in the tropics or at low elevations.

Indications:

Skin test as an aid in the diagnosis of tuberculosis.

The 5TU strength is the standard selected for the routine testing of individuals for tuberculosis, for testing of individuals suspected of having contact with active tuberculosis, and as a follow-up verification test in individuals who have had reactions to skin tests with tuberculin multiple-puncture devices, which are often used as a screening procedure for detection of reactors to tuberculins.

The American Academy of Pediatrics recommends that, if tuberculin screening of children is conducted, skin tests be applied at 12 months, 4 to 6 years, and 14 to 16 years of age.

Contraindications:

Tuberculin positive reactors (see Warnings).

Warnings:

Repeated testing of the uninfected individual does not sensitize to tuberculin, but may have a "booster" effect in persons with low degrees of homologous or heterologous mycobacterial antigens or may even cause an apparent development of sensitivity in some cases.

Tuberculin positive reactors: Do not administer to known tuberculin-positive reactors because of the severity of reactions (eg, vesiculation, ulceration or necrosis) that may occur at the test site.

SC injection should be avoided. If this occurs, a general febrile reaction or acute inflammation around old tuberculous lesions may occur in sensitive individuals.

Immunodeficiency: Skin-test responsiveness may be suppressed during or for as much as 6 weeks following viral infection, live viral vaccination, miliary or pulmonary tuberculosis infection, bacterial infection, severe febrile illness, malnutrition, sarcoidosis, malignancy or immunosuppression (eg, corticosteroids or other immunosuppressive pharmacotherapy). In most patients who are very sick with tuberculosis, a previously negative tuberculin test becomes positive after a few weeks of chemotherapy. When of diagnostic importance, accept a negative test as proof that hypersensitivity is absent only after normal reactivity to common antigens has been demonstrated, such as with an anergy-test panel.

Hypersensitivity: Have epinephrine immediately available. See also Management of Acute Hypersensitivity Reactions.

Elderly: Skin-test responsiveness may be delayed or reduced in magnitude among older persons. Two-step testing is especially important in persons ≥ 35 years old.

TUBERCULIN TESTS

Pregnancy: Category C. The risk of unrecognized tuberculosis and the close postpartum contact between a mother with active disease and her infant leaves the infant in grave danger of tuberculosis and complications such as tuberculous meningitis. No adverse effects upon the fetus recognized as being due to tuberculosis skin testing have been reported.

Lactation: It is unlikely that tuberculin is excreted in breast milk.

Children: A child who has been exposed to a tuberculous adult must not be judged free of infection until there is a negative tuberculin reaction at least 10 weeks after ending contact with the tuberculous person.

Precautions:

Administration site: Do not apply on acneiform skin, hairy areas or areas without adequate subcutaneous tissue.

Active tuberculosis: Perform tuberculin testing with caution in persons with active tuberculosis. However, activation of quiescent lesions is rare.

Altered reactivity: Reactivity to tuberculin may be depressed or suppressed for as long as 4 weeks by viral infections, live virus vaccines (ie, measles, smallpox, polio, rubella and mumps), severe febrile illness, sarcoidosis or malignancy, overwhelming miliary or pulmonary tuberculosis, administration of corticosteroids or immunosuppressive drugs, old age and malnutrition. When of diagnostic importance, accept a negative test as proof that hypersensitivity is absent only after normal reactivity to nonspecific irritants has been demonstrated. In most patients who are very sick with tuberculosis, the previously negative tuberculin test becomes positive after a few weeks of treatment.

Positive reaction does not necessarily signify active disease. Perform further diagnostic procedures such as chest x-ray and bacteriologic examinations of sputa before making a diagnosis of tuberculosis.

Adverse Reactions:

In highly sensitive individuals, strong positive reactions including vesiculation, ulceration or necrosis may occur at the test site. Cold packs or topical steroids may provide symptomatic relief. Minimal bleeding at puncture site occurs infrequently and does not affect test interpretation. Strongly positive reactions may result in scarring at the test site.

Tuberculin Tests

TUBERCULIN PURIFIED PROTEIN DERIVATIVE (Mantoux; PPD; Tuberculin skin test [TST])

For complete prescribing information, refer to the Tuberculin Tests group monograph.

Administration and Dosage:

Aqueous solutions of a purified protein fraction isolated from culture filtrates of human type strains of *Mycobacterium tuberculosis.*

Intradermal (Mantoux) test: For the initial test, use 5 tuberculin units (TU). The 1 TU dose is used for individuals suspected of being highly sensitized, since larger initial doses may result in severe skin reactions. Use the 250 TU test dose exclusively for the testing of individuals who fail to react to a previous injection of either 1 or 5 TU. *Never* use it for the initial injection.

Test method: The preferred test site is the flexor or dorsal surface of the forearm about 4 inches below the elbow. Inject intradermally with a disposable syringe using a 26- or 27-gauge x ½ inch needle.

If the intradermal injection is performed properly, a definite white bleb will rise at the needle point, about 6 to 10 mm (⅜″) in diameter. This will disappear within minutes. No dressing is required.

Avoid SC injection. If injected SC (ie, no bleb will form), or if a significant part of the dose leaks from the injection site, repeat the test immediately at least 5 cm (2″) removed from the first site.

Interpretation: Read 48 to 72 hours after administration. Consider only induration in interpretation. Measure the diameter of induration transversely to the long axis of the forearm and record in millimeters. Disregard erythema of < 10 mm. If the area of erythema is > 10 mm and induration is absent, the injection may have been too deep; retesting is indicated. Interpret reactions as follows:

Positive – Palpable induration measuring ≥ 10 mm. This indicates hypersensitivity to tuberculoprotein; interpret as positive for past or present infection.

Inconclusive – Induration of 5 to 9 mm. Retest using a different injection site. In the case of known contacts, interpret an induration measuring 5 mm or even smaller as positive. Rule out cross-reaction from other mycobacterial infection.

Negative – Induration of < 5 mm. This indicates a lack of hypersensitivity to tuberculoprotein; tuberculous infection is highly unlikely.

Retesting: An individual who does not show a positive reaction to 1 or 5 TU on the first test may be retested with 5 TU, and if negative, with 250 TU. If a second test is employed, repeat on the other forearm.

An individual who does not positively react to 5 TU is considered tuberculin negative although the test may be positive to 250 TU. If negative to 250 TU, this individual is nonreactive.

Rx	**Tubersol** (Connaught)	**Injection:** 1 TU per 0.1 ml	In 1 ml (10 test) vials.[1]
Rx	**Aplisol** (Parke-Davis)	**Injection:** 5 TU per 0.1 ml	In 1 ml (10 test) and 5 ml (50 test) vials.[2]
Rx	**Tubersol** (Connaught)		In 1 ml (10 test) and 5 ml (50 test) vials.[1]
Rx	**Tubersol** (Connaught)	**Injection:** 250 TU per 0.1 ml	In 1 ml (10 test) vials.[3]

[1] In isotonic phosphate buffer saline with 0.28% phenol and polysorbate 80.
[2] With potassium and sodium phosphates, 0.35% phenol and polysorbate 80.
[3] In potassium and sodium phosphate buffered saline with 0.5% phenol and polysorbate 80.

TUBERCULIN PPD MULTIPLE PUNCTURE DEVICE

For complete prescribing information, refer to the Tuberculin Tests group monograph.

Administration and Dosage:

A single use, multiple puncture type device for determining tuberculin sensitivity. Each unit consists of a cylindrical plastic holder bearing four stainless steel tines coated with tuberculin PPD. The units give reactions equivalent to 5 tuberculin units (TU) of PPD-S administered intradermally in the Mantoux test.

Regard all multiple puncture type devices as screening tools; employ appropriate diagnostic procedures for retesting "doubtful" reactors.

Test method: The volar surface of the upper one-third of the forearm, over a muscle belly, is preferred. Avoid hairy areas and areas without adequate subcutaneous tissue.

Grasp the patient's forearm firmly to stretch the skin taut at the site and to prevent any jerking motion of the arm that could cause scratching with the tines. Apply the unit firmly and without twisting to the test area for approximately 1 second.

TUBERCULIN PPD MULTIPLE PUNCTURE DEVICE

Exert sufficient pressure to assure that all 4 tines have penetrated the skin of the test area and a circular depression is visible.

Interpretation: Read tests at 48 to 72 hours after application. Vesiculation or the extent of induration are the determining factors; erythema without induration is of no significance. Determine the size of the induration in millimeters by inspection, measuring and palpation with gentle finger stroking. Measure the diameter of the largest single reaction around one of the puncture sites. With pronounced reactions, the areas of induration around the puncture sites may coalesce.

Positive reaction – If vesiculation is present, the test is positive; manage the patient as if classified positive to the Mantoux test. The test may be interpreted as positive if induration is > 2 mm, but consider further diagnostic procedures.

Inconclusive – Induration < 2 mm, often resulting from either atypical mycobacteria or *Mycobacterium tuberculosis.* Give these patients a Mantoux test, 5 TU/0.1 ml. Base decisions for patient management on response to the Mantoux test.

Negative reaction – Induration < 2 mm or erythema of any size. There is no need for retesting unless the person is a contact of a patient with tuberculosis or there is clinical evidence suggestive of the disease.

Rx	**Aplitest** (Parke-Davis)	**Injection:** 5 TU activity per test	In 25 test packages.[1]
Rx	**Tine Test PPD** (Lederle-Praxis)		In 25 and 100 test packages.[2]

[1] With potassium and sodium phosphate buffers and 0.5% phenol.
[2] With 7% acacia, 30% dextrose and 5% glycerol.

OLD TUBERCULIN, MULTIPLE PUNCTURE DEVICES

For complete prescribing information, refer to the Tuberculin Tests group monograph.

Administration and Dosage:

Tuberculin, Old, Tine Test units give reactions equivalent to or more potent than 5 TU of standard old tuberculin administered intradermally in the Mantoux test. However, regard all multiple puncture-type devices as screening tools and use other appropriate diagnostic procedures such as the Mantoux test for retesting reactors.

Although clinical allergy to acacia is very rare, use Tuberculin, Old, Tine Test with caution in patients with known allergy to this component.

Test method: The volar surface of the upper one-third of the forearm, over a muscle belly, is preferred. Avoid hairy areas and areas without adequate subcutaneous tissue.

Grasp the patient's forearm firmly, since the sharp momentary sting may cause a jerk of the arm, resulting in scratching. Stretch the skin of the forearm tightly and apply the disc with the other hand. Hold at least 1 second. Release tension grip on forearm. Withdraw tine unit. Exert sufficient pressure so that the 4 puncture sites and circular depression of the skin from the plastic base are visible.

Interpretation: Read tests at 48 to 72 hours following administration. Vesiculation or the extent of induration are the determining factors; erythema without induration is not significant. Determine the size of the induration in millimeters by inspection, measuring and palpation with gentle finger stroking. Measure the diameter of the largest single reaction around one of the puncture sites. With pronounced reactions, the areas of induration around the puncture sites may coalesce.

Positive reaction – If vesiculation is present, the test is positive. The management of the patient is the same as that for one classified as positive to the Mantoux test. If induration is ≥ 2 mm, the test may be interpreted as positive, but consider further diagnostic procedures.

Inconclusive – Induration < 2 mm, often resulting from either atypical mycobacteria or *Mycobacterium tuberculosis.* Give these patients a Mantoux test, 5 TU/0.1 ml. Base decisions for patient management on response to the Mantoux test.

Negative reaction – Induration < 2 mm. There is no need to retest unless the person is a contact of a tuberculosis patient or clinical evidence suggests the disease.

Rx	**Mono-Vacc Test (O.T.)** (Connaught)	**Injection:** 5 TU activity per test	In boxes of 25 tests.
Rx	**Tuberculin, Old, Tine Test** (Lederle Praxis)	**Injection:** 5 TU activity per test[1]	Individual test units in sets of 25, 100 and 250.

[1] Solution of Old Tuberculin containing 7% acacia and 8.5% lactose.

COCCIDIOIDIN

Actions:

Pharmacology: Positive skin tests result from activation of sensitized T-lymphocytes, a delayed-hypersensitivity reaction involving cellular immunity. Coccidioidin deposited in the skin reacts with sensitized lymphocytes, causing the release of mediators that induce the inflammatory, edematous reaction recognized as a positive reaction. The reaction depends on the person having been previously sensitized to coccidioidin.

Spherule-derived coccidioidin may detect significantly more infected persons than mycelium-derived coccidioidin. Nonetheless, 50% false-negative rates have occurred in patients with disseminated disease. Coccidioidin tests are highly specific, implying that few healthy test recipients will test falsely positive. Mycelium- and spherule-derived products are probably equally specific.

Indications:

For detection of delayed hypersensitivity to *Coccidioidin immitis*. Serves as an aid in the diagnosis of coccidiodomycosis. The skin test is a valuable diagnostic tool to differentiate coccidioidomycosis from the common cold, influenza and other mycotic or bacterial infections (eg, blastomycosis, histoplasmosis, tuberculosis, sarcoidosis).

Unlabeled uses: In endemic areas (eg, the southwestern US), coccidioidin may be a useful addition to anergy skin-test panels to assess competence of recipients' cell-mediated immunity, but use of mycelial coccidioidin may obscure the results of other fungal assays.

Contraindications:

Hypersensitivity to thimerosal; patients with erythema nodosum.

Warnings:

Immunodeficiency: Persons receiving immunosuppressive therapy or with other immunodeficiencies (especially those involving cell-mediated immunity) may have a diminished skin-test response to this and other diagnostic antigens.

Hypersensitivity: Because of the possibility of an immediate systemic allergic reaction, observe the patient for 15 minutes after the injection. Have epinephrine available in case an acute hypersensitivity reaction occurs. See also Management of Acute Hypersensitivity Reactions.

Pregnancy: Category C. Use only if clearly needed. It is unlikely that coccidioidin crosses the placenta.

Lactation: It is not likely that coccidioidin is excreted in breast milk.

Children: Safety and efficacy of mycelial coccidioidin have not been specifically established in children, but spherule-derived coccidioidin is safe and effective in children, including those < 5 years of age.

Drug Interactions:

Coccidioidin Drug Interactions

Precipitant drug	Object drug*		Description
Immunosuppressants	Coccidioidin	⬆	Reactivity to any delayed-hypersensitivity test may be suppressed in persons receiving corticosteroids or other immunosuppressive drugs, or in persons who were recently immunized with live virus vaccines (eg, measles, mumps, rubella, poliovirus). If delayed-hypersensitivity skin testing is indicated, perform it either preceding or simultaneous with immunization or 4 to 6 weeks after immunization.
Cimetidine	Coccidioidin	⬆	Several weeks of cimetidine therapy may augment or enhance delayed-hypersensitivity responses to skin test antigens, although this effect was not consistently observed. The effect may be mediated through cimetidine binding to suppressor T-lymphocytes.

* ⬆ = Object drug increased

Drug/Lab test interactions: A positive reaction to *BioCox* may cause a rise in titers of complement-fixing antibodies against *Emmonsiella capsulata* (*Histoplasma capsulatum*) and coccidioidin. Unlike *BioCox, Spherulin* does not induce humoral antibodies nor does it affect complement-fixation titers for either histoplasmosis or coccidioidomycosis. Either coccidioidin may boost existing hypersensitivity in recipients, manifested after a subsequent test.

COCCIDIOIDIN

Adverse Reactions:

Systemic: Patients with great sensitivity may rarely develop a systemic reaction consisting of fever or erythema nodosum. There are no reports that skin testing can cause a recrudescence of the disease.

Local: An occasional patient may develop an immediate local wheal reaction. Occasionally, large local reactions may lead to vesiculation, local tissue necrosis and scar formation.

Administration and Dosage:

Test method: Inject 0.1 ml of a 1:100 dilution intradermally on the flexor surface of the forearm. Use a weaker 1:1000 or 1:10,000 dilution if erythema nodosum is evident.

Perform the 1:10 dilution skin test only on persons nonreactive to the 1:100 dilution.

Interpretation: Consider the following points in interpretation: (1) A positive reaction may cause a transitory rise in titer of complement fixation antibody to histoplasma antigens, but not to coccidioidin; (2) coccidioidin may elicit skin test cross-reactions in individuals infected with *Histoplasma, Blastomyces* and possibly other fungi; (3) coccidioidin may boost level of skin sensitivity to coccidioidin in already sensitive individuals; (4) the skin test may be negative in severe forms of disease (anergy) or when prolonged periods of time have passed since infection.

Positive reaction – Induration of ≥ 5 mm. Erythema without induration is considered negative. Read tests both at 24 and 48 hours because some reactions may fade after 36 hours. A positive test reaction indicates present or past infection with *Coccidioides immitis.*

Negative reaction – A negative test (< 5 mm induration) means the individual has not been sensitized to coccidioidin or has lost sensitivity.

Storage/Stability: Store at 2° to 8°C (36° to 46°F). Discard if frozen. Product can tolerate 14 days at room temperature. Refrigerate dilutions after compounding and discard within 24 hours.

Rx	**BioCox** (Iatric)	**Injection:** 1:100 w/v	With 0.01% thimerosal. Mycelial derivative. In 1 ml 10-test multidose vial.
	Spherulin (ALK)		With 0.01% thimerosal. Spherule derivative. In 1 ml 10-test multi dose-vial.
Rx	**BioCox** (Iatric)	**Injection:** 1:10 w/v	With 0.01% thimerosal. Mycelial derivative. 10-test multidose vial.
	Spherulin (ALK)		With 0.01% thimerosal. Spherule derivative. 10-test multidose vial.

HISTOPLASMIN

Actions:

Pharmacology: Positive skin tests result from activation of sensitized T-lymphocytes, a delayed-hypersensitivity reaction involving cellular immunity. Histoplasmin antigens deposited in the skin react with sensitized lymphocytes, causing the release of mediators that induce the inflammatory, edematous reaction recognized as a positive reaction. The reaction depends on the person having been previously sensitized to histoplasmin.

The sensitivity of mycelial histoplasmin is not described, but some infected test recipients will test falsely negative. Yeast-lysate histoplasmin tests are 83% sensitive, implying that 17% of infected test recipients will test falsely negative. Most patients with acute or chronic pulmonary histoplasmosis react positively to the test. However in critically ill people or those with disseminated disease, the frequency of positive reactions falls to about 50%. In epidemic histoplasmosis, the rate of positive reactions may approach 100%.

The specificity of mycelial histoplasmin is not described, but some uninfected test recipients will test falsely positive. Mycelial histoplasmin may cross-react and yield false-positive responses to *Blastomyces, Coccidioides* and related fungi. Yeast-lysate histoplasmin tests are highly specific, implying that few uninfected test recipients will test falsely positive.

Indications:

An aid in diagnosing histoplasmosis, in detecting delayed hypersensitivity to *Histoplasma capsulatum* and in differentiating possible histoplasmosis from coccidioidomycosis, sarcoidosis and other mycotic or bacterial infections, and in interpreting x-rays showing pulmonary infiltration and calcification. It may also be useful in epidemiological studies of persons with exposure to histoplasmosis and other infectious diseases.

Unlabeled uses: In endemic areas (eg, the Ohio and Mississippi River valleys), histoplasmin may be a useful addition to anergy skin test panels to assess competence of recipients' cell-mediated immunity, but use of mycelial histoplasmin may obscure the results of other fungal assays.

Warnings:

Immunodeficiency: Persons receiving immunosuppressive therapy or with other immunodeficiencies (especially those involving cell-mediated immunity) may have a diminished skin-test response to this and other diagnostic antigens.

Hypersensitivity: Have epinephrine immediately available in case an anaphylactoid or acute hypersensitivity reaction occurs. See also Management of Acute Hypersensitivity Reactions.

Do not administer histoplasmin to known histoplasmin-positive reactors because of the severity of reactions (eg, vesiculation, ulceration, necrosis) that may occur at the test site in very highly hypersensitive individuals.

Pregnancy: Category C. Use only if clearly needed. It is unlikely that histoplasmin crosses the placenta.

Lactation: It is unlikely that histoplasmin is excreted in breast milk.

Children: Safety and efficacy of mycelial histoplasmin have not been established, but yeast-lysate histoplasmin has been routinely administered to children with no special safety problems noted.

Precautions:

Monitoring: If serological studies are indicated, draw the blood sample prior to administering the skin test or within 48 to 96 hours following the skin-test injection. After this time period, a rise in titer associated with a positive skin test may occur.

Local reactions: Greater than recommended doses (eg, > 0.1 ml) may produce severe erythema and induration followed by necrosis and ulceration that may last for several weeks.

HISTOPLASMIN

Drug Interactions:

Histoplasmin Drug Interactions

Precipitant drug	Object drug*		Description
Cimetidine	Histoplasmin	↑	Several weeks of cimetidine therapy may augment or enhance delayed-hypersensitivity responses to skin test antigens, although this effect was not consistently observed. The effect may be mediated through cimetidine binding to suppressor T-lymphocytes.
Immunosuppressants Vaccines, virus	Histoplasmin	↓	Reactivity to any delayed-hypersensitivity test may be suppressed in persons receiving corticosteroids or other immunosuppressive drugs, or in persons who were recently immunized with live virus vaccines (eg, measles, mumps, rubella, poliovirus). If delayed-hypersensitivity skin testing is indicated, perform it either preceding or simultaneously with immunization or 4 to 6 weeks after immunization.

* ↑ = Object drug increased. ↓ = Object drug decreased.

Adverse Reactions:

Local: In highly sensitive individuals, vesiculation, ulceration or necrosis may occur at the test site and may result in scarring. Cold packs or topical steroids may provide symptomatic relief of the associated pain, pruritus and discomfort.

Hypersensitivity: Urticaria, angioedema, shortness of breath and excessive perspiration (see Warnings).

Administration and Dosage:

Inject intradermally only.

The two forms of histoplasmin are generically inequivalent. Mycelial histoplasmin is more likely to boost complement-fixing antibody titers than yeast-lysate histoplasmin.

Test method: Inject 0.1 ml intradermally into the flexor surface of the forearm. Use a tuberculin syringe and a 26-gauge x ⅜ inch or 27-gauge x ½ inch needle. If correctly injected, a small bleb will rise over the needle point. Read reactions 48 to 72 hours after injection. The usual delayed skin test reaction appears in 24 hours and reaches a maximum in 48 to 72 hours.

Interpretation: Describe and measure the reaction in terms of millimeters of induration and degree of reaction (from slight induration to vesiculation and necrosis). A reaction of ≥ 5 mm induration is positive. In case of doubt and if clinically indicated, repeat the test only after obtaining serum for antibody titer.

Positive reaction – May indicate a past infection or a mild, subacute or chronic infection with *H capsulatum* or immunologically-related organisms, such as *Blastomyces* or *Coccidioides* species. It may also denote improvement in cases of serious illness of symptomatic histoplasmosis that previously may have been histoplasmin-negative.

Differential diagnosis – Histoplasmin is of little value in diagnosing acute fulminating infections because a negative reaction usually occurs. In mild infections, repeatedly negative reactions may suggest the exclusion of *Histoplasma* as the causative agent. Employ the tuberculin test in conjunction with histoplasmin to exclude the possibility of tuberculosis. The histoplasmin skin test sometimes causes elevation of serum antibody titers to histoplasmin.

To distinguish lesions associated with histoplasmin sensitivity from other causes, consider: (1) Skin sensitivity to histoplasmin but not tuberculin; (2) lesions must persist for 2 months (to exclude transient pneumonic lesions); and (3) laboratory and clinical examinations to exclude tuberculosis, Boeck's sarcoid, sarcoidosis, Hodgkin's disease, etc. These criteria may help interpret roentgenographic findings.

Storage: Store at 2° to 8°C (36° to 46°F).

Rx	**Histoplasmin, Diluted** (Parke-Davis)	**Injection:** 1:100 w/v (P-D) or v/v (ALK). Standardized sterile filtrate from cultures of *Histoplasma capsulatum.*	With 0.5% phenol and polysorbate 80. Controlled yeast lysate. In 1 ml, 10 test multidose vials.
Rx	**Histolyn-CYL** (ALK Labs)		With 0.4% phenol and polysorbate 80, human serum albumin. Mycelial derivative. In 1.3 ml multidose vials.

CANDIDA ALBICANS SKIN TEST ANTIGEN

Actions:

Pharmacology: The potency of *Candida albicans* is measured by dose-response skin tests in healthy adults. The procedure involves concurrent (side-by-side) testing of production lots with an internal reference (IR), using sensitive adults who have been previously screened and qualified to serve as test subjects. The induration response at 48 hours elicited by 0.1 ml of a production lot is measured and compared to the response elicited by 0.1 ml of the IR. The test is satisfactory if the potency of the production lot does not differ more than ± 20% from the potency of the IR, when analyzed by the paired t-test.

Cellular or delayed-type hypersensitivity (DTH) can be assessed by intracutaneous testing with bacterial, viral and fungal antigens to which most healthy persons are sensitized. A positive skin test denotes prior antigenic exposure, T-cell competency and an intact inflammatory response. The reaction usually peaks 48 hours after antigen is introduced into the skin and is manifest as induration at the test site.

Recall antigens may be useful in evaluating DTH by eliciting positive induration reactions 48 to 72 hours after intracutaneous administration. Except for mumps skin test antigen, most commonly used recall antigens were developed for other purposes, and the size of the reaction elicited may not be directly related to cellular immunity because of variablility in antigen source and dose and skin test administration and measurement techniques. Useful antigens are those which elicit a reaction size > 5 mm in > 50% of healthy individuals. The combination of results from skin testing with more than one antigen should result in detection of DTH in at least 95% of healthy subjects.

The inflammatory response associated with the DTH reaction is characterized by an infiltration of lymphocytes and macrophages at the site of antigen deposition. Specific cell types that appear to play a major role in the DTH response include CD4+ and CD8+ T-lymphocytes which leave the recirculating lymphocyte pool in response to exogenous antigen. Both CD4+ and CD8+ lymphocytes have been recovered from DTH reactions elicited by *Candida* antigen.

Clinical trials: The incidence of DTH reactions to unstandardized *Candida* antigens has been reported to vary from 52% to 89%, depending on the strength of the antigen and the mm induration required for a positive test.

In one group of 18 healthy adults, 78% of the individuals reacted to *C albicans* with an induration response of ≥ 5 mm at 48 hours. In a second study of 35 subjects, 60% had induration reactions > 5 mm at 48 hours. In this study, 65% of males tested positive compared to 53% of females; the mean induration in responding males was 12.8 mm and in responding females was 13 mm. When subjects in these studies were tested with two reagents, *C albicans* and mumps skin test antigen, 92% were positive to at least one antigen, a higher response rate than to either antigen used alone.

In another study, the skin test responses of adults with HIV infection were compared to those of healthy control subjects. The responses in HIV-infected patients who did not meet the definition of AIDS were less than in uninfected subjects, but the differences were not statistically significant. A significant difference was found between AIDS patients and uninfected controls in both mean induration and proportion with ≥ 5 mm response.

In a related study involving 20 male patients diagnosed with AIDS, one subject responded to *C albicans*. In this study, 65% of the male control subjects had DTH reactions > 5 mm to *C albicans*. The mean induration response at 48 hours for control subjects was 8.33 mm, compared to 1.78 mm for the AIDS subjects.

In a published study of DTH anergy, 479 subjects (334 males and 145 females) infected with HIV and being screened for tuberculosis were skin tested with several additional antigens, including *C albicans*. Only 12% reacted to tuberculin (≥ 5 mm), 57% reacted to *C albicans* (≥ 3 mm) and 60% reacted to either tuberculin or *C albicans* or both. In this study, a 3 mm induration response to *C albicans* was considered positive. In conclusion, HIV-infected subjects, testing with other DTH antigens, increases the accuracy of interpretation of negative tuberculin reactions.

In another study of 18 patients with lung cancer, *C albicans* elicited a positive induration response in 28%. In a second series of 20 patients with metastatic cancer, no reactions ≥ 5 mm were observed.

CANDIDA ALBICANS SKIN TEST ANTIGEN

Indications:

Reduced cellular hypersensitivity: For use as a recall antigen for detecting DTH by intracutaneous (intradermal) testing. The product may be useful in evaluating the cellular immune response in patients suspected of having reduced cellular hypersensitivity. Because some persons with normal cellular immunity are not hypersensitive to *C albicans*, a response rate < 100% to the antigen is to be expected in healthy individuals. Therefore, the concurrent use of other licensed DTH skin test antigens is recommended.

HIV: Antigens of *C albicans* are useful in the assessment of diminished cellular immunity in persons infected with HIV. Responses to DTH antigens have prognostic value in patients with cancer. Because HIV infection can modify the DTH response to tuberculin, it is advisable to skin test HIV-infected patients at high risk of tuberculosis with antigens in addition to tuberculin, to assess their competency to react to tuberculin. (See Warnings.)

Contraindications:

Following a previous unacceptable adverse reaction to this antigen or to a similar product (eg, extreme hypersensitivity or allergy).

Warnings:

Type I allergy: The product should not be used to diagnose or treat Type I allergy to *C albicans.*

Immunodeficiency: Immunodeficiency states, such as advanced HIV infection or cancer, can modify the DTH response to tuberculin. It may be advisable to skin test patients at high risk of tuberculosis with antigens in addition to tuberculin to confirm the patient's state of cellular immunity.

Local reactions usually subside within hours or days after administration of the skin test. In some patients, skin discoloration may persist for several weeks. Local reactions may be treated with a cold compress and topical steroids. Severe loval reactions may require additional measures as appropriate.

In persons with a bleeding tendency, bruising and non-specific induration may occur due to the trauma of the skin test.

Systemic reactions to C albicans have not been observed. However, all foreign antigens have the remote possibility of causing type I anaphylaxis and even death when injected intradermally. Systemic reactions usually occur within 30 minutes fter the injection of antigen.

Hypersensitivity: As has been observed with other, unstandardized antigens used for DTH skin testing, it is possible that some patients may have exquisite immediate hypersensitivity to *C albicans.* These reactions are characterized by the presence of an edematous hive surrounded by a zone of erythema. They occur ≈ 15 to 20 minutes after the intradermal injection of the antigen. The size of the immediate reaction varies depending on the sensitivity of the individual. Immediate hypersensitivity reactions have been reported in 17% to 22% of patients, with erythema of 10 to 24 mm in diameter, and in another 5% to 13% of patients, with erythema of 5 to 9 mm. When using this product, have available the facilities and medications necessary to treat all potential local and systemic side effects. Refer to Management of Acute Hypersensitivity Reactions.

Elderly: C albicans has not been adequately studied in elderly patients. However, the DTH response to *C albicans* may be diminished in elderly patients, since the aging process is known to alter cell-mediated immunity.

Pregnancy: Category C. It is not known whether *C albicans* can cause fetal harm when administered to a pregnant woman or can affect reproduction capacity. Give to pregnant women only if clearly needed. Problems in pregnancy are unlikely.

Lactation: It is not known whether *C albicans* is excreted in breast milk. Problems in breast-feeding are unlikely.

Children: The safety and efficacy in children has not been established.

Precautions:

Route of administration: Inject the antigen intradermally as superficially as possible causing a distinct, sharply defined bleb at the skin test site. An unreliable reaction may result if the product is injected subcutaneously. It must not be given IV. Do not inject into a blood vessel.

CANDIDA ALBICANS SKIN TEST ANTIGEN

Drug Interactions:

Corticosteroids: Pharmacologic doses of corticosteroids may variably suppress the DTH skin test response after 2 weeks of therapy. The mechanism of suppression is believed to involve a decrease in monocytes and lymphocytes, particularly T-cells. The skin test response usually returns to the pretreatment level within several weeks after steroid therapy is discontinued.

Adverse Reactions:

Systemic: Sneezing, coughing, itching, shortness of breath, abdominal cramps, vomiting, diarrhea, tachycardia, hypotension, respiratory failure. Progression of the delayed reaction to vesiculation, necrosis and ulceration is possible (see Warnings).

Local: Redness; swelling; bruising; pruritus; excoriation; discoloration of the skin; rash; vesiculation; bullae dermal exfoliation; cellulitis (severe). (See Warnings.)

Administration and Dosage:

Approved by the FDA on November 27, 1995.

Test method: C albicans skin test antigen is administered intradermally, on the volar surface of the forearm or on the outer aspect of the upper arm. The test dose is 0.1 ml. Cleanse the skin with 70% alcohol before applying the skin test. (See Precautions.)

Interpretation: A positive DTH reaction consists of induration ≥ 5 mm. The time required for the induration response to reach maximum intensity varies with the individual. The reaction usually begins within 24 hours and peaks between 24 and 48 hours. Read the skin test after 48 hours by visually inspecting the test site and palpating the indurated area. Measure across two diameters. Report the mean of the longest and midpoint diameters of the indurated area as the DTH response. For example, a reaction that is 10 mm (longest diameter) by 8 mm (midpoint orthogonal diameter) has a sum of 18 mm and a mean of 9 mm. The DTH response is therefore 9 mm.

Storage/Stability: Store between 2° to 8°C (35° to 46°F). Do not freeze.

Rx	**Candin** (Allermed)	**Injection**: Prepared from the culture filtrate and cells of two strains of *Candida albicans.*	In 1 ml multidose vial.

MUMPS SKIN TEST ANTIGEN (MSTA)

Actions:

Pharmacology: Positive skin tests result from activation of sensitized T-lymphocytes, a delayed-hypersensitivity reaction involving cellular immunity. MSTA deposited in the skin reacts with sensitized lymphocytes, causing the release of mediators that induce the inflammatory, edematous reaction recognized as a positive reaction. The reaction depends on the person having been previously sensitized to mumps.

When used to assess delayed-hypersensitivity reactivity in a group of 90 cancer patients, MSTA was essentially 100% sensitive (as confirmed by reaction to at least one other delayed-hypersensitivity test antigen), implying that no immunocompetent test recipients would test falsely negative.

Indications:

For detection of delayed hypersensitivity to mumps antigens and assessment of cell-mediated immunity. Since most of the population (except the very young) have had contact or infection with mumps virus, they usually demonstrate a delayed cutaneous hypersensitivity to mumps skin test antigen if the immune system is intact; 67% to 90% of healthy adults demonstrate a delayed hypersensitivity reaction.

Contraindications:

Generally, do not administer this product to anyone with a history of hypersensitivity, especially anaphylactic reactions, to eggs or egg products; hypersensitivity to thimerosal.

Warnings:

Immunodeficiency: Persons receiving immunosuppressive therapy or with other immunodeficiencies (especially those involving cell-mediated immunity) may have a diminished skin-test response to this and other diagnostic antigens. Tuberculosis, bacterial, or viral infection, malnutrition, malignancy and immunosuppression may suppress skin-test responsiveness.

Hypersensitivity: Treatment facilities should be readily available. See also Management of Acute Hypersensitivity Reactions.

Elderly: Skin-test responsiveness may be delayed or reduced in magnitude in older persons.

Pregnancy: Category C. Use only if clearly needed. It is unlikely that MSTA crosses the placenta.

Lactation: It is unlikely that MSTA is excreted into breast milk.

Children: Safety and efficacy in children have not been established.

Precautions:

Mumps: MSTA was initially used to determine susceptibility to mumps. It is no longer considered effective at identifying immunity to mumps virus infection. Safety and efficacy have not been established in young adults who have been immunized with live mumps vaccine.

Drug Interactions:

Mumps Skin-Test Antigen Drug Interactions			
Precipitant drug	Object drug*		Description
Cimetidine	MSTA	↑	Several weeks of cimetidine therapy may augment or enhance delayed-hypersensitivity responses to skin-test antigens, although this effect was not consistently observed. The effect may be mediated through cimetidine binding to suppressor T-lymphocytes.
Immunosuppressants Vaccines, viral	MSTA	↓	Reactivity to any delayed-hypersensitivity test may be suppressed in persons receiving corticosteroids or other immunosuppressive drugs, or in persons who were recently immunized with live virus vaccines (eg, measles, mumps, rubella, poliovirus). If delayed-hypersensitivity skin testing is indicated, perform it either preceding or simultaneously with immunization or 4 to 6 weeks after immunization.

* ↑ = Object drug increased. ↓ = Object drug decreased.

MUMPS SKIN TEST ANTIGEN (MSTA)

Adverse Reactions:

Local reactions may include tenderness, pruritus, vesiculation and rash. Sloughing, necrosis, abscess formation, or regional lymphadenopathy may be associated with unusually large delayed-hypersensitivity reactions. Adverse reactions may include nausea, anorexia, headache, unsteadiness, drowsiness, sweating, sensation of warmth and lymphadenopathy.

Administration and Dosage:

Must be given intradermally. If it is injected SC, no reaction or an unreliable reaction may occur.

Test method: Inject 0.1 ml intradermally on the inner surface of the forearm after suitable preparation of the skin. Examine the reaction in 48 to 72 hours.

Interpretation: Positive reaction consists of a mean diameter of induration > 5 mm (ie, the average of the longest width and the longest length). A positive test implies previous antigenic exposure and, indirectly, T-lymphocyte competence and an intact inflammatory response, and confirms the integrity of the cellular immune response.

Negative reaction: If the test has been given correctly, it probably indicates either anergy or nonsensitivity.

Pseudopositive reactions may develop in persons sensitive to egg protein.

Storage/Stability: Store between 2° and 8°C (36° to 46°F). Discard if frozen. Product can tolerate ≤ 4 days at ≤ 37°C (100°F).

Rx	**MSTA** (Connaught)	**Injection:** 40 complement-fixing units per ml	With 0.012 M glycine, < 1:8000 formaldehyde solution and 1:10,000 thimerosal. In 1 ml vials (10 tests).

SKIN TEST ANTIGENS, MULTIPLE

The skin test for multiple antigens consists of a disposable applicator with eight sterile heads preloaded with the following seven delayed hypersensitivity skin test antigens and glycerin negative control for percutaneous administration: Tetanus Toxoid Antigen, Diphtheria Toxoid Antigen, Streptococcus Antigen, Old Tuberculin, Candida Antigen, Trichophyton Antigen and Proteus Antigen. The delayed cutaneous responses associated with this test appear to be typical cellular hypersensitivity reactions.

Indications:

For detection of anergy (nonresponsiveness to antigens) by means of delayed hypersensitivity skin testing.

Contraindications:

Do not apply on acneiform, infected or inflamed skin. Although severe systemic reactions are rare to diphtheria and tetanus antigens, persons known to have a history of systemic reactions should be tested only after the test heads containing these antigens have been removed.

Warnings:

Hypersensitivity: Epinephrine should be available. See also Management of Acute Hypersensitivity Reactions.

Pregnancy: Category C. Animal reproduction studies have not been conducted. It is not known whether skin test antigens can cause fetal harm when administered to a pregnant woman or can affect reproduction capacity. Give to a pregnant woman only if clearly needed. Pregnancy may result in a decreased level of sensitivity to the test antigens.

Children: Skin testing is recommended only for subjects ≥ 17 years. Safety and efficacy in children below this age have not been established.

Precautions:

Reactivity to delayed hypersensitivity skin test antigens may decrease or disappear temporarily as a result of: Febrile illness; measles and other viral infections; live virus vaccination including measles, mumps, rubella and poliomyelitis vaccines.

Loss of reactivity may occur in patients undergoing treatment with drugs or procedures that suppress immunity such as: Corticosteroids, chemotherapeutic agents, antilymphocyte globulin and irradiation.

Administration and Dosage:

Remove skin test antigens from refrigeration approximately 1 hour before use.

Select only test sites that permit sufficient surface area and subcutaneous tissue to allow adequate penetration of all points on all 8 test heads. Preferred sites are the volar surfaces of the arms and the back; skin of the posterior thighs may be used. If several tests are planned, alternate forearms. Avoid hairy areas when possible because reaction interpretation will be more difficult.

Interpretation: Read test sites at both 24 and 48 hours, if possible, and use the largest reaction recorded from the 2 readings at each test site. If 2 readings are not possible, a single 48 hour reading is recommended.

A positive reaction from any of the 7 antigens is induration of ≥ 2 mm, providing there is no induration at the negative control site.

Periodic testing can determine if anergy persists or if skin reactivity has returned. If periodic testing is done more frequently than every 2 months, rotate the test sites so that retesting is not conducted at the same site sooner than 2 months. Refer to the manufacturer's scoring system for instruction.

Storage: Store at 2° to 8°C (35° to 46°F).

Rx	**Multitest CMI** (Connaught)	In single use, preloaded applicators.
Rx	**T.R.U.E. Test** (Glaxo Wellcome)	In multipack cartons (5s).

PEGADEMASE BOVINE

Actions:

Pharmacology: Pegademase bovine is a modified enzyme used for enzyme replacement therapy for the treatment of severe combined immunodeficiency disease (SCID) associated with a deficiency of adenosine deaminase. The drug will not benefit patients with immunodeficiency due to other causes. It is a conjugate of numerous strands of monomethoxypolyethylene glycol (PEG), covalently attached to the enzyme adenosine deaminase (ADA). ADA, used in the manufacture of pegademase bovine, is derived from bovine intestine.

Pegademase bovine provides specific replacement of the deficient enzyme. In the absence of the enzyme ADA, the purine substrates adenosine, 2'-deoxyadenosine and their metabolites are toxic to lymphocytes. The direct action of pegademase bovine is the correction of these metabolic abnormalities. Improvement in immune function and diminished frequency of opportunistic infections only occurs after metabolic abnormalities are corrected. There is a lag between the correction of the metabolic abnormalities and improved immune function. This period of time is variable, from a few weeks to as long as 6 months. In contrast to the natural history of combined immunodeficiency disease due to ADA deficiency, a trend toward diminished frequency of opportunistic infections and fewer complications of infections has occurred in patients receiving pegademase bovine.

SCID associated with ADA deficiency is a rare, inherited and often fatal disease. In the absence of ADA enzyme, purine substrates adenosine and 2'-deoxyadenosine accumulate, causing metabolic abnormalities that are directly toxic to lymphocytes.

The immune deficiency can be cured by bone marrow transplantation. When a suitable bone marrow donor is unavailable or when bone marrow transplantation fails, non-selective replacement of the ADA enzyme has been provided by periodic irradiated red blood cell transfusions. However, transmission of viral infections and iron overload are serious risks, and relatively few ADA-deficient patients have benefited from chronic transfusion therapy.

In patients with ADA deficiency, rigorous adherence to a schedule of pegademase bovine can eliminate toxic metabolites of ADA deficiency and improve immune function. Carefully monitor by measurement of the level of ADA activity in plasma. Monitoring the level of deoxyadenosine triphosphate (dATP) in erythrocytes is also helpful in determining that the dose is adequate.

Pharmacokinetics: Pharmacokinetics and biochemical effects have been studied in six children ranging in age from 6 weeks to 12 years with SCID associated with ADA deficiency. After IM injection, peak plasma ADA activity levels were reached in 2 to 3 days. ADA plasma elimination half-life of was variable, even for the same child. Range was 3 to > 6 days. Following weekly injections of 15 U/kg, average trough level of ADA activity in plasma was between 20 and 25 mcmol/hr/ml.

The changes in red blood cell deoxyadenosine nucleotide (ie, dATP) and S-adenosylhomocysteine hydrolase (SAHase) have been evaluated. In patients with ADA deficiency, inadequate elimination of 2'-deoxyadenosine caused a marked elevation in dATP and a decrease in SAHase level in red blood cells. Prior to treatment with pegademase bovine, the levels of dATP in the red blood cells ranged from 0.056 to 0.899 mcmol/ml of erythrocytes. After 2 months of maintenance treatment, the levels decreased to 0.007 to 0.015 mcmol/ml. The normal value of dATP is below 0.001 mcmol/ml. In the same period of time, SAHase increased from pretreatment range of 0.09 to 0.22 nmol/hr/mg protein to 2.37 to 5.16 nmol/hr/mg protein. Normal value for SAHase is 4.18 $\pm$ 1.9 nmol/hr/mg protein.

Indications:

For enzyme replacement therapy for ADA deficiency in patients with severe combined immunodeficiency disease who are not suitable candidates for or who have failed bone marrow transplantation. Pegademase bovine is recommended for use in infants from birth or in children of any age at the time of diagnosis. It is not intended as a replacement for HLA identical bone marrow transplant therapy, and it is also not intended to replace continued close medical supervision and the initiation of appropriate diagnostic tests and therapy (eg, antibiotics, nutrition, oxygen, gammaglobulin) as indicated for intercurrent illnesses.

Contraindications:

There is no evidence to support the safety and efficacy of pegademase bovine as preparatory or support therapy for bone marrow transplantation. Since the drug is administered by IM injection, use with caution in patients with thrombocytopenia and do not use if thrombocytopenia is severe.

Warnings:

Product potency testing prior to distribution may not assure the initial and continuing potency of each new lot of pegademase bovine. Report any laboratory or clinical indication of a decrease in potency *immediately* by telephone to Enzon (201-668-1800).

PEGADEMASE BOVINE

Pregnancy: Category C. It is not known whether pegademase bovine can cause fetal harm when administered to a pregnant woman or can affect reproduction capacity. Give to a pregnant woman only if clearly needed.

Lactation: It is not known whether pegademase bovine is excreted in breast milk. Exercise caution when administering to a nursing woman.

Precautions:

Immunodeficiency: Maintain appropriate care to protect immune-deficient patients until improvement in immune function has been documented. The degree of immune function improvement may vary from patient to patient and, therefore, each patient will require appropriate care consistent with immunologic status.

Laboratory test monitoring: Monitor the treatment of SCID associated with ADA deficiency with pegademase bovine by measuring plasma ADA activity and red blood cell dATP levels.

Determine plasma ADA activity and red cell dATP prior to treatment. Once treatment has been initiated, a desirable range of plasma ADA activity (trough level before maintenance injection) should be 15 to 35 mcmol/hr/ml. This minimum trough level will ensure that plasma ADA activity from injection to injection is maintained above the level of total erythrocyte ADA activity in the blood of normal individuals.

Determine plasma ADA activity (pre-injection) every 1 to 2 weeks during the first 8 to 12 weeks of treatment in order to establish an effective dose. After 2 months of maintenance treatment, red cell dATP levels should decrease to a range of ≤ 0.005 to 0.015 mcmol/ml. The normal value of dATP is below 0.001 mcmol/ml. Once the level of dATP has fallen adequately, measure 2 to 4 times during the remainder of the first year and 2 to 3 times a year thereafter, assuming no interruption in therapy.

Between 3 and 9 months, determine plasma ADA twice a month, then monthly until after 18 to 24 months of treatment. In patients who have successfully been maintained on therapy for 2 years, continue to have plasma ADA measured every 2 to 4 months and red cell dATP measured twice yearly. More frequent monitoring would be necessary if therapy were interrupted or if an enhanced rate of clearance of plasma ADA activity develops.

Once effective ADA plasma levels have been established, should a patient's plasma ADA activity level fall below 10 mcmol/hr/ml (which cannot be attributed to improper dosing, sample handling or antibody development) then all patients receiving this lot of pegademase bovine will be required to have a blood sample for plasma ADA determination taken prior to their next injection. The index patient will require retesting for determination of plasma ADA activity prior to their next injection. If this value, as well as the value from one of the other patients from a different site, is < 10 mcmol/hr/ml, then the lot in use will be recalled and replaced with a new clinical lot by Enzon.

Immune function, including the ability to produce antibodies, generally improves after 2 to 6 months of therapy, and matures over a longer period. Compared with the natural history of combined immunodeficiency disease due to ADA deficiency, a trend toward diminished frequency of opportunistic infections and fewer complications of infections has occurred in patients receiving pegademase bovine. However, the lag between the correction of the metabolic abnormalities and improved immune function with a trend toward diminished frequency of infections and complications of infection is variable, and has ranged from a few weeks to ≈ 6 months. Improvement in the general clinical status of the patient may be gradual (as evidenced by improvement in various clinical parameters) but should be apparent by the end of the first year of therapy.

A decline in immune function, with increased risk of opportunistic infections and complications of infection, will result from failure to maintain adequate levels of plasma ADA activity (whether due to the development of antibody, improper calculation of dosage, interruption of treatment or to improper storage with subsequent loss of activity). If a persistent decline in plasma ADA activity occurs, monitor immune function and clinical status closely and take precautions to minimize the risk of infection. If antibody to ADA or pegademase bovine is found to be the cause of a persistent fall in plasma ADA activity, then adjustment in the dosage and other measures may be taken to induce tolerance and restore adequate ADA activity.

Antibody to pegademase bovine may develop in patients and may result in more rapid clearance of the drug. Suspect antibody to pegademase bovine if a persistent fall in pre-injection level of plasma ADA to < 10 mcmol/hr/ml occurs. If other causes for a decline in plasma ADA levels can be ruled out (eg, improper storage of vials [freezing or prolonged storage at temperatures > 4°C], or improper handling of plasma samples [eg, repeated freezing and thawing during transport to laboratory];), then perform a specific assay for antibody to ADA and pegademase bovine (ELISA, enzyme inhibition).

PEGADEMASE BOVINE

One of 12 patients showed an enhanced rate of clearance of plasma ADA activity after 5 months of therapy at 15 U/kg/week. Enhanced clearance was correlated with the appearance of an antibody that directly inhibited both unmodified ADA and pegademase bovine. Subsequently, the patient was treated with twice weekly IM injections at an increased dose of 20 U/kg, or a total weekly dose of 40 U/kg. No adverse effects were observed at the higher dose and effective levels of plasma ADA were restored. After 4 months, the patient returned to a weekly dosage schedule of 20 U/kg and effective plasma levels have been maintained.

Drug Interactions:

Vidarabine is a substrate for ADA and **2′-deoxycoformycin** is a potent inhibitor of ADA. Thus, the activities of these drugs and pegademase bovine could be substantially altered if they are used in combination with one another.

Adverse Reactions:

Clinical experience is limited. The following adverse reactions have occurred: Headache (one patient) and pain at the injection site (two patients).

Overdosage:

An intraperitoneal dose of 50,000 U/kg of pegademase bovine in mice resulted in weight loss up to 9%.

Administration and Dosage:

Before prescribing pegademase bovine, the physician should be thoroughly familiar with the details of this prescribing information. For further information concerning the essential monitoring of therapy, contact Enzon, Inc., 40 Cragwood Road, South Plainfield, NJ 07080 (201-668-1800).

Pegademase bovine is recommended for use in infants from birth or in children of any age at the time of diagnosis.

Administer every 7 days as an IM injection. Individualize the dosage.

First dose – 10 U/kg;
Second dose – 15 U/kg;
Third dose – 20 U/kg;
Usual maintenance dose – 20 U/kg/week. Further increases of 5 U/kg/week may be necessary, but a maximum single dose of 30 U/kg should not be exceeded.

Plasma levels of ADA more than twice the upper limit of 35 mcmol/hr/ml have occurred on occasion in several patients, and have been maintained for several weeks in one patient who received twice weekly injections (20 U/kg per dose). No adverse effects have been observed at these higher levels; there is no evidence that maintaining pre-injection plasma ADA > 35 mcmol/hr/ml produces any additional clinical benefits.

Dose proportionality has not been established; closely monitor patients when the dosage is increased. Pegademase bovine is not recommended for IV administration.

Establish the optimal dosage and schedule of administration for each patient based on monitoring of plasma ADA activity levels (trough levels before maintenance injection), biochemical markers of ADA deficiency (primarily red cell dATP content). Since improvement in immune function follows correction of metabolic abnormalities, maintenance dosage in individual patients should be aimed at achieving the following biochemical goals: 1) Maintain plasma ADA activity (trough levels before maintenance injection) in the range of 15 to 35 mcmol/hr/ml (assayed at 37°C); and 2) decline in erythrocyte dATP to ≤ 0.005 to 0.015 mcmol/ml packed erythrocytes, or ≤ 1% of the total erythrocyte adenine nucleotide (ATP= dATP) content, with a normal ATP level, as measured in a pre-injection sample. In addition, continued monitoring of immune function and clinical status is essential in any patient with a primary immunodeficiency disease and should be continued in patients being treated with pegademase bovine.

Admixture incompatibility: Pegademase bovine should not be diluted nor mixed with any other drug prior to administration.

Storage: Refrigerate. Store between 2°C and 8°C (36°F and 46°F). Do not freeze. Pegademase bovine should not be stored at room temperature. This product should not be used if there are any indications that it may have been frozen.

Rx	**Adagen** (Enzon)	**Injection:** 250 units[1]/ml[2]	In 1.5 ml vials.

[1] One unit of activity is defined as the amount of ADA that converts 1 mcM of adenosine to inosine per minute at 25°C and pH 7.3.

[2] With 1.2 mg monobasic sodium phosphate, 5.58 mg dibasic sodium phosphate, 8.5 mg sodium chloride and water for injection.

INTERFERON GAMMA-1B

Actions:

Pharmacology: Interferon gamma-1b, a biologic response modifier, is a single-chain polypeptide containing 140 amino acids. Production of interferon gamma is achieved by fermentation of a genetically engineered *Escherichia coli* bacterium containing the DNA which encodes for the human protein.

Interferons are a family of functionally related, species-specific proteins synthesized by eukaryotic cells in response to viruses and a variety of natural and synthetic stimuli. The most striking differences between interferon gamma and other classes of interferon concern the immunomodulatory properties of this molecule. While gamma, alpha and beta interferons share certain properties, interferon gamma has potent phagocyte-activating effects not seen with other interferon preparations, including generation of toxic oxygen metabolites within phagocytes, which are capable of mediating the killing of microorganisms such as *Staphylococcus aureus, Toxoplasma gondii, Leishmania donovani, Listeria monocytogenes,* and *Mycobacterium avium intracellulare.*

Clinical studies in patients using interferon gamma have revealed a broad range of biological activities including the enhancement of the oxidative metabolism of tissue macrophages, enhancement of antibody-dependent cellular cytotoxicity and natural killer cell activity. Additionally, effects of Fc receptor expression on monocytes and major histocompatibility antigen expression have been noted.

To the extent that interferon gamma is produced by antigen-stimulated T lymphocytes and regulates activity of immune cells, it is appropriate to characterize it as a lymphokine of the interleukin type. There is growing evidence that interferon gamma interacts functionally with other interleukin molecules such as interleukin-2, and that all interleukins form part of a complex, lymphokine regulatory network. For example, interferon gamma and interleukin-4 appear to reciprocally interact to regulate murine IgE levels; interferon gamma can suppress IgE levels and inhibit collagen production at the transcription level in human systems.

Pharmacokinetics: Following single-dose administration of 100 mcg/m^2, interferon gamma is rapidly cleared after IV use (1.4 L/minute) and slowly absorbed after IM or SC injection. After IM or SC injection, the apparent fraction of dose absorbed was > 89%. The mean elimination half-life after IV administration was 38 minutes. The mean elimination half-lives for IM and SC dosing were 2.9 and 5.9 hours, respectively. Peak plasma concentrations occurred approximately 4 hours (1.5 ng/ml) after IM dosing and 7 hours (0.6 ng/ml) after SC dosing. Multiple-dose SC pharmacokinetic studies were conducted in 38 healthy male subjects. There was no accumulation of drug after 12 consecutive daily injections of 100 mcg/m^2. Use in nephrectomized mice and squirrel monkeys demonstrated reduced clearance of drug from blood; however, prior nephrectomy did not prevent elimination.

Clinical trials: A randomized, double-blind, placebo controlled study in patients (n = 128; 1 to 44 years of age) with chronic granulomatous disease (an inherited disorder characterized by deficient phagocyte oxidative metabolism) was performed to determine whether SC interferon gamma 3 times weekly could decrease the incidence of serious infectious episodes and improve existing infectious and inflammatory conditions. Most patients received prophylactic antibiotics. Serious infection was defined as a clinical event requiring hospitalization and the use of parenteral antibiotics. There was a 67% reduction in relative risk of serious infection in patients receiving interferon gamma (n = 63) compared to placebo (n = 65). Additional supportive evidence of treatment benefit included a twofold reduction in the number of primary serious infections in the interferon gamma group and the total number and rate of serious infections including recurrent events. Placebo patients required three times as many inpatient hospitalization days for treatment of clinical events compared to patients receiving interferon gamma. The beneficial effect of therapy was observed throughout the entire study, in which the mean duration of administration was 8.9 months per patient.

Indications:

For reducing the frequency and severity of serious infections associated with chronic granulomatous disease.

Contraindications:

Hypersensitivity to interferon gamma, *E coli* derived products or any component of the product.

Warnings:

Seizure disorders/compromised CNS function: Exercise caution in patients with these conditions. CNS adverse reactions including decreased mental status, gait disturbance and dizziness have been observed, particularly in patients receiving doses > 250 mcg/m^2/day. Most of these abnormalities were mild and reversible within a few days upon dose reduction or discontinuation of therapy.

INTERFERON GAMMA-1B

Cardiac disease: Use with caution in pre-existing cardiac disease, including symptoms of ischemia, CHF or arrhythmia. No direct cardiotoxic effect has been demonstrated, but it is possible that acute and transient "flu-like" or constitutional symptoms such as fever and chills frequently associated with interferon gamma administration at doses of ≥ 250 mcg/m²/day may exacerbate pre-existing conditions.

Myelosuppression: Exercise caution in patients with myelosuppression. Reversible neutropenia and elevation of hepatic enzymes can be dose-limiting at doses > 250 mcg/m²/day. Thrombocytopenia and proteinuria have also occurred rarely.

Hypersensitivity: Acute serious hypersensitivity reactions have not been observed in patients receiving interferon gamma; however, if such an acute reaction develops, discontinue the drug immediately and institute appropriate medical therapy. Refer to Management of Acute Hypersensitivity Reactions. Transient cutaneous rashes have occurred in some patients following injection but have rarely necessitated treatment interruption.

Fertility impairment: Female monkeys treated with daily SC doses of 150 mcg/kg (approximately 100 times the human dose) exhibited irregular menstrual cycles or absence of cyclicity during treatment.

Pregnancy: Category C. Interferon gamma has shown an increased incidence of abortions in primates when given in doses approximately 100 times the human dose. There are no adequate and well controlled studies in pregnant women. Use during pregnancy only if the potential benefit justifies the potential risk to the fetus. In addition, studies evaluating recombinant murine interferon gamma in pregnant mice revealed increased incidences of uterine bleeding and abortifacient activity and decreased neonatal viability at maternally toxic doses. The clinical significance of this observation is uncertain.

Lactation: It is not known whether interferon gamma is excreted in breast milk. Because of the potential for serious adverse reactions in nursing infants, decide whether to discontinue nursing or to discontinue the drug, depending on the importance of the drug to the mother.

Children: Safety and efficacy in children < 1 year of age has not been established.

Precautions:

Monitoring: In addition to tests normally required for monitoring patients with chronic granulomatous disease, the following laboratory tests are recommended for all patients prior to beginning therapy and at 3 month intervals during treatment: Hematologic tests including complete blood counts, differential and platelet counts; blood chemistries including renal and liver function tests; urinalysis.

Drug Interactions:

Myelosuppressive agents: Exercise caution when administering in combination with potentially myelosuppressive agents (see Warnings).

Preclinical studies in rodents have demonstrated a decrease in hepatic microsomal cytochrome P–450 concentrations. This could potentially lead to a depression of the hepatic metabolism of certain drugs that utilize this degradative pathway.

Adverse Reactions:

The following data on adverse reactions are based on the SC use of 50 mcg/m² interferon gamma 3 times weekly in 63 patients with chronic granulomatous disease.

Interferon Gamma-1B Adverse Reactions (%)

Adverse reaction	Interferon gamma-1b (n = 63)	Placebo (n = 65)	Adverse reaction	Interferon gamma-1b (n = 63)	Placebo (n = 65)
Fever	52	28	Abdominal pain[1]	8	3
Headache	33	9	Weight loss	6	6
Rash	17	6	Myalgia	6	0
Chills	14	0	Anorexia	3	5
Injection site erythema or tenderness	14	2	Depression[1]	3	0
			Arthralgia	2	0
Fatigue	14	11	Back pain[1]	2	0
Diarrhea	14	12	Injection site pain	0	2
Vomiting	13	5			
Nausea	10	2			

[1] May have been related to underlying disease.

INTERFERON GAMMA-1B

Interferon gamma has also been evaluated in additional disease states in studies in which patients have generally received higher doses (> 100 mcg/m^2/day) administered by IM injection or IV infusion. All of the previously described adverse reactions which occurred in patients with chronic granulomatous disease have also been observed in patients receiving higher doses. Adverse reactions not observed in patients with chronic granulomatous disease receiving doses < 100 mcg/m^2/day but seen rarely in patients receiving interferon gamma in other studies include:

Cardiovascular: Hypotension; syncope; tachyarrhythmia; heart block; heart failure; myocardial infarction.

CNS: Confusion; disorientation; gait disturbance; parkinsonian symptoms; seizure; hallucinations; transient ischemic attacks.

GI: Hepatic insufficiency; GI bleeding; pancreatitis.

Hematologic: Deep venous thrombosis; pulmonary embolism.

Pulmonary: Tachypnea; bronchospasm; interstitial pneumonitis.

Metabolic: Hyponatremia; hyperglycemia.

Miscellaneous: Exacerbation of dermatomyositis; reversible renal insufficiency.

Patient Information:

Inform patients of the potential benefits and risks associated with treatment. If home use is determined to be desirable by the physician, give instructions on appropriate use, including a review of the contents of the Patient Information insert. This information is intended to aid in the safe and effective use of the medication; it is not a disclosure of all possible adverse or intended effects.

If home use is prescribed, supply the patients with a puncture resistant container for the disposal of used syringes and needles. Thoroughly instruct patients in the importance of proper disposal and caution against any reuse of needles and syringes. Dispose of the full container according to the directions provided by the physician.

The most common adverse experiences are "flu-like" or constitutional symptoms such as fever, headache, chills, myalgia or fatigue which may decrease in severity as treatment continues. Some of the "flu-like" symptoms may be minimized by bedtime administration. Acetaminophen may be used to prevent or partially alleviate the fever and headache.

Administration and Dosage:

Chronic granulomatous disease: 50 mcg/m^2 (1.5 million U/m^2) for patients whose body surface area is > 0.5 m^2 and 1.5 mcg/kg/dose for patients whose body surface area is ≤ 0.5 m^2. Administer SC 3 times weekly (eg, Monday, Wednesday, Friday). The optimum sites of injection are the right and left deltoid and anterior thigh. Interferon gamma can be administered by a physician, nurse, family member or patient when trained in the administration of SC injections.

The formulation does not contain a preservative. A vial is suitable for a single dose only. Discard the unused portion of any vial.

Higher doses are not recommended. Safety and efficacy have not been established for interferon gamma given in doses greater or less than the recommended dose of 50 mcg/m^2. The minimum effective dose has not been established.

If severe reactions occur, modify the dosage (50% reduction) or discontinue therapy until the adverse reaction abates.

Interferon gamma may be administered using either sterilized glass or plastic disposable syringes.

Storage/Stability: Vials must be placed in a 2° to 8°C (36° to 46°F) refrigerator immediately upon receipt to ensure optimal retention of physical and biochemical integrity; do not freeze. Avoid excessive or vigorous agitation; do not shake. An unentered vial should not be left at room temperature for a total time exceeding 12 hours prior to use. Vials exceeding this time period should not be returned to the refrigerator; discard such vials.

Rx	**Actimmune** (Genentech)	**Injection:** 100 mcg (3 million U)	In single-dose vials.[1]

[1] With 20 mg mannitol, 0.36 mg sodium succinate, 0.05 mg polysorbate 20.

INTERFERON BETA

Actions:

Pharmacology: Interferon beta-1a and 1b are purified, sterile, lyophilized protein products produced by recombinant DNA techniques and formulated for use by injection. Interferon beta-1a is a 166 amino acid glycoprotein. It is produced by mammalian cells (Chinese hamster ovary cells) into which the human interferon beta gene has been introduced. The amino acid sequence of interferon beta-1a is identical to that of natural human interferon beta. Interferon beta-1b is manufactured by bacterial fermentation of a strain of *Escherichia coli* that bears a genetically engineered plasmid containing the gene for human interferon $beta_{ser17}$. Interferon beta-1b is a highly purified protein that has 165 amino acids. It does not include the carbohydrate side chains found in the natural material.

Interferons are a family of naturally occuring proteins and glycoproteins that are produced by eukaryotic cells in response to viral infection and other biological inducers. Interferon beta is produced by various cell types including fibroblasts and macrophages. Three major classes of interferons have been identified: Alfa, beta and gamma; they each have overlapping yet distinct biologic activities.

Interferon beta has both antiviral, antiproliferative and immunoregulatory activities. The mechanisms by which it exerts its actions in multiple sclerosis (MS) are not clearly understood. However, it is known that the biologic response-modifying properties of interferon beta are mediated through its interactions with specific cell receptors found on the surface of human cells. The binding to these receptors induces the expression of a number of interferon-induced gene products that are believed to be the mediators of the biological actions of interferon beta.

Pharmacokinetics:

Interferon beta-1a – Biological response markers (eg, neopterin and β_2—microglobulin) are induced by interferon beta-1a following parenteral doses of 15 to 75 mcg in healthy subjects and treated patients. Biological response marker levels increase within 12 hours of dosing and remain elevated for at least 4 days. Peak biological response marker levels are typically observed 48 hours after dosing.

Pharmacokinetic Parameters Following 60 mcg Administration of Interferon beta-1a

Route	AUC (IU•hr/ml)	C_{max} (IU/ml)	T_{max} (range [hr])	Elimination half-life (hr)
IM	1352	45	9.8 (3-15)	10
SC	478	30	7.8 (3-18)	8.6

Interferon beta-1b – Because serum concentrations of interferon beta-1b are low or not detectable following SC administration of ≤ 0.25 mg (8 mIU), pharmacokinetic information in patients with MS receiving the recommended dose is not available. Following single and multiple daily SC administrations of 0.5 mg (16 mIU) to healthy volunteers (n = 12), serum concentrations were generally < 100 IU/ml. Peak serum concentrations occurred between 1 to 8 hours, with a mean peak serum concentration of 40 IU/ml. Bioavailability, based on a total dose of 0.5 mg given as two SC injections at different sites, was ≈ 50%.

After IV administration (0.006 [0.2 mIU] to 2 mg [64 mIU]), similar pharmacokinetic profiles were obtained from healthy volunteers (n = 12) and from patients with diseases other than MS (n = 142). In patients receiving single IV doses up to 2 mg, increases in serum concentrations were dose-proportional. Mean serum clearance values ranged from 9.4 to 28.9 ml/min/kg and were independent of dose. Mean terminal elimination half-life values ranged from 8 minutes to 4.3 hours and mean steady-state volume of distribution values ranged from 0.25 to 2.88 L/kg. IV dosing 3 times a week for 2 weeks resulted in no accumulation of interferon beta-1b in the serum of patients. Pharmacokinetic parameters after single and multiple IV doses were comparable.

INTERFERON BETA

Clinical trials:

Interferon beta-1a – Patients with relapsing (stable or progressive) MS (n = 301) received either 6 million IU (30 mcg) of interferon beta-1a (n = 158) or placebo (n = 143) by IM injection once weekly. Patients received injections for up to 2 years. There were 144 patients treated for > 1 year, 115 for > 18 months and 82 for 2 years. Time to onset of sustained progression in disability was significantly longer in patients treated with interferon beta-1a than in patients receiving placebo.

Interferon beta-1b – The effectiveness of interferon beta-1b in relapsing-remitting MS was evaluated in MS patients, aged 18 to 50, who were ambulatory, exhibited a relapsing-remitting clinical course, met Poser's criteria for clinically definite or laboratory supported definite MS and had experienced at least two exacerbations over 2 years preceding the trial without exacerbation in the preceding month. Patients were randomized to treatment with either placebo (n = 123), or interferon beta-1b 0.05 (n = 125) or 0.25 mg (n = 124) self-administered SC every other day. Outcome was evaluated after 2 years.

In the 2 year analysis, there was a 31% reduction in annual exacerbation rate, from 1.31 in the placebo group to 0.9 in the 0.25 mg interferon beta-1b group. The proportion of patients free of exacerbations was 16% in the placebo group, compared with 25% in the 0.25 mg interferon beta-1b group. Results from other endpoints measured included the following (placebo vs 0.25 mg interferon beta-1b): Median number of months to first on-study exacerbation, 5 vs 9; rate of moderate or severe exacerbations per year, 0.47 vs 0.23; mean number of moderate or severe exacerbation days per patient, 44.1 vs 19.5; median duration in days per exacerbation, 36 vs 35.5; percent change in mean MRI lesion area at endpoint, 21.4% vs -0.9% (the exact relationship between MRI findings and the clinical status of patients is unknown; changes in lesion area often do not correlate with clinical exacerbations).

Indications:

Multiple sclerosis (MS): Treatment of MS. See individual monographs for specific indications.

Unlabeled uses: Interferon beta is being investigated in the treatment of AIDS, AIDS-related Kaposi's sarcoma, metastatic renal-cell carcinoma, herpes of the lips or genitals, malignant melanoma, cutaneous T-cell lymphoma and acute non-A/non-B hepatitis.

Contraindications:

Hypersensitivity to natural or recombinant interferon beta, albumin human or any other component of the formulations.

Warnings:

Chronic progressive MS: The safety and efficacy of interferon beta in chronic progressive MS have not been evaluated.

Depression: Use interferon beta with caution in patients with depression. Depression and suicide have been reported in patients receiving other interferon compounds. Depression and suicidal ideation are known to occur at an increased frequency in the MS population. A relationship between occurrence of depression or suicidal ideation and the use of interferon beta has not been established. An equal incidence of depression was seen in the placebo-treated and interferon beta-treated patients in the MS study.

Advise patients treated with interferon beta to report immediately any symptoms of depression or suicidal ideation. If a patient develops depression, consider cessation of therapy. Other mental disorders have been observed and can include anxiety, emotional lability, depersonalization and confusion.

Seizures: Exercise caution when administering interferon beta to patients with preexisting seizure disorder. It is not known whether these events were related to the effects of MS alone, to interferon beta or to a combination of both. For patients with no prior history of seizures who develop seizures during therapy with interferon beta, establish an etiologic basis and institute appropriate anticonvulsant therapy prior to considering resumption of treatment.

Cardiac disease: Closely monitor patients with cardiac disease, such as angina, CHF or arrhythmia, for worsening of their clinical condition during initiation. Interferon beta does not have any known direct-acting cardiac toxicity; however, symptoms of flu syndrome seen with interferon beta therapy may prove stressful to patients with severe cardiac conditions.

Pregnancy: Category C. There are no adequate and well controlled studies in pregnant women. Abortifacient activity has been shown in animals. If the patient becomes pregnant or plans to become pregnant while taking interferon beta, apprise the patient of the potential hazards to the fetus and recommend that the patient discontinue therapy.

Lactation: It is not known whether interferon beta is excreted in breast milk. Decide whether to discontinue nursing or discontinue the drug, taking into account the importance of the drug to the mother.

Children: Safety and efficacy in children < 18 years of age have not been established.

Precautions:

Monitoring: The following laboratory tests are recommended prior to initiating therapy and at periodic intervals thereafter: Hemoglobin; complete and differential WBC counts; platelet counts and blood chemistries including liver function tests.

Self-administration: Instruct patients in injection techniques to ensure the safe self-administration of interferon beta. A patient information sheet is provided with the product.

Flu-like symptoms complex was reported in 61% to 76% of the patients treated with interferon beta. A patient was defined as having a flu-like symptom complex if at least two of the following symptoms were concurrently reported: Fever, chills, myalgia, malaise, sweating or flu-like syndrome.

Photosensitivity: Photosensitization (photoallergy or phototoxicity) may occur; therefore, caution patients to take protective measures (ie, sunscreens, protective clothing) against exposure to ultraviolet light or sunlight until tolerance is determined.

INTERFERON BETA

Adverse Reactions:

Interferon Beta Adverse Reactions (%)[1]

Adverse Reaction	Interferon beta-1a	Interferon beta-1b
Body as a whole		
Injection site reaction	4	85
Headache	67	84
Fever	23	59
Flu-like symptoms	61	76
Pain	24	52
Asthenia	21	49
Chills	21	46
Infection	11	-
Abdominal pain	9	32
Chest pain	6	-
Malaise	4	15
Generalized edema	-	8
Pelvic pain	-	6
Injection site necrosis/inflammation	3	5
Cyst/Ovarian cyst	3	4
Suicide attempt	4	2
Goiter	-	2
Hypersensitivity reaction	3	-
Cardiovascular		
Migraine	-	12
Palpitation	-	8
Hypertension	-	7
Tachycardia	-	6
Peripheral vascular disorder	-	5
Hemorrhage	-	3
Syncope	4	-
Vasodilation	4	-
Hemic/Lymphatic		
Lymphocytes $<1500/mm^3$	-	82
ANC $< 1500/mm^3$	-	18
WBC $< 3000/mm^3$	-	16
Lymphadenopathy	-	14
Anemia	8	-
Eosinophils ≥ 10%	5	-
HCT (%) ≤ 37	3	-
Ecchymosis at injection site	2	-
Respiratory		
Sinusitis	18	36
Upper Respiratory tract infection	31	-
Dyspnea	6	8
Laryngitis	-	6
Musculoskeletal		
Myalgia	34	44
Myasthenia	-	13
arthralgia	9	-

Adverse Reaction	Interferon beta-1a	Interferon beta-1b
GI		
Nausea	33	-
Diarrhea	16	35
Constipation	-	24
Vomiting	-	21
Dyspepsia	11	-
Anorexia	7	-
GI disorder	-	6
Metabolic/Nutritional		
ALT > 5 × baseline	-	19
Glucose < 55 mg/dl	-	15
Total bilirubin > 2.5 × baseline	-	6
Urine protein > 1+	-	5
AST > 5 × baseline	-	4
Weight gain	-	4
Weight loss	-	4
AST ≥ 3 × ULN	3	-
CNS		
Mental symptoms	-	29
Hypertonia	-	26
Sleep difficulty	19	-
Dizziness	15	35
Muscle spasm	7	-
Somnolence	-	6
Speech disorder	3	3
Convulsion	3	2
Ataxia	2	-
Hyperkinesia	-	2
Dermatologic		
Sweating	-	23
Urticaria	5	-
Alopecia	4	4
Nevus	3	-
Herpes zoster	3	-
Herpes simplex	2	-
Special senses		
Conjunctivitis	-	12
Abnormal vision	-	7
Otitis media	6	-
Hearing decreased	3	-
GU		
Dysmenorrhea	-	18
Menstrual disorder	-	17
Metrorrhagia	-	15
Cystitis	-	8
Breast pain	-	7
Menorrhagia	-	6
Urinary urgency	-	4
Vaginitis	4	-
Fibrocystic breast	-	3
Breast neoplasm	-	2

[1] Data are pooled from separate studies and are not necessarily comparable.

- = Not reported.

INTERFERON BETA

Other adverse reaction include the following:

Miscellaneous: Abscess; ascites; cellulitis; hernia; hypothyroidism; sepsis; arrhythmia; hypotension; postural hypotension; dry mouth; GI hemorrhage; gingivitis; hepatomegaly; intestinal obstruction; periodontal abscess; proctitis; thirst; arthritis; abnormal gait; depersonalization; facial paralysis; hyperesthesia; neurosis; psychosis; hemoptysis; hiccoughs; hyperventilation; contact dermatitis; furunculosis; seborrhea; skin ulcer; earache; epididymitis; gynecomastia; hematuria; kidney calculus; leukorrhea; nocturia; vaginal hemorrhage.

Interferon beta-1a: Other adverse reactions include the following. Because most of the events were observed in open and uncontrolled studies, the role of interferon beta-1a in their causation cannot be reliably determined.

Body as a whole – Facial edema; injection site fibrosis; injection site hypersensitivity; lipoma; neoplasm; photosensitivity reaction; sinus headache; toothache.

Cardiovascular – Arteritis; heart arrest; hemorrhage; palpitation; pericarditis; peripheral ischemia; peripheral vascular disorder; pulmonary embolus; spider angioma; telangiectasia; vascular disorder.

CNS – Amnesia; Bell's Palsy; clumsiness; drug dependence; increased libido.

Dermatologic – Basal cell carcinoma; blisters; cold clammy skin; erythema; genital pruritus; skin discoloration.

GI – Blood in stool; colitis; constipation; diverticulitis; gallbladder disorder; gastritis; gum hemorrhage; hepatoma; increased appetite; intestinal perforation; periodontitis; tongue disorder.

GU – Breast fibroadenosis; breast mass; dysuria; fibrocystic change of the breast; fibroids; kidney pain; menopause; pelvic inflammatory disease; penis disorder; Peyronie's disease; polyuria; postmenopausal hemorrhage; prostatic disorder; pyelonephritis; testis disorder; urethral pain; urinary urgency; urinary retention; urinary incontinence.

Hematologic/Lymphatic – Coagulation time increased; ecchymosis; lymphadenopathy; petechia.

Metabolic/Nutritional – Abnormal healing; dehydration; hypoglycemia; hypomagnesemia; hypokalemia.

Musculoskeletal – Bone pain; myasthenia; osteonecrosis; synovitis.

Respiratory – Emphysema; laryngitis; pharyngeal edema; pneumonia.

Special Senses – Abnormal vision; conjunctivitis; eye pain; labyrinthitis; vitreous floaters.

Interferon beta-1b: Other adverse reactions include the following:

Body as a whole – Adenoma; anaphylactoid reaction; hydrocephalus; hypothermia; sarcoma; shock.

Cardiovascular – Angina pectoris; atrial fibrillation; cardiomegaly; cardiac arrest; cerebral hemorrhage; cerebral ischemia; endocarditis; heart failure; MI; pericardial effusion; pulmonary embolus; spider angioma; subarachnoid hemorrhage; syncope; thrombophlebitis; thrombosis; varicose veins; vasospasm; venous pressure increased; ventricular extrasystoles/fibrillation.

CNS – Acute/chronic brain syndrome; agitation; apathy; aphasia; ataxia; brain edema; coma; delirium; delusions; dementia; diplopia; dystonia; encephalopathy; euphoria; foot drop; hallucinations; hemiplegia; hypalgesia; incoordination; intracranial hypertension; libido decreased; manic reaction; meningitis; neuralgia; neuropathy; nystagmus; oculogyric crisis; ophthalmoplegia; papilledema; paralysis; paranoid reaction; reflexes decreased; stupor; subdural hematoma; torticollis; tremor.

Dermatologic – Erythema nodosum; exfoliative dermatitis; hirsutism; leukoderma; lichenoid dermatitis; maculopapular rash; photosensitivity; psoriasis; skin benign neoplasm; skin carcinoma; skin hypertrophy; skin necrosis; urticaria; vesiculobulous rash.

Endocrine – Cushing's syndrome; diabetes insipidus; diabetes mellitus; inappropriate ADH.

GI – Aphthous stomatitis; cardiospasm; cheilitis; cholecystitis; cholelithiasis; duodenal ulcer; enteritis; esophagitis; fecal impaction/incontinence; flatulence; gastritis; glossitis; hematemesis; hepatic neoplasia; hepatitis; ileus; increased salivation; melena; nausea; oral leukoplakia; oral moniliasis; pancreatitis; rectal hemorrhage; salivary gland enlargement; stomach ulcer; peritonitis; tenesmus.

GU – Urinary retention; anuria; balanitis; breast engorgement; cervicitis; impotence; kidney failure/tubular disorder; nephritis; oliguria; polyuria; salpingitis; urethritis; urinary incontinence; uterine fibroids enlarged; uterine neoplasm.

Hematologic/Lymphatic – Chronic lymphocytic leukemia; hemoglobin < 9.4 g/dl; petechia; platelets < 75,000/mm^3; splenomegaly.

Metabolic/Nutritional – Alcohol intolerance; alkaline phosphatase > 5 times baseline value; BUN > 40 mg/dl; calcium > 11.5 mg/dl; cyanosis; edema; glucose > 160 mg/dl; glycosuria; hypoglycemic reaction; hypoxia; ketosis.

INTERFERON BETA

Musculoskeletal – Arthrosis; bursitis; leg cramps; muscle atrophy; myopathy; myositis; ptosis; tenosynovitis.

Respiratory – Apnea; asthma; atelectasis; lung carcinoma; hypoventilation; interstitial pneumonia; lung edema; pleural effusion; pneumothorax.

Special Senses – Blepharitis; blindness; deafness; dry eyes; iritis; keratoconjunctivitis; mydriasis; otitis externa; otitis media; parosmia; photophobia; retinitis; taste loss; taste perversion; visual field defect.

Patient Information:

Instruction on self-injection technique and procedures: Instruct patients in the use of aseptic technique when administering interferon beta. Give appropriate instruction for reconstitution of the product and self-injection including careful review of the patient information sheet that is provided. If possible, perform the first injection under the supervision of an appropriately qualified healthcare professional.

Disposal: Caution patients against the re-use of needles or syringes and instruct them in safe disposal procedures. Supply the patient with a puncture resistant container for disposal of used needles/syringes along with instructions for safe disposal of containers.

Injection site reactions: Injection site reactions may occur one or more times during therapy. In general, these are transient and do not require discontinuation of therapy, but carefully assess the nature and severity of all reported reactions. Periodically reevaluate patient understanding and use of aseptic self-injection technique and procedures.

Flu-like symptoms are not uncommon following initiation of therapy. In clinical trials, acetaminophen was permitted for relief of fever or myalgia.

Dosage schedule: Caution patients not to change the dosage or the schedule of administration without medical consultation.

Depression/Suicide: Caution patients to report depression or suicidal ideation.

Abortifacient potential: Advise patients about the abortifacient potential.

Photosensitivity: Avoid prolonged exposure to sunlight or sunlamps; interferon beta may cause photosensitivity.

INTERFERON BETA-1A

Indications:

Multiple sclerosis: For the treatment of relapsing forms of multiple sclerosis to slow the accumulation of physical disability and decrease the frequency of clinical exacerbations.

Administration and Dosage:

Approved by the FDA on May 17, 1996.

Relapsing/Remitting MS: 30 mcg IM once/week.

Preparaton of solution: Reconstitute interferon beta-1a with 1.1 ml of diluent and swirl gently to dissolve.

Storage/Stability: Vials of interferon beta-1a must be stored in a refrigerator at 2° to 8°C (36° to 46°F). Should refrigeration be unavailable, interferon beta-1a can be stored at 25°C (77°F) for a period of up to 30 days. Following reconstitution, use as soon as possible (≤ 6 hours) stored at 2° to 8°C (36° to 46°F).

Rx	**Avonex** (Biogen)	**Powder for Injection, lyophilized:** 33 mcg (6.6 million IU)	Preservative free. With 16.5 mg albumin human. In single use vials with diluent of Sterile Water for Injection or in Administration Dose Packs.

INTERFERON BETA-1B

Indications:

Multiple sclerosis (MS): For use in ambulatory patients with relapsing-remitting MS to reduce the frequency of clinical exacerbations. Relapsing-remitting MS is characterized by recurrent attacks of neurologic dysfunction followed by complete or incomplete recovery.

Administration and Dosage:

Approved by the FDA on July 23, 1993.

Relapsing/Remitting MS: 0.25 mg (8 mIU) SC every other day. The effectiveness of lower doses is undocumented. Evidence of efficacy > 2 years is not known.

Preparation of solution: To reconstitute, inject 1.2 ml of diluent supplied (sodium chloride 0.54% solution) into the vial. Gently swirl the vial to dissolve the drug completely; do not shake. After reconstitution with accompanying diluent, vials contain 0.25 mg/ml of solution.

Administration: Withdraw 1 ml of reconstituted solution from the vial into a sterile syringe fitted with a 27-guage needle and inject the solution SC. Sites for self-injection include arms, abdomen, hips and thighs.

Storage/Stability: Reconstituted product contains no preservative. A vial is suitable for single use only; discard unused portions. Before and after reconstituion with diluent, store at 2° to 8°C (36° to 46°F). Use within 3 hours of reconstitution.

Rx	**Betaseron** (Berlex)	**Powder for Injection, lyophilized** 0.3 mg (9.6 mIU)	With 15 mg albumin human, 15 mg dextrose per vial. In single-use 5 ml capacity vials and 2 ml vial of diluent (sodium chloride 0.54%).

GLATIRAMER ACETATE

Actions:

Pharmacology: Glatiramer, for use in patients with multiple sclerosis (MS) is a random synthetic copolymer of L-alanine, L-glutamic acid, L-lysine and L-tyrosine in a molar ratio of 6:1.9:4.7:1.

The mechanism by which glatiramer exerts its effects in patients with MS is unknown. However, glatiramer is thought to act by modifying immune processes that are currently held to be responsible for the pathogenesis of MS. This view of glatiramer derives from knowledge that it reduces the incidence and severity of experimental allergic encephalomyelitis (EAE), a condition induced in several animal species through immunization against CNS-derived material containing myelin and often used as an experimental animal model of MS.

Pharmacokinetics: Pharmacokinetic studies in humans have not been performed. However, it is assumed based in part on the results of animal studies, that a substantial fraction of SC injection of glatiramer is hydrolyzed locally. Some fraction of injected material is presumed to enter the lymphatic circulation, enabling it to reach regional lymph nodes, and some may enter the systemic circulation intact.

Clinical trials: Fifty patients (glatiramer, 25; placebo, 25) diagnosed with relapsing-remitting multiple sclerosis (RR MS) were randomized to receive daily doses of glatiramer 20 mg SC or placebo. Over the 2-year trial, 56% of patients treated with glatiramer compared with 28% in the control group were relapse-free; the mean frequency of attacks was 0.6/2 years for glatiramer patients and 2.4/2 years for control patients; and the mean time to first relapse was 700 days vs 150 days for glatiramer and control patients, respectively.

Indications:

Relapsing-remitting multiple sclerosis (RR MS): For the reduction of the frequency of relapses in patients with RR MS.

Contraindications:

Hypersensitivity to glatiramer acetate or mannitol.

Warnings:

Administration: Administer SC, not IV.

Immediate post-injection reaction: A constellation of side effects including flushing, chest pain, palpitations, anxiety, dyspnea, laryngeal constriction and urticaria immediately after injection has been reported (≈ 10%). Symptoms were invariably transient and self-limited and did not require specific treatment. In general, these symptoms have their onset several months after the initiation of treatment although they may occur earlier in the course of treatment, and a given patient may experience one or several episodes of these symptoms. Whether or not this constellation of symptoms actually represents a specific syndrome is uncertain.

Whether these episodes are mediated by an immunologic or non-immunologic mechanism, or whether several similar episodes seen in a given patient have identical mechanisms is unknown.

Chest pain: Approximately 26% of glatiramer patients (compared with 10% of placebo patients) experienced at least one episode of what was described as transient chest pain. While some of these episodes occurred in the context of the immediate post-injection reaction, many did not. The temporal relationship of the chest pain to an injection of glatiramer was not always known, although the pain was transient (usually lasting only a few minutes), often unassociated with other symptoms and appeared to have no important clinical sequelae. Some patients experienced more than one such episode, and episodes usually began ≥ 1 month after the initiation of treatment. The pathogenesis of this symptom is unknown.

Pregnancy: Category B. There are no adequate and well-controlled studies in pregnant women. Use glatiramer acetate during pregnancy only if clearly needed.

Lactation: It is not known whether glatiramer is excreted in breast milk. Exercise caution when administering to a nursing woman.

Children: The safety and efficacy have not been established in individuals < 18 years of age.

Precautions:

Immunity: Because glatiramer can modify immune response, consider the possibility that it could interfere with useful immune function. For example, treatment with glatiramer might interfere with the recognition of foreign antigens in a way that would undermine the body's defenses against infections and tumor surveillance. There is no evidence that it does so, but there has as yet been no systematic evaluation of this risk.

Because glatiramer is an antigenic material it is possible that its use may lead to the induction of untoward host responses. Although there is no evidence that this

GLATIRAMER ACETATE

occurs in humans, systematic surveillance for these effects has not been undertaken. However, studies in both the rat and monkey have suggested that immune complexes are deposited in the renal glomeruli. Furthermore, in a controlled trial of 125 patients with RR MS given glatiramer 20 mg SC every day for 2 years, serum IgG levels reached ≈ 3 times baseline values in 80% of patients within 3 to 6 months of initiation of treatment. These values returned to ≈ 50% greater than baseline during the remainder of treatment.

Although glatiramer is intended to minimize the autoimmune response to myelin, there is the possibility that continued alteration of cellular immunity caused by chronic treatment with glatiramer might result in untoward effects.

Drug Interactions:

Interactions between glatiramer and other drugs have not been fully evaluated. Results from existing clinical trials do not suggest any significant interactions of glatiramer with therapies commonly used in MS patients. This includes the concurrent use of corticosteroids for up to 28 days.

Adverse Reactions:

Glatiramer Adverse Reactions (%)

Adverse Reaction	Glatiramer (n = 201)	Placebo (n = 206)
Body as a whole		
Infection	50	48
Asthenia	41	38
Pain	28	25
Chest pain	21	11
Flu syndrome	19	17
Back pain	16	15
Fever	8	7
Neck pain	8	4
Face edema	6	1
Bacterial infection	5	4
Chills	4	1
Cyst	2	0
Cardiovascular		
Vasodilation	27	10
Palpitations	17	8
Tachycardia	5	4
Migraine	5	2
Syncope	5	2
CNS		
Anxiety	23	19
Hypertonia	22	18
Tremor	7	3
Vertigo	6	5
Agitation	4	2
Foot drop	3	2
Nervousness	2	1
Nystagmus	2	1
Speech disorder	2	1
Confusion	2	0
Dermatologic		
Rash	18	15
Pruritus	18	13
Sweating	15	10
Herpes simplex	4	3
Erythema	4	2
Urticaria	4	2
Skin nodule	2	0
GI		
Nausea	22	17
Diarrhea	12	11
Anorexia	8	7
Vomiting	6	4
GI disorder	5	4
Gastroenteritis	3	1
GU		
Urinary urgency	10	8
Vaginal moniliasis	8	4
Dysmenorrhea	6	5
Hematologic		
Ecchymosis	8	6
Lymphadenopathy	12	6
Injection Site		
Pain	73	38
Erythema	66	19
Inflammation	49	11
Pruritus	40	6
Mass	27	10
Induration	13	0
Welt	11	2
Hemorrhage	5	3
Urticaria	5	0
Metabolic and Nutritional		
Peripheral Edema	7	4
Edema	3	0
Weight Gain	3	0
Respiratory System		
Dyspnea	19	7
Rhinitis	14	13
Bronchitis	9	6
Laryngismus	5	3
Special Senses		
Ear Pain	7	6
Eye Disorder	4	0
Miscellaneous		
Arthralgia	24	19

GLATIRAMER ACETATE

Body as a whole: Headache, injection site ecchymosis, accidental injury, abdominal pain, allergic rhinitis, neck rigidity, malaise, injection site edema, injection site atrophy, abscess (≥ 1%); injection site hematoma, injection site fibrosis, moon face, cellulitis, generalized edema, hernia, injection site abscess, serum sickness, suicide attempt, injection site hypertrophy, injection site melanosis, lipoma, photosensitivity reaction (≤ 1%).

Cardiovascular: Hypertension (≥ 1%); hypotension, midsystolic click, systolic murmur, atrial fibrillation, bradycardia, fourth heart sound, postural hypotension, varicose veins (≤ 1%).

CNS: Abnormal dreams, emotional lability, stupor (≥ 1%); ataxia, circumoral paresthesia, depersonalization, hallucinations, hostility, hypokinesia, coma, concentration disorder, facial paralysis, decreased libido, mania reaction, memory impairment, myoclonus, paranoid reaction, paraplegia, psychotic depression, transient stupor (≤ 1%); dizziness, hypesthesia, paresthesia, insomnia, depression, dysesthesia, incoordination, somnolence, abnormal gait, amnesia, emotional lability, Lhermitte's sign, abnormal thinking, twitching, euphoria, sleep disorder.

Dermatologic: Eczema, herpes zoster, pustular rash, skin atrophy and warts (≥ 1%); dry skin, skin hypertrophy, dermatitis, furunculosis, psoriasis, angiodema, contact dermatitis, erythema nodosum, fungal dermatitis, maculopapular rash, pigmentation, benign skin neoplasm, skin carcinoma, skin striae, vesiculobullous rash (≤ 1%); acne; alopecia; nail disorder.

Endocrine: Goiter, hyperthyroidism, hypothyroidism (≤ 1%).

GI: Bowel urgency, oral moniliasis, salivary gland enlargement, tooth caries, ulcerative stomatitis (≥ 1%); dry mouth, stomatitis, burning sensation on tongue, cholecystitis, colitis, esophageal ulcer, esophagitis, carcinoma, gum hemorrhage, hepatomegaly, increased appetite, melena, mouth ulceration, pancreas disorder, pancreatitis, rectal hemorrhage, tenesmus, tongue discoloration, duodenal ulcer (≤ 1%); dyspepsia; constipation; dysphagia; fecal incontinence; flatulence; nausea and vomiting; gastritis; gingivitis; periodontal abscess; dry mouth.

GU: Amenorrhea, hematuria, impotence, menorrhagia, suspicious papanicolaou smear, vaginal hemorrhage (≥ 1%); vaginitis, flank pain (kidney), abortion, breast engorgement, breast enlargement, carcinoma *in situ* cervix, fibrocystic breast, kidney calculus, nocturia, ovarian cyst, priapism, pyelonephritis, abnormal sexual function, urethritis (≤ 1%); urinary tract infection, urinary frequency, urinary incontinence, urinary retention, dysuria, cystitis, metrorrhagia, breast pain, vaginitis.

Hematologic/Lymphatic: Leukopenia, anemia, cyanosis, eosinophilia, hematemesis, lymphedema, pancytopenia, splenomegaly (≤ 1%).

Metabolic/Nutritional: Weight loss, alcohol intolerance, Cushing's syndrome, gout, abnormal healing, xanthoma (≤ 1%).

Musculoskeletal: Myasthenia, myalgia, arthritis, muscle atrophy, bone pain, bursitis, muscle disorder, myopathy, osteomyelitis, tendon pain, and tenosynovitis (≤ 1%).

Respiratory: Hyperventilation (≥ 1%);asthma, pneumonia, epistaxis, hypoventilation, voice alteration (≤ 1%); pharyngitis, sinusitis, increased cough, laryngitis.

Special senses: Dry eyes, otitis externa, ptosis, cataract, corneal ulcer, mydriasis, optic neuritis, photophobia, taste loss (≤ 1%); abnormal vision, diplopia, amblyopia, eye pain, conjunctivitis, tinnitus, taste perversion, deafness.

Patient Information:

Inform your physician if you are pregnant, if you are planning to become pregnant, if you become pregnant or if you are nursing while taking this medication.

Do not stop taking the drug without consulting your physician.

Administration and Dosage:

The recommended dose of glatiramer acetate for the treatment of RR MS is 20 mg/day injected SC. Sites for injection include arms, abdomen, hips and thighs. See the Glatiramer Acetate Patient Information booklet for Self-Injection Procedure.

Reconstitution: Reconstitute with the diluent supplied, Sterile Water for Injection. Gently swirl the vial of glatiramer acetate and let stand at room temperature until the solid material is completely dissolved.

Storage/stability: The reconstituted product contains no preservative; use immediately. Before reconstitution, store at -20° to -10°C (-4° to 14°F, freeze). The diluent may be stored at room temperature.

Rx	**Copaxone** (TEVA)	**Injection**: 20 mg	40 mg mannitol. Single-dose 2 ml vial. Diluent in 1 ml vial. In 32s.

CDC BIOLOGICALS

In addition to the commercially available products, the Centers for Disease Control and Prevention (CDC) in Atlanta, GA can supply various rare immunobiological products for use in certain emergency situations or for special immunization needs. These biological products are available through the CDC Drug Service, Scientific Resources Program, Center for Infectious Diseases, Centers for Disease Control in Atlanta, Georgia. For further information, call 404-639-3356, Monday through Friday, 8 am to 4:30 pm, or refer to the numbers listed below. After working hours, on weekends and holidays, call 404-639-2888 (emergency requests only).

Available CDC Biologicals	
Product	Telephone number
Antitoxins	
Botulism Equine trivalent Antitoxin (ABE) – Licensed	404-639-3356
Diphtheria Equine Antitoxin – (IND*)	404-639-8255
Immune Serum Globulins	
Vaccinia Immune Globulin (VIG) (Human) – Licensed	404-639-3356
Vaccines (for high laboratory risk immunization, nonemergency)	
Botulinum Toxoid, pentavalent (ABCDE) - (IND*)	404-639-3356
Vaccinia (Smallpox Vaccine)	404-639-3356

* Investigational New Drug

chapter 10

topical preparations

TOPICAL OPHTHALMICS

General Considerations in Topical Ophthalmic Drug Therapy: Proper administration is essential to optimal therapeutic response. In many instances, health professionals may be too casual when instructing patients on proper use of ophthalmics. The administration technique used often determines drug safety and efficacy.

- The normal eye retains ≈ 10 mcl of fluid (adjusted for blinking). The average dropper delivers 25 to 50 mcl/drop. The value of more than one drop is questionable.
- Minimize systemic absorption of ophthalmic drops by compressing lacrimal sac for 3 to 5 minutes after instillation. This retards passage of drops via nasolacrimal duct into areas of potential absorption such as nasal and pharyngeal mucosa.
- Because of rapid lacrimal drainage and limited eye capacity, if multiple drop therapy is indicated, the best interval between drops is 5 minutes. This ensures that the first drop is not flushed away by the second or that the second is not diluted by the first.
- Topical anesthesia will increase the bioavailability of ophthalmic agents by decreasing the blink reflex and the production and turnover of tears.
- Factors that may increase absorption from ophthalmic doseforms include lax eyelids of some patients, usually the elderly, which creates a greater reservoir for retention of drops, and hyperemic or diseased eyes.
- Eyecup use is discouraged due to risk of contamination and spreading disease.
- Ophthalmic suspensions mix with tears less rapidly and remain in the cul-de-sac longer than solutions.
- Ophthalmic ointments maintain contact between the drug and ocular tissues by slowing the clearance rate to as little as 0.5% per minute. Ophthalmic ointments provide maximum contact between drug and external ocular tissues.
- Ophthalmic ointments may impede delivery of other ophthalmic drugs to the affected side by serving as a barrier to contact.
- Ointments may blur vision during the waking hours. Use with caution in conditions where visual clarity is critical (eg, operating motor equipment, reading) or use at bedtime.
- Monitor expiration dates closely. Do not use outdated medication.
- Solutions and ointments are frequently misused. Do not assume that patients know how to maximize safe and effective use of these agents. Combine appropriate patient education and counseling with prescribing and dispensing of ophthalmics.

Topical application is the most common route of administration for ophthalmic drugs. Advantages include convenience, simplicity, noninvasive nature and the ability of the patient to self-administer. Because of blood and aqueous losses of drug, topical medications do not typically penetrate in useful concentrations to posterior ocular structures and therefore are of no therapeutic benefit for diseases of retina, optic nerve and other posterior segment structures.

Ingredients: The following inactive agents may be present in ophthalmic products:

PRESERVATIVES destroy or inhibit multiplication of microorganisms introduced into the product by accident.

benzalkonium Cl	mercurial preservatives (phenylmercuric nitrate, phenyl mercuric acetate, thimerosal)	methyl/propylparabens
benzethonium Cl		phenylethyl alcohol
cetylpyridinium Cl		sodium benzoate
chlorobutanol		sodium propionate
EDTA		sorbic acid

VISCOSITY-INCREASING AGENTS slow drainage of the product from the eye, thus increasing retention time of the active drug. Increased bioavailability may result.

carboxymethylcellulose sodium	hydroxyethylcellulose	poloxamer 407
dextran 70	hydroxypropyl methylcellulose	polysorbate 80
gelatin	methylcellulose	propylene glycol
glycerin	PEG	polyvinyl alcohol
		polyvinylpyrrolidone (povidone)

ANTIOXIDANTS prevent or delay deterioration of products by oxygen in the air.

EDTA	sodium metabisulfite	sodium thiosulfate
sodium bisulfite		thiourea

TOPICAL OPHTHALMICS

WETTING AGENTS reduce surface tension, allowing drug solution to spread over eye.

polysorbate 20 and 80
poloxamer 282
tyloxapol

BUFFERS help maintain ophthalmic products in the range of pH 6 to 8, which is the comfortable range for ophthalmic instillation.

acetic acid
boric acid
hydrochloric acid
phosphoric acid
potassium bicarb.
potass. borate and tetraborate
potassium carbonate
potassium citrate
potassium phosphates
sodium acetate
sodium bicarbonate
sodium biphosphate
sodium borate
sodium carbonate
sodium citrate
sodium hydroxide
sodium phosphate

TONICITY AGENTS help the ophthalmic product solutions to be isotonic with natural tears. Products in the sodium chloride equivalence range of 0.9% ± 0.2% are considered isotonic and will help prevent ocular pain and tissue damage. A range of 0.6% to 1.8% is usually comfortable for ophthalmic use.

buffers
dextran 40 and 70
dextrose
glycerin
potassium Cl
propylene glycol
sodium Cl

Packaging Standards: To help reduce confusion in labeling and identification of various topical ocular medications, drug packaging standards have been proposed. When fully implemented by the ophthalmic drug industry, the standard colors for drug labels and bottle caps will include the following:

Ophthalmic Drug Packaging Standards

Therapeutic class	Proposed color
Beta blockers	Yellow, blue or both
Mydriatics and cycloplegics	Red
Miotics	Green
Nonsteroidal anti-inflammatory agents	Grey
Anti-infectives	Brown, tan

Medications:

Solutions and suspensions: Most topical ocular preparations are commercially available as solutions or suspensions that are applied directly to the eye from the bottle, which serves as the eye dropper. Avoid touching the dropper tip to the eye because this can lead to contamination of the medication and may also cause ocular injury. Resuspend suspensions (notably, many ocular steroids) by shaking to provide an accurate dosage of drug.

Recommended procedures for administration of solutions or suspensions:

- Wash hands thoroughly before administration.
- Tilt head backward or lie down and gaze upward.
- Gently grasp lower eyelid below eyelashes and pull the eyelid away from the eye to form a pouch.
- Place dropper directly over eye. Avoid contact of the dropper with the eye, finger or any surface.
- Look upward just before applying a drop.
- After instilling the drop, look downward for several seconds.
- Release the lid slowly and close eyes gently.
- With eyes closed, apply gentle pressure with fingers to the inside corner of eye for 3 to 5 min. This retards drainage of solution from intended solution.
- Do not rub the eye or squeeze the eyelid. Minimize blinking.
- Do not rinse the dropper.
- Do not use eye drops that have changed color or contain a precipitate.
- If more than one type of ophthalmic drop is used, wait ≥ 5 minutes before administering the second agent.
- When the instillation of eye drops is difficult (eg, pediatric patients, adults with particularly strong blink reflex), the close-eye method may be used. This involves lying down, placing the prescribed number of drops on the eyelid in the inner corner of the eye, then opening eye so that drops will fall into the eye by gravity.

Ointments: The primary purpose for an ophthalmic ointment vehicle is to prolong drug contact time with the external ocular surface. This is particularly useful for treating children, who may "cry out" topically applied solutions, and for medicating ocular injuries, such as corneal abrasions, when the eye is to be patched. Administer solutions before ointments. Ointments preclude entry of subsequent drops.

TOPICAL OPHTHALMICS

Recommended procedures for administration of ointments:

- Wash hands thoroughly before administration.
- Holding the ointment tube in the hand for a few minutes will warm the ointment and facilitate flow.
- When opening the ointment tube for the first time, squeeze out and discard the first 0.25 inch of ointment as it may be too dry.
- Tilt head backward or lie down and gaze upward.
- Gently pull down the lower eyelid to form a pouch.
- Place 0.25 to 0.5 inch of ointment with a sweeping motion inside the lower eyelid by squeezing the tube gently and slowly release the eyelid.
- Close the eye for 1 to 2 minutes and roll the eyeball in all directions.
- Temporary blurring of vision may occur. Avoid activities requiring visual acuity until blurring clears.
- Remove excessive ointment around the eye or ointment tube tip with a tissue.
- If using more than one kind of ointment, wait about 10 minutes before applying the second drug.

Gels: Ophthalmic gels are similar in viscosity and clinical usage to ophthalmic ointments. Pilocarpine *(Pilopine HS)* is currently the only ophthalmic preparation available in gel form, and it is intended to serve as a "sustained-release" pilocarpine, requiring only once-daily administration (at bedtime).

Sprays: Although not commercially available, some practitioners use mydriatics or cycloplegics, alone or in combination, administered as a spray to the eye to dilate the pupil or for cycloplegic examination. This is most often used for pediatric patients, and the solution is administered using a sterile perfume atomizer.

Lid scrubs: Commercially available eyelid cleansers or antibiotic solutions or ointments can be applied directly to the lid margin for the treatment of noninfectious blepharitis. This is best accomplished by applying the medication to the end of a cotton-tipped applicator and then scrubbing the eyelid margin several times daily.The gauze pads supplied with commercially available eyelid cleansers are also convenient.

Devices:

Contact lenses: Soft contact lenses can absorb water-soluble drugs and release them to the eye over prolonged periods of time. This has the clinical advantage of promoting sustained-release solutions or suspensions that would otherwise be removed quickly from the external ocular tissues. Soft contact lenses as drug delivery devices are most often used in the management of dry eye disorders, but the technique is occasionally used for the treatment of ocular infections, including corneal ulcers.

Corneal shields: A non-cross-linked, homogenized, porcine scleral collagen shield is available *(Bio-Cor Fyodoror Collagen Corneal Shield)*. This device is placed as a bandage on the cornea following surgery or injury, protecting and lubricating the cornea. Topical antibiotics have been used in conjunction with the shield to promote healing of corneal ulcers.

Cotton pledgets: Small pieces of cotton can be saturated with ophthalmic solutions and placed in the conjunctival sac. These devices allow a prolonged ocular contact time with solutions that are normally administered topically into the eye. The clinical use of pledgets is usually reserved for mydriatic solutions such as cocaine or phenylephrine. This drug delivery method promotes maximum mydriasis in an attempt to break posterior synechiae or to dilate sluggish pupils.

Filter paper strips: Sodium fluorescein and rose bengal dyes are commercially available as drug-impregnated filter paper strips. The strips help ensure sterility of sodium fluorescein which, when prepared in solution, can become easily contaminated with *Pseudomonas aeruginosa*. These dyes are used diagnostically to disclose corneal injuries, infections such as herpes simplex, and dry eye disorders.

Artificial tear inserts: A rod-shaped pellet of hydroxypropyl cellulose without preservative *(Lacrisert)*, is inserted into the inferior conjunctival sac with a specially designed applicator. Following placement, the device absorbs fluid, swells and then releases the nonmedicated polymer to the eye for up to 24 hours. The device is designed as a sustained-release artificial tear for the treatment of dry eye disorders.

Membrane-bound inserts: A membrane-controlled drug delivery system *(Ocusert)* delivers a constant quantity of pilocarpine to the eye for up to 1 week. Placed onto the bulbar conjunctiva under the upper or lower eyelid, it is a useful substitute for pilocarpine drops or gel in glaucoma patients who cannot comply with more frequent instillation or in those with ocular or visual side effects from pilocarpine solutions.

AGENTS FOR GLAUCOMA

Glaucoma is a condition of the eye in which an elevation of the intraocular pressure (IOP) leads to progressive cupping and atrophy of the optic nerve head, deterioration of the visual fields and ultimately, blindness. Primary open-angle glaucoma is the most common type of glaucoma. Angle-closure glaucoma and congenital glaucoma are treated primarily by surgical methods, although short-term drug therapy is used to decrease IOP prior to surgery.

Drugs used in the therapy of primary open-angle glaucoma include a variety of agents with different mechanisms of action.The therapeutic goal in treating glaucoma is reducing the elevated IOP, a major risk factor in the pathogenesis of glaucomatous visual field loss. The higher the level of IOP, the greater the likelihood of glaucomatous visual field loss and optic nerve damage. Reduction of IOP may be accomplished by: 1) Decreasing the rate of production of aqueous humor or 2) increasing the rate of outflow (drainage) of aqueous humor from the anterior chamber of the eye.

The six groups of agents used in therapy of primary open-angle glaucoma are listed in the table, which summarizes their mechanism of decreasing IOP, effects on pupil size and ciliary muscle and duration of action.

Agents for Glaucoma

Drug	Strength	Duration (hrs)	Decrease aqueous production	Increase aqueous outflow	Effect on pupil	Effect on ciliary muscle
Sympathomimetics						
Apraclonidine[1]	0.5%–1%	7–12	+++	NR	NR	NR
Epinephrine	0.1%-2%	12	+	++	mydriasis	NR
Dipivefrin	0.1%	12	+	++	mydriasis	NR
Brimonidine	0.2%	12	++	++	NR	NR
Beta Blockers						
Betaxolol	0.25%–0.5%	12	+++	NR	NR	NR
Carteolol	1%	12	+++	nd	NR	NR
Levobunolol	0.25%–0.5%	12-24	+++	NR	NR	NR
Metipranolol	0.3%	12-24	+++	+	NR	NR
Timolol	0.25%-0.5%	12-24	+++	+	NR	NR
Miotics, Direct-Acting						
Acetylcholine[2]	1%	10-20 min	NR	+++	miosis	accommodation
Carbachol[2]	0.75%-3%	6–8	NR	+++	miosis	accommodation
Pilocarpine[3]	0.25%-10%	4-8	NR	+++	miosis	accommodation
Miotics, Cholinesterase Inhibitors						
Physostigmine	0.25%-0.5%	12-36	NR	+++	miosis	accommodation
Demecarium	0.125%-0.25%	days/wks	NR	+++	miosis	accommodation
Echothiophate	0.03%-0.25%	days/wks	NR	+++	miosis	accommodation
Carbonic Anhydrase Inhibitors						
Dichlorphenamide[4]	50 mg	6-12	+++	NR	NR	NR
Acetazolamide[4]	125-500 mg	8-12	+++	NR	NR	NR
Methazolamide[4]	25-50 mg	10-18	+++	NR	NR	NR
Dorzolamide[5]	2%	≈ 8	+++	NR	NR	NR
Prostaglandin analogue						
Latanoprost	.005%	24	NR	+++	NR	NR

+++ = significant activity ++ = moderate activity + = some activity
NR = no activity reported nd = No data available

[1] 1% used only to decrease IOP in surgery.
[2] Intraocular administration only for miosis during surgery; carbachol also available as a topical agent.
[3] Also available as a gel and an insert; the duration of these doseforms is longer (18 to 24 hours and 1 week, respectively) than the solution.
[4] Systemic agents; for detailed information, see group monograph in Cardiovascular section.
[5] Topical ophthalmic agent.

AGENTS FOR GLAUCOMA

Sympathomimetic agents (adrenergic agonists) have both α and β activity (apraclonidine is a relatively selective alpha adrenergic agonist). They lower IOP mainly by increasing outflow and reducing production of aqueous humor. Epinephrine is used as an adjunct to miotic or beta blocker therapy; however, it is also used as primary therapy, especially in young patients or patients with cataracts.The combination of a miotic and a sympathomimetic will have additive effects in lowering IOP.

Dipivefrin HCl is a prodrug that is metabolized to epinephrine in vivo.The IOP-lowering and intraocular effects are qualitatively and quantitatively similar to epinephrine; however, extraocularly, dipivefrin may be better tolerated and have a lower incidence of adverse effects.

Beta-adrenergic blocking agents may be used alone or in conjunction with other agents. They may be more effective than either pilocarpine or epinephrine alone and have the advantage of not affecting either pupil size or accommodation. They lower IOP by decreasing the rate of aqueous production.

Miotics, direct-acting, were considered the first step in glaucoma therapy. They have now yielded to the β-blockers. Pilocarpine is a useful adjunctive agent that is additive to either the β-blockers, carbonic anhydrase inhibitors or the sympathomimetics. Dosage and frequency of administration must be individualized. Patients with darkly pigmented irides may require higher strengths of pilocarpine.

Miotics, cholinesterase inhibitors, include both reversible/short-acting (eg, physostigmine) and irreversible/long-acting (eg, echothiophate) agents that enhance the effects of endogenous acetylcholine by inactivation of the enzyme acetylcholinesterase. These agents are more potent and longer-acting than the direct-acting cholinergic agents. Side effects and systemic toxicity are more common and of greater significance. Using a direct-acting cholinergic and a cholinesterase inhibitor provides no improvement in response.

Carbonic anhydrase inhibitors are administered systemically, except for the topical agent, dorzolamide. IOP is lowered by suppressing the secretion of aqueous humor (inflow). Systemic carbonic anhydrase inhibitors are used as adjunctive therapy and do not replace topical therapy.

Hyperosmotic agents (mannitol, urea, glycerin and isosorbide) are administered systemically and are useful in lowering IOP in acute situations. These agents lower IOP by creating an osmotic gradient between the ocular fluids and plasma. They are not for chronic use.

Prostaglandin analogues increase uveoscleral outflow through a new mechanism of action; selective prostenoid receptor agonism. Latanoprost, currently the only agent available in this class, can be used concomitantly with other topical ophthalmic drug products to reduce IOP.

Alpha-2 Adrenergic Agonist

BRIMONIDINE TARTRATE

Actions:

Pharmacology: Brimonidine tartrate is an alpha–2 adrenergic receptor agonist. It has a peak, ocular hypotensive effect occurring at 2 hours post-dosing. Fluorophotometric studies in animals and humans suggest that brimonidine tartrate has a dual mechanism of action by reducing aqueous humor production and increasing uveoscleral outflow.

Pharmacokinetics: After ocular administration of a 0.2% solution, plasma concentrations peaked within 1 to 4 hours and declined with a systemic half-life of ≈ 3 hours.

Systemic metabolism of brimonidine is extensive. It is metabolized primarily by the liver. Urinary excretion is the major route of elimination of the drug and its metabolites. Approximately 87% of an orally-administered radioactive dose was eliminated within 120 hours, with 74% found in the urine.

Clinical trials: In comparative clinical studies with timolol 0.5% lasting up to 1 year, the intraocular pressure (IOP) lowering effect of brimonidine tartrate was ≈ 4 to 6 mmHg compared with ≈ 6 mmHg for timolol. In these studies, both patient groups were dosed twice a day. Eight percent of subjects were discontinued from studies because of inadequately controlled IOP which occurred in 30% of patients during the first month of therapy. Approximately 20% were discontinued because of adverse experiences.

Indications:

Intraocular pressure (IOP): Lowering IOP in patients with open-angle glaucoma or ocular hypertension.

Contraindications:

Hypersensitivity to brimonidine tartrate or any component of this medication; patients receiving monoamine oxidase (MAO) inhibitor therapy.

Warnings:

Soft contact lenses: The preservative in brimonidine tartrate, benzalkonium chloride, may be absorbed by soft contact lenses. Instruct patients wearing soft contact lenses to wait at least 15 minutes after instilling brimonidine tartrate to insert soft contact lenses.

Renal/Hepatic function impairment: Use caution when treating patients with hepatic or renal impairment.

Pregnancy: Category B. There are no studies of brimonidine tartrate in pregnant women. However, in animal studies, brimonidine tartrate crossed the placenta and entered into the fetal circulation to a limited extent. Use brimonidine tartrate during pregnancy only if the potential benefit to the mother justifies the potential risk to the fetus.

Lactation: It is not known whether brimonidine tartrate is excreted in breast milk. Decide whether to discontinue the drug, taking into account the importance of the drug to the mother.

Children: Safety and effectiveness in pediatric patients have not been established.

Precautions:

Cardiovascular disease: Although brimonidine tartrate had minimal effect on blood pressure of patients in clinical studies, exercise caution in treating patients with severe cardiovascular disease.

Use with caution in patients with depression, cerebral or coronary insufficiency, Raynaud's phenomenon, orthostatic hypotension or thromboangiitis obliterans.

Loss of effect in some patients may occur. The IOP-lowering efficacy observed with brimonidine tartrate during the first month of therapy may not always reflect the long-term level of IOP reduction. Therefore, routinely monitor IOP.

Alpha-2 Adrenergic Agonist

BRIMONIDINE TARTRATE

Drug Interactions:

Brimonidine Tartrate Drug Interactions			
Precipitant Drug	Object Drug*		Description
Brimonidine	CNS depressants (eg, alcohol, barbiturates, opiates, sedatives or anesthetics)	↑	Consider the possibility of an additive or potentiating effect with CNS depressants.
Brimonidine	Beta blockers, antihypertensives, cardiac glycosides	↑	Because alpha-agonists, as a class, may reduce pulse and blood pressure, use caution with concomitant drugs such as beta-blockers (ophthalmic and systemic), antihypertensives or cardiac glycosides.
Tricyclic antidepressants	Brimonidine	↓	Tricyclic antidepressants can affect the metabolism and uptake of circulating amines.

* ↑ = Object drug increased. ↓ = Object drug decreased.

Adverse Reactions:

Adverse events occurring in ≈ 10% to 30% of patients in descending order included: Oral dryness, ocular hyperemia, burning and stinging, headache, blurring, foreign body senstaion, fatigue/drowsiness, conjunctival follicles, ocular allergic reactions and ocular pruritus.

Adverse events occurring in ≈ 3% to 9% in descending order included: Corneal staining/erosion, photophobia, eyelid erythema, ocular ache/pain, ocular dryness, tearing, upper respiratory symptoms, eyelid edema, conjunctival edema, dizziness, blepharitis, ocular irritation, gastrointestinal symptoms, asthenia, conjunctival blanching, abnormal vision and muscular pain.

Adverse effects occurring in < 3%: Lid crusting, conjunctival hemorrhage, abnormal taste, insomnia, conjunctival discharge, depression, hypertension, anxiety, palpitations, nasal dryness and syncope.

Overdosage:

No information is available on overdosage in humans. Treatment of an oral overdose includes supportive and symptomatic therapy; maintain a patent airway.

Patient Information:

Soft contact lenses: Instruct patients wearing soft contact lenses to wait at least 15 minutes after instilling brimonidine tartrate to insert soft contact lenses.

As with other drugs in this class, brimonidine tartrate may cause fatigue or drowsiness in some patients. Caution patients who engage in hazardous activities of the potential for a decrease in mental alertness.

Administration and Dosage:

The recommended dose is one drop of brimonidine tartrate in the affected eye(s) 3 times daily, ≈ 8 hours apart.

Storage/Stability: Store at or below 25°C (77°F).

Rx	**Alphagan** (Allergan)	**Solution:** 0.2% brimonidine tartrate	Polyvinyl alcohol. In 5 or 10 ml dropper bottles.

Sympathomimetics

EPINEPHRINE

Actions:

Pharmacology: Epinephrine, a direct-acting sympathomimetic agent, acts on α and β receptors. Therefore, topical application causes conjunctival decongestion (vasoconstriction), transient mydriasis (pupillary dilation) and reduction in intraocular pressure (IOP). It is believed IOP reduction is primarily due to reduced aqueous production and increased aqueous outflow. The duration of decrease in IOP is 12 to 24 hours.

Epinephrine is available as hydrochloride and borate salts. These preparations are therapeutically equal when given in equivalent doses of epinephrine base.

Indications:

Glaucoma: Management of open-angle (chronic simple) glaucoma; may be used in combination with miotics, beta blockers, hyperosmotic agents or carbonic anhydrase inhibitors.

Contraindications:

Hypersensitivity to epinephrine or any component of the formulation; narrow- or shallow-angle (angle Y closure) glaucoma; aphakia; patients with a narrow angle but no glaucoma; if the nature of the glaucoma is not clearly established. Do not use while wearing soft contact lenses; discoloration of lenses may occur.

Warnings:

For ophthalmic use only. Not for injection or intraocular use.

Gonioscopy: Because pupil dilation may precipitate an acute attack of narrow-angle glaucoma, evaluate anterior chamber angle by gonioscopy prior to beginning therapy.

Anesthesia: Discontinue use prior to general anesthesia with anesthetics that sensitize the myocardium to sympathomimetics (eg, cyclopropane, halothane).

Aphakic patients: Maculopathy with associated decrease in visual acuity may occur in the aphakic eye; if this occurs, promptly discontinue use.

Elderly: Use with caution.

Pregnancy: Category C. Safety for use during pregnancy has not been established. Use only when clearly needed.

Lactation: It is not known whether this drug is excreted in breast milk. Exercise caution when administering to a nursing woman.

Children: Safety and efficacy for use in children have not been established.

Precautions:

Instillation discomfort: Epinephrine is relatively uncomfortable upon instillation. Discomfort lessens as concentration of epinephrine decreases.

Special risk patients: Use with caution in the presence of or history of: Hypertension; diabetes; hyperthyroidism; heart disease; cerebral arteriosclerosis; bronchial asthma.

Potentially hazardous tasks: Epinephrine may cause temporarily blurred or unstable vision after instillation; observe caution while driving, operating machinery or performing other tasks requiring coordination or physical dexterity.

Sulfite sensitivity: Some of these products contain sulfites that may cause allergic-type reactions (eg, hives, itching, wheezing, anaphylaxis) in certain susceptible persons. Although the overall prevalence of sulfite sensitivity in the general population is probably low, it is seen more frequently in asthmatics or atopic nonasthmatics.

Drug Interactions:

Consider interactions that occur with systemic use of epinephrine (see Epinephrine monograph in the Vasopressors Used in Shock section).

Sympathomimetics

EPINEPHRINE

Adverse Reactions:

Local: Transient stinging and burning; eye pain/ache; browache; headache; allergic lid reaction; conjunctival hyperemia; conjunctival or corneal pigmentation, ocular irritation (hypersensitivity), localized adrenochrome deposits in conjunctiva and cornea (prolonged use); reversible cystoid macular edema may result from use in aphakic patients.

Systemic: Headache; palpitations; tachycardia; extrasystoles; cardiac arrhythmia; hypertension; faintness.

Overdosage:

If ocular overdosage occurs, flush eye(s) with water or normal saline.

Patient Information:

To avoid contamination, do not touch tip of container to any surface. Replace cap after using.

Do not use if solution is brown or contains a precipitate.

Do not use while wearing soft contact lenses.

Transitory stinging may occur upon initial instillation. Headache or browache may occur.

Patients should immediately report any decrease in visual acuity.

Refer to Topical Ophthalmic Drugs introduction for more complete information.

Administration and Dosage:

Instill 1 drop into affected eye(s) once or twice daily. Determine frequency of instillation by tonometry.

More frequent instillation than 1 drop twice daily does not usually elicit any further improvement in therapeutic response.

When used in conjunction with miotics, instill the miotic first.

Storage: Store at 2° to 24°C (36° to 75°F). Keep container tightly sealed. Protect solution from light; store in cool place. Do not freeze. Discard if solution becomes discolored or contains a precipitate.

EPINEPHRINE HCl

Rx	**Epinephrine HCl** (Ciba Vision)	**Solution:** 0.1%	In 1 ml Dropperettes (12s).[1]
Rx	**Epifrin** (Allergan)	**Solution:** 0.5% (as base)	In 15 ml dropper bottles.[2]
Rx	**Epifrin** (Allergan)	**Solution:** 1% (as base)	In 15 ml dropper bottles.[2]
Rx	**Glaucon** (Alcon)	**Solution:** 1%	In 10 ml Drop-Tainers.[3]
Rx	**Epifrin** (Allergan)	**Solution:** 2% (as base)	In 15 ml dropper bottles.[2]
Rx	**Glaucon** (Alcon)	**Solution:** 2%	In 10 ml Drop-Tainers.[3]

[1] With 0.5% chlorobutanol and sodium bisulfite.
[2] With benzalkonium chloride, sodium metabisulfite, EDTA and hydrochloric acid.
[3] With 0.01% benzalkonium chloride, sodium metabisulfite, EDTA, sodium chloride, hydrochloric acid and sodium hydroxide.

EPINEPHRYL BORATE

Rx	**Epinal** (Alcon)	**Solution:** 0.5%	In 7.5 ml.[1]
		1%	In 7.5 ml.[1]

[1] With 0.01% benzalkonium chloride, ascorbic acid, acetylcysteine, boric acid and sodium carbonate.

Sympathomimetics

DIPIVEFRIN HCl (Dipivalyl epinephrine)

Refer to Agents for Glaucoma Introduction for a general discussion of these products.

Actions:

Pharmacology: Dipivefrin is a prodrug of epinephrine formed by diesterification of epinephrine and pivalic acid, enhancing its lipophilic character and, consequently, penetration into anterior chamber. Dipivefrin, converted to epinephrine in the eye by enzymatic hydrolysis, appears to act by decreasing aqueous production and enhancing outflow facility. It has the same therapeutic effects as epinephrine with fewer local and systemic side effects.

Dipivefrin does not produce the miosis or accommodative spasm that cholinergic agents produce. The blurred vision and night blindness often associated with miotic agents do not occur with dipivefrin. In patients with cataracts the inability to see around lenticular opacities caused by constricted pupil is avoided.

Pharmacokinetics: The onset of action with 1 drop occurs about 30 minutes after treatment, with maximum effect seen at about 1 hour.

Clinical trials: In patients with a history of epinephrine intolerance, only 3% of dipivefrin-treated patients exhibited intolerance, while 55% treated with epinephrine again developed an intolerance. Response to dipivefrin twice daily is less than that to 2% epinephrine twice daily and comparable to 2% pilocarpine 4 times daily. Patients using dipivefrin twice daily had mean IOP reductions ranging from 20% to 24%.

Indications:

Glaucoma: Initial therapy or as an adjunct with other antiglaucoma agents for the control of IOP in chronic open-angle glaucoma.

Contraindications:

Hypersensitivity to dipivefrin or any formulation component; narrow-angles (any dilation of pupil may predispose patient to an attack of angle-closure glaucoma).

Warnings:

Pregnancy: Category B. There are no adequate and well controlled studies in pregnant women. Use only when clearly needed.

Lactation: It is not known whether this drug is excreted in breast milk. Use caution in nursing mothers.

Children: Safety and efficacy for use in children have not been established.

Precautions:

Aphakic patients: Macular edema occurs in up to 30% of aphakic patients treated with epinephrine. Discontinuation generally results in reversal of the maculopathy.

Adverse Reactions:

Cardiovascular: Tachycardia, arrhythmias, hypertension (reported with epinephrine).

Local: Burning and stinging (6%); conjunctival injection (6.5%); follicular conjunctivitis, mydriasis, allergic reactions (infrequent). Epinephrine therapy can lead to adrenochrome deposits in the conjunctiva and cornea.

Dipivefrin 0.1% is less irritating than 1% epinephrine HCl. Only 1.8% of dipivefrin patients reported discomfort due to photophobia, glare or light sensitivity.

Sympathomimetics

DIPIVEFRIN HCl (Dipivalyl epinephrine)

Patient Information:

Slight stinging or burning on initial instillation may occur.

Do not try to "catch up" on missed doses by applying more than one dose at a time.

Administration and Dosage:

Initial glaucoma therapy: Instill 1 drop into the eye(s) every 12 hours.

Replacement therapy: When transferring patients to dipivefrin from antiglaucoma agents other than epinephrine, continue the previous medication the first day and add 1 drop of dipivefrin in affected eye(s) every 12 hours. The next day, discontinue the other agent and continue with dipivefrin. Monitor with tonometry.

When transferring patients from conventional epinephrine therapy, discontinue the epinephrine and institute the dipivefrin regimen. Monitor with tonometry.

Concomitant therapy: When patients receiving other antiglaucoma agents require additional therapy, add 1 drop of dipivefrin every 12 hours.

Rx	**Dipivefrin HCl** (Various, eg, Falcon, Schein)	**Solution:** 0.1%	In 5, 10 and 15 ml.
Rx	**Propine** (Allergan)		In 5, 10 & 15 ml C Cap Compliance Cap B.I.D.[1]
Rx	**AKPro** (Akorn)	**Liquid:** 0.1%	In 2, 5, 10 and 15 ml.

[1] With 0.005% benzalkonium chloride, sodium chloride, EDTA and hydrochloric acid.

Sympathomimetics

APRACLONIDINE HCl

Actions:

Pharmacology: Apraclonidine has the action of reducing elevated, as well as normal, intraocular pressure (IOP) whether accompanied by glaucoma or not. Apraclonidine is a relatively selective α-adrenergic agonist that does not have significant membrane stabilizing (local anesthetic) activity. When instilled into the eyes, apraclonidine reduces IOP and has minimal effect on cardiovascular parameters.

Optic nerve head damage and visual field loss may result from an acute elevation in IOP that can occur after argon laser surgical procedures. The higher the peak or spike of IOP, the greater the likelihood of visual field loss and optic nerve damage, especially in patients with previously compromised optic nerves. The onset of action is usually within 1 hour and the maximum IOP reduction occurs 3 to 5 hours after application of a single dose. Apraclonidine's mechanism of action is not completely established, although its predominant action may be related to a reduction of aqueous formation via stimulation of the alpha-adrenergic system.

Pharmacokinetics: Topical use of apraclonidine 0.5% leads to systemic absorption. Studies of apraclonidine ophthalmic solution dosed 1 drop 3 times daily in both eyes for 10 days in healthy volunteers yielded mean peak and trough concentrations of 0.9 and 0.5 ng/ml, respectively. The half-life of apraclonidine 0.5% was calculated to be 8 hours.

Clinical trials: The clinical utility of apraclonidine 0.5% is most apparent for those glaucoma patients on maximally tolerated medical therapy (ie, patients were using combinations of a topical beta blocker, sympathomimetics, parasympathomimetics and oral carbonic anhydrase inhibitors). Patients with advanced glaucoma and uncontrolled IOP scheduled to undergo laser trabeculoplasty or trabeculectomy surgery were enrolled in a study to determine whether apraclonidine dosed 3 times daily could delay the need for surgery for ≤ 3 months. Apraclonidine treatment resulted in a significantly greater percentage of treatment successes compared with patients treated with placebo.

Indications:

1%: To control or prevent post-surgical elevations in IOP that occur in patients after argon laser trabeculoplasty or iridotomy.

0.5%: Short-term adjunctive therapy in patients on maximally tolerated medical therapy who require additional IOP reduction.

Contraindications:

Hypersensitivity to any component of this medication or to clonidine; concurrent monoamine oxidase inhibitor therapy (see Drug Interactions).

Warnings:

Concomitant therapy: The addition of apraclonidine 0.5% to patients already using two aqueous suppressing drugs (eg, beta-blocker plus carbonic anhydrase inhibitor) as part of their maximally tolerated medical therapy may not provide additional benefit. This is because apraclonidine is an aqueous suppressing drug and the addition of a third aqueous suppressant may not significantly reduce IOP.

Tachyphylaxis: The IOP lowering efficacy of apraclonidine 0.5% diminishes over time in some patients. This loss of effect, or tachyphylaxis, appears to be an individual occurrence with a variable time of onset and should be closely monitored. The benefit for most patients is < 1 month.

Hypersensitivity: Apraclonidine can lead to an allergic-like reaction characterized wholly or in part by the symptoms of hyperemia, pruritus, discomfort, tearing, foreign body sensation and edema of the lids and conjunctiva. If ocular allergic-like symptoms occur, discontinue therapy. Refer to Management of Acute Hypersensitivity Reactions.

Renal/Hepatic function impairment: Although the topical use of apraclonidine has not been studied in renal failure patients, structurally related clonidine undergoes a significant increase in half-life in patients with severe renal impairment. Close monitoring of cardiovascular parameters in patients with impaired renal function is advised if they are candidates for topical apraclonidine therapy. Close monitoring of cardiovascular parameters in patients with impaired liver function is also advised as the systemic dosage form of clonidine is partly metabolized in the liver.

Pregnancy: Category C. Apraclonidine has an embryocidal affect in rabbits when given in an oral dose of 3 mg/kg (60 times the maximum recommended human dose). There are no adequate and well controlled studies in pregnant women. Use during pregnancy only if the potential benefit justifies the potential risk to the fetus.

Sympathomimetics

APRACLONIDINE HCl

Lactation: It is not known if topically applied apraclonidine is excreted in breast milk. Exercise caution when apraclonidine is administered to a nursing woman. Consider discontinuing nursing for the day on which apraclonidine is used.

Children: Safety and efficacy for use in children have not been established.

Precautions:

Monitoring: Glaucoma patients on maximally tolerated medical therapy who are treated with apraclonidine 0.5% to delay surgery should have their visual fields monitored periodically. Discontinue treatment if IOP rises significantly.

IOP reduction: Since apraclonidine is a potent depressor of IOP, closely monitor patients who develop exaggerated reductions in IOP. An unpredictable decrease of IOP control in some patients and incidence of ocular allergic responses and systemic side effects may limit the utility of apraclonidine 0.5%. However, patients on maximally tolerated medical therapy may still benefit from the additional IOP reduction provided by the short-term use of apraclonidine 0.5%.

Cardiovascular disease: Acute administration of apraclonidine has had minimal effect on heart rate or blood pressure; however, observe caution in treating patients with severe cardiovascular disease, including hypertension.

Use apraclonidine 0.5% with caution in patients with coronary insufficiency, recent myocardial infarction, cerebrovascular disease, chronic renal failure, Raynaud's disease or thromboangiitis obliterans.

Depression: Caution and monitor depressed patients since apraclonidine has been infrequently associated with depression.

Vasovagal attack: Consider the possibility of a vasovagal attack occurring during laser surgery; use caution in patients with a history of such episodes.

Corneal changes: Topical ocular administration of apraclonidine 1.5% to rabbits 3 times daily for 1 month resulted in sporadic and transient instances of minimal corneal cloudiness. No corneal changes were observed in humans given at least one dose of apraclonidine 1%.

Drug Interactions:

Apraclonidine Drug Interactions

Precipitant drug	Object drug*		Description
Apraclonidine	Cardiovascular agents	⬇	Since apraclonidine may reduce pulse and blood pressure, caution in using cardiovascular drugs is advised. Patients using cardiovascular drugs concurrently with apraclonidine 0.5% should have pulse and blood pressures frequently monitored.
Apraclonidine	MAO inhibitors	⬆	Apraclonidine should not be used in patients receiving MAO inhibitors (see Contraindications).

* ⬆ = Object drug increased. ⬇ = Object drug decreased.

Adverse Reactions:

In clinical studies the overall discontinuation rate related to apraclonidine was 15%. The most commonly reported events leading to discontinuation included (in decreasing order of frequency): Hyperemia; pruritus; tearing; discomfort; lid edema; dry mouth; foreign body sensation.

The following adverse effects were reported with the use of apraclonidine in laser surgery: Upper lid elevation (1.3%); conjunctival blanching (0.4%); mydriasis (0.4%).

The following additional adverse effects were reported:

Ophthalmic:

1% – Conjunctival blanching; upper lid elevation; mydriasis; burning; discomfort; foreign body sensation; dryness; itching; hypotony; blurred or dimmed vision; allergic response; conjunctival microhemorrhage.

0.5% – Hyperemia (13%); pruritus (10%); discomfort (6%); tearing (4%); lid edema, blurred vision, foreign body sensation, dry eye, conjunctivitis, discharge, blanching (< 3%); lid margin crusting, conjunctival follicles, conjunctival edema, edema, abnormal vision, pain, lid disorder, keratitis, blepharitis, photophobia, corneal staining, lid erythema, blepharoconjunctivitis, irritation, corneal erosion, corneal infiltrate, keratopathy, lid scales, lid retraction (< 1%).

Sympathomimetics

APRACLONIDINE HCl

GI:

1% – Abdominal pain; diarrhea; stomach discomfort; emesis; dry mouth.

0.5% – Dry mouth (2%); constipation, nausea (< 1%).

Cardiovascular:

1% – Bradycardia; vasovagal attack; palpitations; orthostatic episode.

0.5% – Asthenia (< 3%); peripheral edema, arrhythmia (< 1%). Although there are no reports of bradycardia, consider the possibility.

CNS:

1% – Insomnia; dream disturbances; irritability; decreased libido; headache; paresthesia.

0.5% – Headache (< 3%); somnolence, dizziness, nervousness, depression, insomnia, paresthesia (< 1%).

Hypersensitivity: Use can lead to an allergic-like reaction (see Warnings).

Respiratory:

0.5% – Dry nose (2%); rhinitis, dyspnea, pharyngitis, asthma (< 1%).

Miscellaneous:

1% – Taste abnormalities; nasal burning or dryness; head cold sensation; chest heaviness or burning; clammy or sweaty palms; body heat sensation; shortness of breath; increased pharyngeal secretion; extremity pain or numbness; fatigue; pruritus not associated with rash.

0.5% – Taste perversion (3%); contact dermatitis, dermatitis, chest pain, abnormal coordination, malaise, facial edema (< 1%); myalgia, parosmia (0.2%)

Patient Information:

Do not touch dropper tip to any surface as this may contaminate the contents.

Apraclonidine can cause dizziness and somnolence. Patients who engage in hazardous activities requiring mental alertness should be warned of the potential for a decrease in mental alertness, physical dexterity or coordination while using apraclonidine.

Administration and Dosage:

0.5%: Instill one to two drops in the affected eye(s) 3 times daily. Since apraclonidine 0.5% will be used with other ocular glaucoma therapies, use an approximate 5 minute interval between instillation of each medication to prevent washout of the previous dose. Not for injection into the eye.

1%: Instill 1 drop in scheduled operative eye 1 hour before initiating anterior segment laser surgery. Instill second drop into same eye immediately upon completion of surgery.

Storage: Store at room temperature. Protect from light and freezing (0.5%).

Rx	**Iopidine** (Alcon)	**Solution:** 1%	0.01% benzalkonium chloride. In 0.1 ml (2s).
		Solution: 0.5%	0.01% benzalkonium chloride. In 5 ml and 10 ml Drop-Tainers.

BETA-ADRENERGIC BLOCKING AGENTS

Refer to the general discussion of these products in the Topical Ophthalmic Introduction for more complete information.

Actions:

Pharmacology: Timolol, levobunolol, carteolol and metipranolol are noncardioselective (β_1 and β_2) β-blockers; betaxolol is a cardioselective (β_1) β-blocker. Topical β-blockers do not have significant membrane-stabilizing (local anesthetic) actions or intrinsic sympathomimetic activity. They reduce elevated and normal intraocular pressure (IOP), with or without glaucoma.

The exact mechanism of ocular antihypertensive action is not established, but it appears to be a reduction of aqueous production. However, some studies show a slight increase in outflow facility with timolol and metipranolol.

These agents reduce IOP with little or no effect on pupil size or accommodation. Blurred vision and night blindness often associated with miotics are not associated with these agents. In addition, in patients with cataracts, the inability to see around lenticular opacities when the pupil is constricted, is avoided. These agents may be absorbed systemically (see Warnings).

Pharmacokinetics:

Pharmacokinetics of Ophthalmic β-Adrenergic Blocking Agents

Drug	β-receptor selectivity	Onset (min)	Maximum effect (hr)	Duration (hr)
Carteolol	β_1 and β_2	nd[1]	nd[1]	12
Betaxolol	β_1	30	2	12
Levobunolol	β_1 and β_2	< 60	2 to 6	12 to 24
Metipranolol	β_1 and β_2	≤ 30	≈ 2	12 to 24
Timolol	β_1 and β_2	30	1 to 2	12 to 24

[1] nd = No data

Clinical trials:

Timolol – In controlled studies of untreated IOP of ≥ 22 mm Hg, timolol 0.25% or 0.5% bid caused greater IOP reduction than 4% pilocarpine solution 4 times daily or 2% epinephrine HCl solution twice daily. In comparative studies, mean IOP reduction was 31% to 33% with timolol, 22% with pilocarpine and 28% with epinephrine.

In ocular hypertension, effects of timolol and acetazolamide are additive. Timolol, generally well tolerated, produces fewer and less severe side effects than pilocarpine or epinephrine. Timolol has been well tolerated in patients wearing conventional (PMMA) hard contact lenses.

Betaxolol ophthalmic was compared to ophthalmic timolol and placebo in patients with reactive airway disease. Betaxolol had no significant effect on pulmonary function as measured by Forced Expiratory Volume (FEV_1), Forced Vital Capacity (FVC) and FEV_1/VC. Also, action of isoproterenol was not inhibited. Timolol significantly decreased these pulmonary functions. No evidence of cardiovascular β-blockade during exercise was observed with betaxolol. Mean arterial blood pressure was not affected by any treatment; however, timolol significantly decreased mean heart rate. Betaxolol reduces mean IOP 25% from baseline. In controlled studies, the magnitude and duration of the ocular hypotensive effects of betaxolol and timolol were clinically equivalent.

Clinical observation of glaucoma patients treated with betaxolol solution for up to 3 years shows that the IOP-lowering effect is well maintained.

Betaxolol has been successfully used in glaucoma patients who have undergone laser trabeculoplasty and have needed long-term antihypertensive therapy. The drug is well tolerated in glaucoma patients with hard or soft contact lenses and in aphakic patients.

Levobunolol effectively reduced IOP in controlled clinical studies from 3 months to over 1 year when given topically twice daily; IOP was well maintained. The mean IOP decrease from baseline was 6.8 and 9 mm Hg with 0.5% levobunolol.

Metipranolol reduced the average intraocular pressure approximately 20% to 26% in controlled studies of patients with IOP > 24 mm Hg at baseline. Clinical studies in patients with glaucoma treated ≤ 2 years indicate that an intraocular pressure lowering effect is maintained.

Carteolol produced a median percent IOP reduction of 22% to 25% when given twice daily in clinical trials ranging from 1.5 to 3 months.

Indications:

Glaucoma: Lowering IOP in patients with chronic open-angle glaucoma.

For specific approved indications, refer to individual drug monographs.

BETA-ADRENERGIC BLOCKING AGENTS

Contraindications:

Bronchial asthma, a history of bronchial asthma or severe chronic obstructive pulmonary disease; sinus bradycardia; second-degree and third-degree AV block; overt cardiac failure; cardiogenic shock; hypersensitivity to any component of the products.

Warnings:

Systemic absorption: These agents may be absorbed systemically. The same adverse reactions found with systemic β-blockers (see group monograph in Cardiovascular section) may occur with topical use. For example, severe respiratory reactions and cardiac reactions, including death due to bronchospasm in asthmatics, and rarely, death associated with cardiac failure, have been reported with topical β-blockers. Levobunolol and metipranolol may decrease heart rate and blood pressure, and betaxolol has had adverse effects on pulmonary and cardiovascular parameters. Detectable, perhaps significant serum timolol levels may be achieved in some patients. Exercise caution with all of these agents.

Cardiovascular: Timolol can decrease resting and maximal exercise heart rate even in healthy subjects.

Cardiac failure – Sympathetic stimulation may be essential for circulation support in diminished myocardial contractility; its inhibition by β-receptor blockade may precipitate more severe failure.

In patients without history of cardiac failure, continued depression of myocardium with β-blockers may lead to cardiac failure. Discontinue at the first sign or symptom of cardiac failure.

Non-allergic bronchospasm patients or patients with a history of chronic bronchitis, emphysema, etc, should receive β-blockers with caution; they may block bronchodilation produced by catecholamine stimulation of β_2-receptors.

Major surgery: Withdrawing β-blockers before major surgery is controversial. Beta-receptor blockade impairs the heart's ability to respond to β-adrenergically mediated reflex stimuli. This may augment the risk of general anesthesia. Some patients on β-blockers have had protracted severe hypotension during anesthesia. Difficulty restarting and maintaining heartbeat has been reported. In elective surgery, gradual withdrawal of β-blockers may be appropriate.

The effects of β-blocking agents may be reversed by β-agonists such as isoproterenol, dopamine, dobutamine or norepinephrine.

Diabetes mellitus: Administer with caution to patients subject to spontaneous hypoglycemia or to diabetic patients (especially labile diabetics). Beta-blocking agents may mask signs and symptoms of acute hypoglycemia.

Thyroid: Beta-adrenergic blocking agents may mask clinical signs of hyperthyroidism (eg, tachycardia). Manage patients suspected of developing thyrotoxicosis carefully to avoid abrupt withdrawal of β-blockers which might precipitate thyroid storm.

Cerebrovascular insufficiency: Because of potential effects of β-blockers on blood pressure and pulse, use with caution in patients with cerebrovascular insufficiency. If signs or symptoms suggesting reduced cerebral blood flow develop, consider alternative therapy.

Carcinogenesis: In female mice receiving oral metipranolol doses of 5, 50 and 100 mg/kg/day, the low dose had an increased number of pulmonary adenomas.

Pregnancy: Category C. There have been no adequate and well controlled studies in pregnant women. Use during pregnancy only if the potential benefits outweigh potential hazards to the fetus.

Carteolol – Increased resorptions and decreased fetal weights occurred in rabbits and rats at maternal doses ≈ 1052 and 5264 times the maximum human dose, respectively. A dose-related increase in wavy ribs was noted in the developing rat fetus when pregnant rats received doses ≈ 212 times the maximum human dose.

Betaxolol – In oral studies with rats and rabbits, evidence of post-implantation loss was seen at dose levels above 12 mg/kg and 128 mg/kg, respectively. Betaxolol was not teratogenic, however, and there were no other adverse effects on reproduction at subtoxic dose levels.

Levobunolol – Fetotoxicity was observed in rabbits at doses 200 and 700 times the glaucoma dose.

Metipranolol – Increased fetal resorption, fetal death and delayed development occurred in rabbits receiving 50 mg/kg orally during organogenesis.

Timolol – Doses 1000 times the maximum recommended human oral dose were maternotoxic in mice and resulted in increased fetal resorptions. Increased fetal resorptions were also seen in rabbits at 100 times the maximum recommended human oral dose.

BETA-ADRENERGIC BLOCKING AGENTS

Lactation: It is not known whether betaxolol, levobunolol or metipranolol are excreted in breast milk. Systemic β-blockers and topical timolol maleate are excreted in milk. Carteolol is excreted in breast milk of animals. Exercise caution when administering to a nursing mother.

Because of the potential for serious adverse reactions from **timolol** in nursing infants, decide whether to discontinue nursing or discontinue the drug taking into account the importance of the drug to the mother.

Children: Safety and efficacy for use in children have not been established.

Precautions:

Angle-closure glaucoma: The immediate objective is to reopen the angle, requiring constriction of the pupil with a miotic. These agents have little or no effect on the pupil. When they are used to reduce elevated IOP in angle-closure glaucoma, use with a miotic.

Muscle weakness: Beta-blockade may potentiate muscle weakness consistent with certain myasthenic symptoms (eg, diplopia, ptosis, generalized weakness). **Timolol** has increased muscle weakness in some patients with myasthenic symptoms.

Long-term therapy: Diminished responsiveness to **betaxolol** and **timolol** after prolonged therapy has been reported. However, in long-term studies (2 and 3 years), no significant differences in mean IOP were observed after initial stabilization.

Sulfite sensitivity: Some of these products contain sulfites which may cause allergic-type reactions (eg, hives, itching, wheezing, anaphylaxis) in certain susceptible persons. Although the overall prevalence of sulfite sensitivity in the general population is probably low, it is seen more frequently in asthmatics or atopic nonasthmatics.

Drug Interactions:

Ophthalmic Beta Blocker Drug Interactions

Precipitant drug	Object drug*		Description
Beta blockers, ophthalmic	Beta blockers, oral	⬆	Use topical β-blockers with caution because of the potential for additive effects on systemic β-blockade.
Beta blockers, ophthalmic	Epinephrine, ophthalmic	⟷	Use of epinephrine with topical β-blockers is controversial. Some reports indicate initial effectiveness decreases over time. In one case verified by rechallenge, combined use of topical epinephrine and topical timolol appeared to result in hypertension from unopposed α-adrenergic stimulation. However, this combination has been used to reduce IOP.
Beta blockers, ophthalmic	Quinidine	⬆	One case of sinus bradycardia has been reported with the coadministration of ophthalmic timolol. The incidence was reaffirmed by a negative rechallenge with the β-blockers alone and positive rechallenge with the combination.
Beta blockers, ophthalmic	Verapamil	⬆	Coadministration of ophthalmic timolol has caused bradycardia and asystole.

* ⬆ = Object drug increased. ⟷ = Undetermined effect.

Other drugs that may interact with systemic β-adrenergic blocking agents may also interact with ophthalmic agents. For further information, refer to the β-blocker group monograph in the Cardiovascular section.

Adverse Reactions:

The following have occurred with ophthalmic β_1 *and* β_2 *(nonselective) blockers:*

CNS – Headache; depression.

Cardiovascular – Arrhythmia; syncope; heart block; cerebral vascular accident; cerebral ischemia; congestive heart failure; palpitation.

GI – Nausea.

Dermatologic – Hypersensitivity, including localized and generalized rash.

Respiratory – Bronchospasm (predominantly in patients with preexisting bronchospastic disease); respiratory failure.

Endocrine – Masked symptoms of hypoglycemia in insulin-dependent diabetics (see Warnings).

Ophthalmic – Keratitis; blepharoptosis; visual disturbances including refractive changes (due to withdrawal of miotic therapy in some cases); diplopia; ptosis.

BETA-ADRENERGIC BLOCKING AGENTS

The following adverse reactions have occurred with each individual agent:

Carteolol –

Ophthalmic: Transient irritation, burning, tearing, conjunctival hyperemia, edema (≈ 25%), blurred/cloudy vision, photophobia, decreased night vision, ptosis, blepharoconjunctivitis, abnormal corneal staining and corneal sensitivity.

Systemic: Bradycardia; decreased blood pressure; arrhythmia; heart palpitation; dyspnea; asthenia; headache; dizziness; insomnia; sinusitis; taste perversion.

Betaxolol –

Ophthalmic: Brief discomfort (> 25%); occasional tearing (5%). Rare: Decreased corneal sensitivity; erythema; itching; corneal punctate staining; keratitis, anisocoria; photophobia.

Systemic: Insomnia; depressive neurosis (rare).

Metipranolol –

Ophthalmic: Transient local discomfort; conjunctivitis; eyelid dermatitis; blepharitis; blurred vision; tearing; browache; abnormal vision; photophobia; edema.

Systemic: Allergic reaction; headache; asthenia; hypertension; myocardial infarction; atrial fibrillation; angina; palpitation; bradycardia; nausea; rhinitis; dyspnea; epistaxis; bronchitis; coughing; dizziness; anxiety; depression; somnolence; nervousness; arthritis; myalgia; rash.

Levobunolol –

Ophthalmic: Transient burning/stinging (25%); blepharoconjunctivitis (5%); iridocyclitis (rare); decreased corneal sensitivity.

Cardiovascular: Effects may resemble timolol.

CNS: Ataxia, dizziness, lethargy (rare).

Dermatologic: Urticaria, pruritus (rare).

Timolol –

Ophthalmic: Ocular irritation including conjunctivitis; blepharitis; keratitis; blepharoptosis; decreased corneal sensitivity; visual disturbances including refractive changes (due, in some cases, to withdrawal of miotics); diplopia; ptosis.

CNS: Dizziness; depression; fatigue; lethargy; hallucinations; confusion.

Cardiovascular: Bradycardia; arrhythmia; hypotension; syncope; heart block; cerebral vascular accident; cerebral ischemia; heart failure; palpitation; cardiac arrest. These generally occur in the elderly or in preexisting cardiovascular problems.

Respiratory: Bronchospasm (mainly in patients with preexisting bronchospastic disease); respiratory failure; dyspnea.

Miscellaneous: Aggravation of myasthenia gravis; alopecia; nail pigmentary changes; nausea; hypersensitivity including localized and generalized rash; urticaria; asthenia; sexual dysfunction including impotence, decreased libido and decreased ejaculation; hyperkalemia; masked symptoms of hypoglycemia in insulin-dependent diabetics; diarrhea; paresthesia.

Causal relationship unknown – Hypertension; chest pain; dyspepsia; anorexia; dry mouth; behavioral changes (eg, anxiety, disorientation, nervousness, somnolence, psychic disturbance); aphakic cystoid macular edema; retroperitoneal fibrosis.

Systemic β-adrenergic blocker-associated reactions: Consider potential effects with ophthalmic use (see Warnings).

Overdosage:

If ocular overdosage occurs, flush eye(s) with water or normal saline. If accidentally ingested, efforts to decrease further absorption may be appropriate (gastric lavage).

The most common signs and symptoms of overdosage from systemic β-blockers are bradycardia, hypotension, bronchospasm and acute cardiac failure. If these occur, discontinue therapy and initiate appropriate supportive therapy.

Patient Information:

Transient stinging/discomfort is relatively common; notify physician if severe.

Administration and Dosage:

Concomitant therapy: If IOP is not controlled with these agents, institute concomitant pilocarpine, other miotics, dipivefrin or systemic carbonic anhydrase inhibitors.

Use of epinephrine with topical β-blockers is controversial. Some reports indicate initial effectiveness of the combination decreases over time (see Drug Interactions).

BETA-ADRENERGIC BLOCKING AGENTS

Monitoring: The IOP-lowering response to betaxolol and timolol may require a few weeks to stabilize. Determine the IOP during the first month of treatment. Thereafter, determine IOP on an individual basis.

Because of diurnal IOP variations in individual patients, satisfactory response to twice-a-day therapy is best determined by measuring IOP at different times during the day. Intraocular pressures ≤ 22 mm Hg may not be optimal to control glaucoma in each patient; therefore, individualize therapy.

LEVOBUNOLOL HCl

For complete prescribing information, refer to the Beta-adrenergic Blocking Agents group monograph.

Indications:

Lowering IOP in chronic open-angle glaucoma or ocular hypertension.

Administration and Dosage:

Usual dose: Instill 1 drop in the affected eye(s) once or twice a day.

Rx	**Levobunolol** (Various, eg, B&L, Pacific Pharma)	**Solution:** 0.25%	In 5 and 10 ml.
Rx	**AKBeta** (Akorn)		In 5 and 10 ml.
Rx	**Betagan Liquifilm** (Allergan)		In 5 and 10 ml dropper bottles with B.I.D. *C Cap.*[1]
Rx	**Levobunolol** (Various, eg, B&L)	**Solution:** 0.5%	In 5, 10 and 15 ml.
Rx	**AKBeta** (Akorn)		In 5, 10 and 15 ml.
Rx	**Betagan Liquifilm** (Allergan)		In 2 ml bottles with B.I.D. and Q.D. *C Cap.*[1]

[1] With 1.4% polyvinyl alcohol, 0.004% benzalkonium chloride, sodium metabisulfite and EDTA.

BETAXOLOL HCl

For complete prescribing information, refer to the Beta-adrenergic Blocking Agents group monograph.

Indications:

Treatment of ocular hypertension and chronic open-angle glaucoma. Betaxolol may be used alone or in combination with other antiglaucoma drugs.

Administration and Dosage:

Usual dose: Instill 1 to 2 drops twice daily.

Replacement therapy (single agent): Continue the agent already used and add 1 drop of betaxolol twice daily. The following day, discontinue the previous agent and continue betaxolol. Monitor with tonometry.

Replacement therapy (multiple agents): When transferring from several concomitant antiglaucoma agents, individualize dosage. Adjust 1 agent at a time at intervals of not less than 1 week. One may continue the agents being used and add 1 drop betaxolol twice daily. The next day, discontinue another agent. Decrease or discontinue remaining antiglaucoma agents according to patient response.

Storage: Store at room temperature 15° to 30°C (59° to 86°F). Shake suspension well.

Rx	**Betoptic** (Alcon)	**Solution:** 5.6 mg (equiv. to 5 mg base) per ml (0.5%)	In 2.5, 5, 10 and 15 ml Drop-Tainer bottles.[1]
Rx	**Betoptic S** (Alcon)	**Suspension:** 2.8 mg (equiv. to 2.5 mg base) per ml (0.25%)	In 2.5, 5, 10 and 15 ml Drop-Tainer bottles.[2]

[1] With 0.01% benzalkonium chloride and EDTA.

[2] With 0.01% benzalkonium chloride, mannitol, poly sulfonic acid, carbomer 934P and EDTA.

Beta-adrenergic Blocking Agents

METIPRANOLOL HCl

For complete prescribing information, refer to the Beta-adrenergic Blocking Agents group monograph.

Indications:

Treatment of ocular conditions in which lowering IOP is likely to be of therapeutic benefit, including ocular hypertension and chronic open angle glaucoma.

Administration and Dosage:

Usual dose: Instill 1 drop in the affected eye(s) twice a day. If the patient's IOP is not at a satisfactory level on this regimen, more frequent administration or a larger dose is not known to be of benefit. Concomitant therapy to lower IOP can be instituted.

Rx	**OptiPranolol** (Bausch & Lomb)	**Solution:** 0.3%	In 5 or 10 ml dropper bottles.[1]

[1] With 0.004% benzalkonium chloride and EDTA.

CARTEOLOL HCl

For complete prescribing information, refer to the Beta-adrenergic Blocking Agents group monograph.

Indications:

Treatment of chronic open-angle glaucoma and intraocular hypertension. It may be used alone or in combination with other intraocular pressure lowering drugs.

Administration and Dosage:

Usual dose: Instill 1 drop in affected eye(s) twice daily. If the patient's IOP is not at a satisfactory level on this regimen, concomitant therapy can be instituted.

Rx	**Ocupress** (Otsuka America)	**Solution:** 1%	In 5 and 10 ml dropper bottles.[1]

[1] With 0.005% benzalkonium chloride.

Beta-adrenergic Blocking Agents

TIMOLOL MALEATE

For complete prescribing information, refer to the Beta-adrenergic Blocking Agents group monograph.

Indications:

Lowering IOP in chronic open-angle glaucoma, aphakic glaucoma patients, some patients with secondary glaucoma and in patients with elevated IOP who need ocular pressure lowering. In patients who respond inadequately to multiple antiglaucoma drug therapy, the addition of timolol may produce further IOP reduction .

Administration and Dosage:

Solution:

Initial therapy – Instill 1 drop of 0.25% twice daily. If clinical response is not adequate, change the dosage to 1 drop of 0.5% solution twice a day. If the IOP is maintained at satisfactory levels, change the dosage to 1 drop once a day. Since the pressure-lowering response may require a few weeks to stabilize, evaluation should include a determination of IOP after approximately 4 weeks of treatment.

Replacement therapy (single agent) – When a patient is transferred from another topical ophthalmic β-adrenergic blocker, discontinue that agent after proper dosing on one day, and start treatment the next day with 1 drop of 0.25% timolol twice daily. Increase to 1 drop of 0.5% solution twice a day if response is inadequate.

When changing from an agent other than an ophthalmic β-blocker, on the first day continue with the agent being used and add 1 drop 0.25% timolol twice daily. The next day, discontinue the previously used agent completely and continue timolol. If a higher dosage is required, substitute 1 drop 0.5% twice daily.

Replacement therapy (multiple agents) – When transferring from several concomitantly administered agents, individualize dosage. If any of the agents is an ophthalmic β-blocker, discontinue it before starting timolol. Adjust 1 agent at a time, at intervals of not less than 1 week. Continue the agents being used and add 1 drop of 0.25% twice a day. The next day, discontinue one of the other agents. Decrease or discontinue remaining agents according to patient response. If a higher dosage is required, use 1 drop of 0.5% twice daily.

Gel: Invert the closed container and shake once before each use; it is not necessary to shake it more than once. Administer other ophthalmics at least 10 minutes before the gel. Dose is 1 drop (0.25% or 0.5%) once daily. Dosages > 1 drop of 0.5% have not been studied. Consider concomitant therapy if IOP is not at a satisfactory level. When patients are switched from timolol solution twice daily to the gel once daily, the ocular hypotensive effect should remain constant.

Rx	**Timolol Maleate Ophthalmic Solution** (Various, eg, Akorn, Alcon, Fougera)	**Solution:** 0.25%	In 2.5, 5, 10 and 15 ml.
Rx	**Betimol** (Ciba Vision)		In 2.5, 5, 10 and 15 ml.[1]
Rx	**Timoptic** (Merck)		In 2.5, 5, 10 & 15 ml Ocumeters[1] & UD 60s Ocudose.[2]
Rx	**Timolol Maleate Ophthalmic Solution** (Various, eg, Akorn, Alcon, Fougera)	**Solution:** 0.5%	In 2.5, 5, 10 and 15 ml.
Rx	**Betimol** (Ciba Vision)		In 2.5, 5, 10 and 15 ml.[1]
Rx	**Timoptic** (Merck)		In 2.5, 5, 10 & 15 ml Ocumeters[1] & UD 60s Ocudose.[2]
Rx	**Timoptic-XE** (Merck)	**Solution, gel-forming:** 0.25%	In 2.5 and 5 ml.[3]
		0.5%	In 2.5 and 5 ml.[3]

[1] With 0.01% benzalkonium chloride.

[2] Preservative free; use immediately after opening; discard remaining contents.

[3] With 0.012% benzododecinium bromide.

MIOTICS, DIRECT-ACTING

Refer to the Agents for Glaucoma introduction for a general discussion of these products-.For information on the oral use of pilocarpine, refer to the monograph in the Mouth and Throat Products section.

Actions:

Pharmacology: The direct-acting miotics are parasympathomimetic (cholinergic) drugs which duplicate the muscarinic effects of acetylcholine. When applied topically, these drugs produce pupillary constriction, stimulate the ciliary muscles and increase aqueous humor outflow facility. Miosis, produced through contraction of the iris sphincter, causes increased tension on the scleral spur (reducing outflow resistance) and opening of the trabecular meshwork spaces facilitating outflow. With the increase in outflow facility, there is a decrease in intraocular pressure (IOP). Topical ophthalmic instillation of acetylcholine causes no discernible response as cholinesterase destroys the molecule more rapidly than it can penetrate the cornea; therefore, acetylcholine is only used intraocularly.

Miosis Induction of Direct-Acting Miotics

Miotic	Onset	Peak	Duration
Acetylcholine, intraocular	seconds	—	10 min
Carbachol			
Intraocular	seconds	2 to 5 min	1 to 2 days
Topical	10 to 20 min	—	4 to 8 hours
Pilocarpine, topical	10 to 30 min	—	4 to 8 hours

Indications:

Carbachol, topical; pilocarpine:

Glaucoma – To decrease elevated IOP in glaucoma.

Acetylcholine; carbachol, intraocular:

Miosis – To induce miosis during surgery.

See individual monographs for specific indications.

Contraindications:

Hypersensitivity to any component of the formulation; where constriction is undesirable (eg, acute iritis, acute or anterior uveitis, some forms of secondary glaucoma, pupillary block glaucoma, acute inflammatory disease of the anterior chamber).

Warnings:

Corneal abrasion: Use carbachol with caution in the presence of corneal abrasion to avoid excessive penetration.

Pregnancy: Category C (carbachol, pilocarpine). Safety for use during pregnancy has not been established. Use only when clearly needed.

Lactation: It is not known whether these drugs are excreted in breast milk; exercise caution when administering to a nursing woman.

Children: Safety and efficacy for use in children have not been established.

Precautions:

Systemic reactions: Caution is advised in patients with acute cardiac failure, bronchial asthma, peptic ulcer, hyperthyroidism, GI spasm, urinary tract obstruction, Parkinson's disease, recent MI, hypertension or hypotension.

Retinal detachment has been caused by miotics in susceptible individuals, in individuals with preexisting retinal disease or in those who are predisposed to retinal tears. Fundus examination is advised for all patients prior to initiation of therapy.

Miosis usually causes difficulty in dark adaptation. Advise patients to use caution while night driving or performing hazardous tasks in poor light.

Angle-closure: Although withdrawal of the peripheral iris from the anterior chamber angle by miosis may reduce the tendency for narrow-angle closure, miotics can occasionally precipitate angle closure by increasing resistance to aqueous flow from posterior to anterior chamber.

Pilocarpine ocular system (Ocusert): Carefully consider and evaluate patients with acute infectious conjunctivitis or keratitis prior to use.

MIOTICS, DIRECT-ACTING

Drug Interactions:

Nonsteroidal anti-inflammatory agents, topical: Although studies with acetylcholine chloride or carbachol revealed no interference, and there is no known pharmacological basis for an interaction, there have been reports that both of these drugs have been ineffective when used in patients treated with topical nonsteroidal anti-inflammatory agents.

Adverse Reactions:

Acetylcholine:

Ophthalmic – Corneal edema; clouding; decompensation.

Systemic – Bradycardia; hypotension; flushing; breathing difficulties; sweating.

Carbachol:

Ophthalmic – Transient stinging and burning; corneal clouding; persistent bullous keratopathy; postoperative iritis following cataract extraction with intraocular use; retinal detachment; transient ciliary and conjunctival injection; ciliary spasm with resultant temporary decrease of visual acuity.

Systemic – Headache; salivation; GI cramps; vomiting; diarrhea; asthma; syncope; cardiac arrhythmia; flushing; sweating; epigastric distress; tightness in bladder; hypotension; frequent urge to urinate.

Pilocarpine:

Ophthalmic – Transient stinging and burning; tearing; ciliary spasm; conjunctival vascular congestion; temporal, peri- or supra-orbital headache; superficial keratitis; induced myopia (especially in younger individuals who have recently started administration); blurred vision; poor dark adaptation; reduced visual acuity in poor illumination in older individuals and in individuals with lens opacity. A subtle corneal granularity has occurred with pilocarpine gel. Lens opacity (prolonged use), retinal detachment (rare; see Precautions).

Systemic – Hypertension, tachycardia, bronchiolar spasm, pulmonary edema, salivation, sweating, nausea, vomiting, diarrhea (rare).

Pilocarpine ocular system (Ocusert): Conjunctival irritation, including mild erythema with or without a slight increase in mucus secretion with first use. These symptoms tend to lessen or disappear after the first week of therapy. Ciliary spasm may occur with pilocarpine usage but is not a contraindication to continued therapy unless the induced myopia is debilitating to the patient. Rarely, a sudden increase in pilocarpine effects has been reported during use.

Irritation from pilocarpine has been infrequently encountered and may require cessation of therapy. True allergic reactions are uncommon, but require discontinuation of therapy. Corneal abrasion and visual impairment have been reported.

Overdosage:

Should accidental overdosage in the eye(s) occur, flush with water.

Treatment: Treatment includes usual supportive measures. Refer to General Management of Acute Overdosage. Observe patients for signs of toxicity (eg, salivation, lacrimation, sweating, nausea, vomiting, diarrhea). If these occur, therapy with anticholinergics (atropine) may be necessary. Bronchial constriction may be a problem in asthmatic patients.

Patient Information:

May sting upon instillation, especially first few doses.

May cause headache, browache and decreased night vision. Use caution while night driving or performing hazardous tasks in poor light.

To avoid contamination, do not touch tip of container to any surface. Replace cap after using. Keep bottle tightly closed when not in use. Discard solution after expiration date.

Miotics, Direct-Acting

ACETYLCHOLINE CHLORIDE, INTRAOCULAR

For complete prescribing information, refer to the Miotics, Direct-Acting group monograph.

Indications:

Miosis: To produce complete miosis in seconds after delivery of the lens in cataract surgery. In penetrating keratoplasty, iridectomy and other anterior segment surgery where rapid, complete miosis may be required.

Administration and Dosage:

Instill the solution into the anterior chamber before or after securing one or more sutures. The pupil is rapidly constricted and the peripheral iris drawn away from the angle of the anterior chamber if there are no mechanical hindrances. Any anatomical hindrance to miosis may require surgery to permit desired effect of drug.

In cataract surgery, use only after delivery of the lens.

Solution: 0.5 to 2 ml produces satisfactory miosis. Solution need not be flushed from the chamber after miosis occurs. Since acetylcholine has a short duration of action, pilocarpine may be applied topically before dressing to maintain miosis.

Preparation of solution: The aqueous solution of acetylcholine chloride is unstable. Prepare solution immediately before use. Do not use solution which is not clear and colorless. Discard any solution that has not been used. Do not gas sterilize.

Storage: Store at room temperature 15° to 30°C (59° to 86°F). Do not freeze.

Rx	**Miochol-E** (Ciba Vision)	**Solution:** 1:100 acetylcholine chloride when reconstituted	In 2 ml dual chamber univial (lower chamber 20 mg lyophilized acetylcholine chloride and 56 mg mannitol; upper chamber 2 ml electrolyte diluent[1] and sterile water for injection).

[1] Sodium chloride, potassium chloride, magnesium chloride hexahydrate, calcium chloride dihydrate.

Miotics, Direct-Acting

CARBACHOL, INTRAOCULAR

For complete prescribing information, refer to the Miotics, Direct-Acting group monograph.

Indications:

Miosis: Intraocular use for miosis during surgery.

Administration and Dosage:

For single-dose intraocular use only. Discard unused portion.

Open under aseptic conditions only.

Gently instill no more than 0.5 ml into the anterior chamber before or after securing sutures. Miosis is usually maximal 2 to 5 minutes after application.

Storage: Store at room temperature 15° to 30°C (59° to 86°F).

Rx	**Carbastat** (Ciba Vision)	**Solution:** 0.01%	In 1.5 ml vials.[1]
Rx	**Miostat** (Alcon)		In 1.5 ml vials.[1]

[1] With 0.64% sodium chloride, 0.075% potassium chloride, 0.048% calcium chloride dihydrate, 0.03% magnesium chloride hexahydrate, 0.39% sodium acetate trihydrate, 0.17% sodium citrate dihydrate, sodium hydroxide, hydrochloric acid.

CARBACHOL, TOPICAL

For complete prescribing information, refer to the Miotics, Direct-Acting group monograph.

Indications:

Glaucoma: For lowering intraocular pressure in the treatment of glaucoma.

Administration and Dosage:

Instill 2 drops into eye(s) up to 3 times daily.

Storage: Store at 8° to 27°C (46° to 80°F).

Rx	**Isopto Carbachol** (Alcon)	**Solution:** 0.75%	In 15 and 30 ml Drop-Tainers.[1]
		1.5%	In 15 and 30 ml Drop-Tainers.[1]
		2.25%	In 15 ml Drop-Tainers.[1]
Rx	**Isopto Carbachol** (Alcon)	3%	In 15 and 30 ml Drop-Tainers.[1]
Rx	**Carboptic** (Optopics)		In 15 ml.[2]

[1] With 0.005% benzalkonium chloride, 1% hydroxypropyl methylcellulose, sodium chloride, boric acid and sodium borate.

[2] With benzalkonium chloride, polyvinyl alcohol and sodium phosphate dibasic and monobasic.

Miotics, Direct-Acting

PILOCARPINE HCl

For complete prescribing information, refer to the Miotics, Direct-Acting group monograph.

Indications:

Chronic simple glaucoma, especially open-angle glaucoma. Patients may be maintained on pilocarpine as long as intraocular pressure (IOP) is controlled and there is no deterioration in the visual fields.

Chronic angle-closure glaucoma.

Acute (angle-dose) glaucoma: Alone, or in combination with other miotics, β-adrendergic blocking agents, epinephrine, carbonic anhydrase inhibitors or hyperosmotic agents to decrease IOP prior to surgery.

Pre- and postoperative intraocular tension.

Mydriasis caused by mydriatic or cycloplegic agents.

Administration and Dosage:

Solution:

Initial – 1 or 2 drops 3 to 4 times a daily. The frequency of instillation and the concentration are determined by patient response. Individuals with heavily pigmented irides may require higher strengths.

Gel: Apply a 0.5 inch ribbon in the lower conjunctival sac of affected eye(s) once daily at bedtime. If other glaucoma medication is also used at bedtime, use drops at least 5 minutes before the gel.

Storage – Do not freeze. Store at room temperature.

Rx	**Isopto Carpine** (Alcon)	**Solution:** 0.25%	In 15 ml.[1]
Rx	**Pilocarpine HCl** (Various, eg, Rugby)	**Solution:** 0.5%	In 15 and 30 ml.
Rx	**Isopto Carpine** (Alcon)		In 15 and 30 ml.[1]
Rx	**Pilocar** (Ciba Vision)		In 15 ml and twin-pack (2 × 15 ml).[2]
Rx	**Piloptic-½** (Optopics)		In 15 ml.[3]
Rx	**Pilostat** (Bausch & Lomb)		In 15 ml.[5]
Rx	**Pilocarpine HCl** (Various, eg, Alcon, Goldline, Rugby)	**Solution:** 1%	In 2, 15 and 30 ml and UD 1 ml.
Rx	**Adsorbocarpine** (Alcon)		In 15 ml.[4]
Rx	**Akarpine** (Akorn)		In 15 ml.
Rx	**Isopto Carpine** (Alcon)		In 15 and 30 ml.[1]
Rx	**Pilocar** (Ciba Vision)		In 15 ml, twin-pack (2 × 15 ml) and 1 ml dropperettes.[2]
Rx	**Piloptic-1** (Optopics)		In 15 ml.[3]
Rx	**Pilostat** (Bausch & Lomb)		In 15 ml and twin-pack (2 × 15 ml).[5]
Rx	**Pilocarbpine HCl** (Various eg, Alcon, Goldline, Rugby)	**Solution:** 2%	In 2, 15, and 30 ml.
Rx	**Adsorbocarpine** (Alcon)		In 15 ml dropper bottles.[4]
Rx	**Akarpine** (Akorn)		In 15 ml dropper bottles.
Rx	**Isopto Carpine** (Alcon)		In 15 and 30 ml.[1]
Rx	**Pilocar** (Ciba Vision)		In 15 ml, twin-pack (2 × 15 ml) and 1 ml dropperettes.[2]
Rx	**Piloptic-2** (Optopics)		In 15 ml.[3]
Rx	**Pilostat** (Bausch & Lomb)		In 15 ml and twin-pack (2 × 15 ml).[5]

Miotics, Direct-Acting

PILOCARPINE HCl			
Rx	**Isopto Carpine** (Alcon)	**Solution:** 3%	In 15 ml and 30 ml.[1]
Rx	**Pilocar** (Ciba Vision)		In 15 ml and twin-pack (2 × 15 ml).[2]
Rx	**Piloptic-3** (Optopics)		In 15 ml.[3]
Rx	**Pilostat** (Bausch & Lomb)		In 15 ml and twin-pack (2 × 15 ml).[5]
Rx	**Pilocarpine HCl** (Various, eg, Alcon, Goldline, Rugby)	**Solution:** 4%	In 2, 15 and 30 ml.
Rx	**Adsorbocarpine** (Alcon)		In 15 ml dropper bottles.[4]
Rx	**Akarpine** (Akorn)		In 15 ml dropper bottles.
Rx	**Isopto carpine** (Alcon)		In 15 and 30 ml.[1]
Rx	**Pilocar** (Ciba Vision)		In 15 ml, twin-pack (2 × 15 ml) and 1 ml dropper-ettes.[2]
Rx	**Piloptic-4** (Optopics)		In 15 ml.[4]
Rx	**Pilopto-Carpine** (Lebeh Pharmacal)		In 15 ml.
Rx	**Pilostat** (Bausch & Lomb)		In 15 ml and twin-pack (2 × 15 ml) ml.[5]
Rx	**Isopto Carpine** (Alcon)	**Solution:** 5%	In 15 ml.[1]
Rx	**Pilocarpine HCl** (Various, eg, Rugby)	**Solution:** 6%	In 15 ml.
Rx	**Isopto Carpine** (Alcon)		In 15 and 30 ml.[1]
Rx	**Pilocar** (Ciba Vision)		In 15 ml and twin-pack (2 × 15 ml).[3]
Rx	**Piloptic-6** (Optopics)		In 15 ml.[3]
Rx	**Pilostat** (Bausch & Lomb)		In 15 ml.[5]
Rx	**Pilocarpine HCl** (Alcon)	**Solution:** 8%	In 2 ml.
Rx	**Isopto Carpine** (Alcon)		In 15 ml.
Rx	**Isopto Carpine** (Alcon)	**Solution:**10%	In 15 ml.[1]
Rx	**Pilopine HS** (Alcon)	**Gel:** 4%	In 3.5 g.[6]

[1] With 0.5% hydroxypropyl methylcellulose and 0.01% benzalkonium chloride.
[2] With dydroxypropyl methylcellulose, benzalkonium chloride and EDTA.
[3] With polyvinyl alcohol, benzalkonium chloride and EDTA.
[4] With 0.004% benzalkonium chloride, EDTA, povidone, PEG and hydroxyethyl cellulose.
[5] With dydroxypropyl methylcellulose, 0.01% benzalkonium chloride and EDTA.
[6] With 0.008% benzalkonium chloride, carbopol 940 and EDTA.

Miotics, Direct-Acting

PILOCARPINE NITRATE

For complete prescribing information, refer to the Miotics, Direct-Acting group monograph.

Indications:

To control IOP in glaucoma.

For emergency relief of mydriasis in an acutely glaucomatous situation.

To reverse mydriasis caused by cycloplegic agents.

Administration and Dosage:

Glaucoma: Instill 1 to 2 drops 2 to 4 times daily. Patient response may vary.

Emergency miosis: Instill 1 to 2 drops of higher concentrations.

Reversal of mydriasis: Dosage and strength required are dependent on the cycloplegic used.

Storage: Shake well before using. Do not freeze. Keep out of reach of children.

Rx	**Pilagan** (Allergan)	**Solution:** 1%	In 15 ml.[1]
		2%	In 15 ml.[1]
		4%	In 15 ml.[1]

[1] With 1.4% polyvinyl alcohol, 0.5% chlorobutanol, menthol, camphor, phenol and eucalyptol.

Miotics, Direct-Acting

PILOCARPINE OCULAR THERAPEUTIC SYSTEM

Refer to the general discussion in the Miotics, Direct-Acting group monograph.

Actions:

Pharmacology: An elliptical unit designed for continuous release of pilocarpine following placement in the cul-de-sac of the eye. Pilocarpine is released from the system as soon as it is placed in contact with the conjunctival surfaces.

Pharmacokinetics: Ocusert initially releases the drug at 3 times the rated value in the first hours and declines to the rated value in approximately 6 hours. A total of 0.3 to 0.7 mg pilocarpine is released during this initial 6 hour period (one drop of 2% pilocarpine ophthalmic solution contains 1 mg pilocarpine). During the remainder of the 7 day period, the release rate is within ± 20% of the rated value.

Ocular hypotensive effect is fully developed within 1.5 to 2 hours after placement in cul-de-sac. A satisfactory ocular hypotensive response is maintained around the clock. IOP reduction for the entire week is achieved with the system from either 3.4 or 6.7 mg pilocarpine (20 or 40 mcg/hr times 24 hrs/day times 7 days, respectively), vs 28 mg given as a 2% ophthalmic solution 4 times daily.

During the first several hours after insertion, induced myopia may occur. In contrast to fluctuating and high levels of induced myopia typical of pilocarpine use, the amount of induced myopia with *Ocusert* decreases after the first several hours to a low baseline level (≤ 0.5 diopters), which persists for the therapeutic life of the system. Pilocarpine-induced miosis approximately parallels induced myopia.

Indications:

IOP reduction: Control of elevated IOP in pilocarpine-responsive patients.

Patient Information:

Patient package insert is available with the product.

Wash hands with soap and water before touching or manipulating the system. If a displaced system contacts unclean surfaces, rinse with cool tap water before replacing. Discard contaminated systems and replace with a fresh unit.

Check for the presence of the system before retiring at night and upon arising.

Administration and Dosage:

Damaged or deformed systems: Do not place or retain in the eye. Remove and replace systems believed to be associated with an unexpected increase in drug action.

Initiation of therapy: There is no direct correlation between the strength of *Ocusert* used and the strength of pilocarpine eyedrop solutions required to achieve a given level of pressure lowering. It has been estimated that *Ocusert* 20 mcg is roughly equal to 0.5% or 1% drops and 40 mcg is roughly equal to 2% or 3% drops. *Ocusert* reduces the amount of drug necessary to achieve adequate medical control; therefore, therapy may be started with the 20 mcg system, regardless of the strength of pilocarpine solution the patient previously required. Because of the patient's age, family history and disease status or progression, however, therapy may be started with the 40 mcg system. The patient should return during the first week of therapy for evaluation of IOP, and as often thereafter as deemed necessary.

If pressure is satisfactorily reduced with the 20 mcg system, the patient should continue its use, replacing each unit every 7 days. If IOP reduction greater than that achieved by 20 mcg is needed, transfer the patient to the 40 mcg system. If necessary, concurrently use epinephrine, a β-blocker or carbonic anhydrase inhibitor; *Ocusert's* release rate is not influenced by other ophthalmic preparations.

Placement and removal of the system: The system is placed in and removed from the eye by the patient. Since pilocarpine-induced myopia may occur during the first several hours of therapy, place the system into the conjunctival cul-de-sac at bedtime. By morning, the myopia is at a stable level (≤ 0.5 diopters).

In those patients in whom retention is a problem, superior cul-de-sac placement is often more desirable. The unit can be manipulated from lower to upper conjunctival cul-de-sac by gentle digital massage through the eyelid. If possible, move the unit before sleep to the upper conjunctival cul-de-sac for best retention. Should the unit slip out during sleep, its ocular hypotensive effect after loss continues for a period comparable to that following instillation of eyedrops.

Ocusert has been used concomitantly with various ophthalmic medications.

Storage: Refrigerate at 2° to 8°C (36° to 46°F).

Rx	**Ocusert Pilo-20** (Alza)	**Ocular Therapeutic System**: Releases 20 mcg pilocarpine per hour for 1 week	In packs of 8 individ. sterile systems.	4.4
Rx	**Ocusert Pilo-40** (Alza)	**Ocular Therapeutic System**: Releases 40 mcg pilocarpine per hour for 1 week	In packs of 8 individ. sterile systems.	4.4

MIOTICS, CHOLINESTERASE INHIBITORS

Refer to the general discussion of these products in the Topical Ophthalmics Introduction.

Actions:

Pharmacology: These indirect-acting agents inhibit the enzyme cholinesterase, potentiating the action of acetylcholine on the parasympathomimetic end organs. Topical application to the eye produces intense miosis and muscle contraction. Intraocular pressure (IOP) is reduced by a decreased resistance to aqueous outflow.

Cholinesterase inhibitors are subdivided into reversible and irreversible agents. Reversible agents (eg, physostigmine, demecarium) quickly combine with cholinesterase; the resulting complex is slowly hydrolyzed and the inhibited enzyme is regenerated. The demecarium-enzyme complex is hydrolyzed more slowly than the physostigmine complex; therefore, its duration of action is longer.

Irreversible agents (eg, echothiophate) also bind to cholinesterase; however, the resulting covalent bond is not hydrolyzed. Therefore, cholinesterase is not regenerated. More cholinesterase must be synthesized or supplied from depots elsewhere in the body before ophthalmic action dependent on cholinesterase returns. Echothiophate will depress both plasma and erythrocyte cholinesterase levels in most patients after a few weeks of eyedrop therapy.

These effects are accompanied by increased capillary permeability of the ciliary body and iris, increased permeability of the blood-aqueous barrier and vasodilation. Myopia may be induced or, if present, may be augmented by the increased refractive power of the lens that results from the accommodative effect of the drug. Demecarium indirectly produces some of the muscarinic and nicotinic effects of acetylcholine as quantities of the latter accumulate.

Cholinesterase-Inhibiting Miotics

Miotics	Miosis		IOP reduction		
	Onset (minutes)	Duration	Onset (hours)	Peak (hours)	Duration
Reversible					
Physostigmine	20 to 30	12 to 36 hrs	—	2 to 6	12 to 36 hrs
Demecarium	15 to 60	3 to 10 days	—	24	7 to 28 days
Irreversible					
Echothiophate	10 to 30	1 to 4 weeks	4 to 8	24	7 to 28 days

Indications:

Glaucoma: Therapy of open-angle glaucoma.

For other specific indications, refer to the individual monographs.

Contraindications:

Hypersensitivity to cholinesterase inhibitors or any component of the formulation; active uveal inflammation or any inflammatory disease of the iris or ciliary body; glaucoma associated with iridocyclitis.

Demecarium: Pregnancy.

Echothiophate: Most cases of angle-closure glaucoma (due to the possibility of increasing angle-block).

Warnings:

Myasthenia gravis: Because of possible additive adverse effects, administer demecarium and echothiophate only with extreme caution to patients with myasthenia gravis who are receiving systemic anticholinesterase therapy. Conversely, exercise extreme caution in the use of anticholinesterase drugs for the treatment of myasthenia gravis patients who are already undergoing topical therapy with cholinesterase inhibitors.

Surgery: In patients receiving cholinesterase inhibitors, administer succinylcholine with extreme caution before and during general anesthesia (see Drug Interactions). Use prior to ophthalmic surgery only as a considered risk because of the possible occurrence of hyphema.

Pregnancy: Category X (demecarium). Contraindicated in women who are or who may become pregnant. If this drug is used during pregnancy, or if the patient becomes pregnant while taking this drug, apprise the patient of the potential hazard to the fetus.

Category C (physostigmine, echothiophate). Safety for use during pregnancy has not been established. Use only when clearly needed and when the potential benefits outweigh the potential hazards to the fetus.

MIOTICS, CHOLINESTERASE INHIBITORS

Lactation: It is not known whether these drugs are excreted in breast milk. Exercise caution when administering to a nursing woman. Because of the potential for serious adverse reactions in nursing infants, decide whether to discontinue nursing or the drug, taking into account the importance of the drug to the mother.

Children: The occurrence of iris cysts is more frequent in children (see Precautions). Exercise extreme caution in children receiving demecarium who may require general anesthesia. Safety and efficacy for use of physostigmine have not been established.

Precautions:

Concomitant therapy: Cholinesterase inhibitors may be used in combination with adrenergic agents, β-blockers, carbonic anhydrase inhibitors or hyperosmotic agents.

Narrow angle glaucoma: Use with caution in patients with chronic angle-closure (narrow-angle) glaucoma or in patients with narrow angles, because of the possibility of producing pupillary block and increasing angle blockage.

Special risk patients: Use caution in patients with marked vagotonia, bronchial asthma, spastic GI disturbances, peptic ulcer, pronounced bradycardia/hypotension, recent MI, epilepsy, parkinsonism and other disorders that may respond adversely to vagotonic effects.Temporarily discontinue if cardiac irregularities occur.

Ophthalmic ointments may retard corneal healing.

Miosis usually causes difficulty in dark adaptation. Use caution while driving at night or performing hazardous tasks in poor light.

Gonioscopy: Use only when shorter-acting miotics have proved inadequate. Gonioscopy is recommended prior to use of medication. Routine examination (eg, slit-lamp) to detect lens opacities should accompany therapy.

Concomitant ocular conditions: When an intraocular inflammatory process is present, breakdown of the blood-aqueous barrier from anticholinesterase therapy requires abstention from, or cautious use of, these drugs. Use with great caution where there is a history of quiescent uveitis. After long-term use, blood vessel dilation and resultant greater permeability increase possibility of hyphema during or prior to ophthalmic surgery. Discontinue 3 to 4 weeks before surgery.

Systemic effects: Repeated administration may cause depression of the concentration of cholinesterase in the serum and erythrocytes, with resultant systemic effects. Discontinue if salivation, urinary incontinence, diarrhea, profuse sweating, muscle weakness, respiratory difficulties, shock or cardiac irregularities occur.

Although systemic effects are infrequent, use digital compression of the nasolacrimal ducts for 1 to 2 minutes after instillation to minimize drainage into the nasopharyngeal area.

Iris cysts: Iris cysts may form, enlarge and obscure vision (more frequent in children). The iris cyst usually shrinks upon discontinuance of the miotic, or following reduction in strength of the drops or frequency of instillation. Rarely, the cyst may rupture or break free into the aqueous humor. Frequent examination for this occurrence is advised.

Sulfite sensitivity: Some of these products contain sulfites which may cause allergic-type reactions (eg, hives, itching, wheezing, anaphylaxis) in certain susceptible persons. Although the overall prevalence of sulfite sensitivity in the general population is probably low, it is seen more frequently in asthmatics or atopic nonasthmatics.

MIOTICS, CHOLINESTERASE INHIBITORS

Drug Interactions:

Ophthalmic Cholinesterase Inhibitor Drug Interactions			
Precipitant drug	Object drug*		Description
Carbamate/ Organophosphate insecticides, pesticides	Cholinesterase inhibitors	⬆	Warn persons on cholinesterase inhibitors who are exposed to these substances (eg, gardeners, organophosphate plant or warehouse workers, farmers) of systemic effects possible from absorption through respiratory tract or skin. Advise use of respiratory masks, frequent washing and clothing changes.
Succinylcholine	Cholinesterase inhibitors	⬆	Use extreme caution before or during general anesthesia to patients on cholinesterase inhibitors because of possible respiratory and cardiovascular collapse.
Anticholinesterases, systemic	Cholinesterase inhibitors	⬆	Additive effects are possible; coadminister topical cholinesterase inhibitors cautiously, regardless of which therapy is added (see Warnings).

* ⬆ = Object drug increased

Adverse Reactions:

Ophthalmic: Iris cysts (see Precautions); burning; lacrimation; lid muscle twitching; conjunctival and ciliary redness; browache; headache; activation of latent iritis or uveitis; induced myopia with visual blurring; retinal detatchment; lens opacities (see Precautions); conjuntival thickening and destruction of nasolacrimal canals (prolonged use).

Paradoxical increase in IOP by pupillary block may follow instillation. Alleviate with pupil-dilating medication.

Systemic: Nausea; vomiting; abdominal cramps; diarrhea; urinary incontinence; fainting sweating; salivation; difficulty in breathing; cardiac irregularities.

Overdosage:

Treatment: If systemic effects occur, give parenteral atropine sulfate (IV if necessary):

Adults – 0.4 to 0.6 mg.

Infants and children up to 12 years – 0.01 mg/kg repeated every 2 hours as needed until the desired effect is obtained, or adverse effects of atropine preclude further usage. The maximum single dose should not exceed 0.4 mg.

Much larger atropine doses for anticholinesterase intoxication in adults have been used. Initially, 2 to 6 mg followed by 2 mg every hour or more often, as long as muscarinic effects continue. Consider the greater possibility of atropinization with large doses, particularly in sensitive individuals.

Pralidoxime chloride (see Antidotes) has been useful in treating systemic effects due to cholinesterase inhibitors. However, use in addition to, not as a substitute for, atropine.

A short-acting barbiturate is indicated for convulsions not relieved by atropine. Promptly treat marked weakness or paralysis of respiratory muscles by maintaining a clear airway and by artificial respiration.

Patient Information:

Local irritation and headache may occur at initiation of therapy.

Notify physician if abdominal cramps, diarrhea or excessive salivation occurs.

Wash hands immediately after administration.

Use caution while driving at night or performing hazardous tasks in poor light.

Refer to the Topical Ophthalmics Introduction for more complete information.

Miotics, Cholinesterase Inhibitors

PHYSOSTIGMINE

For complete prescribing information, refer to the Miotics, Cholinesterase Inhibitors group monograph.

Indications:

Glaucoma: Reduction of IOP in primary glaucoma.

Administration and Dosage:

Ointment: Apply small quantity to lower fornix, up to 3 times daily.

Storage: Keep tightly closed. Protect from heat.

Rx	**Eserine Sulfate** (Ciba Vision)	**Ointment:** 0.25% (as sulfate)	In 3.5 g.

DEMECARIUM BROMIDE

For complete prescribing information, refer to the Miotics, Cholinesterase Inhibitors group monograph.

Indications:

Glaucoma: Treatment of open-angle glaucoma (use only when shorter-acting miotics have proved inadequate).

Aqueous outflow: Conditions affecting aqueous outflow (eg, synechial formation) that are amenable to miotic therapy.

Iridectomy: Following iridectomy procedure.

Accommodative esotripia: Treatment of accomodative esotripia (accomodative convergent stabismus).

Administration and Dosage:

Do not use more often than directed. Caution is necessary to avoid overdosage. Individualize dosage to obtain maximal therapeutic effect.

Closely observe the patient during the initial period. If the response is not adequate within the first 24 hours, consider other measures. Keep frequency of use to a minimum in all patients, especially children, to reduce chance of iris cyst development.

Glaucoma:

Initial – Instill 1 or 2 drops into eye(s). A decrease in IOP should occur within a few hours. During this period, keep patient under supervision and perform tonometric examinations at least hourly for 3 or 4 hours to make sure no immediate rise in pressure occurs.

Usual dose – Instill 1 or 2 drops twice a week to 1 or 2 drops twice a day. The 0.125% strength used twice daily usually results in smooth control of the physiologic diurnal variation in IOP.

Strabismus: Essentially equal visual acuity of both eyes is a prerequisite to successful treatment.

Diagnosis – For initial evaluation, use as a diagnostic aid to determine if an accommodative factor exists. This is especially useful preoperatively in young children and in patients with normal hypermetropic refractive errors. Instill 1 drop daily for 2 weeks, then 1 drop every 2 days for 2 to 3 weeks. If the eyes become straighter, an accommodative factor is demonstrated. This technique may supplement or complement standard testing with atropine and trial with glasses for the accommodative factor.

Therapy – In esotropia uncomplicated by amblyopia or anisometropia, instill not more than 1 drop at a time in both eyes every day for 2 to 3 weeks; too severe a degree of miosis may interfere with vision. Then reduce dosage to 1 drop every other day for 3 to 4 weeks and reevaluate the patient's status. Continue with a dosage of 1 drop every 2 days to 1 drop twice a week (the latter dosage may be maintained for several months). Evaluate the patient's condition every 4 to 12 weeks. If improvement continues, reduce to 1 drop once a week and eventually to a trial without medication. However discontinue therapy after 4 months if control of the condition still requires 1 drop every 2 days.

Storage: Do not freeze. Protect from heat.

Rx	**Humorsol** (Merck)	**Solution:** 0.125%	In 5 ml Ocumeters.[1]
		0.25%	In 5 ml Ocumeters.[1]

[1] With 1:5000 benzalkonium chloride and sodium chloride.

Miotics, Cholinesterase Inhibitors

ECHOTHIOPHATE IODIDE

For complete prescribing information, refer to the Miotics, Cholinesterase Inhibitors group monograph.

Indications:

Glaucoma: Chronic open-angle glaucoma; subacute or chronic angle-closure glaucoma after iridectomy or where surgery is refused or contraindicated; certain nonuveitic secondary types of glaucoma, especially glaucoma following cataract surgery.

Accomodative esotropia: Concomitant esotropias with a significant accommodative component.

Administration and Dosage:

Tolerance may develop after prolonged use; a rest period restores response to the drug.

Glaucoma:

Two doses per day are preferred to maintain as smooth a diurnal tension curve as possible, although 1 dose/day or every other day has been used with satisfactory results. It is unnecessary and undesirable to exceed a schedule of twice a day. Instill the daily dose or 1 of the 2 daily doses just before bedtime to avoid inconvenience due to miosis.

Early chronic simple glaucoma – Instill a 0.03% solution just before retiring and in the morning in cases not controlled with pilocarpine. Control during the night and early morning hours may then be obtained. Change therapy if IOP fails to remain at an acceptable level.

Advanced chronic simple glaucoma and glaucoma secondary to cataract surgery – Instill 0.03% solution twice daily, as above. When transferring a patient to echothiophate because of unsatisfactory control with other miotics, one of the higher strengths will usually be needed. In this case, a brief trial with 0.03% solution will be advantageous because higher strengths will then be more easily tolerated.

Concomitant therapy: May be coadministered with epinephrine, a carbonic anhydrase inhibitor or both.

Accommodative esotropia:

Diagnosis – Instill 1 drop of 0.125% solution once a day into both eyes at bedtime for 2 or 3 weeks. If the esotropia is accommodative, a favorable response may begin within a few hours.

Treatment – Use lowest concentration and frequency which gives satisfactory results. After initial period of treatment for diagnostic purposes, reduce schedule to 0.125% every other day or 0.06% every day. Dosages can often be gradually lowered as treatment progresses. The 0.03% strength has proven effective in some cases. The maximum recommended dose is 0.125% once a day, although more intensive therapy has been used for short periods.

Duration of treatment – In diagnosis, only a short period is required and little time will be lost in instituting other procedures if the esotropia proves to be unresponsive. In therapy, there is no definite limit if the drug is well tolerated. However, if the eyedrops, with or without eyeglasses, are gradually withdrawn after a year or two and deviation recurs, consider surgery.

Storage/Stability: Preparation of solution

Store at room temperature 15° to 30°C (59° to 86°F). After reconstitution, keep eye drops in refrigerator to obtain maximum useful life of 6 months. Use within 1 month if stored at room temperature.

Rx	**Phospholine Iodide** (Wyeth-Ayerst)	**Powder for Reconstitution:** 1.5 mg to make 0.03%	With 5 ml diluent.[1]
		3 mg to make 0.06%	With 5 ml diluent.[1]
		6.25 mg to make 0.125%	With 5 ml diluent.[1]
		12.5 mg to make 0.25%	With 5 ml diluent.[1]

[1] With potassium acetate, 0.55% chlorobutanol and 1.2% mannitol.

Carbonic Anhydrase Inhibitors

DORZOLAMIDE HCl

Actions:

Pharmacology: Dorzolamide is a carbonic anhydrase inhibitor formulated for topical ophthalmic use. Carbonic anhydrase (CA) is an enzyme found in many tissues of the body, including the eye. It catalyzes the reversible reaction involving the hydration of carbon dioxide and the dehydration of carbonic acid. In humans, carbonic anhydrase exists as a number of isoenzymes, the most active being carbonic anhydrase II (CA-II), found primarily in red blood cells (RBCs), but also in other tissues. Inhibition of CA in the ciliary processes of the eye decreases aqueous humor secretion, presumably by slowing the formation of bicarbonate ions with subsequent reduction in sodium and fluid transport. The result is a reduction in intraocular pressure (IOP). Dorzolamide, by inhibiting CA-II, reduces elevated IOP. Elevated IOP is a major risk factor in the pathogenesis of optic nerve damage and glaucomatous visual field loss.

Pharmacokinetics: When topically applied, dorzolamide reaches the systemic circulation. To assess the potential for systemic CA inhibition following topical administration, drug and metabolite concentrations in RBCs and plasma and CA inhibition in RBCs were measured. Dorzolamide accumulates in RBCs during chronic dosing as a result of binding to CA-II. The parent drug forms a single N-desethyl metabolite that inhibits CA-II less potently than the parent drug but also inhibits CA-I. The metabolite also accumulates in RBCs, where it binds primarily to CA-I. Plasma concentrations of parent and metabolite are generally below the assay limit of quantitation. Dorzolamide binds moderately to plasma proteins (≈ 33%). The drug is primarily excreted unchanged in the urine, and the metabolite is also excreted in urine. After dosing is stopped, dorzolamide washes out of RBCs nonlinearly, resulting in a rapid decline of drug concentration initially, followed by a slower elimination phase with a half-life of about 4 months.

To simulate the systemic exposure after long-term topical ocular administration, dorzolamide was given orally to eight healthy subjects for up to 20 weeks. The oral dose of 2 mg twice daily closely approximates the amount of drug delivered by topical ocular administration of 2% 3 times daily. Steady state was reached within 8 weeks. The inhibition of CA-II and total CA activities was below the degree of inhibition anticipated to be necessary for a pharmacological effect on renal function and respiration in healthy individuals.

Clinical trials: The efficacy of dorzolamide was demonstrated in clinical studies in the treatment of elevated IOP in patients with glaucoma or ocular hypertension (baseline IOP ≥ 23 mm Hg). The IOP-lowering effect of dorzolamide was approximately 3 to 5 mm Hg throughout the day, and this was consistent in clinical studies with durations of up to 1 year.

Indications:

Elevated intraocular pressure (IOP): Treatment of elevated IOP in patients with ocular hypertension or open-angle glaucoma.

Contraindications:

Hypersensitivity to any component of this product.

Warnings:

Systemic effects: Dorzolamide is a sulfonamide and, although administered topically, is absorbed systemically. Therefore, the same types of adverse reactions attributable to sulfonamides may occur with topical administration of dorzolamide (refer to the systemic Sulfonamides monograph in the Anti-Infectives section). Fatalities have occurred, although rarely, due to severe reactions to sulfonamides including Stevens-Johnson syndrome, toxic epidermal necrolysis, fulminant hepatic necrosis, agranulocytosis, aplastic anemia and other blood dyscrasias. Sensitization may recur when a sulfonamide is readministered regardless of the route of administration. If signs of serious reactions or hypersensitivity occur, discontinue the use of this preparation.

Renal/Hepatic function impairment: Dorzolamide has not been studied in patients with severe renal impairment (Ccr < 30 ml/min). However, because dorzolamide and its metabolite are excreted predominantly by the kidney, dorzolamide is not recommended in such patients.

Dorzolamide has not been studied in patients with hepatic impairment and should therefore be used with caution in such patients.

Carcinogenesis: In a 2 year study of dorzolamide administered orally to male and female Sprague-Dawley rats, urinary bladder papillomas were seen in male rats in the highest dosage group of 20 mg/kg/day (250 times the recommended human ophthalmic dose); papillomas were not seen in rats given oral doses equivalent to

≈ 12 times the recommended dose. The increased incidence of urinary bladder papillomas is a class effect of CA inhibitors in rats.

Elderly: Of all the patients in clinical studies, 44% were ≥ 65 years of age and 10% were ≥ 75 years of age. No overall differences in efficacy or safety were observed between these patients and younger patients, but greater sensitivity of some older individuals to the product cannot be ruled out.

Pregnancy: Category C. Studies in rabbits at oral doses of ≥ 2.5 mg/kg/day (31 times the recommended human ophthalmic dose) revealed malformations of the vertebral bodies. These malformations occurred at doses that caused metabolic acidosis with decreased body weight gain in dams and decreased fetal weights. There are no adequate and well controlled studies in pregnant women. Use during pregnancy only if the potential benefit justifies the risk to the fetus.

Lactation: In lactating rats, decreases in body weight gain of 5% to 7% were seen in offspring at an oral dose of 7.5 mg/kg/day (94 times the recommended human ophthalmic dose). A slight delay in postnatal development (incisor eruption, vaginal canalization and eye openings), secondary to lower fetal body weight, was noted.

It is not known whether this drug is excreted in breast milk. Because of the potential for serious adverse reactions in nursing infants, decide whether to discontinue nursing or to discontinue the drug, taking into account the importance of the drug to the mother.

Children: Safety and efficacy in children have not been established.

Precautions:

Corneal endothelium effects: Carbonic anhydrase activity has been observed in both the cytoplasm and around the plasma membranes of the corneal endothelium. The effect of continued administration of dorzolamide on the corneal endothelium has not been fully evaluated.

Acute angle-closure glaucoma: The management of patients with acute angle-closure glaucoma requires therapeutic interventions in addition to ocular hypotensive agents. Dorzolamide has not been studied in patients with acute angle-closure glaucoma.

Ocular effects: Local ocular adverse effects, primarily conjunctivitis and lid reactions, were reported with chronic administration of dorzolamide. Many of these reactions had the clinical appearance and course of an allergic-type reaction that resolved upon discontinuation of drug therapy. If such reactions are observed, discontinue dorzolamide and evaluate the patient before considering restarting the drug.

Concomitant oral CA inhibitors: There is a potential for an additive effect on the known systemic effects of CA inhibition in patients receiving an oral CA inhibitor and dorzolamide. The concomitant administration of dorzolamide and oral CA inhibitors is not recommended.

Bacterial keratitis: There have been reports of bacterial keratitis associated with the use of topical ophthalmic products in multiple dose containers . These containers had been inadvertently contaminated by patients who, in most cases, had a concurrent corneal disease or a disruption of the ocular epithelial surface.

Contact lenses: The preservative in dorzolamide solution, benzalkonium chloride, may be absorbed by soft contact lenses. Dorzolamide should not be administered while wearing soft contact lenses.

Drug Interactions:

Although acid-base and electrolyte disturbances were not reported in the clinical trials with dorzolamide, these disturbances have been reported with oral CA inhibitors and have, in some instances, resulted in drug interactions (eg, toxicity associated with high-dose salicylate therapy). Therefore, consider the potential for such drug interactions in patients receiving dorzolamide.

Adverse Reactions:

Ocular burning, stinging or discomfort immediately following administration (≈ 33%); bitter taste following administration (≈ 25%); superficial punctate keratitis (10% to 15%); signs and symptoms of ocular allergic reaction (≈ 10%); blurred vision, tearing, dryness, photophobia (≈ 1% to 5%); headache, nausea, asthenia/fatigue (infrequent); skin rashes, urolithiasis, iridocyclitis (rare).

Overdosage:

Electrolyte imbalance, development of an acidotic state and possible CNS effects may occur. Monitor serum electrolyte levels (particularly potassium) and blood pH levels. Significant lethality was observed in female rats and mice after single oral doses of 1927 and 1320 mg/kg, respectively.

Carbonic Anhydrase Inhibitors

DORZOLAMIDE HCl

Patient Information:

Dorzolamide is a sulfonamide, and, although administered topically, it is absorbed systemically. Therefore, the same types of adverse reactions that are attributable to sulfonamides may occur with topical administration. Advise patients that if serious or unusual reactions or signs of hypersensitivity occur, they should discontinue use of the product.

Advise patients that if they develop any ocular reactions, particularly conjunctivitis and lid reactions, they should discontinue use and seek their physician's advice.

Instruct patients to avoid allowing the tip of the dispensing container to contact the eye or surrounding structures. Ocular solutions, if handled improperly or if the tip of the dispensing container contacts the eye or surrounding structures, can become contaminated by common bacteria known to cause ocular infections. Serious damage to the eye and subsequent loss of vision may result from using contaminated solutions.

Advise patients that if they develop an intercurrent ocular condition (eg, trauma, ocular surgery, infection), they should immediately seek their physician's advice concerning the continued use of the present multidose container.

If more than one topical ophthalmic drug is being used, administer the drugs at least 10 minutes apart.

Administration and Dosage:

Approved by the FDA on December 9, 1994 (1P classification).

Dosage: One drop in the affected eye(s) 3 times daily.

Concomitant therapy: Dorzolamide may be used concomitantly with other topical ophthalmic drug products to lower intraocular pressure. If more than one ophthalmic drug is being used, administer the drugs at least 10 minutes apart.

Rx	**Trusopt** (Merck)	**Solution:** 2%	In 5 and 10 ml.

Prostaglandin Agonist

LATANOPROST

Actions:

Pharmacology: Latanoprost is a prostaglandin $F_{2\alpha}$ analog that is believed to reduce the intraocular pressure (IOP) by increasing the outflow of aqueous humor.

Pharmacokinetics:

Absorption – Latanoprost is absorbed through the cornea where the isopropyl ester prodrug is hydrolyzed by esterases to the biologically active acid. Studies in man indicate that the peak concentration in the aqueous humor is reached ≈ 2 hours after topical administration.

Distribution – The distribution volume in humans is 0.16 L/kg. The acid of latanoprost could be measured in aqueous humor during the first 4 hours and in plasma only during the first hour after local administration.

Metabolism – The active acid of latanoprost reaching systemic circulation is primarily metabolized by the liver to the 1,2–dinor and 1,2,3,4–tetranor metabolites via fatty acid β-oxidation.

Excretion – The elimination of the acid of latanoprost from human plasma was rapid (half-life was 17 min) after both IV and topical administration. Systemic clearance is ≈ 7 ml/min/kg. Following hepatic β-oxidation, the metabolites are mainly eliminated via the kidneys. Approximately 88% to 98% of the administered dose is recovered in the urine after topical and IV dosing, respectively.

Clinical trials: Patients with mean baseline IOP of 24 to 25 mmHg who were treated for 6 months in multicenter, randomized, controlled trials demonstrated 6 to 8 mmHg reductions in IOP. This IOP reduction with 0.005% latanoprost dosed once daily was equivalent to the effect of 0.5% timolol dosed twice daily.

Indications:

Elevated intraocular pressure (IOP): For reduction of elevated IOP in patients with open-angle glaucoma and ocular hypertension who are intolerant of other IOP lowering medications or insufficiently responsive (failed to achieve target IOP determined after multiple measurements over time) to another IOP lowering medication.

Contraindications:

Hypersensitivity to any component of this product.

Warnings:

Eye pigment changes: Latanoprost may gradually change eye color, increasing the amount of brown pigment in the iris by increasing the number of melanosomes (pigment granules) in melanocytes. The long-term effects on the melanocytes and the consequences of potential injury to the melanocytes or deposition of pigment granules to other areas of the eye is currently unknown.

The change in iris color occurs slowly and may not be noticeable for several months to several years. Typically, the brown pigmentation around the pupil spreads concentrically towards the periphery in affected eyes, but the entire iris or parts of it may also become more brownish. Until more information about increased brown pigmentation is available, patients should be examined regularly and, depending on the clinical situation, treatment may be stopped if increased pigmentation ensues. The increase in brown iris pigment has not been shown to progress further upon discontinuation of treatment, but the resultant color change may be permanent. Neither nevi nor freckles of the iris have been affected by treatment.

Pregnancy: Category C. Reproduction studies have been performed in rats and rabbits. In rabbits, 4 out of 16 dams had no viable fetuses at a dose that was ≈ 80 times the maximum human dose, and the highest nonembryocidal dose in rabbits was ≈ 15 times the maximum human dose. There are no adequate and well controlled studies in pregnant women. Use during pregnancy only if the potential benefit justifies the potential risk to the fetus.

Lactation: It is not known whether this drug or its metabolites are excreted in breast milk. Because many drugs are excreted in breast milk, exercise caution when administering latanoprost to a nursing woman.

Children: Safety and effectiveness in children have not been established.

Precautions:

Cornea: Latanoprost is hydrolyzed in the cornea. The effect of continued administration of latanoprost on the corneal endothelium has not been fully evaluated.

Bacterial keratitis: There have been reports of bacterial keratitis associated with the use of multiple-dose containers of topical ophthalmic products. These containers had been inadvertently contaminated by patients who, in most cases, had a concurrent corneal disease or a disruption of the ocular epithelial surface.

Contact lenses: Do not administer latanoprost while wearing contact lenses.

Prostaglandin Agonist

LATANOPROST

Drug Interactions:

In vitro studies have shown that precipitation occurs when eye drops containing thimerosal are mixed with latanoprost. If such drugs are used, administer with an interval of at least 5 minutes between applications.

Adverse Reactions:

Local: The ocular adverse events and ocular signs and symptoms reported in 5% to 15% of the patients on latanoprost in a 6 month controlled trial were blurred vision, burning and stinging, conjunctival hyperemia, foreign body sensation, itching, increased pigmentation of the iris and punctate epithelial keratopathy. Local conjunctival hyperemia was observed; however, < 1% of the latanoprost-treated patients required discontinuation of therapy because of intolerance to conjunctival hyperemia. Also reported were dry eye, excessive tearing, eye pain, lid crusting, lid edema, lid erythema, lid discomfort/pain, photophobia (1% to 4%); conjunctivitis, diplopia, discharge from the eye (<1%); retinal artery embolus, retinal detachment, vitreous hemorrhage from diabetic retinopathy (rare).

Systemic: The most common systemic adverse events seen with latanoprost were upper respiratory tract infection/cold/flu (4%); pain in muscle/joint/back, chest pain/angina pectoris, rash/allergic skin reaction (1% to 2%).

Overdosage:

Symptoms: Apart from ocular irritation and conjunctival or episcleral hyperemia, the ocular effects of latanoprost administered at high doses are not known. IV administration of large doses of latanoprost in monkeys has been associated with transient bronchoconstriction; however, in 11 patients with bronchial asthma treated with latanoprost, bronchoconstriction was not induced. IV infusions of up to 3 mcg/kg in healthy volunteers produced mean plasma concentrations 200 times higher than during clinical treatment, and no adverse reactions were observed. IV dosages of 5.5 to 10 mcg/kg caused abdominal pain, dizziness, fatigue, hot flushes, nausea and sweating.

Treatment: If overdosage occurs, treatment should be symptomatic.

Patient Information:

Inform patients about the possibility of iris color change because of an increase of the brown pigment and resultant cosmetically different eye coloration that may occur. Iris pigmentation changes may be more noticeable in patients with green-brown, blue/gray-brown or yellow-brown irides.

Advise patients to avoid allowing the tip of the dispensing container to contact the eye or surrounding structures because this could cause the tip to become contaminated by common bacteria known to cause ocular infections. Serious damage to the eye and subsequent loss of vision may result from using contaminated solutions.

Advise patients that if they develop any ocular reactions, particularly conjunctivitis and lid reactions, they should immediately seek their physician's advice.

Latanoprost contains benzalkonium chloride, which may be absorbed by contact lenses. Remove contact lenses prior to administration of the solution. Lenses may be reinserted 15 minutes following latanoprost administration.

If more than one topical ophthalmic drug is being used, administer the drugs at least 5 minutes apart.

Administration and Dosage:

The recommended dosage is one drop (1.5 mcg) in the affected eye(s) once daily in the evening. Do not exceed once daily dosage because it has been shown that more frequent administration may decrease the IOP lowering effect. Reduction of the IOP starts ≈ 3 to 4 hours after administration, and the maximum effect is reached after 8 to 12 hours.

Latanoprost may be used concomitantly with other topical ophthalmic drug products to lower IOP. If more than one topical ophthalmic drug is being used, administer the drugs at least 5 minutes apart.

Storage/Stability: Protect from light. Refrigerate unopened bottle at 2° to 8°C (36° to 46°F). Once opened, the container may be stored at room temperature up to 25°C (77°F) for 6 weeks.

Rx	**Xalatan** (Pharmacia)	**Solution:** 0.005% (50 mcg/ml)	0.02% benzalkonium chloride. In 2.5 ml fill dropper bottles.

Combinations

PILOCARPINE AND EPINEPHRINE

Also refer to the general discussion of Miotics, Cholinesterase Inhibitors.

Ingredients:

PILOCARPINE lowers IOP by a direct cholinergic action that improves outflow facility on chronic administration (see Agents for Glaucoma: Miotics, Direct-Acting).

EPINEPHRINE reduces IOP by increasing outflow facility (see Agents for Glaucoma, Sympathomimetics).

The combination of pilocarpine and epinephrine provides additive effects in lowering IOP; opposing actions on the pupil may prevent marked miosis or mydriasis. These fixed combinations do not permit the flexibility necessary to adjust the dosage of each agent.

Administration and Dosage:

Instill 1 or 2 drops into the eye(s) 1 to 4 times daily. Determine concentration and frequency of instillation by severity of the glaucoma and by patient response.

Individuals with heavily pigmented irides may require larger doses.

Storage: Store at 8° to 30°C (46° to 86°F). Keep tightly closed. Do not use solution if it is brown or contains a precipitate. Protect from light and heat.

Rx	**E-Pilo-1** (Ciba Vision)	**Solution**: 1% pilocarpine HCl, 1% epinephrine bitartrate	In 10 ml dropper bottles.[1]
Rx	**P_1E_1** (Alcon)		In 15 ml Drop-Tainers.[2]
Rx	**E-Pilo-2** (Ciba Vision)	**Solution**: 2% pilocarpine HCl, 1% epinephrine bitartrate	In 10 ml dropper bottles.[1]
Rx	**P_2E_1** (Alcon)		In 15 ml Drop-Tainers.[2]
Rx	**P_3E_1** (Alcon)	**Solution**: 3% pilocarpine HCl, 1% epinephrine bitartrate	In 15 ml Drop-Tainers.[2]
Rx	**E-Pilo-4** (Ciba Vision)	**Solution**: 4% pilocarpine HCl, 1% epinephrine bitartrate	In 10 ml dropper bottles.[1]
Rx	**P_4E_1** (Alcon)		In 15 ml Drop-Tainers.[2]
Rx	**E-Pilo-6** (Ciba Vision)	**Solution**: 6% pilocarpine HCl, 1% epinephrine bitartrate	In 10 ml dropper bottles.[1]
Rx	**P_6E_1** (Alcon)		In 15 ml Drop-Tainers.[2]

[1] With benzalkonium chloride, EDTA, mannitol and sodium bisulfite.

[2] With 0.01% benzalkonium chloride, methylcellulose, EDTA, chlorobutanol, polyethylene glycol and sodium bisulfite.

DAPIPRAZOLE HCl

Actions:

Pharmacology: Dapiprazole acts through blocking the alpha-adrenergic receptors in smooth muscle and produces miosis through an effect on the dilator muscle of the iris.

The drug does not have any significant activity on ciliary muscle contraction and, therefore, does not induce a significant change in the anterior chamber depth or the thickness of the lens.

Dapiprazole has demonstrated safe and rapid reversal of mydriasis produced by phenylephrine and, to a lesser degree, tropicamide. In patients with decreased accommodative amplitude due to treatment with tropicamide, the miotic effect of dapiprazole may partially increase the accommodative amplitude.

Eye color affects the rate of pupillary constriction. In individuals with brown irides, the rate of pupillary constriction may be slightly slower than in individuals with blue or green irides. Eye color does not appear to affect the final pupil size.

Dapiprazole does not significantly alter intraocular pressure (IOP) in normotensive eyes or in eyes with elevated IOP.

Indications:

Mydriasis: Treatment of iatrogenically induced mydriasis produced by adrenergic (phenylephrine) or parasympatholytic (tropicamide) agents.

Contraindications:

When constriction is undesirable, such as acute iritis; hypersensitivity to any component of this preparation.

Warnings:

For topical ophthalmic use only. Not for injection.

Frequency of use: Do not use in the same patient more frequently than once a week.

IOP reduction: Not indicated for the reduction of IOP or in the treatment of open-angle glaucoma.

Vision reduction: May cause difficulty in dark adaptation and may reduce field of vision. Patients should exercise caution in night driving or when performing other activities in poor illumination.

Pregnancy: Category B. There are no adequate and well controlled studies in pregnant women. Use during pregnancy only when clearly needed and when potential benefits outweigh the potential hazards to the fetus.

Lactation: It is not known whether this drug is excreted in breast milk. Exercise caution when dapiprazole is administered to a nursing woman.

Children: Safety and efficacy for use in children have not been established.

Adverse Reactions:

Conjunctival injection lasting 20 minutes (> 80%); burning on instillation (≈ 50%); ptosis, lid erythema, lid edema, chemosis, itching, punctate keratitis, corneal edema, browache, photophobia, headaches (10% to 40%); dryness of the eye, tearing, blurring of vision (less frequent).

Patient Information:

May cause difficulty in dark adaptation and may reduce field of vision. Exercise caution when driving at night or performing other activities in poor illumination.

To avoid contamination, do not touch tip of container to any surface.

Do not use in the same patient more frequently than once a week.

Discard any solution that is not clear and colorless.

Administration and Dosage:

Instill 2 drops into the conjunctiva of each eye followed 5 minutes later by an additional 2 drops. Administer after the ophthalmic examination to reverse the diagnostic mydriasis.

Shake container for several minutes to ensure mixing.

Storage/Stability: Store at room temperature 15° to 30°C (59° to 86°F) for 21 days after reconstitution.

Rx	**Rēv-Eyes** (Storz/Lederle)	**Powder, lyophilized:** 25 mg (0.5% solution when reconstituted)	In vial with 5 ml diluent and dropper.[1]

[1] With 2% mannitol, 0.4% hydroxypropyl methylcellulose, 0.01% EDTA, 0.01% benzalkonium chloride and sodium chloride.

OPHTHALMIC VASOCONSTRICTORS/MYDRIATICS

Actions:

Pharmacology: The effects of sympathomimetic agents on the eye include: Pupil dilation, increase in outflow of aqueous humor and vasoconstriction (alpha-adrenergic effects); relaxation of the ciliary muscle and a decrease in the formation of aqueous humor (beta-adrenergic effects). Hydroxyamphetamine dilates the pupil, probably by stimulating the dilator muscles of the iris.

Strong (alpha) vasoconstriction preparations (phenylephrine 2.5% and 10%; hydroxyamphetamine) cause vasoconstriction and pupillary dilation for diagnostic eye exams, during surgery and to prevent synechiae formation in uveitis. Weak sympathomimetic solutions (phenylephrine 0.12%; naphazoline; tetrahydrozoline) are used as ophthalmic decongestants (vasoconstriction of conjunctival blood vessels) for symptomatic relief of minor eye irritations. Epinephrine is used for open-angle glaucoma and is not included in this monograph (see monograph in Agents for Glaucoma section).

Ophthalmic Vasoconstrictors/Mydriatics

Vasoconstrictor/ Mydriatic	Duration of action (hr)	Available concentration	Prescription status
Hydroxyamphetamine	few hours	1%	Rx
Naphazoline	3 to 4	0.012%	otc
		0.02%	otc
		0.03%	otc
		0.1%	Rx
Oxymetazoline	4 to 6	0.025%	otc
Phenylephrine	0.5 to 1.5	0.12%	otc
	—	2.5%	Rx
	—	10%	Rx
Tetrahydrozoline	1 to 4	0.05%	otc

Indications:

Refer to individual product listings for specific indications.

Contraindications:

Hypersensitivity to any of these agents; narrow-angle glaucoma or anatomically narrow (occludable) angle and no glaucoma; prior to peripheral iridectomy in eyes capable of angle closure because mydriatic action may precipitate angle block.

Phenylephrine 10%: Patients with insulin-dependent diabetes; hypertensive patients; generalized arteriosclerosis; aneurysms; preexisting cardiovascular diseases; infants, small children with low body weight; elderly patients.

Warnings:

Anesthetics: Discontinue prior to use of anesthetics which sensitize the myocardium to sympathomimetics (eg, cyclopropane, halothane).

Local anesthetics can increase absorption of topically applied drugs; exercise caution when applying prior to use of phenylephrine. However, use of a local anesthetic prior to phenylephrine 2.5% or 10% may help prevent pain.

Overuse may produce increased redness of the eye.

Pregnancy: Category C. Safety for use during pregnancy is not established. Use only if clearly needed and if the potential benefits outweigh potential hazards to the fetus.

Lactation: Safety for use during breastfeeding has not been established. Use caution when administering to a nursing woman.

Children: Safety and efficacy have not been established. Phenylephrine 10% is contraindicated in infants.

Precautions:

Special risk patients: Use with caution in the presence of hypertension, diabetes, hyperthyroidism, cardiovascular abnormalities, arteriosclerosis.

Narrow-angle glaucoma: Ordinarily, any mydriatic is contraindicated in patients with glaucoma. However, when temporary pupil dilation may free adhesions, or when vasoconstriction of intrinsic vessels may lower intraocular tension, these advantages may temporarily outweigh danger from coincident pupil dilation.

OPHTHALMIC VASOCONSTRICTORS/MYDRIATICS

Rebound congestion may occur with frequent or extended use of ophthalmic vasoconstrictors. This may be of importance when there is retinal detachment or prior to cataract surgery. Rebound miosis has occurred in older persons 1 day after receiving phenylephrine; reinstillation produced a reduction in mydriasis.

Systemic absorption: Exceeding recommended dosages of these agents or applying **phenylephrine** 2.5% to 10% solutions to the instrumented, traumatized, diseased or postsurgical eye or adnexa, or to patients with suppressed lacrimation, as during anesthesia, may result in the absorption of sufficient quantities to produce a systemic vasopressor response.

Pigment floaters: Older individuals may develop transient pigment floaters in the aqueous humor 30 to 45 minutes after instillation of phenylephrine. The appearance may be similar to anterior uveitis or to a microscopic hyphema.

Potentially hazardous tasks: **Phenylephrine** may cause temporary blurred or unstable vision; observe caution while driving or performing other hazardous tasks.

Sulfite sensitivity: Some of these products contain sulfites that may cause allergic-type reactions (eg, hives, itching, wheezing, anaphylaxis) in certain susceptible persons. Although the overall prevalence of sulfite sensitivity in the general population is probably low, it is seen more frequently in asthmatics or in atopic nonasthmatic persons.

Drug Interactions:

Ophthalmic Sympathomimetic Drug Interactions

Precipitant drug	Object drug*		Description
Anesthetics	Ophthalmic sympathomimetics	⬆	Cautiously use anesthetics that sensitize the myocardium to sympathomimetics (eg, cyclopropane, halothane). Local anesthetics can increase absorption of topical drugs; exercise caution when applying prior to use of phenylephrine.
Beta blockers	Ophthalmic sympathomimetics	⬆	Systemic side effects may occur more readily in patients taking these drugs.
MAOIs	Ophthalmic sympathomimetics	⬆	When given with, or up to 21 days after MAOIs, exaggerated adrenergic effects may result. Supervise and adjust dosage carefully.

* ⬆ = Object drug increased.

Also consider drug interactions that may occur with systemic use of the sympathomimetics (see Vasopressors Used for Shock).

Adverse Reactions:

Ophthalmic: Transitory stinging on initial instillation; blurring of vision; mydriasis; increased redness; irritation; discomfort; blurring; punctate keratitis; lacrimation; increased IOP.

Phenylephrine may cause rebound miosis and decreased mydriatic response to therapy in older persons.

Cardiovascular: Palpitation; tachycardia; cardiac arrhythmia; hypertension; ventricular arrhythmias (ie, premature ventricular contractions); reflex bradycardia; coronary occlusion; pulmonary embolism; subarachnoid hemorrhage; myocardial infarction; stroke; death associated with cardiac reactions. Headache or browache may occur.

Phenylephrine 10% – Significant elevation of blood pressure is rare but can occur after conjunctival instillation. Exercise caution with elderly patients and children of low body weight. Carefully monitor the blood pressure of these patients. (See Warnings and Contraindications.) There have been rare reports of the development of serious cardiovascular reactions, including ventricular arrhythmias and myocardial infarctions. These episodes, some fatal, have usually occurred in elderly patients with preexisting cardiovascular diseases.

Miscellaneous: Headache; blanching; tremor; trembling; sweating; dizziness; nausea; nervousness; drowsiness; weakness; hyperglycemia.

OPHTHALMIC VASOCONSTRICTORS/MYDRIATICS

Overdosage:

Hydroxyamphetamine: If ocular overdosage occurs, dilute pilocarpine (1%) may be administered. If accidentally ingested, sedation is indicated. Further treatment is symptomatic.

Patient Information:

Do not use beyond 48 to 72 hours without consulting a physician.

If irritation, blurring or redness persists, or if severe eye pain, headache, vision changes, floating spots, dizziness, decrease in body temperature, drowsiness, acute eye redness or pain with light exposure occur, discontinue use and consult a physician.

Do not use if you have glaucoma except under the advice of a physician.

Refer to the Topical Ophthalmic Introduction for more complete information.

Potentially hazardous tasks: Phenylephrine may cause temporary blurred or unstable vision; observe caution while driving or performing other hazardous tasks.

TETRAHYDROZOLINE HCl

For complete prescribing information, refer to the Vasoconstrictors/Mydriatics group monograph.

Indications:

Redness: For relief of redness of the eye due to minor irritations.

Burning/irritation: For temporary relief of burning and irritation due to dryness of the eye or discomfort due to minor irritations or to exposure to wind or sun.

Administration and Dosage:

Instill 1 or 2 drops into eye(s) up to 4 times a day.

Stability: Do not use if solution changes color or becomes cloudy.

otc	**Tetrahydrozoline HCl** (Various, eg, Moore, Rugby, Steris)	**Solution:** 0.05%	In 15 and 30 ml.
otc	**Collyrium Fresh** (Wyeth-Ayerst)		In 15 ml.[2]
otc	**Eye Drops** (Bausch & Lomb)		In 15 ml.[3]
otc	**Eyesine** (Akorn)		In 15 ml.[3]
otc	**Geneye** (Goldline)		In 15 ml.[5]
otc	**Geneye Extra** (Goldline)		In 15 ml.[6]
otc	**Mallazine Eye Drops** (Roberts Hauck)		In 15 ml.[3]
otc	**Murine Plus** (Ross)		In 15 and 30 ml.[7]
otc	**Optigene 3** (Pfeiffer)		In 15 ml.[5]
otc	**Tetrasine** (Optopics)		In 15 and 22.5 ml.[8]
otc	**Tetrasine Extra** (Optopics)		In 15 ml.[6]
otc	**Visine** (Pfizer)		In 15, 22.5 and 30 ml.[5]
otc	**Visine Moisturizing** (Pfizer)		In 15 and 30 ml.[9]

[1] With 0.01% benzalkonium chloride, 0.1% EDTA and 1% glycerin.
[2] With 0.01% benzalkonium chloride and EDTA.
[3] With 0.01% benzalkonium chloride and 0.1% EDTA.
[4] With benzalkonium chloride, EDTA, 1.4% polyvinyl alcohol and 0.6% povidone.
[5] With benzalkonium chloride and EDTA.
[6] With 1% polyethylene glycol 400, benzalkonium chloride and EDTA.
[7] With 0.013% benzalkonium chloride, 0.1% EDTA and 1% PEG-400.

PHENYLEPHRINE HCl

For complete prescribing information, refer to the Vasoconstrictors/Mydriatics group monograph.

Indications:

2.5% and 10%: Decongestant and vasoconstrictor and for pupil dilation in uveitis (posterior synechiae), open-angle glaucoma, refraction without cycloplegia, prior to surgery, ophthalmoscopic examination, diagnostic procedures (funduscopy).

0.12%: A decongestant to provide relief of minor eye irritations.

Administration and Dosage:

Vasoconstrictors and pupil dilation: Apply a drop of topical anesthetic. Follow in a few minutes by 1 drop of the 2.5% or 10% phenylephrine. The anesthetic prevents stinging and consequent dilution of solution by lacrimation. It may be necessary to repeat the instillation after 1 hour, again preceded by a topical anesthetic.

Uveitis: The formation of synechiae may be prevented by using the 2.5% or 10% solution and atropine to produce wide dilation of the pupil. However, the vasoconstrictor effect of phenylephrine may be antagonistic to the increase of local blood flow in uveal infection.

To free recently formed posterior synechiae, instill 1 drop of the 2.5% or 10% solution to the upper surface of the cornea. Continue treatment the following day, if necessary. In the interim, apply hot compresses for 5 or 10 minutes, 3 times daily using 1 drop of 1% or 2% solution of atropine sulfate and before and after each series of compresses.

Glaucoma: Instill 1 drop of 10% solution on the upper surface of the cornea as often as necessary. The 2.5% and 10% solutions may be used in conjunction with miotics in patients with open-angle glaucoma. Phenylephrine reduces the difficulties experienced by the patient because of the small field produced by miosis, and permits and often supports the effect of the miotic in lowering the IOP in open-angle glaucoma. Hence, there may be marked improvement in visual acuity after using phenylephrine with miotic drugs.

Surgery: When a short-acting mydriatic is needed for wide dilation of the pupil before intraocular surgery, the 2.5% or 10% solution may be instilled from 30 to 60 minutes before the operation.

Refraction: Prior to determination of refractive errors, the 2.5% solution may be used effectively with homatropine HBr, atropine sulfate, cyclopentolate, tropicamide HCl or a combination of homatropine and cocaine HCl.

Adults – Place 1 drop of the preferred cycloplegic in each eye; follow in 5 minutes with 1 drop phenylephrine 2.5% solution and in 10 minutes with another drop of the cycloplegic. In 50 to 60 minutes, the eyes are ready for refraction.

Since adequate cycloplegia is achieved at different time intervals after the necessary number of drops, different cycloplegics will require different waiting periods.

Children – Place 1 drop of atropine sulfate 1% in each eye; follow in 10 to 15 minutes with 1 drop of phenylephrine 2.5% solution and in 5 to 10 minutes with a second drop of atropine sulfate 1%. In 1 to 2 hours, the eyes are ready for refraction.

For a "one application method", combine 2.5% phenylephrine solution with a cycloplegic to elicit synergistic action. The additive effect varies depending on the patient. Therefore, when using a "one application method", it may be desirable to increase the concentration of the cycloplegic.

Ophthalmoscopic examination: Place 1 drop of 2.5% phenylephrine solution in each eye. Sufficient mydriasis is produced in 15 to 30 minutes and lasts 1 to 3 hours.

Diagnostic procedures: Heavily pigmented irides may require larger doses in all the following procedures.

Provocative test for angle block in patients with glaucoma – The 2.5% solution may be used as a provocative test when latent increased IOP is suspected. Measure tension before application and again after dilation. A 3 to 5 mm Hg rise in pressure suggests the presence of angle block in patients with glaucoma; however, failure to obtain such a rise does not preclude the presence of glaucoma from other causes.

Shadow test (retinoscopy) – When dilation of the pupil without cycloplegic action is desired, the 2.5% solution may be used alone.

Blanching test – Instill 1 to 2 drops of the 2.5% solution in the injected eye. After 5 minutes, examine for perilimbal blanching. If blanching occurs, the congestion is superficial and probably does not indicate iritis.

Minor eye irritations: Instill 1 or 2 drops of the 0.12% solution in eye(s) up to 4 times daily as needed.

Stability: Prolonged exposure to air or strong light may cause oxidation and discoloration. Do not use if solution changes color, becomes cloudy or contains a precipitate.

PHENYLEPHRINE HCl

otc	**AK-Nefrin** (Akorn)	**Solution:** 0.12%	In 15 ml.[1]
otc	**Prefrin Liquifilm** (Allergan)		In 20 ml.[2]
otc	**Relief** (Allergan)		Preservative free. In UD 0.3 ml.[3]
Rx	**Phenylephrine HCl** (Various, eg, Steris)	**Solution:** 2.5%	In 15 ml.
Rx	**AK-Dilate** (Akorn)		In 2 and 15 ml.[4]
Rx	**Mydfrin 2.5%** (Alcon)		In 3 and 5 ml Drop-Tainers.[5]
Rx	**Neo-Synephrine** (Sanofi Winthrop)		In 15 ml.[6]
Rx	**Phenoptic** (Optopics)		In 2, 5 and 15 ml.
Rx	**Phenylephrine HCl** (Various, eg, Iolab, Steris)	**Solution:** 10%	In 2 and 5 ml.
Rx	**AK-Dilate** (Akorn)		In 2 and 5 ml.[4]
Rx	**Neo-Synephrine** (Sanofi Winthrop)		In 5 ml.[7]
Rx	**Neo-Synephrine Viscous** (Sanofi Winthrop)		In 5 ml.[8]

[1] With 0.005% benzalkonium chloride, 1.4% polyvinyl alcohol and EDTA.
[2] With 1.4% polyvinyl alcohol, 0.004% benzalkonium chloride and EDTA.
[3] With 1.4% polyvinyl alcohol and EDTA.
[4] With benzalkonium chloride.
[5] With 0.01% benzalkonium chloride, EDTA and sodium bisulfite.
[6] With 1:7500 benzalkonium chloride.
[7] With 1:10,000 benzalkonium chloride.
[8] With 1:10,000 benzalkonium chloride and methylcellulose.

HYDROXYAMPHETAMINE HBr

For complete prescribing information, refer to the Vasoconstrictors/Mydriatics group monograph.

Indications:

Dilation of the pupil.

Administration and Dosage:

Instill 1 or 2 drops into the conjunctival sac(s).

Rx	**Paredrine**[1] (Pharmics)	**Solution:** 1%	In 15 ml.[2]

[1] Paredrine is not currently available from the manufacturer pending FDA manufacturing approval. Availability is expected in 1996.
[2] With 1:50,000 thimerosal and 2% boric acid.

OXYMETAZOLINE HCl

For complete prescribing information, refer to the Vasoconstrictors/Mydriatics group monograph.

Indications:

Redness: For relief of redness of the eye due to minor eye irritations.

Administration and Dosage:

Adults and children ≥ 6 years of age: Instill 1 or 2 drops in the affected eye(s) every 6 hours.

Stability: Do not use if solution changes color or becomes cloudy.

otc	**OcuClear** (Schering-Plough)	**Solution:** 0.025%	In 30 ml.[1]
otc	**Visine L.R.** (Pfizer)		In 15 and 30 ml.[1]

[1] With 0.01% benzalkonium chloride and 0.1% EDTA.

NAPHAZOLINE HCl

For complete prescribing information, refer to the Vasoconstrictors/Mydriatics group monograph.

Indications:

Redness: To soothe, refresh and remove redness due to minor eye irritations such as smoke, smog, sunglare, wearing contact lenses, allergies or swimming.

Administration and Dosage:

Instill 1 or 2 drops into the conjunctival sac of affected eye(s) every 3 to 4 hours, up to 4 times daily.

Storage/Stability: Do not use if solution changes color or becomes cloudy.

otc	**Allerest Eye Drops** (Ciba)	**Solution:** 0.012%	In 15 ml.[1]
otc	**Clear Eyes** (Ross)		In 15 and 30 ml.[2]
otc	**Clear Eyes ACR** (Ross)		In 15 and 30 ml.[3]
otc	**Degest 2** (Akorn)		In 15 ml.[4]
otc	**Naphcon** (Alcon)		In 15 ml.[5]
otc	**Allergy Drops** (Bausch & Lomb)		In 15 ml.[6]
otc	**VasoClear** (Ciba Vision)	**Solution:** 0.02%	In 15 ml.[7]
otc	**Comfort Eye Drops** (Pilkington/Barnes Hind)	**Solution:** 0.03%	In 15 ml.[8]
otc	**Maximum Strength Allergy Drops** (Bausch & Lomb)		In 15 ml.[9]
Rx	**Naphazoline HCl** (Various, eg, Goldline, Rugby)	**Solution:** 0.1%	In 15 ml.
Rx	**AK-Con** (Akorn)		In 15 ml.[5]
Rx	**Albalon** (Allergan)		In 15 ml.[10]
Rx	**Nafazair** (Bausch & Lomb)		In 15 ml.[5]
Rx	**Naphcon Forte** (Alcon)		In 15 ml Drop-Tainers.[5]
Rx	**Vasocon Regular** (Ciba Vision)		In 15 ml.[11]

[1] With benzalkonium chloride, EDTA.
[2] With benzalkonium chloride, EDTA, 0.2% glycerin.
[3] With benzalkonium chloride, EDTA, 0.25% zinc sulfate, 0.2% glycerin.
[4] With 0.0067% benzalkonium chloride, 0.02% EDTA, hydroxyethylcellulose, povidone.
[5] With 0.01% benzalkonium chloride, EDTA.
[6] With 0.2% PEG-300, 0.01% benzalkonium chloride.
[7] With 0.01% benzalkonium chloride, 0.25% polyvinyl alcohol, 1% PEG-400, EDTA.
[8] With 0.005% benzalkonium chloride and 0.02% EDTA.
[9] With 0.01% benzalkonium chloride, 0.5% hydroxypropyl methylcellulose and EDTA.
[10] With 0.004% benzalkonium chloride, EDTA, 1.4% polyvinyl alcohol.
[11] With benzalkonium chloride, polyvinyl alcohol, EDTA, PEG-8000.

OLOPATADINE HCl

Actions:

Pharmacology: Olopatadine is an inhibitor of histamine release from the mast cell and a relatively selective histamine H_1-antagonist that inhibits the in vivo and in vitro type 1 immediate hypersensitivity reaction. Olopatadine is devoid of effects on alpha-adrenergic, dopamine, muscarinic type 1 and 2, and serotonin receptors.

Pharmacokinetics: Olopatadine has low systemic exposure. Plasma concentrations are generally below the quantitation limit of the assay (< 0.5 ng/ml). Samples in which olopatadine is quantifiable are typically found within 2 hours of dosing and range from 0.5 to 1.3 ng/ml. The half-life in plasma is ≈ 3 hours, and elimination is predominantly through renal excretion. Approximately 60% to 70% of the dose is recovered in the urine as parent drug. Two metabolites, the mono-desmethyl and the N-oxide, were detected at low concentrations in the urine.

Indications:

Allergic conjunctivitis: For temporary prevention of itching of the eye due to allergic conjunctivitis.

Contraindications:

Hypersensitivity to any component of this product.

Warnings:

Pregnancy: Category C. Olopatadine was not found to be teratogenic in rats and rabbits. There are no adequate and well controlled studies in pregnant women. Use this drug in pregnant women only if the potential benefit to the mother justifies the potential risk to the embryo or fetus.

Lactation: Olopatadine has been identified in the milk of nursing rats following oral administration. It is not known whether topical ocular administration could result in sufficient systemic absorption to produce detectable quantities in breast milk. Exercise caution when olopatadine is administered to a nursing mother.

Children: Safety and effectiveness in pediatric patients < 3 years old have not been established.

Precautions:

For topical use only. Not for injection. Do not instill olopatadine while wearing contact lenses.

Adverse Reactions:

Ophthalmic: Burning or stinging, dry eye, foreign body sensation, hyperemia, keratitis, lid edema, pruritus (< 5%).

Miscellaneous: Headache (7%); asthenia, cold syndrome, pharyngitis, rhinitis, sinusitis, taste perversion (< 5%).

Patient Information:

To prevent contaminating the dropper tip and solution, do not touch the eyelids and surrounding areas with the dropper tip of the bottle.

Keep bottle tightly closed when not in use.

Administration and Dosage:

The recommended dose is 1 to 2 drops in each affected eye 2 times per day at an interval of 6 to 8 hours.

Storage/Stability: Store at 39° to 86°F (4° to 30°C).

Rx	**Patanol** (Alcon)	**Solution:** 0.1%	Benzalkonium chloride. In 5 ml *Drop-Tainer* dispenser.

OPHTHALMIC DECONGESTANT/ANTIHISTAMINE COMBINATIONS

In these combinations:

PHENYLEPHRINE HCl, NAPHAZOLINE HCl and **TETRAHYDROZOLINE** have decongestant actions. See individual monographs for further information.

HYDROXYPROPYLMETHYLCELLULOSE and **POLYVINYL ALCOHOL** increase the viscosity of the solution, thereby increasing contact time.

ZINC SULFATE is an astringent.

PHENIRAMINE MALEATE and **ANTAZOLINE** are antihistamines.

Indications:

Itching/Redness: Temporary relief of the minor eye symptoms of itching and redness caused by pollen, animal hair, etc.

Warnings:

Antihistamines: Topical antihistamines are potential sensitizers and may produce a local sensitivity reaction. Because they may produce angle closure, use with caution in persons with a narrow angle or a history of glaucoma.

Administration and Dosage:

Recommendations vary. Refer to manufacturer package insert for instructions.

		Decongestant	Antihistamine	
otc	**Zincfrin Solution** (Alcon)	phenylephrine HCl 0.12%		In 15 and 30 ml Drop-Tainers.[1]
otc	**Clear Eyes ACR Solution** (Ross)	naphazoline HCl 0.012%		In 15 and 30 ml.[2]
otc	**VasoClear A Solution** (Ciba Vision)	naphazoline HCl 0.02%		In 15 ml.[3]
otc	**Naphazoline HCl & Pheniramine Maleate Solution** (Various, eg, Moore)	naphazoline HCl 0.025%	pheniramine maleate 0.3%	In 15 ml.
otc	**Naphazoline Plus Solution** (Parmed)			In 15 ml.[4]
otc	**Naphcon-A Solution** (Alcon)			In 15 ml Drop-Tainers.[4]
Rx	**Naphoptic-A Solution** (Optopics)			In 15 ml.[5]
otc	**Opcon-A Solution** (Bausch & Lomb)	naphazoline HCl 0.027%	pheniramine maleate 0.315%	In 15 ml.[6]
otc	**Naphazoline HCl & Antazoline Phosphate Sodium** (Various, eg, Moore, Schein, Steris)	naphazoline HCl 0.05%	antazoline phosphate 0.5%	In 5 and 15 ml.
Rx	**Vasocon-A Solution** (Ciba Vision)			In 15 ml.[7]

OPHTHALMIC DECONGESTANT/ANTIHISTAMINE COMBINATIONS

		Decongestant	Antihistamine	
otc	**Visine Allergy Relief** (Pfizer)	tetrahydrozoline HCl 0.05%		In 15 and 30 ml.[8]
otc	**Geneye AC Allergy Formula** (Goldline)			In 15 ml.[9]

[1] With 0.01% benzalkonium Cl, polysorbate 80, 0.25% zinc sulfate.
[2] With 0.2% glycerin, benzalkonium Cl, EDTA, boric acid, 0.25% zinc sulfate.
[3] With 0.005% benzalkonium Cl, EDTA, 0.25% polyvinyl alcohol, PEG-400, 0.25% zinc sulfate.
[4] With 0.01% benzalkonium Cl, EDTA.
[5] With benzalkonium Cl, boric acid, EDTA, sodium borate.
[6] With 0.5% hydroxypropyl methylcellulose, 0.01% benzalkonium CL, 0.1% EDTA, boric acid.
[7] With 0.01% benzalkonium Cl, PEG-8000, polyvinyl alcohol, EDTA.
[8] With 0.01% benzalkonium Cl, 0.1% EDTA, 0.25% zinc sulfate.
[9] With 0.01% benzalkonium Cl, EDTA, 0.25% zinc sulfate.

CYCLOPLEGIC MYDRIATICS

Actions:

Pharmacology: Anticholinergic agents block the responses of the sphincter muscle of the iris and the muscle of the ciliary body to cholinergic stimulation, producing pupillary dilation (mydriasis) and paralysis of accommodation (cycloplegia).

Cycloplegic Mydriatics

Drug	Mydriasis		Cycloplegia		Solution available
	Peak (minutes)	Recovery (days)	Peak (minutes)	Recovery (days)	
Atropine	30 - 40	7 - 10	60 - 180	6 - 12	0.5% - 2%
Homatropine	40 - 60	1 - 3	30 - 60	1 - 3	2% - 5%
Scopolamine	20 - 30	3 - 7	30 - 60	3 - 7	0.25%
Cyclopentolate	30 - 60	1	25 - 75	0.25 - 1	0.5% - 2%
Tropicamide	20 - 40	0.25	20 - 35	< 0.25	0.5% - 1%

Indications:

Mydriasis/Cycloplegia: For cycloplegic refraction and for dilating the pupil in inflammatory conditions of the iris and uveal tract. See individual monographs for specific indications.

Contraindications:

Primary glaucoma or a tendency toward glaucoma (eg, narrow anterior chamber angle); hypersensitivity to belladonna alkaloids or any component of the products; adhesions (synechiae) between the iris and the lens; children who have previously had a severe systemic reaction to atropine.

Warnings:

For topical ophthalmic use only. Not for injection.

Glaucoma: Determine the intraocular tension and the depth of the angle of the anterior chamber before and during use to avoid glaucoma attacks.

Elderly: Use these products with caution in the elderly and others where increased IOP may be encountered.

Pregnancy: Category C (**atropine, homatropine**). Safety for use during pregnancy has not been established. Give to a pregnant woman only if clearly needed.

Lactation: **Atropine** and **homatropine** may be detectable, in very small amounts, in breast milk. Although this is controversial, according to the American Academy of Pediatrics, these agents are compatible with breastfeeding. It is not known if **cyclopentolate** is excreted in breast milk. Exercise caution when administering to a nursing woman.

Children: Excessive use in children and in certain susceptible individuals may produce systemic toxic symptoms. Use with extreme caution in infants and small children.

Tropicamide and cyclopentolate may cause CNS disturbances, which may be dangerous in infants and children. Keep in mind the possibility of occurrence of psychotic reaction and behavioral disturbance due to hypersensitivity to anticholinergic drugs. Use with extreme caution. Increased susceptibility to cyclopentolate has been reported in infants, young children and in children with spastic paralysis or brain damage. Feeding intolerance may follow ophthalmic use of this product in neonates. It is recommended that feeding be withheld for 4 hours after examination. Do not use in concentrations > 0.5% in small infants.

Precautions:

Systemic effects: Avoid excessive systemic absorption by compressing the lacrimal sac by digital pressure for 1 to 3 minutes after instillation.

Down's syndrome/children with brain damage: Use cycloplegics with caution. These patients may demonstrate a hyperreactive response to topical atropine.

Hazardous tasks: May produce drowsiness, blurred vision or sensitivity to light (due to dilated pupils); observe caution while driving or performing other tasks requiring alertness, coordination or physical dexterity.

Sulfite sensitivity: Some of these products contain sulfites which may cause allergic-type reactions (eg, hives, itching, wheezing, anaphylaxis) in certain susceptible persons. Although the overall prevalence of sulfite sensitivity in the general population is probably low, it is seen more frequently in asthmatics or in atopic nonasthmatic persons. Specific products containing sulfites are identified in the product listings.

CYCLOPLEGIC MYDRIATICS

Adverse Reactions:

Local: Increased intraocular pressure; transient stinging/burning; irritation with prolonged use (eg, allergic lid reactions, hyperemia, follicular conjunctivitis, blepharoconjunctivitis, vascular congestion, edema, exudate, eczematoid dermatitis).

Systemic: Dryness of the mouth and skin; blurred vision; photophobia with or without corneal staining; tachycardia; headache; parasympathetic stimulation; somnolence; visual hallucinations.

Other toxic manifestations of anticholinergic drugs include: Skin rash; abdominal distention in infants; unusual drowsiness; hyperpyrexia; vasodilation; urinary retention; diminished GI motility; decreased secretion in salivary and sweat glands, pharynx, bronchii and nasal passages. Severe manifestations of toxicity include: Coma; medullary paralysis; death. Severe reactions are manifested by hypotension with progressive respiratory depression.

Cyclopentolate and **tropicamide** have been associated with psychotic reactions and behavioral disturbances in children. CNS disturbances have occurred in children on **tropicamide**. Ataxia, incoherent speech, restlessness, hallucinations, hyperactivity, seizures, disorientation as to time and place, and failure to recognize people have occurred with **cyclopentolate**.

Overdosage:

Ocular: If ocular overdosage occurs, flush eye(s) with water or normal saline. Use of a topical miotic may be required. If accidentally ingested, induce emesis or gastric lavage.

Systemic: If symptoms develop (see Adverse Reactions), patients usually recover spontaneously when the drug is discontinued. In cases of severe toxicity, give physostigmine salicylate (see individual monograph). Have atropine (1 mg) available for immediate injection if physostigmine causes bradycardia, convulsions or bronchoconstriction.

Cyclopentolate toxicity may produce exaggerated symptoms (see Adverse Reactions). When administration of the drug product is discontinued, the patient usually recovers spontaneously. In case of severe manifestations of toxicity, the antidote of choice is physostigmine salicylate.

Children – Slowly inject 0.5 mg physostigmine salicylate IV. If toxic symptoms persist and no cholinergic symptoms are produced, repeat at 5 minute intervals to a maximum cumulative dose of 2 mg.

Adults and adolescents – Slowly inject 2 mg physostigmine salicylate IV. A second dose of 1 to 2 mg may be given after 20 minutes if no reversal of toxic manifestations has occurred.

Patient Information:

To avoid contamination, do not touch dropper tip to any surface. Replace cap after using.

May cause blurred vision. Do not drive or engage in any hazardous activities while the pupils are dilated.

May cause sensitivity to light. Protect eyes in bright illumination during dilation.

Keep out of the reach of children. These drugs should not be taken orally. Wash your own hands and the child's following administration.

If eye pain occurs, discontinue use and consult physician immediately.

Refer to the Topical Ophthalmics Introduction for more complete information on administration and use.

ATROPINE SULFATE

For complete prescribing information, refer to the Cycloplegic Mydriatics group monograph.

Indications:

Mydriasis/Cycloplegia: For cycloplegic refraction or pupil dilation in acute inflammatory conditions of iris and uveal tract.

Administration and Dosage:

Solution:

Adults –

Uveitis: Instill 1 or 2 drops into the eye(s) up to 4 times daily.

Refraction: Instill 1 or 2 drops of 1% solution into eye(s) 1 hr before refracting.

Children –

Uveitis: Instill 1 or 2 drops of 0.5% solution into the eye(s) up to 3 times daily.

Refraction: Instill 1 or 2 drops of 0.5% solution into the eye(s) twice daily for 1 to 3 days before examination.

Ointment: Apply a small amount in the conjunctival sac up to 3 times daily.

Compress the lacrimal sac by digital pressure for several minutes after instillation.

Individuals with heavily pigmented irides may require larger doses.

Storage: Keep from heat.

Rx	**Atropine Sulfate Ophthalmic** (Various, eg, Bausch & Lomb, Fougera, Goldline, Pharmafair)	**Ointment:** 1%	In 3.5 and UD 1 g.
Rx	**Isopto Atropine** (Alcon)	**Solution:** 0.5%	In 5 ml Drop-Tainers.[1]
Rx	**Atropine Sulfate** (Various, eg, Alcon, Allergan, Bausch & Lomb, Goldline, Optopics, Pharmafair, Rugby)	**Solution:** 1%	In 2, 5 and 15 ml and UD 1 ml.
Rx	**Atropine Care** (Akorn)		In 2, 5 and 15 ml.[2]
Rx	**Atropine-1** (Optopics)		In 2, 5 and 15 ml.
Rx	**Atropisol** (Ciba Vision)		In 1 ml Dropperettes.[3]
Rx	**Isopto Atropine** (Alcon)		In 5 and 15 ml Drop-Tainers.[1]
Rx	**Atropine Sulfate** (Alcon)	**Solution:** 2%	In 2 ml.

[1] With 0.01% benzalkonium chloride, 0.5% hydroxypropyl methylcellulose and boric acid.
[2] With 0.01% benzalkonium chloride, hydroxypropyl methylcellulose and boric acid.
[3] With benzalkonium chloride, EDTA and boric acid.

SCOPOLAMINE HBr (Hyoscine HBr)

For complete prescribing information, refer to the Cycloplegic Mydriatics group monograph.

Indications:

Mydriasis/Cycloplegia: For cycloplegia and mydriasis in diagnostic procedures.

Iridocyclitis: For preoperative and postoperative states in the treatment of iridocyclitis.

Administration and Dosage:

Uveitis: Instill 1 or 2 drops into the eye(s) up to 4 times daily.

Refraction: Instill 1 or 2 drops into the eye(s) 1 hour before refracting.

Compress the lacrimal sac by digital pressure for several minutes after instillation.

Storage: Protect from light. Store at 8° to 27°C (46° to 80°F)

Rx	**Isopto Hyoscine** (Alcon)	**Solution:** 0.25%	In 5 and 15 ml Drop-Tainers.[1]

[1] With 0.01% benzalkonium chloride and 0.5% hydroxypropyl methylcellulose.

HOMATROPINE HBr

For complete prescribing information, refer to the Cycloplegic Mydriatics group monograph.

Indications:

Mydriasis/Cycloplegia: A moderately long-acting mydriatic and cycloplegic for refraction, and in the treatment of inflammatory conditions of the uveal tract. For preoperative and postoperative states when mydriasis is required.

Lens opacity: As an optical aid in some cases of axial lens opacities.

Administration and Dosage:

Uveitis: Instill 1 or 2 drops into the eye(s) up to every 3 to 4 hours.

Refraction: Instill 1 or 2 drops into the eye(s); repeat in 5 to 10 minutes if necessary.

Individuals with heavily pigmented irides may require larger doses.

Children: Use only the 2% strength.

Compress the lacrimal sac by digital pressure for several minutes after instillation.

Storage: Store at 8° to 24°C (46° to 75°F)

Rx	**Isopto Homatropine** (Alcon)	**Solution:** 2%	In 5 and 15 ml Drop-Tainers.[1]
Rx	**Homatropine HBr** (Various, eg, Alcon, Ciba Vision)	**Solution:** 5%	In 1, 2 and 5 ml.
Rx	**AK-Homatropine** (Akorn)		In 5 ml.
Rx	**Isopto Homatropine** (Alcon)		In 5 and 15 ml Drop-Tainers.[2]

[1] With 0.01% benzalkonium chloride, 0.5% hydroxypropylmethylcellulose and polysorbate 80.
[2] With 0.005% benzethonium chloride and 0.5% hydroxypropylmethylcellulose.

TROPICAMIDE

For complete prescribing information, refer to the Cycloplegic Mydriatics group monograph.

Indications:

Mydriasis/Cycloplegia: For mydriasis and cycloplegia for diagnostic purposes.

Administration and Dosage:

Refraction: Instill 1 or 2 drops of 1% solution into the eye(s); repeat in 5 minutes. If patient is not seen within 20 to 30 minutes, instill an additional drop to prolong mydriatic effect.

For examination of fundus, instill 1 or 2 drops of 0.5% solution 15 to 20 minutes prior to examination. Compress the lacrimal sac by digital pressure for several minutes after instillation to avoid excessive absorption.

Individuals with heavily pigmented irides may require larger doses.

Storage: Store away from heat. Do not refrigerate.

Rx	**Tropicamide** (Various, eg, Bausch & Lomb)	**Solution:** 0.5%	In 2 and 15 ml.
Rx	**Mydriacyl** (Alcon)		In 15 ml Drop-Tainers.[1]
Rx	**Opticyl** (Optopics)		In 2 and 15 ml.
Rx	**Tropicacyl** (Akorn)		In 15 ml.[2]
Rx	**Tropicamide** (Various, eg, Bausch & Lomb)	**Solution:** 1%	In 15 ml.
Rx	**Mydriacyl** (Alcon)		In 3 and 15 ml Drop-Tainers.[1]
Rx	**Opticyl** (Optopics)		In 2 and 15 ml.
Rx	**Tropicacyl** (Akorn)		In 2 and 15 ml.[2]

[1] With 0.01% benzalkonium chloride and EDTA.
[2] With 0.1% benzalkonium chloride and EDTA.

CYCLOPENTOLATE HCl

For complete prescribing information, refer to the Cycloplegic Mydriatics group monograph.

Indications:

Mydriasis/Cycloplegia: For mydriasis and cycloplegia in diagnostic procedures.

Administration and Dosage:

Adults: Instill 1 or 2 drops of 0.5%, 1% or 2% solution into eye(s). Repeat in 5 to 10 minutes, if necessary. Complete recovery usually occurs in 24 hours.

Children: Instill 1 or 2 drops of 0.5%, 1% or 2% solution into each eye. Follow in 5 to 10 minutes with a second application of 0.5% or 1% solution, if necessary.

Small infants: Instill 1 drop of 0.5% solution into each eye. Observe patient closely for at least 30 minutes following instillation.

Compress the lacrimal sac by digital pressure for several minutes after instillation.

Individuals with heavily pigmented irides may require higher strengths.

Storage: Store at 8° to 27°C (46° to 80°F)

Rx	**Cyclogyl** (Alcon)	**Solution**: 0.5%	In 2, 5 and 15 ml Drop-Tainers.[1]
Rx	**Cyclopentolate HCl** (Various, eg, Bausch & Lomb, Schein, Steris)	**Solution**: 1%	In 2, 5 and 15 ml.
Rx	**AK-Pentolate** (Akorn)		In 2 and 15 ml.[1]
Rx	**Cyclogyl** (Alcon)		In 2, 5 and 15 ml.[1]
Rx	**Cyclogyl** (Alcon)	**Solution**: 2%	In 2, 5 and 15 ml Drop-Tainers.[1]
Rx	**Pentolair** (Bausch & Lomb)	**Solution**: 1%	In 2 and 15 ml squeeze bottles.[2]

[1] With 0.01% benzalkonium chloride, EDTA and boric acid.
[2] With 0.01% benzalkonium chloride and EDTA.

MYDRIATIC COMBINATIONS

These combinations induce mydriasis that is greater than that of either drug used alone. See individual monographs for complete prescribing information.

Indications:

Cyclomydril: Production of mydriasis.

Murocoll-2: For mydriasis, cycloplegia and to break posterior synechiae in iritis.

Paremyd: Mydriasis with partial cycloplegia.

Administration and Dosage:

Cyclomydril: Instill 1 drop into each eye every 5 to 10 minutes, not to exceed 3 times.

Murocoll-2:

Mydriasis – Instill 1 or 2 drops into eye(s); repeat in 5 minutes, if necessary.

Postoperatively – Instill 1 or 2 drops into the eye(s) 3 or 4 times daily.

Paremyd: Instill 1 to 2 drops into the conjunctival sac(s).

Rx	**Cyclomydril** (Alcon)	**Solution**: 0.2% cyclopentolate HCl and 1% phenylephrine HCl.	In 2 and 5 ml Drop-Tainers.[1]
Rx	**Murocoll-2** (Bausch & Lomb)	**Drops**: 0.3% scopolamine HBr and 10% phenylephrine HCl.	In 5 ml.[2]
Rx	**Paremyd** (Allergan)	**Solution**: 1% hydroxyamphetamine HBr and 0.25% tropicamide.	In 5 and 15 ml.[3]

[1] With 0.01% benzalkonium chloride, EDTA and boric acid.
[2] With 0.01% benzalkonium chloride, sodium metabisulfite and EDTA.
[3] With 0.005% benzalkonium chloride and 0.015% EDTA.

Enzymes

CHYMOTRYPSIN

Actions:

Pharmacology: Chymotrypsin is a proteolytic enzyme. The principal proteolytic effect is exerted by the splitting of peptide bonds of amino acids in the zonular fibers and ocular tissues.

Pharmacokinetics: Destruction of the equatorial pericapsular membrane of the lens occurs in 5 minutes. Zonular fibers are lysed within 10 to 15 minutes of application; complete lysis of the entire zonular membrane occurs in 30 minutes.

Indications:

Lens extraction: For enzymatic zonulysis for intracapsular lens extraction.

Contraindications:

Congenital cataracts; high vitreous pressure; gaping incisional wound; hypersensitivity to chymotrypsin or any component of the preparation; patients < 20 years old.

Precautions:

Intraocular pressure (IOP): Chymotrypsin may produce an acute rise in IOP.

Synechiae lysis: The enzyme will not lyse the synechiae that may exist between the lens and other eye structures.

Adverse Reactions:

Transient increases in IOP; moderate uveitis; corneal edema; striation. Delayed healing of incisions has been reported, but not confirmed.

Administration and Dosage:

Instruments and syringes must be free of enzyme-inactivating alcohol and other chemicals. Do not use solution if it is cloudy or contains a precipitate.

Reconstitution: Reconstitute immediately prior to use. The 300 unit vial reconstituted with 2 ml of diluent yields a 1:5000 dilution.

Procedure –

1.) Following incision, irrigate the posterior chamber (under the iris) with 1 to 2 ml chymotrypsin solution.
2.) Wait 2 to 4 minutes, then irrigate anterior chamber with suitable irrigating solution, if desired. If zonules are still intact, irrigate the posterior chamber with additional chymotrypsin solution (0.5 to 2 ml). After an additional 2 to 4 minutes, irrigate again with a suitable irrigating solution, if desired. Extract lens.

Rx	**Catarase 1:5000** (Ciba Vision)	**Ophthalmic Solution:** 300 units	With 2 ml sodium chloride diluent per dual chamber univial.

NONSTEROIDAL ANTI-INFLAMMATORY AGENTS (NSAIDs)

Actions:

Pharmacology: Flurbiprofen, suprofen, diclofenac and ketorolac are NSAIDs available as ophthalmic solutions. Flurbiprofen and suprofen are phenylalkanoic acids, diclofenac is a phenylacetic acid and ketorolac tromethamine is a member of the pyrrolo-pyrrolle group; they have analgesic, antipyretic and anti-inflammatory activity. Their mechanism of action is believed to be through inhibition of the cyclooxygenase enzyme that is essential in the biosynthesis of prostaglandins.

In animals, prostaglandins are mediators of certain kinds of intraocular inflammation. Prostaglandins produce disruption of the blood-aqueous humor barrier, vasodilation, increased vascular permeability, leukocytosis and increased intraocular pressure (IOP). These agents have no significant effect on IOP.

Prostaglandins also appear to play a role in the miotic response produced during ocular surgery by constricting the iris sphincter independently of cholinergic mechanisms. These agents inhibit the miosis induced during the course of cataract surgery.

Indications:

Flurbiprofen, suprofen: Inhibition of intraoperative miosis.

Diclofenac: Treatment of postoperative inflammation following cataract extraction.

Ketorolac: Relief of ocular itching caused by seasonal allergic conjunctivitis. Treatment of postoperative inflammation following cataract extraction.

Unlabeled uses:

Flurbiprofen – Topical treatment of cystoid macular edema, inflammation after cataract or glaucoma laser surgery and uveitis syndromes.

Contraindications:

Hypersensitivity to the drugs or any component of the products.

Flurbiprofen, suprofen: Epithelial herpes simplex keratitis (dendritic keratitis).

Diclofenac, ketorolac: Patients wearing soft contact lenses (see Precautions).

Warnings:

Cross-sensitivity: The potential for cross-sensitivity to acetylsalicylic acid and other NSAIDs exists. Use caution when treating individuals who have previously exhibited sensitivities to these drugs.

Bleeding tendencies: Systemic absorption occurs with drugs applied ocularly. With some NSAIDs, there exists the potential for increased bleeding time caused by interference with thrombocyte aggregation. There have been reports that ocularly applied NSAIDs may cause increased bleeding of ocular tissues (including hyphemas) in conjunction with ocular surgery. Use with caution in surgical patients with known bleeding tendencies or in patients taking drugs known to cause bleeding (eg, anticoagulants).

Flank pain/Renal function impairment: Use of oral suprofen has been associated with a syndrome of acute flank pain and generally reversible renal insufficiency, which may present as acute uric acid nephropathy. This syndrome occurs in ≈ 1 in 3500 patients and has been reported with as few as one to two doses of a 200 mg capsule.

Pregnancy: Category C (flurbiprofen, ketorolac, suprofen); Category B (diclofenac). **Flurbiprofen** is embryocidal, delays parturition, prolongs gestation, reduces weight and slightly retards fetal growth in rats at daily oral doses of ≥ 0.4 mg/kg (≈ 185 times the human daily topical dose).

Oral doses of **ketorolac** at 1.5 mg/kg (8.8 mg/m^2), which was half of the human oral exposure, administered after gestation day 17 caused dystocia and higher pup mortality in rats.

Oral doses of **suprofen** of up to 200 mg/kg/day in animals resulted in an increased incidence of fetal resorption associated with maternal toxicity. There was an increase in still-births and a decrease in postnatal survival in pregnant rats treated with ≥ 2.5 mg/kg/day.

Oral **diclofenac** in mice and rats crosses the placental barrier. In rats, maternally toxic doses were associated with dystocia, prolonged gestation and reduced fetal weights, growth and survival. Because of the known effects of prostaglandin-inhibiting drugs on the fetal cardiovascular system, avoid using ophthalmic diclofenac during late pregnancy.

There are no adequate and well controlled studies in pregnant women. Use during pregnancy only if the potential benefits outweigh the potential hazards to the fetus.

NONSTEROIDAL ANTI-INFLAMMATORY AGENTS (NSAIDs)

Lactation: It is not known whether **flurbiprofen** is excreted in breast milk. Because of the potential for serious adverse reactions in nursing infants, decide whether to discontinue nursing or to discontinue the drug, taking into account the importance of the drug to the mother.

Suprofen is excreted in breast milk after a single oral dose. Based on measurements of plasma and milk levels in women taking oral suprofen, the milk concentration is ≈ 1% of the plasma level. Because systemic absorption may occur from topical ocular administration, consider discontinuing nursing while on suprofen; its safety in human neonates has not been established.

Exercise caution while **ketorolac** is administered to a nursing woman.

Children: Safety and efficacy for use in children have not been established.

Precautions:

Wound healing may be delayed with the use of flurbiprofen.

Contact lenses: Patients wearing hydrogel soft contact lenses who have used diclofenac concurrently have experienced ocular irritation manifested by redness and burning.

Drug Interactions:

Acetylcholine chloride and carbachol: Although clinical and animal studies revealed no interference, and there is no known pharmacological basis for an interaction, both of these drugs have reportedly been ineffective when used in patients treated with flurbiprofen or suprofen.

Adverse Reactions:

Most frequent: Transient burning and stinging upon instillation (diclofenac 15%, ketorolac ≈ 40%); other minor symptoms of ocular irritation.

Suprofen – Discomfort; itching; redness; allergy, iritis, pain, chemosis, photophobia, irritation, punctate epithelial staining (< 0.5%).

Diclofenac – Keratitis (28%, although most cases occurred in cataract studies prior to drug therapy); elevated IOP (15%, although most cases occurred post-surgery and prior to drug therapy); anterior chamber reaction; ocular allergy; nausea, vomiting (1%); viral infections (≤ 1%).

Ketorolac – Ocular irritation; allergic reactions; superficial keratitis; superficial ocular infections; eye dryness; corneal infiltrates; corneal ulcer; blurry vision.

Flurbiprofen: Increased bleeding tendency of ocular tissues in conjunction with ocular surgery.

Overdosage:

Overdosage will not ordinarily cause acute problems. If accidentally ingested, drink fluids to dilute.

Nonsteroidal Anti-Inflammatory Agents

FLURBIPROFEN SODIUM

Complete prescribing information begins in the Ophthalmic NSAIDs group monograph.

Administration and Dosage:

Instill 1 drop approximately every 30 minutes, beginning 2 hours before surgery (total of 4 drops).

Rx	**Ocufen** (Allergan)	**Solution:** 0.03%	In 2.5 ml dropper bottles.[1]
Rx	**Flurbiprofen Sodium Ophthalmic** (Various, eg, Bausch & Lomb)		In 2.5 ml.[1]

[1] With 1.4% polyvinyl alcohol, 0.005% thimerosal and EDTA.

SUPROFEN

Complete prescribing information begins in the Ophthalmic NSAIDs group monograph.

Administration and Dosage:

On the day of surgery, instill 2 drops into the conjunctival sac at 3, 2 and 1 hour(s) prior to surgery. Two drops may be instilled into the conjunctival sac every 4 hours while awake the day preceding surgery.

Rx	**Profenal** (Alcon)	**Solution:** 1%	In 2.5 ml Drop-Tainers.[1]

[1] With 0.005% thimerosal, 2% caffeine and EDTA.

DICLOFENAC SODIUM

Complete prescribing information begins in the Ophthalmic NSAIDs group monograph.

Administration and Dosage:

Instill 1 drop to the affected eye 4 times/day beginning 24 hours after cataract surgery and continuing throughout the first 2 weeks of the postoperative period.

Rx	**Voltaren** (Ciba Vision Ophthalmics)	**Solution:** 0.1%	In 2.5 and 5 ml dropper bottles.[1]

[1] With 1 mg/ml EDTA, boric acid, polyoxyl 35 castor oil, 2 mg/ml sorbic acid and tromethamine.

KETOROLAC TROMETHAMINE

Complete prescribing information begins in the Ophthalmic NSAIDs group monograph.

Administration and Dosage:

Ocular itching: Administer 1 drop (0.25 mg) 4 times/day.

Following cataract extraction: Apply 1 drop to the affected eye(s) 4 times/day beginning 24 hours after cataract surgery and continuing through the first 2 weeks of the postoperative period.

Rx	**Acular** (Allergan)	**Solution:** 0.5%	In 3, 5 and 10 ml dropper bottles.[1]

[1] With 0.01% benzalkonium Cl, 0.1% EDTA and octoxynol 40.

CORTICOSTEROIDS

Actions:

Pharmacology: Topical corticosteroids exert an anti-inflammatory action. Aspects of the inflammatory process such as hyperemia, cellular infiltration, vascularization and fibroblastic proliferation are suppressed. Steroids inhibit inflammatory response to inciting agents of mechanical, chemical or immunological nature. Topical corticosteroids are effective in acute inflammatory conditions of the conjunctiva, sclera, cornea, lids, iris, ciliary body and anterior segment of the globe; and in ocular allergic conditions. In ocular disease, route depends on site and extent of disorder.

The mechanism of the anti-inflammatory action is thought to be potentiation of epinephrine vasoconstriction, stabilization of lysosomal membranes, retardation of macrophage movement, prevention of kinin release, inhibition of lymphocyte and neutrophil function, inhibition of prostaglandin synthesis and, in prolonged use, decrease of antibody production.

Inhibiting fibroblastic proliferation may prevent symblepharon formation in chemical and thermal burns. Decreased scarring with clearer corneas after topical corticosteroids is a result of inhibiting fibroblastic proliferation and vascularization.

Indications:

Inflammatory conditions: Treatment of steroid-responsive inflammatory conditions of the palpebral and bulbar conjunctiva, lid, cornea and anterior segment of the globe, such as: Allergic conjunctivitis; nonspecific superficial keratitis; superficial punctate keratitis; herpes zoster keratitis; iritis; cyclitis; and selected infective conjunctivitis when the inherent hazard of steroid use is accepted to obtain a diminution in edema and inflammation.

Corneal injury: For corneal injury from chemical, radiation or thermal burns or penetration of foreign bodies.

Graft rejection: May use to suppress graft reaction after keratoplasty.

Contraindications:

Acute superficial herpes simplex keratitis; fungal diseases of ocular structures; vaccinia, varicella and most other viral diseases of the cornea and conjunctiva; ocular tuberculosis; hypersensitivity; after uncomplicated removal of a superficial corneal foreign body.

Medrysone is not for use in iritis and uveitis; its efficacy has not been demonstrated.

Warnings:

Moderate to severe inflammation: Use higher strengths for moderate to severe inflammations. In difficult cases of anterior segment eye disease, systemic therapy may be required. When deeper ocular structures are involved, use systemic therapy.

Ocular damage: Prolonged use may result in glaucoma, elevated IOP, optic nerve damage, defects in visual acuity and fields of vision, posterior subcapsular cataract formation or secondary ocular infections from pathogens liberated from ocular tissues. Check IOP and lens frequently. In diseases that cause thinning of cornea or sclera, perforation has occurred with topical steroids.

Mustard gas keratitis or Sjögren's keratoconjunctivitis: Topical steroids are not effective.

Infections: Acute, purulent, untreated eye infections may be masked or the activity enhanced by steroids. Fungal infections of the cornea have been reported with long-term local steroid applications. Therefore, suspect fungal invasion in any persistent corneal ulceration where a steroid has been used or is being used.

Stromal herpes simplex keratitis treatment with steroid medication requires great caution; frequent slit-lamp microscopy is mandatory.

Pregnancy: Category C. Use only when clearly needed and when potential benefits outweigh potential hazards.

Lactation: It is not known whether topical steroids are excreted in breast milk. Exercise caution when administering to a nursing mother.

Children: Safety and efficacy have not been established in children.

Precautions:

Sulfite sensitivity: Some of these products contain sulfites that may cause allergic-type reactions (eg, hives, itching, wheezing, anaphylaxis) in certain susceptible persons. Although the overall prevalence of sulfite sensitivity in the general population is probably low, it is seen more frequently in asthmatics or in atopic nonasthmatic persons. Specific products containing sulfites are identified in the product listings.

CORTICOSTEROIDS

Adverse Reactions:

Glaucoma (elevated IOP) with optic nerve damage, loss of visual acuity and field defects; posterior subcapsular cataract formation; secondary ocular infection from pathogens, including herpes simplex liberated from ocular tissues; perforation of globe; exacerbation of viral and fungal corneal infections; transient stinging or burning; blurred vision, discharge, discomfort, ocular pain, foreign body sensation, hyperemia, pruritus (rimexolone). Rarely, filtering blebs have been reported with steroid use after cataract surgery.

Systemic: Systemic side effects may occur with extensive use (see Adrenal Cortical Steroids group monograph).

Patient Information:

Medical supervision during therapy is recommended.

To avoid contamination, do not touch applicator tip to any surface. Replace cap after using.

If improvement in the condition being treated does not occur within several days, or if pain, itching or swelling of the eye occurs, notify the physician. Do not discontinue use without consulting physician. Take care not to discontinue prematurely.

Refer to the Topical Ophthalmics introduction for more complete information on administration and use.

Administration and Dosage:

Treatment duration varies with type of lesion and may extend from a few days to several weeks, depending on therapeutic response. Relapse may occur if therapy is reduced too rapidly; taper over several days. Relapses, more common in chronic active lesions than in self-limited conditions, usually respond to retreatment.

Suspensions and solutions: Instill 1 or 2 drops into the conjunctival sac every hour during the day and every 2 hours during the night. When a favorable response is observed, reduce dosage to 1 drop every 4 hours. Later, 1 drop 3 or 4 times daily may suffice to control symptoms. For postoperative inflammation, instill 1 to 2 drops 4 times daily beginning 24 hours after surgery; continue throughout the first 2 weeks of the postoperative period.

Ointments: Apply a thin coating in the lower conjunctival sac 3 or 4 times a day. When a favorable response is observed, reduce the number of daily applications to twice, and later to once a day as a maintenance dose if sufficient to control symptoms.

Ointments are particularly convenient when an eye pad is used and may be the preparation of choice when prolonged contact of drug with ocular tissues is needed.

FLUOROMETHALONE

Complete prescribing information begins in the Opthalmic Corticosteroids group monograph.

Rx	**Fluor-Op** (Ciba Vision)	**Suspension:** 0.1%	In 5, 10 and 15 ml.[1]
Rx	**FML** (Allergan)		In 1, 5, 10 and 15 ml.[1]
Rx	**Flarex** (Alcon)	**Suspension:** 0.1% fluorometholone acetate	In 2.5, 5 and 10 ml Drop-Tainers.[2]
Rx	**FML Forte** (Allergan)	**Suspension:** 0.25%	In 2, 5, 10 and 15 ml.[3]
Rx	**FML S.O.P.** (Allergan)	**Ointment:** 0.1%	In 3.5 g.[4]

[1] With 0.004% benzalkonium chloride, EDTA, polysorbate 80 and 1.4% polyvinyl alcohol.
[2] With 0.01% benzalkonium chloride, EDTA, hydroxyethylcellulose and tyloxapol.
[3] With 0.005% benzalkonium chloride, EDTA, polysorbate 80 and 1.4% polyvinyl alcohol.
[4] With 0.0008% phenylmercuric acetate, white petrolatum, mineral oil and lanolin alcohol.

MEDRYSONE

Complete prescribing information begins in the Ophthalmic Corticosteroids group monograph.

Rx	**HMS** (Allergan)	**Suspension:** 1%	In 5 and 10 ml.[1]

[1] With 0.004% benzalkonium chloride, EDTA, 1.4% polyvinyl alcohol and hydroxypropyl methylcellulose.

Corticosteroids

PREDNISOLONE

Complete prescribing information begins in the Ophthalmic Corticosteroids group monograph.

Rx	**Pred Mild** (Allergan)	**Suspension:** 0.12% prednisolone acetate	In 5 and 10 ml.[1]
Rx	**Econopred** (Alcon)	**Suspension:** 0.125% prednisolone acetate	In 5 and 10 ml Drop-Tainers.[2]
Rx	**Prednisolone Sodium Phosphate** (Various, eg, Steris)	**Solution:** 0.125% prednisolone sodium phosphate	In 5 and 15 ml.
Rx	**AK-Pred** (Akorn)		In 5 ml.[3]
Rx	**Inflamase Mild** (Iolab)		In 3, 5 and 10 ml.[4]
Rx	**Econopred Plus** (Alcon)	**Suspension:** 1% prednisolone acetate	In 5 and 10 ml Drop-Tainers.[2]
Rx	**Pred Forte** (Allergan)		In 1, 5, 10 and 15 ml.[1]
Rx	**Prednisolone Acetate Ophthalmic** (Falcon)		In 5 and 10 ml.[2]
Rx	**Prednisolone Sodium Phosphate** (Various, eg, Bausch & Lomb, Rugby)	**Solution:** 1% prednisolone sodium phosphate	In 5, 10 and 15 ml.
Rx	**AK-Pred** (Akorn)		In 5 and 15 ml.[3]
Rx	**Inflamase Forte** (Iolab)		In 3, 5, 10 and 15 ml.[4]

[1] With benzalkonium chloride, EDTA, polysorbate 80, hydroxypropyl methylcellulose and sodium bisulfite.
[2] With 0.01% benzalkonium chloride, EDTA, polysorbate 80, hydroxypropyl methylcellulose and glycerin.
[3] With 0.01% benzalkonium chloride, EDTA, hydroxypropyl methylcellulose and sodium bisulfite.
[4] With 0.01% benzalkonium chloride and EDTA.

Corticosteroids

DEXAMETHASONE

Complete prescribing information begins in the Ophthalmic Corticosteroids group monograph.

Rx	**Dexamethasone Sodium Phosphate** (Various, eg, Rugby, Iolab, Steris)	**Solution**: 0.1% dexamethasone phosphate (as sodium phosphate)	In 5 ml.
Rx	**AK-Dex** (Akorn)		In 5 ml.[1]
Rx	**Decadron Phosphate** (Merck)		In 5 ml Ocumeters.[2]
Rx	**Dexamethasone** (Steris)	**Suspension**: 0.1% dexamethasone	In 5 ml.
Rx	**Maxidex** (Alcon)		In 5 and 15 ml Drop-Tainers.[3]
Rx	**Dexamethasone Sodium Phosphate** (Various, eg, Goldline, Major)	**Ointment**: 0.05% dexamethasone phosphate (as sodium phosphate)	In 3.5 g.
Rx	**AK-Dex** (Akorn)		In 3.5 g.[4]
Rx	**Decadron Phosphate** (Merck)		In 3.5 g.[5]
Rx	**Maxidex** (Alcon)		In 3.5 g.[5]

[1] With 0.01% benzalkonium chloride, EDTA and hydroxyethylcellulose.
[2] With polysorbate 80, EDTA, 0.1% sodium bisulfite, 0.25% phenylethanol, 0.02% benzalkonium chloride.
[3] With 0.01% benzalkonium chloride, EDTA, 0.5% hydroxypropylmethylcellulose, polysorbate 80.
[4] With lanolin anhydrous, parabens, PEG-400, white petrolatum and mineral oil.
[5] With white petrolatum and mineral oil.

RIMEXOLONE

Complete prescribing information begins in the Ophthalmic Corticosteroids group monograph.

Rx	**Vexol** (Alcon)	**Suspension**: 1%	In 5 and 10 ml Drop-Tainers.[1]

[1] With 0.01% benzalkonium chloride, polysorbate 80 and EDTA.

Antiallergic

LODOXAMIDE TROMETHAMINE

Actions:

Pharmacology: Lodoxamide is a mast cell stabilizer that inhibits, in vivo, the Type I immediate hypersensitivity reaction. Lodoxamide therapy inhibits the increases in cutaneous vascular permeability that are associated with reagin or IgE and antigen-mediated reactions. In vitro, lodoxamide stabilizes rodent mast cells and prevent mast cell inflammatory mediators (ie, SRS-A, slow-reacting substances of anaphylaxis, also known as the peptidoleukotrienes) and inhibits eosinophil chemotaxis. Although lodoxamide's precise mechanism of action is unknown, the drug may prevent calcium influx into mast cells upon antigen stimulation.

Lodoxamide has no intrinsic vasoconstrictor, antihistaminic, cyclooxygenase inhibition or other anti-inflammatory activity.

Pharmacokinetics: The disposition of lodoxamide was studied in six healthy adult volunteers receiving a 3 mg oral dose. Urinary excretion was the major route of elimination. The elimination half-life was 8.5 hours in urine. In a study in 12 healthy adult volunteers, topical administration of one drop in each eye 4 times per day for 10 days did not result in any measurable lodoxamide plasma levels at a detection limit of 2.5 ng/ml.

Indications:

Treatment of the ocular disorders referred to by the terms vernal keratoconjunctivitis, vernal conjunctivitis and vernal keratitis.

Contraindications:

Hypersensitivity to any component of this product.

Warnings:

For ophthalmic use only. Not for injection.

Contact lenses: As with all ophthalmic preparations containing benzalkonium chloride, instruct patients not to wear soft contact lenses during treatment with lodoxamide.

Pregnancy: Category B. There are no adequate and well controlled studies in pregnant women. Use during pregnancy only if clearly needed.

Lactation: It is not known whether lodoxamide is excreted in breast milk. Exercise caution when administering to a nursing woman.

Children: Safety and efficacy in children < 2 years of age have not been established.

Precautions:

Burning/Stinging: Patients may experience a transient burning or stinging upon instillation of lodoxamide. Should these symptoms persist, advise the patient to contact their physician.

Adverse Reactions:

Ophthalmic: Transient burning, stinging or discomfort upon instillation (≈ 15%); ocular itching/pruritus, blurred vision, dry eye, tearing/discharge, hyperemia, crystalline deposits, foreign body sensation (1% to 5%); corneal erosion/ulcer, scales on lid/lash, eye pain, ocular edema/swelling, ocular warming sensation, ocular fatigue, chemosis, corneal abrasion, anterior chamber cells, keratopathy/keratitis, blepharitis, allergy, sticky sensation, epitheliopathy (< 1%).

Systemic: Headache (1.5%); heat sensation, dizziness, somnolence, nausea, stomach discomfort, sneezing, dry nose, rash (< 1%).

Overdosage:

Overdose of an oral preparation of 120 to 180 mg resulted in a temporary sensation of warmth, profuse sweating, diarrhea, lightheadedness and a feeling of stomach distension; no permanent adverse effects were observed. Side effects reported following oral administration of 0.1 to 10 mg included a feeling of warmth or flushing, headache, dizziness, fatigue, sweating, nausea, loose stools and urinary frequency/urgency. Consider emesis in the event of accidental ingestion.

Administration and Dosage:

Approved by the FDA on September 23, 1993.

Adults and children > 2 years of age: Instill 1 to 2 drops in each affected eye 4 times daily for up to 3 months.

Rx	**Alomide** (Alcon)	**Solution:** 0.1%	In 10 ml Drop-Tainers.

Antiallergic

LEVOCABASTINE HCl

Actions:

Pharmacology: Levocabastine is a potent, selective histamine H_1-receptor antagonist for topical ophthalmic use. Antigen challenge studies performed 2 and 4 hours after initial drug instillation indicated activity was maintained for at least 2 hours.

Pharmacokinetics: After instillation in the eye, levocabastine is systemically absorbed. However, the amount of systemically absorbed levocabastine after therapeutic ocular doses is low (mean plasma concentrations in the range of 1 to 2 ng/ml).

Clinical trials: Levocabastine instilled 4 times daily was significantly more effective than its vehicle in reducing ocular itching associated with seasonal allergic conjunctivitis.

Indications:

Allergic conjunctivitis: For the temporary relief of the signs and symptoms of seasonal allergic conjunctivitis.

Contraindications:

Hypersensitivity to any components of the product; while soft contact lenses are being worn.

Warnings:

For ophthalmic use only: Not for injection.

Carcinogenesis/Mutagenesis/Fertility impairment: In female mice, levocabastine doses of 5000 and 21,500 times the maximum recommended ocular human use level resulted in an increased incidence of pituitary gland adenoma and mammary gland adenocarcinoma possibly produced by increased prolactin levels. The clinical relevance of this finding is unknown with regard to the interspecies differences in prolactin physiology and the very low plasma concentrations of levocabastine following ocular administration.

Pregnancy: Category C. Levocabastine is teratogenic (polydactyly) in rats when given in doses 16,500 times the maximum recommended human ocular dose. Teratogenicity (polydactyly, hydrocephaly, brachygnathia), embryotoxicity and maternal toxicity were observed in rats at 66,000 times the maximum recommended ocular human dose. There are no adequate and well controlled studies in pregnant women. Use during pregnancy only if the potential benefit justifies the potential risk to the fetus.

Lactation: Based on determinations of levocabastine in breast milk after ophthalmic administration of the drug to one nursing woman, it was calculated that the daily dose of levocabastine in the infant was about 0.5 mcg.

Children: Safety and efficacy in children < 12 years of age have not been established.

Adverse Reactions:

Mild, transient stinging and burning (15%); headache (5%); visual disturbances, dry mouth, fatigue, pharyngitis, eye pain/dryness, somnolence, red eyes, lacrimation/discharge, cough, nausea, rash/erythema, eyelid edema, dyspnea (1% to 3%).

Patient Information:

Shake well before using.

To prevent contaminating the dropper tip and suspension, take care not to touch the eyelids or surrounding areas with the dropper tip of the bottle.

Keep bottle tightly closed when not in use. Do not use if the suspension has discolored. Store at controlled room temperature. Protect from freezing.

Administration and Dosage:

Shake well before using.

The usual dose is 1 drop instilled in affected eyes 4 times daily. Treatment may be continued for up to 2 weeks.

Storage/Stability: Keep tightly closed when not in use. Do not use if the suspension has discolored. Store at controlled room temperature of 15° to 30°C (59° to 86°F). Protect from freezing.

Rx	**Livostin** (Ciba Vision)	**Ophthalmic suspension:** 0.05%	With 0.15 mg benzalkonium chloride, propylene glycol, EDTA. In 2.5, 5 and 10 ml dropper bottles.

Antiallergic

CROMOLYN SODIUM

Actions:

Pharmacology: In vitro and in vivo animal studies have shown that cromolyn inhibits the degranulation of sensitized mast cells that occurs after exposure to specific antigens. Cromolyn acts by inhibiting the release of histamine and SRS-A (slow-reacting substance of anaphylaxis) from the mast cell.

Another activity demonstrated in vitro is the capacity of cromolyn to inhibit the degranulation of non-sensitized rat mast cells by phospholipase A and the subsequent release of chemical mediators. In another study, cromolyn did not inhibit the enzymatic activity of released phospholipase A on its specific substrate.

Cromolyn has no intrinsic vasoconstrictor, antihistaminic or anti-inflammatory activity.

Pharmacokinetics: Cromolyn is poorly absorbed. When multiple doses of cromolyn ophthalmic solution are instilled into normal rabbit eyes, < 0.07% of the dose is absorbed into the systemic circulation (presumably by way of the eye, nasal passages, buccal cavity and GI tract). Trace amounts (< 0.01%) of the dose penetrate into the aqueous humor, and clearance from this chamber is virtually complete within 24 hours after treatment is stopped.

In healthy volunteers, analysis of drug excretion indicates that approximately 0.03% of cromolyn is absorbed following administration to the eye.

Indications:

Conjunctivitis: Treatment of vernal keratoconjunctivitis, vernal conjunctivitis and vernal keratitis.

Contraindications:

Hypersensitivity to cromolyn or to any of the other ingredients.

Warnings:

Stinging/Burning: Patients may experience a transient stinging or burning sensation following instillation of cromolyn.

Duration/Frequency of therapy: The recommended frequency of administration should not be exceeded. Symptomatic response to therapy (decreased itching, tearing, redness and discharge) is usually evident within a few days, but longer treatment for up to 6 weeks is sometimes required. Once symptomatic improvement has been established, continue therapy for as long as needed to sustain improvement.

Contact lens use: As with all ophthalmic preparations containing benzalkonium chloride, users of soft (hydrophilic) contact lenses should refrain from wearing lenses while under treatment with cromolyn ophthalmic solution. Wear can be resumed within a few hours after discontinuation of the drug.

Concomitant therapy: If required, corticosteroids may be used concomitantly with cromolyn ophthalmic solution.

Pregnancy: Category B. In animals receiving parenteral cromolyn, adverse fetal effects (increased resorption and decreased fetal weight) were noted only at the very high parenteral doses that produced maternal toxicity. There are no adequate and well controlled studies in pregnant women. Use during pregnancy only if clearly needed.

Lactation: It is not known whether this drug is excreted in breast milk. Exercise caution when cromolyn is administered to a nursing woman.

Children: Safety and efficacy in children < 4 years of age have not been established.

Adverse Reactions:

The most frequently reported adverse reaction is transient ocular stinging or burning upon instillation. Other adverse reactions (infrequent) include: Conjunctival injection; watery eyes; itchy eyes; dryness around the eye; puffy eyes; eye irritation; styes.

Patient Information:

Advise patients that the effect of cromolyn therapy is dependent on its administration at regular intervals, as directed.

Do not wear soft contact lenses while using cromolyn.

Administration and Dosage:

Instill 1 or 2 drops in each eye 4 to 6 times a day at regular intervals. One drop contains approximately 1.6 mg cromolyn sodium.

Rx	**Crolom** (Bausch & Lomb)	**Solution:** 4%	In 2.5 and 10 ml bottles with controlled drop tip.

ANTIBIOTICS

Indications:

Ocular infections: Treatment of superficial ocular infections involving the conjunctiva or cornea (eg, conjunctivitis, keratitis, keratoconjunctivitis, corneal ulcers, blepharitis, blepharoconjunctivitis, acute meibomianitis and dacryocystitis) due to strains of microorganisms susceptible to antibiotics.

Erythromycin: Prophylaxis of ophthalmia neonatorum due to *Neisseria gonorrhoeae* or *Chlamydia trachomatis.*

Chloramphenicol: Use only in those serious infections for which less potentially dangerous drugs are ineffective or contraindicated (see Warnings).

For a list of microorganisms usually susceptible to these agents, refer to systemic monographs in the Anti-infectives chapter.

Topical Ophthalmic Antibiotic Preparations

		Miscellaneous							Quinolones			Aminoglycosides			Sulfonamides	
	Organism/Infection	Bacitracin	Gramicidin	Polymyxin B	Erythromycin	Chloramphenicol	Trimethoprim	Oxytetracycline	Norfloxacin	Ciprofloxacin	Ofloxacin	Neomycin	Gentamicin	Tobramycin	Sodium Sulfacetamide	Sulfisoxazole
Gram-Positive	Staphylococcus sp	✓	✓						✓	✓	✓		✓	✓		
	S aureus	✓	✓		✓	✓	✓		✓	✓	✓	✓	✓[1]	✓	✓	✓
	Streptococcus sp	✓	✓			✓				✓	✓			✓	✓	✓
	S pneumoniae	✓	✓		✓	✓	✓		✓	✓	✓		✓[1]	✓	✓	✓
	α-hemolytic streptococci (viridans group)				✓										✓	✓
	β-hemolytic streptococci	✓											✓[1]	✓		
	S pyogenes	✓			✓		✓			✓	✓		✓		✓	✓
	Corynebacterium sp	✓	✓		✓							✓	✓	✓		
Gram-Negative	Escherichia coli			✓		✓	✓	✓	✓	✓	✓	✓	✓	✓	✓	✓
	Haemophilus aegyptius					✓	✓		✓				✓	✓	✓	✓
	H ducreyi					✓		✓		✓			✓	✓		
	H influenzae or parainfluenzae			✓	✓	✓	✓	✓	✓	✓	✓	✓	✓	✓		
	Klebsiella sp					✓		✓	✓	✓	✓				✓	✓
	K pneumoniae			✓			✓		✓	✓	✓		✓	✓		
	Neisseria sp	✓				✓				✓		✓	✓	✓		
	N gonorrhoeae	✓			✓[2]				✓	✓	✓		✓		✓	
	Proteus sp						✓		✓	✓	✓	✓	✓	✓	✓	✓
	Acinetobacter calcoaceticus								✓	✓	✓		✓	✓		
	Enterobacter aerogenes			✓			✓	✓	✓	✓	✓	✓	✓	✓		
	Enterobacter sp					✓			✓	✓	✓	✓	✓	✓	✓	✓
	Serratia marcescens					✓			✓	✓	✓		✓	✓		
	Moraxella sp					✓					✓		✓	✓		
	Chlamydia trachomatis				✓[2]					✓	✓				✓	✓
	Pasteurella tularensis							✓								
	Pseudomonas aeruginosa			✓					✓	✓	✓		✓[1]	✓		
	Bartonella bacilliformis							✓								
	Bacteroides sp							✓								
	Vibrio sp					✓		✓	✓	✓			✓	✓		
	Providencia sp								✓	✓						

[1] Increasing resistance has been seen.
[2] For prophylaxis.

ANTIBIOTICS

Contraindications:

Hypersensitivity to any component of these products; epithelial herpes simplex keratitis (dendritic keratitis); vaccinia; varicella; mycobacterial infections of the eye; fungal diseases of the ocular structure; use of steroid combinations after uncomplicated removal of a corneal foreign body.

Warnings:

Sensitization from the topical use of an antibiotic may contraindicate the drug's later systemic use in serious infections. For this reason, topical preparations containing antibiotics not ordinarily administered systemically are preferable.

Products with neomycin sulfate may cause cutaneous/conjunctival sensitization.

Cross-sensitivity: Allergic cross-reactions may occur that could prevent future use of any or all of these antibiotics: Kanamycin, neomycin, paromomycin, streptomycin, and possibly, gentamicin.

Hematopoietic toxicity has occurred occasionally with the systemic use of **chloramphenicol** and rarely with topical administration. It is generally a dose-related toxic effect on bone marrow, and is usually reversible on cessation of therapy. Rare cases of aplastic anemia, bone marrow hypoplasia and death have been reported with prolonged (months to years) or frequent intermittent (over months and years) use of ocular chloramphenicol.

Corneal healing: Ophthalmic ointments may retard corneal epithelial healing.

Pregnancy: Category B (erythromycin, tobramycin), Category C (gentamicin, ciprofloxacin, norfloxacin, ofloxacin, polymyxin B). Safety for use during pregnancy has not been established. Use only when clearly needed and when the potential benefits outweigh the potential hazards to the fetus.

Lactation: It is not known whether **ciprofloxacin, norfloxacin** or **ofloxacin** appears in breast milk following ophthalmic use. Exercise caution when administering **ciprofloxacin** to a nursing mother. Because of the potential for adverse reactions in nursing infants from **norfloxacin, ofloxacin, chloramphenicol** and **tobramycin,** decide whether to discontinue nursing or discontinue the drug, taking into account the importance of the drug to the mother.

Children: **Tobramycin** is safe and effective in children. Safety and efficacy of **fluoroquinolones** in infants < 1 year of age, and **polymyxin B/trimethoprim** in infants < 2 months have not been established.

Precautions:

Monitoring: Perform culture and susceptibility testing during treatment.

Systemic antibiotics: In all except very superficial infections, supplement the topical use of antibiotics with appropriate systemic medication. Systemic aminoglycoside antibiotics require monitoring the total serum concentration (peak and trough).

Crystalline precipitate: A white crystalline precipitate located in the superficial portion of the corneal defect was observed in ≈ 17% of patients on **ciprofloxacin**. Onset was within 1 to 7 days after starting therapy. The precipitate resolved in most patients within 2 weeks, and did not preclude continued use nor adversely affect the clinical course or outcome.

Superinfection: Do not use topical antibiotics in deep-seated ocular infections or in those that are likely to become systemic. Use of antibiotics (especially prolonged or repeated therapy) may result in bacterial or fungal overgrowth of nonsusceptible organisms. Such overgrowth may lead to a secondary infection. Take appropriate measures if superinfection occurs.

Sulfite sensitivity: Some of these products contain sulfites which may cause allergic-type reactions (eg, hives, itching, wheezing, anaphylaxis) in certain susceptible persons. Although the overall prevalence of sulfite sensitivity in the general population is probably low, it is seen more frequently in asthmatics or in atopic nonasthmatic persons. Specific products containing sulfites are identified in the product listings.

ANTIBIOTICS

Adverse Reactions:

Sensitivity reactions such as transient irritation, burning, stinging, itching, inflammation, angioneurotic edema, urticaria, vesicular and maculopapular dermatitis have occurred in some patients.

Chloramphenicol: Hematological events (including aplastic anemia) have been reported (see Warnings).

Fluoroquinolones: White crystalline precipitates; lid margin crusting; crystals/scales; foreign body sensation; conjunctival hyperemia; bad/bitter taste in mouth; corneal staining; keratopathy/keratitis; allergic reactions; lid edema; tearing; photophobia; corneal infiltrates; nausea; decreased vision; chemosis.

Aminoglycosides: Localized ocular toxicity and hypersensitivity, lid itching, lid swelling and conjunctival erythema (< 3% with tobramycin); bacterial/fungal corneal ulcers; nonspecific conjunctivitis; conjunctival epithelial defects; conjunctival hyperemia (gentamicin). Similar reactions may occur with the topical use of other aminoglycoside antibiotics.

Overdosage:

Symptoms: Symptoms of tobramycin overdose include punctate keratitis, erythema, increased lacrimation, edema and lid itching. These may be similar to adverse reactions.

Treatment: A topical overdose of **ciprofloxacin** may be flushed from the eyes with warm tap water.

Patient Information:

Tilt head back, place medication in conjunctival sac and close eyes. Apply light finger pressure on lacrimal sac for 1 minute following instillation.

May cause temporary blurring of vision or stinging following administration. Notify physician if stinging, burning or itching becomes pronounced or if redness, irritation, swelling, decreasing vision or pain persists or worsens.

To avoid contamination, do not touch tip of container to any surface. Replace cap after using.

In general, patients being treated for bacterial conjunctivitis should not wear contact lenses; however, if the physician considers contact lens use appropriate, wait at least 15 minutes after using any solutions containing benzalkonium chloride before inserting the lens, as it may be absorbed by the lens.

Quinolones: Discontinue use and notify physician at the first sign of a skin rash or other allergic reaction.

Administration and Dosage:

Administration and dosage varies for the individual products. Refer to the individual manufacturer inserts.

Antibiotics

CHLORAMPHENICOL

Complete prescribing information begins in the OphthalmicAntibiotics group monograph.

Rx	**Chloramphenicol** (Various, eg, Goldline, Schein)	**Solution**[1]: 5 mg/ml	In 7.5 and 15 ml.
Rx	**AK-Chlor** (Akorn)		In 7.5 and 15 ml.[2]
Rx	**Chloroptic** (Allergan)		In 2.5 and 7.5 ml.[3]
Rx	**Chloramphenicol** (Various, eg, Schein)	**Ointment**:10 mg/g	In 3.5 g.
Rx	**AK-Chlor** (Akorn)		In 3.5 g.[4]
Rx	**Chloromycetin** (Parke-Davis)		Preservative free. In 3.5 g.[5]
Rx	**Chloroptic S.O.P.** (Allergan)		In 3.5 g[6].
Rx	**Chloromycetin** (Parke-Davis)	**Powder for solution**: 25 mg/vial.	Preservative free. In 15 ml with diluent.

[1] Refrigerate until dispensed.
[2] With 0.5% chlorobutanol, boric acid, sodium borate, hydroxypropyl methylcellulose, sodium hydroxide and hydrochloric acid.
[3] With 0.5% chlorobutanol, PEG-300, polyoxyl 40 stearate and sodium hydroxide or hydrochloric acid.
[4] With white petrolatum, mineral oil and polysorbate 60.
[5] With liquid petrolatum and polyethylene base.
[6] With 0.5% chlorobutanol, white petrolatum, mineral oil, polyoxyl 40 stearate, petrolatum (and) lanolin alcohol and PEG-300.

ERYTHROMYCIN

Complete prescribing information begins in the OpthalmicAntibiotics group monograph.

Rx	**Erythromycin** (Various, eg, Akorn, Bausch & Lomb, Fougera, Goldline, Rugby)	**Ointment**: 5%	In 3.5 g.
Rx	**Ilotycin** (Dista)		In 3.5 g.[1]

[1] With white petrolatum, mineral oil and parabens.

GENTAMICIN

Complete prescribing information begins in the Ophthalmic Antibiotics group monograph.

Rx	**GentamicinOphthalmic** (Various, eg, Goldline)	**Solution**: 3 mg/ml	In 5 and 15 ml.
Rx	**Garamycin** (Schering)		In 5 ml dropper bottles.[1]
Rx	**Genoptic** (Allergan)		In 1 and 5 ml dropper bottles.[2]
Rx	**Gentacidin** (Ciba Vision)		In 5 ml dropper bottles.[1]
Rx	**Gentak** (Akorn)		In 5 and 15 ml dropper bottles.[1]
Rx	**Gentamicin Ophthalmic** (Various, eg, Major)	**Ointment**: 3 mg/g	In 3.5 g.
Rx	**Garamycin** (Schering)		In 3.5 g.[3]
Rx	**Genoptic S.O.P.** (Allergan)		In 3.5 g.[3]
Rx	**Gentacidin** (Ciba Vision)		In 3.5 g.[4]
Rx	**Gentak** (Akorn)		In 3.5 g.[3]

[1] With 0.1 mg/ml benzalkonium chloride, sodium phosphate and NaCl.
[2] With benzalkonium chloride, 1.4% polyvinyl alcohol, EDTA, sodium phosphate dibasic, NaCl and hydrochloric acid or sodium hydroxide.
[3] With white petrolatum and parabens.
[4] With white petrolatum and mineral oil.

Antibiotics

TOBRAMYCIN

Complete prescribing information begins in the Opthalmic Antibiotics group monograph.

Rx	**Tobramycin** (Various, eg, Bausch & Lomb, Steris)	**Solution**: 0.3% tobramycin	In 5 ml bottle.[1]
Rx	**AKTob** (Akorn)		In 5 ml.[2]
Rx	**Defy** (Akorn)		In 5 ml.
Rx	**Tobrex** (Alcon)		In 5 ml Drop-Tainers.[3]
Rx	**Tobrex** (Alcon)	**Ointment**: 3 mg tobramycin per g	In 3.5 g.[4]

[1] With 0.01% benzalkonium Cl and boric acid.
[2] With 0.01% benzalkonium chloride, boric acid and sodium sulfate.
[3] With 0.01% benzalkonium chloride, tyloxapol and boric acid.
[4] With white petrolatum, mineral oil and 0.5% chlorobutanol.

POLYMYXIN B SULFATE

Complete prescribing information begins in the Opthalmic Antibiotics group monograph.

Rx	**Polymyxin B Sulfate Sterile** (Roerig)	**Powder for solution**: 500,000 units	In 20 ml vials.

BACITRACIN

Complete prescribing information begins in the Ophthalmic Antibiotics group monograph.

Rx	**Bacitracin** (Various, eg, Goldline, Major, Schein, URL)	**Ointment**: 500 units/g	In 3.5 and 3.75 g.
Rx	**AK-Tracin** (Akorn)		Preservative free. In 3.5 g.[1]

[1] With white petrolatum and mineral oil.

CIPROFLOXACIN

Complete prescribing information begins in the Opthalmic Antibiotics group monograph.

Rx	**Ciloxan** (Alcon)	**Solution**: 3.5 mg/ml (equivalent to 3 mg base)	In 2.5 and 5 ml Drop-Tainers.[1]

[1] With 0.006% benzalkonium chloride, 4.6% mannitol and 0.05% EDTA.

NORFLOXACIN

Complete prescribing information is found in the Ophthalmic Antibiotics group monograph.

Rx	**Chibroxin** (Merck)	**Solution**: 3 mg/ml	In 5 ml Ocumeters.[1]

[1] With 0.0025% benzalkonium chloride and EDTA.

OFLOXACIN

Complete prescribing information begins in the Opthalmic Antibiotics group monograph.

Rx	**Ocuflox** (Allergan)	**Solution**: 3 mg/ml	In 1 and 5 ml.[1]

[1] With 0.005% benzalkonium chloride.

COMBINATION ANTIBIOTIC PRODUCTS

Complete prescribing information begins in the Opthalmic Antibiotics group monograph.

	Product and Distributor	**Polymyxin B Sulfate** (units/g or ml)	**Neomycin Sulfate** (mg/g or ml)	**Bacitracin Zinc** (units/g)	Other Antibiotics	How Supplied
Rx	**Triple Antibiotic Ophthalmic Ointment** (Various, eg, Fougera)	10,000	3.5	400		In 3.5 g.
Rx	**Bacitracin Neomycin Polymyxin B Ointment** (Various, eg, Fougera)					In 3.5 g.
Rx	**AK-Spore Ointment** (Akorn)					Preservative free. White petrolatum, mineral oil. In 3.5 g.
Rx	**Neosporin Ophthalmic Ointment** (Glaxo Wellcome)					White petrolatum. In 3.5 g.
Rx	**Ocutricin Ointment** (Bausch & Lomb)					White petrolatum, mineral oil. In 3.5 g.
Rx	**Neomycin Sulfate-Polymyxin B Sulfate-Gramicidin Solution** (Various, eg, Goldline, Rugby, Steris)	10,000	1.75		0.025 mg/ml gramicidin	In 2 and 10 ml.
Rx	**AK-Spore Solution** (Akorn)					In 2 and 10 ml.[1]
Rx	**Neosporin Ophthalmic Solution** (Glaxo Wellcome)					In 10 ml Drop Dose.[1]
Rx	**Bacitracin Zinc and Polymyxin B Ointment** (Bausch & Lomb)	10,000		500		White petrolatum and mineral oil. In 3.5 g.
Rx	**AK-Poly-Bac Ointment** (Akorn)					Preservative free. White petrolatum, mineral oil. In 3.5 g.
Rx	**Polysporin Ophthalmic Ointment** (Glaxo Wellcome)					White petrolatum. In 3.5 g.
Rx	**Terramycin w/Polymyxin B Ointment** (Roerig)	10,000			5 mg/g oxytetracycline HCl	White and liquid petrolatum. In 3.5 g.
Rx	**Terak Ointment** (Akorn)	10,000			5 mg/g oxytetracycline HCl	White and liquid petrolatum. In 3.5 g.
Rx	**Polytrim Ophthalmic Solution** (Allergan)	10,000			1 mg/ml trimethoprim	In 10 ml.[2]

[1] With 0.001% thimerosal, 0.5% alcohol, propylene glycol, polyoxyethylene polyoxypropylene.

[2] With 0.004% benzalkonium chloride and NaCl.

STEROID AND ANTIBIOTIC SOLUTIONS AND SUSPENSIONS

Indications:

Inflammatory conditions: For steroid-responsive inflammatory ocular conditions in which a corticosteroid is indicated and in which bacterial infection or risk of infection exists.

For inflammatory conditions of the palpebral and bulbar conjunctiva, cornea and anterior segment of the globe in which the inherent risk of steroid use in certain infective conjunctivitides is accepted to obtain a diminution in edema and inflammation. For chronic anterior uveitis and corneal injury from chemical, radiation or thermal burns, or penetration of foreign bodies.

Administration and Dosage:

Store suspensions upright and shake well before using.

Instill 1 or 2 drops into the affected eye(s) every 3 or 4 hours, or more frequently as required. Taper to discontinuation as inflammation subsides.

Do not prescribe > 20 ml initially; do not refill without further evaluation. For complete dosage instructions, see individual manufacturer inserts.

	Product & Distributor	Steroid (per ml)	Antibiotic (per ml)	Other Content	How Supplied
Rx	**Chloromycetin/Hydrocortisone for Suspension** (Parke-Davis)	0.5% hydrocortisone acetate[1] (2.5% as powder)	0.25% chloramphenicol[1] (1.25% as powder)	Cholesterol, methylcellulose, 0.01% benzethonium chloride, boric acid	In 5 ml w/diluent and dropper.
Rx	**Neomycin/Polymyxin B Sulfate/Hydrocortisone** (Various, eg, Rugby, Schein)	1% hydrocortisone	Neomycin sulfate equivalent to 0.35% neomycin base and 10,000 units polymyxin B sulfate		In 7.5 and 10 ml.
Rx	**AK-Spore H.C. Ophthalmic Suspension** (Akorn)			0.001% thimerosal, cetyl alcohol, glyceryl monostearate, polyoxyl 40 stearate, propylene glycol, mineral oil, NaCl	In 7.5 ml.
Rx	**Cortisporin Suspension** (Glaxo Wellcome)				In 7.5 ml Drop Dose.
Rx	**Terra-Cortril Suspension** (Roerig)	1.5% hydrocortisone acetate	0.5% oxytetracycline (as HCl)	Mineral oil and aluminum tristearate	In 5 ml.
Rx	**Poly-Pred Suspension** (Allergan)	0.5% prednisolone acetate	Neomycin sulfate equivalent to 0.35% neomycin base, 10,000 units polymyxin B sulfate	1.4% polyvinyl alcohol, 0.001% thimerosal, polysorbate 80, propylene glycol	In 5 and 10 ml.
Rx	**Pred-G Suspension** (Allergan)	1% prednisolone acetate	Gentamicin sulfate equivalent to 0.3% gentamicin base	1.4% polyvinyl alcohol, 0.005% benzalkonium chloride, EDTA, hydroxypropyl methylcellulose, polysorbate 80, NaCl	In 2, 5 and 10 ml.

STEROID AND ANTIBIOTIC SOLUTIONS AND SUSPENSIONS

	Product & Distributor	Steroid (per ml)	Antibiotic (per ml)	Other Content	How Supplied
Rx	**Neomycin Sulfate/ Dexamethasone Sodium Phosphate Solution** (Various, eg, Goldline, Rugby, Schein)	0.1% dexamethasone phosphate (as sodium phosphate)	Neomycin sulfate equivalent to 0.35% neomycin base		In 5 ml.
Rx	**NeoDecadron Solution** (Merck)			Polysorbate 80, EDTA, 0.2% benzalkonium Cl, 0.1% sodium bisulfite	In 5 ml Ocumeters.
Rx	**Neo-Dexameth** (Major)			0.01% benzalkonium Cl, EDTA, polysorbate 80, sodium bisulfite	In 5 ml.
Rx	**AK-Neo-Dex Solution** (Akorn)			0.02% benzalkonium Cl, polysorbate 80, EDTA, 0.1% sodium bisulfite	In 5 ml.
Rx	**TobraDex Suspension** (Alcon)	0.1% dexamethasone	0.3% tobramycin	0.01% benzalkonium Cl, tyloxapol, EDTA, hydroxyethylcellulose, sodium sulfate, NaCl	In 2.5 and 5 ml Drop-Tainers.
Rx	**Neomycin/Polymyxin B Sulfate/Dexamethasone Suspension** (Various, eg, Goldline, Rugby, Schein)	0.1% dexamethasone	Neomycin sulfate equivalent to 0.35% neomycin base and 10,000 units polymyxin B sulfate		In 5 and 10 ml.
Rx	**Dexacidin Suspension** (Ciba Vision)			Hydroxypropyl methylcellulose, polysorbate 20, 0.04% benzalkonium chloride, NaCl	In 5 ml.
Rx	**AK-Trol Suspension** (Akorn)			0.004% benzalkonium chloride, polysorbate 20, 0.5% hydroxypropyl methylcellulose, NaCl	In 5 ml.
Rx	**Maxitrol Suspension** (Alcon)			0.5% hydroxypropyl methylcellulose, polysorbate 20, 0.004% benzalkonium chloride	In 5 ml Drop-Tainers.

[1] As a prepared solution.

STEROID AND ANTIBIOTIC OINTMENTS

Administration and Dosage:

Apply ointment to the affected eye(s) every 3 or 4 hours, depending on the severity of the condition.

Do not prescribe > 8 g initially, and the prescription should not be refilled until further evaluation. For complete dosage instructions, see individual manufacturer inserts.

	Product & Distributor	Steroid (per g)	Antibiotic (per g)	Other Content	How Supplied
Rx	**Ophthocort** (Parke-Davis)	0.5% hydrocortisone acetate	1% chloramphenicol, 10,000 units polymyxin B (as sulfate)	Liquid petrolatum, polyethylene	Preservative free. In 3.5 g.
Rx	**Bacitracin Zinc/Neomycin Sulfate/Polymyxin B Sulfate/Hydrocortisone** (Various, eg, Fougera)	1% hydrocortisone	Neomycin sulfate equivalent to 0.35% neomycin base, 400 units bacitracin zinc, 10,000 units polymyxin B sulfate		In 3.5 g.
Rx	**AK-Spore H.C.** (Akorn)			White petrolatum, mineral oil	Preservative free. In 3.5 g.
Rx	**Cortisporin** (Glaxo Wellcome)			White petrolatum	In 3.5 g.
Rx	**Neotricin HC** (Bausch & Lomb)	1% hydrocortisone acetate	Neomycin sulfate equivalent to 0.35% neomycin base, 400 units bacitracin zinc, 10,000 units polymyxin B sulfate	White petrolatum, mineral oil	In 3.5 g.
Rx	**Pred-G S.O.P.** (Allergan)	0.6% prednisolone acetate	Gentamicin sulfate equivalent to 0.3% gentamicin base	0.5% chlorobutanol, white petrolatum, mineral oil, petrolatum, lanolin alcohol	In 3.5 g.
Rx	**NeoDecadron** (Merck)	0.05% dexamethasone phosphate (as sodium phosphate)	Neomycin sulfate equivalent to 0.35% neomycin base	White petrolatum, mineral oil	In 3.5 g.
Rx	**TobraDex** (Alcon)	0.1% dexamethasone	0.3% tobramycin	0.5% chlorobutanol, white petrolatum, mineral oil	In 3.5 g.

STEROID AND ANTIBIOTIC OINTMENTS

	Product & Distributor	Steroid (per g)	Antibiotic (per g)	Other Content	How Supplied
Rx	**Neomycin/Polymyxin B Sulfate/Dexamethasone** (Various, eg, Fougera, Rugby)	0.1% dexamethasone	Neomycin sulfate equivalent to 0.35% neomycin base, 10,000 units polymyxin B sulfate		In 3.5 g.
Rx	**AK-Trol** (Akorn)			White petrolatum, lanolin oil, mineral oil, parabens	In 3.5 g.
Rx	**Dexacidin** (Ciba Vision)			White petrolatum, mineral oil	In 3.5 g.
Rx	**Dexasporin** (Bausch & Lomb)			White petrolatum, mineral oil	In 3.5 g.
Rx	**Maxitrol** (Alcon)			White petrolatum, anhydrous liquid lanolin, parabens	In 3.5 g.

SULFONAMIDES

Actions:

Pharmacology: Sulfonamides are bacteriostatic against a wide range of susceptible gram-positive and gram-negative microorganisms. Through competition with para-aminobenzoic acid (PABA), they restrict synthesis of folic acid which bacteria require for growth. For complete information, refer to the systemic sulfonamides monograph in the Anti-infectives chapter.

Pharmacokinetics: Sulfonamides do not appear to be appreciably absorbed from mucous membranes.

Microbiology: Topically applied sulfonamides are considered active against susceptible strains of the following common bacterial eye pathogens: *Escherichia coli, Staphylococcus aureus, Streptococcus pneumoniae, Streptococcus* (viridans group), *Haemophilus influenzae, Klebsiella* sp and *Enterobacter* sp.

Topically applied sulfonamides do not provide adequate coverage against *Neisseria* sp, *Serratia marcescens* and *Pseudomonas aeruginosa.* A significant percentage of staphylococcal isolates are completely resistant to sulfa drugs.

Indications:

Ocular infections: For conjunctivitis, corneal ulcer and other superficial ocular infections due to susceptible microorganisms.

Trachoma: As an adjunct to systemic sulfonamide therapy in the treatment of trachoma.

Contraindications:

Hypersensitivity to sulfonamides or any component of the product; infants < 2 months of age; in epithelial herpes simplex keratitis (dendritic keratitis), vaccinia, varicella and many other viral diseases of the cornea and conjunctiva; mycobacterial infection or fungal diseases of the ocular structures; after uncomplicated removal of a corneal foreign body (steroid combinations).

Warnings:

Staphylococcus species: A significant percentage of isolates are resistant to sulfa drugs.

Hypersensitivity: Severe sensitivity reactions have been identified in individuals with no prior history of sulfonamide hypersensitivity (see Adverse Reactions).

Pregnancy: Category C. Safety for use during pregnancy has not been established. Use only when clearly needed and when potential benefits outweigh potential hazards to the fetus.

Lactation: Systemic sulfonamides are excreted in breast milk.

Children: Safety and efficacy not established. Contraindicated in infants < 2 months old.

Precautions:

For topical ophthalmic use only. Not for injection.

Epithelial healing: Ophthalmic ointments may retard corneal wound healing.

Sensitization may occur when a sulfonamide is readministered, regardless of route. Cross-sensitivity between different sulfonamides may occur. If signs of sensitivity or other untoward reactions occur, discontinue use of the preparation.

PABA present in purulent exudates inactivates sulfonamides.

Dry eye: Use with caution in patients with severe dry eye.

Superinfection: Use of antibiotics (especially prolonged or repeated therapy) may result in bacterial or fungal overgrowth of nonsusceptible organisms. Such overgrowth may lead to a secondary infection. Take appropriate measures if this occurs.

Sulfite sensitivity: May cause allergic-type reactions (eg, hives, itching, wheezing, anaphylaxis) in certain susceptible persons. Although overall prevalence in the general population is probably low, it is more common in asthmatics or in atopic nonasthmatics. Specific products containing sulfites are identified in product listings.

Drug Interactions:

Silver preparations are incompatible with these solutions.

Adverse Reactions:

Headache; local irritation; itching; periorbital edema, burning and transient stinging; bacterial and fungal corneal ulcers. As with all sulfonamide preparations, severe sensitivity reactions include rare occurrences of Stevens-Johnson syndrome, exfoliative dermatitis, toxic epidermal necrolysis, photosensitivity, fever, skin rash, GI disturbance and bone marrow depression; fatalities have occurred.

SULFONAMIDES

Patient Information:

For topical use only.

To avoid contamination, do not touch tip of container to any surface.

Keep bottle tightly closed when not in use. Do not use if solution has darkened.

Notify physician if improvement is not seen after several days, if condition worsens, or if pain, increased redness, itching or swelling of the eye occurs or persists for > 48 hours. Do not discontinue use without consulting physician.

Administration and Dosage:

Usual duration of treatment is 7 to 10 days.

Solutions:

Conjunctivitis or other superficial ocular infections – Instill 1 to 2 drops into the lower conjunctival sac(s) every 1 to 4 hours initially according to severity of infection. Dosages may be tapered by increasing the time interval between doses as the condition responds.

Trachoma – 2 drops every 2 hours. Concomitant systemic sulfonamide therapy is indicated.

Storage – Protect from light. On long standing, solutions will darken in color and should be discarded.

Ointments: Apply a small amount (0.5 inch) into the lower conjunctival sac(s) 3 to 4 times daily and at bedtime. Dosages may be tapered by increasing the time interval between doses as the condition responds. Or apply 0.5 to 1 inch into the conjunctival sac(s) at night in conjunction with the use of drops during the day, or before an eye is patched.

Storage – Store away from heat.

SULFACETAMIDE SODIUM

Complete prescribing information begins in the Sulfonamides group monograph.

Rx	**Sulster** (Akorn)	**Solution:** 1%	In 5 and 10 ml.
Rx	**Sulfacetamide Sodium** (Various, eg, Bausch & Lomb, Fougera, Geneva, Goldline, Moore, Optopics, Rugby, Schein, Steris, URL)	**Solution:** 10%	In 15 ml.
Rx	**AK-Sulf** (Akorn)		In 2, 5 and 15 ml.[1]
Rx	**Bleph-10** (Allergan)		In 2.5, 5 and 15 ml.[2]
Rx	**Ocusulf-10** (Optopics)		In 2, 5 and 15 ml.[3]
Rx	**Sodium Sulamyd** (Schering)		In 5 and 15 ml.[1]
Rx	**Storz Sulf** (Lederle)		In 15 ml.
Rx	**Sulf-10** (Iolab)		In 1 ml Dropperettes[4] and 15 ml dropper bottles.[5]
Rx	**Isopto Cetamide** (Alcon)	**Solution:** 15%	In 5 and 15 ml Drop-Tainers.[6]
Rx	**Sulfacetamide Sodium** (Various, eg, Schein, Steris)	**Solution:** 30%	In 15 ml.
Rx	**Sodium Sulamyd** (Schering)		In 15 ml.[7]

Sulfonamides

SULFACETAMIDE SODIUM

Rx	**Sodium Sulfacetamide** (Various, eg, Fougera, Moore, URL)	**Ointment**: 10%	In 3.5 g
Rx	**AK-Sulf** (Akorn)		In 3.5 g.[8]
Rx	**Bleph-10** (Allergan)		In 3.5 g.[9]
Rx	**Cetamide** (Alcon)		In 3.5 g.[10]
Rx	**Sodium Sulamyd** (Schering)		In 3.5 g.[11]

[1] 3.1 mg sodium thiosulfate pentahydrate, 5 mg methylcellulose, 0.5 mg methylparaben and 0.1 mg propylparaben per ml.

[2] With 1.4% polyvinyl alcohol, 0.005% benzalkonium chloride, polysorbate 80, sodium thiosulfate and EDTA.

[3] With parabens, 1.4% polyvinyl alcohol and sodium thiosulfate.

[4] With sodium thiosulfate and 0.005% thimerosal.

[5] With 0.1% hydroxypropyl methylcellulose 2208, sodium thiosulfate and 0.01% thimerosal.

[6] With 0.05% methylparaben, 0.01% propylparaben, 0.5% hydroxypropyl methylcellulose 2910 and 0.3% sodium thiosulfate.

[7] With 1.5 mg sodium thiosulfate pentahydrate, 0.5 mg methylparaben and 0.1 mg propylparaben per ml.

[8] With 0.5 mg methylparaben, 0.1 mg propylparaben, 0.25 mg benzalkonium chloride and petrolatum base per g.

[9] With 0.0008% phenylmercuric acetate, white petrolatum, mineral oil, petrolatum and lanolin alcohol.

[10] With 0.05% methylparaben, 0.01% propylparaben, white petrolatum, anhydrous liquid lanolin and mineral oil.

[11] With 0.5 mg methylparaben, 0.1 mg propylparaben, 0.25 mg benzalkonium chloride and petrolatum base per g.

SULFONAMIDE/DECONGESTANT COMBINATION

Complete prescribing information begins in the Sulfonamides group monograph.

In this combination, phenylephrine HCl, an alpha sympathetic receptor agonist, produces vasoconstriction.

Administration and Dosage:

Instill 1 or 2 drops into the lower conjunctival sac(s) every 2 or 3 hours during the day, less often at night.

Storage: Keep tightly closed. Protect from light.

Rx	**Vasosulf** (Iolab)	**Solution**: 15% sodium sulfacetamide and 0.125% phenylephrine HCl	With sodium thiosulfate, poloxamer 188 and parabens. In 5 and 15 ml.

STEROID AND SULFONAMIDE COMBINATIONS, SUSPENSIONS AND SOLUTIONS

The information for steroid preparations and sulfonamide preparations must be considered when using these products. See individual monographs.

Indications:

Inflammation/Infection: For corticosteroid-responsive inflammatory ocular conditions for which a corticosteroid is indicated and where superficial bacterial ocular infection or a risk of infection exists.

Administration and Dosage:

Solutions/Suspensions: Instill 1 to 3 drops into the conjunctival sac(s) every 1 to 4 hours during the day and at bedtime until a favorable response is obtained.

Do not prescribe > 20 ml initially, and the prescription should not be refilled without further evaluation.

For complete dosage instructions, see individual manufacturer inserts.

Storage – Protect from light. Do not freeze. Shake suspensions well before using. Do not use if solution or suspension has darkened. Clumping may occur on long standing at high temperatures.

Ointments: Apply a small amount (≈ ½ inch ribbon) into the conjunctival sac(s) 3 or 4 times daily and once at bedtime (or once or twice at night) until a favorable response is obtained.

Do not prescribe > 8 g initially, and the prescription should not be refilled without further evaluation.

For complete dosage instructions, see individual manufacturer inserts.

Storage – Keep tightly closed. Store away from heat.

	Product & Distributor	Steroid	Sulfonamide	Other Content	How Supplied
Rx	**FML-S Suspension** (Allergan)	0.1% fluorometholone	10% sodium sulfacetamide	EDTA, 1.4% polyvinyl alcohol, 0.006% benzalkonium chloride, polysorbate 80, povidone, sodium thiosulfate and sodium chloride	In 5 and 10 ml.
Rx	**Blephamide Suspension** (Allergan)	0.2% prednisolone acetate	10% sodium sulfacetamide	EDTA, 1.4% polyvinyl alcohol, polysorbate 80, sodium thiosulfate, benzalkonium chloride	In 2.5, 5 and 10 ml.
Rx	**Isopto Cetapred Suspension** (Alcon)	0.25% prednisolone acetate	10% sodium sulfacetamide	0.5% hydroxypropyl methylcellulose 2910, EDTA, polysorbate 80, sodium thiosulfate, 0.025% benzalkonium chloride, 0.05% methylparaben, 0.01% propylparaben	In 5 and 15 ml Drop-Tainers.

STEROID AND SULFONAMIDE COMBINATIONS, SUSPENSIONS AND SOLUTIONS

	Product & Distributor	Steroid	Sulfonamide	Other Content	How Supplied
Rx	**AK-Cide Suspension** (Akorn)	0.5% prednisolone acetate	10% sodium sulfacetamide	5 mg phenethyl alcohol, tyloxapol, sodium thiosulfate, 0.25 mg benzalkonium chloride and EDTA per ml	In 5 ml dropper bottle
Rx	**Metimyd Suspension** (Schering)			0.5% phenylethyl alcohol, 0.025% benzalkonium chloride, sodium thiosulfate, EDTA, tyloxapol	In 5 ml.
Rx	**Sulfacetamide Sodium and Prednisolone Sodium Phosphate** (Schein)	0.25% prednisolone sodium phosphate	10% sodium sulfacetamide	0.01% mg thimerosal, EDTA, boric acid	In 5 and 10 ml
Rx	**Sulster Solution** (Akorn)			0.01% mg thimerosal, EDTA	In 5 and 10 ml.
Rx	**Vasocidin Solution** (Iolab)			EDTA, 0.01% thimerosal, poloxamer 407	In 5 and 10 ml.

STEROID AND SULFONAMIDE COMBINATIONS, OINTMENTS

	Product & Distributor	Steroid	Sulfonamide	Other Content	How Supplied
Rx	**Blephamide** (Allergan)	0.2% prednisolone acetate	10% sodium sulfacetamide	0.0008% phenylmercuric acetate, mineral oil, white petrolatum, lanolin alcohol	In 3.5 g.
Rx	**Cetapred** (Alcon)	0.25% prednisolone acetate	10% sodium sulfacetamide	Mineral oil, white petrolatum, lanolin oil, 0.05% methylparaben, 0.01% propylparaben	In 3.5 g.
Rx	**AK-Cide** (Akorn)	0.5% prednisolone acetate	10% sodium sulfacetamide	0.5 mg methylparaben, 0.1 mg propylparaben per g, mineral oil, white petrolatum	In 3.5 g applicator tube.
Rx	**Metimyd** (Schering)			Mineral oil, white petrolatum, 0.05% methylparaben, 0.01% propylparaben	In 3.5 g.
Rx	**Vasocidin** (Iolab)			Mineral oil, white petrolatum	In 3.5 g.

Antiseptic Preparations

POVIDONE IODINE

Actions:

Pharmacology: Povidone iodine has broad-spectrum antimicrobial action.

Indications:

Ophthalmic preoperative prep: Used prior to eye surgery to prep the periocular region (lids, brow and cheek) and irrigate the ocular surface (cornea, conjunctiva and palpebral fornices).

Contraindications:

Hypersensitivity to iodine.

Warnings:

For external use only: Not for intraocular injection or irrigation.

Pregnancy: Category C. Safety for use during pregnancy has not been established. Use only when clearly needed.

Lactation: Because of the potential for adverse reactions in nursing infants, decide whether to discontinue nursing or discontinue the drug, taking into account the importance of the drug to the mother.

Children: Safety and efficacy have not been established.

Precautions:

Thyroid disorders: Use caution in patients with thyroid disorders due to the possibility of iodine absorption.

Adverse Reactions:

Local sensitivity has been exhibited by some individuals.

Administration and Dosage:

Transfer solution to a sterile prep cup. Apply to lashes and lid margins with sterile applicator, repeat once. Apply to lids, brow and cheek with sterile applicator, repeat 3 times. Irrigate cornea, conjunctiva and palpebral fornices with solution and leave in for 2 minutes; flush with sterile saline solution.

Rx	**Betadine 5% Sterile Ophthalmic Prep Solution** (Akorn)	**Solution:** 5% povidone iodine	In 50 ml.[1]

[1] Glycerin, sodium chloride, sodium hydroxide and sodium phosphate.

Antiseptic Preparations

SILVER NITRATE

Actions:

Pharmacology: Silver nitrate ophthalmic solution is an anti-infective. In weak solutions, it is used as a germicide and astringent to mucous membranes. The germicidal action is due to precipitation of bacterial proteins by liberated silver ions.

Indications:

Ophthlamic neonatorum: Prevention of gonorrheal ophthalmia neonatorum.

Contraindications:

Hypersensitivity to any component of the formulation.

Warnings:

Neonatal chlamydial conjunctivitis: Silver nitrate has not been effective for the prevention of neonatal chlamydial conjunctivitis.

Cauterization of cornea: A 1% solution is considered optimal. Use with caution, since cauterization of the cornea and blindness may result, especially with repeated applications.

Caustic/Irritant: Silver nitrate is caustic and irritating to the skin and mucous membranes.

Precautions:

Staining: Handle solutions carefully because they tend to stain skin and utensils. Stains may be removed from linen by applications of iodine tincture followed by sodium thiosulfate solution.

Drug Interactions:

Sulfonamide preparations are incompatible with silver preparations.

Adverse Reactions:

A mild chemical conjunctivitis should result from a properly performed Credé prophylaxis using silver nitrate. A more severe chemical conjunctivitis occurs in ≤ 20% of cases.

Overdosage:

When ingested, silver nitrate is highly toxic to the GI tract and CNS. Swallowing can cause severe gastroenteritis that may be fatal. Sodium chloride may be used by gastric lavage to remove the chemical.

When a solution of ≥ 2% silver nitrate concentration is used in the eye, conjunctivits may be produced. Irrigate the eye with an isotonic solution of sodium chloride after solutions of silver nitrate stronger than 1% are instilled.

Administration and Dosage:

Immediately after birth, clean the child's eyelids with steril absorbent cotton or gauze and sterile water. Use a separate pledget for each eye; wash unopened lids from the nose outward until free of blood, mucus or meconium. Next, separate the lids and instill 2 drops of 1% solutions. Elevate lids away from the eyeball so that a lake of silver nitrate may lie for ≥ 30 seconds between them, contacting the entire conjunctival sac.

The American Academy of Pediatrics has endorsed a statement from the Committee on Ophthalmia Neonatorum of the National Society for the prevention of Blindness, which does not recommend irrigation of the eyes following instillation of the silver nitrate.

Storage: Do not freeze. Do not use when cold. Protect from light.

Rx	**Silver Nitrate** (Lilly)	**Solution**: 1%	WIth acetic acid and sodium acetate. In 100s (wax ampules).

Antifungal Agent

NATAMYCIN

Actions:

Pharmacology: Natamycin, a tetraene polyene antibiotic, is derived from *Streptomyces natalensis.* It possesses in vitro activity against a variety of yeast and filamentous fungi, including *Candida, Aspergillus, Cephalosporium, Fusarium* and *Penicillium.* The mechanism of action appears to be through binding of the molecule to the fungal cell membrane. The polyenesterol complex alters membrane permeability, depleting essential cellular constituents. Although activity against fungi is dose-related, natamycin is predominantly fungicidal. It is not effective in vitro against gram-negative or -positive bacteria.

Pharmacokinetics: Topical administration appears to produce effective concentrations within the corneal stroma, but not in intraocular fluid. Absorption from the GI tract is very poor. Systemic absorption should not occur after topical administration.

Indications:

Fungal blepharitis, conjunctivitis and keratitis caused by susceptible organisms. Natamycin is the initial drug of choice in *Fusarium solani* keratitis.

Contraindications:

Hypersensitivity to any component of the formulation.

Warnings:

Pregnancy: Catagory C. Safety for use during pregnancy has not been established. Use only when clearly needed and when potential benefits outweigh potential hazards to the fetus.

Lactation: It is not known if natamycin is excreted in breast milk. Use with caution in nursing women.

Children: Safety and efficacy have not been established

Precautions:

For topical use only. Not for injection.

Fungal endophthalmitis: The effectiveness of topical natamycin as a single agent in fungal endophthalmitis has not been established.

Resistance: Failure of keratitis to improve following 7 to 10 days of administration suggests that the infection may be caused by a microorganism not susceptible to natamycin. Base continuation of therapy on clinical reevaluation and additional laboratory studies.

Toxicity: Adherence of the suspension to areas of epithelial ulceration or retention in the fornices occurs regularly. Should suspicion of drug toxicity occur, discontinue the drug.

Diagnosis/Monitoring: Determine initial and sustained therapy of fungal keratitis by the clinical diagnosis (laboratory diagnosis by smear and culture of corneal scrapings) and by response to the drug. Whenever possible, determine the in vitro activity of natamycin against the responsible fungus. Monitor tolerance to natamycin at least twice weekly.

Adverse Reactions:

One case of conjunctival chemosis and hyperemia, thought to be allergic in nature, was reported.

Patient Information:

Refer to the Topical Ophthalmics introduction.

Administration and Dosage:

Fungal keratitis: Instill 1 drop into the conjunctival sac at 1 or 2 hour intervals. The frequency of application can usually be reduced to 1 drop 6 to 8 times daily after the first 3 to 4 days. Generally, continue therapy for 14 to 21 days, or until there is resolution of active fungal keratitis. In many cases, it may help to reduce the dosage gradually at 4 to 7 day intervals to ensure that the organism has been eliminated.

Fungal blepharitis and conjunctivitis: 4 to 6 daily applications may be sufficient.

Storage: Store at room temperature 8° to 24°C (46° to 75°F) or refrigerate at 2° to 8°C (36° to 46°F). Do not freeze. Avoid exposure to light and excessive heat. Shake well before each use.

Rx	**Natacyn** (Alcon)	**Suspension:** 5%	With 0.02% benzalkonium chloride. In 15 ml.

ANTIVIRAL AGENTS

The topical ophthalmic antiviral preparations appear to interfere with viral reproduction by altering DNA synthesis. Idoxuridine, vidarabine and trifluridine are effective treatment for herpes simplex infections of the conjunctiva and cornea. Ganciclovir is indicated for use in immunocompromised patients with cytomegalovirus (CMV) retinitis and for prevention of CMV retinitis in transplant patients. Foscarnet is indicated for use only in AIDS patients with CMV retinitis.

Agents for Ophthalmic Conditions

Generic name	Trade name (manufacturer)	Preparations	Indications
Foscarnet sodium[1]	*Foscavir* (Astra)	Solution for Injection	Cytomegalovirus (CMV) retinitis
Ganciclovir sodium[1]	*Cytovene* (Syntex)	Reconstituted powder Capsules 250 mg	Cytomegalovirus (CMV) retinitis
Idoxuridine	*Herplex* (Allergan)	Solution 0.1%	Herpes simplex
Vidarabine	*Vira-A* (Parke-Davis)	Ointment 3%	Herpes simplex types 1 and 2; idoxuridine-resistant herpes
Trifluridine	*Viroptic* (Burroughs Wellcome)	Solution 1%	Herpes simplex types 1 and 2; idoxuridine hypersensitivity; vidarabine-resistant keratitis

[1] Refer to specific monograph in the Antivirals section.

Viral infection, especially epidemic keratoconjunctivitis (EKC), is more often associated with a follicular conjunctivitis, a serous conjunctival discharge and preuricular lymphadenopathy. The exceptionally contagious organism causing EKC is not susceptible to antiviral therapy at this time.

IDOXURIDINE (IDU)

Actions:

Pharmacology: Idoxuridine (IDU) blocks reproduction of herpes simplex virus by altering normal DNA synthesis. In chemical structure, IDU closely approximates the configuration of thymidine, one of the four building blocks of DNA. As a result, IDU replaces thymidine in the enzymatic step of viral replication. The consequent production of faulty DNA results in a pseudostructure which cannot infect or destroy tissue.

Indications:

Herpes simplex keratitis: Epithelial infections (especially initial attacks), characterized by the presence of a dendritic figure, respond better than stromal infections.

Contraindications:

Hypersensitivity to IDU or any component of the formulation.

Antiviral Agents

IDOXURIDINE (IDU)

Warnings:

Recurrences may be seen if medication is not continued for 5 to 7 days after the epithelial lesion has apparently healed.

Corticosteroids can accelerate the spread of a viral infection and are usually contraindicated in herpes simplex epithelial infections.

Carcinogenesis: Regard this cytotoxic drug as potentially carcinogenic, although data are inadequate for assessment. It can inhibit DNA synthesis or function, and is incorporated into the DNA of mammalian cells as well as into the genome of DNA viruses. IDU induces RNA tumor virus production from mouse cells and has caused in vitro cell transformation and induction of specific neoplasms (lymphatic leukemias and carcinomas) upon inoculation into syngeneic mice.

Mutagenesis: IDU has caused chromosome aberrations in mice and is mutagenic in mammalian cells in culture.

Pregnancy: Category C. IDU crosses the placental barrier and produces fetal malformations when administered topically to the eyes of pregnant rabbits in clinical doses and when administered by various routes in high doses to other rodents.

Safety for use during pregnancy has not been established. Use only if clearly needed and when the potential benefits outweigh the potential hazards to the fetus.

Lactation: It is not known whether IDU is excreted in breast milk. Because of the potential for tumorigenicity shown for IDU in animal studies, decide whether to discontinue nursing or to discontinue the drug, taking into account the importance of the drug to the mother.

Children: Safety and efficacy have not been established.

Precautions:

Resistance: Some strains of herpes simplex appear to be resistant. If there is no lessening of fluorescein staining in 14 days, undertake another form of therapy.

Frequency/Duration: Do not exceed the recommended frequency and duration of administration.

Drug Interactions:

Boric acid-containing solutions: Coadministration may result in a precipitate formation which may cause irritation.

Adverse Reactions:

Occasional irritation, pain, pruritus, inflammation or edema of the eyes or lids; allergic reactions; photophobia; corneal clouding; stippling; punctate defects in the corneal epithelium.

Overdosage:

Local: Overdose will not ordinarily cause acute problems. Should accidental overdosage in the eye(s) occur, flush with water or normal saline.

Accidental ingestion: Animal data indicate that the minimum systemic dose that will produce toxic effects is many times greater than the quantity in a commercial bottle. Also, metabolic breakdown and excretion take place very rapidly. Thus, no untoward consequences should be expected from accidental ingestion of even an entire bottle of the solution. Drink fluids to dilute.

Patient Information:

May cause sensitivity to bright light; this may be minimized by wearing sunglasses. Notify physician if improvement is not seen after 14 days, if condition worsens, or if pain, decreased vision, itching or swelling of the eye occurs.

Refer to the Topical Ophthalmics introduction.

Administration and Dosage:

For optimal results, keep infected tissues saturated with IDU.

Solution: Initially, instill 1 drop into infected eye(s) every hour during the day and every 2 hours at night. Continue until definite improvement has taken place, usually within 7 days, as evidenced by loss of staining with fluorescein. Then reduce dosage to 1 drop every 2 hours during the day and every 4 hours at night. To minimize recurrences, continue therapy at this reduced dosage for 3 to 7 days after healing appears complete. Maximum treatment period is ≤ 21 days.

Alternate dosing schedule – Instill 1 drop every minute for 5 minutes. Repeat every 4 hours, day and night.

Antiviral Agents

IDOXURIDINE (IDU)

Concomitant therapy: Topical corticosteroids may be used with IDU in some conditions. Use such combined therapy for as long as the condition warrants. It is important to continue IDU therapy a few days after the steroid has been withdrawn (see Warnings).

Storage/Stability: Store at room temperature 15° to 30°C (59° to 86°F). Protect from light.

Rx	**Herplex** (Allergan)	**Solution:** 0.1%	Benzalkonium chloride, EDTA, NaCl, 1.4% polyvinyl alcohol. In 15 ml dropper bottles.

Antiviral Agents

VIDARABINE (Adenine Arabinoside; Ara-A)

Actions:

Pharmacology: The antiviral mechanism of action has not been established. Vidarabine appears to interfere with the early steps of viral DNA synthesis. It is rapidly deaminated to arabinosylhypoxanthine (Ara-Hx), the principal metabolite. Ara-Hx also possesses in vitro antiviral activity less than vidarabine's. In contrast to topical idoxuridine, vidarabine demonstrated less cellular toxicity in regenerating corneal epithelium of rabbits.

Pharmacokinetics:

Absorption – Systemic absorption is not expected to occur following ocular administration and swallowing lacrimal secretions. In laboratory animals, vidarabine is rapidly deaminated in the GI tract to Ara-Hx.

Distribution – Because of its low solubility, trace amounts of both vidarabine and Ara-Hx can be detected in the aqueous humor only if there is an epithelial defect in the cornea. If the cornea is normal, only trace amounts of Ara-Hx can be recovered from the aqueous humor.

Microbiology: Vidarabine possesses in vitro and in vivo antiviral activity against herpes simplex types 1 and 2, varicella-zoster and vaccinia viruses. Except for rhabdovirus and oncornavirus, it does not display antiviral activity against other RNA or DNA viruses, including adenovirus.

Indications:

Acute keratoconjunctivitis and recurrent epithelial keratitis due to herpes simplex virus types 1 and 2.

Superficial keratitis caused by herpes simplex virus which has not responded to topical idoxuridine, or when toxic or hypersensitivity reactions to idoxuridine have occurred.

Contraindications:

Hypersensitivity to vidarabine; sterile trophic ulcers.

Warnings:

Efficacy in other conditions: Vidarabine is not effective against RNA virus, adenoviral ocular infections, bacterial, fungal or chlamydial infections of the cornea, or trophic ulcers. Effectiveness against stromal keratitis and uveitis due to herpes simplex virus has not been established.

Corticosteroids alone are normally contraindicated in herpes simplex virus eye infections. If vidarabine is coadministered with topical corticosteroid therapy, consider corticosteroid-induced ocular side effects such as glaucoma or cataract formation and progression of bacterial or viral infection.

Temporary visual haze may be produced with vidarabine.

Carcinogenesis: In female mice treated with IM vidarabine, there was an increase in liver tumor incidence; some male mice developed kidney neoplasia.

In rats, intestinal, testicular and thyroid neoplasia occurred with greater frequency among the vidarabine-treated animals.

Mutagenesis: In vitro, vidarabine can be incorporated into mammalian DNA and can induce mutation. In vivo studies have not been conclusive; however, vidarabine may be capable of producing mutagenic effects in male germ cells.

Vidarabine has caused chromosome breaks and gaps when added to human leukocytes in vitro. While the significance is not fully understood, there is a well known correlation between the ability of various agents to produce such effects and their ability to produce heritable genetic damage.

Pregnancy: Category C. A 10% ointment applied to 10% of the body surface during organogenesis induced fetal abnormalities in rabbits. The possibility of embryonic or fetal damage in pregnant women is remote. The topical ophthalmic dose is small, and the drug is relatively insoluble. Its ocular penetration is very low. However, a safe dose for a human embryo or fetus has not been established, and there are no adequate and well controlled studies in pregnant women. Therefore, use only if the potential benefit outweighs the potential risk to the fetus.

Lactation: It is not known whether vidarabine is excreted in breast milk. Excretion of vidarabine in breast milk is unlikely because the drug is rapidly deaminated in the GI tract. However, it is still recommended that either nursing or the drug be discontinued, taking into account the importance of the drug to the mother.

Precautions:

Viral resistance to vidarabine has not been observed, although this possibility exists.

Antiviral Agents

VIDARABINE (Adenine Arabinoside; Ara-A)

Adverse Reactions:

Lacrimation; foreign body sensation; conjunctival infection; burning; irritation; superficial punctate keratitis; pain; photophobia; punctal occlusion; sensitivity.

Uveitis, stromal edema, secondary glaucoma, trophic defects, corneal vascularization and hyphema have occurred but may be disease-related.

Overdosage:

The rapid deamination to Ara-Hx should preclude any difficulty. No untoward effects should result from ingestion of the entire contents of a tube. Overdosage by ocular instillation is unlikely because any excess is quickly expelled from the conjunctival sac. Avoid too frequent administration.

Patient Information:

May cause sensitivity to bright light; this may be minimized by wearing sunglasses.

Notify physician if improvement is not seen after 7 days, if condition or pain worsens, decrease in vision, burning or irritation of the eye occurs. Do not discontinue use without consulting physician.

Refer to the Topical Ophthalmics introduction.

Administration and Dosage:

Administer approximately 0.5 inch of ointment into the lower conjunctival sac(s) 5 times daily at 3 hour intervals.

If there are no signs of improvement after 7 days, or if complete re-epithelialization has not occurred in 21 days, consider other forms of therapy. Some severe cases may require longer treatment.

After re-epithelialization has occurred, treat for an additional 7 days at a reduced dosage (such as twice daily) to prevent recurrence.

Concomitant therapy: Topical corticosteroids (prednisolone or dexamethasone) have been administered concurrently with vidarabine without an increase in adverse reactions, although their advantages and disadvantages must be considered (see Warnings).

Rx	**Vira-A** (Parke-Davis)	**Ointment:** 3% vidarabine monohydrate (equivalent to 2.8% vidarabine)	In a liquid petrolatum base. In 3.5 g.

TRIFLURIDINE (Trifluorothymidine)

Actions:

Pharmacology: A fluorinated pyrimidine nucleoside with in vitro and in vivo activity against herpes simplex virus types 1 and 2, and vaccinia virus. Some strains of adenovirus are also inhibited in vitro. Trifluridine interferes with DNA synthesis in cultured mammalian cells. However, its antiviral mechanism of action is not completely known.

Pharmacokinetics:

Absorption – Intraocular penetration occurs after topical instillation. Decreased corneal integrity or stromal or uveal inflammation may enhance the penetration into the aqueous humor. Systemic absorption following therapeutic dosing appears negligible.

Indications:

Primary keratoconjunctivitis and recurrent epithelial keratitis due to herpes simplex virus types 1 and 2.

Epithelial keratitis that has not responded clinically to topical idoxuridine, or when ocular toxicity or hypersensitivity to idoxuridine has occurred. In a smaller number of patients resistant to topical vidarabine, trifluridine was also effective.

Contraindications:

Hypersensitivity reactions or chemical intolerance to trifluridine.

Warnings:

Efficacy in other conditions: The clinical efficacy in the treatment of stromal keratitis and uveitis due to herpes simplex or ophthalmic infections caused by vaccinia virus and adenovirus, or in the prophylaxis of herpes simplex virus keratoconjunctivitis and epithelial keratitis has not been established by well controlled clinical trials. Not effective against bacterial, fungal or chlamydial infections of the cornea or trophic lesions.

Dosage/Frequency: Do not exceed the recommended dosage or frequency of administration.

Antiviral Agents

TRIFLURIDINE (Trifluorothymidine)

Mutagenesis: Trifluridine has exerted mutagenic, DNA-damaging and cell-transforming activities in various standard in vitro test systems. Although the significance of these test results is not clear or fully understood, it is possible that mutagenic agents may cause genetic damage in humans.

Pregnancy: Category C. Fetal toxicity consisting of delayed ossification of portions of the skeleton occurred at dose levels of 2.5 and 5 mg/kg/day in rats and rabbits. In addition, both 2.5 and 5 mg/kg/day produced fetal death and resorption in rabbits. There are no adequate and well controlled studies in pregnant women. Use during pregnancy only if the potential benefit justifies the risk to the fetus.

Lactation: It is unlikely that trifluridine is excreted in breast milk after ophthalmic instillation because of the relatively small dosage (≤ 5 mg/day), its dilution in body fluids and its extremely short half-life (≈ 12 minutes). However, do not prescribe for nursing mothers unless the potential benefits outweigh the potential risks.

Precautions:

Viral resistance, although documented in vitro, has not been reported following multiple exposure to trifluridine; this possibility may exist.

Adverse Reactions:

The most frequent adverse reactions reported are mild, transient burning or stinging upon instillation (4.6%) and palpebral edema (2.8%). Other adverse reactions in decreasing order of reported frequency were: Superficial punctate keratopathy; epithelial keratopathy; hypersensitivity reaction; stromal edema; irritation; keratitis sicca; hyperemia and increased intraocular pressure.

Overdosage:

Local: Overdosage by ocular instillation is unlikely because any excess solution is quickly expelled from the conjunctival sac.

Systemic: No untoward effects are likely to result from ingestion of the entire contents of a bottle. Single IV doses of 15 to 30 mg/kg/day in children and adults with neoplastic disease produce reversible bone marrow depression as the only potentially serious toxic effect and only after three to five courses of therapy.

Patient Information:

Transient stinging may occur upon installation.

Notify physician if improvement is not seen after 7 days, if condition worsens or if irritation occurs. Do not discontinue use without consulting physician.

Refer to the Topical Ophthalmics introduction for more complete information.

Administration and Dosage:

Instill 1 drop onto the cornea of the affected eye(s) every 2 hours while awake for a maximum daily dosage of 9 drops until the corneal ulcer has completely re-epithelialized. Following re-epithelialization, treat for an additional 7 days with 1 drop every 4 hours while awake for a minimum daily dosage of 5 drops.

If there are no signs of improvement after 7 days, or if complete re-epithelialization has not occurred after 14 days, consider other forms of therapy. Avoid continuous administration for periods > 21 days because of potential ocular toxicity.

Storage/Stability: Store under refrigeration, 2° to 8°C (36° to 46°F).

Rx	**Viroptic** (Glaxo Wellcome)	**Solution:** 1%	In aqueous solution with NaCl and 0.001% thimerosal. In 7.5 ml Drop-Dose.

ARTIFICIAL TEAR SOLUTIONS

Actions:

Pharmacology: These products contain: Balanced amounts of salts to maintain ocular tonicity (0.9% NaCl equivalent); buffers to adjust pH; viscosity agents to prolong eye contact time; preservatives for sterility. See the Topical Ophthalmics introduction for a description and listing of these ingredients.

Indications:

Ophthalmic lubricants: These products offer tear-like lubrication for the relief of dry eyes and eye irritation associated with deficient tear production. Also used as ocular lubricants for artificial eyes.

Patient Information:

Do not touch the tip of the container or dropper to any surface. Close container immediately after use.

If headache, eye pain, vision changes, continued redness or irritation occurs, or if condition worsens or persists for > 3 days, discontinue use and consult a physician.

May cause mild stinging or temporary blurred vision.

Some of these products should not be used with soft contact lenses.

Administration and Dosage:

Instill 1 to 2 drops into eye(s) 3 or 4 times daily, as needed.

otc	**Adsorbotear** (Alcon)	**Solution:** 0.4% hydroxyethylcellulose, 1.67% povidone, water soluble polymers, 0.004% thimerosal, 0.1% EDTA	In 15 ml.
otc	**Akwa Tears** (Akorn)	**Solution:** 0.01% benzalkonium Cl, 1.4% polyvinyl alcohol, sodium phosphate, EDTA, NaCl	In 15 ml.
otc	**Tear Drop** (Parmed)	**Solution:** Polyvinyl alcohol, NaCl, EDTA, 0.01% benzalkonium Cl	In 15 ml.
otc	**Puralube Tears** (Fougera)	**Solution:** 1% polyvinyl alcohol, 1% PEG 400, EDTA, benzalkonium Cl	In 15 ml.
otc	**Artificial Tears** (Various, eg, Parmed, Rugby, Schein)	**Solution:** 0.01% benzalkonium chloride. May also contain EDTA, NaCl, polyvinyl alcohol, hydroxypropyl methylcellulose	In 15 and 30 ml.
otc	**Teargen** (Goldline)	**Solution:** 0.01% benzalkonium Cl, EDTA, NaCl, polyvinyl alcohol	In 15 ml.
otc	**AquaSite** (Ciba Vision)	**Solution:** 0.2% PEG-400, 0.1% dextran 70, polycarbophil, NaCl, EDTA, sodium hydroxide	Preservative free. In 0.6 ml (single-use 24s) and 15 ml.
otc	**Artificial Tears Plus** (Various, eg, Rugby, Steris)	**Solution:** 1.4% polyvinyl alcohol, 0.6% povidone, 0.5% chlorobutanol, NaCl	In 15 ml.
otc	**Cellufresh** (Allergan)	**Solution:** 0.5% carboxymethylcellulose sodium, NaCl	Preservative free. In 0.3 ml (single-use 4s and 30s).
otc	**Celluvisc** (Allergan)	**Solution:** 1% carboxymethylcellulose, NaCl, KCl, sodium lactate	Preservative free. In 0.3 ml (UD 30s).
otc	**Comfort Tears** (Pilkington/Barnes Hind)	**Solution:** Hydroxyethylcellulose, 0.005% benzalkonium chloride, 0.02% EDTA	In 15 ml.
otc	**Dakrina** (Dakryon)	**Solution:** Povidone, polyvinyl alcohol, antitoxidant retinyl palmitate, boric acid, 0.09% EDTA, 0.001% WSCP, NaCl, KCl	In 15 ml.
otc	**Dry Eye Therapy** (Bausch & Lomb)	**Solution:** 0.3% glycerin, NaCl, KCl, sodium citrate, sodium phosphate	Preservative free. In 0.3 ml (UD 32s).
otc	**Dry Eyes** (Bausch & Lomb)	**Solution:** 1.4% polyvinyl alcohol, 0.01% benzalkonium chloride, sodium phosphate, EDTA, NaCl	In 15 ml.
otc	**Dwelle** (Dakryon)	**Solution:** 0.09% EDTA, NaCl, KCl, boric acid, povidone, 0.001% NPX	In 15 ml.

ARTIFICIAL TEAR SOLUTIONS

otc	**Eye-Lube-A** (Optopics)	**Solution:** 0.25% glycerin, EDTA, sodium chloride, benzalkonium Cl	In 15 ml.
otc	**HypoTears** (Ciba Vision)	**Solution:** 1% polyvinyl alcohol, PEG-400, 1% dextrose, 0.01% benzalkonium Cl, EDTA	In 15 and 30 ml.
otc	**HypoTears PF** (Ciba Vision)	**Solution:** 1% polyvinyl alcohol, PEG-400, 1% dextrose, EDTA	Preservative free. In 0.6 ml (30s).
otc	**Ultra Tears** (Alcon)	**Solution:** 1% hydroxypropyl methylcellulose 2910, 0.01% benzalkonium chloride, NaCl	In 15 ml.
otc	**Isopto Plain** (Alcon)	**Solution:** 0.5% hydroxypropyl methylcellulose 2910, 0.01% benzalkonium chloride, NaCl, sodium phosphate, sodium citrate	In 15 ml Drop-Tainers.
otc	**Isopto Tears** (Alcon)		In 15 and 30 ml.
otc	**Just Tears** (Blairex)	**Solution:** Benzalkonium chloride, EDTA, 1.4% polyvinyl alcohol, NaCl, KCl	In 15 ml.
otc	**Liquifilm Tears** (Allergan)	**Solution:** 1.4% polyvinyl alcohol, 0.5% chlorobutanol, NaCl	In 15 and 30 ml.
otc	**LubriTears** (Bausch & Lomb)	**Solution:** 0.3% hydroxypropyl methylcellulose 2906, 0.1% dextran 70, EDTA, KCl, NaCl, 0.01% benzalkonium chloride	In 15 ml.
otc	**Moisture Drops** (Bausch & Lomb)	**Solution:** 0.5% hydroxypropyl methylcellulose, 0.1% povidone, 0.2% glycerin, 0.01% benzalkonium chloride, EDTA, NaCl, boric acid, KCl, sodium borate	In 15 and 30 ml.
otc	**Murine** (Ross)	**Solution:** 0.5% polyvinyl alcohol, 0.6% povidone, benzalkonium chloride, dextrose, EDTA, NaCl, sodium bicarbonate, sodium phosphate	In 15 and 30 ml.
otc	**Murocel** (Bausch & Lomb)	**Solution:** 1% methylcellulose, propylene glycol, NaCl, 0.046% methylparaben, 0.02% propylparaben, boric acid, sodium borate	In 15 ml.
otc	**Nature's Tears** (Rugby)	**Solution:** 0.4% hydroxypropyl methylcellulose 2910, KCl, NaCl, sodium phosphate, 0.01% benzalkonium Cl, EDTA	In 15 ml.
otc	**Nu-Tears** (Optopics)	**Solution:** 1.4% polyvinyl alcohol, EDTA, sodium chloride, benzalkonium chloride, KCl	In 15 ml.
otc	**Nu-Tears II** (Optopics)	**Solution:** 1% polyvinyl alcohol, 1% PEG-400, EDTA, benzalkonium chloride	In 15 ml.
otc	**Refresh** (Allergan)	**Solution:** 1.4% polyvinyl alcohol, 0.6% povidone, NaCl	Preservative free. In 0.3 ml (UD 30s, 50s).
otc	**Refresh Plus** (Allergan)	**Solution:** 0.5% carboxymethylcellulose sodium, KCl, NaCl	Preservative free. In 0.3 ml single-use containers (30s and 50s).
otc	**TearGard** (Lee)	**Solution:** 0.25% sorbic acid, 0.1% EDTA, hydroxyethylcellulose	Thimerosal free. In 15 ml.
otc	**Tearisol** (Iolab)	**Solution:** 0.5% hydroxypropyl methylcellulose, 0.01% benzalkonium chloride, EDTA, boric acid, KCl	In 15 ml.
otc	**OcuCoat** (Storz Ophthalmics)	**Solution:** 0.1% dextran 70, 0.8% hydroxypropyl methylcellulose, sodium phosphate, KCl, NaCl, 0.01% benzalkonium chloride, dextrose	In 15 ml.
otc	**OcuCoat PF** (Storz Ophthalmics)	**Solution:** 0.1% dextran 70, 0.8% hydroxypropyl methylcellulose, sodium phosphate, KCl, NaCl, dextrose	Preservative free. In 0.5 ml single-dose containers (28s).

ARTIFICIAL TEAR SOLUTIONS

otc	**Tears Naturale** (Alcon)	**Solution:** 0.1% dextran 70, 0.01% benzalkonium chloride, 0.3% hydroxypropyl methylcellulose, NaCl, EDTA, hydrochloric acid, sodium hydroxide, KCl	In 15 and 30 ml.
otc	**Tears Naturale Free** (Alcon)	**Solution:** 0.3% hydroxypropyl methylcellulose 2910, 0.1% dextran 70, NaCl, KCl, sodium borate	Preservative free. In 0.6 ml single-use containers.
otc	**Tears Naturale II** (Alcon)	**Solution:** 0.1% dextran 70, 0.3% hydroxypropyl methylcellulose 2910, 0.001% polyquaternium-1, NaCl, KCl, sodium borate	In 15 and 30 ml Drop-Tainers.
otc	**Tears Plus** (Allergan)	**Solution:** 1.4% polyvinyl alcohol, NaCl, 0.6% povidone, 0.5% chlorobutanol	In 15 and 30 ml.
otc	**Tears Renewed** (Akorn)	**Solution:** 0.01% benzalkonium chloride, EDTA, 0.1% dextran 70, NaCl, 0.3% hydroxypropyl methylcellulose 2906	In 2, 15 and 30 ml.
otc	**Viva-Drops** (Vision Pharm)	**Solution:** Polysorbate 80, sodium chloride, EDTA, retinyl palmitate, mannitol, sodium citrate, pyruvate	Preservative free. In 10 and 15 ml.
otc	**Bion Tears** (Alcon)	**Solution:** 0.1% dextran 70, 0.3% hydroxypropyl methylcellulose 2910, NaCl, KCl, sodium bicarbonate	Preservative free. In single-use 0.45 ml containers (28s).

ARTIFICIAL TEAR INSERT

Actions:

Pharmacology: The hydroxypropyl cellulose insert acts to stabilize and thicken the precorneal tear film and prolong tear film breakup time, which is usually accelerated in patients with dry eye states. The insert also acts to lubricate and protect the eye.

Signs and symptoms resulting from moderate to severe dry eye syndromes, such as conjunctival hyperemia, corneal and conjunctival staining with rose bengal, exudation, itching, burning, foreign body sensation, smarting, photophobia, dryness and blurred or cloudy vision are reduced. Progressive visual deterioration may be retarded, halted or sometimes reversed.

Pharmacokinetics: Hydroxypropyl cellulose is a physiologically inert substance. Dissolution studies in rabbits showed that the inserts became softer within 1 hour after they were placed in the conjunctival sac. Most dissolved completely in 14 to 18 hours; with a single exception, all had disappeared by 24 hours after insertion. Similar dissolution of inserts was observed during prolonged use (up to 54 weeks).

Clinical trials: In a multicenter crossover study, the 5 mg insert administered into the inferior cul-de-sac once a day during the waking hours was compared to artificial tears used ≥ 4 times daily. There was a prolongation of tear film breakup time and a decrease in foreign body sensation associated with dry eye syndrome in patients during treatment with inserts as compared to artificial tears. Improvement was greater in most patients who used the inserts.

Indications:

Dry eye syndromes, moderate to severe: Keratoconjunctivitis sicca (especially in patients who remain symptomatic after an adequate trial of artificial tear solutions); exposure keratitis; decreased corneal sensitivity; recurrent corneal erosions.

Contraindications:

Hypersensitivity to hydroxypropyl cellulose.

Adverse Reactions:

The following have occurred, but in most instances were mild and transient: Transient blurring of vision; ocular discomfort or irritation; matting or stickiness of eyelashes; photophobia; hypersensitivity; edema of the eyelids; hyperemia.

Patient Information:

May produce transient blurring of vision; exercise caution while operating hazardous machinery or driving a motor vehicle.

If improperly placed in the inferior cul-de-sac, corneal abrasion may result. Patient should practice insertion and removal in physician's office until proficiency is achieved.

Illustrated instructions are included in each package.

If symptoms worsen, remove insert and notify physician.

Administration and Dosage:

Once daily, inserted into inferior cul-de-sac beneath the base of the tarsus, not in apposition to the cornea nor beneath the eyelid at the level of the tarsal plate. Individual patients may require twice-daily use for optimal results.

If not properly positioned, the insert will be expelled into the interpalpebral fissure, and may cause symptoms of a foreign body.

Occasionally, the insert is inadvertently expelled from the eye, especially in patients with shallow conjunctival fornices. Caution the patient against rubbing the eye(s), especially upon awakening, so as not to dislodge or expel the insert. If required, another insert may be used. If transient blurred vision develops, the patient may want to remove the insert a few hours after insertion to avoid this.

Rx	**Lacrisert** (Merck)	**Insert**: 5 mg hydroxpropyl cellulose	Preservative free. In 60s with applicator.

OCULAR LUBRICANTS

Actions:

Pharmacology: These products serve as lubricants and emollients.

Indications:

Ophthalmic lubrication: Protection and lubrication of the eye.

Contraindications:

Hypersensitivity to any component of the products.

Patient Information:

Do not touch tube tip to any surface since this may contaminate the product.

Do not use with contact lenses.

If eye pain, vision changes or continued redness or irritation occurs, or if the condition worsens or persists for > 72 hours, discontinue use and contact a physician.

Refer to the Topical Ophthalmics introduction for more complete information.

Administration and Dosage:

Pull down the lower lid of affected eye(s) and apply a small amount (0.25 inch) of ointment to the inside of the eyelid.

Storage: Store at room temperature 15° to 30°C (59° to 86°F). Store away from heat.

otc	**Akwa Tears** (Akorn)	**Ointment:** White petrolatum, mineral oil, lanolin	Preservative free. In 3.5 g.
otc	**Dry Eyes** (Bausch & Lomb)		Preservative free. In 3.5 g.
otc	**Artificial Tears** (Rugby)	**Ointment:** White petrolatum, anhydrous liquid lanolin, mineral oil	In 3.5 g.
otc	**Duratears Naturale** (Alcon)		Preservative free. In 3.5 g.
otc	**LubriTears** (Bausch & Lomb)	**Ointment:** White petrolatum, mineral oil, lanolin, 0.5% chlorobutanol	In 3.5 g.
otc	**HypoTears** (Ciba Vision)	**Ointment:** White petrolatum, light mineral oil	Preservative and lanolin free. In 3.5 g.
otc	**Puralube** (Fougera)		In 3.5 g.
otc	**Tears Renewed** (Akorn)		Preservative and lanolin free. In 3.5 g.
otc	**Stye** (Del Pharm)	**Ointment:** 55% white petrolatum, 32% mineral oil, boric acid, stearic acid, wheat germ oil	In 3.5 g.
otc	**Lacri-Lube NP** (Allergan)	**Ointment:** 55.5% white petrolatum, 42.5% mineral oil, 2% petrolatum/lanolin alcohol	Preservative free. In 0.7 g (UD 24s).
otc	**Lacri-Lube S.O.P.** (Allergan)	**Ointment:** 56.8% white petrolatum, 42.5% mineral oil, chlorobutanol, lanolin alcohols	In 3.5 and 7 g.
otc	**Refresh PM** (Allergan)	**Ointment:** 56.8% white petrolatum, 41.5% mineral oil, lanolin alcohols, sodium chloride	Preservative free. In 3.5 g.

PUNCTAL PLUGS

Actions:

Pharmacology: These flexible silicone plugs partially block the puncta and horizontal canaliculus and eliminate tear loss by this route.

Indications:

Keratitis sicca (dry eye): Treatment of symptoms of dry eye (eg, redness, burning, reflex tearing, itching, foreign body sensation); after eye surgery to prevent complications due to dry eye; to enhance the efficacy of ocular medications; for patients experiencing dry eye-related contact lens problems.

Contraindications:

Hypersensitivity to silicone; eye infection.

Precautions:

Injection path: If injecting an anesthetic agent in the region of the canaliculus, maintain approximately a 5 mm distance between the injection path and the angular vessels.

Dilation: Do not dilate punctal opening > 1.2 mm.

Irritation: If irritation caused by plug insertion persists longer than several days, reexamine the patient and consider plug removal.

Patient Information:

Do not press fingers on or near the eyelid. Use a cotton-tipped swab to remove "sleep" from the corner of eyes.

Do not attempt to replace a plug that has fallen out.

Relief may not occur immediately after insertion; some discomfort and tearing may occur for a few days.

Administration and Dosage:

Plugs must be inserted by a physician or doctor of optometry.

Rx	**Herrick Lacrimal Plug** (Lacrimedics)	**Plug**: Silicone plug	In 0.3 and 0.5 mm sizes (packs of 2 plugs).
Rx	**Punctum Plug** (Eagle Vision)		In 0.5, 0.6, 0.7 and 0.8 mm sizes (packs of 2 plugs). Contains one inserter tool.

COLLAGEN IMPLANTS

Actions:

Pharmacology: These absorbable implants partially block the puncta and horizontal canaliculus, eliminating tear loss by this route.

Indications:

Dry eyes: For the relief of dry eyes and secondary abnormalities such as conjunctivitis, corneal ulcer, pterygium, blepharitis, keratitis, red lid margins, recurrent chalazion, recurrent corneal erosion, filamentary keratitis and other noninfectious external eye diseases; to enhance the effect of ocular medications; treatment of symptoms of dry eye (eg, redness, burning, reflex tearing, itching, foreign body sensation); after eye surgery to prevent complications; for patients experiencing dry eye-related contact lens problems.

Contraindications:

Tearing secondary to chronic dacryocystitis with mucopurulent discharge; allergy to bovine collagen; inflammation of eyelid; epiphoria.

Patient Information:

Relief may not occur immediately after insertion.

No removal is necessary; implants dissolve within 7 to 10 days.

Reexamination is usually required within 14 days.

Successful treatment may indicate a need for permanent treatment (eg, nondissolvable silicone plugs).

Administration and Dosage:

Implants must be inserted by a physician or doctor of optometry. Placement of implants in all four canaliculi is recommended to prevent a false negative response.

Rx	**Collagen Implant** (Lacrimedics)	**Implant**: Collagen implant	In 0.2, 0.3, 0.4, 0.5 and 0.6 mm sizes (72s).
Rx	**Temporary Punctal/ Canalicular Collagen Implant** (Eagle Vision)		In 0.2, 0.3, 0.4, 0.5 and 0.6 mm sizes (72s).

Ophthalmic Irrigation Solutions

INTRAOCULAR IRRIGATING SOLUTIONS

Actions:

Pharmacology: Sterile irrigating solution is a sterile physiological balanced salt solution, each ml containing sodium chloride 0.64%, potassium chloride 0.075%, calcium chloride dihydrate 0.048%, magnesium chloride hexahydrate 0.03%, sodium acetate trihydrate 0.39%, sodium citrate dihydrate 0.17%, sodium hydroxide or hydrochloric acid (to adjust pH) and water. This solution is isotonic to ocular tissue and contains electrolytes required for normal cellular metabolic functions.

Indications:

Irrigation: For irrigation during various surgical procedures of the eyes. Some products may also be used for the ears, nose and throat (consult specific product labeling).

Warnings:

Route of administration: Not for injection or IV infusion. Use aseptic technique only.

Precautions:

Preservative-free solutions: Do not use for more than one patient.

Corneal clouding and edema have been reported following ocular surgery in which balanced salt solution was used as an irrigating solution. Take appropriate measures to minimize trauma to the cornea and other ocular tissues.

Concomitant medication: Addition of any medication to balanced salt solution may result in damage to intraocular tissue.

Diabetics: Studies suggest that intraocular irrigating solutions which are iso-osmotic with normal aqueous fluids should be used with caution in diabetic patients undergoing vitrectomy as intraoperative lens changes have been observed.

Adverse Reactions:

When corneal endothelium is abnormal, irrigation or any other trauma may result in bullous keratopathy. Postoperative inflammatory reactions and corneal edema and decompensation have occurred. Relationship to balanced salt solution is not established.

Administration and Dosage:

Use balanced salt solution according to the established practices for each surgical procedure. Follow the manufacturer directions for the particular administration set to be used. For products with separate solutions for reconstitution, never use either Part I or Part II alone; this could result in damage to the eye.

Storage/Stability: Store at 8° to 30°C (46° to 86°F). Avoid excessive heat. Do not freeze. Discard prepared solution after 6 hours. Do not use if cloudy or if seal or packaging is damaged. Do not use reconstituted solution if it is discolored or contains a precipitate.

Rx	**Balanced Salt Solution** (Various, eg, Akorn)	**Solution:** 0.64% NaCl, 0.075% KCl, 0.03% magnesium chloride, 0.048% calcium chloride, 0.39% sodium acetate, 0.17% sodium citrate and sodium hydroxide or hydrochloric acid	In 18 and 500 ml.
Rx	**AMO Endosol** (Allergan)		Preservative free. In 500 ml.
Rx	**BSS** (Alcon)		Preservative free. In 15, 30, 250 and 500 ml.
Rx	**Iocare Balanced Salt** (Ciba Vision)		Preservative free. In 15 ml.
Rx	**AMO Endosol Extra** (Allergan)	**Solution:** Mix aseptically just prior to use. **Part** I: 7.14 mg NaCl, 0.38 mg KCl, 0.154 mg calcium chloride dihydrate, 0.2 mg magnesium chloride hexahydrate, 0.92 mg dextrose, hydrochloric acid or sodium hydroxide/ml	Preservative free. In 515 ml.
		Part II: 1081 mg sodium bicarbonate, 216 mg dibasic sodium phosphate (anhydrous) and 95 mg glutathione disulfide (oxidized glutathione)/vial	Preservative free. In 60 ml.

Ophthalmic Irrigation Solutions

INTRAOCULAR IRRIGATING SOLUTIONS

Rx	**BSS Plus** (Alcon)	**Solution:** Mix aseptically just prior to use. **Part I:** 7.44 mg NaCl, 0.395 mg KCl, 0.433 mg dibasic sodium phosphate, 2.19 mg sodium bicarbonate, hydrochloric acid or sodium hydroxide/ml	Preservative free. In 240 ml.
		Part II: 3.85 mg calcium chloride dihydrate, 5 mg magnesium chloride hexahydrate, 23 mg dextrose, 4.6 mg glutathione disulfide/ml	Preservative free. In 10 ml.
Rx	**B-Salt Forte** (Akorn)	**Solution:** Mix aseptically just prior to use. **Part I:** 7.14 mg NaCl, 0.38 mg KCl, 0.154 mg calcium chloride dihydrate, 0.2 mg magnesium chloride hexahydrate, 0.92 mg dextrose, hydrochloric acid or sodium hydroxide/ml	Preservative free. In 515 ml.
		Part II: 1081 mg sodium bicarbonate, 216 mg dibasic sodium phosphate (anhydrous) and 95 mg glutathione disulfide (oxidized glutathione)/vial	Preservative free. In 60 ml.

EXTRAOCULAR IRRIGATING SOLUTIONS

Actions:

Pharmacology: These sterile isotonic solutions are for general ophthalmic use. Office uses include irrigating procedures following tonometry, gonioscopy, foreign body removal or use of fluorescein; they are also used to soothe and cleanse the eye. Because these solutions have a short contact time with the eye, they do not need to provide nutrients to cells. Unlike intraocular irrigants, irrigants for extraocular use contain preservatives which prevent bacteriostatic contamination. However, the preservatives are exceedingly toxic to the corneal endothelium and intraocular use of extraocular irrigating fluids is contraindicated.

Indications:

Irrigation: For irrigating the eye to help relieve irritation by removing loose foreign material, air pollutants (smog or pollen) or chlorinated water.

Contraindications:

Hypersensitivity to any component of the formulation; as a saline solution for rinsing and soaking contact lenses; injection or intraocular surgery.

Patient Information:

If you experience eye pain, changes in vision, continued redness or irritation of the eye, or if the condition worsens or persists, consult a doctor.

Obtain immediate medical treatment for all open wounds in or near the eyes.

If solution changes color or becomes cloudy, do not use. Do not use these products with contact lenses.

To avoid contamination, do not touch tip of the container to any surface. Replace cap after using.

Administration and Dosage:

Solution: Flush the affected eye(s) as needed, controlling the rate of flow of solution by pressure on the bottle.

Eyecup: Fill the sterile eyecup halfway with eye wash. Apply the cup tightly to the affected eye and tilt the head backward. Open eyes wide, rotate eye and blink several times to ensure that the solution completely floods the eye. Discard the wash. Rinse the cup with clean water and repeat the procedure with the other eye, if necessary.

Rinse the eyecup before and after every use. Avoid contamination of the rim or inside surfaces of the cup.

Storage: If solution changes color or becomes cloudy, do not use.

Ophthalmic Irrigation Solutions

EXTRAOCULAR IRRIGATING SOLUTIONS

otc	**AK-Rinse** (Akorn)	**Solution:** Sodium carbonbate, KCl, boric acid, EDTA, 0.01% benzalkonium Cl	In 30 and 118 ml.
otc	**Blinx** (Akorn)	**Solution:** NaCl, KCl, sodium phosphate, 0.005% benzalkonium Cl, 0.02% EDTA	In 120 ml.
otc	**Collyrium for Fresh Eyes Wash** (Wyeth-Ayerst)	**Solution:** Boric acid, sodium borate, benzalkonium Cl	In 120 ml.
otc	**Dacriose** (Ciba Vision)	**Solution:** NaCl, KCl, sodium phosphate, sodium hydroxide, 0.01% benzalkonium Cl, EDTA	In 15 and 120 ml.
otc	**Eye Stream** (Alcon)	**Solution:** 0.64% NaCl, 0.075% KCl, 0.03% magnesium Cl hexahydrate, 0.048% calcium Cl dihydrate, 0.39% sodium acetate trihydrate, 0.17% sodium citrate dihydrate, 0.013% benzalkonium Cl	In 30 and 118 ml.
otc	**Eye Wash** (Bausch & Lomb)	**Solution:** Boric acid, KCl, EDTA, sodium carbonate, 0.01% benzalkonium Cl	In 118 ml.
otc	**Eye Wash** (Goldline)	**Solution:** Boric acid, KCl, EDTA, anhydrous sodium carbonate, 0.01% benzalkonium Cl	In 118 ml.
otc	**Eye Wash** (Lavoptik)	**Solution:** 0.49% NaCl, 0.4% sodium biphosphate, 0.45% sodium phosphate, 0.005% benzalkonium Cl	In 180 ml with eyecup.
otc	**Eye Irrigating Wash** (Roberts Hauck)	**Solution:** Boric acid, KCl, sodium carbonate, EDTA, 0.01% benzalkonium Cl	In 120 ml.
otc	**Eye Irrigating Solution** (Rugby)	**Solution:** NaCl, mono- and dibasic sodium phosphate, benzalkonium Cl, EDTA	In 118 ml.
otc	**Irrigate Eye Wash** (Optopics)	**Solution:** NaCl, mono- and dibasic sodium phosphate, benzalkonium Cl, EDTA	In 118 ml.
otc	**Optigene** (Pfeiffer)	**Solution:** NaCl, mono- and dibasic sodium phosphate, EDTA, benzalkonium Cl	In 118 ml.
otc	**Visual-Eyes** (Optopics)	**Solution:** NaCl, mono- and dibasic sodium phosphate, benzalkonium Cl, EDTA	In 120 ml.

Hyperosmolar Preparations

SODIUM CHLORIDE, HYPERTONIC

Actions:

Pharmacology: A hypertonic (hyperosmolar) solution exerts an osmotic gradient greater than that present in the body tissues and fluids, so that water is drawn from the body tissues and fluids across semipermeable membranes. Applied topically to the eye, a hypertonicity agent creates an osmotic gradient which draws water out of the cornea.

Indications:

Corneal edema: Temporary relief.

Contraindications:

Hypersensitivity to any component of the product.

Adverse Reactions:

May cause temporary burning and irritation upon instillation.

Patient Information:

To avoid contamination, do not touch tip of container to any surface. Replace cap after using.

Do not use this product except under the advice and supervision of a physician. If you experience eye pain, changes in vision, continued redness or irritation of the eye or if the condition worsens or persists, discontinue use and consult a physician.

Product may cause temporary burning and irritation when instilled into the eye.

If solution changes color or becomes cloudy, do not use.

Administration and Dosage:

Solution: Instill 1 or 2 drops in affected eye(s) every 3 or 4 hours, or as directed.

Ointment: Pull down lower eyelid of the affected eye(s) and apply a small amount (≈ ¼ inch) of ointment to the inside of the affected eye(s) every 3 or 4 hours, or as directed.

Storage: Store at 8° to 30°C (46° to 86°F). Keep tightly closed. Protect from light.

otc	**Adsorbonac** (Alcon)	**Solution:** 2%	In 15 ml.[1]
otc	**Muro 128** (Bausch & Lomb)		In 15 ml.[2]
otc	**Adsorbonac** (Alcon)	**Solution:** 5%	In 15 ml.[1]
otc	**AK-NaCl** (Akorn)		In 15 ml.[3]
otc	**Muro 128** (Bausch & Lomb)		In 15 and 30 ml.[4]
otc	**Muroptic-5** (Optopics)		In 15 ml.[5]
otc	**AK-NaCl** (Akorn)	**Ointment:** 5%	Preservative free. In 3.5 g.[6]
otc	**Muro 128** (Bausch & Lomb)		In 3.5 g single and twin packs.[7]

[1] With povidone, hydroxyethylcellulose 2910, PEG-90M, poloxamer 188, 0.004% thimerosal, EDTA.
[2] With hydroxypropyl methylcellulose 2906, 0.046% methylparaben, 0.02% propylparaben, propylene glycol, boric acid.
[3] With hydroxypropyl methylcellulose, propylene glycol, 0.023% methylparaben, 0.01% propylparaben, boric acid.
[4] Boric acid, hydroxypropyl methylcellulose 2910, propylene glycol, 0.023% methylparaben, 0.01% propylparaben.
[5] With benzalkonium chloride, EDTA, polyvinyl alcohol, propylene glycol.
[6] With mineral oil, white petrolatum, lanolin oil.
[7] With mineral oil, white petrolatum, lanolin.

Hyperosmolar Preparations

GLYCERIN, TOPICAL

Actions:

Pharmacology: Glycerin ophthalmic solution is used only for topical application to the cornea. By virtue of its osmotic action (attraction of water through the semipermeable corneal epithelium), it promptly reduces edema and causes clearing of corneal haze. The action is transient and therefore is used primarily for diagnostic purposes.

Indications:

Edematous cornea: To clear an edematous cornea in order to facilitate ophthalmoscopic and gonioscopic examination in acute glaucoma, bullous keratitis and Fuchs' endothelial dystrophy.

Contraindications:

Hypersensitivity to any component of the product.

Warnings:

Pregnancy: Category C. Safety for use during pregnancy has not been established. Use only when clearly needed.

Lactation: It is not known whether glycerin is excreted in breast milk. Exercise caution when administering to a nursing mother.

Children: Safety and efficacy for use in children have not been established.

Precautions:

Irritation: Because glycerin is an irritant and may cause pain, instill a local anesthetic before use.

Adverse Reactions:

Some pain or irritation may occur upon instillation.

Administration and Dosage:

Instill 1 or 2 drops prior to examination. In gonioscopy of an edematous cornea, additional glycerin may be used as a lubricant.

Storage: Keep bottle tightly closed. Store at room temperature 25°C (77°F). Discard product 6 months after dropper is first placed in the drug solution.

Rx	**Ophthalgan** (Wyeth-Ayerst)	**Solution:** Glycerin	0.55% chlorobutanol. In 7.5 ml.

GLUCOSE, TOPICAL

Indications:

Corneal edema: Topical osmotherapy for reducing corneal edema.

Contraindications:

Hypersensitivity to any component of the product.

Precautions:

Irritation: If irritation develops, discontinue use.

Administration and Dosage:

May be used 2 to 6 times daily.

Depress lower lid with index finger while looking upward. Introduce a small amount of ointment behind depressed eyelid into conjunctival sac. Close and open eyes 2 times. Wipe off excess ointment. If eyelids are sticky, clean them before each application with a pledget of cotton and lukewarm boiled water.

Rx	**Glucose-40** (Ciba Vision)	**Ointment:** 40%	White petrolatum, anhydrous lanolin, parabens. In 3.5 g.

CONTACT LENS PRODUCTS

Contact lens guidelines: Inadequate cleaning can lead to lens discoloration and lens surface buildup of protein, lipids, minerals and other environmental contaminants, which can contribute to giant papillary conjunctivitis (GPC), superficial punctate keratitis (SPK) and corneal abrasion. Irregular contact lens disinfection can cause severe ocular infection.

Contact Lens Guidelines
• Proper contact lens care will increase success and decrease complications.
• Cleaning does not disinfect lenses.
• Disinfecting does not clean lenses.
• Enzyme solutions are not a substitute for disinfection.
• Wash and rinse hands thoroughly before handling contact lenses.
• Do not insert contact lenses if eyes are red or irritated. If eyes become painful or vision worsens while wearing lenses, remove lenses and consult an eye-care practitioner immediately.
• Do not wear contact lenses while sleeping unless they have been prescribed for extended wear.
• For soft lens care, use only products designed for soft lenses.
• For rigid lens care, use only products designed for rigid lenses.
• Do not change or substitute products from a different manufacturer without consulting a doctor.
• Do not use non-sterile, home-prepared saline solutions unless recommended by your eye-care practitioner.
• Always follow label directions or doctor's recommendations.
• Do not store lenses in tap water.
• After removal, lenses must be cleaned, rinsed and disinfected before wearing again.
• Lenses that are stored > 12 hours may again require cleaning, rinsing and disinfection; consult package insert or eye care practitioner.
• Never use saliva to wet contact lenses.
• Keep lens care products out of the reach of children.
• Do not instill topical medications while contact lenses are being worn unless directed by a doctor.
• Do not get cosmetic lotions, creams or sprays in your eyes or on lenses. It is best to put on lenses before putting on makeup and remove them before removing makeup. Water-based cosmetics are less likely to damage lenses than oil-based products.
• Schedule and keep follow-up appointments with your eye-care practitioner (approximately every 6 to 12 months or as recommended).
• Contact lenses wear out with time and should be replaced regularly. Throw away disposable lenses after the recommended wearing period.
• Check with your eye-care practitioner regarding wearing lenses during sports activities.

Contact lens materials: Three types of contact lenses are manufactured: Hard, rigid gas permeable and soft.

Hard contact lenses: Hard contact lenses are made from polymethylmethacrylate (PMMA). PMMA does not transmit the oxygen needed for normal corneal integrity. Hard contact lenses have caused chronic corneal edema, corneal distortion, edematous corneal formations, spectacle blur, polymegathism and corneal abrasions. Because of these ocular complications, hard lenses are seldom the lens of choice for a new contact lens patient. Less than 1% of the contact lens population wear hard contact lenses.

Rigid gas permeable lenses: Approximately 20% of contact lens patients wear rigid gas permeable (RGP) lenses. These lenses are oxygen permeable; therefore, the RGP patient does not have the severe physiological complications of the hard lens patient. Several lens polymers with a high degree of oxygen permeability have been approved by the FDA for extended wear. RGP lenses provide the patient with good vision, durability and easy care.

CONTACT LENS PRODUCTS

Soft contact lenses: Soft contact lenses are made of hydroxyethylmethacrylate (HEMA), a plastic compound. The first soft lens was marketed in the US in 1971. Today, most soft lenses manufactured from HEMA contain 30% to 50% water.

Daily wear soft contact lenses are designed to be worn all day (12 to 14 hours), but must be removed nightly to be cleaned and disinfected. Extended wear soft lenses can be worn for ≥ 24 hours. The FDA and most eye care practitioners recommend a maximum wearing period of 7 days. The lenses must then be removed overnight for cleaning and disinfection. The major advantage of extended wear lenses is convenience. Daily wear soft lenses provide the same level of comfort and vision as extended wear soft lenses. The popularity of extended wear soft lenses has decreased in the last few years due to the increased risk of infection.

Disposable soft lenses: Disposable soft lenses are designed to eliminate the complications of lens deposits by planned lens replacement. Lens deposits can interfere with vision, cause corneal irritation and contribute to ocular infection. In addition, disposable lenses offer the patient the convenience of reduced lens care.

Disposable lenses are approved for daily wear and extended wear. It is recommended that the lenses be discarded after a specified length of time; the physician will prescribe the replacement schedule for each patient. If a disposable lens is not discarded immediately after lens removal, it should be cleaned with a surfactant cleaner and stored in a disinfection solution.

Contact Lens Care Products: Products for use with contact lenses possess the same general characteristics of all ophthalmic products (eg, sterile, isotonic, free of particulate matter). Additionally, product formulations contain various components to achieve specific goals of contact lens care.

Although all contact lenses serve similar functions in correcting visual defects, each distinct type of lens material requires a unique lens care program. In selecting appropriate lens care solutions, it is essential to correctly identify the type of lens the patient is using.

Hard and rigid gas permeable lenses: Similar lens care is used for the hard and RGP lenses. Products include *wetting/soaking/disinfecting solutions*, cleaning agents and rewetting solutions.

When a rigid contact lens is removed from the eye, it may be covered with lipids, proteins, eye makeup and other debris. After removal, immediately clean the lens with a *surfactant cleaner*. Improper cleaning can contribute to a lens surface buildup that can interfere with vision and potentially cause corneal irritation.

Soak rigid lenses overnight in a *wetting/soaking/disinfecting solution*. This solution has four major functions:

1. To enhance the lens surface wettability
2. To maintain the lens hydration similar to that achieved during daily contact lens wear
3. To disinfect the lens
4. To act as a mechanical buffer between the lens and the cornea

It is not uncommon for a rigid lens patient to experience dryness after several hours of wear. This is especially true with RGP lens patients because of the hydrophobic nature of the lens material. *Rewetting drops* can provide temporary relief by rinsing some debris off the lens surface and rewetting the eye and the lens.

Many clinicians routinely recommend the weekly use of an enzyme (papain) cleaner with RGP lenses. This weekly cleaning process is very effective in removing protein deposits from the lens surface. A protein film on an RGP lens can decrease vision and cause giant papillary conjunctivitis.

Soft contact lenses: Soft contact lens care systems are designed to clean, disinfect and rewet the lenses. The first step is proper cleaning. Cleaning the lens gently in the palm of the hand with a *daily surfactant cleaner* will remove fresh lipids, oils and other environmental debris. Clean soft lenses thoroughly with a surfactant cleaner each time a lens is removed. After cleaning the lens, thoroughly rinse with a soft lens *rinsing/storage solution*. All *rinsing/storage solutions* contain 0.9% saline. Some are available with no preservatives in unit-dose vials or aerosol containers. Other saline solutions contain preservatives to decrease microorganism growth. Discourage use of saline made with salt tablets because of risk of contamination and infection (see Precautions).

Enzymatic cleaners are generally used on a weekly basis. They more effectively remove protein deposits than surfactant cleaners because they contain proteolytic enzymes (papain, pancreatin or subtilisin). Most enzymes are dissolved directly in saline, but the subtilisin enzyme tablet can be dissolved in a hydrogen peroxide disinfection solution.

CONTACT LENS PRODUCTS

Disinfection: Disinfection is the most important step in soft lens care. Disinfection is achieved by using a thermal (heat) or chemical (cold) system.

Thermal disinfection was the first system approved for soft contact lenses. A heat unit designed for soft lenses is used for 10 min at 80°C (176°F). This procedure will kill most microorganisms that are dangerous to the eye. Recently, *Acanthamoeba* keratitis has become a concern to many clinicians. Heat disinfection is the most effective procedure to successfully kill *Acanthamoeba*; however, heat disinfection cannot be used with all soft lens material. Also, continued use of heat can shorten soft lens life.

Chemical disinfection –

Recommended Disinfection Times For Soft Lenses by Product

System	Manufacturer	Disinfection time (minimum)	Neutralization time (minimum)
Allergan Hydrocare Cleaning and Disinfecting	Allergan	4 hours	none
AOSEPT	Ciba Vision	6 hours[1]	6 hours[1]
Disinfecting Solution	Bausch & Lomb	4 hours	none
Flex-Care	Alcon	4 hours	none
MiraSept System	Alcon	10 minutes	10 minutes
Opti-Free	Alcon	4 hours	none
Opti-Soft	Alcon	4 hours	none
ReNu Multi-Purpose	Bausch & Lomb	4 hours	none
Soft Mate	Pilkington Barnes Hind	4 hours	none
Soft Mate Consept	Pilkington Barnes Hind	10 minutes	10 minutes

[1] One-step method: Disinfection and neutralization occur together for a total of 6 hours.

The original chemical soft lens disinfection systems used thimerosal with either chlorhexidine or a quaternary ammonium compound. These systems had a high incidence of sensitivity reactions. Various hydrogen peroxide care systems are currently available in the US. Most systems require two steps to achieve disinfection and hydrogen peroxide neutralization; one other system combines disinfection and neutralization in a single step. Hydrogen peroxide (3%) is very effective and can be used with all soft lens polymers. However, hydrogen peroxide care systems can be complex and expensive. Do not substitute generic peroxide solutions for solutions formulated for contact lenses. They may be contaminated with heavy metals, have different concentrations of hydrogen peroxide or use stabilizers that may discolor soft lenses.

The two newest chemical soft lens care systems introduced into the US marketplace include *Opti-Free* by Alcon and *ReNu* by Bausch & Lomb. Polyquad (polyquaternium-1) and Dymed (polyammopropylbiguamide) are the disinfection agents utilized in these care systems. Both are simple to use and may therefore increase patient compliance. These two chemical systems have become the care system of choice for the majority of soft lens patients.

Soft lens rewetting solutions permit the lubrication of the soft lens while it is on the eye. Most patients find these rewetting drops minimally effective in reducing the symptoms of dryness. Maximum relief can be achieved by removing the lens, cleaning it with a daily surfactant cleaner and thoroughly rinsing it with a rinsing/storage saline solution.

Precautions:

Acanthamoeba keratitis: Soft contact lens wearers who use homemade saline solution are at risk of developing *Acanthamoeba* keratitis, a serious and painful corneal infection that may cause blindness or impaired vision. Homemade saline solutions (nonsterile) may be used during thermal disinfection but NOT after.

Drug interference with contact lens use: Systemic medications may affect the physiology of the cornea, lids and tear system. In addition, many drugs may discolor soft contact lenses. Pharmacists and eye-care practitioners should be aware of the interaction of systemic medications and contact lenses.

CONTACT LENS PRODUCTS

Drug Interference With Contact Lens Use		
Drug	RGP/Hard/Soft Lens	Action
Anticholinergics	RGP, hard, soft	Tear volume decreased
Antihistamines, sympathomimetics	RGP, hard, soft	Tear volume decreased, blink rate decreased
Chlorthalidone	RGP, hard, soft	Causes lid or corneal edema
Clomiphene	RGP, hard, soft	Causes lid or corneal edema
Diuretics, thiazide	RGP, hard, soft	Tear volume decreased
Dopamine	soft	Discoloration of contact lenses
Epinephrine, topical	soft	Discoloration of contact lenses
Fluorescein, topical	soft	Lens absorbs the yellow dye
Hypnotics, sedatives, muscle relaxants	RGP, hard, soft	Blink rate decreased
Iodine groups	soft	Discoloration of contact lenses
Nitrofurantoin	soft	Discoloration of contact lenses
Oral contraceptives	RGP, hard, soft	Increased stickiness of mucus; corneal lid edema due to fluid retention properties of estrogens
Phenazopyridine	soft	Discoloration of contact lenses
Phenolphthalein	soft	Discoloration of contact lenses
Phenylephrine	soft	Discoloration of contact lenses
Primidone	RGP, hard, soft	Causes lid or corneal edema
Rifampin	soft	Lens absorbs drug, causing orange discoloration
Sulfasalazine	soft	Yellow staining
Tetracycline	soft	Discoloration of contact lenses
Tricyclic antidepressants	RGP, hard, soft	Tear volume decreased

Products are listed on the following pages and are grouped as follows:

Contact Lens Solutions	
Type of lens	Type of solution
Hard	Wetting Cleaning Cleaning/Soaking Wetting/Soaking Cleaning/Soaking/Wetting Rewetting
RGP	Disinfecting/Wetting/Soaking Cleaning Enzymatic Cleaners Cleaning/Disinfecting/Soaking Rewetting
Soft	Rinsing/Storage Chemical Disinfection Surfactant Cleaning Enzymatic Cleaners Rewetting

CONTACT LENS PRODUCTS

HARD (PMMA) CONTACT LENS PRODUCTS

Conventional hard lenses are made of a rigid hydrophobic polymer, polymethylmethacrylate (PMMA). For optimum comfort, these lenses require care with separate wetting, cleaning and soaking solutions. Refer to the general discussion of these products in the Contact Lens Products monograph.

WETTING SOLUTIONS, HARD LENSES

Wetting solutions contain surfactants to facilitate hydration of the hydrophobic hard lens surface. These solutions include methylcellulose and derivatives, polyvinyl alcohol, povidone, some newer polymers, preservatives and buffers. These agents increase solution viscosity and act as a physical cushioning agent between lens and cornea.

otc	**Liquifilm Wetting** (Allergan)	**Solution**: 0.004% benzalkonium chloride, EDTA, hydroxypropyl methylcellulose, NaCl, KCl, polyvinyl alcohol	In 60 ml.
otc	**Sereine** (Optikem)	**Solution**: Buffered. 0.1% EDTA, 0.01% benzalkonium chloride	In 60 and 120 ml.
otc	**Wetting Solution** (Pilkington Barnes Hind)	**Solution**: Polyvinyl alcohol, 0.004% benzalkonium chloride, 0.02% EDTA	In 60 ml.

WETTING/SOAKING SOLUTIONS, HARD LENSES

otc	**Sereine** (Optikem)	**Solution**: Buffered, isotonic. 0.1% EDTA, 0.01% benzalkonium chloride	In 120 ml.
otc	**Soac-Lens** (Alcon)	**Solution**: Buffered. 0.004% thimerosal, 0.1% EDTA, wetting agents	In 118 ml.
otc	**Wetting & Soaking** (Pilkington Barnes Hind)	**Solution**: Buffered, isotonic. 0.005% chlorhexidine gluconate, 0.02% EDTA, NaCl, octylphenoxy (oxyethylene) ethanol, povidone, polyvinyl alcohol, propylene glycol, hydroxyethylcellulose	In 120 ml.
otc	**Wet-N-Soak Plus** (Allergan)	**Solution**: Buffered, isotonic. 0.003% benzalkonium chloride, polyvinyl alcohol, EDTA	In 120 and 180 ml.

REWETTING SOLUTIONS, HARD LENSES

Rewetting solutions are intended for use directly in the eye in conjunction with a contact lens. These products improve wearing time by rehydrating the lens, which may become dry and contaminated during wear, although more benefit is obtained by actually removing and rewetting the lens. The principle components of these solutions are wetting agents.

otc	**Adapettes** (Alcon)	**Solution**: Buffered, isotonic. Povidone and other water-soluble polymers, sorbic acid, EDTA	Thimerosal free. In 15 ml.
otc	**Clerz 2** (Alcon)	**Solution**: Isotonic. Hydroxyethylcellulose, poloxamer 407, NaCl, KCl, sodium borate, boric acid, sorbic acid, EDTA	Thimerosal free. In 5, 15 and 30 ml.
otc	**Lens Lubricant** (Bausch & Lomb)	**Solution**: Buffered, isotonic. 0.004% thimerosal, 0.1% EDTA, povidone, polyoxyethylene	In 15 ml.
otc	**Opti-Tears** (Alcon)	**Solution**: Isotonic. 0.1% EDTA, 0.001% polyquaternium-1, dextran, NaCl, KCl, hydroxymethylcellulose	Thimerosal and sorbic acid free. In 15 ml.
otc	**Lens Drops** (Ciba Vision)	**Solution**: Buffered, isotonic. NaCl, carbamide, poloxamer 407, 0.2% EDTA, 0.15% sorbic acid.	Thimerosal free. In 15 ml.

Contact Lens Products

CLEANING SOLUTIONS, HARD LENSES

Cleaning solutions contain surfactant cleaners to facilitate removal of oleaginous, proteinaceous and other types of debris from the lens surface. To adequately clean, physically rub lens in the palm of the hand or between thumb and finger with solution for about 20 seconds and rinse with water or sterile saline solution.

otc	**LC-65** (Allergan)	**Solution:** Buffered. 0.001% thimerosal, EDTA	In 15 and 60 ml.
otc	**MiraFlow Extra Strength** (Ciba Vision)	**Solution:** 15.7% isopropyl alcohol, poloxamer 407, amphoteric 10	Preservative free. In 12 ml.
otc	**Opti-Clean** (Alcon)	**Solution:** Buffered, isotonic. Tween 21, hydroxyethylcellulose, polymeric cleaners, 0.004% thimerosal, 0.1% EDTA	In 12 and 20 ml.
otc	**Opti-Clean II** (Alcon)	**Solution:** Buffered, isotonic. Tween 21, polymeric cleaners, 0.1% EDTA, 0.001% polyquaternium-1	Thimerosal free. In 12 and 20 ml.
otc	**Resolve/GP** (Allergan)	**Solution:** Buffered. Cocoamphocarboxyglycinate, sodium lauryl sulfate, hexylene glycol, alkyl ether sulfate, fatty acid amide surfactants	Preservative free. In 30 ml.
otc	**Sereine** (Optikem)	**Solution:** Cocoamphodiacetate and glycols, 0.1% EDTA, 0.01% benzalkonium chloride	In 60 ml.
otc	**Titan** (Pilkington Barnes Hind)	**Solution:** Buffered. Nonionic cleaning agents, 2% EDTA, 0.13% potassium sorbate	In 30 ml.

CLEANING AND SOAKING SOLUTIONS, HARD LENSES

otc	**Clean-N-Soak** (Allergan)	**Solution:** Buffered. Surfactant cleaning agent with 0.004% phenylmercuric nitrate	In 120 ml.

CLEANING/SOAKING/WETTING SOLUTIONS, HARD LENSES

otc	**Total** (Allergan)	**Solution:** Buffered, isotonic. Polyvinyl alcohol, benzalkonium chloride, EDTA	In 60 and 120 ml.

Contact Lens Products

RIGID GAS PERMEABLE CONTACT LENS PRODUCTS

Refer to the general discussion of these products in Contact Lens Products monograph.

Actions:

Pharmacology:

Gas permeable hard lenses – Silicone/acrylate and fluoropolymers are used in rigid gas permeable (RGP) contact lenses. Lens care regimens include the use of a surfactant cleaner, enzyme cleaner and storage in a chemical disinfecting solution. Advise patients to follow the lens care protocol provided by the lens manufacturer or the instructions of their doctor.

DISINFECTING/WETTING/SOAKING SOLUTIONS, RGP LENSES

otc	**Boston Advance Comfort Formula** (Polymer Tech)	**Solution:** Buffered, slightly hypertonic. 0.00015% polyaminopropyl biguanide, 0.05% EDTA, cationic cellulose derivative polymer (wetting agent)	In 120 ml.
otc	**Boston Conditioning Solution** (Polymer Tech)	**Solution:** Buffered, slightly hypertonic, low viscosity. 0.05% EDTA, 0.006% chlorhexidine gluconate, cationic cellulose derivative polymer as wetting agent	In 120 ml.
otc	**Flex-Care Especially for Sensitive Eyes** (Alcon)	**Solution:** Buffered, isotonic. 0.1% EDTA, 0.005% chlorhexidine gluconate, NaCl, sodium borate, boric acid	Thimerosal free. In 118, 237 and 355 ml.
otc	**Stay-Wet 3** (Sherman)	**Solution:** 0.02% sodium bisulfite, 0.1% benzyl alcohol, 0.05% sorbic acid, 0.1% EDTA, sodium and potassium chloride salts containing polyvinyl pyrrolidone, polyvinyl alcohol, hydroxyethylcellulose	Thimerosal free. In 30 ml.
otc	**Stay-Wet 4** (Sherman)	**Solution:** 0.15% benzyl alcohol, 0.1% EDTA, NaCl, KCl, polyvinyl alcohol, hydroxyethyl cellulose	Thimerosal free. In 30 ml.
otc	**ComfortCare GP Wetting & Soaking** (Pilkington Barnes Hind)	**Solution:** Buffered, isotonic. 0.005% chlorhexidine gluconate, 0.02% EDTA, octylphenoxy (oxyethylene) ethanol, povidone, polyvinyl alcohol, propylene glycol, hydroxyethylcellulose, NaCl	In 120 and 240 ml.
otc	**Wetting and Soaking Solution** (Bausch & Lomb)	**Solution:** Buffered, hypertonic. 0.006% chlorhexidine gluconate, 0.05% EDTA, cationic cellulose derivative polymer	Thimerosal free. In 118 ml.
otc	**Wet-N-Soak Plus** (Allergan)	**Solution:** Buffered, isotonic. 0.003% benzalkonium chloride, polyvinyl alcohol, EDTA	In 120 and 180 ml.

CLEANING SOLUTIONS, RGP LENSES

otc	**Boston Advance Cleaner** (Polymer Tech)	**Solution:** Concentrated homogenous surfactant. Alkyl ether sulfate, ethoxylated alkyl phenol, tri-quaternary cocoa-based phospholipid, silica gel	In 30 ml.
otc	**Boston Cleaner** (Polymer Tech)	**Solution:** Concentrated homogenous surfactant. Alkyl ether sulfate, silica gel, titanium dioxide	In 30 ml.
otc	**Concentrated Cleaner** (Bausch & Lomb)	**Solution:** Surfactant solution with alkyl ether sulfate and silica gel	Preservative free. In 30 ml.
otc	**Gas Permeable Daily Cleaner** (Pilkington Barnes Hind)	**Solution:** 0.13% potassium sorbate, 2% EDTA, ethoxylated polyoxypropylene glycol, tris (hydroxymethyl) amino methane, hydroxyethylcellulose	Thimerosal free. In 30 ml.
otc	**LC-65** (Allergan)	**Solution:** Buffered cleaning agent. 0.001% thimerosal and EDTA	In 15 and 60 ml.

Contact Lens Products

CLEANING SOLUTIONS, RGP LENSES

otc	**Opti-Clean** (Alcon)	**Solution:** Buffered, isotonic. 0.004% thimerosal, 0.1% EDTA, Tween 21, hydroxyethylcellulose, *Microclens* polymeric cleaners	In 12 and 20 ml.
otc	**Opti-Clean II Especially for Sensitive Eyes** (Alcon)	**Solution:** Buffered, isotonic. 0.1% EDTA, 0.001% polyquaternium-1, *Microclens* polymeric cleaners, Tween 21	Thimerosal free. In 12 and 20 ml.
otc	**Resolve/GP** (Allergan)	**Solution:** Buffered. Cocoamphocarboxyglycinate, sodium lauryl sulfate, hexylene glycol, alkyl ether sulfate, fatty acid amide surfactants	Preservative free. In 30 ml.

ENZYMATIC CLEANERS, RGP LENSES

otc	**Opti-Zyme Enzymatic Cleaner Especially for Sensitive Eyes** (Alcon)	**Tablets:** Highly purified pork pancreatin. *To make solution for soaking, dilute in preserved saline or sterile unpreserved saline solution*	Preservative free. In 8s, 24s, 36s and 56s.
otc	**ProFree/GP Weekly Enzymatic Cleaner** (Allergan)	**Tablets:** Papain, NaCl, sodium carbonate, sodium borate, EDTA	In 16s and 24s with vials.

CLEANING/DISINFECTING/SOAKING SOLUTIONS, RGP LENSES

otc	**de • STAT 3** (Sherman)	**Solution:** 0.1% benzyl alcohol, 0.5% EDTA, lauryl sulfate salt of imidazoline, octylphenoxypolyethoxyethanol	Thimerosal free. In 118 ml.
otc	**de • STAT 4** (Sherman)	**Solution:** 0.3% benzyl alcohol, 0.5% EDTA, lauryl sulfate salt of imidazoline, octylphenoxypolyethoxyethanol	Thimerosal free. In 118 ml.

REWETTING SOLUTIONS, RGP LENSES

otc	**Boston Rewetting Drops** (Polymer Tech)	**Solution:** Buffered, slightly hypertonic. 0.006% chlorhexidine gluconate, 0.05% EDTA, cationic cellulose derivative polymer as wetting agent	In 10 ml.
otc	**Wet-N-Soak** (Allergan)	**Solution:** Borate buffered, isotonic. 0.006% WSCP, hydroxyethylcellulose	In 15 ml.

Contact Lens Products

SOFT (HYDROGEL) CONTACT LENS PRODUCTS

Refer to the general discussion of these products in the Contact Lens Products monograph.

Warning:
Do NOT use conventional (hard) lens solutions on soft contact lenses. Use caution in product selection. Not all products are intended for use on all types of soft lenses.

Actions:

Pharmacology: Soft (hydrogel) contact lenses are made of hydrophilic polymers. Hydrogel lenses must be maintained in a hydrated state in physiological saline to prevent them from becoming brittle. Hydrogel lenses will absorb many substances; therefore, use only solutions specifically formulated for hydrogel lenses. In addition, these lenses must be disinfected either by heating in saline solution or by soaking in a chemical solution. Heating a lens in solutions used for chemical disinfection only may cause the lens to become opaque.

Soft lens solutions are especially formulated to be compatible with, and to meet the particular needs of, soft contact lenses. Of particular importance to soft lens care is the need for thorough cleaning to remove deposits which coat and may discolor the lens, especially when subjected to asepticizing by heating.

RINSING/STORAGE SOLUTIONS, SOFT CONTACT LENSES

Use these solutions for rinsing and storage of hydrogel lenses in conjunction with heat disinfection. Prepared saline solutions may contain chelating agents (EDTA) which prevent calcium deposits from forming. Thimerosal-free preserved saline solutions may be used by patients sensitive to thimerosal or mercury-containing compounds. Preservative-free solutions are for patients intolerant to preservatives. Salt tablets are available to make saline solution; however, these solutions are nonsterile and contain no preservatives; use only with heat disinfection methods. Because cases of *Acanthamoeba* keratitis (a serious eye infection) have occurred in patients using homemade saline solutions, the use of salt tablets for soft contact lens storage/rinsing solution is not recommended.

PRESERVED SALINE SOLUTIONS, SOFT CONTACT LENSES

otc	**Hydrocare Preserved Saline** (Allergan)	**Solution:** Buffered, isotonic. 0.01% EDTA, 0.001% thimerosal, NaCl, sodium hexametaphosphate, boric acid, sodium borate	In 240 and 360 ml.
otc	**Opti-Soft** (Alcon)	**Solution:** Buffered, isotonic. 0.1% EDTA, 0.001% polyquaternium-1, NaCl, borate buffer system. For lenses with ≤ 45% water content	Thimerosal free. In 355 ml.
otc	**ReNu** (Bausch & Lomb)	**Solution:** Buffered, isotonic. 0.00003% polyaminopropyl biguanide, NaCl, boric acid, EDTA	In 355 ml.
otc	**Saline** (Bausch & Lomb)	**Solution:** Buffered, isotonic. 0.001% thimerosal, boric acid, NaCl, EDTA	In 355 ml.
otc	**Sensitive Eyes** (Bausch & Lomb)	**Solution:** Buffered, isotonic. 0.1% sorbic acid, 0.025% EDTA, NaCl, boric acid, sodium borate	Thimerosal free. In 118, 237 and 355 ml.
otc	**Sensitive Eyes Plus** (Bausch & Lomb)	**Solution:** Boric acid, sodium borate, KCl, NaCl, 0.00003% polyaminopropyl biguanide, 0.025% EDTA	In 118 and 355 ml.
otc	**BarnesHind Saline for Sensitive Eyes** (Pilkington Barnes Hind)	**Solution:** Isotonic. 0.13% potassium sorbate, 0.025% EDTA	In 360 ml (2s).
otc	**Your Choice Sterile Preserved Saline Solution** (Amcon)	**Solution:** Isotonic. 0.1% sorbic acid, boric buffer, EDTA, NaCl	In 60 and 360 ml.

Contact Lens Products

PRESERVED SALINE SOLUTIONS, SOFT CONTACT LENSES

otc	**Alcon Saline Especially for Sensitive Eyes** (Alcon)	**Solution:** Buffered, isotonic. NaCl, borate buffer system, sorbic acid, EDTA	Thimerosal free. In 360 ml.
otc	**SoftWear** (Ciba Vision)	**Solution:** Isotonic, NaCl, boric acid, sodium borate, sodium perborate (generating up to 0.006% hydrogen peroxide stabilized with phosphonic acid)	Thimerosal free. In 120, 240 and 360 ml.

PRESERVATIVE FREE SALINE SOLUTIONS, SOFT CONTACT LENSES

otc	**Blairex Sterile Saline** (Blairex)	**Solution:** Buffered, isotonic. NaCl, boric acid, sodium borate	In 90, 240 and 360 ml aerosol.
otc	**Unisol** (Alcon)		Thimerosal free. In 15 ml (25s) and 120 ml (2s, 3s).
otc	**Unisol 4** (Alcon)		Thimerosal free. In 120 ml.
otc	**Unisol Plus** (Alcon)		In 240 and 360 ml aerosol.
otc	**Your Choice Non-Preserved Saline Solution** (Amcon)		In 360 ml.
otc	**Ciba Vision Saline** (Ciba Vision)	**Solution:** Buffered, isotonic. NaCl, boric acid, sodium borate	In 240 and 360 ml aerosol.
otc	**Lens Plus Sterile Saline** (Allergan)	**Solution:** Buffered, isotonic. NaCl, boric acid, nitrogen	In 90, 240 and 360 ml aerosol.
otc	**Oxysept 2** (Allergan)	**Solution:** Buffered, isotonic. NaCl, catalytic neutralizing agent, EDTA, mono- and dibasic sodium phosphates	In 15 ml single-use containers (25s).

SALT TABLETS FOR NORMAL SALINE, SOFT CONTACT LENSES

Actions:

Pharmacology: Reconstitute tablets in container provided with distilled, deionized or purified water; do not use mineral or tap water. These solutions are not sterile and are intended only for use in conjunction with heat disinfection regimens. Use only as a rinse *prior* to heat disinfection and as storage *during* heat disinfection. Not for use as a rinse *after* disinfection (ie, before lens placement in the eye). Not for use in the eye. See Precautions in the Contact Lens Products monograph.

otc	**Marlin Salt System** (Marlin)	**Tablets:** 250 mg NaCl	In 200s with 27.7 ml bottle.

Contact Lens Products

SURFACTANT CLEANING SOLUTIONS, SOFT CONTACT LENSES

Indications:

Cleaning solutions are used for daily prophylactic cleaning to prevent the accumulation of proteinaceous (mucus) deposits and to remove other debris.

otc	**Preflex Daily Cleaning Especially for Sensitive Eyes** (Alcon)	**Solution**: Buffered, isotonic. NaCl, sodium phosphates, tyloxapol, hydroxyethyl cellulose, polyvinyl alcohol, EDTA, sorbic acid	In 30 ml.
otc	**DURAcare** II (Blairex)	**Solution**: Buffered, hypertonic. 0.1% sodium bisulfite, 0.1% sorbic acid, 0.25% EDTA, salt buffers, ethylene/propylene oxide, octylphenoxypolyethoxyethanol, lauryl sulfate salt of imidazoline	Thimerosal free. In 30 ml.
otc	**LC-65** (Allergan)	**Solution**: Buffered. 0.001% thimerosal, EDTA	In 15 and 60 ml.
otc	**Ciba Vision Cleaner for Sensitive Eyes** (Ciba Vision)	**Solution**: Cocoamphorcarboxyglycinate, sodium lauryl sulfate, hexylene glycol, 0.1% sorbic acid, 0.2% EDTA	In 15 ml.
otc	**Lens Plus Daily Cleaner** (Allergan)	**Solution**: Buffered. Cocoamphocarboxyglycinate, sodium lauryl sulfate, hexylene glycol, NaCl, sodium phosphate	Preservative free. In 15 and 30 ml.
otc	**MiraFlow Extra Strength** (Ciba Vision)	**Solution**: 15.7% isopropyl alcohol, poloxamer 407, amphoteric 10	Thimerosal free. In 12 and 20 ml.
otc	**Opti-Clean** (Alcon)	**Solution**: Buffered, isotonic. 0.004% thimerosal, 0.1% EDTA, Tween 21, hydroxyethyl cellulose, *Microclens* polymeric cleaners	In 12 and 20 ml.
otc	**Opti-Clean** II (Alcon)	**Solution**: Buffered, isotonic. 0.1% EDTA, 0.001% polyquaternium-1, *Microclens* polymeric cleaners, *Tween 21*	Thimerosal free. In 12 and 20 ml.
otc	**Opti-Free** (Alcon)	**Solution**: Buffered, isotonic. 0.01% EDTA, 0.001% polyquaternium-1, *Microclens* polymeric cleaners, *Tween 21*	Thimerosal free. In 12 and 20 ml.
otc	**Pliagel** (Alcon)	**Solution**: 0.25% sorbic acid, 0.5% EDTA, NaCl, KCl, poloxamer 407	In 25 ml.
otc	**Sensitive Eyes Daily Cleaner** (Bausch & Lomb)	**Solution**: Buffered, isotonic. 0.25% sorbic acid, 0.5% EDTA, NaCl, hydroxypropyl methylcellulose, poloxamine, sodium borate	In 20 ml.
otc	**Sensitive Eyes Saline/Cleaning** (Bausch & Lomb)	**Solution**: Buffered, isotonic. 0.15% sorbic acid, 0.1% EDTA, boric acid, poloxamine, sodium borate, NaCl	In 237 ml.
otc	**Soft Mate Hands Off Daily Cleaner** (Pilkington Barnes-Hind)	**Solution:** Isotonic. Octylphenoxy ethanol, hydroxyethylcellulose, NaCl, 0.13% potassium sorbate, 0.2% EDTA	In 240 ml.

Contact Lens Products

ENZYMATIC CLEANERS, SOFT CONTACT LENSES

Actions:

Pharmacology: Enzymatic cleaning, by soaking in a solution prepared from enzyme tablets, is recommended once weekly to remove protein and other lens deposits.

otc	**Allergan Enzymatic** (Allergan)	**Tablets:** Papain, NaCl, sodium carbonate, sodium borate, EDTA. *To make solution for soaking, dilute in sterile saline.*	In 12s, 24s, 36s and 48s.
otc	**Enzymatic Cleaner for Extended Wear** (Alcon)	**Tablets:** Highly purified pork pancreatin. *To make solution for soaking, dilute in preserved saline or sterile unpreserved saline.*	In 12s.
otc	**Opti-zyme Enzymatic Cleaner Especially for Sensitive Eyes** (Alcon)		Preservative free. In 8s, 24s, 36s and 56s.
otc	**Vision Care Enzymatic Cleaner** (Alcon)		In 24s.
otc	**Opti-Free** (Alcon)	**Tablets:** Highly purified pork pancreatin. *To make solution for soaking, dilute in* **Opti-Free** *disinfecting solution.*	In 6s, 12s and 18s.
otc	**ReNu Effervescent Enzymatic Cleaner** (Bausch & Lomb)	**Tablets:** Subtilisin, polyethylene glycol, sodium carbonate, NaCl, tartaric acid. *To make solution for soaking, dilute in preserved saline or sterile unpreserved saline solution.*	In 10s, 20s and 30s.
otc	**ReNu Thermal Enzymatic Cleaner** (Bausch & Lomb)	**Tablets:** Subtilisin, sodium carbonate, NaCl, boric acid. *To make solution for heat disinfection directly in lens carrying case.*	In 16s.
otc	**Ultrazyme Enzymatic Cleaner** (Allergan)	**Tablets:** Effervescing, buffering and tableting agents. Subtilisin A. *To make solution for soaking, dilute in 3% hydrogen peroxide disinfecting solution.*	In 5s, 10s, 15s and 20s.
otc	**Complete Weekly Enzymatic Cleaner** (Allergan)	**Tablets:** Effervescing, buffering and tableting agents. Subtilisin A. *To make solution for soaking, dilute in sterile saline.*	In 8s.

REWETTING SOLUTIONS, SOFT CONTACT LENSES

Actions:

Pharmacology: May be used directly in the eye to rehydrate and improve comfort of hydrogel lenses.

otc	**Adapettes Especially For Sensitive Eyes** (Alcon)	**Solution:** Buffered, isotonic. Povidone and other water-soluble polymers, sorbic acid, EDTA	Thimerosal free. In 15 ml.
otc	**Blairex Lens Lubricant** (Blairex)	**Solution:** Isotonic. 0.25% sorbic acid, 0.1% EDTA, borate buffer, NaCl, hydroxypropyl methylcellulose, glycerin	Thimerosal free. In 15 ml.
otc	**Clerz 2** (Alcon)	**Solution:** Isotonic. NaCl, KCl, hydroxyethylcellulose, poloxamer 407, sodium borate, boric acid, sorbic acid, EDTA	Thimerosal free. In 5 (2s), 15 and 30 ml.
otc	**Lens Lubricant** (Bausch & Lomb)	**Solution:** Buffered, isotonic. 0.004% thimerosal, 0.1% EDTA, povidone, polyoxyethylene	In 15 ml.
otc	**Lens Plus Rewetting Drops** (Allergan)	**Solution:** Buffered, isotonic. NaCl, boric acid	Preservative free. In 0.35 ml (30s).
otc	**Opti-Tears** (Alcon)	**Solution:** Isotonic. 0.1% EDTA, 0.001% polyquaternium-1, dextran, NaCl, KCl, hydroxypropyl methylcellulose	Thimerosal free. In 15 ml.

Contact Lens Products

REWETTING SOLUTIONS, SOFT CONTACT LENSES

otc	**Opti-Free** (Alcon)	**Solution:** Isotonic. Citrate buffer, NaCl, 0.05% EDTA, 0.001% polyquaternium-1	In 10 and 20 ml.
otc	**Opti-One** (Alcon)		In 10 ml.
otc	**Sensitive Eyes Drops** (Bausch & Lomb)	**Solution:** Buffered. 0.1% sorbic acid, 0.025% EDTA, NaCl, boric acid, sodium borate	In 30 ml.
otc	**Soft Mate Comfort Drops** (Pilkington Barnes Hind)	**Solution:** Borate buffered. 0.13% potassium sorbate, 0.1% EDTA, NaCl, hydroxyethylcellulose, octylphenoxyethanol	In 15 ml.
otc	**Lens Drops** (Ciba Vision)	**Solution:** Buffered, isotonic. NaCl, borate buffer, poloxamer 407, 0.2% EDTA, 0.15% sorbic acid, carbamide	In 15 ml.
otc	**Complete** (Allergan)	**Solution:** Buffered, isotonic. NaCl, 0.0001% polyhexamethylene biguanide, tromethamine, tyloxapol, EDTA	In 15 ml.

Contact Lens Products

CHEMICAL DISINFECTION SYSTEMS

Actions:

Pharmacology: Chemical disinfection is an alternative to heat. Two-solution systems use separate disinfecting and rinsing solutions. One-solution systems use the same solution for rinsing and storage.

Warnings:

Heat disinfection: Lenses must NOT be disinfected by heating when using these solutions.

HYDROGEN PEROXIDE-CONTAINING SYSTEMS, SOFT LENSES

otc	**MiraSept** (Alcon)	**Disinfecting Solution**: 3% hydrogen peroxide, sodium stannate, sodium nitrate	In 120 ml.
		Rinse and Neutralizer: Isotonic. Boric acid, sodium borate, NaCl, sodium pyruvate, EDTA	In 120 ml (2s).
otc	**Oxysept** (Allergan)	**Disinfecting Solution**: 3% hydrogen peroxide, sodium stannate, sodium nitrate, phosphate buffer	In 240 and 360 ml.
		Neutralizer Tablets: Catalase, buffering agents	In 12s (with Oxy-Tab cup) and 36s.
otc	**Soft Mate Consept** (Pilkington Barnes Hind)	**Consept 1 Cleaning and Disinfecting Solution**: 3% hydrogen peroxide, polyoxyl 40 stearate, sodium stannate, sodium nitrate, phosphate buffer	In 240 ml.
		Consept 2 Neutralizing and Rinsing Spray: Isotonic. 0.5% sodium thiosulfate, borate buffers	Aerosol. In 360 ml.
		Consept 2 Neutralizing and Rinsing Solution: Isotonic. 0.5% sodium thiosulfate, borate buffers, 0.001% chlorhexidine gluconate	In 360 ml.
otc	**Ultra-Care** (Allergan)	**Disinfecting Solution**: 3% hydrogen peroxide, sodium stannate, sodium nitrate, phosphate buffer	In 120 and 360 ml.
		Neutralizer Tablets: Catalase, hydroxypropyl methylcellulose, buffering agents	In 12s and 36s with cup.
otc	**Quick CARE** (Ciba Vision)	**Disinfecting Solution**: Isopropanol, NaCl, polyoxypropylenepolyoxyethylene block copolymer, disodium lauroamphodiacetate	In 15 ml.
		Rinse and Neutralizer: Isotonic. Sodium borate, boric acid, sodium perborate (generating up to 0.006% hydrogen peroxide), phosphonic acid	In 360 ml.
otc	**AOSEPT** (Ciba Vision)	**Disinfecting Solution**: 3% hydrogen peroxide, 0.85% NaCl, phosphonic acid, phosphate buffers	In 120, 240 and 360 ml.
		AODISC Neutralizer: Platinum-coated tablet	Tablet good for 100 uses or 3 months of daily use.[1]

[1] For use only with the AOSEPT system.

Contact Lens Products

NON-HYDROGEN PEROXIDE-CONTAINING SYSTEMS, SOFT LENSES

otc	**Disinfecting Solution** (Bausch & Lomb)	**Solution**: Buffered, isotonic. 0.005% chlorhexidine, 0.1% EDTA, 0.001% thimerosal, NaCl, sodium borate, boric acid	In 355 ml.
otc	**Flex-Care Especially for Sensitive Eyes** (Alcon)	**Solution**: Buffered, isotonic. 0.1% EDTA, 0.005% chlorhexidine gluconate, NaCl, sodium borate, boric acid	In 360 ml.
otc	**Hydrocare Cleaning and Disinfecting** (Allergan)	**Solution**: Buffered, isotonic. 0.002% thimerosal, Tris (2-hydroxyethyl) and bis (2-hydroxyethyl) tallow ammonium Cl, sodium bicarbonate, sodium phosphates, hydrochloric acid, propylene glycol, polysorbate 80, polyhema	In 240 and 360 ml.
otc	**Opti-Free** (Alcon)	**Solution**: Isotonic. 0.05% EDTA, 0.001% polyquaternium-1, citrate buffer, NaCl	Thimerosal free. In 118, 237 and 355 ml.
otc	**Opti-One Multi-Purpose** (Alcon)	**Solution**: Buffered, isotonic. 0.05% EDTA, 0.001% polyquaternium-1, sodium chloride, NaCl	In 118, 237, 355 and 473ml.
otc	**Complete All-In-One Solution** (Allergan)	**Solution**: Buffered, isotonic. NaCl, 0.0001% polyhexamethylene biguanide, EDTA	In 60, 120 and 360 ml.
otc	**ReNu Multi-Purpose** (Bausch & Lomb)	**Solution**: Isotonic. 0.00005% polyaminopropyl biguanide, 0.01% EDTA, NaCl, sodium borate, boric acid, poloxamine	In 118, 237 and 355 ml.
otc	**Soft Mate Disinfecting for Sensitive Eyes** (Pilkington Barnes Hind)	**Solution**: Isotonic. 0.1% EDTA, 0.005% chlorhexidine gluconate, NaCl, povidone, octylphenoxy (oxyethylene) ethanol, borate buffer	Thimerosal free. In 240 ml.

Local Anesthetics

LOCAL ANESTHETICS

Actions:

Pharmacology: Local anesthetics stabilize the neuronal membrane so the neuron is less permeable to ions. This prevents the initiation and transmission of nerve impulses, thereby producing the local anesthetic action.

Studies indicate that local anesthetics influence permeability of the nerve cell membrane by limiting sodium ion permeability by closing the pores through which the ions migrate in the lipid layer of the nerve cell membrane. This limitation prevents the fundamental change necessary for the generation of the action potential.

Pharmacokinetics: Tetracaine and proparacaine are approximately equally potent. They have a rapid onset of anesthesia beginning within 13 to 30 seconds following instillation; the duration of action is 15 to 20 minutes.

Indications:

Corneal anesthesia of short duration (eg, tonometry, gonioscopy, removal of corneal foreign bodies and sutures); short corneal and conjunctival procedures; cataract surgery; conjunctival and corneal scraping for diagnostic purposes; paracentesis of the anterior chamber.

Ophthalmic Uses of Local Anesthetics

Route	Use
Injectable	Facial nerve block
	Retrobulbar anesthesia
	Eyelid infiltration
Topical	Gonioscopy
	Tonometry
	Fundus contact lens biomicroscopy
	Evaluation of corneal abrasions
	Forced duction testing
	Schirmer tear testing
	Electroretinography
	Lacrimal dilation and irrigation
	Contact lens fitting
	Superficial foreign body removal
	Minor surgery of conjunctiva
	Suture removal
	Corneal epithelial debridement

Contraindications:

Hypersensitivity to similar drugs (ester-type local anesthetics), para-aminobenzoic acid or its derivatives or to any other ingredient in these preparations; prolonged use, especially for self-medication (not recommended).

Warnings:

For topical ophthalmic use only. Prolonged use may diminish duration of anesthesia, retard wound healing and cause corneal epithelial erosions (see Adverse Reactions).

Systemic toxicity is rare with topical ophthalmic application of local anesthetics. It usually occurs as CNS stimulation followed by CNS and cardiovascular depression.

Protection of the eye from irritating chemicals, foreign bodies and rubbing during the period of anesthesia is very important. Thoroughly rinse tonometers soaked in sterilizing or detergent solutions with sterile distilled water before use. Advise the patient to avoid touching the eye until anesthesia has worn off. Because the "blink" reflex is temporarily eliminated, it is advised that the eye be covered with a patch following instillation.

Pregnancy: Category C. Safety for use during pregnancy has not been established. Use only when clearly needed and when potential benefits outweigh potential hazards to the fetus.

Lactation: Safety for use during lactation has not been established. Use only when clearly needed and when potential benefits outweigh potential hazards to the infant.

Children: Safety and efficacy for use in children have not been established.

Precautions:

Tolerance varies with the status of the patient; give debilitated, elderly or acutely ill patients doses commensurate with their weight, age and physical status.

Local Anesthetics

LOCAL ANESTHETICS

Reduced plasma esterase: Use caution in patients with abnormal or reduced levels of plasma esterases.

Special risk patients: Use cautiously and sparingly in patients with known allergies, cardiac disease or hyperthyroidism.

Adverse Reactions:

Prolonged ophthalmic use of topical anesthetics has been associated with corneal epithelial erosions, retardation or prevention of healing of corneal erosions and reports of severe keratitis and permanent corneal opacification with accompanying visual loss and scarring or corneal perforation. Inadvertent damage may be done to the anesthetized cornea and conjunctiva by rubbing an eye to which topical anesthetics have been applied.

Tetracaine: Transient stinging, burning and conjunctival redness may occur. A rare, severe, immediate type allergic corneal reaction has been reported characterized by acute diffuse epithelial keratitis with filament formation and sloughing of large areas of necrotic epithelium, diffuse stromal edema, descemetitis and iritis.

Rarely, local reactions including lacrimation, photophobia and chemosis have occurred.

Proparacaine: Local or systemic sensitivity occurs occasionally. At recommended concentration and dosage, proparacaine usually produces little or no initial irritation, stinging, burning, conjunctival redness, lacrimation or increased winking. However, some local irritation and stinging may occur several hours after instillation.

Rarely, a severe, immediate-type, hyperallergic corneal reaction may occur, which includes acute, intense and diffuse epithelial keratitis, a gray, ground-glass appearance, sloughing of large areas of necrotic epithelium, corneal filaments and, sometimes, iritis with descemetitis. Pupillary dilation or cycloplegic effects have been observed rarely.

Allergic contact dermatitis with drying and fissuring of the fingertips and softening and erosion of the corneal epithelium and conjunctival congestion and hemorrhage have been reported.

Patient Information:

Avoid touching or rubbing the eye until the anesthesia has worn off because inadvertent damage may be done to the anesthetized cornea and conjunctiva.

To avoid contamination, do not touch dropper tip to any surface. Replace cap after using.

Do not use if discolored, cloudy or if it contains a precipitate. Protect from light.

Refer to the Topical Ophthalmics introduction for more complete information.

TETRACAINE

Complete prescribing information begins in the Local Anesthetics, Topical group monograph.

Solution: Instill 1 or 2 drops. Not for prolonged use.

Storage: Store at 8° to 27°C (46° to 80°F). Protect from light.

Rx	**Tetracaine HCl** (Various, eg, Alcon, Iolab, Optopics, Schein)	**Solution**: 0.5%	In 1, 2 and 15 ml.
otc	**Pontocaine** (Sanofi Winthrop)		In 15 ml Mono-drop and 59 ml.[1]

[1] With 0.4% chlorobutanol and 0.75% sodium chloride.

Local Anesthetics

PROPARACAINE HCl

For complete prescribing information, refer to the Topical Local Anesthetics general monograph.

Administration and Dosage:

Deep anesthesia as in cataract extraction: 1 drop every 5 to 10 minutes for 5 to 7 doses.

Removal of sutures: Instill 1 or 2 drops 2 or 3 minutes before removal of sutures.

Removal of foreign bodies: Instill 1 or 2 drops prior to operating.

Tonometry: Instill 1 or 2 drops immediately before measurement.

Storage: Store at 8° to 24°C (46° to 75°F). Protect from light.

Rx	**Proparacaine HCl** (Various, eg, Moore, Raway, Rugby)	**Solution:** 0.5%	In 2, 15 ml and UD 1 ml.
Rx	**Alcaine** (Alcon)		In 15 ml Drop-Tainers.[1, 2]
Rx	**Ophthaine** (Apothecon)		In 15 ml.[3, 4]
Rx	**Ophthetic** (Allergan)		In 15 ml.[4, 5]

[1] With glycerin and 0.01% benzalkonium Cl.
[2] Refrigerate after opening.
[3] With glycerin, 0.2% chlorobutanol and benzalkonium Cl.
[4] Refrigerate.
[5] With 0.01% benzalkonium Cl, glycerin and sodium Cl.

MISCELLANEOUS LOCAL ANESTHETIC COMBINATIONS

For complete prescribing information, refer to the Topical Local Anesthetics general monograph.

Indications:

For procedures in which a topical ophthalmic anesthetic agent in conjunction with a disclosing agent is indicated: Corneal anesthesia of short duration (eg, tonometry, gonioscopy, removal of corneal foreign bodies); short corneal and conjunctival procedures.

Administration and Dosage:

Removal of foreign bodies or sutures; tonometry: 1 to 2 drops (in single instillations) in each eye before operating.

Deep ophthalmic anesthesia:

Proparacaine/fluorescein – Instill 1 drop in each eye every 5 to 10 minutes for 5 to 7 doses. Use of an eye patch is recommended.

Benoxinate/fluorescein – Instill 2 drops into each eye at 90 second intervals for 3 instillations.

Storage: Protect from light.

Rx	**Fluoracaine** (Akorn)	**Solution:** 0.5% proparacaine HCl and 0.25% fluorescein sodium	In 5 ml.[1, 2]
Rx	**Fluorescein Sodium with Proparacaine HCl** (Pasadena)		In 5 ml with dropper.[3]
Rx	**Fluress** (Pilkington Barnes Hind)	**Solution:** 0.4% benoxinate HCl and 0.25% fluorescein sodium	In 5 ml with dropper.[4]
Rx	**Flu-Oxinate** (Pasadena)		In 5 ml.[5]
Rx	**Flurate** (Bausch & Lomb)		In 5 ml with dropper.[6]

[1] Refrigerate.
[2] With glycerin, povidone, polysorbate 80 and 0.01% thimerosal.
[3] With povidone, glycerin, EDTA and 0.01% thimerosal.
[4] With povidone, boric acid and 1% chlorobutanol.
[5] Povidone, glycerin, EDTA and 1% chlorobutanol.
[6] 1% chlorobutnol, povidone.

DIAGNOSTIC PRODUCTS

In addition to the following products, the ophthalmic vasoconstrictors, cycloplegic mydriatics and topical local anesthetics are used in diagnostic procedures (see individual monographs).

Vasoconstrictors/Mydriatics with α-sympathomimetic activity cause dilation of the pupil and are used to facilitate ophthalmoscopic examination and other diagnostic procedures.

Cycloplegic Mydriatics (anticholinergics) cause both dilation of the pupil and paralysis of accommodation. These agents are used to facilitate refraction.

Local Anesthetics: Used to facilitate gonioscopy, tonometry and other procedures.

FLUORESCEIN SODIUM

Actions:

Pharmacology: Sodium fluorescein, a yellow water-soluble dibasic acid xanthine dye, produces an intense green fluorescent color in alkaline (pH > 5) solution. Fluorescein demonstrates defects of corneal epithelium. It does not stain tissues, but is a useful indicator dye. Normal precorneal tear film will appear yellow or orange. The intact corneal epithelium resists fluorescein penetration and is not colored. Any break in the epithelial barrier permits rapid penetration. Whether resulting from trauma, infection or other causes, epithelial corneal defects appear bright green and are easily seen. If epithelial loss is extensive, topical fluorescein penetrates into the aqueous humor and is readily visible biomicroscopically as a green flare.

Indications:

Topical: In fitting contact lenses; in applanation tonometry; diagnosis and detection of corneal stippling, abrasions, ulcerations, herpetic lesions, foreign bodies (not epithelialized), contact lens pressure points; making lacrimal drainage test; wound leakage tests (Seidel Test).

Injection: Diagnostic aid in ophthalmic angiography, including examination of the fundus; evaluation of the iris vasculature; distinction between viable and nonviable tissue; observation of the aqueous flow; differential diagnosis of malignant and nonmalignant tumors; determination of circulation time and adequacy.

Contraindications:

Hypersensitivity to fluorescein or any other component of the product; do not use with soft contact lenses (lenses may become discolored).

Topical: Not for injection. Do not use in intraocular surgery.

Warnings:

Topical (drops): Discontinue if sensitivity develops. May stain soft contact lenses. Do not touch dropper tip to any surface, as this may contaminate the solution.

Extravasation: Avoid extravasation during injection. The high pH can result in severe local tissue damage. Complications have occurred from extravasation: Sloughing of skin, superficial phlebitis, SC granuloma and toxic neuritis along the median curve in the antecubital area. Extravasation can cause severe pain in the arm for several hours. When significant extravasation occurs, discontinue injection and use conservative measures to treat damaged tissue and relieve pain (see Warnings).

Hypersensitivity: Exercise caution when administering to patients with a history of hypersensitivity, allergies or asthma. If signs of sensitivity develop, discontinue use.

Pregnancy: Category C. Avoid parenteral fluorescein angiography during pregnancy, especially in first trimester. There are no reports of fetal complications during pregnancy.

Lactation: Fluorescein is excreted in breast milk. Use caution when administering to a nursing woman.

Children: Safety and efficacy for use in children have not been established.

Adverse Reactions:

Injection: Nausea; headache; GI distress; vomiting; syncope; hypotension and other symptoms and signs of hypersensitivity; cardiac arrest; basilar artery ischemia; thrombophlebitis at injection site; severe shock; convulsions; death (rare); temporary yellowish skin discoloration. Hives, itching, bronchospasm, anaphylaxis, pyrexia, transient dyspnea, angioneurotic edema and slight dizziness may occur. A strong taste may develop with use. Urine becomes bright yellow. Skin discoloration fades in 6 to 12 hours, urine fluorescence in 24 to 36 hours. Extravasation at injection site causes intense pain at the site and dull aching pain in the injected arm (see Warnings).

Diagnostic Products

FLUORESCEIN SODIUM

Patient Information:

May cause strong taste with use.

May cause temporary yellowish discoloration of the skin. Urine will turn bright yellow. Discoloration of skin fades in 6 to 12 hours; urine in 24 to 36 hours.

Soft contact lenses may become stained. Do not wear lenses while fluorescein is being used. Whenever fluorescein is used, flush the eyes with sterile normal saline solution and wait at least 1 hour before replacing the lenses.

Administration and Dosage:

Topical: To detect foreign bodies and corneal abrasions, instill 1 or 2 drops of 2% solution; allow a few seconds for staining. Wash out excess with sterile irrigating solution.

Strips: Moisten strip with sterile water. Place moistened strip at the fornix in the lower cul-de-sac close to the punctum. For best results, patient should close lid tightly over strip until desired amount of staining is obtained. The patient should blink several times after application.

Applanation tonometry strips – Anesthetize the eyes. Retract upper lid and touch tip of strip moistened with saline or ocular irrigating solution (eg, *Blinx*) to the bulbar conjunctiva on the temporal side until an adequate amount of stain is available for a clearly defined endpoint reading.

Injection: Inject the contents of the ampule or pre-filled syringe rapidly into the antecubital vein *after taking precautions to avoid extravasation.* A syringe, filled with fluorescein, is attached to transparent tubing and a 25-gauge scalp vein needle for injection. Insert the needle and draw blood to the hub of the syringe so that a *small* air bubble separates the blood in the tubing from the fluorescein. With the room lights on, slowly inject the blood back into the vein while watching the skin over the needle tip. If the needle has extravasated, the patient's blood will bulge the skin, and the injection should be stopped before any fluorescein is injected. When assured that extravasation has not occurred, the room light may be turned off and the fluorescein injection completed. Luminescence appears in the retina and choroidal vessels in 9 to 15 seconds and can be observed by standard viewing equipment.

If potential allergy is suspected, an intradermal skin test may be performed prior to IV administration (ie, 0.05 ml injected intradermally to be evaluated 30 to 60 minutes following injection).

In patients with inaccessible veins where early phases of an angiogram are not necessary, such as cystoid macular edema, 1 g fluorescein has been given orally. Ten to 15 minutes usually pass before evidence of dye appears in the fundus.

Adults – 500 to 750 mg injected rapidly into the antecubital vein.

Children – 7.5 mg/kg (3.5 mg/lb) injected rapidly into the antecubital vein.

Have 0.1% epinephrine IM or IV, an antihistamine, soluble steroid, aminophylline IV and oxygen available.

Storage: Store at 8° to 30°C (46° to 86°F). Do not use if solution contains a precipitate. Discard any unused solution. Keep out of the reach of children.

Rx	**AK-Fluor** (Akorn)	**Injection:** 10%	In 5 ml amps and vials.
Rx	**Fluorescite** (Alcon)		In 5 ml amps with syringes.
Rx	**Funduscein-10** (Ciba Vision)		In 5 ml amps.
Rx	**Ophthifluor** (Deklerht)		In 5 ml amps.
Rx	**AK-Fluor** (Akorn)	**Injection:** 25%	In 2 ml amps and vials.
Rx	**Fluorescite** (Alcon)		In 2 ml amps.
Rx	**Funduscein-25** (Ciba Vision)		In 3 ml amps.
Rx	**Fluorescein Sodium** (Various, eg, Alcon)	**Solution:** 2%	In 1, 2 and 15 ml.
otc	**Ful-Glo** (Sola/Barnes-Hind)	**Strips:** 0.6 mg	In 300s.
otc	**Fluorets** (Akorn)	**Strips:** 1 mg	In 100s.
Rx	**Fluor-I-Strip-A.T.** (W-A)		In 300s.[1]
Rx	**Fluor-I-Strip** (W-A)	**Strips:** 9 mg	In 300s.[1]

[1] With boric acid, polysorbate 80, 0.5% chlorobutanol.

Diagnostic Products

FLUOREXON

Actions:

Pharmacology: Fluorexon is a large molecular weight fluorescent solution for use as a diagnostic and fitting aid for patients with hydrogel (soft) contact lenses. Used with or without lens in place, when fluorescein is contraindicated to avoid staining lenses. It may be used in both soft and hard lenses.

Indications:

Contact lens fitting aid: Assessment of proper fitting characteristics of hydrogel lenses. For quickly and accurately locating the optic zone in aphakic or low-plus lenses.

Evaluation of corneal integrity of patients wearing hydrogel contact lenses. In many instances, arcuate staining will show definite correlation with the edge of the optic zone, indicating improper bearing surfaces.

For use in place of sodium fluorescein when conducting the tear breakup time (B.U.T.) test.

For conducting the applanation tonometry procedure without removing the lens.

For locating the lathe-cut index markings (toric lenses). Use as directed for fitting contact lenses.

Contraindications:

Hypersensitivity to fluorescein sodium.

Warnings:

Contact lenses: When used with lenses with > 55% hydration, some color may remain on lens. Remove by washing repeatedly with washing solution approved for the lens. Rinse with saline or water. Any residual coloring will wash out with the tear flow when the lens is reinserted in the eye. With highly hydrated lenses, the amount of coloring picked up will vary with exposure. Avoid unnecessary delays in examination procedure.

Precautions:

Hydrogen peroxide: Do not use hydrogen peroxide solutions to clean or sterilize lenses until all traces of fluorexon are removed because fluorexon molecules may bind to the lens.

Administration and Dosage:

Place 1 drop on the concave surface of the lens and place the lens immediately on the eye. Alternately place 1 or 2 drops in the lower cul-de-sac and have the patient blink several times.

As the dye passes under the lens, observe a central dark zone of 6 to 9 mm in diameter (ie, a limbal fluorescent ring about 2 mm wide) which forms after each blink. If such staining pattern cannot be observed immediately, slide the lens upward by gently pushing it with a finger, causing the dye to penetrate under the lens as it slides back into normal position. Additional drops may be used if the fluorescence starts to dissipate after prolonged examination. When the examination is completed, rinse the eye and lens with saline. The lens may be reinserted immediately, as opposed to the long waiting period required after the use of fluorescein.

Begin the examination immediately after instillation of fluorexon drops. The material tends to dissipate readily with the tear flow, leading to a progressive reduction in fluorescence. Prolonged examination may require sequential application of drops.

Applanation tonometry (without removing lens): After seating the patient at the slit lamp and instilling a drop of fluorexon along with a drop of proparacaine or similar topical anesthetic, the contact lense is displaced to one side onto the sclera with the finger and the procedure begun.

otc	**Fluoresoft** (Various, eg, Akorn, Holles)	**Solution:** 0.35%	In 0.5 ml pipettes (12s).

Diagnostic Products

ROSE BENGAL

Actions:

Pharmacology: Stains dead or degenerated epithelial cells (corneal and conjunctival) and mucus.

Indications:

Suspected corneal/conjunctival damage: A diagnostic agent when superficial corneal or conjunctival tissue damage is suspected. Effective aid for diagnosis of keratitis, squamous cell carcinomas, keratoconjunctivitis sicca, corrosions or abrasions, and for the detection of foreign bodies.

Contraindications:

Hypersensitivity to rose bengal or any component of the formulation.

Precautions:

Irritation: The solution may be irritating.

Contact lenses: Whenever rose bengal is used in patients with soft contact lenses, flush the eyes thoroughly with sterile normal saline solution and wait at least 1 hour before replacing the lens.

Administration and Dosage:

Strips: Thoroughly saturate tip of strip with sterile irrigating solution. Touch bulbar conjunctiva or lower fornix with moistened strip. The patient should blink several times after application.

otc	**Rose Bengal** (Barnes-Hind)	**Strips**: 1.3 mg per strip	In 100s.
Rx	**Rosets** (Akorn)		In 100s.

INDOCYANINE GREEN

Actions:

Pharmacology: Sterile, water soluble, tricarbocyanine dye with a peak spectral absorption at 800 to 810 nm in blood or blood plasma. Indocyanine green contains ≤ 5% sodium iodide.

Indocyanine green permits recording of indicator-dilution curves for both diagnostic and research purposes independently of fluctuations in oxygen saturation. In the performance of dye dilution curves, a known amount of dye is usually injected as a single bolus as rapidly as possible via a cardiac catheter into selected sites in the vascular system. A recording instrument (oximeter or densitometer) is attached to a needle or catheter for sampling of the blood-dye mixture from a systemic arterial sampling site.

The peak absorption and emission of indocyanine green lie in a region (800 to 850 nm) where transmission of energy by the pigment epithelium is more efficient than in the region of visible light energy. Because indocyanine green is also nearly 98% bound to blood protein, excessive dye extravasation does not take place in the highly fenestrated choroidal vasculature. It is, therefore, useful in both absorption and fluorescence infrared angiography of the choroidal vasculature when using appropriate filters and film in a fundus camera.

Pharmacokinetics: Following IV injection, indocyanine green is rapidly bound to plasma protein, of which albumin is the principle carrier (95%). Indocyanine green undergoes no significant extrahepatic or enterohepatic circulation; simultaneous arterial and venous blood estimations have shown negligible renal, peripheral, lung or cerebrospinal uptake of the dye. Indocyanine green is taken up from the plasma almost exclusively by the hepatic parenchymal cells and is secreted entirely into the bile. After biliary obstruction, the dye appears in the hepatic lymph, independently of the bile, suggesting that the biliary mucosa is sufficiently intact to prevent diffusion of the dye, though allowing diffusion of bilirubin. These characteristics make indocyanine green a helpful index of hepatic function.

Indications:

Angiography: For ophthalmic angiography.

In vivo diagnostics: For determining cardiac output, hepatic function and liver blood flow (see In Vivo Diagnostic Aids).

Warnings:

Pregnancy: Category C. It is not known whether indocyanine green can cause fetal harm when administered to a pregnant woman or can affect reproduction capacity. Give to a pregnant woman only if clearly indicated.

Lactation: It is not known whether this drug is excreted in breast milk. Exercise caution when indocyanine green is administered to a nursing woman.

Diagnostic Products

INDOCYANINE GREEN

Precautions:

Plasma fractional disappearance rate at the recommended 0.5 mg/kg dose has been reported to be significantly greater in women than in men, however there was no significant difference in the calculated value for clearance.

Radioactive iodine uptake studies: Do not perform for at least a week following the use of indocyanine green.

Iodide allergy: Use with caution in individuals who have a history of allergy to iodides.

Drug Interactions:

Drug/Lab test interactions: Heparin preparations containing sodium bisulfite reduce the absorption peak of indocyanine green in blood. Do not use heparin as an anticoagulant for the collection of samples for analysis.

Adverse Reactions:

Indocyanine green contains sodium iodide. Use with caution in patients who have a history of allergy to iodides. Anaphylactic or urticarial reactions have also been reported in patients without history of allergy to iodides. If such reactions occur, treat with appropriate agents (eg, epinephrine, antihistamines and corticosteroids).

Administration and Dosage:

Use 40 mg dye in 2 ml of aqueous solvent. In some patients, half the volume has been found to produce angiograms of comparable resolution. Immediately follow the injected dye bolus with a 5 ml bolus of normal saline. This injection regimen is designed to provide delivery of a spatially limited dye bolus of optimal concentration to the choroidal vasculature following IV injection.

Compatibility: Use only the Aqueous Solvent (pH, 5.5 to 6.5) provided, which is specially prepared Sterile Water for Injection, to dissolve indocyanine green because there have been reports of incompatibility with some commercially available Water for Injection products.

Storage/Stability: Indocyanine green is unstable in aqueous solution and must be used within 10 hours. However, the dye is stable in plasma and whole blood so that samples obtained in discontinuous sampling techniques may be read hours later. Use sterile techniques in handling the dye solution and in the performance of the dilution curves.

Indocyanine green powder may cling to the vial or lump together because it is freeze-dried in the vials. *This is not due to the presence of water.*

Rx	**Cardio-Green (CG)** (Becton-Dickinson)	**Powder for Injection:** 25 mg	In 10 ml amps of aqueous solvent (2s).
		50 mg	In 10 ml amps of aqueous solvent (2s).

Diagnostic Products

TEAR TEST STRIPS

Indications:

Schirmer Tear Test:

Test I – To diagnose dry eye syndrome, to evaluate lacrimal gland function in contact lens wearers, to check tear production prior to eyelid surgery and prior to corneal transplantation and cataract surgery.

Test II – To assess the adequacy of reflex lacrimation.

Sno-Strips: Perform test on eye before any topical medication (especially anesthetic) is administered or other procedures are carried out (eg, manipulation of eyelids).

Administration and Dosage:

Schirmer Tear Test: Strips are placed at the junction of the middle and temporal one-third of the eyelid margin. To avoid increased reflex lacrimation and pain, do not touch the cornea.

Sno-Strips: Apply to lower temporal lid margin of eye. The distance between notch and shoulder of strip is 10 mm, which should be wetted in approximately 3 minutes. Repeat if > 5 minutes; > 10 minutes indicates reduced tear secretion.

otc	**Sno-Strips** (Akorn)	**Strips:** Sterile tear flow test strips	In 100s.
otc	**Schirmer Tear Test** (Various, eg, Alcon)	**Strips:** Sterile test strips	In 250s.

Miscellaneous

SODIUM HYALURONATE

Actions:

Pharmacology: Sodium hyaluronate and sodium chondroitin sulfate are widely distributed in extracellular matrix of connective tissues. They are found in synovial fluid, skin, umbilical cord and vitreous and aqueous humor. The cornea is the ocular tissue having the greatest concentration of sodium chondroitin sulfate; the vitreous and aqueous humor contain the greatest concentration of sodium hyaluronate.

This preparation is a specific fraction of sodium hyaluronate developed for use in anterior segment and vitreous procedures as a viscoelastic agent. It has high molecular weight, is nonantigenic, does not cause inflammatory or foreign body reactions and has a high viscosity. The 1% solution is transparent and remains in the anterior chamber for < 6 days. It protects corneal endothelial cells and other ocular structures. It does not interfere with epithelialization and normal wound healing.

Indications:

Surgical aid: As a surgical aid in cataract extraction (intra- and extracapsular), intraocular lens implantation (IOL), corneal transplant, glaucoma filtration, retinal attachment surgery and posterior segment surgery to gently separate, maneuver and hold tissues.

To maintain a deep anterior chamber in surgical procedures in the anterior segment of the eye, allowing for efficient manipulation with less trauma to the corneal endothelium and other surrounding tissues.

To push back the vitreous face and prevent formation of a postoperative flat chamber.

To create a clear field of vision, facilitating intra- and postoperative inspection of the retina and photocoagulation.

Unlabeled uses: Sodium hyaluronate has been used in the treatment of refractory dry eye syndrome.

Warnings:

Hypersensitivity: Because this preparation is extracted from avian tissues and contains minute amounts of protein, risks of hypersensitivity may exist.

Precautions:

For intraocular use: Use only if solution is clear.

Postoperative intraocular pressure (IOP) may be elevated as a result of preexisting glaucoma, compromised outflow and by operative procedures and sequelae, including enzymatic zonulysis, absence of an iridectomy, trauma to filtration structures and by blood and lenticular remnants in the anterior chamber. Because the exact role of these factors is difficult to predict in any individual case, the following precautions are recommended:

Do not overfill the anterior chamber (except in glaucoma surgery). (See Administration and Dosage.)

Carefully monitor IOP, especially during the immediate postoperative period. Treat significant increases appropriately.

In posterior segment surgery, in aphakic diabetics, exercise special care to avoid using large amounts of the drug.

Remove some of the preparation by irrigation or aspiration at the close of surgery (except in glaucoma surgery). (See Administration and Dosage.)

Avoid trapping air bubbles behind the drug.

Cloudiness/precipitate: Reports indicate that the drug may become cloudy or form a slight precipitate after instillation. The clinical significance is not known because the majority do not indicate any harmful effects on ocular tissues. Be aware of this phenomenon and remove cloudy or precipitated material by irrigation or aspiration. In vitro studies suggest that this phenomenon may be related to interactions with certain concomitantly administered ophthalmic medications.

Miscellaneous

SODIUM HYALURONATE

Adverse Reactions:

Although well tolerated, a transient postoperative increase of IOP has been reported (see Precautions).

Other reactions that have occurred include postoperative inflammatory reactions (iritis, hypopyon); corneal edema; corneal decompensation.

Administration and Dosage:

Cataract surgery - IOL implantation: Slowly introduce a sufficient amount (using cannula or needle) into anterior chamber. Inject either before or after delivery of lens. Injection before lens delivery protects corneal endothelium from possible damage from removal of the cataractous lens. May use to coat surgical instruments and the IOL prior to insertion. May inject additional amounts during surgery to replace any of the drug lost.

Glaucoma filtration surgery: In conjunction with the performance of the trabeculectomy, inject slowly and carefully through a corneal paracentesis to reconstitute the anterior chamber. Further injection can be continued to allow it to extrude into the subconjunctival filtration site through and around the sutured outer scleral flap.

Corneal transplant surgery: After removal of the corneal button, fill the anterior chamber with the drug. Then, suture the donor graft in place. An additional amount may be injected to replace the lost amount as a result of surgical manipulation.

Sodium hyaluronate has also been used in the anterior chamber of the donor eye prior to trepanation to protect the corneal endothelial cells of the graft.

Retinal attachment surgery: Slowly introduce into the vitreous cavity. The injection may be directed to separate membranes from retina for safe excision and release of traction. Also serves to maneuver tissues into desired position (eg, to gently push back a detached retina or unroll a retinal flap); aids in holding retina against the sclera for reattachment.

Storage: Amvisc/Amvisc Plus, Healon/Healon GV: Store at 2° to 8°C (36° to 46°F).

AMO Vitrax – Store at room temperature (15° to 30°C; 59° to 86°F). Do not freeze. Protect from light.

Rx	**Healon** (Kabi Pharmacia)	**Injection**:10 mg/ml[1]	In 0.4, 0.55, 0.85 and 2 ml disp. syringes.
Rx	**Amvisc** (Chiron)	**Injection**: 12 mg/ml[2]	In 0.5 or 0.8 ml disp. syringe.
Rx	**Healon GV** (Kabi Pharmacia)	**Injection**: 14 mg/ml[1]	In 0.55 and 0.85 ml disp. syringes.
Rx	**Amvisc Plus** (Chiron)	**Injection**: 16 mg/ml[2]	In 0.5 or 8 ml disp. syringe.
Rx	**AMO Vitrax** (Allergan)	**Injection**: 30 mg/ml[3]	In 0.65 ml disp. syringe.

[1] With 8.5 mg NaCl per ml.
[2] With 9 mg NaCl per ml.
[3] With 3.2 mg NaCl, 0.75 mg KCl, 0.48 mg calcium chloride, 0.3 mg magnesium chloride, 3.9 mg sodium acetate and 1.7 mg sodium citrate per ml.

Miscellaneous

SODIUM HYALURONATE AND CHONDROITIN SULFATE

Refer to the Sodium Hyaluronate monograph for more complete information.

Indications:

Surgical aid: A surgical aid in anterior segment procedures including cataract extraction and intraocular lens implantation.

Administration and Dosage:

Carefully introduce (using a 27-gauge cannula) into the anterior chamber. May inject prior to or following delivery of the crystalline lens. Instillation prior to lens delivery provides additional protection to corneal endothelium, protecting it from possible damage arising from surgical instrumentation. May also be used to coat intraocular lens and tips of surgical instruments prior to implantation surgery. May inject additional solution during anterior segment surgery to fully maintain the chamber or to replace solution lost during surgery. At the end of surgery, remove solution by thoroughly irrigating the eye with a balanced salt solution. Alternatively, the solution may be left in the eye when used as directed.

Storage: Store at 2° to 8°C (36° to 46°F). Do not freeze.

Rx	**Viscoat** (Alcon)	**Solution:** ≤ 40 mg sodium chondroitin sulfate, 30 mg sodium hyaluronate per ml	0.45 mg sodium dihydrogen phosphate hydrate, 2 mg disodium hydrogen phosphate, 4.3 mg sodium chloride per ml. In 0.5 ml disposable syringes.

Miscellaneous

SODIUM HYALURONATE AND FLUORESCEIN SODIUM

Refer to the Sodium Hyaluronate and Fluorescein Sodium monographs for more complete information.

Indications:

Surgical aid: A surgical aid in anterior segment procedures including cataract extraction, intraocular lens (IOL) implantation and corneal transplant surgery. The fluorescein sodium facilitates visualization of the product during the surgical procedure.

Precautions:

IOP: Do not overfill the anterior segment as it may result in increased intraocular pressure, glaucoma or other ocular damage.

Administration and Dosage:

Cataract surgery/IOL implantation: Carefully introduce (using a 27–gauge cannula) into the anterior chamber. May inject prior to or following delivery of the lens. Instillation prior to lens delivery provides additional protection to corneal endothelium, protecting it from possible damage arising from removal of the cataractous lens. May also be used to coat the intraocular lens and surgical instruments prior to insertion. May inject additional solution during surgery to replace solution lost during surgical manipulation. Remove solution by irrigation or aspiration at the close of surgery.

Corneal transplant surgery: After removal of the corneal button, fill the anterior chamber with the solution. Then, suture the donor graft in place. May inject additional solution to replace solution lost during surgical manipulation. Remove solution by irrigation or aspiration at the close of surgery.

Storage: Store at 2° to 8°C (36° to 46°F). Allow to attain room temperature (approximately 30 min) prior to use. Do not freeze. Protect from light.

Rx	**Healon Yellow** (Pharmacia)	**Solution:** 10 mg sodium hyaluronate, 0.005 mg fluorescein sodium per ml	8.5 mg NaCl, 0.28 mg disodium hydrogen phosphate dihydrate, 0.04 mg sodium dihydrogen phosphate hydrate per ml. In 0.55 or 0.85 ml disposable syringes with cannula.

HYDROXYPROPYL METHYLCELLULOSE

Actions:

Pharmacology: Hydroxypropyl methylcellulose is an isotonic, nonpyrogenic viscoelastic solution with a high molecular weight (> 80,000 daltons). It maintains a deep chamber during anterior segment surgery and allows for more efficient manipulation with less trauma to the corneal endothelium and other ocular tissues. The viscoelasticity helps the vitreous face to be pushed back, preventing formation of a postoperative flat chamber. It is also used as a demulcent agent.

Indications:

Surgical aid:

2% solution – An ophthalmic surgical aid in anterior segment surgical procedures including cataract extraction and intraocular lens implantation.

2.5% solution – For professional use in gonioscopic examinations.

Precautions:

Intraocular pressure (IOP): Transient increased IOP may occur following surgery because of preexisting glaucoma or due to the surgery itself. If the postoperative IOP increases above expected values, administer appropriate therapy.

Adverse Reactions:

Although well tolerated, a transient, postoperative increase in IOP has been reported (see Precautions). Other reactions that have occurred include postoperative inflammatory reactions (iritis, hypopyon), corneal edema and corneal decompensation.

Administration and Dosage:

Anterior segment surgery: Carefully introduce into the anterior chamber using a 20-gauge or smaller cannula. The 2% solution may be used prior to or following delivery of the crystalline lens. Injection of 2% solution prior to lens delivery will provide additional protection to the corneal endothelium and other ocular tissues.

Miscellaneous

HYDROXYPROPYL METHYLCELLULOSE

The 2% solution may also be used to coat an intraocular lens and tips of surgical instruments prior to implantation surgery. May inject during anterior segment surgery to fully maintain the chamber, or to replace fluid lost during the surgical procedure. Remove solution from the anterior chamber at the end of surgery.

Gonioscopic examinations: Fill gonioscopic prism with 2.5% solution, as necessary.

Storage/Stability: If this solution dries on optical surfaces, let them stand in cool water before cleansing. If solution changes color or becomes cloudy, do not use. Not for use with hot laser treatment as solution clouding will occur.

To avoid contamination, do not touch tip of container to any surface. Replace cap after using. Keep container tightly closed. Store at room temperature 15° to 30°C (59° to 86°F). Avoid excessive heat over 60°C (140°F). Protect from light.

Rx	**OcuCoat** (Storz)	**Solution:** 2%	In a balanced salt solution. In 1 ml syringe with cannula.
otc	**Gonak** (Akorn)	**Solution:** 2.5%	In 15 ml.[1]
otc	**Goniosol** (Ciba Vision)		In 15 ml.[1]

[1] With 0.01% benzalkonium chloride and EDTA.

TYLOXAPOL

Actions:

Pharmacology: The cleaning/lubricant solution is a sterile, buffered isotonic solution formulated especially for artificial eye wearers. It contains the antibacterial agent benzalkonium chloride to kill most germs that are commonly found in the eye socket of artificial eye wearers. Tyloxapol, a detergent, liquifies the solid matter so that it is less irritating. Benzalkonium chloride, in addition to its germ-killing action, aids tyloxapol in wetting the artificial eye so that it is completely covered.

Indications:

Cleaner/Lubricant: To lubricate, clean and wet artificial eyes to increase wearing comfort.

Contraindications:

Hypersensitivity to any component of the formulation.

Patient Information:

If irritation persists or increases, discontinue use and consult your physician. Keep container tightly closed. Keep out of the reach of children.

To avoid contamination, do not touch dropper tip to any surface. Replace cap after using.

Administration and Dosage:

Use drops just as ordinary eye drops are used. With the artificial eye in place, apply 1 or 2 drops 3 or 4 times daily. The artificial eye may be removed periodically if advised by your physician, and 2 or 3 drops applied to remove oily or mucous materials. The artificial eye is then rubbed between the fingers and rinsed with tap water. Then 1 or 2 drops may be applied to the artificial eye, either prior to or after reinsertion.

Storage: Store at 8° to 27°C (46° to 80°F).

otc	**Enuclene** (Alcon)	**Solution:** 0.25%	0.02% benzalkonium Cl. In 15 ml Drop-Tainers.

HYDROXYETHYLCELLULOSE

Indications:

Gonioscopic bonding: For use in bonding gonioscopic prisms to the eye.

Administration and Dosage:

Storage: Store at room temperature 15° to 30°C (59° to 86°F).

Rx	**Gonioscopic** (Alcon)	**Solution:** Hydroxyethylcellulose	0.004% thimerosal, 0.1% EDTA. In 15 ml Drop-Tainers.

Miscellaneous

LID SCRUBS

Indications:

Eyelid cleansing: To aid in the removal of oils, debris or desquamated skin.

Precautions:

For external use only. Do not instill directly into eye.

Administration and Dosage:

Close eye(s) and gently scrub on eyelid(s) and lashes using lateral side-to-side strokes; rinse thoroughly.

otc	**Eye Scrub** (Ciba Vision Ophthalmics)	**Solution:** PEG-200 glyceryl monotallowate, disodium laureth sulfosuccinate, cocoamidopropylamine oxide, PEG-78 glyceryl monococoate, benzyl alcohol, EDTA	In 240 ml.
otc	**Lid Wipes-SPF** (Akorn)	**Solution:** PEG-200 glyceryl tallowate, PEG-80 glyceryl cocoate, laureth-23, cocoamidopropylamine oxide, NaCl, glycerin, sodium phosphate, sodium hydroxide	Preservative free. In UD 30s (pads).
otc	**OCuSOFT** (OCuSOFT)	**Solution:** PEG-80 sorbitan laurate, sodium trideceth sulfate, PEG-150 distearate, cocoamidopropyl hydroxysultaine, lauroamphocarboxyglycinate, sodium laureth-13 carboxylate, PEG-15 tallow polyamine, quaternium-15	Alcohol and dye free. In UD 30s (pads), 30, 120 and 240 ml and compliance kit (120 ml and 100 pads).

HAMAMELIS WATER

Indications:

Optic opacity: The manufacturer claims usefulness for the treatment of "optic opacity caused by cataract." Not intended for use in glaucoma.

Administration and Dosage:

Instill 2 drops morning and night into affected eye(s).

Rx	**Succus Cineraria Maritima** (Walker Pharm)	**Solution:** Aqueous and glycerin solution of senecio compositae, hamamelis water, boric acid	In 7 ml.

ZINC SULFATE SOLUTION

Indications:

Astringent: A mild astringent for temporary relief of minor eye irritation.

Warnings:

Irritation/Eye pain: If irritation persists or increases, or if eye pain or a change in vision occurs, discontinue use and consult physician.

Administration and Dosage:

Instill 1 to 2 drops into eye(s) up to 4 times daily. If solution discolors or becomes cloudy, do not use.

otc	**Eye-Sed** (Scherer)	**Solution:** 0.25%	In 15 ml.[1]

[1] With 0.05% tetrahydrozoline HCl, EDTA, benzalkonium Cl and NaCl.

Miscellaneous

BOTULINUM TOXIN TYPE A

Actions:

Pharmacology: Botulinum toxin is a sterile, lyophilized form of purified botulinum toxin type A, produced from a culture of the Hall strain of Clostridium botulinum grown in a medium containing N-Z amine and yeast extract. Botulinum toxin type A blocks neuromuscular conduction by binding to receptor sites on motor nerve terminals, entering the nerve terminals, and inhibiting the release of acetylcholine. When injected IM at therapeutic doses, botulinum toxin type A produces a localized chemical denervation muscle paralysis. When the muscle is chemically denervated, it atrophies and may develop extrajunctional acetylcholine receptors. There is evidence that the nerve can sprout and reinnervate the muscle, with the weakness thus being reversible.

The paralytic effect on muscles injected with botulinum toxin type A is useful in reducing the excessive, abnormal contractions associated with blepharospasm. When used for the treatment of strabismus, the administration of botulinum toxin type A may affect muscle pairs by inducing an atrophic lengthening of the injected muscle and a corresponding shortening of the muscle's antagonist. Following periocular injection of botulinum toxin type A, distant muscles show electrophysiologic changes, but no clinical weakness or other clinical change for a period of several weeks or months, parallel to the duration of local clinical paralysis.

Clinical trials: In one study, botulinum toxin was evaluated in 27 patients with essential blepharospasm; 26 had previously undergone drug treatment utilizing benztropine mesylate, clonazepam or baclofen without adequate clinical results. Three of these patients then underwent muscle stripping surgery still without an adequate outcome. Upon using botulinum toxin, 25 of the 27 patients reported improvement within 48 hours. One of the other patients was later controlled with a higher dosage. The remaining patient reported only mild improvement but remained functionally impaired.

In another study, 12 patients with blepharospasm were evaluated in a double-blind, placebo controlled study. All patients receiving botulinum toxin (n = 8) were improved compared with no improvements in the placebo group (n = 4). The mean dystonia score improved by 72%, the self-assessment score rating improved by 61%, and a videotape evaluation rating improved by 39%. The effects of the treatment lasted a mean of 12.5 weeks.

Patients with blepharospasm (n = 1684) evaluated in an open trial showed clinical improvement lasting an average of 12.5 weeks prior to need for retreatment.

Patients with strabismus (n = 677) treated with one or more injections of botulinum toxin type A were evaluated in an open trial; 55% were improved to an alignment of 10 prism diopters when evaluated ≥ 6 months following injection. These results are consistent with results from additional open label trials.

Indications:

Treatment of strabismus and blepharospasm associated with dystonia, including benign essential blepharospasm or VII nerve disorders in patients ≥ 12 years of age.

Unlabeled uses: Treatment of hemifacial spasms, spasmodic torticollis (ie, cervical dystonia, clonic twisting of the head), oromandibular dystonia, spasmodic dysphonia (laryngeal dystonia) and for other dystonias (eg, writer's cramp, focal task-specific dystonias). Botulinum toxin is being assessed in the treatment of head and neck tremor unresponsive to pharmacologic therapy. Designated an orphan drug for the treatment of dynamic muscle contracture in pediatric cerebral palsy patients.

Contraindications:

Hypersensitivity to any ingredient in the formulation.

Warnings:

Strabismus: The efficacy of botulinum toxin type A in deviations > 50 prism diopters, in restrictive strabismus, in Duane's syndrome with lateral rectus weakness, and in secondary strabismus caused by prior surgical over-recession of the antagonist is doubtful, or multiple injections over time may be required. Botulinum toxin type A is ineffective in chronic paralytic strabismus except to reduce antagonist contracture in conjunction with surgical repair.

Dosage: Do not exceed the recommended dosages and frequencies of administration. There have been no reported instances of systemic toxicity resulting from accidental injection or oral ingestion of botulinum toxin type A. Should accidental injection or oral ingestion occur, medically supervise the person for several days on an outpatient basis for signs or symptoms of systemic weakness or muscle paralysis. The entire contents of a vial is below the estimated dose for systemic toxicity in humans weighing ≥ 6 kg.

BOTULINUM TOXIN TYPE A

Hypersensitivity: As with all biologic products, epinephrine and other precautions should be available should an anaphylactic reaction occur. Refer to General Management of Acute Hypersensitivity Reactions.

Pregnancy: Category C. It is not known whether botulinum toxin type A can cause fetal harm when administered to a pregnant woman or can affect reproduction capacity. Administer to pregnant women only if clearly needed.

Lactation: It is not known whether this drug is excreted in breast milk. Exercise caution when botulinum toxin type A is administered to a nursing woman.

Children: Safety and efficacy in children < 12 years of age have not been established.

Precautions:

Safe and effective use of botulinum toxin type A depends upon proper storage of the product, selection of the correct dose and proper reconstitution and administration techniques. Physicians administering botulinum toxin type A must understand the relevant neuromuscular and orbital anatomy and any alterations to the anatomy due to prior surgical procedures, and standard electromyographic techniques.

Retrobulbar hemorrhages: During the administration of botulinum toxin type A for the treatment of strabismus, retrobulbar hemorrhages sufficient to compromise retinal circulation have occurred from needle penetrations into the orbit. Have appropriate instruments to decompress the orbit accessible. Ocular (globe) penetrations by needles have also occurred. An ophthalmoscope to diagnose this condition should be available.

Reduced blinking from botulinum toxin type A injection of the orbicularis muscle can lead to corneal exposure, persistent epithelial defect and corneal ulceration, especially in patients with VII nerve disorders. One case of corneal perforation in an aphakic eye requiring corneal grafting has occurred because of this effect. Carefully test corneal sensation in eyes previously operated upon, avoid injection into the lower lid area to avoid ectropion and vigorously treat any epithelial defect. This may require protective drops, ointment, therapeutic soft contact lenses, or closure of the eye by patching or other means.

Antibodies: Presence of antibodies to botulinum toxin type A may reduce the effectiveness of therapy. In clinical studies, reduction in effectiveness due to antibody production has occurred in one patient with blepharospasm receiving 3 doses over a 6 week period totaling 92 U and in several patients with torticollis who received multiple doses experimentally, totaling over 300 U in 1 month. For this reason, keep the dose of botulinum toxin type A for strabismus and blepharospasm as low as possible, in any case < 200 U in a 1 month period.

Drug Interactions:

Aminoglycosides: The effect of botulinum toxin may be potentiated by aminoglycoside antibiotics or any other drug that interferes with neuromuscular transmission. Exercise caution when botulinum toxin type A is used in patients taking these drugs.

Adverse Reactions:

Ophthalmic:

Strabismus – Inducing paralysis in one or more extraocular muscles may produce spatial disorientation, double vision or past-pointing. Covering the affected eye may alleviate these symptoms. Extraocular muscles adjacent to the injection site are often affected, causing ptosis or vertical deviation, especially with higher doses. Side effects in 2058 adults who received 3650 injections for horizontal strabismus included ptosis (15.7%) and vertical deviation (16.9%). The incidence of ptosis was much less after inferior rectus injection (0.9%) and much greater after superior rectus injection (37.7%).

Side effects persisting for > 6 months in an enlarged series of 5587 injections of horizontal muscles in 3104 patients included ptosis lasting over 180 days (0.3%) and vertical deviation > 2 prism diopters lasting over 180 days (2.1%).

In these patients, the injection procedure itself caused 9 scleral perforations. A vitreous hemorrhage occurred and later cleared in one case. No retinal detachment or visual loss occurred in any case; 16 retrobulbar hemorrhages occurred. Decompression of the orbit after 5 minutes was done to restore retinal circulation in one case. No eye lost vision from retrobulbar hemorrhage. Five eyes had pupillary change consistent with ciliary ganglion damage (Adies pupil).

Blepharospasm – In 1684 patients who received 4258 treatments (involving multiple injections) for blepharospasm, incidence of adverse reactions per treated eye was: Ptosis (11%); irritation/tearing, includes dry eye, lagophthalmos, and photophobia (10%); ectropion, keratitis, diplopia and entropion occurred rarely (< 1%).

BOTULINUM TOXIN TYPE A

Ecchymosis occurs easily in the soft eyelid tissues. This can be prevented by applying pressure at the injection site immediately after the injection. In two cases of VII nerve disorder (one case of an aphakic eye), reduced blinking from botulinum toxin type A injection of the orbicularis muscle led to serious corneal exposure, persistent epithelial defect and corneal ulceration. Perforation requiring corneal grafting occurred in one case, an aphakic eye (see Precautions).

Two patients previously incapacitated by blepharospasm experienced cardiac collapse attributed to over-exertion within 3 weeks following botulinum toxin type A therapy. Caution sedentary patients to resume activity slowly and carefully following the administration of botulinum toxin type A.

Local: Diffuse skin rash (n = 7) and local swelling of the eyelid skin (n = 2) lasting for several days following eyelid injection have occurred.

Overdosage:

In the event of overdosage or injection into the wrong muscle, additional information may be obtained by contacting Allergan Pharmaceuticals at (800) 347-5063 from 8 am to 4 pm Pacific Time, or at (714) 724-5954 for a recorded message at other times.

Patient Information:

Patients with blepharospasm may have been extremely sedentary for a long time. Caution these patients to resume activity slowly and carefully follow administration.

Administration and Dosage:

Strabismus: Botulinum toxin type A is intended for injection into extraocular muscles utilizing the electrical activity recorded from the tip of the injection needle as a guide to placement within the target muscle. Injection without surgical exposure or electromyographic guidance should not be attempted. Physicians should be familiar with electromyographic technique.

Preparation: An injection of botulinum toxin type A is prepared by drawing into a sterile 1 ml tuberculin syringe an amount of the properly diluted toxin (see Dilution Table) slightly greater than the intended dose. Air bubbles in the syringe barrel are expelled and the syringe is attached to the electromyographic injection needle, preferably a 1½ inch, 27 gauge needle. Injection volume in excess of the intended dose is expelled through the needle into an appropriate waste container to assure patency of the needle and to confirm that there is no syringe-needle leakage. Use a new, sterile needle and syringe to enter the vial on each occasion for dilution or removal of botulinum toxin type A.

To prepare the eye for botulinum toxin type A injection, give several drops of a local anesthetic and an ocular decongestant several minutes prior to injection.

Note: The volume of botulinum toxin type A injected for treatment of strabismus should be between 0.05 to 0.15 ml per muscle.

The initial listed doses of the diluted botulinum toxin type A (see Dilution table) typically create paralysis of injected muscles beginning 1 to 2 days after injection and increasing in intensity during the first week. The paralysis lasts for 2 to 6 weeks and gradually resolves over a similar time period. Overcorrections lasting > 6 months have been rare. About one half of patients will require subsequent doses because of inadequate paralytic response of the muscle to the initial dose, or because of mechanical factors such as large deviations or restrictions, or because of the lack of binocular motor fusion to stabilize the alignment.

1.) Initial doses in units (U). Use the lower listed doses for treatment of small deviations. Use the larger doses only for large deviations.
   a.) For vertical muscles, and for horizontal strabismus of < 20 prism diopters: 1.25 to 2.5 U in any one muscle.
   b.) For horizontal strabismus of 20 prism diopters to 50 prism diopters: 2.5 to 5 U in any one muscle.
   c.) For persistent VI nerve palsy of ≥ 1 month duration: 1.25 to 2.5 U in the medial rectus muscle.
2.) Subsequent doses for residual or recurrent strabismus.
   a.) Re-examine patients 7 to 14 days after each injection to assess the effect of that dose.
   b.) Patients experiencing adequate paralysis of the target muscle who require subsequent injections should receive a dose comparable to the initial dose.
   c.) Subsequent doses for patients experiencing incomplete paralysis of the target muscle may be increased up to twofold the previously administered dose.
   d.) Subsequent injections should not be administered until the effects of the previous dose have dissipated as evidenced by substantial function in the injected and adjacent muscles.

BOTULINUM TOXIN TYPE A

e.) Maximum recommended dose as a single injection for any one muscle is 25 U.

Blepharospasm: Diluted botulinum toxin type A (see Dilution table) is injected using a sterile, 27 to 30 gauge needle without electromyographic guidance. Initially, 1.25 to 2.5 U (0.05 to 0.1 ml volume at each site) injected into the medial and lateral pre-tarsal orbicularis oculi of the upper lid and into the lateral pre-tarsal orbicularis oculi of the lower lid is the initial recommended dose.

In general, the initial effect of the injections is seen within 3 days and reaches a peak at 1 to 2 weeks post-treatment. Each treatment lasts approximately 3 months, following which the procedure can be repeated indefinitely. At repeat treatment sessions, the dose may be increased up to twofold if the response from the initial treatment is considered insufficient (usually defined as an effect that does not last > 2 months). However, there appears to be little benefit obtainable from injecting > 5 U per site. Some tolerance may be found when botulinum toxin type A is used in treating blepharospasm if treatments are given any more frequently than every 3 months, and it is rare to have the effect be permanent.

The cumulative dose of botulinum toxin type A in a 30 day period should not exceed 200 U.

Dilution technique: To reconstitute lyophilized botulinum toxin type A, use sterile normal saline without a preservative; 0.9% sodium chloride injection is the recommended diluent. Draw up the proper amount of diluent in the appropriate size syringe. Since botulinum toxin type A is denatured by bubbling or similar violent agitation, inject the diluent into the vial gently. Discard the vial if a vacuum does not pull the diluent into the vial. Record the date and time of reconstitution on the space on the label. Administer within 4 hours after reconstitution.

During this time period, store reconstituted botulinum toxin type A in a refrigerator (2° to 8°C; 36° to 46°F). Reconstituted botulinum toxin type A should be clear, colorless and free of particulate matter. The use of one vial for more than one patient is not recommended because the product and diluent do not contain a preservative.

Dilution of Botulinum Toxin Type A

Diluent added (0.9% sodium chloride injection)	Resulting dose
1 ml	10 units
2 ml	5 units
4 ml	2.5 units
8 ml	1.25 units

Note: These dilutions are calculated for an injection volume of 0.1 ml. A decrease or increase in the botulinum toxin type A dose is also possible by administering a smaller or larger injection volume – from 0.05 ml (50% decrease in dose) to 0.15 ml (50% increase in dose).

Storage: Store the lyophilized product in a freezer at or below -5°C (23°F). Administer within 4 hours after the vial is removed from the freezer and reconstituted. During these 4 hours, store reconstituted botulinum toxin type A in a refrigerator (2° to 8°C; 36° to 46°F). Reconstituted botulinum toxin type A should be clear, colorless and free of particulate matter.

Rx	**Botox** (Allergan)	**Powder for Injection (lyophilized)**: 100 units of lyophilized *Clostridium botulinum* toxin type A[1]	Preservative free. 0.05 mg albumin (human), 0.9 mg sodium chloride. In vials.

[1] One unit corresponds to the calculated median lethal intraperitoneal dose (LD/50) in mice of the reconstituted drug injected.

Miscellaneous

POLYDIMETHYLSILOXANE (Silicone Oil)

Actions:

Pharmacology: Polydimethylsiloxane, an oil that is injected into the vitreous space of the eye, is used as a prolonged retinal tamponade in select cases of retinal detachment.

Clinical trials:

Anatomic reattachment rates – Successful reattachment of the retina occurred in 64% to 75% of the patients who were treated with polydimethylsiloxane. This rate varied depending on the specific etiology of the disease and the severity of the condition. In AIDS CMV retinitis patients receiving silicone oil as a primary means for reattaching the retina, attachment rates were as high as 90% within an average 6 month follow up period.

Visual acuity outcomes – From 45% to 70% of patients showed improvements in visual acuity at 6 months. In about 15% to 26% of patients, visual acuity did not change and in about 15% to 30%, worsening of visual acuity occurred. Deterioration of visual acuity in treated patients appeared to be related to redetachment of the retina, further progression of retinal disease, or to keratopathy and cataract complications. In AIDS CMV retinitis patients, improvement or maintenance of visual acuity was documented in 57% of the patients within an average 6 month follow-up period. In AIDS patients, further decline in visual acuity was seen due to continuing progression of retinal and optic nerve disease and development of oil related cataracts in 33% of patients within 4 to 5 months of oil instillation.

Indications:

Retinal detachments: Prolonged retinal tamponade in selected cases of complicated retinal detachments where other interventions are not appropriate for patient management. Complicated retinal detachments or recurrent retinal detachments occur most commonly in eyes with proliferative vitreoretinopathy (PVR), proliferative diabetic retinopathy (PDR), cytomegalovirus (CMV) retinitis, giant tears and following perforating injuries.

For primary use in detachments due to AIDS-related CMV retinitis and other viral infections.

Contraindications:

Pseudophakic patients with silicone intraocular lens (silicone oil can chemically interact and opacify silicone elastomers).

Warnings:

Cataract: Approximately 50% to 70% of phakic patients developed a cataract within 12 months of oil instillation. Approximately 33% of phakic AIDS CMV retinitis patients developed some degree of cataract within an average 4 to 5 month time frame from oil instillation.

Anterior chamber oil migration: In 17% to 20% of patients, oil emulsification or migration into the anterior chamber was observed. Migration into the anterior chamber occurred in both phakic and aphakic patients.

Keratopathy: From 8% to 20% of patients developed keratopathy (0.6%, AIDS patients). This complication occurred most frequently in aphakic patients (18% to 21%) and in the patients in whom oil had migrated into the anterior chamber (30%); the keratopathy in these cases was attributed to prolonged physical contact between the corneal endothelium and the silicone oil.

Glaucoma: Approximately 19% to 20% (0.06%, AIDS patients) of patients developed a persistent elevation in intraocular pressure (> 23 to 25 mm Hg). The neovascular glaucoma rate was about 8%. Moderate temporary postoperative increases occurred within the first 3 weeks of treatment. Thereafter, secondary ocular hypertension occurred by several mechanisms. Glaucoma complications occurred in approximately 30% of patients in which anterior chamber oil is noted. Patients with proliferative diabetic retinopathy were at highest risk for development of glaucoma following silicone oil instillation into the vitreous space.

Precautions:

Long-term use: The safety and efficacy of long-term use have not been established.

Adverse Reactions:

Most common: The most common adverse reactions include: Cataract (50% to 70%); anterior chamber oil migration (17% to 20%); keratopathy (8% to 20%); glaucoma (19% to 20%). See Warnings.

Miscellaneous

POLYDIMETHYLSILOXANE (Silicone Oil)

Miscellaneous: Other adverse reactions ranked by frequency of occurrence: Redetachment, optic nerve atrophy, rubeosis iritis, temporary IOP increase, macular pucker, vitreous hemorrhage, phthisis, traction detachment, angle block (> 2%); subretinal strands, retinal rupture, endophthalmitis, subretinal silicone oil, choroidal detachment, aniridia, PVR reproliferation, cystoid macular edema, enucleation (< 2%).

Administration and Dosage:

Approved by the FDA on November 7, 1994.

Polydimethylsiloxane can be used in conjunction with or following standard retinal surgical procedures including scleral buckle surgery, vitrectomy, membrane peeling and retinotomy or relaxing retinectomy.

Avoid introduction of air bubbles into the oil by careful withdrawal or decanting of the oil into the syringe. The oil can be injected into the vitreous from the syringe via a single use cannulated infusion line or syringe needle. Subretinal fluid can be drained with a flute needle concurrent with polydimethylsiloxane infusion. The vitreous space can be filled with the oil to between 80% and 100% while exchanging for fluid or air, taking necessary precautions to avoid high intraocular pressure from developing during the exchange. Because the polydimethylsiloxane is less dense than the eye aqueous fluid, a basal iridectomy at the 6 o'clock meridian (Ando iridectomy) is recommended to minimize oil induced pupillary block and early angle-closure glaucoma. Upon choice of the physician, it may be desirable to have the patient assume a face-down posture during the first 24 hours following surgery.

Monitor the patient closely for development of glaucoma, cataract and keratopathy complications and schedule for follow-up reexamination at regular intervals.

It is recommended that polydimethylsiloxane be removed at an appropriate interval within 1 year following instillation if the retina is stable, attached and without significant remnants of proliferation. Although there is insufficient clinical evidence to support justification for longer term tamponade, whether or not the oil should be removed in patients at high risk for redetachment or the development of phthisis and shrinkage due to hypotony must be determined individually by the physician. In order to minimize the number of invasive traumatic experiences for patients with AIDS and CMV retinitis at high risk for redetachment and who have a shortened expected lifespan, avoid silicone oil removal procedures if the patient concurs.

Polydimethylsiloxane can be removed from the posterior chamber by withdrawal with a normal 10 ml syringe and a wide bore 1 mm cannula. By repeated oil-fluid exchange most of the remaining small silicone oil droplets can subsequently be mobilized and removed from the eye. Alternatively, oil may be passively removed by infusion of an appropriate aqueous solution under the oil bubble, while allowing the oil to effuse out of a sclerotomy incision, or limbal incision in aphakic patients.

As there is a possible correlation between the migration of polydimethylsiloxane into the anterior chamber and the appearance of corneal changes such as edema, hazing or opacification, Descemet folds or decompensation, perform regular monitoring of the patient's corneal status and take early corrective action if necessary, including extraction of the oil from the anterior chamber. Large bubbles or droplets of oil in the anterior chamber can be removed manually by syringe. Further standard practice for medical treatment of the keratopathy is recommended.

Temporary pressure increases > 3 weeks after surgery that can normalize either spontaneously or that can be corrected by surgical treatment are those in which the polydimethylsiloxane causes a mechanical blockage of the pupil or inferior iridectomy or causes chamber angle closure by forcing its way anteriorly. In these situations some of the oil may be withdrawn to relieve the mechanical force of the oil interface. Presence of polydimethylsiloxane droplets in the anterior chamber may also cause a chronic outflow obstruction of the trabecular meshwork. In such situations elevated intraocular pressure can be managed with anti-glaucoma medication in the majority of outflow obstruction patients.

Admixture incompatibility: Do not admix with any other substances prior to injection.

Storage/Stability: Store at room or cool temperature (8° to 24°C; 46° to 75°F). Polydimethylsiloxane is supplied in a sterile vial intended for single use only and contains no preservative. Do not resterilize. Discard unused portions. Product should be discarded following expiration date.

Rx	**AdatoSil 5000** (Escalon Ophthalmics[1])	**Injection**: Polydimethylsiloxane oil	In single-use 10 and 15 ml vials.

[1] Escalon Ophthalmics, Inc., Montgomery Knoll, 182 Tamarack Circle, Skillman, NJ 08558; (800) 486–4848.

OTIC PREPARATIONS

The otic preparations on the following pages are divided into groups as follows:

Steroid and Antibiotic Combinations
Miscellaneous Preparations
Antibiotics

Patient Information: For use in the ear only. Avoid contact with the eyes.

Notify physician if burning or itching occurs or if condition persists.

Perforated tympanic membrane is considered a contraindication to the use of any medication in the external ear canal.

Proper use of ear drops:

- Wash hands thoroughly.
- Avoid touching the dropper to the ear or any other surface. For accuracy and to avoid contamination, have another person insert the ear drops when possible.
- Hold container in the hand for a few minutes to warm to near body temperature if it has been refrigerated.
- If the drops are in a suspension form, shake well for 10 seconds before using.
- Lie on your side or tilt the affected ear up for ease of administration.To allow the drops to run in:
  - *Adults*-Hold the earlobe up and back.
  - *Children*-Hold the earlobe down and back.
- Instill the prescribed number of drops in the ear.
- Do not insert the dropper into the ear.
- Keep the ear tilted for about 2 minutes, or insert a soft cotton plug, whichever is recommended.

Products used to soften, loosen and remove earwax:

- Do not use if ear drainage, discharge, pain, irritation or rash occurs.
- If you become dizzy, consult a physician.
- Do not use if injury or perforation of the ear drum exists or after ear surgery unless directed otherwise.
- Do not use for > 4 days; if excessive earwax remains after use of this product, consult a physician.
- Any wax remaining after treatment may be removed by gently flushing with warm water using a soft rubber bulb ear syringe.

STEROID AND ANTIBIOTIC COMBINATIONS

Refer also to Patient Information in the Otic Product Preparations introduction for instructions on the use of these products.

Actions:

Pharmacology:

In these combinations –

HYDROCORTISONE is used for its antiallergic, antipruritic and anti-inflammatory effects.

ANTIBIOTICS are used for their antibacterial actions.

Indications:

Treatment of superficial bacterial infections of the external auditory canal.

Suspension: Also used to treat infections of mastoidectomy and fenestration cavities.

Contraindications:

Hypersensitivity to any component.

Precautions:

Superinfection: Prolonged treatment may result in overgrowth of nonsusceptible organisms and fungi (eg, herpes simplex, vaccinia, varicella).

Administration and Dosage:

The usual adult dose is 4 drops instilled 3 or 4 times daily.

STEROID AND ANTIBIOTIC COMBINATIONS, SOLUTIONS

Complete prescribing information begins in the Steroid and Antibiotic Combinations monograph.

Rx	**Antibiotic Ear Solution** (Various, eg, Geneva, Rugby, URL)	**Solution:** 1% hydrocortisone, 5 mg neomycin sulfate[1], 10,000 units polymyxin B	In 10 ml.
Rx	**AntibiOtic** (Parnell)		In 10 ml.[2]
Rx	**AK-Spore H.C. Otic** (Akorn)		In 10 ml with dropper.[2]
Rx	**Cortatrigen Modified Ear Drops** (Goldline)		In 10 ml with dropper.[2]
Rx	**Cortisporin Otic** (Glaxo Wellcome)		In 10 ml with dropper.[3]
Rx	**Drotic** (Ascher)		In 10 ml with dropper.[2]
Rx	**Ear-Eze** (Hyrex)		In 10 ml with dropper.[2]
Rx	**LazerSporin-C** (Pedinol)		In 10 ml with dropper.
Rx	**Otic-Care** (Parmed)		In 10 ml.
Rx	**Octicair** (Bausch & Lomb)		In 10 ml with dropper.[2]
Rx	**Otocort** (Lemmon)		In 10 ml with dropper.
Rx	**Otomycin-HPN Otic** (Misemer)		In 10 ml with dropper.[2]
Rx	**Otosporin** (Calmic)		In 10 ml with dropper.
Rx	**Otobiotic Otic** (Schering)	**Solution:** 0.5% hydrocortisone, 10,000 units polymyxin B	In 15 ml with dropper.[4]

[1] 5 mg neomycin sulfate is equivalent to 3.5 mg neomycin base.
[2] With propylene glycol, glycerin and potassium metabisulfite.
[3] With cupric sulfate, propylene glycol, glycerin and potassium metabisulfite.
[4] With propylene glycol, glycerin, EDTA, sodium bisulfite and anhydrous sodium sulfite.

Steroid and Antibiotic Combinations

STEROID AND ANTIBIOTIC COMBINATIONS, SUSPENSIONS

Complete prescribing information begins in the Steroid and Antibiotic Combinations group monograph.

Rx	**Antibiotic Ear Suspension** (Various, eg, Geneva, Rugby, URL)	**Suspension:** 1% hydrocortisone, 5 mg neomycin sulfate[1], 10,000 units polymyxin B**Suspension:** 1% hydrocortisone,	In 10 ml with dropper.
Rx	**AntibiOtic** (Parnell)		In 10 ml with dropper.[2]
Rx	**AK-Spore H.C. Otic** (Akorn)		In 10 ml with dropper.[2]
Rx	**Cortatrigen Ear** (Goldline)		In 10 ml with dropper.[2]
Rx	**Cortisporin Otic** (Glaxo Wellcome)		In 10 ml with dropper.[2]
Rx	**Octicair** (Bausch & Lomb)		In 10 ml with dropper.[3]
Rx	**Otic-Care** (Parmed)		In 10 ml with dropper.[3]
Rx	**OtiTricin** (Bausch & Lomb)		In 7.5 and 10 ml with dropper.[4]
Rx	**Otocort** (Lemmon)		In 10 ml with dropper.
Rx	**Pediotic** (Glaxo Wellcome)		In 7.5 ml with dropper.[5]
Rx	**UAD Otic** (UAD)		In 10 ml.
Rx	**Neomycin/Polymyxin B Sulfates/Hydrocortisone Otic** (Steris)		In 10 ml with dropper.[2]
Rx	**Coly-Mycin S Otic** (Parke-Davis)	**Suspension:** 1% hydrocortisone, 4.71 neomycin sulfate[6]	With 3 mg colistin (as sulfate) and 0.05% thonzonium Br/ml. In 5 and 10 ml with dropper.[7]

[1] 5 mg neomycin sulfate is equivalent to 3.5 mg neomycin base.
[2] With cetyl alcohol, propylene glycol, polysorbate 80 and thimerosal.
[3] With cetyl alcohol, polyoxyl 40 stearate, polysorbate 80, propylene glycol, sulfuric acid and benzalkonium Cl.
[4] With cetyl alcohol, polyoxyl 40 stearate, polysorbate 80, propylene glycol and benzalkonium Cl.
[5] With thimerosal, cetyl alcohol, glyceryl monostearate, mineral oil, polyoxyl 40 stearate and propylene glycol.
[6] 4.71 mg neomycin sulfate is equivalent to 3.3 mg neomycin base.
[7] With polysorbate 80, acetic acid, sodium acetate and thimerosal.

MISCELLANEOUS OTIC PREPARATIONS

In these combinations:

HYDROCORTISONE and DESONIDE are steroids used for their anti-inflammatory and antipruritic effects.

PHENYLEPHRINE is a vasoconstrictor which may be a decongestant.

ACETIC ACID, M-CRESYL ACETATE, BORIC ACID, BENZALKONIUM CHLORIDE, BENZETHONIUM CHLORIDE and ALUMINUM ACETATE (BUROW'S SOLUTION) provide antibacterial or antifungal action.

CARBAMIDE PEROXIDE and TRIETHANOLAMINE emulsify and disperse ear wax.

GLYCERIN is a solvent and vehicle; it has emollient, hygroscopic and humectant properties.

BENZOCAINE is a local anesthetic.

ANTIPYRINE is an analgesic.

Rx	**VoSoL HC Otic** (Wallace)	**Solution:** 1% hydrocortisone, 2% acetic acid, 3% propylene glycol diacetate, 0.015% sodium acetate and 0.02% benzethonium chloride *Dose:* Insert saturated wick into ear; leave in for 24 hours, keeping moist with 3 to 5 drops every 4 to 6 hours. Keep moist for 24 hours. Remove wick and instill 5 drops 3 or 4 times daily	With 0.05% citric acid. In 10 ml with dropper.
Rx	**Acetasol HC** (Barre-National)		With 0.2% citric acid. In 10 ml with dropper.
otc	**EarSol-HC** (Parnell)	**Solution:** 1% hydrocortisone, 44% alcohol, propylene glycol, *Dermprotective Factor* yerba santa, benzyl benzoate *Dose:* Insert 4 to 6 drops into ear ≤ 3 to 4 times/day	In 30 ml.
Rx	**Cortic Ear** (Everett)	**Drops:** 1% hydrocortisone, 1% pramoxine HCl, 0.1% chloroxylenol, 3% propylene glycoldiacetate *Dose:* Insert 4 to 5 drops into affected ear 3 or 4 times/day	In 10 ml.
Rx	**Oti-Med** (Hyrex)	**Drops:** 0.1% chloroxylenol, 1% pramoxine HCl, 1% hydrocortisone, propylene glycol, benzalkonium Cl *Dose:* Adults - Instill 4 to 5 drops into affected ear 3 or 4 times daily. Children and infants - Instill 3 drops into affected ear 3 or 4 times daily.	In 10 ml vials.
Rx	**Tri-Otic** (Pharmics)	**Drops:** 0.1% chloroxylenol, 1% pramoxine HCl; 1% hydrocortisone	In 10 ml vials.
Rx	**AA-HC Otic** (Schein)	**Solution:** 1% hydrocortisone, 2% acetic acid glacial, 3% propylene glycol diacetate, 0.02% benzethonium Cl, 0.015% sodium acetate, 0.2% citric acid *Dose:* Insert saturated wick into ear; leave in for 24 hours, keeping moist with 3 to 5 drops every 4 to 6 hours. Keep moist for 24 hours. Remove wick and instill 5 drops 3 or 4 times daily	In 10 ml.
Rx	**Allergen Ear Drops** (Goldline)	**Solution:** 1.4% benzocaine, 5.4% antipyrine, glycerin *Dose:* Fill ear canal with 2 to 4 drops; insert saturated cotton pledget. Repeat 3 or 4 times daily, or up to once every 1 to 2 hours	In 15 ml with dropper.[1]
Rx	**Antipyrine and Benzocaine Otic** (Various)		In 10 and 15 ml.
Rx	**Auralgan Otic** (Wyeth-Ayerst)		In 10 ml with dropper.
Rx	**Auroto Otic** (Barre-National)		In 15 ml with dropper.[1]
Rx	**Ear Drops** (Rugby)		In 10 ml.[1]
Rx	**Otocalm Ear** (Parmed)		In 15 ml.

MISCELLANEOUS OTIC PREPARATIONS

Rx	**Tympagesic** (Adria)	**Solution:** 5% benzocaine, 5% antipyrine, 0.25% phenylephrine HCl, propylene glycol *Dose:* Fill ear canal; plug with saturated cotton. Repeat every 2 to 4 hours	In 13 ml with dropper.
Rx	**Americaine Otic** (Fisons)	**Solution:** 20% benzocaine, 0.1% benzethonium chloride, 1% glycerin, PEG 300 *Dose:* Instill 4 or 5 drops. Insert cotton pledget. Repeat every 1 to 2 hours	In 15 ml with dropper.
Rx	**Otocain** (Abana)		In 15 ml.
Rx	**Cresylate** (Recsei)	**Solution:** 25% m-cresyl acetate, 25% isopropanol, 1% chlorobutanol, 1% benzyl alcohol, 5% castor oil, propylene glycol *Dose:* 2 to 4 drops as required	In 15 ml with dropper and pt.
Rx	**Acetic Acid Otic** (Various, eg, Geneva, Rugby, Schein)	**Solution:** 2% acetic acid with 3% propylene glycol diacetate, 0.02% benzethonium chloride, 0.015% sodium acetate *Dose:* Insert saturated wick; keep moist 24 hours. Remove wick and instill 5 drops 3 or 4 times daily	In 15 ml.
Rx	**Acetasol** (Barre)		In 15 ml.
Rx	**VoSoL Otic** (Wallace)		In 15 and 30 ml dropper bottles.
Rx	**Acetic Acid 2% and Aluminum Acetate Otic Solution** (Bausch & Lomb)	**Solution:** 2% acetic acid in aluminum acetate solution *Dose:* Insert saturated wick; keep moist for 24 hours. Instill 4 to 6 drops every 2 to 3 hours	In 60 ml.
Rx	**Burow's Otic** (Rugby)		In 60 ml.
Rx	**Otic Domeboro** (Miles Pharm.)		In 60 ml with dropper.
Rx	**Borofair Otic** (Major)	**Solution:** 2% acetic acid, aluminum acetate	In 60 ml.
Rx	**Cerumenex Drops** (Purdue Frederick)	**Solution:** 10% triethanolamine polypeptide oleate-condensate, 0.5% chlorobutanol, propylene glycol *Dose:* Fill ear canal. Insert cotton plug, allow to remain 15 to 30 minutes. Flush ear	In 6 and 12 ml with dropper.
Rx	**Zoto-HC** (Horizon)	**Drops:** 0.1% chloroxylenol, 1% pramoxine HCl, 1% hydrocortisone, 3% propylene glycol *Dose:* Instill 4 to 5 drops into affected ear 3 or 4 times daily	In 10 ml plastic dropper vials.
otc	**Auro-Dri** (Commerce)	**Solution:** 2.75% boric acid, isopropyl alcohol *Dose:* Instill 3 to 8 drops in each ear	In 30 ml with dropper.
otc	**Dri/Ear** (Pfeiffer)		In 30 ml.
otc	**Ear-Dry** (Scherer)		In 30 ml w/ dropper.
otc	**Star-Otic** (Stellar)	**Solution:** Nonaqueous acetic acid, Burow's solution, boric acid, propylene glycol *Dose:* Instill 2 to 3 drops before and after swimming or showering	In 15 ml with dropper.
otc	**Debrox** (Marion Merrell Dow)	**Drops:** 6.5% carbamide peroxide, glycerin, propylene glycol, sodium stannate *Dose:* Instill 5 to 10 drops twice daily for up to 4 days	In 30 ml with dropper.

MISCELLANEOUS OTIC PREPARATIONS

otc	**Murine Ear** (Ross)	**Drops:** 6.5% carbamide peroxide, 6.3% alcohol, glycerin, polysorbate 20 *Dose:* Instill 5 to 10 drops twice daily for up to 4 days	In 15 ml.
otc	**Auro Ear Drops** (Commerce)	**Solution:** 6.5% carbamide peroxide in an anhydrous glycerine base *Dose:* Instill 5 to 10 drops twice daily for up to 4 days	In 15 ml.
otc	**E•R•O Ear** (Scherer)	**Drops:** 6.5% carbamide peroxide, anhydrous glycerin *Dose:* Instill 5 to 10 drops twice daily for up to 4 days	In 15 ml.
otc	**Mollifene Ear Wax Removing Formula** (Pfeiffer)		With propylene glycol and sodium stannate. In 15 ml with dropper.
otc	**Swim-Ear** (Fougera)	**Liquid:** 95% isopropyl alcohol, 5% anhydrous glycerin *Dose:* Instill 4 or 5 drops in affected ear after swimming, showering or bathing	In 30 ml.
otc	**EarSol** (Parnell)	**Drops:** 44% alcohol, propylene glycol, *Dermaprotective Factor* yerba santa, benzyl benzoate *Dose:* Instill 6 to 8 drops twice daily	In 50 ml.

[1] With oxyquinoline sulfate.

CHLORAMPHENICOL

Actions:

Pharmacology: Chloramphenicol is a broad-spectrum antibiotic originally isolated from *Streptomyces venezuelae.* It is primarily bacteriostatic and acts by inhibition of protien synthesis by interfering with the transfer of activated aminio acids from soluble RNA to ribosomes. Development of resistance to chloramphenicol can be regarded as minimal for staphylococci and many other species of bacteria.

Indications:

For treating superficial infections involving the external auditory canal. For inner ear infections, use systemic antibiotic therapy.

Contraindications:

Hypersensitivity to any component; when less potentially dangerous agents would be expected to provide effective treatment; perforated tympanic membrane.

Warnings:

Bone marrow hypoplasia, including aplastic anemia and death, has been reported following local application of chloramphenicol.

Inner ear infections: Use systemic antibiotic therapy.

Sensitization/Irritation: Discontinue promptly if these occur.

Ototoxicity: The possibility of ototoxicity must be considered if medication is allowed to enter the middle ear.

Precautions:

Superinfection: Use of antibiotics (especially prolonged or repeated therapy) may result in bacterial or fungal overgrowth of nonsusceptible organisms. Such overgrowth may lead to secondary infection. Take appropriate measures if superinfection occurs.

Serious infections: Supplement topical chloramphenicol with appropriate systemic medication.

Adverse Reactions:

Signs of local irritation (itching or burning, angioneurotic edema, urticaria, vesicular and maculopapular dermatitis) have occurred in patients sensitive to chloramphenicol and are causes for discontinuation. Blood dyscrasias have occurred with chloramphenicol. Similar sensitivity reactions to other materials in topical preparations may also occur.

Administration and Dosage:

Instill 2 or 3 drops into the ear 3 times daily.

Rx	**Chloromycetin Otic** (Parke-Davis)	**Solution:** 0.5% in propylene glycol	In 15 ml with dropper.

NYSTATIN

Actions:

Pharmacology: Nystatin, an antifungal antibiotic, is both fungistatic and fungicidal in vitro against a wide variety of yeasts and yeast-like fungi. It is a polyene antibiotic of undetermined structural formula that is obtained from *Streptomyces noursei.* It binds to sterols in the cell membrane of the fungus with a resultant change in membrane permeability.

Pharmacokinetics: Following oral administration, nystatin is sparingly absorbed with no detectable blood levels. Most of the orally adminstered drug is passed unchanged in the stool.

Indications:

Candidiasis: Treatment of oral candidiasis.

For information on nystatin for treatment of intestinal candidiasis, refer to the monograph in the Antifungals Agents section.

Contraindications:

Hypersensitivity to nystatin.

Warnings:

Systemic mycoses: Nystatin is not indicated for the treatment of systemic mycoses.

Pregnancy: Category C. Safety for use during pregnancy has not been established. Use only if clearly needed and when the potential benefits outweigh the potential hazards to the fetus.

Adverse Reactions:

GI: Nausea, vomiting, GI distress and diarrhea occur occasionally with large doses.

Overdosage:

Oral doses of nystatin > 5,000,000 units/day have caused nausea and GI upset.

Patient Information:

Retain the drug in the mouth as long as possible.

Continue use at least 2 days after symptoms have subsided.

Administration and Dosage:

Oral suspension:

Adults and children – 400,000 to 600,000 units 4 times daily (one half of dose in each side of mouth, retaining the drug as long as possible before swallowing).

Infants – 200,000 units 4 times daily (100,000 units in each side of mouth).

Premature and low birth weight infants – Limited clinical studies indicate that 100,000 units 4 times daily is effective.

Troches (pastilles):

Adults and children – 200,000 to 400,000 units 4 or 5 times daily , for as long as 14 days, if necessary. Do not chew or swallow whole. To achieve maximum effect from the medication, the roches must be allowed to dissolve slowly in the mouth; therefore, patients, including children and the elderly, must be competent to utilize the dosage form as intended. Discontinue dosage if symptoms persist after the initial 14 day treatment period.

Powder for extemporaneous compounding:

Adults and children – Add ⅛ tsp (≈ 500,000 units) to ≈ ½ cup of water and stir well. Administer 4 times daily. Use immediately after mixing; do not store.

Continue local treatment at least 48 hours after perioral signs and symptoms have disappeared and cultures have returned to normal.

To improve oral retention of the drug, nystatin (250,000 units) has been administered for oral candidiasis in the form of flavored frozen popsicles.

Rx	**Nystatin** (Various, eg, Geneva, Major, NMC, Parmed, Rugby)	**Oral suspension:** 100,000 units/ml	In 5, 60 and 480 ml.
Rx	**Mycostatin** (Apothecon)		< 1% alcohol, saccharin, 50% sucrose. In 60 and 473 ml.
Rx	**Nilstat** (Lederle)		Cherry flavor. In 60 and 473 ml.
Rx	**Nystex** (Savage)		In 60 ml.
Rx	**Mycostatin Pastilles** (Bristol-Myers Oncology)	**Troches:** 200,000 units	In 30s.

NYSTATIN

Rx	**Nystatin** (Paddock)	**Bulk Powder:** 50 million units	
Rx	**Nilstat** (Lederle)	**Bulk Powder:** 150 million units	
Rx	**Nystatin** (Paddock)		
Rx	**Nystatin** (Paddock)	**Bulk Powder:** 500 million units	
Rx	**Nilstat** (Lederle)	**Bulk Powder:** 1 billion units	
Rx	**Nystatin** (Paddock)		
Rx	**Nilstat** (Lederle)	**Bulk Powder:** 2 billion units	
Rx	**Nystatin** (Paddock)		
Rx	**Nystatin** (Paddock)	**Bulk Powder:** 5 billion units	

TANNIC ACID

Actions:

Pharmacology: These products form a thin pliable film over sores or blisters within 60 seconds of application. This protective film, if used in the mouth, normally withstands eating and drinking.

Indications:

For temporary relief of pain, burning and itching caused by cold sores, fever blisters and canker sores.

Precautions:

Do not use in or around eyes: If contact occurs, flush immediately and continuously with clear water for 10 minutes. Consult physician immediately if pain or irritation persists.

Stinging sensation: A slight, temporary stinging sensation may occur when the drug is applied to an open sore or blister.

Infection: If infection persists beyond 10 days, discontinue use and consult a physician.

Administration and Dosage:

At first symptoms, apply every 4 hours for the first three days and then as needed. Wipe affected areas dry before applying.

otc	**Zilactin Medicated** (Zila Pharm.)	**Gel:** 7% suspended in 80% alcohol	In 7.5 g.

CLOTRIMAZOLE

For information on oral and vaginal clotrimazole, refer to individual monographs.

Actions:

Pharmacology: A broad spectrum antifungal agent that inhibits yeast growth by altering cell membrane permeability. It is fungicidal in vitro against *Candida albicans* and other *Candida* sp.

Pharmacokinetics: Following oral administration, long-term concentration in saliva appears related to the slow release of drug from the oral mucosa to which clotrimazole is apparently bound. Dosing every 3 hours maintains effective salivary levels for most strains of *Candida.*

Indications:

Treatment: Local treatment of oropharyngeal candidiasis.

Prophylaxis: To reduce the incidence of oropharyngeal candidiasis in patients immunocompromised by conditions that include chemotherapy, radiotherapy or steroid therapy utilized in the treatment of leukemia, solid tumors or renal transplantation.

Contraindications:

Hypersensitivity to clotrimazole.

Warnings:

Systemic mycoses: Clotrimazole is not indicated for the treatment of systemic mycoses.

Prophylactic use: There are no data to establish safety and efficacy for prophylactic use in patients immunocompromised by etiologies other than those listed in indications.

Pregnancy: Category C. Clotrimazole is embryotoxic in rats and mice given doses 100 times the adult human dose, possibly secondary to maternal toxicity. Doses of 120 times the human dose in mice from 9 weeks before mating through weaning was associated with impairment of mating, decreased number of viable young and

CLOTRIMAZOLE

decreased survival to weaning. There are no adequate and well controlled studies in pregnant women. Use only when clearly needed and when the potential benefits outweight the potential hazards to the fetus.

Children: Safety and efficacy for use in children under 3 years of age have not been established; therefore, use in these patients is not recommended. Safety and efficacy of the prophylactic use of clotrimazole troches in children have not been established.

Precautions:

Abnormal liver function tests: AST levels were minimally elevated in ≈ 15% of patients in clinical trials. It was often impossible to distinguish effects of clotrimazole from other therapy and the underlying disease (malignancy in most cases). Assess hepatic function periodically, particularly in patients with pre-existing hepatic impairment.

Because patients must allow the troche to dissolve slowly in the mouth to achieve maximum effect, they must be of such an age or physical/mental condition to comprehend such instructions.

Adverse Reactions:

Abnormal liver function test; elevated AST levels were reported in ≈ 15% of patients in clinical trials (see Precautions).

Nausea, vomiting, unpleasant mouth sensations, pruritus.

Patient Information:

To achieve maximum effect, allow troche to dissolve slowly in the mouth.

Administration and Dosage:

Dissolve troche slowly in mouth in order to achieve maximum effect.

Treatment: Adminster 1 troche 5 times a day for 14 consecutive days. Only limited data are available on safety and efficacy after prolonged administration; therefore, limit therapy to short-term use if possible.

Prophylaxis: Administer 1 troche 3 times daily of rthe duration of chemotherapy or until steroids are reduced to maintenance levels.

Storage/Stability: Store below 30°C (56°F); avoid freezing.

Rx	**Mycelex** (Bayer)	**Troches:** 10 mg	(Miles 095). White. In 70s and 140s.

CHLORHEXIDINE GLUCONATE

Actions:

Pharmacology: Chlorhexidine provides microbicidal activity during oral rinsing. The clinical significance is not clear. Microbiological sampling of plaque has shown a reduction of aerobic and anaerobic bacteria, ranging from 54% to 97% through 6 months of use.

In a 6–month clinical study, there were no significant changes in bacterial resistance, overgrowth of potentially opportunistic organisms or other adverse changes in the oral microbial ecosystem. The number and resistance of bacteria in plaque had returned to baseline levels 3 months after use was discontinued.

Pharmacokinetics: Approximately 30% of chlorhexidine is retained in the oral cavity following rinsing and is slowly released into the oral fluids. Chlorhexidine is poorly absorbed from teh GI tract. The mean peak plasma level of 0.206 mcg/g was reached 30 minutes after ingestion of 300 mg. Detectable levels were not present in the plasma 12 hours after administration. Excretion occurred primarily through the feces (≈ 90%); < 1% was excreted in the urine.

Indications:

Gingivitis: For the treatment of gingivitis as characterized by gingival redness and swelling, including bleeding upon probing.

Contraindications:

Hypersensitivity to chlorhexidine gluconate.

Warnings:

Necrotizing ulcerative gingivitis: Chlorhexidine gluconate has not been tested in acute nectrotizing ulcerative gingivitis.

Calculus depositis: An increase in supragingival calculus was noted in clinical testing in chlorhexidine users. It is not known if use results in an increase in subgingival calculus. Remove calculus deposits by dental prophylaxis at 6 month intervals.

Hypersensitvity and generalized allergic reactions have been reported rarely. Have epinephrine 1:1000 immediately available. Refer to Management of Acute Hypersensitivity Reactions.

Pregnancy: Category B. Safety for use during pregnancy has not been established. Use only if clearly needed and when the potential benefits outweigh the potential hazards to the fetus.

Lactation: It is not known whether this drug is excreted in breast milk. Exercise caution when administering to a nursing mother.

Children: Efficacy has not been established in children < 18 years of age.

Precautions:

Gingivitis and periodontitis: The presence or absence of gingival inflammation following treatment should not be used as a major indicator of underlying periodonitis.

Staining of oral surfaces, such as tooth surfaces, restorations and the dorsum of the tongue may occur. In clinical testing, 56% of users exhibited a measurable increase in facial anterior stain, compared with 35% of control users after 6 months. Stain will be more pronounced in patients who have heavier accumulations of unremoved plaque.

Stain resulting from use does not adversely affect health of the gingivae or other oral tissues. Stain can be removed from most tooth surfaces by conventional professional prophylactic techniquees. Use discretion when prescribing to patients with anterior facial restorations with rough surfaces or margins. If natural stain cannot be removed from these surfaces by dental prophylaxis, exclude patients from treatment if permanent discoloration is unacceptable. Stain in these areas may be difficult to remove and may rarely necessitate replacement of restorations.

Taste perception alteration may occur while undergoing treatment. Most patients accommodate with continued use. Permanent taste alterations has not been reported.

Adverse Reactions:

Miscellaneous:

Most common – Increase in staining of teeth and other oral surfaces, increase in calculus formation and altered taste perception (see Warnings and Precautions).

Local: Minor irritation and superficial desquamation of the oral mucosa, particularly among children. Transient parotitis.

Overdosage:

Ingestion of 30 to 60 ml by a small child (≈ 10 kg body weight) might result in gastric distress, including nausea, or signs of alcohol intoxication. Seek medical attention if a small child ingest 120 ml or if signs of alcohol intoxication develop.

CHLORHEXIDINE GLUCONATE

Administration and Dosage:

Initiate therapy directly following dental prophylaxis. Reevaluate and give a thorough prophylaxis every 6 months.

Use twice daily as an oral rinse for 30 seconds, morning and evening after toothbrushing. Usual dosage is 15 ml (marked in cap) of undiluted drug. Not intended for ingestion; expectorate after rinsing.

Storage/Stability: Do not freeze.

Rx	**Peridex** (Procter & Gamble)	**Oral Rinse**: 0.12%	In 480 ml.[1]
Rx	**PerioGard** (Colgate Oral)		In 473 ml with 15 ml dose cup.[1]

[1] 11.6% alcohol, saccharin.

CARBAMIDE PEROXIDE (Urea Peroxide)

Actions:

Pharmacology: Releases oxygen on contact with mouth tissues to provide cleansing effects. Helps reduce inflammation, relieve pain and inhibit odor-forming bacteria.

Indications:

Oral inflammation: For relief of minor oral inflammation such as canker sores, denture irritation, post-dental procedure irritation and irritation related to inflamed gums. Used to aid oral hygiene when normal cleansing measures are inadequate or when patient wears orthodontic or dental appliances.

Contraindications:

Children < 3 years of age.

Warnings:

Irritation: Discontinue use and consult physician or dentist promptly if irritation persists or worsens or if inflammation develops.

Children: Do not use in children < 3 years of age unless otherwise directed.

Patient Information:

Severe or persistent oral inflammation, denture irritation or gingivitis may be serious. If these or unexpected side effects occur, consult physician or dentist promptly.

Discontinue use if condition persists or worsens.

Do not use in children < 3 years of age unless directed by physician or dentist.

Administration and Dosage:

Solution: Apply undiluted, 4 times daily after meals and at bedtime, or as directed. Place several drops on affected area (expectorate after 2 to 3 minutes; or place 10 drops on tongue, mix with saliva, swish for several minutes and expectorate).

Gel: Do not dilute. Use 4 times a day, or as directed. Gently massage medication on affected area. Do not drink or rinse mouth for 5 minutes after use.

otc	**Gly-Oxide Liquid** (SKB Consumer Healthcare)	**Solution**: 10% in anhydrous glycerol	In 15 and 60 ml.
otc	**Orajel Perioseptic** (Del Pharm)	**Liquid**: 15% in anhydrous glycerin	Saccharin, EDTA, methylparaben. In 13.3 ml.
otc	**Proxigel** (Reed & Carnrick)	**Gel**: 10% in a water free gel base	In 34 g w/applicator.

PILOCARPINE HCl

For information on the ophthalmic use of pilocarpine, refer to the individual monograph in the Topicals chapter.

Actions:

Pharmacology: Pilocarpine is a cholinergic parasympathomimetic agent exerting a broad spectrum of pharmacologic effects with predominant muscarinic action. Pilocarpine, in appropriate dosage, can increase secretion by the exocrine glands. The sweat, salivary, lacrimal, gastric, pancreatic and intestinal glands and the mucous cells of the respiratory tract may be stimulated. Dose-related smooth muscle stimulation of the intestinal tract may cause increased tone, increased motility, spasm and tenesmus. Bronchial smooth muscle tone may increase. The tone and motility of urinary tract, gallbladder, and biliary duct smooth muscle may be enhanced. Pilocarpine may have paradoxical effects on the cardiovascular system. The expected effect of a muscarinic agonist is vasodepression, but administration of pilocarpine may produce hypertension after a brief episode of hypotension. Bradycardia and tachycardia have both been reported with use of pilocarpine.

Pharmacokinetics: In a study in 12 healthy male volunteers there was a dose-related increase in unstimulated salivary flow following single 5 and 10 mg oral doses. The stimulatory effect was time-related with an onset at 20 minutes and peak at 1 hour with a duration of 3 to 5 hours.

In a multiple-dose pharmacokinetic study in male volunteers following 2 days of 5 or 10 mg oral pilocarpine given at 8 am, noon and 6 pm, the mean elimination half-life was 0.76 and 1.35 hours for the 5 and 10 mg doses, respectively. T_{max} was 1.25 and 0.85 hours and C_{max} was 15 and 41 ng/ml, respectively. The AUC was 33 and 108 hr•ng/ml, respectively, following the last 6 hour dose.

Pharmacokinetics in elderly male volunteers (n = 11) were comparable to those in younger men. In five healthy elderly female volunteers, the mean C_{max} and AUC were approximately twice that of elderly males and young healthy male volunteers.

When taken with a high fat meal, there was a decrease in the rate of absorption of pilocarpine. Mean T_{max} was 1.47 and 0.87 hours and mean C_{max} was 51.8 and 59.2 ng/ml for fed and fasted states, respectively.

Inactivation of pilocarpine is thought to occur at neuronal synapses and probably in plasma. Pilocarpine and its minimally active or inactive degradation products, including pilocarpic acid, are excreted in the urine.

Clinical trials: In a 12 week study in 207 patients, a statistically significant improvement in mouth dryness occurred in the pilocarpine-treated patients compared to placebo. Increases from baseline of whole saliva flow for the 5 mg (63%) and 10 mg (90%) tablets, respectively, were seen 1 hour after the first dose. Increases in unstimulated parotid flow were seen following the first dose. In this study, no correlation existed between the amount of increase in salivary flow and the degree of symptomatic relief. The 5 and 10 mg treated patients could not be distinguished.

In another 12 week study, the effects of placebo were compared to pilocarpine 2.5 mg 3 times/day for 4 weeks followed by titration to 5 mg 3 times/day and 10 mg 3 times/day. Lowering of the dose was necessary because of adverse events in 3 of 67 patients treated with 5 mg and in 7 of 66 patients treated with 10 mg. After 4 weeks of treatment, 2.5 mg 3 times/day was comparable to placebo in relieving dryness. In patients treated with 5 and 10 mg, the greatest improvement in dryness was noted in patients with no measurable salivary flow at baseline.

In both studies, some patients noted improvement in the global assessment of their xerostomia, speaking without liquids, and a reduced need for supplemental oral comfort agents.

Indications:

Xerostomia: Treatment of symptoms of xerostomia from salivary gland hypofunction caused by radiotherapy for cancer of the head and neck.

Contraindications:

Uncontrolled asthma; hypersensitivity to pilocarpine; when miosis is undesirable (eg, in acute iritis and in narrow-angle [angle closure] glaucoma).

Warnings:

Cardiovascular disease: Patients with significant cardiovascular disease may be unable to compensate for transient changes in hemodynamics or rhythm induced by pilocarpine. Pulmonary edema has been reported as a complication of pilocarpine toxicity from high ocular doses given for acute angle-closure glaucoma. Administer pilocarpine with caution and under close medical supervision in patients with cardiovascular disease.

The dose-related cardiovascular effects of pilocarpine include hypotension, hypertension, bradycardia and tachycardia.

PILOCARPINE HCl

Ocular effects: Carefully examine the fundus prior to initiating therapy with pilocarpine. An association of ocular pilocarpine use and retinal detachment in patients with preexisting retinal disease has been reported. The systemic blood level that is associated with this finding is not known.

Ocular formulations of pilocarpine have caused visual blurring which may result in decreased visual acuity, especially at night and in patients with central lens changes, and impairment of depth perception. Advise caution while driving at night or performing hazardous activities in reduced lighting.

Pulmonary disease: Pilocarpine has been reported to increase airway resistance, bronchial smooth muscle tone and bronchial secretions. Administer with caution and under close medical supervision in patients with controlled asthma, chronic bronchitis or chronic obstructive pulmonary disease.

Fertility impairment: Male rats who received pilocarpine at a dosage of 39 mg/kg/day (≈11 times the maximum recommended dose for a 60 kg human) exhibited morphologic evidence of reduced spermatogenesis. The possibility that pilocarpine may impair male fertility in humans cannot be excluded.

Elderly: Adverse events reported by those > 65 and those ≤ 65 years of age were comparable. Of the 15 elderly volunteers (5 women, 10 men), the 5 women had a higher C_{max} and AUC than the men.

Pregnancy: Category C. Pilocarpine was associated with a reduction in the mean fetal body weight and an increase in the incidence of skeletal variations when given to pregnant rats at a dosage of 90 mg/kg/day (≈ 26 times the maximum recommended dose for a 60 kg human). These effects may have been secondary to maternal toxicity. There are no adequate and well controlled studies in pregnant women. Use during pregnancy only if the potential benefit justifies the potential risk to the fetus.

Lactation: It is not known whether this drug is excreted in breast milk. Because of the potential for serious adverse reactions in nursing infants, decide whether to discontinue nursing or to discontinue the drug, taking into account the importance of the drug to the mother.

Children: Safety and efficacy in children have not been established.

Precautions:

Toxicity: Pilocarpine toxicity is characterized by an exaggeration of its parasympathomimetic effects. These may include: Headache; visual disturbance; lacrimation; sweating; respiratory distress; GI spasm; nausea; vomiting; diarrhea; AV block; tachycardia; bradycardia; hypotension; hypertension; shock; mental confusion; cardiac arrhythmia; tremors.

Biliary tract: Administer with caution to patients with known or suspected cholelithiasis or biliary tract disease. Contractions of the gallbladder or biliary smooth muscle could precipitate complications including cholecystitis, cholangitis and biliary obstruction.

Renal colic: Pilocarpine may increase ureteral smooth muscle tone and could theoretically precipitate renal colic (or "ureteral reflux"), particularly in patients with nephrolithiasis.

Psychiatric disorder: Cholinergic agonists may have dose-related CNS effects. Consider this when treating patients with underlying cognitive or psychiatric disturbances.

Drug Interactions:

Pilocarpine (Oral) Drug Interactions

Precipitant drug	Object drug*		Description
Pilocarpine	Beta blockers	↑	Use concurrent administration with caution because of possible conduction disturbances.
Pilocarpine	Anticholinergics	↓	Pilocarpine might antagonize the anticholinergic effects of drugs used concomitantly. Consider these effects when anticholinergic properties may be contributing to the therapeutic effect of concomitant medication (eg, atropine, inhaled ipratropium).

* ↑ = Object drug increased. ↓ = Object drug decreased.

Drug/Food interactions: The rate of absorption of pilocarpine is decreased when taken with a high fat meal. Maximum concentration is decreased and time to reach maximum concentration is increased.

PILOCARPINE HCl

Adverse Reactions:

The most frequent adverse experiences associated with pilocarpine were a consequence of the expected pharmacologic effects.

Pilocarpine Adverse Reactions (%)

Adverse reaction	Placebo (n=152)	Pilocarpine 5 mg tid (n = 141)	10 mg tid (n = 121)	5 or 10 mg tid (n = 212)
Sweating	9	29	68	-
Nausea	4	6	15	-
Rhinitis	7	5	14	-
Chills	<1	3	14	-
Flushing	3	8	13	-
Urinary frequency	7	9	12	-
Dizziness	4	5	12	-
Asthenia	3	6	12	-
Headache	8	-	-	11
Dyspepsia	5	-	-	7
Lacrimation	8	-	-	6
Diarrhea	5	-	-	6
Edema	4	-	-	5
Abdominal pain	4	-	-	4
Amblyopia	2	-	-	4
Vomiting	1	-	-	4
Pharyngitis	8	-	-	3
Hypertension	1	-	-	3
Conjunctivitis	4	-	-	2
Tachycardia	1	-	-	2
Epistaxis	1	-	-	2
Tremor	0	-	-	2
Dysphagia	<1	-	-	2
Voice alteration	0	-	-	2
Rash	4	-	-	1
Taste perversion	2	-	-	1
Sinusitis	2	-	-	1
Abnormal vision	1	-	-	1
Myalgias	1	-	-	1
Pruritus	<1	-	-	1

The following events were also reported (<1%):

Body as a whole – Body odor; hypothermia; mucous membrane abnormality.

Cardiovascular – Bradycardia; ECG abnormality; palpitations; syncope.

GI – Anorexia; increased appetite; esophagitis; GI disorder; tongue disorder.

Hematologic – Leukopenia; lymphadenopathy.

CNS – Anxiety; confusion; depression; abnormal dreams; hyperkinesia; hypesthesia; nervousness; paresthesias; speech disorder; twitching

Respiratory – Increased sputum; stridor; yawning.

Special Senses – Deafness; eye pain; glaucoma.

GU – Dysuria; metrorrhagia; urinary impairment.

Miscellaneous – Seborrhea. In two patients with underlying cardiovascular disease, one experienced a myocardial infarct and the other an episode of syncope.

Overdosage:

Pilocarpine fatal overdosage resulting from poisoning has been reported at doses presumed to be > 100 mg in two hospitalized patients; 100 mg is considered potentially fatal. Treat overdosage with atropine titration (0.5 to 1 mg SC or IM) and use supportive measures to maintain respiration and circulation. Epinephrine (0.3 to 1 mg SC or IV) may also be of value in the presence of severe cardiovascular depression or bronchoconstriction. Refer to General Management of Acute Overdosage. It is not known if pilocarpine is dialyzable.

PILOCARPINE HCl

Patient Information:

Inform patients that pilocarpine may cause visual disturbances, especially at night, that could impair their ability to drive safely.

If a patient sweats excessively while taking pilocarpine and cannot drink enough liquid, the patient should consult a physician. Dehydration may develop.

Administration and Dosage:

The recommended dose for the initiation of treatment is 5 mg 3 times/day. Titration up to 10 mg 3 times/day may be considered for patients who have not responded adequately and who can tolerate lower doses. The incidence of the most common adverse events increases with dose. Use the lowest dose that is tolerated and effective for maintenance.

Rx	**Salagen** (MGI Pharma)	**Tablets:** 5 mg	(MGI 705). White. Film coated. In 100s.

SALIVA SUBSTITUTES

Indications:

These products are used as saliva substitutes for relief of dry mouth and throat in xerostomia and hyposalivation, which may be due to the following: Surgery or radiation near the salivary glands; infection or dysfunction of the salivary glands; inflammation of mouth or throat; fever; emotional factors such as fear or anxiety; obstruction of salivary ducts; Sjogren's syndrome; Bell's Palsy.

Administration and Dosage:

Refer to specific product labeling for dosage guidelines.

otc	**Glandosane** (Kenwood/Bradley)	**Solution:** 0.51 g sodium carboxymethylcellulose, 1.52 g sorbitol, 0.043 g sodium chloride, 0.061 g potassium chloride, 0.007 g calcium chloride, 0.003 g magnesium chloride, 0.017 g dipotassium hydrogen phosphate per 50 ml	Unflavored, lemon and mint flavors. In 50 ml spray.
otc	**Saliva Substitute** (Roxane)	**Solution:** Sorbitol, sodium carboxymethylcellulose	In 5 and 120 ml single-dose vials.
otc	**Optimoist** (Colgate-Palmolive)	**Solution:** Xylitol, calcium phosphate monobasic, citric acid, sodium hydroxide, sodium benzoate, acesulfame potassium, hydroxyethyl cellulose, sodium monofluorophosphate, 2 ppm fluoride	In 60 and 355 ml spray.
otc	**Moi-Stir** (Kingswood)	**Solution:** Dibasic sodium phosphate, magnesium, calcium, sodium and potassium chlorides, sorbitol, sodium carboxymethylcellulose, parabens	Mint flavor. In 120 ml w/pump spray.
otc	**Moi-Stir Swabsticks** (Kingswood)		In packets (3s).
otc	**Entertainer's Secret** (KLI Corp)	**Solution:** Sodium carboxymethylcellulose, potassium chloride, dibasic sodium phosphate, parabens, aloe vera gel, glycerin	In 60 ml spray.
otc	**Salivart** (Gebauer)	**Solution:** 1% sodium carboxymethylcellulose, 3% sorbitol, 0.084% sodium chloride, 0.12% potassium chloride, 0.015% calcium chloride, 0.005% magnesium chloride, 0.034% dibasic potassium phosphate and nitrogen (as propellant)	Preservative free. In 25 and 75 ml spray cans.
otc	**Mouthkote** (Unimed)	**Solution:** Xylitol, sorbitol, mucoprotective factor (MPF), yerba santa, saccharin	Alcohol free. Citrus flavor. In 60 and 240 ml and UD 5 ml.
otc	**Salix** (Scandinavian Natural Health & Beauty[1])	**Lozenges:** Sorbitol, dicalcium phosphate, hydroxypropyl methylcellulose, carboxy methylcellulose, malic acid, hydrogenated cottonseed oil, sodium citrate, citric acid, silicon dioxide	In 100s.

[1] Scandinavian Natural Health & Beauty Products, Inc. 13 North Seventh Street, Perkasie, PA 18944; (215) 453–2505, (800) 288–2844.

TETRACYCLINE HCl

For information on the systemic, topical and ophthalmic use of tetracycline, refer to the individual monographs.

Actions:

Pharmacology: Tetracycline periodontal fiber for periodontal pocket placement consists of a 23 cm (9 inch) monofilament of ethylene/vinyl acetate copolymer, 0.5 mm in diameter, containing 12.7 mg of evenly dispersed tetracycline. The fiber provides continuous release of tetracycline for 10 days. The tetracyclines are primarily bacteriostatic and are thought to exert their antimicrobial effect by inhibiting protein synthesis.

Pharmacokinetics: The fiber releases tetracycline in vitro at a rate of approximately 2 mcg/cm•hr. In the periodontal pocket, the system provides for a per site mean gingival fluid concentration of 1590 mcg/ml tetracycline throughout the 10 day treatment period.

Concentration in saliva immediately after fiber placement (9 teeth) was 50.7 mcg/ml and declined to 7.6 mcg/ml at the end of 10 days.

During fiber treatment of up to 11 teeth per patient (average tetracycline dose of 105 mg), mean tetracycline concentrations in plasma were below the lower limit of assay detection (< 0.1 mcg/ml). This lower assay limit is 20- to 25-fold lower than that expected during a regimen of 250 mg oral capsule every 6 hours.

Microbiology: In vitro, probable periodontal pathogens including *Fusobacterium nucleatum, Porphyromonas (Bacteroides) gingivalis, Prevotella intermedia (Bacteroides intermedius), Eikenella corrodens, Campylobacter rectus (Wolinella recta)*, and *Actinobacillus actinomycetemcomitans*, are susceptible to local 32 mcg/ml tetracycline concentrations achieved in the periodontal pocket with the use of tetracycline periodontal fiber.

Clinical trials: In a controlled 60 day clinical trial, 113 adult patients with periodontitis received supragingival cleaning followed by one of four treatments, randomized to a single tooth per quadrant. The treatments were: 1) tetracycline fiber for 10 ± 2 days, 2) control fiber for 10 ± 2 days, 3) scaling and root planing under local anesthesia, or 4) no treatment. Teeth treated with tetracycline fiber were later found to have significantly reduced probing depth and bleeding on controlled force probing. Both tetracycline fiber and scaling and root planing produced significant reductions in the number of sites infected with probable periodontal pathogens compared to untreated controls.

Indications:

Periodontitis: Adjunct to scaling and root planing for reduction of pocket depth and bleeding on probing in patients with adult periodontitis. Treatment with tetracycline is a component of an intervention program which includes good oral hygiene, scaling and root planing.

Contraindications:

Hypersensitivity to any tetracycline.

Warnings:

Efficacy: Effectiveness of repeated fiber applications in a site has not been studied. The effects of tetracycline on bone loss, tooth mobility or tooth loss from periodontal disease have not been established.

Teeth discoloration: The use of the tetracycline class during tooth development (last half of pregnancy, infancy and childhood to age of 8 years) may cause permanent discoloration of the teeth. Tetracycline drugs should not be used in this age group unless other treatment is not likely to be effective or if alternative therapy is contraindicated.

Renal function impairment: Accumulations of tetracycline associated with renal failure can lead to liver toxicity. These effects have not been studied in the plasma concentration range associated with tetracycline fiber.

Pregnancy: Category C. Administration of tetracycline during pregnancy may cause permanent discoloration of teeth of offspring. Animal studies indicate that tetracyclines can cause retardation of fetal skeletal development. It is not known whether tetracycline fiber can cause fetal harm when administered to a pregnant woman or can affect reproductive capacity. Use in a pregnant woman only if clearly needed.

Lactation: Tetracycline appears in breast milk following oral administration. It is not known whether tetracycline is excreted in breast milk following use of tetracycline fiber. Because of the potential for serious adverse reactions in nursing infants, use in a nursing woman only if clearly needed.

Children: Safety and efficacy in children have not been established. Oral doses of tetracycline in children up to 8 years of age have caused permanent discoloration of teeth.

TETRACYCLINE HCl

Precautions:

Removal of fiber: Tetracycline fibers must be removed after 10 days.

Abscesses: Packing fibers tightly into a draining abscess without allowance for drainage might result in the formation of a lateral fistula. Fibers should not be used in an acutely abscessed periodontal pocket. Their use in chronic abscesses has not been evaluated.

Candidiasis: Use with caution in patients with a history of or predisposition to oral candidiasis. Safety and efficacy of tetracycline fiber have not been established for the treatment of periodontitis in patients with coexistent oral candidiasis.

Resistance: Use of antibiotic preparations may result in the development of resistant bacteria. Resistance has not been observed during 10 days of tetracycline fiber therapy.

Contributing disorders: Management of patients with periodontal disease should include a consideration of potentially contributing medical disorders.

Superinfection: As with other antibiotic preparations, tetracycline fiber therapy may result in overgrowth of nonsusceptible organisms, including fungi.

Photosensitivity: Tetracyclines as a class are associated with photosensitivity. Discontinue treatment at the first sign of cutaneous erythema.

Adverse Reactions:

The most frequently reported adverse reactions in 226 patients in clinical trials were discomfort on fiber placement (10%) and local erythema following removal (11%).

In controlled and open-label trials, the following adverse reactions were reported in <1% of patients: Oral candidiasis; glossitis; possible allergic response; staining of the tongue; severe gingival inflammation; throbbing pain; pain following placement in an abscessed area; minor throat irritation.

Patient Information:

When tetracycline fiber is in place, patients should avoid actions that may dislodge the fiber: Do not chew hard, crusty or sticky foods; do not brush or floss near any treated areas (continue to clean other teeth); do not engage in any other hygienic practices that could potentially dislodge the fibers; do not probe at the treated area with tongue or fingers; notify the dentist promptly if the fiber is dislodged or falls out before the scheduled recall visit, or if pain, swelling or other problems occur.

Photosensitization (photoallergy or phototoxicity) may occur; therefore, caution patients to take protective measures against exposure to ultraviolet or sunlight (ie, sunscreens, protective clothing) until tolerance is determined.

Administration and Dosage:

Approved by the FDA on March 25, 1994.

Insert into the periodontal pocket until the pocket is filled. The length of fiber used will vary with pocket depth and contour. The fiber should be placed to closely approximate the pocket anatomy and should be in contact with the base of the pocket. Use an appropriate cyanoacrylate adhesive to help secure the fiber in the pocket.

When placed within a periodontal pocket, tetracycline fiber provides continuous release of tetracycline for 10 days. At the end of 10 days of treatment, all fibers must be removed. Replace fibers lost before 7 days.

Rx	**Actisite** (Alza)	**Fiber:** 12.7 mg tetracycline HCl per 23 cm.	Yellow. In 10s.

AMLEXANOX

Actions:

Pharmacology: The mechanism of action by which amlexanox accelerates healing of aphthous ulcers is unknown. In vitro, amlexanox is a potent inhibitor of the formation or release of inflammatory mediators (histamine and leukotrines) from mast cells, neutrophils and mononuclear cells. Given orally to animals, amlexanox has demonstrated anti-allergic and anti-inflammatory activities and suppresses both immediate and delayed-type hypersensitivity reactions. The relevance of these activities of amlexanox to its effects on aphthous ulcers has not been established.

Pharmacokinetics:

Absorption – After a single oral application of 100 mg of paste (5 mg amlexanox), maximal serum levels of ≈ 120 ng/ml are observed at 2.4 hours. Most of the systemic absorption of amlexanox is via the GI tract, and the amount absorbed directly through the active ulcer is not a significant portion of the applied dose.

Distribution – With multiple applications 4 times daily, steady-state levels were reached within 1 week and no accumulation was observed with up to 4 weeks.

Metabolism/Excretion – The elimination half-life is 3.5 hours in healthy individuals. Approximately 17% of the dose is eliminated into the urine as unchanged amlexanox, a hydroxylated metabolite and their conjugates.

Clinical trials: The safety of amlexanox oral paste 5%, was established in a study in which 100 patients with aphthous ulcers applied the medication 4 times daily for 28 days with no significant topical or systemic adverse effects. The effectiveness was demonstrated in three controlled clinical studies of patients with mild to moderate aphthous ulcers. Amlexanox oral paste 5% accelerated healing of aphthous ulcers in a statistically significant manner as compared with vehicle and no treatment.

Indications:

Aphthous ulcers: Aphthous ulcer treatment in people with normal immune systems.

Contraindications:

Hypersensitivity to amlexanox or other ingredients in the formulation.

Warnings:

Pregnancy: Category B. There are no adequate and well controlled studies in pregnant women. Use during pregnancy only if clearly needed.

Lactation: Amlexanox was found in the milk of rats; therefore, exercise caution when administering amlexanox oral paste to a nursing woman.

Children: Safety and efficacy in pediatric patients have not been established.

Precautions:

Local irritation: In the event that rash or contact mucositis occurs, discontinue use.

Adverse Reactions:

Transient pain, stinging or burning at the site of application (1% to 2%); contact mucositis, nausea, diarrhea (< 1%).

Patient Information:

Apply the paste as soon as possible after noticing the symptoms of an aphthous ulcer. Continue to use the paste 4 times daily, preferably following oral hygiene after breakfast, lunch, dinner and at bedtime.

Squeeze a dab of paste ≈ 0.25 inch (0.5 cm) onto a fingertip. Dab the paste onto each ulcer in the mouth using gentle pressure.

Wash hands immediately after applying amlexanox oral paste.

Wash eyes promptly if they should come in contact with the paste.

Use the paste until the ulcer heals. If significant healing or pain reduction has not occurred in 10 days, consult your dentist or physician.

Administration and Dosage:

Apply as soon as possible after noticing symptoms of an aphthous ulcer and use 4 times daily, preferably following oral hygiene after breakfast, lunch, dinner and at bedtime. Squeeze a dab of paste ≈ 0.25 inch (0.5 cm) onto a fingertip. With gentle pressure, dab paste onto each ulcer in mouth. Use medication until ulcer heals. If significant healing or pain reduction has not occurred in 10 days, consult your dentist or physician.

Rx	**Aphthasol** (Block)	**Paste:** 5%	Benzyl alcohol, glyceryl monostearate, mineral oil, petrolatum. In 5 g.

MOUTH AND THROAT PRODUCTS

BENZOCAINE and DYCLONINE are local anesthetics.

CETYLPYRIDINIUM CHLORIDE, EUCALYPTUS OIL, THYMOL and HEXYLRESORCINOL have antiseptic activity.

TERPIN HYDRATE is an expectorant.

MENTHOL, CAMPHOR, CAPSICUM, DYCLONINE and PHENOL are used for their antipruritic, local anesthetic and counterirritant activities.

ANTIPYRINE is an analgesic.

HYDROCORTISONE and TRIAMCINOLONE (CORTICOSTEROIDS) are used for their anti-inflammatory activities.

Indications:

These products are indicated in minor sore throat and in minor irritation of the throat or mouth.

Warnings:

Severe/Persistent sore throat: Severe and persistent sore throat or sore throat accompanied by high fever, headache, nausea and vomiting may be serious. Consult physician promptly.

Administration and Dosage:

Do not use for > 2 days or in children < 2 years of age, unless directed by physician. For dosage guidelines, refer to the specific package labeling.

LOZENGES AND TROCHES

otc *sf*	**Cylex** (Pharmakon)	**Lozenges:** 15 mg benzocaine, 5 mg cetylpyridinium chloride	Sorbitol. Cherry flavor. In 12s.
otc *sf*	**Mycinettes** (Pfeiffer)	**Lozenges:** 15 mg benzocaine	Sorbitol, saccharin, menthol. Cherry flavor. In 12s.
otc	**Spec-T** (Apothecon)	**Lozenges:** 10 mg benzocaine	Sucrose. In 10s.
otc	**Trocaine** (Roberts)	**Lozenges:** 10 mg benzocaine	In UD 4s and 500s.
otc	**Vicks Chloraseptic Sore Throat** (Richardson -Vicks)	**Lozenges:** 6 mg benzocaine, 10 mg menthol	Cool mint, cherry, menthol flavors. In 18s.
otc	**Vicks Children's Chloraseptic** (Richardson-Vicks)	**Lozenges:** 5 mg benzocaine	Corn syrup, sucrose. Grape flavor. In 18s.
otc	**Sucrets Children's Sore Throat** (SK-Beecham)	**Lozenges:** 1.2 mg dyclonine HCl	Corn syrup, sucrose. Cherry flavor. In 24s.
otc	**Cēpacol Throat** (J.B. Williams)	**Lozenges:** 0.07% cetylpyridinium chloride, 0.3% benzyl alcohol	Tartrazine. In 27s and 40s.
otc	**Kof-Eze** (Roberts Med)	**Lozenges:** 6 mg menthol	In 4s and 500s.
otc	**Sucrets Maximum Strength** (SK-Beecham)	**Lozenges:** 3 mg dyclonine HCl	Corn syrup, menthol, sucrose. Wintergreen and vapor black cherry flavors. In 24s, 48s and 55s.
otc	**Vapor Lemon Sucrets** (SK-Beecham)	**Lozenges:** 2 mg dyclonine HCl	Sucrose, corn syrup. In 18s.
otc	**Sucrets Sore Throat** (SK-Beecham)	**Lozenges:** 2.4 mg hexylresorcinol	In regular and mentholated flavors. In 24s.
otc *sf*	**Cēpastat Extra Strength** (SK-Beecham)	**Lozenges:** 29 mg phenol, menthol, eucalyptus oil	Sorbitol. In 18s.
otc *sf*	**Cēpastat Cherry** (SK-Beecham)	**Lozenges:** 14.5 mg phenol, menthol	Saccharin, sorbitol. Cherry flavor. In 18s.
otc	**Robitussin Liquid Center Cough Drops** (Robins)	**Lozenges:** 10 mg menthol	Sucrose, corn syrup, eucalyptus oil, high fructose corn syrup, honey, lemon oil, parabens, sorbitol. Honey-lemon with cherry center flavor. In 20s.

LOZENGES AND TROCHES

otc sf	**N'ice** (SK-Beecham)	**Lozenges:** 5 mg menthol	Saccharin, sorbitol. Citrus, cherry, cool peppermint and assorted flavors. In 16s.
otc sf	**N'ice 'n Clear** (SK-Beecham)	**Lozenges:** 5 mg menthol	Sorbitol. Cool peppermint, cherry eucalyptus and menthol eucalyptus flavors. In 16s.
otc	**Vicks Cherry Cough Drops** (Richardson-Vicks)	**Lozenges:** Menthol	Cherry flavor. In 14s and 40s.
otc	**Vicks Menthol Cough Drops** (Richardson-Vicks)	**Lozenges:** Menthol, thymol, eucalyptus oil, camphor, tolu balsam	Benzyl alcohol. Menthol flavor. In 14s and 40s.
otc	**Throat Discs** (SK- Beecham)	**Lozenges:** Capsicum, peppermint oil, mineral oil.	Sucrose. In 60s.
otc	**Maximum Strength Halls-Plus** (Warner-Lambert)	**Lozenges:** 10 mg menthol	Corn syrup, sucrose. In regular, cherry, mentholyptus and honey-lemon flavors. In 10s and 25s.
otc	**Extra Strength Vicks Cough Drops** (Richardson-Vicks)	**Lozenges:** 8.4 mg menthol	Corn syrup, sucrose. Menthol flavor. In 9s and 30s.
otc	**Extra Strength Vicks Cough Drops** (Richardson-Vicks)	**Lozenges:** 10 mg menthol	Corn syrup, sucrose. Cherry and honey lemon flavors. In 9s and 30s.
otc	**Robitussin Cough Drops** (Robins)	**Lozenges:** 7.4 mg menthol	Eucalyptus oil, sucrose, corn syrup. In cherry and menthol eucalyptus flavors. In 9s and 25s.
		10 mg menthol	Eucalyptus oil, sucrose, corn syrup. Honey-lemon flavor. In 9s and 25s.
otc	**Cēpacol Anesthetic** (J. B. Williams)	**Troches:** 10 mg benzocaine, 0.07% cetylpyridinium chloride	Tartrazine. In 18s and 24s.
otc sf	**Hall's Sugar Free Mentho-Lyptus** (Warner-Lambert)	**Tablets:** 6 mg menthol, 2.8 mg eucalyptus oil	Mountain menthol flavor. In 25s.
		Tablets: 5 mg menthol, 2.8 mg eucalyptus oil	Citrus blend and black cherry flavors. In 25s.

MOUTHWASHES AND SPRAYS

otc	**MouthKote O/R** (Unimed)	**Solution:** 1.25% diphenhydramine, cetylpyridinium Cl	EDTA, saccharin. In 40 ml.
otc	**MouthKote P/R** (Unimed)	**Solution:** 1.25% diphenhydramine, cetylpyridinium Cl	EDTA, saccharin. In 40 ml.
otc	**TiSol** (Parnell)	**Solution:** 1% benzyl alcohol, 0.04% menthol, 0.9% isotonic NaCl	EDTA, sorbitol. In 237 ml.
otc	**FreshBurst Listerine** (Glaxo Wellcome)	**Rinse:** 0.064% thymol, 0.092% eucalyptol, 0.06% methyl salicylate, 0.042% menthol, 21.6% alcohol	Sorbitol, saccharin. In 250 ml.
otc	**Scope** (Procter & Gamble)	**Rinse:** Cetylpyridinium chloride, 67.9% SD alcohol 38-F	Tartrazine, saccharin. Original mint and wintergreen flavors. In 90, 180, 360, 720, 1080 and 1440 ml.
otc sf	**MouthKote O/R** (Unimed)	**Rinse:** Benzyl alcohol, menthol	Sorbitol. Cinnamon flavor. In 240 ml.

MOUTHWASHES AND SPRAYS

otc sf	**Sucrets** (SK- Beecham)	**Throat Spray**: 0.1% dyclonine HCl, 10% alcohol	Sorbitol. Mint and cherry flavors. In 90 and 180 ml.
otc	**Cheracol Sore Throat** (Roberts)	**Throat Spray**: 1.4% phenol, 12.5% alcohol	Sorbitol, saccharin. Cherry flavor. In 180 ml.
otc	**Orasept** (Pharmakon)	**Throat Spray**: 0.996% benzocaine, 1.037% methylbenzethonium Cl, menthol	70% sorbitol, saccharin, peppermint oil. In 45 ml.
otc sf	**Mycinette** (Pfeiffer)	**Throat Spray**: 1.4% phenol, 0.3% alum (aluminum ammonium sulfate)	Alcohol free. Regular, cherry, mint and cool blue menthol flavors. In 180 ml.
otc	**N'ice** (SK- Beecham)	**Throat Spray**: 0.12% menthol, 25% glycerin, 23% alcohol	Glucose, saccharin, sorbitol. Peppermint flavor. In 180 ml.
otc	**Children's Vicks Chloraseptic** (Procter & Gamble)	**Throat Spray**: 0.5% phenol	Alcohol free. Saccharin, sorbitol. Grape flavor. In 177 ml.
otc	**Listermint Arctic Mint** (Warner-Wellcome)	**Mouthwash**: Glycerin, poloxamer 335, PEG 600, sodium lauryl sulfate, sodium benzoate, benzoic acid, zinc chloride	Saccharin. In 946 ml.
otc	**Cēpacol** (J. B. Williams)	**Mouthwash**: 0.05% cetylpyridinium chloride, 14% alcohol	Tartrazine, saccharin. In 360, 540, 720, 960 ml.
otc	**Advanced Formula Plax** (Pfizer)	**Mouthwash**: Tetrasodium pyrophosphate, alcohol	Saccharin. Original, peppermint and softmint flavors. In 120, 240, 473, 720 and 1740 ml.
otc	**Listerine** (Warner-Wellcome)	**Mouthwash**: 0.06% thymol, 0.09% eucalyptol, 0.06% methyl salicylate, 0.04% menthol, 26.9% alcohol (regular flavor), 21.6% alcohol (cool mint flavor).	Sorbitol, saccharin (Cool Mint). Regular, cool mint flavors. In 90, 180, 360, 540, 720, 960, 1440 ml.
otc	**Phylorinol** (Schaffer)	**Mouthwash**: 0.6% phenol, methyl salicylate	Alcohol free. Sorbitol. In 240 ml.
otc sf	**Vicks Chloraseptic** (Procter & Gamble)	**Mouthrinse/gargle**: 1.4% phenol	Alcohol free. Saccharin. Menthol flavor. In 355 ml.

MISCELLANEOUS MOUTH AND THROAT PREPARATIONS

otc	**Dent's Extra Strength Toothache Gum** (C.S. Dent)	**Gum**: Benzocaine	In 1 g.
otc	**Maximum Strength Orajel** (Del Pharm)	**Liquid**: 20% benzocaine, 44.2% ethyl alcohol, phenol	Tartrazine, saccharin. In 13.3 ml.
otc sf	**Orajel Mouth-Aid** (Del Pharm)	**Liquid**: 20% benzocaine, 0.1% cetylpyridinium chloride, 70% ethyl alcohol, povidone	Tartrazine, saccharin. In 13.3 ml.
otc	**Tanac** (Del Pharm)	**Liquid**: 10% benzocaine, 0.12% benzalkonium chloride	Saccharin. In 13 ml.
otc	**Anbesol** (Whitehall)	**Liquid**: 6.3% benzocaine, 0.5% phenol, 70% alcohol, menthol, camphor, povidone-iodine	In 9 and 22 ml.
otc	**Orasol** (Goldline)	**Liquid**: 6.3% benzocaine, 0.5% phenol, 70% alcohol, povidone-iodine	In 14.79 ml.
otc sf	**Tanac Roll-On** (Del Pharm)	**Liquid**: 5% benzocaine, 0.12% benzalkonium chloride	Saccharin. In 8.8 ml.
otc	**Dent's Maximum Strength Toothache Drops** (C.S. Dent)	**Liquid**: Benzocaine, 74% alcohol, 0.09% chlorobutanol anhydrous	In 3.7 ml.
otc	**Double-Action Toothache Kit** (C.S. Dent)	**Liquid**: Benzocaine, 74% alcohol, 0.09% chlorobutanol anhydrous	Also contains *Maranox Pain Relief Tablets* containing 325 mg acetaminophen. In 8 tablets with 3.7 ml drops.
otc	**Orasept** (Pharmakon Labs)	**Liquid**: 12.16% tannic acid, 1.53% methylbenzethonium Cl, 53.31% denatured ethyl alcohol, camphor, menthol, benzyl alcohol, spearmint oil and oil of Cassia	In 15 ml.
otc	**Phylorinol** (Schaffer)	**Liquid**: 0.6% phenol, boric acid, strong iodine solution, sodium copper chlorophyll	Sorbitol. In 240 ml.
otc	**ORA5** (McHenry)	**Liquid**: Copper sulfate, iodine, potassium iodide, 1.5% alcohol	In 3.75 and 30 ml.
otc	**Maximum Strength Anbesol** (Whitehall)	**Liquid**: 20% benzocaine, 60% alcohol, polyethylene glycol	Saccharin. In 9 ml.
otc	**Red Cross Toothache** (Mentholatum)	**Liquid**: 85% eugenol, sesame oil	In 3.7 ml with cotton pellets and tweezers.
otc sf	**Ulcerease** (Med-Derm)	**Liquid**: 0.6% liquified phenol, glycerin, sodium bicarbonate, sodium borate	Alcohol free. In 180 ml.
otc	**Mouth Kote P/R** (Unimed)	**Ointment**: 25% diphenhydramine HCl	In 15 g.
otc	**Benzodent** (P & G)	**Ointment**: 20% benzocaine	In 30 g.
otc	**Blistex** (Blistex)	**Ointment**: 0.5% camphor, 0.5% phenol, 1% allantoin, lanolin	Mineral oil base. In 4.2 and 10.5 g.
otc	**Lip Medex** (Blistex)	**Ointment**: Petrolatum, 1% camphor, 0.54% phenol, cocoa butter, lanolin	In 210 g.
otc	**Orabase Lip** (Colgate)	**Cream**: 5% benzocaine, 1.5% allantoin, 0.5% menthol, phenol, camphor, petrolatum, lanolin, parabens	In 10 g.

MISCELLANEOUS MOUTH AND THROAT PREPARATIONS

otc	**Numzit Teething** (Goody's)	**Lotion**: 0.2% benzocaine, 12.1% alcohol, 0.02% saccharin, 2% glycerin, 0.5% kelgin MU, methylparaben	Saccharin. In 15 ml.
otc sf	**Babee Teething** (Pfeiffer)	**Lotion**: 2.5% benzocaine, 0.02% cetalkonium chloride, camphor, eucolyptol, menthol.	Dye free. Alcohol. In 15 ml.
otc	**Pfeiffer's Cold Sore** (Pfeiffer)	**Lotion**: 7% gum benzoin, camphor, menthol, eucalyptol, 85% alcohol	In 15 ml.
otc	**Banadyne-3** (Norstar)	**Solution**: 4% lidocaine, menthol 1%, 45% alcohol	In 7.5 ml.
otc	**Peroxyl Dental Rinse** (Colgate)	**Solution**: 1.5% hydrogen peroxide, 6% alcohol	Mint flavor. In 240 ml and pint.
otc	**MG Cold Sore Formula** (Outdoor Recreations)	**Solution**: 1% menthol, lidocaine	Propylene glycol/alcohol base. In 7.5 ml.
otc	**Amosan** (Oral-B)	**Powder**: Sodium peroxyborate monohydrate (derived from sodium perborate)	Saccharin. Peppermint, menthol and vanilla flavors. In 1.7 g UD packets (20s and 40s).
otc	**Maximum Strength Orajel** (Del Pharm)	**Gel**: 20% benzocaine	Saccharin. In 9.45 g.
otc	**Maximum Strength Anbesol** (Whitehall)	**Gel**: 20% benzocaine, 60% alcohol, carbomer 934P, polyethylene glycol	Saccharin. In 7.2 g.
otc sf	**Orajel Brace-aid** (Del Pharm)	**Gel**: 20% benzocaine	Saccharin. In 14.1 g.
otc sf	**Orajel Mouth-Aid** (Del Pharm)	**Gel**: 20% benzocaine, 0.02% benzalkonium chloride, 0.1% zinc chloride	Saccharin. In 9.45 g.
otc	**SensoGARD** (Block)	**Gel**: 20% benzocaine	Parabens. In 0.5 g.
otc	**Numzident** (Goody's)	**Gel**: 10% benzocaine, 47.86% PEG 400 N.F., 10% PEG 3350 NF	Saccharin. Cherry-vanilla flavor. In 15 g.
otc	**Zilactin-B Medicated** (Zila)	**Gel**: 10% benzocaine, 76% alcohol	In 7.5 g.
otc sf	**Rid-a-Pain** (Pfeiffer)	**Gel**: 10% benzocaine, menthol, eucalyptol	7.5% alcohol. In 10 g.
otc sf	**Orajel/d** (Del Pharm)	**Gel**: 10% benzocaine	Saccharin. In 9.45 g.
otc	**Denture Orajel** (Del Pharm)	**Gel**: 10% benzocaine	Saccharin. In 9.45 g.
otc	**Baby Anbesol** (Whitehall)	**Gel**: 7.5% benzocaine, EDTA	Saccharin. In 7.2 g
otc	**Baby Orajel** (Del Pharm)	**Gel**: 7.5% benzocaine	Alcohol free. Saccharin, sorbitol. In 9.45 g.
otc	**Baby Orajel Nighttime** (Del Pharm)	**Gel**: 10% benzocaine	Alcohol free. Saccharin, sorbitol. Cherry flavor. In 6 g.
otc	**Baby Orajel Tooth & Gum Cleanser** (Del Pharm)	**Gel**: 2% poloxamer 407, 0.12% simethicone	Parabens, saccharin, sorbitol. In 14.2 g.
otc	**Orabase Baby** (Colgate Oral)	**Gel**: 7.5% benzocaine	Alcohol free. Mild fruit flavor. In 7.2 g.

MISCELLANEOUS MOUTH AND THROAT PREPARATIONS

otc	**Numzit Teething** (Goody's)	**Gel:** 7.5% benzocaine, 0.018% peppermint oil, 0.09% clove leaf oil, 66.2% PEG-400, 26.1% PEG-3350	0.036% saccharin. In 14.1 g.
otc sf	**Anbesol** (Whitehall)	**Gel:** 6.3% benzocaine, 0.5% phenol, 70% alcohol, camphor	In 7.5 g.
otc	**Toothache Gel** (Roberts Med)	**Gel:** Benzocaine, oil of cloves, benzyl alcohol, propylene glycol	In 15 g.
otc	**Probax** (Fischer)	**Gel:** 2% propolis, petrolatum, mineral oil, lanolin	In 3.5 g.
otc	**Tanac** (Del Pharm)	**Gel:** 1% dyclonine, HCl 0.5% allantoin, petrolatum. lanolin.	In 9.45 g.
otc	**Peroxyl** (Colgate)	**Gel:** 1.5% hydrogen peroxide	Mint flavor. In 15 g.
otc	**Orabase-B** (Colgate)	**Paste:** 20% benzocaine, mineral oil.	In 5 and 15 g.
Rx	**Orabase HCA** (Colgate)	**Paste:** 0.5% hydrocortisone acetate, 5% polyethylene, mineral oil.	In 5 g.
Rx	**Kenalog in Orabase** (Apothecon)	**Paste:** 0.1% triamcinolone acetonide	In 5 g.
Rx	**Oralone Dental** (Thames)	**Paste:** 0.1% triamcinolone acetonide	In 5 g.
otc	**Orabase-Plain** (Colgate)	**Paste:** Plasticized hydrocarbon gel	In 5 and 15 g.
otc	**Tanac Dual Core** (Del Pharm)	**Stick:** 7.5% benzocaine, 6% tannic acid, 0.75% octyl dimethyl PABA, 0.2% allantoin, 0.12% benzalkonium chloride, cetyl alcohol, butylparaben	In 2.84 g stick.
otc	**Blistex** (Blistex)	**Lip Balm:** SPF 10. 0.5% camphor, 0.5% phenol, 1% allantoin, 2% dimethicone, 6.6% padimate O, 2.5% oxybenzone, parabens, petrolatum	In 4.5 g.
otc	**Herpecin-L** (Campbell Labs)	**Lip Balm:** Allantoin, padimate 0	In 2.8 g.
otc	**Chap Stick Medicated Lip Balm** (Robins)	**Lip Balm:** 1% camphor, 0.6% menthol, 0.5% phenol, petrolatum, mineral oil, cocoa butter, lanolin, parabens	In jars (7 g), squeezable tubes (10 g) and sticks (4.2 g).
otc	**3 in 1 Toothache Relief** (C.S. Dent)	**Gum, Liquid, Lotion/Gel:** Benzocaine	In family first-aid packs.
otc	**Kank-a** (Blistex)	**Liquid/Film:** 20% benzocaine, benzoin compound tincture, SD alcohol 38b, benzyl alcohol, castor oil	Saccharin. In 9.9 ml.
otc	**Ulcerease** (Med-Derm)	**Liquid:** 0.6% liquified phenol, glycerin, sodium borate	In 180 ml.
otc	**Dent's Lotion-Jel** (C.S. Dent)	**Lotion/Gel:** Benzocaine	In 6 g.

PREPARATIONS FOR SENSITIVE TEETH

These toothpastes are specially formulated to replace regular toothpaste for persons with sensitive teeth. Use daily as in regular dental care.

otc	**Denquel Sensitive Teeth** (Procter & Gamble)	**Toothpaste**: 5% potassium nitrate	Mint flavor. In 48, 90 and 135 g.
otc	**Sensodyne Cool Gel** (Block)	**Toothpaste**: Potassium nitrate, sodium fluoride	Saccharin, sorbitol, parabens. In 28.3 g.
otc	**Promise with Fluoride** (Block)	**Toothpaste**: Potassium nitrate, sodium mono fluorophosphate	Saccharin, sorbitol, parabens. Mint flavor. In 48, 90 and 135 g.
otc	**Sensodyne-F** (Block)		Saccharin, sorbitol. In 72 and 138 g.
otc	**Sensodyne-SC** (Block)	**Toothpaste**: 10% strontium Cl hexahydrate	Saccharin, sorbitol, parabens. In 26 g.
otc	**Sensitivity Protection Crest** (Procter & Gamble)	**Toothpaste**: Sodium fluoride, potassium nitrate	Mint flavor. In 175 g.
otc	**Sensodyne Fresh Mint** (Block)	**Toothpaste**: Potassium nitrate, sodium monofluorophosphate	Sorbitol, saccharin. In 26 g.
Rx	**Triamcinolone Acetonide Dental 0.1%** (Various, eg, Qualitest, Taro)	**Paste**: 0.1% triamcinolone acetonide	In 5 g.

VAGINAL ANTIFUNGAL AGENTS

Actions:

Pharmacology: Treatment of vaginal candidiasis (moniliasis) is complicated by a high recurrence rate due to the ubiquitous nature of *Candida albicans* and non-albicans species of *Candida*. Predisposing factors include diabetes, antibiotics, pregnancy, corticosteroids, oral progestin-dominant contraceptives and decreased host immunity.

Agents approved for local treatment of vulvovaginal candidiasis include nystatin (a polyene antibiotic), the imidazoles (butoconazole, clotrimazole, miconazole, tioconazole) and terconazole (a triazole derivative). All these agents are fungicidal against *Candida*. Nystatin and clotrimazole are fungistatic and fungicidal.

Nystatin binds to sterols in the cell membrane of the fungus with a resultant change in membrane permeability allowing leakage of intracellular components. The primary action of imidazoles appears to be alteration of the permeability of the fungus cell membrane which allows leakage of essential intracellular components.

Terconazole's exact pharmacologic mode of action is uncertain. It may exert antifungal activity by disruption of normal fungal cell membrane permeability.

Pharmacokinetics:

Butoconazole – Approximately 5.5% is absorbed after vaginal administration; plasma half-life is 21 to 24 hours.

Terconazole – Following intravaginal administration of suppositories, absorption ranged from 5% to 8% in three hysterectomized subjects and 12% to 16% in two non-hysterectomized subjects with tubal ligations.

Tioconazole – Systemic absorption in nonpregnant patients is negligible.

Clotrimazole – Serum levels of clotrimazole in six healthy volunteers who had one 500 mg vaginal tablet inserted were higher than those in other volunteers given 100 mg and 200 mg vaginal tablets; these levels did not exceed 10 ng/ml. It has been estimated that 3% to 10% of a vaginal dose of clotrimazole may be absorbed, but the drug rapidly and efficiently degrades to microbiologically inactive metabolites. Nearly all the clotrimazole given in the 500 mg vaginal tablet remains in the vagina for 48 hours, and in some cases 72 hours, in fungicidal concentrations.

Microbiology: Terconazole is effective only for vulvovaginitis caused by the genus *Candida*. Tioconazole also exhibits fungicidal activity in vitro against *Torulopsis glabrata*. Other pathogens commonly associated with vulvovaginitis *(Trichomonas* and *Gardnerella vaginalis)* do not respond to these antifungal agents.

Indications:

Candidiasis: Local treatment of vulvovaginal candidiasis (eg, moniliasis, vaginal yeast infection).

Contraindications:

Hypersensitivity to specific drug or component of the product.

Warnings:

Diagnosis: It is important that vaginal infections be differentiated, as bacterial vaginosis, trichomoniasis and vulvovaginal candidiasis may produce common symptoms. The diagnosis of vulvovaginal candidiasis may be confirmed prior to therapy by KOH smears or cultures. This does not apply to otc use of these agents, which requires self-diagnosis by the patient.

OTC products:

Other conditions – If abdominal pain, fever or foul-smelling vaginal discharge is present, do not use these products. If there is no improvement within 3 days, stop using these products. A condition more serious than a yeast infection may be present.

Vaginal itch/discomfort – The patient should consult a physician before using these products if it is their first experience with vaginal itch and discomfort.

Recurrent infections – If the patient has been exposed to HIV and is having recurrent vaginal infections, especially infections that do not clear up easily with proper treatment, consult a physician to determine the cause of the symptoms. If symptoms return within 2 months, the patient could be pregnant or there could be a serious underlying medical cause for the infections, including diabetes or a damaged immune system (including HIV infection).

VAGINAL ANTIFUNGAL AGENTS

Pregnancy: Category A – nystatin; Category B – clotrimazole; Category C – butoconazole, terconazole, tioconazole. No adverse effects or complications are reported in infants born to women treated with these agents. During pregnancy, use of a vaginal applicator may be contraindicated; manual insertion of tablets may be preferred. Use only on advice of physician.

Since small amounts of these drugs may be absorbed from the vagina, use during the first trimester only when essential. Use **butoconazole** only during the second and third trimesters. Possible exposure of the fetus through direct transfer of **terconazole** from an irritated vagina to the fetus by diffusion across amniotic membranes may occur.

Lactation: It is not known whether these drugs are excreted in breast milk. Safety for use during lactation has not been established. Exercise caution or temporarily discontinue nursing during administration.

Terconazole – Because of the potential for adverse reaction in nursing infants from terconazole, decide whether to discontinue nursing or to discontinue the drug, taking into account the importance of the drug to the mother.

Children: Safety and efficacy have not been established.

Precautions:

For vaginal use only: Do not use creams in mouth or eyes.

Irritation: If irritation or sensitization occurs, discontinue use.

Chronic or recurrent candidiasis may be a symptom of unrecognized diabetes mellitus or a damaged immune system (including HIV infection). A persistently resistant infection may actually be due to reinfection; evaluate sources of reinfection.

Refractory patients: If there is lack of response, repeat microbiological studies to confirm diagnosis and rule out other pathogens before reinstituting antifungal therapy.

Adverse Reactions:

Irritation; sensitization; vulvovaginal burning.

Clotrimazole: Skin rash, lower abdominal cramps, bloating, vulval irritation, slight cramping, slight urinary frequency, burning or irritation in the sexual partner (rare); intercurrent cystitis (one case); vaginal soreness with coitus; vaginal irritation; itching; burning; dyspareunia.

Miconazole: Vulvovaginal burning, itching, irritation (2%); pelvic cramps (2%); headache (1.3%); maceration and allergic contact dermatitis; hives, skin rash (< 0.5%).

Butoconazole: Vulvar/vaginal burning (2.3%); vulvar itching (0.9%); discharge, soreness, swelling, itchy fingers (0.2%).

Terconazole: Headache (21% to 30%); dysmenorrhea (6%); pain of the female genitalia (4.2%); body pain (2.1% to 3.9%); abdominal pain (3.4%); fever (1% to 2.8%); chills (0.4% to 1.8%); vulvovaginal burning (5% to 15%); itching (2.3% to 5%); irritation (3.1%). Most frequent reasons for discontinuing therapy were vulvovaginal itching (0.6% to 2.5%); burning (2.5%); pruritus (1.8%).

Photosensitivity reactions may occur following repeated dermal application under conditions of filtered artificial ultraviolet light.

Tioconazole: Burning (6%); itching (5%); irritation, discharge, vulvar edema and swelling, vaginal pain, dysuria, nocturia, dyspareunia, dryness of vaginal secretions, desquamation (< 1%).

Patient Information:

Patient instructions are enclosed with product. Patients should carefully read *otc* product labeling.

Open applicator just prior to administration to prevent contamination. Clean applicator after use with mild soap solution and rinse thoroughly with water.

Insert high into the vagina (except during pregnancy).

Complete full course of therapy. Use continuously, even during menstrual period.

Notify physician if burning or irritation occurs.

Refrain from sexual intercourse.

Use sanitary napkin or minipad to prevent staining of clothing. Do not use a tampon.

The base used in some of these formulations may interact with (weaken) certain latex products such as condoms or diaphragms. Concurrent use (within 72 hours) is not recommended.

Antifungal Agents

CLOTRIMAZOLE

Refer to the general discussion of these products in the Vaginal Antifungal agents group monograph. For information on oral and topical clotrimazole, refer to individual monographs.

Administration and Dosage:

Tablets:

100 mg – Insert 1 tablet intravaginally at bedtime for 7 consecutive days.
500 mg – Insert 1 tablet intravaginally, preferably at bedtime.

Cream:

Intravaginal – Insert 1 applicatorful a day, preferable at bedtime, for 7 consecutive days.
Topical – Apply to affected areas twice daily (morning and evening for 7 consecutive days.

otc	**Clotrimazole** (Various, eg, Goldline, Major, Moore)	**Vaginal tablets:** 100 mg	In 7s with applicator(s).
otc	**Gyne-Lotrimin** (Schering-Plough)		In 7s with 1 applicator.
otc	**Mycelex-7** (Bayer)		Lactose. In 7s with 1 applicator.
otc	**Mycelex-7 Combination Pack** (Bayer)		In 7s with applicator.
otc	**Femcare** (Schering-Plough)		In 7s with 1 applicator.
otc	**Sweet'n fresh Clotrimazole-7** (NutraMax Products)		Lactose. In 7s with applicator.
Rx	**Mycelex-G** (Bayer)	**Vaginal tablets:** 500 mg	Lactose. (Miles 097). White, bullet shape. In 1s with applicator.
otc	**Clotrimazole** (Various, eg, Goldline, Major, Moore, NMC)	**Vaginal cream:** 1%	In 45 g with applicator(s).
otc	**Mycelex-7** (Bayer)		Benzyl alcohol, cetostearyl alcohol. In 45 g with 1 applicator or 45 g with 7 disposable applicators.
otc	**Mycelex-7 Combination Pack** (Bayer)		In 7 g.
otc	**Sweet'n fresh Clotrimazole-7** (NutraMax Products)		Benzyl alcohol, cetostearyl alcohol. In 45 g with applicator.
otc	**Gyne-Lotrimin** (Schering-Plough)		In 45 g with 1 applicator, 45 g with 7 apllicators, 45 g with 7 pre-filled applicators.
otc	**Femcare** (Schering-Plough)		Benzyl alcohol, alcohol. In 45 g with applicator.
Rx	**Mycelex Twin Pack** (Bayer)	**Vaginal tablets:** 500 mg	Lactose. (Miles 097). White, bullet shape. In 1s with applicator.
		Topical cream: 1%	Benzyl alcohol, cetyl stearyl alcohol. In 7 g tube.
otc	**Gyne-Lotrimin Combination Pack** (Schering-Plough)	**Vaginal tablets:** 100 mg	Lactose. In 7s with applicator.
		Topical cream: 1%	Beznyl alcohol, cetostearyl alcohol. In 7 g tubes.

Antifungal Agents

MICONAZOLE NITRATE

Refer to the general discussion of these agents in the Vaginal Antifungal Agents group monograph. For information on systemic and topical miconazole refer to individual monographs.

Administration and Dosage:

Tablets: Insert 1 suppository intravaginally once daily at bedtime for 7 consecutive days (100 mg) or 3 consecutive days (200 mg).

Cream:

Intravaginal – Insert 1 applicatorful intravaginally once daily at bedtime for 7 days.
Topical – Apply to affected areas twice daily (morning and evening) for 7 days.

Repeat course if necessary, after ruling out ohter pathogens.

Sotrage: Refrigerate below 15° to 30°C (59° to 86°F).

Rx	**Monistat 3** (Ortho)	**Vaginal Suppositories**: 200 mg	Hydrogenated vegetable oil. White/off-white, elliptical shape. In 3s with 1 applicator.
otc	**Monistat-7** (Advanced Care)	**Vaginal Suppositories**: 100 mg	Hydrogenated vegetable oil. In 7s with 1 applicator and blister-pack 7s with 1 applicator.
Rx	**Monistat-Derm** (Ortho)	**Topical Cream**: 2%	Mineral oil. In 15, 30 and 90 g tubes.
otc	**Miconazole Nitrate** (Various, eg, Copley, Goldline, Major, Moore)	**Vaginal Cream**: 2%	In 45 g with applicator(s).
otc	**Femizol-M** (Lake Consumer Products)		In 45 g with applicator.
otc	**Monistat 7** (Advanced Care)		Mineral oil. In 45 g with 1 applicator or with 7 disposable applicators and blister-pack 7s with 1 applicator or 7 disposable applicators.
Rx	**Monistat Dual-Pak** (Ortho)	**Vaginal Suppositories**: 200 mg	Hydrogenated vegetable oil. White/off-white, elliptical shape. In 3s with 1 applicator.
		Topical Cream: 2%	Pegoxol 7 stearate, peglicol 5 oleate, mineral oil, benzoic acid, butylated hydroxyanisole. In 15, 30 and 90 g tubes.
otc	**Monistat 7 Combination Pack** (Advanced Care)	**Vaginal Suppositories**: 100 mg	Hydrogenated vegetable oil. In 7s with 1 applicator and blister-pack 7s with 1 applicator.
		Topical Cream: 2%	In 9 g.

TIOCONAZOLE

Refer to the general discussion of these products in the Vaginal Antifungal Agents group monograph.

Administration and Dosage:

Single dose: Insert 1 applicatorful (≈ 4.6 g) intravaginally just prior to bedtime.

otc	**Vagistat-1** (Bristol-Myers Squibb)	**Vaginal Ointment**: 6.5%	In 4.6 g prefilled single-dose applicator.

Antifungal Agents

NYSTATIN

Refer to the general discussion of these products in the Vaginal Antifungal Agents group monograph. For information on oral and topical nystatin, refer to the individual monographs.

Administration and Dosage:

The usual dosage is 1 tablet intravaginally daily for 2 weeks.

Symptomatic relief may occur in a few days; continue full course of treatment.

Storage: Refrigerate below 15°C (59°F).

Rx	**Nystatin** (Various, eg, Goldline, Harbor, Major, Moore, Rugby, Schein)	**Vaginal Tablets:** 100,000 units	In 15s and 30s with or without applicator(s).
Rx	**Mycostatin** (Apothecon)		Lactose. (457). Diamond shape. In 15s and 30s w/applicators.

TERCONAZOLE

Refer to the general discussion of these products in the Vaginal Antifungal Agents group monograph.

Administration and Dosage:

Tablets: Administer one suppository (2.5 g) intravaginally once daily at bedtime for 3 consecutive days.

Cream:

0.4% – Administer one applicatorful (5 g) intravaginally once daily at bedtime for 7 consecutive days.

0.8% – Administer one applicatorful (5 g) intravaginally once daily at bedtime for 3 consecutive days.

Before prescribing another course of therapy, reconfirm diagnosis by smears or cultures and rule out other pathogens commonly associated with vulvovaginitis. The therapeutic effect of terconazole is not affected by menstruation.

Rx	**Terazol 7** (Ortho)	**Vaginal Cream:** 0.4%	Cetyl alcohol, stearyl alcohol. In 45 g tube with 1 measured-dose applicator.
Rx	**Terazol 3** (Ortho)	**Vaginal Cream:** 0.8%	In 20 g tube with 1 measured-dose applicator.
		Vaginal Suppositories: 80 mg	Coconut oil, palm kernal oil. White, elliptical shape. In 3s with 1 measured-dose applicator.

BUTOCONAZOLE NITRATE

Refer to the general discussion of these products in the Vaginal Antifungal Agents group monograph.

Administration and Dosage:

Pregnant patients: (2nd and 3rd trimesters only) — 1 applicatorful (≈ 5 g) intravaginally at bedtime for 6 days (see Warnings).

Nonpregnant patients: 1 applicatorful (≈ 5 g) intravaginally at bedtime for 3 days. May be extended to 6 days, if necessary.

Storage: Do not store above 40° C (104° F). Avoid freezing.

otc	**Femstat 3** (Syntex)	**Vaginal Cream:** 2%	Parabens, mineral oil, cetyl alcohol, stearyl alcohol. In 5 g pre-filled applicators (3s) and 20 g with applicators.

Miscellaneous Anti-infectives

SULFONAMIDES

For complete prescribing information for the systemic sulfonamides, refer to the monograph in the Anti-infectives section.

Actions:

Pharmacology: Sulfonamides exert a bacteriostatic action by competitive antagonism of para-aminobenzoic acid (PABA), an essential component of folic acid synthesis.

Indications:

Triple sulfa: Treatment of *Gardnerella vaginalis* vaginitis.

Sulfanilamide: Treatment of *Candida albicans* vulvovaginitis only.

Contraindications:

Hypersensitivity to any component of the product; kidney disease; pregnancy at term; lactation.

Warnings:

Diagnosis: Standard office diagnostic procedures for vaginitis are usually sufficient to establish the diagnosis of *Gardnerella vaginalis* and to rule out a trichomonal or monilial infection.

Systemic effects: Because sulfonamides may be absorbed from the vaginal mucosa, the usual precautions for oral sulfonamides apply. If skin rash or evidence of systemic toxicity develops, discontinue treatment.

Pregnancy: Category C. Safe use in pregnancy has not been established. It is not known whether these agents can cause fetal harm when administered during pregnancy. Use only if clearly needed.

Lactation: Sulfonamides appear in maternal milk and have caused kernicterus in the newborn. Because of the potential for serious adverse reactions in the nursing infant, decide whether to discontinue nursing or discontinue the drug, taking into account the importance of the drug to the mother.

Children: Safety and efficacy have not been established.

Precautions:

For vaginal use only: Avoid contact of the cream with the eyes.

Applicators: Use vaginal applicators and inserters with caution after the seventh month of pregnancy.

Adverse Reactions:

Local irritations (increased discomfort; burning); allergic reactions; Stevens Johnson syndrome (rare); agranulocytosis (one case).

Patient Information:

Patient instructions are included with product.

Insert high into vagina (with applicator provided). Use of an applicator may not be recommended during pregnancy.

Complete full course of therapy.

Notify physician if burning, irritation, itching or signs of a systemic allergic reaction occur.

Do not engage in vaginal intercourse during treatment.

Miscellaneous Anti-infectives

SULFONAMIDES

Administration and Dosage:

Triple sulfa:

Tablets – One tablet intravaginally morning and evening for 10 days; repeat if necessary.

Cream – One applicatorful intravaginally twice daily for 4 to 6 days; treatment may then be reduced 50% to 25%. Repeat if necessary.

Sulfanilamide:

Cream – One applicatorful intravaginally once or twice daily continued through one complete menstrual cycle.

Suppository – One suppository intravaginally once or twice daily; continue for 30 days.

TRIPLE SULFA

For complete prescribing information, refer to the Vaginal Sulfonamides group monograph.

Rx	**Sultrin Triple Sulfa** (Ortho)	**Vaginal Tablets**: 172.5 mg sulfathiazole, 143.75 mg sulfacetamide, 184 mg sulfabenzamide, urea	Lactose. (Ortho). White, capsule shape. In 20s with applicator.
Rx	**Triple Sulfa** (Various, eg, Fougera, Goldline, Major, NMC, Rugby, Schein)	**Vaginal Cream**: 3.42% sulfathiazole, 2.86% sulfacetamide, 3.7% sulfabenzamide	In 78, 80, 82.5, 90 and 120 g with applicator(s).
Rx	**Dayto Sulf** (Dayton)		0.64% urea. In 78 g with 8 disposable applicators.
Rx	**Gyne-Sulf** (G & W)		In 82.5 g with applicator.
Rx	**Sultrin Triple Sulfa** (Ortho)		2% cetyl alcohol, lanolin, parabens, peanut oil. In 78 g with measured-dose applicator.
Rx	**Trysul** (Savage)		Cetyl alcohol, peanut oil, parabens. In 78 g with measured-dose applicator.
Rx	**V.V.S.** (Econo Med)		In 90 g with applicator.

SULFANILAMIDE

For complete prescribing information, refer to the Vaginal Sulfonamides group monograph.

Rx	**Sulfanilamide** (Various, eg, Lemmon)	**Vaginal Cream:** 15% sulfanilamide	In 120 g with applicator.
Rx	**AVC** (Hoechst Marion Roussel)		Lactose, parabens. In 120 g with applicator
Rx	**AVC** (Hoechst Marion Roussel)	**Vaginal Suppositories:** 1.05 g sulfanilamide	Lactose, parabens. White. In 16s with inserter.

Miscellaneous Anti-infectives

CLINDAMYCIN PHOSPHATE

Actions:

Pharmacology: Clindamycin phosphate is a water soluble ester of the semi-synthetic antibiotic produced by a 7(S)-chloro-substitution of the 7(R)-hydroxyl group of the parent antibiotic lincomycin. The 2% cream is for intravaginal use only. Clindamycin inhibits bacterial protein synthesis by its action at the bacterial ribosome. The antibiotic binds preferentially to the 50S ribosomal subunit and affects the process of peptide chain initiation. Although clindamycin phosphate is inactive in vitro, rapid in vivo hydrolysis converts this compound to the antibacterially active clindamycin.

Pharmacokinetics: Following a once a day intravaginal dose of 100 mg clindamycin vaginal cream administered to 6 healthy female volunteers for 7 days, approximately 5% (range, 0.6% to 11%) of the administered dose was absorbed systemically. The peak serum clindamycin concentration observed on the first day averaged 18 ng/ml (range, 4 to 47 ng/ml) and averaged 25 ng/ml (range, 6 to 61 ng/ml) on day 7. These peak concentrations were attained in approximately 10 hours post-dosing (range, 4 to 24 hours).

Following a once a day intravaginal dose of 100 mg clindamycin vaginal cream administered for 7 consecutive days to 5 women with bacterial vaginosis, absorption was slower and less variable than that observed in healthy females. Approximately 5% (range, 2% to 8%) of the dose was absorbed systemically. The peak serum clindamycin concentration observed on the first day averaged 13 ng/ml (range, 3 to 34 ng/ml) and averaged 16 ng/ml (range 7 to 26 ng/ml) on day 7. These peak concentrations were attained in approximately 16 hours post-dosing (range, 8 to 24 hours).

There was little or no systemic accumulation of clindamycin after repeated vaginal dosing of clindamycin vaginal cream. The systemic half-life was 1.5 to 2.6 hours.

Microbiology: Clindamycin is active in vitro against most strains of the following organisms that have been reported to be associated with bacterial vaginosis: *Bacteroides* sp, *Gardnerella vaginalis; Mobiluncus* sp; *Mycoplasma hominis; Peptostreptococcus* sp.

Indications:

Treatment of bacterial vaginosis (formerly referred to as Haemophilus vaginitis, *Gardnerella* vaginitis, nonspecific vaginitis, *Corynebacterium* vaginitis or anaerobic vaginosis).

Contraindications:

Hypersensitivity to clindamycin, lincomycin, or any of the components of the vaginal cream; regional enteritis; ulcerative colitis; "antibiotic-associated" colitis.

Warnings:

Pseudomembranous colitis has been reported with nearly all antibacterial agents, including clindamycin, and may range in severity from mild to life-threatening. Orally and parenterally administered clindamycin has been associated with severe colitis which may end fatally. Diarrhea, bloody diarrhea and colitis (including pseudomembranous colitis) have been reported with the use of orally and parenterally administered clindamycin as well as with topical (dermal) formulations of clindamycin. Therefore, it is important to consider this diagnosis in patients who present with diarrhea subsequent to the administration of clindamycin, even when administered by the vaginal route, because approximately 5% of the clindamycin dose is systemically absorbed from the vagina.

Treatment with antibacterial agents alters the normal flora of the colon and may permit overgrowth of clostridia. Studies indicate that a toxin produced by Clostridium difficile is a primary cause of "antibiotic-associated" colitis.

After the diagnosis of pseudomembranous colitis has been established, initiate therapeutic measures. Mild cases of pseudomembranous colitis usually respond to a discontinuation of the drug alone. In moderate to severe cases, give consideration to management with fluids and electrolytes, protein supplementation and treatment with an antibacterial drug clinically effective against *Clostridium difficile* colitis.

Onset of pseudomembranous colitis symptoms may occur during or after antimicrobial treatment.

Mineral oil: This cream contains mineral oil. Mineral oil may weaken latex or rubber products such as condoms or vaginal contraceptive diaphragms; therefore, use of such products within 72 hours following treatment with clindamycin vaginal cream is not recommended.

Miscellaneous Anti-infectives

CLINDAMYCIN PHOSPHATE

Diagnosis: A clinical diagnosis of bacterial vaginosis is defined by the presence of a homogeneous vaginal discharge that (a) has a pH of > 4.5, (b) emits a "fishy" amine odor when mixed with 10% KOH solution, and (c) contains clue cells on microscopic examination. Gram's stain results consistent with a diagnosis of bacterial vaginosis include (a) markedly reduced or absent *Lactobacillus* morphology, (b) predominance of *Gardnerella* morphotype, and (c) absent or few white blood cells.

Rule out other pathogens commonly associated with vulvovaginitis (eg, *Trichomonas vaginalis, Chlamydia trachomatis, N gonorrhoeae, Candida albicans* and herpes simplex virus).

Pregnancy: Category B. There are no adequate and well controlled studies in pregnant women. Use during pregnancy only if clearly needed.

Lactation: It is not known if clindamycin is excreted in breast milk following the use of vaginally administered clindamycin. However, after oral or parenteral administration, clindamycin has been detected in breast milk. Because of the potential for serious adverse reactions in nursing infants from clindamycin phosphate, decide whether to discontinue nursing or to discontinue the drug, taking into account the importance of the drug to the mother.

Children: Safety and efficacy in children have not been established.

Precautions:

For intravaginal use only. Avoid contact with the eyes. Clindamycin vaginal cream contains ingredients that will cause burning and irritation of the eye. In the event of accidental contact with the eye, rinse the eye with copious amounts of cool tap water.

Overgrowth of nonsusceptible organisms: The use of clindamycin vaginal cream may result in the overgrowth of nonsusceptible organisms, particularly yeasts, in the vagina. Approximately 16% of patients treated with clindamycin vaginal cream developed symptomatic cervicitis/vaginitis with 11% of patients developing cervicitis/vaginitis secondary to C albicans.

Adverse Reactions:

In clinical trials, approximately 4% of patients discontinued therapy due to drug-related adverse events.

Genital tract: Cervicitis/vaginitis, symptomatic (16%; Candida albicans 11%, *Trichomonas vaginalis* 1%); vulvar irritation 6%.

GI: Heartburn, nausea, vomiting, diarrhea, constipation, abdominal pain (< 1%).

CNS: Dizziness, headache, vertigo (< 1%).

Body as a whole: Urticaria, rash.

Other clindamycin formulations: Other effects that have been reported in association with the use of topical (dermal) formulations of clindamycin include severe colitis (including pseudomembranous colitis), contact dermatitis, skin irritation (eg, erythema, peeling, burning), oily skin, gram-negative folliculitis, abdominal pain and GI disturbances.

Clindamycin vaginal cream affords minimal peak serum levels and systemic exposure of clindamycin compared to 100 mg oral dosing. Although these lower levels of exposure are less likely to produce the common reactions seen with oral clindamycin, the possibility of these and other reactions cannot be excluded presently. Refer to the Clindamycin and Lincomycin monographs in the Anti-infectives chapter.

Overdosage:

Vaginally applied clindamycin cream could be absorbed in sufficient amounts to produce systemic effects.

Patient Information:

Instruct patients not to engage in vaginal sexual intercourse during treatment with this product.

Administration and Dosage:

Recommended dose is one applicatorful (5 g containing approximately 100 mg clindamycin phosphate) intravaginally, preferably at bedtime, for 7 consecutive days.

Rx	**Cleocin** (Upjohn)	**Cream:** 2%	With mineral oil, benzyl alcohol, propylene glycol, polysorbate 60, sorbitan monostearate. In 40 g tube with 7 disposable applicators.

Miscellaneous Anti-infectives

METRONIDAZOLE

Metronidazole is also available for topical and systemic use. For further information, refer to the individual monographs in the Anti-infectives chapter and the Acne Products section in the Topical chapter.

Actions:

Pharmacology: Metronidazole an imidazole, is classified therapeutically as an antiprotozoal and antibacterial agent. The intracellular targest of action of metronidazole on anaerobes are largely unkown. The 5–nitro group of metronidazole is reduced by metabolically active anaerobes and the reduced form of the drug interacts with bacterial DNA. However, it is not clear whether interaction with DNA alone is an important component in the bactericidal action of metronidazole.

Pharmacokinetics:

Healthy subjects – A single, intravaginal 5 g dose of metronidazole vaginal gel (equivalent to 37 .5 mg metronidazole) to 12 healthy subjects resulted in a mean maximum serum metronidazole concentration of 237 ng/ml (range, 152 to 368 ng/ml). This is approximately 2% of the mean maximum serum metronidazole concentration reported in the same subjects administered a single oral 500 mg dose of metronidazole (mean C_{max} = 12,785 ng/ml; range, 10,013 to 17, 400 ng/ml). These peak concentrations were obtained in 6 to 12 hours after dosing with metronidzaole vaginal gel and 1 to 3 hours after dosing with oral metronidazole.

The extent of exposure (area under the curve; AUC) of metronidazole, when administered as a single intravaginal 5 g dose was approximately 4% of the AUC of a single oral 500 mg dose (4977 ng•hr/ml and ≈ 125,000 ng•hr/ml, respectively). When administered vaginally, absorption was ≈ 50% that of an oral dose.

Patients with bacterial baginosis – Single and multiple 5 g doses of metonidazole vaginal gel to 4 patietns with bacterial vaginosis resulted in a mean maximum serum metronidazole concentation of 214 ng/ml on day 1 and 294 ng/ml (range, 228 to 349 ng/ml) on day 5. Steady-state metronidazole serum concentrations following oral dosages of 400 to 500 mg twice dialy range from 6000 to 20,000 ng/ml.

Microbiology: Metronidazole is active in vitro against most strains of the following organisms that are associated with bacterial vaginosis: *Bacteroides sp; Gardnerella vaginalis; Mobiluncus sp; Peptostreptococcus sp.*

Indications:

Treatment of bacterial vaginosis (formerly referred to as *Hemophilus* vaginitis, *Gardnerella* vaginitis, nonspecific vaginitis, *Corynebacterium* vaginitis, anaerobic vaginosis).

Contraindications:

Hypersensitivity to metronidazole, parabens or other ingredients of the formulation or other nitroimidazole derivatives.

Warnings:

Convulsive seizures and peripheral neuropathy: Convulsive seizures and peripheral neuropathy, the latter characterized mainly by numbness or paresthesia of an extremity, have occurred in patients treated with oral metronidazole. The appearance of abnormal neurologic signs demands the prompt discontinuation of metronidazole vaginal gel therapy. Administer with caution to patients with CNS diseases.

Psychotic reactions: Psychotic reactions have occurred in alcoholic patients who were using oral metronidazole and disulfiram concurrently. Do not administer metronidazole vaginal gel to patients who have taken disulfiram within the last 2 weeks.

Diagnosis: A clinical diagnosis of bacterial vaginosis is usually defined by the presence of a homogeneous vaginal discharge that (a) has a pH of > 4.5, (b) emits a "fishy" amine odor when mixed with a 10% KOH solution, and (c) contains clue cells on microscopic examination. Gram's stain results consistent with a diagnosis of bacterial vaginosis include (a) markedly reduced or absent *Lactobacillus* morphology, (b) predominance of *Gardnerella* morphotype, and (c) absent/few white blood cells.

Rule out other pathogens commonly associated with vulvovaginitis (eg, *Trichomonas vaginalis, Chlamydia trachomatis, Neisseria gonorrheae, Candida albicans, Herpes simplex* virus).

Hepatic function impairment: Patients with severe hepatic disease metabolize metronidazole slowly. This results in the accumulation of metronidazole and its metabolites in the plasma. Accordingly, for such patients, administer metronidazole vaginal gel cautiously.

Carcinogenesis: Metronidazole has shown evidence of carcinogenic activity in a number of studies involving chronic, oral administration in mice and rats.

Pregnancy: Category B. There are no adequate and well controlled studies in pregnant women. Use during pregnancy only if clearly needed.

Miscellaneous Anti-infectives

METRONIDAZOLE

Lactation: Specific studies of metronidazole levels in breast milk following intravaginal metronidazole have not been performed. However, metronidazole is secreted in breast milk in concentrations similar to those found in plasma following oral administration. Decide whether to discontinue nursing or to discontinue the drug, taking into account the importance of the drug to the mother.

Children: Safety and efficacy in children have not been established.

Precautions:

Vaginal candidiasis: Known or previously unrecognized vaginal candidiasis may present more prominent symptoms during metronidazole vaginal gel therapy; ≈ 6% of patients developed symptomatic *Candida* vaginitis during or immediately after therapy.

For intravaginal use only: Avoid contact with the eyes. Metronidazole vaginal gel contains ingredients that may cause burning and irritation of the eye. In the event of accidental contact with the eye, rinse with copious amounts of cool tap water.

Drug Interactions:

Metronidazole Interactions (Vaginal Gel)			
Precipitant drug	Object drug*		Description
Metronidazole	Anticoagulants	↑	Oral metronidazole may potentiate the anticoagulant effect of warfarin, resulting in a prolongation of prothrombin time. Consider this possibility with the vaginal gel.
Metronidazole	Disulfiram	↑	Disulfiram-like reaction to alcohol has occurred with oral metronidazole. Consider the possibility with the vaginal gel.
Metronidazole	Ethanol	↑	A disulfiram-like reaction may occur with concurrent use. Although the risk for most patients may be slight, caution is advised.

* ↑ = Object drug increased.

Drug/Lab test interactions: Metronidazole may interfere with certain types of determinations of serum chemistry values, such as AST, ALT, LDH, triglycerides and glucose hexokinase; values of zero may be observed.

METRONIDAZOLE

Adverse Reactions:

GU: Candida cervicitis/vaginitis, symptomatic (6.1%); vaginal, perineal or vulvar itching (1.4%); urinary frequency, vaginal or vulvar burning or irritation, vaginal discharge (not *Candida*), vulvar swelling (< 1%).

GI: Cramps/pain (abdominal/uterine) (3.4%); nausea (2%); metallic or bad taste (1.7%); constipation, decreased appetite, diarrhea (< 1%).

CNS: Dizziness, headache, lightheadedness (< 1%).

Miscellaneous: Increased/decreased white blood cell counts (1.7%); rash (< 1%).

Other metronidazole formulations: Other effects that have been reported in association with the use of topical (dermal) formulations of metronidazole include skin irritation, transient skin erythema, and mild skin dryness and burning (≤ 2%).

Metronidazole vaginal gel affords minimal peak serum levels and systemic exposure of metronidazole compared to 500 mg oral dosing. Although these lower levels of exposure are less likely to produce the common reactions seen with oral metronidazole, the possibility of these and other reactions cannot be excluded presently. Refer to the Metronidazole Oral monograph in the Anti-infectives chapter.

Overdosage:

Vaginally applied metronidazole could be absorbed in sufficient amounts to produce systemic effects (see Warnings).

Patient Information:

Do not drink alcohol while being treated with metronidazole vaginal gel. While blood levels are significantly lower than with usual doses or oral metronidazole, a possible interaction with alcohol cannot be excluded.

Instruct patient not to engage in vaginal intercourse during treatment with this product.

Administration and Dosage:

Recommended dose is one applicatorful (≈ 5 g containing ≈ 37.5 mg metronidazole) intravaginally twice daily for 5 days. Apply once in the morning and evening.

Rx	**MetroGel-Vaginal** (Curatek)	**Gel:** 0.75%	With carbomer 934P, EDTA, parabens and propylene glycol. In 70 g tube with applicator.

VAGINAL ANTI-INFECTIVE COMBINATIONS

Ingredients:

In these combinations:

SULFONAMIDES are used for infections due to susceptible organisms (see specific monograph).

AMINACRINE is an antiseptic.

ALLANTOIN may aid in debriding necrotic tissue and in tissue regeneration.

POLYOXYETHYLENE NONYL PHENOL and *DOCUSATE SODIUM* are wetting agents.

Rx	**Vagisec Plus** (Schmid)	**Vaginal Suppositories:** 6 mg aminacrine HCl, 5.25 mg polyoxyethylene nonyl phenol, 0.66 mg EDTA and 0.07 mg docusate sodium. *Dose:* 1 twice daily. Continue through 2 menstrual cycles.	In 28s with applicator.
Rx	**Alasulf** (Major)	**Vaginal cream:** 15% sulfanilamide, 0.2% aminacrine HCl and 2% allantoin *Dose:* 1 applicatorful once or twice daily. Continue through 1 complete menstrual cycle.	In 120 g.
Rx	**Deltavac** (Trimen)		In 113.4 g with applicator.
Rx	**D.I.T.I-2** (Dunhall)		In 142 g.
Rx	**Aci-jel** (Ortho)	**Vaginal jelly:** 0.921% glacial acetic acid, 0.025% oxyquinolone sulfate, 0.7% ricinoleic acid, 5% glycerin, propylparaben	In 85 g with applicator.

DOUCHE PRODUCTS

Vaginal douches are for general cleansing of the vaginal and perineal areas; for deodorizing; for relief of itching, burning and edema; for removing vaginal secretions or discharge or for altering vaginal acidity.

POVIDONE-IODINE, CETYLPYRIDINIUM CHLORIDE, EUCALYPTOL, MENTHOL, OXYQUINOLINE SULFATE, PHENOL, SODIUM PERBORATE and THYMOL may have antiseptic or germicidal activity.

Povidine-iodine also relieves minor irritation. It may be absorbed from the vagina; advise patients with thyroid disorders and pregnant patients to avoid iodine-containing douches.

EUCALYPTOL, MENTHOL, PHENOL, METHYL SALICYLATE and THYMOL are counterirritants used for their anesthetic or antipruritic effects.

AMMONIUM ALUM is an astringent that reduces local edema and inflammation; high concentrations can be irritating.

DOCUSATE SODIUM, OCTOXYNOL 9, ALKYL ARYL SULFONATE, SODIUM LAURYL SULFATE and BENZALKONIUM CHLORIDE are surfactants that facilitate douche spread over vaginal mucosa.

SODIUM PERBORATE, SODIUM BICARBONATE, LACTIC ACID, SODIUM ACETATE and CITRIC ACID affect pH.

Patient Information:

Consult manufacturers' recommendations for proper dilution and use of these products.

Vaginal douches are not contraceptive agents.

Douche no sooner than 6 hours after use of a vaginal spermicide.

If irritation occurs, discontinue use.

If infection or disease is suspected, consult physician.

otc	**Triva Douche** (Boyle)	**Powder**: 2% oxyquinoline sulfate, 35% alkyl aryl sulfonate, 0.33% EDTA, 53% sodium sulfate, 9.67% lactose	In 3 g packets (24s).
otc	**Massengill Douche** (Beecham Products)	**Powder**: Ammonium alum, phenol, methyl salicylate, eucalyptus oil, menthol, thymol, PEG-8	In 120, 240, 480 and 660 g jar and UD Packettes (10s and 12s).
otc	**Trichotine Douche** (Reed & Carnrick)	**Powder**: Sodium lauryl sulfate, sodium perborate, monohydrate silica	In 150 and 360 g.
Rx	**Vagisec Douche** (Schmid)	**Solution**: Polyoxyethylene nonyl phenol, EDTA	In 120 ml.
otc	**Trichotine Douche** (Reed & Carnrick)	**Solution**: Sodium lauryl sulfate, sodium borate, 8% SD alcohol 23-A, EDTA	In 120 and 240 ml.
otc	**Zonite Douche** (Menley & James)	**Solution concentrate**: 0.1% benzalkonium chloride, EDTA, menthol, thymol	In 240 and 360 ml.
otc	**Massengill Douche** (Beecham Products)	**Solution concentrate**: Lactic acid, sodium bicarbonate, SD alcohol 40, octoxynol 9	In 120 ml.
otc	**Feminique Disposable Douche** (Schmid)	**Solution**: Sodium benzoate, sorbic acid, lactic acid, octoxynol 9	Baby powder or wildflower scents. In 120 ml twin-packs.
otc	**Massengill Baking Soda Freshness** (Beecham)	**Solution**: Sodium bicarbonate	In 180 ml.
otc	**Acu-dyne Douche** (Acme United)	**Concentrate**: Povidone-iodine	In 240 ml care kits.
otc	**Operand Douche** (Redi Products)		In 60, 240 and UD 15 ml.

DOUCHE PRODUCTS

otc	**Yeast-Gard Medicated Douche** (Lake Pharm)	**Concentrate**: 10% povidone-iodine	In 240 ml.
otc	**Massengill Medicated Douche w/Cepticin** (SK-Beecham)	**Liquid concentrate**: 12% povidone-iodine	In 120 and 240 ml.
otc	**Betadine Medicated Douche** (Purdue Frederick)	**Solution**: 10% povidone-iodine (0.30% when diluted)	In 15 ml (6s) packettes and 240 ml.
otc	**Yeast-Gard Medicated Disposable Douche Premix** (Lake Pharm)	**Solution**: Octoxynol-9, lactic acid, sodium lactate, sodium benzoate, aloe vera	In 180 ml twin-pack.
otc	**Betadine Medicated Disposable Douche** (Purdue Frederick)	**Solution**: 10% povidone-iodine (0.30% when diluted)	In 5.4 ml medicated douche concentrate w/180 ml bottle sanitized water. In 1 and 2 packs.
otc	**Betadine Premixed Medicated Disposable Douche** (Purdue Frederick)		In 180 ml (1s and 2s).
otc	**Massengill Medicated Disposable Douche w/Cepticin** (SK-Beecham)		In 5 ml vial w/180 ml bottle of sanitized water.
otc	**Summer's Eve Medicated Disposable Douche** (Fleet)	**Solution**: 0.30% povidone-iodine when reconstituted	In 135 ml (1s and 2s).
otc	**Yeast-Gard Medicated Disposable Douche** (Lake Pharm)		In 180 ml twin-pack w/two 5.4 ml medicated douche concentrate packets.
otc	**Massengill Disposable Douche** (SK-Beecham)	**Solution**: SD alcohol 40, lactic acid, sodium lactate, octoxynol-9, cetylpiridinium chloride, propylene glycol, diazolidinyl urea, parabens, EDTA	In Belle-Mai, country flowers, spring flowers and fresh mountain breeze scents. In 180 ml.
otc	**Summer's Eve Disposable Douche** (Fleet)	**Solution, regular**: Citric acid, sodium benzoate	In 135 ml (1s, 2s and 4s).
		Solution, scented: Citric acid, octoxynol 9, sodium benzoate, EDTA	In herbal, musk and white flowers scents. In 135 ml (1s, 2s and 4s).
otc	**Summer's Eve Post-Menstrual Disposable Douche** (Fleet)	**Solution**: Sodium lauryl sulfate, parabens, monosodium and disodium phosphates, EDTA	In 135 ml (2s).
otc	**Feminique Disposable Douche** (Schmid)	**Solution**: Vinegar	In 180 ml (2s).
otc	**Massengill Disposable Douche** (SK-Beecham)		In 180 ml.
otc	**Massengill Vinegar & Water Extra Mild** (SK-Beecham)		Preservative free. In 180 ml.
otc	**Summer's Eve Disposable Douche** (Fleet)		In 135 ml (1s and 2s).
otc	**Summer's Eve Disposable Douche Extra Cleansing** (Fleet)	**Solution**: Vinegar, sodium chloride, benzoic acid	In 135 ml (1s, 2s and 4s).
otc	**Massengill Vinegar & Water Extra Cleansing with Puraclean** (SK-Beecham)	**Solution**: Vinegar, cetylpyridinium chloride, diazolidinyl urea, EDTA	In 180 ml.

SPERMICIDES

Actions:

Pharmacology: Topical contraceptive agents provide spermicidal action which is generally reliable when properly used, either in conjunction with a vaginal diaphragm or as the sole method of contraception. These agents are generally less effective than oral contraceptives. To minimize the potential for conception, follow directions for use carefully.

Condom use and STD – The CDC advises the use of condoms to prevent sexually transmitted diseases (STD). If used properly, condoms help prevent infection by *Chlamydia trachomatis, Ureaplasma urealyticum, Trichomonas vaginalis, Candida albicans,* herpes simplex 1 and 2 (when lesions are on penis or female genital area), human papilloma virus, *Treponema pallidum, Haemophilus ducreyi* and AIDS.

Nonoxynol 9 helps to inhibit a variety of sexually transmissible organisms, including those responsible for gonorrhea, chlamydial infection, candidiasis, genital herpes, syphilis, trichomoniasis and AIDS.

The following table gives ranges of pregnancy rates reported for various means of contraception. Efficacy in most cases depends greatly upon degree of compliance and user reliability. No other contraceptive drug or device except levonorgestrel implant and medroxyprogesterone injection approaches the efficacy of the combined oral contraceptives.

Pregnancy Rates for Various Means of Contraception (%)[1]

Method of contraception	Lowest expected[2]	Typical[3]
Oral Contraceptives		3
Combined	0.1	nd
Progestin only	0.5	nd
Mechanical/Chemical		
Levonorgestrel implant	0.2	0.2
Medroxyprogesterone injection	0.3	0.3
IUD		
Progesterone	2	nd
Copper T 380A	0.8	nd
Condom		
Without spermicide	2	12
With spermicide[4]	1.8	4-6
Spermicide alone	3	21
Diaphragm (with spermicidal cream or gel)	6	18
Female condom	2-4	12-25
Periodic abstinence (ie, rhythm; all methods)	1-9	20
Sterility		
Vasectomy	0.1	0.15
Tubal ligation	0.2	0.4
No contraception	85	85

nd = no data.

[1] During first year of continuous use.

[2] Best guess of percentage expected to experience an accidental pregnancy among couples who initiate a method and use it consistently and correctly.

[3] A "typical" couple who initiate a method and experience an accidental pregnancy.

[4] Used as a separate product (not in condom package).

Warnings:

Sensitivity: Should sensitivity to the ingredients or irritation of the vagina or penis develop, discontinue use and consult your physician.

Pregnancy: Controversy surrounds the relationship between the use of vaginal spermicides during pregnancy and congenital malformations. One 1981 study has suggested an association between vaginal spermicides and congenital anomalies (eg, limb-reduction deformities, neoplasms, chromosomal abnormalities). However, many other studies do not support these findings and several of the authors of the 1981 study agree that a causal association is unlikely.The FDA concurs with the Advisory Committee on Fertility and Maternal Health Drugs that there is currently no need for a labeling revision of spermicidal products.

SPERMICIDES

Patient Information:

Consult manufacturers' recommendations for proper use of these products. The following general principles should be noted:

Apply at least 10 minutes, but not more than 1 hour before intercourse to ensure effectiveness.

Apply high in the vagina, near the cervix.

Reapply prior to each time intercourse takes place.

Allow suppositories adequate time to disperse.

Do not douche for 6 to 8 hours after intercourse. Premature douching may dilute the spermicide, remove few sperm and may propel sperm into the uterus.

MISCELLANEOUS SPERMICIDES

For complete prescribing information, see the Spermicides group monograph.

otc	**Delfen Contraceptive** (Advanced Care)	**Vaginal Foam:** 12.5% nonoxynol 9	In 20 g w/applicator and 42 g refills.
otc	**Koromex** (Schmid)		In 40 g.
otc	**Because** (Schering)	**Vaginal Foam:** 8% nonoxynol 9	In 10 g (6 dose contraceptor unit).
otc	**Emko** (Schering)		In 40 g w/applicator and 40 & 90 g refills.
otc	**Emko Pre-Fil** (Schering)		In 30 g w/applicator and 60 g refills.
otc	**Ramses** (Schmid)	**Vaginal Jelly:** 5% nonoxynol 9	In 150 g.
otc	**Koromex** (Schmid)	**Vaginal Jelly:** 3% nonoxynol 9	In 126 g.
otc	**Conceptrol Disposable Contraceptive** (Advanced Care)	**Vaginal Gel:** 4% nonoxynol 9	In 2.7 g prefilled applications (6s and 10s).
otc	**Encare** (Thompson Medical)	**Suppositories:** 2.27% nonoxynol 9	In 12s.
otc	**Semicid** (Whitehall)	**Suppositories:** 100 mg nonoxynol 9	Methylparaben. In 9s and 18s.
otc	**Conceptrol Contraceptive Inserts** (Advanced Care)	**Suppositories:** 150 mg nonoxynol-9	In 10s.
otc	**VCF** (Apothecus)	**Vaginal Film:** 28% nonoxynol 9	Glycerin, alcohol. In 3s, 6s and 12s.

SPERMICIDES USED WITH A VAGINAL DIAPHRAGM

For complete prescribing information, see the Spermicides group monograph.

The following products are for use in conjunction with a vaginal diaphragm.

otc	**Koromex** (Schmid)	**Cream:** 3% octoxynol	In 115 g w/applicator.
otc	**Ortho-Gynol Contraceptive** (Advanced Care)	**Gel:** 1% octoxynol 9	In 75 g w/applicator and 75 and 114 g refills.
otc	**Gynol II Contraceptive** (Advanced Care)	**Gel:** 2% nonoxynol 9	In 75 g w/applicator and 75 and 114 g refills.
otc	**Shur-Seal** (Milex)	**Gel:** 2% nonoxynol 9	In 24 UD gel paks.
otc	**Koromex Crystal Clear** (Schmid)	**Gel:** 2% nonoxynol 9	In 126 g with or without applicator.
otc	**K-Y Plus** (Johnson & Johnson)	**Gel:** 2.2% nonoxynol-9	Methylparaben. In 113 g.
otc	**Advantage 24** (Women's Health Institute)	**Gel:** 3.5% nonoxynol-9	Mineral oil, glycerin, parabens, palm oil, sorbic acid. In 3s and 6s (1.5 g each) with applicators.
otc	**Gynol II Extra Strength Contraceptive** (Advanced Care)	**Jelly:** 3% nonoxynol-9	In 75 g and 114 g.

SPERMICIDE-CONTAINING CONDOMS

For complete prescribing information, see the Spermicides group monograph.

A latex condom with a lubricant containing the spermicide nonoxynol 9. The combination of barrier protection combined with the spermicide improves contraceptive effectiveness over traditional condoms.

otc	**Excita Extra** (Schmid)	**Condom:** 8% nonoxynol 9	Ribbed. In 3s, 12s and 36s.
otc	**Sheik Elite** (Schmid)		In 3s, 12s. 24s and 36s
otc	**Ramses Extra** (Schmid)	**Condom:** 15% nonoxynol-9	In 3s, 12s, 24s and 36s.

MISCELLANEOUS VAGINAL PREPARATIONS

otc	**Betadine Medicated** (Purdue Frederick)	**Gel**: 10% povidone-iodine	In 18 and 85 g w/applicator.
		Suppositories: 10% povidone-iodine *Indication*: Relief of irritation and itching. *Dosage*: 1 applicator of gel or 1 suppository at night for 7 days.	In 7s w/applicator.
otc	**Lubrin** (Kenwood/Bradley)	**Inserts**: Caprylic/capric trigylceride, glycerin *Indication*: Prolonged lubrication for sexual intercourse. *Dosage*: 1 intravaginally 5 to 30 minutes before intercourse. Allow 5 to 10 minutes for insert to dissolve.	In 5s, 12s and 40s.
otc	**Vaginex** (Schmid)	**Cream**: Tripelennamine HCl *Indication*: Temporary relief of external vaginal irritation. *Dosage*: Apply externally 3 or 4 times a day.	In 30 g.
otc	**Replens** (Warner Lambert)	**Gel**: Glycerin, mineral oil, methylparaben *Indication*: Replenishes vaginal moisture. *Dosage*: Apply intravaginally.	In 3 and 8 pre-filled applicators.
otc	**Astroglide** (BioFilm)	**Gel**: Glycerin, propylene glycol, parabens *Indications*: Vaginal lubricant. *Dosage*: Apply externally or internally.	In 70.5 ml bottle and 5 ml travel packets.
otc	**Lubricating Jelly** (Taro)	**Jelly**: Glycerin, propylene glycol *Indication*: Provides additional vaginal moisture.	In 60 and 125 g.
otc	**K-Y** (Johnson & Johnson)	**Jelly**: Glycerin, hydroxyethyl cellulose, methylparaben *Indication:* Lubricant *Dosage:* Apply as needed.	Sterile or regular. In 2.7 g, 5 g, 12 g (3s), 60 g and 120 g.
otc	**Maxilube** (Mission)	**Jelly**: Water, silicone oil, glycerin, carbomer 934, triethanolamine, sodium lauryl sulfate, parabens. *Indication:* Lubricant.	In 3 or 5 oz tubes.
otc	**Surgel** (Ulmer)	**Gel**: Propylene glycol, glycerin *Indications*: Vaginal lubricant.	In 120, 240 and 480 ml and gal.
otc	**Gyne-Moistrin** (Schering-Plough)	**Gel**: Propylene glycol, parabens *Indication*: Vaginal lubricant. *Dosage*: Apply externally or internally as needed.	In 45 and 75 g.

MISCELLANEOUS VAGINAL PREPARATIONS

otc	**Trimo-San** (Milex)	**Jelly**: 0.025% oxyquinoline sulfate, 1% boric acid, 0.7% sodium borate, 0.1% sodium lauryl sulfate, glycerin, methylparaben *Indication*: Controls odor-causing bacteria. *Dosage*: ⅕ to 1 full applicator no more than twice a week.	In 120 g w/applicator and 120 g refill.
Rx	**Amino-Cerv pH 5.5** (Milex)	**Cream**: 8.34% urea, 0.5% sodium propionate, 0.83% methionine, 0.35% cystine, 0.83% inositol, benzalkonium Cl *Indications*: Treatment of mild cervicitis and postpartum cervicitis/cervical tears, postconization and for postsurgical procedures. *Dosage*: See manufacturer's information for complete information.	Water miscible base. In 82.5 g w/applicator and 82.5 g refill.
otc	**Summer's Eve Feminine Wash** (Fleet)	**Wipes**: Octoxynol-9, EDTA	In 16s.
		Liquid: Ammonium laureth sulfate, PEG-75, lanolin, EDTA *Indication*: Vaginal cleansing. *Dosage*: Apply externally.	In 120 ml mist, 240 and 450 ml.
otc	**Summer's Eve Feminine Bath** (Fleet)	**Liquid**: Ammonium laureth sulfate, EDTA *Indication*: Gentle vaginal cleansing. *Dosage*: Apply externally.	In 340 ml.
otc	**Summer's Eve Feminine Powder** (Fleet)	**Powder**: Cornstarch, octoxynol-9, benzethonium chloride *Indications*: Absorbs vaginal moisture. *Dosage*: Apply externally.	In 198 g.
otc	**Yeast X** (Fleet)	**Powder**: Cornstarch, zinc oxide *Indication*: Relieves external vaginal irritation and itching. *Dosage*: Apply externally as needed.	In 196 g.
		Suppositories: Pulsatilla 28× *Indication*: Relieves vaginal irritation, itching and burning. *Dosage*: One suppository daily as needed.	In 12s w/applicator.

MISCELLANEOUS VAGINAL PREPARATIONS

otc	**Norforms** (Fleet)	**Powder**: Cornstarch, zinc oxide *Indications*: Relieves external vaginal irritation and itching. *Dosage*: One suppository daily as needed.	In 120 g.
		Suppositories: PEG-18, PEG-32, PEG-20 stearate, methylparaben *Indication*: Feminine deodorant. *Dosage*: One suppository daily as needed.	In 6s, 12s and 24s w/applicator.
otc	**Moist Again** (Lake)	**Gel**: Aloe vera, EDTA, methylparaben, glycerin *Indication*: Vaginal lubricant. *Dosage*: Apply as needed.	In 70.8 g.
otc	**H-R Lubricating Jelly** (Carter-Wallace)	**Jelly**: Hydroxypropyl, methylcellulose, parabens *Indication*: Vaginal lubricant. *Dosage*: Apply as needed.	In 150 g.
otc	**Yeast-Gard Maximum Strength** (Lake)	**Cream**: 20% benzocaine, 3% resorcinol, methylparaben, sodium sulfite, EDTA, mineral oil *Indicaions*: Relieves external vaginal irritation, itching and burning. *Dosage*: Apply externally 3 to 4 times/day.	In 28.35 g.
otc	**Yeast-Gard Sensitive Formula** (Lake)	**Cream**: 5% benzocain, 2% resorcinol, methylparaben, sodium sulfite, EDTA, mineral oil *Indication*: Relieves external vaginal irritation, itching and burning. *Dosage*: Apply externally 3 to 4 times/day.	In 28.35 g.
otc	**Yeast-Gard** (Lake)	**Suppositories**: Pulsatilla 28×, *Candida albicans* 28× *Indication*: Relieves vaginal irrigation, itching and burning. *Dosage*: One suppository daily for 7 days.	In 10s and 15s w/applicator.
otc	**Lubricating Gel** (Lake)	**Gel**: Chlorhexidine gluconate, methylparaben, glycerin *Indication*: Relieves vaginal dryness. *Dosage*: Apply as needed.	In 113.4 g tube and 3 g individual packets.

MISCELLANEOUS VAGINAL PREPARATIONS

otc	**Femicine** (Lake)	**Suppositories**: Pulsatilla 28×, mercurius vivus 28×, sulphur 28×, polythylene glycol *Indications*Relieves vaginal irritaion and itching and removes vaginal discharge. *Dosage*: One suppository daily for 7 days.	In 10s and 15s w/applicator.
otc	**Massengill Feminine Cleansing Wash** (SmithKline Beecham)	**Liquid**: Sodium laureth sulfate, sodium oleth sulfate, magnesium oleth sulfate, PEG-120 methyl glucose dioleate, parabens *Indication*: Vaginal cleansing *Dosage*: Apply externally.	In 240 ml.
otc	**Vagisil** (Combe)	**Powder**: Cornstarch, aloe, mineral oil, benzethonium chloride	In 198 and 312 g.

ANORECTAL PREPARATIONS

The anorectal preparations are used primarily for the symptomatic relief of the discomfort associated with hemorrhoids and perianal itching or irritation. In addition to the products specifically listed in this section, many of the Topical Local Anesthetics and Topical Corticosteroids may also be used locally in anorectal therapy (see specific monographs in the Topicals section).

Ingredients:

The various components of these products are briefly discussed below. For complete information on specific indications, contraindications, precautions and adverse effects of ingredients, refer to the appropriate monographs as indicated.

HYDROCORTISONE (see additional monographs in Hormones and Topicals sections) reduces inflammation, itching and swelling.

LOCAL ANESTHETICS (benzocaine, pramoxine) temporarily relieve pain, itching and irritation. The most frequent adverse effects of topical local anesthetic use are allergic reactions (eg, burning, itching). Their safety and efficacy when used intrarectally require further evaluation. (See additional monographs in the Topicals section).

VASOCONSTRICTORS (ephedrine, phenylephrine) reduce swelling and congestion of anorectal tissues. They relieve local itching by a slight anesthetic effect. These agents are not effective in stopping bleeding from venous tissues.

ASTRINGENTS (witch hazel, zinc oxide) coagulate the protein in skin cells, protecting the underlying tissue and decreasing the cell volume. They lessen mucus and other secretions, and relieve anorectal irritation and inflammation.

ANTISEPTICS (benzalkonium chloride, phenylmercuric nitrate) are not of therapeutic value when applied to the anorectal area. There is no convincing evidence that they prevent infection in the anorectal area. Many are present as preservatives.

EMOLLIENTS/PROTECTANTS (glycerin, lanolin, mineral oil, petrolatum, zinc oxide, cocoa butter, shark liver oil, bismuth salts) form a physical barrier on the skin and lubricate tissues, preventing irritation of the anorectal area and water loss from the stratum corneum. Many of these substances are used as bases and carriers of pharmacologically active compounds.

COUNTERIRRITANTS (camphor) evoke a feeling of comfort, cooling, tingling or warmth and distract the perception of pain and itching.

KERATOLYTICS (resorcinol) cause desquamation and sloughing of epidermal surface cells and may help to expose underlying tissue to therapeutic agents.

WOUND-HEALING AGENTS (balsam Peru, skin respiratory factor or SRF, yeast cell derivative) are claimed to promote wound healing or tissue repair. Effectiveness of these compounds has not been conclusively demonstrated.

ANTICHOLINERGIC AGENTS inhibit the action of acetylcholine. Because these agents produce their action systemically, they are not effective in ameliorating local symptoms of anorectal disease.

Patient Information:

Maintain normal bowel function by proper diet, adequate fluid intake and regular exercise.

Products for external use only are not to be used intrarectally. Apply external products sparingly after, rather than before, a bowel movement. If possible, wash, rinse and dry the area before use.

Avoid excessive laxative use.

Stool softeners or bulk laxatives may be useful adjunctive therapy.

In general, patients with conditions such as diabetes, hypertension, hyperthyroidism or cardiovascular disease should not use products containing vasoconstrictors.

Products containing resorcinol should not be used on open wounds.

If anorectal symptoms do not improve in 7 days, or if bleeding, protrusion, seepage or pain occurs, consult a physician.

STEROID-CONTAINING PRODUCTS

Refer to the general discussion of these products in the Anorectal Preparations Introduction.

Rx	**Proctocort** (Monarch Pharmaceuticals)	**Cream:** 1% hydrocortisone	Stearyl and benzyl alcohols. In 30 g with applicator.
Rx	**Dermol HC** (Dermol)		Mineral oil, lanolin and cetyl alcohols, parabens. In 30 g.
Rx	**Analpram-HC** (Ferndale)	**Cream:** 1% hydrocortisone acetate, 1% pramoxine HCl	Cetyl alcohol, 0.1% potassium sorbate, 0.1% sorbic acid. In 30 g.
Rx	**ProctoCream-HC** (Schwarz Pharma)		In 30 g.
Rx	**Analpram-HC** (Ferndale)	**Cream:** 2.5% hydrocortisone acetate, 1% pramoxine HCl	0.1% potassium sorbate, 0.1 % sorbic acid, cetyl alcohol. In 30 g.
Rx	**Anusol-HC** (Parke-Davis)	**Cream:** 2.5% hydrocortisone	Petrolatum, EDTA, benzyl and stearyl alcohols. In 30 g.
Rx	**ProctoCream-HC** (Schwarz Pharma)	**Cream:** 2.5% hydrocortisone	Glycerin, stearyl alcohol, benzyl alcohol. In 30 g.
Rx	**Dermol HC** (Dermol)	**Cream:** 2.5% hydrocortisone	Mineral oil, lanolin and cetyl alcohols, parabens. In 30 g.
Rx	**Dermol HC** (Dermol)	**Ointment:** 1% hydrocortisone	Mineral oil, white petrolatum. In 30 g.
Rx	**Proctofoam-HC** (Schwarz Pharma)	**Aerosol Foam:** 1% hydrocortisone acetate, 1% pramoxine HCl	Parabens, cetyl alcohol, stearyl alcohol. In 10 g (≥ 14 applications) w/applicator.
Rx	**Pramoxine HC** (Rugby)		Parabens, cetyl alcohol. In 10 g with applicator.
Rx	**Anucort-HC** (G & W)	**Suppositories:** 25 mg hydrocortisone acetate	Vegetable oil. In 12, 24s and 100s.
Rx	**Anusol-HC** (Parke-Davis)		In 12s and 24s.
Rx	**Cort-Dome High Potency** (Bayer)		In 12s.
Rx	**Hemril-HC Uniserts** (Upsher-Smith)		Vegetable oil. In 12s.
Rx	**Hemorrhoidal HC** (Various, eg, Schein, Geneva, Goldline)		In 12s, 24s, 50s, 100s & UD 12s.
Rx	**Anumed HC** (Major)	**Suppositories:** 10 mg hydrocortisone acetate	In 12s.
Rx	**Rectacort** (Century)		In 12s.

LOCAL ANESTHETIC-CONTAINING PRODUCTS

Refer to the general discussion of these products in the Anorectal Preparations Introduction.

otc	**Tronolane** (Ross)	**Cream:** 1% pramoxine HCl	Zinc oxide, parabens. In 30 and 60 g
otc	**Americaine** (Ciba)	**Ointment:** 20% benzocaine	In 22.5 g
otc	**Medicone** (EE Dickinson)	**Ointment:** 20% benzocaine	Mineral oil, white petrolatum. In 30 g
otc	**Anusol** (Parke-Davis)	**Ointment:** 1% pramoxine HCl	12.5% zinc oxide, mineral oil and cocoa butter. In 30 g with applicator.
otc	**ProctoFoam NS** (Schwarz Pharma)	**Aerosol Foam:** 1% pramoxine HCl	In 15 g with applicator.
otc	**Fleet Pain Relief** (Fleet)	**Pads:** 1% pramoxine HCl, 12% glycerin	In 100s.

PERIANAL HYGIENE PRODUCTS

Refer to the general discussion of these products in the Anorectal Preparations Introduction.

otc	**Balneol Perianal Cleansing** (Solvay)	**Lotion:** Mineral oil, lanolin oil and methylparaben	In 120 ml.
otc	**Tucks Clear** (Warner Wellcome)	**Gel:** 50% hamamelis water, 10% glycerin, benzyl alcohol, EDTA	In 19.8 g.
otc	**Aloe Vesta Perineal** (Calgon Vestal)	**Solution:** Sodium C_{14-16} olefin sulfonate, propylene glycol, aloe vera gel and hydrolyzed collagen	In 118 and 236 ml and gal.
otc	**Preparation H Cleansing** (Whitehall)	**Tissues:** Propylene glycol, phenoxyethanol, parabens, citric acid	Alcohol free. In 15s and 40s.
otc	**Tucks** (Parke-Davis)	**Pads:** 50% witch hazel and 10% glycerin with 0.003% benzalkonium Cl	In 40s & 100s.
otc	**Tucks Take-Alongs** (Parke-Davis)		In 12s.
otc	**Hygienic Cleansing** (Rugby)	**Pads:** 50% witch hazel, glycerin, benzalkonium chloride and methylparaben, sodium hydroxide	In 100s
otc	**Fleet Medicated Wipes** (Fleet)	**Pads:** 50% hamamelis water, 7% alcohol, 10% glycerin, benzalkonium chloride and methylparaben	In 100s.

MISCELLANEOUS ANORECTAL COMBINATION PRODUCTS

Refer to the general discussion of these products in the Anorectal Preparations Introduction.

otc	**Preparation H** (Whitehall)	**Cream:** 78% petrolatum, 12% glycerin, 3% shark liver oil, 0.25% phenylephrine HCl, cetyl and stearyl alcohols, EDTA, parabens, lanolin, tocopherol	In 27 and 54 g.
		Ointment: 71.9% petrolatum, 14% mineral oil, 3% shark liver oil, 0.25% phenylephrine HCl, corn oil, glycerin, lanolin, lanolin alcohol, parabens, tocopherol	In 30 and 60 g.
otc	**Rectagene Medicated Rectal Balm** (Pfeiffer)	**Ointment:** Live yeast cell derivative supplying 2000 units Skin Respiratory Factor per ounce, 3% shark liver oil, 1:10,000 phenylmercuric nitrate, lanolin, white petrolatum and thyme oil.	In 56.7 g
otc	**Pazo Hemorrhoid** (Bristol-Myers)	**Ointment:** 0.2% ephedrine sulfate, 2% camphor, 5% zinc oxide, lanolin, petrolatum	In 28 g

MISCELLANEOUS ANORECTAL COMBINATION PRODUCTS

otc	**Hem-Prep** (G&W)	**Ointment**: 0.025% phenylephrine HCl, 11% zinc oxide, white petrolatum	In 42.5 g
otc	**Preparation H** (Whitehall)	**Suppositories**: 3% shark liver oil, 79% cocoa butter, corn oil, EDTA, parabens and tocopherol	In 12s, 24s, 36s and 48s.
otc	**Calmol 4** (Mentholatum)	**Suppositories**: 80% cocoa butter, 10% zinc oxide, parabens	In 12s and 24s.
otc	**Wyanoids Relief Factor** (Wyeth)	**Suppositories**: 79% cocoa butter, 3% shark liver oil, corn oil, EDTA, parabens and tocopherol	In 12s.
otc	**Nupercainal** (Ciba Consumer)	**Suppositories**: 2.1 g cocoa butter, 0.25 g zinc oxide and sodium bisulfite	In 12s and 24s.
otc	**Anusol** (Glaxo Wellcome)	**Suppositories**: 51% topical starch, benzyl alcohol, soy bean oil, tocopheryl acetate	In 12s.
otc	**Anumed** (Major)	**Suppositories**: 2.25% bismuth subgallate, 1.75% bismuth resorcin compound, 1.2% benzyl benzoate, 11% zinc oxide, 1.8% balsam Peru in hydrolyzed vegetable oil base	In 12s.
otc	**Hemril Uniserts** (Upsher-Smith)		In 12s and 50s.
otc	**Rectagene** (Pfeiffer)	**Suppositories**: Live yeast cell derivative supplying 2000 units Skin Respiratory Factor per ounce and shark liver oil in a cocoa butter base	In 12s.
otc	**Rectagene II** (Pfeiffer)	**Suppositories**: 2.25% bismuth subgallate, 1.75% bismuth resorcin compound, 1.2% benzyl benzoate, 1.8% peruvian balsam, 11% zinc oxide, bismuth subiodide, calcium phosphate in a hydrogenated vegetable oil base	In 12s.
otc	**Medicone** (EE Dickinson)	**Suppositories**: 0.25% phenylephrine HCl, 88.7% hard fat, parabens	In 12s and 24s.
otc	**Pazo Hemorrhoid** (Bristol-Myers)	**Suppositories**: 3.8 mg ephedrine sulfate, 96.5 mg zinc oxide, vegetable oil	In 12s and 24s.
otc	**Hem-Prep** (G & W)	**Suppositories**: 0.25% phenylephrine HCl, 11% zinc oxide	In 12s.
otc	**Tronolane** (Ross)	**Suppositories**: 11% zinc oxide and 95% hard fat	In 10s and 20s.
otc	**Hemorid For Women** (Thompson Medical)	**Lotion**: Mineral oil, petrolatum, glycerin, parabens, diazolidinyl urea, cetyl alcohol	In 118 ml.
		Cream: 30% white petrolatum, 20% mineral oil, 1% pramoxine HCl, 0.25% phenylephrine HCl, aloe vera gel, parabens, cetyl and stearyl alcohols	In 28.3 g.
		Suppositories: 11% zinc oxide, 0.25% phenylephrine HCl, 88.25% hard fat, aloe vera	In 12s.

ADAPALENE

Actions:

Pharmacology: Adapalene is a retinoid-like compound. It is a modulator of cellular differentiation, keratinization and inflammatory processes, all of which represent important features in the pathology of acne vulgaris.

Adapalene binds to specific retinoic acid nuclear receptors but does not bind to the cytosolic receptor protein. Although the exact mode of action of adapalene is unknown, it is suggested that topical adapalene may normalize the differentiation of follicular epithelial cells resulting in decreased microcomedone formation.

Pharmacokinetics:

Absorption – Absorption of adapalene through human skin is low. Only trace amounts (< 0.25 ng/ml) of parent substance has been found in the plasma of acne patients following chronic topical application of adapalene.

Excretion – Excretion appears to be primarily by the biliary route.

Indications:

Acne vulgaris: Topical treatment of acne vulgaris.

Contraindications:

Hypersensitivity to adapalene or any of the components in the vehicle gel.

Warnings:

Sunburn: Advise patients with sunburn not to use the product until fully recovered.

Minimize exposure to sunlight, including sunlamps, during the use of adapalene. Warn patients who normally experience high levels of sun exposure and those with inherent sensitivity to sun, to exercise caution. Use of sunscreen products and protective clothing over treated areas is recommended when exposures cannot be avoided. Weather extremes, such as wind or cold, also may be irritating to patients under treatment with adapalene.

Hypersensitivity: Discontinue use of adapalene if hypersensitivity to any of the ingredients is noted.

Pregnancy: Category C. No teratogenic effects were seen in rats at oral doses of adapalene 0.15 to 5 mg/kg/day topically. There are no adequate and well controlled studies in pregnant women. Use adapalene during pregnancy only if the potential benefit justifies the potential risk to the fetus.

Lactation: It is not known whether this drug is excreted in breast milk. Exercise caution when administering adapalene to a nursing mother.

Children: Safety and effectiveness in pediatric patients < 12 years of age have not been established.

Precautions:

Mucous membranes: Avoid contact with the eyes, lips, angles of the nose and other mucous membranes. Do not apply to cuts, abrasions, eczematous skin or sunburned skin.

Local adverse reactions: Certain cutaneous signs and symptoms such as erythema, dryness, scaling, burning or pruritus may occur during treatment. These are most likely to occur during the first 2 to 4 weeks and will usually lessen with continued use of the medication. Depending upon the severity of adverse events, instruct patients to reduce the frequency of application or discontinue use.

Local irritants: As adapalene has the potential to produce local irritation in some patients, concomitant use of other potentially irritating topical products (medicated or abrasive soaps and cleansers; soaps and cosmetics that have a strong drying effect; products with high concentrations of alcohol, astringents, spices or lime) should be approached with caution. Exercise particular caution in using preparations containing sulfur, resorcinol or salicylic acid in combination with adapalene. If these preparations have been used, it is advisable not to start therapy with adapalene until the effects of such preparations in the skin have subsided.

Adverse Reactions:

These adverse reactions are most commonly seen during the first month of therapy and decrease in frequency and severity thereafter. All adverse effects with use of adapalene during clinical trials were reversible upon discontinuation of therapy.

Erythema, scaling, dryness, pruritus, burning (10% to 40%); pruritus or burning immediately after application (20%); skin irritation, stinging sunburn, acne flares (≤ 1%).

ADAPALENE

Overdosage:

Adapalene is intended for cutaneous use only. If the medication is applied excessively, no more rapid or better results will be obtained and marked redness, peeling or discomfort may occur. The acute oral toxicity of adapalene in mice and rats is > 10 ml/kg. Chronic ingestion of the drug may lead to the same side effects as those associated with excessive oral intake of vitamin A.

Administration and Dosage:

Apply once a day to affected areas after washing in the evening before retiring. Apply a thin film of the gel, avoiding eyes, lips and mucous membranes.

During the early weeks of therapy, an apparent exacerbation of acne may occur. This is because of the action of the medication on previously unseen lesions and should not be considered a reason to discontinue therapy. Therapeutic results should be noticed after 8 to 12 weeks of treatment.

Storage/Stability: Store at controlled room temperature 20° to 25°C (68° to 77°F).

Rx	**Differin** (Galderma)	**Gel:** 0.1% adapalene	EDTA, methylparaben. In 15 and 45 g tubes.

TRETINOIN (trans-Retinoic Acid; Vitamin A Acid)

Actions:

Pharmacology: Although the exact mode of action of tretinoin is unknown, current evidence suggests that topical tretinoin decreases cohesiveness of follicular epithelial cells with decreased microcomedone formation. Additionally, tretinoin stimulates mitotic activity and increases turnover of follicular epithelial cells, causing extrusion of the comedones.

Indications:

Acne: Topical treatment of acne vulgaris.

Unlabeled uses: Tretinoin has been used to treat several different forms of skin cancer, and various dermatologic conditions including lamellar ichthyosis, mollusca contagiosa, verrucae plantaris, verrucae planae juvenilis, hyperpigmented lesions in blacks, ichthyosis vulgaris, bullous congenital ichthyosiform and pityriasis rubra pilaris.

Tretinoin appears to enhance the percutaneous absorption of topical minoxidil.

Tretinoin 0.025% to 0.1% appears to significantly improve photoaged skin, especially wrinkles and liver spots. Long-term consequences are unknown.

Contraindications:

Hypersensitivity to any component of the product.

Warnings:

For external use only: Keep tretinoin away from the eyes, mouth, angles of the nose and mucous membranes.

Pregnancy: Category C. Oral tretinoin is teratogenic. There are no adequate and well controlled studies in pregnant women. However, tretinoin does not appear to be teratogenic when used topically. One study showed no increased risk of major congenital disorders associated with topical tretinoin. Use during pregnancy only if the potential benefit justifies the potential risk.

Lactation: It is not known whether this drug is excreted in breast milk. Exercise caution when tretinoin is administered to a nursing mother.

Precautions:

Irritation: Tretinoin may induce severe local erythema and peeling at the application site. If the degree of local irritation warrants, use medication less frequently, discontinue use temporarily or completely. Tretinoin may cause severe irritation to eczematous skin; use with caution in patients with this condition.

Excessive application: Applying medication excessively will not improve the results and may cause redness, peeling or discomfort.

Photosensitivity: Studies in mice suggest that tretinoin may accelerate the tumorigenic potential of ultraviolet radiation. Although the significance to humans is not clear, avoid or minimize exposure to the sun.

It is advisable to "rest" a patient's skin until effects of keratolytic agents subside before beginning tretinoin. Minimize exposure to sunlight and sunlamps, and advise patients with sunburn not to use tretinoin until fully recovered because of heightened susceptibility to sunlight as a result of tretinoin use. Patients who undergo considerable sun exposure due to occupation and those with inherent sun sensitivity should exercise particular caution. Use sunscreen products and wear protective clothing over treated areas. Weather extremes, such as wind and cold, also may irritate treated areas.

Drug Interactions:

Sulfur, resorcinol, benzoyl peroxide or salicylic acid: Cautiously use concomitant topical medications because of possible interactions with tretinoin. Significant skin irritation may result.

Soaps: Cautiously use medicated or abrasive soaps and cleansers, soaps and cosmetics that have a strong drying effect and products with high concentrations of alcohol, astringents, spices or lime because of possible interactions with tretinoin.

Adverse Reactions:

Sensitive skin may become excessively red, edematous, blistered or crusted. If these effects occur, discontinue medication until skin integrity is restored or adjust to a tolerable level. True contact allergy is rare.

Temporary hyperpigmentation or hypopigmentation has been reported with repeated application. Some individuals have a heightened susceptibility to sunlight while under treatment.

All adverse effects have been reversible upon discontinuation.

TRETINOIN (trans-Retinoic Acid; Vitamin A Acid)

Overdosage:

Oral ingestion of tretinoin may lead to the same side effects as those associated with excessive oral intake of vitamin A.

Patient Information:

Patient instructions are available with the product.

Before application, thoroughly cleanse the area to be treated.

Keep away from eyes, mouth, angles of the nose and mucous membranes.

Avoid excessive exposure to sunlight and sunlamps.

Application may cause a transitory feeling of warmth and slight stinging. Redness and peeling may occur with excessive application; if excessive redness or discomfort occurs, decrease or discontinue use temporarily.

Normal use of cosmetics is permissible.

Administration and Dosage:

Apply once a day, before bedtime. Cover the entire affected area lightly. Thoroughly wash hands immediately after applying tretinoin.

Liquid: Apply with fingertip, gauze pad or cotton swab. Do not oversaturate gauze or cotton to the extent that liquid will run into unaffected areas.

Gel: Excessive application results in "pilling" of the gel, which minimizes the likelihood of overapplication by the patient.

Closely monitor alterations of vehicle, drug concentration or dose frequency. During the early weeks of therapy, an apparent exacerbation of inflammatory lesions may occur due to the action of the medication on deep, previously undetected lesions; this is not a reason to discontinue therapy.

Therapeutic results should be seen after 2 to 3 weeks, but may not be optimal until after 6 weeks. Once lesions have responded satisfactorily, maintain therapy with less frequent applications or other dosage forms.

Patients may use cosmetics, but thoroughly cleanse area to be treated before applying medication.

Rx	**Retin-A** (Ortho)	**Cream:** 0.025%	Hydrophilic vehicle. In 20 and 45 g.
		0.05%	Hydrophilic vehicle. In 20 and 45 g.
		0.1%	Hydrophilic vehicle. In 20 and 45 g.
		Gel: 0.025%	With 90% alcohol. In 15 and 45 g.
		0.01%	With 90% alcohol. In 15 and 45 g.
		Liquid: 0.05%	With PEG-400, butylated hydroxytoluene and 55% alcohol. In 28 ml.
Rx	**Retin-A Micro** (Ortho)	**Gel:** 0.1%	With glycerin, propylene glycol, benzyl alcohol. In 20 and 45 g tubes.
🍁	**Vesanoid** (Roche)	**Gelatin capsule:** 10 mg[1]	Oval, red-brown and brown- yellow. In 100s.
🍁	**Vitinoin** (Pharmascience)	**Gel:** 0.025%	In emollient, topical alcoholic vehicle. In 20 g.
		Cream: 0.025%, 0.05%, 0.1%	In emollient, topical vehicle. In 20 g.
🍁	**Retin-A** (McNeil)	**Gel:** 0.01%, 0.025%	In 30 g tubes.
		Cream: 0.01%, 0.025%, 0.05%, 0.1%	Hydrophilic base. In 30 g tubes.

[1] With mannitol, soybean oil and sorbitol.

ISOTRETINOIN (13-cis-Retinoic Acid)

Warning:

Pregnant women or those who may become pregnant must not use isotretinoin. There is an extremely high risk that a deformed infant will result if pregnancy occurs while taking this drug in any amount even for short periods. Potentially, all exposed fetuses can be affected.

Contraindicated in women of childbearing potential unless the patient meets all of the following conditions:

- Has severe disfiguring cystic acne that is recalcitrant to standard therapies
- Is reliable in understanding and carrying out instructions
- Is capable of complying with the mandatory contraceptive measures
- Has received both oral and written warnings of the hazards of taking isotretinoin during pregnancy and the risk of possible contraception failure and has acknowledged her understanding of these warnings in writing
- Has had a negative *serum* pregnancy test within 2 weeks prior to beginning therapy (it is also recommended that pregnancy testing and contraception counseling be repeated on a monthly basis)
- Will begin therapy only on the second or third day of the next normal menstrual period

Major human fetal abnormalities related to use of the drug have included hydrocephalus, microcephaly, external ear abnormalities (micropinna, small or absent external auditory canals), microphthalmia, facial dysmorphia, cleft palate, cardiovascular abnormalities, thymus gland abnormalities, parathyroid hormone deficiency and cerebellar malformation. There is also an increased risk of spontaneous abortion.

Effective contraception must be used for at least 1 month before beginning therapy, during therapy and for 1 month following discontinuation of therapy. It is recommended that two reliable forms of contraception be used simultaneously unless abstinence is the chosen method.

In 47 patients treated chronically with **etretinate**, another retinoid, five had detectable serum drug levels 2.1 to 2.9 years after therapy was discontinued.

Counsel women fully on the serious risk to the fetus if they become pregnant during treatment. If pregnancy occurs, discuss continuing the pregnancy.

Actions:

Pharmacology: Isotretinoin is an isomer of all-trans retinoic acid, a metabolite of retinol (vitamin A). The exact mechanism of action is unknown. Clinical improvement in cystic acne patients is associated with reduction in sebum secretion. This temporary decrease is related to dose and treatment duration; it reflects a reduction in sebaceous gland size and inhibition of sebaceous gland differentiation. Isotretinoin and other retinoids may also prevent abnormal keratinization.

Sebum lipid production and composition is altered during isotretinoin therapy, but returns to pretreatment composition upon discontinuation, even though sebum production may not return to pretreatment levels.

Pharmacokinetics:

Absorption/Distribution – Oral bioavailability from oil-filled capsules is ≈ 23% to 25%. Plasma levels may be better maintained if the drug is taken with meals. After oral administration of 80 mg, peak plasma concentrations of 98 to 535 ng/ml (mean, 256 to 262 ng/ml) were measured at 2.9 to 3.2 hours. The minimum steady-state blood concentration of isotretinoin averaged 160 ng/ml with 40 mg twice daily administration. The drug is 99.9% bound to plasma albumin. Maximum concentrations of 4-oxo-isotretinoin, the major metabolite, were 87 to 399 ng/ml, and were reached in 6 to 20 hours.

Metabolism/Excretion – The major metabolite in blood, 4-oxo-isotretinoin, generally exceeds the concentration of isotretinoin after 6 hours. Terminal elimination half-life of isotretinoin is 10 to 20 hours. Elimination half-life of 4-oxo-isotretinoin ranges from 17 to 50 hours (average, 25 hours). Relatively equal amounts were recovered in the urine and feces with 65% to 83% of the dose recovered.

Indications:

Severe recalcitrant cystic acne: Adverse effects are significant; reserve treatment for patients unresponsive to conventional therapy, including systemic antibiotics. A single course has resulted in complete, prolonged remission in many patients. Patients may continue to improve while not receiving the drug.

ISOTRETINOIN (13-cis-Retinoic Acid)

Unlabeled uses: Isotretinoin has been used in the treatment of keratinization disorders such as keratosis follicularis (Darier-White disease), pityriasis rubra pilaris, lamellar ichthyosis, keratosis palmaris et plantaris, rosacea, psoriasis and other ichthyotic conditions.

Success has been reported in the treatment of cutaneous T-cell lymphoma (mycosis fungoides) and leukoplakia.

In patients who have been treated for squamous-cell carcinoma of the head and neck, high-dose isotretionoin (50 to 100 mg/m^2) appears to be effective in preventing second primary tumors.

Contraindications:

Pregnancy (see boxed Warning); hypersensitivity to parabens (used as preservatives in the formulation).

Warnings:

Pseudotumor cerebri (benign intracranial hypertension) has occurred with isotretinoin. Early signs and symptoms include papilledema, headache, nausea, vomiting and visual disturbances. Screen patients with these symptoms for papilledema; if present, discontinue drug immediately and consult a neurologist. **Minocycline** and **tetracycline** have been associated with pseudotumor cerebri or papilledema in isotretinoin patients.

Corneal opacities have appeared in patients receiving isotretinoin for acne and more frequently in patients on higher dosages for keratinization disorders. If visual difficulties occur, discontinue the drug and perform an ophthalmological examination. Corneal opacities have either completely resolved or were resolving at follow-up 6 to 7 weeks after discontinuation.

Decreased night vision has occurred during therapy. Because the onset in some patients was sudden, advise patients of this potential problem and warn them to be cautious when driving or operating any vehicle at night. Carefully monitor visual problems.

Inflammatory bowel disease (including regional ileitis) has been temporally associated with isotretinoin in patients with no history of intestinal disorders. Discontinue treatment immediately if abdominal pain, rectal bleeding or severe diarrhea occurs.

Hypertriglyceridemia occurs in ≈ 25% of patients; 15% develop a *decrease* in high density lipoproteins (HDL) and ≈ 7% show an *increase* in cholesterol. Alcohol consumption may potentiate serum triglyceride elevations. Obtain baseline values, then perform tests weekly or biweekly until lipid response is established (usually 4 weeks).

These effects are reversible after cessation of therapy. Patients with increased tendency to develop hypertriglyceridemia include those with diabetes mellitus, obesity, increased alcohol intake and a familial history.

Cardiovascular consequences of hypertriglyceridemia are not well understood, but may increase risk status. Serum triglycerides > 800 mg/dl have been associated with acute pancreatitis. Control significant triglyceride elevation. Reduction of weight, dietary fat, alcohol intake and dose may lower serum triglycerides, allowing patients to continue therapy.

An obese male patient with Darier's disease developed elevated triglycerides and subsequent eruptive xanthomas.

Musculoskeletal symptoms (including arthralgia) develop in ≈ 16% of patients. In general, these are mild to moderate and occasionally require discontinuation. They generally clear rapidly after discontinuing isotretinoin and rarely persist.

In clinical trials of keratinization, a high prevalence of skeletal hyperostosis was noted with a mean dose of 2.24 mg/kg/day. Two children showed x–ray findings suggestive of premature closure of the epiphysis. Additionally, skeletal hyperostosis was noted in six of eight patients in a prospective study of keratinization disorders.

Minimal skeletal hyperostosis has been observed by x–ray in prospective studies of cystic acne patients treated with a single course of therapy at recommended doses.

Hepatotoxicity: Several cases of clinical hepatitis are possibly or probably related to isotretinoin therapy. Additionally, mild to moderate elevations of liver enzymes have been seen in ≈ 15% of patients, some of which normalized with dosage reduction or continued administration of the drug. If normalization does not readily occur, or if hepatitis is suspected, stop the drug and further investigate etiology.

Pregnancy: Category X. See boxed Warning.

Lactation: It is not known whether this drug is excreted in breast milk. Because of the potential for adverse effects, do not give to a nursing mother.

ISOTRETINOIN (13-cis-Retinoic Acid)

Children: Safety and efficacy have not been established.

One study showed x-ray findings suggestive of premature closure of the epiphyses in two children; another study suggested potential benefits in children 2 to 76 months of age with juvenile chronic myelogenous leukemia.

Precautions:

Healing response: As may be seen with healing cystic acne lesions, an occasional exaggerated healing response, manifested by exuberant granulation with crusting, has occurred.

Bleeding: Isotretinoin may increase fibrinolysis in patients with pre-existing bleeding disorders; tissue plasminogen activator production may also be stimulated.

Exacerbation of acne (transient) has occurred, generally during initial therapy period.

Contact lens tolerance may decrease.

Diabetes: Certain patients have experienced problems in the control of their blood sugar. In addition, new cases of diabetes have been diagnosed during therapy, although no causal relationship has been established.

Blood donation: Due to isotretinoin's teratogenic potential, patients receiving the drug should not donate blood for transfusion for 30 days after discontinuing therapy.

Photosensitivity: Photosensitization (photoallergy or phototoxicity) may occur; caution patients to take protective measures (eg, sunscreens, protective clothing) against exposure to ultraviolet light or sunlight until tolerance is determined.

Drug Interactions:

Vitamin A: To avoid additive toxic effects, do not take concomitantly with isotretinoin.

Tetracycline and minocycline have been associated with pseudotumor cerebri or papilledema in isotretinoin patients.

Carbamazepine: Coadministration has resulted in reduced carbamazepine plasma levels.

Drug/Food interactions: When taken with food or milk, the absorption of isotretinoin is increased.

Adverse Reactions:

Most adverse reactions are reversible upon discontinuation; however, some have persisted after cessation of therapy. Many are similar to those described in patients taking high doses of vitamin A.

CNS: Fatigue, headache (5%); pseudotumor cerebri, including headache, visual disturbances and papilledema. Depression has occurred and has subsided with discontinuation of therapy and recurred upon reinstitution.

Dermatologic: Cheilitis, usually dose-related (> 90%); dry skin, pruritus, skin fragility (≤ 80%); facial skin desquamation, drying of mucous membranes (30%); petechiae (25%); nail brittleness (10%); rash (including erythema, seborrhea and eczema), thinning of hair that has rarely persisted (< 10%); peeling of palms and soles, skin infections, photosensitivity (5%); erythema nodosum, paronychia, hypo- or hyperpigmentation, urticaria, hirsutism, hair problems other than thinning, nail dystrophy (< 1%); exaggerated healing response manifested by exuberant granulation tissue with crusting; pyogenic granuloma; bruising.

GI: Dry mouth (≤ 80%); nausea, vomiting, abdominal pain (20%); nonspecific GI symptoms (5%); anorexia (4%); inflammatory bowel disease including regional enteritis (see Warnings), weight loss, bleeding and inflammation of the gums (< 1%).

GU: White cells in urine (10% to 20%); proteinuria, microscopic or gross hematuria (< 10%); nonspecific urogenital findings (5%); abnormal menses (< 1%).

Musculoskeletal: Mild to moderate musculoskeletal symptoms which occasionally require drug discontinuation and rarely persist after discontinuation (16%); arthralgia, bone, joint and muscle pain and stiffness (16% to 17%); skeletal hyperostosis. (See Warnings.)

Ophthalmic: Conjunctivitis (40%); optic neuritis, photophobia, eyelid inflammation (< 1%); corneal opacities (see Warnings); cataracts; visual disturbances. Dry eyes and decreased night vision have occurred and, in rare instances, have persisted.

Miscellaneous: Epistaxis, dry nose (≤ 80%); transient chest pain (rarely persists after discontinuation); vasculitis (including Wegener's granulomatosis); flushing, anemia, palpitation, tachycardia, lymphadenopathy, disseminated herpes simplex, edema, respiratory infections occurred in < 1% and may bear no relationship to therapy.

Lab test abnormalities: Elevated sedimentation rate (40%); changes in serum lipids such as reversible dose-related triglyceride elevation (25%; ≈ 4% to 11% showed triglyceride elevation > 500 mg/dl); reversible mild to moderate decrease in HDL (16%);

ISOTRETINOIN (13-cis-Retinoic Acid)

decreased red blood cell parameters and white blood cell counts, elevated platelet counts, increased alkaline phosphatase, AST, ALT, GGTP and LDH (10% to 20%); increased fasting blood sugar, hyperuricemia, thrombocytopenia, elevated CPK levels in patients who undergo vigorous physical activity (< 10%); reversible minimal elevation of cholesterol (7%).

Overdosage:

Overdosage has been associated with transient headache, vomiting, facial flushing, cheilosis, abdominal pain, headache, dizziness and ataxia. All symptoms quickly resolved without apparent residual effects.

Patient Information:

Patient information leaflet available with product.

Prior to use, have patients complete a consent form included with package insert.

Take with meals. Do not take vitamin supplements containing vitamin A. Avoid alcohol consumption.

Women of childbearing potential should practice contraception during therapy and for 1 month before and after therapy. A pregnancy test 2 weeks prior to starting therapy is advised. Notify physician immediately if pregnancy is suspected.

A transient exacerbation of acne may occur during the initial period of therapy.

May cause photosensitivity; avoid prolonged exposure to sunlight or sunlamps.

Report visual disturbances, abdominal pain, rectal bleeding, severe diarrhea, difficulty in controlling blood sugar and decreased tolerance to contact lens wear to physician immediately.

Do not donate blood for transfusion for 30 days after stopping therapy.

Administration and Dosage:

Individualize dosage. Adjust the dose according to side effects and disease response.

Recommended course of therapy: Initial dose is 0.5 to 1 mg/kg/day (range, 0.5 to 2 mg/kg/day) divided into 2 doses, for 15 to 20 weeks. Patients whose disease is very severe or is primarily manifest on the body may require up to the maximum recommended dose, 2 mg/kg/day. If the total cyst count decreases by > 70% prior to completing 15 to 20 weeks of treatment, the drug may be discontinued. After ≥ 2 months off therapy, and if warranted by persistent or recurring severe cystic acne, a second course of therapy may be initiated.

In studies comparing 0.1, 0.5 and 1 mg/kg/day, all doses provided initial clearing of disease, but there was a greater need for retreatment with the lower doses.

Doses as low as 0.05 mg/kg/day have been effective with minimal toxicity; however, relapses were more frequent.

Dosing Isotretinoin by Body Weight

Body weight		Total mg/day		
kg	lbs	0.5 mg/kg	1 mg/kg	2 mg/kg
40	88	20	40	80
50	110	25	50	100
60	132	30	60	120
70	154	35	70	140
80	176	40	80	160
90	198	45	90	180
100	220	50	100	200

Rx	**Accutane** (Roche)	**Capsules:**[1] 10 mg	(Accutane 10 Roche). Light pink. In UD 100s.
		20 mg	(Accutane 20 Roche). Maroon. In UD 100s.
		40 mg	(Accutane 40 Roche). Yellow. In UD 100s.
	Accutane (Roche)	**Gelatin Capsule:** 10 mg[2]	(Accutane 10 Roche). Light pink. Opaque, oval. In blister pack 30s.
		40 mg[2]	(Accutane 40 Roche). Yellow. Opaque, oval. In blister pack 30s.

[1] Capsule contains suspension of drug in soybean oil; also contains EDTA, glycerin and parabens.

[2] With glycerin, methyl- and propylparaben, palm oil and soybean oil.

AZELAIC ACID

Actions:

Pharmacology: The exact mechanism of action of azelaic acid is not known. In vitro, azelaic acid possesses anitmicrobial activity against *Propionibacterium acnes* and *Staphylococcus epidermidis*. The antimicrobial action may be attributable to inhibition of microbial cellular protein synthesis. A normalization of keratinization leading to an anticomedonal effect of azelaic acid may also contribute to its clinical activity. Evaluation of skin biopsies from human subjects treated with azelaic acid demonstrated a reduction in the thickness of the stratum corneum, a reduction in number and size of keratohyalin granules and a reduction in the amount and distribution of filaggrin (a protein component of kertohyalin) in epidermal layers. This is suggestive of the ability to decrease micromedo formation.

Pharmacokinetics: Following a single application to human skin in vitro, azelaic acid penetrates into the stratum corneum (≈ 3% to 5% of the applied dose) and other viable skin layers (up to 10% of the dose is found in the epidermis and dermis). Negligible cutaneous metabolism occurs after topical application. Approximately 4% of the topically applied azelaic acid is systemically absorbed. Azelaic acid is mainly excreted unchanged in the urine but undergoes some β-oxidation to shorter chain dicarboxylic acids. The observed half-lives in healthy subjects are ≈ 45 minutes after oral dosing and 12 hours after topical dosing, indicating percutaneous absorption rate-limited kinetics.

Azelaic acid is a dietary constituent (whole grain cereals and animal products), and can be formed endogenously from longer-chain dicarboxylic acids, metabolism of oleic acid and co-oxidation of monocarboxylic acids. Endogenous plasma concentration (20 to 80 ng/ml) and daily urinary excretion (4 to 28 mg) of azelaic acid are highly dependent on dietary intake. After topical treatment, plasma concentration and urinary excretion are not significantly different from baseline levels.

Indications:

Acne vulgaris: Topical treatment of mild to moderate inflammatory acne vulgaris.

Contraindications:

Hypersensitivity to any component of the product.

Warnings:

For external dermatologic use only: Not for ophthalmic use.

Hypopigmentation: There have been isolated reports of hypopigmentation after use of azelaic acid. Because azelaic acid has not been well studied in patients with dark complexions, monitor these patients for early signs of hypopigmentation.

Pregnancy: Category B. Embryotoxic effects were observed in rats receiving 2500 mg/kg/day of azelaic acid. Similar effects were observed in rabbits given 150 to 500 mg/kg/day and in monkeys given 500 mg/kg/day. The doses at which these effects were noted were all within toxic dose ranges for the dams. No teratogenic effects were observed. There are no adequate and well controlled studies in pregnant women. Use during pregnancy only if clearly needed.

Lactation: In vitro, at an azelaci acid concentration of 25 mcg/ml, the milk/plasma distribution coefficient was 0.7 and the milk/buffer distribution was 1, indicating that passage of drug into breast milk may occur. Because < 4% of a topically applied dose is systemically absorbed, the uptake of azelaic acid into breast milk is not expected to cause a significant change from baseline azelaic acid leves in the milk. However, exercise caution when administering to a nursing mother.

Children: Safety and efficacy in children < 12 years of age have not been established.

Precautions:

Sensitivity/Irritation: If sensitivity or severe irritation develops, discontinue treatment and institute appropriate therapy.

Adverse Reactions:

In clinical trials, adverse reactions were generally mild and transient and included: Pruritus, burning, stinging, tingling (1% to 5%); erythema, dryness, rash, peeling, irrritation, dermatitis, contact dermatitis (< 1%); worsening of asthma, vitiligo depigmentation, small depigmented spots, hypertrichosis, reddening (signs of keratosis pilaris), exacerbation of recurrent herpes labialis (rare); potential for allergic reactions.

Patient Information:

Use for the full prescribed treatment period.

Avoid the use of occlusive dressings or wrappings.

Keep away from the mouth, eyes and other mucous membranes. If it does come in contact with the eyes, patients should wash their eyes with large amounts of water and consult a physician if eye irritation persists.

AZELAIC ACID

If patients have dark complexions, they should report abnormal changes in skin color to their physician (see Warnings).

Due in part to the low pH of azelaic acid, temporary skin irritation (pruritus, burning or stinging) may occur when azelaic acid is applied to broken or inflamed skin, usually at the start of treatment. However, this irritation commonly subsides if treatment is continued. If it continues, apply only once a day, or stop the treatment until these effects have subsided. If troublesome irritation persists, discontinue use and consult the physician (see Adverse Reactions).

Administration and Dosage:

After the skin is thoroughly washed and patted dry, gently but thoroughly massage a thin film of azelaic acid cream in to the affected areas twice daily, in the morning and evening. Wash the hands following application. The duration of use of azelaic acid cream can vary from person to person and depends on the severity of the acne. In the majority of patients with inflammatory lesions, improvement of the condition occurs within 4 weeks.

Storage/Stability: Protect from freezing. Store between 15° to 30°C (59° to 86°F).

Rx	**Azelex** (Allergan Herbert)	**Cream:** 20%	With glycerin, cetearyl alcohol and benzoic acid. In 30 g.

BENZOYL PEROXIDE

Actions:

Pharmacology: Effectiveness of benzoyl peroxide is primarily attributable to its antibacterial activity, especially against *Propionibacterium acnes,* the predominant organism in sebaceous follicles and comedones. This activity is presumably due to the release of active or free-radical oxygen capable of oxidizing bacterial proteins. Resolution of the acne (ie, reduction in comedones and acne lesions) usually coincides with reduction in the levels of *P acnes* and of lipids and free fatty acids in the follicle. This is aided by a drying action, removal of excess sebum, mild desquamation (drying and peeling) and sebostatic effects.

Pharmacokinetics: Benzoyl peroxide is absorbed by the skin, where it is metabolized to benzoic acid and then excreted as benzoate in the urine.

Indications:

Acne: Treatment of mild to moderate acne vulgaris and oily skin.

May be used in more severe cases as an adjunct in therapeutic regimens including benzoyl peroxide gels, antibiotics, retinoic acid products and sulfur/salicylic acid-containing preparations. Improvement of the treated condition depends on degree and type of acne, frequency of product use and nature of other therapies.

Contraindications:

Hypersensitivity to benzoyl peroxide. Cross-sensitivity may occur with benzoic acid derivatives (see Precautions).

Warnings:

Carcinogenesis: In August 1991, the FDA downgraded benzoyl peroxide from Category I (safe and effective) to Category III (data insufficient to permit classification) in the tentative final monograph for *otc* topical antiacne drugs based on reports that the drug was a tumor promoter in rodents. There is no evidence that the drug is carcinogenic in humans. It will remain on the market while additional tests are conducted in animals.

Pregnancy: Category C. It is not known whether benzoyl peroxide can cause fetal harm when administered to a pregnant woman or can affect reproductive capacity. However, topical application is generally considered safe for use in pregnancy. Use in pregnant women only if clearly needed.

Lactation: It is not known whether this drug is excreted in breast milk. Administer with caution to nursing mothers.

Children: Safety and efficacy in children < 12 years of age have not been established.

Precautions:

External use only. Avoid contact with eyelids, lips, mucous membranes and highly inflamed or damaged skin. If accidental contact occurs, rinse with water.

Irritation: If severe irritation develops, discontinue use and institute appropriate therapy. After the reaction clears, treatment may often be resumed with less frequent application.

Bleaching effect: Benzoyl peroxide is an oxidizing agent; it may bleach hair and colored fabric.

BENZOYL PEROXIDE

Cross-sensitization with benzoic acid derivatives (eg, cinnamon and certain topical anesthetics) may occur.

Sulfite sensitivity: Some of these products contain sulfites, which may cause allergic-type reactions including anaphylactic symptoms and life-threatening/less severe asthmatic episodes in susceptible persons. The overall prevalence in the general population is unknown and probably low. It is seen more frequently in asthmatic persons.

Drug Interactions:

Tretinoin: Concomitant use may cause significant skin irritation.

Adverse Reactions:

Excessive drying, manifested by marked peeling, erythema and possible edema (≈ 4%); allergic contact sensitization/dermatitis (1% to 5%).

Overdosage:

Symptoms: Excessive scaling, erythema or edema.

Treatment: Discontinue use. If reaction is due to excessive use and not allergy, cautiously reinstate at reduced dosage after signs and symptoms subside. To hasten resolution of adverse effects, use emollients, cool compresses or topical corticosteroids.

Patient Information:

Keep away from eyes, mouth, inside of nose and mucous membranes. If contact occurs, rinse with water.

May cause transitory feeling of warmth or slight stinging. Expect dryness and peeling; if excessive redness or discomfort occurs, decrease or discontinue use temporarily. If excessive irritation develops, discontinue use and contact a physician.

Avoid other sources of skin irritation (eg, sunlight, sun lamps, other topical acne medications) unless directed by a physician.

Avoid contact with hair or colored fabric; bleaching may occur.

Use with PABA-containing sunscreens may cause transient skin discoloration.

Normal use of water-based cosmetics is permissible.

Administration and Dosage:

Cleansers: Wash once or twice daily. Wet skin areas to be treated prior to administration. Rinse thoroughly and pat dry. Control amount of drying or peeling by modifying dose frequency or concentration.

Other doseforms: Apply once daily; gradually increase to two or three times daily if needed. After cleansing skin, smooth small amount over affected area. If bothersome dryness or peeling occurs, reduce dosage. If excessive stinging or burning occurs after any single application, remove with mild soap and water; resume use the next day.

Rx	**Benzac AC Wash 2½** (Galderma)	**Liquid**: 2.5%	Glycerin. In 240 ml.
Rx	**Benzac AC Wash 5** (Galderma)	**Liquid**: 5%	Glycerin. In 240 ml.
Rx	**Benzac W Wash 5** (Galderma)		In 120 and 240 ml.
Rx	**Benzoyl Peroxide 5% Wash** (Glades)		Cetyl alcohol. In 120, 150 and 240 ml.
Rx	**Desquam-X 5 Wash** (Westwood-Squibb)		EDTA. In 150 ml.
otc	**Dryox Wash 5** (C & M)		In 240 ml.

BENZOYL PEROXIDE

Rx	**Benzac AC Wash 10** (Galderma)	**Liquid:** 10%	Glycerin. In 240 ml.
Rx	**Benzac W Wash 10** (Galderma)		In 240 ml.
Rx	**Benzoyl Peroxide 10% Wash** (Glades)		Cetyl alcohol. In 150 and 240 ml.
Rx	**Desquam-X 10 Wash** (Westwood-Squibb)		EDTA. In 150 ml.
otc	**Dryox Wash 10** (C & M)		In 240 ml.
otc	**Fostex 10% Wash** (Bristol-Myers)		EDTA. In 150 ml.
otc	**Oxy 10 Wash** (SK Beecham)		Parabens, diazolidinyl urea. In 120 ml.
otc	**PanOxyl** (Stiefel)	**Bar:** 5%	Cetostearyl alcohol, EDTA, glycerin, castor oil, mineral oil. In 113 g.
otc	**Fostex** (Bristol-Myers)	**Bar:** 10%	EDTA, urea. In 106 g.
otc	**PanOxyl** (Stiefel)		Cetostearyl alcohol, castor oil, mineral oil. Soap free. In 113 g.
otc	**Neutrogena Acne Mask** (Neutrogena)	**Mask:** 5%	SD alcohol 40, glycerin, titanium dioxide. In 60 g.
otc	**Benzoyl Peroxide** (Various, eg, IDE, Moore, Rugby)	**Lotion:** 5%	In 30 ml.
otc	**Acne 5** (Various, eg, Goldline)		In 30 ml.
otc	**Benoxyl 5** (Stiefel)		Parabens. Greaseless. In 30 and 60 ml.
otc	**Vanoxide** (Dermik)		35% benzoyl peroxide, 64% Ca phosphate, 1% silica (before mixing). Cetyl alcohol, EDTA, parabens, mineral oil, lanolin alcohol. Dye free. Vanishing. In 25 and 50 ml.
otc	**Oxy 5 Tinted** (SmithKline-Beecham)		Cetyl alcohol, probpylene glycol, parabens. In 30 ml.
otc	**Loroxide** (Dermik)	**Lotion:** 5.5%	35% benzoyl peroxide, 64% Ca phosphate, 1% silica (before mixing). Cetyl alcohol, EDTA, parabens, mineral oil, lanolin alcohol. Tinted. In 25 ml.
otc	**Benzoyl Peroxide** (Various, eg, IDE, Moore, Rugby)	**Lotion:** 10%	In 30 ml.
otc	**Acne-10** (Various, eg, Goldline, Major)		In 30 ml.
otc	**Benoxyl 10** (Stiefel)		Parabens. Greaseless. In 30 and 60 ml.
otc	**BlemErase** (Young)		Parabens. In 12 ml with dispensing tip.
otc	**Clearasil Maximum Strength** (P & G)		Cetyl alcohol, parabens. Vanishing. In 29 ml.
Rx	**Benzashave** (Medicis)	**Cream:** 5%	Mineral oil, aloe vera, parabens. In 113.4 g.
otc	**Exact** (Premier)		Cetyl alcohol, stearyl alcohol, parabens. Tinted or vanishing. In 18 g.

BENZOYL PEROXIDE

otc	**Ambi 10** (Kiwi Brands)	**Cream:** 10%	Parabens. In 28.3 g.
Rx	**Benzashave** (Medicis)		Mineral oil, aloe vera, parabens. In 113.4 g.
otc	**Clearasil Maximum Strength** (P & G)		Parabens. Tinted or vanishing In 18 and 28 g.
Rx	**Benzac AC 2½** (Galderma)	**Gel:** 2.5%	Water base. Glycerin, EDTA. In 60 and 90 g.
otc	**Clear By Design** (SK Beecham)		Greaseless, invisible base. EDTA. In 45 g.
otc	**Dermoxyl** (ICN)		In 30 g.
Rx	**Desquam-E** (Westwood-Squibb)		Water base. EDTA. In 42.5 g.
otc	**Dryox 2.5** (C & M Pharm.)		Alcohol-free. Methylparaben. In 30 and 60 g.
otc	**Advanced Formula Oxy Sensitive** (SK Beecham)		Vanishing. Diazolidinyl urea, EDTA. In 30 g.
Rx	**PanOxyl AQ 2½** (Stiefel)		EDTA, methylparaben. In 57 and 113 g.
Rx	**Brevoxyl** (Stiefel)	**Gel:** 4%	Cetyl alcohol, stearyl alcohol. In 42.5 and 90 g.
Rx[1]	**Benzoyl Peroxide** (Various, eg, Bausch & Lomb, Glades, Moore, Rugby)	**Gel:** 5%	In 45 g.
Rx	**Benzac AC 5** (Galderma)		EDTA. In 60 and 90 g.
Rx	**Benzac 5** (Galderma)		12% alcohol. In 60 g.
Rx	**Benzac W 5** (Galderma)		EDTA. In 60 and 90 g.
Rx	**5-Benzagel** (Dermik)		14% alcohol. In 42.5 and 85 g.
Rx	**Del Aqua-5** (Del-Ray)		6% laureth-4. In 42.5 g.
Rx	**Desquam-E 5** (Westwood-Squibb)		Water base. EDTA. In 42.5 g.
Rx	**Desquam-X 5** (Westwood-Squibb)		Water base. EDTA. In 42.5 and 85 g.
otc	**Perfectoderm** (Treblu Labs)		Water base. EDTA. In 45 g.
otc	**Dryox 5** (C & M)		Alcohol-free. Methylparaben. In 30 and 60 g.
Rx	**PanOxyl 5** (Stiefel)		20% alcohol. In 56.7 and 113.4 g.
Rx	**PanOxyl AQ 5** (Stiefel)		Methylparaben, EDTA. In 56.7 and 113.4 g.
Rx	**Peroxin A 5** (Dermal)		EDTA. In 45 g.
Rx	**Persa-Gel** (Ortho Derm)		In 45 and 90 g.
Rx	**Persa-Gel W 5%** (Ortho Derm)		Water base. In 45 and 90 g.
Rx	**Triaz** (Medicus Dermatologics)	**Gel:** 6%	EDTA. IN 42.5 g.

BENZOYL PEROXIDE

Rx[1]	**Benzoyl Peroxide** (Various, eg, Bausch & Lomb, Glades, Moore, Rugby)	**Gel**: 10%	In 45 and 90 g.
Rx	**Benzac AC 10** (Galderma)		Water base. Glycerin, EDTA. In 60 and 90 g.
Rx	**Benzac 10** (Galderma)		12% alcohol. In 60 g.
Rx	**Benzac W 10** (Galderma)		Water base. In 60 and 90 g.
Rx	**Benzox-10** (Treblu Labs)		12% alcohol, EDTA. In 45 and 90 g.
Rx	**10-Benzagel** (Dermik)		14% alcohol, 6% laureth 4. In 42.5 and 85 g.
Rx	**Del Aqua-10** (Del-Ray)		6% laureth-4, EDTA. In 42.5 g.
Rx	**Desquam-E 10** (Westwood-Squibb)		Water base. EDTA. In 42.5 g.
Rx	**Desquam-X 10** (Westwood-Squibb)		Water base. EDTA. In 42.5 and 85 g.
otc	**Dryox 10** (C & M Pharm.)		Alcohol-free. Methylparaben. In 30 and 60 g.
otc	**Fostex 10% BPO** (Westwood-Squibb)		EDTA. In 42.5 g.
Rx	**Peroxin A 10** (Dermal)		EDTA. In 45 g.
Rx	**PanOxyl 10** (Stiefel)		20% alcohol. In 56.7 and 113.4 g.
Rx	**PanOxyl AQ 10** (Stiefel)		Methylparaben, EDTA. In 56.7 and 113.4 g.
Rx	**Persa-Gel** (Ortho Derm)		In 45 and 90 g.
Rx	**Persa-Gel W 10%** (Ortho Derm)		Water base. In 45 and 90 g.
otc	**Oxy 10 Maximum Strength Advanced Formula** (SK Beecham)		EDTA. Vanishing and tinted. In 30 g.
Rx	**Triaz** (Medicus Dermatologics)		EDTA. In 42.5 g
otc	**Dryox 20** (C & M Pharm.)	**Gel: 20%**	Alcohol-free. Methylparaben. In 30 and 60 g.
Rx	**Triaz** (Medicus Dermatologics)	**Cleanser**: 10%	Menthol. In 85.1 g.

[1] Product available *otc* or *Rx*, depending on product labeling.

BENZOYL PEROXIDE COMBINATIONS

Rx	**Sulfoxyl Regular** (Stiefel)	**Lotion**: 5% benzoyl peroxide, 2% sulfur	In 60 ml.
Rx	**Sulfoxyl Strong** (Stiefel)	**Lotion**: 10% benzoyl peroxide, 5% sulfur	In 60 ml.
otc	**Dryox 10S 5** (C & M Pharm.)	**Gel**: 10% benzoyl peroxide, 5% sulfur, methylparaben	Alcohol-free. In 30 and 60 g.
otc	**Dryox 20S 10** (C & M Pharm.)	**Gel**: 20% benzoyl peroxide, 10% sulfur, methylparaben	Alcohol-free. In 30 and 60 g.

SULFUR PREPARATIONS

Actions:

Pharmacology: Sulfur, a keratolytic, provides peeling and drying actions. Although it may help to resolve comedones, it may also promote the development of new ones by increasing horny cell adhesion.

Indications:

Acne: An aid in the treatment of mild acne and oily skin.

Precautions:

For external use only. Avoid contact with eyes. Certain individuals may be sensitive to one or more components. If undue skin irritation develops or increases, discontinue use and consult physician.

Concomitant treatment: Using other topical acne medications at the same time or immediately following sulfur products may increase dryness or irritation of the skin. If this occurs, use only one medication unless otherwise directed.

Patient Information:

Keep away from the eyes.

May cause irritation of the skin; discontinue use and notify physician if this occurs.

Administration and Dosage:

Apply a thin layer. Use 1 to 3 times daily. For best results, wash skin thoroughly with a mild cleanser prior to application.

otc	**Sulpho-Lac Acne Medication** (Doak)	**Cream:** 5% sulfur	27% zinc sulfate, 53% Vleminckx's solution base. Greaseless. In 28.35 and 50 g.
otc	**Acne Lotion 10** (C & M)	**Lotion:** 10% colloidal sulfur	22.5% isopropyl alcohol. Tinted. Aqueous. In 60 ml.
otc	**Liquimat** (Galderma)	**Lotion:** 4% sulfur	22% SD alcohol 40, cetyl alcohol. Assorted tints. In 45 ml.
otc	**Sulpho-Lac** (Doak)	**Soap:** 5% sulfur	In a coconut and tallow oil soap base. In 85 g.
otc	**Sulmasque** (C & M)	**Mask:** 6.4% sulfur	With 15% isopropyl alcohol, methylparaben. In 150 g.

METRONIDAZOLE

For information on the systemic and vaginal use of metronidazole, refer to the individual monographs in the Anti-infectives chapter.

Actions:

Pharmacology: Metronidazole is classified therapeutically as an antiprotozoal and antibacterial agent. The mechanisms by which topical metronidazole acts in reducing inflammatory lesions of acne rosacea are unknown, but may include an antibacterial or an anti-inflammatory effect.

Pharmacokinetics: Bioavailability studies on administration of 1 g topical metronidazole (≈ 7.5 mg metronidazole) to the faces of 10 rosacea patients showed a maximum serum concentration of 66 ng/ml. This is ≈ 100 times less than concentrations afforded by a single 250 mg oral tablet. Three patients had no detectable serum concentrations of metronidazole. The mean dose of gel applied during clinical studies was 600 mg (≈ 4.5 mg metronidazole) per application. Therefore, under normal usage levels, the formulation affords minimal serum concentrations.

Indications:

Rosacea: Topical application in the treatment of inflammatory papules, pustules and erythema of rosacea.

Unlabeled uses: Topical metronidazole has been used for the treatment of infected decubitus ulcers. However, a 1% solution prepared from the oral tablets, not the gel formulation, was used.

Contraindications:

History of hypersensitivity to metronidazole, parabens or other ingredients.

Warnings:

Pregnancy: Category B. There has been no experience to date with the use of topical metronidazole in pregnant patients. Metronidazole crosses the placental barrier and enters the fetal circulation rapidly. Since oral metronidazole is a carcinogen in some rodents, use during pregnancy only if clearly needed.

Lactation: After oral administration, metronidazole is excreted in breast milk in concentrations similar to those in plasma. Even though metronidazole blood levels are significantly lower than those achieved after oral metronidazole, discontinue nursing or the drug, taking into account the importance of the drug to the mother.

METRONIDAZOLE

Children: Safety and efficacy in children have not been established.

Precautions:

For external use only: Tearing of the eyes has occurred; avoid eye contact. If a reaction suggesting local irritation occurs, direct patients to use the medication less frequently, discontinue use temporarily or discontinue use until further instructions.

Blood dyscrasia: Metronidazole is a nitroimidazole; use with care in patients with evidence of, or history of, blood dyscrasia.

Drug Interactions:

Anticoagulants: Drug interactions are less likely with topical administration but should be kept in mind when topical metronidazole is prescribed for patients who are receiving anticoagulant treatment. Oral metronidazole may potentiate the anticoagulant effect of warfarin and coumarin resulting in a prolongation of prothrombin time.

Adverse Reactions:

Because of the minimal absorption of metronidazole and its insignificant plasma concentration after topical administration, the adverse experiences reported with the oral form of the drug have not been reported with topical metronidazole.

Watery (tearing) eyes if the gel is applied too closely to this area, transient redness, mild dryness, burning and skin irritation (≤ 2%).

Overdosage:

The acute oral toxicity of the topical metronidazole formulation was determined to be > 5 g/kg (the highest dose given) in albino rats.

Patient Information:

For external use only. Avoid contact with the eyes.

Administration and Dosage:

Apply and rub in a thin film twice daily, morning and evening, to entire affected areas after washing. Significant therapeutic results should be noticed within 3 weeks. Clinical studies have demonstrated continuing improvement through 9 weeks of therapy.

Cleanse areas to be treated before application of topical metronidazole. Patients may use cosmetics after application of topical metronidazole.

Rx	**MetroGel** (Galderma)	**Gel:** 0.75%	In 28.4 g tube.

TETRACYCLINES, TOPICAL

For information on the systemic and periodontal use of tetracycline, refer to the individual monographs in the Anti-infectives, oral , and Topical, periodontal sections.

Actions:

Pharmacology: These agents deliver the drug to the pilosebaceous apparatus and adjacent tissues.The mechanism of action by which they improve acne is unknown. Systemic tetracycline seems to decrease the amount of free fatty acids present in acne lesions, which may play a role in the case of inflammation. It appears that these drugs possess a localized effect since they are not absorbed through the skin in sufficient quantities to be detected systemically.

Indications:

Acne: Treatment of acne vulgaris.

Contraindications:

Hypersensitivity to any of the tetracyclines or to any component of the products.

Warnings:

Renal/Hepatic function impairment: Significant percutaneous absorption may result from prolonged use. Use with caution in patients with hepatic/renal dysfunction.

Pregnancy: Category B. Safety for use during pregnancy has not been established. Use only when clearly needed and when the potential benefits outweigh the potential hazards to the fetus. Oral tetracycline is not recommended for use during pregnancy (refer to the systemic monograph).

Lactation: It is not known whether topical tetracycline is excreted in breast milk. Exercise caution when giving the drug to a nursing woman.

Children: Safety and efficacy for use in children < 11 years have not been established.

Precautions:

For external use only. Keep out of eyes, nose and mouth.

Formaldehyde allergy: Use meclocycline with caution in patients allergic to formaldehyde.

TETRACYCLINES, TOPICAL

Sulfite sensitivity: Some of these products contain sulfites or sodium formaldehyde sulfoxylate, a sulfite-producing agent, both of which may cause allergic-type reactions including anaphylactic symptoms and life-threatening/less severe asthmatic episodes in susceptible persons. The overall prevalence in the general population is unknown and probably low. It is seen more frequently in asthmatic persons.

Adverse Reactions:

Tetracycline: There is one report of severe dermatitis. About one third of patients may experience a stinging or burning sensation upon application. A slight yellowing of the skin in the areas of application may be noticed. This condition is superficial, and the color can be eliminated by washing. However, *Topicycline* has been formulated to greatly reduce or eliminate this effect. Treated areas of skin may also fluoresce under an ultraviolet light source.

Meclocycline: There is one report of acute contact dermatitis and isolated reports of skin irritation. Temporary follicular staining may occur with excessive application. The cream has demonstrated no photosensitivity or contact allergy potential.

Topical administration results in low serum levels; systemic side effects are unlikely.

Patient Information:

Apply solution generously until skin is thoroughly wet. Avoid eyes, nose and mouth.

Stinging or burning may occur, but will subside in a few minutes.

Yellowing of the skin may occur; this may be removed by washing (tetracycline).

Tetracycline: Normal use of cosmetics is permissible.

Administration and Dosage:

Apply to affected areas twice daily, morning and evening. Less frequent application of cream may be used depending on patient response. Apply solution generously until skin is thoroughly wet. Excessive cream use may cause fabric staining.

TETRACYCLINE HCl

Complete prescribing information begins in the Antibiotics group monograph.

Rx	**Topicycline** (Roberts)	**Topical solution:** 2.2 mg/ml	Sodium bisulfite, 40% ethanol. With powder/diluent for 70 ml.

MECLOCYCLINE SULFOSALICYLATE

For complete prescribing information, refer to the Tetracyclines, Topical group monograph.

Rx	**Meclan** (Ortho Derm)	**Cream:** 1%	Formaldehyde sulfoxylate. In 20 and 45 g.

CLINDAMYCIN, TOPICAL

For information on the systemic and vaginal use of clindamycin, refer to the specific monographs in the Anti-infectivesand Topicals chapters.

Actions:

Pharmacology: Clindamycin demonstrates in vitro activity against isolates of *Propionibacterium acnes* which may account for its usefulness in acne. Free fatty acids on the skin surface decrease from approximately 14% to 2% following application. In vitro, clindamycin inhibits all *P acnes* cultures tested.

Pharmacokinetics: Following multiple topical applications at a concentration equivalent to 10 mg/ml, very low levels (0 to 3 ng/ml) are present in the serum and < 0.2% of the dose is recovered in urine as clindamycin. The mean concentration of activity in comedonal extracts from acne patients was 597 mcg/g (range 0 to 1490).

Indications:

Acne: Treatment of acne vulgaris.

Unlabeled uses: Clindamycin lotion has been used in the treatment of rosacea.

Contraindications:

Hypersensitivity to clindamycin or lincomycin; history of regional enteritis or ulcerative colitis; history of antibiotic-associated colitis.

Warnings:

Colitis: Diarrhea, bloody diarrhea and colitis (including pseudomembranous colitis) have occurred with topical and systemic clindamycin. Symptoms can occur after a few days, weeks or months after therapy initiation, but have also begun up to several weeks after cessation of therapy. Toxin(s) produced by *Clostridium difficile* is one primary cause of antibiotic-associated colitis, which is usually characterized by severe persistent diarrhea, severe abdominal cramps and the passage of blood and mucus. When significant diarrhea occurs, stop the drug. Consider large bowel endoscopy in severe diarrhea.

CLINDAMYCIN, TOPICAL

Treatment – Mild cases of colitis may respond to drug discontinuation. Manage moderate to severe cases promptly with fluid, electrolyte and protein supplementation as indicated. Vancomycin is effective in the treatment of antibiotic-associated pseudomembranous colitis produced by *C difficile* (see individual monograph).

Cholestyramine and colestipol resins bind the toxin in vitro. Systemic steroids and steroid retention enemas may help relieve colitis. Antiperistaltic agents such as opiates and diphenoxylate with atropine may prolong or worsen the condition.

Pregnancy: Category B. There are no adequate and well-controlled studies in pregnant women.Use only when clearly needed and when the potential benefits outweigh the unknown potential hazards to the fetus.

Lactation: It is not known whether topical clindamycin is excreted in breast milk, although oral and parenteral clindamycin appear in breast milk. Because of the potential for serious adverse reactions in nursing infants, discontinue nursing or discontinue the drug, taking into account the importance of the drug to the mother.

Children: Safety and efficacy in children < 12 years old have not been established.

Precautions:

For external use only: Avoid contact with the eyes. Clindamycin topical solution has an alcohol base which will cause burning and irritation of the eye. In case of accidental contact with eyes, abraded skin or mucous membranes, bathe with copious amounts of cool tap water. Use caution when applying medication around the mouth.

Atopic patients: Prescribe with caution in atopic individuals.

Drug Interactions:

Erythromycin: Antagonism has been demonstrated with clindamycin.

Adverse Reactions:

Dermatologic: Dryness (15%); erythema (13%); burning (9%); peeling (8%); oiliness/oily skin (7%); itching (6%).

GI: Diarrhea, bloody diarrhea, abdominal pains and colitis (including pseudomembranous colitis); GI disturbance.

Overdosage:

Topical clindamycin can be absorbed enough to produce systemic effects.

Patient Information:

Notify physician if abdominal pain or diarrhea occurs.

Avoid contact with eyes, abraded skin or mucous membranes; clindamycin may cause burning and irritation.

Administration and Dosage:

Apply a thin film to affected area twice daily; a pledget may also be used. More than one pledget may be used. Use each pledget only once, then discard.

Lotion: Shake well immediately before using.

Pledget: Remove from foil just before use. Discard after single use.

Rx	**Clindamycin Phosphate** (Various, eg, Geneva, Greenstone)	**Gel:** 10 mg (as phosphate)/ml	In 30 g.
Rx	**Cleocin T** (Upjohn)		Methylparaben. In 7.5 and 30 g.
Rx	**Clindamycin Phosphate** (Various, eg, Geneva, Greenstone)	**Lotion:** 10 mg (as phosphate)/ml	In 60 ml.
Rx	**Cleocin T** (Upjohn)		In 60 ml.[1]

CLINDAMYCIN, TOPICAL

Rx	**Cleocin T** (Upjohn)	**Topical Solution**: 10 mg (as phosphate)/ml	In 30 and 60 ml and pledget applicator.[2]
Rx	**Clinda-Derm** (Paddock)		51.5% isopropyl alcohol. In 60 ml.
	Clindamycin Phosphate (Various, eg, Geneva, Greenstone)		In 30 and 60 ml.
Rx	**C/T/S** (Hoechst Marion Roussel)		In 30 and 60 ml with applicator.

[1] With 2.5% cetostearyl alcohol, 2.5% isostearyl alcohol, 0.3% methylparaben.
[2] With 50% isopropyl alcohol.

ERYTHROMYCIN, TOPICAL

For information on the systemic and ophthalmic use of erythromycin, refer to the specific monographs in the Anti-infectives and Topicals chapters.

Actions:

Pharmacology: Erythromycin is a bacteriostatic macrolide antibiotic, but may be bactericidal in high concentrations. Although the mechanism by which topical erythromycin acts in reducing inflammatory lesions of acne vulgaris is unknown, it is presumably due to its antibiotic action.

Indications:

Acne: Topical control of acne vulgaris.

Contraindications:

Hypersensitivity to erythromycin or to any component of these products.

Warnings:

Pregnancy: (Category B: Eryderm 2%, Erygel; Category C: A/T/S, Erymax, T-Stat, Staticin). Safety for use during pregnancy has not been established. Use only when clearly needed and when the potential benefits outweigh potential hazards to the fetus.

Lactation: Erythromycin is excreted in breast milk. Exercise caution when administering to a nursing mother.

Children: Safety and efficacy in children < 12 years of age have not been established.

Precautions:

For external use only. Keep away from eyes, nose, mouth and other mucous membranes.

Superinfection: Use of antibiotics (especially prolonged or repeated therapy) may result in bacterial or fungal overgrowth of nonsusceptible organisms. Such overgrowth may lead to a secondary infection. Take appropriate measures if superinfection occurs.

Drug Interactions:

Topical Erythromycin Drug Interactions			
Precipitant drug	Object drug*		Description
Acne therapy	Erythromycin, topical	⬆	Use concomitant topical acne therapy with caution because a cumulative irritant effect may occur.
Clindamycin	Erythromycin, topical	⬇	Antagonism has occurred between clindamycin and erythromycin.

* ⬆ = Object drug increased. ⬇ = Object drug decreased.

Adverse Reactions:

Erythema; desquamation; burning sensation; eye irritation; tenderness; dryness; pruritus; oily skin; generalized urticarial reaction which required the use of systemic steroids (one case).

Overdosage:

Symptoms: Ingestion may cause nausea and vomiting.

Treatment: Based on amount ingested and time elapsed since ingestion, treatment methods include general supportive measures. Refer to General Management of Acute Overdosage.

Patient Information:

Wash, rinse and dry affected areas before application.

Keep away from the eyes, nose, mouth and other mucous membranes.

Administration and Dosage:

Apply morning and evening to affected areas. Before applying, thoroughly wash with warm water and soap, rinse and pat dry all areas to be treated. Apply with fingertips or applicator. Wash hands after use.

Preparation of gel: The topical gel is supplied in a package containing 20 g benzoyl peroxide gel and a plastic vial containing 0.8 g erythromycin powder. Prior to dispensing, add 3 ml of ethyl alcohol (to the mark) to vial and immediately shake to dissolve erythromycin. Add this solution to gel and stir until homogenous in appearance (1 to 1.5 minutes). Refrigerate.

Storage/Stability – Prior to reconstitution, store at room temperature. After reconstitution, store under refrigeration. Do not freeze. Expiration date is 3 months.

ERYTHROMYCIN, TOPICAL

Rx	**Staticin** (Westwood Squibb)	**Solution:** 1.5%	55% alcohol. In 60 ml with optional applicator.
Rx	**Erythromycin** (Various, eg, Barre-National, Bausch & Lomb, Goldline, Major, Rugby, Schein, URL)	**Solution:** 2%	In 60 ml.
Rx	**Akne-mycin** (Hermal)		68% alcohol. In 60 ml with applicator.
Rx	**A/T/S** (Hoechst Marion Roussel)		66% alcohol. In 60 ml.
Rx	**Del-Mycin** (Del-Ray)		66% ethyl alcohol. In 60 ml with applicator.
Rx	**Erycette** (Ortho)		66% alcohol. In 60 pledgets.
Rx	**Eryderm 2%** (Abbott)		77% alcohol. In 60 ml with applicator.
Rx	**Erymax** (Allergan Herbert)		66% SD alcohol 40-2. In 59 and 118 ml.
Rx	**Erythra-Derm** (Paddock)		66% alcohol. In 60 ml.
Rx	**Theramycin Z** (Medicis)		81% SD alcohol 40B. In 60 ml with applicator.
Rx	**T-Stat** (Westwood Squibb)		71.2% alcohol. In pads (60s) and 60 ml with optional applicator.
Rx	**A/T/S** (Hoechst Marion Roussel)	**Gel:** 2%	92% alcohol. In 30 g.
Rx	**Erygel** (Allergan Herbert)		92% alcohol. In 30 and 60 g and as *Erygel 6* in 5 g (6s).
Rx	**Erythromycin** (Glades)		95% alcohol. In 30 & 60 g.
Rx	**Akne-Mycin** (Hermal)	**Ointment:** 2%	Cetostearyl alcohol, petrolatum, mineral oil. In 25 g.
Rx	**Erythromycin Pledgets** (Glades)	**Pledgets:** 2%	68.5% alcohol. In 60s.

ERYTHROMYCIN TOPICAL COMBINATIONS

Rx	**Benzamycin** (Dermik)	**Gel:** 30 mg erythromycin and 50 mg benzoyl peroxide per g	16% alcohol. In 23.3 g after reconstitution.

Creams, Lotions and Gels

ACNE PRODUCTS, CREAMS, LOTION AND GELS

The following products contain keratolytics and astringents to aid in removing keratin and to dry the skin. Many products also have hydroalcoholic or organic solvent bases to aid in removal of sebum. Individual components include:

ANTIMICROBIAL: Parachlorometaxylenol, sodium thiosulfate and sodium sulfacetamide.

ANTISEPTIC: Benzalkonium Cl, oxyquinoline, methylbenzethonium Cl, ethanol, isopropyl alcohol, phenol, triclosan, thymol, sulfur and acetone.

ASTRINGENTS: Zinc oxide, and calamine.

COUNTERIRRITANT (local anesthetic): Methylsalicylate.

KERATOLYTICS: Salicylic acid, resorcinol and sulfur.

PROTECTIVES and ADSORBANTS: Titanium dioxide and zinc oxide.

Hydrocortisone-containing acne products are listed under Topical Corticosteroid Combinations.

		Sulfur	Salicylic Acid	Resorcinol	Other Content	How Supplied
otc	**Finac Lotion** (C & M Pharm.)		2%		22.5% isopropyl alcohol, propylene glycol, acetone	In 60 ml.
otc	**PROPApH Cleansing Lotion for Normal/Combination Skin**(Del)		0.5%		SD alcohol 40, menthol, EDTA	In 180 ml (lotion) and 45s (pads).
otc	**PROPApH Cleansing Pads** (Del)		0.5%		SD alcohol 40, EDTA, menthol	In 45s.
otc	**PROPApH Cleansing for Oily Skin Lotion**(Del)		0.6%		SD alcohol 40, EDTA, menthol	In 180 ml.
Rx	**Sodium Sulfacetamide 10% and Sulfur 5%** (Glades)	5%			10% sodium sulfacetamide, cetyl alcohol, benzyl alcohol, EDTA	In 30 ml tube and 25 ml.
Rx	**Sulfacet-R Lotion** (Dermik)	5%			10% sodium sulfacetamide, parabens	Tinted. In 25 ml.
Rx	**Novacet Lotion** (Genderm)	5%			10% sodium sulfacetamide, cetyl alcohol, benzyl alcohol, EDTA, sodium thiosulfate	In 30 ml.
otc	**Seale's Lotion Modified** (C & M)	6.4%				In 60 and 480 ml.
otc	**Acno Lotion** (Baker Cummins)	3%				Greaseless. In 120 ml.
otc	**Therac Lotion** (C & M)	10%[2]				In 60 ml.
otc	**Acnotex Lotion** (C & M)	8%		2%	20% isopropyl alcohol	In 60 ml.
otc	**Acnomel Cream** (Menley & James)	8%		2%	11% alcohol	In 28 g.
otc	**Bensulfoid Cream** (ECR)	8%[2]		2%	12% alcohol	In 15 g.
otc	**Medicated Acne Cleanser** (C & M)	4%		2%		In 129 g.
otc	**Sulforcin Lotion** (Galderma)	5%		2%	11.65% SD alcohol 40, methylparaben	In 120 ml.
otc	**Rezamid Lotion** (Summers)	5%		2%	28% alcohol	In 56.7 ml.
otc	**R/S Lotion** (Summers)					In 56.7 ml.

Creams, Lotions and Gels

ACNE PRODUCTS, CREAMS, LOTION AND GELS

		Sulfur	Salicylic Acid	Resorcinol	Other Content	How Supplied
otc	**Clearasil Clearstick Maximum Strength** (Procter & Gamble)		2%		39% alcohol, menthol, EDTA	For regular and sensitive skin. In 35 ml.
otc	**Clearasil Double Clear Maximum Strength Pads** (Procter & Gamble)		2%		40% alcohol, witch hazel distillate, menthol	In 32s.
otc	**Fostex Acne Cleansing Cream** (Westwood)		2%		Stearyl alcohol, EDTA	In 118 g.
otc	**Oxy Night Watch Maximum Strength Lotion** (SK-Beecham)		2%		Cetyl alcohol, EDTA, parabens, stearyl alcohol.	In 60 ml.
otc	**PROPApH Acne Maximum Strength Cream** (Del)		2%		Lanolin alcohol, cetearyl alcohol, EDTA, menthol, stearyl alcohol	In 19.5 g.
otc	**Sal-Clens Acne Cleanser Gel** (C & M Pharm)		2%			In 240 g.
otc	**Sebasorb Lotion** (Summers)		2%		10% attapulgite	In 45 ml.
otc	**Stridex Clear Gel** (Sterling Health)		2%		9.3% SD alcohol	In 30 g.
otc	**Clearasil Clearstick Regular Strength** (Procter & Gamble)		1.25%		39% alcohol, aloe vera gel, menthol, disodium EDTA	In 35 ml.
otc	**Clearasil Double Clear Pads Regular Strength** (Procter & Gamble)		1.25%		40% alcohol, witch hazel distillate, menthol	In 32s.
otc	**Oxy Night Watch Sensitive Skin Lotion** (SK-Beecham)		1%		Cetyl alcohol. EDTA, stearyl alcohol, parabens	In 60 ml.
otc	**RA Lotion** (Medco Lab)			3%	43% alcohol	In 120, 240 and 480 ml.
otc	**Clearasil Adult Care Cream** (P & G)				Sulfur, resorcinol, 10% alcohol, parabens	In 17 g.
otc	**Fostril Lotion** (Westwood-Squibb)				Sulfur, zinc oxide, parabens, EDTA	In 28 ml.
Rx	**Klaron** (Dermik)				10% sodium sulfacetamide. Propylene glycol, polyethylene glycol 400, methylparaben, EDTA.	In 59 ml.
otc	**Neutrogena Drying Gel** (Neutrogena)				Witch hazel, isopropyl alcohol, EDTA, parabens, tartrazine	In 22.5 g.

[1] As precipitated sulfur.
[2] As colloidal sulfur.

Medicated Bar Cleansers

MEDICATED BAR CLEANSERS			
otc	**Clearasil Antibacterial Soap** (Procter & Gamble)	**Bar**: Triclosan	In 92 g.
otc	**Oxy Medicated Soap** (SmithKline Beecham)	**Bar**: 1% triclosan, EDTA	In 97.5 g.
otc	**Stri-Dex Cleansing Bar** (Sterling Health)	**Bar**: 1% triclosan, lanolin alcohol, EDTA	In 105 g.
otc	**Salicylic Acid Cleansing** (Stiefel)	**Bar**: 2% salicylic acid, EDTA	In 113 g.
otc	**Sulfur Soap** (Stiefel)	**Bar**: 10% precipitated sulfur, EDTA	In 116 g.
otc	**Buf-Puf Acne Cleansing** (3M Personal Care)	**Bar**: 2% salicylic acid, vitamin E acetate, EDTA	In 99 g.
otc	**Fostex Acne Medication Cleansing** (Westwood)	**Bar**: 2% salicylic acid, EDTA	In 106 g.
otc	**Salicylic Acid and Sulfur Soap** (Stiefel)	**Bar**: 10% precipitated sulfur, 3% salicylic acid, EDTA	In 116 g.
otc	**SAStid Soap** (Stiefel)	**Bar**: 10% precipitated sulfur, EDTA	In 116 g.
otc	**Aveeno Cleansing for Acne-Prone Skin** (Rydelle)	**Bar**: Salicylic acid, colloidal oatmeal, glycerin and titanium dioxide.	Soap free. In 90 g.

Abrasive Cleansers

ABRASIVE CLEANSERS

otc	**Pernox Lathering Abradant Scrub** (Westwood-Squibb)	**Lotion**: Sulfur, salicylic acid	In 141 g.
otc	**Pernox Scrub for Oily Skin** (Westwood-Squibb)	**Cleanser**: Sulfur, salicylic acid, EDTA	Regular or lemon scent. In 56 and 113 g.
otc	**Brasivol** (Stiefel)	**Cleanser**: Aluminum oxide particles in a surfactant cleansing base.	In fine (153 g), medium (180 g) and rough (195 g) textures.
otc	**Ionax** (Galderma)	**Scrub**: Benzalkonium chloride, SD alcohol 40	Lemon scented. In 60 and 120 g.
otc	**Seba-Nil Cleansing Mask** (Galderma)	**Scrub**: SD alcohol-40, castor oil, methylparaben	In 105 g.
otc	**PROPApH Peel-off Acne Mask** (Del Pharm.)	**Mask**: 2% salicylic acid, polyvinyl alcohol, parabens, SD alcohol 40, vitamin E acetate	In 60 ml.

Liquid Cleansers

LIQUID CLEANSERS

otc	**SalAc Cleanser** (GenDerm)	2% salicylic acid, benzyl alcohol, glyceryl cocoate.	In 177 ml.
otc	**Clearasil Medicated Deep Cleanser** (Procter & Gamble)	0.5% salicylic acid and 42% alcohol, menthol, EDTA, aloe vera gel, hydrogenated castor oil	In 229 ml.
otc	**Clearasil Double Textured Pads** (Procter & Gamble)	**Regular Strength**: 2.0% salicylic acid, 40% alcohol, glycerin, aloe vera gel, disodium EDTA	In 32s and 40s.
		Maximum Strength: 2.0% salicylic acid, 40% alcohol, aloe vera gel, menthol, disodium EDTA	In 32s and 40s.
otc	**Stri-Dex Pads** (Sterling Health)	**Regular Strength**: 0.5% salicylic acid, 28% SD alcohol, citric acid, menthol	In 55s.
		Maximum Strength: 2% salicylic acid, 44% SD alcohol, citric acid, menthol.	In 55s and 90s. Dual textured in 32s.
		Oil Fighting Formula: 2% salicylic acid, citric acid, menthol, 54% SD alcohol	In 55 Super Scrub pads.
		Sensitive Skin: 0.5% salicylic acid, citric acid, aloe vera gel, menthol, 28% SD alcohol	In 55s.
otc	**Oxy Medicated Cleanser and Pads** (SK Beecham)	**Cleanser and Regular Strength Pads**: 0.5% salicylic acid, 40% alcohol, citric acid, menthol, propylene glycol	**Cleanser**: In 120 ml. **Pads**: In 50s and 90s.
		Maximum Strength Pads: 2% salicylic acid, 50% alcohol, citric acid, menthol, propylene glycol	In 50s and 90s.
		Sensitive Skin Pads: 0.5% salicylic acid, 22% alcohol, disodium lauryl sulfosuccinate, menthol, trisodium EDTA	In 50s and 90s.
otc	**Ionax Astringent Cleanser** (Galderma)	Salicylic acid, EDTA, isopropyl alcohol	In 240 ml.
otc	**Drytex Lotion** (C & M)	Salicylic acid, 10% acetone, 40% isopropyl alcohol, tartrazine	In 240 ml.
otc	**Seba-Nil Oily Skin Cleanser** (Galderma)	SD alcohol 40, acetone	In 240 and 473 ml.
otc	**Tyrosum Cleanser** (Summers)	50% isopropanol, 10% acetone, 2% polysorbate 80	**Liquid**: In 120 ml and pt. **Packets**: In 24s and 50s.
otc	**Acno Cleanser** (Baker Cummins)	60% isopropyl alcohol, EDTA	In 240 ml.
Rx	**Xerac AC** (Person & Covey)	6.25% aluminum chloride-hexahydrate in 96% anhydrous ethyl alcohol	In 35 and 60 ml.

Liquid Cleansers

LIQUID CLEANSERS

otc	**Exact** (Premier)	2.0% salicylic acid, propylene glycol, aloe vera gel, disodium EDTA, menthol, parabens, glycerin, diazolidinyl urea	In 118 ml.
otc	**Neutrogena Oil-free Acne Wash** (Neutrogena)	2% salicylic acid, EDTA, propylene glycol, tartrazine, aloe extract	In 180 ml.
otc	**Neutrogena Antiseptic Cleanser for Acne-Prone Skin** (Neutrogena)	Benzethonium chloride, butylene glycol, methylparaben, menthol, peppermint oil, eucalyptus oil, cornmint oil, rosemary oil, witch hazel extract, camphor	In 135 ml.
otc	**PROPApH Cleansing for Sensitive Skin** (Del Pharm.)	**Pads**: 0.5% salicylic acid, SD alcohol 40, EDTA, menthol, aloe vera gel	In 45s.
otc	**PROPApH Cleansing Maximum Strength** (Del Pharm)	**Pads**: 2.0% salicylic acid, SD alcohol 40, propylene glycol, EDTA, menthol, aloe vera gel	In 45s.
otc	**PROPApH Foaming Face Wash**(Del Pharm.)	2.0% salicylic acid, EDTA, menthol, aloe vera gel	Alcohol-, oil-,and soap-free. In 180 ml.
otc	**Ionax Foam** (Galderma)	Benzalkonium chloride, propylene glycol	Lemon scented and unscented. In 150 ml aerosol.
otc	**Oil of Olay Foaming Face Wash Liquid** (Procter & Gamble)	Potassium cocoyl hydrolyzed collagen, glycerin, EDTA	Regular and sensitive skin formulas: In 90 ml tubes and 210 ml pump.
otc	**Oxy ResiDON'T Medicated Face Wash** (SK Beecham)	Cocamidopropyl betaine, sodium laureth sulfate sodium cocoyl isethionate, triclosan, diazolidinyl urea	In 240 ml.

THERAPEUTIC SKIN CLEANSERS

These products are recommended for patients with sensitive, dry or irritated skin, who may react adversely to common soap products. Some products may be useful for patients with atopic dermatitis, diaper dermatitis and other eczematous skin conditions. Therapeutic cleansers include "soap free" cleansers, which may be adjusted to a neutral pH and are less irritating to sensitive skin, and "modified" soap products, which may contain emollient components or may be adjusted to a neutral or slightly acidic pH.

SOAP FREE CLEANSERS

otc	**Aquanil Cleanser** (Person & Covey)	**Lotion**: Lipid free. Glycerin, cetyl, stearyl and benzyl alcohol, sodium laureth sulfate, xanthan gum	In 240 and 480 ml.
otc	**Aveeno Cleansing** (Rydelle)	**Bar, combination skin formula**: Soap free. 51% colloidal oatmeal, sodium cocoyl isethionate, glycerin, lactic acid, sodium lactate, petrolatum, magnesium aluminum silicate, potassium sorbate, titanium dioxide, PEG-14M	In 90 g.
otc	**Aveeno Cleansing** (Rydelle)	**Bar, dry skin formula**: Soap free. 51% colloidal oatmeal, sodium cocoyl isethionate, vegetable oil and shortening, glycerin, PEG-75, lauramide DEA, lactic acid, sodium lactate, sorbic acid, titanium dioxide	In 90 g.
otc	**Bacti-Cleanse** (Pedinol)	**Lotion**: Benzalkonium chloride, mineral oil, isopropyl palmitate, cetyl alcohol, glycerine, glyceryl stearate, PEG 100 stearate, dimethicone, diazolidinyl urea, parabens, DMDM hydantoin, EDTA	In 453.6 ml.
otc	**Derm-Cleanse** (Yers Pharm)	**Liquid**: Soap free. Sodium lauryl sulfate, mineral oil, propylene glycol, hydroxyethylcellulose, EDTA	In 240 ml.
otc	**Drytergent** (C&M)	**Liquid**: TEA-dodecylbenzenesulfonate, boric acid, lauramide DEA, propylene glycol, tartrazine	In 240 and 480 ml.
otc	**Duplex** (C&M)	**Liquid**: 15% sodium lauryl sulfate, lauramide DEA	In 480 ml.
otc	**Free & Clear** (Pharmaceutical Specialties)	**Shampoo**: Ammonium laureth sulfate, disodium cocamido MEA sulfsosuccinate, cocamidopropyl hydroxysultaine, cocamide DEA, PEG-120 methyl glucose dioleate, EDTA, potassium sorbate, citric acid.	Dye free. In 240 ml
otc	**Green Soap** (Paddock)	**Liquid**: Soybean oil, potassium salt, ethanol.	For skin and hair. In 3780 ml.
otc	**Lowila Cake** (Westwood Squibb)	**Bar**: Soap free. Dextrin, sodium lauryl sulfoacetate, boric acid, urea, sorbitol, mineral oil, PEG-14 M, lactic acid, cellulose gum, DSS	In 112.5 g.
otc	**Cetaphil** (Galderma)	**Cream**: Lipid free. Cetyl alcohol, stearyl alcohol, sodium lauryl sulfate, propylene glycol, parabens	In 480 g.
		Lotion: Cetyl alcohol, propylene glycol, sodium lauryl sulfate, stearyl alcohol, parabens	In 120, 240, 480 ml.
otc	**Ancet** (C & M Pharm)	**Liquid**: Sodium lauryl sulfate, lauramide DEA, propylene glycol, hydroxyethyl ethylcellulose, PCMX	In 240 ml.
otc	**Ceta** (C & M Pharm)	**Liquid**: Soap free. Propylene glycol, hydroxyethylcellulose, cetyl and cetearyl alcohols, sodium lauryl sulfate, parabens	In 240 ml.

SOAP FREE CLEANSERS

otc	**pHisoDerm** (Chattem)	**Liquid**: Soap free. Sodium octoxynol-2 ethane sulfonate solution, petrolatum, octoxynol-3, mineral oil (with lanolin alcohol and oleyl alcohol), cocamide MEA, imidazolidinyl urea, sodium benzoate, tetrasodium EDTA and methylcellulose	Regular formula: Scented and unscented. In 150, 270, 480 ml and gal. Oily Skin formula: In 150 and 480 ml.
otc	**pHisoDerm For Baby** (Chattem)	**Liquid**: Sodium octoxynol-2 ethane sulfonate solution, petrolatum, octoxynol-3, mineral oil (with lanolin alcohol and oleyl alcohol), cocamide MEA, imidazolidinyl urea, sodium benzoate, tetrasodium EDTA and methylcellulose. pH adjusted with hydrochloric acid.	In 150 and 270 ml.
otc	**Spectro-Jel** (Recsei)	**Gel**: Soap free. Iodo-methyl-cellulose, carboxypolymethylene, cetyl alcohol, sorbitan monooleate, fumed silica, triethanolamine stearate, glycol polysiloxane, propylene glycol, glycerine and 5% isopropyl alcohol	In 127.5 ml, pt and gal.
otc	**Lobana Body Shampoo** (Ulmer)	**Liquid**: Chloroxylenol in a mild sudsing base with conditioners and emollients	In 240 ml and gal.
otc	**Sulfoil** (C & M Pharm)	**Liquid**: Soap free. Neutral pH. Sulfonated castor oil	For skin and hair. In pt and gal.
otc	**Tersaseptic** (Doak)	**Shampoo/Liquid**: DEA-lauryl sulfate, lauramide DEA, propylene glycol, ethoxydiglycol, PEG-12 distearate, EDTA, triclosan, citric acid	In 475 ml.
otc	**Lobana Liquid Lather** (Ulmer)	**Body wash**: Sodium laureth sulfate, sodium lauroyl sarcosinate, sodium myristyl sarcosonate, lauramide DEA, linoleamide DEA, octyl hydroxystearate, polyquarternium 7, tetrasodium EDTA, quaternium 15, sodium chloride, citric acid	In 240 ml and gal.
otc	**Neutrogena Non-Drying Cleansing** (Neutrogena)	**Lotion**: Glycerin, caprylic/capric triglyceride, PEG-20 almond glycerides, cetyl recinoleate, isohexadecane, TEA-cocoyl glutamate, PEG-20 methyl glucose sesquistearate, methyl glucose sesquistearate, stearyl alcohol, cetyl alcohol, EDTA, dipotassium glycyrrhizate, stearyl glycyrrhetinate, bisabolol, parabens, acrylates/C 10-30 alkyl acrylate crosspolymer, triethanolamine, diazolidinyl urea	In 165 ml.
otc	**SFC** (Stiefel)	**Lotion**: Soap free. PEG-75, stearyl alcohol, sodium cocoyl isethionate, parabens	In 237 and 480 ml.

MODIFIED BAR SOAPS

otc	**pHisoDerm Cleansing Bar** (Chattem)	**Bar**: Sodium tallowate, sodium cocoate, petrolatum, glycerin, lanolin, sodium chloride, BHT, EDTA, titanium dioxide	Scented or unscented. In 99 g.
otc	**Oilatum Soap** (Stiefel)	**Bar**: Sodium tallowate, sodium cocoate, peanut oil, octyl hydroxystearate, lecithin, NaCl, PEG-14M, titanium dioxide, o-tolyl biguanide, EDTA, sodium borohydride, glyceryl oleate, corn oil, t-butyl hydroquinone, propylene glycol	Scented or unscented. In 120 and 240 g.

MODIFIED BAR SOAPS

otc	**Neutrogena Baby Cleansing Formula Soap** (Neutrogena Corp.)	**Bar:** TEA-stearate, triethanolamine, glycerin, sodium tallowate, sodium cocoate, TEA-oleate, sodium ricinoleate, cocamide DEA, laneth-10 acetate, nonoxynol-12 , PEG-5 octanoate, tocopherol	Transparent. Scented. In 105 g.
otc	**Neutrogena Dry Skin Soap** (Neutrogena Corp.)	**Bar:** TEA-stearate, triethanolamine, sodium tallowate, glycerin, sodium cocoate, sodium ricinoleate, TEA-oleate, laneth-10 acetate, cocamide DEA, nonoxynol 12, PEG-5 octanoate, tocopherol	Transparent. Scented or unscented. In 105 and 165 (scented only) g.
otc	**Neutrogena Oily Skin Soap** (Neutrogena Corp.)	**Bar:** TEA-stearate, triethanolamine, sodium tallowate, glycerin, sodium lauroyl sarcosinate, sodium cocoate, sodium ricinoleate, witch hazel, tocopherol	Transparent. Scented. In 105 g.
otc	**Neutrogena Soap** (Neutrogena Corp.)	**Bar:** TEA-stearate, triethanolamine, glycerin, sodium tallowate, sodium cocoate, sodium ricinoleate, TEA-oleate, cocamide DEA, tocopherol	Transparent. Scented or unscented. In 105 and 165 g.
otc	**Neutrogena Cleansing for Acne-Prone Skin** (Neutrogena Corp.)	**Bar:** TEA-stearate, triethanolamine, glycerin, sodium tallowate, sodium cocoate, TEA-oleate, sodium ricinoleate, acetylated lanolin alcohol, cocamide DEA, TEA lauryl sulfate, tocopherol	Transparent, nonmedicated. In 105 g.
otc	**Ambi 10** (Kiwi Brands)	**Bar:** Triclosan, sodium tallowate, PEG-20, titanium dioxide	In 99 g.
otc	**Alpha Keri Moisturizing Soap** (Bristol-Myers)	**Bar:** Sodium tallowate, sodium cocoate, mineral oil, lanolin oil, PEG-75, glycerin, titanium dioxide, sodium chloride, BHT, EDTA	Nondetergent, emollient. In 120 g.
otc	**Purpose Soap** (Johnson & Johnson)	**Bar:** Sodium tallowate, sodium cocoate, glycerin, NaCl, BHT, EDTA	In 108 and 180 g.
otc	**Nivea Moisturizing Creme Soap** (Beiersdorf)	**Bar:** Sodium tallowate, sodium cocoate, glycerin, petrolatum, titanium dioxide, NaCl, octyldodecanol, macadamia nut oil, aloe, sodium thiosulfate, lanolin alcohol, pentasodium pentetate, EDTA, BHT, beeswax	In 90 and 150 g.
otc	**Cuticura Medicated Soap** (DEP Corp.)	**Bar:** 1% triclocarban, sodium tallowate, sodium cocoate, glycerin, mineral oil, petrolatum, sodium chloride, tetra sodium EDTA, sodium bicarbonate, magnesium silicate and iron oxides	Phosphorus free. Emollient. Mildly antibacterial. In 97.5 and 142 g.
otc	**Formula 405** (Doak)	**Bar:** Sodium tallowate, sodium cocoate, Doak Additive A, PPG-20 methyl glucose ether, titanium dioxide, trochlorocarbanilide, pentasodium pentetate, EDTA	Fragrance free. In 100 g.

ANTIPSORIATICS, TOPICAL

In addition to the products described here, other products for treatment of psoriasis include: Coal tar; corticosteroids; salicylic acid. Refer to individual monographs.

ANTHRALIN (Dithranol)

Actions:

Pharmacology: Anthralin reduces the mitotic rate; in vitro evidence suggests that anthralin's antimitotic effect results from inhibition of DNA synthesis. Additionally, the chemically reducing properties of anthralin may upset oxidative metabolic processes, providing a further slowing down of epidermal mitosis.

Indications:

Psoriasis: Quiescent or chronic psoriasis.

Contraindications:

Hypersensitivity to anthralin or any component of the product; use on the face; acutely or actively inflamed psoriatic eruptions.

Warnings:

For external use only: Avoid contact with the eyes (severe conjunctivitis may occur) or mucous membranes. Anthralin should not normally be applied to intertriginous skin areas and high strengths should not be used on these sites. Do not apply to face or genitalia. Remove any unintended residue which may be deposited behind the ears. Avoid applying to the folds and creases of the skin. Discontinue use if a sensitivity reaction occurs or if excessive irritation develops on uninvolved skin areas. Wash hands thoroughly after using.

Renal/Hepatic function impairment: Although no renal or hepatic abnormalities have occurred with topical application, use caution in patients with renal disease and in those having extensive and prolonged applications. Perform periodic urine tests for albuminuria. Discontinue use if sensitivity reactions occur.

Carcinogenesis: In long-term studies with mice, anthralin demonstrated carcinogenic and tumorigenic activity.

Pregnancy: Category C. It is not known whether anthralin can cause fetal harm when administered to a pregnant woman or can affect reproduction capacity. Administer only if clearly needed.

Lactation: It is not known whether this drug is excreted in breast milk. Because of the potential for tumorigenicity in animal studies, discontinue nursing or the drug, taking into account the importance of the drug to the mother.

Children: Safety and efficacy have not been established.

Precautions:

Staining: May stain fabrics, skin or hair; apply sparingly and carefully to psoriatic lesions only. To prevent the possibility of staining clothing or bed linen while gaining experience in using anthralin, it may be advisable to use protective dressings. To prevent the possibility of discoloration, especially when using higher strengths, always rinse the bath/shower with hot water immediately after washing/showering and then use a suitable cleanser to remove any deposit on the surface of the bath or shower. Contact with fabrics, plastics and other materials may cause staining and should be avoided.

Drug Interactions:

Corticosteroids, topical: As long-term use of topical corticosteroids may destabilize psoriasis, and withdrawal may also give rise to a "rebound" phenomenon, allow an interval of at least 1 week between the discontinuance of such steroids and the commencement of therapy. Petrolatum or a suitably bland emollient may be applied during the intervening period.

Adverse Reactions:

Very few instances of contact allergic reactions to anthralin have been reported. However, transient primary irritation of normal skin or uninvolved skin surrounding the treated lesions is more frequently seen and may occasionally be severe. Application must be restricted to the psoriatic lesions. If the initial treatment produces excessive soreness or if the lesions spread, reduce frequency of application and, in extreme cases, discontinue use and consult physician.

Some temporary discoloration of hair and fingernails may arise during the period of treatment but should be minimized by careful application. Anthralin may stain skin, hair or fabrics. Staining of fabrics may be permanent; avoid contact. See Precautions.

Patient Information:

Patient instructions are available with products.

ANTHRALIN (Dithranol)

Administration and Dosage:

Generally, apply once a day or as directed. Anthralin is known to be a potential skin irritant. The irritant potential of anthralin is directly related to the strength being used and each patient's individual tolerance. Therefore, where the response to treatment has not previously been established, always commence treatment for at least 1 week using the lowest strength possible. Increase strengths when directed. Apply as directed and remove by washing or showering. The optimal period of contact will vary according to the strength used and the patient's response to treatment. Continue treatment until the skin is entirely clear (ie, when there is nothing to feel with fingers and the texture is normal).

Skin application: Apply sparingly only to the psoriatic lesions and rub gently and carefully into the skin until absorbed. It is most important to avoid applying an excessive quantity which may cause unnecessary soiling and staining of the clothing or bed linen. At the end of each treatment period, take a bath or shower to remove any surplus (cream may have become red/brown in color). The margins of the lesions may gradually become stained purple/brown as treatment progresses, but this will disappear after treatment cessation.

Scalp application: Comb the hair to remove scalar debris and, after suitably parting, rub the cream well into the lesions, taking care to prevent the cream from spreading onto the forehead. Keep away from the eyes. Take care to avoid application to uninvolved scalp margins. Remove any unintended residue which may be deposited behind the ears. At the end of each period of contact, wash the hair and scalp to remove any surplus (cream may have become red/brown in color).

Short-contact regimens have been used preferably for stable plaque-type psoriasis. Initial contact time is 0.1% to 2% for 15 to 20 minutes, followed by thorough removal of the anthralin with an appropriate solvent (soap or petrolatum) and application of an emollient. Short-contact therapy plus other treatments (eg, ultraviolet light, retinoids, topical steroids, psoralens plus UV light) may improve the response.

Rx	**Anthra-Derm** (Dermik)	**Ointment:** 0.1%	In 42.5 g
		0.25%	In 42.5 g.
Rx	**Anthra-Derm** (Dermik)	**Ointment:** 0.5%	In 42.5 g.
		1%	In 42.5 g.
Rx	**Drithocreme** (Dermik)	**Cream:** 0.1%	White petrolatum, cetostearyl alcohol. In 50 g.
Rx	**Drithocreme** (Dermik)	**Cream:** 0.25%	White petrolatum, cetostearyl alcohol. In 50 g.
Rx	**Dritho-Scalp** (Dermik)		White petrolatum, mineral oil, cetostearyl alcohol. In 50 g w/applicator.
Rx	**Dritho-Scalp** (Dermik)	**Cream:** 0.5%	White petrolatum, mineral oil, cetostearyl alcohol. In 50 g w/applicator.
Rx	**Drithocreme** (Dermik)		White petrolatum, cetostearyl alcohol. In 50 g.
Rx	**Drithocreme HP 1%** (Dermik)	**Cream:** 1%	White petrolatum, cetostearyl alcohol. In 50 g.
Rx	**Micanol** (Bioglan Pharma)		In 50 g.

CALCIPOTRIENE

Actions:

Pharmacology: Calcipotriene is a synthetic vitamin D_3 analog for the treatment of moderate plaque psoriasis. In humans, the natural supply of vitamin D depends mainly on exposure to the ultraviolet rays of the sun for conversion of 7-dehydrocholesterol to vitamin D_3 (cholecalciferol) in the skin. After entering the bloodstream, it is metabolized in the liver and kidneys to its active form, the hormone calcitriol. Vitamin D_3 receptors, proteins that bind chemically to calcitriol, occur in many parts of the body, including the skin cells known as keratinocytes. The scaly red patches of psoriasis are caused by the abnormal growth and production of the keratinocytes. Calcipotriene regulates skin cell production and development.

Pharmacokinetics: Approximately 6% of an applied dose is absorbed systemically when the ointment is applied topically to psoriasis plaques or 5% when applied to normal skin; much of the absorbed active drug is converted to inactive metabolites within 24 hours of application.

Vitamin D and its metabolites are transported in the blood, bound to specific plasma proteins. The active form of the vitamin, 1,25-dihydroxy vitamin D_3 (calcitriol), is known to be recycled via the liver and excreted in the bile. Calcipotriene metabolism following systemic uptake is rapid, and occurs via a similar pathway to the natural hormone. The primary metabolites are much less potent than the parent compound. The systemic disposition of calcipotriene is expected to be similar to that of the naturally occurring vitamin.

Clinical trials: Patients treated with calcipotriene have demonstrated improvement usually beginning after 2 weeks of therapy. This improvement continued with approximately 70% of patients showing at least marked improvement after 8 weeks of therapy, but only approximately 10% showing complete clearing.

Indications:

Psoriasis: Treatment of moderate plaque psoriasis.

Contraindications:

Hypersensitivity to any components of the preparation; patients with demonstrated hypercalcemia or evidence of vitamin D toxicity; use on the face.

Warnings:

Dermatoses: The safety and efficacy of topical calcipotriene in dermatoses other than psoriasis have not been established.

For external use only. Not for ophthalmic, oral or intravaginal use.

Elderly: Of the total number of patients in clinical studies of calcipotriene ointment, approximately 12% were ≥ 65 years of age, while approximately 4% were ≥ 75. The results of an analysis of severity of skin-related adverse events showed a statistically significant difference for subjects > 65 years of age (more severe) compared to those < 65 (less severe).

Pregnancy: Category C. Doses of calcipotriene up to 36 mcg/kg/day in the rabbit did not result in teratogenic effects; however, increased maternal and fetal toxicity was observed at ≥ 12 mcg/kg/day. In the rat, oral doses of 54 mcg/kg/day resulted in a significantly higher incidence of skeletal abnormalities consisting primarily of enlarged fontanelles and extra ribs. The enlarged fontanelles is most likely due to calcipotriene's effect upon calcium metabolism. There is evidence that maternal calcitriol may enter the fetal circulation. There are no adequate and well controlled studies in pregnant women. Use during pregnancy only if the potential benefit justifies the potential risk to the fetus.

Lactation: It is not known whether calcipotriene is excreted in breast milk. Exercise caution when administering to a nursing woman.

Children: Safety and efficacy have not been established. Because of a higher ratio of skin surface area to body mass, children are at greater risk than adults of systemic adverse effects when they are treated with topical medication.

Precautions:

Irritation: Use of calcipotriene may cause irritation of lesions and surrounding uninvolved skin. If irritation develops, discontinue the drug.

Hypercalcemia: Transient, rapidly reversible elevation of serum calcium has occurred with use of calcipotriene. If elevation in serum calcium occurs outside the normal range, discontinue treatment until normal calcium levels are restored.

Adverse Reactions:

Burning, itching, skin irritation (≈ 10% to 15%); erythema, dry skin, peeling, rash, worsening of psoriasis (including development of facial/scalp psoriasis), dermatitis (1% to 10%); skin atrophy, hyperpigmentation, hypercalcemia, folliculitis (< 1%).

CALCIPOTRIENE

Overdosage:

Topically applied calcipotriene can be absorbed in sufficient amounts to produce systemic effects. Elevated serum calcium has been observed with excessive use.

Patient Information:

Use as directed. It is for external use only; avoid contact with the face or eyes. As with any topical medication, wash hands after application.

Do not use for any disorder other than that for which it was prescribed.

Patients should report any signs of local adverse reactions.

Administration and Dosage:

Approved by the FDA on December 29, 1993 (1S classification).

Apply a thin layer to the affected skin twice daily and rub in gently and completely. Safety and efficacy have been demonstrated in patients treated for 8 weeks.

Rx	**Dovonex** (Westwood-Squibb)	**Ointment:** 0.005% calcipotriene	In 30, 60 and 100 g.
		Cream: 0.005% calcipotriene	In 30, 60 and 100 g.

AMMONIATED MERCURY

Indications:

Psoriasis: Treatment of psoriasis of the scalp, isolated psoriatic lesions and seborrheic dermatitis.

Contraindications:

Hypersensitivity to mercurials.

Warnings:

Efficacy: Since more effective and less toxic therapies are available, the use of ammoniated mercury is not recommended.

Mercury poisoning: Frequent or prolonged application to large areas or to broken skin or mucous membranes may cause mercury poisoning.

Children: Avoid use of ammoniated mercury in infants; it may cause acrodynia (pink disease).

Precautions:

For external use only. Do not apply to eyes, mouth, extensive areas or open wounds. If redness, swelling or pain persists or increases, or if infection, rash or irritation occurs, discontinue use and consult physician.

Adverse Reactions:

Ammoniated mercury is a potential sensitizer, capable of evoking allergic reactions following topical application.

Administration and Dosage:

Apply 1 or 2 times daily.

Storage: Protect from light.

Rx	**Emersal** (Medco Lab)	**Lotion:** 5% with 2.5% salicylic acid	In 120 ml.

METHOTREXATE (Amethopterin; MTX)

This is an abbreviated monograph. For complete prescribing information and use of methotrexate as an antineoplastic or antirheumatic agent, see monographs in the antineoplastic and antirheumatic sections.

> **Warning:**
>
> Due to the possibility of fatal or severe toxic reactions, inform patient of risks involved; keep under constant supervision. Deaths have occurred. Restrict use to severe, recalcitrant, disabling psoriasis not adequately responsive to other therapy when diagnosis is established by biopsy or after dermatologic consultation.
>
> May produce marked bone marrow depression with resultant anemia, leukopenia or thrombocytopenia.
>
> Methotrexate has caused fetal death or congenital anomalies. Therefore, it is not recommended for women of childbearing potential unless there is clear medical evidence that the benefits can be expected to outweigh the considered risks. Pregnant patients with psoriasis should not receive methotrexate.
>
> Diarrhea and ulcerative stomatitis require interruption of therapy; otherwise, hemorrhagic enteritis and death from intestinal perforation may occur.
>
> Periodic monitoring for toxicity, including CBC with differential and platelet counts, and liver and renal function tests is a mandatory part of methotrexate therapy. Periodic liver biopsies may be indicated in some situations. Monitor patients at increased risk for impaired methotrexate elimination (eg, renal dysfunction, pleural effusions, ascites) more frequently.
>
> Methotrexate causes hepatotoxicity, fibrosis and cirrhosis, but generally only after prolonged use. Acutely, liver enzyme elevations are frequently seen, these are usually transient and asymptomatic and also do not appear predictive of subsequent hepatic disease. Liver biopsy after sustained use often shows histologic changes, and fibrosis and cirrhosis have been reported; these latter lesions often are not preceded by symptoms or abnormal liver function tests.
>
> Methotrexate-induced lung disease is a potentially dangerous lesion, which may occur acutely at any time during therapy and which has been reported at doses as low as 7.5 mg per week. It is not always fully reversible. Pulmonary symptoms (especially a dry, nonproductive cough) may require interruption of treatment and careful investigation.
>
> Use with extreme caution, and at reduced dosages, in patients with impaired renal function because renal dysfunction will prolong methotrexate elimination.
>
> Unexpectedly severe (sometimes fatal) marrow suppression and GI toxicity have occurred with concomitant administration of methotrexate (usually in high dosage) along with some nonsteroidal anti-inflammatory drugs.
>
> Methotrexate formulations and diluents containing preservatives must not be used for intrathecal or high-dose methotrexate therapy.

Actions:

Pharmacology: Actively proliferating tissues are generally more sensitive to the effect of methotrexate. In psoriasis, the rate of production of epithelial cells in the skin is greatly increased over normal skin. This differential in proliferation rates is the basis for the use of this drug to control the psoriatic process.

Indications:

Psoriasis: For the symptomatic control of severe, recalcitrant, disabling psoriasis which is not adequately responsive to other therapy. Use only when the diagnosis has been established by biopsy or after dermatologic consultation. It is important to ensure that a psoriasis "flare" is not due to an undiagnosed concomitant disease affecting immune responses.

Methotrexate is also used as an antineoplastic agent and in the management of rheumatoid arthritis (see individual monographs).

Unlabeled uses: Methotrexate has shown potential value in the treatment of psoriatic arthritis and Reiter's disease.

Administration and Dosage:

Assess hematologic, hepatic, renal and pulmonary function before beginning, periodically during, and before reinstituting therapy.

Severe, recalcitrant, disabling psoriasis: Individualize dosage. A test dose may be given prior to therapy to detect extreme sensitivity to adverse effects.

Weekly single oral, IM or IV dosage schedule – 10 to 25 mg/week until adequate response is achieved. Do not exceed 30 mg per week.

Divided oral dose schedule – 2.5 mg at 12 hour intervals for 3 doses. Do not exceed 30 mg per week.

METHOTREXATE (Amethopterin; MTX)

Once optimal clinical response is achieved, reduce to lowest possible amount of drug with the longest possible rest period. Methotrexate may permit return to conventional topical therapy, which should be encouraged.

Rx	**Methotrexate** (Various, eg, Barr, Geneva, Goldline, Lederle, Major, Qualitest, Rugby, Schein, UDL,)	**Tablets:** 2.5 mg	In 36s, 100s and UD 20s.
Rx	**Rheumatrex** (Lederle)		In 5, 7.5, 10, 12.5 and 15 mg/week dose packs.
Rx	**Methotrexate** (Immunex)	**Powder for injection, lyophilized:** 1 g/vial	Preservative free. In single-use vials.
		20 mg (as sodium)/vial	Freeze dried, preservative free. In single-use vials.[1]
Rx	**Methotrexate** (Lederle)	**Injection:** 25 mg (as sodium) per ml	Preservative protected in 2 and 10 ml vials.[2]

[1] Contains ≈ 0.14, ≈ 0.33, and 7 mEq sodium, respectively.
[2] Contains 0.9% benzyl alcohol, sodium chloride 0.26% and water for injection.

ETRETINATE

Warning:

Etretinate must not be used by females who are pregnant, who intend to become pregnant or who are unreliable or may not use reliable contraception while undergoing treatment. The period of time during which pregnancy must be avoided after treatment has not been determined. Blood levels of 0.5 to 12 ng/ml have been reported in 5 of 47 patients 2.1 to 2.9 years after treatment was concluded.

Major human fetal abnormalities related to administration have been reported, including meningomyelocoele, meningoencephalocoele, multiple synostoses, facial dysmorphia, syndactylies, absence of terminal phalanges, malformations of hip, ankle and forearm, low set ears, high palate, decreased cranial volume and alterations of the skull and cervical vertebrae on x-ray.

Women of childbearing potential must not be given etretinate until pregnancy is excluded. Perform a pregnancy test within 2 weeks prior to initiating therapy. Start therapy on the second or third day of the next normal menstrual period. An effective form of contraception must be used for at least 1 month before, during and following discontinuation of therapy for an indefinite period of time.

Counsel women on the serious risks to the fetus should they become pregnant while undergoing treatment or after discontinuation of therapy. If pregnancy does occur, the physician and patient should discuss the desirability of continuing the pregnancy.

Actions:

Pharmacology: Etretinate is related to retinoic acid and retinol (vitamin A). The mechanism of action is unknown.However, it is possible that it reduces cell proliferation by inhibiting ornithine decarboxylase, the rate-limiting enzyme in polyamine production, which is responsible for regulating cell growth, proliferation and differentiation. It may also inhibit migration of neutrophils into the epidermis. The drug has anti-keratinizing and anti-inflammatory effects. Improvement in psoriatic patients occurs in association with a decrease in scale, erythema and thickness of lesions, as well as histological evidence of normalization of epidermal differentiation, decreased stratum corneum thickness and decreased inflammation in the epidermis and dermis.

Pharmacokinetics: The pharmacokinetic profile is linear. The absorption of etretinate is increased by whole milk or a high-lipid diet. Etretinate is extensively metabolized following oral dosing, with significant first-pass metabolism to the acid form, which is pharmacologically active. Subsequent metabolism results in conjugates that are ultimately excreted in the bile and urine.

C_{max} values range from 102 to 389 ng/ml and occur at T_{max} values of 2 to 6 hours. In 47 patients treated chronically with etretinate, five had detectable serum drug levels (0.5 to 12 ng/ml) 2.1 to 2.9 years after therapy was discontinued. In one study, the apparent terminal half-life after 6 months of therapy was approximately 120 days. The long half-life appears to be due to storage of etretinate in adipose tissue.

Etretinate is > 99% bound to plasma proteins, predominantly lipoproteins; its active metabolite is predominantly bound to albumin. Concentrations of etretinate in blister fluid after 6 weeks of dosing were approximately one-tenth those observed in plasma. Concentrations of etretinate and its metabolite in epidermal specimens obtained after 1 to 36 months were a function of location; subcutis >> serum > epidermis > dermis. Similarly, liver concentrations of etretinate in patients receiving therapy for 6 months were generally higher than concomitant plasma concentrations.

Clinical trials: Etretinate resulted in clinical improvement in most patients. Complete clearing of the disease was observed after 4 to 9 months of therapy in 13% of all patients treated for severe psoriasis. This included complete clearing in 16% with erythrodermic psoriasis and 37% with generalized pustular psoriasis. After discontinuation, most patients experienced some degree of relapse by the end of 2 months. After relapse, subsequent 4 to 9 month courses of therapy resulted in a similar clinical response as experienced during initial therapy.

Indications:

Psoriasis: Treatment of severe recalcitrant psoriasis, including the erythrodermic and generalized pustular types.

Unlabeled uses: Etretinate may be beneficial in the following conditions: Bronchial metaplasia; mycosis fungoides; actinic keratoses; arsenical keratoses; basal cell carcinomas; genodermatosis; pustular bacterids; hyperkeratotic eczemas of palms/soles; cutaneous lupus erythematosus.

ETRETINATE

Contraindications:

Pregnancy (see boxed Warning).

Warnings:

> *Pseudotumor cerebri:* Retinoids have been associated with pseudotumor cerebri (benign intracranial hypertension). Early signs and symptoms include papilledema, headache, nausea, vomiting and visual disturbances. If present, discontinue the drug immediately and refer the patient for neurologic diagnosis and care.
>
> *Hepatotoxicity:* Of 652 patients treated in US clinical trials, 10 had clinical or histologic hepatitis possibly related to etretinate treatment. Liver function tests returned to normal in eight patients after the drug was discontinued; one patient had histologic changes resembling chronic active hepatitis 6 months off therapy, and one patient had no follow-up available. There have been four reports of hepatitis-related deaths worldwide; two had received etretinate for ≤ 1 month before hepatic symptom occurrence.
>
> Elevations of AST, ALT or LDH have occurred in 18%, 23% and 15%, respectively, of individuals treated. Pathology findings of hepatic fibrosis, necrosis or cirrhosis possibly related to etretinate therapy have occurred. If hepatotoxicity is suspected during treatment, discontinue the drug and investigate the etiology. Perform these tests prior to initiation of therapy, at 1 to 2 week intervals for the first 1 to 2 months of therapy, and thereafter at intervals of 1 to 3 months, depending on the response to etretinate.

Severe psoriasis: Because of its significant adverse effects, etretinate should be prescribed only by physicians knowledgeable in the systemic use of retinoids and reserved for patients with severe recalcitrant psoriasis who are unresponsive to or intolerant of standard therapies (eg, topical tar plus UVB light; psoralens plus UVA light; systemic corticosteroids; methotrexate).

Ophthalmic effects: Corneal erosion, abrasion, irregularity and punctate staining have occurred, although these effects were absent or improved in follow-up examinations after therapy was stopped. Corneal opacities have occurred in patients receiving isotretinoin; they had either completely resolved or were resolving at follow-up 6 to 7 weeks after discontinuation of the drug. Other ophthalmic effects that have occurred include decreased visual acuity and blurring of vision, decreased night vision, minimal posterior subcapsular cataract, iritis, blot retinal hemorrhage, scotoma and photophobia. Because the onset in some patients was sudden, advise patients of this potential problem and to be cautious when driving or operating any vehicle at night. Any patient experiencing visual difficulties should discontinue the drug and have an ophthalmological examination.

Hyperostosis: In clinical trials, 45 patients (mean age, 40 years) were retrospectively evaluated. They received a mean dose of 0.8 mg/kg for a mean duration of 33 months at time of x–ray. Eleven patients had psoriasis, while 34 patients had a keratinization disorder. Of 38 of these patients who continued to receive etretinate for an average of 60 months, 32 (84%) had radiographic evidence of extraspinal tendon and ligament calcification. The most common sites of involvement were the ankles (76%), pelvis (53%) and knees (42%); spinal changes were uncommon. Involvement tended to be bilateral and multifocal. There were no bone or joint symptoms in 47% of the affected patients.

Lipids: Perform blood lipid determinations before etretinate is administered, and then at intervals of 1 or 2 weeks until the lipid response is established; this usually occurs within 4 to 8 weeks. Approximately 45% of patients experienced an elevation of plasma triglycerides (46% had elevations > 250 mg/dl), 37% developed a decrease in high density lipoproteins (HDL; 54% had decreases < 36 mg/dl) and about 16% showed an increase in cholesterol levels (19% had elevations > 300 mg/dl). They were reversible after discontinuation of therapy. Some patients have been able to reverse triglyceride and cholesterol elevations or HDL decrease by weight reduction or restriction of dietary fat and alcohol while continuing therapy. Increased triglycerides have also occurred (25% to 50% of patients).

Patients with a tendency to develop hypertriglyceridemia include those with diabetes mellitus, obesity, increased alcohol intake or a familial history of these conditions.

Cardiovascular effects: Two cases of myocardial infarction have been reported, one possibly related to etretinate therapy.

Pregnancy: Category X. See Warning Box.

ETRETINATE

Lactation: Etretinate is excreted in the milk of lactating rats; however, it is not known whether this drug is excreted in human breast milk. Because of the potential for adverse effects, nursing mothers should not receive etretinate.

Children: Ossification of interosseous ligaments and tendons of the extremities has been reported. Two children showed x-ray changes suggestive of premature epiphyseal closure during treatment. Skeletal hyperostosis has also been reported after treatment with isotretinoin. It is not known if any of these effects occur more commonly in children, but concern is greater because of the growth process. Pretreatment x-rays for bone age including x-rays of the knees, followed by yearly monitoring, are advised. Evaluate pain or limitation of motion with appropriate radiological examination. Because of the lack of data and the possibility of children being more sensitive to effects of the drug, use only when all alternative therapies have been exhausted.

Drug Interactions:

Vitamin A: To avoid additive toxic effects, do not take concomitantly with etretinate.

Drug/Food interactions: Milk consumption and food, especially high lipid diets, increase the absorption of etretinate.

Adverse Reactions:

Adverse events generally resemble those of the hypervitaminosis A syndrome.

Mucocutaneous: Dry nose, chapped lips (> 75%); thirst, sore mouth (50% to 75%); nosebleed (25% to 50%); cheilitis, sore tongue (10% to 25%); dry eyes, mucous membrane abnormalities, dry mouth, gingival bleeding/inflammation (1% to 10%); decreased mucus secretion, rhinorrhea (< 1%).

GU: WBC in urine (10% to 25%), proteinuria, glycosuria, microscopic hematuria, casts, acetonuria, hemoglobinuria (1% to 10%); abnormal menses, atrophic vaginitis, dysuria, polyuria, urinary retention (< 1%).

Dermatologic: Hair loss, palm/sole/fingertip peeling (> 75%); dry skin, itching, rash, red scaly face, skin fragility (50% to 75%); bruising, sunburn (25% to 50%); nail disorder, skin peeling (10% to 25%); hair abnormalities, bullous eruption, cold/clammy skin, onycholysis, paronychia, pyogenic granuloma, changes in perspiration (1% to 10%); abnormal skin odor, granulation tissue, healing impairment, herpes simplex, hirsutism, increased pore size, sensory skin changes, skin atrophy/fissures/infection/nodules/ulceration, urticaria (< 1%).

Musculoskeletal: Hyperostosis (> 75%); bone/joint pain (50% to 75%); muscle cramps (25% to 50%); myalgia (1% to 10%); gout, hyperkinesia, hypertonia (< 1%).

CNS: Fatigue (50% to 75%); headache (25% to 50%); fever (10% to 25%); dizziness, lethargy, sensation change, pain, rigors (1% to 10%); abnormal thinking, amnesia, anxiety, depression, pseudotumor cerebri (see Warnings), emotional lability, faint feeling (< 1%).

Special senses: Eye irritation (50% to 75%); eyeball pain, eyelid abnormalities (25% to 50%); conjunctivitis, decreased visual acuity, double vision, abnormalities of conjunctiva, cornea, lens and retina (10% to 25%); earache, otitis externa, abnormalities of lacrimation, vision, extraocular musculature, ocular tension, pupil and vitreous (1% to 10%); equilibrium change, ear drainage/infection, hearing change, decreased night vision, photophobia, visual change, scotoma (< 1%).

GI: Abdominal pain, appetite change (25% to 50%); nausea (10% to 25%); hepatitis (see Warnings) (1% to 10%); constipation, diarrhea, melena, flatulence, weight loss, oral ulcers, taste perversion, tooth caries (< 1%).

Cardiovascular: Cardiovascular thrombotic or obstructive events, edema (1% to 10%); atrial fibrillation, chest pain, coagulation disorder, phlebitis, postural hypotension, syncope (< 1%).

Respiratory: Dyspnea (1% to 10%); coughing, increased sputum, dysphonia, pharyngitis (< 1%).

Hematologic: Increased MCHC (60%); increased MCH, reticulocytes, PTT or ESR (25% to 50%). Decreased hemoglobin/HCT, RBC or MCV; increased platelets; increased or decreased WBC and components or prothrombin time (10% to 25%); decreased platelets, MCH, MCHC or PTT and increased hemoglobin/HCT or RBC (1% to 10%).

Hepatic: Increased triglycerides (25% to 50%); increased AST, ALT, alkaline phosphatase, GGTP, globulin, cholesterol (10% to 25%); increased bilirubin, increased or decreased total protein or albumin (1% to 10%). See Warnings.

Renal: Increased BUN or creatinine (1% to 10%); kidney stones (< 1%).

Electrolyte Disturbance: Increased or decreased potassium, calcium or phosphorus (25% to 50%); increased or decreased venous CO_2, sodium or chloride (10% to 25%).

ETRETINATE

Miscellaneous: Increased or decreased FBS (10% to 25%); increased CPK and malignant neoplasms (1% to 10%); flu-like symptoms (< 1%).

Patient Information:

Advise women of childbearing potential that they must not be pregnant when therapy is initiated; they should use effective contraception for 1 month prior to therapy, while taking etretinate and after it has been discontinued. Etretinate has been found in the blood of some patients 2 to 3 years after its discontinuation. See Warning Box.

Patients should not take vitamin A supplements because of possible additive toxic effects.

Transient exacerbation of psoriasis is common during the initial period of therapy.

Patients may experience decreased tolerance to contact lenses during and after therapy.

Administer with food. Milk and food, especially high-lipid diets, increase absorption of etretinate.

Administration and Dosage:

Individualize dosage. Initiate at 0.75 to 1 mg/kg/day in divided doses; do not exceed 1.5 mg/kg/day. Erythrodermic psoriasis may respond to lower initial doses of 0.25 mg/kg/day increased by 0.25 mg/kg/day each week until optimal initial response is attained.

Maintenance doses of 0.5 to 0.75 mg/kg/day generally begin after 8 to 16 weeks of therapy. Therapy is usually terminated in patients whose lesions have sufficiently resolved. Relapses may be treated as outlined for initial therapy.

Rx	**Tegison** (Roche)	**Capsules:** 10 mg	(Tegison 10 Roche). Brown and green. In 30s.
		25 mg	(Tegison 25 Roche). Brown and caramel. In 30s.

NITROFURAZONE

Actions:

Pharmacology: Nitrofurazone, a synthetic nitrofuran with a broad antibacterial spectrum, is bactericidal against a number of gram-negative and -positive bacteria commonly causing surface infections, including *Staphylococcus aureus, Streptococcus, Escherichia coli, Clostridium perfringens, Aerobacter aerogenes* and *Proteus* sp.

Indications:

Burn treatment: Adjunctive therapy of patients with second and third degree burns when bacterial resistance to other agents is a real or potential problem.

Skin grafting where bacterial contamination may cause graft rejection or donor site infection, particularly in hospitals with historical resistant bacteria epidemics.

Contraindications:

Hypersensitivity to nitrofurazone or any component of the product.

Warnings:

Minor burns/infections: There is no evidence of effectiveness in treatment of minor burns or surface bacterial infections involving wounds, cutaneous ulcers or the various pyodermas.

Renal function impairment: Use the soluble burn dressing with caution in patients with known or suspected renal impairment. The polyethylene glycol present in the base can be absorbed through denuded skin and may not be excreted normally by a compromised kidney, leading to symptoms of progressive renal impairment including increased BUN, anion gap and metabolic acidosis.

Pregnancy: Category C. There are no adequate and well controlled studies in pregnant women. Use only when potential benefits outweigh risk to the fetus.

Lactation: It is not known whether this drug is excreted in breast milk. Decide whether to discontinue nursing or to discontinue the drug, taking into account the importance of the drug to the mother.

Children: Safety and efficacy have not been established.

Precautions:

For external use only. Avoid contact with eyes.

Superinfection: Use may result in bacterial or fungal overgrowth of nonsusceptible organisms, including fungi and *Pseudomonas.* Such overgrowth may lead to a secondary infection. If this occurs, or if irritation, sensitization or superinfection develops, discontinue treatment and institute appropriate therapy.

Adverse Reactions:

Varying degrees of contact dermatitis such as rash, pruritus and local edema (≈1%). Treat allergic reactions symptomatically.

Patient Information:

Notify physician if condition worsens or if rash or irritation occurs.

Administration and Dosage:

For the treatment of burns, apply directly to the lesion or place on gauze. Reapply once daily or every few days, depending on dressing technique. Flushing dressing with sterile saline facilitates removal.

Storage:

Cream – Avoid exposure to direct sunlight, excessive heat (> 40°C; 104°F), strong fluorescent lighting and alkaline materials.

Rx	**Nitrofurazone** (Various, eg, Clay-Park, Thames)	**Topical Solution:** 0.2%	In pt and gal.
Rx	**Furacin** (Roberts)		In 480 ml.
Rx	**Nitrofurazone** (Various, eg, Clay-Park, Rugby)	**Ointment (soluble):** 0.2%	In 480 g.
Rx	**Furacin Soluble Dressing** (Roberts)		In a polyethylene glycol base. In 28, 56 and 454 g.
Rx	**Furacin** (Roberts)	**Cream:** 0.2%	Cetyl alcohol, mineral oil, parabens. Water-miscible base. In 28 g.

MAFENIDE

Actions:

Pharmacology: Mafenide, a sulfonamide, is bacteriostatic against many gram-negative and gram-positive organisms, including *Pseudomonas aeruginosa* and certain strains of anaerobes. It is active in the presence of pus and serum; its activity is not altered by changes in the acidity of the environment.

Mafenide reduces the bacterial population present in the avascular tissues of second and third degree burns. This permits spontaneous healing of deep partial-thickness burns and prevents conversion of burn wounds from partial thickness to full thickness. However, delayed eschar separation has occurred in some cases.

Pharmacokinetics: Applied topically, mafenide diffuses through devascularized areas and is absorbed and rapidly metabolized to p-carboxybenzenesulfonamide which is cleared through the kidneys. The metabolite has no antibacterial activity but retains the ability to inhibit carbonic anhydrase.

Indications:

Burn treatment: Adjunctive therapy of second and third degree burns.

Contraindications:

Hypersensitivity to the drug. It is a not known whether there is cross-sensitivity to other sulfonamides.

Warnings:

Renal function impairment: Use with caution in patients with acute renal failure.

Pregnancy: Category C. It is not known whether mafenide can cause fetal harm when administered to a pregnant woman or can affect reproduction capacity. Not recommended for the treatment of women of childbearing potential unless the burned area covers > 20% of the total body surface or benefit is greater than the possible risk to the fetus.

Lactation: It is not known whether mafenide is excreted in breast milk. Because of the potential for serious adverse reactions in nursing infants, decide whether to discontinue nursing or discontinue the drug, taking into account the importance of the drug to the mother.

Children: Use the same administration and dosage as for adults.

Precautions:

For external use only: Avoid contact with eyes.

Metabolic acidosis: Mafenide and its metabolite inhibit carbonic anhydrase, which may result in metabolic acidosis, usually compensated by hyperventilation. In the presence of renal function impairment, high blood levels of mafenide and its metabolite may exaggerate the carbonic anhydrase inhibition. Therefore, close monitoring of acid-base balance is necessary, particularly in patients with extensive second degree or partial thickness burns and in those with pulmonary and renal dysfunction. Some burn patients treated with mafenide have also manifested an unexplained syndrome of marked hyperventilation with resulting respiratory alkalosis (slightly alkaline blood pH, low arterial pCO_2 and decreased total CO_2); change in arterial pO_2 is variable. The etiology and significance of these findings are unknown.

If acidosis occurs and becomes difficult to control, particularly in patients with pulmonary dysfunction, discontinuing therapy for 24 to 48 hours while continuing fluid therapy may aid in restoring acid-base balance.

Superinfection: Use may result in bacterial or fungal overgrowth of nonsusceptible organisms. Such overgrowth may lead to a secondary infection. Appropriate measures should be taken if superinfection occurs.

Fungal colonization in and below the eschar may occur concomitantly with reduction of bacterial growth in the burn wound. However, fungal dissemination through the infected burn wound is rare.

Sulfite sensitivity: Some of these products contain sulfites that may cause allergic-type reactions (including anaphylactic symptoms and life-threatening or less severe asthmatic episodes) in certain susceptible people. The overall prevalence of sulfite sensitivity in the general population is unknown and probably low. It is seen more frequently in asthmatic or atopic nonasthmatic people. Specific products containing sulfites are identified in the product listings.

MAFENIDE

Adverse Reactions:

It is difficult to distinguish a reaction to mafenide from the effect of a severe burn.

Allergic: Rash; itching; facial edema; swelling; hives; blisters; erythema; eosinophilia.

Dermatologic: Pain on application or a burning sensation (most frequent); excoriation of new skin, bleeding of skin (rare).

Respiratory: Tachypnea or hyperventilation; decrease in arterial pCO_2.

Metabolic: Acidosis; increase in serum chloride.

Miscellaneous: Bone marrow depression, acute attack of porphyria (one case each); fatal hemolytic anemia with disseminated intravascular coagulation, presumably related to a glucose-6-phosphate dehydrogenase deficiency; diarrhea due to accidental ingestion.

Patient Information:

Notify physician if condition worsens, if irritation occurs or if hyperventilation occurs.

Bathe burned area daily; a whirlpool bath is particularly helpful.

Continue treatment until healing occurs or until site is ready for grafting.

Administration and Dosage:

Application: Apply to the clean and debrided wound with a sterile gloved hand, once or twice daily, to a thickness of approximately 1⁄16 inch; thicker application is not recommended. Cover the burned areas with mafenide at all times. Reapply to any areas from which it has been removed (eg, by patient activity). Dressings are usually not required, but if necessary, use only a thin layer of dressing.

Bathing: When feasible, bathe the patient daily to aid in debridement. A whirlpool bath is particularly helpful, but the patient may be bathed in bed or in a shower.

Duration of therapy: Continue treatment until healing is progressing well or until the site is ready for grafting. Do not withdraw mafenide while infection is still possible. However, if allergic manifestations occur, consider discontinuing treatment.

Storage: Avoid exposure to excessive heat (> 40°C; 104°F).

Rx	**Sulfamylon** (Dow B. Hickam)	**Cream:** 85 mg (as acetate) per g	EDTA, cetyl alcohol, stearyl alcohol, parabens. sodium metabisulfite. In 37, 114 and 411 g.

SILVER SULFADIAZINE

Actions:

Pharmacology: Silver sulfadiazine acts only on the cell membrane and cell wall to produce its bactericidal effect. Silver is slowly released from the preparation in concentrations that are selectively toxic to bacteria. It is not a carbonic anhydrase inhibitor.

Reduction in bacterial growth after application of topical antibacterial agents has been reported to permit spontaneous healing of deep partial thickness burns by preventing conversion of the partial thickness to full thickness by sepsis. However, reduction in bacterial colonization has caused delayed separation, in some cases necessitating escharotomy in order to prevent contracture.

Pharmacokinetics: While ≤ 1% of the silver content is absorbed, up to 10% of the sulfadiazine may be absorbed. Serum concentrations of 10 to 20 mcg/ml have been reported when extensive areas were involved.

Microbiology: Silver sulfadiazine is bactericidal for many gram-negative and gram-positive bacteria and is effective against yeast. Silver sulfadiazine will inhibit bacteria resistant to other antimicrobial agents and is superior to sulfadiazine.

Organisms Generally Susceptible to Silver Sulfadiazine		
Pseudomonas aeruginosa	*Proteus mirabilis*	*Staphylococcus epidermidis*
Pseudomonas maltophilia	*Morganella morganii*	*β-hemolytic streptococcus*
Enterobacter species	*Providencia rettgeri*	*Enterococcus* species
Enterobacter cloacae	*Proteus vulgaris*	*Candida albicans*
Klebsiella species	*Providencia* species	*Corynebacterium diphtheriae*
Escherichia coli	*Citrobacter* species	*Clostridium perfringens*
Serratia species	*Acinetobacter calcoaceticus*	
	Staphylococcus aureus	

Indications:

Burn treatment: As an adjunct for prevention and treatment of sepsis in second and third degree burns.

Contraindications:

Hypersensitivity to the contents of the preparation; pregnant women at or near term, premature infants, infants ≤ 2 months old (sulfonamides may increase the possibility of kernicterus).

Warnings:

G-6–PD deficiency: Use in glucose-6-phosphate dehydrogenase-deficient individuals may be hazardous, as hemolysis may occur.

Fungal colonization in and below the eschar may occur; however, incidence of fungal superinfection is low.

Serum sulfonamide concentrations: In the treatment of burn wounds involving extensive areas of the body, the serum sulfa concentration may approach adult therapeutic levels (8 to 12 mg/dl). Therefore, in these patients, monitor serum sulfa concentrations. Monitor renal function carefully and check the urine for sulfa crystals.

Leukopenia (< 5000 WBC/mm^3) has been reported which reverted to normal upon drug discontinuation or recovered spontaneously. Leukopenia associated with silver sulfadiazine administration is primarily characterized by decreased neutrophil count. Maximal WBC depression occurs within 2 to 4 days of initiation of therapy. Rebound to normal leukocyte levels follows onset within 2 to 3 days. Recovery is not influenced by continuation of silver sulfadiazine therapy. The incidence of leukopenia averages about 20%. An increased incidence of leukopenia has been reported in patients treated concurrently with cimetidine.

Hypersensitivity: There is potential cross-sensitivity between silver sulfadiazine and other sulfonamides. If allergic reactions attributable to silver sulfadiazine occur, continuation of therapy must be weighed against the potential hazards of the particular allergic reaction. Refer to Management of Acute Hypersensitivity Reactions.

Renal/Hepatic function impairment: If hepatic or renal function becomes impaired and drug elimination decreases, accumulation may occur. Weigh discontinuation against the therapeutic benefit being achieved.

*Pregnancy: Category B.*There are no adequate and well controlled studies in pregnant women. Use during pregnancy only if clearly justified, especially in pregnant women approaching or at term.

Lactation: It is not known whether silver sulfadiazine cream is excreted in breast milk. However, sulfonamides are excreted in breast milk and all sulfonamide derivatives increase the possibility of kernicterus. Decide whether to discontinue nursing or to discontinue the drug, taking into acccount the importance of the drug to the mother.

Children: Safety and efficacy have not been established.

SILVER SULFADIAZINE

Precautions:

For external use only: Avoid contact with eyes.

Reduction in bacterial colonization has caused delayed separation, in some cases necessitating escharotomy to prevent contracture.

Absorption of silver sulfadiazine varies depending upon the percent of the body surface area and the extent of the tissue damage. Although few have been reported, since significant quantities of sulfadiazine are absorbed, it is possible that any of the adverse reactions attributable to sulfonamides may occur (see monograph in Anti-Infectives chapter).

Drug Interactions:

Topical proteolytic enzymes: Silver may inactivate such enzymes if these agents are used in conjunction with silver sulfadiazine.

Drug/Lab test interactions: Absorption of the propylene glycol vehicle, affecting serum osmolality, has occurred.

Adverse Reactions:

Leukopenia (20%; see Warnings); skin necrosis, erythema multiforme, skin discoloration, burning sensation, rashes, interstitial nephritis (infrequent).

Administration and Dosage:

Application: Apply under sterile conditions once or twice daily to a thickness of approximately 1/16 inch to the clean and debrided wound. Cover the burn areas with silver sulfadiazine at all times. Whenever necessary, reapply the cream to any areas from which it has been removed by patient activity. Reapply immediately after hydrotherapy. Dressings are not required, but may be used if individual patient requirements make them necessary.

Bathing: When feasible, bathe patient daily to aid in debridement. A whirlpool bath is particularly helpful, but the patient may be bathed in bed or in a shower.

Duration of therapy: Continue treatment until satisfactory healing occurs or until the site is ready for grafting. Do not withdraw the drug while the possibility of infection remains, unless a significant adverse reaction occurs.

Rx	**SSD Cream** (Boots)	**Cream**: 10 mg per g in a water-miscible base[1]	Cetyl alcohol. In 25, 50, 85, 400 and 1000 g.
Rx	**Silvadene** (Hoescht Marion Roussel)		In 20, 50, 85, 400 and 1000 g.
Rx	**Thermazene** (Sherwood)		In 50, 400 and 1000 g.
Rx	**SSD AF Cream** (Boots)		In 50, 400 and 1000 g.

[1] Contains white petrolatum, stearyl alcohol, 0.3% methylparaben.

SUNSCREENS

Actions:

Pharmacology: Sunscreens provide either a chemical or a physical barrier to sunlight. These agents help to prevent sunburn, actinic keratosis, premature aging, photosensitivity reactions, and to reduce incidences of skin cancer. Chemical sunscreens act by absorbing ultraviolet (UV) radiation in the medium wavelength range of 290 to 320 nm (UVB range). This is the spectrum of UV radiation primarily responsible for sunburning and inducing skin cancer. UVA may augment the carcinogenic effects of UVB. Long wavelength UV radiation in the 320 to 400 nm (UVA range) can cause tanning and is responsible for most photosensitivity reactions that occur with many drugs, plants, soaps and cosmetics; it is also a major risk factor for serious skin damage. UVA irradiation can exceed that of UVB by 10 to 1000 fold. UVA deeply penetrates into the dermis; UVB is primarily absorbed in the epidermis.There has been discussion of dividing UVA into UVA I (340 to 400 nm) and UVA II (320 to 340 nm); besides UVB, UVA II may cause the most skin damage. Physical sunscreens reflect or scatter light in both the visible and UV spectrum (290 to 700 nm), preventing penetration of the skin.

UV radiation in the 200 to 290 nm band is known as UVC; although little reaches the earth from the sun, some artificial sources emit UVC. UVC is thought to cause some erythema of the skin.

Sunscreen effectiveness is dependent on UV absorption spectrum, concentration, vehicle and ability to withstand swimming or sweating.

Sunscreen Ingredients

	Sunscreens	UV spectrum (nm)	Concentrations (%)
Chemical	*Benzophenones*	UVA and UVB	
	Oxybenzone	270-350	2-6
	Dioxybenzone	260-380[1]	3
	PABA and PABA esters	UVB	
	p-aminobenzoic acid	260-313	5-15
	Ethyl dihydroxy propyl PABA	280-330	1-5
	Padimate O (octyl dimethyl PABA)	290-315	1.4-8
	Glyceryl PABA	264-315	2-3
	Cinnamates	UVB[2]	
	Cinoxate	270-328	1-3
	Ethylhexyl p-methoxycinnamate	290-320	2-7.5
	Octocrylene	250-360	7-10
	Octyl methoxycinnamate	290-320	—
	Salicylates	UVB[3]	
	Ethylhexyl salicylate	280-320	3-5
	Homosalate	295-315	4-15
	Octyl salicylate	280-320	3-5
	Miscellaneous	UVB	
	Menthyl anthranilate	260-380[4]	3.5-5
	Digalloyl trioleate	270-320	2-5
	Avobenzone (butyl-methoxy-dibenzoylmethane; Parsol 1789)	UVA 320-400	3
Physical	Titanium dioxide	290-700	2-25
	Red petrolatum	290-365[5]	30-100
	Zinc oxide	290-700	—

[1] Values available when used in combination with other screens.
[2] Some UVA spectrum.
[3] Primarily UVB, but has about ⅓ the absorbency of PABA.
[4] Values are for concentrations higher than normally found in nonprescription drugs.
[5] At 334 nm, 16% UV radiation is transmitted; at 365 nm, 58% is transmitted.

Indications:

Sunburn prevention. Overexposure to the sun may cause premature skin aging and skin cancer. The liberal and regular use of these products may help reduce the occurrence of these harmful effects.

For persons with conditions such as systemic lupus erythematosus, solar urticaria, erythropoietic protoporphyria or those taking photosensitizing drugs. Following is a partial list of drugs that may cause photosensitivity:

Antihistamines (eg, cyproheptadine, diphenhydramine)
Anti-infectives (eg, tetracyclines, nalidixic acid, sulfonamides)
Antineoplastic agents (eg, fluorouracil, methotrexate, procarbazine)
Antipsychotic agents (eg, phenothiazines, haloperidol)
Diuretics (eg, thiazides, acetazolamide, amiloride)
Hypoglycemic agents (eg, sulfonylureas)
Nonsteroidal anti-inflammatory drugs (eg, phenylbutazone, ketoprofen, naproxen)
Miscellaneous (eg, bergamot oils, etc, used in cosmetics; coal tar; psoralens; amiodarone; oral contraceptives; quinidine; disopyramide; gold salts; isotretinoin; captopril; carbamazepine)

Precautions:

Sensitivity: Avoid prolonged exposure to sun and to tanning lamps. Sun-sensitive persons particularly should exercise caution. If irritation or sensitization occurs, discontinue use.

Do not use sunscreens containing PABA or its derivatives if sensitive to benzocaine, procaine, sulfonamides, thiazides, PABA or PABA esters.

For external use only: Avoid contact with eyes.

Vehicle: Do not use sunscreens in highly alcoholic vehicles on eczematous or inflamed skin.

PABA may cause a permanent yellow stain on clothing.

Vitamin D deficiency may occur in elderly patients; sunscreens that block UV-B may block cutaneous vitamin D synthesis.

UV exposure: The amount of UV exposure is influenced by many factors (eg, time of day, season, latitude, altitude, atmospheric conditions). UVB radiation is strongest between 10 am and 2 pm; UVA is relatively constant. Each 1000 foot increase in altitude adds 4% to UV light intensity. Reflectance from water depends on the angle of exposure, with almost 100% when the sun is directly overhead. Fresh snow reflects approximately 85% to 100% of UV light, and sand reflects 20% to 25%.

Adverse Reactions:

Contact dermatitis may develop with PABA or its esters (especially glyceryl PABA), benzophenones and cinnamates. Physical sunscreens are occlusive; miliaria or folliculitis may occur.

Patient Information:

Follow directions on product container concerning frequency of application; reapply after swimming or sweating. Reapplication does not extend the protection period.

For external use only. Do not swallow. Avoid contact with the eyes.

Discontinue use if signs of irritation or rash appear.

PABA may permanently stain clothing yellow.

Wear protective eye coverings or sunglasses; UV light can cause corneal damage.

Administration and Dosage:

Apply liberally to all exposed areas (2 mg/cm^2 is recommended) at least 30 minutes prior to sun exposure (up to 2 hours for aminobenzoic acid and its esters) to allow for penetration and binding to the skin. Reapply after swimming or excessive sweating.

Children: Do not use sunscreens on infants < 6 months old. Do not use SPFs as low as 2 or 3 on children < 2 years of age.

Sun protection factor (SPF): Sunscreen products include SPF ratings. This factor indicates the amount of increased resistance to sunburning the product provides, relative to unprotected skin. The SPF value is based on a numerical index designed to tell how much protection from the sun a product will provide. The SPF value is defined as the ratio of the amount of energy required to produce a minimal erythema dose (MED) or minimal sunburn through a film of a sunscreen drug product to the amount of energy required to produce the same MED without any treatment. (Example: Using a product with an SPF value of 6 would permit 6 times as much sun exposure.) Base product selection on the patient's history of response to sun exposure.

SUNSCREENS

Recommended Sunscreen Product Guide[1]

Skin type	Patient characteristics[2]	Suggested product SPF
I	Always burns easily; rarely tans	20 to 30
II	Always burns easily; tans minimally	12 to < 20
III	Burns moderately; tans gradually	8 to < 12
IV	Burns minimally; always tans well	4 to < 8
V	Rarely burns; tans profusely	2 to < 4
VI[3]	Never burns; deeply pigmented (insensitive)	None indicated

[1] Based on the FDA's tentative final monograph (TFM) for sunscreen products.
[2] Based on first 45 to 60 minutes sun exposure after winter season or no sun exposure.
[3] This skin type not included in TFM.

Waterproof formulas maintain sunburn protection after being in the water up to 80 minutes.

Water resistant formulas maintain sunburn protection after being in the water up to 40 minutes.

Sweat resistant formulas maintain protection after ≤ 30 minutes of continuous heavy perspiration.

SPFs > 15 were not recommended by the 1978 FDA advisory panel on sunscreens. However, the agency issued a tentative final monograph on this product class in May 1993, and is proposing an upper limit for SPF values of 30. Scientific evidence shows a point of diminishing returns at levels > SPF 30; any benefits that might be derived from using sunscreens with SPFs > 30 are negligible. An SPF of at least 15 for most individuals is recommended by the Skin Cancer Foundation.

In addition to the products listed on the following pages, there are other sunscreens available from various cosmetic manufacturers.

		SPF		
otc	**Hawaiian Tropic Baby Faces Sunblock** (Tanning Research)	50	**Lotion**: Titanium dioxide, octyl methoxycinnamate, octocrylene, benzophenone-3, octyl salicylate	PABA free. Waterproof. In 120 ml.
otc	**SolBar PF** (Person & Covey)	50	**Cream**: Oxybenzone, octyl methoxycinnamate, octocrylene	PABA free. Waterproof. In 120 g.
otc	**Presun Moisturizing** (Bristol-Myers)	46	**Lotion**: Octyl dimethyl PABA, oxybenzone, cetyl alcohol, diazolidinyl urea	Waterproof. In 120 ml.
otc	**Hawaiian Tropic Sunblock** (Tanning Research)	45+	**Lotion**: Titanium dioxide, octyl methoxycinnamate, benzophenone-3, octyl salicylate, octocrylene	PABA free. Waterproof. In 120 and 300 ml.
otc	**Coppertone Moisturizing Sunblock** (Schering-Plough)	45	**Lotion**: Ethylhexyl p-methoxycinnamate, 2-ethylhexyl salicylate, octocrylene, oxybenzone	PABA free. Waterproof. In 120 and 300 ml.
otc	**Shade Sunblock** (Schering-Plough)	45	**Lotion**: Ethylhexyl p–methoxycinnamate, octocrylene, oxybenzone, 2–ethylhexyl salicylate	Waterproof. In 120 ml.
otc	**Water Babies UVA/UVB Sunblock** (Schering-Plough)	45	**Lotion**: Ethylhexyl p–methoxycinnamate, 2–ethylhexyl salicylate, octocrylene, oxybenzone	PABA free. Waterproof. In 120 ml.
otc	**Hawaiian Tropic Just For Kids Sunblock** (Tanning Research)	45	**Lotion**: Octyl methoxycinnamate, benzophenone-3, octyl salicylate, octocrylene, titanium dioxide	PABA free. Waterproof, all day protection. In 88.7 ml.
otc	**Vaseline Intensive Care Blockout** (Chesebrough Pond's)	40	**Lotion**: Padimate, ethylhexyl p-methoxycinnamate, oxybenzone, 2-ethylhexyl salicylate, titanium dioxide.	Waterproof. In 120 ml.

SUNSCREENS

		SPF		
otc	**Bullfrog Sunblock** (Chattem)	36	**Gel**: Benzophenone-3, octocrylene, octyl methoxycinnamate, aloe, vitamin E, isostearyl alcohol	PABA free. Waterproof, all day protection. In 120 g.
otc	**Hawaiian Tropic Baby Faces Sunblock** (Tanning Research)	35	**Lotion:** Octyl methoxycinnamate, benzophenone-3, octyl salicylate, titanium dioxide, octocrylene	PABA free. Waterproof, all day protection. In 60, 120 and 300 ml.
otc	**Hawaiian Tropic Sunblock** (Tanning Research)	30+	**Lotion:** Homosalate, octyl methoxycinnamate, benzophenone-3, menthyl anthranilate, octyl salicylate	PABA free. Waterproof, all day protection. In 120 ml.
otc	**Vaseline Intensive Care Baby 30+ Moisturizing Sunblock** (Chesebrough Pond's)	30+	**Lotion:** Ethylhexyl p-methoxycinnamate, oxybenzone, 2-ethylhexyl salicylate, titanium dioxide, C12-15 alkyl benzoate, glycerin, aloe vera gel, vitamin E, cetyl alcohol, parabens, EDTA	PABA free. Waterproof. In 180 ml.
otc	**DuraScreen** (Schwarz Pharma)	30	**Lotion:** Octyl methoxycinnamate, octyl salicylate, oxybenzone, 2-phenylbenzimidazole-5-sulfonic acid, titanium dioxide, cetearyl alcohol, diazolidinyl urea, shea butter	PABA free. Waterproof. In 105 ml.
otc	**Neutrogena No-Stick Sunscreen** (Neutrogena)	30	**Cream:** 15% homosalate, 7.5% octyl methoxycinnamate, 6% benzophenone-3, 5% octyl salicylate	EDTA, parabens, diazolidinyl urea. In 118 g.
otc	**Johnson's Baby Sunblock Extra Protection** (Johnson & Johnson)	30	**Lotion:** Octyl methoxycinnamate, octyl salicylate, titanium dioxide, oxybenzone, C12-15 alcohols benzoate, cetyl alcohol, EDTA, vitamin E	PABA free. Waterproof. In 120 ml.
otc	**TI·Screen** (Pedinol)	30	**Lotion:** 7.5% octyl methoxycinnamate, 6% oxybenzone, 5% octyl salicylate, 7.5% octocrylene	PABA free. Waterproof. In 120 ml.
otc	**PreSun Active** (Bristol-Myers)	30	**Gel:** Octyl methoxycinnamate, oxybenzone, octyl salicylate, 69% SD alcohol 40	PABA free. Waterproof, non-greasy. In 120 ml.
otc	**Sundown Sunblock** (Johnson & Johnson)	30	**Lotion:** Octyl methoxycinnamate, octyl salicylate, oxybenzone, titanium dioxide	PABA free. Waterproof, non-greasy. In 120 ml.
otc	**Bain de Soleil All Day for Kids** (Procter & Gamble)	30	**Lotion:** Ethylhexyl p-methoxycinnamate, 2-ethylhexyl 2-cyano-3, 3-diphenylacrylate, oxybenzone, titanium dioxide, stearyl alcohol, vitamin E, EDTA	PABA free. Waterproof. In 120 ml.
otc	**Bain de Soleil All Day Waterproof Sunblock** (Procter & Gamble)	30	**Lotion:** Ethylhexyl p-methoxycinnamate, 2-ethylhexyl 2-cyano-3, 3-diphenylacrylate, oxybenzone, titanium dioxide, stearyl alcohol, vitamin E, EDTA	PABA free. Waterproof, non-greasy, all day protection. In 120 ml.
otc	**Coppertone Moisturizing Sunblock** (Schering-Plough)	30	**Lotion:** Ethylhexyl p-methoxycinnamate, oxybenzone, 2-ethylhexyl salicylate, homosalate	PABA free. Waterproof. In 120 and 240 ml.
otc	**Coppertone Sport** (Schering-Plough)	30	**Lotion:** Ethylhexyl p-methoxycinnamate, oxybenzone, 2-ethylhexyl salicylate	PABA free. Waterproof. In 120 ml.

SUNSCREENS

		SPF		
otc	**Shade Sunblock** (Schering-Plough)	30	**Stick:** Ethylhexyl p–methoxy-cinnamate, oxybenzone, 2-ethylhexyl salicylate, homosalate	Waterproof. In 18 g.
otc	**Shade Sunblock** (Schering-Plough)	30	**Lotion:** Ethylhexyl p–methoxy-cinnamate, 2–ethylhexyl salicylate, homosalate, oxybenzone	Waterproof. In 120 ml.
otc	**Shade Sunblock** (Schering-Plough)	30	**Gel:** Ethylhexyl p-methoxy-cinnamate, homosalate, oxybenzone, 73% SD alcohol 40	Waterproof. Oil free. In 120 g.
otc	**Tropical Gold Sunblock** (Goldline)	30	**Lotion:** Ethylhexyl p-methoxycinnamate, 2-ethylhexyl salicylate, homosalate, oxybenzone, aloe extract, vitamin E, vegetable and jojoba oils, benzyl alcohol, imidazolidinyl urea, parabens, EDTA	PABA free. Waterproof. In 118 ml.
otc	**Water Babies UVA/ UVB Sunblock** (Schering-Plough)	30	**Lotion:** Ethylhexyl p–methoxy-cinnamate, 2–ethylhexyl salicylate, homosalate, oxybenzone	PABA free. Waterproof. In 120 and 240 ml.
otc	**Hawaiian Tropic Just For Kids Sunblock** (Tanning Research)	30	**Lotion:** Homosalate, octyl methoxy-cinnamate, benzophenone-3, menthyl anthranilate, octyl salicylate	PABA free. Waterproof, all day protection. In 88.7 ml.
otc	**Hawaiian Tropic Sport Sunblock** (Tanning Research)	30	**Lotion:** Octyl methoxycinnamate, octocrylene, benzophenone-3, octyl salicylate, titanium dioxide	PABA free. Waterproof, all day protection. In 88.7 ml.
otc	**SolBar PF** (Person & Covey)	30	**Liquid:** 10% octocrylene, 7.5% octyl methoxycinnamate, 6% oxybenzone, 77% SD alcohol 40	PABA free. In 114 ml.
otc	**Bain de Soleil SPF 30 + Color** (Procter & Gamble)	30	**Lotion:** Octocrylene, octyl methoxy-cinnamate, oxybenzone, mineral oil, cetyl alcohol, EDTA	Waterproof. In 118 ml.
otc	**Coppertone Kids Sunblock** (Schering-Plough)	30	**Lotion:** Octocrylene, ethylhexyl p-methoxycinnamate, oxybenzone, 2-ethylhexyl salicylate	PABA free. Waterproof. In 120 and 240 ml.
otc	**Neutrogena Sunblock** (Neutrogena)	30	**Cream:** Octocrylene, octyl methoxy-cinnamate, menthyl anthranilate, zinc oxide, mineral oil, vitamin E	PABA free. Waterproof. In 67.5 g.
otc	**Tréo** (Biopharm Lab[1])	30	**Lotion:** Octocrylene, octyl methoxy-cinnamate, benzophenone-3, octyl salicylate, isostearyl alcohol, diazolidinyl urea, propylparabens. Also contains 0.05% citronella oil as an insect repellent	PABA free. Waterproof. In 118 ml.
otc	**PreSun Sensitive Skin Sunscreen** (Bristol-Myers)	29	**Lotion:** Octyl methoxycinnamate, oxybenzone, octyl salicylate, cetyl alcohol, diazolidinyl urea	PABA free. Waterproof. In 120 ml.
otc	**PreSun for Kids** (Bristol-Myers)	29	**Lotion:** Octyl methoxycinnamate, oxybenzone, octyl salicylate, cetyl alcohol, diazolidinyl urea	PABA free. Waterproof. In 120 ml.
otc	**Coppertone Moisturizing Sunblock** (Schering-Plough)	25	**Lotion:** Ethylhexyl p-methoxy-cinnamate, oxybenzone, 2-ethylhexyl salicylate, homosalate	PABA free, Waterproof. In 120 ml.

SUNSCREENS

		SPF		
otc	**Vaseline Intensive Care Moisturizing Sunblock** (Chesebrough Pond's)	25	**Lotion:** Ethylhexyl p-methoxycinnamate, oxybenzone, 2-ethylhexyl salicylate, glycerin, aloe vera gel, C12-15 alkyl benzoate, cetyl alcohol, petrolatum, vitamin E, parabens, EDTA	PABA free, Waterproof. In 118 ml.
otc	**Neutrogena Sunblock Stick** (Neutrogena)	25	**Stick:** Octyl methoxycinnamate, benzophenone-3, octyl salicylate, castor oil, cetearyl alcohol, propylparaben, shea butter	PABA free. Waterproof. In 12.6 g.
otc	**PreSun Moisturizing Sunscreen with Keri** (Bristol-Myers)	25	**Lotion:** Octyl methoxycinnamate, oxybenzone, octyl salicylate, petrolatum, cetyl alcohol, diazolidinyl urea	Waterproof. In 120 ml.
otc	**PreSun Spray Mist** (Bristol-Myers)	23	**Spray Mist:** Octyl dimethyl PABA, octyl methoxycinnamate, oxybenzone, octyl salicylate, 19% SD alcohol 40, C12-15 alcohols benzoate	Waterproof. In 105 ml.
otc	**PreSun for Kids Spray Mist** (Bristol-Myers)			Waterproof. In 105 ml.
otc	**TI-Screen Sunless** (Pedinol)	23	**Creme:** 7.5% octyl methoxycinnamate, 3% benzophenone-3.	Mineral oil, alcohols, PEG-100, parabens. In 188 ml.
otc	**TI •Screen** (Pedinol)	20+	**Gel:** 7.5% ethylhexyl p-methoxycinnamate, 5% oxybenzone, 5% 2-ethylhexyl salicylate, 71% SD alcohol 40	PABA free. In 120 g.
otc	**Eucerin Dry Skin Care Daily Facial** (Beiersdorf)	20	**Lotion:** Ethylhexyl p-methoxycinnamate, titanium dioxide, 2-phenylbenzimidazole-5-sulfonic acid, 2-ethylhexyl salicylate, mineral oil, cetearyl alcohol, castor oil, lanolin alcohol, EDTA	In 120 ml.
otc	**Hawaiian Tropic Baby Faces** (Tanning Research)	20	**Gel:** Octyl methoxycinnamate, octocrylene, benzophenone-3, menthyl anthranilate	PABA free. Waterproof. In 120 g.
otc	**Bullfrog Sunblock** (Chattem)	18	**Gel:** Octocrylene, benzophenone-3, octyl methoxycinnamate, isostearyl alcohol, vitamin E, aloe	PABA free. Waterproof, all day protection. In 120 g.
otc	**Bullfrog** (Chattem)	18	**Stick:** Benzophenone-3, octyl methoxycinnamate, isostearyl alcohol, aloe, hydrogenated vegetable oil, vitamin E	Waterproof. In 16.5 g.
otc	**Bullfrog Extra Moisturizing Gel** (Chattem)	18	**Gel:** Benzophenone-3, octocrylene, octyl methoxycinnamate, vitamin E, aloe	PABA free. Waterproof, all day protection. In 90 g.
otc	**Bullfrog Sport Lotion** (Chattem)	18	**Lotion:** Benzophenone-3, octocrylene, octyl methoxycinnamate, octyl salicylate, titanium dioxide, diazolidinyl urea, EDTA, parabens, vitamin E, aloe	Waterproof, all day protection. In 120 ml.
otc	**Bullfrog for Kids** (Chattem)	18	**Gel:** Octocrylene, octyl methoxycinnamate, octyl salicylate, vitamin E, aloe, C12-15 alcohols benzoate	Waterproof, non-greasy, all day protection. In 60 g.

SUNSCREENS

		SPF		
otc	**TI-Screen Sunless** (Pedinol)	17	**Creme:** 7.5% octyl methoxycinnamate, 3% benzophenone-3.	Mineral oil, alcohols, PEG-100, parabens. In 118 ml.
otc	**Neutrogena Chemical-Free Sunblocker** (Neutrogena)	17	**Lotion:** Titanium dioxide, parabens, diazolidinyl urea, shea butter	PABA free. In 120 ml.
otc	**SUNPRuF 17** (C&M)	17	**Gel:** 7.8% octyl methoxycinnamate, 5.2% octyl salicylate	Oil free, water-resistant. In 120 g.
otc	**TI•Baby Natural** (Pedinol)	16	**Lotion:** 5% titanium dioxide	PABA free. Waterproof. In 120 ml.
otc	**TI•Screen Natural** (Pedinol)	16	**Lotion:** 5% titanium dioxide	PABA free. Waterproof. In 120 ml.
otc	**Hawaiian Tropic 15 Plus Sunblock** (Tanning Research)	15+	**Lotion:** Menthyl anthranilate, octyl methoxycinnamate, benzophenone-3	PABA free. Waterproof, all day protection. In 7.5, 15, 60, 120, 240 and 300 ml.
otc	**Hawaiian Tropic 15 Plus** (Tanning Research)	15+	**Gel:** Octyl methoxycinnamate, octocrylene, benzophenone-3, menthyl anthranilate	PABA free. Waterproof, all day protection. In 120 g.
otc	**TI•Screen** (Pedinol)	15+	**Lotion:** 7.5% ethylhexyl p-methoxycinnamate, 5% oxybenzone	PABA free. Water resistant. In 120 ml.
otc	**Sundown Sport Sunblock** (Johnson & Johnson)	15	**Lotion:** Titanium dioxide, zinc oxide	PABA free. Waterproof. In 90 ml.
otc	**Vaseline Intensive Care Baby Sunblock** (Chesebrough Pond's)	15	**Lotion:** Titanium dioxide, zinc oxide, mineral oil, glycerin, EDTA	PABA free. Waterproof. In 177 ml.
otc	**TI•Lite** (Pedinol)	15	**Cream:** 7.5% ethylhexyl p-methoxycinnamate, 2% titanium dioxide, cetyl alcohol, phenethyl alcohol, parabens, EDTA	In 60 g.
otc	**Aquaderm** (Baker Cummins)	15	**Cream:** 7.5% octyl methoxycinnamate, 6% oxybenzone	In 105 g.
otc	**SolBar PF Sunscreen** (Person & Covey)	15	**Liquid:** 7.5% octyl methoxycinnamate, 5% oxybenzone, 76% SD alcohol 40	PABA free. In 120 ml.
otc	**SUNPRuF 15** (C&M)	15	**Lotion:** 7.5% octyl methoxycinnamate, 5% benzophenone-3	PABA free. Water-resistant. In 240 ml.
otc	**Bain de Soleil SPF 15 + Color** (Procter & Gamble)	15	**Lotion:** Octyl methoxycinnamate, octocrylene, oxybenzone, mineral oil, cetyl alcohol, EDTA	Waterproof. In 118 ml.
otc	**Catrix Correction** (Donell DerMedex)	15	**Cream:** Octyl methoxycinnamate, menthyl anthranilate, benzophenone 3, titanium dioxide, sesame oil, cetearyl alcohol, urea, EDTA, imidazolidinyl urea, parabens	PABA free. In 39 g.

SUNSCREENS

		SPF		
otc	**Oil of Olay Daily UV Protectant** (Procter & Gamble)	15	**Cream:** Octyl methoxycinnamate, phenylbenzimidazole sulfonic acid, glycerin, cetyl alcohol, titanium dioxide, imidazolidinyl urea, parabens, EDTA, castor oil	Scented or unscented. In 51g.
otc	**Bain de Soleil All Day Waterproof Sunblock** (Procter & Gamble)	15	**Lotion:** Ethylhexyl p-methoxycinnamate, 2-ethylhexyl 2-cyano-3, 3-diphenylacrylate, oxybenzone, titanium dioxide, stearyl alcohol, vitamin E, EDTA	PABA free. Waterproof, non-greasy, all day protection. In 120 ml.
otc	**Coppertone Sport** (Schering-Plough)	15	**Lotion:** Ethylhexyl p-methoxycinnamate, oxybenzone	PABA free. Waterproof. In 120 ml.
otc	**DuraScreen** (Schwarz Pharma)	15	**Lotion:** Ethylhexyl p-methoxycinnamate, 2-ethylhexyl salicylate, oxybenzone, cetyl alcohol, parabens	Waterproof. In 105 ml.
otc	**Shade Sunblock** (Schering-Plough)	15	**Gel:** Ethylhexyl p–methoxycinnamate, oxybenzone, 75% SD alcohol 40	Waterproof. Oil free. In 120 g.
otc	**Tropical Gold Sport Sunblock** (Goldline)	15	**Lotion:** Ethylhexyl p-methoxycinnamate, oxybenzone, diazolidinyl urea, parabens, aloe extract, jojoba oil, vitamin E, EDTA	PABA free. Perspiration proof. In 180 ml.
otc	**Tropical Gold Sunblock** (Goldline)	15	**Lotion:** Ethylhexyl p-methoxycinnamate, oxybenzone, vegetable oil, benzyl alcohol, parabens, imidazolidinyl urea, vitamin E, aloe extract, jojoba oil, EDTA	PABA free. Waterproof. In 118 ml.
otc	**Vaseline Intensive Care Moisturizing Sunblock** (Chesebrough Pond's)	15	**Lotion:** Ethylhexyl p-methoxycinnamate, oxybenzone, glycerin, aloe vera gel, cetyl alcohol, petrolatum, vitamin E, parabens, EDTA	PABA free. Waterproof. In 118 ml.
otc	**Vaseline Intensive Care Sport Sunblock** (Chesebrough Pond's)	15	**Lotion:** Ethylhexyl p-methoxycinnamate, oxybenzone, C12-15 alkyl benzoate, aloe vera gel, vitamin E, EDTA	PABA free. Waterproof, non-greasy. In 118 ml.
otc	**Coppertone Kids Sunblock** (Schering-Plough)	15	**Lotion:** Ethylhexyl p-methoxycinnamate, oxybenzone, 2-ethylhexyl salicylate, homosalate	PABA free. Waterproof. In 120 and 240 ml.
otc	**Coppertone Moisturizing Sunblock** (Schering-Plough)	15	**Lotion:** Ethylhexyl p-methoxycinnamate, oxybenzone	PABA free. Waterproof. In 120, 240 and 300 ml.
otc	**Faces Only Moisturizing Sunblock by Coppertone** (Schering-Plough)	15	**Lotion:** Ethylhexyl p-methoxycinnamate, oxybenzone	PABA free. In 55.5 ml.
otc	**Oil of Olay Daily UV Protectant** (Procter & Gamble)	15	**Lotion:** Ethylhexyl p-methoxycinnamate, 2-phenylbenzimidazole-5-sulfonic acid, titanium dioxide, cetyl alcohol, imidazolidinyl urea, parabens, EDTA, castor oil, tartrazine	PABA free. Greaseless. Scented or unscented. In 105 and 157.7 ml.
otc	**Vaseline Intensive Care Ultra Violet Daily Defense** (Chesebrough Pond's)	15	**Lotion:** Ethylhexyl p-methoxycinnamate, oxybenzone, vitamin E, cetyl alcohol, acetylated lanolin alcohol, parabens, EDTA	PABA free. Non-greasy. In 120 and 300 ml.

SUNSCREENS

		SPF		
otc	**Hawaiian Tropic Sport Sunblock** (Tanning Research)	15	**Lotion**: Octyl methoxycinnamate, benzophenone-3, octocrylene	PABA free. Waterproof, all day protection. In 88.7 ml.
otc	**Neutrogena Intensified Day Moisture** (Neutrogena)	15	**Cream**: Octyl methoxycinnamate, 2-phenylbenzimidazole sulfonic acid, titanium dioxide, cetyl alcohol, diazolidinyl urea, parabens, EDTA	PABA free. In 67.5 g.
otc	**Ray Block** (Del Ray)	15	**Lotion**: 5% octyl dimethyl PABA, 3% benzophenone-3, SD alcohol	In 118.3 ml.
otc	**Solex A15 Clear Lotion** (Dermol)	15	**Lotion**: 5% octyl dimethyl PABA, 33% benzophenone, SD alcohol	Non-oily. In 120 ml.
otc	**PreSun Sensitive Skin Sunscreen** (Bristol-Myers)	15	**Lotion**: Octyl methoxycinnamate, oxybenzone, octyl salicylate, cetyl alcohol, diazolidinyl urea	PABA free. Waterproof. In 120 ml.
otc	**Johnson's Baby Sunblock** (Johnson & Johnson)	15	**Lotion**: Hydrogenated castor oil, EDTA, hydroxylated lanolin, zinc oxide, mineral oil, titanium dioxide	PABA free. Waterproof. In 120 ml.
otc	**Total Eclipse Oily and Acne Prone Skin Sunscreen** (Triangle Labs)	15	**Lotion**: Padimate O, oxybenzone, glyceryl PABA, 77% alcohol	In 120 ml.
otc	**Total Eclipse Moisturizing** (Triangle Labs)	15	**Lotion**: Padimate O, oxybenzone, octyl salicylate	In 120 ml.
otc	**Shade UVAGuard** (Schering-Plough)	15	**Lotion**: 7.5% octyl methoxycinnamate, 3% avobenzone, 3% oxybenzone	Waterproof. In 120 ml.
otc	**SolBar Plus 15** (Person & Covey)	15	**Cream**: 4% oxybenzone, 2% dioxybenzone, 6% octyl dimethyl PABA	In 113 g.
otc	**PreSun Moisturizing Sunscreen with Keri** (Bristol-Myers)	15	**Lotion**: Octyl dimethyl PABA, oxybenzone, cetyl alcohol, diazolidinyl urea	Waterproof. In 120 ml.
otc	**SolBar PF** (Person & Covey)	15	**Cream**: 7.5% octyl methoxycinnamate, 5% oxybenzone	PABA free. In 222 g.
otc	**Sundown Sunblock** (Johnson & Johnson)	15	**Lotion**: Octyl methoxycinnamate, oxybenzone, octyl salicylate, titanium dioxide	PABA free. Waterproof, non-greasy. In 120 ml.
otc	**Water Babies UVA/UVB Sunblock** (Schering-Plough)	15	**Lotion**: Ethylhexyl p-methoxycinnamate, oxybenzone	PABA free. Waterproof. In 120 ml.
otc	**DML Facial Moisturizer** (Person & Covey)	15	**Cream**: 8% octyl methoxycinnamate, 4% oxybenzone, benzyl alcohol, petrolatum, EDTA	In 45 g.
otc	**Hawaiian Tropic Self Tanning Sunblock** (Tanning Research)	15	**Cream**: Octyl methoxycinnamate, benzophenone-3, aloe, cetyl alcohol, stearyl alcohol, cocoa butter, parabens, vitamin E	PABA free. In 93.75 ml.
otc	**Nivea Sun** (Beiersdorf)	15	**Lotion**: Octyl methoxycinnamate, octyl salicylate, benzophenone-3, 2-phenylbenzimidazole-5-sulfonic acid	PABA free. Waterproof. In 120 ml.
otc	**Neutrogena Moisture** (Neutrogena)	15	**Lotion**: Octyl methoxycinnamate, benzophenone-3, parabens, diazolidinyl urea	PABA free. In sheer tint and untinted. In 120 ml.

SUNSCREENS

		SPF		
otc	**Neutrogena Sunblock** (Neutrogena)	15	**Cream:** Octyl methoxycinnamate, octyl salicylate, menthyl anthranilate, mineral oil, titanium dioxide, propylparaben	PABA free. Waterproof. In 67.5 g.
otc	**PreSun Active** (Bristol-Myers)	15	**Gel:** Oxybenzone, octyl methoxycinnamate, octyl salicylate, SD alcohol 40	PABA free. Waterproof, non-greasy. In 120 g.
otc	**Tréo** (Biopharm Lab[1])	15	**Lotion:** Octocrylene, octyl methoxycinnamate, benzophenone-3, octyl salicylate, isostearyl alcohol, diazolidinyl urea, propylparabens. Also contains 0.05% citronella oil as an insect repellent	PABA free. Waterproof. In 118 ml.
otc	**Hawaiian Tropic 10 Plus** (Tanning Research)	10+	**Lotion:** Octyl methoxycinnamate, benzophenone-3, menthyl anthranilate	PABA free. Waterproof, all day protection. In 120 ml.
otc	**Original Eclipse Sunscreen** (Triangle Labs)	10	**Lotion:** Padimate O, glyceryl PABA	In 120 ml.
otc	**Hawaiian Tropic 8 Plus** (Tanning Research)	8+	**Gel:** Octyl methoxycinnamate, benzophenone-3, menthyl anthranilate	PABA free. Waterproof, all day protection. In 120 g.
otc	**Vaseline Intensive Care No Burn No Bite** (Chesebrough Pond's)	8	**Lotion:** Ethylhexyl p-methoxycinnamate, oxybenzone	PABA free. Waterproof. In 180 ml.
otc	**TI•Screen** (Pedinol)	8	**Lotion:** 6% ethylhexyl p–methoxycinnamate, 2% oxybenzone	PABA free. Water resistant. In 120 ml.
otc	**Bain de Soleil All Day Waterproof Sunfilter** (Procter & Gamble)	8	**Lotion:** 2-ethylhexyl 2-cyano-3, 3-diphenylacrylate, ethylhexyl p-methoxycinnamate, titanium dioxide, stearyl alcohol, vitamin E, EDTA	PABA free. Waterproof, non-greasy, all day protection. In 120 ml.
otc	**Coppertone Moisturizing Sunscreen** (Schering-Plough)	8	**Lotion:** Ethylhexyl p–methoxycinnamate, oxybenzone	PABA free. Waterproof. In 120 and 240 ml.
otc	**Coppertone Sport** (Schering-Plough)	8	**Lotion:** Ethylhexyl p–methoxycinnamate, oxybenzone	PABA free. Waterproof. In 120 ml.
otc	**Tropical Gold Sunscreen** (Goldline)	8	**Lotion:** Ethylhexyl p-methoxycinnamate, oxybenzone, benzyl alcohol, parabens, aloe extract, jojoba oil, vitamin E, EDTA	PABA free. Waterproof. In 118 ml.
otc	**Vaseline Intensive Care Active Sport** (Chesebrough Pond's)	8	**Lotion:** Ethylhexyl p-methoxycinnamate, oxybenzone	PABA free. In 120 ml.
otc	**Vaseline Intensive Care Moisturizing Sunscreen** (Chesebrough Pond's)	8	**Lotion:** Ethylhexyl p-methoxycinnamate, oxybenzone, C12-15 alkyl octanoate, glycerin, aloe vera gel, cetyl alcohol, petrolatum, vitamin E, parabens, EDTA	PABA free. Waterproof. In 118 ml.
otc	**Bain de Soleil SPF 8 + Color** (Procter & Gamble)	8	**Lotion:** Octyl methoxycinnamate, octocrylene, mineral oil, cetyl alcohol, EDTA	Waterproof. In 118 ml.

SUNSCREENS

		SPF		
otc	**Neutrogena Glow Sunless Tanning** (Neutrogena)	8	**Lotion:** Octyl methoxycinnamate, cetyl alcohol, diazolidinyl urea, parabens, EDTA	PABA free. In 120 ml.
otc	**Neutrogena Sunblock** (Neutrogena)	8	**Cream:** Octyl methoxycinnamate, menthyl anthranilate, titanium dioxide, mineral oil	PABA free. Waterproof. In 67.5 g.
otc	**Sundown Sunscreen** (Johnson & Johnson)	8	**Lotion:** Octyl methoxycinnamate, octyl salicylate, oxybenzone, titanium dioxide	PABA free. Waterproof. In 120 ml.
otc	**Tréo** (Biopharm Lab[1])	8	**Lotion:** Octocrylene, octyl methoxycinnamate, benzophenone-3, octyl salicylate, isostearyl alcohol, diazolidinyl urea, propylparabens. Also contains 0.05% citronella oil as an insect repellent	PABA free. Waterproof. In 118 ml.
otc	**Hawaiian Tropic Protective Tanning** (Tanning Research)	6	**Lotion:** Titanium dioxide	PABA free. Waterproof. In 240 ml.
otc	**Coppertone Moisturizing Sunscreen** (Schering-Plough)	6	**Lotion:** Ethylhexyl p–methoxycinnamate, oxybenzone	PABA free. Waterproof. In 120 ml.
otc	**Faces Only Clear Sunscreen by Coppertone** (Schering-Plough)	6	**Gel:** Ethylhexyl p-methoxycinnamate, oxybenzone	PABA free. In 55.5 g.
otc	**Hawaiian Tropic Protective Tanning Dry** (Tanning Research)	6	**Oil:** 2-ethylhexyl p-methoxycinnamate, homosalate, menthyl anthranilate	Waterproof. In 180 ml.
			Gel: Phenylbenzimidazole, sulfonic acid, benzophenone-4	In 180 g.
otc	**Neutrogena Moisture** (Neutrogena)	5	**Lotion:** Octyl methoxycinnamate, petrolatum, cetyl alcohol, parabens, diazolidinyl urea, EDTA, cetyl alcohol	PABA free. In 60 and 120 ml.
otc	**Bain de Soleil Mega Tan** (Procter & Gamble)	4	Lotion: Ethylhexyl p-methoxycinnamate, 2-ethylhexyl salicylate, lanolin, cocoa butter, palm oil, aloe, DMDM hydantoin, xanthan gum, shea butter, EDTA	Waterproof. In 120 ml.
otc	**Bain de Soleil Orange Gelée** (Procter & Gamble)	4	**Gel:** Ethylhexyl p-methoxycinnamate, 2-ethylhexyl salicylate	PABA free. In 93.75 g.
otc	**Bain de Soleil Tropical Deluxe** (Procter & Gamble)	4	**Lotion:** Ethylhexyl p-methoxycinnamate, 2-ethylhexyl salicylate, cetyl alcohol, EDTA	PABA free. Waterproof. In 240 ml.
otc	**Coppertone Moisturizing Suntan** (Schering-Plough)	4	**Lotion:** Ethylhexyl p-methoxycinnamate, oxybenzone	PABA free. Waterproof. In 120 and 240 ml.
otc	**Hawaiian Tropic Dark Tanning with Sunscreen** (Tanning Research)	4	**Oil:** Ethylhexyl p–methoxycinnamate, octyl dimethyl PABA	Waterproof. In 240 ml.
			Gel: Phenylbenzimidazole, sulfonic acid	PABA free. In 240 g.
otc	**Tropical Gold Dark Tanning** (Goldline)	4	**Lotion:** Ethylhexyl p-methoxycinnamate, oxybenzone, benzyl alcohol, parabens, aloe extract, jojoba oil, vitamin E, EDTA	PABA free. Waterproof. In 240 ml.

SUNSCREENS

		SPF		
otc	**Vaseline Intensive Care Moisturizing Suncreen** (Chesebrough Pond's)	4	**Lotion:** Ethylhexyl p-methoxycinnamate, oxybenzone, C12-15 alkyl octanoate, glycerin, aloe vera gel, cetyl alcohol, petrolatum, vitamin E, parabens, EDTA	PABA free. Waterproof. In 177 ml.
otc	**Tropical Blend Dark Tanning** (Schering-Plough)	4	**Lotion:** Ethylhexyl p-methoxycinnamate, oxybenzone	Waterproof. In 240 ml.
			Oil: Padimate O, oxybenzone	Waterproof. In 240 ml.
otc	**Coppertone Sport** (Schering-Plough)	4	**Lotion:** Ethylhexyl p-methoxycinnamate, oxybenzone	PABA free. Waterproof. In 120 ml.
otc	**Coppertone Tan Magnifier Suntan** (Schering-Plough)	4	**Lotion:** Ethylhexyl p-methoxycinnamate	PABA free. In 120 ml.
			Gel: 2-phenylbenzimidazole-5-sulfonic acid	PABA free. In 120 g.
otc	**Bain de Soleil All Day** (Procter & Gamble)	4	**Lotion:** 2-ethylhexyl 2-cyano-3, 3-diphenylacrylate, ethylhexyl p-methoxycinnamate, titanium dioxide, stearyl alcohol, vitamin E, EDTA	PABA free. Waterproof. In 120 ml.
otc	**Tropical Blend Dry Oil** (Schering-Plough)	4	**Oil:** Homosalate, oxybenzone	Non-greasy. In 180 ml.
otc	**Tropical Blend Tan Magnifier** (Schering-Plough)	4	**Oil:** Triethanolmine salicylate	Waterproof. In 240 ml.
otc	**Q.T. Quick Tanning Suntan by Coppertone** (Schering-Plough)	2	**Lotion:** Ethylhexyl p-methoxycinnamate, dihydroxyacetone	PABA free. In 120 ml.
otc	**Tropical Gold Dark Tanning** (Goldline)	2	**Oil:** Ethylhexyl p-methoxycinnamate, octyldimethyl PABA, mineral oil, coconut oil, cocoa butter, aloe, lanolin, eucalyptus oil, oils of plumeria, manako (mango), kuawa (guava), mikana (papaya), lilikol (passion fruit), taro, kukui	In 240 ml.
otc	**Coppertone Moisturizing Suntan** (Schering-Plough)	2	**Oil:** Homosalate	PABA free. Waterproof. In 120 ml.
otc	**Tropical Blend Dark Tanning** (Schering-Plough)	2	**Lotion/Oil:** Homosalate	Waterproof. In 240 ml.
otc	**Tropical Blend Dry Oil** (Schering-Plough)	2	**Oil:** Homosalate	Non-greasy. In 180 ml.
otc	**Hawaiian Tropic Dark Tanning** (Tanning Research)	2	**Gel:** Phenylbenzimidazole sulfonic acid	In 240 ml.
			Oil: 2-ethylhexyl methoxycinnamate, octyl dimethyl PABA	Waterproof. In 240 ml.
otc	**Coppertone Tan Magnifier Suntan** (Schering-Plough)	2	**Oil:** Triethanolamine salicylate	PABA free. In 120 ml.
otc	**Tropical Blend Tan Magnifier** (Schering-Plough)	2	**Oil:** Triethanolamine salicylate	Waterproof. In 240 ml.
otc	**A-Fil** (GenDerm)	*	**Cream:** 5% menthyl anthranilate, 5% titanium dioxide	In 45 g.

SUNSCREENS

		SPF		
otc	**RVPaque** (ICN Pharm)	*	**Cream:** Red petrolatum, zinc oxide, cinoxate	Water resistant. Greaseless. Tinted. In 15 and 37.5 g.
otc	**Hawaiian Tropic 45 Plus Sunblock Lip Balm** (Tanning Research)	45+	**Lip balm:** Octyl methoxycinnamate, benzophenone-3, octyl salicylate, titanium dioxide, menthyl anthranilate	PABA free. Waterproof. Tropical, mint and cherry flavors. In 4.2 g.
otc	**Blistex Ultra Protection** (Blistex)	30	**Lip balm:** Octyl methoxycinnamate, oxybenzone, octyl salicylate, menthyl anthranilate, homosalate, dimethicone	PABA free. Water resistant. In 4.2 g.
otc	**Water Babies Little Licks by Coppertone** (Schering-Plough)	30	**Lip Balm:** Ethylhexyl p-methoxycinnamate, oxybenzone, 2-ethylhexyl salicylate	PABA free. Waterproof. In 4.5 g.
otc	**Stay Moist Lip Conditioner** (Stanback)	15+	**Lip balm:**	Padimate O, oxybenzone, aloe vera, vitamin E. Tropical fruit flavor. In 4.8 g.
otc	**TI·Screen** (Pedinol)	15+	**Lip balm:** 7.5% ethylhexyl p-methoxycinnamate, 5% oxybenzone, petrolatum	PABA free. In 4.5 g.
otc	**Catrix Lip Saver** (Donell DerMedex)	15	**Lip Balm:** Allantoin, ethylhexyl p-methoxycinnamate, oxybenzone, mineral oil, castor oil, petrolatum, vitamin E, propylparaben	PABA free. In 4.5 g.
otc	**ChapStick Sunblock 15 Petroleum Jelly Plus** (Robins)	15	**Ointment:** 89% white petrolatum, 7% padimate O, 3% oxybenzone, aloe, lanolin	In 10 g.
otc	**Chapstick Sunblock 15** (Robins)	15	**Lip balm:** 7% padimate O, 3% oxybenzone, 0.5% cetyl alcohol, 44% petrolatums, 0.5% lanolin, 0.5% isopropyl myristate, parabens, mineral oil, titanium dioxide	In 4.25 g.
otc	**Eclipse Lip and Face Protectant** (Triangle Labs)	15	**Stick:** Padimate O, oxybenzone	In 4.5 g.
otc	**Neutrogena Lip Moisturizer** (Neutrogena)	15	**Lip balm:** Octyl methoxycinnamate, benzophenone-3, corn oil, castor oil, mineral oil, lanolin oil, petrolatum, lanolin, stearyl alcohol	PABA free. In 4.5 g.
otc	**Coppertone Lipkote** (Schering-Plough)	15	**Lip balm:** Ethylhexyl p-methoxycinnamate, oxybenzone	PABA free. In 4.5 g.
otc	**Daily Conditioning Treatment** (Blistex)	15	**Lip balm:** 7.5% padimate O, 3.5% oxybenzone, cetyl alcohol, aloe, cocoa butter, lanolin, vitamins A and E, petrolatum	In 7 g.
otc	**Daily Lip Protector** (Retsews Corp)			In 7.5 g.
otc	**Blistex** (Blistex)	10	**Lip balm:** 6.6% padimate O, 2.5% oxybenzone, 2% dimethicone, cocoa butter, lanolin, parabens, mineral oil, petrolatum	Regular, mint and berry flavors. In 4.5 g.

[1] Biopharm Lab, Inc., 990 Station Road, Bellport, NY 11713; (516) 286–5983.
* SPF data not provided by distributor.

METHIONINE

Actions:

Pharmacology: The acid-producing effect of methionine on urine pH creates an ammonia free urine.

Indications:

Treatment of diaper rash in infants and for control of odor, dermatitis and ulceration caused by ammoniacal urine in incontinent adults.

Contraindications:

A history of liver disease; large doses of methionine may exaggerate the toxemia of the disease.

Precautions:

Protein intake: Excessive methionine added alone to the diet over extended periods may result in a less than normal weight gain in infants when protein intake is insufficient. Maintain adequate protein intake during therapy and do not exceed the recommended dosage.

Patient Information:

Take with food, milk or other liquid.

Administration and Dosage:

Diaper rash caused by ammoniacal urine: 75 mg in warm formula or other liquid, 3 or 4 times daily or 3 to 5 days. In severe cases or when the infant is > 1 year old it may be necessary to double the dosage the first two days of treatment.

Control of odor in incontinent adults: 200 to 500 mg, 3 or 4 times daily after meal

Rx	**Pedameth** (Forest)	**Capsules:** 200 mg	In 50s and 500s.
Rx	**M-Caps** (Pal-Pak)		In 1000s.
Rx	**Uracid** (Wesley)		In 1000s.
Rx[1]	**Methionine** (Various, eg, Mason, Tyson & Assoc.)	**Tablets:** 500 mg	In 30s and 60s.
Rx	**Pedameth** (Forest)	**Liquid:** 75 mg per 5 ml	Fruit flavor. In pt.

[1] Products available *otc* or *Rx*, depending on product labeling.

TOPICAL DIAPER RASH PRODUCTS

These products are intended for use in diaper rash or ammonia dermatitis. The principal active components of these formulations include:

ANTIMICROBIAL AGENTS (triclosan and eucalyptol) to minimize bacterial proliferation.

ZINC OXIDE for drying.

CAMPHOR is a local anesthetic. Relieves pain, itching and irritation.

BALSAM PERU is claimed to promote wound healing or tissue repair, but effectiveness has not been conclusively demonstrated.

CALCIUM CARBONATE and *KAOLIN*are used for their moisture absorbing abilities.

PROTECTANTS and LUBRICANTS to minimize chafing and irritation.

otc	**Diaper Rash** (Various, eg, Goldline, Rugby, Schein)	**Ointment**: Zinc oxide, cod liver oil, lanolin, methylparaben, petrolatum, talc	In 113 g.
otc	**A and D Medicated** (Schering-Plough)	**Ointment**: White petrolatum, zinc oxide, benzyl alcohol, cod liver oil, light mineral oil, propylparabens, vitamins A and D	In 113 g.
otc	**Bottom Better** (InnoVisions)	**Ointment**: 49% petrolatum, 15.5% lanolin, lanolin alcohols, EDTA, parabens	In 3.75 g packets (18).
otc	**Desitin** (Leeming)	**Ointment**: 40% zinc oxide, cod liver oil, talc, petrolatum, lanolin, methylparaben	In 30, 60, 120, 240 and 270 g.
otc	**Diaper Guard** (Del)	**Ointment**: 1% dimethicone, 66% white petrolatum, cocoa butter, parabens, vitamins A, D_3 and E, zinc oxide	In 49.6 and 99.2 g.
otc	**Diaparene Diaper Rash** (Lehn & Fink)	**Ointment**: Zinc oxide, petrolatum, parabens, imidazolidinyl urea	In 60 g.
otc	**Flanders Buttocks** (Flanders Inc.)	**Ointment**: Zinc oxide, castor oil, balsam peru	In 60 g.
otc	**Daily Care** (Pfizer)	Ointment: 10% zinc oxide, mineral oil, white petrolatum, parabens.	In 57 g.
otc	**Diaparene Baby** (Lehn & Fink)	**Cream**: Mineral oil, petrolatum, aloe, EDTA, diazolidinyl urea, parabens	In 60 g.
otc	**Dyprotex** (Blistex)	**Pads**: 40% micronized zinc oxide, 37.6% petrolatum, 2.5% dimethicone, cod liver oil, aloe	In 3 pads (9 applications) and 8 pads (24 applications).
otc	**Balmex Baby** (Macsil)	**Powder**: Zinc oxide, balsam peru, corn starch, calcium carbonate	In 240 g.
otc	**Diaparene Cornstarch Baby** (Lehn & Fink)	**Powder**: Corn starch, aloe	In 120, 270 and 420 g.
otc	**Mexsana Medicated** (Schering-Plough)	**Powder**: Kaolin, eucalyptus oil, camphor, corn starch, lemon oil, zinc oxide	In 90, 187.5 and 330 g.
otc	**ZBT Baby** (Glenwood)	**Powder**: Talc, mineral oil	In 120 g.
otc	**Desitin with Zinc Oxide** (Pfizer)	Powder: 88.2% cornstarch, 10% zinc oxide	In 28 and 397 g.

TOPICAL POISON IVY TREATMENT PRODUCTS

For other products used for relief of symptoms associated with contact dermatoses, see also: Antihistamine-Containing Products, Topical; Local Anesthetics, Topical; Corticosteroids, Topical.

Indications:

Relief of itching, pain and discomfort of ivy, oak and sumac poisoning. Some products are also recommended for insect bites and other minor skin irritations.

Precautions:

For external use only. Do not use in the eyes. If the condition for which these preparations are used persists or recurs, or if rash, irritation or sensitivity develops, discontinue use and consult physician.

The principal active components of these products include:

ANTIMICROBIAL: Phenylcarbinol (benzyl alcohol).

ANTISEPTIC: Phenol, isopropyl alcohol, benzalkonium chloride, camphor, menthol.

ASTRINGENTS: Calamine, zinc oxide.

COUNTERIRRITANTS: Camphor, methyl salicylate.

LOCAL ANESTHETICS: Benzocaine, pramoxine, phenol, menthol, phenylcarbinol (benzyl alcohol).

ANTIPRURITICS: Phenylcarbinol (benzyl alcohol), camphor, phenol, menthol.

MISCELLANEOUS: Polyvinylpyrrolidone (povidone).

Administration and Dosage:

Apply to affected area 3 to 4 times daily.

otc	**Ivarest** (Blistex)	**Cream & Lotion:** 14% calamine and 5% benzocaine	**Cream:** In 3.75 & 60 g. **Lotion:** In 120 ml.
otc	**Caladryl for Kids** (Parke-Davis)	**Cream:** 8% calamine, 1% pramoxine HCl	Camphor, cetyl alcohol, diazolidinyl urea, parabens. In 45 g.
otc	**Calamine** (Various, eg, Barre, Goldline, Major, Moore, Paddock, Purepac, Rugby)	**Lotion:** 8% calamine, 8% zinc oxide, 2% glycerin and bentonite magma in calcium hydroxide solution	In 120, 240 and 480 ml.
otc	**Phenolated Calamine** (Humco)	**Lotion:** 8% calamine, 8% zinc oxide, 2% glycerin, bentonite magma and 1% phenol in calcium hydroxide solution	In 120 and 240 ml.
otc	**Caladryl** (Parke-Davis)	**Lotion:** 8% calamine, 1% pramoxine HCl	2.2% alcohol,camphor, diazolidinyl urea, parabens. In 180 ml.
otc	**Caladryl Clear** (Parke-Davis)	**Lotion:** 1% pramoxine HCl, 0.1% zinc acetate	2% alcohol, camphor, diazolidinyl urea, parabens. In 180 ml.
otc	**Resinol** (Mentholatum)	**Ointment:** 6% calamine, 12% zinc oxide, 2% resorcinol, lanolin, petrolatum, starch	In 35.4 g.
otc	**Calamox** (Hauck)	**Ointment:** Each 100 g contains 17 g prepared calamine	In 60 g and lb.
otc	**Calamatum** (Blair)	**Spray:** Calamine, zinc oxide, menthol, camphor, 1% benzocaine and isopropyl alcohol	In 85 g aerosol.
otc	**Rhuli Spray** (Rydelle)	**Spray:** 13.8% calamine, 0.7% camphor, and 5% benzocaine in a base of benzyl alcohol, hydrated silica, isobutane, 70% isopropyl alcohol, oleyl alcohol, sorbitan trioleate	In 120 ml.

TOPICAL POISON IVY TREATMENT PRODUCTS

otc	**Aveeno Anti-Itch** (Rydelle)	**Cream & Lotion**: 3% calamine, 1% pramoxine HCl, 0.3% camphor in a base of glycerin, distearyldimonium chloride, petrolatum, oatmeal flour, isopropyl palmitate, cetyl alcohol, dimethicone	**Cream**: In 30 g. **Lotion**: In 120 ml.
otc	**Rhuli Gel** (Rydelle)	**Gel**: 2% benzyl alcohol, 0.3% menthol, 0.3% camphor and 31% SD alcohol 23A in a base of propylene glycol, carbomer 940, triethanolamine, benzophenone-4, EDTA	In 60 g.
otc	**Ivy-Chex** (JMI)	**Spray**: Polyvinylpyrrolidone vinylacetate copolymers, methyl salicylate, benzalkonium chloride and 89.5% SD alcohol 40	In 120 g.
otc	**Ivy-Rid** (Roberts)	**Spray**: Polyvinylpyrrolidone vinylacetate copolymers, isobutane, methyl chloride, benzalkonium chloride, SDA alcohol and isopropul myristate	In 82.5 ml aerosol.

TOPICAL POISON IVY PREVENTATIVES

Indications:

Protection from effects of poisonous foliage, plants and grasses.

Administration and Dosage:

Apply to skin before exposure.

otc	**Stoko Gard** (Stockhausen[1])	**Cream:** PPG-3 diamine dilinoleate, mineral oil, petroleum wax, PEG-7 hydrogenated castor oil, glycerin, petrolatum, aluminum distearate	In 100 g.
otc	**Poison Oak-N-Ivy Armor** (Tec Labs)	**Lotion:** Trioctyl citrate, mineral oil, monostearyl citrate, beeswax, 4-chloro-3, 5-xylenol	In 59.1 ml
otc	**Tecnu Poison Oak -N-Ivy Armor** (Tec Labs)	Liquid: Deodorized mineral spirits, propylene glycol, polyethylene glycol, octylphenoxy-polyethoxyethanol, mixed fatty acid soap.	In 118.3 and 355 ml.

[1] Stockhausen Inc., Greensboro, NC 27406, 1-800-328-2935.

SELENIUM SULFIDE

Actions:

Pharmacology: Selenium sulfide appears to have a cytostatic effect on cells of the epidermis and follicular epithelium, thus reducing corneocyte production.

Indications:

Treatment of dandruff, seborrheic dermatitis of the scalp and tinea versicolor.

Contraindications:

Allergy to any component of the product.

Warnings:

Pregnancy: Category C (tinea versicolor). It is not known whether this drug can cause fetal harm or can affect reproduction capacity. Use only if clearly needed. Under ordinary circumstances, do not use for tinea versicolor in pregnant women.

Children: Safety and efficacy in infants have not been established.

Precautions:

Hypersensitivity: If sensitivity reactions occur, discontinue use.

Treatment of tinea versicolor: Selenium sulfide may irritate the skin, especially in the genital area and in skin folds. Rinse these areas thoroughly after application.

For external use only. Avoid contact with the eyes.

Acute inflammation/exudation: Do not use when present; absorption may be increased.

Adverse Reactions:

Skin irritation; greater than normal hair loss; hair discoloration (avoid or minimize by thorough rinsing after treatment); oiliness or dryness of hair and scalp.

Overdosage:

Accidental oral ingestion:

Symptoms – Selenium sulfide shampoos have generally low toxicity if ingested. Nausea, vomiting and diarrhea usually occur after oral ingestion. There may also be a burning sensation in the mouth and a garlic-like taste/smell to the breath. The detergents found in selenium sulfide shampoos may act as emetics, thereby preventing significant GI absorption of selenium.

Treatment includes usual supportive measures. Refer to General Management of Acute Overdosage.

Patient Information:

For external use only. Avoid contact with the eyes. Do not use on acutely inflamed skin.

If irritation occurs, discontinue use. Thoroughly rinse after application.

If using before or after bleaching, tinting or permanent waving, rinse hair for at least 5 minutes in cool running water.

May damage jewelry; remove before using.

Administration and Dosage:

Massage 5 to 10 ml into wet scalp. Allow to remain on scalp 2 to 3 min. Rinse thoroughly. Repeat application and rinse thoroughly. Wash hands after treatment.

Usually, 2 applications each week for 2 weeks will afford control. After this, it may be used at less frequent intervals-weekly, every 2 weeks or even every 3 or 4 weeks in some cases. Do not apply more frequently than required to maintain control.

Tinea versicolor: Apply to affected areas and lather with a small amount of water. Allow to remain on skin for 10 min; rinse body thoroughly. Repeat once a day for 7 days.

otc	**Selenium Sulfide** (Various, eg, Barre-National, Moore, Rugby)	**Lotion/Shampoo**: 1%	In 120, 210 and 240 ml
otc	**Head & Shoulders Intensive Treatment Dandruff Shampoo** (Procter & Gamble)		In regular and conditioning formulas. In 120, 210 and 330 ml.
otc	**Selsun Blue** (Ross)		In dry, normal, oily, extra conditioning and extra medicated formulas. In 120, 210 and 330 ml.
otc	**Selsun Gold for Women** (Ross)	**Shampoo**: 1% selenium sulfide	In 120, 210 and 330 ml.

SELENIUM SULFIDE

otc	**Selenium Sulfide** (Various, eg, Dixon-Shane, Geneva Marsam, IDE, Lannett, PBI, Rugby, Schein)	**Lotion/Shampoo:** 2.5%	In 120 ml.
Rx	**Exsel** (Herbert)		In 120 ml.
Rx	**Selsun** (Abbott)		In 120 ml.

TAR DERIVATIVES, SHAMPOOS

Actions:

Pharmacology: Tar derivatives help correct keratinization abnormalities by decreasing epidermal proliferation and dermal infiltration; also antipruritic and antibacterial.

Indications:

For treatment of scalp psoriasis, eczema, seborrheic dermatitis, dandruff, cradle-cap and other oily, itchy conditions of the body and scalp.

Contraindications:

Acute inflammation; open or infected lesions.

Warnings:

Children: Use on children < 2 years of age only as directed by a physician.

Precautions:

For external use only. Avoid contact with eyes.

Irritation: Discontinue if irritation develops.

If condition worsens or does not improve after regular use as directed, or if excessive dryness or any undesirable effect occurs, discontinue use and contact physician.

Adverse Reactions:

Minor dermatologic side effects include rash or burning sensation. Photosensitivity may occur. May discolor skin.

Patient Information:

For external use only. Avoid contact with the eyes.

Use caution in the sunlight after applying; it may increase the tendency to sunburn up to 24 hours after application.

Do not use for prolonged periods (> 6 months) without consulting physician.

Administration and Dosage:

Refer to specific product labeling. Rub shampoo liberally into wet hair and scalp. Rinse thoroughly. Repeat; leave on 5 minutes. Rinse thoroughly. Depending on product, use from once daily to at least twice a week. For severe scalp problems, use daily.

otc	**DHS Tar** (Person & Covey)	**Shampoo:** 0.5% coal tar	**Liquid:** In 120, 240 & 480 ml.
			Gel: In 240 ml.
otc	**TVC-2 Dandruff Shampoo** (Dermol)	**Shampoo:** 2% zinc pyrithione.	In 120 ml.
otc	**Doctar** (Savage)	**Shampoo:** 0.5% coal tar w/conditioner	In 100 ml.
otc	**Theraplex T** (Medicis)	**Shampoo:** 1% coal tar, benzyl alcohol	In 240 ml.
otc	**Zetar** (Dermik)	**Shampoo:** 1% whole coal tar	In 180 ml.
otc	**Ionil T Plus** (Owen/Galderma)	**Shampoo:** 2% coal tar	In 120 and 240 ml.
otc	**Neutrogena T/Gel** (Neutrogena Corp.)	**Shampoo:** 2% coal tar extract	In 132, 255, 480 ml.
		Conditioner: 1.5% coal tar extract in a conditioner base	In 132 ml.
otc	**Doak Tar** (Doak)	**Shampoo:** 3% Doak tar distillate	In 237 ml.
otc	**Pentrax Gold** (GenDerm)	**Shampoo:** 4% solubilized coal tar extract	In 168 ml.
otc	**Pentrax** (GenDerm)	**Shampoo:** 4.3% coal tar w/conditioner	In 118 and 237 ml.
otc	**Protar Protein** (Dermol)	**Shampoo:** 5% coal tar	Odor free. In 120 ml.

TAR DERIVATIVES, SHAMPOOS

otc	**Tegrin Medicated** (Block)	**Shampoo:** 5% coal tar solution, 4.6% alcohol	**Gel:** In 71 g.
			Lotion: In 110 and 198 ml.
otc	**Creamy Tar** (C&M)	**Shampoo:** 6.65% coal tar solution, 0.67% crude coal tar	In 240 ml.
otc	**Advanced Formula Tegrin** (Block)	**Shampoo:** 7% coal tar solution USP, 7% alcohol	7% alcohol,hydroxypropyl methylcellulose, parabens. In 207 ml.
otc	**Tegrin Medicated Extra Conditioning** (Block)	**Shampoo:** 7% coal tar solution, 6.4% alcohol	In 110 and 198 ml.
otc	**Denorex** (Whitehall)	**Shampoo:** 9% coal tar solution, 1.5% menthol and 7.5% alcohol	In 120, 240 & 360 ml.
otc	**Extra Strength Denorex** (Whitehall)	**Shampoo:** 12.5% coal tar solution, 1.5% menthol, 10.4% alcohol	In regular and w/conditioner. In 120, 240, 360 ml.
otc	**High Potency Tar** (C&M)	**Shampoo, gel:** 25% coal tar solution	In 240 ml.
otc	**MG 217 Medicated** (Triton)	**Shampoo:** 5% coal tar solution, 2% salicyclic acid, 1.5% colloidal sulfur	In 120 and 240 ml.
		Conditioner: 2% coal tar solution	In 120 ml.
otc	**Duplex T** (C & M Pharm.)	**Shampoo:** 10% coal tar soln., 15% sodium lauryl sulfate, 8.3% alcohol	In pt and gal.
otc	**Iocon** (Owen/Galderma)	**Shampoo, gel:** Coal tar solution and 2.1% alcohol	In 105 g.
otc	**Polytar** (Stiefel)	**Shampoo:** 2.5% polytar (coal tar solution, solubilized crude coal tar equivalent to 0.5% coal tar)	In 180 and 360 ml.
otc	**Packer's Pine Tar** (Rydelle)	**Shampoo:** Pine tar	In 180 ml.

PYRITHIONE ZINC

Actions:

Pharmacology: Pyrithione zinc, a cytostatic agent, reduces cell turnover rate. Its action is thought to be due to a nonspecific toxicity for epidermal cells. The compound strongly binds to both hair and external skin layers.

Indications:

Helps control dandruff and seborrheic dermatitis of the body *(ZNP Bar Soap)* and of the scalp, and for effective control of dry scalp and dry scalp symptoms.

Precautions:

For external use only. Keep out of eyes; if contact occurs, rinse thoroughly with water.

Overdosage:

Oral: Refer to General Management of Acute Overdosage.

Administration and Dosage:

Apply shampoo; lather, rinse and repeat. Use once or twice weekly.

otc	**Danex** (Herbert)	**Shampoo:** 1%	In 120 ml.
otc	**Zincon** (Lederle)		In 118 and 240 ml.
otc	**Head & Shoulders** (Procter & Gamble)		In "normal to oily" and "normal to dry" formulas.
			Cream: In 165 g.
			Lotion: In 120, 210, 330 and 450 ml.
otc	**Head & Shoulders Dry Scalp** (Procter & Gamble)		In regular and conditioning formulas. In 210, 330 and 450 ml.
otc	**DHS Zinc** (Person & Covey)	**Shampoo:** 2%	In 180 and 360 ml.
otc	**Sebulon** (Westwood Squibb)		In 120 and 240 ml.
otc	**Theraplex Z** (Medicis)		In 240 ml.
otc	**TVC-2 Dandruff** (Dermol)		In 120 ml.
otc	**ZNP Bar** (Stiefel)	**Soap:** 2%	In 119 g.

POVIDONE-IODINE SHAMPOO

Actions:

Pharmacology: A broad spectrum antimicrobial agent. Liberates free iodine.

Indications:

Temporary relief of scaling and itching due to dandruff.

Precautions:

For external use only. Avoid contact with eyes.

Irritation/Inflammation: Discontinue if signs of irritation or inflammation develop.

Administration and Dosage:

Apply 2 tsp to hair and scalp; use warm water to lather. Rinse. Repeat application. Massage gently into scalp. Allow to remain on scalp for at least 5 minutes. Work up lather to a golden color, using warm water. Rinse scalp thoroughly. Repeat twice weekly until improvement is noted. Thereafter, shampoo weekly.

otc	**Betadine** (Purdue Frederick)	**Shampoo:** 7.5%	In 118 ml.

SULFACETAMIDE SODIUM

For complete information on sulfonamides, see monograph in Anti-Infectives Section.

Actions:

Pharmacology: Has bacteriostatic effect against gram-positive and -negative microorganisms commonly isolated from secondary cutaneous pyogenic infections.

Indications:

Topical application in the following scaling dermatoses: Seborrheic dermatitis; seborrhea sicca (dandruff). Also indicated in secondary bacterial infections of the skin.

Contraindications:

Hypersensitivity to sulfonamides or to any of the components of the product.

Warnings:

Stevens-Johnson syndrome has occurred with topical sulfacetamide sodium use.

Drug-induced systemic lupus erythematosus from topical sulfacetamide has occurred; one case was fatal.

Pregnancy: Category C. Safety for use is not established. Use only when clearly needed and when potential benefits outweigh potential hazards to the fetus.

Lactation: It is not known whether this drug is excreted in breast milk. Exercise caution when administering to a nursing woman.

Children: Safety and efficacy in children < 12 years of age are not established.

Precautions:

For external use only.

Systemic absorption of topical sulfonamides is greater following application to large, infected, abraded, denuded or severely burned areas.

Hypersensitivity reactions may recur when a sulfonamide is readministered, regardless of the route of administration; cross hypersensitivity between sulfonamides may occur. If signs of hypersensitivity or other untoward reactions occur, discontinue use. Refer to Management of Acute Hypersensitivity Reactions.

Superinfection: Use of antibiotics (especially prolonged or repeated therapy) may result in bacterial or fungal overgrowth of nonsusceptible organisms. Such overgrowth may lead to secondary infection. Take appropriate measures if superinfection occurs.

Overdosage:

Oral ingestion:

Symptoms – Nausea; vomiting. Large doses may cause hematuria, crystalluria and renal shutdown due to precipitation of sulfa crystals in renal tubules and urinary tract.

Treatment – Refer to General Management of Acute Overdosage.Observe kidney function for up to 1 week; have the patient ingest copious amounts of fluid. Mannitol infusions may be helpful at the first sign of oliguria. Alkalinization of urine by bicarbonate ingestion may prevent crystallization of sulfa drug in the kidney.

Patient Information:

For external use only. If irritation occurs or continues, or if rash develops, discontinue use and notify physician. Discontinue promptly if arthritis, fever or mouth sores develop.

Administration and Dosage:

Seborrheic dermatitis: In mild cases involving the scalp and adjacent skin areas, including noninflammatory types with scaling (dandruff), apply at bedtime and allow to remain overnight. Precede application by a shampoo if the hair and scalp are oily or greasy or if there is considerable debris. In severe cases with crusting, heavy scaling and inflammation involving the scalp, apply twice daily. Initially, and as frequently as necessary thereafter, cleanse the hair and scalp with a nonirritating shampoo to ensure complete contact of the medication with the affected skin.

The plastic tube is convenient for applying the lotion, especially for patients with thick hair. Part hair a section at a time; squeeze small amount on scalp from inverted tube. Completely moisten scalp and gently rub in with fingertips. Brush hair thoroughly for 2 to 3 minutes. The next morning wash hair and scalp if desired. Wash hair at least once a week. (Rinsing with plain water or thorough brushing will remove any excess medication.) Repeat application at bedtime, as described, for 8 to 10 nights. As eruption subsides, lengthen interval between applications. Applications once or twice weekly or every other week may prevent recurrence. Should the eruption recur after stopping therapy, reinitiate as at the beginning of treatment.

Secondary cutaneous bacterial infections: Apply 2 to 4 times daily until infection clears.

Sulfacetamide sodium is incompatible with silver preparations.

Rx	**Sebizon** (Schering)	**Lotion:** 10%	In 85 g.

CHLOROXINE

Actions:

Pharmacology: A synthetic antibacterial compound; also has antifungal activity. Chloroxine reduces excess scaling in patients with scaling or seborrheic dermatitis.

Indications:

Treatment of dandruff and mild to moderately severe seborrheic dermatitis of the scalp.

Contraindications:

Hypersensitivity to any of the ingredients. Do not use on acutely inflamed lesions.

Warnings:

Pregnancy: Category C. Safety for use during pregnancy has not been established. Use only when clearly needed and when the potential benefits outweigh the potential hazards to the fetus.

Lactation: It is not known whether the drug is excreted in breast milk. Exercise caution when administering to a nursing woman.

Children: Safety and efficacy for use in children have not been established.

Precautions:

For external use only. Avoid contact with eyes; if contact occurs, flush with cool water.

Adverse Reactions:

Irritation and burning of the scalp and adjacent areas have occurred. Discoloration of light colored hair has occurred.

Patient Information:

For external use only. Avoid contact with eyes.

If irritation, burning or rash occurs, discontinue use.

May discolor blond, gray or bleached hair.

Administration and Dosage:

Massage thoroughly into wet scalp. Allow lather to remain on scalp for 3 minutes; rinse. Repeat application and rinse. Two treatments per week are usually sufficient.

Rx	**Capitrol** (Westwood Squibb)	**Shampoo**: 2%	In 120 ml.

ANTISEBORRHEIC COMBINATIONS

Ingredients:

SALICYLIC ACID and SULFUR (see individual monographs) are used for antiseborrheic and keratolytic/keratoplastic actions.

TAR PREPARATIONS, PYRITHIONE ZINC (see individual monographs) and MYRISTYLTRIMETHYLAMMONIUM BROMIDE are used for their antipruritic, antibacterial or antiseborrheic actions.

MENTHOL is used as an antipruritic.

BENZALKONIUM CHLORIDE, ISOPROPYL ALCOHOL, PHENOL and MENTHOL are used as antiseptics.

IODOQUINOL, METHYLBENZETHONIUM CHLORIDE and BENZYL ALCOHOL are antimicrobial agents.

Precautions:

For external use only. Avoid contact with eyes; in case of contact, flush with water.

If undue skin irritation develops or increases, discontinue use and consult physician. Preparations containing tar may temporarily discolor blond, bleached or tinted hair. Slight staining of clothing may also occur.

ANTISEBORRHEIC SHAMPOOS

Complete prescribing information begins in the Antiseborrheic Combinations introduction.

otc	**Maximum Strength Meted** (GenDerm)	**Shampoo**: 5% sulfur and 3% salicylic acid	In 118 ml.
otc	**MG400** (Triton)	**Shampoo**: 3% salicylic acid, 5% colloidal sulfur in Guy-Base II.	In 240 ml and pt.
otc	**Sebex** (Rugby)	**Shampoo**: 2% sulfur and 2% salicylic acid	In 118 ml.
otc	**Sebulex** (Westwood Squibb)		Regular and with conditioners. In 120 and 240 ml.

ANTISEBORRHEIC SHAMPOOS

otc	**Ionil Plus** (Owen/Galderma)	**Shampoo:** 2% salicylic acid	In 120 and 240 ml.
otc	**P & S** (Baker Cummins)		In 120 ml.
otc	**Sulfoam** (Bradley)		In 118, 236 and 465 ml.
otc	**Neutrogena T/Sal** (Triton)	**Shampoo:** 2% salicyclic acid, 2% solubilized coal tar extract	In 135 ml.
otc	**Ionil** (Owen/Galderma)	**Shampoo:** Salicylic acid, benzalkonium chloride, EDTA	In 120 and 240 ml, pt and qt.
otc	**X•Seb** (Baker Cummins)	**Shampoo:** 4% salicylic acid	In 120 ml.
otc	**Tarsum** (Summers)	**Shampoo/Gel:** 10% crude coal tar and 5% salicylic acid	In 120 and 240 ml.
otc	**X•Seb T** (Baker Cummins)	**Shampoo:** 10% coal tar solution, 4% salicylic acid	In 120 ml.
otc	**X•Seb T Plus** (Baker Cummins)	**Shampoo:** 10% coal tar solution, 3% salicylic acid and 1% menthol	In 120 ml.
otc	**Sebutone** (Westwood Squibb)	**Shampoo:** 0.5% coal tar, 2% sulfur, 2% salicylic acid	**Cream:** In 120 g. **Liquid:** In 120 and 240 ml.
otc	**Sebex-T** (Rugby)	**Shampoo:** 5% coal tar solution, 2% colloidal sulfur and 2% salicylic acid	Soapless. In 118 ml.
otc	**Ionil T** (Owen/Galderma)	**Shampoo:** Coal tar solution, salicylic acid, benzalkonium chloride	In 120 and 240 ml, pt and qt.
otc	**Sebaquin** (Summers)	**Shampoo:** 3% iodoquinol, lanolin	In 120 ml.
otc	**X•Seb Plus** (Baker Cummins)	**Shampoo:** 1% pyrithione zinc and 2% salicylic acid	In 120 ml.

MEDICATED HAIR DRESSINGS

Complete prescribing information begins in the Antiseborrheic Combinations introduction.

Rx	**Sal-Oil-T** (Syosset)	**Solution:** 10% crude coal tar, 6% salicylic acid, vegetable oil	In 59.14 ml.
otc	**SLT Lotion** (C & M Pharm.)	**Lotion:** 2% coal tar solution, 3% salicylic acid, 5% lactic acid, 65% isopropyl alcohol, 1.6% benzyl alcohol and benzalkonium chloride	In 129 ml.
otc	**Tarlene** (Medco Lab)	**Lotion:** 2% refined coal tar, 2.5% salicylic acid	In 60 ml.
otc	**Sebucare** (Westwood Squibb)	**Lotion:** 1.8% salicylic acid with 61% alcohol	In 120 ml.
otc	**Scadan** (Miles Inc.)	**Lotion:** 1% myristyltrimethylammonium bromide and 0.1% stearyl dimethyl benzyl ammonium chloride	In 120 ml.
otc	**P & S** (Baker Cummins)	**Liquid:** Phenol, mineral oil and glycerin	In 120 and 240 ml.

Antiviral Agents

PENCICLOVIR

Actions:

Pharmacology: Penciclovir is an antiviral agent active against herpes viruses. It has in vitro inhibitory activity against herpes simplex virus types 1 (HSV-1) and 2 (HSV-2). In cells infected with HSV-1 or HSV-2, viral thymidine kinase phosphorylates penciclovir to a monophosphate form which, in turn, is converted to penciclovir triphosphate by cellular kinases. In vitro studies demonstrate that penciclovir triphosphate inhibits HSV polymerase competitively with deoxyguanosine triphosphate. Consequently, herpes viral DNA synthesis and replication are selectively inhibited.

Drug resistance – Penciclovir-resistant mutants of HSV can result from qualitative changes in viral thymidine kinase or DNA polymerase. The most commonly encountered acyclovir-resistant mutants that are deficient in viral thymidine kinase are also resistant to penciclovir.

Pharmacokinetics: Measurable penciclovir concentrations were not detected in plasma or urine of healthy male volunteers following single or repeat application of the 1% cream at a dose of 180 mg penciclovir daily (≈ 67 times the estimated usual clinical dose).

Clinical trials: Penciclovir was studied in two double-blind, placebo controlled trials for the treatment of recurrent herpes labialis in which otherwise healthy adults were randomized to either penciclovir or placebo. Therapy was to be initiated by the subjects within 1 hour of noticing signs or symptoms and continued for 4 days, with application of study medication every 2 hours while awake. In both studies, the mean duration of lesions was ≈ ½ day shorter in the subjects treated with penciclovir (n = 1516) compared with subjects treated with placebo (n = 1541) (≈ 4.5 days vs 5 days, respectively). The mean duration of lesion pain was also ≈ ½ day shorter in the penciclovir group compared with the placebo group.

Indications:

Herpes labialis: For the treatment of recurrent herpes labialis (cold sores) in adults.

Contraindications:

Hypersensitivity to the product or any of its components.

Warnings:

Fertility impairment: Testicular toxicity was observed in multiple animal species (rats and dogs) following repeated IV administration of penciclovir at doses ≈ 1155 and 3255, respectively, times the human dose. Testicular changes seen in both species included atrophy of the seminiferous tubules and reductions in epididymal sperm counts or an increased incidence of sperm with abnormal morphology or reduced motility. Adverse testicular effects were related to an increasing dose or duration of exposure to penciclovir.

There was no evidence of any clinically significant effects on sperm count, motility or morphology in 2 placebo-controlled clinical trials of famciclovir (the oral prodrug of penciclovir [250 mg bid; n = 66]) in immunocompetent men with recurrent genital herpes, when dosing and follow-up were maintained for 13 and 8 weeks, respectively (≈ 2 and 1 spermatogenic cycles in the human).

Elderly: In patients ≥ 65 years of age, the adverse events profile was comparable with that observed in younger patients.

Pregnancy: Category B. No adverse effects on the course and outcome of pregnancy or on fetal development were noted in rats and rabbits following the IV administration of penciclovir. There are no adequate and well-controlled studies in pregnant women. Use during pregnancy only if clearly needed.

Lactation: There is no information on whether penciclovir is excreted in breast milk after topical administration. However, following oral administration of famciclovir (the oral prodrug of penciclovir) to lactating rats, penciclovir was excreted in breast milk at concentrations higher than those seen in the plasma. Therefore, a decision should be made whether to discontinue the drug or discontinue nursing, taking into account the importance of the drug to the mother. There are no data on the safety of penciclovir in newborns.

Children: Safety and effectiveness in pediatric patients have not been established.

Precautions:

Mucous membranes: Use penciclovir on herpes labialis on the lips and face only. Because no data are available, application to human mucous membranes is not recommended. Take particular care to avoid application in or near the eyes because it may cause irritation.

Antiviral Agents

PENCICLOVIR

Immunocompromised patients: Penciclovir's effect in immunocompromised patients has not been established.

Adverse Reactions:

Penciclovir Adverse Reactions		
Adverse Reaction	Penciclovir n = 1516 (%)	Placebo n = 1541 (%)
Application site reaction	1.3	1.8
Hypesthesia/local anesthesia	0.9	1.4
Taste perversion	0.2	0.3
Pruritus	0.0	0.3
Pain	0.0	0.1
Rash (erythematous)	0.1	0.1
Allergic Reaction	0.0	0.1
Headache	5.3	5.8
Mild erythema[1]	≈ 50	-

[1] A 5% penciclovir cream was applied.

Overdosage:

Because penciclovir is poorly absorbed following oral administration, adverse reactions related to penciclovir ingestion are unlikely. There is no information on overdose.

Administration and Dosage:

Apply penciclovir every 2 hours while awake for 4 days. Start treatment as early as possible (eg, during the prodrome or when lesions appear).

Rx	**Denavir** (SmithKline Beecham)	**Cream:** 10mg/g	In 2 g tubes.

Antiviral Agents

ACYCLOVIR (Acycloguanosine)

For information on systemic acyclovir, refer to monograph in Anti-infectives section.

Actions:

Pharmacology: Acyclovir, a synthetic acyclic purine nucleoside analog, has in vitro inhibitory activity against herpes simplex types 1 and 2 (HSV-1, HSV-2), varicella-zoster, Epstein-Barr and cytomegalovirus. Acyclovir is activated by herpesvirus thymidine kinase, resulting in phosphorylation to produce acyclovir triphosphate. Acyclovir triphosphate interferes with herpes simplex virus DNA polymerase and inhibits viral DNA replication. It inhibits cellular alpha-DNA polymerase to a lesser degree. In vitro, acyclovir triphosphate can be incorporated into growing DNA chains by viral DNA polymerase. When incorporation occurs, the DNA chain is terminated. Acyclovir is preferentially taken up and selectively converted to active triphosphate form by herpesvirus infected cells. Thus, acyclovir is much less toxic in vitro for normal uninfected cells. The relationship between in vitro susceptibility of herpes simplex virus to antiviral drugs and clinical response is not established.

Pharmacokinetics: Systemic absorption after topical application is minimal.

Clinical trials: In clinical trials of initial herpes genitalis, acyclovir decreased healing time and, in some cases, decreased duration of viral shedding and pain. Studies in immunocompromised patients with mainly herpes labialis showed decreased duration of viral shedding and slight decrease in pain duration. In contrast, studies of recurrent herpes genitalis and herpes labialis in nonimmunocompromised patients showed no clinical benefit; there was some decrease in duration of viral shedding.

Indications:

Management of initial episodes of herpes genitalis and in limited non-life-threatening mucocutaneous herpes simplex virus infections in immunocompromised patients.

Contraindications:

Hypersensitivity or chemical intolerance to the components of the formulation.

Warnings:

For cutaneous use only. Do not use in eyes.

Pregnancy: Category C. There are no adequate and well controlled studies in pregnant women. Use during pregnancy only if the potential benefits outweigh the potential hazards to the fetus.

Lactation: It is not known whether this drug is excreted in breast milk. Exercise caution when applying on a nursing mother.

Precautions:

Do not exceed the recommended administration and dosage. No data demonstrate that acyclovir will either prevent transmission of infection to other persons or prevent recurrent infections when applied in the absence of signs and symptoms. Do not use to prevent recurrent HSV infections. Although clinically significant viral resistance associated with acyclovir use has not been observed, this possibility exists.

Adverse Reactions:

Mild pain with transient burning/stinging (28.3%); pruritus (4%); rash, vulvitis (0.3%).

In all studies, there was no significant difference between the drug and placebo groups in the rate or type of reported adverse reactions.

Patient Information:

For external use only. Apply ointment every 3 hours 6 times daily for 1 week.

Ointment must thoroughly cover all lesions. Use a finger cot or rubber glove to apply ointment to prevent spread of infection.

May cause transient burning, stinging, itching and rash; notify physician if these become pronounced or persist.

Acyclovir ointment is not a cure for herpes simplex infections and it is of little benefit in treating recurrent attacks.

Administration and Dosage:

Initiate therapy as early as possible following onset of signs and symptoms.

Apply sufficient quantity to adequately cover all lesions every 3 hours 6 times daily for 7 days. The dose size per application will vary depending upon the total lesion area; a 0.5 inch ribbon of ointment covers approximately 4 square inches of surface area. Use a finger cot or rubber glove when applying acyclovir to prevent autoinoculation of other body sites and transmission of infection to other persons.

Rx	**Zovirax** (Burroughs Wellcome)	**Ointment:** 5% (50 mg per g)	In a polyethylene glycol base. In 3 and 15 g.

Antibiotics

MUPIROCIN (Pseudomonic Acid A)

Actions:

Pharmacology: Mupirocin, a topical antibacterial structurally unrelated to other agents, inhibits bacterial protein synthesis by reversibly and specifically binding to bacterial isoleucyl transfer-RNA synthetase. Therefore, mupirocin shows no cross-resistance with chloramphenicol, erythromycin, fusidic acid, gentamicin, lincomycin, methicillin, neomycin, novobiocin, penicillin, streptomycin and tetracycline.

Pharmacokinetics: Mupirocin has shown no measurable systemic absorption.

Microbiology: The aerobic isolates of *Staphylococcus aureus* (including methicillin-resistant and β-lactamase producing strains), *S. epidermidis, S. saprophyticus* and *Streptococcus pyogenes* are susceptible to mupirocin in vitro.

Indications:

Topical: Impetigo due to *S. aureus*, beta-hemolytic *Streptococcus* and *S. pyogenes*.

Nasal: Eradication of nasal colonization with methicillin-resistant *S. aureus* in adult patients and healthcare workers as part of a comprehensive infection control program to reduce infection risk among patients at high risk of methicillin-resistant *S. aureus* infection during institutional outbreaks of infections with this pathogen.

Contraindications:

Hypersensitivity reactions to any components of the products.

Warnings:

Topical:

For external use only. Avoid contact with the eyes.

Pregnancy: Category B. There are no adequate and well controlled studies in pregnant women. Use during pregnancy only if clearly needed.

Lactation: It is not known whether mupirocin is excreted in breast milk. Temporarily discontinue nursing while using mupirocin.

Children: Safety in children < 12 years old has not been established for mupirocin nasal.

Precautions:

Open wounds: Polyethylene glycol can be absorbed from open wounds and damaged skin and is excreted by the kidney. Do not use if absorption of large quantities of polyethylene glycol is possible, especially if there is evidence of moderate or severe renal impairment.

Prophylaxis: There are insufficient data at this time to recommend use of mupirocin nasal for general prophylaxis or to establish that this product is safe and effective as part of an intervention program to prevent autoinfection of high-risk patients from their own nasal colonization.

Sensitivity reaction: If a reaction suggesting sensitivity or chemical irritation occurs, discontinue treatment and institute appropriate alternative therapy.

Superinfection: Use of antibiotics may result in bacterial or fungal overgrowth of nonsusceptible organisms.

Drug Interactions:

Do not use mupirocin nasal concurrently with any other nasal products.

Antibiotics

MUPIROCIN (Pseudomonic Acid A)

Adverse Reactions:

Topical: Burning, stinging or pain (1.5%); itching (1%); rash, nausea, erythema, dry skin, tenderness, swelling, contact dermatitis and increased exudate (< 1%).

Nasal: Headache (9%); rhinitis (6%); respiratory disorder including upper respiratory tract congestion (5%); pharyngitis (4%); taste perversion (3%); burning/stinging, cough (2%); pruritus (1%); blepharitis, diarrhea, dry mouth, ear pain, epistaxis, nausea, rash (< 1%).

Administration and Dosage:

Topical: Apply a small amount to the affected area 3 times daily. The area may be covered with gauze dressing. Reevaluate those not showing a response in 3 to 5 days.

Nasal: Divide ≈ ½ of the ointment from the single-use tube between the nostrils and apply twice daily (morning and evening) for 5 days.

After application, close nostrils by pressing together and releasing sides of the nose repeatedly for ≈ 1 minute.

Storage/Stability: Store the topical ointment between 15° and 30°C (59° to 86°F), and store the nasal ointment at or below 25°C (77°F).

Rx	**Bactroban** (SmithKline Beecham)	**Ointment**: 2% (20 mg/g) in a polyethylene glycol base	In 15 and 30 g.
Rx	**Bactroban Nasal** (SmithKline Beecham)	**Ointment**: 2% mupirocin calcium	In 1 g single use tubes.

ANTIBIOTICS

Actions:

Pharmacology: The topical anti-infectives may be either bactericidal or bacteriostatic. Most inhibit protein synthesis.

Bacitracin inhibits the cell wall synthesis.

The mechanism by which **erythromycin** acts in reducing the inflammatory lesions of acne vulgaris are unknown. **Erythromycin** is active against *Propionibacterium acnes. P. acnes* produces free fatty acids, which may lead to microcomedo formation and induce acne inflammation.

Gentamicin is a bactericidal agent that is not effective against viruses or fungi in skin infections. **Gentamicin** is active against strains of streptococci (group A beta-hemolytic, alpha-hemolytic), *Staphylococcus aureus* (coagulase-positive, coagulase-negative and some penicillinase-producing strains) and the gram-negative bacteria, *Pseudomonas aeruginosa, Aerobacter aerogenes, Escherichia coli, Proteus vulgaris* and *Klebsiella pneumoniae.*

Indications:

Infection: These antibiotic preparations are used for infection treatment or prophylaxis in minor cuts, wounds, burns and skin abrasions, as an aid to healing and for the treatment of superficial infections of the skin due to susceptible organisms amenable to local treatment.

Erythromycin is indicated for control of acne vulgaris.

Gentamicin is indicated for the relief of primary skin infections (impetigo contagiosa, superficial folliculitis, ecthyma, furunculosis, sycosis barbae, pyoderma gangrenosum) and secondary skin infections (infectious eczematoid dermatitis, pustular acne, pustular psoriasis, infected seborrheic dermatitis, infected contact dermatitis, infected excoriations and bacterial superinfections of fungal or viral infections). **Gentamicin** is useful in the treatment of infected skin cysts and certain other skin abscesses when preceded by incision and drainage to permit adequate contact between the antibiotic and the infecting bacteria, infected stasis and other skin ulcers, infected superficial burns, paronychia, infected insect bites and stings, infected lacerations and abrasions and wounds from minor surgery.

Contraindications:

Prior sensitization to any of the ingredients; use in eyes.

Warnings:

External use: For external use only. Do not use in or near the eyes, nose, mouth or any mucous membrane.

Systemic therapy: Deeper cutaneous infections may require systemic antibiotic therapy in addition to local treatment. Use caution when applying over large areas of the body for deep puncture wounds, animal bites or serious burns.

Concomitant topical acne therapy with **erythromycin** should be used with caution because a possible cumulative irritancy effect may occur, especially with the use of peeling, desquamating or abrasive agents.

Neomycin toxicity: Due to the potential nephrotoxicity and ototoxicity of **neomycin**, use with care in treating extensive burns, trophic ulceration or other extensive conditions where absorption is possible. Do not apply more than once daily in burn cases where > 20% of body surface is affected, especially if the patient has impaired renal function or is receiving other aminoglycoside antibiotics concurrently.

Pregnancy: Category C. It is not known whether **erythromycin** can cause fetal harm when administered to a pregnant woman. Use **erythromycin** only if clearly needed.

Lactation: **Erythromycin** is excreted in breast milk. Caution should be exercised when **erythromycin** is administered to a nursing woman.

Children: Safety and effectiveness in children have not been established.

Gentamicin has been used successfully in infants over one year of age.

Precautions:

Neomycin hypersensitivity: Chronic application of **neomycin sulfate** to inflamed skin of individuals with allergic contact dermatitis and chronic dermatoses (eg, chronic otitis externa or stasis dermatitis) increases the possibility of sensitization. Low grade reddening with swelling, dry scaling and itching or a failure to heal are usually manifestations of this hypersensitivity. During long-term use of **neomycin**-containing products, perform periodic examinations and discontinue use if symptoms appear. These symptoms regress upon withdrawal of medication, but avoid **neomycin**-containing products thereafter. Patients sensitive to **neomycin** can be treated with **gentamicin**.

Antibiotics

ANTIBIOTICS

Superinfection: Prolonged use of antibiotics may result in overgrowth of nonsusceptible organisms, particularly fungi. Such overgrowth may lead to a secondary infection. Discontinue the drug and take appropriate measures if superinfection occurs.

Adverse Reactions:

Gentamicin: Possible photosensitization has been reported.

Bacitracin ointment: Allergic contact dermatitis has occurred.

Neomycin: Ototoxicity and nephrotoxicity have occurred (see Warnings).

Erythromycin: Isolated cases of skin irritation such as dryness, tenderness, pruritus, desquamation, erythema, peeling, oiliness and burning sensations have occurred.

Patient Information:

For external use only. Cleanse affected area of skin prior to application (unless directed otherwise).

Notify physician if condition worsens or if rash or irritation develops.

ERYTHROMYCIN

Complete prescribing information begins in the Antibiotics group monograph.

Rx	**Akne-mycin** (Hermal)	**Ointment**: 2%	Petrolatum, mineral oil. In 25 g.
Rx	**Emgel** (Glaxo)	**Ointment and Gel**: 2%	In 27 g.
Rx	**Erygel** (Herbert)	**Gel**: 2%	92% alcohol. In 30 and 60 g w/5 g travel size.

GENTAMICIN

Complete prescribing information begins in the Antibiotics group monograph.

Rx	**Gentamicin** (Various, eg, Geneva, Major, NMC, Schein)	**Ointment**: 0.1% (as 1.7 mg sulfate per g) in a bland, unctuous petrolatum base	In 15 g.
Rx	**Garamycin** (Schering)		Parabens. In 15 g.
Rx	**Gentamicin** (Various, eg, Geneva , Major, NMC, Rugby, Schein)	**Cream**: 0.1% (as 1.7 mg sulfate per g) in a bland emulsion-type base	In 15 g.
Rx	**Garamycin** (Schering)		Parabens. In 15 g.
Rx	**G-myticin** (Pedinol)	**Ointment**: Gentamicin sulfate equiv. to 1 mg base	In 15 g.
		Cream: Gentamicin sulfate equiv. to 1 mg base	In 15 g.

BACITRACIN

Complete prescribing information begins in the Antibiotics group monograph.

otc	**Bacitracin** (Various, eg, Geneva, NMC, Parmed, Rugby, Schein, URL)	**Ointment**: 500 units per g	In 0.94, 15 and 30 g and lb.
otc	**Baciguent** (Upjohn)		Anhydrous lanolin, mineral oil, white petrolatum. In 15 and 30 g.

NEOMYCIN SULFATE

Complete prescribing information begins in the Antibiotics group monograph.

otc	**Neomycin** (Various, eg, Rugby, Schein)	**Ointment**: 3.5 mg neomycin (as sulfate) per g	In 15 and 30 g.
otc	**Myciguent** (Upjohn)		Lanolin, mineral oil, white petrolatum. In 15, 30 g.
otc	**Myciguent** (Upjohn)	**Cream**: 3.5 mg neomycin (as sulfate) per g	Methylparaben. In 15 g.

Antibiotics, Multiple

COMBINATION ANTI-INFECTIVE PRODUCTS

Complete prescribing information begins in the Antibiotics group monograph.

	Product and Distributor	Polymyxin B Sulfate (units/g or ml)	Neomycin (mg/g or ml)[1]	Bacitracin (units/g or ml)	Other (g or ml)	How Supplied
otc	**Betadine First Aid Antibioitics + Moisturizer** (Purdue Frederick)	10,000		500		In 14 g.
otc	**Polysporin Ointment** (Glaxo Wellcome)					White petrolatum base. In 15, 30 and UD 0.94 g (144s).
otc	**Polysporin Powder** (Glaxo Wellcome)					Lactose base. In 10 g.
otc	**Neosporin Cream** (Glaxo Wellcome)	10,000	3.5			0.25% parabens, mineral oil, white petrolatum. Non-greasy. In 15 g and UD 0.94 g (144s).
otc	**Neosporin Plus** (Glaxo Wellcome)				40 mg lidocaine/g	0.25% methylparaben, mineral oil, white petrolaum. In 15 g.
otc	**Maximum Strength Neosporin Ointment** (Glaxo Wellcome)	10,000	3.5	500		White petrolatum. In 15 g.
otc	**Neosporin Plus Ointment** (Glaxo Wellcome)				40 mg lidocaine	White petrolatum base. In 15 g,
otc	**Lanabiotic Ointment** (Combe)					Lanolin, mineral oil and petrolatum. In 15 and 30 g.
otc	**Neopsorin Plus** (Glaxo Wellcome)				40 mg lidocain/g	In a white petrolatum base. In 15 g.
otc	**Neosporin Plus Cream** (Glaxo Wellcome)	10,000	3.5		40 mg lidocaine	0.25% methylparaben, mineral oil, white petrolatum. In 15 g.
otc	**Triple Antibiotic Ointment** (Various, eg, Dixon-Shane, Geneva Marsam, Goldline, Parmed, Rugby, Schein)	5000	3.5	400		In 2.4, 9.6, 15 and 30 g.
otc	**Medi-Quick Ointment** (Mentholatum)					Mineral oil and petrolatum. In 14.2 g.
otc	**Neomixin Ointment** (Hauck)					Petrolatum base. In 15 g and 1 g (144s).
otc	**Neosporin Ointment** (Glaxo Wellcome)					White petrolatum. In 15 & 30 g, UD 0.94 g (144s).
otc	**Septa Ointment** (Circle)					In 28.3 g.
otc	**Spectrocin Plus Ointment** (Numark Labs)				5 mg lidocaine	Mineral oil, white petrolatum. In 15, 30 g.
otc	**Bactine First Aid Antibiotic Plus Anesthetic Ointment** (Miles)				10 mg diperodon HCl	Mineral oil and white petrolatum. In 15 g.
otc	**Clomycin** (Roberts)				40 mg lidocaine/g.	Yellow petrolatum, anhydrous lanolin, light mineral oil. In 28.35 g.

Antibiotics, Multiple

COMBINATION ANTI-INFECTIVE PRODUCTS

	Product and Distributor	Polymyxin B Sulfate (units/g or ml)	Neomycin (mg/g or ml)[1]	Bacitracin (units/g or ml)	Other (g or ml)	How Supplied
otc	**Maximum Strength Mycitracin Triple Antibiotic Ointment** (Upjohn)	5000	3.5	500		Parabens, mineral oil, white petrolatum. In 15 and 30 g and UD 0.94 g (144s).
otc	**Campho-Phenique Antibiotic Plus Pain-Reliever Ointment** (Winthrop)				40 mg lidocaine	White petrolatum. In 15 g.
otc	**Clomycin** (Roberts)					Yellow petrolatum, anhydrous lanolin, light mineral oil. In 28.35 g.
otc	**Mycitracin Plus Ointment** (Upjohn)					Mineral oil, parabens and white petrolatum. In 14.2 and 30 g.
otc	**Tribiotic Plus** (Thompson)				40 mg lidocaine/g	Lanolin, light mineral oil, petrolatum. In 28.35 g.
otc	**Polysporin Spray** (Glaxo Wellcome)	2222		111		In 90 g.

[1] As base; equivalent to 5 mg neomycin sulfate.

Antifungal Agents

UNDECYLENIC ACID AND DERIVATIVES

Indications:

Antifungal and antibacterial agents for tinea pedis (athlete's foot), exclusive of the nails and hairy areas. Also recommended for the relief and prevention of diaper rash, itching, burning and chafing, prickly heat, tinea cruris (jock itch), excessive perspiration and irritation in the groin area and bromhidrosis.

Warnings:

For external use only. Avoid inhaling and contact with the eyes or other mucous membranes. Patients with impaired circulation, including diabetics, should consult a physician before using. Do not use in children < 2 years old except on advice of physician.

Administration and Dosage:

Cleanse and dry area well; smooth or spray on. Apply as needed or as directed.

The choice of vehicle is important for these products. Ointments, creams and liquids are used as primary therapy. In general, powders are used as adjunctive therapy, but they may be acceptable as primary therapy in very mild conditions.

otc	**Protectol Medicated** (Daniels)	**Powder:** 15% calcium undecylenate	Starch. In 56.7 g.
otc	**Caldesene** (Fisons)	**Powder:** 10% calcium undecylenate	In 60 and 120 g.
otc	**Cruex** (Ciba Consumer)		Talc. In 45 g.
otc	**Cruex Aerosol** (Ciba Consumer)	**Powder:** 19% total undecylenate as undecylenic acid and zinc undecylenate	Menthol, talc. In 54, 105 and 165 g.
otc	**Desenex** (Ciba)	**Powder:** 25% total undecylenate as undecylenic acid and zinc undecylenate	Talc. In 45g.
otc	**Phicon F** (T.E. Williams)	**Cream:** 8% undecylenic acid, 0.05% pramoxine HCl	In 60 g.
otc	**Breezee Mist Aerosol** (Pedinol)	**Powder:** Undecylenic acid, menthol and aluminum chlorhydrate	Talc. In 113 g.
Rx	**Blis-To-Sol** (Chattem)	**Powder:** 12% zinc undecylenate	Talc, zinc oxide. In 60 g.
Rx	**Pedi-Dri** (Pedinol)	**Powder:** Zinc undecylenate, aluminum chlorhydroxide, menthol and formaldehyde	Cornstarch. In 60 g.
otc	**Pedi-Pro** (Pedinol)	**Powder:** Zinc undecylenate, aluminum chlorhydroxide, menthol, chloroxylenol	Starch. In 60 g.
otc	**Desenex** (Ciba)	**Ointment:** 25% total undecylenate (as undecylenic acid and zinc undecylenate)	Lanolin, parabens, white petrolatum. In 14 g.
otc	**Decylenes** (Rugby)	**Ointment:** Undecylenic acid and zinc undecylenate	In 30 g and 1 lb.
otc	**Cruex** (Ciba Consumer)	**Cream:** 20% total undecylenate as undecylenic acid and zinc undecylenate	Lanolin, parabens, white petrolatum. In 15 g.
otc	**Desenex** (Ciba)	**Cream:** 25% total undecylenate (as undecylenic acid and zinc undecylenate)	Lanolin, parabens, white petrolatum. In 15 g.
otc	**Fungoid AF** (Pedinol)	**Solution:** 25% undecylenic acid	In 30 ml.
otc	**Desenex** (Ciba)	**Foam:** 10% total undecylenate (undecylenic acid)	29.2% isopropyl alcohol. In 45 g.
otc	**Desenex** (Ciba)	**Soap:** Undecylenic acid	In 97.5 g.
otc	**Desenex** (Ciba)	**Aerosol spray powder:** 25% total undecylenate (as undecylenic acid and zine undecylenate)	Menthol, talc. In 81 g.

Antifungal Agents

CLIOQUINOL (Iodochlorhydroxyquin)

Actions:

Pharmacology: Has antibacterial and antifungal properties.

Indications:

Inflamed conditions of skin (eg, eczema, athlete's foot, other fungal infections).

Precautions:

For external use only. Avoid contact with the eyes.

Sensitivity: In rare cases, may irritate sensitized skin. If itching, redness, irritation, stinging or swelling persists or increases, discontinue use.

May stain fabric, skin or hair.

Administration and Dosage:

Apply to affected areas 2 or 3 times daily. Not for use > 1 week.

otc	**Vioform** (Ciba)	**Cream:** 3%	Water washable base. In 30 g.
		Ointment: 3%	Petrolatum base. In 30 g.

MICONAZOLE NITRATE

For information on systemic and vaginal miconazole, refer to individual monographs.

Actions:

Pharmacokinetics: Miconazole alters cellular membrane permeability and interferes with mitochondrial and peroxisomal enzymes, resulting in intracellular necrosis. It inhibits growth of the common dermatophytes, *Trichophyton rubrum, T mentagrophytes, Epidermophyton floccosum, Candida albicans* and the active organism in tinea versicolor, *Malassezia furfur.*

Indications:

Rx and otc: Tinea pedis (athlete's foot), tinea cruris (jock itch) and tinea corporis (ringworm) caused by *T rubrum, T mentagrophytes* and *E floccosum.*

Rx only: Cutaneous candidiasis (moniliasis); tinea versicolor.

Warnings:

For external use only. Avoid contact with the eyes.

Sensitivity: If a reaction occurs suggesting sensitivity or chemical irritation, discontinue use.

Adverse Reactions:

Isolated reports of irritation, burning, maceration and allergic contact dermatitis.

Patient Information:

For external use only.

If condition persists or worsens, or if irritation (burning, itching, stinging, redness) occurs, discontinue use and notify physician.

Use for full treatment time, even if symptoms improve. Notify physician if there is no improvement after 2 weeks (*Candida* infections, tinea cruris and corporis) or 4 weeks (tinea pedis).

Administration and Dosage:

Cream and lotion: Cover affected areas twice daily, morning and evening (once daily in patients with tinea versicolor). Lotion is preferred in intertriginous areas; if cream is used, apply sparingly to avoid maceration effects.

Powder: Spray or sprinkle liberally over affected area morning and evening.

Early relief of symptoms (2 to 3 days) occurs in most patients; clinical improvement may be seen fairly soon after treatment. However, treat candida, tinea cruris and tinea corporis for 2 weeks, and tinea pedis for 1 month, to reduce chance of recurrence. If no clinical improvement after 1 month, reevaluate diagnosis. Patients with tinea versicolor usually exhibit clinical and mycological clearing in 2 weeks.

Antifungal Agents

MICONAZOLE NITRATE

otc	**Miconazole Nitrate** (Taro)	**Cream:** 2%	Benzoic acid, mineral oil, apricot kernal oil. In 15 and 30 g.
otc	**Micatin** (Ortho)		Mineral oil. In 15 and 30 g.
Rx	**Monistat-Derm** (Ortho)		Water miscible, mineral oil base. In 15, 30 and 90 g.
otc	**Maximum Strength Desenex Antifungal** (Ciba)		EDTA. In 14 g.
Rx	**Fungoid Creme** (Pedinol)		Mineral oil. In 56.7 g.
otc	**Micatin** (Ortho)	**Powder:** 2%	In 90 g.
otc	**Lotrimin AF** (Schering-Plough)		Talc. In 90 g.
otc	**Zeasorb-AF** (Stiefel)		In 70 g.
otc	**Breezee Mist Antfungal** (Pedinol)		Isobutane, talc, aluminum chlorhydrate, cyclomenticone, isopropyl myristate, propylene carbonate, menthol
otc	**Absorbine Antifungal Foot Powder** (W.F. Young)		10% alcohol. In 85 g.
otc	**Ony-Clear** (Pedinol)	**Spray:** 2%	Benzyl alcohol. In 42.5 g.
otc	**Lotrimin AF** (Schering-Plough)	**Spray Powder:** 2%	10% SD alcohol 40. In 100 g.
otc	**Micatin** (Ortho)		Alcohol. Available with and without deodorant. In 90 g.
otc	**Prescription Strength Desenex** (Ciba)		10% SD alcohol 40-B, aloe vera gel. In 90 ml.
otc	**Micatin** (Ortho)	**Spray Liquid:** 2%	Alcohol. In 105 ml.
otc	**Lotrimin AF** (Schering-Plough)		17% SD alcohol 40. In 113 ml.
otc	**Prescription Strength Desenex** (Ciba)		15% SD alcohol 40-B. In 105 ml.
otc	**Fungoid Tincture** (Pedinol)	**Solution:** 2%	Alcohol. In 7.39 and 29.57 ml with brush applicator.

Antifungal Agents

ECONAZOLE NITRATE

Actions:

Pharmacokinetics: After topical application to the skin, systemic absorption is extremely low. Although most of the applied drug remains on the skin surface, drug concentrations were found in the stratum corneum which exceeded, by far, the minimum inhibitory concentration for dermatophytes. Inhibitory concentrations were achieved in the epidermis and as deep as the middle region of the dermis. Less than 1% of the applied dose was recovered in the urine and feces.

Microbiology: In vitro studies revealed econazole nitrate's broad spectrum antifungal activity against the dermatophytes, *Trichophyton rubrum, T mentagrophytes, T tonsurans, Microsporum canis, M audouini, M gypseum* and *Epidermophyton floccosum,* the yeasts, *Candida albicans* and *Malassezia furfur* (the organism responsible for tinea versicolor) and certain gram-positive bacteria.

Indications:

Treatment of tinea pedis (athlete's foot), tinea cruris (jock itch) and tinea corporis (ringworm) caused by *T rubrum, T mentagrophytes, T tonsurans, M canis, M audouini, M gypseum* and *E floccosum;* cutaneous candidiasis; tinea versicolor.

Contraindications:

Hypersensitivity to econazole nitrate or any ingredients of the product.

Warnings:

Pregnancy: Category C. Fetotoxic or embryotoxic effects were observed in animal studies with oral doses 10 to 40 times the human dermal dose.

Do not use in the first trimester of pregnancy, unless essential to the patient's welfare. Use during the second and third trimesters only if clearly needed.

Lactation: It is not known whether econazole is excreted in breast milk. Following oral administration to lactating rats, econazole or its metabolites were excreted in milk. Exercise caution when applying on a nursing mother.

Precautions:

Sensitivity: If sensitivity or chemical irritation occurs, discontinue use.

For external use only. Avoid contact with the eyes.

Adverse Reactions:

Local: Burning, itching, stinging, erythema (3%); pruritic rash (one case).

Patient Information:

For external use only. Avoid contact with the eyes.

Cleanse skin with soap and water and dry thoroughly.

For athlete's foot, wear well-fitting and ventilated shoes and change shoes and socks at least once a day.

If condition persists or worsens, or if irritation (burning, itching, stinging, redness) occurs, discontinue use and notify physician.

Use medication for the full treatment time, even though symptoms may have improved. Notify physician if there is no improvement after 2 weeks (tinea cruris and corporis) or 4 weeks (tinea pedis).

Apply after cleansing affected area (unless directed otherwise).

Administration and Dosage:

Tinea pedis, tinea cruris, tinea corporis and tinea versicolor: Apply sufficient quantity to cover affected areas once daily.

Cutaneous candidiasis: Apply twice daily (morning and evening).

Early relief of symptoms is experienced by most patients, and clinical improvement may be seen fairly soon after treatment is begun. However, treat candidal infections and tinea cruris and corporis for 2 weeks and tinea pedis for 1 month, to reduce the possibility of recurrence. If no clinical improvement occurs after the treatment period, reevaluate diagnosis. Patients with tinea versicolor usually exhibit clinical and mycological clearing after 2 weeks of treatment.

Rx	**Spectazole** (Ortho)	**Cream:** 1%	Water miscible base. Mineral oil. In 15, 30 and 85 g.

Antifungal Agents

CICLOPIROX OLAMINE

Actions:

Pharmacology: A broad spectrum, antifungal agent. The primary site of action is the cell membrane. At concentrations < 20 mg/L, ciclopirox blocks transmembrane transport of amino acids into the fungal cell. At higher concentrations, the fungal cell membrane integrity is altered, allowing leakage of intracellular material.

Pharmacokinetics: An average of 1.3% was absorbed when applied topically, followed by occlusion for 6 hours. The half-life was 1.7 hours and excretion occurred via the kidney. Fecal excretion was negligible.

Studies in human cadaverous skin from the back with ciclopirox cream 1% showed 0.8% to 1.6% of the dose in stratum corneum 1.5 to 6 hours after application. Levels in the dermis were still 10 to 15 times above the minimum inhibitory concentrations.

Ciclopirox penetrates into the hair and through the epidermis and hair follicles into the sebaceous glands and dermis, while a portion of the drug remains in the stratum corneum.

Microbiology: Ciclopirox inhibits the growth of pathogenic dermatophytes, yeasts and Malassezia furfur. It exhibits fungicidal activity in vitro against isolates of *Trichophyton rubrum, T mentagrophytes, Epidermophyton floccosum, Microsporum canis* and *Candida albicans.*

Indications:

Tinea pedis (athlete's foot), tinea cruris (jock itch) and tinea corporis (ringworm) due to *T rubrum, T mentagrophytes, E floccosum* and *M canis;* candidiasis (moniliasis) due to *C albicans;* tinea (pityriasis) versicolor due to *M furfur.*

Contraindications:

Hypersensitivity to ciclopirox olamine or any of its components.

Warnings:

Pregnancy: Category B. There are no adequate or well controlled studies in pregnant women. Use during pregnancy only if clearly needed.

Lactation: It is not known whether this drug is excreted in breast milk. Exercise caution when applying on a nursing woman.

Children: Safety and efficacy in children < 10 years old have not been established.

Precautions:

For external use only. Avoid contact with the eyes.

Sensitivity: If sensitivity or chemical irritation occurs, discontinue treatment.

Adverse Reactions:

Local reactions consist of irritation, pruritus at applicaiton site, redness, pain, burning, worsening of clinical signs and symptoms.

Patient Information:

For external use only. Avoid contact with the eyes.

Cleanse skin with soap and water and dry thoroughly.

For athlete's foot, wear well-fitting, ventilated shoes and change shoes and socks at least once a day.

Use the medication for the full treatment time, even though symptoms may have improved. Notify the physician if no improvement occurs after 4 weeks.

Inform physician if the area of application shows signs of increased irritation (eg, redness, itching, burning, blistering, swelling, oozing) indicative of possible sensitization.

Avoid the use of occlusive wrappings or dressings.

Administration and Dosage:

Gently massage cream into the affected and surrounding skin areas twice daily, morning and evening. Clinical improvement usually occurs within the first week of treatment. If no improvement occurs after 4 weeks of treatment, reevaluate the diagnosis. Patients with tinea versicolor usually exhibit clinical and mycological clearing after 2 weeks of treatment.

Rx	**Loprox** (Hoechst Marion Roussel)	**Cream:** 1%	Water miscible base. 1% benzyl alcohol, mineral oil. In 15, 30 and 90 g.
		Lotion: 1%	Water miscible base. 1% benzyl alcohol, mineral oil. In 30 ml.

Antifungal Agents

CLOTRIMAZOLE

For information on oral and vaginal clotrimazole, refer to individual monographs.

Actions:

Microbiology: Clotrimazole, a broad spectrum antifungal agent, inhibits growth of pathogenic dermatophytes, yeasts and *Malassezia furfur.* Exhibits fungistatic and fungicidal activity in vitro against isolates of *Trichophyton rubrum, T mentagrophytes, Epidermophyton floccosum, Microsporum canis* and *Candida* sp, including *C albicans.* No single step or multiple step resistance to clotrimazole has developed during successive passages of *C albicans* and *T mentagrophytes.*

Indications:

Otc products: Topical treatment of tinea pedis (athlete's foot), tinea cruris (jock itch) and tinea corporis (ringworm) due to *T rubrum, T mentagrophytes, E floccosum* and *M canis.*

Mycelex (Rx): Same as *otc* products plus candidiasis due to *C albicans* and tinea versicolor due to *M furfur.*

Lotrimin (Rx): Candidiasis due to *C albicans* and tinea versicolor due to *M furfur.*

Contraindications:

Hypersensitivity to clotrimazole or any product component.

Warnings:

Pregnancy: Category B. In clinical trials, vaginal use in pregnant women in their second and third trimesters has not been associated with ill effects.

There are, however, no adequate and well controlled studies in pregnant women during the first trimester of pregnancy. Use only if clearly indicated during the first trimester.

Lactation: It is not known whether this drug is excreted in breast milk. Exercise caution when applying on a nursing mother.

Precautions:

For external use only. Avoid contact with the eyes.

If irritation or sensitivity develops, discontinue use and institute appropriate therapy.

Adverse Reactions:

Erythema; stinging; blistering; peeling; edema; pruritus; urticaria; burning; general skin irritation.

Patient Information:

For external use only. Avoid contact with the eyes.

Apply after cleansing affected area (unless directed otherwise).

If condition persists or worsens, or if irritation occurs, discontinue use and notify physician.

Use the medication for the full treatment time even though the symptoms may have improved. Notify physician if no improvement after 4 weeks of treatment.

Inform the physician if the area of application shows signs of increased irritation (eg, redness, itching, burning, blistering, swelling, oozing) indicative of possible sensitization.

Administration and Dosage:

Gently massage into affected and surrounding skin areas twice daily, morning and evening. Clinical improvement, with relief of pruritus, usually occurs within the first week of treatment. If patient shows no clinical improvement after 4 weeks, reevaluate the diagnosis.

Antifungal Agents

CLOTRIMAZOLE

Rx	**Clotrimazole** (Taro)	**Cream:** 1%	1% benzyl alcohol, cetostearyl alcohol. Vanishing base. In 15, 30, 45 and 2 x 45 g.
Rx	**Lotrimin** (Schering)		In 15, 30, 45 and 90 g.
otc	**Lotrimin AF** (Schering-Plough)		In 12 g.
Rx	**Mycelex** (Miles)		In 15, 30 and 45 g.
otc	**Mycelex OTC** (Miles)		1% benzyl alcohol. In 15 g.
otc	**Prescription Strength Desenex** (Ciba)		1% benzyl alcohol, cetostearyl alcohol. In 15 g.
Rx	**Clotrimazole** (Lemmon)	**Solution:** 1%	In 10 and 30 ml.
Rx	**Fungoid** (Pedinol)		PEG 400. In 30 ml.
Rx	**Lotrimin** (Schering)		PEG 400. In 10 and 30 ml.
otc	**Lotrimin AF** (Schering-Plough)		Polyethylene glycol. In 10 ml.
Rx	**Mycelex** (Miles)		In 10 and 30 ml.
otc	**Mycelex OTC** (Miles)		PEG 400. In 10 ml.
Rx	**Lotrimin** (Schering)	**Lotion:** 1%	In 30 ml.
Rx	**Lotrimin AF** (Schering-Plough)		1% benzyl alcohol, cetearyl alcohol. In 20 ml.

Antifungal Agents

TRIACETIN (Glyceryl Triacetate)

Actions:

Pharmacology: Triacetin, broad spectrum antifungal and antimicrobial agent, inhibits growth of fungus, yeast and bacterial infections of skin, intertriginous areas and topical mycoses. Effective against the following organisms:

Microbiology:

Fungus, yeasts – Aureobasidium mansonii (Cladosporium werneckii and *mansonii); Alternaria solani; Aspergillus niger; Candida albicans; Epidermophyton floccosum; Microsporum audouinii, canis* and *gypseum; Penicillium chrysogenum; Piedraia hortae; Rhizopus (nigricans) arrhizus; Saccharomyces (pastorianus) bayanus; Torula roseus (Candida* sp); *Trichophyton mentagrophytes,* and *rubrum, schoenleinii, tonsurans* and *violaceum; Trichosporon beigelii.*

Gram positive – Bacillus ammoniagenes (Brevibacterium ammoniagenes), cereus (subsp. *mycoides)* and *subtilis; Staphylococcus aureus; Streptococcus faecalis.*

Gram negative – Enterobacter aerogenes; Escherichia coli; Pseudomonas aeruginosa; Proteus vulgaris.

When used for onychomycosis, it facilitates removal of hyperkeratotic or mycotic tissue before debriding nail groove due to its apparent softening effect.

Indications:

Treatment of onychomycosis (nail fungus), tinea pedis (athlete's foot), tinea cruris (jock itch), tinea corporis (ringworm), monilial impetigo and dermatitis.

Spray and tincture: Only for treatment of onychomycosis.

Contraindications:

Sensitivity to any components of the products.

Precautions:

Irritation or sensitivity: Discontinue treatment and notify physician.

For external use only. Not for ophthalmic use.

Diabetics or patients with impaired blood circulation: Use spray with caution.

Patient Information:

For external use only. Avoid contact with the eyes.

Apply after cleansing affected area (unless directed otherwise).

Notify the physician if there is no improvement after 4 weeks of treatment (except when treating nail fungus, which may take several months).

Inform the physician if the area of application shows signs of increased irritation indicative of possible sensitization.

Administration and Dosage:

Cream, solution: Cleanse and dry affected areas. Gently massage sufficient amount into affected and surrounding skin areas 3 times daily. Clinical improvement usually occurs within the first week of therapy. If no clinical improvement occurs after 4 weeks of treatment, review the diagnosis.

Tincture: Cleanse and dry affected areas. Use brush to apply twice daily to affected areas of nail surface, beds, edges and under surface of the nail. Continued use may be necessary for several months before results are seen.

Spray: Shake well. Dry affected areas. Spray onto affected nails, holding actuator down 1 to 2 seconds.

Rx	**Fungoid Tincture** (Pedinol)	**Solution:** Triacetin, cetylpyridinium chloride, chloroxylenol, benzyl alcohol, acetone, benzalkonium chloride	In 30 ml and pt.
Rx	**Fungoid** (Pedinol)	**Solution:** Triacetin, PEG-8, cetylpyridinium chloride, chloroxylenol and benzalkonium chloride	In 15 ml.
Rx	**Fungoid Creme** (Pedinol)	**Cream:** Triacetin, cetylpyridinium chloride, chloroxylenol, mineral oil, lanolin, propylene glycol, parabens in a vanishing cream base	In 30 g.
Rx	**Ony-Clear Nail** (Pedinol)	**Spray, Aerosol:** Triacetin, cetylpyridinium chloride, chloroxylenol, benzalkonium chloride, alcohol	In 45 and 60 ml.

Antifungal Agents

TOLNAFTATE

Actions:

Pharmacology: Effective in the treatment of superficial fungus infections of the skin.

Indications:

Treatment of tinea pedis (athlete's foot), cruris (jock itch) or corporis (ringworm) due to infection with *Trichophyton rubrum, T mentagrophytes, T tonsurans, Microsporum canis, M audouini* and *Epidermophyton floccosum* and for tinea versicolor due to *Malassezia furfur.*

In onychomycosis, in chronic scalp infections in which fungi are numerous and widely distributed in skin and hair follicles, where kerion has formed and in fungus infections of palms and soles, use tolnaftate concurrently for adjunctive local benefit in these lesions.

Powder and powder aerosol: Also effective prophylactically against athlete's foot.

Warnings:

Sensitization or irritation: Discontinue treatment.

Nail/Scalp infections: Not recommended for these infections except as adjunctive therapy to systemic treatment.

If symptoms do not improve after 10 days of use as recommended by the labeling, discontinue use unless otherwise directed.

Precautions:

For external use only. Keep out of eyes.

Reevaluate patient if no improvement occurs after 4 weeks.

Adverse Reactions:

A few cases of sensitization have been confirmed; mild irritation has occurred.

Patient Information:

For external use only. Avoid contact with the eyes.

Cleanse skin with soap and water and dry thoroughly before applying product.

For athlete's foot, wear well-fitting, ventilated shoes; change shoes and socks at least once a day.

Administration and Dosage:

Only small quantities are required. Treatment twice a day for 2 or 3 weeks is usually adequate, although 4 to 6 weeks may be required if the skin has thickened. Continue treatment to maintain remission.

The choice of vehicle is important for these products. Ointments, creams and liquids are used as primary therapy. In general, powders are used as adjunctive therapy, but they may be acceptable as primary therapy in very mild conditions.

Antifungal Agents

TOLNAFTATE

otc	**Tolnaftate** (Various, eg, Fougera, Goldline, IDE, Major, Moore, Parmed, NMC, Rugby, UDL)	**Cream:** 1%	In 15 g.
otc	**Absorbine Antifungal** (W.F. Young)		Glyceryl monostearate, PPG, diazolidinyl urea, parabens. In 21.3 g.
otc	**Genaspor** (Goldline)		In 15 g.
otc	**NP • 27** (Thompson Med)		In 15 and 30 g.
otc	**Tinactin** (Schering-Plough)		In 15 and 30 g.
otc	**Tinactin for Jock Itch** (Schering-Plough)		Petrolatum, mineral oil. In 15 g.
otc	**Ting** (Fisons)		In 15 g.
otc	**Abosrbine Athlete's Foot Care** (W.F. Young)	**Liquid:** 1% tolnaftate	Menthol. In 59.2 ml.
otc	**Tolnaftate** (Various, eg, Copley, Fougera, Goldline, IDE, Major, Moore, NMC, Parmed, Rugby)	**Solution:** 1%	In 10 ml.
otc	**Blis-To-Sol** (Chattem)		In 30 and 55.5 ml.
otc	**NP • 27** (Thompson Med)		In 15 ml.
otc	**Tinactin** (Schering-Plough)		In 10 ml.
otc	**Aftate for Athlete's Foot** (Schering-Plough)	**Gel:** 1%	In 15 g.
otc	**Aftate for Jock Itch** (Schering-Plough)		In 15 g.
otc	**Tolnaftate** (Various)	**Powder:** 1%	In 45 g.
otc	**Absorbine Antifungal** (W.F. Young)		Corn starch, parabens, zinc stearate. In 56.7 g.
otc	**Absorbine Jock Itch** (W.F. Young)		Corn starch, parabens, zinc stearate. In 56.7 g.
otc	**Aftate for Athlete's Foot** (Schering-Plough)		Starch, talc. In 67.5 g.
otc	**Aftate for Jock Itch** (Schering-Plough)		14% alcohol, talc. In 75 g.
otc	**Breezee Mist Antifungal** (Pedinol)		Talc, menthol crystals. In 113 g.
otc	**NP • 27** (Thompson Med)		Cornstarch, talc. In 45 g.
otc	**Quinsana Plus** (Mennen)		Cornstarch, talc. In 90 g.
otc	**Tinactin** (Schering-Plough)		Cornstarch, talc. In 45, 90 g.
otc	**Ting** (Fisons)		Cornstarch, talc. In 45 g.
otc	**Zeasorb-AF** (Stiefel)		Talc. In 70.9 g.
otc	**Dr. Scholl's Maximum Strength Tritin** (Schering-Plough)		Talc. In 56 g.
otc	**Dr. Scholl's Athlete's Foot** (Schering-Plough)		Talc. In 63 g.

Antifungal Agents

TOLNAFTATE

otc	**Tolnaftate** (Various)	**Spray Powder:** 1%	In 105 g.
otc	**Aftate for Athlete's Foot** (Schering-Plough)		14% alcohol and talc. In 105 g.
otc	**Aftate for Jock Itch** (Schering-Plough)		36% alcohol. In 105 g.
otc	**NP • 27** (Thompson Medical)		14.9% alcohol, talc. In 105 g.
otc	**Tinactin** (Schering-Plough)		14% alcohol and talc. **Deodorant:** In 100 g. **Regular:** In 100, 150 g.
otc	**Tinactin for Jock Itch** (Schering-Plough)		14% alcohol and talc. In 100 g.
otc	**Ting** (Fisons)		14% alcohol, talc. In 90 g.
otc	**Dr. Scholl's Athlete's Foot** (Schering-Plough)		14% SD alcohol 40. In 99 g.
otc	**Dr. Scholl's Maximum Strength Tritin** (Schering-Plough)		14% SD alcohol 40. In 85 g.
otc	**Absorbine Jr. Antifungal** (W.F. Young)	**Spray Liquid:** 1%	Acetone, chloroxylenol, menthol, wormwood oil. In 59.2 and 118.3 ml.
otc	**Aftate for Athlete's Foot** (Schering-Plough)		36% alcohol. In 120 ml.
otc	**Desenex** (Fisons)		With PEG 400 and 41% SD alcohol 40-B. In 90 ml.
otc	**Tinactin** (Schering-Plough)		36% alcohol. In 120 ml.
otc	**Ting** (Fisons)		41% alcohol. In 90 ml.
otc	**Dr. Scholl's Athlete's Foot** (Schering-Plough)		36% alcohol. In 113 ml.

GENTIAN VIOLET (Methylrosaniline chloride; Crystal Violet)

Actions:

Pharmacology: An antibacterial and antifungal dye. It is bactericidal to gram-positive organisms in very high dilutions. It inhibits the growth of *Monilia, Torula, Epidermophyton* and *Trichophyton.* Because of its cosmetic effects and staining of clothing, gentian violet has generally been replaced in practice by other topical agents.

Indications:

Topical anti-infective.

Precautions:

For external use only. Avoid contact with the eyes.

Patient Information:

For external use only. Avoid contact with the eyes.

Gentian violet will stain skin and clothing.

Do not apply to an ulcerative lesion; may result in "tattooing" of the skin.

Administration and Dosage:

Apply locally 2 times daily or as directed.

otc	**Gentian Violet** (Various)	**Solution:** 1%	In 30 ml.
		2%	In 30 ml.

OXICONAZOLE NITRATE

Actions:

Pharmacology: Oxiconazole is a broad spectrum antifungal for topical dermatologic use. The fungicidal activity of oxiconazole results primarily from the inhibition of ergosterol synthesis, which is needed for cytoplasmic membrane integrity. It has in vitro activity against a wide range of organisms. Five hours after application of 2.5 mg/cm^2 of oxiconazole cream, the concentration of oxiconazole nitrate in the epidermis, upper corium and deeper corium was 16.2, 3.64 and 1.29 mcmol, respectively. Systemic absorption of oxiconazole appears to be low. Less than 0.3% of the applied dose was recovered in the urine of subjects up to 5 days after application.

Microbiology: Oxiconazole is active against most strains of the following organisms both in vitro and in clinical infections: *Epidermophyton floccosum, Trichophyton rubrum* and *T mentagrophytes.*

Oxiconazole is active against the following microorganisms in vitro; however, clinical significance is unknown. However, safety and efficacy in treating clinical infections due to these organisms have not been established in adequate and well controlled trials: *Trichophyton tonsurans, T violaceum, Microsporum canis, M audouini, M gypseum, Candida albicans* and *Malassezia furfur.*

Indications:

Topical treatment of the following dermal infections: Tinea pedis (athlete's foot), tinea cruris (jock itch) and tinea corporis (ringworm) due to *T rubrum,T mentagrophytes* and *Epidermophyton floccosum.*

Contraindications:

Hypersensitivity to oxiconazole or any of the components of the product.

Warnings:

Fertility impairment: At doses 3 mg/kg/day in female rats and 15 mg/kg/day in male rats, the following effects were observed: Reduction in the fertility parameters; reduction in the number of sperm in vaginal smears; extended estrus cycle; decrease in mating frequency.

Pregnancy: Category B. There are no adequate and well controlled studies in pregnant women. Use during pregnancy only if clearly needed.

Lactation: Since oxiconazole is excreted in breast milk, exercise caution when the drug is applied on a nursing woman.

Precautions:

Sensitivity: If a reaction suggesting sensitivity or chemical irritation should occur with the use of oxiconazole nitrate, discontinue treatment and institute appropriate therapy.

For external use only. Avoid contact with the eyes or vagina.

Adverse Reactions:

Pruritus (0.4% to 1.6%); burning (0.7% to 1.4%); stinging (0.7%); irritation, contact dermatitis, scaling, tingling, pain, dyshidrotic eczema (0.4%); folliculitis (0.3%); erythema (0.2%); papules, rash, stinging, nodules, maceration, fissuring (0.1%).

Patient Information:

For external use only. Avoid contact with the eyes or vagina.

Administration and Dosage:

Apply to cover affected areas once to twice daily in patients with tinea pedis, tinea corporis and tinea cruris. Treat tinea corporis and tinea cruris for 2 weeks and tinea pedis for 1 month to reduce the possibility of recurrence. If a patient shows no clinical improvement after the treatment period, review the diagnosis.

Rx	**Oxistat** (Glaxo Wellcome)	**Cream:** 1%	White petrolatum, propylene glycol, 0.2% benzoic acid. In 15, 30 and 60 g tubes.
		Lotion: 1%	White petrolatum, propylene glycol, 0.2% benzoic acid. In 30 ml.

Antifungal Agents

SULCONAZOLE NITRATE

Actions:

Pharmacology: Sulconazole nitrate, a broad spectrum antifungal agent for topical use, is an imidazole derivative with antifungal and antiyeast activity. It inhibits growth of the common pathogenic dermatophytes including *Trichophyton rubrum* (cream only), *T mentagrophytes, Epidermophyton floccosum* and *Microsporum canis.* It also inhibits the organism responsible for tinea versicolor, *(Malassezia furfur), Candida albicans* (cream only) and certain gram-positive bacteria.

A maximization test showed no evidence of irritation or contact sensitization. A modified Draize test showed no allergic contact dermatitis and a phototoxicity study showed no phototoxic or photoallergic reaction to sulconazole nitrate cream.

Indications:

Treatment of tinea pedis (athlete's foot; cream only), tinea cruris (jock itch) and tinea corporis (ringworm) caused by *T rubrum, T mentagrophytes, E floccosum* and *M canis;* tinea versicolor.

Solution: Efficacy has not been proven in tinea pedis (athlete's foot).

Contraindications:

Hypersensitivity to any of the components of the product.

Warnings:

Pregnancy: Category C. There are no adequate and well controlled studies in pregnant women. Use during pregnancy only if clearly needed. Sulconazole is embryotoxic in rats when given in doses 125 times the adult human dose. Sulconazole given orally to rats at a dose 125 times the human dose resulted in prolonged gestation and dystocia. Several females died during the perinatal period, most likely due to labor complications.

Lactation: Use with caution in nursing mothers since it is not known if sulconazole appears in breast milk.

Children: Safety and efficacy for use in children have not been established.

Precautions:

For external use only. Avoid contact with the eyes.

If irritation develops, discontinue the solution and institute appropriate therapy.

Adverse Reactions:

Local: Itching, burning, stinging (3%); redness (1%).

Patient Information:

Use only as directed.

For external use only. Avoid contact with the eyes.

Administration and Dosage:

Gently massage a small amount into the affected and surrounding skin areas once or twice daily, except in tinea pedis, where administration should be twice daily.

Early relief of symptoms is experienced by the majority of patients and clinical improvement may be seen fairly soon after treatment is begun. To reduce the possibility of recurrence, treat tinea cruris, tinea corporis and tinea versicolor for 3 weeks and tinea pedis for 4 weeks.

If significant clinical improvement is not seen after 4 to 6 weeks of treatment, consider an alternate diagnosis.

Rx	**Exelderm** (Westwood Squibb)	**Cream:** 1%	In 15, 30 and 60 g tubes.
		Solution: 1%	In 30 ml.

Antifungal Agents

NYSTATIN

For information on oral and vaginal nystatin, refer to the individual monographs.

Actions:

Pharmacology: An antifungal antibiotic which is both fungistatic and fungicidal in vitro against a wide variety of yeasts and yeast-like fungi. It probably acts by binding to sterols in the cell membrane of the fungus with a resultant change in membrane permeability allowing leakage of intracellular components. It provides specific therapy for all localized forms of candidiasis, and cure is effected both clinically and mycologically in most localized cases. Symptomatic relief is rapid, often occurring within 24 to 72 hours after initiation of treatment.

Indications:

Treatment of cutaneous or mucocutaneous mycotic infections caused by *Candida (Monilia) albicans* and other *Candida* species.

Contraindications:

Hypersensitivity to any component; not for ophthalmic use.

Precautions:

For external use only. Avoid contact with the eyes.

Hypersensitivity: Should a hypersensitivity reaction occur, withdraw drug and take appropriate measures.

Adverse Reactions:

Virtually nontoxic and nonsensitizing; well tolerated by all age groups including debilitated infants, even on prolonged administration. If irritation occurs, discontinue use.

Patient Information:

For external use only. Avoid contact with the eyes.

Apply after cleansing affected area (unless directed otherwise).

If irritation occurs, discontinue use and notify physician.

Administration and Dosage:

Apply to affected areas 2 to 3 times daily, or as indicated, until healing is complete. For fungal infection of the feet caused by *Candida,* dust the powder freely on the feet as well as in shoes and socks. The cream is usually preferred in candidiasis involving intertriginous areas; very moist lesions, however, are best treated with powder.

Rx	**Nystatin** (Various, eg, Geneva, Major, NMC, Parmed, Rugby)	**Cream:** 100,000 units per g	In 15 and 30 g.
Rx	**Mycostatin** (Westwood Squibb)		Aqueous vanishing cream base. In 15 and 30 g.
Rx	**Nilstat** (Lederle)		Aqueous vanishing cream base. In 15 and 240 g.
Rx	**Nystex** (Savage)		Aqueous vanishing cream base. White petrolatum, parabens. In 15 & 30 g.
Rx	**Nystatin** (Various, eg, Genetco, Goldline, Major, Moore, NMC, Rugby, Schein, URL)	**Ointment:** 100,000 units per g	In 15 and 30 g.
Rx	**Mycostatin** (Westwood Squibb)		Polyethylene and mineral oil gel base. In 15 and 30 g.
Rx	**Nilstat** (Lederle)		Light mineral oil and plastibase 50W. In 15 g.
Rx	**Nystex** (Savage)		Polyethylene and mineral oil base. In 15 g.
Rx	**Mycostatin** (Westwood Squibb)	**Powder:** 100,000 units per g	Dispersed in talc. In 15 g.
Rx	**Pedi-Dri** (Pedinol)		Cornstarch, aluminum chlorhydroxide, menthol. In 56.7 g.

Antifungal Agents

BUTENAFINE HCl

Actions:

Pharmacology:

Mechanism of action – Butenafine is a benzylamine derivative with a mode of action similar to that of the allylamine class of antifungal drugs. Butenafine is hypothesized to act by inhibiting the epoxidation of squalene, thus blocking the biosynthesis of ergosterol, an essential component of fungal cell membranes. The benzylamine derivatives, like the allylamines, act at an earlier step in the ergosterol biosynthesis pathway than the azole class of antifungal drugs. Depending on the concentration of the drug and the fungal species tested in vitro, butenafine may be antifungal.

Pharmacokinetics: Following daily application for 14 days of 6 grams of butenafine cream 1% to the dorsal skin (3000 cm^2), the mean (± SD) maximum plasma concentration of butenafine was 1.4 ng/ml. The mean time to peak plasma concentration, T_{max}, was 15 hours. After daily dosing to the arms, trunk and groin areas (10,000 cm^2) for 14 days with 20 grams of butenafine cream 1%, the mean maximum plasma concentration of butenafine was 5 ng/ml at a mean T_{max} of 6 hours. The total amount of butenafine absorbed through the skin into the systemic circulation has not been quantitated. The primary urine metabolite was formed through hydroxylation at the terminal γ-butyl side cjain.

Microbiology: Butenafine has been shown to be active against most strains of the following microorganisms, both in vitro and in clinical infections: *Epidermophyton floccosum, Trichophyton mentagrophytes* and *Trichophyton rubrum.*

Indications:

Treatment of interdidgital tinea pedis (athelete's foot) due to *E. floccosum, T. mentagrophytes* or *T. rubrum.*

Contraindications:

Known hypersensitivity to butenafine or any of its components.

Warnings:

Irritation: If irritation or sensitivity develops with the use of butenafine, discontinue treatment and institute appropriate therapy.

Diagnosis of the disease should be confirmed either by direct microscopic examination of a mounting of infected tissue in a solution of potassium hydroxide or by culture in an appropriate medium.

Hypersensitivity: Patients who are known to be sensitive to allylamine antifungals should use butenafine with caution, because it is possible that these drugs may be cross-reactive.

Pregnancy: Category B. There are no adequate and well controlled studies of topically applied butenafine in pregnant women. Use during pregnancy only if clearly needed.

Lactation: It is not known if this drug is excreted in breast milk. Exercise caution when administering to a breastfeeding woman.

Children: Safety and efficacy in pediatric patients < 12 years of age have not been established.

Adverse Reactions:

Contact dermatitis, burning/stinging, worsening of the condition (≈ 2%); erythema, irritation and itching (< 2%). No patient treated with butenafine discontinued treatment due to an adverse event. In the vehicle-treated patients, 1 of 132 patients discontinued because of severe burning/stinging and itching at the site of application.

Patient Information:

Use as directed by physician. Wash hands after applying medication to the affected area(s). Avoid contact with the eyes, nose, mouth and other mucous membranes.

Butenafine is for external use only.

If the patient wishes to apply the medication after bathing, dry the feet thoroughly, especially between the toes, before application.

Use the medication for the full treatjment time recommended by the physician, even though symptoms may have improved. Notify the physician if the condition worsens or if there is no improvement after 4 weeks.

Inform the physician if the area of application shows signs of increased irritation, redness, itching, burning, blistering, swelling or oozing.

Avoid the use of occlusive dressings unless otherwise directed by the physician.

Do not use this medication for any disorder except that for which it is prescribed.

Antifungal Agents

BUTENAFINE HCl

Administration and Dosage:

For external use only.

Butenafine is not for ophthalmic, oral or intravaginal use. Apply butenafine to cover the affected area and immediately surrounding skin once daily for 4 weeks. If a patient shows no clinical signs of improvement after the treatment period, review the disgnosis.

Storage/Stability: Store between 5° and 30°C (41° and 86°F).

Rx	**Mentax** (Penederm)	**Cream:** 1% butenafine HCl	Benzyl and cetyl alcohol. In 2, 15 and 30 g tubes.

AMPHOTERICIN B

For information on the systemic use of amphotericin B, refer to the individual monograph in the Anti-infectives section.

Actions:

Pharmacology: An antibiotic with antifungal activity produced by a strain of *Streptomyces nodosus.* It exhibits greater in vitro activity than nystatin against *Candida (Monilia) albicans.* Topical amphotericin B was comparable to nystatin in similar formulations.

Although amphotericin B exhibits some in vitro activity against the superficial dermatophytes (ringworm organisms), it has not demonstrated an effectiveness in vivo on topical application.

Indications:

Treatment of cutaneous and mucocutaneous mycotic infections caused by *Candida* sp.

Contraindications:

Hypersensitivity to any of the components.

Precautions:

For external use only. Avoid contact with the eyes.

Hypersensitivity: If a hypersensitivity reaction occurs, discontinue use; initiate appropriate measures.

Adverse Reactions:

These preparations have only a slight sensitizing potential.

Cream: May have a "drying" effect on some skin. Local irritation (erythema, pruritus or a burning sensation) may occur, particularly in intertriginous areas.

Lotion: Rare local intolerance has included increased pruritus with or without other evidence of local irritation or exacerbation of preexisting candidal lesions. Allergic contact dermatitis is rare.

Ointment: May occasionally irritate when applied to moist, intertriginous areas.

Antifungal Agents

AMPHOTERICIN B

Patient Information:

For external use only. Avoid contact with the eyes.

Cleanse affected area(s) of skin prior to application (unless directed otherwise).

Apply liberally to lesions and rub in gently.

The cream may cause drying and slight discoloration of the skin. The lotion and ointment may cause staining of nail lesions, but not skin, if thoroughly rubbed in. Redness, itching or burning may also occur, particularly in skin folds; notify physician if these effects become bothersome, if skin rash develops or if the condition being treated worsens.

Any discoloration of fabrics from the cream or lotion may be removed by hand washing the fabric with soap and warm water. Any fabric discoloration from the ointment may be removed by applying a standard cleaning fluid.

Administration and Dosage:

Apply liberally to candidal lesions 2 to 4 times daily. Therapy duration depends on patient response. Intertriginous lesions usually respond in a few days; treatment may be complete in 1 to 3 weeks. Similarly, candidiasis of the diaper area, perleche and glabrous skin lesions usually clear in 1 to 2 weeks. Interdigital lesions may require 2 to 4 weeks intensive therapy; paronychias also require relatively prolonged therapy, and onychomycoses that respond may require several months or more of treatment. Relapses are frequent in the last 3 conditions.

Rx	**Fungizone** (Apothecon)	**Cream:** 3%	In an aqueous vehicle. In 20 g.
		Lotion: 3%	In an aqueous vehicle. In 30 ml.
		Ointment: 3%	In a polyethylene and mineral oil gel base with titanium dioxide. In 20 g.

Antifungal Agents

KETOCONAZOLE

Actions:

Pharmacology: Ketoconazole is a broad spectrum antifungal agent. In vitro studies suggest it impairs ergosterol synthesis, which is a vital component of fungal cell membranes. The therapeutic effect in seborrheic dermatitis and dandruff may be due to reduction of *Pityrosporum ovale (Malassezia ovale)*.

Pharmacokinetics: In animal and human studies, there were no detectable plasma levels following the use of the shampoo.

Microbiology: Ketoconazole inhibits the growth of the following common dermatophytes and yeasts by altering the permeability of the cell membrane. Dermatophytes: *Trichophyton rubrum, T mentagrophytes, T tonsurans, Microsporum canis, M audouini, M gypseum* and *Epidermophyton floccosum*. Yeasts: *Candida albicans, C tropicalis, P ovale (M ovale);* and *P orbiculare (M furfur,* the organism responsible for tinea versicolor). Development of resistance to the drug has not been reported.

Clinical trials: In a 4 week, double-blind, placebo controlled trial, the decrease in *P ovale* on the scalp was significantly greater with ketoconazole shampoo than with placebo and was comparable to selenium sulfide. Ketoconazole and selenium sulfide reduced the severity of adherent dandruff significantly more than placebo.

Indications:

Cream: Tinea corporis (ringworm), tinea cruris (jock itch) and tinea pedis (athlete's foot) caused by *Trichophyton rubrum, T mentagrophytes* and *E floccosum;* tinea (pityriasis) versicolor caused by *P orbiculare (M furfur);* cutaneous candidiasis caused by *Candida* sp; seborrheic dermatitis.

Shampoo: Reduction of scaling due to dandruff.

Contraindications:

Hypersensitivity to any component of the product.

Warnings:

Pregnancy: Category C. There are no adequate and well controlled studies in pregnant women. Use during pregnancy only if the potential benefits outweigh the potential hazards to the fetus.

Lactation: Safety for use in the nursing mother has not been established; however, exercise caution when applying on a nursing woman.

Children: Safety and efficacy in children have not been established.

Precautions:

For external use only. Avoid contact with the eyes.

Sensitivity: Discontinue if sensitivity or chemical irritation occurs.

Sulfite sensitivity: The cream contains sulfites that may cause allergic-type reactions including anaphylactic symptoms and life-threatening or less severe asthmatic episodes in certain susceptible persons. The overall prevalence of sulfite sensitivity in the general population is unknown and probably low. It is seen more frequently in asthmatic or atopic nonasthmatic persons.

Adverse Reactions:

Cream: Severe irritation, pruritus, stinging (≈ 5%); painful allergic reaction (one patient).

Shampoo: Increase in normal hair loss, irritation (< 1%); abnormal hair texture; scalp pustules; mild dryness of skin; itching; oiliness/dryness of hair and scalp.

Overdosage:

Shampoo: In the event of ingestion, employ supportive measures, including gastric lavage with sodium bicarbonate. Refer to General Management of Acute Overdosage.

Patient Information:

For external use only. Avoid contact with the eyes.

Shampoo: Removal of the curl from permanently waved hair may occur.

Administration and Dosage:

Cream:

Cutaneous candidiasis, tinea corporis, tinea cruris and tinea (pityriasis) versicolor – Apply once daily to cover the affected and immediate surrounding area. Clinical improvement may be seen fairly soon after treatment is begun; however, treat candidal infections and tinea cruris and corporis for 2 weeks in order to reduce the possibility of recurrence. Patients with tinea versicolor usually require 2 weeks of treatment. Patients with tinea pedis require 6 weeks of treatment.

Antifungal Agents

KETOCONAZOLE

Seborrheic dermatitis – Apply to the affected area twice daily for 4 weeks or until clinical clearing.

If a patient shows no clinical improvement after the treatment period, redetermine the diagnosis.

Shampoo:

Dandruff – Moisten hair and scalp thoroughly with water. Apply sufficient shampoo to produce enough lather to wash scalp and hair and gently massage it over the entire scalp area for ≈ 1 minute. Rinse hair thoroughly with warm water. Repeat, leaving shampoo on scalp for an additional 3 minutes. After the second thorough rinse, dry hair with towel or warm air flow.

Shampoo twice a week for 4 weeks with at least 3 days between each shampooing, and then intermittently as needed to maintain control.

Storage – Do not store above room temperature (25°C; 77°F); protect from light.

Rx	**Nizoral** (Janssen)	**Cream:** 2% in an aqueous vehicle[1]	In 15, 30 and 60 g.
		Shampoo: 2% in an aqueous suspension	In 120 ml.

[1] With sodium sulfite.

HALOPROGIN

Actions:

Pharmacology: A synthetic antifungal agent for treatment of superficial fungal infections of the skin.

Indications:

Treatment of tinea pedis (athlete's foot), tinea cruris (jock itch), tinea corporis (ringworm) and tinea manuum due to *Trichophyton rubrum, T tonsurans, T mentagrophytes, Microsporum canis* and *Epidermophyton floccosum.* Also useful in the topical treatment of tinea versicolor due to *Malassezia furfur.*

Contraindications:

Hypersensitivity to any of the components.

Warnings:

Pregnancy: Category B. There are no adequate and well controlled studies in pregnant women. Use only when clearly needed.

Lactation: It is not known whether this drug is excreted in breast milk. Exercise caution when applying on a nursing woman.

Children: Safety and efficacy for use in children have not been established.

Precautions:

Sensitization or irritation: Discontinue treatment and institute appropriate therapy.

Reevaluate the diagnosis if no improvement occurs after 4 weeks of treatment. In mixed infections where bacteria or nonsusceptible fungi are present, supplementary systemic anti-infective therapy may be indicated.

For external use only. Keep out of eyes.

Adverse Reactions:

Local irritation; burning sensation; vesicle formation; erythema; scaling; itching; folliculitis; pruritus.

Patient Information:

For external use only. Avoid contact with eyes.

If condition worsens, or if irritation, redness, swelling, stinging or burning persists, discontinue use and notify physician.

Complete full course of therapy.

Administration and Dosage:

Apply liberally to the affected area twice daily for 2 to 3 weeks. Intertriginous lesions may require up to 4 weeks of therapy.

Rx	**Halotex** (Westwood-Squibb)	**Cream:** 1% in a water dispersible base	In 15 and 30 g.
		Solution: 1% with 75% alcohol	In 10 and 30 ml.

Antifungal Agents

NAFTIFINE HCl

Actions:

Pharmacology: Naftifine, a broad spectrum antifungal agent, is a synthetic allylamine derivative. Although the exact mechanism of action against fungi is not known, naftifine appears to interfere with sterol biosynthesis by inhibiting the enzyme squalene 2,3-epoxidase. This inhibition of enzyme activity results in decreased amounts of sterols, especially ergosterol, and a corresponding accumulation of squalene in the cells.

Pharmacokinetics: Naftifine penetrates the stratum corneum to inhibit the growth of dermatophytes. Following a single topical application of 1% naftifine to the skin of healthy subjects, systemic absorption was ≈ 6% (cream) and ≤ 4.2% (gel). Naftifine or its metabolites are excreted via the urine and feces with a half-life of ≈ 2 to 3 days.

Microbiology: Naftifine exhibits fungicidal activity in vitro against a broad spectrum of organisms including *Trichophyton rubrum, T mentagrophytes, T tonsurans, Epidermophyton floccosum, Microsporum canis, M audouini* and *M gypseum,* and fungistatic activity against *Candida* sp, including *C albicans.*

Indications:

Topical treatment of tinea pedis (athlete's foot), tinea cruris (jock itch) and tinea corporis (ringworm) caused by the organisms *T rubrum, T mentagrophytes, T tonsurans** and *E floccosum.*

Contraindications:

Hypersensitivity to naftifine or any component of the product.

Warnings:

Pregnancy: Category B. There are no adequate studies in pregnant women. Use only when clearly needed and when potential benefits outweigh potential hazards to the fetus.

Lactation: It is not known whether naftifine is excreted in breast milk. Exercise caution when applying on a nursing woman.

Children: Safety and efficacy for use in children have not been established.

Precautions:

For external use only. Avoid contact with the eyes.

If irritation or sensitivity develops, discontinue treatment and institute appropriate therapy.

Adverse Reactions:

Local:

Cream – Burning/stinging (6%); dryness (3%); erythema, itching, local irritation (2%).

Gel – Burning/stinging (5%); itching (1%); erythema, rash, tenderness (0.5%).

Patient Information:

Avoid the use of occlusive dressings or wrappings unless otherwise directed by the physician.

For external use only. Keep away from the eyes, nose, mouth and other mucous membranes.

Administration and Dosage:

Gently massage a sufficient quantity into the affected area and surrounding skin once a day with the cream, twice a day (morning and evening) with the gel. Wash hands after application.

If no clinical improvement is seen after 4 weeks of treatment, re-evaluate the patient.

Rx	**Naftin** (Allergan Herbert)	**Cream:** 1%	In 15, 30 and 60 g.
		Gel: 1%	In 20, 40 and 60 g.

* Gel; efficacy studied in < 10 infections.

TERBINAFINE HCl

Actions:

Pharmacology: Terbinafine HCl is a synthetic allylamine derivative, which exerts its antifungal effect by inhibiting squalene epoxidase, a key enzyme in sterol biosynthesis in fungi. This action results in a deficiency in ergosterol and a corresponding accumulation of squalene within the fungal cell and causes fungal cell death.

Pharmacokinetics: Following a single application of 100 mcl (1 mg) to a 30 cm^2 area of the ventral forearm of six healthy subjects, the recovery in urine and feces averaged 3.5% of the administered dose.

In a study of 16 healthy subjects (eight of whose skin was artificially compromised by stripping the stratum corneum to the viable layer), single and multiple applications (average, 0.1 mg/cm^2 twice daily for 5 days) of terbinafine were made to various sites. Systemic absorption was highly variable. The maximum measured plasma concentration of terbinafine was 11.4 ng/ml, and the maximum measured plasma concentration of the demethylated metabolite was 11 ng/ml. In many patients, there were no detectable plasma levels of either parent compound or metabolite. Urinary excretion accounted for ≤ 9% of the topically applied dose; the majority excreted < 4%.

In a study of 10 patients with tinea cruris, once daily application for 7 days resulted in plasma concentrations of 0 to 11 ng/ml on day 7. Plasma concentrations of the metabolites of terbinafine ranged from 11 to 80 ng/ml in these patients.

Approximately 75% of cutaneously absorbed terbinafine is eliminated in the urine, predominantly as metabolites.

Microbiology: Terbinafine is active against most strains of the following organisms both in vitro and in clinical infections: *Epidermophyton floccosum; Trichophyton mentagrophytes; Trichophyton rubrum.* Terbinafine exhibits satisfactory in vitro MICs against most strains of the following organisms; however, safety and efficacy of terbinafine in treating clinical infections due to these organisms have not been established: *Microsporum canis, gypseum and nanum; Trichophyton verrucosum.*

Clinical trials: In the following tables, the term "successful outcome" refers to those patients evaluated at a specific time point who had both negative mycological results (culture and KOH preparation) and a total clinical score of < 2 graded on a scale from 0 = absent to 3 = severe for each sign and symptom. Mean clinical scores at entry ranged from 8 to 11.

Terbinafine Therapy: Successful Outcomes for Tinea Pedis

Therapy	1 week therapy			4 week therapy	
	At 1 week	At 4 weeks	At 6 weeks	At 4 weeks	At 6 weeks
Terbinafine	14%	51%	65%	71%	73%
Vehicle	6%	13%	12%	nd	nd
Active control	nd	nd	nd	63%	59%

nd = no data

Terbinafine Therapy: Successful Outcomes for Tinea Corporis/Cruris after 1 Week of Therapy

Disease	Drug	At 1 week	At 4 weeks
Tinea corporis	Terbinafine	21%	83%
	Vehicle	0	31%
Tinea cruris	Terbinafine	43%	92%
	Vehicle	9%	25%

Indications:

Topical treatment of the following dermatologic infections: Interdigital tinea pedis (athlete's foot), tinea cruris (jock itch) or tinea corporis (ringworm) due to *E. floccosum, T. mentagrophytes* or *T. rubrum.*

Unlabeled uses: Terbinafine is effective in the treatment of cutaneous candidiasis and pityriasis (tinea) versicolor.

Contraindications:

Hypersensitivity to terbinafine or any component of the product.

Warnings:

Diagnosis: Confirm diagnosis of the disease either by direct microscopic examination of scrapings from infected tissue mounted in a solution of potassium hydroxide or by culture.

TERBINAFINE HCl

For external use only. Not for oral, ophthalmic or intravaginal use.

Pregnancy: Category B. There are no adequate and well controlled studies in pregnant women.

Lactation: After administering a single oral dose of 500 mg to two volunteers, the total dose of terbinafine secreted in breast milk during the 72 hour post-dosing period was 0.65 mg in one person and 0.15 mg in the other. The total excretion of terbinafine in the breast milk was 0.13% and 0.03% of the administered dose, respectively. The concentrations of the one metabolite measured in breast milk of these two volunteers were below the detection limit of the assay used (150 ng/ml of milk).

Decide whether to discontinue nursing or the drug, taking into account the importance of the drug to the mother. Nursing mothers should not apply to the breast.

Children: Safety and efficacy in children < 12 years of age have not been established.

Precautions:

Irritation/Sensitivity: If irritation or sensitivity develops, discontinue treatment and institute appropriate therapy.

Adverse Reactions:

In clinical trials, 0.2% of patients discontinued therapy because of adverse events and 2.3% reported adverse reactions. These reactions included: Irritation (1%); burning (0.8%); itching, dryness (0.2%).

Overdosage:

Acute overdosage with topical application is unlikely because of the limited absorption and would not be expected to lead to a life-threatening situation.

Overdosage in rats and mice by the oral and IV routes of drug administration has produced sedation, drowsiness, ataxia, dyspnea, exophthalmos and piloerection. The majority of deaths in animals occurred following oral administration of doses exceeding 3 g/kg or following 200 mg/kg administered IV. In rabbits, overdosage produced edema, erythema and scale formation following topical doses > 1.5 g/kg.

Patient Information:

Use as directed; avoid contact with eyes, nose, mouth or other mucous membranes.

Use the medication for the recommended treatment time.

Inform the physician if the area of application shows signs of increased irritation or possible sensitization (redness, itching, burning, blistering, swelling or oozing).

Avoid the use of occlusive dressings unless otherwise directed.

Administration and Dosage:

Approved by the FDA on December 30, 1992.

Interdigital tinea pedis (athlete's foot): Apply to cover the affected and immediate surrounding areas twice daily until clinical signs and symptoms are significantly improved. In many patients, this occurs by day 7. Duration should be for a minimum of 1 week and should not exceed 4 weeks.

Tinea cruris (jock itch) or tinea corporis (ringworm): Apply to cover the affected and immediate surrounding areas once or twice daily until clinical signs and symptoms are significantly improved. In many patients, this occurs by day 7 of therapy. Therapy should be for a minimum of 1 week and should not exceed 4 weeks.

Many patients treated with shorter durations of therapy (1 to 2 weeks) continue to improve during the 2 to 4 weeks after drug therapy has been completed. As a consequence, patients should not be considered therapeutic failures until they have been observed for a period of 2 to 4 weeks off therapy.

If successful outcome is not achieved during the post-treatment observation period, review the diagnosis.

Storage: Store cream between 5° and 30°C (41° and 86°F).

Rx	**Lamisil** (Sandoz)	**Cream:** 1%	With benzyl alcohol, cetyl alcohol and stearyl alcohol. In 15 and 30 g.

ANTIFUNGAL COMBINATIONS

The principal active components of these formulations include:

Antifungal agents:

UNDECYLENIC ACID (see individual monograph), *SODIUM PROPIONATE, BENZOIC ACID, SODIUM THIOSULFATE.*

Other components include:

SALICYLIC ACID for its topical keratolytic action (see individual monograph).

BORIC ACID as an astringent and antiseptic.

CHLOROXYLENOL as an antiseptic.

BENZOCAINE as an anesthetic (see individual monograph).

MENTHOL and PHENOL for their antipruritic, anesthetic and antiseptic effects.

RESORCINOL as an antipruritic and antiseptic.

CHLOROPHYLL DERIVATIVES to promote healing, although there is no evidence to support this effect. These agents do have a deodorant action.

BASIC FUCHSIN for its antifungal and antibacterial activity.

Note: The choice of vehicle is important for these products. Ointments, creams and liquids are used as primary therapy. In general, powders are used as adjunctive therapy, but they may be acceptable as primary therapy in very mild conditions.

otc	**Prophyllin** (Rystan)	**Ointment**: 5% sodium propionate and 0.0125% chlorophyllin derivatives	In 30 g.
otc	**Dermasept Antifungal** (Pharmakon)	**Liquid**: 6.098% tannic acid, 5.081% zinc Cl, 2.032% benzocaine, 3.049% methylbenzethonium HCl, 1.017% tolnaftate, 5.081% undecylenic acid, 58.539% ethanol 38B, phenol, benzyl alcohol, benzoic acid, coal tar, camphor, menthol	In 30 ml bottle w/spray dispenser.
Rx	**Gordochom** (Gordon)	**Solution**: 25% undecylenic acid, 3% chloroxylenol in an oil base	In 6ml, 30 ml bottles w/applicator and pints.
otc	**SteriNail** (Dr. Nordyke's Labs)	**Solution**: Undecylenic acid tolnaftate, propylene glycol, acetone, acetic acid, pripionic acid, benzyl alcohol, eucalyptol and benzyl acetate	In 30 ml. 3-step kit includes SteriScrub (28.35 g) and SteriBrush.
otc	**Blis-To-Sol** (Chattem)	**Liquid**: 1% tolnaftate	In 30 ml.
otc	**Whitfield's** (Various, eg, Dixon-Shane, Fougera, Goldline, Lannett, Lilly, Moore, NMC, Rugby, Schein, URL)	**Ointment**: 6% benzoic acid and 3% salicylic acid	In 30 g and 1 lb.

ANTIFUNGAL COMBINATIONS

otc	**Blis-To-Sol** (Chattem)	**Powder:** 12% zinc undecylenate.	Talc, zinc oxide. In 60 g.
Rx	**Tinver** (Sola/Barnes-Hind)	**Lotion:** 25% sodium thiosulfate, 1% salicylic acid, 10% isopropyl alcohol, menthol, propylene glycol, EDTA and colloidal alumina	In 120 and 180 ml.
Rx	**Versiclear** (Hope Pharmaceuticals)		In 120 ml.
Rx	**Castellani Paint Modified** (Pedinol)	**Liquid:** Basic fuchsin, phenol, resorcinol and acetone.	In 30 and 480 ml.
		Also available as a colorless solution with alcohol and without basic fuchsin.	In 30 and 480 ml.
otc	**Castel Minus** (Syosset)	**Liquid:** Resorcinol, acetone, 0.0001% basic fuchsin, hydroxyethylcelluose and 11.5% alcohol	In 29.57 ml.
otc	**Castel Plus** (Syosset)	**Liquid:** Resorcinol, acetone, 0.3% basic fuchsin, hydroxyethylcellulose and 11.5% alcohol	In 29.57 ml.
otc	**Fungi-Nail** (Kramer)	**Liquid:** 1% resorcinol, 2% salicylic acid, 2% chloroxylenol, 0.5% benzocaine, 50% isopropyl alcohol	In 30 ml.
otc	**Castaderm** (Lannett)	**Liquid:** Resorcinol, boric acid, acetone, basic fuchsin, phenol and 9% alcohol	In 30, 120 and 480 ml.

ANTIHISTAMINE-CONTAINING PREPARATIONS, TOPICAL

Other ingredients used with the antihistamines include:

BENZOCAINE as a local anesthetic.

CHLOROXYLENOL, BENZALKONIUM CHLORIDE, EUCALYPTOL as bacteriostatic agents.

BENZYL ALCOHOL, CAMPHOR, MENTHOL and **PHENOL** for antipruritic effects.

CALAMINE and **ZINC OXIDE** as astringents.

DIMETHYL POLYSILOXANE as a skin protectant.

CHLOROPHYLLIN SODIUM promotes healing.

ISOPROPYL ALCOHOL as an antiseptic.

CHLOROBUTANOL for antipruritic and antiseptic effects.

Actions:

Pharmacology: Topical antihistamines have some local anesthetic activity and are used to relieve itching. Some transdermal absorption may occur, but not in sufficient quantities to produce systemic side effects. They may cause local irritation and sensitization, especially with prolonged use. Refer to Antihistamine monograph in Respiratory Drugs section for further information on systemic antihistamines.

Indications:

Temporary relief of itching due to minor skin disorders, ivy, sumac and oak poisoning, sunburn, insect bites (nonpoisonous) and stings.

Warnings:

Do not apply to blistered, raw or oozing areas of the skin, or around the eyes or other mucous membranes (eg, nose, mouth).

Precautions:

For external use only. Avoid contact with the eyes.

If the condition persists, recurs after a few days or irritation develops, discontinue use.

Avoid prolonged use (> 7 days) or use on extensive skin areas.

otc	**Maximum Strength Benadryl 2%** (Parke-Davis)	**Cream**: 2% diphenhydramine HCl and parabens in a greaseless base	In 15 g.
		Spray, non-aerosol: 2% diphenhydramine HCl, 85% alcohol	In 60 ml.
otc	**Dermamycin** (Pfeiffer)	**Cream**: 2% diphenhydramine HCl, parabens, polyethylene glycol monostearate, propylene glycol	In 28.35 g.
otc	**Maximum Strength Benadryl Itch Relief** (Pfeiffer)	**Cream**: 2% diphenhydramine HCl, 0.1% zinc acetate, parabens, aloe vera	In 14.2 g.
		Stick: 2% diphenhydramine HCl, 0.1% zinc acetate, 73.5% alcohol, aloe vera	In 14 ml.
otc	**Ziradryl** (Parke-Davis)	**Lotion**: 1% diphenhydramine HCl, 2% zinc oxide, 2% alcohol, camphor, parabens	In 180 ml.
otc	**Caladryl Clear** (Warner-Lambert)	**Lotion**: 1% diphenhydramine HCl, 2% zinc oxide, 2% alcohol, camphor, chlorophyllin sodium, parabens	In 180 ml.
otc	**Benadryl** (Parke-Davis)	**Cream**: 1% diphenhydramine HCl, parabens in a greaseless base	In 15 g.
		Spray, non-aerosol: 1% diphenhydramine HCl, 85% alcohol	In 60 ml.
otc	**Caladryl** (Parke-Davis)	**Cream**: 1% diphenhydramine HCl, 8% calamine, parabens, camphor	In 45 g.
		Lotion: 1% diphenhydramine HCl, 8% calamine, camphor, 2% alcohol	In 75 and 180 ml.
otc	**Di-Delamine** (Commerce)	**Gel and Spray, non-aerosol**: 1% diphenhydramine HCl, 0.5% tripelennamine HCl, 0.12% benzalkonium Cl, menthol, EDTA	Gel: In 37.5 g. Spray: In 120 ml.
otc	**Cala-gen** (Goldline)	**Lotion**: 1% diphenhydramine HCl, camphor, 2% alcohol	In 178 ml.
otc	**Sting-Eze** (Wisconsin Pharm.)	**Concentrate**: Diphenhydramine HCl, camphor, phenol, benzocaine, eucalyptol	In 15 ml.

ANTIHISTAMINE-CONTAINING PREPARATIONS, TOPICAL

otc	**Medacote** (Dal-Med)	**Lotion:** 1% pyrilamine maleate, dimethyl polysiloxane, zinc oxide, menthol and camphor in a greaseless base	In 120 ml.
otc	**Derma-Pax** (Recsei Labs)	**Lotion:** 0.44% pyrilamine maleate, 0.06% chlorpheniramine, 1% benzyl alcohol, 35% isopropanol, chlorobutanol	In 120 ml and pt.
otc	**Calamycin** (Pfeiffer)	**Lotion:** Zinc oxide and 10% calamine, benzocaine, chloroxylenol, pyrilamine maleate, 2% isopropyl alcohol	In 120 ml.
otc	**Benadryl Itch Stopping Children's Formula** (Warner Wellcome)	**Gel:** 1% diphenhydramine HCl, 1% zinc acetate, camphor, parabens	In 118 g.
otc	**Benadryl Itch Stopping Maximum Strength** (Warner Wellcome)	**Gel:** 2% diphenhydramine HCl, 1% zinc acetate, camphor, parabens	In 118 g.
otc	**Dermarest** (Del)	**Gel:** 2% diphenhydramine HCl, 2% resorcinol, aloe vera gel, benzalkonium chloride, EDTA, menthol, methylparaben, propylene glycol	In 29.25 and 56.25 g.
otc	**Dermarest Plus** (Del)	**Gel:** 2% diphenhydramine HCl, 1% menthol, aloe vera gel, benzalkonium chloride, isopropyl alcohol, methylparaben propylene glycol	In 15 and 30 g.
		Spray: 2% diphenhydramine HCl, 1% menthol, aloe vera gel, benzalkonium chloride, methylparaben, propylene glycol, SD alcohol 40, EDTA	In 15 and 30 g.
otc	**Clearly Cala-gel** (Tec Labs)	**Gel:** Diphenhydramine HCl, zinc acetate, menthol, EDTA	Clear. In 180 g.
otc	**Benadryl Itch Relief** (Glaxo Wellcome)	**Spray:** 2% diphenhydramine HCl, 0.1% zinc acetate, 73.6% alcohol, aloe vera	In 59 ml.
otc	**Benadryl Itch Relief Children's** (Glaxo Wellcome	**Cream:** 1% diphendydramine HCl, 0.1% zinc acetate, aloe vera, cetyl alcohol, parabens	In 14.2 g.
		Spray: 1% diphendydramine HCl, 0.1% zinc acetate, 73.6% alcohol, aloe vera, providone	In 59 ml.

DOXEPIN HCl

For information on the systemic use of doxepin, refer to the individual monographs in the CNS Drugs chapter.

Actions:

Pharmacology: Doxepin cream, a dibenzoxepin tricyclic compound, is a topical antipruritic. The exact mechanism by which doxepin exerts its antipruritic effect is unknown. However, it does have potent H_1 and H_2 receptor blocking actions. Histamine-blocking drugs appear to compete at histamine receptor sites and inhibit the biological activation of histamine receptors. In addition, doxepin produces drowsiness in significant numbers of patients. Sedation may have an effect on certain pruritic symptoms.

Pharmacokinetics: In 19 pruritic eczema patients treated with doxepin cream, plasma doxepin concentrations ranged from nondetectable to 47 ng/ml from percutaneous absorption. Target therapeutic plasma levels of oral doxepin for the treatment of depression range from 30 to 150 ng/ml.

Once absorbed into the systemic circulation, doxepin undergoes hepatic metabolism that results in conversion to pharmacologically active desmethyldoxepin. Further glucuronidation results in urinary excretion of the parent drug and its metabolites. Desmethyldoxepin has a half-life that ranges from 28 to 52 hours and is not affected by multiple dosing. Plasma levels of both doxepin and desmethyl-

DOXEPIN HCl

doxepin are highly variable and are poorly correlated with dosage. Renal disease, genetic factors, age and other medications affect the metabolism and subsequent elimination of doxepin.

Indications:

Pruritus: Short-term (up to 8 days) management of moderate pruritus in adults with the following forms of eczematous dermatitis: Atopic dermatitis; lichen simplex chronicus.

Contraindications:

Untreated narrow angle glaucoma, tendency to urinary retention (since doxepin has an anticholinergic effect and because significant plasma levels are detectable after topical application); hypersensitivity to any components of the product.

Warnings:

For external use only: Do not use ophthalmically, orally or intravaginally.

Drowsiness occurs in > 20% of patients treated with doxepin cream, especially in patients receiving treatment to > 10% of their body surface area. Warn patients of this possibility and caution them against driving a motor vehicle or operating hazardous machinery while being treated with doxepin cream. Also warn patients that the effects of alcoholic beverages can be potentiated when using doxepin cream. If excessive drowsiness occurs it may be necessary to reduce the number of applications, the amount of cream applied or the percentage of body surface area treated, or discontinue the drug.

Pregnancy: Category B. There are no adequate and well controlled studies in pregnant women. Use during pregnancy only if clearly needed.

Lactation: Doxepin is excreted in breast milk after oral administration. Significant systemic levels of doxepin are obtained after topical administration; therefore, it is possible that doxepin could be secreted in breast milk following topical administration. One case of apnea and drowsiness occurred in a nursing infant whose mother was taking an oral dosage form of doxepin. Because of the potential for serious adverse reactions in nursing infants, decide whether to discontinue nursing or to discontinue the drug, taking into account the importance of the drug to the mother.

Children: Safety and efficacy in children have not been established.

Drug Interactions:

Drugs metabolized by P450IID6: A subset (3% to 10%) of the population has reduced activity of certain drug metabolizing enzymes such as the cytochrome P450 isozyme P450IID6. Such individuals are referred to as "poor metabolizers" and may have higher than expected plasma concentrations of tricyclic antidepressants (TCAs) when given usual doses. In addition, certain drugs that are metabolized by this isozyme may inhibit its activity, and thus may make normal metabolizers resemble poor metabolizers, leading to drug interactions. Concomitant use of TCAs with other drugs metabolized by cytochrome P450IID6 may require lower doses than usually prescribed for either the TCA or the other drug. Therefore, coadministration of TCAs with other drugs that are metabolized by this isoenzyme should be approached with caution.

Since plasma levels of doxepin similar to therapeutic ranges for antidepressant use can be obtained following topical application of the cream, it would not be unexpected for the following drug interactions to be possible following topical application.

Topical Doxepin Drug Interactions

Precipitant drug	Object drug*		Description
Alcohol	Doxepin	⬆	Alcohol ingestion may exacerbate the potential sedative effects of doxepin cream.
Cimetidine	Doxepin	⬆	Cimetidine produces clinically significant fluctuations in steady-state serum concentrations of various tricyclic antidepressants (TCAs). Serious anticholinergic symptoms have occurred with elevated TCA levels.
MAO inhibitors	Doxepin	⬆	Serious side effects and even death have been reported following the concomitant use of MAOIs and other drugs chemically related to doxepin. Therefore, discontinue MAOIs at least 2 weeks prior to the initiation of treatment with doxepin cream.

* ⬆ = Object drug increased.

DOXEPIN HCl

Adverse Reactions:

Systemic: The most common systemic effect was drowsiness (22%); ≈ 5% discontinued therapy. Other effects included: Dry mouth/lips, thirst, headache, fatigue, dizziness, emotional changes, taste changes (1% to 10%); nausea, anxiety, fever (< 1%).

Local: The most common local effect was burning or stinging at the application site (21%; ≈ 25% reported the reaction as "severe"); four patients withdrew from therapy. Other effects included: Pruritus or eczema exacerbation, dryness/tightness of skin, paresthesias, edema (1% to 10%); irritation, tingling, scaling, cracking (< 1%).

Overdosage:

Symptoms:

Mild – Drowsiness, stupor, blurred vision, excessive dryness of mouth.

Severe – Respiratory depression, hypotension, coma, convulsions, cardiac arrhythmias, tachycardias, urinary retention (bladder atony), decreased GI motility (paralytic ileus), hyperthermia, hypothermia, hypertension, dilated pupils, hyperactive reflexes.

Treatment:

Mild – Observation and supportive therapy is all that is usually necessary. It may be necessary to reduce the percent of body surface area treated or the frequency of application or apply a thinner layer of cream.

Severe – Management consists of aggressive supportive therapy. Thoroughly wash the area covered with cream. Establish an adequate airway in comatose patients and use assisted ventilation if necessary. ECG monitoring may be required for several days because relapse after apparent recovery has been reported with oral doxepin. Treat arrhythmias with the appropriate antiarrhythmic agent. Many of the cardiovascular and CNS symptoms of TCA poisoning in adults may be reversed by the slow IV administration of 1 to 3 mg of physostigmine salicylate. Because physostigmine is rapidly metabolized, repeat the dosage as required. Convulsions may respond to standard anticonvulsant therapy; however, barbiturates may potentiate any respiratory depression. Dialysis and forced diuresis generally are not of value due to high tissue and protein binding of doxepin.

Patient Information:

Caution patients about operating hazardous machinery, including automobiles, until they are reasonably certain that doxepin therapy does not adversely affect their ability to engage in such activities.

Do not use occlussive dressings since absorption may be increased.

Administration and Dosage:

Approved by the FDA on April 1, 1994.

Apply a thin film of cream 4 times each day with at least a 3 to 4 hour interval between applications. There are no data to establish the safety and efficacy when used for > 8 days. Chronic use beyond 8 days may result in higher systemic levels.

Drowsiness is significantly more common in patients applying doxepin cream to > 10% of body surface area. If excessive drowsiness occurs it may be necessary to do one or more of the following: Reduce the body surface area treated, reduce the number of applications per day, reduce the amount of cream applied or discontinue the drug. Occlusive dressings may increase the absorption of most topical drugs; therefore, occlusive dressings with doxepin cream should not be utilized.

Rx	**Zonalon** (GenDerm)	**Cream:** 5%	Cetyl alcohol, petrolatum, benzyl alcohol, titanium dioxide. In 30 g.

SCABICIDES/PEDICULICIDES

The following section discusses the various agents used as scabicides and pediculicides. Malathion is used only as a pediculicide; crotamiton is used only as a scabicide; permethrin and lindane are both scabicides and pediculicides. Pyrethrins, available only in combination with piperonyl butoxide, are used only as a pediculicide; piperonyl butoxide is used as a synergist for the pyrethrins.

Malathion acts via cholinesterase inhibition. In contrast, lindane and pyrethrins are nervous system stimulants and permethrin disrupts neuronal repolarization and causes paralysis.

These agents differ in kill time, ovicidal and residual activity. This information is summarized in the table below. Crotamiton is not included since it is not a pediculicide.

Activity of Various Pediculicides

Pediculicide	Kill time (min)	Ovicidal activity	Residual activity	Application time
Lindane	190	45% to 70%	none	4 minutes
Malathion	4.4	95%	up to 4 weeks	8 to 12 hours
Permethrin	10 to 15	70% to 80%	up to 10 days	10 minutes
Pyrethrins and piperonyl butoxide[1]	10.5 to 18.6	≈ 75%	none	10 minutes

[1] Products used for data included *A-200 Pyrinate* and *R & C*.

LINDANE (Gamma Benzene Hexachloride)

Actions:

Pharmacology: An ectoparasiticide and ovicide.

Indications:

Treatment of *Pediculus capitis* (head lice) and *Pediculus pubis* (crab lice) and their ova. The cream and lotion forms are also indicated for *Sarcoptes scabiei* (scabies).

Contraindications:

Premature neonates, because their skin may be more permeable than that of full-term infants and their liver enzymes may not be sufficiently developed; patients with known seizure disorders; hypersensitivity to lindane or any component of the products.

Warnings:

Absorption: Simultaneous application of creams, ointments or oils may enhance absorption.

Carcinogenesis: In mice, 600 ppm of lindane was associated with a significant increase in the incidence of hepatomas. Although other derivatives of hexachlorocyclohexane have demonstrated carcinogenicity, lindane has not.

Pregnancy: Category B. There are no adequate and well controlled studies in pregnant women. Do not exceed the recommended dosage; treat no more than twice during a pregnancy.

Lactation: Lindane is secreted in breast milk in low concentrations. The levels of lindane found in blood after topical application make it unlikely that amounts of lindane sufficient to cause serious adverse reactions will be excreted in the milk of nursing mothers. If there is any concern, use an alternate method of feeding for 2 days.

Children: Lindane penetrates human skin and has the potential for CNS toxicity. Studies indicate that potential toxic effects of topically applied lindane are greater in the young. Seizures have occurred after excessive use or ingestion of lindane. No residual effects have been demonstrated; do not use prophylactically.

Precautions:

For external use only. Avoid contact with eyes; if this occurs, immediately flush eyes with water.

Irritation or sensitization: Consult physician.

Oils may enhance absorption. If an oil-based hair dressing is used, shampoo, rinse and dry hair before applying lindane shampoo.

Adverse Reactions:

Adverse reactions occur in < 0.001% of patients.

CNS: Stimulation ranging from dizziness to convulsions. Cases of convulsions have been reported, although these incidents were almost always associated with accidental oral ingestion or misuse of the product.

Dermatologic: Eczematous eruptions due to irritation.

LINDANE (Gamma Benzene Hexachloride)

Overdosage:

Symptoms: Overdosage or oral ingestion can cause CNS excitation and, if taken in sufficient quantities, seizures may occur. A blood level of 290 ng/ml was associated with convulsions following the accidental ingestion of a lindane-containing product. Analysis of blood taken from subjects before and after the lindane shampoo showed a mean peak blood level of only 3 ng/ml at 6 hours which disappeared 2 hours later.

Treatment: If accidental ingestion occurs, institute prompt gastric emptying. However, since oils favor absorption, give saline cathartics for intestinal evacuation rather than oil laxatives. If CNS manifestations occur, administer pentobarbital, phenobarbital or diazepam. Refer to General Management of Acute Overdosage.

Patient Information:

Patient instructions and information are available with product. Do not exceed prescribed dosage.

For external use only (oral ingestion can lead to serious CNS toxicity). Do not apply to face. Avoid eyes; if there is contact, flush well with water for several minutes. Avoid unnecessary skin contact or contact with mucous membranes (eg, nose, mouth). Wear rubber gloves, particularly when applying to more than one person.

Notify physician if condition worsens or if itching, redness, swelling, burning or skin rash occurs.

Avoid use on open cuts and extensive excoriations.

Treat sexual contacts simultaneously.

Administration and Dosage:

Cream and lotion:

Scabies – Apply a thin layer to dry skin and rub in thoroughly. If crusted lesions are present, a tepid bath preceding the medication is helpful. Allow the skin to dry before application. Usually 2 oz are sufficient for an adult. Make total body application from the neck down. Scabies rarely affects the head of children or adults, but may occur in infants. Leave on 8 to 12 hours; remove by thorough washing. One application is usually curative. Many patients exhibit persistent pruritus after treatment; this does not indicate reapplication unless living mites can be demonstrated.

Lotion:

Pediculosis pubis – Apply sufficient quantity only to thinly cover hair and skin of pubic area and, if infested, thighs, trunk and axillary regions. Rub into skin and hair, leave in place for 12 hours, then wash thoroughly. Reapplication is usually unnecessary unless there are living lice after 7 days. Treat sexual contacts concurrently.

Pediculosis capitis – Apply sufficient quantity to cover only affected and adjacent hairy areas. Rub into scalp and hair and leave in place 12 hours; follow by thorough washing. Reapplication is usually not necessary unless there are living lice after 7 days.

Shampoo:

Pediculosis capitis and pubis – Apply a sufficient quantity to dry hair (1 oz for short, 1½ oz for medium and 2 oz for long hair). Work thoroughly into the hair and allow to remain in place 4 minutes. Add small quantities of water until a good lather forms. Rinse hair thoroughly and towel briskly. Comb with a fine toothed comb or use tweezers to remove any remaining nits or nit shells.

Pediculosis pubis – Reapplication is usually not necessary. Reapply if there are demonstrable living lice after 7 days. Treat sexual contacts concurrently.

Do not use as a routine shampoo.

Rx	**Lindane** (Various, eg, Barre-National, Geneva, Major, Moore, Parmed, PBI, Rugby, Schein, URL)	**Lotion:** 1%	In 30 and 60 ml, pt and gal.
Rx	**G-well** (Goldline)		In 60 and 480 ml.
Rx	**Scabene** (Stiefel)		In 59 and 480 ml.
Rx	**Lindane** (Various, eg, Barre-National, Geneva , Major, Moore, Parmed, PBI, Rugby, Schein, URL)	**Shampoo:** 1%	In 30 and 60 ml, pt and gal.
Rx	**G-well** (Goldline)		In 60 ml, pt and gal.
Rx	**Scabene** (Stiefel)		In 59 and 480 ml.

PERMETHRIN

Actions:

Pharmacology: Permethrin is a synthetic pyrethroid, active against lice, ticks, mites and fleas. It acts on the parasites' nerve cell membranes to disrupt the sodium channel current, resulting in delayed repolarization and paralysis of the pests.

In vitro data indicate permethrin has pediculicidal and ovicidal activity against *Pediculus humanus* var. *capitis.* The high cure rate (97% to 99%) in patients with head lice demonstrated at 14 days following a single application is attributable to a combination of its pediculicidal and ovicidal activities and its residual persistence on the hair which may also prevent reinfestation.

Pharmacokinetics: Permethrin is rapidly metabolized by ester hydrolysis to inactive metabolites which are excreted primarily in the urine. Although the amount of permethrin absorbed after a single application of the 5% cream has not been determined precisely, preliminary data suggest it is < 2% of the amount applied. Residual persistence is detectable on the hair for at least 10 days following a single application.

Indications:

Cream: For the single-application treatment of Sarcoptes scabiei (scabies).

Liquid: For the single-application treatment of infestation with *Pediculus humanus* var. *capitis* (the head louse) and its nits (eggs). Treatment for recurrences is required in < 1% of patients since the ovicidal activity may be supplemented by residual persistence in the hair. If live lice are observed ≥ 7 days following the initial application, give a second application.

Contraindications:

Hypersensitivity to any synthetic pyrethroid or pyrethrin, to chrysanthemums or to any component of the product. If hypersensitivity develops, discontinue use.

Warnings:

Carcinogenesis: Species-specific increases in pulmonary adenomas, a common benign tumor of mice, were seen in the mouse studies. In one study, incidence of pulmonary alveolar-cell carcinomas and benign liver adenomas increased only in female mice when permethrin was given in their food at a concentration of 5000 ppm.

Pregnancy: Category B. There are no adequate and well controlled studies in pregnant women. Use during pregnancy only if clearly needed.

Lactation: It is not known whether this drug is excreted in breast milk. Because of the evidence for tumorigenic potential of permethrin in animal studies, consider discontinuing nursing temporarily or withholding the drug while the mother is nursing.

Children: Safety and efficacy for use in children < 2 months of age or < 2 years (liquid) have not been established.

Precautions:

For external use only.

Pruritus, erythema and edema often accompany scabies and head lice infestation. Treatment with permethrin may temporarily exacerbate these conditions.

Adverse Reactions:

The most frequent adverse reaction is pruritus. Usually a consequence of scabies or head lice infestation itself, it may be temporarily aggravated following treatment.

Cream: Mild transient burning/stinging (10%); mild temporary itching (7%); tingling, numbness, mild transient erythema, edema or rash (≤ 2%).

Liquid: Mild temporary itching (5.9%); mild transient burning/stinging, tingling, numbness, discomfort (3.4%); mild transient erythema, edema or rash (2.1%).

Overdosage:

If ingested, perform gastric lavage and employ general supportive measures.

Patient Information:

For external use only. Avoid contact with the mucous membranes (eg, nose, mouth).

Itching, redness or swelling of the scalp may occur; notify physician if irritation persists.

Elimite: May be very mildly irritating to the eyes. Avoid contact with the eyes; flush with water immediately if eye contact with the drug occurs.

Patient instructions and information are available with the product. Do not exceed the prescribed dosage.

PERMETHRIN

Administration and Dosage:

Sarcoptes scabiei: Thoroughly massage into the skin from the head to the soles of the feet. Treat infants on the hairline, neck, scalp, temple and forehead. Remove the cream by washing after 8 to 14 hours. Usually 30 g is sufficient for the average adult. One application is curative.

Pediculus capitis: Use after the hair has been washed with shampoo, rinsed with water and towel dried. Apply a sufficient volume to saturate the hair and scalp. Allow to remain on the hair for 10 minutes before rinsing off with water.

A single treatment eliminates head lice infestation. Combing of nits is not required for therapeutic efficacy, but may be done for cosmetic reasons.

Rx	**Elimite** (Herbert)	**Cream:** 5%	In 60 g tubes.
otc	**Nix** (Glaxo Wellcome)	**Liquid (creme rinse):** 1%[1]	In 60 ml with comb.

[1] With 20% isopropyl alcohol, 0.2% imidazolidinyl urea, parabens.

CROTAMITON

Actions:

Pharmacology: Scabicidal and antipruritic; the mechanisms of action are not known.

Indications:

Eradication of scabies (*Sarcoptes scabiei*) and symptomatic treatment of pruritic skin.

Contraindications:

Do not administer to patients who develop a sensitivity to or are allergic to crotamiton or who manifest a primary irritation response.

Warnings:

For external use only. Do not apply to acutely inflamed skin, raw weeping surfaces, eyes or mouth. Defer use until acute inflammation has subsided.

Irritation/sensitization: If severe irritation or sensitization develops, discontinue use.

Pregnancy: Category C. It is not known whether crotamiton can cause fetal harm when applied topically to a pregnant woman or if it can affect reproduction capacity. Use on a pregnant woman only if clearly needed.

Children: Safety and efficacy for use in children have not been established.

Adverse Reactions:

Allergic sensitivity or primary irritation reactions may occur.

Overdosage:

Signs and symptoms of ingestion include burning sensation in mouth, irritation of the buccal, esophageal and gastric mucosa, nausea, vomiting and abdominal pain.

Treatment: There is no specific antidote. General measures to eliminate the drug and reduce its absorption, combined with symptomatic treatment, are recommended. Refer to General Management of Acute Overdosage.

Patient Information:

Patient instructions available with product.

Shake well before using.

Patients with scabies should take a routine bath or shower.

Change clothing and bed linen the next day. Contaminated clothing and bed linen may be dry cleaned or washed in the hot cycle of the washing machine.

For external use only. Keep away from the eyes and mucous membranes (eg, nose, mouth); do not apply to inflamed skin.

Discontinue use and notify physician if irritation or sensitization occurs.

Administration and Dosage:

Scabies: Thoroughly massage into the skin of the whole body from the chin down, paying particular attention to all folds and creases. A second application is advisable 24 hours later. Change clothing and bed linen the next morning. Take a cleansing bath 48 hours after the last application.

Pruritus: Massage gently into affected areas until medication is completely absorbed. Repeat as necessary.

Rx	**Eurax** (Westwood Squibb)	**Cream:** 10% in a vanishing base	In 60 g.
		Lotion: 10% in an emollient base	In 60 and 454 ml.

MALATHION

Actions:

Pharmacology: Malathion is an organophosphate pediculicide liquid for topical application to the hair and scalp. Malathion acts via cholinesterase inhibition and exerts both lousicidal and ovicidal actions in vitro. This activity is selective to insects because malathion is rapidly hydrolyzed and detoxified in mammals.

When in contact with the hair, malathion slowly bonds to the hair shaft via bonding between its own sulfur atoms and the sulfur in structural amino cids of the hair. This can give a residual protective effect against reinfestation. This chemical reaction is slow. No useful protection is sufficiently developed before about 6 hours of continuous exposure and the effect takes about 12 hours to maximize.

Pharmacokinetics: Malathion in an acetone vehicle is absorbed through human skin only to the extent of 8% of the applied dose. However, percutaneous absorption from the *Ovide* lotion formulation has not been studied and the parameters of distribution and excretion after absorption are not known.

Indications:

Treatment of head lice and their ova.

Contraindications:

Sensitivity to malathion or any components of the product.

Warnings:

Pregnancy: Category B. Use during pregnancy only if clearly needed.

Lactation: It is not known whether malathion is excreted in breast milk. However, because malathion is systemically absorbed, exercise caution when using on a nursing mother.

Children: The majority of the subjects participating in clinical trials with malathion lotions ranged from 2 to 11 years of age; no pediatric-related problems have been documented to date. Safety and efficacy in children < 2 years of age have not been established.

Precautions:

Contains flammable alcohol. The lotion and wet hair should not be exposed to open flame or electric heat, including hair dryers. Do not smoke while applying lotion, or while hair is wet. Allow hair to dry naturally and uncovered after application.

For external use only. Avoid contact with the eyes; if accidentally placed in the eye, flush immediately with water.

Systemic toxicity: Although topical malathion used in recommended dosage has not been reported to cause systemic toxicity, the remote possibility exists. Daily application of 10% malathion dust to adult human skin for 3 weeks produces little or no inhibition of blood cholinesterase.

Carbamate or organophosphate-type insecticides or pesticides: Exposure of patients using malathion to these preparations may increase the possibility of systemic effects due to absorption of the insecticide or pesticide through the respiratory tract or skin; advise patients to protect themselves from contact with such insecticides or pesticides during therapy with malathion.

Drug Interactions:

No drug interactions have been reported with malathion lotion. However, since malathion inhibits cholinesterase, interaction with the following medications could theoretically occur if percutaneous malathion absorption was unexpectedly large.

Aminoglycosides, parenteral: Additive respiratory depression because of the neuromuscular blocking action of the parenteral aminoglycosides may occur.

Anesthetics, local (ester-derivative): Inhibition of the metabolism of ester-derivative local anesthetics, including those topically applied and absorbed in significant amounts, leading to increased risk of systemic toxicity.

Antimyasthenics or cholinesterase inhibitors (including ophthalmic agents): Additive toxicity may result.

Edrophonium: Caution is recommended in administering edrophonium to patients with myasthenic weakness who are also using topical malathion, since symptoms of cholinergic crisis (overdosage) may be similar to symptoms occurring with myasthenic crisis (underdosage) and the patient's condition may be worsened by use of edrophonium.

Succinylcholine: Plasma concentrations or activity of pseudocholinesterase, the enzyme that metabolizes succinylcholine, may be decreased, thereby enhancing the neuromuscular blockade of succinylcholine.

Adverse Reactions:

Irritation of the scalp has occurred.

MALATHION

Overdosage:

Oral:

Symptoms – Malathion, although a weaker cholinesterase inhibitor and therefore safer than other organophosphates, may be expected to exhibit the same symptoms of cholinesterase depletion after accidental ingestion orally. The symptoms of systemic toxicity may be delayed for up to 12 hours and can include: Abdominal cramps; anxiety; unsteadiness; confusion; diarrhea; labored breathing; dizziness; drowsiness; increased sweating; watery eyes; muscle twitching; pinpoint pupils; seizures; slow heartbeat.

Treatment – Induce vomiting promptly or lavage the stomach with 5% sodium bicarbonate solution.

Severe respiratory distress is the major and most serious symptom of organophosphate poisoning requiring artificial respiration and large doses of IM or IV atropine. The usual starting dose of atropine is 1 to 4 mg with supplementation hourly as needed to counteract the symptoms of cholinesterase depletion. Repeat analyses of serum and RBC cholinesterase assist in establishing the diagnosis and formulating a long-range prognosis.

IV pralidoxime chloride may be used to reverse muscle paralysis. It appears to be most effective if administered within a few hours after poisoning occurs; it is usually not effective if initially administered after 48 hours have elapsed.

A short-acting barbiturate may be given to control seizures.

Give consideration, as a part of the treatment program, to the high concentration of isopropyl alcohol in the vehicle.

Observe the patient for signs of deterioration due to delayed absorption.

Patient Information:

For external use only (serious toxicity may occur if ingested). Avoid contact with the eyes.

Administration and Dosage:

1) Sprinkle lotion on dry hair and rub gently until the scalp is thoroughly moistened. Pay special attention to the back of the head and neck.
2) Allow to dry naturally; use no heat and leave uncovered.
3) After 8 to 12 hours, wash the hair with a nonmedicated shampoo.
4) Rinse and use a fine toothed comb to remove dead lice and eggs.
5) If required, repeat with second application in 7 to 9 days.

Further treatment is generally not necessary. Evaluate other family members to determine if infested; if so, treat.

Rx	**Ovide** (GenDerm)	**Lotion:** 0.5%[1]	In 59 ml.

[1] In a vehicle of 78% isopropyl alcohol, terpineol, dipentene and pine needle oil.

NIT REMOVAL SYSTEM

Actions:

Pharmacology: Appears to loosen the bond which continues to hold both live and dead lice eggs to the hair shaft after pediculicide treatment. Surviving nits can cause reinfestation if not removed. Does not kill head lice or lice eggs.

Indications:

For use following a pediculicide to aid in cleansing lice eggs from the hair shaft.

Patient Information:

For external use only. Avoid contact with the eyes, eyelashes and eyebrows.

Administration and Dosage:

Shake well before using. Protect eyes with a dry towel. Apply to wet hair after rinsing out the pediculicide. Apply enough to saturate each hair shaft and cover the entire scalp, making sure to cover the area around the ears and back of the neck. Do not apply to eyelashes or eyebrows.

Allow to remain on the hair for approximately 10 minutes. Rinse with lukewarm water and dry with a hair dryer. Avoid contact with eyes.

otc	**Step 2** (GenDerm)	**Creme rinse:** Benzyl alcohol, cetyl alcohol, 8% formic acid, glyceryl stearate, PEG-100 stearate, polyquaternium-10	In 60 ml.

MISCELLANEOUS PEDICULICIDES

Indications:

Treatment of infestations of head lice, body lice and pubic (crab) lice and their eggs.

Contraindications:

Hypersensitivity to ingredients; ragweed sensitized persons (pyrethrins and permethrins).

Precautions:

For external use only: Harmful if swallowed or inhaled. May be irritating to the eyes and mucous membranes. In case of contact with eyes, flush with water. Discontinue use and notify physician if irritation or infection occurs.

Infestation of eyelashes or eyebrows: Do not use in these areas. Consult physician.

Reinfestation: To prevent, sterilize or treat all clothing and bedding concurrently.

Administration and Dosage:

Administration and Dosage varies. Refer to individual package inserts for information.

otc	**End Lice** (Thompson)	**Liquid**: 0.3% pyrethrins, 3% piperonyl butoxide technical	In 177 ml.
otc	**Pyrinyl II** (Barre)		In 59, 120 and 237 ml.[1]
otc	**Triple X Kit**[1] (Carter)		With shampoo.
otc	**Tisit** (Pfeiffer)	**Liquid**: 0.3% pyrethrins, 2% piperonyl butoxide technical	In 60 and 118 ml.
otc	**Pyrinyl** (Various)	**Liquid**: 0.2% pyrethrins, 2% piperonyl butoxide technical, 0.8% deodorized kerosene	In 60 and 120 ml.
otc	**Barc** (Del)	**Liquid**: 0.18% pyrethrins, 2.2% piperonyl butoxide technical, 5.52% petroleum distillate	In 60 ml.
otc	**Blue** (Various, eg, Ambix, Moore)	**Gel**: 0.3% pyrethrins, 3% piperonyl butoxide technical, 1.2% petroleum distillate	In 30 g.
otc	**Tisit Blue** (Pfeiffer)		In 30 g.
otc	**InnoGel Plus** (Hogil Pharm)	**Gel**: 0.3% pyrethrins, 3% piperonyl butoxide technical	In kits containing 3 pre-dosed gel paks and a comb.
otc	**A-200** (Hogil)	**Shampoo**: 0.33% pyrethrins, 4% piperonyl butoxide technical	In 60 and 120 ml.
otc	**Pronto** (Del)		In 60 and 120 ml and 60 ml with creme rinse packet.
otc	**Lice•Enz Foam Kit** (Copley)	**Shampoo**: 0.3% pyrethrins, 3% piperonyl butoxide technical	In 60 g aerosol.
otc	**Pyrinyl Plus** (Rugby)		In 59 and 118 ml.
otc	**R & C** (Reed & Carnrick)		In 60 and 120 ml.
otc	**RID**[2] (Pfizer)		In 60, 120 & 240 ml.
otc	**Tisit** (Pfeiffer)		In 118 ml.
otc	**Clear Total Lice Elimination System** (Care Technologies)		In kits containing shampoo (2 and 4 ml), egg remover and nit comb.
otc	**Pyrinex Pediculicide** (Ambix)	**Shampoo**: 0.2% pyrethrins, 2% piperonyl butoxide technical, 0.8% deodorized kerosene	In 118 ml.
otc	**Tegrin-LT** (Block)	**Shampoo/Conditioner**: 0.33% pyrethrins, 3.15% piperonyl butoxide technical	In 118 ml.

[1] Contains petroleum distillate.

[2] With 1.2% petroleum distillate and 2.4% benzyl alcohol.

CORTICOSTEROIDS, TOPICAL

Actions:

Pharmacology: Topical corticosteroids are adrenocorticosteroid derivatives incorporated into a vehicle suitable for application to skin or external mucous membranes. Modifications of the essential 4-ring steroid structure such as hydroxylation, methylation, fluorination or esterification are often made to increase lipid solubility and potency and decrease mineralocorticoid effects.

The primary therapeutic effects of the topical corticosteroids are due to their anti-inflammatory activity which is non-specific (ie, they act against most causes of inflammation including mechanical, chemical, microbiological and immunological).

Topically applied corticosteroids diffuse across cell membranes to interact with cytoplasmic receptors located in both the dermal and intradermal cells. The intracellular effects are similar to those that occur with systemically administered corticosteroids.

At the cellular level, corticosteroids appear to induce phospholipase A_2 inhibitory proteins (lipocortins), thus depressing formation, release and activity of the endogenous mediators of inflammation such as prostaglandins, kinins, histamine, liposomal enzymes and the complement system.

When corticosteroids are applied to inflamed skin, they inhibit the migration of macrophages and leukocytes into the area by reversing vascular dilation and permeability. The clinical result is a decrease in edema, erythema and pruritus.

By suppressing DNA synthesis, topically applied corticosteroids have an antimitotic effect on epidermal cells. This property is useful in proliferative disorders such as psoriasis, but also can be demonstrated in normal skin.

Pharmacokinetics: The amount of corticosteroid absorbed from the skin depends on the intrinsic properties of the drug itself, the vehicle used, the duration of exposure and the surface area and condition of the skin to which it is applied. In general, absorption will be enhanced by increased skin temperature, hydration, application to inflamed or denuded skin, intertriginous areas (eg, eyelids, groin, axilla) or skin surfaces with a thin stratum corneum layer (eg, face, scrotum). Palms, soles and crusted surfaces are less permeable. Occlusive dressings greatly enhance skin penetration and, therefore, increase drug absorption.

Infants and children have a higher total body surface to body weight ratio that decreases with age. Therefore, proportionately more topically applied medications will be absorbed systemically in this population, putting them at a greater risk for systemic effects.

Following topical absorption, corticosteroids enter the systemic circulation and are metabolized and excreted via pathways described for systemically administered corticosteroids.

Vehicles – Ointments are more occlusive and are preferred for dry scaly lesions. Use creams on oozing lesions or in intertriginous areas where the occlusive effects of ointments may cause maceration and folliculitis. Creams are often preferred by patients for aesthetic reasons even though their water content makes them more drying than ointments. Gels, aerosols, lotions and solutions are useful on hairy areas. Urea enhances the penetration of hydrocortisone and selected steroids by hydrating the skin. As a general rule, ointments and gels are more potent than creams or lotions. However, optimized vehicles that have been formulated for some products have demonstrated equal potency in cream, gel and ointment forms. Steroid impregnated tapes are useful for occlusive therapy in small areas.

Occlusive dressings – Occlusive dressings such as a plastic wrap increase skin penetration approximately tenfold by increasing the moisture content of the stratum corneum. Occlusion can be beneficial in resistant cases but it may also lead to sweat retention and increased bacterial and fungal infections. Additionally, increased absorption of the corticosteroid may produce systemic side effects. Therefore, do not use occlusive dressings > 12 hours per day and when using very potent topical corticosteroids.

Relative potency – The relative potency of a product depends on several factors including the characteristics and concentration of the drug and the vehicle used. Vasoconstrictor assays are used to measure the relative potency of the commercially available products. The estimated relative potency of selected topical corticosteroid preparations is given in the following table. Ranking is based on vasoconstrictor assays of brand name products. In some cases, generic "equivalents" have less vasoconstrictive activity.

CORTICOSTEROIDS, TOPICAL

Relative Potency of Selected Topical Corticosteroid Products

Drug	Dosage Form	Strength
I. *Very high potency*		
Augmented betamethasone dipropionate	Ointment	0.05%
Clobetasol propionate	Cream, Ointment	0.05%
Diflorasone diacetate	Ointment	0.05%
Halobetasol propionate	Cream, Ointment	0.05%
II. *High potency*		
Amcinonide	Cream, Lotion, Ointment	0.1%
Augmented betamethasone dipropionate	Cream	0.05%
Betamethasone dipropionate	Cream, Ointment	0.05%
Betamethasone valerate	Ointment	0.1%
Desoximetasone	Cream, Ointment	0.25%
	Gel	0.05%
Diflorasone diacetate	Cream, Ointment (emollient base)	0.05%
Fluocinolone acetonide	Cream	0.2%
Fluocinonide	Cream, Ointment, Gel	0.05%
Halcinonide	Cream, Ointment	0.1%
Triamcinolone acetonide	Cream, Ointment	0.5%
III. *Medium potency*		
Betamethasone benzoate	Cream, Gel, Lotion	0.025%
Betamethasone dipropionate	Lotion	0.05%
Betamethasone valerate	Cream	0.1%
Clocortolone pivalate	Cream	0.1%
Desoximetasone	Cream	0.05%
Fluocinolone acetonide	Cream, Ointment	0.025%
Flurandrenolide	Cream, Ointment	0.025%
	Cream, Ointment, Lotion	0.05%
	Tape	4 mcg/cm^2
Fluticasone propionate	Cream	0.05%
	Ointment	0.005%
Hydrocortisone butyrate	Ointment, Solution	0.1%
Hydrocortisone valerate	Cream, Ointment	0.2%
Mometasone furoate	Cream, Ointment, Lotion	0.1%
Triamcinolone acetonide	Cream, Ointment, Lotion	0.025%
	Cream, Ointment, Lotion	0.1%
IV. *Low potency*		
Aclometasone dipropionate	Cream, Ointment	0.05%
Desonide	Cream	0.05%
Dexamethasone	Aerosol	0.01%
	Aerosol	0.04%
Dexamethasone sodium phosphate	Cream	0.1%
Fluocinolone acetonide	Cream, Solution	0.01%
Hydrocortisone	Lotion	0.25%
	Cream, Ointment, Lotion, Aerosol	0.5%
	Cream, Ointment, Lotion, Solution	1%
	Cream, Ointment, Lotion	2.5%
Hydrocortisone acetate	Cream, Ointment	0.5%
	Cream, Ointment	1%

CORTICOSTEROIDS, TOPICAL

Indications:

Relief of inflammatory and pruritic manifestations of corticosteroid-responsive dermatoses.

Some of the conditions in which topical corticosteroids have been proven effective include: Contact dermatitis, atopic dermatitis, nummular eczema, stasis eczema, asteatotic eczema, lichen planus, lichen simplex chronicus, insect and arthropod bite reactions, first- and second-degree localized burns and sunburns.

Alternative/Adjunctive treatment: Psoriasis, seborrheic dermatitis, severe diaper rash, disidrosis, nodular prurigo, chronic discoid lupus erythematosus, alopecia areata, lymphocytic infiltration of the skin, mycosis fungoides and familial benign pemphigus of Hailey-Hailey.

Possibly effective in the following conditions: Bullous pemphigoid, cutaneous mastocytosis, lichen sclerosus et atrophicus and vitiligo.

Topical corticosteroids relieve inflammatory symptoms associated with dermatophyte and yeast infections of the skin and may be used concomitantly with antifungal agents for initial treatment.

The use of topical corticosteroids in combination with antibiotics in secondary infected dermatoses remains controversial.

Nonprescription hydrocortisone preparations: Temporary relief of itching associated with minor skin irritations, inflammation and rashes due to eczema, insect bites, poison ivy, poison oak, poison sumac, soaps, detergents, cosmetics, jewelry, seborrheic dermatitis, psoriasis and external genital and anal itching.

Contraindications:

Hypersensitivity to any component; monotherapy in primary bacterial infections such as impetigo, paryonchia, erysipelas, cellulitis, angular cheilitis, erythrasma (clobetasol), treatment of rosacea, perioral dermatitis or acne; use on the face, groin or axilla (very high or high potency agents); ophthalmic use (prolonged ocular exposure may cause steroid-induced glaucoma and cataracts). When applied to the eyelids or skin near the eyes, the drug may enter the eyes.

Warnings:

Pregnancy: Category C. Corticosteroids are teratogenic in animals when administered systemically at relatively low dosages. The more potent corticosteroids are teratogenic after dermal application in animals. There are no adequate and well controlled studies in pregnant women. Therefore, use during pregnancy only if the potential benefits outweigh the potential hazards to the fetus. In pregnant patients, do not use extensively; do not use in large amounts or for prolonged periods of time.

Lactation: It is not known whether topical corticosteroids could result in sufficient systemic absorption to produce detectable quantities in breast milk. Systemic corticosteroids are secreted into breast milk in quantities not likely to have a deleterious effect on the infant. Nevertheless, exercise caution when administering topical corticosteroids to a nursing mother.

Children: Children may be more susceptible to topical corticosteroid-induced hypothalamic-pituitary-adrenal (HPA) axis suppression and Cushing's syndrome than adults because of a larger skin surface area to body weight ratio.

HPA axis suppression, Cushing's syndrome and intracranial hypertension have occurred in children receiving topical corticosteroids. Manifestations of adrenal suppression include linear growth retardation, delayed weight gain, low plasma cortisol levels and absence of response to ACTH stimulation. Manifestations of intracranial hypertension include bulging fontanelles, headaches and bilateral papilledema.

Limit administration to the least amount compatible with effective therapy. Chronic corticosteroid therapy may interfere with the growth and development of children.

Do not use potent topical corticosteroids to treat diaper dermatoses in infants.

Safety and efficacy of augmented betamethasone dipropionate, clobetasol, fluticasone propionate, desoximetasone and halobetasol propionate are not established.

Precautions:

Systemic effects: Systemic absorption of topical corticosteroids has produced reversible HPA axis suppression, Cushing's syndrome, hyperglycemia and glycosuria. Conditions that augment systemic absorption include the application of the more potent steroids, use over large surface areas, prolonged use and the addition of occlusive dressings.

Periodically evaluate patients for evidence of HPA axis suppression by using morning plasma cortisol, urinary free cortisol and ACTH stimulation tests. If HPA axis suppression is noted, attempt to withdraw the drug, reduce the frequency of application, substitute a less potent steroid or use a sequential approach with the occlusive technique. Also test for impairment of thermal homeostasis.

Recovery of HPA axis function and thermal homeostasis are generally prompt and complete upon discontinuation of the drug. Infrequently, signs and symptoms of steroid withdrawal may occur, requiring supplemental systemic corticosteroids.

Clobetasol suppresses the HPA axis at doses as low as 2 g per day.

Children may absorb proportionally larger amounts of topical corticosteroids and may be more susceptible to systemic toxicity (see Warnings).

As a general rule, little effect on the HPA axis will occur with use of a potent topical corticosteroid in amounts of < 50 g weekly for an adult and 15 g weekly for a small child, without occlusion. To cover the adult body one time requires 12 to 26 g.

For information regarding systemic corticosteroids, refer to the Adrenal Cortical Steroids, Glucocorticoids group monograph in the Hormones section.

Local irritation: If local irritation develops, discontinue use and institute appropriate therapy. Medications containing alcohol may produce dry skin or burning sensations/irritation in open lesions. Allergic contact dermatitis is usually diagnosed by observing failure to heal rather than noting clinical exacerbation as with most topical products not containing corticosteroids. Corroborate such an observation with diagnostic patch testing.

Skin atrophy is common and may be clinically significant in 3 to 4 weeks with potent preparations. Atrophy occurs most readily at sites where percutaneous absorption is high.

Take care when using periorbitally or in the genital area. Avoid use of high potency topical corticosteroids on the face and in intertriginous areas because of resulting striae.

Psoriasis: Do not use topical corticosteroids as sole therapy in widespread plaque psoriasis.

In rare instances, treatment (or withdrawal of treatment) of psoriasis with corticosteroids is thought to have provoked the pustular form of the disease.

Atrophic changes: Certain areas of the body, such as the face, groin and axillae, are more prone to atrophic changes than other areas of the body following treatment with corticosteroids. Frequent observation of the patient is important if these areas are to be treated.

Infections: In the presence of an infection, institute therapy with an antifungal or antibacterial agent. If a favorable response does not occur promptly, discontinue the corticosteroid until the infection has been controlled. Treating skin infections with topical corticosteroids can extensively worsen the infection.

For external use only: Avoid inhalation of aerosols, ingestion or contact with eyes.

Vehicles: Many topical corticosteroids are in specially formulated bases designed to maximize their release and potency. Mixing with other bases or vehicles may affect potency far beyond that normally expected from the dilution. Exercise caution before mixing; if necessary, contact the manufacturer to determine if there may be an incompatibility.

Occlusive therapy: Discontinue the use of occlusive dressings if infection develops, and institute appropriate antimicrobial therapy.

Occasionally, a patient may develop a sensitivity reaction to a particular occlusive dressing material or adhesive; a substitute material may be necessary.

Do not use occlusive dressings in **augmented betamethasone dipropionate, betamethasone dipropionate, clobetasol, halobetasol propionate** and **mometasone** treatment regimens.

Adverse Reactions:

Local: Burning; itching; irritation; erythema; dryness; folliculitis; hypertrichosis; pruritus; acneiform eruptions; hypopigmentation; perioral dermatitis; allergic contact dermatitis; numbness of fingers; stinging and cracking/tightening of skin; maceration of the skin; secondary infection; skin atrophy; striae; miliaria; telangiectasia. These may occur more frequently with occlusive dressings.

Also, there have been reports of development of pustular psoriasis from chronic plaque psoriasis following reduction or discontinuation of potent topical corticosteroids.

Sensitivity to a particular dressing material or adhesive may occur occasionally.

Systemic: Systemic absorption of topical corticosteroids has produced reversible HPA axis suppression, manifestations of Cushing's syndrome, hyperglycemia and glycosuria (see Precautions). This is more likely to occur with occlusive dressings and with the more potent steroids. Patients with liver failure or children (see Warnings) may be at at higher risk. Lightheadedness and hives have been reported rarely.

CORTICOSTEROIDS, TOPICAL

Following prolonged application around the eyes, cataracts and glaucoma may develop. In diffusely atrophied skin, blood vessels may become visible on the skin surface; telangiectasia and purpura may occur at the site of trauma.

The risk of adverse reactions may be minimized by changing to a less potent agent, reducing the dosage or using intermittent therapy.

Overdosage:

Topical corticosteroids can be absorbed in sufficient amounts to produce systemic effects (see Precautions).

Patient Information:

Apply ointments, creams or gels sparingly in a light film; rub in gently. Washing or soaking the area before application may increase drug penetration.

To use a lotion, solution or gel on your scalp, part your hair, apply a small amount of the medicine on the affected area and rub it in gently. Protect the area from washing, clothing, rubbing, etc until the lotion dries. You may wash your hair as usual but not right after applying the medicine.

To apply aerosols, shake well and spray on affected area holding container about 3 to 6 inches away. Spray for about 2 seconds to cover an area the size of your hand. Take care not to inhale the vapors. If you are spraying your face or near your face, cover your eyes.

Use only as directed. Do not put bandages, dressing, cosmetics or other skin products over the treated area unless directed by your physician.

Notify your physician if the condition being treated gets worse, or if burning, swelling or redness develop.

Avoid prolonged use around the eyes, in the genital and rectal areas, on the face, armpits and in skin creases unless directed by your physician. Avoid contact with the eyes.

If you forget a dose, apply it as soon as you remember and continue on your regular schedule. If it is almost time for the next application, wait and continue on your regular schedule. Do not apply double doses.

For parents of pediatric patients: Do not use tight-fitting diapers or plastic pants on a child treated in the diaper area; these garments may work like occlusive dressings and cause more of the drug to be absorbed into your child's body.

Administration and Dosage:

Usual dose: Apply sparingly to affected areas 2 to 4 times daily.

General considerations: Topical corticosteroids have a repository effect; with continuous use, one or two applications per day may be as effective as three or more. Many clinicians advise applying twice daily until clinical response is achieved, and then only as frequently as needed to control the condition.

Short term or intermittent therapy using high potency agents (eg, every other day, 3 to 4 consecutive days per week, or once per week) may be more effective and cause fewer adverse effects than continuous regimens using lower potency products.

Do not discontinue treatment abruptly. After long-term use or after using a potent agent, in order to prevent a rebound effect, switch to a less potent agent or alternate use of topical corticosteroids and emollient products.

Use low potency agents in children, on large areas, and on body sites especially prone to steroid damage such as the face, scrotum, axilla, flexures and skin folds. Reserve higher potency agents for areas and conditions resistant to treatment with milder agents; they may be alternated with milder agents.

Perform appropriate clinical and laboratory tests if a topical corticosteroid is used for long periods or over large areas of the body.

Treatment with very high potency topical corticosteroids should not exceed 2 consecutive weeks and the total dosage should not exceed 50 g per week because of the potential for these drugs to suppress the HPA axis.

Occlusive dressing technique:

1.) Soak the area in water or wash it well.
2.) While the skin is still moist, gently rub medication into the affected areas.
3.) Cover the area with a plastic wrap (eg, Saran Wrap, Handi Wrap;). Alternatively, plastic gloves may be used for hands, plastic bags for feet, or a bathing cap for scalp.
4.) Seal edges with tape or bandage, ensuring that the wrap adheres closely to the skin.
5.) Leave in place overnight or at least 6 hours. Do not use for > 12 hours in a 24 hour period. Do not use this technique with very high potency topical corticosteroids.

ALCLOMETASONE DIPROPIONATE

Complete prescribing information begins in the Topical Corticosteroids group monograph.

Rx	**Aclovate** (Glaxo Wellcome)	**Ointment:** 0.05%	Hexyleneglycol, white wax, propylene glycol stearate, white petrolatum. In 15 and 45 g.
		Cream: 0.05%	Hydrophilic, emollient base. Propylene glycol, white petrolatum glyceryl stearate, PEG-100 stearate, chlorocresol. In 15 and 45 g.

AMCINONIDE

Complete prescribing information begins in the Topical Corticosteroids group monograph.

Rx	**Cyclocort** (Fujisawa)	**Ointment:** 0.1%	White petrolatum. 2% benzyl alcohol. In 15, 30 and 60 g.
		Cream: 0.1%	Hydrophilic base. 2% benzyl alcohol, glycerin. In 15, 30 and 60 g.
		Lotion: 0.1%	Hydrophilic base. 1% benzyl alcohol, glycerin. In 20 and 60 ml.

AUGMENTED BETAMETHASONE DIPROPIONATE

Complete prescribing information begins in the Topical Corticosteroids group monograph.

Rx	**Diprolene** (Schering)	**Ointment:** 0.05%	In an optimized vehicle. Propylene glycol, propylene glycol stearate, white wax, white petrolatum. In 15 and 45 g.
Rx	**Diprolene AF** (Schering)	**Cream:** 0.05%	Emollient base. Chlorocresol, propylene glycol, white petrolatum, white wax. In 15 and 45 g.
Rx	**Diprolene** (Schering)	**Gel:** 0.05%	Propylene glycol. In 15 and 45 g.
Rx	**Diprolene** (Schering)	**Lotion:** 0.05%	30% isopropyl alcohol, hydroxypropylcellulose, propylene glycol. In 30 and 60 ml.

BETAMETHASONE BENZOATE

Complete prescribing information begins in the Topical Corticosteroids group monograph.

Rx	**Uticort** (Parke-Davis)	**Cream:** 0.025%	Emollient base. Light mineral oil, propylene glycol. In 60 g.
		Lotion: 0.025%	Water-miscible. Propylene glycol, sodium lauryl sulfate, parabens. In 60 ml.
		Gel: 0.025%	Greaseless. 13.8% alcohol, EDTA, propylene glycol, dusopropanolamine. In 15 and 60 g.

BETAMETHASONE DIPROPIONATE

Complete prescribing information begins in the Topical Corticosteroids group monograph.

Rx	**Betamethasone Dipropionate** (Various, eg, NMC)	**Ointment**: 0.05%	In 15 and 45 g.
Rx	**Alphatrex** (Savage)		Mineral oil, white petrolatum. In 15 and 45 g.
Rx	**Diprosone** (Schering)		Mineral oil, white petrolatum. In 15 and 45 g.
Rx	**Maxivate** (Westwood-Squibb)		Mineral oil, white petrolatum.
Rx	**Betamethasone Dipropionate** (Various, eg, Geneva, NMC, Schein)	**Cream**: 0.05%	In 15 and 45 g.
Rx	**Alphatrex** (Savage)		Hydrophilic. Mineral oil, white petrolatum, polyethylene glycol, chlorocresol. In 15 and 45 g.
Rx	**Diprosone** (Schering)		Hydrophilic, emollient. Mineral oil, white petrolatum, chlorocresol, propylene glycol. In 15 and 45 g.
Rx	**Maxivate** (Westwood-Squibb)		Hydrophilic base. Mineral oil, white petrolatum, polyethylene glycol, chlorocresol. In 15 and 45 g.
Rx	**Teladar** (Dermol)		Mineral oil, white petrolatum, polyethylene glycol, 4 chloro-m-cresol, propylene glycol. In 15 and 45 g.
Rx	**Betamethasone Dipropionate** (Various, eg, Goldline, Major, Moore, Rugby)	**Lotion**: 0.05%	In 20 and 60 ml.
Rx	**Alphatrex** (Savage)		Isopropyl alcohol. In 60 ml.
Rx	**Diprosone** (Schering)		46.8% alcohol. In 30 and 60 ml.
Rx	**Maxivate** (Westwood-Squibb)		Isopropyl alcohol. In 60 ml.
Rx	**Diprosone** (Schering)	**Aerosol**: 0.1%	10% isopropyl alcohol, mineral oil. In 85 g.

BETAMETHASONE VALERATE

Complete prescribing information begins in the Topical Corticosteroids group monograph.

Rx	**Betamethasone Valerate** (Various, eg, Genetco, Goldline, Major, Taro)	**Ointment**: 0.1%	In 15 and 45 g.
Rx	**Betatrex** (Savage)		Mineral oil, white petrolatum. In 15 and 45 g.
Rx	**Valisone** (Schering)		Mineral oil, white petrolatum, hydrogenated lanolin. In 15 and 45 g.
Rx	**Valisone Reduced Strength** (Schering)	**Cream**: 0.01%	Aqueous, hydrophilic, emollient base. Mineral oil, white petrolatum, chlorocresol. In 15 and 60 g.
Rx	**Psorion Cream** (ICN)	**Cream**: 0.05%	Mineral oil, white petrolatum, propylene glycol. In 15 and 45 g.
Rx	**Betamethasone Valerate** (Various, eg, Genetco, Geneva, Major, Moore, Taro)	**Cream**: 0.1%	In 15 and 45 g.
Rx	**Betatrex** (Savage)		Hydrophilic. Mineral oil, white petrolatum, chlorocresol. In 15 and 45 g.
Rx	**Beta-Val** (Lemmon)		Aqueous, vanishing base. Mineral oil, white petrolatum, 4-chloro-m-cresol. In 15 and 45 g.
Rx	**Valisone** (Schering)		Hydrophilic, emollient base. Mineral oil, white petrolatum, chlorocresol. In 15, 45, 110 and 430 g.
Rx	**Betamethasone Valerate** (Various, eg, Major, Moore)	**Lotion**: 0.1%	In 60 ml.
Rx	**Betatrex** (Savage)		Isopropyl alcohol. In 60 ml.
Rx	**Beta-Val** (Lemmon)		47.5% isopropyl alcohol. In 60 ml.
Rx	**Valisone** (Schering)		47.5% isopropyl alcohol. In 20 and 60 ml.
Rx	**Betamethasone Valerate** (Paddock)	**Powder for Compounding**	In micronized 5 and 10 g.

CLOBETASOL PROPIONATE

Complete prescribing information begins in the Topical Corticosteroids group monograph.

Rx	**Clobetasol Propionate** (Various, eg, Copley, NMC Labs)	**Ointment**: 0.05%	In 15, 30 and 45 g.
Rx	**Temovate** (Glaxo Wellcome)		White petrolatum, sorbitan sesquioleate. In 15, 30 and 45 g.
Rx	**Cormax** (Oclassen)		White petrolatum, sorbitan sesquioleate. In 15 and 45 g.
Rx	**Clobetasol Propionate** (Various, eg, Copley, NMC Labs)	**Cream**: 0.05%	In 15, 30 and 45 g.
Rx	**Temovate** (Glaxo Wellcome)		Chlorocresol. In 15, 30 and 45 g.
Rx	**Temovate Emollient** (Glaxo Wellcome)		Emollient base. In 15, 30 and 60 g.
Rx	**Temovate** (Glaxo Wellcome)	**Scalp application**: 0.05%	39.3% isopropyl alcohol. In 25 and 50 ml.
Rx	**Temovate** (Glaxo Wellcome)	**Gel**: 0.05% clobetasol propionate	In 15, 30 and 60 g.

CLOCORTOLONE PIVALATE

Complete prescribing information begins in the Topical Corticosteroids group monograph.

Rx	**Cloderm** (Hermal)	**Cream**: 0.1%	Water-washable, emollient base. White petrolatum, mineral oil, EDTA, parabens. In 15 and 45 g.

DESONIDE

Complete prescribing information begins in the Topical Corticosteroids group monograph.

Rx	**Desonide** (Various, eg, Copley, Goldline, Major, Moore, Rugby, Taro)	**Ointment**: 0.05%	In 15 and 60 g.
Rx	**DesOwen** (Owen/Galderma)		Mineral oil. In 15 and 60 g.
Rx	**Tridesilon** (Bayer)		White petrolatum. In 15 and 60 g.
Rx	**Desonide** (Taro)	**Cream**: 0.05%	White petrolatum, mineral oil, methylparaben. In 15 and 60 g.
Rx	**DesOwen** (Owen/Galderma)		In 15 and 60 g.
Rx	**Tridesilon** (Miles Inc.)		White petrolatum, glycerin, mineral oil, methylparaben. In 15 and 60 g.
Rx	**DesOwen** (Owen/Galderma)	**Lotion**: 0.05%	Light mineral oil, parabens, EDTA. In 60 and 120 ml.

DESOXIMETASONE

Complete prescribing information begins in the Topical Corticosteroids group monograph.

Rx	**Topicort** (Hoechst Marion Roussel)	**Ointment**: 0.25%	White petrolatum, sorbitan sesquioleate. In 15 and 60 g.
Rx	**Desoximetasone** (Various, eg, Taro)	**Cream**: 0.05%	Emollient base. White petrolatum, lanolin alcohols, mineral oil, EDTA. In 15 and 60 g.
Rx	**Topicort LP** (Hoechst Marion Roussel)		Emollient. White petrolatum, mineral oil, lanolin alcohols, EDTA. In 15 and 60 g.
Rx	**Desoximetasone** (Various, eg, Taro)	**Cream**: 0.25%	Emollient base. White petrolatum, lanolin alcohols, mineral oil. In 15 and 60 g.
Rx	**Topicort** (Hoechst Marion Roussel)		Emollient. White petrolatum, mineral oil, lanolin alcohols. In 15, 60, 120 g.
Rx	**Topicort** (Hoechst Marion Roussel)	**Gel**: 0.05%	20% SD alcohol 40, EDTA, docusate sodium, trolamine. In 15 and 60 g.

DEXAMETHASONE

Complete prescribing information begins in the Topical Corticosteroids group monograph.

Rx	**Aeroseb-Dex** (Herbert)	**Aerosol**: 0.01%	59% SD alcohol 40-2. In 58 g.
Rx	**Decaspray** (Merck)	**Aerosol**: 0.04%	In 25 g.

DEXAMETHASONE SODIUM PHOSPHATE

Complete prescribing information begins in the Topical Corticosteroids group monograph.

Rx	**Decadron Phosphate** (Merck)	**Cream**: 0.1%	Greaseless base. Mineral oil, EDTA, 0.15% methylparabens, 0.1% sorbic acid. In 15 and 30 g.

DIFLORASONE DIACETATE

Complete prescribing information begins in the Topical Corticosteroids group monograph.

Rx	**Florone** (Dermik)	**Ointment**: 0.05%	Emollient, occlusive base. Lanolin alcohol, white petrolatum. In 15, 30 and 60 g.
Rx	**Maxiflor** (Herbert)		Emollient, occlusive base. Lanolin alcohol, white petrolatum. In 15, 30 and 60 g.
Rx	**Psorcon** (Dermik)		White petrolatum. In 15, 30, 60 g.
Rx	**Florone** (Dermik)	**Cream**: 0.05%	Emulsified, hydrophilic base. Propylene glycol. In 15, 30 and 60 g.
Rx	**Florone E** (Dermik)		Emollient, hydrophilic vanishing base. Mineral oil. In 15, 30 and 60 g.
Rx	**Maxiflor** (Herbert)		Emulsified, hydrophilic base. 15% propylene glycol. In 15, 30 and 60 g.
Rx	**Psorcon** (Dermik)		Mineral oil, lanolin alcohol, vegetable oil, cetyl alcohol. In 15, 30 and 60 g.

FLUOCINOLONE ACETONIDE

Complete prescribing information begins in the Topical Corticosteroids group monograph.

Rx	**Fluocinolone** (Various, eg, Fougera, Goldline, Major, Moore)	**Ointment**: 0.025%	In 15 and 60 g.
Rx	**Flurosyn** (Rugby)		In 15 and 60 g.
Rx	**Synalar** (Syntex)		White petrolatum. In 15, 30 and 425 g.
Rx	**Fluocinolone** (Various, eg, Fougera, Geneva, Goldline, Major, Moore, NMC, URL)	**Cream**: 0.01%	In 15 and 60 g.
Rx	**Flurosyn** (Rugby)		Washable. Parabens. In 15, 60, 425 g.
Rx	**Synalar** (Syntex)		Water-washable, aqueous base. Mineral oil, EDTA, parabens. In 30 and 425 g.
Rx	**Fluocinolone** (Various, eg, Fougera, Geneva, Goldline, Major, Moore, NMC, URL)	**Cream**: 0.025%	In 15 and 60 g.
Rx	**Flurosyn** (Rugby)		Washable. Parabens. In 15, 60, 425 g.
Rx	**Synalar** (Syntex)		Water-washable, aqueous base. Mineral oil, EDTA, parabens. In 30, 60 and 425 g.
Rx	**Synalar-HP** (Syntex)	**Cream**: 0.2%	Water-washable, aqueous base. Mineral oil, parabens. In 12 g.
Rx	**Fluocinolone** (Various, eg, Fougera, Geneva, Goldline, Major, Moore, Rugby, URL)	**Solution**: 0.01%	In 20 and 60 ml.
Rx	**Fluonid** (Herbert)		In 20 and 60 ml.
Rx	**Synalar** (Syntex)		Water-washable base. In 20, 60 ml.
Rx	**FS Shampoo** (Hill)	**Shampoo**: 0.01%	In 12 mg capsule with shampoo base to be mixed by pharmacist before dispensing. 5.48 mg dibasic calcium phosphate dihydrate. In 180 ml.
Rx	**Derma-Smoothe/FS** (Hill)	**Oil**: 0.01%	A blend of oils, including mineral oil and peanut oil. In 120 ml

FLUOCINONIDE

Complete prescribing information begins in the Topical Corticosteroids group monograph.

Rx	**Fluocinonide** (Various, eg, Geneva, Goldline, Lemmon, Taro, URL)	**Cream**: 0.05%	In 15, 30, 60 and 120 g.
Rx	**Fluocinonide "E" Cream** (Various, eg, Goldline, Major, Taro, URL)		In 15, 30, 60 and 120 g.
Rx	**Fluonex** (ICN)		Greaseless, anhydrous, water-washable. In 15 and 30 g.
Rx	**Lidex** (Syntex)		Water-miscible, emollient, hydrophilic, anhydrous, greaseless. In 15, 30, 60, 120 g.
Rx	**Lidex-E** (Syntex)		Water-washable, aqueous emollient base. Mineral oil. In 15, 30 and 60 g.
Rx	**Fluocinonide** (Various, eg, Lemmon, Rugby, Taro)	**Ointment**: 0.05%	In 15, 30 and 60 g.
Rx	**Lidex** (Syntex)		Occlusive, emollient. White petrolatum. In 15, 30, 60 and 120 g.
Rx	**Fluocinonide** (Various, eg, Fougera, Geneva, Goldline, Lemmon, Major, Moore)	**Solution**: 0.05%	In 60 ml.
Rx	**Lidex** (Syntex)		35% alcohol. In 20 and 60 ml.
Rx	**Fluocinonide** (Various, eg, Fougera, Lemmon, Moore)	**Gel**: 0.05%	In 60 g.
Rx	**Lidex** (Syntex)		Water-miscible, greaseless. EDTA. In 15, 30, 60 and 120 g.

FLURANDRENOLIDE

Complete prescribing information begins in the Topical Corticosteroids group monograph.

Rx	**Cordran** (Oclassen)	**Ointment:** 0.025%	White petrolatum. In 30 and 60 g.
Rx	**Cordran** (Oclassen)	**Ointment:** 0.05%	White petrolatum. In 15, 30 and 60 g.
Rx	**Cordran SP** (Oclassen)	**Cream:** 0.025%	Emulsified base. Mineral oil. In 30 and 60 g.
Rx	**Cordran SP** (Oclassen)	**Cream:** 0.05%	Emulsified base. Mineral oil. In 15, 30 and 60 g.
Rx	**Flurandrenolide** (Various, eg, Barre-National)	**Lotion:** 0.05%	In 60 ml.
Rx	**Cordran** (Oclassen)		Oil-in-water base. Mineral oil, glycerin, menthol, benzyl alcohol. In 15 and 60 ml.
Rx	**Cordran** (Oclassen)	**Tape:** 4 mcg per square cm	In 24″ x 3″ and 80″ x 3″ rolls.

FLUTICASONE PROPIONATE

Complete prescribing information begins in the Topical Corticosteroids group monograph.

Rx	**Cutivate** (Glaxo Wellcome)	**Cream:** 0.05%	Mineral oil base. Imidurea. In 15, 30 and 60 g.
Rx	**Cutivate** (Glaxo Wellcome)	**Ointment:** 0.005%	In 15 and 60 g.

HALCINONIDE

Complete prescribing information begins in the Topical Corticosteroids group monograph.

Rx	**Halog** (Princeton)	**Ointment:** 0.1%	Polyethylene and mineral oil gel base. In 15, 30, 60 and 240 g.
Rx	**Halog** (Princeton)	**Cream:** 0.025%	In 15 and 60 g.
Rx	**Halog** (Princeton)	**Cream:** 0.1%	Titanium dioxide. In 15, 30, 60 and 240 g.
Rx	**Halog-E** (Princeton)		Water-washable, greaseless, hydrophilic, vanishing, emollient. White petrolatum. In 15, 30 and 60 g.
Rx	**Halog** (Princeton)	**Solution:** 0.1%	EDTA. In 20 and 60 ml.

HALOBETASOL PROPIONATE

Complete prescribing information begins in the Topical Corticosteroids group monograph.

Rx	**Ultravate** (Westwood-Squibb)	**Ointment:** 0.05%	Petrolatum. In 15 and 45 g.
		Cream: 0.05%	Glycerin, diazolidinyl urea. In 15 and 45 g.

HYDROCORTISONE

Complete prescribing information begins in the Topical Corticosteroids group monograph.

Rx[1]	**Hydrocortisone** (Various, eg, Carolina Medical, Fougera, Parmed, Rugby[2], URL)	**Ointment**: 0.5%	In 30 g.
otc	**Cortizone•5** (Thompson)		White petrolatum. In 30 g.
Rx[1]	**Hydrocortisone** (Various, eg, Carolina Medical[3], Fougera, Major, Parmed, Rugby, URL)	**Ointment**: 1%	In 20, 30 and 120 g and lb.
otc	**Cortizone•10** (Thompson)		White petrolatum. In 30 g.
Rx	**Hycort** (Everett)		White petrolatum and mineral oil base. In 30 g.
Rx	**Hytone** (Dermik)		Mineral oil, white petrolatum. Emollient base. In 30 g.
otc	**Tegrin-HC** (Block)		Mineral oil, white petrolatum. In 28 g.
Rx	**1% HC** (C & M Pharmacal)		Washable. Petrolatum base. In 15, 20, 30, 60, 120 and 240 g and lb.
Rx	**Hydrocortisone** (Various, eg, Major, Parmed, Rugby, URL)	**Ointment**: 2.5%	In 20 g.
Rx	**Hytone** (Dermik)		Emollient base. Mineral oil, white petrolatum. In 30 g.
Rx[1]	**Hydrocortisone** (Various, eg, Fougera, Geneva, Major, Roberts Hauck, Rugby[2], URL)	**Cream**: 0.5%	In 15, 30 and 120 g and lb.
otc	**Bactine Hydrocortisone** (Miles Inc.)		Glycerin, lanolin alcohol, mineral oil, EDTA, corn oil, parabens. In 15 g.
Rx	**Cort-Dome** (Miles Inc.)		Glycerin, white petrolatum, light mineral oil, methylparaben. In 30 g.
otc	**Cortizone•5** (Thompson)		Glycerin, mineral oil, white petrolatum, parabens. In 60 g.
otc	**Delcort** (Roberts Med)		In 1 g packets.
otc	**Dermolate** (Schering-Plough)		Greaseless, vanishing. Petrolatum, mineral oil, chlorocresol. In 15 and 30 g.
otc	**Dermtex HC with Aloe** (Pfeiffer)		Aloe vera gel, glycerin, white petrolatum, lt. mineral oil, parabens. In 30 g.
otc	**HydroTex** (Syosset)		In 30 and 60 g.

HYDROCORTISONE

Rx[1]	**Hydrocortisone** (Various, eg, Fougera, Geneva, Goldline, Major, Moore, Parmed, Roberts Hauck, Rugby, Schein, URL[2])	**Cream**: 1%	In 20, 30 and 120 g and lb.
Rx	**Ala-Cort** (Del-Ray)		Glycerin. In 30 and 90 g.
otc	**Maximum Strength Bactine** (Miles Inc.)		Glycerin, lt. mineral oil, methylparaben, white petrolatum. In 30 g.
otc	**Cortaid Intensive Therapy** (Pharmacia and Upjohn)		Alcohols, parabens. In 58 g tubes.
Rx	**Cort-Dome** (Miles Inc.)		Glycerin, white petrolatum, lt. mineral oil, methylparaben. In 30 g.
Rx	**Delcort** (Roberts Med)		In 1 g packets.
Rx	**Dermacort** (Solvay)		Benzyl alcohol. In lb.
Rx	**Hi-Cor 1.0** (C & M Pharm.)		Washable. Petrolatum, glycerin. In 15, 20, 30, 60, 120 & 240 g & lb.
Rx	**Hycort** (Everett)		In 30 g.
Rx	**Hytone** (Dermik)		Water-washable. Cholesterol. In 30 and 120 g.
Rx	**Nutracort** (Owen/Galderma)		In 30, 60 and 120 g.
Rx	**Penecort** (Herbert)		Petrolatum, benzyl alcohol, EDTA. In 30 g.
otc	**Procort** (Roberts)		In 30 g.
Rx	**Synacort** (Syntex)		Mineral oil. In 15, 30 and 60 g.
otc	**Maximum Strength KeriCort-10** (Bristol-Myers Squibb)		Parabens, cetyl alcohol, stearyl alcohol. In 56.7 g.
Rx	**Hydrocortisone** (Various, eg, Geneva, Goldline, Major, Moore, NMC, Rugby, Schein, URL)	**Cream**: 2.5%	In 20 and 30 g and lb.
Rx	**Anusol-HC 2.5%** (Parke-Davis)		Water-washable. Benzyl alcohol, petrolatum, EDTA. In 30 g.
Rx	**Eldecort** (ICN)		Light mineral oil, propylene glycol, allantoin. In 15 and 30 g.
Rx	**Hi-Cor 2.5** (C & M Pharm.)		Washable. Petrolatum, glycerin. In 15, 20, 30, 60, 120 & 240 g & lb.
Rx	**Hydrocort** (Parmed)		In 20 and 30 g and lb.
Rx	**Hytone** (Dermik)		Water-washable base. Cholesterol. In 30 and 60 g.
Rx	**Synacort** (Syntex)		Mineral oil. In 30 g.
Rx	**Cetacort** (Owen/Galderma)	**Lotion**: 0.25%	Parabens. In 120 ml.

HYDROCORTISONE

Rx[1]	**Hydrocortisone** (Various, eg, Goldline, Mericon, Parmed, Rugby, Schein, URL)	**Lotion**: 0.5%	In 30, 60 and 120 ml.
Rx	**Cetacort** (Owen/Galderma)		Parabens. In 60 ml.
Rx	**S-T Cort** (Scot-Tussin)		Water-washable base. Lanolin alcohol, mineral oil, parabens. In 120 ml.
otc[1]	**Hydrocortisone** (Various, eg, Geneva, Mericon)	**Lotion**: 1%	In 120 ml.
Rx	**Acticort 100** (Baker Cummins)		In 60 ml.
Rx	**Ala-Cort** (Del-Ray)		Light mineral oil, glycerin. In 118 ml.
Rx	**Dermacort** (Solvay)		Benzyl alcohol. In 118 ml.
Rx	**Hytone** (Dermik)		Cholesterol, triethanolamine. In 120 ml.
Rx	**LactiCare-HC** (Stiefel)		Light mineral oil, lactic acid. In 120 ml.
Rx	**Ala-Scalp** (Del-Ray)	**Lotion**: 2%	Isopropyl alcohol. Benzalkonium chloride. In 30 ml.
Rx	**Hytone** (Dermik)	**Lotion**: 2.5%	Cholesterol, triethanolamine. In 60 ml.
Rx	**LactiCare-HC** (Stiefel)		Light mineral oil, lactic acid. In 60 ml.
otc	**Scalpicin** (Combe)	**Liquid**: 1%	Menthol. SD alcohol 40. In 45, 75 and 120 ml.
otc	**T/Scalp** (Neutrogena)		Greaseless. In 60 and 600 ml.
otc	**Extra Strength CortaGel** (Norstar)	**Gel**: 1%	Greaseless. EDTA. In 15 and 30 g.
Rx	**Penecort** (Allergan)	**Solution**: 1%	Alcohol, petrolatum, propylene glycol. In 30 and 60 ml.
Rx	**Texacort** (GenDerm)		Lipid free. 33% SD alcohol 40-2. In 30 ml.
otc	**Maximum Strength Cortaid** (Pharmacia & Upjohn)	**Pump Spray**: 1%	55% alcohol. Glycerin, methylparaben. In 45 ml.
otc	**Procort** (Roberts)	**Spray**: 1%	In 45 ml.
otc	**Maximum Strength Cortaid Faststick** (Pharmacia & Upjohn)	**Stick, roll-on**: 1%	55% alcohol. Glycerin, methylparaben. In 14 g.

[1] Products are available *otc* or *Rx* depending on product labeling.

HYDROCORTISONE ACETATE

Complete prescribing information begins in the Topical Corticosteroids group monograph.

otc	**Cortaid with Aloe** (Pharmacia & Upjohn)	**Ointment**: 0.5%	Aloe vera, cholesterol, mineral oil, white petrolatum, parabens. In 15 and 30 g.
otc	**Lanacort-5** (Combe)		Acetylated lanolin alcohols, aloe, petrolatum. In 15 g.

HYDROCORTISONE ACETATE

otc	**Corticaine** (UCB)	**Cream**: 0.5%	Greaseless. Glycerin, EDTA, menthol, parabens. In 30 g.
otc	**Cortaid with Aloe** (Pharmacia & Upjohn)		Aloe vera, parabens. In 15 and 30 g.
otc	**Cortef Feminine Itch** (Pharmacia & Upjohn)		Vanishing. Aloe vera, parabens. In 15 g.
otc	**Lanacort-5 Creme** (Combe)		Aloe, parabens. In 15 and 22.5 g.
otc	**Anusol HC-1** (Parke-Davis)	**Ointment**: 1%	Diazolidinyl urea, parabens, mineral oil, sorbitan sesquioleate, white petrolatum. In 21 g.
otc	**Maximum Strength Cortaid** (Pharmacia & Upjohn)		Mineral oil, parabens, cholesterol, white petrolatum. In 30 g.
Rx[1]	**Hydrocortisone Acetate** (Various, eg, Clay-Park, Thames)	**Cream**: 1%	Mineral oil, parabens. In 20, 30 and 120 g.
otc	**Gynecort Female Creme** (Combe)		Parabens, sorbitol, zinc pyrithione. In 15 g.
otc	**Lanacort 10 Creme** (Combe)		Parabens. In 15 and 30 g.
otc	**Maximum Strength Cortaid** (Pharmacia & Upjohn)		Parabens, glycerin, white petrolatum. In 15 g.

[1] Products are available *otc* or *Rx* depending on product labeling.

HYDROCORTISONE BUTEPRATE

Complete prescribing information begins in the Topical Corticosteroids group monograph.

Administration and Dosage:

Apply a thin film to the affected area once or twice a day depending on the severity of the condition. Massage gently until the medication disappears. Use occlusive dressings only under the advice of a physician for the management of refractory lesions of psoriasis and other deep-seated dermatoses. Do not apply in the diaper area, as diapers or plastic pants may constitute occlusive dressings.

Storage: Store at controlled room temperature 15° to 30°C (59° to 86°F).

Rx	**Pandel** (Savage)	**Cream**: 1%	Alcohol, glyceryls, mineral oil, parabens, white petrolatum. In 15 and 45 g.

HYDROCORTISONE BUTYRATE

Complete prescribing information begins in the Topical Corticosteroids group monograph.

Administration and Dosage:

Cream and ointment: Apply to the affected area as a thin film 2 or 3 times daily depending on the severity of the condition. Use occlusive dressings under the direction of a physician for the management of psoriasis or recalcitrant conditions. Do not use tight-fitting diapers or plastic pants on a child being treated in the diaper area, as these garments may constitute occlusive dressings. If an infection develops, discontinue occlusive dressings and institute appropriate antimicrobial therapy.

Solution: Apply to the affected area as a thin film 2 or 3 times daily depending on the severity of the condition. Use occlusive dressings only under the advice of a physician. Do not use tight-fitting diapers or plastic pants on a child being treated in the diaper area, as these garments may constitute occlusive dressing.

Rx	**Locoid** (Ferndale)	**Ointment**: 0.1%	Mineral oil. In 15 and 45 g.
Rx	**Locoid** (Ferndale)	**Cream**: 0.1%	Alcohol, mineral oil, parabens, white petrolatum. In 15 and 45 g.
Rx	**Locoid** (Ferndale)	**Solution**: 0.1%	Alcohol (50%), glycerin. In 20 and 60 ml.

HYDROCORTISONE VALERATE

Complete prescribing information begin in the Topical Corticosteroids group monograph.

Rx	**Westcort** (Westwood-Squibb)	**Ointment:** 0.2%	Hydrophilic base. White petrolatum, mineral oil. In 15, 45 and 60 g.
Rx	**Westcort** (Westwood-Squibb)	**Cream:** 0.2%	Hydrophilic base. White petrolatum. In 15, 45, 60 and 120 g.

MOMETASONE FUROATE

Complete prescribing information begins in the Topical Corticosteroids group monograph.

Rx	**Elocon** (Schering)	**Ointment:** 0.1%	White petrolatum. In 15 and 45 g.
Rx	**Elocon** (Schering)	**Cream:** 0.1%	White petrolatum. In 15 and 45 g.
Rx	**Elocon** (Schering)	**Lotion:** 0.1%	40% isopropyl alcohol. In 27.5 and 55 ml.

PREDNICARBATE

Complete prescribing information begins in the Topical Corticosteroids group monograph.

Rx	**Dermatop** (Hoechst Marion Roussel)	**Cream:** 0.1% prednicarbate	Preservative free. White petrolatum, mineral oil, EDTA. In 15 and 60 g.

TRIAMCINOLONE ACETONIDE

Complete prescribing information begins in the Topical Corticosteroids group monograph.

Rx	**Triamcinolone Acetonide** (Various, eg, Fougera, Goldline, Major, Moore, Rugby, URL)	**Ointment:** 0.025%	In 15, 80 and 454 g.
Rx	**Flutex** (Syosset)		White petrolatum, mineral oil. In 28, 57 and 113 g.
Rx	**Kenalog** (Westwood-Squibb)		In *Plastibase* (polyethylene, mineral oil gel base). In 15, 80 and 240 g.
Rx	**Triamcinolone Acetonide** (Various, eg, Fougera, Geneva, Goldline, Major, Moore, NMC, Rugby, URL)	**Ointment:** 0.1%	In 15 and 80 g and lb.
Rx	**Aristocort** (Fujisawa)		White petrolatum. In 15, 60 and 240 g.
Rx	**Aristocort A** (Fujisawa)		White petrolatum. In 15 and 60 g.
Rx	**Flutex** (Syosset)		White petrolatum, mineral oil. In 28, 57 and 113 g.
Rx	**Kenalog** (Westwood-Squibb)		In *Plastibase* (polyethylene, mineral oil gel base). In 15, 60, 80 and 240 g.
Rx	**Triamcinolone Acetonide** (Various, eg, Rugby, URL)	**Ointment:** 0.5%	In 15 g.
Rx	**Aristocort** (Fujisawa)		White petrolatum base. In 15 and 240 g.
Rx	**Flutex** (Syosset)		White petrolatum, mineral oil. In 28, 57 and 113 g.
Rx	**Kenalog** (Westwood-Squibb)		In *Plastibase* (polyethylene, mineral oil gel base). In 20 g.

TRIAMCINOLONE ACETONIDE

Rx	**Triamcinolone Acetonide** (Various, eg, Geneva, Goldline, Major, Moore, Rugby, Schein, URL)	**Cream:** 0.025%	In 15, 80 and 454 g.
Rx	**Aristocort** (Fujisawa)		In 15 & 60 g & lb.
Rx	**Aristocort A** (Fujisawa)		Water-washable. 2% benzyl alcohol. In 15 & 60 g.
Rx	**Flutex** (Syosset)		Mineral oil, lanolin alcohol, sodium bisulfite. In 15, 30, 60, 120 and 240 g.
Rx	**Kenalog** (Westwood-Squibb)		Vanishing base. White petrolatum. In 15, 80, 240 g.
Rx	**Triamcinolone Acetonide** (Various, eg, Fougera, Geneva, Goldline)	**Cream:** 0.1%	In 15, 80 and 454 g.
Rx	**Aristocort** (Fujisawa)		In 15, 60 and 240 g and lb.
Rx	**Aristocort A** (Fujisawa)		Water-washable base. Glycerin, 2% benzyl alcohol. In 15, 60 and 240 g.
Rx	**Delta-Tritex** (Dermol)		In 30 and 80 g.
Rx	**Flutex** (Syosset)		Mineral oil, lanolin alcohol, sodium bisulfite. In 15, 30, 60, 120 and 240 g.
Rx	**Kenalog** (Westwood-Squibb)		Vanishing base. White pet. In 15, 60, 80 & 240 g.
Rx	**Kenalog-H** (Westwood-Squibb)		Hydrophilic, vanishing. White petrolatum, castor oil. In 15 and 60 g.
Rx	**Kenonel** (Marnel)		In 20 g.
Rx	**Triacet** (Lemmon)		Vanishing base. In 15 and 80 g.
Rx	**Triderm** (Del-Rey)		Mineral oil. In 30 and 90 g.
Rx	**Triamcinolone Acetonide** (Various, eg, Fougera, Geneva, Goldline, Moore, Rugby, URL)	**Cream:** 0.5%	In 15 g.
Rx	**Aristocort** (Fujisawa)		In 15 and 240 g.
Rx	**Aristocort A** (Fujisawa)		Water-washable base. 2% benzyl alcohol. In 15 g.
Rx	**Flutex** (Syosset)		Mineral oil, lanolin alcohol, sodium bisulfite. In 15, 30, 60, 120 and 240 g.
Rx	**Kenalog** (Westwood-Squibb)		Vanishing base. White petrolatum. In 20 g.
Rx	**Triamcinolone Acetonide** (Various, eg, Major, Morton Grove, Rugby)	**Lotion:** 0.025%	In 60 ml.
Rx	**Kenalog** (Westwood-S)		In 60 ml.
Rx	**Triamcinolone Acetonide** (Various, eg, Geneva, Goldline, Morton Grove, Moore, PBI)	**Lotion:** 0.1%	In 60 ml.
Rx	**Kenalog** (Westwood-S)		In 15 and 60 ml.
Rx	**Delta-Tritex** (Dermol)	**Ointment:** 0.1%	In 30 g.
Rx	**Kenalog** (Westwood-Squibb)	**Aerosol:** (2 sec. spray)	10.3% alcohol. In 23 and 63 g.

CORTICOSTEROID COMBINATIONS, TOPICAL

The following products contain corticosteroids in combination with various other components.They are indicated for a variety of specific and nonspecific dermatoses. For further information see individual monographs. Components of these formulations include:

CORTICOSTEROID, used for their anti-inflammatory, antipruritic and vasoconstrictive effects.

CLIOQUINOL, IODOQUINOL, TRIACETIN, CLOTRIMAZOLE, NYSTATIN, POLYMYXIN B SULFATE, BACITRACIN ZINC, CETYLPYRIDINIUM Cl and *CHLOROXYLENOL*are used for their antifun gal, antibacterial and anti-eczematous effects.

LIDOCAINE is used as a local anesthetic.

UREA is a mild keratolytic and hydrates dry skin.

PYRILAMINE, CHLORPHENIRAMINE and *CHLORCYCLIZINE* are antihistamines.

BENZOYL PEROXIDE is used for its peeling and drying effects.

	Product & Distributor	Hydrocortisone (%)	Clioquinol (%)	Pramoxine (%)	Other Content and How Supplied
Rx	**Hydrocortisone with Clioquinol Cream** (Various, eg, Moore, Rugby)	0.5	3		In 30 g.
Rx	**Ala-Quin Cream** (Del-Ray)				Glycerin. In 30 g.
Rx	**Hydrocortisone with Clioquinol Cream** (Various, eg, Goldline, Moore, Rugby, Schein, URL)	1	3		In 20, 30 and 300 g.
Rx	**Corque Cream** (Geneva)				In 20 g.
Rx	**Hysone Cream** (Roberts Med)				In 20 g tube.
Rx	**Pedi-Cort V Creme** (Pedinol)				In 20 g.
Rx	**Hydrocortisone with Clioquinol Ointment** (Various, eg, Moore, Rugby)	1	3		In 20 and 30 g.
Rx	**1 + 1-F Creme** (Dunhall)	1	3	1	Mineral oil, lanolin alcohol, parabens. In 30 g.
Rx	**Analpram-HC Cream** (Ferndale)	1[1]		1	0.1% potassium sorbate, 0.1% sorbic acid. In 30 g.
Rx	**Enzone Cream** (UAD)				Hydrophilic. 0.1% K sorbate, 0.1% sorbic acid. In 30 g.
Rx	**Pramosone Cream** (Ferndale)				Hydrophilic base. 0.1% potassium sorbate, 0.1% sorbic acid. In 30, 60 and 120 g.
Rx	**ProctoCream-HC Cream** (Reed & Carnrick)				Hydrophilic base. Propylene glycol. In 30 g.
Rx	**Pramosone Ointment** (Ferndale)				Emollient base. White petrolatum. In 30 and 120 g.
Rx	**Pramosone Lotion** (Ferndale)				Hydrophilic. Glycerin, 0.1% potassium sorbate, 0.1% sorbic acid. In 60, 120, 240 ml.
Rx	**Epifoam Aerosol Foam** (Schwarz Pharma)				Parabens, propylene glycol. In 10 g.
Rx	**ProctoFoam-HC Aerosol Foam** (Reed & Carnrick)				Hydrophilic base. Parabens. In 10 g.
Rx	**Carmol HC Cream** (Doak)	1[1]			Water-washable, vanishing. 10% urea, sodium metabisulfite. In 30 and 120 g.

CORTICOSTEROID COMBINATIONS, TOPICAL

	Product & Distributor	Hydrocortisone (%)	Clioquinol (%)	Pramoxine (%)	Other Content and How Supplied
Rx	**Vytone Cream** (Dermik)	1			Greaseless. 1% iodoquinol, propylene glycol. In 30 g.
Rx	**Analpram-HC Cream** (Ferndale)	2.5[1]		1	In 30 g.
Rx	**Pramosone Cream** (Ferndale)				Hydrophilic. 0.1% K sorbate, 0.1% sorbic acid. In 30, 120 g.
Rx	**Pramosone Ointment** (Ferndale)				Emollient base. White petrolatum. In 30 and 120 g.
Rx	**Pramosone Lotion** (Ferndale)				Hydrophilic. Glycerin, 0.1% potassium sorbate, 0.1% sorbic acid. In 60 and 120 ml.
Rx	**Zone-A Forte Lotion** (UAD)				Hydrophilic. Glycerin, triethanolamine, 0.1% K sorbate, 0.1% sorbic acid. In 60 ml.
Rx	**Lida-Mantle-HC Cream** (Miles Inc.)	0.5[1]			3% lidocaine, glycerin, parabens. In 30 g.
Rx	**Mantadil Cream** (Burroughs Wellcome)				Vanishing. 2% chlorcyclizine HCl, 0.25% parabens, petrolatum. In 15 g.
otc	**HC Derma-Pax Liquid** (Recsei)	0.5[1]			0.44% pyrilamine maleate, 0.06% chlorpheniramine maleate, 1% benzyl alcohol, 35% isopropanol, 25% chlorobutanol. In 60 and 120 ml.
otc	**Massengill Medicated Towelettes** (SK-Beecham)				Diazolidinyl urea, parabens, propylene glycol. In 10 and 16 softcloth towelettes.
Rx	**Vanoxide-HC Lotion** (Dermik)				Water-washable. 5% benzoyl peroxide, mineral oil, propylene glycol, EDTA, parabens. In 25 ml.

[1] Hydrocortisone acetate.

CORTICOSTEROID AND ANTIBIOTIC COMBINATIONS, TOPICAL

Consider the information for Topical Corticosteroids, Antibiotics and Antifungals when using these products (see individual monographs).

		Dosage form	Corticosteroid	Neomycin sulfate	Other	Base/ How Supplied
Rx	**Neo-Cortef** (Upjohn)	Cream	1% hydrocortisone	0.5%	0.1% methyl- and 0.4% butyl parabens	Water-soluble, non-greasy, vanishing base. In 20 g.
Rx	**Neodecadron** (Merck)		0.1% dexamethasone phosphate		Greaseless. Mineral oil, 0.15% methylparaben, 0.18% sodium bisulfite, EDTA	In 15 and 30 g.
Rx	**Cortisporin** (Glaxo Wellcome)		0.5% hydrocortisone acetate		10,000 units polymyxin B sulfate per g; white, liquid petrolatum; 0.25% methylparaben	In 7.5 g.
Rx	**Myco-Biotic II** (Moore)		0.1% triamcinolone acetonide		Aqueous vanishing. 100,000 units nystatin per g, white petrolatum.	In 15, 30 and 60 g and lb.
Rx	**Neo-Cortef** (Upjohn)	Ointment	0.5% hydrocortisone acetate	0.5%	White petrolatum, mineral oil, parabens	In 20 g.
Rx	**Hydrocortisone-Neomycin** (Various, eg, Rugby)		1% hydrocortisone		White petrolatum, mineral oil	In 20 g.
Rx	**Neo-Cortef** (Upjohn)		1% hydrocortisone acetate		White petrolatum, mineral oil, parabens	In 20 g.
Rx	**Cortisporin** (Glaxo Wellcome)		1% hydrocortisone		400 units bacitracin zinc, white petrolatum, and 5000 units polymyxin B sulfate per g	In 15 g.

CORTICOSTEROID AND ANTIFUNGAL COMBINATIONS, TOPICAL

Consider the information given for Topical Corticosteroids and for Topical Antifungals when using these products.

		Dosage form	Corticosteroid	Antifungal	Base/How Supplied
Rx	**Fungoid-HC** (Pedinol)	Cream	0.5% hydrocortisone	triacetin, cetyl pyridinium Cl, chloroxylenol	Vanishing base. In 30 g.
Rx	**Lotrisone** (Schering)		0.05% betamethasone (as dipropionate)	1% clotrimazole	Hydrophilic. Mineral oil, white petrolatum, benzyl alcohol. In 15 and 45 g.
Rx	**Nystatin-Triamcinolone Acetonide** (Various, eg, Fougera, Taro)		0.1% triamcinolone acetonide	100,000 units nystatin per g	In 15, 30 and 60 g and UD 1.5 g.
Rx	**Mycogen II** (Goldline)				In 15, 30, 60 and 120 g.
Rx	**Mycolog-II** (B-M Squibb)				Vanishing base. White petrolatum. In 15, 30, 60 and 120 g.
Rx	**Myconel** (Marnel)				In 20 g.
Rx	**Myco-Triacet II** (Lemmon)				Aqueous, vanishing base. White petrolatum, parabens. In 15, 30 and 60 g.
Rx	**Mytrex** (Savage)				White petrolatum, propylene glycol, benzyl alcohol, polyoxyethylene fatty alcohol ether. In 15, 30 and 60 g and UD 1.5 g.
Rx	**N.G.T.** (Geneva)				In 15, 30 and 60 g.
Rx	**Tri-Statin II** (Rugby)				Vanishing base. White petrolatum. In 15, 30 and 60 g.
Rx	**Nystatin-Triamcinolone Acetonide** (Various, eg, Fougera)	Ointment	0.1% triamcinolone acetonide	100,000 units nystatin per g	In 15, 30 and 60 g.
Rx	**Mycogen II** (Goldline)				In 15, 30 and 60 g.
Rx	**Mycolog-II** (B-M Squibb)				Mineral oil, gel base. In 15, 30, 60 and 120 g.
Rx	**Myco-Triacet II** (Lemmon)				Vanishing base. White petrolatum and mineral oil. In 15 and 30 g.
Rx	**Mytrex** (Savage)				Mineral oil. In 15, 30 and 60 g.
Rx	**Fungoid HC Creme** (Pedinol)	Cream	1% hydrocortisone	2% miconazole nitrate	In 56.7 g and 1 g dual packets (30s).

LOCAL ANESTHETICS, TOPICAL

Since topical anesthetics are available in various forms, products are grouped according to their intended site of application: Topical Anesthetics for Skin Disorders and Topical Anesthetics for Mucous Membranes.

In addition to the single entity products listed in this section, other products containing topical local anesthetics are listed in other sections, based on their specific uses. These include: Anorectal Preparations and Ophthalmic Local Anesthetics (see individual monographs).

Because of the diversity of uses of these products, the following is a general discussion. For information on specific applications of individual products, consult the manufacturer's package literature.

Actions:

Pharmacology: Local anesthetics inhibit conduction of nerve impulses from sensory nerves. This action results from an alteration of the cell membrane permeability to ions. Although poorly absorbed through the intact epidermis (except for the lidocaine/prilocaine mixture; penetration and subsequent systemic absorption is enhanced over use of each agent alone), these agents are readily absorbed from mucous membranes. When skin permeability has been increased by abrasions or ulcers, the absorption and, subsequently, the efficacy of local anesthetics improves; however, the incidence of side effects also increases. Onset, depth and duration of dermal analgesia provided by the lidocaine/prilocin mixture depends primarily on duration of application.

Topical Local Anesthetics: Indications, Dose, Strength, Peak Effect and Duration

Local anesthetics, topical	Indications: Skin	Indications: Mucous membrane	Maximum adult dose (mg)	Available or recommended strengths (%)	Peak[1] effect (minutes)	Duration[1] of effect (minutes)
Amides						
Dibucaine	✓		25	0.5-1	< 15	15-45
Lidocaine	✓	✓	†[2]	2-5	2-5	15-45
Esters						
Benzocaine	✓	✓		0.5-20	< 5	15-45
Butamben picrate	✓			1		
Cocaine		✓	50-200	4-10	1-5	30-60
Tetracaine	✓	✓	50	0.5-2	3-8	30-60
Miscellaneous						
Dyclonine		✓	100	0.5-1	< 10	< 60
Pramoxine	✓		200	1	3-5	
Lidocaine/Prilocaine	✓			2.5/2.5	60-120	60-120

[1] Based primarily on application to mucous membranes.
[2] Variable depending on doseform.

Indications:

Skin disorders: For topical anesthesia in local skin disorders, including: Pruritus and pain due to minor burns, skin manifestations of systemic disease (eg, chickenpox), prickly heat, abrasions, sunburn, plant poisoning, insect bites, eczema; local analgesia on normal, intact skin (EMLA).

Mucous membranes: For local anesthesia of accessible mucous membranes, including: Oral, nasal and laryngeal mucous membranes; respiratory or urinary tracts. Also for the treatment of pruritus ani, pruritus vulvae and hemorrhoids.

Contraindications:

Hypersensitivity to any component of these products; ophthalmic use.

Warnings:

Systemic effects: Use the lowest dose effective for anesthesia to avoid high plasma levels and serious adverse effects. Repeated doses of **lidocaine** and **dyclonine** may cause significant increases in blood levels with each repeated dose because of slow accumulation of the drug or its metabolites. Have resuscitative equipment available for immediate use. Lidocaine/prilociane is not recommended for use on mucous membranes because of its much greater absorption through this area than through intact skin, potentially resulting in serious adverse effects.

Methomoglobinemia: **Benzoacaine, lidocaine** and **prilocaine** should not be used in those rare patients with congenital or idiopathic methemoglobinemia and in infants < 12 months of age who are receiving treatment with methemoglobin-inducing agents. Very young patients or patients with glucose-6–phosphate deficiencies are more susceptible to methemoglobinemia.

LOCAL ANESTHETICS, TOPICAL

Ototoxic effects: **Lidocaine/prilocaine** has an ototoxic effect when instilled into the middle ear of animals, but not when used in the external auditory canal. Do not use this combination in any situation where penetration or migration beyond the tympanic membrane into the middle ear is possible.

Hepatic function impairment: Patients with severe hepatic disease, because of their inability to metabolize local anesthetics normally, are at greater risk of developing toxic plasma concentrations of lidocaine and prilocaine.

Pregnancy: Category B (lidocaine); *Category C* (benzocaine, cocaine, dyclonine, tetracaine). Safety for use during pregnancy has not been established. Use in women of childbearing potential, and particularly in early pregnancy, only when the potential benefits outweigh the potential hazards to the fetus.

Lactation: Lidocaine, and probably prilocaine, are excreted in breast milk. Exercise caution when administering any of these drugs to a nursing woman.

Children: Safety and efficacy of dyclonine and tetracaine have not been established in children < 12 years of age. Do not use benzocaine in infants < 1 year of age. Dosages in children should be reduced commensurate with age, body weight and physical condition.

Precautions:

For external or mucous membrane use only. Do not use in the eyes.

Minimal effective dose: Reactions and complications are best averted by using the minimal effective dose. Not for prolonged use. Give debilitated or elderly patients, acutely ill patients and children dosages commensurate with their age, size and physical condition.

Severe shock/heartblock: Use **lidocaine** and **dyclonine** with caution.

Traumatized mucosa: Use cautiously in persons with known drug sensitivities or in patients with severely traumatized mucosa and sepsis in the region of the application. If irritation or rash occurs, discontinue treatment and institute appropriate therapy.

Oral use: Topical anesthetics may impair swallowing and enhance danger of aspiration. Do not ingest food for 1 hour after anesthetic use in mouth or throat. This is particularly important in children because of their frequency of eating.

Tartrazine sensitivity: Some of these products contain tartrazine, which may cause allergic-type reactions (including bronchial asthma) in susceptible individuals. Although the incidence of tartrazine sensitivity in the general population is low, it is frequently seen in patients who also have aspirin hypersensitivity. Specific products containing tartrazine are identified in the product listings.

Sulfite sensitivity: Some of these products contain sulfites which may cause allergic-type reactions including anaphylactic symptoms and life-threatening or less severe asthmatic episodes in certain susceptible persons. The overall prevalence of sulfite sensitivity in the general population is unknown and probably low. Sulfite sensitivity is seen more frequently in asthmatic or atopic non-asthmatic persons. Specific products containing sulfites are identified in the product listings.

Drug Interactions:

Class I antiarrhythmic agents: Use with caution in patients receiving Class I antiarrhythmic drugs (such as tocainide and mexiletine) because the toxic effects are additive and potentially synergistic.

Drug/Lab test interactions: Dyclonine topical solutions should not be used in cystoscopic procedures folliwng intravenous pyelography because an iodine precipitate occurs which interferes with visualization.

Adverse Reactions:

Adverse reactions are, in general, dose-related and may result from high plasma levels due to excessive dosage or rapid absorption, hypersensitivity, idiosyncrasy or diminished tolerance. (See Overdosage.)

Hypersensitivity: Cutaneous lesions; urticaria; edema; contact dermatitis; bronchospasm; shock; anaphylactoid reactions. The detection of sensitivity by skin testing is of doubtful value.

Miscellaneous: Urethritis with and without bleeding. In a few case reports, methemoglobinemia characterized by cyanosis has followed topical application of **benzocaine** or **lidocaine/prilocaine** and may be more common with prilocaine (see Warnings). Seizures in children have occurred from overuse of **oral lidocaine**.

Local: Burning; stinging; tenderness; sloughing.

Overdosage:

Symptoms: Reactions due to overdosage (high plasma levels) are systemic and involve the CNS (convulsions) or the cardiovascular system (hypotension).

LOCAL ANESTHETICS, TOPICAL

CNS – Reactions are excitatory or depressant, and may be characterized by: Nervousness; apprehension; euphoria; confusion; dizziness; lightheadedness; tinnitus; blurred vision; vomiting; sensations of heat, cold or numbness; twitching; tremors; drowsiness; convulsions; unconsciousness; respiratory depression or arrest. Excitatory reactions may be very brief or not occur at all; in this case, first sign of toxicity may be drowsiness, merging into unconsciousness and respiratory arrest.

Cardiovascular – Reactions are depressant, and may be characterized by: Hypotension; myocardial depression; bradycardia; cardiac arrest; cardiovascular collapse.

Treatment: Maintain airway and support ventilation. Cardiovascular support consists of vasopressors, preferably those that stimulate the myocardium, IV fluids and perhaps blood transfusions. Control convulsions by slow IV of 0.1 mg/kg diazepam or 10 to 50 mg succinylcholine, with continued use of oxygen. Refer to General Management of Acute Overdosage.

Methemoglobinemia may be treated with methylene blue 1%, 0.1 ml/kg IV over 10 minutes (refer to individual monograph).

Patient Information:

Do not ingest food for 1 hour following use of oral topical anesthetic preparations in the mouth or throat. Topical anesthesia may impair swallowing, thus enhancing the danger of aspiration.

Numbness of the tongue or buccal mucosa may increase the danger of biting trauma. Do not eat or chew gum while the mouth or throat area is anesthetized.

When lidocaine/prilocaine is used, the patient should be aware that the production of dermal analgesia may be accompanied by the block of all senstions in the treated skin. For this reason, the patient should avoid inadvertent trauma to the treated area by scratching, rubbing, or exposure to extreme hot or cold temperatures until complete sensation has returned.

Administration and Dosage:

Topical: Apply to the affected area as needed. Ointments and creams can be applied to gauze or to a bandage prior to applying to the skin.

Mucous membranes: Dosage varies and depends upon the area to be anesthetized, vascularity of tissues, individual tolerance and technique of anesthesia. Administer the lowest dose possible that still provides adequate anesthesia. Apply to affected areas using the proper technique (see individual manufacturer inserts).

In debilitated, elderly patients or children, administer lower concentrations.

A combination of tetracaine 0.5%, epinephrine 1:2000 and cocaine 11.8% (also known as TAC) in a liquid topical formulation has been used for minor skin lacerations, especially of the face and scalp. Other preparations include cocaine 11.8% and epinephrine 1:1000, and lidocaine 4%, epinephrine 1:1000 and tetracaine 0.5%, both utilizing mehtylcellulose for a more viscous gel formulation. Use results in decreased pain on application, allowing for better compliance and tolerance of repair procedure. This may be beneficial in patients who cannot tolerate injection anesthesia or those who are difficult to control (eg, children). A commercial preparation of lidocaine and prilocaine (EMLA) was developed for a similar purpose (increased absorption in children) on intact skin. However, toxic effects are also more likely to occur in infants and children with all of these preparations.

The use of the lidocaine/prilocaine combination appears to be beneficial as a pretreatment in decreasing the pain of DPT vaccinations (and presumably other vaccinations) in infants. The cream is applied at the injection site with occlusive dressing for at least 60 minutes prior to the vaccination.

Topical Anesthetics for Skin Disorders

BENZOCAINE (Ethyl Aminobenzoate)

Complete prescribing information begins in the Local Anesthetics, Topical group monograph.

otc	**Americaine Anesthetic** (Fisons)	**Spray:** 20%	In 60 ml.
otc	**Boil-Ease** (Del)	**Ointment:** 20% with camphor, lanolin, eucalyptus oil, menthol, petrolatum, phenol	In 30 g.
otc	**Dermoplast** (Whitehall-Robins)	**Spray:** 20% with 0.5% menthol, methylparaben, aloe, lanolin	In 82.5 ml.
otc	**Lanacane** (Combe)	**Spray:** 20% with 0.1% benzethonium Cl, 36% ethanol, aloe extract	In 113 ml.
otc	**Dermoplast** (Whitehall-Robins)	**Lotion:** 8% with 0.5% menthol, aloe, glycerin, parabens, lanolin	In 90 ml.
otc	**Solarcaine** (Schering-Plough)	**Aerosol:** 20% with 0.13% triclosan, 35% SD alcohol 40, tocopheryl acetate	In 90 and 120 ml.
otc	**Bicozene** (Sandoz)	**Cream:** 6% with 1.67% resorcinol, castor oil, glycerin	In 30 g.
otc	**Foille Plus** (Blistex)	**Aerosol:** 5% with 0.6% chloroxylenol, 57.33% alcohol	In 105 ml.
otc	**Foille** (Blistex)	**Spray:** 5% with 0.63% chloroxylenol	In 97.5 ml.
otc	**Benzocaine** (Various, eg, IDE)	**Cream:** 5%	In 480 g.
otc	**Foille Medicated First Aid** (Blistex)	**Ointment:** 5% with 0.1% chloroxylenol, benzyl alcohol, EDTA in corn oil base	In 3.5 and 28 g.
		Aerosol: 5% with 0.6% chloroxylenol, benzyl alcohol in corn oil base	In 92 ml.
otc	**Chigger-Tox** (Scherer)	**Liquid:** Benzocaine with benzyl benzoate and green soap in an isopropanol base	In 30 ml.
otc	**Solarcaine** (Schering-Plough)	**Lotion:** Benzocaine with triclosan, mineral oil, alcohol, aloe extract, tocopheryl acetate, menthol, camphor, parabens, EDTA	In 120 ml.
otc	**Lanacane** (Combe)	**Cream:** 6% with 0.1% benzethonium Cl, aloe, parabens, castor oil, glycerin, isopropyl alcohol	In 28 and 56 g.

Topical Anesthetics for Skin Disorders

DIBUCAINE

Complete prescribing information begins in the Local Anesthetics, Topical group monograph.

otc	**Dibucaine** (Various, eg, IDE, Moore, NMC)	**Ointment:** 1%	In 30 g.
otc	**Nupercainal** (Ciba)		Acetone sodium bisulfite, lanolin, mineral oil, white petrolatum. In 30 and 60 g.
otc	**Nupercainal** (Ciba)	**Cream:** 0.5%	Acetone sodium bisulfite, glycerin. In 42.5 g.

LIDOCAINE

Complete prescribing information begins in the Local Anesthetics, Topical group monograph.

otc	**Zilactin-L** (Zila)	**Liquid:** 2.5%	79.3% alcohol. In 10 ml.
Rx	**Lidocaine HCl** (Moore)	**Ointment:** 5%	In 50 g.
otc	**Xylocaine** (Astra)	**Ointment:** 2.5%	In water soluble carbowaxes. In 37.5 g.
otc	**Solarcaine ALoe Extra Burn Relief** (Schering-Plough)	**Cream:** 0.5%	Aloe, lanolin oil, lanolin, camphor, propylparaben, eucalyptus oil, EDTA, menthol, tartrazine. In 120 g.
otc	**SolarcaineAloe Extra Burn Relief** (Schering-Plough)	**Gel:** 0.5%	Aloe vera gel, glycerin, EDTA, isopropyl alcohol, menthol, diazolidinyl urea, tartrazine. In 120 and 240 g.
otc	**DermaFlex** (Zila)	**Gel:** 2.5%	79% alcohol. In 15 g.
otc	**Solarcaine Aloe Extra Burn Relief** (Schering-Plough)	**Spray:** 0.5%	Aloe vera gel, glycerin, EDTA, diaolidinyl urea, vitamin E, parabens. In 135 mg.

BUTAMBEN PICRATE

Complete prescribing information begins in the Local Anesthetics, Topical group monograph.

otc	**Butesin Picrate** (Abbott)	**Ointment:** 1%	Lanolin, parabens, mineral oil. In 28.4 g.

TETRACAINE

Complete prescribing information begins in the Local Anesthetics, Topical group monograph.

otc	**Pontocaine** (Winthrop)	**Ointment:** 0.5% tetracaine base	White petrolatum, light mineral oil. In 30 g.
		Cream: 1% (as HCl)	Water miscible base with light mineral oil, paraben, sodium metabisulfite. In 28.35 g.

Topical Anesthetics for Skin Disorders

PRAMOXINE HCl

Complete prescribing information begins in the Local Anesthetics, Topical group monograph.

otc	**Tronothane HCl** (Abbott)	**Cream:** 1%	Water miscible base with cetyl alcohol, glycerin, parabens. In 28.4 g.
otc	**PrameGel** (GenDerm)	**Gel:** 1%	Emollient base with 0.5% menthol, benzyl alcohol, SD alcohol 40. In 118 g.
otc	**Prax** (Ferndale)	**Lotion:** 1%	Hydrophilic base with mineral oil, cetyl alcohol, glycerin, lanolin, 0.1% potassium sorbate, 0.1% sorbic acid. In 15, 120 and 240 ml.
		Cream: 1%	Hydrophilic base with glycerin, cetyl alcohol, white petrolatum. In 30, 113.4 g and 1 lb.
otc	**Itch-X** (Ascher & Co.)	**Gel:** 1%	10% benzyl alcohol, aloe vera gel, diazolidinyl urea, SD alcohol 40, parabens. In 35.4 g.
		Spray: 1%	10% benzyl alcohol, aloe vera gel, SD alcohol 40. In 60 ml.

MISCELLANEOUS TOPICAL ANESTHETICS

Complete prescribing information begins in the Local Anesthetics, Topical group monograph.

Rx	**Ethyl Chloride** (Gebauer)	**Spray**: Chloroethane **Indications:** Topical vapo-coolant to control pain associated with minor surgical procedures (eg, lancing boils, incision and drainage of small abscesses), athletic injuries, injections and for treatment of myofascial pain, restricted motion and muscle spasm	In 100 g metal tubes, 105 ml "Spra-Pak" and 120 ml bottles (fine, medium and coarse spray).
Rx	**Fluro-Ethyl** (Gebauer)	**Aerosol spray**: 25% ethyl chloride and 75% dichlorotetrafluoroethane **Indications**: Topical refrigerant anesthetic to control pain associated with minor surgical procedures, dermabrasion, injections, contusions and minor strains	In 270 ml.
Rx	**Fluori-Methane** (Gebauer)	**Spray**: 15% dichlorodifluoromethane and 85% trichloromonofluoromethane **Indications**: Vapo-coolant for topical application in management of myofascial pain, restricted motion and muscle spasm, and for control of pain associated with injections	In 105 ml glass bottles (fine or medium spray).
otc	**Aerofreeze** (Graham-Field)	**Spray**: Trichloromonofluoromethane and dichlorodifluoromethane **Indications:** Topical anesthesia for pre-injection, skin planing, dermabrasion and minor surgical procedures; for treatment of strains, sprains and muscle spasms	In 240 ml.
otc	**PretzPak** (Parnell)	**Ointment**: 3.5% benzyl alcohol, polyethylene glycols, carboxymethylcellulose, urea, poloxamer, *Mucoprotective Factor* (MPF), yerba santa, allantoin, aluminum chlorhydroxy allantoin **Indications**: For operative and postoperative care in intranasal and endoscopic surgery	In 15 g.

Topical Anesthetics for Mucous Membranes

LIDOCAINE HCl

Complete prescribing information begins in the Local Anesthetics, Topical group monograph.

Rx	**Xylocaine 10% Oral** (Astra)	**Spray**: 10% *For* topical anesthesia of the mucous membranes of the mouth and oropharynx.	Saccharin, cetylpyridinium Cl, absolute alcohol. Flavored. In 30 ml aerosol and 1 ml disposable cannula (50s).
Rx	**Xylocaine** (Astra)	**Ointment**: 5% For anesthesia of accessible mucous membranes of the oropharynx; anesthetic lubricant for intubation; for temporary relief of pain of minor burns, skin abrasions and insect bites.	Saccharin (flavored only). Flavored and unflavored. In 3.5 and 35 g.
Rx	**Xylocaine** (Astra)	**Liquid**: 5% For relief of painful, irritated or inflamed mucous membranes of the mouth; far anesthesia for minor dental surgical procedures.	Saccharin, glycerin. Flavored. In 30 ml.
Rx	**Lidocaine HCl Topical**[1] (Various, eg, Moore, Roxane)	**Solution**: 4% *For* topical anesthesia of accessible mucous membranes of the oral and nasal cavities and proximal portions of the digestive tract.	In 50 ml.[1]
Rx	**Xylocaine** (Astra)		Parabens. In 50 ml.

Topical Anesthetics for Mucous Membranes

LIDOCAINE HCl

Rx	**Lidocaine 2% Viscous**[2] (Various, eg, Moore, Roxane)	**Solution**: 2% *For* topical anesthesia of irritated or inflamed mucous membranes of the mouth and pharynx. Also used to reduce gagging during the taking of x-rays or dental impressions.	In 50 and 100 ml and UD 20 ml.[1,2,3]
Rx	**Xylocaine Viscous** (Astra)		Sodium carboxymethylcellulose, parabens, saccharin. In 100 and 450 ml & UD 20 ml (25s).
Rx	**Xylocaine** (Astra)	**Jelly**: 2% *For* prevention and control of pain in procedures involving the male and female urethra, for topical treatment of painful urethritis and as an anesthetic lubricant for endotracheal intubation.	Hydroxypropylmethylcellulose base, parabens. In 30 ml.
Rx	**Anestacon** (PolyMedica)		1% hydroxypropylmethylcellulose, 0.01% benzalkonium chloride. In 15 and 240 ml disposable units.
Rx	**Dentipatch** (Noven)	**Patch**:23/2 cm² patch For production of mild topical anesthesia of accessible muous membranes of the mouth prior to superficial dental procedures.	Aspartame. In 50s or 100s.
		46.1/2 cm² patch For production of mild topical anesthesia of accessible mucous membranes of the mouth prior to superficial dental procedures.	Aspartame. In 50s and 100s.

[1] May contain parabens.
[2] May contain sodium carboxymethylcellulose.
[3] May contain saccharin.

BENZOCAINE (Ethyl Aminobenzoate)

Complete prescribing information begins in the Local Anesthetics, Topical group monograph.

otc	**Maximum Strength Anbesol** (Whitehall)	**Liquid**: 20%	50% alcohol, saccharin. In 9 ml.
otc	**Hurricane** (Beutlich)	**Gel**: 20%	60% alcohol, saccharin. In 7 g.
		Spray: 20% For oral and mucosal anesthesia to conrol pain and suppress the gag reflex.	Cherry flavor. In 60 ml.
Rx	**Americaine Anesthetic Lubricant** (Fisons)	**Gel**: 20% For use as a lubricant and anesthetic on inratracheal catheters and pharyngeal and nasal airways; on nasogastric and endoscopic tubes; urinary catheters; laryngoscopes; proctoscopes; sigmoidoscopes; vaginal specula.	0.1% benzethonium chloride. In 30 g and UD 2.5 g.

Topical Anesthetics for Mucous Membranes

BENZOCAINE (Ethyl Aminobenzoate)

otc	**Orajel Mouth-Aid** (Del)	**Liquid:** 20%	0.1% cetylpyridinium Cl, 70% ethyl alcohol, tartrazine, saccharin. in 13.5 ml.
		Gel: 20%	0.02 benzalkonium Cl, 0.1% zinc Cl, EDTA, saccharin. In 5.6 and 10 g.
otc	**Orabase Gel** (Colgate-Palmolive)	**Gel:** 15%	Ethyl alcohol, saccharin. In 7 g.

TETRACAINE HCl

Complete prescribing information begins in the Local Anesthetics, Topical group monograph.

Rx	**Pontocaine HCl** (Winthrop)	**Solution:** 2% *For anesthesia of nose and throat; also when the laryngeal and esophageal reflexes are to be abolished prior to performing bronchoscopy, bronchography and esophagoscopy.*	0.4% chlorobutanol. In 30 and 118 ml.

DYCLONINE HCl

Complete prescribing infomratin begins in the Local Anesthetics, Topical group monograph.

Rx	**Dyclone** (Astra)	**Solution:** 0.5%	Chlorobutanol. In 30 ml.
		1% *For anesthetizing mucous membranes (eg, the mouth, pharynx, larynx, trachea, esophagus and urethra) prior to endoscopic procedures. The 0.5% solution may be used to block the gag reflex and relieve pain associated with oral or anogenital lesions.*	Chlorobutanol. In 30 ml.

Topical Anesthetics for Mucous Membranes

COCAINE

Actions:

Pharmacology: Cocaine is an alkaloid derived from the plant *Erythroxylon coca;* chemically, it is benzoylmethylecgonine. Following local application, cocaine blocks the initiation or conduction of the nerve impulse and causes intense vasoconstriction. It not only lessens sensibility to pain and touch but, when applied to the nose or mouth, diminishes the acuity of taste and smell. Its most striking systemic effect is general CNS stimulation, manifested in descending order of frequency as euphoria, stimulation, reduced fatigue, loquacity, sexual stimulation, increased mental ability, alertness and increased sociality. As the dose is increased, tremors and tonic-clonic convulsions may occur. In addition, vomiting centers may also be stimulated. Central stimulation is soon followed by depression. The medullary centers are eventually depressed; death results from respiratory failure.

Small doses of cocaine may slow the heart as a result of central sympathetic stimulation, but after moderate doses, the heart rate increases. Although blood pressure may finally fall, there is at first a prominent rise in blood pressure due to sympathetically mediated tachycardia and vasoconstriction.

Cocaine is markedly pyrogenic. It increases muscular activity which augments heat production; vasoconstriction decreases heat loss. Cocaine may also have a direct action on central heat regulating centers.

Cocaine interferes with the uptake of norepinephrine and dopamine by the presynaptic adrenergic nerve terminals; therefore, it may produce sensitization to catecholamines, causing vasoconstriction and mydriasis.

Pharmacokinetics:

Absorption/Distribution – Cocaine is rapidly absorbed from all sites of application and absorption is enhanced in the presence of inflammation. When it is applied to mucous membranes, maximum local anesthesia occurs within 5 minutes. A 10% cocaine solution (1.5 mg/kg) applied to nasal mucosa yielded peak plasma levels in 15 to 60 minutes that declined over 3 to 5 hours. Peak effects occur in 2 to 5 minutes, persisting for 30 minutes. Absorption from mucous membranes may exceed the rate of metabolism and excretion.

Metabolism/Excretion – Cocaine is degraded in the liver to its principal metabolite, benzoylecgonine, which is then excreted in the urine. Cocaine is also metabolized by plasma cholinesterase. At therapeutic doses, < 20% is excreted unchanged in the urine. Half-life is approximately 1 to 2.5 hours.

For comparative data of cocaine with other local anesthetics, refer to the Topical Local Anesthetics group monograph.

Indications:

Topical anesthesia for mucous membranes.

Contraindications:

Systemic use; hypersensitivity to cocaine; ophthalmologic anesthesia (see Warnings).

Warnings:

Dependence: Although cocaine does not produce true physical dependence with definite withdrawal symptoms, continual exposure creates an excessively strong psychological dependence, and sometimes depression, as an indirect effect. Chronic use may cause progression from euphoria to paranoid psychosis; included may be perceptual changes (halo lights) and intense pruritus ("cocaine bugs"). This drug produces the highest degree of psychic dependence seen among recreationally abused drugs; thus, cocaine does produce an addictive syndrome.

"Crack" is a form of cocaine that is prepared with ammonia to alkalinize the solution and precipitate alkaloidal cocaine, thereby making it suitable for smoking. This form of cocaine is widely abused, highly addictive and potentially lethal.

Treatment of dependence – In addition to behavior modification and supportive psychotherapy, several agents may help decrease withdrawal symptoms associated with cocaine abuse or dependence, including: Amantadine; bromocriptine; desipramine; mazindol; carbamazepine.

Systemic effects: Concentrations > 4% are not advisable because of the potential for increasing the incidence and severity of systemic toxic reactions.

Ophthalmic use: Cocaine causes sloughing of the corneal epithelium, causing clouding, pitting and occasionally, ulceration of the cornea. Ophthalmic use is contraindicated.

Elderly: Because elderly patients with vascular disease may be sensitive to the vasoconstrictive effects of the drug and may have slowed cocaine metabolism, a lower dosage is recommended.

Topical Anesthetics for Mucous Membranes

COCAINE

Pregnancy: Category C. Cocaine use/abuse can lead to major toxicity in the mother, fetus and neonate. Consider cocaine abuse by a pregant woman as possibly teratogenic. Cocaine causes placental vasoconstriction, decreasing blood flow to the fetus. An increase in uterine contractility has occurred. A study compared 23 women who used cocaine only (n = 12) or cocaine plus narcotics (n = 11) during pregnancy with a group of women who were on methadone (n = 15) and a control group (n = 15). There was a higher rate of spontaneous abortion in the cocaine group. In addition, infants exposed to cocaine had depression of interactive behavior and a poor organizational response to environmental stimuli. In one retrospective trial, pregnant women who used "crack" delivered infants who were more likely to have a birth weight and head circumference under the tenth percentile for their gestational age. Other fetal effects noted following maternal cocaine use include growth retardation, fetal distress, cerebrovascular accidents and congential anomalies. Abnormal mild neurobehavioral signs (eg, irritability, muscular rigidity, tremulousness) were also more prevalent after birth, and GI symptoms (eg, nausea, vomiting) have occurred.

Women who use cocaine during pregnancy are at significant risk for shorter gestations, premature delivery, spontaneous abortions, abruptio placentae and death. Use only when clearly needed.

Lactation: Safety for use in the nursing mother has not been established. In one report, benzoylecgonine was detected in breast milk for up to 36 hours after the mother's last dose. Cocaine and its metabolite have been found in the urine of an infant following breastfeeding. Several case reports indicated that infants exposed via breastfeeding may develop symptoms of cocaine toxicity (eg, irritability, tremulousness, increased startle responese).

Because of the potential for serious adverse reactions in nursing infants from cocaine, it is recommended that nursing be discontinued during cocaine use. Strongly discourage cocaine use during breastfeeding. The American Academy of Pediatrics considers cocaine to be contraindicated during breastfeeding.

Children: Safety and efficacy for use in children have not been established. See Lactation.

Convulsions have occurred in infants, who may be especially susceptible to cocaine-induced toxicity.

Precautions:

Limit administration to office and surgical procedures. Safety and efficacy depends on proper dosage, correct technique, adequate precautions and readiness for emergencies.

Traumatized mucosa: Use with caution in patients with severely traumatized mucosa and sepsis in the region of the proposed application.

Adverse Reactions:

CNS: Reactions are excitatory or depressant. Nervousness, restlessness, euphoria, excitement, tremors and tonic-clonic convulsions may result. Central stimulation is followed by depression, with death resulting from respiratory failure.

Cardiovascular: Small doses of cocaine slow the heart rate; after moderate doses, the rate is increased due to central sympathetic stimulation. Hypertension, tachycardia, tachypnea and myocardial ischemia may occur.

Topical Anesthetics for Mucous Membranes

COCAINE

Overdosage:

Symptoms: Toxicity may occur following ingestion, parenteral administration, inhalation or absorption from topical administration to mucous membranes. Initial symptoms of acute poisoning are anxiety, restlessness, excitability, hallucinations, tachycardia, dilated pupils, chills or fever, abdominal pain, nausea, vomiting, numbness and muscular spasm, followed by irregular respirations, convulsions, coma and circulatory failure. If acute poisoning ends in death, it occurs quickly, from minutes to a maximum of 3 hours.

Chronic poisoning may be similar, but long-term changes involve mental deterioration, weight loss, change of character and perhaps, perforated nasal septum from chronic sniffing of cocaine.

Fatal dose – 500 mg to 1.2 g orally. Severe toxic effects have occurred with doses as low as 20 mg.

Treatment: Maintain airway and respiration. If drug was ingested, attempt delay of absorption with activated charcoal, gastric lavage or emesis. Limit absorption from an injection site by tourniquet or ice pack. Control convulsions with diazepam (0.1 mg/kg orally or slow IV) or 2.5% thiopental sodium slowly IV; in severe cases, use pancuronium bromide or succinylcholine with mechanical ventilation. The drug of choice for tachycardia and other arrhythmias is propranolol (1 mg slowly IV, every 5 minutes, up to a dose of 5 to 8 mg) or lidocaine 1 mg/minute IV.

Maintain blood pressure with fluids (vasopressors are hazardous). For hypertensive reactions, give phentolamine, 5 mg slowly IV. Treat hyperthermia if it occurs.

Refer to General Management of Acute Overdosage. If the patient survives the first 3 hours after acute poisoning, recovery is likely.

Administration and Dosage:

Reduce dosages for children and for elderly and debilitated patients. Cocaine solution can be given by means of cotton applicators or packs, instilled into a cavity or as a spray.

For topical application (ear, nose, throat, bronchoscopy), concentrations of 1% to 4% are used. As a general guide, the maximum single dose should be 1 mg/kg. Concentrations > 4% are not advisable because of the potential for increased incidence and severity of systemic toxic reactions.

C-II	**Cocaine HCl** (Roxane)	**Topical Solution**: 4%	In 10 ml multi-dose and UD 4 ml.
		10%	In 10 ml multi-dose and UD 4 ml.
C-II	**Cocaine Viscous** (Roxane)	**Topical Solution**: 4%	In 10 ml multidose and UD 4 ml.
		10%	In 10 ml multi-dose bottles and UD 4 ml.
C-II	**Cocaine HCl** (Mallinckrodt)	**Powder:**	In 5 and 25 g.

LOCAL ANESTHETICS, TOPICAL COMBINATIONS

Refer to the general discussion of these products beginning in the Local Anesthetics, Topical group monograph.

otc	**Americaine First Aid** (Fisons)	**Ointment**: 20% benzocaine with benzethonium chloride	In 22.5 g.
otc	**Detane** (Del)	**Gel**: 7.5% benzocaine, carbomer 940, PEG 400	In 15 g.
otc	**Sting-Kill** (Kiwi)	**Swabs**: 18.9% benzocaine, 0.9% menthol	In 0.5 & 14 ml.
Rx	**Cetacaine** (Cetylite)	14% benzocaine, 2% tetracaine HCl, 2% butamben and 0.5% benzalkonium chloride with 0.005% cetyl dimethyl ethyl ammonium bromide in a bland water soluble base	**Gel**: In 29 g. **Liquid**: In 56 ml. **Ointment**: In 37 g. **Aerosol**: In 56 g.
otc	**Aerocaine** (Aeroceuticals)	**Aerosol**: 13.6% benzocaine with 0.5% benzethonium Cl	In 15 and 75 ml.
otc	**Aerotherm** (Aeroceuticals)		In 150 ml.
otc	**Anbesol** (Whitehall)	**Liquid**: 6.3% benzocaine with 0.5% phenol, povidone-iodine, 70% alcohol, camphor, menthol	In 9.3 & 22.2 ml.
		Gel: 6.3% benzocaine, 0.5% phenol, 70% alcohol	In 7.5 g.
Rx	**EMLA** (Astra)	**Cream**: 2.5% lidocaine, 2.5% prilocaine	In 5 g with *Tegaderm* dressings and 30 g.
otc	**Vagisil** (Combe)	**Cream**: Benzocaine and resorcin with lanolin alcohol, parabens, trisodium HEDTA, mineral oil and sodium sulfite	In 30 and 60 g.
otc	**Chiggerex** (Scherer)	**Ointment**: Benzocaine with camphor, menthol	In 50 g.
otc	**Dermacoat** (Century)	**Aerosol**: Benzocaine with p-chloro-m-xylenol, menthol, 20% isopropyl alcohol	In 210 g.
otc	**Skeeter Stik** (Triton)	**Liquid**: 4% lidocaine with 2% phenol in an isopropyl alcohol base	In 14 ml.
otc	**Bactine Antiseptic Anesthetic** (Miles)	2.5% lidocaine HCl, 0.13% benzalkonium chloride, EDTA, 3.17% alcohol	**Aerosol**: In 90 g. **Liquid**: In pt. **Spray**: In 60, 120 and 480 ml.
otc	**Unguentine Plus** (Mentholatum)	**Cream**: 2% lidocaine HCl with 2% chloroxylenol and 0.5% phenol, parabens, mineral oil	In 30 g.
otc	**Medi-Quik** (Mentholatum)	**Aerosol**: Lidocaine HCl and benzalkonium chloride	In 90 ml.
		Spray: 2% lidocaine, 0.13% benzalkonium chloride, 0.2% camphor, benzyl alcohol	In 85 ml.
otc	**Dr. Scholl's Cracked Heel Relief** (Schering-Plough)	**Cream**: 2% lidocaine, 0.13% benzethonium Cl	Aloe. In 89 ml.
otc	**ProTech First-Aid Stik** (Triton)	**Liquid**: 2.5% lidocaine HCl, 10% povidone iodine	In 14 ml dab-on applicator.

DEXPANTHENOL

Indications:

Relieves itching and aids healing of skin in mild eczemas and dermatoses; itching skin, minor wounds, stings, bites, poison ivy, poison oak (dry stage) and minor skin irritations. Also used in infants and children for diaper rash, chafing and mild skin irritations.

Administration and Dosage:

For external use only. Avoid contact with the eyes.

Apply to affected areas once or twice daily.

otc	**Panthoderm** (Jones Med)	**Cream:** 2% in a water miscible base	In 30 and 60 g.

UREA (Carbamide)

Indications:

Promote hydration, remove excess keratin in dry skin and hyperkeratotic conditions.

40% urea: Treatment of nail destruction and dissolution. It removes dystrophic and potentially disabling nails without local anesthesia and surgery.

Administration and Dosage:

For external use only. Avoid contact with the eyes.

Apply 2 to 4 times daily to affected area or as directed. Rub in completely.

40% urea: Cover surrounding surfaces. Generously apply directly to the diseased nail surface and cover with plastic film, wrap and anchor with adhesive tape. Cover with a "finger" cut from plastic or vinyl glove and anchor with more tape. Keep completely dry. Remove treated nails in either 3, 7 or 14 days. Nail bed usually hardens in 12 to 36 hours when left open to the air.

otc	**Aquacare** (Menley & James)	**Cream:** 10%	Petrolatum, glycerin, lanolin oil, mineral oil, lanolin alcohol, benzyl alcohol. In 75 g.
otc	**Nutraplus** (Owen/Galderma)		Mineral oil, parabens. In lb.
otc	**Carmol 20** (Doak)	**Cream:** 20%	Nonlipid vanishing cream base. In 90 g and lb.
otc	**Gormel Creme** (Gordon)		Mineral oil, parabens. In 75, 120 g, lb.
otc	**Lanaphilic** (Medco)		Petrolatum, lanolin oil, PPG, lactic acid, parabens. In lb.
otc	**Ureacin-20** (Pedinol)		Lactic acid, glycerin, mineral oil, parabens, EDTA. In 75 g.
Rx	**Gordon's Urea 40%** (Gordon)	**Cream:** 40%	Petrolatum base. In 30 g.
otc	**Aquacare** (Menley & James)	**Lotion:** 10%	Mineral oil, petrolatum, parabens. In 240 ml.
otc	**Nutraplus** (Owen/Galderma)		Lanolin alcohol, petrolatum, parabens. In 240, 480 ml.
otc	**Carmol 10** (Doak)		In 180 ml.
otc	**Ureacin-10** (Pedinol)		EDTA, parabens, lactic acid. In 240 ml.
otc	**Ultra Mide 25** (Baker Cummins)	**Lotion:** 25%	Mineral oil, glycerin, lanolin, EDTA. In 240 ml.

VITAMINS A, D and E, TOPICAL

Indications:

For temporary relief of discomfort due to minor burns, sunburn, windburn, abrasions, chapped or chafed skin and other minor non-infected skin irritations including diaper rash and irritations associated with ileostomy and colostomy skin drainage.

Warnings:

For external use only. Avoid contact with the eyes.

Worsened condition: If the condition for which these preparations is used worsens or does not improve within 7 days, consult a physician.

Administration and Dosage:

Apply locally to affected skin with gentle massage.

VITAMINS A, D and E, TOPICAL

otc	**Vitamin A & D** (Various, eg, Goldline, Rugby)	**Ointment**	In 60 g and lb.
otc	**A and D** (Schering-Plough)	**Ointment:** Fish liver oil, cholecalciferol, lanolin, petrolatum, mineral oil	In 45, 120, 480 g, 75 g pump dispenser.
otc	**Caldesene** (Fisons)	**Ointment:** Cod liver oil (vitamins A and D), 15% zinc oxide, lanolin oil, 54% petrolatum, parabens, talc	In 37.5 g.
otc	**Comfortine** (Dermik)	**Ointment:** Vitamins A and D, lanolin, zinc oxide, chloroxylenol, iron oxides, lanolin alcohol, mineral oil, triethanolamine, vegetable oil	In 45 and 120 g.
otc	**Desitin** (Pfizer)	**Ointment:** Cod liver oil (vit A & D), 40% zinc oxide, talc, petrolatum-lanolin base	In 30, 60, 120, 240 and 270 g.
otc	**Lobana Peri-Garde** (Ulmer)	**Ointment:** Vitamins A, D and E and chloroxylenol in an emollient base	In 240 g.
otc	**Clocream** (Roberts)	**Cream:** Cod liver oil (vitamins A and D), cholecalciferol, vitamin A palmitate, cottonseed oil, glycerin, parabens, mineral oil	In a vanishing base. In 30 g.
otc	**Lazer Creme** (Pedinol)	**Cream:** Vitamins A (3333.3 units/g) and E (116.67 units/g)	In 60 g.
otc	**Lobana Derm-Ade** (Ulmer)	**Cream:** Vitamins A, D and E, moisturizers, emollients, silicone	In a vanishing base. In 270 g.
otc	**Retinol** (Nature's Bounty)	**Cream:** 100,000 IU vitamin A, glycol stearate, mineral oil, propylene glycol, lanolin oil, propylene glycol stearate SE, lanolin alcohol, retinol, parabens, EDTA	In 60 g.
otc	**Retinol-A** (Young Again Products)	**Cream:** 300,000 IU vitamin A palmitate per 30 g.	In 60 g.
otc	**Aloe Grande** (Gordon)	**Lotion:** Vitamins A (3333.3 units/g) and E (50 units/g), petrolatum, mineral oil, sodium lauryl sulfate, oleic acid, parabens, triethanolamine, aloe	In 240 ml.

VITAMIN E

Indications:

Temporary relief of minor skin disorders such as diaper rash, burns, sunburn and chapped or dry skin.

Administration and Dosage:

For external use only. Avoid contact with the eyes.

Apply a thin layer over affected area.

otc	**Vitamin E** (Various, eg, Nature's Bounty)	**Cream**	In 60 g.
otc	**Vitec** (Pharmaceutical Specialities)	**Cream:** dl-alpha tocopheryl acetate in a vanishing cream base, cetearyl alcohol, sorbitol, propylene glycol, simethicone, glyceryl monostearate, PEG monostearate	In 120 g.
otc	**Vite E Creme** (Gordon)	**Cream:** 50 mg dl-alpha tocopheryl acetate per g	In lb.
otc	**Vitamin E** (Various, eg, Nature's Bounty)	**Lotion**	In 120 ml.
otc	**Vitamin E** (Various, eg, Mission, Nature's Bounty)	**Oil**	In 30 and 60 ml.[1]

[1] May or may not contain aloe.

EMOLLIENTS

These preparations lubricate and moisturize the skin, counteracting dryness and itching.

otc	**Balmex** (Macsil)	**Ointment:** Bismuth subnitrate, zinc oxide, Balsam Peru, benzoic acid, beeswax, mineral oil, silicone, synthetic white wax	In 30, 60, 120 and 480 g.
otc	**Allercreme Ultra Emollient** (Carme[1])	**Cream:** Mineral oil, petrolatum, lanolin, lanolin alcohol, lanolin oil, glycerin, glyceryl stearate, PEG-100 stearate, squalane, parabens	Unscented. In 60 g.
otc	**Aveeno Moisturizing** (Rydelle)	**Cream:** 1% colloidal oatmeal, glycerin, petrolatum, dimethicone, phenylcarbinol	In 120 g.
otc	**Catrix Correction** (Donell DerMedex)	Cream: Dipentaerythrityl, hexacaprylate/hexacaprate, sesame oil, *Catrix* (bovine derived complex mucopolysaccharide), ceteareth-20, glycerin, caprylic/capric triglyceride, glycereth-7, dimethicone, xanthan gum, tocopheryl linoleate, alanine, glycine, urea, EDTA, imidazolidinyl urea, parabens, phenoxyethanol, orange oil, cardamon oil, titanium dioxide	In 36.9 g.
otc	**Complex 15 Face** (Schering-Plough)	**Cream:** Caprylic/capric triglyceride, squalane, glycerin, glyceryl stearate, lecithin, PEG-50 stearate, propylene glycol, dimethicone, diazolidinyl urea, carbomer-934P, EDTA	In 75 g.
otc	**Complex 15 Hand & Body** (Schering-Plough)	**Cream:** Mineral oil, glycerin, squalane, caprylic/capric triglyceride, glycol stearate, PEG-50, carboxylic acid sterol ester, glyceryl stearate, lecithin, dimethicone, diazolidinyl urea, carbomer-934, EDTA	In 120 g.
otc	**Curel Moisturizing** (Bausch & Lomb)	**Cream:** Glycerin, petrolatum, dimethicone, parabens	In 90 g.
otc	**Cutemol** (Summers)	**Cream:** Allantoin, mineral oil, acetylated lanolin, lanolin alcohols extract, mineral wax, beeswax, sorbitan sesquioleate, parabens	In 60 and 240 g.
otc	**DML Forte** (Person & Covey)	**Cream:** Petrolatum, PPG-2 myristyl ether propionate, glyceryl stearate, glycerin, simethicone, benzyl alcohol, silica, EDTA, sodium carbomer 1342	In 113 g.
otc	**Hydrisinol** (Pedinol)	**Cream:** Sulfonated hydrogenated castor oil, hydrogenated vegetable oil	In 120 g and lb.
otc	**Keri Creme** (Westwood)	**Cream:** Mineral oil, lanolin alcohol, talc, sorbitol, ceresin, propylene glycol, magnesium stearate, glyceryl oleate, parabens	In 75 g.
otc	**Lanolor** (Squibb)	**Cream:** Lanolin oil, glyceryl stearates, propylene glycol, sodium lauryl sulfate, simethicone, polyoxyl 40 stearate, cetyl esters wax, methylparaben	In 60 and 240 g.
otc	**Lubriderm** (Warner-Lambert)	**Cream:** Mineral oil, petrolatum, lanolin, lanolin alcohol, lanolin oil, glycerin, glyceryl stearate, PEG-100 stearate, sorbitan laurate, parabens	Scented and unscented. In 81 g.
otc	**Massé Breast** (Advanced Care)	**Cream:** Glyceryl stearate, glycerin, peanut oil, sorbitan stearate, sodium benzoate, parabens. For care of the nipples of pregnant and nursing women	In 60 g.

EMOLLIENTS

otc	**Nephro-Derm** (R&D Labs)	**Cream:** Camphor, menthol, *Eucerin*, glyceryl stearate, petrolatum, paraffin wax, mineral oil, vitamin B_{12}, polysorbate, parabens	In 113.6 g.
otc	**Neutrogena Norwegian Formula Hand** (Neutrogena)	**Cream:** Glycerin, sodium cetearyl sulfate, sodium sulfate, parabens	Scented and unscented. In 56.7 g.
Rx	**Lactinol-E Creme** (Pedinol)	**Cream:** 10% lactic acid, 3500 IU/30 g vitamin E	In 56.7
otc	**Lady Esther** (Menley & James)	Cream: Mineral oil	In 120 g
otc	**Nivea Ultra Moisturizing Creme** (Beiersdorf)	**Cream:** Mineral oil, petrolatum, glycerin, isohexadecane, microcrystalline wax, citric acid, paraffin, lanolin alcohol, magnesium sulfate, decyl oleate, octyldodecanol	In 60 and 120 g.
otc	**Nutraderm** (Owen/Galderma)	**Cream:** Mineral oil, sorbitan stearate, stearyl alcohol, sorbitol, citric acid, cetyl esters wax, sodium lauryl sulfate, dimethicone, parabens, diazolidinyl urea	In 90, 240 and 480 g.
otc	**Penecare** (Reed & Carnrick)	**Cream:** Lactic acid, mineral oil, imidurea	In 120 g.
otc	**Pedi-Vit-A Creme** (Pedinol)	**Cream:** 100,000 units vitamin A/30 g	In 60 g.
otc	**Pen•Kera** (B.F. Ascher)	**Cream:** Glycerin, mineral oil, sorbitan stearate, urea, wheat germ glycerides, carbomer 940, triethanolamine, DMDM hydantoin, diazolidinyl urea	Dye and fragrance free. In 237 ml.
otc	**Phicon** (T.E. Williams)	**Cream:** 250 IU vitamin A and 66.7 IU E per g, aloe vera, 5% pramoxine HCl	In 60 g.
otc	**Polysorb Hydrate** (Fougera)	**Cream:** Sorbitan sesquioleate in a wax and petrolatum base	In 56.7 g and lb.
otc	**Purpose Dry Skin** (J&J-Merck)	**Cream:** Mineral oil, white petrolatum, sweet almond oil, propylene glycol, glyceryl stearate, xanthan gum, steareth-2, steareth-20, sodium lactate, cetyl esters wax, lactic acid	In 85 g.
otc	**Shepard's Skin** (Dermik)	**Cream:** Glycerin, glyceryl stearate, ethoxydiglycol, propylene glycol, urea, lecithin, parabens	Unscented. In 113.4 g.
otc	**Xeroderm Lotion** (Dermol Pharm)	**Lotion:** Mineral oil, acetylate lanolin alcohol, cetyl alcohol, parabens, imidazolidinyl urea.	In 267 ml.
otc	**Soft Sense** (Bausch & Lomb)	Lotion: Petrolatum, vitamin E, parabens	Aloe (Hand lotion). Non-greasy. In 444 ml.
otc	**Allercreme Skin** (Carme[1])	**Lotion:** Mineral oil, sorbitol, triethanolamine, parabens	In 240 ml.
otc	**Penecare** (Reed & Carnrick)	**Lotion:** Lactic acid, imidurea	In 240 ml.
otc	**Aquanil** (Person & Covey)	**Lotion:** Glycerin, benzyl alcohol, sodium laureth sulfate, stearyl alcohol, xanthan gum	In 240 and 480 ml.
otc	**Aveeno** (Rydelle)	**Lotion:** 1% colloidal oatmeal, glycerin, phenylcarbinol, petrolatum, dimethicone, benzyl alcohol	In 240 ml.
otc	**Balmex Emollient** (Macsil)	**Lotion:** Lanolin oil, silicone, Balsam Peru, glycerol monostearate	In 180 ml.

EMOLLIENTS

otc	**Complex 15 Hand & Body** (Schering-Plough)	**Lotion:** Caprylic/capric triglyceride, PEG-50 stearate, squalane, carboxylic acid sterol ester, diazolidinyl urea, glycerin, glyceryl stearate, lecithin, dimethicone, glycol stearate, carbomer-934P, EDTA	Unscented. In 30 ml.
otc	**Corn Huskers** (Warner-Lambert)	**Lotion:** 6.7% glycerin, 5.7% SD alcohol 40, algin, guar gum, methylparaben	In 120 and 210 ml.
otc	**Curel Moisturizing** (Bausch & Lomb)	**Lotion:** Glycerin, petrolatum, dimethicone, parabens	Regular and fragrance free. In 180, 300 and 390 ml.
otc	**Derma Viva** (Rugby)	**Lotion:** Mineral oil, glyceryl stearate, laureth-4, lanolin oil, PEG-100 stearate, PEG-40 stearate, PEG-4 dilaurate, trolamine, DSS, parabens	In 237 ml.
otc	**DML** (Person & Covey)	**Lotion:** Petrolatum, glycerin, dimethicone, benzyl alcohol, volatile silicone, glyceryl stearate, palmitic acid, carbomer 941, xanthan gum	Unscented. In 240 and 480 ml.
otc	**Emollia** (Gordon Labs)	**Lotion:** Mineral oil, propylene glycol, white wax, sodium lauryl sulfate, oleic acid, parabens	In 120 and 240 ml and gal.
otc	**Epilyt** (Stiefel)	**Lotion concentrate:** Propylene glycol, glycerin, oleic acid, lactic acid	In 118 ml.
otc	**Esotérica Dry Skin Treatment** (SK-Beecham)	**Lotion:** Propylene glycol, dicaprylate/dicaprate, mineral oil, glyceryl stearate, cetyl esters wax, hydrolyzed animal protein, dimethicone, TEA-carbomer-941, parabens	In 37.5 ml.
otc	**Eucerin Moisturizing** (Beiersdorf)	**Lotion:** Mineral oil, PEG-40 sorbitan peroleate, lanolin acid glycerin ester, sorbitol, propylene glycol, cetyl palmitate, lanolin alcohol	Unscented. In 52.5, 120 and 240 ml, pt and gal.
otc	**Hydrisea** (Pedinol)	**Lotion:** 8% Dead Sea salts concentrate, NaCl, MgCl, KCl, CaCl, mineral oil, propylene glycol, sorbitan stearate, glyceryl stearate, PEG-75 lanolin, EDTA, imidazolidinyl urea, tartrazine, parabens	In 120 ml.
otc	**Hydrisinol** (Pedinol)	**Lotion:** Sulfonated castor oil, hydrogenated vegetable oil, propylene glycol stearate SE, mineral oil, lanolin, lanolin alcohol, sesame oil, sunflower oil, aloe, triethanolamine, sorbitan stearate, parabens, hydroxyethyl cellulose	In 240 ml.
otc	**Keri** (Westwood)	**Lotion:** Mineral oil, lanolin oil, propylene glycol, glyceryl stearate, PEG–100 stearate, PEG–40 stearate, PEG-4 dilaurate, laureth–4, carbomer-934, triethanolamine, docusate sodium, parabens	Scented and unscented. In 195, 390 and 600 ml.
otc	**Keri Light** (Westwood)	**Lotion:** Glycerin, stearyl alcohol, ceteareth–20, cetearyl octanoate, stearyl heptanoate, squalane, parabens, carbomer-934	In 195 and 390 ml.
Rx	**Lac-Hydrin** (Westwood-Squibb)	**Lotion:** 12% ammonium lactate (12% lactic acid neutralized with ammonium hydroxide), light mineral oil, cetyl alcohol, parabens	In 150 and 360 ml.

EMOLLIENTS

otc	**Lac-Hydrin Five** (Westwood)	**Lotion:** Lactic acid, glycerin, petrolatum, squalane, steareth-2, PCE-21-stearyl ether, propylene glycol dioctanoate, dimethicone, cetyl palmitate, diazolidinyl urea	Unscented. In 120 and 240 ml.
otc	**LactiCare** (Stiefel)	**Lotion:** Lactic acid, mineral oil, sodium hydroxide, glyceryl stearate, PEG-100 stearate, carbomer-940, DMDM hydantoin	In 222 and 345 ml.
otc	**Lobana Body** (Ulmer)	**Lotion:** Mineral oil, triethanolamine stearate, lanolin, propylene glycol and parabens	In 120 and 240 ml and gal.
otc	**Lubriderm** (Warner-Lambert)	**Lotion:** Mineral oil, petrolatum, sorbitol, lanolin, lanolin alcohol, triethanolamine and parabens	Scented and unscented. In 75, 120, 240, 360, 480 ml.
otc	**Moisturel** (Westwood)	**Lotion:** 3% dimethicone, petrolatum, glycerin, steareth-2, benzyl alcohol, laureth-23, carbomer-934	In 360 and 480 ml.
otc	**Neutrogena Body** (Neutrogena)	**Lotion:** Glyceryl stearate, PEG–100 stearate, imidazolidinyl urea, carbomer-954, parabens, sodium lauryl sulfate, triethanolamine	Scented and unscented. In 240 ml.
otc	**Nivea After Tan** (Beiersdorf)	**Lotion:** SD alcohol 40B, mineral oil, PEG-40 castor oil, glyceryl stearate, parabens, aloe extract, lanolin alcohol, imidazolidinyl urea, phenoxyethanol, triethanolamine, chamomile extract, carbomer, simethicone	In 120 ml.
otc	**Nivea Moisturizing** (Beiersdorf)	**Lotion:** Mineral oil, glycerin, lanolin alcohol, glyceryl stearate, simethicone	In 120, 240 and 360 ml.
otc	**Nivea Moisturizing Extra Enriched** (Beiersdorf)	**Lotion:** Mineral oil, PEG-40 sorbitan peroleate, glycerin, polyglyceryl-3 diisostearate, petrolatum, glyceryl lanolate, lanolin alcohol, phenoxyethanol	In 120, 240 and 360 ml.
otc	**Nutraderm** (Owen/Galderma)	**Lotion:** Mineral oil, sorbitan stearate, stearyl alcohol, sodium lauryl sulfate, carbomer 940, diazolidinyl urea, parabens, triethanolamine	In 240 and 480 ml.
otc	**Pro-Cute** (Ferndale)	**Lotion:** Glycerin, silicone, triethanolamine, P.V.P., menthol	In 240 ml.
otc	**Shepard's Cream** (Dermik)	**Lotion:** Glycerin, sesame oil, vegetable oil, SD alcohol 40-B, propylene glycol, ethoxydiglycol, triethanolamine, glyceryl stearate, simethicone, monoglyceride citrate, parabens	Unscented. In 240 and 480 ml.
otc	**Sofenol 5** (C & M Pharm.)	**Lotion:** Glycerin, petrolatum, allantoin, dimethicone, soluble collagen, PEG-40-stearate, carbomer 940, kaolin	Unscented. In 240 ml.
otc	**Therapeutic Bath** (Goldline)	**Lotion:** Mineral oil, glyceryl stearate, PEG-100 stearate, propylene glycol, PEG-40 stearate, laureth-4, PEG-4 dilaurate, lanolin oil, parabens, carbomer 934, trolamine, DSS	In 236 ml.
otc	**Ultra Derm** (Baker Cummins)	**Lotion:** Mineral oil, petrolatum, lanolin oil, glycerin, propylene glycol, glyceryl stearate, PEG–50 stearate, propylene glycol stearate SE, sorbitan laurate, potassium sorbate, phosphoric acid, EDTA	In 240 ml.

EMOLLIENTS

otc	**Wibi** (Owen/Galderma)	**Lotion:** Glycerin, SD alcohol 40, PEG–4, PEG–6–32 stearate, PEG–6–32, carbomer–940, PEG–75, parabens, triethanolamine, menthol	In 240 and 480 ml.
otc	**Wondra** (Richardson-Vicks)	**Lotion:** Petrolatum, lanolin acid, glycerin, EDTA, hydrogenated vegetable glycerides phosphate, carbomer, dimethicone, imidazolidinyl urea, EDTA, titanium dioxide, parabens	Scented and unscented. In 300 ml.
otc	**Xeroderm** (Dermol Pharm.)	**Lotion:** Mineral oil, acetylate lanolin alcohol, cetyl alcohol, glycerin, triethanolamine, parabens, imidazolidinyl urea	In 267 ml.
otc	**Collastin Oil Free Moisturizer** (Dermol)	**Lotion:** Solluble collagen, hydrolyzed elastin	In 60 ml.
otc	**Eucerin Plus** (Beiersdorf)	**Lotion:** Mineral oil, hydrogenated castor oil, 5% sodium lactate, 5% urea, glycerin, lanolin alcohol	In 177 ml.
Rx	**Lactinol** (Pedinol)	**Lotion:** 10% lactic acid.	In 237 ml.
otc	**Hawaiian Tropic Cool Aloe With I.C.E.** (Tanning Research)	**Gel:** Lidocaine, menthol,	Aloe, SD alcohol 40, diazolidinyl urea, EDTA, vitamins A and E, tartrazine. In 360 g.
otc	**Neutrogena Body** (Neutrogena)	**Oil:** Sesame oil, PEG-40 sorbitan peroleate	In 240 ml.
otc	**Nivea Moisturizing** (Beiersdorf)	**Oil:** Mineral oil, PEG-40 sorbitan peroleate, lanolin acid glycerin ester, sorbitol, propylene glycol, lanolin alcohol	In 120 ml.
otc	**Nivea Skin** (Beiersdorf)	**Oil:** Mineral oil, lanolin, petrolatum, glyceryl lanolate, lanolin alcohol	In 240 ml.
otc	**Sardoettes** (Schering-Plough)	**Towelettes:** Mineral oil, tocopherol, beta-carotene.	In 25s.

[1] Carme, Inc., 84 Galli, Novato, CA, 94949, (800) 447-6758.

SKIN PROTECTANTS

Indications:

To protect skin against contact irritants.

Contraindications:

Do not use silicone on wet, exudative lesions or inflamed or abraded skin.

otc	**Hydropel** (C&M Pharm.)	**Ointment**: 30% silicone, 10% hydrophobic starch derivative, petrolatum	In 60 g and lb.
otc	**Silicone No. 2** (C&M Pharm)	**Ointment**: 10% silicone in petrolatum, hydrophobic starch derivative, methylparaben	In 30 and 480 g.
otc	**White Cloverine** Salve (Medtech)	**Ointment**: 97% white petrolatum, rectified turpentine oil, white wax	In 30 g.
otc	**Kerodex** (Whitehall)	**Cream**: #51-Bentonite, calcium carbonate, cellulose gum, chloroxylenol, glycerin, iron oxides, isopropyl alcohol, kaolin, parabens, petrolatum, sodium lauryl sulfate, spermaceti. Nongreasy invisible barrier for dry or oily work	In 113 g.
		Cream: #71-Calcium carbonate, cetrimonium bromide, iron oxide, isopropyl alcohol, kaolin, parabens, mineral oil, paraffin, petrolatum, sodium hexametaphosphate, sodium lauryl sulfate, zinc oxide. Nongreasy invisible water repellent barrier for wet work	In 113 g.
otc	**BlisterGard** (Medtech)	**Liquid**: 6.7% alcohol, pyroxylin solution, oil of cloves, 8-hydroxyquinoline	In 30 ml.
otc	**New-Skin** (Medtech)		In 10 and 30 ml bottle and 3.5 ml tube.
otc	**Skin Shield** (Del)	**Liquid**: 0.75% dyclonine HCl, 0.2% benzethonium chloride, acetone, castor oil, 10% SD alcohol 40. Waterproof.	In 13.3 ml.
otc	**New-Skin Antiseptic** (Medtech)	**Spray Liquid**: Pyroxylin solution, acetone ACS, oil of cloves, 8-hydroxyquinoline, 4.2% alcohol	In 28.5 g.
otc	**Aerozoin** (Graham Field)	**Spray**: 30% tincture of benzoin compound, 44.8% isopropyl alcohol	In 105 ml.
otc	**Benzoin** (Various, eg, Humco, Lannett)	**Tincture**	In 60 and 120 ml, pt and gal.
otc	**Benzoin Compound** (Various, eg, Century, Humco, Lannett, Paddock, Purepac)	**Tincture**: Benzoin, aloe, storax, tolu balsam, 74% to 80% alcohol	In 30, 60 and 120 ml, pt and gal.
otc	**TinBen** (Ferndale)	**Tincture**: Benzoin, 75% to 83% alcohol	In 120 ml.
otc	**TinCoBen** (Ferndale)	**Tincture**: Benzoin, aloe, tolu balsam, storax, 77% alcohol	In 120 ml.

OINTMENT AND LOTION BASES

Uses: These products are used as bases for incorporation of various active ingredients in extemporaneously compounded dermatological prescriptions.

otc	**Lanaphilic** (Medco Labs)	**Ointment:** Stearyl alcohol, white petrolatum, isopropyl palmitate, lanolin oil, propylene glycol, sorbitol, sodium lauryl sulfate, parabens	In lb.
otc	**Lanaphilic w/Urea 10%** (Medco Labs)	**Ointment:** Urea, stearyl alcohol, white petrolatum, isopropyl palmitate, lanolin oil, sorbitol, propylene glycol, sodium lauryl sulfate, lactic acid, parabens	In lb.
otc	**Petrolatum** (Carolina Medical)	**Ointment:** Petrolatum, mineral oil, ceresin wax, woolwax alcohol	In 430 g.
otc	**Absorbase** (Carolina Medical)	**Ointment:** Petrolatum, mineral oil, ceresin wax, woolwax alcohol, potassium sorbate	Unscented. In 114 and 454 g.
otc	**Hydrophilic** (Rugby)	**Ointment:** White petrolatum, stearyl alcohol, propylene glycol, sodium lauryl sulfate, parabens	In 454 g.
otc	**Aquabase** (Paddock)	**Ointment:** Petrolatum, mineral oil, mineral wax, woolwax alcohol, sorbitan sesquioleate	Unscented. Dye free. In 454 g.
otc	**Aquaphilic** (Medco Labs)	**Ointment:** Stearyl alcohol, white petrolatum, isopropyl palmitate, sorbitol, propylene glycol, sodium lauryl sulfate, parabens	In lb.
otc	**Aquaphilic w/Carbamide 10% and 20%** (Medco Labs)	**Ointment:** Urea, stearyl alcohol, white petrolatum, isopropyl palmitate, propylene glycol, sorbitol, sodium lauryl sulfate, lactic acid, parabens	In lb.
otc	**Aquaphor Natural Healing** (Beiersdorf)	**Ointment:** Petrolatum, mineral oil, mineral wax, woolwax alcohol, panthenol, glycerin, chamomile essence	In 52.5 g.
otc	**Polyethylene Glycol** (Medco)	**Ointment:** Water soluble greaseless base with PEG-8 and PEG-75	In lb.
otc	**Solumol** (C&M Pharm.)	**Ointment:** Petrolatum, mineral oil, cetearyl alcohol, sodium lauryl sulfate, glycerin, propylene glycol	In lb.
otc	**Unibase** (Warner Chilcott)	**Ointment:** Nongreasy, water removable base with white petrolatum, glycerin, sodium lauryl sulfate, propylparaben. Will absorb 30% of its weight in water	In lb.
otc	**Acid Mantle** (Doak)	**Cream:** Water, cetearyl alcohol, sodium lauryl sulfate, sodium cetearyl sulfate, petrolatum, glycerin, synthetic beeswax, mineral oil, methylparaben, aluminum sulfate, calcium acetate, white potato dextrin.	In 120 g.
otc	**Velvachol** (Owen/Galderma)	**Cream:** Water miscible vehicle containing petrolatum, mineral oil, stearyl alcohol, sodium lauryl sulfate, cholesterol, parabens	In lb.
otc	**Dermabase** (Paddock)	**Cream:** Mineral oil, petrolatum, cetostearyl alcohol, propylene glycol, sodium lauryl sulfate, isopropyl palmitate, imidazolidinyl urea, parabens	In 454 g.
otc	**Dermovan** (Owen/Galderma)	**Cream:** Nonionic, water miscible vanishing cream vehicle containing glyceryl stearate, stearamidoethyl diethylamine, glycerin, mineral oil, cetyl esters, parabens	In lb.

OINTMENT AND LOTION BASES

otc	**Heb Cream Base** (Sola Barnes/Hind)	**Cream:** Self-emulsifying base containing mineral oil, white petrolatum, stearyl alcohol, sodium lauryl sulfate, parabens	In 454 g.
otc	**Hydrocream Base** (Paddock)	**Cream:** Petrolatum, mineral oil, mineral wax, woolwax alcohol, cholesterol, imidazolidinyl urea, parabens	In 454 g.
otc	**Eucerin** (Beiersdorf)	**Cream:** Petrolatum, mineral oil, mineral wax, woolwax alcohol	In 60, 120, 240 and 480 g.
otc	**Vanicream** (Pharmaceutical Specialties)	**Cream:** White petrolatum, cetearyl alcohol, ceteareth-20, sorbitol solution, propylene glycol, simethicone, glyceryl monostearate, polyethylene glycol monostearate	In 120 g and lb.
otc	**Nutraderm** (Owen/Galderma)	**Lotion:** Mineral oil, sorbitan stearate, stearyl alcohol, sodium lauryl sulfate, cetyl alcohol, carbomer-940, parabens, triethanolamine	In 240 and 480 ml.
otc	**E-Solve** (Syosset)	**Lotion:** 85% absolute alcohol, propylene glycol, lauramide-DEA, hydroxypropyl cellulose, titanium dioxide, polysorbate 20, polyvinylpyrrolidone, polysorbate 80, talc, iron oxides	In 50 ml.
otc	**C-Solve** (Syosset)	**Lotion:** SD alcohol 40B, glycerin, polysorbate 20 and 80, hydroxyethyl cellulose, polyvinylpyrrolidone, hydrolyzed animal protein, collagen, imidazolidinyl urea	In 50 ml with applicator.
otc	**Vehicle/N** (Neutrogena)	**Solution:** 45% SD alcohol 40, laureth-4, propylene glycol, 4% isopropyl alcohol	In 50 ml with applicator.
otc	**Vehicle/N Mild** (Neutrogena)	**Solution:** 37.5% SD alcohol 40, laureth-4, 5% isopropyl alcohol	In 50 ml with applicator.
otc	**Solvent-G** (Syosset)	**Liquid:** 55% SD alcohol 40B, laureth-4, isopropyl alcohol, propylene glycol	In 50 ml.

EMOLLIENT PREPARATIONS

Indications:

These products contain colloidal solids and various oils which act as emollients. They are recommended for relief of minor skin irritations and pruritus associated with common dermatoses and dry skin conditions.

Precautions:

For external use only. Avoid contact with the eyes; if this occurs, flush with clear water.
Use caution when using bath oils to avoid slipping in tub.
Do not use on acutely inflamed areas.

otc	**Aveeno Regular Bath** (Rydelle)	100% natural colloidal oatmeal	In 30 g packets (8).
otc	**Aveeno Oilated Bath** (Rydelle)	43% colloidal oatmeal, mineral oil	In 30 g packets (8).
otc	**ActiBath Effervescent Tablets** (Jergens)	20% colloidal oatmeal	In 4s.
otc	**Aveeno Shave Gel** (Rydelle)	Oatmeal flour	In 210 g.
otc	**Nutra•Soothe** (Pertussin)	Colloidal oatmeal, light mineral oil	In individual oil (9) & oatmeal powder packets (9).
otc	**Pedi-Bath Salts** (Pedinol)	Colloidal sulfur, potassium iodide, Balsam Peru, sodium hyposulfate, sodium bicarbonate, pine needle oil	In 170 g.
otc	**Nutraderm Bath Oil** (Owen/Galderma)	Mineral oil, lanolin oil, PEG-4 dilaurate, benzophenone-3, butylparaben	In 240 ml.
otc	**Sardo Bath & Shower** (Schering-Plough)	**Oil**: Mineral oil, tocopherol	In 112.5 ml.
otc	**Ultra Derm Bath Oil** (Baker Cummins)	Mineral oil, lanolin oil, octoxynol–3	In 240 ml.
otc	**Alpha Keri Therapeutic Bath Oil** (Westwood)	Mineral oil, lanolin oil, PEG-4 dilaurate, benzophenone-3	In 120 and 240 ml and pt.
otc	**Therapeutic Bath Oil** (Goldline)		In 473 ml.
otc	**LubraSol Bath Oil** (Pharmaceutical Specialties)	Mineral oil, lanolin oil, PEG-200 dilaurate, oxybenzone	In 240 ml.
otc	**Domol Bath & Shower Oil** (Miles)	Di-isopropyl sebacate, mineral oil	In 240 ml.
otc	**Alpha Keri Spray** (Westwood)	Mineral oil, lanolin oil, 28% SD alcohol 40, PPG-15 stearyl ether, C12-15 alcohols benzoate, PEG-4 dilaurate, polysorbate 85	In 150 g.
otc	**Lubriderm Bath Oil** (Warner-L)	Mineral oil, PPG-15, stearyl ether oleth-2, nonoxynol-5	In 480 ml.
otc	**Surfol Post-Immersion Bath Oil** (Stiefel)	Mineral oil, isostearic acid, PEG-40 sorbitan peroleate, drometrizole	In 237 ml.
otc	**Cameo Oil** (Medco)	Mineral oil, PEG-8 dioleate, lanolin oil	Unscented. In 240, 480 and 960 ml.
otc	**RoBathol Bath Oil** (Pharmaceutical Specialties)	Cottonseed oil and alkyl aryl polyether alcohol	Lanolin free. Dye free. In 240 ml, pt and gal.

EMOLLIENT PREPARATIONS

otc	**Esoterica Soap** (Medicis)	Sodium tallowate, sodium cocoate, mineral oil, acacia, sodium cocoyl isethionate, lauramide DEA, potassium oleate, titanium dioxide, pentasodium pentetate, tetra sodium etidronate	In 85 g.
otc	**Dermasil** (Chesebrough -Ponds)	**Lotion**: Glycerin, dimethicone, sunflower seed oil, petrolatum, borage seed oil, vitamin E acetate, vitamin A palmitate, vitamin D_3, corn oil, EDTA, methylparaben.	In 120 and 240 ml.
otc	**Aveeno Shower & Bath** (Rydelle)	**Oil**: 5% colloidal oatmeal, mineral oil, glyceryl stearate, PEG 100 stearate, laureth-4, benzyl alcohol, silica benzaldehyde	In 240 ml.

TAR-CONTAINING PRODUCTS

Indications:

These products contain tar derivatives which have keratoplastic, antieczematous, emollient and antipruritic effects. They are used as adjuncts in a wide range of pruritic dermatoses including: Psoriasis, seborrheic dermatitis, atopic dermatitis and eczematoid dermatitis.

Contraindications:

Open or infected lesions; when acute inflammation is present.

Warnings:

Pregnancy: Category C. It is not known whether coal tar can cause fetal harm when administered to a pregnant woman or can affect reproduction capacity. Use on a pregnant woman only if clearly needed.

Lactation: It is not known whether this drug is excreted in breast milk. Therefore, decide whether to discontinue nursing or discontinue the drug, taking into account the importance of coal tar to the mother.

Precautions:

For external use only. Avoid contact with the eyes.

Use caution to avoid slipping in the bathtub.

Staining of plastic or fiberglass tubs may occur.

Irritation: If irritation persists, discontinue use. In rare cases, coal tar may cause allergic irritation.

Photosensitivity: Coal tar is photosensitizing; for 72 hours after use, avoid exposure to direct sunlight or sunlamps.

Adverse Reactions:

Dermatitis; allergic sensitization; folliculitis; photosensitization (see Precautions).

Administration and Dosage:

Directions: Add to bath water. Soak 10 to 20 minutes and then pat dry.

otc	**Doak Tar Oil** (Doak)	**Liquid:** 2% Doak tar distillate	In 237 ml.
otc	**Balnetar** (Westwood)	**Liquid:** 2.5% coal tar in mineral oil, laureth-4, lanolin oil, PEG-4 dilaurate, docusate sodium	In 225 ml.
otc	**Cutar Bath Oil Emulsion** (Summers)	**Liquid:** 7.5% coal tar in mineral oil, isopropyl myristate, polysorbate 80, sorbitan sesquioleate, lanolin alcohols extract, parabens, xanthan gum, carbomer	In 180 ml and gal.
otc	**Polytar Bath** (Stiefel)	**Liquid:** 25% polytar (juniper tar, pine tar, coal tar solution, vegetable oil and solubilized crude coal tar) in a water miscible base	In 240 ml.
Rx	**Zetar Emulsion** (Dermik)	**Liquid:** 30% whole coal tar in polysorbates	In 177 ml.

TAR-CONTAINING PREPARATIONS, TOPICAL

For other tar-containing preparations, refer to the Antiseborrheic and Bath Dermatologicals sections.

COAL TAR (or derivatives) is used for its antipruritic, anti-eczematous and keratoplastic actions. Used in psoriasis and other chronic skin disorders.

PRECIPITATED SULFUR is a keratolytic, antifungal and antiparasitic agent. See monograph in Acne Products section.

BENZOCAINE is an anesthetic. See Local Anesthetics, Topical.

SALICYLIC ACID is a keratolytic agent. See individual monograph.

ZINC OXIDE is an astringent, antiseptic and protective agent. See individual monograph.

Contraindications:

Do not use on patients sensitive to any component.

Warnings:

Children: Do not use in children < 2 years of age.

Precautions:

For external use only. Avoid contact with the eyes.

Photosensitivity: Avoid exposure to sunlight for up to 24 hours. Do not use on patients who have a disease characterized by photosensitivity (eg, lupus erythematosus, sunlight allergy).

Do not apply to acutely inflamed or broken skin or to the genital or rectal areas. If the condition covers a large area of the body, consult a physician before using.

Discoloration/Staining – Light-colored, bleached or tinted hair may become temporarily discolored. Slight staining of clothes may also occur; standard laundry procedures will remove most stains.

Psoriasis – Do not use with other forms of psoriasis therapy (eg, ultraviolet radiation, drug therapy) unless directed to do so.

otc	**Medotar** (Medco Lab.)	**Ointment**: 1% coal tar, 0.5% polysorbate 80, octoxynol–5, zinc oxide, white petrolatum	In 480 g.
otc	**Taraphilic** (Medco)	**Ointment**: 1% coal tar, 0.5% polysorbate 20, stearyl alcohol, white petrolatum, sorbitol, propylene glycol, sodium lauryl sulfate, parabens	In lb.
otc	**MG217 Medicated** (Triton)	**Ointment**: 2% coal tar solution, 1.1% colloidal sulfur, 1.5% salicylic acid	In 108 and 480 g.
otc	**Fototar** (ICN Pharm)	**Cream**: 2% coal tar in an emollient moisturizing base	In 85 and 454 g.
otc	**Tegrin for Psoriasis** (Reedco)	**Cream**: 5% coal tar solution, acetylated lanolin alcohol, 4.6% alcohol, carbomer 934P, glyceryl tribehenate, mineral oil, potassium hydroxide, lanolin alcohol, petrolatum, titanium dioxide, stearyl alcohol	In 60 and 124 g.
Rx	**Unguentum Bossi** (Doak)	**Cream**: 5% tar distillate "Doak", 5% ammoniated mercury, 2% methenamine sulfosalicylate, 40% Doak oil, petrolatum, sorbitol sesquioleate, cholesterol derivatives, beeswax	In 60 and 480 g.
otc	**Doak Tar** (Doak)	**Lotion**: 5% Doak tar distillate (equiv. to 2% coal tar)	In 118 ml.
otc	**MG217 Dual Treatment** (Triton)	**Lotion**: 5% coal tar solution in a light greaseless moisturizing base with jojoba	In 120 ml.
otc	**Tegrin for Psoriasis** (Reedco)	**Lotion**: 5% coal tar solution, 4.6% alcohol, carbomer-940, parabens, PEG-40 stearate, polysorbate-60, propylene glycol, squalane, propylene glycol dipelargonate, titanium dioxide, triethanolamine	In 177 ml.
otc	**Doak Tar Distillate** (Doak)	**Liquid**: 40% coal tar distillate	In 59 ml.

TAR-CONTAINING PREPARATIONS, TOPICAL

otc	**Oxipor VHC** (Whitehall)	**Lotion**: 25% coal tar solution, 79% alcohol	In 56 ml.
otc	**Coal Tar or Carbonis Detergens** (Various, eg, Lannett)	**Solution**: 20% coal tar	In 120 ml, pt and gal.
otc	**AquaTar** (Allergan Herbert)	**Gel**: 2.5% coal tar extract, glycerin, imidurea, parabens, mineral oil, poloxamer 407, polysorbate 80	In 90 g.
otc	**Estar** (Westwood)	**Gel**: Coal tar extract equivalent to 5% coal tar, benzyl alcohol, carbomer 940, glycereth-7 coconate, laureth-4, polysorbate 80, 15.6% SD alcohol 40, simethicone, sorbitol	In 90 g.
otc	**P & S Plus** (Baker Cummins)	**Gel**: 8% coal tar solution (1.6% crude coal tar, 6.4% ethyl alcohol), 2% salicylic acid	In 105 g.
otc	**PsoriGel** (Owen/Galderma)	**Gel**: 7.5% coal tar solution, 33% alcohol	In 120 g.
otc	**Packer's Pine Tar** (GenDerm)	**Soap**: Soap base. Pine tar, pine oil, iron oxide, PEG-75	In 99 g.
otc	**Polytar** (Stiefel)	**Soap**: 1% polytar (juniper tar, pine tar, coal tar solution, solubilized crude coal tar, octoxynol-9, povidone, sodium borohydride, sodium cocoate, sodium tallowate, trisodium HEDTA)	In 99 g.
otc	**Tegrin Medicated for Psoriasis** (Reedco)	**Soap**: 5% coal tar solution, chromium hydroxide green, glycerin, titanium dioxide	In 127 g.
otc	**Neutrogena T/Derm** (Neutrogena)	**Oil**: 5% solubilized coal tar extract in an oil base	In 120 ml.

ALUMINUM ACETATE SOLUTION (Burow's or Modified Burow's Solution)

Indications:

An astringent wet dressing for relief of inflammatory conditions of the skin, such as insect bites, poison ivy, swelling, allergy, bruises and athlete's foot.

Precautions:

Discontinue use if intolerance, irritation or extension of inflammatory condition being treated occurs. If symptoms persist > 7 days, discontinue use and consult physician.

Do not use plastic or other impervious material to prevent evaporation.

For external use only. Avoid contact with the eyes.

Drug Interactions:

Collegenase: The enzyme activity of topical collagenase may be inhibited by aluminum acetate solution because of the metal ion and low pH. Cleanse the site of the solution with repeated washings of normal saline before applying the enzyme ointment.

otc	**Buro-Sol** (Doak)	**Powder**: 0.23% aluminum acetate	In 12 packets.
otc	**Burow's Solution** (Various, eg, Paddock)	Aluminum acetate solution	In 480 ml.
otc	**Bluboro Powder** (Allergan Herbert)	Aluminum sulfate and calcium acetate. One packet or tablet in a pint of water produces a modified 1:40 Burow's solution. Apply every 15 to 30 minutes for 4 to 8 hours.	**Powder packets**: 1.8 g. In 12s and 100s.
otc	**Boropak Powder** (Glenwood)		**Powder packets**: 2.4 g. In 12s and 100s.
otc	**Domeboro Powder and Tablets** (Miles)		**Effervescent tablets**: In 12s and 100s.
			Powder packets: In 12s and 100s.
otc	**Pedi-Boro Soak Paks** (Pedinol)		**Powder packets**: 2.7 g. In 12s and 100s.

RUBS AND LINIMENTS

Indications:

These products are used for relief of pain of muscular aches, neuralgia, rheumatism, arthritis, sprains and like conditions, when skin is intact.

Individual components include:

COUNTERIRRITANTS: Cajuput oil, camphor, capsicum preparations (capsicum oleoresin, capsaicin), eucalyptus oil, menthol, methyl nicotinate, methyl salicylate, mustard oil, wormwood oil.

ANTISEPTICS: Chloroxylenol, thymol.

LOCAL ANESTHETIC: Benzocaine (see Local Anesthetics, Topical).

ANALGESICS: Trolamine salicylate.

Contraindications:

Allergy to components of any formulation or to salicylates.

Warnings:

For external use only. Avoid contact with eyes and mucous membranes.

Precautions:

Apply to affected parts only. Do not apply to irritated skin; if excessive irritation develops, discontinue use. If pain persists for more than 7 to 10 days, or if redness is present, or in conditions affecting children < 10 years of age, consult a physician.

Heat therapy: Do not use an external source of heat (eg, heating pad) with these agents since irritation or burning of the skin may occur.

Protective covering: Applying a tight bandage or wrap over these agents is not recommended since increased absorption may occur.

Drug Interactions:

Anticoagulants: An enhanced anticoagulant effect (eg, increased prothrombin time) occurred in several patients receiving an anticoagulant and using topical methylsalicylate concurrently.

Adverse Reactions:

If applied to large skin areas, salicylate side effects may occur, such as tinnitus, nausea or vomiting. Toxic if ingested.

Counterirritants may cause local irritation, especially in patients with sensitive skin.

otc	**Analgesia Creme** (Rugby)		In 85 g.
otc	**Aspercreme Cream** (Thompson)		In 37.5, 90 and 150 g.
otc	**Mobisyl Creme** (Ascher)		In 35.4, 100 and 227 g.
otc	**Myoflex Creme** (Fisons)		In 60, 120 and 240 g and lb.
otc	**Sportscreme** (Thompson)		In 37.5 and 90 g.
otc	**infraRUB Cream** (Whitehall)	35% methyl salicylate, 10% menthol	In 37.5 and 90 g.
otc	**Panalgesic Cream** (E.C. Robins/Poythress)	35% methyl salicylate, 4% menthol	In 120 g.
otc	**Icy Hot Cream** (Chattem)	30% methyl salicylate, 10% menthol, carbomer, cetyl esters wax, emulsifying wax, trolamine	In 37.5 and 90 g.
otc	**ArthriCare Triple-Medicated Gel** (Commerce)	30% methyl salicylate, 1.25% menthol, 0.7% methyl nicotinate, isopropyl alcohol, propylene glycol, hydroxypropylmethylcellulose, DSS	In 90 g.
otc	**Musterole Deep Strength Rub** (Schering-Plough)	30% methyl salicylate, 0.5% methyl nicotinate and 3% menthol	In 37 and 90 g.

RUBS AND LINIMENTS

otc	**Ben-Gay Ultra Strength Cream** (Pfizer)	30% methyl salicylate, 10% menthol, 4% camphor, EDTA, glyceryl stearate SE, anhydrous lanolin, polysorbate 80, potassium carbomer and stearate, triethanolamine carbomer and stearate	In 35 g.
otc	**Ben-Gay Extra Strength Cream** (Pfizer)	30% methyl salicylate, 8% menthol, glyceryl stearate SE, anhydrous lanolin, polysorbate 85, potassium stearate, sorbitan tristearate, xanthan gum	In 35 g.
otc	**Exocaine Plus Rub** (Commerce Drug)	30% methyl salicylate	In 39 and 120 g.
otc	**Icy Hot Stick** (Chattem)	30% methyl salicylate, 10% menthol, ceresin, cyclomethicone, hydrogenated castor oil, microcrystalline wax, paraffin, PEG-150 distearate, propylene glycol	In 52.5 g.
otc	**Icy Hot Balm** (Chattem)	29% methyl salicylate, 7.6% menthol, paraffin, white petrolatum	In 105 g.
otc	**Exocaine Medicated Rub** (Commerce)	25% methyl salicylate	In 39 and 120 g.
otc	**Improved Analgesic Ointment** (Rugby)	18.3% methyl salicylate, 16% menthol	In 36, 85 and 454 g.
otc	**Ben-Gay Original Ointment** (Pfizer)	18.3% methyl salicylate, 16% menthol, anhydrous lanolin, microcrystalline wax, synthetic bees wax	In 35 and 90 g.
otc	**Pain Bust•RII** (Continental)	17% methyl salicylate, 12% menthol	In 90 g.
otc	**Arthritis Hot Creme** (Thompson)	15% methyl salicylate, 10% menthol, glyceryl stearate, carbomer 934, lanolin, PEG-100 stearate, propylene glycol, trolamine, parabens	In 90 g.
otc	**Ben-Gay Regular Strength Cream** (Pfizer)	15% methyl salicylate, 10% menthol, glyceryl stearate SE, anhydrous lanolin, polysorbate 85, sorbitan tristearate, triethanolamine stearate	In 35, 85 and 142 g.
otc	**Muscle Rub Ointment** (Schein)	15% methyl salicylate, 10% menthol, glyceryl stearate, lanolin, parabens, propylene glycol, trolamine	In 85 g.
otc	**Deep-Down Rub** (SK-Beecham)	15% methyl salicylate, 5% menthol, 0.5% camphor, 40.5% SD alcohol	In 37.5 and 90 g.
otc	**Minit-Rub** (Bristol-Myers)	15% methyl salicylate, 3.5% menthol, 2.3% camphor, anhydrous lanolin	In 45 and 90 g.

RUBS AND LINIMENTS

otc	**Thera-gesic Cream** (Mission)	15% methyl salicylate, menthol, dimethylpolysiloxane, glycerin, carbopol, triethanolamine, parabens	In 90 and 150 g.
otc	**Gordogesic Creme** (Gordon)	10% methyl salicylate, propylene glycol, mineral oil, white wax, triethanolamine, parabens	In 75 g and lb.
otc	**Methagual** (Gordon)	8% methyl salicylate, 2% guaiacol, petrolatum, white wax, parabens	In 60 g and lb.
otc	**Blue Gel Muscular Pain Reliever** (Rugby)	Menthol	In 240 g.
otc	**Eucalyptamint Maximum Strength Ointment** (Ciba)	16% menthol, lanolin, eucalyptus oil.	In 60 ml.
otc	**Maximum Strength Flex-all 454** (Chattem)	16% menthol, aloe vera gel, eucalyptus oil, methylsalicylate, peppermint oil, SD alcohol 38-B, thyme oil	In 90 g.
otc	**Eucalyptamint Gel** (Ciba)	8% menthol, eucalyptus oil, SD 3A alcohol	In 60 g.
otc	**Wonder Ice Gel** (Pedinol)	5.25% menthol	In 113 and 473 g.
otc	**Double Ice ArthriCare Gel** (Commerce)	4% menthol, 3.1% camphor, aloe vera gel, carbomer 940, dioctylsodium sulfosuccinate, isopropyl alcohol, propylene glycol, triethanolamine	In 90 g.
otc	**Absorbine Power Gel** (W.F. Young)	4% menthol	In 88 g.
otc	**Pain Gel Plus** (Mentholatum Co.)	4% menthol, aloe, vitamin E	In 57 g.
otc	**Odor Free ArthriCare Rub** (Commerce)	1.25% menthol, 0.25% methyl nicotinate, 0.025% capsaicin, aloe vera gel, carbomer 940, DMDM hydantoin, emulsifying wax, glyceryl stearate SE, isopropyl alcohol, myristyl propionate, propylparaben, triethanolamine	In 90 g.
otc	**Iodex w/Methyl Salicylate** (Medtech)	4.7% iodine with oleic acid and 4.8% oil of wintergreen in a petrolatum base	In 30 and 480 g.
otc	**Soltice Quick-Rub** (Chattem)	Methyl salicylate, camphor, menthol, eucalyptus oil, glycerin, oleic acid	In 40 and 112 g.
otc	**Dermal-Rub Balm** (Hauck)	Methyl salicylate, camphor, racemic menthol, cajuput oil	In 30 g and lb.
otc	**Analgesic Balm** (Various, eg, Goldline, Major, Schein, URL)	Methyl salicylate, menthol	In 30 and 454 g.
otc	**Argesic Cream** (Econo Med)	Methyl salicylate, triethanolamine	Vanishing base. In 60 g.
otc	**Musterole Extra Strength** (Schering-Plough)	5% camphor, 3% menthol, methyl salicylate, lanolin, oil of mustard, petrolatum	In 27, 30 and 67.5 g.

RUBS AND LINIMENTS

otc	**Vicks VapoRub** (Richardson-Vicks)	**Cream**: 4.7% camphor, 2.6% menthol, 1.2% eucalyptus oil, cedarleaf oil, EDTA, glycerin, imidazolidinyl urea, cetyl and stearyl alcohols, parabens, nutmeg oil, titanium dioxide, spirits of turpentine	In 45, 60, 90 and 180 g.
otc	**Methalgen Cream** (Alra)	Camphor, menthol, methyl salicylate, oil of mustard	In 60 and 480 g.
otc	**Therapeutic Mineral Ice Exercise Formula Gel** (Bristol-Myers)	4% menthol, ammonium hydroxide, carbomer 934P or 934, cupric sulfate, isopropyl alcohol, thymol	In 90 g.
otc	**Ben-Gay Vanishing Scent Gel** (Pfizer)	3% menthol, benzophenone-4, camphor, diazolidinyl urea, EDTA, isopropyl alcohol, potassium carbomer 940	In 35 g.
otc	**Sportscreme Ice Gel** (Thompson)	2% menthol, carbomer 934, styrene/acrylate copolymer, triethanolamine, 38% SD alcohol 40	In 227 g.
otc	**Therapeutic Mineral Ice Gel** (Bristol-Myers)	2% menthol, ammonium hydroxide, carbomer 934, cupric sulfate, isopropyl alcohol, thymol	In 105, 240 and 480 g.
otc	**Flex-all 454 Gel** (Chattem)	Menthol in an aloe vera gel, methyl salicylate, alcohol, allantoin, boric acid, carbomer 940, diazolidinyl urea, iodine, polysorbate 60, propylene glycol, potassium iodide, triethanolamine, eucalyptus oil, glycerin, parabens	In 60, 120 and 240 g.
otc	**MenthoRub Ointment** (Schein)	2.6% menthol, 4.73% camphor, eucalyptus oil, rectified oil of turpentine, cedarleaf oil, nutmeg oil, petrolatum, thymol	In 100 g.
otc	**Eucalyptamint** (Ciba)	**Gel**: 8% menthol	
otc	**Extra Strength Absorbine Jr. Liquid** (W.F. Young)	4% menthol	In 59 and 118 ml.
otc	**Sports Spray** (Mentholatum)	35% methyl salicylate, 10% menthol, 5% camphor, 58% alcohol	In 85 g.
otc	**Aspercreme Rub Lotion** (Thompson)	10% trolamine salicylate, cetyl alcohol, glyceryl stearate, lanolin, parabens, potassium phosphate, propylene glycol, sodium lauryl sulfate, stearic acid	In 180 ml.
otc	**Panalgesic Gold Liniment** (ECR Pharm)	55% methyl salicylate, 3.1% camphor, 1.25% menthol, 18.6% emollient oils, 22% alcohol	In 120 ml.

RUBS AND LINIMENTS

otc	**Gordobalm** (Gordon)	Menthol, camphor, methyl salicylate, 16% isopropyl alcohol, tragacanth, thymol, acetone, eucalyptus oil, tartrazine	In 120 ml and gal.
otc	**Heet Liniment** (Whitehall)	15% methyl salicylate, 3.6% camphor, capsicum oleoresin (as 0.025% capsaicin), acetone, 70% alcohol	In 68.5 and 150 ml.
otc	**Banalg Hospital Strength Lotion** (Forest)	14% methyl salicylate, 3% menthol	In 60 ml.
otc	**Banalg Lotion** (Forest)	4.9% methyl salicylate, 2% camphor, 1% menthol	In 60 and 480 ml.
otc	**Extra Strength Absorbine Jr.** (W.F. Young)	4% natural menthol	In 60 ml.
otc	**Absorbine Jr. Liniment** (W.F. Young)	1.27% menthol, plant extracts of calendula, echinacea and wormwood, iodine, potassium iodide, thymol, acetone, chloroxylenol	In 60 and 120 ml.
otc	**Betuline Lotion** (Ferndale)	Methyl salicylate, camphor, menthol, peppermint oil in a water soluble base	In 30, 60 and 480 ml.
otc	**Dermolin Liniment** (Roberts)	Methyl salicylate, camphor, racemic menthol, mustard oil, 8% isopropyl alcohol	In 45 and 120 ml and pt.

SALICYLIC ACID

Actions:

Pharmacology: Salicylic acid is the only *otc* product considered safe and effective by the FDA for use as a keratolytic for corns, calluses and warts. Salicylic acid produces desquamation of the horny layer of skin, while not affecting the structure of the viable epidermis, by dissolving intercellular cement substance. The keratolytic action causes the cornified epithelium to swell, soften, macerate and then desquamate.

Salicylic acid is keratolytic at concentrations of ≈ 2% to 6%. These concentrations are generally used for treatment of dandruff, seborrhea and psoriasis. Concentrations of 5% to 17% in collodion are safe and effective for the removal of common and plantar warts; up to 40% in plasters is used to remove warts, corns and calluses.

Salicylic acid preparations, alone or in combination, have also been used to treat dandruff, seborrheic dermatitis, acne, tinea infections and psoriasis.

Pharmacokinetics: In a study of the percutaneous absorption of salicylic acid in four patients with extensive active psoriasis, peak serum salicylate levels never exceeded 5 mg/dl even though > 60% of the applied salicylic acid was absorbed. Systemic toxic reactions are usually associated with much higher serum levels (30 to 40 mg/dl). Peak serum levels occurred within 5 hours of the topical application under occlusion.

The major urinary metabolites identified after topical administration differ from those after oral salicylate administration; those derived from percutaneous absorption contain more salicylate glucuronides (42%) and less salicyluric (52%) and salicylic acid (6%).

Indications:

A topical aid in the removal of excessive keratin in hyperkeratotic skin disorders, including common and plantar warts, psoriasis, calluses and corns.

Unlabeled uses: The use of a 40% salicylic acid disk covered with an adhesive strip has been used to aid in the removal of inaccessible splinters in children.

Contraindications:

Sensitivity to salicylic acid; prolonged use, especially in infants, diabetics and patients with impaired circulation; use on moles, birthmarks or warts with hair growing from them, genital or facial warts or warts on mucous membranes, irritated skin or any area that is infected or reddened.

Warnings:

Salicylate toxicity: Prolonged use over large areas, especially in young children and those patients with significant renal or hepatic impairment, could result in salicylism. Limit the area to be treated and be aware of signs of salicylate toxicity (eg, nausea, vomiting, dizziness, loss of hearing, tinnitus, lethargy, hyperpnea, diarrhea, psychic disturbances). In the event of salicylic acid toxicity, discontinue use.

Refer to the Salicylates monograph in the CNS Drugs chapter for additional information on the systemic effects of salicylates.

Special risk patients: Do not use if diabetic or poor blood circulation exists.

Pregnancy: Category C. There are no adequate and well controlled studies in pregnant women. Use during pregnancy only if the potential benefit justifies the potential risk to the fetus.

Precautions:

For external use only: Avoid contact with eyes, mucous membranes and normal skin surrounding warts. If contact with eyes or mucous membranes occurs, immediately flush with water for 15 minutes. Avoid inhaling vapors.

Drug Interactions:

Interactions have been reported with both topical and oral salicylates. Refer to the Salicylates monograph for a complete listing.

Adverse Reactions:

Local irritation may occur from contact with normal skin surrounding the affected area. If irritation occurs, temporarily discontinue use and take care to apply only to wart site when treatment is resumed.

Patient Information:

For external use only. Avoid contact with eyes, face, genitals, mucous membranes and normal skin surrounding warts.

Medication may cause reddening or scaling of skin when used on open skin lesions.

Contact with clothing, fabrics, plastics, wood, metal or other materials may cause damage; avoid contact.

SALICYLIC ACID

Administration and Dosage:

For specific instructions for use of these products, refer to individual product labeling.

Apply to affected area. May soak in warm water for 5 minutes prior to use to hydrate skin and enhance the effect. Remove any loose tissue with brush, wash cloth or emery board and dry thoroughly.

In general, for treatment of warts, improvement should occur in 1 to 2 weeks; maximum resolution may be expected after 4 to 6 weeks, although application for up to 12 weeks may be necessary. If skin irritation develops or there is no improvement after several weeks, contact a physician.

Storage/Stability: Some products are flammable; keep away from fire or flame. Keep bottle tightly capped and store at room temperature away from heat.

otc	**Panscol** (Baker Cummins)	**Ointment:** 3%	In 90 g.
otc	**Fostex** (Bristol Products)	**Cream:** 2% with etetic acid, stearyl alcohol	In 118 g.
otc	**Panscol** (Baker Cummins)	**Lotion:** 3%	In 120 ml.
otc	**Mosco** (Medtech)	**Liquid:** 17.6% in a flexible collodion base with 33% alcohol and 65.5% ether	In 10 ml.
otc	**Dr Scholl's Wart Remover Kit** (Schering-Plough)	**Liquid:** 17% in a flexible collodion with 17% alcohol, 52% ether, acetone	In 10 ml with brush and cushions.
otc	**Occlusal-HP** (GenDerm)	**Liquid:** 17% in a polyacrylic vehicle with isopropyl alcohol	In 10 ml with brush applicator.
otc	**Compound W** (Whitehall)	**Liquid:** 17% with collodion, 21.2% alcohol, 63.6% ether, camphor, castor oil, menthol	In 9 ml.
otc	**DuoFilm** (Schering-Plough)	**Liquid:** 17% in flexible collodion with 15.8% alcohol, castor oil, 42.6% ether	In 15 ml with brush applicator.
otc	**Maximum Strength Wart Remover** (Glades)	**Liquid:** 17% with 29% alcohol, castor oil in a flexible collodion	In 13.3 ml with applicator.
otc	**Off-Ezy Wart Remover Kit** (Del Pharm)	**Liquid:** 17% in collodion-like vehicle with 21% alcohol and 65% ether, acetone	In 13.5 ml with skin buffer and applicator.
otc	**Off-Ezy Corn & Callus Remover Kit** (Del Pharm)	**Liquid:** 17% in collodion-like vehicle with 21% alcohol and 65% ether, acetone	In 13.5 ml with callus smoother and corn cushions.
otc	**Wart-Off** (Pfizer)	**Liquid:** 17% in flexible collodion with 26.35% alcohol, propylene glycol dipelargonate	In 15 ml with applicator.
otc	**Salactic Film** (Pedinol)	**Liquid:** 17% in collodion-like vehicle	In 15 ml with brush applicator.
otc	**Wart Remover** (Rugby)	**Liquid:** 17% in a flexible collodion with isopropyl alcohol	In 14.8 ml with applicator.
otc	**Gordofilm** (Gordon)	**Liquid:** 16.7% in flexible collodion	In 15 ml with brush applicator.
otc	**Freezone** (Whitehall)	**Liquid:** 13.6% in a collodion-like vehicle, 20.5% alcohol, 64.8% ether, castor oil	In 9 ml.
otc	**Dr Scholl's Corn/Callus Remover** (Schering-Plough)	**Liquid:** 12.6% in flexible collodion with 18% alcohol, 55% ether, acetone, hydrogenated vegetable oil	In 10 ml with 3 cushions.
otc	**Sal-Plant** (Pedinol)	**Gel:** 17% in collodion-like vehicle	In 14 g.
otc	**Compound W** (Whitehall)	**Gel:** 17% with 67.5% alcohol, camphor, castor oil, collodion, colloidal silicon dioxide, hydroxypropyl cellulose, hypophosphorous acid, polysorbate 80	In 7 g.

SALICYLIC ACID

otc	**DuoPlant** (Schering-Plough)	**Gel:** 17% in flexible collodion with 57.6% alcohol, 16.42% ether, ethyl lactate, hydroxypropyl cellulose, polybutene	In 14.2 g.
otc	**Psor-a-set** (Hogil)	**Soap:** 2%	In 97.5 g.
otc	**DuoFilm** (Schering-Plough)	**Transdermal Patch:** 40% in a rubber-based vehicle	In 18s (containing 3 sizes).
otc	**Trans-Ver-Sal PlantarPatch** (Doak)	**Transdermal Patch:** 15% with karaya, PEG-300, propylene glycol, quaternium-15	20 mm patches in 25s with 25 securing tapes and one emery file.
otc	**Trans-Ver-Sal PediaPatch** (Doak)	**Transdermal Patch:** 15% in karaya gum base	In 6 mm (20s) with bandage tapes.
otc	**Trans-Ver-Sal AdultPatch** (Doak)	**Transdermal Patch:** 15% with karaya, PEG-300, propylene glycol, quaternium-15	6 or 12 mm patches in 40s with 42 securing tapes and one emery file.
otc	**Sal-Acid** (Pedinol)	**Plaster:** 40% in a collodion-like vehicle	In 14s.
otc	**Mediplast** (Beiersdorf)	**Plaster:** 40%	2″ x 3″ patches in 2s and 25s.
otc	**Dr Scholl's Advanced Pain Relief Corn Removers** (Schering-Plough)	**Disk:** 40% in a rubber-based vehicle	In 6s with cushions.
otc	**Dr Scholl's Callus Removers** (Schering-Plough)		In 4s with 6 pads and 4s with 4 pads (extra-thick).
otc	**Dr Scholl's Clear Away Plantar** (Schering-Plough)		In 24s with cushions.
otc	**Dr Scholl's Clear Away** (Schering-Plough)		In 18s with cover-up disks.
otc	**Dr Scholl's Corn Removers** (Schering-Plough)		In 9s (pads and disks) as regular, extra-thick, soft, small, waterproof and ultra-thin and 6s (pads and disks) as wrap-around.
otc	**Dr Scholl's Moisturizing Corn Remover Kit** (Schering-Plough)		In 6s with moisturizing cream and cushions.
otc	**Dr Scholl's Clear Away OneStep** (Schering-Plough)	**Strips:** 40% in a rubber-based vehicle	In 14s.
otc	**Dr Scholl's OneStep Corn Removers** (Schering-Plough)		In 6s.

PODOPHYLLUM RESIN (Podophyllin)

Actions:

Pharmacology: Podophyllum resin is the powdered mixture of resins removed from the May apple or Mandrake (*Podophyllum peltatum* Linne'), a perennial plant of the northern and middle US. Podophyllum is a cytotoxic agent that has been used topically in the treatment of genital warts. It arrests mitosis in metaphase, an effect it shares with other cytotoxic agents such as the vinca alkaloids. The active agent is podophyllotoxin, whose concentration varies with the type of podophyllum resin used; American podophyllum typically has a reduced level of podophyllotoxin and normally contains one-fourth the amount of the Indian source.

Indications:

Wart removal: For the removal of soft genital (venereal) warts (condylomata acuminata) and other papillomas; for multiple superficial epitheliomatosis and keratoses.

The CDC recommends podophyllum resin as an alternative regimen to cryotherapy for the treatment of external genital/perianal warts, vaginal warts and urethral meatus warts (CDC 1989 Sexually Transmitted Diseases Treatment Guidelines. Morbidity and Mortality Weekly Report 1989 Sept 1;38[No.S-8]:20-21).

Contraindications:

Diabetics; patients using steroids or with poor blood circulation; use on bleeding warts, moles, birthmarks or unusual warts with hair growing from them; pregnancy, lactation (see Warnings).

Warnings:

For external use only: Podophyllum is a powerful caustic and severe irritant. Keep away from the eyes; if eye contact occurs, flush with copious amounts of warm water and consult physician or poison control center immediately for advice.

Physician use (application) only: Podophyllum resin is to be applied only by a physician. It is not to be dispensed to the patient.

Pregnancy: There have been reports of complications associated with the topical use of podophyllum on condylomas of pregnant patients including birth defects, fetal death and stillbirth. Do not use on pregnant patients or patients who plan to become pregnant.

Lactation: It is not known whether podophyllum is excreted in breast milk following topical application. Do not use on nursing patients.

Precautions:

Inflamed/Irritated tissue: Do not use if wart or surrounding tissue is inflamed or irritated. Do not use on bleeding warts, moles, birthmarks or unusual warts with hair growing from them.

Adverse Reactions:

Paresthesia; polyneuritis; paralytic ileus; pyrexia; leukopenia; thrombocytopenia; nausea; vomiting; diarrhea; abdominal pain; confusion; dizziness; stupor; convulsions; coma; death.

Significant neuropathy and death are generally related to large amounts used for multiple and widespread lesions. Onset of neuropathy may occur within hours of application and duration may range from months to years with some neurologic deficit.

Patient Information:

To be applied only by a physician.

For external use only. Avoid contact with eyes and healthy tissue.

Administration and Dosage:

Podophyllum is to be applied only by a physician. It is not to be dispensed to the patient. Thoroughly cleanse affected area. Use applicator to apply sparingly to lesion. Avoid contact with healthy tissue. Allow to dry thoroughly. Treat only intact (non-bleeding) lesions. As podophyllum is a powerful caustic and severe irritant, it is recommended the first application be left in contact for only a short time (30 to 40 minutes) to determine patient's sensitivity. To avoid systemic absorption, use the minimum time of contact necessary to produce the desired result (1 to 4 hours, depending on condition of lesion and of patient), with the physician developing their own experience and technique. Do not treat large areas or numerous warts at once. After treatment time has elapsed, remove dried podophyllum resin thoroughly with alcohol or soap and water.

Rx	**Podocon-25** (Paddock)	**Liquid:** 25% podophyllum resin in tincture of benzoin	In 15 ml.
Rx	**Podofin** (Syosset)		In 15 ml.

CANTHARIDIN

Actions:

Pharmacology: Effectiveness against warts is presumed to result from the "exfoliation" of the tumor as a consequence of its acantholytic action. The lytic action of cantharidin does not go beyond the epidermal cells, the basal layer remains intact and there is minimal effect on the corium; as a result, there is no scarring from topical application.

Indications:

A vesicant for removal of benign epithelial growths: Warts (including ordinary, periungual, subungual and plantar) and molluscum contagiosum.

Contraindications:

Diabetics or persons with impaired peripheral circulation; use on eyes, mucous membranes, ano-genital or intertriginous areas, moles, birthmarks or unusual warts with hair growing from them, or if lesion is being treated with other agents; if growth or surrounding tissue is inflamed or irritated.

Warnings:

Vesicant properties: Cantharidin is a strong vesicant. Use sparingly. Do not use in ano-genital area. Keep away from eyes and mucosal tissue. Avoid use in intertriginous sites due to problems with spreading and body occlusion which often lead to more intense, painful reactions.

Cantharidin may produce blisters on normal skin or mucous membranes. If spilled on skin, wipe off at once, using acetone, alcohol or tape remover; wash with warm soapy water and rinse well. If spilled on mucous membranes or in eyes, flush with water, remove precipitated collodion; flush with water for an additional 15 minutes.

Physician use (application) only: Cantharidin is a potent vesicant and should be applied only by a physician. It is not to be dispensed to the patient.

Sensitivity: Patients vary in sensitivity to cantharidin; tingling, burning or extreme tenderness may develop rarely. In these cases, remove tape and soak the area in cool water for 10 to 15 minutes; repeat as required for relief. If soreness persists, puncture blister aseptically, apply antiseptic and cover with bandage. Treat only one or two lesions on the first visit, until the sensitivity of the patient is known. Expect a more intense reaction in patients with fair skin and blue eyes. Do not reapply to the same lesion more than once per week. Defer second treatment if inflammation is intense.

Palpebral warts: Use great care if treating palpebral warts. Make certain film is thoroughly dry; warn patient not to touch the eyelid.

Pigmentation: Although rare, use care in the selection of site application since residual pigmentation changes may occur.

Pregnancy: There have been no adequate and well controlled studies in pregnant women; therefore, the use of cantharidin during pregnancy is not recommended.

Lactation: Use in nursing mothers is not recommended.

Adverse Reactions:

Annular warts have occurred in some patients. These are superficial and present little problem, although they may alarm patients. Reassure patient and treat again.

There have been several reports of chemical lymphangitis following use of cantharidin, one in combination with salicylic acid plaster. A case of extreme, painful blistering occurred after treatment of multiple axillary lesions.

Patient Information:

May cause tingling, itching or burning within a few hours after application; site may be extremely tender for 2 to 6 days.

If spilled on skin, wipe off at once with acetone, alcohol or tape remover and wash with soap and water.

For external use only. If spilled in the eyes, flush with water and contact physician.

Administration and Dosage:

Ordinary and periungual warts: No cutting or prior treatment is required. Apply directly to the lesion and cover the growth completely, extending beyond by about 1 mm. Allow a few minutes for a thin membrane to form. Cover completely with nonporous tape. Remove tape in 24 hours and replace with a loose bandage. On next visit (1 to 2 weeks), remove necrotic tissue and reapply to any remaining growth. Defer second treatment if inflammation is intense. A single treatment frequently suffices.

CANTHARIDIN

Plantar warts: Pare away keratin covering the wart; avoid cutting viable tissue. Apply to wart and 1 to 3 mm around the wart. Allow to dry, secure with nonporous tape; application of a protective cut-out cushion over the tape may be helpful. After 24 hours, the patient may bathe and replace dressing. Debride 1 to 2 weeks after treatment. If any viable wart tissue remains, reapply as above; ≥ 3 treatments may be required for large lesions. For large mosaic warts, treat a portion of the wart at a time. Applying cantharidin to open tissue will result in stinging from the solvent. Avoid by paring carefully and scheduling treatments 2 weeks apart.

Molluscum contagiosum: Apply a very small amount of solution to only the top of each lesion. Let dry completely. No occlusive tape or dressing is needed. Alert patient that blistering is the desired result and that temporary hypopigmentation may occur. The patient may bathe after 4 to 6 hours; sooner if discomfort occurs. Blisters are usually formed by about 24 hours and crust up in about 4 days. Mild discomfort or itching can usually be controlled with bathing and night sedation. In 1 week, treat new or remaining lesions the same way and re-treat any resistant lesions. This time, cover with a small piece of occlusive tape. Remove tape in 4 to 6 hours, sooner if discomfort occurs.

Note: Use of a mild antibacterial is recommended until the tissue re-epithelializes.

Rx	**Verr-Canth** (Palisades)	**Liquid**: 0.7% cantharidin in an adherent film-forming base of ethylcellulose, cellosolve, castor oil, penederm (octylphenylpolyethylene glycol), acetone	In 7.5 ml.

KERATOLYTIC COMBINATIONS

Rx	**Verrex** (Palisades)	**Liquid**: 30% salicylic acid and 10% podophyllum in an adherent film-forming vehicle of penederm (octylphenylpo-lyethylene glycol), ethylcellulose, cello-solve, collodion, castor oil, acetone	In 7.5 ml with applicator.
otc	**Gets-It** (Oakhurst)	**Liquid**: Salicylic acid, zinc chloride and collodion in ≈35% ether and ≈28% alcohol	In 12 ml.

CHLOROACETIC ACIDS

Actions:

Pharmacology: Rapidly penetrates and cauterizes skin, keratin and other tissues. Monochloroacetic acid is more deeply destructive than trichloroacetic acid.

Indications:

Dichloroacetic acid: Verrucae (warts); calluses; hard and soft corns; xanthoma palpebrarum; seborrheic keratoses; ingrown nails; cysts and benign erosion of the cervix; endocervicitis; epistaxis.

Monochloroacetic and trichloroacetic acid: Removal of verrucae.

The CDC recommends trichloroacetic acid as an alternative regimen to cryotherapy for treatment of external genital/perianal warts and vaginal and anal warts.

Contraindications:

Treatment of malignant or premalignant lesions; hypersensitivity to any component.

Warnings:

Cauterant properties: These acids are powerful keratolytics and cauterants. Restrict use to areas where these effects are desired. May cause severe burning, inflammation or tenderness of skin.

Cervical lesions: A careful diagnosis and possibly a biopsy is required to rule out malignancy; treatment is contraindicated in the event of positive findings.

Normal tissue: Apply only to the lesion being treated. To prevent acid from spreading onto normal skin, apply petrolatum around the area to be treated. If any acid is spilled on normal tissue or if too much acid is applied, remove immediately and wash with water. Sodium bicarbonate may be applied as a local antidote.

MONOCHLOROACETIC ACID

Complete prescribing information begins in the Chloroacetic Acids group monograph.

Administration and Dosage:

Remove callus tissue. Apply to verruca. Apply bandage and allow to remain in place for 5 to 6 days. Remove verruca tissue and reapply as needed. If crystallization of liquid occurs, place capped bottle in hot water to redissolve.

Rx	**Mono-Chlor** (Gordon)	**Liquid:** 80%	In 15 ml.

DICHLOROACETIC ACID

Complete prescribing information begins in the Chloroacetic Acids group monograph.

Administration and Dosage:

Amount applied varies with the nature of the lesion. Dense horny lesions (corns, warts, calluses, plantar warts) require repeated intensive treatment. Lesions of light density (pedunculated warts, xanthoma palpebrarum, soft corns, seborrheic keratoses, condyloma acuminata) receive lighter applications.

Application technique depends on type of lesion. Treat dense growths by rubbing the acid into the lesion with a pointed wooden or cotton-tipped applicator; 3 or 4 treatments may be necessary. Lesions of light density should receive a lighter application at each visit. Usually 1 or 2 such treatments are sufficient.

Apply thin layer of petrolatum to normal tissue surrounding the lesion. Use microdropper to transfer some acid to small-stemmed acid receptacle. The acid should not contact the microdropper's neoprene bulb. Use microdropper upright; fill no more than halfway. Moisten a sharpened applicator stick in acid and draw over flared lip to remove excess. There should never be a large excess drop on applicator.

When applying very small amounts, hold applicator level or with the point up so that a tiny fraction of one drop can be transferred to small lesions. To follow cauterization progress, observe change in color of treated area to gray-white, using a magnifying lens if necessary. It is sometimes advantageous to apply by rolling applicator over surface of lesion, using the point only at the edges. To avoid contamination, do not return any remaining acid from receptacle to bottle. Keep bottle tightly capped except when removing acid. Discard applicators after use.

See manufacturer's package insert for treatment of specific lesions.

Rx	**Bichloracetic Acid** (Glenwood)	**Liquid:** 10 ml dichloroacetic acid	In treatment kit with 16 g petrolatum, applicators, acid receptacles, microdropper and holder.

TRICHLOROACETIC ACID

Complete prescribing information begins in the Chloroacetic Acids group monograph.

Administration and Dosage:

Debride callus tissue. Apply to verruca. Cover with bandage for 5 to 6 days. Remove verruca. Reapply as needed. If crystallization of liquid occurs, place capped bottle in hot water to redissolve.

Rx	**Tri-Chlor** (Gordon)	**Liquid:** 80%	In 15 ml.	452

SILVER NITRATE

For prevention of gonorrheal ophthalmia neonatorum, see monograph in Ophthalmics.

Actions:

Pharmacology: Silver nitrate is a strong caustic and escharotic providing antisepetic, astringent, germicidal, local (epithelial) stimulant or caustic action externally.

The attachment of silver to a reactive group of a protein sharply decreases the protein's solubility; the protein's conformation may also be altered and denaturation may occur. Precipitation of the protein generally results. At low concentrations of silver, precipitation is confined to proteins in the interstices and an astringent action occurs. At high concentrations, membrane and intracellular structures are damaged and there is a casutic or corrosive effect.

Because silver ions attach so readily to the various groups of proteins, the ions are captured before they diffuse far into tissues. Precipitation of silver as silver chloride also limits extent of ion movement. Thus, local effects of silver are self-limiting and spread of damage occurs only when the dose overwhelms the capacity of tissues to fix the ion at the application site. Antiseptic effects of silver may derive in part from the reaction with bacterial and viral proteins.

Indications:

To treat indolent wounds, destroy exuberant granulations, freshen the edges of ulcers and fissures, touch the bases of vesicular, bullous or aphthous lesions and provide styptic action.

10% Ointment: Podiatry - To treat neurovascular helomas; to cauterize and destroy small nerve endings and blood vessels. It forms a protective covering after the removal of corns and calluses.

10% Solution: Impetigo vulgaris. *Podiatry* - Helomas.

25% Solution: Pruritus. *Podiatry* - Plantar warts.

50% Solution: Podiatry - Plantar warts; granulation tissue; papillomatous growths; granuloma pyogenicum.

Unlabeled uses: Concentrations of 0.1% to 0.5% are used as wet dressings in burns and on lesions.

Contraindications:

Application on wounds, cuts or broken skin.

Warnings:

Skin discoloration: Prolonged or frequent use may permanently discolor skin due to deposition of reduced silver. However, topical silver nitrate for local application to suppress granulation tissue apparently does not produce argyria.

Staining of clothes: Will stain clothing and linens.

Electrolyte abnormalities: If wet dressings are used over extensive areas or prolonged periods, electrolyte abnormalities can result. Sodium and chloride leach into the dressing and hyponatremia or hypochloremia can occur. Absorbed nitrate can cause methemoglobinemia.

Precautions:

Irritation: Discontinue use if redness or irritation occurs.

For external use only: Avoid contact with the eyes.

Overdosage:

Symptoms: The fatal dose of silver nitrate may be as low as 2 g. Oral intake of silver nitrate causes a local corrosive effect including pain and burning of mouth, salivation, vomiting, diarrhea progressing to anuria, shock, coma, convulsions and death. Blackening of skin and mucous membranes occurs (sometimes permanent).

Treatment: Give NaCl in water, 10 g/L, to precipitate silver Cl. Follow with catharsis, including NaCl solution. Also attend to shock and methemoglobinemia if present.

If splashed in eyes, wash with copious amounts of water and see a physician.

Administration and Dosage:

Ointment: Apply in apertured pad on affected area for ≈ 5 days, as needed.

Solution: Apply a cotton applicator dipped in solution on the affected area or lesion 2 or 3 times a week for 2 or 3 weeks, as needed.

Rx	**Silver Nitrate** (Gordon Labs)	**Ointment**: 10%	Petrolatum base. In 30 g.
		Solution: 10%	In 30 ml.
		25%	In 30 ml.
		50%	In 30 ml.
Rx	**Silver Nitrate** (Graham-Field)	**Applicators**: 75% with 25% potassium nitrate	In 100s.

SUTILAINS

Actions:

Pharmacology: Selectively digests necrotic soft tissues by proteolytic action. It dissolves and facilitates removal of necrotic tissues and purulent exudates that otherwise impair formation of granulation tissue and delay wound healing.

Indications:

As an adjunct to wound care for biochemical debridement of the following lesions: Second and third degree burns; decubitus ulcers; incisional, traumatic and pyogenic wounds; ulcers secondary to peripheral vascular disease.

Contraindications:

Wounds communicating with major body cavities; wounds containing exposed major nerves or nerve tissue; fungating neoplastic ulcers.

Warnings:

For external use only: Do not permit ointment to come into contact with the eyes. If this inadvertently occurs, rinse immediately with copious amounts of sterile water.

Pregnancy: Category B. There are no adequate or well controlled studies in pregnant women. Use during pregnancy only if no adequate alternatives are available.

Children: Safety and efficacy for use in children have not been established.

Precautions:

A moist environment is essential for optimal enzyme activity.

Systemic therapy: In cases where there is existent or threatening invasive infection, institute systemic antibiotic therapy.

Antibody response: Although there have been no reports of systemic allergic reactions in humans, there may be an antibody response to absorbed enzyme material.

Impairment of enzyme activity: Enzyme activity may be impaired by certain agents. In vitro, several detergents and antiseptics (benzalkonium chloride, hexachlorophene, iodine and **nitrofurazone**) render the substrate indifferent to the action of the enzyme. Compounds such as **thimerosal**, which contain metallic ions, interfere directly with enzyme activity to a slight degree, whereas, **neomycin, mafenide, streptomycin** and **penicillin** do not affect enzyme activity. If adjunctive topical therapy has been used and no dissolution of slough occurs after treatment for 24 to 48 hours, further application, because of interference by adjunctive agents, is unlikely to be successful.

Adverse Reactions:

Systemic toxicity has not been observed as a result of topical application.

Local: Mild, transient pain; paresthesias; bleeding; transient dermatitis. If bleeding or dermatitis occurs, discontinue therapy. Pain can usually be controlled with mild analgesics. Side effects severe enough to warrant discontinuation of therapy have occurred.

Administration and Dosage:

Thoroughly cleanse and irrigate wound area with sodium chloride or water solutions. Wound must be cleansed of antiseptics or heavy-metal antibacterials which may denature enzyme or alter substrate characteristics (see Precautions).

Thoroughly moisten wound area through bathing, showering or wet soaks (eg, sodium chloride or water solutions).

Apply ointment in a thin layer (⅛ inch), assuring intimate contact with necrotic tissue and complete wound coverage extending ½ to ¼ inch beyond the area to be debrided.

Apply moist dressings.

Repeat entire procedure 3 to 4 times per day for best results.

Storage: Ointment must be refrigerated at 2° to 8°C (36° to 46°F).

Rx	**Travase** (Boots)	**Ointment:** 82,000 casein units per g in a hydrophobic base of 95% mineral oil and 5% polyethylene	In 14.2 g.

COLLAGENASE

Actions:

Pharmacology: Since collagen accounts for 75% of the dry weight of skin tissue, the ability of collagenase to digest collagen in the physiological pH range and temperature makes it effective in the removal of tissue debris. Complete debridement occurs in 10 to 14 days. Collagenase thus contributes to the formation of granulation tissues and subsequent epithelialization of dermal ulcers and severely burned areas. Collagen in healthy tissue or in newly formed granulation tissue is not attacked.

Indications:

For debriding chronic dermal ulcers and severely burned areas.

Contraindications:

Local or systemic hypersensitivity to collagenase.

Precautions:

For external use only. Avoid contact with the eyes.

Optimal pH range of the enzyme is 6 to 8.

Systemic bacterial infections: Monitor debilitated patients for systemic bacterial infections because debriding enzymes may increase the risk of bacteremia.

Slight transient erythema has been noted occasionally in surrounding tissue, particularly when the ointment was not confined to the lesion. Therefore, apply carefully within the area of the lesion. Irritation may be prevented by applying a protectant (eg, zinc oxide paste) to the surrounding tissue.

Inhibition of enzymatic activity: Enzymatic activity is inhibited by **detergents, benzalkonium chloride, hexachlorophene, nitrofurazone, tincture of iodine** and **heavy metal ions** such as **mercury** and **silver** which are used in some antiseptics. When such materials have been used, carefully cleanse the site by repeated washings with normal saline before ointment is applied. Avoid soaks containing metal ions or acidic solutions such as **Burow's solution** because of the metal ion and low pH. Cleansing materials such as hydrogen peroxide, Dakin's solution or normal saline do not interfere with enzyme activity.

Adverse Reactions:

No allergic sensitivity or toxic reactions have been noted in clinical investigations. However, one case of systemic manifestations of hypersensitivity to collagenase in a patient treated for > 1 year with a combination of collagenase and cortisone has been reported.

Overdosage:

Action of the enzyme may be stopped by the application of Burow's solution (pH 3.6 to 4.4) to the lesion.

Administration and Dosage:

Apply once daily (more frequently if the dressing becomes soiled).

Prior to application, cleanse the lesion of debris and digested material by gently rubbing with a gauze pad saturated with hydrogen peroxide or Dakin's solution, followed by sterile normal saline.

When infection is present, use an appropriate topical antibacterial agent. Neomycin-bacitracin-polymyxin B is compatible with collagenase ointment; apply to the lesion prior to the application of collagenase ointment. Should the infection not respond, discontinue therapy until remission of the infection occurs.

Apply ointment (using a wooden tongue depressor or spatula) directly to deep wounds; with shallow wounds, use a sterile gauze pad, apply to wound and secure properly.

Crosshatching thick eschar with a #10 blade allows collagenase more surface contact with necrotic debris. Remove as much loosened tissue debris as possible with forceps and scissors.

Remove all excess ointment each time dressing is changed.

Terminate use of the ointment when debridement of necrotic tissue is complete and granulation tissue is well established.

Rx	**Santyl** (Knoll)	**Ointment**: 250 units collagenase enzyme per g. In white petrolatum.	In 15 and 30 g.

FIBRINOLYSIN AND DESOXYRIBONUCLEASE

Actions:

Pharmacology: Combination of these enzymes is based on the observation that purulent exudates consist largely of fibrinous material and nucleoprotein. Desoxyribonuclease attacks the deoxyribonucleic acid (DNA) and fibrinolysin attacks principally fibrin of blood clots and fibrinous exudates.

The activity of desoxyribonuclease is limited principally to the production of large polynucleotides, which are less likely to be absorbed than the more diffusible protein fractions liberated by enzyme preparations obtained from bacteria. Fibrinolytic action is directed mainly against denatured proteins, such as those found in devitalized tissue, while protein elements of living cells remain relatively unaffected.

Indications:

Topical: Debriding agent in general surgical wounds; ulcerative lesions (trophic, decubitus, stasis, arteriosclerotic); second- and third-degree burns; circumcision; episiotomy.

In infected lesions such as burns, ulcers and wounds where a topical antibiotic is desired, the product containing the enzymes plus chloramphenicol is indicated. Except in very superficial infections, systemic medication is also indicated.

Intravaginal: Cervicitis (benign, postpartum and postconization) and vaginitis.

Irrigating agent: Infected wounds (abscesses, fistulae and sinus tracts); otorhinolaryngologic wounds; superficial hematomas (except when the hematoma is adjacent to or within adipose tissue).

Contraindications:

Hypersensitivity reactions to any component; parenteral use (bovine fibrinolysin may be antigenic).

Warnings:

Bone marrow hypoplasia, aplastic anemia and death have been reported following the local application of chloramphenicol (present in Elase-Chloromycetin;).

Precautions:

Hypersensitivity: Observe precautions against allergic reactions, particularly in persons with a history of sensitivity to bovine material. Have epinephrine 1:1000 immediately available. Refer to Management of Acute Hypersensitivity Reactions.

Superinfection:

Chloramphenicol – Use of antibiotics (especially prolonged or repeated therapy) may result in bacterial or fungal overgrowth of nonsusceptible organisms and may lead to a secondary infection. Take appropriate measures if superinfection occurs.

Adverse Reactions:

Side effects have not been a problem for the indications and dose recommended. With higher concentrations, local hyperemia may occur.

Administration and Dosage:

After application, these products become rapidly and progressively less active; only insignificant activity remains after 24 hours.

Individualize dosage. Successful use of enzymatic debridement depends on several factors: (1) Remove any dense, dry eschar surgically before enzymatic debridement is attempted; (2) the enzyme must be in constant contact with the substrate; (3) periodically remove accumulated necrotic debris; (4) replenish the enzyme at least once daily; and (5) employ secondary closure or skin grafting as soon as possible after optimal debridement. Administer appropriate systemic antibiotics if indicated.

General topical uses: Repeat local application for as long as enzyme action is desired.

Procedure – Clean wound with water, peroxide or normal saline and dry area gently. Surgically remove dense, dry eschar before applying ointment. Apply a thin layer of ointment and cover with petrolatum gauze or other nonadhering dressing.

Change dressing at least once a day, preferably 2 or 3 times daily. Frequency of application is more important than amount of ointment used. Flush away the necrotic debris and fibrinous exudates with saline, peroxide or warm water so that newly applied ointment is in direct contact with the substrate.

The solution may be applied topically as a liquid, wet dressing or spray by using a conventional atomizer.

Wet dressing – Mix 1 vial of powder with 10 to 50 ml saline and saturate strips of fine-mesh gauze or unfolded sterile gauze sponge with solution. Pack ulcerated area with gauze so that it remains in contact with the necrotic substrate. Allow gauze to dry in contact with ulcerated lesion (approximately 6 to 8 hours). Remove dried gauze; this mechanically debrides the area. Repeat wet-to-dry procedure 3 or 4 times daily since frequent dressing changes enhance results. After 2 to 4 days, the area will be clean and will begin to fill in with granulation tissue.

FIBRINOLYSIN AND DESOXYRIBONUCLEASE

Intravaginal use: In mild to moderate vaginitis and cervicitis, apply 5 g of ointment deep into the vagina at bedtime for approximately 5 applications. In more severe cases, instill 10 ml of solution intravaginally, wait 1 or 2 minutes for enzyme to disperse, then insert a cotton tampon in the vaginal canal. Remove tampon the next day. Continue therapy with the ointment.

Abscesses, empyema cavities, fistulae, sinus tracts or SC hematomas: Despite contraindications against parenteral use, the solution has been used to irrigate these conditions. Drain and replace solution at intervals of 6 to 10 hours to reduce amount of by–product accumulation and minimize loss of enzyme activity. Traces of blood in discharge usually indicate active filling in of the cavity.

Preparation of solution: Reconstitute contents of each vial with 10 ml isotonic NaCl solution. Prepare higher or lower concentrations by varying amount of diluent.

To be maximally effective, solutions must be freshly prepared before use. The loss in activity is reduced by refrigeration; however, do not use solution ≥ 24 hours after reconstitution, even when refrigerated.

Rx	**Elase** (Fujisawa)	**Powder, lyophilized:** 25 units (Loomis) fibrinolysin and 15,000 units (modified Christensen method) desoxyribonuclease[1] per vial	In 30 ml vials.
		Ointment: 1 unit fibrinolysin and 666.6 units desoxyribonuclease[1] per g in liquid petrolatum and polyethylene	In 10 and 30 g tubes.
Rx	**Elase-Chloromycetin** (Fujisawa)	**Ointment:** 10 mg chloramphenicol, 1 unit fibrinolysin & 666.6 units desoxyribonuclease[1] per g in liquid petrolatum and polyethylene	In 10 and 30 g tubes.

[1] From bovine pancreas.

TOPICAL ENZYME COMBINATIONS

TRYPSIN and *PAPAIN* are used for the enzymatic debridement and promotion of normal healing, especially where healing is retarded by eschar, necrotic tissue and debris.

BALSAM PERU is an effective capillary bed stimulant intended to improve circulation to the wound site. It may have a mildly antiseptic action.

CASTOR OIL (also refer to Laxative monograph) is used to improve epithelialization by reducing premature epithelial desiccation and cornification, and as protective cover.

UREA (see monograph in Emollients section) is an emollient and keratolytic.

CHLOROPHYLL DERIVATIVES (see individual monograph) aid wound healing and control wound odor.

Warnings:

Arterial clots: Do not spray trypsin products on fresh arterial clots.

For external use only. Avoid contact with the eyes.

Transient burning may be associated with initial application.

Administration and Dosage:

Apply medication once or twice daily.

Clean wound prior to application (hydrogen peroxide solution may inactivate papain) and at each redressing.

Rx	**Dermuspray** (Warner Chilcott)	**Aerosol:** 0.1 mg trypsin, 72.5 mg Balsam Peru and 650 mg castor oil per 0.82 ml	In 120 g.
Rx	**Granulderm** (Copley)		In 113.4 g.
Rx	**Granulex** (Hickam)		In 60 and 120 g.
Rx	**GranuMed** (Rugby)		In 113 g.
Rx	**Panafil** (Rystan)	**Ointment:** 10% papain, 10% urea and 0.5% chlorophyllin copper complex in a hydrophilic base with white petrolatum, PPG, sorbitan monostearate, polyoxy-40 stearate, boric acid, sodium borate, chlorobutanol	In 30 g and lb.
Rx	**Panafil White** (Rystan)	**Ointment:** 10% papain and 10% urea in hydrophilic base w/white petrolatum, PPG, sorbitan monostearate, polyoxy-40 stearate, boric acid, sodium borate, chlorobutanol	In 30 g.

Antimitotics

PODOFILOX

Actions:

Pharmacology: Podofilox is a topical antimitotic drug which can be chemically synthesized or purified from the plant families *Coniferae* and *Berberidaceae* (eg, species of *Juniperus* and *Podophyllum*). Treatment of anogenital warts with podofilox results in necrosis of visible wart tissue. The exact mechanism of action is unknown. Condylomas, or genital warts, are caused by the human papillomavirus. In males the warts appear on the penis, anus and perineum; in females they are found on the vagina, cervix, perineum and anus. The number of warts increases in immunosuppressed patients and in those with AIDS and other immunologic deficiencies. Genital warts are epidemiologically associated with cervical carcinoma. Distinguishing between these conditions can be difficult. Obtain histopathologic confirmation if there is any doubt of the diagnosis.

Pharmacokinetics: In 52 patients, topical application of 0.05 ml of 0.5% podofilox solution to external genitalia did not result in detectable serum levels. Applications of 0.1 to 1.5 ml resulted in peak serum levels of 1 to 17 ng/ml 1 to 2 hours after application. The elimination half-life ranged from 1 to 4.5 hours. The drug did not accumulate after multiple treatments.

Clinical trials:

Solution – In double-blind clinical studies, patients were treated for 2 to 4 weeks and reevaluated at a 2 week follow-up examination. Although the number of patients and warts evaluated at each time period varied, the results among investigators were relatively consistent.

Patient Response to Podofilox Treatment[1]

	Initially cleared	Recurred after clearing	Cleared at 2 week follow-up
Warts (n = 524)	79%	35%	60%
Patients (n = 70)	50%	60%	25%

[1] Cleared and clearing mean no visible wart tissue remained at the treated sites.

Gel – In 326 patients with anogenital warts, podofilox and its vehicle were applied in a double-blind fashion to comparable patient groups; 176 were treated with podofilox. Patients applied podofilox twice daily for 3 consecutive days followed by a 4–day rest period. At the end of 4 weeks, 38.4% of the patients had complete clearing of the wart tissue when treated with podofilox.

In another trial in 108 evaluable patients with anogenital warts, podofilox solution was compared with podofilox gel for efficacy. Patients applied podofilox gel twice daily for 3 consecutive days followed by a 4–day rest period. Similar clearance rates were observed. At the end of 4 weeks, 25.6% of the patients had complete clearing of the wart tissue when treated with podofilox gel.

Indications:

Gel: Topical treatment of anogenital warts (external genital and perianal warts). Not indicated in treatment of mucous membrane warts.

Solution: Topical treatment of external warts (Condyloma acuminatum). Not indicated in the treatment of perianal or mucous membrane warts.

Contraindications:

Hypersensitivity or intolerance to any component of the formulation.

Warnings:

Diagnosis: Correct diagnosis of the lesions to be treated is essential. Although anogenital warts have a characteristic appearance, obtain histopathologic confirmation if there is any doubt of the diagnosis. Differentiating warts from squamous cell carcinoma (so-called "Bowenoid papulosis") is of particular concern. Squamous cell carcinoma may also be associated with human papillomavirus but should not be treated with podofilox.

The gel is not indicated for treatment of mucous membrane warts; the solution is not indicated for perianal or mucous membrane warts.

External use only: Podofilox is intended for cutaneous use only. Avoid contact with the eyes. If eye contact occurs, immediately flush the eye with copious quantities of water and seek medical advice.

Carcinogenesis/Mutagenesis: In mouse studies, crude podophyllum resin (containing podofilox) applied topically to the cervix produced changes resembling carcinoma in situ. These changes were reversible at 5 weeks after treatment cessation. In one report, epidermal carcinoma of the vagina and cervix was found in 1 of 18 mice after 120 applications of podophyllin (applied twice weekly over 15 months).

Results from the mouse micronucleus in vivo assay using podofilox 0.5% solution in concentrations up to 25 mg/kg indicate that podofilox should be considered a potential clastogen (a chemical that induces disruption and breakage of chromosomes).

Pregnancy: Category C. Podofilox is embryotoxic in rats when administered at ≈ 250 times the recommended maximum human dose systemically or ≈19 times the recommended maximum human dose intraperitoneally. There are no adequate and well controlled studies in pregnant women. Use in pregnancy only if the potential benefit justifies the potential risk to the fetus.

Lactation: It is not known whether this drug is excreted in breast milk. Decide whether to discontinue nursing or to discontinue the drug, taking into account the importance of the drug to the mother.

Children: Safety and efficacy in children have not been established.

Precautions:

Perianal/Mucous membrane warts: Data are not available on the safe and effective use of this product for treatment of warts occurring on mucous membranes of the genital area (including the urethra, rectum and vagina). Data are not available on the safe and effective use of podofilox **solution** for treatment of warts occurring in the perianal area. Do not exceed the recommended method of application, frequency of application or duration of usage (see Administration and Dosage).

Adverse Reactions:

In clinical trials, the following local adverse reactions occurred at some point during treatment. Reports of burning and pain were more frequent and of greater severity in women than in men treated with the solution. The severity of local adverse reactions in gel-treated patients were predominantly mild or moderate and did not increase during the treatment period; severe reactions were most frequent within the first 2 weeks of treatment.

Podofilox Adverse Reactions (%)

Adverse Reaction	Solution	Gel
Burning	64-78	12-37
Pain	50-72	12-24
Inflammation	63-71	9-32
Erosion	67	9-27
Itching	50-65	8-32
Bleeding	N/A	1-19

Miscellaneous (< 5%):

Solution – Pain with intercourse; insomnia; tingling; bleeding; tenderness; chafing; malodor; dizziness; scarring; vesicle formation; crusting edema; dryness/peeling; foreskin irretraction; hematuria; vomiting; ulceration.

Gel – Headache, stinging, and erythema; less commonly reported local adverse events included desquamation, scabbing, discoloration, tenderness, dryness, crusting, fissures, soreness, ulceration, swelling/edema, tingling, rash and blisters.

Overdosage:

Symptoms: Topically applied podofilox may be absorbed systemically. Toxicity reported following systemic administration of podofilox in investigational use for cancer treatment included: Nausea; vomiting; fever; diarrhea; bone marrow depression; oral ulcers. Following 5 to 10 daily IV doses of 0.5 to 1 mg/kg/day, significant hematological toxicity occurred but was reversible. Other toxicities occurred at lower doses.

Toxicity reported following systemic administration of podophyllum resin included: Nausea; vomiting; fever; diarrhea; peripheral neuropathy; altered mental status; lethargy; coma; tachypnea; respiratory failure; leukocytosis; pancytosis; hematuria; renal failure; seizures.

Treatment of topical overdosage should include washing the skin free of any remaining drug and symptomatic and supportive therapy. Refer to General Management of Acute Overdosage.

Patient Information:

Provide the patient with a Patient Information leaflet when a podofilox prescription is filled.

Antimitotics

PODOFILOX

Use only as directed by the health care provider. Instruct patients to wash their hands thoroughly before and after each application. It is for external use only. Avoid contact with the eyes.

Advise patients not to use this medication for any disorder other than for which it was prescribed.

Patients should report any signs of adverse reactions to the health care provider.

If no improvement is observed after 4 weeks of treatment, discontinue the medication and consult the health care provider.

Administration and Dosage:

Solution: Apply twice daily morning and evening (every 12 hours) to the warts with a cotton-tipped applicator supplied with the drug. Touch the drug-dampened applicator to the wart to be treated, applying the minimium amount of solution necessary to cover the lesion. Limit treatment to < 10 cm^2 of wart tissue and to ≤ 0.5 ml of the solution per day. There is no evidence to suggest that more frequent application will increase efficacy, but additional applications would be expected to increase the rate of local adverse reactions and systemic absorption. Allow the solution to dry before allowing the return of opposing skin surfaces to their normal positions. After each treatment, dispose of the used applicator and wash hands.

Gel: Apply twice daily to the warts with the applicator tip or finger. Minimize application on the surrounding normal tissue. Limit to ≤ 10 cm^2 of wart tissue and to ≤ 0.5 g of the gel per day. Allow the gel to dry before allowing the return of opposing skin surfaces to their normal positions. Instruct patients to wash their hands thoroughly before and after each application.

The prescriber should ensure that the patient is fully aware of the correct method of therapy and identify which specific warts should be treated. If there is incomplete response after 4 treatment weeks, consider alternate treatment. Safety and effectiveness of > 4 treatment weeks have not been established. Apply twice daily for 3 consecutive days, then withhold use for 4 consecutive days. This 1–week cycle of treatment may be repeated up to 4 times until there is no visible wart tissue.

Storage/Stability: Store at room temperature between 15° to 30°C (59° to 86°F). Avoid excessive heat. Do not freeze.

Rx	**Condylox** (Oclassen)	**Topical Gel:** 0.5% podofilox	Alcohol. In 3.5 ml aluminum tubes.
Rx	**Condylox** (Oclassen)	**Topical Solution:** 0.5% podofilox	Alcohol. In 3.5 ml bottles.

FLUOROURACIL

For information on the systemic use of fluorouracil, refer to the monograph in the Antineoplastic chapter.

Actions:

Pharmacology: Fluorouracil appears to inhibit the synthesis of deoxyribonucleic acid (DNA); to a lesser extent, ribonucleic acid (RNA) is inhibited. These effects are most marked on rapidly growing cells which take up fluorouracil at a rapid pace.

When applied to a lesion, response occurs as follows:

1.) Early inflammation – Minimal reaction, erythema for several days.
2.) Severe inflammation – Burning, stinging, vesiculation.
3.) Disintegration – Erosion, ulceration, necrosis, pain, crusting, reepithelialization.
4.) Healing – Complete, with residual erythema and occasional, temporary hyperpigmentation, over 1 to 2 weeks.

Pharmacokinetics: Fluorouracil is not significantly absorbed (≈ 6%).

Indications:

Multiple actinic or solar keratoses.

Superficial basal cell carcinomas: The 5% strength is useful when conventional methods are impractical (ie, multiple lesions, difficult treatment sites). Establish diagnosis prior to treatment.

Unlabeled uses: A 1% solution of fluorouracil in 70% ethanol and the 5% cream have been used in the treatment of condylomata acuminata.

Contraindications:

Hypersensitivity to any component; pregnancy (see Warnings).

Warnings:

Occlusive dressings may increase the incidence of inflammatory reactions in the adjacent normal skin. A porous gauze dressing may be applied for cosmetic reasons without increase in reaction.

Inflammation: There is a possibility of increased absorption through ulcerated or inflamed skin.

Photosensitivity: Avoid prolonged exposure to ultraviolet rays while under treatment with fluorouracil because the intensity of the reaction may be increased.

Hypersensitivity: The potential for a delayed hypersensitivity reaction to fluorouracil exists. Patch testing to prove hypersensitivity may be inconclusive.

Pregnancy: Category X. Fluorouracil may cause fetal harm when administered to a pregnant woman. In animal studies, fluorouracil is both teratogenic and embryolethal. The drug is contraindicated in women who are or who may become pregnant. If fluorouracil is used during pregnancy, or if the patient becomes pregnant while taking this drug, apprise her of the potential hazard to the fetus.

Lactation: It is not known whether this drug is excreted in breast milk. Because there is some systemic absorption of the drug after topical administration, mothers should not breast feed while receiving this drug.

Children: Safety and efficacy have not been established.

Precautions:

Biopsies: To rule out the presence of a frank neoplasm, biopsy those areas failing to respond to treatment or recurring after treatment. Perform follow-up biopsies as indicated in the management of superficial basal cell carcinoma.

Adverse Reactions:

Local reactions include: Pain; pruritus; hyperpigmentation; irritation; inflammation; burning at site of application; allergic contact dermatitis; scarring; soreness; tenderness; suppuration; scaling; swelling.

Other reactions include: Alopecia; insomnia; irritability; stomatitis; medicinal taste; photosensitivity (see Warnings); lacrimation; telangiectasia; urticaria; toxic granulation.

Lab test abnormalities: Leukocytosis; thrombocytopenia; eosinophilia.

FLUOROURACIL

Overdosage:

Ordinarily overdosage will not cause acute problems. If fluorouracil accidently comes in contact with the eye, flush the eye with water or normal saline. If fluorouracil is accidentally ingested, induce emesis and gastric lavage. Administer symptomatic and supportive care as needed.

Patient Information:

Avoid prolonged exposure to ultraviolet rays or other forms of ultraviolet irradiation while under treatment; intensity of reaction may be increased.

If applied with fingers, wash hands immediately afterward. Apply with care near the eyes, nose and mouth.

Reaction in the treated areas may be unsightly during therapy and, in some cases, for several weeks following cessation of therapy.

Administration and Dosage:

Actinic or solar keratoses: Apply twice daily to cover lesions. Continue until inflammatory response reaches erosion, necrosis and ulceration stage, then discontinue use. Usual duration of therapy is from 2 to 6 weeks. Complete healing may not be evident for 1 to 2 months following cessation. Increasing the frequency of application and a longer period of administration may be required on areas other than the head and neck.

Superficial basal cell carcinomas: Only the 5% strength is recommended. Apply twice daily in an amount sufficient to cover the lesions. Continue treatment for at least 3 to 6 weeks. Therapy may be required for as long as 10 to 12 weeks.

Rx	**Efudex** (Roche)	**Cream:** 5%	In a white petrolatum base. In 25 g.
Rx	**Fluoroplex** (Allergan Herbert)	**Cream:** 1%	In a base of benzyl alcohol, emulsifying wax and mineral oil. In 30 g.
Rx	**Efudex** (Roche)	**Solution:** 2%	With propylene glycol, EDTA and parabens. In 10 ml with dropper.
		5%	With propylene glycol, EDTA and parabens. In 10 ml with dropper.
Rx	**Fluoroplex** (Allergan Herbert)	**Solution:** 1%	With propylene glycol. In 30 ml.

MINOXIDIL

Actions:

Pharmacology: Minoxidil topical solution stimulates vertex hair growth in individuals with alopecia androgenetica, expressed in males as baldness of the vertex of the scalp and in females as diffuse hair loss or thinning of the frontoparietal areas. There is no effect in patients with predominantly frontal hair loss. The mechanism is not known, but like minoxidil, some other arterial dilating drugs also stimulate hair growth when given systemically.

In placebo controlled trials involving > 3500 male patients given topical minoxidil for 4 months (longer treatment was given after the placebo group was discontinued), and in > 300 female patients given topical minoxidil for 8 months, typical systemic effects of oral minoxidil (weight gain, edema, tachycardia, fall in blood pressure and their more serious consequences) did not occur more frequently in patients given topical minoxidil than in those given topical placebo.

To study the potential for systemic effects of topical minoxidil, three concentrations (1%, 2% and 5%) applied twice daily were compared to low oral doses (2.5 and 5 mg given once daily) and placebo in hypertensive patients in a double-blind controlled trial. The 5 mg oral dose had readily detectable effects, including a fall in diastolic pressure of about 5 mm Hg and an increase in heart rate of 7 bpm. No other group had a clear effect, although there was some evidence of a weak and inconsistent effect in the 2.5 mg oral, and possibly the 5% topical, treatments.

Pharmacokinetics: Topical minoxidil has poor absorption, averaging ≈ 1.4% (range 0.3% to 4.5%) from normal intact scalp, and about 2% in the hypertensive patients, whose scalps were shaved.

In a comparison of topical and oral absorption, peak serum levels of unchanged drug after 1 ml twice a day of 2% solution (the maximum recommended dose) averaged 5.8% (range, 1.4% to 12.7%) of the level observed after 2.5 mg orally twice a day. Similarly, in the hypertension study where patients had shaved scalps, mean concentrations after 1 ml twice a day of 2% topical solution (1.7 ng/ml) were 1/20 the concentrations seen after daily oral doses of 2.5 mg (32.8 ng/ml) or 5 mg (59.2 ng/ml). Blood levels obtained in the large controlled hair growth trials averaged < 2 ng/ml for the 2% solution (range, up to 30 ng/ml). If more than the recommended dose is applied to inflamed skin in an individual with relatively high absorption, blood levels with systemic effects might rarely be obtained.

Serum levels resulting from topical administration are governed by the drug's percutaneous absorption rate. Following cessation of topical dosing, ≈ 95% of systemically absorbed minoxidil is eliminated within 4 days.

Clinical trials:

Males – Three main parameters of efficacy were used: Hair counts in a 1 inch diameter circle on the vertex of the scalp; investigator evaluation of terminal hair regrowth; and patient evaluation of hair regrowth. At the end of 4 month placebo controlled portions of 12 month clinical studies (ie, baseline to month 4), topical minoxidil (20 mg/ml) demonstrated the following efficacy:

Hair counts: Topical minoxidil was significantly more effective than placebo in producing hair regrowth as assessed by hair counts. Patients using topical minoxidil had a mean increase from baseline of 72 nonvellus hairs in the 1 inch diameter circle compared with a mean increase of 39 nonvellus hairs in patients on placebo.

Investigator evaluation: Of patients on topical minoxidil, 8% demonstrated moderate to dense terminal hair regrowth compared with 4% on placebo. During the initial 4 months of treatment, however, very little regrowth of terminal hair can be expected. Although most patients did not demonstrate cosmetically significant hair regrowth, 26% of the patients showed minimal terminal hair regrowth using topical minoxidil compared with 16% of those using placebo.

Patient evaluation: 26% using topical minoxidil demonstrated moderate to dense hair regrowth compared with 11% using placebo.

Patients who continued on topical minoxidil during the remaining 8 months of the 12 month clinical studies (ie, the non-placebo controlled portion of the studies) continued to sustain a regrowth response. At the end of the 8 months, the following results were obtained:

Hair counts – Patients using topical minoxidil had a mean increase of 112 nonvellus hairs in the same 1 inch diameter circle as compared to month 4.

Investigator evaluation – 39% of the patients achieved moderate to dense terminal hair regrowth by month 12.

Patient evaluation – 48% felt they had achieved moderate to dense hair regrowth at month 12.

Trends in the data suggest that those patients who are older, who have been balding for a longer period of time, or who have a larger area of baldness, may do less well.

MINOXIDIL

Females (18 to 45 years of age; 90% Caucasian) – In females with Ludwig grade I and II diffuse frontoparietal hair thinning, the main parameters of efficacy were: Nonvellus hair counts in a designated 1 cm^2 site on the frontoparietal areas of the scalp; investigator evaluation of hair regrowth; and patient evaluation of hair regrowth. Data demonstrate that 44% to 63% of women with androgenetic alopecia will have discernible growth of nonvellus hair when treated with minoxidil for 32 weeks vs 29% to 39% for vehicle control treated women.

Two 8 month placebo controlled studies produced the following results:

Hair counts – Minoxidil was significantly more effective than placebo in producing hair regrowth as assessed by hair counts in both studies. Patients using minoxidil had a mean increase from baseline of 22.7 and 33.2 nonvellus hairs, respectively, in the same 1 cm^2 site compared with a mean increase of 11 and 19.1 nonvellus hairs, respectively, in patients using placebo.

Investigator evaluation – Based on the investigators' evaluation, 63% (13% moderate and 50% minimal) and 44% (12% moderate and 32% minimal), respectively, of the patients using minoxidil in the two studies achieved hair regrowth at week 32, compared with 39% (6% moderate and 33% minimal) and 29% (5% moderate and 24% minimal), respectively, of those using placebo.

Patient evaluation – Based on the patients' self evaluation, 59% (19% moderate and 40% minimal) and 55% (1% dense, 24% moderate and 30% minimal), respectively, of the patients using minoxidil reported hair regrowth at week 32, compared with 40% (7% moderate and 33% minimal) and 41% (12% moderate and 29% minimal), respectively, of those using placebo.

Hair growth was defined as follows:

Investigator evaluation of growth – No visible new hair growth; minimal growth (definite growth but no substantial covering of thinning areas); moderate growth (new growth partially covering thinning areas, less dense than non-thinning areas; readily discernible); dense growth (full covering of thinning areas; hair density similar to non-thinning areas).

Patient evaluation of growth – No visible hair growth; minimal hair growth (barely discernible); moderate new hair growth (readily discernible); dense new hair growth.

Indications:

Treatment of androgenetic alopecia, expressed in males as baldness of the vertex of the scalp and in females as diffuse hair loss or thinning of the frontoparietal areas. At least 4 months of twice daily applications are generally required before evidence of hair growth can be expected.

Unlabeled uses: Although further study is needed, topical minoxidil may be useful in the treatment of alopecia areata (a systemic disease in which patches of hair fall out over a period of a few days; any part of the body may be involved).

Contraindications:

Hypersensitivity to any component of the preparation.

Warnings:

Cardiac lesions: Minoxidil produces several cardiac lesions in animals. The significance of these lesions for humans is not clear, as they have not been recognized in patients treated with oral minoxidil at systemically active doses (see the systemic Minoxidil monograph in the Antihypertensive Vasodilators section).

Need for normal scalp: The majority of clinical studies included only healthy patients with normal scalps and no cardiovascular disease. Before starting a patient on topical minoxidil, ascertain that the patient has a healthy, normal scalp. Local abrasion or dermatitis may increase absorption and, hence, increase the risk of side effects.

Systemic effects: Although extensive use has not revealed evidence that enough topical drug is absorbed to cause systemic effects, greater absorption because of misuse, individual variability or unusual sensitivity could lead to a systemic effect.

As is the case with other topically applied drugs, decreased integrity of the epidermal barrier caused by inflammation or disease processes in the skin (eg, excoriations of the scalp, scalp psoriasis, severe sunburn) may increase percutaneous absorption. Also, do not use in conjunction with other topical agents (eg, corticosteroids, retinoids, petrolatum) or agents that are known to enhance cutaneous drug absorption.

Heart disease: Adverse effects might be especially serious in patients with a history of underlying heart disease. Be alert for tachycardia and fluid retention and watch for increased heart rate, weight gain or other systemic effects.

Pregnancy: Category C. Adequate and well controlled studies have not been conducted in pregnant women. Do not administer to a pregnant woman.

Lactation: Because of the potential for adverse effects in nursing infants from minoxidil absorption, do not apply on a nursing woman.

Children: Safety and efficacy in patients < 18 years of age have not been established.

Precautions:

Monitoring: Patients being considered for topical minoxidil should have a history and physical examination. Advise of the potential risk; the patient and physician should decide that the benefits outweigh the risks.

Monitor patients at least 1 month after starting topical minoxidil and at least every 6 months thereafter. If systemic effects occur, discontinue use.

Alcohol base: This product contains an alcohol base which will cause burning and irritation of eyes. In the event of accidental contact with sensitive surfaces (eg, eyes, abraded skin, mucous membranes), bathe the area with large amounts of cool tap water.

Avoid inhalation of the spray mist.

For topical use only. Accidental ingestion could lead to adverse systemic effects.

Adverse Reactions:

Hypersensitivity: Non-specific allergic reactions, hives, allergic rhinitis, facial swelling, sensitivity (1.3%; placebo 1%).

Respiratory: Bronchitis, upper respiratory infection, sinusitis (7.2%; placebo 8.6%).

Dermatologic: Irritant dermatitis, allergic contact dermatitis (7.4%; placebo 5.4%); eczema; hypertrichosis; local erythema; pruritus; dry skin/scalp flaking; exacerbation of hair loss; alopecia.

GI: Diarrhea, nausea, vomiting (4.3%; placebo 6.6%).

CNS: Headache, dizziness, faintness, lightheadedness (3.4%; placebo 3.5%).

Musculoskeletal: Fractures, back pain, tendinitis, aches and pains (2.6%; placebo 2.2%).

Cardiovascular: Edema, chest pain, blood pressure increases/decreases, palpitations, pulse rate increases/decreases (1.5%; placebo 1.6%).

Special senses: Conjunctivitis, ear infections, vertigo (1.2%; placebo 1.2%); visual disturbances including decreased visual acuity.

Metabolic: Edema, weight gain (1.2%; placebo 1.3%).

GU: Urinary tract infections, renal calculi, urethritis, prostatitis, epididymitis, vaginitis, vulvitis, vaginal discharge, itching (0.9%; placebo 0.8% to 1.1%); sexual dysfunction.

Psychiatric: Anxiety, depression, fatigue (0.4%; placebo 1%).

Hematologic: Lymphadenopathy, thrombocytopenia, anemia (0.3%; placebo 0.6%).

Endocrine: Menstrual changes, breast symptoms (0.5%; placebo 0.5%).

Overdosage:

Topical: Increased systemic absorption of minoxidil may potentially occur if more frequent or larger doses than directed are used or if the drug is applied to large surface areas of the body or areas other than the scalp. There are no known cases of minoxidil overdosage resulting from topical administration.

In a 14 day controlled clinical trial, 1 ml of 3% minoxidil solution was applied 8 times daily (6 times the recommended dose) to the scalp of 11 healthy male volunteers and to the chest of 11 other volunteers. No significant systemic effects were observed in these subjects when compared with a similar number of placebo-treated subjects.

Systemic: Because of the high concentration of minoxidil in the topical solution, accidental ingestion has the potential of producing systemic effects related to the pharmacologic action of the drug (5 ml contains 100 mg minoxidil, the maximum adult dose for oral minoxidil administration when used to treat hypertension).

Symptoms – Signs and symptoms of minoxidil overdosage would most likely be cardiovascular effects associated with fluid retention and tachycardia.

Treatment – Manage fluid retention with appropriate diuretic therapy. Control clinically significant tachycardia by administration of a β-adrenergic blocking agent. If encountered, control hypotension by IV administration of normal saline. Avoid sympathomimetic drugs, such as norepinephrine and epinephrine, because of their excessive cardiac-stimulating activity.

MINOXIDIL

Patient Information:

Evidence of hair growth usually will take ≥ 4 months.

First hair growth may be soft, downy, colorless hair that is barely visible. After further treatment, the new hair should be the same color and thickness as the other hair on the scalp.

If there is no response to treatment after a reasonable period of time (≥ 4 months), consult physician as to whether to discontinue use.

If treatment is stopped, new hair will probably be shed within a few months.

If one or two daily applications are missed, restart twice-daily application and return to the usual schedule. Do not attempt to make up for missed applications.

More frequent applications or use of larger doses (> 1 ml twice a day) will not speed up the process of hair growth and may increase the possibility of side effects.

Minoxidil topical solution contains alcohol, which could cause burning or irritation of the eyes, mucous membranes or sensitive skin areas. If accidental contact occurs, bathe the area with large amounts of cool tap water. Consult physician if irritation persists.

Because absorption of minoxidil may be increased and the risk of side effects may become greater, apply only to the scalp; do not use on other parts of the body. Do not use if scalp becomes irritated or is sunburned; do not use along with other topical medication on scalp.

Administration and Dosage:

Dry the hair and scalp prior to application. Apply 1 ml to the total affected areas of the scalp twice daily, once in the morning and at night. The total daily dosage should not exceed 2 ml. If finger tips are used to facilitate drug application, wash hands afterwards. Twice daily application for ≥ 4 months may be required before evidence of hair regrowth is observed. Onset and degree of hair regrowth may be variable among patients. If hair regrowth is realized, twice daily applications are necessary for additional and continued hair regrowth. Some anecdotal patient reports indicate that regrown hair and the balding process return to their untreated state 3 to 4 months following cessation of the drug.

Other topical agents: Do not use in conjunction with other topical agents including topical corticosteroids, retinoids and petrolatum or agents that are known to enhance cutaneous drug absorption.

otc	**Rogaine** (Pharmacia & Upjohn)	**Solution:** 2%	In 60 ml bottle with multiple applicators.
otc	**Minoxidil for Men** (Lemmon)	**Topical solution:** 2%	60% alcohol. In 60 ml single and twin pouches.

MASOPROCOL

Actions:

Pharmacology: The mechanism of action of masoprocol in the treatment of actinic keratoses is unknown. In tissue culture, masoprocol has antiproliferative activity against keratinocytes. However, the relevance of this activity to its therapeutic effect has not been established.

Pharmacokinetics: A study in 6 male patients with a single topical application of masoprocol cream demonstrated low absorption (< 1%) as measured by plasma, urine and feces over the 96 hour period after application. In a separate study, 6 patients who were treated twice daily for 28 days demonstrated up to 2% absorption over the 96 hour period after application.

Indications:

Topical treatment of actinic (solar) keratoses.

Contraindications:

Hypersensitivity to masoprocol or any other ingredients of the formulation.

Warnings:

Occlusive dressings: Do not use occlusive dressings with this product.

Mutagenesis: Masoprocol produced mutagenic results in the Ames assay. It was negative with three strains of Salmonella and positive with one.

Pregnancy: Category B. There are no adequate and well controlled studies in pregnant women. Use during pregnancy only if clearly needed.

Lactation: It is not known whether this drug is excreted in breast milk. Exercise caution when the drug is applied to a nursing woman.

Children: Safety and efficacy have not been established.

MASOPROCOL

Precautions:

Allergic contact dermatitis: Masoprocol frequently induces sensitization (allergic contact dermatitis). When patients treated with 5% or 10% masoprocol cream in clinical trials were patch tested with a 1% cream, 9% had reactions indicative of sensitization. In patients rechallenged with 10% cream, dermal reactions were more frequent and more severe. Discontinue use of masoprocol if sensitivity is noted. Masoprocol does not appear to cause photosensitization. However, because solar keratoses are related to exposure to sunlight, the patient should avoid undue sun exposure.

For external use only: Avoid contact with the eyes. If applying the product near the eyes, nose or mouth, advise patients to do so with special care. If masoprocol comes into contact with the eyes (conjunctiva), itching, irritation or transient pain may occur; wash the eye with water promptly. If masoprocol is applied with fingers, wash the hands immediately after use.

Staining: Masoprocol cream may stain clothing or fabrics.

Sulfite sensitivity: This product contain sulfites which may cause allergic-type reactions (eg, hives, itching, wheezing, anaphylaxis) in certain susceptible persons. Although the overall prevalence of sulfite sensitivity is probably low, it is seen more frequently in asthmatics or in atopic nonasthmatic persons.

Adverse Reactions:

Erythema, flaking (46%); itching (32%); dryness (27%); edema (14%); burning (12%); soreness (5%); bleeding, crusting, eye irritation, oozing, rash, skin irritation, soreness, stinging, tightness, tingling (1% to 5%); blistering, eczema, excoriation, fissuring, leathery feeling to the skin, skin roughness, wrinkling (< 1%).

While local skin reactions are frequent, they usually resolve within 2 weeks of discontinuation. The presence or absence of local skin reactions does not correlate with successful ultimate therapeutic outcome.

Overdosage:

In animals receiving high oral doses of masoprocol, the commonly affected systems were the GI and hepatic systems. If ingested, evacuate stomach contents, taking care to prevent aspiration.

Patient Information:

For external use only. Take special care if masoprocol cream is to be applied near the eyes, nose or mouth. In case of contact with the eye, wash the eye with water promptly.

If masoprocol cream is applied with fingers, wash the hands immediately after use.

Contact physician immediately if a severe reaction occurs, including, for example, oozing or blistering.

While using this product, do not use other skin care products or make-up without the advice of a physician.

Administration and Dosage:

Approved by the FDA on September 4, 1992.

Wash and dry areas where actinic keratoses are present. Gently massage masoprocol into the area where actinic keratoses are present until it is evenly distributed, avoiding the eyes and mucous membranes of the nose and mouth. Repeat application each morning and evening for 28 days.

Do not use occlusive dressings.

Immediately after applying masoprocol, the patient might experience a transient local burning sensation.

Rx	**Actinex** (Schwarz Pharma)	**Cream:** 10%	With isostearyl and stearyl alcohol, light mineral oil, parabens, polyethylene glycol 400, propylene glycol and sodium metabisulfite. In 30 g tubes.

TRETINOIN

Topical tretinoin is also used as a treatment for acne vulgaris. Refer to the monograph in the Acne Products section.

Actions:

Pharmacology: The exact mechanism of action of tretinoin is unknown, although retinoids are believed to exert an effect on the growth and differentiation of various epithelial cells. However, when applied topically there is no noted increase in desmosine, hydroxyproline or elastin mRNA in human skin. In addition, the role of the irritative nature of this product in bringing out its positive effects is not fully determined.

Pharmacokinetics: The transdermal absorption of tretinoin from various topical formulations ranged from 1% to 31% of applied dose, depending on whether it was applied to healthy skin or dermatatic skin.

Clinical trials: Two trials were conducted involving 161 patients treated with tretinoin and 154 patients treated with the vehicle emollient cream on the face for 24 weeks as an adjunct to a comprehensive skin care and sun avoidance program, to assess the effects on the wrinkling, mottled hyperpigmentation and tactile skin roughness.

The results of these assessments are as follows:

Tretinoin Effects on Various Dermatologic Conditions

Condition/Treatment	No improvement	Minimal improvement	Moderate improvement
Fine wrinkling			
Tretinoin + CSP[1]	36%	40%	24%
Vehicle + CSP	62%	30%	8%
Mottled hyperpigmentation			
Tretinoin + CSP	35%	27%	38%
Vehicle + CSP	53%	21%	27%
Tactile skin roughness			
Tretinoin + CSP	49%	35%	16%
Vehicle + CSP	67%	23%	10%

[1] CSP = Comprehensive skin protection and sun avoidance programs including use of sunscreens, protective clothing and emollient cream.

Most of the improvement was noted during the first 24 weeks of therapy. Thereafter, therapy primarily maintained the improvement noticed during the first 24 weeks.

Indications:

Dermatologic conditions: Adjuntive agent for use in the mitigation (palliation) of the fine wrinkles, mottled hyperpigmentation and tactile roughness of facial skin in patients who do not achieve such palliation using comprehensive skin care and sun avoidance programs alone.

Contraindications:

Sensitivity reactions to any of the drug's components; discontinue if hypersensitivity to any ingredient is noted.

Warnings:

Mitigating effects: Tretinoin has shown no mitigating effects on significant signs of chronic sun exposure (eg, coarse or deep wrinkling, skin yellowing, lentigines, telangiectasia, skin laxity, keratinocytic atypia, melanocytic atypia or dermal elastosis).

Tretinoin does not eliminate wrinkles, repair sun damaged skin, reverse photoaging or restore a more youthful or younger dermal histologic pattern.

Many patients achieve desired palliative effect on fine wrinkling, mottled hyperpigmentation and tactile roughness of facial skin with the use of comprehensive skin care and sun avoidance programs including sunscreens, protective clothing and emollient creams containing tretinoin.

Long-term use: Tretinoin is a dermal irritant, and the results of continued irritation of the skin for > 48 weeks are not known. There is evidence of atypical changes in melanocytes and keratinocytes and of increased dermal elastosis in some patients treated with tretinoin for > 48 weeks.

Photosensitivity: Because of heightened burning susceptibility, avoid or minimize exposure to sunlight (including sunlamps) during use of tetinoin. Warn patients to use sunscreens (minimum SPF of 15) and protective clothing when using tretinoin. Advise patients with sunburn not to use tretinoin until fully recovered. Patients who may have considerable sun exposure due to their occupations and those with inherent sensitvity to sunlight should exercise particular caution when using tretinoin.

Local reactions: Topical use may cause severe erythema, pruritus, burning, stinging and peeling at the site of application. These signs and symptoms were usually of mild to moderate severity and generally occurred early in therapy. In most patients,

TRETINOIN

the dryness, peeling and redness recurred after the initial (24 weeks) decline. If the degree of local irritation warrants, direct patients to use less medication, decrease the freuqncy of application, discontinue use temporarily or dicontinue use altogether. Four percent of patients had to discontinue use of tretinoin because of adverse reactions.

Eczematous skin: Tretinoin has been reported to cause severe irritation on eczematous skin and should only be used with utmost caution in patients with this condition.

Carcinogenesis: In a lifetime dermal study in CD-1 mice, at 100 and 200 times the average recommended human topical clinical dose, a few skin tumors in the female mice and liver tumors in the male mice were observed. The biological significance of these findings is not clear beacue they occurred at doses that exceeded the dermal maximally tolerated dose of tretinoin and because they were within the background natural occurrence rats for these tumors in this strain of mice.

Pregnancy: Category C. Thirty cases of temporally-associated congential malformations have been reported during two decades of clinical use of another formulation of topical tretinoin (acne preparation). Although no definite pattern of teratogenicity and no causal association has been established from these cases, five of the reports describe the rare birth defect category holoprosencephaly (defects associated with incomplete midline development of the forebrain). The significance of these spontaneous reports in terms of risk to the fetus is unknown.

Lactation: It is not known whether this drug is excreted in breast milk. Exercise caution when administering to a nursing woman.

Children: Safety and efficacy in patients < 18 years of age have not been established.

Drug Interactions:

Topical preparations: Use caution with concomitatnt topcial medications, medicated or abrasive soaps, shampoos, cleansers, cosmetics with a strong drying effect, products with high concentrations of alcohol, astringents, spices or lime, permanent wave solutions, electrolysis, hair depilatories or waxes, and products that may irritate the skin in patients being treated with tretinoin because they may increase irritation.

Photosensitizers: Do not use tretinoin if the patient is also taking drugs known to be photosensitizers (eg, thiazides, tetracyclines, fluoroquinolones, phenothiazines, sulfonamides) because of the possibility of augmented phototoxicity.

Adverse Reactions:

Dermatologic: Peeling, dry skin, burning, stinging, erythema and pruritus (see Warnings).

CNS: Neurotoxicity (one report; the patient was using a large amount of topical tretinoin and had hepatic dysfunction).

Overdosage:

Application of larger amounts of medication than recommended will not lead to more rapid or better results, and marked redness, peeling or discomfort may occur. Oral ingestion of the drug may lead to the same side effects as those assocaited with excessive oral intake of vitamin A.

Patient Information:

Tretinoin is not a cosmetic preparation. Apply only as an adjunct to a comprehensive skin care and sun avoidance program. Use a sunscreeen with minimun SPF of 15 during the day when being treated with tretinoin. Following discontinuation of tretinoin, continued avoidance of the sun and use of a sunscreen with a minimum SPF of 15 is recommended. Avoid direct sun exposure as much as possible and avoid sunlamps totally while using tretinoin. Do not use if sunburned or if eczema or other chronic skin conditions exist. Do not use if inherently sensitive to sunlight or if also taking other drugs that increase senstivity to sunlight.

Never use tretinoin more often than instructed as application of larger amounts of medication than recommended will not lead to more rapid or better results, and redness, peeling or discomfort may occur (see Overdosage). Only apply tretinoin at bedtime.

Do not use if pregnant, attempting to become pregnant or at high risk of pregnancy.

Use tretinoin with caution. If also using other agents with a strong skin drying effect, products with high concentrations of alcohol, astringents, spices or lime, medicated soaps or shampoos, permanent wave solutions, electrolysis, hair depilatories or waxes, or other preparations or processes that might dry or irritate the skin, unless otherwise instructed by a healthcare practitioner.

Discontinue use and consult doctor if sensitivity or increased irritaiton occurs.

TRETINOIN

A majority of patients will lose most mitigating effects on fine wrinkles, mottled hyperpigmentation and tactile roughness of facial skin with discontinuation of a comprehensive skin care and sun avoidance program including tretinoin; however, the safety and efficacy of tretinoin daily use for > 48 weeks have not been established.

Administration and Dosage:

Apply tretinoin to the face once a day at bedtime, using only enough to cover the entire affected area lightly. Gently wash face with a mild soap, pat the skin dry, and wait 20 to 30 minutes before applying. Apply a pea-sized amount of cream to cover the entire face. Take caution to avoid contact with eyes, ears, nostrils and mouth.

Mitigation (palliation) of fine facial wrinkling, mottled hyperpigmentation and tactile roughness may occur gradually over the course of therapy. Up to 6 months of therapy may be required before the effects are seen. Most of the improvement noted with tretinoin is seen during the first 24 weeks of therapy. Thereafter, therapy primarily maintains the improvement noticed during the first 24 weeks.

Patients treated with tretinoin may use cosmetics, but the areas to be treated should be cleansed thoroughly before the medication is applied.

Storage/Stability: Store between 15° and 25°C (59° and 77°F). Do not freeze.

Rx	**Renova** (Ortho)	**Cream:** 0.05%	In a water in oil emulsion. In 40 and 60 g.

DEXTRANOMER

Actions:

Pharmacology: Dextranomer's ability to remove exudates rapidly and continuously from the surface of the wound results in a reduction of inflammation and edema. In vitro evidence suggests that the suction forces created by the drug may remove bacteria and inflammatory exudates from the surface of the wound.

Dextranomer is a hydrophilic dextran polymer in the form of tiny beads or paste. The hydrophilic beads absorb approximately 4 ml of fluid per 1 g of beads. The beads swell to approximately 4 times their original size. This swelling causes significant suction forces and capillary action in the spaces between the beads. This action continues as long as unsaturated beads or paste are in proximity to the wound.

When applied to the surface of wet ulcers or wounds, dextranomer removes various exudates and particles that impede tissue repair. Low molecular weight components of wound exudates are drawn up within the beads or paste, while higher molecular weight components (plasma proteins and fibrinogen) are found between the swollen beads. Removal of these latter components (particularly fibrin and fibrinogen) retards eschar formation.

Indications:

For use in cleaning wet ulcers and wounds such as venous stasis ulcers, decubitus ulcers, infected traumatic and surgical wounds and infected burns.

Precautions:

For external use only. Avoid contact with the eyes.

Wound packing: When treating cratered decubitus ulcers, do not pack wound tightly. Allow for expansion of beads. Maceration of surrounding skin may result if occlusive dressings are used.

Removal of dextranomer: Do not use dextranomer in deep fistulas, sinus tracts or any body cavity where complete removal is not assured.

Remove the beads or paste once they are saturated. This avoids encrustation which makes removal more difficult. All dextranomer must be removed before any surgical procedures to close the wound (ie, graft or flap).

Edema reduction: Wounds may appear larger during the first few days of treatment due to reduction of edema.

Dry wounds: Not effective in cleansing dry wounds.

Complete healing: Not all wounds require treatment with dextranomer to complete healing. When the wound is no longer wet and a healthy granulation base is established, discontinue dextranomer.

Treatment of the underlying condition (eg, venous or arterial flow, pressure) should proceed concurrently with the use of dextranomer.

Adverse Reactions:

Upon application or removal of beads, transitory pain, bleeding, blistering and erythema have occurred. Severe infections have been associated with administration in both diabetic and immunosuppressed patients.

Patient Information:

For external use only. Avoid contact with the eyes.

DEXTRANOMER

Administration and Dosage:

Application: Debride and clean the wound (dextranomer is not an enzyme and will not debride). Leave cleansed area moist. Apply to at least a thickness of ¼ inch to achieve desired suction effects. Cover area with a dry dressing and close on all sides.

Removal: When saturated, dextranomer changes colors and should be removed. Removal should be as complete as possible and is best achieved by irrigation. Vigorous irrigation (ie, soaking or whirlpool) may be necessary to remove patches that adhere to the wound surface.

Paste may be needed for hard to reach areas or irregular body surfaces.

Mix beads with glycerin either on the dry dressing or in a receptacle or use premixed paste. Do not mix with any substance but glycerin. (See package insert for complete procedure.) Dress wound in the usual manner. Mix a fresh paste for each application. Do not reuse.

Reapply dextranomer beads or paste every 12 hours or more frequently if necessary. Reduce number of applications as exudate diminishes. Discontinue applications when the area is free of exudate and edema, or when a healthy granulation base is present. Consult physician if condition worsens or persists beyond 14 to 21 days.

otc	**Debrisan** (Johnson & Johnson)	**Beads**	In 25, 60 and 120 g containers and 4 g packets (in 7s and 14s).
		Paste	Premixed, sterile. In 10 g packets (6s).

FLEXIBLE HYDROACTIVE DRESSINGS AND GRANULES

Actions:

Pharmacology: The dressings interact with wound exudate producing a soft moist gel at the wound surface enabling removal of the dressing with little or no damage to newly formed tissues. They are designed to remain in place from 1 to 7 days.

Indications:

Dressings: For the local management of: Dermal ulcers; pressure ulcers; leg ulcers; superficial wounds (eg, minor abrasions, donor sites, second-degree burns); protective dressings; postoperative wounds.

Granules: For use in the local management of exudating dermal ulcers in association with the dressings.

Paste: For use in association with *DuoDerm* dressings for local management of exudating dermal ulcers.

Contraindications:

Dermal ulcers involving muscle, tendon or bone; ulcers resulting from infection, such as tuberculosis, syphilis and deep fungal infections; lesions in patients with active vasculitis, such as periarteritis nodosa, systemic lupus erythematosus and cryoglobulinemia; third-degree burns; clinically infected wounds.

Precautions:

Excess exudate: In the presence of excess exudate, the ability of the dressings to remain in place with less frequent leakage may be improved by applying the granules directly into the wound site. Used in this way, with the dressings, the granules may reduce the frequency of dressing change.

Odor: Wounds often have a characteristic disagreeable odor. The odor usually disappears following wound cleansing.

Wound deterioration: When using any occlusive dressing, the wound will increase in size and depth during the initial phase as the necrotic debris is cleaned away.

Infection: If clinical infection develops, discontinue DuoDerm and institute appropriate treatment. Restart *DuoDerm* when the infection has been eradicated.

Administration and Dosage:

Clean and prepare the wound site before application. See package labeling for wound management and application/removal instructions for the dressing and granules. Dressings are designed to remain in place from 1 to 7 days.

otc	**IntraSite** (Smith & Nephew)	**Gel:** 2% graft T starch copolymer, 78% water, 20% propylene glycol. Sterile amorphous hydrogel dressing	In UD 25 g (10s).
otc	**Shur-Clens** (Calgon Vestal)	**Solution:** 20% poloxamer 188	In UD 100 and 200 ml.

FLEXIBLE HYDROACTIVE DRESSINGS AND GRANULES

otc	**DuoDerm** (ConvaTec)	**Dressings, sterile**: 4″ x 4″, 6″ x 8″, 8″ x 8″ and 8″ x 12″	In 3s (8″ x 12″ only), 5s and 20s
		Dressing, adhesive border: 4″ x 4″	In 5s.
		8″ x 8″	In 3s.
		Granules, sterile: 5 g per tube	In 5s.
		Paste, sterile	In 30 g tube.
otc	**DuoDerm CGF** (ConvaTec)	**Control gel formula dressing, sterile:** 4″ x 4″, 6″ x 6″, 8″ x 8″	In 5s.
		Control gel formula border dressing, sterile: 2.5″ x 2.5″, 4″ x 4″, 6″ x 6″, 4″ x 5″, 6″ x 7″ with adhesive borders	In 5s.
otc	**DuoDerm Extra Thin** (ConvaTec)	**Control gel formula dressing, extra thin, sterile:** 4″ x 4″, 6″ x 6″	In 10s.
otc	**Sorbsan** (Dow B. Hickam)	**Pads, sterile**: Calcium alginate fiber 2″ x 2″, 3″ x 3″, 4″ x 4″ and 4″ x 8″	In 1s.
		Wound packing fibers, sterile: Calcium alginate fiber. 12″ (2 g)	In 1s.
otc	**Kaltostat** (Calgon Vestal)	**Dressing, sterile:** Calcium-sodium alginate fiber, 3″x 4¾″	In 1s.
otc	**Kaltostat Fortex** (Calgon Vestal)	**Dressing, sterile:** Calcium-sodium alginate fiber, 4″x 4″	In 1s.

HYDROQUINONE

Actions:

Pharmacology: Hydroquinone depigments hyperpigmented skin by inhibiting the enzymatic oxidation of tyrosine and suppressing other melanocyte metabolic processes, thereby inhibiting melanin formation. Hydroquinone may also act on the essential subcellular metabolic processes of melanocytes with resultant cytolysis (ie, nonenzyme-mediated depigmentation). Skin color diminution usually occurs after 3 or 4 weeks of treatment. Because the rate of depigmentation varies among individuals, a positive response may require 3 weeks to 6 months.

Exposure to sunlight or UV light will cause repigmentation; prevent by using sunblocking agents. In addition to hydroquinone, some products contain sunscreens (eg, octyl dimethyl PABA, ethyl dihydroxypropyl PABA, dioxybenzone, oxybenzone).

Indications:

Temporary bleaching of hyperpigmented skin conditions (eg, freckles, senile lentigines, chloasma and melasma, and other forms of melanin hyperpigmentation).

Contraindications:

Hypersensitivity to hydroquinone or any of the other ingredients of the products.

Warnings:

Sunscreen use is an essential aspect of hydroquinone therapy because minimal sun exposure sustains melanocytic activity. Therefore, avoid sun exposure by using a sunscreen, a sun block or protective clothing to prevent repigmentation.

Sensitivity testing: Test for skin sensitivity before using. Apply small amount to unbroken skin and check in 24 hours. If vesicle formation, itching or excessive inflammation occurs, do not use. Minor redness is not a contraindication.

Discontinue use if no bleaching or lightening effect is noted after 2 months of use.

Pregnancy: Category C. Safety for use during pregnancy has not been established. It is not known whether hydroquinone can cause fetal harm when used topically on a pregnant woman or affect reproductive capacity. It is also not known to what degree, if any, systemic absorption occurs. Use only if clearly needed.

Lactation: It is not known whether topical hydroquinone is absorbed or excreted in breast milk. Caution is advised when used by a nursing mother.

Children: Safety and efficacy in children ≤ 12 years of age have not been established.

Precautions:

Lips: A bitter taste and anesthetic effect may occur if applied to lips.

For external use only. If rash or irritation develops, discontinue treatment. Do not use near eyes. Use in paranasal and infraorbital areas increases the chance of irritation.

Peroxide: Concurrent use of peroxide may result in transient dark staining of skin areas due to oxidation of hydroquinone. Staining can be removed by discontinuing concurrent use and by normal soap cleansing.

Sulfite sensitivity: Some of these products contain sulfites which may cause allergic-type reactions (eg, hives, itching, wheezing, anaphylaxis) in certain susceptible persons. Although the overall prevalence of sulfite sensitivity in the general population is probably low, it is seen more frequently in asthmatics or atopic nonasthmatics.

Adverse Reactions:

Dryness and fissuring of paranasal and infraorbital areas; erythema; stinging; irritation; sensitization and contact dermatitis in susceptible individuals.

Overdosage:

There have been no systemic reactions from the use of topical hydroquinone. However, limit treatment to relatively small areas of the body at one time, since some patients experience a transient skin reddening and a mild burning sensation which does not preclude treatment.

Patient Information:

For external use only. Avoid contact with the eyes.

Protection from the sun (eg, sunscreens, clothing) is an essential aspect of therapy.

Do not use on irritated, denuded or damaged skin.

Discontinue use and consult physician if rash or irritation develops.

Administration and Dosage:

Hydroquinone bleaching is faster, more dependable and easier if the treated area is protected from ultraviolet light. Therefore, preparations with a sunscreen may be preferred for use during the day.

Apply to affected skin twice daily.

HYDROQUINONE

otc	**Esoterica Sensitive Skin Formula** (Medicis)	**Cream:** 1.5%	With mineral oil, sodium bisulfite, parabens, EDTA. In 85 g.
otc	**Eldopaque** (ICN)	**Cream:** 2%	With sunblock. In 14.2 and 28.4 g.
otc	**Eldoquin** (ICN)		In 14.2 and 28.4 g.
otc	**Esoterica Facial** (Medicis)		With 3.3% padimate O, 2.5% oxybenzone, sodium bisulfites, parabens, EDTA. In 85 g.
otc	**Esoterica Regular** (Medicis)		With parabens, sodium bisulfite, EDTA. In 85 g.
otc	**Esoterica Sunscreen** (Medicis)		With 3.3% padimate O, 2.5% oxybenzone, mineral oil, parabens, sodium bisulfite, EDTA. In 85 g.
otc	**Porcelana** (DEP)		In 60 and 120 g.
otc	**Porcelana with Sunscreen** (DEP)		With 2.5% padimate O. In 120 g.
otc	**Solaquin** (ICN)		With sunscreens. In 28.4 g.
Rx	**Eldopaque-Forte** (ICN)	**Cream:** 4%	In a sunblock base. With talc, iron oxides, mineral oil, EDTA, sodium metabisulfite. In 14.2 and 28.4 g.
Rx	**Eldoquin-Forte Sunbleaching** (ICN)		In a vanishing cream base. With mineral oil, propylparaben, sodium metabisulfite. In 14.2 and 28.4 g.
Rx	**Solaquin Forte** (ICN)		With 5% ethyl dihydroxypropyl PABA, 3% dioxybenzone, 2% oxybenzone, EDTA, sodium metabisulfite. In 14.2 and 28.4 g.
Rx	**Nuquin HP** (Stratus)		30 mg dioxybenzone, 20 mg oxybenzone per g. Stearyl alcohol, EDTA, sodium metabisulfite. Vanishing base. In 14.2, 28.4 and 56.7 g.
Rx	**Melquin HP** (Stratus)		Mineral oil, propylparaben, sodium metabisulfite. Vanishing base. In 14.2 and 28.4 g.
Rx	**Melpaque HP** (Stratus)		EDTA, sodium metabisulfite, talc. Tinted, sunblocking base. In 14.2 and 28.4 g.
Rx	**Viquin Forte** (ICN)		80 mg padimate O, 30 mg dioxybenzone, 20 mg oxybenzone/g, stearyl alcohol, cetearly alcohol, EDTA, sodium metabisulfite. PABA-free. In 28.4 g.
otc	**Ambi Skin Tone** (Kiwi Brands)	**Cream**	Dry, oily and normal skin formulas. With padimate O, sodium metabisulfite, parabens, EDTA, vitamin E. In 57 and 114 g.
Rx	**Melanex** (Neutrogena)	**Solution:** 3%	With 45% SD alcohol 40, propylene glycol. In 30 ml.
Rx	**Hydroquinone** (Glades)		With 45% SD alcohol 40, proylene glycol, 4% isopropyl alcohol. In 30 ml with applicator.
Rx	**Hydroquinone** (Glades)	**Gel:** 3%	With 5% padimate O, 3% dioxybenzone, EDTA, sodium metabisulfite. Hydroalcoholic base. In 30 g.
otc	**NeoStrata AHA Gel for Age Spots and Skin Lightening** (NeoStrata)	**Gel:** 2%	SD alcohol 40, glycolic acid, propylene glycol, polyquaternuim-10, sodium bisulfite, citric acid, sodium sulfite, EDTA, BHT

HYDROQUINONE

Rx	**Solaquin Forte** (ICN)	**Gel:** 4%	With 5% ethyl dihydroxypropyl PABA, 3% dioxybenzone, EDTA, sodium metabisulfite. Hydroalcoholic base. In 14.2 and 28.4 g.
Rx	**Nuquin HP** (Stratus)		Alcohol, sodium metabisulfite, EDTA. In 14.2 and 28.4 g

FORMALDEHYDE

Indications:

Antiperspirant for treatment of hyperhidrosis and bromidrosis. Drying agent for pre- and post-surgical removal of warts or nonsurgical laser treatment of warts.

Contraindications:

Hypersensitivity to any ingredients of the product.

Precautions:

For external use only. Avoid contact with eyes or mucous membranes.

Irritation/Sensitivity: May be irritating and sensitizing to the skin of some patients; check skin for sensitivity prior to application. If redness or irritation persists, consult physician.

Administration and Dosage:

Apply once a day to affected areas as directed.

Rx	**Formalyde-10** (Pedinol)	**Spray:** 10%	In 60 ml.
Rx	**Lazer Formalyde** (Pedinol)	**Solution:** 10%	In 90 ml.

IMIQUIMOD

Actions:

Pharmacology: Imiquimod is an immune response modifier. The mechanism of action of imiquimod in treating genital/perianal warts is unknown. Imiquimod has no direct antiviral activity in cell culture. Mouse skin studies suggest that imiquimod induces cytokines, including interferon-alpha and others, in humans and animals. However, the clinical relevance of these findings is unknown.

Pharmacokinetics: Percutaneous absorption of imiquimod was minimal in a study involving six healthy subjects treated with a single topical application (5 mg) of imiquimod cream. Less than 0.9% of the dose was excreted in the urine and feces following topical application.

Clinical trials: In a double-blind placebo controlled clinical trial, 209 otherwise healthy patients ≥ 18 years of age with genital/perianal warts were treated with imiquimod 5% cream or vehicle control 3 times a week for a maximum of 16 weeks. The median baseline wart area was 69 mm^2 (range 8 to 5525 mm^2). Fifty percent of patients experienced complete clearance of warts.

Indications:

Genital and perianal warts: Treatment of external genital and perianal warts/condyloma acuminata in adults.

Contraindications:

None known.

Warnings:

Other conditions: Imiquimod has not been evaluated for the treatment of urethral, intravaginal, cervical, rectal or intra-anal human papilloma viral disease and is not recommended for these conditions.

Pregnancy: Category B. There are no adequate and well controlled studies in pregnant women.

Lactation: It is not known whether imiquimod is excreted in breast milk.

Children: Safety and efficacy in patients < 18 years of age have not been established.

Precautions:

Skin reactions: The most frequently reported adverse reactions were local skin and application site reactions. These reactions were usually mild to moderate in intensity. These reactions were more frequent and more intense with daily application than with 3 times a week application. In the 3 times a week application clinical studies, 1.2% (4/327) of the patients discontinued because of local skin/application site reactions.

Local skin reactions such as erythema, erosion, excoriation/flaking and edema are common. Should severe local skin reaction occur, remove the cream by washing the treatment area with mild soap and water. Treatment with imiquimod cream can be resumed after the skin reaction has subsided. There is no clinical experience with imiquimod cream therapy immediately following the treatment of genital/perianal warts with other cutaneously applied drugs; therefore, imiquimod cream administration is not recommended until genital/perianal tissue is healed from any previous drug or surgical treatment. Imiquimod has the potential to exacerbate inflammatory conditions of the skin.

Adverse Reactions:

Imiquimod Adverse Reactions (3 Times a Week Application) (%)				
Adverse reaction	Mild/moderate		Severe	
	Females	Males	Females	Males
Local				
Erythema	61	54	4	4
Itching	32	22	-	-
Erosion	30	29	1	1
Burning	26	9	-	-
Excoriation/flaking	18	25	0	1
Edema	17	12	1	0
Pain	8	2	-	-
Induration	5	7	0	0
Ulceration	5	4	3	0
Scabbing	4	13	0	0
Vesicles	3	2	0	0
Soreness	3	0	-	-

Imiquimod Adverse Reactions (3 Times a Week Application) (%)				
	Mild/moderate		Severe	
Adverse reaction	Females	Males	Females	Males
Systemic				
Headache	4	5	-	-
Influenza-like symptoms	3	1	-	-
Myalgia	1	1	-	-

Females: Fungal infection (11%); erythema (3%); ulceration (2%); edema (1%).

Males: Erosion, fungal infection (2%); erythema, edema, induration, excoriation/flaking (1%).

Other adverse reactions (> 1%) include: Application site disorders; wart site reactions (eg, burning, hypopigmentation, irritation, itching, pain, rash, sensitivity, soreness, stinging, tenderness); remote site reactions (eg, bleeding, burning, itching, pain, tenderness, tinea cruris); fatigue; fever; influenza-like symptoms; headache; diarrhea; myalgia.

Overdosage:

Overdosage of imiquimod in humans is unlikely because of minimal percutaneous absorption. Animal studies reveal a rabbit dermal lethal imiquimod dose of > 1600 mg/m^2. Persistent topical overdosing of imiquimod could result in severe local skin reactions. The most clinically serious adverse event reported following multiple oral imiquimod doses of > 200 mg was hypotension that resolved following oral or IV fluid administration.

Patient Information:

Imiquimod may weaken condoms and vaginal diaphragms. Therefore, concurrent use is not recommended.

This medication is for external use only. Avoid contact with eyes.

Do not occlude the treatment area with bandages or other covers or wraps.

Avoid sexual (genital, anal, oral) contact while the cream is on the skin.

Wash the treatment area with mild soap and water 6 to 10 hours following application of imiquimod.

Patients commonly experience local skin reactions such as erythema, erosion, excoriation/flaking and edema at the site of application or surrounding areas. Most skin reactions are mild to moderate. Severe skin reactions can occur; promptly report severe reactions to the physician.

Uncircumcised males treating warts under the foreskin should retract the foreskin and clean the area daily.

Imiquimod is not a cure; new warts may develop during therapy.

Administration and Dosage:

Apply imiquimod 3 times per week, prior to normal sleeping hours, and leave on the skin for 6 to 10 hours. Following the treatment period, remove cream by washing the treated area with mild soap and water. Examples of 3 times per week application schedules are: Monday, Wednesday, Friday; or Tuesday, Thursday, Saturday. Continue imiquimod treatment until there is total clearance of the genital/perianal warts or for ≤ 16 weeks. A rest period of several days may be taken if required by the patient's discomfort or severity of the local skin reaction. Treatment may resume once the reaction subsides.

Non-occlusive dressings such as cotton gauze or cotton underwear may be used in the management of skin reactions. Handwashing before and after cream application is recommended. Imiquimod is packaged in single-use packets that contain sufficient cream to cover a wart area of up to 20 cm^2; avoid use of excessive amounts of cream. Instruct patients to apply imiquimod to external or perianal warts. Apply a thin layer to the wart area and rub in until the cream is no longer visible. Do not occlude the application site.

Storage/Stability: Do not store at > 30°C (86°F). Avoid freezing.

Rx	**Aldara** (3M)	**Cream:** 5%	In 250 mg single-use packets. In boxes of 12.

CAPSAICIN

Actions:

Pharmacology: Capsaicin is a natural chemical derived from plants of the solanaceae family. Although the precise mechanism of action is not fully understood, evidence suggests that the drug renders skin and joints insensitive to pain by depleting and preventing reaccumulation of substance P in peripheral sensory neurons. Substance P is thought to be the principle chemomediator of pain impulses from the periphery to the central nervous system.

Indications:

Temporary relief of pain from rheumatoid arthritis, osteoarthritis and relief of neuralgias such as the pain following shingles (herpes zoster) or painful diabetic neuropathy.

Unlabeled uses: Capsaicin is being investigated for use in other disorders including psoriasis, vitiligo and intractable pruritus, as well as postmastectomy and postamputation neuroma (phantom limb syndrome), vulvar vestibulitis, apocrine chromhidrosis and reflex sympathetic dystrophy.

Warnings:

For external use only. Avoid getting in eyes or on broken or irritated skin. Use care when handling contact lenses following application of capsaicin; irritation and burning may occur following lens insertion. Washing hands or using gloves or an applicator may alleviate this problem.

Bandage use: Do not bandage tightly.

Worsened condition: If condition worsens or if symptoms persist 14 to 28 days, discontinue use and consult physician.

Adverse Reactions:

Burning (≥ 30%; usually diminishes with repeated use); stinging; erythema; cough; respiratory irritation

Patient Information:

For external use only. Avoid contact with the eyes. Use caution when handling contact lens following application; washing hands or using gloves or an applicator is recommended.

Do not bandage tightly.

If condition worsens or symptoms persist 14 to 28 days, contact a physician.

Administration and Dosage:

Adults and children ≥ 2 years of age: Apply to affected area not more than 3 or 4 times daily. May cause transient burning on application. This is observed more frequently when application schedules of < 3 or 4 times daily are used. If applied with the fingers, wash hands immediately after application.

otc	**Capsin** (Flemming)	**Lotion:** 0.025% capsaicin	Benzyl alcohol, propylene glycol, denatured alcohol. In 59 ml.
otc	**Capsin** (Flemming)	**Lotion:** 0.075% capsaicin	Benzyl alcohol, propylene glycol, denatured alcohol. In 59 ml.
otc	**Capzasin•P** (Thompson Medical)	**Cream:** 0.025% capsaicin	Benzyl and cetyl alcohol. In 42.5 g.
otc	**Pain Doctor** (Fougera)	**Cream:** 0.025% capsaicin	25% methyl salicylate, 10% menthol, propylene glycol, parabens. In 60 g.
otc	**Zostrix** (GenDerm)	**Cream:** 0.025% in an emollient base	In 45 and 90 g.
otc	**Zostrix-HP** (GenDerm)	**Cream:** 0.075% in an emollient base	In 30 and 60 g.
otc	**Dolorac** (GenDerm)	**Cream:** 0.25% in an emollient base.	Benzyl alcohol and cetyl alcohol. In 28 g tubes.
otc	**R-Gel** (Healthline Labs)	**Gel:** 0.025%	EDTA. In 15 and 30 g.

CAPSAICIN

otc	**Pain-X** (BF Ascher)	**Gel:** 0.05% capsaicin, 5% menthol, 4% camphor	Alcohols, parabens. In 42.5 g.
otc	**No Pain-HP** (Young Again Products)	**Roll-on:** 0.075%	In 60 ml.

ALUMINUM CHLORIDE HEXAHYDRATE

Indications:

An astringent used as an aid in the management of hyperhidrosis.

Warnings:

For external use only. Avoid contact with the eyes.

Discontinue use if irritation or sensitization occurs.

Metals/fabrics: Aluminum chloride hexahydrate may be harmful to certain metals and fabrics.

Precautions:

Burning or prickling sensation may occur. Do not apply to broken, irritated or recently shaved skin.

Administration and Dosage:

Apply to the affected area once a day, only at bedtime. To help prevent irritation, completely dry area prior to application.

For maximum effect cover the treated area with plastic wrap, held in place by a snug fitting "T" or body shirt, mitten or sock. (Never hold plastic wrap in place with tape.) Wash the treated area the following morning. Excessive sweating may stop after ≥ 2 treatments. Thereafter, apply once or twice weekly or as needed.

Rx	**Drysol** (Person & Covey)	**Solution:** 20% in 93% SD alcohol 40	In 37.5 ml or 35 ml with Dab-O-Matic applicator.

MONOBENZONE

Indications:

Final depigmentation in extensive vitiligo.

Contraindications:

Freckling; hyperpigmentation due to photosensitization following use of certain perfumes or following inflammation of the skin; melasma (chloasma) of pregnancy; cafe-au-lait spots; pigmented nevi; malignant melanoma; pigment resulting from pigments other than melanin, including bile, silver and artificial pigments; hypersensitivity to monobenzone or any ingredients of the product.

Warnings:

Extensive vitiligo: Monobenzone is a potent depigmenting agent, not a mild cosmetic bleach; do not use except for final depigmentation in extensive vitiligo.

Pregnancy: Category C. It is not known whether the drug can cause fetal harm when used topically on a pregnant woman. Use only when clearly needed.

Lactation: It is not known whether monobenzone is absorbed or excreted in breast milk. Use with caution in nursing mothers.

Children: Safety and efficacy in children ≤ 12 years of age have not been established.

Adverse Reactions:

Irritation; burning sensation; dermatitis.

Administration and Dosage:

For external use only. Avoid contact with the eyes.

Apply and rub into the pigmented areas to be treated, 2 or 3 times daily. Depigmentation is usually observed after 1 to 4 months of therapy. If satisfactory results have not been obtained within 4 months, discontinue treatment.

Rx	**Benoquin** (ICN)	**Cream:** 20% in a water washable base	In 35.4 g.

HAMAMELIS WATER (Witch Hazel)

Actions:

Pharmacology: Hamamelis water is a mild astringent prepared from twigs of *Hamamelis virginiana*; the distillate is then adjusted with an appropriate amount of alcohol.

Indications:

Temporary relief of anal or vaginal irritation and itching, hemorrhoids, postepisiotomy discomfort and hemorrhoidectomy discomfort.

Warnings:

Worsened conditions: If condition worsens or does not improve within 7 days consult a physician.

Bleeding: In case of bleeding, consult physician promptly.

Precautions:

For external use only. Avoid contact with eyes.

Administration and Dosage:

Apply locally up to 6 times daily or after each bowel movement.

otc	**Witch Hazel** (Various, eg, Humco, Lannett, Purepac)	**Liquid**	In 120 and 240 ml, pt and gal.
otc	**Tucks Hemorrhoidal** (Parke-Davis)	**Cream:** 50%. White petrolatum, 7% alcohol, lanolin	In 42 g.
otc	**A•E•R** (Birchwood)	**Pads:** 50%. 12.5% glycerin, methylparaben, benzalkonium chloride	In 40s.

ARNICA

Indications:

Relief of pain from sprains and bruises; of doubtful value.

Precautions:

For external use only. Avoid getting into eyes or mucous membranes.

Irritation: Do not apply to irritated skin or if excessive irritation develops.

Adverse Reactions:

Arnica is an irritant to mucous membranes; when ingested, it has produced severe gastroenteritis, nervous disturbances, tachycardia, bradycardia and collapse.

Arnica may cause dermatitis in sensitive persons.

Administration and Dosage:

Apply locally with massage 2 or 3 times daily.

otc	**Arnica** (Various, eg, Humco)	**Tincture:** 20%	In 30, 60, 120 ml, pt, gal.

ZINC OXIDE

Indications:

Minor skin irritations, burns, abrasions, chafed skin and diaper rash.

Administration and Dosage:

For external use only. Avoid contact with the eyes.

Apply to affected areas as required.

otc	**Zinc Oxide** (Various, eg, Major, Moore, Paddock, Rugby, Schein)	**Ointment:** 20%	In 30 and 60 g and lb.
otc	**Borofax Skin Protectant** (Warner-Wellcome)	**Ointment:** 15%. 68.6% petrolatum, lanolin, mineral oil	In 50 g.

DIHYDROXYACETONE

Indications:

For vitiligo and hypopigmented skin.

Precautions:

For external use only. Do not apply to hair, eyelids and around eyes.

Sun exposure: Does not protect skin from sunlight; use a sunblock on affected areas.

Administration and Dosage:

Use applicator top to apply evenly to areas of skin to be darkened. Allow to remain on the skin at least 30 minutes before washing. The first effects appear a few hours after initial application. To avoid overapplication, use once at bedtime and allow color to develop overnight. If more color is desired, apply once an hour until proper shade is obtained. The coloration will last 3 to 6 days with gradual and even fading. Any initial overuse will be remedied by natural fading acelerated by gently scrubbing the affected area. Maintenance applications of once a day or less should be sufficient.

otc	**Chromelin Complexion Blender** (Summers)	5% in isopropanol	In 30 ml.

CHLOROPHYLL DERIVATIVES

Actions:

Pharmacology: Aids wound healing by helping to produce a clean, granulating wound base for epithelialization or skin grafting. It also soothes inflamed, painful tissues and controls wound odor, even in malignant lesions. This is a true deodorizing, not a masking, action.

Indications:

Arteriosclerotic, diabetic and varicose ulcers; trophic decubitus ulcers and chronic ulcers of nonspecific origin; malignant lesions (where deodorization is desired); traumatic injuries; skin grafting and skin defects; thermal, chemical and irradiation injuries; a wide variety of dermatoses.

Adverse Reactions:

Sensitivity reactions (rare); itching; irritation.

Administration and Dosage:

Ointment: Apply generously and cover with gauze, linen or other appropriate dressing. For best results, do not change dressings more often than every 48 to 72 hours.

Solution: Apply full strength as continuous wet dressing, or instill directly into sinus tracts, fistulae, deep ulcers or cavities.

otc	**Chloresium** (Rystan)	**Ointment:** 0.5% chlorophyllin copper complex in a hydrophilic base	In 30 and 120 g and lb.
		Solution: 0.2% chlorophyllin copper complex in isotonic saline	In 240 and 960 ml.

BORIC ACID OINTMENT

Indications:

A soothing application for chafed skin, abrasions, burns and other skin irritations.

Administration and Dosage:

For external use only. Avoid contact with the eyes.

Apply directly to affected area once or twice daily.

otc	**Boric Acid** (Various, eg, Ambix, Clay-Park, Fougera, IDE, Major, Moore, NMC, Rugby, URL)	**Ointment:** 10%	In 30 and 60 g and lb.

TOPICAL COMBINATIONS, MISCELLANEOUS

Principal active ingredients of these formulations include:

BORIC ACID, OXYQUINOLINE and BENZALKONIUM Cl are used as antiseptics.

ZINC OXIDE, CALAMINE, ALUMINUM and ALUMINUM ACETATE provide astringent and topical protectant actions.

CAMPHOR, EUCALYPTOL, MENTHOL and PHENOL are used as antipruritics, mild local anesthetics and counterirritants.

BENZOCAINE and LIDOCAINE are local anesthetics.

PYRILAMINE MALEATE is an antihistamine.

CASTOR OIL (RICINUS OIL), GLYCERIN and MINERAL OIL are used as emollients.

BENZYL ALCOHOL is used as an antipruritic.

BISMUTH SUBNITRATE is used as a skin protectant.

BALSAM PERU is used to stimulate tissue growth.

BIEBRICH SCARLET RED is used to promote wound healing.

ICHTHAMMOL is used as an anti-infective.

JUNIPER TAR is used as an antieczematic.

SULFUR provides antibacterial, peeling and drying action.

otc	**Boyol Salve** (Pfeiffer)	**Salve:** 10% ichthammol, benzocaine, lanolin, petrolatum	In 30 g.
otc	**Dr. Dermi-Heal** (Quality)	**Ointment:** 1% allantoin, zinc oxide, Balsam Peru, castor oil, petrolatum *For relief of diaper rash, chafing, minor burns, bed sores, external vaginal itching and irritation, ostomy irritation and heat rash.*	In 75 g.
otc	**Ichthammol** (Various, eg, NMC)	**Ointment:** 10% or 20% ichthammol, lanolin-petrolatum base *For relief of minor skin irritations.*	In 28.4g.
otc	**Mammol** (Abbott)	**Ointment:** 40% bismuth subnitrate, 30% castor oil, 22% anhydrous lanolin, 7% ceresin wax and 1% Balsam Peru *For prevention of sore, cracked nipples during lactation.*	In 25 g.
otc	**Saratoga** (Blair)	**Ointment:** Zinc oxide, boric acid, eucalyptol, acetylated lanolin alcohols, white petrolatum, white beeswax *For temporary relief of itching and minor skin irritations, chapped and chafed skin, diaper rash, bed sores, mild burns.*	In 28 and 60 g.
otc	**Unguentine** (Mentholatum)	**Ointment:** 1% phenol, petrolatum, oleostearine, zinc oxide, eucalyptus oil, thyme oil *For pain relief in minor burns.*	In 30 g.
otc	**Ostiderm** (Pedinol)	**Lotion:** Aluminum sulfate, zinc oxide For foot odor/excessive moisture.	In 42.5 ml.
		Roll-On: Aluminum chlorohydrate, camphor, alcohol, EDTA, diazolidinyl urea, Safeguards against offensive odor and dries excessive moisture of the feet.	In 88.7 ml.
otc	**Sarna Anti-Itch** (Stiefel)	**Lotion:** 0.5% camphor, 0.5% menthol, carbomer 940, DMDM hydantoin, glyceryl stearate, PEG-8 stearate, PEG-100 stearate, petrolatum *For relief of dry, itching skin, sunburn, poison ivy and poison oak.*	In 222 ml.
otc	**Schamberg** (Paddock)	**Lotion:** 8.25% zinc oxide, 0.25% menthol, 1.5% phenol, 30% cottonseed oil, 15% olive oil and lime water *For pruritic eczema.*	In 480 ml.

TOPICAL COMBINATIONS, MISCELLANEOUS

otc	**Schamberg's** (C & M)	**Lotion:** Zinc oxide, 0.15% menthol, 1% phenol, peanut oil and lime water *For the temporary relief of itching.*	In 480 ml.
otc	**Soothaderm** (Pharmakon)	**Lotion:** 2.07 mg pyrilamine maleate, 2.08 mg benzocaine and 41.35 mg zinc oxide per ml, simethicone, parabens, propylene glycol, camphor, menthol *For relief of itching due to chicken pox, diaper rash, insect bites, poison ivy/oak, prickly heat and sunburn.*	In 118 ml.
otc	**Florida Sunburn Relief** (Pharmacel)	**Lotion:** 3% benzyl alcohol, 0.4% phenol, 0.2% camphor, 0.15% menthol *For relief of pain due to sunburn.*	In 60 ml.
otc	**Outgro** (Whitehall)	**Solution:** 25% tannic acid, 5% chlorobutanol, 83% isopropyl alcohol *For temporary pain relief of ingrown toenails.*	In 9.3 ml.
otc	**Stypto-Caine** (Pedinol)	**Solution:** 250 mg aluminum chloride, 2.5 mg tetracaine HCl, 1 mg oxyquinoline sulfate per g with glycerin *To stop bleeding in minor cuts.*	In 59 ml.
otc	**Campho-Phenique** (Sterling Health)	**Liquid:** 10.8% camphor, 4.7% phenol, eucalyptus oil, light mineral oil *To relieve pain and combat infections.*	In 22.5, 45 and 120 ml.
otc	**Oxyzal Wet Dressing** (Gordon)	**Liquid:** Oxyquinoline sulfate, benzalkonium Cl 1:2000 *For minor infections.*	In 30, 120 and 480 ml.
otc	**Campho-Phenique** (Sterling Health)	**Gel:** 4.7% phenol, 10.8% camphor, colloidal silicon dioxide, eucalyptus oil, glycerin, light mineral oil *Pain relief in cold sores, fever blisters, cuts, scrapes, burns and insect bites.*	In 6.9 and 15 g.
otc	**Topic** (Syntex)	**Gel:** 5% benzyl alcohol, camphor, menthol, 30% isopropyl alcohol *For temporary relief of itching from poison oak/ivy, insect bites, eczema, minor skin allergies and heat rash.*	In 60 g.
otc	**Aluminum Paste** (Paddock)	**Ointment:** 10% metallic aluminum *An occlusive skin protectant.*	White petrolatum base. In lb.
otc	**Sarna Anti-Itch** (Stiefel)	**Foam:** 0.5% camphor, 0.5% menthol, carbomer 940, DMDM hydantoin, glyceryl stearate, PEG-8 and PEG-100 stearate, petrolatum *For relief of dry, itching skin.*	In 99 g.
otc	**ProTech First-Aid Stik** (Triton)	**Liquid:** 10% povidone iodine, 2.5% lidocaine HCl *For cleaning and pain relief of cuts, scrapes and burns.*	In 14 ml.
otc	**Proderm Topical** (Dow B. Hickam)	**Dressing:** 650 mg castor oil and 72.5 mg Balsam Peru per 0.82 ml *For prevention and management of decubitus ulcers.*	In 113.4 g.
otc	**Dome-Paste** (Miles)	**Wound dressing:** Zinc oxide, calamine, gelatin *For conditions of extremities (eg, varicose ulcers) requiring protection.*	3″ by 10 yd or 4″ by 10 yd bandages.
Rx	**Scarlet Red Ointment Dressings** (Sherwood Medical)	**Wound dressings:** 5% scarlet red, lanolin, olive oil and petrolatum in fine mesh absorbent gauze *For epithelialization of donor sites, burns and wounds.*	In 5″ x 9″ strips.

Iodine Compounds

IODINE

Indications:

Iodine preparations are used externally for their broad microbicidal spectrum against bacteria, fungi, viruses, spores, protozoa and yeasts. Iodine may be used to disinfect intact skin preoperatively. Potassium iodide is added to increase the solubility of the iodine. Sodium iodide is present to stabilize the tincture and make it miscible with water in all proportions.

Contraindications:

Hypersensitivity to iodine.

Warnings:

For external use only: Avoid contact with the eyes and mucous membranes.

Highly toxic if ingested. Sodium thiosulfate is the most effective chemical antidote.

Staining: Iodine preparations stain skin and clothing.

Occlusive dressings: Do not use.

otc	**Iodine Topical** (Various, eg, AA–Spectrum)	**Solution:** 2% iodine and 2.4% sodium iodide in purified water	In 500 and 4000 ml.
otc[1]	**Strong Iodine (Lugol's Solution)** (Various, eg, Lannett)	**Solution:** 5% iodine and 10% potassium iodide in water	In pt and gal.
otc	**Iodine Tincture** (Various, eg, Century, Lannett, Purepac)	**Solution:** 2% iodine and 2.4% sodium iodide in 47% alcohol, purified water	In pt and gal.
otc	**Strong Iodine Tincture** (Various, eg, A-A Spectrum)	**Solution:** 7% iodine and 5% potassium iodide in 83% alcohol	In 500 and 4000 ml.

[1] Some of these products may be available *Rx,* depending on distributor discretion.

Iodine Compounds

POVIDONE IODINE

Actions:

Pharmacology: Water soluble complex of iodine with povidone. Povidone-iodine contains 9% to 12% available iodine. It retains the bactericidal activity of iodine but is less potent, therefore causes less irritation to skin and mucous membranes. In vitro, HIV appears to be completely inactivated by povidone-iodine preparations; further study is needed.

Warnings:

Hypothyroidism: A 6–week-old infant developed low serum total thyroxine concentration and high thyroid stimulating hormone concentration following maternal use of topical povidone-iodine during pregnancy and lactation. In one study, the use of povidone-iodine solution on very-low birthweight infants resulted in neonatal hypothyroidism. In contrast, women who used povidone-iodine douche daily for 14 days did not develop overt hypothyroidism; however, there was a significant increase in serum total iodine concetration and urine iodine excretion. Use with caution during pregnancy and lactation and in infants.

Open wounds: Avoid solutions containing a detergent if treating open wounds with povidone-iodine. The value of povidone-iodine on open wounds has not been established.

Administration and Dosage:

Unlike iodine tincture, treated areas may be bandaged.

otc	**Povidone-Iodine** (Various, eg, Humco, IDE, Major, NMC, Qualitest, Schein, URL)	**Ointment**: 10%	In 30 g and lb.
		Solution: 10%	In pt and gal.
		Liquid	In pt.
otc	**ACU-dyne** (Acme United)	**Ointment**	In 1, 1.2 and 2.7 g packets (100s).
		Perineal was concetrate: 1% available iodine	In 240 ml.
		Prep solution	In 240 ml, pt, qt, gal and 30 and 60 ml packets.
		Skin cleanser	In 60 and 240 ml, pt, qt and gal.
		Solution, prep swabs: 1% available iodine	In 100s.
		Solution, swabsticks	1 or 3/packet in 25s.
otc	**Aerodine** (Graham-Field)	**Aerosol**	In 90 ml.

Iodine Compounds

POVIDONE IODINE

otc	**Betadine** (Purdue-Frederick)	**Aerosol**: 5%. Glycerin, dibasic sodium phosphate	In 88.7 ml.
		Antiseptic gauze pads (viscous formula): 10%. Emusifying wax, poloxamer, polyethylene glyccol, proylene glycol, white petrolatum	In 12s (3″ × 9″).
		Antiseptic gauze pads: 10%. Citric acid, dibasic sodium phosphate, glycerin, polyethelne glycols	In 12s (3″ × 9″).
		Antiseptic lubricating gel: 5%. Citric acid, dibasic sodium phosphate, glycerin, hydroxypropyl methylcellulsoe, propylene glycol	In 5 g.
		Cream: 5%. Glycerin, mineral oil, polyoxyethylene, stearate, polysorbate, sorbitan monostearate, white petrolatum	In 14 g.
		Gel (vaginal): 10%. Polyehtylene glycols.	In 18 and 90 g w/vaginal applicator.
		Mouthwas/Gargle: 0.5%. 8% alcohol, glycerin, saccharin	In 177 ml.
		Ointment: 10%. Polyethylene glycols.	In 28 g tube, lb jar and 0.94 and 3.8 g packets.
		Perineal wash concentrate: 10%. Citric acid, dibasic sodium phosphate	In 236 ml with empty dispenser bottle.
		Skin cleanser: 7.5%. Ammonium nonoxynol-4-sulfate, lauramide DEA	In 30 and 118 ml.
		Skin cleanser, foam: 7.5%. Ammonium nonoxynol-4-sulfate, lauramide DEA	In 170 g.
		Solution: 10%. Citric acid, dibasic sodium phosphate, glycerin	In 15, 120 and 237 ml, pt, qt, gal and 30 ml packets.
		Solution, swab aid: 10%. Citric acid, dibasic sodium phosphate, glycerin	In 100s.
		Solution, swabsticks: 10%. Citric acid, dibasic sodium phosphate, glycerin	In packets of 1 (200s) or 3 (50s).
		Surgical scrub: 7.5%. Ammonium nonoxynol-4-sulfate, lauramide DEA	In pt with or without pump, qt, gal and 15 ml packets.
		Surgi-Prep sponge brush: 7.5%. Nonoxynol-4-sulfate, lauramide DEA	In 1s with nail pick.
		Vaginal suppositories: 10%. Polyethylene glycol	In 7s w/applicator.

Iodine Compounds

POVIDONE IODINE			
otc	**Betagen** (Goldline)	**Ointment:** 1/5 available iodine. PEG-8 and PEG-75	In 28.35 g and lb.
		Solution: 10%	In pt and gal.
		Surgical scrub: 7.5%	In pt.
otc	**Biodine Topical 1%** (Major)	**Solution:** 1% iodine	In pt and gal.
otc	**Efodine** (Fougera)	**Ointment:** 1% available iodine	In 30 g, lb and 0.94 g (144s).
otc	**Iodex** (Lee)	**Ointment:** 4.7% iodine wiht oleic acid, petrolatum	In 30 g and lb.
otc	**Iodex-p** (Lee)	**Ointment:** 10%	In 30 g.
otc	**Mallisol** (Hauck)	**Ointment**	In 1 g packets.
otc	**Minidyne** (Pedinol)	**Solution:** 10%. Citric acid and sodium phosphate dibasic	In 15 ml.
otc	**Operand** (Redi-Products)	**Aerosol:** 0.5% iodine	In 90 ml.
		Iofoam skin cleanser: 1% iodine	In 90 ml.
		Ointment: 1% iodine	In 30 g, 1 lb and 1.2 an d2.7 g packets.
		Perineal wash concetrate: 1 % iodine	In 240 ml.
		Prep solution: 1% iodine	In 60, 120 and 240 ml, pt, and qt.
		Solution, prep pads	In 100s.
		Solution, swab sticks	In 25s.
		Surgical scrub: 7.5%	In 60, 120 and 240 ml, pt, qt, gal and 22.5 ml packets.
otc	**Polydine** (Century)	**Ointment**	In 30 and 120 g & lb.
		Scrub	In 30, 120 and 240 ml, pt and gal.
		Solution	In 30, 120 and 240 ml, pt and gal.
otc	**Povidine** (Various, eg, Barre-National, Moore, Rugby)	**Ointment:** 10%	In 28.4 g and lb.
		Solution: 10%	In pt and gal.
		Surgical scrub: 5.5	In pt and gal.

[1] Glycerin, sodium chloride, sodium hydroxide and sodium phosphate.

Mercury Compounds

THIMEROSAL (49% mercury)

Actions:

Pharmacology: An organomercurial antiseptic with sustained bacteriostatic and fungistatic activity against common pathogens.

Indications:

Tincture/Solution: For antisepsis of the skin prior to surgery and for first aid treatment.

Spray: For cuts, scratches, wounds, lacerations and abrasions; as a pre- and post-operative antiseptic.

Contraindications:

Hypersensitivity to thimerosal.

Precautions:

For external use only. Avoid contact with the eyes.

Prolonged repeated applications: Frequent or prolonged use or application to large areas may cause serious mercury poisoning.

Incompatibilities: Thimerosal is incompatible with strong acids, salts of heavy metals, potassium permanganate and iodine; do not use in combination with or immediately following their application.

Discontinue and consult physician if redness, swelling, pain, infection, rash or irritation persists or increases.

Adverse Reactions:

Some individuals are hypersensitive to the thio or mercuri radicals. Symptoms include erythematous, papular and vesicular eruptions over the application area.

Overdosage:

For ingestion of the tincture, consider alcohol and acetone content.

Treatment: Supportive therapy. Refer to General Management of Acute Overdosage.

Administration and Dosage:

Apply locally 1 to 3 times a day.

otc	**Thimerosal** (Lannett)	**Solution**: 1:1000	Stainless. In pt and gal.
otc	**Mersol** (Century Pharm.)		Colorless. In 120 ml, pt and gal.
otc	**Mersol** (Century Pharm.)	**Tincture**: 1:1000 with 50% alcohol	In 120 ml, pt and gal.
otc	**Aeroaid** (Graham-Field)	**Antiseptic spray**: 1:1000 with 72% alcohol	In 90 ml.

Mercury Compounds

TRICLOSAN (Irgasan)

Actions:

Pharmacology: Triclosan, a bis-phenol disinfectant, is a bacteriostatic agent with activity against a wide range of gram-positive and gram-negative bacteria.

Indications:

Septi-Soft: Skin cleanser. May use as hand/body wash, shampoo, bed or towel bath.

Septisol: Healthcare personnel handwash and skin degermer.

Contraindications:

Use on burned or denuded skin or mucous membranes; routine prophylactic total body bathing.

Septi-Soft: Not a surgical scrub; do not use in preparation for surgery.

Precautions:

For external use only. Avoid contact with the eyes.

Administration and Dosage:

Dispense a small amount (5 ml) on hands, rub thoroughly for 30 seconds, rinse thoroughly, dry.

Septi-Soft may also be used as hand/body wash, shampoo, bed or towel bath.

otc	**Oxy ResiDon't** (SK Beecham)	**Liquid**: 0.6%, diazolidinyl urea	In 240 ml
otc	**Septi-Soft** (Calgon Vestal)	**Solution**: 0.25%. With glycerin, emollients	In 240 ml, qt, gal.
otc	**Septisol** (Calgon Vestal)		In 240 ml, qt, gal.
otc	**Stridex Face Wash** (Sterling Health)	**Solution**: 1% triclosan	Glycerin, EDTA. Alcohol free. In 237 ml.
otc	**Clearasil Daily Face Wash** (Procter & Gamble)	Liquid: 0.3% triclosan	Aloe vera gel, glycerin, EDTA. In 135 ml.

HEXACHLOROPHENE

Actions:

Pharmacology: Hexachlorophene is a bacteriostatic agent with activity against staphylococci and other gram-positive bacteria. Cumulative antibacterial action develops with repeated use.

Indications:

Surgical scrub and bacteriostatic skin cleanser; control of an outbreak of gram-positive infection when other procedures are unsuccessful.

Contraindications:

Use on burned or denuded skin; as an occlusive dressing, wet pack or lotion; routine prophylactic total body bathing; as a vaginal pack or tampon or on any mucous membrane; sensitivity to any component; primary light sensitivity to halogenated phenol derivatives because of the possibility of cross sensitivity to hexachlorophene.

Warnings:

Rinse thoroughly after use, especially from sensitive areas (eg, scrotum, perineum).

Rapid absorption of hexachlorophene may occur with resultant toxic blood levels when applied to skin lesions such as ichthyosis congenita, the dermatitis of Letterer-Siwe's syndrome, or other generalized dermatological conditions. Application to burns has produced neurotoxicity and death.

Cerebral irritability: Discontinue promptly if signs and symptoms of cerebral irritability occur.

Fertility impairment: Topical exposure of neonatal rats to 3% hexachlorophene solution caused reduced fertility in 7-month-old males, due to inability to ejaculate.

Pregnancy: Category C. Placental transfer occurs in rats. There are no adequate and well controlled studies in pregnant women. Use during pregnancy only if the potential benefit justifies the risk to the fetus. Hexachlorophene is not recommended as an antiseptic lubricant for vaginal exams during labor because appreciable amounts have been detected in maternal and cord serum.

Lactation: It is not known whether this drug is excreted in breast milk. Decide whether to discontinue nursing or discontinue the drug, taking into account the importance of the drug to the mother.

Children: Infants, especially those who weigh < 1200 g and those with a gestational age of < 35 weeks, or those with dermatoses, are particularly susceptible to hexachlorophene absorption. Systemic toxicity may manifest as CNS stimulation (irritation), sometimes with convulsions.

Infants have developed dermatitis, irritability, generalized clonic muscular contractions and decerebrate rigidity following application of 6% hexachlorophene powder. Examination of brain stems revealed vacuolization. Moreover, histologic sections of premature infants who died of unrelated causes have shown a correlation between hexachlorophene baths and white matter brain lesions.

Precautions:

For external use only. Avoid contact with the eyes. If contact occurs, rinse out promptly and thoroughly with water.

Adverse Reactions:

Dermatitis; photosensitivity. Sensitivity to hexachlorophene is rare; however, persons who have developed photoallergy to similar compounds may also become sensitive to hexachlorophene.

Persons with highly sensitive skin may develop a reaction characterized by redness or mild scaling or dryness, especially when combined with mechanical factors such as excessive rubbing or exposure to heat or cold.

Overdosage:

Symptoms: Ingestion of 30 to 120 ml has caused anorexia, vomiting, abdominal cramps, diarrhea, dehydration, convulsions, hypotension, shock and fatalities.

Treatment: If patients are seen early, evacuate the stomach by emesis or gastric lavage. Administer olive oil or vegetable oil (60 ml) to delay absorption, followed by a saline cathartic to hasten removal. Treatment is symptomatic and supportive; may give IV fluids (5% dextrose in physiologic saline solution) for dehydration. Correct electrolyte imbalance. If marked hypotension occurs, vasopressor therapy is indicated. Consider use of opiates if GI symptoms (eg, cramping, diarrhea) are severe.

Patient Information:

For external use only.

Avoid getting suds in eyes; if this occurs, rinse promptly and thoroughly with water.

Rinse skin thoroughly after washing.

Do not use on burns or mucous membranes.

HEXACHLOROPHENE

Administration and Dosage:

Surgical wash or scrub: As indicated.

Bacteriostatic cleansing: Wet hand with water and squeeze ≈ 5 ml into palm; add water; work up lather; apply to area to be cleansed. Rinse thoroughly after each washing.

Infant care: Do not use routinely for bathing infants (see Warnings). Use of baby skin products containing alcohol may decrease the antibacterial action.

Storage: Prolonged direct exposure to strong light may cause brownish surface discoloration, but this does not affect its action. Shaking disperses the color.

Rx	**pHisoHex** (Winthrop Pharm.)	**Liquid**: 3%. With petrolatum, lanolin, PEG	In 150 ml, pt and gal and UD 8 ml (50s).
Rx	**Septisol** (Calgon Vestal)	**Foam**: 0.23%. With 56% alcohol	In 180 and 600 ml.

CHLORHEXIDINE GLUCONATE

Actions:

Pharmacology: Provides a persistent antimicrobial effect against a wide range of microorganisms, including gram-positive and gram-negative bacteria such as *Pseudomonas aeruginosa.*

Indications:

Surgical scrub; skin cleanser; preoperative skin preparation; skin wound cleanser; preoperative showering and bathing (Hibiclens liquid).

Hand rinse: Healthcare personnel germicidal hand rinse; when hands are physically clean, but need degerming, and when routine handwashing is inconvenient or undesirable.

Chlorhexidine gluconate 0.12% is also indicated for the treatment of gingivitis. See monograph in the Mouth and Throat Products section.

Unlabeled uses: Chlorhexidine gluconate 4% skin cleanser twice daily appears effective in the treatment of acne vulgaris (significant reduction of papules plus pustules count).

Contraindications:

Hypersensitivity to chlorhexidine gluconate or any component of the product.

Warnings:

Hypersensitivity: There have been several case reports of anaphylaxis following disinfection with 0.05% to 1% chlorhexidine. Symptoms included generalized urticaria, bronchospasm, cough, dyspnea, wheezing and malaise. Symptoms resolved following therapy with various agents including oxygen, aminophylline, epinephrine, corticosteroids or antihistamines. Refer to Management of Acute Hypersensitivity Reactions.

Lactation: In one case report, a mother sprayed chlorhexidine gluconate on her breasts to prevent mastitis. Her 2-day-old infant developed bradycardia episodes after breastfeeding; symptoms resolved when the chlorhexidine was discontinued.

Precautions:

For external use only. Keep out of eyes, ears and mouth; if this accidentally occurs, rinse out promptly and thoroughly with water. Do not use as a preoperative skin preparation of the face or head (except Hibiclens liquid;). Serious and permanent eye injury has occurred when it enters and remains in the eye during surgery (see Adverse Reactions).

Meninges: Avoid contact with meninges (see Adverse Reactions).

Excessive heat: Avoid exposing the drug to excessive heat (> 40°C; 104°F).

Do not use routinely on wounds involving more than the superficial layers of skin, or for repeated general skin cleansing of large body areas except in those patients whose underlying condition makes it necessary to reduce the bacterial population of the skin.

Deafness: May cause deafness when instilled in the middle ear. Take particular care in the presence of a perforated eardrum to prevent exposure of inner ear tissues.

Adverse Reactions:

Irritation; dermatitis; photosensitivity (rare); deafness (see Precautions). Sensitization and generalized allergic reactions have occurred, especially in the genital areas. If adverse reactions occur, discontinue use immediately. If severe, contact physician.

CHLORHEXIDINE GLUCONATE

Administration and Dosage:

Cleanser:

Surgical scrub – Wet hands and forearms with warm water. Apply about 5 ml and scrub 3 minutes using a wet brush, paying particular attention to the nails, cuticles and interdigital spaces. Rinse thoroughly. Wash for an additional 3 minutes with 5 ml and rinse under running water. Dry thoroughly.

Preoperative skin preparation – Apply liberally to surgical site and swab for ≥ 2 minutes. Dry with sterile towel. Repeat for an additional 2 minutes and dry with sterile towel.

Preoperative showering and whole-body bathing (Hibiclens liquid): Instruct patient to wash the entire body, including the scalp, on two consecutive occasions immediately prior to surgery. Each procedure should consist of two consecutive thorough applications followed by thorough rinsing. If the patient's condition allows, showering is recommended for whole-body bathing. The recommended procedure is: Wet the body, including hair. Wash the hair using 25 ml and the body with another 25 ml. Rinse. Repeat. Rinse thoroughly after second application.

Hand wash – Wet hands with water. Apply about 5 ml into cupped hands and wash vigorously for 15 seconds. Rinse and dry thoroughly.

Skin wound and general skin cleanser – Thoroughly rinse affected area with water. Apply a sufficient amount to cover skin or wound area and wash gently. Rinse again thoroughly.

Hand rinse/wipe: Dispense about 5ml into cupped hand or use one towelette and rub vigorously until dry (about 15 seconds), paying particular attention to nails and interdigital spaces. Rinse dries rapidly; no water or toweling are necessary.

Sponge/Brush for surgical hand scrub: Wet hands. Use nail cleaner under fingernails and to clean cuticles. Wet hands and forearms to the elbow with warm water. Wet sponge side of sponge/brush. Squeeze and pump immediately to work up adequate lather. Apply lather to hands and forearms using sponge side of the product. Start 3 minute scrub by using the brush side of the product to scrub *only* nails, cuticles and interdigital areas. Use sponge side for scrubbing hands and forearms (avoid using brush on these more sensitive areas). Rinse thoroughly with warm water. Scrub for an additional 3 minutes *using sponge side* only. To produce additional lather, add a small amount of water and pump the sponge. (While scrubbing, do not use excessive pressure to produce lather – a small amount of lather is all that is required to adequately cleanse skin.) Rinse and dry thoroughly, blotting hands and forearms with a soft sterile towel.

CHLORHEXIDINE GLUCONATE

otc	**BactoShield 2** (Amsco)	**Solution**: 2% with 4% isopropyl alcohol	In 960 ml.
otc	**Exidine-2 Scrub** (Baxter)		In 120 ml.
otc	**Bactoshield** (AMSCO)	**Solution**: 4% with 4% isopropyl alcohol	In 960 ml.
otc	**Exidine-4 Scrub** Care (Baxter)		In 120, 240, 480 and 887 ml and gal.
otc	**Dyna-Hex 2 Skin Cleanser** (Western Medical)	**Liquid**: 2% with 4% isopropyl alcohol	In 120, 240, 480 and 960 ml and gal.
otc	**Betasept** (Purdue Frederick)	**Liquid**: 4% with 4% isopropyl alcohol	In 946 ml.
otc	**Dyna-Hex Skin Cleanser** (Western Medical)		In 120, 240 and 480 ml and gal.
otc	**Exidine Skin Cleanser** (Baxter Health Care)		In 120 and 240 ml, qt and gal.
otc	**Hibiclens Antiseptic/ Antimicrobial Skin Cleanser** (Stuart)		In 120 and 240 ml, pt,½ gal and gal and UD 15ml.
otc	**Hibistat** Germicidal Hand Rinse (Stuart)	**Rinse**: 0.5% with 70% isopropanol and emollients	In 120 and 240 ml.
otc	**Hibistat Towelettes** (Stuart)	**Wipes**: 0.5% with 70% isopropanol	In 50s.
otc	**Hibiclens** (Stuart)	**Sponge/Brush**: 4% with 4% isopropyl alcohol	In unit-of-use 22 ml.
otc	**Bactoshield** (AMSCO)	**Foam**: 4% with 4% isopropyl alcohol	In 180 ml aerosol.

BENZALKONIUM CHLORIDE (BAC)

Actions:

Pharmacology: Benzalkonium chloride (BAC), a cationic surface-active agent, is also a rapidly acting anti-infective agent with a moderately long duration of action. It is active against bacteria and some viruses, fungi and protozoa. Bacterial spores are resistant. Solutions are bacteriostatic or bactericidal according to their concentration. The exact mechanism of bactericidal action is unknown, but may be due to enzyme inactivation. Solutions also have deodorant, wetting, detergent, keratolytic and emulsifying activity.

Indications:

Aqueous solutions in appropriate dilutions: Antisepsis of skin, mucous membranes and wounds; preoperative preparation of the skin; surgeons' hand and arm soaks; treatment of wounds; preservation of ophthalmic solutions; irrigations of the eye, body cavities, bladder and urethra; vaginal douching.

Tinctures and sprays: Preoperative preparation of the skin and treatment of minor skin wounds and abrasions.

Sterile storage of instruments and hospital utensils.

Contraindications:

Use in occlusive dressings, casts and anal or vaginal packs because irritation or chemical burns may result.

Warnings:

Diluents: Use Sterile Water for Injection as a diluent for aqueous solutions intended for deep wounds or for irrigation of body cavities. Otherwise, use freshly distilled water. Tap water containing metallic ions and organic matter may reduce antibacterial potency. Do not use resin deionized water since it may contain pathogenic bacteria.

Storage: Organic, inorganic and synthetic materials and surfaces may adsorb sufficient quantities to significantly reduce the antibacterial potency in solutions, resulting in serious contamination of solutions with viable pathogenic bacteria. Do not use corks to stopper bottles containing BAC solution. Do not store cotton, wool, rayon or other materials in solutions. Use sterile gauze sponges and fiber pledgets to apply solutions to the skin, and store in separate containers; immerse in BAC solutions immediately prior to application.

Soaps: BAC solutions are inactivated by soaps and anionic detergents; therefore, rinse thoroughly if these agents are employed prior to BAC use.

Sterilization: Do not rely upon antiseptic solutions to achieve complete sterilization; they do not destroy bacterial spores and certain viruses, including the etiologic agent of infectious hepatitis, and may not destroy Mycobacterium tuberculosis and other bacteria. In addition, when applied to the skin, BAC may form a film under which bacteria remain viable.

Flammable solvents: The tinted tincture and spray contain flammable organic solvents; do not use near an open flame or cautery.

Eyes/Mucous membranes: If solutions stronger than 1:3000 enter the eyes, irrigate immediately and repeatedly with water; obtain medical attention promptly. Do not use concentrations > 1:5000 on mucous membranes, except the vaginal mucosa (see recommended dilutions). Keep the tinted tincture and spray, which contain irritating organic solvents, away from the eyes or other mucous membranes.

Precautions:

Prolonged contact: In preoperative antisepsis, do not prolong solution contact with the patient's skin. Avoid pooling of the solution on the operating table.

Inflamed/Irritated tissues: Solutions used must be more dilute than those used on normal tissues (see recommended dilutions).

Corrosion of instruments: To prevent corrosion of metal instruments, sodium nitrite (Anti-Rust Tablets) is added to the BAC solution. See Administration and Dosage.

Adverse Reactions:

Solutions in concentrations normally used have low systemic and local toxicity and are generally well tolerated, although a rare individual may exhibit hypersensitivity.

BENZALKONIUM CHLORIDE (BAC)

Overdosage:

Symptoms: Marked local GI tract irritation (eg, nausea, vomiting) may occur after ingestion. Signs of systemic toxicity include restlessness, apprehension, weakness, confusion, dyspnea, cyanosis, collapse, convulsions and coma. Death occurs as a result of respiratory muscle paralysis.

Treatment: Immediately administer several glasses of mild soap solution, milk or egg whites beaten in water. This may be followed by gastric lavage with a mild soap solution. Avoid alcohol as it promotes absorption.

To support respiration, clear airway and administer oxygen; employ artificial respiration if necessary. If convulsions occur, a short-acting parenteral barbiturate may be given with caution.

Administration and Dosage:

Thoroughly rinse anionic detergents and soaps from the skin or other areas prior to use of solutions because they reduce the antibacterial activity of BAC.

Incompatibilities: The following are incompatible with BAC solutions: Iodine; silver nitrate; fluorescein; nitrates; peroxide; lanolin; potassium permanganate; aluminum; caramel; kaolin; pine oil; zinc sulfate; zinc oxide; yellow oxide of mercury.

Recommended dilutions for specific applications of BAC solutions:

Bladder retention lavage – 1:20,000 to 1:40,000 aqueous solution.
Bladder and urethral irrigation – 1:5000 to 1:20,000 aqueous solution.
Breast/nipple hygiene – 1:1000 to 1:2000 aqueous solution.
Catheters and other adsorbent articles – 1:500 aqueous solution (replenish frequently).
Deep infected wounds – 1:3000 to 1:20,000 aqueous solution.
Denuded skin and mucous membranes – 1:5000 to 1:10,000 aqueous solution.
Eye irrigation – 1:5000 to 1:10,000 aqueous solution.
Hospital disinfection – 1:750 aqueous solution.
Metallic instruments, ampuls and thermometers – 1:750 aqueous solution (replenish frequently).
Minor wounds/lacerations – 1:750 tincture or spray.
Oozing and open infections – 1:2000 to 1:5000 aqueous solution.
Postepisiotomy care – 1:5000 to 1:10,000 aqueous solution.
Preoperative disinfection of skin – 1:750 tincture, aqueous solution or spray.
Preservation of ophthalmic solutions – 1:5000 to 1:7500 aqueous solution.
Surgeons' hand and arm soaks – 1:750 aqueous solution.
Vaginal douche/irrigation – 1:2000 to 1:5000 aqueous solution.
Wet dressings – 1:5000 or less aqueous solution.
Preoperative prep – Perform preoperative periorbital skin or head prep only before the patient or eye is anesthetized.

Prevention of rust: To protect metal instruments stored in BAC solution, add crushed Anti-Rust Tablets (eg, Sanofi Winthrop, Lannett). Add 4 tablets/quart to the antiseptic solution. Change solution at least once a week. Not for storage of aluminum or zinc instruments, instruments with lenses fastened by cement (such as cystoscopes or optical instruments), lacquered catheters or some synthetic rubber goods.

otc	**Benzalkonium Chloride** (Various, eg, A-A Spectrum)	**Concentrate**: 17%	In 500 ml and 4 L.
otc	**Benza** (Century)	**Solution**: 1:750	In 60 and 120 ml.
otc	**Zephiran** (Sanofi Winthrop)	**Solution, aqueous**: 1:750	In 240 ml and gal.
		Disinfectant concentrate: 17%	In 120 ml and gal.
		Tincture: 1:750	In gal.
		Tincture spray: 1:750	In 30 and 180 g and gal.
		Tissue: 1:750. With chlorothymol, iso-propyl alcohol and alcohol (20%)	In individual single use packets.
otc	**Mycocide NS** (Woodward)	**Solution**: Benzalkonium chloride, propylene glycol, diazolidinyl urea, methylparaben	In 30 ml.

GLUTARALDEHYDE

Actions:

Pharmacology: Glutaraldehyde (pH 3 to 4) is a mildly acidic dialdehyde. Following alkalinization to a pH of 7.5 to 8.5 with sodium bicarbonate or aqueous potassium salt, it becomes a highly effective antimicrobial agent with potent bactericidal, tuberculocidal, fungicidal, sporicidal and virucidal activity. A high degree of effectiveness is retained even in the presence of organic material (eg, blood, tissue, mucus).

Indications:

Germicidal agent for disinfection and sterilization of rigid and flexible fiberoptic endoscopes, plastic and rubber respiratory and anesthesia equipment, surgical and dental instruments and thermometers.

Precautions:

Avoid contact with eyes, skin and mucous membranes. If contact with skin or mucous membranes occurs, wash promptly with water. Should accidental contact with the eye occur, promptly irrigate with water and report to a physician.

Fumes from the solution may be irritating to the respiratory tract, therefore keep solutions covered and use only in a well ventilated area.

Directions: To remove debris from equipment thoroughly brush clean with a mild detergent solution that does not contain an emollient; rinse and rough dry equipment prior to placement in the solution.

Place clean, dry instruments or equipment in perforated pail or tray and immerse in container of alkalinized glutaraldehyde solution. Cover container to minimize odor and prevent evaporation.

Disinfection – Follow specific label directions for immersion to destroy vegetative pathogens on inanimate surfaces. Rinse equipment thoroughly before use.

Sterilization – Immerse completely for a minimum of 10 hours to destroy resistant pathogenic spores. Use sterile technique to remove instruments from solution. Rinse thoroughly with sterile water. Carefully flush all lumens and cannulas. Dry prior to use.

Preparation of solution – Add activator to the solution. The activator contains a rust inhibitor; do not add any other such agent. Upon mixing, the colorless solution changes to a nonstaining green.

otc	**Cidex**[1] (J & J Medical)	**Solution:** 2%	In qt, gal and 2.5 gal.[3]
otc	**Cidex-7**[2] (J & J Medical)		In qt, gal and 5 gal.[4]
otc	**Cidex Plus 28**[2] (J & J Medical)	**Solution:** 3.2%	In qt, gal and 2.5 gal.[5]

[1] Activated dialdehyde is stable for 14 days after activation.
[2] Long-life activated dialdehyde is stable for 28 days after activation.
[3] Vial of activator contains solid sodium salts as buffer to adjust pH to 8.2 to 8.9.
[4] Vial of activator contains aqueous potassium salts as buffer to adjust pH to 7.5 to 8.1.
[5] Vial of activator contains aqueous potassium salts as buffer to adjust pH to 7.2 to 7.8.

SODIUM HYPOCHLORITE

Actions:

Pharmacology: Sodium hypochlorite has germicidal, deodorizing and bleaching properties. It is effective against vegetative bacteria and viruses, and also, to some degree, against spores and fungi.

Indications:

Applied topically to the skin as an antiseptic.

Precautions:

Chemical burns may be produced; avoid skin or eye contact with this solution.

otc	**Dakin's** (Century Pharm.)	**Solution:** 0.25%	In pt.
		0.5%	In pt and gal.

OXYCHLOROSENE SODIUM

Actions:

Pharmacology: Oxychlorosene is a complex of the sodium salt of dodecylbenzenesulfonic acid and hypochlorous acid. Its action is markedly cidal, rapid and complete against both gram-negative and gram-positive bacteria, fungi, yeast, mold, viruses and spores.

Indications:

Used for treating localized infections, particularly when resistant organisms are present; to remove necrotic debris in massive infections or from radiation necrosis; to counteract odorous discharges; as a preoperative and postoperative irrigant and for the cleansing and disinfection of fistulae, sinus tract, empyemas and wounds.

Contraindications:

Infection sites not exposed to direct contact with the solution; systemic use.

Precautions:

Bladder/Eye instillation: Instillation of 0.2% solution, particularly into the bladder or into the eye, may cause severe discomfort. Pretreat the eye with a topical anesthetic. In the bladder, use a 0.1% concentration for the first treatment, instilling the solution to the capacity of the bladder without over-distention.

Administration and Dosage:

Apply by irrigation, instillation, spray, soaks or wet compresses, preferably thoroughly cleansing with gravity flow irrigation or syringe to provide copious quantities of fresh solution to remove organic wastes and debris. Also for preoperative skin preparation and postoperative protection. Apply topically as the 0.4% solution in water or isotonic saline. Use dilutions of 0.1% to 0.2% in urology and ophthalmology.

otc	**Clorpactin WCS-90** (Guardian)	**Powder for Solution:** 2 g sodium oxychlorosene	In 2 g bottles (5s).

SILVER PROTEIN, MILD

Indications:

For use on mucous membranes, especially the eye, nose and throat.

Precautions:

Prolonged or frequent use of silver products may produce argyria.

otc	**Argyrol S.S. 10%** (Iolab)	**Solution:** 10% stabilized solution of mild silver protein (20 mg/ml of silver) with 10 mg EDTA	In 15 and 30 ml.

MISCELLANEOUS ANTISEPTICS

otc	**Stat•One Isopropyl Rubbing Alcohol** (Continental)	**Gel:** 70% isopropyl rubbing alcohol	In 28.4 g.
otc	**Stat•One Hydrogen Peroxide** (Continental)	**Gel:** 3% hydrogen peroxide	In 28.4 g.
otc	**S.T. 37** (Menley & James)	**Solution:** 0.1% hexylresorcinol, 28% glycerin	In 165 and 360 ml.
otc	**Mercurochrome** (Purepac)	**Solution:** 2% merbromin	In 30 ml.
otc	**Tincture of Green Soap** (Paddock)	**Liquid:** With 28% to 32% alcohol	In gal.
otc	**Stat•One Hydrogen Peroxide** (Continental)	**Gel:** 3% hydrogen peroxide	In 28.4 g.
otc	**Stat•One Isopropyl Rubbing Alcohol** (Continental)	**Gel:** 70% isopropyl rubbing alcohol	In 28.4 g.
otc	**B.F.I. Antiseptic** (Menley & James)	**Powder:** 16% bismuth-formic-iodide, zinc phenol sulfonate, potassium alum, bismuth subgallate, boric acid, menthol, eucalyptol, thymol	In 7.5, 37.5 and 240 g.
otc	**Alcare** (Calgon Vestal)	**Foam:** 62% ethyl alcohol	In 210, 330 and 600 ml.
otc	**Alco-Gel** (Tweezerman)	**Gel:** 60% ethyl alcohol	In 60 and 480 g.

PHYSIOLOGICAL IRRIGATING SOLUTION

Indications:

For general irrigation, washing and rinsing purposes which permit use of a sterile, nonpyrogenic electrolyte solution.

Contraindications:

Irrigation during electrosurgical procedures.

Warnings:

For irrigation only, not for injection.

Absorption: Irrigating fluids enter the systemic circulation in relatively large volumes and must be regarded as a systemic drug. Absorption of large amounts can cause fluid or solute overloading resulting in dilution of serum electrolyte concentrations, overhydration, congested states or pulmonary edema.

Dilutional states: The risk of dilutional states is inversely proportional to the electrolyte concentrations of administered parenteral solutions. The risk of solute overload causing congested states with peripheral and pulmonary edema is directly proportional to the electrolyte concentrations of such solutions.

Do not heat to > 66°C (> 150°F).

Pregnancy: Category C. It is not known whether these solutions can cause fetal harm when administered to a pregnant woman or can affect reproduction capacity. Give to a pregnant woman only if clearly needed.

Precautions:

Continuous irrigation: Observe caution when solution is used for continuous irrigation or allowed to "dwell" inside body cavities because of possible absorption into the blood stream and circulatory overload.

Aseptic technique is essential for irrigation of body cavities, wounds and urethral catheters or for wetting dressings that come in contact with body tissues.

Accidental contamination from careless technique may transmit infection.

Containers: When used as a "pour" irrigation, do not allow any part of the contents to contact the surface below the outer protected thread area of the semi-rigid wide mouth container. When used via irrigation equipment, attach the administration set promptly. Discard unused portions and use a fresh container for the start-up of each cycle or repeat procedure. For repeated irrigations of urethral catheters, use a separate container for each patient.

Displaced catheters/drainage tubes can lead to irrigation or infiltration of unintended structures or cavities.

Additives may be incompatible. When introducing additives, use aseptic technique, mix thoroughly and do not store.

Tissue distention/disruption: Excessive volume or pressure during irrigation of closed cavities may cause undue distention or disruption of tissues.

Adverse Reactions:

Should any adverse reaction occur, discontinue the irrigant, evaluate the patient, institute appropriate countermeasures and save the remainder of the fluid for examination.

Overdosage:

In overhydration or solute overload, reevaluate and institute corrective measures.

Administration and Dosage:

The dose depends on the capacity or surface area of the structure to be irrigated and the nature of the procedure. When used as a vehicle for other drugs, follow manufacturer's recommendations.

Storage/Stability: Avoid excessive heat. Do not freeze. Store at 25°C (77°F); however, brief exposure to 40°C (104°F) does not cause adverse effects.

PHYSIOLOGICAL IRRIGATING SOLUTION

Rx	**0.45% Sodium Chloride Irrigation** (Abbott)	**Solution:** 450 mg sodium chloride per 100 ml	In 250 and 500 ml and 1, 1.5, 2 and 3 L.
Rx	**0.9% Sodium Chloride Irrigation** (Abbott)	**Solution:** 900 mg sodium chloride per 100 ml	In 100, 250 and 500 ml and 1, 1.5, 2 and 3 L.
Rx	**Ringer's Irrigation** (Various, eg, McGaw)	**Solution:** 860 mg sodium chloride, 30 mg potassium chloride, 33 mg calcium chloride per 100 ml	In 1 L.
Rx	**AMO Endosol** (Allergan)	**Solution:** 0.64% sodium chloride, 0.075% potassium chloride, 0.048% calcium chloride dihydrate, 0.03% magnesium chloride hexahydrate, 0.39% sodium acetate trihydrate, 0.17% sodium citrate dihydrate.	Preservative free. In 18 and 500 ml.
Rx	**Tis-U-Sol** (Baxter)	**Solution:** 800 mg NaCl, 40 mg KCl, 20 mg magnesium sulfate, 8.75 mg dibasic sodium phosphate heptahydrate and 6.25 mg monobasic potassium phosphate per 100 ml	In 1 L.
Rx	**Lactated Ringer's Irrigation** (Abbott)	**Solution:** 600 mg sodium chloride, 310 mg sodium lactate, anhydrous, 30 mg potassium chloride, 20 mg calcium chloride, dihydration per 100 ml.	In 300 ml.
Rx	**Physiolyte** (American McGaw)	**Solution:** 530 mg NaCl, 370 mg sodium acetate, 500 mg sodium gluconate, 37 mg KCl and 30 mg magnesium Cl per 100 ml	In 1 L.
Rx	**PhysioSol** (Abbott)	**Solution:** 526 mg NaCl, 222 mg sodium acetate, 502 mg sodium gluconate, 37 mg KCl and 30 mg magnesium chloride hexahydrate per 100 ml	In 250 and 500 ml and 1 L.
Rx	**Cytosol** (Cytosol Ophthalmics)	**Solution:** 48 mg calcium chloride, 30 mg magnesium chloride, 75 mg potassium chloride, 390 mg sodium acetate, 640 mg sodium chloride, 170 mg sodium citrate per 100 ml	In 200 and 500 ml.
Rx	**Saf-Clens** (Calgon Vestal)	**Spray:** Meroxapol 105, NaCl, potassium sorbate NF, DMDM hydantoin	In 177 ml.

chapter 11

antineoplastic agents

ANTINEOPLASTICS INTRODUCTION

The chemotherapeutic agents include a wide range of compounds which work by various mechanisms. Although development has been directed toward agents capable of selective actions on neoplastic tissues, those presently available manifest significant toxicity on normal tissues as a major complication of therapy. Thoroughly consider the risks vs benefits of therapy when using these agents.

Because of the complexities and dangers in cancer chemotherapy, use should be restricted to, or under the direct supervision of, physicians experienced in their use. In addition to drug therapy, surgical excision and radiation therapy also are employed when appropriate.

Handling of cytotoxic agents: Most antineoplastics are toxic compounds known to be carcinogenic, mutagenic or teratogenic. Direct contact may cause irritation of the skin, eyes and mucous membranes. Safe and aseptic handling of parenteral chemotherapeutic drugs by medical personnel involved in preparation and administration of these agents is mandatory. Potential risks from repeated contact with parenteral antineoplastics can be controlled by a combination of specific containment equipment and proper work techniques. The NIH Division of Safety brochure outlines recommendations for safe handling of these agents.

Mechanisms of action: The mechanism of action by which these agents suppress proliferation of neoplasms is not fully understood. Generally, they affect one or more stages of cell growth or replication. Those more active at one specific phase of cellular growth are referred to as *cell cycle specific* agents; those that are active on both proliferating and resting cells are *cell cycle nonspecific* agents. The selectivity of cytotoxic agents inversely follows cell cycle specificity. Rapidly dividing normal tissues including bone marrow, blood components, hair follicles and mucous membranes of the GI tract may also experience major adverse effects.

Alkylating agents form highly reactive carbonium ions which react with essential cellular components, thereby altering normal biological function. Alkylating agents replace hydrogen atoms with an alkyl radical causing cross-linking and abnormal base pairing in deoxyribonucleic acid (DNA) molecules. They also react with sulfhydryl, phosphate and amine groups resulting in multiple lesions in both dividing and nondividing cells. The resultant defective DNA molecules are unable to carry out normal cellular reproductive functions. Examples of alkylating agents are:

Busulfan
Carboplatin
Carmustine
Chlorambucil
Cisplatin
Cyclophosphamide
Dacarbazine
Estramustine
Ifosfamide
Lomustine
Mechlorethamine
Melphalan
Pipobroman
Streptozocin
Thiotepa
Uracil mustard

Antimetabolites include a diverse group of compounds which interfere with various metabolic processes, thereby disrupting normal cellular functions. These agents may act by two general mechanisms: By incorporating the drug, rather than a normal cellular constituent, into an essential chemical compound; or by inhibiting a key enzyme from functioning normally. Their primary benefit is the ability to disrupt nucleic acid synthesis. These agents work only on dividing cells during the S phase of nucleic acid synthesis and are most effective on rapidly proliferating neoplasms. Examples of antimetabolites are:

Cytarabine
Floxuridine
5–Fluorouracil
Fludarabine
Gemcitabine
Hydroxyurea
Mercaptopurine
Methotrexate
Thioguanine

Hormones have been used to treat several types of neoplasms. Hormonal therapy interferes at the cellular membrane level with growth stimulatory receptor proteins. The mechanism of action, however, is still unclear. Adrenocortical steroids are used primarily for their suppressant effect on lymphocytes in leukemias and lymphomas and as a component in many combination regimens. The counterbalancing effect of androgens, estrogens and progestins has been used to advantage in the therapy of malignancies of tissues dependent upon these sex-related hormones (eg, tumors of the breast, endometrium and prostate). These agents have the advantage of greater specificity for tissues responsive to their effects, thus inhibiting proliferation without a direct cytotoxic action.

ANTINEOPLASTICS INTRODUCTION

Examples of hormone agents are:

Aminoglutethimide	Leuprolide
Anastrozole	Medroxyprogesterone
Bicalutamide	Megestrol
Diethylstilbestrol	Mitotane
Estramustine	Polyestradiol
Flutamide	Tamoxifen
Goserelin	Testolactone

Antibiotic type agents, unlike their anti-infective relatives, are capable of disrupting cellular functions of host (mammalian) tissues. Their primary mechanisms of action are to inhibit DNA-dependent RNA synthesis and to delay or inhibit mitosis. The antibiotics are cell cycle nonspecific. Examples of antineoplastic antibiotics are:

Bleomycin	Mitomycin
Dactinomycin	Mitoxantrone
Daunorubicin	Pentostatin
Doxorubicin	Plicamycin
Idarubicin	

Mitotic inhibitors have mechanisms that are not fully understood. Podophyllotoxin derivatives inhibit DNA synthesis at specific phases of the cell cycle. Vinca alkaloids bind to tubulin, the subunits of the microtubules that form the mitotic spindle. This complex inhibits microtubule assembly causing metaphase arrest. In contrast, paclitaxel enhances the polymerization of tubulin and induces the production of stable, nonfunctional microtubules, thus inhibiting cell replication. Podophyllotoxin derivatives include etoposide and teniposide. Vinca alkaloids include vinblastine, vincristine and vinorelbine. A new class of agents called taxanes include paclitaxel and docetaxel.

Radiopharmaceuticals exert direct toxic effects on exposed tissue via radiation emission. Primary activity is against metastatic disease. Examples include strontium-89, sodium iodide I 131 and chromic phosphate P 32.

Biological response modifiers have complex antineoplastic, antiviral and immunomodulating activities. It is believed that the antitumor activity of interferons is a result of a direct antiproliferative action against tumor cells and modulation of the host immune response. Examples of biological agents are:

Aldesleukin (human interleukin-2)	Interferon alfa-n3 (human leukocyte)
Interferon alfa-2a (recombinant DNA)	Interferon gamma-1B (recombinant DNA)
Interferon alfa-2b (recombinant DNA)	

Miscellaneous: Metabolism of **altretamine** is required for cytotoxicity, although the mechanisms are not clear. **Asparaginase** is an enzyme that inhibits protein synthesis of malignant cells by inhibiting asparagine, which is required for protein synthesis. Intravesical **BCG** is a suspension of *Mycobacterium bovis* which promotes a local inflammatory reaction in the urinary bladder and reduces cancerous lesions. **Cladribine** inhibits DNA synthesis and repair through a complex mechanism. **Levamisole** is an immunomodulator with complex effects. **Procarbazine** produces toxic metabolites which induce chromosomal breakage. **Tretinoin** is a retinoid related to retinol (vitamin A) which induces cytodifferentiation. **Porfimer** is a photosensitivity agent. **Topotecan** and **irinotecan** are topoisomerase I inhibitors.

Extravasation occurs when IV fluid and medication leak into interstitial tissue. Damage resulting from extravasation of certain antineoplastic agents can range from painful erythematous swelling to full-thickness injury with deep necrotic lesions requiring surgical debridement and skin grafting.

Prevention of extravasation injury is based on careful, accurate IV drug administration. Avoid areas of previous irradiation and extremities with poor venous circulation for IV cannula placement. Dilute drugs properly and give at an appropriate rate.

Treatment of extravasation includes immediate discontinuation of infusion and appropriate antidote administration. Goals of treatment are palliation and prevention of severe tissue damage. For further information regarding the instillation of a specific antidote, refer to individual product monographs. Consider surgical evaluation if an open wound occurs. Some practitioners recommend leaving the IV cannula in place to aspirate some of the chemotherapeutic agent and administering an antidote to the injured site. Others recommend immediate removal of the cannula and administration of the antidote by intradermal or SC injections. Immediate removal of the cannula followed by application of ice has also been recommended for all agents except etoposide, vinblastine and vincristine (warm compresses are recommended for these agents). Apply the ice for 15 to 20 minutes every 4 to 6 hours for the first 72 hours. Elevate the affected area.

Hydrocortisone sodium succinate or dexamethasone sodium phosphate have been used on the extravasated site for their anti-inflammatory activity. However, these agents as well as other drugs (sodium bicarbonate, DMSO) are unproven for antidote use.

ANTINEOPLASTICS INTRODUCTION

Specific antidotes that are recommended include sodium thiosulfate for mechlorethamine and hyaluronidase for vincristine and vinblastine.

Drugs associated with severe local necrosis (vesicants) –

Dacarbazine
Dactinomycin
Daunorubicin
Doxorubicin
Idarubicin
Mechlorethamine
Mitomycin
Streptozocin
Vinblastine
Vincristine
Vinorelbine

Nausea and vomiting may be the most prominent adverse reactions of cancer chemotherapy from the patient's perspective, with 30% or more of patients experiencing some degree of emesis. Therefore, effective management of these effects is an important aspect of therapy.

Antineoplastics can be categorized according to their emetogenic potential based on the frequency of emesis (Level 1, least emetogenic).

Emetogenic Potential of Antineoplastics

Level	Frequency of emesis	Agent
1	< 10%	Vincristine Bleomycin Fludarabine 2-Chlorodeoxyadenosine 6-Thioguanine (po) Chlorambucil (po) Cyclophosphamide (po) L-phenylalanine mustard (po)
2	10% to 30%	Methotrexate < 250 mg/m^2 Mitomycin Vinblastine Vinorelbine 5-Fluorouracil Paclitaxel Etoposide
3	30% to 60%	Methotrexate 250 to 1000 mg/m^2 Cyclophosphamide ≤ 750 mg/m^2 Doxorubicin 20 to 60 mg/m^2 Mitoxantrone Idarubicin Ifosfamide Hexamethylmelamine (po)
4	60% to 90%	Cisplatin < 50 mg/m^2 Dacarbazine Cyclophosphamide > 750 mg/m^2 to ≤ 1500 mg/m^2 Doxorubicin > 60 mg/m^2 Procarbazine (po) Carboplatin Methotrexate > 1000 mg/m^2 Carmustine ≤ 250 mg/m^2 Cytarabine > 1 g/m^2
5	> 90%	Cisplatin ≥ 50 mg/m^2 Cyclophosphamide > 1500 mg/m^2 Carmustine > 250 mg/m^2 Streptozocin Mechlorethamine

However, the incidence of emesis with these and other agents varies greatly among individuals. Dose, schedule, concomitant therapy, other medical complications and psychologic parameters may affect the incidence as well.

Treatment of nausea and vomiting should include measures such as dietary adjustment, restriction of activity and positive support. However, if pharmacologic management is necessary, several agents or groups of agents may prove useful. Some drugs that have been used with varying degrees of success, either alone or in combination, *include 5–HT$_3$ receptor antagonists (such as ondansetron and granisetron)*, phenothiazines, butyrophenones, cannabinoids, corticosteroids, antihistamines, benzodiazepines, metoclopramide, ACTH and scopolamine.

CHEMOTHERAPY REGIMENS

Combinations of antineoplastic agents are frequently superior to single drug therapy in the management of many diseases, leading to higher response rates and increased duration of remissions. Improved response may be due to the use of agents that work by differing mechanisms. Neoplastic cells that acquire rapid resistance to a single agent by random mutation develop resistance less rapidly when treated with a combination of agents.

Selection of agents for combination chemotherapeutic regimens is based on: Mechanism of drug action; cell-cycle specificity of action; responsiveness to dosage schedules; and drug toxicity.

A number of commonly used combination chemotherapeutic regimens are listed below:

ABV

Use:	Kaposi's. *Cycle*: 28 days
Regimen:	Doxorubicin 40 mg/m^2 IV, day 1 Bleomycin 15 units/m^2 IV, days 1 and 15 Vinblastine 6 mg/m^2 IV, day 1

ABVD

Use:	Lymphoma (Hodgkin's).
Regimen:	Doxorubicin 25 mg/m^2 IV, days 1 and 15 Bleomycin 10 units/m^2 IV, days 1 and 15 Vinblastine 6 mg/m^2 IV, days 1 and 15 *with* Dacarbazine 350-375 mg/m^2 IV, days 1 and 15 *or* Dacarbazine 150 mg/m^2 IV, days 1 through 5

AC

Use:	Breast cancer. *Cycle*: 21 days
Regimen:	Doxorubicin 45-60 mg/m^2 IV, day 1 Cyclophosphamide 400-600 mg/m^2 IV, day 1
Use:	Sarcoma (bony). *Cycle*: 28 days
Regimen:	Doxorubicin 75-90 mg/m^2 total dose continuous infusion (CI) over 96 hours Cisplatin 90-120 mg/m^2 IV or IA, day 6

ACE - see CAE

ACe

Use:	Breast cancer. *Cycle*: 21 to 28 days
Regimen:	Cyclophosphamide 200 mg/m^2/day PO, days 1 through 3 or 3 through 6 Doxorubicin 40 mg/m^2 IV, day 1

A-DIC

Use:	Sarcoma (soft tissue). *Cycle*: 21 days
Regimen:	Doxorubicin 45-60 mg/m^2 IV, day 1 Dacarbazine 200-250 mg/m^2 IV, days 1 through 5

AP

Use:	Ovarian, endometrial cancer. *Cycle*: 21 days
Regimen:	Doxorubicin 50-60 mg/m^2 IV, day 1 Cisplatin 50-60 mg/m^2 IV, day 1

BCVPP

Use:	Lymphoma (Hodgkin's). *Cycle*: 28 days
Regimen:	Carmustine 100 mg/m^2 IV, day 1 Cyclophosphamide 600 mg/m^2 IV, day 1 Vinblastine 5 mg/m^2 IV, day 1 Procarbazine 50 mg/m^2/day PO, day 1 Procarbazine 100 mg/m^2/day PO, days 2 through 10 Prednisone 60 mg/m^2/day PO, days 1 through 10

BEP

Use:	Testicular cancer. *Cycle*: 21 days
Regimen:	Bleomycin 30 units IV, days 2, 9, 16 Etoposide 100 mg/m^2 IV, days 1 through 5 Cisplatin 20 mg/m^2 IV, days 1 through 5

BIP

Use: Cervical cancer. *Cycle*: 21 days

Regimen: Bleomycin 30 units CI, day 1
Ifosfamide 5 g/m^2 CI, day 2
Cisplatin 50 mg/m^2 IV, day 2
Mesna 8 g/m^2 CI over 36 hours, day 2 (with ifosfamide)

BOMP

Use: Cervical cancer. *Cycle*: 6 weeks

Regimen: Bleomycin 10 units IM, weekly
Vincristine 1 mg/m^2 IV, days 1, 8, 22, 29
Cisplatin 50 mg/m^2 IV, days 1 and 22
Mitomycin 10 mg/m^2 IV, day 1

CAE (ACE)

Use: Lung cancer (non-small cell). *Cycle*: 21 days

Regimen: Cyclophosphamide 1 g/m^2 IV, day 1
Doxorubicin 45 mg/m^2 IV, day 1
Etoposide 50 mg/m^2 IV, days 1 through 5

CAF

Use: Breast cancer. *Cycle*: 21 days

Regimen: Cyclophosphamide 400-600 mg/m^2 IV, day 1
or
Cyclophosphamide 100 mg/m^2/day PO, days 1 through 14
with
Doxorubicin 40-60 mg/m^2 IV, day 1
Fluorouracil 400-600 mg/m^2 IV, day 1

CAL-G

Use: Acute lymphocytic leukemia (ALL).

Regimen: Cyclophosphamide 1.2 g IV, day 1
Daunorubicin 45 mg/m^2 IV, days 1 through 3
Vincristine 2 mg IV, days 1, 8, 15, 22
Prednisone 60 mg/m^2/day PO, days 1 through 21
with
Asparaginase 6000 units/m^2 IV, days 5, 8, 11, 15, 18, 22
or
Pegaspargase 2500 units/m^2 IM or IV every other week

CAMP

Use: Lung cancer (non-small cell). *Cycle*: 28 days

Regimen: Cyclophosphamide 300 mg/m^2/day IV, days 1 and 8
Doxorubicin 20 mg/m^2 IV, days 1 and 8
Methotrexate 15 mg/m^2 IV, days 1 and 8
Procarbazine 100 mg/m^2/day PO, days 1 through 10

CAP

Use: Lung cancer (non-small cell). *Cycle*: 28 days

Regimen: Cyclophosphamide 400 mg/m^2 IV, day 1
Doxorubicin 40 mg/m^2 IV, day 1
Cisplatin 60 mg/m^2 IV, day 1

CAV (VAC)

Use: Lung cancer (small cell). *Cycle*: 21 days

Regimen: Cyclophosphamide 750-1000 mg/m^2 IV, day 1
Doxorubicin 40-50 mg/m^2 IV, day 1
Vincristine 1.4 mg/m^2 (2 mg maximum dose) IV, day 1

CAVE

Use: Lung cancer (small cell). *Cycle*: 21 to 28 days

Regimen: Add to CAV:
Etoposide 60-100 mg/m^2 IV, days 1 through 5

CC

Use: Ovarian cancer. *Cycle*: 28 days

Regimen:
Carboplatin 300-350 mg/m^2 IV, day 1
Cyclophosphamide 600 mg/m^2 IV, day 1

CDDP/VP

Use: Brain tumors (pediatric).

Regimen:
Cisplatin 90 mg/m^2 IV, day 1
Etoposide 150 mg/m^2 IV, days 2 and 3

CEV

Use: Lung cancer (small cell). *Cycle*: 21 to 28 days

Regimen:
Cyclophosphamide 1 g/m^2 IV, day 1
Etoposide 50 mg/m^2 IV, day 1
Etoposide 100 mg/m^2/day PO, days 2 through 5
Vincristine 1.4 mg/m^2 (2 mg maximum dose) IV, day 1

CF

Use: Adenocarcinoma, head and neck cancer. *Cycle*: 21 to 28 days

Regimen:
Cisplatin 100 mg/m^2 IV, day 1
Fluorouracil 1 g/m^2/day CI, days 1 through 4 or 5

CF*

Use: Head and neck cancer. *Cycle*: 21 to 28 days

Regimen:
Carboplatin 400 mg/m^2 IV, day 1
Fluorouracil 1 g/m^2/day CI, days 1 through 4 or 5

CFM (CNF/FNC)

Use: Breast cancer. *Cycle*: 21 days

Regimen:
Cyclophosphamide 500 mg/m^2 IV, day 1
Fluorouracil 500 mg/m^2 IV, day 1
Mitoxantrone 10 mg/m^2 IV, day 1

CHAP

Use: Ovarian cancer. *Cycle*: 28 days

Regimen:
Cyclophosphamide 150 mg/m^2/day PO, days 2 through 8
or
Cyclophosphamide 300-500 mg/m^2/day PO, day 1
with
Altretamine 150 mg/m^2/day PO, days 2 through 8
Doxorubicin 30 mg/m^2 IV, day 1
Cisplatin 50-60 mg/m^2 IV, day 1

ChIVPP

Use: Lymphoma (Hodgkin's). *Cycle*: 28 days

Regimen:
Chlorambucil 6 mg/m^2/day (10 mg/day maximum dose) PO, days 1 through 14
Vinblastine 6 mg/m^2 (10 mg/day maximum dose) IV, days 1 and 8
Procarbazine 100 mg/m^2/day (150 mg/day max dose) PO, days 1 through 14
Prednisone 40 mg/m^2/day (25 mg/m^2 - pediatrics) PO, days 1 through 14

ChIVPP/EVA

Use: Lymphoma (Hodgkin's). *Cycle*: 21 to 28 days

Regimen:
See ChIVPP, except Chlorambucil, Procarbazine and Prednisone days 1 through 7 and Vinblastine day 1 only
with
Etoposide 200 mg/m^2 IV, day 8
Vincristine 2 mg IV, day 8
Doxorubicin 50 mg/m^2 IV, day 8

CHOP

Use: Lymphoma (non-Hodgkin's). *Cycle*: 21 days

Regimen:
Cyclophosphamide 750 mg/m^2 IV, day 1
Doxorubicin 50 mg/m^2 IV, day 1
Vincristine 1.4 mg/m^2 (2 mg maximum dose) IV, day 1
Prednisone 100 mg/day PO, days 1 through 5

CHOP-BLEO

Use: Lymphoma (non-Hodgkin's). *Cycle*: 14 to 21 days

Regimen: Add to CHOP:
Bleomycin 15 units/day IV, days 1 through 5

CISCA

Use: Bladder cancer. *Cycle*: 21 to 28 days

Regimen: Cyclophosphamide 650 mg/m^2 IV, day 1
Doxorubicin 50 mg/m^2 IV, day 1
Cisplatin 70-100 mg/m^2 IV, day 2

CISCA$_{II}$/VB$_{IV}$

Use: Germ cell tumors.

Regimen: Cyclophosphamide 1 g/m^2 IV, days 1 and 2
Doxorubicin 80-90 mg/m^2 IV, days 1 and 2
Cisplatin 100-120 mg/m^2 IV, day 3
alternating with
Vinblastine 3 mg/m^2/day CI, days 1 through 5
Bleomycin 30 units/day CI, days 1 through 5

CMF

Use: Breast cancer. *Cycle*: 21 to 28 days

Regimen: Cyclophosphamide 400-600 mg/m^2 IV, day 1
or
Cyclophosphamide 100 mg/m^2/day PO, days 1 through 14
with
Methotrexate 40-60 mg/m^2 IV, day 1
Fluorouracil 400-600 mg/m^2 IV, day 1

CMFP

Use: Breast cancer. *Cycle*: 28 days

Regimen: Cyclophosphamide 100 mg/m^2/day PO, days 1 through 14
Methotrexate 30-60 mg/m^2/day IV, days 1 and 8
Fluorouracil 400-700 mg/m^2/day IV, days 1 and 8
Prednisone 40 mg/m^2/day PO, days 1 through 14

CMFVP

Use: Breast cancer. *Cycle*: 21 to 28 days

Regimen: Add to CMF:
Vincristine 1 mg IV, days 1 and 8
Prednisone 20-40 mg/day PO, days 1 through 7 or 14

CMV

Use: Bladder cancer. *Cycle*: 21 days

Regimen: Cisplatin 100 mg/m^2 IV, day 2 (at least 12 hours after MTX)
Methotrexate 30 mg/m^2 IV, days 1 and 8
Vinblastine 4 mg/m^2 IV, days 1 and 8

COB

Use: Head and neck cancer. *Cycle*: 21 days

Regimen: Cisplatin 100 mg/m^2 IV, day 1
Vincristine 1 mg IV, days 2 and 5
Bleomycin 30 units/day CI, days 2 through 5

CODE

Use: Lung cancer (small cell).

Regimen: Cisplatin 25 mg/m^2 IV, every week for 9 weeks
Vincristine 1 mg/m^2 (2 mg maximum dose) IV, weeks 1, 2, 4, 6, 8
Doxorubicin 25 mg/m^2 IV, weeks 1, 3, 5, 7, 9
Etoposide 80 mg/m^2 IV, weeks 1, 3, 5, 7, 9

COMLA

Use: Lymphoma (non-Hodgkin's). *Cycle*: 13 weeks

Regimen:
Cyclophosphamide 1.5 g/m^2 IV, day 1
Vincristine 1.4 mg/m^2 (2 mg maximum dose) IV, days 1, 8 and 15
Methotrexate 120 mg/m^2 IV, days 22, 29, 36, 43, 50, 57, 64 and 71
Leucovorin 25 mg/m^2 PO every 6 hours for 4 doses, 24 hours after MTX
Cytarabine 300 mg/m^2 IV, days 22, 29, 36, 43, 50, 57, 64 and 71

COMP

Use: Lymphoma (Hodgkin's - pediatric).

Regimen:
Cyclophosphamide 500 mg/m^2 IV, days 1 and 15
Vincristine 1.4 mg/m^2 (2 mg maximum dose) IV, days 1 and 8
Methotrexate 40 mg/m^2 IV, days 1 and 2
Prednisone 40 mg/m^2/day PO, days 1 through 15

COP

Use: Lymphoma (non-Hodgkin's). *Cycle*: 21 days

Regimen:
Cyclophosphamide 400 to 1000 mg/m^2 IV, day 1
Vincristine 1.4 mg/m^2 (2 mg maximum dose) IV, day 1
Prednisone 60 mg/m^2/day PO, days 1 through 5

COPE

Use: Lung cancer (small cell). *Cycle*: 21 days

Regimen:
Cyclophosphamide 750 mg/m^2 IV, day 1
Vincristine 1.4 mg/m^2 (2 mg maximum dose) IV, day 3
Cisplatin 20 mg/m^2 IV, days 1 through 3
Etoposide 100 mg/m^2 IV, days 1 through 3

COPP ("C" MOPP)

Use: Lymphoma (non-Hodgkin's or Hodgkin's). *Cycle*: 28 days

Regimen:
Cyclophosphamide 500-650 mg/m^2 IV, days 1 and 8
Vincristine 1.4 mg/m^2 (2 mg maximum dose) IV, days 1 and 8
Procarbazine 100 mg/m^2/day PO, days 1 through 14
Prednisone 40 mg/m^2/day PO, days 1 through 14

CP

Use: Chronic lymphocytic leukemia (CLL).

Regimen:
Chlorambucil 0.4 mg /kg/day PO, day 1
Prednisone 100 mg/day PO, days 1 through 7

Use: Ovarian cancer. *Cycle*: 21 days

Regimen:
Cyclophosphamide 600-1000 mg/m^2 IV, day 1
Cisplatin 50-100 mg/m^2 IV, day 1

CT

Use: Ovarian cancer. *Cycle*: 21 days

Regimen:
Cisplatin 75 mg/m^2 IV, day 1
Paclitaxel 135 mg/m^2 IV, day 1

CVD

Use: Malignant melanoma. *Cycle*: 21 days

Regimen:
Cisplatin 20 mg/m^2 IV, days 1 through 5
Vinblastine 1.6 mg/m^2 IV, days 1 through 3
Dacarbazine 800 mg/m^2 IV, day 1

CVI (VIC)

Use: Lung cancer (non-small cell). *Cycle*: 28 days

Regimen:
Carboplatin 300 mg/m^2 IV, day 1
Etoposide 60-100 mg/m^2 IV, days 1, 3, 5
Ifosfamide 1.5 g/m^2 IV, days 1, 3, 5
Mesna 400 mg IV bolus, then 1600 mg over 24 hours, days 1, 3, 5

CVP

Use: Lymphoma (non-Hodgkin's), chronic lymphocytic leukemia (CLL). *Cycle*: 21 days

Regimen:
Cyclophosphamide 400 mg/m²/day PO, days 1 through 5
Vincristine 1.4 mg/m² (2 mg maximum dose) IV, day 1
Prednisone 100 mg/m²/day PO, days 1 through 5

CVPP

Use: Lymphoma (Hodgkin's). *Cycle*: 28 days

Regimen:
Lomustine 75 mg/m²/day PO, day 1
Vinblastine 4 mg/m² IV, days 1 and 8
Procarbazine 100 mg/m²/day PO, days 1 through 14
Prednisone 30 mg/m²/day PO, days 1 through 14 (cycles 1 and 4 only)

CYVADIC

Use: Sarcoma (bony or soft tissue). *Cycle*: 21 days

Regimen:
Cyclophosphamide 400-600 mg/m² IV, day 1
Vincristine 1.4 mg/m² (2 mg maximum dose) IV, days 1 and 5
Doxorubicin 40-50 mg/m² IV, day 1
Dacarbazine 200-250 mg/m² IV, days 1 through 5

DA

Use: Acute myelocytic leukemia (AML; induction, pediatrics).

Regimen:
Daunorubicin 45-60 mg/m²/day CI, days 1 through 3
Cytarabine 100 mg/m² IV every 12 hours for 5 to 7 days

DAL

Use: Acute myelocytic leukemia (AML; induction, pediatrics).

Regimen:
Cytarabine 3 g/m² IV every 12 hours, days 1 through 3
Daunorubicin 45 mg/m² IV, days 1 and 2
Asparaginase 6000 units/m² IV, day 3 (usually alternated with DAT)

DAT

Use: Acute myelocytic leukemia (AML; induction, pediatrics).

Regimen:
Daunorubicin 45 mg/m²/day CI, days 1 through 3
Cytarabine 100 mg/m²/day CI, days 1 through 7
Thioguanine 100 mg/m²/day PO, days 1 through 7

DAV

Use: Acute myelocytic leukemia (AML; induction, pediatrics).

Regimen:
Daunorubicin 30 mg/m²/day CI, days 1 through 3
Cytarabine 250 mg/m²/day CI, days 1 through 5
Etoposide 200 mg/m²/day CI, days 5 through 7

DCT (DAT, TAD)

Use: Acute myelocytic leukemia (AML; adult induction).

Regimen:
Daunorubicin 60 mg/m² IV, days 1 through 3
Cytarabine 200 mg/m²/day CI, days 1 through 5
Thioguanine 100 mg/m² PO every 12 hours, days 1 through 5

DHAP

Use: Lymphoma (non-Hodgkin's). *Cycle*: 21 to 28 days

Regimen:
Cisplatin 100 mg/m² CI over 24 hours, day 1
Cytarabine 2 g/m² IV every 12 hours for 2 doses (total dose 4 g/m²), day 2
Dexamethasone 40 mg/day PO or IV, days 1 through 4

DI

Use: Sarcoma (soft-tissue). *Cycle*: 21 days

Regimen:
Doxorubicin 50 mg/m² CI, day 1
Ifosfamide 5 g/m² CI, day 1
Mesna 600 mg/m² IV bolus, then 2.5 g/m²/day CI

DVP

Use: Acute lymphocytic leukemia (ALL; adult induction).

Regimen:
Daunorubicin 45 mg/m^2 IV, days 1 through 3 and 14
Vincristine 2 mg IV, weekly for 4 weeks
Prednisone 45 mg/m^2/day PO for 28 to 35 days

Use: Acute lymphocytic leukemia (ALL; pediatric induction).

Regimen:
Daunorubicin 25 mg/m^2 IV, days 1 and 8
Vincristine 1.5 mg/m^2 (2 mg maximum dose) IV, days 1, 8, 15, 22
Prednisone 40 mg/m^2/day PO, days 1 through 29

EAP

Use: Gastric, small bowel cancer. *Cycle*: 21 to 28 days

Regimen:
Etoposide 120 mg/m^2 IV, days 4 through 6
Doxorubicin 20 mg/m^2 IV, days 1 and 7
Cisplatin 40 mg/m^2 IV, days 2 and 8

EC

Use: Lung cancer (small cell). *Cycle*: 28 days

Regimen:
Etoposide 60-100 mg/m^2 IV, days 1 through 3
with
Carboplatin 400 mg/m^2 IV, day 1
or
Carboplatin 100-125 mg/m^2 IV, days 1 through 3

EFP

Use: Gastric, small bowel cancer. *Cycle*: 24 to 28 days

Regimen:
Etoposide 90 mg/m^2 IV, days 1, 3, 5
Fluorouracil 900 mg/m^2/day CI, days 1 through 5
Cisplatin 20 mg/m^2 IV, days 1 through 5

ELF

Use: Gastric cancer. *Cycle*: 21 to 28 days

Regimen:
Etoposide 120 mg/m^2 IV, days 1 through 3
Leucovorin 150-300 mg/m^2 IV, days 1 through 3
Fluorouracil 500 mg/m^2 IV, days 1 through 3

EMA 86

Use: Acute myelocytic leukemia (AML; adult induction).

Regimen:
Mitoxantrone 12 mg/m^2 IV, days 1 through 3
Etoposide 200 mg/m^2/day CI, days 8 through 10
Cytarabine 500 mg/m^2/day CI, days 1 through 3 and 8 through 10

EP

Use: Adenocarcinoma. *Cycle*: 21 days

Regimen:
Etoposide 75-100 mg/m^2 IV, days 1 through 3
Cisplatin 75-100 mg/m^2 IV, day 1

ESHAP

Use: Lymphoma (non-Hodgkin's). *Cycle*: 21 to 28 days

Regimen:
Methylprednisolone 500 mg/day IV, days 1 through 4
Etoposide 40-60 mg/m^2 IV, days 1 through 4
Cytarabine 2 g/m^2 IV, day 5
Cisplatin 25 mg/m^2/day CI, days 1 through 4

EVA

Use: Lymphoma (Hodgkin's). *Cycle*: 28 days

Regimen:
Etoposide 100 mg/m^2 IV, days 1 through 3
Vinblastine 6 mg/m^2 IV, day 1
Doxorubicin 50 mg/m^2 IV, day 1

FAC

Use: Breast cancer. *Cycle*: 21 days

Regimen:
Fluorouracil 500 mg/m^2 IV, day 1 and bolus on day 4, 5 or 8
Doxorubicin 50 mg/m^2 total dose CI over 48 to 96 hours starting on day 1
Cyclophosphamide 500 mg/m^2 IV, day 1

FAM

Use: Adenocarcinoma, gastric cancer. *Cycle*: 8 weeks

Regimen: Fluorouracil 600 mg/m^2/day IV, days 1, 8, 29 and 36
Doxorubicin 30 mg/m^2/day IV, days 1 and 29
Mitomycin 10 mg/m^2 IV, day 1

FAMe

Use: Gastric cancer. *Cycle*: 10 weeks

Regimen: Fluorouracil 350 mg/m^2 IV, days 1 through 5 and 36 through 40
Doxorubicin 40 mg/m^2 IV, days 1 and 36
Semustine 150 mg/m^2/day PO, day 1

FAMTX

Use: Gastric cancer. *Cycle*: 28 days

Regimen: Fluorouracil 1.5 g/m^2 IV, day 1
Doxorubicin 30 mg/m^2 IV, day 15
Methotrexate 1.5 g/m^2 IV, day 1
Leucovorin 20-25 mg PO every 6 hours for 8 doses, 24 hours after MTX

FAP

Use: Gastric cancer. *Cycle*: 5 weeks

Regimen: Fluorouracil 300 mg/m^2 IV, days 1 through 5
Doxorubicin 40 mg/m^2 IV, day 1
Cisplatin 60 mg/m^2 IV, day 1

F-CL (FU/LV)

Use: Colorectal cancer. *Cycle*: 4 to 8 weeks

Regimen: Fluorouracil 600 mg/m^2 IV, weekly for 6 weeks
Leucovorin 500 mg/m^2 IV, weekly for 6 weeks
or
Fluorouracil 370-600 mg/m^2/day IV or CI, days 1 through 5
Leucovorin 20 mg/m^2/day IV or CI, days 1 through 5

FED

Use: Lung cancer (non-small cell). *Cycle*: 21 days

Regimen: Fluorouracil 960 mg/m^2/day CI, days 2 through 4
Etoposide 80 mg/m^2 IV, days 2 through 4
Cisplatin 100 mg/m^2 IV, day 1

FL

Use: Prostate cancer. *Cycle*: 28 days

Regimen: Flutamide 250 mg PO every 8 hours
with
Leuprolide acetate 1 mg SC daily
or
Leuprolide depot 7.5 mg IM every 28 days

FLe

Use: Colorectal cancer.

Regimen: Fluorouracil 450 mg/m^2 IV, days 1 through 5 and day 28; weekly thereafter
Levamisole 50 mg PO every 8 hours, days 1 through 3 every 2 weeks for 1 year

FU/LV - see F-CL

FZ

Use: Prostate cancer.

Regimen: Flutamide 250 mg PO every 8 hours
Goserelin acetate 3.6 mg implant SC every 28 days

HDMTX

Use: Sarcoma (bony). *Cycle*: 2 to 4 weeks

Regimen: Methotrexate 8-12 g/m^2 (20 g maximum dose) IV, day 1
Leucovorin 15 mg/m^2 PO or IV every 6 hours for 10 doses, 30 hours after beginning of 4 hour methotrexate infusion

ICE - see MICE

IE

Use:	Sarcoma (soft-tissue). *Cycle*: 21 days
Regimen:	Ifosfamide 1.8 g/m² IV, days 1 through 5 Etoposide 100 mg/m² IV, days 1 through 5 Mesna 20% of ifosfamide prior to, then 4 and 8 hours after ifosfamide

IfoVP

Use:	Sarcoma (osteo, pediatric).
Regimen:	Ifosfamide 2 g/m² IV, days 1 through 3 Etoposide 100 mg/m² IV, days 1 through 3 Mesna 2 g/m² IV, days 1 through 3

M-2

Use:	Multiple myeloma. *Cycle*: 5 weeks
Regimen:	Vincristine 0.03 mg/kg (2 mg maximum dose) IV, day 1 Carmustine 0.5-1 mg/kg IV, day 1 Cyclophosphamide 10 mg/kg IV, day 1 Melphalan 0.25 mg/kg/day PO, days 1 through 4 Prednisone 1 mg/kg/day PO, days 1 through 7, tapered over next 14 days

MACOP-B

Use:	Lymphoma, (non-Hodgkin's).
Regimen:	Methotrexate 400 mg/m² IV, weeks 2, 6, 10 Leucovorin 15 mg PO every 6 hours for 6 doses, 24 hours after MTX Doxorubicin 50 mg/m² IV, weeks 1, 3, 5, 7, 9, 11 Cyclophosphamide 350 mg/m² IV, weeks 1, 3, 5, 7, 9, 11 Vincristine 1.4 mg/m² (2 mg maximum dose) IV, weeks 2, 4, 6, 8, 10, 12 Bleomycin 10 units/m² IV, weeks 4, 8, 12 Prednisone 75 mg/day PO for 12 weeks, tapered over last 2 weeks

MAID

Use:	Sarcoma (soft-tissue). *Cycle*: 21 to 28 days
Regimen:	Mesna 1.5-2.5 g/m²/day CI, days 1 through 4 Doxorubicin 15-20 mg/m²/day CI, days 1 through 3 Ifosfamide 1.5-2.5 g/m²/day CI, days 1 through 3 Dacarbazine 250-300 mg/m²/day CI, days 1 through 3

m-BACOD

Use:	Lymphoma (non-Hodgkin's). *Cycle*: 21 days
Regimen:	Methotrexate 200 mg/m² IV, days 8 and 15 Leucovorin 10 mg/m² PO every 6 hours for 8 doses, 24 hours after MTX Bleomycin 4 units/m² IV, day 1 Doxorubicin 45 mg/m² IV, day 1 Cyclophosphamide 600 mg/m² IV, day 1 Vincristine 1 mg/m² (2 mg maximum dose) IV, day 1 Dexamethasone 6 mg/m²/day PO, days 1 through 15

M-BACOD

See m-BACOD, except methotrexate 3 g/m² IV, day 14

MBC

Use:	Head and neck cancer. *Cycle*: 21 days
Regimen:	Methotrexate 40 mg/m² IV, days 1 and 15 Bleomycin 10 units/m² IM or IV, days 1, 8, 15 Cisplatin 50 mg/m² IV, day 4

MC

Use:	Acute myelocytic leukemia (AML; adult induction). *Cycle*: 28 days
Regimen:	Mitoxantrone 12 mg/m² IV, days 1 through 3 Cytarabine 100-200 mg/m²/day CI, days 1 through 7

MF

Use:	Breast cancer. *Cycle*: 28 days
Regimen:	Methotrexate 100 mg/m² IV, days 1 and 8 Fluorouracil 600 mg/m² IV, days 1 and 8, given 1 hour after MTX Leucovorin 10 mg/m² IV or PO every 6 hours for 6 doses, 24 hours after MTX

MICE (ICE)

Use: Sarcoma, lung cancer. *Cycle*: 28 days

Regimen: Mesna 20% ifosfamide dose IV before, 4 and 8 hours after ifosfamide
Ifosfamide 2 g/m^2 IV, days 1 through 3
Carboplatin 300-600 mg/m^2 IV, day 1 or 3
Etoposide 60-100 mg/m^2 IV, days 1 through 3

MINE-ESHAP

Use: Lymphoma (Hodgkin's). *Cycle*: 21 days

Regimen: Mesna 1.33 g/m^2 IV, days 1 through 3
Mesna 500 mg PO, 4 hours after ifosfamide
Ifosfamide 1.33 g/m^2 IV, days 1 through 3
Mitoxantrone 8 mg/m^2 IV, day 1
Etoposide 65 mg/m^2 IV, days 1 through 3
Repeat for 6 cycles, then give ESHAP for 3 to 6 cycles

mini-BEAM

Use: Lymphoma (Hodgkin's). *Cycle*: 4 to 7 weeks

Regimen: Carmustine 60 mg/m^2 IV, day 1
Etoposide 75 mg/m^2 IV, days 2 through 5
Cytarabine 100 mg/m^2 IV every 12 hours, days 2 through 5
Melphalan 30 mg/m^2 IV, day 6

MIV

Use: Lymphoma (non-Hodgkin's). *Cycle*: 21 days

Regimen: Mitoxantrone 10 mg/m^2 IV, day 1
Ifosfamide 1.5 g/m^2 IV, days 1 through 3 with mesna
Etoposide 150 mg/m^2 IV, days 1 through 3

MOP

Use: Brain tumors, pediatrics.

Regimen: See MOPP without prednisone

MOPP

Use: Lymphoma (Hodgkin's). *Cycle*: 28 days

Regimen: Mechlorethamine 6 mg/m^2 IV, days 1 and 8
Vincristine 1.4 mg/m^2 (2 mg maximum dose) IV, days 1 and 8
Procarbazine 100 mg/m^2/day PO, days 1 through 14
Prednisone 40 mg/m^2/day PO, days 1 through 14

MOPP/ABV

Use: Lymphoma (Hodgkin's). *Cycle*: 28 days

Regimen: Mechlorethamine 6 mg/m^2 IV, day 1
Vincristine 1.4 mg/m^2 (2 mg maximum dose) IV, day 1
Procarbazine 100 mg/m^2/day PO, days 1 through 7
Prednisone 40 mg/m^2/day PO, days 1 through 14
Bleomycin 10 units/m^2 IV, day 8
Vinblastine 6 mg/m^2 IV, day 8
Doxorubicin 35 mg/m^2 IV, day 8

MOPP/ABVD

Use: Lymphoma (Hodgkin's).

Regimen: Alternate MOPP and ABVD regimens every month

MP

Use: Multiple myeloma. *Cycle*: 28 days

Regimen: Melphalan 8-10 mg/m^2/day PO, days 1 through 4
Prednisone 40-60 mg/m^2/day PO, days 1 through 7

MTXCP-PDAdr

Use: Osteosarcoma (pediatrics).

Regimen: Methotrexate 12 g/m^2 IV, days 1 and 8
Leucovorin 15 mg/m^2 PO or IV every 6 hours for 10 doses, 30 hours after beginning of 4 hour methotrexate infusion
Cisplatin 100 mg/m^2 IV, day 1
Doxorubicin 37.5 mg/m^2 IV, days 2 and 3
(MTX + leucovorin alternating every 2 weeks with cisplatin + doxorubicin)

MV

Use: Breast cancer. *Cycle*: 6 to 8 weeks

Regimen: Mitomycin 20 mg/m^2 IV, day 1
Vinblastine 0.15 mg/kg IV, days 1 and 21

M-VAC

Use: Bladder cancer. *Cycle*: 28 days

Regimen: Methotrexate 30 mg/m^2 IV, days 1, 15 and 22
Vinblastine 3 mg/m^2 IV, days 2, 15 and 22
Doxorubicin 30 mg/m^2 IV, day 2
Cisplatin 70 mg/m^2 IV, day 2

MVP

Use: Lung cancer (non-small cell).

Regimen: Mitomycin 8 mg/m^2 IV, days 1, 29, 71
Vinblastine 4.5 mg/m^2 IV, days 15, 22, 29, then every 2 weeks
Cisplatin 120 mg/m^2 IV, days 1 and 29, then every 6 weeks

MVPP

Use: Lymphoma (Hodgkin's). *Cycle*: 4 to 6 weeks

Regimen: Mechlorethamine 6 mg/m^2 IV, days 1 and 8
Vinblastine 6 mg/m^2 IV, days 1 and 8
Procarbazine 100 mg/m^2/day PO, days 1 through 14
Prednisone 40 mg/m^2/day PO, days 1 through 14

NFL

Use: Breast cancer. *Cycle*: 21 days

Regimen: Mitoxantrone 12 mg/m^2 IV, day 1
Fluorouracil 350 mg/m^2 IV, days 1 through 3 after leucovorin
Leucovorin 300 mg IV, days 1 through 3
or
Mitoxantrone 10 mg/m^2 IV, day 1
Fluorouracil 1 g/m^2/day CI, days 1 through 3
Leucovorin 100 mg/m^2 IV, days 1 through 3

NOVP

Use: Lymphoma (Hodgkin's). *Cycle*: 21 days

Regimen: Mitoxantrone 10 mg/m^2 IV, day 1
Vincristine 2 mg IV, day 8
Vinblastine 6 mg/m^2 IV, day 1
Prednisone 100 mg/day PO, days 1 through 5

OPA

Use: Lymphoma (Hodgkin's - pediatrics).

Regimen: Vincristine 1.5 mg/m^2 (2 mg maximum dose) IV, days 1, 8, 15
Prednisone 60 mg/m^2 PO, days 1 through 15
Doxorubicin 40 mg/m^2 IV, days 1 and 15

OPPA

Use: Lymphoma (Hodgkin's - pediatrics).

Regimen: Add to OPA:
Procarbazine 100 mg/m^2/day PO, days 1 through 15

PAC

Use: Ovarian, endometrial cancer. *Cycle*: 21 to 28 days

Regimen: Cisplatin 50-60 mg/m^2 IV, day 1
Doxorubicin 45-50 mg/m^2 IV, day 1
Cyclophosphamide 600 mg/m^2 IV, day 1

PC

Use: Lung cancer (non-small cell). *Cycle*: 21 days

Regimen: Paclitaxel 135 mg/m^2/day CI, day 1
Carboplatin dose by Calvert equation to AUC 7.5, day 1

PCV

Use: Brain tumor. *Cycle*: 6 to 8 weeks

Regimen: Lomustine 110 mg/m^2/day PO, day 1
Procarbazine 60 mg/m^2/day PO, days 8 through 21
Vincristine 1.4 mg/m^2 (2 mg maximum dose) IV, days 8 and 29

PFL

Use: Head and neck, gastric cancer. *Cycle*: 28 days

Regimen: Cisplatin 25 mg/m^2/day CI, days 1 through 5
Fluorouracil 800 mg/m^2/day CI, days 2 through 5 or 6
Leucovorin 500 mg/m^2/day CI, days 1 through 5 or 6

POC

Use: Brain tumors (pediatrics). *Cycle*: 6 weeks

Regimen: Prednisone 40 mg/m^2/day PO, days 1 through 14
Methyl-CCNU 100 mg/m^2/day PO, day 2
Vincristine 1.5 mg/m^2 (2 mg maximum dose), days 1, 8, 15

ProMACE/cytaBOM

Use: Lymphoma (non-Hodgkin's).

Regimen: Prednisone 60 mg/m^2 PO, days 1 through 14
Doxorubicin 25 mg/m^2 IV, day 1
Cyclophosphamide 650 mg/m^2 IV, day 1
Etoposide 120 mg/m^2 IV, day 1
Cytarabine 300 mg/m^2 IV, day 8
Bleomycin 5 units/m^2 IV, day 8
Vincristine 1.4 mg/m^2 (2 mg maximum dose) IV, day 8
Mitoxantrone 120 mg/m^2 IV, day 8
Leucovorin 25 mg/m^2 PO every 6 hours for 6 doses, 24 hours after MTX

ProMACE

Use: Lymphoma (Hodgkin's).

Regimen: Prednisone 60 mg/m^2/day PO, days 1 through 14
Methotrexate 1.5 mg/m^2 IV, day 14
Leucovorin 50 mg/m^2 IV every 6 hours for 6 doses, 24 hours after MTX
Doxorubicin 25 mg/m^2 IV, days 1 and 8
Cyclophosphamide 650 mg/m^2 IV, days 1 and 8
Etoposide 120 mg/m^2 IV, days 1 and 8

ProMACE/MOPP

Use: Lymphoma (Hodgkin's).

Regimen: Repeat ProMACE for prescribed cycles, then begin MOPP cycles

PVB

Use: Testicular cancer, adenocarcinoma. *Cycle*: 21 to 28 days

Regimen: Cisplatin 20 mg/m^2 IV, days 1 through 5
Vinblastine 0.15-0.4 mg/kg IV, day 1 (± day 2)
Bleomycin 30 units IV, day 1 or day 2 weekly

PVDA

Use: Acute lymphocytic leukemia (ALL; induction, pediatrics).

Regimen: Add to VDA:
Prednisone 40 mg/m^2/day PO, days 1 through 29

PVP-16

Use: Lung (non-small cell). *Cycle*: 21 to 28 days

Regimen:
Cisplatin 60-120 mg/m^2 IV, day 1
Etoposide 50-120 mg/m^2 IV, days 1 through 3

Stanford V

Use: Lymphoma (Hodgkin's).

Regimen:
Mechlorethamine 6 mg/m^2 IV, weeks 1, 5, 9
Doxorubicin 25 mg/m^2 IV, weeks 1, 3, 5, 7, 9, 11
Vinblastine 6 mg/m^2 IV, weeks 1, 3, 5, 7, 9, 11
Vincristine 1.4 mg/m^2 (2 mg maximum dose) IV, weeks 2, 4, 6, 8, 10, 12
Bleomycin 5 units/m^2 IV, weeks 2, 4, 6, 8, 10, 12
Etoposide 60 mg/m^2 IV, days 1 and 2 in weeks 3, 7, 11
Prednisone 40 mg/m^2/day PO every other day, tapered over last 15 days

VAC Pulse

Use: Sarcomas.

Regimen:
Vincristine 2 mg/m^2 (2 mg maximum dose) IV, weekly for 12 weeks
Dactinomycin 0.015 mg/kg IV, days 1 through 5, weeks 1 and 13
Cyclophosphamide 10 mg/kg/day IV or PO for 7 days, repeat every 6 weeks

VAC Standard

Use: Sarcoma (soft-tissue).

Regimen:
Vincristine 2 mg/m^2 (2 mg/week maximum dose) IV, weekly for 12 weeks
Dactinomycin 0.015 mg/kg/day (0.5 mg/day maximum dose) IV, days 1 through 5, every 3 months
Cyclophosphamide 2.5 mg/kg/day PO, daily for 2 years

VACAdr-IfoVP

Use: Sarcoma (bony and soft-tissue - pediatrics).

Regimen:
Vincristine 1.5 mg/m^2 (2 mg maximum dose) IV, days 1, 8, 15
Dactinomycin 1.5 mg/m^2 (2 mg maximum dose) IV, every other week
Doxorubicin 60 mg/m^2 CI, day 1
Cyclophosphamide 1-1.5 g/m^2 IV, day 1
Ifosfamide 1.6-2 g/m^2 IV, days 1 through 5
Etoposide 150 mg/m^2 IV, days 1 through 5
(vincristine + dactinomycin alternating with either doxorubicin + cyclophosphamide or ifosfamide + etoposide)

VAdrC

Use: Sarcoma (bony and soft-tissue - pediatrics).

Regimen:
Vincristine 1.5 mg/m^2 (2 mg maximum dose) IV, days 1, 8, 15
Doxorubicin 35-60 mg/m^2 IV, day 1
Cyclophosphamide 500-1500 mg/m^2 IV, day 1

VAD

Use: Wilm's tumor (pediatrics).

Regimen:
Vincristine 1.5 mg/m^2 (2 mg maximum dose) IV, weekly for 10 weeks
with
Dactinomycin 0.45 mg/kg every 3 weeks
alternating with
Doxorubicin 30 mg/m^2 every 3 weeks

Use: Multiple myeloma, leukemia. *Cycle*: 4 to 5 weeks

Regimen:
Vincristine 0.4 mg/m^2/day (2 mg maximum dose) CI, days 1 through 4
Doxorubicin 9-12 mg/m^2/day CI, days 1 through 4
Dexamethasone 20 mg/m^2/day PO, days 1–4, 9–12, 17–20

VATH

Use: Breast cancer. *Cycle*: 21 days

Regimen:
Vinblastine 4.5 mg/m^2 IV, day 1
Doxorubicin 45 mg/m^2 IV, day 1
Thiotepa 12 mg/m^2 IV, day 1
Fluoxymesterone 30 mg/day PO, daily

VBAP

Use: Multiple myeloma. *Cycle*: 21 days

Regimen:
Vincristine 1 mg/m^2 (2 mg maximum dose) IV, day 1
Carmustine 30 mg/m^2 IV, day 1
Doxorubicin 30 mg/m^2 IV, day 1
Prednisone 60 mg/m^2/day PO, days 1 through 4

VC

Use: Lung cancer (non-small cell). *Cycle*: 6 weeks

Regimen:
Vinorelbine 30 mg/m^2 IV, weekly
Cisplatin 120 mg/m^2 IV, days 1 and 29

VCAP

Use: Multiple myeloma. *Cycle*: 28 days

Regimen:
Vincristine 1 mg/m^2 (2 mg maximum dose) IV, day 1
Cyclophosphamide 100-125 mg/m^2/day PO, days 1 through 4
Doxorubicin 25-30 mg/m^2 IV, day 2
Prednisone 60 mg/m^2/day PO, days 1 through 4

VDA

Use: Acute lymphocytic leukemia (ALL; induction, pediatrics).

Regimen:
Vincristine 1.5 mg/m^2 (2 mg maximum dose) IV, days 1, 8, 15, 22
Daunorubicin 25 mg/m^2 IV, days 1 and 8
Asparaginase 10,000 units/m^2 IM, days 2, 4, 6, 8, 10, 12, 15, 17, 19

VDP

Use: Malignant melanoma. *Cycle*: 21 to 28 days

Regimen:
Vinblastine 5 mg/m^2 IV, days 1 and 2
Dacarbazine 150 mg/m^2 IV, days 1 through 5
Cisplatin 75 mg/m^2 IV, day 5

VIP

Use: Testicular cancer. *Cycle*: 21 days

Regimen:
Vinblastine 0.11 mg/kg IV, days 1 through 2
or
Etoposide 75 mg/m^2 IV, days 1 through 5
with
Ifosfamide 1.2 g/m^2/day CI, days 1 through 5
Cisplatin 20 mg/m^2 IV, days 1 through 5
Mesna 400 mg/m^2 IV, 15 min pre-ifosfamide, day 1
Mesna 1.2 g/m^2/day CI, days 1 through 5

VIP-1

Use: Lung cancer (small cell). *Cycle*: 28 days

Regimen:
Ifosfamide 1.2 g/m^2 IV, days 1 through 4, with mesna
Cisplatin 20 mg/m^2 IV, days 1 through 4
Etoposide 37.5 mg/m^2/day PO, days 1 through 21

VIP-2

Use: Lung cancer (non-small cell). *Cycle*: 28 days

Regimen:
Ifosfamide 1-1.2 g/m^2 IV, day 1, with mesna
Cisplatin 100 mg/m^2 IV, days 1 and 8
Etoposide 60-75 mg/m^2 IV, days 1 through 3

VM

Use: Breast cancer. *Cycle*: 6 to 8 weeks

Regimen:
Mitomycin 10 mg/m^2 IV, days 1 and 28 for 2 cycles, then day 1 only
Vinblastine 5 mg/m^2 IV, days 1, 14, 28, 42 for 2 cycles, then days 1 and 21 only

V-TAD

Use: Acute myelocytic leukemia (AML; induction).

Regimen:
Etoposide 50 mg/m^2 IV, days 1 through 3
Thioguanine 75 mg/m^2 PO every 12 hours, days 1 through 5
Daunorubicin 20 mg/m^2 IV, days 1 and 2
Cytarabine 75 mg/m^2/day CI, days 1 through 5

5 + 2

Use:	Acute myelocytic leukemia (AML; reinduction).
Regimen:	Cytarabine 100-200 mg/m^2/day CI, days 1 through 5 *with* Daunorubicin 45 mg/m^2 IV, days 1 and 2 *or* Mitoxantrone 12 mg/m^2 IV, days 1 and 2

7 + 3

Use:	AML (induction).
Regimen:	Cytarabine 100-200 mg/m^2/day CI, days 1 through 7 *with* Daunorubicin 30-45 mg/m^2 IV, days 1 through 3 *or* Idarubicin 12 mg/m^2 IV, days 1 through 3 *or* Mitoxantrone 12 mg/m^2 IV, days 1 through 3

"8 in 1"

Use:	Brain tumors (pediatrics).
Regimen:	Methylprednisolone 300 mg/m^2, day 1 Vincristine 1.5 mg/m^2 (2 mg maximum dose) IV, day 1 Methyl-CCNU 75 mg/m^2/day PO, day 1 Procarbazine 75 mg/m^2/day PO, day 1 Hydroxyurea 1.5-3 g/m^2/day PO, day 1 Cisplatin 60-90 mg/m^2 IV, day 1 Cytarabine 300 mg/m^2 IV, day 1 Cyclophosphamide 300 mg/m^2 IV, day 1 or Dacarbazine 150 mg/m^2 IV, day 1

VIC - see CVI

Nitrogen Mustards

MECHLORETHAMINE HCl (Nitrogen Mustard; HN_2)

Warning:
Extravasation of the drug into subcutaneous tissues results in painful inflammation and induration; sloughing may occur. If leakage of drug is obvious, promptly infiltrate the area with sterile isotonic sodium thiosulfate (1/6 molar), and apply an ice compress for 6 to 12 hours.

Actions:

Pharmacology: An alkylating agent with cytotoxic, mutagenic and radiomimetic actions that inhibits rapidly proliferating cells. In water or body fluids, mechlorethamine rapidly undergoes chemical transformation and reacts with various cellular compounds so the active drug is no longer present within a few minutes. Less than 0.01% of the active drug is recovered in the urine; however, > 50% of inactive metabolites are excreted in the urine in the first 24 hours.

Indications:

IV: Palliative treatment of Hodgkin's disease (Stages III and IV); lymphosarcoma; chronic myelocytic or chronic lymphocytic leukemia; polycythemia vera; mycosis fungoides; bronchogenic carcinoma.

Intrapleurally, intraperitoneally or intrapericardially: Palliative treatment of metastatic carcinoma resulting in effusion.

Unlabeled uses: A topical mechlorethamine solution or ointment has been used to treat patients with cutaneous mycosis fungoides.

Contraindications:

Patients with infectious disease; previous anaphylactic reactions to the drug.

Warnings:

Extravasation: See Warning Box.

Inoperable neoplasms or terminal stage: Balance the potential risk and discomfort from use in patients with inoperable neoplasms or in the terminal stage of the disease against the limited gain obtainable. Routine use in cases of widely disseminated neoplasms is discouraged.

Hematologic: The usual course of treatment (total dose, 0.4 mg/kg) produces lymphocytopenia within 24 hours after the first injection; significant granulocytopenia occurs within 6 to 8 days and lasts for 10 days to 3 weeks. Agranulocytosis is infrequent and recovery from leukopenia is usually complete within 2 weeks. Thrombocytopenia is variable, but the time course of appearance and recovery generally parallels the sequence of granulocyte levels. Severe thrombocytopenia may lead to bleeding from the gums and GI tract, petechiae and small subcutaneous hemorrhages; these symptoms appear transient and, in most cases, disappear with return to a normal platelet count. However, a severe and uncontrollable hematopoietic depression occasionally may follow the usual dose, particularly in patients with widespread disease and debility and in patients previously treated with other antineoplastic agents or radiation. In rare instances, hemorrhagic complications may be caused by hyperheparinemia. Erythrocyte and hemoglobin levels may decline, but rarely significantly, during the first 2 weeks after therapy. Depression of the hematopoietic system may occur ≥ 50 days after starting therapy.

Use extreme caution when exceeding the average recommended dose. With total doses exceeding 0.4 mg/kg for a single course, severe leukopenia, anemia, thrombocytopenia and hemorrhagic diathesis with subsequent delayed bleeding may develop. Death may follow. The only treatment for excessive dosage appears to be repeated blood product transfusions, antibiotic treatment of complicating infections and general supportive measures.

Chronic lymphatic leukemia: Drug toxicity, especially sensitivity to bone marrow failure, appears to be more common in chronic lymphatic leukemia than in other conditions; administer in this condition with great caution, if at all.

Tumors of bone and nervous tissue respond poorly to therapy. Results are unpredictable in desseminated and malignant tumors of different types.

Amyloidosis: Nitrogen mustard therapy may contribute to extensive and rapid development of amyloidosis; use only if foci of acute and chronic suppurative inflammation are absent.

Herpes zoster, common with lymphomas, may first appear after therapy is instituted and may be precipitated by treatment. Discontinue further treatment during the acute phase of this illness to avoid progression to generalized herpes zoster.

Nitrogen Mustards

MECHLORETHAMINE HCl (Nitrogen Mustard; HN_2)

Hypersensitivity: Reactions, including anaphylaxis, have occurred. Refer to Management of Acute Hypersensitivity Reactions.

Carcinogenesis/Fertility impairment: Therapy with nitrogen mustard may be associated with an increased incidence of a second malignant tumor, especially when it is combined with other antineoplastic agents or radiation therapy.

Impaired spermatogenesis, azoospermia and total germinal aplasia have occurred in male patients, especially those receiving combination therapy. Spermatogenesis may return in patients in remission, but this may occur several years after chemotherapy has been discontinued. Warn patients of the potential risks to their reproductive capacity.

Pregnancy: Category D. Mechlorethamine can cause fetal harm when administered to a pregnant woman. The drug has been used in pregnancy, usually in combination with other antineoplastic drugs. Most reports have not shown an adverse effect in the fetus; however, two malformed infants have resulted following first trimester use. There are no adequate and well controlled studies in pregnant women. If this drug is used during pregnancy or if the patient becomes pregnant while taking this drug, apprise her of the potential hazard to the fetus. Advise women of childbearing potential to avoid becoming pregnant.

Lactation: It is not known whether this drug is excreted in breast milk. Because of the potential for serious adverse reactions from nitrogen mustards in breastfeeding infants, decide whether to discontinue breastfeeding or to discontinue the drug, taking into account the importance of the drug to the mother.

Children: Safety and efficacy in children have not been established by well controlled studies. Use in children has been limited. Nitrogen mustards have been used in Hodgkin's disease (Stages III and IV) in combination with other oncolytic agents (MOPP schedule). The MOPP chemotherapy combination includes mechlorethamine, vincristine, procarbazine and prednisone or prednisolone.

Precautions:

Monitoring: Many renal, hepatic and bone marrow function abnormalities occur in patients with neoplastic disease who receive mechlorethamine. Check renal, hepatic and bone marrow functions frequently.

Local toxicity: This drug is highly toxic and is a powerful vesicant. Should skin contact occur, immediately irrigate the affected part with large amounts of water for ≥ 15 minutes and then apply 2% sodium thiosulfate solution.

Concomitant therapy: Hematopoietic function is characteristically depressed by x-ray therapy or other chemotherapy in alternating courses. Do not give mechlorethamine following X-ray or X-ray subsequent to the drug until bone marrow function has recovered. In particular, irradiation of such areas as sternum, ribs and vertebrae shortly after a nitrogen mustard course may lead to hematologic complications.

Immunosuppressive activity has occurred with nitrogen mustard. Use may predispose the patient to bacterial, viral or fungal infection.

Hyperuricemia: Urate precipitation may develop during therapy, particularly in the treatment of lymphomas; institute adequate methods to hyperuricemia and maintain adequate fluid intake before treatment.

Intercavitary administration: Pain occurs rarely with intrapleural use; it is common with intraperitoneal injection and is often associated with nausea, vomiting and diarrhea of 2 to 3 days duration. Transient cardiac irregularities may occur with intrapericardial injection. Death, possibly accelerated by nitrogen mustard, has occurred following intracavitary use. Although absorption by the intracavitary route is probably not complete because of its rapid deactivation by body fluids, the systemic effect is unpredictable. The acute side effects such as nausea and vomiting are usually mild. Bone marrow depression is generally milder than when the drug is given IV. Avoid use by the intracavitary route when other agents that may suppress bone marrow function are being used systemically.

GI: Nausea and vomiting usually begins 1 to 3 hours after use. Vomiting may persist for the first 8 hours, nausea for 24 hours. Vomiting may be so severe as to precipitate vascular accidents in patients with a hemorrhagic tendency. Premedication with antiemetics and sedatives may be beneficial.

Nitrogen Mustards

MECHLORETHAMINE HCl (Nitrogen Mustard; HN_2)

Adverse Reactions:

Dermatologic: Herpes zoster (see Warnings); maculopapular skin eruption; alopecia; erythema multiforme.

GI: Nausea, vomiting (see Precautions); diarrhea.

GU: Impaired spermatogenesis, azoospermia, total germinal aplasia (see Warnings); delayed menses; oligomenorrhea; temporary or permanent amenorrhea.

Hematologic: Lymphocytopenia, granulocytopenia, agranulocytosis, thrombocytopenia, hematopoietic depression, hyperheparinemia (see Warnings); persistent pancytopenia; hemolytic anemia (rare).

Local toxicity: Thrombosis; thrombophlebitis; extravasation (see Warning Box).

Miscellaneous: Anorexia; weakness; vertigo, tinnitus, jaundice, diminished hearing (infrequent); chromosomal abnormalities; hyperuricemia; depression; hypersensitivity (see Warnings).

Administration and Dosage:

IV: Individualize dosage. Give a total dose of 0.4 mg/kg for each course either as a single dose or in divided doses of 0.1 to 0.2 mg/kg/day. Base dosage on ideal dry body weight. Administration at night is preferred, in case sedation for side effects is required.

Do not give subsequent courses until the patient has recovered hematologically from the previous course; determine by studies of the peripheral blood elements awaiting their return to normal levels. This is a mandatory guide to subsequent therapy. It is possible to give repeated courses of mechlorethamine as early as 3 weeks after treatment.

The margin of safety is narrow; exercise considerable care with dosage.

It is preferable to inject into the rubber or plastic tubing of a flowing IV infusion set. This reduces the possibility of extravasation or high drug concentration; it also minimizes a chemical reaction between the drug and the solution. The rate of injection is not critical provided it is completed within a few minutes.

Intercavitary administration has been used with varying success for the control of pleural, peritoneal and pericardial effusions caused by malignant cells.

Consult product labeling for details of intracavitary administration. The technique and dose used by any of these routes varies. The usual dose is 0.4 mg/kg, although 0.2 mg/kg (or 10 to 20 mg) has been used intrapericardially.

Preparation of solution: Each vial contains 10 mg of mechlorethamine HCl triturated with 100 mg sodium chloride. In neutral or alkaline aqueous solution, it undergoes rapid chemical transformation and is highly unstable. Prepare solutions immediately before each injection because they will decompose on standing.

Reconstitute with 10 ml of Sterile Water for Injection or Sodium Chloride Injection. The resultant solution contains 1 mg/ml mechlorethamine HCl.

Decontamination: To clean rubber gloves, tubing, glassware, etc, after administration, soak them in an aqueous solution containing equal volumes of sodium thiosulfate (5%) and sodium bicarbonate (5%) for 45 minutes. Excess reagents and reaction products are washed away easily with water. Neutralize any unused injection solution by mixing with an equal volume of sodium thiosulfate/sodium bicarbonate solution. Allow the mixture to stand for 45 minutes. Treat contaminated vials in the same way with thiosulfate/bicarbonate solution before disposal.

Storage/Stability: Store at controlled room temperature 15° to 30°C (59° to 86°F). Protect from light and humidity. Prepare immediately before use.

Rx	**Mustargen** (Merck)	**Powder for injection:** 10 mg	In sets of 4 vials.
🍁	**Mustargen** (MSD)		

Nitrogen Mustards

CHLORAMBUCIL

> **Warning:**
> *Chlorambucil* can severely suppress bone marrow function; is carcinogenic in humans; is probably mutagenic and teratogenic in humans; affects human fertility. (see Warnings).

Actions:

Pharmacology: Chlorambucil is a bifunctional alkylating agent of the nitrogen mustard type. A cell cycle nonspecific drug, chlorambucil interacts with cellular DNA to produce a cytotoxic cross-linkage.

Pharmacokinetics:

Absorption/Distribution – Chlorambucil is rapidly and completely absorbed from the GI tract following oral administration. Peak plasma levels of chlorambucil and phenyacetic acid mustard are similar, ≈ 1 mcg/ml and are reached in 1 hour.

Chlorambucil and its metabolites are extensively bound to plasma and tissue proteins. In vitro, it is 99% bound to plasma proteins, specifically albumin.

Metabolism/Excretion – The terminal half-life is ≈ 1.5 hours; however, the metabolite's half-life is 1.6 times greater than that of the parent drug.

Chlorambucil is extensively metabolized in the liver, primarily to phenylacetic acid mustard which has antineoplastic activity. Chlorambucil and its major metabolite spontaneously degrade in vivo, forming monohydroxy and dihydroxy derivatives. Approximately 15% to 60% of the dose appears in the urine after 24 hours; less than 1% is in the form of chlorambucil or phenylacetic acid mustard.

Indications:

Leukemia/Lymphomas: Palliation for chronic lymphocytic leukemia, malignant lymphomas including lymphosarcoma, giant follicular lymphoma and Hodgkin's disease. It is not a curative in any of these disorders, but it may produce clinically useful palliation.

Unlabeled uses: Chlorambucil (0.1 mg/kg/day) has been used in the treatment of uveitis and meningoencephalitis associated with Behcet's disease. A chlorambucil dosage of 0.1 to 0.2 mg/kg/day every other month alternating with a corticosteroid for 6 months duration has been successful in the treatment of idiopathic membranous nephropathy. Chlorambucil 0.1 to 0.3 mg/kg/day has been used for rheumatoid arthritis with mixed results. Toxicity is a limiting factor although it may be useful at a lower dosage when combined with other antirheumatic agents. Possible alternative to MOPP in combination with vinblastine, procarbazine and prednisone.

Contraindications:

Resistance to the agent; hypersensitivity. There may be cross-hypersensitivity (skin rash) between chlorambucil and other alkylating agents.

Warnings:

Seizures: Rare, focal or generalized seizures have occurred in adults and children at therapeutic daily doses, pulse dosing regimens and in acute overdosage.

Children with nephrotic syndrome and patients receiving high pulse doses of the drug may have an increased risk of seizures. Exercise caution when administering chlorambucil to patients with a history of seizure disorders, head trauma or to patients receiving other potentially epileptogenic drugs.

Bone marrow damage: Observe patients carefully to avoid life-threatening damage to the bone marrow.

A slowly progressive lymphopenia may develop during treatment. The lymphocyte count usually rapidly returns to normal levels upon completion of drug therapy. Most patients have some neutropenia after the third week of treatment which may continue for up to 10 days after the last dose. Subsequently, the neutrophil count usually rapidly returns to normal. Severe neutropenia appears to be dose-related and usually occurs only in patients who have received a total dose of ≥ 6.5 mg/kg in one course. About one fourth of all patients receiving this dosage, and one third of those receiving this dosage in ≤ 8 weeks, develop severe neutropenia.

It is not necessary to discontinue chlorambucil at the first evidence of a fall in neutrophil count. Decreases may continue for 10 days after the last dose is given. As the total dose approaches 6.5 mg/kg, irreversible bone marrow damage may occur. Most patients who receive benefit from chlorambucil require a smaller dosage than this amount. Decrease dosage if leukocyte or platelet counts fall below normal values; discontinue if more severe depression occurs. Persistently low neutrophil and platelet counts or peripheral lymphocytosis suggest bone marrow infiltration. If confirmed by bone marrow examination, do not exceed a daily dosage of 0.1 mg/kg.

CHLORAMBUCIL

Carcinogenesis: Because of its carcinogenic properties, do not give to patients with conditions other than chronic lymphatic leukemia or malignant lymphomas. Convulsions, infertility, leukemia and secondary malignancies are observed when chlorambucil is used in the therapy of malignant and non-malignant diseases.

There are many additional reports of acute leukemia arising in patients with both malignant and nonmalignant diseases following chlorambucil treatment. Patients often received additional chemotherapeutic agents or radiation therapy. Risk of leukemogenesis apparently increases with both chronicity of treatment and with large cumulative doses. However, it is impossible to define a cumulative dose below which there is no risk of inducing secondary malignancy. Weigh the potential benefits of therapy against the risk of inducing a secondary malignancy.

Fertility impairment: Chlorambucil has caused chromatid or chromosome damage in males. Reversible and permanent sterility have occurred in both sexes.

A high incidence of sterility occurs when chlorambucil is administered to prepubertal and pubertal males. Prolonged or permanent azoospermia has also occurred in adult males. While most reports of gonadal dysfunction secondary to chlorambucil are related to males, the induction of amenorrhea in females with alkylating agents is well documented, and chlorambucil can produce amenorrhea. Autopsy studies of the ovaries from women with malignant lymphoma treated with combination chemotherapy including chlorambucil show varying degrees of fibrosis, vasculitis and depletion of primordial follicles.

Pregnancy: Category D. Chlorambucil can cause fetal harm when administered to a pregnant woman. Unilateral renal agenesis has been observed in two offspring whose mothers received chlorambucil during the first trimester. Urogenital malformations including absence of a kidney were found in fetuses of rats given chlorambucil. There are no adequate and well controlled studies in pregnant women. If this drug is used during pregnancy, or if the patient becomes pregnant while taking this drug, apprise her of the potential hazard to the fetus. Advise women of childbearing potential to avoid becoming pregnant.

Lactation: It is not known whether this drug is excreted in breast milk. Because of the potential for serious adverse reactions in breastfeeding infants, decide whether to discontinue breastfeeding or to discontinue the drug, taking into account the importance of the drug to the mother.

Children: Safety and efficacy in children have not been established.

Precautions:

Monitoring: Determine weekly hemoglobin levels, total and differential leukocyte counts and quantitative platelet counts. Also, during the first 3 to 6 weeks of therapy, perform white blood cell (WBC) counts 3 to 4 days after each of the weekly complete blood counts. It is dangerous to allow a patient to go > 2 weeks without hematological and clinical examinations.

Radiation and chemotherapy: Do not give at full dosage before 4 weeks after a full course of radiation therapy or chemotherapy because of the vulnerability of the bone marrow to damage under these conditions. If the pretherapy leukocyte or platelet counts are depressed from bone marrow disease process prior to institution of therapy, institute treatment at a reduced dosage.

Adverse Reactions:

CNS: Tremors; muscular twitching; confusion; agitation; ataxia; flaccid paresis; seizures (see Warnings); hallucinations (rare).

Dermatologic: Skin rash progressing to erythema multiforme, toxic epidermal necrolysis or Stevens-Johnson syndrome (rare). Discontinue promptly in patients who develop skin reactions.

GI: Nausea; vomiting; diarrhea; oral ulceration (infrequent).

Pulmonary: Pulmonary fibrosis.

Reproductive: Sterility; prolonged or permanent azoospermia; amenorrhea. (see Warnings.)

Miscellaneous: Drug fever; hepatotoxicity with jaundice; peripheral neuropathy; interstitial pneumonia; sterile cystitis; keratitis; bone marrow depression (see Warnings).

CHLORAMBUCIL

Overdosage:

Reversible pancytopenia was the main finding. Neurological toxicity ranging from agitated behavior and ataxia to multiple grand mal seizures has also occurred. As there is no known antidote, closely monitor the blood picture and institute general supportive measures, together with appropriate blood transfusions if necessary. Chlorambucil is not dialyzable. Refer to General Management of Acute Overdosage.

Patient Information:

Inform patients that the major toxicities of chlorambucil are related to hypersensitivity, drug fever, myelosuppression, hepatotoxicity, infertility, seizures, GI toxicity and secondary malignancies.

Notify physician of unusual bleeding or bruising, fever, nausea, vomiting, skin rash, chills, sore throat, cough, shortness of breath, seizures, amenorrhea, unusual lumps or masses, flank or stomach pain, joint pain, sores in the mouth or on the lips or yellow discoloration of the skin or eyes.

Contraceptive measures are recommended during therapy.

Administration and Dosage:

Initial and short courses of therapy: Usual dose is 0.1 to 0.2 mg/kg/day for 3 to 6 weeks as required (average, 4 to 10 mg/day). The entire daily dose may be given at one time. Adjust carefully to response of the patient and reduce immediately if there is an abrupt fall in the WBC count. Patients with Hodgkin's disease usually require 0.2 mg/kg/day; patients with other lymphomas or chronic lymphocytic leukemia usually require only 0.1 mg/kg/day. When lymphocytic infiltration of bone marrow is present, or bone marrow is hypoplastic, do not exceed 0.1 mg/kg/day (average, 6 mg/day).

An alternate schedule for the treatment of chronic lymphocytic leukemia using intermittent, bi-weekly or monthly pulse doses of chlorambucil consists of an initial single dose of 0.4 mg/kg. Doses are increased by 0.1 mg/kg until control of lymphocytosis or toxicity is observed. Subsequent doses are modified to produce mild hematologic toxicity. The response rate of chronic lymphocytic leukemia to biweekly or monthly administration is similar to or better than that reported with daily administration, and hematologic toxicity was ≤ that encountered using daily chlorambucil.

Radiation and cytotoxic drugs render the bone marrow more vulnerable to damage. Therefore, use chlorambucil with particular caution within 4 weeks of a full course of radiation therapy or chemotherapy. However, small doses of palliative radiation over isolated foci remote from the bone marrow will not usually depress neutrophil and platelet count; chlorambucil may be given in the customary dosage.

Short courses of treatment are safer than continuous maintenance therapy, although both methods have been effective. It must be recognized that continuous therapy may give the appearance of "maintenance" in patients who are actually in remission and have no immediate need for further drug. It may be desirable to withdraw drug after maximal control has been achieved, because intermittent therapy reinstituted at time of relapse may be as effective as continuous treatment.

Maintenance therapy: Do not exceed 0.1 mg/kg/day; may be as low as 0.03 mg/kg/day (usually 2 to 4 mg/day or less depending on blood counts).

Storage/Stability: Store at 15° to 25°C (59° to 77°F) in a dry place.

Rx	**Leukeran** (Glaxo Wellcome)	**Tablets:** 2 mg	(635). White, sugar coated. In 50s.
🍁	**Leukeran** (Glaxo Wellcome)		(635). White, sugar coated. In 25s.

Nitrogen Mustards

MELPHALAN (L-PAM; L-Phenylalanine Mustard; L-Sarcolysin)

> **Warning:**
> Severe bone marrow suppression with resulting infection or bleeding may occur. Controlled trials comparing IV with oral melphalan have shown more myelosuppression with the IV formulation. Hypersensitivity reactions, including anaphylaxis, have occurred in ≈ 2% of patients who received the IV formulation. Melphalan is leukemogenic in humans. It produces chromosomal aberrations in vitro and in vivo; therefore, it is potentially mutagenic in humans (see Warnings).

Actions:

Pharmacology: Melphalan is a bifunctional, alkylating agent of the bischloroethylamine type. Its cytotoxicity appears to be related to the extent of its interstrand cross-linking with DNA, probably by binding at the N^7 position of guanine. Like other bifunctional alkylating agents, it is active against both resting and rapidly dividing tumor cells.

Pharmacokinetics:

Absorption/Distribution – Plasma melphalan levels vary after oral dosing with respect to the time of first detectable levels (0 to 336 minutes) and to the peak concentrations achieved (0.166 to 3741 mcg/ml). These results may be due to incomplete intestinal absorption, a variable "first-pass" hepatic metabolism, or to rapid hydrolysis. Mean AUCs after an oral dose of 0.6 mg/kg were found to be 61% (range, 25% to 89%) of those of the same IV dose. Following injection, mean peak plasma levels were 1.2 and 2.8 ng/ml after 10 and 20 mg/m^2 doses, respectively. The steady-state volume of distribution is 0.5 L/kg. Plasma protein binding of melphalan ranges from 60% to 90%, with ≈ 30% being covalently (irreversibly) bound. Melphalan binds primarily to albumin with alpha$_1$-acid glycoprotein accounting for ≈ 20% of plasma binding.

Metabolism/Excretion – Plasma half-life after oral dosing is ≈ 90 minutes. Following injection, drug plasma concentrations decline rapidly in a bi-exponential manner with distribution phase and terminal elimination phase half-lives of ≈ 10 and 75 minutes, respectively. Total body clearance is ≈ 7 to 9 ml/min/kg. Melphalan is eliminated from plasma primarily by chemical hydrolysis to monohydroxy and dihydroxy melphalan; no other metabolites have been seen. The contribution of renal elimination to melphalan clearance appears to be low; ≈ 10% is excreted unchanged in urine within 24 hours.

Clinical trials: A randomized trial compared prednisone plus IV melphalan with prednisone plus oral melphalan in the treatment of myeloma. Overall response rates at week 22 were comparable (38% IV and 44 oral). An association between poor renal function and myelosuprression required changes in protocol design after week 22, which prevented further comparison of efficacy parameters. The amendment required a 50% reduction in IV melphalan if BUN was ≥ 30 mg/dl.

The rate of severe leukopenia in the IV treatment arm decreased from 50% to 11% after the protocol amendment; the incidence of drug-related death in the IV arm also decreased (10% to 3%). Severe myelotoxicity was more common in the IV group (28%) than in the oral group (11%).

Indications:

Palliative treatment of multiple myeloma and non-resectable epithelial ovarian carcinoma. Use the IV formulation in patients with multiple myeloma when oral therapy is not appropriate.

Contraindications:

Hypersensitivity to melphalan; demonstrated prior resistance to the drug.

Warnings:

Bone marrow suppression: As with other nitrogen mustard drugs, excessive dosage will produce marked bone marrow suppression, which is the most significant toxicity associated with IV melphalan in most patients. Therefore, perform the following tests at the start of therapy and prior to each subsequent dose: Platelet count, hemoglobin, WBC count and differential. Thrombocytopenia or leukopenia are indications to withhold further therapy until the blood counts have sufficiently recovered. Frequent blood counts are essential to determine optimal dosage and to avoid toxicity. Discontinue the drug or decrease the dosage upon evidence of bone marrow suppression. Consider dose adjustment on the basis of blood counts at the nadir and day of treatments. If leukocyte count falls to < 3000/mm^3 or platelet count to < 100,000/mm^3, discontinue drug until peripheral blood cell counts have recovered.

Nitrogen Mustards

MELPHALAN (L-PAM; L-Phenylalanine Mustard; L-Sarcolysin)

Hypersensitivity reactions including anaphylaxis have occurred with both oral and injection. Acute hypersensitivity reactions including anaphylaxis occurred in 2.4% of patients on IV melphalan. These were characterized by urticaria, pruritus, edema, tachycardia, bronchospasm, dyspnea and hypotension. These usually occur after multiple courses. Treatment is symptomatic. Terminate melphalan immediately; follow with volume expanders, pressor agents, corticosteroids or antihistamines. If a hypersensitivity reaction occurs, do not readminister melphalan. Refer to Management of Acute Hypersensitivity Reactions.

Renal function impairment:

IV – Consider dose reduction in patients with renal insufficiency receiving IV melphalan. In one trial, increased bone marrow suppression was seen in patients with BUN levels ≥ 30 mg/dl. A 50% reduction in IV dose decreased incidence of severe bone marrow suppression in the latter portion of this study.

Oral – Whether routine dosage reductions are needed in impaired creatinine clearance is unknown; only a small amount of a dose appears as parent drug in urine of patients with normal renal function. Closely observe azotemics to make dosage reductions, if required, at the earliest possible time.

Determine hemoglobin levels, total and differential leukocyte counts and platelet enumeration weekly. Patients may develop symptoms of anemia if hemoglobin falls below 9 to 10 g/dl; they are at risk of severe infection if absolute neutrophil count is < 1000/mm^3 and may bleed if platelet count is < 50,000/mm^3.

Carcinogenesis: Secondary malignancies, including acute nonlymphocytic leukemia, myeloproliferative syndrome and carcinoma, occurred in cancer patients following therapy with alkylating agents (including melphalan). According to one study, melphalan is 2 to 3 times more likely to induce leukemia than cyclophosphamide. Reports strongly suggest that melphalan is leukemogenic in patients with multiple myeloma. Risk of leukemogenesis increases with chronicity of treatment and large cumulative doses. However, it is unknown if there is a cumulative dose below which there is no risk of the induction of secondary malignancy. Evaluate the potential benefits and the risk of carcinogenesis.

Fertility impairment: Melphalan causes chromatid or chromosome damage in humans. Suppression of ovarian function may occur in premenopausal women, resulting in amenorrhea in many patients. Reversible and irreversible testicular suppression has also occurred.

Elderly: Clinical experience has not identified differences in responses between elderly and younger patients. In general, use caution in dose selection for elderly patients.

Pregnancy: Category D. May cause fetal harm when administered to a pregnant woman, but there have been no reports linking melphalan to congenital defects. If this drug is used during pregnancy, or if the patient becomes pregnant while taking it, apprise her of the potential hazard to the fetus. Advise women of childbearing potential to avoid becoming pregnant.

Lactation: It is not known whether this drug is excreted in breast milk. Do not give to nursing mothers.

Children: Safety and efficacy in children have not been established.

Precautions:

Monitoring: Perform periodic CBCs with differential during the course of treatment. Obtain at least one determination prior to each dose. Observe patients closely for consequences of bone marrow suppression, which include severe infections, bleeding and symptomatic anemia (see Warnings).

Prior radiation and chemotherapy: Use with extreme caution in patients whose bone marrow reserve may have been compromised by prior irradiation or chemotherapy or whose marrow function is recovering from previous cytotoxic therapy.

Nitrogen Mustards

MELPHALAN (L-PAM; L-Phenylalanine Mustard; L-Sarcolysin)

Drug Interactions:

Melphalan Drug Interactions			
Precipitant drug	Object drug*		Description
Cisplatin	Melphalan	⬆	Cisplatin may affect melphalan kinetics by inducing renal dysfunction and subsequently altering melphalan clearance.
Interferon alfa	Melphalan	⬇	Serum melphalan concentrations may be decreased.
Nalidixic acid	Melphalan	⬆	Incidence of severe hemorrhagic necrotic enterocolitis may increase in pediatric patients.
Melphalan	Carmustine	⬆	Carmustine lung toxicity threshold may be reduced.
Melphalan	Cyclosporine	⬆	An increase in the toxicity of cyclosporine, particularly nephrotoxicity, has been observed following coadministration.

* ⬆ = Object drug increased. ⬇ = Object drug decreased.

Adverse Reactions:

Dermatologic: Skin hypersensitivity; alopecia; skin ulceration at injection site; skin necrosis (rarely requiring skin grafting).

GI: Nausea, vomiting, diarrhea, oral ulceration (infrequent); hepatotoxicity (including veno-occlusive disease) (rare).

Miscellaneous: Pulmonary fibrosis; interstitial pneumonitis; vasculitis; hemolytic anemia; allergic reaction; bone marrow suppression (see Warnings).

Overdosage:

Symptoms: Overdoses resulting in death have occurred. Overdoses, including doses up to 290 mg/m^2 (IV) and 50 mg/day for 6 days (oral), have produced the following symptoms: Severe nausea and vomiting; decreased consciousness; convulsions; muscular paralysis; cholinomimetic effects; severe mucositis, stomatitis, colitis, diarrhea and hemorrhage of the GI tract at high doses (> 100 mg/m^2, IV); elevations in liver enzymes and veno-occlusive disease (infrequent). Significant hyponatremia caused by an associated inappropriate secretion of ADH syndrome; nephrotoxicity and adult respiratory distress syndrome (rare). The principal toxic effect is bone marrow suppression. A pediatric patient survived a 254 mg/m^2 overdose treated with standard supportive care.

Treatment: Closely follow hematologic parameters for 3 to 6 weeks. An uncontrolled study suggests that administration of autologous bone marrow or hematopoietic growth factors (eg, sargramostim, filgrastim) may shorten the period of pancytopenia. Institute general supportive measures together with appropriate blood transfusions and antibiotics as deemed necessary. This drug is not removed from plasma to any significant degree by hemodialysis or hemoperfusion.

Patient Information:

Inform patients that the major toxicities are related to myelosuppression, hypersensitivity, GI toxicity, pulmonary toxicity, infertility and non-lymphocytic leukemia. Do not take without close medical supervision.

Notify physician of unusual bleeding or bruising, fever, chills, sore throat, shortness of breath, yellow discoloration of skin or eyes, persistent cough, flank or stomach pain, joint pain, mouth sores, black tarry stools, skin rash, vasculitis, amenorrhea, nausea, vomiting, weight loss or unusual lumps or masses.

Contraceptive measures are recommended during therapy.

Administration and Dosage:

Multiple myeloma:

Oral – The usual dose is 6 mg/day. May give entire daily dose at one time. Adjust, as required, on the basis of weekly blood counts. After 2 to 3 weeks of treatment, discontinue drug for up to 4 weeks, and carefully monitor blood count. When WBC and platelet counts are rising, institute a maintenance dose of 2 mg/day. Because of patient-to-patient variations in melphalan plasma levels following oral use, some recommend a cautious dosage increase until myelosuppression is observed, to ensure therapeutic drug levels have been reached.

Alternative regimens: Initial course of 10 mg/day for 7 to 10 days. Maximal suppression of the leukocyte and platelet counts occurs within 3 to 5 weeks and recovery within 4 to 8 weeks. Institute maintenance therapy with 2 mg/day when the WBC count is > 4000/mcl and the platelet count is > 100,000/mcl. Adjust dosage to

MELPHALAN (L-PAM; L-Phenylalanine Mustard; L-Sarcolysin)

between 1 and 3 mg/day depending on hematological response. Maintain a significant degree of bone marrow depression to keep the leukocyte count in the range of 3000 to 3500 cells/mcl.

Other investigators start treatment with 0.15 mg/kg/day for 7 days, followed by a rest period of at least 2 weeks (up to 5 to 6 weeks). Begin maintenance therapy at ≤ 0.05 mg/kg/day when the WBC and platelet counts are rising; adjust according to the blood count. About 33% to 50% of patients with multiple myeloma show a favorable response to oral administration of the drug. In one study, melphalan in combination with prednisone significantly improved the percentage of patients with multiple myeloma who achieved palliation. One regimen is to administer melphalan at
0.25 mg/kg/day for 4 consecutive days (or 0.2 mg/kg/day for 5 consecutive days) for a total dose of 1 mg/kg/course. These 4- to 5-day courses are then repeated every 4 to 6 weeks if the granulocyte and platelet counts have returned to normal.

Response may be very gradual over many months; it is important to give repeated courses or continuous therapy, because improvement may continue slowly over many months, and the maximum benefit may be missed if treatment is abandoned too soon.

In patients with moderate to severe renal impairment, current pharmacokinetic data does not justify an absolute recommendation on dosage reduction, but it may be prudent to use a reduced dose initially.

IV – The usual dose is 16 mg/m^2. Consider reduction of up to 50% in patients with renal insufficiency (BUN ≥ 30 mg/dl). Administer as a single infusion over 15 to 20 min. Give at 2-week intervals for 4 doses, then, after adequate recovery from toxicity, at 4-week intervals. Experience suggests that repeated courses should be given because improvement may continue slowly over many months, and the maximum benefit may be missed if treatment is abandoned prematurely. Consider dose adjustment on the basis of blood cell counts at the nadir and day of treatment.

Preparation for administration:

1.) Reconstitute with 10 ml of the supplied diluent and shake vigorously until a clear solution is obtained. This provides a 5 mg/ml solution.
2.) Immediately dilute the dose to be administered in 0.9% sodium chloride injection to a concentration ≤ 0.45 mg/ml.
3.) Administer the diluted product over a minimum of 15 minutes.
4.) Complete administration within 60 minutes of reconstitution.

Keep the time between reconstitution/dilution and administration to a minimum because reconstituted and diluted solutions are unstable. Over as short a time as 30 minutes, a citrate derivative of melphalan has been detected in reconstituted material from the reaction of melphalan with the sterile diluent. Upon further dilution with saline, nearly 1% label strength of melphalan hydrolyzes every 10 minutes.

Epithelial ovarian cancer: 0.2 mg/kg/day for 5 days as a single course. Repeat courses every 4 to 5 weeks depending on hematologic tolerance.

Storage/Stability:

Tablets – Store at 15° to 25°C (59° to 77°F). Protect from light. Dispense in glass.

IV – Store at 15° to 30°C (59° to 86°F). Protect from light. A precipitate forms if the reconstituted solution is stored at 5°C (41°F). Do not refrigerate the reconstituted product.

Rx	**Alkeran** (Glaxo Wellcome)	**Tablets:** 2 mg	(Alkeran A2A). Lactose. White, scored. In 50s.
🍁	**Alkeran** (Glaxo Wellcome)		
Rx	**Alkeran** (Glaxo Wellcome)	**Powder for injection:** 50 mg	In single-use vials[1] with 10 ml vial of sterile diluent.[2]
🍁	**Alkeran** (Glaxo Wellcome)		

[1] With 20 mg povidone.

[2] Water for injection with 0.2 g sodium citrate, 6 ml propylene glycol and 0.52 ml ethanol.

IFOSFAMIDE

Warning:

Urotoxic side effects, especially hemorrhagic cystitis, as well as CNS toxicities such as confusion and coma have been associated with ifosfamide. When they occur, they may require cessation of ifosfamide therapy (see Warnings).

Severe myelosuppression has occurred (see Warnings).

Actions:

Pharmacology: Ifosfamide is a chemotherapeutic agent chemically related to the nitrogen mustards and a synthetic analog of cyclophosphamide. Ifosfamide requires metabolic activation by microsomal liver enzymes to produce biologically active metabolites. Activation occurs by hydroxylation to form the unstable intermediate 4-hydroxyifosfamide. This metabolite rapidly degrades to the stable urinary metabolite 4-ketoifosfamide. Formation of the stable urinary metabolite, 4-carboxyifosfamide also occurs. These urinary metabolites are not cytotoxic. Ifosphoramide and acrolein are also found. Enzymatic oxidation of the chloroethyl side chains and subsequent dealkylation produces the major urinary metabolites, dechloroethyl ifosfamide and dechloroethyl cyclophosphamide. The alkylated metabolites of ifosfamide interact with DNA.

Pharmacokinetics:

Absorption/Distribution – Ifosfamide exhibits dose-dependent pharmacokinetics. Small quantities (nmole/ml) of ifosfamide mustard and 4-hydroxyifosfamide are detectable in plasma.

Metabolism/Excretion – At single doses of 3.8 to 5 g/m^2, the plasma concentrations decay biphasically, and the mean terminal elimination half-life is ≈ 15 hours. At doses of 1.6 to 2.4 g/m^2/day, the plasma decay is monoexponential, and the terminal elimination half-life is ≈ 7 hours. Ifosfamide is extensively metabolized, and the metabolic pathways appear to be saturated at high doses. Metabolism of ifosfamide is required for the generation of the biologically active species and while metabolism is extensive, it varies among patients. After administration of doses of 5 g/m^2, 70% to 86% of the dose was recovered in the urine, with about 61% of the dose excreted as parent compound. At doses of 1.6 to 2.4 g/m^2, only 12% to 18% of the dose was excreted in the urine as unchanged drug within 72 hours.

Clinical trials: In one study, 50 fully evaluable patients with germ cell testicular cancer were given ifosfamide and cisplatin and either vinblastine or etoposide after failing (47 of 50) at least two prior chemotherapy regimens consisting of cisplatin/vinblastine/bleomycin (PVB), cisplatin/vinblastine/actinomycin D/bleomycin/cyclophosphamide (VAB6) or the combination of cisplatin and etoposide. Patients were selected for remaining cisplatin sensitivity because they had previously responded to a cisplatin-containing regimen and had not progressed while on the regimen or within 3 weeks of stopping it. Patients served as their own control based on the premise that long-term complete responses could not be achieved by retreatment with a regimen to which they had previously responded and subsequently relapsed.

Ten of 50 patients were still alive 2 to 5 years after treatment. Four of the 10 long-term survivors were rendered free of cancer by surgical resection after the ifosfamide regimen; median survival for the entire group of 50 patients was 53 weeks.

Indications:

Germ cell testicular cancer: In combination with certain other approved antineoplastics for third-line chemotherapy of germ cell testicular cancer.

Ordinarily used in combination with a prophylactic agent for hemorrhagic cystitis, such as mesna (see individual monograph).

Unlabeled uses: Ifosfamide has shown activity in lung, breast, ovarian, pancreatic and gastric cancer, sarcomas, acute leukemias (except AML) and malignant lymphomas. Further studies are needed with ifosfamide alone and with other agents.

Contraindications:

Continued use in patients with severely depressed bone marrow function (see Warnings and Precautions); hypersensitivity to ifosfamide.

Warnings:

Urotoxic side effects, especially hemorrhagic cystitis, have been frequently associated with ifosfamide. Obtain a urinalysis prior to each dose. If microscopic hematuria (> 10 RBCs per high power field) is present, then withhold subsequent administration until complete resolution. Use ifosfamide with a protector, such as mesna, to prevent hemorrhagic cystitis.

IFOSFAMIDE

Myelosuppression: When given in combination with other chemotherapeutic agents, severe myelosuppression is frequent. In studies, this was dose-related and dose-limiting. It consisted mainly of leukopenia and, to a lesser extent, thrombocytopenia. A WBC count < 3000/mm^3 is expected in 50% of patients given ifosfamide alone at 1.2 g/m^2/day for 5 consecutive days. At this dose level, thrombocytopenia (platelets < 100,000/mm^3) occurred in ≈ 20% of patients. At higher dosages, leukopenia was almost universal; at total dosages of 10 to 12 g/m^2/cycle, half of the patients had a WBC count < 1000/mm^3 and 8% had platelet counts < 50,000/mm^3. Myelosuppression is usually reversible, and treatment can be given every 3 to 4 weeks. When used in combination with other myelosuppressive agents, dose adjustments may be necessary. Patients who experience severe myelosuppression are potentially at increased risk for infection.

Close hematologic monitoring is recommended. Obtain a WBC count, platelet count and hemoglobin prior to each administration and at appropriate intervals. Unless clinically essential, do not administer to patients with a WBC count < 2000/mm^3 or a platelet count < 50,000/mm^3.

Neurologic manifestations consisting of somnolence, confusion, hallucinations and in some instances, coma, have occurred. The occurrence of these symptoms requires discontinuing ifosfamide therapy. The symptoms have usually been reversible; maintain supportive therapy until their complete resolution.

Hematuria: At doses of 1.2 g/m^2/day for 5 consecutive days without a protector, microscopic hematuria is expected in ≈ 50% of the patients and gross hematuria in ≈ 8% of patients. Dose fractionation, vigorous hydration and a protector (eg, mesna) can significantly reduce hematuria incidence, especially gross hematuria, associated with hemorrhagic cystitis. At 1.2 g/m^2/day for 5 consecutive days, leukopenia, if it occurs, is usually mild to moderate.

Renal function impairment: Use with caution. Clinical signs (eg, elevation in BUN or serum creatinine or decrease in creatinine clearance) were usually transient and most likely related to tubular damage.

Carcinogenesis: Ifosfamide is carcinogenic in rats, with female rats showing a significant incidence of leiomyosarcomas and mammary fibroadenomas. The mutagenic potential is documented in bacterial systems in vitro and mammalian cells in vivo. In vivo, ifosfamide has induced mutagenic effects in mice and *Drosophila melanogaster* germ cells and has induced a significant increase in dominant lethal mutations in male mice as well as recessive sex-linked lethal mutations in *Drosophila*.

Ifosfamide has caused resorptions, fetal anomalies, embryolethality and embryotoxicity in various rodent species in doses ranging from 18 to 88 mg/m^2.

Pregnancy: Category D. Animal studies indicate that the drug can cause gene mutations and chromosomal damage in vivo. Embryotoxic and teratogenic effects have been observed in mice, rats and rabbits at doses 0.05 to 0.075 times the human dose. Ifosfamide can cause fetal damage when administered to a pregnant woman. If ifosfamide is used during pregnancy or if the patient becomes pregnant while taking this drug, apprise the patient of the potential hazard to the fetus.

Lactation: Ifosfamide is excreted in breast milk. Because of the potential for serious adverse events and the tumorigenicity shown in animal studies, discontinue nursing or the drug, taking into account the importance of the drug to the mother.

Children: Safety and efficacy in children have not been established.

Precautions:

Monitoring: During treatment, monitor the patient's hematologic profile (particularly neutrophils and platelets) regularly to determine the degree of hematopoietic suppression. Examine regularly for red cells that may precede hemorrhagic cystitis. Closely monitor serum and urine chemistries including phosphorus, potassium, alkaline phosphatase and other appropriate laboratory studies is recommended. Administer appropriate replacement therapy as indicated.

Compromised bone marrow reserve: Administer cautiously to patients with compromised bone marrow reserve, as indicated by: Leukopenia, granulocytopenia, extensive bone marrow metastases, prior therapy with radiation or other cytotoxic agents.

Wound healing: Ifosfamide may interfere with normal wound healing.

Adverse Reactions:

GI: Nausea and vomiting (58%); anorexia, diarrhea, constipation (< 1%).

GU: Hematuria (6% to 92%, see Warnings); hemorrhagic cystitis; dysuria; urinary frequency; metabolic acidosis (31%); proteinuria and acidosis (rare); renal tubular acidosis that progressed into chronic renal failure (one episode).

IFOSFAMIDE

CNS: Somnolence, confusion, depressive psychosis, hallucinations (12%); dizziness, disorientation, cranial nerve dysfunction, seizures, coma (less frequent); encephalopathy (rare). CNS toxicity incidence may be higher with altered renal function.

Body as a whole: Alopecia (≈ 83%); myelosuppression (50%); infection (8%); liver dysfunction (3%); phlebitis (2%); fever of unknown origin (1%); allergic reactions, cardiotoxicity, coagulopathy, dermatitis, fatigue, hypertension, hypotension, malaise, polyneuropathy, pulmonary symptoms, salivation, stomatitis (< 1%); acute pancreatitis (rare).

Lab test abnormalities: Increases in liver enzymes or bilirubin (3%).

Overdosage:

No specific antidote for ifosfamide is known. Management includes general supportive measures to sustain patient through any toxicity that might occur. Refer to General Management of Acute Overdosage.

Patient Information:

Notify physician of unusual bleeding/bruising, fever, chills, sore throat, cough, shortness of breath, seizures, lack of menstrual flow, unusual lumps or masses, flank, stomach or joint pain, sores in mouth or on lips, yellow discoloration of skin or eyes.

Contraceptive measures are recommended during therapy for men and women.

Administration and Dosage:

Administer IV at a dose of 1.2 g/m^2/day for 5 consecutive days. Repeat every 3 weeks or after recovery from hematologic toxicity (platelets ≥ 100,000/mm^3, WBC ≥ 4,000/mm^3). To prevent bladder toxicity, give with extensive hydration consisting of ≥ 2 L of oral or IV fluid per day. Use a protector, such as mesna, to prevent hemorrhagic cystitis. Administer ifosfamide as slow IV infusion lasting ≥ 30 minutes. Ifosfamide has been used in a small number of patients with compromised hepatic or renal function.

Preparation: Add Sterile Water for Injection or Bacteriostatic Water for Injection (benzyl alcohol or parabens preserved) to the vial and shake to dissolve. Use the quantity of diluent shown below to reconstitute the product:

Reconstitution of Ifosfamide

Dosage strength	Quantity of diluent	Final concentration
1 g	20 ml	50 mg/ml
3 g	60 ml	50 mg/ml

Storage/Stability: Reconstituted solutions are chemically and physically stable for 1 week at 30°C (86°F) or 3 weeks at 5°C (41°F).

Solutions of ifosfamide may be diluted further to concentrations of 0.6 to 20 mg/ml in the following fluids: 5% Dextrose Injection; 0.9% Sodium Chloride Injection; Lactated Ringer's Injection; Sterile Water for Injection. Such admixtures, when stored in large volume parenteral glass bottles, Viaflex bags or *PAB* bags, are physically and chemically stable for ≥ 1 week at 30°C (86°F) or 6 weeks at 5°C (41°F).

Because essentially identical stability results were obtained for Sterile Water admixtures as for the other admixtures, the use of large volume parenteral glass bottles, Viaflex bags or *PAB* bags that contain intermediate concentrations or mixtures of excipients (eg, 2.5% Dextrose Injection, 0.45% Sodium Chloride Injection or 5% Dextrose and 0.9% Sodium Chloride Injection) is also acceptable.

Refrigerate dilutions not prepared by constitution with Bacteriostatic Water for Injection (benzyl alcohol or parabens preserved), and use within 6 hours.

May store dry powder at room temperature. Avoid storage > 40°C (104°F).

Rx	**Ifex** (Mead Johnson Oncology)	**Powder for Injection:** 1 g	In single dose vials.[1]
🍁	**Ifex** (Bristol)		
Rx	**Ifex** (Mead Johnson Oncology)	3 g	In single dose vials.[2]
🍁	**Ifex** (Bristol)		

[1] Includes 200 mg amps *Mesnex* (mesna).

[2] Includes 400 mg amps *Mesnex* (mesna).

CYCLOPHOSPHAMIDE

Actions:

Pharmacology: Cyclophosphamide is an alkylating agent chemically related to the nitrogen mustards.

Cyclophosphamide is first hydroxylated by hepatic microsomal (P450 mixed-function oxidase) enzymes to the intermediate metabolites 4-hydroxycyclophosphamide and aldophosphamide. These are oxidized to the active antineoplastic alkylating compounds acrolein and phosphoramide mustard. The mechanism of action of the active metabolites is thought to involve cross-linking of DNA, which interferes with growth of susceptible neoplasms and normal tissues. It has not been demonstrated that any single metabolite is responsible for either the therapeutic or toxic effects of cyclophosphamide.

Pharmacokinetics:

Absorption/Distribution – Cyclophosphamide is well absorbed after oral administration with a bioavailability > 75%. Several cytotoxic and noncytotoxic metabolites have been identified in urine and in plasma. Concentrations of metabolites reach a maximum in plasma 2 to 3 hours after an IV dose. Plasma protein binding of unchanged drug is low, but some metabolites are > 60% bound.

Metabolism/Excretion – The drug is activated and inactivated to alkylating and nonalkylating metabolites respectively, by the P450 system in the liver. It is eliminated primarily in the form of metabolites; 5% to 25% of a dose is excreted as unchanged cyclophosphamide which has an elimination half-life of 3 to 12 hours. Although elevated levels of metabolites have occurred in patients with renal failure, increased clinical toxicity has not been demonstrated.

Indications:

Frequently used concurrently or sequentially with other antineoplastics. The following malignancies are often susceptible to cyclophosphamide treatment:

Malignant disease: Malignant lymphomas (Stages III and IV, Ann Arbor Staging System): Hodgkin's disease; lymphocytic lymphoma (nodular or diffuse); mixed-cell type lymphoma; histiocytic lymphoma; Burkitt's lymphoma; multiple myeloma; neuroblastoma (disseminated disease); adenocarcinoma of the ovary; retinoblastoma; carcinoma of the breast.

Leukemias: Chronic lymphocytic leukemia; chronic granulocytic leukemia (usually ineffective in acute blastic crisis); acute myelogenous and monocytic leukemia; acute lymphoblastic (stem-cell) leukemia in children (given during remission, cyclophosphamide is effective in prolonging remission duration).

Mycosis fungoides : Advanced disease.

Nonmalignant disease:

Biopsy proven "minimal change" nephrotic syndrome in children – Cyclophosphamide is useful in carefully selected cases but should not be used as primary therapy. In children whose disease fails to respond adequately to appropriate corticosteroid therapy or in whom the corticosteroid therapy produces or threatens to produce intolerable side effects, cyclophosphamide may induce a remission. Cyclophosphamide is not indicated for the nephrotic syndrome in adults or for any other renal disease.

Unlabeled uses: Variety of severe rheumatologic conditions: Wegener's granulomatosis, other steroid-resistant vasculidites and in some cases of severe progressive rheumatoid arthritis and systemic lupus erythematosus. Toxicity is limiting.

Cyclophosphamide (total dose 1 to 12 g) has been used to halt the progression of multiple sclerosis or decrease the frequency and duration of episodes. It has also been used in the treatment of polyarteritis nodosa using an initial dose of 2 mg/kg/day orally or 4 mg/kg/day IV. Cyclophosphamide (500 mg over 1 hour every 1 to 3 weeks), alone or in combination with corticosteroids, may be useful in the treatment of polymyositis.

Possible treatment for severe neuropsychiatric systemic lupus erythematosus (NPSLE).

CYCLOPHOSPHAMIDE

Contraindications:

Previous hypersensitivity to the drug; continued use in severely depressed bone marrow function.

Warnings:

Hematologic: Leukopenia is an expected effect and is used as a guide to dosage. Leukopenia of < 2000 cells/mm^3 develops commonly in patients treated with an initial loading dose of the drug, and less frequently in patients maintained on smaller doses. The degree of neutropenia is particularly important because it correlates with a reduction in resistance to infections. Thrombocytopenia or anemia develop occasionally. These effects are usually reversible when therapy is interrupted. Recovery from leukopenia usually begins in 7 to 10 days after cessation of therapy.

Cardiac toxicity: Although a few instances of cardiac dysfunction have occurred following use of recommended doses of cyclophosphamide, no causal relationship has been established. Cardiotoxicity has been observed in some patients receiving high doses of cyclophosphamide ranging from 120 to 270 mg/kg administered over a period of a few days, usually as a portion of an intensive antineoplastic multidrug regimen or in conjunction with transplantation procedures. In a few instances with high doses of cyclophosphamide, severe, and sometimes fatal, congestive heart failure has occurred within a few days after the first cyclophosphamide dose. Histopathologic examination has primarily shown hemorrhagic myocarditis.

No residual cardiac abnormalities as evidenced by electrocardiogram or echocardiogram appear to be present in the patients surviving episodes of apparent cardiac toxicity associated with high doses of cyclophosphamide.

Adrenalectomy patients: Adjustment of the doses of both replacement steroids and cyclophosphamide may be necessary for the adrenalectomized patient.

Wound healing: Cyclophosphamide may interfere with normal wound healing.

GU: Acute hemorrhagic cystitis occurs in 7% to 12% of patients, although some report an occurrence of up to 40%. Hemorrhagic cystitis can be severe, even fatal, and is probably caused by urinary metabolites. Nonhemorrhagic cystitis and bladder fibrosis have also been reported. Ample fluid intake and frequent voiding help to prevent cystitis, but when it occurs, it is usually necessary to interrupt therapy. Hematuria usually resolves spontaneously within a few days after therapy is discontinued, but may persist. In protracted cases, medical or surgical supportive treatment may be required.

A formalin (37% formaldehyde solution diluted to a 1% solution) bladder instillation has successfully controlled the cystitis. Complications may occur with the 10% solution; there appears to be no additional value in using > 4% solutions. The use of mesna has reduced the incidence of cyclophosphamide-induced cystitis (see individual monograph).

Treatment with cyclophosphamide may cause significant suppression of immune responses. Serious, sometimes fatal, infections may develop in severely immunosuppressed patients. Cyclophosphamide treatment may not be indicated, should be interrupted or the dose reduced in patients who have or who develop viral, bacterial, fungal, protozoan or helminthic infections.

Hypersensitivity reactions (type I) have occurred, mediated through increased B-cell activity and production of IgE. Refer to Management of Acute Hypersensitivity Reactions.

Rare instances of anaphylactic reaction including one death have occurred. One instance of possible cross sensitivity with other alkylating agents has occurred.

Renal/Hepatic function impairment: Use cautiously. Patients with compromised renal function may show some measurable changes in pharmacokinetic parameters of cyclophosphamide metabolism, but there is no evidence indicating a need for modified dosage in these patients.

Carcinogenesis: Secondary neoplasia has developed with cyclophosphamide alone or with other antineoplastic drugs or radiation therapy. These most frequently have been urinary bladder, myeloproliferative and lymphoproliferative malignancies. Secondary malignancies have developed most frequently in patients with primary myeloproliferative and lymphoproliferative malignancies and nonmalignant diseases in which immune processes are pathologically involved. In some cases, the secondary malignancy was detected several years after drug discontinuance. Secondary urinary bladder malignancies generally have occurred in patients who previously developed hemorrhagic cystitis. One case of carcinoma of the renal pelvis occurred with long-term therapy for cerebral vasculitits. Consider the possibility of secondary malignancy in any benefit-to-risk assessment for use of the drug.

Fertility impairment: Cyclophosphamide interferes with oogenesis and spermatogenesis. It may cause sterility in both sexes. Development of sterility appears to depend on the dose, duration of therapy, and the state of gonadal function at the time of treatment. Cyclophosphamide-induced sterility may be irreversible in some patients.

Amenorrhea associated with decreased estrogen and increased gonadotropin secretion develops in a significant proportion of women treated with cyclophosphamide. Affected patients generally resume regular menses within a few months after cessation of therapy. Girls treated during prepubescence generally develop secondary sexual characteristics normally and have regular menses. Ovarian fibrosis with apparently complete loss of germ cells after prolonged cyclophosphamide treatment in late prepubescence has occurred. Girls treated with cyclophosphamide during prepubescence subsequently have conceived.

Men treated with cyclophosphamide may develop oligospermia or azoospermia associated with increased gonadotropin but normal testosterone secretion. Sexual potency and libido are unimpaired in these patients. Boys treated during prepubescence develop secondary sexual characteristics normally, but may have oligospermia or azoospermia and increased gonadotropin secretion. Some degree of testicular atrophy may occur. Cyclophosphamide-induced azoospermia is reversible in some patients, though the reversibility may not occur for several years after cessation of therapy. Men temporarily rendered sterile by cyclophosphamide have subsequently fathered normal children.

Pregnancy: Category D. Both normal and malformed newborns have been reported following the use of cyclophosphamide in pregnancy. Malformations have included limb abnormalities (missing fingers and toes), cardiac anomalies and hernias. In addition, 40% of infants exposed to anticancer drugs (timing of exposure not considered) were of low birth weight. However, use of cyclophosphamide in the second and third trimesters does not seem to place the infant at risk for congenital defects; this does not include the possibility of physical and mental growth abnormalities.

Also, *paternal* use of combination chemotherapy, including cyclophosphamide prior to conception, has been associated with cardiac and limb abnormalities in an infant.

If this drug is used during pregnancy, or if the patient becomes pregnant while taking this drug, apprise the patient of the potential hazard to the fetus. Advise women of childbearing potential to avoid becoming pregnant.

Lactation: Cyclophosphamide is excreted in breast milk. Because of the potential for serious adverse reactions and the potential for tumorigenicity decide whether to discontinue breastfeeding or to discontinue the drug, taking into account the importance of the drug to the mother.

Children: See Administration and Dosage.

Precautions:

Monitoring: During treatment, monitor the patient's hematologic profile (particularly neutrophils and platelets) regularly to determine the degree of hematopoietic suppression. Examine urine regularly for red cells which may precede hemorrhagic cystitis.

Special risk patients: Give cautiously to patients with: Leukopenia; thrombocytopenia; tumor cell infiltration of bone marrow; previous radiation therapy; previous cytotoxic therapy.

Immunosuppression: Treatment with cyclophosphamide may cause significant suppression of immune responses. Serious, sometimes fatal, infections may develop in severely immunosuppressed patients. Treatment may not be indicated or should be interrupted or the dose reduced in patients who have or who develop viral, bacterial, fungal, protozoan or helminthic infections.

Renal effects: A syndrome of inappropriate antidiuretic hormone (SIADH) has occurred with IV doses > 50 mg/kg. It is both a limitation to and consequence of fluid loading. Hemorrhagic ureteritis and renal tubular necrosis have occurred. Such lesions usually resolve following cessation of therapy.

CYCLOPHOSPHAMIDE

Drug Interactions:

Cyclophosphamide Drug Interactions			
Precipitant Drug	Object Drug*		Description
Allopurinol	Cyclophosphamide	⬆	The myelosuppressive effects of cyclophosphamide may be enhanced, possibly increasing the risk of bleeding or infection.
Chloramphenicol	Cyclophosphamide	⬇	Cyclophosphamide half-life may increase and metabolite concentrations may be decreased.
Phenobarbital	Cyclophosphamide	⬇	The rate of metabolism and the leukopenic activity of cyclophsphamide reportedly are increased by chronic administration of high doses of phenobarbital.
Thiazide diuretics	Cyclosphosphamide[1]	⬆	Antineoplastic-induced leukopenia may be prolonged.
Cyclophosphamide	Anticoagulants	⬆	Anticoagulant effect is increased.
Cyclophosphamide[1]	Digoxin	⬇	Digoxin serum levels may be reduced.
Cyclophosphamide	Doxorubicin	⬆	Doxorubicin-induced cardiotoxicity is potentiated.
Cyclophosphamide	Quinolone	⬇	The antimicrobial effects of quinolones may be decreased.
Cyclophosphamide	Succinylcholine	⬆	Neuromuscular blockade may be prolonged, because of inhibition of cholinesterase activity.

* ⬆ = Object drug increased. ⬇ = Object drug decreased.
[1] Cyclophosphamide used in combination with other antineoplastics.

Adverse Reactions:

Cardiovascular: Cardiotoxicity (hemorrhagic cardiac necrosis, transmural hemorrhages, coronary artery vasculitis) (See Warnings).

Dermatologic: Alopecia (frequent); regrowth of hair can be expected, although it may be of a different color or texture; skin rash (occasionally); pigmentation of the skin and changes in nails.

GI: Anorexia; nausea; vomiting; diarrhea; stomatitis; abdominal discomfort or pain; hemorrhagic colitis; oral mucosal ulceration.

GU: Acute hemorrhagic cystitis; amenorrhea, oligospermia, azoospermia, sterility (see Warnings); urinary bladder fibrosis; hematuria; hemorrhagic ureteritis; renal tubular necrosis.

Hematologic: Leukopenia, thrombocytopenia, anemia (see Warnings).

Pulmonary: Interstitial pulmonary fibrosis.

Miscellaneous: Secondary neoplasia; anaphylactic reactions; infections (see Warnings); jaundice; interferance with normal wound healing; interstitial pulmonary fibrosis with prolonged high dosage.

Overdosage:

No specific antidote for cyclophosphamide is known. Use general supportive measures. Cyclophosphamide and its metabolites are dialyzable although there are probably quantitative differences depending upon the dialysis system being used. Refer to General Management of Acute Overdosage. Cyclophosphamide and its metabolites are dialyzable.

Patient Information:

Take tablets preferably on an empty stomach. If GI upset is severe, take with food.

Notify your doctor of unusual bleeding or bruising, fever, chills, sore throat, cough, shortness of breath, seizures, lack of menstrual flow, unusual lumps or masses, flank or stomach pain, joint pain, sores in the mouth or on the lips, or yellow discoloration of the skin or eyes.

Contraceptive measures are recommended during therapy for both men and women.

CYCLOPHOSPHAMIDE

Administration and Dosage:

Malignant diseases (adults and children):

IV – When used as the only oncolytic drug therapy, the initial IV dose for patients with no hematologic deficiency is 40 to 50 mg/kg, usually given in divided doses over 2 to 5 days. Other IV regimens include 10 to 15 mg/kg every 7 to 10 days or 3 to 5 mg/kg twice weekly.

Oral – Usual range of 1 to 5 mg/kg/day for initial and maintenance dosing.

When cyclophosphamide is included in combined cytotoxic regimens, it may be necessary to reduce the dose of cyclophosphamide as well as that of the other drugs.

Dosages must be adjusted in accord with evidence of antitumor activity or leukopenia. The total leukocyte count is a good, objective guide for regulating dosage.

Nonmalignant diseases:

Biopsy proven "minimal change" nephrotic syndrome in children – An oral dose of 2.5 to 3 mg/kg daily for a period of 60 to 90 days is recommended. In males, the incidence of oligospermia and azoospermia increases if the duration of treatment exceeds 60 days. Treatment beyond 90 days increases the probability of sterility. Corticosteroid therapy may be tapered and discontinued during the course of cyclophosphamide therapy. See Precautions section concerning hematologic monitoring.

Preparation of parenteral solution: Add Sterile Water for Injection to the vial and shake to dissolve. Use the quantity of diluent shown in the following table to reconstitute the product.

Reconstitution of Cyclophosphamide	
	Quantity of diluent (ml)
Vial strength	Powder for Injection
100 mg	5
200 mg	10
500 mg	25
1 g	50
2 g	100

Prepared solutions may be injected IV, IM, intraperitoneally or intrapleurally, or they may be infused IV in 5% Dextrose Injection or 5% Dextrose and 0.9% Sodium Chloride Injection, 5% Dextrose and Ringer's Injection, Lactated Ringer's Injection, 0.45% Sodium Chloride Injection or ⅙ molar Sodium Lactate Injection.

Preparation of oral solution: Dissolve injectable cyclophosphamide in Aromatic Elixir; store under refrigeration in glass containers and use within 14 days.

Storage/Stability: Use solutions prepared with Bacteriostatic Water for Injection (paraben preserved) within 24 hours if stored at room temperature or within 6 days if stored under refrigeration. If cyclophosphamide is not prepared with Bacteriostatic Water for Injection use the solution promptly (preferably within 6 hours). Cyclophosphamide does not contain an antimicrobial agent; take care to ensure the sterility of prepared solutions.

Rx	**Cytoxan** (Mead Johnson Oncology)	**Tablets:** 25 mg	White with blue flecks. In 100s.
		50 mg	White with blue flecks. In 100s and 1000s.
Rx	**Cytoxan Lyophilized** (Mead Johnson Oncology)	**Powder for Injection:** 75 mg mannitol/100 mg cyclophosphamide	In 100, 200 and 500 mg and 1 and 2 g vials.
Rx	**Neosar** (Pharmacia and Upjohn)	**Powder for Injection:** 82 mg sodium bicarbonate/100 mg cyclophosphamide	In 100, 200 and 500 mg and 1 and 2 g vials.

Nitrosoureas

LOMUSTINE (CCNU)

Warning:

Bone marrow suppression, notably thrombocytopenia and leukopenia, which may contribute to bleeding and overwhelming infections in an already compromised patient, is the most common and severe of the toxic effects of lomustine.

Because the major toxicity is delayed bone marrow suppression, monitor blood counts weekly for ≥ 6 weeks after a dose. At the recommended dosage, do not give courses of lomustine more frequently than every 6 weeks.

Bone marrow toxicity is cumulative. Consider dosage adjustments on the basis of nadir blood counts from prior dosage (see Administration and Dosage and Warnings).

Actions:

Pharmacology: Lomustine acts as an alkylating agent, but like other nitrosoureas, it may also inhibit several key enzymatic processes. Its mechanism of action involves the inhibition of both DNA and RNA synthesis through DNA alkylation. Lomustine has been shown to affect a number of cellular processes including RNA, protein synthesis and the processing of ribosomal and nucleoplasmic messenger RNA; DNA base component structure; the rate of DNA synthesis and DNA polymerase activity. It is cell cycle non-specific.

Pharmacokinetics:

Absorption – The lipid soluble nitrosoureas are rapidly and completely absorbed when given orally; appearance in plasma occurs ≈ 10 minutes postadministration and peak levels of metabolites appear in ≈ 3 hours.

Distribution – The lipid solubility of lomustine results in extensive tissue distribution. Blood-brain penetration is good; cerebrospinal fluid levels of 15% to 50% of those in plasma have been noted.

Metabolism – Lomustine is rapidly degraded, apparently in the liver, to several cytotoxic metabolites. The serum half-life of the metabolites ranges from 16 hours to 2 days. Tissue levels are comparable with plasma levels at 15 minutes after IV administration.

Excretion – About half of the dose is excreted in the form of degradation products within 24 hours. Small amounts are excreted via the feces and lungs.

Indications:

As a single agent in addition to other treatment modalities, or in established combination therapy with other agents in the following:

Brain tumors: Both primary and metastatic in patients who have already received appropriate surgical or radiotherapeutic procedures.

Hodgkin's disease: Secondary therapy in combination with other drugs in patients who relapse while on primary therapy, or who fail to respond to primary therapy.

Contraindications:

Hypersensitivity to lomustine.

Warnings:

Hematologic: The most frequent and most serious toxicity is delayed myelosuppression. It usually occurs 4 to 6 weeks after drug administration and is dose-related. Thrombocytopenia occurs ≈ 4 weeks after a dose and persists for 1 to 2 weeks. Leukopenia occurs ≈ 5 to 6 weeks after a dose and persists for 1 to 2 weeks. About 65% of patients develop white blood cell (WBC) counts < 5000/mm^3, and 36% of patients develop WBC counts < 3000/mm^3. Thrombocytopenia is generally more severe than leukopenia; however, both may be dose-limiting toxicities. Anemia also occurs, but is less frequent and less severe than thrombocytopenia or leukopenia. Cumulative myelosuppression may occur, manifested by more depressed indices or longer duration of suppression after repeated doses.

Hepatic toxicity: A reversible type of hepatic toxicity, manifested by increased transaminase, alkaline phosphatase and bilirubin levels, has occurred in a small percentage of patients.

Renal toxicity: Decrease in kidney size, progressive azotemia and renal failure have occurred in patients who received large cumulative doses after prolonged therapy. Kidney damage has occurred occasionally in patients receiving lower total doses.

Pulmonary toxicity: Pulmonary toxicity characterized by pulmonary infiltrates or fibrosis occurs rarely and appears to be dose-related. Onset of toxicity has occurred after an interval of ≥ 6 months from start of therapy with cumulative doses usually > 1100 mg/m^2. There is one report of pulmonary toxicity at a cumulative dose of 600 mg.

LOMUSTINE (CCNU)

Delayed onset pulmonary fibrosis occurring ≤ 15 years after treatment has been reported in patients who received related nitrosoureas in childhood and early adolescence combined with cranial radiotherapy for intracranial tumors.

Carcinogenesis: Carcinogenic in rats and mice in approximately clinical doses. Acute leukemia and bone marrow dysplasias have occurred after long term nitrosourea therapy.

Fertility impairment: There have been reports of persistent testicular damage causing infertility.

Pregnancy: Category D. Lomustine can cause fetal harm when administered to a pregnant woman. There are no adequate and well controlled studies in pregnant women. Advise patient of the potential hazard to the fetus if patient becomes pregnant while taking lomustine. Advise women of childbearing potential to avoid becoming pregnant while on lomustine.

Lactation: It is not known whether lomustine is excreted in breast milk. Because of the potential for serious adverse reactions, decide whether to discontinue breastfeeding or to discontinue the drug, taking into account the importance of the drug to the mother.

Children: See Administration and Dosage.

Precautions:

Monitoring: Major toxicity is delayed bone marrow suppression; monitor blood counts weekly for 6 weeks after a dose. Monitor liver and renal function periodically.

Also conduct baseline pulmonary function studies during treatment. Patients with a baseline < 70% of the predicted Forced Vital Capacity (FVC) or Carbon Monoxide Diffusing Capacity (DL_{CO}) are particularly at risk.

GI: Nausea and vomiting may occur 3 to 6 hours after an oral dose and usually last < 24 hours. Antiemetics prior to dosing may diminish and sometimes prevent these effects. May also be reduced by administration to fasting patients.

Adverse Reactions:

Most adverse reactions are reversible if detected early. When adverse reactions occur, reduce dosage or discontinue drug and take appropriate corrective measures.

Secondary malignancies: Long-term use of nitrosoureas may be associated with development of secondary malignancies (see Warnings).

GI: Nausea, vomiting (see Precautions); sore mouth, lips and throat; bleeding.

Hematologic: Delayed myelosuppression, leukopenia, anemia (see Warnings).

Renal: Decrease in kidney size, progressive azotemia, renal failure (see Warnings).

Miscellaneous: Alopecia; stomatitis (infrequent); disorientation, lethargy, ataxia, dysarthria (the relationship to medication is unclear); hepatic toxicity, pulmonary toxicity, pulmonary fibrosis (see Warnings).

Overdosage:

There are no proven antidotes for lomustine overdosage. Refer to General Management of Acute Overdosage.

Patient Information:

Notify physician if fever, chills, sore throat, unusual bleeding or bruising, shortness of breath, dry cough, swelling of feet or lower legs, yellowing of eyes and skin, confusion, sores on the mouth or lips or unusual tiredness occurs.

Medication may cause loss of appetite, nausea and vomiting; hair loss, skin rash or itching (infrequent); notify physician if these reactions become pronounced.

Take on an empty stomach to reduce nausea.

Avoid alcohol for short periods after taking a dose of lomustine.

Contraceptive measures are recommended during therapy.

Administration and Dosage:

Adults and children: 130 mg/m^2 as a single oral dose every 6 weeks. In compromised bone marrow function, reduce dose to 100 mg/m^2 every 6 weeks. Do not give a repeat course until circulating blood elements have returned to acceptable levels (platelets > 100,000/mm^3; leukocytes > 4000/mm^3). Monitor blood counts weekly and do not give repeat courses before 6 weeks; hematologic toxicity is delayed and cumulative.

Adjust doses subsequent to the initial dose according to the hematologic response of the patient to the preceding dose as follows:

Nitrosoureas

LOMUSTINE (CCNU)

Suggested Lomustine Dose Following Initial Dose		
Nadir after prior dose		Percentage of prior dose to be given
Leukocytes/mm^3	Platelets/mm^3	
> 4000	> 100,000	100%
3000-3999	75,000-99,999	100%
2000-2999	25,000-74,999	70%
< 2000	< 25,000	50%

Concomitant therapy: With other myelosuppressive drugs, adjust dosage accordingly.

Storage/Stability: Avoid excessive heat (over 40°C; 104°F).

Rx	**CeeNu** (Bristol-Myers Oncology)	**Capsules:** 10 mg	Two-tone white. In 20s.
		40 mg	White/green. In 20s.
		100 mg	Two-tone green. In 20s.
		Dose Pack: Two 100 mg capsules, two 40 mg capsules and two 10 mg capsules.	

Nitrosoureas

CARMUSTINE (BCNU)

Warning:

Because delayed bone marrow suppression is the major toxic effect of injectable carmustine, monitor complete blood counts weekly for at least 6 weeks after a dose. Do not give repeat doses more frequently than every 6 weeks. Bone marrow toxicity is cumulative; therefore, adjust dosage on the basis of nadir blood counts from prior dose (see dosage adjustment table under Administration and Dosage).

Bone marrow suppression, notably thrombocytopenia and leukopenia, which may contribute to bleeding and overwhelming infections in an already compromised patient, is the most common and severe of the toxic effects of injectable carmustine.

Pulmonary toxicity from injectable carmustine appears to be dose-related. Patients receiving > 1400 mg/m^2 cumulative dose are at significantly higher risk than those receiving less. Other risk factors include history of lung disease and duration of treatment. Cases of fatal pulmonary toxicity have occurred.

Additionally, delayed onset pulmonary fibrosis occurring up to 15 years after treatment has been reported in patients who received injectable carmustine in childhood and early adolescence.

Actions:

Pharmacology: Carmustine alkylates deoxyribonucleic acid (DNA) and ribonucleic acid (RNA) and also inhibits several enzymes by carbamoylation of amino acids in proteins. Carmustine is not cross resistant with other alkylators. Antineoplastic and toxic activities may be caused by metabolites.

Pharmacokinetics:

Injection – Because of the high lipid solubility and the lack of ionization at physiological pH, carmustine crosses the blood-brain barrier effectively. Levels of radioactivity in the CSF are ≥ 50% of those in plasma.

Following IV administration, it is rapidly degraded. The average terminal half-life, clearance and steady-state volume of distribution were 22 minutes, 56 ml/min/kg and 3.25 L/kg, respectively. Approximately 60% to 70% of the total dose is excreted in the urine in 96 hours, and 6% is expired as CO_2. The fate of the remainder is undetermined.

Wafer – Wafers are biodegradable in the human brain when implanted into the cavity after tumor resection. The carmustine released from the wafer diffuses into the surrounding brain tissue. The rate of biodegradation is variable from patient to patient. A wafer remnant may be observed on brain imaging scans or at re-operation even though extensive degradation of all components has occurred. The absorption, distribution, metabolism and excretion of the copolymer in humans is unknown.

Indications:

Injection: Palliative therapy as a single agent or combined with other approved chemotherapeutic agents in the following:

Brain tumors: Glioblastoma, brainstem glioma, medulloblastoma, astrocytoma, ependymoma and metastatic brain tumors.

Wafer: An adjunct to surgery to prolong survival in patients with recurrent glioblastoma multiforme for whom surgical resection is indicated.

Multiple myeloma: In combination with prednisone.

Hodgkin's disease and non-Hodgkin's lymphomas: As secondary therapy in combination with other approved drugs in patients who relapse with, or who fail to respond to, primary therapy.

Unlabeled uses: Mycosis fungoides (0.5 to 3 mg/ml topical solution).

Contraindications:

Hypersensitivity to carmustine or to any components of the wafer formulation.

Warnings:

Hematologic: The most frequent and serious toxic effect of injectable carmustine is delayed myelosuppression which usually occurs 4 to 6 weeks after administration and is dose-related (see Warning Box). Thrombocytopenia occurs at ≈ 4 weeks postadministration and persists for 1 to 2 weeks. Leukopenia occurs at 5 to 6 weeks after a dose and persists for 1 to 2 weeks. Thrombocytopenia is generally more severe than leukopenia; however, both may have dose-limiting toxicities. Anemia is generally less severe. The occurrence of acute leukemia and bone marrow dysplasias have been reported in patients following long-term nitrosourea therapy.

CARMUSTINE (BCNU)

Renal toxicity: Decrease in kidney size, progressive azotemia and renal failure have occurred in patients who received large cumulative doses of injectable carmustine after prolonged therapy; occasionally reported in patients receiving lower total doses.

Hepatic toxicity: Reversible hepatic toxicity, manifested by increased transaminase, alkaline phosphatase and bilirubin levels, has occurred in a small percentage of patients using injectable carmustine.

Pulmonary infiltrates or fibrosis have occurred with injectable carmustine (see Warning Box).

Ocular: Toxicity manifested as nerve fiber-layer infarcts and retinal hemorrhages has been associated with high dose injectable carmustine therapy. Carmustine administration through an intra-arterial intracarotid route is investigational and has been associated with ocular toxicity.

Brain herniation: Cases of intracerebral mass effect unresponsive to corticosteroids have been described in patients treated with the wafer, including one case leading to brain herniation.

Seizures: The majority of seizures in the placebo vs wafer study were mild or moderate in severity. The incidence of new or worsened seizures was the same for the treatment group and placebo (19%). Of the 22 patients with new or worsened seizures post-operatively, 54% of wafer-treated patients and 9% of placebo patients experienced the first new or worsened seizure within the first 5 post-operative days; the median time to onset was 3.5 days and 61 days, respectively. The occurrence of seizures did not reduce the survival benefit.

Brain edema: Brain edema was noted in 4% of patients treated with the wafer and in 1% of placebo patients. Development of brain edema with mass effect (caused by tumor recurrence, intracranial infection or necrosis) may necessitate re-operation and, in some cases, removal of wafer or its remnants.

Intracranial infection: Intracranial infection (meningitis or abscess) occurred in 4% of patients treated with the wafer and in 1% of patients receiving placebo. In wafer-treated patients, there were two cases of bacterial meningitis, one case of chemical menigitis and one case of meningitis, which was not further specified. A brain abscess developed in one placebo-treated patient. The rate of deep wound infection (infection of subgaleal space, bone, meninges or neural parenchyma) was 6% in both the wafer and placebo treated patients.

Obstructive hydrocephalus: Avoid communication between the surgical resection cavity and the ventricular system to prevent the wafers from migrating into the ventricular system and causing obstructive hydrocephalus. If a communication exists, close it prior to wafer implantation.

Mutagenesis: Long-term use of nitrosoureas has been reported to be associated with the development of secondary malignancies.

Fertility impairment: There have been reports of persistent testicular damage causing infertility with injectable carmustine.

Pregnancy: Category D. Carmustine is embryotoxic and teratogenic in rats and embryotoxic in rabbits at dose levels equivalent to the human dose. Carmustine may cause fetal harm when administered to a pregnant woman. There are no adequate and well controlled studies in pregnant women. If this drug is used during pregnancy, or if the patient becomes pregnant while taking this drug, advise her of the potential hazard to the fetus. Advise women of childbearing potential to avoid becoming pregnant.

Lactation: It is not known whether this drug is excreted in breast milk. Because of the potential for serious adverse reactions in breastfeeding infants from carmustine, decide whether to discontinue breastfeeding or to discontinue the drug, taking into account the importance of the drug to the mother.

Children: Safety and efficacy for use in children have not been established.

Precautions:

Monitoring:

Injection – Because of delayed bone marrow suppression, monitor blood counts weekly for at least 6 weeks after a dose.

Conduct baseline pulmonary function studies and frequent pulmonary function tests during treatment. Patients with a baseline < 70% of predicted Forced Vital Capacity (FVC) or Carbon Monoxide Diffusing Capacity (DL_{CO}) are at particular risk. Monitor liver and renal function tests periodically.

CARMUSTINE (BCNU)

Wafer – Monitor patients undergoing craniotomy for malignant glioma and implantation of the wafer closely for known complications of craniotomy, including seizures, intracranial infections, abnormal wound healing and brain edema.

Healing abnormalities: The majority of these events were mild to moderate in severity. Healing abnormalities occurred in 14% of wafer-treated patients compared with 5% of placebo recipients. These events included CSF leaks, subdural fluid collections, subgaleal or wound effusions and wound break-downs.

GI: Nausea and vomiting after IV administration. This dose-related toxicity appears within 2 hours of dosing and lasts 4 to 6 hours. Prior administration of antiemetics is effective in diminishing or preventing these side effects.

Drug Interactions:

Carmustine Drug Interactions			
Preciptant drug	Object drug*		Description
Cimetidine	Carmustine	⬆	Cimetidine may enhance the myelosuppressive effects of carmustine, possibly to the point of toxity.
Mitomycin	Carmustine	⬆	Qualitative and quantitative changes in tear films, with corneal and conjunctival epithelial damage.
Carmustine	Digoxin	⬇	Digoxin serum levels may be reduced, and its actions may be decreased by a combination chemotherapy regimen including carmustine.
Carmustine	Phenytoin	⬇	Phenytoin serum concentrations may be decreased by a combination chemotherapy regimen including carmustine.

* ⬆ = Object drug increased. ⬇ = Object drug decreased.

Adverse Reactions:

Most adverse reactions are reversible if detected early. When toxic effects or adverse reactions occur, reduce dosage or discontinue injectable carmustine and take appropriate corrective measures. Reinstitute injectable carmustine therapy with caution.

GI: Nausea, vomiting (see Precautions).

Hematologic: Myelosuppression, thrombocytopenia, leukopenia, anemia, leukemia, bone marrow dysplasias (see Warnings).

Local: Burning at the injection site may occur; thrombosis is rare.
Accidental contact of reconstituted carmustine with the skin has caused burning and hyperpigmentation of the affected areas.

Miscellaneous: Renal hepatic toxicity, pulmonary infiltrater or fibrosis, ocular toxicity (see Warnings); neuroretinitis.

Other: Rapid IV infusion may produce intensive flushing of the skin and suffusion of the conjunctiva within 2 hours, lasting ≈ 4 hours.

The following post-operative adverse events were observed in ≥ 4% of the patients receiving the wafer in the placebo-controlled clinical trial. Except for nervous system effects, only events more common in the wafer group are listed.

Nitrosoureas

CARMUSTINE (BCNU)

Adverse Reactions: Carmustine Wafer vs Placebo (≥ 4%)		
Adverse reaction	Wafer with carmustine (n=110; %)	Wafer without carmustine (n=112; %)
Body as a whole		
Urinary tract infection	21	17
Healing abnormal	14	5
Fever	12	8
Nausea and vomiting	8	6
Pain	7	1
Rash	5	4
CNS		
Convulsion	19	19
Hemiplegia	19	20
Headache	15	13
Somnolence	14	11
Confusion	10	8
Aphasia	9	11
Stupor	6	6
Brain edema	4	1
Intracranial hypertension	4	8
Meningitis or absess	4	1

Overdosage:
No proven antidotes have been established for carmustine overdosage.

Patient Information:
Contraceptive measures are recommended during therapy.

Administration and Dosage:
Wafer: It is recommended that eight wafers be placed in the resection cavity if the size and shape of cavity allows. Should the size and shape not accommodate eight wafers, the maximum number of wafers as allowed should be used. Slight overlapping of the wafer is acceptable. Wafers broken in half may be used, but discard wafers broken in more than two pieces. Oxidized regenerated cellulose may be placed over the wafers to secure them against the cavity surface. After placement of the wafers, the resection cavity should be irrigated and the dura closed in a water tight fashion.

Injection: As a single agent in previously untreated patients, 150 to 200 mg/m^2 IV every 6 weeks. Give as a single dose or divided daily injections (eg, 75 to 100 mg/m^2 on 2 successive days).

When used in combination with other myelosuppressive drugs or in patients in whom bone marrow reserve is depleted, adjust doses accordingly.

Do not give a repeat course until circulating blood elements have returned to acceptable levels (platelets > 100,000/mm^3; leukocytes > 4000/mm^3). Adequate number of neutrophils should be present on a peripheral blood smear. Monitor blood counts weekly; do not give repeat courses before 6 weeks because of delayed and cumulative toxicity.

The following schedule is suggested as a guide to dosage adjustment based on the patient's hematologic response to the previous dose:

Suggested Carmustine Dose Following Initial Dose		
Nadir after prior dose		Percentage of prior dose to be given
Leukocytes/mm^3	Platelets/mm^3	
> 4000	> 100,000	100%
3000-3999	> 75,000-99,999	100%
2000-2999	> 25,000-74,999	70%
< 2000	< 25,000	50%

Preparation/Handling of solutions:
Wafer – Use of double gloves is recommended. Use surgical instrument dedicated to the handling of the wafers for implantation. Deliver the aluminum foil laminate pouches containing the wafer to the operating room and leave unopened until ready to implant the wafers.

Nitrosoureas

CARMUSTINE (BCNU)

Injection – Dissolve with 3 ml of the supplied sterile diluent, then add 27 ml of Sterile Water for Injection to the alcohol solution. The resulting solution contains 3.3 mg/ml of carmustine in 10% ethanol; pH is 5.6 to 6.

Reconstitution as recommended results in a clear colorless to yellowish solution that may be further diluted with 0.9% Sodium Chloride for Injection or 5% Dextrose for Injection.

Administer the reconstituted solution by IV drip over 1 to 2 hours. Shorter infusion times may produce intense pain and burning at the injection site.

The lyophilized dosage formulation contains no preservatives and is not intended as a multiple dose vial.

Storage/Stability:

Wafer – Unopened foil pouches may be kept at ambient room temperature for a maximum of 6 hours at a time. Store at or below -20°C (-4°F).

Injection – Store unopened vials of the dry powder in a refrigerator (2° to 8°C; 36° to 46°F).The recommended storage of unopened vials provides a stable product for 2 years. After reconstitution as recommended, carmustine is stable for 8 hours at room temperature (25° C; 77° F) or 24 hours under refrigeration (4°C; 39°F). Protect from light.

Vials reconstituted as directed and further diluted to a concentration of 0.2 mg/ml in 5% Dextrose Injection or 0.9% Sodium Chloride Injection are stable for 48 hours under refrigeration (4°C; 39°F) and an additional 8 hours at room temperature (25°C; 77°F) under normal room fluorescent light.

Only use glass containers.

Carmustine has a low melting point (≈ 30.5° to 32°C; ≈ 87° to 90°F). Exposure of the drug to this temperature or above will cause it to liquefy and appear as an oil film on the bottom of the vials. This is a sign of decomposition; discard the vial. If there is a question of adequate refrigeration upon receipt of this product, immediately inspect the larger vial in each individual carton. Hold the vial to a bright light for inspection. The carmustine will appear as a very small amount of dry flakes or dry congealed mass. If this is evident, the carmustine is suitable for use; refrigerate immediately.

Rx	**BiCNU** (Bristol-Myers Oncology)	**Powder for Injection:** 100 mg	In vials with 3 ml sterile diluent.
Rx	**Gliadel** (Rhone-Poulenc Rorer)	**Wafer**: 7.7 mg of carmustine	In single dose treatment box with 8 individually pouched wafers.

STREPTOZOCIN

> **Warning:**
> A patient need not be hospitalized but should have access to a facility with laboratory and supportive resources sufficient to monitor drug tolerance and to protect and maintain a patient compromised by drug toxicity. Renal toxicity is dose-related and cumulative and may be severe or fatal. Other major toxicities are nausea and vomiting, which may be severe and, at times, treatment limiting. In addition, liver dysfunction, diarrhea and hematological changes have been observed.
> Judge the possible benefit against the known toxic effects of this drug.

Actions:

Pharmacology: Streptozocin is a naturally occurring nitrosourea that contains a glucose moiety not present in the other compounds. The glucose moiety is believed to contribute to reduced myelotoxicity, specificity for pancreatic islet cells and the drug's much slower reactivity toward DNA compared with other nitrosoureas.

Streptozocin inhibits DNA synthesis without significantly affecting RNA or protein synthesis in bacterial and mammalian cells. The biochemical mechanism leading to mammalian cell death has not been established but is at least partially caused by DNA alkylation causing intrastrand crosslinks; streptozocin inhibits cell proliferation at a considerably lower level than that needed to inhibit precursor incorporation into DNA or to inhibit several of the enzymes involved in DNA synthesis. The drug is cell cycle nonspecific.

Pharmacokinetics: After rapid IV injection, unchanged drug is rapidly cleared from the plasma (half-life, 35 minutes). Two hours after administration, metabolites are detected in spinal fluid in equivalent concentration to plasma. Metabolites persist in plasma over 24 hours and concentrate in the liver and kidney. Approximately 60% to 72% of an administered dose can be detected in the urine within 4 hours; 10% to 20% as parent drug. Most excretion is completed in 24 hours.

Indications:

Metastatic islet cell carcinoma of the pancreas (functional and nonfunctional carcinomas). Because of its inherent renal toxicity, limit therapy with this drug to patients with symptomatic or progressive metastatic disease.

Warnings:

Hematologic: Hematologic toxicity has been rare, most often involving mild decreases in hematocrit. However, fatal hematologic toxicity with substantial reductions in leukocyte and platelet counts has been observed.

GI: Nausea and vomiting usually begins 1 to 4 hours after administration and lasts 24 hours; occasionally requiring discontinuation of drug therapy.

Hypoglycemia: Mild to moderate abnormalities of glucose tolerance have generally been reversible, but insulin shock with hypoglycemia has occurred.

Hydration: Because of renal toxicity, keep the patient well hydrated. Increase fluid intake for sore lips, mouth or throat, diarrhea or jaundice.

Renal toxicity occurs in up to ⅔ of all patients treated with streptozocin, as evidenced by azotemia, anuria, hypophosphatemia, glycosuria and renal tubular acidosis. *Such toxicity is dose-related and cumulative and may be severe or fatal.* Monitor renal function before and after each course of therapy. Obtain serial urinalysis, BUN, plasma creatinine, serum electrolytes and creatinine clearance prior to, at least weekly during, and for 4 weeks after drug administration. Serial urinalysis is particularly important for the early detection of proteinuria; quantitate with a 24 hour collection when proteinuria is detected. Mild proteinuria is one of the first signs of renal toxicity and may herald further deterioration of renal function. Reduce the dose or discontinue treatment in the presence of significant renal toxicity. In patients with preexisting renal disease, judge potential benefit of streptozocin against known risk of serious renal damage.

Do not use in combination or concomitantly with other potential nephrotoxins.

Carcinogenesis/Mutagenesis/Fertility impairment: When administered parenterally, streptozocin induces renal tumors in rats, and liver and other tumors in hamsters. Stomach and pancreatic tumors were observed in rats treated orally with streptozocin. Streptozocin is mutagenic in mammalian cells. It has also been carcinogenic in mice and has adversely affected fertility in rats.

Pregnancy: Category C. Streptozocin is teratogenic in rats and has abortifacient effects in rabbits. There are no studies in pregnant women. Use during pregnancy only if the potential benefit outweighs the potential risks.

STREPTOZOCIN

Lactation: It is not known whether streptozocin is excreted in breast milk. Because of the potential for serious adverse reactions in breastfeeding infants, discontinue breastfeeding in patients receiving streptozocin.

Precautions:

Monitoring: Closely monitor for evidence of renal (see Warnings), hepatic and hematopoietic toxicity. Perform complete blood counts and liver function tests at least weekly. Dosage adjustments or discontinuance of the drug may be indicated, depending upon the degree of toxicity.

Topical exposure: When exposed dermally, some rats developed benign tumors at the site of application. Consequently, streptozocin may pose a carcinogenic hazard following topical exposure if not properly handled.

Adverse Reactions:

CNS: Confusion, lethargy and depression have occurred with a 5 day continuous infusion regimen that may have facilitated these effects.

GI: Nausea, vomiting (> 90%; see Warnings); diarrhea; sore mouth, lips and throat; bleeding; duodenal ulcer.

Hepatic: Chemical liver dysfunction (≈ 25%); hepatic toxicity characterized by elevated liver enzymes (AST and LDH); hypoalbuminemia; jaundice.

Miscellaneous: Nephrogenic diabetes insipidus (two cases: One had spontaneous recovery; the second responded to indomethacin); hematological toxicity (rare); glucose intolerance (see Warnings).

Overdosage:

No specific antidote for streptozocin is known. Refer to General Management of Acute Overdosage.

Administration and Dosage:

Administer IV. Intra-arterial administration is not recommended because adverse renal effects may be evoked more rapidly.

Dosage schedules: The following two different dosage schedules have been used successfully. The ideal duration of maintenance therapy has not been established for either schedule:

Daily schedule – 500 mg/m² of body surface area (BSA) for 5 consecutive days every 6 weeks until maximum benefit or until treatment limiting toxicity is observed. Dosage increases are not recommended.

Weekly schedule – Initial dose is 1000 mg/m² BSA at weekly intervals for the first 2 courses (weeks). In subsequent courses, increase drug doses in patients who have not achieved a therapeutic response and have not experienced significant toxicity with the previous course of treatment. However, do not exceed a single dose of 1500 mg/m² BSA, as a greater dose may cause azotemia. On this schedule, the median time to onset of response is ≈ 17 days and the median time to maximum response is ≈ 35 days. The median total dose to onset of response is ≈ 2000 mg/m² BSA and the median total dose to maximum response is ≈ 4000 mg/m² BSA.

For patients with functional tumors, serial monitoring of fasting insulin levels allows a determination of biochemical response to therapy. For patients with either functional or nonfunctional tumors, response to therapy can be determined by measurable reductions of tumor size (reduction of organomegaly, masses or lymph nodes).

Reconstitute with 9.5 ml of Dextrose Injection or 0.9% Sodium Chloride Injection. The resulting pale gold solution contains 100 mg/ml streptozocin. Where more dilute infusion solutions are desirable, further dilution in the above vehicles is recommended.

Storage/Stability: The total storage time for reconstituted streptozocin is 12 hours. This product contains no preservatives and is not intended as a multiple dose vial. Refrigerate unopened vials at 2° to 8°C (35° to 46°F) and protect from light.

Rx	**Zanosar** (Pharmacia & Upjohn)	**Powder for Injection:** 1 g (100 mg/ml)	In vials.

THIOTEPA (Triethylenethiophosphoramide; TSPA; TESPA)

Actions:

Pharmacology: Thiotepa is a cell cycle nonspecific alkylating agent related to nitrogen mustard. Its radiomimetic action is believed to occur through the release of ethylenimine radicals, which disrupt the bonds of deoxyribonucleic acid (DNA). The drug has no apparent differential affinity for neoplasms.

Pharmacokinetics: TEPA, which possesses cytotoxic activity, appears to be the major metabolite of thiotepa found in the serum and urine. Urinary excretion of thiotepa and metabolites was 63% in a 34-year-old patient with metastatic carcinoma of the cecum who received a dose of 0.3 mg/kg IV. Thiotepa and TEPA in urine each accounts for < 2% of the dose.

Thiotepa pharmacokinetics are essentially the same in children as in adults at conventional doses.

Select IV Thiotepa Pharmacokinetics

	Thiotepa		TEPA	
Parameters	60 mg	80 mg	60 mg	80 mg
Peak serum concentration (ng/ml)	1331	1828	273	353
Elimination half-life (hr)	2.4	2.3	17.6	15.7
AUC (ng/hr/ml)	2832	4127	4789	7452
Total body clearance (ml/min)	446	419	-	-

Indications:

Carcinomas: Adenocarcinoma of the breast or ovary.

Controlling intracavitary effusions secondary to diffuse or localized neoplastic disease of various serosal cavities.

Treatment of superficial papillary carcinoma of the urinary bladder.

Lymphomas: While now largely superseded by other treatments, this drug has been effective against lymphomas, such as lymphosarcoma and Hodgkin's disease.

Contraindications:

Hypersensitivity to thiotepa; existing hepatic, renal or bone marrow damage (see Warnings).

Warnings:

Hematopoietic toxicity: This drug is highly toxic to the hematopoietic system. A rapidly falling white blood cell (WBC) or platelet count indicates a need to discontinue or reduce dosage. Perform weekly blood and platelet counts during therapy and for ≥ 3 weeks after therapy discontinuation.

The most serious complication of excessive therapy or sensitivity is bone marrow depression, causing leukopenia, thrombocytopenia and anemia. Death from septicemia and hemorrhage has occurred as a result of hematopoietic depression.

The most reliable guide to toxicity is the WBC count; if this falls to ≤ 3000/mm^3, discontinue use. If the platelet count falls to 150,000/mm^3, discontinue therapy. Red blood cell (RBC) count is a less accurate indicator of toxicity.

Death has occurred after intravesical administration. This was caused by bone marrow depression from systemically absorbed drug.

Hypersensitivity: Allergic reactions have occurred (see Adverse Reactions). Refer to Management of Acute Hypersensitivity Reactions.

Renal/Hepatic function impairment: If the benefits outweigh the potential risks, use in low doses and monitor hepatic and renal function.

Carcinogenesis/Mutagenesis/Fertility impairment: Like many alkylating agents, this drug has been shown to be carcinogenic.

Thiotepa is mutagenic. In vitro, it causes chromatid-type chromosomal aberrations. The frequency of induced aberrations increases with the patient's age.

Thiotepa impaired fertility in male mice at oral or IP doses ≥ 0.7 mg/kg (≈ 12-fold less than the maximum recommended human therapeutic dose). Thiotepa (0.5 mg) inhibited implantation in female rats when instilled into the uterine cavity. Thiotepa interfered with spermatogenesis in male mice at IP doses ≥ 0.5 mg/kg.

Pregnancy: Category D. Thiotepa can cause fetal harm when administered to a pregnant woman. Thiotepa given by the IP route was teratogenic in mice and rats at doses ≥ 1 and 3 mg/kg, respectively (≈ 8-fold less than and ≈ equal to the maximum recommended human therapeutic dose [0.8 mg/kg]) and lethal to rabbit fetuses at a dose of 3 mg/kg.

Use effective contraception during therapy if either the patient or partner is of childbearing potential. There are no adequate and well controlled studies in pregnant women. If thiotepa is used during pregnancy, or if pregnancy occurs during therapy, apprise the patient and partner of the potential hazard to the fetus.

THIOTEPA (Triethylenethiophosphoramide; TSPA; TESPA)

Lactation: It is not known whether thiotepa is excreted in breast milk. Because of the potential for tumorigenicity in animals, decide whether to discontinue breastfeeding or to discontinue the drug, taking into account the importance of the drug to the mother.

Children: Safety and efficacy have not been established.

Precautions:

Monitoring: Because of hematopoietic toxicity, perform weekly blood and platelet counts during therapy and for ≥ 3 weeks after therapy discontinuation.

Concomitant therapy: Do not combine therapeutic modalities having the same mechanism of action. Thiotepa combined with other alkylating agents, such as nitrogen mustard or cyclophosphamide, or with irradiation, would intensify toxicity rather than enhance therapeutic response. If these agents must follow each other, it is important that recovery from the first, as indicated by WBC count, be complete before therapy with the second agent is instituted.

Lymphomas: Thiotepa is now largely superseded by other treatments.

Drug Interactions:

Neuromuscular blocking agents: Coadministration of thiotepa and **pancuronium** resulted in prolonged muscular paralysis and respiratory depression.

Avoid other drugs that are known to produce bone-marrow depression.

Adverse Reactions:

Dermatologic: Contact dermatitis; pain at injection site; alopecia; dermatitis; skin depigmentation (following topical use).

GI: Nausea; vomiting; abdominal pain; anorexia.

GU: Dysuria; urinary retention; chemical or hemorrhagic cystitis (rare, following intravesical but not parenteral use); amenorrhea; interference with spermatogenesis (see Warnings).

CNS: Dizziness; headache; blurred vision.

Hypersensitivity: Allergic reactions have occurred (eg, rash, urticaria, laryngeal edema, asthma, anaphylactic shock, wheezing).

Miscellaneous: Conjunctivitis; fatigue; weakness; febrile reaction and discharge from a subcutaneous lesion (result of tumor tissue breakdown); hematopoietic toxicity (see Warnings).

Overdosage:

Hematopoietic toxicity can occur, manifested by a decrease in the white cell count or platelets. RBC count is a less accurate indicator of toxicity. Bleeding manifestations may develop. The patient may become more vulnerable to infection and less able to combat such infection. Dosages within and minimally above the recommended therapeutic doses have been associated with potentially life-threatening hematopoietic toxicity. Thiotepa has a toxic effect on the hematopoietic system that is dose-related. Thiotepa is dialyzable. There is no known antidote for thiotepa overdosage. Transfusions of whole blood or platelets have proven beneficial for hematopoietic toxicity.

Patient Information:

Notify the physician in the case of any sign of bleeding (epistaxis, easy bruising, change in color of urine, black stool) or infection (fever, chills).

Notify the physician for possible pregnancy to patient or partner. Use effective contraception during thiotepa therapy if either the patient or the partner is of childbearing potential.

Administration and Dosage:

Do not administer orally because GI absorption is variable.

Individualize dosage. A slow response may be deceptive and may lead to unwarranted frequency of administration with subsequent toxicity. After maximum benefit is obtained by initial therapy, continue with maintenance therapy (1- to 4–week intervals). In order to sustain optimal effect, do not give maintenance doses more frequently than weekly to preserve correlation between dose and blood counts.

Initial and maintenance doses: Usually, the higher dose in the given range is administered initially. Adjust the maintenance dose weekly based on pretreatment control blood counts and subsequent blood counts.

IV administration: 0.3 to 0.4 mg/kg at 1- to 4–week intervals by rapid administration.

Intracavitary administration: Administer 0.6 to 0.8 mg/kg through the same tubing used to remove fluid from the cavity.

THIOTEPA (Triethylenethiophosphoramide; TSPA; TESPA)

Intravesical administration: Dehydrate patients with papillary carcinoma of the bladder for 8 to 12 hours prior to treatment. Then instill 60 mg in 30 to 60 ml of sodium chloride injection into the bladder by catheter. For maximum effect, retain the solution for 2 hours. If the patient finds it impossible to retain 60 ml for 2 hours, give the dose in a volume of 30 ml. If desired, the patient may be repositioned every 15 minutes for maximum area contact. The usual course of treatment is once a week for 4 weeks. Repeat if necessary, but give second and third courses with caution because bone marrow depression may be increased. Deaths have occurred after intravesical use caused by bone marrow depression from systemically absorbed drug.

Reconstitute with Sterile Water for Injection.

Withdrawable Quantities and Concentration of Thiotepa

Label claim (mg/vial)	Actual content (mg/vial)	Amount of diluent to be added (ml)	Approximate withdrawable volume (ml)	Approximate withdrawable amount (mg/vial)	Approximate reconstituted concentration (mg/ml)
15	15.6	1.5	1.4	14.7	10.4

The reconstituted solution is hypotonic and should be further diluted with Sodium Chloride Injection before use. In order to eliminate haze, filter solutions through a 0.22 micron filter prior to administration. Filtering does not alter potency. Do not use solutions that remain opaque or precipitate after filtration.

Storage/Stability: Store the powder in the refrigerator at 2° to 8°C (36° to 46°F). Protect from light. When reconstituted with Sterile Water for Injection, store in a refrigerator and use within 8 hours. Use reconstituted solutions further diluted with Sodium Chloride Injection immediately.

Rx	**Thioplex** (Immunex)	**Powder for Injection, lyophilized:** 15 mg	In vials.

BUSULFAN

> **Warning:**
> Busulfan can induce severe bone marrow hypoplasia. Reduce or discontinue dosage immediately at the first sign of any unusual depression of bone marrow function as reflected by an abnormal decrease in any of the formed elements of the blood. Perform a bone marrow examination if bone marrow status is uncertain (see Warnings).

Actions:

Pharmacology: An alkylsulfonate, busulfan's predominant effect is against cells of the granulocytic series. Although a polyfunctional alkylating agent, it appears to interact with cellular thiol groups. Little crosslinking of nucleoproteins is observed. The drug is cell cycle-phase nonspecific.

The biochemical basis for acquired resistance to busulfan is speculative; altered transport of busulfan into the cell and increased intracellular inactivation before it reaches DNA are possibilities. Resistance to these compounds may reflect an acquired ability of the cell to repair alkylation damage more effectively.

Pharmacokinetics:

Absorption/Distribution – Busulfan is well absorbed following oral administration. There is a lag period of 0.6 to 2 hours prior to detection in blood. It is well distributed into the spinal fluid with a cerebrospinal fluid: plasma ratio of 1.3:1; distribution into saliva is equivalent to that of plasma. Plasma protein binding is only 7.4%.

Metabolism/Excretion – The plasma elimination half-life is 2.5 hours and is similar for cerebrospinal fluid. The drug appears to be extensively metabolized and renally excreted with little unchanged drug (1%) found in the urine. The clearance of busulfan is more rapid in children than adults.

Indications:

Palliative treatment of chronic myelogenous leukemia (myeloid, myelocytic, granulocytic): Approximately 90% of adults with previously untreated chronic myelogenous leukemia (CML) will obtain hematologic remission with regression or stabilization of organomegaly following busulfan. It is superior to splenic irradiation with respect to survival times and maintenance of hemoglobin levels and equivalent to irradiation at controlling splenomegaly.

Busulfan is less effective in patients with CML who lack the Philadelphia (Ph^1) chromosome. Juvenile CML, associated with the absence of a Philadelphia chromosome, responds poorly to busulfan. The drug is of no benefit if the disease has entered a "blastic" phase.

Contraindications:

Patients whose disease has demonstrated prior resistance to this drug without a diagnosis of chronic myelogenous leukemia.

Busulfan is of no value in chronic lymphocytic leukemia, acute leukemia or in the "blastic crisis" of chronic myelogenous leukemia.

Warnings:

Adrenal insufficiency: A clinical syndrome closely resembling adrenal insufficiency and characterized by weakness, severe fatigue, anorexia, weight loss, nausea, vomiting and melanoderma has developed after prolonged therapy. The symptoms have sometimes been reversible when busulfan was withdrawn. Adrenal responsiveness to exogenously administered ACTH is usually normal. However, pituitary function testing with metyrapone revealed a blunted urinary 17-hydroxycorticosteroid excretion in two patients. Following the discontinuation of busulfan (which was associated with clinical improvement), rechallenge with metyrapone revealed normal pituitary-adrenal function.

Hyperuricemia and hyperuricosuria –

They may occur in patients with chronic myelogenous leukemia. Additional rapid destruction of granulocytes may accompany chemotherapy and increase the urate pool. Minimize adverse effects by increased hydration, urine alkalinization and the prophylactic administration of allopurinol.

Hematopoietic toxicity: The most frequent and serious side effect is bone marrow failure (which may or may not be anatomically hypoplastic), resulting in severe pancytopenia that may be more prolonged than that induced with other alkylating agents. The usual cause is the failure to stop administration of the drug soon enough; individual idiosyncrasy appears unimportant. Use with extreme caution in patients whose bone marrow reserve or function may be compromised by or recovering from prior irradiation or chemotherapy. Although recovery from busulfan-induced pancytopenia may take from 1 month to 2 years, it is potentially reversible; vigorously support the patient through any period of severe pancytopenia.

The most consistent dose-related toxicity is bone marrow suppression. This may be manifested by anemia, leukopenia, thrombocytopenia or any combination of these. Instruct patients to report promptly the development of fever, sore throat, signs of local infection, bleeding from any site or symptoms suggestive of anemia. Any one of these findings may indicate busulfan toxicity or transformation of the disease to an acute "blastic" form. Because busulfan may have a delayed effect, it is important to withdraw the medication temporarily at the first sign of an abnormally large or exceptionally rapid fall in any of the formed elements of the blood.

Evaluate the hemoglobin or hematocrit, white blood cell (WBC) count, differential count and platelet count weekly. If the cause of fluctuation in the formed element of the peripheral blood is obscure, bone marrow examination may be useful. Individualize therapy based not only on the absolute hematologic values, but also on the rapidity with which changes are occurring. The dosage of busulfan may need to be reduced if the agent is combined with other myelosuppressive drugs. Occasionally, patients may be unusually sensitive to busulfan administered at standard dosage and suffer neutropenia or thrombocytopenia after relatively short exposure to the drug. Do not use busulfan where facilities for complete blood counts, including quantitative platelet counts, are not available at weekly (or more frequent) intervals. Never allow patients to take the drug without supervision.

Busulfan may cause additive myelosuppression when used with other myelosuppressive agents.

Pulmonary: A rare, but important complication of busulfan therapy is the development of bronchopulmonary dysplasia with pulmonary fibrosis. Symptoms have occurred within 8 months to 10 years after initiation of therapy (the average duration of therapy being 4 years). Histologic findings associated with "busulfan lung" mimic those seen following pulmonary irradiation. Clinically, patients report the insidious onset of cough, dyspnea and low-grade fever. Pulmonary function studies reveal diminished diffusion capacity and decreased pulmonary compliance. Exclude more common conditions (such as opportunistic infections or leukemic infiltration of the lungs). If sputum cultures, virologic studies and exfoliative cytology fail to establish an etiology for the pulmonary infiltrates, lung biopsy may be necessary.

Treatment is unsatisfactory; most patients have died within 6 months after diagnosis. There is no specific therapy other than the immediate discontinuation of busulfan. Corticosteroid administration has been suggested, but the results have not been impressive or uniformly successful.

Seizures: Seizures have been reported in patients receiving very high, investigational doses of busulfan. As with any potentially epileptogenic drug, exercise caution when administering very high doses of busulfan to patients with a history of seizure disorder, head trauma, or receiving other potentially epileptogenic drugs. Some investigators have used prophylactic anticonvulsant therapy in this setting.

Cellular dysplasia: Busulfan may cause cellular dysplasia in many organs in addition to the lung. Giant, hyperchromatic nuclei have been reported in lymph nodes, pancreas, thyroid, adrenal glands, bone marrow and liver. This cytologic dysplasia may be severe enough to cause difficulty in interpretation of exfoliative cytologic examinations from the lung, bladder, breast and the uterine cervix.

Hepatotoxicity: Hepatic veno-occlusive disease, which may be life-threating, has been reported following the investigational use of very high doses of busulfan in combinatin with cyclophosphamide or other chemotherapeutic agents prior to bone marrow transplantation. Possible risk factors include: Total busulfan dose > 16 mg/kg based on ideal body weight and concurrent use of multiple alkylating agents. A clear cause and effect relationship with busulfan has not been demonstrated.

Carcinogenesis/Mutagenesis: Malignant tumors have occurred in patients on busulfan therapy; this drug may be a human carcinogen. Four cases of acute leukemia occurred among 243 patients treated with busulfan for 5 to 8 years as adjuvant chemotherapy following surgical resection of bronchogenic carcinoma. Busulfan is mutagenic in mice and, possibly, in humans. Chromosome aberrations have been reported in cells from patients receiving busulfan.

Fertility impairment: Ovarian suppression and amenorrhea with menopausal symptoms commonly occur during busulfan therapy in premenopausal patients. There have been clinical reports of sterility, azoospermia and testicular atrophy in males.

Pregnancy: Category D. Busulfan may cause fetal harm when administered to a pregnant woman. Although healthy children have been born after busulfan treatment during pregnancy, one malformed baby was delivered by a mother treated with busulfan. During this pregnancy, the mother received x-ray therapy early in the first trimester, mercaptopurine until the third month, then busulfan until delivery.

BUSULFAN

There are reports of small infants being born after the mothers received busulfan during pregnancy; in particular, during third trimester administration. In one case, an infant had mild anemia and neutropenia at birth after busulfan was administered to the mother from the eighth week of pregnancy to term.

There are no adequate and well controlled studies in pregnant women. If this drug is used during pregnancy or if the patient becomes pregnant while taking this drug, apprise her of the potential hazard to the fetus. Advise women of childbearing potential to avoid becoming pregnant.

Lactation: It is not known whether this drug is excreted in breast milk. Because of the potential for tumorigenicity, decide whether to discontinue breastfeeding or to discontinue the drug, taking into account the importance of the drug to the mother.

Children: See Administration and Dosage.

Precautions:

Monitoring: Periodic measurement of serum transaminases, alkaline phosphatase, and bilirubin is indicated for early detection of hepatotoxicity. It is recommended that evaluation of the hemoglobin or hematocrit, total white blood cell count and differential count and quantitative platelet count be obtained weekly while the patient is on busulfan therapy. In cases where the cause of fluctuation in the formed elements of the peripheral blood is obscure, bone marrow examination may be useful for evaluation of marrow status. Do not use busulfan where facilities for complete blood counts, including quantitative platelet counts, are not available at weekly (or more frequent) intervals.

Cardiovascular: Cardiac tamponade has been reported in a small number of patients with thalassemia (2% in one series) who received high doses of busulfan and cyclophosphamide as the preparatory regimen for bone marrow transplantation and was often fatal. Abdominal pain and vomiting preceded the tamponade in most patients.

Drug Interactions:

Busulfan Drug Interactions			
Precipitant drug	Object drug*		Description
Cyclophosphamide	Busulfan	⬆	Cardiac tamponade has been reported in a small number of patients with thalassemia (2% in one series) who received high doses of busulfan and cyclophosphamide as the preparatory regimen for bone marrow transplantation and was often fatal. Abdominal pain and vomiting preceded the tamponade in most patients.
Thioguanine	Busulfan	⬆	In one study, ≈ 3.6% of 330 patients receiving continuous (6 to 45 months) concomitant therapy for treatment of CML had esophageal varices associated with abnormal liver function tests. Liver biopsies performed in 33% of these patients all showed evidence of nodular regenerative hyperplasia. Use with caution in long-term continous therapy.

* ⬆ = Object drug increased.

Adverse Reactions:

Dermatologic: Hyperpigmentation (5 to 10%, particularly in those with a dark complexion); urticaria; erythema multiforme; erythema nodosum; alopecia; porphyria cutanea tarda; excessive dryness and fragility of the skin with anhidrosis; dryness of the oral mucous membranes; cheilosis.

Hematologic: See Warnings.

Metabolic: Adrenal insufficiency, hyperuricemia, hyperuricosuria (see Warnings).

Pulmonary: Interstitial pulmonary fibrosis (see Warnings).

Miscellaneous: Cataracts (0% to 10%) occurred only after prolonged administration of the drug. Gynecomastia, cholestatic jaundice, myasthenia gravis, (a clear cause and effect relationship has not been demonstrated); endocardial fibrosis (see Precautions); seizures; sterility (80% to 100%, see Warnings).

Overdosage:

Symptoms: Two distinct types of toxic responses are seen at median lethal doses given intraperitoneally. Within hours, there are signs of stimulation of the CNS with convulsions and death on the first day. With doses at the LD_{50}, there is also delayed death because of bone marrow damage. The principal toxic effect is on the bone marrow. Survival after a single 140 mg dose has been reported in an 18 kg, 4-year-old child, but hematologic toxicity is likely to be more profound with chronic overdosage.

Treatment: Closely monitor hematologic status and institute vigorous supportive measures if necessary. Induce vomiting or gastric lavage, and follow by administration of charcoal if ingestion is recent. It is not known if busulfan is dialyzable. Refer to General Management of Acute Overdosage.

Patient Information:

Notify physician if unusual bleeding or bruising, fever, cough, shortness of breath, flank, stomach or joint pain, abrupt weakness, unusual fatigue, anorexia or weight loss occurs.

Inform patients that some toxicities to busulfan include fertility, amenorrhea, skin hyperpigmentation, drug hypersensitivity, dryness of the mucous membranes and cataract formation (rare).

Medication may cause darkening of skin, diarrhea, dizziness, fatigue, appetite loss, mental confusion, nausea, vomiting; notify physician if these become pronounced.

Take medication at the same time each day.

Extra fluid intake may be recommended.

Contraceptive measures are recommended during therapy.

If nausea or vomiting occurs, take the drug on an empty stomach.

Administration and Dosage:

Remission induction: 4 to 8 mg/day total dose. Dosing on a weight basis is the same for both children and adults, ≈ 60 mcg of body weight or 1.8 mg/m^2 of body surface daily. Because the rate at which the leukocyte count falls is dose-related, reserve daily doses exceeding 4 mg/day for patients with the most compelling symptoms; the greater the total daily dose, the greater the possibility of inducing bone marrow aplasia.

A decrease in the leukocyte count is not usually seen during the first 10 to 15 days of treatment; the leukocyte count may actually increase during this period and should not be interpreted as drug resistance, nor should the dose be increased. Because the leukocyte count may continue to fall for > 1 month after discontinuing the drug, discontinue busulfan before the total leukocyte count falls into the normal range. When the total leukocyte count has declined to ≈ 15,000/mcl, withdraw the drug.

With a constant dose of busulfan, the total leukocyte count declines exponentially; a weekly plot of the leukocyte count on semilogarithmic graph paper aids in predicting the time when therapy should be discontinued. A normal leukocyte count is usually achieved in 12 to 20 weeks with the recommended dose of busulfan,.

Maintenance therapy: During remission, examine the patient monthly and resume treatment with the induction dosage when total leukocyte count reaches ≈ 50,000/mcl. When remission is < 3 months, maintenance therapy of 1 to 3 mg/day may keep the hematological status under control and prevent rapid relapse.

Rx	**Myleran** (Glaxo Wellcome)	**Tablets:** 2 mg	(Myleran K2A). White, scored. In 25s.

> **Warning:**
> *Cumulative renal toxicity* associated with cisplatin is severe (see Warnings). Other major dose-related toxicities are myelosuppression, nausea and vomiting.
> *Ototoxicity,* which may be more pronounced in children, is manifested by tinnitus or loss of high frequency hearing and, occasionally, deafness.
> *Anaphylactic-like reactions* have occurred (see Warnings).

Actions:

Pharmacology: Cisplatin is an inorganic heavy metal coordination complex containing a central atom of platinum surrounded by two chloride atoms and two ammonia molecules in the cis position that produces DNA-protein crosslinks in DNA, like alkylating agents, but these do not correlate with antitumor activity. The antitumor effect of cisplatin has been correlated with binding to DNA, production of intrastrand crosslinks and formation of DNA adducts.

Pharmacokinetics:

Absorption/Distribution – Plasma concentrations of the parent compound, cisplatin, have a half-life of ≈ 20 to 30 minutes; the total body clearance and volume of distribution at steady-state are ≈ 15 $L/hr/m^2$ and ≈ 11 L/m^2, respectively. The ratios of cisplatin to total free platinum in the plasma vary considerably between patients and range from 0.5 to 1.1. Cisplatin does not undergo binding to plasma proteins; however, platinum is 90% bound to several plasma proteins including albumin, transferrin and gamma globulin. The albumin-platinum complexes do not dissociate significantly and are slowly eliminated with a minimum half-life of ≥ 5 days.

Maximum red blood cell concentrations of platinum are reached within 90 to 150 minutes and have a terminal half-life of 36 to 47 days. Concentrations of platinum are highest in liver, prostate and kidney, somewhat lower in bladder, muscle, testicle, pancreas and spleen and lowest in bowel, adrenal, heart, lung, cerebrum and cerebellum. Platinum is present in tissues for ≤ 180 days after the last administration.

Metabolism/Excretion – 90% of the drug is removed by renal mechanisms whereas < 10% is removed by biliary excretion. The parent compound, cisplatin, is excreted in the urine and accounts for 13% to 17% of the administered dose excreted within 1 hour of administration. The renal clearance of cisplatin and platinum exceed creatinine clearance indicating active secretion by the kidney. The mean renal clearance of cisplatin is ≈ 56 $ml/min/m^2$; platinum clearance is non-linear, variable and is dependent on dose, urine flow rate and individual variability of active secretion and possible tubular reabsorption. Approximately 10% to 40% of the administreed platinum is excreted in the urine within 24 hours with a mean of 35% to 51% excreted in the urine over 5 days.

Indications:

For palliative therapy in:

Metastatic testicular tumors: In combination therapy in patients who have received appropriate surgical or radiotherapeutic procedures.

Metastatic ovarian tumors: In combination therapy (eg, cyclophosphamide) in patients who have received appropriate surgical or radiotherapeutic procedures. Cisplatin, as a single agent, is indicated as secondary therapy in patients refractory to standard chemotherapy who have not previously received cisplatin.

Advanced bladder cancer: As a single agent for patients with transitional cell bladder cancer no longer amenable to local treatments (eg, surgery or radiotherapy).

Contraindications:

Preexisting renal impairment; myelosuppression; hearing impairment; history of allergic reactions to platinum-containing compounds.

Warnings:

Hematologic: The nadirs in circulating platelets and leukocytes occur between days 18 and 23 (range 7.5 to 45); most patients recover by day 39 (range, 13 to 62). Leukopenia and thrombocytopenia are more pronounced at doses > 50 mg/m^2. Anemia (decrease of 2 g hemoglobin/dl) occurs at the same frequency and with the same timing as leukopenia and thrombocytopenia.

Hepatotoxicity: Transient elevations of liver enzymes, especially AST, as well as bilirubin, have been reported to be associated with cisplatin administration at the recommended doses.

Vascular toxicities coincident with use of cisplatin in combination with other antineoplastic agents have occurred rarely. The events are clinically heterogeneous and may include myocardial infarction, cerebrovascular accident, thrombotic microangiopathy or cerebral arteritis. Various mechanisms have been proposed for these vascular complications. There are also reports of Raynaud's phenomenon occurring in patients treated with the combination of bleomycin and vinblastine with or without cisplatin. Hypomagnesemia developing coincident with use of cisplatin may be an added, although not essential, factor associated with this event. However, it is currently unknown if the cause of Raynaud's phenomenon in these cases is the disease, underlying vascular compromise, bleomycin, vinblastine, hypomagnesemia or a combination of any of these factors.

Hyperuricemia occurs at ≈ the same frequency as increases in BUN and serum creatinine. It is more pronounced after doses > 50 mg/m^2, and peak uric acid levels generally occur 3 to 5 days after the dose. Allopurinol is effective.

Electrolyte disturbance: Hypomagnesemia, hypocalcemia, hyponatremia, hypokalemia and hypophosphatemia have occurred and are probably related to renal tubular damage. Tetany has occasionally occurred in those patients with hypocalcemia and hypomagnesemia. Generally, normal serum electrolyte levels are restored by administering supplemental electrolytes and discontinuing cisplatin.

Increased plasma iron levels and inappropriate antidiuretic hormone syndrome have also been reported.

Ophthalmic effects: Optic neuritis, papilledema and cerebral blindness have occurred infrequently in patients receiving standard recommended cisplatin doses. Improvement or total recovery usually occurs after drug discontinuation. Steroids with or without mannitol have been used; however, efficacy has not been established.

Blurred vision and altered color perception have occurred after the use of regimens with higher doses or greater dose frequencies than those recommended. The altered color perception manifests as a loss of color discrimination, particularly in the blue-yellow axis. The only finding on funduscopic exam is irregular retinal pigmentation of the macular area.

Renal toxicity: Dose-related and cumulative renal insufficiency is the major dose-limiting toxicity. Renal toxicity has been noted in 28% to 36% of patients treated with a single dose of 50 mg/m^2. First noted during the second week after a dose, it is manifested by elevations in BUN and creatinine, serum uric acid or a decrease in creatinine clearance. Renal toxicity becomes more prolonged and severe with repeated courses of the drug. Renal function must return to normal before another dose can be given.

Amifostine can be used to reduce cumulative renal toxicity in patients with advanced ovarian cancer receiving repeated cisplatin administration. Refer to the individual monograph in the Antineoplastic Adjuncts section.

Impairment of renal function is associated with renal tubular damage. The administration of cisplatin using a 6 to 8 hour infusion with IV hydration and mannitol has been used to reduce nephrotoxicity. However, renal toxicity can still occur (see Precautions).

Neuropathies: Severe neuropathies have occurred in patients receiving higher doses of cisplatin or greater dose frequencies than those recommended or after prolonged therapy (4 to 7 months) however, neurologic symptoms have been reported to occur after a single dose. Although symptoms and signs of cisplatin neuropathy usually develop during treatment, symptoms of neuropathy may begin 3 to 8 weeks after the last dose of cisplatin (rare). These neuropathies may be irreversible and are seen as paresthesias in a stocking-glove distribution, areflexia and loss of proprioception and vibratory sensation. Loss of motor function has also occurred. Discontinue therapy when symptoms are first observed.

Ototoxicity has occurred in ≤ 31% of patients given a single 50 mg/m^2 dose. It is manifested by tinnitus or hearing loss in the high frequency range (4000 to 8000 Hz); decreased ability to hear normal conversational tones occurs occasionally. Ototoxic effects may be more severe in children. Hearing loss can be unilateral or bilateral and is more frequent and severe with repeated doses. It is unclear whether ototoxicity is reversible. Because ototoxicity of cisplatin is cumulative, perform audiometry before starting therapy and prior to subsequent doses. Vestibular toxicity has occurred. Deafness after the initial dose of cisplatin has been reported rarely. Coadministration with loop diuretics may have an additive ototoxic effect.

High/cumulative doses: Muscle cramps, defined as localized, painful, involuntary skeletal muscle contractions of sudden onset and short duration, have been reported and were usually associated in patients receiving a relatively high cumulative dose of cisplatin and with a relatively advanced symptomatic stage of peripheral neuropathy.

Hypersensitivity: Anaphylactic-like reactions have occurred. Facial edema, wheezing, tachycardia and hypotension may occur within minutes of use in patients with prior drug exposure. They are alleviated by use of epinephrine, corticosteroids and antihistamines. Refer to Management of Acute Hypersensitivity Reactions.

Mutagenesis: The drug is mutagenic in bacteria and produces chromosome aberrations in animal cell tissue cultures.

Pregnancy: Of five reported pregnancy cases, one infant developed profound leukopenia with neutropenia, which resolved after 10 days. The mother had developed profound neutropenia just prior to delivery. By 12 weeks of age, the child was developing normally, except for moderate bilateral hearing loss.

Precautions:

Monitoring: Monitor peripheral blood counts weekly and liver function periodically. Perform neurologic and auditory examinations regularly. Measure serum creatinine, BUN, creatinine clearance, magnesium, sodium, calcium and potassium levels prior to initiating therapy and prior to each subsequent course. Do not give more frequently than once every 3 to 4 weeks. Perform audiometry before starting therapy and prior to subsequent doses.

GI: Marked nausea and vomiting occur in almost all patients, and are occasionally so severe that the drug must be discontinued. Nausea and vomiting usually begin 1 to 4 hours after treatment and last up to 24 hours; nausea and anorexia may persist for up to 1 week after treatment. Metoclopramide in high doses has been used in the prophylaxis of vomiting associated with cisplatin therapy.

Drug Interactions:

Cisplatin Drug Interactions

Precipitant drug	Object drug*		Description
Aminoglycosides	Cisplatin	⬆	Cisplatin produces cumulative nephrotoxicity that is potentiated by aminoglycosides (see Warnings).
Cisplatin	Phenytoin	⬇	Combination chemotherapy (including cisplatin) may reduce phenytoin plasma levels.

* ⬆ = Object drug increased. ⬇ = Object drug decreased.

Adverse Reactions:

Body as a whole:

Infrequent – Cardiac abnormalities, hiccups, alopecia, rash, serum amylase and elevated ALT.

CNS: Peripheral neuropathies; seizures; loss of taste; Lhermitte's sign; autonomic neuropathy (see Warnings).

Electrolyte Disturbance: Hypomagnesemia, hypocalcemia, hyponatremia, hypokalemia, hypophosphatemia, increased plasma iron levels, antidiuretic hormone syndrome (see Warnings).

GI: Nausea, vomiting (see Precautions).

Hematologic: Myelosuppression (25% to 30%); leukopenia, thrombocytopenia, anemia (see Warnings).

Ophthalmic: Optic neuritis, papilledema, cerebral blindness, blurred vision, altered color perception (infrequent, see Warnings).

Renal: Renal insufficiency, renal tubular damage (see Warnings).

Special senses: Tinnitus, high frequency hearing loss, vestibular toxicity (see Warnings).

Miscellaneous: Vascular toxicities (rare); hyperuricemia, ototoxicity, anaphlactic-like reactions (see Warnings); cardiac abnormalities; anorexia; rash; elevated ALT.

Overdosage:

System: Acute overdosage with this drug may result in kidney failure, liver failure, deafness, ocular toxicity (including detachment of the retina), significant myelosuppression, intractable nausea and vomiting or neuritis. In addition, death can occur following overdosage.

Treatment: No proven antidotes have been established for cisplatin overdosage. Hemodialysis, even when initiated 4 hours after the overdosage, appears to have little effect on removing platinum from the body because of cisplatin's rapid and high degree of protein binding. Management of overdosage should include general supportive measures to sustain the patient through any period of toxicity that may occur. Refer to General Management of Acute Overdosage.

Administration and Dosage:

For IV use only.

Metastatic testicular tumors: 20 mg/m^2/day IV for 5 days/cycle.

CISPLATIN (CDDP)

Metastatic ovarian tumors:

Cisplatin – 75 to 100 mg/m² IV once every 4 weeks/cycle.

Cyclophosphamide – 600 mg/m² IV once every 4 weeks, (Day 1).

In combination therapy, administer cisplatin and cyclophosphamide sequentially.

Administer cisplatin as a single agent at a dose of 100 mg/m² IV/cycle once every 4 weeks.

Advanced bladder cancer: Administer as a single agent. Give 50 to 70 mg/m² IV/cycle once every 3 to 4 weeks, depending on prior radiation therapy or chemotherapy. For heavily pretreated patients, give an initial dose of 50 mg/m²/cycle repeated every 4 weeks.

Repeat courses: Do not give a repeat course until the serum creatinine is < 1.5 mg/dl, or the BUN is < 25 mg/dl or until circulating blood elements are at an acceptable level (platelets ≥ 100,000/mm³, WBC ≥ 4000/mm³). Do not give subsequent doses until an audiometric analysis indicates that auditory acuity is within normal limits.

Note: Do not use needles or IV sets containing aluminum parts for preparation. Aluminum reacts with cisplatin, causing precipitation and a loss of potency.

Skin reactions associated with accidental exposure may occur. Use gloves. If powder or solution contacts skin or mucosa, wash immediately with soap and water.

Hydration: Perform pretreatment hydration with 1 to 2 L fluid infused for 8 to 12 hours prior to dose. Then dilute the drug in 2 L of 5% Dextrose in ½ or ⅓ Normal Saline containing 37.5 g mannitol and infuse over 6 to 8 hours. Maintain adequate hydration and urinary output during the following 24 hours.

Admixture compatibility: Cisplatin and fluorouracil admixtures are stable in 0.9% Normal Saline for 1 hour.

Storage/Stability: Store at 15°C to 25°C. Do not refrigerate. The cisplatin remaining in the amber vial following initial entry is stable for 28 days protected from light or for 7 days under fluorescent room light.

Rx	**Platinol-AQ** (Bristol-Myers Oncology)	**Injection:** 1 mg/ml	In 50 and 100 mg vials.

CARBOPLATIN

Warning:
Bone marrow suppression is dose-related and may be severe, resulting in infection or bleeding. Anemia may be cumulative and require transfusion support (see Warnings).
Vomiting is a frequent drug-related side effect (see Warnings).
Anaphylactic-like reactions may occur within minutes of administration. Epinephrine, corticosteroids and antihistamines may alleviate symptoms (see Warnings).

Actions:

Pharmacology: Carboplatin is a platinum coordination compound that is used as a cancer chemotherapeutic agent. Carboplatin, like cisplatin, produces predominantly interstrand DNA cross-links rather than DNA-protein cross-links. This effect is apparently cell-cycle nonspecific. The aquation of carboplatin, which is thought to produce the active species, occurs at a slower rate than cisplatin. Despite this difference, both carboplatin and cisplatin induce equal numbers of drug-DNA cross-links, causing equivalent lesions and biological effects. Differences in potencies for carboplatin and cisplatin appear to be directly related to the difference in aquation rates.

Pharmacokinetics:

Absorption/Distribution – Carboplatin exhibits linear pharmacokinetics over the dosing range 300 to 500 mg/m^2. When creatinine clearance (Ccr) is ≥ 60 ml/min, the initial plasma half-life (alpha) is 1.1 to 2 hours, and the postdistribution plasma half-life (beta) is 2.6 to 5.9 hours. The apparent volume of distribution and mean residence time is 16 L and 3.5 hours, respectively. Carboplatin is not bound to plasma proteins. However, platinum from carboplatin becomes irreversibly bound to plasma proteins and is slowly eliminated with a minimum half-life of 5 days.

Metabolism/Excretion – Plasma levels of intact carboplatin decay in a biphasic manner after a 30 minute IV infusion of 300 to 500 mg/m^2. The total body clearance is 4.4 L/hour. The major route of elimination is renal excretion. When Ccr is ≥ 60 ml/min, 65% of the dose is excreted in the urine within 12 hours and 71% within 24 hours. All of the platinum in the 24 hour urine is present as carboplatin. Only 3% to 5% of the administered platinum is excreted in the urine between 24 and 96 hours.

Clinical trials:

Initial treatment – Two randomized controlled studies with carboplatin vs cisplatin, both in combination with cyclophosphamide every 28 days for six courses before surgical re-evaluation, demonstrated equivalent overall survival between the two groups.

Secondary treatment – In two prospective randomized controlled studies in patients with advanced ovarian cancer previously treated with chemotherapy, carboplatin achieved six clinical complete responses in 47 patients. Response duration ranged from 45 to ≥ 71 weeks.

Among patients previously treated with cisplatin, those developing progressive disease while receiving cisplatin may have a decreased response rate.

Indications:

Ovarian carcinoma:

Initial treatment of advanced ovarian carcinoma in established combination with other approved chemotherapeutic agents. One established combination regimen consists of carboplatin and cyclophosphamide.

Secondary treatment – Palliative treatment of patients with ovarian carcinoma recurrent after prior chemotherapy, including patients who have been previously treated with cisplatin.

Unlabeled uses: Carboplatin has shown activity as a single agent in previously treated and untreated patients with small cell lung cancer, but is most effective when combined with other agents (eg, etoposide). It is useful either alone or in combination (usually with fluorouracil) in the treatment of advanced or recurrent squamous cell carcinoma of the head and neck. Activity has also been demonstrated in advanced endometrial cancer, in relapsed and refractory acute leukemia and for seminoma of testicular cancer, but further studies are needed.

Contraindications:

History of severe allergic reactions to cisplatin or other platinum compounds or mannitol; severe bone marrow depression (see Warnings); significant bleeding.

Warnings:

Bone marrow suppression (leukopenia, neutropenia and thrombocytopenia) is dose-dependent and is also the dose-limiting toxicity. Frequently monitor peripheral blood counts during carboplatin treatment and, when appropriate, until recovery. Median nadir occurs at day 21 in patients receiving single-agent carboplatin. By day 28, 90%

of patients have platelet counts > 100,000/mm^3; 74% have neutrophil counts > 2,000/mm^3; 67% have leukocyte counts > 4,000/mm^3. In general, do not repeat single intermittent courses until leukocyte, neutrophil and platelet counts recover.

Because anemia is cumulative, transfusions may be needed during treatment with carboplatin, particularly in patients receiving prolonged therapy.

Bone marrow suppression is increased in patients who have received prior therapy, especially regimens including cisplatin. Bone marrow suppression is also increased in impaired kidney function. Patients with poor performance status have also had a higher incidence of severe leukopenia and thrombocytopenia. Bone marrow depression may be more severe when carboplatin is combined with other bone marrow suppressing drugs or with radiotherapy. Appropriately reduce initial carboplatin dosages in these patients (see Administration and Dosage) and carefully monitor blood counts between courses. If used in combination with other bone marrow suppressing therapies, carefully manage with respect to dosage and timing to minimize additive effects.

Renal toxicity is limited, but concomitant treatment with aminoglycosides has resulted in increased renal or audiologic toxicity. Exercise caution when a patient receives both drugs. Development of abnormal renal function test results is uncommon, despite the fact that carboplatin, unlike cisplatin, has usually been administered without high-volume fluid hydration or forced diuresis. Most of the reported abnormalities have been mild and ≈ 50% of them were reversible.

Creatinine clearance has been the most sensitive measure of kidney function in carboplatin patients, and it appears to be the most useful test for correlating drug clearance and bone marrow suppression. Of the patients who had a baseline value of ≥ 60 ml/min, 27% demonstrated a reduction below this value during therapy.

Emesis can be induced which can be more severe in patients previously receiving emetogenics. Carboplatin is significantly less emetogenic than cisplatin. Nausea and vomiting usually cease within 24 hours of treatment, and the incidence and intensity of emesis have been reduced by using antiemetic premedication. Although no conclusive efficacy data exist with the following schedules of carboplatin, lengthening the duration of single IV administration to 24 hours or dividing the total dose over 5 consecutive daily pulse doses has reduced emesis.

Peripheral neurotoxicity is infrequent, but its incidence is increased in patients > 65 years old and in patients previously treated with cisplatin. Carboplatin produces significantly fewer and less severe neurologic side effects than cisplatin. Preexisting cisplatin-induced neurotoxicity does not worsen in ≈ 70% of patients receiving carboplatin as secondary treatment. Although overall incidence of peripheral neurologic side effects induced by carboplatin is low, prolonged treatment, particularly in cisplatin-pretreated patients, may result in cumulative neurotoxicity.

Hypersensitivity to carboplatin has occurred and may occur within minutes of administration; manage with appropriate supportive therapy. Refer to Management of Acute Hypersensitivity Reactions.

Renal function impairment: Patients with impaired kidney function (Ccr < 60 ml/min) are at increased risk of severe bone marrow suppression. In renally impaired patients who received single-agent carboplatin therapy, the incidence of severe leukopenia, neutropenia or thrombocytopenia was ≈ 25% with dosage modifications. (See Administration and Dosage). In patients with Ccr < 60 ml/min, total body and renal clearances of carboplatin decreases as Ccr decreases. Reduce dosages (see Administration and Dosage).

Carcinogenesis: The carcinogenic potential has not been studied, but compounds with similar mechanisms of action and mutagenicity profiles have been carcinogenic. Carboplatin is mutagenic both in vitro and in vivo. It is also embryotoxic and teratogenic in rats receiving the drug during organogenesis.

Pregnancy: Category D. Carboplatin may cause fetal harm when administered to a pregnant woman. It is embryotoxic and teratogenic in rats. There are no adequate and well controlled studies in pregnant women. If used during pregnancy, or if the patient becomes pregnant while receiving this drug, apprise her of the potential hazard to the fetus. Advise women of childbearing potential to avoid pregnancy.

Lactation: It is not known whether carboplatin is excreted in breast milk. Because there is a possibility of toxicity in nursing infants secondary to carboplatin treatment of the mother, discontinue breastfeeding if the mother is treated with carboplatin.

Precautions:

Aluminum can react with carboplatin, causing precipitate formation and potency loss. Do not use needles or IV administration sets containing aluminum parts that may come in contact with carboplatin for the preparation or administration of the drug.

CARBOPLATIN

Lab test abnormalities: High dosages of carboplatin (more than four times the recommended dose) have resulted in severe abnormalities of liver function tests, which have generally been mild and reversible in ≈ 50% of the cases; however, the role of metastatic tumor in the liver may complicate the assessment in many patients. In a limited series of patients receiving very high doses of carboplatin and autologous bone marrow transplantation, severe abnormalities of liver function tests occurred.

Drug Interactions:

Phenytoin: Serum concentrations may be decreased, resulting in a loss of therapeutic effect.

Adverse Reactions:

Carboplatin Adverse Reactions in Patients with Ovarian Cancer (%)		
Adverse reaction	First line combination therapy [1] (n = 393)	Second line single agent therapy (n = 553)
Bone marrow		
Thrombocytopenia		
< 100,000/mm^3	66	62
< 50,000/mm^3	33	35
Neutropenia		
< 2000 cells/mm^3	96	67
< 1000 cells/mm^3	82	21
Leukopenia		
< 4000 cells/mm^3	97	85
< 2000 cells/mm^3	71	26
Anemia		
< 11 g/dl	90	90
< 8 g/dl	14	21
Transfusions	35	44
Infections	16	5
Bleeding	8	5
GI		
Nausea and vomiting	93	92
Vomiting	83	81
Other GI side effects	46	21
CNS		
Central neurotoxicity	26	5
Peripheral neuropathies	15	6
Ototoxicity	12	1
Other sensory side effects	5	1
Renal/Hepatic		
Alkaline phosphatase elevations	29	37
AST elevations	20	19
Blood urea elevations	17	22
Serum creatinine elevations	6	10
Bilirubin elevations	5	5
Electrolyte loss		
Magnesium	61	43
Calcium	16	31
Potassium	16	28
Sodium	10	47
Miscellaneous		
Alopecia	49	2
Pain	44	23
Asthenia	41	11
Cardiovascular	19	6
Allergic	11	2
Respiratory	10	6
GU	10	2
Mucositis	8	1

[1] Combination therapy with cyclophosphamide in NCIC and SWOG studies. Combination therapy as well as treatment duration may be responsible for the differences noted with single agent therapy.

CARBOPLATIN

The following incidences of adverse events are based on data from 1,893 patients with various types of tumors who received carboplatin as single-agent therapy.

Allergic reactions: Hypersensitivity (2%), including rash, urticaria, erythema, pruritus, and rarely bronchospasm and hypotension (see Warnings).

Body as a whole: Pain; asthenia; alopecia (3%); cardiovascular, respiratory, genitourinary and mucosal side effects (≤ 6%); cardiovascular events (cardiac failure, embolism, cerebrovascular accidents) (fatal in < 1%); cancer-associated hemolytic uremic syndrome (rare).

Electrolyte Disturbance: Abnormally decreased serum electrolyte values (rarely associated with symptoms): Sodium (29%); magnesium (29%); calcium (22%); potassium (20%).

GI: Vomiting (65%), severe in about ⅓ of these patients (see Warnings); nausea alone (additional 10% to 15%); pain (17%); diarrhea, constipation (6%).

Hematologic: Bone marrow suppression is the dose-limiting toxicity of carboplatin: Thrombocytopenia, platelet count < 50,000/mm^3 (25%); neutropenia, granulocyte count < 1,000/mm^3 (16%); leukopenia, WBC count < 2,000/mm^3 (15%). See Warnings; infectious or hemorrhagic complications (5%); drug-related death (< 1%); anemia (hemoglobin < 11 g/dl), (71% see Warnings); transfusions (26%).

Lab test abnormalities: Alkaline phosphatase (24%); AST (15%); total bilirubin (5%). See Precautions.

Neurologic: Peripheral neuropathies (4%) with mild paresthesias occurring most frequently (see Warnings); ototoxicity and other sensory abnormalities such as visual disturbances and change in taste (1%); central nervous system symptoms (5%) appear to be most often related to the use of antiemetics.

Renal:

Nephrotoxicity (see Warnings): Abnormal renal function tests - Blood urea nitrogen (14%); serum creatinine (6%).

Comparative toxicity, carboplatin vs cisplatin: In the studies when cisplatin and carboplatin were used in combination with cyclophosphamide, the pattern of toxicity exerted by the carboplatin-containing regimen was significantly different from that of the cisplatin-containing combinations. The carboplatin regimens induced significantly more thrombocytopenia and, in one study, significantly more leukopenia and more need for transfusional support. In one study of the cisplatin regimen produced significantly more anemia. Non-hematologic toxicities (eg, emesis, neurotoxicity, ototoxicity, renal toxicity, hypomagnesemia, alopecia) were significantly more frequent with cisplatin in both studies.

Overdosage:

There is no known antidote for carboplatin overdosage. The anticipated complications would be secondary to bone marrow suppression or hepatic toxicity.

Administration and Dosage:

Note: Aluminum reacts with carboplatin; (see Precautions).

Carboplatin as a single agent: 360 mg/m^2 IV on day 1 every 4 weeks (see Formula Dosing for alternative dose). In general, however, do not repeat single intermittent courses of carboplatin until the neutrophil count is at ≥ 2,000/mm^3 and the platelet count is ≥ 100,000/mm^3.

Combination therapy with cyclophosphamide: Carboplatin 300 mg/m^2 IV (see Formula Dosing for alternative dose) plus cyclophosphamide 600 mg/m^2 IV, both on day 1 every 4 weeks for six cycles. Do not repeat intermittent courses of the combination until the neutrophil count is ≥ 2000/mm^3 and the platelet count is ≥ 100,000/mm^3.

Dose adjustment: The dose adjustments in the table below for single agent or combination therapy are modified from controlled trials in previously treated and untreated patients with ovarian carcinoma. Blood counts were done weekly; recommendations are based on the lowest post-treatment platelet or neutrophil value.

Carboplatin Dose Adjustments

Platelets/mm^3	Neutrophils/mm^3	Adjusted dose[1] from prior course
> 100,000	> 2,000	125%
50,000-100,000	500-2,000	No adjustment
<50,000	< 500	75%

[1] Percentages apply to carboplatin as a single agent or to both carboplatin and cyclophosphamide in combination.

CARBOPLATIN

Doses > 125% of the starting dose are not recommended.

Carboplatin is usually administered by an infusion lasting ≥ 15 minutes. No pretreatment or post-treatment hydration or forced diuresis is required.

Renal function impairment: These dosing recommendations apply to the initial course of treatment. Adjust subsequent dosages according to the patient's tolerance based on degree of bone marrow suppression.

Carboplatin in Renal Insufficiency	
Baseline Ccr (ml/min)	Recommended dose on day 1
41 to 59	250 mg/m^2
16 to 40	200 mg/m^2
≤ 15	†

† Data too limited to permit a recommendation for treatment.

Formula dosing: Another approach for determining the initial dose of the drug is the use of mathematical formulae, which are based on a patients's pre-existing renal function or renal function and desired platelet nadir. The use of dosing formulae, as compared to empirical dose calculation based on body surface area, allows compensation for patient variations in pretreatment renal function that might otherwise result in underdosing (in patients with impaired renal function).

A simple formulae for calculating dosage, based upon a patient's glomerular filtration rate (GFR in ml/min) and carboplatin's target area under the concentration versus time curve (AUC in mg/ml•min), has been proposed by Calvert. In these studies, GFR was measured by Cr-EDTA, which has a good correlation with creatinine clearance. Total dose (mg)=(target AUC) x (GFR + 25), note: with the Calvert formula, the total dose of carboplatin is calculated in mg, not mg/m^2.

The target AUC of 4 to 6 mg/ml • min using single agent carboplatin appears to provide the most appropriate dose range in previously treated patients.

Preparation of IV solutions: Immediately before use, the content of each vial must be reconstituted with either Sterile Water for Injection, 5% Dextrose in Water or 0.9% Sodium Chloride Injection, according to the following schedule:

Preparation of Carboplatin Solutions		
Vial strength (mg)	Diluent volume (ml)	Concentration (mg/ml)
50	5	10
150	15	10
450	45	10

Carboplatin can be further diluted to concentrations ≥ 0.5 mg/ml with 5% Dextrose in Water or 0.9% Sodium Chloride Injection.

Storage/Stability: Store the unopened vials at controlled room temperature (15° to 30°C; 59° to 86°F). Protect from light. When prepared as directed, solutions are stable for 8 hours at room temperature (25°C; 77°F). Because no antibacterial preservative is contained in the formulations, discard solutions 8 hours after dilution.

Rx	**Paraplatin** (Bristol-Myers Oncology)	**Powder for Injection, lyophilized:** 50 mg[1]	In vials.
		150 mg[1]	In vials.
		450 mg[1]	In vials.

[1] With mannitol.

METHOTREXATE (Amethopterin; MTX)

Warning:

The high dose regimens recommended for osteosarcoma require meticulous care.

Deaths have occurred with the use of methotrexate (MTX) in malignancy, psoriasis and rheumatoid arthritis.

Marked bone marrow depression may occur with resultant anemia, leukopenia or thrombocytopenia.

Unexpectedly severe (sometimes fatal) marrow suppression and GI toxicity have occurred with coadministration of MTX (usually in high dosage) along with some NSAIDs (see Precautions, Drug Interactions).

Periodic monitoring for toxicity, including CBC with differential and platelet counts, and liver and renal function tests is mandatory. Periodic liver biopsies may be indicated in some situations. Monitor patients at increased risk for impaired MTX elimination (eg, renal dysfunction, pleural effusions, ascites) more frequently (see Precautions).

Liver: MTX causes hepatotoxicity, fibrosis and cirrhosis, but generally only after prolonged use. Acutely, liver enzyme elevations are frequent, usually transient and asymptomatic, and also do not appear predictive of subsequent hepatic disease. Liver biopsy after sustained use often shows histologic changes, and fibrosis and cirrhosis have occurred; these latter lesions often are not preceded by symptoms or abnormal liver function tests (see Precautions).

MTX-induced lung disease is a potentially dangerous lesion that may occur acutely at any time during therapy and has occurred at doses as low as 7.5 mg/week. It is not always fully reversible. Pulmonary symptoms (especially a dry, nonproductive cough) may require interruption of treatment and careful investigation.

Pregnancy: Fetal death or congenital anomalies have occurred; do not use in women of childbearing potential unless benefits outweigh possible risks.

Renal use: Use MTX in patients with impaired renal function with extreme caution, and at reduced dosages, because renal dysfunction will prolong elimination.

GI: Diarrhea and ulcerative stomatitis require interruption of therapy; hemorrhagic enteritis and death from intestinal perforation may occur.

MTX has been administered in very high dosage followed by leucovorin rescue for certain neoplastic diseases. This procedure is investigational.

Do not use MTX formulations and diluents containing preservatives for intrathecal or experimental high dose MTX therapy.

Severe reactions: Because of the possibility of severe toxic reactions, fully inform patient of the risks involved and assure constant supervision.

Actions:

Pharmacology: Methotrexate (MTX) competitively inhibits dihydrofolic acid reductase. Dihydrofolates must be reduced to tetrahydrofolic acid by this enzyme in the process of deoxyribonucleic acid (DNA) synthesis and cellular replication.

Actively proliferating tissues such as malignant cells, bone marrow, fetal cells, buccal and intestinal mucosa, and cells of the urinary bladder are generally more sensitive to this effect of MTX. Cellular proliferation in malignant tissue is greater than in most normal tissue; thus, MTX may impair malignant growth without irreversibly damaging normal tissues.

The original rationale for high dose MTX therapy was based on the concept of selective rescue of normal tissues by leucovorin. More recent evidence suggests that high-dose MTX may also overcome MTX resistance caused by impaired active transport, decreased affinity of dihydrofolic acid reductase for MTX, increased levels of dihydrofolic acid reductase resulting from gene amplification, or decreased polyglutamation of MTX. The actual mechanism of action is unknown.

Pharmacokinetics:

Absorption/Distribution – In adults, oral absorption appears to be dose-dependent. After oral doses ≤ 30 mg/m^2, MTX is generally well absorbed with a mean bioavailability of about 60%. The absorption of doses > 80 mg/m^2 is significantly less, possibly due to a saturation effect. Peak serum levels are usually reached in 1 to 2 hours. In leukemic children, oral absorption reportedly varies widely (23% to 95%). A 20-fold difference between highest and lowest peak levels was reported. Significant interindividual variability was also noted in time-to-peak concentration and fraction of dose absorbed. Food delayed absorption and reduced peak concentration.

METHOTREXATE (Amethopterin; MTX)

After injection, the drug is generally completely absorbed, and peak serum levels are seen in 30 to 60 minutes. After IV administration, the initial volume of distribution is ≈ 0.18 L/kg (18% of body weight) and steady-state volume of distribution is ≈ 0.4 to 0.8 L/kg (40% to 80% of body weight). MTX competes with reduced folates for active transport across cell membranes by means of a single carrier-mediated active transport process. At serum concentrations >100 micromolar, passive diffusion becomes a major pathway by which effective intracellular concentrations can be achieved. Approximately 50% of the absorbed drug is bound to serum protein. MTX does not penetrate the blood-cerebrospinal fluid barrier in therapeutic amounts. High CSF drug concentrations may be attained by direct intrathecal administration.

Metabolism/Excretion – After absorption, MTX undergoes hepatic and intracellular metabolism to polyglutamated forms which can be converted back to MTX by hydrolase enzymes. These polyglutamates act as inhibitors of dihydrofolate reductase and thymidylate synthetase. Small amounts of MTX polyglutamates may remain in tissues for extended periods. The retention and prolonged drug action of these active metabolite(s) vary among different cells, tissues and tumors. A small amount of metabolism to 7-hydroxymethotrexate may occur at doses commonly prescribed. Accumulation of this metabolite may become significant at the high doses used in osteogenic sarcoma. The aqueous solubility of 7-hydroxymethotrexate is threefold to fivefold lower than the parent compound. MTX is partially metabolized by intestinal flora after oral administration.

The terminal half-life is approximately 3 to 10 hours for patients receving low-dose antineoplastic therapy (< 30 mg/m^2). For patients on high doses, the terminal half-life is 8 to 15 hours.

Renal excretion is the primary route of elimination and is dependent upon dosage and route of administration. With IV administration, 80% to 90% of the administered dose is excreted unchanged in the urine within 24 hours. There is limited biliary excretion of ≤ 10%. Enterohepatic recirculation of MTX has been proposed. Renal excretion occurs by glomerular filtration and active tubular secretion. Impaired renal function, as well as concurrent use of drugs such as weak organic acids that also undergo tubular secretion, can markedly increase serum levels. Excellent correlation has been reported between MTX clearance and endogenous creatinine clearance.

Clearance rates vary widely and are generally decreased at higher doses. Delayed drug clearance is one of the major factors responsible for toxicity because the toxicity for normal tissues appears more dependent upon the duration of exposure to the drug rather than the peak level achieved. When a patient has delayed drug elimination due to compromised renal function or other causes, MTX serum concentrations may remain elevated for prolonged periods.

The potential for toxicity from high-dose regimens or delayed excretion is reduced by leucovorin calcium during the final phase of MTX plasma elimination. Guidelines for monitoring serum MTX levels, and for adjustment of leucovorin dosing to reduce the risk of toxicity, are provided in Administration and Dosage.

Indications:

Antineoplastic chemotherapy: Treatment of gestational choriocarcinoma, chorioadenoma destruens and hydatidiform mole.

Acute lymphocytic leukemia: Treatment and prophylaxis of meningeal leukemia and maintenance therapy in combination with other chemotherapeutic agents.

MTX alone or in combination with other anticancer agents for treatment of breast cancer, epidermoid cancers of the head and neck, advanced mycosis fungoides and lung cancer, particularly squamous cell and small cell types; in combination therapy in the treatment of advanced-stage non-Hodgkin's lymphomas.

MTX in high doses followed by leucovorin rescue in combination with other chemotherapeutic agents for prolonging relapse-free survival in patients with non-metastatic osteosarcoma who have undergone surgical resection or amputation for the primary tumor.

Psoriasis: Symptomatic control of severe, recalcitrant, disabling psoriasis (see specific monograph).

Rheumatoid arthritis: Management of severe, active, classical or definite rheumatoid arthritis (see specific monograph).

Unlabeled uses: High-dose regimen followed by leucovorin rescue for adjuvant therapy of non-metastatic osteosarcoma (orphan drug designation granted in 1985); to reduce corticosteroid requirements in patients with severe corticosteroid-dependent asthma.

Contraindications:

Hypersensitivity to the drug; nursing mothers.

METHOTREXATE (Amethopterin; MTX)

Warnings:

Toxic effects, potentially serious, may be related in frequency and severity to dose or frequency of administration, but have been seen at all doses. These effects can occur at any time during therapy; follow patients closely. Most adverse reactions are reversible if detected early. When reactions occur, reduce dosage or discontinue drug and take appropriate corrective measures; this could include use of leucovorin calcium. Use caution if therapy is reinstituted. Consider further need for the drug and possibility of recurrence of toxicity. Pharmacists should dispense no more than a 7 day supply of the drug at one time. Refill of such prescriptions should be by direct order (written or oral) of the physician only.

Renal function impairment: MTX is excreted principally by the kidneys. Its use in impaired renal function may result in accumulation of toxic amounts or additional renal damage. Determine the patient's renal status prior to and during therapy. Exercise caution should significant renal impairment occur. Reduce or discontinue drug dosage until renal function improves or is restored.

Mutagenesis: Although there is evidence that the drug causes chromosomal damage to animal somatic cells and human bone marrow cells, the clinical significance remains uncertain. Weigh benefit against this potential risk before using MTX alone or in combination with other drugs, especially in children or young adults.

The drug causes embryotoxicity, abortion and fetal defects in humans. It has also caused impairment of fertility, oligospermia and menstrual dysfunction during and for a short period after cessation of therapy.

Elderly: Clinical pharmacology has not been well studied in these patients. Due to diminished hepatic and renal function and increased folate stores in this population, consider relatively low doses. Closely monitor for early signs of toxicity.

Pregnancy: Category D. MTX has caused fetal death and congenital anomalies. Do not use unless benefits outweigh risks. Women of childbearing potential should not receive MTX until pregnancy is excluded and they should be fully counseled on the serious risk to the fetus should they become pregnant while undergoing treatment. Avoid pregnancy if either partner is receiving MTX, during and for a minimum of 3 months after therapy for males, and during and for at least one ovulatory cycle after therapy for females.

Category X. Do not administer to pregnant psoriatic or rheumatoid arthritis patients.

Lactation: Contraindicated in nursing mothers. MTX is excreted in breast milk in low concentrations with a milk:plasma ratio of 0.08. The significance of this small amount is unknown. Since the drug may accumulate in neonatal tissues, breast-feeding is not recommended. Decide whether to discontinue nursing, or to discontinue the drug, taking into account the importance of the drug to the mother.

Children: Safety and efficacy in children have not been established, other than in cancer chemotherapy.

Precautions:

Monitoring: Complete blood count with differential and platelet counts; hepatic enzymes; renal function tests; chest x-ray. During initial or changing doses, or during periods of increased risk of elevated MTX blood levels (eg, dehydration), more frequent monitoring may be indicated.

A relationship between abnormal liver function tests and fibrosis or cirrhosis of the liver has not been established. Transient liver function test abnormalities are observed frequently after MTX administration and are usually not cause for modification of MTX therapy. Persistent liver function test abnormalities just prior to dosing, or depression of serum albumin, may indicate serious liver toxicity; they require evaluation.

Pulmonary function tests may be useful if MTX-induced lung disease is suspected, especially if baseline measurements are available.

Intrathecal therapy: Large doses may cause convulsions. Untoward side effects may occur with any intrathecal injection and are commonly neurological. Intrathecal MTX appears significantly in systemic circulation and may cause systemic toxicity; therefore, adjust systemic antileukemic therapy appropriately. Focal leukemic involvement of the CNS may not respond to intrathecal chemotherapy and is best treated with radiotherapy.

Organ system toxicity:

GI – If vomiting, diarrhea or stomatitis occur, which may result in dehydration, discontinue MTX until recovery occurs. Use with extreme caution in the presence of peptic ulcer disease or ulcerative colitis.

Hematologic – MTX can suppress hematopoiesis and cause anemia, leukopenia or thrombocytopenia. Use with caution, if at all, in patients with malignancy and preexisting hematopoietic impairment. Continue MTX only if potential benefit war-

METHOTREXATE (Amethopterin; MTX)

rants risk of severe myelosuppression. Evaluate those with profound granulocytopenia and fever immediately; they usually require parenteral broad-spectrum antibiotics. In severe bone marrow depression, blood or platelet transfusions may be needed.

Hepatic – MTX has the potential for acute (elevated transaminases) and chronic (fibrosis and cirrhosis) hepatotoxicity. Chronic toxicity is potentially fatal; it generally occurs after prolonged use (generally ≥ 2 years) and after a total dose of at least 1.5 g. An accurate incidence rate is undetermined; the rate of progression and reversibility of lesions is not known. Special caution is indicated in the presence of preexisting liver damage or impaired hepatic function.

Periodically perform liver function tests, including serum albumin, prior to dosing. They are often normal in the face of developing fibrosis or cirrhosis. These lesions may be detectable only by biopsy.

Infection or immunologic states – Use with extreme caution in the presence of active infection; usually contraindicated in patients with overt or laboratory evidence of immunodeficiency syndromes. Immunization may be ineffective when given during MTX therapy. Immunization with live virus vaccines is generally not recommended. Disseminated vaccinia infections after smallpox immunization have occurred in patients receiving MTX. Hypogammaglobulinemia occurs rarely.

Neurologic – There have been reports of leukoencephalopathy following IV administration of MTX to patients who have had craniospinal irradiation. Chronic leukoencephalopathy has also occurred in patients with osteosarcoma who received repeated doses of high-dose MTX with leucovorin rescue even without cranial irradiation. Discontinuation of MTX does not always result in complete recovery.

A transient acute neurologic syndrome has been observed in patients treated with high dosage regimens. Manifestations may include behavioral abnormalities, focal sensorimotor signs and abnormal reflexes. The exact cause is unknown.

After intrathecal use of MTX, the CNS toxicity that may occur can be classified as follows: Chemical arachnoiditis manifested by headache, back pain, nuchal rigidity and fever; paresis, usually transient, manifested by paraplegia associated with involvement with one or more spinal nerve roots; leukoencephalopathy manifested by confusion, irritability, somnolence, ataxia, dementia and convulsions.

Pulmonary symptoms (especially a dry, nonproductive cough) or a non-specific pneumonitis occurring during therapy indicate a potentially dangerous lesion and require interruption of treatment and careful investigation. The typical patient presents with fever, cough, dyspnea, hypoxemia and an infiltrate on chest x-ray; infection needs to be excluded. This lesion can occur at all dosages.

Renal – High doses used in the treatment of osteosarcoma may cause renal damage leading to acute renal failure. Nephrotoxicity is due primarily to the precipitation of MTX and 7-hydroxymethotrexate in the renal tubules. Close attention to renal function including adequate hydration, urine alkalinization and measurement of serum MTX and creatinine levels are essential for safe administration.

Other precautions – Use with extreme caution in the presence of debility.

MTX exits slowly from third space compartments (eg, pleural effusions or ascites). This results in a prolonged terminal plasma half-life and unexpected toxicity. In patients with significant third space accumulations, evacuate the fluid before treatment and monitor plasma MTX levels.

Lesions of psoriasis may be aggravated by concomitant exposure to ultraviolet radiation. Radiation dermatitis and sunburn may be "recalled" by the use of MTX.

Drug Interactions:

Aminoglycosides, oral may decrease the absorption and AUC of concurrent oral MTX, although the effect is unpredictable. Consider parenteral MTX.

Charcoal lowers the plasma levels of both oral and IV MTX and may be particularly significant with high dose therapies. Depending on the clinical situation, this will reduce the effectiveness or toxicity of MTX.

Etretinate: Hepatotoxicity occurred in two patients receiving etretinate and MTX for psoriasis, and MTX plasma levels increased in another patient.

Folic acid or its derivatives contained in some vitamins may decrease response to MTX.

Nonsteroidal anti-inflammatory drugs: Concurrent MTX caused fatal interactions in four patients (three with **ketoprofen** , one with **naproxen**). **Indomethacin** and **phenylbutazone** increased MTX plasma levels. The mechanism of action is not known, but may involve inhibition of renal prostaglandin synthesis or competitive renal secretion. Excessive MTX levels did not result when **ketoprofen** was given at least 12 hours after completion of therapy. The possibility of a similar interaction exists with the other NSAIDs. Administer concomitantly with extreme caution, if at all.

Phenytoin serum concentrations may be decreased by a combination chemotherapy regimen including MTX.

Probenecid, salicylates and **sulfonamides** (including **TMP-SMZ**):The therapeutic as well as toxic effects of MTX may be increased by these agents. Inhibition of renal tubular secretion, competition for a common elimination pathway or protein displacement may be the mechanisms involved. However, if protein displacement is the mechanism, it may involve displacement of the highly bound metabolic 7-hydroxymethotrexate since the parent drug is only 50% bound.

Procarbazine may increase the nephrotoxicity of MTX.

Thiopurines: MTX may increase AUC and plasma levels of thiopurines.

Drug/Food interactions: Food may delay the absorption and reduce the peak concentration of MTX.

Adverse Reactions:

The incidence and severity of acute side effects are generally related to dose and dosing frequency. See also Precautions section under "Organ System Toxicity."

The most common adverse reactions are: Ulcerative stomatitis; leukopenia; nausea; abdominal distress; malaise; fatigue; chills; fever; dizziness; decreased resistance to infection.

Dermatologic: Erythematous rashes; pruritus; urticaria; photosensitivity; pigmentary changes; alopecia; ecchymosis; telangiectasia; acne; furunculosis. Lesions of psoriasis may be aggravated by concomitant exposure to ultraviolet radiation.

Hematologic: Bone marrow depression; leukopenia; thrombocytopenia; anemia; hypogammaglobulinemia; hemorrhage; septicemia.

GI: Gingivitis; stomatitis; pharyngitis; anorexia; nausea; vomiting; diarrhea; hematemesis; melena; GI ulceration and bleeding; enteritis.

GU: Renal failure; azotemia; cystitis; hematuria; severe nephropathy; defective oogenesis or spermatogenesis; transient oligospermia; menstrual dysfunction and vaginal discharge; infertility; abortion; fetal defects.

Pulmonary: Deaths from interstitial pneumonitis; chronic interstitial obstructive pulmonary disease.

CNS: Headaches; drowsiness; blurred vision; aphasia; hemiparesis; paresis; convulsions. Leukoencephalopathy following IV use in patients who have had craniospinal irradiation.

After intrathecal use, the CNS toxicity that may occur can be classified as follows:

(1) Chemical arachnoiditis (headache, back pain, nuchal rigidity, fever);
(2) transient paresis (paraplegia with involvement of spinal nerve roots);
(3) leukoencephalopathy (confusion, irritability, somnolence, ataxia, dementia, occasionally major convulsions).

Miscellaneous: Rarer reactions related to the use of MTX include arthralgia/myalgia, diabetes, osteoporosis and sudden death. A few cases of anaphylactoid reactions have occurred.

Overdosage:

Leucovorin (citrovorum factor) is used to neutralize toxic effects. Administer leucovorin as promptly as possible. As the time interval between administration and leucovorin rescue increases, leucovorin's effectiveness in counteracting hematologic toxicity diminishes. Leucovorin may be administered as follows: 10 mg/m^2 orally or parenterally initially, followed by 10 mg/m^2 orally every 6 hours for 72 hours. Leucovorin rescue is usually begun within 24 hours of antifolate administration. If, after 24 hours following MTX administration, the serum creatinine is 50% or greater than the pre-methotrexate serum creatinine, immediately increase the leucovorin dose to 100 mg/m^2 every 3 hours until the serum MTX level is $< 5 \times 10^{-8}$ M.

Charcoal hemoperfusion can lower serum MTX levels, and ventriculolumbar perfusion was used in one patient who received an overdose of intrathecal MTX.

In cases of massive overdosage, hydration and urinary alkalinization may be necessary to prevent the precipitation of MTX and its metabolites in the renal tubules. Neither hemodialysis nor peritoneal dialysis improves MTX elimination.

METHOTREXATE (Amethopterin; MTX)

Patient Information:

Avoid alcohol, salicylates and prolonged exposure to sunlight or sunlamps (particularly patients with psoriasis).

May cause nausea, vomiting, loss of appetite, hair loss, skin rash, boils or acne. Notify physician if these effects persist.

Use contraceptive measures during and for at least 3 months (males) or 1 ovulatory cycle (females) after cessation of therapy.

Notify physician if any of the following occurs: Diarrhea; abdominal pain; black tarry stools; fever and chills; sore throat; unusual bleeding or bruising; sores in or around the mouth; cough or shortness of breath; yellow discoloration of the skin or eyes; darkened urine; bloody urine; swelling of the feet or legs; joint pain.

Administration and Dosage:

Oral administration is often preferred. Preservative free MTX preparations may be given IM, IV, intra-arterially or intrathecally. If desired, the solution may be further diluted immediately prior to use with an appropriate sterile preservative free medium such as 5% Dextrose Solution or Sodium Chloride Injection. The preserved formulation contains benzyl alcohol and must not be used for intrathecal or high dose therapy.

Intrathecal use: Reconstitute immediately prior to use. Use preservative free medium such as 0.9% Sodium Chloride Injection. Concentration should be 1mg/ml.

Powder for injection: Reconstitute 20 and 50 mg vials with an appropriate sterile preservative free medium such as 5% Dextrose Solution or Sodium Chloride Injection to a concentration no greater than 25 mg/ml. Reconstitute the 1g vial with 19.4 ml to a concentration of 50mg/ml.

Choriocarcinoma and similar trophoblastic diseases: 15 to 30 mg orally or IM daily for a 5 day course. Repeat courses 3 to 5 times, as required, with rest periods of ≥ 1 weeks between courses, until any toxic symptoms subside. Evaluate the effectiveness of therapy by 24 hour quantitative analysis of urinary chorionic gonadotropin hormone (hCG), which should return to normal or < 50 IU/24 hr usually after the third or fourth course and is usually followed by a complete resolution of measurable lesions in 4 to 6 weeks. One to two courses of MTX after normalization of hCG is usually recommended. Careful clinical assessment is essential before each course. Cyclic combination therapy with other antitumor drugs may be useful.

Since hydatidiform mole may precede choriocarcinoma, prophylaxis with MTX has been recommended. Chorioadenoma destruens is an invasive form of hydatidiform mole. Administer MTX in doses similar to those for choriocarcinoma.

Leukemia: Acute lymphatic (lymphoblastic) leukemia in children and young adolescents is most responsive. In young adults and older patients, clinical remission is more difficult to obtain and early relapse is more common.

When used for induction, MTX in doses of 3.3 mg/m^2 in combination with prednisone 60 mg/m^2 given daily, produced remission in 50% of patients, usually within 4 to 6 weeks. MTX in combination with other agents is the drug of choice for maintenance of remissions. When remission is achieved and supportive care has produced general clinical improvement, initiate maintenance therapy as follows: Give MTX orally or IM 2 times weekly in total weekly doses of 30 mg/m^2 or 2.5 mg/kg IV every 14 days. If relapse occurs, repeat initial induction regimen.

Meningeal leukemia: Administer 12 mg/m^2 intrathecally or an empirical dose of 15 mg. Dilute preservative-free MTX to a concentration of 1 mg/ml with a sterile, preservative-free medium such as 0.9% Sodium Chloride Injection. Administer at intervals of 2 to 5 days, and repeat until the cell count of the CSF returns to normal, then give one additional dose. Administration at intervals of < 1 week may result in increased subacute toxicity. For prophylaxis against meningeal leukemia, the dosage is the same as for treatment, except for the intervals of administration.

CSF volume is dependent on age and not body surface area (BSA). The CSF is at 40% of the adult volume at birth and reaches adult volume in several years.

Intrathecal MTX 12 mg/m^2 (max, 15 mg) has resulted in low CSF MTX concentrations and reduced efficacy in children and high concentrations and neurotoxicity in adults. The following dosage regimen is based on age instead of BSA and appears to result in more consistent CSF MTX concentrations and less neurotoxicity:

Intrathecal MTX Dose Based on Age

Age (years)	Dose (mg)
< 1	6
1	8
2	10
≥ 3	12

METHOTREXATE (Amethopterin; MTX)

Because the CSF volume and turnover may decrease with age, a dose reduction may be indicated in elderly patients.

Lymphomas: Burkitt's Tumor, Stages I and II: 10 to 25 mg/day orally for 4 to 8 days. In Stage III, give MTX concomitantly with other antitumor agents. Treatment in all stages generally consists of several courses with 7 to 10 day rest periods. Lymphosarcomas in Stage III may respond to combined drug therapy with MTX 0.625 to 2.5 mg/kg/day.

Mycosis fungoides: MTX therapy produces clinical remissions in 50% of cases. Dosage - 2.5 to 10 mg daily orally for weeks or months. Dose levels of drug are guided by patient response and hematologic monitoring. MTX has also been given IM in doses of 50 mg once weekly or 25 mg twice weekly.

Osteosarcoma: Effective therapy requires several cytotoxic chemotherapeutic agents. In addition to high-dose MTX with leucovorin rescue, these agents may include doxorubicin, cisplatin and the combination of bleomycin, cyclophosphamide and dactinomycin (BCD) in the doses and schedule shown in the table below. The starting dose for high dose MTX treatment is 12 g/m^2. If this dose is not sufficient to produce a peak serum concentration of 1000 micromolar (10^{-3} mol/L) at the end of the MTX infusion, the dose may be increased to 15 g/m^2 in subsequent treatments. If the patient is vomiting or is unable to tolerate oral medication, give leucovorin IV or IM at the same dose and schedule.

Chemotherapy Regimens for Osteosarcoma

Drug[1]	Dose[1]	Treatment week after surgery
Methotrexate	12 g/m^2 IV as 4 hour infusion (starting dose)	4, 5, 6, 7, 11, 12, 15, 16, 29, 30, 44, 45
Leucovorin	15 mg orally every 6 hours for 10 doses starting at 24 hours after start of MTX infusion	
Doxorubicin[2] as a single drug	30 mg/m^2 /day IV x 3 days	8, 17
Doxorubicin[2] Cisplatin[2]	50 mg/m^2 IV 100 mg/m^2 IV	20, 23, 33, 36 20, 23, 33, 36
Bleomycin[2] Cyclophosphamide[2] Dactinomycin[2]	15 units/m^2 IV x 2 days 600 mg/m^2 IV x 2 days 0.6 mg/m^2 IV x 2 days	2, 13, 26, 39, 42 2, 13, 26, 39, 42 2, 13, 26, 39, 42

[1] Link MP, Goorin AM, Miser AW, et al. The effect of adjuvant chemotherapy on relapse-free survival in patients with osteosarcoma of the extremity. *N Engl J Med* 1986;314(25):1600-6.

[2] See each respective monograph for more complete information. Dosage modifications may be necessary because of drug-induced toxicity.

When administering high doses of MTX, closely observe the following guidelines.

Guidelines for methotrexate therapy with leucovorin rescue: Delay MTX administration until recovery if:

- the WBC count is < 1500/mm^3
- the neutrophil count is < 200/mm^3
- the platelet count is < 75,000/mm^3
- the serum bilirubin level is > 1.2 mg/dl
- the ALT level is > 450 U
- mucositis is present, until there is evidence of healing
- persistent pleural effusion is present; drain dry prior to infusion.

Adequate renal function must be documented: Serum creatinine must be normal, and creatinine clearance must be > 60 ml/min, before initiation of therapy.

Serum creatinine must be measured prior to each subsequent course of therapy. If serum creatinine has increased by ≥ 50% compared to a prior value, the creatinine clearance must be measured and documented to be > 60 ml/min (even if serum creatinine is still within the normal range).

Patients must be well hydrated, and must be treated with sodium bicarbonate for urinary alkalinization.

Administer 1 L/m^2 of IV fluid over 6 hours prior to initiation of the MTX infusion. Continue hydration at 125 ml/m^2 /hr (3 L/m^2 /day) during MTX infusion, and for 2 days after the infusion has been completed.

Alkalinize urine to maintain pH above 7 during MTX infusion and leucovorin calcium therapy by giving sodium bicarbonate orally or by incorporation into a separate IV solution.

METHOTREXATE (Amethopterin; MTX)

Repeat serum creatinine and serum MTX 24 hours after starting MTX and at least once daily until the level is $< 5 \times 10^{-8}$ mol/L (0.05 micromolar).

Guidelines for leucovorin calcium dosage based upon serum MTX levels:

Leucovorin Rescue Schedules Following Treatment With Higher Doses of Methotrexate		
Clinical situation	Laboratory findings	Leucovorin dosage and duration
Normal MTX elimination	Serum MTX level ≈ 10 micromolar at 24 hrs after administration, 1 micromolar at 48 hrs, and < 0.2 micromolar at 72 hrs	15 mg po, IM or IV q 6 hrs for 60 hrs (10 doses starting at 24 hrs after start of MTX infusion)
Delayed late MTX elimination	Serum MTX level remaining > 0.2 micromolar at 72 hrs, and > 0.05 micromolar at 96 hrs after administration	Continue 15 mg po, IM or IV q 6 hrs, until MTX level is < 0.05 micromolar
Delayed early MTX elimination or evidence of acute renal injury	Serum MTX level of ≥ 50 micromolar at 24 hrs, or ≥ 5 micromolar at 48 hrs after administration, or; a ≥ 100% increase in serum creatinine level at 24 hours after MTX administration (eg, an increase from 0.5 mg/dl to a level of ≥1 mg/dl)	150 mg IV q 3 hrs, until MTX level is < 1 micromolar; then 15 mg IV q 3 hrs until MTX level is < 0.05 micromolar

Patients who experience delayed early MTX elimination are likely to develop nonreversible oliguric renal failure. In addition to appropriate leucovorin therapy, these patients require continuing hydration and urinary alkalinization, and close monitoring of fluid and electrolyte status, until serum MTX level has fallen to < 0.05 micromolar and the renal failure has resolved.

Some patients will have abnormalities in MTX elimination, or abnormalities in renal function following MTX administration, which are significant but less severe than those described in the table; they may or may not be associated with significant clinical toxicity. If significant clinical toxicity is observed, extend leucovorin rescue for an additional 24 hours (total 14 doses over 84 hours) in subsequent courses of therapy. Consider the possibility that the patient is taking other medications which interact with MTX when laboratory abnormalities or clinical toxicities are observed.

Hepatic function impairment: If the bilirubin is between 3 and 5, or AST > 180, reduce dose by 25%. If bilirubin is > 5, omit the dose.

Consider procedures for proper handling and disposal of anticancer drugs.

Rx	**Rhumatrex Dose Pack** (Lederle)	**Tablets:** 2.5 mg (as sodium)	(LLM1). Yelow, scored. 4 cards, each w/2, 3, 4, 5 or 6 tablets.
Rx	**Methotrexate** (Lyphomed[1])	**Injection:** 2.5 mg (as sodium) per ml	In 2 ml vials.
Rx	**Methotrexate** (Various, eg, Americal, Astra, Cetus, Dupont[1], Lederle[2], Lyphomed[1], Quad[2], VHA Supply)	**Injection:** 25 mg (as sodium) per ml	In 2, 4, 8 and 10 ml vials.
Rx	**Methotrexate** (Various, eg, Lederle[1], Quad, VHA Supply)	**Powder for injection, lyophilized:** 20 mg per vial (as sodium) 50 mg per vial (as sodium) 1 g per vial (as sodium)	In single-use vials.
Rx	**Methotrexate LPF** (Lederle)	**Preservative Free Injection:** 25 mg (as sodium) per ml	In 2, 4, 8 and 10 ml vials.[1]
Rx	**Folex PFS** (Adria)		In 2, 4, 8 and 10 ml vials.[1]

[1] Contains no preservative. For single use only.

[2] Contains benzyl alcohol.

FLUOROURACIL AND FLOXURIDINE

Actions:

Pharmacology: There is evidence that the metabolism of fluorouracil in the anabolic pathway blocks the methylation reaction of deoxyuridylic acid to thymidylic acid. In this manner, fluorouracil interferes with the synthesis of deoxyribonucleic acid (DNA) and to a lesser extent inhibits the formation of ribonucleic acid (RNA). Since DNA and RNA are essential for cell division and growth, the effect of fluorouracil may be to create a thymine deficiency provoking unbalanced growth and death of the cell. DNA and RNA deprivation most effect those cells that grow rapidly and take up fluorouracil at a more rapid pace.

Pharmacokinetics: Following IV injection, fluorouracil distributes into tumors, intestinal mucosa, bone marrow, liver and other body tissues. In spite of its limited lipid solubility, fluorouracil diffuses readily across the blood-brain barrier and distributes into CSF and brain tissue.

The parent drug is excreted unchanged (7% to 20%) in the urine in 6 hours; of this, > 90% is excreted in the first hour. The remaining percentage is metabolized, primarily in the liver. The catabolic metabolism of fluorouracil results in inactive degradation products (eg, CO_2, urea, α-fluoro-β-alanine). The inactive metabolites are excreted in the urine over the next 3 to 4 hours. Approximately 90% is excreted in expired CO_2. Following IV use, 90% of the dose is accounted for during the first 24 hours; the mean half-life of elimination from plasma is ≈ 16 minutes (range, 8 to 20 minutes) and is dose-dependent. No intact drug can be detected in the plasma 3 hours after an IV injection.

Floxuridine is rapidly catabolized to 5-fluorouracil. Thus, the same toxic and antimetabolic effects as 5-fluorouracil occur.

Indications:

See individual product listings.

Contraindications:

Poor nutritional status; depressed bone marrow function; potentially serious infections; hypersensitivity to fluorouracil.

Warnings:

Hospitalize patients during initial course due to possible severe toxic reactions.

Use with extreme caution in poor-risk patients who have had high-dose pelvic irradiation or previous use of alkylating agents, or who have widespread involvement of bone marrow by metastatic tumors or impaired hepatic or renal function. These drugs are not intended as adjuvants to surgery.

Combination therapy: Any form of therapy which adds to the stress of the patient, interferes with nutrition or depresses bone marrow function will increase toxicity.

Mutagenesis: A positive effect was observed in the micronucleus test on bone marrow cells of the mouse, and fluorouracil at very high concentrations produced chromosomal breaks in hamster fibroblasts in vitro.

Fertility impairment: Intraperitoneal doses of 125 or 250 mg/kg induce chromosomal aberrations and changes in chromosomal organization of spermatogonia in rats. Spermatogonial differentiation was also inhibited by fluorouracil, resulting in transient infertility. In female rats, intraperitoneal fluorouracil 25 or 50 mg/kg/week for 3 weeks during the pre-ovulatory phase of oogenesis, significantly reduced the incidence of fertile matings, delayed pre- and postimplantation embryo development, increased preimplantation lethality incidence and induced chromosomal anomalies in these embryos.

Pregnancy: Category D (fluorouracil). Fluorouracil crosses the placenta and enters into fetal circulation in the rat, resulting in increased resorptions and embryolethality. In monkeys, maternal doses > 40 mg/kg resulted in abortion of all embryos exposed to fluorouracil. Compounds which inhibit DNA, RNA and protein synthesis might be expected to have adverse effects on peri- and postnatal development.

Fluorouracil may cause fetal harm when administered to a pregnant woman; it is teratogenic and mutagenic in laboratory animals. Malformations included cleft palates, skeletal defects and deformed appendages, paws and tails. Teratogenic dosages in animals are 1 to 3 times the maximum recommended human therapeutic dose. There are no adequate and well controlled studies in pregnant women. Advise women of childbearing potential to avoid pregnancy. If the drug is used during pregnancy, or if the patient becomes pregnant while taking the drug, tell her of the potential hazard to the fetus. Do not use during pregnancy (particularly in the first trimester) unless the potential benefit justifies the potential risk to the fetus.

Lactation: It is not known whether fluorouracil is excreted in breast milk. Because fluorouracil inhibits DNA, RNA and protein synthesis, do not nurse while using it.

Children: Safety and efficacy of fluorouracil in children have not been established.

FLUOROURACIL AND FLOXURIDINE

Precautions:

Discontinue if signs of toxicity occur: Stomatitis or esophagopharyngitis (at first visible sign); rapidly falling WBC count; leukopenia (WBC < $3500/mm^3$); intractable vomiting; diarrhea or frequent bowel movements; GI ulceration and bleeding; thrombocytopenia (platelets < $100,000/mm^3$); hemorrhage.

These are highly toxic drugs with a narrow margin of safety. Therapeutic response is unlikely to occur without some toxicity. Inform patients of toxic effects, particularly oral manifestations. Measure WBC count with differential before each dose. Severe hematological toxicity, GI hemorrhage and death may result, despite meticulous patient selection and dosage adjustment. Although severe toxicity and fatalities are more likely in poor-risk patients, these effects may occur in patients in relatively good condition.

Angina: Coronary vasospasm with episodes of angina may occur in patients receiving fluorouracil. The angina appears to occur ≈ 6 hours (range, minutes to 7 days) after the third dose (range, 1 to 13 doses). Patients with preexisting coronary artery disease may be at increased risk. Nitrates or morphine appear effective in relieving the pain; pretreatment with a calcium channel blocker may also be successful.

Drug Interactions:

Leucovorin calcium may enhance the toxicity of fluorouracil.

Drug/Lab test interactions: Elevations in **alkaline phosphatase, serum transaminase, serum bilirubin** and **lactic dehydrogenase** may occur.

Adverse Reactions:

Hypersensitivity: Anaphylaxis; generalized allergic reactions.

Hematologic: Leukopenia; thrombocytopenia; pancytopenia; agranulocytosis; anemia; thrombophlebitis. Low WBC counts are usually observed between days 9 and 14 after the first course of treatment. The count usually normalizes by day 30.

Ophthalmic: Photophobia; lacrimation; decreased vision; nystagmus; diplopia; lacrimal duct stenosis; visual changes.

Miscellaneous: Fever; epistaxis.

Regional arterial infusion complications – Arterial aneurysm; arterial ischemia; arterial thrombosis; bleeding at catheter site; catheter blocked, displaced or leaking; embolism; fibromyositis; abscesses; infection at catheter site; thrombophlebitis.

Cardiovascular: Myocardial ischemia; angina (see Precautions).

GI: Stomatitis and esophagopharyngitis (which may lead to sloughing and ulceration), diarrhea, anorexia, nausea, vomiting, enteritis (common); cramps; duodenal ulcer; watery stools; duodenitis; gastritis; glossitis; pharyngitis; possible intra- and extrahepatic biliary sclerosis; acalculus cholecystitis; GI ulceration; bleeding.

Dermatologic: Alopecia; dermatitis, often as a pruritic maculopapular rash on the extremities or trunk (usually reversible and responsive to symptomatic treatment); nonspecific skin toxicity; photosensitivity as manifested by erythema or increased skin pigmentation; nail changes including loss of nails; dry skin; fissuring; vein pigmentation.

CNS: Lethargy, malaise, weakness, acute cerebellar syndrome (may persist following discontinuation of treatment); headache.

Psychiatric: Disorientation; confusion; euphoria.

Lab test abnormalities: BSP; prothrombin; total proteins; sedimentation rate; thrombocytopenia.

Overdosage:

The possibility of overdosage with fluorouracil is unlikely in view of the mode of administration. Nevertheless, the anticipated manifestations would be nausea, vomiting, diarrhea, GI ulceration and bleeding, bone marrow depression (including thrombocytopenia, leukopenia and agranulocytosis). No specific antidotal therapy exists. Patients who have been exposed to an overdose of fluorouracil should be monitored hematologically for at least 4 weeks. Should abnormalities appear, utilize appropriate therapy.

Patient Information:

Transient alopecia may occur with fluorouracil; alert the patient to this possibility.

Contraceptive measures are recommended for men and women during therapy.

Notify doctor if chills, nausea, vomiting, unusual bleeding or bruising, yellowing of skin or eyes, abdominal pain, flank or joint pain, or swelling of feet or legs occurs.

May cause diarrhea, fever and weakness. Notify doctor if these become pronounced.

Drink plenty of liquids while taking this drug.

FLUOROURACIL (5-Fluorouracil; 5-FU)

For complete prescribing information, refer to the Fluorouracil and Floxuridine group monograph.

Indications:

Palliative management of carcinoma of the colon, rectum, breast, stomach and pancreas.

Also used in combination with levamisole (see individual monograph) after surgical resection in patients with Dukes' stage C colon cancer.

In patients with metastatic colorectal carcinoma, IV leucovorin 200 mg/m^2/day for 5 days followed by fluorouracil 370 mg/m^2/day for 5 days and repeated every 28 days significantly increased response rate, decreased time to disease progression and prolonged overall survival compared to fluorouracil alone.

Administration and Dosage:

Individualize dosage. Give IV; avoid extravasation. No dilution required. Individualize dosage based on actual weight. Use lean body weight (dry weight) if patient is obese or has had spurious weight gain due to edema, ascites or other abnormal fluid retention.

Although not FDA approved, fluorouracil has been administered orally in a small number (< 5%) of patients when more acceptable methods are not possible. Absorption is erratic and plasma concentrations are variable. If given orally, do not dilute the dose in orange or grape juice; mix with water only.

Initial dosage: 12 mg/kg IV once daily for 4 days. Do not exceed 800 mg/day. If no toxicity is observed, give 6 mg/kg on days 6, 8, 10 and 12. No therapy is given on days 5, 7, 9 or 11. Discontinue at end of day 12, even with no apparent toxicity.

Poor-risk patients or those not in an adequate nutritional state receive 6 mg/kg/day for 3 days. If no toxicity is observed, give 3 mg/kg on days 5, 7 and 9. Give no therapy on days 4, 6 or 8. Do not exceed 400 mg/day.

A sequence of injections on either schedule constitutes a "course of therapy." Discontinue therapy promptly when any signs of toxicity appear.

Maintenance therapy: Where toxicity has not been a problem, continue therapy using either of the following schedules: (1) Repeat dosage of first course every 30 days after last day of previous course; (2) when toxic signs from the initial course of therapy have subsided, administer a maintenance dosage of 10 to 15 mg/kg/week as a single dose. Do not exceed 1 g/week. Use reduced doses for poor risk patients. Consider the patient's reaction to the previous course and adjust dosage accordingly. Some patients have received from 9 to 45 courses over 12 to 60 months.

Storage: Solution may discolor during storage; potency and safety are not adversely affected. Store at room temperature, 15° to 30°C (59° to 86°F) and protect from light. If precipitate forms due to exposure to low temperatures, heat to 60°C (140°F) with vigorous shaking; cool to body temperature before using.

Rx	**Fluorouracil** (Various, eg, Americal, Cetus, Fujisawa, Quad, VHA Supply)	**Injection:** 50 mg/ml	In 10, 20 and 100 ml vials and 10 ml amps.
Rx	**Fluorouracil** (Roche)		In 10 ml vials.
Rx	**Fluorouracil** (Solopak)		In 10 ml amps, 10 and 50 ml vials and 100 ml bulk vials.
Rx	**Adrucil** (Adria)		In 10 ml amps.

FLOXURIDINE

For complete prescribing information, refer to the Fluorouracil and Floxuridine group monograph.

Indications:

Palliative management of GI adenocarcinoma metastatic to the liver, given by continuous regional intra-arterial infusion in selected patients considered incurable by surgery or other means. Patients with disease extending beyond an area capable of infusion via a single artery should, except in unusual circumstances, be considered for systemic therapy with other agents.

Administration and Dosage:

For intra-arterial infusion only: Continuous arterial infusion of 0.1 to 0.6 mg/kg/day. The higher dose ranges (0.4 to 0.6 mg) are usually employed for hepatic artery infusion because the liver metabolizes the drug, thus reducing the potential for systemic toxicity. Administer until adverse reactions appear. When side effects have subsided, resume therapy. Maintain therapy as long as response continues. Use an infusion pump to overcome pressure in large arteries and to ensure a uniform infusion rate.

Reconstitution/Storage:

Powder for injection – Reconstitute with 5 ml sterile water. Refrigerate reconstituted vials at 2° to 8°C (36° to 46°F) for not more than 2 weeks.

Rx	**Floxuridine** (Quad)	**Powder for Injection:** 500 mg	In 10 ml vials.
Rx	**FUDR** (Roche)		In 5 ml vials.

CYTARABINE (Cytosine Arabinoside; ARA-C)

Warning:

For induction therapy, treat patients in a facility with laboratory and supportive resources sufficient to monitor drug tolerance and protect and maintain a patient compromised by drug toxicity.

The main toxic effect is bone marrow suppression with leukopenia, thrombocytopenia and anemia. Less serious toxicity includes nausea, vomiting, diarrhea, abdominal pain, oral ulceration and hepatic dysfunction.

Actions:

Pharmacology: Cytarabine exhibits cell phase specificity, primarily killing cells undergoing deoxyribonucleic acid (DNA) synthesis (S-phase) and under certain conditions blocking the progression of cells from the G_1 phase to the S-phase. Although the mechanism of action is not completely understood, it appears that cytarabine inhibits DNA polymerase. Incorporation of cytarabine into both DNA and ribonucleic acid (RNA) has also been reported. Chromosomal damage has been produced in rodent cell cultures. Deoxycytidine prevents or delays (but does not reverse) the cytotoxic activity.

Cell culture studies have shown that cytarabine has an antiviral effect. However, efficacy against herpes zoster or smallpox could not be demonstrated in clinical trials.

Cellular resistance and sensitivity – Cytarabine is metabolized by deoxycytidine kinase and other nucleotide kinases to the nucleotide triphosphate, an effective inhibitor of DNA polymerase; it is inactivated by a pyrimidine nucleoside deaminase, which converts it to the nontoxic uracil derivative. It appears that the balance of kinase and deaminase levels may be an important factor in determining sensitivity or resistance of the cell to cytarabine.

Pharmacokinetics: When given orally, cytarabine is rapidly metabolized by the GI mucosa and liver, resulting in < 20% systemic availability. After SC or IM use, peak plasma levels are achieved in 20 to 60 minutes and are considerably lower than after IV use.

Following rapid IV injection, the disappearance from plasma is biphasic; the distributive phase half-life is about 10 minutes, and the elimination phase half-life is about 1 to 3 hours. Cytarabine is eliminated by enzymatic deamination to nontoxic uracil arabinoside (ara-U). Within 24 hours, about 80% of a dose is recovered in the urine, approximately 90% of which is ara-U.

Relatively constant plasma levels can be achieved by continuous IV infusion.

Cerebrospinal fluid (CSF) levels of cytarabine are lower than plasma levels after single IV injection. However, in one patient in whom CSF levels were examined after 2 hours of constant IV infusion, levels approached 40% of the steady-state plasma level. With intrathecal administration, CSF levels declined with a first order half-life of about 2 hours. Because CSF levels of deaminase are low, little conversion to ara-U was observed.

Immunosuppressive action – Cytarabine may obliterate immune responses with little or no accompanying toxicity. Suppression of antibody responses to E-coli-VI antigen and tetanus toxoid have been demonstrated. This suppression was obtained during both primary and secondary antibody responses. Following 5 days of therapy, the immune response is suppressed as indicated by the following parameters: Macrophage ingress into skin windows; circulating antibody response following primary antigenic stimulation; lymphocyte blastogenesis with phytohemagglutinin. A few days after termination of therapy there was a rapid return to normal.

Cytarabine also suppresses cell-mediated immune responses such as delayed hypersensitivity skin reaction to dinitrochlorobenzene. However, it had no effect on already established delayed hypersensitivity reactions.

Indications:

Induction and maintenance of remission in acute myelocytic leukemia (AML) of both adults and children. It has also been useful in the treatment of other leukemias, such as acute lymphocytic leukemia (ALL) and chronic myelocytic leukemia (blast phase).

Acute myelocytic leukemia (AML): Response rates are higher in children than in adults with similar treatment schedules. With induction and initial drug responsiveness, childhood AML appears to be more similar to childhood acute lymphocytic leukemia (ALL) than to its adult variant.

Acute lymphocytic leukemia (adults and children): Has been effective singly or in combination in patients relapsed on other therapy. When used with other antineoplastic agents as part of a total therapy program, results were equal to or better than those reported with such programs which did not include cytarabine.

CYTARABINE (Cytosine Arabinoside; ARA-C)

Intrathecal use in meningeal leukemia: Cytarabine has been used intrathecally in acute leukemia. Dosage schedule is usually governed by type and severity of CNS manifestations and response to previous therapy. Focal leukemic involvement of the CNS may not respond to intrathecal cytarabine and may be better treated with radiotherapy. Prophylactic triple therapy following the successful treatment of the acute meningeal episode may be useful.

Unlabeled uses: Cytarabine has been used experimentally in a variety of neoplastic diseases. In general, few patients with solid tumors have benefited.

Contraindications:

Hypersensitivity to cytarabine.

Warnings:

Myelosuppression: Cytarabine is a potent bone marrow suppressant. Start therapy cautiously in patients with preexisting drug-induced bone marrow suppression. Keep patients under close medical supervision and, during induction therapy, perform leukocyte and platelet counts daily. Perform bone marrow examinations frequently after blasts have disappeared from the peripheral blood. Have facilities available for management of bone marrow complications, possibly fatal (infection resulting from granulocytopenia and other impaired body defenses, and hemorrhage secondary to thrombocytopenia).

Experimental doses: Severe and sometimes fatal CNS, GI and pulmonary toxicity (different from that seen with conventional cytarabine regimens) have occurred. These reactions include reversible corneal toxicity and hemorrhagic conjunctivitis, which may be prevented or diminished by prophylaxis with local corticosteroid eye drops; cerebral and cerebellar dysfunction, usually reversible, including personality changes, dysarthria, ataxia, confusion, somnolence and coma; severe GI ulceration, including pneumatosis cystoides intestinalis leading to peritonitis; sepsis and liver abscess; pulmonary edema; liver damage with increased hyperbilirubinemia; bowel necrosis; and necrotizing colitis. Rarely, severe skin rash leading to desquamation may occur. Complete alopecia is more common with experimental high-dose therapy than with standard cytarabine treatment programs. If experimental high-dose therapy is used, do not use a diluent containing benzyl alcohol. In one report, the CNS toxicity occurred only in those patients greater than 55 years of age.

An increase in cardiomyopathy with subsequent death has occurred following experimental high-dose therapy with cytarabine in combination with cyclophosphamide when used for bone marrow transplant preparation.

A syndrome of sudden respiratory distress, rapidly progressing to pulmonary edema and radiographically pronounced cardiomegaly, has been reported following experimental high-dose therapy with cytarabine used for the treatment of relapsed leukemia from one institution in 16 of 72 patients. The outcome of this syndrome can be fatal.

Ten patients treated with experimental intermediate doses of cytarabine (1 g/m^2) with and without other chemotherapeutic agents (meta-AMSA, daunorubicin, etoposide) at various dose regimens developed a diffuse interstitial pneumonitis without clear cause that it may be related to cytarabine.

Benzyl alcohol is contained in the diluent for this product. Benzyl alcohol has been reported to be associated with a fatal "Gasping Syndrome" in premature infants.

Hypersensitivity: Cases of anaphylaxis have occurred resulting in acute cardiopulmonary arrest which required resuscitation. Refer to Management of Acute Hypersensitivity Reactions.

Pregnancy: Category D. Cytarabine can cause fetal harm when administered to a pregnant woman. There are no adequate and well controlled studies in pregnant women. If cytarabine is used during pregnancy, or if the patient becomes pregnant while taking cytarabine, apprise the patient of the potential hazard to the fetus. Advise women of childbearing potential to avoid becoming pregnant.

The potential for abnormalities exists, particularly during the first trimester. Inform patient of potential risk to the fetus and advisability of pregnancy continuation. There is a lesser risk if therapy is initiated during the second or third trimester. Normal infants have been delivered to patients treated in all three trimesters of pregnancy; however, follow-up of such infants is advisable.

In 32 reported cases where cytarabine was given during pregnancy, either alone or in combination with other cytotoxic agents; 18 normal infants were delivered. Four infants had first trimester exposure, and five were premature or of low birth weight. Twelve of the 18 normal infants were followed up at ages ranging from 6 weeks to 7 years, and showed no abnormalities. One apparently normal infant died of gastroenteritis at 90 days. Two cases of congenital abnormalities have been reported, one with upper and lower distal limb defects, and the other with extremity and ear deformities. Both of these cases had first trimester exposure.

CYTARABINE (Cytosine Arabinoside; ARA-C)

There were seven infants with various problems in the neonatal period, which included: Pancytopenia; transient depression of WBC, hematocrit or platelets; electrolyte abnormalities; transient eosinophilia; increased IgM levels and hyperpyrexia possibly due to sepsis (one case). Six of the seven infants were also premature. The child with pancytopenia died of sepsis at 21 days.

Therapeutic abortions were done in five cases. Four fetuses were grossly normal, but one had an enlarged spleen and another showed Trisomy C chromosomal abnormality in the chorionic tissue.

Lactation: It is not known whether this drug is excreted in breast milk. Because of the potential for serious adverse reactions in nursing infants from cytarabine, decide whether to discontinue nursing or discontinue the drug, taking into account the importance of the drug to the mother.

Precautions:

Monitoring: Monitor patients closely. Frequent platelet and leukocyte counts and bone marrow examinations are mandatory. Suspend or modify therapy when drug-induced marrow depression results in a platelet count < 50,000/mm^3 or a polymorphonuclear granulocyte count < 1000/mm^3. Counts of formed elements in the peripheral blood may continue to fall after the drug is stopped and reach lowest values after drug free intervals of 12 to 24 days. Restart therapy when definite signs of marrow recovery appear (on successive bone marrow studies). Patients whose drug is withheld until "normal" peripheral blood values are attained may escape from control.

Perform periodic checks of liver and kidney functions.

Rapid administration: When large IV doses are given rapidly, patients are frequently nauseated and may vomit for several hours. This tends to be less severe when the drug is infused slowly.

Hepatic function impairment: The liver detoxifies much of an administered dose. Use the drug with caution and at reduced doses in patients with poor liver function.

Hyperuricemia may be induced due to lysis of neoplastic cells. Monitor patient's blood uric acid level; use supportive and pharmacologic measures as necessary.

Acute pancreatitis has occurred in patients being treated with cytarabine who have had prior treatment with L-asparaginase.

Two other cases of pancreatitis have occurred following experimental doses of cytarabine and numerous other drugs. Cytarabine could have been the causative agent.

Peripheral motor and sensory neuropathies have occurred in two patients with adult acute non-lymphocytic leukemia after consolidation with high dose cytarabine, daunorubicin and asparaginase. Observe patients on high dose cytarabine for neuropathy since dose schedule alterations may be needed to avoid irreversible neurologic disorders.

Intrathecal cytarabine may cause systemic toxicity; carefully monitor the hematopoietic system. Modification of other antileukemia therapy may be necessary. Major toxicity is rare. The most frequent reactions after intrathecal administration are nausea, vomiting and fever; these reactions are mild and self-limiting. Paraplegia and neurotoxicity have occurred. Necrotizing leukoencephalopathy occurred in five children who had also been treated with intrathecal methotrexate and hydrocortisone and CNS radiation. Blindness occurred in 2 patients in remission whose treatment had consisted of combination systemic chemotherapy, prophylactic CNS radiation and intrathecal cytarabine. Focal leukemic involvement of the CNS may not respond to intrathecal cytarabine and may be better treated with radiotherapy.

If used intrathecally, do not use a diluent with benzyl alcohol. Two patients with childhood acute myelogenous leukemia who received intrathecal and IV cytarabine at conventional doses (in addition to a number of other coadministered drugs) developed delayed progressive ascending paralysis resulting in death in one patient.

Drug Interactions:

Digoxin: Combination chemotherapy (including cytarabine) may decrease digoxin absorption even several days after stopping chemotherapy. **Digoxin capsules** and **digitoxin** do not appear to be affected.

Adverse Reactions:

Infection: Viral, bacterial, fungal, parasitic or saprophytic infections in any location in the body may be associated with the use of cytarabrine alone or in combination with other immunosuppressive agents following immunosuppressant doses that affect cellular or humoral immunity. These infections may be mild, but can be severe and sometimes fatal.

A cytarabine syndrome characterized by fever, myalgia, bone pain, occasional chest pain, maculopapular rash, conjunctivitis and malaise has been described. It usually

CYTARABINE (Cytosine Arabinoside; ARA-C)

occurs 6 to 12 hours following drug administration. Corticosteroids have been beneficial in treating or preventing this syndrome. If the symptoms are treatable, consider use of corticosteroids as well as continuation of cytarabine therapy.

Most frequent: Anorexia; nausea and vomiting (following rapid IV injection); diarrhea; oral and anal inflammation or ulceration; hepatic dysfunction; fever; rash; thrombophlebitis; bleeding (all sites).

Less frequent: Sepsis; pneumonia; cellulitis at injection site; skin ulceration; urinary retention; renal dysfunction; neuritis or neural toxicity; sore throat; esophageal ulceration; esophagitis; chest pain; bowel necrosis; abdominal pain; freckling; jaundice; conjunctivitis (may occur with rash); dizziness; alopecia; anaphylaxis (see Warnings); allergic edema; pruritus; shortness of breath; urticaria; headache.

Experimental doses: Severe and sometimes fatal CNS, GI and pulmonary toxicity (different from that seen with conventional therapy regimens of cytarabine) have occurred. Cardiomyopathy and a syndrome of sudden respiratory distress are other possibly fatal reactions to experimental doses of cytarabine (see Warnings).

Hematologic: Because cytarabine is a bone marrow suppressant, anemia, leukopenia, thrombocytopenia, megaloblastosis and reduced reticulocytes can be expected. The severity of these reactions is dose and schedule dependent. Expect cellular changes in the morphology of bone marrow and peripheral smears.

Following a 5 day constant infusion or acute injections of 50 to 600 mg/m^2, white cell depression follows a biphasic course. Regardless of initial count, dosage level or schedule, there is an initial fall starting the first 24 hours with a nadir at days 7 to 9. A brief rise follows which peaks around day 12. A second and deeper fall reaches nadir at days 15 to 24, then there is rapid rise to above baseline in the next 10 days. Platelet depression is noticeable at 5 days with a peak depression occurring between days 12 to 15. A rapid rise to above baseline occurs in the next 10 days.

Overdosage:

There is no antidote for cytarabine overdosage. Doses of 4.5 g/m^2 by IV infusion over 1 hour every 12 hours for 12 doses has caused an unacceptable increase in irreversible CNS toxicity and death.

Single doses as high as 3 g/m^2 have been administered by rapid IV infusion without apparent toxicity.

Administration and Dosage:

Cytarabine is not active orally; give SC or intrathecally or by IV infusion or injection. Thrombophlebitis has occurred at the injection or infusion site and, rarely, pain and inflammation occur at SC injection sites. The drug is generally well tolerated.

Patients can tolerate higher total doses when the drug is given by rapid IV injection as compared with slow infusion, due to the drug's rapid inactivation and brief exposure of susceptible normal and neoplastic cells to significant levels after rapid injection. There is no distinct clinical advantage demonstrated for either.

Acute non-lymphocytic leukemia: In combination with other anti-cancer drugs, give 100 mg/m^2 /day by continuous IV infusion (days 1 to 7) or 100 mg/m^2 IV every 12 hours (days 1 to 7).

Acute lymphocytic leukemia: Consult the literature for current recommendations.

Refractory acute leukemia: High-dose cytarabine 3 g/m^2 IV every 12 hou.rs for 4 to 12 doses (repeated at 2 to 3 week intervals) has been used. Remission rates in one study were similar for patients with AML and ALL. Therapies using 4 to 6 doses every 2 weeks or 9 doses every 3 weeks appear equally effective and less toxic.

Intrathecal use in meningeal leukemia: Doses range from 5 to 75 mg/m^2 once daily for 4 days or once every 4 days. The most common dose is 30 mg/m^2 every 4 days until CSF findings are normal, followed by one additional treatment.

CYTARABINE (Cytosine Arabinoside; ARA-C)

Preparation of solutions:

Preparation of Cytarabine Solutions		
Vial size	Amount of Bacteriostatic Water 0.9% to add	Resultant solution
100 mg	5 ml	20 mg/ml
500 mg	10 ml	50 mg/ml
1 g	10 ml	100 mg/ml
2 g	20 ml	100 mg/ml

If used intrathecally, do not use a diluent containing benzyl alcohol. Reconstitute with preservative free 0.9% Sodium Chloride for Injection; use immediately.

Many investigators prefer to use a special diluent for intrathecal use which is physiologically similar to spinal fluid (Elliott's B Solution).

Storage: Store solutions at controlled room temperature 15° to 30°C (59° to 86°F) for 48 hours. Discard if a slight haze develops. When repackaged in glass or plastic, maximum stability appears to be provided by glass stored at 5°C (41°F); however, storage of cytarabine in plastic disposable syringes stored at 5°C is an acceptable alternative.

Chemical stability in infusion solutions: When the reconstituted cytarabine was added to Water for Injection, 5% Dextrose in Water or Sodium Chloride Injection, 94% to 96% of the cytarabine was present after 192 hours storage at room temperature.

Rx	**Tarabine PFS** (Adria)	**Injection:** 20 mg/ml	Preservative free. In 5 ml single vials and 50 ml bulk package vials.
Rx	**Cytarabine** (Various, eg, Cetus, Quad, Schein)	**Powder for Injection**[1]: 100 mg	In vials.
Rx	**Cytosar-U** (Upjohn)		In vials.
Rx	**Cytarabine** (Various, eg, Cetus, Quad, Schein)	**Powder for Injection**[1]: 500 mg	In vials.
Rx	**Cytosar-U** (Upjohn)		In vials.
Rx	**Cytarabine** (Quad)	**Powder for Injection**[1]: 1 g	In 30 ml vials.
Rx	**Cytosar-U** (Upjohn)		In vials.
Rx	**Cytosar-U** (Upjohn)	**Powder for Injection**[1]: 2 g	In vials.

[1] Supplied with ampul of Bacteriostatic Water for Injection with benzyl alcohol.

MERCAPTOPURINE (6-Mercaptopurine; 6-MP)

Actions:

Pharmacology: Mercaptopurine (6-MP) competes with hypoxanthine and guanine for the enzyme hypoxanthine-guanine phosphoribosyltransferase and is converted to thioinosinic acid (TIMP). This intracellular nucleotide inhibits several reactions involving inosinic acid (IMP). In addition, 6-methylthioinosinate (MTIMP) is formed by the methylation of TIMP. Both TIMP and MTIMP inhibit de novo purine ribonucleotide synthesis. Radiolabeled 6-MP may be recovered from deoxyribonucleic acid (DNA) in the form of deoxythioguanosine. Some mercaptopurine is converted to nucleotide derivatives of 6-thioguanine.

Animal tumors resistant to mercaptopurine often have lost the ability to convert mercaptopurine to TIMP. Resistance may be acquired by other means as well, particularly in human leukemias. It is not known which biochemical effects of mercaptopurine and its metabolites are directly or predominantly responsible for cell death.

Pharmacokinetics:

Absorption/Distribution – The absorption of oral mercaptopurine is incomplete and variable, averaging 50%. Recent reports using a more sensitive assay indicate bioavailability may be less (range from 5% to 37%). There is negligible entry of mercaptopurine into cerebrospinal fluid. Plasma protein binding averages 19% over the concentration range 10 to 50 mcg/ml.

Metabolism/Excretion – There are two major pathways for hepatic drug metabolism: Methylation of the sulfhydryl group and oxidation by the enzyme xanthine oxidase. Allopurinol inhibits xanthine oxidase and retards catabolism of mercaptopurine and its active metabolites. Plasma half-life averages 21 and 47 minutes in children and adults, respectively. Metabolites appear in urine within 2 hours. After 24 hours, > 50% of a dose is recovered in urine as intact drug and metabolites.

Indications:

For remission induction and maintenance therapy of acute lymphatic leukemia. Response to mercaptopurine depends upon the subclassification of acute lymphatic leukemia and age of patient (child or adult).

Acute lymphatic (lymphocytic, lymphoblastic) leukemia (ALL): Given as a single agent, mercaptopurine induces complete remission in ≈ 25% of children and 10% of adults. Reliance upon mercaptopurine alone is not justified for initial remission induction of ALL since combination chemotherapy with vincristine, prednisone and L-asparaginase more frequently induces complete remission induction than mercaptopurine alone or in combination. The induced complete remission in acute lymphatic leukemia is so brief without use of maintenance therapy that some form of drug therapy is considered essential. Mercaptopurine, as a single agent, can significantly prolong complete remission duration; however, combination therapy has produced remission longer than mercaptopurine alone.

Acute myelogenous (and acute myelomonocytic) leukemia: As a single agent, mercaptopurine will induce complete remission in approximately 10% of children and adults. These results are inferior to those achieved with combination chemotherapy.

Contraindications:

Prior resistance to this drug. There is usually complete cross-resistance between mercaptopurine and thioguanine.

Mercaptopurine is not effective for prophylaxis or treatment of CNS leukemia, chronic lymphatic leukemia, the lymphomas (including Hodgkin's disease) or solid tumors.

Warnings:

Bone marrow toxicity: The most consistent dose-related toxicity is bone marrow suppression. It may be manifested by anemia, leukopenia or thrombocytopenia. This may also indicate progression of the underlying disease. Patients should report any fever, sore throat, signs of local infection, bleeding from any site or symptoms suggestive of anemia. Since mercaptopurine may have a delayed effect, withdraw medication temporarily at the first sign of an abnormally large fall in any formed blood elements. Toxic effects are often unavoidable during the induction phase of adult acute leukemia if remission induction is to be successful. Whether these effects demand modifying or ceasing dosage depends upon both the response of the underlying disease and availability of supportive facilities. Life-threatening infections and bleeding have occurred as a result of granulocytopenia and thrombocytopenia. Supportive therapy with platelet transfusions for bleeding, and antibiotics and granulocyte transfusions for sepsis, may be required.

The induction of complete remission of acute lymphatic leukemia frequently is associated with marrow hypoplasia. Maintenance of remission generally involves multiple drug regimens whose component agents cause myelosuppression. Anemia, leukopenia and thrombocytopenia are frequently observed. Dosages and schedules are adjusted to prevent life-threatening cytopenias.

MERCAPTOPURINE (6-Mercaptopurine; 6-MP)

If it is not the intent to induce bone marrow hypoplasia, discontinue the drug temporarily at the first evidence of any abnormally large fall in white blood cell (WBC) count, platelet count or hemoglobin concentration. With severe depression of the formed elements of the blood due to mercaptopurine, the bone marrow may appear hypoplastic or normocellular on aspiration or biopsy.

Evaluate hemoglobin or hematocrit, total WBC, differential counts and platelet counts weekly during therapy. Where the cause of fluctuation in the formed elements in the peripheral blood is obscure, bone marrow examination may help evaluate marrow status. Base the decision to continue mercaptopurine on the absolute hematologic values and the rate at which changes occur in these values, particularly during the induction phase of acute leukemia. Perform complete blood counts more frequently than once a week to evaluate therapeutic effect. Dosage may need to be reduced when combined with other drugs whose primary or secondary toxicity is myelosuppression.

Hepatotoxicity occurs with greatest frequency when doses of 2.5 mg/kg/day are exceeded. Deaths have occurred from hepatic necrosis. The histologic pattern includes both intrahepatic cholestasis and parenchymal cell necrosis, either of which may predominate. It is not clear how much hepatic damage is due to direct toxicity from the drug and how much may be due to a hypersensitivity reaction.

Published reports cite widely varying incidences of overt hepatotoxicity. In patients with various neoplastic diseases, mercaptopurine was given orally in doses ranging from 2.5 to 5 mg/kg without any hepatotoxicity. No definite clinical evidence of liver damage could be ascribed to the drug, although an occasional case of serum hepatitis occurred in patients receiving 6-MP who previously had transfusions. In smaller cohorts of adult and pediatric leukemic patients, the incidence of hepatotoxicity ranged from 0% to 6%. In one report, jaundice occurred more frequently (40%), especially when doses exceeded 2.5 mg/kg.

Usually, clinically detectable jaundice appears early in treatment (1 to 2 months), but has occurred from 1 week to 8 years after the start of treatment. In some patients, jaundice cleared following drug withdrawal and reappeared with reintroduction.

Monitoring of serum transaminase, alkaline phosphatase and bilirubin levels may allow early detection of hepatotoxicity. Monitor weekly when beginning therapy and monthly thereafter. More frequent liver function tests may be advisable in patients receiving other hepatotoxic drugs or with known preexisting liver disease. Approach all combination therapy involving mercaptopurine with caution. Use of mercaptopurine with doxorubicin was hepatotoxic in 19 of 20 patients undergoing remission induction therapy for leukemia resistant to previous therapy.

Hepatotoxicity has been associated with anorexia, jaundice, diarrhea and ascites. Hepatic encephalopathy has occurred. The onset of clinical jaundice, hepatomegaly or anorexia with tenderness in the right hypochondrium are immediate indications for withholding mercaptopurine until the exact etiology can be identified. Upon any evidence of deterioration in liver function, toxic hepatitis or biliary stasis, promptly discontinue drug and search for an etiology of hepatotoxicity.

Immunosuppression may be manifested by decreased cellular hypersensitivities and impaired allograft rejection. Immunity to infectious agents or vaccines will be subnormal. The degree of immunosuppression depends on antigen dose and temporal relationship to drug. Carefully consider with regard to intercurrent infections and risk of subsequent neoplasia.

Renal function impairment: Start with smaller doses due to the possibility of slower drug elimination and a greater cumulative effect.

Carcinogenesis/Mutagenesis: Mercaptopurine causes chromosomal aberrations in humans. Carcinogenic potential exists in humans, but risk is unknown.

Pregnancy: Category D. Mercaptopurine can cause fetal harm when administered to a pregnant woman. Women receiving the drug in the first trimester of pregnancy have an increased incidence of abortion; the risk of malformation in offspring surviving first trimester exposure is not known. In a series of 28 women receiving mercaptopurine after the first trimester, three mothers died undelivered, one delivered a stillborn child and one aborted; there were no cases of macroscopically abnormal fetuses. Use during pregnancy, especially the first trimester, only if the benefit justifies the risk to the fetus. The drug's effect on fertility is unknown. There are no adequate and well controlled studies in pregnant women. Inform patient of potential hazard to the fetus. Advise women of childbearing potential to avoid pregnancy.

Lactation: It is not known whether mercaptopurine is excreted in breast milk. Because of potential for serious adverse reactions in nursing infants, decide whether to discontinue nursing or the drug, taking into account the drug's importance to the mother.

MERCAPTOPURINE (6-Mercaptopurine; 6-MP)

Precautions:

Pancreatitis: An increased risk of pancreatitis may be associated with the investigational use of mercaptopurine in inflammatory bowel disease.

Drug Interactions:

Allopurinol: When administered concomitantly with mercaptopurine, reduce mercaptopurine to ⅓ to ¼ the usual dose. Failure to observe this dosage reduction will delay catabolism of mercaptopurine and increase likelihood of severe toxicity.

Trimethoprim-sulfamethoxazole: When coadministered with mercaptopurine, enhanced marrow suppression has occurred.

Adverse Reactions:

Bone marrow toxicity and hepatotoxicity: See Warnings.

Oral lesions are rare and resemble thrush rather than antifolic ulcerations.

Hyperuricemia occurs as a consequence of rapid cell lysis accompanying the antineoplastic effect. Minimize adverse effects by increasing hydration, urine alkalinization and the prophylactic administration of allopurinol (see Drug Interactions).

Drug fever has occurred rarely with mercaptopurine. Exclude the more common causes of pyrexia, such as sepsis, in patients with acute leukemia.

GI: GI ulceration has occurred. Nausea, vomiting and anorexia are uncommon during initial administration. Mild diarrhea and sprue-like symptoms have been noted, but it is difficult to attribute these to the medication.

Dermatologic: Dermatologic reactions can occur as a consequence of disease; however, mercaptopurine may cause skin rashes and hyperpigmentation.

Overdosage:

Discontinue the drug immediately when toxicity develops. If a patient is seen immediately following overdosage of the drug, induced emesis may be useful.

Signs and symptoms of overdosage may be immediate (anorexia, nausea, vomiting, diarrhea) or delayed (myelosuppression, liver dysfunction and gastroenteritis). Dialysis cannot be expected to clear mercaptopurine. Hemodialysis is of marginal use due to the rapid intracellular incorporation of mercaptopurine into active metabolites with long persistence. There is no known pharmacologic antagonist.

Patient Information:

Contraceptive measures are recommended during therapy for men and women.

Notify physician if fever, sore throat, chills, nausea, vomiting, unusual bleeding or bruising, yellow discoloration of the skin or eyes, abdominal pain, flank or joint pain, swelling of the feet or legs, or symptoms suggestive of anemia occurs.

May cause diarrhea, fever and weakness; notify physician if these become pronounced.

Maintain adequate fluid intake.

Administration and Dosage:

Induction therapy: Individualize dosage.

Usual initial dose is 2.5 mg/kg/day (100 to 200 mg in the average adult and 50 mg in an average 5-year-old). Children with acute leukemia tolerate this dose without difficulty in most cases. Continue daily for several weeks or more. If, after 4 weeks on this dosage there is no clinical improvement and no definite evidence of leukocyte or platelet depression, increase dosage up to 5 mg/kg/day.

A dosage of 2.5 mg/kg/day may result in a rapid fall in leukocyte count within 1 to 2 weeks in some adults with ALL and high total leukocyte counts.

Daily dosage may be given at one time. Calculate to the closest multiple of 25 mg.

Monitor the leukocyte count closely; because the drug may have a delayed action, discontinue treatment at the first sign of an abnormally large or rapid fall in leukocyte count or platelet count. If the leukocyte count or platelet count subsequently remains constant for 2 or 3 days, or rises, resume treatment.

Maintenance therapy: If complete hematologic remission is obtained with mercaptopurine alone or in combination with other agents, maintenance therapy is essential. Maintenance doses vary from patient to patient. Usual daily dose - 1.5 to 2.5 mg/kg/day as a single dose. In children with acute lymphatic leukemia in remission, superior results have been obtained when mercaptopurine has been combined with other agents (most frequently with methotrexate) for remission maintenance. Mercaptopurine should rarely be relied upon as a single agent for maintenance of remissions induced in acute leukemia.

Rx	**Purinethol** (Glaxo Wellcome)	**Tablets** : 50 mg	(Purinethol O4A). Off-white, scored. In 25s and 250s.

THIOGUANINE (TG; 6-Thioguanine)

Actions:

Pharmacology: Thioguanine, an analog of the nucleic acid constituent guanine, is closely related structurally and functionally to 6-mercaptopurine.

Thioguanine competes with hypoxanthine and guanine for the enzyme hypoxanthine-guanine phosphoribosyltransferase (HGPRTase) and is converted to 6-thioguanylic acid (TGMP). TGMP interferes at several points with the synthesis of guanine nucleotides. It inhibits de novo purine biosynthesis by inhibiting glutamine-5-phosphoribosylpyrophosphate amidotransferase. Thioguanine nucleotides are incorporated into both RNA and DNA by phosphodiester linkages and incorporation of such fraudulent bases may contribute to the cytotoxicity of thioguanine.

Thioguanine has multiple metabolic effects. Its tumor inhibitory properties may be due to one or more of its effects on feedback inhibition of *de novo* purine synthesis; inhibition of purine nucleotide interconversions; incorporation into DNA and RNA. The net consequence of its actions is a sequential blockade of the synthesis and utilization of the purine nucleotides.

Resistance may result from the loss of HGPRTase activity (inability to convert thioguanine to TGMP) or increased catabolism of TGMP by a nonspecific phosphatase. Although variable, cross-resistance with mercaptopurine usually occurs.

Pharmacokinetics: Oral absorption averages 30% (14% to 46%). Following oral administration of ^{35}S-6-thioguanine, total plasma radioactivity reached a maximum at 8 hours and declined slowly thereafter.

Intravenous administration of ^{35}S-6-thioguanine disclosed a median plasma half-life of 80 minutes (25 to 240 minutes) when the compound was given in single doses of 65 to 300 mg/m^2. There was no correlation between the plasma half-life and the dose. Thioguanine does not appear to reach therapeutic concentrations in the CSF.

The catabolism of thioguanine and its metabolites is complex. Only trace quantities of parent drug are excreted in the urine. However, a methylated metabolite unaffected by allopurinol, MTG, appeared very early, rose to a maximum 6 to 8 hours after drug administration, and was still being excreted after 12 to 22 hours. Radiolabeled sulfate appeared somewhat later than MTG, but was the principal metabolite after 8 hours. Thiouric acid and some unidentified products were found in the urine in small amounts.

Indications:

Acute nonlymphocytic leukemias: Remission induction, consolidation and maintenance therapy of acute nonlymphocytic leukemias. Response depends upon the age of the patient (younger patients faring better than older) and previous treatment. Reliance upon thioguanine alone is seldom justified for initial remission induction of acute nonlymphocytic leukemias because combination chemotherapy including thioguanine results in more frequent remission induction and longer duration of remission than thioguanine alone.

Other neoplasms: Thioguanine is not effective in chronic lymphocytic leukemia, Hodgkin's lymphoma, multiple myeloma or solid tumors. Although thioguanine is one of several agents with activity in the treatment of the chronic phase of chronic myelogenous leukemia, more objective responses are observed with busulfan; therefore busulfan is usually regarded as the preferred drug.

Contraindications:

Prior resistance to this drug. There is usually complete cross-resistance between mercaptopurine and thioguanine.

Warnings:

Bone marrow suppression may be manifested by anemia, leukopenia or thrombocytopenia. Any of these may also reflect progression of the underlying disease. Instruct patients to report promptly any fever, sore throat, jaundice, nausea, vomiting, signs of local infection, bleeding from any site or symptoms suggestive of anemia. Since thioguanine may have a delayed effect, withdraw the medication temporarily at the first sign of an abnormally large fall in any of the formed elements of the blood.

THIOGUANINE (TG; 6-Thioguanine)

Evaluate hemoglobin concentration or hematocrit, total white blood cell (WBC) and differential counts and quantitative platelet count frequently during therapy. Where the cause of fluctuation in the formed elements in the peripheral blood is obscure, bone marrow examination may help evaluate marrow status. Base the decision to change thioguanine dosage on the absolute and rate of change of hematologic values. During the induction phase of acute leukemia, perform CBCs more frequently to evaluate therapeutic effect. The thioguanine dosage may need to be reduced when combined with other myelosuppressive drugs.

Myelosuppression is often unavoidable during the induction phase of adult acute leukemia if remission response is to be successful. Whether this demands modification or cessation of dosage depends upon both the response of the underlying disease and availability of supportive facilities. Life-threatening infections and bleeding have occurred as a result of thioguanine-induced granulocytopenia and thrombocytopenia.

Carcinogenesis: Thioguanine is potentially mutagenic and carcinogenic; consider risk of carcinogenesis when administering thioguanine.

Pregnancy: Category D. Drugs such as thioguanine are potential mutagens and teratogens. Thioguanine may cause fetal harm when administered to a pregnant woman. Thioguanine is teratogenic in rats at doses 5 times the human dose. When given to the rat on the 4th and 5th days of gestation, 13% of surviving placentas did not contain fetuses; 19% of offspring were malformed or stunted. Malformations included generalized edema, cranial defects and general skeletal hypoplasia, hydrocephalus, ventral hernia, situs inversus and incomplete limb development. There are no adequate and well controlled studies in pregnant women. Inform patient of the potential hazard to the fetus. Advise women of childbearing potential to avoid becoming pregnant.

Lactation: It is not known whether this drug is excreted in breast milk. Because of the potential for tumorigenicity, decide whether to discontinue nursing or to discontinue the drug, taking into account the importance of the drug to the mother.

Precautions:

Although the primary toxicity of thioguanine is myelosuppresion, other toxicities occasionally occur, particularly when thioguanine is used in combination with other cancer chemotherapeutic agents.

Hepatotoxicity: Jaundice has occurred. Among these were two adult males and four children with acute myelogenous leukemia, and an adult male with acute lymphocytic leukemia who developed veno-occlusive hepatic disease while receiving chemotherapy. Six patients had received cytarabine prior to treatment with thioguanine, and some were receiving other chemotherapy in addition to thioguanine when they became symptomatic. Withhold thioguanine if there is evidence of toxic hepatitis, biliary stasis, clinical jaundice, hepatomegaly or anorexia with tenderness in the right hypochondrium. Initiate appropriate clinical and laboratory investigations to establish the etiology of the hepatic dysfunction.

Monitor liver function tests (serum transaminases, alkaline phosphatase, bilirubin) at weekly intervals when first beginning therapy and at monthly intervals thereafter. More frequent liver function tests may be advisable in patients with preexisting liver disease or who are receiving other hepatotoxic drugs. Instruct patients to discontinue thioguanine immediately if clinical jaundice is detected. If deterioration in liver function studies during thioguanine therapy occurs promptly discontinue treatment and search for an explanation of the hepatotoxicity.

Adverse Reactions:

Bone marrow toxicity and hepatotoxicity: See Warnings and Precautions.

Myelosuppression is the most frequent adverse reaction to thioguanine. Induction of complete remission of acute myelogenous leukemia usually requires combination chemotherapy in dosages which produce marrow hypoplasia. Since consolidation and maintenance of remission are also affected by multiple drug regimens whose component agents cause myelosuppression, pancytopenia is observed in nearly all patients.

GI: Nausea, vomiting, anorexia and stomatitis may occur. Intestinal necrosis and perforation have also occurred in patients who received multiple drug chemotherapy including thioguanine.

Renal:

Hyperuricemia frequently occurs as a consequence of rapid cell lysis accompanying the antineoplastic effect. Minimize adverse effects by increasing hydration, urine alkalinization and the prophylactic administration of allopurinol. Unlike mercaptopurine and azathioprine, continue thioguanine in the usual dosage when allopurinol is used concurrently to inhibit uric acid formation.

THIOGUANINE (TG; 6-Thioguanine)

Overdosage:

Discontinue immediately if unintended toxicity occurs during treatment. Severe hematologic toxicity may require supportive therapy with platelet transfusions for bleeding, and granulocyte transfusions and antibiotics if sepsis is documented.

If a patient is seen immediately following an acute overdosage, induced emesis may be useful. Signs and symptoms of overdosage may be immediate (nausea, vomiting, malaise, hypertension, diaphoresis) or delayed (myelosuppression and azotemia). Hemodialysis is of marginal use due to the rapid intracellular incorporation of active thioguanine metabolites with long persistence. Symptoms of overdosage may occur after a single dose of as little as 2 to 3 mg/kg thioguanine. As much as 35 mg/kg has been given in a single oral dose with reversible myelosuppression observed. There is no known pharmacologic antagonist of thioguanine.

Patient Information:

Notify physician if fever, chills, nausea, vomiting, sore throat, unusual bleeding or bruising, yellow discoloration of the skin or eyes, swelling of the feet or legs, or abdominal pain or joint or flank pain occurs.

May cause diarrhea, fever and weakness. Notify physician if these become pronounced.

Drink plenty of liquids while taking this drug.

Contraceptive measures are recommended during therapy for men and women.

Administration and Dosage:

Individualize dosage.

Initial dosage for children and adults: 2 mg/kg/day orally. If after 4 weeks, there is no clinical improvement and no leukocyte or platelet depression, the dosage may be cautiously increased to 3 mg/kg/day. The total daily dose may be given at one time.

Combination therapy: Of 163 children with previously untreated acute nonlymphocytic leukemia, 96 (59%) obtained complete remission with a multiple-drug protocol including thioguanine, prednisone, cytarabine, cyclophosphamide and vincristine. Remission was maintained with daily thioguanine, 4 day pulses of cytarabine and cyclophosphamide, and a single dose of vincristine every 28 days. The median duration of remission was 11.5 months. Of previously untreated adults with acute nonlymphocytic leukemias, 53% attained remission following use of the combination of thioguanine and cytarabine. A median duration of remission of 8.8 months was achieved with the multiple-drug maintenance which included thioguanine.

Concomitant therapy: In contrast to mercaptopurine or azathioprine, the dosage of thioguanine does not need to be reduced during coadministration of allopurinol. See Adverse Reactions.

Rx	**Thioguanine** (Glaxo Wellcome)	**Tablets:** 40 mg	(Wellcome U3B). Greenish-yellow, scored. In 25s.

FLUDARABINE PHOSPHATE

> **Warning:**
> Administer fludarabine under the supervision of a qualified physician experienced in the use of antineoplastic therapy. Fludarabine can severely suppress bone marrow function. When used at high doses in dose-ranging studies in patients with acute leukemia, fludarabine was associated with severe neurologic effects, including blindness, coma and death. This severe CNS toxicity occurred in 36% of patients treated with doses approximately four times greater (96 mg/m^2 /day for 5 to 7 days) than the recommended dose. Similar severe CNS toxicity has rarely occurred (≤ 0.2%) in patients treated at doses in the range of the dose recommended for chronic lymphocytic leukemia.

Actions:

Pharmacology: Fludarabine is a fluorinated nucleotide analog of the antiviral agent vidarabine that is relatively resistant to deamination by adenosine deaminase. Fludarabine is rapidly dephosphorylated to 2-fluoro-ara-A and then phosphorylated intracellularly by deoxycytidine kinase to the active triphosphate, 2-fluoro-ara-ATP. This metabolite appears to act by inhibiting DNA polymerase alpha, ribonucleotide reductase and DNA primase, thus inhibiting DNA synthesis. The mechanism of action of this antimetabolite is not completely characterized and may be multi-faceted.

Pharmacokinetics: Fludarabine is rapidly converted to the active metabolite, 2-fluoro-ara-A, within minutes after IV infusion. Consequently, clinical pharmacology studies have focused on 2-fluoro-ara-A pharmacokinetics. In a study with 4 patients treated with 25 mg/m^2 /day for 5 days, the half-life of 2-fluoro-ara-A was ≈ 10 hours. The mean total plasma clearance was 8.9 L/hr/m^2 and the mean volume of distribution was 98 L/m^2 . Approximately 23% of the dose was excreted in the urine as unchanged 2-fluoro-ara-A. The mean maximum concentration after the day 1 dose was 0.57 mcg/ml and after the day 5 dose was 0.54 mcg/ml. Total body clearance of 2-fluoro-ara-A is inversely correlated with serum creatinine, suggesting renal elimination of the compound. A correlation was noted between the degree of absolute granulocyte count nadir and increased area under the concentration-time curve (AUC).

Clinical trials: Two single-arm open-label studies have been conducted in patients with chronic lymphocytic leukemia (CLL) refractory to at least one prior standard alkylating agent-containing regimen.

Fludarabine Efficacy in Refractory CLL Patients

Parameter	Studies	
	MDAH[1] (n = 48)	SWOG[2] (n = 31)
Overall objective response	48%	32%
Complete response	13%	13%
Partial response	35%	19%
Median time to response	7 weeks (range, 1 to 68)	21 weeks (range, 1 to 53)
Median duration of disease control	91 weeks	65 weeks
Median survival	43 weeks	52 weeks

[1] M.D. Anderson Cancer Center. Dosage: 22 to 40 mg/m^2 /day for 5 days every 28 days.

[2] Southwest Oncology Group. Dosage: 15 to 25 mg/m^2 /day for 5 days every 28 days.

The ability of fludarabine to induce a significant rate of response in refractory patients suggests minimal cross-resistance with commonly used anti-CLL agents.

Rai stage improved to Stage II or better in 7 of 12 MDAH responders (58%) and in 5 of 7 SWOG responders (71%) who were Stage III or IV at baseline. In the combined studies, mean hemoglobin concentration improved from 9 g/dl at baseline to 11.8 g/dl at the time of response in a subgroup of anemic patients. Similarly, average platelet count improved from 63,500/mm^3 to 103,300/mm^3 at the time of response in a subgroup of patients who were thrombocytopenic at baseline.

FLUDARABINE PHOSPHATE

Indications:

Chronic lymphocytic leukemia (CLL): Treatment of patients with B-cell CLL who have not reponded to or have progressed during treatment with at least one standard alkylating agent-containing regimen.

The safety and efficacy in previously untreated or non-refractory patients with CLL have not been established.

Unlabeled uses: Fludarabine may also be useful in the treatment of non-Hodgkin's lymphoma, macroglobulinemic lymphoma, prolymphocytic leukemia or prolymphocytoid variant of CLL, mycosis fungoides, hairy-cell leukemia and Hodgkin's disease. Further study is needed to determine efficacy and dosage.

Contraindications:

Hypersensitivity to this drug or its components.

Warnings:

Dose-dependent toxicity (see boxed Warning): There are clear dose-dependent toxic effects seen with fludarabine. Dose levels ≈ 4 times greater (96 mg/m^2 /day for 5 to 7 days) than those recommended for CLL (25 mg/m^2 /day for 5 days) were associated with a syndrome characterized by delayed blindness, coma and death. Symptoms appeared from 21 to 60 days following the last dose. Thirteen of 36 patients (36%) who received high doses (96 mg/m^2 /day for 5 to 7 days) developed this severe neurotoxicity. This syndrome has been reported rarely in patients treated with doses in the range of the recommended CLL dose of 25 mg/m^2 /day for 5 days every 28 days. The effect of chronic administration on the CNS is unknown; however, patients have received the recommended dose for up to 15 courses of therapy.

Severe bone marrow suppression, notably anemia, thrombocytopenia and neutropenia, has occurred in patients treated with fludarabine. In solid tumor patients, the median time to nadir counts was 13 days (range, 3 to 25 days) for granulocytes and 16 days (range, 2 to 32) for platelets. Most patients had hematologic impairment at baseline either as a result of disease or as a result of prior myelosuppressive therapy. Cumulative myelosuppression may be seen. While chemotherapy-induced myelosuppression is often reversible, administration of fludarabine requires careful hematologic monitoring.

Renal function impairment: Administer cautiously. The total body clearance of 2-fluoro-ara-A is inversely correlated with serum creatinine, suggesting renal elimination of the compound.

Mutagenesis: Chromosomal aberrations were seen in an in vitro assay. Fludarabine was also determined to increase sister chromatid exchanges in vitro.

Fertility impairment: Studies in mice, rats and dogs have demonstrated dose-related adverse effects on the male reproductive system. Observations consisted of a decrease in mean testicular weights in mice and rats with a trend toward decreased testicular weights in dogs and degeneration and necrosis of spermatogenic epithelium of the testes in mice, rats and dogs.

Pregnancy: Category D . Fludarabine may cause fetal harm when administered to a pregnant woman. Fludarabine was teratogenic in rats and rabbits. At 10 and 30 mg/kg/day in rats, there was an increased incidence of various skeletal malformations; dose-related teratogenic effects manifested by external deformities and skeletal malformations were observed in rabbits at 5 and 8 mg/kg/day. There are no adequate and well controlled studies in pregnant women. If fludarabine is used during pregnancy, or if the patient becomes pregnant while taking this drug, apprise her of the potential hazard to the fetus. Advise women of childbearing potential to avoid becoming pregnant.

Lactation: It is not known whether this drug is excreted in breast milk. Decide whether to discontinue nursing or to discontinue the drug, taking into account the importance of the drug to the mother.

Children: Safety and efficacy have not been established.

Precautions:

Monitoring: During treatment, monitor the patient's hematologic profile (particularly neutrophils and platelets) regularly to determine the degree of hematopoietic suppression.

Hematologic toxicity: Fludarabine is a potent antineoplastic with potentially significant toxic side effects. Closely observe patients for signs of hematologic and nonhematologic toxicity. Periodic assessment of peripheral blood counts is recommended to detect the development of anemia, neutropenia and thrombocytopenia.

FLUDARABINE PHOSPHATE

Tumor lysis syndrome associated with fludarabine treatment has occured in CLL patients with large tumor burdens. Since fludarabine can induce a response as early as the first week of treatment, take precautions in patients at risk of developing this complication.

Adverse Reactions:

Fludarabine Adverse Reactions in the MDAH and SWOG Studies (%)

Adverse reaction	MDAH (n = 101)	SWOG (n = 32)	Adverse reaction	MDAH (n = 101)	SWOG (n = 32)
Any adverse reaction	88	91	Esophagitis	3	0
Body as a whole	72	84	Mucositis	2	0
Fever	60	69	Liver failure	1	0
Chills	11	19	Abnormal liver function test	1	3
Fatigue	10	38			
Infection	33	44	Cholelithiasis	0	3
Pain	20	22	Constipation	1	3
Malaise	8	6	Dysphagia	1	0
Diaphoresis	1	13	*Cutaneous*	17	18
Alopecia	0	3	Rash	15	15
Anaphylaxis	1	0	Pruritus	1	3
Hemorrhage	1	0	Seborrhea	1	0
Hyperglycemia	1	6	*GU*	12	22
Dehydration	1	0	Dysuria	4	3
Neurological	21	69	Urinary infection	2	15
Weakness	9	65	Hematuria	2	3
Paresthesia	4	12	Renal failure	1	-
Headache	3	0	Abnormal renal function test	1	0
Visual disturbance	3	15			
Hearing loss	2	6	Proteinuria	1	0
Sleep disorder	1	3	Hesitancy	0	3
Depression	1	0	*Cardiovascular*	12	38
Cerebellar syndrome	1	0	Edema	8	19
			Angina	0	6
Impaired mentation	1	0	CHF	0	3
			Arrhythmia	0	3
Pulmonary	35	69	Supraventricular tachycardia	0	3
Cough	10	44			
Pneumonia	16	22	Myocardial infarction	0	3
Dyspnea	9	22			
Sinusitis	5	0	Deep venous thrombosis	1	3
Pharyngitis	0	9			
Upper resp infection	2	16	Phlebitis	1	3
Allergic pneumonitis	0	6	Transient ischemic attack	1	0
Epistaxis	1	0			
Hemoptysis	1	6	Aneurysm	1	0
Bronchitis	1	0	Cerebrovascular accident	0	3
Hypoxia	1	0			
GI	46	63	*Musculoskeletal*	7	16
Nausea/Vomiting	36	31	Myalgia	4	16
Diarrhea	15	13	Osteoporosis	2	0
Anorexia	7	34	Arthralgia	1	0
Stomatitis	9	0	*Tumor lysis syndrome*	1	0
GI bleeding	3	13			

The most common adverse events include myelosuppression (neutropenia, thrombocytopenia, anemia), fever, chills, infection, nausea and vomiting. Common adverse events also include malaise, fatigue, anorexia, weakness. Serious opportunistic infections occurred in CLL patients treated with fludarabine. Frequently reported, clearly drug-related adverse events appear below.

Hematologic: Hematologic events (neutropenia, thrombocytopenia or anemia) were reported in the majority of CLL patients (see Warnings). During treatment of 133 patients with CLL, the absolute neutrophil count decreased to < 500/mm^3 in 59% of patients, hemoglobin decreased from pretreatment values by at least 2 g% in 60%,

FLUDARABINE PHOSPHATE

and platelet count decreased from pretreatment values by at least 50% in 55% of patients. Myelosuppression may be severe and cumulative. Bone marrow fibrosis occurred in one CLL patient.

Metabolic: Tumor lysis syndrome, which may include hyperuricemia, hyperphosphatemia, hypocalcemia, metabolic acidosis, hyperkalemia, hematuria, urate crystalluria and renal failure. The onset of this syndrome may be heralded by flank pain and hematuria. See Precautions.

CNS: See Warnings. Objective weakness, agitation, confusion, visual disturbances, coma (at the recommended dose); peripheral neuropathy; wrist-drop (one case).

Pulmonary: Pneumonia (16% to 22%; a frequent manifestation of infection in CLL patients); pulmonary hypersensitivity reactions characterized by dyspnea, cough and interstitial pulmonary infiltrate.

GI: Nausea; vomiting; anorexia; diarrhea; stomatitis; GI bleeding.

Cardiovascular: Edema (frequent); pericardial effusion (one patient).

Dermatologic: Skin toxicity, consisting primarily of skin rashes.

Overdosage:

High doses are associated with an irreversible CNS toxicity characterized by delayed blindness, coma and death (see Warnings). High doses are also associated with severe thrombocytopenia and neutropenia due to bone marrow suppression. There is no known specific antidote for fludarabine overdosage. Treatment consists of drug discontinuation and supportive therapy. Refer to General Management of Acute Overdosage.

Administration and Dosage:

Fludarabine was approved by the FDA in April 1991.

Usual dose: 25 mg/m^2 administered IV over a period of ≈ 30 minutes daily for 5 consecutive days. Commence each 5 day course of treatment every 28 days. Dosage may be decreased or delayed based on evidence of hematologic or nonhematologic toxicity. Physicians should consider delaying or discontinuing the drug if neurotoxicity occurs.

A number of clinical settings may predispose to increased toxicity including advanced age, renal insufficiency and bone marrow impairment. Monitor such patients closely for excessive toxicity and modify the dose accordingly.

Duration – The optimal duration of treatment has not been clearly established. It is recommended that three additional cycles be administered following the achievement of a maximal response and then discontinue the drug.

Preparation of solution – When reconstituted with 2 ml of Sterile Water for Injection, USP, the solid cake should fully dissolve in ≤ 15 seconds; each ml of the resulting solution will contain 25 mg fludarabine phosphate, 25 mg mannitol and sodium hydroxide to adjust the pH to 7.7. The pH range for the final product is 7.2 to 8.2. In clinical studies, the product has been diluted in 100 or 125 ml of 5% Dextrose Injection, USP or 0.9% Sodium Chloride, USP. Reconstituted fludarabine contains no antimicrobial preservative; use within 8 hours of reconstitution.

Handling and disposal – Consider procedures for proper handling and disposal according to guidelines issued for cytotoxic drugs. If the solution contacts the skin or mucous membranes, wash thoroughly with soap and water; rinse eyes thoroughly with plain water. Avoid exposure by inhalation or by direct contact of the skin or mucous membranes.

Storage – Store under refrigeration, between 2° to 8°C (36° to 46°F).

Rx	**Fludara** (Berlex)	**Powder for reconstitution (lyophilized)**: 50 mg[1]	In single dose vial (6 ml capacity).

[1] With 50 mg mannitol and sodium hydroxide.

Androgens

TESTOLACTONE

This is an abbreviated monograph. For complete information on Androgens, see the group monograph in the Hormones chapter.

Actions:

Pharmacology: The precise mechanism by which testolactone produces a clinical antineoplastic effect is unknown. Testolactone's principal action appears to be inhibition of steroid aromatase activity and consequent reduction in estrone synthesis from adrenal androstenedione, the major source of estrogen in postmenopausal women. Based on in vitro studies, the aromatase inhibition may be noncompetitive and irreversible. This phenomenon may account for the persistence of testolactone's effect on estrogen synthesis after drug withdrawal.

Testolactone is effective in 15% of patients with advanced or disseminated mammary cancer.

Testolactone is well absorbed from the GI tract. It is metabolized to several derivatives in the liver, all of which preserve the lactone D-ring. These metabolites, as well as some unmetabolized drug, are excreted in the urine. Additional pharmacokinetic data in humans are unavailable.

Indications:

Adjunctive therapy in the palliative treatment of advanced disseminated breast carcinoma in postmenopausal women when hormonal therapy is indicated.

Premenopausal women with disseminated breast carcinoma in whom ovarian function has been subsequently terminated.

Contraindications:

Carcinoma of the male breast; hypersensitivity to the drug.

Warnings:

Pregnancy: Category C. Testolactone is intended for use in postmenopausal women and is not indicated for use during pregnancy.

Lactation: It is not known whether this drug is excreted in breast milk. Decide whether to discontinue nursing or to discontinue the drug, taking into account the importance of the drug to the mother.

Children: Safety and efficacy have not been established.

Precautions:

Monitoring: Routinely monitor plasma calcium levels in any patient receiving therapy for mammary cancer, particularly during periods of active remission of bony metastases. If hypercalcemia occurs, institute appropriate measures.

The usual precautions pertaining to use of androgens apply (see the Androgen group monograph in the Hormones chapter).

Consult the physician regarding missed doses.

Drug Interactions:

Anticoagulants, oral: Pharmacologic effects may be increased by testolactone; monitor and adjust the anticoagulant dose accordingly.

Drug/Lab test interactions: Physiologic effects of testolactone may result in decreased estradiol concentrations with radioimmunoassays for estradiol, increased plasma calcium concentrations and increased 24 hour urinary excretion of creatine and 17-ketosteroids.

Adverse Reactions:

GI: Glossitis; anorexia; nausea; vomiting.

CNS: Paresthesia.

Miscellaneous: Maculopapular erythema; aches and edema of the extremities; alopecia; nail growth disturbances (rare); increase in blood pressure.

Patient Information:

Notify physician if numbness or tingling of fingers, toes or face occurs.

Contraceptive measures are recommended during treatment.

Medication may cause diarrhea, loss of appetite, nausea, vomiting, loss of hair, swelling or redness of the tongue; notify physician if these become pronounced.

Administration and Dosage:

Administer 250 mg 4 times daily. To evaluate response, continue therapy for a minimum of 3 months, unless there is active disease progression.

c-III	**Teslac** (Bristol Myers)	**Tablets:** 50 mg	Lactose. (690). White. Round, biconvex. In 100s.

BICALUTAMIDE

Actions:

Pharmacology: Bicalutamide is a nonsteroidal antiandrogen. it competitively inhibits the action of androgens by binding to cytosol androgen receptors in the target tissue. Protastic carcinoma is known to be androgen sensitive and responds to treatment that counteracts the effect of androgen or removes the source of androgen.

In clinical trials with bicalutamide as a single agent for prostate cancer, rises in serum testosterone and estradiol have been noted. When bicalutamide is combined with luteinizing hormone-releasing hormone (LHRH) analog therapy, bicalutamide does not affect the suppression of serum testosterone induced by the LHRH analog.

Pharmacokinetics:

Absorption – Bicalutamide is well absorbed following oral administration, although the absolute bioavailability is unknown. Coadministration with food has no clinically significant effect on rate or extent of absorption.

Metabolism/Excretion – Bicalutamide undergoes stereospecific metabolism. The S-(inactive) isomer is metabolized primarily by glucuronidation. The R-(active) isomer also undergoes glucuronidation but is predominantly oxidized to an inactive metabolite followed by glucuronidation. Both the parent and metabolite glucuronides are eliminated in the urine and feces. The S-enantiomer is rapidly cleared relative to the R-enantiomer, with the R-enantiomer accounting for ≈ 99% of toal steady-state plasma levels. In healthy males, apparent oral clearance of the active enantiomer is 0.32 L/hr, peak concentration (single-dose) is 0.77 mcg/ml, time to peak concentration (single-dose) is 31.3 hours and half-life is 5.8 days. Mean steady-state concentration of the active enantiomer in patients with prostate cancer is 8.9 mcg/ml.

Clinical trials: In a large multicenter, double-blind, controlled clinical trial, 813 patients with previously untreated prostate cancer were randomized to receive bicalutamide 50 mg once daily (404 patients) or flutamide 250 mg (409 patients) three times a day, each in combination with LHRH analogs (either goserelin acetate implant or leuprolide acetate depot). At a meadian follow-up of 95 weeks, time to treament failure with bicalutamide-LHRH analog therapy was not dissimilar when compared with flutamide-LHRH analog therpay. At the same timepoint, 130 (32%) patients treated with bicalutamide-LHRH analog therapy and 145 (35%) patients treated with flutamide-LHRH analog therapy had died.

Indications:

Prostate cancer: For use in combination therapy with a luteinizing hormone-releasing hormone (LHRH) analog for the treatment of advanced prostate cancer.

Contraindications:

Hypersensitivity to the drug or any of the components of the product; pregnancy (see Warnings).

Warnings:

Gynecomastia/Breast pain: In clinical trails with bicalutamide as a single agent for prostate cancer, gynecomastia and breast pain were reported in up to 38% and 39% of patients, respectively.

Renal function impairment: Renal impairment (as measured by creatinine clearance) had no significant effect on the elimination of total bicalutamide or the active R-enantiomer. No dosage adjustment is necessary.

Hepatic function impairment: No clinically significant difference in the pharmacokinetics of either enantiomer of bicalutamide was noted in patients with mild-to-moderate hepatic disease as compared with healthy controls. Patients with severe liver disease have significantly longer half-life values for the R-enantiomer. Bicalutamide is extensively metabolized by the liver. Limited data in subjects with severe hepatic impairment suggest that excretion of bicalutamide may be delayed and could lead to further accumulation. Consider periodic liver function tests for patients on long-term therapy. Use with caution in patients with moderate-to-severe hepatic impairment.

Carcinogenesis/Fertility impairment: Two-year oral carcinogenicity studies were conducted in both male and female rats and mice. A variety of tumor target organ effects were identified and were attributed to the antiandrogenicity of bicalutamide, namely, testicular benign interstitial (Leydig) cell tumors in male rats and uterine adenocarcinoma in female rats. There is no evidence of Leydig cell hyperplasia in humans; uterine tumors are not releveant to the indicated patient population. A small increase in the incidence of hepatocellular carcinoma in male mice and an increased incidence of benign thyroid follicular cell adenomas in rats were recorded.

Antiandrogens

BICALUTAMIDE

Administration of bicalutamide may lead to inhibition o f spermatogenesis. In male rats the precoital interval and time to successful mating were increased in the first pairing, but no effects on fertility following successful mating were seen. These effects were reversed by 7 weeks after the end of an 11–week period of dosing. Administration of bicalutamide to pregnant females resulted in feminization of the male offspring, leading to hypospadias at all dose levels. Affected male offspring were also impotent.

Elderly: In two studies in patients given 50 or 150 mg daily, no significant relationship between age and steady-state levels of total bicalutamide or the active R-enantiomer has been shown.

Pregnancy: Category X. Bicalutamide may cause fetal harm when administered to pregnant women. The male offspring of rats receiving doses of ≥ 10 mg/kg/day (plasma drug concentrations in rats equal to ≈ ⅔ human therapeutic concentrations) were observed to have reduced anogenital distance and hypospdias in reproductive toxicology studies. These pharmacological effects have been observed with other antiandrogens. Bicalutamide is contraindicated in women who are or may become pregnant. If this drug is used during pregnancy, or if the patient becomes pregnant while taking this drug, apprise the patient of the potential hazard to the fetus.

Lactation: It is not known whether this drug is excreted in breast milk. Exercise caution when administering to a nursing woman.

Children: Safety and efficacy in children have not been established. Because of the mechanism of action and the indication, bicalutamide has not been studied in women or pediatric subjects.

Precautions:

Monitoring: Regular assessments of serum Prostate Specific Antigen (PSA) may be helpful in monitoring the patient's response. If PSA levels rise during therapy, evaluate the patient for clinical progression. For patients who have objective progression of disease together with an elevated PSA, consider a treatment-free period of antiandrogens whlie continuing the LHRH analog.

Because transaminase abnormalities and rarely, jaundice have been reported with the use of bicalutamide, consider periodic liver function tests. If clinically indicated (eg, when the patient has jaundice or laboratory evidence of liver injury in the absence of live metastases), discontinue therapy. If transaminases increase over 2 times the upper limit of normal, discontinue treatment. Abnormalities are usually reversible upon discontinuation.

Drug Interactions:

Anticoagulants: In vitro bicalutamide can displace coumarin anticoagulants (eg, warfarin), from their protein-binding sites. It is recommended that if bicalutamide is started in patients already receiving coumarin anticoagulants, closely monitor prothrombin times and adjust the anticoagulant dose if necessary.

Adverse Reactions:

In patients with advanced prostate cancer treated with bicalutamide in combination with an LHRH analog, the most frequent adverse reaction was hot flashes (49%). Diarrhea was the adverse event most frequently leading to treatment withdrawal: 6% with flutamide-LHRH analog and 0.5% with bicalutamide-LHRH analog.

BICALUTAMIDE

Adverse Reactions: Bicalutamide vs Flutamide (%)

Adverse reactions	Bicalutamide plus LHRH analog (n = 401)	Flutamide plus LHRH analog (n = 407)	Adverse reactions	Bicalutamide plus LHRH analog (n = 401)	Flutamide plus LHRH analog (n = 407)
Body as a whole			*CNS*		
Pain (general)	27	23	Dizziness	7	7
Back pain	15	17	Paresthesia	6	7
Asthenia	15	17	Insomnia	5	7
Pelvic pain	13	11	*Dermatologic*		
Abdominal pain	8	8	Rash	6	5
Chest pain	6	5	Sweating	6	4
Flu syndrome	4	5	*GU*		
Cardiovascular			Nocturia	9	11
Hot flashes	49	50	Hematuria	7	5
Hypertension	5	4	Urinary tract infection	6	6
GI			Impotence	5	7
Constipation	17	12	Gynecomastia	5	6
Nausea	11	11	Urinary incontinence	2	5
Diarrhea	10	24	*Miscellaneous*		
Increased liver enzyme test[1]	6	10	Infection	10	9
Vomiting	3	5	Anemia[2]	7	9
Metabolic/Nutritional			Dyspnea	7	6
Peripheral edema	8	7	Bone pain	4	6
Hyperglycemia	5	4	Headache	4	5
Weight loss	4	5			

[1] Increased liver enzyme test includes increases in AST, ALT or both.
[2] Anemia includes anemia, hypochromic and iron deficiency anemia.

Other adverse reactions (≥ 2 to < 5%) reported in the bicalutamide-LHRH analog treatment group are listed below in order of decreasing frequency within each body system.

Body as a whole: Edema; neoplasm; fever; neck pain; chills; sepsis.

Cardiovascular: Angina pectoris; congestive heart failure.

GI: Anorexia; dyspepsia; rectal hemorrhage; dry mouth; melena.

Endocrine: Breast pain; diabetes mellitus.

Metabolic/Nutritional: Alkaline phosphatase increased; weight gain; creatinine increased; dehydration; gout.

Musculoskeletal: Myasthenia; arthritis; myalgia; leg cramps; pathological fracture.

CNS: Anxiety; depression; libido decreased; hypertonia; confusion; neuropathy; somnolence; nervousness.

Respiratory: Cough increased; pharyngitis; bronchitis; pneumonia; rhinitis; lung disorder.

Dermatologic: Dry skin; pruritus; alopecia.

GU: Urinary frequency; urination impaired; dysuria; urinary retention; urinary urgency.

Lab test abnormalities: Elevated AST, ALT, bilirubin, BUN and creatinine and decreased hemoglobin and white cell count have been reported in both bicalutamide-LHRH analog treated and flutamide-LHRH analog treated patients. Increased liver enzyme tests and decreases in hemoglobin were reported less frequently with bicalutamide-LHRH analog therapy.

Overdosage:

Long-term clinical trials have been conducted with dosages of ≤ 200 mg daily, and these dosages have been well tolerated. A single dose of bicalutamide that results in symptoms of an overdose considered life-threatening has not been established. There is no specific antidote.

In the management of an overdose with bicalutamide, vomiting may be induced if the patient is alert. It should be remembered that, in this patient population, multiple drugs may have been taken. Dialysis is not likely to be helpful because bicalutamide

Antiandrogens

BICALUTAMIDE

is highly protein bound and is extensively metabolized. General supportive care, including frequent monitoring of vital signs and close observation of the patient is indicated.

Patient Information:

Inform patients that therapy with bicalutamide and the LHRH analog should be initiated concomitantly (eg, at the same time), and that they should not interrupt or stop taking these medications without consulting their physician.

Administration and Dosage:

Approved by the FDA on October 4, 1995 (1SE classification).

The recommended dose for bicalutamide therapy in combination with an LHRH analog is one 50 mg tablet once daily (morning or evening), with or without food. It is recommended that bicalutamide be taken at the same time each day. Start treatment with bicalutamide at the same time as treatment with an LHRH analog.

Rx	**Casodex** (Zeneca)	**Tablets**: 50 mg	Lactose. (CDX50/Casodex). White. Film-coated. In 30s, 100s and UD 30s.

Antiandrogens

FLUTAMIDE

Actions:

Pharmacology: Flutamide, a nonsteroidal agent, demonstrates potent antiandrogenic effects in animal studies. It exerts its antiandrogenic action by inhibiting androgen uptake or by inhibiting nuclear binding of androgen in target tissues. Prostatic carcinoma is androgen-sensitive and responds to treatment that counteracts the effect of androgen or removes the source of androgen (eg, castration).

Pharmacokinetics: Analysis of plasma, urine and feces following a single oral 200 mg dose of tritium-labeled flutamide to human volunteers showed that the drug is rapidly and completely absorbed. It is excreted mainly in the urine with only 4.2% of the dose excreted in the feces over 72 hours. Flutamide is rapidly and extensively metabolized, with flutamide comprising only 2.5% of plasma radioactivity 1 hour after administration. At least six metabolites have been identified in plasma. The major plasma metabolite is a biologically active alpha-hydroxylated derivative that accounts for 23% of the plasma tritium 1 hour after drug administration.

Following a single 250 mg oral dose to healthy adult volunteers, low plasma levels of varying amounts of flutamide were detected. The biologically active alpha-hydroxylated metabolite reaches maximum plasma levels in about 2 hours, indicating that it is rapidly formed from flutamide. The plasma half-life for this metabolite is about 6 hours.

Following multiple oral dosing of 250 mg 3 times a day in healthy geriatric volunteers, flutamide and its active metabolite approached steady-state plasma levels (based on pharmacokinetic simulations) after the fourth flutamide dose. The half-life of the active metabolite in geriatric volunteers after a single flutamide dose is about 8 hours and at steady state is 9.6 hours.

Flutamide is 94% to 96% bound to plasma proteins at steady-state plasma concentrations of 24 to 78 ng/ml. The active metabolite of flutamide at steady-state plasma concentrations of 1556 to 2284 ng/ml is 92% to 94% bound to plasma proteins.

In male rats, neither flutamide nor any of its metabolites are preferentially accumulated in any tissue except the prostate after an oral 5 mg/kg dose. Total drug levels were highest 6 hours after drug administration in all tissues. Levels declined at roughly similar rates to low levels at 18 hours. The major metabolite was present at higher concentrations than flutamide in all tissues studied.

Elevations of plasma testosterone and estradiol levels have been noted following flutamide administration.

Clinical trials: Flutamide interferes with testosterone at the cellular level. This can complement medical castration achieved with leuprolide, which suppresses testicular androgen production by inhibiting luteinizing hormone secretion.

To study the effects of combination therapy, 617 patients (311 leuprolide= flutamide; 306 leuprolide= placebo) with previously untreated advanced prostatic carcinoma were enrolled in a large multicenter, controlled clinical trial.

Median survival had been reached 3.5 years after the study was initiated. The median actuarial survival time is 34.9 months for patients treated with leuprolide and flutamide versus 27.9 months for patients treated with leuprolide alone (a 25% improvement in overall survival with the flutamide therapy). Analysis of progression-free survival showed a 2.6 month improvement in patients who received leuprolide plus flutamide (a 19% increment over leuprolide and placebo).

Indications:

In combination with LHRH agonistic analogs (such as leuprolide acetate) for the treatment of metastatic prostatic carcinoma (stage D_2). To achieve the benefit of the adjunctive therapy, treatment must be started simultaneously using both drugs.

Contraindications:

Hypersensitivity to flutamide or any component of the preparation.

Antiandrogens

FLUTAMIDE

Warnings:

Carcinogenesis/Fertility impairment: Daily use of flutamide to rats for 52 weeks at doses of 30, 90 or 180 mg/kg/day (≈ 3, 8 or 17 times the human dose) produced testicular interstitial cell adenomas at all doses.

Reduced sperm counts were observed during a 6–week study of flutamide monotherapy in healthy volunteers. Male rats treated with 150 mg/kg/day (30 times the minimum effective antiandrogenic dose) failed to mate; mating behavior returned to normal after dosing was stopped. Conception rates were decreased in all dosing groups. Suppression of spermatogenesis was observed in animals dosed for 52 to 78 weeks at 1.4 to 17 times the human dose.

Pregnancy: Category D. Flutamide may cause fetal harm when administered to a pregnant woman. There was decreased 24–hour survival in the offspring of rats treated with flutamide at doses of 30, 100 or 200 mg/kg/day (≈ 3, 9 and 19 times the human dose) during pregnancy. A slight increase in minor variations in development of the sternebra and vertebra was seen in the fetuses of rats at the two higher doses. Feminization of the males also occurred at the two higher dose levels. There was a decreased survival rate in the offspring of rabbits receiving the highest dose (15 mg/kg/day; equal to 1.4 times the human dose.

Precautions:

Monitoring: Consider periodic liver function tests in patients on long-term treatment because transient abnormalities of transaminases have occurred; however, < 1% of the patients treated with the combination had transaminases > 5 to 10 times the normal values.

Inform patients that flutamide and the drug used for medical castration should be administered concomitantly, and that they should not interrupt their dosing or stop taking these medications without consulting their physician.

Adverse Reactions:

The following occurred during treatment with flutamide in combination with LHRH-agonists: Hot flashes (61%); loss of libido (36%); impotence (33%); diarrhea (12%); nausea/vomiting (11%); gynecomastia (9%); other GI disturbances (6%).

The most frequently occurring adverse experiences (hot flashes, impotence, loss of libido) were those associated with low serum androgen levels and that occur with LHRH-agonists alone. The only notable difference was the higher incidence of diarrhea in the flutamide plus LHRH-agonist group (12%), which was severe in 5% as opposed to the placebo plus LHRH agonist (4%), which was severe in < 1%.

Other reactions:

CNS – Drowsiness, confusion, depression, anxiety, nervousness (1%).

GI – Diarrhea (12%); nausea/vomiting (11%); other GI reactions (6%).

Hematologic – Anemia (6%); leukopenia (3%); thrombocytopenia (1%); hemolytic and macrocytic anemia.

Hepatic – Hepatitis, jaundice (< 1%); cholestatic jaundice; hepatic encephalopathy; hepatic necrosis. These conditions were usually reversible after stopping therapy.

Dermatologic – Injection site irritation, rash (3%); photosensitivity (five patients).

Body as a whole – Gynecomastia (9%); edema, anorexia (4%); neuromuscular, GU symptoms (2%); hypertension (1%); pulmonary symptoms (< 1%).

Lab test abnormalities – Elevated AST, ALT and bilirubin values; elevated creatinine values; elevated alpha-glutamyl transferase values.

Overdosage:

Symptoms: In animals, signs of overdose included: Hypoactivity; piloerection; slow respiration; ataxia; lacrimation; anorexia; tranquilization; emesis.

Clinical trials have been conducted with flutamide in doses up to 1500 mg/day for periods up to 36 weeks with no serious adverse effects reported. Those adverse reactions reported included gynecomastia, breast tenderness and some increases in AST. The single dose of flutamide ordinarily associated with symptoms of overdose or considered to be life-threatening has not been established.

Treatment: Because flutamide is highly protein bound, dialysis may not be of any use. If it does not occur spontaneously, induce vomiting if the patient is alert. Use general supportive care, including frequent monitoring of the vital signs and close observation of the patient. Refer to General Management of Acute Overdosage.

Administration and Dosage:

Two capsules 3 times a day at 8–hour intervals for a total daily dosage of 750 mg.

Rx	**Eulexin** (Schering)	**Capsules:** 125 mg	(Schering 525). Brown. In 100s, 500s and UD 100s.

NILUTAMIDE

Actions:

Pharmacology:

Mechanism of action – Nilutamide is nonsteroidal with antiandrogen activity. In animal studies, nilutamide has demonstrated antiandrogenic activity without other hormonal (estrogen, progesterone, mineralocorticoid and glucocorticoid) effects. In vitro, nilutamide blocks the effects of testosterone at the androgen receptor level. In vivo, nilutamide interacts with the androgen receptor and prevents the normal androgenic response.

Pharmacokinetics:

Absorption – Analysis of blood, urine and feces samples following a single oral 150 mg dose of nilutamide in patients with metastatic prostate cancer showed that the drug is rapidly and completely absorbed and that it yields high and persistent plasma concentrations.

Distribution – After absorption of the drug, there is a detectable distribution phase with moderate binding of the drug to plasma proteins and low binding to erythrocytes. The binding is nonsaturable except in the case of alpha-1–glycoprotein, which makes a minor contribution to the total concentration of proteins in the plasma. The results of binding studies do not indicate any effects that would cause nonlinear pharmacokinetics.

Metabolism – Nilutamide is extensively metabolized and < 2% of the drug is excreted unchanged in the urine after 5 days. Five metabolites have been isolated from human urine. Two metabolites display an asymmetric center, because of oxidation of a methyl group, resulting in the formation of D- and L-isomers. One of the metabolites was shown, in vitro, to possess 25% to 50% of the pharmacological activity of the parent drug, and the D-isomer of the active metabolite showed equal or greater potency compared with the L-isomer. However, the pharmacokinetics and pharmacodynamics of the metabolites have not been fully investigated.

Excretion – The majority (62%) of orally administered nilutamide is eliminated in the urine during the first 120 hours after a single 150 mg dose. Fecal elimination is negligible, ranging from 1.4% to 7% of the dose after 4 to 5 days. Excretion of radioactivity in urine likely continues beyond 5 days. The mean elimination half-life of nilutamide determined in studies in which subjects received a single dose of 100 to 300 mg ranged from 38 to 59.1 hours with most values between 41 and 49 hours. The elimination of at least one metabolite is generally longer than that of unchanged nilutamide (59 to 126 hours). During multiple dosing of 3 × 50 mg twice a day, steady-state was reached within 2 to 4 weeks for most patients, and mean steady-state AUC_{0-12} was 110% higher than the AUC obtained from the first dose of 3 × 50 mg.

These data and in vitro metabolism data suggest that, upon multiple dosing, metabolic enzyme inhibition may occur for this drug.

Indications:

Metastatic prostate cancer: For use in combination with surgical castration for the treatment of metastatic prostate cancer (Stage D_2).

For maximum benefit, nilutamide treatment must begin on the same day as or on the day after surgical castration.

Contraindications:

Severe hepatic impairment; severe respiratory insufficiency; hypersensitivity to nilutamide or any component of this preparation.

Warnings:

Interstitial pneumonitis has been reported in 2% of patients in controlled clinical trials in patients exposed to nilutamide. Patients typically presented with progressive exertional dyspnea, and possibly with cough, chest pain and fever. X-rays showed interstitial or alveolo-interstitial changes. The suggestive signs of pneumonitis most often occurred within the first 3 months of nilutamide treatment.

Perform routine chest x-rays before treatment, and tell patients to report immediately any dyspnea or aggravation of pre-existing dyspnea.

At the onset of dyspnea or worsening of pre-existing dyspnea at any time during the treatment, interrupt nilutamide until it can be determined if respiratory symptoms are drug-related. Obtain a chest x-ray, and if there are findings suggestive of interstitial pneumonitis, discontinue treatment with nilutamide. The pneumonitis is almost always reversible when treatment is discontinued.

If the chest x-ray appears normal, perform pulmonary function tests including DL_{CO} (diffusing capacity of the lung for carbon monoxide). If a significant decrease in DL_{CO} or a restrictive pattern is observed on pulmonary function testing, terminate nilutamide treatment. In the absence of chest x-ray and pulmonary function test

NILUTAMIDE

findings consistent with interstitial pneumonitis, treatment with nilutamide can be restarted under close monitoring of pulmonary symptoms.

Because interstitial pneumonitis was reported in 8 of 47 patients (17%) in a small study performed in Japan, observe specific caution in the treatment of Asian patients.

Hepatitis: Hepatitis or marked increases in liver enzymes leading to drug discontinuation occurred in 1% of nilutamide patients.

Measure serum hepatic enzyme levels at baseline and at regular intervals (3 months); if transaminases increase over 2 to 3 times the upper limit of normal, discontinue treatment.

Perform appropriate laboratory testing at the first symptom/sign of liver injury (eg, jaundice, dark urine, fatigue, abdominal pain or unexplained GI symptoms) and nilutamide treatment must be discontinued immediately if transaminases exceed 3 times the upper limit of normal.

There has been a report of elevated hepatic enzymes followed by death in a 65 year old patient being treated with nilutamide.

Aplastic anemia: Foreign postmarketing surveillance has revealed isolated cases of aplastic anemia in which a causal relationship with nilutamide could not be ascertained.

Carcinogenesis: Administration of nilutamide to rats for 18 months at doses of 0, 5, 15 or 45 mg/kg/day produced benign Leydig cell tumors in 35% of male rats. The increased incidence of Leydig cell tumors is secondary to elevated luteinizing hormone (LH) concentrations resulting from loss of feedback inhibition at the pituitary. Elevated LH and testosterone concentrations are not observed in castrated men receiving nilutamide. Nilutamide had no effect on the incidence, size or time of onset of any spontaneous tumor in rats.

Pregnancy: Category C. Animal reproduction studies have not been conducted with nilutamide. It is also not known whether nilutamide can cause fetal harm when administered to a pregnant woman or can affect reproductive capacity. Give nilutamide to a pregnant woman only if clearly needed.

Children: Safety and effectiveness in pediatric patients have not been established.

Precautions:

Delay in adaptation to the dark: Thirteen percent to 57% of patients receiving nilutamide reported a delay in adaptation to the dark, ranging from seconds to a few minutes, when passing from a lighted area to a dark area. This effect sometimes does not abate as drug treatment is continued. Caution patients who experience this effect about driving at night or through tunnels. This effect can be alleviated by wearing tinted glasses.

Drug Interactions:

In vitro, nilutamide has been shown to inhibit the activity of liver cytochrome P450 isoenzymes and, therefore, may reduce the metabolism of compounds requiring these systems. Drugs with a low therapeutic margin, such as vitamin K antagonists, phenytoin and theophylline, could have a delayed elimination and increases in their serum half-life leading to a toxic level. The dosage of these drugs or others with a similar metabolism may need to be modified if they are administered concomitantly with nilutamide.

Adverse Reactions:

Adverse Reactions for Nilutamide + Leuprolide vs Nilutamide + Surgical Castration

Adverse experience	Nilutamide + leuprolide (%; n = 209)	Nilutamide + surgical castration (%; n = 225)
Body as a whole		
Pain	26.8	—
Headache	13.9	—
Asthenia	19.1	—
Back pain	11.5	—
Abdominal pain	10	—
Chest pain	7.2	—
Flu syndrome	7.2	—
Fever	5.3	—

Antiandrogens

NILUTAMIDE

Adverse experience	Nilutamide + leuprolide (%; n = 209)	Nilutamide + surgical castration (%; n = 225)
Cardiovascular		
Hypertension	9.1	5.3
GI		
Nausea	23.9	9.8
Constipation	19.6	7.1
Anorexia	11	—
Dyspepsia	6.7	—
Vomiting	5.7	—
Endocrine		
Hot flushes	66.5	28.4
Impotence	11	—
Libido decrease	11	—
Hemic/Lymphatic		
Anemia	7.2	—
Metabolic/Nutritional		
Increased AST	12.9	8
Peripheral edema	12.4	—
Increased ALT	9.1	7.6
Musculoskeletal		
Bone pain	6.2	—
CNS		
Insomnia	16.3	—
Dizziness	10	7.1
Depression	8.6	—
Hypesthesia	5.3	—
Respiratory		
Dyspnea	10.5	6.2
Upper respiratory infection	8.1	—
Pneumonia	5.3	—
Dermatologic		
Sweating	6.2	—
Alopecia	5.7	—
Dry skin	5.3	—
Rash	5.3	—
Special senses		
Impaired adaptation to dark	56.9	12.9
Chromatopsia	8.6	—
Impaired adaptation to light	7.7	—
Abnormal vision	6.2	6.7
GU		
Testicular atrophy	16.3	—
Gynecomastia	10.5	—
Urinary tract infection	8.6	8
Hematuria	8.1	—
Urinary tract disorder	7.2	—
Nocturia	6.7	—

The following adverse experiences were reported in 2% to 5% of patients treated with nilutamide in combination with leuprolide or orchiectomy.

Cardiovascular: Heart failure (3%); angina, syncope (2%).

GI: Diarrhea, GI disorder, GI hemorrhage, melena (2%).

Metabolic/Nutritional: Alcohol intolerance (5%); edema, weight loss (2%).

CNS: Paresthesia (3%); dry mouth, nervousness (2%).

NILUTAMIDE

Respiratory: Lung disorder (4%); cough increased, interstitial lung disease, rhinitis (2%).

Special senses: Cataract, photophobia (2%).

Lab test abnormalities: Hyperglycemia (4%); alkaline phosphatase increased, leukopenia (3%); haptoglobin increased, BUN creatinine increased (2%).

Miscellaneous: Malaise, pruritis, arthritis (2%).

Overdosage:

One case of massive overdosage has been published. A 79 year old man attempted suicide by ingesting 13 g of nilutamide. Despite immediate gastric lavage and oral administration of activated charcoal, plasma nilutamide levels peaked at 6 times the normal range 2 hours after ingestion. There were no clinical signs or symptoms or changes in parameters such as transaminases or chest x-ray. Maintainence treatment (150 mg/day) was resumed 30 days later.

In repeated-dose tolerance studies, doses of 600 mg/day and 900 mg/day were administered to 9 and 4 patients, respectively. The ingestion of these doses was associated with GI disorders, including nausea and vomiting, malaise, headache and dizziness. In addition, a transient elevation in hepatic enzyme levels was noted in one patient.

Because nilutamide is protein bound, dialysis may not be useful as treatment for overdose. As in the management of overdosage with any drug, bear in mind that multiple agents may have been taken. If vomiting does not occur spontaneously, induce if the patient is alert. General supportive care, including frequent monitoring of the vital signs and close observation of the patient, is indicated. (Refer to Management of Acute Overdose)

Administration and Dosage:

The recommended dosage is six tablets (50 mg each) once a day for a total daily dose of 300 mg for 30 days followed thereafter by three tablets (50 mg each) once a day for a total daily dosage of 150 mg. Nilutamide tablets can be taken with or without food.

Storage/Stability: Store at room temperature between 15° and 30°C (59° and 86°F). Protect from light.

Rx	**Nilandron** (Hoechst Marion Roussel)	**Tablets:** 50 mg	Lactose. (168). White, biconvex. In 90s.
	Anandron (Hoescht Marion Roussel	**Tablet:** 50 mg	(ANANDRON 50). Biconvex, white. Lactose. Bottles of 90.
		100 mg	(Anandron 100). Biconvex, white, scored. Lactose. Bottles of 90.

MEGESTROL ACETATE

This is an abbreviated monograph. For complete information, see the Progestins group monograph in the Hormones chapter.

> **Warning:**
> The use of megestrol is not recommended during the first 4 months of pregnancy.

Actions:

Pharmacology: The exact mechanism by which megestrol acetate produces its antineoplastic effects is unknown. An antiluteinizing effect mediated via the pituitary has been postulated. Evidence also suggests a local effect as a result of the marked changes from direct instillation of progestational agents into the endometrial cavity.

Indications:

Palliative treatment of advanced carcinoma of the breast or endometrium (ie, recurrent, inoperable or metastatic disease). Do not use in place of surgery, radiation or chemotherapy.

Unlabeled uses: Megestrol is currently being studied for and appears effective as an appetite stimulant in HIV-related cachexia. The dosage used has been 80 mg 4 times daily; average weight gain was 0.5 kg/week.

Contraindications:

As a diagnostic test for pregnancy.

Warnings:

The use of megestrol acetate in other types of neoplastic disease is not recommended.

Pregnancy: The use of progestational agents during the first 4 months of pregnancy is not recommended. Reports suggest an association between intrauterine exposure to female sex hormones and congenital anomalies.

If the patient is exposed to megestrol acetate during the first 4 months of pregnancy or becomes pregnant while taking this drug, apprise her of risks to the fetus.

Precautions:

Use with caution in patients with a history of thrombophlebitis.

Adverse Reactions:

Weight gain is a frequent side effect of megestrol acetate. This effect has been associated with increased appetite, not necessarily with fluid retention.

Thromboembolic phenomena, including thrombophlebitis and pulmonary embolism have occurred rarely.

Other: Nausea/vomiting; edema; breakthrough bleeding; dyspnea; tumor flare (with or without hypercalcemia); hyperglycemia; alopecia; carpal tunnel syndrome; rash.

No serious side effects resulted from megestrol acetate studies using doses as high as 800 mg/day.

Patient Information:

Medication may cause back or abdominal pain, headache, nausea, vomiting or breast tenderness; notify physician if these effects become pronounced.

Contraceptive measures are recommended during therapy.

Administration and Dosage:

Breast cancer: 160 mg/day (40 mg 4 times daily).

Endometrial carcinoma: 40 to 320 mg/day in divided doses.

At least 2 months of continuous treatment is adequate for determining efficacy.

Rx	**Megestrol Acetate** (Various, eg, Balan, Bioline, Geneva, Goldline, Major, Moore, Parmed, PBI, Rugby, Schein)	**Tablets:** 20 mg	In 100s and UD 100s.
Rx	**Megace** (Mead Johnson Onc)		Blue. In 100s.
Rx	**Megestrol Acetate** (Various, eg, Balan, Bioline, Geneva, Goldline, Major, Moore, Parmed, Rugby, Schein, URL)	**Tablets:** 40 mg	In 100s, 250s, 500s and UD 100s.
Rx	**Megace** (Mead Johnson Onc)		Blue, scored. In 100s, 250s, 500s.

Progestins

MEDROXYPROGESTERONE ACETATE

This is an abbreviated monograph. For complete information, see the Progestins group monograph in the Hormones chapter.

> **Warning:**
> Use is not recommended during the first 4 months of pregnancy.

Actions:

Pharmacology: Recommended parenteral doses to women with adequate endogenous estrogen, it transforms proliferative endometrium into secretory endometrium. Medroxyprogesterone inhibits (in the usual dose range) the secretion of pituitary gonadotropin which, in turn, prevents follicular maturation and ovulation.

Indications:

Adjunctive therapy and palliative treatment of inoperable, recurrent and metastatic endometrial carcinoma or renal carcinoma.

Unlabeled uses: Depot medroxyprogesterone acetate has been used as a long-acting contraceptive (150 mg IM every 3 months or 450 mg every 6 months) and in the treatment of advanced breast cancer.

Contraindications:

Thrombophlebitis, thromboembolic disorders, stroke or patients with past history of these conditions; breast carcinoma; undiagnosed vaginal bleeding; missed abortion; sensitivity to medroxyprogesterone acetate; as a diagnostic test for pregnancy.

Warnings:

Hepatic function impairment: Upon earliest manifestations of impaired liver function, discontinue the drug and re-evaluate the patient's status.

Pregnancy: The use of progestational agents during the first 4 months of pregnancy is not recommended. Several reports suggest an association between intrauterine exposure to female sex hormones and congenital anomalies. The risk of hypospadias, 5 to 8 per 1,000 male births in the general population, may be approximately doubled with exposure to progestational agents. There are insufficient data to quantify the risk to exposed female fetuses, but because some of these drugs induce mild virilization of the external genitalia of the female fetus, and because of the increased association of hypospadias in the male fetus, it is prudent to avoid the use of these drugs during the first trimester of pregnancy.

If the patient is exposed to medroxyprogesterone acetate during the first 4 months of pregnancy or if she becomes pregnant while taking this drug, she should be apprised of the potential risks to the fetus.

Lactation: Medroxyprogesterone does not adversely affect lactation; if breastfeeding is desired, it may be used safely. Milk production and duration of lactation may be increased if given in the puerperium.

Adverse Reactions:

Following repeated injections, amenorrhea and infertility may persist for up to 18 months and occasionally longer.

In a few instances there have been undesirable sequelae at the site of injection, such as residual lump, change in color of skin or sterile abscess.

Thromboembolic phenomena: Thrombophlebitis; pulmonary embolism.

Skin and mucous membranes: Angioneurotic edema; pruritus; urticaria; generalized rash; acne; alopecia; hirsutism.

CNS: Nervousness; insomnia; somnolence; fatigue; dizziness; headache (rare).

GI: Nausea (rare); jaundice, including neonatal jaundice.

Body as a whole: Hyperpyrexia (rare); anaphylaxis.

Administration and Dosage:

For IM administration only.

Endometrial or renal carcinoma: Initially, 400 to 1000 mg IM per week. If improvement occurs within a few weeks or months and the disease appears stabilized, it may be possible to maintain improvement with as little as 400 mg/month.

Rx	**Depo-Provera** (Upjohn)	**Injection:** 400 mg per ml[2]	In 2.5 and 10 ml vials and 1 ml U-ject.

[1] With polyethylene glycol 3350, polysorbate 80 and parabens.
[2] With polyethylene glycol 3350, sodium sulfate anhydrous, myristyl-gamma-picolinium Cl.

Estrogens

For complete information on Estrogens, see the group monograph in the Hormones chapter.

DIETHYLSTILBESTROL DIPHOSPHATE

Actions:

Pharmacology: Diethylstilbestrol is a synthetic estrogen.

Putative receptor proteins for estrogens have been detected in estrogen-responsive tissues. Estrogens are first bound to a cytoplasmic receptor protein. Following modification, the estrogen-containing complex is translocated to the nucleus where ultimate binding of the estrogen-containing complex occurs. As a result of such binding charactersitics metabolic alterations ensue. In the male patient with androgenic hormone dependent conditions such as metastatic carcinoma of the prostrate gland, estrogens counter the androgenic influence by competing for receptor sites. Metastatic bone lesions may also show improvement.

Pharmacokinetics: Metabolism and inactivation occur primarily in the liver. Some estrogens are excreted into the bile; however, they are reabsorbed from the intestine and returned to the liver through the portal venous system. Water soluble estrogen conjugates are strongly acidic and are ionized in body fluids, which favor excretion through the kidneys since tubular reabsorption is minimal.

Indications:

Inoperable, progressing prostatic cancer. Not indicated in the treatment of any disorder in women.

Estrogens should not be used in men with any of the following conditions:

Known or suspected cancer of the breast except in appropriately selected patients being treated for metastatic disease.

Known or suspected estrogen-dependent neoplasia.

Active thrombophlebitis or thromboembolic disorders.

Adverse Reactions:

Estrogen use has been associated with thrombophlebitis, pulmonary embolism, cerebral thrombosis and possibly coronary thrombosis.

Diethylstilbestrol has been associated with hepatic cutaneous porphyria, erythema nodosum and erythema multiforme.

Patient Information:

Medication may cause nausea, vomiting, headache, abdominal pain, painful swelling of breasts; notify physician if these become pronounced.

Diethylstilbestrol diphosphate should not be used by women.

Promptly report the following side effects: Bloating, loss of appetite, skin rash, mood changes, depression, nervousness, dizziness, chest pain, shortness of breath, numbness or tingling about the nose or mouth, fluid accumulation, disturbance in vision, frequent or painful urination, painful swelling of extremities.

Consult a physician regularly for evaluation of blood pressure and heart rate.

Diabetic patients should monitor urine very carefully. Test of blood sugar may be necessary as well.

Administration and Dosage:

Oral: Initially, 50 mg 3 times daily; increase to ≥ 200 mg 3 times daily, depending on patient tolerance. Maximum daily dose not to exceed 1 g. If relief is not obtained with high oral doses, administer IV.

Parenteral: On the first day, give 0.5 g IV, dissolved in 250 ml of saline or 5% dextrose. On subsequent days give 1 g dissolved in ≈ 250 to 500 ml of saline or dextrose. Administer slowly (20 to 30 drops per minute) during the first 10 to 15 minutes and then adjust the flow rate so that the entire amount is given in 1 hour. Follow this procedure for ≥ 5 days, depending upon patient response. Following this first intensive course of therapy, administer 0.25 to 0.5 g in a similar manner once or twice weekly, or obtain maintenance with oral administration.

Stability of solution: After reconstitution, keep the solution at room temperature and away from direct light. Under these conditions the solution is stable for about 5 days, as long as cloudiness or evidence of a precipitate has not occurred.

Rx	**Stilphostrol** (Miles Inc.)	**Tablets:** 50 mg	(Miles 132). White to off-white with gray/tan mottling, scored. In 50s.
		Injection: 0.25 g (as sodium salt)	In 5 ml amps.

Estrogen/Nitrogen Mustard

ESTRAMUSTINE PHOSPHATE SODIUM

Actions:

Pharmacology: Estramustine phosphate combines estradiol and nornitrogen mustard by a carbamate link. The molecule is phosphorylated to make it water soluble.

Mechanism of action – Estramustine appears to act as a relatively weak alkylating agent and imparts a weak estrogenic activity. The estrogenic portion of the molecule acts as a carrier to facilitate selective uptake of the drug into estrogen receptor-positive cells. Due to the selective steroidal uptake, the alkylating effect of the nitrogen mustard is enhanced in these cells.

Pharmacokinetics:

Absorption/Distribution – Estramustine phosphate is readily dephosphorylated during absorption, and the major metabolites in plasma are estromustine, the estrone analog, estradiol and estrone.

Prolonged treatment produces elevated total plasma concentrations of estradiol that are within ranges similar to the elevated estradiol levels found in prostatic cancer patients given conventional estradiol therapy. Estrogenic effects, as demonstrated by changes in circulating levels of steroids and pituitary hormones, are similar in patients treated with either estramustine phosphate or conventional estradiol.

Metabolism/Excretion – Estromustine (17-keto analog) is the major metabolite. Estrone and estradiol are also present, as a result of cleavage of the nitrogen mustard from the steroid. Terminal half-life of estramustine phosphate is ≈ 20 hours.

The metabolic urinary patterns of estradiol and the estradiol moiety of estramustine phosphate are very similar, although the metabolites derived from estramustine phosphate are excreted at a slower rate. The majority of the drug is excreted in the stool.

Indications:

Palliative treatment of metastatic or progressive carcinoma of the prostate.

Contraindications:

Hypersensitivity to estradiol or nitrogen mustard.

Active thrombophlebitis or thromboembolic disorders, except where the actual tumor mass is the cause of the thromboembolic phenomenon and the benefits of therapy outweigh the risks.

Warnings:

Thrombosis: The risk of thrombosis, including nonfatal myocardial infarction, increases in men receiving estrogens for prostatic cancer. Use with caution in patients with a history of thrombophlebitis, thrombosis or thromboembolic disorders, especially if they were associated with estrogen therapy. Use with caution in patients with cerebral vascular or coronary artery disease.

Glucose tolerance may be decreased; observe diabetic patients receiving this drug.

Elevated blood pressure may occur; monitor blood pressure periodically during therapy.

Hepatic function impairment: Estramustine may be poorly metabolized in patients with impaired liver function. Administer with caution.

Carcinogenesis/Mutagenesis/Fertility impairment: Long-term continuous administration of estrogens in certain animal species increases frequency of carcinomas of the breast and liver. Compounds structurally similar to estramustine are carcinogenic in mice.

Although testing by the Ames method failed to demonstrate mutagenicity for estramustine, both estradiol and nitrogen mustard are mutagenic. For this reason, and because some patients who had been impotent while on estrogen therapy have regained potency while taking the drug, advise use of contraceptive measures.

Precautions:

Fluid retention: Exacerbation of preexisting or incipient peripheral edema or congestive heart disease may occur in some patients. Other conditions potentially influenced by fluid retention, such as epilepsy, migraine or renal dysfunction, require careful observation.

Calcium/Phosphorus metabolism may be influenced by estramustine; use with caution in patients with metabolic bone diseases associated with hypercalcemia or in patients with renal insufficiency.

Laboratory tests: Abnormalities of hepatic enzymes and of bilirubin have occurred, but have seldom required cessation of therapy. Perform such tests at appropriate intervals during therapy and repeat after the drug has been withdrawn for 2 months.

ESTRAMUSTINE PHOSPHATE SODIUM

Drug Interactions:

Drug/Food interactions: Milk, milk products and calcium-rich foods or drugs may impair the absorption of estramustine phosphate sodium.

Adverse Reactions:

Cardiovascular/Respiratory: Cerebrovascular accident; myocardial infarction; thrombophlebitis; pulmonary emboli; congestive heart failure; edema; dyspnea; leg cramps; upper respiratory discharge; hoarseness.

GI: Nausea; vomiting; diarrhea; anorexia; flatulence; GI bleeding; burning throat; thirst; minor GI upset.

Dermatologic: Rash; pruritus; dry skin; peeling skin of fingertips; easy bruising; flushing; thinning hair.

Miscellaneous: Lethargy; emotional lability; insomnia; headache; anxiety; chest pain; tearing of eyes; breast tenderness; mild to moderate breast enlargement.

Lab test abnormalities: Laboratory test abnormalities in hematologic tests for leukopenia and thrombocytopenia. Also abnormalities of bilirubin, LDH and AST.

Overdosage:

Although there has been no experience with overdosage, it may produce pronounced manifestations of the adverse reactions. In the event of overdosage, evacuate gastric contents by gastric lavage and initiate symptomatic therapy. Monitor hematologic and hepatic parameters for at least 6 weeks after overdosage.

Patient Information:

Because of the possibility of mutagenic effects, use contraceptive measures.

Take with water at least 1 hour before or 2 hours after meals.

Milk, milk products and calcium-rich foods or drugs (such as calcium-containing antacids) must not be taken simultaneously with estramustine phosphate sodium.

Administration and Dosage:

Recommended daily dosage: 14 mg/kg/day (ie, one 140 mg capsule for each 10 kg or 22 lb) in 3 or 4 divided doses (dosage range, 10 to 16 mg/kg/day).

Treat for 30 to 90 days before assessing the possible benefits of continued therapy. Continue therapy as long as response is favorable. Some patients have been maintained on therapy for > 3 years at doses ranging from 10 to 16 mg/kg/day.

Storage: Refrigerate at 2° to 8°C (36° to 46°F). Capsules may be left out of the refrigerator for 24 to 48 hours without affecting potency.

Rx	**Emcyt** (Pharmacia)	**Capsules**: Estramustine phosphate sodium equivalent to 140 mg estramustine phosphate (12.5 mg sodium/capsule)	White. In 100s.

Antiestrogen

TAMOXIFEN CITRATE

Actions:

Pharmacology: Tamoxifen is a nonsteroidal agent with potent antiestrogenic properties due to its ability to compete with estrogen for binding sites in target tissues such as the breast. Tumor hormone receptors may help predict which patients will benefit from the adjuvant therapy, but not all breast cancer adjuvant tamoxifen studies have shown a clear relationship between hormone receptor status and treatment effect. Tamoxifen competes with estradiol for estrogen receptor protein.

Pharmacokinetics: Tamoxifen is extensively metabolized after oral administration. Studies in women receiving 20 mg of tamoxifen have shown that ≈ 65% of the administered dose was excreted from the body over a period of 2 weeks with fecal excretion as the primary route of elimination. The drug was excreted mainly as polar conjugates, with unchanged drug and unconjugated metabolites accounting for < 30% of the total fecal radioactivity.

N-desmethyl tamoxifen was the major metabolite found in patients' plasma. The biological activity of N-desmethyl tamoxifen appears to be similar to tamoxifen. 4-hydroxytamoxifen and a side chain primary alcohol derivative of tamoxifen have been identified as minor metabolites in plasma.

Chronic administration of 10 mg tamoxifen given twice daily for three months to patients results in average steady-state plasma concentrations of 120 ng/ml (range, 67 to 183 ng/ml) for tamoxifen and 336 ng/ml (range, 148 to 654 ng/ml) for N-desmethyl tamoxifen. After initiation of therapy, steady-state concentrations for tamoxifen are achieved in about 4 weeks and steady-state concentrations for N-desmethyl tamoxifen are achieved in about 8 weeks, suggesting a half-life of ≈ 14 days for this metabolite.

Clinical trials: In a meta-analysis of 40 clinical trials of adjuvant therapy with tamoxifen involving ≈ 30,000 women with breast cnacer who were followed up for 10 years, tamoxifen reduced the risk of death by 17% per year in node-negative patients and 18% annually among node-positive patients compared with controls. The statistically significant overall survival benefit increased steadily with the length of follow-up. The analysis concluded that long-term tamoxifen (2 to 5 years) is significantly more effective than short-term use. The greatest difference appears to be node-positive, estrogen receptor-positive patients.

Indications:

Breast cancer:

Adjuvant therapy – For treatment of axillary node-negative breast cancer in women following total mastectomy or segmental mastectomy, axillary dissection and breast irradiation. Data are insufficient to predict which women are most likely to benefit and to determine if tamoxifen provides any benefit in women with tumors < 1 cm.

For treatment of node-positive breast cancer in postmenopausal women following total mastectomy or segmental mastectomy, axillary dissection, and breast irradiation. In some tamoxifen adjuvant studies, most of the benefit to date has been in the subgroup with 4 or more positive axillary nodes.

The estrogen and progesterone receptor values may help to predict whether adjuvant tamoxifen therapy is likely to be beneficial.

Advanced disease therapy – Effective in the treatment of metastatic breast cancer in women and men. In premenopausal women with metastatic breast cancer, tamoxifen is an alternative to oophorectomy or ovarian irradiation. Estrogen receptor positive tumors are most likely to benefit.

Unlabeled uses: Treatment of mastalgia (10 mg/day for 4 months) and for decreasing the size and pain of gynecomastia.

Studies are currently being considered for use of tamoxifen as chemosuppressive (preventive) therapy in women at high risk for primary breast cancer. Tamoxifen may also be useful in pancreatic, and advanced/recurrent endometrial and hepatocellular carcinoma.

Contraindications:

Hypersensitivity to the drug.

Warnings:

Visual disturbances, including corneal changes, cataracts and retinopathy, have occurred with tamoxifen use.

Hypercalcemia has occurred in some breast cancer patients with bone metastases within a few weeks of starting therapy with tamoxifen. If hypercalcemia occurs, institute appropriate measures and, if severe, discontinue use.

Hepatic effects: Tamoxifen has been associated with changes in liver enzyme levels and, on rare occasions, a spectrum of more severe liver abnormalities including fatty liver, cholestasis, hepatitis and hepatic necrosis. A few of these serious cases included fatalities. In most cases the relationship to tamoxifen was uncertain; however, some positive rechallenges and dechallenges have been reported. Perform periodic liver function tests.

Disease of the bone: Increased bone and tumor pain and local disease flare are sometimes associated with a good tumor response shortly after starting tamoxifen, and generally subside rapidly. Lesion size may increase suddenly in soft tissue disease, sometimes with new lesions or with erythema in or around the lesion.

Carcinogenesis/Mutagenesis/Fertility impairment: A study in rats revealed hepatocellular carcinomas at doses of 5 to 35 mg/kg/day for up to 2 years; incidence was significantly higher using doses of 20 and 35 mg/kg/day (69%) vs 5 mg/kg/day (14%). In addition, preliminary data from two independent reports revealed liver tumors that one study classified as malignant. Also, in a trial using 40 mg/day for 2 to 5 years in humans, three cases of liver cancer were reported vs one case in the control group.

Granulosa cell ovarian tumors and interstitial cell testicular tumors were found in mice.

An increased frequency of endometrial changes including hyperplasia, polyps and endometrial cancer has been reported with tamoxifen. The incidence and pattern suggest that the underlying mechanism is related to the estrogenic properties.

An increased incidence of uterine cancer was noted in 23 of 1372 patients receiving tamoxifen 40 mg/day for 2 to 5 years vs 4 of 1357 control patients. In addition, after ≈ 6.8 years of follow-up in an ongoing trial, 15 of 1419 women receiving tamoxifen 20 mg/day for 5 years developed uterine cancer vs 2 of 1424 controls. Most of the uterine cancers were diagnosed at an early stage, but deaths have occurred.

Tamoxifen is genotoxic in rodent and human MCL-5 cells.

Fertility in female rats decreased following 0.04 mg/kg for 2 weeks prior to mating through day 7 of pregnancy. There was a decreased number of implantations, and all fetuses were found dead.

Pregnancy: Category D. Tamoxifen may cause fetal harm when administered to a pregnant woman. Patients should not become pregnant while taking tamoxifen and should use barrier or nonhormonal contraceptive measures. Effects on reproductive functions are expected from the antiestrogenic properties of the drug. In reproductive studies in rats at dose levels equal to or below the human dose, nonteratogenic developmental skeletal changes were seen and were found to be reversible. In fertility and teratology studies in rats and rabbits using doses at or below those in humans, a lower incidence of embryo implantation and a higher incidence of fetal death or retarded in utero growth were observed, with slower learning behavior in some rat pups.

In studies of reproductive tract development in rodents, tamoxifen (at doses 0.3– to 2.4–fold the human maximum recommended dose on a mg/m^2 basis) caused changes in both sexes that are similar to those caused by estradiol, ethynylestradiol and diethylstilbestrol. Although the clinical relevance of these changes is unknown, some of these changes, especially vaginal adenosis, are similar to those seen in young women exposed to diethylstilbestrol in utero and who have a 1 in 1000 risk of developing clear-cell adenocarcinoma of the vagina or cervix. To date, in utero exposure to tamoxifen has not been shown to cause vaginal adenosis, or clear-cell adenocarcinoma of the vagina or cervix in young women. However, only a small number of young women have been exposed to tamoxifen in utero, and a smaller number have been followed long enough (to age 15 to 20) to determine whether vaginal or cervical neoplasia could occur as a result of this exposure.

There are no adequate and well controlled studies in pregnant women. There have been reports of spontaneous abortions, birth defects, fetal deaths and vaginal bleeding. If this drug is used during pregnancy or if the patient becomes pregnant while taking this drug or within ≈ 2 months of discontinuing therapy, apprise her of the potential hazard to the fetus, including potential long-term risk of a DES-like syndrome.

Lactation: It is not known whether this drug is excreted in breast milk. Because there is potential for serious adverse reactions in nursing infants, decide whether to discontinue nursing or discontinue the drug.

Precautions:

Monitoring: Perform periodic complete blood counts, including platelet counts, and liver function tests.

Leukopenia/Thrombocytopenia: Use cautiously in patients with existing leukopenia or thrombocytopenia. Leukopenia and thrombocytopenia have occurred occasionally. Decreases in platelet counts (usually to 50,000 to 100,000/mm^3, but infrequently lower) have occurred. In patients with significant thrombocytopenia, rare hemorrhagic episodes have occurred but it is uncertain if these episodes are due to tamoxifen therapy.

Hyperlipidemias have occurred infrequently. However, total cholesterol and LDL levels have also decreased during therapy. Periodic monitoring of plasma triglycerides and cholesterol may be indicated in patients with pre-existing hyperlipidemias.

Drug Interactions:

Tamoxifen Drug Interactions			
Precipitant drug	Object drug*		Description
Tamoxifen	Anticoagulants	⬆	The hypoprothrombinemic effect may be increased by concurrent tamoxifen.
Bromocriptine	Tamoxifen	⬆	Bromocriptine may elevate serum tamoxifen and N-desmethyl tamoxifen.

* ⬆ = Object drug increased.

Drug/Lab test interactions: T_4 elevations occurred in a few postmenopausal patients but were not accompanied by clinical hyperthyroidism. An increase in thyroid-binding globulin in postmenopausal women on tamoxifen may explain T_4 elevations during treatment. Variations in the karyopyknotic index on vaginal smears and various degrees of estrogen effect on Pap smears have been infrequently seen in postmenopausal patients.

Adverse Reactions:

Adverse reactions to tamoxifen are relatively mild and rarely require discontinuation of therapy. If adverse reactions are severe, it is sometimes possible to control severe adverse reactions by dosage reduction without losing control of the disease.

Females:

Most frequent – Hot flashes, nausea, vomiting (up to 25%, rarely severe).

Less frequent – Vaginal bleeding; vaginal discharge; menstrual irregularities; skin rash. Usually not severe enough to require dosage reduction or discontinuation.

Infrequent – Hypercalcemia; peripheral edema; food distaste; pruritus vulvae; depression; dizziness; lightheadedness; headache; retinopathy; thrombocytopenia; leukopenia; hair thinning or partial loss.

Ovarian cysts have been observed in a small number of premenopausal patients with advanced breast cancer who have been treated with tamoxifen. There have also been reports of endometriosis and uterine fibroids.

Changes in liver enzyme levels (see Warnings).

Tamoxifen Adverse Reactions: 5 Year Therapy (%)		
Adverse reaction	Tamoxifen (n = 1424)	Placebo (n = 1440)
Hot flashes	63.9	47.6
Weight gain (> 5%)	38.1	40.1
Fluid retention	32.4	29.7
Vaginal discharge	29.6	15.2
Nausea	25.7	23.9
Irregular menses	24.6	18.8
Weight loss (> 5%)	22.6	18
Skin changes	18.7	15.3
Increased BUN	18.1	20.2
Diarrhea	11.2	14
Increased AST	4.8	2.8
Increased alkaline phosphatase	3	4.6
Vomiting	2.1	1.7
Increased bilirubin	1.8	1.2
Increased creatinine	1.7	1
Thrombocytopenia (platelets < 100,000/mm^3)	1.5	1.2
Deep vein thrombosis	0.8	0.3
Leukopenia (WBC < 3000/mm^3)	0.4	1.1
Pulmonary embolism	0.4	0.1
Superficial phlebitis	0.3	0

TAMOXIFEN CITRATE

Tamoxifen vs Ovarian Ablation: Adverse Reactions (%)		
Adverse reactions	Tamoxifen (n = 104)	Ovarian ablation (n = 100)
Flush	32.7	46
Amenorrhea	16.3	69
Altered menses	12.5	5
Oligomenorrhea	8.7	1
Bone pain	5.7	6
Menstrual disorder	5.7	4
Nausea	4.8	4
Coughing	3.8	1
Edema	3.8	1
Fatigue	3.8	1
Musculoskeletal pain	2.8	0
Pain	2.8	4
Ovarian cyst(s)	2.8	2
Depression	1.9	2
Abdominal cramps	1	2
Anorexia	1	2

Males: Tamoxifen is well tolerated in males with breast cancer. The safety profile appears to be similar to that in females. Loss of libido and impotence have resulted in discontinuation of therapy. Also, in oligospermic males treated with tamoxifen, LH, FSH, testosterone and estrogen levels were elevated.

Overdosage:

Symptoms: In animals, respiratory difficulties and convulsions occurred at high doses. In advanced metastatic cancer patients receiving loading doses of > 400 mg/m^2, followed by maintenance doses of 150 mg/m^2 twice daily, acute neurotoxicity manifested by tremor, hyperreflexia, unsteady gait and dizziness was noted. Symptoms occurred within 3 to 5 days of beginning therapy and cleared within 2 to 5 days after stopping therapy. One patient experienced a seizure several days after discontinuation and after neurotoxic symptoms had resolved. The causal relationship to tamoxifen therapy is unknown. Prolongation of the QT interval was also noted in patients given doses > 250 mg/m^2 loading dose followed by 80 mg/m^2 twice daily. Minimal loading dose and maintenance doses given at which neurological symptoms and QT changes occurred were at least sixfold higher than the maximum recommended dose.

Treatment: Treatment includes usual supportive measures. Refer to General Management of Acute Overdosage.

Antiestrogen

TAMOXIFEN CITRATE

Patient Information:

Advise women who are receiving or who have previously received tamoxifen to have regular gynecologic examinations and promptly inform their physician of menstrual irregularities, abnormal vaginal bleeding, change in vaginal discharge or pelvic pain or pressure.

Advise women not to become pregnant during therapy. Barrier or nonhormonal contraceptive measures are recommended during treatment if sexually active.

Notify physician if marked weakness, sleepiness, mental confusion, pain/swelling of legs, shortness of breath, blurred vision, bone pain, hot flashes, nausea, vomiting, weight gain, dizziness, headache or loss of appetite occurs.

Administration and Dosage:

10 or 20 mg twice daily (morning and evening) or 20 mg daily.

Some studies have used dosages of 10 mg 2 or 3 times a day for 2 years, and 10 mg twice daily for 5 years. The reduction in recurrence and mortality was greater in those studies that used the drug for ≥ 2 years than in those that used it for < 2 years. There was no indication that doses > 20 mg/day were more effective. However, optimal duration of adjuvant therapy is not known.

Rx	**Nolvadex** (Zeneca)	**Tablets:** 10 mg (as citrate)	(Nolvadex 600). White. In 60s and 250s.
Rx	**Tamoxifen** (Barr)		In 60s and 250s.
Rx	**Nolvadex** (Zeneca)	**Tablets:** 20 mg (as citrate)	(Nolvadex 604). White In 30s.

Gonadotropin-Releasing Hormone Analog

LEUPROLIDE ACETATE

Actions:

Pharmacology: Leuprolide, an LH-RH agonist , is a synthetic nonapeptide analog of naturally occurring gonadotropin-releasing hormone (GnRH or LH-RH) with greater potency than the natural hormone. It occupies pituitary GnRH receptors and desensitizes them ; thus, it inhibits gonadotropin secretion when given continuously and in therapeutic doses. After initial stimulation, chronic leuprolide suppresses ovarian and testicular steroidogenesis, which is reversible upon discontinuation.

Advanced prostatic cancer – Leuprolide initially increases circulating levels of luteinizing hormone (LH) and follicle stimulating hormone (FSH), leading to a transient increase in gonadal steroids (testosterone and dihydrotestosterone in males; estrone and estradiol in premenopausal females). However, continuous daily administration results in decreased LH and FSH in all patients . In males, testosterone is reduced to castrate levels. In premenopausal females, estrogens are reduced to postmenopausal levels. These decreases occur within 2 to 4 weeks after initiation. Castrate levels of testosterone in prostatic cancer have been seen for up to 5 years . Leuprolide also inhibits growth of certain hormone-dependent tumors and atrophy of the reproductive organs.

Central precocious puberty (CPP) – In children with CPP, stimulated and basal gonadotropins are reduced to prepubertal levels. Testosterone and estradiol are reduced to prepubertal levels in males and females, respectively. Reduction of gonadotropins will allow for normal physical and psychological growth and development. Natural maturation occurs when gonadotropins return to pubertal levels following discontinuation of leuprolide acetate.

The following physiologic effects have been noted with the chronic administration of leuprolide acetate in this patient population:

Skeletal growth – A measurable increase in body length can be noted since the epiphyseal plates will not close prematurely;

Organ growth – Reproductive organs will return to a prepubertal state;

Menses – If present, will cease.

Pharmacokinetics:

Leuprolide injection has a plasma half-life of approximately 3 hours when used for the treatment of prostatic cancer.

Depot –

Monthly formulation: Following a single depot injection, mean peak leuprolide plasma concentration was almost 20 ng/ml at 4 hours and 0.36 ng/ml at 4 weeks. Nondetectable leuprolide acetate plasma concentrations have been seen during chronic use, but testosterone levels appear to be maintained at castrate levels.

3 month formulation: Following a single injection, mean peak plasma levels of 48.9 ng/ml were seen at 4 hours and then declined to 0.67 ng/ml at 12 weeks. Leuprolide appeared to be released at a constant rate after onset of steady state levels during the third week of dosing, providing steady plasma concentrations through the 12 week dosing interval. The initial burst, followed by rapid decline to a steady-state level, was similar to the release pattern seen with the monthly formulation.

The mean steady-state volume of distribution of leuprolide following IV bolus administration to healthy male volunteers was 27 L. In vitro binding to human plasma proteins ranged from 43% to 49%.

In healthy male volunteers, a 1 mg bolus of leuprolide administered IV revealed that the mean systemic clearance was 7.6 L/hr.

Following administration to 3 patients, < 5% of the dose was recovered as parent and the M-I metabolite in the urine.

Clinical trials:

Advanced prostatic cancer – In a controlled study comparing leuprolide 1 mg/day SC to diethylstilbestrol (DES) 3 mg/day, the survival rate for the 2 groups was comparable after 2 years of treatment. The objective response to treatment was also similar for the 2 groups. In clinical trials, the safety and efficacy of monthly leuprolide depot did not differ from that of the SC injection.

In clinical studies with the 3 month depot formulation, 85% of patients had no progression during the first 24 weeks of treatment. A decrease from baseline in serum prostate specific antigen (PSA) of ≥ 90% occurred in 71% and a change to within normal range (≥ 3.99 ng/ml) occurred in 63%.

Endometriosis – Leuprolide depot 3.75 mg monthly for 6 months was comparable to danazol 800 mg/day in relieving clinical symptoms (eg, pelvic pain, dysmenorrhea, dyspareunia, pelvic tenderness, induration) and in reducing the size of endometrial implants.

Gonadotropin-Releasing Hormone Analog

LEUPROLIDE ACETATE

Uterine leiomyomata (fibroids) – Administration of leuprolide depot 3.75 mg for 3 or 6 months decreased uterine and fibroid volume, thus allowing for relief of clinical symptoms (eg, abdominal bloating, pelvic pain, pressure). Excessive vaginal bleeding (eg, menorrhagia menometrorrhagia) decreased (in one study, 80% of the patients experienced relief), resulting in improvement in hematologic parameters.

Indications:

Advanced prostatic cancer (injection or depot): Palliative treatment alternative when orchiectomy or estrogen administration are not indicated or are unacceptable.

Leuprolide is also used with flutamide (see individual monograph) to treat metastatic prostatic carcinoma. This combination may be superior to leuprolide alone.

Endometriosis (leuprolide depot 3.75 mg only): Management of endometriosis, including pain relief and reduction of endometriotic lesions. Experience is limited to women ≥ 18 years of age treated for 6 months.

Central precocious puberty (injection or depot): Treatment of children with CPP.

Uterine leiomyomata (fibroids) (leuprolide depot 3.75 mg only): Leuprolide depot 3.75 mg and iron therapy are indicated for the preoperative hematologic improvement of patients with anemia caused by uterine leiomyomata. The clinician may want to consider a 1 month trial period on iron alone in as much as some patients will respond to iron alone. Leuprolide may be added if the response to iron alone is considered inadequate. Recommended therapy duration with leuprolide is up to 3 months. Experience with leuprolide depot in females has been limited to women ≥18 years old.

Patients Achieving Hemoglobin ≥ 12 g/dl: Leuprolide with Iron vs Iron alone (%)

Treatment	Week 4	Week 8	Week 12
Leuprolide 3.75 mg with iron	41	71	79
Iron alone	17	40	56

Unlabeled uses: Leuprolide may be useful in the treatment of breast, ovarian and endometrial cancer; infertility; prostatic hypertrophy.

Contraindications:

Depot: Pregnancy, lactation (see Warnings); hypersensitivity to GnRH, GnRH agonist analogs or product excipients; undiagnosed abnormal vaginal bleeding .

Injection: Pregnancy (see Warnings); hypersensitivity to GnRH, GnRH agonist analogs and excipients.

Warnings:

Worsening of signs and symptoms:

Prostatic cancer – There are isolated cases of worsening of signs and symptoms during the first few weeks of treatment with LH-RH analogs. It may contribute to paralysis with or without fatal complications. For patients at risk, consider initiating therapy with daily injections for the first 2 weeks to facilitate withdrawal of treatment if necessary. Worsening of symptoms may occur during the first 2 weeks of treatment and is usually manifested by an increase in bone pain. In a few cases, a temporary worsening of existing hematuria and urinary tract obstruction occurred during the first week. Temporary weakness and paresthesia of the lower limbs have occurred, which may have contributed to a rapid fatal outcome in 2 cases with another LH-RH analog. Closely observe patients with metastatic vertebral lesions or urinary tract obstruction during the first few weeks of therapy. Potential exacerbations of signs and symptoms during the first few weeks of treatment is a concern in patients with vertebral metastases or urinary obstruction or hematuria which, if aggravated, may lead to neurological problems such as temporary weakness or paresthesia of the lower limbs or worsening of urinary symptoms.

CPP – During the early phase of therapy, gonadotropins and sex steroids rise above baseline because of the natural stimulatory effect of the drug. Therefore, an increase in clinical signs and symptoms may be observed. Noncompliance with drug regimen or inadequate dosing may result in inadequate control of the pubertal process. The consequences of poor control include the return of pubertal signs such as menses, breast development and testicular growth. The long-term consequences of inadequate control of gonadal steroid secretion are unknown, but may include a further compromise of adult stature.

Hypersensitivity: Anaphylaxis has occurred with synthetic GnRH. Patients allergic to benzyl alcohol, a component of the leuprolide injection vehicle, may present symptoms of hypersensitivity, usually local, in the form of erythema and induration at the injection site. Leuprolide depot is preservative free.

Carcinogenesis: In rats, a dose-related increase in benign pituitary hyperplasia and benign pituitary adenomas was noted after 2 years with high daily doses . There was a significant, but not dose-related, increase of pancreatic islet cell adenomas in females and of testes interstitial cell adenomas in males (highest incidence in the low dose group).

Studies with leuprolide and similar analogs have shown full reversibility of fertility suppression when the drug is stopped after continuous use for up to 24 weeks.

Pregnancy: Category X. Leuprolide is contraindicated in women who are or may become pregnant while receiving the drug. When given on day 6 of pregnancy (1/600 to 1/6 the adult human dose) to rabbits, monthly leuprolide produced a dose-related increase in major fetal abnormalities. There was increased fetal mortality and decreased fetal weights in rabbits and rats. The effects on fetal mortality are logical consequences of the alterations in hormonal levels brought about by this drug. Therefore, the possibility exists that spontaneous abortion may occur if the drug is given during pregnancy.

Before starting therapy, pregnancy must be excluded. When used monthly at the recommended dose, leuprolide depot usually inhibits ovulation and stops menstruation; however, contraception is not ensured (see Patient information).

Lactation: It is not known whether leuprolide depot is excreted in breast milk. Do not use during nursing.

Children: Indicated for treatment of children with CPP.

Precautions:

CPP, selection for use: Select children for treatment of CPP based on the following criteria: 1) Clinical diagnosis of CPP (idiopathic or neurogenic) with onset of secondary sexual characteristics earlier than 8 years old in females and in 9 years old in males; 2) confirmed diagnosis by a pubertal response to a GnRH stimulation test, bone age advanced 1 year beyond chronological age; 3) baseline evaluation including height, weight, sex steroid levels, adrenal steroid level to exclude congenital adrenal hyperplasia, beta human chorionic gonadotropin level to rule out a chorionic gonadotropin secreting tumor, computerized tomography of head to rule out intracranial tumor.

Bone density changes: The induced hypoestrogen state results in small loss in bone density over the course of treatment, some of which may not be reversible for a period of up to 6 months. This bone loss should not be important. In patients with major risk factors for decreased bone mineral content (eg, chronic alcohol or tobacco use, strong family history of osteoporosis, chronic use of drugs that can reduce bone mass [eg, anticonvulsants, corticosteroids], leuprolide may pose additional risk; weigh the risks and benefits before starting therapy. Repeated courses of therapy beyond 6 months are not recommended, particularly in patients with major risk factors for loss of bone mineral content.

Monitoring:

Prostatic cancer – Monitor response by measuring serum levels of testosterone, prostatic acid phosphatase and PSA levels. In the majority of patients, testosterone levels increased above baseline during the first week, declining thereafter to baseline levels or below by the end of the second week. Castrate levels were reached within 2 to 4 weeks and were maintained for as long as drug administration was maintained on time. Occasional transient increases in acid phosphatase levels may occur early in treatment. By the fourth week, the elevated levels usually decreased to values at or near baseline.

Endometriosis/Uterine leiomyomata – During the early phase of therapy, sex steroids temporarily rise above baseline because of the physiologic effect of the drug. Therefore, an increase in clinical signs and symptoms may occur during the initial days of therapy, but these will dissipate with continued therapy.

CPP – Monitor response to leuprolide acetate 1 to 2 months after the start of therapy with a GnRH stimulation test and sex steroid levels. Measurement of bone age for advancement should be done every 6 to 12 months.

Sex steroids may increase or rise above prepubertal levels if the dose is inadequate. Once a therapeutic dose has been established, gonadotropin and sex steroid levels will decline to prepubertal levels.

Gonadotropin-Releasing Hormone Analog

LEUPROLIDE ACETATE

Drug Interactions:

Drug/Lab test interactions: Since leuprolide suppresses the pituitary-gonadal system, diagnostic tests of pituitary gonadotropic and gonadal functions during treatment and up to 12 weeks after discontinuing leuprolide depot may be misleading.

Adverse Reactions:

Leuprolide Acetate Adverse Reactions (%)								
	Prostatic cancer				Endometriosis[1]		CPP	Uterine leiomyomata
Adverse Reaction	Leuprolide injection (n = 98)	DES (n = 101)	Leuprolide depot (monthly) (n = 56)	Leuprolide depot (3 month) (n = 94)	Leuprolide depot (n = 166)	Danazol (n = 136)	Leuprolide (n = 395)	Leuprolide depot (n = 66)
Cardiovascular								
ECG changes/ischemia	19.4	22	—	—	—	—	—	—
High blood pressure	8.2	5	—	< 5	—	—	—	—
Murmur	3.1	7.9	—	—	—	—	—	—
CHF/Heart failure	1	5	—	< 5	—	—	—	—
Thrombosis/phlebitis	2	9.9	—	—	—	—	—	—
Edema	12.2	29.7	12.5	< 5	7	14	< 2	5.4
CNS								
Depression/emotional lability	< 5	—	—	< 5	21	18	< 2	10.8
Insomnia/sleep disorders	7.1	5	< 5	8.5	2	4	—	< 5
Pain	13.3	12.9	7.1	26.6	19	18	2	8.4
Headache	7.1	4	—	6.4	31	22	< 2	25.9
Dizziness/lightheadedness	5.1	6.9	—	6.4	11	4	—	< 5
Nervousness	< 5	—	—	< 5	7	9	< 2	< 5
Paresthesias	< 5	—	< 5	< 5	8	9	—	< 5
Endocrine								
Androgen-like effects	—	—	—	—	15	32	—	< 5
↓ testicular size/atrophy	7.1	10.9	5.4	20.2	—	—	—	—
Impotence/↓libido	< 5	11.9	5.4	< 5	12	5	—	< 5
Gynecomastia/breast tenderness/changes	7.1	62.4	< 5	< 5	7	9	< 2	< 5
Hot flashes/sweats	56.1	11.9	58.9	58.5	81	57	—	72.9
GI								
GI disturbances	< 5	—	—	16	8	6	—	< 5
Anorexia	6.1	5	< 5	< 5	—	—	—	—
Constipation	7.1	8.9	—	—	—	—	—	—
Nausea/vomiting	5.1	16.8	5.4	—	13	13	< 2	< 5
Musculoskeletal								
Joint disorder/pain	< 5	—	—	11.7	8	8	—	7.8
Myalgia	3.1	8.9	< 5	—	2	6	—	< 5
Bone pain	5.1	2	< 5	—	—	—	—	—
Neuromuscular disorders	—	—	—	9.6	8	12	—	< 5
GU								
Vaginitis/bleeding/discharge	—	—	—	—	28	18	2	11.4
Urinary frequency/urgency/disorders	6.1	7.9	< 5	14.9	—	—	—	✓[2]
Hematuria	6.1	4	< 5	—	—	—	—	—
Urinary tract infection	3.1	6.9	—	—	—	—	—	—
Miscellaneous								
Dyspnea	2	7.9	5.4	—	—	—	—	—
Sinus congestion	5.1	5.9	—	—	—	—	—	—
Weight gain/loss	—	—	< 5	—	12	28	< 2	< 5
Anemia	5.1	5	—	< 5	—	—	—	—
Dermatitis/skin reactions/acne/seborrhea	5.1	7.9	< 5	8.5	10	15	2	< 5
Asthenia	10.2	9.9	5.4	7.4	4	8	—	8.4

[1] Percentages approximate.

[2] Occurred; no incidence given.

Gonadotropin-Releasing Hormone Analog

LEUPROLIDE ACETATE

Leuprolide injection and depot:

Cardiovascular – Angina, cardiac arrhythmias (< 5%) ; hypotension (< 5%, 3 month depot); vasodilation (< 2% in CPP); TIA/stroke.

CNS – Anxiety (< 5%); peripheral neuropathy, memory disorder (< 5%, injection); syncope (< 2% in CPP; < 5%, injection); personality disorder, somnolence (< 2% in CPP); hearing disorder, spinal fracture/paralysis.

Dermatologic – Injection site reactions including abscess (13.8%, 3 month depot; 5% in CPP); hair growth (< 5%, depot); ecchymosis (< 5%, injection); hair loss (< 5%, injection; < 2% in CPP); skin striae, rash including erythema multiforme (2% in CPP).

GI – Diarrhea, taste disorders/perversion (< 5%); dysphagia (< 5%, injection; < 2% in CPP); gingivitis (< 2% in CPP); hepatic dysfunction.

GU – Testicular pain, dysuria (< 5%); incontinence (< 5%, injection; < 2% in CPP); cervix disorder (< 2% in CPP); penile swelling, prostate pain, increased libido.

Musculoskeletal – Pelvic fibrosis, ankylosing spondylosis.

Respiratory – Respiratory disorders (6.4%, 3 month depot); pneumonia (< 5%); hemoptysis (< 5%, depot); epistaxis (< 5%, 3 month depot; < 2% in CPP); pulmonary infiltrates.

Miscellaneous – Ophthalmic disorder /abnormal vision, diabetes, fever, chills (< 5%); hard nodule in throat (< 5%, depot); tinnitus (< 5%, 3 month depot); infection (< 5%, injection; < 2% in CPP); body odor (< 5%, depot; < 2% in CPP); accelerated sexual maturity (< 2% in CPP).

Lab test abnormalities – Increased BUN (≥ 5%, 3 month depot; < 5%, injection); increased calcium (< 5%); increased uric acid (< 5%, depot); hypoproteinemia, decreased WBC.

Leuprolide depot:

Cardiovascular – Tachycardia (< 5%); bradycardia, heart failure, varicose vein (< 5%, 3 month depot); palpitations.

CNS – Delusions, hypesthesia (< 5%, 3 month depot); confusion.

Endocrine – Menstrual disorder (< 5%); lactation.

GI – Duodenal ulcer, dry mouth, appetite changes (< 5%); thirst (< 5%, 3 month depot); glossitis.

GU – Penis disorder, testis disorder (< 5%, 3 month depot); pyelonephritis.

Respiratory – Rhinitis (< 5%); pharyngitis, pleural effusion (< 5%, 3 month depot).

Miscellaneous – Conjunctivitis, nail disorder, flu syndrome (< 5%); enlarged abdomen, lymphedema, amblyopia, dehydration, dry eyes (< 5%, 3 month depot); lymphadenopathy.

Lab test abnormalities – LDH (> 2 N) (19.6%); SGOT (> 2 N), alkaline phosphatase (> 1.5 N) (5.4%); hyperglycemia, hyperlipidemia (total cholesterol, LDL cholesterol, triglycerides), hyperphosphatemia, abnormal liver function tests, increased PT, increased PTT, decreased platelets, decreased potassium, increased WBC (≥ 5%, 3 month depot).

Endometriosis: In clinical trials, SGOT (AST) was > 2 x the ULN in 1 patient. There was no other clinical or laboratory evidence of abnormal liver function.

Uterine leiomyomata: Post-treatment transaminase levels were ≥ 2 x the baseline value and ULN in 5 (3%) patients. There were no other clinical symptoms.

Leuprolide injection (< 5%):

Cardiovascular – Myocardial infarction, pulmonary embolism.

CNS – Lethargy, mood swings, numbness, blackouts, fatigue.

Dermatologic – Carcinoma of skin/ear, dry skin, itching, pigmentation, skin lesions.

GI – GI bleeding, peptic ulcer, rectal polyps.

GU – Bladder spasms, urinary obstruction.

Respiratory – Cough, pleural rub, pulmonary fibrosis.

Miscellaneous – Thyroid enlargement, hypoglycemia, increased creatinine, inflammation, swelling (temporal bone), blurred vision.

Overdosage:

In rats, SC administration of 250 to 500 times the recommended human dose, resulted in dyspnea, decreased activity and local irritation at the injection site.

Patient Information:

Patient package insert is available with each injection kit. Patient information is available from the manufacturer (1-800-622-2011).

Do not discontinue medication except on advice of physician.

Patients should use nonhormonal methods of contraception. Advise patients to see their physician if they believe they may be pregnant. If the patient becomes pregnant during treatment, discontinue the drug and apprise the patient of the potential risk to fetus.

Gonadotropin-Releasing Hormone Analog

LEUPROLIDE ACETATE

Prostatic cancer: May cause increased bone pain and increased difficulty in urinating during the first few weeks of treatment. May cause hot flashes, injection site irritation (eg, burning, itching, swelling) and may cause or aggravate nerve symptoms; notify physician if these become pronounced.

CPP: Prior to starting therapy the parent or guardian must be aware of the importance of continuous therapy. Adherence to 4 week drug administration schedules must be accepted if therapy is to be successful.

During the first 2 months of therapy, a female may experience menses or spotting. If bleeding continues beyond the second month, notify the physician.

Report any irritation at the injection site to the physician immediately.

Report any unusual signs or symptoms to the physician.

Endometriosis/Uterine leiomyomata: Effective doses of leuprolide depot should stop menstruation; notify physician if it persists. Successive missed doses may cause breakthrough bleeding or ovulation with the potential for conception. Do not use if pregnant, breastfeeding or in the presence of undiagnosed abnormal vaginal bleeding. Nonhormonal methods of birth control should be used during treatment. Adverse reactions associated with hypoestrogenism include: Hot flashes, headaches, emotional lability, decreased libido, acne, myalgia, decreased breast size, vaginal dryness. Estrogen levels return to normal after treatment discontinuation. (Also see Bone Density Changes in Precautions.)

Administration and Dosage:

Advanced prostate cancer:

Injection – 1 mg SC daily. Use the syringes included in the kit.

Depot –

Monthly: 7.5 mg IM monthly . Do not use needles smaller than 22 gauge. Reconstitute only with the diluent provided.

3 month depot: 22.5 mg every 3 months (84 days). Due to different release characteristics, a fractional dose of the 3 month depot formulation is not equivalent to the same dose of the monthly formulation and should not be given.

Central precocious puberty (CPP): Individualize dosage on a mg/kg basis. Younger children require higher doses on a mg/kg ratio:

Injection – May be administered by a patient/parent or healthcare professional. Recommended starting dose is 50 mcg/kg/day as a single SC injection. If total downregulation is not achieved, titrate upward by 10 mcg/kg/day, which will be considered the maintenance dose.

Depot – Must be administered under physician supervision. Recommended starting dose is 0.3 mg/kg/4 weeks (minimum, 7.5 mg) as a single IM injection. Determine the starting dose as follows:

Leuprolide Depot Starting Dose for CPP	
Weight (kg)	Dose (mg)
≤ 25	7.5
> 25 to 37.5	11.25
> 37.5	15

If total downregulation is not achieved, titrate upward in 3.75 mg increments every 4 weeks, which will be considered the maintenance dose.

Injection/Depot – After 1 to 2 months of initiating therapy or changing doses, monitor to confirm downregulation. Monitor measurements of bone age for advancement every 6 to 12 months. Titrate the dose upwards until no progression of the condition is noted either clinically or by lab parameters. The first dose to result in adequate downregulation can probably be maintained for duration of therapy in most children. However, there are insufficient data to guide dosage adjustment as patients move into higher weight categories. Verify adequate downregulation in patients whose weight has increased significantly while on therapy. Vary the injection site periodically. Before age 11 in females and before age 12 in males, consider discontinuation of therapy.

Endometriosis/Uterine leiomyomata (depot only): 3.75 mg as a single monthly intramuscular injection.

Endometriosis – Recommended duration is 6 months. Retreatment cannot be recommended since safety data are not available. If the symptoms of endometriosis recur after a course of therapy and further treatment is contemplated, it is recommended that bone density be assessed before retreatment begins to ensure that values are within normal limits.

Gonadotropin-Releasing Hormone Analog

LEUPROLIDE ACETATE

Uterine leiomyomata (fibroids) – Recommended duration of therapy is up to 3 months. The symptoms associated with uterine leiomyomata will recur following discontinuation of therapy. If additional treatment is contemplated, assess bone density prior to initiation of therapy to ensure that values are within normal limits.

Depot preparation:

Monthly formulation – For a single IM injection, reconstitute the lyophilized microspheres. Using a 22 gauge needle, withdraw 1 ml diluent from amp; inject into vial. Shake well to obtain uniform suspension. It will appear milky. Withdraw entire contents into syringe and inject immediately.

3 month formulation – For a single IM injection, reconstitute the lyophilized microspheres. Using a 23 gauge needle, withdraw 1.5 ml diluent from amp; inject into vial. Shake well to obtain uniform suspension. It will appear milky. Withdraw entire contents into syringe and inject immediately.

Storage/Stablility:

Injection – Refrigerate until dispensed. Patients may store at room temperature ≤ 30°C (86°F). Avoid freezing. Protect from light; store vial in carton until use.

Depot – May be stored at room temperature. The suspension is stable for 24 hours following reconstitution; however, since the product does not contain a preservative, discard if not used immediately.

Rx	**Lupron** (TAP Pharm.)	**Injection:** 5 mg/ml	In 2.8 ml multiple-dose vials supplied with 14 (2 week kit) or 28 (4 week kit) syringes, or 6-pack vials only.
Rx	**Lupron Depot** (TAP Pharm.)	**Lyophilized microspheres for injection:**[1] 3.75 mg	Preservative free. Single-dose vial with diluent.
		7.5 mg	Preservative free. Single-dose vial with diluent and syringe.
Rx	**Lupron Depot-Ped** (TAP Pharm.)	**Lyophilized microspheres for injection:**[1] 7.5 mg	Preservative free. Single-dose kit containing 7.5 mg vial leuprolide, 1.5 ml amp diluent, syringe and needle.
		11.25 mg	Preservative free. Single-dose kit containing 3.75 mg and 7.5 mg vials leuprolide, 1.5 ml amp diluent, syringe and needle.
		15 mg	Preservative free. Single-dose kit containing two 7.5 mg vials leuprolide, 1.5 ml amp diluent, syringe and needle.
Rx	**Lupron Depot - 3 Month** (TAP Pharm)	**Lyophilized microspheres for injection:**[1] 22.5 mg	Preservative free. Single use kit containing 22.5 mg vial leuprolide with 1.5 ml diluent.

[1] Listed as total dose; vials are combined to provide proper strength.

Gonadotropin-Releasing Hormone Analog

GOSERELIN ACETATE

Actions:

Pharmacology: Goserelin acetate is a synthetic decapeptide analog of luteinizing hormone-releasing hormone (LHRH or GnRH). It acts as a potent inhibitor of pituitary gonadotropin secretion when administered in the biodegradable formulation. Following initial administration in males, the drug causes an initial increase in serum luteinizing hormone (LH) and follicle stimulating hormone (FSH) values with subsequent increases in serum levels of testosterone. Chronic administration leads to sustained suppression of pituitary gonadotropins; serum levels of testosterone consequently fall into the range normally seen in surgically castrated men approximately 2 to 4 weeks after initiation of therapy. This leads to accessory sex organ regression. In clinical trials with follow-up of > 2 years, suppression of serum testosterone to castrate levels has been maintained for the duration of therapy.

In females, a similar down-regulation of the pituitary gland by chronic exposure to goserelin leads to suppression of gonadotropin secretion, a decrease in serum estradiol to levels consistent with the postmenopausal state, and would be expected to lead to a reduction of ovarian size and function, reduction in the size of the uterus and mammary gland, as well as a regression of sex hormone-responsive tumors, if present. Serum estradiol is suppressed to levels similar to those observed in postmenopausal women within 3 weeks following initial administration; however, after this suppression was attained, isolated estradiol elevations were seen in 10% of patients in the clinical trials. Serum LH and FSH are suppressed to follicular phase levels within 4 weeks after initial administration and are usually maintained in that range with continued use of goserelin. In ≤ 5% of women treated with goserelin, FSH and LH levels may not be suppressed to follicular phase levels on day 28 post-treatment with use of a single 3.6 mg depot injection. In certain individuals, suppression of these hormones to such levels may not be achieved with goserelin. With the 3.6 mg implant, estradiol, LH and FSH levels return to pretreatment values within 12 weeks following the last implant administration in all but rare cases.

Pharmacokinetics: In the 3.6 mg implant, peak serum concentrations are achieved 12 to 15 days after SC administration in males; mean peak serum concentrations are ≈ 2.84 and 1.46 ng/ml in males and females, respectively.

Goserelin 3.6 mg implant is absorbed at a much slower rate initially for the first 8 days, and then there is more rapid and continuous absorption for the remainder of the 28 day dosing period. Despite the change in the releasing rate of goserelin, administration every 28 days resulted in testosterone levels that were suppressed to and maintained in the range normally seen in surgically castrated men. Administration of 3.6 mg results in measurable concentrations of the drug in serum throughout the 28 day dosing period.

In clinical trials with the 3.6 mg solution formulation, male subjects with impaired renal function (creatinine clearance < 20 ml/min) had a serum elimination half-life of 12.1 hours compared to 4.2 hours for subjects with normal renal function. However, in clinical trials with the 3.6 mg formulation of goserelin, the incidence of adverse events is unknown in patients with impaired renal function.

Clearance of goserelin following SC administration of the 3.6 mg solution formulation is very rapid and occurs via a combination of hepatic metabolism and urinary excretion.

Clinical trials:

Prostatic carcinoma –

3.6 mg implant: In controlled studies of patients with advanced prostatic cancer comparing goserelin to orchiectomy, the long-term endocrine responses and objective responses were similar between the two treatments. Additionally, duration of survival was similar between the two treatments in a major comparative trial.

10.8 mg implant: In studies iwth advanced prostatic cancer, the 10.8 mg implant produced a pharmacodynamically similar effect in terms of suppression of serum testosterone to that achieved with the 3.6 mg implant. Clinical outcome similar to that produced with the use of goserelin 3.6 mg implant administered every 28 days is predicted with the 10.8 mg implant administered every 12 weeks.

Endometriosis – In controlled clinical studies using the 3.6 mg formulation every 28 days for 6 months, goserelin was as effective as danazol in relieving clinical symptoms (eg, dysmenorrhea, dyspareunia, pelvic pain) and signs (eg, pelvic tenderness, pelvic induration) of endometriosis and decreasing the size of endometrial lesions as determined by laparoscopy. The clinical significance of a decrease in endometriotic lesions is not known at this time; goserelin led to amenorrhea in 80% to 92% of all treated women within 8 weeks after initial administration. Menses usually resumed within 8 weeks following completion of therapy. Within 4 weeks fol-

Gonadotropin-Releasing Hormone Analog

GOSERELIN ACETATE

lowing initial administration, clinical symptoms were significantly reduced, and at the end of treatment were reduced by ≈ 84%.

Indications:

Prostatic carcinoma: Palliative treatment of advanced carcinoma of the prostate. Goserelin offers an alternative treatment of prostatic cancer when orchiectomy or estrogen administration are either not indicated or unacceptable to the patient.

3.6 mg only:

Endometriosis – Management of endometriosis, including pain relief and reduction of endometriotic lesions for the duration of therapy.

Advanced breast cancer – Palliative treatment of advanced breast cancer in pre- and perimenopausal women. Estrogen and progesterone receptor values may help to predict whether goserelin therapy is likely to be beneficial.

The 10.8 mg implant is not indicated in women as the data are insufficient to support reliable suppression of serum estradiol.

Contraindications:

Pregnancy, lactation, nondiagnosed vaginal bleeding (see Warnings); hypersensitivity to LHRH, LHRH agonist analogs or any component of the product.

Warnings:

Prostatic cancer worsening: Initially, goserelin, like other LHRH agonists, transiently increases serum levels of testosterone in men with prostate cancer of estrogen in women with breast cancer. Transient worsening of symptoms, or the occurrence of additional signs and symptoms of prostatic cancer, may occasionally develop during the first few weeks of treatment. Some patients may experience a temporary increase in bone pain, which can be managed symptomatically.

As with other LHRH agonists, isolated cases of exacerbation of disease symptoms, either ureteral obstruction or spinal cord compression, have been observed in prostate cancer patients. Monitor closely during first month of therapy. If spinal cord compression or renal impairment due to ureteral obstruction develops, institute standard treatment of these complications; in extreme cases, consider an immediate orchiectomy.

Hypercalcemia has occurred in some prostate and breast cancer patients with bone metastases after starting goserelin treatment. If hypercalcemia does occur, initiate appropriate treatment.

Lipids: In a controlled trial in women, 3.6 mg goserelin resulted in a minor but statistically significant effect on serum lipids. In patients treated for endometriosis, at 6 months following therapy initiation, goserelin increased LDL and HDL cholesterol by 21.3 and 2.7 mg/dl, respectively (vs. 33.3 mg/dl increase in LDL and a 21.3 mg/dl decrease in HDL with danazol). Triglycerides increased by 8 mg/dl with goserelin vs an 8.9 mg/dl decrease with danazol.

In endometriosis treatment, goserelin increased total cholesterol and LDL cholesterol during 6 months of treatment. However, goserelin resulted in HDL cholesterol levels that were significantly higher relative to danazol therapy. At the end of 6 months of treatment, HDL cholesterol fractions (HDL_2 and HDL_3) were decreased by 13.5 and 7.7 mg/dl, respectively, for danazol-treated patients compared with treatment increases of 1.9 and 0.8 mg/dl, respectively, for goserelin-treated patients.

Bone mineral density changes: After 6 months of treatment, 109 female patients treated with goserelin showed an average 4.3% decrease of vertebral trabecular bone mineral density (BMD) compared to pretreatment values. Patients (n = 66) were assessed for BMD loss 6 months after the completion of the 6-month therapy. Data from these patients showed an average 2.4% BMD loss compared to pretreatment values. Data from 28 patients at 12 months post-therapy showed an average decrease of 2.5% in BMD compared to pretreatment values. These data suggest a possibility of partial reversibility.

In patients with a history of treatment that may have resulted in bone mineral density loss or in patients with major risk factors for decreased bone mineral density such as chronic alcohol abuse or tobacco abuse, significant family history of osteoporosis, or chronic use of drugs that can reduce bone density such as anticonvulsants or corticosteroids, therapy may pose an additional risk. In these patients the risks and benefits must be weighed carefully before therapy is instituted.

Antibody formation: Among 115 goserelin-treated patients tested for development of binding to goserelin following treatment with goserelin, one patient showed low-titer binding to goserelin. On further testing of this patient's plasma obtained after treatment, her goserelin binding component was found not to be precipitated with rabbit antihuman immunoglobulin polyvalent sera. These findings suggest the possiblity of antibody formation.

Vaginal bleeding: During the first two months of goserelin use, some women experience vaginal bleeding of variable duration and intensity. In all likelihood, the bleeding represents estrogen withdrawal bleeding and is expected to stop spontaneously.

Carcinogenesis: Subcutaneous implant of goserelin in male and female rats once every 4 weeks for 1 year and recovery for 23 weeks at doses of about 3 to 9 times the recommended human dose resulted in an increased incidence of pituitary adenomas. An increased incidence of pituitary adenomas was also observed following SC implant of goserelin in rats at similar dose levels for a period of 72 weeks. The relevance of the rat pituitary adenomas to humans has not been established. SC implant of goserelin every 3 weeks for 2 years delivered to mice at doses of about 70 times the recommended human dose resulted in an increased incidence of histiocytic sarcoma of the vertebral column and femur.

Fertility impairment: Administration of goserelin led to gonadal suppression in both male and female rats as a result of its endocrine action. In male rats treated at 30 to 60 times the recommended monthly dose for a 70 kg human, a decrease in weight and atrophic histological changes were observed in the testes, epididymis, seminal vesicle and prostate gland with complete suppression of spermatogenesis. In female rats treated with 3 to 60 times the recommended monthly dose for a 70 kg human, suppression of ovarian function led to decreased size and weight of ovaries and secondary sex organs, follicular development was arrested at the antral stage and the corpora lutea were reduced in size and number. Except for the testes, almost complete histologic reversal of these effects in males and females was observed several weeks after dosing was stopped; however, fertility and general reproductive performance were reduced in those that became pregnant after the drug was discontinued. Fertile matings occurred within 2 weeks after cessation of dosing, even though total recovery of reproductive function may not have occurred before mating took place; ovulation rate, corresponding implantation rate and number of live fetuses were reduced.

In male and female dogs, the suppression of fertility was fully reversible when drug treatment was stopped after continuous administration for 1 year.

Pregnancy: Category D (breast cancer); Category X (endometriosis). Studies in both rats and rabbits at doses 2 to 100 times the maximum recommended dose given during organogenesis have confirmed that this drug will increase pregnancy loss in a dose-related manner. Goserelin increased preimplantation loss, resorptions, abortions and decreased fetus and pup survival in rats. In rats and dogs, the drug suppressed ovarian function, decreased ovarian weight and size and led to atrophic changes in secondary sex organs. Further evidence suggests that fertility was reduced in female rats that became pregnant after goserelin was stopped. These effects are an expected consequence of the hormonal alterations produced by goserelin in humans. Also, in rats the incidence of umbilical hernia was significantly increased.

Before starting treatment with goserelin, pregnancy must be excluded. Its safe use during pregnancy has not been established; goserelin can cause fetal harm when administered to a pregnant woman. Do not use in women who are or who may become pregnant while receiving the drug. If goserelin is used during pregnancy or if pregnancy occurs while taking this drug, apprise the patient of the potential hazard to the fetus or potential risk for loss of the pregnancy due to possible hormonal imbalance as a result of the expected pharmacologic action of goserelin treatment. Advise women of childbearing potential to avoid becoming pregnant. Effective nonhormonal contraception must by used by all premenopausal women during goserelin therapy and for 12 weeks following discontinuation of therapy. There are no adequate and well controlled studies in pregnant women using goserelin.

When used every 28 days, goserelin usually inhibits ovulation and stops menstruation. Contraception is not ensured.

Lactation: It is not known if goserelin is excreted in breast milk. Because of the potential for serious adverse reactions in nursing infants from goserelin, discontinue the drug prior to breastfeeding.

Children: Safety and efficacy have not been established. Goserelin use for endometriosis has been limited to women ≥ 18 years old and treated for 6 months.

Drug Interactions:

Drug/Lab test interactions: Goserelin suppresses the pituitary-gonadal system. Therefore, diagnostic tests of pituitary-gonadotropic and gonadal functions conducted dur-

Gonadotropin-Releasing Hormone Analog

GOSERELIN ACETATE

ing treatment and until resumption of menses may show misleading results. Normal function is usually restored within 12 weeks of treatment discontinuation.

Adverse Reactions:

Goserelin Adverse Reactions in Males (%)			
Adverse Reaction	Goserelin 3.6 mg (n = 242)	Orchiectomy (n = 254)	Goserelin 10.8 mg (n = 157)
Hot flashes	62	53	64
Sexual dysfunction	21	15	-
Decreased erections	18	16	-
Lower urinary tract symptoms	13	8	-
Lethargy	8	4	-
Pain (may have worsened in the first 30 days)	8	3	14
Edema	7	8	-
Upper respiratory infection	7	2	-
Rash	6	1	-
Sweating	6	4	-
Anorexia	5	2	-
Chronic obstructive pulmonary disease	5	3	-
Congestive heart failure	5	1	
Dizziness	5	4	1 to < 5%
Insomnia	5	1	-
Nausea	5	2	-
Complications of surgery	0	18	-

Goserelin Adverse Reactions in Endometriosis (%)					
Adverse Reaction	Goserelin (n = 411)	Danazol (n = 207)	Adverse Reaction	Goserelin (n = 411)	Danazol (n = 207)
Hot flashes	96	67	Nausea	8	14
Vaginitis	75	43	Hirsutism	7	15
Headache	75	63	Breast pain	7	4
Libido decreased	61	44	Abdominal pain	7	7
Emotional lability	60	56	Back pain	7	13
Depression	54	48	Dizziness	6	4
Sweating	45	30	Application site reaction	6	-
Acne	42	55			
Breast atrophy	33	42	Flu syndrome	5	5
Seborrhea	26	52	Pharyngitis	5	2
Peripheral edema	21	34	Hair disorders	4	11
Breast enlargement	18	15	Voice alterations	3	8
Pelvic symptoms	18	23	Myalgia	3	11
Pain	17	16	Nervousness	3	5
Dyspareunia	14	5	Weight gain	3	23
Infection	13	11	Leg cramps	2	6
Libido increased	12	19	Increased appetite	2	5
Asthenia	11	13	Pruitus	2	6
Insomnia	11	4	Hypertonia	1	10

Goserelin Adverse Reactions in Advanced Breast Cancer (%)		
Adverse reaction	Goserelin (n = 57)	Oophorectomy (n = 55)
Hot flashes	70	47
Tumor flare	23	4
Nausea	11	7
Malaise/fatigue/lethargy	5	2
Vomiting	4	7

Males: Goserelin is generally well tolerated; withdrawal from treatment was rare. As seen with other hormonal therapies, the most commonly observed adverse events were due to the expected physiological effects from decreased testosterone levels, including hot flashes, sexual dysfunction and decreased erections.

Metabolic/Nutritional – Gout, hyperglycemia, weight increase (> 1% to < 5% in 3.6 mg); diabetes mellitus (> 1% to < 5% in 10.8 mg).

Cardiovascular – Cerebrovascular accident (> 1% to < 5%); arrhythmia, hypertension, myocardial infarction, peripheral vascular disorder, chest pain (> 1% to < 5% in 3.6 mg); angina pectoris, cerebral ischemia, heart failure, pulmonary embolus, varicose veins (> 1% to < 5% in 10.8 mg).

CNS – Asthenia (5% in 10.8 mg); anxiety, depression, headache (> 1% to < 5% in 3.6 mg); paresthesia (> 1% to < 5% in 10.8 mg).

GI – Diarrhea (> 1% to < 5%); constipation, diarrhea, ulcer, vomiting (> 1% to < 5% in 3.6 mg); hematemesis (> 1% to < 5% in 10.8 mg).

GU – Gynecomastia (8% in 10.8 mg); renal insufficiency, urinary obstruction, urinary tract infection (> 1% to < 5% in 3.6 mg); bladder neoplasm, hematuria, impotence, urinary frequency/incontinence, urinary tract disorder, impaired urination, urinary tract infection (> 1% to < 5% in 10.8 mg).

Respiratory – Cough increased, dyspnea, pneumonia (> 1% to < 5% in 10.8 mg).

Miscellaneous – Pelvic/bone pain (6% in 10.8 mg; see Warnings); anemia (> 1% to < 5%); chills, fever, breast pain/swelling/tenderness (> 1% to < 5% in 3.6 mg); abdominal/back pain, flu syndrome, sepsis, aggravation reaction, herpes simplex, pruritus, peripheral edema (> 1% to < 5% in 10.8 mg); injection site reaction (< 1% in 3.6 mg).

Females (3.6 mg implant only):

Body as a whole – Allergic reaction, chest pain, fever, malaise, edema, ecchymosis (≥ 1%).

Cardiovascular – Hemorrhage, hypertension, migraine, palpitations, tachycardia (≥ 1%).

GI – Anorexia, constipation, diarrhea, dry mouth, dyspepsia, flatulence (≥ 1%).

Musculoskeletal – Arthralgia, joint disorder (≥ 1%); bone mineral density changes (see Warnings).

CNS – Anxiety, paresthesia, somnolence, abnormal thinking (≥ 1%).

Respiratory – Bronchitis, cough increased, epistaxis, rhinitis, sinusitis (≥ 1%).

Dermatologic – Alopecia, dry skin, rash, skin discoloration (≥ 1%).

Special Senses – Amblyopia, dry eyes (≥ 1%).

GU – Dysmenorrhea, urinary frequency, urinary tract infection, vaginal hemorrhage (see Warnings).

Lab test abnormalities – Elevation of liver enzymes (AST, ALT; < 1%) with no other evidence of abnormal liver function; changes in serum lipids (see Warnings).

Miscellaneous – Acne, hair disorders, osteoporosis and voice alterations have also occurred with the 3.6 mg implant.

Overdosage:

There is no experience of overdosage. If overdosage occurs, manage symptomatically. Refer to General Management of Acute Overdosage.

Patient Information:

Females (3.6 mg only): Since menstruation should stop with effective doses of goserelin, the patient should notify her physician if regular menstruation persists. Patients missing one or more successive doses may experience breakthrough menstrual bleeding. As with other hormonal interventions that disrupt the pituitary-gonadal axis, some patients may have delayed return to menses. The rare patient, however, may experience persistent amenorrhea.

Use of goserelin in pregnancy is contraindicated in women being treated for endometriosis. Therefore, use a nonhormonal method of contraception during treatment. Advise patients that if they miss one or more successive doses, breakthrough menstrual bleeding or ovulation may occur with the potential for conception. If a patient becomes pregnant during treatment of endometriosis, discontinue treatment and advise the patient of the possible risks to the pregnancy and fetus. (See Warnings.)

Adverse events occurring most frequently are associated with hypoestrogenism. The most frequently reported are hot flashes (flushes), headache, vaginal dryness, emotional lability, change in libido, depression, sweating and change in breast size.

Treatment induces a hypoestrogenic state which results in a loss of bone mineral density over the course of treatment, some of which may not be reversible.

Males: Carefully consider the use of goserelin in patients at particular risk of developing ureteral obstruction or spinal cord compression, and monitor the patients closely

Gonadotropin-Releasing Hormone Analog

GOSERELIN ACETATE

during the first month of therapy. Patients with ureteral obstruction or spinal cord compression should have appropriate treatment prior to iniation of goserelin.

Administration and Dosage:

Monthly (3.6 mg) implant: Administer SC every 28 days into the upper abdominal wall. Local anesthesia may be used prior to injection. While a delay of a few days is permissible, attempt to adhere to the 28 day schedule.

3 Month (10.8 mg) implant: Administer SC every 12 weeks into the upper abdominal wall. Local aneshthesia may be used prior to injection. While a delay of a few days is permissible, attempt to adhere to the 12–week schedule.

Prostatic carcinoma: Intended for long-term administration unless clinically inappropriate.

Endometriosis: Recommended duration is 6 months. Currently, there are no clinical data on the effect of treatment of benign gynecological conditions with goserelin for periods > 6 months. Retreatment cannot be recommended since safety data are not available. If symptoms recur after a course of therapy, and further treatment is contemplated, consider monitoring bone mineral density.

Renal/Hepatic function impairment: No dosage adjustment is necessary.

Administration technique: 1) Do not remove the sterile syringe until immediately before use. Examine syringe for damage and make sure the drug is visible in the translucent chamber. 2) After cleaning with an alcohol swab, a local anesthetic may be used on an area of skin on the upper abdominal wall. 3) Stretch the patient's skin with one hand, and grip the needle with fingers around the barrel of the syringe. Insert the hypodermic needle into the SC fat. Do not aspirate. If the hypodermic needle penetrates a large vessel, blood will be seen instantly in the syringe chamber. If a vessel is penetrated, withdraw the needle and inject elsewhere with a new syringe. 4) Change the direction of the needle so it parallels the abdominal wall. Push the needle in until the barrel hub touches the patient's skin. Withdraw the needle 1 cm to create a space to discharge the drug; fully depress the plunger to discharge. 5) Withdraw needle and bandage the site. Confirm discharge by ensuring tip of the plunger is visible within the tip of the needle.

In the unlikely event of the need to surgically remove goserelin, it can be localized by ultrasound.

Rx	**Zoladex** (Zeneca)	**Implant:** 3.6 mg	In preloaded syringes (16 gauge needle).
		10.8 mg	In preloaded syringes (14 gauge needle).

Aromatase Inhibitor

ANASTROZOLE

Actions:

Pharmacology: Anastrozole is a potent and selective non-steroidal aromatase inhibitor. It significantly lowers serum estradiol concentrations and has no detectable effect on formation of adrenal corticosteroids or aldosterone.

Many breast cancers have estrogen receptors, and growth of these tumors can be stimulated by estrogens. In post-menopausal women, the principal source of circulating estrogen (primarily estradiol) is conversion of adrenally generated androstenedione to estrone by aromatase in peripheral tissues, such as adipose tissue, with further conversion of estrone to estradiol.

Treatment of breast cancer has included efforts to decreased estrogen levels by ovariectomy premenopausally and by use of anti-estrogens and progestational agents both pre- and post-menopausally, and these interventions lead to decreased tumor mass or delayed progression of tumor growth in some women.

Clinically significant suppression of serum estradiol was seen with all doses. The recommended daily dose (1 mg) reduced estradiol by ≈ 70% within 24 hours and by ≈ 80% after 14 days of daily dosing. Suppression of serum estradiol was maintained for up to 6 days after cessation of daily dosing with 1 mg.

Anastrozole did not affect cortisol or aldosterone secretion at baseline or in response to ACTH. No glucocorticoid or mineralocorticoid replacement therapy is necessary with anastrozole.

Pharmacokinetics: Inhibition of aromatase activity is primarily due to anastrozole, the parent drug. Orally administered anastrozole is well absorbed into the systemic circulation with 83% to 85% of the dose recovered in urine or feces. Food does affect the extent of absorption. Elimination of anastrozole is primarily via hepatic metabolism (≈ 85%) and to a lesser extent, renal excretion (≈ 11%). Anastrozole has a mean terminal elimination half-life of ≈ 50 hours in postmenopausal women. The major circulating metabolite of anastrozole, triazole, lacks pharmacologic activity. The pharmacokinetic parameters are similar in patients and in healthy postmenopausal volunteers. Consistent with the ≈ 2–day terminal elimination half-life, plasma concentrationsn approach steady-state levels at ≈ 7 days of once daily dosing and steady-state levels are ≈ 3– to 4–fold higher than levels observed after a single dose of anastrozole. Anastrozole is 40% bound to plasma proteins.

Studies in postmenopausal women demonstrated that anastrozole is extensively metabolized with ≈ 10% of the dose excreted in the urine as unchanged drug within 72 hours of dosing, and the remainder (≈ 60% of the dose) excreted in the urine as metabolites. Metabolism of anastrozole occurs by N-dealkylation, hydroxylation and glucuronidation. Three metabolites of anastrozole have been identified in human plasma and urine. The known metabolites are triazole, a glucuronide conjugate of hydroxyanastrozole and a glucuronide of anastrozole itself. Several minor metabolites have not been identified.

Clinical trials: Anastrozole was studied in two well controlled clinical trials in postmenopausal women with advanced breast cancer who had disease progression following tamoxifen therapy for either advanced or early breast cancer. Some of the patients had also received previous cytotoxic treatment. Most patients were ER (estrogen receptor)-positive. Patients were randomized to receive either a single daily dose of 1 or 10 mg anastrozole or 40 mg megestrol acetate 4 times a day.

Both trials included > 375 patients. Approximately 33% of the patients in each treatment group had either an objective response or stabilization of their disease for > 24 weeks. Of the 263 patients who received anastrozole 1 mg, there were six complete responders and 21 partial responders. In those who had an objective response, > 60% responded for > 6 months and > 15% responded for > 12 months. Both anastrozole 1 and 10 mg were similar in efficacy to megestrol acetate.

Indications:

Breast cancer, advanced: Treatment of advanced breast cnacer in postmenopausal women with disease progression following tamoxifen therapy.

Patients with ER-negative disease and patients who did not respond to tamoxifen therapy rarely responded to anastrozole.

Warnings:

Endocrine effects: Anastrozole does not possess direct progestogenic, androgenic or estrogenic activity in animals, but does perturb the circulating levels of progesterone, androgens and estrogens.

Lipid profile: Mean serum total cholesterol levels increased by 0.5 mmol/L among patients receiving anastrozole. Increases in LDL cholesterol have been shown to contribute to these changes.

Aromatase Inhibitor

ANASTROZOLE

Renal function impairment: Anastrozole renal clearance decreased proportionally with creatinine clearance (Ccr) and was ≈ 50% lower in volunteers with severe renal impairment (Ccr < 30 ml/min/1.73m^2) compared with controls. Because only about 10% of anastrozole is excreted unchanged in the urine, the reduction in renal clearance did not influence the total body clearance. Dosage adjustment in patients with renal insufficiency is not necessary.

Hepatic function impairment: Hepatic metabolism accounts for ≈ 85% of anastrozole elimination. Anastrozole pharmacokinetics have been investigated in subjects with hepatic cirrhosis related to alcohol abuse. The apparent oral clearance (CL/F) of anastrozole was ≈ 30% lower in subjects with stable hepatic cirrhosis than in control subjects with normal liver function. However, plasma anastrozole concentrations in subjects with hepatic cirrhosis were within the range concentrations seen in normal subjects across all clinical trials. Therefore no dosage adjustment is needed.

Fertility impairment: Hypertrophy of the ovaries and the presence of follicular cysts in rats administered doses ≥ 1 mg/kg/day were found. In addition, hyperplastic uteri were observed in chronic studies of female dogs administered doses ≥ 1 mg/kg/day. It is not known whether these effects on the reproductive organs of animals are associated with impaired fertility in humans.

Elderly: In postmenopausal female volunteers and patients with breast cancer, no age-related effects were seen over the range < 50 to > 80 years of age. Fifty percent of patients were ≥ 65 years of age. Response rates and time to progression were similar for patients of all ages.

Pregnancy: Category C. Anastrozole can cause fetal harm when administered to a pregnant woman. Anastrozole has been found to cross the placenta following oral administration of 0.1 mg/kg in rats and rabbits (about ¾ and 1.5 times the recommended human dose, respectively). Administration during organogenesis showed anastrozole to increase pregnancy loss, increase resorption and decrease the number of live fetuses; these effects were dose-related.

There are no adequte and well-controlled studies in pregnant women. If anastrozole is used during pregnancy or if the patient becomes pregnant while receiving this drug, apprise the patient of the potential hazard to the fetus and risk for loss of the pregnancy.

Lactation: It is not known whether anastrozole is excreted in breast milk. Exercise caution when administering to a nursing woman.

Children: Safety and efficacy for use in children have not been established.

Precautions:

Laboratory tests: Three-fold elevations of mean serum gamma glutamyl transferase (GGT) levels have been observed among patients with liver metastases receiving anastrozole or megestrol acetate. These changes were likely related to the progression of liver metastases in these patients, although other contributing factors could not be ruled out.

Drug Interactions:

Anastrozole inhibited in vitro metabolic reactions catalyzed by cytochromes P450 1A2, 2C8/9 and 3A4, but only at relatively high concentrations. It is unlikely that coadministration of anastrozole with other drugs will result in clinically significant inhibition of cytochrome P450–mediated metabolism of the other drugs.

Adverse Reactions:

Anastrozole was generally well tolerated, with < 3.3% of the anastrozole-treated patients and 4% of the megestrol acetate-treated patients withdrawing because of an adverse reaction. The principal adverse reaction more common with anastrozole than megestrol acetate was diarrhea.

Adverse Reactions with Anastrozole vs Megestrol Acetate (%)

Adverse reaction	1 mg anastrozole (n = 262)	10 mg anastrozole (n = 246)	160 mg megestrol acetate (n = 253)
Asthenia	16	13.4	18.6
Nausea	15.6	19.5	11.1
Headache	13	17.9	9.5
Hot flushes	12.2	10.6	8.3
Pain	10.7	15.4	11.5
Back pain	10.7	10.6	7.5

Adverse Reactions with Anastrozole vs Megestrol Acetate (%)			
Adverse reaction	1 mg anastrozole (n = 262)	10 mg anastrozole (n = 246)	160 mg megestrol acetate (n = 253)
Dyspnea	9.2	11	20.9
Vomiting	9.2	10.6	6.3
Cough increased	8.4	7.3	7.5
Diarrhea	8.4	7.3	2.8
Constipation	6.9	7.3	8.3
Abdominal pain	6.9	5.7	7.1
Anorexia	6.9	7.7	4.3
Bone pain	6.5	11.8	7.5
Pharyngitis	6.1	9.3	5.9
Dizziness	6.1	4.9	5.9
Rash	5.7	6.1	7.5
Dry mouth	5.7	4.5	5.1
Peripheral edema	5.3	8.5	11.1
Pelvic pain	5.3	6.9	5.1
Depression	5.3	2.4	2
Chest pain	5	7.3	5.1
Paresthesia	4.6	6.1	3.6
Vaginal hemorrhage	2.3	1.6	5.1
Weight gain	1.5	3.7	11.9
Sweating	1.5	1.2	6.3
Increased appetite	0	0.4	5.1

Less frequent (2% to 5%) adverse reactions are listed below by decreasing frequency:

Body as a whole: Flu syndrome; fever; neck pain; malaise; accidental injury; infection; weight loss.

Cardiovascular: Hypertension; thrombophlebitis.

CNS: Somnolence; confusion; insomnia; anxiety; nervousness.

Dermatologic: Hair thinning; pruritus.

GU: Urinary tract infection; breast pain.

Hematologic: Anemia; leukopenia.

Lab test abnormalities: GGT, AST, ALT, alkaline phosphatase, total cholesterol and LDL cholesterol increased.

Musculoskeletal: Myalgia; arthralgia; pathalogical fracture.

Respiratory: Sinusistis; bronchitis; rhinitis.

Aromatase Inhibitor

ANASTROZOLE

Overdosage:

Single doses of ≤ 60 mg given to healthy male volunteers and ≤ 10 mg given to postmenopausal women with advanced breast cancer were well tolerated.

There is no specific antidote to overdosage. Treatment must by symptomatic. Vomiting may be induced if the patient is alert. Dialysis may be helpful because anastrozole is not highly protein bound. General supportive care, including frequent monitoring of all vital signs and close observation, is indicated. Refer to General Management of Acute Overdosage.

Administration and Dosage:

Approved by the FDA on December 27, 1995.

Breast cancer: 1 mg once daily.

Renal/Hepatic function imipairment: No changes in dose are recommended.

Rx	**Arimidex** (Zeneca)	**Tablets:** 1 mg	Lactose. (A/Adx 1). Biconvex. Film coated. In 30s.

Topoisomerase Inhibitors

TOPOTECAN HCl

Warning:

Do not give topotecan therapy to patients with baseline neutrophil counts of < 1500 cells/mm^3. In order to monitor the occurrence of bone marrow suppression, primarily neutropenia, which may be severe and result in infection and death, perform frequent peripheral blood cell counts on all patients receiving topotecan.

Actions:

Pharmacology: Topotecan HCl is a semi-synthetic derivative of camptothecin and is and anti-tumor drug with topoisomerase I-inhibitory activity. Topoisomerase I relieves torsional strain in DNA by inducing reversible single-strand breaks. Topotecan binds to the topoisomerase I-DNA complex and prevents religation of these single-strand breaks. The cytotoxicity of topotecan is thought to be due to double-strand DNA damage produced during DNA synthesis when replication enzymes interact with the ternary complex formed by topotecan, topoisomerase I and DNA.

Pharmacokinetics:

Metabolism/Excretion – Topotecan undergoes a reversible pH-dependent hydrolysis of its lactone moiety; it is the lactone form that is pharmacologically active. In vitro studies in human liver microsomes indicate that metabolism of topotecan to an N-demethylated metabolite represents a minor metabolic pathway.

About 30% of the dose is excreted in the urine and renal clearance is an important determinant of topotecan elimination.

Topotecan exhibits multiexponential pharmacokinetics with a terminal half-life of 2 to 3 hours. Total exposure (AUC) is approximately dose-proportional. Binding of topotecan to plasma proteins is ≈ 35%.

Renal impairment: In patients with mild renal impairment (creatinine clearance of 40 to 60 ml/min), topotecan plasma clearance was decreased to ≈ 67% of the value in patients with normal renal function. In patients with moderate renal impairment (Ccr of 20 to 39 ml/min), topotecan plasma clearance was reduced to ≈ 34% of the value in control patients, with an increase in half-life. Mean half-life, estimated in three renally impaired patients, was ≈ 5 hours (see Administration and Dosage).

Hepatic impairment: Plasma clearance in patients with hepatic impairment (serum bilirubin levels between 1.7 and 15 mg/dl) was decreased to ≈ 67% of the value in patients without hepatic impairment. Topotecan half-life increased slightly, from 2 to 2.5 hours, but these hepatically impaired patients tolerated the usual recommended topotecan dosage regimen.

Elderly: Topotecan pharmacokinetics have not been specifically studied in an elderly population, but population pharmacokinetic analysis in female patients did not identify age as a significant factor. Decreased renal clearance, common in the elderly, is a more important determinant of topotecan clearance.

Gender: The overall mean topotecan plasma clearance in male patients was ≈24% higher than in female patients, largely reflecting difference in body size.

Clinical trials: Two studies involving 223 patients given topotecan are mature enough for evaluation (although survival results are incomplete). Topotecan was compared with paclitaxel in a randomized trial involving 112 patients treated with topotecan (1.5 mg/m^2/day × 5 days starting on day 1 of a 21–day course) and 114 patients treated with paclitaxel (175 mg/m^2 over 3 hours on day 1 of a 21–day course). All patients had recurrent ovarian cancer after a platinum-containing regimen or had not responded to at least one prior platinum-containing regimen.

The time to response was longer with topotecan therapy compared with paclitaxel with a mean of 10 weeks (range, 3.1 to 24.1) vs 7 weeks (range, 2.4 to 12.3). Consequently, the efficacy of topotecan may not be achieved if patients are withdrawn from treatment prematurely.

In the crossover phase, 5 of 53 (9.4%) patients who received topotecan after paclitaxel had a partial response and 1 of 37 (2.7%) patients who received paclitaxel after topotecan had a complete response.

Topotecan was active in patients who had developed resistance to platinum-containing therapy, defined as tumor progression while on, or tumor relapse within 6 months after completion of, a platinum-containing regimen. One complete and seven partial responses were seen in 60 patients, for a response rate of 13%. In the same study, there were no complete responders and four partial responders on the paclitaxel arm, for a response rate of 7%.

Indications:

Ovarian cancer: Treatment of patients with metastatic carcinoma of the ovary after failure of initial or subsequent chemotherapy.

Topoisomerase Inhibitors

TOPOTECAN HCl

Contraindications:

Hypersensitivity to topotecan or to any of its ingredients; patients who are pregnant or breastfeeding; those with severe bone marrow depression.

Warnings:

Bone marrow suppression (primary neutropenia) is the dose-limiting toxicity of topotecan. Neutropenia is not cumulative over time. Administer topotecan only to patients with adequate bone marrow reserves, including baseline neutrophil counts of at least 1500 cells/mm^3 and platelet counts of at least 100,000/mm^3.

Neutropenia: Severe (< 500 cells/mm^3) neutropenia was most common during course 1 of treatment (60%) and occurred in 40% of all courses, with a median duration of 7 days. The nadir neutrophil count occurred at a median of 11 days. Prophylactic G-CSF was given in 27% of courses after the first cycle. Therapy-related sepsis or febrile neutropenia occurred in 26% of patients and sepsis was fatal in 0.7%.

Thrombocytopenia: Grade 4 thrombocytopenia (< 25,000/mm^3) occurred in 26% of patients and in 9% of courses, with a median duration of 5 days and a platelet nadir at a median of 15 days. There were no episodes of serious bleeding. Platelet transfusions were given to 13% of patients and in 4% of courses.

Anemia: Severe anemia (grade 3/4, < 8 g/dl) occurred in 40% of patients and in 16% of courses. Median nadir was at day 15. Transfusions were needed in 56% of patients and in 23% of courses.

Pregnancy: Category C. Topotecan may cause fetal harm when administered to a pregnant woman. The effects of topotecan on pregnant women have not been studied. If topotecan is used during pregnancy, or if a patient becomes pregnant while taking topotecan, warn her of the potential hazard to the fetus. Warn patients to avoid becoming pregnant.

Lactation: It is not known whether this drug is excreted in breast milk. Breastfeeding should be discontinued when administering topotecan.

Children: Safety and effectiveness in pediatric patients have not been established.

Precautions:

Monitoring: Institute frequent monitoring of peripheral blood cell counts during treatment with topotecan. Do not treat patients with subsequent courses of topotecan until neutrophils recover to > 1000 cells/mm^2, platelets recover to > 100,000 cells/mm^3 and hemoglobin levels recover to 9 mg/dl (with transfusion if necessary).

Extravasation with topotecan has been associated with only mild local reactions such as erythema and bruising.

Drug Interactions:

Pharmacokinetic studies of the interaction of topotecan with concomitantly administered medications have not been formally investigated. In vitro inhibition studies using marker substrates known to be metabolized by human P450 CYP1A2, CYP2A6, CYP2C8/9, CYP2C19, CYP2D6, CYP2E, CYP3A9 or CYP4A or dihydropyrimidine dehydrogenase indicate that the activities of these enzymes were not altered by topotecan. Enzyme inhibition by topotecan has not been evaluated in vivo.

Topotecan Drug Interactions

Precipitant drug	Object drug*		Description
G-CSF	Topotecan	⬆	Concomitant administration can prolong the duration of neutropenia. If G-CSF is used, do not initiate until day 6 of the course of therapy, 24 hours after completion of treatment with topotecan.
Cisplatin	Topotecan	⬆	Myelosuppression is more severe when topotecan was given in combination with cisplatin. There are no adequate data to define a safe and effective regimen for topotecan and cisplatin in combination.

* ⬆ = Object drug increased.

Adverse Reactions:

Data in this section are based on the experiences of 452 patients with metastatic ovarian carcinoma treated with topotecan.

Topoisomerase Inhibitors

TOPOTECAN HCl

Hemotologic Adverse Events in Patients Receiving Topotecan (%)	
Hematologic adverse events	Incidence (n = 452)
Neutropenia	
< 1500 cells/mm^3	98
< 500 cells/mm^3	81
Leukopenia	
< 3000 cells/mm^3	98
< 1000 cells/mm^3	32
Thrombocytopenia	
< 75,000 cells/mm^3	63
< 25,000 cells/mm^3	26
Anemia	
< 10 g/dl	95
< 8 g/dl	40
Sepsis or fever/infection with grade 4 neutropenia	26
Platelet transfusions	13
RBC transfusions	56

Comparative Toxicity Profiles for Ovarian Cancer Patients Randomized to Receive Topotecan or Paclitaxel				
	Topotecan		Paclitaxel	
Adverse event	Patients (n=112) %	Courses (n=555) %	Patients (n=114) %	Courses (n=550) %
Hematologic Grade 4				
Grade 4 neutropenia (< 500 cells/mm^3)	79.5	36.7	21.9	8.5
Grade 3/4 anemia (Hgb < 8 g/dl)	40.5	16	6.3	2
Grade 4 thrombocytopenia (< 25, 000 plts/ml)	25.3	9.6	1.8	0.4
Fever/Grade 4 neutropenia	23.2	5.4	2.6	0.5
Documented sepsis	5.4	1.1	1.8	0.4
Death related to sepsis	1.8	0.4	0	0
Non-Hematologic Grade 3/4				
GI				
Abdominal pain	5.4	1.1	3.5	0.9
Constipation	5.4	1.1	0	0
Diarrhea	6.3	1.6	0.9	0.2
Intestinal obstruction	4.5	1.1	4.4	0.9
Nausea	8.9	3.1	1.8	0.4
Stomatitis	0.9	0.2	0.9	0.2
Vomiting	9.8	2	2.6	0.5

Topoisomerase Inhibitors

TOPOTECAN HCl

Comparative Toxicity Profiles for Ovarian Cancer Patients Randomized to Receive Topotecan or Paclitaxel				
	Topotecan		Paclitaxel	
Adverse event	Patients (n=112) %	Courses (n=555) %	Patients (n=114) %	Courses (n=550) %
Body as a Whole				
Anorexia	3.6	0.2	0	0
Dyspnea	6.3	1.8	5.3	1.3
Fatigue	8	2.2	5.3	2
Malaise	1.8	0.5	1.8	0.4
CNS				
Arthralgia	0.9	0.2	3.5	0.5
Asthenia	5.4	1.8	3.5	1.3
Headache	0.9	0.2	1.8	0.9
Myalgia	0	0	2.6	1.6
Pain	5.4	1.1	10.5	2.2

GI: Nausea (77%); vomiting (58%); diarrhea (42%); constipation (3%); abdominal pain (3.3%).

Dermatologic: Total alopecia (42%).

CNS: Headache (21%) was the most frequently reported neurologic toxicity. Paresthesia occurred in 9% of patients but was generally Grade 1.

Hepatic: Grade 1 transient elevations in AST and ALT occurred in 5% of patients. Greater elevations, Grade 3/4, occurred in < 1%. Grade 3/4 elevated bilirubin occurred in < 3% of patients.

Respiratory: Dyspnea (20%); Grade 3/4 dyspnea (4%).

Overdosage:

There is no known antidote for overdosage with topotecan. The primary complication of overdosage would consist of bone marrow suppression.

Administration and Dosage:

The recommended dose of topotecan is 1.5 mg/m^2 by IV infusion over 30 minutes daily for 5 consecutive days, starting on day 1 of a 21–day course. A minimum of four courses is recommended because median time to response in three clinical trials was 9 to 12 weeks. In the event of severe neutropenia during any course, reduce the dose by 0.25 mg/m^2 for subsequent courses. Alternatively, in the event of severe neutropenia, G-CSF may be administered following the subsequent course (before resorting to dosage reduction) starting from day 6 of the course (24 hours after completion of topotecan administration).

Renal function impairment: No dosage adjustment appears to be required for treating patients with mild renal impairment (Ccr 40 to 60 ml/min). Dosage adjustment to 0.75 mg/m^2 is recommended for patients with moderate renal impairment (Ccr 20 to 39 ml/min). Insufficient data are available in patients with severe renal impairment to provide a dosage recommendation.

Preparation of IV infusion: Reconstitute each topotecan 4 mg vial with 4 ml Sterile Water for Injection. Then dilute the appropriate volume of the reconstituted solution either in 0.9% Sodium Chloride IV infusion or 5% Dextrose IV infusion.

Storage/Stability: Store the vials protected from light in the original cartons at controlled room temperature between 20° and 25°C (68° and 77°F). Reconstituted vials of topotecan diluted for infusion are stable at ≈ 20° to 25°C (68° to 77°F) and ambient lighting conditions for 24 hours.

Rx	**Hycamtin** (SmithKline Beecham)	**Powder for injection (lyophilized)**: 4 mg (free base) topotecan HCl	48 mg mannitol. In single-dose vials.

IRINOTECAN HCl

Actions:

Pharmacology: Irinotecan is a derivative of camptothecin. Camptothecins interact specifically with the enzyme topoisomerase I, which relieves torsional strain in DNA by inducing reversible single-strand breaks. Irinotecan and its active metabolite SN-38 bind to the topoisomerase I-DNA complex and prevent religation of these single-strand breaks. Current research suggests that the cytotoxicity of irinotecan is due to double-strand DNA damage produced during DNA synthesis when replication enzymes interact with the ternary complex formed by topoisomerase I, DNA and either irinotecan or SN-38. Mammalian cells cannot efficiently repair these double-strand breaks.

In vitro cytotoxicity assays show that the potency of SN-38 relative to irinotecan varies from 2- to 2000-fold. The precise contribution of SN-38 to the activity of irinotecan is thus unknown.

Pharmacokinetics:

Metabolism/Excretion – The metabolic conversion of irinotecan to the active metabolite SN-38 is mediated by carboxylesterase enzymes and primarily occurs in the liver. SN-38 subsequently undergoes conjugation to form a glucuronide metabolite. SN-38 glucuronide had 1/50 to 1/100 the activity of SN-38 in cytotoxicity assays using two cell lines in vitro. The disposition of irinotecan has not been fully elucidated in humans. The urinary excretion of irinotecan is 11% to 20%; SN-38, < 1%; and SN-38 glucuronide, 3%. The cumulative biliary and urinary excretion of irinotecan and its metabolites (SN-38 and SN-38 glucuronide) over a period of 48 hours following irinotecan administration in two patients ranged from ≈ 25% (100 mg/m²) to 50% (300 mg/m²).

After IV infusion of irinotecan in humans, plasma concentrations decline in a multiexponential manner, with a mean terminal elimination half-life of ≈ 6 hours. The mean terminal elimination half-life of the active metabolite SN-38 is ≈ 10 hours. The half-lives of the lactone (active) forms of irinotecan and SN-38 are similar to those of total irinotecan and SN-38, as the lactone and hydroxy acid forms are in equilibrium.

Over the dose range of 50 to 350 mg/m², the AUC of irinotecan increases linearly with dose; the AUC of SN-38 increases less than proportionally with dose. Maximum concentrations of the active metabolite SN-38 are generally seen within 1 hour following the end of a 90-minute infusion of irinotecan.

Irinotecan exhibits moderate plasma protein binding (30% to 68% bound). SN-38 is highly bound to human plasma proteins (≈ 95% bound). The plasma protein to which irinotecan and SN-38 predominantly binds is albumin.

Mean Irinotecan and SN-38 Pharmacokinetic Parameters in Patients with Metastatic Carcinoma of the Colon and Rectum (n = 64)

Dose (mg/m²)	Irinotecan C_{max}[1] (ng/ml)	Irinotecan AUC_{0-24}[2] (ng•hr/ml)	Irinotecan $t_{1/2}$[3] (hr)	Irinotecan V_{area}[4] (L/m²)	Irinotecan CL[5] (L/hr/m²)	SN-38 C_{max} (ng/ml)	SN-38 AUC_{0-24} (ng•hr/ml)	SN-38 $t_{1/2}$ (hr)
125	1660	10200	5.8	110	13.3	26.3	229	10.4

[1] C_{max} = Maximum plasma concentration.
[2] AUC_{0-24} = Area under the plasma concentration-time curve from time 0 to 24 hours after the end of the 90-minute infusion.
[3] $t_{1/2}$ = Terminal elimination half-life.
[4] V_{area} = Volume of distribution of terminal elimination phase.
[5] CL = Total systemic clearance.

Elderly: The terminal half-life of irinotecan was 6 hours in patients who were ≥65 years of age and 5.5 hours in patients < 65 years of age. Dose-normalized AUC_{0-24} for SN-38 in patients who were ≥ 65 years of age was 11% higher than in patients < 65 years. No change in dosage and administration is recommended.

Clinical trials: In the intent-to-treat analysis of the pooled data from three studies, 193 of 304 patients began therapy at the recommended starting dose of 125 mg/m². Among 193 patients, 2 complete and 27 partial responses were observed, for an overall response rate of 15% at this starting dose. A considerably lower response rate was seen with a starting dose of 100 mg/m². The majority of responses were observed within the first two courses of therapy, and all but one of the responses were observed by the fourth course of therapy (one response was seen after the eighth course). The response duration (median) for patients beginning therapy at 125 mg/m² was 5.8 months.

IRINOTECAN HCl

Indications:

Metastatic carcinoma of the colon or rectum: Irinotecan injection is indicated for the treatment of metastatic carcinoma of the colon or rectum in patients whose disease has recurred or progressed following 5–FU-based therapy.

Contraindications:

Hypersensitivity to irinotecan.

Warnings:

Diarrhea: Irinotecan injection can induce early and late forms of diarrhea that appear to be mediated by different mechanisms. Early diarrhea (occurring during or within 24 hours of irinotecan administration) is cholinergic in nature. It can be severe but is usually transient. It may be preceded by complaints of diaphoresis and abdominal cramping. Early diarrhea may be ameliorated by atropine 0.25 to 1 mg IV.

Late diarrhea (occurring more than 24 hours after irinotecan administration) can be prolonged, may lead to dehydration and electrolyte imbalances, and can be life-threatening. Treat late diarrhea promptly with loperamide. Carefully monitor patients with severe diarrhea and give fluid and electrolyte replacement if they become dehydrated. National Cancer Institute (NCI) grade 3 diarrhea is defined as an increase of 7 to 9 stools daily, or incontinence or severe cramping. NCI grade 4 diarrhea is defined as an increase of ≥ 10 stools daily, or grossly bloody stool, or need for parenteral support. If grade 3 or 4 late diarrhea occurs, delay administration until patient recovers and decrease subsequent doses. (See Administration and Dosage.)

Irradiation: Patients who have previously received pelvic/abdominal irradiation are at an increased risk of severe myelosuppression following irinotecan administration. The concurrent administration of irinotecan with irradiation has not been adequately studied and is not recommended.

Myelosuppression: Deaths due to sepsis following severe myelosuppression have been reported in patients treated with irinotecan. Temporarily discontinue therapy if neutropenic fever occurs or if the absolute neutrophil count drops below 500/mm^3. Reduce the irinotecan dose if there is a clinically significant decrease in the total white blood cell count (< 2000/mm^3), neutrophil count (< 1000/mm^3), hemoglobin (< 8 g/dl) or platelet count (< 100,000/mm^3) (see Administration and Dosage). Routine administration of a colony-stimulating factor (CSF) is not necessary, but physicians may consider CSF use in patients experiencing significant neutropenia.

Orthostatic hypotension: Dizziness may sometimes have represented symptomatic evidence of orthostatic hypotension in patients with dehydration.

Elderly: Exercise particular caution in monitoring the effects of irinotecan in the elderly (≥ 65 years).

Pregnancy: Category D. Irinotecan may cause fetal harm when administered to a pregnant woman. There are no adequate and well controlled studies in pregnant women. If the drug is used during pregnancy, or if the patient becomes pregnant while receiving the drug, apprise the patient of the potential hazard to the fetus. Advise women of childbearing potential to avoid becoming pregnant while receiving treatment with irinotecan.

Lactation: Because many drugs are excreted in breast milk and because of the potential for serious adverse reactions in nursing infants, discontinue nursing when receiving therapy with irinotecan.

Children: The safety and efficacy of irinotecan in children have not been established.

Precautions:

Monitoring: Careful monitoring of the white blood cell count with differential, hemoglobin and platelet count is recommended before each irinotecan dose.

Extravasation: Irinotecan is administered by IV infusion. Take care to avoid extravasation and monitor the infusion site for signs of inflammation. Should extravasation occur, flush the site with sterile water and apply ice.

Premedication with antiemetics: Irinotecan is emetigenic. It is recommended that patients receive premedication with antiemetic agents. In clinical studies, the majority of patients received 10 mg of dexamethasone given in conjunction with another type of antiemetic agent, such as a 5–HT$_3$ blocker (eg, ondansetron or granisetron). Give antiemetic agents on the day of treatment, starting at least 30 minutes before administration of irinotecan. Consider providing patients with an antiemetic regimen (eg, prochlorperazine) for subsequent use as needed.

Topoisomerase Inhibitors

IRINOTECAN HCl

Drug Interactions:

Irinotecan Drug Interactions			
Precipitant drug	Object drug*		Description
Antineoplastics	Irinotecan	⬆	The adverse effects of irinotecan, such as myelosuppression and diarrhea, would be expected to be exacerbated by other antineoplastic agents having similar adverse effects.
Dexamethasone	Irinotecan	⬆	Lymphocytopenia has been reported in patients receiving irinotecan, and it is possible that the administration of dexamethasone as an antiemetic prophylaxis may have enhanced the likelihood of this effect. Hyperglycemia has also been reported in patients receiving irinotecan. It is probable that dexamethasone given as emetic prophylaxis contributed to hyperglycemia in some patients.
Prochlorperazine	Irinotecan	⬆	The incidence of akathisia in clinical trials was greater (8.5%) when prochlorperazine was administered on the same day as irinotecan than when these drugs were given on separate days (1.3%). The 8.5% incidence of akathisia, however, is within the range reported for use of prochlorperazine when given as a premedication for other chemotherapeutics.
Laxatives	Irinotecan	⬆	It would be expected that laxative use during therapy with irinotecan would worsen the incidence or severity of diarrhea, but this has not been studied.
Irinotecan	Diuretics	⬆	In view of the potential risk of dehydration secondary to vomiting and diarrhea induced by irinotecan, the physician may wish to withhold diuretics during dosing with irinotecan and during periods of active vomiting or diarrhea.

* ⬆ = Object drug increased.

Adverse Reactions:

Adverse Events Occurring in > 10% of Previously Treated Irinotecan Patients with Metastatic Carcinoma of the Colon or Rectum (n = 304)		
	% of patients reporting	
Body system and event	NCI grades 1 to 4	NCI grades 3 and 4
GI		
Diarrhea (late)[1]	87.8	30.6
7 to 9 stools/day (grade 3)	—	16.4
≥ 10 stools/day (grade 4)	—	14.1
Nausea	86.2	16.8
Vomiting	66.8	12.5
Anorexia	54.9	5.9
Diarrhea (early)[2]	50.7	7.9
Constipation	29.9	2
Flatulence	12.2	0
Stomatitis	11.8	0.7
Dyspepsia	10.5	0
Hematologic		
Leukopenia	63.2	28
Anemia	60.5	6.9
Neutropenia	53.9	26.3
500 to < 1000/mm^3 (grade 3)	—	14.8
< 500/mm^3 (grade 4)	—	11.5
Body as a whole		
Asthenia	75.7	12.2
Abdominal cramping/pain	56.9	16.4
Fever	45.4	0.7

Topoisomerase Inhibitors

IRINOTECAN HCl

Adverse Events Occurring in > 10% of Previously Treated Irinotecan Patients with Metastatic Carcinoma of the Colon or Rectum (n = 304)		
	% of patients reporting	
Body system and event	NCI grades 1 to 4	NCI grades 3 and 4
Pain	23.7	2.3
Headache	16.8	0.7
Back pain	14.5	1.6
Chills	13.8	0.3
Minor infections[3]	14.5	0
Edema	10.2	1.3
Abdominal enlargement	10.2	0.3
Metabolic and nutritional		
Decreased body weight	30.3	0.7
Dehydration	14.8	4.3
Increased alkaline phosphatase	13.2	3.9
Increased AST	10.5	1.3
Dermatologic		
Alopecia	60.5	na[4]
Sweating	16.4	0
Rash	12.8	0.7
Respiratory		
Dyspnea	22	3.6
Increased coughing	17.4	0.3
Rhinitis	15.5	0
CNS		
Insomnia	19.4	0
Dizziness	14.8	0
Cardiovascular		
Vasodilation (flushing)	11.2	0

[1] Occurring > 24 hours after irinotecan administration.
[2] Occurring ≤ 24 hours after irinotecan administration.
[3] Primarily upper respiratory infections.
[4] Not applicable: Complete hair loss = NCI grade 2.

Hematologic: Serious thrombocytopenia was uncommon. Neutropenic fever (concurrent NCI grade 4 neutropenia and fever of grade 2 or greater; 3%); NCI grade 3 or 4 anemia (6.9%); blood transfusions (9.9%). The frequency of grade 3 and 4 neutropenia was significantly higher in patients who received previous pelvic/abdominal irradiation then in those who had not received irradiation (48.1% vs 24.1%).

Hepatic: NCI grade 3 or 4 liver enzyme abnormalities (< 10%). These events occurred in patients with known hepatic metastases.

Dermatologic: Alopecia; rashes.

Respiratory: Severe pulmonary events were infrequent; NCI grade 3 or 4 dyspnea was reported in 3.6% of patients. Over half of the patients with dyspnea had lung metastases, the extent to which malignant pulmonary involvement or other preexisting lung disease may have contributed to dyspnea in these patients is unknown.

Overdosage:

Single doses of up to 750 mg/m^2 of irinotecan have been given. The adverse events in these patients were similar to those reported with the recommended dose and regimen. There is no known antidote for overdosage of irinotecan. Institute maximum supportive care to prevent dehydration due to diarrhea and to treat any infectious complications.

Administration and Dosage:

Approved by the FDA on June 14, 1996.

Starting dose and dose modifications: The recommended starting dose of irinotecan injection is 125 mg/m^2. Administer all doses as an IV infusion over 90 minutes. The recommended treatment regimen (one treatment course) is 125 mg/m^2 administered once weekly for 4 weeks, followed by a 2–week rest period. Thereafter, additional courses of treatment may be repeated every 6 weeks (4 weeks on therapy, 2 weeks off therapy). Adjust subsequent doses to as high as 150 mg/m^2 or to as low as 50 mg/m^2 in 25 to 50 mg/m^2 increments depending upon individual tolerance of

Topoisomerase Inhibitors

IRINOTECAN HCl

treatment. Provided intolerable toxicity does not develop, treatment with additional courses of irinotecan may be continued indefinitely in patients who attain a response or in patients whose disease remains stable. Monitor patients for toxicity.

At the start of a subsequent course of therapy, decrease the dose of irinotecan by 25 mg/m², compared to the initial dose of the previous course, for other NCI grade 2 or by 50 mg/m² for other grade 3 or 4 nonhematologic toxicities. Base all dose modifications on the worst preceding toxicity. Do not begin a new course of therapy until the granulocyte count has recovered to ≥ 1500/mm³ and the platelet count has recovered to ≥ 100,000/mm³ and treatment-related diarrhea is fully resolved. Delay treatment 1 to 2 weeks to allow for recovery from toxicity. Consider discontinuing irinotecan if the patient has not recovered after a 2-week delay.

Irinotecan Recommended Dose Modifications[1]

Toxicity NCI grade[2](value)	During a course of therapy[1]	At the start of the next course of therapy[1]
No toxicity	Maintain dose level	↑ 25 mg/m² up to a maximum dose of 150 mg/m²
Neutropenia		
1 (1500 to 1900/mm³)	Maintain dose level	Maintain dose level
2 (1000 to 1400/mm³)	↓ 25 mg/m²	Maintain dose level
3 (500 to 900/mm³)	Omit dose, then ↓ 25 mg/m² when resolved to ≤ grade 2	↓ 25 mg/m²
4 (< 500/mm³)	Omit dose, then ↓ 50 mg/m² when resolved to ≤ grade 2	↓ 50 mg/m²
Neutropenic fever (grade 4 neutropenia and ≥ grade 2 fever)	Omit dose, then ↓ 50 mg/m² when resolved	↓ 50 mg/m²
Other toxicities		
Diarrhea		
1 (2 to 3 stools/day > pretreatment)	Maintain dose level	Maintain dose level
2 (4 to 6 stools/day > pretreatment)	↓ 25 mg/m²	Maintain, if the only grade 2 toxicity
3 (7 to 9 stools/day > pretreatment)	Omit dose, then ↓ 25 mg/m² when resolved to ≤ grade 2	↓ 25 mg/m², if the only grade 3 toxicity
4 (≥ 10 stools/day > pretreatment)	Omit dose, then ↓ 50 mg/m² when resolved to ≤ grade 2	↓ 50 mg/m²
Grade 1 toxicity	Maintain dose level	Maintain dose level
Grade 2 toxicity	↓ 25 mg/m²	↓ 25 mg/m²
Grade 3 toxicity	Omit dose, then ↓ 25 mg/m² when resolved to ≤ grade 2	↓ 50 mg/m²
Grade 4 toxicity	Omit dose, then ↓ 50 mg/m² when resolved to ≤ grade 2	↓ 50 mg/m²

[1] Base all dose modifications upon the worst preceding toxicity.

[2] National Cancer Institute Common Toxicity Criteria

Patients should receive premedication with antiemetic agents.

Preparation of infusion solution: Dilute in 5% Dextrose Injection (preferred), or 0.9% Sodium Chloride Injection to a final concentration of 0.12 to 1.1 mg/ml.

Storage/Stability: Solutions diluted in 5% Dextrose Injection, stored at refrigerated temperatures (≈ 2° to 8°C; 36° to 46°F) and protected from light are physically and chemically stable for 48 hours. Do not refrigerate admixtures using 0.9% Sodium Chloride Injection due to a low and sporadic incidence of visible particulate freezing. Freezing irinotecan and admixtures of irinotecan may result in precipitation of the drug. Because of possible microbial contamination during dilution, use the admixture within 24 hours if refrigerated (2° to 8°C; 36° to 46°F) or within 6 hours if kept at room temperature (15° to 30°C; 59° to 86°F). Store vials at controlled room temperature 15° to 30°C (59° to 86°F). Protect from light.

Rx	**Camptosar** (Pharmacia & Upjohn)	**Injection:** 20 mg/ml	Sorbitol. In 5 ml vials.

BLEOMYCIN SULFATE (BLM)

Warning:

Pulmonary fibrosis is the most severe toxicity. It is most frequently seen as pneumonitis, which occasionally progresses to pulmonary fibrosis. Incidence is higher in elderly patients and in those receiving > 400 units total dose, but pulmonary toxicity has occurred in young patients and those treated with low doses (see Warnings).

A severe idiosyncratic reaction consisting of hypotension, mental confusion, fever, chills and wheezing has occurred in ≈ 1% of lymphoma patients.

Actions:

Pharmacology: Bleomycin sulfate is a mixture of cytotoxic glycopeptide antibiotics isolated from a strain of *Streptomyces verticillus.* The exact mechanism of action is unknown; however, the main mode of action appears to be inhibition of deoxyribonucleic acid (DNA) synthesis with lesser inhibition of ribonucleic acid (RNA) and protein synthesis. Bleomycin is cell cycle phase specific, with major effects in G_2 and M phases.

When administered intrapleurally for the treatment of malignant pleural effusion, bleomycin acts as a sclerosing agent.

Pharmacokinetics:

Absorption/Distribution – Following IV administration, bleomycin has a rapid initial distribution half-life of 10 to 20 minutes. IM injection produces peak blood levels in 30 to 60 minutes that are ≈ ⅓ of those produced IV.

Metabolism/Excretion – 60% to 70% of an administered dose is recovered in the urine as active bleomycin. Only 20% to 40% of this amount is active drug. In patients with a creatinine clearance of > 35 ml/min, the plasma terminal elimination half-life is ≈ 2 hours. At creatinine clearances of < 35 ml/min, the plasma terminal elimination half-life increases exponentially as the creatinine clearance decreases.

Indications:

Palliative treatment in the following neoplasms as either a single agent or in combination with other chemotherapeutic agents:

Squamous cell carcinoma: Head and neck including mouth, tongue, tonsil, nasopharynx, oropharynx, sinus, palate, lip, buccal mucosa, gingiva, epiglottis, skin and larynx. Response is poorer in patients with head and neck cancer previously irradiated. Bleomycin is also indicated in carcinoma of the skin, penis, cervix and vulva.

Lymphomas: Hodgkin's and non-Hodgkin's.

Testicular carcinoma: Embryonal cell, choriocarcinoma and teratocarcinoma.

Malignant pleural effusion: Effective as a sclerosing agent for the treatment of malignant pleural effusion and prevention of recurrent pleural effusions.

Contraindications:

Hypersensitivity or idiosyncratic reaction to bleomycin sulfate (see Warnings).

Warnings:

Idiosyncratic reactions similar to anaphylaxis occur in ≈ 1% of lymphoma patients. These reactions (hypotension, confusion, fever, chills and wheezing) may be immediate or delayed for several hours and usually occur after the first or second dose; careful monitoring is essential. Refer to Management of Acute Hypersensitivity Reactions.

Skin toxicity, a relatively late manifestation, appears to be related to the cumulative dose; it usually develops in the second and third week of treatment after administration of 150 to 200 units of the drug.

Pulmonary toxicities, the most serious side effect, occur in 10% of treated patients. In ≈ 1%, the drug-induced nonspecific pneumonitis progresses to pulmonary fibrosis and death. Although this is age- and dose-related, it is unpredictable. It is more common in patients > 70 years of age and in those receiving > 400 units total dose. However, pulmonary toxicity has been seen in young patients receiving low doses.

Identifying pulmonary toxicity is extremely difficult because of lack of specificity of the clinical syndrome. The earliest symptom is dyspnea; the earliest sign is fine rales.

Radiographically, the pneumonitis produces nonspecific patchy opacities, usually of the lower lung field. Pulmonary function tests show a decrease in total lung volume and vital capacity. These changes do not predict fibrosis development.

The nonspecific microscopic tissue changes include bronchiolar squamous metaplasia, reactive macrophages, atypical alveolar epithelial cells, fibrinous edema and interstitial fibrosis. The acute stage may involve capillary changes and subsequent

BLEOMYCIN SULFATE (BLM)

fibrinous exudation into alveoli, producing a change similar to hyaline membrane formation and progressing to a diffuse interstitial fibrosis resembling the Hamman-Rich syndrome.

Take chest x-rays every 1 to 2 weeks to monitor the onset of pulmonary toxicity. If changes are noted, discontinue treatment until it is determined if they are drug-related. Sequential measurements of the pulmonary diffusion capacity for carbon monoxide (DL_{co}) may indicate subclinical pulmonary toxicity. Monitor the DL_{co} monthly; discontinue the drug when the DL_{co} falls below 30% to 35% of the pretreatment value. Because of bleomycin's sensitization of lung tissue, patients are at greater risk of developing pulmonary toxicity when oxygen is given in surgery. Long exposure to very high oxygen concentrations is a known cause of lung damage; however, after bleomycin administration, lung damage can occur at concentrations usually considered safe. Suggested preventive measures are to maintain FIO_2 at concentrations approximating that of room air (25%) during surgery and the postoperative period and to carefully monitor fluid replacement, focusing more on colloid administration rather than crystalloid.

Renal/Hepatic function impairment: At creatinine clearances of < 35 ml/min, the plasma terminal elimination half-life increases exponentially as the creatinine clearance decreases. Renal or hepatic toxicity, beginning as a deterioration in renal or liver function tests, has occurred infrequently. These toxicities may occur at any time.

Carcinogenesis: Bleomycin has caused an increased incidence of nodular hyperplasia, fibrosarcomas and various renal tumor in rats.

Pregnancy: Category D. Bleomycin can cause fetal harm when administered to a pregnant woman but there have been no reports linking the use of bleomycin with congenital defects in humans. If bleomycin is used during pregnancy, or if the patient becomes pregnant while receiving this drug, apprise the patient of the potential hazard to the fetus. Advise women of childbearing age to avoid becoming pregnant during therapy.

Lactation: It is not known whether this drug is excreted in breast milk. Because of the potential for serious adverse reactions in breastfeeding infants, it is recommended that breastfeeding be discontinued by women receiving therapy.

Children: Safety and efficacy of bleomycin have not been established.

Precautions:

Monitoring: Frequent roentgenograms are recommended.

Chest tube drainage: It is generally accepted that chest tube drainage should be < 100 ml in a 24-hour period prior to sclerosis. However, bleomycin instillation may be appropriate when drainage is between 100 and 300 ml under clinical conditions that necessitate sclerosis therapy.

Drug Interactions:

Digoxin serum levels may be decreased by combination chemotherapy (including bleomycin). Digitoxin and digoxin capsules do not appear to be affected.

Phenytoin serum concentrations may be decreased by combination chemotherapy.

Adverse Reactions:

Pulmonary: Pneumonitis, pulmonary fibrosis (see Warnings).

Integument and mucous membranes: Erythema, rash, striae, vesiculation, hyperpigmentation, skin tenderness, hyperkeratosis, nail changes, alopecia, pruritus, stomatitis (≈ 50%). Drug therapy was stopped in 2% of patients because of these toxicities.

Miscellaneous: Fever, chills, vomiting (frequent); anorexia, weight loss (common, may persist long after termination of the drug); pain at tumor site, phlebitis (infrequent).

Combination therapy: Vascular toxicities coincident with the use of bleomycin in combination with other antineoplastics occur rarely. The events are clinically heterogeneous and may include myocardial infarction, cerebrovascular accident, thrombotic microangiopathy or cerebral arteritis. There are also reports of Raynaud's phenomenon with bleomycin alone or with vinblastine with or without cisplatin.

Sudden onset of an acute chest pain syndrome suggestive of pleuropericarditis has occurred rarely during bleomycin sulfate infusions. Evaluate each patient individually, but further courses of bleomycin do not appear to be contraindicated.

Administration and Dosage:

May administer IM, IV, SC or intrapleurally.

Because of the possibility of anaphylactoid reaction, treat lymphoma patients with ≤ 2 units for the first 2 doses. If no acute reaction occurs, follow the regular dosage schedule. The following schedule is recommended:

Squamous cell carcinoma, non-Hodgin's lymphoma, testicular carcinoma: 0.25 to 0.5 units/kg (10 to 20 units/m^2) IV, IM or SC once or twice/week.

BLEOMYCIN SULFATE (BLM)

Hodgkin's disease: 0.25 to 0.5 units/kg (10 to 20 units/m^2) IV, IM or SC once or twice weekly. After a 50% response, give a maintenance dose of 1 unit daily or 5 units/week IV or IM. Improvement of Hodgkin's disease and testicular tumors is prompt (≤ 2 weeks). If no improvement is seen by this time, it is unlikely to occur. Squamous cell cancers respond more slowly, sometimes requiring 3 weeks for improvement.

Pulmonary toxicity of bleomycin appears dose-related with a striking increase when total dose is > 400 units. Give total doses > 400 units with great caution.

When bleomycin is used in combination with other antineoplastic agents, pulmonary toxicities may occur at lower doses.

Malignant pleural effusion: 60 units of bleomycin are dissolved in 50 to 100 ml sodium chloride injection 0.9% and administered through a thoracostomy tube following drainage of excess pleural fluid and confirmation of complete lung expansion. The amount of drainage from the chest tube should be as minimal as possible prior to installation of bleomycin. The thoracostomy tube is clamped after bleomycin instillation. The patient is moved from the supine to the left and right lateral positions several times during the next four hours. The clamp is then removed and suction reestablished.

Preparation of solutions:

IM or SC – Reconstitute the 15 unit vial with 1 to 5 ml or the 30 unit vial with 2 to 10 ml Sterile Water for Injection, 0.9% NaCl for Injection or Bacteriostatic Water for Injection.

IV solution – Dissolve contents of 15 unit or 30 unit vial with 5 or 10 ml, respectively, of 0.9% NaCl for injection; administer slowly over 10 minutes.

Intrapleural: Dissolve 60 units of bleomycin in 50 to 100 ml of 0.9% NaCl injection.

Stability: Bleomycin demonstrates a loss of potency and should not be reconstituted or diluted with D_5W or other dextrose-containing diluents.

Bleomycin is stable for 24 hours at room temperature in NaCl. Store the powder under refrigeration (2° to 8°C; 36° to 46°F).

Rx	**Blenoxane** (Bristol-Myers Oncology)	**Powder for Injection:** 15 units	In vials.
		30 units	In vials.
🍁	**Blenoxane** (MSD)	**Powder for Injection:** 15 units	In vials.

PENTOSTATIN (2'-deoxycoformycin; DCF)

Warning:

Administer under the supervision of a physician qualified and experienced in the use of cancer chemotherapeutic agents. The use of higher doses than those specified is not recommended. Dose-limiting severe renal, liver, pulmonary and CNS toxicities occurred in Phase I studies that used pentostatin at higher doses than recommended (20 to 50 mg/m^2 in divided doses over 5 days).

In a clinical investigation in patients with refractory chronic lymphocytic leukemia using pentostatin at the recommended dose in combination with fludarabine phosphate, four of six patients had severe or fatal pulmonary toxicity. The use of pentostatin in combination with fludarabine phosphate is not recommended.

Actions:

Pharmacology: Pentostatin is a potent transition state inhibitor of the enzyme adenosine deaminase (ADA) and is isolated from fermentation cultures of Streptomyces antibioticus. The greatest activity of ADA is found in cells of the lymphoid system with T-cells having higher activity than B-cells and T-cell malignancies having higher ADA activity than B-cell malignancies. Pentostatin inhibition of ADA, particularly in the presence of adenosine or deoxyadenosine, leads to cytotoxicity due to elevated intracellular levels of d;ATP which can block DNA synthesis through inhibition of ribonucleotide reductase. Pentostatin can also inhibit RNA synthesis as well as cause increased DNA damage. In addition to elevated dATP, these mechanisms may contribute to the overall cytotoxic effect of pentostatin. However, the precise mechanism of pentostatin's antitumor effect in hairy cell leukemia is not known.

Pharmacokinetics: In rats pentostatin concentrations were highest in the kidneys with very little CNS penetration.

In man, following a single dose of 4 mg/m^2 pentostatin infused over 5 minutes, the distribution half-life was 11 minutes, the mean terminal half-life was 5.7 hours, the mean plasma clearance was 68 $ml/min/m^2$, and ≈ 90% of the dose was excreted in the urine as unchanged pentostatin or metabolites as measured by adenosine deaminase inhibitory activity. The plasma protein binding of pentostatin is low, ≈ 4%.

A positive correlation was observed between pentostatin clearance and creatinine clearance (Ccr) in patients with Ccr values ranging from 60 to 130 ml/min. Pentostatin half-life in patients with renal impairment (Ccr < 50 ml/min) was 18 hours, which was much longer than that observed in patients with normal renal function (Ccr > 60 ml/min), which was about 6 hours.

Clinical trials: Patients with hairy cell leukemia (n = 133) previously treated with alpha-interferon were treated with pentostatin in five clinical studies. Forty-four of these patients were refractory to alpha-interferon and were evaluable for response to pentostatin. Pentostatin was administered at a dose of 4 mg/m^2 every other week for 3 months; responding patients received 3 additional months (M.D. Anderson Hospital study). Another group of patients received 4 mg/m^2 pentostatin every other week for 3 months; responding patients were treated monthly for up to 9 additional months (Cancer and Leukemia Group B study; CALGB). A complete response required clearing of the peripheral blood and bone marrow of hairy cells, normalization of organomegaly and lymphadenopathy, and recovery of the hemoglobin to at least 12 g/dl, platelet count to at least 100,000/mm^3 and granulocyte count to at least 1500/mm^3. A partial response required that the percentage of hairy cells in the blood and bone marrow decrease by > 50%, enlarged organs and lymph nodes had to decrease by > 50%, and hematologic parameters had to meet the same criteria as for a complete response. For those patients who were clearly refractory to alpha-interferon, the complete response rate was 58% and the partial response rate was 28% giving a total response rate (complete plus partial responses) of 86%. Median time to achieve a response was 4.7 months (range, 2.9 to 24.1 months). Duration of response ranged from 1.4 to 35.1+ months in the CALGB study (median > 7.7 months) and from 1.3+ to 31.2+ months for the M.D. Anderson study (median > 15.2 months). Median duration of follow-up ranged from 3.9 months in the CALGB study to 19.3 months in the M.D. Anderson study. Only 4 of 20 and 2 of 13 responding patients had relapsed, respectively.

Responding patients with abnormal peripheral blood counts at the start of therapy showed increases in their hemoglobin, granulocyte count and platelet count in response to treatment with pentostatin.

Indications:

Single agent for adult patients with alpha-interferon-refractory hairy cell leukemia, defined as progressive disease after a minimum of 3 months of alpha-interferon treatment or no response after a minimum of 6 months of alpha-interferon.

PENTOSTATIN (2′-deoxycoformycin; DCF)

Contraindications:

Hypersensitivity to pentostatin.

Warnings:

Myelosuppression: Patients with hairy cell leukemia may experience myelosuppression, primarily during the first few courses of treatment. Patients with infections prior to pentostatin treatment have in some cases developed worsening of their condition leading to death, whereas others have achieved complete response. Treat patients with infection only when the potential benefit justifies the potential risk to the patient. Attempt to control the infection before treatment is initiated or resumed.

In patients with progressive hairy cell leukemia, the initial courses of pentostatin treatment were associated with worsening of neutropenia. Therefore, frequent monitoring of complete blood counts during this time is necessary. If severe neutropenia continues beyond the initial cycles, evaluate patients for disease status, including a bone marrow examination.

Renal toxicity was observed at higher doses in early studies; however, in patients treated at the recommended dose, elevations in serum creatinine were usually minor and reversible. There were some patients who began treatment with normal renal function who had evidence of mild to moderate toxicity at a final assessment.

Rashes, occasionally severe, were commonly reported and may worsen with continued treatment. Withholding of treatment may be required.

Mutagenesis: Pentostatin was nonmutagenic when tested with various Salmonella typhimurium strains; however, when tested with strain TA-100, a repeatable statistically significant response trend was observed with and without metabolic activation. Formulated pentostatin was clastogenic in the in vivo mouse bone marrow micronucleus assay at 20, 120 and 240 mg/kg.

Fertility impairment: In a 5 day IV toxicity study in dogs, mild seminiferous tubular degeneration was observed with doses of 1 and 4 mg/kg. The possible adverse effects on fertility in humans have not been determined.

Pregnancy: Category D. Pentostatin can cause fetal harm when administered to a pregnant woman. Pentostatin was administered IV to pregnant rats on days 6 through 15 of gestation; drug-related maternal toxicity occurred at doses of 0.1 and 0.75 mg/kg/day (0.6 and 4.5 mg/m^2). Teratogenic effects were observed at 0.75 mg/kg/day manifested by increased incidence of various skeletal malformations. In another study, fetal malformations that occurred were an omphalocele at 0.05 mg/kg (0.3 mg/m^2), gastroschisis at 0.75 and 1 mg/kg/day (4.5 and 6 mg/m^2), and a flexure defect of the hind limbs at 0.75 mg/kg/day (4.5 mg/m^2). Pentostatin was also teratogenic in mice when administered as a single 2 mg/kg (6 mg/m^2) intraperitoneal injection on day 7 of gestation. Pentostatin was not teratogenic in rabbits when administered IV on days 6 through 18 of gestation; however, maternal toxicity, abortions, early deliveries and deaths occurred in all drug-treated groups. There are no adequate and well controlled studies in pregnant women. If pentostatin is used during pregnancy, or if the patient becomes pregnant while taking this drug, apprise her of the potential hazard to the fetus. Advise women of childbearing potential to avoid becoming pregnant while taking this drug.

Lactation: It is not known whether pentostatin is excreted in breast milk. Decide whether to discontinue nursing or discontinue the drug, taking into account the importance of the drug to the mother.

Children: Safety and efficacy in children or adolescents have not been established.

Precautions:

Monitoring: Therapy with pentostatin requires regular patient observation and monitoring of hematologic parameters and blood chemistry values. If severe adverse reactions occur, withhold the drug and take appropriate corrective measures.

Prior to initiating therapy, assess renal function with a serum creatinine or a Ccr assay. Perform complete blood counts and serum creatinine before each dose and at other appropriate periods during therapy. Severe neutropenia has been observed following the early courses of treatment; therefore, frequent monitoring of complete blood counts is recommended during this time. If hematologic parameters do not improve with subsequent courses, evaluate patients for disease status, including a bone marrow examination. Perform periodic monitoring of the peripheral blood for hairy cells to assess the response to treatment.

In addition, bone marrow aspirates and biopsies may be required at 2 to 3 month intervals to assess the response to treatment.

CNS toxicity: Withhold or discontinue therapy in those with evidence of CNS toxicity.

PENTOSTATIN (2′-deoxycoformycin; DCF)

Drug Interactions:

Allopurinol and pentostatin are both associated with skin rashes. Based on clinical studies in 25 refractory patients, combined use did not appear to produce a higher incidence of skin rashes than observed with pentostatin alone. One patient experienced a hypersensitivity vasculitis that resulted in death. It was unclear whether this adverse event and subsequent death resulted from the drug combination.

Fludarabine: Concurrent use with pentostatin is not recommended because it may be associated with an increased risk of fatal pulmonary toxicity (see Warning box).

Vidarabine: Pentostatin enhances the effects of vidarabine. The combined use may result in an increase in adverse reactions associated with each drug. The therapeutic benefit of the drug combination has not been established.

Adverse Reactions:

Pentostatin Adverse Reactions (%)

Adverse reaction	Incidence	Adverse reaction	Incidence
Hematologic/Lymphatic		*Hepatic*	
Leukopenia	60	Hepatic disorder/elevated	
Anemia	35	liver function tests	19
Thrombocytopenia	32	*Respiratory*	
Ecchymosis	3-10	Cough	17
Lymphadenopathy	3-10	Upper respiratory infection	16
Petechia	3-10	Lung disorder	12
GI		Bronchitis	3-10
Nausea/Vomiting	22-53	Dyspnea	3-10
Anorexia	16	Epistaxis	3-10
Diarrhea	15	Lung edema	3-10
Constipation	3-10	Pneumonia	3-10
Flatulence	3-10	Pharyngitis	3-10
Stomatitis	3-10	Rhinitis	3-10
Dermatologic		Sinusitis	3-10
Rash	26	*GU*	
Skin disorder	17	Genitourinary disorder	15
Eczema	3-10	Hematuria	3-10
Dry skin	3-10	Dysuria	3-10
Herpes simplex/zoster	3-10	Increased BUN	3-10
Maculopapular rash	3-10	Increased creatinine	3-10
Vesiculobullous rash	3-10	*CNS*	
Pruritus	3-10	Headache	13
Seborrhea	3-10	Neurologic, CNS	11
Skin discoloration	3-10	Anxiety	3-10
Sweating	3-10	Confusion	3-10
Body as a whole		Depression	3-10
Fever	42	Dizziness	3-10
Infection	36	Insomnia	3-10
Fatigue	29	Nervousness	3-10
Pain	20	Paresthesia	3-10
Allergic reaction	11	Somnolence	3-10
Chills	11	Abnormal thinking	3-10
Death	3-10	*Musculoskeletal*	
Sepsis	3-10	Myalgia	11
Chest pain	3-10	Arthralgia	3-10
Abdominal pain	3-10	*Cardiovascular*	
Back pain	3-10	Arrhythmia	3-10
Flu syndrome	3-10	Abnormal ECG	3-10
Asthenia	3-10	Thrombophlebitis	3-10
Malaise	3-10	Hemorrhage	3-10
Neoplasm	3-10	*Special senses*	
Metabolic/Nutritional		Abnormal vision	3-10
Weight loss	3-10	Conjunctivitis	3-10
Peripheral edema	3-10	Ear pain	3-10
Increased LDH	3-10	Eye pain	3-10

PENTOSTATIN (2′-deoxycoformycin; DCF)

The adverse events listed in the preceding table were reported during clinical studies with pentostatin in patients with hairy cell leukemia who were refractory to alpha-interferon therapy. Most patients experienced an adverse event. The drug association is uncertain since the adverse reactions may be associated with the disease itself (eg, fever, infection, anemia), but other events, such as the GI symptoms, hematologic suppression, rashes and abnormal liver function tests, can in many cases be attributed to the drug. Most adverse events that were assessed for severity were either mild (52%) or moderate (26%) and diminished in frequency with continued therapy; 11% of patients withdrew from treatment due to an adverse event.

The remaining adverse events occurred in < 3% of patients; their relationship to pentostatin is uncertain:

Body as a whole: Abscess; enlarged abdomen; ascites; cellulitis; cyst; face edema; fibrosis; granuloma; hernia; injection-site hemorrhage or inflammation; moniliasis; neck rigidity; pelvic pain; photosensitivity reaction; anaphylactoid reaction; immune system disorder; mucous membrane disorder; neck pain.

Cardiovascular: Aortic stenosis; arterial anomaly; cardiomegaly; congestive heart failure; cardiac arrest; flushing; hypertension; myocardial infarct; palpitation; shock; varicose vein.

GI: Colitis; dysphagia; eructation; gastritis; GI hemorrhage; gum hemorrhage; hepatitis; hepatomegaly; intestinal obstruction; jaundice; leukoplakia; melena; periodontal abscess; proctitis; abnormal stools; dyspepsia; esophagitis; gingivitis; hepatic failure; mouth disorder.

Hematologic/Lymphatic: Abnormal erythrocytes; leukocytosis; pancytopenia; purpura; splenomegaly; eosinophilia; hematologic disorder; hemolysis; lymphoma-like reaction; thrombocythemia.

Metabolic/Nutritional: Acidosis; increased creatine phosphokinase; dehydration; diabetes mellitus; increased gamma globulins; gout; abnormal healing; hypocholesterolemia; weight gain; hyponatremia.

Musculoskeletal: Arthritis; bone pain; osteomyelitis; pathological fracture.

CNS: Agitation; amnesia; apathy; ataxia; CNS depression; coma; convulsions; abnormal dreams; depersonalization; emotional lability; facial paralysis; abnormal gait; hyperesthesia; hypesthesia; hypertonia; incoordination; decreased libido; neuropathy; postural dizziness; decreased reflexes; stupor; tremor; vertigo.

Respiratory: Asthma; atelectasis; hemoptysis; hyperventilation; hypoventilation; laryngitis; larynx edema; lung fibrosis; pleural effusion; pneumothorax; pulmonary embolus; increased sputum.

Dermatologic: Acne; alopecia; contact dermatitis; exfoliative dermatitis; fungal dermatitis; psoriasis; benign skin neoplasm; subcutaneous nodule; skin hypertrophy; urticaria.

Special senses: Blepharitis; cataract; deafness; diplopia; exophthalmos; lacrimation disorder; optic neuritis; otitis media; parosmia; retinal detachment; taste perversion; tinnitus. One patient developed unilateral uveitis with vision loss.

GU: Albuminuria; fibrocystic breast; glycosuria; gynecomastia; hydronephrosis; kidney failure; oliguria; polyuria; pyuria; toxic nephropathy; urinary frequency/retention/urgency; urinary tract infection; impaired urination; urolithiasis; vaginitis.

Lab test abnormalities: Liver function test elevations occurred during treatment and were generally reversible.

Overdosage:

Symptoms: Pentostatin administered at higher doses than recommended (20 to 50 mg/m^2 in divided doses over 5 days) was associated with deaths due to severe renal, hepatic, pulmonary and CNS toxicity.

Treatment: Management would include general supportive measures through any period of toxicity that occurs. Refer to General Management of Acute Overdosage.

Administration and Dosage:

Hydrate with 500 to 1000 ml of 5% Dextrose in 0.5 Normal Saline or equivalent before pentostatin administration. Administer an additional 500 ml of 5% Dextrose or equivalent after pentostatin is given.

Alpha-interferon-refractory hairy cell leukemia: 4 mg/m^2 every other week. Pentostatin may be administered IV by bolus injection or diluted in a larger volume and given over 20 to 30 minutes. (See Preparation of IV Solution.)

Higher doses are not recommended.

No extravasation injuries were reported in clinical studies.

PENTOSTATIN (2′-deoxycoformycin; DCF)

Duration/Response: The optimal duration of treatment has not been determined. In the absence of major toxicity and with observed continuing improvement, treat the patient until a complete response has been achieved. Although not established, the administration of two additional doses has been recommended following the achievement of a complete response.

Assess all patients receiving pentostatin at 6 months for response to treatment. If the patient has not achieved a complete or partial response, discontinue treatment.

If the patient has achieved a partial response, continue treatment in an effort to achieve a complete response. At any time that a complete response is achieved thereafter, two additional doses of pentostatin are recommended; then stop treatment. If the best response to treatment at the end of 12 months is a partial response, stop treatment with pentostatin.

Therapy/Dose discontinuation: Withholding or discontinuing individual doses may be needed when severe adverse reactions occur. Withhold drug treatment in patients with severe rash, and withhold or discontinue in patients showing evidence of CNS toxicity.

Withhold treatment in patients with active infection occurring during the treatment; may resume treatment when the infection is controlled.

Patients who have elevated serum creatinine should have their dose withheld and a Ccr determined. There are insufficient data to recommend a starting or a subsequent dose for patients with impaired renal function (Ccr < 60 ml/min).

Renal function impairment: Treat patients only when potential benefit justifies potential risk. Two patients with impaired renal function (Ccr 50 to 60 ml/min) achieved complete response without unusual adverse events when treated with 2 mg/m^2.

Hematologic effects: No dosage reduction is recommended at the start of therapy in patients with anemia, neutropenia or thrombocytopenia. In addition, dosage reductions are not recommended during treatment in patients with anemia and thrombocytopenia if patients can be otherwise supported hematologically. Temporarily withhold pentostatin if the absolute neutrophil count falls below 200 cells/mm^3 during treatment in a patient who had an initial neutrophil count > 500 cells/mm^3; treatment may be resumed when the count returns to predose levels.

Preparation of IV solution: 1. Follow procedures for proper handling and disposal of anticancer drugs. Treat spills and wastes with 5% sodium hypochlorite solution prior to disposal.

2. Protective clothing including polyethylene gloves must be worn.

3. Transfer 5 ml Sterile Water for Injection, USP to the vial containing pentostatin and mix thoroughly to obtain complete dissolution of a solution yielding 2 mg/ml.

4. Pentostatin may be given IV by bolus injection or diluted in a larger volume (25 to 50 ml) with 5% Dextrose Injection, USP or 0.9% Sodium Chloride Injection, USP. Dilution of the entire contents of a reconstituted vial with 25 or 50 ml provides a pentostatin concentration of 0.33 or 0.18 mg/ml, respectively, for the diluted solutions.

5. Pentostatin solution, when diluted for infusion with 5% Dextrose Injection, USP or 0.9% Sodium Chloride Injection, USP does not interact with PVC infusion containers or administration sets at concentrations of 0.18 to 0.33 mg/ml.

Storage/Stability: Pentostatin vials are stable when stored at refrigerated temperatures (2° to 8°C; 36° to 46°F) for the period stated on the package. Vials reconstituted or reconstituted and further diluted as directed may be stored at room temperature and ambient light; however, use within 8 hours because pentostatin contains no preservatives.

Rx	**Nipent** (Parke-Davis)	**Powder for Injection:** 10 mg/vial[1]	In single dose vials.

[1] With 50 mg mannitol per vial.

IDARUBICIN HCl

Warning:

Give idarubicin slowly into a freely flowing IV infusion. It must never be given IM or SC. Severe local tissue necrosis can occur if there is extravasation during administration.

Idarubicin can cause myocardial toxicity leading to congestive heart failure. Cardiac toxicity is more common in patients who have received prior anthracyclines or who have pre-existing cardiac disease.

Severe myelosuppression occurs when idarubicin is used at therapeutic doses.

The physician and institution must be capable of responding rapidly and completely to severe hemorrhagic conditions or overwhelming infection.

Reduce dosage in patients with impaired hepatic or renal function. (See Administration and Dosage.)

Actions:

Pharmacology: Idarubicin HCl is a synthetic antineoplastic anthracycline for IV use; it is a DNA-intercalating analog of daunorubicin which has an inhibitory effect on nucleic acid synthesis and interacts with the enzyme topoisomerase II. The compound has a high lipophilicity which results in an increased rate of cellular uptake compared with other anthracyclines.

Pharmacokinetics: Following IV administration of 10 to 12 mg/m^2 daily for 3 to 4 days (as a single agent or combined with cytarabine) to adult leukemia patients with normal renal and hepatic function, there is a rapid distributive phase with a very high volume of distribution presumably reflecting extensive tissue binding. The plasma clearance is twice the expected hepatic plasma flow indicating extensive extrahepatic metabolism. The drug is eliminated predominantly by biliary and to a lesser extent by renal excretion, mostly in the form of the primary metabolite, 13-dihydroidarubicin (idarubicinol).

The estimated mean terminal half-life is 22 hours (range, 4 to 46 hours) when used as a single agent and 20 hours (range, 7 to 38 hours) when used in combination with cytarabine. The elimination of idarubicinol is considerably slower with an estimated mean terminal half-life that exceeds 45 hours; hence, its plasma levels are sustained for a period > 8 days. As idarubicinol has cytotoxic activity, it presumably contributes to the effects of idarubicin.

The extent of drug and metabolite accumulation predicted in leukemia patients for days 2 and 3 of dosing is 1.7- and 2.3-fold, respectively, and suggests no change in kinetics following a 3 times daily regimen.

In patients with moderate or severe hepatic dysfunction, the metabolism of idarubicin may be impaired and lead to higher systemic drug levels. See Warnings.

Peak cellular idarubicin concentrations are reached a few minutes after injection. Idarubicin and idarubicinol concentrations in nucleated blood and bone marrow cells are > 100 times the plasma concentrations. Idarubicin disappearance rates in plasma and cells were comparable with a terminal half-life of about 15 hours. The terminal half-life of idarubicinol in cells was about 72 hours.

The percentages of idarubicin and idarubicinol bound to human plasma proteins averaged 97% and 94%, respectively. The binding is concentration-independent.

Idarubicin studies in pediatric leukemia patients, at doses of 4.2 to 13.3 mg/m^2/day for 3 days, suggest dose-independent kinetics. There is no difference between the half-lives of the drug following 3 times daily or 3 times weekly administration.

Cerebrospinal fluid (CSF) levels of idarubicin and idarubicinol were measured in pediatric leukemia patients. Idarubicin was detected in 2 of 21 CSF samples (0.14 and 1.56 ng/ml), while idarubicinol was detected in 20 of these 21 CSF samples obtained 18 to 30 hours after dosing (mean, ≈ 0.51 ng/ml, range, 0.22 to 1.05 ng/ml). The clinical relevance of these findings is currently being evaluated.

Clinical trials: Four prospective randomized studies have been conducted to compare the safety and efficacy of idarubicin (IDR) to that of daunorubicin (DNR), each in combination with cytarabine (Ara-C) as induction therapy in previously untreated adult patients with acute myeloid leukemia (AML). These data are summarized in the following table and demonstrate significantly greater complete remission rates and significantly longer overall survival for the IDR regimen in two of the studies.

IDARUBICIN HCl

Efficacy of Idarubicin vs Daunorubicin in AML

Studies	Induction[1] regimen dose in mg/m² daily x 3 days		Complete remission rate		Median survival (days)	
	IDR	DNR	IDR	DNR	IDR	DNR
1. Age ≤ 60 years	12[2]	50[2]	51/65[4] (78%)	38/65 (58%)	508[4]	435
2. Age ≥ 15 years	12[3]	45[3]	76/111[4] (69%)	65/119 (55%)	328	277
3. Age ≥ 18 years	13[3]	45[3]	68/101 (67%)	66/113 (58%)	393[4]	281
4. Age ≥ 55 years	12[3]	45[3]	49/124 (40%)	49/125 (39%)	87	169

[1] Patients who had persistent leukemia after the first induction course received a second course

[2] Ara-C 25 mg/m² bolus IV followed by 200 mg/m² daily x 5 days by continuous infusion

[3] Ara-C 100 mg/m² daily x 7 days by continuous infusion

[4] Overall $p < 0.05$, unadjusted for prognostic factors or multiple endpoints

The following consolidation regimens were used in US controlled trials: Patients received the same anthracycline for consolidation as was used for induction.

Studies 1 and 3 utilized 2 courses of consolidation therapy consisting of IDR 12 or 13 mg/m² daily for 2 days, respectively (or DNR 50 or 45 mg/m² daily for 2 days), and Ara-C, either 25 mg/m² daily by IV bolus followed by 200 mg/m² daily by continuous infusion for 4 days (Study 1), or 100 mg/m² daily for 5 days by continuous infusion (Study 3). A rest period of 4 to 6 weeks is recommended prior to initiation of consolidation and between the courses; hematologic recovery is mandatory prior to initiation of each consolidation course.

Study 2 utilized 3 consolidation courses, administered at intervals of 21 days or upon hematologic recovery. Each course consisted of IDR 15 mg/m² IV for 1 dose (or DNR 50 mg/m² IV for 1 dose), Ara-C 100 mg/m² every 12 hours for 10 doses and 6-thioguanine 100 mg/m² for 10 doses. If severe myelosuppression occurred, subsequent courses were given with 25% reduction in the doses of all drugs. In addition, this study included 4 courses of maintenance therapy (2 days of the same anthracycline as was used in induction and 5 days of Ara-C).

Toxicities and duration of aplasia were similar during induction except for an increase in mucositis on the IDR arm in one study. During consolidation, duration of aplasia on the IDR arm was longer in all three studies and mucositis was more frequent in two studies. During consolidation, transfusion requirements were higher on the IDR arm in the two studies in which they were tabulated, and patients on the IDR arm in Study 3 spent more days on IV antibiotics (Study 3 used a higher dose of IDR).

The benefit of consolidation and maintenance therapy in prolonging the duration of remission and survival is not proven.

Intensive maintenance with IDR is not recommended in view of the considerable toxicity (including deaths in remission) experienced by patients during the maintenance phase of Study 2.

Indications:

In combination with other approved antileukemic drugs for the treatment of AML in adults. This includes French-American-British (FAB) classifications M1 through M7.

Warnings:

Bone marrow suppression: Idarubicin is a potent bone marrow suppressant. Do not give to patients with pre-existing bone marrow suppression induced by previous drug therapy or radiotherapy unless the benefit warrants the risk.

Severe myelosuppression will occur in all patients given a therapeutic dose of this agent for induction, consolidation or maintenance. Careful hematologic monitoring is required. Deaths due to infection or bleeding have occurred during the period of severe myelosuppression. Facilities with laboratory and supportive resources adequate to monitor drug tolerability and protect and maintain a patient compromised by drug toxicity should be available. It must be possible to treat rapidly and completely a severe hemorrhagic condition or a severe infection.

Cardiotoxicity: Pre-existing heart disease and previous therapy with anthracyclines at high cumulative doses or other potentially cardiotoxic agents are co-factors for

IDARUBICIN HCl

increased risk of idarubicin-induced cardiac toxicity; weigh the benefit-to-risk ratio of idarubicin therapy in such patients before starting treatment.

Myocardial toxicity, as manifested by potentially fatal congestive heart failure, acute life-threatening arrhythmias or other cardiomyopathies, may occur following therapy with idarubicin. Appropriate therapeutic measures for the management of congestive heart failure or arrhythmias are indicated.

Carefully monitor cardiac function during treatment in order to minimize the risk of cardiac toxicity of the type described for other anthracycline compounds. The risk of such myocardial toxicity may be higher following concomitant or previous radiation to the mediastinal-pericardial area or in patients with anemia, bone marrow depression, infections, leukemic pericarditis or myocarditis. While there are no reliable means for predicting congestive heart failure, cardiomyopathy induced by anthracyclines is usually associated with a decrease of the left ventricular ejection fraction (LVEF) from pretreatment baseline values.

Hepatic and renal function impairment can affect the disposition of idarubicin. Evaluate liver and kidney function with conventional clinical laboratory tests (using serum bilirubin and serum creatinine as indicators) prior to and during treatment. Consider dose reduction if the bilirubin or creatinine levels are above the normal range. (See Administration and Dosage.)

Carcinogenesis: Idarubicin and related compounds have mutagenic and carcinogenic properties when tested in experimental models (including bacterial systems, mammalian cells in culture and female Sprague-Dawley rats).

In male dogs given ≥ 1.8 mg/m^2 /day idarubicin (3 times per week for 13 weeks), testicular atrophy was observed with inhibition of spermiogenesis and sperm maturation, and few or no mature sperm. Effects were not readily reversible after an 8 week recovery period.

Pregnancy: Category D. Idarubicin was embryotoxic and teratogenic in the rat at a dose of 1.2 mg/m^2 /day or one-tenth the human dose, which was nontoxic to dams. Idarubicin was embryotoxic but not teratogenic in the rabbit. Even at a dose of 2.4 mg/m^2 /day or two-tenths the human dose, which was toxic to dams. There is no conclusive information about idarubicin adversely affecting human fertility or causing teratogenesis. There are no adequate and well controlled studies in pregnant women. If idarubicin is to be used during pregnancy, or if the patient becomes pregnant during therapy, apprise the patient of the potential hazard to the fetus. Advise women of childbearing potential to avoid pregnancy.

Lactation: It is not known whether this drug is excreted in breast milk. Because of the potential for serious adverse reactions in nursing infants from idarubicin, mothers should discontinue nursing prior to taking this drug.

Children: Safety and efficacy in children have not been established.

Precautions:

Monitoring: Therapy with idarubicin requires close observation of the patient and careful laboratory monitoring. Frequent complete blood counts and monitoring of hepatic and renal function tests are recommended.

Hyperuricemia secondary to rapid lysis of leukemic cells may be induced. Take appropriate measures to prevent hyperuricemia and to control any systemic infection before beginning therapy.

Administer slowly (over 10 to 15 minutes) into the tubing of a freely running IV infusion of 0.9% Sodium Chloride Injection, USP or 5% Dextrose Injection, USP. Attach the tubing to a Butterfly needle or other suitable device and insert preferably into a large vein.

Extravasation of idarubicin can cause severe local tissue necrosis. Extravasation may occur with or without an accompanying stinging or burning sensation even if blood returns well on aspiration of the infusion needle. If signs or symptoms of extravasation occur, terminate the injection or infusion immediately and restart in another vein.

Care in the administration of idarubicin will reduce the chance of perivenous infiltration. It may also decrease the chance of local reactions such as urticaria and erythematous streaking. If it is known or suspected that SC extravasation has occurred, it is recommended that intermittent ice packs (½ hour immediately, then ½ hour 4 times per day for 3 days) be placed over the area of extravasation and that the affected extremity be elevated. Because of the progressive nature of extravasation reactions, frequently examine the area of injection and obtain plastic surgery consultation early if there is any sign of a local reaction such as pain, erythema, edema

IDARUBICIN HCl

or vesication. If ulceration begins or there is severe persistent pain at the site of extravasation, consider early wide excision of the involved area.

Adverse Reactions:

The table below lists the adverse experiences reported in one US study and is representative of the experiences in other studies.

Adverse Reactions: Idarubicin vs Daunorubicin		
Adverse Reactions	IDR (n = 110)	DNR (n = 118)
Infection	95%	97%
Nausea and vomiting	82%	80%
Hair loss	77%	72%
Abdominal cramps/Diarrhea	73%	68%
Hemorrhage	63%	65%
Mucositis	50%	55%
Dermatologic	46%	40%
Mental status	41%	34%
Pulmonary-clinical	39%	39%
Fever	26%	28%
Headache	20%	24%
Cardiac-clinical	16%	24%
Neurologic-peripheral nerves	7%	9%
Seizure	4%	5%
Cerebellar	4%	5%
Pulmonary allergy	2%	4%

The duration of aplasia and incidence of mucositis were greater on the IDR arm than the DNR arm, especially during consolidation in some US controlled trials (see Clinical studies).

The following information reflects experience based on US controlled clinical trials.

Hepatic and renal: Changes in hepatic and renal function tests have been observed. These changes were usually transient and occurred in the setting of sepsis and while patients were receiving potentially hepatotoxic and nephrotoxic antibiotics and antifungal agents. Severe changes in renal function occurred in no more than 1% of patients, while severe changes in hepatic function occurred in < 5% of patients.

Myelosuppression: Severe myelosuppression is the major toxicity associated with idarubicin therapy, but this effect of the drug is required in order to eradicate the leukemic clone. During the period of myelosuppression, patients are at risk of developing infection and bleeding which may be life-threatening or fatal. (See Warnings.)

GI: Nausea or vomiting, mucositis, abdominal pain and diarrhea occurred frequently, but were severe in < 5% of patients. Severe enterocolitis with perforation has occurred rarely. The risk of perforation may be increased by instrumental intervention. Consider the possibility of perforation in patients who develop severe abdominal pain and take appropriate steps for diagnosis and management.

Dermatologic: Alopecia occurred frequently and dermatologic reactions including generalized rash, urticaria and a bullous erythrodermatous rash of the palms and soles have occurred. The dermatologic reactions were usually attributed to concomitant antibiotic therapy. Local reactions including hives at the injection site have occurred.

Cardiovascular: Congestive heart failure (frequently attributed to fluid overload), serious arrhythmias including atrial fibrillation, chest pain, myocardial infarction and asymptomatic declines in LVEF have occurred in patients undergoing induction therapy for AML. Myocardial insufficiency and arrhythmias were usually reversible and occurred in the setting of sepsis, anemia and aggressive IV fluid administration. The events were reported more frequently in patients > 60 years old and in those with pre-existing cardiac disease. (See Warnings.)

IDARUBICIN HCl

Overdosage:

Two cases of fatal overdosage in patients receiving therapy for AML have been reported. The doses were 135 mg/m^2 over 3 days and 45 mg/m^2 of idarubicin and 90 mg/m^2 of daunorubicin over a 3 day period.

It is anticipated that overdosage with idarubicin will result in severe and prolonged myelosuppression and possibly in increased severity of GI toxicity. Adequate supportive care including platelet transfusions, antibiotics and symptomatic treatment of mucositis is required. The effect of acute overdose on cardiac function is not fully known, but severe arrhythmia occurred in one of the two patients exposed. It is anticipated that very high doses of idarubicin may cause acute cardiac toxicity and may be associated with a higher incidence of delayed cardiac failure.

The profound multicompartment behavior, extensive extravascular distribution and tissue binding, coupled with the low unbound fraction available in the plasma pool make it unlikely that therapeutic efficacy or toxicity would be altered by conventional peritoneal or hemodialysis.

Administration and Dosage:

Induction therapy in adult patients with AML: 12 mg/m^2 daily for 3 days by slow (10 to 15 min) IV injection in combination with Ara-C, 100 mg/m^2 daily given by continuous infusion for 7 days or as a 25 mg/m^2 IV bolus followed by 200 mg/m^2 daily for 5 days by continuous infusion. In patients with unequivocal evidence of leukemia after the first induction course, a second course may be administered. Delay administration of the second course in patients who experience severe mucositis until recovery from this toxicity has occurred; a dose reduction of 25% is recommended.

Renal/Hepatic function impairment: In patients with hepatic or renal impairment, consider a dose reduction of idarubicin. Do not administer if the bilirubin level is > 5 mg/dl (see Warnings).

Preparation of solution: Reconstitute 5, 10 and 20 mg vials with 5, 10 and 20 ml, respectively, of 0.9% Sodium Chloride Injection, USP to give a final concentration of 1 mg/ml. Bacteriostatic diluents are not recommended.

The vial contents are under a negative pressure to minimize aerosol formation during reconstitution; therefore, take particular care when the needle is inserted. Avoid inhalation of any aerosol produced during reconstitution.

IV incompatibility: Unless specific compatability data are available, idarubicin should not be mixed with other drugs. Precipitation occurs with heparin. Prolonged contact with any solution of any alkaline pH will result in degradation of the drug.

Storage/Stability: Reconstituted solutions are physicially and chemically stable for at least 168 hours (7 days) under refrigeration (2° to 8° C; 36° to 46°F) and 72 hours (3 days) at controlled room temperature (15° to 30°C; 59° to 86°F). Discard unused solutions in an appropriate manner.

Rx	**Idamycin** (Adria)	**Powder for Injection (lyophilized):** 5 mg	50 mg lactose. In single-dose vials.
		10 mg	100 mg lactose. In single-dose vials.

Anthracyclines

DOXORUBICIN HCl (ADR)

Warning:

Severe local tissue necrosis will result if extravasation occurs. Do not give IM or SC.

Serious irreversible myocardial toxicity with delayed congestive failure often unresponsive to supportive therapy may occur as total dosage approaches 550 mg/m^2.

Acute infusion-associated reactions (flushing, shortness of breath, facial swelling, headache, chills, back pain, tightness in the chest or throat and hypertension) have occurred in ≈ 7% of patients treated with liposomal doxorubicin. In most patients, these reactions resolve over the course of several hours to a day once the infusion is terminated. In some patients, the reaction resolves by slowing the infusion rate.

Reduce dosage in patients with impaired hepatic function (see Administration and Dosage).

Severe myelosuppression may occur.

Actions:

Pharmacology: Doxorubicin is a cytotoxic anthracycline antibiotic isolated from cultures of *Streptomyces peucetius* var. *caesius*. Its mechanism is related to its ability to bind to DNA and inhibit nucleic acid synthesis. Cell culture studies have shown rapid cell penetration, perinucleolar chromatin binding, rapid inhibition of mitotic activity and nucleic acid synthesis, mutagenesis and chromosomal aberrations.

Liposomal doxorubicin is encapsulated in long-circulating liposomes. Liposomes are microscopic vesicles composed of a phospholipid bilayer that are capable of encapsulating active drugs. The liposomes of liposomal doxorubicin are formulated with surface-bound methoxypolyethylene glycol (MPEG), a process often referred to as pegylation, to protect liposomes from detection by the mononuclear phagocyte system (MPS) and to increase blood circulation time.

The liposomes have a half-life of ≈ 55 hours in humans. They are stable in blood, and direct measurement of liposomal doxorubicin shows that at least 90% of the drug (the assay used cannot quantify < 5% to 10% free doxorubicin) remains liposome-encapsulated during circulation.

It is hypothesized that because of their small size (≈ 1000 nm) and persistence in the circulation to pegylated doxorubicin, liposomes are able to penetrate the altered and often compromised vasculature of tumors. This hypothesis is supported by studies using colloidal gold-containing liposomes, which can be visualized microscopically. Evidence of penetration of the liposomes from blood vessels and their entry and accumulation in tumors have been seen in mice with C-26 colon carcinoma tumors and in transgenic mice with Kaposi's sarcoma-like lesions. Once the liposomes distribute to the tissue compartment, the encapsulated doxorubicin becomes available. The exact mechanism of release is not understood.

Liposomal encapulation or incorporation in a lipid complex can substantially affect a drug's functional properties relative to those of the unencapsulated or nonlipid-associated drug. In addition, different liposomal or lipid-complexed products with a common active ingredient may vary from one another in the chemical composition and physical form of the lipid component. Such differences may affect functional properties of these drug products.

Pharmacokinetics:

Absorption/Distribution –

Conventional doxorubicin undergoes rapid and extensive binding to tissue and plasma proteins after IV use. It does not cross blood-brain barrier.

Liposomal doxorubicin: In contrast to original doxorubicin, the steady-state volumne of distribution of liposomal doxorubicin indicates that it is confined mostly to the vascular fluid volume. Plasma protein binding has not been determined.

Metabolism/Excretion –

Conventional doxorubicin: Plasma disappearance follows a triphasic pattern with mean half-lives of 12 minutes, 3.3 hours and 29.6 hours. Doxorubicin is metabolized by carbonyl reduction to the active alcohol, doxorubicinol and inactive aglycones. Other inactive metabolites have been identified in urine and bile.

Liver function impairment, as reflected by elevated serum bilirubin, results in slower excretion and increased retention and accumulation of drug and metabolites in plasma and tissues. Other liver function abnormalities are not predictive. Urinary excretion accounts for ≈ 4% to 5% of the dose in 5 days. Biliary excretion is the major excretion route; 40% to 50% is recovered in bile or feces in 7 days.

DOXORUBICIN HCl (ADR)

Liposomal doxorubicin: Doxorubicinol, the major metabolite of doxorubicin, was detected at very low levels (range, 0.8 to 26.2 ng/ml) in the plasma of patients who received 10 or 20 mg/m^2 liposomal doxorubicin.

The plasma clearance of liposomal doxorubicin was slow, with a mean clearance value of 0.041 L/hr/m^2. This is in contrast to original doxorubicin.

Because of its slower clearance, the AUC of liposomal doxorubicin, primarily representing the circulation of liposome-encapsulated doxorubicin, is ≈ two to three orders of magnitude larger than the AUC for a similar dose of conventional doxorubicin as reported.

Indications:

Conventional doxorubicin: To produce regression in the following: Acute lymphoblastic leukemia, acute myeloblastic leukemia, Wilms' tumor, neuroblastoma, soft tissue and bone sarcomas, breast carcinoma, ovarian carcinoma, transitional cell bladder carcinoma, thyroid carcinoma, Hodgkin's and non-Hodgkin's lymphomas, bronchogenic carcinoma (the small cell histologic type is the most responsive) and gastric carcinoma.

Liposomal doxorubicin: Treatment of AIDS-related Kaposi's sarcoma in patients with disease that has progressed on prior combination chemotherapy or in patients who are intolerant to such therapy.

Contraindications:

Malignant melanoma, kidney carcinoma, large bowel carcinoma, brain tumors and metastases to the CNS are not significantly responsive to doxorubicin therapy.

Do not initiate therapy in patients with marked myelosuppression induced by previous treatment with other antitumor agents or by radiotherapy.

Conclusive data are not available on preexisting heart disease as a cofactor of increased risk of drug-induced cardiac toxicity. In such cases cardiac toxicity may occur at doses lower than recommended cumulative limit. Do not use doxorubicin in such cases.

A history of hypersensitivity reactions to conventional or liposomal doxorubicin or their components.

Previous treatment with complete cumulative doses of doxorubicin or daunorubicin.

Warnings:

Myelosuppression (60% to 84% of patients), primarily of leukocytes, requires careful monitoring. With the recommended dosage schedule, leukopenia is usually transient, reaching its nadir 10 to 14 days after treatment, with recovery usually by the 21st day. Expect white blood cell counts as low as 1000/mm^3 during treatment. Hematologic toxicity may require dose reduction, suspension or delay of therapy. Persistent, severe myelosuppression may result in superinfection or hemorrhage.

Necrotizing colitis manifested by typhlitis (cecal inflammation), bloody stools and severe and sometimes fatal infections have occurred with doxorubicin given by IV push daily for 3 days with cytarabine continuous infusion daily for ≥ 7 days.

Cardiac toxicity must be given special attention. Although uncommon, acute left ventricular failure has occurred, particularly in patients who have received total dosage exceeding the recommended limit of 550 mg/m^2. Dose-related incidences range from < 2% at total doses of ≤ 400 mg/m^2 to > 20% at total doses of > 700 mg/m^2. This limit appears to be lower (400 mg/m^2) in patients who received radiotherapy to the mediastinal area. The total dose of drug should also take into account any previous or concomitant therapy with other potentially cardiotoxic agents such as cyclophosphamide or daunorubicin. Cardiomyopathy or CHF may occur several weeks after drug discontinuation and is often unresponsive to medical or physical therapy.

Early diagnosis of drug-induced heart failure is essential for successful treatment with digitalis, diuretics, low salt diet and bed rest. Severe cardiac toxicity may occur precipitously without antecedent ECG changes. Perform an ECG at and prior to each dose or after 300 mg/m^2 cumulative dose. Transient ECG changes (eg, T wave flattening, ST depression, arrhythmias) lasting up to 2 weeks after a dose are not indications for therapy suspension. Doxorubicin cardiomyopathy is associated with persistent reduction in voltage of the QRS wave, prolongation of the systolic time interval and reduction of ejection fraction. None of these tests have consistently identified patients approaching their maximally tolerated cumulative dose. If test results indicate cardiac function change, carefully evaluate benefit of continued therapy against risk of producing irreversible cardiac damage. Some clinicians recommend discontinuing therapy if ejection fraction is < 0.45 with a drop of 0.15 from baseline. Acute life-threatening arrhythmias occurred during or within a few hours of use.

DOXORUBICIN HCl (ADR)

Preliminary evidence suggests cardiotoxicity may be reduced and total dosage safely increased by giving the drug on a weekly schedule or as a prolonged (48 to 96 hrs) continuous infusion.

The most definite test for anthracycline myocardial injury is endomyocardial biopsy. Other methods such as echocardiography or gated radionuclide scans have been used to monitor cardiac function during anthracycline therapy. If these test results indicate possible cardiac injury associated with doxorubicin or liposomal doxorubicin therapy, weigh the benefit of continued therapy against the risk of myocardial injury. Dexrazoxane, a cardioprotective agent, may be effective in preventing doxorubicin-induced cardiotoxicity (see individual monograph).

Extravasation at injection site with or without a stinging or burning sensation may occur, even if blood returns well on aspiration of the infusion needle. Consider liposomal doxorubicin an irritant. If any signs of extravasation occur, terminate the infusion immediately and restart in another vein. For management, see the Antineoplastic Introduction.

The application of ice over the site of extravasation for ≈ 30 minutes may be helpful in alleviating the local reaction. Do not give IM or SC.

Infusion reactions appear to occur with the first infusion and do not appear to occur with later infusions if not present initially. In most patients, these reactions resolve over the course of several hours to a day once the infusion is terminated. In some patients, the reaction resolves by slowing the rate of infusion. Similar reactions have not been reported with conventional doxorubicin, and they presumably represent a reaction to liposomal doxorubicin or one of its surface components.

Many patients were able to tolerate futher infusions without complications; however, six patients were terminated from therapy because of an infusion reaction to liposomal doxorubicin.

Palmar-plantar erythrodysesthesia: Among 705 patients with AIDS-related Kaposi's sarcoma treated with liposomal doxorubcin, 24 (3.4%) developed palmar-plantar skin eruptions characterized by swelling, pain, erythema and desquamation of the skin on the hands and feet. The syndrome was generally seen after ≥ 6 weeks of treatment but may occur earlier. The incidence of this reaction may be higher when liposomal doxorubicin is administered at doses that are higher or at intervals that are shorter than those recommended. In most patients, the reaction is mild and resolves in 1 to 2 weeks so that prolonged delay of therapy need not occur. However, the reaction can be severe and debilitating in some patients and may require discontinuation of treatment.

Mucositis may occur 5 to 10 days after administration, leading to ulceration, and represent a site or origin for severe infections. Incidence and severity of mucositis is greater with the 3 successive daily dosage regimen. Ulceration and necrosis of the colon, especially the cecum, may occur leading to bleeding or severe infections that can be fatal. This reaction has occurred in patients with acute non-lymphocytic leukemia treated with 3 days of doxorubicin plus cytarabine.

Hepatic function impairment: Doxorubicin is excreted primarily via the bile and toxicity is enhanced by hepatic impairment. Prior to dosing, evaluate hepatic function using clinical laboratory tests such as AST, ALT, alkaline phosphatase and bilirubin. Reduction of dose is recommended (see Administration and Dosage).

Carcinogenesis/Mutagenesis: Doxorubicin and related compounds have mutagenic and carcinogenic properties in experimental models.

Elderly: Patients > 65 years of age tolerate acute side effects as well as the younger age group.

Pregnancy: Category D. Safety for use during pregnancy is not established. Use only when the potential benefits outweigh the potential hazards to the fetus. Doxorubicin is embryotoxic and teratogenic in rats and embryotoxic and abortifacient in rabbits. Doxorubicin has been given during pregnancy without adverse fetal effect and has been detected in fetal tissue; however, its effect on the human fetus is unknown.

Children: Children treated with doxorubicin during childhood are more likely to have abnormal cardiac function. Females may be at more risk.

Precautions:

Monitoring: Initial treatment requires close patient observation and extensive laboratory monitoring. Hospitalize patients at least during the first phase of treatment.

Hyperuricemia may be induced by doxorubicin secondary to rapid lysis of neoplastic cells. Monitor patient's blood uric acid level.

Urine discoloration: Doxorubicin imparts a red color to the urine for 1 to 2 days after administration; advise patients to expect this during active therapy.

DOXORUBICIN HCl (ADR)

Drug Interactions:

Doxorubicin Drug Interactions			
Precipitant drug	Object drug*		Description
Barbiturates	Doxorubicin	⬇	The toal plasma clearance of doxorubicin may be increased.
Doxorubicin	Cyclophosphamide Mercaptopurine	⬆	Exacerbation of cyclophosphamide-induced hemorrhagic cystitis and enhancement of 6-mercaptopurine have occurred.
Doxorubicin	Digoxin	⬇	Serum levels may be decreased by combination chemotherapy (including doxorubicin). Digitoxin and digoxin capsules do not appear to affected.
Doxorubicin	Radiation	⬆	Radiation-induced toxicity to the myocardium, mucosa, skin and liver have been increased by doxorubicin administration.

* ⬆ = Object drug increased. ⬇ = Object drug decreased.

Adverse Reactions:

Infusion reactions: Acute infusion-associated reactions characterized by flushing, shortness of breath, facial swelling, headache, chills, back pain, tightness in the chest and throat and hypotension have occurred in ≈ 6.8% of patients treated with liposomal doxorubicin (see Warnings).

Dermatologic: Reversible complete alopecia (85% to 100%); hyperpigmentation of nailbeds and dermal creases (primarily in children); onycholysis; recall of skin reaction due to prior radiotherapy; palmar-plantar erythrodysesthesia (see Warnings).

Vascular: Phlebosclerosis, especially when small veins or a single vein is used for repeated administration. Facial flushing may occur if injection is too rapid.

GI: Acute nausea and vomiting (21% to 55%) may be severe and may be alleviated by antiemetic therapy. Mucositis (stomatitis and esophagitis; see Warnings); anorexia, diarrhea (occasionally).

Local: Severe cellulitis, vesication and tissue necrosis occur if drug is extravasated (see Warnings). Erythematous streaking along the vein next to the injection site has occurred.

Hypersensitivity: Fever; chills; urticaria; anaphylaxis; lincomycin cross-sensitivity.

Ophthalmic: Conjunctivitis and lacrimation (rare).

Overdosage:

Acute overdosage enhances the toxic effects of mucositis, leukopenia, pancytopneia and thrombocytopenia. Treat the severely myelosuppressed patient by hospitalization, antibiotics, platelet and granulocyte transfusions and give symptomatic treatment of mucositis.

Chronic overdosage with cumulative doses exceeding 550 mg/m^2 increases the risk of cardiomyopathy and resultant CHF. Vigorously manage CHF with digitalis preparations and diuretics. Use of peripheral vasodilators is recommended.

Administration and Dosage:

For IV use only.

Conventional doxorubicin:

Recommended dosage schedule – 60 to 75 mg/m^2, as a single IV injection administered at 21 day intervals. Give the lower dose to patients with inadequate marrow reserves due to old age, prior therapy or neoplastic marrow infiltration.

Alternative dose schedules – 30 mg/m^2 on each of 3 successive days, repeated every 4 weeks. Another alternative dose schedule is weekly doses of 20 mg/m^2 which may produce a lower incidence of CHF.

Dosage in patients with elevated bilirubin – Serum bilirubin 1.2 to 3 mg/dl, give 50% of normal dose; > 3 mg/dl, give 25% of normal dose.

Liposomal doxorubicin:

Recommended dosage schedule – Administer IV at a dose of 20 mg/m^2 (conventional doxorubicin equivalent) over 30 minutes, once every 3 weeks, for as long as the patient responds satisfactorily and tolerates treatment.

Do not administer as a bolus injection or an undiluted solution. Rapid infusion may increase the risk of infusion-related reactions.

Alternative dose schedules –

DOXORUBICIN HCl (ADR)

Liposomal Doxorubicin Dosing in Palmar-Plantar Erythrodysesthesia			
Toxicity grade	Symptoms	Weeks since last dose	
		3	4
0	No symptoms	Redose at 3-week interval	Redose at 3-week interval
1	Mild erythema, swelling or desquamation not interfering with daily activities	Redose unless patient has experienced a previous grade 3 or 4 skin toxicity, in which case, wait an additional week.	Redose at 25% dose reduction; return to 3-week interval.
2	Erythema, desquamation or swelling interfering with, but not precluding, normal physical activities; small blisters or ulcerations < 2 cm in diameter	Wait an additional week.	Redose at 50% dose reduction; return to 3-week interval.
3	Blistering, ulceration or swelling interfering with walking or normal daily activities; cannot wear regular clothing	Wait an additional week.	Discontinue liposomal doxorubicin.
4	Diffuse or local process causing infectious complications, or a bedridden state or hospitalization		

Liposomal Doxorubicin Dosing in Hematological Toxicity			
Grade	ANC (cells/mm^3)	Platelets (cells/mm^3)	Modification
1	1500 - 1900	75,000 - 150,000	None
2	1000 - < 1500	50,000 - < 75,000	None
3	500 - 999	25,000 - < 50,000	Wait until ANC is ≥ 1000 or platelets are ≥ 50,000, then redose at 25% dose reduction.
4	< 500	< 25,000	Wait until ANC is ≥ 1000 or platelets are ≥ 50,000, then redose at 50% dose reduction.

Liposomal Doxorubicin Dosing in Stomatitis		
Grade	Symptoms	Modification
1	Painless ulcers, erythema or mild soreness	None.
2	Painful erythema, edema or ulcers, but can eat	Wait 1 week and if symptoms improve, redose at 100% dose.
3	Painful erythema, edema or ulcers, and cannot eat	Wait 1 week and if symptoms improve, redose at 25% dose reduction.
4	Requires parenteral or enteral support	Wait 1 week and if symptoms improve, redose at 50% dose reduction.

Patients with impaired hepatic function – Limited clinical experience exists in treating hepatically impaired patients with liposomal doxorubicin. Therefore, based on experience with conventional doxorubicin, it is recommended that liposomal doxorubicin dosage be reduced if the bilirubin is elevated as follows: Serum bilirubin 1.2 to 3 mg/dl, give ½ normal dose, > 3 mg/dl, give ¼ normal dose.

IV infusion: Administer slowly into the tubing of a freely running IV infusion of NaCl Injection or 5% Dextrose Injection. Attach the tubing to a butterfly needle inserted into a large vein. Avoid veins over joints or in extremities with compromised venous or lymphatic drainage. Rate depends on size of vein and dosage; however, do not administer in < 3 to 5 minutes. Local erythematous streaking along the vein as well as facial flushing may indicate too rapid administration.

DOXORUBICIN HCl (ADR)

Extravasation – A burning or stinging sensation may indicate perivenous infiltration; perivenous infiltration may occur painlessly (see Warnings).

Preparation/storage of solution:

Conventional doxorubicin – Dilute the 10 mg vial with 5 ml, the 20 mg vial with 10 ml, the 50 mg vial with 25 ml, the 100 mg vial with 50 ml, and the 150 mg vial with 75 ml of 0.9% NaCl for a final concentration of 2 mg/ml. Bacteriostatic diluents are not recommended.

Liposomal doxorubicin – Dilute the appropriate dose of liposomal doxorubicin, up to a maximum of 90 mg, in 250 ml of 5% Dextrose Injection, USP prior to administration. Do not use with in-line filters.

IV compatibilities/incompatibilities:

Conventional doxorubicin – Incompatible with **heparin, cephalothin** and **dexamethasone sodium phosphate**; a precipitate will form. A color change in doxorubicin from red to blue-purple which denotes decomposition occurs with **aminophylline** and **5-fluorouracil.** Until specific data are available, do not mix doxorubicin with other drugs. One study reported that a solution of doxorubicin and vinblastine in 0.9% Sodium Chloride is compatible and relatively stable for at least 5 days.

Liposomal doxorubicin – Do not mix with other drugs. Do not use with any diluent other than 5% Dextrose Injection. Do not use any bacteriostatic agent, such as benzyl alcohol. Liposmal doxorubicin is not a clear solution but a translucent, red liposomal dispersion.

Storage/Stability:

Conventional doxorubicin – Reconstituted solution is stable for 24 hrs at room temperature and 48 hrs at 2° to 8°C (36° to 46°F). Protect from sunlight; discard unused solution.

Liposomal doxorubicin – Refrigerate diluted liposomal doxorubicin at 2° to 8°C (36° to 46°F) and administer within 24 hours. Avoid freezing. Prolonged freezing may adversely affect liposomall drug products; however, short-term freezing (< 1 month) does not appear to have a deleterious effect on liposomal doxorubicin.

Rx	**Doxorubicin HCl** (Cetus)	**Powder for Injection (lyophilized)**: 10 mg	With 50 mg lactose. In vials.
Rx	**Rubex** (Bristol-Myers Oncology)		With 50 mg lactose. In vials
Rx	**Doxorubicin HCl** (Cetus)	**Powder for Injection (lyophilized)**: 20 mg	With 100 mg lactose. In vials.
Rx	**Doxorubicin HCl** (Cetus)	**Powder for Injection (lyophilized)**: 50 mg	With 250 mg lactose. In vials.
Rx	**Rubex** (Bristol-Myers Oncology)		With 250 mg lactose. In vials.
Rx	**Rubex** (Bristol-Myers Oncology)	**Powder for Injection (lyophilized)**: 100 mg	With 500 mg lactose. In vials.
Rx	**Adriamycin RDF** (Pharmacia)	**Powder for Injection (lyophilized)**: 10, 20, 50 and 150[1] mg	In vials.[2] *Rapid dissolution formula.*
Rx	**Doxorubicin HCl** (Cetus)	**Injection, aqueous**: 2 mg/ml	0.9% NaCl. In 5, 10 and 25 ml vials.
Rx	**Adriamycin PFS** (Pharmacia)	**Preservative Free Injection**: 2 mg/ml	In 5, 10, 25 and 100 ml vials.
Rx	**Doxil** (Sequus)	**Injection**: 20 mg	Sucrose. In 10 ml vials.

[1] Multiple-dose vial.
[2] With methylparaben and 50, 100, 250 and 750 mg lactose, respectively.

DAUNORUBICIN CITRATE LIPOSOMAL

Actions:

Pharmacology: Liposomal daunorubicin contains an aqueous solution of the citrate salt of daunorubicin encapsulated within lipid vesicles (liposomes) composed of a lipid bilayer of distearoylphosphatidylcholine and cholesterol (2:1 molar ratio). Daunorubicin is an anthracycline antibiotic with antineoplastic activity, which is originally obtained from *Streptomyces peucetius.* It may also be isolated from *Streptomyces coeruleorubidus.* Daunorubicin has a 4–ring anthracycline moiety linked by a glycosidic bond to daunosamine, an amino sugar.

DAUNORUBICIN CITRATE LIPOSOMAL

Liposomal daunorubicin is a liposomal preparation of daunorubicin formulated to maximize the selectivity of daunorubicin for solid tumors in situ. In the circulation, the liposomal daunorubicin formulation helps to protect the entrapped daunorubicin from chemical and enzymatic degradation, minimizes protein binding and generally decreases uptake by normal (non-reticuloendothelial system) tissues. The specific mechanism by which liposomal daunorubicin is able to deliver daunorubicin to solid tumors in situ is not known. However, it is believed to be a function of increased permeability of the tumor neovasculature to some particles in the size range of liposmal daunorubicin. Once within the tumor environment, daunorubicin is released over time enabling it to exert its antineoplastic activity.

Pharmacokinetics:

Absorption/Distribution – Following IV injection, plasma clearance shows monoexponential decline. Plasma clearance is 17.3 ml/min, volume of distribution is 6.4 L, distribution half-life is 4.41 hrs, steady-state is 6.4 L and elimination half-life is 4.4 hrs. Daunorubicinol, the major active metabolite of daunorubiciin, was detected at low levels in the plasma.

Clinical trials: In advanced HIV-related Kaposi's sarcoma, two treatment regimens were compared as first-line cytotoxic therapy: Liposomal daunorubicin 40 mg/m^2 and ABV (doxorubicin 10 mg/m^2, bleomycin 15 U and vincristine 1 mg). Twenty of 33 ABV patients and 11 of 27 liposomal daunorubicin patients responded to therapy by criteria more stringent than flattening of lesions. Photographic evidence of tumor response to liposomal daunorubicin and ABV was comparable across all anatomic sities (eg, face, oral cavity, trunk, legs and feet).

Indications:

Advanced HIV-associated Kaposi's sarcoma: First-line cytotoxic therapy for advanced HIV-associated Kaposi's sarcoma.

Contraindications:

Hypersensitivity reaction to previous doses or to any constituents of the product.

Warnings:

Myelosuppression: The primary toxicity of daunorubicin is myelosuppression, especially of the granulocytic series, which may be severe, with much less marked effects on the platelets and erythroid series.

Potential cardiac toxicity, particularly in patients who have received prior anthracyclines or who have pre-existing cardiac disease, may occur. Although there is no reliable means of predicting CHF, cardiomyopathy induced by anthracyclines is usually associated with a decrease of the left ventricular ejection fraction (LVEF). Certain ECG chages and a descrease in the systolic ejection fraction from pretreatment baseline may aid in recognizing those patients at greatest risk. A decrease of ≥ 30% in limb lead QRS voltage has been associated with significant risk of drug-induced cardiomyopathy. Weigh the benefits of continued therapy against the risk. Early clinical diagnosis of drug induced CHF is essential for successful treatment with digitalis, diuretics, sodium restriction and bed rest.

Back pain, flushing and chest tightness has been reported in 13.8% of the patients. This generally occurs during the first 5 minutes of the infusion, subsides with interruption of the infusion and generally does not recur if the infusion is then resumed at a slower rate. This combination of symptoms appears to be related to the lipid component of liposomal daunorubicin, as a similar set of signs and symptons has been observed with other liposomal products not containing daunorubicin.

Extravasation at injection site: Conventional daunorubicin has been associated with local tissue necrosis at the site of drug extravasaion. Although grade 3 to 4 injection site inflammation was reported in two patients treated with liposomal daunorubicin, no instances of local tissue necrosis were observed with extravasation. Ensure that there is no extravasation of the drug.

Hepatic function impairment: Reduce dosage in patients with impaired hepatic function (see Adminstration and Dosage).

Elderly: Safety and efficacy in the elderly have not been established.

Pregnancy: Category D. Daunorubicin can cause fetal harm when administered to a pregnant woman. If liposomal daunorubicin is used during pregnancy, or if the patient becomes pregnant while taking liposomal daunorubicin, the patient must be warned of the potential hazard to the fetus.

Children: Safety and efficacy in children have not been established.

DAUNORUBICIN CITRATE LIPOSOMAL

Precautions:

Monitoring: Observe patient closely and monitor chemical and laboratory tests extensively. Evaluate cardiac, renal and hepatic function prior to each course of treatment. Repeat blood counts prior to each dose and withhold if the absoute granulocyte count is < 750 cells/mm^3. Monitor serum uric acid levels.

Hyperuricemia may be induced secondary to rapid lysis of leukemic cells. As a precaution, administer allopurinol prior to initiating antileukemic therapy.

Infection: Control any systemic infections before beginning therapy.

Drug Interactions:

No systemic studies of interaction have been conducted.

Adverse Reactions:

Adverse Reactions of Liposomal Daunorubicin Compared with ABV (Doxorubicin, Bleomycin and Vincristine) (%)

	Liposomal daunorubicin (n=116)		ABV (n = 111)	
Adverse effects	Mild/Moderate	Severe	Mild/Moderate	Severe
CNS				
Depression	7	3	6	-
Dizziness	8	-	9	-
Fatigue	43	6	44	7
Headache	22	3	23	2
Insomnia	6	-	14	-
Malaise	9	1	11	1
Neuropathy	12	1	38	3
GI				
Abdominal pain	20	3	23	4
Anorexia	21	2	26	2
Constipation	7	-	18	-
Diarrhea	34	4	29	6
Nausea	51	3	45	5
Stomatitis	9	1	8	-
Vomiting	20	3	26	2
Musculoskeletal				
Arthralgia	7		6	-
Back pain	16	-	8	-
Myalgia	7		12	-
Rigors	19		23	-
Respiratory				
Cough	26	2	19	-
Dyspnea	23	3	17	3
Rhinitis	12	-	6	-
Sinusitis	8	-	5	1
Dermatologic				
Alopecia	8		36	-
Pruritus	7	-	14	-
Miscellaneous				
Abnormal vision	3	2	3	-
Alleric reactions	21	3	19	2
Chest pain	9	1	7	-
Edema	9	2	8	1
Fever	42	5	49	5
Sweating	12	2	12	-
Tenesmus	4	1	1	

Other adverse events (liposomal daunorubicin vs ABV): Neutropenia (< 1000 cells/mm^3), 36% vs 35% of patients; neutropenia (< 500 cells/mm^3), 15% vs 5%; opportunistic infections/illnesses, 40% vs 27%; median time to first opportunistic infection/illness, 214 vs 412 days; number of cases with absolute reduction in ejection fraction of 20% to 25%, 3 vs 1 case; known number of cases removed from therapy due to cardiac causes, 2 vs 0; influenza-like symptoms, 5% each.

DAUNORUBICIN CITRATE LIPOSOMAL

Other (≤ 5%):

Cardiovascular – Hot flushes, hypertension, palpitation, syncope, tachycardia.

CNS – Amnesia, anxiety, ataxia, confusion, convulsions, emotional lability, abnormal gait, hallucinations, hyperkinesia, hypertonia, meningitis, somnolence, abnormal thinking, tremors.

Dermatologic – Folliculitis, seborrhea, dry skin.

GI – Increased appetite, dysphagia, GI hemorrhage, gastritis, gingival bleeding, hemorrhoids, hepatomegaly, melena, dry mouth, tooth caries.

GU – Dysuria, nocturia, polyuria.

Respiratory – Hemoptysis, hiccoughs, pulmonary infiltration, increased sputum.

Special Senses – Conjunctivitis, deafness, ear/eye pain, taste perversion, tinnitus.

Miscellaneous – Infection site inflammation; lympadenopathy; splenomegaly; dehydration; thirst.

Overdosage:

Symptoms of acute overdosage are increased severities of the observed dose-limiting toxicities of therpeutic doses, myelosuppression (especially granulocytopenia), fatigue, nausea and vomiting.

Administration and Dosage:

Approved by the FDA on April 8, 1996

Administer IV over 1 hour at a dose of 40 mg/m^2. Repeat every 2 weeks. Continue treatment until there is evidence of progressive disease (eg, based on best response achieved; new visceral sites of involvement progression of visceral disease; development of 10 or more new, cutaneous lesions or a 25% increase in the number of lesions compared to baseline; a change in the character of ≥ 25% of all previously counted flat lesions to raised; increase in surface area of the indicator lesions) or until other complications of HIV disease preclude continuation of therapy.

Hepatic or renal function impairment: Reduce dosage.

Liposomal Daunorubicin Dosage in Hepatic or Renal Function Impairment		
Serum bilirubin	Serum creatinine	Recommended dose
1.2 to 3 mg/dl		¾ normal dose
> 3 mg mg/dl	> 3 mg/dl	½ normal dose

Preparation and storage: Liposomal daunorubicin should be diluted 1:1 with 5% Dextrose Injection before administration. Do not use an in-line filter for IV infusion.

Storage/Stability: Refrigerate at 2° to 8°C (36° to 46°F). Store reconstituted solution for a maximum of 6 hours. Do not freeze. Protect from light.

Rx	**DaunoXome** (NeXstar)	**Injection:** 2 mg/ml (equivalent to 50 mg daunorubicin base)	In vials. 1, 4 and 10 unit packs.

MITOXANTRONE HCl

> **Warning:**
> When used in doses indicated for the treatment of leukemia, severe myelosuppression will occur. Therefore, it is recommended that the drug be administered only by physicians experienced in the chemotherapy of this disease. Laboratory and supportive services must be available for hematologic and chemistry monitoring and adjunctive therapies, including antibiotics. Blood and blood products must be available to support patients during the expected period of medullary hypoplasia and severe myelosuppression. Give particular care to assuring full hematologic recovery before undertaking consolidation therapy (if this treatment is used); monitor patients closely during this phase.

Actions:

Pharmacology: Mitoxantrone is a synthetic antineoplastic anthracenedione for IV use.

Although its mechanism of action is not fully elucidated, mitoxantrone is a DNA-reactive agent. It has a cytocidal effect on both proliferating and nonproliferating cultured human cells, suggesting lack of cell cycle phase specificity.

Pharmacokinetics:

Absorption/Distribution – Pharmacokinetic studies in adults following a single IV administration have demonstrated multi-exponential plasma clearance. Distribution to tissues is rapid and extensive. Multiple IV doses in dogs daily for 5 days resulted in a fourfold accumulation in plasma and tissue. The apparent steady-state volume of distribution exceeds 1000 L/m^2. Elimination is slow with an apparent mean terminal plasma half-life of 5.8 days (range, 2.3 to 13). The half-life in tissues may be longer. Mitoxantrone is 78% bound to plasma proteins in the concentration range of 26 to 455 ng/ml.

Metabolism/Excretion – Excretion is via the renal and hepatobiliary systems. Renal excretion is limited; only 6% to 11% of the dose is recovered in the urine within 5 days after administration. Of the material recovered in the urine, 65% is unchanged drug; the remaining 35% is comprised of two inactive metabolites and their glucuronide conjugates (mono- and dicarboxylic acid derivatives). Hepatobiliary elimination of drug appears to be of greater significance; 25% of the dose is recovered in the feces within 5 days of IV dosing. No significant difference in pharmacokinetics was observed in seven patients with moderately impaired liver function (serum bilirubin 1.3 to 3.4 mg/dl) as compared with 16 patients without hepatic dysfunction. Results of pharmacokinetic studies on four patients with severe hepatic dysfunction (bilirubin > 3.4 mg/dl) suggest that these patients have a lower total body clearance and a larger area under curve than other patients at a comparable dose.

Clinical trials: The benefit of consolidation therapy in acute nonlymphocytic leukemia (ANLL) patients who achieve a complete remission remains controversial. However, in the only well controlled prospective, randomized multicenter trials with mitoxantrone in ANLL, consolidation therapy was given to all patients who achieved a complete remission. During consolidation in the US study, two myelosuppression-related deaths occurred in mitoxantrone patients and one in daunorubicin patients. However, in the foreign study, there were eight deaths in mitoxantrone patients during consolidation that were related to the myelosuppression, and none in daunorubicin patients where less myelosuppression occurred.

Indications:

ANLL in adults: In combination with other approved drug(s) in the initial therapy of ANLL in adults. This includes myelogenous, promyelocytic, monocytic and erythroid acute leukemias.

Unlabeled uses: Mitoxantrone may be beneficial, alone or in combination with other agents, in the treatment of breast cancer and refractory lymphomas. Response rates for breast cancer have been as high as 40% when used as a single agent. For non-Hodgkin's lymphoma, a high-dose intermittent dosage schedule appears to be more effective than a lower-dose weekly schedule.

Contraindications:

Hypersensitivity to mitoxantrone.

Warnings:

Myelosuppression: Patients with preexisting myelosuppression as the result of prior drug therapy should not receive mitoxantrone unless it is felt that the possible benefit from such treatment warrants the risk of further medullary suppression.

Cardiac: Functional cardiac changes including congestive heart failure (CHF) and decreases in left ventricular ejection fraction (LVEF) occur. Cardiac toxicity may be more common in patients with prior treatment with anthracyclines, prior mediastinal radiotherapy, or with preexisting cardiovascular disease. Such patients should have regular cardiac monitoring of LVEF from the initiation of therapy. In investigational trials of intermittent single doses in other tumor types, patients who received up to the cumulative dose of 140 mg/m^2 had a cumulative 2.6% probability of clinical CHF. The overall cumulative probability rate of moderate or serious decreases in LVEF at this dose was 13% in comparative trials.

Acute CHF may occasionally occur in patients treated for ANLL. In first-line comparative trials of mitoxantrone plus cytosine arabinoside in adult patients with previously untreated ANLL, therapy was associated with CHF in 6.5% of patients. A causal relationship between drug therapy and cardiac effects is difficult to establish in this setting since myocardial function is frequently depressed by the anemia, fever, infection and hemorrhage which often accompany the underlying disease.

Carcinogenesis: Mitoxantrone can result in chromosomal aberrations in animals and it is mutagenic in bacterial systems. Mitoxantrone caused DNA damage and sister chromatid exchanges in vitro.

Pregnancy: Category D. May cause fetal harm when administered to a pregnant woman. In treated rats, low fetal birth weight and retarded development of the fetal kidney were seen in greater frequency. In rabbits, an increased incidence of premature delivery was observed. Mitoxantrone was not teratogenic in rabbits. There are no adequate and well controlled studies in pregnant women. If this drug is used during pregnancy, or if the patient becomes pregnant while taking this drug, apprise her of the potential hazard to the fetus. Advise women of childbearing potential to avoid becoming pregnant.

Lactation: It is not known whether this drug is excreted in breast milk. Because of the potential for serious adverse reactions in infants, discontinue breastfeeding before starting treatment.

Children: Safety and efficacy for use in children have not been established.

Precautions:

Monitoring: Accompany therapy by close and frequent monitoring of hematologic and chemical laboratory parameters, as well as frequent patient observation. Serial complete blood counts and liver function tests are necessary for appropriate dose adjustments.

For IV use only: Safety for use by routes other than IV administration has not been established. Do not use intrathecally.

Hyperuricemia may occur as a result of rapid lysis of tumor cells. Monitor serum uric acid levels and institute hypouricemic therapy prior to initiation of antileukemic therapy.

Systemic infections: Treat concomitantly with or just before starting mitoxantrone.

Hepatotoxicity: Patients have developed transient elevations of AST and ALT following mitoxantrone administration (4 to 24 days after treatment).

Adverse Reactions:

Mitoxantrone has been studied in approximately 600 patients with ANLL. The following table summarizes adverse reactions occurring in patients treated with mitoxantrone plus cytosine arabinoside for therapy of ANLL in a large multicenter randomized prospective US trial. Adverse reactions are presented as major categories and selected examples of clinically significant subcategories. Experience in the large foreign study was similar. A much wider experience in a variety of other tumor types revealed no additional important reactions other than cardiomyopathy. Note that the listed adverse reaction categories include overlapping clinical symptoms related to the same condition (eg, dyspnea, cough, pneumonia). In addition, the listed adverse reactions cannot all necessarily be attributed to chemotherapy as it is often impossible to distinguish effects of the drug from effects of the underlying disease. It is clear, however, that the combination of mitoxantrone plus cytosine arabinoside was responsible for nausea and vomiting, alopecia, mucositis/stomatitis and myelosuppression.

MITOXANTRONE HCl

Mitoxantrone Adverse Reactions	Induction (%)	Consolidation (%)
Cardiovascular	26	11
CHF	5	0
Arrhythmias	3	4
Bleeding	37	20
GI bleeding	16	2
Petechiae/Ecchymosis	7	11
GI	88	58
Nausea/Vomiting	72	31
Diarrhea	47	18
Abdominal pain	15	9
Mucositis/Stomatitis	29	18
Hepatic	10	14
Jaundice	3	7
Infections	66	60
UTI	7	7
Pneumonia	9	9
Sepsis	34	31
Fungal infections	15	9
Pulmonary	43	24
Cough	13	9
Dyspnea	18	6
CNS	30	34
Seizures	4	2
Headache	10	13
Eye	7	2
Conjunctivitis	5	0
Other		
Renal failure	8	0
Fever	78	24
Alopecia	37	22

Other adverse reactions include: Chest pain; asymptomatic decreases in LVEF; tachycardia; ECG changes; myelosuppression; hypotension, urticaria, dyspnea, rashes (occasionally); phlebitis at infusion site (infrequent); tissue necrosis following extravasation (rare).

Overdosage:

There is no known specific antidote. Accidental overdoses have occurred. Four patients receiving 140 to 180 mg/m^2 as a single bolus injection died as a result of severe leukopenia with infection. Hematologic support and antimicrobial therapy may be required during prolonged periods of medullary hypoplasia.

Although patients with severe renal failure have not been studied, mitoxantrone is extensively tissue bound and it is unlikely that the therapeutic effect or toxicity would be mitigated by peritoneal or hemodialysis.

Patient Information:

Mitoxantrone may impart a blue-green color to the urine for 24 hours after administration; advise patients to expect this during therapy. Bluish discoloration of the sclera may also occur. Advise patients of the signs and symptoms of myelosuppression.

MITOXANTRONE HCl

Administration and Dosage:

Mitoxantrone solution must be diluted prior to use.

Combination initial therapy for ANLL in adults: For induction, 12 mg/m^2 /day on days 1 to 3 given as an IV infusion, and 100 mg/m^2 of cytosine arabinoside for 7 days given as a continuous 24 hour infusion on days 1 to 7.

Most complete remissions will occur following the initial course of induction therapy. In the event of an incomplete antileukemic response, a second induction course may be given. Give mitoxantrone for 2 days and cytosine arabinoside for 5 days using the same daily dosage levels.

If severe or life-threatening nonhematologic toxicity is observed during the first induction course, withhold the second induction course until toxicity clears.

Consolidation therapy used in two large randomized multicenter trials consisted of mitoxantrone 12 mg/m^2 given by IV infusion daily for days 1 and 2, and cytosine arabinoside 100 mg/m^2 for 5 days given as a continuous 24 hour infusion on days 1 to 5. The first course was given ≈ 6 weeks after the final induction course, the second was generally administered 4 weeks after the first. Severe myelosuppression occurred.

Preparation of solution – Dilute solution to at least 50 ml with either 0.9% Sodium Chloride Injection or 5% Dextrose Injection. Introduce this solution slowly into the tubing as a freely running IV infusion of 0.9% Sodium Chloride Injection or 5% Dextrose Injection over a period of not less than 3 minutes. Discard unused infusion solutions in an appropriate fashion. If extravasation occurs, stop administration immediately and restart in another vein. The nonvesicant properties of mitoxantrone minimize the possibility of severe local reactions following extravasation. However, take care to avoid extravasation at the infusion site and to avoid contact with the skin, mucous membranes or eyes.

Mitoxantrone may be further diluted into Dextrose 5% in Water, Normal Saline or Dextrose 5% with Normal Saline and used immediately.

If skin is accidentally exposed to mitoxantrone, rinse copiously with warm water; if the eyes are involved, use standard irrigation techniques immediately. The use of goggles, gloves and protective gowns is recommended during preparation and administration of the drug. Spills on equipment and environmental surfaces may be cleaned using an aqueous solution of calcium hypochlorite (5.5 parts calcium hypochlorite in 13 parts by weight of water for each 1 part of mitoxantrone). Absorb the solution with gauze or towels and dispose of these in a safe manner. Wear appropriate safety equipment such as goggles and gloves while working with calcium hypochlorite.

IV incompatibility – Do not mix in the same infusion as heparin; a precipitate may form. Because specific compatibility data are not available, it is recommended that mitoxantrone not be mixed in the same infusion with other drugs.

Storage – Do not freeze.

Rx	**Novantrone** (Immunex)	**Injection**: 2 mg mitoxantrone base per ml	In 5, 10, 12.5 and 15 ml vials.

MITOMYCIN (Mitomycin-C; MTC)

> **Warning:**
>
> *Bone marrow suppression,* notably thrombocytopenia and leukopenia, which may contribute to overwhelming infection in an already compromised patient, is the most common and severe toxic effect (see Warnings and Adverse Reactions).
>
> *Hemolytic uremic syndrome,* a serious syndrome of microangiopathic hemolytic anemia, thrombocytopenia and irreversible renal failure has occurred (see Warnings).

Actions:

Pharmacology: Mitomycin is an antibiotic with antitumor activity isolated from Streptomyces caespitosus. It selectively inhibits the synthesis of deoxyribonucleic acid (DNA). The guanine and cytosine content correlates with the degree of mitomycin-induced cross-linking. At high concentrations, cellular ribonucleic acid (RNA) and protein synthesis are also suppressed.

Pharmacokinetics:

Absorption/Distribution – IV mitomycin is rapidly cleared from the serum. Maximal serum concentrations were 2.4 mcg/ml after IV injection of 30 mg; 1.7 mcg/ml after a 20 mg dose, and 0.52 mcg/ml after 10 mg. Serum half-life after a 30 mg bolus injection is 17 minutes.

Metabolism/Excretion – Clearance is effected primarily by hepatic metabolism, but metabolism occurs in other tissues as well. Clearance rate is inversely proportional to maximal serum concentration due to saturation of degradative pathways. About 10% of a dose is excreted unchanged in urine. Because of saturable metabolic pathways, the percent excreted in urine increases with increasing dose.

Indications:

Therapy of disseminated adenocarcinoma of stomach or pancreas with other chemotherapeutic agents, and as palliative treatment when other modalities fail.

Unlabeled uses: Mitomycin has been given by the intravesical route for the management of superficial bladder cancer. Mitomycin as an ophthalmic solution appears beneficial as an adjunct to surgical excision in primary or recurrent pterygia.

Contraindications:

Primary therapy as a single agent; to replace surgery or radiotherapy; hypersensitivity or idiosyncratic reaction to mitomycin; patients with thrombocytopenia, coagulation disorder or an increase in bleeding tendency due to other causes.

Warnings:

Bone marrow suppression, particularly thrombocytopenia and leukopenia, occurring in 64% of patients, is the most serious toxicity and is cumulative. Thrombocytopenia or leukopenia may occur any time within 8 weeks (average 4 weeks) of therapy; recovery after therapy is within 10 weeks. About 25% of the patients did not recover.

Perform the following during and for at least 8 weeks following therapy: Platelet count, WBC, differential and hemoglobin. A platelet count < 100,000/mm^3 or a WBC < 4,000/mm^3, or a progressive decline in either, is an indication to interrupt therapy. Observe patients frequently during and after therapy. Advise patients of potential toxicity, particularly bone marrow suppression. Deaths have occurred due to septicemia as a result of leukopenia.

Renal function impairment: Observe patients for evidence of renal toxicity. Do not give to patients with a serum creatinine > 1.7 mg/dl.

Carcinogenesis: At doses approximating the recommended clinical dose in man, mitomycin produces a 50% to 100% increase in tumor incidence in rats and mice.

Pregnancy: Safety for use during pregnancy has not been established. Teratological changes have been noted in animal studies.

Precautions:

Adult respiratory distress syndrome: A few cases have occurred in patients receiving mitomycin in combination with other chemotherapy and maintained at FIO_2 concentrations > 50% perioperatively. Exercise caution to use only enough oxygen to provide adequate arterial saturation since oxygen itself is toxic to the lungs. Pay careful attention to fluid balance; avoid overhydration.

Drug Interactions:

Vinca alkaloids: Acute shortness of breath and severe bronchospasm have occurred following use of vinca alkaloids in patients who had previously or simultaneously received mitomycin. Onset of this acute respiratory distress occurs within minutes to hours after the vinca alkaloid injection. Total number of doses for each drug varies considerably. Bronchodilators, steroids or oxygen produce symptomatic relief.

MITOMYCIN (Mitomycin-C; MTC)

Adverse Reactions:

Bone marrow toxicity: (64%): Thrombocytopenia and leukopenia (see Warnings).

Integument and mucous membrane: (4%): Cellulitis at injection site is occasionally severe; stomatitis; alopecia. Rashes occur rarely.

Extravasation – The most important dermatological problem with this drug is necrosis and consequent tissue sloughing if the drug is extravasated during injection, which may occur with or without stinging or burning and even if there is adequate blood return when the needle is aspirated. Delayed erythema or ulceration may occur either at or distant from injection site, weeks to months after use, even when no evidence of extravasation was seen during use. For management, see Antineoplastics Introduction.

Renal: 2% of 1281 patients had a significant rise in serum creatinine. There was no correlation between total dose or duration of therapy and degree of renal impairment.

Pulmonary toxicity: Infrequent, but can be severe or life-threatening. Dyspnea with nonproductive cough and radiographic evidence of pulmonary infiltrates may indicate pulmonary toxicity. If other etiologies are eliminated, discontinue therapy. Steroids have been used to treat this toxicity, but therapeutic value is not determined. Adult respiratory distress syndrome may also occur (see Precautions).

Hemolytic uremic syndrome (HUS): This serious complication of chemotherapy, consisting primarily of microangiopathic hemolytic anemia (hematocrit $\le$ 25%), thrombocytopenia ($\le$ 100,000/mm^3) and irreversible renal failure (serum creatinine $\ge$ 16 mg/dl) has occurred in patients receiving mitomycin. Microangiopathic hemolysis with fragmented red blood cells on peripheral blood smears has occurred in 98% of patients with the syndrome. Other less frequent complications may include: Pulmonary edema (65%); neurologic abnormalities (16%); hypertension. Exacerbation of the symptoms associated with HUS has occurred in some patients receiving blood product transfusions. A high mortality rate (52%) has been associated with HUS.

The syndrome may occur at any time during therapy with mitomycin as a single agent or in combination with other cytotoxic drugs. Closely monitor patients receiving $\ge$ 60 mg for unexplained anemia with fragmented cells on peripheral blood smear, thrombocytopenia and decreased renal function.

Acute side effects (14%): Fever; anorexia; nausea; vomiting.

Other: Headache; blurred vision; confusion; drowsiness; syncope; fatigue; edema; thrombophlebitis; hematemesis; diarrhea; pain. These did not appear to be dose-related and were not unequivocally drug-related.

MITOMYCIN (Mitomycin-C; MTC)

Administration and Dosage:

Give IV only. If extravasation occurs, cellulitis, ulceration and sloughing may result.

After hematological recovery (see dosage adjustment guide) from previous chemotherapy use 20 mg/m^2 IV as a single dose at 6 to 8 week intervals.

Because of cumulative myelosuppression, reevaluate patients after each course of therapy; reduce dose if patient experiences any toxicity. Doses > 20 mg/m^2 are not more effective, and are more toxic than lower doses. Do not repeat dosage until leukocyte count has returned to 4000/mm^3 and platelet count to 100,000/mm^3. If disease continues to progress after two courses, discontinue; chances of response are minimal. When used with other myelosuppressives, adjust dosage appropriately.

Dosage Adjustment for Mitomycin

Nadir after prior dose per mm^3		% of prior dose to be given
Leukocytes	Platelets	
> 4000	> 100,000	100
3000-3999	75,000-99,999	100
2000-2999	25,000-74,999	70
< 2000	< 25,000	50

Preparation of solution: Reconstitute 5, 20 or 40 mg vial with 10, 40 or 80 ml Sterile Water for Injection, respectively. If product does not dissolve immediately, allow to stand at room temperature until solution is obtained.

Stability: Avoid excessive heat (> 40°C). Reconstituted with Sterile Water for Injection to 0.5 mg/ml, solution is stable for 14 days under refrigeration, 7 days at room temp.

Diluted in various IV fluids at room temperature to a concentration of 20 to 40 mcg/ml, stability is as follows: 5% Dextrose Injection, 3 hours; 0.9% NaCl Injection, 12 hours; Sodium Lactate Injection, 24 hours.

The combination of mitomycin (5 to 15 mg) and heparin (1,000 to 10,000 units) in 30 ml of 0.9% NaCl Injection is stable for 48 hours at room temperature.

Rx	**Mutamycin** (Bristol-Myers Oncology)	**Powder for Injection:** 5, 20 and 40 mg	In vials. With 10, 40 and 80 mg mannitol, respectively.

DACTINOMYCIN (Actinomycin D; ACT)

> **Warning:**
> Dactinomycin is extremely corrosive to soft tissue. If extravasation occurs during IV use, severe damage to soft tissues will occur. In at least one instance, this has led to contracture of the arms.

Actions:

Pharmacology: Dactinomycin is the principal component of the mixture of actinomycins produced by *Streptomyces parvullus.* Dactinomycin exerts an inhibitory effect on gram-positive and gram-negative bacteria and on some fungi. However, its toxic properties preclude its use as an antibiotic in treating infectious diseases.

Dactinomycin anchors into a purine-pyrimidine (DNA) base pair by intercalation, inhibiting messenger RNA synthesis. Although maximal cell-kill is noted in G_1 phase, the cytotoxic action is primarily cell cycle nonspecific. Actively proliferating cells are more sensitive.

Pharmacokinetics: Very little active drug can be detected in circulating blood 2 minutes after IV injection. It concentrates in nucleated cells and does not cross the blood-brain barrier. Dactinomycin is minimally metabolized. Plasma half-life is ≈ 36 hours.

Indications:

Wilms' tumor: Combinations with vincristine, radiotherapy and surgery.

Rhabdomyosarcoma: Combinations with vincristine, cyclophosphamide and doxorubicin.

Metastatic and nonmetastatic choriocarcinoma: Combination with methotrexate.

Nonseminomatous testicular carcinoma.

Ewing's sarcoma: Palliative treatment alone, with other antineoplastics or x-ray.
Nonmetastatic Ewing's – Cyclosphosphamide and radiotherapy.

Sarcoma botryoides: Palliative treatment alone, with other antineoplastics or radiotherapy.

Radiation therapy effects may be potentiated by dactinomycin; the converse also appears likely. Dactinomycin may be tried in radiosensitive tumors not responding to x-ray therapy. Objective improvement in tumor size and activity may be observed when lower, better tolerated doses of both types of therapy are employed.

Perfusion technique: Dactinomycin alone or with other antineoplastics has been given by the isolation-perfusion technique, either as palliative treatment or as an adjunct to tumor resection; some tumors resistant to chemotherapy and radiation therapy may respond. Neoplasms in which dactinomycin has been tried using this technique include various types of sarcoma, carcinoma and adenocarcinoma. This technique offers advantages, provided drug leakage into the general circulation is minimal. By this technique the drug is in continuous contact with the tumor for the duration of treatment. The dose may be increased well over that used by the systemic route, usually without added toxicity.

Contraindications:

If given at or about the time of infection with chicken pox or herpes zoster, a severe generalized disease may occur, which could result in death.

Warnings:

Radiation: With combined dactinomycin-radiation therapy, the normal skin, as well as the buccal and pharyngeal mucosa, show early erythema. A smaller than usual x-ray dose, when given with dactinomycin, causes erythema and vesiculation which progress more rapidly through the tanning and desquamation stages. Healing may occur in 4 to 6 weeks rather than 2 to 3 months. Erythema from previous x-ray therapy may be reactivated by dactinomycin alone, even when irradiation occurred many months earlier, and especially when the interval between the two forms of therapy is brief. When the nasopharynx is irradiated, the combination may produce severe oropharyngeal mucositis. Severe reactions may appear if high doses are used or if the patient is particularly sensitive to such combined therapy.

Increased incidence of GI toxicity and marrow suppression has occurred when dactinomycin was given with x-ray therapy. Use particular caution in the first 2 months after irradiation for the treatment of right-sided Wilms' tumor, since hepatomegaly and elevated AST levels have been noted.

Reports indicate an increased incidence of second primary tumors following treatment with radiation and dactinomycin.

Carcinogenesis/Mutagenesis: The International Agency on Research on Cancer has judged that dactinomycin is a positive carcinogen in animals. Local sarcomas were produced in mice and rats after repeated SC or intraperitoneal injection. Mesenchymal tumors occurred in male rats given intraperitoneal injections of 0.05 mg/kg, 2 to 5 times per week for 18 weeks. The first tumor appeared at 23 weeks.

Dactinomycin has been mutagenic in a number of test systems in vitro and in vivo including human fibroblasts and leukocytes, and HELA cells. DNA damage and cytogenetic effects have been demonstrated in the mouse and the rat.

Pregnancy: Category C. The drug has caused malformations and embryotoxicity in the rat, rabbit and hamster in doses 3 to 7 times the maximum recommended human dose. There are no adequate and well controlled studies in pregnant women. Safety for use during pregnancy has not been established. Use only when clearly needed and when potential benefits outweigh potential hazards to the fetus.

Lactation: It is not known whether this drug is excreted in breast milk. Because of the potential for serious adverse reactions in nursing infants decide whether to discontinue nursing or to discontinue the drug, taking into account the importance of the drug to the mother.

Infants – Do not give to infants < 6 to 12 months of age because of greater frequency of toxic effects.

Precautions:

Reactions may involve any body tissue; anaphylactoid reactions may occur.

Nausea and vomiting due to dactinomycin necessitates intermittent administration. Observe the patient daily for toxic side effects when multiple chemotherapy is used; a full course of therapy occasionally is not tolerated. If stomatitis, diarrhea or severe hematopoietic depression appear, discontinue use until the patient has recovered.

Renal, hepatic and bone marrow function: Many abnormalities have occurred.

This drug is highly toxic. Handle and administer both powder and solution with care. Avoid inhalation of dust or vapors and contact with skin or mucous membranes, especially those of the eyes. Should accidental eye contact occur, immediately institute copious irrigation with water, followed by prompt ophthalmologic consultation. Should accidental skin contact occur, immediately irrigate the affected part with copious amounts of water for at least 15 minutes.

Extravasation: Dactinomycin is extremely corrosive. Extravasation during IV administration causes severe damage to soft tissues. This has led to contracture of the arms in at least one instance. If extravasation occurs, immediately discontinue the infusion. Apply cold compresses to the area. Local infiltration with an injectable corticosteroid may lessen the local reaction. Dilute the drug by infusing saline injection through the line into the infiltrated area.

Drug Interactions:

Drug/Lab test interactions: Dactinomycin may interfere with bioassay procedures for the determination of antibacterial drug levels.

Adverse Reactions:

Toxic effects usually do not become apparent until 2 to 4 days after a course of therapy and may not be maximal before 1 to 2 weeks. Adverse reactions are usually reversible with discontinuation of therapy.

Oral: Cheilitis; dysphagia; esophagitis; ulcerative stomatitis; pharyngitis.

GI: Anorexia; abdominal pain; diarrhea; GI ulceration; proctitis; liver toxicity (including ascites, hepatomegaly, hepatitis and liver function test abnormalities). Alleviate nausea and vomiting occurring during the first few hours after use by giving antiemetics.

Hematologic: Anemia (including aplastic anemia); agranulocytosis; leukopenia; thrombocytopenia; pancytopenia; reticulopenia. Perform platelet and white cell counts daily. If either count markedly decreases, withhold drug until marrow recovery occurs; this often takes up to 3 weeks.

Dermatologic: Alopecia; skin eruptions; acne; flare-up of erythema; increased pigmentation of previously irradiated skin.

Miscellaneous: Malaise; fatigue; lethargy; fever; myalgia; hypocalcemia; death.

Perfusion technique complications may consist of hematopoietic depression, absorption of toxic products from massive destruction of neoplastic tissue, increased susceptibility to infection, impaired wound healing and superficial ulceration of the gastric mucosa. Other side effects may include edema of the extremity involved, damage to soft tissues of the perfused area and (potentially) venous thrombosis.

DACTINOMYCIN (Actinomycin D; ACT)

Administration and Dosage:

Toxic reactions are frequent and may limit the amount of drug that may be given. Severity of toxicity varies and is only partly dependent on dose. Administer the drug in short courses.

IV: Individualize dosage. Do not exceed 15 mcg/kg or 400 to 600 mcg/m^2 daily IV for 5 days. Calculate the dosage for obese or edematous patients on the basis of surface area in an effort to relate dosage to lean body mass.

Adults – 0.5 mg/day IV for a maximum of 5 days.

Children – 0.015 mg/kg/day IV for 5 days. Alternative schedule is a total dosage of 2.5 mg/m^2 IV over 1 week.

In both adults and children, administer a second course after at least 3 weeks, provided all signs of toxicity have disappeared.

Isolation-perfusion technique: 0.05 mg/kg for lower extremity or pelvis; 0.035 mg/kg for upper extremity. Use lower doses in obese patients, or when previous therapy has been employed. Complications are related to amount of drug that escapes into systemic circulation.

Use "two-needle technique" if given directly into the vein without use of an infusion. Reconstitute and withdraw dose from vial with one sterile needle. Use another needle for direct injection into vein.

Preparation of solution: Reconstitute by adding 1.1 ml Sterile Water for Injection (without preservative). The resulting solution contains approximately 0.5 mg/ml. Add directly to infusion solutions of 5% Dextrose or Sodium Chloride Injection or to the tubing of a running IV infusion. Although chemically stable after reconstitution, the product does not contain a preservative; discard any unused portion. Use of water that contains preservatives (benzyl alcohol or parabens) to reconstitute the drug for injection results in precipitate formation.

Partial removal of dactinomycin from IV solutions by cellulose ester membrane filters used in some IV in-line filters has been reported.

Storage: Protect from light.

Rx	**Cosmegen** (MSD)	**Lyophilized Powder for Injection:** 0.5 mg	In vials.[1]

[1] With 20 mg mannitol.

PLICAMYCIN (Mithramycin)

> **Warning:**
> Severe thrombocytopenia, hemorrhagic tendency and even death may result from use. Although severe toxicity is more apt to occur in patients with advanced disease or patients otherwise considered poor risks for therapy, serious toxicity may also occasionally occur in patients who are in relatively good condition.

Actions:

Pharmacology: Plicamycin is a compound produced by the organism *Streptomyces plicatus*. The exact mechanism of tumor inhibition is unknown; the drug forms a complex with deoxyribonucleic acid (DNA) and inhibits cellular ribonucleic acid (RNA) and enzymatic RNA synthesis. The binding to DNA in the presence of Mg^{++} (or other divalent cations) is responsible for the inhibition of DNA-dependent or DNA-directed RNA synthesis. This presumably accounts for plicamycin's biological properties.

Plicamycin demonstrates a consistent calcium-lowering effect not related to its tumoricidal activity. It may block the hypercalcemic action of pharmacologic doses of vitamin D. It also acts on osteoclasts and blocks the action of parathyroid hormone. Plicamycin's inhibition of DNA-dependent RNA synthesis appears to render osteoclasts unable to fully respond to parathyroid hormone with the biosynthesis necessary for osteolysis. Decreases in serum phosphate levels and urinary calcium excretion accompany the lowering of serum calcium concentrations.

Pharmacokinetics: Rapidly cleared from blood within the first 2 hrs; excretion is also rapid. Of measured excretion, 67% occurs within 4 hrs, 75% within 8, and 90% in the first 24 hours after injection. Crosses the blood-brain barrier; the concentration in brain tissue is low, but persists longer than in other tissues.

Clinical pharmacology: Inoperable testicular tumors – In a combined series of 305 patients with inoperable testicular tumors treated with plicamycin, 33 (11%) had a complete disappearance of tumor masses; 80 (26%) had significant partial regression. Longest duration of a continuing complete response is > 8.5 yrs.

Plicamycin may be useful in testicular tumors resistant to other chemotherapeutic agents. Prior radiation or chemotherapy did not alter response rate, suggesting no significant cross-resistance between plicamycin and other antineoplastics.

Hypercalcemia/Hypercalciuria: A limited number of plicamycin patients with hypercalcemia (range: 12 - 25.8 mg/dl) and hypercalciuria (range: 215 - 492 mg/day) associated with malignant disease had reversal of these abnormal levels. In some patients, the primary malignancy was of nontesticular origin.

Indications:

Malignant testicular tumors when surgery or radiation is impossible.

Hypercalcemia and hypercalciuria in symptomatic patients (NOT responsive to conventional treatment) associated with advanced neoplasms.

Contraindications:

Thrombocytopenia, thrombocytopathy, coagulation disorders or increased susceptibility to bleeding due to other causes; impairment of bone marrow function; pregnancy (see Warnings).

PLICAMYCIN (Mithramycin)

Warnings:

Hemorrhagic syndrome, the most important form of toxicity, usually begins with epistaxis. It may only consist of a single or several episodes of epistaxis and progress no further. It can start with hematemesis progressing to more widespread GI hemorrhage or to a more generalized bleeding tendency. It is most likely due to abnormalities in multiple clotting factors and is dose-related. With doses of ≤ 30 and >30 mcg/kg/day for ≤ 10 doses, the incidence of bleeding episodes has been 5.4% and 11.9% with a mortality rate of 1.6% and 5.7%, respectively.

Renal function impairment: Use extreme caution. Monitor renal function carefully before, during and after treatment.

Mutagenesis: Histologic evidence of inhibition of spermatogenesis occurs in some male rats receiving doses of ≥ 0.6 mg/kg/day.

Pregnancy: Category X. Use only when clearly needed and when benefits outweigh potential toxicity to the embryo or fetus. Plicamycin may cause fetal harm when given to a pregnant woman, and is contraindicated in women who are or may become pregnant. If used during pregnancy or if patient becomes pregnant while taking this drug, inform her of the potential hazard to the fetus.

Lactation: It is not known whether plicamycin is excreted in breast milk. Because of the potential for serious adverse reactions in nursing infants, discontinue nursing or the drug, taking into account the importance of the drug to the mother.

Precautions:

Monitoring: Obtain platelet count, prothrombin and bleeding times frequently during therapy and for several days following the last dose. Discontinue therapy if thrombocytopenia or a significant prolongation of prothrombin or bleeding times occurs.

Electrolyte imbalance (especially hypocalcemia, hypokalemia and hypophosphatemia): Correct with appropriate therapy prior to treatment.

Adverse Reactions:

Most common: GI symptoms (anorexia, nausea, vomiting, diarrhea and stomatitis).

Less frequent: Fever; drowsiness; weakness; lethargy; malaise; headache; depression; phlebitis; facial flushing; skin rash; hepatotoxicity (mild, reversible).

Lab test abnormalities: Generally reversible following cessation of treatment.

Hematologic: Depression of platelet count, white count, hemoglobin and prothrombin; elevation of clotting and bleeding times; abnormal clot retraction. Thrombocytopenia may have rapid onset and occur at any time during therapy or within several days after the last dose. Infusion of platelet concentrates of platelet-rich plasma may help elevate platelet count. Leukopenia is relatively uncommon (≈ 6%).

Abnormalities in clotting time or clot retraction are not commonly demonstrated prior to the onset of an overt bleeding episode. Perform these tests periodically; abnormalities may serve as a warning of impending serious toxicity.

Hepatic: Increased AST, ALT, isocritic and lactic dehydrogenases, alkaline phosphatase, serum bilirubin, ornithine carbamyl transferase, bromsulphalein retention.

Renal: Increased BUN and serum creatinine; proteinuria.

Electrolyte Disturbance: Depression of serum calcium, phosphorus and potassium.

Overdosage:

Expect exaggeration of usual adverse effects. Closely monitor hematologic picture including factors involved in clotting mechanism, hepatic and renal functions and serum electrolytes. No specific antidote is known. Management includes general supportive measures.

Patient Information:

Notify physician of any of these: Fever; sore throat; rashes; chills; unusual bleeding or bruising; bloody nose; black tarry stools; dark urine; yellowing of skin/eyes.

Nausea, vomiting and stomach upset are common. Avoid sweet, fried or fatty foods. Eat smaller light meals several times a day. Dry foods (eg, toast, crackers) and liquids (eg, soups, unsweetened apple juice) may be more easily digested. Do not lie down after eating. If this does not help, antinausea drugs may be prescribed.

Contraceptive measures are recommended during treatment.

Calcium supplements are sometimes needed during plicamycin therapy.

Administration and Dosage:

Base dose on body weight. Use ideal weight if patient has abnormal fluid retention.

Testicular tumors: 25 to 30 mcg/kg/day for 8 to 10 days unless significant side effects or toxicity occurs. Do not use > 10 daily doses. Do not exceed 30 mcg/kg/day.

PLICAMYCIN (Mithramycin)

In responsive tumors, some degree of regression is usually evident within 3 or 4 weeks following the initial course of therapy. If tumor masses remain unchanged, additional courses at monthly intervals are warranted.

When significant tumor regression is obtained, give additional courses of therapy at monthly intervals until complete regression is obtained or until definite tumor progression or new tumor masses occur, in spite of continued therapy.

Hypercalcemia and hypercalciuria (associated with advanced malignancy): 25 mcg/kg/day for 3 or 4 days. If desired degree of reversal is not achieved with initial course of therapy, repeat at intervals of ≥ 1 week to achieve desired result or to maintain serum and urinary calcium excretion at normal levels. It may be possible to maintain normal calcium balance with single, weekly doses or with 2 or 3 doses per week.

Administer IV only. Dilute daily dose in 1 L of 5% Dextrose Inj or NaCl Inj; infuse slowly IV over 4 to 6 hrs. Avoid rapid direct IV injection; it may cause a higher incidence and greater severity of GI side effects. Extravasation may cause local irritation and cellulitis at injection sites. If thrombophlebitis or perivascular cellulitis occur, stop infusion and restart at another site. Moderate heat on the site may help disperse the compound and minimize discomfort and local tissue irritation. Antiemetics may help relieve nausea and vomiting.

Preparation of solution: Reconstitute with 4.9 ml of Sterile Water for Injection to make 500 mcg plicamycin per ml. Discard unused solution. Prepare fresh solutions daily.

Storage: Refrigerate unreconstituted vials at 2° to 8°C (36° to 46°F).

Rx	**Mithracin** (Miles)	**Powder for Injection:** 2500 mcg	100 mg mannitol. In vials.

PODOPHYLLOTOXIN DERIVATIVES

Warning:

Severe myelosuppression with resulting infection or bleeding may occur.

Hypersensitivity reactions, including anaphylaxis-like symptoms, may occur with initial dosing or at repeated exposure to teniposide. Epinephrine, with or without corticosteroids and antihistamines, has been used to alleviate symptoms.

Actions:

Pharmacology: These drugs are semisynthetic derivatives of podophyllotoxin.

Etoposide – Its main effect appears to be at the G_2 portion of the cell cycle. Two dose-dependent responses occur: At high concentrations (≥ 10 mcg/ml), lysis of cells entering mitosis is seen; at low concentrations (0.3 to 10 mcg/ml), cells are inhibited from entering prophase. The predominant macromolecular effect appears to be DNA synthesis inhibition.

Teniposide is a phase-specific cytotoxic drug, acting in the late S or early G_2 phase of the cell cycle, thus preventing cells from entering mitosis. Teniposide causes dose-dependent single- and double-stranded breaks in DNA and DNA:protein cross-links. The mechanism of action appears to be related to the inhibition of type II topoisomerase activity since teniposide does not intercalate into DNA or bind strongly to DNA. The cytotoxic effects of teniposide are related to the relative number of double-stranded DNA breaks produced in cells, which are a reflection of the stabilization of a topoisomerase II-DNA intermediate. Teniposide has a broad spectrum of in vivo antitumor activity against murine tumors, including hematologic malignancies and various solid tumors. Notably, it is active against sublines of certain murine leukemias with acquired resistance to cisplatin, doxorubicin, amsacrine, daunorubicin, mitoxantrone or vincristine.

Pharmacokinetics: The pharmacokinetic characteristics of teniposide differ from those of etoposide. Teniposide is more extensively bound to plasma proteins and its cellular uptake is greater. Teniposide also has a lower systemic clearance, a longer elimination half-life and is excreted in the urine as parent drug to a lesser extent than etoposide.

Various Pharmacokinetic Parameters for Etoposide and Teniposide

Parameter	Etoposide	Teniposide
Total body clearance (ml/min)	33-48	10.3
Terminal half-life (hrs)	4-11	5
Volume of distribution (L)	18-29	3-11 (children) 8-44 (adults)
Protein binding (%)	97	> 99
Elimination	Renal (35%) and nonrenal (ie, mostly metabolism, ≤ 6% bile)	Renal (44%) and fecal (≤ 10%)
Excreted unchanged in urine (%)	< 50	4-12

Etoposide –

Absorption/Distribution: The mean oral bioavailability is approximately 50% (range, 25% to 75%). There is no evidence of a first-pass effect for etoposide. On IV administration, the disposition of etoposide is a biphasic process with a distribution half-life of about 1.5 hours. The areas under the plasma concentration-time curves (AUC) and maximum plasma concentration (Cmax) values increase linearly with dose. Etoposide does not accumulate in the plasma following daily administration of 100 mg/m^2 for 4 to 5 days. After either IV infusion or oral administration, Cmax and AUC values exhibit marked intra- and intersubject variability. These values for oral etoposide consistently fall in the same range as the Cmax and AUC values for an IV dose of half the size of the oral dose.

PODOPHYLLOTOXIN DERIVATIVES

Although detectable in CSF and intracerebral tumors, the concentrations are lower than in extracerebral tumors and plasma. Concentrations are higher in normal lung than in lung metastases and are similar in primary tumors and normal tissues of the myometrium. An inverse relationship between plasma albumin levels and renal clearance is found in children.

Metabolism/Excretion: The major urinary metabolite is the hydroxy acid. Glucuronide or sulfate conjugates of etoposide are excreted in human urine and represent 5% to 22% of the dose.

In adults, total body clearance is correlated with creatinine clearance, serum albumin concentration and nonrenal clearance. In children, elevated serum ALT levels are associated with reduced drug total body clearance. Prior use of cisplatin may also result in a decrease of etoposide total body clearance in children.

Teniposide – Plasma drug levels decline biexponentially following IV infusion in children. In adults, plasma levels increase linearly with dose. Drug accumulation did not occur after daily administration for 3 days. In children, Cmax after infusions of 137 to 203 mg/m^2 over a period of 1 to 2 hours exceeded 40 mcg/ml; by 20 to 24 hours after infusion plasma levels were generally < 2 mcg/ml.

The blood-brain barrier appears to limit diffusion of teniposide into the brain, although in a study in patients with brain tumors, CSF levels were higher than in patients without brain tumors.

Clinical trials:

Teniposide – Nine children with acute lymphocytic leukemia (ALL) failing induction therapy with a cytarabine-containing regimen were treated with teniposide plus cytarabine. Three of these patients were induced into complete remission with durations of remission of 30 weeks, 59 weeks and 13 years. In another study, 16 children with ALL refractory to vincristine/prednisone-containing regimens were treated with teniposide plus vincristine and prednisone. Three patients were induced into complete remission with durations of remission of 5.5, 37 and 73 weeks.

Indications:

Etoposide:

Refractory testicular tumors in combination with other chemotherapeutic agents in patients who have received surgery, chemotherapy and radiotherapy. Adequate data on the use of oral etoposide are not available.

Small cell lung cancer in combination with other agents as first line treatment.

Teniposide: In combination with other approved anticancer agents for induction therapy in patients with refractory childhood acute lymphoblastic leukemia (ALL). Available under a Treatment IND since 1988 for relapsed or refractory ALL.

Unlabeled uses:

Etoposide has been used alone or in combination in acute nonlymphocytic leukemias (monocytic), Hodgkin's disease, non-Hodgkin's lymphomas, Kaposi's sarcoma and neuroblastoma. Other tumors with a response rate of 5% to 20% to etoposide as a single agent include: Choriocarcinoma; rhabdomyosarcoma; hepatocellular carcinoma; epithelial ovarian, non-small and small cell lung, testicular, gastric, endometrial and breast cancers; acute lymphocytic leukemia; soft tissue sarcoma.

Contraindications:

Hypersensitivity to etoposide, teniposide or Cremophor EL (polyoxyethylated castor oil, present in the teniposide preparation).

PODOPHYLLOTOXIN DERIVATIVES

Warnings:

Myelosuppression: Observe patients for myelosuppression during and after therapy. Dose-limiting bone marrow suppression is the most significant toxicity.

Laboratory studies – Perform at the start of therapy and prior to each subsequent dose: Platelet count, hemoglobin, white blood cell count and differential. A platelet count < 50,000/mm^3 or an absolute neutrophil count < 500/mm^3 is an indication to withhold further therapy until the blood counts have sufficiently recovered.

Anaphylaxis manifested by chills, fever, tachycardia, bronchospasm, dyspnea, facial flushing, hypertension or hypotension may occur (etoposide, 0.7% to 2%; teniposide, ≈ 5%). The reactions usually respond to cessation of infusion and institution of appropriate therapy. Refer to Management of Acute Hypersensitivity Reactions.

This reaction may occur with the first dose of teniposide and may be life threatening if not treated promptly with antihistamines, corticosteroids, epinephrine, IV fluids and other supportive measures as clinically indicated. The exact cause of these reactions is unknown; they may be due to the polyoxyethylated castor oil component of the vehicle or to teniposide itself. The incidence appears to be increased in patients with brain tumors and neuroblastoma. Patients who have experienced prior hypersensitivity reactions to teniposide are at risk for recurrence of symptoms and should only be retreated if the antileukemic benefit already demonstrated clearly outweighs the risk of a probable hypersensitivity reaction for that patient. When a decision is made to retreat a patient, pretreat with corticosteroids and antihistamines and carefully observe during and after the infusion. To date, there is no evidence to suggest cross-sensitization between teniposide and etoposide.

Monitoring: In addition to hematologic tests, carefully monitor renal and hepatic function tests prior to and during therapy.

Hypotension: Administer by slow IV infusion (30 to 60 minutes or longer) since hypotension may occur with rapid IV injection. With teniposide, it may also be due to a direct effect of the polyoxyethylated castor oil component. If hypotension occurs, stop infusion and give fluids or other supportive therapy, as appropriate. When restarting infusion, use a slower rate.

Benzyl alcohol: Teniposide contains benzyl alcohol, which has been associated with a fatal "gasping" syndrome in premature infants.

CNS depression: Acute CNS depression and hypotension have occurred in patients receiving investigational infusions of high-dose teniposide who were pretreated with antiemetic drugs. The depressant effects of the antiemetic agents and the alcohol content of the teniposide formulation may place patients receiving higher than recommended doses at risk for CNS depression.

Down's syndrome patients: Patients with both Down's syndrome and leukemia may be especially sensitive to myelosuppressive chemotherapy; therefore, reduce initial dosing with teniposide in these patients. It is suggested that the first course be given at half the usual dose. Subsequent courses may be administered at higher dosages depending on the degree of myelosuppression and mucositis encountered in earlier courses in an individual patient.

Hepatic function impairment: There appears to be some association between an increase in serum alkaline phosphatase or gamma glutamyl-transpeptidase and a decrease in plasma clearance of teniposide. Therefore, exercise caution if teniposide is administered to patients with hepatic dysfunction. In children, elevated serum ALT levels are associated with reduced drug total body clearance of etoposide.

PODOPHYLLOTOXIN DERIVATIVES

Carcinogenesis: These agents are possible carcinogens. Mutagenic and genotoxic potential has been established in mammalian cells.

Children with ALL in remission who received maintenance therapy with teniposide at weekly or twice weekly doses (plus other chemotherapeutic agents) had a relative risk of developing secondary acute nonlymphocytic leukemia (ANLL) approximately 12 times that of patients treated according to other less intensive schedules. A short course of teniposide for remission-induction or consolidation therapy was not associated with an increased risk of secondary ANLL, but the number of patients assessed was small. The potential benefit must be weighed on a case by case basis against the potential risk of the induction of a secondary leukemia.

Pregnancy: Category D. Etoposide and teniposide may cause fetal harm. They are teratogenic and embryotoxic in animals. There are no adequate and well controlled studies in pregnant women. If used during pregnancy, or if the patient becomes pregnant while receiving this drug, apprise her of the potential hazard to the fetus. Avoid becoming pregnant.

Lactation: It is not known whether this drug is excreted in breast milk. Because of the potential for serious adverse reactions in nursing infants, decide whether to discontinue nursing or the drug, accounting for the importance of the drug to the mother.

Children: Safety and efficacy for use of etoposide in children have not been established. Teniposide is indicated for use in children.

Drug Interactions:

Etoposide/Teniposide Drug Interactions			
Precipitant drug	Object drug*		Description
Etoposide	Warfarin	↑	Prolongation of the prothrombin time may occur.
Teniposide	Methotrexate	↑	Plasma clearance of methotrexate may be slightly increased. In vitro, increased intracellular levels were observed.
Sodium salicylate Sulfamethizole Tolbutamide	Teniposide	↑	Teniposide was displaced from protein-binding sites by these agents to a small but significant extent. Because of the extremely high binding of teniposide to plasma proteins, these small decreases in binding could cause substantial increases in free drug levels, resulting in potentiation of toxicity.

* ↑ = Object drug increased.

Adverse Reactions:

Most adverse reactions are reversible if detected early. If severe reactions occur, reduce or discontinue dosage and institute corrective measures. Reinstitute therapy with caution, consider further need for the drug and be alert to recurrence of toxicity.

Etoposide/Teniposide Adverse Reactions (%)		
Adverse reaction	Etoposide	Teniposide
Hematologic		
Myelosuppression, nonspecified	✓	75
Leukopenia (WBC/mm^3)		
<4000	60-91	—
<3000	—	89
<1000	3-17	—
Neutropenia (ANC/mm^3)		
<2000	—	95
Thrombocytopenia (platelets/mm^3)		
<100,000	22-41	85
<50,000	1-20	—
Anemia	≤ 33	88

PODOPHYLLOTOXIN DERIVATIVES

Etoposide/Teniposide Adverse Reactions (%)		
Adverse reaction	Etoposide	Teniposide
GI		
Mucositis	—	76
Nausea/Vomiting	31-43	29
Anorexia	10-13	—
Diarrhea	1-13	33
Abdominal pain	≤ 2	—
Stomatitis	1-6	—
Hepatic dysfunction/toxicity	≤ 3	< 1
Dysphagia	✓	—
Constipation	✓	—
Dermatologic		
Alopecia (reversible)[1]	≤ 66	9
Rash	✓	3
Pigmentation	✓	—
Pruritus	✓	—
Cardiovascular		
Hypotension[2]	1-2	2
Hypertension	✓	—
Miscellaneous		
Hypersensitivity/Anaphylactic reactions[2]	0.7-2 (< 1 oral)	≈ 5
Peripheral neurotoxicity	1-2	< 1
Aftertaste	✓	—
Fever	✓	3
Transient cortical blindness	✓	—
Infection		12
Bleeding	—	5
Renal dysfunction	—	< 1
Metabolic abnormalities	—	< 1

[1] Sometimes progressing to total baldness.
[2] See Warnings.
✓ = Adverse reaction observed, incidence not reported.
– = Not reported.

Overdosage:

Symptoms: The anticipated complications of overdosage are secondary to bone marrow suppression.

Treatment: There is no known antidote for overdosage. Treatment should consist of supportive care including blood products and antibiotics as indicated.

Patient Information:

Contraceptive measures are recommended during treatment.

Notify physician of any of these: Fever; chills; rapid heartbeat; difficult breathing.

Podophyllotoxin Derivatives

ETOPOSIDE (VP-16-213)

For complete prescribing information, refer to the Podophyllotoxin Derivatives group monograph.

Administration and Dosage:

Approved by the FDA in 1983.

Modify the dosage, by either route, to account for the myelosuppressive effects of other drugs in combination, the effects of prior x–ray therapy or chemotherapy which may have compromised bone marrow reserve.

Administer solution over 30 to 60 minutes or longer. Do not give by rapid IV injection.

Testicular cancer:

Parenteral – Usual dose is 50 to 100 mg/m²/day on days 1 to 5 to 100 mg/m²/day on days 1, 3 and 5.

Small cell lung cancer:

Parenteral – 35 mg/m²/day for 4 days to 50 mg/m²/day for 5 days. Courses are repeated at 3 to 4 week intervals after recovery from toxicity.

Oral – 2 times the IV dose rounded to the nearest 50 mg.

Preparation for IV administration: Dilute with either 5% Dextrose Injection or 0.9% Sodium Chloride Injection to give a final concentration of 0.2 or 0.4 mg/ml.

Plastic devices made of acrylic or ABS have cracked and leaked when used with undiluted etoposide. This has not been reported with diluted solutions.

Handling: Skin reactions may occur with accidental exposure. Use gloves. If solution contacts the skin or mucosa, immediately wash the area thoroughly with soap and water.

Storage/Stability: Unopened vials are stable for 2 years at room temperature (25°C; 77°F). Diluted solutions (concentration of 0.2 or 0.4 mg/ml) are stable for 96 and 48 hours, respectively, at room temperature under normal room fluorescent light in both glass and plastic containers. Capsules must be stored at 2° to 8°C (36° to 46°F). Stable for 2 years under refrigeration, 3 months at room temperature. Do not freeze.

Rx	**VePesid** (Bristol-Myers Oncology)	**Capsules:** 50 mg	Sorbitol. (Bristol 3091). Pink. In blisterpack 20s.
Rx	**Etoposide** (Various, eg, Gensia)	**Injection:** 20 mg/ml	In 5, 12.5 and 25 ml vials.[1]
Rx	**VePesid** (Bristol-Myers Oncology)		In 5 ml vials.[2]
Rx	**Toposar** (Pharmacia)		In 5, 10 and 25 ml.[3]
Rx	**Etopophos** (Bristol-Myers Oncology)	**Powder for injection, lyophilized:** 100 mg	In single dose vials.

[1] May contain alcohol, benzyl alcohol, 80 mg polysorbate 80, polyethylene glycol or citric acid.

[1] With 30 mg/ml benzyl alcohol, 80 mg polysorbate 80, 650 mg polyethylene glycol 300, 30.5% alcohol.

[2] With 30 mg/ml benzyl alcohol, 30.5% alcohol.

TENIPOSIDE (VM-26)

For complete prescribing information, refer to the Podophyllotoxin Derivatives group monograph.

Administration and Dosage:

Approved by the FDA on July 14, 1992.

Teniposide must be administered as an IV infusion. Take care to ensure that the IV catheter or needle is in the proper position and functional prior to infusion. Improper administration may result in extravasation causing local tissue necrosis or thrombophlebitis. In some instances, occlusion of central venous access devices has occurred during 24-hour infusion at a concentration of 0.1 to 0.2 mg/ml. Frequent observation during these infusions is necessary to minimize this risk.

Administer over 30 to 60 minutes or longer. Do not give by rapid IV injection. Hypotension has been reported following rapid IV administration.

In one study, childhood ALL patients failing induction therapy with a cytarabine-containing regimen were treated with the combination of teniposide 165 mg/m² and cytarabine 300 mg/m² IV twice weekly for 8 to 9 doses. In another study, patients with childhood ALL refractory to vincristine/prednisone-containing regimens were treated with the combinationn of teniposide 250 mg/m² and vincristine 1.5 mg/m² IV weekly for 4 to 8 weeks and prednisone 40 mg/m² orally for 28 days.

Podophyllotoxin Derivatives

TENIPOSIDE (VM-26)

Hepatic/Renal function imipairment: Adequate data in patients with hepatic or renal insufficiency are lacking, but dose adjustments may be necessary for patients with significant renal or hepatic impairment.

Down's syndrome patients: Reduce initial dosing; give the first course at half the usual dose (see Warnings).

Preparation for IV administration: Teniposide must be diluted with either 5% Dextrose Injection, USP, or 0.9% Sodium Chloride Injection, USP, to give final teniposide concentrations of 0.1, 0.2, 0.4 or 1 mg/ml.

Contact of undiluted teniposide with plastic equipment or devices used to prepare solutions for infusion may result in softening or cracking and possible drug product leakage. This effect has not been reported with diluted solutions.

In order to prevent extraction of the plasticizer DEHP, prepare and administer solutions in non-DEHP-containing LVP containers such as glass or polyolefin plastic bags or containers. The use of PVC containers is not recommended.

Lipid administration sets or low DEHP containing nitroglycerin sets will keep patients' exposure to DEHP at low levels and are suitable for use. The diluted solutions are chemically and physically compatible with the recommended IV administration sets and LVP containers for up to 24 hours at ambient room temperature and lighting conditions.

Teniposide is a cytotoxic anticancer drug; use caution in handling and preparing the solution. Skin reactions associated with accidental exposure may occur. The use of gloves is recommended. If teniposide solution contacts the skin, immediately wash the skin thoroughly with soap and water. If the drug contacts mucous membranes, flush thoroughly with water.

Admixture incompatibilities: Heparin solution can cause precipitation of teniposide, therefore, flush the administration apparatus thoroughly with 5% Dextrose Injection or 0.9% Sodium Chloride Injection, USP before and after administration of teniposide. Because of the potential for precipitation, compatibility with other drugs, infusion materials or IV pumps cannot be assured.

Storage/Stability: Unopened amps are stable until the date indicated on the package when stored under refrigeration (2° to 8°C; 36° to 46°F) in the original package (to protect from light). Freezing does not adversely affect the product. Reconstituted solutions are stable at room temperature for up to 24 hours after preparation. Administer 1 mg/ml solutions within 4 hours of preparation to reduce the potential for precipitation. Refrigeration of solutions is not recommended. Stability and use times are identical in glass and plastic containers.

Although solutions are chemically stable under the conditions indicated, precipitation of teniposide may occur at the recommended concentrations, especially if the diluted solution is subjected to more agitation than is recommended to prepare the drug solution for parenteral administration. In addition, minimize storage time prior to administration and take care to avoid contact of the diluted solution with other drugs or fluids. Precipitation has been reported during 24-hour infusions of teniposide concentrations of 0.1 to 0.2 mg/ml, resulting in occlusion of central venous access catheters in several patients.

Rx	**Vumon** (Bristol-Myers Oncology)	**Injection**[1]: 50 mg (10 mg/ml)	In 5 ml amps.[2]

[1] Must be diluted prior to administration.

[2] With 30 mg benzyl alcohol and 500 mg *Cremophor EL* (polyoxyethylated castor oil) per ml, with 42.7% dehydrated alcohol.

VINORELBINE TARTRATE

Warning:

Vinorelbine should be administered under the supervision of a physician experienced in the use of cancer chemotherapeutic agents. This product is for IV use only. Intrathecal administration of other vinca alkaloids has resulted in death. Syringes containing this product should be labeled, "Warning: Vinorelbine for intravenous use only."

Severe granulocytopenia resulting in increased susceptibility to infection may occur. Granulocyte counts should be ≥ 1000 cells/mm^3 prior to the administration of vinorelbine. Adjust dosage according to complete blood counts with differentials obtained on the day of treatment.

It is extremely important that the IV needle or catheter be properly positioned before vinorelbine is injected. Improper administration of vinorelbine may result in extravasation causing local tissue necrosis or thrombophlebitis (see Administration and Dosage).

Actions:

Pharmacology: Vinorelbine is a semi-synthetic vinca alkaloid with antitumor activity that interferes with microtubule assembly. The vinca alkaloids are structurally similar compounds comprised of two multi-ringed units, vindoline and catharanthine. Unlike other vinca alkaloids, the catharanthine unit is the site of structural modification for vinorelbine. The antitumor activity of vinorelbine is thought to be due primarily to inhibition of mitosis at metaphase through its interaction with tubulin. Like other vinca alkaloids, vinorelbine may also interfere with: 1) amino acid, cyclic AMP and glutathione metabolism, 2) calmodulin-dependent Ca^{++} -transport ATPase activity, 3) cellular respiration and 4) nucleic acid and lipid biosynthesis. In intact tectal plates from mouse embryos, vinorelbine, vincristine and vinblastine inhibited mitotic microtubule formation at the same concentration (2 mcM), inducing a blockade of cells at metaphase. Vincristine produced depolymerization of axonal microtubules at 5 mcM, but vinblastine and vinorelbine did not have this effect until concentrations of 30 mcM and 40 mcM, respectively. These data suggest relative selectivity of vinorelbine for mitotic microtubules.

Pharmacokinetics: Following IV administration, vinorelbine concentration in plasma decays in a triphasic manner. The initial rapid decline primarily represents distribution of the drug to peripheral compartments followed by metabolism and excretion of the drug during subsequent phases. The prolonged terminal phase is due to relatively slow efflux of vinorelbine from peripheral compartments. The terminal phase half-life averages 27.7 to 43.6 hours and the mean plasma clearance ranges from 0.97 to 1.26 L/hr/kg. Steady-state volume of distribution values range from 25.4 to 40.1 L/kg.

Vinorelbine demonstrated high binding to human platelets and lymphocytes. The binding to plasma constituents in cancer patients ranged from 79.6% to 91.2%. Vinorelbine binding was not altered in the presence of cisplatin, 5-fluorouracil or doxorubicin.

Vinorelbine undergoes substantial hepatic elimination, with large amounts recovered in feces. One metabolite, deacetylvinorelbine, possesses antitumor activity. This metabolite has been detected but not quantified in human plasma. The effects of renal or hepatic dysfunction on the disposition of vinorelbine have not been assessed, but based on experience with other anticancer vinca alkaloids, dose adjustments are recommended for patients with impaired hepatic function (see Administration and Dosage).

Approximately 18% of an administered dose was recovered in urine and 46% in feces; 10.9% ± 0.7% of a 30 mg/m^2 IV dose was excreted unchanged in the urine.

Clinical trials: Patients (n = 612) were randomized to treatment with single-agent vinorelbine (30 mg/m^2 /week), vinorelbine (30 mg/m^2 /week) plus cisplatin (120 mg/m^2 days 1 and 29, then every 6 weeks) and vindesine (3 mg/m^2 /week for 7 weeks, then every other week) plus cisplatin (120 mg/m^2 days 1 and 29, then every 6 weeks). Vinorelbine plus cisplatin produced longer survival times than vindesine plus cisplatin (median survival 40 weeks vs 32 weeks). The median survival time for patients receiving single-agent vinorelbine was similar to that of vindesine plus cisplatin (31 vs 32 weeks). The 1 year survival rates were 35% for vinorelbine plus cisplatin, 27% for vindesine plus cisplatin and 30% for single-agent vinorelbine. The overall objective response rate (all partial responses) was significantly higher with vinorelbine plus cisplatin (28%) than with vindesine plus cisplatin (19%) and with single-agent vinorelbine (14%). The response rates for vindesine plus cisplatin and single-agent vinorelbine were not significantly different. Significantly less nausea, vomiting, alopecia and neurotoxicity were observed in patients receiving single-agent vinorelbine compared to vindesine and cisplatin.

In another study, patients were treated with vinorelbine (n = 143; 30 mg/m^2) weekly or 5-fluorouracil (5-FU; n = 68; 425 mg/m^2 IV bolus) plus leucovorin (LV; 20 mg/m^2 IV bolus) daily for 5 days every 4 weeks. Vinorelbine showed improved survival time compared to 5-FU/LV. The median survival time for patients receiving vinorelbine was 30 weeks and for those receiving 5-FU/LV was 22 weeks. The 1 year survival rates were 24% for vinorelbine and 16% for the 5-FU/LV group. The median survival time with 5-FU/LV was similar to, or slightly better than, that usually observed in untreated patients with advanced NSCLC, suggesting that the difference was not related to some unknown detrimental effect of 5-FU/LV therapy. The response rates (all partial responses) for vinorelbine and 5-FU/LV were 12% and 3%, respectively. Quality-of-life was not adversely affected by vinorelbine when compared to control.

Indications:

Non-small cell lung cancer (NSCLC): Single agent or in combination with cisplatin for the first-line treatment of ambulatory patients with unresectable, advanced NSCLC. In patients with Stage IV NSCLC, vinorelbine is indicated as a single agent or in combination with cisplatin. In Stage III NSCLC, vinorelbine is indicated in combination with cisplatin.

Unlabeled uses:

Breast cancer – 30 mg/m^2/week; response rates of 30% to 53% (single agent) and 46% to 74% (combination therapy).

Ovarian carcinoma (cisplatin-resistant) – Response rates of 16% (single agent) to 35% (combination therapy).

Hodgkin's disease – 30 mg/m^2/week; response rates of 34% to 90%.

Contraindications:

Patients with pretreatment granulocyte counts < 1000 cells/mm^3 (see Warnings).

Warnings:

Granulocytopenia: Frequently monitor patients treated with vinorelbine for myelosuppression both during and after therapy. Granulocytopenia is dose-limiting. Granulocyte nadirs occur between 7 and 10 days after dosing with granulocyte count recovery usually within the following 7 to 14 days. Perform complete blood counts with differentials and review results prior to giving each dose. Do not administer to patients with granulocyte counts < 1000 cells/mm^3. Carefully monitor patients developing severe granulocytopenia for evidence of infection or fever. See Administration and Dosage for recommended dose adjustments for granulocytopenia.

Prophylactic hematologic growth factors have not been routinely used with vinorelbine. If medically necessary, growth factors may be administered at recommended doses no earlier than 24 hours after the administration of cytotoxic chemotherapy. Growth factors should not be given within 24 hours before the administration of chemotherapy.

Hepatic function impairment: There is no evidence that the toxicity of vinorelbine is enhanced in patients with elevated liver enzymes. However, exercise caution when administering vinorelbine to patients with severe hepatic injury or impairment (see Administration and Dosage).

Mutagenesis/Fertility impairment: In vivo, vinorelbine affects chromosome number and possibly structure.

Biweekly administration for 13 or 26 weeks in rats at 2.1 and 7.2 mg/m^2 (approximately one-fifteenth and one-fourth the human dose) resulted in decreased spermatogenesis and prostate/seminal vesicle secretion.

Elderly: In patients ≥ 65 years of age, no overall differences in effectiveness or safety were observed between these patients and younger patients. However, greater sensitivity of some older individuals cannot be ruled out.

Pregnancy: Category D. Vinorelbine may cause fetal harm if administered to a pregnant woman. A single dose of vinorelbine was embryo- or fetotoxic in mice and rabbits at doses of 9 mg/m^2 and 5.5 mg/m^2, respectively (one-third and one-sixth the human dose). At nonmaternotoxic doses, fetal weight was reduced and ossification was delayed. There have been no studies in pregnant women. If vinorelbine is used during pregnancy, or if the patient becomes pregnant while receiving this drug, apprise the patient of the potential hazard to the fetus. Advise women of childbearing potential to avoid becoming pregnant during therapy with vinorelbine.

Lactation: It is not known whether the drug is excreted in breast milk. Because of the potential for serious adverse reactions in nursing infants from vinorelbine, nursing should be discontinued in women who are receiving vinorelbine therapy.

Children: Safety and efficacy in children have not been established.

Precautions:

Monitoring: Since dose-limiting clinical toxicity is the result of depression of the white blood cell count, it is imperative that complete blood counts with differentials be obtained and reviewed on the day of treatment prior to each dose of vinorelbine (see Warnings).

Bone marrow: Use with extreme caution in patients whose bone marrow reserve may have been compromised by prior irradiation or chemotherapy or whose marrow function is recovering from the effects of previous chemotherapy (see Administration and Dosage).

Bronchospasm: Acute shortness of breath and severe bronchospasm have been reported infrequently following the administration of vinorelbine and other vinca alkaloids, most commonly when the vinca alkaloid was used in combination with mitomycin. These adverse reactions may require treatment with supplemental oxygen, bronchodilators or corticosteroids, particularly when there is pre-existing pulmonary dysfunction.

Eye contact: Avoid contamination of the eye with concentrations of vinorelbine used clinically. Severe irritation of the eye has been reported with accidental exposure to another vinca alkaloid. If exposure occurs, immediately flush the eye(s) with water.

Drug Interactions:

Vinorelbine Drug Interactions			
Precipitant drug	Object drug*		Description
Cisplatin	Vinorelbine	↑	Although the pharmacokinetics of vinorelbine are not influenced by the concurrent administration of cisplatin, the incidence of granulocytopenia with vinorelbine used in combination with cisplatin is significantly higher than with single-agent vinorelbine.
Mitomycin	Vinorelbine	↑	Acute pulmonary reactions have been reported with vinorelbine and other anticancer vinca alkaloids used in conjunction with mitomycin.

* ↑ = Object drug increased.

Adverse Reactions:

Most drug-related adverse reactions are reversible. If severe adverse reactions occur, reduce dosage or discontinue and take appropriate corrective measures. Reinstitution of therapy with vinorelbine should be carried out with caution and alertness as to possible recurrence of toxicity.

Vinorelbine (Single-Agent Use) Adverse Reactions (%)[1]						
	All grades		Grade 3		Grade 4	
Adverse reaction	All patients (n = 365)	NSCLC (n = 143)	All patients	NSCLC	All patients	NSCLC
Bone marrow						
Granulocytopenia (cells/mm³)						
< 2000	90	80	-	-	-	-
< 500	36	29	-	-	-	-
Leukopenia (cells/mm³)						
< 4000	92	81	-	-	-	-
< 1000	15	12	-	-	-	-
Thrombocytopenia (cells/mm³)						
< 100,000	5	4	-	-	-	-
< 50,000	1	1	-	-	-	-
Anemia (g/dl)						
< 11	83	77	-	-	-	-
< 8	9	1	-	-	-	-
Hospitalizations due to granulocytopenic complications	9	8	-	-	-	-

Vinorelbine (Single-Agent Use) Adverse Reactions (%)[1]						
	All grades		Grade 3		Grade 4	
Adverse reaction	All patients (n = 365)	NSCLC (n = 143)	All patients	NSCLC	All patients	NSCLC
Lab test abnormalities						
Total bilirubin elevation (n = 351)	13	9	4	3	3	2
AST elevation (n = 346)	67	54	5	2	1	1
GI						
Nausea	44	34	2	1	0	0
Vomiting	20	15	2	1	0	0
Constipation	35	29	3	2	0	0
Diarrhea	17	13	1	1	0	0
Miscellaneous						
Asthenia	36	27	7	5	0	0
Injection site reactions	28	38	2	5	0	0
Injection site pain	16	13	2	1	0	0
Phlebitis	7	10	< 1	1	0	0
Peripheral neuropathy	25	20	1	1	< 1	0
Dyspnea	7	3	2	2	1	0
Alopecia	12	12	≤ 1	1	0	0

[1] Grade based on modified criteria from the National Cancer Institute. Patients with NSCLC had not received prior chemotherapy, the majority of the remaining patients had received prior chemotherapy.

Hematologic: Granulocytopenia was the major dose-limiting toxicity; it was generally reversible and not cumulative over time. Granulocyte nadirs occurred 7 to 10 days after the dose, with granulocyte recovery usually within the following 7 to 14 days. Granulocytopenia resulted in hospitalizations for fever or sepsis in 8% of patients; septic deaths occurred in approximately 1% of patients.

Grade 3 or 4 anemia occurred in 1%, although blood products were administered to 18% of patients who received vinorelbine; grade 3 or 4 thrombocytopenia has occurred in 1% of patients.

CNS: Mild to moderate peripheral neuropathy manifested by paresthesia and hypesthesia were the most frequently reported neurologic toxicities. Loss of deep tendon reflexes (< 5%); development of severe peripheral neuropathy (1%; generally reversible).

Dermatologic: Alopecia (12%; was usually mild).

Like other anticancer vinca alkaloids, vinorelbine is a moderate vesicant. Injection site reactions, including erythema, pain at injection site and vein discoloration occurred in ≈ one-third of patients; 5% were severe. Chemical phlebitis along the vein proximal to the site of injection was reported in 10% of patients.

GI: Mild or moderate nausea (34%); severe nausea (< 2%). Prophylactic antiemetics were not routine in patients treated with single-agent vinorelbine. Due to the low incidence of severe nausea and vomiting with single-agent vinorelbine, the use of serotonin antagonists is generally not required. Constipation (29%); paralytic ileus (1%); vomiting, diarrhea, anorexia, stomatitis (< 20%; usually mild or moderate).

Hepatic: Transient liver enzyme elevations occurred without clinical symptoms.

Cardiovascular: Chest pain (5%). Most reports of chest pain were in patients who had either a history of cardiovascular disease or tumor within the chest. There have been rare reports of myocardial infarction.

Pulmonary: Shortness of breath (3%); it was severe in 2% (see Precautions). Interstitial pulmonary changes were documented in a few patients.

Miscellaneous: Fatigue (27%), usually mild or moderate but tended to increase with cumulative dosing; jaw pain, myalgia, arthralgia, rash (< 5%); hemorrhagic cystitis, syndrome of inappropriate ADH secretion (< 1%).

VINORELBINE TARTRATE

Combination use: In a randomized study, 206 patients received treatment with vinorelbine plus cisplatin and 206 patients received single-agent vinorelbine. The incidence of severe nausea and vomiting was 30% for vinorelbine/cisplatin compared to < 2% for single-agent vinorelbine. Cisplatin did not appear to increase the incidence of neurotoxicity observed with single-agent vinorelbine. However, myelosuppression, specifically Grade 3 and 4 granulocytopenia, was greater with the combination of vinorelbine/cisplatin (79%) than with single-agent vinorelbine (53%). The incidence of fever and infection may be increased with the combination.

Overdosage:

There is no known antidote for overdoses of vinorelbine. The primary anticipated complications of overdosage would consist of bone marrow suppression and peripheral neurotoxicity. If overdosage occurs, institute general supportive measures together with appropriate blood transfusions and antibiotics as deemed necessary by the physician. Refer to General Management of Acute Overdosage.

Patient Information:

Inform patients that the major acute toxicities of vinorelbine are related to bone marrow toxicity, specifically granulocytopenia with increased susceptibility to infection. Advise them to report fever or chills immediately.

Advise women of childbearing potential to avoid pregnancy during treatment.

Administration and Dosage:

Approved by the FDA on December 23, 1994.

The usual initial dose is 30 mg/m^2 administered weekly. The recommended method of administration is an IV injection over 6 to 10 minutes. In controlled trials, single-agent vinorelbine was given weekly until progression or dose-limiting toxicity. Vinorelbine was used at the same dose in combination with 120 mg/m^2 of cisplatin, given on days 1 and 29, then every 6 weeks.

Hematologic toxicity: Granulocyte counts should be ≥ 1000 cells/mm^3 prior to the administration of vinorelbine. Base dosage adjustments on granulocyte counts obtained on the day of treatment as follows:

Vinorelbine Dose Adjustments Based on Granulocyte Counts	
Granulocytes (cells/mm^3) on days of treatment	Dose (mg/m^2)
≥ 1500	30
1000 to 1499	15
< 1000	Do not administer. Repeat granulocyte count in 1 week. If 3 consecutive weekly doses are held because granulocyte count is < 1000 cells/mm^3, discontinue vinorelbine.
Note: For patients who, during treatment, have experienced fever or sepsis while granulocytopenic or had 2 consecutive weekly doses held due to granulocytopenia, subsequent doses of vinorelbine should be: 22.5 mg/m^2 for granulocytes ≥ 1500 cells/mm^3 11.25 mg/m^2 for granulocytes 1000 to 1499 cells/mm^3	

Renal function impairment: No dose adjustments are required for renal insufficiency. If moderate or severe neurotoxicity develops, discontinue vinorelbine. Adjust the dosage according to hematologic toxicity or hepatic insufficiency, whichever results in the lower dose.

Hepatic function impairment: Administer with caution to patients with hepatic insufficiency. In patients who develop hyperbilirubinemia during treatment with vinorelbine, adjust the dose for total bilirubin as follows.

Vinorelbine Dose Modification Based on Total Bilirubin	
Total bilirubin (mg/dl)	Dose (mg/m^2)
≤ 2	30
2.1 - 3	15
> 3	7.5

Concurrent hematologic toxicity and hepatic insufficiency: In patients with both hematologic toxicity and hepatic insufficiency, administer the lower of the doses determined from the previous tables.

VINORELBINE TARTRATE

Administration precautions: Vinorelbine must be administered intravenously. It is extremely important that the IV needle or catheter be properly positioned before any vinorelbine is injected. Leakage into surrounding tissue during IV administration may cause considerable irritation, local tissue necrosis or thrombophlebitis. If extravasation occurs, discontinue the injection immediately and introduce any remaining portion of the dose into another vein. Since there are no established guidelines for the treatment of extravasation injuries with vinorelbine, institutional guidelines may be used. The ONS Chemotherapy Guidelines provide additional recommendations for the prevention of extravasation injuries.*

As with other toxic compounds, exercise caution in handling and preparing the solution of vinorelbine. Skin reactions may occur with accidental exposure. The use of gloves is recommended. If the solution of vinorelbine contacts the skin or mucosa, immediately wash the skin or mucosa thoroughly with soap and water. Severe irritation of the eye has been reported with accidental contamination of the eye with another vinca alkaloid. If this happens with vinorelbine, flush the eye with water immediately and thoroughly. Use procedures for proper handling and disposal of anticancer drugs.

Preparation for administration: Vinorelbine must be diluted in either a syringe or IV bag using one of the recommended solutions. Administer the diluted vinorelbine over 6 to 10 minutes into the side port of a free-flowing IV closest to the IV bag followed by flushing with at least 75 to 125 ml of one of the solutions. Diluted vinorelbine may be used for up to 24 hours under normal room light when stored in polypropylene syringes or polyvinyl chloride bags at 5° to 30° C (41° to 86° F).

Syringe – Dilute the calculated dose of vinorelbine to a concentration between 1.5 and 3 mg/ml. These solutions may be used for dilution: 5% Dextrose Injection, USP; 0.9% Sodium Chloride Injection, USP.

IV bag – Dilute the calculated dose of vinorelbine to a concentration between 0.5 and 2 mg/ml. These solutions may be used for dilution: 5% Dextrose Injection, USP; 0.45% or 0.9% Sodium Chloride Injection, USP; 5% Dextrose and 0.45% Sodium Chloride Injection, USP; Ringer's Injection, USP; Lactated Ringer's Injection, USP.

Storage/Stability: Unopened vials of vinorelbine are stable until the date indicated on the package when stored under refrigeration at 2° to 8° C (36° to 46° F) and protected from light in the carton. Unopened vials of vinorelbine are stable at temperatures up to 25° C (77° F) for up to 72 hours. Protect from light. Do not freeze. If particulate matter is seen, do not administer.

Rx	**Navelbine** (Glaxo Wellcome)	**Injection**: 10 mg/ml	Preservative free. In 1 and 5 ml single-use vials.

* ONS Clinical Practice Committee. Cancer Chemotherapy Guidelines: Recommendations for the management of vesicant extravasation, hypersensitivity, and anaphylaxis. Pittsburgh, PA: Oncology Nursing Society;1992:1-4.

VINCRISTINE SULFATE (VCR; LCR)

Warning:

It is extremely important that the IV needle or catheter be properly positioned before injection. Leakage into surrounding tissue may cause considerable irritation.

This preparation is for IV use only. Intrathecal use usually results in death.

Actions:

Pharmacology: Vincristine sulfate is an alkaloid obtained from the periwinkle (Vinca rosea Linn). Mode of action is unknown. In vitro, it arrests mitotic division at metaphase. Antineoplastic effects are related to interference with intracellular tubulin function. It reversibly binds to microtubule and spindle proteins in the S phase.

Pharmacokinetics:

Absorption/Distribution – Within 15 to 30 minutes following IV administration, > 90% of the drug is distributed from blood into tissue where it remains tightly, but not irreversibly, bound. Penetration across the blood-brain barrier is poor.

Metabolism/Excretion – Studies in cancer patients show a triphasic serum decay pattern following rapid IV injection. Initial, middle and terminal half-lives are 5 min, 2.3 hrs and 85 hrs, respectively; the range of the terminal half-life is 19 to 155 hrs. The liver is the major excretory organ; ≈ 80% of a dose appears in feces and 10% to 20% in urine. Hepatic dysfunction may alter elimination kinetics and augment toxicity.

Combination cancer chemotherapy involves simultaneous use of several agents. Generally, each agent has a unique toxicity and mechanism so that therapeutic enhancement occurs without additive toxicity. It is rarely possible to achieve equally good results with single agent treatment. Vincristine is often chosen as part of polychemotherapy because of lack of significant bone marrow suppression (at recommended doses) and of unique clinical toxicity (neuropathy). See Administration and Dosage for possible increased toxicity when used in combination therapy.

Indications:

Acute leukemia.

Combination therapy in Hodgkin's disease, non-Hodgkin's malignant lymphomas (lymphocytic, mixed-cell, histiocytic, undifferentiated, nodular and diffuse types), rhabdomyosarcoma, neuroblastoma and Wilms' tumor.

Unlabeled uses: Vincristine has been used in the treatment of idiopathic thrombocytopenic purpura, Kaposi's sarcoma, breast cancer and bladder cancer.

Contraindications:

Do not give to patients with demyelinating form of Charcot-Marie-Tooth syndrome.

Warnings:

Administer IV only; intrathecal administration is uniformly fatal.

Hypersensitivity, temporally related to vincristine therapy, has occurred. Refer to Management of Acute Hypersensitivity Reactions. See Adverse Reactions.

Carcinogenesis/Mutagenesis/Fertility impairment: Patients who received vincristine with anticancer drugs known to be carcinogenic have developed secondary malignancies. Vincristine's contributing role in this development has not been determined.

Laboratory tests failed to conclusively demonstrate mutagenicity. Reports of both males and females who received multiple agent chemotherapy that included vincristine indicate azoospermia and amenorrhea can occur in postpubertal patients. Recovery occurred many months after chemotherapy completion in some. It is much less likely to cause permanent azoospermia and amenorrhea in prepubertal patients.

Pregnancy: Category D. Vincristine can cause fetal harm when administered to a pregnant woman. In several animal species, it induces teratogenic effects and embryolethality with doses that are nontoxic to the mother. There are no adequate and well controlled studies in pregnant women. If this drug is used during pregnancy or if the patient becomes pregnant while receiving it, apprise her of the potential hazard to the fetus. Advise women of childbearing potential to avoid becoming pregnant.

Lactation: It is not known whether this drug is excreted in breast milk. Because of the potential for serious adverse reactions in nursing infants, decide whether to discontinue nursing or the drug, taking into account importance of the drug to the mother.

Precautions:

Monitoring: Dose-limiting clinical toxicity is manifested as neurotoxicity; clinical evaluation (history, physical examination) is necessary to detect need for dosage modification. Following vincristine, some patients may have a fall in WBC or platelet counts, particularly when previous therapy or the disease has reduced bone marrow function. Perform complete blood count before each dose. Acute serum uric acid elevation may occur during induction of remission in acute leukemia; thus deter-

VINCRISTINE SULFATE (VCR; LCR)

mine such levels frequently during the first 3 to 4 treatment weeks or take appropriate measures to prevent uric acid nephropathy.

Acute uric acid nephropathy has occurred.

CNS leukemia has occurred in patients undergoing otherwise successful therapy with vincristine. If CNS leukemia is diagnosed, additional agents may be required, since this drug does not adequately cross the blood-brain barrier.

Leukopenia or complicating infection: In the presence of these conditions, administration of the next dose warrants careful consideration.

Neuromuscular disease: Pay particular attention to dosage and neurological side effects if administered to patients with preexisting neuromuscular disease or when other neurotoxic drugs are used.

Eye contamination should be avoided with concentrations used clinically. If accidental contamination occurs, severe irritation (or, if drug was delivered under pressure, even corneal ulceration) may result. Wash eyes immediately and thoroughly.

Pulmonary reactions: Acute shortness of breath and severe bronchospasm have followed administration of vinca alkaloids, most frequently when the drug was used with mitomycin-C. The onset may be within minutes or several hours after the vinca is injected and may occur up to 2 weeks following the dose of mitomycin.

Concomitant radiation therapy: Do not give to patients receiving radiation therapy through ports that include the liver.

Drug Interactions:

Digoxin: Combination chemotherapy (including vincristine) may decrease digoxin plasma levels and renal excretion.

L-asparaginase: Administering L-asparaginase first may reduce hepatic clearance of vincristine. Give vincristine 12 to 24 hrs before L-asparaginase to minimize toxicity.

Mitomycin-C: Acute pulmonary reactions may occur (see Precautions).

Phenytoin: Combination chemotherapy (including vincristine) may reduce phenytoin plasma levels, requiring increased dosage to maintain therapeutic plasma levels.

Adverse Reactions:

Adverse reactions are generally reversible and dose-related. With single weekly doses, leukopenia, neuritic pain and constipation may occur and are usually of short duration (ie, < 7 days). When dosage is reduced, reactions may lessen or disappear. They seem to increase when the drug is given in divided doses. Other adverse reactions, such as hair loss, sensory loss, paresthesia, difficulty in walking, slapping gait, loss of deep tendon reflexes and muscle wasting, may persist for at least as long as therapy is continued. Generalized sensorimotor dysfunction may become progressively more severe with continued treatment. Neuromuscular difficulties usually disappear by the sixth week after treatment is discontinued, but they may persist for prolonged periods in some patients. Hair regrowth may occur while maintenance therapy continues.

SIADH: The syndrome of inappropriate antidiuretic hormone secretion (SIADH), including high urinary sodium excretion in the presence of hyponatremia, occurs rarely. Renal or adrenal disease, hypotension, dehydration, azotemia and clinical edema are absent. With fluid deprivation, hyponatremia and renal sodium loss improve.

CNS: Loss of deep-tendon reflexes, ataxia, footdrop and paralysis have been seen with continued use. Cranial nerve manifestations, including isolated paresis or paralysis of muscles may occur; extraocular and laryngeal muscles are most commonly involved. Severe pain may occur in the jaw, pharynx, parotid gland, bones, back and limbs. Myalgias have occurred. Reduced intestinal motility results in constipation. Convulsions, often with hypertension, have occurred in a few patients. Convulsions followed by coma have been seen in children. Frequently, there is a sequence in the development of neuropathy: Initially, sensory impairment and paresthesias, then neuritic pain may appear and later, motor difficulties. Neurotoxicity is dose-related and cumulative to where therapy must be stopped after a cumulative dose of 30 to 50 mg. It is reversible upon discontinuation, but recovery takes several months.

In one study, the administration of glutamic acid (500 mg 3 times daily) decreased the neurotoxicity induced by vincristine.

GI: Oral ulceration; abdominal cramps; nausea; vomiting; diarrhea; anorexia; intestinal necrosis or perforation.

Constipation may take the form of upper colon impaction, and, on examination, the rectum may be empty. Colicky abdominal pain may accompany an empty rectum. A flat film of the abdomen demonstrates this condition. Cases respond to high enemas and laxatives. Use routine prophylaxis for constipation.

VINCRISTINE SULFATE (VCR; LCR)

Paralytic ileus which mimics the "surgical abdomen" may occur, particularly in young children. The ileus will reverse itself upon temporary discontinuation of vincristine and with symptomatic care.

Hematologic: Serious bone marrow depression (usually not dose-limiting); anemia; leukopenia; thrombocytopenia. Thrombocytopenia, if present when therapy is begun, may improve before the appearance of marrow remission.

Hypersensitivity: Rare cases of allergic type reactions, such as anaphylaxis, rash and edema, that are temporally related to vincristine therapy have occurred in patients receiving vincristine as a part of multi-drug chemotherapy regimens. See Warnings.

GU: Polyuria; dysuria; urinary retention due to bladder atony. Discontinue other drugs known to cause urinary retention (particularly in the elderly), if possible, for the first few days following administration.

Ophthalmic: Optic atrophy with blindness; transient cortical blindness; ptosis; diplopia; photophobia.

Pulmonary: Acute shortness of breath, severe bronchospasm (see Precautions).

Miscellaneous: Hyper- or hypotension; weight loss; fever; alopecia; rash; headache.

Overdosage:

Symptoms: Side effects are dose-related. After an overdose, expect exaggerated side effects. In children < 13 years of age, death has occurred after doses 10 times those recommended; severe symptoms may occur with 3 to 4 mg/m^2. Adults may experience severe symptoms after single doses ≥ 3 mg/m^2.

Treatment: Supportive care should include prevention of side effects resulting from SIADH (ie, fluid intake restriction and perhaps a diuretic affecting function of Henle's loop and distal tubule); phenobarbital (anticonvulsant); enemas or cathartics to prevent ileus (in some instances, GI tract decompression may be necessary); monitor cardiovascular system; determine daily blood counts to guide transfusion requirements.

Folinic acid, 100 mg IV every 3 hrs for 24 hrs, then every 6 hrs for at least 48 hrs, may help treat overdose. Folinic acid does not eliminate need for supportive measures.

Most of an IV dose is excreted into the bile after rapid tissue binding. Hemodialysis is not likely to be helpful. Patients with liver disease sufficient to decrease biliary excretion may experience increased severity of side effects.

Administration and Dosage:

Cautiously calculate and administer dose; overdosage may be serious or fatal.

Administer IV only, at weekly intervals. Inject solution either directly into a vein or into the tubing of a running IV infusion. Injection may be completed in about 1 minute.

Adults: 1.4 mg/m^2.

Children: 2 mg/m^2. For children weighing ≤ 10 kg or having a body surface area < 1 m^2, give 0.05 mg/kg once a week.

Hepatic function impairment: A 50% reduction in the dose is recommended for patients having a direct serum bilirubin value > 3 mg/dl.

Extravasation: Properly position needle in vein before injecting. Leakage into surrounding tissue may cause considerable irritation. Discontinue immediately; finish dose in another vein. Locally inject hyaluronidase; apply moderate heat to the area to disperse drug and minimize discomfort and possibility of cellulitis.

Compatibility: Do not dilute in solutions that raise or lower the pH outside the range of 3.5 to 5.5. Do not mix with anything other than normal saline or glucose in water.

Consider procedures for proper handling and disposal of anticancer drugs.

Rx	**Vincristine Sulfate** (Various, eg, Americal, Balan, Lyphomed, Moore, Quad, VHA Supply)	**Injection:** 1 mg/ml	In 1, 2 and 5 ml vials.
Rx	**Oncovin** (Lilly)		In 1, 2 and 5 ml vials and 1 and 2 ml Hyporets.[1]
Rx	**Vincasar PFS** (Adria)		In 1, 2, 5 ml flip-top vials.[2]

[1] With 100 mg mannitol, 1.3 mg methylparaben and 0.2 mg propylparaben per ml. Refrigerate.
[2] With 100 mg mannitol. Refrigerate.

VINBLASTINE SULFATE (VLB)

Warning:

It is extremely important the needle be properly positioned in the vein before this product is injected. If leakage into surrounding tissue should occur during IV administration of vinblastine sulfate, it may cause considerable irritiation. The injection should be discontinued immediately, and any remaining portion of the dose should then be introduced into another vein. Local injection of hyaluronidase and the application of moderate heat to the area of leakage will help disperse the drug and are thought to minimize the discomfort and the possibiliity of cellulitis.

Fatal if given intrathecally. For IV use only.

See Warnings for the treatment of patients given intrathecal vinblastine sulfate injection.

Actions:

Pharmacology: Vinblastine sulfate, an alkaloid extracted from Vinca rosea Linn, interferes with metabolic pathways of amino acids leading from glutamic acid to the citric acid cycle and urea. Studies have demonstrated an stathmokinetic effect and various atypical mitotic figures. However, therapeutic responses are not fully explained by the cytologic changes, since these changes are sometimes observed clinically and experimentally in the absence of any oncolytic effects.

Vinblastine has an effect on cell energy production required for mitosis and interferes with nucleic acid synthesis. In vitro, the drug arrests growing cells in metaphase.

Reversal of the antitumor effect by glutamic acid or tryptophan has occurred.

Pharmacokinetics:

Absorption/Distribution – Similar to vincristine, vinblastine undergoes rapid distribution and extensive tissue binding following IV injection. Vinblastine also localizes in platelets and leukocyte fractions of whole blood.

Metabolism/Excretion – Vinblastine is partially metabolized to deacetyl vinblastine which is more active than the parent drug. Plasma decline follows a triphasic pattern. The initial, middle and terminal half-lives are 3.7 minutes, 1.6 hours and 24.8 hours, respectively. Toxicity may be increased if liver disease is present.

Vinblastine is metabolized by the hepatic P–450IIIA cytochromes, and the major route of excretion may be through the biliary system.

Indications:

Palliative treatment of the following:

Frequently responsive malignancies: Generalized Hodgkin's disease (stages III and IV, Ann Arbor modification of Rye staging system), lymphocytic lymphoma (nodular and diffuse, poorly and well differentiated); histiocytic lymphoma; mycosis fungoides (advanced stages); advanced testicular carcinoma; Kaposi's sarcoma and Letterer-Siwe disease (histiocytosis X).

Less frequently responsive malignancies: Choriocarcinoma resistant to other chemotherapy; breast cancer unresponsive to endocrine surgery and hormonal therapy.

Multiple drug protocols: Vinblastine, effective as a single agent, is usually administered with other antineoplastics. Combination therapy enhances therapeutic effect without additive toxicity when agents with different dose-limiting toxicities and mechanisms of action are selected.

Hodgkin's disease: Vinblastine used as a single agent; advanced Hodgkin's disease has also been successfully treated with multiple-drug regimens that included vinblastine.

Advanced testicular germinal-cell cancers (embryonal carcinoma, teratocarcinoma and choriocarcinoma) are sensitive to vinblastine alone, but better clinical results are achieved with combination therapy. Vinblastine enhances the effect of bleomycin if given 6 to 8 hours prior to bleomycin administration; this schedule permits more cells to be arrested during metaphase, the stage in which bleomycin is active.

Contraindications:

Leukopenia; presence of bacterial infection (infections must be under control prior to initiating therapy); significant granulocytopenia unless it is a result of the disease being treated.

VINBLASTINE SULFATE (VLB)

Warnings:

This product is for IV use only: The intrathecal administration of vinblastine has resulted in death. Syringes containing this product should be labeled "Vinblastine Sulfate for Intravenous Use Only."

Extemporaneously prepared syringes containing this product must be packaged in an overwrap that is labeled "Do Not Remove Covering Until Moment of Injection. Fatal if Given Intrathecally. For Intravenous Use Only."

The following treatment successfully arrested progressive paralysis in a single patient mistakenly given the related vinca alkaloid, vincristine sulfate intrathecally. If vinblastine is mistakenly administered intrathecally, this treatment is recommended and should be initiated immediately after the intrathecal injection.

1.) Remove as much spinal fluid as can be safely done through the lumbar access.
2.) Insert a catheter in a lateral cerebral ventricle for the purpose of flushing the subarachnoid space from above with removal through a lumbar access.
3.) Initiate flushing through the cerebral catheter with Lactated Ringer's Solution infused at the rate of 150 mg/dl.
4.) As soon as fresh frozen plasma becomes available, infuse 25 ml diluted in 1L of Lactated Ringer's Solution through the cerebral ventricular catheter at the rate of 75 ml/hr with removal through the lumbar access. The rate of infusion should be adjusted to maintain a protein level in the spinal fluid of 150 mg/dl.
5.) Administer 10 g of glutamic acid IV over 24 hours followed by 500 mg 3 times daily by mouth for 1 month or until neurological dysfunction stabilizes. The role of glutamic acid in this treatment is not certain and may not be essential.

The use of this treatment has not been reported following intrathecal vinblastine.

Hematologic effects: Leukopenia is expected; leukocyte count is an important guide to therapy. In general, the larger the dose, the more profound and longer lasting the leukopenia will be. If the WBC count returns to normal after drug-induced leukopenia, the white cell-producing mechanism is not permanently depressed. Usually, WBC count has completely returned to normal after virtual disappearance of white cells from peripheral blood. The nadir in WBC count occurs 5 to 10 days after the last dose of drug is given. Recovery of the WBC count is fairly rapid and usually complete within 7 to 14 days. With smaller doses employed for maintenance therapy, leukopenia may not occur.

Although the thrombocyte count ordinarily is not significantly lowered by therapy, recently impaired bone marrow by prior therapy with radiation or with other oncolytic drugs may show thrombocytopenia (< 200,000 platelets/mm^3). When other chemotherapy or radiation has not been previously employed, thrombocytopenia is rare, even when vinblastine may be causing significant leukopenia. Rapid recovery (within a few days) from thrombocytopenia is the rule.

The effect on red blood cell count and hemoglobin is usually insignificant in the absence of other therapy; however, patients with malignant disease may exhibit anemia in the absence of any therapy.

If leukopenia (< 2000 WBC/mm^3) occurs following a dose of this drug, carefully watch the patient for evidence of infection until a safe WBC count has returned.

When cachexia or ulcerated skin surface occur, a more profound leukopenic response may occur; avoid use in older persons suffering from these conditions.

In patients with malignant cell infiltration of bone marrow, leukocyte and platelet counts have sometimes fallen precipitously after moderate doses, making further use of the drug inadvisable.

Leukopenia (granulocytopenia) may reach dangerously low levels following use of the higher recommended doses. Follow recommended dosage technique. Stomatitis and neurologic toxicity, although not common or permanent, can be disabling.

Hepatic function impairment: Toxicity may be enhanced in the presence of hepatic insufficiency. A dose reduction is recommended (see Administration and Dosage).

Fertility impairment: Aspermia has been reported. Amenorrhea has occurred in some patients treated with a combination of an alkylating agent, procarbazine, prednisone and vinblastine. Its occurrence was related to the total dose of these agents. Recovery of menses was frequent. The same combination of drugs given to male patients produced azoospermia; if spermatogenesis did return, it was not likely to do so with less than 2 years of unmaintained remission.

Pregnancy: Category D. Information is very limited. Animal studies suggest teratogenicity may occur. Animals given the drug early in pregnancy suffer resorption of the conceptus; surviving fetuses demonstrate gross deformities. There are no adequate and well controlled studies in pregnant women, but the drug can cause fatal harm. If the drug is used during pregnancy, or if the patient becomes pregnant while receiving this drug, apprise her of the potential hazard to the fetus. Advise women of childbearing potential to avoid becoming pregnant.

Lactation: It is not known whether this drug is excreted in breast milk. Because of the potential for serious adverse reactions in nursing infants, decide whether to discontinue nursing or to discontinue the drug, taking into account the importance of the drug to the mother.

Precautions:

Long-term use: Using small amounts of drug daily for long periods is not advised, even though the resulting total weekly dose may be similar to that recommended. Strict adherence to the recommended dosage schedule is very important. When amounts equal to several times the recommended weekly dosage were given in 7 daily installments for long periods, convulsions, severe and permanent CNS damage and death occurred.

Avoid eye contamination: Severe irritation or corneal ulceration (if the drug was delivered under pressure) may result. Thoroughly wash the eye with water immediately.

Pulmonary reactions: Acute shortness of breath and severe bronchospasm have occurred following use of vinca alkaloids. These reactions occur most frequently when the vinca alkaloid is used with mitomycin. Onset may be within minutes or several hours after the vinca is injected and may occur up to 2 weeks after the dose of mitomycin. (See Drug Interactions.)

Benzyl alcohol, contained in some of these products as a preservative, has been associated with a fatal "gasping syndrome" in premature infants.

Drug Interactions:

Vinblastine Drug Interactions

Precipitant drug	Object drug*		Description
Vinblastine	Mitomycin	↑	Acute shortness of breath and severe bronchospasm have occurred following use of vinca alkaloids in patients who had prevoiusly or simultaneously recived mitomycin. Onset may be within minutes or several hours after the vinca alkaloid is injected and may occur up to 2 weeks after the dose of mitomycin.
Vinblastine	Phenytoin	↓	Combination chemotherapy (including vinblastine) may reduce phenytoin plasma levels and increase seizure activity. Adjust the dosage based on serial blood level monitoring.
Erythromycin	Vinblastine	↑	May cause toxicity of vinblastine. Severe myalgia, neutropenia and constipation have been reported.
Agents that inhibit the cytochrome P-450 pathway	Vinblastine	↑	Vinblastine is metabolized by the P-450IIIA enzyme. Use caution when coadministering drugs that inhibit P-450 enzymes.

* ↑ = Object drug increased. ↓ = Object drug decreased.

Adverse Reactions:

Incidence of adverse reactions is dose-related. Except for epilation, leukopenia and neurologic side effects, adverse reactions have not usually persisted for longer than 24 hours. Neurologic side effects are not common; when they occur, they often last for more than 24 hours. Leukopenia, the most common adverse reaction, is usually the dose-limiting factor.

Hematologic: Leukopenia (granulocytopenia), anemia, thrombocytopenia (myelosuppression). See Warnings.

Cardiovascular: Hypertension. Cases of unexpected myocardial infarction and cerebrovascular accidents have occurred in patients undergoing combination chemotherapy with vinblastine, bleomycin and cisplatin.

GI: Nausea and vomiting (may be controlled by antiemetics); pharyngitis; vesiculation of the mouth; ileus; diarrhea; constipation; anorexia; abdominal pain; rectal bleeding; hemorrhagic enterocolitis; bleeding from an old peptic ulcer.

CNS: Numbness of digits; paresthesias; peripheral neuritis; mental depression; loss of deep tendon reflexes; headache; convulsions.

Dermatologic: Alopecia is common. Total epilation infrequently develops. In some cases, hair regrows during maintenance therapy. Vesiculation of the skin may occur. A single case of light sensitivity has been associated with this drug.

VINBLASTINE SULFATE (VLB)

Miscellaneous: Malaise; weakness; dizziness; pain in tumor site; bone and jaw pain. The syndrome of inappropriate secretion of antidiuretic hormone has occurred with higher than recommended doses.

Extravasation during IV injection may lead to cellulitis and phlebitis; sloughing may occur (see Administration and Dosage).

There are isolated reports of Raynaud's phenomenon occurring in patients with testicular carcinoma treated with bleomycin, cisplatin and vinblastine sulfate. It is unknown whether the cause was the disease, the drugs or a combination of these.

Overdosage:

Symptoms: Side effects are dose-related. After an overdose, expected exaggerated effects. In addition, neurotoxicity similar to that with vincristine may occur.

Treatment: Supportive care should include prevention of side effects that result from the syndrome of inappropriate secretion of antidiuretic hormone (ie, restriction of the volume of daily fluid intake to that of the urine output plus insensible loss and perhaps use of a diuretic affecting the function of the loop of Henle and the distal tubule); administration of an anticonvulsant; prevention of ileus; monitoring the cardiovascular system; and determining daily blood counts for guidance in transfusion requirements and assessing the risk of infection. The major effect of excessive doses will be myelosuppression, which may be life-threatening. There is no information regarding the effectiveness of dialysis nor of cholestyramine for the treatment of overdosage.

In the dry state, the drug is irregularly and unpredictably absorbed from the GI tract following oral administration. Absorption of the solution has not been studied. If vinblastine is swallowed, oral activated charcoal in a water slurry may be given along with a cathartic. The use of cholestyramine in this situation has not been reported.

Patient Information:

Immediately report sore throat, fever, chills or sore mouth to the physician.

The following may occur: Alopecia, jaw pain, pain in the organs containing tumor tissue, nausea and vomiting. Scalp hair will regrow to its pretreatment extent, even with continued treatment. Report any other serious medical event to the physician.

Avoid constipation.

Administration and Dosage:

Leukopenic responses vary following therapy. For this reason, do not administer drug more than once weekly. Initiate therapy for adults with a single IV dose of 3.7 mg/m^2 of body surface. Thereafter, measure WBC counts to determine patient's sensitivity. A 50% dose reduction is recommended for patients having a direct serum bilirubin value > 3 mg/dl. Since metabolism and excretion are primarily hepatic, no modification is recommended for patients with impaired renal function.

Incremental Dosage Weekly Intervals		
	Adult Dose (mg/m^2)	Pediatric Dose (mg/m^2)
First dose	3.7	2.5
Second dose	5.5	3.75
Third dose	7.4	5
Fourth dose	9.25	6.25
Fifth dose	11.1	7.5

Use the same increments until a max. dose not exceeding 18.5 mg/m^2 for adults and 12.5 mg/m^2 for children is reached. Do not increase dose after WBC count is reduced to ≈ 3000 $cells/mm^3$. For most adults the weekly dosage range is 5.5 to 7.4 mg/m^2

Maintenance therapy: When the dose produces the above degree of leukopenia, administer a dose one increment smaller at weekly intervals for maintenance. Even though 7 days have elapsed, do not give the next dose until the WBC count has returned to at least $4000/mm^3$. In some cases, oncolytic activity may be encountered before leukopenic effect but do not increase the size of subsequent doses.

Duration of maintenance therapy varies according to the disease and the combination of antineoplastics used. Prolonged chemotherapy for maintaining remission involves several risks: Life-threatening infections, sterility, secondary cancers through suppression of immune surveillance. In some disorders, survival following complete remission may not be as prolonged as that achieved with shorter periods of maintenance therapy. Conversely, failure to provide maintenance therapy may lead to unnecessary relapse; complete remission in patients with testicular cancer, unless maintained for at least 2 years, often results in early relapse.

VINBLASTINE SULFATE (VLB)

IV: Inject into either the tubing of a running IV infusion or directly into a vein over 1 minute. Secure the needle within the vein so that no solution extravasates, to prevent cellulitis or phlebitis. To further minimize extravasation, rinse syringe and needle with venous blood before withdrawal of needle. Do not dilute the dose in large volumes of diluent (ie, 100 to 250 ml) or give IV for prolonged periods (30 to 60 min. or more), since this often results in vein irritation and increases the chance of extravasation.

Because of the enhanced possibility of thrombosis, do not inject solution into an extremity in which circulation is impaired or potentially impaired by conditions such as compressing or invading neoplasm, phlebitis or varicosity.

Powder for injection:

Preparation of solution – Add 10 ml of Bacteriostatic Sodium Chloride Injection (preserved with phenol or benzyl alcohol) to the vial for a concentration of 1 mg/ml. The drug dissolves instantly to give a clear solution. A preservative-containing solvent is unnecessary if unused portions are discarded immediately.

Compatability – Do not dilute with solvents that raise or lower the pH of the resulting solution from between 3.5 and 5. Solutions should be made with either Normal Saline or 0.9% Sodium Chloride Injection (each with or without preservative) and should not be combined in the same container with any other chemical.

Storage – After reconstitution and removal of a portion from the vial, refrigerate the remainder for 28 days without loss of potency. Refrigerate unopened vials at 2° to 8°C (36° to 46°F).

Rx	**Vinblastine Sulfate** (Various, eg, Cetus, LyphoMed, VHA Supply)	**Powder for Injection:** 10 mg	In vials.
Rx	**Velban** (Lilly)		In vials.
Rx	**Vinblastine Sulfate** (LyphoMed, Quad)	**Injection:** 1 mg/ml	In 10 and 25 ml vials[1].

[1] With 0.9% benzyl alcohol.

STRONTIUM-89 CHLORIDE

Actions:

Pharmacology: Strontium-89 is an injectable radioisotope for metastatic bone pain. Following IV injection, soluble strontium compounds behave like their calcium analogs, clearing rapidly from blood and selectively localizing in bone mineral. Uptake of strontium by bone occurs preferentially in sites of active osteogenesis; primary bone tumors and areas of metastatic involvement (blastic lesions) can accumulate significantly greater concentrations of strontium than surrounding normal bone.

Strontium-89 is retained in metastatic bone lesions much longer than in normal bone, where turnover is about 14 days. In patients with extensive skeletal metastases, well over half of the injected dose is retained in the bones.

The drug, a pure beta emitter, selectively irradiates sites of primary metastatic bone involvement with minimal effect on soft tissues distant from bone lesions.

Pharmacokinetics: Strontium-89 decays by beta emission with a physical half-life of 50.5 days. Excretion pathways are two-thirds urinary and one-third fecal in patients with bone metastases. Urinary excretion, which is higher in people without bone lesions, is greatest in the first 2 days following injection.

Clinical trials:

Clinical trials have examined relief of pain in cancer patients who have received external radiation therapy for bone metastases but in whom persistent pain recurred.

Comparison of Effects of Strontium-89 vs Placebo (%)

	Months post-treatment						
Parameter	1	2	3	4	5	6	9
Reduced pain, no increase in analgesic/radiotherapy retreatment							
Strontium-89	71.4	78.9	60.6	59.3	36.4	63.6	—
Placebo	61.4	57.1	55.9	25	31.8	35	—
Pain free without analgesic							
Strontium-89	14.3	13.2	15.2	11.1	18.2	18.2	18.2
Placebo	6.8	8.6	5.9	0	4.5	5	0

Indications:

Painful skeletal metastases: Relief of bone pain in patients with painful skeletal metastases.

Warnings:

Bone marrow toxicity: Use of strontium-89 in patients with evidence of seriously compromised bone marrow from previous therapy or disease infiltration is not recommended unless the potential benefit of the treatment outweighs its risks. Bone marrow toxicity is to be expected following administration, particularly white blood cells (WBCs) and platelets. The extent of toxicity is variable. It is recommended that the patient's peripheral blood cell counts be monitored at least once every other week. Typically, platelets will be depressed by about 30% compared to pre-administration levels. The nadir of platelet depression in most patients is found between 12 and 16 weeks following administration of strontium-89. WBCs are usually depressed to a varying extent compared to pre-administration levels. Therefore, recovery occurs slowly, typically reaching pre-administration levels 6 months after treatment unless the patient's disease or additional therapy intervenes.

In considering repeat administration, carefully evaluate hematologic response to initial dose, current platelet level and other evidence of marrow depletion.

Patient identification: Verification of dose and patient identification is necessary prior to use because strontium-89 delivers a relatively high dose of radioactivity.

Renal function impairment: Strontium-89 is excreted primarily by the kidneys. In patients with renal dysfunction, weigh the possible risks of administering strontium-89 against the possible benefits.

Carcinogenesis: Strontium-89 is a potential carcinogen. Of 40 rats injected with strontium-89 in 10 consecutive monthly doses of either 250 or 350 mcCi/kg, 33 developed malignant bone tumors after a latency period of ≈ 9 months. No neoplasia was observed in control animals. Restrict treatment to patients with well documented metastatic bone disease.

Pregnancy: Category D. Strontium-89 may cause fetal harm when administered to a pregnant woman. There are no adequate and well controlled studies in pregnant women. If this drug is used during pregnancy, or if the patient becomes pregnant while receiving this drug, apprise the patient of the potential hazard to the fetus. Advise women of childbearing potential to avoid becoming pregnant.

STRONTIUM-89 CHLORIDE

Lactation: Because strontium acts as a calcium analog, secretion into breast milk is likely; however, it is not known whether this drug is excreted in breast milk. It is recommended that nursing be discontinued by mothers about to receive IV strontium-89.

Children: Safety and efficacy in children < 18 years of age have not been established.

Precautions:

Bone metastases: Strontium-89 is not indicated for use in patients with cancer not involving bone. Confirm presence of bone metastases prior to therapy. Use with caution in patients with platelet counts < 60,000 and white cell counts < 2400.

Radiopharmaceuticals should only be used by physicians who are qualified by training and experience in the safe use and handling of radionuclides and whose experience and training have been approved by the appropriate government agency authorized to license the use of radionuclides. Like other radioactive drugs, handle with care and take safety measures to minimize radiation to clinical personnel.

Onset: In view of the delayed onset of pain relief, typically 7 to 20 days post-injection, administration to patients with very short life expectancy is not recommended.

Flushing sensation: A calcium-like flushing sensation has been observed in patients following a rapid (< 30 second injection) administration.

Incontinence: Take special precautions, such as urinary catheterization, following administration to patients who are incontinent to minimize the risk of radioactive contamination of clothing, bed linen and the patient's environment.

Adverse Reactions:

One case of fatal septicemia following leukopenia was reported during clinical trials. Most severe reactions of marrow toxicity can be managed by conventional means.

A small number of patients have reported a transient increase in bone pain at 36 to 72 hours after injection. This is usually mild and self-limiting, and controllable with analgesics. One patient reported chills and fever 12 hours after injection without long-term sequelae.

Patient Information:

The patient may feel a slight increase in pain for 2 or 3 days beginning 2 or 3 days after injection. The physician may suggest a temporary increase in the dose of pain medication until the pain is under control. After about 1 to 2 weeks, the pain should begin to diminish.

The patient can eat and drink normally and there is no need to avoid alcohol or caffeine unless already advised to do so. The physician may want to carry out periodic, routine blood tests.

Advise patients to tell any health practitioner who is giving them medical treatment that they have received strontium-89.

During the first week after injection, strontium-89 will be present in the blood and urine. It is therefore important to consider the following common sense precautions for 1 week: 1) Where a normal toilet is available, use in preference to a urinal. Flush the toilet twice; 2) Wipe up any spilled urine with a tissue and flush it away; 3) Always wash hands after using the toilet; 4) Immediately wash any linen or clothes that become stained with urine or blood. Wash them separately from other clothes, and rinse thoroughly; 5) If any urine collection device is used, follow instructions on its use; 6) Wash away any spilled blood if a cut occurs.

In many people who receive Strontium-89, the effect lasts for several months. If pain returns, consult the physician.

Administration and Dosage:

Approved by the FDA on June 18, 1993.

The recommended dose is 148 MBq, 4 mCi given by slow IV injection (1 to 2 minutes). Alternatively, a dose of 1.5 to 2.2 MBq/kg, 40 to 60 mcCi/kg may be used.

Base repeated administrations on an individual patient's response to therapy, current symptoms and hematologic status; repeat doses are generally not recommended at intervals of < 90 days.

Measure dose by suitable radioactivity calibration system immediately prior to use.

Storage/Stability: The vial is shipped in a transportation shield with an ≈ 3 mm lead wall thickness. Store the vial and its contents inside its transportation container at room temperature (15° to 25°C; 59° to 77°F).

Rx	**Metastron** (Medi-Physics/Amersham)	**Injection**: 148MBq, 4mCi (10.9 to 22.6 mg/ml)	Preservative free. In 10 ml vials with Water for Injection.

SODIUM IODIDE I 131

Sodium Iodide I 131 is also used for treatment of hyperthyroidism. Refer to the monograph in the Hormones chapter.

Actions:

Pharmacology: After rapid GI absorption, iodine 131 is primarily distributed within extracellular fluid. It is trapped and rapidly converted to protein-bound iodine by the thyroid; it is concentrated, but not protein bound, by the stomach and salivary glands. It is promptly excreted by kidneys.

About 90% of the local irradiation is caused by beta radiation and 10% is caused by gamma radiation. Iodine 131 has a physical half-life of 8.04 days.

Indications:

Thyroid carcinoma: Selected cases of thyroid carcinoma. Palliative effects may occur in patients with papillary or follicular thyroid carcinoma. Stimulation of radioiodide uptake may be achieved by giving thyrotropin. (Radioiodide will not be taken up by giant cell and spindle cell carcinoma of the thyroid or by amyloid solid carcinomas.)

Hyperthyroidism: Treatment of hyperthyroidism (see monograph in Hormones chapter).

Contraindications:

Preexisting vomiting and diarrhea; women who are or may become pregnant (see Warnings).

Warnings:

Pregnancy: Category X. Do not give to pregnant women (see Contraindications). Do not use in women who are or may become pregnant. Iodine 131 may cause fetal harm (eg, permanent damage to thyroid). If used during pregnancy or if patient becomes pregnant while taking this drug, inform her of the hazard to the fetus.

Lactation: Iodine 131 is excreted in breast milk; discontinue nursing during therapy. Do not resume nursing until all radiation is absent from breast milk (≈ 14 days).

Children: Safety and efficacy in children have not been established.

Precautions:

Radiation exposure: Ensure minimum radiation exposure to patients and occupational workers consistent with proper patient management.

Sulfite sensitivity: Some of these products contain sulfites that may cause allergic-type reactions including anaphylactic symptoms and life-threatening or less severe asthmatic episodes in susceptible persons. The overall prevalence in the general population is unknown and probably low. It is seen more frequently in asthmatic or atopic nonasthmatic persons.

Drug Interactions:

Iodine, thyroid and antithyroid agents: Uptake of iodine 131 will be affected by recent intake of stable iodine in any form, or by use of *thyroid, antithyroid* and certain other drugs. Question the patient regarding previous medication and procedures involving radiographic contrast media.

Adverse Reactions:

Hematologic: Depression of hematopoietic system with large doses; bone marrow depression; acute leukemia; anemia; blood dyscrasia; leukopenia; thrombocytopenia; death.

Endocrine: Acute thyroid crises.

Miscellaneous: Radiation sickness (nausea, vomiting); severe sialoadenitis; increased clinical symptoms; chest pain, tachycardia, rash, hives, chromosomal abnormalities; tenderness and swelling of neck, pain on swallowing, sore throat and cough may occur around third day after treatment (usually amenable to analgesics); temporary hair thinning (may occur 2 to 3 months after treatment). Allergic reactions (infrequently).

Overdosage:

Symptoms: Overdosage may result in hypothyroidism.

Treatment: Give appropriate replacement therapy.

Administration and Dosage:

Measure dose by a suitable radioactivity calibration system immediately prior to use.

Carcinoma of the thyroid: Individualize dosage.

Usual dose for ablation of normal thyroid tissue – 50 mCi, with subsequent therapeutic doses usually 100 to 150 mCi.

Preparation of oral solution: To prepare a stock solution use Purified Water with 0.2% sodium thiosulfate as a reducing agent. Acidic diluents may cause pH to drop below

SODIUM IODIDE I 131

7.5 and stimulate volatilization of iodine 131-hydriodic acid. Equipment used to prepare the stock solution must be thoroughly rinsed and free of acidic cleaning agents.

Storage/Stability: Store at room temperature (< 30°C; < 86°F).

Physical characteristics: See product literature for specific calibration and dosimetry.

Rx	**Iodotope** (Bracco Diagnostics)[1]	**Capsules:** Radioactivity ranging from 1 to 50 mCi per capsule at time of calibration.	Blue/bluff.
		Oral solution: Radioactivity concentration of 7.05 mCi/ml at time of calibration.	1 mg/ml EDTA. In vials containing ≈ 7, 14, 28, 70 or 106 mCi at time of calibration.
Rx	**Sodium Iodide I 131** (Mallinckrodt)	**Capsules:** Radioactivity ranging from 0.75 to 100 mCi per capsule.	Various strengths.
		Oral solution: Radioactivity ranging from 3.5 to 150 mCi/vial.	With 0.1% sodium bisulfite and 0.2% EDTA. In vials.

[1] Bracco Diagnostics, 1 Squibb Drive, Building 124, New Brunswick, NJ 08903, (800) 447–6883.

SAMARIUM SM 153 LEXIDRONAM

Actions:

Pharmacology: Samarium Sm 153 lexidronam is a therapeutic agent consisting of radioactive samarium and a tetraphosphonate chelator, ethylenediaminetetramethylenephosphonic acid (EDTMP). It has an affinity for bone and concentrates in areas of bone turnover in association with hydroxyapatite. In clinical studies employing planar imaging techniques, more samarium accumulates in osteoblastic lesions than in normal bone with a lesion-to-bone ratio of ≈ 5. The mechanism of action of samarium in relieving the pain of bone metastases is not known.

Principle Radiation Emission Data of Samarium-153

Particle	Radiation Energy (keV)[1]	Abundance
Beta	640	30%
Beta	710	50%
Beta	810	20%
Gamma	103	29%

[1] Maximum energies are listed for the beta emissions, the average beta particle is 233 keV.

Pharmacokinetics:

Absorption – The greater the number of metastatic lesions, the more skeletal uptake of samarium radioactivity. The relationship between skeletal uptake and the size of the metastatic lesions has not been studied. The total skeletal uptake of radioactivity is ≈ 65.5% of the injected dose. The percent of the injected dose (% ID) taken up by bone ranged from 56.3% in a patient with 5 metastatic lesions to 76.7% in a patient with 52 metastatic lesions. If the number of metastatic lesions is fixed, over the range of 0.1 to 3 mCi/kg, the % ID taken up by bone is the same regardless of the dose.

Distribution – At physiologic pH, > 90% of the complex is present as $^{153}Sm[EDTMP]^{-5}$ and < 10% as $^{153}SmH[EDTMP]^{-4}$. The beta particle of ^{153}Sm-EDTMP travels an average of 3.1 mm in soft tissue and 1.7 mm in bone.

Metabolism – The complex formed by samarium and EDTMP is excreted as an intact, single species that consists of one atom of samarium and one molecule of EDTMP. Metabolic products of samarium Sm-153 EDTMP were not detected.

Excretion –

Blood: Clearance of radioactivity from the blood demonstrated biexponential kinetics after IV injection. During the first 30 minutes, the radioactivity in the blood decreased to 15% of the injected dose with a half-life of 5.5 minutes. After 30 minutes, the radioactivity cleared from the blood more slowly with a half-life of 65.4 minutes. Less than 1% of the injected dose remained in the blood 5 hours after injection.

Urine: Samarium Sm-153 EDTMP radioactivity was excreted in the urine after IV injection. During the first 6 hours, 34.5% was excreted. Overall, the greater the number of metastatic lesions, the less radioactivity was excreted.

SAMARIUM SM 153 LEXIDRONAM

Hepatic function impairment: Accumulation of activity was not detected in the liver or the intestine; this suggests that hepatobiliary excretion did not occur.

Clinical trials: Samarium was evaluated in 580 patients. Eligible patients had painful metastatic bone lesions that had failed other treatments, had ≥ 6–month expected survival and had a positive radionuclide bone scan.

The mean area under the pain curve (AUPC) decreased significantly from baseline with samarium than with placebo.

Indications:

Bone lesions: Relief of pain in patients with confirmed osteoblastic metastatic bone lesions that enhance on radionuclide bone scan.

Unlabeled uses: Ankylosing spondylitis; Paget's disease; rheumatoid arthritis.

Contraindications:

Hypersensitivity to EDTMP or similar phosphonate compounds.

Warnings:

Bone marrow suppression: Samarium causes bone marrow suppression. Use with caution in patients with compromised bone marrow reserves. In clinical trials, white blood cell counts and platelet counts decreased to a nadir of ≈ 40% to 50% of baseline in 123 (95%) of patients within 3 to 5 weeks after samarium and tended to return to pretreatment levels by 8 weeks.

Before administering samarium, give consideration to the patient's current clinical and hematologic status and bone marrow response history to treatment with myelotoxic agents. Metastatic prostate and other cancers can be associated with disseminated intravascular coagulation (DIC); exercise caution in treating cancer patients whose platelet counts are falling or who have other clinical or laboratory findings suggesting DIC. Because of the unknown potential for additive effects on bone marrow, do not give concurrently with chemotherapy or external beam radiation therapy unless clinical benefits outweigh the risks. Use of samarium in patients with evidence of compromised bone marrow reserve from previous therapy or disease involvement is not recommended unless the potential benefits of treatment outweigh the risks. Monitor blood counts weekly for at least 8 weeks or until recovery of adequate bone marrow function.

Radioactivity: Verify the dose of radioactivity to be administered to the patient before administering samarium. Do not release patients until their radioactivity levels and exposure rates comply with federal and local regulations.

Elderly: The pharmacokinetics of samarium Sm-153 EDTMP did not change with age.

Pregnancy: Category C. As with other radiopharmaceutical drugs, samarium can cause fetal harm when administered to a pregnant woman. Adequate and well controlled studies have not been conducted in pregnant women. Women of childbearing age should have a negative pregnancy test before administration of samarium. If this drug is used during pregnancy or if a patient becomes pregnant after taking this drug, apprise her of the potential hazard to the fetus. Advise women of childbearing potential to avoid becoming pregnant soon after receiving samarium. Advise male and female patients to use an effective method of contraception after the administration of samarium.

Lactation: It is not known whether samarium is excreted in breast milk. Because of the potential for serious adverse reactions from samarium in breastfeeding infants, make a decision to discontinue breastfeeding or discontinue the drug, taking into account the importance of the drug to the mother. If samarium is administered, it is recommended to discontinue breastfeeding.

Children: Safety and efficacy in pediatric patients < 16 years old have not been established.

Precautions:

Monitoring: Because of the potential for bone marrow suppression, beginning 2 weeks after samarium administration, monitor blood counts weekly for at least 8 weeks or until recovery of adequate bone marrow function.

ECG changes: EDTMP is a chelating agent. Although the chelating effects have not been evaluated thoroughly in humans, dogs that received non-radioactive samarium EDTMP (6 times the human dose based on body weight, 3 times based on surface area) developed a variety of ECG changes (with or without the presence of hypocalcemia). Use caution and appropriate monitoring when administering samarium to patients.

Skeletal effects: Spinal cord compression frequently occurs in patients with known metastases to the cervical, thoracic or lumbar spine. In clinical studies of samarium, spinal cord compression was reported in 7% of patients who received placebo and in 8.3% of patients who received 1 mCi/kg samarium. Samarium is not indicated for treatment of spinal cord compression. Samarium administration for pain relief of metastatic bone cancer does not prevent the development of spinal cord compression. When there is a clinical suspicion of spinal cord compression, appropriate diagnostic and therapeutic measures must be taken immediately to avoid permanent disability.

Incontinence: Take special precautions with bladder catheterization in incontinent patients to minimize the risk of radioactive contamination of clothing, bed linen and the patient's environment. Urinary excretion of radioactivity occurs within ≈ 12 hours (with 35% occurring during the first 6 hours).

Hypocalcemia: Exercise caution when administering samarium to patients at risk for developing hypocalcemia.

Flare reactions: Some patients have reported a transient increase in bone pain shortly after injection (flare reaction). This is usually mild and self-limiting and occurs within 72 hours of injection. Such reactions are usually responsive to analgesics.

Drug Interactions:

Chemotherapy: The potential for additive bone marrow toxicity of samarium with chemotherapy or external beam radiation has not been studied. Do not give samarium concurrently with chemotherapy or external beam radiation therapy unless the benefit outweighs the risks. Do not give samarium after either of these treatments until there has been time for adequate marrow recovery (see Warnings).

Adverse Reactions:

In a subgroup of 399 patients who received samarium 1 mCi/kg, there were 23 deaths and 46 serious adverse events. The deaths occurred an average of 67 days (range, 9 to 130) after samarium. Serious events occurred an average of 46 days (range, 1 to 118) after samarium. Although most of the patient deaths and serious adverse events appear to be related to the underlying disease, the relationship of end stage disease, marrow invasion by cancer cells, previous myelotoxic treatment and samarium toxicity cannot be easily distinguished. In clinical studies, two patients with rapidly progressive prostate cancer developed thrombocytopenia and died 4 weeks after receiving samarium. One of the patients showed evidence of disseminated intravascular coagulation (DIC); the other patient experienced a fatal cerebrovascular accident, with a suspicion of DIC. The relationship of the DIC to the bone marrow suppressive effect of samarium is not known.

Samarium Adverse Reactions (%)

Adverse Event	Samarium 1 mCi/kg n = 199 (%)	Placebo n = 90 (%)	Adverse Event	Samarium 1 mCi/kg n = 199 (%)	Placebo n = 90 (%)
Cardiovascular			*Infection*		
Arrhythmias	5	2.2	Fever/Chills	8.5	11.1
Chest pain	4	4.4	Infection, not specified	7	4.4
Hypertension	3	0	Oral moniliasis	2	1.1
Hypotension	2	2.2	Pneumonia	1.5	1.1
GI			*CNS*		
Abdominal pain	6	7.8	Dizziness	4	1.1
Diarrhea	6	3.3	Paresthesia	2	7.8
Nausea/Vomiting	32.7	41.1	Spinal cord compression	6.5	5.5
Hematologic/Lymphatic			Cerebrovascular accident/stroke	1	0
Coagulation disorder	1.5	0	*Dermatologic*		
Hemoglobin decreased	40.7	23.3	Purpura	1	0
Leukopenia	59.3	6.7	Rash	1	2.2
Lymphadenopathy	2	0	*Miscellaneous*		
Thrombocytopenia	69.3	8.9	Pain flare reaction[2]	7	5.6
Bleeding Manifestations[1]			Myasthenia	6.5	8.9
Ecchymosis	3	1.1	Pathologic fracture	2.5	2.2
Epistaxis	2	1.1	Bronchitis/Cough increased	4	2.2
Hematuria	5	3.3			

[1] Includes hemorrhage (GI, ocular) reported in < 1%.

[2] See Warnings.

Other adverse reactions include: Bone marrow toxicity (47%); sinus bradycardia, vasodilation (≥ 1%); alopecia, angina, congestive heart failure.

SAMARIUM SM 153 LEXIDRONAM

Overdosage:

Overdosage with samarium has not been reported. An antidote for samarium overdosage is not known. The anticipated complications of overdosage would likely be secondary to bone marrow suppression from the radioactivity of ^{153}Sm or secondary to hypocalcemia and cardiac arrhythmias related to EDTMP.

Patient Information:

Advise patients who receive samarium that for several hours following administration, radioactivity will be present in excreted urine. To help protect themselves and others in their environment, precautions need to be taken for 12 hours following administration. Whenever possible, use a toilet rather than a urinal and flush the toilet several times after each use. Clean up spilled urine completely and wash hands thoroughly. If blood or urine gets onto clothing, wash the clothing separately or store for 1 to 2 weeks to allow for decay of the samarium.

Women of childbearing age should have a negative pregnancy test before administration of samarium. If this drug is used during pregnancy, or if a patient becomes pregnant after taking this drug, apprise her of the potential hazard to the fetus. Advise women of childbearing potential to avoid becoming pregnant soon after receiving samarium. Advise male and female patients to use an effective method of contraception after the administration of samarium.

Administration and Dosage:

Approved by the FDA on March 28, 1997.

The recommended dose of samarium is 1 mCi/kg, administered IV over a period of 1 minute through a secure indwelling catheter and followed with a saline flush. Dose adjustment in patients at the extremes of weight have not been studied. Exercise caution when determining the dose in very thin or very obese patients.

Measure the dose by a suitable radioactivity calibration system, such as a radioisotope dose calibrator, immediately before administration.

Have the patient ingest (or receive by IV administration) a minimum of 500 ml (2 cups) of fluids prior to injection and void as often as possible after injection to minimize radiation exposure to the bladder.

Samarium contains calcium and may be incompatible with solutions that contain molecules that can complex with and form calcium precipitates.

Do not dilute or mix samarium with other solutions.

SAMARIUM SM 153 LEXIDRONAM

Radiation dosimetry: The dosimetry estimates are based on clinical biodistribution studies using methods developed for radiation dose calculations by the Medical Internal Radiation Dose (MIRD) Committee of the Society of Nuclear Medicine.

Radiation exposure is based on a urinary voiding interval of 4.8 hours. Radiation dose estimates for bone and marrow assume that radioactivity is deposited on bone surfaces, as noted in autoradiograms of biopsy bone samples in 7 patients who received samarium. Although electron emissions from ^{153}Sm are abundant, with energies up to 810 keV, rapid blood clearance of samarium and low energy and abundant photon emissions generally result in low radiation doses to those parts of the body where the complex does not localize.

When blastic osseous lesions are present, significantly enhanced localization of the radiopharmaceutical will occur, with correspondingly higher doses to the lesions compared with normal bones and other organs.

Estimated Absorbed Radiation Doses of Samarium to an Average 70 kg Adult Patient

Target organ	Rad/mCi	mGy/MBq
Bone surfaces	25	6.76
Red marrow	5.7	1.54
Urinary bladder wall	3.6	0.097
Kidneys	0.065	0.018
Whole body	0.04	0.011
Lower large intestine	0.037	0.01
Ovaries	0.032	0.0086
Muscle	0.028	0.0076
Small intestine	0.023	0.0062
Upper large intestine	0.02	0.0054
Testes	0.02	0.0054
Liver	0.019	0.0051
Spleen	0.018	0.0049
Stomach	0.015	0.0041

Storage/Stability: Thaw at room temperature before administration and use within 8 hours. Store frozen at –20° to –10°C (–4° to 14°F) in a lead shielded container.

Rx	**Quadramet** (Du Pont Pharma)	**Injection:** 1850 MBq/ml (50 mCi/ml) at calibration	Frozen, single-dose 10 ml vials. In 2 ml fill (3700 MBq) and 3 ml fill (5550 MBq).

SODIUM PHOSPHATE P 32

Actions:

Pharmacology: Phosphorus is necessary to the metabolic and proliferative activity of cells. Radioactive phosphorus concentrates to a very high degree in rapidly proliferating tissue.

Sodium phosphate P 32 decays by beta emission with a physical half-life of 14.3 days. The mean energy of the sodium phosphate P 32 beta particle is 695 keV.

Indications:

Leukemia: Treatment of polycythemia vera, chronic myelocytic leukemia and chronic lymphocytic leukemia.

Skeletal metastases: Palliative treatment of selected patients with multiple areas of skeletal metastases.

Contraindications:

Sequential therapy: Do not use as part of sequential treatment with a chemotherapeutic agent.

Polycythemia vera: Do not administer when the leukocyte count is < 5,000/mm^3 or platelet count is < 150,000/mm^3.

Chronic myelocytic leukemia: Do not administer when the leukocyte count is < 20,000/mm^3.

Bone metastases: Usually not administered when the leukocyte count is < 5,000/mm^3 and the platelet count is < 100,000/mm^3.

Warnings:

Pregnancy: Category C. Safey for use during pregnancy has not been established. It is not known if the drug causes fetal harm or affects reproductive ability. Use only when clearly needed and when the potential benefits outweigh the potential hazards to the fetus.

Perform examinations using radiopharmaceuticals (especially elective examinations) to women of childbearing capacity during the first 10 days following the onset of menses.

Lactation: It is not known whether sodium phosphate is excreted in breast milk. Discontinue nursing during therapy.

Children: Safety and efficacy in children have not been established.

Precautions:

Monitoring: Monitor blood and bone marrow at regular intervals.

Minimum exposure: Ensure minimum radiation exposure to patients and occupational workers consistent with proper patient management.

Retinoblastomas: Sodium phosphate P 32 does not usually localize in retinoblastomas.

Overdosage:

May produce serious effects on the hematopoietic system.

Administration and Dosage:

Administer IV. Do not administer as an intracavity injection. Oral administration of high-specific-activity sodium phosphate P 32 in the fasting state may equal IV administration.

Measure dose by a suitable radioactivity calibration system immediately before use.

Polycythemia vera: 1 to 8 mCi IV are given, depending upon the stage of disease and size of the patient. Individualize repeat doses.

Chronic leukemia: 6 to 15 mCi usually with concomitant hormone manipulation.

Storage/Stability: Store at room temperature, 15° to 30°C (59° to 86°F).

Rx	**Sodium Phosphate P 32** (Mallinckrodt)	**Injection**: 0.67 mCi/ml	5mCi per vial.

CHROMIC PHOSPHATE P 32

Actions:

Pharmacology: Local irradiation by beta emission.

P 32 decays by beta emission with a physical half-life of 14.3 days. The mean energy of the beta particle is 695 keV.

Indications:

Intracavitary instillation: Treatment of peritoneal or pleural effusions caused by metastatic disease.

Interstitial injection: Treatment of cancer.

Contraindications:

Presence of ulcerative tumors; administration in exposed cavities or where there is evidence of loculation unless its extent is determined.

Warnings:

Radiopharmaceuticals: Restrict use to physicians qualified in the safe use and handling of radionuclides produced by nuclear reactor or particle accelerator and whose experience and training have been approved by the appropriate government agency.

Benzyl alcohol: This product contains benzyl alcohol, which has been associated with fatal "gasping syndrome" in preterm infants.

Pregnancy: Category C. Use only when clearly needed and when the potential benefits outweigh the potential hazards to the fetus.

Lactation: Use only when clearly needed and when the potential benefits outweigh the potential hazards to the nursing infant.

Precautions:

Radioactive material: Ensure minimum radiation exposure to the patient and occupational workers consistent with proper patient management.

Intracavitary use: Not for intravascular use.

Careful intracavitary instillation is required to avoid placing the dose of chromic phosphate P 32 into intrapleural or intraperitoneal loculations, bowel lumen or the body wall. Intestinal fibrosis or necrosis and chronic fibrosis of the body wall have resulted from unrecognized misplacement of the therapeutic agent.

Large tumor masses indicate the need for other forms of treatment; however, when other forms of treatment fail to control the effusion, chromic phosphate P 32 may be useful. In bloody effusion, treatment may be less effective.

Adverse Reactions:

Transitory radiation sickness, bone marrow depression, pleuritis, peritonitis, nausea and abdominal cramping.

Radiation damage may occur if injected interstitially or into a loculation.

Administration and Dosage:

For interstitial or intracavitary use only.

Measure dose by suitable radioactivity calibration system immediately prior to use.

The suggested dose range in the average patient (70 kg) is:

Intraperitoneal instillation – 10 to 20 mCi.

Intrapleural instillation – 6 to 12 mCi.

Interstitial use – 0.1 to 0.5 mCi/g of estimated weight of tumor.

Physical characteristics – Consult product literature for specific calibration and dosimetry information.

Rx	**Phosphocol P 32** (Mallinckrodt)	**Suspension** : 15 mCi with a concentration of up to 5 mCi/ml and specific activity of up to 5 mCi/mg at time of standardization.	In 10 ml vials.[1]

[1] With 2% benzyl alcohol, NaCl and sodium acetate.

INTERFERON ALFA-2a (rIFN-A; IFLrA)

> **Warning:**
> Depression and suicidal behavior including suicidal ideation, suicidal attempts and suicides have been reported in association with alfph interferon treatment. Patients to be treated with interferon alfa-2a should be informed that depression and suicidal ideation may be side effects of treatment and should be advised to report these side effects immediately to the prescribing physician. Monitor patients receiving interferon alfa-2a therapy closely for the occurrence of depressive symptoms. Consider cessation of treatment for patients experiencing depression. Although dose reduction or treatment cessation may lead to resolution of depressive symptoms, depression may persist and suicides have occurred after withdrawal of therapy.

Actions:

Pharmacology: Interferon alfa-2a is a sterile protein product manufactured by recombinant DNA technology that employs a genetically engineered *Escherichia coli* bacterium. Interferon alfa-2a is a highly purified protein containing 165 amino acids.

The mechanism by which interferons exert antitumor activity is not clearly understood. However, direct antiproliferative action against tumor cells and modulation of the host immune response may play important roles.

Using human cells in culture, interferon alfa-2a has antiproliferative and immunomodulatory activities that are very similar to those of the mixture of interferon alfa subtypes produced by human leukocytes. In vivo, interferon alfa-2a inhibits the growth of several human tumors growing in immunocompromised mice.

Pharmacokinetics:

Absorption/Distribution – In healthy people, interferon alfa-2a exhibited an elimination half-life of 3.7 to 8.5 hours (mean, 5.1 hours), volume of distribution at steady state of 0.223 to 0.748 L/kg (mean, 0.4 L/kg) and a total body clearance of 2.14 to 3.62 ml/min/kg (mean, 2.79 ml/min/kg) after a 36 million IU (2.2×10^8 pg) IV infusion. After IM and SC administrations of 36 million IU, peak serum concentrations ranged from 1500 to 2580 pg/ml (mean, 2020 pg/ml) at a mean time to peak of 3.8 hours and from 1250 to 2320 pg/ml (mean, 1730 pg/ml) at a mean time to peak of 7.3 hours, respectively. The serum concentrations of interferon alfa-2a reflected a large intersubject variation. Dose proportional increases in serum concentrations were observed after single doses up to 198 million IU. There were no changes in the distribution or elimination of interferon alfa-2a during twice daily (0.5 to 36 million IU), once daily (1 to 54 million IU) or 3 times weekly (1 to 136 million IU) dosing regimens up to 28 days of dosing. Multiple IM doses resulted in accumulation of 2 to 4 times the single dose serum concentrations. The apparent fraction of the dose absorbed after IM injection was > 80%.

Metabolism/Excretion – Alpha interferons are filtered through the glomeruli and undergo rapid proteolytic degradation during tubular reabsorption, rendering a negligible reappearance of intact alpha interferon in the systemic circulation, suggesting near complete reabsorption of interferon alfa-2a catabolites. Liver metabolism and subsequent biliary excretion are minor pathways of elimination.

Clinical trials:

Hairy cell leukemia – During the first 1 to 2 months of treatment, significant depression of hematopoiesis was likely to occur. Subsequently, there was improvement in circulating blood cell counts.

Of the 75 patients evaluated for at least 16 weeks of therapy, 46 (61%) achieved complete or partial response. Twenty-one patients (28%) had a minor remission, eight (11%) remained stable and none had worsening of disease. All patients who achieved either a complete or partial response had complete or partial normalization of all peripheral blood elements with a concomitant decrease in peripheral blood and bone marrow hairy cells. Responding patients also exhibited a marked reduction in red blood cell and platelet transfusion requirements, a decrease in infectious episodes, and improvement in performance status. The probability of survival for 2 years in patients receiving interferon alfa-2a (94%) was statistically increased compared with a historical control group (75%).

AIDS-related Kaposi's sarcoma – Doses of 3 to 54 million IU daily were evaluated in more than 350 patients. An additional 91 patients received interferon alfa-2a in combination with vinblastine. The best response rate associated with acceptable toxicity was observed when interferon alfa-2a was administered as a single agent at a dose of 36 million IU daily. The escalating regimen of 3 to 36 million IU provided equivalent therapeutic benefit with some amelioration of acute toxicity in some patients. Lower doses were less effective in inducing tumor regression and doses higher than 36 million IU daily were associated with unacceptable toxicity.

INTERFERON ALFA-2a (rIFN-A; IFLrA)

The likelihood of response to interferon alfa-2a varies with the clinical manifestations of human immunodeficiency virus (HIV) infection but not to extent of tumor involvement. Patients with prior opportunistic infection or B symptoms (eg, night sweats, weight loss > 10% of body weight or 15 lbs, fever > 100°F without identifiable source of infection) are unlikely to respond to treatment.

Patients who were otherwise asymptomatic, with no prior opportunistic infection and near-normal levels of CD4 lymphocytes, experienced higher response rates. Responding patients with a baseline CD4 lymphocyte count > 200 cells/mm^3 had a distinct survival advantage over both responding patients with a baseline CD4 lymphocyte count of ≤ 200 cells/mm^3 and nonresponding patients regardless of their baseline CD4 lymphocyte count.

The median time to response was 2.7 months. The median duration of response for patients achieving a partial or complete response was 6.3 and 20.7 months, respectively. Complete and partial responses lasting > 3 years have been observed.

Indications:

Hairy cell leukemia: In select patients 18 years of age and older.

AIDS-related Kaposi's sarcoma: In select patients 18 years of age and older.

Chronic myelogenous leukemia (CML): In chrnic phase, Philadelphia chromosome (Ph) positive CML patients who are minimally pretreated (within 1 year of diagnosis).

Unlabeled uses: Alfa interferons have been used for a variety of conditions. Clinical trials are in progress to further determine clinical efficacy, optimal dosage and length of treatment.

Interferon Alfa Unlabeled Uses		
Neoplastic Diseases		
Significant activity	*Limited activity*	*No activity*
Bladder tumors (local use for superficial tumors) Carcinoid tumor Chronic myelogenous leukemia Cutaneous T-cell lymphoma Essential thrombocythemia Non-Hodgkin's lymphoma (low-grade)	Acute leukemias Cervical carcinoma Chronic lymphocytic leukemia Hodgkin's disease Malignant gliomas Melanoma Multiple myeloma Mycosis fungoides/Se'zary syndrome Nasopharyngeal carcinoma Osteosarcoma Ovarian carcinoma Renal carcinoma	Breast cancer Colorectal carcinoma Gastric carcinoma Lung carcinoma Pancreatic carcinoma Prostatic carcinoma Soft tissue carcinoma
Viral Infections		**Miscellaneous**
Chronic non-A, non-B hepatitis Condyloma acuminatum Cutaneous warts Cytomegaloviruses Herpes keratoconjunctivitis	Herpes simplex Papillomaviruses Rhinoviruses Vaccinia virus Varicella zoster Viral hepatitis B[1]	Hemangiomas of infancy (life-threatening) Multiple sclerosis

[1] May be more effective following prednisone withdrawal (immunologic priming).

Contraindications:

Hypersensitivity to alfa interferon or any component of the product.

Warnings:

GI hemorrhage: Infrequently, severe or fatal GI hemorrhage has been reported in association with alfa interferon therapy.

Exercise caution in the following: In patients with severe renal or hepatic disease, seizure disorders, compromised CNS function or myelosuppression.

Administer with caution to patients with cardiac disease or with any history of cardiac illness. No direct cardiotoxic effect has been demonstrated, but it is likely that acute, self-limited toxicities (ie, fever, chills) frequently associated with interferon alfa administration may exacerbate preexisting cardiac conditions. Rarely, myocardial infarction has occurred.

CNS reactions have occurred in a number of patients and included decreased mental status, exaggerated CNS function and dizziness. More severe obtundation and coma have been rarely observed. Most of these were mild and reversible within a few days to 3 weeks upon dose reduction or drug discontinuation. Careful periodic neuropsychiatric monitoring of all patients is recommended.

INTERFERON ALFA-2a (rIFN-A; IFLrA)

Leukopenia and elevation of hepatic enzymes occurred frequently but were rarely dose-limiting. Thrombocytopenia occurred less frequently. Proteinuria and increased cells in urinary sediment were also seen infrequently. Rarely, significant hepatic, renal and myelosuppressive toxicities were noted.

Anemia: In CML patients, a severe or life-threatening anemia was seen in 15% of patients. A severe life-threatening leukopenia and thrombocytopenia were seen in up to 27% of patients. Changes were usually reversible when therapy was discontinued. One case of aplastic anemia and one case of Coomb's positive hemolytic anemia were seen in 310 patients treated with interferon alfa-2a in clinical studies. Severe cytopenias led to discontinuation of therapy in 4% of patients.

Neutralizing antibodies were detected in ≈ 27% of all patients (3.4% for patients with hairy cell leukemia). No clinical sequelae have been documented. Antibodies to human leukocyte interferon may occur spontaneously in certain clinical conditions (cancer, systemic lupus erythmatosus, herpes zoster) in patients who have never received exogenous interferon.

Renal/Hepatic function impairment: Transient increases in liver transaminases or alkaline phosphatase of any intensity were seen in up to 50% of patients during treatment with interferon alfa-2a. Only 5% of patients had a severe or life-threatening increase in AST. In clinical studies, such abnormalities required termination of therapy in < 1% of patients.

Dose-limiting hepatic or renal toxicities are unusual. Severe renal toxicities, sometimes requiring renal dialysis, are infrequent.

Pregnancy: Category C. Safety in pregnancy has not been established. Use during pregnancy only if the potential benefit justifies the potential risk to the fetus. Fertile women should not receive interferon alfa-2a unless they are using effective contraception during therapy.

Lactation: It is not known whether this drug is excreted in breast milk. Because of the potential for serious adverse reactions in nursing infants, decide whether to discontinue nursing or to discontinue the drug, taking into account the importance of the drug to the mother.

Children: Safety and efficacy in children < 18 years of age have not been established.

Precautions:

Monitoring: Prior to initiation of therapy, perform tests to quantitate peripheral blood hemoglobin, platelets, granulocytes, hairy cell and bone marrow hairy cells. Monitor periodically (eg, monthly) during treatment to determine response to treatment. If a patient does not respond within 6 months, discontinue treatment. If a response occurs, continue treatment until no further improvement is observed and these laboratory parameters have been stable for about 3 months. It is not known whether continued treatment after that time is beneficial.

Perform periodic complete blood counts and liver function tests during the course of treatment. Perform prior to therapy and at appropriate periods during therapy. Because responses of hairy cell leukemia are not generally observed for 1 to 3 months after initiation of treatment, very careful monitoring for severe depression of blood cell counts is warranted during the initial phase of treatment.

Cardiac ECG – Those patients who have preexisting cardiac abnormalities or who are in advanced stages of cancer should have ECGs taken prior to and during the course of treatment.

Depression: Depression and suicidal ideation may be side effects of treatment (see Warning Box).

INTERFERON ALFA-2a (rIFN-A; IFLrA)

Drug Interactions:

Interferon alfa-2a Drug Interactions			
Precipitant drug	Object drug*		Description
Interferon alfa-2a	Theophylline	↑	Reduced clearance of theophylline following concomitant administration has been reported.
Interferon alfa-2a	Neurotoxic, hematotoxic or cardiotoxic drugs	↑	Effects of previously or concurrently administered drugs may be decreased by interferons.
Interferon alfa-2a	Interleukin-2	↑	Potential risk of renal failure.
Interferon alfa-2a	CNS drugs	↔	Interactions could occur following concurrent administration of centrally-acting drugs.
Interferon alfa-2a	Aminophylline	↑	In one study, a single IM injection of interferon alfa-2a significantly reduced the clearance of aminophylline 33% to 81% in 8 of 9 subjects, probably due to inhibition of the cytochrome P-450 enzyme system.

↑ = Object drug increased. ↔ = Undetermined effect.

Other interactions: Alfa-interferons may affect the oxidative metabolic process by reducing the activity of hepatic microsomal cytochrome enzymes in the P-450 group. Although the clinical relevance is still unclear, take into account when prescribing concomitant therapy with drugs metabolized by this route.

Adverse Reactions:

Most adverse reactions are reversible if detected early. If severe reactions occur, reduce dosage or discontinue the drug; take appropriate corrective measures according to physician's clinical judgment. Reinstitute therapy with caution; consider further need for the drug, and be alert to possible recurrence of toxicity.

Hairy cell leukemia:

Flu-like syndrome – Fever (92%); fatique (86%); myalgias (71%); headache, chills (64%); weight loss (33%); dizziness (21%).

Dermatologic – Skin rash (44%); diaphoresis (22%); partial alopecia, dry skin (17%); pruritus (13%).

Musculoskeletal – Joint or bone pain (25%); arthritis or polyarthritis (5%).

GI – Anorexia (43%); nausea/vomiting (39%); diarrhea (34%); throat irritation (21%).

Respiratory – Coughing (16%); dyspnea, rhinorrhea (12%); pneumonia, sinusitis (11%).

CNS – Depression (16%); paresthesia, numbness (12%); sleep disturbance, decreased mental status (10%); anxiety, lethargy, visual disturbance (6%); confusion (5%).

Cardiovascular – Chest pain, edema, hypertension (11%).

Miscellaneous – Generalized pain (24%); back pain (16%).

Other (< 5%): Gait disturbance; nervousness; syncope; vertigo; cardiac murmur; thrombophlebitis; hypotension; ecchymosis; epistaxis; bleeding gums; petechiae; urticaria; inflammation at injection site.

AIDS-related Kaposi's sarcoma:

Flu-like symptoms – Fatique (95%); fever (74%); myalgia (69%); headache (66%); chills (41%); arthralgia (24%).

GI – Anorexia (65%); nausea (51%); diarrhea (42%); emesis (17%); abdominal pain (15%).

CNS – Dizzines (40%); decreased mental status (17%); depression (16%); paresthesia, confusion (8%); diaphoresis (7%); sleep disturbance, visual disturbance (5%); numbness (3%).

Respiratory – Coughing (27%); dryness or inflammation of oropharynx (14%); dyspnea (11%); chest pain, rhinorrhea (4%).

Dermatologic – Partial alopecia (22%); rash (11%); dry skin or pruritus (5%).

Miscellaneous – Weight loss, taste perversion (25%); edema (9%); night sweats (8%); hypotension (4%).

Other (< 3%): Anxiety; nervousness; emotional lability; vertigo; forgetfulness; cardiac palpitations; arrhythmia; sinusitis; constipation; chest congestion; pneumonia; urticaria; flatulence; ataxia; seizures; cyanosis; gastric distress; bronchospasm; pain at injection site; earache; eye irritation; rhinitis; poor coordination; lethargy; muscle contractions; neuropathy; tremor; involunatry movements; syncope; aphasia; aphonia; dysarthria; amnesia; weakness; flushing of skin; cardiomyopathy.

INTERFERON ALFA-2a (rIFN-A; IFLrA)

CML:

Flu-like syndrome – Fever (92%); asthenia or fatigue (88%); myalgia (68%); chills (63%); arthralgia/bone pain (47%); headache (44%).

GI – Anorexia (48%); nausea, vomiting, diarrhea (37%).

CNS – Headahce (44%); depression (28%); decreased mental status (16%); dizziness, sleep disturbancs (11%); paresthesia (8%); involuntary movements (7%); visual disturbances (6%).

Dermatologic – Hair changes (including alopecia), skin rash (18%); sweating (15); dry skin, pruritus (7%).

Miscellaneous – Coughing (19%); dypnea (8%); dysarrhythmia (7%).

Other (< 4%): Chest pain; syncope; hypotension; impotence; alterations in taste or hearing; confusion; seizures; memory loss; disturbances of libido; bruising; coagulopathy; Coomb's positive hemolytic anemia; aplastic anemia; hypothyroidism; cardiomyopathy; hypertriglyceridemia; bronchospasm.

Abnormal laboratory test values:

Hematologic – Leudopenia (3% to 49%); neutropenia (≤ 68%); thrombocytopenia (5% to 62%); decreased hemoglobin (4% to 31%); severe anemia (15%); severe cytopenias (4%) (see Warnings).

Hepatic – AST (≤ 46%); alkaline phosphatase (≤ 11%) (see Warnings); LDH (≤ 10%); bilirubin (< 1 %).

Renal/Urinary: Proteinuria (≤ 10%); uric acid (< 5%); serum creatinine, BUN (< 1%).

Other (< 5%): Hypocalcemia; elevated fasting serum glucose and elevated serum phosphorus.

Patient Information:

Patient package insert available with product.

Warn patients not to change brands of interferon; changes in dosage may result.

Patients should be well hydrated, especially during initial treatment.

Administration and Dosage:

Approved by the FDA in 1986.

Give SC or IM. Subcutaneous administration is suggested for, but not limited to, patients who are thrombocytopenic (platelet count < 50,000/mm^3) or who are at risk for bleeding.

Hairy cell leukemia:

Induction dose – 3 million IU daily for 16 to 24 weeks, SC or IM.

Maintenance dose – 3 million IU 3 times per week. Dosage reduction by one-half or withholding of individual doses may be needed when severe adverse reactions occur.

The use of doses higher than 3 million IU is not recommended.

Treat patients for approximately 6 months before determining whether to continue therapy. Patients with hairy cell leukemia have been treated for up to 20 consecutive months. The optimal duration of treatment for this disease has not been determined.

AIDS-related Kaposi's sarcoma:

Induction dose – 36 million IU daily for 10 to 12 weeks, administered IM or SC.

Maintenance dose – 36 million IU, 3 times per week. Dose reductions by one-half or withholding of individual doses may be required when severe adverse reactions occur. An escalating schedule of 3, 9 and 18 million IU daily for 3 days followed by 36 million IU daily for the remainder of the 10 to 12 week induction period has also produced equivalent therapeutic benefit with some amelioration of the acute toxicity in some patients.

When disease stabilization or a response to treatment occurs, treatment should continue until there is no further evidence of tumor or until discontinuation is required because of a severe opportunistic infection or adverse effects. The optimal duration of treatment for this disease has not been determined.

If severe reactions occur, modify dosage (50% reduction) or temporarily discontinue therapy until the adverse reactions abate. The need for dosage reduction should take into account the effects of prior x-ray therapy or chemotherapy that may have compromised bone marrow reserve. Minimum effective doses have not been established.

CML:

Chronic phase Ph positive CML – Prior to initiation of therapy, make a diagnosis of Ph positive CML in chronic phase by the appropriate peripheral blood, bone marrow and other diagnostic testing. Regularly monitor hematologic parameters (eg, monthly). Because significant cytogenic changes are not readily apparent until after hematologic response has occurred, and usually not until several months of therapy

INTERFERON ALFA-2a (rIFN-A; IFLrA)

have elapsed, cytogenic monitoring may be performed at less frequent intervals. Achievement of complete cytogenic response has been observed up to 2 years following the start of interferon alfa-2a treatment.

Induction dose – 9 million units daily administered SC or IM. Based on clinical experience, short-term tolerance may be improved by gradually increasing the dose of interferon alfa-2a over the first week of administration from 3 million IU daily for 3 days to 6 million IU daily for 3 days to the target dose of 9 million IU daily for the duration of the treatment period.

Maintenance – Optimal dose and duration of therapy have not been determined.

Even though the median time to achieve a complete hematologic response was 5 months in clinical studies, hematologic responses have been observed up to 18 months after starting treatment. Continue therapy until disease progression. If severe side effects occur, a treatment interruption or reduction in either the dose or the frequence of injections may be necessary to achieve the individual maximally tolerated dose.

Children – Limited data are available on the use of interferon alfa-2a in children with CML. In one report of 15 children with Ph positive, adult-type CML, doses between 2.5 to 5 million IU/m²/day given IM were tolerated. In another study, severe adverse effects including death were noted in children with previously untreated, Ph negative juvenile CML, who received interferon doses of 30 million IU/m²/day.

Storage: Refrigerate 2° to 8°C (36° to 46°F). Do not freeze; do not shake. Once the powder is reconstituted, use within 30 days.

Rx	**Roferon-A** (Roche)	**Injection Solution**: 3 million IU/ml	In 1 ml vials (3 million IU per vial).[1]
		6 million IU/ml	In 3 ml vials (18 million IU per vial).[1]
		36 million IU/ml[2]	In 1 ml vials (36 million IU per vial).[2]
		Powder for Injection: 6 million IU/ml when reconstituted	In vials (18 million IU) with diluent.[1]

[1] With NaCl, human serum albumin and phenol.

[2] Do not use this strength for the treatment of hairy cell leukemia.

INTERFERON ALFA-2b (IFN-alpha 2; rIFN-α2; α-2-interferon)

Actions:

Pharmacology: Interferon alfa is a protein produced by recombinant DNA techniques. It is obtained from a strain of *Escherichia coli* bearing a genetically engineered plasmid containing an interferon alfa-2b gene from human leukocytes.

The interferons are naturally occurring small protein molecules. They are produced and secreted by cells in response to viral infections or synthetic and biological inducers. Three major classes of interferons have been identified: Alpha, beta and gamma. These classes are not homogenous; each may contain several different molecular species. At least 14 genetically distinct human alpha interferons have been identified thus far.

Interferons exert their cellular activities by binding to specific membrane receptors on the cell surface. Once bound to the cell membrane, interferon initiates a complex sequence of intracellular events that includes the induction of certain enzymes. This process, at least in part, may be responsible for the various cellular responses to interferon, including inhibition of virus replication in virus-infected cells, suppression of cell proliferation and such immunomodulating activities as enhancement of the phagocytic activity of macrophages and augmentation of the specific cytotoxicity of lymphocytes for target cells.

Pharmacokinetics: Maximum serum concentrations obtained were ≈ 18 to 116 IU/ml and occurred 3 to 12 hours after administration. Elimination half-lives were approximately 2 to 3 hours. Serum concentrations were below the detection limit by 16 hours after the injections.

After IV use, serum concentrations peaked (135 to 273 IU/ml) by the end of infusion, then declined at a slightly more rapid rate than after IM or SC administration, becoming undetectable 4 hours after infusion. Elimination half-life was ≈ 2 hours.

Interferon could not be detected in urine; the kidney may be the main site of interferon catabolism.

Clinical trials:

Malignant melanoma – In a randomized, controlled trial in 280 patients, 143 patients received interferon alfa-2b therapy at 20 million IU/m^2 IV 5 times/week for 4 weeks (induction phase), followed by 10 million IU/m^2 SC 3 times/week for 48 weeks (maintenance phase). Interferon alfa-2b therapy was begun ≤ 56 days after surgical resection. The remaining 137 patients were observed.

Interferon alfa-2b therpay produced a significant increase in relapse-free and overall survival. Median time to relapse for the interferon alfa-2b treated patients vs observation patients was 1.72 years vs 0.98 years. The estimated 5–year , relapse-free survival rate was 37% for interferon alfa-2b patients vs observation patients was 3.82 years vs 2.78 years. The estimated 5–year overall survival rate was 46% for interferon alfa-2b patients vs 37% for observation patients.

Condylomata acuminata – A total of 192 patients were injected intralesionally with 1 million IU interferon alfa-2b per lesion. Up to five lesions per patient were treated 3 times a week for 3 weeks, and the patients were then observed for up to 16 weeks after the full treatment course. Interferon alfa-2b was significantly more effective than placebo in the treatment of condylomata, as measured by disappearance of lesions, decreases in lesion size and by an overall change in disease status. In the 192 patients evaluated, 42% experienced clearing of all treated lesions, while 24% experienced marked and 18% experienced moderate reduction in lesion size, and 10% of patients had a slight reduction in lesion size.

AIDS-related Kaposi's sarcoma – A total of 144 patients were treated in three clinical trials with various dosage regimens. Significantly greater activity occurred in asymptomatic (afebrile and without weight loss) patients than systemic symptom patients (57% vs 23%) in one study. In another study, a 44% response rate occurred in asymptomatic patients vs 7% in symptomatic patients. Median time to response was ≈ 2 months and median duration of response ≈ 3 months for asymptomatic patients. For symptomatic patients, median time to response and median duration of response were both 1 month.

Chronic hepatitis non-A, non-B/C (NANB/C) – A total of 332 patients were given interferon alfa-2b SC at doses of 1, 2 or 3 million IU 3 times a week for 6 months in four controlled studies. Interferon alfa-2b produced a statistically significant improvement in serum alanine aminotransferase (ALT) levels in all studies.

Chronic hepatitis B – A total of 86 patients received either 5 million IU every day (n = 38) or 10 million IU 3 times a week (n = 48) for 16 weeks. Compared to untreated controls, a significantly greater proportion of interferon alfa-2b-treated patients exhibited a virologic response (7% vs 39% to 48%). No patient responding to therapy relapsed during a follow-up period of 2 to 6 months. Loss of serum HBeAg and HBV-DNA (indicators of HBV replication) was maintained in 100% of 19 responding patients for 3.5 to 36 months of follow-up.

INTERFERON ALFA-2b (IFN-alpha 2; rIFN-α2; α-2-interferon)

Indications:

Hairy cell leukemia: In select patients ≥ 18 years of age, both previously splenectomized and nonsplenectomized.

Malignant melanoma: Adjuvant to surgical treatment in patients ≥ 18 years with malignant melanoma who are free of disease but at high risk for systemic recurrence within 56 days of surgery.

Condylomata acuminata: Intralesional treatment of genital or venereal warts in patients who do not respond to other treatment modalities or whose lesions are more readily treatable by interferon alfa-2b.

AIDS-related Kaposi's sarcoma: In select patients ≥ 18 years of age.

Chronic hepatitis non-A, non-B/C: In patients ≥ 18 years of age with compensated liver disease and a history of blood or blood product exposure or are HCV antibody positive.

Chronic hepatitis B: In patients ≥ 18 years of age with compensated liver disease and HBV replication. Patients must be serum HBsAg positive for at least 6 months and have HBV replication (serum HBeAg positive) with elevated serum ALT.

Unlabeled uses: Alpha interferons have been used for a variety of conditions, a list of which follows. Clinical trials are currently in progress to further determine clinical efficacy, optimal dosage and length of treatment.

Interferon Alfa Unlabeled Uses		
Neoplastic Diseases		
Significant activity	Limited activity	No activity
Bladder tumors (local use for superficial tumors) Carcinoid tumor Chronic myelogenous leukemia Cutaneous T-cell lymphoma Essential thrombocythemia Non-Hodgkin's lymphoma (low-grade)	Acute leukemias Cervical carcinoma Chronic lymphocytic leukemia Hodgkin's disease Malignant gliomas Melanoma Multiple myeloma Nasopharyngeal carcinoma Osteosarcoma Ovarian carcinoma Renal carcinoma	Breast cancer Colorectal carcinoma Gastric carcinoma Lung carcinoma Pancreatic carcinoma Prostatic carcinoma Soft tissue carcinoma
Viral Infections		**Miscellaneous**
Cutaneous warts Cytomegaloviruses Herpes keratoconjunctivitis Herpes simplex	Papillomaviruses Rhinoviruses Vaccinia virus Varicella zoster	Multiple sclerosis

Contraindications:

Hypersensitivity to interferon alfa-2b or any components of the product.

Warnings:

Hairy cell leukemia:

Monitoring – Before initiating therapy, perform tests to quantitate peripheral blood hemoglobin, platelets, granulocytes and hairy cells and bone marrow hairy cells. Monitor periodically to determine response. If no response within 6 months, discontinue treatment. If response does occur, continue treatment until no further improvement is observed and these laboratory parameters have been stable for ≈ 3 months. It is not known if continued treatment after that point is beneficial.

Do not give IM to patients with platelet counts < 50,000/mm³. Instead, give SC.

Cardiovascular adverse experiences such as significant hypotension, arrhythmia or tachycardia (≥ 150 beats/min), were observed in ≈ 3% of patients studied with various malignancies who were treated at doses higher than those for hairy cell leukemia. Incidence in patients with preexisting heart disease is unknown. Hypotension may occur during use, or for up to 2 days post-therapy, and may require supportive therapy, including fluid replacement, to maintain intravascular volume. Supraventricular arrhythmias, rare, appeared to be correlated with preexisting conditions and prior therapy with cardiotoxic agents. These events were controlled by modifying dose or discontinuing drug, but may require specific additional therapy. Closely monitor patients with recent MI or previous or current arrhythmic disorder.

CNS effects (eg, depression, confusion, other alterations of mental status) were seen in ≈ 2% of hairy cell leukemia patients. Overall incidence in a larger patient population with other malignancies treated with higher doses was 10%. More significant obtundation and coma may occur in some patients, usually elderly, treated at higher doses for other malignant diseases. These effects are usually rapidly revers-

INTERFERON ALFA-2b (IFN-alpha 2; rIFN-α2; α-2-interferon)

ible. In a few severe episodes, full resolution takes up to 3 weeks. Closely monitor until these effects resolve. Discontinuation of therapy may be required. Narcotics, hypnotics or sedatives may be used concurrently with caution.

Condylomata acuminata:

Do not use 3, 5 and 25 million IU strengths intralesionally; the dilution would result in a hypertonic solution. Do not use 50 million IU strength for condylomata.

AIDS-related Kaposi's sarcoma:

Monitoring – Perform lesion measurements and blood counts prior to initiation of therapy; monitor periodically during treatment.

Rapidly progressive visceral disease – Do not use.

Chronic hepatitis - NANB/C:

Monitoring – Perform a liver biopsy to establish diagnosis. Test for presence of antibody to HCV. Exclude patients with other causes of chronic hepatitis, including autoimmune hepatitis. Establish that the patient has compensated liver disease. Before treatment, establish and consider the following criteria: Bilirubin ≤ 2 mg/dl; albumin stable and within normal limits; prothrombin time (PT) < 3 seconds prolonged; WBC ≥ 3000/mm^3; platelets > 70,000/mm^3; serum creatinine normal or near normal. Evaluate CBC and platelet counts; repeat at weeks 1 and 2 after therapy initiation, monthly thereafter. Evaluate ALT levels after 2, 16 and 24 weeks.

Preexisting psychiatric condition/history of severe psychiatric disorder – Do not treat; discontinue therapy in any patient developing severe depression.

Preexisting thyroid abnormalities – Patients whose thyroid function cannot be maintained in the normal range by medication should not be treated. Discontinue therapy in patients developing thyroid abnormalities during treatment.

Chronic hepatitis B:

Monitoring – Perform a liver biopsy to establish presence of chronic hepatitis and extent of liver damage. Establish that the patient has compensated liver disease. Before treatment, establish and consider the following criteria: Bilirubin normal; albumin stable and within normal limits; PT < 3 seconds prolonged; WBC ≥ 4000/mm^3; platelets ≥ 100,000/mm^3 . Evaluate CBC and platelet counts, then repeat at weeks 1, 2, 4, 8, 12 and 16. Evaluate liver function tests, including serum ALT, albumin and bilirubin at treatment weeks 1, 2, 4, 8, 12 and 16. Evaluate HBeAg, HBsAg and ALT at the end of therapy and 3 and 6 months post-therapy.

ALT increase – A transient increase in ALT ≥ 2 times baseline (flare) can occur, generally 8 to 12 weeks after therapy initiation, and is more frequent in responders. Continue therapy unless signs and symptoms of hepatic failure occur. During the ALT flare, monitor clinical symptomatology and liver function tests (including ALT, PT, alkaline phosphatase, albumin and bilirubin) at ≈ 2 week intervals.

Hepatic function impairment – Chronic hepatitis B patients with evidence of decreasing hepatic synthetic functions (eg, decreasing albumin levels, prolongation of PT) may be at increased risk of clinical decompensation in association with a flare of aminotransferases.

Fever/"flu-like" symptoms: Because of fever and other "flu-like" symptoms associated with this drug, use cautiously in debilitating medical conditions, such as those with a history of cardiovascular disease (eg, unstable angina, uncontrolled CHF), pulmonary disease (eg, chronic obstructive pulmonary disease) or diabetes mellitus prone to ketoacidosis. Observe caution in coagulation disorders (eg, thrombophlebitis, pulmonary embolism) or severe myelosuppression.

Pulmonary infiltrates, pneumonitis and pneumonia, including fatality, have been observed rarely. The etiologic explanation for these pulmonary findings has not been established. Take chest X-rays of any patient developing fever, cough, dyspnea or other respiratory symptoms. If X-ray shows pulmonary infiltrates or there is evidence of pulmonary function impairment, closely monitor the patient and, if appropriate, discontinue therapy. While this has been reported more often in patients with chronic hepatitis NANB/C treated with interferon alfa, it has also been reported in patients with oncologic diseases treated with interferon alfa.

Retinal hemorrhages, cotton wool spots and retinal artery or vein obstruction have been observed rarely. The etiologic explanation for this has not been established. These events appear to occur after use of the drug for several months, but also have been reported after short treatment periods. Diabetes mellitus or hypertension have been present in some patients. Examine the eyes of any patient complaining of changes in visual acuity or visual fields or reporting any other ophthalmologic symptoms during treatment with interferon alfa-2b.

A baseline ocular examination is recommended prior to treatment with interferon alfa-2b in patients with diabetes mellitus or hypertension because the retinal events may have to be differentiated from those seen with diabetic or hypertensive retinopathy.

INTERFERON ALFA-2b (IFN-alpha 2; rIFN-α2; α-2-interferon)

Hypersensitivity reactions (eg, urticaria, angioedema, bronchoconstriction, anaphylaxis) have not been observed in patients receiving interferon alfa-2b; however, if such an acute reaction develops, discontinue the drug immediately and institute appropriate medical therapy. Have epinephrine 1:1000 immediately available. Refer to Management of Acute Hypersensitivity Reactions. Transient cutaneous rashes have occurred following injection, but have not necessitated treatment interruption.

Hepatic function impairment: Do not treat patients with decompensated liver disease, autoimmune hepatitis, history of autoimmune disease, or immunosuppressed transplant recipients. In these patients, worsening liver disease, including jaundice, hepatic encephalopathy, hepatic failure and death have occurred following therapy. Discontinue therapy for any patient developing signs and symptoms of liver failure.

Fertility impairment: Interferon may impair fertility. In non-human primates, abnormalities of the menstrual cycle have been observed. Decreases in serum estradiol and progesterone concentrations have occurred in women treated with human leukocyte interferon. Fertile women should not receive interferon alfa-2b unless they are using effective contraception. Use with caution in fertile men.

Pregnancy: Category C. Another interferon alfa preparation has abortifacient effects in rhesus monkeys when given at 20 to 500 times the human dose. Therefore, use during pregnancy only if the potential benefit justifies the potential risk to the fetus.

Lactation: It is not known if this drug is excreted in breast milk. Because of the potential for serious reactions in nursing infants, decide whether to stop nursing or to stop the drug, taking into account the importance of the drug to the mother.

Children: Safety and efficacy in children < 18 years of age have not been established.

Precautions:

Monitoring: In addition to tests normally required for monitoring patients, the following are recommended for all patients on interferon therapy, prior to beginning treatment and periodically thereafter: Standard hematologic tests with complete blood counts and differential, platelet counts, blood chemistries, electrolytes and liver function tests. Patients with preexisting cardiac abnormalities, or in advanced stages of cancer, should have ECGs taken before and during treatment. Refer also to the monitoring sections under Warnings for each indication.

Baseline chest X-rays are suggested; repeat if clinically indicated.

For malignant melanoma patients, monitor differential WBC count and liver function tests weekly during the induction phase of therapy and monthly during the maintenance phase of therapy.

Photosensitivity may occur; therefore, caution patients to take protective measures (ie, sunscreens, protective clothing) against exposure to ultraviolet light or sunlight until tolerance is determined.

Drug Interactions:

Interferon Alfa-2b Drug Interactions			
Precipitant drug	Object drug*		Description
Interferon alfa-2b	Aminophylline	↑	IM injection of interferon alfa-2a significantly reduced the clearance of aminophylline by 33% to 81% in 8 of 9 subjects, probably due to inhibition of the cytochrome P-450 enzyme system.
Interferon alfa-2b	Zidovudine	↑	There may be synergistic adverse effects between interferon alfa-2b and zidovudine. Patients have had a higher incidence of neutropenia than that expected with zidovudine alone. Carefully monitor WBC count.

* ↑ = Object drug increased.

Adverse Reactions:

Adverse reactions are dose-related. Most are mild to moderate in severity. Some are transient and most diminish with continued therapy. The most frequently reported reactions are flu-like symptoms, particularly fever, headache, chills, myalgia and fatigue.

INTERFERON ALFA-2b (IFN-alpha 2; rIFN-α2; α-2-interferon)

Interferon Alfa-2b Adverse Reactions Based on Indication (%)

	Adverse reaction	Hairy cell leukemia (n = 145)	Condylomata acuminata (n = 352)	AIDS-related Kaposi's sarcoma[1] (n = 103)	Chronic hepatitis non-A non-B/C (n = 159)	Chronic hepatitis B[1] (n = 179)
Flu-like symptoms	Fever	68	56	47-55	43	66-86
	Fatigue	61	18	48-84	19	69-75
	Chills	46	45	—	—	—
	Headache	39	47	21-36	43	44-61
	Myalgia	39	44	28-34	42	40-59
Central and peripheral nervous systems	Dizziness	12	9	7-24	9	10-13
	Paresthesia	6	1	3-21	1	3-6
	Depression	6	3	9-28	8	6-17
	Anxiety	5	<1	1-3	1	2
	Confusion	< 5	4	10-12	1	—
	Hypoesthesia	< 5	1	10	—	—
	Amnesia	< 5	—	14	—	—
	Impaired concentra tion	—	< 1	3-14	4	5-8
	Nervousness	—	1	3	—	3
	Irritability	—	—	—	4	12-16
	Somnolence	< 5	3	3	1	9-14
	Decreased libido	< 5	—	—	1	1-5
GI	Nausea	21	17	21-28	23	33-50
	Diarrhea	18	2	18-45	13	8-19
	Vomiting	6	2	11-14	3	7-10
	Anorexia	19	1	38-41	13	43-53
	Dyspepsia	—	2	4	3	3-8
	Constipation	< 1	—	1-10	< 1	5
	Loose stools	—	<1	10	3	2
	Abdominal pain	< 5	1	5-21	6	4-5
Respiratory	Pharyngitis	< 5	1	1-31	1	1-7
	Nasal congestion	—	1	10	—	4
	Dyspnea	< 1	—	1-34	< 1	5
	Coughing	< 1	—	14-31	< 1	1-4
	Sinusitis	—	—	21	—	—
	Dry mouth/thirst	19	< 5	22-28	< 5	5-6
Bone, joint, muscle	Arthralgia	8	9	3	19	8-19
	Asthenia	7	—	11	24	5-15
	Rigors	—	—	14-30	27	38-42
	Back pain	19	6	1-3	3	—
	Muscle pain/ weakness	<5	< 5	< 5	< 5	≤ 9
Dermatologic	Rash	25	—	9-10	6	1-8
	Pruritus	11	1	7	6	4-6
	Dry skin	9	—	9-10	< 1	3
	Dermatitis	8	—	—	—	1
	Alopecia	8	—	12-31	17	26-38
	Moniliasis	—	< 1	17	—	—
	Edema/facial edema	—	< 1	10	1	1-3
	Injection site reaction (eg, inflammation, burning, pain, bleeding)	20	< 5	< 5	7	3-< 5

INTERFERON ALFA-2b (IFN-alpha 2; rIFN-α2; α-2-interferon)

Interferon Alfa-2b Adverse Reactions Based on Indication (%)

	Adverse reaction	Hairy cell leukemia (n = 145)	Condylomata acuminata (n = 352)	AIDS-related Kaposi's sarcoma[1] (n = 103)	Chronic hepatitis non-A non-B/C (n = 159)	Chronic hepatitis B[1] (n = 179)
Miscellaneous	Pain	18	3	3	—	—
	Chest pain	< 1	< 1	1-28	1	4
	Increased sweating	8	2	4-21	3	1
	Malaise	—	14	5	3	6-9
	Taste alteration	13	< 1	5-7	1	10
	Insomnia	—	< 1	3	4	6-11
	Weight loss	< 1	< 1	3-5	< 1	2-5
	Herpes simplex	—	1	3	—	5
	Gingivitis	—	—	14	—	1
Lab test abnormalities	Hemoglobin	na	—	1-15	15	23-32
	WBC count	na	17	10-22	18	34-68
	Platelet count	na	—	8	9	5-12
	Serum creatinine	0	—	—	2	3
	Alkaline phosphatase	4	—	—	3	4-8
	Serum urea nitrogen	0	—	—	1	—
	AST	4	12	11-41	—	—
	ALT	13	—	10-15	—	—
	Granulocyte count					
	Total	na	—	31-39	37	61-71
	1000-< 1500/mm^3	—	—	—	—	31-32
	750-< 1000/mm^3	—	—	—	—	18-23
	500-< 750/mm^3	—	—	—	—	9-15
	<500/mm^3	—	—	—	—	2

[1] Incidence related to dosage.

Additional reactions reported for all indications and occurring at an incidence of < 5% are as follows:

Body as a whole: Abscess; cachexia; dehydration; fungal infection; herpes zoster; hypercalcemia; lymphadenopathy; peripheral edema; sepsis; stye; substernal chest pain; trichomoniasis; viral infection; weakness.

Cardiovascular: Arrhythmia; atrial fibrillation; bradycardia; cardiac failure; cardiomyopathy; extrasystoles; hypertension; hypotension; palpitations; postural hypotension; tachycardia.

CNS: Abnormal coordination, dreaming, gait and thinking; aggravated depression; aggressive reaction; agitation; apathy; aphasia; ataxia; CNS dysfunction; coma; convulsions; dysphonia; emotional lability; extrapyramidal disorder; feeling of ebriety; flushing; hot flashes; hyperesthesia; hyperkinesia; hypertonia; hypokinesia; impaired consciousness; migraine; neuropathy; neurosis; paresis; paroniria; parosmia; personality disorder; polyneuropathy; suicide attempt; syncope; tremor.

Dermatologic: Abnormal hair texture; acne; cyanosis of the hand; cold/clammy skin; dermatitis lichenoides; epidermal necrolysis; erythema; folliculitis; furunculosis; increased hair growth; lipoma; melanosis; nail disorders; nonherpetic cold sores; peripheral ischemia; photosensitivity (see Precautions); psoriasis; purpura; skin depigmentation; skin discoloration; urticaria; vitiligo.

Endocrine: Aggravation of diabetes mellitus; gynecomastia; thyroid disorder; virilism.

GI: Abdominal distention; ascites; dysphagia; eructation; esophagitis; flatulence; gallstones; gastric ulcer; gastroenteritis; GI hemorrhage; GI mucosal discoloration; gingival bleeding; gum hyperplasia; halitosis; increased appetite; increased saliva; melena; oral leukoplakia; rectal bleeding after stool; rectal hemorrhage; stomatitis; ulcerative stomatitis.

GU: Albumin/protein in urine; amenorrhea; impotence; incontinence; increased BUN; hematuria; leukorrhea; menorrhagia; micturition disorder/frequency; nocturia; pelvic pain; polyuria; uterine bleeding.

Hematologic: Anemia; granulocytopenia; hemolytic anemia; leukopenia; thrombocytopenia.

Hepatic: Abnormal hepatic function tests; bilirubinemia; increased transaminases; jaundice; right upper quadrant pain; hepatic encephalopathy; hepatic failure.

Musculoskeletal: Arthritis; arthrosis; bone pain; carpal tunnel syndrome; leg cramps; muscle weakness.

Respiratory: Bronchitis; bronchospasm; cyanosis; epistaxis; lung fibrosis; pleural pain; pneumonia; rhinitis; rhinorrhea; sneezing; wheezing.

Special senses: Abnormal/Blurred vision; conjunctivitis; diplopia; dry eyes; earache; eye pain; hearing disorder; lacrimal gland disorder; periorbital edema; photophobia; speech disorder; taste loss; tinnitus; vertigo.

Patient Information:

Patient package insert available with product.

Do not change brands of interferon; changes in dosage may result.

The most common adverse effects are "flu-like" symptoms, such as fever, headache, fatigue, anorexia, nausea and vomiting. These appear to decrease in severity as treatment continues. Some of these "flu-like" symptoms may be minimized by bedtime doses. Use acetaminophen to prevent or partially alleviate fever and headache.

Patients should be well hydrated, especially during the initial stages of treatment.

Administration and Dosage:

Hairy cell leukemia: 2 million IU/m^2, IM or SC 3 times/week. Normalization of one or more hematologic variables usually begins within 2 months of initiation. Improvement in all 3 hematologic variables may require ≥ 6 months of therapy.

Maintain this dosage regimen unless the disease progresses rapidly, or severe intolerance occurs. If severe adverse reactions develop, modify dosage (50% reduction) or discontinue therapy until reactions abate. Discontinue if intolerance persists or recurs following adequate dosage adjustment, or if disease progresses.

The patient may self-administer the dose at bedtime.

Malignant melanoma: 20 million IU/m^2 IV on 5 consecutive days/week for 4 weeks. Maintnenance dosage is 10 million IU/m^2 SC 3 times/week for 48 weeks.

Perform regular laboratory testing to monitor abnormalities for the purposes of dose modification. If adverse reactions develop during interferon alfa-2b treatment, particularly if granulocytes decrease to < 500/mm^3 or ALT/AST rises to > 5 x upper limit of normal, temporarily discontinue treatment until adverse reactions abate.

Restart interferon alfa-2b at 50% of the previous dose. If intolerance persists or if granulocytes decreased to < 250/mm^3 or ALT/AST rises to > 10 x upper limit of normal, discontinue interferon alfa-2b therapy.

Maintain therapy for 1 year unless there is progression of disease.

Condylomata acuminata: 1 million IU/lesion 3 times/wk for 3 weeks intralesionally. Use only 10 million IU vial since dilution of other strengths required for intralesional use results in a hypertonic solution. Do not reconstitute 10 million IU vial with > 1 ml diluent. Use tuberculin or similar syringe and 25 to 30 gauge needle. Do not go beneath lesion too deeply or inject too superficially. As many as 5 lesions can be treated at one time. To alleviate side effects, give in evening with acetaminophen.

Maximum response usually occurs 4 to 8 weeks after therapy initiation. If results are not satisfactory after 12 to 16 weeks, a second course may be instituted. Patients with six to ten condylomata may receive a second sequential course. Patients with > 10 condylomata may receive additional sequences.

Drug delivery – Direct the needle at the center of the base of the wart and at an angle almost parallel to the plane of the skin. This will deliver the interferon to the dermal core of the lesion, infiltrating the lesion and causing a small wheal.

AIDS-related Kaposi's sarcoma: 30 million IU/m^2 3 times a week administered SC or IM. Use only 50 million IU vial. Maintain the selected dosage regimen unless the disease progresses rapidly or severe intolerance occurs. If severe adverse reactions develop, modify dosage (50% reduction) or temporarily discontinue therapy until adverse reactions abate. When patients initiate therapy at 30 million IU/m^2 3 times a week, average dose tolerated at end of 12 weeks therapy is 110 million IU/week and 75 million IU/week at end of 24 weeks therapy.

When disease stabilization or response to treatment occurs, continue treatment until there is no further evidence of tumor or until discontinuation is required by evidence of a severe opportunistic infection or adverse effect.

INTERFERON ALFA-2b (IFN-alpha 2; rIFN-α2; α-2-interferon)

Chronic hepatitis NANB/C: 3 million IU 3 times/week SC or IM. Normalization of ALT levels may occur in some patients as early as 2 weeks after treatment initiation; however, current experience suggests completing a 6 month course of therapy in responding patients. Consider discontinuing therapy in nonresponders after 16 weeks. If severe adverse reactions develop, modify the dose (50% reduction) or temporarily discontinue therapy until reactions abate. Patients who relapse may be retreated with the same dosage regimen to which they had previously responded.

Chronic hepatitis B: 30 to 35 million IU per week SC or IM, either as 5 million IU daily or 10 million IU 3 times a week for 16 weeks. If serious adverse reactions or lab abnormalities develop during therapy, decrease the dose by 50% or discontinue if appropriate until adverse reactions abate. If intolerance persists after dose adjustment, discontinue the drug.

Decreased granulocyte or platelet counts – Use the following guidelines:

Interferon Alfa-2b Dose with Decreased Granulocyte or Platelet Counts

Granulocyte count	Platelet count	Interferon alfa-2b dose
< 750/mm³	< 50,000/mm³	Reduce by 50%
< 500/mm³	< 30,000/mm³	Interrupt

When platelet or granulocyte counts return to normal or baseline values, reinstitute therapy at up to 100% of initial dose.

Preparation of solution: Inject diluent (Bacteriostatic Water for Injection) amount stated in chart below into vial. Agitate gently, withdraw with sterile syringe, give IM or SC.

Preparation of Interferon Alfa-2b Powder for Injection Based on Indication

Vial strength	Amount of diluent	Final concentration
Hairy cell leukemia		
3 million IU	1 ml	3 million IU/ml
5 million IU	1 ml	5 million IU/ml
10 million IU	2 ml	5 million IU/ml
18 million IU[1]	3.8 ml	6 million IU/ml
25 million IU	5 ml	5 million IU/ml
Malignant melanoma		
Induction:		
3 million IU	1 ml	3 million IU/ml
5 million IU	1 ml	5 million IU/ml
10 million IU	1 ml	10 million IU/ml
18 million IU	1 ml	18 million IU/ml
25 million IU	5 ml	5million IUml
50 million IU	1 ml	50 million IU/ml
Maintenance		
3 million IU	1 ml	3 million IU/ml
5 million IU	1 ml	5 million IU/ml
10 million IU	1 ml	10 million IU/ml
18 million IU	1 ml	18 million IU/ml
50 milion IU	1 ml	50 million IU/ml
Condylomata acuminata		
10 million IU	1 ml	10 million IU/ml
AIDS-related Kaposi's sarcoma		
50 million IU	1 ml	50 million IU/ml
Chronic hepatitis - NANB/C		
3 million IU	1 ml	3 million IU/ml
18 million IU[1]	3.8 ml	6 million IU/ml
Chronic hepatitis B		
5 million IU	1 ml	5 million IU/ml
10 million IU	1 ml	10 million IU/ml

[1] Multi-dose vial.

INTERFERON ALFA-2b (IFN-alpha 2; rIFN-α2; α-2-interferon)

Preparation of Interferon Alfa-2b Solution Based on Indication		
Vial strength	Amount of diluent	Final concentration
Hairy cell leukemia		
10 million IU	2 ml	5 million IU/ml
18 million IU[1]	3.8 ml	6 million IU/ml
25 million IU	5 ml	5 million IU/ml
Chronic hepatitis NANB/C		
10 million IU	2 ml	5 million IU/ml
18 million IU[1]	3.8 ml	6 million IU/ml
25 million IU	5 ml	5 million IU/ml
Chronic hepatitis B		
10 million IU	2 ml	5 million IU/ml
25 million IU	5 ml	5 million IU/ml

[1] Multi-dose vial.

Stability and storage: After reconstitution, solution is stable for 1 month at 2° to 8°C (36° to 46°F). Store solution before and after reconstitution between 2° and 8°C.

Rx	**Intron A** (Schering)	**Powder for Injection, lyophilized:**[1] 3 million IU/vial	In vials with 1 ml diluent vial or syringe.
		5 million IU/vial	In vials with 1 ml diluent vial or syringe.
		10 million IU/vial	In vials with 2 ml diluent vial or 1 ml diluent syringe.
		18 million IU/vial	In multi-dose vial with 3.8 ml diluent vial.
		25 million IU/vial	In vials with 5 ml diluent vial.
		50 million IU/vial[2]	In vials with 1 ml diluent vial.
		Solution for Injection[3]: 10 million IU/vial	In 2 ml vials.
		18 million IU/vial	In 3.8 ml multi-dose vials.
		25 million IU/vial	In 5 ml vials.

[1] Forumulation includes human albumin.
[2] To be used *only* for treatment of AIDS-related Kaposi's sarcoma.
[3] 20 mg glycine, 2.3 mg sodium phosphate dibasic, 0.55 mg sodium phosphate monobasic, 1 mg human albumin, parabens.

INTERFERON ALFA-n3

Actions:

Pharmacology: Interferon alfa-n3 (Human Leukocyte Derived) is a sterile aqueous formulation of purified, natural, human interferon alpha proteins for use by injection comprising approximately 166 amino acids. It is manufactured from pooled units of human leukocytes induced by incomplete infection with an avian virus (Sendai virus) to produce interferon alfa-n3.

Since interferon alfa-n3 is manufactured using human leukocytes, donors are screened to minimize the risk that the leukocytes could contain infectious agents including hepatitis B surface antigen (HBsAg) and antibodies to human immunodeficiency virus (HIV-1) and human T lymphotropic virus-I (HTLV-I). In addition, the manufacturing process contains steps which inactivate viruses, and there has been no evidence of infection transmission to recipients in clinical trials.

Interferons are naturally occurring proteins with both antiviral and antiproliferative properties. They are produced and secreted in response to viral infections and to a variety of other synthetic and biological inducers. Three major families of interferons have been identified: alpha, beta, and gamma. The interferon alpha family contains at least 15 different molecular species.

Interferons bind to specific membrane receptors on cell surfaces. Interferon alfa-n3 binds to the same receptors as interferon alfa-2b with high species specificity.

Binding of interferon to membrane receptors initiates a series of events including induction of protein synthesis. These actions are followed by a variety of cellular responses, including inhibition of virus replication and suppression of cell proliferation. Immunomodulation, including enhancement of phagocytosis by macrophages, augmentation of the cytotoxicity of lymphocytes and enhancement of human leukocyte antigen expression occurs in response to exposure to interferons.

Pharmacokinetics: In a study of intralesional use of interferon alfa-n3 injection for the treatment of condylomata acuminata, plasma concentrations of interferon were below the detection limit of the assay (≤ 3 IU/ml). Minor systemic effects (eg, myalgias, fever, headaches) were noted, indicating that some of the injected interferon entered the systemic circulation (see Adverse Reactions).

Clinical trials:

Condylomata acuminata (venereal or genital warts) are associated with infections of human papilloma virus (HPV), especially HPV type-6 and possibly type-11.

In a multicenter randomized double-blind, placebo controlled clinical trial, intralesional administration of interferon alfa-n3 was an effective treatment for condylomata acuminata. Patients (n = 81) had a mean of five warts (range: 2 to 14) and were injected intralesionally with a mean of 225,000 IU per wart 2 times a week for up to 8 weeks.

Overall, 80% of patients treated had a complete or partial resolution of warts compared with 44% (n = 75) of placebo-treated patients. Interferon alfa-n3 was significantly more effective than placebo in producing a complete resolution of warts, as shown by the following table:

Degree of Wart Resolution with Interferon Alfa-n3

	Complete Resolution	Partial (≥ 50%) Resolution	Minor (< 50%) Resolution	Progression/ No Change
Interferon alfa-n3 (n = 81)	54%	26%	15%	5%
Placebo (n = 75)	20%	24%	13%	43%

Of the patients who had a complete resolution of warts, approximately 50% of patients had complete resolution by the end of treatment, and 50% had complete resolution during the 3 months after treatment cessation. Patients with complete resolution were followed for a median of 48 weeks. Overall, 76% of interferon alfa-n3-treated patients remained clear of all treated lesions during follow-up.

A total of 762 evaluable warts were injected in this trial. Of the 407 interferon alfa-n3-treated warts, 73% completely resolved, as compared to 35% of the placebo-treated warts. Interferon alfa-n3 was effective in treating lesions of all sizes, and there was no difference in resolution for perianal, penile or vulvar lesions. Among patients with recalcitrant warts, 82% of patients had complete or partial resolution of warts due to intralesional administration of interferon alfa-n3 compared to 43% of placebo patients.

In an open clinical trial using a once-a-week treatment schedule for up to 16 weeks, 28 patients were evaluable for efficacy; 89% had a complete or partial resolution of warts following treatment with interferon alfa-n3. The condylomata acuminata resolved completely in 46% of the patients. Of the 154 warts treated, 77% resolved completely.

INTERFERON ALFA-n3

Antigenicity – To date, no antibodies to interferon alfa-n3 have been detected in tested patients. No hypersensitivity reactions to the components of interferon alfa-n3 have been observed. Interferon alfa-n3 uses a murine monoclonal antibody in one of the purification procedures. A possibility exists that patients treated with interferon alfa-n3 may develop hypersensitivity to the mouse proteins. However, none of the patients developed antibodies or hypersensitivity to mouse proteins (see Contraindications).

Although no egg protein (ovalbumin) has been detected in the initial stage of interferon manufacture, a possibility exists that patients treated with interferon alfa-n3 may develop hypersensitivity to egg protein (see Contraindications).

The leukocyte nutrient medium contains the antibiotic neomycin sulfate at a concentration of 35 mg/L; however, neomycin sulfate is not detectable in the final product.

Indications:

Condylomata acuminata: For the intralesional treatment of refractory or recurring external condylomata acuminata in patients ≥ 18 years of age.

Select patients for treatment after consideration of a number of factors: Locations and sizes of the lesions, past treatment and response, and the patient's ability to comply with the treatment regimen. Interferon alfa-n3 is particularly useful for patients who have not responded satisfactorily to other treatment modalities (eg, podophyllin resin, surgery, laser or cryotherapy).

Unlabeled uses: Alpha interferons have been used for a variety of conditions, a list of which follows. Clinical trials are currently in progress to further determine clinical efficacy, optimal dosage and length of treatment.

Interferon Alpha Unlabeled Uses		
Neoplastic Diseases		
Significant Activity	*Limited Activity*	*No Activity*
Bladder tumors (local use for superficial tumors)	Acute leukemias	Breast cancer
Carcinoid tumor	Cervical carcinoma	Colorectal carcinoma
Chronic myelogenous leukemia	Chronic lymphocytic leukemia	Gastric carcinoma
Cutaneous T-cell lymphoma	Hodgkin's disease	Lung carcinoma
Essential thrombocythemia	Malignant gliomas	Pancreatic carcinoma
Hairy cell leukemia[1];	Melanoma	Prostatic carcinoma
Non-Hodgkin's lymphoma (low-grade)	Multiple myeloma	Soft tissue carcinoma
	Nasopharyngeal sarcoma	
	Osteosarcoma	
	Ovarian carcinoma	
	Renal carcinoma	
Viral Infections		
	AIDS-related Kaposi's sarcoma[1]	
	Chronic non-A, non-B hepatitis	
	Cutaneous warts	
	Cytomegaloviruses	
	Herpes keratoconjunctivitis	
	Herpes simplex	
	Papillomaviruses	
	Rhinoviruses	
	Vaccinia virus	
	Varicella zoster	
	Viral hepatitis B	

[1] Interferon alfa-2a and -2b indicated for this use.

Contraindications:

Hypersensitivity to human interferon alpha or any component of the product; patients who have anaphylactic sensitivity to mouse immunoglobulin (IgG), egg protein or neomycin (see Actions).

Warnings:

Debilitating medical conditions: Because of the fever and other "flu-like" symptoms associated with interferon alfa-n3, use cautiously in patients with debilitating medical conditions such as cardiovascular disease (eg, unstable angina and uncontrolled congestive heart failure), severe pulmonary disease (eg, chronic obstructive pulmonary disease), diabetes mellitus with ketoacidosis, coagulation disorders (eg, thrombophlebitis, pulmonary embolism and hemophilia), severe myelosuppression or seizure disorders.

INTERFERON ALFA-n3

Hypersensitivity: Acute, serious hypersensitivity reactions (eg, urticaria, angioedema, bronchoconstriction, anaphylaxis) have not been observed in patients receiving interferon alfa-n3. However, if such reactions develop, discontinue administration immediately and institute appropriate medical therapy. Refer to Management of Acute Hypersensitivity Reactions.

Fertility impairment: In studies with adult females, interferon alpha affects the menstrual cycle and decreases serum estradiol and progesterone levels. Caution fertile women to use effective contraception while being treated with interferon alfa-n3. Use caution in fertile men.

Changes in the menstrual cycle and abortions have occurred in primates given extremely high doses of recombinant interferon alpha. When given at daily IM doses 326 times the average intralesional dose (120 times the maximum recommended dose), this recombinant interferon formulation produced menstrual cycle changes in monkeys. In human clinical trials of 51 women, there was no significant difference between interferon alfa-n3 and placebo treatment groups with regard to menstrual cycle changes.

Pregnancy: Category C. It is not known whether interferon alfa-n3 can cause fetal harm when administered to a pregnant woman or can affect reproductive capacity. Use in pregnant women only if clearly needed.

Changes in the menstrual cycle and abortions occurred in primates given extremely high doses of recombinant interferon alpha. Abortifacient effects were noted when the recombinant interferon alpha was given daily during early to mid-gestation at IM doses of 978 times the average intralesional dose of interferon alfa-n3 (360 times the maximum recommended dose).

Lactation: It is not known whether interferon alfa-n3 is excreted in breast milk. Studies in mice have shown that mouse interferons are excreted in milk. Because of the potential for serious adverse reactions in nursing infants, decide whether to discontinue nursing or to not initiate drug treatment, taking into account the importance of the drug to the mother and the potential risks to the infant.

Children: Safety and efficacy have not been established in patients < 18 years of age.

Precautions:

Product interchange: Because the manufacturing process, strength, and type of interferon (eg, natural, human leukocyte interferon vs single-subspecies recombinant interferon) may vary for different interferon formulations, changing brands may require a change in dosage. Therefore, physicians are cautioned not to change from one interferon product to another without considering these factors.

Adverse Reactions:

In the double-blind efficacy trial for the treatment of condylomata acuminata, 104 patients were treated with doses of interferon alfa-n3 of 0.05 to 2.5 million IU per treatment session (average dose = 0.92 million IU/treatment session) by intralesional injection. In open trials, an additional 98 patients received a dose range of 0.05 to 4.6 million IU of interferon alfa-n3/treatment session (average dose = 1.12 million IU/treatment session). Patients with cancer were given doses of interferon alfa-n3 injection of 3, 9, or 15 million IU/day for 10 days by IM injection.

In a total of 104 patients with condylomata acuminata, adverse reactions consisted primarily of "flu-like" symptoms (myalgias, fever or headache) which were in most cases mild or moderate and transient, and did not interfere with treatment.

The "flu-like" adverse reactions, consisting of fever, myalgias, or headache, occurred primarily after the first treatment session and were reported by 30% of the patients. The frequency of "flu-like" adverse reactions abated with repeated dosing so that the incidences due to interferon alfa-n3 and placebo were similar after 3 to 4 weeks of treatment (after six to eight treatment sessions). "Flu-like" symptoms were relieved by acetaminophen.

Adverse Reactions of Interferon Alfa-n3

Adverse Reactions	Condylomata acuminata: Interferon alfa-n3 (n = 104)	Condylomata acuminata: Placebo (n = 85)	Cancer: Interferon alfa-n3 (n = 31)
Autonomic Nervous System			
Sweating	2%	1%	0.3%
Vasovagal reaction	2%	0%	
Body as a Whole			
Fever	40%	19%	81%
Chills	14%	2%	87%
Fatigue	14%	6%	6%
Malaise	9%	9%	65%
Central & Peripheral Nervous System			
Dizziness/Lightheadedness	9%	4%	0.3%
Insomnia	2%	1%	
Sleepiness			10%
GI System			
Nausea	4%	7%	48%
Vomiting	3%	0%	29%
Dyspepsia/Heartburn	3%	1%	0.3%
Diarrhea	2%	2%	6%
Constipation			0.3%
Anorexia			68%
Sore mouth/Stomatitis			0.3-6%
Dry mouth/Mucositis			
Musculoskeletal System			
Myalgias	45%	15%	16%
Headache	31%	15%	10%
Arthralgia	5%	1%	10%
Back pain	4%	1%	0.3%
Miscellaneous			
Depression	2%	1%	0.3%
Nose/Sinus drainage	2%	2%	
Generalized pruritis	2%	0%	
Sore injection site			10%
Blurred vision/Ocular rotation pain			0.3-6%
Chest pains			10%
Low blood pressure			6%

Most of the systemic adverse reactions were mild or moderate. Severe systemic adverse reactions were reported by 18% of interferon alfa-n3-treated patients and 13% of placebo-treated patients. Most of the severe systemic adverse reactions reported were "flu-like". Other severe systemic adverse reactions included back pain, insomnia and sensitivity to allergens.

Adverse reactions reported by 1% of patients treated with interferon alfa-n3 in the double-blind and open clinical trials included: Left groin lymph node swelling; tongue hyperesthesia; thirst; tingling of legs/feet; hot sensation on bottom of feet; strange taste in mouth; increased salivation; heat intolerance; visual disturbances; pharyngitis; sensitivity to allergens; muscle cramps; nose bleed; throat tightness and papular rash on neck; herpes labialis; hot flashes; nervousness; decrease in concentration; dysuria; photosensitivity; swollen lymph nodes.

Lab test abnormalities: Decreased WBC (11%).

Adverse reactions in patients with cancer: Thirty-one patients with cancer were treated with a maximum of 10 IM injections of interferon alfa-n3 in doses of 3, 9, or 15 million IU/treatment session. The occurrence of adverse reactions was judged to be unrelated to the dose of interferon alfa-n3. See table for major adverse reactions. Those adverse reactions which were each reported by only one patient treated with interferon alfa-n3 included: Face flushed; edema; coughing; numbness; numbness in hands or fingers; ringing in ears; cramps; confusion.

INTERFERON ALFA-n3

Abnormal Laboratory Test Values with Interferon Alfa-n3	
Laboratory Test	Cancer Patients (n = 31)
Hemoglobin Level	2 (7%)
WBC Count	1 (3%)
Platelet Count	1 (3%)
GGT	1 (6%)
AST	1 (3%)
Alkaline Phosphatase	2 (8%)
Total Bilirubin	1 (4%)

Patient Information:

Inform patients of the early signs of hypersensitivity reactions including hives, generalized urticaria, tightness of the chest, wheezing, hypotension and anaphylaxis, and advise them to contact their physician if these symptoms occur.

Inform patients of benefits and risks associated with treatment.

Caution patients not to change brands of interferon without medical consultation, as a change in dosage may occur.

Administration and Dosage:

Condylomata acuminata: 0.05 ml (250,000 IU) per wart. Administer twice weekly for up to 8 weeks. The maximum recommended dose/treatment session is 0.5 ml (2.5 million IU). Inject into the base of each wart, preferably using a 30 gauge needle. For large warts, interferon alfa-n3 may be injected at several points around the periphery of the wart, using a total dose of 0.05 ml per wart.

The minimum effective dose for the treatment of condylomata acuminata has not been established. Moderate to severe adverse experiences may require modification of the dosage regimen or, in some cases, termination of therapy.

Genital warts usually begin to disappear after several weeks of treatment. Continue treatment for a maximum of 8 weeks. In clinical trials, many patients who had partial resolution of warts during treatment experienced further resolution of their warts after treatment cessation. Of the patients who had complete resolution of warts due to treatment, half the patients had complete resolution by the end of the treatment and half had complete resolution during the 3 months after cessation of treatment. Thus, it is recommended that no further therapy (interferon alfa-n3 or conventional therapy) be administered for 3 months after the initial 8 week course of treatment unless the warts enlarge or new warts appear. Studies to determine the safety and efficacy of a second course of treatment with interferon alfa-n3 have not been conducted.

Storage: Store at 2° to 8°C (36° to 46°F). Do not freeze. Do not shake.

Rx	**Alferon N** (Purdue Frederick)	**Injection:** 5 mIU/vial	In 1 ml vials.[1]

[1] With 3.3 mg phenol and 1 mg albumin.

LEVAMISOLE HCl

Actions:

Pharmacology: Levamisole is an immunomodulator. The mechanism of action of levamisole in combination with fluorouracil is unknown. The effects of levamisole on the immune system are complex. The drug appears to restore depressed immune function rather than to stimulate response to above normal levels. Levamisole can stimulate formation of antibodies to various antigens, enhance T-cell responses by stimulating T-cell activation and proliferation, potentiate monocyte and macrophage functions including phagocytosis and chemotaxis, and increase neutrophil mobility adherence and chemotaxis. Other drugs have similar short-term effects, and the clinical relevance is unclear.

Besides its immunomodulatory function, levamisole also inhibits alkaline phosphatase and has cholinergic activity.

Pharmacokinetics: The pharmacokinetics of levamisole have not been studied in the dosage regimen recommended with fluorouracil nor in patients with hepatic insufficiency. It appears that levamisole is rapidly absorbed from the GI tract. Mean peak plasma concentrations of 0.13 mcg/ml are attained within 1.5 to 2 hours. The plasma elimination half-life is between 3 to 4 hours. Levamisole 150 mg is extensively metabolized by the liver, and the metabolites are excreted mainly by the kidneys (70% over 3 days). The elimination half-life of metabolite excretion is 16 hours. Approximately 5% is excreted in the feces; < 5% is excreted unchanged in the urine and < 0.2% in the feces. Approximately 12% is recovered in urine as the glucuronide of p-hydroxy-levamisole.

Clinical trials: Two clinical trials having essentially the same design have demonstrated an increase in survival and a reduction in recurrence rate in patients with resected Dukes' C colon cancer treated with levamisole plus fluorouracil. After surgery patients were randomized to no further therapy, levamisole alone, or levamisole plus fluorouracil.

In one clinical trial, 262 Dukes' C colorectal cancer patients were evaluated for a minimum follow-up of 5 years. The estimated reduction in death rate was 27% for levamisole plus fluorouracil and 28% for levamisole alone. The estimated reduction in recurrence rate was 36% for levamisole plus fluorouracil and 28% for levamisole alone. In another clinical trial designed to confirm these results, 929 Dukes' C colon cancer patients were evaluated for a minimum follow-up of 2 years. The estimated reduction in death rate and recurrence rate was 33% and 41%, respectively for levamisole plus fluorouracil. The group on levamisole alone did not show advantage over the group receiving no treatment on improving recurrence or survival rates. There are presently insufficient data to evaluate the effect of the combination of levamisole plus fluorouracil in Dukes' B patients. There are also insufficient data to evaluate the effect of levamisole plus fluorouracil in patients with rectal cancer.

Indications:

Only as adjuvant treatment in combination with fluorouracil after surgical resection in patients with Dukes' stage C colon cancer.

Contraindications:

Hypersensitivity to the drug or its components.

Warnings:

Agranulocytosis: Levamisole has been associated with agranulocytosis, sometimes fatal. The onset of agranulocytosis is frequently accompanied by a flu-like syndrome (eg, fever, chills); however, in a small number of patients, it is asymptomatic. A flu-like syndrome may also occur in the absence of agranulocytosis. It is essential that appropriate hematological monitoring be done routinely during therapy with levamisole and fluorouracil. Neutropenia is usually reversible following discontinuation of therapy. Instruct patients to report immediately any flu-like symptoms.

Higher than recommended doses of levamisole may be associated with an increased incidence of agranulocytosis, so do not exceed the recommended dose.

The combination of levamisole and fluorouracil has been associated with frequent neutropenia, anemia and thrombocytopenia.

Fertility impairment: In rats given 20, 60 and 180 mg/kg, copulation period was increased, duration of pregnancy was slightly increased, and fertility, pup viability and weight, lactation index and number of fetuses were decreased at 60 mg/kg.

Pregnancy: Category C. In rats, embryotoxicity was present at 160 mg/kg; in rabbits, at 180 mg/kg. There are no adequate and well controlled studies in pregnant women. Do not be administer levamsiole unless the potential benefits outweigh the risks. Advise women taking the combination of levamisole and fluorouracil not to become pregnant.

Lactation: It is not known whether levamisole is excreted in breast milk; it is excreted in cows' milk. Because of the potential for serious adverse reactions in nursing infants from levamisole, decide whether to discontinue nursing or discontinue the drug, taking into account the importance of the drug to the mother.

Children: Safety and efficacy of levamisole in children have not been established.

Precautions:

Monitoring: On the first day of therapy with levamisole and fluorouracil, perform a CBC with differential and platelets, electrolytes and liver function tests performed. Thereafter, perform a CBC with differential and platelets weekly prior to each fluorouracil treatment; perform electrolyte and liver function tests every 3 months for a total of 1 year. Institute dosage modifications (see Administration and Dosage).

Drug Interactions:

Alcohol: Levamisole may produce disulfiram-like effects with concomitant alcohol.

Phenytoin: Coadministration with levamisole and fluorouracil has led to increased phenytoin plasma levels. Monitor phenytoin plasma levels and decrease the dose if necessary.

Adverse Reactions:

Levamisole and Levamisole/Fluorouracil Adverse Reactions (%)

Adverse Reaction	Levamisole (n = 440)	Levamisole plus fluorouracil (n = 599)
Hematological		
Leukopenia		
< 2,000/mm^3	< 1	1
≥ 2,000 to <4,000/mm^3	4	19
≥4,000/mm^3	2	33
unscored category	0	< 1
Thrombocytopenia		
< 50,000/mm^3	0	0
≥ 50,000 to < 130,000/mm^3	1	8
≥ 130,000/mm^3	1	10
Anemia	0	6
Granulocytopenia	< 1	2
Epistaxis	0	1
Skin and appendages		
Dermatitis	8	23
Alopecia	3	22
Pruritus	1	2
Skin discoloration	0	2
Urticaria	< 1	0
Body as a whole		
Fatigue	6	11
Fever	3	5
Rigors	3	5
Chest pain	< 1	1
Edema	1	1
GI		
Nausea	22	65
Diarrhea	13	52
Stomatitis	3	39
Vomiting	6	20
GI (Cont.)		
Anorexia	2	6
Abdominal pain	2	5
Constipation	2	3
Flatulence	< 1	2
Dyspepsia	< 1	1
Special senses		
Taste perversion	8	8
Altered sense of smell	1	1
Musculoskeletal system		
Arthralgia	5	4
Myalgia	3	2
Central and peripheral nervous system		
Dizziness	3	4
Headache	3	4
Paresthesia	2	3
Ataxia	0	2
Psychiatric		
Somnolence	3	2
Depression	1	2
Nervousness	1	2
Insomnia	1	1
Anxiety	1	1
Forgetfulness	0	1
Vision		
Abnormal tearing	0	4
Blurred vision	1	2
Conjunctivitis	< 1	2
Other		
Infection	5	12
Hyperbilirubinemia	< 1	1

Less frequent adverse experiences included: Exfoliative dermatitis; periorbital edema; vaginal bleeding; anaphylaxis; confusion; convulsions; hallucinations; impaired concentration; renal failure; elevated serum creatinine; increased alkaline phosphatase. An encephalopathy-like syndrome has occurred.

LEVAMISOLE HCl

Almost all patients receiving levamisole and fluorouracil reported adverse experiences. In a clinical trial, 66 of 463 patients (14%) discontinued the combination of levamisole plus fluorouracil because of adverse reactions; 43 (9%) developed isolated or a combination of GI toxicities (eg, nausea, vomiting, diarrhea, stomatitis, anorexia). Ten patients developed rash or pruritus. Five patients discontinued therapy because of flu-like symptoms or fever with chills; 10 patients developed CNS symptoms such as dizziness, ataxia, depression, confusion, memory loss, weakness, inability to concentrate and headache. Two patients developed reversible neutropenia and sepsis: One because of thrombocytopenia, one because of hyperbilirubinemia. One patient in the levamisole plus fluorouracil group developed agranulocytosis and sepsis, and died.

In the levamisole alone arm of the trial, 15 of 310 patients (4.8%) discontinued therapy because of adverse experiences. Six of these (2%) discontinued because of rash, six because of arthralgia/myalgia, and one each for fever and neutropenia, urinary infection and cough.

Overdosage:

Fatalities have occurred in a 3-year-old child who ingested 15 mg/kg and in an adult who ingested 32 mg/kg. No further clinical information is available. In cases of overdosage, gastric lavage is recommended together with symptomatic and supportive measures. Refer to General Management of Acute Overdosage.

Patient Information:

Immediately notify the physician if flu-like symptoms or malaise occurs.

Administration and Dosage:

Adjuvant use of levamisole and fluorouracil is limited to the following schedule:

Initial therapy: Levamisole - 50 mg orally every 8 hours for 3 days (starting 7 to 30 days post-surgery).
Fluorouracil - 450 mg/m^2 /day IV for 5 days concomitant with a 3 day course of levamisole (starting 21 to 34 days post-surgery).

Maintenance: Levamisole - 50 mg orally every 8 hours for 3 days every 2 weeks.
Fluorouracil - 450 mg/m^2 /day IV once a week beginning 28 days after the initiation of the 5 day course.

Treatment: Initiate levamisole no earlier than 7 and no later than 30 days post-surgery at a dose of 50 mg every 8 hours for 3 days repeated every 14 days for 1 year. Initiate fluorouracil therapy no earlier than 21 days and no later than 35 days after surgery providing the patient is out of the hospital, ambulatory, maintaining normal oral nutrition, has well healed wounds and is fully recovered from any postoperative complications. If levamisole has been initiated from 7 to 20 days after surgery, initiate fluorouracil therapy coincident with the second course of levamisole, ie, at 21 to 34 days. If levamisole is initiated from 21 to 30 days after surgery, initiate fluorouracil simultaneously with the first course of levamisole.

Administer fluorouracil by rapid IV push at a dosage of 450 mg/m^2 /day for 5 consecutive days. Dosage is based on actual weight (estimated dry weight). If the patient develops any stomatitis or diarrhea (≥ 5 loose stools), discontinue this course before the full 5 doses are administered. Twenty-eight days after initiation of this course, institute weekly fluorouracil at 450 mg/m^2 /week and continue for a total treatment time of 1 year. If stomatitis or diarrhea develop during weekly therapy, defer the next dose of fluorouracil until these side effects have subsided. If these side effects are moderate to severe, reduce the fluorouracil dose 20% when it is resumed.

Institute dosage medications as follows: If WBC is 2500 to 3500/mm^3 defer the fluorouracil dose until WBC is > 3500/mm^3 . If WBC is < 2500/mm^3 , defer the fluorouracil dose until WBC is > 3500/mm^3 , then resume the fluorouracil dose reduced by 20%. If WBC remains < 2500/mm^3 for > 10 days despite deferring fluorouracil, discontinue administration of levamisole. Defer both drugs unless platelets are adequate (≥ 100,000/mm^3).

Levamisole should not be used at doses exceeding the recommended dose or frequency. Clinical studies suggest a relationship between levamisole adverse experiences and increasing dose, and some of these (eg, agranulocytosis) may be life-threatening (see Warnings).

Before beginning this combination adjuvant treatment, the physician should become familiar with the labeling for fluorouracil.

Rx	**Ergamisol** (Janssen)	**Tablets:** 50 mg levamisole base	(Janssen L 50). White. In blister pack 36s.

ALTRETAMINE (Hexamethylmelamine)

Warning:

Administer only under the supervision of a physician experienced in the use of antineoplastic agents.

Monitor peripheral blood counts at least monthly, prior to the initiation of each course of altretamine therapy and as clinically indicated (see Adverse Reactions).

Because of the possibility of altretamine-related neurotoxicity, perform neurologic examination regularly during administration (see Adverse Reactions).

Actions:

Pharmacology: Altretamine, formerly known as hexamethylmelamine, is a synthetic cytotoxic antineoplastic s-triazine derivative. The precise mechanism by which altretamine exerts its cytotoxic effect is unknown, although a number of theoretical possibilities have been studied. Structurally, altretamine resembles the alkylating agent triethylenemelamine, yet in vitro tests for alkylating activity of altretamine and its metabolites have been negative. Altretamine is efficacious for certain ovarian tumors resistant to classical alkylating agents. Metabolism of altretamine is a requirement for cytotoxicity. Synthetic monohydroxymethylmelamines and products of altretamine metabolism in vitro and in vivo can form covalent adducts with tissue macromolecules including DNA, but the relevance of these reactions to antitumor activity is unknown.

Pharmacokinetics: Altretamine is well absorbed following oral administration, but undergoes rapid and extensive demethylation in the liver, producing variations in altretamine plasma levels. The principal metabolites are pentamethylmelamine and tetramethylmelamine. After oral administration to 11 patients with advanced ovarian cancer in doses of 120 to 300 mg/m^2, peak plasma levels were reached between 0.5 and 3 hours, varying from 0.2 to 20.8 mg/L. Half-life of the β-phase of elimination ranged from 4.7 to 10.2 hours. Altretamine and metabolites show binding to plasma proteins. The free fractions of altretamine, pentamethylmelamine and tetramethylmelamine are 6%, 25% and 50%, respectively.

Following oral administration of 4 mg/kg, urinary recovery was 61% at 24 hours and 90% at 72 hours. Human urinary metabolites were N-demethylated homologues of altretamine with < 1% unmetabolized altretamine excreted at 24 hours. After intraperitoneal administration to mice, tissue distribution was rapid in all organs, reaching a maximum at 30 minutes. The excretory organs (liver and kidney) and the small intestine showed high concentrations, whereas relatively low concentrations were found in other organs, including the brain.

Clinical trials: In two studies in patients with persistent or recurrent ovarian cancer following first-line treatment with cisplatin or alkylating agent-based combinations, altretamine was administered as a single agent for 14 or 21 days of a 28 day cycle. In the 51 patients with measurable or evaluable disease, there were 6 clinical complete responses, 1 pathologic complete response, and 2 partial responses for an overall response rate of 18%. The duration of these responses ranged from 2 months in a patient with a palpable pelvic mass to 36 months in a patient who achieved a pathologic complete response. In some patients, tumor regression was associated with improvement in symptoms and performance status.

Indications:

For use as a single agent in the palliative treatment of patients with persistent or recurrent ovarian cancer following first-line therapy with a cisplatin- or alkylating agent-based combination.

Contraindications:

Hypersensitivity to altretamine.

Pre-existing severe bone marrow depression or severe neurologic toxicity; however, altretamine has been administered safely to patients heavily pretreated with cisplatin or alkylating agents including patients with pre-existing cisplatin neuropathies. Careful monitoring of neurologic function in these patients is essential.

Warnings:

Neurotoxicity: Altretamine causes mild to moderate neurotoxicity. Peripheral neuropathy and CNS symptoms (eg, mood disorders, disorders of consciousness, ataxia, dizziness, vertigo) have occurred. They are more likely to occur in patients receiving continuous high-dose daily altretamine than moderate-dose altretamine administered on an intermittent schedule. Neurologic toxicity appears to be reversible when therapy is discontinued. It has been suggested that the incidence and severity of neurotoxicity may be decreased by concomitant administration of pyridoxine, but this remains unproven. Perform a neurologic examination prior to the initiation of each course of therapy.

ALTRETAMINE (Hexamethylmelamine)

Hematologic: Altretamine causes mild to moderate dose-related myelosuppression. Leukopenia < 3000 WBC/mm^3 occurred in < 15% of patients on a variety of intermittent or continuous dose regimens; < 1% had leukopenia < 1000 WBC/mm^3. Thrombocytopenia < 50,000 platelets/mm^3 was seen in < 10% of patients. When given in doses of 8 to 12 mg/kg/day over a 21 day course, nadirs of leukocyte and platelet counts were reached by 3 to 4 weeks, and normal counts were regained by 6 weeks. With continuous administration at doses of 6 to 8 mg/kg/day, nadirs are reached in 6 to 8 weeks (median). Monitor peripheral blood counts prior to the initiation of each course of therapy, monthly, and as clinically indicated. Adjust the dose as necessary (see Administration and Dosage).

Carcinogenesis/Mutagenesis/Fertility impairment: Drugs with similar mechanisms of action are carcinogenic. Altretamine was weakly mutagenic when tested in strain TA100 of Salmonella typhimurium. Altretamine administered to female rats 14 days prior to breeding through the gestation period had no adverse effect on fertility but decreased postnatal survival at 120 mg/m^2 /day and was embryocidal at 240 mg/m^2 /day. Administration of 120 mg/m^2 /day to male rats for 60 days prior to mating resulted in testicular atrophy, reduced fertility and a possible dominant lethal mutagenic effect. Male rats treated with 450 mg/m^2 /day for 10 days had decreased spermatogenesis and atrophy of testes, seminal vesicles and ventral prostate.

Pregnancy: Category D. Altretamine is embryotoxic and teratogenic in rats and rabbits when given at doses 2 and 10 times the human dose, and it may cause fetal damage when administered to a pregnant woman. If altretamine is used during pregnancy, or if the patient becomes pregnant while taking the drug, apprise the patient of the potential hazard to the fetus. Advise women to avoid becoming pregnant.

Lactation: It is not known whether altretamine is excreted in breast milk. Because there is a possibility of toxicity in nursing infants secondary to altretamine treatment of the mother, it is recommended that breastfeeding be discontinued if the mother is treated with altretamine.

Children: Safety and efficacy in children have not been established.

Precautions:

Nausea and vomiting: With continuous high-dose daily altretamine, nausea and vomiting of gradual onset occur frequently. In most instances, these symptoms are controllable with antiemetics; at times, however, the severity requires dose reduction or, rarely, discontinuation of therapy. In some instances, a tolerance of these symptoms develops after several weeks of therapy. The incidence and severity of nausea and vomiting are reduced with moderate-dose administration of altretamine. In two clinical studies of single-agent altretamine utilizing a moderate, intermittent dose and schedule, only 1 patient (1%) discontinued altretamine due to severe nausea and vomiting.

Drug Interactions:

Cimetidine, an inhibitor of microsomal drug metabolism, increased altretamine's half-life and toxicity in a rat model.

Monoamine oxidase inhibitors and concurrent altretamine may cause severe orthostatic hypotension. Four patients, all > 60 years of age, experienced symptomatic hypotension after 4 to 7 days of concomitant therapy.

Adverse Reactions:

The most common adverse reactions are: Nausea and vomiting (see Precautions); peripheral neuropathy, CNS symptoms and myelosuppression (see Warnings).

Data in the following table are based on the experience of 76 patients with ovarian cancer previously treated with a cisplatin-based combination regimen who received single-agent altretamine. In one study, altretamine 260 mg/m^2 /day was administered for 14 days of a 28 day cycle. In another study, altretamine 6 to 8 mg/kg/day was administered for 21 days of a 28 day cycle.

ALTRETAMINE (Hexamethylmelamine)

Altretamine Adverse Reactions in Previously Treated Ovarian Cancer Patients (n = 76)

Adverse reaction	Incidence (%)
GI	
Nausea and vomiting	
Mild to moderate	32
Severe	1
Increased alkaline phosphatase	9
Neurologic	
Peripheral sensory neuropathy	
Mild	22
Moderate to severe	9
Anorexia and fatigue	1
Seizures	1
Hematologic	
Leukopenia	
WBC 2000 to 2999/mm^3	4
WBC < 2000/mm^3	1
Thrombocytopenia	
Platelets 75,000 to 99,000/mm^3	6
Platelets < 75,000/mm^3	3
Anemia	
Mild	20
Moderate to severe	13
Renal	
Serum creatinine 1.6 to 3.75 mg/dl	7
BUN	
25-40 mg/dl	5
41-60 mg/dl	3
> 60 mg/dl	1

Additional adverse reaction information is available from 13 single-agent altretamine studies (total of 1014 patients). The treated patients had a variety of tumors and many were heavily pretreated with other chemotherapies; most of these trials utilized high, continuous daily doses of altretamine (6 to 12 mg/kg/day). In general, adverse reaction experiences were similar in the two trials described above. Additional toxicities not reported in the above table included hepatic toxicity, skin rash, pruritus and alopecia, each occurring in < 1% of patients.

Administration and Dosage:

Altretamine is administered orally. Calculate doses on the basis of body surface area.

Altretamine may be administered either for 14 or 21 consecutive days in a 28 day cycle at a dose of 260 mg/m^2 /day. Give the total daily dose as 4 divided oral doses after meals and at bedtime.

Temporarily discontinue altretamine (for ≥ 14 days) and subsequently restart at 200 mg/m^2 /day for any of the following situations: GI intolerance unresponsive to symptomatic measures; WBC < 2000/mm^3 or granulocyte count < 1000/mm^3 ; platelet count < 75,000/mm^3 ; progressive neurotoxicity.

If neurologic symptoms fail to stabilize on the reduced dose schedule, discontinue altretamine indefinitely.

Rx	**Hexalen** (US Bioscience)	**Capsules:** 50 mg	Lactose. (USB001 Hexalen 50 mg). Clear. In 100s.

CLADRIBINE (2-chlorodeoxyadenosine; CdA)

Warning:

Administer under the supervision of a qualified physician experienced in the use of antineoplastic therapy. Anticipate suppression of bone marrow function. This is usually reversible and appears to be dose-dependent. High doses (4 to 9 times the recommended dose for hairy cell leukemia) in conjunction with cyclophosphamide and total body irradiation as preparation for bone marrow transplantation, have been associated with severe, irreversible, neurologic toxicity (paraparesis/quadriparesis) or acute renal insufficiency in 45% of patients treated for 7 to 14 days.

Actions:

Pharmacology: Cladribine is a synthetic antineoplastic agent for continuous IV infusion. The selective toxicity of cladribine towards certain normal and malignant lymphocyte and monocyte populations is based on the relative activities of deoxycytidine kinase, deoxynucleotidase and adenosine deaminase. In cells with a high ratio of deoxycytidine kinase to deoxynucleotidase, cladribine, a purine nucleoside analog, passively crosses the cell membrane. It is phosphorylated by deoxycytidine kinase to 2-chloro-2'deoxy-β-D-adenosine mono-phosphate (2-CdAMP). Since cladribine is resistant to deamination by adenosine deaminase and there is little deoxynucleotide deaminase in lymphocytes and monocytes, 2-CdAMP accumulates intracellularly and is subsequently converted into the active triphosphate deoxynucleotide, 2-CdATP. It is postulated that cells with high deoxycytidine kinase and low deoxynucleotidase activities will be selectively killed by cladribine as toxic deoxynucleotides accumulate intracellularly.

Cells containing high concentrations of deoxynucleotides are unable to properly repair single-strand DNA breaks. The broken ends of DNA activate the enzyme poly (ADP-ribose) polymerase resulting in NAD and ATP depletion and disruption of cellular metabolism. There is also evidence that 2-CdATP is incorporated into the DNA of dividing cells, resulting in impairment of DNA synthesis. Thus, cladribine can be distinguished from other chemotherapeutic agents affecting purine metabolism in that it is cytotoxic to both actively dividing and quiescent lymphocytes and monocytes, inhibiting both DNA synthesis and repair.

Pharmacokinetics: Seventeen patients with hairy cell leukemia (HCL) and normal renal function were treated for 7 days with the recommended treatment regimen (0.09 mg/kg/day) by continuous IV infusion. The mean steady-state serum concentration was estimated to be 5.7 ng/ml with an estimated systemic clearance of 663.5 ml/hr/kg. Accumulation over the 7 day treatment period was not noted. In HCL patients, there does not appear to be a relationship between serum concentrations and ultimate clinical outcome.

Eight patients with hematologic malignancies received a 2 hour infusion (0.12 mg/kg). The mean end-of-infusion plasma concentration was 48 $\pm$ 19 ng/ml. For five of these patients, the disappearance of cladribine could be described by either a biphasic or triphasic decline. For patients with normal renal function, the mean terminal half-life was 5.4 hours. Mean value for clearance and steady-state volume of distribution were 978 $\pm$ 422 ml/hr/kg and 4.5$\pm$ 2.8 L;/kg, respectively. Cladribine is bound approximately 20% to plasma proteins.

In rats, approximately 41% to 44% of cladribine was recovered in the urine in the first 6 hours from 1 mg/kg bolus or infusion. Only small amounts were recovered after 6 hours; $\leq$ 1% was excreted in the feces following a bolus dose.

Clinical trials: Two single-center open label studies were conducted in patients with HCL with evidence of active disease requiring therapy. In one study, 89 patients were treated with a single course of cladribine (0.09 mg/kg/day) given by continuous IV infusion for 7 days. In a second study, 35 patients were treated with a 7 day continuous IV infusion at a comparable dose of 3.6 mg/m^2 /day.

A complete response (CR) required clearing of the peripheral blood and bone marrow of hairy cells and recovery of the hemoglobin to 12 g/dl, platelet count to 100 $\times$ 10^9 / L, and absolute neutrophil count to 1500 $\times$ 10^6 /L. A good partial response (GPR) required the same hematologic parameters as a complete response, and that < 5% of hairy cells remain in the bone marrow. A partial response (PR) required that hairy cells in the bone marrow be decreased by at least 50% from baseline and the same response for hematologic parameters as for complete response. A pathologic relapse was defined as an increase in bone marrow hairy cells to 25% of pretreatment levels. A clinical relapse was defined as the recurrence of cytopenias, specifically, decreases in hemoglobin $\geq$ 2 g/dl, ANC $\geq$ 25% or platelet counts $\geq$ 50,000.

CLADRIBINE (2-chlorodeoxyadenosine; CdA)

Response Rates to Cladribine Treatment in Patients with Hairy Cell Leukemia		
Patient population	CR[1]	Overall[2]
Evaluable patients (n = 106)	66%	88%
Intent-to-treat population (n = 123)	54%	89%

[1] Complete response
[2] Complete + good partial+ partial responses.

In these studies, 60% of the patients had not received prior chemotherapy for HCL or had undergone splenectomy as the only prior treatment and were receiving cladribine as a first-line treatment. The remaining 40% of patients received cladribine as a second-line treatment, having been previously treated with other agents, including interferon alfa or pentostatin. The overall response rate for patients without prior chemotherapy was 92% compared with 84% for previously treated patients. Cladribine is active in previously treated patients; however, retrospective analysis suggests that the overall response rate is decreased in patients previously treated with splenectomy or pentostatin and in patients refractory to interferon alfa.

Overall Response Rates[1] To Cladribine Treatment in Patients with Hairy Cell Leukemia		
	Overall response (n = 123)	NR[2] + relapse
No prior chemotherapy	92%	6 + 4 (14%)
Any prior chemotherapy	84%	8 + 3 (22%)
Previous splenectomy	78%	9 + 1 (24%)
Previous interferon	83%	8 + 3 (23%)
Interferon refractory	55%	5 + 2 (64%)
Previous pentostatin	50%	3 + 1 (66%)

[1] CR + GPR + PR
[2] No response.

After a reversible decline, normalization of peripheral blood counts (hemoglobin > 12 g/dl, platelets > 100 x 10^9 / L, absolute neutrophil count [ANC] > 1500 x 10^6 / L) was achieved by 92% of evaluable patients. The median time to normalization of peripheral counts was 9 weeks from the start of treatment (range, 2 to 72). With normalization of platelet count and hemoglobin, requirements for platelet and RBC transfusions were abolished after months 1 and 2, respectively, in those patients with complete response. Platelet recovery may be delayed in a minority of patients with severe baseline thrombocytopenia. Corresponding to normalization of ANC, a trend toward a reduced incidence of infection was seen after the third month, when compared to the months immediately preceding the therapy.

Time to Normalization of Peripheral Blood Counts Following Cladribine in HCL Patients	
Parameter	Median time to normalization of count[1]
Platelet count	2 weeks
Absolute neutrophil count	5 weeks
Hemoglobin	8 weeks
ANC, hemoglobin and platelet count	9 weeks

[1] Day 1 = First day of infusion

CLADRIBINE (2-chlorodeoxyadenosine; CdA)

For patients achieving a complete response, the median time to response (absence of hairy cells in bone marrow and peripheral blood together with normalization of peripheral blood parameters), measured from treatment start, was ≈ 4 months. Since bone marrow aspiration and biopsy were frequently not performed at the time of peripheral blood normalization, the median time to complete response may actually be shorter than that which was recorded. At the time of data cut-off, the median duration of complete response was > 8 months and ranged to 25 + months. Among 93 responding patients, seven had evidence of disease progression at the time of the data cut-off. In four of these patients, disease was limited to the bone marrow without peripheral blood abnormalities (pathologic progression), while in three patients there were also peripheral blood abnormalities (clinical progression). Seven patients who did not respond to a first course received a second course of therapy. In the five patients who had adequate follow-up, additional courses did not appear to improve their overall response.

Indications:

Hairy cell leukemia (HCL): Treatment of active HCL as defined by clinically significant anemia, neutropenia, thrombocytopenia or disease-related symptoms.

Unlabeled uses: Cladribine (generally 0.1 mg/kg/day for 7 days) appears to be beneficial in the following conditions: Advanced cutaneous T-cell lymphomas; chronic lymphocytic leukemia; non-Hodgkins lymphomas; acute myeloid leukemia; autoimmune hemolytic anemia; mycosis fungoides or the Sezary syndrome.

Contraindications:

Hypersensitivity to the drug or any of its components.

Warnings:

Bone marrow suppression: Severe bone marrow suppression, including neutropenia, anemia and thrombocytopenia, has been commonly observed in patients treated with cladribine, especially at high doses. At initiation of treatment, most patients in the clinical studies had hematologic impairment as a manifestation of active HCL. Following treatment, further hematologic impairment occurred before recovery of peripheral blood counts began. During the first 2 weeks after treatment initiation, mean platelet count, ANC and hemoglobin concentration declined and subsequently increased with normalization of mean counts by day 12, week 5 and week 8, respectively. The myelosuppressive effects were most notable during the first month following treatment. Forty-four percent of patients received transfusions with RBCs and 14% received transfusions with platelets during month 1. Careful hematologic monitoring, especially during the first 4 to 8 weeks after treatment, is recommended.

Nephrotoxicity/Neurotoxicity: In a study using high-dose cladribine (4 to 9 times the recommended dose for HCL) as part of a bone marrow transplant conditioning regimen, which also included high-dose cyclophosphamide and total body irradiation, acute nephrotoxicity and delayed onset neurotoxicity were observed. Thirty-one poor-risk patients with drug-resistant acute leukemia in relapse (29 cases) or non-Hodgkins lymphoma (two cases) received cladribine for 7 to 14 days prior to bone marrow transplantation. During infusion, eight patients experienced GI symptoms. While the bone marrow was initially cleared of all hematopoietic elements, including tumor cells, leukemia eventually recurred in all treated patients. Within 7 to 13 days after starting treatment, six patients (19%) developed manifestations of renal dysfunction (eg, acidosis, anuria, elevated serum creatinine) and five required dialysis. Several of these patients were also being treated with other medications having known nephrotoxic potential. Renal dysfunction was reversible in two of these patients. In the four patients whose renal function had not recovered at the time of death, autopsies were performed; in two of these, evidence of tubular damage was noted. Eleven patients (35%) experienced delayed onset neurologic toxicity. In the majority, this was characterized by progressive irreversible motor weakness (paraparesis/quadriparesis) of the upper or lower extremities, first noted 35 to 84 days after starting high-dose therapy. Non-invasive testing (electromyography and nerve conduction studies) was consistent with demyelinating disease.

In patients with HCL treated with the recommended treatment regimen (0.09 mg/kg/day for 7 consecutive days), there have been no reports of similar nephro- or neurologic toxicities. Mild neurologic toxicities, specifically paresthesias and dizziness, have been reported rarely.

CLADRIBINE (2-chlorodeoxyadenosine; CdA)

Fever 37.8°C (≥100°F) was associated with the use of cladribine in ≈ 66% of patients in the first month of therapy. Virtually all patients were treated empirically with parenteral antibiotics. Overall, 47% of patients had fever in the setting of neutropenia (ANC ≤ 1000), including 32% with severe neutropenia (ANC ≤ 500). Since the majority of fevers occurred in neutropenic patients, closely monitor patients during the first month of treatment and initiate empiric antibiotics as clinically indicated. Although 69% of patients developed fevers, < 33% of febrile events were associated with documented infection. Given the known myelosuppressive effects of cladribine, carefully evaluate the risks and benefits of administering this drug to patients with active infections.

Death: Of the 196 HCL patients entered in the trials, there were eight deaths following treatment. Of these, six were of infectious etiology (including three pneumonias), and 2 occurred in the first month following therapy. Of the eight deaths, six occurred in previously treated patients who were refractory to interferon alfa.

Benzyl alcohol, a constituent of the recommended diluent for the 7 day infusion solution, has been associated with a fatal "Gasping Syndrome" in premature infants.

Renal function impairment: The kidney has not been established as the pathway of excretion for cladribine. There are inadequate data on dosing of patients with renal or hepatic insufficiency. Development of acute renal insufficiency in some patients receiving high doses of cladribine has been described. Until more information is available, use caution when administering the drug to patients with known or suspected renal or hepatic insufficiency.

Mutagenesis: As expected for compounds in this class, the actions of cladribine yield DNA damage. In mammalian cells in culture, cladribine caused an imbalance of intracellular deoxyribonucleotide triphosphate pools. This imbalance results in the inhibition of DNA synthesis and DNA repair, yielding DNA strand breaks and subsequently cell death. Inhibition of thymidine incorporation into human lymphoblastic cells was 90% at concentrations of 0.3 mcM. Cladribine was also incorporated into DNA of these cells.

Fertility impairment: When administered IV to Cynomolgus monkeys, cladribine caused suppression of rapidly generating cells, including testicular cells. The effect on human fertility is unknown.

Pregnancy: Category D. Cladribine is teratogenic in mice and rabbits and consequently has the potential to cause fetal harm when administered to a pregnant woman. A significant increase in fetal variations was observed in mice receiving 1.5 mg/kg/day, and increased resorptions, reduced litter size and increased fetal malformations were observed when mice received 3 mg/kg/day. Fetal death and malformations were observed in rabbits that received 3 mg/kg/day.

Although there is no evidence of teratogenicity in humans due to cladribine, other drugs that inhibit DNA synthesis (eg, methotrexate) are teratogenic in humans. Cladribine is embryotoxic in mice when given in doses equivalent to the recommended dose. If cladribine is used during pregnancy, or if the patient becomes pregnant while taking this drug, apprise the patient of the potential hazard to the fetus. Advise women of childbearing age to avoid becoming pregnant. Use during pregnancy only if the potential benefit justifies the potential risk to the fetus.

Lactation: It is not known whether this drug is excreted in breast milk. Because of the potential for serious adverse reactions in nursing infants, decide whether to discontinue nursing or discontinue the drug, taking into account the importance of the drug to the mother.

Children: Safety and efficacy in children have not been established. In a Phase I study involving patients 1 to 21 years old with relapsed acute leukemia, cladribine was given by continuous IV infusion in doses ranging from 3 to 10.7 mg/m^2 /day for 5 days (one-half to twice the dose recommended in HCL). In this study, the dose-limiting toxicity was severe myelosuppression with profound neutropenia and thrombocytopenia. At the highest dose (10.7 mg/m^2 /day), three of seven patients developed irreversible myelosuppression and fatal systemic bacterial or fungal infections. No unique toxicities were noted in this study.

Precautions:

Monitoring: Cladribine is a potent antineoplastic agent with potentially significant toxic side effects. Administer only under the supervision of a physician experienced with the use of cancer chemotherapeutic agents. Closely observe patients undergoing therapy for signs of hematologic and non-hematologic toxicity. Periodic assessment of peripheral blood counts, particularly during the first 4 to 8 weeks post-treatment, is recommended to detect the development of anemia, neutropenia and thrombocytopenia and for early detection of any potential sequelae (eg, infection, bleeding). As with other potent chemotherapeutic agents, monitor renal and hepatic function, especially in patients with underlying kidney or liver dysfunction.

CLADRIBINE (2-chlorodeoxyadenosine; CdA)

During and following treatment, monitor the patient's hematologic profile regularly to determine the degree of hematopoietic suppression. In the clinical studies, following reversible declines in all cell counts, the mean platelet count reached 100 x 10^9 /L by day 12, the mean ANC reached 1500 x 10^6 /L by week 5 and the mean hemoglobin reached 12 g/dl by week 8. After peripheral counts have normalized, perform bone marrow aspiration and biopsy to confirm response to treatment. Investigate febrile events with appropriate laboratory and radiologic studies. Perform periodic assessment of renal and hepatic function as clinically indicated.

Hyperuricemia/Tumor lysis syndrome: While hyperuricemia and tumor lysis syndrome is always possible in patients with large tumor burdens, patients in these studies were treated empirically with allopurinol and no episodes of tumor lysis were reported.

Administration: Cladribine must be diluted in designated IV solutions prior to administration (see Administration and Dosage).

Adverse Reactions:

In month 1 of the HCL clinical trials, the following occurred: Severe neutropenia (70%); fever (69%); infection (28%). Other adverse experiences reported frequently during the first 14 days after initiating treatment included: Fatigue (45%); nausea (28%); rash (27%); headache (22%); injection site reactions (19%). Most non-hematologic adverse experiences were mild to moderate in severity.

Myelosuppression was frequently observed during the first month after starting treatment. Neutropenia (ANC < 500 <8dh> 10;^{6} /L) was noted in 70% of patients, compared with 26% in whom it was present initially. Severe anemia (hemoglobin < 8.5 g/dl) developed in 37% of patients, compared with 10% initially and thrombocytopenia (platelets < 20 <8dh> 10;^{9} /L) developed in 12% of patients, compared to 4% in whom it was noted initially.

Infection: During the first month, 28% exhibited documented evidence of infection. Serious infections (eg, septicemia, pneumonia) were reported in 6% of all patients; the remainder were mild or moderate. Several deaths were attributable to infection or complications related to the underlying disease. During the second month, the overall rate of documented infection was 6%; these infections were mild to moderate and no severe systemic infections were seen. After the third month, the monthly incidence of infection was either less than or equal to that of the months immediately preceding therapy.

Fever: During the first month, 11% of patients experienced severe fever (≥ 40°C; 104°F). Documented infections were noted in < 33% of febrile episodes. Of the 196 patients studied, 19 were noted to have a documented infection in the month prior to treatment. In the month following treatment, there were 54 episodes of documented infection: 42% were bacterial, 20% were viral and 20% were fungal. Seven of 8 documented episodes of herpes zoster occurred during the month following treatment. Fourteen of 16 episodes of documented fungal infections occurred in the first 2 months following treatment. Virtually all of these patients were treated empirically with antibiotics.

CD4 count suppression: Analysis of lymphocyte subsets indicates that treatment with cladribine is associated with prolonged depression of the CD4 counts. Prior to treatment, the mean CD4 count was 766/mcl. The mean CD4 count nadir, which occurred 4 to 6 months following treatment, was 272/mcl. Fifteen months after treatment, mean CD4 counts remained < 500/mcl. CD8 counts behaved similarly, though increasing counts were observed after 9 months. There were no associated opportunistic infections reported during this time.

Bone marrow hypocellularity: Another event of unknown clinical significance includes the observation of prolonged bone marrow hypocellularity. Bone marrow cellularity of < 35% was noted after 4 months in 34% of patients treated in two trials. This hypocellularity was noted 2.8 years later. It is not known whether the hypocellularity is the result of disease-related marrow fibrosis or if it is the result of cladribine toxicity. There was no apparent clinical effect on the peripheral blood counts.

Rash: The vast majority of rashes were mild and occurred in patients who were receiving or had recently been treated with other medications (eg, allopurinol, antibiotics) known to cause rash.

Nausea: Most episodes of nausea were mild, not accompanied by vomiting, and did not require treatment with antiemetics. In patients requiring antiemetics, nausea was easily controlled, most frequently with chlorpromazine.

Other adverse reactions reported during the first 2 weeks following treatment initiation by > 5% of patients included:

Body as a whole: Fever (69%); fatigue (45%); chills, asthenia, diaphoresis (9%); malaise (7%); trunk pain (6%).

CLADRIBINE (2-chlorodeoxyadenosine; CdA)

GI: Nausea (28%); decreased appetite (17%); vomiting (13%); diarrhea (10%); constipation (9%); abdominal pain (6%).

Hematologic/Lymphatic: Purpura (10%); petechiae (8%); epistaxis (5%).

CNS: Headache (22%); dizziness (9%); insomnia (7%).

Cardiovascular: Edema, tachycardia (6%).

Respiratory: Abnormal breath sounds (11%); cough (10%); abnormal chest sounds (9%); shortness of breath (7%).

Dermatologic: Rash (27%); injection site reactions (19%); pruritus, pain, erythema (6%).

Musculoskeletal: Myalgia (7%); arthralgia (5%).

IV administration: Injection site infections (redness, swelling, pain; 9%); thrombosis, phlebitis (2%); broken catheter (1%). These appear to be related to the infusion procedure or indwelling catheter rather than the medication or the vehicle.

From day 15 to the last follow-up visit, the only events reported by > 5% of patients were: Fatigue (11%); rash (10%); headache, cough (7%); malaise (5%).

Overdosage:

Symptoms: High doses of cladribine have been associated with: Irreversible neurologic toxicity (paraparesis/quadriparesis), acute nephrotoxicity, severe bone marrow suppression resulting in neutropenia, anemia and thrombocytopenia (see Warnings). There is no known specific antidote.

Treatment: of overdosage consists of discontinuation of cladribine, careful observation and appropriate supportive measures. Refer to General Management of Acute Overdosage. It is not known whether the drug can be removed from the circulation by dialysis or hemofiltration.

Administration and Dosage:

Approved by the FDA on February 26, 1993.

Usual dose: The recommended dose and schedule for active HCL is a single course given by continuous infusion for 7 consecutive days at a dose of 0.09 mg/kg/day. Deviations from this dosage regimen are not advised. Consider delaying or discontinuing the drug if neurotoxicity or renal toxicity occurs (see Warnings).

Specific risk factors predisposing to increased toxicity from cladribine have not been defined. In view of the known toxicities of agents of this class, it would be prudent to proceed carefully in patients with known or suspected renal insufficiency or severe bone marrow impairment of any etiology. Monitor patients closely for hematologic and non-hematologic toxicity. (See Warnings and Precautions.)

Preparation/Administration of IV solutions: Cladribine must be diluted with the designated diluent prior to administration. Since the drug product does not contain any anti-microbial preservative or bacteriostatic agent, aseptic technique and proper environmental precautions must be observed in preparation of solutions.

Preparation of a single daily dose – Add the calculated dose (0.09 mg/kg or 0.09 ml/kg) to an infusion bag containing 500 ml 0.9% Sodium Chloride Injection, USP. Infuse continuously over 24 hours. Repeat daily for a total of 7 consecutive days. The use of 5% dextrose as a diluent is not recommended because of increased degradation of cladribine. Admixtures of cladribine are chemically and physically stable for at least 24 hours at room temperature under normal room fluorescent light in Baxter Viaflex PVC infusion containers. Since limited compatibility data are available, adherence to the recommended diluents and infusion systems is advised.

Preparation of Single Daily Cladribine Doses

Method	Dose	Recommended diluent	Quantity of diluent
24 hour infusion	1 (day) + 0.09 mg/kg	0.9% sodium chloride	500 ml

Preparation of a 7 day infusion – Only prepare the 7 day infusion solution with Bacteriostatic 0.9% Sodium Chloride Injection, USP (0.9% benzyl alcohol preserved). In order to minimize the risk of microbial contamination, pass both cladribine and the diluent through a sterile 0.22 micron disposable hydrophilic syringe filter as each solution is being introduced into the infusion reservoir. First add the calculated dose of cladribine (7 days x 0.09 mg/kg or ml/kg) to the infusion reservoir through the sterile filter, then add a calculated amount of Bacteriostatic 0.9% Sodium Chloride Injection (also through the filter) to bring the total volume of the solution to 100 ml. After completing solution preparation, clamp off the line, disconnect and discard the filter. Aseptically aspirate air bubbles from the reservoir as necessary using the syringe and a dry second sterile filter or a sterile vent filter assembly. Reclamp the line and discard the syringe and filter assembly. Infuse continuously over 7 days. Solutions prepared with Bacteriostatic Sodium Chloride Injection for individuals weighing > 85 kg may have reduced preservative effectiveness due to greater dilution of the benzyl alcohol preservative. Admixtures for the 7 day infusion have demonstrated acceptable chemical and physical stability for at least 7 days in Pharmacia *Deltec* medication cassettes.

Preparation of 7 Day Cladribine Infusion

Method	Dose	Recommended diluent	Quantity of diluent
7 day infusion method	7 days x 0.09 mg/kg	Bacteriostatic 0.9% Sodium Chloride	qs to 100 ml

IV admixture incompatibility: Since limited compatibility data are available, adherence to the recommended diluents and infusion systems is advised. Solutions containing cladribine should not be mixed with other IV drugs or additives or infused simultaneously via a common IV line, since compatability testing has not been performed. Do not use preparations containing benzyl alcohol in neonates (see Warnings).

Handling and disposal: The use of disposable gloves and protective garments is recommended. If cladribine injection contacts the skin or mucous membranes, wash the involved surface immediately with copious amounts of water.

Storage/Stability: Refrigerate unopened vials (2° to 8° C; 36° to 46° F); protect from light. When stored in refrigerated conditions and protected from light, unopened vials are stable until the expiration date indicated on the package. Freezing does not adversely affect the solution. However, a precipitate may form during the exposure of cladribine to low temperatures; it may be resolubilized by allowing the solution to warm naturally to room temperature and by shaking vigorously. Do not heat or microwave. Once thawed, the vial is stable until expiration date if refrigerated. Do not refreeze. Once diluted, administer solutions containing cladribine injection promptly or store in the refrigerator for no more than 8 hours prior to administration. Vials of cladribine are for single use only. Discard any unused portion in an appropriate manner.

Rx	**Leustatin** (Ortho Biotech)	**Solution:** 1 mg/ml	Preservative free. In 10 ml or 10 ml fill in 20 ml single-use vials.

HYDROXYUREA

Actions:

Pharmacology: The precise mechanism of cytotoxic action is unknown. Hydroxyurea causes an immediate inhibition of deoxyribonucleic acid (DNA) synthesis without interfering with the synthesis of ribonucleic acid (RNA) or protein. It may also inhibit the incorporation of thymidine into DNA.

Three mechanisms have been postulated for the effectiveness of hydroxyurea with irradiation on squamous cell (epidermoid) carcinomas of the head and neck. In vitro, hydroxyurea is lethal to normally radioresistant S-stage cells, and holds other cells in the G-1 or pre-DNA synthesis stage where they are most susceptible to the irradiation effects. Also, hydroxyurea, by inhibiting DNA synthesis, hinders the normal repair process of cells damaged but not killed by irradiation, decreasing their survival rate; RNA and protein synthesis have shown no alteration.

Pharmacokinetics:

Absorption/Distribution – Hydroxyurea is readily absorbed from the GI tract, reaching peak serum concentrations within 2 hours; by 24 hours the serum concentration is essentially zero. Hydroxyurea readily crosses the blood-brain barrier with peak CSF levels at 3 hours.

Metabolism/Excretion – About 50% of an oral dose is degraded in the liver and excreted into the urine as urea and as respiratory carbon dioxide; the remainder is excreted intact in the urine. Approximately 80% may be recovered in the urine within 12 hours.

Indications:

Melanoma; resistant chronic myelocytic leukemia; recurrent, metastatic or inoperable carcinoma of the ovary.

Concomitant administration with irradiation therapy in the local control of primary squamous cell (epidermoid) carcinomas of the head and neck, excluding the lip.

Contraindications:

Marked bone marrow depression (leukopenia < 2500/mm^3 WBC or thrombocytopenia < 100,000/mm^3 platelets); severe anemia.

Warnings:

Erythema: Patients who have received prior irradiation therapy may have an exacerbation of post-irradiation erythema.

Bone marrow suppression may occur, and leukopenia is generally the first and most common manifestation. Thrombocytopenia and anemia occur less often, seldom without a preceding leukopenia. Recovery from myelosuppression is rapid when therapy is interrupted. Bone marrow depression is more likely in patients who have previously received radiotherapy or cytotoxic antineoplastics. Correct severe anemia with whole blood replacement before initiating hydroxyurea therapy.

Erythrocytic abnormalities: Self-limiting megaloblastic erythropoiesis is often seen early in hydroxyurea therapy. The morphologic changes resemble pernicious anemia but are not related to vitamin B-12 or folic acid deficiency. Hydroxyurea may delay plasma iron clearance and reduce the rate of iron utilization by erythrocytes, but it does not alter the RBC survival time.

Renal function impairment: Hydroxyurea is excreted by the kidneys; therefore, use with caution in patients with marked renal dysfunction.

Elderly patients may be more sensitive to the effects of hydroxyurea and may require a lower dosage regimen.

Pregnancy: Drugs that affect DNA synthesis may be mutagenic. Hydroxyurea is a known teratogen in animals. Do not use in women who are or who may become pregnant, unless the potential benefits outweigh the possible hazards.

Children: Dosage regimens for children have not been established.

Precautions:

Monitoring: Therapy requires close supervision. Determine the complete status of the blood, including bone marrow examination if indicated, as well as renal and liver function prior to and during treatment.

Hematology – Monitor hemoglobin, total leukocyte counts and platelet counts at least once a week throughout therapy. If WBC decreases to less than 2500/mm^3 or the platelet count to less than 100,000/mm^3, interrupt therapy until values rise significantly toward normal. Treat anemia with whole blood replacement; do not interrupt therapy.

Drug Interactions:

Drug/Lab test interactions: **Serum uric acid, BUN** and **creatinine** levels may be increased by hydroxyurea.

HYDROXYUREA

Adverse Reactions:

Neurological: Headache, dizziness, disorientation, hallucinations and convulsions are extremely rare. Large doses may produce moderate drowsiness.

Other: Fever, chills, malaise and elevation of hepatic enzymes have been reported. Abnormal BSP retention has been reported. Dysuria occurs rarely.

Combination therapy: Adverse reactions observed with combined hydroxyurea and irradiation therapy are similar to those reported using either one alone, primarily bone marrow depression (anemia and leukopenia) and gastric irritation. Combined therapy may cause an increase in the incidence and severity of these side effects. Almost all patients receiving an adequate course of combined therapy will demonstrate concurrent leukopenia. Platelet depression (< 100,000 cells/mm^3;) has occurred rarely and only in the presence of marked leukopenia.

Mucositis at the site is attributed to irradiation, although more severe cases may be due to combination therapy. Control pain or discomfort with topical anesthetics and oral analgesics. If the reaction is severe, temporarily interrupt hydroxyurea therapy; if it is extremely severe, irradiation dosage may be temporarily postponed. This is rarely necessary.

Control severe gastric distress by temporary interruption of hydroxyurea administration; interruption of irradiation is rarely necessary.

Most frequent: Primarily bone marrow depression (leukopenia, anemia and occasionally thrombocytopenia).

Less frequent:

GI – Stomatitis, anorexia, nausea, vomiting, diarrhea, and constipation.

Dermatologic – Maculopapular rash, facial erythema. Alopecia occurs very rarely.

Renal: May temporarily impair renal tubular function accompanied by elevated serum uric acid, BUN and creatinine levels.

Patient Information:

Notify physician if fever, chills, sore throat, nausea, vomiting, loss of appetite, diarrhea, sores in the mouth and on the lips, unusual bleeding or bruising occur.

Medication may cause drowsiness, constipation, redness of the face, skin rash, itching and loss of hair; notify physician if these become pronounced.

Extra fluid intake is recommended.

Contraceptive measures are recommended during therapy.

Administration and Dosage:

Base dosage on the patient's actual or ideal weight, whichever is less. If the patient prefers, or is unable to swallow capsules, empty the contents of the capsules into a glass of water and take immediately. Some inert material may not dissolve.

An adequate trial period to determine effectiveness is 6 weeks. When there is regression in tumor size or arrest in tumor growth, continue therapy indefinitely. Interrupt therapy if the WBC drops below 2500/mm^3 or the platelet count below 100,000/mm^3. In these cases, recheck counts after 3 days, and resume therapy when the counts rise significantly toward normal. Since the hematopoietic rebound is prompt, it is usually necessary to omit only a few doses. If prompt rebound has not occurred during combined hydroxyurea and irradiation therapy, irradiation may also be interrupted. However, this is rare. Correct anemia with whole blood replacement; do not interrupt hydroxyurea therapy.

Because hematopoiesis may be compromised, administer cautiously to patients who have recently received extensive radiation therapy or cytotoxic chemotherapy.

Solid tumors: Patients on intermittent therapy rarely require complete discontinuation of therapy because of toxicity.

Intermittent therapy – 80 mg/kg as a single dose every third day.

Continuous therapy – 20 to 30 mg/kg as a single daily dose.

Concomitant irradiation therapy (carcinoma of head and neck): 80 mg/kg as a single dose every third day. Begin hydroxyurea at least 7 days before initiation of irradiation and continue during radiotherapy and indefinitely afterwards, provided the patient is adequately observed and exhibits no unusual or severe reactions. Administer maximum irradiation dose appropriate for the therapeutic situation; adjustment of irradiation dosage is not usually necessary with concomitant hydroxyurea.

Resistant chronic myelocytic leukemia: Continuous therapy (20 to 30 mg/kg as a single daily dose) is recommended.

Children: Dosage regimens have not been established.

Storage: Avoid excessive heat.

Rx	**Hydrea** (Immunex)	**Capsules:** 500 mg	(830). In 100s.

BCG, INTRAVESICAL

Actions:

Pharmacology: BCG is a freeze-dried suspension of an attenuated strain of *Mycobacterium bovis* (Bacillus Calmette and Guerin) used in the non-specific active therapy of carcinoma in situ of the urinary bladder. BCG live *(TheraCys)* is used only for carcinoma in situ of the urinary bladder; BCG Vaccine *(TICE BCG)* is also used for immunization against tuberculosis (see individual monograph in Biologicals section).

BCG promotes a local inflammatory reaction with histiocytic and leukocytic infiltration in the urinary bladder. The local inflammatory effects are associated with an apparent elimination or reduction of superficial cancerous lesions of the urinary bladder. The exact mechanism is unknown.

Clinical trials:

TheraCys – In a randomized, actively controlled multicenter study, *TheraCys* was compared to doxorubicin HCl in the treatment of carcinoma in situ of the urinary bladder. The response of 114 patients is given in the following table. Among the 54 patients receiving *TheraCys*, 74% had a complete response. The estimated median time to treatment failure (recurrence, progression or death) was 48.2 months.

Response of Patients with Carcinoma In Situ to Treatment with TheraCys (n = 54) or Doxorubicin (n = 60)

Response	*TheraCys*	Doxorubicin
Complete response[1]	74%	42%
No response[2]	11%	10%
Progressive disease[3]	13%	42%
No evaluation	2%	7%
Number of failures	27	46
Median time to treatment failure (TTF)	48.2 months	5.9 months

[1] Confirmed by cytology and cystoscopic examination.
[2] Less than a CR or stable disease.
[3] Increase of stage or grade.

The effect of chemotherapy (other than *TheraCys* or doxorubicin) prior to entry into the controlled study was analyzed.

Prior vs No Prior Treatment for Carcinoma In Situ of the Urinary Bladder

Prior treatment	Study arm	Response rate	Median TTF (# events/n)
Yes	BCG live	81%	Not reached (11/26)
Yes	Doxorubicin	53%	7 months (22/30)
No	BCG live	68%	32.8 months (16/28)
No	Doxorubicin	30%	3.7 months (24/30)

No survival advantage for *TheraCys* therapy over that for doxorubicin was demonstrated after a 40 to 72 month follow-up. The median time to death for each group was 23 and 21 months for *TheraCys* and doxorubicin, respectively.

The clinical trials carried out with *TheraCys* included percutaneous administration of 0.5 ml, which was reconstituted in the diluent provided and further diluted in 50 ml sterile preservative-free saline with each intravesical dose. Some studies have suggested that this may not be necessary. If severe reactions (eg, ulceration) occurred, the percutaneous treatment was discontinued.

TICE BCG – In 119 evaluable patients, 54 (45.4%) had a complete histological response and 36 (30.2%) had a complete clinical response without cytology. Of the 54 patients classified as complete histological response, 30 remained without evidence of disease after a median follow-up of 47 months. Of the 90 (75.6%) overall responders, 36.7% relapsed; 13.3% died of other diseases, and 50% remained in complete response. In addition, two who relapsed were reinduced in complete response by a second course of *TICE BCG*. Among the 119 evaluable patients there was no significant difference in response rates between patients with or without prior intravesical chemotherapy. Median duration of response is estimated at ≥ 4 years.

Indications:

Intravesical use in the treatment of primary and relapsed carcinoma in situ of the urinary bladder to eliminate residual tumor cells and to reduce the frequency of tumor recurrence *(TheraCys)*; primary or secondary treatment in absence of invasive cancer for patients with medical contraindications to radical surgery *(TICE BCG)*.

Treatment of carcinoma in situ with or without associated papillary tumors. Not indicated for the treatment of papillary tumors occurring alone.

Therapy for patients with carcinoma in situ of the bladder following failure to respond to other treatment regimens.

BCG, INTRAVESICAL

BCG vaccines for tuberculosis prevention are discussed in the Biologicals section.

Contraindications:

Patients on immunosuppressive or corticosteroid therapy, with compromised immune systems, or asymptomatic carriers with a positive HIV serology due to the risk of overwhelming systemic mycobacterial sepsis.

Fever, unless the cause of the fever is determined and evaluated. If the fever is due to an infection, withhold therapy until the patient is afebrile and off all therapy.

Urinary tract infection because administration may result in the risk of disseminated BCG infection or in an increased severity of bladder irritation.

Not a vaccine for the prevention of cancer.

TheraCys: As an immunizing agent for the prevention of tuberculosis.

TICE BCG: Positive Mantoux test, only if there is evidence of an active TB infection.

Warnings:

Tuberculosis prevention: TheraCys should not be administered as an immunizing agent to prevent TB. These agents may cause TB sensitivity. Since this is a valuable aid in TB diagnosis, it may be useful to determine tuberculin reactivity by PPD skin testing before treatment.

Cancer prevention: These agents are not vaccines for cancer prevention.

Urinary status monitoring: Since administration of intravesical BCG causes an inflammatory response in the bladder and has been associated with hematuria, urinary frequency, dysuria and bacterial urinary tract infection, careful monitoring of urinary status is required. If there is an increase in the patient's existing symptoms, if symptoms persist, or if any of these symptoms develop, evaluate and manage the patient for urinary tract infection or BCG toxicity.

BCG infection, systemic: Death has occurred due to systemic BCG infection; closely monitor for symptoms of such infection. Withhold BCG upon any suspicion of systemic infection (eg, granulomatous hepatitis). If such infection is suspected (ie, fever > 39°C [103°F], persistent fever > 38°C [101°F] over 2 days or severe malaise), consult an infectious disease specialist and initiate fast-acting antituberculosis therapy. These infections are rarely evidenced by positive cultures.

Antimicrobial therapy: Evaluate patients undergoing antimicrobial therapy for other infections to assess whether the therapy will obviate the effects of BCG actions.

Small bladder capacity: Consider increased risk of severity of local irritation when deciding to treat with these agents.

Hypersensitivity: Allergic reactions are possible in individuals sensitive to the product components. Refer to Management of Acute Hypersensitivity Reactions.

Pregnancy: Category C. It is not known whether BCG can cause fetal harm when administered to a pregnant woman. Give to a pregnant woman only if clearly needed. Advise women not to become pregnant while on therapy.

Lactation: It is not known whether BCG is excreted in breast milk. Exercise caution when BCG is administered to a nursing woman.

Children: Safety and efficacy for use in children have not been established.

Precautions:

Contains viable attenuated mycobacteria. Handle as infectious. Use aseptic technique.

Instillation equipment disposal: After usage, immediately place all equipment and materials (eg, syringes, catheters and containers that may have come into contact with BCG) used for instillation of the product into the bladder into plastic bags labeled "Infectious Waste" and dispose of accordingly as biohazardous waste.

Aseptic technique must be used during administration so as not to introduce contaminants into the urinary tract or to unduly traumatize the urinary mucosa.

Urine disinfection: Disinfect urine voided for 6 hours after instillation with an equal volume of 5% hypochlorite solution (undiluted household bleach) and allow to stand for 15 minutes before flushing.

Transurethral resection: Do not give intravesical BCG any sooner than 1 to 2 weeks following transurethral resection. Fatalities due to disseminated BCG infection have occurred with BCG use after traumatic catheterization.

If the physician believes that the bladder catheterization has been traumatic (eg, associated with bleeding or possible false passage), then BCG should not be administered, and there must be a treatment delay of at least 1 to 2 weeks. Resume subsequent treatment as if no interruption in the schedule had occurred. That is, administer all doses even after a temporary halt in administration.

BCG, INTRAVESICAL

Drug Interactions:

Bone marrow depressants, immunosuppressants or **radiation** may impair response to BCG or increase the risk of osteomyelitis or disseminated BCG infection.

Adverse Reactions:

BCG therapy can affect several organs (or parts) of the body in addition to the cancer cells. Most local adverse reactions occur following the third intravesical instillation. Symptoms usually begin 2 to 4 hours after instillation and persist 24 to 72 hours. Systemic reactions usually last for 1 to 3 days after each intravesical instillation.

BCG Adverse Reactions (≥ 1% of patients)[1]

Local			Systemic		
Adverse Reaction	Total (%)	Severe[2] %	Adverse Reaction	Total (%)	Severe[2] %
Dysuria	51.8-59.5	3.6-10.7	Malaise/Fatigue	7.4-40.2	2
Urinary frequency	≈ 40.4	1.8-7.4	Fever (> 38°C)	19.9-38.4	2.6-7.6
Hematuria	26-39.3	7.4-17	Chills	3.3-33.9	1-2.6
Cystitis	5.9-29.5	0-1.9	Anemia	1.3-20.5	0-0.4
Urinary urgency	5.8-17.9	0-1.3	Nausea/Vomiting	3-16.1	0-0.3
Urinary tract infection	1.5-17.9	0.9-1	Anorexia	2.2-10.7	0-0.1
Urinary incontinence	2.4-6.3	0	Renal toxicity	0-9.8	0-2
Cramps/Pain	4-6.3	0-0.9	Genital pain	0-9.8	0
Decreased bladder capacity	0-5.4	0	Myalgia/Arthralgia/Arthritis	2.7-7.1	0.4-1
Nocturia	0-4.5	0-0.6	Diarrhea	1.2-6.3	0-0.1
Urinary debris	0.9-2.2	0-0.4	Leukopenia	0.3-5.4	0
Genital inflammation/Abscess	0-1.8	0-0.4	Mild liver involvement/Hepatitis/Hepatic granuloma	0.2-2.7	0-0.4
Urethritis	0-1.2	0	Mild abdominal pain	1.5-2.7	0-0.6
			Systemic infection[3]	0.4-2.7	0.4-2
			Pulmonary infection[3]	0-2.7	0
			Cardiac	1.9-2.7	0-1.3
			Coagulopathy	0.3-2.7	0-0.3
			Headache/Dizziness	2.4-2.7	0
			Allergic	1.8-2.1	0-0.4
			Respiratory	0-1.6	0-0.2
			Pneumonitis	0-1.2	0-0.6

[1] Pooled data from two products: *TheraCys* (n = 112); *TICE BCG* (n = 674).
[2] Severe is defined as grade 3 (severe) or grade 4 (life-threatening).
[3] Includes both BCG and other infections.

Manage irritative bladder symptoms associated with BCG administration with phenazopyridine HCl, propantheline bromide or oxybutynin and acetaminophen or ibuprofen.

Systemic side effects (such as malaise, fever and chills) may represent hypersensitivity reactions and can be treated with antihistamines. Systemic infection as a result of the spread of BCG organisms has occasionally occurred with intravesical BCG administration (see Warnings). At least two deaths occurred as a result of systemic BCG infection and sepsis. There have been two cases of nephrogenic adenoma, a benign lesion of bladder epithelium, associated with intravesical BCG therapy.

Overdosage:

Overdosage occurs if > 1 amp of TICE BCG is given per instillation. Closely monitor for signs of systemic BCG infection; treat with anti-tuberculous medication.

Patient Information:

Advise patients to check with their doctor as soon as possible if there is an increase in their existing symptoms, or if their symptoms persist even after receiving a number of treatments, or if any of the following symptoms develop: Blood in the urine, fever, chills, increased urinary frequency, joint pain, nausea, vomiting, painful urination (more common); cough, skin rash (rare).

A cough that develops after administration of BCG could indicate a BCG systemic infection that is life-threatening. Notify the physician immediately.

All patients should sit while voiding following instillation of solution.

Disinfect urine voided for 6 hours after instillation with an equal volume of 5% hypochlorite solution (undiluted household bleach); allow to stand 15 min; flush.

BCG, INTRAVESICAL

Administration and Dosage:

Intravesical treatment and prophylaxis for carcinoma in situ of the urinary bladder:

TheraCys – Begin between 7 to 14 days after biopsy or transurethral resection. Give a dose of 3 vials intravesically under aseptic conditions once weekly for 6 weeks (induction therapy). Each dose (3 reconstituted vials) is further diluted in an additional 50 ml sterile, preservative free saline for a total of 53 ml. Follow the induction therapy by one treatment given 3, 6, 12, 18 and 24 months after initial treatment.

TICE BCG – Allow 7 to 14 days to elapse after bladder biopsy or transurethral resection before administration. Patients should not drink fluids for 4 hours before treatment and should empty their bladder prior to administration. The dose consists of one amp suspended in 50 ml preservative free saline. A standard treatment schedule consists of one instillation per week for 6 weeks. This may be repeated once if tumor remission has not been achieved and if the clinical circumstances warrant. Thereafter, continue approximately monthly for at least 6 to 12 months.

TheraCys and TICE BCG – A urethral catheter is inserted into the bladder under aseptic conditions, the bladder is drained, and then the suspension is instilled slowly by gravity, following which the catheter is withdrawn.

During the first hour following instillation, the patient should lie for 15 minutes each in the prone and supine positions and also on each side. The patient is then allowed to be up but should retain the suspension for another 60 minutes for a total of 2 hours. All patients may not be able to retain the suspension 2 hours and should be instructed to void in less time if necessary. At the end of 2 hours, all patients should void in a seated position for safety reasons. Maintain adequate hydration.

If the bladder catheterization has been traumatic (eg, associated with bleeding or possible false passage), BCG should not be administered, and there must be a treatment delay of at least 1 week. Resume subsequent treatment as if no interruption in the schedule had occurred (ie, administer all doses even after a temporary halt in administration).

Preparation of TheraCys solution: Do not remove the rubber stopper from the vial.

Reconstitute and dilute immediately prior to use.

Persons handling product should be masked and gloved.

TheraCys should not be handled by persons with a known immunologic deficiency.

TheraCys should be handled as infectious material.

Reconstitute only with the diluent provided to ensure proper dispersion of the organisms.

The reconstituted material from three vials (1 dose) is further diluted in an additional 50 ml sterile, preservative free saline to a final volume of 53 ml for intravesical instillation (and percutaneous injection if it is given).

Preparation of TICE BCG solution: Draw 1 ml of sterile, preservative free saline into a small (eg, 3 ml) syringe and add to one amp of *TICE BCG*. Draw the mixture into the syringe and gently expel back into the amp three times to ensure thorough mixing and minimize clumping of the mycobacteria. Dispense the cloudy BCG suspension into the top end of a catheter-tip syringe which contains 49 ml saline diluent bringing the total volume to 50 ml. Gently rotate the syringe. Do not filter the contents. Perform all mixing operations in sterile glass or thermosetting plastic containers and syringes.

Stability/Storage: Keep BCG and any accompanying diluent in a refrigerator at a temperature between 2° and 8°C (36° and 46°F). It should not be used after the expiration date marked on the vial, otherwise it may be inactive. Use immediately after reconstitution. Do not use after 2 hours. Any reconstituted product which exhibits flocculation or clumping that cannot be dispersed with gentle shaking should not be used. At no time should the freeze-dried or reconstituted BCG be exposed to sunlight, direct or indirect. Exposure to artificial light should be kept to a minimum.

Rx	**TICE BCG** (Organon)	**Freeze-dried suspension for reconstitution**: 1 to 8 x 10^8 CFU (equivalent to approximately 50 mg)	In 2 ml amps.
Rx	**TheraCys** (Connaught)	**Freeze-dried suspension for reconstitution**: 27 mg (3.4 ± 3 x 10^8 CFU)/vial	In 3 vials with 3 vials diluent (1 ml/vial).

ALDESLEUKIN (Interleukin-2; IL-2)

> **Warning:**
>
> Administer aldesleukin only in a hospital setting under the supervision of a qualified physician experienced in the use of anti-cancer agents. An intensive care facility and specialists skilled in cardiopulmonary or intensive care medicine must be available.
>
> Aldesleukin administration has been associated with capillary leak syndrome (CLS). CLS results in hypotension and reduced organ perfusion which may be severe and can result in death (see Warnings).
>
> Restrict therapy to patients with normal cardiac and pulmonary functions as defined by thallium stress testing and formal pulmonary function testing. Use extreme caution in patients with normal thallium stress tests and pulmonary function tests who have a history of prior cardiac or pulmonary disease.
>
> Hold aldesleukin administration in patients developing moderate to severe lethargy or somnolence; continued administration may result in coma.

Actions:

Pharmacology: Aldesleukin, a human recombinant interleukin-2 product, is a highly purified protein (lymphokine) produced by recombinant DNA technology using a genetically engineered *Eschericia coli* strain containing an analog of the human interleukin-2 gene. The human IL-2 gene is modified, and the resulting expression clone encodes a modified human interleukin-2. This recombinant form differs from native interleukin-2 in the following ways: 1) Aldesleukin is not glycosylated; 2) the molecule has no N-terminal alanine; 3) the molecule has serine substituted for cysteine at amino acid position 125; and 4) the aggregation state of aldesleukin is likely to be different from that of native interleukin-2. Aldesleukin exists as biologically active, non-covalently bound microaggregates with an average size of 27 recombinant IL-2 molecules.

Aldesleukin possesses the biological activity of human native interleukin-2. In vitro, the immunoregulatory properties of aldesleukin include: 1) Enhancement of lymphocyte mitogenesis and stimulation of long-term growth of human interleukin-2 dependent cell lines; 2) enhancement of lymphocyte cytotoxicity; 3) induction of killer cell (lymphokine-activated [LAK] and natural [NK]) activity; and 4) induction of interferon-gamma production.

Administration produces multiple immunological effects in a dose-dependent manner. These effects include activation of cellular immunity with profound lymphocytosis, eosinophilia and thrombocytopenia, the production of cytokines (including tumor necrosis factor, IL-1 and gamma interferon) and inhibition of tumor growth. The exact mechanism by which aldesleukin mediates its antitumor activity is unknown.

Pharmacokinetics: The solubilizing agent, sodium dodecyl sulfate, may affect the kinetic properties of this product. The pharmacokinetic profile of aldesleukin is characterized by high plasma concentrations following a short IV infusion, rapid distribution to extravascular, extracellular space and elimination from the body by metabolism in the kidneys with little or no bioactive protein excreted in the urine. Approximately 30% of the dose initially distributes to the plasma. This is consistent with studies in rats that demonstrate a rapid (< 1 minute) and preferential uptake of approximately 70% of an administered dose into the liver, kidney and lung.

The serum distribution and elimination half-lives in 52 cancer patients following a 5 minute IV infusion were 13 and 85 minutes, respectively.

The relatively rapid clearance rate of aldesleukin has led to dosage schedules characterized by frequent, short infusions. Observed serum levels are proportional to the dose.

Following the initial rapid organ distribution, the primary route of clearance of circulating aldesleukin is the kidney; it is cleared from the circulation by both glomerular filtration and peritubular extraction. This may account for the preservation of clearance in patients with rising serum creatinine values. Greater than 80% of the amount distributed to plasma, cleared from the circulation and presented to the kidney is metabolized to amino acids in the cells lining the proximal convoluted tubules. The mean clearance rate in cancer patients is 268 ml/min.

Microbiology:

Immunogenicity – Of 76 renal cancer patients, 58 (76%) treated with the every 8 hour regimen developed low titers of non-neutralizing anti-interleukin-2 antibodies. Neutralizing antibodies were not detected in this group of patients, but have been detected in < 1% treated with IV aldesleukin using a wide variety of schedules and doses. The clinical significance of anti-interleukin-2 antibodies is unknown.

ALDESLEUKIN (Interleukin-2; IL-2)

Clinical trials: Patients with metastatic renal cell cancer (n = 255) were treated with single agent aldesleukin. Patients were required to have bidimensionally measurable disease, Eastern Cooperative Oncology Group (ECOG) Performance Status (PS) of 0 or 1 (see table), and normal organ function; 218 (85%) patients had undergone nephrectomy prior to treatment. All patients were treated with 28 doses or until dose-limiting toxicity occurred requiring ICU-level support. Patients received a median of 20 of 28 scheduled doses.

Objective response was seen in 37 patients (15%) with 9 (4%) complete and 28 (11%) partial responders. Onset of tumor regression has been observed as early as 4 weeks after completion of the first course of treatment and tumor regression may continue for up to 12 months after the start of treatment. Median duration of objective (partial or complete) response was 23.2 months (1 to 50 months); the median duration of objective partial response was 18.2 months. The proportion of responding patients who will have response durations of ≥ 12 months is projected to be 85% for all responders and 79% for patients with partial responses. Response was observed in both lung and non-lung sites (eg, liver, lymph node, renal bed recurrences, soft tissue). Patients with individual bulky lesions as well as large cumulative tumor burden achieved durable responses.

An analysis of prognostic factors showed that performance status as defined by the ECOG (see table) was a significant predictor of response. In addition, the frequency of toxicity was related to the performance status. As a group, PS 0 patients, when compared with PS 1 patients, had lower rates of adverse events with fewer on-study deaths (4% vs 6%), less frequent intubations (8% vs 25%), gangrene (0% vs 6%), coma (1% vs 6%), GI bleeding (4% vs 8%) and sepsis (6% vs 18%).

Eastern Cooperative Oncology Group (ECOG) Performance Status (PS) Scale

Performance status equivalent		
ECOG	Karnofsky	Performance status definitions
0	100	Asymptomatic
1	80-90	Symptomatic; fully ambulatory
2	60-70	Symptomatic; in bed < 50% of day
3	40-50	Symptomatic; in bed > 50% of day
4	20-30	Bedridden

Aldesleukin Response Analyzed by ECOG Performance Status

Pretreatment ECOG PS	Patients treated (n = 255)	Response		Patients responding (%)	On-study death rate
		Complete	Partial		
0	166	9	21	18	4%
1	80	0	7	9	6%
≥ 2	9	0	0	0	0%

Indications:

Metastatic renal cell carcinoma in adults (≥ 18 years of age).

Careful patient selection is mandatory prior to administration. Patients with more favorable ECOG performance status (ECOG PS 0) at treatment initiation respond better to aldesleukin with a higher response rate and lower toxicity. Experience in patients with PS > 1 is extremely limited.

Unlabeled uses: Aldesleukin is being investigated in the treatment of Kaposi's sarcoma in combination with zidovudine. Aldesleukin may be beneficial for metastatic melanoma; 20% to 30% response rates have been reported in combination with low-dose cyclophosphamide. Aldesleukin has been used with some success in the treatment of colorectal cancer and non-Hodgkin's lymphoma, often in combination with lymphokine activated killer (LAK) cells.

Contraindications:

Hypersensitivity to interleukin-2 or any component of the formulation; abnormal thallium stress test or pulmonary function tests; organ allografts.

Retreatment is contraindicated in patients who experienced the following toxicities while receiving an earlier course of therapy: Sustained ventricular tachycardia (≥ 5 beats); cardiac rhythm disturbances uncontrolled or unresponsive; recurrent chest pain with ECG changes, consistent with angina or myocardial infarction (MI); intubation required > 72 hours; pericardial tamponade; renal dysfunction requiring dialysis > 72 hours; coma or toxic psychosis lasting > 48 hours; repetitive or difficult to control seizures; bowel ischemia/perforation; GI bleeding requiring surgery.

Warnings:

Capillary leak syndrome (CLS): Aldesleukin has been associated with CLS which begins immediately after treatment starts and results from extravasation of plasma pro-

ALDESLEUKIN (Interleukin-2; IL-2)

teins and fluid into the extravascular space and loss of vascular tone. This usually results in a concomitant drop in mean arterial blood pressure within 2 to 12 hours after the start of treatment and reduced organ perfusion which may be severe and can result in death. With continued therapy, clinically significant hypotension (systolic blood pressure < 90 mm Hg or a 20 mm Hg drop from baseline systolic pressure) and hypoperfusion will occur. In addition, extravasation will lead to edema and effusions. The CLS may be associated with cardiac arrhythmias (supraventricular and ventricular), angina, MI, respiratory insufficiency requiring intubation, GI bleeding or infarction, renal insufficiency and mental status changes.

Medical management of CLS begins with careful monitoring of the patient's fluid and organ perfusion status. Frequently determine blood pressure and pulse, and monitor organ function, including assessment of mental status and urine output. Assess hypovolemia by catheterization and central pressure monitoring.

Flexibility in fluid and pressor management is essential for maintaining organ perfusion and blood pressure. Consequently, use extreme caution in treating patients with fixed requirements for large volumes of fluid (eg, patients with hypercalcemia).

Patients with hypovolemia are managed by administering IV fluids, either colloids or crystalloids. IV fluids are usually given when the central venous pressure (CVP) is < 3 to 4 mm H_2O. Correction of hypovolemia may require large volumes of IV fluids but use caution because unrestrained fluid administration may exacerbate problems associated with edema or effusions.

With extravascular fluid accumulation, edema is common and some patients may develop ascites or pleural effusions. Carefully balance the effects of fluid shifts so that neither the consequences of hypovolemia (eg, impaired organ perfusion) nor the consequences of fluid accumulations (eg, pulmonary edema) exceeds the patient's tolerance.

Early administration of dopamine (1 to 5 mcg/kg/min) to patients manifesting CLS, before the onset of hypotension, can help maintain organ perfusion particularly to the kidney and thus preserve urine output. Carefully monitor weight and urine output. If organ perfusion and blood pressure are not sustained by dopamine therapy, the dose of dopamine may be increased to 6 to 10 mcg/kg/min or phenylephrine HCl (1 to 5 mcg/kg/min) may be added to low-dose dopamine. Prolonged use of pressors, either in combination or as individual agents at relatively high doses, may be associated with cardiac rhythm disturbances.

Failure to maintain organ perfusion, demonstrated by altered mental status, reduced urine output, a fall in the systolic blood pressure < 90 mm Hg or onset of cardiac arrhythmias, should lead to holding the subsequent doses until recovery of organ perfusion and a return of systolic blood pressure > 90 mm Hg are observed.

Recovery from CLS begins soon after cessation of therapy, within a few hours. If there has been excessive weight gain or edema formation, particularly if associated with shortness of breath from pulmonary congestion, use of diuretics, once blood pressure has normalized, hastens recovery. Oxygen is given if pulmonary function monitoring confirms that P_aO_2 is decreased.

Clinical evaluation: Because of the severe adverse events which generally accompany therapy at the recommended dosages, perform thorough clinical evaluation to exclude from treatment patients with significant cardiac, pulmonary, renal, hepatic or CNS impairment. Patients who have had a nephrectomy are still eligible for treatment if they have serum creatinine levels ≤ 1.5 mg/dl.

CNS metastases: Aldesleukin may exacerbate disease symptoms in patients with clinically unrecognized or untreated CNS metastases. Thoroughly evaluate all patients and treat CNS metastases prior to therapy. Patients should be neurologically stable with a negative CT scan. In addition, exercise extreme caution in treating patients with a history of seizure disorder because aldesleukin may cause seizures.

Bacterial infections: Intensive treatment is associated with impaired neutrophil function (reduced chemotaxis) and with an increased risk of disseminated infection, including sepsis and bacterial endocarditis. Consequently, adequately treat preexisting bacterial infections prior to initiation of therapy. Additionally, give all patients with indwelling central lines antibiotic prophylaxis effective against *Staphylococcus aureus*. Antibiotic prophylaxis which has been associated with a reduced incidence of staphylococcal infections in aldesleukin studies includes the use of oxacillin, nafcillin, ciprofloxacin or vancomycin. Disseminated infections acquired in the course of treatment are a major contributor to treatment morbidity; use of antibiotic prophylaxis and aggressive treatment of suspected and documented infections may reduce the morbidity.

Renal/Hepatic function impairment: Occurs during treatment. Use of concomitant medications known to be nephrotoxic or hepatotoxic may further increase toxicity to the kidney or liver. In addition, reduced kidney and liver function secondary to treatment may delay elimination of concomitant medications and increase their risk of adverse events.

Fertility impairment: It is recommended that this drug not be administered to fertile persons of either sex not practicing effective contraception.

Pregnancy: Category C. It is not known whether aldesleukin can cause fetal harm when administered to a pregnant woman or can affect reproduction capacity. In view of the known adverse effects of aldesleukin, only give to a pregnant woman with extreme caution, weighing the potential benefit with the risks associated with therapy.

Lactation: It is not known whether this drug is excreted in breast milk. Because of the potential for serious adverse reactions in nursing infants, decide whether to discontinue nursing or to discontinue the drug, taking into the account the importance of the drug to the mother.

Children: Safety and efficacy in children < 18 years of age have not been established.

Precautions:

Monitoring: The following clinical evaluations are recommended for all patients prior to beginning treatment and then daily during drug administration: Standard hematologic tests, including CBC, differential and platelet counts; blood chemistries, including electrolytes, renal and hepatic function tests; chest x-rays.

All patients should have baseline pulmonary function tests with arterial blood gases. Document adequate pulmonary function (FEV_1 > 2 L or ≥ 75% of predicted for height and age) prior to initiating therapy. Screen all patients with a stress thallium study. Document normal ejection fraction and unimpaired wall motion. If a thallium stress test suggests minor wall motion abnormalities of questionable significance, a stress echocardiogram to document normal wall motion may be useful to exclude significant coronary artery disease.

Daily monitoring during therapy should include vital signs (temperature, pulse, blood pressure and respiration rate) and weight. In a patient with a decreased blood pressure, especially < 90 mm Hg, conduct constant cardiac monitoring for rhythm. If an abnormal complex or rhythm is seen, perform an ECG. Take vital signs in these hypotensive patients hourly and check CVP.

During treatment monitor pulmonary function on a regular basis by clinical examination, assessment of vital signs and pulse oximetry. Further assess patients with dyspnea or clinical signs of respiratory impairment (tachypnea or rales) with arterial blood gas determination. Repeat these tests as often as clincally indicated.

Cardiac function is assessed daily by clinical examination and assessment of vital signs. Further assess patients with signs or symptoms of chest pain, murmurs, gallops, irregular rhythm or palpitations with an ECG examination and CPK evaluation. If there is evidence of cardiac ischemia or CHF, perform a repeat thallium study.

Anemia/Thrombocytopenia may occur. Packed red blood cell transfusions have been given both for relief of anemia and to ensure maximal oxygen carrying capacity. Platelet transfusions have been given to resolve absolute thrombocytopenia and to reduce the risk of GI bleeding. In addition, leukopenia and neutropenia have been observed.

Mental status changes including irritability, confusion or depression may occur and may be indicators of bacteremia or early bacterial sepsis. Mental status changes due solely to aldesleukin are generally reversible when drug administration is discontinued. However, alterations in mental status may progress for several days before recovery begins.

Thyroid function impairment has occurred following treatment. Some patients went on to require thyroid replacement therapy. This impairment of thyroid function may be a manifestation of autoimmunity; consequently, exercise extra caution when treating patients with known autoimmune disease.

Allograft rejection: Aldesleukin enhancement of cellular immune function may increase the risk of allograft rejection in transplant patients.

ALDESLEUKIN (Interleukin-2; IL-2)

Drug Interactions:

Aldesleukin Drug Interactions

Precipitant drug	Object drug*		Description
Antihypertensives	Aldesleukin	⬆	Antihypertensives may potentiate the hypotension seen with aldesleukin.
Corticosteroids	Aldesleukin	⬇	Although glucocorticoids reduce the side effects of aldesleukin including fever, renal insufficiency, hyperbilirubinemia and dyspnea, concomitant use may reduce the antitumor effectiveness of aldesleukin; avoid concurrent use.
Cardiotoxic agents (eg, doxorubicin) Hepatotoxic agents (eg, methotrexate, asparaginase) Myelotoxic agents (eg, cytotoxic chemotherapy) Nephrotoxic agents (eg, aminoglycosides, indomethacin)	Aldesleukin	⬆	Increased toxicity in these organ systems may occur during concomitant administration.
Aldesleukin	Psychotropic agents	⟷	Aldesleukin may affect CNS function. Therefore, interactions could occur following concurrent use of these agents.

* ⬆ = Object drug increased. ⬇ = Object drug decreased. ⟷ = Undetermined effect.

Adverse Reactions:

Adverse events are frequent, often serious and sometimes fatal. Administration results in fever, chills, rigors, pruritus and GI side effects in most patients treated at recommended doses. The rate of drug-related deaths in the 255 metastatic renal cell carcinoma patients who received single-agent aldesleukin was 4% (11/255). Frequency and severity of adverse reactions have generally been dose-related and schedule-dependent. Most adverse reactions are self-limiting and are usually, but not invariably, reversible within 2 or 3 days of discontinuation of therapy. The incidence of these events has been higher in PS 1 patients than in PS 0 patients. Examples of adverse reactions with permanent sequelae include MI, bowel perforation/infarction and gangrene. Should adverse events occur which require dose modification, withhold rather than reduce dosage.

ALDESLEUKIN (Interleukin-2; IL-2)

Aldesleukin Adverse Reactions (n = 373[1])

Adverse reaction	Incidence (%)
Cardiovascular	
Hypotension	85
(requiring pressors)	71
Sinus tachycardia	70
Arrhythmias	22
Atrial	8
Supraventricular	5
Ventricular	3
Junctional	1
Bradycardia	7
PVCs	5
Premature atrial contractions	4
Myocardial ischemia	3
Myocardial infarction	2
Cardiac arrest	2
CHF	1
Myocarditis/Endocarditis	1
Stroke	1
Gangrene	1
Pericardial effusion	1
Thrombosis	1
Pulmonary	
Pulmonary congestion	54
Dyspnea	52
Pulmonary edema	10
Respiratory failure	9
Tachypnea	8
Pleural effusion	7
Wheezing	6
Apnea	1
Pneumothorax	1
Hemoptysis	1
Hepatic	
Jaundice	11
Ascites	4
Hepatomegaly	1
Hematologic	
Anemia	77
Thrombocytopenia	64
Leukopenia	34
Coagulation disorders	10
Leukocytosis	9
Eosinophilia	6
Lab test abnormalities	
Elevated bilirubin	64
BUN ↑	63
Serum creatinine ↑	61
Transaminase ↑	56
Alkaline phosphatase ↑	56
Hypomagnesemia	16
Acidosis	16
Hypocalcemia	15
Hypophosphatemia	11
Hypokalemia	9
Hyperuricemia	9
Hypoalbuminemia	8
Hypoproteinemia	7
Hyponatremia	4
Hyperkalemia	4
Alkalosis	4
Hypo/Hyperglycemia	2
Hypocholesterolemia	1
Hypercalcemia	1
Hypernatremia	1
Hyperphosphatemia	1
GI	
Nausea and vomiting	87
Diarrhea	76
Stomatitis	32
Anorexia	27
GI bleeding	13
(requiring surgery)	2
Dyspepsia	7
Constipation	5
Intestinal perforation/ileus	2
Pancreatitis	< 1
CNS	
Mental status changes	73
Dizziness	17
Sensory dysfunction	10
Disorders of vision, speech, taste	7
Syncope	3
Motor dysfunction	2
Coma	1
Seizure (grand mal)	1
Renal	
Oliguria/Anuria	76
Proteinuria	12
Hematuria	9
Dysuria	3
Renal impairment requiring dialysis	2
Urinary retention	1
Urinary frequency	1
Dermatologic	
Pruritus	48
Erythema	41
Rash	26
Dry skin	15
Exfoliative dermatitis	14
Purpura/Petechiae	4
Urticaria	2
Alopecia	1
Musculoskeletal	
Arthralgia	6
Myalgia	6
Arthritis	1
Muscle spasm	1
Miscellaneous	
Fever/Chills	89
Pain (all sites)	54
Abdominal	15
Chest	12
Back	9
Fatigue/Weakness/Malaise	53
Edema	47
Infection (including urinary tract, injection site, catheter tip, phlebitis, sepsis)	23
Weight gain (≥ 10%)	23
Headache	12
Weight loss (≥ 10%)	5
Conjunctivitis	4
Injection site reactions	3
Allergic reactions	1
Hypothyroidism	< 1

[1] 255 patients with renal cell cancer, 118 with other tumors receiving the recommended every 8 hour, 15 minute infusion dosing regimen.

ALDESLEUKIN (Interleukin-2; IL-2)

Other serious adverse events were derived from trials involving > 1800 patients treated with aldesleukin-based regimens. These events each occurred with a frequency of < 1% and included: Liver or renal failure resulting in death; duodenal ulceration; fatal intestinal perforation; bowel necrosis; fatal cardiac arrest, myocarditis and supraventricular tachycardia; permanent or transient blindness secondary to optic neuritis; fatal malignant hyperthermia; pulmonary edema resulting in death; respiratory arrest; fatal respiratory failure; fatal stroke; transient ischemic attack; meningitis; cerebral edema; pericarditis; allergic interstitial nephritis; tracheo-esophageal fistula; fatal pulmonary emboli; severe depression leading to suicide.

Overdosage:

Symptoms: Side effects following the use of aldesleukin are dose-related. Administration of more than the recommended dose has been associated with a more rapid onset of expected dose-limiting toxicities.

Treatment: Adverse reactions generally will reverse when the drug is stopped, particularly because its serum half-life is short. Treat any continuing symptoms supportively. Refer to General Management of Acute Overdosage. Life-threatening toxicities have been ameliorated by the IV administration of dexamethasone, which may result in loss of therapeutic effect of aldesleukin.

Administration and Dosage:

Approved by the FDA on May 5, 1992.

Administer by a 15 minute IV infusion every 8 hours. Before initiating treatment, carefully review the prescribing information, particularly regarding patient selection, possible serious adverse events, patient monitoring and withholding dosage.

Metastatic renal cell carcinoma in adults: Each course of treatment consists of two 5 day treatment cycles separated by a rest period:

1) 600,000 IU/kg (0.037 mg/kg) administered every 8 hours by a 15 minute IV infusion for a total of 14 doses. Following 9 days of rest, repeat the schedule for another 14 doses, for a maximum of 28 doses per course.

2) Patients treated with this schedule received a median of 20 of the 28 doses during the first course of therapy due to toxicity.

Retreatment: Evaluate patients for response approximately 4 weeks after completion of a course of therapy and again immediately prior to the scheduled start of the next treatment course. Additional courses of treatment may be given to patients only if there is some tumor shrinkage following the last course and retreatment is not contraindicated (see Contraindications). Separate each treatment course by a rest period of at least 7 weeks from the date of hospital discharge. Tumors have continued to regress up to 12 months following the initiation of therapy.

Dose modification: Accomplish dose modification for toxicity by holding or interrupting a dose rather than reducing the dose to be given. Decisions to stop, hold or restart therapy must be made after a global assessment of the patient with use the following guidelines:

Guidelines for Discontinuation of Aldesleukin Therapy

Organ system	Permanently discontinue treatment for the following toxicities:
Cardiovascular	Sustained ventricular tachycardia (≥ 5 beats) Cardiac rhythm disturbances not controlled or unresponsive Recurrent chest pain with ECG changes, documented angina or MI Pericardial tamponade
Pulmonary	Intubation required > 72 hours
Renal	Renal dysfunction requiring dialysis > 72 hours
CNS	Coma or toxic psychosis lasting > 48 hours Repetitive or difficult to control seizures
GI	Bowel ischemia/perforation/GI bleeding requiring surgery

ALDESLEUKIN (Interleukin-2; IL-2)

Guidelines for Held Doses and Subsequent Doses of Aldesleukin		
Organ system	Hold dose for:	Subsequent doses may be given if:
Cardiovascular	Atrial fibrillation, supraventricular tachycardia or bradycardia that requires treatment or is recurrent or persistent.	Patient is asymptomatic with full recovery to normal sinus rhythm.
	Systolic bp < 90 mm Hg with increasing needs for pressors.	Systolic bp ≥ 90 mm Hg and stable or improving needs for pressors.
	Any ECG change consistent with MI or ischemia with/without chest pain; suspicion of cardiac ischemia.	Patient is asymptomatic. MI has been ruled out, clinical suspicion of angina is low.
Pulmonary	O_2 saturation < 94% on room air or < 90% w/2 L O_2 by nasal prongs.	O_2 saturation ≥ 94% on room air or ≥90% w/2 L O_2 by nasal prongs.
CNS	Mental status changes, including moderate confusion or agitation.	Mental status changes completely resolved.
Systemic	Sepsis syndrome, patient is clinically unstable.	Sepsis syndrome has resolved, patient is clinically stable, infection is under treatment.
Renal	Serum creatinine ≥ 4.5 mg/dl or a serum creatinine of 4 mg/dl in the presence of severe volume overload, acidosis or hyperkalemia.	Serum creatinine < 4 mg/dl and fluid and electrolyte status is stable.
	Persistent oliguria, urine output of ≤ 10 ml/hr for 16 to 24 hours with rising serum creatinine.	Urine output > 10 ml/hour with a decrease of serum creatinine ≥ 1.5 mg/dl or normalization of serum creatinine.
Hepatic	Signs of hepatic failure including encephalopathy, increasing ascites, pain, hypoglycemia.	All signs of hepatic failure have resolved[1].
GI	Stool guaiac repeatedly 3 to 4+.	Stool guaiac negative.
Skin	Bullous dermatitis or marked worsening of preexisting skin condition (avoid topical steroid therapy).	Resolution of all signs of bullous dermatitis.

[1] Discontinue all further treatment for that course. Consider starting a new course of treatment at least 7 weeks after cessation of adverse event and hospital discharge.

Reconstitution and dilutions: Reconstitute and dilute only as recommended since the delivery or pharmacology of aldesleukin may be altered.

1) Each vial contains 22 million IU (1.3 mg) aldesleukin; reconstitute aseptically with 1.2 ml Sterile Water for Injection, USP. When reconstituted as directed, each ml contains 18 million IU (1.1 mg). The resulting solution should be a clear, colorless to slightly yellow liquid. The vial is for single-use only; discard unused portion.

2) During reconstitution, direct the Sterile Water for Injection, USP at the side of the vial and swirl the contents gently to avoid excess foaming. Do not shake.

3) Dilute the dose of aldesleukin reconstituted in Sterile Water for Injection, USP (without preservative) in 50 ml of 5% Dextrose Injection, USP and infuse over 15 minutes. Although glass bottles and plastic (polyvinyl chloride) bags have been used in clinical trials with comparable results, use plastic bags as the dilution container since experimental studies suggest that use of plastic containers results in more consistent drug delivery. Do not use in-line filters when administering aldesleukin.

4) Avoid reconstitution or dilution with Bacteriostatic Water for Injection, USP or 0.9% Sodium Chloride Injection, USP because of increased aggregation. Dilution with albumin can alter the pharmacology of aldesleukin. Do not mix with other drugs.

Storage/Stability: Before and after reconstitution and dilution, store vials in a refrigerator at 2° to 8°C (36° to 46°F). Do not freeze. Administer within 48 hours of reconstitution. Bring the solution to room temperature prior to infusion in the patient. This product contains no preservative; discard unused portion.

Rx	**Proleukin** (Chiron)	**Powder for Injection, lyophilized:** 22 x 10^6 IU per vial (18 million IU [1.1 mg] per ml when reconstituted).	In single-use vials (10s).[1]

[1] Preservative free. With 50 mg mannitol, 0.18 mg sodium dodecyl sulfate and 0.17 mg monobasic and 0.89 mg dibasic sodium phosphate.

PACLITAXEL

Warning:

Administer under the supervision of a physician experienced in the use of cancer chemotherapeutic agents. Appropriate management of complications is possible only when adequate diagnostic and treatment facilities are readily available.

Severe hypersensitivity reactions characterized by dyspnea and hypotension requiring treatment, angioedema and generalized urticaria have occurred in 2% of patients. One of these reactions was fatal in a patient treated without premedication in a Phase I study. Pretreat patients receiving paclitaxel with corticosteroids, diphenhydramine and H_2 antagonists to prevent these reactions (see Administration and Dosage). Patients who experience severe hypersensitivity reactions to paclitaxel should not be rechallenged with the drug.

Do not give paclitaxel therapy to patients with baseline neutrophil counts of < 1500 cells/mm^3. In order to monitor the occurrence of bone marrow suppression, primarily neutropenia, which may be severe and result in infection, perform frequent peripheral blood cell counts on all patients receiving paclitaxel.

Actions:

Pharmacology: Paclitaxel is a natural product with antitumor activity. It is a novel antimicrotubule agent that promotes the assembly of microtubules from tubulin dimers and stabilizes microtubules by preventing depolymerization. This stability results in the inhibition of the normal dynamic reorganization of the microtubule network that is essential for vital interphase and mitotic cellular functions. In addition, paclitaxel induces abnormal arrays or "bundles" of microtubules throughout the cell cycle and multiple esters of microtubules during mitosis.

Pharmacokinetics: Following IV administration, the drug exhibits a biphasic decline in plasma concentrations. The initial rapid decline represents distribution to the peripheral compartment and significant elimination of the drug. The later phase is due, in part, to a relatively slow efflux of paclitaxel from the peripheral compartment. Following 1, 3, 6 and 24 hour infusions at dosing levels of 15 to 275 mg/m^2, mean terminal half-life ranges from 513.1 to 52.7 hours, mean values for total body clearance range from 12.2 to 23.8 L/hr/m^2, and the mean steady-state volume of distribution ranges from 227 to 688 L/m^2, indicating extensive extravascular distribution or tissue binding of paclitaxel. The drug is 89% to 98% protein bound. With a 24–hour infusion, a 30% increase in dose increased the C_{max} by 87%; with a 3–hour infusion, a 30% dose increase resulted in a 68% increase in C_{max}.

The disposition of paclitaxel has not been fully elucidated. After IV administration of 15 to 275 mg/m^2 doses as 1, 6 and 24 hour infusions, mean values for cumulative urinary recovery of unchanged drug range from 1.3% to 12.6% of the dose, indicating extensive non-renal clearance. Paclitaxel is metabolized in the liver in animals and there is evidence suggesting hepatic metabolism in humans. High paclitaxel concentrations have occurred in the bile of patients treated with paclitaxel. The effect of renal or hepatic dysfunction on the disposition of paclitaxel has not been investigated.

Clinical trials:

Ovarian carcinoma – Two studies (n = 92) utilized an initial dose of 135 to 170 mg/m^2 in most patients (> 90%) administered over 24 hours by continuous infusion. Response rates in these two studies were 22% and 30% with a total of six complete and 18 partial responses in 92 patients. The median duratio of overall response in these two studies measured from the first day of treatment was 7.2 months and 7.5 months, respectively. The median survival was 8.1 months and 15.9 months.

Breast carcinoma – In data from several trials utilizing either a 3 or 24 hour infusion of 135 to 175 mg/m^2 or 200 to 250 mg/m^2, respectively, response rates were 26% and 30% to 57%, respectively. In the 3–hour infusion study, median duration of response was 8.1 months; median survival was 11.7 monhts.

In general, the results of the studies performed at initial doses of 135 to 170 mg/m^2 were similar to results from three other studies in patients with ovarian carcinoma using higher initial doses and, in two of the studies, concomitant administration of filgrastim.

The effect of paclitaxel was similar in the subset of patients who had developed resistance to platinum-containing therapy (defined as tumor progression while on, or tumor relapse within 6 months from completion of, a platinum-containing regimen) to the effect in patients overall.

Indications:

Ovarian carcinoma: Treatment of metastatic carcinoma of the ovary after failure of first-line or subsequent chemotherapy.

Breast carcinoma: Treatment of breast cancer after failure of combination chemotherapy for metastatic disease or relapse within 6 months of adjuvant chemotherapy. Prior therapy should have included an anthracycline unless clinically contraindicated.

Unlabeled uses: Paclitaxel, alone or in combination with other chemotherapy agents, is being investigated for use in the following conditions: Advanced head and neck cancer; previously untreated extensive-stage small-cell lung cancer; adenocarcinoma of the upper GI tract; hormone-refractory prostate cancer; advanced non-small-cell lung cancer; leukemias. Further study is needed.

Contraindications:

Hypersensitivity reactions to paclitaxel or other drugs formulated in Cremophor EL (polyoxyethylated castor oil) (see Warnings); patients with baseline neutropenia of < 1500 cells/mm^3 (see Warnings).

Warnings:

Bone marrow suppression (primarily neutropenia) is dose-dependent and is the major dose-limiting toxicity. Neutropenia is generally rapidly reversible. Neutrophil nadirs occurred at a median of 11 days. Do not administer to patients with baseline neutrophil counts of < 1500 cells/mm^3. Institute frequent monitoring of blood counts during treatment. Do not retreat with subsequent cycles of paclitaxel until neutrophils recover to a level of > 1500 cells/mm^3 and platelets recover to a level > 100,000 cells/mm^3. In the case of severe neutropenia (< 500 cells/mm^3 for ≥ 7 days) during a course of therapy, a 20% reduction in dose for subsequent courses of therapy is recommended.

Cardiac effects: Severe conduction abnormalities have been documented in (< 1%) patients during therapy. If patients develop significant conduction abnormalities during administration, administer appropriate therapy and perform continuous cardiac monitoring during subsequent therapy.

Hypersensitivity: Do not use in patients with a history of severe hypersensitivity reactions to products containing Cremophor EL. Pretreat all patients with corticosteroids, diphenhydramine and H_2 antagonists before administering paclitaxel to avoid the occurrence of severe hypersensitivity reactions. Severe hypersensitivity reactions characterized by dyspnea and hypotension requiring treatment, angioedema and generalized urticaria have occurred in 2% of patients and require immediate discontinuation of paclitaxel and aggressive symptomatic therapy. Refer to Management of Acute Hypersensitivity Reactions.These reactions are probably histamine-mediated. One of these reactions was fatal in a patient with pulmonary metastases. This patient received no premedication; the first course of paclitaxel, which was uneventful, was administered at 190 mg/m^2 infused over 3 hours. Within a few minutes from the beginning of a second course, the patient developed severe hypotension and died. Patients who experience severe hypersensitivity reactions to paclitaxel should not be rechallenged with the drug. Minor symptoms such as flushing, skin reactions, dyspnea, hypotension or tachycardia do not require interruption of therapy.

Hepatic function impairment: There is no evidence that the toxicity of paclitaxel is enhanced in patients with elevated liver enzymes. However, evidence suggests that the liver plays an important role in the metabolism of paclitaxel. Therefore, exercise caution when administering to patients with severe hepatic impairment.

Mutagenesis/Fertility impairment: Paclitaxel is mutagenic in vitro (chromosome aberrations in human lymphocytes) and in vivo (micronucleus test in mice) mammalian test systems; however, it did not induce mutagenicity in the Ames test of the CHO/HGPRT gene mutation assay.

At an IV dose of 1 mg/kg (6 mg/m^2), paclitaxel produced low fertility and fetal toxicity in rats.

Pregnancy: Category D. Paclitaxel may cause fetal harm when administered to a pregnant woman. It is embryo- and fetotoxic in rats and rabbits and decreases fertility in rats. In these studies, paclitaxel resulted in abortions, decreased corpora lutea, decreased implantations and live fetuses, and increased resorptions and embryo-fetal deaths. No gross external, soft tissue or skeletal alterations occurred. There are no studies in pregnant women. If paclitaxel is used during pregnancy, or if the patient becomes pregnant while receiving this drug, apprise the patient of the potential hazard. Advise women of childbearing potential to avoid becoming pregnant during therapy with paclitaxel.

Lactation: It is not known whether the drug is excreted in breast milk. Because of the potential for serious adverse reactions in nursing infants, discontinue nursing when receiving paclitaxel therapy.

Children: Safety and efficacy of paclitaxel in children have not been established.

Precautions:

PVC equipment: Contact of the undiluted concentrate of paclitaxel with plasticized polyvinyl chloride (PVC) equipment or devices used to prepare solutions for infusion is not recommended (see Administration and Dosage).

Cardiovascular: Hypotension and bradycardia have been observed during paclitaxel administration, but generally do not require treatment. Frequently monitor vital signs, particularly during the first hour of infusion. Continuous cardiac monitoring is not required except for patients with serious conduction abnormalities (see Warnings).

CNS: Although the occurrence of peripheral neuropathy is frequent, the development of severe symptomatology is unusual and requires a dose reduction of 20% for all subsequent courses of paclitaxel.

Drug Interactions:

Paclitaxel Drug Interactions

Precipitant drug	Object drug*		Description
Paclitaxel	Cisplatin	⬆	In a Phase I trial using escalating doses of paclitaxel (110 to 200 mg/m^2) and cisplatin (50 or 75 mg/m^2) given as sequential infusions, myelosuppression was more profound when paclitaxel was given after cisplatin than with paclitaxel before cisplatin. Pharmacokinetic data from these patients demonstrated a decrease in paclitaxel clearance of ≈ 33% when paclitaxel was administered following cisplatin.
Ketoconazole	Paclitaxel	⬇	Based on in vitro data, there is the possibility of an inhibition of paclitaxel metabolism in patients treated with ketoconazole. As a result, use caution when treating patients with paclitaxel when they are receiving concurrent ketoconazole.

* ⬆ = Object drug increased. ⬇ = Object drug decreased.

Adverse Reactions:

Data in the following table are based on the experience of patients with carcinoma of the ovary and of the breast.

Paclitaxel Adverse Reactions

Adverse reactions	Incidence (n = 812)
Bone marrow	
Neutropenia < 2000/mm^3	90%
< 500/mm^3	52%
Leukopenia < 4000/mm^3	90%
< 1000/mm^3	17%
Thrombocytopenia < 100,000/mm^3	20%
< 50,000/mm^3	7%
Anemia < 11 g/dl	78%
< 8 g/dl	16%
Infections	30%
Bleeding	14%
Red cell transfusions	25%
Platelet transfusions	2%
Hypersensitivity reaction	
All	41%
Severe	2%

Paclitaxel Adverse Reactions

Adverse reactions	Incidence (n = 812)
Cardiovascular	
Bradycardia[1]	3%
Hypotension[1]	12%
Severe cardiovascular events	1%
Abnormal ECG	
All patients	23%
Patients with normal baseline (n = 559)	14%
Peripheral neuropathy	
Any symptoms	60%
Severe symptoms	3%
Myalgia/Arthralgia	
Any symptoms	60%
Severe symptoms	8%
GI	
Nausea and vomiting	52%
Diarrhea	38%
Mucositis	31%
Hepatic (Patients with normal base line and on study data)	
Bilirubin elevations (n = 765)	7%
Alkaline phosphatase elevations (n = 575)	22%
AST elevations (n = 591)	19%
Miscellaneous	
Alopecia	87%
Injection site reaction	13%

[1] During first 3 hours of infusion.

Hematologic: Bone marrow suppression was the major dose limiting toxicity. Neutropenia, the most important hematologic toxicity, was dose- and schedule-dependent and was generally rapidly reversible. Among patients treated with a 3–hour infusion, neutrophil counts declinced below 500 cells/mm^3 in 13% of the patients treated with a dose of 135 mg/m^2 compared with 27% at a dose of 175 mg/m^2. Severe neutropenia (< 500/mm^3) was more frequent with the 24–hour than with the 3–hour infusion; infusion duration had a greater impact on myelosuppression than dose. Neutropenia did not appear to increase with cumulative exposure and did not appear to be more frequent nor more severe for patients previously treated iwht radiation therapy.

Fever was frequent (12% of all treatment courses). Infectious episodes occurred in 30% of all patients and 9% of all courses; these episodes were fatal in 1% of all patients, and included sepsis, pneumonia and peritonitis. Infectious episodes were reported in 19% of the patients given either 135 or 175 mg/m^2 dose by a 3–hour infusion. Urinary tract infections and upper respiratory tract infections were the most frequently reported infectious complications.

Thrombocytopenia was uncommon, and almost never severe (< 50,000 cells/mm^3); 20% of the patients experienced a drop in their platelet count below 100,000 cells/mm^3 at least once while on treatment; 7% had a platelet count < 50,000 cells/mm^3 at the time of their worst nadir. Among the 812 patients, bleeding episodes were reported in 4% of all courses and by 14% of all patients but most of the hemorrhagic episodes were localized and the frequency of these events was unrelated to the dose and schedule. Bleeding episodes were reported in 10% of the patients receiving either the 135 or 175 mg/m^2 dose given by a 3–hour infusion; no patients treated with the 3–hour infusion received platelet transfusions.

Anemia (Hgb < 11 g/dl) was observed in 78% of all patients and was severe (Hgb < 8 g/dl) in 16% of cases. No consistent relationship between dose or schedule and the frequency of anemia was observed. Among all patients with normal baseline hemoglobin, 69% became anemic on study but only 7% had severe anemia. Red cell transfusions were required in 25% of all patients and in 12% of those with normal baseline hemoglobin levels.

Hypersensitivity: (See Warnings.) The frequency and severity werwe not affected by the dose or schedule. The 3–hour infusion was not associated with a greater increase in reactions when compared with the 24–hour infusion. Hypersensitivity reactions were observed in 20% of all courses and in 41% of all patients. These reactions were severe in < 2% of the patients and 1% of the courses. No severe reactions were observed after course 3 and severe symptoms occurred generally within the first hour of infusion. The most frequent symptoms observed during these severe reactions were dyspnea, flushing, chest pain and tachycardia.

The minor hypersensitivity reactions consisted mostly of flushing (28%), rash (12%), hypotension(4%), dyspnea, tachycardia (2%) and hypertension (1%). The frequency of hypersensitivity reactions remained relatively stable during the entire treatment period.

Cardiovascular:

Hypotension during the first 3 hours of infusion occurred in 12% of all patients and 3% of all courses administered. Bradycardia during the first 3 hours of infusion occurred in 3% of all patients and 1% of all courses. Neither dose nor schedule had an effect on the frequency of hypotension and bradycardia. These vital sign changes most often caused no symptoms and required niether specific therapy nor treatment discontinuation. The frequency of hypotension and bradycardia were not influenced by prior anthracycline therapy.

Significant cardiovascular events occurred in ≈ 1% of all patients. These events included syncope, rhythm abnormalities, hypertension and venous thrombosis. One of the patients with syncope treated with 175 mg/m^2 over 24 hours had progressive hypotension and died. The arrhythmias included asymptomatic ventricular tachycardia, bigeminy and complete AV block requiring pacemaker placement.

ECG abnormalities were common among patients at baseline. ECG abnormalities on study did not usually result in symptoms, were not dose-limiting, and required no intervention. ECG abnormalities were noted in 23% of all patients. Among patients with a normal ECG prior to study entry, 14% of all patients developed an abnormal tracing while on study. The most frequently reported ECG modifications were non-specific repolarization abnormalities, sinus bradycardia, sinus tachycardia and premature beats. Among patients with normal ECG at baseline, prior therapy with anthracyclines did not influence the frequency of ECG abnormalities.

CNS: The frequency and severity of neurologic manifestations were dose-dependent, but were not influenced by infusion duration. Peripheral neuropathy was observed in 60% of all patients (3% severe) and in 52% (2% severe) of the patients without pre-existing neuropathy.

The frequency of peripheral neuropathy increased with cumulative dose. Neurologic symptoms were observed in 27% of the patients after the first course of treatment and in 34% to 51% from course 2 to 10.

Peripheral neuropathy was the cause of discontinuation in 1% of all patients. Sensory symptoms have usually improved or resolved within several months of discontinuation. The incidence of neurologic symptoms did not increase in the subset of patients previously treated with cisplatin. Pre-existing neuropathies resulting from prior therapies are not a contraindication for therapy.

Other than peripheral neuropathy, serious neurologic events following administration have been rare (< 1%), and have included grand mal seizures, syncope, ataxia, neuroencephalopathy and autonomic neuropathy resulting in paralytic ileus.

Musculoskeletal: There was no consistent relationship between dose or schedule and the frequency or severity of arthralgia/myalgia; 60% of all patients treated experienced arthralgia/myalgia; 8% experienced severe symptoms. The symptoms were usually transient, occurred 2 or 3 days after administration, and resolved within a few days. The frequency and severity of musculoskeletal symptoms remained unchanged throughout the treatment period.

Hepatic: No relationship was observed between liver function abnormalities and either dose or schedule of administration. Among patients with normal baseline liver function 7%, 22% and 19% had elevations in bilirubin, alkaline phosphatase and AST, respectively. Prolonged exposure was not associated with cumulative hepatic toxicity. Hepatic necrosis/encephalopathy leading to death have occurrerd (rare).

GI: Nausea/vomiting (52%), diarrhea (38%) and mucositis (31%). These manifestations were usually mild to moderate. Mucositis was schedule-dependent and occurred more frequently with the 24–hour than with the 3–hour infusion. Rare reports of intestinal obstruction, intestinal perforation and ischemic colitis have occurred.

Local: Injection site reactions, including reactions secondary to extravasation, were usually mild and consisted of erythema, tenderness, skin discoloration or swelling at the injection site. These reactions have been observed more frequently with 24–hour infusion than with 3–hour infusion. A specific treatment for extravasation reactions is unknown at this time. Rare reports of more severe events such as phlebitis and cellulitis have occurred.

PACLITAXEL

Miscellaneous: Alopecia was observed in almost all (87%) of the patients. Transient skin changes due to paclitaxel-related hypersensitivity reactions have been observed, but no other skin toxicities were significantly associated with administration. Nail changes (changes in pigmentation or discoloration of nail bed) were uncommon (2%). Edema was reported in 21% of all patients (17% of those without baseline edema); only 1% had severe edema and none of these patients required treatment discontinuation. Edema was observed in 5% of all courses for patients with normal baseline and did not increase with time on study. Rare reports of skin abnormalities related to radiation recall have occurred.

Overdosage:

There is no known antidote for paclitaxel overdosage. The primary anticipated complications of overdosage would consist of bone marrow suppression, peripheral neurotoxicity and mucositis.

Administration and Dosage:

Approved by the FDA on December 29, 1992.

Premedicate all patients prior to administration in order to prevent severe hypersensitivity reactions. Such premedication may consist of oral dexamethasone 20 mg administered approximately 12 and 6 hours before paclitaxel, diphenhydramine (or its equivalent) 50 mg IV 30 to 60 minutes prior to paclitaxel, and cimetidine (300 mg) or ranitidine (50 mg) IV 30 to 60 minutes before paclitaxel.

Dosage:

Ovarian carcinoma – 135 mg/m^2 administered IV over 24 hours every 3 weeks is effective in patients with metastatic carcinoma of the ovary after failure of first-line or subsequent chemotherapy. Larger doses, with or without filgrastim, have so far produced responses similar to 135 mg/m^2.

Breast carcinoma: 175 mg/m^2 IV over 3 hours every 3 weeks is effective after failure of chemotherapy for metastatic disease or relapse within 6 months of adjuvant chemotherapy.

Do not repeat courses of paclitaxel until the neutrophil count is at least 1500 cells/mm^3 and the platelet count is at least 100,000 cells/mm^3. Reduce dosage by 20% for subsequent courses in patients who experience severe neutropenia (neutrophils < 500 cells/mm^3 for ≥ 1 week) or severe peripheral neuropathy during therapy. The incidence and severity of neurotoxicity and hematologic toxicity increase with dose, especially > 190 mg/m^2.

Preparation and administration precautions: Paclitaxel is a cytotoxic anticancer drug and, as with other potentially toxic compounds, exercise caution in handling the drug. The use of gloves is recommended. If paclitaxel solution contacts the skin, wash the skin immediately and thoroughly with soap and water. If paclitaxel contacts mucous membranes, thoroughly flush the membranes with water.

Preparation for IV administration: Paclitaxel concentrate must be diluted prior to infusion in 0.9% Sodium Chloride Injection, USP; 5% Dextrose Injection, USP; 5% Dextrose and 0.9% Sodium Chloride Injection, USP; or 5% Dextrose in Ringer's Injection to a final concentration of 0.3 to 1.2 mg/ml. The solutions are physically and chemically stable for up to 24 hours at ambient temperature (≈ 25°C; 77°F) and room lighting conditions.

Upon preparation, solutions may show haziness, which is attributed to the formulation vehicle. No significant losses in potency have been noted following simulated delivery of the solution through IV tubing containing an in-line (0.22 micron) filter.

Administer through an in-line filter with a microporous membrane not greater than 0.22 microns. Use of filter devices such as Ivex-2 filters, which incorporate short inlet and outlet PVC-coated tubing, has not resulted in significant leaching of DEHP (di-[2–ethylhexyl]phthalate).

PACLITAXEL

Contact of the undiluted concentrate with plasticized PVC equipment or devices used to prepare solutions for infusion is not recommended. In order to minimize patient exposure to the plasticizer DEHP [di-(2-ethylhexyl)phthalate], which may be leached from PVC infusion bags or sets, store diluted paclitaxel solutions in bottles (glass, polypropylene) or plastic bags (polypropylene, polyolefin) and administer through polyethylene-lined administration sets.

Storage/Stability: Unopened vials of paclitaxel for injection concentrate are stable until the date indicated on the package when stored under refrigeration (2° to 8°C; 36° to 46°F) in the original package. Upon refrigeration, components in the vial may precipitate, but will redissolve upon reaching room temperature with little or no agitation. There is no impact on product quality. If the solution remains cloudy or if an insoluble precipitate is noted, discard the vial. Retain in the original package to protect from light. Freezing does not adversely affect the product. Solutions for infusion prepared as recommended are stable at ambient temperature (≈ 25°C; 77°F) and lighting conditions for up to 27 hours.

Rx	**Taxol** (Bristol-Myers Squibb)	**Injection:** 30 mg/5 ml	In single-dose vials.[1]

[1] With 527 mg/ml polyoxyethylated castor oil *(Cremophor EL)* and 49.7% dehydrated alcohol, USP.

DOCETAXEL

Warning:

The incidence of treatment-related mortality associated with docetaxel is increased in patients with abnormal liver function and in patients receiving higher doses.

Docetaxel should generally not be given to patients with bilirubin > upper limit of normal (ULN), or to patients with AST or ALT > 1.5 × ULN concomitant with alkaline phosphatase (AP) > 2.5 × ULN. Patients with elevations of bilirubin or abnormalities of transminases concurrent with alkaline phosphatase are at increased risk for the development of grade 4 neutropenia, febrile neutropenia, infections, severe thrombocytopenia, severe stomatitis, severe skin toxicity and toxic death. Patients with isolated elevations of transaminases > 1.5 × ULN also had a higher rate of febrile neutropenia grade 4 but did not have an increased incidence of toxic death.

Do not give to patients with neutrophil counts of < 1500 cells/mm^3.

Severe hypersensitivity reactions characterized by hypotension or bronchospasm or generalized rash/erythema occurred in 0.9% of patients who received the recommended dexamethasone premedication. Hypersensitivity reactions requiring discontinuation of the docetaxel infusion were reported in five patients who did not receive premedication. These reactions resolved after discontinuation of the infusion and the administration of appropriate therapy. Docetaxel must not be given to patients who have a history of severe hypersensitivity reactions to docetaxel or other drugs formulated with polysorbate 80.

Severe fluid retention occurred in 6% of patients despite use of a 5–day dexamethasone premedication regimen. It was characterized by one or more of the following events: Poorly tolerated peripheral edema, generalized edema, pleural effusion requiring urgent drainage, dyspnea at rest, cardiac tamponade or pronounced abdominal distention (due to ascites).

Actions:

Pharmacology: Docetaxel is an antineoplastic agent belonging to the taxoid family. It is prepared by semisynthesis beginning with a precursor extracted from the renewable needle biomass of the yew plant. It acts by disrupting the microtubular network in cells that is essential for mitotic and interphase cellular functions. Docetaxel binds to free tubulin and promotes the assembly of tubulin into stable microtubules while simultaneously inhibiting their disassembly. This leads to the production of microtubules bundles without normal function and to the stabilization of microtubules, which results in teh inhibition of mitosis in cells. Docetaxel's binding to microtubules does not alter the number of protofilaments in the bound microtubules, a feature which differs from most spindle poisons currently in clinical use.

Pharmacokinetics: The area under the curve (AUC) was dose proportional following doses of 70 to 115 mg/m^2 with infusion times of 1 to 2 hours. Docetaxel's pharmacokinetic profile is consistent with a three compartment pharmacokinetic model, with half-lives for the α, β, and γ phases of 4 min, 36 min and 11.1 hr, respectively. The initial rapid decline represents distribution to the peripheral compartments and the late (terminal) phase is due, in part, to a relatively slow efflux of docetaxel from the peripheral compartment. Mean values for total body clearance and steady-state volume of distribution were 21 L/hr/m^2 and 113 L, respectively.

Docetaxel is eliminated in both the urine and feces following oxidative metabolism of the tert-butyl ester group, but fecal excretion was the main elimination route. Within 7 days, urinary and fecal excretion accounted for ≈ 6 % and 75% of the administered radioactivity, respectively. About 80% of the radioactivity recovered iin feces is excreted during the first 48 hours as one major and three minor metabolites with very small amounts (< 8%) of unchanged drug. Based on in vitro studies, isoenzymes of the cytochrome P4503A (CYP 3A) subfamily appear to be involved in docetaxel metabolism. In vitro studies showed that docetaxel is ≈ 94% protein bound, mainly to α_1-acid glycoprotein, albumin and lipoproteins.

Hepatic function impairment – In patients with clinical chemistry data suggestive of mild to moderate liver function impairment (AST or ALT > 1.5 × ULN concomitant with alkaline phosphatase > 2.5 × ULN), total body clearance was lowered by an average of 27%, resulting in a 38% increase in systemic exposure (AUC). However, this average includes a substantial range and there is, at present, no measurement that would allow recommendation for dose adjustment in such patients.

Clinical trials: Docetaxel was evaluated in 134 patients with anthracycline-resistant, locally advanced or metastatic breast carcinoma. Anthracycline resistance was defined as progressive disease on anthracyclines for advanced disease or relapse on anthracycline adjuvant therapy. Docetaxel was administered at a 100 mg/m^2 dose given as a 1–hour infusion every 3 weeks. The overall response rate (ORR) considering all patients (intent-to-treat) was 41% and the complete response (CR) was 2%. The median survival time was 43 weeks. In the evaluable patients, the ORR was 47% and the CR was 2.8%.

Indications:

Breast cancer: For the treatment of patients with locally advanced or metastatic breast cancer who have progressed during anthracycline-based therapy or have relapsed during anthracycline-based adjuvant therapy.

Contraindications:

History of severe hypersensitivity reactions to docetaxel or to other drugs formulated with polysorbate 80; neutrophil counts of < 1500 cells/mm^3.

Warnings:

Toxic deaths: Docetaxel administered as 100 mg/m^2 was associated with deaths considered possibly or probably related to treatment in 2.4% of patients with normal liver function and in 11% of patients with abnormal liver function (AST or ALT > 1.5 × ULN together with AP < 2.5 × ULN). Among patients dosed at 60 mg/m^2, mortality related to treatment occurred in 0.6% of patients with normal liver function and in 3 of 7 patients with abnormal liver function. Approximately half of these deaths occurred during the first cycle. Sepsis accounted for the majority of the deaths.

Fluid retention: Premedicate patients with oral corticosteroids such as dexamethasone 16 mg/day for 5 days starting 1 day prior to docetaxel to reduce the severity of fluid retention and hypersensitivity reactions (see Warning Box).

Neutropenia: Neutropenia (< 2000 neutrophils/mm^3) occurs in virtually all patients given 60 to 100 mg/m^2 of docetaxel and grade 4 neutropenia (< 500 cells/mm^3) occurs in nearly all patients given 100 mg/m^2 and 75% to 80% of patients given 60 to 75 mg/m^2. Frequent monitoring of blood counts is, therefore, essential so that dose can be adjusted. Do not administer to patients with neutrophils < 1500 cells/mm^3. Febrile neutropenia occurred in about 12% of patients given 100 mg/m^2 but was very uncommon in patients given 60 to 75 mg/m^2.

Cutaneous reactions: Reversible cutaneous reactions characterized by a rash including localized eruptions, mainly on the feet or hands, but also on the arms, face or thorax, usually associated with pruritus, have been observed. Eruptions generally occurred within 1 week after infusion, recovered before the next infusion and were not disabling. Severe symptoms, such as eruptions followed by desquamation, occurred in 5.6% of patients and rarely led to interruption of discontinuation.

Hypersensitivity: Observe patients closely for hypersensitivity reactions. Hypersensitivity reactions may occur within a few minutes following initiation of a docetaxel infusion. If minor reactions such as flushing or localized skin reactions occur, interruption of therapy is not required. All patients should be premedicated with an oral corticosteroid prior to the initiation of the infusion of docetaxel (see Warning Box).

Hepatic function impairment: Three breast cancer patients with severe liver impairment (bilirubin > 1.7 × ULN) developed fatal GI bleeding associated with severe drug-induced thrombocytopenia (see Warning Box).

Pregnancy: Category D. Docetaxel can cause fetal harm when administered to pregnant women. There are no adequate and well controlled studies in pregnant women using docetaxel. If docetaxel is used during pregnancy, or if the patient becomes pregnant while receiving this drug, apprise the patient of the potential hazard to the fetus or potential risk for loss of the pregnancy. Advise women of childbearing potential to avoid becoming pregnant during therapy.

Lactation: It is not known whether docetaxel is excreted in breast milk. Because of the potential for serious adverse reactions in nursing infants from docetaxel, mothers should discontinue nursing prior to taking the drug.

Children: Safety and efficacy in children < 16 years of age have not been established.

Precautions:

Monitoring: To monitor the occurrence of myelotoxicity, it is recommended that frequent peripheral blood cell counts be performed on all patients (see Warnings).

Obtain bilirubin, AST or ALT and alkaline phosphatase values prior to each cycle of docetaxel therapy.

Neurologic: Severe neurosensory symptoms (paresthesia, dysesthesia, pain) were observed among 7% of patients with anthracycline-resistant breast cancer. When these occur, dosage must be adjusted. If symptoms persist, discontinue treatment.

Asthenia: Severe asthenia has been reported in 11.1% of the patients but has led to treatment discontinuation in only 2.6%. It was reported in 23% of patients with anthracycline-resistant breast cancer and 5.5% of cycles received. Fatigue and weakness may last from a few days to several weeks and may be associated with deterioration of performance status in patients with progressive disease.

DOCETAXEL

Drug Interactions:

In vitro studies have shown that the metabolism of docetaxel may be modified by concomitant administration of compounds that induce, inhibit or are metabolized by cytochrome P450 3A4, such as cyclosporine, terfenadine, ketoconazole, erythromycin and troleandomycin. Exercise caution with these drugs when treating patients receiving docetaxel as there is a potential for a significant interaction.

Adverse Reactions:

Docetaxel Adverse Reactions (%)_		
Adverse reactions	Normal LFTs[1] at baseline (n = 1435)	Elevated LFTs at baseline (n = 55)
Hematologic[2]		
Neutropenia		
<2000 cells/mm³	96.3	96
< 500 cells/mm³	76	86
Leukopenia		
< 4000 cells/mm³	96.5	98.1
< 1000 cells/mm³	31	44.2
Thrombocytopenia		
< 100,000 cells/mm³	7.5	27.3
Anemia		
< 11 g/dl	89.5	92.7
< 8g/dl	8.4	30.9
Febrile neutropenia	11.8	26.4
GI [2]		
Nausea	40.4	40
Diarrhea	40.4	32.7
Vomiting	24	25.5
Stomatitis		
any	42.3	47.3
severe	5.3	14.5
Musculoskeletal		
Myalgia		
any	19.4	18.2
severe	1.4	1.9
Arthralgia	8.6	7.3
Dermatologic		
Cutaneous[2]		
any	58.5	61.8
severe	5.6	10.9
Nail changes		
any	28.2	18.2
severe	2.6	4.6
Miscellanous		
Septic death	1.8	3.6
Nonseptic death	0.6	7.3
Infections		
any	21.7	32.7
severe	5.6	16.4
Fever in absence of infection		
any	30.2	50.9
severe	1.7	9.1
Hypersensitivity reaction[2] w/premedication	(n = 229)	(n = 6)
any	15.7	0
severe	0.9	0
Fluid retention [2]w/premedication	(n = 229)	(n = 6)
any	48.5	66.7
severe	5.2	33.3
Neurosensory[2]		
any	53.7	41.8
severe	3.9	0

DOCETAXEL

Docetaxel Adverse Reactions (%)_		
Adverse reactions	Normal LFTs[1] at baseline (n = 1435)	Elevated LFTs at baseline (n = 55)
Neuromotor (eg, distal extremity weakness)		
any	13.4	5.5
severe	3.7	1.8
Alopecia	80	61.8
Asthenia		
any	61.5	54.5
severe	11.1	23.6
Infusion site reacions	5.6	3.6

[1] Liver function tests.
[2] See Warnings.

Cardiovascular: Hypotension (3.6%, 3.4% required treatment); atrial fibrillation, deep vein thrombosis, ECG abnormalities, thrombocytopenia, pulmonary embolism, syncope, tachycardia, heart failure, sinus tachycardia, atrial flutter, dysrhythmia, unstable angina, pulmonary edem,a, hypertension (rare).

Infusion site reactions: Hyperpigmentation, inflammation, redness or dryness of the skin, phlebitis, extravasation, swelling of the vein (mild).

Hepatic: Increased ALT and AST (see Warnings).

GI: Constipation, ulcer, esophagitis, GI hemorrhage, intestinal obstruction, ileus.

Respiratory: Dyspnea, acute pulmonary edema, acute respiratory distress syndrome.

Miscellaneous: Abdominal pain, diffuse pain, chest pain, confusion, renal insufficiency.

Overdosage:

In case of overdosage, keep patient in a specialized unit where vital functions can be closely monitored. Anticipated complications of overdosage include: Bone marrow suppression, peripheral neurotoxicity and mucositis.

There were two reports of overdose. One patient received 150 mg/m^2 as 1–hour infusions. Both patients experienced severe neutropenia, mild asthenia, cutaneous reactions and mild paresthesia and recovered.

Administration and Dosage:

Approved by the FDA on May 14, 1996.

Recommended dose: 60 to 100 mg/m^2 administered IV over 1 hour every 3 weeks.

Premedication regimen: Premedicate patients with oral corticosteroids (see Warnings).

Dosage adjustment during treatment: Patients who are dosed initially at 100 mg/m^2 and who experience either febrile neutropenia, neutrophils < 500 cells/mm^3 for > 1 week, severe or cumulative cutaneous reactions or severe peripheral neuropathy during docetaxel therapy should have the dosage adjusted from 100 to 75 mg/m^2. If the patient continues to experience these reactions, either decrease the dosage from 75 to 55 mg/m^2 or discontinue treatment. Patients who are dosed at 60 mg/m^2 and do not experience these symptoms may tolerate higher doses.

Preparation of solution: Dilution is required prior to administration. Dilute with 0.9% Sodium Chloride Injection or 5% Dextrose Injection.

Storage/Stability: Refrigerate at 2° to 8°C (36° to 46°F) and protect from light. Stand vials at room temperature for ≈ 5 minutes before using. Do not store in PVC bags. The premixed solution is stable for 8 hours either at room temperature, 15° to 25°C (59° to 77°F), or stored refrigerated, 2° to 8°C (36° to 46°F).

Rx	**Taxotere** (Rhone-Poulenc Rorer)	**Injection:** 20 mg	In 0.5 ml polysorbate 80. In single dose vials with diluent.
		80 mg	In 2 ml polysorbate 80. In single dose vials with diluent.

TRETINOIN

Warning:

Experienced physician and institution: Patients with acute promyelocytic leukemia (APL) are at high risk in general and can have severe adverse reactions to tretinoin. Therefore, administer under the supervision of a physician who is experienced in the management of patients with acute leukemia and in a facility with laboratory and supportive services sufficient to monitor drug tolerance and to protect and maintain a patient compromised by drug toxicity, including respiratory compromise. Use of tretinoin requires that the physician concludes that the possible benefit to the patient outweighs the following adverse effects.

Retinoic acid-APL syndrome: About 25% of APL patients treated with tretinoin have experienced a syndrome called the retinoic acid-APL (RA-APL) syndrome characterized by fever, dyspnea, weight gain, radiographic pulmonary infiltrates and pleural or pericardial effusions. This syndrome has occasionally been accompanied by impaired myocardial contractility and episodic hypotension. It has been observed with or without concomitant leukocytosis. Endotracheal intubation and mechanical ventilation have been required in some cases due to progressive hypoxemia, and several patients have expired with multi-organ failure. The syndrome generally occurs during the first month of treatment, with some cases reported following the first dose.

The management of the syndrome has not been defined rigorously, but high-dose steroids given at the first suspicion of the RA-APL syndrome appear to reduce morbitity and mortality. At the first signs suggestive of the syndrome (unexplained fever, dyspnea or weight gain, abnormal chest auscultatory findings or radiographic abnormalities), immediately initiate high-dose steroids (dexamethasone 10 mg IV) every 12 hours for 3 days or until the resolution of symptoms, regardless of the leukocyte count. The majority of patients do not require termination of tretinoin therapy during treatment of the RA-APL syndrome.

Leukocytosis: During treatment, ≈ 40% of patients will develop rapidly evolving leukocytosis. Patients who present with high WBC at diagnosis ($> 5 \times 10^9$/L) have an increased risk of a further rapid increase in WBC counts. Rapidly evolving leukocytosis is associated with a higher risk of life-threatening complications.

If signs and symptoms of the RA-APL syndrome are present together with leukocytosis, initiate treatment with high-dose steroids immediately. Some investigators routinely add chemotherapy to tretinoin treatment in the case of patients presenting with a WBC count of $> 5 \times 10^9$/L or in the case of a rapid increase in WBC count for patients leukopenic start of treatment, and have reported a lower incidence of the RA-APL syndrome. Consider adding full-dose chemotherapy (including an anthracycline, if not contraindicated) to the tretinoin therapy on day 1 or 2 for patients presenting with a WBC count of $> 5 \times 10^9$/L or immediately, for patients presenting with a WBC count of $< 5 \times 10^9$/L, if the WBC count reaches $\geq 6 \times 10^9$/L by day 5, or $\geq 10 \times 10^9$/L by day 10 or $\geq 15 \times 10^9$/L by day 28.

Teratogenic effects:

Pregnancy Category D (see Warnings) – There is a high risk that a severely deformed infant will result if tretinoin is administered during pregnancy. If, nonetheless, it is determined that tretinoin represents the best available treatment for a pregnant woman or a woman of childbearing potential, it must be assured that the patient has received full information and warnings of the risk to the fetus if she were pregnant and of the risk of possible contraception failure. She must be instructed in the need to use two reliable forms of contraception simultaneously during therapy and for 1 month following discontinuation of therapy, unless abstinence is the chosen method.

Within 1 week prior to the institution of tretinoin therapy, the patient should have blood or urine collected for a serum or urine pregnancy test with a sensitivity of at least 50 mIU/L. When possible, delay tretinoin therapy until a negative result from this test is obtained. When a delay is not possible, place the patient on two reliable forms of contraception. Repeat pregnancy testing and contraception counseling monthly throughout the period of treatment.

Actions:

Pharmacology: Tretinoin is a retinoid that induces maturation of acute promelocytic leukemia (APL) cells in culture. Chemically, tretinoin is all-trans retinoic acid and is related to retinol (vitamin A). Tretinoin is not a cytolytic agent but instead induces cytodifferentiation and decreased [rp;oferatopm pf APL cells. In APL patients, tretinoin produces an initial maturation of the primitive promyelocytes derived from the leukemic clone, followed by a repopulation of the bone marrow and peripheral blood by normal, polyclonal hematopoietic cells in patients achieving complete remission (CR). The exact mechanism of action of tretinoin in APL is unknown.

Pharmacokinetics:

Absorption/Distribution – A single 45 mg/m^2 (≈ 80 mg) oral dose to APL patients resulted in a mean peak concentration of 347 ng/ml. Time to reach peak concentration was between 1 and 2 hours. Tretinoin is > 95% bound in plasma, predominately to albumin.

Metabolism – Tretinoin metabolites have been identified in plasma and urine. Cytochrome P450 (CYP) enzymes have been implicated in the oxidative metabolism of tretinoin. Metabolites include 13–cis retinoic acid, 4–oxo trans retinoic acid, 4–oxo cis retinoinc acid and 4–oxo trans retinoic acid glucuronide. In APL patients, daily administration of a 45 mg/m^2 dose resulted in an ≈ 10–fold increase in the urinary excretion of 4–oxo trans retinoic acid glucuronide after 2 to 6 weeks of continuous dosing when compared with baseline values.

Excretion – Studies with radiolabeled drug have demonstrated that after the oral administration of 2.75 and 50 mg, > 90% of the radioactivity was recovered in the urine and feces; ≈ 63% of radioactivity was recovered in the urine with 72 hours and 31% appeared in the feces within 6 days.

Tretinoin activity is primarily due to the parent drug. In studies, orally administered drug was well absorbed into the systemic circulation, with ≈ 66% recovered in the urine. The terminal elimination half-life following initial dosing is 0.5 to 2 hours in patients with APL. There is evidence that tretinoin induces its own metabolism. Plasma concentrations decrease on average to ⅓ of their day 1 values during 1 week of continuous therapy. Mean peak concentrations decreased from 394 to 138 ng/ml, while area under the curve (AUC) values decreased from 537 to 249 ng•hr/ml during 45 mg/m^2 daily dosing in seven APL patients. Increasing the dose to "correct" for this change has not increased response.

Clinical trials: In 114 previously treated APL patients and in 67 previously untreated ("de novo") patients, tretinoin 45 mg/m^2/day was given for up to 90 days or 30 days beyond the day that CR was reached. Complete remission occurred in 50% to 80% of relapsed patients and in 36% to 73% of de novo patients. Median survival was 5.8 to 10.8 months (relapsed) and 0.55 months (de novo).

The median time to CR was between 40 and 50 days (range, 2 to 120 days). Most patients in these studies received cytotoxic chemotherapy during the remission phase. These results compare with the 30% to 50% CR rate and ≤ 6 month median survival reported for cytotoxic chemotherapy of APL in the treatment of relapse. Ten of 15 pediatric cases achieved CR.

Indications:

Acute promyelocytic leukemia (APL): Induction of remission in patients with APL, French American British (FAB) classification M3 (including the M3 variant), characterized by the presence of the t(15;17) translocation or the presence of the PML/RARα gene who are refractory to or who have relapsed from anthracycline chemotherapy, or for whom anthracycline-based chemotherapy is contraindicated. Tretinoin is for the induction of remission only. All patients should receive an accepted form of remission consolidation or maintenance therpay for APL after completion of induction therapy with tretinoin.

Contraindications:

Hypersensitivity to retinoids; patients sensitive to parabens, which are used as preservatives in the gelatin capsule.

Warnings:

Patients without the t(15:17) translocation: Initiation of therapy with tretinoin may be based on the morphological diagnosis of APL. Confirm the diagnosis of APL by detection of the t(15:17) genetic marker by cytogenetic studies. If these are negative, PML/RARα fusion should be sought using molecular diagnostic techniques. The response rate of other AML subtypes to tretinoin has not been demonstrated; therefore, consider alternative treatment for patients who lack the genetic marker.

Retinoic acid-APL (RA-APL) syndrome: In up to 25% of APL patients treated with tretinoin, a syndrome occurs which can be fatal (see Warning Box).

Leukocytosis: See Warning Box.

Pseudotumor cerebri: Retinoids, including tretinoin, have been associated with pseudotumor cerebri (benign intracranial hypertension), especially in children. Early signs and symptoms include papilledema, headache, nausea, vomiting and visual disturbances. Evaluate patients with these symptoms for pseudotumor cerebri, and, if present, institute appropriate care with neurological assessment.

Lipids: Up to 60% of patients experienced hypercholesterolemia or hypertriglyceridemia, which were reversible upon completion of treatment. The clinical consequences of temporary elevation of triglycerides and cholesterol are unknown, but venous thrombosis and myocardial infarction have been reported in patients who ordinarily are at low risk for such complications.

Carcinogenesis/Mutagenesis/Fertility impairment: In short-term carcinogenicity studies, tretinoin at a dose of 30 mg/kg/day (about 2 times the human dose) increased the rate of diethylnitrosamine (DEN)-induced mouse liver adenomas and carcinoms. A 2–fold increase in the sister chromatid exchange (SCE) has been demonstrated in human diploid fibroblasts. In a 6–week toxicology study in dogs, minimal to marked testicular degeneration, with increased numbers of immature spermatozoa, were observed at 10 mg/kg/day (about 4 times the equivalent human dose).

Pregnancy: Category D. (see Warning Box). Tretinoin has teratogenic and embryotoxic effects in animals, and may be expected to cause fetal harm when administered to a pregnant woman. Tretinoin causes fetal resorptions and a decrease in live fetuses in all animals studied. Gross external, soft tissue and skeletal alterations occurred at doses ranging from 1/20 to 4 times the human dose.

There are no adequate and well controlled studies in pregnant women. Although experience with humans is extremely limited, increased spontaneous abortions and major human fetal abnormalities related to the use of other retinoids have been documented. Reported defects include abnormalities of the CNS, musculoskeletal system, external ear, eye, thymus and great vessels; and facial dysmorphia, cleft palate and parathyroid hormone deficiency. Some of these abnormalities were fatal. Cases of IQ scores < 85, with or without obvious CNS abnormalities, have also have been reported. All fetuses exposed during pregnancy can be affected, and there is no antepartum means of determining which fetuses are and are not affected.

Effective contraception must be used by all females during tretinoin therapy and for 1 month following discontinuation of therapy. Contraception must be used even when there is a history of infertility or menopause, unless a hysterectomy has been performed. Whenever contraception is required, it is recommended that two reliable forms of contraception be used simultaneously, unless abstinence is the chosen method. If pregnancy does occur during treatment, the physician and patient should discuss the desirability of continuing or terminating the pregnancy.

Lactation: It is not known whether this drug is excreted in breast milk. Because of the potential for serious adverse reactions from tretinoin in nursing infants, mothers should discontinue nursing prior to taking this drug.

Children: There are limited clinical data on the pediatric use of tretinoin. Of 15 pediatric patients (age range, 1 to 16 years) treated with tretinoin, the incidence of complete remission was 67%. Safety and efficacy in pediatric patients < 1 year of age have not been established. Some pediatric patients experience severe headache and pseudotumor cerebri, requiring analgesic treatment and lumbar puncture for relief. Increased caution is recommended. Consider dose reduction in children experiencing serious or intolerable toxicity; however, the efficacy and safety of tretinoin at doses < 45 mg/m^2/day have not been evaluated.

Precautions:

Monitoring: Monitor the patient's hematologic profile, coagulation profile, liver function test results and triglyceride and cholesterol levels frequently.

Lab test abnormalities: Elevated liver function test results occur in 50% to 60% of patients during treatment. Carefully monitor liver function test results during treatment and give consideration to a temporary withdrawal of tretinoin if test results reach > 5 times the upper limit of normal. However, the majority of these abnormalities resolve without interruption of or after completion of treatment.

Toxic side effects: Tretinoin has potentially significant toxic side effects in APL patients. Closely observe patients undergoing therapy for signs of respiratory compromise or leukocytosis (see Warning Box). Maintain supportive care appropriate for APL patients (eg, prophylaxis for bleeding, prompt therapy for infection) during therapy.

Drug Interactions:

Ketoconazole: In 13 patients, ketoconazole (400 to 1200 mg) 1 hour prior to tretinoin led to a 72% increase in tretinoin mean plasma AUC.

As tretinoin is metabolized by the hepatic CYP system, there is a potential for alteration of pharmacokinetics in patients administered concomitant medications that are also inducers or inhibitors of this system.

Drug/Food interactions: The absorption of retinoids as a class has been shown to be enhanced when taken together with food.

Adverse Reactions:

Virtually all patients experience some drug-related toxicity, especially headache, fever, weakness and fatigue. These adverse effects are seldom permanent or irreversible nor do they usually require therapy interruption.

TRETINOIN

Typical retinoid toxicity: The most frequently reported adverse events were similar to those described in patients taking high doses of vitamin A and included headache (86%); fever (83%); skin/mucous membrane dryness, bone pain (77%); nausea/vomiting (57%); rash (54%); mucositis (26%); pruritus, increased sweating (20%); visual disturbances, ocular disorders (17%); alopecia, skin changes (14%); changed visual acuity (6%); bone inflammation, viual field defects (3%).

Ear disorders: Earache or feeling of fullness in the ears (23%); hearing loss and other unspecified auricular disorders (6%); irreversible hearing loss (< 1%).

Body as a whole: Malaise (66%); shivering (63%); hemorrhage (60%); infections (58%); peripheral edema (52%); pain (37%); chest discomfort (32%) edema (29%); disseminated intravascular coagulation (26%); weight increase (23%); injection site reactions, anorexia, weight decrease (17%); myalgia (14%); flank pain (9%); cellulitis (8%); face edema, fluid imbalance, pallor, lymph disorders (6%); acidosis, hypothermia, ascites (3%).

Respiratory: The majority of these events are symptoms of the RA-APL syndrome (see Warning Box): Upper respiratory tract disorders (63%); dyspnea (60%); respiratory insufficiency (26%); pleural effusion (20%); pneumonia, rales, expiratory wheezing (14%); lower respiratory tract disorders (9%); pulmonary infiltration (6%); bronchial asthma, pulmonary/larynx edema, unspecified pulmonary disease (3%).

GI: GI hemorrhage (34%); abdominal pain (31%); other GI disorders (26%); diarrhea (23%); constipation (17%); dyspepsia (14%); abdominal distention (11%); hepatosplenomegaly (9%); hepatitis, ulcer, unspecified liver disorder (3%).

Cardiovascular: Arrhythmiaa, flushing (23%); hypotension (14%); hypertension, phlebitis (11%); cardiac failure (6%); cardiac arrest, myocardial infarction, enlarged heart, heart murmur, ischemia, stroke, myocarditis, pericarditis, pulmonary hypertension, secondary cardiomyopathy (3%).

CNS: Dizziness (20%); paresthesias, anxiety (17%); insomnia, depression (14%); confusion (11%); cerebral hemorrhage, intracranial hypertension, agitation (9%); hallucinations (6%); abnormal gain, agnosia, aphasia, asterixis, cerebellar edema, cerebellar disorders, convulsions, coma, CNS depression, dysarthria, encephalopathy, facial paralysis, hemiplegia, hyporeflexia, hypotaxia, no light reflex, neurologic reaction, spinal cord disorder, tremor, leg weakness, unconsciousness, dementia, forgetfulness, somnolence, slow speech (3%).

GU: Renal insufficiency (11%); dysuria (9%); acute renal failure, micturition frequency, renal tubular necrosis, enlarged prostate (3%).

Miscellaneous: Erythema nodosum, basophilia, hyperhistaminemia, Sweet's syndrome, organomegaly, hypercalcemia, pancreatitis, myositis (isolated cases).

Overdosage:

The maximal tolerated dose in patients with myelodysplastic syndrome or solid tumors was 195 mg/m^2/day. The maximal tolerated dose in pediatric patients was lower (60 mg/m^2/day). Overdosage with other retinoids has been associated with transient headache, facial flushing, cheilosis, abdominal pain, dizziness and ataxia. These symptoms have quickly resolved without appaprent residual effects.

Administration and Dosage:

Approved by the FDA on November 22, 1995.

The recommended dose is 45 mg/m^2/day administered as two evenly divided doses until complete remission is documented. Discontinue therapy 30 days after achievement of complete remission or after 90 days of treatment, whichever occurs first. If after initiation of treatment the presence of the t(15:17) translocation is not confirmed by cytogenetics or by polymerase chain reaction studies and the patient has not responded to tretinoin, consider alternative therapy.

Tretinoin is for the induction of remission only. Optimal consolidation or maintenance regimens have not been determined. All patients should therefore receive a standard consolidation or maintenance chemotherapy regimen for APL after induction therapy with tretinoin unless otherwise contraindicated.

Rx	**Vesanoid** (Hoffmann-La Roche)	**Capsules**: 10 mg	(Vesanoid 10 Roche). Orange-yellow/reddish-brown. In 100s.

PROCARBAZINE HCl (N-Methylhydrazine; MIH)

Actions:

Pharmacology: The mode of cytotoxic action is not clear; procarbazine may inhibit protein, ribonucleic acid (RNA) and deoxyribonucleic acid (DNA) synthesis. Procarbazine may inhibit transmethylation of methyl groups of methionine into t-RNA. The absence of functional t-RNA could cause the cessation of protein synthesis and consequently DNA and RNA synthesis. In addition, procarbazine may directly damage DNA. Hydrogen peroxide, formed during the auto-oxidation of the drug, may attack protein sulfhydryl groups contained in residual protein which is tightly bound to DNA. Procarbazine is metabolized primarily in the liver and kidneys. No cross-resistance with other agents, radiotherapy or steroids has been demonstrated.

Pharmacokinetics:

Absorption/Distribution – Procarbazine is rapidly and completely absorbed from the GI tract and quickly equilibrates between plasma and cerebrospinal fluid (CSF). Peak CSF levels occur in 30 to 90 minutes. Following oral administration, maximum peak plasma concentrations occur within 60 minutes.

Metabolism/Excretion – Procarbazine is metabolized in the liver and kidneys to cytotoxic products. The major portion of drug is excreted in the urine as N-isopropylterephthalamic acid (≈ 70% within 24 hours following oral and IV administration). Less than 5% is excreted in urine unchanged.

After IV injection, the plasma half-life is ≈ 10 minutes. Procarbazine crosses the blood-brain barrier.

Indications:

Hodgkin's disease: In combination with other antineoplastics for treatment of Stage III and IV Hodgkin's disease. Use procarbazine as part of the MOPP (nitrogen mustard, vincristine, procarbazine, prednisone) regimen. It has also been used as part of the ChlVPP (chlorambucin, vinblastine, procarbazine, prednisone) regimen.

Contraindications:

Hypersensitivity to procarbazine. Inadequate marrow reserve demonstrated by bone marrow aspiration (consider in any patient with leukopenia, thrombocytopenia or anemia).

Warnings:

Toxicity, common to many hydrazine derivatives, includes hemolysis and the appearance of Heinz-Ehrlich inclusion bodies in erythrocytes.

Discontinue if any of the following occurs: CNS signs or symptoms; leukopenia (WBC < $4000/mm^3$); thrombocytopenia (platelets < $100{,}000/mm^3$); hypersensitivity reaction; stomatitis (the first small ulceration or persistent spot soreness); diarrhea; hemorrhage or bleeding tendencies.

Resume therapy after side effects clear; adjust to a lower doage schedule.

Renal/Hepatic function impairment: Undue toxicity may occur if used in patients with known impairment of renal or hepatic function. Consider hospitalization for the initial treatment course.

Carcinogenesis/Mutagenesis/Fertility impairment: Carcinogenesis in mice, rats and monkeys has been reported including: Instances of a second non-lymphoid malignancy, including acute myelocytic leukemia, (in patients with Hodgkin's disease treated with procarbazine in combination with other chemotherapy or radiation). The International Agency for Research on Cancer (IARC) considers that there is "sufficient evidence" for the human carcinogenicity of procarbazine HCl when it is given in intensive regimens which include other antineoplastic agents but there is inadequate evidence of carcinogenicity in humans given procarbazine HCl alone.

Procarbazine is mutagenic in a variety of bacterial and mammalian test systems.

Azoospermia and antifertility effects associated with procarbazine coadministered with other antineoplastics for treating Hodgkin's disease have been reported in human clinical studies. Since these patients received multicombination therapy, it is difficult to determine to what extent procarbazine alone was involved in the male germ-cell damage. Compounds which inhibit DNA, RNA or protein synthesis might be expected to have adverse effects on gametogenesis. Unscheduled DNA synthesis in the testis of rabbits and decreased fertility in male mice treated with procarbazine HCl have been reported.

Pregnancy: Category D. Procarbazine can cause fetal harm when administered to a pregnant woman. There are no adequate and well controlled studies in pregnant women. If this drug is used during pregnancy, inform patient of the potential hazard to the fetus. Advise women of childbearing potential to avoid pregnancy.

Administration in first trimester of pregnancy has been described in five patients; congenital malformations were observed in four. The other pregnancy was electively terminated. When combined with other antineoplastics, procarbazine may produce

PROCARBAZINE HCl (N-Methylhydrazine; MIH)

gonadal dysfunction in males and females. Use only when clearly needed and when the potential benefits outweigh the potential hazards.

Procarbazine is teratogenic in the rat when given at doses approximately 4 to 13 times the maximum recommended human therapeutic dose of 6 mg/kg/day.

Lactation: It is not known whether procarbazine is excreted in human milk. Because of the potential for tumorigenicity shown in animal studies, mothers should not nurse while receiving this drug.

Children: Close clinical monitoring is mandatory. Toxicity, evidenced by tremors, convulsions and coma, has occurred. (See Administration and Dosage.)

Precautions:

Monitoring: Obtain baseline laboratory data prior to initiation of therapy. Monitor hemoglobin, hemtocrit, WBC, differential, reticulocytes and platelets at least every 3 or 4 days. Bone marrow depression often occurs 2 to 8 weeks after the start of infection.

Evaluate hepatic and renal function prior to initiation of therapy.

Repeat urinalysis, transaminases, alkaline phosphatase and BUN at least weekly.

Drug Interactions:

Procarbazine Drug Interactions

Precipitant drug	Object drug*		Description
Procarbazine	Digitalis glycosides	⬇	May result in a decrease in digoxin plasma levels, even several days after stopping chemotherapy.
Procarbazine	Levodopa	⬆	Flushing and a significant rise in blood pressure may result within 1 hour of levodopa administration.
Procarbazine	Narcotics	⬆	Concomitant use may result in depressant effects on the CNS leading to deep coma and death.
Procarbazine	Sympathomimetics (indirect acting)	⬆	May cause an abrupt increase in blood pressure, resulting in a potentially fatal hypertensive crisis.
Procarbazine	Tricyclic antidepressants	⬆	Severe toxic and fatal reactions including excitability, flucuations in blood pressure, convulsions and coma may occur. However, some studies report uneventful concurrent use with MAO inhibitors.
Procarbazine	Radiation or other chemotherapy	⬆	Use following radiation or other chemotherapy is known to have marrow depressant activity. Wait ≥ 1 month before starting procarbazine. Interval length may also be determined by evidence of bone marrow recovery based on successive bone marrow studies.

* ⬆ = Object drug increased. ⬇ = Object drug decreased.

Drug/Food interactions: Ingestion of foods with high tyramine content (see the Monamine Oxidase Inhibitors monograph) may cause an abrupt increase in blood pressure, resulting in a potentially fatal hypertensive crisis.

Adverse Reactions:

GI: Nausea, vomiting (frequent); anorexia; stomatitis; dry mouth; dysphagia; abdominal pain; hematemesis; melena; diarrhea; constipation.

Hematologic: Leukopenia, anemia, thrombocytopenia (frequent); pancytopenia; eosinophilia; hemolytic anemia; bleeding tendencies such as petechiae; purpura; epistaxis; hemoptysis.

Cardiovascular: Hypotension; tachycardia; syncope.

GU: Hematuria, urinary frequency, nocturia.

Endocrine: Gynecomastia in prepubertal and early pubertal boys.

Dermatologic: Dermatitis; pruritus; rash; urticaria; herpes; hyperpigmentation; flushing; alopecia.

CNS: Paresthesias and neuropathies; headache; dizziness; depression; apprehension; nervousness; insomnia; nightmares; hallucinations; falling; weakness; fatigue; lethargy; drowsiness; unsteadiness; ataxia; foot drop; decreased reflexes; tremors; coma; confusion; convulsions.

Ophthalmic: Retinal hemorrhage; nystagmus; photophobia; diplopia; inability to focus; papilledema.

Respiratory: Pleural effusion; pneumonitis; cough.

Miscellaneous: Pain, including myalgia and arthralgia; pyrexia; diaphoresis; chills; intercurrent infections; edema; hoarseness; generalized allergic reactions; hearing loss; slurred speech.

Second nonlymphoid malignancies, including acute myelocytic leukemia and malignant myelosclerosis and azoospermia have been reported in patients with Hodgkin's disease treated with procarbazine in combination with other chemotherapy or radiation.

Overdosage:

The major manifestations of overdosage with procarbazine would be anticipated to be nausea, vomiting, enteritis, diarrhea, hypotension, tremors, convulsions and coma. Treatment consists of either the administration of an emetic or gastric lavage. Use general supportive measures such as IV fluids. Since the major toxicity of procarbazine is hematologic and hepatic, perform frequent complete blood counts and liver function tests throughout recovery period and for a minimum of 2 weeks thereafter. Should abnormalities appear in any of these determinations, immediately undertake appropriate measures for correction and stabilization.

Patient Information:

May produce drowsiness and dizziness; patients should observe caution while driving or performing other tasks requiring alertness.

Consumption of alcoholic beverages while taking procarbazine may cause a disulfiram-like reaction.

Avoid ingestion of the following: Tyramine-containing foods (see see the Monamine Oxidase Inhibitors monograph), certain cold, hay fever or weight-reducing preparations containing sympathomimetics (see Drug Interactions).

Notify physician if cough, shortness of breath, thickened bronchial secretions, fever, chills, sore throat, unusual bleeding or bruising, black tarry stools or vomiting of blood occurs.

Medication may cause muscle or joint pain, nausea, vomiting, sweating, tiredness, weakness, constipation, headache, difficulty swallowing, loss of appetite, loss of hair, and mental depression; notify physician if these become pronounced.

Avoid prolonged exposure to sunlight; photosensitivity may occur. Wear protective clothing and use sunscreens until tolerance is determined.

Contraceptive measures are recommended during therapy for both men and women.

Administration and Dosage:

Base dosages on the patient's actual weight. Use estimated lean body mass (dry weight) if patient is obese or if there has been a spurious weight gain due to edema, ascites or other forms of abnormal fluid retention.

The following doses are for administration of procarbazine as a single agent. When used in combination with other anticancer drugs, appropriately reduce procarbazine dosage (eg, in the MOPP regimen, the procarbazine dose is 100 mg/m^2 daily for 14 days).

Adults: To minimize nausea and vomiting, give single or divided doses of 2 to 4 mg/kg/day for the first week. Maintain daily dosage at 4 to 6 mg/kg/day until the WBC falls below 4,000/cu mm or the platelets fall below 100,000/cu mm, or until maximum response is obtained. Upon evidence of hematologic toxicity, discontinue the drug until there has been satisfactory recovery. Resume treatment at 1 to 2 mg/kg/day. When maximum response is obtained, maintain the dose at 1 to 2 mg/kg/day.

Children: Close clinical monitoring is mandatory. Toxicity, evidenced by tremors, coma and convulsions, has occurred. Individualize dosage. This dosage schedule is a guideline only: 50 mg/m^2 daily for the first week. Maintain daily dosage at 100 mg/m^2 until leukopenia or thrombocytopenia occurs or maximum response is obtained. Upon evidence of hematologic toxicity, discontinue drug until there has been satisfactory response. When maximum response is attained, maintain the dose at 50 mg/m^2 /day.

Rx	**Matulane** (Roche)	**Capsules:** 50 mg	Parabens. (Roche Matulane). Ivory. In 100s.

DACARBAZINE (DTIC; Imidazole Carboxamide)

Warning:
Hemopoietic depression is the most common toxicity (see Warnings).
Hepatic necrosis has been reported (see Warnings).

Actions:

Pharmacology: The exact mechanism of action is unknown. There is some evidence for activity via three mechanisms: Alkylation through an activated carbonium ion; inhibition of DNA synthesis by acting as a purine analog; and interaction with sulfhydryl groups in proteins. Both deoxyribonucleic acid (DNA) and ribonucleic acid (RNA) synthesis are inhibited. Although dacarbazine appears to be more active on cells in late G_2 phase, it is considered cell cycle phase nonspecific.

Pharmacokinetics:

Absorption/Distribution – After IV administration of dacarbazine, the volume of distribution exceeds total body water content suggesting tissue localization, probably in the liver. There is relatively little distribution into the cerebrospinal fluid (CSF). At therapeutic concentrations, the drug is not appreciably bound to plasma protein.

Metabolism/Excretion – Plasma disappearance is biphasic with an initial half-life of 19 minutes and a terminal half-life of 5 hours. In renal and hepatic dysfunction, half-lives increase to 55 minutes and 7.2 hours.

An average of 40% of dacarbazine is excreted unchanged in the urine in 6 hours. Dacarbazine is subject to renal tubular secretion rather than glomerular filtration. Besides unchanged dacarbazine, 5-aminoimidazole-4 carboxamide (AIC) is a major metabolite in the urine.

Indications:

Metastatic malignant melanoma.

Hodgkin's disease: Second-line therapy in Hodgkin's disease in combination with other agents.

Unlabeled uses: In combination with cyclophosphamide and vincristine for malignant pheochromocytoma; coadministration with tamoxifen for metastatic malignant melanoma (more effective than dacarbazine alone).

Contraindications:

Hypersensitivity to dacarbazine.

Warnings:

Hemopoietic depression is the most common toxicity and involves primarily the leukocytes and platelets, although anemia sometimes occurs. Leukopenia and thrombocytopenia may be severe enough to cause death. Possible bone marrow depression requires careful monitoring of WBC, RBC and platelet levels. Hemopoietic toxicity may warrant temporary suspension or cessation of therapy.

GI symptoms: Anorexia, nausea and vomiting occur in over 90% of patients with the initial few doses. The vomiting lasts 1 to 12 hours and is incompletely and unpredictably palliated with phenobarbital or prochlorperazine. Rarely, intractable nausea and vomiting have necessitated discontinuation of therapy. Diarrhea occurs rarely. Restricting the patient's oral intake of fluids and food for 4 to 6 hours prior to treatment may be beneficial. Rapid tolerance to these symptoms suggests that a CNS mechanism may be involved; symptoms usually subside after the first 1 or 2 days.

Hepatotoxicity, accompanied by hepatic vein thrombosis and hepatocellular necrosis resulting in death, has been reported in approximately 0.01% of patients treated. This toxicity has been observed mostly when dacarbazine was coadministered with other antineoplastics, but it has also been reported with dacarbazine alone.

Hypersensitivity: Anaphylaxis can occur following the administration of dacarbazine.

Carcinogenesis: Angiosarcomas of the spleen and proliferative endocardial lesions, including fibrosarcomas and sarcomas, were induced in small animals after administration.

Pregnancy: Category C. Teratogenicity has been demonstrated in animals given 7 to 20 times the human dose. There are no adequate and well controlled studies in pregnant women. Use during pregnancy only if the potential benefit justifies the potential risk to the fetus.

Lactation: It is not known if this drug is excreted in breast milk. Because of the potential for tumorigenicity, decide whether to discontinue nursing or to discontinue the drug, taking into account the importance of the drug to the mother.

DACARBAZINE (DTIC; Imidazole Carboxamide)

Adverse Reactions:

GI: Anorexia, nausea and vomiting occur in over 90% of patients with the initial few doses. The vomiting lasts 1 to 12 hours and is incompletely and unpredictably palliated with phenobarbital or prochlorperazine. Rarely, intractable nausea and vomiting have necessitated discontinuation of therapy. Diarrhea occurs rarely. Restricting the patient's oral intake of fluids and food for 4 to 6 hours prior to treatment may be beneficial. Rapid tolerance to these symptoms suggests that a CNS mechanism may be involved; symptoms usually subside after the first 1 or 2 days.

Dermatologic: Erythematous and urticarial rashes (infrequent) and alopecia. Photosensitivity reactions may occur rarely (see Precautions).

Miscellaneous:

A flu-like syndrome of fever to 39°C, myalgia and malaise has been reported. Symptoms usually occur after large single doses, may last for several days and may occur with successive treatments.

Lab test abnormalities: Significant liver or renal function test abnormalities have been few.

Overdosage:

Give supportive treatment and monitor blood cell counts.

Administration and Dosage:

Administer IV only. Extravasation of the drug subcutaneously during IV administration may result in tissue damage and severe pain.

Malignant melanoma: 2 to 4.5 mg/kg/day IV for 10 days. Repeat at 4 week intervals.

Alternatively, administer 250 mg/m^2 /day IV for 5 days. Repeat every 3 weeks.

Hodgkin's disease: 150 mg/m^2 /day for 5 days, in combination with other effective drugs. Repeat every 4 weeks.

Alternatively, administer 375 mg/m^2 on day 1, in combination with other effective drugs; repeat every 15 days.

Preparation of the solution: Reconstitute the 100 mg vials with 9.9 ml and the 200 mg vials with 19.7 ml of Sterile Water for Injection. The resulting solution contains 10 mg/ml of dacarbazine with a pH of 3 to 4. The reconstituted solution may be further diluted with 5% Dextrose Injection or Sodium Chloride Injection, and administered as an IV infusion.

Storage/Stability: After reconstitution, store the solution in the vial at 4°C up to 72 hours or at normal room conditions (temperature and light) up to 8 hours. If the reconstituted solution is further diluted in 5% Dextrose Injection or Sodium Chloride Injection, store the resulting solution at 4°C up to 24 hours or at normal room conditions up to 8 hours. A white flocculent precipitate was observed when IV tubing containing dacarbazine (25 mg/ml) in 0.9% Sodium Chloride was flushed with heparin sodium. However, no precipitate was observed when 10 mg/ml of dacarbazine was used.

Rx	**DTIC-Dome** (Bayer)	**Injection:** 10 mg/ml	Mannitol. In 10 and 20 ml vials.

GEMCITABINE HCl

Actions:

Pharmacology: Gemcitabine is a nucleoside analog that exhibits antitumor activity. Gemcitabine exhibits cell phase specificity, primarily killing cells undergoing DNA synthesis (S-phase), and also blocking the progression of cells through the G1/S-phase boundary. Gemcitabine is metabolized intracellularly by nucleoside kinases to the active diphosphate (dFdCDP) and triphosphate (dFdCTP) nucleosides. The cytotoxic effect of gemcitabine is attributed to a combination of two actions of the diphosphate and the triphosphate nucleosides, which leads to inhibition of DNA synthesis. First, gemcitabine diphosphate inhibits ribonucleotide reductase, which is responsible for catalyzing the reactions that generate the deoxynucleoside triphosphates for DNA synthesis. Inhibition of this enzyme by diphosphate nuclioside causes a reduction in the concentrations of deoxynucliotides, including dCTP. Second, gemcitabine triphosphate competes with dCTP for incorporation into DNA. After the gemcitabiine nucleotide is incorporated into DNA, only one additional nucleotide is added to the growing DNA strands. After this addition, there is inhibition of further DNA synthesis. DNA polymerase epsilon is unable to remove the gemcitabine nucleotide and repair the growing DNA strands (masked chain termination).

Pharmacokinetics: Gemcitabine pharmacokinetics are linear and are described by a 2–compartment model. Population pharmacokinetic analyses of combined single and multiple dose studies showed that the volume of distribution of gemcitabine was significantly influenced by duration of infusion and gender. Clearance was affected by age and gender. Differences in either clearance or volume of distribution based on patient characteristics or the duration of infusion result in changes in half-life and plasma concentrations.

Gemcitabine Clearance and Half-Life for the "Typical" Patient

Age	Clearance Men (L/hr/m²)	Clearance Women (L/hr/m²)	Half-life[1] Men (min)	Half-life[1] Women (min)
29	92.2	69.4	42	49
45	75.7	57	48	57
65	55.1	41.5	61	73
79	40.7	30.7	79	94

[1] Half-life for patients receiving a short infusion (< 70 min).

The volume of distribution was increased with infusion length. Volume of distribution of gemcitabine was 50 L/m² following infusions lasting < 70 minutes, indicating that gemcitabine, after short infusions, is not extensively distributed into tissues. For long infusions, the volume of distribution rose to 370 L/m², reflecting slow equilibration of gemcitabine within the tissue compartment.

The maximum plasma concentrations of dFdU (inactive metabolite) were achieved up to 30 minutes after discontinuation of the infusions and the metabolite is excreted in urine without undergoing further biotransformation. The metabolite did not accumulate with weekly dosing, but its elimination is dependent on renal excretion and could accumulate with decreased renal function.

Clinical trials:

No prior treatment – In a multicenter prospective, single-blinded, two-arm, randomized, comparison of gemcitabine and 5–FU in patients with locally advanced or metastatic pancreatic cancer who had received no prior treatment with chemotherapy, 5–FU was administered IV at a weekly dose of 600 mg/m² for 30 minutes. Patients treated with gemcitabine had statistically significant increases in clinical benefit response, survival and time to progressive disease compared with 5–FU. No confirmed objective tumor responses were observed with either treatment.

Prior treatment – The second trial was a multicenter, open-label study in 63 patients with advanced pancreatic cancer previously treated with 5–FU or a 5–FU-containing regimen. The study showed a clinical benefit response rate of 27% and median survival of 3.9 months.

Indications:

Adenocarcinoma of the pancreas: First-line treatment for patients with locally advanced (nonresectable Stage II or Stage III) or metastatic (Stage IV) adenocarcinoma of the pancreas. Gemcitabine is indicated for patients previously treated with 5–FU.

Contraindications:

Known hypersensitivity to the drug.

Warnings:

Infusion: Prolongation of the infusion time beyond 60 minutes and more frequent than weekly dosing have been shown to increase toxicity.

Myelosuppression: Gemcitabine can suppress bone marrow function as manifested by leukopenia, thrombocytopenia and anemia, and myelosuppression is usually the dose-limiting toxicity.

Fever: The overall incidence of fever was 41%. This is in contrast to the incidence of infection (16%) and indicates that gemcitabine may cause fever in the absence of clinical infection. Fever was frequently associated with other flu-like symptoms and was usually mild and clinically manageable.

Rash: Rash was reported in 30% of patients. The rash was typically a macular or finely granular maculopapular pruritic eruption of mild to moderate severity involving the truck and extremities. Pruritus was reported for 13% of patients.

Renal/Hepatic function impairment: Gemcitabine should be used with caution in patients with pre-existing renal impairment or hepatic insufficiency. Gemcitabine has not been studied in patients with significant renal or hepatic impairment.

Hepatic – Gemcitabine was associated with transient elevations of serum transaminases in ≈ ⅔ of patients, but there was no evidence of increasing hepatic toxicity with either longer duration of exposure to gemcitabine or with greater total cumulative dose.

Renal – Mild proteinuria and hematuria were commonly reported. Hemolytic uremic syndrome (HUS) on gemcitabine therapy or immediately post-therapy has been reported in 0.25% of patients. Renal failure may not be reversible even with discontinuation of therapy, and dialysis may be required.

Elderly: Gemcitabine clearance is affected by age. However, there is no evidence that unusual dose adjustments are necessary in patients > 65 years of age, and, in general adverse reactions rates were similar in patients ≥ 65 years of age. Grade 3/4 thrombocytopenia was more common in the elderly.

Gender – Older woomen were more likely not to proceed to a subsequent cycle and to experience grade 3/4 neutropenia and thrombocytopenia.

Pregnancy: Category D. Gemcitabine can cause fetal harm when administered to a pregnant woman. There are no studies of gemcitabine in pregnant women. If gemcitabine is used during pregnancy, or if the patient becomes pregnant while taking gemcitabine, the patient should be apprised of the potential hazard to the fetus.

Lactation: It is not known whether gemcitabine or its metabolites are excreted in breast milk. Because many drugs are excreted in human milk and because of the potential for serious adverse reactions from gemcitabine in nursing infants, the mother should be warned and a decision should be made whether to discontinue nursing or to discontinue the drug, taking into account the importance of the drug to the mother and the potential risk to the infant.

Children: Gemcitabine has not been studied in pediatric patients. Safety and effectiveness in pediatric patients have not been established.

Precautions:

Monitoring: Patients receiving gemcitabine should be monitored prior to each dose with a complete blood count (CBC), including differential and platelet count. Suspension or modification of therapy should be considered when marrow suppression is detected (see Administration and Dosage).

Hepatic and renal – Laboratory evaluation of renal and hepatic function should be performed prior to initiation of therapy and periodically thereafter.

GEMCITABINE HCl

Adverse Reactions:

Myelosuppression is the principal dose-limiting factor with gemcitabine therapy.

Gemcitabine Adverse Reactions (%)					
	All patients (n = 699 to 974)	Pancreatic cancer patients (n = 161 to 241)	Discontinuations (n = 979)	Gemcitabine vs 5-FU: Gemcitabine (n = 58 to 63)	Gemcitabine vs 5-FU: 5-FU (n = 61 to 63)
Laboratory					
Hematologic					
Anemia	68	73	< 1	65	45
Leukopenia	62	64	< 1	71	15
Neutropenia	63	61		62	18
Thrombocytopenia	24	36	< 1	47	15
Hepatic			< 1		
ALT	68	72		72	38
AST	67	78		72	52
Alkaline phosphatase	55	77		71	64
Bilirubin	13	26		16	25
Renal			< 1		
Proteinuria	45	32		10	2
Hematuria	35	23		13	0
BUN	16	15		8	10
Creatinine	8	6		2	0
Nonlaboratory					
Nausea and Vomiting	69	71	< 1	64	58
Pain	48	42	< 1	10	7
Fever	41	38	< 1	30	16
Rash	30	28	< 1	24	13
Dyspnea	23	10	< 1	6	3
Constipation	23	31	0	10	11
Diarrhea	19	30	0	24	31
Hemorrhage	17	4	< 1	0	2
Infection	16	10	< 1	8	3
Alopecia	15	16	0	18	16
Stomatitis	11	10	< 1	14	15
Somnolence	11	11	< 1	5	7
Paresthesias	10	10	0	2	2

Cardiovascular: Two percent of patients discontinued therapy with gemcitabine due to cardiovascular events such as myocardial infarction, cerebrovascular accident, arrhythmia and hypertension. Many of these patients had a prior history of cardiovascular disease.

CNS: Mild paresthesias (10%); severe paresthesias (< 1%).

Dermatologic: Rash (30%; see Warnings); hair loss, usually minimal (15%).

GI: Nausea and vomiting (69%); transeient elevations of serum transaminases (≈ 67%; see Warnings); diarrhea (19%); stomatitis (11%).

Hematologic: Red blood cell transfusions (19%); petechiae or mild blood loss (hemorrhage) (16%); sepsis, platelet transfusions (< 1%).

Pulmonary: Dyspnea (23%); severe dyspnea (3%); dyspnea may be due to underlying disease such as lung cancer (40%) or pulmonary manifestations of other malignancies. Dyspnea was occasionally accompanied by bronchospasm (< 2 %); parenchymal lung toxicity consistent with drug-induced pneumonitis (rare).

Renal: Mild proteinuria, hematuria, hemolytic uremic syndrome (see Warnings).

Miscellaneous: Peripheral edema (20%); "flu syndrome" (19%; including fever [41%; see Warnings]; asthenia, anorexia, headache, cough, chills, myalgia [common]; insomnia, rhinitis, sweating, malaise [infrequent]; < 1% discontinued due to flu-like symptoms); infections (16%); edema (13%); injection site related events (4%; there were no reports of injection site necrosis as gemcitabine is not a vesicant); bronchospasm (< 2%); sepsis, generalized edema (< 1% [< 1% of patients discontinued due to edema]); anaphylactoid reaction (rare).

GEMCITABINE HCl

Overdosage:

There is no known antidote for overdoses of gemcitabine. Myelosuppression, paresthesias and severe rash were the principal toxicities seen when a single dose as high as 5700 mg/m^2 was administered IV infusion over 30 minutes every 2 weeks.

Treatment: In the event of suspected overdose, the patient should be monitored with appropriate blood counts and should receive supportive therapy, as necessary.

Administration and Dosage:

IV use only.

Gemcitabine may be administered on an outpatient basis.

Adults: Administered IV at a dose of 1000 mg/m^2 over 30 minutes once weekly for up to 7 weeks (or until toxicity necessitates reducing or holding a dose), followed by a week of rest from treatment. Subsequent cycles should consist of infusions once weekly for 3 consecutive weeks out of every 4 weeks.

Gemcitabine Dosage Reduction Guidelines			
Absolute granulocyte count ($\times 10^6$/L)		Platelet count ($\times 10^6$/L)	% of full dose
≥ 1000	and	≥ 100,000	100
500 to 999	or	50,000 to 99,000	75
< 500	or	< 50,000	hold

Patients who complete an entire 7–week initial cycle of gemcitabine therapy or a subsequent 3–week cycle at a dose of 1000 mg/m^2 may have the dose for subsequent cycles increased by 25% (to 1250 mg/m^2), provided that the absolute granulocyte count (AGC) and platelet nadirs exceed 1500 $\times 10^6$/L and 100,000 $\times 10^6$, respectively, and if nonhematologic toxicity has not been greater than World Health Organization Grade 1 (see Adverse Reactions). If patients tolerate the susequent course at a dose of 1250 mg/m^2, the dose for the next cycle can be increased to 1500 mg/m^2, provided that the ACG and platelet nadirs exceed 1500 $\times 10^6$/L and 100,00 $\times 10^6$/L, respectively, and again, if nonhematologic toxicity has not been greater than WHO Grade 1.

Dilution: Diluent for reconstition of gemcitabine is 0.9% Sodium Chloride Injection without preservatives. Due to solubility considerations, the maximum concentration for gemcitabine upon reconstitution is 40 mg/ml. Reconstitution at concentrations greater than 40 mg/ml may result in incomplete dissolution and should be avoided.

To reconstitute, add 5 ml of 0.9% Sodium Chloride Injection to the 200 mg vial or 25 ml of 0.9% Sodium Chloride Injection to the 1 g vial. Shake to dissolve. These dilutions each yield a gemcitabine concentration of 40 mg/ml. The appropriate amount of drug may be administered as prepared of further diluted with 0.9% Sodium Chloride Injection to concentrations as low as 0.1 mg/ml.

Storage/Stability: Solutions of reconstituted gemcitabine should not be refrigerated, as crystallization may occur. Store at controlled room temperature 20° to 25°C (68° to 77°F). Gemcitabine solutions are stable for 24 hours at controlled room temperature.

Rx	**Gemzar** (Lilly)	**Powder, lyophilized:** 20 mg/ml	Mannitol. In 10 and 50 ml vials.

MITOTANE (o, p'-DDD)

Warning:
Discontinue temporarily following shock or severe trauma since the prime action of mitotane is adrenal suppression. Administer exogenous steroids in such circumstances, since the depressed adrenal may not immediately start to function.

Actions:

Pharmacology: Mitotane is an adrenal cytotoxic agent, although it can cause adrenal inhibition without cellular destruction. The primary action is upon the adrenal cortex. The production of adrenal steroids is reduced. The biochemical mechanism of action is unknown. Data suggest that the drug modifies the peripheral metabolism of steroids and directly suppresses the adrenal cortex.

Use of mitotane alters the peripheral metabolism of cortisol, leading to a reduction in measurable 17-hydroxycorticosteroids, even though plasma levels of corticosteroids do not fall. The drug causes increased formation of 6-β-hydroxycortisol.

Pharmacokinetics:

Absorption/Distribution – Approximately 40% of oral mitotane is absorbed; it can be found in all body tissues but is primarily stored in fat. Blood levels detectable for up to 10 weeks after discontinuation of therapy may be related to a slow persistent release of drug from lipid storage sites. Blood levels do not appear to correlate with therapeutic or toxic effects.

Metabolism/Excretion – The primary metabolites of mitotane are oxidation products; several polar metabolites are also produced. Approximately 10% to 25% of the drug is excreted in the urine as an unidentified water soluble metabolite. Up to 60% is excreted unchanged in the stool.

No unchanged mitotane has been found in the urine or bile.

Clinical trials: A number of patients have been treated intermittently, restarting treatment when severe symptoms reappeared. Patients often do not respond after the third or fourth such course. Continuous treatment with the maximum possible dosage may be the best approach.

A substantial percentage of patients show signs of adrenal insufficiency. Watch for this condition and institute steroid therapy if necessary. The metabolism of exogenous steroids is modified with mitotane; somewhat higher doses than just replacement therapy may be required.

Clinical effectiveness can be shown by reductions in tumor mass, pain, weakness or anorexia and steroid symptoms.

Indications:
Treatment of inoperable adrenal cortical carcinoma (functional and nonfunctional).

Contraindications:
Hypersensitivity to mitotane.

Warnings:

Shock or severe trauma: Temporarily discontinue mitotane immediately following shock or severe trauma, since adrenal suppression is its prime action. Use exogenous steroids in such circumstances, since the depressed adrenal may not immediately start to secrete steroids.

Tumor tissue: Surgically remove all possible tumor tissue from large metastatic masses before administration to minimize the possibility of infarction and hemorrhage in the tumor due to a rapid, cytotoxic effect of the drug.

Long-term therapy: Continuous administration of high doses may lead to brain damage and impairment of function. Conduct behavioral and neurological assessments at regular intervals when continuous treatment exceeds 2 years.

Hepatic function impairment: Administer with care to patients with liver disease other than metastatic lesions of the adrenal cortex. Interference with mitotane metabolism may occur, causing drug accumulation.

Carcinogenesis: The carcinogenic and mutagenic potential is unknown. However, the mechanism of action suggests that the drug probably has less carcinogenic potential than other cytotoxic chemotherapeutic drugs.

Pregnancy: Category C. Safety for use during pregnancy has not been established. Use only when clearly needed and when the potential benefits outweigh the potential hazards to the fetus.

Lactation: It is not known whether this drug is excreted in breast milk. Because of the potential for adverse reactions in nursing infants, decide whether to discontinue nursing or discontinue the drug.

MITOTANE (o, p'-DDD)

Precautions:

Adrenal insufficiency may develop; consider adrenal steroid replacement in these patients.

Drug Interactions:

Use mitotane with caution in patients receiving drugs susceptible to the influence of hepatic enzyme induction.

Mitotane Drug Interactions			
Precipitant drug	Object drug*		Description
Mitotane	Corticosteroids	↓	Corticosteroid metabolism may be altered by mitotane; higher dosages may be required.
Mitotane	Warfarin	↓	The metabolism of warfarin may be accelerated by the mechanism of hepatic microsomal enzyme induction, leading to an increase in dosage requirements of warfarin. Monitor patients for a change in anticoagulant dosage requirements when admininstering mitotane to patients on coumarin-type anticoagulants.

* ↓ = Object drug decreased.

Adverse Reactions:

GI: Anorexia, nausea or vomiting and diarrhea (80%).

CNS: 40%. Primarily depression as manifested by lethargy and somnolence (25%), and dizziness or vertigo (15%).

Dermatologic: Primarily transient skin rashes. In some instances, this side effect subsided while patients were maintained on the drug.

Infrequent:

Ophthalmic – Visual blurring, diplopia, lens opacity and toxic retinopathy.

GU – Hematuria, hemorrhagic cystitis and albuminuria.

Cardiovascular – Hypertension, orthostatic hypotension and flushing.

Miscellaneous – Generalized aching, hyperpyrexia and lowered PBI.

Patient Information:

Notify physician if nausea, vomiting, loss of appetite, diarrhea, mental depression, skin rash or darkening of the skin occurs.

Medication may cause aching muscles, fever, flushing or muscle twitching; notify physician if these become pronounced.

May produce drowsiness, dizziness and tiredness; patients should observe caution when driving or performing other tasks requiring alertness.

Contraceptive measures are recommended during therapy.

Administration and Dosage:

Start at 2 to 6 g/day in divided doses, 3 or 4 times daily. Increase dose incrementally to 9 to 10 g per day. If severe side effects appear, reduce to the maximum tolerated dose. If the patient can tolerate higher doses, and if improved clinical response appears possible, increase the dose until adverse reactions interfere. Maximum tolerated dose varies from 2 to 16 g/day (usually 9 to 10 g). The highest doses used in studies were 18 to 19 g/day.

Continue treatment as long as clinical benefits are observed (ie, maintenance of clinical status or slowing of growth of metastatic lesions). If no clinical benefits are observed after 3 months at the maximum tolerated dose, consider the case a clinical failure. However, 10% of the patients who showed a measurable response required more than 3 months at the maximum tolerated dose. Early diagnosis and prompt institution of treatment improve the probability of a positive clinical response.

Storage/Stability: Store at room temperature (15° to 30°C; 59° to 86°F).

Rx	**Lysodren** (Bristol-Myers Oncology)	**Tablets:** 500 mg	Scored. In 100s.

ASPARAGINASE

Warning:

Because of possible severe reactions, including anaphylaxis and sudden death, administer only in a hospital setting under the supervision of a physician qualified by training and experience in antineoplastic agents. Be prepared to treat anaphylaxis at each administration.

Actions:

Pharmacology: Asparaginase contains the enzyme L-asparagine amidohydrolase, type EC-2, derived from *Escherichia coli*.

In a significant number of patients with acute (particularly lymphocytic) leukemia, the malignant cells depend on exogenous asparagine for survival. Normal cells are able to synthesize asparagine and thus are affected less by the rapid depletion produced by treatment. Administration of asparaginase hydrolyzes serum asparagine to nonfunctional asparatic acid and ammonia, depriving tumor cells of a required amino acid. Tumor cell proliferation is blocked due to interruption of asparagine-dependent protein synthesis. The inhibitory activity is maximal in the postmitotic (G_1) phase of the cell cycle.

Pharmacokinetics:

Absorption/Distribution – Initial plasma levels of L-asparaginase following IV administration are correlated to dose. Daily administration results in a cumulative increase in plasma levels. Asparaginase serum levels following IM use are approximately one-half those achieved with IV administration. Apparent volume of distribution is approximately 70% to 80% of estimated plasma volume. There is some slow movement from vascular to extravascular, extracellular space. L-asparaginase is detected in the lymph. Cerebrospinal fluid levels usually are less than 1% of concurrent plasma levels.

Metabolism/Excretion – Plasma half-life varied from 8 to 30 hours and is not influenced by dosage. Only minimal urinary and biliary excretion occurs.

Indications:

Acute lymphocytic leukemia, primarily in combination with other chemotherapeutic agents, in the induction of remissions of disease in children. Do not use as the sole induction agent unless combination therapy is deemed inappropriate.

Contraindications:

Anaphylactic reactions to asparaginase; pancreatitis or a history of pancreatitis.

Warnings:

Hematologic: Bone marrow depression, leukopenia, thrombosis and clotting factors depressed; increase in blood ammonia during the conversion of asparagine to asparatic acid by the enzyme.

Bone marrow depression: Rarely, transient bone marrow depression has been seen as evidenced by a delay in return of hemoglobin or hematocrit levels to normal in patients undergoind hematologic remission of leukemia. Marked leukopenia has been reported.

Bleeding: In addition to hypogibrinogemia, other clotting factors may be depressed. Most marked has been a decrease in factors V and VIII with a variable decrease in factors VII and IX. A decrease in circulating platelets has occurred in low incidence, which, with the increased levels of fibrin degradation products in the serum, may indicate consumption coagulopathy. Bleeding has been a problem in only a few patients; however, intracranial hemorrhage and fatal bleeding associated with low fibrinogen levels have been reported. Increased compensatory fibrinolytic activity has also occurred.

Hyperglycemia with glucosuria and polyuria has been reported in low incidence. Serum and urine acetone are usually absent or negligible; this syndrome thus resembles hyperosmolar, nonketotic hyperglycemia. It usually responds to drug discontinuation and judicious use of IV fluid and insulin, but it may be fatal.

Hepatotoxicity occurs in the majority of patients. Therapy may increase preexisting liver impairment caused by prior therapy or underlying disease; asparaginase may increase the toxicity of other medications.

Hypersensitivity: Reactions are frequent and may occur during the primary course of therapy. They are not completely predictable based on the intradermal skin test. Anaphylaxis and death have occurred.

Once a patient has received asparaginase, there is an increased risk of hypersensitivity reactions with retreatment. In patients found to be hypersensitive by skin testing, and in any patient previously under therapy with asparaginase, administer the drug only after successful desensitization. Even then, the possible benefit should

ASPARAGINASE

be judged as greater than the increased risk since desensitization may also be hazardous (see Administration and Dosage).

In children with advanced leukemia, a lower incidence of anaphylaxis has occurred with IM use, although there was a higher incidence of milder hypersensitivity reactions than with IV use.

Anaphylactic reactions require the immediate use of epinephrine, oxygen and IV steroids. Refer to Management of Acute Hypersensitivity Reactions.

Pregnancy: Category C. Asparaginase has been shown to retard the weight gain of mothers and fetuses, has caused resorptions, and has resulted in dose-dependent embryotoxicity and gross abnormalities in various rodent species when given in doses ranging from 0.05 to 1 times the human dose. There are no adequate and well controlled studies in pregnant women. Use during pregnancy only if the potential benefit justifies the potential risk to the fetus.

Lactation: It is not known whether this drug is excreted in breast milk. Because of potential serious adverse reactions in nursing infants, discontinue nursing or discontinue the drug, considering the importance of the drug to the mother.

Children: Asparaginase toxicity is reported to be greater in adults than in children.

Precautions:

Monitoring: The fall in circulating lymphoblasts is often quite marked; normal or below normal leukocyte counts are noted frequently several days after initiating therapy and may be accompanied by a marked rise in serum uric acid. Uric acid nephropathy may develop; take appropriate preventive measures (eg, allopurinol, increased fluid intake, alkalinization of urine). Monitor peripheral blood count and bone marrow frequently.

Obtain frequent serum amylase determinations to detect early evidence of pancreatitis. If pancreatitis occurs, discontinue therapy.

Monitor blood sugar during therapy because hyperglycemia may occur (see Warnings).

Infection: Asparaginase has immunosuppressive activity in animals; consider the possibility of predisposition to infection.

Drug Interactions:

Asparaginase Drug Interactions

Precipitant drug	Object drug*		Description
Asparaginase	Methotrexate	⬇	Asparaginase may diminish or abolish methotrexate's effect on malignant cells; this effect persists as long as plasma asparagine levels are suppressed. Do not use methotrexate with, or following asparaginase, while asparagine levels are below normal.
Vincristine and prednisone	Asparaginase	⬆	IV administration of asparaginase concurrently with or immediately before a course of these drugs may be associated with increased toxicity.

* ⬆ = Object drug increased. ⬇ = Object drug decreased.

Drug/Lab test interactions: L-asparaginase may interfere with the interpretation of **thyroid function tests** by producing a rapid and marked reduction in serum concentrations of thyroxine-binding globulin within 2 days after the first dose. Serum concentrations of thyroxine-binding globulin returned to pretreatment values within 4 weeks of the last dose of L-asparaginase.

Adverse Reactions:

Hypersensitivity: Skin rashes, urticaria, arthralgia, respiratory distress, and acute anaphylaxis (see Warnings).

CNS: Depression, somnolence, fatigue, coma, confusion, agitation and hallucinations (mild to severe); headache, irritability (mild); Parkinson-like syndrome with tremor and a progressive increase in muscular tone (rare). These effects usually reversed spontaneously after stopping treatment. No clear correlation exists between elevated blood ammonia levels and CNS changes.

Renal: Azotemia, usually prerenal, occurs frequently. Acute renal shut-down and fatal renal insufficiency have been reported. Proteinuria has occurred infrequently.

ASPARAGINASE

Hepatic: Elevations of serum glutamic-oxaloacetic transaminase (SGOT), serum glutamic-pyruvic transaminase (SGPT), alkaline phosphatase, bilirubin (direct and indirect), and depression of serum albumin, cholesterol (total and esters) and plasma fibrinogen. Increases and decreases of total lipids; marked hypoalbuminemia associated with peripheral edema. These abnormalities usually are reversible on discontinuation of therapy and some reversal may occur during the course of therapy. Fatty changes in the liver and malabsorption syndrome have been reported (see Warnings).

GI: Nausea, vomiting, anorexia, abdominal cramps (usually mild). Pancreatitis, sometimes fulminant, and acute hemorrhagic pancreatitis have occurred; both may be fatal.

Miscellaneous: Chills, fever, weight loss (usually mild); fatal hyperthermia, hypoglycemia (see Warning Box).

Administration and Dosage:

Maintenance: Not recommended for maintenance therapy.

Because of the unpredictability of adverse reactions, use only in a hospital (see Warning Box).

IV: Give over 30 minutes through the side arm of an already running infusion of Sodium Chloride Injection or 5% Dextrose Injection. The drug has little tendency to cause phlebitis when given IV.

IM: Limit the volume at a single injection site to 2 ml. For a volume greater than 2 ml, use 2 injection sites.

Induction regimens: One of the following combination regimens is recommended for acute lymphocytic leukemia in *children*. (Day 1 is considered the first day of therapy.)

Regimen I –

Prednisone 40 mg/m² /day orally in 3 divided doses for 15 days, followed by tapering of the dosage as follows: 20 mg/m² for 2 days, 10 mg/m² for 2 days, 5 mg/m² for 2 days, 2.5 mg/m² for 2 days and then discontinue.

Vincristine sulfate 2 mg/m² IV once weekly on days 1, 8 and 15. The maximum single dose should not exceed 2 mg.

Asparaginase 1,000 IU/kg/day IV for 10 successive days beginning on day 22.

Regimen II –

Prednisone 40 mg/m² /day orally in 3 divided doses for 28 days (the total daily dose to the nearest 2.5 mg), then gradual discontinuation over 14 days.

Vincristine sulfate 1.5 mg/m² IV weekly for 4 doses, on days 1, 8, 15 and 22. The maximum single dose should not exceed 2 mg.

Asparaginase 6000 IU/m² IM on days 4, 7, 10, 13, 16, 19, 22, 25 and 28.

When remission is obtained with either of the above regimens, institute appropriate maintenance therapy. Do not use asparaginase as part of a maintenance regimen.

The above regimens do not preclude the need for special therapy to prevent CNS leukemia.

Asparaginase has been used in other combination regimens. Administering the drug IV concurrently with or immediately before a course of vincristine and prednisone may be associated with increased toxicity.

Single agent induction therapy: Use asparaginase as the sole induction agent only when a combined regimen is inappropriate because of toxicity or other specific patient-related factors, or in cases refractory to other therapy.

Children or adults – 200 IU/kg/day IV for 28 days. Complete remissions are of short duration, 1 to 3 months. Asparaginase has been used as the sole induction agent in other regimens.

Dosage adjustments: Carefully monitor patients undergoing induction therapy; individualize dosage according to response and toxicity. Adjustments always involve decreasing dosages of one or more agents or discontinuation. Patients who have received a course of therapy, if treated again, have an increased risk of hypersensitivity reactions. Therefore, repeat treatment only when the benefit of such therapy is weighed against the increased risk.

ASPARAGINASE

Intradermal skin test: Perform an intradermal skin test prior to initial administration of asparaginase and when it is given after a week or more has elapsed between doses.

Prepare the skin test solution as follows – Reconstitute a 10,000 IU vial with 5 ml of diluent. From this solution (2000 IU/ml), withdraw 0.1 ml and inject it into another vial containing 9.9 ml of diluent, yielding a skin test solution of approximately 20 IU/ml. Use 0.1 ml of this solution (about 2 IU) for the intradermal skin test. Observe the skin test site for at least 1 hour for a wheal or erythema that indicates a positive reaction. An allergic reaction even to the skin test dose may occur rarely. A negative skin test reaction does not preclude possible development of an allergic reaction.

Desensitization: Perform desensitization before giving the first treatment dose of asparaginase in positive reactors, and on retreatment of any patient. Attempt rapid desensitization of the patient by progressively increasing amounts of the drug IV. Take adequate precautions to treat an acute allergic reaction. One schedule begins with 1 IU given IV and doubles the dose every 10 minutes if no reaction has occurred, until the accumulated total amount given equals the planned doses for that day. For convenience, the following table is included to calculate the number of doses necessary to reach the patient's total dose for that day:

Asparaginase Dosing Based on Total Daily Requirements

Injection Number[1]	Dose (IU)	Accumulated Total Dose (IU)
1	1	1
2	2	3
3	4	7
4	8	15
5	16	31
6	32	63
7	64	127
8	128	255
9	256	511
10	512	1,023
11	1,024	2,047
12	2,048	4,095
13	4,096	8,191
14	8,192	16,383
15	16,384	32,767
16	32,768	65,535
17	65,536	131,071
18	131,072	262,143

[1] For example: A patient weighing 20 kg who is to receive 200 IU/kg (total dose 4000 IU) would receive injections 1 through 12 during desensitization.

Preparation of solutions:

IV – Reconstitute the 10,000 unit vial with 5 ml Sterile Water for Injection or with Sodium Chloride Injection. Ordinary shaking during reconstitution does not inactivate the enzyme. This solution may be used for direct IV administration within 8 hours following reconstitution. For administration by infusion, dilute solutions with Sodium Chloride Injection or 5% Dextrose Injection. Infuse within 8 hours and only if clear.

Occasionally, gelatinous fiber-like particles may develop on standing. Filtration through a 5 micron filter during administration will remove the particles with no loss of potency. Some loss of potency has been observed with the use of a 0.2 micron filter.

IM – Reconstitute by adding 2 ml Sodium Chloride Injection to the 10,000 unit vial. Use the resulting solution within 8 hours and only if clear.

Storage: Store at 2° to 8°C (36° to 46°F). Because it is preservative-free, store reconstituted solution at 2° to 8°C (36° to 46°F); discard after 8 hours or sooner if cloudy.

Rx	**Elspar** (Merck)	**Powder for Injection, lyophilized:** 10,000 IU	80 mg mannitol. Preservative free. In 10 ml vials.

PEGASPARGASE (PEG-L-asparaginase)

Actions:

Pharmacology: Pegaspargase is a modified version of the enzyme L-asparaginase. It is an oncolytic agent used in combination chemotherapy for the treatment of patients with acute lymphoblastic leukemia (ALL) who are hypersensitive to native forms of L-asparaginase. L-asparaginase is modified by covalently conjugating units of monomethoxypolyethylene glycol (PEG), molecular weight of 5000, to the enzyme, forming the active ingredient PEG-L-asparaginase. The L-asparaginase used in the manufacture of pegaspargase is derived from *Escherichia coli*.

Leukemic cells are unable to synthesize asparagine due to a lack of asparagine synthetase and are dependent on an exogenous source of asparagine for survival. Rapid depletion of asparagine, which results from treatment with the enzyme L-asparaginase, kills the leukemic cells. Normal cells, however, are less affected by the rapid depletion due to their ability to synthesize asparagine. This is an approach to therapy based on a specific metabolic defect in some leukemic cells which do not produce asparagine synthetase.

Pharmacokinetics: In a study in predominately L-asparaginase-naive adult patients with leukemia and lymphoma, initial plasma levels of L-asparaginase following IV administration were determined. Plasma half-life did not appear to be influenced by dose levels, and it could not be correlated with age, sex, surface area, renal or hepatic function, diagnosis or extent of disease. Apparent volume of distribution was equal to estimated plasma volume. L-asparaginase was measurable for at least 15 days following the initial treatment with pegaspargase. The enzyme could not be detected in the urine.

In a study of newly diagnosed pediatric patients with ALL who received either a single IM injection of pegaspargase (2500 IU/m^2), *E coli* L-asparaginase (25,000 IU/m^2), or *Erwinia* L-asparaginase (25,000 IU/m^2), the plasma half-lives for the three forms of L-asparaginase were 5.73, 1.24 and 0.65 days, respectively.

The in vivo early leukemic cell kill after a single IM injection of pegaspargase (2500 IU/m^2), native *E coli* L-asparaginase (25,000 IU/m^2) and *Erwinia* L-asparaginase (25,000 IU/m^2) was studied. Bone marrow aspirates were taken before and 5 days after a single dose of one of the three different forms of L-asparaginase. The percent reduction of viable lymphoblasts at day 5 for each group was 55.7%, 57.8% and 57.9%, respectively.

In three pharmacokinetic studies, 37 relapsed ALL patients received pegaspargase at 2500 IU/m^2 every 2 weeks. The plasma half-life was 3.24 ± 1.83 days in nine patients who were previously hypersensitive to native L-asparaginase and 5.69 ± 3.25 days in 28 non-hypersensitive patients. The area under the curve was 9.5 ± 3.95 IU/ml/day in the previously hypersensitive patients, and 9.83 ± 5.94 IU/ml day in the non-hypersensitive patients.

Clinical trials: In four open-label studies, 42 previously hypersensitive acute leukemia patients (39 [93%] with ALL) with multiple relapses received pegaspargase at a dose of 2000 or 2500 IU/m^2 administered IM or IV every 14 days during induction combination chemotherapy. The reinduction response rate was 50% (36% complete remissions and 14% partial remissions). This response rate is comparable to that reported in the literature for relapsed patients treated with native L-asparaginase as part of combination chemotherapy.

Pegaspargase was also shown to have some activity as a single agent in multiply relapsed hypersensitive ALL patients, the majority of whom were pediatric. Treatment resulted in three responses (one complete remission and two partial remissions) in nine previously hypersensitive patients who would not have been able to receive any further L-asparaginase treatment.

Pegaspargase was also studied in non-hypersensitive, relapsed ALL patients who were randomized to receive two doses of pegaspargase at 2500 IU/m^2 every 14 days or twelve doses of *E coli* L-asparaginase at 10,000 IU/m^2 3 times a week during a 28 day induction combination chemotherapy regimen (which included vincristine and prednisone). Although the enrollment in this study was too small to be conclusive, the data showed that for 20 patients there was no significant difference between the overall response rates of 60% and 50%, respectively, or the complete remission rates of 50% and 50%, respectively.

Pegaspargase was administered during maintenance therapy regimens to 33 previously hypersensitive patients. The average number of doses received during maintenance therapy was 5.8 (range, 1 to 24) and the average duration of maintenance therapy was 126 days (range, 1 to 513).

PEGASPARGASE (PEG-L-asparaginase)

Indications:

Acute lymphoblastic leukemia (ALL): For patients with ALL who require L-asparaginase in their treatment regimen, but have developed hypersensitivity to the native forms of L-asparaginase. Pegaspargase, like native L-asparaginase, is generally used in combination with other chemotherapeutic agents, such as vincristine, methotrexate, cytarabine, daunorubicin and doxorubicin. Use of pegaspargase as a single agent should only be undertaken when multi-agent chemotherapy is judged to be inappropriate for the patient.

Contraindications:

Pancreatitis or a history of pancreatitis; patients who have had significant hemorrhagic events associated with prior L-asparaginase therapy; previous serious allergic reactions, such as generalized urticaria, bronchospasm, laryngeal edema, hypotension, or other unacceptable adverse reactions to pegaspargase.

Warnings:

Hypersensitivity: Hypersensitivity reactions to pegaspargase, including life-threatening anaphylaxis, may occur during therapy, especially in patients with known hypersensitivity to the other forms of L-asparaginase. As a routine precaution, keep patients under observation for 1 hour with resuscitation equipment and other agents necessary to treat anaphylaxis (eg, epinephrine, oxygen, IV steroids) available.

Hypersensitivity reactions to *E coli* L-asparaginase have been reported in the literature in 3% to 73% of patients. Patients in pegaspargase clinical studies were considered to be previously hypersensitive if they experienced a systemic rash, urticaria, bronchospasm, laryngeal edema or hypotension following administration of any form of native L-asparaginase. Patients were also considered to be previously hypersensitive it they experienced local erythema, urticaria, or swelling > 2 cm for at least 10 minutes following administration of any form of native L-asparaginase. The National Cancer Institute Common Toxicity Criteria (CTC) were used to classify the severity of the hypersensitivity reactions. These are: Grade 1 - transient rash (mild); grade 2 - mild bronchospasm (moderate); grade 3 - moderate bronchospasm or serum sickness (severe); grade 4 - hypotension or anaphylaxis (life-threatening). Additionally most transient local urticaria were considered grade 2 hypersensitivity reactions, while most sustained urticaria distant from the injection site were considered grade 3 hypersensitivity reactions. In general, the moderate to life-threatening hypersensitivity reactions were considered dose-limiting; that is, they required L-asparaginase treatment to be discontinued.

In separate studies, pegaspargase was administered IV to 48 patients and IM to 126 patients. The incidence of hypersensitivity reactions when pegaspargase was administered IM was 30% in patients who were previously hypersensitive to native L-asparaginase and 11% in non-hypersensitive patients. The incidence of hypersensitivity reactions when pegaspargase was administered IV was 60% in patients who were previously hypersensitive to native L-asparaginase and 12% in non-hypersensitive patients. Since only five previously hypersensitive patients received pegaspargase IV, no meaningful analysis of the incidence of hypersensitivity reactions was possible between either the previously hypersensitive and non-hypersensitive patients, or between the IV and IM routes of administration.

Incidence of Pegaspargase Hypersensitivity Reactions						
		CTC grade of hypersensitivity reaction				
Patient status	No.	1	2	3	4	Total
Previously hypersensitive patients	62	7	8	4	1	20 (32%)
Non-hypersensitive patients	112	5	4	1	1	11 (10%)
Total patients	174	12	12	5	2	31 (18%)

The probability of previously hypersensitive and non-hypersensitive patients completing 8 doses of therapy without developing a dose-limiting hypersensitivity reaction was 77% and 95%, respectively.

All of the 62 hypersensitive patients treated with pegaspargase in five clinical studies had previous hypersensitivity reactions to one or more of the native forms of L-asparaginase. Of the 35 patients who had previous hypersensitivity reactions to *E coli* L-asparaginase, only 5 (14%) had dose-limiting hypersensitivity reactions. Of the 27 patients who had hypersensitivity reactions to both *E coli* and *Erwinia* L-asparaginase, 7 (26%) had pegaspargase dose-limiting hypersensitivity reactions. The overall incidence of dose-limiting hypersensitivity reactions in 174 patients treated with pegaspargase was 9% (19% in 62 hypersensitive and 3% in 112 non-hypersensitive patients). Of the total of 9% dose-limiting hypersensitivity reactions, 1% were anaphylactic (CTC grade 4) and the other 8% were ≤ CTC grade 3.

PEGASPARGASE (PEG-L-asparaginase)

Pregnancy: Category C. It is not known whether pegaspargase can cause fetal harm when administered to a pregnant woman or can affect reproduction capacity. Give to a pregnant woman only if clearly needed.

Lactation: It is not known whether pegaspargase is excreted in breast milk. Because of the potential for serious adverse reactions in nursing infants, decide whether to discontinue nursing or discontinue the drug, taking into account the importance of the drug to the mother.

Precautions:

Monitoring: Carefully monitor and adjust the therapeutic regimen according to response and toxicity.

A fall in circulating lymphoblasts is often noted after initiating therapy. This may be accompanied by a marked rise in serum uric acid. As a guide to the effects of therapy, monitor the patient's peripheral blood count and bone marrow. Obtain frequent serum amylase determinations to detect early evidence of pancreatitis. Monitor blood sugar during therapy because hyperglycemia may occur. When using pegaspargase in conjunction with hepatotoxic chemotherapy, monitor patients for liver dysfunction. Pegaspargase may affect a number of plasma proteins; therefore, monitoring of fibrinogen, PT and PTT may be indicated.

Handling: This drug may be a contact irritant, and the solution must be handled and administered with care. Gloves are recommended. Inhalation of vapors and contact with skin or mucous membranes, especially those of the eyes, must be avoided. In case of contact, wash with copious amounts of water for at least 15 minutes.

Bleeding: Patients taking pegaspargase are at higher than usual risk for bleeding problems, especially with simultaneous use of other drugs that have anticoagulant properties, such as aspirin and non-steroidal anti-inflammatories (see Drug Interactions).

Infection: Pegaspargase may have immunosuppressive activity. Therefore, it is possible that use of the drug may predispose patients to infection.

Hepatic/CNS toxicity: Severe hepatic and CNS toxicity following multi-agent chemotherapy that includes pegaspargase may occur. Caution appears warranted when treating patients with pegaspargase in combination with hepatotoxic agents, particularly when liver dysfunction is present.

Drug Interactions:

Depletion of serum proteins by pegaspargase may increase the toxicity of other drugs which are protein bound. Additionally, during the period of its inhibition of protein synthesis and cell replication, pegaspargase may interfere with the action of drugs such as methotrexate, which require cell replication for their lethal effects. Pegaspargase may interfere with the enzymatic detoxification of other drugs, particularly in the liver.

Imbalances in coagulation factors have been noted with the use of pegaspargase, predisposing to bleeding or thrombosis. Use caution when administering any concurrent anticoagulant therapy, such as warfarin, heparin, dipyridamole, aspirin or nonsteroidal anti-inflammatory agents.

Adverse Reactions:

Adverse reactions have occurred in adults and pediatric patients. Overall, the adult patients had a somewhat higher incidence of known L-asparaginase toxicities, except for hypersensitivity reactions, than the pediatric patients.

Excluding hypersensitivity reactions, the most frequently occurring known L-asparaginase related toxicities and adverse experiences were chemical hepatotoxicities and coagulopathies, the majority of which did not result in any significant clinical events. The incidence of significant clinical events included clinical pancreatitis (1%), hyperglycemia requiring insulin therapy (3%) and thrombosis (4%).

The following adverse reactions were reported for 174 patients in five clinical studies: Allergic reactions (which may have included rash, erythema, edema, pain, fever, chills, urticaria, dyspnea or bronchospasm), ALT increase, nausea or vomiting, fever, malaise (> 5%).

Anaphylactic reactions, dyspnea, injection site hypersensitivity, lip edema, rash, urticaria, abdominal pain, chills, pain in the extremities, hypotension, tachycardia, thrombosis, anorexia, diarrhea, jaundice, abnormal liver function test, decreased anticoagulant effect, disseminated intravascular coagulation, decreased fibrinogen, hemolytic anemia, leukopenia, pancytopenia, thrombocytopenia, increased thromboplastin, injection site pain/reaction, bilirubinemia, hyperglycemia, hyperuricemia, hypoglycemia, hypoproteinemia, peripheral edema, increased AST, arthralgia, myalgia, convulsion, headache, night sweats, paresthesia (> 1% but < 5%).

PEGASPARGASE (PEG-L-asparaginase)

Bronchospasm, petechial rash, face edema, lesional edema, sepsis, septic shock, chest pain, endocarditis, hypertension, constipation, flatulence, GI pain, hepatomegaly, increased appetite, liver fatty deposits, coagulation disorder, increased coagulation time, decreased platelet count, purpura, increased amylase, edema, excessive thirst, hyper-ammonemia, hyponatremia, weight loss, bone pain, joint disorder, confusion, dizziness, emotional lability, somnolence, increased cough, epistaxis, upper respiratory infection, erythema simplex, pruritus, hematuria, increased urinary frequency, abnormal kidney function (< 1%).

The following pegaspargase-related adverse reactions have been observed in patients with hematologic malignancies, primarily ALL (≈ 75%), non-Hodgkins lymphoma (≈ 13%), acute myelogenous leukemia (≈ 3%), and a variety of solid tumors (≈ 9%):

Hypersensitivity – These reactions may be acute or delayed, and include acute anaphylaxis, bronchospasm, dyspnea, urticaria, arthralgia, erythema, induration, edema, pain, tenderness, hives, swelling, lip edema, chills, fever and skin rashes (see Warnings).

Pancreatic: Pancreatitis, (sometimes fulmitant and fatal); increased serum amylase and lipase.

Hepatic – Elevations of AST, ALT and bilirubin (direct and indirect); jaundice, ascites and hypoalbuminemia, which may be associated with peripheral edema (usually are reversible on discontinuance of therapy, and some reversal may occur during the course of therapy); fatty changes in the liver; liver failure.

Hematologic – Hypofibrinogenemia; prolonged prothrombin times; prolonged partial thromboplastin times; decreased antithrombin III; superficial and deep venous thrombosis; sagittal sinus thrombosis; venous catheter thrombosis; atrial thrombosis; leukopenia; agranulocytosis; pancytopenia; thrombocytopenia; disseminated intravascular coagulation; severe hemolytic anemia; anemia; clinical hemorrhage (may be fatal); easy bruisability; ecchymosis.

Metabolic – Mild to severe hyperglycemia (low incidence, usually responds to discontinuation of pegaspargase and the judicious use of IV fluid and insulin); hypoglycemia; increased thirst; hyponatremia; uric acid nephropathy; hyperuricemia; hypoproteinemia; peripheral edema; hypoalbuminemia; proteinuria; weight loss; metabolic acidosis; increase in blood ammonia during the conversion of L-asparagine to aspartic acid by the enzyme.

CNS – Status epilepticus; temporal lobe seizures; somnolence; coma; malaise; mental status changes; dizziness; emotional lability; headache; lip numbness; finger paresthesia; mood changes; night sweats; a Parkinson-like syndrome; mild to severe confusion; disorientation; paresthesia. These side effects usually have reversed spontaneously after treatment was stopped.

Renal – Increased BUN; increased creatinine; increased urinary frequency; hematuria due to thrombopenia; severe hemorrhagic cystitis; renal dysfunction; renal failure.

Cardiovascular – Chest pain; subacute bacterial endocarditis; hypertension; severe hypotension; tachycardia.

GI – Anorexia; constipation; decreased appetite; diarrhea; indigestion; flatulence; gas; GI pain; mucositis; hepatomegaly; elevated gamma-glutamyltranspeptidase; increased appetite; mouth tenderness; severe colitis; nausea; vomiting.

Musculoskeletal – Diffuse and local musculoskeletal pain; arthralgia; joint stiffness; cramps.

Respiratory – Cough; epistaxis; severe bronchospasm; upper respiratory infection.

Dermatologic – Itching; alopecia; fever blister; purpura; hand whiteness; fungal changes; nail whiteness and ridging; erythema simplex; jaundice; petechial rash.

Miscellaneous – Localized edema; injection site reactions (including pain, swelling or redness); malaise; infection; sepsis; fatigue; septic shock.

Overdosage:

Three patients received 10,000 IU/m^2 as an IV infusion. One patient experienced a slight increase in liver enzymes. A second patient developed a rash 10 minutes after the start of the infusion, which was controlled with the administration of an antihistamine and by slowing down the infusion rate. A third patient did not experience any adverse reactions.

Patient Information:

Inform patients of the possibility of hypersensitivity reactions, including immediate anaphylaxis.

Pegaspargase patients are at higher than usual risk for bleeding problems. Instruct patients that the simultaneous use of pegaspargase with other drugs that may increase the risk of bleeding should be avoided (see Drug Interactions).

PEGASPARGASE (PEG-L-asparaginase)

Pegaspargase may affect the ability of the liver to function normally in some patients. Therapy with pegaspargase may increase the toxicity of other medications (see Drug Interactions).

Pegaspargase may have immunosuppressive activity. Therefore, it is possible that use of the drug in patients may predispose the patient to infection. Patients should notify their physicians of any adverse reactions that occur.

Administration and Dosage:

Approved by the FDA on February 1, 1994.

As a component of selected multiple-agent regimens, the recommended dose is 2500 IU/m^2 every 14 days by either the IM or IV route of administration. The preferred route of administration, however, is the IM route because of the lower incidence of hepatotoxicity, coagulopathy, and GI and renal disorders compared to the IV route.

Do not administer if there is any indication that the drug has been frozen. Although there may not be an apparent change in the appearance of the drug, pegaspargase's activity is destroyed after freezing.

Dosage: The safety and efficacy of pegaspargase have been established in patients with known previous hypersensitivity to L-asparaginase whose ages ranged from 1 to 21 years old. The recommended dose for children with a body surface area ≥ 0.6 m^2 is 2500 IU/m^2 administered every 14 days. The recommended dose for children with a body surface area < 0.6 m^2 is 82.5 IU/kg administered every 14 days.

Administration:

IM – When administering IM, limit the volume at a single injection site to 2 ml. If the volume to be administered is > 2 ml, use multiple injection sites.

IV – When administered IV, give over a period of 1 to 2 hours in 100 ml of Sodium Chloride or Dextrose Injection 5%, through an infusion that is already running.

Use as a single agent – Use of pegaspargase as the sole induction agent should be undertaken only in an unusual situation when a combined regimen, which uses other chemotherapeutic agents such as vincristine, methotrexate, cytarabine, daunorubicin or doxorubicin, is inappropriate because of toxicity or other specific patient-related factors, or in patients refractory to other therapy. When pegaspargase is to be used as the sole induction agent, the recommended dosage regimen is also 2500 IU/m^2 every 14 days.

Maintenance – When a remission is obtained, appropriate maintenance therapy may be instituted. Pegaspargase may be used as part of a maintenance regimen.

Storage/Stability: Avoid excessive agitation; do NOT shake. Keep refrigerated at 2° to 8°C (36° to 46°F). Do not use if cloudy or if precipitate is present. Do not use if stored at room temperature for > 48 hours. Do NOT freeze. Do not use product if it is known to have been frozen. Freezing destroys activity, which cannot be detected visually. Use only one dose per vial; do not re-enter the vial. Discard unused portions. Do not save unused drug for later administration.

Rx	**Oncaspar** (Enzon)	**Injection**: 750 IU/ml in a phosphate buffered saline solution	Preservative free. In single-use vials.

PORFIMER SODIUM

Actions:

Pharmacology: Porfirmer is a photosensitizing agent used in the photodynamic therapy (PDT) of tumors. The cytotoxic and antitumor actions of porfimer are light and oxygen dependent. Photodynamic therapy with porfimer is a two-stage process. The first stage is the IV injection of porfimer. Clearance from a variety of tissues occurs over 40 to 72 hours, but tumors, skin and organs of the reticuloendothelial system (including liver and spleen) retain porfimer for a longer period. Illumination with 630 nm wavelength laser light constitutes the second stage of therapy. Tumor selectivity in treatment occurs through a combination of selective retention of porfimer sodium and selective delivery of light. Cellular damage caused by porfimer PDT is a consequence of the propagation of radical reactions. Radical initiation may occur after porfimer absorbs light to form a porphyrin excited state. Spin transfer from porfimer to molecular oxygen may then generate singlet oxygen. Subsequent radical reactions can form superoxide and hydroxyl radicals. Tumor death also occurs through ischemic necrosis secondary to vascular occlusion that appears to be partly mediated by thromboxane A_2 release. The laser treatment induces a photochemical, not a thermal, effect.

Pharmacokinetics: Following a 2 mg/kg dose to four male cancer patients, the average peak plasma concentration was 15 mcg/ml, the elimination half-life was 250 hours, the steady-state volume of distribution was 0.49 L/kg and the total plasma clearance was 0.051 ml/min/kg. The mean plasma concentration at 48 hours was 2.6 mcg/ml.

Porfimer was ≈ 90% protein bound in human serum in vitro. The binding was independent of concentration over the range of 20 to 100 mcg/ml.

Clinical trials: PDT with porfimer was utilized in a study of 17 patients with completely obstructing esophageal carcinoma. After a single course of therapy, 94% of patients obtained an objective tumor response and 76% experienced some palliation of their dysphagia. On average, before treatment these patients had difficulty swallowing liquids, even saliva. After one course of therapy, there was a statistically significant improvement in mean dysphagia grade, and 13 of 17 patients could swallow liquids without difficulty 1 week or 1 month after treatment. Based on all courses, three patients achieved a complete tumor response (CR). In two of these patients, the CR was documented only at week 1 as they had no further assessments. The third patient achieved a CR after a second course of therapy, which was supported by negative histopathology and maintained for the entire follow-up of 6 months.

Of the 17 treated patients, 11 (65%) received clinically important benefit from PDT. Clinically important benefit was defined hierarchically as a complete tumor response (3 patients), achievement of normal swallowing (two patients went from Grade 5 dysphagia to Grade 1) or achievement of a marked improvement of two or more grades of dysphagia with minimal adverse reactions (six patients). The median duration of benefit in these patients was 69+ days. All of these patients were still in response at their last assessment and, therefore, the estimate of 69 days is conservative. The median survival for these 11 patients was 115 days.

Indications:

Esophageal cancer: Photodynamic therapy with porfimer for palliation of patients with completely obstructing esophageal cancer, or of patients with partially obstructing esophageal cancer who cannot be satisfactorily treated with Nd:YAG laser therapy.

Contraindications:

Porfimer: Porphyria or in patients with known allergies to porphyrins.

PDT: Existing tracheoesophageal or bronchoesophageal fistula; tumors eroding into a major blood vessel.

Warnings:

Fistula: If the esophageal tumor is eroding into the trachea or bronchial tree, the likelihood of tracheoesophageal or bronchoesophageal fistula resulting from treatment is sufficiently high that PDT is not recommended.

Photosensitivity: All patients who receive porfimer sodium will be photosensitive and must observe precautions to avoid exposure of skin and eyes to direct sunlight or bright indoor light (eg, examination lamps, including dental lamps, operating room lamps, unshaded light bulbs at close proximity) for 30 days. The photosensitivity is due to residual drug which will be present in all parts of the skin. Exposure of the skin to ambient indoor light is beneficial because the remaining drug will be inactivated gradually and safely through a photobleaching reaction. Therefore, patients should not stay in a darkened room during this period and should be encouraged to expose their skin to ambient indoor light.

The level of photosensitivity will vary for different areas of the body, depending on the extent of previous exposure to light. Before exposing any area of skin to direct sunlight or bright indoor light the patient should test it for residual photosensitivity. Expose a small area of skin to sunlight for 10 minutes. If no photosensitivity reaction (erythema, edema, blistering) occurs within 24 hours, the patient can gradually resume normal outdoor activities, initially continuing to exercise caution and gradually allowing increased exposure. If some photosensitivity reaction occurs with the limited skin test, the patient should continue precautions for another 2 weeks before retesting. The tissue around the eyes may be more sensitive, and therefore, it is not recommended that the face be used for testing. If patients travel to a different geographical area with greater sunshine, they should retest their level of photosensitivity. UV (ultraviolet) sunscreens are of no value in protecting against photosensitivity reactions, because photoactivation is caused by visible light.

Mutagenesis: Porfimer caused less than 2-fold, but significant, increases in sister chromatid exchange in CHO cells irradiated with visible light and a 3-fold increase in Chinese hamster lung fibroblasts irradiated with near UV light. Porfimer-PDT caused an increase in thymidine kinase mutants and DNA-protein cross-links in mouse L5178Y cells, and caused a light-dose dependent increase in DNA-strand breaks in malignant human cervical carcinoma cells, but not in normal cells.

Elderly: Almost 80% of patients treated with PDT using porfimer in clinical trials were > 60 years of age. There was no apparent difference in effectiveness or safety in these patients compared with younger people. Dose modification based on age is not required.

Pregnancy: Category C. Women of childbearing potential should practice an effective method of contraception during therapy.

In rats, porfimer (8 mg/kg/day; 0.64 time the clinical dose) for 10 days caused maternal and fetal toxicity resulting in increased resorptions, decreased litter size, delayed ossification and reduced fetal weight. When given to rabbits during organogenesis at 4 mg/kg/day for 13 days, maternal toxicity occurred, resulting in increased resportions, decreased litter size and reduced fetal body weight. Porfimer given to rats during late pregnancy through lactation for at least 42 days caused a reversible decrease in growth of offspring. There are no adequate and well-controlled studies in pregnant women. Use during pregnancy only if the potential benefit justifies the potential risk to the fetus.

Lactation: It is not known whether this drug is excreted in breast milk. Because of the potential for serious adverse reactions in nursing infants, women receiving porfimer must not breastfeed.

Children: Safety and efficacy in children have not been established.

Precautions:

Ocular sensitivity: Ocular discomfort, commonly described as sensitivity to sun, bright lights or car headlights has been reported in patients who received porfimer. For 30 days, when outdoors, patients should wear dark sunglasses which have an average white light transmittance of < 4%.

Chest pain: As a result of PDT treatment, patients may complain of substernal chest pain because of inflammatory responses within the area of treatment. Such pain may be of sufficient intensity to warrant the short-term prescription of opiate analgesics.

Drug Interactions:

Photosensitizing agents: It is possible that concomitant use of other photosensitizing agents (eg, tetracyclines, sulfonamides, phenothiazines, sulfonylureas, thiazide diuretics, griseofulvin) could increase the photosensitivity reaction.

PDT causes direct intracellular damage by initiating radical chain reactions that damage intracellular membranes and mitochondria. Tissue damage also results from ischemia secondary to vasoconstriction, platelet activation and aggregation and clotting. Research in animals and in cell culture has suggested that many drugs could influence the effects of PDT.

Compounds that quench active oxygen species or scavenge radicals, such as dimethyl sulfoxide, β-carotene, ethanol and mannitol would be expected to decrease PDT activity. Preclinical data also suggest that tissue ischemia, allopurinol, calcium channel blockers and some prostaglandin synthesis inhibitors could interfere with porfimer. Drugs that decrease clotting, vasoconstriction or platelet aggregation (eg, thromboxane A_2 inhibitors) could decrease the efficacy of PDT. Glucocorticoid hormones given before or concomitantly with PDT may decrease the efficacy of the treatment.

Adverse Reactions:

Systemically induced affects associated with PDT with porfimer consist of photosensitivity and mild constipation. All patients who receive porfimer will be photosensitive and must observe precautions to avoid sunlight and bright indoor light (see Warnings). Photosensitivity reactions (mostly mild erythem on the face and hands)

PORFIMER SODIUM

occurred in ≈ 20% of patients treated with porfimer. Most toxicities associated with this therapy are local effects seen in the region of illumination and occasionally in surrounding tissues. The local adverse reactions are characteristic of an inflammatory response induced by the photodynamic effect.

Porfimer-PDT Adverse Reactions (≥ 5%)

Adverse reaction	PDT with Porfimer (n = 88)	Adverse reaction	PDT with Porfimer (n = 88)
Patients with ≥ 1 adverse reaction	95	Nausea	24
Autonomic Nervous System		Vomiting	17
Hypertension	6	*Cardiovascular*	
Hypotension	7	Atrial fibrillation	10
Body as a whole		Cardiac failure	7
Asthenia	6	Tachycardia	6
Back pain	11	*Metabolic/Nutritional*	
Chest pain	22	Dehydration	7
Chest pain (substernal)	5	Weight decrease	9
Edema generalized	5	*CNS*	
Edema peripheral	7	Anorexia	8
Fever	31	Anxiety	7
Pain	22	Confusion	8
Surgical complication	5	Insomnia	14
GI		*Respiratory*	
Abdominal pain	20	Coughing	7
Constipation	24	Dyspnea	20
Diarrhea	5	Pharyngitis	11
Dyspepsia	6	Pleural effusion	32
Dysphagia	10	Pneumonia	18
Eructation	5	Respiratory insufficiency	10
Esophageal edema	8	Tracheoesophageal fistula	6
Esophageal tumor bleeding	8	*Miscellaneous*	
Esophageal stricture	6	Anemia	32
Esophagitis	5	Photosensitivity reaction	19
Hematemesis	8	Moniliasis	9
Melena	5	Urinary tract infection	7

Location of the tumor was a prognostic factor for three adverse events: Upper-third of the esophagus (esophageal edema), middle-third (atrial fibrillation) and lower-third, the most vascular region (anemia). Also, patients with large tumors (> 10 cm) were more likely to experience anemia. Two of 17 patients with complete esophageal obstruction from tumor experienced esophageal perforations which were possibly treatment associated; these perforations occurred during subsequent endoscopies.

Serious and other notable adverse events observed in < 5% of patients include:

GI: Esophageal perforation, gastric ulcer, ileus, jaundice, peritonitis.

Cardiovascular: Angina pectoris, bradycardia, myocardial infarction, sick sinus syndrome, supraventricular tachycardia.

Respiratory: Bronchitis, bronchospasm, laryngotracheal edema, pneumonitis, pulmonary hemorrhage, pulmonary edema, respiratory failure, stridor.

Miscellaneous: Sepsis has been recorded occasionally. The temporal relationship of some GI, cardiovascular and respiratory events to the administration of light was suggestive of mediastinal inflammation in some patients. Vision-related events of abnormal vision, diplopia, eye pain and photophobia have been reported. PDT with porfimer may result in anemia due to tumor bleeding.

Overdosage:

Effects of overdosage on the duration of photosensitivity are unknown. Laser treatment should not be given if an overdose of porfimer is administered. In the event of an overdose, patients should protect their eyes and skin from direct sunlight or bright indoor lights for 30 days. At this time, patients should test for residual photosensitivity. Porfimer is not dialyzable.

PORFIMER SODIUM

Overdose of laser light following porfimer injeciton: Increased symptoms and damage to normal tissue might be expected following an overdose of light.

Administration and Dosage:

Approved by the FDA on December 27, 1995.

Photodynamic therapy with porfimer is a two-stage process requiring administration of both drug and light. Practitioners should be trained in the safe and efficacious treatment of esophageal cancer using photodynamic therapy with porfimer and associated light delivery devices. The first stage of PDT is the IV injection of porfimer at 2 mg/kg. Illumination with laser light 40 to 50 hours following injection with porfimer constitutes the second stage of therapy. A second laser light application may be given 96 to 120 hours after injection, preceded by gentle debridement of residual tumor (see Administration of laser light). In clinical studies, debridement via endoscopy was required 2 days after the initial light application. More recently, experienced investigators have indicated that mandatory debridement may not be necessary because of the natural sloughin action in the esophagus, and may needlessly traumatize the area.

Patients may receive a second course of PDT a minimum of 30 days after the initial therapy; up to three courses of PDT (each separated by a minimum of 30 days) can be given. Before each course of treatment, evaluate patients for the presence of a tracheoesophageal or bronchoesophageal fistula (see Contraindications).

Porfimer: Administer porfimer as single slow IV injection over 3 to 5 minutes at 2 mg/kg. Reconstitute each vial of porfimer with 31.8 ml of either 5% Dextrose Injection or 0.9% Sodium Chloride Injection resulting in a final concentration of 2.5 mg/ml and a pH in the range of 7 to 8. Shake well until dissolved. Do not mix porfimer with other drugs in the same solution. Porfimer has been formulated wiht an over-age to deliver th 75 mg labeled quantity. Protect the reconstituted product from bright light and use immediately. Reconstituted porfimer is an opaque solution in which detection of particulate matter by visual inspection is extremely difficult.

Extravasation: Take precautions to prevent extravasation at the injection site. If extravasation occurs, take care to protect the area from light. There is no known benefit from injecting the extravasation site with another substance.

Administration of laser light: Initiate 630 nm wavelength laser light delivery to the patient 40 to 50 hours following injection with porfimer. A second laser light treatment may be given as early as 96 hours or as late as 120 hours after the initial injection with porfimer. No further injection of porfimer should be given for such retreatment with laser light. Before providing a second laser light treatment, debride the residual tumor. Vigourous debridement may cause tumor bleeding.

The laser system must be approved for delivery of a stable power output at a wavelength of 630 nm. Light is delivered to the tumor by cylindrical *Optiquide* fiber optic duffusers passed through the operating channel of an endoscope. Carefully read instructions for use of the fiber optic and the selected laser system before use. Photoactivation of porfimer is controlled by the total light dose delivered. In the treatment of esophageal cancer, deliver a light dose of 300 joules/cm of tumor length. *Optiguide* cylindrical diffusers are available in several lengths. The choice of diffuser tip length depends on the length of the tumor. Size diffuser length to avoid exposure of nonmalignant tissue to light and to prevent overlapping of previously treated malignant tissue. The total power output at the fiber tip is set to deliver the appropriate light dose using exposure times of 12 minutes and 30 seconds. Refer to the *Optiguide* instructions for complete instructions concering the fiber optic diffuser.

Handling spills and disposal: Wipe up spills of porfimer with a damp cloth. Avoid skin and eye contact due to the potential for photosensitivity reactions upon exposure to light; use of rubber gloves and eye protection is recommended. Dispose of all contaminated materials in a polyethylene bag in a manner consistent with local regulations.

Storage/Stability: Store at a controlled room temperature of 20° to 25°C (68° to 77°F).

Rx	**Photofrin** (QLT Photo)	**Cake or Powder (freeze-dried) for Injection:** 75 mg	In vials.

Cytoprotective Agents

MESNA

Actions:

Pharmacology: Mesna is used to reduce the incidence of ifosfamide-induced hemorrhagic cystitis. In the kidney, the mesna disulfide is reduced to the free thiol compound, mesna, which reacts chemically with the urotoxic ifosfamide metabolites (acrolein and 4-hydroxy-ifosfamide), resulting in their detoxification. The first step in the detoxification process is the binding of mesna to 4-hydroxy-ifosfamide, forming a nonurotoxic 4-sulfoethylthioifosfamide. Mesna also binds to the double bonds of acrolein and other urotoxic metabolites.

Pharmacokinetics: Analogous to the physiological cysteine-cystine system, following IV administration mesna is rapidly oxidized to its only metabolite, mesna disulfide (dimesna). Mesna disulfide remains in the intravascular compartment and is rapidly eliminated by the kidneys.

After administration of 800 mg, the half-lives of mesna and dimesna in the blood are 0.36 and 1.17 hours, respectively. Approximately 32% and 33% of the administered dose is eliminated in the urine in 24 hours as mesna and dimesna, respectively. The majority of the dose recovered is eliminated within 4 hours. Mesna has a volume of distribution of 0.652 L/kg and a plasma clearance of 1.23 L/kg/hour.

Ifosfamide has dose-dependent pharmacokinetics. At doses of 2 to 4 g, its terminal elimination half-life is about 7 hours. As a result, repeated doses of mesna are required to maintain adequate levels of mesna in the urinary bladder during the course of elimination of the urotoxic ifosfamide metabolites.

Clinical trials: Mesna was given as bolus doses prior to ifosfamide and at 4 and 8 hours after ifosfamide administration. The hemorrhagic cystitis produced by ifosfamide is dose dependent. At a dose of 1.2 g/m^2 ifosfamide administered daily for 5 days, 16% to 26% of the patients who received conventional uroprophylaxis (high fluid intake, alkalinization of the urine and the administration of diuretics) developed hematuria (> 50 rbc/hpf or macrohematuria). In contrast, none of the patients who received mesna together with this dose of ifosfamide developed hematuria. Higher doses of ifosfamide (from 2 to 4 g/m^2 administered for 3 to 5 days) produced hematuria in 31% to 100% of the patients. When mesna was administered together with these doses of ifosfamide, the incidence of hematuria was < 7%.

Indications:

Ifosfamide-induced hemorrhagic cystitis: Prophylactic agent to reduce the incidence of ifosfamide-induced hemorrhagic cystitis (see ifosfamide monograph).

Unlabeled uses: Mesna may be useful in reducing the incidence of cyclophosphamide-induced hemorrhagic cystitis.

Contraindications:

Hypersensitivity to mesna or other thiol compounds.

Warnings:

Ifosfamide toxicities: Mesna prevents ifosfamide-induced hemorrhagic cystitis. It will not prevent or alleviate other adverse reactions or toxicities associated with ifosfamide therapy.

Hematuria: Mesna does not prevent hemorrhagic cystitis in all patients. Up to 6% of patients treated with mesna have developed hematuria (> 50 rbc/hpf or WHO grade 2 and above). As a result, examine a morning specimen of urine for hematuria (red blood cells) each day prior to ifosfamide therapy. If hematuria develops when mesna is given with ifosfamide according to the dosage schedule, depending on the severity of the hematuria, dosage reductions or discontinuation of ifosfamide therapy may be initiated.

Mesna must be administered with each dose of ifosfamide (see Administration and Dosage). Mesna is not effective in preventing hematuria due to other pathological conditions such as thrombocytopenia.

Hypersensitivity: Allergic reactions were reported in patients with autoimmune disorders. The symptoms ranged from mild hypersensitivity to systemic anaphylactic reactions. Pretreatment with an antihistamine, a corticosteroid or both may be indicated when there has been a previous allergic reaction to mesna.

Pregnancy: Category B. It is not known whether mesna can cause fetal harm when administered to a pregnant woman or can effect reproductive capacity. Give to a pregnant woman only if the benefits clearly outweigh any risks.

Lactation: It is not known whether mesna or dimesna is excreted in breast milk. Because of the potential for adverse reactions in nursing infants, decide whether to discontinue nursing or to discontinue the drug, taking into account the importance of the drug to the mother.

Cytoprotective Agents

MESNA

Precautions:

Benzyl alcohol: Benzyl alcohol, contained in this product as a preservative, has been associated with a fatal "gasping syndrome" in premature infants.

Drug Interactions:

Drug/Lab test interactions: A false positive test for urinary ketones may arise in patients treated with mesna. In this test, a red-violet color develops that, with the addition of glacial acetic acid, will return to violet.

Adverse Reactions:

Because mesna is used in combination with ifosfamide and other chemotherapeutic agents with documented toxicities, it is difficult to distinguish which adverse reactions may be due to mesna.

In one study, a bad taste in the mouth (100%) and soft stools (70%) were reported. At IV and oral bolus 10 times the recommended clinical doses (0.24 g/m^2), diarrhea (83%), limb pain (50%), headache (50%), fatigue (33%), nausea (33%), hypotension (17%) and allergy (17%; see Warnings) occurred in six patients.

In controlled clinical studies, adverse reactions were vomiting, diarrhea and nausea.

Overdosage:

There is no known antidote for mesna.

Administration and Dosage:

For the prophylaxis of ifosfamide-induced hemorrhagic cystitis, mesna is given as IV bolus injections in a dosage equal to 20% of the ifosfamide dosage (w/w) at the time of ifosfamide administration and 4 and 8 hours after each dose of ifosfamide. The total daily dose of mesna is 60% of the ifosfamide dose.

Dosing Schedule for Mesna

	0 hours	4 hours	8 hours
Ifosfamide	1.2 g/m^2	—	—
Mesna	240 mg/m^2	240 mg/m^2	240 mg/m^2

To maintain adequate protection, repeat this dosing schedule on each day that ifosfamide is administered. When the dosage of ifosfamide is adjusted (either increased or decreased), modify the dose of mesna accordingly.

Preparations of IV solutions: For IV administration, the drug can be diluted with any of the following fluids obtaining final concentrations of 20 mg/ml: 5% Dextrose Injection, 5% Dextrose and 0.2% Sodium Chloride Injection, 5% Dextrose and 0.33% Sodium Chloride Injection, 5% Dextrose and 0.45% Sodium Chloride Injection, 0.92% Sodium Chloride Injection or Lactated Ringer's Injection.

Admixture incompatibility/compatibility: Mesna is not compatible with cisplatin. Mesna and ifosfamide are compatible in the same infusion fluid.

Storage/Stability:

Diluted solutions are chemically and physically stable for 24 hours at 25°C (77°F), but it is recommended that solutions of mesna be refrigerated, and they should be used within 6 hours of reconstitution.

The mesna multidose vials may be stored and used for up to 8 days.

When exposed to oxygen, mesna is oxidized to the disulfide, dimesna. As a result, any unused drug remaining in the ampules after dosing should be discarded and a new ampule used for each administration.

Rx	**Mesnex** (Mead Johnson Oncology)	**Injection:** 100 mg/ml	With 0.25 mg/ml EDTA. In 2 ml ampules[1] and 10 ml multidose vials.[2]

[1] Available in compassionate use cases only.
[2] With 10.4 mg benzyl alcohol as a preservative.

Cytoprotective Agents

AMIFOSTINE

Actions:

Pharmacology: Amifostine is an organic thiophosphate cytopreotective agent. It is a pro-drug that is dephosphorylated by alkaline phosphatase in tissues to a pharmacologically active free thiol metabolite that can reduce the toxic effects of cisplatin. The ability to differentially protect normal tissues is attributed to the higher capillary alkaline phosphatase activity, higher pH and better vascularity of normal tissues relative to tumor tissue, which results in a more rapid generation of the active thiol metabolite as well as higher rate constant for uptake. The higher concentration of free thiol in normal tissues is available to bind to, and thereby detoxify, reactive metabolites of cisplatin, and also, it can act as a scavenger of free radicals that may be generated in tissues exposed to cisplatin.

Pharmacokinetics: Amifostine is rapidly cleared from the plasma with a distribtion half-life of < 1 minute and an elimination half-life of ≈ 8 minutes. Less than 10% of amifostine remains in the plasma 6 minutes after drug administration. Amifostine is rapidly metabolized to an active free thiol metabolite. A disulfide metabolite is produced subsequently and is less active than the free thiol. After a 10 second bolus dose of 150 mg/m² of amifostine, renal excretion of the parent drug and its two metabolites was low during the hour following drug administration, averaging 0.69%, 2.64% and 2.22% of the adminstered dose for the parent, thiol and disulfide, respectively. Measureable levels of the free thiol metabolite have been found in bone marrow cells 5 to 8 minutes after IV infusion of amifostine.

Clinical trials: A randomized controlled trial compared six cycles of cyclophosphamide 1000 mg/m² and cisplatin 100 mg/m² with or without amifostine pretreatment at 910 mg/m², in 121 patients with advanced ovarian cancer. Pretreatment with amifostine significantly reduced the cumulative renal toxicity associated with cisplatin as assessed by the proportion of patients who had ≥ 40% decrease in creatinine clearance from pretreatment values, protracted elevations in serum creatinine (> 1.5 mg/dl) or severe hypomagnesemia.

Indications:

Renal toxicity: Reduction of cumulative renal toxicity associated with repeated administration of cisplatin in patients with advanced ovarian cancer.

Unlabeled uses: Protects lung fibroblasts from the damaging effects of paclitaxel.

Contraindications:

Sensitivity to aminothiol compounds or mannitol.

Warnings:

Effectiveness of the cytotoxic regimen: Limited data are currently available regarding the preservation of antitumor efficacy when amifostine is administered prior to cisplatin chemotherapy in settings other than advanced ovarian cancer. Although some animal data suggest interference is possible, in most tumor models the antitumor effects of chemotherapy are not altered by amifostine. The possibility of interference with the efficacy of cancer treatment would be of particular concern in those settings where chemotherapy is potentially curative. Amifostine should therefore not be used in patients receiving chemotherapy for malignancies that are potentially curable (eg, certain malignancies of germ cell origin).

Hypotension: A transient reduction in blood pressure has occurred in 62% of patients treated with amifostine. Mean time of onset was 14 minutes into the infusion; mean duration was 6 minutes. In some cases, the infusion had to be terminated because of a more pronounced drop in systolic pressure. In general, blood pressure returns to normal within 5 to 15 minutes. Patients who hare hypotensive or in a state of dehydration should not receive amifostine. Patients receiving antihypertensive therapy that cannot be stopped for 24 hours preceding amifostine treatment also should not receive amifostine. Adequately hydrate patients prior to amifostine infusion and keep in a supine position during the infusion. If hypotension requiring interruption of therapy occurs, place patients in the Trendelenburg position and give an infusion of Normal Saline using a separate IV line.

Nausea and vomiting: Administer antiemetic medication prior to and in conjunction with amifostine. When amifostine is administered with highly emetogenic chemotherapy, carefully monitor the fluid balance of the patient.

Hypocalcemia: Reports of clinically relevant hypocalcemia are rare, but monitor serum calcium levels in patients at risk of hypocalcemia, such as those with nephrotic syndrome. If necessary, calcium supplements can be administered.

Elderly: Safety has not been established in elderly patients > 70 years of age.

Cytoprotective Agents

AMIFOSTINE

Pregnancy: Category C. Amifostine is embryotoxic in rabbits at doses of 50 mg/kg, ≈ 60% of the recommended dose in humans on a body surface area basis. There are no adequate and well-controlled studies in pregnant women. Amifostine should not be used during pregnancy unless the potential benefit justifies the potential risk to the fetus.

Lactation: No information is available on teh excretion of amifostine or its metabolites into breast milk. It is recommended that breastfeeding be discontinued if the mother is treated with amifostine.

Precautions:

Monitoring: Monitor serum calcium levels in patients at risk of hypocalcemia, such as those with nephrotic syndrome. Monitor blood pressure every 5 minutes during the infusion.

Cardiovascular or cerebrovascular disease: Safety has not been established in patients with pre-existing cardiovascular or cerebrovascular conditions such as ischemic heart disease, arrhythmias, congestive heart failure or history of stroke or transient ischemic attacks.

Drug Interactions:

Antihypertensives: Give special consideration to the administration of amifostine in patients receiving antihypertensive medications or other drugs that could potentiate hypotension.

Adverse Reactions:

Flushing/feeling of warmth; chills/feeling of coldness; dizziness; somnolence; hiccoughs; sneezing; hypotension (62%; see Warnings); severe nausea and vomiting (19%); hypocalcemia (< 1%; see Warnings); short-term, reversible loss of consciousness (rare).

Hypersensitivity: Mild skin rash, rigors (< 1%).

Overdosage:

In clinical trials, the maximum single dose of amifostine was 1300 mg/m^2. No information is available on single doses higher than this in adults. Children have received single doses of up to 2700 mg/m^2 with no unexpected effects. Multiple infusions (up to three) of 740 to 910 mg/m^2 doses have been administered within a 24–hour period without unexpected effects. Administration of amifostine at 2 and 4 hours after the initial dose has not led to increased or cumulative side effects.

Administration and Dosage:

Starting dose: 910 mg/m^2 administered once daily as a 15–minute IV infusion, starting within 30 minutes prior to chemotherapy. The 15–minute infusion is better tolerated than more extended infusions.

Interrupt the infusion of amifostine if the systolic blood pressure decreases significantly from the baseline value as listed in the guideline below.

Guideline for Interrupting Amifostine Infusion Due to Decrease in Systolic Blood Pressure					
	Baseline Systolic Blood Pressure (mmHg)				
	< 100	100 to 119	120 to 139	140 to 179	≥ 180
Decrease in systolic blood pressure during infusion of amifostine (mmHg)	20	25	30	40	50

If the blood pressure returns to normal within 5 minutes and the patient is asymptomatic, the infusion may be restarted so that the full dose of amifostine may be administered. If the full dose of amifostine cannot be administered, the dose of amifostine for subsequent cycles should be 740 mg/m^2.

Coadministration: It is recommended that antiemetic medication, including dexamethasone 20 mg IV and a serotonin 5HT$_3$ receptor antagonist, be administered prior to and in conjunction with amifostine. Additional antiemetics may be required based on the chemotherapy drugs administered.

Reconstitue with 9.5 ml of 0.9% Sodium Chloride Injection.

Storage/Stability: Store vial in the refrigerator (2° to 8°C; 36° to 46°F). The reconstituted solution is chemically stable for up to 5 hours at room temperature (≈ 25°C; 77°F) or up to 24 hours under refrigeration (2° to 8°C; 36° to 46°F).

Rx	**Ethyol** (Alza/US Bioscience)	**Powder for Injection, lyophilized:** 500 mg (anhydrous basis)	500 mg mannitol. In 10 ml single use vials.

Cytoprotective Agents

DEXRAZOXANE

Actions:

Pharmacology: Dexrazoxane, a derivative of EDTA, is a cardioprotective agent for use in conjunction with doxorubicin. It is a potent intracellular chelating agent. The mechanism by which dexrazoxane exerts its cardioprotective activity is not fully understood. Dexrazoxane is a cyclic derivative of EDTA that readily penetrates cell membranes. Dexrazoxane appears to be converted intracellularly to a ring-opened chelating agent that interferes with iron-mediated free radical generation thought to be responsible, in part, for anthracycline-induced cardiomyopathy.

Pharmacokinetics:

Mean Dexrazoxane Pharmacokinetic Parameters					
Doxorubicin dose (mg/m^2)	Dexrazoxane dose (mg/m^2)	Elimination half-life (hr)	Plasma clearance ($L/hr/m^2$)	Renal clearance ($L/hr/m^2$)	Volume of distribution (L/m^2)
50	500	2.5	7.88	3.35	22.4
60	600	2.1	6.25	—	22.0

The mean peak plasma concentration of dexrazoxane was 36.5 mcg/ml at the end of the 15 minute infusion of a 500 mg/m^2 dose administered 15 to 30 minutes prior to the 50 mg/m^2 doxorubicin dose. Following a rapid distributive phase, dexrazoxane reaches post-distributive equilibrium within 2 to 4 hours. Metabolism studies have confirmed the presence of unchanged drug, a diacid-diamide cleavage product and two monoacid-monoamide ring products in the urine. Urinary excretion plays an important role in elimination; of the 500 mg/m^2 dose of dexrazoxane, 42% was excreted in the urine. Dexrazoxane is not bound to plasma proteins.

Clinical trials: The ability of dexrazoxane to prevent/reduce the incidence and severity of doxorubicin-induced cardiomyopathy was demonstrated in three studies. In these studies, patients were treated with a doxorubicin-containing regimen and either dexrazoxane or placebo starting with the first course of chemotherapy. There was no restriction on the cumulative dose of doxorubicin. Patients receiving dexrazoxane had significantly smaller mean decreases from baseline in left ventricular ejection fraction and lower incidences of CHF than the control group.

Retrospective historical analyses were performed to compare the likelihood of heart failure in patients when dexrazoxane was added to the fluorouracil, doxorubicin and cyclophosphamide (FAC) regimen after they had received six courses of FAC (and who then continued treatment with FAC therapy) with the heart failure rate in patients who had received six courses of FAC and continued to receive this regimen without added dexrazoxane. These analyses showed that the risk of experiencing a cardiac event at a given cumulative dose of doxorubicin > 300 mg/m^2 was substantially greater in the patients who did not receive dexrazoxane beginning with their seventh course of FAC than in the patients who did receive dexrazoxane.

In an analysis of the risk of developing CHF by cumulative dose of doxorubicin in patients who received dexrazoxane starting with their seventh course of FAC compared with patients who did not, patients unprotected by dexrazoxane had a 13 times greater risk of developing CHF. Overall, 3% treated with dexrazoxane developed CHF vs 22% not receiving the drug.

Indications:

Cardiomyopathy: Reduction of the incidence and severity of cardiomyopathy associated with doxorubicin administration in women with metastatic breast cancer who have received a cumulative doxorubicin dose of 300 mg/m^2 and who would benefit from continuing therapy with doxorubicin. It is not recommended for use with the initiation of doxorubicin therapy (see Warnings).

Contraindications:

Do not use with chemotherapy regimens that do not contain an anthracycline.

Warnings:

Myelosuppression: Dexrazoxane may add to the myelosuppression caused by chemotherapeutic agents.

Antitumor interference: There is some evidence that the use of dexrazoxane concurrently with the initiation of FAC therapy interferes with the antitumor efficacy of the regimen, and this use is not recommended. In the largest of three breast cancer trials, patients who received dexrazoxane starting with their first cycle of FAC therapy had a lower response rate (48% vs 63%) and shorter time to progression than patients who did not receive dexrazoxane. Therefore, dexrazoxane should only be used in those patients who have received a cumulative doxorubicin dose of 300 mg/m^2 and are continuing with doxorubicin therapy.

Anthracycline-induced cardiac toxicity: Although clinical studies have shown that patients receiving FAC with dexrazoxane may receive a higher cumulative dose of doxorubicin before experiencing cardiac toxicity than patients receiving FAC without dexrazoxane, the use of dexrazoxane in patients who have already received a cumulative dose of doxorubicin of 300 mg/m^2 without dexrazoxane does not eliminate the potential for anthracycline-induced cardiac toxicity. Therefore, carefully monitor cardiac function.

Carcinogenesis/Mutagenesis/Fertility impairment: Secondary malignancies (primarily acute myeloid leukemia) have been reported in patients treated chronically with razoxane (razoxane is the racemic mixture, of which dexrazoxane is the S(+)-enantiomer). One case of T-cell lymphoma, one case of B-cell lymphoma and six to eight cases of cutaneous basal cell or squamous cell carcinoma have also been reported in patients treated with razoxane.

Dexrazoxane was clastogenic to human lymphocytes in vitro and to mouse bone marrow erythrocytes in vivo (micronucleus test).

Testicular atrophy was seen with dexrazoxane administration at doses as low as 30 mg/kg weekly for 6 weeks in rats (1/3 the human dose) and as low as 20 mg/kg weekly for 13 weeks in dogs (approximately equal to the human dose).

Pregnancy: Category C. Dexrazoxane was maternotoxic at doses of 2 mg/kg (1/40 the human dose) and embryotoxic and teratogenic at 8 mg/kg when given daily to pregnant rats during the period of organogenesis. Teratogenic effects in the rat included imperforate anus, microphthalmia and anophthalmia. In rabbits, doses of 5 mg/kg/day during the period of organogenesis were maternotoxic and dosages of 20 mg/kg were embryotoxic and teratogenic. Teratogenic effects in the rabbit included several skeletal malformations such as short tail, rib and thoracic malformations; soft tissue variations including subcutaneous, eye and cardiac hemorrhagic areas; and agenesis of the gallbladder and of the intermediate lobe of the lung. There are no adequate and well controlled studies in pregnant women. Use during pregnancy only if the potential benefit justifies the potential risk to the fetus.

Lactation: It is not known whether dexrazoxane is excreted in breast milk. Because of the potential for serious adverse reactions in nursing infants exposed to dexrazoxane, advise mothers to discontinue nursing during dexrazoxane therapy.

Children: Safety and efficacy in children have not been established.

Precautions:

Monitoring: Because dexrazoxane will always be used with cytotoxic drugs, and because it may add to the myelosuppressive effects of cytotoxic drugs, frequent complete blood counts are recommended.

Administration: Doxorubicin should not be given prior to the IV injection of dexrazoxane. Give dexrazoxane by slow IV push or rapid drip IV infusion from a bag. Give doxorubicin within 30 minutes after beginning the infusion with dexrazoxane. (See Administration and Dosage).

DEXRAZOXANE

Adverse Reactions:

Dexrazoxane Adverse Reactions in Patients Receiving FAC (%)				
	FAC + Dexrazoxane		FAC + Placebo	
Adverse reaction	Courses 1 - 6 (n = 413)	Courses ≥ 7 (n = 102)	Courses 1 - 6 (n = 458)	Courses ≥ 7 (n = 99)
Alopecia	94	100	97	98
Nausea	77	51	84	60
Vomiting	59	42	72	49
Fatigue/ Malaise	61	48	58	55
Anorexia	42	27	47	38
Stomatitis	34	26	41	28
Fever	34	22	29	18
Infection	23	19	18	21
Diarrhea	21	14	24	7
Pain on injection	12	13	3	0
Sepsis	17	12	14	9
Neurotoxicity	17	10	13	5
Streaking/ Erythema	5	4	4	2
Phlebitis	6	3	3	5
Esophagitis	6	3	7	4
Dysphagia	8	0	10	5
Hemorrhage	2	3	2	1
Extravasa- tion	1	3	1	2
Urticaria	2	2	2	0
Recall skin reaction	1	1	2	0

The adverse experiences listed above are likely attributable to the FAC regimen, with the exception of pain on injection that was observed mainly with dexrazoxane.

Hematologic: Patients receiving FAC with dexrazoxane experienced more severe leukopenia, granulocytopenia and thrombocytopenia at nadir than patients receiving FAC without dexrazoxane, but recovery counts were similar for the two groups.

Lab test abnormalities: Patients receiving FAC plus dexrazoxane or FAC plus placebo experienced marked abnormalities in hepatic or renal function tests.

Overdosage:

Retention of a significant dose fraction of the unchanged drug in the plasma pool, minimal tissue partitioning or binding and availability of > 90% of the systemic drug levels in the unbound form suggest that dexrazoxane could be removed using conventional peritoneal or hemodialysis. Manage instances of suspected overdose with good supportive care until resolution of myelosuppression, and related conditions, is complete. Management of overdose should include treatment of infections, fluid regulation and maintenance of nutritional requirements. Refer to General Management of Acute Overdosage.

Administration and Dosage:

Approved by the FDA on May 26, 1995 (1P classification).

The recommended dosage ratio of dexrazoxane:doxorubicin is 10:1 (eg, 500 mg/m^2 dexrazoxane:50 mg/m^2 doxorubicin). Dexrazoxane must be reconstituted with 0.167 Molar (M/6) Sodium Lactate Injection to give a concentration of 10 mg dexrazoxane for each ml of sodium lactate. Administer the reconstituted solution by slow IV push or rapid drip IV infusion from a bag. After completing the infusion, and prior to a total elapsed time of 30 minutes (from the beginning of the dexrazoxane infusion), give the IV injection of doxorubicin.

Cytoprotective Agents

DEXRAZOXANE

Dilution: The reconstituted dexrazoxane solution may be diluted with either 0.9% Sodium Chloride Injection or 5% Dextrose Injection to a concentration range of 1.3 to 5 mg/ml in IV infusion bags.

Admixture incompatibility: Dexrazoxane should not be mixed with other drugs.

Handling and disposal: Exercise caution in the handling and preparation of the reconstituted solution; the use of gloves is recommended. If dexrazoxane powder or solutions contact the skin or mucosae, immediately wash with soap and water.

Storage/stability: Store at controlled room temperature, 15° to 30°C (59° to 86°F). Reconstituted and diluted solutions are stable for 6 hours at controlled room temperature or under refrigeration, 2° to 8°C (36° to 46°F). Discard unused solutions.

Rx	**Zinecard** (Pharmacia)	**Powder for injection (lyophilized):** 250 mg (10 mg/ml reconstituted)	In single-dose vials with 25 ml vial sodium lactate injection.
		500 mg (10 mg/ml reconstituted)	In single-dose vials with 50 ml vial sodium lactate injection.

NCI INVESTIGATIONAL AGENTS

The National Cancer Institute (NCI), Division of Cancer Treatment (DCT), is involved in the development and research of antineoplastic drugs. Certain agents under investigation may be categorized as Group C drugs. To be designated a Group C drug, an investigational agent must be effective in the treatment of a specific neoplasm and those results supported by multiple studies. Such drugs have altered or are likely to alter the pattern of treatment of a specific disease and can be distributed to any properly trained physician for use without specialized supportive care facilities.

Use of Group C agents: Physicians desiring to use Group C investigational agents must: (1) register as an investigator with NCI by submitting FD-form 1572; (2) submit a request for the drugs, indicating the disease to be treated; (3) follow NCI established protocol; (4) report all adverse reactions to the NCI Investigational Drug Branch. For further information contact: Pharmaceutical Management Branch, National Cancer Institute, EPN, Room 804, 6130 Executive Blvd., Rockville, MD 20852, (301) 496-5725.

The following Group C agents are available from NCI for the conditions indicated:

Amsacrine

Other names:	NSC-249992, m-AMSA, Acridinyl Anisidide
Use:	Refractory adult acute myelogenous leukemia (AML)

Azacitidine

Other names:	NSC-102816, 5-Azacytidine, AZA-CR, 5-AZC, Ladakamycin
Use:	Refractory acute myelogenous leukemia

Erwinia Asparaginase

Other names:	NSC-106977, Porton Asparaginase
Use:	Acute lymphocytic leukemia (ALL) in patients sensitive to *E coli* L-asparaginase

chapter 12

miscellaneous products

LOCAL ANESTHETICS, INJECTABLE

This information on local anesthetics is not intended to be comprehensive. Consult standard textbooks for further discussion of techniques and applications.

Actions:

Pharmacology: These agents prevent generation and conduction of nerve impulses by inhibiting ionic fluxes, increasing electrical excitation threshold, slowing nerve impulse propagation and reducing rate of rise of action potential. Progression of anesthesia is related to the diameter, myelination and conduction velocity of affected nerve fibers. The order of loss of nerve function is: Pain, temperature, touch, proprioception and skeletal muscle tone.

Systemic absorption of local anesthetics affects the cardiovascular system and CNS. At blood concentrations achieved with normal therapeutic doses, changes in cardiac conduction, excitability, refractoriness, contractility and peripheral vascular resistance are minimal. However, toxic blood concentrations depress cardiac conduction and excitability, which may lead to atrioventricular block and ultimately to cardiac arrest. In addition, with toxic blood concentrations, myocardial contractility may be depressed and peripheral vasodilation may occur, leading to decreased cardiac output and arterial blood pressure.

Following systemic absorption, toxic blood concentrations can produce CNS stimulation, depression or both. Apparent central stimulation may manifest as restlessness, tremors and shivering, which may progress to convulsions. Depression and coma may occur, possibly progressing ultimately to respiratory arrest. Local anesthetics have a primary depressant effect on the medulla and on higher centers. The depressed stage may occur without a prior stage of CNS stimulation.

The use of vasoconstrictors (eg, epinephrine) with local anesthetics promotes local hemostasis, decreases systemic absorption and prolongs duration of action.

Pharmacokinetics: Various pharmacokinetic parameters can be significantly altered by presence of hepatic or renal disease, addition of epinephrine, factors affecting urinary pH, renal blood flow, administration route and age of patient.

Injectable Local Anesthetics Pharmacokinetics

Anesthetic	Onset (minutes)	Duration (hours)	Equivalent anesthetic concentration (%)	pKa	Partition[1] coefficient	Systemic protein binding (%)
ESTERS						
Procaine[2]	2-5	0.25-1	2	9.1	0.02	5.8[3]
(w/Epinephrine)	nd	0.5-1.5				
(Epidural)[4]	15-25	0.5-1.5				
Chloroprocaine[2]	6-12	0.5	2	9	0.14	nd
(w/Epinephrine)	nd	0.5-1.5				
(Epidural)[4]	5-15	0.5-1.5				
Tetracaine[2]	≤ 15	2-3	0.25	8.5	4.1	75.6[5]
(Epidural)[4]	20-30	3-5				
(Spinal)	nd	1.25-3				
AMIDES						
Lidocaine[2]	< 2	0.5-1	1	7.9	2.9	64.3
(w/Epinephrine)	< 2	2-6				
(Epidural)[4]	5-15	1-3				
(Spinal)	nd	0.5-1.5				
Prilocaine[2]	< 2	≥ 1	1	7.9	0.9	55
(w/Epinephrine)	< 2	2.25				
(Epidural)[4]	5-15	1-3				
Mepivacaine[2]	3-5	0.75-1.5	1	7.8	0.8	77.5[5]
(w/Epinephrine)	nd	2-6				
(Epidural)[4]	5-15	1-3				
(Spinal)	nd	0.5-1.5				
Bupivacaine[2]	5	2-4	0.25	8.2	27.5	95.6[5]
(w/Epinephrine)	nd	3-7				
(Epidural)[4]	10-20	3-5				
(Spinal)	nd	1.25-2.5				
Etidocaine[2]	3-5	5 to 10	0.5	7.7	141	94[5]
(w/Epinephrine)	nd	3-7				
(Epidural)[4]	5-15	3-5				

[1] n-Heptane/Buffer, pH 7.4.
[2] Values in this line are for infiltrative anesthesia.
[3] Nerve homogenate binding.
[4] With epinephrine 1:200,000.
[5] Plasma protein binding.

nd – No data.

LOCAL ANESTHETICS, INJECTABLE

Rate of systemic absorption depends on total dose and concentration of drug, vascularity of administration site and presence of vasoconstrictors. Depending on route, local anesthetics are distributed to some extent to all body tissues. High concentrations are found in highly perfused organs (eg, liver, lungs, heart, brain). Rate and extent of placental diffusion are determined by plasma protein binding, ionization and lipid solubility. The nonionized form of the drug crosses cellular membranes to site of action. Fetal/maternal ratios are inversely related to degree of protein binding. Only free, unbound drug is available for placental transfer. Drugs with the highest protein binding capacity may have the lowest fetal/maternal ratios. Lipid soluble, nonionized drugs readily enter fetal blood from maternal circulation.

The onset of local anesthesia is dependent on the dissociation constant (pKa), lipid solubility, pH at the injection site, protein binding and molecular size. In general, local anesthetics with high lipid solubility or low pKa have a faster onset.

Local anesthetics are divided into two groups: **Esters**, which are derivatives of para-aminobenzoic acid, and **amides**, which are derivatives of aniline. The "ester" local anesthetics are metabolized by hydrolysis of the ester linkage by plasma esterase, probably plasma cholinesterase. The "amide" local anesthetics are metabolized primarily in the liver, then excreted primarily in the urine as metabolites, with a small fraction of unchanged drug. Hypersensitivity reactions may occur with local anesthetics of the ester type (see Warnings).

Indications:

Refer to individual product listings.

Contraindications:

Hypersensitivity to local anesthetics, para-aminobenzoic acid (amides only) or parabens; congenital or idiopathic methemoglobinemia (**prilocaine**); spinal and caudal anesthesia in septicemia, existing neurologic disease, spinal deformities and severe hypertension; subarachnoid administration (**chloroprocaine**).

Bupivacaine: Obstetrical paracervical block anesthesia (such use has resulted in fetal bradycardia and death); IV regional anesthesia (Bier block; cardiac arrest and death have occurred). (See Warnings.)

Warnings:

> *Obstetrical anesthesia:* The 0.75% concentration of **bupivacaine** is not recommended for obstetrical anesthesia. Cardiac arrest with difficult resuscitation or death has occurred during use for epidural anesthesia in obstetrical patients. Resuscitation has been difficult or impossible despite adequate preparation and appropriate management. Cardiac arrest has occurred after convulsions resulting from systemic toxicity, presumably following unintentional intravascular injection. Reserve the 0.75% concentration for surgical procedures where a high degree of muscle relaxation and prolonged effect are necessary.
>
> Have resuscitative equipment and drugs immediately available when any local anesthetic is used.
>
> Do NOT use preparations containing preservatives for caudal epidural anesthesia. When using preparations without preservatives, discard any unused drug remaining in vial.

Head and neck area: Small doses of local anesthetics injected into the head and neck area, including retrobulbar, dental and stellate ganglion blocks, may produce adverse reactions similar to systemic toxicity seen with unintentional intravascular injections of larger doses. The injection procedures require the utmost care. Confusion, convulsions, respiratory depression or arrest and cardiovascular stimulation or depression have been reported. These reactions may be due to intra-arterial injection of the local anesthetic with retrograde flow to cerebral circulation. They may also be due to puncture of the dural sheath of the optic nerve during retrobulbar block with diffusion of any local anesthetic along the subdural space to the midbrain. Observe patient carefully. Monitor respiration and circulation. Do not exceed dosage recommendations.

Ophthalmic – When local anesthetic solutions are used for retrobulbar block, complete corneal anesthesia usually precedes onset of clinically acceptable external ocular muscle akinesia. Therefore, presence of akinesia rather than anesthesia alone should determine readiness of the patient for surgery.

LOCAL ANESTHETICS, INJECTABLE

Dentistry – Because of the long duration of anesthesia of **bupivacaine with epinephrine**, caution patients about the possibility of inadvertent trauma to tongue, lips and buccal mucosa and advise against chewing solid foods or testing anesthetized area by biting or probing.

Cardiovascular reactions are depressant. They may be the result of direct drug effect, the result of vasovagal reaction, particularly if the patient is in the sitting position. Failure to recognize premonitory signs such as sweating, feeling of faintness, changes in pulse or sensorium may result in progressive cerebral hypoxia and seizure, or serious cardiovascular catastrophe. Place patient in recumbent position and administer oxygen. Vasoactive drugs such as ephedrine or methoxamine may be administered IV.

Hypersensitivity reactions, including anaphylaxis, may occur in a small segment of the population allergic to para-aminobenzoic acid derivatives (eg, procaine, tetracaine, benzocaine). The amide-type local anesthetics have not shown cross-sensitivity with the esters. Hypersensitivity reactions and anaphylaxis have occurred rarely with lidocaine. (See Management of Acute Hypersensitivity Reactions.)

Administer ester-type local anesthetics cautiously to patients with abnormal or reduced levels of plasma esterases.

Renal function impairment: Use **mepivacaine** with caution in patients with renal disease.

Hepatic function impairment: Because amide-type local anesthetics are metabolized primarily in the liver, patients with hepatic disease, especially severe hepatic disease, may be more susceptible to potential toxicity. Use cautiously in such patients.

Elderly: Repeated doses may cause accumulation of the drug or its metabolites or slow metabolic degradation. Give reduced doses.

Pregnancy: Category B (etidocaine, lidocaine, prilocaine). *Category C* (bupivacaine, chloroprocaine, mepivacaine, tetracaine). Safety for use in pregnant women, other than those in labor, has not been established. Local anesthetics rapidly cross the placenta. When used for epidural, caudal, paracervical or pudendal block, they can cause varying degrees of maternal, fetal and neonatal toxicity involving alterations of the CNS, peripheral vascular tone and cardiac function. The incidence and degree of toxicity depend upon the procedure, type and amount of drug used and technique of administration.

Labor, delivery and abortion – Fetal bradycardia may occur in 10% to 30% of patients receiving amide-type anesthetics for paracervical block and may be associated with fetal acidosis. Always monitor fetal heart rate during paracervical anesthesia. Added risk appears to be present in prematurity, toxemia of pregnancy and fetal distress. Weigh the possible advantages against dangers when considering paracervical block in these conditions. The use of some local anesthetics during labor and delivery may be followed by diminished muscle strength and tone for the infant's first day or two of life.

Careful adherence to recommended dosage is extremely important. Failure to achieve adequate analgesia via intended paracervical or pudendal block or both with these doses may indicate intravascular or fetal intracranial injection. Babies so affected present with unexplained neonatal depression at birth and usually manifest seizures within 6 hours. Prompt use of supportive measures and forced urinary excretion of the local anesthetic have been used successfully.

Maternal hypotension has resulted from regional anesthesia. Local anesthetics produce vasodilation by blocking sympathetic nerves. Elevating the patient's legs and positioning her on her left side will help prevent decreases in blood pressure. Continuously monitor fetal heart rate; electronic monitoring is advisable. It is extremely important to avoid aortocaval compression by the gravid uterus during administration of regional block.

Epidural, caudal or pudendal anesthesia may alter the forces of parturition through changes in uterine contractility or maternal expulsive efforts. Epidural anesthesia has been reported to prolong the second stage of labor by removing the parturient's reflex urge to bear down or by interfering with motor function. The use of obstetrical anesthesia may increase the need for forceps assistance.

Maternal convulsions and cardiovascular collapse following use of some local anesthetics for paracervical block in early pregnancy (as anesthesia for elective abortion) suggest that systemic absorption may be rapid. Therefore, do not exceed the recommended maximum dose per side. Inject slowly, with frequent aspirations. Allow a 5 minute interval between sides.

Lactation: Safety for use in the nursing mother has not been established. It is not known whether local anesthetic drugs are excreted in breast milk.

Children: Due to lack of clinical experience, the administration of **bupivacaine** to children < 12 years of age is not recommended.

Safety and efficacy of **tetracaine** in children have not been established.

Dosages in children should be reduced, commensurate with age, body weight and physical condition.

Precautions:

Dosage: Use the lowest dosage that results in effective anesthesia to avoid high plasma levels and serious adverse effects. Inject slowly, with frequent aspirations before and during the injection, to avoid intravascular injection. Perform syringe aspirations before and during each supplemental injection in continuous (intermittent) catheter techniques. During the administration of epidural anesthesia, it is recommended that a test dose be administered initially and that the patient be monitored for CNS toxicity and cardiovascular toxicity, as well as for signs of unintended intrathecal administration, before proceeding.

Inflammation or sepsis: Use local anesthetic procedures with caution when there is inflammation or sepsis in the region of proposed injection.

CNS toxicity: Monitor cardiovascular and respiratory vital signs and state of consciousness after each injection. Restlessness, anxiety, incoherent speech, lightheadedness, numbness and tingling of the mouth and lips, metallic taste, tinnitus, dizziness, blurred vision, tremors, twitching, depression or drowsiness may be early signs of CNS toxicity.

Special risk patients: Debilitated patients, acutely ill patients, children, obstetric delivery patients and patients with increased intra-abdominal pressure: Repeated doses may cause accumulation of the drug or its metabolites or slow metabolic degradation. Give reduced doses. Use anesthetics with caution in patients with severe disturbances of cardiac rhythm, hypotension, shock or heart block. Local anesthetics should also be used with caution in patients with impaired cardiovascular function because they may be less able to compensate for functional changes associated with the prolongation of A-V conduction produced by these drugs.

Malignant hyperthermia: Many drugs used during anesthesia are considered potential triggering agents for familial malignant hyperthermia. It is not known whether amide-type local anesthetics may trigger this reaction and the need for supplemental general anesthesia cannot be predicted in advance; therefore, have a standard protocol for management available.

Vasoconstrictors: Use solutions containing a vasoconstrictor with caution and in carefully circumscribed quantities in areas of the body supplied by end arteries or having otherwise compromised blood supply (eg, digits, nose, external ear, penis). Use with extreme caution in patients whose medical history and physical evaluation suggest the existence of hypertension, peripheral vascular disease, arteriosclerotic heart disease, cerebral vascular insufficiency or heart block: These individuals may exhibit exaggerated vasoconstrictor response.

Intravenous regional anesthesia: Cardiac arrest and death are reported with the use of **bupivacaine** for IV regional anesthesia (Bier block). Bupivacaine is not recommended for this technique.

Sulfite sensitivity: Some of these products contain sulfites. Sulfites may cause allergic-type reactions (eg, hives, itching, wheezing, anaphylaxis) in certain susceptible persons. Although the overall prevalence of sulfite sensitivity in the general population is probably low, it is seen more frequently in asthmatics or in atopic nonasthmatic persons.

Drug Interactions:

Intercurrent use: Mixtures of local anesthetics are sometimes employed to compensate for the slower onset of one drug and the shorter duration of action of the second drug. Toxicity is probably additive with mixtures of local anesthetics, but some experiments suggest synergisms. Exercise caution regarding toxic equivalence when mixtures of local anesthetics are employed.

Prior use of **chloroprocaine** may interfere with subsequent use of **bupivacaine**. Because of this, and because safety of intercurrent use of bupivacaine and chloroprocaine has not been established, such use is not recommended.

Some preparations contain vasoconstrictors. Keep this in mind when using concurrently with other drugs that may interact with vasoconstrictors (refer to the Vasopressors Used in Shock monographs).

LOCAL ANESTHETICS, INJECTABLE

Injectable Local Anesthetic Drug Interactions			
Precipitant drug	Object drug*		Description
Local anesthetics	Sedatives	↑	If employed to reduce patient apprehension during dental procedures, use reduced doses, since local anesthetics used in combination with CNS depressants may have additive effects. Give young children minimal doses of each agent.
Local anesthetics	Sulfonamides	↓	The para-aminobenzoic acid metabolite of procaine, chloroprocaine and tetracaine inhibits the action of sulfonamides. Therefore, do not use procaine, chloroprocaine or tetracaine in any condition in which a sulfonamide drug is employed.

* ↑ = Object drug increased. ↓ = Object drug decreased.

Adverse Reactions:

The most common acute adverse reactions are related to the CNS and cardiovascular systems. These are generally dose-related and may result from rapid absorption from the injection site, from diminished tolerance or from unintentional intravascular injection.

Dermatologic: Cutaneous lesions, urticaria, pruritus, erythema, angioneurotic edema (including laryngeal edema), sneezing, syncope, excessive sweating, elevated temperature and anaphylactoid symptoms (including severe hypotension). Skin testing is of limited value.

CNS: Restlessness, anxiety, dizziness, tinnitus, blurred vision, nausea, vomiting, chills, pupil constriction or tremors may occur, possibly proceeding to convulsions (≈ 0.1% of local anesthetic epidural administrations). Excitement may be transient or absent, with depression being the first manifestation. This may quickly be followed by drowsiness merging into unconsciousness and respiratory arrest.

Postspinal headache, meningismus, arachnoiditis, palsies, apprehension, double vision, euphoria, sensation of heat, cold, numbness and spinal nerve paralysis (spinal anesthesia) have also occurred.

Cardiovascular: Myocardial depression, hypotension (with spinal anesthesia due to vasomotor paralysis and pooling of blood in the venous bed), decreased cardiac output, heart block, syncope, bradycardia, ventricular arrhythmias (including tachycardia and fibrillation), cardiac arrest and fetal bradycardia (see Warnings).

Respiratory: Respiratory impairment or paralysis due to level of anesthesia (spinal) extending to upper thoracic and cervical segments. (See Warnings.)

Miscellaneous: Occasional unintentional penetration of the subarachnoid space by the catheter may occur. Subsequent adverse effects may depend partially on amount of drug administered intrathecally. These may include: High or total spinal block; hypotension secondary to spinal block; urinary retention; fecal or urinary incontinence; loss of perineal sensation and sexual function; persistent anesthesia; paresthesia, weakness and paralysis of the lower extremities and loss of sphincter control; headache and backache; septic meningitis; meningismus; slowing of labor and increased incidence of forceps delivery; cranial nerve palsies due to traction on nerves from loss of cerebrospinal fluid; arachnoiditis; persistent motor, sensory or autonomic deficit of some lower spinal segments with slow (several months) or incomplete recovery.

Methemoglobinemia – **Prilocaine** may produce dose-dependent methemoglobinemia due to the metabolite O-toluidine. Administration of prilocaine in doses > 400 mg has been associated with methemoglobinemia in adult patients and with proportionately lower doses in children. While methemoglobin values of < 20% do not generally produce any clinical symptoms, evalute the appearance of cyanosis at 2 to 4 hours following administration in terms of the patient's status.

Treat methemoglobinemia with 1 to 2 mg/kg of methylene blue administered IV over 5 minutes. (See Methylene Blue monograph in the Antidotes section.)

There have been rare reports of trismus in patients who have received etidocaine for dental anesthesia. Onset of symptoms occurs within hours or days upon resolution of blockade. In most patients, symptoms resolved within days to weeks, although some reports have suggested that symptoms were present for many months. Symptomatic treatment with analgesics, moist heat and physiotherapy was helpful in some cases.

LOCAL ANESTHETICS, INJECTABLE

Overdosage:

Acute emergencies from local anesthetics are generally related to high plasma levels encountered during therapeutic use or to unintended subarachnoid injection.

Management: The first consideration is prevention.

Convulsions, as well as underventilation or apnea, are due to unintentional subarachnoid injection; maintain patent airway and assist or control ventilation with oxygen and a delivery system capable of permitting immediate positive airway pressure by mask. Evaluate circulation. If convulsions persist despite respiratory support, and if the status of the circulation permits, give small increments of an ultra short-acting barbiturate (eg, thiopental) or a benzodiazepine (eg, diazepam) IV. Circulatory depression may require administration of IV fluids and a vasopressor.

If not treated immediately, convulsions and cardiovascular depression can result in hypoxia, acidosis, bradycardia, arrhythmias and cardiac arrest. Underventilation or apnea may produce these same signs and also lead to cardiac arrest if ventilatory support is not instituted. If cardiac arrest occurs, institute standard cardiopulmonary resuscitative measures.

Endotracheal intubation may be indicated.

Patient Information:

When appropriate, inform patients in advance that they may experience temporary loss of sensation and motor activity, usually in the lower half of the body, following proper administration of caudal or epidural anesthesia.

Administration and Dosage:

The dose of local anesthetic administered varies with the procedure, vascularity of the tissues, depth of anesthesia, degree of required muscle relaxation, duration of anesthesia desired and the physical condition of the patient. Reduce dosages for children, elderly and debilitated patients and patients with cardiac or liver disease.

Buffering lidocaine solution with sodium bicarbonate may help reduce the pain associated with injection. Some reports used a 1% lidocaine solution with sodium bicarbonate in a 9:1 or 10:1 ratio by volume. Use immediately after preparation.

Infiltration or regional block anesthesia: Always inject slowly, with frequent aspirations, to prevent intravascular injection.

For detailed Administration and Dosage, refer to specific manufacturers' labeling.

ETIDOCAINE HCl

For complete prescribing information, refer to the Local Anesthetics, Injectable group monograph.

Indications:

Peripheral nerve block, central nerve block or lumbar peridural: 1% solution.

Intra-abdominal/pelvic/lower limb surgery or caesarean section: 1% or 1.5% solution.

Caudal: 1% solution.

Retrobulbar: 1% or 1.5% solution.

Maxillary infiltration or inferior alveolar nerve block: 1.5% solution.

Rx	**Duranest MPF** (Astra)	**Injection:** 1%	In 30 ml single dose vials.
		1% with 1:200,000 epinephrine	In 30 ml single dose vials.[1]
		1.5% with 1:200,000 epinephrine	In 20 ml amps.[1]
Rx	**Duranest** (Astra)		In 1.8 dental cartridge.[1]

[1] With sodium metabisulfite.

PROCAINE HCl

For complete prescribing information, refer to the Local Anesthetics, Injectable group monograph.

Indications:

Infiltration anesthesia: 0.25% to 0.5% solution.

Peripheral nerve block: 0.5%, 1% and 2% solution.

Spinal anesthesia: 10% solution.

Dilution instructions: To prepare 60 ml of a 0.5% solution (5 mg/ml), dilute 30 ml of the 1% solution with 30 ml 0.9% sodium chloride injection. To prepare 60 ml of a 0.25% solution (2.5 mg/ml), dilute 15 ml of the 1% solution with 45 ml 0.9% sodium chloride injection. Add 0.5 to 1 ml of epinephrine 1:1000 per 100 ml anesthetic solution for vasoconstrictive effect (1:200,000 to 1:100,000).

Rx	**Procaine HCl** (Various, eg, Abbott)	**Injection:** 1%	In 30 ml vials.
Rx	**Novocain** (Sanofi Winthrop)		In 2 and 6 ml amps[1] and 30 ml vials.[2]
Rx	**Procaine HCl** (Various, eg, Abbott, IDE, Schein)	**Injection:** 2%	In 30 ml vials.
Rx	**Novocain** (Sanofi Winthrop)		In 30 ml vials.[2]
Rx	**Novocain** (Sanofi Winthrop)	**Injection:** 10%	In 2 ml amps.[1]

[1] With ≤ 1 mg acetone sodium bisulfite per ml.
[2] With ≤ 2 mg acetone sodium bisulfite and ≤ 2.5 mg chlorobutanol per ml.

CHLOROPROCAINE HCl

For complete prescribing information, refer to the Local Anesthetics, Injectable group monograph.

Indications:

Infiltration and peripheral nerve block: 1% to 2% solution.

Mandibular – 2% solution.
Infraorbital – 2% solution.
Brachial Plexus – 2% solution.
Digital (without epinephrine) – 1% solution.
Pudendal block – 2% solution.
Paracervical block – 1% solution.

Infiltration, peripheral and central nerve block, including caudal and epidural block: 2% or 3% solution (without preservatives).

Rx	**Nesacaine** (Astra)	**Injection:** 1%	In 30 ml vials.[1]
		2% (Not for epidural or caudal block.)	In 30 ml vials.[1]
Rx	**Nesacaine-MPF** (Astra)	**Injection:** 2%	In 30 ml vials.[2,3]
		3%	In 30 ml vials.[2,3]

[1] With 1 mg methylparaben and EDTA per ml.
[2] Preservative free.
[3] With EDTA.

TETRACAINE HCl

For complete prescribing information, refer to the Local Anesthetics, Injectable group monograph.

Indications:

Spinal anesthesia (high, median, low and saddle blocks): 0.2% to 0.3% solution.

Spinal anesthesia, prolonged (2 to 3 hours): 1% solution.

Storage: Store under refrigeration.

Rx	**Pontocaine HCl** (Sanofi Winthrop)	**Injection:** 1%	In 2 ml amps.[1]
		0.2%	With 6% dextrose. In 2 ml amps.
		0.3%	With 6% dextrose. In 5 ml amps.
		Powder for reconstitution:	In 20 mg Niphanoid (instantly soluble) amps.

[1] With acetone sodium bisulfite.

PROPOXYCAINE HCl and PROCAINE HCl

For complete prescribing information, refer to the Local Anesthetics, Injectable group monograph.

Indications:

For local anesthesia by nerve block or infiltration in dental procedures.

Rx	**Ravocaine and Novocain with Levophed** (Cook-Waite)	**Injection:** 7.2 mg propoxycaine HCl, 36 mg procaine with norepinephrine 0.12 mg per 1.8 ml dental cartridge.[1]

[1] With ≤ 3.6 mg acetone sodium bisulfite.

LIDOCAINE HCl

For complete prescribing information, refer to the Local Anesthetics, Injectable group monograph.

Indications:

Infiltration:
- *Percutaneous* – 0.5% or 1% solution.
- *IV regional* – 0.5% solution.

Peripheral nerve block:
- *Brachial* – 1.5% solution.
- *Dental* – 2% solution.
- *Intercostal or paravertebral* – 1% solution.
- *Pudendal or paracervical obstetrical (each side)* – 1% solution.

Sympathetic nerve blocks:
- *Cervical (stellate ganglion) or lumbar* – 1% solution.

Central neural blocks:
- *Epidural –*
  - *Thoracic:* 1% solution.

Lumbar:
- *Analgesia* – 1% solution.
- *Anesthesia* – 1.5% or 2% solution.

Caudal:
- *Obstetrical analgesia* – 1% solution.
- *Surgical anesthesia* – 1.5% solution.
- *Spinal anesthesia* – 5% solution with glucose.

Low spinal or "saddle block" anesthesia: 1.5% solution with dextrose.

Retrobulbar or transtracheal injection: 4% solution.

Rx	**Xylocaine** (Astra)	**Injection:** 0.5%	In 50 ml multiple dose vials.[1]
Rx	**Xylocaine MPF** (Astra)		In 50 ml single dose vials.
Rx	**Lidocaine HCl** (Various, eg, Abbott, American Regeant, Forest, Goldline, Moore, Schein)	**Injection:** 1%	In 2 and 5 ml amps, 2, 20, 30 and 50 ml vials and 5 ml syringes.
Rx	**Dilocaine** (Hauck)		In 50 ml vials.
Rx	**Lidoject-1** (Mayrand)		In 50 ml vials.
Rx	**Nervocaine 1%** (Keene)		In 50 ml vials.
Rx	**Xylocaine** (Astra)		In 10, 20 and 50 ml multiple dose vials[1] and 2, 5, 10 and 30 ml single dose vials.
Rx	**Xylocaine MPF** (Astra)		In 2, 5 and 30 ml amps.
Rx	**Lidocaine HCl** (Various, eg, Abbott)	**Injection:** 1.5%	In 20 ml amps.
Rx	**Xylocaine MPF** (Astra)		In 20 ml amps and 10 and 20 ml single dose vials.

LIDOCAINE HCl

Rx	**Lidocaine HCl** (Various, eg, Abbott, American Regeant, Forest, Goldline, Keene, Moore, Schein)	**Injection:** 2%	In 20, 30 and 50 ml vials and 5 ml syringes.
Rx	**Dilocaine** (Hauck)		In 50 ml vials.[1]
Rx	**Lidoject-2** (Mayrand)		In 50 ml vials.
Rx	**Xylocaine** (Astra)		In 10, 20 and 50 ml vials[1] and 1.8 ml cartridge.
Rx	**Xylocaine MPF** (Astra)		In 2 and 10 ml amps and 2, 5 and 10 single dose vials.
Rx	**Xylocaine MPF** (Astra)	**Injection:** 4%	In 5 ml amps and 5 ml disp. syringe with laryngo-tracheal cannula.
Rx	**Duo-Trach Kit** (Astra)		In 5 ml pre-filled syringe with cannula.
Rx	**Xylocaine HCl** (Astra)	**Injection:** 0.5% with 1:200,000 epinephrine	In 50 ml vials.[1]
Rx	**Xylocaine HCl** (Astra)	**Injection:** 1% with 1:100,000 epinephrine	In 10, 20 and 50 ml vials.[1]
Rx	**Xylocaine HCl** (Astra)	**Injection:** 1% with 1:200,000 epinephrine	In 30 ml amps.[2]
Rx	**Xylocaine MPF** (Astra)		In 5, 10 and 30 ml vials.[2]
Rx	**Lidocaine HCl** (Abbott)	**Injection:** 1.5% with 1:200,000 epinephrine	In 5 ml amps.
Rx	**Xylocaine MPF** (Astra)		In 5 and 30 ml amps[2] and 5, 10 and 30 ml single dose vials.[2]
Rx	**Octocaine HCl** (Novocol)[4]	**Injection:** 2% with 1:50,000 epinephrine	In 1.8 ml *Needleject* pre-filled cartridge.
Rx	**Xylocaine HCl** (Astra)		In 1.8 ml dental cartridge.[2]
Rx	**Octocaine HCl** (Novocol)[4]	**Injection:** 2% with 1:100,000 epinephrine	In 1.8 ml *Needleject* pre-filled cartridge.
Rx	**Xylocaine HCl** (Astra)		In 10[1], 20[3] and 50 ml vials[1] and 1.8 ml cartridge.[2]
Rx	**Xylocaine HCl** (Astra)	**Injection:** 2% with 1:200,000 epinephrine	In 20 ml amps.[2]
Rx	**Xylocaine MPF** (Astra)		In 5, 10 and 20 ml single dose vials.[2]
Rx	**Xylocaine HCl** (Astra)	**Injection:** 1.5% with 7.5% dextrose	In 2 ml amps.
Rx	**Xylocaine MPF** (Astra)	**Injection:** 5% with 7.5% glucose	In 2 ml amps.

[1] With methylparaben and sodium metabisulfite.
[2] With sodium bisulfite.
[3] With sodium metabisulfite.
[4] Novocol Pharmaceutical, 25 Wolseley Court, Cambridge, Ontario N1R 6X3.

PRILOCAINE HCl

For complete prescribing information, refer to the Local Anesthetics, Injectable group monograph.

Indications:

For local anesthesia by nerve block or infiltration in dental procedures: 4% solution.

Rx	**Citanest HCl** (Astra)	**Injection, Plain:** 4%	In 1.8 ml cartridge.
		Injection, Forte: 4% with 1:200,000 epinephrine	In 1.8 ml cartridge.[1]

[1] With sodium metabisulfite.

MEPIVACAINE HCl

For complete prescribing information, refer to the Local Anesthetics, Injectable group monograph.

Indications:

Peripheral nerve block (eg, cervical, brachial, intercostal, pudendal): 1% or 2% solution.

Transvaginal block (paracervical plus pudendal): 1% solution.

Paracervical block in obstetrics: 1% solution.

Caudal and epidural block: 1%, 1.5% or 2% solution.

Infiltration: 0.5% (via dilution) or 1% solution

Therapeutic block: 1% or 2% solution.

Dental procedures (infiltration or nerve block): 3% solution or 2% solution with levonordefrin.

Rx	**Carbocaine** (Sanofi Winthrop)	**Injection:** 1%	In 30 ml vials and 50 ml vials.[1]
Rx	**Mepivacaine HCl** (Various, eg, Goldline, Schein)		In 50 ml vials.
Rx	**Polocaine** (Astra)		In 50 ml vials.
Rx	**Polocaine MPF** (Astra)		In 30 ml vials.
Rx	**Carbocaine** (Sanofi Winthrop)	**Injection:** 1.5%	In 30 ml vials.
Rx	**Polocaine MPF** (Astra)		In 30 ml vials.
Rx	**Carbocaine** (Sanofi Winthrop)	**Injection:** 2%	In 20 ml vials and 50 ml vials.[1]
Rx	**Polocaine** (Astra)		In 50 ml vials.
Rx	**Polocaine MPF** (Astra)		In 20 ml vials.
Rx	**Mepivacaine** (Various, eg, Goldline, IDE, Moore, Schein)		In 50 ml vials.
Rx	**Carbocaine** (Cook-Waite)	**Injection:** 3%	In 1.8 ml dental cartridge.
Rx	**Isocaine HCl** (Novocol)[4]		In 1.8 ml dental cartridge.
Rx	**Polocaine** (Astra)		In 1.8 ml dental cartridge.
Rx	**Carbocaine with Neo-Cobefrin** (Cook-Waite)	**Injection:** 2% with 1:20,000 levonordefrin	In 1.8 ml dental cartridge.[2]
Rx	**Isocaine HCl** (Novocol)[4]		In 1.8 ml dental cartridge.[3]
Rx	**Polocaine** (Astra)		In 1.8 ml cartridge.[3]

[1] With methylparaben.

[2] With acetone sodium bisulfite.

[3] With sodium bisulfite.

[4] Novocol Pharmaceutical, 25 Wolseley Court, Cambridge, Ontario N1R 6X3.

BUPIVACAINE HCl

For complete prescribing information, refer to the Local Anesthetics, Injectable group monograph.

Indications:

Local infiltration and sympathetic block: 0.25% solution.

Lumbar epidural: 0.25%, 0.5% and 0.75% solutions (0.75% nonobstetrical).

Subarachnoid block: 0.75% solution.

Caudal block: 0.25% and 0.5% solutions.

Peripheral nerve block: 0.25% and 0.5% solutions.

Retrobulbar block: 0.75% solution.

Dental block: 0.5% solution with epinephrine.

Rx	**Bupivacaine HCl** (Abbott)	**Injection:** 0.25%	In 20 ml amps and 50 ml *Abboject*.
Rx	**Marcaine HCl** (Sanofi Winthrop)		In 50 ml amps and 10, 30 and 50[1] ml vials.
Rx	**Sensorcaine** (Astra)		In 50[1] ml vials.
Rx	**Sensorcaine MPF** (Astra)		In 30 ml amps and 10 and 30 ml vials.
Rx	**Bupivacaine HCl** (Abbott)	**Injection:** 0.5%	In 20 ml amps and *Abboject* and 30 ml *Abboject*.
Rx	**Marcaine HCl** (Sanofi Winthrop)		In 30 ml amps and 10, 30 and 50[1] ml vials.
Rx	**Sensorcaine** (Astra)		In 50[1] ml vials.
Rx	**Sensorcaine MPF** (Astra)		In 30 ml amps and 10 and 30 ml vials.
Rx	**Bupivacaine HCl** (Abbott)	**Injection:** 0.75%	In 20 ml amps and 20 ml *Abboject*.
Rx	**Marcaine HCl** (Sanofi Winthrop)		In 30 ml amps and 10 and 30 ml vials.
Rx	**Marcaine Spinal** (Sanofi Winthrop)		In 2 ml single dose amps.[2]
Rx	**Sensorcaine MPF** (Astra)		In 30 ml amps and 10 and 30 ml vials.
Rx	**Sensorcaine MPF Spinal** (Astra)		In 2 ml amps.[2]
Rx	**Marcaine HCl** (Sanofi Winthrop)	**Injection:** 0.25% with 1:200,000 epinephrine	In 50 ml amps[3] and 10,[3] 30[3] and 50[1,3] ml vials.
		0.5% with 1:200,000 epinephrine	In 3 and 30 ml amps[3] and 10,[3] 30[3] and 50[1,3] ml vials.
		0.75% with 1:200,000 epinephrine	In 30 ml amps.[3]
Rx	**Sensorcaine** (Astra)	**Injection:** 0.25% with 1:200,000 epinephrine	In 50 ml vials.[1]
		0.5% with 1:200,000 epinephrine	In 50 ml vials.[1]
Rx	**Sensorcaine MPF** (Astra)	**Injection:** 0.25% with 1:200,000 epinephrine	In 10 and 30 ml vials.[4]
		0.5% with 1:200,000 epinephrine	In 5 and 30 ml amps and 10 and 30 ml vials.[4]
		0.75% with 1:200,000 epinephrine	In 30 ml amps and 10 and 30 ml vials.[4]

[1] With 1 mg methylparaben per ml.
[2] With 8.25% dextrose per ml.
[3] With 0.5 mg sodium metabisulfite and 0.1 mg EDTA per ml.
[4] With 0.5 mg sodium metabisulfite per ml.

ROPIVACAINE HCl

Indications:

For the production of local or regional anesthesia for surgery, postoperative pain management and obstetrical procedures.

Administration and Dosage:

Avoid the rapid administration of a large volume of local anesthetic solution and use fractional (incremental) doses. Administer the smallest dose and concentration required to produce the desired result.

Use an adequate test dose (3 to 5 ml of a short-acting local anesthetic containing epinephrine) prior to induction of complete block. Repeat this test dose if patient movement potentiates epidural catheter displacement. Ropivacaine epidural infusions can be used for up to 24 hours.

Ropivacaine Dosage Recommendations

Procedures	Conc. mg/ml (%)	Volume ml	Dose mg	Onset min	Duration hours
Surgical anesthesia					
Lumbar epidural administration					
Surgery	5 (0.5%)	15 - 30	75 - 150	15 - 30	2 - 4
	7.5 (0.75%)	15 - 25	119 - 188	10 - 20	3 - 6
	10 (1%)	15 - 20	150 - 200	10 - 20	4 - 8
Cesarean section	5 (0.5%)	20 - 30	100 - 150	15 - 25	2 - 4
Thoracic epidural administration					
To establish block for postoperative pain relief	5 (0.5%)	5 - 15	25 - 75	10 - 20	na
Major nerve block					
(eg, brachial plexus block)	5 (0.5%)	35 - 50	175 - 250	15 - 30	5 - 8
Field block					
(eg, minor nerve blocks and infiltration)	5 (0.5%)	1 - 10	5 - 200	1 - 15	2 - 6
Labor pain management					
Lumbar epidural administration					
Initial dose	2 (0.2%)	10 - 20	20 - 40	10 - 15	0.5 - 1.5
Continuous infusion[1]	2 (0.2%)	6 - 14 ml/hr	12 - 28 mg/hr	na	na
Incremental injections (top-up)[1]	2 (0.2%)	10 - 15 ml/hr	20 - 30 mg/hr	na	na
Postoperative pain management					
Lumbar epidural administration					
Continuous infusion[2]	2 (0.2%)	6 - 1 ml/hr	12 - 20 mg/hr	na	na
Thoracic epidural administration					
Continuous infusion[2]	2 (0.2%)	4 - 8 ml/hr	8 - 16 mg/hr	na	na
Infiltration					
(eg, minor nerve block)	2 (0.2%)	1 - 100	2 - 200	1 - 5	2 - 6
	5 (0.5%)	1 - 10	5 - 200	1 - 5	2 - 6

[1] Median dose of 21 mg/hour was administered by continuous infusion or incremental injections (top-ups) over a median delivery time of 5.5 hours.

[2] Cumulative doses up to 770 mg of ropivacaine over 24 hours for postoperative pain management have been well tolerated in adults.

Rx	**Naropin** (Astra)	**Injection:** 2, 5, 7.5 and 10 mg/ml concentrations	Preservative free. In single dose amps, vials and infusion bottles.

ADENOSINE PHOSPHATE (A_5MP)

Actions:

Pharmacology: Adenosine is converted to adenosin monophosphate (A_5MP) which is associated with many normal biochemical processes. The mechanism of action is not understood. Clinical benefits may result from correction of underlying biochemical imbalances or deficiences at the cellular level. The drug may also be a neurotransmitter.

Indications:

Varicose veins: Symptomatic relief of complications with stasis dermatitis.

Unlabeled uses: Adenosine monophosphate has been used to treat herpes infections. Adenosine is currently being investigaed for use in increasing blood flow to brain tumors and in porphyria cutanea tarda.

Contraindications:

History of myocardial infarction; cerebral hemorrhage.

Warnings:

Anaphylactoid reactions: If a patient complains of dyspnea and chest tightness following an injection, do not administer further injections. Immediately institute treatment for allergic reactions. Refer to Management of Acute Hypersensitivity Reactions.

Pregnancy: Category C. Safe use has not been established with respect to adverse effects upon fetal development. Do not use in women of childbearing potential or during early pregnancy unless the benefits outweight the potential hazards.

Children: Not recommended for use in children. Clinical experience has been insufficient to establish safety or a suitable dosage regimen.

Adverse Reactions:

Flushing, dizziness, palpitations, hypotension, dyspnea, epigastric discomfort, nausea, occasional local rash and diureses, increase in symptoms of bursitis and tendinitis.

Administration and Dosage:

Administer IM only. Not for IV use.

Initial: Administer 25 to 50 mg once or twice daily until symptoms subside.

Maintenance: 25 mg 2 or 3 times weekly.

Storage/Stability: Store at room temperature 15° to 30°C (59° to 86°F).

Rx	**Adenosine Phosphate** (Various, eg, Pasadena, Steris)	**Injection:** 25 mg per ml in an aqueous solution	In 10 and 30 ml vials.[1]

[1] May contain benzyl alcohol.

LIVER DERIVATIVE COMPLEX

Actions:

Pharmacology: Claimed to enhance the resolution of inflammation and edema.

Indications:

Skin: Management of acne vulgaris, herpes zoster, "poison ivy" dermatitis, pityriasis rosea, seborrheic dermatitis, urticaria and eczema, severe sunburn, rosacea.

Contraindications:

Hypersensitivity or intolerance to liver or pork products.

Warnings:

Hypersensitivity: Use caution in suspected hypersensitivity to liver or other allergic diatheses.

Lactation: It is not known whether liver derivative is excreted in breast milk. Use caution when administering to a nursing woman.

Drug Interactions:

MAO inhibitors: This product contains tyramine and therefore can cause a hypertensive crisis.

Adverse Reactions:

Local reactions include: Pain, rash, stinging, swelling and erythema.

Administration and Dosage:

The usual dose is 2 ml SC or IM daily or as indicated.

Storage/Stability: Store at controlled room temperature 15° to 30°C (59° to 86°F).

Rx	**Kutapressin** (Schwarz Pharma)	**Injection:** 25.5 mg/ml. Liver derivative complex composed of peptides and amino acids	0.5% phenol. In 20 ml vials.

CHLOROPHYLL DERIVATIVES (Chlorophyllin)

Indications:

Oral: To control fecal odors in colostomy, ileostomy or incontinence; also for certain breath and body odors.

Topical: To promote normal healing, relieve pain and inflammation, and reduce malodors in wounds, burns, surface ulcers, cuts, abrasions and skin irritations.

Warnings:

Diarrhea: If cramping or diarrhea occur, reduce the dosage.

Adverse Reactions:

Oral: No toxic effects have been reported. A temporary mild laxative effect may occur; the stool is commonly stained dark green.

Topical: Sensitivity reactions are extremely rare; only a few instances of slight itching or irritation have been reported.

Administration and Dosage:

Topical:

Ointment – Apply generously and cover with gauze, linen or other appropriate dressing. Change no more often than every 48 to 72 hours.

Solution – Apply full strength as continuous wet dressing.

Oral:

Adults and children (> 12 years of age) – 1 to 2 tablets/day; may be increased to 3 tablets/day.

Children (< 12 years of age) – Consult physician.

Ostomies: In ostomies, take tablets orally or place in the appliance.

otc *sf*	**Chlorophyll** (Freeda)	**Tablets:** 20 mg chlorophyll	In 100s, 250s and 500s.
otc	**Derifil** (Rystan)	**Tablets:** 100 mg water-soluble chlorophyll derivatives	In 30s, 100s and 1000s.
otc	**PALS** (Palisades)	**Tablets:** 100 mg chlorophyllin copper complex	In 100s.
otc	**Chloresium** (Rystan)	**Tablets:** 14 mg chlorophyllin copper complex	In 100s and 1000s.
otc	**Chloresium** (Rystan)	**Solution:** 0.2% chlorophyllin copper complex in an isotonic saline solution	In 240 ml and qt.
otc	**Chloresium** (Rystan)	**Ointment:** 0.5% water-soluble chlorophyllin copper complex in a hydrophilic base	In 30 and 120 g and lb.

BISMUTH SUBGALLATE

Indications:

To control fecal odors in colostomy, ileostomy or incontinence.

Adverse Reactions:

A temporary darkening of the tonge or stool may occur.

Administration and Dosage:

Take 1 or 2 tablets 3 times daily with meals. Chew or swallow whole.

otc	**Devrom** (Parthenon)	**Tablets:** 200 mg	Lactose, sugar. Chewable. In 100s.

PERITONEAL DIALYSIS SOLUTIONS

Indications:

Acute or chronic renal failure; acute poisoning by dialyzable toxins; intractable edema; hyperkalemia, hypercalcemia, azotemia and uremia; hepatic coma. Refer to manufacturer's package literature for specific prescribing information.

Electrolyte content given in mEq/liter.

	Product and Distributor	Dextrose (g/liter)	Na+	Ca++	Mg++	Cl–	Lactate	Osmolarity (mOsm/liter)	How Supplied
Rx	**Dialyte Pattern LM w/1.5% Dextrose** (Gambro)	15	131	3.5	0.5	94	40	345	In 1000, 2000 and 4000 ml.
Rx	**Dialyte Pattern LM w/2.5% Dextrose** (Gambro)	25	131.5	3.5	0.5	94	40	395	In 1000, 2000 and 4000 ml.
Rx	**Dialyte Pattern LM w/4.25% Dextrose** (Gambro)	42.5	131.5	3.5	0.5	94	40	485	In 1000, 2000 and 4000 ml.

EMERGENCY KITS

Some of these products contain sulfites that may cause allergic-type reactions (including anaphylactic symptoms and life-threatening or less severe asthmatic episodes) in certain susceptible people. The overall prevalence of sulfite sensitivity in the general population is unknown and probably low. It is seen more frequently in asthmatic or atopic nonasthmatic people. Specific products containing sulfites are identified in the product listings.

Rx **Cyanide Antidote Package** (Various)
For the treatment of cyanide poisoning.
Sodium nitrite, 300 mg in 10 ml (2 amps)
Sodium thiosulfate, 12.5 g in 50 ml (2 amps)
Amyl nitrite inhalant, 0.3 ml (12 aspirols)
Also disposable syringes, stomach tube, tourniquet and instructions.

Rx **AtroPen Auto-Injector** (Survival Technology)
For toxic exposure to organophosphorus or carbamate insecticides.
Atropine sulfate with 2 mg phenol. In prefilled automatic injection device.

Rx **LidoPen Auto-Injector** (Survival Technology)
For cardiac arrhythmias.
Lidocaine HCl, 10% solution. In 3 ml (300 mg) disposable, prefilled automatic injection device for self-administration.

Rx **EpiPen Auto-Injector** (Center Labs)[1]
For emergency treatment of severe allergic reactions in adults.
Delivers 0.3 mg IM dose of 1:1000 epinephrine.[2] In 2 ml disposable injectors.

Rx **EpiPen Jr. Auto-Injector** (Center Labs)[1]
For emergency treatment of severe allergic reactions in children.
Delivers 0.15 mg IM dose of 1:2000 epinephrine.[2]
In 2 ml disposable injectors.

Rx **Ana-Guard Epinephrine** (Bayer)
For emergency treatment of severe allergic reactions.
1:1000 epinephrine and ≤ 5 mg chlorobutanol per ml.[3]
In 1 ml syringes designed to deliver 2 doses of 0.3 ml each.

Rx **Ana-Kit** (Bayer)
Emergency insect sting treatment.
Epinephrine, 1:1000 in 1 ml (1 sterile syringe)[3]
Chlorpheniramine maleate, 2 mg (4 chewable tablets)
Sterile alcohol pads (2 each)
Tourniquet (1 each)

Rx **Emergent-Ez Kit** (Healthfirst Corp.)
Aminophylline (1 amp)
Ammonia Inhalants (3 each)
Amyl Nitrite Inhalants (2 each)
Atropine (2 amps)
Benadryl (2 amps)
Diazepam (2 amps)
Epinephrine (2 amps)
Nitroglycerin (1 bottle)
Solu-Cortef (1 Mix-o-vial)
Talwin (1 amp)
Tigan (1 amp)
Wyamine (2 amps)
Plastic Airway (1 each)
Disposable Syringes
Tracheotomy Needle (1 each)
Tourniquet (1 each)

Rx **Glucagon Emergency Kit** (Lilly)
For treatment of severe insulin reactions (low blood glucose).
1 mg glucagon and 49 mg lactose with diluent.
In 1 ml Hyporets for injection.

---

otc **Poison Antidote Kit** (JMI-Canton)
Emergency poison treatment.
Syrup of ipecac in 30 ml (1 bottle)
Charcoal suspension in 60 ml (4 bottles)

---

otc **Potable Aqua** (Wisconsin)
For emergency disinfection of drinking water.
Tablets for solution: 16.7% tetraglycine hydroperiodide (6.68% titrable iodine).
In 50s.

---

[1] Center Labs., 35 Channel Dr., Port Washington, NY 11050-0110.
[2] With sodium metabisulfite.
[3] With sodium bisulfite.

ANTIDOTES

Various Antidotes and Their Uses	
Drug (trade name)	Toxic/Overdosed Substance
Dimercaprol (**BAL In Oil**)	Arsenic, gold, mercury, lead
Deferoxamine mesylate (**Desferal**)	Iron
Edetate Calcium disodium (**Calcium Disodium Versenate**)	Lead
Sodium thiosulfate (Various)	Cyanide
Narcotic Antagonists Naloxone (**Narcan**) Nalmefene (**Revex**) Naltrexone (**ReVia**)	Opioids
Flumazenil (**Romazicon**)	Benzodiazepines
Physostigmine salicylate (**Antilirium**)	Anticholinergics (including tricyclic antidepressants) Diazepam (CNS depression)
Pralidoxime Cl (**Protopam Cl**)	Organophosphates Anticholinesterases
Digoxin immune fab (**Digibind**)	Digoxin, digitoxin
Mesna (**Mesnex**)	Ifosfamide-induced hemorrhagic cardiomyopathy
Dexrazoxane (**Zinecard**)	Doxorubicin-induced cardiomyopathy
Methylene blue (Various)	Cyanide
Other agents used additionally as antidotes	
Leucovorin calcium (**Wellcovorin**)	Folic acid antagonists (eg, methotrexate)
Hydroxocobalamin (Various)	Cyanide poisoning from nitroprusside
Vitamin K (Various)	Oral anticoagulants
Protamine Sulfate (Various)	Heparin
Glucagon	Insulin-induced hypoglycemia
Edetate disodium (Various)	Hypercalcemia Digitalis toxicity
Acetylcysteine (**Mucomyst, Mucosil**)	Acetaminophen
Atropine (Various)	Cholinergic agents: Organophosphates, carbamates, pilocarpine, physostigmine, isofluorophate or choline esters.
Amyl nitrite, Na Nitrite, Na Thiosulfate (**Cyanide antidote kit**)	Cyanide
Anticholinesterases Pyridostigmine Br (**Mestinon, Regonol**) Neostigmine Br (**Prostigmin**) Edrophonium Cl (**Tensilon**)	Nondepolarizing muscle relaxants
Nonspecific therapy of overdoses include:	
Osmotic diuretics Cathartics	Nonspecific, supportive therapies of overdoses. See also General Management of Acute Overdosage
Peritoneal dialysis solutions	
Emetics Syrup of ipecac (Various)	
Activated charcoal (Various)	
Urinary Alkalinizers	
Urinary Acidifiers	

DIMERCAPROL

Actions:

Pharmacology: Dimercaprol promotes excretion of arsenic, gold and mercury by chelation. The dimercaprol sulfhydryl groups form complexes with metals. This increases urinary and fecal elimination of the metals. Dimercaprol is most effective at preventing sulfhydryl enzyme inhibition when administered 1 to 2 hours after exposure. Dimercaprol may reactivate affected enzymes.

Pharmacokinetics: After IM use, peak concentrations occur in 30 to 60 minutes. It has a short half-life; metabolism and excretion are complete within 4 hours.

Indications:

Poisoning: Treatment of arsenic, gold and mercury poisoning; acute lead poisoning when used with calcium edetate disodium; acute mercury poisoning if therapy is begun within 1 or 2 hours. Not effective for chronic mercury poisoning.

Contraindications:

Hepatic or renal insufficiency, except postarsenical jaundice (see Warnings).

Iron, cadmium or selenium poisoning; the resulting dimercaprol-metal complexes are more toxic than the metal alone, especially to the kidneys.

Warnings:

Other metal poisonings: Dimercaprol is of questionable value in metal poisonings other than those listed in Indications (eg, antimony, bismuth).

Renal/Hepatic function impairment: Do not use in hepatic insufficiency. Discontinue or use only with extreme caution if acute renal insufficiency develops during therapy.

Pregnancy: Category C. Do not use unless necessary.

Lactation: It is not known if dimercaprol is excreted in breast milk. Use caution when administering to a nursing woman.

Children: Fever may persist during therapy (≈ 30%). A transient reduction of the percentage of polymorphonuclear leukocytes may also occur.

Precautions:

Urinary alkalinization is recommended because the dimercaprol-metal complex breaks down easily in an acid medium. Alkaline urine protects the kidney during therapy.

G–6–PD deficiency: Use with caution in these patients, especially in the presence of infection or other stressful situations; hemolysis may occur.

Drug Interactions:

Iron: Do not administer to patients under therapy with dimercaprol.

Adverse Reactions:

A consistent response to dimercaprol is a rise in blood pressure accompanied by tachycardia, proportional to the dose. Larger than recommended doses may cause other transitory signs and symptoms in order of frequency as follows: Nausea; vomiting; headache; burning sensation in the lips, mouth and throat; feeling of constriction or pain in the throat, chest or hands; conjunctivitis, lacrimation, blepharal spasm, rhinorrhea, salivation; tingling of the hands; burning sensation in the penis; sweating of the forehead, hands and other areas; abdominal pain; local pain at injection site; occasional appearance of painful sterile abscesses. These may be accompanied by anxiety, weakness and unrest, and may be relieved by an antihistamine.

Overdosage:

Dosage exceeding 5 mg/kg will usually be followed by vomiting, convulsions and stupor beginning within 30 minutes and subsiding within 6 hours following injection.

Administration and Dosage:

Give by deep IM injection only. Begin therapy as early as possible along with other supportive measures.

Mild arsenic or gold poisoning: 2.5 mg/kg 4 times daily for 2 days, then 2 times on the third day, and once daily thereafter for 10 days.

Severe arsenic or gold poisoning: 3 mg/kg every 4 hours for 2 days, then 4 times on the third day, then twice daily thereafter for 10 days.

Mercury poisoning: 5 mg/kg initially, then 2.5 mg/kg 1 to 2 times/day for 10 days.

Acute lead encephalopathy: 4 mg/kg alone in the first dose and thereafter at 4 hour intervals in combination with calcium edetate disodium administered at a separate site. For less severe poisoning, the dose can be reduced to 3 mg/kg after the first dose. Maintain treatment for 2 to 7 days, depending on clinical response.

Storage/Stability: Store at 15° to 30°C (59° to 86°F).

Rx	**BAL In Oil** (Becton Dickinson)	**Injection:** 100 mg per ml	In peanut oil with benzyl benzoate. In 3 ml ampuls.

DEFEROXAMINE MESYLATE

Actions:

Pharmacology: Chelates iron and prevents it from chemically reacting. Binds free serum iron, iron of ferritin and hemosiderin, but minimally affects iron of transferrin. The iron of cytochromes and hemoglobin is inaccessible. One hundred parts by weight can bind 8.5 parts of ferric iron. Does not demonstrably increase electrolyte/trace metal excretion.

Pharmacokinetics: Parenteral use required for systemic activity. Rapidly metabolized by plasma enzymes; excreted in urine. Iron chelate is excreted renally, giving urine a reddish color. Some is excreted in feces via bile.

Indications:

Acute iron intoxication: An adjunct to standard treatment measures.

Chronic iron overload can promote iron excretion in patients with secondary iron overload from transfusions. Deferoxamine slows hepatic iron accumulation; retards or eliminates hepatic fibrosis progression.

Unlabeled uses: Management of aluminum accumulation in bone in renal failure patients, and in aluminum-induced dialysis encephalopathy.

May be helpful in some cancers and Alzheimer's disease.

Contraindications:

Severe renal disease or anuria; primary hemochromatosis.

Warnings:

Cataracts occur rarely with prolonged therapy. Perform periodic slit-lamp exams on patients treated for chronic iron overload. Other ocular disturbances (rare) include: Decreased visual acuity; impaired peripheral, color and night vision; retinal pigmentary abnormalities. Disturbances were usually reversible on treatment cessation.

Auditory disturbances: Neurotoxicity-related auditory abnormalities have been reported including high-frequency sensorineural hearing loss. Younger patients are more affected than older patients.

Pregnancy: Category C. Skeletal anomalies were seen in animal fetuses at doses just above those recommended for humans. Do not use unless clearly needed.

Children: Iron mobilization by deferoxamine is relatively poor in patients < 3 years old with relatively small degrees of iron overload. Withhold the drug in such patients unless significant iron mobilization (eg, ≥ 1 mg of iron/day) is demonstrated.

Precautions:

Rapid infusion: Flushing of the skin, urticaria, hypotension and shock have occurred with rapid IV injection.

Adverse Reactions:

Occasional pain and induration at injection site.

Acute iron intoxication: Red urine; generalized erythema (rapid IV use; see Precautions).

Long-term therapy: Allergic-type reactions (cutaneous wheal formation, generalized itching, rash, anaphylactic reaction), blurred vision, cataracts, auditory disturbances (see Warnings); dysuria; abdominal discomfort; diarrhea; leg cramps; tachycardia; fever.

SC therapy: Localized pain, pruritus, erythema, skin irritation and swelling, which might also occur in a patient treated for acute intoxication.

Administration and Dosage:

May administer IM, by continuous SC mini-infusion or by slow IV infusion. Net iron excretion with SC use is greater than with equal IM doses because the labile (chelatable) intracellular iron pool is constantly exposed to the drug.

Acute iron intoxication: IM - Preferred route; use for all patients not in shock. Initially, 1 g; then 0.5 g every 4 hrs for 2 doses. Subsequently, give 0.5 g every 4 to 12 hrs based on clinical response. Do not exceed 6 g/day.

IV – Use only in cardiovascular collapse by slow infusion (≤ 15 mg/kg/hr). Dosage is same as with IM use. As soon as possible, stop IV and give IM. In most cases, IV use is preferred assuring the slow infusion rate.

DEFEROXAMINE MESYLATE

Chronic iron overload: Individualize dosage.

IM – 0.5 to 1 g daily. Give 2 g IV with, but separate from, each unit of blood. The rate of IV infusion must not exceed 15 mg/kg/hour.

SC – 1 to 2 g/day (20 to 40 mg/kg/day) over 8 to 24 hrs with continuous mini-infusion pump. Individualize infusion duration. In some patients, iron excretion will be as great after a short infusion (8 to 12 hrs) as if same dose is given over 24 hrs.

Oral use is controversial and unlabeled (binding iron in the GI tract) and appears to be generally discouraged.

Children: A maximum of 6 g/24 hr or 2 g/dose.

Preparation: Add 2 ml Sterile Water for Injection to each vial. For IV use, add to saline, glucose in water or Ringer's Lactate solution.

Storage/Stability: Do not store solutions reconstituted with sterile water longer than 1 week. Protect from light. Do not store above 25°C (77°F).

Rx	**Desferal** (Ciba)	**Powder for Injection:** 500 mg	In vials.

EDETATE CALCIUM DISODIUM (Calcium EDTA)

Actions:

Pharmacology: The calcium in edetate calcium disodium is readily displaced by heavy metals, such as lead, to form stable complexes which are excreted in the urine.

Pharmacokinetics: Edetate calcium disodium is poorly absorbed (< 5%) from the GI tract. The elimination half-life of the injection is 20 to 60 minutes. About 50% is excreted in the urine in 1 hour; 95% in 24 hours. 5%) from the GI tract. The elimination half-life of the injection is 20 to 60 minutes. About 50% is excreted in the urine in 1 hour; 95% in 24 hours.

Indications:

Lead poisoning: Acute and chronic lead poisoning and lead encephalopathy.

Contraindications:

Anuria.

Warnings:

Do not exceed recommended dosage. EDTA can produce toxic and potentially fatal effects. In lead encephalopathy, avoid rapid infusion; the IM route is preferred.

Renal effects: Severe acute lead poisoning may cause proteinuria and microscopic hematuria. EDTA may produce the same signs of renal damage. Perform urinalysis daily during therapy to monitor for progression of renal tubular damage. The presence of large renal epithelial cells, increasing numbers of red blood cells in the urinary sediment or greater proteinuria call for immediate discontinuation. Perform periodic BUN determinations before and during each course of therapy.

Hepatic effects: Mild increases in ALT and AST are common but return to normal within 48 hours after discontinuing therapy.

Pregnancy: Category B. Safety for use during pregnancy has not been established; do not use during pregnancy unless potential benefits outweigh potential hazards to the fetus.

Precautions:

Hydration: Avoid excess fluids in patients with lead encephalopathy and increased intracranial pressure. In such cases, mix a 20% solution with procaine to give a final concentration of 0.5% procaine and administer IM.

Acutely ill individuals may be dehydrated from vomiting. Since EDTA is excreted in the urine, establish urine flow by IV infusion before administering the first dose. Once urine flow is established, restrict further IV fluid to basal water and electrolyte requirements. Stop EDTA when urine flow ceases.

Adverse Reactions:

Body as a whole: Pain at IM injection site (see Administration and Dosage); fever; chills; malaise; fatigue; myalgia; arthralgia.

Cardiovascular: Hypotension; cardiac rhythm irregularities.

CNS: Tremors; headache; numbness; tingling.

GI: Cheilosis; nausea; vomiting; anorexia; excessive thirst.

GU: Glycosuria; proteinuria; microscopic hematuria and large epithelial cells in urinary sediment.

Hematologic: Transient bone marrow depression; anemia.

Hypersensitivity: Histamine-like reactions (sneezing, nasal congestion, lacrimation); rash.

Metabolic: Zinc deficiency; hypercalcemia.

EDETATE CALCIUM DISODIUM (Calcium EDTA)

Renal: Acute necrosis of proximal tubules which may result in fatal nephrosis (see Warnings).

Lab test abnormalities: Increasing AST and ALT (see Warnings).

Administration and Dosage:

Effective IV, SC or IM; however, because of convenience and greater safety in treating symptomatic children, the IM route is preferred and is recommended in patients with overt or incipient lead encephalopathy. Rapid IV infusion may be lethal by suddenly increasing intracranial pressure in this group of patients with cerebral edema.

Do not administer larger than recommended doses.

IV: Dilute the 5 ml amp with 250 to 500 ml normal saline or 5% dextrose solution. In asymptomatic adults, administer this dilution over at least 1 hour twice daily for up to 5 days. Interrupt therapy for 2 days; follow with another 5 days of treatment, if indicated.

IM administration results in good absorption, but pain occurs at the injection site.

Young children – Give total daily dose in divided doses every 8 or 12 hours for 3 to 5 days; give a second course after a rest period of ≥ 4 days. Add procaine to produce a concentration of 0.5% to minimize pain at injection site.

Lead encephalopathy is relatively rare in adults, but is common in children and has a high mortality rate. Though some investigators have employed a combination of EDTA and dimercaprol, EDTA alone has been used over a longer period of time. When administered concurrently, inject dimercaprol and EDTA at separate deep IM sites.

Storage/Stability: Store at controlled room temperature: 15° to 30°C (59° to 86°F).

Rx	**Calcium Disodium Versenate** (3M Pharm.)	**Injection:** 200 mg per ml	In 5 ml amps.

SODIUM THIOSULFATE

Actions:

Pharmacology: The primary mechanism of cyanide detoxification involves conversion of cyanide to the relatively nontoxic thiocyanate ion. This reaction involves the enzyme rhodanese (thiosulfate cyanide sulfurtransferase) found in many body tissues, but with major activity in the liver. The body has the capability to detoxify cyanide; however, the rhodanese enzyme system responds slowly to large amounts of cyanide. The rhodanese enzyme reaction can be accelerated by supplying an exogenous source of sulfur, accomplished by administering sodium thiosulfate.

Pharmacokinetics: Following IV injection, sodium thiosulfate is distributed throughout the extracellular fluid and excreted unchanged in the urine. The biological half-life is 0.65 hours.

Indications:

Cyanide poisoning: It may be used alone or as adjunctive therapy with sodium nitrite or amyl nitrite in cyanide toxicity.

Warnings:

Pregnancy: Category C. Safety for use during pregnancy has not been established. Use only when clearly needed and when the potential benefits outweigh the potential hazards to the fetus.

Administration and Dosage:

Death from cyanide poisoning occurs rapidly; avoid delays in administering sodium thiosulfate.

Sodium thiosulfate injection is meant for slow IV use only.

Cyanide poisoning:

Adults – 12.5 g IV over ≈ 10 minutes, whether used alone or in combination with other cyanide antidotes.

Children – 7 g/m^2; maximum dose 12.5 g.

Monitoring – Closely monitor patients for 24 to 48 hours for symptoms to reappear. If symptoms recur, repeat administration at one-half the original dose.

Rx	**Sodium Thiosulfate** (Various, eg, Pasadena)	**Injection:** 25% (250 mg/ml)	4.4 mg potassium chloride, 2.8 mg boric acid. In 50 ml single-dose vials.

Narcotic Antagonists

NALMEFENE HCl

Actions:

Pharmacology: Nalmefene, an opioid antagonist, is a 6-methylene analog of naltrexone. Nalmefene prevents or reverses the effects of opioids, including respiratory depression, sedation and hypotension. It has a longer duration of action than naloxone at fully reversing doses. Nalmefene has no opioid agonist activity; it does not produce respiratory depression, psychotomimetic effects or pupillary constriction, and no pharmacological activity was observed when it was administered in the absence of opioid agonists. Nalmefene can produce acute withdrawal symptoms in individuals who are opioid—dependent.

Pharmacokinetics:

Absorption – Nalmefene was completely bioavailable following IM or SC administration in 12 male volunteers relative to IV use (relative bioavailabilities were 101.5% and 99.7%, respectively). Nalmefene will be administered primarily as an IV bolus, however, it can be given IM or SC if venous access cannot be established. While the time to maximum plasma concentration was 2.3 hours following IM and 1.5 hours following SC administrations, therapeutic plasma concentrations are likely to be reached within 5 to 15 minutes after a 1 mg dose in an emergency. Because of the variability in the speed of absorption for IM and SC dosing, and the inability to titrate to effect, take great care if repeated doses must be given by these routes.

Distribution – Following a 1 mg parenteral dose, nalmefene was rapidly distributed. A 1 mg dose blocked > 80% of brain opioid receptors within 5 minutes after administration. The apparent volumes of distribution centrally and at steady state are 3.9 and 8.6 L/kg, respectively. Over a concentration range of 0.1 to 2 mcg/ml, 45% is bound to plasma proteins. In vitro, nalmefene distributed 67% into red blood cells and 39% into plasma.

Metabolism – Nalmefene is metabolized by the liver, primarily by glucuronide conjugation, and excreted in the urine; < 5% is excreted in the urine unchanged, and 17% is excreted in the feces. It is also metabolized to trace amounts of an N-dealkylated metabolite. Nalmefene glucuronide is inactive; the N-dealkylated metabolite has minimal activity. Nalmefene may undergo enterohepatic recycling.

Excretion – After IV administration of 1 mg to healthy males (age, 19 to 32 years), plasma concentrations declined biexponentially with a redistribution and a terminal elimination half-life of 41 ± 34 minutes and 10.8 ± 5.2 hours, respectively. The systemic clearance of nalmefene is 0.8 L/hr/kg and the renal clearance is 0.08 L/hr/kg.

Nalmefene Pharmacokinetic Parameters in Adult Males (1 mg IV dose)

Parameter	Young (n = 18)	Elderly (n = 11)
Age (years)	19-32	62-80
C_p at 5 min (ng/ml)	3.7	5.8
Vd_{ss} (L/kg)	8.6	8.6
V_c (L/kg)	3.9	2.8
$AUC_{o\text{-}inf}$ (ng•hr/ml)	16.6	17.3
Terminal $t_{1/2}$ (hr)	10.8	9.4
Cl_{plasma} (L/hr/kg)	0.8	0.8

Clinical trials:

Reversal of postoperative opioid depression – In five controlled trials, patients received nalmefene following morphine or fentanyl intraoperatively. Five minutes after administration, initial single doses of 0.1, 0.25, 0.5 or 1 mcg/kg had effectively reversed respiratory depression in a dose-dependent manner. Twenty minutes after initial administration, respiratory depression had been effectively reversed in most patients receiving cumulative doses within the recommended range (0.1 to 1 mcg/kg). Total doses > 1 mcg/kg did not increase the therapeutic response. The postoperative administration of nalmefene at the recommended doses did not prevent the analgesic response to subsequently administered opioids.

Reversal of the effect of intrathecally administered opioids – IV nalmefene doses of 0.5 and 1 mcg/kg were administered to 47 patients given intrathecal morphine. One to two doses reversed respiratory depression in most patients. The administration of nalmefene at the recommended doses did not prevent the analgesic response to subsequently administered opioids.

Management of known or suspected opioid overdose – Nalmefene doses of 0.5 to 2 mg were studied in four trials of patients who were presumed to have taken an opioid overdose. Doses of 0.5 to 1 mg effectively reversed respiratory depression within 2 to 5 minutes in most patients subsequently confirmed to have opioid overdose. A total dose > 1.5 mg did not increase the therapeutic response.

NALMEFENE HCl

Indications:

Reversal of opioid effects: Complete or partial reversal of opioid drug effects, including respiratory depression, induced by either natural or synthetic opioids.

Opioid overdose: Management of known or suspected opioid overdose.

Contraindications:

Hypersensitivity to the product.

Warnings:

Emergency use: Nalmefene, like all drugs in this class, is not the primary treatment for ventilatory failure. In most emergency settings, treatment with nalmefene should follow, not precede, the establishment of a patent airway, ventilatory assistance, administration of oxygen and establishment of circulatory access.

Respiratory depression: Accidental overdose with long acting opioids (eg, methadone, levomethadyl) may result in prolonged respiratory depression. Respiratory depression in both the postoperative and overdose setting may be complex and involve the effects of anesthetic agents, neuromuscular blockers and other drugs. While nalmefene has a longer duration of action than naloxone in fully reversing doses, be aware that a recurrence of respiratory depression is possible, even after an apparently adequate initial response to nalmefene treatment. Observe patients until there is no reasonable risk of recurrent respiratory depression.

Renal function impairment: There was a statistically significant 27% decrease in plasma clearance of nalmefene in the end-stage renal disease (ESRD) population during interdialysis (0.57 L/hr/kg) and a 25% decreased plasma clearance in the ESRD population during intradialysis (0.59 L/hr/kg) compared to controls (0.79 L/hr/kg). The elimination half-life was prolonged in ESRD patients from 10.2 (controls) to 26.1 hr.

Hepatic function impairment: Subjects with hepatic disease had a 28.3% decrease in plasma clearance of nalmefene compared to controls (0.56 vs 0.78 L/hr/kg, respectively). Elimination half-life increased from 10.2 to 11.9 hours in the hepatically impaired. No dosage adjustment is recommended since nalmefene will be administered as an acute course of therapy.

Elderly: Dose proportionality was observed in nalmefene AUC following 0.5 to 2 mg IV administration to elderly male subjects. Following a 1 mg IV dose, there were no significant differences between young and elderly adult male subjects with respect to plasma clearance, steady-state volume of distribution or half-life. There was an apparent age-related decrease in the central volume of distribution that resulted in a greater initial nalmefene concentration in the elderly group. While initial plasma concentrations were transiently higher in the elderly, it would not be anticipated that this population would require dosing adjustment.

Pregnancy: Category B. There are no adequate and well controlled studies in pregnant women. Use this drug during pregnancy only if clearly needed.

Lactation: Nalmefene and its metabolites were secreted into rat milk, reaching concentrations approximately three times those in plasma at 1 hour and decreasing to about half the corresponding plasma concentrations by 24 hours following bolus administration. Exercise caution when nalmefene is administered to a nursing woman.

Children: Safety and efficacy have not been established. Only use nalmefene in the resuscitation of the newborn when the expected benefits outweigh the risks.

Precautions:

Cardiovascular risks: Pulmonary edema, cardiovascular instability, hypotension, hypertension, ventricular tachycardia and ventricular fibrillation have been reported in connection with opioid reversal in both postoperative and emergency department settings. In many cases, these effects appear to be the result of abrupt reversal of opioid effects. Although nalmefene has been used safely in patients with preexisting cardiac disease, use all drugs of this class with caution in patients at high cardiovascular risk or who have received potentially cardiotoxic drugs.

Risk of precipitated withdrawal: Nalmefene is known to produce acute withdrawal symptoms and, therefore, should be used with extreme caution in patients with known physical dependence on opioids or following surgery involving high uses of opioids. Imprudent use or excessive doses of opioid antagonists in the postoperative setting has been associated with hypertension, tachycardia and excessive mortality in patients at high risk for cardiovascular complications.

NALMEFENE HCl

Incomplete reversal of buprenorphine: In animals, nalmefene doses up to 10 mg/kg (437 times the maximum recommended human dose) produced incomplete reversal of buprenorphine-induced analgesia. This appears to be a consequence of a high affinity and slow displacement of buprenorphine from the opioid receptors. Hence, nalmefene may not completely reverse buprenorphine-induced respiratory depression.

Drug Interactions:

Flumazenil: Both flumazenil and nalmefene can induce seizures in animals. Coadministration of these agents produced fewer seizures than expected in a study in rodents, based on the expected effects of each drug alone. Based on these data, an adverse interaction from the coadministration of the two drugs is not expected, but remain aware of the potential risk of seizures from agents in these classes.

Adverse Reactions:

Nalmefene is well tolerated and shows no serious toxicity during experimental administration to healthy individuals, even when given at 15 times the highest recommended dose. In a small number of subjects, at doses exceeding the recommended dose, nalmefene produced symptoms suggestive of reversal of endogenous opioids, such as those that have been reported for other narcotic antagonist drugs. These symptoms (eg, nausea, chills, myalgia, dysphoria, abdominal cramps, joint pain) were usually transient and occurred at very low frequency.

Symptoms of precipitated opioid withdrawal at the recommended clinical doses were seen in both postoperative and overdose patients who were later found to have had histories of covert opioid use. Symptoms of precipitated withdrawal similar to those seen with other opioid antagonists, were transient following the lower doses used in the postoperative setting and more prolonged following the administration of the larger doses used in the treatment of overdose.

Tachycardia and nausea following the use of nalmefene in the postoperative setting were reported at the same frequencies as for naloxone at equivalent doses. The risk of both of these adverse events was low at doses giving partial opioid reversal and increased with increases in dose. Thus, total doses > 1 mcg/kg in the postoperative setting and 1.5 mg/70 kg in the treatment of overdose are not recommended.

Nalmefene Adverse Reactions (> 1%)			
Adverse reaction	Nalmefene (n = 1127)	Naloxone (n = 369)	Placebo (n = 77)
Nausea	18%	18%	4%
Vomiting	9%	7%	6%
Tachycardia	5%	8%	-
Hypertension	5%	7%	-
Postoperative pain	4%	4%	N/A
Fever	3%	4%	-
Dizziness	3%	4%	1%
Headache	1%	1%	4%
Chills	1%	1%	-
Hypotension	1%	1%	-
Vasodilation	1%	1%	-

Other adverse reactions include the following:

Cardiovascular: Bradycardia, arrhythmia (< 1%).

GI: Diarrhea, dry mouth (< 1%).

CNS: Somnolence, depression, agitation, nervousness, tremor, confusion, withdrawal syndrome, myoclonus (< 1%).

Lab test abnormalities: Transient increases in CPK (0.5%; these increases were believed to be related to surgery and not believed to be related to the administration of nalmefene); increases in AST (0.3% with either nalmefene or naloxone).

Miscellaneous: Pharyngitis, pruritus, urinary retention (< 1%).

NALMEFENE HCl

Overdosage:

IV doses of up to 24 mg administered to healthy volunteers in the absence of opioid agonists produced no serious adverse reactions, severe signs or symptoms or clinically significant laboratory abnormalities. As with all opioid antagonists, use in patients physically dependent on opioids can result in precipitated withdrawal reactions that may result in symptoms that require medical attention. Treatment of such cases should be symptomatic and supportive. Refer to General Management of Acute Overdosage. Administration of large amounts of opioids to patients receiving opioid antagonists in an attempt to overcome a full blockade has resulted in adverse respiratory and circulatory reactions.

Administration and Dosage:

Approved by the FDA on April 17, 1995 (1S classification).

IMPORTANT INFORMATION— Dosage strengths: Nalmefene is supplied in two concentrations which are packaged in ampules of different appearance: An amp with a blue label containing one (1) ml at a concentration suitable for postoperative use (100 mcg/ml) and an amp with a green label containing two (2) ml suitable for the management of overdose (1 mg/ml, 10 times as concentrated, 20 times as much drug). Take proper steps to prevent use of the incorrect dosage strength.

Administration: Titrate nalmefene to reverse the undesired effects of opioids. Once adequate reversal has been established, additional administration is not required and may actually be harmful due to unwanted reversal of analgesia or precipitated withdrawal.

Duration of action: The duration of action of nalmefene is as long as most opioid analgesics. The apparent duration of action will vary, however, depending on the half-life and plasma concentration of the narcotic being reversed, the presence or absence of other drugs affecting the brain or muscles of respiration and the dose of nalmefene administered. Partially reversing doses of nalmefene (1 mcg/kg) lose their effect as the drug is redistributed through the body, and the effects of these low doses may not last more than 30 to 60 minutes in the presence of persistent opioid effects. Fully reversing doses (1 mg/70 kg) last many hours, but may complicate the management of patients who are in pain, at high cardiovascular risk or who are physically dependent on opioids.

The recommended doses represent a compromise between a desirable controlled reversal and the need for prompt response and adequate duration of action. Using higher dosages or shorter intervals between incremental doses is likely to increase the incidence and severity of symptoms related to acute withdrawal such as nausea, vomiting, elevated blood pressure and anxiety.

Patients tolerant to or physically dependent on opioids: Nalmefene may cause acute withdrawal symptoms in individuals who have some degree of tolerance to and dependence on opioids. Closely observe these patients for symptoms of withdrawal following administration of the initial and subsequent injections of nalmefene. Administer subsequent doses with intervals of at least 2 to 5 minutes between doses to allow the full effect of each incremental dose of nalmefene to be reached.

Reversal of postoperative opioid depression: Use 100 mcg/ml dosage strength (blue label); refer to the following table for initial doses. The goal of treatment with nalmefene in the postoperative setting is to achieve reversal of excessive opioid effects without inducing a complete reversal and acute pain. This is best accomplished with an initial dose of 0.25 mcg/kg followed by 0.25 mcg/kg incremental doses at 2 to 5 minute intervals, stopping as soon as the desired degree of opioid reversal is obtained. A cumulative total dose > 1 mcg/kg does not provide additional therapeutic effect.

Nalmefene Dosage for Reversal of Postoperative Opioid Depression

Body weight (kg)	Amount of nalmefene 100 mcg/ml solution (ml)
50	0.125
60	0.15
70	0.175
80	0.2
90	0.225
100	0.25

Narcotic Antagonists

NALMEFENE HCl

Cardiovascular risk patients: In cases where the patient is known to be at increased cardiovascular risk, it may be desirable to dilute nalmefene 1:1 with saline or sterile water and use smaller initial and incremental doses of 0.1 mcg/kg.

Management of known/suspected opioid overdose: Use 1 mg/ml dosage strength (green label). The recommended initial dose of nalmefene for nonopioid dependent patients is 0.5 mg/70 kg. If needed, this may be followed by a second dose of 1 mg/70 kg, 2 to 5 minutes later. If a total dose of 1.5 mg/70 kg has been administered without clinical response, additional nalmefene is unlikely to have an effect. Patients should not be given more nalmefene than is required to restore the respiratory rate to normal, thus minimizing the likelihood of cardiovascular stress and precipitated withdrawal syndrome.

If there is a reasonable suspicion of opioid dependency, initially administer a challenge dose of 0.1 mg/70 kg. If there is no evidence of withdrawal in 2 minutes, follow the recommended dosing. Nalmefene had no effect in cases where opioids were not responsible for sedation and hypoventilation. Therefore, patients should only be treated with nalmefene when the likelihood of an opioid overdose is high, based on a history of opioid overdose or the clinical presentation of respiratory depression with concurrent pupillary constriction.

Repeated dosing: Nalmefene is the longest acting of the currently available parenteral opioid antagonists. If recurrence of respiratory depression does occur, the dose should again be titrated to clinical effect using incremental doses to avoid over-reversal.

Hepatic and renal disease: Hepatic disease and renal failure substantially reduce the clearance of nalmefene (see Warnings). For single episodes of opioid antagonism, adjustment of nalmefene dosage is not required. However, in patients with renal failure, slowly administer the incremental doses (over 60 seconds) to minimize the hypertension and dizziness reported following the abrupt administration of nalmefene to such patients.

Loss of IV access: Should IV access be lost or not readily obtainable, a single dose of nalmefene should be effective within 5 to 15 minutes after 1 mg IM or SC doses (see Pharmacokinetics).

Rx	**Revex** (Ohmeda)	**Injection:** 100 mcg/ml nalmefene base	Blue label.[1] In 1 ml amps.
		1 mg/ml nalmefene base	Green label.[2] In 2 ml amps.

[1] The blue labeled product is for postoperative use.

[2] The green labeled product is for management of overdose.

Narcotic Antagonists

NALOXONE HCl

Actions:

Pharmacology: The narcotic antagonist naloxone is clinically useful in the reversal of narcotic-induced respiratory depression. Naloxone, a pure narcotic antagonist, will precipitate abstinence syndrome in the presence of narcotic addiction. Because it is devoid of undesirable agonist properties, naloxone is preferred for reversal of narcotic-induced respiratory depression. Naloxone prevents or reverses opioid effects including respiratory depression, sedation and hypotension; it can reverse psychotomimetic and dysphoric effects of agonist-antagonists (eg, pentazocine).

Mechanism – The mechanism of action is not fully understood; evidence suggests that it antagonizes the opioid effects by competing for the same receptor sites. Nalozone is an essentially pure narcotic antagonis, ie, it does not possess "agonistic" or morphine-like properties.

Effects – Nalozone does not produce respiratory depression, psychotomimetic effects or pupillary constriction. In the absence of narcotics or agonistic effects of other narcotic antagonists, naloxone exhibits essentially no pharmacologic activity.

Pharmacokinetics:

Distribution – After parenteral use, naloxone is rapidly distributed in the body. Onset of action of IV naloxone is generally apparent within 2 min; it is only slightly less rapid when give SC or IM. Duration of action depends upon dose and route. IM use produces a more prolonged effect than IV use. The requirement for repeat doses will also depend upon amount, type and route of the narcotic being antagonized.

Metabolism – Naloxone is metabolized in the liver, primarily by glucuronide conjugation. It is excreted in the urine. The serum of half-life in adults ranged from 30 to 81 minutes (mean 64 ± 12 minutes); in neonates, 3.1 ± 0.5 hours.

Indications:

Reversal of opioid effects: For the complete or partial reversal of narcotic depression, including respiratory depression, induced by opioid including natural and synthetic narcotics, propoxyphene, methadone, nabuphine, butorphanol and pentaxocine.

Opioid overdose: For the diagnosis of suspected acute opioid overdosage.

Unlabeled uses: Naloxone has been used to improve circulation in refractory shock. Naloxone has also been used for the reversal of alcoholic coma, dementia of the Alzheimer type and schizophrenia.

Contraindications:

Hypersensitivity to these agents.

Warnings:

Drug dependence: Administer cautiously to persons who are known or suspected to be physically dependent on opioids, including newborns of mothers with narcotic dependence. Reversal of narcotic effect will precipitate acute abstinence syndrome.

Repeat administration: The patient who has satisfactorily responded should be kept under continued surveillance. Administer repeated doses as necessary, because the duration of action of some narcotics may exceed that of the narcotic antagonist.

Respiratory depression: Not effective against respiratory depression dute to nonopioid drugs. Reversal of buprenorphine-induced respiratory depression may be incomplete; if an incomplete response occurs, mechanically assist respiration.

Pregnancy: Category B. No adequate and well controlled studies in pregnant women. Use during pregnancy only when clearly needed.

Lactation: It is not known whether the drug is excreted in breast milk. Use caution when administering to a nursing woman.

Precautions:

Other supportive therapy: Maintain a free airway and provide artificial respiration, cardiac masage and vasopressor agents; employ when necessary to counteract acute narcotic overdosage.

Cardiovascular effects: Several instances of hypotension, hypertension, pulmonary edema, ventricular tachycardia and fibrillation have been reported in post-operative patients, most of whom had pre-existing cardiovascular disoders or had received other drugs that may have similar adverse cardiovascular effects. A direct cause and effect relationship is not established; use caution in patients with pre-existing cardiac disease or who have received potentially cardiotoxic drugs.

Adverse Reactions:

Abrupt reversal of narcotic depression may result in nausea, vomiting, sweating, tachycardia, increased blood pressure and tremulousness.

Narcotic Antagonists

NALOXONE HCl

In post-operative patients, excessive dosage may result in excitement and significant reversal of analgesia, hypotension, hypertension, pulmonary edema and ventricular tachycardia and fibirllation. Seizures have bee reported infrequently.

Administration and Dosage:

Give IV, IM or SC. The most rapid onset of action is achieved iwth IV use, which is recommended in emergency situations. Duration of actionn of some narcotics may exceed that of naloxone. Keep patient sunder continued surveillance and give repeat doses as necessary.

Adults:

Narcotic overdose (known or suspected) – Initial dose is 0.4 to 2 mg IV; may repeat IV at 2 to 3 minute intervals. If no response is observed after 10 mg has been administered, question the diagnosis of narcotic-induced or partial narcotic-induced toxicity. IM or SC administration may be necessary if the IV route is not available.

Post-operative narcotic depression (partial reversal) – Small doses are usually sufficient. Titrate dose according to the patient's response. Excessive dosage may result in significant reversal of analgesia and increase in blood pressure. Similarly, too rapid reversal may iduce nausea, vomiting, sweating or circulatory stress.

Initial dose: Inject in increments of 0.1 to 0.2 mg IV at 2 to 3 minute intervals to the desired degree of reversal (ie, adequate ventialtion and alertness without significant pain or discomfort).

Repeat dose: Repeat doses may be required within 1 or 2 hr intervals depending on the amount, type (ie, short- or long-acting) and time interval since last administration. Supplemental IM doses have produced a longer lasting effect.

Children:

Narcotic overdose (known or suspected) – Initial dose is 0.01 mg/kg IV; give a subsequent dose of 0.1 mg/kg if needed. If an IV route is not available, may be given IM or SC in divided doses. If necessary, dilute with Sterile Water for Injection.

Post-operative narcotic depression – Follow the recommendations and cautions under adult administration guidelines. For initial reversal of respiratory depression, inject in increments of 0.005 to 0.01 mg IV at 2 to 3 minute intervals to desired degree of reversal.

Neonates:

Narcotic-induced depression – Initial dose is 0.01 mg/kg IV, IM or SC; may be repeated in accordance with adult administration guidelines.

Intravenous infusion: Dilute in normal saline or 5% dextrose solutions. The addition of 2 mg in 500 ml of either solution provides a concentration of 0.004 mg/ml. Titrate the administration rate in accordance with the patient's response.

Incompatibilities – Do not mix naloxone with preparations containing bisulfite, metabisulfite, long-chain or high molecular weight anions, or any solution having an alkaline pH. Do not add any drug or chemical agent unless its effect on the chemical and physical stability of the solution has first been established.

Stability – Use mixtures within 24 hrs. After 24 hrs, discard unused solution.

Rx	**Naloxone HCl** (Various, eg, Abbot, Astra, Elkins-Sinn, SoloPak)	**Injection**: 0.4 mg/ml	In 1 ml amps, 1 ml syringes and 1, 2 and 10 ml vials.
Rx	**Narcan** (DuPont Pharm.)		In 1 ml amps and 10 ml vials.[1]
Rx	**Naloxone HCl** (Various, eg, Astra)	**Injection**: 1 mg/ml	In 1 and 5 ml vials.
Rx	**Narcan** (DuPont Pharm)		In 2 ml amps and 10 ml vials.[1]
Rx	**Naloxone HCl** (Various, eg, Abbott, Astra)	**Neonatal Injection**: 0.02 mg/ml	In 2 ml vials.
Rx	**Narcan** (DuPont Pharm.)		In 2 ml amps.

[1] Available with or without parabens.

NALTREXONE HCl

Actions:

Pharmacology: Naltrexone, a pure opioid antagonist, markedly attenuates or completely reversibly blocks the subjective effects of IV opioids. When coadministered with morphine on a chronic basis, it blocks the physical dependence to morphine, heroin and other opioids. Naltrexone is a synthetic congener of oxymorphone with no opioid agonist properties, and it is related to naloxone. It has few other, if any, intrinsic actions. However, it does produce some pupillary constriction. Administration is not associated with the development of tolerance or dependence. In subjects physically dependent on opioids, naltrexone will precipitate withdrawal symptomatology.

Naltrexone 50 mg will block the pharmacologic effects of 25 mg IV heroin for as long as 24 hours. Data suggest that doubling the dose of naltrexone provides blockade for 48 hours and tripling the dose provides blockade for about 72 hours.

Naltrexone blocks the effects of opioids by competitive binding at opioid receptors. This makes the blockade potentially surmountable, but administration of very high doses of opiates has resulted in excessive symptoms of histamine release in subjects.

The mechanism of action in alcoholism is not understood; however, involvement of the endogenous opioid system is suggested. Naltrexone competitively binds to opioid receptors and may block the effects of endogenous opioids. Opioid antagonists reduce alcohol consumption by animals, and naltrexone reduces alcohol consumption. Naltrexone is not aversive therapy and does not cause a disulfiram-like reaction either as a result of opiate use or ethanol ingestion.

Pharmacokinetics:

Absorption – Although well absorbed orally, naltrexone is subject to significant first pass metabolism with oral bioavailability estimates ranging from 5% to 40%. Following oral administration, naltrexone undergoes rapid and nearly complete absorption with ≈ 96% of the dose absorbed from the GI tract. Peak plasma levels of both naltrexone and 6–β-naltrexol occur within 1 hour of dosing.

Distribution – The volume of distribution for naltrexone after IV administration is estimated to be 1350 L. In vitro, naltrexone is 21% bound to plasma proteins.

Metabolism/Excretion – The major metabolite of naltrexone is 6–β-naltrexol. The activity of naltrexone is believed to be due to both parent and the 6–β-naltrexol metabolite. Two other minor metabolites are 2–hydroxy-3–methoxy-6–β-naltrexol and 2–hydroxy-3–methyl-naltrexone. Naltrexone and its metabolites are also conjugated to form additional metabolic products. The mean elimination half-life values for naltrexone and 6–β-naltrexol are 4 and 13 hours, respectively. The systemic clearance (after IV administration) of naltrexone is ≈ 3.5 L/min, which exceeds liver blood flow (≈ 1.2 L/min). This suggests both that naltrexone is a highly extracted drug (> 98% metabolized) and that extra-hepatic sites of drug metabolism exist.

The renal clearance for naltrexone ranges from 30 to 127 ml/min and suggests that renal elimination is primarily by glomerular filtration. In comparison, the renal clearance for 6–β-naltrexol ranges from 230 to 369 ml/min, suggesting an additional renal tubular secretory mechanism. Both parent drug and metabolites are excreted primarily by the kidney (53% to 79% of the dose), however, urinary excretion of unchanged naltrexone accounts for < 2% of an oral dose and fecal excretion is a minor elimination pathway. The urinary excretion of unchanged and conjugated 6–β-naltrexone accounts for 43% of an oral dose. Naltrexone and its metabolites may undergo enterohepatic recycling.

Clinical trials:

Alcoholism – In one study, 104 alcohol-dependent patients were randomized to receive either naltrexone 50 mg once daily or placebo. Naltrexone proved superior to placebo in measures of drinking including abstention rates (51% vs 23%), number of drinking days and relapse (31% vs 60%). In a second study with 82 alcohol-dependent patients, the group of patients receiving naltrexone had lower relapse rates (21% vs 41%), less alcohol craving and fewer drinking days compared with patients who received placebo, but these results depended on the specific analysis used.

In the clinical studies, treatment with naltrexone supported abstinence, prevented relapse and decreased alcohol consumption. In an uncontrolled study, the patterns of abstinence and relapse were similar to those observed in the controlled studies. Naltrexone was not uniformly helpful to all patients and the expected effect of the drug is a modest improvement in the outcome of conventional treatment.

NALTREXONE HCl

Treatment of narcotic addiction – Naltrexone produces complete blockade of the euphoric effects of opioids in both volunteer and addict populations. When administered by means that enforce compliance, it will produce an effective opioid blockade, but has not been shown to affect the use of cocaine or other non-opioid drugs of abuse.

The drug is reported to be of greatest use in good prognosis narcotic addicts who take the drug as part of a comprehensive occupational rehabilitative program, behavioral contract or other compliance-enhancing protocol. Unlike methadone or levomethadyl, naltrexone does not reinforce medication compliance and is expected to have a therapeutic effect only when given under external conditions that support continued use of the medication.

Indications:

Narcotic addiction: Blockade of the effects of exogenously administered opioids.

Alcoholism: Treatment of alcohol dependence.

Unlabeled uses: Naltrexone has been used in eating disorders and in the treatment of postconcussional syndrome unresponsive to other treatments. To increase patient compliance, an SC implant is being studied.

Contraindications:

Patients receiving opioid analgesics; opioid-dependent patients; patients in acute opioid withdrawal; failed naloxone challenge; positive urine screen for opioids; history of sensitivity to naltrexone (it is not known if there is any cross-sensitivity with naloxone or other phenanthrene-containing opioids); acute hepatitis or liver failure.

Warnings:

Hepatotoxicity: Naltrexone has the capacity to cause hepatocellular injury when given in excessive doses. It is contraindicated in acute hepatitis or liver failure, and its use in patients with active liver disease must be carefully considered in light of its hepatotoxic effects.

The margin of separation between the apparently safe dose of naltrexone and the dose causing hepatic injury appears to be only fivefold or less. Naltrexone does not appear to be a hepatotoxin at the recommended doses.

Warn patients of the risk of hepatic injury and advise them to stop naltrexone and seek medical attention if they experience symptoms of acute hepatitis.

Evidence of its hepatotoxic potential is derived primarily from a placebo controlled study in which naltrexone was administered to obese subjects at a dose approximately fivefold that recommended (300 mg/day). Five of 26 naltrexone recipients developed elevations of serum transaminases 3 to 19 times their baseline values after 3 to 8 weeks of treatment. The patients involved were generally clinically asymptomatic and the transaminase levels of all patients on whom follow-up was obtained returned to (or toward) baseline values in a matter of weeks. The lack of any transaminase elevations of similar magnitude in any of the 24 placebo patients indicates that naltrexone is a direct hepatotoxin.

This is also supported by evidence from other placebo controlled studies in which exposure to naltrexone at doses above the amount recommended for the treatment of alcoholism or opiate blockade (50 mg/day) consistently produced more numerous and more significant elevations of serum transaminases than did placebo. Transaminase elevations in 3 of 9 patients with Alzheimer's disease who received naltrexone (at doses up to 300 mg/day) for 5 to 8 weeks in an open clinical trial have been reported.

Although no cases of hepatic failure have ever been reported, consider this as a possible risk of treatment.

Abstinence precipitation/syndrome: Unintended precipitation of abstinence or exacerbation of a preexisting subclinical abstinence syndrome may occur; therefore, patients should remain opioid-free for a minimum of 7 to 10 days before starting naltrexone. The absence of opioid in urine is not sufficient proof that a patient is opioid-free. Perform a naloxone challenge to exclude the possibility of precipitating a withdrawal reaction (see Administration and Dosage).

Severe opioid withdrawal syndromes precipitated by accidental naltrexone ingestion have occurred in opioid-dependent individuals. Withdrawal symptoms usually appear within 5 minutes of ingestion and may last up to 48 hours. Mental status changes, including confusion, somnolence and visual hallucinations have occurred. Significant fluid losses from vomiting and diarrhea have required IV fluids.

NALTREXONE HCl

Surmountable blockade: While naltrexone is a potent antagonist with a prolonged pharmacologic effect (24 to 72 hours), the blockade produced by naltrexone is surmountable. This poses a potential risk to individuals who attempt to overcome the blockade by self-administering large amounts of opioids. Any attempt by a patient to overcome the antagonism by taking opioids is very dangerous and may lead to fatal overdose. Also, lesser amounts of exogenous opioids are dangerous if they are taken in a manner (ie, relatively long after the last dose of naltrexone) and in an amount that persists in the body longer than effective concentrations of naltrexone and its metabolites.

When reversal of blockade is required – In an emergency situation in patients receiving full blocking doses of naltrexone, a suggested plan of management is regional analgesia, conscious sedation with a benzodiazepine, use of non-opioid analgesics or general anesthesia.

In a situation requiring opioid analgesia, the amount of opioid required may be greater than usual and resulting respiratory depression may be deeper and more prolonged. A rapid-acting analgesic which minimizes respiratory depression is preferred. Individualize dosage; monitor closely.

Additionally, nonreceptor-mediated actions may occur (eg, facial swelling, itching, generalized erythema presumably due to histamine release).

Use with narcotics: Patients taking naltrexone may not benefit from opioid-containing medicines, such as cough and cold preparations, antidiarrheal preparations and opioid analgesics. Use a nonopioid-containing alternative, if available.

Carcinogenesis/Fertility impairment: In a 2 year carcinogenicity study in rats, there were small increases in the numbers of mesotheliomas in males and tumors of vascular origin in both sexes. The number of tumors were within the range seen in historical control groups, except for the vascular tumors in females, where the 4% incidence exceeded the historical maximum of 2%.

Naltrexone (100 mg/kg, ≈ 140 times the human therapeutic dose) caused a significant increase in pseudo-pregnancy in the rat. A decrease in the pregnancy rate of mated female rats also occurred.

Pregnancy: Category C. Naltrexone is embryocidal in rats and rabbits when given in doses ≈ 140 times the human therapeutic dose. There are no adequate and well controlled studies in pregnant women. Use naltrexone in pregnancy only when the potential benefit justifies the risk to the fetus.

Lactation: It is not known if naltrexone is excreted in breast milk. Exercise caution when naltrexone is administered to a nursing mother.

Children: Safety for use in children < 18 years of age has not been established.

Precautions:

Monitoring: A high index of suspicion for drug-related hepatic injury is critical if the occurrence of liver damage induced by naltrexone is to be detected at the earliest possible time. Evaluations, using appropriate batteries of tests to detect liver injury, are recommended at a frequency appropriate to the clinical situation and the dose of naltrexone.

Suicide: The risk of suicide is increased in patients with substance abuse with or without concomitant depression. This risk is not abated by treatment with naltrexone.

Drug Interactions:

Naltrexone Drug Interactions

Precipitant drug	Object drug*		Description
Naltrexone	Opioid-containing products	⬇	Patients taking naltrexone may not benefit from opioid-containing products such as cough/cold and antidiarrheal preparations and opioid analgesics (see Warnings).
Naltrexone	Thioridazine	⬆	Lethargy and somnolence have occurred with concurrent use.

* ⬆ = Object drug increased. ⬇ = Object drug decreased.

Narcotic Antagonists

NALTREXONE HCl

Adverse Reactions:

Alcoholism: Nausea (10%); headache (7%); dizziness, nervousness, fatigue (4%); insomnia, vomiting (3%); anxiety, somnolence (2%). Depression (5% to 7%), suicidal ideation (2%) and attempted suicide (< 1%) have been reported in individuals on naltrexone, placebo and in concurrent control groups undergoing treatment for alcoholism. Although no causal relationship with naltrexone is suspected, be aware that treatment with naltrexone does not reduce the risk of suicide in these patients (see Precautions).

A small fraction of patients may experience an opioid withdrawal-like symptom complex of tearfulness, mild nausea, abdominal cramps, restlessness, bone/joint pain, myalgia and nasal symptoms. This may represent the unmasking of occult opioid use, or it may represent symptoms attributable to naltrexone.

Narcotic addiction:

CNS – Difficulty sleeping, anxiety, nervousness, headache, low energy (> 10%); irritability, increased energy, dizziness (< 10%); depression, paranoia, fatigue, drowsiness, disorientation, restlessness, confusion, hallucinations, nightmares, bad dreams (< 1%).

Cardiovascular – Phlebitis, edema, increased blood pressure, nonspecific ECG changes, palpitations, tachycardia (< 1%).

GI – Abdominal cramps/pain, nausea, vomiting (> 10%); loss of appetite, diarrhea, constipation (< 10%); excess gas, hemorrhoids, ulcer, dry mouth (< 1%); hepatotoxicity (see Warnings).

Respiratory – Nasal congestion, rhinorrhea, sneezing, sore throat, excess mucus or phlegm, sinus trouble, heavy breathing, hoarseness, cough, shortness of breath (< 1%).

Musculoskeletal – Joint/muscle pain (> 10%); painful shoulders/legs/knees, tremors, twitching (< 1%).

GU – Delayed ejaculation, decreased potency (< 10%); increased frequency/ discomfort during urination, increased or decreased sexual interest (< 1%).

Dermatologic – Skin rash (< 10%); itching, oily skin, pruritus, acne, athlete's foot, cold sores, alopecia (< 1%).

Special Senses – Blurred vision, burning/light-sensitive/swollen/aching/strained eyes, "clogged" or aching ears, tinnitus (< 1%).

Lab test abnormalities – Liver test abnormalities, lymphocytosis.

Miscellaneous – Chills, increased thirst (< 10%); increased appetite, weight loss/ gain, yawning, nose bleeds, fever, inguinal pain, swollen glands, "side" pains, head "pounding", cold feet, hot spells (< 1%). Idiopathic thrombocytopenic purpura was reported in one patient but cleared without sequelae after discontinuation of naltrexone and corticosteroid treatment.

Overdosage:

Symptoms: In one study, subjects who received 800 mg/day for up to 1 week showed no evidence of toxicity. In acute toxicity studies in animals, death was due to clonic-tonic convulsions or respiratory failure.

Treatment: Treat symptomatically (see also General Management of Acute Overdosage).

Patient Information:

Patients should wear identification indicating naltrexone use.

If patients attempt self-administration of heroin or any other opiate in small doses, they will perceive no effect. However, self-administration of large doses of heroin or other narcotics can overcome the blockade and may cause coma, serious injury or death.

Naltrexone is well tolerated in the recommended doses, but may cause liver injury when taken in excess or in people who develop liver disease from other causes. If patients develop abdominal pain lasting more than a few days, white bowel movements, dark urine or yellowing of eyes, they should stop taking naltrexone immediately and see their physician as soon as possible.

Narcotic Antagonists

NALTREXONE HCl

Administration and Dosage:

If there is any question of occult opioid dependence, perform a naloxone challenge test. Do not attempt treatment until naloxone challenge is negative.

Alcoholism: A dose of 50 mg once daily is recommended for most patients.

The placebo controlled studies that demonstrated the efficacy of naltrexone as an adjunctive treatment of alcoholism used a dose regimen of 50 mg once daily for up to 12 weeks. Of patients taking naltrexone for alcoholism, 5% to 15% will complain of non-specific side effects, chiefly GI upset. An initial 25 mg dose, splitting the daily dose and adjusting the time of dosing have met with limited success. No dose or pattern of dosing has been shown to be more effective than any other in reducing these complaints for all patients.

Consider naltrexone as only one of many factors determining the success of treatment of alcoholism. Factors associated with a good outcome in the clinical trials with naltrexone were the type, intensity and duration of treatment; appropriate management of comorbid conditions; use of community-based support groups; and good medication compliance. To achieve the best possible treatment outcome, implement appropriate compliance-enhancing techniques for all components of the treatment program, especially medication compliance.

Narcotic dependence: Initiate treatment using the following guidelines:

1. Do not attempt treatment until the patient has remained opioid-free for 7 to 10 days. Verify by analyzing urine for opioids. The patient should not be manifesting withdrawal signs or reporting withdrawal symptoms.

2. Administer a naloxone challenge test (see below). If signs of opioid withdrawal are still observed following challenge, do not treat with naltrexone. The naloxone challenge can be repeated in 24 hours.

3. Initiate treatment carefully, slowly increasing the dose. Administer 25 mg initially; observe patient for 1 hour. If no withdrawal signs occur, give the rest of the daily dose.

Naloxone challenge test: Do not perform in a patient showing clinical signs of opioid withdrawal or in a patient whose urine contains opioids. Administer the challenge test either IV or SC.

IV challenge – Draw 2 ampuls of naloxone, 2 ml (0.8 mg) into a syringe. Inject 0.5 ml (0.2 mg); while the needle is still in the patient's vein, observe for 30 seconds for withdrawal signs or symptoms. If there is no evidence of withdrawal, inject the remaining 1.5 ml (0.6 mg) and observe for an additional 20 minutes for signs and symptoms of withdrawal.

SC challenge – Administer 2 ml (0.8 mg) SC, and observe the patient for signs and symptoms of withdrawal for 45 minutes.

Monitor the patient's vital signs and watch for signs and symptoms of opioid withdrawal. Question the patient carefully. The signs and symptoms of opioid withdrawal include, but are not limited to, the following: Stuffiness or runny nose, tearing, yawning, sweating, tremor, vomiting or piloerection, feeling of temperature change, joint or bone and muscle pain, abdominal cramps, skin crawling.

Interpretation of the challenge – The elicitation of the enumerated signs or symptoms indicates a potential risk for the subject, and naltrexone should not be administered. If there are no signs or symptoms of withdrawal, naltrexone may be administered. If there is any doubt in the observer's mind that the patient is not opioid-free, or is in continuing withdrawal, readminister naloxone as follows:

Confirmatory rechallenge – Inject 4 ml (1.6 mg) of naloxone IV and observe the patient again for signs and symptoms of withdrawal. If none are present, naltrexone may be given. If signs and symptoms of withdrawal are present, delay naltrexone until repeated naloxone challenge indicates the patient is no longer at risk.

Maintenance treatment: Once patient has started naltrexone, 50 mg every 24 hours will produce adequate clinical blockade of the actions of parenterally administered opioids (ie, this dose will block the effects of a 25 mg IV heroin challenge). Flexible dosing may be used. Thus, patients may receive 50 mg every weekday with a 100 mg dose on Saturday, 100 mg every other day, or 150 mg every third day. While the degree of opioid blockade may be somewhat reduced by using higher doses at longer dosing intervals, improved patient compliance may result from dosing every 48 to 72 hours. Several studies have employed the following dosing regimen with success: 100 mg Monday, 100 mg Wednesday and 150 mg Friday.

Rx	**ReVia** (DuPont)	**Tablets:** 50 mg	Sugar. (DuPont NTR). Scored. In 50s.

FLUMAZENIL

Actions:

Pharmacology: Flumazenil is a benzodiazepine receptor antagonist available for IV administration. Flumazenil, an imidazobenzodiazepine derivative, antagonizes the actions of benzodiazepines on the CNS and competitively inhibits the activity at the benzodiazepine recognition site on the GABA/benzodiazepine receptor complex. It is a weak partial agonist in some animal models, but has little or no agonist activity in man. The drug does not antagonize the CNS effects of drugs affecting the GABA-ergic neurons by means other than the benzodiazepine receptor (including ethanol, barbiturates or general anesthetics) and does not reverse the effects of opioids.

Flumazenil antagonizes sedation, impairment of recall, psychomotor impairment and ventilatory depression produced by benzodiazepines in healthy volunteers. The duration and degree of reversal of benzodiazepine effects are related to the dose and plasma concentrations of flumazenil. Generally, doses of ≈ 0.1 to 0.2 mg (corresponding to peak plasma levels of 3 to 6 ng/ml) produce partial antagonism, whereas higher doses of 0.4 to 1 mg (peak plasma levels of 12 to 28 ng/ml) usually produce complete antagonism in patients who have received the usual sedating doses of benzodiazepines. The onset of reversal is usually evident within 1 to 2 minutes after the injection is completed. Within 3 minutes, 80% response will be reached, with the peak effect occurring at 6 to 10 minutes. The duration and degree of reversal are related to the plasma concentration of the sedating benzodiazepine as well as the dose of flumazenil given.

Pharmacokinetics: After IV administration, plasma concentrations of flumazenil follow a 2 compartment open pharmacokinetic model with an initial distribution half-life of 7 to 15 minutes and a terminal half-life of 41 to 79 minutes. Peak concentrations are proportional to dose, with an apparent initial volume of distribution (Vd) of 0.5 L/kg. After redistribution the apparent Vd ranges from 0.77 to 1.6 L/kg. Protein binding is ≈ 50%.

Flumazenil is a highly extracted drug. Clearance of flumazenil occurs primarily by hepatic metabolism and is dependent on hepatic blood flow. In healthy volunteers, total clearance ranges from 0.7 to 1.3 L/hr/kg, with < 1% of the administered dose eliminated unchanged in the urine. The major metabolites of flumazenil identified in urine are in the de-ethylated free acid and its glucuronide conjugate. In preclinical studies there was no evidence of pharmacologic activity exhibited by the de-ethylated free acid. Elimination of drug is essentially complete within 72 hours, with 90% to 95% appearing in urine and 5% to 10% in the feces.

Pharmacokinetic Parameters of Flumazenil Following a 5 min 1 mg Infusion

Parameter	Mean (Range)
Maximum concentration	24 ng/ml (38%, 11-43)
AUC	15 ng • hr/ml (22%, 10-22)
Volume of distribution	1 L/kg (24%, 0.8-1.6)
Clearance	1 L/hr/kg (20%, 0.7-1.4)
Half-life	54 min (21%, 41-79)

The pharmacokinetics of flumazenil are not significantly affected by gender, age, renal failure (creatinine clearance < 10 ml/min) or hemodialysis beginning 1 hour after drug administration. Mean total clearance is decreased to 40% to 60% of normal in patients with moderate liver dysfunction and to 25% of normal in patients with severe liver dysfunction compared with age-matched healthy subjects. This results in a prolongation of the half-life from 0.8 hours in healthy subjects to 1.3 hours in patients with moderate hepatic impairment and 2.4 hours in severely impaired patients.

Clinical trials: Flumazenil has been administered to reverse the effects of benzodiazepines in conscious sedation, general anesthesia and the management of suspected benzodiazepine overdose.

Conscious sedation – In 4 trials in 970 patients who received an average of 30 mg diazepam or 10 mg midazolam for sedation (with or without a narcotic) flumazenil was effective in reversing the sedating and psychomotor effects of the benzodiazepine; however, amnesia was less completely and less consistently reversed. Of patients receiving flumazenil, 78% responded by becoming completely alert. Of those patients, ≈ 50% responded to doses of 0.4 to 0.6 mg, while the other half responded to doses of 0.8 to 1 mg. Reversal of sedation was not associated with any increase in the frequency of inadequate analgesia or increase in narcotic demand in these studies. While most patients remained alert throughout the 3 hour post-procedure observation period, resedation occurred in 3% to 9% of the patients, and was most common in patients who had received high doses of benzodiazepines (see Precautions).

General anesthesia – In 4 trials, 644 patients received midazolam as an induction or maintenance agent in both balanced and inhalational anesthesia. Flumazenil was effective in reversing sedation and restoring psychomotor function, but did not completely restore memory as tested by picture recall. Flumazenil was not as effective in reversal of sedation in patients who had received multiple anesthetics in addition to benzodiazepines. Of patients sedated with midazolam, 81% responded to flumazenil by becoming completely alert or just slightly drowsy. Of those patients, 36% responded to doses of 0.4 to 0.6 mg, while 64% responded to doses of 0.8 to 1 mg.

Resedation in patients who responded to flumazenil occurred in 10% to 15% and was more common with larger doses of midazolam (> 20 mg), long procedures (> 60 minutes) and use of neuromuscular blocking agents (see Precautions).

Management of suspected benzodiazepine overdose – In 2 trials, 497 patients were presumed to have taken an overdose of a benzodiazepine, either alone or in combination with a variety of other agents. In these trials, 299 patients were proven to have taken a benzodiazepine as part of the overdose, and 80% of the 148 who received flumazenil responded by an improvement in level of consciousness. Of the patients who responded to flumazenil, 75% responded to a total dose of 1 to 3 mg. Reversal of sedation was associated with an increased frequency of symptoms of CNS excitation. Of the patients treated with flumazenil, 1% to 3% were treated for agitation or anxiety.

Indications:

Reversal of benzodiazepine sedation: For the complete or partial reversal of the sedative effects of benzodiazepines in cases where general anesthesia has been induced or maintained with benzodiazepines, where sedation has been produced with benzodiazepines for diagnostic and therapeutic procedures, and for the management of benzodiazepine overdose.

Contraindications:

Hypersensitivity to flumazenil or to benzodiazepines; benzodiazepine use for control of a potentially life-threatening condition (eg, control of intracranial pressure or status epilepticus); signs of serious cyclic antidepressant overdose (see Warnings).

Warnings:

Seizures: The use of flumazenil has been associated with the occurrence of seizures. These are most frequent in patients who have been on benzodiazepines for long-term sedation or in overdose cases where patients are showing signs of serious cyclic antidepressant overdose. Individualize the dosage of flumazenil and be prepared to manage seizures.

Seizure risk: The reversal of benzodiazepine effects may be associated with the onset of seizures in certain high-risk populations. Possible risk factors for seizures include: Concurrent major sedative-hypnotic drug withdrawal; recent therapy with repeated doses of parenteral benzodiazepines; myoclonic jerking or seizure activity prior to flumazenil administration in overdose cases; concurrent cyclic antidepressant poisoning.

Flumazenil is not recommended in cases of serious cyclic antidepressant poisoning, as manifested by motor abnormalities (twitching, rigidity, focal seizure), dysrhythmia (wide QRS, ventricular dysrhythmia, heart block), anticholinergic signs (mydriasis, dry mucosa, hypoperistalsis) and cardiovascular collapse at presentation. In such cases, withhold flumazenil and allow the patient to remain sedated (with ventilatory and circulatory support as needed) until the signs of antidepressant toxicity have subsided. Treatment with flumazenil has no known benefit to the seriously ill mixed-overdose patient other than reversing sedation and should not be used in cases where seizures (from any cause) are likely.

Most convulsions associated with flumazenil administration require treatment and have been successfully managed with benzodiazepines, phenytoin or barbiturates. Because of the presence of flumazenil, higher than usual doses of benzodiazepines may be required.

Hypoventilation: Monitor patients who have received flumazenil for the reversal of benzodiazepine effects (after conscious sedation or general anesthesia) for resedation, respiratory depression or other residual benzodiazepine effects for an appropriate period (up to 120 minutes) based on the dose and duration of effect of the benzodiazepine employed, because flumazenil has not been established as an effective treatment for hypoventilation due to benzodiazepine administration. The availability of flumazenil does not diminish the need for prompt detection of hypoventilation and the ability to effectively intervene by establishing an airway and assisting ventilation.

Flumazenil may not fully reverse postoperative airway problems or ventilatory insufficiency induced by benzodiazepines. In addition, even if flumazenil is initially effective, such problems may recur because the effects of flumazenil wear off before the effects of many benzodiazepines. Always monitor overdose cases for resedation until the patients are stable and resedation is unlikely.

Hepatic function impairment: The clearance of flumazenil is reduced to 40% to 60% of normal in patients with mild to moderate hepatic disease and to 25% of normal in patients with severe hepatic dysfunction (see Pharmacokinetics). While the dose of flumazenil used for initial reversal of benzodiazepine effects is not affected, reduce the size and frequency of repeat doses of the drug in liver disease.

Elderly: The pharmacokinetics of flumazenil have been studied in the elderly and are not significantly different from younger patients. Several studies in patients > 65 years of age and one study in patients > 80 years of age suggest that while the doses of benzodiazepines used to induce sedation should be reduced, ordinary doses of flumazenil may be used for reversal.

Pregnancy: Category C. In rabbits, embryocidal effects (as evidenced by increased pre- and post-implantation losses) were observed at 50 mg/kg (200 times the human exposure from a maximum recommended IV dose of 5 mg). In rats at oral dosages of 5, 25 and 125 mg/kg/day, pup survival was decreased during the lactating period, pup liver weight at weaning was increased for the high-dose group (125 mg/kg/day) and incisor eruption and ear opening in the offspring were delayed; the delay in ear opening was associated with a delay in the appearance of the auditory startle response. There are no adequate and well controlled studies in pregnant women. Use during pregnancy only if potential benefits justify potential risks to the fetus.

Labor and delivery – The use of flumazenil to reverse the effects of benzodiazepines used during labor and delivery is not recommended because the effects of the drug in the newborn are unknown.

Lactation: Exercise caution when deciding to administer flumazenil to a nursing woman because it is not known whether flumazenil is excreted in breast milk.

Children: Flumazenil is not recommended for use in children (either for reversal of sedation, management of overdose or resuscitation of the newborn); no clinical studies have been performed to determine the risks, benefits and dosage to be used.

Precautions:

Monitoring: Flumazenil may be expected to improve the alertness of patients recovering from a procedure involving sedation or anesthesia with benzodiazepines, but should not be substituted for an adequate period of post-procedure monitoring. The availability of flumazenil does not reduce the risks associated with the use of large doses of benzodiazepine for sedation. Monitor patients for resedation, respiratory depression (see Warnings) or other persistent or recurrent agonist effects for an adequate period of time after administration of flumazenil.

Return of sedation: Resedation is least likely in cases where flumazenil is administered to reverse a low dose of a short-acting benzodiazepine (< 10 mg midazolam). It is most likely in cases where a large single or cumulative dose of a benzodiazepine has been given in the course of a long procedure along with neuromuscular blocking agents and multiple anesthetic agents.

Profound resedation was observed in 1% to 3% of patients in the clinical studies. In clinical situations where resedation must be prevented, physicians may wish to repeat the initial dose (up to 1 mg given at 0.2 mg/min) at 30 minutes and possibly again at 60 minutes. This dosage schedule, although not studied in clinical trials, was effective in preventing resedation in healthy volunteers.

Intensive Care Unit (ICU): Use with caution in the ICU because of the increased risk of unrecognized benzodiazepine dependence in such settings. Flumazenil may produce convulsions in patients physically dependent on benzodiazepines (see Administration and Dosage and Warnings).

The use of flumazenil to diagnose benzodiazepine-induced sedation in the ICU is not recommended due to the risk of adverse events as described above. In addition, the prognostic significance of a patient's failure to respond to flumazenil in cases confounded by metabolic disorder, traumatic injury, drugs other than benzodiazepines or any other reasons not associated with benzodiazepine receptor occupancy is not known.

Overdose situations: Flumazenil is intended as an adjunct to, not a substitute for, proper management of airway, assisted breathing, circulatory access and support, internal decontamination by lavage and charcoal, and adequate clinical evaluation. Institute necessary measures to secure airway, ventilation and IV access prior to administering flumazenil. Upon arousal patients may try to withdraw endotracheal tubes or IV lines as the result of confusion and agitation following awakening.

Head injury: Use with caution in patients with head injury as flumazenil may be capable of precipitating convulsions or altering cerebral blood flow in patients receiving benzodiazepines.

Neuromuscular blocking agents: Do not use flumazenil until the effects of neuromuscular blockade have been fully reversed.

Psychiatric patients: Flumazenil may provoke panic attacks in patients with a history of panic disorder.

Drug and alcohol dependent patients: Use with caution in patients with alcoholism and other drug dependencies due to the increased frequency of benzodiazepine tolerance and dependence observed in these patient populations. Flumazenil is not recommended either as a treatment for benzodiazepine dependence or for the management of protracted benzodiazepine abstinence syndromes, as such use has not been studied.

The administration of flumazenil can precipitate benzodiazepine withdrawal in humans. This has been seen in healthy volunteers treated with therapeutic doses of oral lorazepam for up to 2 weeks who exhibited effects such as hot flushes, agitation and tremor when treated with cumulative doses of up to 3 mg flumazenil.

Similar adverse experiences suggestive of flumazenil precipitation of benzodiazepine withdrawal have occurred in some patients in clinical trials. Such patients had a short-lived syndrome characterized by dizziness, mild confusion, emotional lability, agitation (with signs and symptoms of anxiety) and mild sensory distortions. This response was dose-related, most common at doses > 1 mg, rarely required treatment other than reassurance and was usually short-lived. When required (5 to 10 cases), these patients were successfully treated with usual doses of a barbiturate, a benzodiazepine or other sedative drug.

Assume that flumazenil administration may trigger dose-dependent withdrawal syndromes in patients with established physical dependence on benzodiazepines and may complicate the management of withdrawal syndromes for alcohol, barbiturates and cross-tolerant sedatives.

Tolerance to benzodiazepines: Flumazenil may cause benzodiazepine withdrawal symptoms in individuals who have been taking benzodiazepines long enough to have some degree of tolerance. Patients who had been taking benzodiazepines prior to entry into the flumazenil trials who were given flumazenil in doses > 1 mg experienced withdrawal-like events 2 to 5 times more frequently than patients who received < 1 mg.

In patients who may have tolerance to benzodiazepines, as indicated by clinical history or by the need for larger than usual doses of benzodiazepines, slower titration rates of 0.1 mg/min and lower total doses may help reduce the frequency of emergent confusion and agitation. In such cases, take special care to monitor the patients for resedation because of the lower doses of flumazenil used.

Pain on injection: To minimize the likelihood of pain or inflammation at the injection site, administer flumazenil through a freely flowing IV infusion into a large vein. Local irritation may occur following extravasation into perivascular tissues.

Respiratory disease: Appropriate ventilatory support is the primary treatment of patients with serious lung disease who experience serious respiratory depression due to benzodiazepines rather than the administration of flumazenil. Flumazenil is capable of partially reversing benzodiazepine-induced alterations in ventilatory drive in healthy volunteers, but is not clinically effective.

Ambulatory patients: Effects may wear off before a long-acting benzodiazepine is completely cleared from the body. In general, if a patient shows no signs of sedation within 2 hours after a 1 mg dose, serious resedation at a later time is unlikely. Provide an adequate observation period for any patient in whom either long-acting benzodiazepines (eg, diazepam) or large doses of short-acting benzodiazepines (eg, > 10 mg midazolam) have been used (see Administration and Dosage).

Because of the increased risk of adverse reactions in patients who have been taking benzodiazepines on a regular basis, it is particularly important to carefully query about benzodiazepine, alcohol and sedative use as part of the history prior to any procedure in which the use of flumazenil is planned (see Drug and Alcohol Dependent Patients).

Drug abuse and dependence: Flumazenil acts as a benzodiazepine antagonist, blocks benzodiazepine effects in animals and man, antagonizes benzodiazepine reinforcement in animals, produces dysphoria in healthy subjects and has had no reported abuse in foreign marketing. It has a benzodiazepine-like structure, but does not act as a benzodiazepine agonist in man and is not a controlled substance.

Drug Interactions:

Mixed drug overdosage: Particular caution is necessary when using flumazenil in cases of mixed drug overdosage; toxic effects (eg, convulsions, cardiac dysrhythmias) of other drugs taken in overdose (especially cyclic antidepressants) may emerge with reversal of the benzodiazepine effect by flumazenil (see Warnings).

Benzodiazepine pharmacokinetics are unaltered in the presence of flumazenil.

Drug/Food interactions: Ingestion of food during an IV infusion of flumazenil results in a 50% increase in flumazenil clearance, most likely due to the increased hepatic blood flow that accompanies a meal.

Adverse Reactions:

Serious adverse reactions: Deaths have occurred in patients who received flumazenil in a variety of clinical settings. The majority of deaths occurred in patients with serious underlying disease or in patients who had ingested large amounts of non-benzodiazepine drugs (usually cyclic antidepressants) as part of an overdose.

Serious adverse events have occurred in all clinical settings, and convulsions are the most common serious adverse event reported. Flumazenil administration has been associated with the onset of convulsions in patients who are relying on benzodiazepine effects to control seizures, are physically dependent on benzodiazepines or who have ingested large doses of other drugs (see Warnings).

Two of the 446 patients who received flumazenil in controlled clinical trials for the management of a benzodiazepine overdosage had cardiac dysrhythmias (1 ventricular tachycardia, 1 junctional tachycardia).

Body as a whole: Headache, injection site pain, increased sweating (3% to 9%); injection site reaction (thrombophlebitis, skin abnormality, rash), fatigue (asthenia, malaise) (1% to 3%); rigors, shivering (< 1%).

Cardiovascular: Cutaneous vasodilation (sweating, flushing, hot flushes) (1% to 3%); arrhythmia (atrial, nodal, ventricular extrasystoles), bradycardia, tachycardia, hypertension, chest pain (< 1%).

GI: Nausea, vomiting (11%); hiccups (< 1%).

CNS: Dizziness (vertigo, ataxia) (10%); agitation (anxiety, nervousness), dry mouth, tremors, palpitations, insomnia, dyspnea, hyperventilation (3% to 9%); emotional lability (abnormal crying, depersonalization, euphoria, increased tears, depression, dysphoria, paranoia) (1% to 3%); confusion (difficulty concentrating, delirium), convulsions (see Warnings), somnolence (stupor), speech disorder (dysphonia, thick tongue) (< 1%).

Special senses: Abnormal vision (visual field defect, diplopia), blurred vision (3% to 9%); paresthesia (sensation abnormal, hypoesthesia) (1% to 3%); abnormal hearing (transient hearing impairment, hyperacusis, tinnitus) (< 1%).

Overdosage:

Large IV doses of flumazenil, when administered to healthy volunteers in the absence of a benzodiazepine agonist, produced no serious adverse reactions. In clinical studies, most adverse reactions to flumazenil were an extension of the pharmacologic effects of the drug in reversing benzodiazepine effects.

Reversal with an excessively high dose of flumazenil may produce anxiety, agitation, increased muscle tone, hyperesthesia and possibly convulsions. Convulsions have been treated with barbiturates, benzodiazepines and phenytoin, generally with prompt resolution of the seizures (see Warnings).

Patient Information:

Flumazenil does not consistently reverse amnesia. Patients cannot be expected to remember information told to them in the post-procedure period; reinforce instructions given to patients in writing or give to a responsible family member. Discuss with patients, both before surgery and at discharge, that although they may feel alert at the time of discharge, the effects of the benzodiazepine may recur. Instruct the patient, preferably in writing, that their memory and judgment may be impaired and specifically advise patients:

1. Not to engage in any activities requiring complete alertness, and not to operate hazardous machinery or a motor vehicle until at least 18 to 24 hours after discharge, and it is certain no residual sedative effects of the benzodiazepine remain.
2. Not to take any alcohol or non-prescription drugs for 18 to 24 hours after flumazenil administration or if the effects of the benzodiazepine persist.

Administration and Dosage:

Approved by the FDA in December 1991.

For IV use only. To minimize the likelihood of pain at the injection site, administer flumazenil through a freely running IV infusion into a large vein (see Precautions).

Individualization of dosage: The serious adverse effects of flumazenil are related to the reversal of benzodiazepine effects. Using more than the minimally effective dose of flumazenil is tolerated by most patients but may complicate the management of patients who are physically dependent on benzodiazepines or patients who are depending on benzodiazepines for therapeutic effect (such as suppression of seizures in cyclic antidepressant overdose).

In high-risk patients, it is important to administer the smallest amount of flumazenil that is effective. The 1 minute wait between individual doses in the dose-titration recommended for general clinical populations may be too short for high-risk patients because it takes 6 to 10 minutes for any single dose of flumazenil to reach full effects. Slow the rate of administration of flumazenil administered to high-risk patients.

Reversal of conscious sedation or in general anesthesia: For the reversal of the sedative effects of benzodiazepines administered for conscious sedation or general anesthesia, the recommended initial dose is 0.2 mg (2 ml) administered IV over 15 seconds. If the desired level of consciousness is not obtained after waiting an additional 45 seconds, a further dose of 0.2 mg (2 ml) can be injected and repeated at 60 second intervals where necessary (up to a maximum of 4 additional times) to a maximum total dose of 1 mg (10 ml). Individualize the dose based on the patient's response, with most patients responding to doses of 0.6 to 1 mg.

The major risk will be resedation because the duration of effect of a long-acting (or large dose of a short-acting) benzodiazepine may exceed that of flumazenil. In the event of resedation, repeated doses may be administered at 20 minute intervals as needed. For repeat treatment, administer ≤ 1 mg (given as 0.2 mg/min) at any one time, and give ≤ 3 mg in any 1 hour.

It is recommended that flumazenil be administered as the series of small injections described (not as a single bolus injection) to allow the practitioner to control the reversal of sedation to the approximate endpoint desired and to minimize the possibility of adverse effects.

Suspected benzodiazepine overdose: For initial management of a known or suspected benzodiazepine overdose, the recommended initial dose is 0.2 mg (2 ml) administered IV over 30 seconds. If the desired level of consciousness is not obtained after waiting 30 seconds, a further dose of 0.3 mg (3 ml) can be administered over another 30 seconds. Further doses of 0.5 mg (5 ml) can be administered over 30 seconds at 1 minute intervals up to a cumulative dose of 3 mg.

The risk of confusion, agitation, emotional lability and perceptual distortion with the doses recommended in patients with benzodiazepine overdose (3 to 5 mg administered as 0.5 mg/min) may be greater than that expected with lower doses and slower administration. The recommended doses represent a compromise between a desirable slow awakening and the need for prompt response and a persistent effect in the overdose situation. If circumstances permit, the physician may elect to use the 0.2 mg/min titration rate to slowly awaken the patient over 5 to 10 minutes, which may help to reduce signs and symptoms on emergence.

Do not rush the administration of flumazenil. Patients should have a secure airway and IV access before administration of the drug and be awakened gradually (see Precautions).

Most patients with benzodiazepine overdose will respond to a cumulative dose of 1 to 3 mg, and doses > 3 mg do not reliably produce additional effects. On rare occasions, patients with a partial response at 3 mg may require additional titration up to a total dose of 5 mg (administered slowly in the same manner).

If a patient has not responded 5 minutes after receiving a cumulative dose of 5 mg, the major cause of sedation is likely not to be due to benzodiazepines, and additional flumazenil is likely to have no effect.

In the event of resedation, repeated doses may be given at 20 minute intervals if needed. For repeat treatment, give ≤ 1 mg (given as 0.5 mg/min) at any one time and give ≤ 3 mg in any 1 hour.

FLUMAZENIL

Admixture compatibility: Flumazenil is compatible with 5% Dextrose in Water, Lactated Ringer's and normal saline solutions. If flumazenil is drawn into a syringe or mixed with any of these solutions, it should be discarded after 24 hours. For optimum sterility, flumazenil should remain in the vial until just before use.

Flumazenil 20 mcg/ml, in 5% Dextrose Injection, was physically compatible and chemically stable for 24 hours at 23° C (73° F) with aminophylline 2 mg/ml, dobutamine 2 mg/ml, cimetidine 2.4 mg/ml, famotidine 0.08 mg/ml, ranitidine 0.3 mg/ml, heparin sodium 50 units/ml, lidocaine HCl 4 mg/ml or procainamide HCl 4 mg/ml. Flumazenil 20 mcg/ml, in 5% Dextrose Injection, was physically compatible and chemically stable for 12 hours at 23° C (73° F) with dopamine HCl 3.2 mg/ml.

Rx	**Romazicon** (Hoffman-La Roche)	**Injection:** 0.1 mg/ml	With parabens and EDTA. In 5 and 10 ml vials.

PHYSOSTIGMINE SALICYLATE

Actions:

Pharmacology: The action of acetylcholine is transient because of hydrolysis by acetylcholinesterase. Physostigmine, a reversible anticholinesterase drug, increases the concentration of acetylcholine at the sites of cholinergic transmission and prolongs and exaggerates the effect of acetylcholine.

Physostigmine reverses these central and peripheral anticholinergic effects –

Central toxic effects: Anxiety, delirium, disorientation, hallucinations, hyperactivity and seizures. Severe poisoning due to anticholinergics may produce coma, medullary paralysis and death.

Peripheral toxic effects: Tachycardia, hyperpyrexia, mydriasis, vasodilation, urinary retention, decreased GI motility, decreased secretion in salivary and sweat glands, loss of secretions in the pharynx, bronchi and nasal passages.

Pharmacokinetics: Physostigmine, a tertiary amine, is readily absorbed and freely crosses the blood-brain barrier following IM or IV administration. Peak effects are seen within minutes and persist for 45 to 60 minutes following IV administration if the patient has not suffered anoxia or other trauma. Physostigmine is rapidly hydrolyzed by cholinesterase. Plasma half-life is ≈ 1 to 2 hours. Renal impairment does NOT require dosage alteration.

Indications:

Anticholinergic toxicity: To reverse toxic CNS effects caused by anticholinergic drugs (including tricyclic antidepressants).

Unlabeled uses: Physostigmine has been used to treat delirium tremens and Alzheimer's disease. It may also antagonize diazepam's CNS-depressant effects.

Contraindications:

Asthma; gangrene; diabetes; cardiovascular disease; GI or GU tract obstruction; any vagotonic state; patients receiving choline esters or depolarizing neuromuscular blocking agents (decamethonium, succinylcholine).

Warnings:

Discontinue drug if symptoms of excessive salivation or emesis, frequent urination or diarrhea occur. If excessive sweating or nausea occurs, reduce dosage.

Administration rate: Rapid administration can cause bradycardia, hypersalivation leading to respiratory difficulties and seizures (see Administration and Dosage).

Hypersensitivity: Because of the possibility of hypersensitivity, atropine sulfate should be available as an antagonist and antidote for physostigmine.

Pregnancy: Category C. Transient muscular weakness noted in neonates whose mothers were treated with other cholinesterase inhibitors for myasthenia gravis. Use only if clearly needed and potential benefits outweigh hazards to the fetus.

Lactation: Safety for use has not been established.

Children: Reserve for life-threatening situations only.

Precautions:

Benzyl alcohol, contained in this product as a preservative, has been associated with a fatal "gasping syndrome" in premature infants.

Sulfite sensitivity: This product contains sulfites that may cause allergic-type reactions (including anaphylactic symptoms and life-threatening or less severe asthmatic episodes) in certain susceptible people. The overall prevalence of sulfite sensitivity in the general population is unknown and probably low. It is seen more frequently in asthmatic or atopic nonasthmatic people.

Adverse Reactions:

Nausea, vomiting, salivation; bradycardia and convulsions (see Warnings).

Overdosage:

Can cause cholinergic crisis. Atropine sulfate is an appropriate antidote.

Administration and Dosage:

Post-anesthesia: 0.5 to 1 mg IM or IV. Administer IV slowly, ≤ 1 mg/min. Repeat at 10 to 30 minute intervals if desired response is not obtained.

Anticholinergic toxicity: 2 mg IM or IV. Administer IV slowly, ≤ 1 mg/min. Repeat if life-threatening signs such as arrhythmia, convulsions or coma occur.

Pediatric: Recommended dosage is 0.02 mg/kg IM or by slow IV injection, ≤ 0.5 mg/min. If necessary, repeat at 5 to 10 minute intervals until a therapeutic effect or a maximum dose of 2 mg is attained.

Rx	**Antilirium** (Forest)	**Injection:** 1 mg/ml	With 2% benzyl alcohol and 0.1% sodium bisulfite. In 2 ml ampules.

PRALIDOXIME CHLORIDE (2-PAM)

Actions:

Pharmacology: Pralidoxime reactivates cholinesterase (mainly outside the CNS) inactivated by phosphorylation due to an organophosphate pesticide or related compound. Destruction of accumulated acetylcholine can then proceed, allowing neuromuscular junctions to function normally. It also slows the "aging" of phosphorylated cholinesterase to a nonreactive form and detoxifies certain organophosphates by direct chemical reaction. The drug's most critical effect is relieving respiratory muscle paralysis. Because pralidoxime is less effective in relieving depression of the respiratory center, concomitant atropine is required to block the effect of accumulated acetylcholine at this site. Pralidoxime relieves muscarinic signs and symptoms (salivation, bronchospasm), but this is relatively unimportant because atropine is adequate for this purpose. Pralidoxime also enhances the effect of atropine.

Pralidoxime does not antagonize the effects on the neuromuscular junction of the carbamate anticholinesterases, neostigmine, pyridostigmine and ambenonium used in treatment of myasthenia gravis. It is relatively ineffective in the treatment of poisoning by carbamate pesticides.

Pharmacokinetics: Pralidoxime is slowly absorbed from the GI tract; blood concentrations are more rapidly achieved with IM or IV use. It is distributed throughout extracellular water. It is not bound to plasma protein, and it does not readily pass into CNS. Pralidoxime is rapidly excreted in urine, partly unchanged and partly as a metabolite produced by the liver. Average half-life is 74 to 77 minutes. It is relatively short-acting; repeated doses may be needed, especially when poison absorption continues. Renal dysfunction will increase drug blood levels.

Indications:

Organophosphate poisoning: Antidote in poisoning due to organophosphate pesticides and chemicals with anticholinesterase activity (eg, azodrin, diazinon, dichlorvos, dioxathion, disulfoton, dursban, echothiophate iodide, endothion, EPN, fenthion, formothion, guthion, isoflurophate, malathion, Metasystox I and fenthion, methyldemeton, methyl parathion, mevinphos, parathion, parathion and mevinphos, phosdrin, phosphamidon, sarin, Systox, TEPP).

Anticholinesterase drug overdosage: Control of overdosage by anticholinesterase drugs used to treat myasthenia gravis.

Adjunct to atropine in poisoning by nerve agents having anticholinesterase activity.

Contraindications:

Hypersensitivity to any component of the product.

Warnings:

Carbamate pesticides: Until further information is available, no recommendation is made for use in intoxication by pesticides of the carbamate class.

Dermal exposure: If dermal exposure has occurred, remove clothing and thoroughly wash hair and skin with sodium bicarbonate or alcohol as soon as possible.

Convulsions: If convulsions interfere with respiration, carefully give 2.5% IV sodium thiopental or diazepam.

Renal function impairment: A decrease in renal function will result in increased drug blood levels; reduce dosage in the presence of renal insufficiency.

Pregnancy: Category C. It is not known whether pralidoxime can cause fetal harm when administered to a pregnant woman or can affect reproduction capacity. Give to a pregnant woman only if clearly needed.

Lactation: It is not known whether this drug is excreted in breast milk. Exercise caution when pralidoxime is administered to a nursing woman.

Children: Safety and efficacy in children have not been established.

Precautions:

Monitoring: Institute treatment of organophosphate poisoning without waiting for laboratory test results. Red blood cell, plasma cholinesterase and urinary paranitrophenol measurements (for parathion exposure) may help confirm diagnosis and follow course of the illness. A reduction in red blood cell cholinesterase concentration to < 50% of normal has been seen only with organophosphate ester poisoning.

Benzyl alcohol, contained in pralidoxime chloride auto-injector as a preservative, has been associated with a fatal "gasping syndrome" in premature infants.

Pralidoxime is generally well tolerated; however, the desperate condition of the organophosphate-poisoned patient will mask minor signs and symptoms noted in healthy subjects.

PRALIDOXIME CHLORIDE (2-PAM)

Injection rate: Administer slowly by IV infusion, because tachycardia, laryngospasm and muscle rigidity have occurred with a too rapid rate of injection. (See Administration and Dosage.)

Auto-injector users must understand the indications and use. Review symptoms of poisoning and operation instructions of the mechanism.

Myasthenia gravis: Use with caution in treating organophosphate overdosage in cases of myasthenia gravis, because it may precipitate a myasthenic crisis.

Drug Interactions:

Barbiturates are potentiated by the anticholinesterases; therefore, use with caution in the treatment of convulsions.

Adverse Reactions:

Mild to moderate pain at the injection site 40 to 60 minutes after IM injection; AST and ALT elevations, which return to normal in 2 weeks; transient elevations in CPK; dizziness; blurred vision; diplopia and impaired accommodation; headache; drowsiness; nausea; tachycardia; increased systolic and diastolic blood pressure; hyperventilation; muscular weakness.

When atropine and pralidoxime are used together, atropinization may occur earlier than expected, especially if the total dose of atropine has been large and the administration of pralidoxime has been delayed. Excitement and manic behavior immediately following recovery of consciousness have been reported. However, similar behavior has occurred in cases of organophosphate poisoning that were not treated with pralidoxime.

Overdosage:

Symptoms: Dizziness, headache, blurred vision, diplopia, impaired accommodation, nausea, slight tachycardia. In therapy, it has been difficult to differentiate side effects due to the drug from those due to the poison.

Treatment: Administer artificial respiration and other supportive therapy as needed.

Administration and Dosage:

Organophosphate poisoning: Initial measures include removal of secretions, maintenance of a patent airway and artificial ventilation. Give atropine 2 to 4 mg IV. Repeat every 5 to 10 minutes until signs of atropine toxicity appear. Maintain atropinization for at least 48 hours. Begin pralidoxime concomitantly with atropine.

Adults – Initial dose of 1 to 2 g IV, preferably as a 15 to 30 minute infusion in 100 ml of saline. If this is not practical or if pulmonary edema is present, give slowly IV as a 5% solution in water over ≥ 5 minutes. After about an hour, give a second dose of 1 to 2 g if muscle weakness is not relieved. Give additional doses cautiously if muscle weakness persists. If IV use is not feasible, give IM or SC.

Children – 20 to 40 mg/kg/dose, given as above.

Treatment is most effective if begun immediately after poisoning. Usually, the drug is ineffective if first administered > 36 to 48 hours after exposure. However, it is indicated in severe poisoning as patients may still respond. In severe cases, especially after ingestion of the poison, monitor the effect of therapy by ECG because of possible heart block due to the anticholinesterase. Where the poison has been ingested, consider the likelihood of continuing absorption from the lower bowel; additional doses of pralidoxime may be needed every 3 to 8 hours or continued for several days.

Anticholinesterase overdosage (eg, neostigmine, pyridostigmine and ambenonium used in the treatment of myasthenia gravis): 1 to 2 g IV followed by increments of 250 mg every 5 minutes.

Exposure to nerve agents: Administer atropine and pralidoxime as soon as possible after exposure. Depending on the severity of symptoms, immediately administer 1 atropine-containing auto-injector, followed by 1 pralidoxime-containing auto-injector. Atropine must be given first until its effects become apparent; then administer pralidoxime. If nerve agent symptoms are present after 15 minutes, repeat injections. If symptoms exist after an additional 15 minutes, repeat injections. If symptoms remain after the third set of injections, seek medical help.

Rx	**Protopam Chloride** (Wyeth-Ayerst)	**Injection (cake):** 1 g	Hospital package containing six 20 ml vials without diluent or syringe.
Rx	**Pralidoxime Chloride**[1] (Survival Technology)	**Injection:** 600 mg	With benzyl alcohol and aminoacetic acid. One 2 ml auto-injector.

[1] For military and civilian emergency responders use only.

DIGOXIN IMMUNE FAB (Ovine)

Actions:

Pharmacology: Digoxin immune fab (ovine) are antigen binding fragments (fab) derived from specific antidigoxin antibodies produced in sheep. Production involves conjugation of digoxin as a hapten to human albumin. Sheep are immunized with this material to produce antibodies specific for the digoxin molecule. The antibody is papain digested, and digoxin-specific fab fragments are isolated and purified.

Ingestion of > 10 mg digoxin by healthy adults, 4 mg by healthy children or steady-state serum concentrations > 10 ng/ml often results in cardiac arrest. Digitalis-induced progressive elevation of serum potassium concentration also suggests imminent cardiac arrest. If the potassium concentration exceeds 5 mEq/L in the setting of severe digitalis intoxication, digoxin fab therapy is indicated.

Pharmacokinetics: After IV injection in subjects with normal renal function, the half-life appears to be 15 to 20 hours. Studies in animals indicate that these antibody fragments have a large volume of distribution in the extracellular space. Improvement in signs and symptoms of digitalis intoxication begins in < 30 minutes.

Fab fragments bind molecules of digoxin, making them unavailable for binding at their site of action. The fab fragment-digoxin complex accumulates in the blood and is excreted by the kidneys.

Indications:

Digitalis intoxication: Treatment of potentially life-threatening digoxin intoxication. It has also been used successfully to treat life-threatening digitoxin overdose.

Manifestations of life-threatening toxicity include severe arrhythmias (eg, ventricular tachycardia or ventricular fibrillation) or progressive bradyarrhythmias (eg, severe sinus bradycardia or second- or third-degree heart block not responsive to atropine).

Contraindications:

None known.

Warnings:

Hypersensitivity: Allergic reactions have occurred rarely, but consider the possibility of anaphylactic, hypersensitivity or febrile reactions. If an anaphylactoid reaction occurs, discontinue the drug infusion and initiate appropriate therapy. Refer to Management of Acute Hypersensitivity Reactions.

Patients allergic to ovine proteins are at risk, as are individuals who have previously received antibodies or fab fragments raised in sheep or who are allergic to antibiotics.

Skin testing for allergy was performed during the clinical investigation of this agent. Only one patient developed erythema at the site of skin testing. The patient had no adverse reaction to systemic treatment. Allergy testing is not routinely required before treatment of life-threatening digitalis toxicity.

Skin testing may be appropriate for high risk individuals, especially patients with known allergy to sheep proteins or those previously treated with digoxin immune fab. The intradermal skin test can be performed by: 1) Diluting 0.1 ml of reconstituted drug (9.5 mg/ml) in 9.9 ml sterile isotonic saline; 2) injecting 0.1 ml of the 1:100 dilution (9.5 mcg) intradermally and observing for an urticarial wheal surrounded by a zone of erythema. Read the test at 20 minutes.

The scratch test procedure is performed by placing 1 drop of a 1:100 dilution on the skin and making a ¼-inch scratch through the drop with a needle. The area is inspected at 20 minutes for an urticarial wheal surrounded by erythema.

If skin testing causes a systemic reaction, apply a tourniquet above the site of testing and treat anaphylaxis. Avoid further administration of the drug unless its use is absolutely essential; in this case, pretreat the patient with corticosteroids and diphenhydramine and make preparations for treating anaphylaxis.

Renal function impairment: The elimination half-life in renal failure has not been clearly defined. Several patients with mild to moderate renal dysfunction have been successfully treated. There is no evidence to suggest any difference between these patients and patients with normal renal function, but excretion of the fab fragment-digoxin complex from the body is probably delayed. In patients who are functionally anephric, anticipate failure to clear the fab fragment-digoxin complex from the blood by glomerular filtration and renal excretion; the reticuloendothelial system might eliminate the complex. Whether this would lead to detoxification or to reintoxication by release of newly unbound digoxin into the blood is not known. Monitor such patients for a prolonged period for possible recurrence of digitalis toxicity.

Pregnancy: Category C. It is not known whether this agent can cause fetal harm or affect reproduction capacity. Use only if clearly needed and if the potential benefits outweigh the potential hazards to the fetus.

Lactation: It is not known whether this drug is excreted in breast milk. Exercise caution when administering to a nursing mother.

DIGOXIN IMMUNE FAB (Ovine)

Children: This agent has been used successfully in infants with no apparent adverse sequelae. Digoxin immune fab is best used when ≥ 0.3 mg of digoxin/kg has been ingested, there is underlying heart disease or serum digoxin concentrations are ≥ 6.4 nmol/L. Use in infants only if the potential benefits outweigh the hazards.

Precautions:

Monitoring: Obtain serum concentrations before administration. These measurements may be difficult to interpret if drawn soon after the last digitalis dose, because at least 6 to 8 hours are required for equilibration of digoxin between serum and tissue. Closely monitor the patient's temperature, blood pressure, ECG and potassium concentration during and after drug administration. The total serum digoxin concentration may rise precipitously following administration, but this will be almost entirely bound to the fab fragment. Fab fragments will interfere with digitalis immunoassay measurements. The standard serum digoxin concentration measurement can be clinically misleading until the fab fragment is eliminated from the body, which may require several days. Patients with impaired renal function may require at least a week before obtaining reliable results.

Potassium – Severe digitalis intoxication can cause life-threatening elevation in serum potassium concentration by shifting potassium from inside to outside the cell. This can lead to increased renal excretion of potassium. These patients may have hyperkalemia with a total body deficit of potassium. When the effect of digitalis is reversed, potassium shifts back inside the cell with a resulting decline in serum potassium concentration. Hypokalemia may develop rapidly. Monitor serum potassium concentration repeatedly, especially over the first several hours after the drug is given, and cautiously treat when necessary.

Withdrawal: Standard therapy for digitalis intoxication includes withdrawal of the drug and correction of factors that may contribute to toxicity such as electrolyte disturbances, hypoxia, acid-base disturbances and agents such as catecholamines. In a few instances, those with low cardiac output states, congestive heart failure or atrial fibrillation may develop a rapid ventricular response from withdrawal of the effects of digitalis on the AV node.

Patients may deteriorate from withdrawal of digoxin. Additional support can be provided by use of IV inotropes (eg, dopamine or dobutamine) or vasodilators. With catecholamines, take care not to aggravate digitalis toxic rhythm disturbances. Do not use other types of digitalis glycosides or redigitalize until the fab fragments have been eliminated from the body; this may require several days. Patients with impaired renal function may require a week or longer.

Adverse Reactions:

Low cardiac output, congestive heart failure, hypokalemia or atrial fibrillation (see Precautions).

Administration and Dosage:

Administer IV over 15 to 30 minutes and infuse through a 0.22 micron membrane filter. If cardiac arrest is imminent, give as a bolus injection.

Dosage varies according to the amount of digoxin to be neutralized. Refer to dosing guidelines in this section. If, after several hours, toxicity has not reversed or appears to recur, readministration may be required. If a patient presents with digitalis toxicity from an acute ingestion, and neither a serum digitalis concentration nor an estimated ingestion amount is available, administer 20 vials (760 mg). This will be adequate to treat most life-threatening ingestions in adults and children.

Children: Same dosing guidelines as for adults. However, in small children, it is important to monitor for volume overload.

Dosage estimates: The dose need not be exactly equimolar. In general, a large dose has a faster onset but enhances the possibility of an allergic or febrile reaction. The following tables give approximate doses.

Approximate Dose for Reversal of a Single Ingestion Digoxin Overdose

Number of digoxin tablets or capsules ingested[1]	Dose	
	mg	# of vials
25	380	10
50	760	20
75	1140	30
100	1520	40
150	2280	60
200	3040	80

[1] 0.25 mg tablets (80% bioavailability); 0.2 mg *Lanoxicaps* capsules (100% bioavailability).

DIGOXIN IMMUNE FAB (Ovine)

Because infants and small children can have much smaller dosage requirements, reconstitute 38 mg vial as directed and administer with tuberculin syringe. For very small doses, dilute reconstituted vial with 34 ml sterile isotonic saline to achieve 1 mg/ml concentration.

Estimates of Fab Fragments From Serum Digoxin Concentration								
	Weight	Serum digoxin concentration (ng/ml)						
Patient	(kg)	1	2	4	8	12	16	20
Infants/Children (dose given in mg)	1	0.4 mg[1]	1 mg[1]	1.5 mg[1]	3 mg[1]	5 mg	6 mg	8 mg
	3	1 mg[1]	2 mg[1]	5 mg	9 mg	14 mg	18 mg	23 mg
	5	2 mg[1]	4 mg	8 mg	15 mg	23 mg	30 mg	38 mg
	10	4 mg	8 mg	15 mg	30 mg	46 mg	61 mg	76 mg
	20	8 mg	15 mg	30 mg	61 mg	91 mg	122 mg	152 mg
Adults (dose given in vials [v])	40	0.5 v	1 v	2 v	3 v	5 v	7 v	8 v
	60	0.5 v	1 v	3 v	5 v	7 v	10 v	12 v
	70	1 v	2 v	3 v	6 v	9 v	11 v	14 v
	80	1 v	2 v	3 v	7 v	10 v	13 v	16 v
	100	1 v	2 v	4 v	8 v	12 v	16 v	20 v

[1] Dilution of reconstituted vial to 1 mg/ml may be desirable.

Exact dosage calculation: The equimolar dose required is calculated from the total amount of digoxin (or digitoxin) in the patient's body. An estimate of total body load is based either on the known acutely ingested dose or is estimated by using a steady-state serum concentration. For toxicity from an acute ingestion, the total body load of digoxin (mg) will be approximately equal to the dose ingested (mg); multiply by 0.8 to correct for incomplete absorption of tablets. Total body load of digitoxin (mg) is equal to the dose ingested (mg). To estimate total load from the steady-state serum concentration, the patient's serum digoxin concentration (SDC) in ng/ml is multiplied by the mean volume of distribution of digoxin (5.6 L/kg times patient weight in kg) to give total body load in mcg. Divide by 1000 to obtain the estimated mg amount of digoxin in the body.

Digoxin: Body load in mg = (SDC) (5.6) (weight in kg) ÷ 1000.

For patients toxic from digitoxin, estimate total body load by using the value 0.56 L/kg volume of distribution in place of the 5.6 L/kg for digoxin.

Digitoxin: Body load in mg = (SDC) (0.56) (weight in kg) ÷ 1000.

Each vial contains 38 mg purified digoxin-specific fab fragments which will bind approximately 0.5 mg digoxin (or digitoxin). Calculate the total number of vials required by dividing the total body load in mg by 0.5 mg/vial.

$$\text{Dose (in \# of vials)} = \frac{\text{Body load (mg)}}{\text{0.5 (mg/vial)}}$$

If the calculation based on ingested dose differs substantially from the calculation based on serum digoxin or digitoxin concentration, it may be preferable to administer an amount based on the higher calculation. Inaccurate serum digitalis concentration measurements are a source of error, especially for very high values.

Chronic therapy:

Adults – Six vials (228 mg) usually is adequate to reverse most cases of toxicity. This dose can be used in patients who are in acute distress or for whom a serum digoxin or digitoxin concentration is not available.

Children – For those weighing ≤ 20 kg, a single vial usually should suffice.

Reconstitution: Dissolve the contents in each vial with 4 ml of Sterile Water for Injection. Mix gently to give an approximately isosmotic solution with a protein concentration of 9.5 mg/ml. Use reconstituted product promptly. If it is not used immediately, store at 2° to 8°C (36° to 46°F) for up to 4 hours. The reconstituted product may be diluted with sterile isotonic saline to a convenient volume.

Rx	**Digibind** (Glaxo Wellcome)	**Powder for injection, lyophilized:** 38 mg per vial. Each vial will bind ≈ 0.5 mg digoxin or digitoxin.	With 75 mg sorbitol. In vials.

IPECAC SYRUP

Actions:

Pharmacology: Ipecac produces vomiting by a local irritant effect on GI mucosa and a central medullary effect (stimulation of chemoreceptor trigger zone). The central effect is caused by emetine and cephaeline, the two alkaloids. An adequate dose causes vomiting within 30 min in > 90% of patients (average time is < 20 min).

Indications:

Overdose/Poisoning: Treatment of drug overdose and in certain poisonings.

Contraindications:

Semiconscious or unconscious patients. Do not use if strychnine, corrosives such as alkalies and strong acids, or petroleum distillates have been ingested.

Warnings:

Syrup/Fluid extract: Do not confuse ipecac syrup with ipecac fluid extract, which is 14 times stronger and has caused some deaths.

Call an emergency room, poison control center or physician before using; if vomiting does not occur within 30 to 45 minutes after the second dose, perform gastric lavage.

Ipecac syrup abuse may occur in bulimic and anorexic patients. It has been implicated as the causative factor of severe cardiomyopathies, and even death, in several persons with eating disorders who used it regularly to induce vomiting.

Pregnancy: Category C. It is not known whether the drug can cause harm when administered to a pregnant woman. Minimal systemic absorption is expected when used as directed (see Administration and Dosage).

Lactation: It is not known whether ipecac alkaloids are excreted in breast milk. Exercise caution if ipecac syrup is used for treatment of a nursing woman.

Precautions:

Absorption: Ipecac syrup can be cardiotoxic if not vomited and allowed to be absorbed. Absorption of emetine may occur and cause heart conduction disturbances, atrial fibrillation or fatal myocarditis.

Drug Interactions:

Activated charcoal will adsorb ipecac syrup. If both are to be used, give the activated charcoal only after vomiting has been produced by the ipecac syrup.

Adverse Reactions:

Reactions are generally not significant if the dose is not exceeded. Diarrhea (25% in children < 3 years); drowsiness (20% in children < 3 years); coughing or choking in association with emesis (< 4%); mild CNS depression; GI upset (may last several hours after emesis).

Overdosage:

Symptoms: Ipecac is cardiotoxic if absorbed and may cause cardiac conduction disturbances, bradycardia, atrial fibrillation, hypotension or fatal myocarditis.

Treatment: Activated charcoal may be given to adsorb ipecac syrup; perform gastric lavage. Support cardiovascular system by symptomatic treatment.

Patient Information:

Always consult a physician or poison control center in cases of accidental ingestion.

Give with adequate amounts of water; do not use milk or carbonated beverages. Do not exceed recommended dosage.

Administration and Dosage:

Ipecac syrup may not work on an empty stomach. Have patient sit upright with head forward before administering dose.

Children (< 1 yr): 5 to 10 ml, then ½ to 1 glass water. Should *probably* give only with medical supervision. There is controversy over giving to children < 1 year, although it appears to be safe and effective.

Children (> 1 year to 12 years): 15 ml followed by 1 to 2 glasses of water.

Adults: 15 to 30 ml followed by 3 to 4 glasses of water.

Repeat dosage (15 ml) once, in persons older than one year, if vomiting does not occur within 20 to 30 min. If vomiting does not occur within 30 to 45 min after the second dose, perform gastric lavage.

otc	**Ipecac** (Various, eg, Barre-National, Roxane)	**Syrup**	1.5% to 1.75% alcohol. In 15 and 30 ml.
Rx	**Ipecac** (Various, eg, Paddock)	**Syrup**	2% alcohol. In 15 and 30 ml.

CHARCOAL, ACTIVATED

Actions:

Pharmacology: Activated charcoal is a carbon residue derived from organic material by exposing it to an oxidizing gas compound of steam, oxygen and acids at high temperatures resulting in the production of increased surface area through the creation of external and internal pores. Activation (to make a fine network of pores) of the charcoal surface increases adsorptive properties. The maximum amount of drug adsorbed by such charcoal is approximately 100 to 1000 mg/g charcoal. Activated charcoal is insoluble in water.

Sorbitol may be added to some activated charcoal products because it improves the taste, and it does not have a gritty oral residue. Sorbitol also reduces intestinal transit time from 25 hours to ≈ 1 hour.

Activated charcoal adsorbs toxic substances by forming an effective barrier between any remaining particulate material and the GI mucosa, thus inhibiting GI adsorption. The adsorptive properties of the activated charcoal in a liquid base are slightly decreased during its shelf life but are still capable of adsorbing at least 99% of the substances tested.

Indications:

Poisoning: For use as an emergency treatment in poisoning by most drugs and chemicals.

Contraindications:

Ineffective for poisoning or overdosage of mineral acids and alkalies.

Although not necessarily contraindicated, activated charcoal is not particularly effective in poisonings of ethanol, methanol and iron salts.

Warnings:

Emesis: Induce emesis before giving activated charcoal. After ipecac-induced vomiting, the patient may be intolerant of activated charcoal for 1 to 2 hours.

Gastric lavage: Activated charcoal can be administered in the early stages of gastric lavage. Use activated charcoal without sorbitol. The gastric lavage returns will be black.

Children: Not recommended in children < 1 year of age.

Drug Interactions:

Syrup of ipecac: Do not administer concomitantly. Activated charcoal will adsorb and inactivate this agent.

The effectiveness of other medication may be decreased when used concurrently because of adsorption by the activated charcoal.

Drug/Food interactions: Do not mix charcoal with milk, ice cream or sherbet since it will decrease the adsorptive capacity of the activated charcoal.

Adverse Reactions:

GI: Rapid ingestion of high doses may cause vomiting. Constipation or diarrhea may occur. Stools will be black.

Sorbitol may cause loose stools, vomiting and dehydration.

Respiratory: Aspiration of activated charcoal has been reported to produce airway obstruction and a limited number of fatalities have occurred. *Bronchiolitis obliterans* resulting in death has developed several weeks after the aspiration of activated charcoal.

Overdosage:

Bowel obstruction.

Administration and Dosage:

Administer to conscious persons only.

Acute intoxication:

Adult initial dose – 25 to 100 g (or 1 g/kg or approximately 10 times the amount of poison ingested) as a suspension (4 to 8 ounces water). For maximum effect, administer activated charcoal solution within 30 minutes after ingestion of poison.

GI dialysis: Multiple administration may be used in severe poisonings to prevent desorption from the charcoal; also promoted to increase GI clearance and rate of elimination of drugs that undergo an enteral recirculation pattern.

Storage/Stability: Activated charcoal adsorbs gases from the air; therefore, store in closed containers.

CHARCOAL, ACTIVATED

otc	**Activated Charcoal,** (Various)	**Powder**	In 15, 30, 40, 120 and 240 g and UD 30 g.
otc	**Activated Charcoal** (Various)	**Liquid:** 208 mg/ml	12.5 g with propylene glycol. In 60 ml bottle. 25 g with propylene glycol. In 120 ml bottle.
otc	**Actidose-Aqua** (Paddock)		25 g in 120 ml suspension. 50 g in 240 ml suspension.
otc	**Actidose with Sorbitol** (Paddock)		25 g in 120 ml suspension with sorbitol. 50 g in 240 ml suspension with sorbitol.
otc	**Liqui-Char** (Jones Medical)		12.5 g in 60 ml bottle, 15 g in 75 ml bottle, 25 g in 120 ml squeeze container, 30 g in 120 ml squeeze container, 50 g in 240 ml squeeze container.
otc	**CharcoAid** (Requa)	**Suspension:** 15 g	Sorbitol. In 120 ml.
		30 g	Sorbitol. In 150 ml.
otc	**CharcoAid 2000** (Requa)	**Liquid:** 15 g	With and without sorbitol. In 120 ml.
		50 g	With and without sorbitol. In 240 ml.
		Granules: 15 g	In 120 ml.

METHYLENE BLUE

Actions:

Pharmacology: This compound has an oxidation-reduction action and a tissue staining property. In high concentrations, methylene blue converts the ferrous iron of reduced hemoglobin in the ferric form; as a result, methemoglobin is produced. This action is the basis for the antidotal action of methylene blue in cyanide poisoning. In contrast, low concentrations of methylene blue are capable of hastening the conversion of methemoglobin to hemoglobin.

Methylene blue is a dye that is a weak germicide and is used as a mild GU antiseptic. It is primarily bacteriostatic.

Indications:

Oral:

Cyanide poisoning – For treatment of idiopathic and drug-induced methemoglobinemia and as an antidote for cyanide poisoning.

Urinary tract calculi – May be useful in the management of patients with oxalate urinary tract calculi.

Genitourinary antiseptic: A mild GU antiseptic and stimulant for mucous surfaces.

Unlabeled uses:

Glutaricaciduria – Methylene blue may be of benefit in neonatal glutaricaciduria type II unresponsive to riboflavin.

Contraindications:

Renal insufficiency; patients allergic to methylene blue; intraspinal injection.

Warnings:

Aniline-induced methemoglobulinemia: Methylene blue should be used with caution in the treatment of aniline-induced methemoglobulinemia because it may precipitate Heinz body formation and hemolytic anemia.

Alkaline urine: Restrict drugs or foods which produce an alkaline urine.

Pregnancy: Category C. Safety for use in pregnancy has not been established. Use only if the potential benefits outweigh the risks.

Precautions:

Photosensitization (photoallergy or phototoxicity) may occur; therefore, caution patients to take protective measures against exposure to ultraviolet or sunlight (eg, sunscreens, protective clothing) until tolerance is determined.

G-6–PD deficiency: Methylene blue may induce hemolysis in glucose-6–phosphate dehydrogenase (G-6–PD) deficient patients.

Anemia: Continued administration may cause a marked anemia due to accelerated destruction of erythrocytes. Therefore, perform frequent hemoglobin checks.

Cyanosis and cardiovascular abnormalities have accompanied treatment in humans.

Additional methemoglobin: Inject IV slowly over a period of several minutes to prevent local high concentrations of the compound from producing additional methemoglobin.

Adverse Reactions:

Oral: Turns the urine and sometimes the stool blue-green. May cause bladder irritation and, in some cases, nausea, vomiting and diarrhea. Large doses may cause fever.

Overdosage:

Oral: Symptoms include vomiting, headache and diarrhea.

Patient Information:

Take after meals with a glass of water.

May discolor the urine or stool blue-green.

Administration and Dosage:

Oral: Take 65 to 130 mg, 3 times daily after meals with a full glass of water.

Parenteral: 1 to 2 mg/kg (0.1 to 0.2 ml/kg) (see Precautions).

Storage/Stability:

Tablets – Store in a dry place at room temperature (15° to 30°C; 59° to 86°F).

Injection – Store below 40°C (104°F), preferably between 15° and 30°C (59° and 86°F).

Rx	**Methblue 65** (Manne Co)	**Tablets:** 65 mg	In 100s and 1000s.
Rx	**Urolene Blue** (Star)		In 100s and 1000s.
Rx	**Methylene Blue** (Various, eg, Pasadena)	**Injection:** 10 mg/ml	In 1 and 10 ml amps.

TRIENTINE HCl

Actions:

Pharmacology: Wilson's disease (hepatolenticular degeneration) is a metabolic defect resulting in excess copper accumulation, possibly because the liver lacks the mechanism to excrete free copper into the bile. Hepatocytes store excess copper, but when their capacity is exceeded copper is released into the blood and is taken up into extrahepatic sites. Treat this condition with a low copper diet and with chelating agents that bind copper to facilitate its excretion from the body. Trientine is a chelating compound for removal of excess copper from the body.

Clinical trials: Forty-one patients (aged 6 to 54) with Wilson's disease who were intolerant of penicillamine were treated in two separate studies with trientine. The average dosage required to achieve an optimal clinical response varied between 1000 and 2000 mg/day (range, 450 to 2400 mg). The mean duration of therapy was 48.7 months (range, 2 to 164 months). Thirty-four patients improved, four had no change in clinical global response, two were lost to follow-up and one showed deterioration in clinical condition.

Thirteen patients were treated with trientine following their development of intolerance to penicillamine. Retrospectively, patients were compared to an additional group of 12 patients with Wilson's disease who were both tolerant of, and controlled with, penicillamine therapy, but who failed to continue copper chelation therapy. In the patients treated with trientine, previous symptoms and signs relating to penicillamine intolerance disappeared in eight patients, improved in four patients and remained unchanged in one. The neurological status in the trientine group was unchanged or improved over baseline, whereas in the untreated group, six patients remained unchanged and six worsened. Kayser-Fleischer rings improved significantly during trientine treatment. Of the 13 patients on therapy with trientine (mean duration, 4.1 years; range, 1 to 13 years), all were alive at the data cutoff date, and in the non-treated group (mean years with no therapy, 2.7 years; range, 3 months to 9 years), 9 of the 12 died of hepatic disease.

Renal clearance studies were carried out with penicillamine and trientine on separate occasions in selected patients treated with penicillamine for at least 1 year. Six hour excretion rates of copper were determined off treatment, and after a single dose of 500 mg penicillamine or 1.2 g trientine. Results demonstrated that trientine is effective as a cupriuretic agent in patients with Wilson's disease, although on a molar basis, the drug appears to be less potent or less effective than penicillamine.

Indications:

Wilson's disease: Treatment of patients with Wilson's disease who are intolerant of penicillamine.

Contraindications:

Hypersensitivity to trientine; cystinuria; rheumatoid arthritis; biliary cirrhosis.

Warnings:

Patient supervision: Patients should remain under regular medical supervision throughout the period of drug administration.

Iron deficiency anemia: Closely monitor patients (especially women) for evidence of iron deficiency anemia.

Pregnancy: Category C. Trientine was teratogenic in rats at doses similar to the human dose. The frequencies of both resorptions and fetal abnormalities, including hemorrhage and edema, increased while fetal copper levels decreased. There are no adequate and well controlled studies in pregnant women. Use during pregnancy only when the potential benefits outweigh the potential hazards to the fetus.

Lactation: It is not known whether this drug is excreted in breast milk. Exercise caution when administering to a nursing woman.

Children: Safety and efficacy for use in children have not been established. Trientine has been used clinically in children as young as 6 years of age with no reported adverse effects.

TRIENTINE HCl

Precautions:

Monitoring: The most reliable index for monitoring treatment is the determination of free copper in the serum, which equals the difference between quantitatively determined total copper and ceruloplasmin-copper. Adequately treated patients will usually have less than 10 mcg free copper/dl of serum.

Therapy may be monitored with a 24 hour urinary copper analysis periodically (ie, every 6 to 12 months). Urine must be collected in copper free glassware. Since a low copper diet should keep copper absorption down to less than 1mg/day, the patient probably will be in the desired state of negative copper balance if 0.5 to 1 mg of copper is present in a 24 hour collection of urine.

Hypersensitivity: There are no reports of hypersensitivity in patients given trientine for Wilson's disease. However, there have been reports of asthma, bronchitis and dermatitis occurring after prolonged environmental exposure in workers who use trientine HCl as a hardener of epoxy resins. Observe patients closely for signs of possible hypersensitivity. Refer to Management of Hypersensitivity Reactions.

Drug Interactions:

Iron: In general, do not give mineral supplements; they may block the absorption of trientine. However, iron deficiency may develop, especially in children and menstruating or pregnant women, or as a result of the low copper diet recommended for Wilson's disease. If necessary, iron may be given in short courses, but since iron and trientine each inhibit absorption of the other, allow 2 hours to elapse between administration of trientine and iron.

Adverse Reactions:

Iron deficiency and systemic lupus erythematosus have occurred in patients with Wilson's disease who were on therapy with trientine.

Trientine is not indicated for treatment of biliary cirrhosis, but in one study of four patients treated with trientine for primary biliary cirrhosis, the following adverse reactions were reported: Heartburn; epigastric pain and tenderness; thickening, fissuring and flaking of the skin; hypochromic microcytic anemia; acute gastritis; aphthoid ulcers; abdominal pain; melena; anorexia; malaise; cramps; muscle pain; weakness; rhabdomyolysis. A causal relationship to drug therapy could not be rejected or established.

Overdosage:

There is a report of an adult woman who ingested 30 g trientine without apparent ill effects.

Patient Information:

Take on an empty stomach, at least 1 hour before meals or 2 hours after meals and at least 1 hour apart from any other drug, food or milk.

Swallow capsules whole with water. Do not open or chew.

Because of the potential for contact dermatitis, any site of exposure to the capsule contents should be promptly washed with water.

Take temperature nightly, and report any symptoms such as fever or skin eruption for the first month of treatment.

Administration and Dosage:

Adults: Initially, 750 mg to 1.25 g/day, in divided doses, 2, 3 or 4 times daily. May increase to a maximum of 2 g/day.

Children ≤ 12 years: Initially, 500 to 750 mg/day, in divided doses, 2, 3 or 4 times daily. May increase to a maximum of 1.5 g/day.

Increase the daily dose only when the clinical response is not adequate or the concentration of free serum copper is persistently above 20mcg/dl. Determine optimal long-term maintenance dosage at 6 to 12 month intervals.

Storage: Store at 2° to 8°C (36° to 46°F).

Rx	**Syprine** (Merck)	**Capsules:** 250 mg	(MSD 661). Light brown. In 100s.

SUCCIMER

Actions:

Pharmacology: Succimer is an orally active, heavy metal chelating agent; it forms water soluble chelates and, consequently, increases the urinary excretion of lead.

Toxicology – In oral toxicity studies up to 28 days, doses up to 200mg/kg/day did not produce significant overt toxicity in rats and dogs. However, in 6 and 28 day oral toxicity studies, doses ≥ 300 mg/kg/day were toxic and lethal to some dogs. The kidney and GI tract were the major target organs for toxicity. Toxicity was manifested by anorexia; emesis; mucoid or bloody diarrhea; increased BUN concentration, AST, ALT and alkaline phosphatase levels; renal tubular necrosis; purulent nephritis; severe GI bleeding and ulceration. Deaths were due to renal failure.

Pharmacokinetics: In a study in healthy adult volunteers, after a single dose of 16, 32 or 48 mg/kg, absorption was rapid but variable, with peak blood levels between 1 and 2 hours. Approximately 49% of the dose was excreted: 39% in the feces, 9% in the urine and 1% as carbon dioxide from the lungs. Since fecal excretion probably represented non-absorbed drug, most of the absorbed drug was excreted by the kidneys. The apparent elimination half-life was about 2 days.

In other studies of healthy adult volunteers receiving a single oral dose of 10 mg/kg, succimer was rapidly and extensively metabolized. Approximately 25% of the dose was excreted in the urine with the peak blood level and urinary excretion occurring between 2 and 4 hours. Of the total amount of drug eliminated in the urine, approximately 90% was eliminated in altered form as mixed succimer-cysteine disulfides; the remaining 10% was eliminated unchanged.

Clinical trials: Studies were performed in 18 men with blood lead levels of 44 to 96 mcg/dl. Three groups of 6 patients received either 10, 6.7 or 3.3 mg/kg every 8 hours for 5 days. After 5 days mean blood levels of the three groups decreased 72.5%, 58.3% and 35.5%, respectively. Mean urinary lead excretions in the initial 24 hours were 28.6, 18.6 and 12.3 times the pretreatment 24 hour urinary lead excretion. As the chelatable pool was reduced during therapy, urinary lead output decreased. A mean of 19 mg lead was excreted during a 5 day course of 30 mg/kg/day. Clinical symptoms, such as headache and colic, and biochemical indices of lead toxicity also improved. Decrease in urinary excretion of d-aminolevulinic acid (ALA) and coproporphyrin paralleled the improvement in erythrocyte ALA dehydratase. Three control patients with lead poisoning of similar severity received edetate calcium disodium (EDTA) IV at a dose of 50 mg/kg/day for 5 days. Mean blood lead level decreased 47.4% and mean urinary lead excretion was 21 mg in controls.

Effect on essential minerals – In the above studies, succimer had no significant effect on the urinary elimination of iron, calcium or magnesium. Zinc excretion doubled during treatment. The effect of succimer on the excretion of essential minerals was small compared to that of EDTA, which can induce more than a tenfold increase in urinary excretion of zinc and doubling of copper and iron excretion.

Succimer vs EDTA: A study was performed in 15 children ages 2 to 7 years with blood lead levels of 30 to 49 mcg/dl and positive EDTA lead mobilization tests. Each group of five patients received 350, 233 or 116 mg/m^2 succimer every 8 hours for 5 days. These doses corresponded to 10, 6.7 and 3.3 mg/kg. Six control patients received 1000 mg/m^2/day EDTA IV for 5 days. Following therapy, the mean blood lead levels decreased 78%, 63% and 42%, respectively, in the three groups treated with succimer. The response of the 350 mg/m^2 every 8 hours (10 mg/kg every 8 hrs) group was significantly better than that of the other succimer-treated groups as well as that of the control group, whose mean blood lead level fell 48%. No adverse reactions or changes in essential mineral excretion were reported in the succimer-treated groups. In the EDTA-treated group, the cumulative amount of urinary lead excreted was slightly but significantly greater than in the succimer group. After EDTA, the urinary excretion of copper, zinc, iron and calcium were significantly increased.

As with other chelators, both adults and children experienced a rebound in blood lead levels after discontinuing succimer. In these studies, after treatment with 350 mg/m^2 (10 mg/kg) every 8 hours for 5 days, the mean lead level rebounded and plateaued at 80% to 85% of pretreatment levels 2 weeks after therapy. The rebound plateau was somewhat higher with lower doses of succimer and with IV EDTA.

In an attempt to control rebound of blood lead levels, 19 children, ages 1 to 7 years, with blood lead levels of 42 to 67 mcg/dl were treated with 350 mg/m^2 every 8 hours for 5 days and then divided into three groups. One group was followed for 2 weeks with no further therapy, the second group was treated for 2 weeks with 350 mg/m^2 daily, and the third with 350 mg/m^2 every 12 hours. After the initial 5 days of therapy, the mean blood lead level in all subjects declined 61%, while the untreated group and the group treated with 350 mg/m^2 daily experienced rebound during the ensuing 2 weeks, the group who received the 350 mg/m^2 every 12 hours experienced no such rebound during the treatment period and less rebound following cessation of therapy.

In another study, ten children, ages 21 to 72 months old, with blood lead levels of 30 to 57 mcg/dl, were treated with succimer 350 mg/m^2 every 8 hours for 5 days, followed by an additional 19 to 22 days of therapy at a dose of 350 mg/m^2 every 12 hours. The mean blood lead levels decreased and remained stable at under 15 mcg/dl during the extended dosing period.

In addition to the controlled studies, approximately 250 patients with lead poisoning have been treated with succimer either orally or parenterally in open US and foreign studies with similar results reported. Succimer has been used to treat lead poisoning in one patient with sickle cell anemia and in five with glucose-6-phosphodehydrogenase (G-6-PD) deficiency without adverse reactions.

Lead encephalopathy: Three adults with lead encephalopathy have improved with succimer therapy. However, data are not available for the use of succimer for treatment of this rare and sometimes fatal complication of lead poisoning in children.

Other heavy metal poisoning: A limited number of patients have received succimer for mercury or arsenic poisoning. These patients showed increased urinary excretion of the heavy metal and varying degrees of symptomatic improvement.

Indications:

Treatment of lead poisoning in children with blood lead levels > 45 mcg/dl. Not indicated for prophylaxis of lead poisoning in a lead-containing environment; always accompany succimer use with identification and removal of lead exposure.

Unlabeled uses: Succimer may be beneficial in the treatment of other heavy metal poisonings (eg, mercury, arsenic); further study is needed.

Contraindications:

History of allergy to the drug.

Warnings:

Keep out of reach of children.

Not a substitute for effective abatement of lead exposure.

Pregnancy: Category C. Succimer is teratogenic and fetotoxic in pregnant mice when given SC in a dose range of 410 to 1640 mg/kg/day during the period of organogenesis. There are no adequate and well controlled studies in pregnant women. Use during pregnancy only if the potential benefit justifies the potential risk to the fetus.

Lactation: It is not known whether this drug is excreted in breast milk. Discourage mothers requiring therapy from nursing their infants.

Children: Refer to the Indications and Administration and Dosage sections. There is no therapeutic experience with succimer in children < 1 year of age.

Precautions:

Carefully observe patients during treatment due to limited clinical experience with succimer.

Elevated blood lead levels and associated symptoms may return rapidly after discontinuation of succimer because of redistribution of lead from bone stores to soft tissues and blood. After therapy, monitor patients for rebound of blood lead levels by measuring the levels at least once weekly until stable. However, use the severity of lead intoxication (as measured by initial blood lead level and rate and degree of rebound of blood lead) as a guide for more frequent blood lead monitoring.

Renal function: Adequately hydrate all patients undergoing treatment. Exercise caution in using succimer therapy in patients with compromised renal function. Limited data suggest that succimer is dialyzable, but that the lead chelates are not.

Hepatic function: Transient mild elevations of serum transaminases have been observed in 6% to 10% of patients during the course of therapy. Monitor serum transaminases before the start of therapy and at least weekly during therapy. Closely monitor patients with a history of liver disease. No data are available regarding the metabolism of succimer in patients with liver disease.

Repeated courses: Clinical experience is limited. The safety of uninterrupted dosing > 3 weeks has not been established and is not recommended.

Allergic reactions: The possibility of allergic or other mucocutaneous reactions must be borne in mind on readministration (and during initial courses). Monitor patients requiring repeated courses during each treatment course. One patient experienced recurrent mucocutaneous vesicular eruptions of increasing severity affecting oral mucosa, external urethral meatus and perianal area on third, fourth and fifth courses. The reaction resolved between courses and on discontinuation of therapy.

SUCCIMER

Drug Interactions:

Chelation therapy (eg, EDTA): Coadministration of succimer with other chelation therapy is not recommended.

Drug/Lab test interactions: Succimer may interfere with serum and urinary laboratory tests. In vitro, succimer caused false-positive results for ketones in urine using nitroprusside reagents such as Ketostix and falsely decreased measurements of serum uric acid and CPK.

Adverse Reactions:

The most common events attributable to succimer (ie, GI symptoms or increases in serum transaminases) have been observed in about 10% of patients (see Precautions). Rashes, some necessitating discontinuation of therapy, have occurred in about 4% of patients. If rash occurs, consider other causes (eg, measles) before ascribing the reaction to succimer. Rechallenge with succimer may be considered if lead levels are high enough to warrant retreatment. One allergic mucocutaneous reaction has occurred on repeated administration of the drug (see Precautions). The following table presents adverse events reported with the administration of succimer for the treatment of lead and other heavy metal intoxication.

Succimer Adverse Reactions (%)[1]

Body system/adverse reaction	Children (n = 191)	Adults (n = 134)
Digestive:		
Nausea; vomiting; diarrhea; appetite loss; hemorrhoidal symptoms; loose stools; metallic taste in mouth	12	20.9
Body as a whole:		
Back, stomach, head, rib, flank pain; abdominal cramps; chills; fever; flu-like symptoms; heavy head/tired; head cold; headache; moniliasis	5.2	15.7
Metabolic:		
Elevated AST, ALT, alkaline phosphatase, serum cholesterol	4.2	10.4
CNS:		
Drowsiness; dizziness; sensorimotor neuropathy; sleepiness; paresthesia	1	12.7
Skin and appendages:		
Papular rash; herpetic rash; rash; mucocutaneous eruptions; pruritus	2.6	11.2
Special senses:		
Cloudy film in eye; ears plugged; otitis media; watery eyes	1	3.7
Respiratory:		
Sore throat; rhinorrhea; nasal congestion; cough	3.7	0.7
GU:		
Decreased urination; voiding difficulty; proteinuria increased	0	3.7
Other:		
Arrhythmia	0	1.8
Increased platelet count; intermittent eosinophilia	0.5	1.5
Kneecap pain; leg pains	0	3

[1] Incidence regardless of attribution or dosage.

SUCCIMER

Overdosage:

Doses of 2300 to 2400 mg/kg in the rat and mouse produced ataxia, convulsions, labored respiration and frequently death. Induction of vomiting or gastric lavage followed by administration of an activated charcoal slurry and appropriate supportive therapy are recommended. Refer to General Management of Acute Overdosage.

Limited data indicate that succimer is dialyzable.

Patient Information:

Instruct patients to maintain adequate fluid intake. If rash occurs, patients should consult their physician.

In young children unable to swallow capsules, the contents of the capsule can be administered in a small amount of food (see Administration and Dosage).

Administration and Dosage:

Succimer was approved by the FDA in February 1991.

Start dosage at 10 mg/kg or 350 mg/m^2 every 8 hours for 5 days; initiation of therapy at higher doses is not recommended (see table). Reduce frequency of administration to 10 mg/kg or 350 mg/m^2 every 12 hours (two-thirds of initial daily dosage) for an additional 2 weeks of therapy. A course of treatment lasts 19 days. Repeated courses may be necessary if indicated by weekly monitoring of blood lead concentration. A minimum of 2 weeks between courses is recommended unless blood lead levels indicate the need for more prompt treatment.

Succimer Pediatric Dosing Chart

Weight		Dose (mg)[1]	Number of capsules[1]
lbs	kg		
18-35	8-15	100	1
36-55	16-23	200	2
56-75	24-34	300	3
76-100	35-44	400	4
> 100	> 45	500	5

[1] To be administered every 8 hours for 5 days, followed by dosing every 12 hours for 14 days.

In young children who cannot swallow capsules, succimer can be administered by separating the capsule and sprinkling the medicated beads on a small amount of soft food or putting them in a spoon and following with a fruit drink.

Identification of the lead source in the child's environment and its abatement are critical to successful therapy. Chelation therapy is not a substitute for preventing further exposure to lead and should not be used to permit continued exposure to lead.

Patients who have received EDTA with or without BAL may use succimer for subsequent treatment after an interval of 4 weeks. Data on the concomitant use of succimer with EDTA with or without BAL are not available, and such use is not recommended.

Rx	**Chemet** (Bock)	**Capsules:** 100 mg	Sucrose. (Chemet 100.) White. In 100s.

PENICILLAMINE

Actions:

Pharmacology:

Rheumatoid arthritis – The mechanism of action of penicillamine in rheumatoid arthritis is unknown. Penicillamine markedly lowers IgM rheumatoid factor, but produces no significant depression in absolute levels of serum immunoglobulins; it dissociates macroglobulins (rheumatoid factor). The drug may decrease cell-mediated immune response by selectively inhibiting T–lymphocyte function. Penicillamine may also act as an anti-inflammatory agent by inhibiting release of lysosomal enzymes and oxygen radicals protecting lymphocytes from the harmful effects of hydrogen peroxide formed at inflammatory sites.

The onset of therapeutic response may not be seen for 2 or 3 months in those patients who respond. The optimum duration of therapy has not been determined. If remissions occur, they may last from months to years, but usually require continued treatment (see Administration and Dosage).

Wilson's disease: Penicillamine is a chelating agent that removes excess copper in patients with Wilson's disease. From in vitro studies which indicate that one atom of copper combines with two molecules of penicillamine, it would appear that 1 g penicillamine should be followed by the excretion of about 200 mg of copper; however, the actual amount excreted is about 1% of this. Noticeable improvement may not occur for 1 to 3 months. Occasionally, neurologic symptoms become worse during initiation of therapy.

Two types of patients require treatment for Wilson's disease:

1.) The symptomatic and
2.) the asymptomatic in whom it can be assumed the disease will develop in the future if the patient is not treated.

Cystinuria: Penicillamine reduces excess cystine excretion in cystinuria. Penicillamine with conventional therapy decreases crystalluria and stone formation and may decrease the size of or dissolve existing stones. This is done, at least in part, by disulfide interchange between penicillamine and cystine, resulting in a substance more soluble than cystine and readily excreted.

Poisoning: Penicillamine also forms soluble complexes with iron, mercury, lead and arsenic which are readily excreted by the kidneys. The drug may be used to treat poisoning by these metals.

Pharmacokinetics: It is well absorbed from the GI tract after oral administration (40% to 70%); peak plasma levels occur in 1 to 3 hours. Take on an empty stomach, at least 1 hour before meals or 2 hours after meals, and at least 1 hour apart from any other drug, food or milk. This permits maximum absorption and reduces the likelihood or inactivation by metal binding in the GI tract.

Most (80%) of the plasma penicillamine is protein bound, primarily to albumin. Penicillamine is rapidly excreted in the urine (42.1 ± 6.2% in 24 hours); 50% is excreted in the feces. Metabolites may be detected in the urine for up to 3 months after stopping the drug. Half-life ranges are 1.7 to 3.2 hours (average 2.1 hours).

Indications:

Rheumatoid arthritis: Because penicillamine can cause severe adverse reactions, restrict its use in rheumatoid arthritis to patients who have severe, active disease and who have failed to respond to an adequate trial of conventional therapy. Carefully consider the benefit-to-risk ratio. Use other measures, such as rest, physiotherapy, salicylates and corticosteroids, when indicated in conjunction with the drug.

Wilson's disease (hepatolenticular degeneration) is an abnormality in copper metabolism. As a result, copper is deposited in several organs and produces pathologic effects most prominently seen in brain, liver, kidneys and eyes. Penicillamine is a copper chelating agent intended to promote excretion of copper deposited in tissues.

Cystinuria: Cystinuria is characterized by excessive urinary excretion of dibasic amino acids, including arginine, lysine, ornithine and cystine. Stone formation is the only known pathology in cystinuria.

Penicillamine may be used as additional therapy, when conventional measures (ie, dilution and alkalinization of the urine, methionine restricted diet) are inadequate to control recurrent stone formation.

Unlabeled uses: The benefits of penicillamine's copper chelating and immunological effects have been investigated for use in the treatment of primary biliary cirrhosis. Doses of 600 to 900 mg/day have been used with both success and failure. Some data suggest that penicillamine may be beneficial in scleroderma.

Contraindications:

History of penicillamine-related aplastic anemia or agranulocytosis; rheumatoid arthritis patients with a history or other evidence of renal insufficiency (because of the potential for causing renal damage); pregnancy (see Warnings); breastfeeding.

PENICILLAMINE

Warnings:

Fatalities: Penicillamine has been associated with fatalities due to aplastic anemia, agranulocytosis, thrombocytopenia, sideroblastic anemia, Goodpasture's syndrome and myasthenia gravis.

Hematologic: Leukopenia (2%) and thrombocytopenia (4%) have occurred. A reduction in WBC below 3500, neutrophils $< 2000/mm^3$, or monocytes $> 500/mm^3$ mandate permanent withdrawal of therapy. Thrombocytopenia may be idiosyncratic, with decreased or absent megakaryocytes in marrow, when it is part of an aplastic anemia. In other cases, thrombocytopenia is presumably on an immune basis since the number of megakaryocytes in the marrow has been normal or sometimes increased. Platelet count below 100,000, even in the absence of clinical bleeding, or a progressive fall in either platelet count or WBC in three successive determinations, even though values are still in the normal range, requires at least temporary cessation of therapy.

Hepatotoxicity: Penicillamine has been associated with a mild elevation of hepatic enzymes that usually returns to normal even with continuation of the drug.

Lupus erythematosus: Certain patients will develop a positive antinuclear antibody (ANA) test and some may show a lupus erythematosus-like syndrome similar to other drug-induced lupus, but it is not associated with hypocomplementemia and may be present without nephropathy. A positive ANA test does not mandate drug discontinuance; however, a lupus erythematosus-like syndrome may develop later.

Oral ulcerations may develop which may have the appearance of aphthous stomatitis; it usually recurs on rechallenge but often clears on a lower dosage. Although rare, cheilosis, glossitis and gingivostomatitis have been reported. They are frequently dose-related and may preclude further increase in dosage or require drug discontinuation.

Hypogeusia occurs in 25% to 33% of patients, except for a lesser incidence in Wilson's disease (4%). Most cases are established within 6 weeks, but most commonly resolve in 2 to 6 months despite continued treatment. Total loss of taste has occurred.

Hypoglycemia has been reported in 4 patients receiving penicillamine therapy for rheumatoid arthritis. The mechanism of hypoglycemia is unknown. Two insulin dependent diabetic patients experienced nighttime hypoglycemia after the addition of penicillamine. Both patients required a reduction in their insulin dosage.

Two nondiabetic patients who had never received insulin or oral hypoglycemics developed anti-insulin antibodies. In these patients, penicillamine was suspected to be responsible for the antibody formation because it has been known to induce autoimmune complexes (see Warnings).

Autoimmune syndromes which may be caused by penicillamine include *polymyositis, diffuse alveolitis* and *dermatomyositis* and the following:

Goodpasture's syndrome is rare. Development of abnormal urinary findings associated with hemoptysis and pulmonary infiltrates on x-ray requires immediate drug cessation.

Obliterative bronchiolitis has been reported rarely. Caution the patient to report immediately pulmonary symptoms such as exertional dyspnea or unexplained cough or wheezing. Consider pulmonary function studies at this time.

Myasthenic syndrome sometimes progressing to myasthenia gravis has been reported. Ptosis and diplopia, with weakness of the extraocular muscles, are often early signs of myasthenia. In most cases, symptoms have receded after withdrawal of the drug.

Pemphigus vulgaris and pemphigus foliaceous are reported most frequently, usually as a late complication of therapy. The seborrhea-like characteristics of pemphigus foliaceous may obscure an early diagnosis. When pemphigus is suspected, discontinue pencillamine. Treatment has consisted of high doses of corticosteroids alone or, in some cases, concomitantly with an immunosuppressant. Treatment may be required for only a few weeks or months but may need to be continued for more than a year.

Sensitivity reactions: Once instituted for Wilson's disease or cystinuria, continue treatment with penicillamine on a daily basis. Interruptions for even a few days have been followed by sensitivity reactions after reinstitution of therapy.

Cross-sensitivity may theoretically appear in patients allergic to penicillin. Reactions from contamination of penicillamine by trace amounts of penicillin have been eliminated now that penicillamine is produced synthetically rather than as a degradation product of penicillin.

PENICILLAMINE

Hypersensitivity: Allergic reactions occur in ≈ ⅓ of patients. They are more common at the start of treatment, and occur as generalized rashes or drug fever. Discontinue treatment and reinstitute at a low dosage such as 250 mg/day, with gradual increases. Administering prednisolone 20 mg/day for the first few weeks of penicillamine therapy reduces the severity of these reactions. Antihistamines may control pruritus.

Drug fever may appear in some patients, usually in the second to third week of therapy; it is sometimes accompanied by a macular cutaneous eruption.

In patients with Wilson's disease or cystinuria, because no alternative treatment is available, temporarily discontinue penicillamine until the reaction subsides. Reinstitute therapy with a small dose and gradually increase until the desired dosage is attained. Systemic steroid therapy may be necessary, and is usually helpful, in patients who develop toxic reactions a second or third time.

In rheumatoid arthritis patients, discontinue penicillamine and try another therapeutic alternative since the febrile reaction will recur in a high percentage of patients upon readministration.

Dermatologic: Observe the skin and mucous membranes for allergic reactions. Skin rashes (44% to 50%) are the most frequent adverse reactions. Early rash occurs during the first few months of treatment and is more common. It is usually a generalized pruritic, erythematous, maculopapular or morbilliform rash and resembles the allergic rash seen with other drugs. It usually disappears within days after stopping penicillamine and seldom recurs when the drug is restarted at a lower dosage. Pruritus and early rash are often controlled by antihistamine coadministration.

A late rash is less commonly seen, usually after 6 months or more of treatment, and requires drug discontinuation. It usually appears on the trunk, is accompanied by intense pruritus, and is usually unresponsive to topical corticosteroids. It may take weeks to disappear after penicillamine is stopped and usually recurs if the drug is restarted.

Pemphigoid rash, the most serious dermatologic adverse reaction occurs most often after 6 to 9 months of penicillamine. From 1 to 2 months may be required for resolution. Do not rechallenge patient.

The appearance of a drug eruption accompanied by fever, arthralgia, lymphadenopathy, or other allergic manifestations usually requires drug discontinuation.

Renal function impairment: Proteinuria or hematuria may develop and may be a warning sign of membranous glomerulopathy which can progress to a nephrotic syndrome. In some patients, proteinuria disappears with continued therapy; in others, penicillamine must be discontinued. When proteinuria or hematuria develops, ascertain whether it is a sign of drug-induced glomerulopathy or is unrelated to penicillamine. History of proteinuria secondary to gold therapy may be a risk factor for penicillamine proteinuria.

Cautiously continue penicillamine in rheumatoid arthritis patients developing moderate degrees of proteinuria; obtain quantitative 24 hour urinary protein determinations at 1 to 2 week intervals. Do not increase dosage. If proteinuria exceeds 1 g/24 hours, or progressively increases, discontinue drug or reduce dosage. Proteinuria has cleared after dosage reduction. One year or more may be required for any urinary abnormalities to disappear after penicillamine has been discontinued.

In patients with Wilson's disease or cystinuria, the risks of continued penicillamine therapy in patients manifesting potentially serious urinary abnormalities must be weighed against the expected therapeutic benefits.

Pregnancy: In 89 known pregnancies, penicillamine was given throughout and three infants had birth defects deemed attributable to the drug. All infants exhibited cutis laxia; one had hypotonia, hyperflexion of hips and shoulders, pyloric stenosis, vein fragility and varicosities; another showed growth retardation, hernia, perforated bowel and simian crease. The latter two died.

Use only when clearly needed and when the potential benefits outweigh the potential hazards to the fetus. Inform women of childbearing potential or who are pregnant of the possible hazards of penicillamine to the developing fetus and advise them to report promptly any missed menstrual periods or other indications of possible pregnancy.

Lactation: Safety has not been established. See Contraindications.

Children: The efficacy of penicillamine in juvenile rheumatoid arthritis has not been established.

PENICILLAMINE

Precautions:

Dietary supplementation: Because of their dietary restriction, give patients with Wilson's disease, cystinuria and rheumatoid arthritis whose nutrition is impaired 25 mg/day of pyridoxine during therapy, since penicillamine increases the requirement for this vitamin. In Wilson's disease, multivitamin preparations must be copper free. Do not give mineral supplements; they may block response to penicillamine.

Iron deficiency may develop, especially in children and in menstruating women. If necessary, give iron in short courses. A period of 2 hours should elapse between administration of penicillamine and iron, since orally administered iron reduces the effects of penicillamine.

Collagen and elastin: Effects of penicillamine on collagen and elastin make it advisable to consider a reduction in dosage to 250 mg/day when surgery is contemplated. Delay full therapy until wound healing is complete.

Penicillamine causes an increase in the amount of soluble collagen. This may cause increased skin friability at sites subject to pressure or trauma, such as shoulders, elbows, knees, toes and buttocks. Extravasations of blood may occur and may appear as purpuric areas, with external bleeding if the skin is broken, or as vesicles containing dark blood. Neither type is progressive. Therapy with penicillamine may be continued in the presence of the lesions. They may not recur if dosage is reduced. Other related effects are excessive wrinkling of the skin and development of small, white papules at venipuncture and surgical sites.

Monitoring: When indicated, monitor drug toxicity or efficacy through urinalysis. In rheumatoid arthritis patients, discontinue the drug if unexplained gross hematuria or persistent microscopic hematuria develops. Perform liver function tests every 6 months for the duration of therapy because of rare reports of intrahepatic cholestasis and toxic hepatitis, and an annual x–ray for renal stones.

Because of the potential for serious adverse hematological and renal reactions, monitor white and differential blood cell count, hemoglobin determination, and direct platelet count every 2 weeks for the first 6 months of penicillamine therapy and monthly thereafter.

Drug Interactions:

Penicillamine Drug Interactions

Precipitant drug	Object drug*		Description
Penicillamine	Gold therapy, antimalarial or cytotoxic drugs, oxyphenbutazone or pheylbutazone	↑	These drugs should not be used in patients who are concurrently receiving penicillamine. These drugs are associated with similar serious hematologic and renal reactions.
Penicillamine	Gold salts	↑	Patients who have had **gold salt** therapy discontinued due to a major toxic reaction may be at greater risk of serious adverse reactions with penicillamine, but not necessarily of the same type. However, this is controversial.
Iron salts	Penicillamine	↓	The absorption of penicillamine is decreased by 35% with coadministration of iron salts.
Antacids	Penicillamine	↓	The absorption of penicillamine is decreased by 66% with coadminstration of antacids.
Penicillamine	Digoxin	↓	Digoxin serum levels may be reduced, possibly decreasing its pharmacological effects. The digoxin dose may need to be increased.

* ↑ = Object drug increased. ↓ = Object drug decreased.

Drug/Food interactions: The absorption of penicillamine is decreased by 52% when taken with food.

Adverse Reactions:

Penicillamine has a high incidence (over 50%) of untoward reactions, some of which are potentially fatal. Medical supervision throughout administration is mandatory.

PENICILLAMINE

Hypersensitivity: Generalized pruritus, early and late rashes (5% to 50%); lupus erythematosus-like syndrome (2%), similar to other drug-induced lupus; pemphigoid-type reactions; drug eruptions (may be accompanied by fever, arthralgia or lymphadenopathy); urticaria and exfoliative dermatitis; thyroiditis and hypoglycemia (extremely rare); migratory polyarthralgia, often with objective synovitis; polymyositis (some fatal); Goodpasture's syndrome (a severe and ultimately fatal glomerular nephritis associated with intra-alveolar hemorrhage); allergic alveolitis; obliterative bronchiolitis.

CNS: Tinnitus; myashenia gravis; polyradiculopathy (rare); peripheral sensory and motor neuropathies (including polyradiculoneuropathy). Muscular weakness may or may not occur with the peripheral neuropathies. Reversible optic neuritis with racemic penicillamine (may be related to pyridoxine deficiency).

GI: Anorexia, epigastric pain, nausea, vomiting or occasional diarrhea (17%); blunting, diminution or total loss of taste perception (12%); intrahepatic cholestasis and toxic hepatitis (rare); cheilosis, glossitis and gingivostomatitis (rare); stomatitis; reactivated peptic ulcer; hepatic dysfunction; pancreatitis; increased serum alkaline phosphatase and lactic dehydrogenase (LDH), positive cephalin flocculation and thymol turbidity tests; oral ulcerations; colitis; altered taste perception.

Hematologic: Thrombocytopenia (4%); leukopenia (2%); bone marrow depression; sideroblastic anemia.

Thrombotic thrombocytopenic purpura, hemolytic anemia, red cell aplasia, monocytosis, leukocytosis, eosinophilia and thrombocytosis (see Warnings).

There have been reports associating penicillamine with leukemia; a cause and effect relationship has not been established.

Renal: Proteinuria (6%) or hematuria which may progress to the nephrotic syndrome as a result of an immune complex membranous glomerulopathy.

Miscellaneous:

Rare – Thrombophlebitis; hyperpyrexia; falling hair or alopecia; lichen planus; myasthenia gravis; dermatomyositis; mammary hyperplasia; elastosis perforans serpiginosa; toxic epidermal necrolysis; anetoderma (cutaneous macular atrophy); fatal renal vasculitis; interstitial pneumonitis and pulmonary fibrosis; bronchial asthma; hot flashes.

Increased skin friability, excessive wrinkling of skin and development of small white papules at venipuncture and surgical sites have been reported. Penicillamine toxicity may be twice as common in elderly patients. The drug's chelating action may cause increased excretion of other heavy metals (eg, zinc, mercury, lead).

Patient Information:

Take on an empty stomach, 1 hour before or 2 hours after meals and at least 1 hour apart from any other drug, food or milk.

Patients with cystinuria should drink copious amounts of water.

Notify physician if skin rash, unusual bruising or bleeding, sore throat, exertional dyspnea, unexplained coughing/wheezing, fever, chills, or other unusual effects occur.

Administration and Dosage:

Give penicillamine on an empty stomach at least 1 hour before meals or 2 hours after meals and at least 1 hour apart from any other drug, food or milk.

Wilson's disease: Initial dosage is 1 g/day for children or adults. This may be increased, as indicated by the urinary copper analyses, but it is seldom necessary to exceed 2 g/day. In patients who cannot tolerate 1 g/day initially, initiating dosage with 250 mg/day and increasing gradually allows closer control of the drug.

Determine optimal dosage by measuring urinary copper excretion. Quantitatively analyze for copper before and soon after initiating therapy. Perform 24 hour urinary copper analysis every 3 months for duration of therapy. The patient probably will be in a negative copper balance of 0.5 to 1 mg copper present in a 24–hour urine collection.

Cystinuria: Adult dosage – 2 g/day (range 1 to 4 g/day).

Pediatric dosage – 30 mg/kg/day in 4 divided doses. If 4 equal doses are not feasible, give the larger portion at bedtime. If adverse reactions necessitate a reduction in dosage, it is important to retain the bedtime dose. Initiating dosage with 250 mg/day, and increasing gradually, allows closer control of the drug and may reduce the incidence of adverse reactions.

Patients should drink about a pint of fluid at bedtime and another pint once during the night when urine is more concentrated and more acid than during the day. The greater the fluid intake, the lower the dosage of penicillamine required.

PENICILLAMINE

Individualize dosage to limit cystine excretion to 100 to 200 mg/day in those with no history of stones, and below 100 mg/day in those who have had stone formation or pain. Consider the inherent tubular defect and the patient's size, age and rate of growth, as well as diet and water intake.

Rheumatoid arthritis – 2 or 3 months may be required before a clinical response is noted.

When treatment has been interrupted because of adverse reactions or other reasons, cautiously reintroduce the drug at a lower dosage and increase slowly.

Initial therapy – A single daily dose of 125 or 250 mg. Thereafter, increase dose at 1 to 3 month intervals by 125 or 250 mg/day as patient response and tolerance indicate. If satisfactory remission is achieved, continue the dose. If there is no improvement and if there are no signs of potentially serious toxicity after 2 to 3 months with doses of 500 to 750 mg/day, continue increases of 250 mg/day at 2 to 3 month intervals until satisfactory remission occurs or toxicity develops. If there is no discernible improvement after 3 to 4 months of treatment with 1 to 1.5 g/day, assume the patient will not respond and discontinue the drug.

Maintenance therapy – Individualize dosage. Many patients respond to 500 to 750 mg/day or less. Changes in dosage level may not be reflected clinically or in the erythrocyte sedimentation rate for 2 to 3 months after each adjustment. Some patients will subsequently require an increase in dosage to achieve maximal disease suppression. In patients who respond but who evidence incomplete disease suppression after the first 6 to 9 months of treatment, increase daily dosage by 125 or 250 mg/day at 3 month intervals. Dosage above 1 g/day is unusual, but up to 1.5 g/day has been required.

Management of exacerbations – Following an initial good response, some patients may experience a self-limited exacerbation of disease activity which can subside within 12 weeks. They are usually controlled by adding nonsteroidal anti-inflammatory drugs. Consider an increase in maintenance dose only if the patient has demonstrated a true "escape" phenomenon (as evidenced by failure of the flare to subside within this time period).

Migratory polyarthralgia due to penicillamine is extremely difficult to differentiate from an exacerbation of the rheumatoid arthritis. Discontinuation or substantial reduction in dosage for several weeks will usually determine which of these processes is responsible for the arthralgia.

Duration of therapy has not been determined. If the patient has been in remission for 6 months or more, attempt a gradual, stepwise dosage reduction in decrements of 125 or 250 mg/day at approximately 3 month intervals.

Concomitant drug therapy – See Drug Interactions. Salicylates, other nonsteroidal anti-inflammatory drugs or systemic corticosteroids may be continued when penicillamine is initiated. After improvement begins, analgesic and anti-inflammatory drugs may be discontinued slowly as symptoms permit. Months of penicillamine treatment may be required before steroids can be completely eliminated.

Dosage frequency – Dosages ≤ 500 mg/day can be given as a single daily dose. Dosages > 500 mg/day should be administered in divided doses.

Alternative dosage forms:

Elixir 50 mg/ml – Dissolve 48 capsules in 100 ml of water. Filter and stir in 100 ml of cherry syrup and 30 ml of alcohol. Bring the volume up to 240 ml with water. Shake well and store in the refrigerator.

Suppositories 750 mg – Melt 51 g of cocoa butter. Dissolve 150 capsules in the cocoa butter. Pour the mixture into a pre-lubricated suppository mold. Freeze, then store in the refrigerator.

Storage/Stability: Store at room temperature 15° to 30°C (59° to 86°F). Protect from moisture.

Rx	**Cuprimine** (Merck)	**Capsules:** 125 mg	Lactose. (MSD 672). Opaque yellow and gray. In 100s.
	Cuprimine (MSD)		Lactose. (MSD 672). Opaque yellow and gray. In 100s.
Rx	**Cuprimine** (Merck)	250 mg	Lactose. (MSD 602). Ivory. In 100s.
	Cuprimine (MSD)		Lactose. (MSD 602). Ivory. In 100s.
Rx	**Depen** (Wallace)	**Tablets, titratable:** 250 mg	Lactose, EDTA. (37-4401). White. Oval. Scored. In 100s.

BETAINE ANHYDROUS

Actions:

Pharmacology: Betaine acts as a methyl group donor in the remethylation of homocysteine to methionine in patients with homocystinuria. As a result, toxic blood levels of homocysteine are reduced in these patients, usually 20% to 80% or less of pretreatment levels.

Elevated homocysteine blood levels are associated with clinical problems such as cardiovascular thrombosis, osteoporosis, skeletal abnormalities and optic lens dislocation. Plasma levels of homocysteine were decreased in nearly all patients treated with betaine. In observational studies without concurrent controls, clinical improvement was reported by physicians in ≈ ¾ of patients taking betaine. Many of these patients were also taking other therapies such as vitamin B_6 (pyridoxine), vitamin B_{12} (cyanocobalamin) and folate with variable biochemical responses. In most cases, adding betaine resulted in a further reduction in homocysteine.

Betaine lowers plasma homocysteine levels in the three types of homocystinuria: Cystathionine beta-synthase (CBS) deficiency; 5,10–methylenetetrahydrofolate reductase (MTHFR) deficiency; and cobalamin cofactor metabolism (cbl) defect.

Betaine has also increased low plasma methionine and S-adenosylmethionine (SAM) levels in patients with MTHFR deficiency and cbl defect.

In CBS-deficient patients, large increases in methionine levels have been observed. However, the increased methionine levels do not appear to have been associated with adverse clinical consequences.

Betaine occurs naturally in the body. It is a metabolite of choline and is present in small amounts in foods (eg, beets, spinach, cereals and seafood).

Pharmacokinetics: The onset of action is within several days and a steady state in response to dosage is achieved within several weeks. Patients have taken betaine for many years without evidence of tolerance.

Indications:

Homocystinuria: Betaine is indicated for the treatment of homocystinuria to decrease elevated homocysteine blood levels. Included within the category of homocystinuria are deficiencies or defects in: 1) Cystathionine beta-synthase (CBS); 2) 5,10–methylenetetrahydrofolate reductase (MTHFR); and 3) cobalamin cofactor metabolism (cbl).

Betaine has been administered concomitantly with vitamin B_6 (pyridoxine), vitamin B_{12} (cyanocobalamin) and folate.

Warnings:

Pregnancy: Category C. It is not known whether betaine can cause fetal harm when administered to a pregnant woman or can affect reproductive capacity. Give to a pregnant woman only if clearly needed.

Lactation: It is not known whether betaine is excreted in breast milk. Its metabolic precursor, choline, occurs at high levels in breast milk. Exercise caution when administering to a nursing woman.

Children: The majority of case studies of homocystinuria patients treated wih betaine have been pediatric patients. The disorder, in its most severe form, can be manifested within the first months or years of life by lethargy, failure to thrive, developmental delays, seizures or optic lens displacement. Patients have been treated successfully without adverse effects within the first months or years of life with dosages ≥ 6 g/day with resultant biochemical and clinical improvement. However, dosage titration may be preferable in pediatric patients (see Dosage and Administration).

BETAINE ANHYDROUS

Adverse Reactions:

Betaine Anhydrous Adverse Reactions	
Adverse reaction	n = 111
Nausea	2
GI distress	2
Diarrhea	1
Aspirated the powder	1
Caused odor	1
Questionable psychological changes	1
Unspecified problem	1

Overdosage:

In an acute toxicology study in rats, death frequently occurred at doses ≥ 10,000 mg/kg.

Patient Information:

Shake bottle lightly before removing cap.

Measure with the scoop provided.

One level scoop (1.7 ml) is equivalent to 1 g of betaine anhydrous powder. Measure the number of scoops your physician has prescribed.

Mix with 120 to 180 ml (4 to 6 oz) of water until completely dissolved, then drink immediately.

Always replace the cap tightly after using. Protect from moisture. Do not use if powder does not completely dissolve or gives a colored solution.

Administration and Dosage:

The usual dosage used in adult and pediatric patients is 6 g/day administered orally in divided doses of 3 g twice daily. Dosages of up to 20 g/day have been necessary to control homocysteine levels in some patients. In pediatric patients < 3 years of age, dosage may be started at 100 mg/kg/day and then increased weekly by 100 mg/kg increments. Dosage in all patients can be gradually increased until plasma homocysteine is undetectable or present only in small amounts.

Measure prescribed amount with the measuring scoop provided (one level 1.7 ml scoop is equal to 1 g of betaine anhydrous powder) and then dissolve in 120 to 180 ml (4 to 6 oz) of water for immediate ingestion.

Storage/Stability: Store at room temperature, 15° to 30°C (59° to 86°F).

Rx	**Cystadane** (Orphan Medical)	**Powder:** 1 g/1.7 ml	White, granular. In 180 g bottles.

TIOPRONIN

Actions:

Pharmacology: Tiopronin is an active reducing and complexing thiol compound for the prevention of cystine (kidney) stone formation. It undergoes thiol-disulfide exchange with cystine to form a mixed disulfide of tiopronin-cysteine; a water-soluble mixed disulfide is formed and the amount of sparingly soluble cystine is reduced.

Cystine stones typically occur in ≈ 10,000 persons in the US who are homozygous for cystinuria. These persons excrete abnormal amounts of cystine in urine, as well as excessive amounts of other dibasic amino acids (eg, lysine, arginine, ornithine). They also show varying intestinal transport defects for these same amino acids. Stone formation is the result of poor aqueous solubility of cystine and is determined primarily by the urinary supersaturation of cystine. Thus, cystine stones, theoretically, form whenever urinary cystine concentration exceeds the solubility limit. Cystine solubility in urine is pH-dependent and ranges from 170 to 300 mg/L at pH 5, 190 to 400 mg/L at pH 7, and 220 to 500 mg/L at pH 7.5.

The goal of therapy is to reduce urinary cystine concentration below its solubility limit. It may be accomplished by dietary means to reduce cystine synthesis and by a high fluid intake to increase urine volume and thereby lower cystine concentration. These conservative measures alone may be ineffective. In some homozygous patients with severe cystinuria, d-penicillamine has been used as an additional therapy. However, d-penicillamine treatment is frequently accompanied by adverse reactions.

Pharmacokinetics: Up to 48% of a dose appears in urine during the first 4 hours and up to 78% by 72 hours. Thus, in patients with cystinuria, a sufficient amount of tiopronin or its active metabolites could appear in urine to react with cystine, lowering cystine excretion.

The decrement in urinary cystine produced by tiopronin is generally proportional to the dose. A reduction in urinary cystine of 250 to 350 mg/day and 500 mg/day at a dosage of 1 and 2 g/day, respectively, might be expected. Tiopronin causes a sustained reduction in cystine excretion without loss of effectiveness. It has a rapid onset and offset ofaction, showing a fall in cystine excretion on the first day of administration and a rise on the first day of drug withdrawal.

Clinical trials:

Versus penicillamine – A multiclinic trial involving 66 cystinuric patients indicated that tiopronin is associated with fewer or less severe adverse reactions than d-penicillamne. Among those stopping d-penicillamine because of toxicity, 64.7% could take tiopronin. In those without a history of d-penicillamine treatment, only 5.9% developed reactions of sufficient severity to require tiopronin withdrawal.

Indications:

Kidney stones Prevention of cystine (kidney) stone formation in patients with severe homozygous cystinuria with urinary cystine > 500 mg/day, who are resistant to treatment with conservative measures of high fluid intake, alkali and diet modification or who have adverse reactions to d-penicillamine.

Contraindications:

History of agrnulocytosis, aplastic anemia or thrombocytopenia on this medication; pregnancy, lactation (see Warnings).

Warnings:

Fatalities from tiopronin are possible (but not reported), as has been reported with d-penicillamine from such complications as aplastic anemia, agranulocytosis, thrombocytopenia, Goodpasture's syndrome or myasthenia gravis.

Hepatotoxicity: Jaundice and abnormal liver function tests have been reported during tiopronin therapy for non-cystinuric conditions. A direct cause and effect relationship, based upon these foreign reports, has not been established. Monitor patients carefully. If any abnormalities are noted, discontinue the drug and treat the patient with appropriate measures.

Hematologic Leukopenia of the granulocytic series may develop without eosinophilia. Thrombocytopenia may be immunologic in origin or idiosyncratic. The reduction in peripheral blood white count to < 3500/mm³ or in platelet count to < 100,000/mm³ mandates cessation of therapy. Instruct patients to report promptly any symptom or sign of these hematological abnormalities, such as fever, sore throat, chills, bleeding or easy bruisability.

Proteinuria, sometimes sufficiently severe to cause nephrotic syndrome, may develop from membranous glomerulopathy. Closely observe patients is mandatory.

TIOPRONIN

Complications (rare) have occurred during d-penicillamine therapy and could occur during tiopronin treatment. Stop therapy if the following occurs: Abnormal urinary findings with hemoptysis and pulmonary infiltrates suggestive of Goodpasture's syndrome; appearance of myasthenic syndrome or myasthenia gravis; development of pemphigus-type reactions. Steroid treatment may be necessary.

Drug fever may develop, usually during the first month of therapy; discontinue until the fever subsides. Treatment may be reinstated at a small dose, with a gradual increase in dosage until the desired level is achieved.

Rash: Generalized rash (erythematous, maculopapular or morbilliform) accompanied by pruritis may develop during the first few months of treatment. It may be controlled by antihistamine therapy, typically recedes when tiopronin is discontinued and seldom recurs when tiopronin is restarted at a lower dosage. Less commonly, rash may appear late in treatment (after > 6 months). Usually located on the trunk, the late rash is associated with intense pruritis, recedes slowly after discontinuing treatment and usually recurs upon resumption of treatment.

Lupus erythematous-like reaction manifested by fever, arthralgia and lymphadenopathy may develop. It may be associated with a positive antinuclear antibody test, but not necessarily with nephropathy. It may require discontinuance of treatment.

Pregnancy: Category C. Skeletal defects and cleft palates occur in the fetus when d-penicillamine is given to pregnant rats at 10 times the dose recommended for humans. A similar teratogenicity might be expected for tiopronin. There are no adequate and well controlled studies in pregnant women. Use during pregnancy is contraindicated except in those with severe cystinuria.

Lactation: Because tiopronin may be excreted in breast milk and because of potential serious adverse reactions of nursing infants, advise mothers taking tiopronin not to nurse.

Children: Safety and effectiveness in children < 9 years old have not been established.

Precautions:

Monitoring tests are recommended, including: Peripheral blood counts, direct platelet count, hemoglobin, serum albumin, liver function tests, 24-hour urinary protein and routine urinalysis at 3 to 6 month intervals during treatment. In order to assess the effect on stone disease, monitor urinary cystine frequently during the first 6 months when the optimum dose schedule is being determined and at 6 month intervals thereafter. Abdominal roentgenogram (KUB) is advised yearly to monitor the size and appearance of stone(s).

Wrinkling and friability of skin usually occurs after long-term treatment and results from the effect of tiopronin on collagen.

Hypoguesia, often self-limiting, may develop as the result of trace metal chelation by tiopronin.

Vitamin B_6 deficiency is uncommonly associated with tiopronin treatment, unlike during d-penicillamine therapy.

Adverse Reactions:

Dermatologic: Rash, lupus erythematous-like reaction, pruritis, wrinkling, friability (see Precautions and Warnings).

Miscellaneous: Drug fever (see Warnings), hypoguesia, vitamin B_6 deficiency (rare) (see Precautions), jaundice, abnormal liver function tests, myasthenic syndrome (≈ 2%); impairment in taste and smell (≈ 4%).

GI: Nausea, emesis, diarrhea or soft stools, anorexia, abdominal pain, bloating or flatus (≈ 17%).

Hypersensitivity: Laryngeal edema, dyspnea, respiratory distress, fever, chills, arthralgia, weakness, fatigue, myalgia, adenopathy (≈ 4%).

Hematologic: Increased bleeding, anemia, leukopenia, thrombocytopenia, eosinophilia (≈ 4%).

Renal: Proteinuria, nephrotic syndrome, hematuria (≈ 1%).

Respiratory: Bronchiolitis, hemoptysis, pulmonary infiltrates, dyspnea (≈ 2%).Despite this apparent reduced toxicity to tiopronin relative to d-penicillamine, tiopronin treatment may potentially be associated with all adverse reactions reported with d-penicillamine.

These reactions are more likely to develop during tiopronin therpy among patients who have previously shown toxicity to d-penicillamine.

TIOPRONIN

Administration and Dosage:

Attempt a conservative treatment program first. Provide at least 3 L of fluid, including two glasses with each meal and at bedtime. Advise the patient to awake at night to urinate and to drink two more glasses of fluids before returning to bed. Consume additional fluids if there is excessive sweating or intestinal fluid loss. Seek a minimum urine output of 2 L/day on a consistent basis. Provide a modest amount of alkali in order to maintain urinary pH at a high normal range (6.5 to 7).

Adverse reactions to d-penicillamine: Patients who previously manifested adverse reactions to d-penicillamine, are more likely to experience adverse reactions to tiopronin than patients who take tiopronin for the first time. A close supervision with a careful monitoring of potential side effects is mandatory during tiopronin treatment. Advise patients to report promptly any symptoms suggesting toxicity. Discontinue treatment if severe toxicity develops.

Excessive alkali therapy is not advisable. When urinary pH increases > 7 with alkali therapy, calcium phosphate nephrolithiasis may ensue because of the enhanced urinary supersaturation of hydroxyapatite in an alkaline environment. Potassium alkali are advantageous over sodium alkali because they do not cause hypercalciuria and are less likely to cause the complication of calcium stones.

In patients who continue to form cystine stones on the above conservative program, tiopronin may be added. Tiopronin may also be substituted for d-penicillamine in patients who have developed toxicity to the latter drug. In both situations, continue the conservative treatment program.

Base tiopronin dosage on the amount required to reduce urinary cystine concentration to below its solubility limit (generally < 250 mg/L). The extent of the decline in cystine excretion is generally dosage dependent.

Initial adult dosage: 800 mg/day in adults with cystine stones; average dose is 1000 mg/day. However, some patients require less.

Children: Initial dosage may be based on 15 mg/kg/day. Measure urinary cystine 1 month after treatment and every 3 months thereafter. Readjust dosage depending on urinary cystine value. Whenever possible, give in divided doses 3 times/day at least 1 hour before or 2 hours after meals.

In patients with severe toxicity to d-penicillamine, initiate tiopronin at a lower dosage.

Rx	**Thiola** (Mission)	**Tablets:** 100 mg	White, sugar coated. In 100s.

ANTICHOLINESTERASE MUSCLE STIMULANTS

Actions:

Pharmacology: These drugs facilitate transmission of impulses across the myoneural junction by inhibiting the destruction of acetylcholine by cholinesterase. They differ in duration of action and in adverse effects. Equivalent doses, onset and duration of action are summarized below.

Drug	Route	Equivalent Dosage (mg)	Onset (min)	Duration (hours)	Indications
Pyridostigmine	PO	60	20-30	3-6	Myasthenia gravis
	IM	2	< 15	2-4	Myasthenia gravis
	IV	2	2-5	2-4	Myasthenia gravis; Nondepolarizing muscle relaxant antagonist
Ambenonium	PO	5-10	20-30	3-8	Myasthenia gravis
Neostigmine	PO	15	45-75	2-4	Myasthenia gravis
	IM	1.5	20-30	2-4	Myasthenia gravis
	IV	0.5	4-8	2-4	Diagnosis myasthenia gravis; Nondepolarizing muscle relaxant antagonist
Edrophonium	IM	10	2-10	0.17-0.67	Diagnosis myasthenia gravis
	IV	10	< 1	0.08-0.33	Diagnosis myasthenia gravis;[1] Nondepolarizing muscle relaxant antagonist

[1] Also used to evaluate treatment requirements in myasthenia gravis.

Indications:

Myasthenia gravis: Treatment of myasthenia gravis.

Urinary retention: The prevention and treatment of postoperative distention and urinary retention after mechanical obstruction has been excluded.

Reversal of nondepolarizing muscle relaxants (**pyridostigmine** and **neostigmine**).

Unlabeled uses: Diagnosis of myasthenia gravis (0.022 mg/kg/dose IM × 1).

Contraindications:

Hypersensitivity to anticholinesterases; mechanical intestinal and urinary obstructions; peritonitis (**neostigmine**); history of reaction to bromides (**neostigmine** and **pyridostigmine**).

Warnings:

Use with caution in patients with bronchial asthma, epilepsy, bradycardia, recent coronary occlusion, vagotonia, hyperthyroidism, cardiac arrhythmias or peptic ulcer. Treat transient bradycardia with atropine sulfate. Isolated instances of cardiac and respiratory arrest, believed to be vagotonic effects, have occurred. When large doses are given, prior or simultaneous injection of atropine sulfate may be advisable. Use separate syringes.

Cholinergic/Masthenic crisis: Overdosage may result in cholinergic crisis, characterized by increasing muscle weakness that, through involvement of the respiratory muscles, may lead to death. Myasthenic crisis because of an increase in disease severity is also accompanied by extreme muscle weakness and may be difficult to distinguish from cholinergic crisis. Differentiation is extremely important; use **edrophonium** and clinical judgment.

Treatment of the two conditions differs radically: Myasthenic crisis requires more intensive anticholinesterase therapy; cholinergic crisis calls for withdrawal of all drugs of this type and immediate use of atropine. Have a syringe containing 1 mg of atropine sulfate immediately available to be given IV to counteract severe cholinergic reactions. Use atropine to abolish or blunt GI side effects or other muscarinic reactions; however, such use may lead to inadvertent induction of cholinergic crisis by masking signs of overdosage.

Used as antagonists to nondepolarizing muscle relaxants: Obtain adequate recovery of voluntary respiration and neuromuscular transmission prior to discontinuing respiratory assistance. Observe continuously. If there is doubt concerning adequacy of recovery from the nondepolarizing muscle relaxant, continue artificial ventilation.

Supervision: Great care and supervision are required with **ambenonium**. Because ambenonium has a more prolonged action than other antimyasthenic drugs, simultaneous use with other cholinergics is contraindicated except under strict supervision. Therefore, when a patient is to be given the drug, suspend use of all other cholinergics until the patient has been stabilized.

Hypersensitivity: Because of possible hypersensitivity in an occasional patient, have atropine and epinephrine readily available when using parenteral therapy.

ANTICHOLINESTERASE MUSCLE STIMULANTS

Pregnancy: (*Category C* – **neostigmine.**) Safety for use during pregnancy has not been established. Transient muscular weakness occurred in ≈ 20% of infants born to mothers treated with these drugs during pregnancy. Use only when clearly needed and when the potential benefits outweigh the potential hazards to the fetus.

Anticholinesterase drugs may cause uterine irritability and induce premature labor when given IV to pregnant women near term.

Lactation: **Pyridostigmine** is excreted in breast milk. Because they are ionized at physiologic pH, **ambenonium** and **neostigmine** would not be expected to be excreted in breast milk.

Children: Safety and efficacy for use of **neostigmine** in children are not established.

Precautions:

Anticholinesterase insensitivity may develop for brief or prolonged periods. Carefully monitor the patient; respiratory assistance may be needed. Reduce or withhold dosages until the patient again becomes sensitive.

Drug Interactions:

Anticholinesterase Muscle Stimulants Drug Interactions

Precipitant drug	Object drug *		Description
Anticholinesterase muscle stimulants	Anticholinesterase drugs	⬆	Exercise caution in patients with myasthenic symptoms who are receiving other anticholinesterase muscle stimulants. Because symptoms of anticholinesterase overdose (cholinergic crisis) may mimic underdosage (myasthenic weakness), the condition may be worsened.
Anticholinesterase muscle stimulants	Succinylcholine	⬆	Neuromuscular blocking effects may be increased. Prolonged respiratory depression with extended periods of apnea may occur. Provide respiratory support as needed.
Aminoglycoside antibiotics (eg, neomycin, streptomycin, kenamycin)	Anticholinesterase muscle stimulants	⬆	Aminoglycoside antibiotics have a mild but definite nondepolarizing blocking action which may accentuate neuromuscular block.
Local and general anesthetics, Antiarrhythmics	Anticholinesterase muscle stimulants	⬇	Use cautiously, if at all, in patients with myasthenia gravis. The neostigmine dose may have to be increased accordingly.
Atropine Belladonna derivatives	Anticholinesterase muscle stimulants	⬆	Routine administration of these agents may suppress the parasympathomimetic (muscarinic) symptoms of excessive GI stimulation leaving only the more serious symptoms of fasciculation and paralysis of voluntary muscles as signs of overdosage.
Corticosteroids	Anticholinesterase muscle stimulants	⬇	May decrease the anticholinesterase effects of these agents. Conversely, anticholinesterase effects may increase after stopping corticosteroids. Provide respiratory support as needed.
Depolarizing muscle relaxants (eg, succinylcholine, decamethonium)	Anticholinesterase muscle stimulants	⬆	Neostigmine may prolong the Phase I block of these drugs. Use these drugs in myasthenic patients only when definitely indicated. Carefully adjust the anticholinesterase dosage.
Magnesium	Anticholinesterase muscle stimulants	⬇	Magnesium has a direct depressant effect on skeletal muscle, and it may antagonize the beneficial effects of anticholinesterase therapy.
Mecamylamine	Anticholinesterase muscle stimulants	⬆	Do not administer to patients receiving this ganglionic blocking agent.
Methocarbamol	Anticholinesterase muscle stimulants	⬇	A single case report indicates this drug may have impaired the effect of **pyridostigmine** in a patient with myasthenia gravis.

* ⬆ = Object drug increased. ⬇ = Object drug decreased.

ANTICHOLINESTERASE MUSCLE STIMULANTS

Adverse Reactions:

Cardiovascular: Arrhythmias (especially bradycardia); fall in cardiac output leading to hypotension; tachycardia; AV block; nodal rhythm; nonspecific EKG changes; cardiac arrest; syncope.

CNS: Convulsions; dysarthria; dysphonia; dizziness; loss of consciousness; drowsiness; headache.

Dermatologic: Skin rash (**pyridostigmine** and **neostigmine**; subsides upon discontinuance); thrombophlebitis (IV).

GI: Increased salivary, gastric and intestinal secretions; nausea; vomiting; dysphagia; increased peristalsis; diarrhea; abdominal cramps; flatulence.

Hypersensitivity: Allergic reactions and anaphylaxis.

Musculoskeletal: Weakness; fasciculations; muscle cramps and spasms; arthralgia.

Respiratory: Increased tracheobronchial secretions; laryngospasm; bronchiolar constriction; respiratory muscle paralysis; central respiratory paralysis; dyspnea; respiratory depression; respiratory arrest; bronchospasm.

Miscellaneous: Urinary frequency and incontinence; urinary urgency; diaphoresis; rash; urticaria; flushing; alopecia (**pyridostigmine**).

Overdosage:

Symptoms: When the drug produces overstimulation, the clinical picture is one of increasing parasympathomimetic action that is more or less characteristic when not masked by the use of atropine. Signs and symptoms of overdosage, including cholinergic crises, vary considerably. They are usually manifested by increasing GI stimulation with epigastric distress, abdominal cramps, diarrhea and vomiting, excessive salivation, pallor, cold sweating, urinary urgency, blurring of vision and eventually fasciculation and paralysis of voluntary muscles, including those of the tongue (thick tongue and difficulty in swallowing), shoulder, neck and arms. Miosis, increase in blood pressure with or without bradycardia and subjective sensations of internal trembling, and often severe anxiety and panic may complete the picture. A cholinergic crisis is usually differentiated from the weakness and paralysis of myasthenia gravis insufficiently treated by cholinergic drugs by the fact that myasthenic weakness is not accompanied by any of the above signs and symptoms, except the last two subjective ones (anxiety and panic).

Treatment: Because the warning of overdosage is minimal, the existence of a narrow margin between the first appearance of side effects and serious toxic effects must be borne in mind constantly. If signs of overdosage occur (excessive GI stimulation, excessive salivation, miosis and more serious fasciculations of voluntary muscles), discontinue temporarily all cholinergic medication and administer from 0.5 to 1 mg (1/120 to 1/60 grain) of atropine IV. A total atropine dose of 5 to 10 mg or more may be required. Give other supportive treatment as indicated (artificial respiration, tracheotomy, oxygen, etc).

Patient Information:

Notify physician if nausea, vomiting, diarrhea, sweating, increased salivary secretions, irregular heartbeat, muscle weakness, severe abdominal pain or difficulty in breathing occurs.

Anticholinesterase Muscle Stimulants

PYRIDOSTIGMINE BROMIDE

For complete prescribing information, refer to the Cholinergic Muscle Stimulants group monograph.

Indications:

Myasthenia gravis: Treatment of myasthenia gravis.

Reversal of nondepolarizing muscle relaxants such as curariform drugs and gallamine triethiodide (IV).

Administration and Dosage:

Myasthenia gravis:

Oral – Individualize dosage.

Adults: 600 mg/day (range, 60 to 1500 mg), spaced to provide maximum relief.

Children: 7 mg/kg/24 hours orally divided into 5 or 6 doses; 0.05 to 0.15 mg/kg/dose IM or IV.

Sustained release tablets: 180 to 540 mg once or twice daily. Individual needs vary markedly. Use dosage intervals of ≥ 6 hours. Do not crush or chew. For optimum control, rapidly acting regular tablets or syrup may also be needed.

Parenteral – To supplement oral dosage preoperatively and postoperatively, during labor and postpartum, during myasthenic crisis or when oral therapy is impractical, give ≈ 1/30 the oral dose, either IM or very slowly IV. Observe patient closely for cholinergic reactions, particularly if the IV route is used.

Neonates of myasthenic mothers may have transient difficulty in swallowing, sucking and breathing. Injectable pyridostigmine may be indicated (by symptoms and use of the edrophonium test) until syrup can be taken. Dosage requirements range from 0.05 to 0.15 mg/kg IM. It is important to differentiate between cholinergic and myasthenic crises in neonates.

Pyridostigmine, given parenterally 1 hour before second stage labor is complete, enables patients to have adequate strength during labor and provides protection to infants in the immediate postnatal state.

Reversal of nondepolarizing muscle relaxants: Give atropine sulfate (0.6 to 1.2 mg) IV immediately prior to pyridostigmine to minimize side effects. Reversal dosages range from 0.1 to 0.25 mg/kg. Pyridostigmine 10 or 20 mg IV is usually sufficient. Full recovery usually occurs ≤ 15 minutes, but ≥ 30 minutes may be required. Satisfactory reversal is evident by adequate voluntary respiration, respiratory measurements and use of a peripheral nerve stimulator device. Keep patient well ventilated and maintain a patent airway until complete recovery of normal respiration.

Once satisfactory reversal has been attained, recurarization has not been reported. Failure of pyridostigmine injection to provide prompt (≤ 30 minutes) reversal may occur (eg, extreme debilitation, carcinomatosis, or with concomitant use of certain broad-spectrum antibiotics or anesthetic agents, notably ether).

Rx	**Mestinon** (ICN)	**Tablets:** 60 mg	(Mestinon 60 Roche). In 100s and 500s.
		Tablets, sustained release 180 mg	(Roche 34). In 100s.
		Syrup: 60 mg/5 ml	5% alcohol. Sorbitol. Raspberry flavor. In 480 ml.
Rx	**Mestinon** (ICN)	**Injection:** 5 mg/ml	In 2 ml amps.[1]
Rx	**Regonol** (Organon)		In 2 ml amps[2] and 5 ml vials.[2]

[1] With 0.2% methyl and propyl parabens.
[2] With 1% benzyl alcohol.

Anticholinesterase Muscle Stimulants

AMBENONIUM CHLORIDE

For complete prescribing information, refer to the Cholinergic Muscle Stimulants group monograph.

Indications:

Myasthenia gravis: Treatment of myasthenia gravis.

Administration and Dosage:

Individualize dosage. The amount of medication necessary to control symptoms may fluctuate in each patient. Because maximum therapeutic effectiveness (optimal muscle strength and no GI disturbances) is highly critical, closely supervise.

Ambenonium has a longer duration of action than other agents and requires administration only every 3 or 4 hours, depending on clinical response. Medication is usually not required throughout the night.

Moderately severe myasthenia: 5 to 25 mg 3 or 4 times daily (range, 5 mg to 75 mg/dose). Start with 5 mg and increase gradually to determine optimum dose. Adjust at 1 to 2 day intervals to avoid drug accumulation and overdosage.

A few patients require greater doses for adequate control, but increasing dosage > 200 mg daily requires exacting supervision to avoid overdosage.

Edrophonium may be used to evaluate adequacy of maintenance dose. See the edrophonium monograph.

Rx	**Mytelase** (Sanofi Winthrop)	**Tablets:** 10 mg	Scored. In 100s.

NEOSTIGMINE

For complete prescribing information, refer to the Cholinergic Muscle Stimulants group monograph.

Indications:

Symptomatic control of myasthenia gravis: In acute myasthenic crisis where difficulty in breathing and swallowing is present, use the parenteral form.

Antidote for nondepolarizing neuromuscular blocking agents (eg, tubocurarine, metocurine, gallamine or pancuronium) after surgery.

Urinary retention: Prevention and treatment of postoperative distention and urinary retention after mechanical obstruction has been excluded.

For additional indications refer to Neostigmine Methylsulfate monograph.

Administration and Dosage:

Symptomatic control of myasthenia gravis:

Oral – 15 to 375 mg/day. Consider possibility of cholinergic crisis before exceeding dosage. The average dosage is 150 mg given over 24 hours; for children, 2 mg/kg/day orally divided every 3 to 4 hours. The interval between doses is of paramount importance; it must be individualized. Frequently, therapy is required day and night. Larger portions of the total daily dose may be given at times of greater fatigue (afternoon, mealtimes, etc).

Parenteral – Inject 1 ml of the 1:2000 solution (0.5 mg) SC or IM. Individualize subsequent doses. For children, 0.01 to 0.04 mg/kg/dose IM, IV or SC every 2 to 3 hours as needed.

Antidote for nondepolarizing neuromuscular blocking agents: When administered IV, also give atropine sulfate (0.6 to 1.2 mg) IV several minutes before the neostigmine. Give 0.5 to 2 mg neostigmine by slow IV injection and repeat as required; however, only in exceptional cases should total dose exceed 5 mg.

Infants – 0.025 to 0.1 mg/kg/dose (doses at low end of range probably are adequate), with atropine (0.01 to 0.04 mg/kg; 0.4 mg for each mg of neostigmine) or glycopyrrolate (0.004 to 0.02 mg/kg; 0.2 mg for each mg of neostigmine).

Children – 0.025 to 0.08 mg/kg/dose, with atropine (0.01 to 0.03 mg/kg; 0.4 mg for each mg of neostigmine) or glycopyrrolate (0.004 to 0.015 mg/kg; 0.2 mg for each mg of neostigmine).

Keep the patient well ventilated and maintain a patent airway until complete recovery. Administer drug when patient is being hyperventilated and the carbon dioxide level of blood is low.

Never administer in the presence of high concentrations of halothane or cyclopropane. In cardiac cases and severely ill patients, titrate the exact dose of neostigmine required using a peripheral nerve stimulator. With bradycardia, increase pulse rate to ≈ 80/minute with atropine before administering neostigmine.

Prevention of postoperative distention and urinary retention: One ml of the 1:4000 solution (0.25 mg) SC or IM as soon as possible after operation; repeat every 4 to 6 hours for 2 or 3 days.

Treatment of postoperative distention: One ml of the 1:2000 solution (0.5 mg) SC or IM as required.

Treatment of urinary retention: One ml of the 1:2000 solution (0.5 mg) SC or IM. If urination does not occur within an hour, catheterize. After the patient has voided, or the bladder has been emptied, continue the 0.5 mg injections every 3 hours for at least 5 injections.

Anticholinesterase Muscle Stimulants

NEOSTIGMINE

Rx	**Prostigmin** (ICN)	**Tablets:** 15 mg	(Prostigmin 15 ICN). White, scored. In 100s.
Rx	**Neostigmine Methylsulfate** (Various)	**Injection:** 1:1000	In 10 ml vials.
Rx	**Prostigmin** (ICN)		In 10 ml vials.[1]
Rx	**Neostigmine Methylsulfate** (Various)	**Injection:** 1:2000	In 1 ml amps and 10 ml vials.
Rx	**Prostigmin** (ICN)		In 1 ml amps[2] and 10 ml vials.
Rx	**Neostigmine Methylsulfate** (Various)	**Injection:** 1:4000	In 1 ml amps.
Rx	**Prostigmin** (ICN)		In 1 ml amps.[2]

[1] With 0.45% phenol.
[2] With 0.2% methyl and propyl parabens.

EDROPHONIUM CHLORIDE

Complete prescribing information for these products begins in the Anticholinesterase Muscle Stimulants group monograph.

Indications:

Differential diagnosis of myasthenia gravis; adjunct in evaluating treatment requirements in myasthenia gravis; evaluate emergency treatment in myasthenic crises. Because of its brief duration of action, it is not useful in maintenance therapy.

Curare antagonist to reverse neuromuscular block produced by curare, tubocurarine or gallamine; adjunct in treating respiratory depression caused by curare overdose.

Administration and Dosage:

Differential diagnosis of myasthenia gravis:

Adults, IV – Prepare tuberculin syringe of 10 mg edrophonium with IV needle. Inject 2 mg IV in 15 to 30 sec. Leave needle in situ. If no reaction occurs after 45 sec, inject remaining 8 mg. If cholinergic reaction (muscarinic side effects, skeletal muscle fasciculations, increased muscle weakness) occurs after 2 mg injection, discontinue test; give atropine sulfate 0.4 to 0.5 mg IV. After 30 min, test may be repeated.

Adults, IM – In adults with inaccessible veins, inject 10 mg IM. Retest subjects who demonstrate hyperreactivity (cholinergic reaction) after 30 minutes with 2 mg IM to rule out false-negative reactions.

Children, IV – Up to 34 kg (75 lbs), 1 mg; > 34 kg (> 75 lbs), 2 mg. If no response after 45 seconds, may titrate up to 5 mg in children < 34 kg (< 75 lbs), and up to 10 mg in heavier children, given in 1 mg increments every 30 to 45 seconds. In infants, give 0.5 mg. Alternatively, the following schedule is recommended: Total dose is 0.2 mg/kg. Give 0.04 mg/kg initially as a test dose, then in 1 mg increments if no reaction occurs within 1 minute. Maximum dose is 10 mg total.

Children, IM – Up to 34 kg (75 lbs), 2 mg; > 34 kg (> 75 lbs), 5 mg. There is a 2 to 10 minute delay in reaction.

Evaluation of treatment requirements in myasthenia gravis: 1 to 2 mg IV 1 hour after oral intake of the treatment drug. Responses are summarized below:

Response to Edrophonium Test in Myasthenia Gravis

Response to edrophonium test	Myasthenic[1]	Adequate[2]	Cholinergic[3]
Muscle strength (ptosis, diplopia, dysphonia, dysphagia, dysarthria, respiration, limb strength)	Increased	No change	Decreased
Fasciculations (orbicularis oculi, facial muscles, limb muscles)	Absent	Present or absent	Present or absent
Side effects (lacrimation, diaphoresis, salivation, abdominal cramps, nausea, vomiting, diarrhea)	Absent	Minimal	Severe

[1] *Myasthenic response:* Occurs in untreated myasthenics and may establish diagnosis; in patients under treatment, it indicates inadequate therapy.
[2] *Adequate response:* Observed in stabilized patients; a typical response in normal individuals. In addition, forced lid closure is often observed in psychoneurotics.
[3] *Cholinergic response:* Seen in myasthenics overtreated with anticholinesterases.

Anticholinesterase Muscle Stimulants

EDROPHONIUM CHLORIDE

Edrophonium test in crisis: When a patient is apneic, secure controlled ventilation immediately. Do not test with edrophonium until respiration is adequate. If patient is *cholinergic,* edrophonium will increase oropharyngeal secretions and further weaken respiratory muscles. If crisis is *myasthenic,* the test clearly improves respiration and the patient can receive a longer acting IV anticholinesterase. Do not have > 2 mg in syringe. Give 1 mg IV initially; carefully observe cardiac response. If, after 1 min, this dose does not further impair the patient, inject the remaining 1 mg. If no clear improvement of respiration occurs after 2 mg, discontinue all anticholinesterase therapy and control ventilation by tracheostomy and assisted respiration.

Curare antagonist: Give 10 mg slowly IV over 30 to 45 seconds to detect onset of cholinergic reaction. Repeat when necessary. Maximal dose is 40 mg. Do not give before use of curare, tubocurarine or gallamine triethiodide; use when needed. When given to counteract curare overdosage, carefully observe the effect of each dose on respiration before repeating, and employ assisted ventilation.

Rx	**Enlon** (Ohmeda)	**Injection:** 10 mg per ml	In 15 ml vials.[1]
Rx	**Reversol** (Organon)		In 10 ml vials (25s).[1]
Rx	**Tensilon** (ICN)		In 1 ml amps,[2] 10 ml vials.[1]

[1] With 0.45% phenol and 0.2% sodium sulfite.
[2] With 0.2% sodium sulfite.

EDROPHONIUM CHLORIDE/ATROPINE SULFATE

Complete prescribing information for these products begins in the Anticholinesterase Muscle Stimulants monograph.

Actions:

Pharmacology: Atropine is added to edrophonium to counteract the unavoidable muscarinic side effects (eg, bradycardia, bronchoconstriction, increased secretions) of edrophonium.

Indications:

As a reversal agent or antagonist of nondepolarizing neuromuscular blocking agents.

Adjunctively in the treatment of respiratory depression caused by curare overdosage.

Not effective against depolarizing neuromuscular blocking agents. Not recommended for use in the differential diagnosis of myasthenia gravis.

Administration and Dosage:

Approved by the FDA on November 6, 1991.

Dosages of edrophonium and atropine injection range from 0.05 to 0.1 ml/kg given slowly over 45 seconds to 1 minute at a point of at least 5% recovery of twitch response to neuromuscular stimulation (95% block). The dosage delivered is 0.5 to 1 mg/kg edrophonium and 0.007 to 0.014 mg/kg atropine. A total dosage of 1 mg/kg edrophonium should rarely be exceeded. Monitor response carefully and secure assisted or controlled ventilation. Satisfactory reversal permits adequate voluntary respiration and neuromuscular transmission (as tested with a peripheral nerve stimulator). Recurarization has not been reported after satisfactory reversal has been attained.

Storage: Store between 15° to 26°C (59° to 78°F).

Rx	**Enlon-Plus** (Ohmeda)	**Injection:** 10 mg edrophonium chloride and 0.14 mg atropine sulfate	In 5 ml amps[1] and 15 ml multidose vials.[2]

[1] With 2 mg sodium sulfite.
[2] With 2 mg sodium sulfite and 4.5 mg phenol.

GUANIDINE HCl

Actions:

Pharmacology: Guanidine enhances the release of acetylcholine following a nerve impulse. It appears to slow the rates of depolarization and repolarization of muscle cell membranes.

Indications:

Myasthenic syndrome of Eaton-Lambert: To reduce symptoms of muscle weakness and easy fatigability associated with myasthenic syndrome of Eaton-Lambert. Not indicated for myasthenia gravis.

Contraindications:

Intolerance or allergy to guanidine.

Warnings:

Fatal bone marrow suppression, apparently dose-related, can occur. Follow baseline blood studies by frequent complete blood cell count (CBC) and differential counts. Discontinue use if bone marrow suppression occurs. Do not continue treatment longer than necessary. Avoid concurrent therapy with other drugs that may cause bone marrow suppression.

Pregnancy: Safety for use during pregnancy has not been established. Use only when clearly needed and when potential benefits outweigh potential hazards to the fetus.

Lactation: Guanidine is excreted in breast milk; discontinue breastfeeding.

Children: Safety for use in children has not been established.

Precautions:

Renal effects: Renal function may be affected in some patients. Perform regular urine examinations and serum creatinine determinations.

Adverse Reactions:

Hematologic: Bone marrow depression with anemia (see Warnings); leukopenia; thrombocytopenia.

CNS: Paresthesia of lips, face, hands, feet; cold sensations in hands, feet; nervousness; lightheadedness; increased irritability; jitteriness; tremor; trembling sensations; ataxia; emotional lability; psychotic state; confusion; mood changes; hallucinations.

GI: Dry mouth; anorexia; gastric irritation; nausea; diarrhea; abdominal cramping. GI side effects may preclude use.

Dermatologic: Rash; flushing or pink complexion; folliculitis; petechiae; purpura; ecchymoses; sweating; skin eruptions; dryness and scaling of the skin.

Renal: Creatinine elevation; uremia; chronic interstitial nephritis; renal tubular necrosis.

Hepatic: Abnormal liver function tests.

Cardiovascular: Palpitations; tachycardia; atrial fibrillation; hypotension.

Miscellaneous: Sore throat; fever; rash.

Overdosage:

Symptoms: Mild GI disorders (anorexia, increased peristalsis or diarrhea) are early warnings that tolerance is being exceeded. These symptoms may be relieved by atropine, but consider dosage reduction. Slight numbness or tingling of the lips and fingertips has occurred shortly after taking a guanidine dose; this is not an indication to discontinue treatment or reduce dosage.

Severe intoxication is characterized by nervous hyperirritability, fibrillary tremors and convulsive contractions of muscle, salivation, vomiting, diarrhea, hypoglycemia and circulatory disturbances.

Treatment: Calcium gluconate IV may control the neuromuscular and convulsive symptoms and relieve other toxic manifestations. Atropine relieves the GI symptoms, circulatory disturbances and changes in blood sugar.

Patient Information:

Notify physician if sore throat, fever, skin rash, flushing, GI upset (nausea, diarrhea), nervousness or tremor occurs.

Administration and Dosage:

Initial dosage is 10 to 15 mg/kg/day in 3 or 4 divided doses; gradually increase to 35 mg/kg/day or up to the development of side effects. As individual tolerance is highly variable, the dosage must be carefully titrated. Continue the tolerable dose. Occasionally, removal of the primary neoplastic lesion may result in improvement of symptoms, permitting drug discontinuation.

Rx	**Guanidine HCl** (Key)	**Tablets:** 125 mg	In 100s.

CYSTEAMINE BITARTRATE

Actions:

Pharmacology: Cysteamine is a cystine depleting agent that lowers the cystine content of cells in patients with cystinosis, an inherited defect of lysosomal transport. Cysteamine is an aminothiol that participates within lysosomes in a thiol-disulfide interchange reaction converting cystine into cysteine and cysteine-cysteamine mixed disulfide, both of which can exit the lysosome in patients with cystinosis.

Cystinosis is an autosomal recessive inborn error of metabolism in which the transport of cystine out of lysosomes is abnormal; in the nephropathic form, accumulation of cystine and formation of crystals damage various organs, especially the kidney, leading to renal tubular Fanconi syndrome and progressive glomerular failure, with end-stage renal failure by the end of the first decade of life. In four studies of cystinosis patients, renal death (need for transplant or dialysis) occurred at a median age of < 10 years. Patients with cystinosis also experience growth failure, rickets and photophobia due to cystine deposits in the cornea. With time, most organs are damaged, including the retina, muscles and CNS. There are approximately 200 pre-transplant cystinosis patients in the US with nephropathic cystinosis.

Healthy individuals and persons heterozygous for cystinosis have white cell cystine levels of < 0.2 and usually < 1 nmol/½cystine/mg protein, respectively. Individuals with nephropathic cystinosis have elevations of white cell cystine > 2 nmol/½ cystine/mg protein. White cell cystine is monitored in these patients to determine adequacy of dosing. In the Long Term Study (see Clinical trials) entry white cell cystine levels were 3.73 nmol/½ cystine/mg protein (range, 0.13 to 19.80) and were maintained close to 1 nmol/½ cystine/mg protein with a cysteamine dose range of 1.3 to 1.95 g/m^2/day. There are approximately 200 pre-transplant cystinosis patients in the US with nephropathic cystinosis.

Clinical trials: The National Collaborative Cysteamine Study (NCCS) treated 94 children with nephropathic cystinosis with increasing doses of cysteamine HCl (mean dose, 54 mg/kg/day) to attain white cell cystine levels of < 2 nmol/½ cystine/mg protein 5 to 6 hours post-dose, and compared their outcome with a historical control group (n = 17). The principal measures of effectiveness were serum creatinine, calculated creatinine clearance (Ccr) and growth (height).

The average median white cell cystine level attained during treatment was 1.7 ± 0.2 nmol/½ cystine/mg protein. Twelve of the 94 cysteamine-treated patients required early dialysis or renal transplant. Median follow-up of cysteamine patients was > 32 months and 20% were followed > 5 years. Among cysteamine patients, glomerular function was maintained over time despite the longer period of treatment and follow-up. Placebo treated patients, in contrast, experienced a gradual rise in serum creatinine. Patients on treatment maintained growth (did not show increasing growth failure compared to healthy individuals) although growth velocity did not increase enough to allow patients to catch up to age norms. Calculated Ccr was evaluated for two groups, one with poor and one with good white cell cystine depletion. The final mean Ccr of the good depletion group was 20.8 ml/min/1 .73 m^2 greater than the mean for the poor depletion group.

The Long Term Study, initiated in 1988, utilized both cysteamine HCl and phosphocysteamine in 46 patients who completed the NCCS (averaging 6.5 years of treatment) and 93 new patients. Patients had cystinosis diagnosed by elevated white cell cystine (mean, 3.63 nmol/½ cystine/mg protein). New patients and 46 continuing patients were required to have serum creatinine < 3 and 4 mg/dl, respectively. Patients were randomized to doses of 1.3 or 1.95 g/m^2/day. Doses could be increased if white cell cystine levels were ≈ 2 nmol/½ cystine/mg protein and lowered due to intolerance.

White cell cystine levels averaged 1.72 ± 1.65 and 1.86 ± 0.92 nmol/½ cystine/mg protein in the 1.3 and 1.95 g/m^2/day groups, respectively. In new patients, serum creatinine was essentially unchanged over the period of follow-up (≈ 50% followed for 24 months) and phosphocysteamine and cysteamine HCl had similar effects. The long-term follow-up group (almost 80% were followed at least 2 years) had essentially no change in renal function. Both groups maintained height (although they did not catch up from baseline). There was no apparent difference between the two doses.

Indications:

Nephropathic cystinosis: Management in children and adults.

Contraindications:

Hypersensitivity to cysteamine or penicillamine.

Warnings:

Rash: If a skin rash develops, withhold cysteamine until the rash clears. Cysteamine may be restarted at a lower dose under close supervision, then slowly titrated to

CYSTEAMINE BITARTRATE

the therapeutic dose. If a severe skin rash develops such as erythema multiforme bullosa or toxic epidermal necrolysis, cysteamine should not be readministered.

CNS symptoms such as seizures, lethargy, somnolence, depression and encephalopathy have been associated with cysteamine. If CNS symptoms develop, carefully evaluate the patient and adjust the dose as necessary. Neurological complications have been described in some cystinotic patients not on cysteamine treatment. This may be a manifestation of the primary disorder. Patients should not engage in hazardous activities until the effects of cysteamine on mental performance are known.

Fertility impairment: At an oral dose of 375 mg/kg/day (1.7 times the recommended human dose), cysteamine reduced the fertility of rats and offspring survival.

Pregnancy: Category C. It is not known whether cysteamine can cause fetal harm when administered to a pregnant woman. Use only when clearly needed and when the potential benefits outweigh the potential hazards to the fetus.

Lactation: It is not known whether cysteamine is excreted in breast milk. Because of the manifested potential of cysteamine for developmental toxicity in suckling rat pups when it was administered to their lactating mothers at an oral dose of 375 mg/kg/day, decide whether to discontinue nursing or to discontinue the drug, taking into account the importance of the drug to the mother.

Children: The safety and efficacy of cysteamine for cystinotic children have been established. Initiate therapy as soon as the diagnosis of nephropathic cystinosis has been confirmed.

Precautions:

Monitoring: Cysteamine has occasionally been associated with reversible leukopenia and abnormal liver function studies. Therefore, monitor blood counts and liver function studies.

Leukocyte cystine measurements are useful to determine adequate dosage and compliance. When measured 5 to 6 hours after cysteamine administration, the goal should be a level < 1 nmol/½ cystine/mg protein. In some patients with poorer tolerability for cysteamine, patients may still receive benefit with a white cell cystine level of < 2 nmol/½ cystine/mg protein. Measurements should be done every 3 months, more frequently when patients are transferred from cysteamine HCl or phosphocysteamine solutions to cysteamine bitartrate.

GI symptoms, including nausea, vomiting, anorexia and abdominal pain (sometimes severe), have been associated with cysteamine. If these develop, therapy may have to be interrupted and the dose adjusted. A dose of 1.95 g/m^2/day (≈ 80 to 90 mg/kg/day) was associated with an increased number of withdrawals from treatment due to intolerance and an increased incidence of adverse events.

Concurrent therapy: Cysteamine can be administered with electrolyte and mineral replacements necessary for management of the Fanconi syndrome as well as vitamin D and thyroid hormone.

Adverse Reactions:

In three clinical trials, cysteamine or phosphocysteamine have been administered to 246 children with cystinosis. Causality of side effects is sometimes difficult to determine because adverse effects may result from the underlying disease.

Adverse reactions or intolerance leading to cessation of treatment occurred in 8% of patients in the US studies. Withdrawals due to intolerance, vomiting associated with medication, anorexia, lethargy and fever appeared dose-related, occurring more frequently in those patients receiving 1.95 vs 1.3 g/m^2/day.

The most frequent adverse reactions seen involve the GI (see Precautions) and central nervous systems (see Warnings). These are especially prominent at the initiation of therapy. Temporarily suspending treatment, then gradual reintroduction may be effective in improving tolerance. The most common events (> 5%) were vomiting (35%), anorexia (31%), fever (22%), diarrhea (16%), lethargy (11%) and rash (7%).

Other adverse reactions are as follows:

GI: Nausea; bad breath; abdominal pain; dyspepsia; constipation; gastroenteritis; duodenitis; duodenal ulceration.

CNS: Somnolence; encephalopathy; headache; seizures; ataxia; confusion; tremor; hyperkinesia; decreased hearing; dizziness; jitteriness.

Psychiatric: Nervousness; abnormal thinking; depression; emotional lability; hallucinations; nightmares.

Miscellaneous: Abnormal liver function; anemia; leukopenia; dehydration; hypertension; urticaria.

CYSTEAMINE BITARTRATE

Overdosage:

Symptoms: A single oral dose of 660 mg/kg was lethal to rats. Symptoms of acute toxicity were reduction of motor activity and generalized hemorrhage in the GI tract and kidneys. One case of massive human overdosage has been reported. The patient immediately vomited the drug and did not develop any symptoms.

Treatment: Should overdose occur, appropriately support the respiratory and cardiovascular systems. No specific antidote is known. Refer to General Management of Acute Overdosage. Hemodialysis may be considered since cysteamine is poorly bound to plasma proteins.

Administration and Dosage:

Approved by the FDA on August 15, 1994.

Initial dose: For the management of nephropathic cystinosis, initiate therapy promptly once the diagnosis is confirmed (ie, increased white cell cystine). Start new patients on ¼ to ⅙ of the maintenance dose of cysteamine. The dose should then be raised gradually over 4 to 6 weeks to avoid intolerance.

Maintenance: The recommended cysteamine maintenance dose for children up to age 12 years is 1.3 g/m²/day of the free base, given in 4 divided doses. Intact cysteamine capsules should not be administered to children under the age of ≈ 6 years due to the risk of aspiration. Cysteamine capsules may be administered to children under the age of ≈ 6 years by sprinkling the capsule contents over food. Patients > 12 years of age and > 110 lbs should receive 2 g/day, in 4 divided doses.

When cysteamine is well tolerated, the goal of therapy is to keep leukocyte cystine levels < 1 nmol/½ cystine/mg protein 5 to 6 hours following administration of cysteamine. Patients with poorer tolerability still receive significant benefit if white cell cystine levels are < 2 nmol/½ cystine/mg protein. The cysteamine dose can be increased to a maximum of 1.95 g/m²/day to achieve this level. The dose of 1.95 g/m²/day has been associated with an increased rate of withdrawal from treatment due to intolerance and an increased incidence of adverse events.

Cystinotic patients taking cysteamine HCl or phosphocysteamine solutions may be transferred to equimolar doses of cysteamine bitartrate capsules.

The recommended maintenance dose of 1.3 g/m²/day can be approximated by administering cysteamine according to the following table, which takes surface area as well as weight into consideration.

Cysteamine Maintenance Dose	
Weight (lbs)	Cysteamine free base every 6 hours (mg)
0-10	100
11-20	150
21-30	200
31-40	250
41-50	300
51-70	350
71-90	400
91-110	450
> 110	500

Patients > 12 years of age and > 110 lbs should receive 2 g/day given in 4 divided doses as a starting maintenance dose. This dose should be reached after 4 to 6 weeks of incremental dosage increases as stated above. The dose should be raised if the leukocyte cystine level remains > 2 nmol/½ cystine/mg/protein.

Obtain leukocyte cystine measurements, taken 5 to 6 hours after dose administration, for new patients after the maintenance dose is achieved. Patients being transferred from cysteamine HCl or phosphocysteamine solutions to capsules should have their white cell cystine levels measured in 2 weeks, and thereafter every 3 months to assess optimal dosage as described above.

If cysteamine is poorly tolerated initially due to GI tract symptoms or transient skin rashes, temporarily stop therapy, then reinstitute at a lower dose and gradually increase to the proper dose.

Rx	**Cystagon** (Mylan)	**Capsules:** 50 mg (as cysteamine bitartrate)	(Cysta 50 Mylan). White. In 100s and 500s.
		150 mg (as cysteamine bitartrate)	(Cystagon 150 Mylan). White. In 100s and 500s.

Alkalinizers

ALKALINIZERS

Urinary alkalinizing agents are bases or salts of bases that increase the excretion of free base in the urine, effectively raising the urinary pH.

Used to correct acidosis in renal tubular disorders and to minimize uric acid crystallization as adjuvants to uricosuric agents in gout. Urine alkalinization increases solubility of sulfonamides and the renal elimination of phenobarbital.

SODIUM BICARBONATE

For information on parenteral sodium bicarbonate, refer to the monograph in the Nutritionals chapter.

One gram of sodium bicarbonate provides 11.9 mEq of sodium and bicarbonate.

Contraindications:

Use cautiously in edema, CHF, liver cirrhosis and low-salt diets.

Precautions:

Use cautiously in toxemia of pregnancy or renal impairment.

Prolonged therapy may lead to systemic alkalosis.

Administration and Dosage:

325 mg to 2 g, up to 4 times daily. The maximum daily intake is 15 g (240 mEq) in patients < 60 years old and 8 g (120 mEq) in those ≥ 60 years old.

otc	**Sodium Bicarbonate** (Various eg, Rugby, URL)	**Tablets:** 325 mg	In 1000s.
		650 mg	In 1000s.
		Powder	In 120.

POTASSIUM CITRATE

For complete prescribing information on citrate and citric acid, see monograph in the Nutritionals chapter.

Administration and Dosage:

Severe hypocitruria: 60 mEq/day (20 mEq 3 times/day or 15 mEq 4 times/day with meals or ≤ 30 minutes after meals).

Mild to moderate hypocitruria: 30 mEq/day (10 mEq 3 times/day with meals).

Do not exceed 100 mEq/day.

Rx	**Urocit-K** (Mission)	**Tablets:** 5 mEq	In 100s.
		10 mEq	In 100s.

POTASSIUM CITRATE COMBINATIONS

For complete prescribing information on citrate and citric acid, see monograph in the Nutritionals chapter.

Administration and Dosage:

Liquids: 15 to 20 ml 4 times daily usually maintains a urinary pH of 7 to 7.6 for 24 hours; 10 to 15 ml 4 times daily usually maintains a urinary pH of 6.5 to 7.4.

Adults – 15 to 30 ml 4 times daily, after meals and at bedtime, diluted with water.

Children – 5 to 15 ml 4 times daily, after meals and at bedtime, diluted with water.

Tablets: 1 to 4 tablets with a full glass of water, after meals and at bedtime.

Rx	**Citrolith** (Beach Pharm.)	**Tablets:** 50 mg potassium citrate and 950 mg sodium citrate	(Beach 1136). In 100s & 500s.	11
Rx	**Polycitra** (Willen)	**Syrup:** 550 mg potassium citrate, 500 mg sodium citrate, 334 mg citric acid/5 ml. (1 mEq K, 1 mEq Na per ml; equiv. to 2 mEq bicarbonate)	Alcohol free. In 120 and 480 ml.	4
Rx *sf*	**Polycitra-LC** (Willen)	**Solution:** 550 mg K citrate, 500 mg sodium citrate, 334 mg citric acid/5 ml. (1 mEq K, 1 mEq Na per ml; equiv. to 2 mEq bicarbonate)	Alcohol free. In 120 and 480 ml.	4
Rx *sf*	**Polycitra-K** (Willen)	**Solution:** 1100 mg potassium citrate, 334 mg citric acid/5 ml. (2 mEq K/ml; equiv. to 2 mEq bicarbonate)	Alcohol free. In 120 and 480 ml.	4
		Crystals for Reconstitution: 3300 mg K citrate, 1002 mg citric acid per UD packet (equiv. to 30 mEq bicarb.)	Alcohol free. In single dose packets.	NA

Alkalinizers

SODIUM CITRATE AND CITRIC ACID SOLUTION (Shohl's Solution, Modified)

Administration and Dosage:

Systemic alkalinization:

Adults – 10 to 30 ml diluted in 30 to 90 ml water, after meals and at bedtime.

Children (> 2 years old) – 5 to 15 ml diluted in 30 to 90 ml water, after meals and at bedtime. Consult physician for use in children < 2 years old.

Neutralizing buffer: 15 ml diluted in 15 ml water, as a single dose.

Rx *sf*	**Bicitra** (Baker Norton)	**Solution:** 500 mg sodium citrate/334 mg citric acid per 5 ml (1 mEq sodium equiv. to 1 mEq bicarbonate/ml)	Grape flavored. In 120 and 473 ml and UD 15 and 30 ml.
Rx	**Oracit** (Carolina Medical Products)	**Solution:** 490 mg sodium citrate/640 mg citric acid per 5 ml (1 mEq sodium equiv. to 1 mEq bicarbonate/ml)	In 500 ml and UD 15 and 30 ml.
	PMS-Dicitrate (Pharmascience)	**Solution:** 500 mg sodium citrate/334 mg citric acid per 5 ml (1 mEq sodium equiv. to 1 mEq bicarbonate/ml)	In 500 ml and UD 30 ml.

Acidifiers

AMMONIUM CHLORIDE

For information on parenteral ammonium chloride, refer to the monograph in the Nutritionals chapter.

Indications:

Used as a diuretic or systemic and urinary acidifying agent.

Contraindications:

Markedly impaired renal or hepatic function.

Adverse Reactions:

Gastric irritation; nausea; vomiting; acidosis with large doses.

Overdosage:

Symptoms: Nausea, vomiting, thirst, headache, hyperventilation and progressive drowsiness leading to profound acidosis and hypokalemia.

Treatment: Correct acidosis and electrolyte loss by administering IV sodium bicarbonate or sodium lactate. Hypokalemia may be treated by oral potassium salts.

Administration and Dosage:

Usual dose is 1 to 2 g every four to six hours.

otc	**Ammonium Cl** (Various)	**Tablets:** 500 mg	In 100s and 1000s.
		Tablets, enteric coated: 486 mg	In 1008s.

ASCORBIC ACID

Ascorbic acid is frequently used as a urinary acidifier; its efficacy is controversial. Refer to the "Actions" section of the ascorbic acid monograph for dosage guidelines.

ACID PHOSPHATES

Indications:

To acidify the urine and lower urinary calcium concentration.

Increases the antibacterial activity of methenamine.

Reduces odor and rash caused by ammoniacal urine.

Contraindications:

Renal insufficiency (< 30% of normal), infected magnesium ammonium phosphate stones, hyperphosphatemia and hyperkalemia. Also use with caution if potassium regulation is desired. Use sodium acid phosphate cautiously in patients on sodium restriction.

Warnings:

Concurrent potassium supplementation: Consider potassium content of these products. Decrease supplemental potassium dosage to avoid hyperkalemia.

Pregnancy: Category C. Safe use during pregnancy is not established. Use only when clearly needed and when potential benefits outweigh potential hazards to the fetus.

Lactation: Safety for use in the nursing mother has not been established. It is not known whether this drug is excreted in breast milk. Exercise caution when administering to a nursing woman.

Precautions:

Exercise caution in following conditions: Cardiac disease (particularly digitalized patients), Addison's disease, acute dehydration, severe renal insufficiency or chronic renal disease, extensive tissue breakdown (such as severe burns), myotonia congenita, cardiac failure, cirrhosis of the liver or severe hepatic disease, peripheral and pulmonary edema, hypernatremia, hypertension, toxemia of pregnancy, hypoparathyroidism, acute pancreatitis and rickets.

Laboratory tests: Carefully monitor renal function and serum electrolytes (calcium, phosphorus, potassium) at periodic intervals during phosphate therapy if required. High serum phosphate levels increase incidence of extraskeletal calcification.

Drug Interactions:

Acid Phosphate Drug Interactions

Precipitant drug	Object drug*		Description
Acid phosphates	Salicylates	⬆	Acidified urine reduces excretion of salicylates and may lead to salicylate toxicity.
Antacids	Acid phosphates	⬇	Antacids containing magnesium, calcium or aluminum in conjunction with phosphate preparations may bind the phosphate and prevent absorption.

Acidifiers

ACID PHOSPHATES

Acid Phosphate Drug Interactions

Precipitant drug	Object drug*		Description
Antihypertensives; corticosteroids	Acid phosphates	↑	Antihypertensives, especially diazoxide, guanethidine, hydralazine, methyldopa or rauwolfia alkaloids; or corticosteroids, especially mineralocorticoids or corticotropin; used concurrently with sodium phosphate may result in hypernatremia.
Potassium-containing medications	Acid phosphates	↑	Potassium-containing medications or potassium-sparing diuretics may cause hyperkalemia when used concurrently with potassium salts. Perform periodic serum potassium level determinations.

* ↑ = Object drug increased. ↓ = Object drug decreased.

Adverse Reactions:

Mild laxation may occur; it usually subsides with dosage reduction. If it persists, discontinue use. Abdominal discomfort, diarrhea, nausea and vomiting may occur.

Less frequent: Fast or irregular heartbeat, dizziness, headache, mental confusion, seizures, weakness or heaviness of legs, unusual tiredness, muscle cramps, numbness, tingling, pain or weakness in hands or feet, numbness or tingling around lips, shortness of breath or troubled breathing, swelling of feet or legs, unusual weight gain, low urine output, thirst, bone and joint pain.

Patient Information:

Notify physician if abdominal pain, nausea or vomiting occurs.

Warn patients with kidney stones of the possibility of passing old stones when phosphate therapy is started.

Advise patients to avoid antacids containing aluminum, calcium or magnesium which may prevent phosphate absorption.

To assure against GI injury associated with oral ingestion of concentrated potassium salt preparations, instruct patients to dissolve tablets completely in an appropriate amount of water before taking.

POTASSIUM ACID PHOSPHATE

For complete prescribing information, refer to the Acid Phosphates group monograph.

Administration and Dosage:

1 g dissolved in 180 to 240 ml water 4 times daily with meals and at bedtime. For best results, soak tablets in water for 2 to 5 minutes. Stir vigorously and swallow.

Rx	**K-Phos Original** (Beach)	**Tablets:** 500 mg (contains 3.7 mEq potassium)	Sodium free. (Beach 1111). White, scored. In 100s and 500s.

POTASSIUM ACID PHOSPHATE AND SODIUM ACID PHOSPHATE

For complete prescribing information, refer to the Acid Phosphates group monograph.

Administration and Dosage:

1 to 2 tablets 4 times daily with a full glass of water. When the urine is difficult to acidify, administer 1 tablet every 2 hours. Do not exceed 8 tablets in 24 hours.

Rx	**K-Phos Neutral** (Beach)	**Tablets:** 852 mg dibasic sodium phosphate anhydrous, 155 mg monobasic potassium phosphate and 130 mg monobasic sodium phosphate monohydrate (contains 1.1 mEq potassium and 13.0 mEq sodium)	(Beach 1125). White, film coated. In 100s and 500s.
Rx	**K-Phos M.F.** (Beach)	**Tablets:** 155 mg potassium acid phosphate and 350 mg sodium acid phosphate (contains 1.1 mEq potassium and 2.9 mEq sodium)	(Beach 1135). White, scored. In 100s and 500s.
Rx	**K-Phos No. 2** (Beach)	**Tablets:** 305 mg potassium acid phosphate and 700 mg sodium acid phosphate (contains 2.3 mEq potassium and 5.8 mEq sodium)	(Beach 1134). Brown. In 100s and 500s.

ANTISPASMODICS

In addition to the GI antispasmodics (refer to the Gastrointestinal chapter), many of which are recommended for urologic conditions, the following agents are indicated specifically for urologic disorders. Urinary antispasmodics in combination with urinary anti-infective agents are listed in the Anti-Infectives chapter. Urinary antispasmodics in combination with urinary analgesics are also available.

FLAVOXATE HCl

Actions:

Pharmacology: Counteracts smooth muscle spasm of the urinary tract. Flavoxate relaxes smooth muscle by cholinergic blockade. It also exerts a direct effect on the muscle. It has anticholinergic, local anesthetic and analgesic properties.

Indications:

For the symptomatic relief of dysuria, urgency, nocturia, suprapubic pain, frequency and incontinence as may occur in cystitis, prostatitis, urethritis, urethrocystitis/urethrotrigonitis.

NOT indicated for definitive treatment but is compatible with drugs used to treat urinary tract infections.

Contraindications:

Pyloric or duodenal obstruction; obstructive intestinal lesions or ileus; achalasia; GI hemorrhage; obstructive uropathies of the lower urinary tract.

Warnings:

Glaucoma: Give cautiously in patients with suspected glaucoma.

Pregnancy: There are no well controlled studies in pregnant women. Use during pregnancy only when clearly needed.

Lactation: It is not known whether this drug is excreted in breast milk. Use caution when flavoxate is administered to a nursing woman.

Children: Safety and efficacy in children < 12 years of age have not been established.

Adverse Reactions:

Nausea; vomiting; dry mouth; nervousness; vertigo; headache; drowsiness; mental confusion (especially in the elderly patient); hyperpyrexia; blurred vision; increased ocular tension; disturbance in eye accommodation; urticaria and other dermatoses; dysuria; tachycardia; palpitations; eosinophilia; leukopenia.

Patient Information:

These agents may cause drowsiness or blurred vision; observe caution while driving or performing other tasks requiring alertness, coordination or physical dexterity.

May cause dry mouth.

Administration and Dosage:

Adults and children > 12 years of age: 100 or 200 mg 3 or 4 times daily. Reduce the dose when symptoms improve.

In one study, investigators used doses ≤ 1200 mg/day for treatment of urinary urgency following pelvic radiotherapy. The 1200 mg/day dose was superior to the 600 mg/day dose.

Rx	**Urispas** (SmithKline Beecham)	**Tablets:** 100 mg	(Urispas SKF). White. Film coated. In 100s and UD 100s.
	Urispas (Pharmascience)	**Tablets:** 200 mg	In 100s.

Antispasmodics

OXYBUTYNIN CHLORIDE

Actions:

Pharmacology: Oxybutynin exerts direct antispasmodic effect on smooth muscle and inhibits the muscarinic action of acetylcholine on smooth muscle. It exhibits one-fifth of the anticholinergic activity of atropine but 4 to 10 times the antispasmodic activity. No blocking effects occur at skeletal neuromuscular junctions or autonomic ganglia (antinicotinic effects).

In patients with conditions characterized by involuntary bladder contractions, oxybutynin increases vesical capacity, diminishes frequency of uninhibited contractions of the detrusor muscle and delays initial desire to void. These effects are more consistently improved in patients with uninhibited neurogenic bladder. Oxybutynin thus decreases urgency and the frequency of both incontinent episodes and voluntary urination.

Oxybutynin is well tolerated in patients administered the drug from 30 days to 2 years.

Indications:

Bladder instability: For the relief of symptoms of bladder instability associated with voiding in patients with uninhibited and reflex neurogenic bladder (eg, urgency, frequency, urinary leakage, urge incontinence, dysuria).

Contraindications:

Glaucoma (angle closure); GI obstruction; paralytic ileus; intestinal atony of the elderly or debilitated; megacolon; toxic megacolon complicating ulcerative colitis; severe colitis; myasthenia gravis; obstructive uropathy; unstable cardiovascular status in acute hemorrhage; hypersensitivity to the product.

Warnings:

Heat prostration: When administered in the presence of high environmental temperature, heat prostration (fever and heat stroke) may occur due to decreased sweating.

Diarrhea may be an early symptom of incomplete intestinal obstruction, especially in patients with ileostomy or colostomy; discontinue treatment.

Pregnancy: Category B. Safety for use during pregnancy has not been established. Use only when clearly needed and when the potential benefits outweigh the potential hazards to the fetus.

Lactation: It is not known whether this drug is excreted in breast milk. Exercise caution when administering to a nursing woman.

Children: Safety and efficacy in children < 5 years of age have not been established.

Precautions:

Use with caution in the elderly and patients with autonomic neuropathy and hepatic or renal disease. Doses administered to patients with ulcerative colitis may suppress GI motility and produce paralytic ileus and precipitate or aggravate toxic megacolon.

Cardiac effects: Symptoms of hyperthyroidism, coronary heart disease, congestive heart failure, cardiac arrhythmias, tachycardia, hypertension, hiatal hernia and prostatic hypertrophy may be aggravated.

Potentially hazardous tasks: May produce drowsiness or dizziness; patients should observe caution while driving or performing other tasks requiring alertness, coordination or physical dexterity.

Drug Interactions:

Oxybutynin Drug Interactions

Precipitant Drug	Object Drug*		Description
Oxybutynin	Acetaminophen	⬇	A slight delay in the absorption of oral acetaminophen from the GI tract is apparently due to decreased GI motility induced by anticholinergics.
Oxybutynin	Atenolol	⬆	The bioavailability of atenolol may be increased by the administration of anticholinergics.
Oxybutynin	Digoxin	⬆	Serum levels of digoxin (administered as slow dissolution tablets) may be increased.
Oxybutynin	Haloperidol	⬇	Worsening of schizophrenic symptoms, decreased serum concentration of haloperidol, development of tardive dyskinesia.
Oxybutynin	Levodopa	⬇	The therapeutic utility of levodopa may be reduced.

Antispasmodics

OXYBUTYNIN CHLORIDE

Oxybutynin Drug Interactions

Precipitant Drug	Object Drug*		Description
Oxybutynin	Nitrofurantoin	↑	Anticholinergics may increase plasma concentration of nitrofurantoin, possibly increasing adverse effects. Delayed gastric emptying by anticholinergics may increase nitrofurantoin bioavailability.
Oxybutynin	Phenothiazines	↔	Increased incidence of anticholinergic side effects, and decreased or increased phenothiazine levels may occur.
Amantadine	Oxybutynin	↑	The anticholinergic side effects may be increased, probably caused by additive or synergistic toxicity.

* ↑ = Object drug increased. ↓ = Object drug decreased. ↔ = Undetermined effect.

Adverse Reactions:
Dry mouth; decreased sweating; rash; urinary hesitancy and retention; decreased lacrimation; mydriasis; amblyopia; cycloplegia; tachycardia; palpitations; vasodilatation; drowsiness; hallucinations; insomnia; restlessness; asthenia; dizziness; nausea; vomiting; constipation; decreased GI motility; impotence; suppression of lactation.

Overdosage:
Symptoms: Signs of CNS excitation (eg, restlessness, tremor, irritability, convulsions, delirium, hallucinations); flushing; fever; nausea; vomiting; tachycardia; hypotension or hypertension; respiratory failure; paralysis; coma.

Treatment should be symptomatic and supportive. Maintain respiration and induce emesis or perform gastric lavage (emesis is contraindicated in a precomatose, convulsive or psychotic state). Activated charcoal may be administered as well as a cathartic. Physostigmine may be considered to reverse symptoms of anticholinergic intoxication. Treat hyperpyrexia symptomatically with ice bags or other cold applications and alcohol sponges. Refer to General Management of Acute Overdosage.

Patient Information:
May cause drowsiness, dizziness or blurred vision; alcohol or sedatives may enhance drowsiness. Observe caution while driving or performing other tasks requiring alertness, coordination or physical dexterity.

May cause dry mouth.

Administration and Dosage:
Adults: 5 mg 2 or 3 times daily. Maximum dose is 5 mg 4 times daily.

Children (> 5 years): 5 mg twice a day. Maximum dose is 5 mg 3 times daily.

Storage/Stability: Store at controlled room temperature 15° to 30°C (59° to 86°F). Dispense in a tight light-resistant container.

Rx	**Oxybutynin Chloride** (Various, eg, Geneva, Goldline, Major, Moore, Parmed, Rugby, Schein, URL)	**Tablets:** 5 mg	In 100s, 500s and 1000s and UD 100s.
Rx	**Ditropan** (Hoechst Marion Roussel)		Lactose. (Marion 1375). Blue, scored. Biconvex. In 100s, 1000s and UD 100s.
Rx	**Ditropan** (Hoechst Marion Roussel)	**Syrup:** 5 mg/5 ml	Sorbitol, sucrose. In 473 ml.
Rx	**Oxybutynin** (Silarx)	**Syrup:** 1 mg/ml	Methylparaben, sorbitol, surcrose. Raspberry flavor. In 473 ml.

Cholinergic Stimulants

BETHANECHOL CHLORIDE

Actions:

Pharmacology: Bethanechol is an ester of a choline-like compound. It acts principally by stimulating the parasympathetic nervous system. It increases the tone of the detrusor urinae muscle, usually producing a contraction strong enough to initiate micturition and empty the bladder. It stimulates gastric motility, increases gastric tone and often restores impaired rhythmic peristalsis.

When spontaneous stimulation of the parasympathetic system is reduced and therapeutic intervention is necessary, acetylcholine can be given, but it is rapidly hydrolyzed by cholinesterase and its effects are transient. Bethanechol is not destroyed by cholinesterase and its effects are more prolonged than those of acetylcholine.

It has prominent muscarinic action and slight or no nicotinic action. Doses that stimulate micturition and defecation and increase peristalsis do not ordinarily stimulate ganglia or voluntary muscles. Therapeutic test doses in healthy human subjects have little effect on heart rate, blood pressure or peripheral circulation.

Pharmacokinetics: Effects appear ≤ 30 to 90 minutes after oral administration. Usual duration is 1 hour, although large doses (eg, 300 to 400 mg) may persist for ≤6 hours. Administration SC is usually effective in 5 to 15 minutes.

A clinical study was conducted on the relative efficacy of oral and SC bethanechol on the stretch response of bladder muscle in patients with urinary retention. A 5 mg SC dose stimulated a response that was more rapid in onset and of larger magnitude than an oral dose of 50, 100 or 200 mg. However, the oral doses had a longer duration of effect than the SC dose. Although the 50 mg oral dose caused little change in intravesical pressure, this dose is effective in the rehabilitation of patients with decompensated bladders.

Indications:

Urinary retention: Acute postoperative and postpartum nonobstructive (functional) urinary retention and neurogenic atony of the urinary bladder with retention.

Unlabeled uses: Bethanechol has been used in adults for treatment (25 mg 4 times/day) and diagnosis (two 50 mcg/kg SC doses 15 minutes apart) of reflux esophagitis. In infants and children, an oral dosage of 3 mg/m^2/dose 3 times/day has been used for gastroesophageal reflux.

Contraindications:

Hypersensitivity to bethanechol; hyperthyroidism; peptic ulcer; latent or active bronchial asthma; pronounced bradycardia; atrio-ventricular conduction defects; vasomotor instability; coronary artery disease; epilepsy; parkinsonism; coronary occlusion; hypotension; hypertension; when the strength or integrity of the GI or bladder wall is in question or in the presence of mechanical obstruction; when increased muscular activity of the GI tract or urinary bladder might prove harmful, as following recent urinary bladder surgery, GI resection and anastomosis, or when there is possible GI obstruction; bladder neck obstruction; spastic GI disturbances; acute inflammatory lesions of the GI tract; peritonitis; marked vagotonia.

Warnings:

Parenteral dosage form: For SC injection only; do not give IM or IV. Violent symptoms of cholinergic overstimulation, such as circulatory collapse, fall in blood pressure, abdominal cramps, bloody diarrhea, shock or sudden cardiac arrest are likely if given IM or IV. These symptoms occur rarely after SC injection and may occur in cases of hypersensitivity or overdosage.

Pregnancy: Category C. It is not known whether bethanechol can cause fetal harm when administered to a pregnant woman or can affect reproduction capacity. Give to a pregnant woman only if clearly needed.

Lactation: It is not known whether this drug is excreted in breast milk. Because of the potential for serious adverse reactions, decide whether to discontinue nursing or discontinue the drug, taking into account the importance of the drug to the mother.

Children: Safety and efficacy have not been established. See Unlabeled uses.

Precautions:

Reflux infection: In urinary retention, if the sphincter fails to relax as bethanechol contracts the bladder, urine may be forced up the ureter into the kidney pelvis. If there is bacteriuria, this may cause reflux infection.

Tartrazine sensitivity: Some of these products contain tartrazine, which may cause allergic-type reactions (including bronchial asthma) in susceptible individuals.

Cholinergic Stimulants

BETHANECHOL CHLORIDE

Although the incidence of sensitivity is low, it is frequently seen in patients who also have aspirin hypersensitivity. Specific products containing tartrazine are identified in the product listing.

Drug Interactions:

Bethanechol Chloride			
Precipitant drug	Object drug*		Description
Cholinergic drugs	Bethanechol	↑	Additive effects may occur, particularly with cholinesterase inhibitors.
Ganglionic blocking compounds	Bethanechol	↑	A critical fall in blood pressure may occur that is usually preceded by severe abdominal symptoms.
Quinidine; procainamide	Bethanechol	↑	Quinidine or procainamide may antagonize cholinergic effects of bethanechol.

* ↑ = Object drug increased.

Adverse Reactions:

Adverse reactions are rare following oral administration of bethanechol but are more common following SC injection. Adverse reactions are more likely to occur when dosage is increased.

GI: Abdominal cramps or discomfort; colicky pain; nausea; belching; diarrhea; borborygmi (rumbling/gurgling of stomach); salivation.

Cardiovascular: Fall in blood pressure with reflex tachycardia; vasomotor response.

Dermatologic: Flushing producing a feeling of warmth; sensation of heat about the face; sweating.

Respiratory: Bronchial constriction; asthmatic attacks.

Special senses: Lacrimation; miosis.

Miscellaneous: Malaise; urinary urgency; headache.

Overdosage:

Symptoms: Early signs of overdosage are abdominal discomfort, salivation, flushing of the skin ("hot feeling"), sweating, nausea and vomiting.

Treatment: Atropine is a specific antidote. The recommended dose for adults is 0.6 mg. Repeat doses may be given every 2 hours according to clinical response.

The recommended dosage in infants and children ≤ 12 years of age is 0.01 mg/kg repeated every 2 hours as needed until the desired effect is obtained or adverse effects of atropine preclude further usage. The maximum single dose should not exceed 0.4 mg.

Subcutaneous injection of atropine is preferred except in emergencies when the IV route may be used. When administering bethanechol SC, always have a syringe containing atropine available.

Patient Information:

To avoid nausea and vomiting, take 1 hour before or 2 hours after meals. If taken soon after eating, nausea and vomiting may occur.

May cause abdominal discomfort, salivation, sweating or flushing; notify physician if these effects are pronounced.

Dizziness, lightheadedness or fainting may occur, especially when getting up from a lying or sitting position.

Administration and Dosage:

Individualize dose and route. Preferably, administer when the stomach is empty. If taken soon after eating, nausea and vomiting may occur.

Oral:

Adults – 10 to 50 mg 3 to 4/day. The minimum effective dose is determined by giving 5 or 10 mg initially; repeat the same amount hourly to a maximum of 50 mg until satisfactory response occurs.

SC: Do not give IV or IM (see Warnings). Usual dose is 5 mg; some patients respond to as little as 2.5 mg. The minimum effective dose is determined by injecting 2.5 mg initially and repeating the same amount at 15 to 30 minute intervals to a maximum of 4 doses until satisfactory response is obtained, unless disturbing reactions appear. The minimum effective dose may be repeated 3 or 4 times/day as required.

Rarely, single doses up to 10 mg are required. Such large doses may cause severe reactions; use only after determining that single doses of 2.5 to 5 mg are not sufficient.

Cholinergic Stimulants

BETHANECHOL CHLORIDE

If necessary, drug effects can be abolished promptly by atropine.

Storage/Stability – Store tablets in a tightly-closed container at room temperature 15° to 30°C (59° to 86°F). Avoid storage > 40°C (104°F). Avoid storage of injection < -20°C (-4°F) and > 40°C (104°F).

Rx	**Bethanechol Chloride** (Various, eg, Danbury, Goldline, Major, Sidmak, Vangard)	**Tablets:** 5 mg	In 100s, 1000s and UD 100s.
Rx	**Urecholine** (Merck)		Lactose. (MSD 403). White, scored. In 100s.
Rx	**Bethanechol Chloride** (Various, eg, Danbury, Geneva, Goldline, Major, Moore, Parmed, Rugby, Schein, Sidmak, URL, Vangard)	**Tablets:** 10 mg	In 100s, 250s, 1000s and UD 100s.
Rx	**Duvoid** (Roberts)		(Roberts 101/10). Pale orange, scored. In 100s.
Rx	**Myotonachol** (Glenwood)		Tartrazine. Blue. In 100s.
Rx	**Urecholine** (Merck)		Lactose. (MSD 412). Pink, scored. In 100s.
🍁	**Duvoid** (Roberts)		(10). Pale orange. In 100s.
🍁	**Myotonachol** (Glenwood)		White. In 100s.
🍁	**PMS-Bethanechol Chloride** (Glenwood)		(PMS 10). Peach. Semi-scored. In 100s.
🍁	**Urecholine** (Frosst)		Lactose. (FROSST 412). White. Quadrisected. In 100s.
Rx	**Bethanechol Chloride** (Various, eg, Danbury, Geneva, Goldline, Major, Moore, Parmed, Rugby, Schein, Sidmak, URL, Vangard)	**Tablets:** 25 mg	In 100s, 250s, 1000s and UD 100s.
Rx	**Duvoid** (Roberts)		(Roberts 102/25). White, scored. In 100s.
Rx	**Myotonachol** (Glenwood)		Tartrazine. In 100s.
Rx	**Urecholine** (Merck)		Lactose. (MSD 457). Yellow, scored. In 100s.
🍁	**Duvoid** (Roberts)		(25). White. In 100s.
🍁	**PMS-Bethanechol Chloride** (Glenwood)		(PMS 25). White. Semi-scored. In 50s and 100s.
🍁	**Urecholine** (Frosst)		Lactose. Yellow. Scored. In 50s.

Cholinergic Stimulants

BETHANECHOL CHLORIDE

Rx	**Bethanechol Chloride** (Various, eg, Danbury, Goldline, Major, Moore, Parmed, Rugby, Schein, Sidmak, URL)	**Tablets:** 50 mg	In 100s, 500s, 1000s and UD 100s.
Rx	**Duvoid** (Roberts)		(Roberts 103/50). Tan, scored. In 100s.
Rx	**Urecholine** (Merck)		Lactose. (MSD 460). Yellow, scored. In 100s.
🍁	**Duvoid** (Roberts)		(50). Tan. In 100s.
🍁	**PMS-Bethanechol Chloride** (Pharmascience)		(PMS 25). Beige. Semi-scored. In 100s.
Rx	**Urecholine** (Merck)	**Injection:** 5 mg/ml	In 1 ml vials.
🍁	**Urecholine** (Frosst)		In 1 ml amps.

NEOSTIGMINE METHYLSULFATE

Neostigmine is also used in the diagnosis and treatment of myasthenia gravis and as an antidote for nondepolarizing neuromuscular blockers; refer to Anticholinesterase Muscle Stimulants.

Actions:

Pharmacology: Neostigmine inhibits acetylcholine hydrolysis by competing for attachment to acetylcholinesterase at sites of cholinergic transmission. It enhances cholinergic action by facilitating the transmission of impulses across neuromuscular junctions. It also has a direct cholinomimetic effect on skeletal muscle and possibly on autonomic ganglion cells and neurons of the CNS.

Pharmacokinetics:

Absorption/Distribution – Neostigmine is poorly absorbed orally. Following IM administration, the drug is rapidly absorbed and eliminated. Serum albumin binding ranges from 15% to 25%.

Metabolism/Excretion – Neostigmine undergoes hydrolysis by cholinesterase and is metabolized by microsomal enzymes in the liver. Approximately 80% is eliminated in the urine ≤ 24 hours, ≈ 50% as the unchanged drug and 30% as metabolites. Following IV administration, plasma half-life is 47 to 60 minutes (mean, 53 minutes).

Onset/Duration: Clinical effects usually begin ≤ 20 to 30 minutes after IM injection and last 2.5 to 4 hours.

Indications:

Urinary retention: Prevention and treatment of postoperative distention and urinary retention.

Contraindications:

Hypersensitivity to neostigmine; peritonitis; mechanical obstruction of the intestinal or urinary tract.

Warnings:

Use with caution in patients with epilepsy, bronchial asthma, bradycardia, recent coronary occlusion, vagotonia, hyperthyroidism, cardiac arrhythmias or peptic ulcer.

Concomitant atropine administration: When large doses are administered, the prior or simultaneous injection of atropine sulfate may be advisable. Use separate syringes for neostigmine and atropine.

Hypersensitivity: Have atropine and antishock medication immediately available. Refer to Management of Acute Hypersensitivity Reactions.

Pregnancy: Category C. There are no adequate or well controlled studies. It is not known whether neostigmine can cause fetal harm when administered to a pregnant woman or can affect reproductive capacity. Anticholinesterase drugs may cause uterine irritability and induce premature labor when given IV to pregnant women near term. Give to a pregnant woman only if clearly needed.

Lactation: It is not known whether neostigmine is excreted in breast milk. Because of the potential for serious adverse reactions in nursing infants, decide whether to discontinue nursing or to discontinue the drug, taking into account the importance of the drug to the mother.

Cholinergic Stimulants

NEOSTIGMINE METHYLSULFATE

Children: Safety and efficacy for use in children have not been established.

Adverse Reactions:

Side effects are generally caused by exaggerated pharmacological effects; salivation and fasciculation are the most common.

CNS: Dizziness; convulsions; loss of consciousness; drowsiness; headache; dysarthria; miosis; visual changes.

Cardiovascular: Cardiac arrhythmias (bradycardia, tachycardia, AV block and nodal rhythm); nonspecific EKG changes; cardiac arrest; syncope; hypotension.

Respiratory: Increased oral, pharyngeal and bronchial secretions; dyspnea; respiratory depression; respiratory arrest; bronchospasm.

Dermatologic: Rash; urticaria.

GI: Nausea; emesis; flatulence; increased peristalsis; bowel cramps; diarrhea.

Musculoskeletal: Muscle cramps and spasms; arthralgia.

Body as a whole: Diaphoresis; flushing; allergic reactions; anaphylaxis; urinary frequency; weakness.

Overdosage:

Symptoms: Overdosage may result in cholinergic crisis, characterized by increasing muscle weakness. This, through involvement of respiratory muscles, may lead to death.

Treatment: Cholinergic crisis calls for the prompt withdrawal of all drugs of this type and the immediate use of atropine (see Anticholinergics/Antispasmodics in the Gastrointestinal chapter).

Atropine may also be used to abolish or minimize GI side effects or other muscarinic reactions; such use can lead to inadvertent induction of cholinergic crisis by masking signs of overdosage.

Administration and Dosage:

Prevention of postoperative distention and urinary retention: 1 ml of the 1:4000 solution (0.25 mg) SC or IM as soon as possible after operation; repeat every 4 to 6 hours for 2 or 3 days.

Treatment of postoperative distention: 1 ml of the 1:2000 solution (0.5 mg) SC or IM, as required.

Treatment of urinary retention: 1 ml of the 1:2000 solution (0.5 mg) SC or IM. If urination does not occur in ≤ 1 hour, catheterize the patient. After the patient has voided or the bladder is emptied, continue 0.5 mg injections every 3 hours for at least 5 injections.

Rx	**Prostigmin** (ICN)	**Injection:** 1:4000 (0.25 mg/ml) solution	In 1 ml amps.[1]
Rx	**Neostigmine Methylsulfate** (Various, eg, Elkins-Sinn, Schein)	**Injection:** 1:2000 (0.5 mg/ml) solution	In 10 ml vials and 10 ml multi-dose vials.
Rx	**Prostigmin** (ICN)		In 1 ml amps[1] and 10 ml multi-dose vials.[2]
🍁	**Prostigmin** (ICN)		In 1 ml amps[1] and 10 ml multi-dose vials.[2]
Rx	**Neostigmine Methylsulfate** (Various, eg, Elkins-Sinn)	**Injection:** 1:1000 (1 mg/ml) solution	In 10 ml vials.
Rx	**Prostigmin** (ICN)		In 10 ml multi-dose vials.[2]
🍁	**Prostigmin** (ICN)		In 10 ml vials.[2]
🍁	**Prostigmin** (ICN)	**Injection:** 1:400 (2.5 mg/ml) solution	In 5 ml vials.

[1] With 0.2% methyl and propyl parabens.
[2] With 0.45% phenol.

Analgesics

PENTOSAN POLYSULFATE SODIUM

Actions:

Pharmacology: Pentosan polysulfate sodium is a low molecular weight heparin-like compound. It has anticoagulant and fibrinolytic effects. The mechanism of action of pentosan polysulfate sodium in interstitial cystitis is not known. Pentosan polysulfate adheres to the bladder wall mucosal membrane and may act as a buffer to control cell permeability preventing irritating solutes in the urine from reaching the cells.

Pharmacokinetics:

Absorption – Pentosan polysulfate sodium absorption is ≈ 3% of the administered dose.

Distribution – Pentosan polysulfate sodium distributes to the uroepithelium of the GU tract with lesser amounts found in the liver, spleen, lung, skin, periosteum and bone marrow. Erythrocyte penetration is low in animals.

Metabolism – Sixty-eight percent of the dose at ≈ 1 hour after IV administration undergoes partial desulfation in the liver and spleen. Partial depolymerization occurs in the kidney. Both the desulfation and depolymerization can be saturated with continued dosing.

Excretion – The elimination half-life of pentosan polysulfate sodium has a mean value at 24 hours after IV injection of 40 mg. The elimination half-life in urine following oral pentosan polysulfate sodium is 4.8 hours for the unchanged drug. Urinary excretion averages 3.5% of the administered dose. After multiple doses of pentosan polysulfate sodium, urine excretion of radioactivity averaged 11% of the administered dose.

Clinical trials: Unblinded evaluations of 2499 patients were made every 3 months for the patients' rating of overall change in pain in comparison to baseline and for the difference calculated in "pain/discomfort" scores. At baseline, pain/discomfort scores for the 2499 patients were severe or unbearable in 60%, moderate in 33% and mild or none in 7% of patients. At 3 months, 722/2499 (29%) of the patients originally in the study had pain scores that improved by one or two categories. By 6 months, in the 892 patients who continued taking pentosan polysulfate sodium, an additional 116/2499 (5%) of patients had improved pain scores. After 6 months, the percent of patients who reported the first onset of pain relief was < 1.5% of patients who originally entered in the study.

Indications:

Interstitial cystitis: The relief of bladder pain or discomfort associated with interstitial cystitis.

Contraindications:

Hypersensitivity to the drug, structurally related compounds or excipients.

Warnings:

Alopecia is associated with pentosan polysulfate sodium and with heparin products. Alopecia may begin within the first 4 weeks of treatment. Ninety-seven percent of the cases of alopecia reported were alopecia areata, limited to a single area on the scalp.

Anticoagulant effects: Pentosan polysulfate sodium is a weak anticoagulant (1/15 the activity of heparin). It inhibits the generation of factor Xa in plasma and inhibits thrombin-induced platelet aggregation in human platelet-rich plasma ex vivo. Bleeding complications of ecchymosis, epistaxis and gum hemorrhage have been reported. Evaluate patients undergoing invasive procedures or having signs/symptoms of underlying coagulopathy or other increased risk of bleeding (because of other therapies such as coumarin anticoagulants, heparin, t-PA, streptokinase or high dose aspirin) for hemorrhage. Also evaluate patients with diseases such as aneurysms, thrombocytopenia, hemophilia, gastrointestinal ulcerations, polyps or diverticula before starting pentosan polysulfate sodium.

Hepatic/Splenic function impairment: Pentosan is desulfated by both the liver and the spleen. The extent to which hepatic insufficiency or splenic disorders may increase the bioavailability of the parent or active metabolites of pentosan polysulfate sodium is not known. Exercise caution when using pentosan polysulfate sodium in these patients. (Increases in PTT and PT [< 1% for both] or thrombocytopenia [0.2%] were noted).

Hepatotoxicity: Mildly (< 2.5 × normal) elevated transaminase, alkaline phosphatase, γ-glutamyl transpeptidase and lactic dehydrogenase occurred in 1.2% of patients. The increases usually appeared 3 to 12 months after the start of pentosan polysulfate sodium therapy and were not associated with jaundice or other clinical signs

PENTOSAN POLYSULFATE SODIUM

or symptoms. These abnormalities are usually transient, may remain essentially unchanged or may rarely progress with continued use.

Pregnancy: Category B. Animal studies did not reveal evidence of impaired fertility or harm to the fetus from pentosan polysulfate sodium. Adequate and well controlled studies have not been performed in pregnant women. Because animal studies are not always predictive of human response, use this drug in pregnancy only if clearly needed.

Lactation: It is not known whether this drug is excreted in breast milk. Exercise caution when pentosan polysulfate sodium is administered to a nursing woman.

Children: Safety and effectiveness in patients < 16 years old have not been established.

Precautions:

Monitoring: Reassess patients after 3 months. If improvement has not occurred and if limiting adverse events are not present, pentosan polysulfate sodium may be continued for another 3 months.

Thrombocytopenia: A similar product that was given subcutaneously, sublingually or intramuscularly (and not initially metabolized by the liver) is associated with delayed immunoallergic thrombocytopenia with symptoms of thrombosis and hemorrhage. Exercise caution when using pentosan polysulfate sodium in patients who have a history of heparin-induced thrombocytopenia.

Adverse Reactions:

CNS: Headache (3%); severe emotional liability/depression (2%); dizziness (1%); insomnia (≤ 1%).

Dermatologic: Alopecia (4%); rash (3%); pruritus, urticaria (≤ 1%).

GI: Diarrhea, nausea (4%); abdominal pain, dyspepsia (2%); anorexia, colitis, constipation, esophagitis, flatulence, gastritis, gum hemorrhage, mouth ulcer, vomiting (≤ 1%).

Hematologic: Increased partial thromboplastin time, increased prothrombin time, anemia, ecchymosis, leukopenia, thrombocytopenia (≤ 1%).

Hypersensitivity: Allergic reaction, photosensitivity (≤ 1%).

Respiratory: Epistaxis, dyspnea, pharyngitis, rhinitis (≤ 1%).

Special senses: Amblyopia, conjunctivitis, optic neuritis, retinal hemorrhage, tinnitus (≤ 1%).

Miscellaneous: Liver function abnormalities (1%; see Warnings).

Overdosage:

Overdose has not been reported. Based upon the pharmacodynamics of the drug, toxicity is likely to be reflected as anticoagulation, bleeding, thrombocytopenia, liver function abnormalities and gastric distress. In the event of acute overdosage, give the patient gastric lavage if possible, carefully observe and give symptomatic and supportive treatment.

Patient Information:

Patients should take the drug as prescribed, in the dosage prescribed and no more frequently than prescribed. Remind patients that pentosan polysulfate sodium has a weak anticoagulant effect. This effect may increase bleeding times.

Administration and Dosage:

The recommended dose of pentosan polysulfate sodium is 300 mg/day taken as one 100 mg capsule orally 3 times daily. Take with water at least 1 hour before or 2 hours after meals.

Storage/Stability: Store at controlled room temperature 15° to 30°C (59° to 86°F).

Rx	**Elmiron** (Baker Norton)	**Capsule:** 100 mg	(BNP7600). White. In 100s.
🍁	**Elmiron** (Baker Cummins)		(BNP7600). White. In 100s.

Analgesics

PHENAZOPYRIDINE HCl (Phenylazo Diamino Pyridine HCl)

Urinary analgesics in combination with urinary anti-infectives are listed in the Anti-Infectives chapter.

Actions:

Pharmacology: Phenazopyridine, an azo dye, is excreted in the urine where it exerts a topical analgesic effect on urinary tract mucosa; therefore, use only for relief of symptoms. Its mechanism of action is unknown. Phenazopyridine is compatible with antibacterial therapy and can help relieve pain and discomfort before antibacterial therapy controls the infection.

Pharmacokinetics: Phenazopyridine is rapidly excreted by the kidneys; 65% is excreted unchanged in urine.

Indications:

Symptomatic relief of pain, burning, urgency, frequency and other discomforts arising from irritation of the lower urinary tract mucosa caused by infection, trauma, surgery, endoscopic procedures or passage of sounds or catheters. Its analgesic action may reduce or eliminate the need for systemic analgesics or narcotics.

Contraindications:

Hypersensitivity to phenazopyridine; renal insufficiency.

Warnings:

Carcinogenesis: Long-term administration of phenazopyridine has induced neoplasia in rats (large intestine) and mice (liver).

Pregnancy: Category B. There are no adequate and well controlled studies in pregnant women. Use during pregnancy only if clearly needed.

Lactation: No information is available on the appearance of this drug or its metabolites in breast milk.

Children: Do not give to children < 12 years of age unless directed by physician.

Precautions:

Skin/sclera discoloration: A yellowish tinge of the skin or sclera may indicate accumulation because of impaired renal excretion; discontinue therapy if this occurs.

Duration of therapy: Treatment of a urinary tract infection (UTI) with phenazopyridine should not exceed 2 days because there is a lack of evidence that the combined administration of phenazopyridine and an antibacterial provides greater benefit than administration of the antibacterial alone after 2 days.

Drug Interactions:

Drug/Lab test interactions: As an azo dye, phenazopyridine may interfere with urinalysis based on spectrometry or color reactions.

Adverse Reactions:

Headache; rash; pruritus; occasional GI disturbances; anaphylactoid-like reaction; methemoglobinemia; hemolytic anemia; renal and hepatic toxicity (usually at overdosage levels); staining of contact lenses.

Overdosage:

Symptoms: Exceeding the recommended dose in patients with good renal function or administering the usual dose to patients with impaired renal function (common in elderly patients), may lead to increased serum levels and toxic reactions. Methemoglobinemia generally follows a massive, acute overdose. Oxidative Heinz body hemolytic anemia may occur, and "bite cells" (degmacytes) may be present in chronic overdosage. Red blood cell G–6–PD deficiency may predispose the patient to hemolysis. Renal and hepatic impairment and failure, usually because of hypersensitivity, may also occur.

Treatment: Methylene blue 1 to 2 mg/kg IV (see individual monograph) or 100 to 200 mg ascorbic acid orally should cause prompt reduction of methemoglobinemia and disappearance of cyanosis. Refer to General Management of Acute Overdosage.

Patient Information:

May cause GI upset; take after meals.

May cause a reddish-orange discoloration of the urine and may stain fabric. This is not abnormal and represents no cause for alarm. Staining of contact lenses has also occurred.

Do not use long-term to treat undiagnosed urinary tract pain. This product treats painful symptoms but not the source or cause of the pain.

Analgesics

PHENAZOPYRIDINE HCl (Phenylazo Diamino Pyridine HCl)

Administration and Dosage:

Do not use chronically to treat undiagnosed pain of the urinary tract. Such use could lead to serious delays in appropriate diagnosis and treatment. This product treats painful symptoms but does not treat the source or cause of the disorder causing the pain.

Adults: 200 mg 3 times/day after meals. Do not administer for > 2 days when used concomitantly with an antibacterial agent for the treatment of UTI.

Children (6 to 12 years): 12 mg/kg/day divided into three oral doses for 2 days.

Storage/Stability: Store at controlled room temperature 15° to 30°C (59° to 86°F).

otc	**Azo-Standard** (Alcon)	**Tablets:** 95 mg	(W). In 30s.
otc	**Prodium** (Breckenridge)		In 12s and 30s.
Rx	**Phenazopyridine HCl** (Various, eg, Moore, Parmed, URL)	**Tablets:** 100 mg	In 100s, 1000s and UD 100s.
otc	**Baridium** (Pfeiffer)		In 32s.
Rx	**Geridium** (Goldline)		Burgundy. Sugar coated. In 100s and 1000s.
Rx	**Pyridiate** (Rugby)		In 100s.
Rx	**Pyridium** (Parke-Davis)		Sucrose, lactose. (P-D 180). Maroon. In 100s, 1000s and UD 100s.
Rx	**Urodine** (Various, eg, IDE, Schein)		In 100s and 1000s.
Rx	**Urogesic** (Edwards)		In 100s.
Rx	**Phenazopyridine HCl** (Various, eg, Moore, Parmed, URL)	**Tablets:** 200 mg	In 100s, 1000s and UD 100s.
Rx	**Geridium** (Goldline)		Burgundy. Sugar coated. In 100s.
Rx	**Pyridium** (Parke-Davis)		Sucrose, lactose. (P-D 181). Maroon. In 100s, 1000s and UD 100s.
Rx	**Urodine** (Schein)		In 100s and 1000s.

DIMETHYL SULFOXIDE (DMSO)

Dimethyl sulfoxide (DMSO) is available in a variety of forms not intended for human use (eg, veterinary and industrial solvents). Discourage human use of such products because of their unknown purity. Because of its cutaneous transport characteristics, impurities and contaminants may be systemically absorbed from topical use.

Actions:

Pharmacology: DMSO is a clear, colorless liquid that is miscible with water and most organic solvents. Its broad range of pharmacological properties include: Anti-inflammatory action, membrane penetration, antifungal activity, cryoprotective effects for living cells and tissues, dissolution of collagen, nerve blockade, diuresis, cholinesterase inhibition, vasodilation and muscle relaxation.

Pharmacokinetics: Following topical application, DMSO is absorbed and widely distributed in tissue and body fluids. It is metabolized to dimethyl sulfone and dimethyl sulfide; DMSO and dimethyl sulfone are excreted in the urine and feces. DMSO is eliminated through the breath and skin and is responsible for the characteristic garlic odor. Unchanged DMSO has a half-life of 12 to 15 hours. Dimethyl sulfone can persist in serum > 2 weeks after a single intravesical instillation. No residual accumulation of DMSO has occurred after treatment for protracted periods of time.

Indications:

Symptomatic relief of interstitial cystitis.

Unlabeled uses: DMSO has been used in the topical treatment of musculoskeletal injuries and collagen diseases and the enhancement of percutaneous absorption of other drugs.

Other topical systemic uses include: Scleroderma; arthritis; tendinitis; bursitis; breast and prostate malignancies; retinitis pigmentosa; herpes virus infections; head and spinal cord injury; stroke. Some reports claim limited extravasation injury and enhanced antineoplastic activity when DMSO is used with some chemotherapy agents. It has been used in renal amyloidosis.

Warnings:

Urinary tract infections, bacterial: There is no clinical evidence of effectiveness in the treatment of bacterial urinary tract infections.

Ocular lens: In monkeys, dogs and rats, chronic administration of DMSO produces changes in the refractive index of the ocular lens and causes opacities. Although no ophthalmic changes have been observed in patients receiving therapy for cystitis, eye examinations are advisable before and after therapy.

Hypersensitivity: DMSO can liberate histamine; hypersensitivity reactions may occur with topical administration. If anaphylactoid symptoms develop, institute appropriate therapy. Refer to Management of Acute Hypersensitivity Reactions.

Pregnancy: Category C. Safety for use during pregnancy has not been established. Use only when clearly needed and when the potential benefits outweigh the potential hazards to the fetus.

High intraperitoneal doses of DMSO caused teratogenesis in small animals, but oral or topical doses did not. Two studies in rabbits using large topical doses produced conflicting reproductive results.

Lactation: It is not known whether this drug is excreted in breast milk. Exercise caution when administering to a nursing woman.

Children: Safety and efficacy for use in children have not been established.

DIMETHYL SULFOXIDE (DMSO)

Precautions:

Monitoring: Perform liver and renal function tests and complete blood counts every 6 months.

Ophthalmic effects: Lens opacities and changes in the refractive index have been seen in animals given chronic high doses of DMSO. Perform full eye evaluations, including slit-lamp examinations, prior to and periodically during treatment.

Intravesical instillation may be harmful to patients with urinary tract malignancy because of DMSO-induced vasodilation.

Garlic-like taste may occur within a few minutes after instillation. This taste may last several hours; odor on the breath and skin may remain for 72 hours.

Transient chemical cystitis has followed instillation of DMSO. Moderately severe discomfort on administration usually becomes less prominent with repeated use.

Drug Interactions:

DMSO administration may decrease the formation of the active metabolite of **sulindac**, possibly resulting in a decreased therapeutic effect. A severe peripheral neuropathy has also occurred when topical **DMSO** was used concurrently with **sulindac**.

Adverse Reactions:

Sedation (52%); nausea (32%); headache (42%); dizziness (18%); burning or aching eyes (9%); vomiting (6%); local dermatitis (3.5%); garlic-like breath, transient chemical cystitis (see precautions); erythema; itching; burning; discomfort; blistering; maceration; scaling; dermatitis; burning on urination; transient disturbance of color perception; photophobia; flu syndrome; diarrhea; weight loss and gain; sore throat; cough; anorexia.

Overdosage:

In case of accidental oral ingestion, induce emesis. Additional measures that may be considered are gastric lavage, activated charcoal and forced diuresis. Refer to General Management of Acute Overdosage.

Patient Information:

A garlic-like taste may be noted within a few minutes of administration; odor on the breath and skin may be present and remain for up to 72 hours.

Administration and Dosage:

Not for IM or IV injection.

Instill 50 ml DMSO solution directly into the bladder by catheter or asepto syringe and allow to remain for 15 minutes. Apply an analgesic lubricant gel, such as lidocaine jelly, to the urethra prior to inserting the catheter to avoid spasm. The medication is expelled by spontaneous voiding. Repeat every 2 weeks until maximum symptomatic relief is obtained. Thereafter, increase time intervals between treatments.

To reduce bladder spasm, administer oral analgesics or suppositories containing belladonna and opium prior to instillation. In patients with severe interstitial cystitis and very sensitive bladders, perform the initial treatment, and possibly the second and third (depending on patient response), under anesthesia (saddle block has been suggested).

Storage/Stability: Protect from strong light. Store at room temperature 15° to 30°C (59° to 86°F).

Rx	**Rimso-50** (Research Industries)	**Solution:** 50% aqueous solution	In 50 ml.
	Rimso-50 (Roberts)	**Solution:** 50% aqueous solution	In 50 ml.
	Kemsol (Horner	**Solution:** 70% solution	Alcohol free. In 250 ml.

CELLULOSE SODIUM PHOSPHATE

Actions:

Pharmacology: Cellulose Sodium Phosphate (CSP), a synthetic compound made by phosphorylation of cellulose, is insoluble in water and is nonabsorbable. CSP has excellent ion exchange properties, the sodium ion exchanging for calcium. When taken orally, CSP binds calcium; the complex of calcium and cellulose phosphate is then excreted in feces.

CSP alters urinary composition of calcium, magnesium (Mg), phosphate and oxalate by affecting their absorption in the intestinal tract. When given orally with meals, CSP binds dietary and secreted calcium and reduces urinary calcium by ≈ 50 mg/5 g of CSP. It also binds dietary magnesium and lowers urinary magnesium. Oral magnesium supplementation given separately from CSP partially overcomes this effect.

CSP administration increases urinary phosphorus and oxalate. The usual rise in urinary phosphorus of 150 to 250 mg/15 g of CSP largely reflects the hydrolysis of 7% to 30% of CSP in the intestinal tract and absorption of released phosphorus. An increase in urinary oxalate occurs. Because CSP binds divalent cations, the cations are not available to complex oxalate and limit its absorption. The rise in urinary oxalate may be largely prevented by moderate dietary oxalate restriction and a modest dose of CSP (10 to 15 g/day).

The marked reduction in urinary calcium, with only slightly increased urinary phosphorus and oxalate, leads to a reduction in urinary saturation and propensity for spontaneous nucleation of calcium oxalate and calcium phosphate (brushite).

CSP apparently does not alter the metabolism of trace metals because it does not significantly change the serum concentration of copper (Cu), zinc (Zn) or iron (Fe).

Indications:

Absorptive hypercalciuria Type I with recurrent calcium oxalate or calcium phosphate nephrolithiasis. Appropriate use of CSP substantially reduces the incidence of new stone formation. Do not expect causes of hypercalciuria other than hyperabsorption to respond to CSP.

Characteristics of absorptive hypercalciuria Type I – Recurrent passage or formation of calcium oxalate or calcium phosphate renal stones; no evidence of bone disease; normal serum calcium and phosphorus; increased intestinal calcium absorption; hypercalciuria; normal urinary calcium during fasting; normal parathyroid function; and lack of renal "leak" or excessive skeletal mobilization of calculi.

Absorptive hypercalciuria Type II is identical, except it can be eliminated by a low calcium diet.

Contraindications:

Primary or secondary hyperparathyroidism, including renal hypercalciuria (renal calcium leak); hypomagnesemic states (serum Mg < 1.5 mg/dl); osteoporosis, osteomalacia, osteitis; hypocalcemic states (eg, hypoparathyroidism, intestinal malabsorption); normal or low intestinal absorption and renal excretion of calcium; enteric hyperoxaluria.

Do not use in patients with high fasting urinary calcium or hypophosphatemia, unless a high skeletal mobilization of calcium can be excluded.

Warnings:

Congestive Heart Failure (CHF) or ascites: The sodium contained in CSP (35 to 48 mEq exchangeable sodium per 15 g CSP) may represent a hazard.

Pregnancy: Category C. Safety for use during pregnancy has not been established. Because of the increased dietary calcium requirement in pregnant women, use only when clearly needed and when the potential benefits outweigh potential hazards to the fetus.

Children: Because of the increased requirement for dietary calcium in growing children, the use of CSP in children < 16 years of age is not recommended.

CELLULOSE SODIUM PHOSPHATE

Precautions:

Parathyroid effects: By inhibiting intestinal calcium absorption, CSP may stimulate parathyroid function, leading to hyperparathyroid hormone levels. Monitor parathyroid hormone levels. CSP treatment can maintain parathyroid function within normal limits if it is used only in absorptive hypercalciuria Type I at a dosage just sufficient to restore normal calcium absorption but not sufficient to cause subnormal absorption.

Long-term use: Complications may potentially develop during long-term use include hyperoxaluria and hypomagnesiuria, which would negate the beneficial effect of hypocalciuria on new stone formation; magnesium depletion; depletion of trace metals (Cu, Zn, Fe). Minimize effects by restricting the use of CSP to only absorptive hypercalciuria Type I; take precautionary measures by monitoring serum Ca, Mg, Cu, Zn, Fe and parathyroid hormone, and perform complete blood counts every 3 to 6 months.

Repeat borderline values for parathyroid hormone and calcium promptly. Obtain serum PTH at least once between the first 2 weeks to 3 months; adjust or stop treatment if serum PTH rises above normal. If there is an inadequate hypocalciuric response to CSP treatment (a reduction in urinary calcium of < 30 mg/5 g of CSP) while patients are maintained on moderate calcium and sodium restriction, discontinue treatment. Consider cessation of treatment if urinary oxalate exceeds 55 mg/day on moderate dietary oxalate restriction.

Dietary measures: Moderate calcium intake; avoid dairy products. Moderately restrict dietary oxalate by avoiding spinach (and similar dark greens), rhubarb, chocolate and brewed tea. Avoid vitamin C supplementation because of its potential metabolism to oxalate. Discourage a high sodium intake to achieve an intake of < 150 mEq/day. Encourage fluid intake to achieve a minimum urine output of 2 L/day.

Adverse Reactions:

GI: Poor taste of the drug; loose bowel movements; diarrhea; dyspepsia.

Administration and Dosage:

Initial dose of CSP is 15 g/day (5 g with each meal) in patients with urinary calcium > 300 mg/day (on moderate calcium-restricted diet). When urinary calcium declines to < 150 mg/day, reduce to 10 g/day (5 g with supper, 2.5 g with each remaining meal). Begin patients with controlled urinary calcium on moderate calcium-restricted diet < 300 mg/day (but > 200 mg/day) on 10 g/day.

Suspend each dose of CSP (powder) in a glass of water, soft drink or fruit juice; ingest within 30 minutes of a meal. Do not take with magnesium gluconate. The amount of bound dietary calcium is considerably reduced when CSP is administered > 1 hour after a meal. Base the initial and maintenance doses of CSP on measurements of 24-hour urinary calcium excretion.

Concomitant magnesium supplements: The dose of oral magnesium supplements, given as magnesium gluconate, depends upon the dose of CSP. Those receiving 15 g of CSP/day should take 1.5 g of magnesium gluconate before breakfast and again at bedtime (separately from CSP). Those taking 10 g of CSP/day should take 1 g of magnesium gluconate twice a day. To avoid binding of magnesium by CSP, give supplemental magnesium at least 1 hour before or after a dose of CSP.

Storage/Stability: Store in a dry place at room temperature 15° to 30°C (59° to 86°F).

Rx	**Calcibind** (Mission)	**Powder:** Inorganic phosphate content 31% to 36% and sodium content ≈ 11%	In 300 g bulk powder.

ACETOHYDROXAMIC ACID (AHA)

Actions:

Pharmacology: Acetohydroxamic acid (AHA) reversibly inhibits the bacterial enzyme urease, thereby inhibiting the hydrolysis of urea and production of ammonia in urine infected with urea-splitting organisms. The reduced ammonia levels and decreased pH enhance the effectiveness of antimicrobial agents and increase the cure rate of these infections. AHA does not acidify urine directly, nor does it have a direct antibacterial effect.

In patients with urea-splitting urinary infections (often accompanied by struvite stone disease) that are recalcitrant to other management, AHA reduces the pathologically elevated urinary ammonia and pH levels.

Pharmacokinetics:

Absorption/Distribution – AHA is well absorbed from the GI tract after oral administration; peak blood levels occur 0.25 to 1 hour after a given dose; it is distributed throughout body water. AHA chelates with dietary iron. Treat concomitant hypochromic anemia with intramuscular iron.

Excretion – From 36% to 65% of the drug is excreted unchanged in the urine and provides the therapeutic effect, but the concentration of AHA in urine that is necessary to inhibit urease is incompletely delineated. Concentrations as low as 8 mcg/ml may be beneficial; expect higher concentrations (eg, 30 mcg/ml) to provide more complete urease inhibition. Plasma half-life of AHA is ≈ 5 to 10 hours with normal renal function and is prolonged in patients with reduced renal function.

Indications:

Adjunctive therapy in chronic urea-splitting urinary infection: Do not use in lieu of curative surgical treatment (for patients with stones) or antimicrobial treatment. Long-term treatment may be warranted to maintain urease inhibition as long as urea-splitting infection is present.

Contraindications:

In patients whose physical state and disease are amenable to surgery or antimicrobial agents, whose urine is infected by nonurease-producing organisms and whose renal function is poor (eg, serum creatinine > 2.5 mg/dl or Ccr < 20 ml/min) and in females without a satisfactory method of contraception whose urinary infections can be controlled by culture-specific oral antimicrobial agents; pregnancy.

Warnings:

Coombs-negative hemolytic anemia has occurred. GI upset characterized by nausea, vomiting, anorexia and generalized malaise have accompanied the most severe forms of hemolytic anemia. Approximately 3% of patients developed hemolytic anemia of sufficient magnitude to interrupt treatment. Approximately 15% of patients on AHA have had only laboratory findings of an anemia. However, most patients developed a mild reticulocytosis. The untoward reactions have reverted to normal following treatment cessation. A complete blood count, including reticulocytes, is recommended after 2 weeks of treatment. If reticulocyte count is > 6%, reduce dosage. Perform a CBC and reticulocyte count at 3-month intervals for the treatment duration.

Hematologic effects: Bone marrow depression (leukopenia, anemia and thrombocytopenia) has occurred in animals receiving large doses of AHA but has not been seen in man. Its bone marrow suppression is probably related to its ability to inhibit DNA synthesis, but anemia could also be related to depletion of iron stores. Hemolysis, with a decrease in the circulating RBCs, hemoglobin and hematocrit, has been noted. Platelet or white blood cell abnormalities have not been noted, but clinical monitoring is recommended.

Renal function impairment: Because AHA is eliminated primarily by the kidneys, closely monitor patients and reduce daily dose to avoid excessive drug accumulation.

Hepatic function impairment: Abnormalities have not been reported, but close monitoring is recommended because a derivative of AHA has caused significant liver dysfunction.

Carcinogenesis/Mutagenesis/Fertility impairment: Acetamide, a metabolite of AHA, caused hepatocellular carcinoma in rats at doses 1500 times the human dose. AHA is cytotoxic and was positive for mutagenicity in the Ames test.

Pregnancy: Category X. May cause fetal harm when administered to a pregnant woman. AHA was teratogenic (retarded or clubbed rear leg at ≥ 750 mg/kg and exencephaly and encephalocele at 1500 mg/kg) when given to rats. Do not use in women who are or who may become pregnant. If a patient becomes pregnant while taking this drug, inform her of the potential hazard to the fetus.

ACETOHYDROXAMIC ACID (AHA)

Lactation: It is not known if AHA is secreted in breast milk. Discontinue nursing or the drug, taking into account the importance of the drug to the mother.

Children: Children with chronic, recalcitrant, urea-splitting urinary infection may benefit from AHA. Dosage has not been established; although, 10 mg/kg/day, taken in 2 or 3 divided doses for up to 1 year, has been tolerated. Monitor patients.

Drug Interactions:

Alcoholic beverages taken with AHA have caused rash.

Heavy metals: AHA chelates heavy metals, notably iron. The absorption of iron and AHA from the intestinal lumen may be reduced when both drugs are taken concomitantly. When iron is indicated, administer IM.

Adverse Reactions:

Of 150 patients treated, most for > 1 year, adverse reactions have occurred in ≤ 30%. Adverse reactions seem more prevalent in patients with preexisting thrombophlebitis, phlebothrombosis or advanced degrees of renal insufficiency. The risk of adverse reactions is highest during the first year of treatment. Chronic treatment does not seem to increase risk or severity of adverse reactions.

CNS: Mild headaches (≈ 30%) during the first 48 hours of treatment respond to oral salicylate analgesics and usually disappear spontaneously.

Depression, anxiety, nervousness, malaise and tremulousness (20% to 25%). In most patients, the symptoms were mild and transitory; however, in ≈ 6%, symptoms warranted interruption or discontinuation of treatment.

GI: Nausea, vomiting, anorexia (20% to 25%). In most, symptoms were mild, transitory and did not interrupt treatment.

Hematologic: A mild reticulocytosis (5% to 6%) without anemia is even more prevalent than anemia. The laboratory findings are occasionally accompanied by malaise, lethargy, fatigue and GI symptoms that improve following cessation of treatment. Hematological abnormalities are more prevalent in patients with advanced renal failure (see Warnings).

Cardiovascular: Superficial phlebitis involving the lower extremities. One patient developed deep vein thrombosis of the lower extremities. All resolved following therapy.

Embolic phenomena were reported in three patients taking AHA; this resolved following discontinuation of AHA and implementation of medical therapy. Several patients have resumed AHA treatment without ill effect. Palpitations have also been reported.

Dermatologic: Nonpruritic, macular skin rash in the upper extremities and on the face have occurred when AHA has been taken long-term and usually concomitantly with alcohol. The rash commonly appears 30 to 45 minutes after ingestion of alcohol, may be associated with a general sensation of warmth and disappears spontaneously in 30 to 60 minutes. In some patients, the rash may warrant drug discontinuation. Alopecia has been reported.

Overdosage:

Symptoms: Mild overdosages resulting in hemolysis have occurred occasionally with reduced renal function after several weeks or months of continuous treatment.

Acute deliberate overdosage has not occurred, but would be expected to induce the following: Anorexia, malaise, lethargy, diminished sense of well being, tremulousness, anxiety, nausea and vomiting. Laboratory findings are likely to include an elevated reticulocyte count and a severe hemolytic reaction requiring hospitalization, symptomatic treatment and possibly blood transfusions. Anticipate concomitant reduction in platelets or white blood cells.

Treatment: Cessation of treatment, monitoring of hematologic status, symptomatic treatment and blood transfusions as required. The drug is probably dialyzable but has not been clinically tested. Refer to General Management of Acute Overdosage.

Administration and Dosage:

Adults: 250 mg, 3 to 4 times a day for a total dose of 10 to 15 mg/kg/day. The recommended starting dose is 12 mg/kg/day, administered at 6- to 8-hour intervals on an empty stomach. The maximum daily dose is ≤ 1.5 g.

Children: Initial dose is 10 mg/kg/day. Monitor clinical condition and hematologic status; dosage titration may be required.

Renal function impairment: Patients with serum creatinine of > 1.8 mg/dl should take no more than 1 g/day, dosed at 12–hour intervals. Further dosage reductions to prevent accumulation may be desirable. Do not treat patients with advanced (eg, serum creatinine > 2.5 mg/dl) renal insufficiency.

Rx	**Lithostat** (Mission)	**Tablets:** 250 mg	White. In unit-of-use 100s.

ALPROSTADIL (Prostaglandin E_1; PGE_1)

For information on the use of alprostadil for patent ductus arteriosus, refer to the specific monograph in the Miscellaneous section.

Actions:

Pharmacology: Alprostadil has a wide variety of pharmacological actions; vasodilation and inhibition of platelet aggregation are among the most notable of these effects. In animals, alprostadil relaxed retractor penis and corpus cavernosum urethrae. Alprostadil also relaxed isolated preparations of human corpus cavernosum and spongiosum, as well as cavernous arterial segments contracted by either noradrenaline or $PGF_{2\alpha}$ in vitro. In pigtail monkeys, alprostadil increased cavernous arterial blood flow. The degree and duration of cavernous smooth muscle relaxation in this animal was dose-dependent.

Alprostadil induces erection by relaxation of trabecular smooth muscle and by dilation of cavernosal arteries. This leads to expansion of lacunar spaces and entrapment of blood by compressing the venules against the tunica albuginea, a process referred to as the corporal veno-occlusive mechanism.

Pharmacokinetics:

Absorption – For the treatment of erectile dysfunction, alprostadil is administered by injection into the corpora cavernosa or inserted intraurethrally. It is absorbed from the urethra, transported throughout the erectile bodies by communicating vessels between the corpus spongiosum and corpora cavernosa and is able to induce vasodilation of the targeted vascular beds.

Intraurethral administration is preceded by urination, and the residual urine disperses the medicated pellet, permitting alprostadil to be absorbed by the urethral mucosa. The transurethral absorption of alprostadil after administration is biphasic. Initial absorption is rapid, with ≈ 80% of an administered dose absorbed within 10 minutes. The mean time to the maximum plasma PGE_1 concentration after a 1000 mcg intraurethral dose is ≈ 16 minutes.

In ten volunteers, endogenous PGE_1 levels in the ejaculate averaged 31 mcg (range, 0 to 161 mcg). In these same volunteers, an average of 123 mcg of additional PGE_1 (range, 30 to 369 mcg) was present in the ejaculate obtained 10 minutes after the highest dose (1000 mcg) of alprostadil. The mean total endogenous PGE content (PGE_1, PGE_2, 19-OH-PGE_1 and 19-OH-PGE_2) of the ejaculate in these subjects was 444 mcg (range, 0 to 1423 mcg).

Distribution –

Intracavernosal: Following intracavernosal injection of 20 mcg, mean peripheral plasma concentrations at 30 and 60 minutes after injection (89 and 102 pcg/ml, respectively) were not significantly greater than baseline levels of endogenous alprostadil (96 pcg/ml). Alprostadil is bound in plasma primarily to albumin (81%) and to a lesser extent to α-globulin IV-4 fraction (55%).

Intraurethral: Following intraurethral administration, alprostadil is absorbed from the urethral mucosa into the corpus spongiosum. A portion of the administered dose is transported to the corpora cavernosa through collateral vessels, while the remainder passes into the pelvic venous circulation through veins draining the corpus spongiosum. The half-life is short, varying between 30 seconds and 10 minutes. Peripheral venous plasma levels of PGE_1 are low or undetectable (< 2 pg/ml) after administration. The mean maximum plasma PGE_1 concentration following intraurethral administration of the highest dose of alprostadil (1000 mcg) was barely detectable (11.4 pg/ml). In a study of 14 subjects, the plasma PGE_1 level was shown to be undetectable within 60 minutes of alprostadil administration in most subjects.

Metabolism – Alprostadil is rapidly converted to compounds that are further metabolized prior to excretion. Following administration, 60% to 90% of circulating alprostadil is metabolized in one pass through the lungs by enzymatic oxidation of the 15-hydroxyl group to 15-keto-PGE_1. The near-complete pulmonary first-pass metabolism of PGE_1 is the primary factor influencing the systemic pharmacokinetics of alprostadil and is a reason that peripheral venous plasma levels of PGE_1 are low or undetectable (< 2 pg/ml) following alprostadil administration. The enzyme catalyzing this process has been isolated from many tissues in the lower GU tract including the urethra, prostate and corpus cavernosum. 15-keto-PGE_1 retains little (1% to 2%) of the biological activity of PGE_1. 15-keto-PGE_1 is rapidly reduced to form the most abundant metabolite in plasma, 13,14-dihydro,15-keto PGE_1 (DHK-PGE_1), which is biologically inactive. The majority of DHK-PGE_1 is further metabolized to smaller prostaglandin remnants that are cleared primarily by the kidney and liver.

Excretion – The metabolites of alprostadil are excreted primarily by the kidney, with almost 90% of an administered IV dose excreted in urine within 24 hours postdose. The remainder of the dose is excreted in the feces. There is no evidence of tissue retention of alprostadil or its metabolites following IV use.

ALPROSTADIL (Prostaglandin E_1; PGE_1)

Indications:

Erectile dysfunction: Treatment of erectile dysfunction due to neurogenic, vasculogenic, psychogenic or mixed etiology.

Intracavernosal alprostadil may be a useful adjunct to other diagnostic tests in the diagnosis of erectile dysfunction.

Unlabeled uses: Diagnostic peripheral arteriography (0.7 mcg/min for 10 min); treatment of atherosclerosis, gangrene and pain due to peripheral vascular disease.

Contraindications:

Hypersensitivity to the drug; conditions that might predispose patients to priapism (eg, sickle cell anemia or trait, multiple myeloma, leukemia); patients with anatomical deformation of the penis (eg, angulation, cavernosal fibrosis, Peyronie's disease); patients with penile implants (intracavernosal); use in women, children or newborns (see Warnings); use in men for whom sexual activity is inadvisable or contraindicated; for sexual intercourse with a pregnant woman unless the couple uses a condom barrier.

Warnings:

Priapism (erection lasting > 6 hours) is known to occur following intracavernosal administration of vasoactive substances, including alprostadil. To minimize the chances of prolonged erection or priapism, titrate slowly to the lowest effective dose. Instruct the patient to immediately report to his physician or, if unavailable, to seek immediate medical assistance for any erection that persists for > 6 hours. Treat priapism according to established medical practice. In the majority of cases, spontaneous detumescence occurs. If priapism is not treated immediately, penile tissue damage and permanent loss of potency may result.

Penile fibrosis: The overall incidence of penile fibrosis, including Peyronie's disease, was 3%. In one self-injection clinical study where duration of use was up to 18 months, the incidence of fibrosis was 7.8%. Regular follow-up of patients, with careful examination of the penis, is strongly recommended to detect signs of penile fibrosis. Discontinue treatment in patients who develop penile angulation, cavernosal fibrosis or Peyronie's disease.

Penile pain after intracavernosal administration was reported by 37% of patients at least once in clinical studies of up to 18 months in duration. In the majority of the cases, penile pain was rated mild or moderate in intensity; 3% discontinued treatment because of penile pain. The frequency of penile pain was 2% in 294 patients who received 1 to 3 injections of placebo. Inject alprostadil slowly to decrease penile pain.

Hematoma/Ecchymosis: In most cases, hematoma/ecchymosis was judged to be a complication of a faulty injection technique. Accordingly, proper instruction of the patient in self-injection is of importance to minimize the potential for this.

Hemodynamic changes, manifested as decreases in blood pressure and increases in pulse rate, principally at doses > 20 mcg, were observed during clinical studies, and appeared to be dose-dependent. However, these changes were usually clinically unimportant; only 3 patients discontinued the treatment because of it.

Erectile dysfunction: Diagnose and treat underlying treatable medical causes of erectile dysfunction prior to initiation of therapy.

Pulmonary disease: The pulmonary extraction of alprostadil following intravascular administration was reduced by 15% in patients with acute respiratory distress syndrome (ARDS) compared with a control group of patients with normal respiratory function who were undergoing cardiopulmonary bypass surgery. Pulmonary clearance was found to vary as a function of cardiac output and pulmonary intrinsic clearance in a group of 14 patients with ARDS or at risk of developing ARDS following trauma or sepsis. In this study, the extraction efficiency of alprostadil ranged from subnormal (11%) to normal (90%), with an overall mean of 67%.

Renal/Hepatic function impairment: Pulmonary first-pass metabolism is the primary factor influencing the systemic clearance of alprostadil. Alterations in renal or hepatic function would not be expected to have a major influence on pharmacokinetics.

Elderly: In patients with ARDS, the mean pulmonary extraction of alprostadil was 72% in 11 elderly patients ≥ 65 years of age and 65% in six young patients ≤ 35 years.

Pregnancy: These products are not indicated for use in women. Do not use for sexual intercourse with a pregnant woman unless the couple uses a condom barrier.

Children: Not indicated for use in newborns or children. However, alprostadil (*Prostin VR Pediatric*) is used in newborns to maintain the patency of the ductus arteriosus in neonates with congenital heart defects (see specific monograph).

Precautions:

Monitoring: During in-clinic dosing, monitor for symptoms of hypotension.

ALPROSTADIL (Prostaglandin E_1; PGE_1)

Drug Interactions:

Alprostadil Drug Interactions			
Precipitant drug	Object drug*		Description
Alprostadil	Anticoagulants	↑	Patients on anticoagulants, such as warfarin or heparin, may have increased propensity for bleeding after intracavernosal injection.
Alprostadil	Cyclosporine	↓	Alprostadil may decrease cyclosporine's blood concentration.
Alprostadil	Vasoactive agents	↔	The safety and efficacy of combinations of alprostadil and other vasoactive agents have not been systematically studied. Therefore, the use of such combinations is not recommended.

* ↑ = Object drug increased. ↓ = Object drug decreased. ↔ = Undetermined effect.

Adverse Reactions:

Local:

Local Adverse Reactions with Alprostadil		
Adverse reaction	Intracavernosal	Intraurethral
Penile pain[1,2]	37%	36%
Urethral pain	-	13%
Urethral burning	< 1%	12%
Urethral bleeding/spotting	-	3%
Testicular pain	< 1%	5%
Prolonged erection[2]	4%	-
Penile fibrosis[2]	3%	-
Injection site hematoma	3%	-
Penis disorder[3]	3%	-
Injection site ecchymosis	2%	-
Penile rash	1%	-
Penile edema	1%	-
Priapism[2]	0.4%	-
Hematoma[2]	3%	-
Ecchymosis[2]	2%	-

[1] Except for penile pain (2%), no significant local adverse reactions were reported by 294 patients who received 1 to 3 injections of placebo.
[2] See Warnings.
[3] Includes numbness, yeast infection, irritation, sensitivity, phimosis, pruritus, erythema, venous leak, penile skin tear, strange feeling of penis, discoloration of penile head, itch at tip of penis.

Other reactions – The following local adverse reactions were reported by < 1% of patients after injection of alprostadil: Balanitis; injection site hemorrhage/inflammation/itching/swelling/edema; penile warmth; numbness; yeast infection; irritation; sensitivity; phimosis; pruritus; erythema; venous leak; painful erection; abnormal ejaculation.

Systemic:

Systemic Adverse Reactions with Alprostadil		
Adverse reaction	Intracavernosal	Intraurethral
CNS		
Headache	2%	3%
Dizziness	1%	4%
Fainting	-	0.4%
Respiratory		
Respiratory infection	4%	3%
Flu syndrome	2%	4%
Sinusitis/Rhinitis	2%	2%
Nasal congestion	1%	-
Cough	1%	-

ALPROSTADIL (Prostaglandin E_1; PGE_1)

Systemic Adverse Reactions with Alprostadil

Adverse reaction	Intracavernosal	Intraurethral
Miscellaneous		
Hypertension	2%	-
Hypotension	< 1%	3%
Localized pain[1]	2%	-
Trauma[2]	2%	-
Prostatic disorder[3]	2%	-
Back pain	1%	2%
Pain	-	3%
Pelvic pain	< 1%	2%
Accidental injury	-	3%

[1] Pain in various anatomical structures other than injection site.
[2] Injuries, fractures, abrasions, lacerations, dislocations.
[3] Prostatitis, pain, hypertrophy, enlargement.

Other reactions – The following systemic events were reported by < 1% of patients in clinical studies: Scrotal disorder/edema; hematuria; impaired urination; urinary frequency/urgency; vasodilation; peripheral vascular disorder; supraventricular extrasystoles; vasovagal reactions; hypesthesia; non-generalized weakness; diaphoresis; rash; non-application site pruritus; skin neoplasm; nausea; dry mouth; increased serum creatinine; leg cramps; mydriasis.

Female – Vaginal burning/itching (5.8%, intraurethral administration only).

Overdosage:

If overdose of alprostadil occurs, the patient should be under medical supervision until any systemic effects have resolved or until penile detumescence has occurred. Symptomatic treatment of any systemic symptoms would be appropriate.

Patient Information:

Patient instructions for administration are included in each package of alprostadil.

The patient should not change the dose of alprostadil established in the physician's office without consulting the physician. The patient may expect an erection to occur within 5 to 20 minutes.

Do not use alprostadil if the female partner is pregnant, unless the couple uses a condom barrier.

Administration and Dosage:

Individualize the dose for each patient by careful titration under supervision by the physician. In general, always employ the lowest possible effective dose. For specific administration techniques, refer to the Patient Information material provided with each product.

Intracavernosal: A ½-inch, 27- to 30-gauge needle is generally recommended.

The first injections of alprostadil must be done at the physician's office by medically trained personnel. Self-injection therapy by the patient can be started only after the patient is properly instructed and well trained in the self-injection technique. The physician should make a careful assessment of the patient's skills and competence with this procedure. The site of injection is usually along the dorso-lateral aspect of the proximal third of the penis. Avoid visible veins. The side of the penis that is injected and the site of injection must be alternated.

The dose of alprostadil that is selected for self-injection treatment should provide the patient with an erection that is satisfactory for sexual intercourse and that is maintained for no longer than 1 hour. If the duration of erection is > 1 hour, reduce the dose. Initiate self-injection therapy for use at home at the dose that was determined in the physician's office; however, make dose adjustments, if required (up to 57% of patients in one clinical study), only after consultation with the physician. Adjust the dose in accordance with the titration guidelines described above. The effectiveness for long-term use of up to 6 months has been documented in an uncontrolled, self-injection study. The mean dose at the end of 6 months was 20.7 mcg.

Exercise careful and continuous follow-up of the patient while in the self-injection program. This is especially true for the initial self-injections, because adjustments in the dose of alprostadil may be needed. The recommended frequency of injection is no more than 3 times weekly, with at least 24 hours between each dose. The reconstituted vial of alprostadil is intended for single use only; discard after use. Instruct the user in the proper disposal of the syringe, needle and vial.

While on self-injection treatment, it is recommended that the patient visit the prescribing physician's office every 3 months. At that time, assess the efficacy and safety of the therapy, and adjust the dose if needed.

ALPROSTADIL (Prostaglandin E_1; PGE_1)

Initial titration – The patient must stay in the physician's office until complete detumescence occurs. If there is no response, then the next higher dose may be given within 1 hour. If there is a response, then wait at least 1 day before the next dose is given.

Erectile dysfunction of vasculogenic, psychogenic or mixed etiology: Initiate dosage titration at 2.5 mcg. If there is a partial response, the dose may be increased by 2.5 mcg to a dose of 5 mcg and then in increments of 5 to 10 mcg, depending on erectile response, until the dose that produces an erection suitable for intercourse and not exceeding a duration of 1 hour is reached. If there is no response to the initial 2.5 mcg dose, the second dose may be increased to 7.5 mcg, followed by increments of 5 to 10 mcg.

Erectile dysfunction of pure neurogenic etiology (spinal cord injury): Initiate dosage titration at 1.25 mcg. The dose may be increased by 1.25 mcg to a dose of 2.5 mcg, followed by an increment of 2.5 mcg to a dose of 5 mcg, and then in 5 mcg increments until the dose that produces an erection suitable for intercourse and not exceeding a duration of 1 hour is reached.

Adjunct to the diagnosis of erectile dysfunction – In the simplest diagnostic test for erectile dysfunction (pharmacologic testing), patients are monitored for the occurrence of an erection after an intracavernosal injection of alprostadil. Extensions of this testing are the use of alprostadil as an adjunct to laboratory investigations, such as duplex or Doppler imaging, ^{133}Xenon washout tests, radioisotope penogram and penile arteriography to allow visualization and assessment of penile vasculature. For these tests, use a single dose of alprostadil that induces a rigid erection.

Solution preparation – Alprostadil is packaged in a 5 ml glass vial. Bacteriostatic Water or Sterile Water for Injection, both preserved with benzyl alcohol 0.945% w/v, must be used as the diluent for reconstitution. After reconstitution, immediately use the solution and do not store or freeze.

Storage/Stability – Store at or below 25°C (77°F). Use the reconstituted solution immediately; do not store or freeze. Use only the diluent supplied.

Intraurethral: Administer as needed to achieve an erection. The onset of effect is within 5 to 10 minutes after administration. The duration of effect is ≈ 30 to 60 minutes. A medical professional should instruct each patient on proper technique for administering alprostadil prior to self-administration. The maximum frequency of use is no more than two systems per 24-hour period.

Initiation of therapy – Titrate dose under the supervision of a physician to test a patient's responsiveness to alprostadil, to demonstrate proper administration technique and to monitor for evidence of hypotension. Individually titrate patients to the lowest dose that is sufficient for sexual intercourse. If necessary, increase the dose (or decrease) on separate occasions in a stepwise manner until the patient achieves an erection that is sufficient for sexual intercourse.

Storage/Stability – Store unopened foil pouches in a refrigerator at 2° to 8°C (36° to 46°F). It may be kept at room temperature (below 30°C or 86°F).

Rx	**Caverject** (Pharmacia & Upjohn)	**Powder for injection (lyophilized)**: 6.15 mcg (5 mcg/ml)	Lactose. In vials with diluent syringes.
		11.9 mcg (10 mcg/ml)	Lactose. In vials with diluent syringes.
		23.2 mcg (20 mcg/ml)	Lactose. In vials with diluent syringes.
Rx	**Muse** (Vivus)	**Pellet**: 125 mcg	PEG 1450. One system consisting of applicator containing pellet (6s).
		250 mcg	PEG 1450. One system consisting of applicator containing pellet (6s).
		500 mcg	PEG 1450. One system consisting of applicator containing pellet (6s).
		1000 mcg	PEG 1450. One system consisting of applicator containing pellet (6s).

YOHIMBINE HCl

Actions:

Pharmacology: Yohimbine, an indolalkylamine alkaloid, has chemical similarity to reserpine. It is the principal alkaloid of the bark of the West African *Corynanthe yohimbe* tree and is also found in Rauwolfia Serpentina (L) Benth. It is believed to have properties similar to rauwolfia alkaloids.

Yohimbine is primarily an α_2-adrenergic blocker. It blocks presynaptic α_2-adrenoreceptors causing release of norepinephrine. Its peripheral autonomic nervous system effect is to increase parasympathetic (cholinergic) and decrease sympathetic (adrenergic) activity. In male sexual performance, erection is linked to cholinergic activity, which theoretically results in increased penile blood inflow, decreased outflow or both, causing erectile stimulation without increasing sexual desire. Yohimbine exerts a stimulating action on mood and may increase anxiety. Such actions appear to require high doses. Yohimbine has a mild antidiuretic action, probably via stimulation of hypothalmic centers and release of posterior pituitary hormone. It may also have a local anesthetic effect.

Its action on peripheral blood vessels resembles that of reserpine, though it is weaker and of short duration. The drug reportedly exerts no significant influence on cardiac stimulation. Its effect on blood pressure, if any, would be to lower it; however, no adequate studies quantitate this effect and some reports indicate that it may increase blood pressure.

Indications:

Yohimbine has no FDA sanctioned indications.

Unlabeled uses: Sympatholytic and mydriatic. It may have activity as an aphrodisiac.

Impotence has been successfully treated with yohimbine in patients with vascular or diabetic origins (18 mg/day), but data are sparse. Urologists have used yohimbine experimentally for the treatment and the diagnostic classification of certain types of male erectile impotence. In some males with sexual dysfunction caused by the use of a selective serotonin reuptake inhibitor, yohimbine may be beneficial in improving sexual function/desire.

Orthostatic hypotension may be favorably affected by yohimbine 12.5 mg/day, but much more research is needed.

Contraindications:

Renal disease; hypersensitivity to any component.

Warnings:

Special risk patients: Not for use in geriatric, psychiatric or cardio-renal patients with a history of gastric or duodenal ulcer. Generally not for use in females.

Pregnancy: Do not use during pregnancy.

Children: Do not use in children.

Drug Interactions:

Antidepressants: Do not use with yohimbine.

Adverse Reactions:

CNS: Yohimbine readily penetrates the CNS and produces a complex pattern of responses in lower doses than those required to produce peripheral α-adrenergic blockade. These include antidiuresis and central excitation including elevated blood pressure and heart rate, increased motor activity, nervousness, irritability and tremor. Dizziness, headache and skin flushing have been reported.

Overdosage:

Doses of 20 to 30 mg/day may produce increases in heart rate and blood pressure, piloerection and rhinorrhea. More severe symptoms may include paresthesias, incoordination, tremulousness and a dissociative state (higher doses). Death occurs via respiratory paralysis. Refer to General Management of Acute Overdosage.

Administration and Dosage:

Male erectile impotence: Experimental dosage has been 1 tablet (5.4 mg) 3 times/day. If side effects occur, reduce to ½ tablet 3 times/day, followed by gradual increases to 1 tablet 3 times/day. Results of therapy > 10 weeks are not known.

Rx	**Yohimbine HCl** (Various, eg, Royce)	**Tablets:** 5.4 mg	In 100s, 500s and 1000s.
Rx	**Aphrodyne** (Star)		Aqua. In 100s and 1000s.
Rx	**Dayto Himbin** (Dayton)		In 60s.
Rx	**Yocon** (Palisades)		In 100s and 1000s.
Rx	**Yohimex** (Kramer)		Pink. In 100s.

SODIUM BENZOATE AND SODIUM PHENYLACETATE

Actions:

Pharmacology: Sodium benzoate and sodium phenylacetate are metabolically active compounds that decrease elevated blood ammonia concentrations in patients with inborn errors of ureagenesis. The mechanisms for this action are conjugation reactions involving acylation of amino acids, which results in decreased ammonia formation. Benzoate and phenylacetate activate conjugation pathways that substitute for or supplement the defective ureagenic pathway in patients with urea cycle enzymopathies (UCE), preventing the accumulation of ammonia.

The therapeutic regimens of sodium benzoate and sodium phenylacetate, which also included dietary manipulation and amino acid supplementation, were effective in long-term management of UCE patients. Survival rate in patients with complete enzyme deficiencies was ≈ 80% with this combined regimen in what was previously an almost universally fatal disease within the first year of life. The survival rate for each complete enzyme deficiency studied was: Carbamylphosphate synthetase, 75%; ornithine transcarbamylase (males), 59%; argininosuccinate synthetase, 96%. Survival in heterozygous females with partial ornithine transcarbamylase deficiency was 95%; for patients with other partial deficiencies, 86%. Early diagnosis and treatment are important in minimizing developmental disabilities. Reversal of preexisting neurologic impairment is not likely to occur with treatment, and neurologic deterioration may continue in some patients.

Pharmacokinetics: Studies have not been conducted in the primary patient population (neonates, infants and children). Preliminary pharmacokinetic data were obtained from only three healthy adult subjects and the overall disposition of sodium benzoate, sodium phenylacetate and their metabolites has not been fully characterized. Peak blood levels of benzoate or phenylacetate occur within 1 hour after a single oral dose of sodium benzoate or sodium phenylacetate. A majority of the administered compound (approximately 80% to 100%) was excreted by the kidneys within 24 hours as the respective conjugation product, hippurate or phenylacetylglutamine. The major sites for metabolism of benzoate and phenylacetate are the liver and kidneys.

Indications:

Hyperammonemia: Adjunctive therapy for the prevention and treatment of hyperammonemia in the chronic management of patients with UCE involving partial or complete deficiencies of carbamylphosphate synthetase, ornithine transcarbamylase or argininosuccinate synthetase.

Warnings:

Sodium: Because of the sodium content of this product, consider the possibility of hypernatremia. Use with great care, if at all, in patients with CHF, severe renal insufficiency and in clinical states in which there is sodium retention with edema. In patients with diminished renal function, administration of solutions containing sodium ions may result in sodium retention.

Benzyl alcohol: Some of these products contain benzyl alcohol, which has been associated with fatal "gasping syndrome" in premature infants.

Hypersensitivity: Do not administer to patients with known hypersensitivities to sodium benzoate or sodium phenylacetate. No such cases of hypersensitivities have been reported.

Pregnancy: Category C. Safety for use during pregnancy has not been established. Use only when clearly needed and when the potential benefits outweigh the hazards to the fetus.

Lactation: It is not known whether this drug is excreted in breast milk. Use caution when administering to a nursing woman.

Precautions:

Adjunctive therapy: Not intended as sole therapy for UCE patients. Combine as adjunctive therapy with dietary management (low protein diet) and amino acid supplementation for optimal results.

Hyperbilirubinemia: Use with caution in neonates with hyperbilirubinemia, as in vitro experiments suggest that benzoate competes for bilirubin binding sites on albumin.

Neonatal hyperammonemic coma: The benefits of treating neonatal hyperammonemic coma with this drug have not been established. The treatment of choice in neonatal hyperammonemic coma is hemodialysis. Peritoneal dialysis may be helpful if hemodialysis is not available.

SODIUM BENZOATE AND SODIUM PHENYLACETATE

Drug Interactions:

Sodium Benzoate/Phenylacetate Drug Interactions			
Precipitant drug	Object drug*		Description
Penicillin	Sodium benzoate/ phenylacetate	⬇	Penicillin may compete with conjugated products of sodium benzoate and sodium phenylacetate for active secretion by renal tubules.
Probenecid	Sodium benzoate/ phenylacetate	⬇	Probenecid inhibits the renal transport of many organic compounds, including amino hippuric acid and may affect renal excretion of the conjugation products of sodium benzoate and sodium phenylacetate.
Valproic acid	Sodium benzoate/ phenylacetate	⬇	Valproic acid may induce hyperammonemia. Therefore, administration of valproic acid to UCE patients may exacerbate their condition and be antagonistic to the effficacy of sodium benzoate/phenylacetate.

* ⬇ = Object drug decreased.

Adverse Reactions:

Nausea and vomiting.

Side effects associated with salicylates such as exacerbation of peptic ulcers, mild hyperventilation and mild respiratory alkalosis may occur due to structural similarities between benzoate and salicylates.

If an adverse reaction does occur, discontinue administration, evaluate the patient and institute appropriate therapeutic countermeasures.

Overdosage:

Four overdoses of sodium phenylacetate or sodium benzoate in UCE patients have been reported, two cases following the use of an IV infusion. Two patients became irritable and vomited after receiving three-fold overdoses of oral sodium benzoate. Both patients recovered without treatment within 24 hours after the drug was discontinued.

Treatment: Discontinue the drug and institute supportive measures for metabolic acidosis and circulatory collapse. Hemodialysis or peritoneal dialysis may be beneficial.

Administration and Dosage:

For oral use only. Must be diluted before use.

The usual total daily dose for adjunctive therapy of UCE patients is 2.5 ml/kg/day (250 mg sodium benzoate and 250 mg sodium phenylacetate) in 3 to 6 equally divided doses. Total daily dose should not exceed 100 ml (10 g each of sodium benzoate and sodium phenylacetate).

Dilute each dose in 4 to 8 ounces of infant formula or milk and administer with meals. If other beverages are used, particularly acidic beverages, precipitation of the drug may occur depending on pH and the final concentration. Inspect the mixture for compatibility before administration.

Because this is a concentrated solution, exercise care in calculating the dose to avoid the possibility of overdosage.

Not intended as sole therapy for UCE patients. Combine as adjunctive therapy with dietary management (low protein diet) and amino acid supplementation for optimal results.

Because sodium phenylacetate has a lingering odor, exercise care in mixing and administering the drug to minimize contact with skin and clothing.

Storage: Store at room temperature. Avoid excessive heat.

Rx	**Ucephan** (McGaw)	**Solution:** 10 g sodium benzoate and 10 g sodium phenylacetate per 100 ml	In 100 ml multiple unit bottles.

ALPROSTADIL (Prostaglandin E_1; PGE_1)

Warning:

Apnea occurs in about 10% to 12% of neonates with congenital heart defects treated with alprostadil. Apnea is most often seen in neonates weighing less than 2 kg at birth and usually appears during the first hour of drug infusion. Monitor respiratory status throughout treatment; have ventilatory assistance immediately available.

Actions:

Pharmacology: Alprostadil (prostaglandin E_1) produces vasodilation, inhibits platelet aggregation and stimulates intestinal and uterine smooth muscle; IV doses of 1 to 10 mcg/kg lower the blood pressure in mammals by decreasing peripheral resistance. Reflex increases in cardiac output and rate accompany the reduction in blood pressure.

Smooth muscle of the ductus arteriosus, especially sensitive to alprostadil, relaxes in the presence of the drug. These effects are beneficial in infants who have congenital defects which restrict the pulmonary or systemic blood flow and who depend on a patent ductus arteriosus for adequate blood oxygenation and lower body perfusion.

In infants with restricted pulmonary blood flow, about 50% responded to alprostadil infusion with at least 10 mm Hg increase in blood pO_2 (mean increase about 14 mm Hg and mean increase in oxygen saturation about 23%). In general, patients who responded best had low pretreatment blood pO_2 and were 4 days old or less. The increase in blood oxygenation is inversely proportional to pretreatment pO_2 values; patients with a low pO_2 respond best, and patients with a $pO_2 \geq 40$ mm Hg usually have little response.

In infants with restricted systemic blood flow, alprostadil often increased pH in those with acidosis. It also increased systemic blood pressure and decreased the ratio of pulmonary artery pressure to aortic pressure.

Pharmacokinetics: Alprostadil is rapidly metabolized. As much as 80% may be metabolized in one pass through the lungs, primarily by oxidation. Metabolites are excreted primarily by the kidneys, and excretion is essentially complete within 24 hours. No unchanged alprostadil has been found in the urine, and there is no evidence of tissue retention.

Indications:

For palliative, not definitive, therapy to temporarily maintain the patency of the ductus arteriosus until corrective or palliative surgery can be performed in neonates who have congenital heart defects and who depend upon the patent ductus for survival. Such defects include pulmonary atresia or stenosis, tricuspid atresia, tetralogy of Fallot, interruption of the aortic arch, coarctation of the aorta or transposition of the great vessels with or without other defects.

Contraindications:

None known.

Warnings:

Administer only by trained personnel in facilities that provide pediatric intensive care.

Precautions:

Skeletal effects: Cortical proliferation of the long bones has been observed in infants during long-term infusions of alprostadil. This regressed after drug withdrawal.

Duration of infusion: Infuse for the shortest time and at the lowest dose that will produce the desired effects. Weigh the risks of long-term infusion against the possible benefits that critically ill infants may derive from its administration.

Hemostatic effects: Because alprostadil inhibits platelet aggregation, use cautiously in neonates with bleeding tendencies.

Respiratory distress syndrome: Do not use alprostadil in respiratory distress syndrome. Make a differential diagnosis between respiratory distress syndrome (hyaline membrane disease) and cyanotic heart disease (restricted pulmonary blood flow). If full diagnostic facilities are not immediately available, cyanosis (pO_2 less than 40 mm Hg) and restricted pulmonary blood flow apparent on an X-ray are appropriate indicators of congenital heart defects.

Monitor arterial pressure intermittently by umbilical artery catheter, auscultation or with a Doppler transducer. If arterial pressure falls significantly, decrease the infusion rate immediately.

In infants with restricted pulmonary blood flow, measure efficacy of alprostadil by monitoring blood oxygenation. To measure efficacy in infants with restricted systemic blood flow, monitor systemic blood pressure and blood pH.

ALPROSTADIL (Prostaglandin E_1; PGE_1)

Adverse Reactions:

CNS: Fever (14%); seizures (4%); cerebral bleeding, hyperextension of the neck, hyperirritability, hypothermia, jitteriness, lethargy and stiffness (< 1%).

Cardiovascular: Flushing (10%, more common after intra-arterial dosing); bradycardia (7%); hypotension (4%); tachycardia (3%); cardiac arrest, edema (1%); congestive heart failure, hyperemia, second degree heart block, shock, spasm of the right ventricle infundibulum, supraventricular tachycardia and ventricular fibrillation (< 1%).

Respiratory: Apnea (12%); bradypnea, bronchial wheezing, hypercapnia, respiratory depression, respiratory distress and tachypnea (< 1%).

GI: Diarrhea (2%); gastric regurgitation and hyperbilirubinemia (< 1%).

Hematologic: Disseminated intravascular coagulation (1%); anemia, bleeding and thrombocytopenia (< 1%).

Renal: Anuria and hematuria (< 1%).

Musculoskeletal: Cortical proliferation of the long bones.

Body as a whole: Sepsis (2%); hypokalemia (1%); peritonitis, hypoglycemia and hyperkalemia (< 1%).

Overdosage:

Symptoms: Apnea, bradycardia, pyrexia, hypotension and flushing.

Treatment: If apnea or bradycardia occurs, discontinue infusion and provide appropriate medical treatment. Use caution in restarting the infusion. If pyrexia or hypotension occurs, reduce the infusion rate until symptoms subside. Flushing is usually a result of incorrect intra-arterial catheter placement; reposition catheter.

Administration and Dosage:

The preferred administration route is continuous IV infusion into a large vein. Alternatively, the drug may be administered through an umbilical artery catheter placed at the ductal opening. Increases in blood pO_2 have been the same by either route.

Begin infusion with 0.05 to 0.1 mcg/kg/minute. A starting dose of 0.1 mcg/kg/min is recommended; however, adequate clinical response has been reported using a starting dose of 0.05 mcg/kg/min. After a therapeutic response is achieved (increased pO_2 in infants with restricted pulmonary blood flow or increased systemic blood pressure and blood pH in infants with restricted systemic blood flow), reduce the infusion rate to the lowest dosage that maintains the response. This may be accomplished by reducing the dosage from 0.1 to 0.05 to 0.025 to 0.01 mcg/kg/minute. If response to 0.05 mcg/kg/minute is inadequate, dosage can be increased up to 0.4 mcg/kg/minute, although in general, higher infusion rates do not produce greater effects.

Preparation of solution: Dilute 500 mcg alprostadil with Sodium Chloride Injection or Dextrose Injection. Dilute to volumes appropriate for the pump delivery system available. Discard and prepare fresh infusion solutions every 24 hours.

Sample Dilutions and Infusion Rates to Provide a Dosage of 0.1 mcg/kg/min

Add 500 mcg alprostadil to:	Approximate concentration of resulting solution (mcg/ml)	Infusion rate (ml/min/kg)
250 ml	2	0.05
100 ml	5	0.02
50 ml	10	0.01
25 ml	20	0.005

Storage: Refrigerate at 2° to 8°C (35° to 46°F).

Rx	**Prostin VR Pediatric** (Upjohn)	**Injection:** 500 mcg/ml[1]	In 1 ml amps.

[1] In 1 ml dehydrated alcohol.

INDOMETHACIN SODIUM TRIHYDRATE

Actions:

Pharmacology: Indomethacin sodium trihydrate is an injectable formulation of indomethacin used for closure of a patent ductus arteriosus in premature infants. Indomethacin is a potent inhibitor of prostaglandin synthesis, both in vitro and in vivo. The exact mechanism of action through which indomethacin causes closure of a patent ductus arteriosus is unknown, but it is believed to be through inhibition of prostaglandin synthesis.

In double-blind, placebo controlled studies of 460 preterm infants who weighed < 1750 g, those treated with IV indomethacin had a 75% to 80% closure rate, thus avoiding surgery.

Pharmacokinetics: Plasma half-life is variable among premature infants and varies inversely with postnatal age and weight. In a study of 28 infants, the plasma half-life of those less than 7 days old averaged 20 hours; in infants older than 7 days, the mean plasma half-life was 12 hours. The mean plasma half-life was 21 hours in infants weighing < 1000 g and 15 hours in those weighing > 1000 g.

Following IV administration in adults, indomethacin is eliminated via renal excretion, metabolism and biliary excretion, and it undergoes appreciable enterohepatic circulation. The mean plasma half-life of indomethacin is 4.5 hours; in the absence of enterohepatic circulation, it is 90 minutes.

Indications:

For closure of a hemodynamically significant patent ductus arteriosus in premature infants weighing between 500 and 1750 g if, after 48 hours, usual medical management is ineffective. Clinical evidence of a hemodynamically significant patent ductus arteriosus should be present (ie, respiratory distress, a continuous murmur, a hyperactive precordium, cardiomegaly and pulmonary plethora on chest x–ray).

Unlabeled uses: Indomethacin IV has been used prophylactically to reduce the incidence of symptomatic patent ductus arteriosus in premature infants with a high probability of developing this condition; a single dose of 0.2 mg/kg 24 hours after birth has been used. However, no study has shown a significant decrease in neonatal morbidity.

Contraindications:

Proven or suspected untreated infection; bleeding, especially active intracranial hemorrhage or GI bleeding; thrombocytopenia; coagulation defects; necrotizing enterocolitis; significant renal impairment; congenital heart disease patients in whom patency of the ductus arteriosus is necessary for satisfactory pulmonary or systemic blood flow (eg, pulmonary atresia, severe tetralogy of Fallot, severe coarctation of aorta).

Warnings:

GI effects: Minor GI bleeding (ie, chemical detection of blood in the stool) has been reported.

Hemorrhage: Prematurity per se is associated with an increased incidence of spontaneous intraventricular hemorrhage. Indomethacin may inhibit platelet aggregation and increase the potential for intraventricular bleeding.

Electrolyte balance: Indomethacin may suppress water excretion to a greater extent than sodium excretion. Perform serum electrolyte determinations and monitor renal function during therapy.

Renal function impairment: Indomethacin may cause significant reduction in urine output (50% or more) with concomitant elevations of BUN and creatinine and reductions in glomerular filtration rate and creatinine clearance. In most infants, these effects are transient and disappear with cessation of therapy. Indomethacin may precipitate renal insufficiency, including acute renal failure, especially in infants with other conditions that may adversely affect renal function during therapy.

When significant suppression of urine volume occurs after a dose, do not give additional doses until the urine output returns to normal levels.

Precautions:

Infection: Indomethacin may mask the usual signs and symptoms of infection. Use with extra care in the presence of existing controlled infection.

Hepatic effects: Severe hepatic reactions have been reported in adults treated chronically with oral indomethacin. If clinical signs and symptoms consistent with liver disease develop in the neonate, or if systemic manifestations occur, discontinue the drug.

Avoid extravascular injection or leakage; the solution may irritate tissue.

Drug Interactions:

Aminoglycosides: In one study of premature infants treated with indomethacin IV and also receiving either gentamicin or amikacin, both peak and trough levels of these aminoglycosides were significantly elevated.

INDOMETHACIN SODIUM TRIHYDRATE

Digitalis: In premature infants, the half-life of digitalis may be further prolonged, due to reduced renal function during therapy with indomethacin.

Frequent ECGs and serum digitalis levels may be required to prevent or detect digitalis toxicity early.

Furosemide: Indomethacin may blunt furosemide's natriuretic effect; this is attributed to inhibition of prostaglandin synthesis. In 19 premature infants with patent ductus arteriosus, infants receiving both agents had significantly higher urinary output, higher levels of sodium and chloride excretion and higher glomerular filtration rates than did infants receiving indomethacin alone. Data suggest furosemide helped to maintain renal function in the premature infant when indomethacin was added.

Adverse Reactions:

Coagulation: Decreased platelet aggregation. There was greater incidence of bleeding problems (ie, gross or microscopic bleeding into the GI tract, oozing from skin after needle stick, pulmonary hemorrhage, disseminated intravascular coagulopathy).

Renal: Renal dysfunction in 41% of infants, including one or more of the following: Oliguria; reduced urine sodium, chloride or potassium, urine osmolality, free water clearance or glomerular filtration rate; elevated serum creatinine or BUN; uremia.

Cardiovascular: Pulmonary hypertension.

GI: GI bleeding (3% to 9%); vomiting, abdominal distention, transient ileus, localized perforation of small or large intestines (1% to 3%).

Metabolic: Hyponatremia; elevated serum potassium (3% to 9%); hypoglycemia, fluid retention (1% to 3%).

The following adverse reactions have also been reported in infants treated with indomethacin; however, a causal relationship has not been established:

Cardiovascular – Intracranial bleeding (3% to 9%); bradycardia (< 3%).
Respiratory – Apnea; exacerbation of preexisting pulmonary infection.
Metabolic – Acidosis/alkalosis.
GI – Necrotizing enterocolitis.
Ophthalmic – Retrolental fibroplasia (3% to 9%).

Additional adverse reactions have been reported with oral indomethacin. Relevance to the preterm neonate receiving indomethacin IV is unknown.

Administration and Dosage:

For IV use only.

A course of therapy is defined as 3 IV doses given at 12 to 24 hour intervals.

Renal impairment: If anuria or marked oliguria (urinary output < 0.6 ml/kg/hr) is evident at the scheduled time of the second or third dose, do not give additional doses until laboratory studies indicate that renal function has returned to normal.

Dosage According to Age

Age at 1st dose	Dose (mg/kg) 1st	2nd	3rd
< 48 hours	0.2	0.1	0.1
2-7 days	0.2	0.2	0.2
> 7 days	0.2	0.25	0.25

If the ductus arteriosus closes or is significantly reduced in size after 48 hours or more from completion of the first course, no further doses are necessary. If the ductus arteriosus reopens, a second course of 1 to 3 doses may be given, each dose separated by a 12 to 24 hour interval as described above.

If the infant remains unresponsive to therapy after 2 courses, surgery may be necessary. If severe adverse reactions occur, stop the drug.

Preparation of solution: Prepare with 1 to 2 ml of Sodium Chloride Injection 0.9% or Water for Injection. All diluents should be preservative free (ie, without benzyl alcohol). If 1 ml of diluent is used, the concentration of indomethacin ≈ 0.1 mg/0.1 ml; if 2 ml of diluent are used, the concentration of the solution ≈ 0.05 mg/0.1 ml. Discard any unused portion of the solution. Prepare a fresh solution just prior to each administration. Once reconstituted, inject IV over 5 to 10 seconds.

Further dilution with IV infusion solutions is not recommended.

Rx	**Indocin I.V.** (Merck)	**Powder for injection:** 1 mg (as sodium trihydrate)	In single dose vials.

ETHANOLAMINE OLEATE

Actions:

Pharmacology: Ethanolamine oleate is a mild sclerosing agent. When injected IV, it acts primarily by irritation of the intimal endothelium of the vein and produces a sterile dose-related inflammatory response. This results in fibrosis and occlusion of the vein. Ethanolamine oleate also rapidly diffuses through the venous wall and produces a dose-related extravascular inflammatory reaction.

The oleic acid component of ethanolamine oleate is responsible for the inflammatory response, and may also activate coagulation in vivo by release of tissue factor and activation of Hageman factor. The ethanolamine component, however, may inhibit fibrin clot formation by chelating calcium, so that a procoagulant action of ethanolamine oleate has not been demonstrated.

Pharmacokinetics: Ethanolamine oleate disappears from the injection site within 5 minutes via the portal vein. When volumes larger than 20 ml are injected, some ethanolamine oleate also flows into the azygos vein through the periesophageal vein. Within 4 days after injection, there is neutrophil infiltration of the esophageal wall and hemorrhage within 6 days. Granulation tissue is first seen at 10 days, red thrombi obliterating the varices by 20 days, and sclerosis of the varices by 2 months. Sclerosis of esophageal varices will be a delayed rather than an immediate effect of the drug.

In dogs, ethanolamine oleate 1 ml/kg injected into the right atrium over 1 minute increases extravascular lung water. The concentration of ethanolamine oleate reaching the lung in human treatment will be less than in the dog studies, but pleural effusions, pulmonary edema, pulmonary infiltration and pneumonitis have occurred. Minimize the total per session dose, especially in those with concomitant cardiopulmonary disease.

Indications:

Treatment of patients with esophageal varices that have recently bled, to prevent rebleeding.

Not indicated for the treatment of patients with esophageal varices that have not bled.

Contraindications:

Hypersensitivity to ethanolamine, oleic acid or ethanolamine oleate.

Warnings:

Sclerotherapy with ethanolamine oleate has no beneficial effect upon portal hypertension, the cause of esophageal varices, so that recanalization and collateralization may occur, necessitating reinjection.

Varicosities of the leg: Use of ethanolamine oleate injection is not supported by adequately controlled clinical trials and is not recommended.

Hypersensitivity: Fatal anaphylactic shock was reported following injection of a larger than normal volume of ethanolamine oleate injection into a male who had a known allergic disposition. There are only three reports of anaphylaxis. Be prepared to treat anaphylaxis appropriately. In emergencies, administer 0.25 ml of a 1:1000 IV solution of epinephrine (0.25 mg); control allergic reactions with antihistamines. Have epinephrine 1:1000 immediately available. Refer to Management of Acute Hypersensitivity Reactions.

Pregnancy: Category C. It is not known whether ethanolamine oleate injection can cause fetal harm when administered to a pregnant woman or can affect reproduction capacity. Give to pregnant women only if clearly needed.

Lactation: It is not known whether this drug is excreted in breast milk. Exercise caution when ethanolamine oleate is administered to a nursing woman.

Children: Safety and efficacy in children have not been established. In one study, 21 children with esophageal varices were treated with ethanolamine oleate via an endotracheal tube using 2 to 5 ml injection per varix to a maximum of 20 ml. Variceal obliteration occurred in 18 of the children.

ETHANOLAMINE OLEATE

Precautions:

Acute renal failure with spontaneous recovery followed injections of 15 to 20 ml in two women.

Severe injection necrosis may result from direct injection of sclerosing agents, especially if excessive volumes are used. At least one fatal case of extensive esophageal necrosis and death has occurred. The drug should be administered by physicians who are familiar with an acceptable injection technique.

Child Class C patients are more likely to develop esophageal ulceration than those in Classes A and B. Complications of ulceration, necrosis and delayed esophageal perforation appear to occur more frequently when ethanolamine oleate is injected submucosally. This route is not recommended.

Concomitant cardiorespiratory disease: Careful monitoring and minimization of the total dose per session is recommended.

Fatal aspiration pneumonia has occurred in elderly patients undergoing esophageal variceal sclerotherapy with ethanolamine oleate. It appears to be procedure-related rather than drug-related, but as aspiration of blood or stomach contents is not uncommon in patients with bleeding esophageal varices, take special precautions to prevent its occurrence, especially in the elderly and critically ill subjects.

Adverse Reactions:

The frequency of complications/adverse events per injection session was 13%.

Most common: Pleural effusion/infiltration (2.1%); esophageal ulcer (2.1%); pyrexia (1.8%); retrosternal pain (1.6%); esophageal stricture (1.3%); pneumonia (1.2%).

Local esophageal reactions: Pleural effusion/infiltration (2.1%); esophageal ulcer (2.1%); esophageal stricture (1.3%); esophagitis, tearing of the esophagus, sloughing of the mucosa overlying the injected varix, necrosis, periesophageal abscess and perforation (0.1% to 0.4%) (see Precautions). These complications appear to be dependent upon the dose and the patient's clinical state.

Other: Pyrexia (1.8%); retrosternal pain (1.6%); fatal aspiration pneumonia (see Precautions); pneumonia (1.2%); bacteremia; anaphylactic shock (see Warnings); acute renal failure with spontaneous recovery (see Precautions). Spinal cord paralysis due to occlusion of the anterior spinal artery has been reported in one child 8 hours after ethanolamine oleate sclerotherapy.

Overdosage:

Overdosage of ethanolamine oleate injection can result in severe intramural necrosis of the esophagus; complications have resulted in death. The minimum lethal dose of ethanolamine oleate injection administered IV to rabbits is 130 mg/kg.

Administration and Dosage:

Local ethanolamine oleate injection sclerotherapy of esophageal varices should be performed by physicians who are familiar with an acceptable technique.

Usual IV dose is 1.5 to 5 ml per varix.

Maximum total dose per treatment session should not exceed 20 ml or 0.4 ml/kg for a 50 kg patient. Patients with significant liver dysfunction (Child Class C) or concomitant cardiopulmonary disease should usually receive less than the recommended maximum dose.

Submucosal injections are not recommended as they are reportedly more likely to result in ulceration at the site of injection.

To obliterate the varix, injections may be made at the time of the acute bleeding espisode and then after 1 week, 6 weeks, 3 months and 6 months as indicated.

Storage: Store at controlled room temperature 15° to 30°C (59° to 86°F). Protect from light.

Rx	**Ethamolin** (Schwarz Pharma)	**Injection:** 5%	In 2 ml amps.[1]

[1] With 2% benzyl alcohol.

SCLEROSING AGENTS

Actions:

Pharmacology: These agents are mild sclerosing drugs used in the treatment of varicose veins. They produce their effect by irritation and inflammation of the venous intimal endothelium and formation of a thrombus. This blood clot occludes the injected vein and fibrous tissue develops, resulting in the obliteration of the vein.

Sodium tetradecyl is an anionic surface active agent. Morrhuate sodium is a mixture of the sodium salts of the saturated and unsaturated fatty acids of cod liver oil.

Indications:

Treatment of small, uncomplicated varicose veins of the lower extremities.

Sclerosing agents may be useful as a supplement to venous ligation to obliterate residual varicosed veins or in patients who have conditions which increase the risk of surgery. Ineffective sclerotherapy may decrease the potential success of later surgery.

Morrhuate sodium has been used for the treatment of internal hemorrhoids; there is no substantial evidence for this indication.

Unlabeled uses: Sclerosing agents have been used to treat esophageal varices, introduced via a flexible fiberoptic esophagoscope.

Contraindications:

Hypersensitivity to any component of these drugs; acute superficial thrombophlebitis; underlying arterial disease; varicosities caused by abdominal and pelvic tumors; uncontrolled diabetes mellitus; sepsis; blood dyscrasia; thyrotoxicosis; tuberculosis; neoplasms; asthma; acute respiratory or skin diseases; any condition which causes the patient to be bedridden; extensive injection treatment in patients who are severely debilitated or senile; an unusual local reaction at the injection site or any systemic reaction; persistent occlusion of deep veins.

Delay treatment if there is any acute local or systemic infection, including infected ulcers.

Do not use if there is significant valvular or deep venous incompetence.

Warnings:

Anaphylactoid and allergic reactions have occurred. Anaphylactoid reactions may occur within a few minutes after the injection and are most likely to occur when therapy is reinstituted after several weeks. Refer to Management of Acute Hypersensitivity Reactions.

Pregnancy: (Category C – sodium tetradecyl sulfate). Safety for use during pregnancy has not been established. Use only when clearly needed and when the potential benefits outweigh the potential hazards to the fetus.

Precautions:

Do not undertake sclerotherapy for the treatment of varicosities unless valvular competency and deep vein patency and competency are determined. Perform the Trendelenburg test, Perthes' test and angiography. Because of the danger of extension of thrombosis into the deep veins, perform a thorough preinjection evaluation for valvular competence and slowly inject a small amount (not more than 2 ml) of the preparation into the varicosity. Necrosis may result from direct injection of sclerosing agents.

Initially treat most patients with symptomatic primary varicosed veins with compression stockings. If this treatment is inadequate, surgery may be required.

For IV use only. Inadvertent intra-arterial injection may result in severe ischemic damage.

Adverse Reactions:

Local: Burning; cramping sensations; urticaria; tissue sloughing and necrosis may occur with extravasation (morrhuate).

A permanent discoloration, usually small and barely noticeable, can occur at the injection site with sodium tetradecyl sulfate and may be cosmetically objectionable.

Hypersensitivity: Dizziness; weakness; vascular collapse; asthma; respiratory depression; GI disturbances (ie, nausea and vomiting); urticaria (see Warnings) (rare).

Body as a whole: Postoperative sloughing can occur.

Pulmonary embolism has occurred. Drowsiness and headache may occur rarely with morrhuate.

SODIUM TETRADECYL SULFATE

Complete prescribing information for these products begins in the Sclerosing Agents group monograph.

Administration and Dosage:

For IV use only. Do not use if precipitated. The strength of solution required depends on the size and degree of varicosity. In general, the 3% solution will be most useful, with the 1% solution preferred for small varicosities. The dosage should be small, using 0.5 to 2 ml for each injection; do not exceed 10 ml of a 3% solution.

As a precaution against anaphylactic shock, give 0.5 ml; observe patient for several hours before administering a larger injection.

Rx	**Sotradecol** (Elkins-Sinn)	**Injection:** 1%	In 2 ml Dosette amps.[1]
Rx	**Sotradecol** (Elkins-Sinn)	**Injection:** 3%	In 2 ml Dosette amps.[1]

[1] With 0.02 ml benzyl alcohol per ml.

MORRHUATE SODIUM

Complete prescribing information for these products begins in the Sclerosing Agents group monograph.

Administration and Dosage:

For IV use only. Avoid extravasation. Dosage depends on the size and degree of varicosity.

To determine possible sensitivity: 0.25 to 1 ml of 5% injection into a varicosity 24 hours before administration of a large dose.

Usual adult dose for obliteration of small or medium veins: 50 to 100 mg (1 to 2 ml). *For large veins:*150 to 250 mg (3 to 5 ml). The drug may be given as multiple injections at one time or in single doses. Therapy may be repeated at 5 to 7 day intervals, according to the patient's response.

Following injection, the vein promptly becomes hard and swollen for 2 to 4 inches, depending on the size and response of the vein. After 24 hours, the vein is hard and slightly tender to the touch (with little or no periphlebitis). The skin around the injection becomes light-bronze; this color usually disappears quickly. An aching sensation and feeling of stiffness usually occurs and lasts approximately 48 hours.

When small veins are injected, or the injection solution is cold, or when solid matter has separated in the solution, warm the ampul or vial by immersing in hot water. The solution should become clear on warming; use only a clear solution that contains no solid matter. Because the solution froths easily, use a large bore needle to fill the syringe; however, use a small bore needle for the injection.

Storage: Store below 40°C (104°F); refrigerate preferably between 15° and 30°C (59° and 86°F).

Rx	**Morrhuate Sodium** (Pasadena Research Labs)	**Injection:** 50 mg/ml	In 30 ml multiple use vials.
Rx	**Scleromate** (Palisades Pharm.)		In 5 ml amps, 10 ml vials, 10 ml fill in 20 ml vials.

CHYMOPAPAIN

Warning:

Use chymopapain only in a hospital setting by physicians experienced and trained in the diagnosis of lumbar disc disease and all acceptable treatment modalities, including surgery and in the management of all potential complications from chymopapain. Anaphylaxis has occurred in about 0.5% of patients (0.4% under local anesthesia versus 0.5% under general anesthesia); it can be fatal.

Paraplegia or paraparesis, central nervous system hemorrhage and other serious neurologic adverse events have been observed within hours or days after chymopapain injection at a rate of about 1 in 2,000. Acute transverse myelitis/acute transverse myelopathy has been observed 2 to 3 weeks following chymopapain injection at a rate of about 1 in 18,000. A cause and effect relationship between these neurologic events and chymopapain when properly injected has not been established.

Chymopapain is extremely toxic when injected intrathecally, as are some radiopaque contrast media used for discography. Therefore, take great care to assure that the dura is not penetrated and that chymopapain, or contrast medium if used, does not enter the subarachnoid space. If there is any question regarding needle tip location within the nucleus of the disc or if contrast medium is used and it extravasates into the subarachnoid space, abandon the procedure and do not inject chymopapain.

Discography at the time of chemonucleolysis is not recommended unless it is determined that the benefits outweigh the risks. Limit chemonucleolysis to the disc producing the patient's signs and symptoms and use supplemented local anesthesia whenever possible.

Actions:

Pharmacology: Chymopapain is a nonpyrogenic proteolytic enzyme derived from the crude latex of *Carica papaya.* Sodium L-cysteinate hydrochloride is added as a reducing agent for this sulphur-containing enzyme to maintain the sulphur in the sulphydryl form. The pH of the reconstituted drug is 5.5 to 6.5.

When injected into the nucleus pulposus of the lumbar intervertebral disc, chymopapain rapidly hydrolyzes the noncollagenous polypeptides or proteins that maintain the tertiary structure of the chondromucoprotein. This degradation lessens the intradiscal osmotic activity, thereby decreasing fluid absorption, reducing intradiscal pressure and relieving compressive symptoms.

Pharmacokinetics: Although the mechanism of action has not been directly established, operative findings in patients undergoing surgery following injection usually revealed the nucleus pulposus to be absent from its former site. A temporary increase in urinary mucopolysaccharide occurs following intradiscal injection of chymopapain, and it appears the inhibitory activity of the alpha$_2$-macroglobulin prevents expression of any significant proteolytic activity outside the disc. Also, due to the inhibitory activity of the plasma alpha$_2$-macroglobulin and the low concentration of chymopapain's reactive fragments (CIP), it is unlikely that any proteolytic activity is expressed outside the disc. Chymopapain and CIP are detectable in plasma at 30 minutes and decline at 24 hours. Small amounts of CIP are also detected in the urine. The liquified nucleus diffuses into the circulation, where the enzyme is inactivated. However, because chymopapain is injected directly into the herniated lumbar intervertebral disc, absorption, distribution and metabolism are not necessary for it to achieve its intended purpose.

Clinical trials: Approximately 75% of patients responded successfully to the drug, compared to approximately 45% for placebo. When the placebo failures were then treated with drug, 90% of them responded with partial or total relief of their symptoms. In open studies success rates ranged from 80% to 89%.

Indications:

For the treatment of documented herniated lumbar intervertebral discs, whose symptoms and signs, particularly sciatica, have not responded to adequate conservative therapy. The drug has not been studied in treatment of herniated discs in areas other than the lumbar spine.

Contraindications:

Known sensitivity to chymopapain, papaya or papaya derivatives (eg, papain-containing contact lens cleaner); severe spondylolisthesis; significant spinal stenosis; severe progressing paralysis, as indicated by rapidly progressing neurologic dysfunction; evidence of spinal cord tumor or other lesions producing spinal motor or sensory dysfunction (eg, a cauda equina lesion); previous injection of chymopapain; any spinal region other than the lumbar area.

CHYMOPAPAIN

Warnings:

Proper selection of patients is mandatory since nerve root compression resulting from conditions other than herniated disc can produce similar signs and symptoms.

Anaphylaxis (severe to mild) occurs in about 0.5% of patients and may be life threatening if not treated promptly and correctly. Females, particularly those with an elevated erythrocyte sedimentation rate, may be prone to develop such a reaction (approximately tenfold more common).

Data obtained from surveillance of over 71,000 patients demonstrate the incidence of anaphylaxis secondary to chymopapain injection varies by gender and type of anesthesia:

Anaphylaxis Incidence with Chymopapain			
	Local	General	Overall
Male	0.3%	0.3%	0.3%
Female	0.6%	0.9%	0.8%
Overall	0.4%	0.5%	0.5%

The anaphylaxis rate is significantly higher for females (0.8% v. 0.3% for males) and for patients who received general anesthesia (0.5% v. 0.4% for local anesthesia). In the population where race has been reported, the incidence is significantly higher in black females.

Preoperative pretreatment regimens to prevent anaphylactic reactions have been used, although there are no clinical studies demonstrating efficacy. Recommended regimens include cimetidine with either diphenhydramine or chlorpheniramine (see Administration and Dosage), diphenhydramine and dexamethasone with prednisone, and doxepin and terbutaline with an optional long-acting corticosteroid. Allergy testing to determine chymopapain-sensitive patients is available; however, the radioallergosorbent test and chymopapain fluorescence assay sensitivity test have excessively high false negative rates, and the skin test may be likely to produce false positives. Also, skin testing itself may sensitize patients.

Symptoms can be immediate or delayed up to 2 hours after injection and can last for minutes to several hours or longer. The patient may have almost immediate hypotension (more common) or bronchospasm and may proceed to laryngeal edema, cardiac arrhythmia, cardiac arrest, coma and death. Instruct patients to anticipate any delayed reactions (rash, urticaria or itching), which may occur for up to 15 days after injection.

Treatment – Clinical judgment, speed of therapy, and choice of agents all enter into treatment. The use of a preoperative screening test for chymopapain-specific IgE antibody should be considered to identify patients at risk for anaphylaxis. Keep at least one open IV line in place to permit rapid management. Epinephrine is indicated for immediate treatment. Beta-blocker therapy may inhibit the action of epinephrine. Reserve other agents such as steroids for cases where epinephrine is not appropriate. Refer to Management of Acute Hypersensitivity Reactions.

Fatalities such as those due to anaphylaxis or complications of anaphylaxis (see Warnings), disc space infection, or central nervous system hemorrhage, may be associated with either the drug or the procedure. Others appear to be coincidental. The overall mortality rate following chymopapain injection is approximately 1 in 5,000 patients (0.02%). In comparison, mortality associated with laminectomy ranges from 0.02% to 0.1%.

CHYMOPAPAIN

Neurological events: Paraplegia, paraparesis (eg, as are seen in the cauda equina syndrome), other serious neurologic adverse events, subarachnoid and intracerebral hemorrhage, and seizures have been observed soon after (within hours or days) chymopapain injection at a rate of about 1 in 2,000. Causal relationships to the drug when properly injected have not been established. Needle trauma or injection of chymopapain and contrast media into the spinal fluid may be causes in some of these reported cases. Other less severe neurologic reactions have included burning sacral pain, leg pain, hypalgesia, leg weakness, foot drop, cramping in both calves, pain in the opposite leg, paresthesia, tingling in legs and numbness of legs/toes.

Acute transverse myelitis/myelopathy has been associated with chymopapain, injection at a rate of about 1 in 18,000, although cause and effect relationship to the injection of chymopapain itself has not been established. These patients are characterized clinically by the delayed (2 to 3 weeks) onset of paraplegia or paraparesis without prior signs or symptoms.

In nearly all cases of serious neurologic adverse events, discography was performed as part of the procedure. Injection of contrast agent and chymopapain into the spinal fluid may be a cause in some cases. Additionally, several patients experiencing neurologic adverse events who did not have discography performed prior to the procedure experienced only transient problems. Therefore, it is recommended that discography not be performed as part of the chemonucleolysis procedure unless, in the judgment of the surgeon, the benefits outweigh the risks for a particular patient. A water or saline acceptance test may be used as an alternative to discography to indicate that the disc is abnormal and to attempt reproduction of sciatic pain in the patient receiving local anesthesia.

Patients receiving injections at two or more disc spaces appear to be at increased risk of serious neurologic adverse events. Therefore, limit chemonucleolysis to the one disc producing the patient's symptoms unless definitive signs, symptoms, and diagnostic procedures indicate that more than one disc is at fault.

Nearly all patients experiencing a serious neurologic adverse event had the procedure performed under general anesthesia. Local anesthesia provides an awake patient, more likely to experience pain and complain if the needle impinges on the nerve tissue. Also, it is unlikely that a patient under local anesthesia will tolerate an excessive number of attempts to place the needle. Although the final choice of anesthetic rests with the patient's physician, it is recommended that local or supplemented local anesthesia be used for chemonucleolysis whenever possible.

Patients who have had prior surgery of the lumbar spine appear to be at increased risk of experiencing a serious neurologic adverse event. Therefore, it is recommended that such patients be selelcted for chemonucleolysis only after careful consideration of the risk/benefit ratio.

Several patients with a history of hypertension, known or suspected cerebrovascular anomaly, previous cerebrovascular accident or a strong family history of cerebrovascular accident have experienced extensive, severe or fatal central nervous system hemorrhage following chemonucleolysis.

Immunological response: Chymopapain, a foreign protein, has the potential to cause an immunological response. Therefore, do not reinject patients who have already received any form of chymopapain injection.

Toxicity: The drug is extremely toxic when injected intrathecally in animals. Exercise caution to assure that chymopapain is not intrathecally injected into the dural canal; avoid transdural or posterior needle placement.

Certain radiopaque contrast media used for discography are neurotoxic when injected intrathecally. Toxicity may be enhanced by intrathecal bleeding. If chymopapain is inadvertently administered intrathecally, disruption of the capillaries may occur resulting in intrathecal bleeding.

Pregnancy: Category C. Safety for use during pregnancy has not been established. Use only when clearly needed and when the potential benefits outweigh the potential hazards to the fetus.

Children: Safety and efficacy for use in children have not been established.

Precautions:

Determine if the patient has multiple allergies, especially papaya, papaya derivatives or iodine. Do not use absorbable iodine during myelography or discography in patients allergic to iodine.

Postinjection pain: Patients may experience pain or involuntary muscle spasm in the lower back for several days. A residual stiffness or soreness may persist for several months.

CHYMOPAPAIN

Adverse Reactions:

Allergic reactions: Erythema; pilomotor erection; rash; pruritic urticaria; conjunctivitis; vasomotor rhinitis; angioedema; various GI disturbances; anaphylaxis (see Warnings).

Frequent: Back pain, stiffness, soreness (≈ 50%); back spasm (≈ 30%).

Less frequent (< 1%): Itching; nausea; paralytic ileus; urinary retention; headache; dizziness; sacral burning; leg pain; hypalgesia; leg weakness; cramping in both calves; pain in the opposite leg; paresthesia; foot drop; tingling and numbness of legs/toes.

Discitis, both bacterial and aseptic.

Causal relationship unknown: Transverse myelitis/myelopathy (see Warning Box and Warnings).

Overdosage:

In animal studies, doses up to 100 times greater than that required to remove the nucleus pulposus were well tolerated when injected IV, intradiscally and epidurally.

Administration and Dosage:

Pretreatment: Prior to injection of chymopapain, pretreat with histamine receptor (H_1 and H_2) antagonists to lessen the severity of an anaphylactic reaction. One widely used regimen is cimetidine 300 mg orally every 6 hours and diphenhydramine 50 mg orally every 6 hours for 24 hours prior to chemonucleolysis.

Because of the abrupt decrease in intravascular volume during anaphylaxis, patients should be well hydrated by oral or IV fluids prior to chemonucleolysis. Always have at least one open IV line in place to permit rapid and adequate management of anaphylaxis.

Note: The unit of chymopapain activity is the nanoKatal (nKat). In general, 1 mg of chymopapain contains at least 0.5 nKat units. Each 2 ml vial of chymopapain contains 4 nKat units of enzyme for reconstitution with 2 ml Sterile Water for Injection, USP. Each 5 ml vial contains 10 nKat units of the enzyme for reconstitution with 5 ml Sterile Water for Injection, USP. The concentration of solution in the reconstituted vial is 2 nKat units of drug per ml.

Dosage is 2 to 4 nKat units per disc, usually 3 nKat units per disc, or a volume injection of 1 to 2 ml, usually 1.5 ml per disc. Maximum dose in a single patient with multiple disc herniation (see Warnings) is 8 nKat units.

Intradiscal administration: Treat each herniated disc with a single injection of chymopapain. Refer to package literature for detailed administration procedure.

Preparation of solution: Use alcohol to cleanse the vial stopper prior to insertion of needles into the vial. However, since alcohol inactivates the enzyme, allow to air dry before continuing the reconstitution process. The manufacturing process results in a residual vacuum in the vial; therefore, do not use automatic filling syringes.

Reconstitution – Reconstitute with 5 ml Sterile Water for Injection, which is supplied with each vial of chymopapain. (Use only 2 ml Sterile Water solution when reconstituting 4 nKat unit vial.) Do not use Bacteriostatic Water for Injection because it may inactivate the enzyme.

Stability and storage: Although it can be shipped unrefrigerated, store chymopapain at 2° to 8°C (36° to 46°F) until reconstitution.

Chymopapain must be used within 2 hours of its reconstitution; promptly discard unused drug.

Rx	**Chymodiactin** (Boots-Flint)	**Powder for Injection**: 4 nKat units and 1.4 mg sodium L–cysteinate HCl per vial w/diluent. (2 nKat units/ml after reconstitution)	In 2 ml vials.

[1] Contains no preservatives.

DISULFIRAM

Warning:
Never give to a patient in a state of alcohol intoxication, or without the patient's full knowledge. Instruct the patient's relatives accordingly.

Actions:

Pharmacology: Disulfiram produces an intolerance to alcohol which results in a highly unpleasant reaction when the patient under treatment ingests even small amounts of alcohol. Disulfiram blocks oxidation of alcohol at the acetaldehyde stage by inhibiting aldehyde dehydrogenase. The concentration of acetaldehyde in the blood may be 5 to 10 times higher than that achieved during normal alcohol metabolism. Accumulation of acetaldehyde produces the disulfiram-alcohol reaction (see Warnings). This reaction persists as long as alcohol is being metabolized. Disulfiram does not influence alcohol elimination.

Pharmacokinetics: Disulfiram is rapidly absorbed from the GI tract and eliminated slowly from the body. About 12 hours are required for its full action. Disulfiram is metabolized to diethyldithiocarbamate, which is oxidized to carbon disulfide and diethylamine. Approximately 20% of the drug remains after 1 week. Ingestion of alcohol may produce unpleasant symptoms for 1 to 2 weeks after the last dose of disulfiram. Prolonged administration of disulfiram does not produce tolerance; the longer a patient remains on therapy, the more sensitive he becomes to alcohol.

Indications:

An aid in the management of selected chronic alcoholics who want to remain in a state of enforced sobriety.

Effectiveness in promoting abstinence is limited. Compliance with the disulfiram regimen and regular follow-ups correlate with abstinence.

Contraindications:

Severe myocardial disease or coronary occlusion; psychoses; hypersensitivity to disulfiram or to other thiuram derivatives used in pesticides and rubber vulcanization; patients receiving or who have recently received metronidazole, paraldehyde, alcohol, or alcohol-containing preparations (eg, cough syrups, tonics).

Warnings:

Never administer to an intoxicated patient or without the patient's knowledge (see Warning box).

Disulfiram-alcohol reaction: Disulfiram plus alcohol, even small amounts, produces flushing, throbbing in head and neck, throbbing headaches, respiratory difficulty, nausea, copious vomiting, sweating, thirst, chest pain, palpitations, dyspnea, hyperventilation, tachycardia, hypotension, syncope, marked uneasiness, weakness, vertigo, blurred vision and confusion. In severe reactions there may be respiratory depression, cardiovascular collapse, arrhythmias, myocardial infarction, acute congestive heart failure, unconsciousness, convulsions and death. The intensity of the reaction is proportional to the amounts of disulfiram and alcohol ingested. Mild reactions may occur in the sensitive individual when the blood alcohol concentration is as low as 5 to 10 mg/dl. Symptoms are fully developed at 50 mg/dl, and unconsciousness usually results at 125 to 150 mg/dl. The duration of the reaction varies from 30 to 60 minutes to several hours.

Concomitant conditions: Because of the possibility of an accidental reaction, use with caution in patients with diabetes mellitus, hypothyroidism, epilepsy, cerebral damage, chronic and acute nephritis, hepatic cirrhosis or insufficiency.

Hypersensitivity: Evaluate patients with a history of rubber contact dermatitis for hypersensitivity to thiuram derivatives before administering disulfiram. Refer to General Management of Acute Hypersensitivity Reactions.

Pregnancy: Safety for use during pregnancy has not been established.

Precautions:

Monitoring: Perform baseline and follow-up transaminase tests (10 to 14 days) to detect hepatic dysfunction resulting from therapy. Perform a CBC and SMA-12 test every 6 months.

Dependence and addiction: Alcoholism may accompany or be followed by dependence on narcotics or sedatives. Barbiturates have been coadministered with disulfiram without untoward effects, but consider the possibility of initiating a new abuse.

Ethylene dibromide: Patients should not be exposed to ethylene dibromide or its vapors. This precaution is based on preliminary results of animal research which suggest a toxic interaction between inhaled ethylene dibromide and ingested disulfiram resulting in higher incidence of tumors and mortality in rats.

DISULFIRAM

Drug Interactions:

Alcohol: Disulfiram causes a severe alcohol-intolerance reaction. Avoid alcohol in all forms. See Warnings.

Benzodiazepines: Disulfiram decreases the plasma clearance of benzodiazepines metabolized by oxidation, possibly resulting in increased CNS depressant actions. When benzodiazepine therapy is indicated, use oxazepam, alprazolam or lorazepam since they are metabolized by glucuronidation.

Caffeine: Cardiovascular and CNS stimulation effects of caffeine may be increased by disulfiram.

Hydantoins: Serum hydantoin levels may be increased by disulfiram, resulting in an increase in the pharmacologic and toxic effects. Monitor hydantoin levels and adjust the dosage as needed.

Isoniazid: Observe patients receiving isoniazid and disulfiram for the appearance of unsteady gait or marked changes in behavior; discontinue disulfiram or reduce the dose if such signs appear.

Metronidazole: Patients may exhibit acute toxic psychosis or confusional state when taking metronidazole in combination with disulfiram, requiring discontinuation of one or both of the agents.

Tricyclic antidepressants and disulfiram coadministration may result in acute organic brain syndrome. The bioavailability of the antidepressant may also be increased.

Warfarin: Disulfiram may increase the anticoagulant effect of warfarin. Monitor prothrombin time and adjust the warfarin dosage as necessary.

Adverse Reactions:

Neurologic: Peripheral neuropathy (with axonal degeneration); polyneuritis; optic or retrobulbar neuritis (with impaired vision, color perceptions and blindness).

CNS: Drowsiness (most common); fatigability; headache; restlessness. Psychotic reactions have been noted, often attributable to high dosage, combined toxicity (metronidazole or isoniazid), or to the unmasking of underlying psychoses.

Dermatologic: Occasional skin eruptions are, as a rule, readily controlled by antihistamines; acneiform eruptions; allergic dermatitis.

GI: Metallic or garlic-like aftertaste, usually during the first 2 weeks of therapy.

Hepatotoxicity resembling viral or alcoholic hepatitis; probably due to hypersensitivity, but toxic metabolite formation has also been proposed.

Multiple cases of both cholestatic and fulminant hepatitis have been associated with disulfiram use.

Miscellaneous: Arthropathy; acetonemia; impotence.

Patient Information:

Never use in intoxicated individuals or without an individual's knowledge.

Do not take for at least 12 hours after drinking alcohol. A reaction may occur for up to 2 weeks after disulfiram has been stopped.

Avoid alcohol in all forms. This includes: Alcoholic beverages, vinegars, many liquid medications (including prescription and nonprescription products), some sauces, aftershave lotions, colognes, liniments, etc.

Always read product labels or ask your pharmacist about alcohol content of all liquid medications before choosing one.

Tablets can be crushed or mixed with liquid.

May cause drowsiness. Use caution while driving or performing other tasks requiring alertness.

The alcohol-disulfiram reaction can have serious effects on the heart and respiratory systems.

Always carry identification indicating you are taking disulfiram. Include the phone numbers of your doctor or the medical facility that should be contacted in case of reaction.

DISULFIRAM

Administration and Dosage:

Do NOT administer until the patient has abstained from alcohol for at least 12 hours.

Initial dosage schedule: Administer a maximum of 500 mg daily in a single dose for 1 to 2 weeks. If a sedative effect is experienced, take at bedtime or decrease dosage.

Maintenance regimen: The average maintenance dose is 250 mg daily (range, 125 to 500 mg), not to exceed 500 mg daily. NOTE: Occasional disulfiram patients report that they are able to drink alcoholic beverages with impunity and without any symptomatology. Such patients must be presumed to be disposing of their tablets without actually taking them. Until such patients are observed reliably taking their daily tablets (preferably crushed and well mixed with liquid), do not assume that disulfiram is ineffective.

Duration of therapy: Continue use until the patient is fully recovered socially and a basis for permanent self-control is established. Maintenance therapy may be required for months or even years.

Trial with alcohol: The test reaction has been largely abandoned. Do not administer a test reaction to a patient > 50 years of age. A clear, detailed and convincing description of the reaction is felt to be sufficient in most cases.

Where a test reaction is deemed necessary, the suggested procedure is: After the first 1 to 2 weeks of therapy with 500 mg daily, a drink of 15 ml of 100 proof whiskey or equivalent is taken slowly. This test dose may be repeated once only so that total dose does not exceed 30 ml (1 g) whiskey. Once a reaction develops, no more alcohol should be consumed. Only perform such tests when the patient is hospitalized and facilities are available.

Management of disulfiram-alcohol reaction: In severe reactions, institute supportive measures to restore blood pressure and treat shock. Other recommendations include: Oxygen or carbogen (95% oxygen and 5% carbon dioxide), vitamin C IV in massive doses (1 g) and ephedrine sulfate. Antihistamines have also been used IV. Monitor potassium levels, particularly in patients on digitalis, since hypokalemia has been reported.

Extemporaneous aqueous suspensions of disulfiram powder or tablets (2.5 g, with 2 g acacia and 100 mg sodium benzoate, with water to make 100 ml) have been reported stable up to 295 days when stored at 24°C (room temperature) in amber-colored bottles under fluorescent light.

Rx	**Disulfiram** (Various, eg, Danbury, Geneva, Goldline, Major, Moore, Qualitest, Rugby, Schein, Sidmak, URL)	**Tablets:** 250 mg	In 100s and 1000s.
Rx	**Antabuse** (Wyeth-Ayerst)		Scored. In 100s.
Rx	**Disulfiram** (Various, eg, Danbury, Geneva, Goldline, Major, Qualitest, Rugby, Schein, Sidmak)	**Tablets:** 500 mg	In 50s, 100s and 500s.
Rx	**Antabuse** (Wyeth-Ayerst)		Scored. In 50s and 1000s.

NICOTINE

Actions:

Pharmacology: Nicotine polacrilex contains nicotine bound to an ion exchange resin in a chewing gum base. The nicotine transdermal system is a multilayered unit containing nicotine as the active agent that provides systemic delivery of nicotine for 24 hours following its application to intact skin.

Nicotine, the chief alkaloid in tobacco products, binds stereoselectively to acetylcholine receptors at the autonomic ganglia, in the adrenal medulla, at neuromuscular junctions and in the brain. Two types of CNS effects are believed to be the basis of nicotine's positively reinforcing properties. A stimulating effect, exerted mainly in the cortex via the locus ceruleus, produces increased alertness and cognitive performance. A "reward" effect via the "pleasure system" in the brain is exerted in the limbic system. At low doses the stimulant effects predominate, while at high doses the reward effects predominate. Intermittent IV administration of nicotine activates neurohormonal pathways, releasing acetylcholine, norepinephrine, dopamine, serotonin, vasopressin, beta-endorphin, growth hormone and ACTH.

The cardiovascular effects of nicotine include peripheral vasoconstriction, tachycardia and elevated blood pressure. Acute and chronic tolerance to nicotine develops from smoking tobacco or ingesting nicotine preparations. Acute tolerance (a reduction in reponse for a given dose) develops rapidly (< 1 hour), but at distinct rates for different physiologic effects (skin temperature, heart rate, subjective effects). Withdrawal symptoms, such as cigarette craving, can be reduced in some individuals by plasma nicotine levels lower than those for smoking.

Withdrawal from nicotine in addicted individuals is characterized by craving, nervousness, restlessness, irritability, mood lability, anxiety, drowsiness, sleep disturbances, impaired concentration, increased appetite, minor somatic complaints (headache, myalgia, constipation, fatigue) and weight gain. Nicotine toxicity is characterized by nausea, abdominal pain, vomiting, diarrhea, diaphoresis, flushing, dizziness, disturbed hearing/vision, confusion, weakness, palpitations, altered respiration and hypotension.

Nicotine's effects are generally dose-dependent. In nonsmokers, CNS-mediated symptoms of hiccoughs, nausea and emesis are commonly associated with the use of even small doses of inhaled smoke or nicotine gum. However, in smokers these symptoms occur only with much larger doses. If nicotine gum (2 mg/piece) is used by smokers at a rate not exceeding 1 piece/hour or if transdermal nicotine is used (21 mg/day), the cardiovascular effects do not differ from those seen with placebo.

Pharmacokinetics:

Nicotine gum –

Absorption/Distribution: The nicotine is bound to an ion exchange resin and is released only during chewing; nicotine will not be released in significant amounts if the gum is swallowed. The blood level of nicotine will depend upon the vigor, rapidity and duration of chewing. The trough level of nicotine obtained by smoking one cigarette/hr is approximately twice that of chewing one 2 mg piece of gum/hr.

Metabolism/Excretion – Nicotine is metabolized mainly by the liver, and to a lesser extent, by the kidney and lung. There is no significant skin metabolism of nicotine. More than 20 metabolites of nicotine have been identified, all of which are believed to be less active than the parent compound. The half-life of nicotine ranges from 1 to 2 hours. The primary metabolite of nicotine in plasma, cotinine, has a half-life of 15 to 20 hours and concentrations that exceed nicotine by 10-fold. Plasma protein binding of nicotine is < 5%. The primary urinary metabolites are cotinine (15% of the dose) and trans-3-hydroxycotinine (45% of the dose). About 10% of nicotine is excreted unchanged in the urine. As much as 30% may be excreted in the urine with high urine flow rates and urine acidification below pH5.

Nicotine transdermal system: All systems are labeled by the actual amount of nicotine absorbed by the patient.

Nicoderm – Following application, ≈ 68% of the nicotine released from the system enters the systemic circulation. The remainder of the nicotine released from the system is lost via evaporation from the edge. After application, plasma concentrations rise rapidly, plateau within 2 to 4 hours, and then slowly decline until the system is removed, after which they decline more rapidly. Nicotine in the adhesive layer is absorbed into and then through the skin, causing the initial rapid rise in plasma concentrations. The nicotine from the reservoir is released slowly through the membrane with a release rate constant approximately 20 times smaller than the skin absorption rate constant. Therefore, the slow decline of plasma nicotine concentrations during 4 to 24 hours is determined primarily by the release of nicotine from the system.

Habitrol – Following an initial lag time of 1 to 2 hours, nicotine levels increase to a broad peak between 6 and 12 hours and then decrease gradually.

NICOTINE

Habitrol/Nicoderm – Following the second daily system application (or within 2 days of initiating treatment), steady-state plasma nicotine concentrations are achieved and are on average 25% to 30% higher compared with single-dose applications. Plasma nicotine concentrations are proportional to dose for the three dosages of the transdermal systems. Nicotine kinetics are similar for all sites of application on the upper body and upper outer arm. Plasma nicotine concentrations from the 21 mg/day system are the same as those from simultaneous use of 14 and 7 mg/day systems.

Following system removal, plasma nicotine concentrations decline in an exponential fashion with an apparent mean half-life of 3 to 4 hours vs 1 to 2 hours for IV use, due to continued absorption from the skin depot. Most nonsmoking patients will have nondetectable nicotine concentrations in 10 to 12 hours.

Half-hourly smoking of cigarettes produces average plasma nicotine concentrations of approximately 44 ng/ml. In comparison, average plasma nicotine concentrations from transdermal nicotine 21 mg/day are about 17 ng/ml.

Obese men using transdermal systems had significantly lower AUC and C_{max} values than normal weight men. Men and women having low body weight are expected to have higher AUC and C_{max} values.

Clinical trials –

Nicotine gum: In the varied controlled trials conducted, the success rate of smoking cessation has been approximately doubled using nicotine gum.

Nicoderm: In two trials of transdermal nicotine vs placebo, treatment with 21 mg/day for 6 weeks provided significantly higher quit rates than the 14 mg/day and placebo treatments at 6 weeks (32% to 92%, 30% to 61% and 15% to 46%, respectively). Quit rates were still significantly different after an additional 6 week weaning period (18% to 63%, 15% to 52% and 0% to 38%, respectively) and at follow-up 3 months later (3% to 50%, 0% to 48% and 0% to 35%, respectively).

Habitrol: In two trials in otherwise healthy smokers with concomitant support, transdermal therapy resulted in higher quit rates than placebo after 7 weeks (19% to 54% vs 9% to 30%). Quit rates were still significantly different after an additional 3 week weaning period (8% to 43% vs 8% to 30%). When transdermal nicotine was used without concomitant support, greater variability and decreased quit rates were demonstrated with both treatment and placebo after 7 weeks (4% to 28% vs 0% to 24%) as well as after a 3 week weaning period (4% to 20% vs 0% to 22%).

Indications:

As an aid to smoking cessation for the relief of nicotine withdrawal symptoms. Use as part of a comprehensive behavioral smoking-cessation program.

In general, smokers who have a high "physical" type of nicotine dependence are most likely to benefit from the use of nicotine gum or transdermal systems. The following characteristics correlate with a "physical" type of nicotine dependence: (1) Smoke > 15 cigarettes per day, (2) prefer brands of cigarettes with nicotine levels > 0.9 mg, (3) usually inhale the smoke frequently and deeply, (4) smoke the first cigarette within 30 minutes of arising, (5) find the first cigarette in the morning the hardest to give up, (6) smoke most frequently during the morning, (7) find it difficult to refrain from smoking in places where it is forbidden, or (8) smoke even when they are so ill they are confined to bed most of the day.

The benefits of use beyond 3 months have not been demonstrated.

Unlabeled uses: In two children, use of nicotine polacrilex gum and haloperidol improved symptoms (eg, tics) of Tourette's syndrome. Further study is needed.

Contraindications:

Hypersensitivity to nicotine or any components of the transdermal system; nonsmokers; during the immediate postmyocardial infarction period; life-threatening arrhythmias; severe or worsening angina pectoris; active temporomandibular joint disease (nicotine polacrilex); pregnancy (see Warnings).

Warnings:

Cardiovascular: Weigh the benefits against the risks of nicotine in patients with certain cardiovascular diseases. Specifically, screen and evaluate patients with coronary heart disease (history of myocardial infarction or angina pectoris), serious cardiac arrhythmias or vasospastic diseases (Buerger's disease, Prinzmetal variant angina) before nicotine is prescribed. There have been occasional reports of tachyarrhythmias associated with nicotine use; therefore, if an increase in cardiovascular symptoms occurs, discontinue the drug. Generally, do not use during the immediate post-myocardial infarction period, with serious arrhythmias or with severe or worsening angina pectoris.

Cigarette smoking may play a perpetuating role in hypertension. Therefore, use nicotine in patients with systemic hypertension only when the benefits of such a smoking cessation program outweigh the risks.

Endocrine: Because of the action of nicotine on the adrenal medulla (release of catecholamines), use with caution in patients with hyperthyroidism, pheochromocytoma or insulin-dependent diabetes.

Renal/Hepatic function impairment: Since nicotine is extensively metabolized and its total system clearance is dependent on liver blood flow, anticipate some influence of hepatic impairment on drug kinetics (reduced clearance). Only severe renal impairment should affect clearance of nicotine or its metabolites from circulation.

Fertility impairment: A decrease of litter size in rats treated with nicotine during the time of fertilization has occurred. Rare reports of miscarriages have been received. A relationship to drug therapy as a contributing factor cannot be excluded.

Elderly: Transdermal nicotine therapy appeared to be as effective in elderly patients > 60 years of age as in younger smokers. However, asthenia, various body aches and dizziness occurred slightly more often in elderly patients.

Pregnancy: Category X (nicotine polacrilex), *Category D* (transdermal nicotine). Nicotine may cause fetal harm when used in a pregnant woman. Use of cigarettes or nicotine gum during the last trimester has been associated with decreased fetal breathing movements. This may result from decreased placental perfusion caused by nicotine. Rare reports of miscarriages have been received, and a relationship to drug therapy as a contributing factor cannot be excluded. Nicotine is contraindicated in women who are or may become pregnant; advise patients to use contraceptive measures. If this drug is used during pregnancy, or if the patient becomes pregnant while taking it, apprise her of the potential hazard to the fetus.

The specific effects of transdermal nicotine on fetal development are unknown. Therefore, encourage pregnant smokers to attempt cessation before using pharmacological approaches. Use during pregnancy only if the likelihood of smoking cessation justifies the potential risk of use of nicotine replacement by the patient who may continue to smoke.

Lactation: Nicotine passes freely into breast milk and has the potential for serious adverse reactions in nursing infants. Nicotine concentrations in milk can be expected to be lower with transdermal nicotine therapy when used as directed than with cigarette smoking, as maternal plasma nicotine concentrations are generally reduced with nicotine replacement. Decide whether to discontinue nursing or to discontinue the drug, weighing the risk of exposure of the infant to nicotine from replacement therapy against the risks associated with the infant's exposure to nicotine from continued smoking by the mother and from nicotine therapy alone or in combination with continued smoking.

Children: Safety and efficacy in children/adolescents who smoke are not evaluated.

The amounts of nicotine that are tolerated by adult smokers can produce symptoms of poisoning and could prove fatal if the transdermal nicotine system is applied or ingested by children or pets. Used 21 mg/day *Nicoderm* and *Habitrol* systems contain about 73% (83 mg) and 60% (32 mg) of their initial drug content, respectively. Therefore, caution patients to keep both the used and unused systems out of the reach of children and pets.

Precautions:

Oral/GI: Use caution in patients with oral or pharyngeal inflammation and in those with history of esophagitis or peptic ulcer. Since nicotine delays healing in peptic ulcer disease, use in patients with active or inactive peptic ulcer only when benefits of including nicotine in a smoking cessation program outweigh risks.

Skin disease: Systems are usually well tolerated by patients with normal skin, but may be irritating for patients with some skin disorders (atopic or eczematous dermatitis).

Allergic reactions: In two studies, 29 of 450 patients exhibited definite erythema at 24 hours after application of the transdermal system. Upon rechallenge, 7 patients exhibited mild to moderate contact allergy. Caution patients with contact sensitization that a serious reaction could occur from exposure to other nicotine-containing products or smoking. Erythema following system removal was typically seen in 14% to 17% of patients, some edema in 3% to 4% and dropouts due to skin reactions in 2% to 6%.

Instruct patients to promptly discontinue the use of nicotine systems and contact their physicians if they experience severe or persistent local skin reactions (eg, severe erythema, pruritus, edema) at the site of application or a generalized skin reaction (eg, urticaria, hives, generalized rash).

Patients using transdermal nicotine concurrently with other transdermal products may exhibit local reactions at both application sites. Reactions were seen in 2 of 7 patients using concomitant estradiol transdermal system. In such patients, use of one or both systems may have to be discontinued.

Dental problems might be exacerbated by chewing nicotine gum.

Drug abuse and dependence: Urge patients to stop smoking completely when initiating therapy. If patients smoke while using nicotine, they may experience adverse effects due to peak nicotine levels higher than those due to smoking alone.

Transference of nicotine dependence is possible. Transdermal nicotine or nicotine gum use beyond 3 months is not shown to increase smoking cessation rate. To minimize risk of dependence, encourage patients to gradually withdraw or stop gum usage at 3 months, transdermal nicotine after 4 to 8 weeks (progressively decrease dose every 2 to 4 weeks). Chronic consumption is toxic and addicting. Weigh relative risks of possible return to smoking and continued, long-term gum use.

Drug Interactions:

Smoking cessation, with or without nicotine substitutes, may alter response to concomitant medication in ex-smokers. Smoking is considered to increase metabolism and lower blood levels of the following drugs through enzyme induction (smoking cessation may reverse these actions).

Acetaminophen
Caffeine
Imipramine
Oxazepam
Pentazocine
Propranolol
Theophylline

Catecholamines and cortisol: Smoking and nicotine can increase circulating cortisol and catecholamines. Therapy with **adrenergic agonists** or **adrenergic blockers** may need to be adjusted upon changes in nicotine therapy or smoking status.

Furosemide: Smoking may reduce diuretic effects of furosemide and decrease cardiac output. Smoking cessation may reverse these actions.

Glutethimide absorption may be decreased with smoking cessation.

Insulin: Increase in subcutaneous insulin absorption with smoking cessation may occur.

Propoxyphene: The first-pass metabolism of propoxyphene may be decreased by smoking cessation.

Drug/Food interactions: Effective absorption of nicotine polacrilex relies on a mildly alkaline saliva (produced from release of buffering agents). Therefore, since coffee, cola and other drinks or food may reduce salivary pH, it may be beneficial to not ingest food or drink during or immediately before the use of nicotine gum.

Adverse Reactions:

Nicotine polacrilex:

Local – Mechanical effects of gum chewing include traumatic injury to oral mucosa or teeth, jaw ache and eructation secondary to air swallowing. Minimize by modifying chewing technique. Oral mucosal changes such as stomatitis, glossitis, gingivitis, pharyngitis and aphthous ulcers, in addition to changes in taste perception, can occur during smoking cessation efforts with or without nicotine gum.

Systemic – Although the systemic effects seen in trials were generally similar, the reported frequency of adverse drug effects was highly variable.

Nicotine Polacrilex Adverse Reactions (%)				
	US studies		British studies	
	Drug (n = 94)	Placebo (n = 95)	Drug (n = 58)	Placebo (n = 58)
CNS				
Insomnia	1.1	1.1		
Dizziness/Lightheadedness	2.1	2.1	19	13.8
Irritability/Fussiness	1.1	1.1		
Headache	1.1	5.3	24.1	29.3
GI				
Nonspecific GI distress	9.6	6.3		
Eructation	6.4	1.1		
Indigestion			41.4	20.7
Nausea/Vomiting	18.1	4.2	31	15.5
Oropharyngeal				
Mouth or throat soreness	37.2	31.6	56.9	53.4
Jaw muscle ache	18.1	9.5	44.8	44.8
Other				
Anorexia	1.1	1.1		
Excess salivation	2.1	0		
Hiccoughs	14.9	0	22.4	3.4

NICOTINE

Cardiovascular – Edema; flushing; hypertension; palpitations; tachyarrhythmias; tachycardia. One patient displayed what may have been nicotine-induced, but reversible, atrial fibrillation. Cardiac irritability is a well known consequence of cigarette smoking.

Deaths, myocardial infarction, congestive heart failure, cerebrovascular accident and cardiac arrest have occurred (a cause and effect relationship has not been established).

CNS – Confusion; convulsions; depression; euphoria; numbness; paresthesia; syncope; tinnitus; weakness.

Dermatologic – Erythema; itching; rash; urticaria.

GI – Alteration of liver function tests; constipation; diarrhea.

Respiratory – Breathing difficulty; cough; hoarseness; sneezing; wheezing.

Miscellaneous – Dry mouth; systemic nicotine intoxication.

Transdermal nicotine: The most common adverse event associated with topical nicotine is a short-lived erythema, pruritus or burning at the application site, which was seen at least once in 35% to 47% of patients in the clinical trials. Local erythema after system removal was noted at least once in 14% to 17% of patients and local edema in 3% to 4%. Erythema generally resolved within 24 hours. Cutaneous hypersensitivity (contact sensitization) occurred in 2% of patients (see Precautions).

Body as a whole – Asthenia, back pain, pain (3% to 9%); chest pain, allergy (1% to 3%).

GI – Diarrhea, dyspepsia, constipation, nausea (3% to 9%); abdominal pain, vomiting, dry mouth (1% to 3%).

CNS – Headache (17% to 29%); insomnia (3% to 23%); abnormal dreams, nervousness, dizziness (3% to 9%); paresthesia, somnolence, impaired concentration (1% to 3%).

Respiratory – Increased cough, pharyngitis (3% to 9%); sinusitis (1% to 3%).

Dermatologic – Rash (3% to 9%).

Musculoskeletal – Myalgia, arthralgia (3% to 9%).

Miscellaneous – Taste perversion, dysmenorrhea (3% to 9%); sweating, hypertension (1% to 3%).

Overdosage:

Symptoms: Overdose will probably be minimized by the early nausea and vomiting that occur with excessive nicotine intake. Signs and symptoms of acute nicotine poisoning include: Nausea; salivation; abdominal pain; vomiting; diarrhea; cold sweat; headache; dizziness; disturbed hearing and vision; mental confusion; marked weakness. Faintness and prostration will ensue and hypotension may occur; breathing is difficult; the pulse may be rapid, weak and irregular; respiratory collapse may be followed by terminal convulsions. Death may result within a few minutes from paralysis of respiratory muscles. The oral minimum lethal dose for nicotine in adults is 40 to 60 mg.

Treatment:

Nicotine polacrilex – If emesis has not occurred, induce with ipecac syrup in conscious patients. A saline cathartic will speed GI passage of the gum. In unconscious patients with a secure airway, gastric lavage followed by suspension of activated charcoal will aid in nicotine removal. Mechanical ventilation for respiratory paralysis may be necessary. Hypotension or cardiovascular collapse may occur; treat vigorously. Refer to General Management of Acute Overdosage.

Transdermal nicotine – Topical exposure – Remove the transdermal system immediately if the patient shows signs of overdosage and seek immediate medical care. The skin surface may be flushed with water and dried. Do not use soap, since it may increase nicotine absorption. Nicotine will continue to be delivered into the bloodstream for several hours after removal of the system because of a depot of nicotine in the skin.

Ingestion – Refer patients to a health care facility for management. Due to the possibility of nicotine-induced seizures, administer activated charcoal. In unconscious patients with a secure airway, instill activated charcoal via a nasogastric tube. A saline cathartic or sorbitol added to the first dose of activated charcoal may speed GI passage of the system. Administer repeated doses of activated charcoal as long as the system remains in the GI tract since it will continue to release nicotine for many hours.

Other supportive measures include diazepam or barbiturates for seizures, atropine for excessive bronchial secretions or diarrhea, respiratory support for respiratory failure and vigorous fluid support for hypotension and cardiovascular collapse.

NICOTINE TRANSDERMAL SYSTEM

For complete prescribing information, refer to the Nicotine group monograph.

Patient Information:

A patient instruction sheet, included in the package dispensed to the patient, contains important information and instructions on proper use and disposal of the transdermal system. Encourage patients to ask questions of physician and pharmacist.

Advise patients to keep used and unused systems out of reach of children and pets.

Administration and Dosage:

Approved by the FDA in November 1991.

Patients must desire to stop smoking. Instruct them to stop smoking immediately as they begin using therapy, to read the patient instruction sheet and to ask questions. Initiate treatment according to recommended dosing schedule (see table).

Once the appropriate dosage is selected, the patient should begin 4 to 12 weeks of therapy at that dosage (refer to specific product guidelines for duration). The patient should stop smoking cigarettes completely during this period. If the patient is unable to stop cigarette smoking within 4 weeks, therapy probably should be stopped, since few additional patients in clinical trials were able to quit after this time. Use beyond 3 months (5 months for *Nicotrol*) has not been studied.

Recommended Dosing Schedule of Transdermal Nicotine for Healthy Patients

Dose	Duration: Per strength of patch	Duration: Entire course of therapy
Habitrol[1]		
21 mg/day	First 6 weeks	8 to 12 weeks
14 mg/day	Next 2 weeks[2]	
7 mg/day	Last 2 weeks[3]	
Nicoderm[1]		
21 mg/day	First 6 weeks	8 to 12 weeks
14 mg/day	Next 2 weeks[2]	
7 mg/day	Last 2 weeks	
Nicotrol		
15 mg/day	First 12 weeks	14 to 20 weeks
10 mg/day	Next 2 weeks[2]	
5 mg/day	Last 2 weeks	
ProStep[3]		
22 mg/day	4 to 8 weeks	6 to 12 weeks
11 mg/day[4]	2 to 4 weeks	

[1] Start with 14 mg/day for 6 weeks for patients who: Have cardiovascular disease; weigh < 100 lbs; smoke < ½ pack of cigarettes/day. Decrease dose to 7 mg/day for the final 2 to 4 weeks.

[2] Patients who have successfully abstained from smoking should have their dose reduced after each 2 to 4 weeks of treatment until the 7 mg/day dose *(Habitrol; Nicoderm)* or 5 mg/day dose *(Nicotrol)* has been used for 2 to 4 weeks.

[3] Start with 22 mg/day except for patients who weigh < 100 lbs; they may start with 11 mg/day with the dose increased as appropriate.

[4] Optional weaning dose.

Application of system: Apply the system promptly upon its removal from the protective pouch to prevent evaporative loss of nicotine from the system. Use only when the pouch is intact to ensure that the product has not been tampered with. Apply only once a day to non-hairy, clean, dry skin site on upper body or upper outer arm.

Habitrol, Nicoderm, ProStep – After 24 hours, remove the used system and apply a new system to an alternate skin site. Skin sites should not be reused for at least a week. Caution patients not to continue to use the same system for > 24 hours.

Nicotrol – Each day apply a new system upon waking and remove at bedtime.

Individualization of dosage: Patients who fail to quit on any attempt may benefit from interventions to improve their chances for success on subsequent attempts. These patients should be counseled to determine why they failed and then probably be given a "therapy holiday" before the next attempt. Encourage a new quit attempt when the factors that contributed to failure can be eliminated or reduced, and conditions are more favorable.

NICOTINE TRANSDERMAL SYSTEM

Safety/Handling: The transdermal nicotine system can be a dermal irritant and can cause contact sensitization. Instruct patients in the proper use of the systems by using demonstration systems. Although exposure of healthcare workers to nicotine from the systems should be minimal, take care to avoid unnecessary contact with active systems. If you do handle active systems, wash with water alone, since soap may increase nicotine absorption. Do not touch your eyes.

Disposal: When the used system is removed from the skin, fold it over and place in the protective pouch that contained the new system. Immediately dispose of the used system in such a way to prevent its access by children or pets.

Storage/Stability: Do not store above 30°C (86°F) because the transdermal systems are sensitive to heat. A slight discoloration of the system is not significant. Do not store out of the pouch. Once removed from the protective pouch, apply promptly since nicotine is volatile and the system may lose strength.

	Product/Distributor	Dose absorbed in 24 hours (mg/day)	Surface area (cm^2)	Total nictine content (mg)	How supplied
Rx	**Habitrol** (Basel Pharm.)	21[1]	30	52.5	30 systems per box.
		14	20	35	
		7	10	17.5	
Rx	**Nicoderm** (Hoechst Marion Roussel)	21	22	114	14 systems per box.
		14	15	78	
		7	7	36	
otc	**Nicotrol** (McNeil)	15[2]	30	24.9	14 systems per box.
		10[2]	20	16.6	
		5[2]	10	8.3	
Rx	**ProStep** (Lederle)	22	7	30	7 systems per box.
		11	3.5	15	

[1] Pouch contains patch labeled 23 mg/24 hr, which delivers 21 mg/day.
[2] Dose absorbed in 16 hours (mg/day).

NICOTINE POLACRILEX (Nicotine resin complex)

For complete prescribing information, refer to the Nicotine group monograph.

Patient Information:

A patient instruction sheet is included in the package dispensed to the patient.

Administration and Dosage:

Approved by the FDA in January 1984.

A candidate for nicotine therapy must desire to stop smoking and should stop smoking immediately. Give the patient an instruction sheet on nicotine gum chewing, and allow patient to read the insturction sheet and ask any questions. Individualize initial dosage on the basis of each patient's nicotine dependence. Highly dependent smokers (Fagerstrom Tolerance Questionnaire Score ≥ 7, or > 25 cigarettes/day) should receive the 4 mg dosage initially. Other patients should begin treatment with the 2 mg dosage strength. Increasing to the 4 mg dose may be considered for patients who fail to stop smoking with the 2 mg dose, or for those whose nicotine withdrawal symptoms remain so strong as to threaten relapse.

Recommended Nicotine Polacrilex Dosing Schedule for Healthy Patients

Nicotine polacrililex	Patient dependency (FTQ)	Number of pieces to be used per day	Maximum pieces per day
4 mg	≥ 7	9 -12	20
2 mg	> 7	9 -12	30

It is important for the patients to learn to chew slowly and to self-titrate the nicotine dose in order to minimize side effects. Chew each piece intermittently for about 30 minutes. The aim of this chewing procedure is to promote slow buccal absorption of the nicotine released from the gum. Chewing too quickly can rapidly release the nicotine which leads to effects similar to oversmoking: Nausea, hiccups or irritation to the throat. Since adverse effects without relieving withdrawal. Proper chewing technique (slow paced chewing and intermittent parking) is designed to minimize swallowed nicotine.

Acidic beverages (eg, coffee, juices, wine, soft drinks) interfere with the buccal absorption before and during chewing of nicotine gum. Therefore, avoid eating and drinking for 15 minutes before and during chewing of nicotine gum.

NICOTINE POLACRILEX (Nicotine resin complex)

Clinical experience suggests that abstinence (quit) rates may be higher when patients chew nicotine gum on a fixed schedule (one piece every 1 to 2 hours) than when allowed to chew it as needed.

Patients using the 2 mg strength should not exceed 30 pieces per day, whereas those using the 4 mg strength should not exceed 20 pieces per day.

When used for smoking cessation, initiate gradual weaning from treatment after 2 to 3 months and complete by 4 to 6 months. Some ex-smokers may need treatment longer to avoid returning to smoking.

Gradual reduction procedures for use in smoking cessation: Initiate gradual withdrawals of treatment to avoid the recurrence of symptoms which may lead to a return to smoking. Suggested procedures for gradually reducing dosage include:

1. Decrease the total number of pieces used per day by ≥ 1 piece every 4 to 7 days.
2. Decrease the chewing time with each piece from the normal 30 minutes to 10 to 15 minutes for 4 to 7 days. Then gradually decrease the total number of pieces used per day.
3. Others may want to chew each piece for > 30 minutes and reduce the number of pieces used per day.
4. Substitute one or more pieces of sugarless gum for an equal number of pieces of nicotine gum. Increase the number of pieces of sugarless gum substituted for nicotine chewing pieces every 4 to 7 days.
5. Replace nocotine gum 4 mg with with 2 mg and apply any of the above suggested procedures.

Withdrawal of treatment may be individualized by modifying or combining the above procedures. Treatment may be stopped when usage has been reduced to one or two pieces per day. The use of nicotine beyond 6 months is not recommended.

Disposal – Place used chewing pieces in a wrapper and dispose of in such a way to prevent its access by children or pets.

Rx sf	**Nicorette** (SK-Beecham)	**Chewing gum**: 2 mg nicotine (as polacrilex) per square	Sorbitol. Beige. In 96s (12 x 8s).
Rx sf	**Nicorette DS** (SK-Beecham)	**Chewing gum**: 4 mg nicotine (as polacrilex) per square.	Sorbitol. Yellow. In 96s (12 x 8s).
Rx	**Nicotrol NS** (McNeil-CPC)	**Spray pump:** 0.5 mg nicotine/actuation	Methylparaben, propylparaben, EDTA. In 10 ml bottles.

LOBELINE

Actions:

Pharmacology: Lobeline, an alkaloid of Lobelia inflata, produces pharmacologic effects similar to, yet weaker than, those produced by nicotine on the peripheral circulation, neuromuscular junctions and the CNS. The majority of controlled studies show that lobeline has only a placebo effect in decreasing the physical craving for cigarettes.

Indications:

A temporary aid to break the cigarette habit. The FDA OTC Advisory Panel has classified it as Category III (ie, safety, but not efficacy, has been established).

Warnings:

Pregnancy: Neither smoking nor lobeline is recommended during pregnancy.

Children: Not intended for use by children.

Precautions:

A single dose of 8 mg can cause epigastric pain, heartburn, belching, nausea, vomiting and faintness. These effects may be lessened by an antacid.

Because of the lack of data, do not use lobeline for longer than 6 weeks.

Adverse Reactions:

GI: Epigastric pain, severe heartburn, nausea and vomiting in higher doses.

Miscellaneous: Coughing; dizziness.

Overdosage:

Symptoms: Sinus arrhythmia; tachycardia; extrasystoles; partial bundle branch block. Profuse diaphoresis, hypotension, muscular twitching, convulsions, paresis, hypothermia and coma may occur. Death has occurred from paralysis of the respiratory center.

Treatment: Empty the stomach. Employ supportive therapy, including ventilatory support, as required. Refer to General Management of Acute Overdosage.

Patient Information:

Do not exceed recommended dosage. Do not use this product longer than 6 weeks.

Notify physician if any of the following occurs: Nausea, vomiting, palpitations, convulsions.

Administration and Dosage:

One tablet after each meal with a half glass of water. Do not use longer than 6 weeks.

otc	**Bantron** (DEP Corp.)	**Tablets:** 2 mg lobeline sulfate alkaloids, 130 mg tribasic calcium phosphate and 130 mg magnesium carbonate	In 18s and 36s.

BUPROPION HCl

Bupropion is also used as an antidepressant. Refer to the Antidepressants section for complete prescribing information.

Actions:

Pharmacology: Bupropion is a non-nicotine aid to smoking cessation. It is a relatively weak inhibitor of the neuronal uptake of norepinephrine, serotonin and dopamine, and does not inhibit monoamine oxidase. The mechanism by which bupropion enhances the ability of patients to abstain from smoking is unknown. However, it is presumed that this action is mediated by noradrenergic or dopaminergic mechanisms.

Pharmacokinetics:

Absorption – Bupropion and its metabolites exhibit linear kinetics following chronic administration. Following oral administration of bupropion to healthy volunteers, mean peak plasma concentrations of 91 and 143 ng/ml were achieved within 3 hours. At steady state, the mean C_{max} was 136 ng/ml following a 150 mg dose every 12 hours.

Food: Food increased the C_{max} by 11%, the extent of absorption (AUC) by 17% and the mean time to peak concentration of bupropion. This effect was of no clinical significance.

Distribution – Bupropion is 84% bound to human plasma proteins in vitro. The extent of protein binding of the hydroxybupropion metabolite is similar to that for bupropion, whereas the extent of protein binding of the threohydrobupropion metabolite is about half that seen with bupropion. The volume of distribution estimated from a single 150 mg dose is 1950 L.

Metabolism – Bupropion is extensively metabolized with a mean elimination half-life of ≈ 21 hours. There are three active metabolites: Hydroxybupropion and the amino-alcohol isomers threohydrobupropion and erythrohydrobupropion. Estimates of the half-lives of the metabolites are 20 hours for hydroxybupropion, 37 hours for threohydrobupropion and 30 hours for erythrohydrobupropion. Steady-state plasma concentrations of bupropion and metabolites are reached within 5 and 8 days, respectively. In mice, hydroxybupropion is comparable in potency with bupropion while the other metabolites are 1/10 to 1/2 as potent. In vitro findings suggest that cytochrome P450 2B6 (CYP2B6) is the principal isoenzyme involved in the formation of hydroxybupropion while cytochrome P450 isoenzymes are not involved in the formation of threohydrobupropion.

Peak plasma concentrations of hydroxybupropion occur ≈ 6 hours after administration and are ≈ 10 times the peak level of the parent drug at steady state. The AUC at steady state is ≈ 17 times that of bupropion. The times to peak concentrations for the erythrohydrobupropion and threohydrobupropion metabolites are similar to that of the hydroxybupropion metabolite, and steady-state AUCs are 1.5 and 7 times that of bupropion, respectively.

Excretion – Following chronic dosing of 150 mg of bupropion every 12 hours for 14 days, the mean apparent clearance at steady state was 160 L/hr. Following oral administration of 200 mg, 87% and 10% of the dose are recovered in the urine and feces, respectively. The fraction of the dose excreted unchanged is only 0.5%.

Bupropion is a racemic mixture. Bupropion follows biphasic pharmacokinetics best described by a two-compartment model; the terminal phase has a mean half-life of ≈ 21 hours while the distribution phase has a mean half-life of 3 to 4 hours.

Hepatic function impairment: The half-life of hydroxybupropion was significantly prolonged in subjects with alcoholic liver disease (32 hours vs 21 hours). The differences in half-life for bupropion and the other metabolites were minimal.

Clinical trials: The efficacy of bupropion as an aid to smoking cessation was demonstrated in two placebo controlled, double-blind trials in nondepressed chronic cigarette smokers (n = 1508, ≥ 15 cigarettes/day). In these studies, bupropion was used in conjunction with individual smoking cessation counseling.

Patients in one study were treated for 7 weeks with one of three doses of bupropion (100, 150 or 300 mg/day) or placebo; quitting was defined as total abstinence during the last 4 weeks of treatment (weeks 4 through 7). A significant dose-dependent increase in the percentage of patients able to achieve 4–week abstinence was demonstrated in the 150 and 300 mg/day treatment groups.

In addition, treatment with bupropion (7 weeks at 300 mg/day) was more effective than placebo in helping patients maintain continuous abstinence through week 26 (6 months) of the study.

In a study, four treatments were evaluated: Bupropion 300 mg/day, nicotine transdermal system (NTS) 21 mg/day, combination of bupropion 300 mg/day plus NTS 21 mg/day, and placebo. Patients were treated for 9 weeks.

Patients treated with either bupropion or NTS achieved greater 4–week abstinence rates than patients treated with placebo. In addition, patients treated with the combination of bupropion and NTS achieved higher abstinence rates than patients treated with either of the individual active treatments alone, although only the comparison with NTS achieved statistical significance.

Treatment with bupropion reduced withdrawal symptoms compared with placebo. Reductions on the following withdrawal symptoms were most pronounced: Irritability; frustration or anger; anxiety; difficulty concentrating; restlessness; depressed mood or negative affect. Depending on the study and the measure used, treatment with bupropion showed evidence of reduction in craving for cigarettes or urge to smoke compared with placebo.

Indications:

Smoking cessation: An aid to smoking cessation treatment.

Contraindications:

Coadministration with a monoamine oxidase (MAO) inhibitor, *Wellbutrin, Wellbutrin SR* or any medications that contain bupropion (see Drug Interactions); current or prior diagnosis of bulimia or anorexia nervosa, seizure disorders (see Warnings); patients who have shown an allergic response to bupropion or other ingredients in the formulation.

Warnings:

Antidepressants: Bupropion is the active ingredient found in *Wellbutrin* and *Wellbutrin SR* used to treat depression. Do not use this product in combination with *Wellbutrin, Wellbutrin SR* or any other medications that contain bupropion.

Anorexia nervosa/bulimia: Do not give with current or prior diagnosis of bulimia or anorexia nervosa because of a higher incidence of seizures noted in patients treated for bulimia with the immediate-release formulation of bupropion.

Seizures: Because the use of bupropion is associated with a dose-dependent risk of seizures, do not prescribe doses > 300 mg/day for smoking cessation. The seizure rate associated with doses of sustained-release bupropion ≤ 300 mg/day is ≈ 0.1%. Data for the immediate-release formulation of bupropion revealed a seizure incidence of ≈ 0.4% in depressed patients treated at doses in a range of 300 to 450 mg/day. In addition, the estimated seizure incidence increases almost 10–fold between 450 and 600 mg/day.

Predisposing factors that may increase the risk of seizure with bupropion use include history of head trauma or prior seizure, CNS tumor and concomitant medications that lower seizure threshold.

Circumstances associated with an increased seizure risk include, among others: Excessive use of alcohol; abrupt withdrawal from alcohol or other sedatives; addiction to opiates, cocaine or stimulants; use of otc stimulants and anorectics; diabetes treated with oral hypoglycemics or insulin.

Reducing the risk of seizures – Retrospective analysis suggests that the risk of seizures may be minimized if the total daily dose of bupropion does not exceed 300 mg (the maximum recommended dose for smoking cessation) and no single dose exceeds 150 mg.

Administer with extreme caution to patients with a history of seizures, cranial trauma or other predisposition(s) toward seizures or patients treated with other agents (eg, antipsychotics, antidepressants, theophylline, systemic steroids) or treatment regimens (eg, abrupt discontinuation of a benzodiazepine) that lower seizure threshold.

Drug abuse and dependence: Bupropion is likely to have a low abuse potential. There have been a few reported cases of drug dependence and withdrawal symptoms associated with the immediate-release formulation of bupropion. In studies of abuse liability, individuals experienced with drugs of abuse reported that bupropion produced a feeling of euphoria and desirability. In these subjects, a single dose of 400 mg (1.33 times the recommended daily dose) of bupropion produced mild, amphetamine-like effects compared with placebo.

Keep in mind that bupropion may induce dependence when evaluating the desirability of including the drug in smoking cessation programs of individual patients.

Hepatotoxicity: An increase in incidence of hepatic hyperplastic nodules, hepatocellular hypertrophy and various histologic changes suggesting mild hepatocellular injury were noted in animals receiving chronic, large doses of bupropion.

Hypersensitivity: Anaphylactoid reactions characterized by symptoms such as pruritus, urticaria, angioedema and dyspnea requiring medical treatment have been reported at a rate of ≈ 1 to 3 per thousand in clinical trials of bupropion. In addition, there have been rare spontaneous postmarketing reports of erythema multiforme, Stevens-Johnson syndrome and anaphylactic shock associated with bupropion.

BUPROPION HCl

Hepatic function impairment: The half-life of hydroxybupropion was significantly prolonged in subjects with alcoholic liver disease (32 hours vs 21 hours). The differences in half0life for bupropion and the other metabolites were minimal.

Carcinogenesis/Mutagenesis: In rats, there was an increase in nodular proliferative lesions of the liver at doses of 100 to 300 mg/kg/day (≈ 3 to 10 times the MRHD on a mg/m^2 basis).

Elderly: Of the ≈ 5600 patients who participated in clinical trials with bupropion sustained-release tablets (depression and smoking cessation studies), the experience with patients ≥ 60 years of age was similar to that in younger patients.

Pregnancy: Category B. There are no adequate and well controlled studies in pregnant women. Use during pregnancy only if clearly needed. Encourage pregnant smokers to attempt cessation using educational and behavioral interventions before pharmacological approaches are used.

Lactation: Bupropion and its metabolites are secreted in breast milk. Because of the potential for serious adverse reactions in breastfeeding infants from bupropion, decide whether to discontinue breastfeeding or discontinue the drug, taking into account the importance of the drug to the mother.

Children: Clinical trials with bupropion did not include individuals < 18 years old. Therefore, the safety and efficacy in the pediatric smoking population have not been established.

Precautions:

Insomnia: In one trial, 29% of patients treated with 150 mg/day and 35% of patients treated with 300 mg/day experienced insomnia vs 21% with placebo. Symptoms were sufficiently severe to require discontinuation of treatment in 0.6% of patients treated with bupropion and none of the placebo patients.

In another trial, 40% of the patients treated with 300 mg/day of bupropion, 28% of the patients treated with 21 mg/day NTS and 45% of the patients treated with the combination of bupropion and NTS experienced insomnia vs 18% with placebo. Symptoms were sufficiently severe to require discontinuation of treatment in 0.8% of patients treated with bupropion and 0% of the patients in the other three treatment groups.

Insomnia may be minimized by avoiding bedtime doses and, if necessary, reduction in dose.

Neuropsychiatric phenomena: The incidence of neuropsychiatric side effects was generally comparable with placebo. Depressed patients treated with bupropion show a variety of neuropsychiatric signs and symptoms including delusions, hallucinations, psychosis, concentration disturbance, paranoia and confusion. In some cases, these symptoms abated upon dose reduction or withdrawal of treatment.

Cardiac effects: Use caution in patients with a recent history of myocardial infarction or unstable heart disease. Bupropion was well-tolerated in depressed patients who had previously developed orthostatic hypotension while receiving tricyclic antidepressants and was generally well tolerated in depressed patients with stable CHF. Bupropion was associated with a rise in supine blood pressure in the study of patients with CHF, resulting in discontinuation of treatment in two patients (5.6%) for exacerbation of baseline hypertension.

In one trial, 6.1% of patients treated with the combination of bupropion and NTS had treatment-emergent hypertension compared with 2.5%, 1.6% and 3.1% of patients treated with bupropion, NTS and placebo, respectively. The majority of these patients had evidence of pre-existing hypertension. Three patients (1.2%) treated with the combination of bupropion and NTS and one patient (0.4%) treated with NTS had study medication discontinued because of hypertension compared with none of the patients treated with bupropion or placebo. Monitor for treatment-emergent hypertension in patients receiving the combination of bupropion and NTS.

Dry mouth: The incidence of dry mouth may be related to the dose of bupropion. Avoid bedtime doses to minimize the occurrence of this adverse event.

Drug Interactions:

In vitro studies indicate that bupropion is primarily metabolized to hydroxybupropion by the CYP2B6 isoenzyme. Therefore, the potential exists for a drug interaction between bupropion and drugs that affect the CYP2B6 isoenzyme metabolism (eg, orphenadrine, cyclophosphamide). The threohydrobupropion metabolite does not appear to be produced by the cytochrome P450 isoenzymes.

Because bupropion is extensively metabolized, the coadministration of other drugs may affect its clinical activity. In particular, certain drugs may induce the metabolism of bupropion (eg, carbamazepine, phenobarbital, phenytoin) while other drugs may inhibit the metabolism of bupropion (eg, cimetidine).

BUPROPION HCl

Physiological changes resulting from smoking cessation itself, with or without treatment with bupropion, may alter the pharmacokinetics of some concomitant medications, which may require dosage adjustment.

Bupropion Drug Interactions			
Precipitant drug	Object drug*		Description
Carbamazepine	Bupropion	⬇	Serum concentrations of bupropion may be decreased.
Levodopa	Bupropion	⬆	A higher incidence of adverse experiences may occur during concurrent administration. Use small initial doses and gradual dose increases of bupropion.
MAO inhibitors	Bupropion	⬆	In animals, the acute toxicity of bupropion is enhanced by the MAO inhibitor phenelzine.
Ritonavir	Bupropion	⬆	Large increases in serum bupropion concentrations may occur, increasing the risk of bupropion toxicity.

* ⬆ = Object drug increased. ⬇ = Object drug decreased.

Drug/Food interactions: Food increased bupropion C_{max} by 11%, extent of absorption (AUC) by 17% and t_{max} by 1 hour, but this was of no clinical significance.

Adverse Reactions:

Adverse Reactions: Bupropion vs NTS vs Placebo (%)				
Adverse reaction	Bupropion 300 mg/day (n = 243)	Nicotine Transdermal System (NTS) 21 mg/day (n = 243)	Bupropion and NTS (n = 244)	Placebo (n = 159)
Body as a whole				
Abdominal pain	3	4	1	1
Accidental injury	2	2	1	1
Chest pain	< 1	1	3	1
Neck pain	2	1	<1	0
Facial edema	< 1	0	1	0
Cardiovascular				
Hypertension	1	< 1	2	0
Palpitations	2	0	1	0
CNS				
Insomnia	40	28	45	18
Dream abnormality	5	18	13	3
Anxiety	8	6	9	6
Disturbed concentration	9	3	9	4
Dizziness	10	2	8	6
Nervousness	4	< 1	2	2
Tremor	1	< 1	2	0
Dysphoria	< 1	1	2	1
Dermatologic				
Application site reaction	11	17	15	7
Rash	4	3	3	2
Pruritus	3	1	5	1
Urticaria	2	0	2	0
GI				
Nausea	9	7	11	4
Dry mouth	10	4	9	4
Constipation	8	4	9	3
Diarrhea	4	4	3	1

BUPROPION HCl

Adverse Reactions: Bupropion vs NTS vs Placebo (%)

Adverse reaction	Bupropion 300 mg/day (n = 243)	Nicotine Transdermal System (NTS) 21 mg/day (n = 243)	Bupropion and NTS (n = 244)	Placebo (n = 159)
GI (Cont.)				
Anorexia	3	1	5	1
Mouth ulcer	2	1	1	1
Thirst	< 1	< 1	2	0
Musculoskeletal				
Myalgia	4	3	5	3
Arthralgia	5	3	3	2
Respiratory				
Rhinitis	12	11	9	8
Increased cough	3	5	< 1	1
Pharyngitis	3	2	3	0
Sinusitis	2	2	2	1
Dyspnea	1	0	2	1
Epistaxis	2	1	1	0
Special senses				
Taste perversion	3	1	3	2
Tinnitus	1	0	< 1	0

Other adverse reactions with both the sustained-release and immediate-release formulations:

Body as a whole: Asthenia, fever, headache (1%); back pain, chills, inguinal hernia, musculoskeletal chest pain, pain, photosensitivity (0.1% to 1%); malaise (rare).

Cardiovascular: Flushing, migraine, postural hypotension, hot flashes, stroke, tachycardia, vasodilation (1%); syncope (rare); cardiovascular disorder; complete AV block; extrasystoles; hypotension; myocardial infarction; phlebitis; pulmonary embolism.

GI: Increased appetite (≥ 1%); dyspepsia, flatulence, vomiting (1%); abnormal liver function, bruxism, dysphagia, gastric reflux, gingivitis, glossitis, jaundice, stomatitis (0.1% to 1%); edema of the tongue (rare); colitis; esophagitis; GI hemorrhage; gum hemorrhage; hepatitis; increased salivation; intestinal perforation; liver damage; pancreatitis; stomach ulcer; stool abnormality.

Hematologic/Lymphatic: Ecchymosis (0.1% to 1%); anemia; leukocytosis; leukopenia; lymphadenopathy and pancytopenia.

Metabolic/Nutritional: Edema, increased weight and peripheral edema (0.1% to 1%); glycosuria.

Musculoskeletal: Leg cramps, twitching (0.1% to 1%); arthritis; muscle rigidity/fever/rhabdomyolysis.

CNS: Somnolence, abnormal thinking, agitation, depression, irritability (≥ 1%); abnormal coordination, CNS stimulation, confusion, decreased libido, decreased memory, depersonalization, emotional lability, hostility, hyperkinesia, hypertonia, hypesthesia, paresthesia, suicidal ideation, vertigo (0.1% to 1%); amnesia, ataxia, derealization, hypomania (rare); abnormal electroencephalogram (EEG); akinesia; aphasia; coma; delirium; delusions; dysarthria; dyskinesia; dystonia; euphoria; extrapyrimidal syndrome; hypokinesia; increased libido; manic reaction; neuralgia; neuropathy; paranoid reaction; unmasking tardive dyskinesia.

Dermatologic: Dry skin, sweating, urticaria (≥ 1%); acne, dry skin (0.1% to 1%); maculopapular rash (rare); angioedema; exfoliative dermatitis; hirsutism.

Special senses: Amblyopia (1%); accommodation abnormality, dry eye (0.1% to 1%); deafness; diplopia; mydriasis.

GU: Urinary frequency (≥ 1%); impotence, polyuria, urinary urgency (0.1% to 1%); abnormal ejaculation; cystitis; dyspareunia; dysuria; gynecomastia; menopause; painful erection; prostate disorder; salpingitis; urinary incontinence; urinary retention; urinary tract disorder; vaginitis.

BUPROPION HCl

Miscellaneous: Bronchitis (≥ 1%); syndrome of inappropriate antidiuretic hormone, allergic reaction, bronchospasm (rare); pneumonia.

Discontinuation of treatment: Adverse events were sufficiently troublesome to cause discontinuation of treatment in 8% of the 706 patients treated with bupropion and 5% of the 313 patients treated with placebo. The more common events leading to discontinuation of treatment with bupropion included nervous system disturbances (3.4%), primarily tremors and skin disorders (2.4%) primarily rashes.

Overdosage:

Symptoms: There has been limited experience with overdosage of the sustained-release formulation of bupropion; three such cases were reported during clinical trials in depressed patients. One patient ingested 3000 mg of bupropion sustained-release tablets and vomited quickly after the overdose; the patient experienced blurred vision and lightheadedness. A second patient ingested a "handful" of bupropion sustained-release tablets and experienced confusion, lethargy, nausea, jitteriness and seizure. A third patient ingested 3600 mg of bupropion sustained-release tablets and a bottle of wine; the patient experienced nausea, visual hallucinations and "grogginess." None of the patients experienced further sequelae.

There has been extensive experience with overdosages of the immediate-release formulation of bupropion. Thirteen overdoses occurred during clinical trials in depressed patients. Twelve patients ingested 850 to 4200 mg and recovered without significant sequelae. Another patient who ingested 9000 mg of the immediate-release formulation of bupropion and 300 mg of tranylcypromine experienced a grand mal seizure and recovered without further sequelae.

Since introduction, overdoses of up to 17,500 mg of the immediate-release formulation of bupropion have been reported. Seizure was reported in ≈ ⅓ of all cases. Other serious reactions reported with the immediate-release formulation of bupropion alone included hallucinations, loss of consciousness and sinus tachycardia. Fever, muscle rigidity, rhabdomyolosis, hypotension, stupor, coma and respiratory failure have been reported when the immediate-release formulation of bupropion was part of multiple drug overdoses.

Although most patients recovered without sequelae, deaths associated with overdoses of the immediate-release formulation of bupropion alone have been reported rarely in patients ingesting massive doses of the drug. Multiple uncontrolled seizures, bradycardia, cardiac failure and cardiac arrest prior to death were reported in these patients.

Treatment: Following suspected overdose, hospitalization is advised. If the patient is conscious, induce vomiting by syrup of ipecac. Activated charcoal also may be administered every 6 hours during the first 12 hours after ingestion. Obtain baseline laboratory values. Monitor ECG and EEG for the next 48 hours. Provide adequate fluid intake.

If the patient is stuporous, comatose or convulsing, airway intubation is recommended prior to undertaking gastric lavage. Although there is little clinical experience with lavage following an overdose of bupropion, it is likely to be of benefit within the first 12 hours after ingestion because absorption of the drug may not yet be complete.

While diuresis, dialysis or hemoperfusion are sometimes used to treat drug overdosage, there is no experience with their use in the management of overdoses of bupropion. Because diffusion of bupropion and its metabolites from tissue to plasma may be slow, dialysis may be of minimal benefit.

Based on studies in animals, it is recommended that seizures be treated with an IV benzodiazepine preparation and other supportive measures, as appropriate. Refer to Management of Acute Overdosage.

Patient Information:

Read all the patient information provided on a separate leaflet for patients. Physicians are advised to review the leaflet with their patients.

Administration and Dosage:

Approved by the FDA on May 14, 1997.

The recommended and maximum dose of bupropion is 300 mg/day, given as 150 mg twice daily. Begin dosing at 150 mg/day given every day for the first 3 days, followed by a dose increase for most patients to the recommended usual dose of 300 mg/day. There should be an interval of ≥ 8 hours between successive doses. Do not give doses > 300 mg/day (see Warnings).

Initiate treatment with bupropion while the patient is still smoking because ≈ 1 week of treatment is required to achieve steady-state blood levels of bupropion. Patients should set a "target quit date" within the first 2 weeks of treatment with bupropion, generally in the second week. Continue treatment for 7 to 12 weeks; base duration of treatment on the relative benefits and risks for individual patients. If a patient has not made significant progress towards abstinence by week 7 of therapy with bupropion, it is unlikely that he or she will quit during that attempt; discontinue treatment. Dose tapering of bupropion is not required when discontinuing treatment. It is important that patients continue to receive counseling and support throughout treatment with bupropion and for a period of time thereafter.

Maintenance: Although clinical data are not available regarding the long-term use (> 12 weeks) of bupropion for smoking cessation, bupropion has been used for longer periods of time in the treatment of depression. Whether to continue treatment with bupropion for periods > 12 weeks for smoking cessation must be determined for individual patients.

Combination treatment: Combination treatment with bupropion and nicotine transdermal system (NTS) may be prescribed for smoking cessation.

Rx	**Zyban** (Glaxo Wellcome)	**Tablets, sustained-release:** 100 mg	(ZYBAN 100). Blue, round, biconvex. Film coated. In 60s.
		150 mg	(ZYBAN 150). Purple, round, biconvex. Film coated. In 60s.

AZATHIOPRINE

Warning:
Chronic immunosuppression with azathioprine increases the risk of neoplasia. Physicians using this drug should be familiar with this risk as well as with the mutagenic potential to both men and women and with possible hematologic toxicities.

Actions:

Pharmacology: Azathioprine, an imidazoyl derivative of 6–mercaptopurine (6–MP), has many biological effects similar to those of the parent compound.

Homograft survival – Although the use of azathioprine for inhibition of renal homograft rejection is well established, the mechanism(s) for this action are obscure. The drug suppresses cell-mediated hypersensitivities and alters antibody production. Suppression of T-cell effects, including ablation of T-cell suppression, depends on the temporal relationship to antigenic stimulus or engraftment. This agent has little effect on established graft rejections or secondary responses.

Alterations in specific immune responses or immunologic functions in transplant recipients are difficult to relate specifically to immunosuppression by azathioprine. These patients have subnormal responses to vaccines, low numbers of T-cells and abnormal phagocytosis by peripheral blood cells, but their mitogenic responses, serum immunoglobulins and secondary antibody responses are usually normal.

Immunoinflammatory response – The severity of adjuvant arthritis is reduced by azathioprine. The mechanisms whereby it affects autoimmune diseases are not known. Azathioprine is immunosuppressive; delayed hypersensitivity and cellular cytotoxicity tests are suppressed to a greater degree than are antibody responses. In the rat model of adjuvant arthritis, azathioprine inhibits the lymph node hyperplasia that precedes the onset of the signs of the disease. Both the immunosuppressive and therapeutic effects in animal models are dose-related. Azathioprine is a slow-acting drug and effects may persist after the drug has been discontinued.

Pharmacokinetics: Azathioprine is well absorbed following oral administration. Maximum serum radioactivity occurs at 1 to 2 hours after oral radioactive azathioprine and decays with a half-life of 5 hours. This is not an estimate of the half-life of azathioprine itself but is the decay rate for all radioactive metabolites of the drug. Because of extensive metabolism, only a fraction of the radioactivity is present as azathioprine. Usual doses produce blood levels of < 1 mcg/ml azathioprine and 6–MP. Blood levels are of little value for therapy since the magnitude and duration of clinical effects correlate with thiopurine nucleotide levels in tissues rather than with plasma drug levels. Azathioprine and 6-MP are 30% bound to serum proteins.

Azathioprine is cleaved in vivo to 6-MP. Both compounds are rapidly eliminated from blood and are oxidized or methylated in erythrocytes and liver; no azathioprine or 6-MP is detectable in urine after 8 hours. Conversion to inactive 6-thiouric acid by xanthine oxidase is an important degradative pathway. Proportions of metabolites are different in individual patients, and this presumably accounts for variable magnitude and duration of drug effects. Renal clearance is probably not important in predicting effectiveness or toxicity, although dose reduction is practiced in patients with poor renal function. Azathioprine and 6-MP are partially dialyzable.

Indications:

Renal homotransplantation: As an adjunct for the prevention of rejection in renal homotransplantation. Experience with > 16,000 transplants shows a 5 year patient survival rate of 35% to 55%, but this is dependent on donor and many other variables.

Rheumatoid arthritis: Indicated only in adult patients meeting criteria for classic or definite rheumatoid arthritis as specified by the American Rheumatism Association. Restrict use to patients with severe, active and erosive disease not responsive to conventional management. Continue rest, physiotherapy and salicylates while azathioprine is given, but it may be possible to reduce the dose of corticosteroids.

Unlabeled uses: Azathioprine has been used in the treatment of chronic ulcerative colitis; however, serious adverse effects may offset its limited value.

Azathioprine 2 to 3 mg/kg/day has been used for the treatment of generalized myasthenia gravis; however, adverse reactions may occur in > 35% of patients.

Azathioprine 2.5 mg/kg/day may be effective in controlling the progression of Behcet's syndrome, especially eye disease, the most serious manifestation.

Although controversial, low-dose azathioprine (75 to 100 mg) may be effective in treating Crohn's disease.

AZATHIOPRINE

Contraindications:

Hypersensitivity to azathioprine; pregnancy in rheumatoid arthritis patients.

Warnings:

Hematologic effects: Severe leukopenia or thrombocytopenia, macrocytic anemia, severe bone marrow depression and selective erythrocyte aplasia may occur in patients on azathioprine. Hematologic toxicities are dose-related, may occur late in the course of therapy and may be more severe in renal transplant patients whose homograft is undergoing rejection. Perform complete blood counts, including platelet counts, weekly during the first month, twice monthly for the second and third months of treatment, then monthly or more frequently if dosage alterations or other therapy changes are necessary. Delayed hematologic suppression may occur. Prompt reduction in dosage or temporary withdrawal of the drug may be necessary if there is a rapid fall in, or persistently low leukocyte count or other evidence of bone marrow depression. Leukopenia does not correlate with therapeutic effect; do not increase the dose intentionally to lower the white blood cell count. Drugs that affect leukocyte production (eg, TMP-SMZ) may lead to exaggerated leukopenia when used concurrently with azathioprine.

Infections: Serious infections are a constant hazard for patients on chronic immunosuppression, especially for homograft recipients. The incidence of infection in renal homotransplantation is 30 to 60 times that in rheumatoid arthritis. Fungal, viral, bacterial and protozoal infections may be fatal and should be treated vigorously. Infection may occur as a secondary manifestation of bone marrow suppression or leukopenia. Consider reduction of azathioprine dosage or use of other drugs.

GI toxicity: A GI hypersensitivity reaction characterized by severe nausea and vomiting has been reported (12% of 676 rheumatoid arthritis patients). These symptoms may also be accompanied by diarrhea, rash, fever, malaise, myalgias, elevations in liver enzymes, and occasionally hypotension. Symptoms of GI toxicity most often develop within the first several weeks of therapy and are reversible upon discontinuation of the drug. The reaction can recur within hours after rechallenge with a single azathioprine dose. The frequency of gastric disturbance can be reduced by administration in divided doses or after meals. Vomiting with abdominal pain may occur rarely with a hypersensitivity pancreatitis. Diarrhea and steatorrhea have been reported (< 1%).

Hepatotoxicity with elevated serum alkaline phosphatase and bilirubin may occur primarily in allograft recipients. This is generally reversible after interruption of azathioprine. Hepatotoxicity has been uncommon in rheumatoid arthritis patients (< 1%). Hepatotoxicity following transplantation most often occurs within 6 months of transplantation and is generally reversible after interruption of azathioprine. A rare, but life-threatening hepatic veno-occlusive disease associated with chronic administration of the drug has occurred in transplant patients and in one patient with panuveitis. Periodically measure serum transaminases, alkaline phosphatase and bilirubin for early detection of hepatotoxicity. If hepatic veno-occlusive disease is suspected, permanently withdraw azathioprine.

Carcinogenesis/Mutagenesis/Fertility impairment: Azathioprine is carcinogenic in animals and may increase the patient's risk of neoplasia. Renal transplant patients have an increased risk of malignancy, predominantly skin cancer and reticulum cell or lymphomatous tumors. The risk of post-transplant lymphomas may be increased in patients who receive aggressive treatment with immunosuppressive drugs. The degree of immunosuppression is determined not only by the immune suppression regimen but also by a number of other patient factors. The number of immunosuppressive agents may not necessarily increase the risk of post-transplant lymphomas. However, transplant patients who receive multiple immunosuppressive agents may be at risk for over-immunosuppression; therefore, maintain immunosuppressive drug therapy at the lowest effective levels. The precise risk of neoplasia due to azathioprine has not been defined, but the risk is lower for rheumatoid arthritis patients than for transplant recipients. However, acute myelogenous leukemia as well as solid tumors have occurred in patients with rheumatoid arthritis receiving azathioprine. Also, rheumatoid arthritis patients previously treated with alkylating agents (eg, cyclophosphamide, chlorambucil, melphalan) may have a prohibitive risk of neoplasia if treated with azathioprine.

Azathioprine is mutagenic in animals and humans.

Temporary depression in spermatogenesis and reduction in sperm viability and sperm count have occurred in mice at doses 10 times the therapeutic human dose. A reduced percentage of fertile matings occurred in animals receiving 5 mg/kg.

AZATHIOPRINE

Pregnancy: Category D. Azathioprine can cause fetal harm when administered to a pregnant woman. Whenever possible, avoid use of this drug in pregnant patients. Do not use for treatment of rheumatoid arthritis in pregnant women.

Limited immunologic and other abnormalities have occurred in a few infants born of renal allograft recipients on azathioprine. In one report, documented lymphopenia, diminished IgG and IgM levels, CMV infection and a decreased thymic shadow were noted in an infant born to a mother receiving 150 mg azathioprine and 30 mg prednisone daily throughout pregnancy. Most of the infants' features had normalized at 10 weeks old. Another case reported pancytopenia and severe immune deficiency in a premature infant whose mother received 125 mg azathioprine daily. One infant was born with preaxial polydactyly; another infant whose father received long-term azathioprine had a large myelomeningocele in the upper lumbar region, bilateral dislocated hips and bilateral talipes equinovarus.

Carefully weigh the benefits vs the risks of azathioprine therapy in women of reproductive potential. There are no adequate and well controlled studies in pregnant women. If this drug is used during pregnancy, or if the patient becomes pregnant while taking it, apprise the patient of the potential hazard to the fetus. Advise women of childbearing age to avoid becoming pregnant.

Lactation: Use in nursing mothers is not recommended. The drug or its metabolites are transferred at low levels, both transplacentally and in breast milk. Because of potential tumorigenicity shown for azathioprine, decide whether to discontinue nursing or drug, taking into account the importance of the drug to the mother.

Children: Safety and efficacy in children have not been established. However, it has been used in children (see Administration and Dosage).

Drug Interactions:

Azathioprine Drug Interactions			
Precipitant drug	Object drug*		Description
ACE inhibitors	Azathioprine	⬆	Concurrent use may induce severe leukopenia.
Allopurinol	Azathioprine	⬆	Allopurinol may increase the pharmacologic and toxic effects of azathioprine.
Methotrexate	Azathioprine	⬆	Plasma levels of the 6-MP metabolite may be increased.
Azathioprine	Anticoagulants	⬇	Azathioprine may decrease the action of the anticoagulants.
Azathioprine	Cyclosporine	⬇	Cyclosporine plasma levels may be decreased.
Azathioprine	Nondepolarizing neuromuscular blockers	⬇	Pharmacologic actions of the neuromuscular blockers may be decreased or reversed.

* ⬆ = Object drug increased. ⬇ = Object drug decreased.

Adverse Reactions:

The principal and potentially serious toxic effects are hematologic and GI (see Warnings). The risks of secondary infection and neoplasia are also important. The frequency and severity of adverse reactions depend on the dose and duration, as well as on the patient's underlying disease or concomitant therapies. The incidence of hematologic toxicities and neoplasia encountered in groups of renal homograft recipients is significantly higher than that in rheumatoid arthritis patients.

Incidence of Hematologic Toxicities and Neoplasia with Azathioprine		
Toxicity	Renal homograft	Rheumatoid arthritis
Leukopenia		
Any degree	> 50%	28%
< $2500/mm^3$	> 16%	5.3%
Infections	> 20%	< 1%
Neoplasia		†[1]
Lymphoma	> 0.5%	
Others	> 2.8%	

[1] 1.8 cases per 1000 patient years of follow-up (one study).

Miscellaneous: Skin rashes (≈ 2%); alopecia, fever, arthralgias, negative nitrogen balance (< 1%).

AZATHIOPRINE

Overdosage:

Very large doses may lead to marrow hypoplasia, bleeding, infection and death. About 30% is bound to serum proteins, but ≈ 45% is removed by 8 hour hemodialysis. A single case of azathioprine overdosage has been reported in a renal transplant patient who ingested a single dose of 7500 mg. The immediate toxic reactions were nausea, vomiting and diarrhea, followed by mild leukopenia and mild abnormalities in liver function. The WBC count, AST and bilirubin returned to normal 6 days after the overdose.

Patient Information:

If GI upset occurs, administer in divided doses or take with food.

Notify physician if any of the following occurs: Unusual bleeding or bruising, fever, sore throat, mouth sores, signs of infection, abdominal pain, pale stools or darkened urine. Inform patients of the necessity of periodic blood counts

May cause nausea, vomiting, skin rash, fever, arthralgias and diarrhea; notify physician if these persist or become bothersome.

Advise patients of the potential risks of therapy during pregnancy and breastfeeding.

Administration and Dosage:

Renal homotransplantation: The dose required to prevent rejection and minimize toxicity varies. Initial dose is usually 3 to 5 mg/kg/day, given as a single daily dose on the day of transplantation, and in a minority of cases, 1 to 3 days before transplantation. It is often initiated IV, with subsequent use of tablets (at the same dose level) after the postoperative period. Reserve IV administration for patients unable to tolerate oral medications. Maintenance levels are 1 to 3 mg/kg/day. Do not increase the dose to toxic levels because of threatened rejection. Discontinuation may be necessary for severe hematologic or other toxicity, even if homograft rejection may be a consequence.

Children – An initial dose of 3 to 5 mg/kg/day IV or orally followed by a maintenance dose of 1 to 3 mg/kg/day has been recommended.

Rheumatoid arthritis: Usually given daily. Initial dose is approximately 1 mg/kg (50 to 100 mg) given as a single dose or twice daily. The dose may be increased, beginning at 6 to 8 weeks and thereafter by steps at 4 week intervals, if there are no serious toxicities and if initial response is unsatisfactory. Use dose increments of 0.5 mg/kg/day, up to a maximum dose of 2.5 mg/kg/day.

Therapeutic response occurs after 6 to 8 weeks of treatment; an adequate trial should be a minimum of 12 weeks. Patients not improved after 12 weeks are refractory. Continue the drug in patients with clinical response, but monitor carefully, and attempt gradual dosage reduction to reduce risk of toxicity. Optimum duration of therapy has not been determined. Use the lowest effective dose for maintenance therapy; lower decrementally with changes of 0.5 mg/kg or approximately 25 mg/day every 4 weeks while other therapy is kept constant. Azathioprine can be discontinued abruptly, but delayed effects are possible.

Renal function impairment: Relatively oliguric patients, especially those with tubular necrosis in the immediate postcadaveric transplant period, may have delayed clearance of azathioprine or its metabolites. They may be particularly sensitive to this drug and may require lower doses.

Use with allopurinol: Reduce dose of azathioprine to approximately 25% to 33% of the usual dose.

Parenteral administration: For IV use only. Add 10 ml Sterile Water for Injection and swirl until a clear solution results; use within 24 hours. Further dilution into sterile saline or dextrose is usually made for infusion. The final volume depends on the infusion time; it is usually 30 to 60 minutes, but ranges from 5 minutes to 8 hours for the daily dose.

Rx	**Imuran** (Glaxo Wellcome)	**Tablets**: 50 mg	(Imuran 50). Yellow to off-white, scored. In 100s and UD 100s.
Rx	**Azathioprine Sodium** (Various, eg, Bedford)	**Injection**: 100 mg (as sodium) per vial	In 20 ml vials.
Rx	**Imuran** (Glaxo Wellcome)		In 20 ml vials.

Warning:
Increased susceptibility to infection and the possible development of lymphoma may result from immunosuppression. Only physicians experienced in immunosuppressive therapy and management of organ transplant patients should prescribe tacrolimus. Manage patients receiving the drug in facilities equipped and staffed with adequate laboratory and supportive medical resources. The physician responsible for maintenance therapy should have complete information necessary for the follow-up of the patient.

Actions:

Pharmacology: Tacrolimus, previously known as FK506, is a macrolide immunosuppressant produced by *Streptomyces tsukubaensis*. Tacrolimus prolongs the survival of the host and transplanted graft in animal transplant models of liver, kidney, heart, bone marrow, small bowel and pancreas, lung and trachea, skin, cornea and limb.

In animals, tacrolimus suppresses some humoral immunity and, to a greater extent, cell-mediated reactions such as allograft rejection, delayed-type hypersensitivity, collagen-induced arthritis, experimental allergic encephalomyelitis, and graft vs host disease.

Tacrolimus inhibits T-lymphocyte activation, although the exact mechanism of action is not known. Evidence suggests that the drug binds to an intracellular protein, FKBP-12. A complex of tacrolimus-FKBP-12, calcium, calmodulin and calcineurin is then formed, and the phosphatase activity of calcineurin inhibited. This effect may prevent the generation of nuclear factor of activated T-cells (NF-AT), a nuclear component thought to initiate gene transcription for the formation of lymphokines (interleukin-2, gamma interferon). The net result is the inhibition of T-lymphocyte activation (ie, immunosuppression).

Pharmacokinetics: Absorption from the GI tract after oral administration is variable. The absorption half-life in 16 liver transplant patients averaged 5.7 hours. Peak concentrations (C_{max}) in blood and plasma were achieved at ≈ 1.5 to 3.5 hours. Mean pharmacokinetic parameters of tacrolimus in whole blood after oral administration were as follows:

Pharmacokinetic Parameters of Tacrolimus in Whole Blood After Oral Administration

Population	Dose (mg/kg/12h)	C_{max} (ng/ml)	T_{max} (hr)	AUC (ng/ml•hr)	Absolute bioavailability
Healthy volunteers (n = 27)	0.07	28.6	1.4	271	14.4
	0.07	36.2	1.3	329	17.4
Liver transplant patients (n = 17)	0.15	68.5	2.3	519	21.8
Food	0.15	27.1	3.2	223	—
Fasting	0.15	52.4	1.5	290	—

The disposition of tacrolimus from whole blood was biphasic with a terminal elimination half-life of 11.7 hours in liver transplant patients and 21.2 hours in healthy volunteers.

Pharmacokinetics of IV Tacrolimus

Population	Dose (mg/kg/12 h)	Volume of distribution (L/kg)	Total body clearance (L/hr/kg)
Healthy volunteers (n = 27)	0.01	0.88	0.042
Liver transplant patients (n = 17)	0.05	0.85	0.053

Absolute bioavailability of the 5 mg capsule was 14.4% and that of five 1 mg capsules was 17.4%. This study failed to establish the bioequivalence of these two formulations.

The presence of food reduces the absorption and bioavailability of tacrolimus. See Drug Interactions.

Tacrolimus is bound to proteins, mainly albumin and alpha-1-acid glycoprotein, and is highly bound toerythrocytes. The protein-binding was 75% and 99% over a range of concentrations of 0.1 to 100 ng/ml. The distribution of tacrolimus between whole blood and plasma depends on several factors such as hematocrit, temperature of separation of plasma, drug concentration and plasma protein concentration. The ratio of whole blood concentration to plasma concentration ranged from 12 to 67 (mean, 35).

Trough concentrations from 10 to 60 ng/ml measured at 10 to 12 hours postdose (C_{min}) correlated well with the area under the plasma or whole blood concentration-time curve (AUC).

Children – Trough concentrations obtained from 30 children (< 12 years old) showed that children need higher doses than adults to achieve similar trough concentrations (see Administration and Dosage).

Tacrolimus is extensively metabolized by the mixed-function oxidase system, primarily cytochrome P-450 (P-450 IIIA). Less than 1% of the dose administered is excreted unchanged in the urine. The major metabolic pathway has not been determined; demethylation and hydroxylation were identified as primary mechanisms in vitro. The major metabolite identified is 13-demethyl tacrolimus. Ten possible metabolites have been identified in human plasma. Two metabolites, a demethylated and a double-demethylated tacrolimus, retain 10% and 7%, respectively, of the inhibitory effect of tacrolimus on T-lymphocyte activation.

Clinical trials: The safety and efficacy of tacrolimus-based immunosuppression following orthotopic liver transplantation were assessed in two prospective, randomized, non-blinded multicenter studies. The active control groups were treated with a cyclosporine-based immunosuppressive regimen (CBIR). Both studies used concomitant adrenal corticosteroids as part of the immunosuppressive regimens. These studies were designed to evaluate whether the two regimens were therapeutically equivalent, with patient and graft survival at 12 months following transplantation as the primary endpoints. The tacrolimus-based immunosuppressive regimen was found to be equivalent to the cyclosporine-based immunosuppressive regimens.

The overall 1-year patient survival (CBIR and tacrolimus-based treatment groups combined) was 78% to 88%. The overall 1-year graft survival (CBIR and tacrolimus-based treatment groups combined) was 73% to 81%. Median time to convert from IV to oral tacrolimus dosing was 2 days.

Indications:

Organ (liver) rejection prophylaxis: Prophylaxis of organ rejection in patients receiving allogeneic liver transplants. It is recommended that tacrolimus be used concomitantly with adrenal corticosteroids. Because of the risk of anaphylaxis, reserve the injection for patients unable to take the capsules orally.

Unlabeled uses: Tacrolimus is being investigated for kidney, bone marrow, cardiac, pancreas, pancreatic island cell and small bowel transplantation. It may be beneficial for the treatment of autoimmune disease and severe recalcitrant psoriasis.

Contraindications:

Hypersensitivity to tacrolimus; hypersensitivity to HCO-60 polyoxyl 60 hydrogenated castor oil (used in vehicle for injection).

Warnings:

Nephrotoxicity: Tacrolimus can cause nephrotoxicity, particularly when used in high doses. Nephrotoxicity has been noted in 33% to 40% of liver transplantation patients receiving the drug. More overt nephrotoxicity is seen early after transplantation, characterized by increasing serum creatinine and a decrease in urine output. Closely monitor patients with impaired renal function; the dosage may need to be reduced. In patients with persistent elevations of serum creatinine who are unresponsive to dosage adjustments, consider changing to another immunosuppressive therapy. Take care in using tacrolimus with other nephrotoxic drugs; in particular, to avoid excess nephrotoxicity, do not use simultaneously with cyclosporine. Discontinue tacrolimus or cyclosporine at least 24 hours prior to initiating the other. In the presence of elevated tacrolimus or cyclosporine concentrations, usually delay further dosing with the other drug. See Drug Interactions.

Hyperkalemia: Mild to severe hyperkalemia has been noted in 10% to 44% of liver transplant recipients treated with tacrolimus, which may require treatment. Monitor serum potassium levels and do not use potassium-sparing diuretics therapy.

Neurotoxicity Neurotoxicity, including tremor, headache and other changes in motor function, mental status and sensory function occurred in ≈ 55% of liver transplant recipients. Tremor and headache have been associated with high whole-blood concentrations of tacrolimus and may respond to dosage adjustment. Seizures have occurred in adult and pediatric patients. Coma and delirium also have been associated with high plasma concentrations of tacrolimus.

TACROLIMUS (FK506)

Lymphomas: As with other immunosuppressants, patients receiving tacrolimus are at increased risk of developing lymphomas and other malignancies, particularly of the skin. The risk appears to be related to the intensity and duration of immunosuppression rather than to the use of any specific agent. A lymphoproliferative disorder (LPD) related to Epstein-Barr Virus (EBV) infection has been reported in immunosuppressed organ transplant recipients. The risk of LPD appears greatest in young children who are at risk for primary EBV infection while immunosuppressed or who are switched to tacrolimus following long-term immunosuppression therapy. Because of the danger of oversuppression of the immune system, which can increase susceptibility to infection, do not administer tacrolimus with other immunosuppressive agents except adrenal corticosteroids. The efficacy and safety of the use of tacrolimus in combination with other immunosuppressive agents has not been determined.

Hypersensitivity: A few patients receiving the injection have experienced anaphylactic reactions. Although the exact cause of these reactions is not known, other drugs with castor oil derivatives in the formulation have been associated with anaphylaxis in a small percentage of patients. Because of this potential risk of anaphylaxis, reserve the injection for patients who are unable to take capsules.

Continuously observe patients receiving the injection for at least the first 30 minutes following the start of the infusion and at frequent intervals thereafter. If signs or symptoms of anaphylaxis occur, stop the infusion. Have an aqueous solution of epinephrine 1:1000 available at the bedside as well as a source of oxygen. Refer to Management of Acute Hypersensitivity Reactions.

Renal/Hepatic function impairment: Use lower doses for patients with renal insufficiency (see Administration and Dosage).

The use of tacrolimus in liver transplant recipients experiencing post-transplant hepatic impairment may be associated with increased risk of developing renal insufficiency related to high whole-blood levels of tacrolimus. Monitor these patients closely and consider dosage adjustments. Use lower doses in these patients (see Administration and Dosage).

Carcinogenesis/Fertility impairment: An increased incidence of malignancy is a recognized complication of immunosuppression in recipients of organ transplants. The most common forms of neoplasms are non-Hodgkin's lymphomas and carcinomas of the skin. As with other immunosuppressive therapies, the risk of malignancies in tacrolimus recipients may be higher than in the healthy population. Lymphoproliferative disorders associated with Epstein-Barr Virus infection have been seen. It has been reported that reduction or discontinuation of immunosuppression may cause the lesions to regress. See also Lymphomas.

Tacrolimus, given orally at 1 mg/kg (0.5 times the recommended human clinical dose) to male and female rats, prior to and during mating, as well as to dams during gestation and lactation, was associated with embryolethality and with adverse effects on female reproduction. Effects on female reproductive function (parturition) and embryolethal effects were indicated by a higher rate of pre-implantation loss and increased numbers of undelivered and nonviable pups. When given at 3.2 mg/kg, tacrolimus was associated with maternal and paternal toxicity as well as reproductive toxicity including marked adverse effects on estrus cycles, parturition, pup viability and pup malformations.

Pregnancy: Category C. In reproduction studies in rats and rabbits, adverse effects on the fetus were observed mainly at dose levels that were toxic to dams. Tacrolimus at oral doses of 0.32 and 1 mg/kg during organogenesis in rabbits was associated with maternal toxicity as well as an increase in incidence of abortions; these doses are equivalent to 0.33 and 1 times the recommended human clinical dose (0.3 mg/kg). At the higher dose only, an increased incidence of malformations and developmental variations was also seen. Tacrolimus, at oral doses of 3.2 mg/kg during organogenesis in rats, was associated with maternal toxicity and caused an increase in late resorptions, decreased numbers of live births, and decreased pup weight and viability. Oral tacrolimus (1 and 3.2 mg/kg) to pregnant rats after organogenesis and during lactation was associated with reduced pup weights.

There are no adequate and well controlled studies in pregnant women. Tacrolimus is transferred across the placenta. The use of tacrolimus during pregnancy has been associated with neonatal hyperkalemia and renal dysfunction. Use during pregnancy only if the potential benefit to the mother justifies potential risk to the fetus.

Lactation: Since tacrolimus is excreted in breast milk, avoid nursing.

Children: Successful liver transplants have been performed in pediatric patients (< 12 years of age) using tacrolimus. Pediatric patients generally require higher doses to maintain blood trough levels of tacrolimus similar to adult patients (see Administration and Dosage).

TACROLIMUS (FK506)

Precautions:

Monitoring: Regularly assess serum creatinine and potassium. Perform routine monitoring of metabolic and hematologic systems as clinically warranted.

Hypertension is a common adverse effect of tacrolimus therapy. Mild or moderate hypertension is more frequently reported than severe hypertension. Antihypertensive therapy may be required; the control of blood pressure can be accomplished with any of the common antihypertensive agents. Since tacrolimus may cause hyperkalemia, avoid potassium-sparing diuretics. While calcium-channel blocking agents can be effective in treating tacrolimus-associated hypertension, take care since interference with tacrolimus metabolism may require a dosage reduction (see Drug Interactions).

Hyperglycemia was associated with the use of tacrolimus in 29% to 47% of liver transplant recipients, and may require treatment.

Drug Interactions:

Tacrolimus Drug Interactions

Precipitant drug	Object drug*		Description
Nephrotoxic agents Aminoglycosides Amphotericin B Cisplatin Cyclosporine	Tacrolimus	↑	Due to the potential for additive or synergistic impairment of renal function, take care when administering tacrolimus with drugs that may be associated with renal dysfunction. Coadministration with cyclosporine resulted in additive/synergistic nephrotoxicity; tacrolimus blood levels may also be increased. Give the first tacrolimus dose no sooner than 24 hours after the last cyclosporine dose.
Antifungals Bromocriptine Calcium channel blockers Cimetidine Clarithromycin Danazol Diltiazem Erythromycin Methylprednisolone Metoclopramide	Tacrolimus	↑	These agents may increase tacrolimus blood levels.
Carbamazepine Phenobarbital Phenytoin Rifamycins	Tacrolimus	↓	These agents may decrease tacrolimus blood levels.
Tacrolimus	Vaccines	↓	Immunosuppressants may affect vaccination. Therefore, during treatment with tacrolimus, vaccination may be less effective. Avoid the use of live vaccines (eg, measles, mumps, rubella, oral polio, BCG, yellow fever, TY 21a typhoid).

* ↑ = Object drug increased. ↓ = Object drug decreased.

Since tacrolimus is metabolized mainly by the cytochrome P-450 IIIA enzyme systems, substances known to inhibit or induce these enzymes may affect the metabolism of tacrolimus with resultant increases or decreases in whole blood or plasma levels. Monitoring of blood levels and appropriate dosage adjustments are essential when such drugs are used concomitantly.

Drug/Food interactions: Tacrolimus was administered in the fasting state or 15 minutes after a breakfast of measured fat content (34% of 400 total calories) to 11 liver transplant patients. The presence of food reduced the absorption of tacrolimus (decrease in AUC and C_{max} and increase in T_{max}). The relative oral bioavailability (whole blood) was reduced by 27% compared to the fasting state.

TACROLIMUS (FK506)

Adverse Reactions:

The principal adverse reactions of tacrolimus are tremor, headache, diarrhea, hypertension, nausea and renal dysfunction. These occur with oral and IV administration and may respond to a reduction in dosing. Diarrhea was sometimes associated with other GI complaints such as nausea and vomiting.

Hyperkalemia, hypomagnesemia and hyperuricemia have occurred. Hyperglycemia has been noted in many patients; some may require insulin therapy. See Warnings and Precautions.

Tacrolimus Adverse Reactions (%)[1]

Adverse reactions	Tacrolimus (n=250)	CBIR[2] (n=250)
CNS		
Headache[3]	31-64	20-60
Tremor[3]	44-56	30-46
Insomnia	29-64	21-68
Paresthesia	15-40	13-30
GI		
Diarrhea	32-72	23-47
Nausea	30-46	22-37
Constipation	19-24	20-27
LFT Abnormal	5-36	2-30
Anorexia	6-34	4-24
Vomiting	12-27	9-15
GU		
Kidney function abnormal	33-40	18-27
Creatinine increased[3]	19-39	16-25
BUN increased[3]	8-30	7-22
Urinary tract infection	16-19	18
Oliguria	16-18	8-15
Hemic/ Lymphatic		
Anemia	4-47	1-38
Leukocytosis	8-32	7-26
Thrombocytopenia	10-24	14-20
Metabolic/Nutritional		
Hyperkalemia[3]	10-45	7-26
Hypokalemia	11-29	14-34
Hyperglycemia[3]	29-47	16-38
Hypomagnesemia	15-48	8-45
Respiratory		
Pleural effusion	30-32	29-32
Atelectasis	5-28	4-30
Dyspnea	3-29	2-23
Skin/Appendages		
Pruritus	11-36	5-20
Rash	8-24	3-19
Miscellaneous		
Abdominal pain	26-59	20-54
Hypertension	31-47	35-56
Pain	19-63	14-57
Fever	15-48	18-56
Asthenia	7-52	4-48
Back pain	13-30	14-29
Ascites	5-27	6-22
Peripheral edema	10-26	11-26

[1] Data are pooled from separate US and European studies and are not necessarily comparable.
[2] CBIR = Cyclosporine-based regimen.
[3] See Precautions or Warnings.

The following adverse events were reported in > 3% of tacrolimus-treated patients.

CNS: Abnormal dreams; agitation; anxiety; confusion; convulsion; depression; dizziness; emotional lability; hallucinations; hypertonia; incoordination; myoclonus nervousness; neuropathy; psychosis; somnolence; thinking abnormal.

TACROLIMUS (FK506)

Special senses: Abnormal vision; amblyopia; tinnitus.

GI: Cholangitis; cholestatic jaundice; dyspepsia; dysphasia; flatulence; GI hemorrhage; GGT increase; GI perforation; hepatitis; ileus; increased appetite; jaundice; liver damage; oral moniliasis.

Cardiovascular: Chest pain; abnormal ECG; hemorrhage; hypotension; tachycardia.

GU: Hematuria; kidney failure.

Metabolic/Nutritional: Acidosis; alkaline phosphatase increased; alkalosis; bilirubinemia; healing abnormal; hyperlipemia; hyperphosphatemia; hyperuricemia; hypocalcemia; hypophosphatemia; hyponatremia; hypoproteinemia; AST increased; ALT increased.

Endocrine: Diabetes mellitus (see Precautions).

Hematologic/Lymphatic: Coagulation disorder; ecchymosis; hypochromic anemia; leukopenia; prothrombin decreased.

Miscellaneous: Abdomen enlarged; abscess; chills; hernia; peritonitis; photosensitivity reaction.

Musculoskeletal: Arthralgia; generalized spasm; leg cramps; myalgia; myasthenia; osteoporosis.

Respiratory: Asthma; bronchitis; cough increased; lung disorder; pulmonary edema; pharyngitis; pneumonia; respiratory disorder; rhinitis; sinusitis; voice alteration.

Dermatologic: Alopecia; herpes simplex; hirsutism; skin disorder; sweating.

Overdosage:

There is minimal experience with overdosage. In patients who have received inadvertent overdosage of tacrolimus, no adverse reactions different from those reported in patients receiving therapeutic doses have been described. Follow general supportive measures and systemic treatment in all cases of overdosage. Refer to General Management of Acute Overdosage.Based on the poor aqueous solubility and extensive erythrocyte and plasma protein binding, it is anticipated that tacrolimus is not dialyzable to any significant extent.

Patient Information:

Inform patients of the need for repeated appropriate lab tests while they are receiving tacrolimus. Give patients complete dosage instructions, advise them of potential risks during pregnancy and inform them of the increased risk of neoplasia.

Administration and Dosage:

Approved by the FDA on April 8, 1994 (1P,E classification).

Injection: For IV infusion only.

In patients unable to take the capsules, therapy may be initiated with the injection. Administer the initial dose no sooner than 6 hours after transplantation. The recommended starting dose is 0.05 to 0.1 mg/kg/day as a continuous IV infusion. Give adult patients doses at the lower end of the dosing range. Concomitant adrenal corticosteroid therapy is recommended early post-transplantation. Continue continuous IV infusion only until the patient can tolerate oral administration.

Preparation for administration – Tacrolimus must be diluted with 0.9% Sodium Chloride Injection or 5% Dextrose Injection to a concentration between 0.004 and 0.02 mg/ml prior to use.

Storage/Stability – Store diluted infusion solution in glass or polyethylene containers and discard after 24 hours. Do not store the diluted infusion solution in a PVC container due to decreased stability and the potential for extraction of phthalates.

Oral: It is recommended that patients be converted from IV to oral therapy as soon as oral therapy can be tolerated. This usually occurs within 2 to 3 days. Give the first dose of oral therapy 8 to 12 hours after discontinuing the IV infusion. The recommended starting oral dose is 0.15 to 0.3 mg/kg/day administered in 2 divided daily doses every 12 hours. Administer the initial dose no sooner than 6 hours after transplantation. Give adult patients doses at the lower end of the dosing range.

Titrate dosing based on clinical assessments of rejection and tolerability. Lower dosages may be sufficient as maintenance therapy. Adjunct therapy with adrenal corticosteroids is recommended early post-transplant.

Children: Pediatric patients without pre-existing renal or hepatic dysfunction have required and tolerated higher doses than adults to achieve similar blood concentrations. Therefore, it is recommended that therapy be initiated in pediatric patients at the high end of the recommended adult IV and oral dosing ranges (0.1 mg/kg/day IV and 0.3 mg/kg/day oral). Dose adjustments may be required.

TACROLIMUS (FK506)

Hepatic/Renal function impairment: Due to the potential for nephrotoxicity, give patients with renal or hepatic impairment doses at the lowest value of the recommended IV and oral dosing ranges. Further reductions in dose below these ranges may be required. Usually delay therapy up to 48 hours or longer in patients with postoperative oliguria.

Conversion from one immunosuppressive regimen to another: Do not use tacrolimus simultaneously with cyclosporine. Discontinue either agent at least 24 hours before initiating the other. In the presence of elevated tacrolimus or cyclosporine concentrations, dosing with the other drug usually should be further delayed.

Blood concentration monitoring: Most study centers have found tacrolimus blood-concentration monitoring helpful in patient management. While no fixed relationship has been established, such blood monitoring may assist in the clinical evaluation of rejection and toxicity, dose adjustments and assessment of compliance.

Various assays have been used to measure blood concentrations of tacrolimus. Comparison of the concentrations in published literature to patient concentrations using current assays must be made with detailed knowledge of the assay methods employed.

US clinical trials show that tacrolimus whole blood concentrations, as measured by ELISA, were most variable during the first week post-transplantation. After this early period, median trough blood concentrations, measured at intervals from the second week to 1 year post-transplantation, ranged from 9.8 to 19.4 ng/ml.

Rx	**Prograf** (Fujisawa)	**Capsules:** 1 mg	Lactose. (1 mg 617). White. In 100s.
		5 mg	Lactose. (5 mg 657). Grayish/red. In 100s.
		Injection: 5 mg/ml	Preservative free. In 1 ml amps.[1]

[1] Contains 200 mg/ml polyoxyl 60 hydrogenated castor oil (HCO-60) and dehydrated alcohol.

MYCOPHENOLATE MOFETIL

Warning:

Increased susceptibility to infection and the possible development of lymphoma may result from immunosuppression. Only physicians experienced in immunosuppressive therapy and management of renal transplant patients should use mycophenolate. Patients receiving the drug should be managed in facilities equipped and staffed with adequate laboratory and supportive medical resources. The physician responsible for maintenance therapy should have complete information requisite for the follow-up of the patient.

Actions:

Pharmacology: Mycophenolate prolongs the survival of allogeneic transplants in animals (kidney, heart, liver, intestine, limb, small bowel, pancreatic islets, and bone marrow). It also reverses ongoing acute rejection in the canine renal and rat cardiac allograft models, and inhibits proliferative arteriopathy in experimental models of aortic and heart allografts in rats, as well as in primate cardiac xenografts. Mycophenolate was used alone or in combination with other immunosuppressive agents in these studies. The drug inhibits immunologically mediated inflammatory responses in animal models, inhibits tumor development and prolongs survival in murine tumor transplant models.

Mycophenolate is rapidly absorbed following oral administration and hydrolyzed to form MPA, which is the active metabolite. MPA is a potent, selective, uncompetitive and reversible inhibitor of inosine monophosphate dehydrogenase (IMPDH), and therefore inhibits the de novo pathway of guanosine nucleotide synthesis without incorporation into DNA. Because T- and B-lymphocytes are critically dependent for their proliferation on de novo synthesis of purines whereas other cell types can utilize salvage pathways, MPA has potent cytostatic effects on lymphocytes. MPA inhibits proliferative responses of T- and B-lymphocytes to both mitogenic and allospecific stimulation. Addition of guanosine or deoxyguanosine reverses the cytostatic effects of MPA on lymphocytes. MPA also suppresses antibody formation by B-lymphocytes. MPA prevents the glycosylation of lymphocyte and monocyte glycoproteins that are involved in intercellular adhesion to endothelial cells and may inhibit recruitment of leukocytes into sites of inflammation and graft rejection.

Pharmacokinetics:

Absorption/Distribution – Following oral administration, mycophenolate undergoes rapid and extensive absorption and complete presystemic metabolism to MPA, the active metabolite. MPA is metabolized to form the phenolic glucuronide of MPA (MPAG), which is not pharmacologically active. Mycophenolate is not measurable systemically in plasma following oral administration. MPA C_{max} was decreased by 40% in the presence of food (see Drug Interactions). In 12 healthy volunteers, the mean absolute bioavailability of oral mycophenolate relative to IV mycophenolate (based on MPA AUC) was 94%. The AUC for MPA appears to increase in a dose-proportional fashion in renal transplant patients receiving multiple doses of mycophenolate up to a daily dose of 3 g.

Immediately post-transplant (< 40 days), mean AUC and C_{max} are ≈ 50% lower in renal transplant patients than that observed in healthy volunteers or in stable renal transplant patients.

The mean apparent volume of distribution of MPA in 12 healthy volunteers is ≈ 3.6 and 4 L/kg following IV and oral administration, respectively. MPA, at clinically relevant concentrations, is 97% bound to plasma albumin. MPAG is 82% bound to plasma albumin at MPAG concentration ranges normally seen in stable renal transplant patients; however, at higher MPAG concentrations (observed in patients with renal impairment or delayed graft function), the binding of MPA may be reduced as a result of competition between MPAG and MPA for protein binding.

Metabolism – In addition to MPA, the following metabolites of the 2-hydroxyethyl-morpholino moiety are also recovered in the urine following oral administration to healthy subjects: N-(2-carboxymethyl)-morpholine, N-(2-hydroxyethyl)-morpholine and the N-oxide of N-(2-hydroxyethyl)-morpholine. Secondary peaks in the plasma MPA concentration-time profile are usually observed 6 to 12 hours post-dose. It appears that enterohepatic recirculation contributes to MPA plasma concentrations.

Excretion – Negligible amount of drug is excreted as MPA (< 1% of dose) in the urine. Oral administration resulted in complete recovery of the administered dose; 93% was recovered in the urine and 6% recovered in feces. Most (about 87%) of the administered dose is excreted in the urine as MPAG. MPA and MPAG are usually not removed by hemodialysis. However, at high MPAG plasma concentrations (> 100 mcg/ml), small amounts of MPAG are removed.

MYCOPHENOLATE MOFETIL

Mean apparent half-life and plasma clearance of MPA are 17.9 hours and 193 ml/min following oral administration and 16.6 hours and 177 ml/min following IV administration, respectively.

Mean Pharmacokinetic Parameters for MPA Following Mycophenolate

Parameter	Dose	T_{max} (hr)	C_{max} (mcg/ml)	AUC (mcg•hr/ml)
Healthy volunteers (n = 129)	1 g	0.8	24.5	63.9 (n = 117)
Renal transplant patients				
Time after renal transplantation				
Early (< 40 days; n = 25)	1 g bid	1.31	8.16	27.3[1]
Early (< 40 days; n = 27)	1.5 g bid	1.21	13.5	38.4[1]
Late (> 3 months; n = 23)	1.5 g bid	0.9	24.1	65.3[1]
Renal impairment (GFR, ml/min/1.73 m²)				
Healthy volunteers (GFR > 80; n = 6)	1 g	0.75	25.3	45[2]
Mild renal impairment (GFR 50 to 80; n = 6)	1 g	0.75	26	59.9[2]
Moderate renal impairment (GFR 25 to 49; n = 6)	1 g	0.75	19	52.9[2]
Severe renal impairment (GFR < 25; n = 7)	1 g	1	16.3	78.6[2]
Hepatic impairment				
Healthy volunteers (n = 6)	1 g	0.63	24.3	29[3]
Alcoholic cirrhosis (n = 18)	1 g	0.85	22.4	29.8[3]

[1] Interdosing interval AUC_{0-12}
[2] Interdosing interval AUC_{0-96}
[3] Interdosing interval AUC_{0-48}

Renal insufficiency: In a single-dose study (6 volunteers per group), plasma MPA AUCs observed in volunteers with severe chronic renal impairment (GFR < 25 ml/min/1.73 m^2) were about 75% higher relative to those observed in healthy volunteers (GFR > 80). In addition, the single-dose plasma MPAG AUC was three- to sixfold higher in volunteers with severe renal impairment than in volunteers with mild renal impairment or healthy volunteers, consistent with the known renal elimination of MPAG.

In patients with delayed graft function post-transplant, mean MPA AUC_{0-12} was comparable to that seen in post-transplant patients without delayed graft function. Mean plasma MPAG AUC_{0-12} was two- to threefold higher than in post-transplant patients without delayed graft function.

Hemodialysis usually does not remove MPA or MPAG. At high concentrations of MPAG (> 100 mcg/ml), hemodialysis removes only small amounts of MPAG.

Pediatrics:

Mean Pharmacokinetic Parameters for MPA Following Multiple Doses of Mycophenolate in Pediatric Renal Transplant Patients

Age range	Dose	T_{max} (hr)	C_{max} (mcg/ml)	AUC_{0-12} (mcg•hr/ml)
≥ 3 mo to < 6 yr (n = 4)	15 mg/kg bid	1.25	3.7	13.6
≥ 6 yr to < 12 yr (n = 4)	15 mg/kg bid	0.5	13.5	23.4
≥ 12 yr to 18 yr (n = 5)	15 mg/kg bid	0.5	13.2	30
≥ 12 yr to 18 yr (n = 7)	23 mg/kg bid	1.14	10.6	28.3

Clinical trials: The safety and efficacy of mycophenolate for the prevention of organ rejection following allogeneic renal transplants were assessed in three randomized, double-blind, multicenter trials. These studies compared two dose levels of mycophenolate (1 and 1.5 g twice daily) with azathioprine (two studies) or placebo (one study) when administered in combination with cyclosporine and corticosteroids to prevent acute rejection episodes. The primary efficacy endpoint was the proportion of patients in each treatment group who experienced treatment failure within the first 6 months after transplantation. Mycophenolate, in combination with corticosteroids and cyclosporine, reduced the incidence of treatment failure within the first 6 months following transplantation.

MYCOPHENOLATE MOFETIL

Incidence of Treatment Failure (%)[1]					
Parameters	Mycophenolate 2 g/day	Mycophenolate 3 g/day	Azathioprine 1 to 2 mg/kg/day	Azathioprine 100 to 150 mg/day	Placebo
All treatment failures	30.3 to 38.2	31.3 to 38.8	47.6	50	56
Early termination without prior acute rejection	9.6 to 13.9	12.7 to 22.5	6	10.2	7.2
Biopsy-proven rejection episode on treatment	17 to 19.8	13.8 to 17.5	38	35.5	46.4

[1] Data from the three studies are pooled.

Cumulative incidence of 12 month graft loss and patient death are as follows: Mycophenolate 2 g/day, 8.5% to 11.7%; mycophenolate 3 g/day, 10% to 11.5%; control (azathioprine or placebo), 11.5% to 13.6%. No advantage of mycophenolate with respect to graft loss and patient death was established. Numerically, patients receiving mycophenolate 2 g/day and 3 g/day experienced a better outcome than controls in all three studies; patients receiving mycophenolate 2 g/day experienced a better outcome than mycophenolate 3 g/day in two of the three studies. Patients in all treatment groups who terminated treatment early were found to have a poor outcome with respect to graft loss and patient death at one year.

Indications:

Organ rejection: For the prophylaxis of organ rejection in patients receiving allogeneic renal transplants. Mycophenolate should be used concomitantly with cyclosporine and corticosteroids.

Contraindications:

Allergic reactions to mycophenolate have been observed; therefore, mycophenolate is contraindicated in patients with a hypersensitivity to the drug, mycophenolic acid or any component of the drug product.

Warnings:

Lymphomas/Malignancies: Patients receiving immunosuppressive regimens involving combinations of drugs, including mycophenolate, as part of an immunosuppressive regimen are at increased risk of developing lymphomas and other malignancies, particularly of the skin. Lymphoproliferative disease or lymphoma developed in ≈ 1% of patients in the controlled studies of prevention of rejection. The risk appears to be related to the intensity and duration of immunosuppression rather than to the use of any specific agent. Oversuppression of the immune system can also increase susceptibility to infection.

Neutropenia: Up to 2% of patients receiving mycophenolate developed severe neutropenia (absolute neutrophil count [ANC] < 0.5 x 10^3/mcl). Monitor patients receiving mycophenolate for neutropenia (see Monitoring in Precautions). The development of neutropenia may be related to mycophenolate itself, concomitant medications, viral infections or some combination of these causes. If neutropenia develops (ANC < 1.3 x 10^3/mcl), interrupt dosing or reduce the dose, perform appropriate diagnostic tests and manage the patient appropriately (see Administration and Dosage). Neutropenia has been observed most frequently in the period from 31 to 180 days post-transplant in patients treated for prevention of rejection.

Renal function impairment: Subjects with severe chronic renal impairment (GFR < 25 ml/min/1.73 m^2) who have received single doses of mycophenolate showed higher plasma MPA and MPAG AUCs relative to subjects with lesser degrees of renal impairment or normal healthy volunteers (see Pharmacokinetics). Avoid mycophenolate doses > 1 g administered twice a day and carefully observe patients.

Pregnancy: Category C. In teratology studies in rats and rabbits, fetal resorptions and malformations occurred in rats at 6 mg/kg/day and in rabbits at 90 mg/kg/day, in the absence of maternal toxicity. These levels are equivalent to 0.03 to 0.92 times the recommended clinical dose. In a female fertility and reproduction study in rats, oral doses of 4.5 mg/kg/day caused malformations (principally of the head and eyes) in the first generation offspring in the absence of maternal toxicity. Adverse effects on fetal development (including malformations) occurred when pregnant rats and rabbits were dosed during organogenesis. These responses occurred at doses lower than those associated with maternal toxicity, and at doses below the recommended clinical dose.

MYCOPHENOLATE MOFETIL

There are no adequate and well controlled studies in pregnant women. Do not use in pregnant women unless the potential benefit justifies the potential risk to the fetus. Women of childbearing potential should have a negative serum or urine pregnancy test within 1 week prior to beginning therapy. It is recommended that mycophenolate therapy should not be initiated until a report of a negative pregnancy test has been obtained.

Effective contraception must be used before beginning mycophenolate therapy, during therapy and for 6 weeks following discontinuation of therapy, even where there has been a history of infertility, unless due to hysterectomy. Two reliable forms of contraception must be used simultaneously unless abstinence is the chosen method. If pregnancy does occur during treatment, the physician and patient should discuss the desirability of continuing the pregnancy.

Lactation: Studies in rats treated with mycophenolate have shown mycophenolic acid to be excreted in milk. It is not known whether this drug is excreted in human milk. Because of the potential for serious adverse reactions in nursing infants from mycophenolate, decide whether to discontinue nursing or to discontinue the drug, taking into account the importance of the drug to the mother.

Children: Safety and efficacy have not been established.

Precautions:

Monitoring: Perform complete blood counts weekly during the first month, twice monthly for the second and third months of treatment, then monthly through the first year.

GI hemorrhage: GI tract hemorrhage has been observed in ≈ 3% of patients treated with mycophenolate. GI tract perforations have rarely been observed. Most patients receiving mycophenolate were also receiving other drugs known to be associated with these complications. Because mycophenolate has been associated with an increased incidence of digestive system adverse events, including infrequent cases of GI tract ulceration, hemorrhage and perforation, administer with caution in patients with active serious digestive system disease.

Delayed graft function: In patients with delayed graft function post-transplant, mean MPA AUC was comparable, but MPAG AUC was two- to threefold higher, compared to that seen in post-transplant patients without delayed graft function. In the three controlled studies of prevention of rejection, 20% of patients had delayed graft function. Although patients with delayed graft function have a higher incidence of certain adverse events (eg, anemia, thrombocytopenia, hyperkalemia) than patients without delayed graft function, these events were not more frequent in patients receiving mycophenolate than azathioprine or placebo. No dose adjustment is recommended for these patients, however, they should be carefully observed.

Drug Interactions:

Drugs that alter the GI flora may interact with mycophenolate by disrupting enterohepatic recirculation. Interference of MPAG hydrolysis may lead to less MPA available for absorption.

Mycophenolate Drug Interactions			
Precipitant drug	Object drug*		Description
Acyclovir Ganciclovir	Mycophenolate	⬆	MPAG and acyclovir plasma AUCs were increased 10.6% and 21.9%, respectively. Because MPAG plasma concentrations are increased in the presence of renal impairment, as are acyclovir and ganciclovir concentrations, the potential exists for the two drugs to compete for tubular secretion further increasing the concentrations of both drugs.
Mycophenolate	Acyclovir		
Antacids	Mycophenolate	⬇	Absorption of a single mycophenolate dose was decreased when coadministered with an aluminum/magnesium hydroxide antacid. The C_{max} and AUC for MPA were 33% and 17% lower, respectively, than when mycophenolate was given alone. It is recommended to avoid simultaneous administration.
Azathioprine	Mycophenolate	⬌	It is recommended to avoid concomitant use due to a lack of clinical studies.
Cholestyramine	Mycophenolate	⬇	Following coadministration, MPA AUC decreased ≈ 40%. Mycophenolate should not be given with cholestyramine or other agents that may interfere with enterohepatic recirculation.

MYCOPHENOLATE MOFETIL

Mycophenolate Drug Interactions			
Precipitant drug	Object drug*		Description
Probenecid	Mycophenolate	↑	In animals, coadministration resulted in a threefold increase in plasma MPAG AUC and a twofold increase in plasma MPA AUC.
Salicylates	Mycophenolate	↑	Coadministration increased the free fraction of MPA.
Mycophenolate	Phenytoin	↓	MPA decreased the binding of phenytoin from 90% to 87%.
Mycophenolate	Theophylline	↓	MPA decreased the binding of theophylline from 53% to 45%.

* ↑ = Object drug increased. ↓ = Object drug decreased. ↔ = Undetermined effect.

Drug/Food interactions: Food (27 g fat, 650 calories) had no effect on the extent of absorption (MPA AUC) of mycophenolate when administered at doses of 1.5 g twice daily to renal transplant patients. However, MPA C_{max} was decreased by 40% in the presence of food.

Adverse Reactions:

The principal adverse reactions associated with mycophenolate include diarrhea, leukopenia, sepsis and vomiting, and there is evidence of a higher frequency of certain types of infections.

Mycophenolate Adverse Reactions (> 10%)[1]				
Adverse reaction	Mycophenolate 2 g/day	Mycophenolate 3 g/day	Azathioprine 1 to 2 mg/kg/day or 100 to 150 mg/day	Placebo
Body as a whole				
Pain	33	31.2	32.2	—
Abdominal pain	12.1-24.7	11.9-27.6	23	11.4
Fever	21.4	23.3	23.3	—
Headache	21.1	16.1	21.2	—
Infection	12.7-18.2	15.6-20.9	19.9	13.3
Sepsis	17.6-21.8	17.5-19.7	15.6	13.9
Asthenia	13.7	16.1	19.9	—
Chest pain	13.4	13.3	14.7	—
Back pain	11.6	12.1	14.1	—
Hypertension	17.6-32.4	16.9-28.2	32.2	19.3
Hemic/Lymphatic				
Anemia	25.6	25.8	23.6	—
Leukopenia	11.5-23.2	16.3-34.5	24.8	4.2
Thrombocytopenia	10.1	8.2	13.2	—
Hypochromic anemia	7.4	11.5	9.2	—
Leukocytosis	7.1	10.9	7.4	—
GU				
Urinary tract infection	37.2-45.5	37-44.4	33.7	37.3
Hematuria	14	12.1	11.3	—
Kidney tubular necrosis	6.3	10	5.8	—
Urinary tract disorder	6.7	10.6	—	4.2
Metabolic/Nutritional				
Peripheral edema	28.6	27	28.2	—
Hypercholesteremia	12.8	8.5	11.3	—
Hypophosphatemia	12.5	15.8	11.7	—
Edema	12.2	11.8	13.5	—
Hypokalemia	10.1	10	8.3	—
Hyperkalemia	8.9	10.3	16.9	—
Hyperglycemia	8.6	12.4	15	—

MYCOPHENOLATE MOFETIL

Mycophenolate Adverse Reactions (> 10%)[1]				
Adverse reaction	Mycophenolate 2 g/day	Mycophenolate 3 g/day	Azathioprine 1 to 2 mg/kg/day or 100 to 150 mg/day	Placebo
GI				
Diarrhea	16.4-31	18.8-36.1	20.9	13.9
Constipation	22.9	18.5	22.4	—
Nausea	19.9	23.6	24.5	—
Dyspepsia	17.6	13.6	13.8	—
Vomiting	12.5	13.6	9.2	—
Nausea and vomiting	10.4	9.7	10.7	—
Oral moniliasis	10.1	12.1	11.3	—
Respiratory				
Infection	15.8-22	13.1-23.9	19.6	9
Dyspnea	15.5	17.3	16.6	—
Cough increased	15.5	13.3	15	—
Pharyngitis	9.5	11.2	8	—
Bronchitis	8.5	11.9	—	8.4
Pneumonia	3.6	10.6	—	10.8
Dermatologic				
Acne	10.1	9.7	6.4	—
Rash	7.7	6.4	10.4	—
CNS				
Tremor	11	11.8	12.3	—
Insomnia	8.9	11.8	10.4	—
Dizziness	5.7	11.2	11	—

[1] Data pooled from three separate studies.

Patients receiving mycophenolate 2 g/day had an overall better safety profile than did patients receiving 3 g/day. Sepsis, which was generally CMV viremia, was slightly more common in patients treated with mycophenolate; diarrhea was most clearly increased in patients receiving mycophenolate. Up to 2% of patients have developed severe neutropenia (see Warnings).

The incidence of malignancies among the 1483 patients enrolled in controlled trials for the prevention of rejection who were followed for ≥ 1 year was similar to the incidence reported in the literature for renal allograft recipients. There was a slight increase in the incidence of lymphoproliferative disease in the mycophenolate treatment groups compared to the placebo and azathioprine groups (see Warnings).

Malignancies Observed with Mycophenolate in Prevention of Renal Rejection Trials (%)				
Malignancy	Mycophenolate 2 g/day (n = 501)	Mycophenolate 3 g/day (n = 490)	Placebo (n = 166)	Azathioprine 1 to 2 mg/kg/day or 100 to 150 mg/day (n = 326)
Lymphoma/Lymphoproliferative disease	0.6	1	0	0.3
Nonmelanoma skin carcinoma	4	1.6	0	2.4
Other malignancy	0.8	1.4	1.8	1.8

Opportunistic Infections in Prevention of Renal Rejection with Mycophenolate (%)[1]				
Infection	Mycophenolate 2 g/day	Mycophenolate 3 g/day	Azathioprine 1 to 2 mg/kg/day or 100 to 150 mg/day	Placebo
Herpes simplex	15.2-16.7	12.5-20	19	6
CMV				
Viremia/Syndrome	13.4-15.2	12.4-15	13.8	13.3
Tissue invasive disease	3.6-8.3	7.5-11.5	6.1	2.4
Herpes zoster	6-6.7	6.9-7.6	5.8	2.4
Candida				
Fungemia/disseminated	0.6	0.6	0.3	0
Tissue invasive	0.6	0.6	0.3	0
Aspergillus/Mucor invasive disease	0.3	0.9	0.3	
Pneumocystis carinii	0.3	0	1.2	2.4

[1] Data pooled from three separate studies.

In the three controlled studies for prevention of rejection, similar rates of fatal infections/sepsis (< 2%) occurred in patients while receiving mycophenolate or control therapy in combination with other immunosuppressive agents (see Warnings).

Other adverse reactions are as follows:

GU: Albuminuria, dysuria, hydronephrosis, impotence, pain, pyelonephritis, urinary frequency, urinary tract disorder (≥ 3%).

Cardiovascular: Angina pectoris, atrial fibrillation, cardiovascular disorder, hypotension, palpitation, peripheral vascular disorder, postural hypotension, tachycardia, thrombosis, vasodilatation (≥ 3%).

GI: Anorexia, esophagitis, flatulence, gastritis, gastroenteritis, GI hemorrhage, GI moniliasis, gingivitis, gum hyperplasia, hepatitis, ileus, infection, mouth ulceration, rectal disorder. (≥ 3%)

Respiratory: Asthma, lung disorder, lung edema, pleural effusion, rhinitis, sinusitis (≥ 3%).

Dermatologic: Alopecia, fungal dermatitis, hirsutism, pruritus, benign skin neoplasm, skin disorder, skin hypertrophy, skin ulcer, sweating (≥ 3%).

CNS: Anxiety, depression, hypertonia, paresthesia, somnolence (≥ 3%).

Endocrine: Diabetes mellitus, parathyroid disorder (≥ 3%).

Musculoskeletal: Arthralgia, joint disorder, leg cramps, myalgia, myasthenia (≥ 3%).

Special senses: Amblyopia, cataract, conjunctivitis (≥ 3%).

Miscellaneous: Abdomen enlarged, accidental injury, chills and fever, cyst, face edema, flu syndrome, hemorrhage, hernia, malaise, pelvic pain, ecchymosis, polycythemia (≥ 3%).

Lab test abnormalities: Increased alkaline phosphatase, creatinine, gamma glutamyl transpeptidase, lactic dehydrogenase, AST and ALT, hypercalcemia, hyperlipemia, hyperuricemia, hypervolemia, hypocalcemia, hypoglycemia, hypoproteinemia, weight gain, dehydration, acidosis (≥ 3%).

Overdosage:

The highest dose administered to renal transplant patients has been 4 g/day. In limited experience with cardiac and hepatic transplant patients, the highest doses used were 4 or 5 g/day. At doses of 4 or 5 g/day, there appears to be a higher rate, compared to the use of ≤ 3 g/day, of GI intolerance (nausea, vomiting or diarrhea), and occasional hematologic abnormalities, principally neutropenia, leading to a need to reduce or discontinue dosing.

MPA and MPAG are usually not removed by hemodialysis. However, at high MPAG plasma concentrations (>100 mcg/ml), small amounts of MPAG are removed. By increasing excretion of the drug, MPA can be removed by bile acid sequestrants, such as cholestyramine.

Patient Information:

Inform patients of the need for repeated appropriate laboratory tests while they are receiving mycophenolate.

Give patients complete dosage instructions and inform them of the increased risk of lymphoproliferative disease and certain other malignancies.

MYCOPHENOLATE MOFETIL

Inform women of childbearing potential of the potential risks during pregnancy, and instruct them to use effective contraception before beginning mycophenolate therapy, during therapy and for 6 weeks after mycophenolate has been stopped (see Pregnancy).

Administration and Dosage:

Approved by the FDA on May 9, 1995.

Give the initial dose of mycophenolate within 72 hours following transplantation. A dose of 1 g administered twice a day (daily dose of 2 g) is recommended for use in combination with corticosteroids and cyclosporine in renal transplant patients. Although a dose of 1.5 g administered twice daily (daily dose of 3 g) was used in clinical trials and was shown to be safe and effective, no efficacy advantage could be established. Patients receiving 2 g/day demonstrated an overall better safety profile than did patients receiving 3 g/day. Food had no effect on MPA AUC, but decreased MPA C_{max} by 40%. It is recommended that mycophenolate be administered on an empty stomach.

Dosage adjustments: In patients with severe chronic renal impairment (GFR < 25 ml/min/1.73 m^2) outside of the immediate post-transplant period, avoid doses > 1 g administered twice a day; carefully observe these patients. No dose adjustments are needed in patients experiencing delayed graft function post-operatively.

If neutropenia develops (ANC < 1.3 x 10^3/mcl), interrupt dosing or reduce the dose, perform appropriate diagnostic tests and appropriately manage the patient (see Warnings and Precautions).

Handling/Disposal: Because mycophenolate has demonstrated teratogenic effects in rats and rabbits, do not open or crush the capsules. Avoid inhalation or direct contact with skin or mucous membranes of the powder contained in mycophenolate capsules. If such contact occurs, wash thoroughly with soap and water; rinse eyes with plain water.

Rx	**CellCept** (Roche)	**Capsules:** 250 mg mycophenolate mofetil	(CellCept 250 Roche). Blue/brown. In 100s, 500s and UD 100s.

CYCLOSPORINE (Cyclosporin A)

Warning:

Only physicians experienced in immunosuppressive therapy and managing organ transplant patients should prescribe cyclosporine. Manage patients in facilities equipped and staffed with adequate lab and supportive medical resources. The physician responsible for maintenance therapy should have complete information requisite for the follow-up of the patient.

Administer *Sandimmune* with adrenal corticosteroids but not with other immunosuppressants. Increased susceptibility to infection and the possible development of lymphoma may result from immunosuppression. Cyclosporine for microemulsion (*Neoral*) may be given with other immunosuppressants.

Sandimmune capsules and oral solution have decreased bioavailability compared to *Neoral*. *Sandimmune* and *Neoral* are not bioequivalent and cannot be used interchangeably without physician supervision.

Cyclosporine absorption during chronic *Sandimmune* use is erratic. Monitor blood levels at repeated intervals and make dose adjustments to avoid toxicity (high levels) or possible organ rejection (low absorption). This is of special importance in liver transplants (see Warnings). For a given trough concentration, cyclosporine exposure will be greater with *Neoral* than with *Sandimmune*. If a patient who is receiving exceptionally high doses of *Sandimmune* is converted to *Neoral*, use particular caution. Comparison of blood concentrations in the published literature with blood concentrations obtained using current assays must be done with detailed knowledge of the assay methods used. Numerous assays are being developed to measure blood levels of cyclosporine. Comparison of levels in published literature to patient levels using current assays must be done with detailed knowledge of the assay methods used. (See Precautions.)

Actions:

Pharmacology: Cyclosporine is a cyclic polypeptide immunosuppressant consisting of 11 amino acids. It is produced as a metabolite by the fungus species *Tolypocladium inflatum Gams* (*Sandimmune*) or *Beauveria nivea* (*Neoral*). It is a potent immunosuppressant which prolongs survival of allogeneic transplants involving skin, heart, kidneys, pancreas, bone marrow, small intestine, liver and lungs in animals. Cyclosporine suppresses some humoral immunity and, to a greater extent, cell-mediated immune reactions such as allograft rejection, delayed hypersensitivity, experimental allergic encephalomyelitis, Freund's adjuvant arthritis and graft vs host disease in many animal species for a variety of organs.

The exact mechanism of action is unknown. Experimental evidence suggests it is due to specific, reversible inhibition of immunocompetent lymphocytes in the G_0- or G_1-phase of the cell cycle. T–lymphocytes are preferentially inhibited. The T–helper cell is the main target, but the T–suppressor cell may also be suppressed. Cyclosporine inhibits lymphokine production and release including interleukin–2 or T–cell growth factor (TCGF). It does not cause bone marrow suppression.

Pharmacokinetics:

Absorption – The absorption from the GI tract is incomplete and variable. The extent of absorption is dependent on the individual patient, patient population and the formulation. Peak concentrations (C_{max}) in blood and plasma are achieved at about 3.5 hours. C_{max} and area under the plasma or blood concentration-time curve (AUC) increase with administered dose; for blood, the relationship is curvilinear (parabolic) between 0 and 1400 mg. As determined by a specific assay, C_{max} is ≈ 1 ng/ml/mg of dose for plasma and 2.7 to 1.4 ng/ml/mg of dose for blood (for low to high doses). Compared to an IV infusion, the absolute bioavailability of *Sandimmune* oral solution is ≈ 30% based on results in two patients. The bioavailability of *Sandimmune* capsules is equivalent to the oral solution.

The relationship between administered dose and exposure AUC is linear within the therapeutic dose range. The intersubject variability of cyclosporine exposure (AUC) when *Neoral* or *Sandimmune* is administered ranges from ≈ 20% to 50% in renal transplant patients. This intersubject variability contributes to the need for individualization of the dosing regimen for optimal therapy. Intrasubject variability of AUC in renal transplant recipients was 9% to 21% for *Neoral* and 19% to 26% for *Sandimmune*. In the same studies, intrasubject variability of trough concentrations was 17% to 30% for *Neoral* and 16% to 38% for *Sandimmune*.

Neoral has increased bioavailability compared to *Sandimmune*. The absolute bioavailability of cyclosporine administered as *Sandimmune* is dependent on the patient population, estimated to be < 10% in liver transplant patients and as great as 89% in renal patients. The increased bioavailability of *Neoral* relative to *Sandimmune* varies across patient populations; however, the absolute bioavailability of *Neoral* has yet to be determined in adults. In crossover studies where stable renal transplant patients received both *Neoral* and *Sandimmune*, the mean relative AUC of *Neoral* to *Sandimmune* ranged from 1.24 to 1.51. The dose normalized AUC in renal transplant patients taking *Neoral* 28 days after transplantation was 50% greater than in those patients administered *Sandimmune*. The increase in AUC is accompanied by an increase in peak blood cyclosporine concentration in the range of 40% to 106% in renal transplant patients and ≈ 90% in liver transplant patients. AUC and C_{max} are also increased (*Neoral* to *Sandimmune*) in heart transplant patients, but data are very limited. Although the AUC and C_{max} values are higher with *Neoral* relative to *Sandimmune*, the pre-dose trough concentrations (dose-normalized) are similar for the 2 formulations.

Absolute bioavailability of cyclosporine oral solution or capsules shows wide patient variability. Factors which may affect bioavailability include: 1) Food that may delay and impair absorption, 2) enterohepatic recirculation, 3) radioimmunoassay (RIA) vs high pressure liquid chromatography (HPLC) assay (RIA cross-reacts with metabolites), 4) whole blood vs plasma specimen.

Following oral administration of *Neoral*, the time to peak blood cyclosporine concentrations (T_{max}) ranged from 1.5 to 2 hours in renal transplant patients. The administration of food decreases the AUC and C_{max} of cyclosporine (see Drug Interactions).

Distribution – Largely outside the blood volume; ≈ 33% to 47% is in plasma, 4% to 9% in lymphocytes, 5% to 12% in granulocytes and 41% to 58% in erythrocytes. At high concentrations, the binding capacity of leukocytes and erythrocytes becomes saturated. In plasma, ≈ 90% is bound to proteins, primarily lipoproteins. The steady state volume of distribution during IV dosing has been reported as 3 to 5 L/kg in solid organ transplant recipients. In blood, the distribution is concentration dependent.

Blood level monitoring is useful in patient management (see Precautions).

Metabolism – Cyclosporine is extensively metabolized to at least 25 metabolites. The disposition of cyclosporine from blood is biphasic with a terminal half-life of ≈19 hours (*Sandimmune*; range, 10 to 27 hours) or 8.4 hours (*Neoral*; range, 5 to 18 hours). Following IV administration, cyclosporine blood clearance (assay: HPLC) is ≈ 5 to 7 ml/min/kg in adult renal allograft recipients. Blood cyclosporine clearance appears to be slightly slower in cardiac transplant patients.

Cyclosporine is extensively metabolized by the cytochrome P450 III-A enzyme system in the liver and, to a lesser degree, in the GI tract and the kidney. At least 25 metabolites have been identified from human bile, feces, blood and urine. The biological activity of the metabolites and their contributions to toxicity are considerably less than those of the parent compound. At steady state following the oral administration of *Sandimmune*, the mean AUCs for blood concentrations of the major metabolites M1, M9 and M4N are about 70%, 21% and 7.5% of the AUC for blood cyclosporine concentrations, respectively. Based on blood concentration data from stable renal transplant patients and bile concentration data from de novo liver transplant patients, the percentage of dose present as M1, M9 and M4N metabolites is similar when either *Neoral* or *Sandimmune* is administered.

Excretion – Only 0.1% of a dose is excreted unchanged in the urine. Excretion is primarily biliary with only 6% of the dose (parent drug and metabolites) excreted in urine. Neither dialysis nor renal failure alter cyclosporine clearance significantly.

Children: Children often need a larger oral dose of cyclosporine than adults. This may be due to the limited absorptive surface area of their intestines. The IV dose is not significantly related to age, weight, height or bowel length.

Indications:

Immunosuppression: Prophylaxis of organ rejection in kidney, liver and heart allogeneic transplants. *Sandimmune* is always to be taken in conjunction with adrenal corticosteroids; *Neoral* has been used in combination with azathioprine and corticosteroids. *Sandimmune* may also be used to treat chronic rejection in patients previously treated with other immunosuppressants. Because of the risk of anaphylaxis, reserve the injection for patients unable to take the capsule or oral solution.

Unlabeled uses: Cyclosporine has had limited, but successful use in other procedures including pancreas, bone marrow and heart/lung transplantation.

The following conditions have been treated with cyclosporine (oral dosages have ranged from 1 to 10 mg/kg/day): Alopecia areata; aplastic anemia; atopic dermatitis; Behcet's disease; biliary cirrhosis; corneal transplantation or other diseases of the eye which have an autoimmune component (compounded into ophthalmic drops; see Administration and Dosage. Cyclosporine currently has orphan drug status for ophthalmic use; see Orphan Drug section); Crohn's disease; dermatomyositis; Graves' ophthalmopathy; insulin-dependent diabetes mellitus (see Glucose Metabolism in Warnings); lichen planus (topical preparation); lupus nephritis; multiple sclerosis; myasthenia gravis; nephrotic syndrome; pemphigus and pemphigoid; polymyositis; psoriatic arthritis; pulmonary sarcoidosis; pyoderma gangrenosum; rheumatoid arthritis; severe psoriasis; ulcerative colitis; uveitis.

CYCLOSPORINE (Cyclosporin A)

Contraindications:

Hypersensitivity to polyoxyethylated castor oil (injection only; see Warnings), cyclosporine or any component of the products.

Warnings:

Elevated BUN and serum creatinine: It is not unusual for serum creatinine and BUN levels to be elevated during therapy. These elevations in renal transplant patients do not necessarily indicate rejection and each patient must be fully evaluated before dosage adjustment is initiated.

Nephrotoxicity: Based on *Sandimmune* oral solution experience, nephrotoxicity has been noted in 25%, 38% and 37% of renal, cardiac and liver transplantation cases, respectively, especially with high doses. Mild nephrotoxicity was generally noted 2 to 3 months after transplant and consisted of an arrest in the fall of preoperative elevations of BUN and creatinine at a range of 35 to 45 mg/dl and 2 to 2.5 mg/dl, respectively. These elevations were often responsive to dosage reduction.

More overt nephrotoxicity was seen early after transplantation and was characterized by a rapidly rising BUN and creatinine. Since these events are similar to rejection episodes, care must be taken to differentiate between them. This form of nephrotoxicity is usually responsive to *Sandimmune* dosage reduction. In one study, the use of transdermal clonidine before and after surgery decreased the frequency of nephrotoxicity.

Although specific diagnostic criteria which reliably differentiate renal graft rejection from drug toxicity have not been found, a number of parameters have been significantly associated to one or the other. It should be noted, however, that up to 20% of patients may have simultaneous nephrotoxicity and rejection.

A form of chronic progressive cyclosporine-associated nephrotoxicity is characterized by serial deterioration in renal function and morphologic changes in the kidneys. From 5% to 15% of transplant recipients will fail to show a reduction in a rising serum creatinine despite a decrease or discontinuation of cyclosporine therapy. Renal biopsies from these patients will demonstrate an interstitial fibrosis with tubular atrophy. In addition, toxic tubulopathy, peritubular capillary congestion, arteriolopathy and a striped form of interstitial fibrosis with tubular atrophy may be present. Though none of these morphologic changes is entirely specific, a histologic diagnosis of chronic progressive cyclosporine-associated nephrotoxicity requires evidence of these.

When considering the development of chronic nephrotoxicity, it is noteworthy that several authors have reported an association between the appearance of interstitial fibrosis and higher cumulative doses or persistently high circulating trough levels of cyclosporine. This is particularly true during the first 6 post-transplant months when the dosage tends to be highest and when, in kidney recipients, the organ appears to be most vulnerable to the toxic effects of cyclosporine. Among other contributing factors to the development of interstitial fibrosis in these patients are prolonged perfusion time, warm ischemia time, as well as episodes of acute toxicity, and acute and chronic rejection. The reversibility of interstitial fibrosis and its correlation to renal function have not yet been determined. Reversibility of arteriopathy has been reported after stopping cyclosporine or lowering the dosage.

Diagnostic Criteria Differentiating Nephrotoxicity From Rejection

Parameter	Nephrotoxicity	Rejection
History	• Donor > 50 years old or hypotensive, • Prolonged kidney preservation, • Prolonged anastomosis time, • Concomitant nephrotoxic drugs	• Antidonor immune response, • Retransplant patient
Clinical	• Often > 6 weeks postop, • Prolonged initial nonfunction (acute tubular necrosis)	• Fever > 37.5° C, • Decrease in daily urine volume > 500 ml (or 50%), • Graft swelling and tenderness, • Weight gain > 0.5 kg
Laboratory	• CyA serum trough level > 200 ng/ml, • Gradual rise in Cr (< 0.15 mg/dl/day), • Cr plateau < 25% above baseline, • BUN/Cr ≥ 20	• CyA serum trough level < 150 ng/ml, • Rapid rise in Cr (> 0.3 mg/dl/day), • Cr > 25% above baseline, • BUN/Cr < 20

CYCLOSPORINE (Cyclosporin A)

Diagnostic Criteria Differentiating Nephrotoxicity From Rejection

Parameter	Nephrotoxicity	Rejection
Biopsy	• Arteriolopathy (medial hypertrophy, hyalinosis, nodular deposits, intimal thickening, endothelial vacuolization, progressive scarring), • Tubular atrophy, isometric vacuolization, isolated calcifications, • Minimal edema, • Mild focal infiltrates, • Diffuse interstitial fibrosis, often striped form	• Endovasculitis (proliferation, intimal arteritis, necrosis, sclerosis), • Tubulitis with RBC and WBC casts, some irregular vacuolization, • Interstitial edema and hemorrhage, • Diffuse moderate to severe mononuclear infiltrates, • Glomerulitis (mononuclear cells)
Aspiration cytology	• CyA deposits in tubular and endothelial cells, • Fine isometric vacuolization of tubular cells	• Inflammatory infiltrate with mononuclear phagocytes, macrophages, lymphoblastoid cells and activated T-cells, • These strongly express HLA-DR antigens
Urine cytology	• Tubular cells with vacuolization and granularization	• Degenerative tubular cells, plasma cells and lymphocyturia > 20% of sediment
Manometry	• Intracapsular pressure < 40 mm Hg	• Intracapsular pressure > 40 mm Hg
Ultrasonography	• Unchanged graft cross sectional area	• Increase in graft cross sectional area, • AP diameter ≥ transverse diameter
Magnetic resonance imagery	• Normal appearance	• Loss of distinct corticomedullary junction, swelling image intensity of parachyma approaching that of psoas, loss of hilar fat
Radionuclide scan	• Normal or generally decreased perfusion, • Decrease in tubular function, • (^{131}I-hippuran) > decrease in perfusion (^{99m}Tc DTPA)	• Patchy arterial flow, • Decrease in perfusion > decrease in tubular function, • Increased uptake of indium 111 labeled platelets or Tc-99m in colloid
Therapy	• Responds to decreased cyclosporine	• Responds to increased steroids or antilymphocyte globulin

Hepatotoxicity has been noted in 4%, 7% and 4% of renal, cardiac and liver transplantation cases, respectively. This usually occurred in the first month of therapy when high doses of cyclosporine were used, and consisted of elevated hepatic enzymes and bilirubin. Chemistry elevations usually decreased with reduced dosage.

Glomerular capillary thrombosis, which may result in graft failure, occasionally develops. The vasculopathy can occur in the absence of rejection and is accompanied by avid platelet consumption within the graft. The pathologic changes resemble those seen in the hemolytic-uremic syndrome and include thrombosis of the renal microvasculature, with platelet-fibrin thrombi occluding glomerular capillaries and afferent arterioles, microangiopathic hemolytic anemia, thrombocytopenia and decreased renal function. Neither pathogenesis nor management of this syndrome is clear. Though resolution has occurred after reduction or discontinuation of cyclosporine and 1) administration of streptokinase and heparin or 2) plasmapheresis, this appears to depend upon early detection with indium 111 labeled platelet scans.

Convulsions have occurred in adult and pediatric patients receiving cyclosporine, particularly in combination with high-dose methylprednisolone.

Bioequivalency: Sandimmune is not bioequivalent to *Neoral.*

CNS toxicity may include: Headache; flushing; confusion; seizures; ataxia; hallucinations; mania; depression; encephalopathy; sleep problems; blurred vision. Various studies have associated these symptoms with low cholesterol, low magnesium, aluminum overload, high-dose methylprednisolone, nephrotoxicity and hypertension.

Lipids: In one study, cyclosporine significantly increased total cholesterol, LDL and apolipoprotein B levels. It is not known if these changes persist over long periods.

Glucose metabolism: There are conflicting reports of the drug's effects on glucose metabolism. Kidney transplant patients have developed insulin-dependent diabetes mellitus after treatment with cyclosporine and prednisolone. The diabetes caused by β–cell toxicity appears dose-related and reversible. Conversely, cyclosporine preserved β–cell function and produced an insulin-independent state in many newly diagnosed insulin-dependent diabetics.

Hypersensitivity: Anaphylactic reactions are rare (≈ 1 in 1000) in patients on cyclosporine injection. Although the exact cause of these reactions is unknown, it is believed to be due to the polyoxyethylated castor oil used as a vehicle for IV formulation. Reactions have consisted of flushing of face and upper thorax, acute respiratory distress with dyspnea and wheezing, blood pressure changes and tachycardia. One patient died after respiratory arrest and aspiration pneumonia. In some cases, the reaction subsided after infusion was stopped.

Continuously observe patients on IV cyclosporine for at least the first 30 minutes after start of infusion and frequently thereafter. If anaphylaxis occurs, stop infusion. Refer to Management of Acute Hypersensitivity Reactions.

Reserve cyclosporine injection for patients unable to take the oral form. Anaphylactic reactions have not been reported with oral doseforms of *Sandimmune* which lack polyoxyethylated castor oil. Patients experiencing anaphylactic reactions were treated subsequently with capsules or with oral solution without incident.

Renal function impairment: Requires close monitoring and possibly frequent dosage adjustment. In patients with persistent high elevations of BUN and creatinine who are unresponsive to dosage adjustments, consider switching to other immunosuppressive therapy. In the event of severe and unremitting rejection, when rescue therapy with pulse steroids and monoclonal antibodies fails to reverse the rejection episode, it is preferable to allow the kidney transplant to be rejected and removed rather than increase the dosage to a very high level in an attempt to reverse the rejection.

Carcinogenesis: The risk of malignancies in cyclosporine recipients is higher than in the healthy population but similar to that in patients receiving other immunosuppressive therapies.

With cyclosporine, some patients have developed a lymphoproliferative disorder, which regresses when the drug is discontinued. Patients receiving cyclosporine are at increased risk for development of lymphomas and other malignancies, particularly those of the skin. The increased risk appears related to the intensity and duration of immunosuppression rather than to the use of specific agents. Because of the danger of oversuppression of the immune system, which can also increase susceptibility to infection, *Sandimmune* should not be given with other immunosuppressive agents except adrenal corticosteroids. Because of the danger of oversuppression of the immune system resulting in increased risk of infection or malignancy due to *Neoral*, use a treatment regimen containing multiple immunosuppressants with caution. The efficacy and safety of cyclosporine in combination with other immunosuppressive agents have not been determined.

Pregnancy: Category C. Sandimmune oral solution is embryotoxic and fetotoxic in rats and rabbits when given in doses 2 to 5 times the human dose. It readily crosses the placenta. Safety for use is not established; however, based on a relatively small number of cases, use during pregnancy does not pose a major fetal risk, and limited experience indicates it is an unlikely teratogen in humans. Use during pregnancy only if the potential benefit justifies the potential risk to the fetus.

The following data represent the reported outcomes of 116 pregnancies in women receiving cyclosporine during pregnancy, 90% of whom were transplant patients and most of whom received cyclosporine throughout the entire gestational period. The only consistent patterns of abnormality were premature birth (gestational period of 28 to 36 weeks) and low birth weight for gestational age. It is not possible to separate the following effects of *Sandimmune* on these pregnancies from the effects of the other immunosuppressants, the underlying maternal disorders or other aspects of the transplantation milieu: Fetal losses, pre-eclampsia, eclampsia, abruptio placentae, oligohydramnios, Rh incompatibility, fetoplacental dysfunction, malformations and neonatal complications.

Lactation: Avoid nursing; cyclosporine is excreted in breast milk.

Children: Patients as young as 6 months of age have received *Sandimmune* with no unusual adverse effects.

Precautions:

Monitoring:

Blood levels – Blood level monitoring of cyclosporine is a useful and essential component in patient management. While no fixed relationships have yet been established, blood concentration monitoring may assist in the clinical evaluation of rejection and toxicity, dose adjustments and the assessment of compliance. In cadaveric renal transplant recipients, dosage was adjusted to achieve specific whole blood 24 hour trough levels of 100 to 200 ng/ml as determined by HPLC.

CYCLOSPORINE (Cyclosporin A)

Of major importance to blood level analysis is the type of assay used, the transplanted organ and other immunosuppressant agents being administered. The above levels are specific to the parent cyclosporine molecule and correlate directly to the new monoclonal specific radioimmunoassays (mRIA-sp). Nonspecific assays are also available which detect the parent compound molecule and various of its metabolites. Older studies often cited levels using a nonspecific assay which were roughly twice those of specific assays, thus comparison of the concentrations in published literature to patient concentrations using current assays must be made with detailed knowledge of the assay methods used. Assay results are not interchangeable and their use should be guided by their approved labeling. If plasma specimens are employed, levels will vary with the temperature at the time of separation from whole blood. Plasma levels may range from ½ to ⅕ of whole blood levels. Refer to individual assay labeling for complete instructions.

While several assays and assay matrices are available, there is a consensus that parent-compound-specific assays correlate best with clinical events. Of these, HPLC is the standard reference, but the monoclonal antibody RIAs and the monoclonal antibody FPIA offer sensitivity, reproducibility and convenience. Most clinicians base their monitoring on trough cyclosporine concentrations. Blood level monitoring is not a replacement for renal function monitoring or tissue biopsies.

Repeatedly assess renal and liver functions by measurement of BUN, serum creatinine, serum bilirubin and liver enzymes.

Malabsorption: Patients with malabsorption may have difficulty achieving therapeutic levels with oral *Sandimmune* use.

Hypertension is a common side effect of cyclosporine therapy. Mild or moderate hypertension, which may occur in ≈ 50% of patients following renal transplantation and in most cardiac transplant patients, is more frequently encountered than severe hypertension and the incidence decreases over time. Control of blood pressure can be accomplished with any of the common antihypertensive agents. However, since cyclosporine may cause hyperkalemia, potassium-sparing diuretics should not be used. While calcium antagonists can be effective agents in treating cyclosporine-associated hypertension, use care since interference with cyclosporine metabolism may require a dosage adjustment.

Hypertension appears to be most severe in children. It is not consistently associated with dose, concentration, duration or prior history of hypertension. Although no specific antihypertensive treatment has been shown to be more effective, angiotensin converting enzyme inhibitors do not appear to be effective.

Drug Interactions:

Monitoring of circulating cyclosporine levels and appropriate dosage adjustment are essential when drugs that affect hepatic microsomal enzymes, particularly the cytochrome P450 III-A enzymes, are used concomitantly.

Nephrotoxic drugs: Use with caution in patients receiving cyclosporine.

Pharmacokinetic Interactions with Cyclosporine		
Drug	Effects on cyclosporine	Mechanism
Carbamazepine Phenobarbital Phenytoin Rifampin Rifabutin	Decreased half-life and blood levels; possible rejection of transplanted organ	Increased cyclosporine metabolism; induction of P450 enzyme system; decreased absorption (phenytoin)
Sulfamethazine/ Trimethoprim IV	Decreased serum levels and possible rejection of transplanted organ	Unknown
Diltiazem Erythromycin Fluconazole Ketoconazole[1] Nicardipine	Increased half-life, blood levels and immunosuppression; possible nephrotoxicity	Inhibition of cyclosporine metabolism; inhibition of biliary excretion and increased absorption (erythromycin); unknown (fluconazole)
Imipenem-cilastatin	Increased blood levels and CNS toxicity	Possible inhibition of cyclosporine metabolism
Methylprednisolone (high-dose) Prednisolone	Increased plasma levels (RIA); decreased blood levels (HPLC)	Inhibition of cyclosporine metabolism (inhibition of P450 enzyme system)
Metoclopramide	Increased bioavailability and plasma levels	Increased absorption

CYCLOSPORINE (Cyclosporin A)

Pharmacokinetic Interactions with Cyclosporine		
Drug	Effects on cyclosporine	Mechanism
Amiodarone	Increase in blood concentrations and possibly nephrotoxicity	Unknown; however, inhibition of cyclosporine metabolism by amiodarone is suspected
Danazol Methyltestosterone	Increased blood concentrations with possible toxicity (eg, nephrotoxicity)	Unknown
Nicardipine	Increased trough blood levels and possibly nephrotoxicity	Unknown; however, nicardipine is suspected to inhibit the hepatic metabolism of cyclosporine
Probucol	Whole blood concentrations may be reduced producing a decrease in clinical effect	Reduced bioavailability is suspected

[1] Since the effect on cyclosporine levels is consistent and predictable, this interaction has been used beneficially to decrease cyclosporine dosage in some patients.

Pharmacologic Interactions with Cyclosporine		
Drug	Effects	Mechanism
Aminoglycosides Amphotericin B NSAIDs TMP-SMZ	Nephrotoxicity	Interacts at tubular or glomerular level; possible effect on prostaglandins (NSAIDs)
Cimetidine Ketoconazole Melphalan Quinolones Ranitidine Vancomycin	Nephrotoxicity	Unknown
Methylprednisolone	Convulsions	Unknown
Azathioprine Corticosteroids Cyclophosphamide	Increased immunosuppression; possible infection; malignancy (see Warning box)	Lymphocytes suppressed
Verapamil	Increased immunosuppression	Lymphocytes suppressed
Digoxin	Elevated digoxin levels with toxicity may occur	Unknown; most likely pharmacokinetic in origin
Nondepolarizing muscle relaxants	Prolonged neuromuscular blockade	Unknown; however, possible inhibition of metabolism by cyclosporine may be involved
Colchicine	Severe adverse clinical symptoms including GI, hepatic, renal and neuromuscular toxicity may occur	Unknown
Vaccines	Vaccination may be less effective and the use of live vaccines should be avoided	Unknown
Lovastatin	Elevated levels of myositis may occur	Unknown
Nifedipine	Gingival hyperplasia	Unknown
Potassium-sparing diuretics	Hyperkalemia	Unknown (see Precautions)

Drug/Food interactions: Administration of food with *Neoral* decreases the AUC and C_{max} of cyclosporine. A high fat meal (669 kcal, 45 g fat) consumed within 30 minutes of *Neoral* administration decreased the AUC by 13% and C_{max} by 33%. The effects of a low fat meal (667 kcal, 15 g fat) were similar. In addition, do not take cyclosporine simultaneously with grapefruit juice unless specifically instructed to do so; trough cyclosporine concentrations may be increased.

CYCLOSPORINE (Cyclosporin A)

Adverse Reactions:

Sandimmune: Principal adverse reactions are renal dysfunction, tremor, hirsutism, hypertension, gum hyperplasia.

Hypersensitivity – Anaphylactic reactions have occurred with cyclosporine injection (see Warnings).

Cardiovascular – Hypertension, usually mild to moderate (see Precautions); myocardial infarction (rare).

Renal – Glomerular capillary thrombosis (see Warnings).

Dermatologic – Brittle finger nails (≤ 2%); hair breaking, pruritus (rare).

GI – Anorexia, gastritis, peptic ulcer, hiccups (≤ 2%); mouth sores, swallowing difficulty, upper GI bleeding, pancreatitis, constipation (rare).

CNS – Hypomagnesemia (see CNS toxicity in Warnings); confusion (≤ 2%); anxiety, depression, lethargy, weakness (rare).

Miscellaneous – Allergic reactions, anemia, conjunctivitis, edema, fever, hearing loss, hyperglycemia, muscle pain, thrombocytopenia, tinnitus (≤ 2%); chest pain, hematuria, joint pain, night sweats, *Pneumocystis carinii* pneumonia, tingling, visual disturbance, weight loss (rare).

Infectious complications developed in approximately 74% of patients taking *Sandimmune*, compared to 94% receiving standard therapy.

Polyoxyethylated castor oil, found in the injectable doseform, is known to cause hyperlipemia and electrophoretic abnormalities of lipoproteins. These effects are reversible upon discontinuation of treatment but are usually not a reason to stop treatment.

Cyclosporine (*Sandimmune*) Adverse Reactions (%)			
	Randomized kidney patients		All *Sandimmune* patients (n = 892) (kidney, heart, liver transplants)
Adverse reactions	*Sandimmune* (n = 227)	Azathioprine (n = 228)	
GU			
Renal dysfunction	32%	6%	25%-38%
Cardiovascular			
Hypertension	26%	18%	13%-53%
Cramps	4%	< 1%	≤ 2%
Dermatologic			
Hirsutism	21%	< 1%	21%-45%
Acne	6%	8%	1%-2%
CNS			
Tremor	12%	0	21%-55%
Convulsions	3%	1%	1%-5%
Headache	2%	< 1%	2%-15%
GI			
Gum hyperplasia	4%	0	5%-16%
Diarrhea	3%	< 1%	3%-8%
Nausea/vomiting	2%	< 1%	4%-10%
Hepatotoxicity	< 1%	< 1%	4%-7%
Abdominal discomfort	< 1%	0	≤ 7%
Autonomic nervous system			
Paresthesia	3%	0	1%-2%
Flushing	< 1%	0	≤ 4%
Hematopoietic			
Leukopenia	2%	19%	≤ 6%
Lymphoma	< 1%	0	1%-6%
Miscellaneous			
Gynecomastia	< 1%	0	≤ 4%
Sinusitis	< 1%	0	3%-7%

Neoral: The nature, severity and incidence of the adverse events that were observed with *Neoral* were comparable with *Sandimmune* when the dosage of the two drugs were adjusted to achieve the same cyclosporine blood trough concentrations.

Overdosage:

Oral: Sandimmune is slowly absorbed; forced emesis is of value ≤ 2 hours after ingestion. Transient hepatotoxicity/nephrotoxicity may occur (should resolve after drug withdrawal). Follow general supportive measures and symptomatic treatment. See

CYCLOSPORINE (Cyclosporin A)

General Management of Acute Overdosage. Cyclosporine is not dialyzable to a great extent, nor cleared well by charcoal hemoperfusion.

Patient Information:

To improve the flavor of the oral solution, dilute with milk, chocolate milk, orange juice or apple juice, preferably at room temperature. Avoid grapefruit and grapefruit juice which affect metabolism of cyclosporine (see Drug Interactions). The combination of *Neoral* with milk can be unpalatable. Use a glass container when taking this medication. Do not allow it to stand before drinking. Stir oral solution well and drink all at once. Rinse glass with the same liquid and drink again to assure that the entire dose was taken.

See your physician regularly to assure that the drug is working properly and that no serious side effects are developing. Do not stop taking this medication unless advised to do so. Contact your physician if fever, sore throat, tiredness or unusual bleeding or bruising occurs.

Inform patients of the necessity of repeated laboratory tests while they are receiving the drug. Also give them careful dosage instructions, advise them of the potential risks during pregnancy, and inform them of the increased risk of neoplasia.

Any change in cyclosporine formulation should be made cautiously and only under physician supervision because it may result in the need for a change in dosage.

Caution patients using cyclosporine oral solution with its accompanying syringe for dosage measurement not to rinse the syringe either before or after use. Introduction of water into the product by any means will cause variation in dose.

Use mechanical contraceptive measures (eg, diaphragm, condom) during cyclosporine treatment. Do not use oral contraceptives.

Advise patients to take cyclosporine on a consistent schedule with regard to time of day and relation to meals.

Administration and Dosage:

Bioequivalency: Sandimmune capsules and oral solution have decreased bioavailability compared to *Neoral. Sandimmune* and *Neoral* are NOT bioequivalent and cannot be used interchangeably without physician supervision.

Because *Sandimmune* is not bioequivalent to *Neoral*, conversion from *Neoral* to *Sandimmune* using a 1:1 ratio (mg/kg/day) may result in a lower cyclosporine blood concentration. Conversion from *Neoral* to *Sandimmune* should be made with increased blood concentration monitoring to avoid the potential of underdosing. *Neoral* capsules and oral solution are bioequivalent.

Adjunct therapy with adrenal corticosteroids is recommended. Different tapering dosage schedules of prednisone appear to achieve similar results. A dosage schedule based on the patient's weight started with 2 mg/kg/day for the first 4 days tapered to 1 mg/kg/day by 1 week, 0.6 mg/kg/day by 2 weeks, 0.3 mg/kg/day by 1 month and 0.15 mg/kg/day by 2 months and thereafter as a maintenance dose. Another center started with an initial dose of 200 mg tapered by 40 mg/day until reaching 20 mg/day. After 2 months at this dose, a further reduction to 10 mg/day was made. Prednisone dosage adjustments must be made according to the clinical situation.

Compounding ophthalmic solution: Using the oral solution, clean the container thoroughly with alcohol, open it and allow evaporation of the alcohol for 24 hours. Add 4 volumes of corn oil or olive oil. Filter through a 0.2 micron filter into a sterile, dry, empty ophthalmic bottle (see Unlabeled Uses).

Sandimmune:

Oral – Initially, a single 15 mg/kg dose 4 to 12 hours prior to transplantation. Although a single daily dose of 14 to 18 mg/kg was used in most clinical trials, few centers continue to use the highest dose, most favoring the lower end of the scale. There is a trend towards use of even lower initial doses for renal transplantation in the ranges of 10 to 14 mg/kg/day. Continue dose postoperatively for 1 to 2 weeks, then taper by 5% per week to a maintenance level of 5 to 10 mg/kg/day. Some centers successfully tapered the maintenance dose to as low as 4 mg/kg/day in selected renal transplant patients without an apparent rise in rejection rate.

Children: In children, the same dose and dosing regimen may be used as in adults although in several studies children have required and tolerated higher doses than those used in adults.

Preparation of oral solution: Solution may be mixed with milk, chocolate milk or orange juice, preferably at room temperature. When taking *Sandimmune*, patients should avoid switching diluents frequently. Administer *Sandimmune* on a consistent schedule with regard to time of day and relation to meals.

Take the prescribed amount of *Sandimmune* from the container using the dosage syringe supplied after removal of the protective cover and transfer the solution to a glass of milk, chocolate milk or orange juice. Stir well and drink at once.

CYCLOSPORINE (Cyclosporin A)

Do not allow it to stand before drinking. Use a glass container and rinse with more diluent to ensure that the total dose is taken.

After use, replace the dosage syringe in the protective cover. Do not rinse the dosage syringe with water or other cleaning agents either before or after use. If the dosage syringe requires cleaning, it must be completely dry before resuming use. Introduction of water into the product by any means will cause variation in dose.

Parenteral – For infusion only. Patients unable to take the oral solution or capsules preoperatively or postoperatively may be given the IV concentrate. Use the IV form at ⅓ the oral dose.

Initial dose: 5 to 6 mg/kg/day given 4 to 12 hours prior to transplantation as a single IV dose. Continue this daily single dose postoperatively until the patient can tolerate the oral doseforms. Switch patients to oral therapy as soon as possible after surgery.

Dilution: Immediately before use, dilute 1 ml concentrate in 20 to 100 ml of 0.9% Sodium Chloride Injection or 5% Dextrose Injection; give in a slow IV infusion over approximately 2 to 6 hours. Discard infusion solutions after 24 hours.

The polyoxyethylated castor oil in the concentrate for IV infusion can cause phthalate stripping from PVC. Discard diluted infusion solutions after 24 hours.

Children: In children, the same dose and dosing regimen as adults although in several studies, children have required and tolerated higher doses than those used in adults. (See Actions.)

Storage/Stability: Store at < 30°C (86°F). Protect IV solution from light. Do not store oral solution in refrigerator; use within 2 months once opened. Do not freeze.

Admixture compatibility/incompatibility –

Magnesium sulfate and cyclosporine in 5% dextrose stored in glass bottles at room temperature is only stable for 6 hours.

Lipid emulsion: After being shaken vigorously, cyclosporine and lipid emulsion is stable for 24 hours.

Neoral:

Initial dose – The initial dose of *Neoral* can be given 4 to 12 hours prior to transplantation or postoperatively. The initial dose varies depending on the transplanted organ and the other immunosuppressive agents included in the protocol. In newly transplanted patients, the initial dose of *Neoral* is the same as the initial oral dose of *Sandimmune*. The mean doses were 9 mg/kg/day for renal transplant patients, 8 mg/kg/day for liver transplant patients and 7 mg/kg/day for heart transplant patients. Divide total daily dose into two equal daily doses. The *Neoral* dose is subsequently adjusted to achieve a pre-defined cyclosporine blood concentration. If cyclosporine trough blood concentrations are used, the target range is the same for *Neoral* as for *Sandimmune*. Using the same trough concentration target range as for *Sandimmune* results in greater cyclosporine exposure when *Neoral* is administered. Titrate dosing based on clinical assessments of rejection and tolerability. Lower *Neoral* doses may be sufficient as maintenance therapy.

Conversion from Sandimmune to Neoral – In transplanted patients who are considered for conversion to *Neoral* from *Sandimmune*, start *Neoral* with the same daily dose as was previously used with *Sandimmune* (1:1 dose conversion). Subsequently adjust *Neoral* to attain the pre-conversion cyclosporine blood trough concentration. Using the same trough concentration target range for *Neoral* as for *Sandimmune* results in greater cyclosporine exposure when *Neoral* is administered. Patients with suspected poor absorption of *Sandimmune* require different dosing strategies. In some patients, the increase in blood trough concentration is more pronounced and may be of clinical significance.

Until the blood trough concentration attains the pre-conversion value, it is strongly recommended that the cyclosporine blood trough concentration be monitored every 4 to 7 days after conversion to *Neoral*. In addition, monitor clinical safety parameters such as serum creatinine and blood pressure every 2 weeks during the first 2 months after conversion. If the blood trough concentrations are outside the desired range or if the clinical safety parameters worsen, the *Neoral* dosage must be adjusted accordingly.

Poor Sandimmune absorption – Patients with lower than expected cyclosporine blood trough concentrations in relation to the oral dose of *Sandimmune* may have poor or inconsistent absorption. After conversion to *Neoral*, patients tend to have higher cyclosporine concentrations. Due to the increase in bioavailability following conversion to *Neoral*, the cyclosporine blood trough concentration may exceed the target range. Exercise particular caution when converting patients to *Neoral* at doses > 10 mg/kg/day. Individually titrate the *Neoral* dose based on cyclosporine trough concentrations, tolerability and clinical response. In this population measure the cyclosporine blood trough concentration more frequently, at least twice a week (daily, if initial dose exceeds 10 mg/kg/day) until the concentration stabilizes within the desired range.

CYCLOSPORINE (Cyclosporin A)

Oral solution – To make *Neoral* oral solution more palatable, dilute preferably with orange or apple juice that is at room temperature. Grapefruit juice affects metabolism of cyclosporine and should be avoided. The combination of *Neoral* with milk can be unpalatable. Take the prescribed amount of oral solution from the container using the dosing syringe supplied, after removal of the protective cover, and transfer the solution to a glass of orange or apple juice. Stir well and drink at once. Do not allow diluted solution to stand before drinking. Use a glass container (not plastic). Rinse the glass with more diluent to ensure that the total dose is consumed. After use, dry the outside of the dosing syringe with a clean towel and replace the protective cover. Do not rinse the dosing syringe with water or other cleaning agents. If the syringe requires cleaning, it must be completely dry before resuming use. It is recommended that *Neoral* be given on a consistent schedule with regard to time of day and meals.

Storage/Stability:

Sandimmune and Neoral oral solutions – Do not store in the refrigerator. Once opened, contents must be used within 2 months. At temperatures < 20° C (68° F), the *Neoral* solution may gel; light flocculation or the formation of a light sediment may also occur. There is no impact on product performance or dosing using the syringe provided. Allow to warm to room temperature (25° C; 77° F) to reverse these changes.

Rx	**Sandimmune** (Sandoz)	**Capsules, soft gelatin:** 25 mg	Sorbitol, ≤ 12.7% dehydrated alcohol. (78/240). Pink. Oblong. In UD 30s.
Rx	**Neoral** (Sandoz)	**Capsules, soft gelatin, for microemulsion:** 25 mg	9.5% dehydrated alcohol. (Neoral 25 mg). Blue-gray. Oval. In UD 30s.
Rx	**Sandimmune** (Sandoz)	**Capsules, soft gelatin:** 50 mg	Sorbitol, ≤ 12.7% dehydrated alcohol. (78/242). Yellow, oblong. In UD 30s.
Rx	**Sandimmune** (Sandoz)	**Capsules, soft gelatin:** 100 mg	Sorbitol, ≤ 12.7% dehydrated alcohol. (78/241). Rose. Oblong. In UD 30s.
Rx	**Neoral** (Sandoz)	**Capsules, soft gelatin, for microemulsion:** 100 mg	9.5% dehydrated alcohol. (Neoral 100 mg). Blue-gray. Oblong. In UD 30s.
Rx	**Sandimmune** (Sandoz)	**Oral Solution:** 100 mg/ml	12.5% alcohol. In 50 ml with syringe.
Rx	**Neoral** (Sandoz)	**Oral Solution for microemulsion:** 100 mg/ml	9.5% dehydrated alcohol. In 50 ml with syringe.
Rx	**Sandimmune** (Sandoz)	**IV Solution:** 50 mg/ml	650 mg polyoxyethylated castor oil per ml and 32.9% alcohol. In 5 ml amps.

MUROMONAB-CD3

Warning:

Only physicians experienced in immunosuppressive therapy and management of renal transplant patients should use muromonab-CD3.

Anaphylactic or anaphylactoid reactions may occur following administration of any dose or course of muromonab-CD3. Serious and occasionally life-threatening systemic, cardiovascular and CNS reactions have been reported. These have included: Pulmonary edema, especially in patients with volume overload; shock; cardiovascular collapse; cardiac or respiratory arrest; seizures; coma. Hence, a patient being treated with muromonab-CD3 must be managed in a facility equipped and staffed for cardiopulmonary resuscitation.

Actions:

Pharmacology: Muromonab-CD3 is a murine monoclonal antibody to the T3 (CD3) antigen of human T cells which functions as an immunosuppressant. Muromonab-CD3 is for IV use only. The antibody is a biochemically purified IgG_{2a} immunoglobulin. It reverses graft rejection, probably by blocking the T cell function, which plays a major role in acute allograft rejection. The drug reacts with, and blocks the function of, a molecule (CD3) in the membrane of human T cells that is associated with the antigen recognition structure of T cells and is essential for signal transduction. Muromonab-CD3 blocks all known T cell functions, and it reacts with most peripheral T cells in blood and in body tissues. Following termination of therapy, T cell function usually returns to normal within 1 week.

A rapid concomitant decrease in the number of circulating CD2, CD3, CD4 and CD8 positive T cells was observed within minutes after administration. This decrease in the number of CD3 positive T cells results from the specific interaction between muromonab-CD3 and the CD3 antigen on the surface of all T lymphocytes. T cell activation results in the release of numerous cytokines/lymphokines, which are thought to be responsible for many of the acute clinical manifestations seen following muromonab-CD3 therapy (see Warnings).

Between days 2 and 7, increasing numbers of circulating CD4 and CD8 positive cells have been observed, although CD3 positive cells are not detectable. CD3 positive cells reappear rapidly and reach pretreatment levels within a week after therapy termination. Increasing numbers of CD3 positive cells have been observed in patients prior to termination of therapy, possibly due to the development of neutralizing antibodies.

Antibodies have occurred (incidence of 21% for IgM, 86% for IgG and 29% for IgE). Mean time of appearance of IgG antibodies was 20 days. Early IgG antibodies occur towards the end of the second week of treatment in 3% of patients.

Pharmacokinetics: Serum levels are measured with an enzyme-linked immunosorbent assay (ELISA). During treatment with 5 mg/day for 14 days, mean serum trough levels rose over the first 3 days and then averaged 0.9 mcg/ml on days 3 to 14. Circulating serum levels $\geq$ 0.8 mcg/ml block the function of cytotoxic T cells in vitro and in vivo.

Clinical trials:

Acute renal allograft rejection – In a controlled randomized clinical trial muromonab-CD3 was significantly more effective than conventional high-dose steroid therapy in reversing acute renal allograft rejection. Patients undergoing acute rejection of cadaveric renal transplants were treated either with muromonab-CD3 daily for a mean of 14 days, with concomitant lowering of the dosage of azathioprine and maintenance steroids (62 patients), or with conventional high-dose steroids (60 patients). Muromonab-CD3 reversed 94% of the rejections compared to a 75% reversal rate obtained with conventional high-dose steroid treatment. The one year Kaplan-Meier (actuarial) estimates of graft survival rates for these patients who had acute rejection were 62% and 45% for muromonab-CD3 and steroid-treated patients, respectively; at 2 years, the rates were 56% and 42%, respectively. One and 2 year patient survivals were not significantly different between the two groups (85% and 75% for muromonab-CD3 treated patients and 90% and 85% for steroid-treated patients).

In additional open clinical trials, the observed rate of reversal of acute renal allograft rejection was 92% for muromonab-CD3 therapy. The drug was also effective in reversing acute renal allograft rejections in 65% of cases where steroids and lymphocyte immune globulin preparations were contraindicated or were not successful (rescue).

Acute cardiac or hepatic allograft rejection – The rate of reversal in acute cardiac allograft rejection and in hepatic allograft rejection in patients unresponsive to treatment with steroids was 90% and 83%, respectively.

MUROMONAB-CD3

Indications:

Renal allograft rejection: Treatment of acute allograft rejection in renal transplant patients.

Cardiac/Hepatic allograft rejection: Treatment of steroid-resistant acute allograft rejection in cardiac and hepatic transplant patients.

Contraindications:

Hypersensitivity to this or any product of murine origin; anti-mouse antibody titers ≥ 1:1000; patients in fluid overload or uncompensated heart failure, as evidenced by chest x-ray or > 3% weight gain within the week prior to treatment; history of seizures or predisposition to seizures; pregnancy, breastfeeding (see Warnings).

Warnings:

Cytokine release syndrome (CRS): Temporally associated with the administration of the first few doses of muromonab-CD3 (particularly, the first two to three doses), most patients have developed an acute clinical syndrome (CRS) that has been attributed to the release of cytokines by activated lymphocytes or monocytes. This clinical syndrome has ranged from a more frequently reported mild, self-limited, "flu-like" illness to a less frequently reported severe, life-threatening shock-like reaction, which may include serious cardiovascular and CNS manifestations. The syndrome typically begins approximately 30 to 60 minutes after administration of a dose (but may occur later) and may persist for several hours. The frequency and severity of this symptom complex is usually greatest with the first dose. With each successive dose, both the frequency and severity of the CRS tend to diminish. Increasing the amount of a dose or resuming treatment after a hiatus may result in a reappearance of the CRS.

Common clinical manifestations – High fever (often spiking, up to 107°F); chills/rigors; headache; tremor; nausea/vomiting; diarrhea; abdominal pain; malaise; muscle/joint aches and pains; generalized weakness. Less frequently reported adverse experiences include minor dermatologic reactions (eg, rash, pruritus) and a spectrum of often serious, occasionally fatal, cardiorespiratory and neuro-psychiatric adverse experiences.

Cardiorespiratory findings may include: Dyspnea; shortness of breath; bronchospasm/wheezing; tachypnea; respiratory arrest/failure/distress; cardiovascular collapse; cardiac arrest; angina/myocardial infarction (MI); chest pain/tightness; tachycardia (including ventricular); hypertension; hemodynamic instability; hypotension, including profound shock; heart failure; pulmonary edema (cardiogenic and non-cardiogenic); adult respiratory distress syndrome; hypoxemia; apnea; arrhythmias.

Pulmonary edema – In the initial renal rejection studies, potentially fatal, severe pulmonary edema, the most serious post-dose reaction, occurred in 4.7% of the initial 107 patients. Fluid overload was present before treatment in all of these cases. However, it occurred in none of the subsequent 311 patients treated with first-dose volume/weight restrictions. In subsequent trials and in post-marketing experience, severe pulmonary edema has occurred in patients who appeared to be euvolemic. The pathogenesis of pulmonary edema may involve all or some of the following: Volume overload; increased pulmonary vascular permeability; reduced left ventricular compliance/contractility.

Serum creatinine – During the first 1 to 3 days of therapy, some patients have experienced an acute and transient decline in the glomerular filtration rate and diminished urine output with a resulting increase in the level of serum creatinine. Massive release of cytokines appears to lead to reversible renal function impairment or delayed renal allograft function. Similarly, transient elevations in hepatic transaminases have been reported following administration of the first few doses.

Patients at risk for more serious complications of the CRS may include those with the following conditions: Unstable angina; recent MI or symptomatic ischemic heart disease; heart failure of any etiology; pulmonary edema of any etiology; any form of chronic obstructive pulmonary disease; intravascular volume overload or depletion of any etiology (eg, excessive dialysis, recent intensive diuresis, blood loss); cerebrovascular disease; patients with advanced symptomatic vascular disease or neuropathy; history of seizures; septic shock. Make efforts to correct or stabilize background conditions prior to the initiation of therapy.

Fluid status – Prior to administration, assess the patient's volume (fluid) status carefully. It is imperative, especially prior to the first few doses, that there be no clinical evidence of volume overload or uncompensated heart failure, including a clear chest X-ray and weight restriction of ≤ 3% above the patient's minimum weight during the week prior to injection.

MUROMONAB-CD3

Prevention/Minimization of CRS – Manifestations of the CRS may be prevented or minimized by pretreatment with 8 mg/kg methylprednisolone (ie, high-dose steroids), given 1 to 4 hours prior to administration of the first dose of muromonab-CD3 and by closely following recommendations for dosage and treatment duration. If any of the more serious presentations of the CRS occur, intensive treatment including oxygen, IV fluids, corticosteroids, pressor amines, antihistamines and intubation may be required.

Neuro-Psychiatric events: Seizures, encephalopathy, cerebral edema, aseptic meningitis and headaches have occurred during therapy with muromonab-CD3, even following the first dose, resulting in part from T cell activation and subsequent systemic release of cytokines.

Seizures, some accompanied by loss of consciousness or cardiorespiratory arrest, or death, have occurred independently or in conjunction with any of the neurologic syndromes described below. Patients predisposed to seizures may include those with the following conditions: Acute tubular necrosis/uremia; fever; infection; a precipitous fall in serum calcium; fluid overload; hypertension; hypoglycemia, history of seizures and electrolyte imbalances; those who are taking a medication concomitantly that may, by itself, cause seizures. The number and regularity of seizure reports indicate that this hazard appears not to be rare. Anticipate convulsions clinically with appropriate patient monitoring.

Encephalopathy – Manifestations may include: Impaired cognition; confusion; obtundation; altered mental status; auditory/visual hallucinations; psychosis (delirium, paranoia); mood changes (eg, mania, agitation, combativeness); diffuse hypotonus; hyperreflexia; myoclonus; tremor; asterixis; involuntary movements; major motor seizures; lethargy/stupor/coma; diffuse weakness. Approximately one-third of patients with a diagnosis of encephalopathy may have had coexisting aseptic meningitis syndrome.

Cerebral edema and other signs of increased vascular permeability (eg, otitis media, nasal and ear stuffiness) have been seen in patients treated with muromonab-CD3 and may accompany some of the other neurologic manifestations.

Aseptic meningitis syndrome – The incidence of this syndrome was 6%. Fever (89%), headache (44%), meningismus (ie, neck stiffness; 14%) and photophobia (10%) were the most commonly reported symptoms; a combination of these four symptoms occurred in 5% of patients. Diagnosis is confirmed by CSF analysis demonstrating leukocytosis with pleocytosis, elevated protein and normal or decreased glucose, with negative viral, bacterial and fungal cultures. In any immunosuppressed transplant patient with clinical findings suggesting meningitis, evaluate the possibility of infection. Approximately one-third of the patients with a diagnosis of aseptic meningitis had coexisting signs and symptoms of encephalopathy. Most patients with the aseptic meningitis syndrome had a benign course and recovered without any permanent sequelae during therapy or subsequent to its completion or discontinuation.

Headache is frequently seen after any of the first few doses and may occur in any of the aforementioned neurologic syndromes or by itself.

The following additional neurologic events have each been reported occasionally: Irreversible blindness; impaired vision; quadri- or paraparesis/plegia; cerebrovascular accident (hemiparesis/plegia); aphasia; transient ischemic attack; subarachnoid hemorrhage; palsy of the VI cranial nerve; hearing loss.

Signs or symptoms of encephalopathy, meningitis, seizures and cerebral edema, with or without headache, have typically been reversible. Headache, aseptic meningitis, seizures and less severe forms of encephalopathy resolved in most patients despite continued treatment. However, some events have been irreversible.

Patients who may be at greater risk for CNS adverse experiences include: Known or suspected CNS disorders (eg, history of seizure disorder); cerebrovascular disease (small or large vessel); conditions having associated neurologic problems (eg, head trauma, uremia); underlying vascular diseases; concomitant medication that may, by itself, affect the CNS.

Infections: Muromonab-CD3 is usually added to immunosuppressive therapeutic regimens, thereby augmenting the degree of immunosuppression. This increase in the total burden of immunosuppression may alter the spectrum of infections observed and increase the risk, the severity and the potential gravity (morbidity) of infectious complications. Approximately 1 to 6 months post-transplant, patients are at risk for viral infections (eg, cytomegalovirus, Epstein-Barr virus, herpes simplex virus), which produce serious systemic disease and also increase the overall state of immunosuppression. Multiple or intensive courses of any anti-T cell antibody preparation, including muromonab-CD3, which produce profound impairment of cell-mediated immunity, further increase the risk of (opportunistic) infection, especially with the herpes viruses and fungi. Anti-infective prophylaxis may reduce the morbidity associated with certain potential pathogens and should be considered for high-risk patients.

MUROMONAB-CD3

Hypersensitivity: Serious and occasionally fatal, immediate (usually within 10 minutes) hypersensitivity (anaphylactic) reactions have occurred. Manifestations of anaphylaxis may appear similar to manifestations of the CRS. It may be impossible to determine the mechanism responsible for any systemic reaction(s). Reactions attributed to hypersensitivity have been reported less frequently than those attributed to cytokine release. Acute hypersensitivity reactions may be characterized by: Cardiovascular collapse; cardiorespiratory arrest; loss of consciousness; hypotension/shock; tachycardia; tingling; angioedema (including laryngeal, pharyngeal or facial edema); airway obstruction; bronchospasm; dyspnea; urticaria; pruritus.

Serious allergic events, including anaphylactic or anaphylactoid reactions, have been reported in patients re-exposed to muromonab-CD3 subsequent to their initial course of therapy. Pretreatment with antihistamines or steroids may not reliably prevent anaphylaxis in this setting. Weigh the possible allergic hazards of retreatment against expected therapeutic benefits and alternatives. If retreatment is employed, have epinephrine and other emergency life-support equipment available, and monitor the patient closely.

If hypersensitivity is suspected, discontinue the drug immediately and do not resume therapy or re-expose the patient to muromonab-CD3. Serious acute hypersensitivity reactions may require emergency treatment with 0.3 to 0.5 ml aqueous epinephrine (1:1000 dilution) SC and other resuscitative measures. Refer to Management of Acute Hypersensitivity Reactions.

Carcinogenesis: As a result of depressed cell-mediated immunity, organ transplant patients have an increased risk of developing malignancies. This risk is evidenced almost exclusively by the occurrence of lymphoproliferative disorders (LPD), lymphomas and skin cancers. Following the initiation of muromonab-CD3 therapy, continuously monitor patients for evidence of LPD. Vigilant surveillance is advised, as early detection with subsequent reduction of total immunosuppression may result in regression of some of these lymphoproliferative disorders.

Because the potential for the development of LPD is related to the duration and extent (intensity) of total immunosuppression, it is advisable to adhere to the recommended dosage and duration of muromonab-CD3 and other anti-T lymphocyte antibody preparations administered within a short period of time. If appropriate, reduce the dosage(s) of immunosuppressive drugs used concomitantly to the lowest level compatible with an effective therapeutic response.

Pregnancy: Category C. It is not known whether muromonab-CD3 can cause fetal harm when administered to a pregnant woman or can affect reproduction capacity. However, it is an IgG antibody and may cross the placenta. If this drug is used during pregnancy, or the patient becomes pregnant while taking this drug, apprise the patient of the potential hazard to the fetus.

Lactation: It is not known whether muromonab-CD3 is excreted in breast milk. Because of the potential for serious adverse reactions/oncogenesis, decide whether to discontinue nursing or to discontinue the drug, taking into account the importance of the drug to the mother.

Children: Safety and efficacy in children have not been established. Muromonab-CD3 has been used in infants/children, beginning with a dose of ≤ 5 mg. Based on immunologic monitoring, the dosage has been adjusted accordingly. Pediatric recipients may be significantly immunosuppressed for a prolonged period of time and therefore require close monitoring post-therapy for opportunistic infection, particularly varicella (VZV), which poses an infectious complication unique to this population. GI fluid loss secondary to diarrhea or vomiting resulting from the CRS may be significant when treating small children and may require parenteral hydration. It is unknown whether there may be significant long-term sequelae (eg, neurodevelopmental language difficulties in infants < 1 year of age) related to the occurrence of seizures, high fever, CNS infections or aseptic meningitis following muromonab-CD3 treatment. In cases where administration would be deemed medically appropriate, more vigilant and frequent monitoring is required for children than in adults.

Precautions:

Monitoring: Monitor the following tests prior to and during therapy:

- *Renal* – BUN, serum creatinine;
- *Hepatic* – Transaminases, alkaline phosphatase, bilirubin;
- *Hematopoietic* – WBCs and differential, platelet count;
- *Chest X-ray* within 24 hours before initiating treatment, which should be free of any evidence of heart failure or fluid overload.

MUROMONAB-CD3

Monitor one of the following immunologic tests during therapy:

- Plasma levels determined by an ELISA (target levels should be ≥ 800 ng/ml); or
- Quantitative T lymphocyte surface phenotyping (CD3, CD4, CD8); target CD3 positive T cells < 25 cells/mm^3.

Testing for human-mouse antibody titers is strongly recommended; a titer ≥ 1:1000 is a contraindication for use.

Intravascular thrombosis: As with other immunosuppressive therapies, arterial or venous thrombosis of allografts and other vascular beds (eg, heart, lungs, brain, bowel) have been reported. Consider these findings when deciding to use muromonab-CD3 in patients with a history of thrombotic events or underlying vascular disease. Consider concomitant use of prophylactic anti-thrombotic interventions (eg, mini-dose heparin).

Drug Interactions:

Indomethacin: Encephalopathy and other CNS effects have occurred with concurrent use.

Adverse Reactions:

Cytokine release syndrome: See Warnings. In trials, the majority of patients experienced pyrexia (90%), of which 19% were ≥ 40°C (104°F), and chills (59%). Other adverse experiences occurring in ≥ 8% during the first 2 days included: Dyspnea (21%); nausea, vomiting (19%); chest pain, diarrhea (14%); tremor, wheezing (13%); headache (11%); tachycardia (10%); rigor, hypertension (8%).

Infections: See Warnings.

Renal rejection trial – The most common infections during the first 45 days of therapy were due to herpes simplex (27%) and cytomegalovirus (CMV; 19%). Other severe and life-threatening infections were *Staphylococcus epidermidis* (4.8%), *Pneumocystis carinii* (3.1%), *Legionella, Cryptococcus, Serratia* and gram-negative bacteria (1.6%).

Hepatic rejection trial – The most common infections during the first 45 days of treatment were CMV (15.7%), fungal infections (14.9%) and herpes simplex (7.5%). Other severe and life-threatening infections were gram-positive (9%), gram-negative (7.5%), viral (1.5%), *Legionella* (0.7%). In another hepatic rejection trial, incidence of fungal infections was 34% and of herpes simplex virus infections was 31%.

Cardiac rejection trial – The most common infections reported during the first 45 days of treatment were herpes simplex (5%), fungal (4%) and CMV (3%).

Neoplasia: See Warnings.

Neuro-Psychiatric: See Warnings.

Hypersensitivity: See Warnings.

Other: Pancytopenia; aplastic anemia; neutropenia; leukopenia; thrombocytopenia; lymphopenia; leukocytosis; lymphadenopathy; arterial and venous thrombosis of allografts and other vascular beds (eg, heart, lung, brain, bowel); disturbances of coagulation.

Body as a whole – Fever (including spiking temperatures as high as 107°F); chills/rigors; flu-like syndrome; fatigue/malaise; generalized weakness; anorexia.

Cardiovascular – Cardiac arrest; hypotension/shock; heart failure; cardiovascular collapse; angina/MI; tachycardia; bradycardia; hemodynamic instability; hypertension; left ventricular dysfunction; arrhythmias; chest pain/tightness.

Respiratory – Respiratory arrest; adult respiratory distress syndrome (ARDS); respiratory failure; pulmonary edema (cardiogenic or noncardiogenic); apnea; dyspnea; bronchospasm; wheezing; shortness of breath; hypoxemia; tachypnea/hyperventilation; abnormal chest sounds; pneumonia/pneumonitis.

Dermatologic – Rash; Stevens-Johnson syndrome; urticaria; pruritus; erythema; flushing; diaphoresis.

GI – Diarrhea; nausea/vomiting; abdominal pain; bowel infarction; GI hemorrhage.

Hepatic – Increases in transaminases (eg, AST, ALT); hepato/splenomegaly or hepatitis, usually secondary to viral infection or lymphoma.

Musculoskeletal – Arthralgia; arthritis; myalgia; stiffness/aches/pains.

Special Senses – Blindness; blurred vision; diplopia; hearing loss; otitis media; tinnitus; vertigo; VI cranial nerve palsy; photophobia; conjunctivitis; nasal/ear stuffiness.

Renal – Anuria/oliguria; delayed graft function; transient and reversible increases in BUN and serum creatinine; abnormal urinary cytology, including exfoliation of damaged lymphocytes, collecting duct cells and cellular casts.

MUROMONAB-CD3

Overdosage:

Symptoms of overdose may include hyperthermia, severe chills, myalgia, vomiting, diarrhea, edema, oliguria, pulmonary edema and acute renal failure. A high incidence (5%) of microangiopathic hemolytic anemia/HUS syndrome in patients receiving 10 mg per day was also reported. In the event of acute overdosage, carefully observe the patient and give symptomatic and supportive treatment.

Patient Information:

Advise patients of the signs and symptoms associated with the cytokine release syndrome, including the potentially serious nature of this symptom complex (eg, systemic, cardiovascular, neuro-psychiatric events).

Advise patients to seek medical attention at the first sign of skin rash, urticaria, rapid heartbeat, difficulty in swallowing and breathing, or any swelling that may suggest angioedema or other allergic reaction.

Patients should know how they might react before operating an automobile or machinery, or engaging in activities requiring mental alertness, coordination or physical dexterity.

Administration and Dosage:

Approved by the FDA in 1986.

Administer as an IV bolus in < 1 minute. Do not give by IV infusion or in conjunction with other drug solutions.

Renal allograft rejection, acute: 5 mg/day for 10 to 14 days. Begin treatment once acute renal rejection is diagnosed.

Cardiac/hepatic allograft rejection, steroid resistant: 5 mg/day for 10 to 14 days. Begin treatment when it is determined that a rejection has not been reversed by an adequate course of corticosteroid therapy.

Monitor patients closely for the first few doses. Methylprednisolone sodium succinate 8 mg/kg IV given 1 to 4 hours prior to muromonab-CD3 administration is strongly recommended to decrease the incidence of reactions to the first dose. Acetaminophen and antihistamines, given concomitantly, may reduce early reactions. Patient temperature should not exceed 37.8°C (100°F) prior to first administration.

Other immune-suppressive drugs: Reduce the dose of concomitant immunosuppressive drugs during muromonab-CD3 administration to the lowest level compatible with an effective therapeutic response. Resume maintenance immunosuppression ≈ 3 days prior to cessation of muromonab-CD3.

Preparation of solution: Draw solution into a syringe through a low protein-binding 0.2 or 0.22 micrometer (μm) filter.

Admixture incompatibility: Do not add or infuse other drugs simultaneously through the same IV line. If the same IV line is used for sequential infusion of several different drugs, flush with saline before and after infusion of muromonab-CD3.

Storage/Stability: Refrigerate at 2° to 8°C (36° to 46°F). Do not freeze or shake. Because this drug is a protein solution, it may develop a few fine translucent particles which do not affect its potency. Since no bacteriostatic agent is present in this product, use the amp immediately once opened and discard the unused portion.

Rx	**Orthoclone OKT3** (Ortho Biotech)	**Injection:** 5 mg per 5 ml	With 1 mg polysorbate 80. In 5 ml amps.

BROMOCRIPTINE MESYLATE

Bromocriptine is also used for Parkinson's disease; refer to the monograph in the Antiparkinson Agents section for further information.

Actions:

Pharmacology: Bromocriptine mesylate is a semisynthetic ergot alkaloid derivative which inhibits prolactin secretion with no effect on other pituitary hormones, except in acromegaly, where it lowers elevated blood levels of growth hormone.

It is a dopamine receptor agonist that activates postsynaptic dopamine receptors. The dopaminergic neurons in the tuberoinfundibular process modulate the secretion of prolactin from the anterior pituitary by secreting a prolactin inhibitory factor (thought to be dopamine) in the corpus striatum; the dopaminergic neurons are involved in the control of motor function. Bromocriptine significantly reduces plasma levels of prolactin in patients with physiologically elevated prolactin and in patients with hyperprolactinemia.

Amenorrhea/galactorrhea/female infertility – In about 75% of cases of galactorrhea and amenorrhea, bromocriptine suppresses the galactorrhea and reinitiates normal ovulatory menstrual cycles, usually in 6 to 8 weeks. However, some patients respond within a few days. Others may take up to 8 months. Menses are usually reinitiated prior to complete suppression of galactorrhea.

Galactorrhea may take longer to control, depending on the degree of stimulation of mammary tissue prior to therapy. A ≥ 75% reduction in secretion usually occurs after 8 to 12 weeks. Some patients fail to respond, even after 12 months.

Acromegaly – Bromocriptine produces a prompt and sustained reduction in circulating levels of serum growth hormone. Since the effects of external pituitary radiation may not become maximal for several years, adjunctive therapy with bromocriptine offers potential benefit before the effects of irradiation are manifested (see Precautions).

Pharmacokinetics:

Absorption/Distribution – Twenty-eight percent of an oral dose is absorbed from the GI tract. Blood levels following a 2.5 mg dose range from 2 to 3 ng equivalents/ml. Plasma levels range from 4 to 6 ng equivalents/ml. The drug undergoes first-pass metabolism and only 6% of the absorbed dose reaches the systemic circulation unchanged. Plasma half-life is 6 to 8 hours. Bromocriptine is 90% to 96% bound to serum albumin.

Metabolism/Excretion – Bromocriptine is completely metabolized prior to excretion; 84.6% of the dose is excreted in the feces. Only 2.5% to 5.5% is excreted in the urine. The major route of excretion of absorbed drug is via the bile.

Indications:

Hyperprolactinemia-associated dysfunctions: Amenorrhea with or without galactorrhea, infertility or hypogonadism. Indicated in patients with prolactin-secreting adenomas, which may be the basic underlying endocrinopathy contributing to above clinical presentations. Reduction in tumor size has been demonstrated in both male and female patients with macroadenomas. In cases where adenectomy is elected, bromocriptine therapy may be used to reduce tumor mass prior to surgery.

Acromegaly: Bromocriptine, alone or as adjunctive therapy with pituitary irradiation or surgery, reduces serum growth hormone by ≥ 50% in ≈ 50% of patients treated, although not usually to normal levels.

Parkinson's disease: See monograph in the Antiparkinson Agents section.

Unlabeled uses: Bromocriptine has been used to treat hyperprolactinemia associated with pituitary adenomas; it has caused elevated prolactin levels to normalize, causing shrinkage of macroprolactinomas. Maintenance doses of 0.625 to 10 mg/day have been used for 6 to 52 months.

Neuroleptic malignant syndrome.

Cocaine addiction.

Cyclical mastalgia.

Bromocroptine was previously indicated for prevention of physiological lactation (secretion, congestion, engorgement) occurring after parturition when the mother does not breastfeed, or after stillbirth or abortion. However, this indication has been withdrawn by the manufacturer; it should no longer be used for this condition.

Contraindications:

Sensitivity to ergot alkaloids; severe ischemic heart disease or peripheral vascular disease; withdraw in patients being treated for hyperprolactinemia when pregnancy is diagnosed (see Warnings).

BROMOCRIPTINE MESYLATE

Warnings:

Pituitary tumors: Since hyperprolactinemia with amenorrhea/galactorrhea and infertility has been found in patients with pituitary tumors, perform evaluation of pituitary before treatment.

Symptomatic hypotension: In postpartum studies, hypotension (decrease in supine systolic and diastolic pressures of > 20 and 10 mm Hg, respectively) was observed in almost 30% of patients. On occasion, the drop in supine systolic pressure was as great as 50 to 59 mm Hg. However, since bromocriptine causes hypotension and, rarely, hypertension, do not initiate therapy until the vital signs are stabilized and no sooner than 4 hours after delivery.

Give particular attention to patients with preeclampsia and to those who have received within the preceding 24 hours other ergot alkaloids or drugs which can alter blood pressure. Monitor blood pressure, particularly during the first few weeks of therapy. Exercise care when bromocriptine is administered concomitantly with other medications known to lower blood pressure.

Rhinorrhea: A few cases of cerebrospinal fluid rhinorrhea occurred in patients receiving bromocriptine for treatment of large prolactinomas. This has occurred rarely, usually only in patients who have received previous transsphenoidal surgery, pituitary radiation, or both, and who were receiving bromocriptine for tumor recurrence. It may also occur in previously untreated patients whose tumor extends into the sphenoid sinus.

Pregnancy: Category B. Since pregnancy is often the therapeutic objective in many hyperprolactinemic patients presenting with amenorrhea/galactorrhea and infertility, assess pituitary to detect the presence of a prolactin secreting adenoma. Advise patients not seeking pregnancy, or those harboring large adenomas, to use contraceptive measures other than oral contraceptives during treatment. Since pregnancy may occur prior to reinitiation of menses, perform a pregnancy test at least every 4 weeks during the amenorrheic period and once menses are reinitiated, every time a patient misses a menstrual period. Discontinuation of bromocriptine treatment in patients with known macroadenomas has been associated with rapid regrowth of tumor and increase in serum prolactin in most cases.

Safe use of bromocriptine has not been demonstrated in pregnancy and use in pregnancy is contraindicated. If pregnancy occurs, discontinue treatment immediately and carefully observe these patients throughout pregnancy for signs and symptoms which may develop if a previously undetected prolactin-secreting tumor enlarges.

Prolactin-secreting adenomas may expand and compression of optic or other cranial nerves may occur and emergency pituitary surgery may be necessary. In most cases, compression resolves following delivery. Reinitiation of bromocriptine has produced improvement in visual fields of patients in whom nerve compression has occurred during pregnancy. The relative efficacy of bromocriptine vs surgery in preserving visual fields is not known. Evaluate patients with rapidly progressive visual field loss to decide on the most appropriate therapy.

Of 1276 reported pregnancies in women who took bromocriptine during early pregnancy, there were 1109 live born infants and 4 stillborn infants.

The total incidence of malformations (3.3%) and spontaneous abortions (11%) does not exceed that of the population at large. There were three hydatidiform moles, two in the same patient.

Lactation: Since bromocriptine prevents lactation, do not administer to mothers who will breastfeed.

Children: Safety and efficacy in children < 15 years of age have not been established.

Precautions:

Acromegaly: Cold sensitive digital vasospasm has occurred in some acromegalic patients treated with bromocriptine. The response can be reversed by reducing the dosage and may be prevented by keeping the fingers warm. Cases of severe GI bleeding from peptic ulcers have been reported, some fatal. Although there is no evidence that bromocriptine increases the incidence of peptic ulcers in acromegalic patients, thoroughly investigate symptoms suggestive of peptic ulcer and treat appropriately.

Possible tumor expansion during therapy has occurred. The natural history of growth hormone secreting tumors is unknown; monitor patients. If evidence of tumor expansion develops, discontinue treatment and consider alternative procedures.

BROMOCRIPTINE MESYLATE

Pulmonary effects: Long-term treatment (6 to 36 months) in doses of 20 to 100 mg/day is associated with pulmonary infiltrates, pleural effusion and pleural thickening. When treatment was terminated, the changes slowly reverted toward normal.

Drug Interactions:

Bromocriptine Drug Interactions			
Precipitant drug	Object drug*		Description
Erythromycin	Bromocriptine	⬆	Bromocriptine levels may be increased, possibly increasing pharmacologic and toxic effects.
Phenothiazines	Bromocriptine	⬇	Efficacy of bromocriptine, when used for prolactin-secreting tumors, may be inhibited.
Sympathomimetics Isometheptene Phenylpropanolamine	Bromocriptine	⬆	In several case reports, bromocriptine side effects were exacerbated during concurrent use of these agents, including ventricular tachycardia and cardiac dysfunction.

* ⬆ = Object drug increased. ⬇ = Object drug decreased.

Adverse Reactions:

Hyperprolactinemic indications: The incidence of adverse effects is high (69%), but they are generally mild to moderate. Therapy was discontinued in approximately 5% of patients. Adverse reactions include: Nausea (49%); headache (19%); dizziness (17%); fatigue (7%); lightheadedness, vomiting (5%); abdominal cramps (4%); nasal congestion, constipation, diarrhea, drowsiness (3%); psychosis; hypotension; cerebrospinal fluid rhinorrhea (see Warnings). Occurrence of these effects may be lessened by temporarily reducing dosage to ½ tablet 2 to 3 times daily.

Acromegaly:

Cardiovascular – Postural/orthostatic hypotension (6%); arrhythmias, ventricular tachycardia (< 1%).

CNS – Digital vasospasm, drowsiness/tiredness (3%); dizziness, headache, syncope, Raynaud's syndrome (< 2%); faintness, lightheadedness, decreased sleep requirement, visual hallucinations, lassitude, vertigo, paresthesia, delusional psychosis (< 1%).

GI – Nausea (18%); constipation (14%); anorexia; dry mouth, indigestion/dyspepsia (4%); vomiting (2%); GI bleeding (< 2%).

Respiratory – Nasal stuffiness (4%); shortness of breath (< 1%).

Miscellaneous – Sluggishness, paranoia, insomnia, heavy headedness, reduced tolerance to cold, tingling of ears, facial pallor, muscle cramps, hair loss, alcohol potentiation (< 1%).

Lab test abnormalities: Elevations in BUN, AST, ALT, GGPT, CPK, alkaline phosphatase and uric acid are usually transient and not clinically significant.

Patient Information:

Take with meals or food.

Dizziness or fainting may occur, particularly following the first dose; take the first dose while lying down. Avoid sudden changes in posture, such as rising from a sitting position. Observe caution while driving or performing other tasks requiring alertness, coordination or physical dexterity.

Advise patients receiving bromocriptine for hyperprolactinemic states associated with macroadenoma or those who have had previous transsphenoidal surgery to report any persistent watery nasal discharge to a physician. Advise patients receiving bromocriptine for treatment of a macroadenoma that discontinuation of drug may be associated with rapid regrowth of the tumor and recurrence of original symptoms.

Use contraceptive measures (other than oral contraceptives) during treatment.

Administration and Dosage:

Hyperprolactinemic indications:

Initial – 0.5 to 2.5 mg daily with meals; 2.5 mg may be added as tolerated every 3 to 7 days or until optimal therapeutic response is achieved. Therapeutic dosage usually is 5 to 7.5 mg (range, 2.5 to 15 mg/day).

BROMOCRIPTINE MESYLATE

Acromegaly: Virtually all patients receiving therapeutic benefit show reductions in circulating levels of growth hormone. Periodically assess growth hormone levels. If no significant reduction in hormone levels has occurred after a brief trial, consider dosage adjustment or discontinue the drug.

Initial – 1.25 to 2.5 mg for 3 days (with food) on retiring. Add an additional 1.25 to 2.5 mg as tolerated every 3 to 7 days until the patient obtains optimal therapeutic benefit. Evaluate patients monthly and adjust the dosage based on reductions of growth hormone. The usual optimal therapeutic dosage range varies from 20 to 30 mg/day. Maximal dosage should not exceed 100 mg/day.

Withdraw patients treated with pituitary irradiation from bromocriptine therapy on a yearly basis to assess both the clinical effects of radiation on the disease process as well as the effects of bromocriptine. Usually, a 4 to 8 week withdrawal period is adequate. Recurrence of symptoms or growth hormone increases indicate the disease process is still active. Consider further courses of bromocriptine.

Rx	**Parlodel** (Sandoz)	**Tablets**: 2.5 mg (as mesylate)	Lactose. (Parlodel 2½). White, scored. In 30s and 100s.
		Capsules: 5 mg (as mesylate)	Lactose. (Parlodel 5 mg). Caramel and white. In 30s and 100s.

CABERGOLINE

Actions:

Pharmacology: The secretion of prolactin by the anterior pituitary is mainly under hypothalmic inhibitory control, likely exerted through release of dopamine by tuberoinfundibular neurons. Cabergoline is a synthetic ergot derivative long-acting dopamine receptor agonist with a high affinity for D_2 receptors. Cabergoline inhibits basal and metoclopramide-induced prolactin secretion. Receptor-binding studies indicate that cabergoline has low affinity for dopamine D_1, alpha$_1$- and alpha$_2$-adrenergic and 5-HT$_1$- and 5-HT$_2$-serotonin receptors.

Pharmacodynamics – Dose response with inhibition of plasma prolactin, onset of maximal effect and duration of effect has been documented following single cabergoline doses to healthy volunteers (0.05 to 1.5 mg) and hyperprolactinemic patients (0.3 to 1 mg). Prolactin inhibition was evident at doses > 0.2 mg, while doses ≥ 0.5 mg caused maximal suppression in most subjects. Higher doses produce prolactin suppression in a greater proportion of subjects and with an earlier onset and longer duration of action. In 12 healthy volunteers, 0.5, 1 and 1.5 mg doses resulted in complete prolactin inhibition, with a maximum effect within 3 hours in 92% to 100% of subjects after the 1 and 1.5 mg doses compared with 50% of subjects after the 0.5 mg dose.

In hyperprolactinemic patients, the maximal prolactin decrease after a 0.6 mg single dose of cabergoline was comparable with 2.5 mg bromocriptine; however, the duration of effect was markedly longer (14 days vs 24 hours). The time to maximal effect was shorter for bromocriptine than cabergoline (6 hours vs 48 hours).

In 72 healthy volunteers, single or multiple doses (≤ 2 mg) of cabergoline resulted in selective inhibition of prolactin with no apparent effect on other anterior pituitary hormones (GH, FSH, LH, ACTH and TSH) or cortisol.

Pharmacokinetics:

Absorption – Following single oral doses of 0.5 mg to 1.5 mg given to 12 healthy adult volunteers, mean peak plasma levels of 30 to 70 picograms of cabergoline were observed within 2 to 3 hours. The absolute bioavailability of cabergoline is unknown. A significant fraction of the administered dose undergoes a first-pass effect. Absorption is not affected by food.

Distribution – Cabergoline is moderately bound (40% to 42%) to human plasma proteins in a concentration-independent manner. Concomitant dosing of highly protein-bound drugs is unlikely to affect its disposition. Over the 0.5 to 7 mg dose range, cabergoline plasma levels appeared to be dose-proportional in 12 healthy adult volunteers and nine adult parkinsonian patients. A repeat-dose study in 12 healthy volunteers suggests that steady-state levels following a once-weekly dosing schedule are expected to be 2– to 3–fold higher than after a single dose.

Metabolism – Cabergoline is extensively metabolized, predominantly via hydrolysis of the acylurea bond or the urea moiety. Cytochrome P-450 mediated metabolism appears to be minimal. Hydrolysis of the acylurea or urea moiety abolishes the prolactin-lowering effect of cabergoline, and major metabolites identified thus far do not contribute to the therapeutic effect. Cytochrome P-450 mediated metabolism appears to be minimal.

Excretion – After oral dosing of radioactive cabergoline to five healthy volunteers, ≈ 22% and 60% of the dose was excreted within 20 days in the urine and feces, respectively. Less than 4% of the dose was excreted unchanged in the urine. Nonrenal and renal clearances for cabergoline are ≈ 3.2 L/min and 0.08 L/min, respectively. Urinary excretion in hyperprolactinemic patients was similar. The elimination half-life is estimated to be 63 to 69 hours. The prolonged prolactin-lowering effect of cabergoline may be related to its slow elimination and long half-life.

Special Populations:

Renal function impairment – The pharmacokinetics of cabergoline were not altered in 12 patients with moderate to severe renal insufficiency as assessed by creatinine clearance.

Cabergoline Pharmacokinetic Parameters in Patients with Renal Insufficiency

Type of Patients	C_{max} (pg/ml)	T_{max}* (hr)	$AUC_{(0-168\ hr)}$ (pg-hr/ml)	CL_R (ml/min)	Ae*$_{(0-168\ hr)}$ (mcg)
Healthy	59.1	2.5	2861	76.7	11.9
Renal insufficiency (moderate)	86.7	1.5	3778	38.9	12.6
Renal insufficiency (severe)	55.7	2.5	2834	34.2	4.4

* Total urinary excretion of unchanged drug.

CABERGOLINE

Hepatic function impairment – In 12 patients with mild to moderate hepatic dysfunction, no effect on mean cabergoline C_{max} or area under the plasma concentration curve (AUC) was observed. However, patients with severe insufficiency show a substantial increase in the mean cabergoline C_{max} and AUC, which necessitates caution.

Clinical trials: In the 8–week, double-blind period of the comparative trial with bromocriptine (cabergoline n = 223; bromocriptine n = 236), prolactin was normalized in 77% of the patients treated with cabergoline at 0.5 mg twice weekly compared with 59% of those treated with bromocriptine at 2.5 mg twice daily. Restoration of menses occurred in 77% of the women treated with cabergoline, compared with 70% of those treated with bromocriptine. Among patients with galactorrhea, this symptom disappeared in 73% of those treated with cabergoline compared with 56% of those treated with bromocriptine.

Indications:

Hyperprolactinemia: The treatment of hyperprolactinemic disorders, either idiopathic or because of pituitary adenomas.

Unlabeled uses: Cabergoline has caused tumor shrinkage in patients with microprolactinoma or macroprolactinoma, but more studies are needed; Parkinson's disease (7.5 mg/day); normalize androgen levels and improve menstrual cyclicity in polycystic ovary syndrome (0.5 mg/week).

Contraindications:

Uncontrolled hypertension or known hypersensitivity to ergot derivatives.

Warnings:

Hepatic function impairment: Because cabergoline is extensively metabolized by the liver, use caution and careful monitoring when administering cabergoline to patients with hepatic function impairment.

Carcinogenesis: There was a slight increase in the incidence of cervical and uterine leiomyomas and uterine leiomyosarcomas in mice. In rats, there was a slight increase in malignant tumors of the cervix and uterus and interstitial cell adenomas.

Fertility impairment: In female rats, a dose of 0.003 mg/kg/day for 2 weeks prior to mating and throughout the mating period inhibited conception.

Pregnancy: Category B. There were 24 out of 204 miscarriages and three abortions induced because of major malformations. Two of the 148 single live-born infants had significant malformations: one megaureter, one scaphocephaly. Follow-up of babies indicates normal physical and mental development. Use this drug during pregnancy only if clearly needed.

Pregnancy-induced hypertension – Do not use dopamine agonists in patients with pregnancy-induced hypertension, for example, preeclampsia and eclampsia, unless the potential benefit is judged to outweigh the possible risk.

Lactation: It is not known whether this drug is excreted in breast milk. Decide whether to discontinue nursing or to discontinue the drug, taking into account the importance of the drug to the mother. Use of cabergoline for the inhibition or suppression of physiologic lactation is not recommended.

The prolactin-lowering action of cabergoline suggests that it will interfere with lactation. Because of this interference with lactation, do not give to women postpartum who are breastfeeding or who are planning to breastfeed.

Postpartum lactation inhibition or suppression – Cabergoline is not indicated for the inhibition or suppression of physiologic lactation. Use of bromocriptine, another dopamine agonist for this purpose, has been associated with cases of hypertension, stroke and seizures.

Children: Safety and effectiveness of cabergoline in pediatric patients have not been established.

Precautions:

Monitoring: Monitor prolactin levels monthly until prolactin levels are normalized (< 20 mcg/L in women and < 15 mcg/L in men).

Orthostatic hypotension: Initial doses > 1 mg may produce orthostatic hypotension. Exercise caution when administering cabergoline with other medications known to lower blood pressure.

CABERGOLINE

Drug Interactions:

Cabergoline Drug Interactions

Precipitant drug	Object drug*		Description
Cabergoline	Antihypertensives	↑	Additive hypotensive effects may occur when cabergoline is administered with other hypotensive medications. In addition, antihypertensive dosage adjustments may be necessary if antihypertensive medications are administered concurrently with cabergoline.
Dopamine (D_2) antagonists (eg, phenothiazines, butyrophenones, thioxanthenes or metoclopramide)	Cabergoline	↓	Dopamine (D_2) antagonists may reduce the therapeutic effects of cabergoline. Do not administer with cabergoline.

* ↑ = Object drug increased. ↓ = Object drug decreased.

Adverse Reactions:

Cabergoline Adverse Reactions Compared with Bromocriptine (%)

Adverse Reaction	Cabergoline	Bromocriptine
Body as a whole		
Asthenia	6	6
Fatigue	5	8
Syncope	1	1
Influenza-like symptoms	1	-
Malaise	1	-
Periorbital edema	1	1
Peripheral edema	1	4
Hot flashes	1	-
CNS		
Headache	26	27
Dizziness	17	18
Somnolence	5	-
Vertigo	4	4
Paresthesia	2	3
Depression	3	-
Nervousness	2	-
Anxiety	+	-
Insomnia	+	-
GU		
Breast pain	1	-
Dysmenorrhea	1	-
Increased libido	+	-

Adverse Reaction	Cabergoline	Bromocriptine
Cardiovascular		
Postural hypotension	4	6
Hypotension	+	6
Palpitations	+	-
GI		
Nausea	29	48
Constipation	7	9
Abdominal pain	5	8
Dyspepsia	5	7
Vomiting	4	7
Dry mouth	2	1
Diarrhea	2	3
Flatulence	2	1
Throat irritation	1	-
Toothache	1	-
Anorexia	+	4
Weight loss/gain	+	-
Miscellaneous		
Nasal stuffiness	+	4
Abnormal vision	1	-
Acne	+	-
Epistaxis	+	-
Pruritus	+	-

+ Occurs, but percentage is unknown.

Compared with bromocriptine, cabergoline was discontinued because of an adverse event in 4 of 221 patients (2%), while bromocriptine was discontinued in 14 of 231 patients (6%). The most common reasons for discontinuation from cabergoline were headache, nausea and vomiting; the most common reasons for discontinuation from bromocriptine were nausea, vomiting, headache, and dizziness or vertigo.

Overdosage:

Overdosage might be expected to produce nasal congestion, syncope or hallucinations. Take measures to support blood pressure if necessary.

Patient Information:

Notify physician if pregnancy occurs or is suspected, or if patient intends to become pregnant during therapy. Perform a pregnancy test if there is any suspicion of pregnancy and discuss discontinuation of treatment.

Inform patients that dizziness or lightheadedness may occur if they stand up too fast. If this occurs, have them get up slowly and avoid sudden changes in posture.

CABERGOLINE

Administration and Dosage:

Approved by the FDA on December 23, 1996.

The recommended dosage of cabergoline for initiation of therapy is 0.25 mg twice a week. Dosage may be increased by 0.25 mg twice weekly to ≤ 1 mg twice a week according to the patient's serum prolactin level.

Dosage increases should not occur more rapidly than every 4 weeks. If the patient does not respond adequately and no additional benefit is observed with higher doses, use the lowest dose that achieved maximal response and consider other therapeutic approaches.

After a normal serum prolactin level has been maintained for 6 months, cabergoline may be discontinued. Periodically monitor the serum prolactin level to determine if or when treatment with cabergoline should be reinstituted. The durability of efficacy beyond 24 months of therapy with cabergoline has not been established.

Rx	**Dostinex** (Pharmacia & Upjohn)	**Tablets:** 0.5 mg	(PU 700). White, scored. Capsule shaped. In bottles of 8.

HYALURONIDASE

Actions:

Pharmacology: Hyaluronidase, a protein enzyme, is a preparation of highly purified bovine testicular hyaluronidase. The exact chemical structure of this enzyme is unknown. Hyaluronidase is available in two dosage forms.

Hyaluronidase is a spreading or diffusing substance which modifies the permeability of connective tissue through the hydrolysis of hyaluronic acid, a polysaccharide found in the intracellular ground substance of connective tissue, and of certain specialized tissues. This temporarily decreases the viscosity of the cellular cement and promotes diffusion of injected fluids or of localized transudates or exudates, thus facilitating their absorption.

The rate of diffusion is proportionate to the amount of enzyme, and the extent is proportionate to the volume of solution.

Studies have demonstrated that hyaluronidase is antigenic; repeated injections of relatively large amounts of this enzyme may result in the formation of neutralizing antibodies. The reconstitution of the dermal barrier removed by intradermal injection of hyaluronidase (20, 2, 0.2, 0.02 and 0.002 U/ml) to adult humans indicated that at 24 hours the restoration of the barrier is incomplete and inversely related to the dosage of enzyme; at 48 hours, the barrier is completely restored in all treated areas.

Indications:

Absorption facilitators: Adjuvant to increase the absorption and dispersion of other injected drugs.

Hypodermoclysis.

Urography: Adjunct in SC urography for improving resorption of radiopaque agents. When IV administration cannot be successfully accomplished, particularly in infants and small children.

Contraindications:

Hypersensitivity to hyaluronidase. Conduct a preliminary test for sensitivity; injection into or around an infected or acutely inflamed area that is known or suspected to be cancerous (because of the danger of spreading a localized infection).

Warnings:

Concomitant therapy: When considering the administration of any other drug with hyaluronidase, consult appropriate references to determine the usual precautions for the use of the other drug (eg, when epinephrine is injected along with hyaluronidase, observe the precautions for the use of epinephrine in cardiovascular disease, thyroid disease, diabetes, digital nerve block, ischemia of the fingers and toes).

Skin test: Perform a preliminary skin test for sensitivity to hyaluronidase with an intradermal injection of ≈ 0.02 ml of the solution. A positive reaction consists of a wheal with pseudopods appearing within 5 minutes, persisting for 20 to 30 minutes and accompanied by localized itching. Transient vasodilation at the site of the test (ie, erythema) is not a positive reaction.

Pregnancy: Category C. It is not known whether hyaluronidase can cause fetal harm when administered to a pregnant woman. Use only if clearly needed.

Human studies on the effect of intravaginal hyaluronidase in sterility due to oligospermia indicated that hyaluronidase may aid conception. Thus, it appears that hyaluronidase may not adversely affect fertility in females. Administration of hyaluronidase during labor has caused no complications. No increase in blood loss or differences in cervical trauma were seen.

Lactation: It is not known whether hyaluronidase is excreted in breast milk. Exercise caution when hyaluronidase is administered to a nursing woman.

Children: Hyaluronidase may be added to small volumes of solution (up to 200 ml), such as a small clysis for infants or solutions of drugs for SC injection. Remember the potential for chemical or physical incompatibilities.

Drug Interactions:

Local anesthetics: When hyaluronidase is added to a local anesthetic agent, it hastens the onset of analgesia and tends to reduce the swelling caused by local infiltration, but the wider spread of the local anesthetic solution increases its absorption; this shortens its duration of action and tends to increase the incidence of systemic reaction.

Adverse Reactions:

The SC administration of hyaluronidase has been associated with very few adverse reactions. Allergic reactions (urticaria) are rare. Anaphylactic-like reactions following retrobulbar block or IV injections have occurred in isolated cases. Cardiac fibrillation has been encountered once.

HYALURONIDASE

Overdosage:

Symptoms: Local edema or urticaria, erythema, chills, nausea, vomiting, dizziness, tachycardia and hypotension.

Treatment: Discontinue enzyme and initiate supportive measures immediately. Agents such as epinephrine, corticosteroids and antihistamines should always be available for emergency treatment. Refer to General Management of Acute Overdosage.

Administration and Dosage:

Lyophilized powder for injection: Add 1 ml of 0.9% sodium chloride to a vial containing 150 U of hyaluronidase, and 10 ml of 0.9% sodium chloride to a vial containing 1,500 U of hyaluronidase, respectively, to provide a solution containing approximately 150 U/ml.

Absorption and dispersion of injected drugs: Add 150 U hyaluronidase to the injection solution. To prepare a solution containing epinephrine, add 0.5 ml epinephrine HCl injection (1:1000) to the above solution. Before adding hyaluronidase to a solution containing another drug, consult appropriate references regarding physical or chemical incompatibilities.

Hypodermoclysis: Insert needle with tip lying free and movable between skin and muscle; begin clysis. Fluid should start in readily without pain or lump. Then inject hyaluronidase solution into rubber tubing close to needle. An alternate method is to inject the solution under skin prior to clysis. 150 U will facilitate absorption of 1000 ml or more of solution. Observe same precautions for restoring fluid and electrolyte balance as in IV injections. Individualize dosage, administration, and type of solution (saline, glucose, Ringer's, etc). When solutions devoid of inorganic electrolytes are given by hypodermoclysis, hypovolemia may occur. This may be prevented by using solutions containing adequate amounts of inorganic electrolytes or controlling the volume and speed of administration.

Hyaluronidase may be added to small volumes of solution (up to 200 ml), such as small clysis for infants or solutions of drugs for SC injection.

For children less than 3 years old. Limit the volume of a single clysis to 200 ml.

Premature infants or during the neonatal period. Do not exceed 25 ml/kg/day. The rate of administration should not be greater than 2 ml/minute.

Older patients – Do not exceed the rate and volume of administration employed for IV infusion.

Subcutaneous urography: With the patient prone, 75 U of hyaluronidase is injected SC over each scapula, followed by injection of the contrast medium at the same sites.

Not recommended for IV use.

Storage/Stability: Keep lyophilized hyaluronidase in a dry place. Sterile reconstituted solution may be stored below 30°C (86°F) for 2 weeks without significant loss of potency. Hyaluronidase solution must be refrigerated.

Rx	**Wydase** (Wyeth-Ayerst)	Purified bovine testicular hyaluronidase. **Injection, lyophilized powder:** 150 units per vial	In 1 ml vials.[1]
		1500 units per vial	In 10 ml vials.[1]
		Injection, stabilized solution: 150 units per ml	In 1 and 10 ml vials.[2]

[1] With lactose and thimerosal.

[2] With sodium chloride, EDTA and thimerosal.

PSORALENS

Warning:

Methoxsalen with ultraviolet (UV) radiation should be used only by physicians with competence in diagnosis and treatment of psoriasis and vitiligo, and with special training and experience in photochemotherapy. Constantly supervise such therapy. For psoriasis, restrict photochemotherapy to patients with severe, recalcitrant, disabling psoriasis not adequately responsive to other therapies, and only when diagnosis is supported by biopsy. Because of possible ocular damage, skin aging and skin cancer (including melanoma), inform patient of risks.

Never dispense methoxsalen lotion to a patient.

These are potent drugs, capable of producing severe burns if improperly used. Read entire monograph before prescribing or dispensing these medications.

Caution:

Oxsoralen-Ultra should not be used interchangeably with regular *Oxsoralen*. This new dosage form of methoxsalen exhibits significantly greater bioavailability and earlier photosensitization onset time than previous dosage forms. Treat patients in accordance with dosimetry specifically recommended for this product. Determine minimum phototoxic dose (MPD) and phototoxic peak time after drug administration prior to onset of photochemotherapy with this dosage form.

Actions:

Pharmacology: Normal skin pigmentation is due to melanin formed by the oxidation of tyrosine to dopa (dihydroxyphenylalanine). Melanin must be activated by radiant energy in the form of UV light, preferably between 290 and 380 nm. The combination treatment regimen of psoralen (P) and UV radiation of 320 to 400 nm wavelength (UVA) is known by the acronym PUVA. Skin reactivity to UVA radiation is markedly enhanced by the ingestion of methoxsalen.

Orally administered methoxsalen reaches the skin via the blood and UVA penetrates well into the skin. If sufficient cell injury occurs in the skin, an inflammatory reaction occurs. The most obvious manifestation of this reaction is delayed erythema, which may not begin for several hours and peaks at 48 to 72 hours. The inflammation is followed over several days to weeks by repair which is manifested by increased melanization of the epidermis and thickening of the stratum corneum.

The exact mechanism of action of psoralens in the process of melanogenesis is not known. The action of these drugs depends upon the presence of functional melanocytes and their proliferation (mitotic activation) by the photoactivated psoralen. One belief is that exposure of methoxsalen-treated patients to UV light thickens the stratum corneum, induces an inflammatory reaction and increases the amount of melanin in exposed areas. The exact mechanism of action of methoxsalen with the epidermal melanocytes and keratinocytes is not known.

Methoxsalen acts as a photosensitizer; subsequent exposure to UVA can lead to cell injury. In the treatment of psoriasis, the mechanism is assumed to be DNA photodamage and resulting decrease in cell proliferation, but other vascular, leukocyte or cell regulatory mechanisms may also be involved. The best known biochemical reaction of methoxsalen is with DNA. Methoxsalen, upon photoactivation, conjugates and forms covalent bonds with DNA which leads to the formation of both monofunctional (addition to a single strand of DNA) and bifunctional (crosslinking of psoralen to both strands of DNA) adducts. Reactions with proteins have also been described.

Pharmacokinetics: Oral psoralen is more than 95% absorbed from the GI tract. Concomitant administration with food increases peak serum concentrations.

Oxsoralen-Ultra Capsules reach peak drug levels in 0.5 to 1 hour (mean = 1.8 hours) vs to 1.5 to 6 hours (mean = 3 hours) for regular *Osxoralen* when given with 8 ounces of milk. Maximum bioavailability of *8-MOP* is reached in 1.5 to 3 hours (mean 2 hours). Peak drug levels were twofold to threefold greater when overall extent of drug absorption was approximately twofold greater for *Oxsoralen-Ultra Capsules* vs *Oxsoralen Capsules*. Detectable methoxsalen levels were observed up to 12 hours post-dose. Half-life is ≈ 2 hours. Photosensitivity studies demonstrate a shorter time of peak photosensitivity of 1.5 to 2.1 hours vs 3.9 to 4.25 hours for *Oxsoralen*. In addition, the mean minimal erythema dose for *Oxsoralen-Ultra* is substantially less than that required for *Oxsoralen*.

Methoxsalen is reversibly bound to serum albumin and is preferentially taken up by epidermal cells. Methoxsalen is rapidly metabolized. Accumulation does not occur during continuous use; metabolism occurs in hepatic microsomal enzymes. About 95% is excreted in urine within 24 hours; 4% to 10% is excreted in feces.

Trioxsalen possesses greater activity than methoxsalen, yet its median lethal dose is 6 times that of methoxsalen.

PSORALENS

Indications:

Oxsoralen, Oxsoralen-Ultra, 8-MOP: Symptomatic control of severe recalcitrant disabling psoriasis not responsive to other therapy when the diagnosis has been supported by biopsy. Administer only in conjunction with a schedule of controlled doses of long wave UV radiation.

Oxsoralen (oral and topical), 8-MOP, trioxsalen: With long wave UV radiation for repigmentation of idiopathic vitiligo.

8-MOP: With long wave UV radiation of white blood cells (photopheresis) and the UVAR System in the palliative treatment of the skin manifestations of cutaneous T–cell lymphoma (CTCL) in persons who have not been responsive to other forms of treatment. Refer to the UVAR System Operator's Manual for specific warnings, cautions, indications and instructions related to photopheresis.

Trioxsalen: For increasing tolerance to sunlight and for enhancing pigmentation.

Contraindications:

Idiosyncratic reactions to psoralen compounds; melanoma or a history of melanoma; invasive squamous cell carcinomas; aphakia (increased risk of retinal damage due to the absence of lenses). Diseases associated with photosensitivity, such as porphyria, acute lupus erythematosus, porphyria cutanea tarda, erythropoietic protoporphyria, variegate porphyria, xeroderma pigmentosum, leukoderma of infectious origin and in albinism.

Do not use with any preparation having internal or external photosensitizing capacity.

Oral trioxsalen and methoxsalen lotion are contraindicated in children ≤ 12 years old.

Warnings:

Skin burning: Serious burns from either UVA or sunlight (even through window glass) can result if recommended drug dosage or exposure schedules are not maintained.

Carcinoma: A 5 year prospective study of 1380 patients revealed an ≈ ninefold increase in risks of squamous cell carcinoma among PUVA patients. This appears greatest among patients who are fair skinned or who had pre-PUVA exposure to prolonged tar and UVB treatment, ionizing radiation or arsenic. An ≈ twofold increase in risk of basal cell carcinoma was also noted. Two patients developed malignant melanoma, and more than developed macular pigmented lesions on buttocks. Observe patients with a history of previous grenz or x-ray therapy, basal cell carcinoma and arsenic therapy for signs of carcinoma.

A study in 690 patients for up to 4 years showed no increase in risk of non-melanoma skin cancer. However, patients had significantly less PUVA exposure. There is no evidence of an increased risk of melanoma in PUVA patients, but there is a need for continued evaluation of melanoma risk in these patients.

In a study in Indian patients treated for 4 years for vitiligo, 12% developed keratoses, but not cancer, in the depigmented, vitiliginous areas.

Cataracts: The concentration of methoxsalen in the lens is proportional to the serum level. If the lens is exposed to UVA during the presence of methoxsalen in the lens, photochemical action may lead to irreversible binding of methoxsalen to proteins and the DNA components of the lens. However, if the lens is shielded from UVA, the methoxsalen will diffuse out of the lens in a 24 hour period. Emphatically instruct patients to wear UVA-absorbing, wrap-around sunglasses for the 24 hours following ingestion of methoxsalen, whether exposed to direct or indirect sunlight in the open, or through window glass.

Among patients using proper eye protection, there is no evidence for a significantly increased risk of cataracts in association with PUVA therapy. Of 1380 patients, 35 have developed cataracts in the 5 years since their first PUVA treatment, an incidence comparable to that expected in a population of this size and age distribution. No relationship between PUVA dose and cataract risk has been noted.

Actinic degeneration: Exposure to sunlight or UV radiation may prematurely age skin.

Cardiac disease: Do not treat patients with cardiac disease or who may be unable to tolerate prolonged standing or exposure to heat stress in a vertical UVA chamber.

Total cumulative safe UVA dosage over long periods of time is not established.

Do not increase the dosage of **trioxsalen** and exposure time. To prevent harmful effects, instruct patient to adhere to prescribed dosage schedule and procedure.

Hepatic function impairment: Since hepatic biotransformation is necessary for drug urinary excretion, treat patients with hepatic insufficiency with caution.

Pregnancy: Category C. It is not known whether psoralens can cause fetal harm when administered to a pregnant woman or can affect reproduction capacity. Use only if clearly needed.

PSORALENS

Lactation: It is not known whether these agents are excreted in breast milk. Exercise caution when administering to a nursing woman.

Children: Safety of methoxsalen use has not been established. Potential hazards include possible carcinogenicity and cataractogenicity, and probable actinic degeneration. Oral trioxsalen and methoxsalen lotion are contraindicated in children ≤ 12 years of age.

Precautions:

Monitoring: Perform the following before therapy, retest in 6 to 12 months and conduct additional tests at more extended time periods as indicated: CBC (hemoglobin or hematocrit; WBC, if abnormal, a differential count), antinuclear antibodies, liver and renal function tests and ophthalmologic examination.

Vitiligo therapy: Do not increase the dosage of methoxsalen above 0.6 mg/kg; overdosage may result in serious burning of the skin. Provide eye and skin sun protection.

Furocoumarin-containing foods: No clinical reports or tests verify that more severe reactions may result from concomitant ingestion, but warn the patient that eating limes, figs, parsley, parsnips, mustard, carrots and celery might be dangerous.

Photosensitivity: Exercise special care in treating patients who are receiving concomitant therapy (either topically or systemically) with known photosensitizing agents such as **anthralin, coal tar** or **coal tar derivatives, griseofulvin, phenothiazines, nalidixic acid, halogenated salicylanilides** (bacteriostatic soaps), **sulfonamides, tetracyclines, thiazides** and certain organic staining dyes such as **methylene blue, toluidine blue, rose bengal** and **methyl orange.**

Tartrazine sensitivity: Some of these products contain tartrazine, which may cause allergic-type reactions (including bronchial asthma) in susceptible individuals. Although the incidence of tartrazine sensitivity in the general population is low, it is frequently seen in patients who also have aspirin hypersensitivity. Specific products containing tartrazine are identified in the product listings.

Adverse Reactions:

Severe burns can result from excessive sunlight or sunlamp UV exposure.

Basal cell epitheliomas have been removed from exposed and unexposed areas.

Nausea is common (10%).

Other effects of **methoxsalen** include nervousness; insomnia; psychological depression; edema; dizziness; headache; malaise; hypopigmentation; vesiculation and bullae formation; nonspecific rash; herpes simplex; miliaria; urticaria; folliculitis; GI disturbances; cutaneous tenderness; leg cramps; hypotension; extension of psoriasis and depression.

Combined methoxsalen/UVA therapy:

Pruritus (approximately 10%) – Alleviate with frequent application of bland emollients or other topical agents; severe pruritus may require systemic treatment. If pruritus is unresponsive, shield pruritic areas from further UVA exposure until the condition resolves. If intractable pruritus is generalized, discontinue UVA treatment until pruritus disappears.

Erythema – Mild, transient erythema 24 to 48 hours after PUVA therapy is expected; it indicates a therapeutic interaction between methoxsalen and UVA. Shield any area showing moderate erythema during subsequent UVA exposures until the erythema has resolved. Erythema greater than Grade 2 which appears within 24 hours after UVA treatment may signal a potentially severe burn. Erythema may worsen progressively over the next 24 hours since peak erythemal reaction characteristically occurs 48 hours or later after methoxsalen ingestion. Protect the patient from further UVA exposures and sunlight; monitor closely.

Overdosage:

Induce emesis within the first 2 to 3 hours after ingestion of methoxsalen, since maximum blood levels are reached by this time. Follow accepted procedures for treatment of severe burns. Keep the individual in a darkened room for 8 to 24 or more hours or until cutaneous reactions subside.

Patient Information:

Use **topical methoxsalen** only on small, well defined lesions which can be protected by clothing from subsequent exposure to radiant energy. If used to treat vitiligo of face or hands, keep the treated area protected from light by use of protective clothing or sunscreens. The area of application may be highly photosensitive for several days and may result in severe burns if exposed to additional UV or sunlight.

Before methoxsalen ingestion: Do not sunbathe during the 24 hours prior to methoxsalen ingestion and UV exposure. Sunburn may prevent an accurate evaluation of the patient's response to photochemotherapy.

PSORALENS

After methoxsalen ingestion: Wear UVA-absorbing wrap-around sunglasses during daylight for 24 hours to prevent cataracts (see Warnings). The protective eyewear must prevent entry of stray radiation to the eyes, including that which may enter from the sides of the eyewear. Visual discrimination should be permitted by the eyewear for patient well-being and comfort.

Avoid sun exposure, even through window glass or cloud cover, for at least 8 hours after methoxsalen ingestion. If sun exposure cannot be avoided, wear protective devices such as a hat and gloves, or apply sunscreens that filter out UVA radiation (eg, sunscreens with SPF ≥ 15). Apply sunscreens to all areas that might be exposed to the sun (including lips). Do not apply sunscreens to areas affected by psoriasis until after treatment in the UVA chamber.

During PUVA therapy, wear total UVA-absorbing/blocking goggles mechanically designed to give maximal ocular protection. Failure to do so may increase the risk of cataract formation. A radiometer can verify elimination of UVA transmission through the goggles.

Protect abdominal skin, breasts, genitalia and other sensitive areas for approximately one-third of the initial exposure time until tanning occurs. Unless affected by disease, shield male genitalia.

After combined methoxsalen/UVA therapy: Wear UVA-absorbing wrap-around sunglasses during the daylight for 24 hrs after therapy. Do not sunbathe for 48 hrs after therapy. Erythema or burning due to photochemotherapy and sunburn are additive.

Minimize or avoid nausea by taking the drug with milk or food, or by dividing into two doses, taken ½ hour apart.

Do not exceed prescribed dosage or exposure time.

Avoid furocoumarin-containing foods (eg, limes, figs, parsley, parsnips, mustard, carrots, celery).

METHOXSALEN (8-Methoxypsoralen, 8-MOP), ORAL

Complete prescribing information begins in the Psoralens group monograph.

Indications:

Oxsoralen, Oxsoralen-Ultra, 8-MOP: Symptomatic control of severe, recalcitrant disabling psoriasis not responsive to other therapy when the diagnosis has been supported by biopsy. Administer only in conjunction with a schedule of controlled doses of long wave UV radiation.

Oxsoralen, 8-MOP: With long wave UV radiation for repigmentation of idiopathic vitiligo.

8-MOP: With long wave UV radiation of white blood cells (photopheresis) and the UVAR System in the palliative treatment of the skin manifestations of cutaneous T–cell lymphoma (CTCL) in persons who have not been responsive to other forms of treatment. Refer to the UVAR System Operator's Manual for specific warnings, cautions, indications and instructions related to photopheresis.

Administration and Dosage:

Caution: Oxsoralen-Ultra represents a new methoxsalen dose form. It exhibits significantly greater bioavailability and earlier photosensitization onset time than previous forms. Evaluate patients by determining minimum phototoxic dose (MPD) and phototoxic peak time after administration prior to onset of photochemotherapy with this dosage form. Human bioavailability studies indicate the following dosage and administration directions are to be used as a guideline only.

Vitiligo (Oxsoralen, 8-MOP): 20 mg daily in one dose with milk or food, taken 2 to 4 hours before UV exposure. Therapy should be on alternate days, and never on consecutive days.

Limit exposure time to sunlight according to the following table:

SUGGESTED SUN EXPOSURE GUIDE

Exposure	Basic Skin Color		
	Light	Medium	Dark
Initial Exposure	15 min	20 min	25 min
Second Exposure	20 min	25 min	30 min
Third Exposure	25 min	30 min	35 min
Fourth Exposure	30 min	35 min	40 min
Subsequent Exposure	Gradually increase exposure based on erythema and tenderness of amelanotic skin.		

METHOXSALEN (8-Methoxypsoralen, 8-MOP), ORAL

Psoriasis: Initial therapy: Take dose 2 hours before UVA exposure (*Oxsoralen-Ultra* 1 to 2 hours with low fat food or milk), according to the following table:

METHOXSALEN DOSING							
	Patient Weight						
kg lb	< 30 < 65	30-50 65-100	51-65 101-145	66-80 146-175	81-90 176-200	91-115 201-250	> 115 > 250
Oxsoralen, 8-MOP: mg	10	20	30	40	50	60	70
Oxsoralen-Ultra							
Low dose: mg	10	10	20	20	30	30	40
mg/kg	0.33	0.33	0.39	0.30	0.37	0.33	0.35
High-dose: mg	10	20	30	40	50	60	70
mg/kg	0.33	0.67	0.59	0.61	0.62	0.66	0.61

Weight change: If the patient's weight changes during treatment and falls into an adjacent weight range/dose category, no dose change is usually required. If a weight change is sufficiently great to modify dose, adjust UVA exposure.

Doses/week: Determine the number of doses per week of methoxsalen capsules by the patient's schedule of UVA exposures. Never give treatments more often than once every other day (*Oxsoralen-Ultra* once every day), because the full extent of phototoxic reactions may not be evident until 48 hours after each exposure.

Dosage increase: If there is no response, or only minimal response, after 15 treatments, increase dosage by 10 mg (a one-time increase). Continue this increased dosage for the remainder of the course of treatment, but do not exceed it.

Cutaneous T–cell lymphoma: Two hours after 8-MOP administration, a pint of blood is withdrawn from the patient and infused into the UVAR system. The red cells and plasma are immediately returned to the patient; before the leukocyte fraction is returned to the patient, it is exposed to UV radiation, which activates the methoxsalen. The methoxsalen becomes an alkylating agent that deactivates when no longer exposed to light. The treated white cells (unable to reproduce) are then returned to the patient. Refer to the UVAR Photopheresis System (by Therakos) for further details.

For UVA source specifications/PUVA protocols, see manufacturer information.

Rx	**Oxsoralen-Ultra**[1] (ICN Pharm)	**Capsules:** 10 mg (soft capsules)	In 50s and 100s.
Rx	**8-MOP** (ICN Pharm)	**Capsules:** 10 mg	Tartrazine. In 8s.

[1] Not interchangeable with *Oxsoralen*. Refer to manufacturer's literature for complete information.

METHOXSALEN (8-Methoxypsoralen, 8-MOP), TOPICAL

Note: Never dispense this product to the patient.

Complete prescribing information for these products begins in the Psoralens group monograph.

Indications:

Repigmenting agent in vitiligo, used in conjunction with controlled doses of UVA (320 to 400 nm) or sunlight.

Patient Information:

Protect treated areas from light by use of a bandage, gloves or a sunscreen (particularly when treating vitiligo of the face or hands).

Administration and Dosage:

Apply lotion to a small, well defined, vitiliginous lesion, then expose this area to UVA light. Initial exposure time must not exceed one-half the minimal erythema dose.

Regulate treatment intervals by erythema response (once a week or less, depending on the results).

Pigmentation may begin after a few weeks; significant repigmentation may take up to 6 to 9 months. Periodic treatment may be needed to retain the new pigment.

Essentially, idiopathic vitiligo is reversible, but not equally in every patient. Repigmentation varies in completeness, time of onset and duration; it occurs more rapidly on fleshy regions such as the face, abdomen and buttocks, and less rapidly over bony areas such as the dorsum of the hands and feet.

Rx	**Oxsoralen** (ICN Pharm)	**Lotion:** 1%	In 30 ml.

TRIOXSALEN, ORAL

Complete prescribing information for these products begins in the Psoralens group monograph.

Indications:

Taken 2 hours before measured periods of exposure to UV light, trioxsalen facilitates:

Repigmentation of idiopathic vitiligo, not equally reversible in every patient, will vary in completeness, time of onset and duration. Repigmentation occurs more rapidly on fleshy regions (face, abdomen and buttocks), and less rapidly over bony areas (dorsum of the hands and feet). Repigmentation may begin after a few weeks; however, significant results may take 6 to 9 months, and repigmentation at the optimum level may require maintenance dosage. If follicular repigmentation is not apparent after 3 months of daily treatment, discontinue treatment.

Increasing tolerance to sunlight: In blond persons and those with fair complexions who suffer painful reactions when exposed to sunlight, trioxsalen aids in increasing resistance to solar damage. Persons who are allergic to sunlight or who exhibit sun sensitivity may benefit from the protective action. In albinism, trioxsalen will increase tolerance to sunlight, although no pigment is formed. This protective action seems to be related to the thickening of the horny layer and retention of melanin which produces a thickened melanized stratum corneum and formation of a stratum lucidum.

Enhancing pigmentation: Use of trioxsalen accelerates pigmentation only when followed by exposure to sunlight or UV irradiation. The increase in pigmentation occurs gradually within a few days of repeated exposure and may become equivalent in degree to that achieved by a full summer of sun exposure. Since sufficient pigment will have been formed within 2 weeks of continuous therapy, discontinue use beyond this period. Maintain pigmentation by periodic exposure to sunlight.

Administration and Dosage:

Wear sunglasses during exposure and protect lips with a light-screening lipstick. May be taken with food or milk.

Adults and children over 12 years of age:

Vitiligo – 10 mg daily, 2 to 4 hours before measured periods of exposure.

To increase tolerance to sunlight or to enhance pigmentation – 10 mg daily, 2 hours before measured periods of exposure to sun or UV irradiation; do not continue for longer than 14 days. Do NOT increase the dosage, as severe burning may occur.

Limit exposure time according to the following:

SUGGESTED SUN EXPOSURE GUIDE

Exposure	Basic Skin Color	
	Light	Medium
Initial Exposure	15 min	20 min
Second Exposure	20 min	25 min
Third Exposure	25 min	30 min
Fourth Exposure	30 min	35 min
Subsequent Exposure	Gradually increase exposure based on erythema and tenderness.	

Rx	**Trisoralen** (ICN Pharm)	**Tablets:** 5 mg	Tartrazine. In 28s and 100s.

BETA-CAROTENE

Actions:

Pharmacology: Beta-carotene, a vitamin A precursor, is a carotenoid pigment occurring naturally in green and yellow vegetables. In terms of vitamin activity, 0.6 mcg of dietary beta-carotene is equivalent to 0.3 mcg of vitamin A (retinol). Bioavailability of beta-carotene depends on fat in the diet to act as a carrier, and on bile in the intestinal tract for its absorption. Beta-carotene is metabolized, primarily in the intestine, to vitamin A at a rate of approximately 50% to 60% of normal dietary intake. The rate falls off rapidly as intake goes up. In humans, an appreciable amount of unchanged beta-carotene is absorbed and stored in various tissues, especially the depot fat. Small amounts may be converted to vitamin A in the liver. The vitamin A derived from beta-carotene follows the same metabolic pathway as that from dietary sources. The major route of elimination is fecal excretion.

Indications:

To reduce severity of photosensitivity reactions in patients with erythropoietic protoporphyria.

Contraindications:

Hypersensitivity to beta-carotene.

Warnings:

Beta-carotene has not been proven effective as a sunscreen.

Renal/Hepatic function impairment: Give with caution to patients with impaired renal or hepatic function, because safety in these conditions has not been established.

Beta-carotene fulfills normal vitamin A requirements; do not prescribe additional vitamin A.

Pregnancy: Category C. Beta-carotene caused an increase in resorption rate but was not teratogenic when given to rats at higher than recommended human doses. There are no adequate and well controlled studies in pregnant women. Use only when clearly needed and when potential benefits outweigh potential hazards to the fetus.

Lactation: It is not known whether this drug is excreted in breast milk. Exercise caution when beta-carotene is administered to a nursing mother.

Adverse Reactions:

Some patients may have occasional loose stools; this is sporadic and may not require drug discontinuation. Ecchymoses and arthralgia (rare) have also been reported.

Patient Information:

Take with meals.

The skin may appear slightly yellow while receiving beta-carotene therapy.

Do not increase exposure to sunlight until carotenemic (first seen as yellowness of palms and soles), usually after 2 to 6 weeks of therapy. Then increase sun exposure gradually. The protective effect is not total; patients must establish their own limits of exposure. Continue sun protection.

Administration and Dosage:

Adjust dosage depending on severity of the symptoms and patient response. Several weeks of therapy are necessary to accumulate enough beta-carotene in the skin to exert its effect. Administer either as a single daily dose or in divided doses, preferably with meals.

Adults: 30 to 300 mg/day.

Children (< 14 years of age): 30 to 150 mg/day. Capsules may be opened and contents mixed in orange or tomato juice to aid administration.

otc	**Provatene** (Solgar)	**Soft Gel Perles:** 15 mg	In 60s and 180s.

RILUZOLE

Actions:

Pharmacology: The etiology and pathogenesis of amyotrophic lateral sclerosis (ALS; Lou Gehrig's disease) are not known, although a number of hypotheses have been advanced. One hypothesis is that motor neurons, made vulnerable through either genetic predisposition or environmental factors, are injured by glutamate. In some cases of familial ALS the enzyme superoxide dismutase has been defective.

The mode of action of riluzole, a benzathiazole, is unknown. Its pharmacological properties include the following, some of which may be related to its effect: 1) an inhibitory effect on glutamate release; 2) inactivation of voltage-dependent sodium channels; and 3) ability to interfere with intracellular events that follow transmitter binding at excitatory amino acid receptors.

In a single study, riluzole delayed median time to death in a transgenic mouse model of ALS. These mice express human superoxide dismutase bearing one of the mutations found in one of the familial forms of human ALS.

It is also neuroprotective in in vivo models of neuronal injury involving excitotoxic mechanisms. It protected cultured rat motor neurons from the excitotoxic effects of glutamic acid and prevented death of cortical neurons induced by anoxia.

Due to its blockade of glutamatergic neurotransmission, riluzole also exhibits myorelaxant and sedative properties in animals at doses of 30 mg/kg (about 20 times the recommended human daily dose), and anticonvulsant properties at 2.5 mg/kg.

Pharmacokinetics:

Absorption/Distribution – Riluzole is well absorbed (≈ 90%), with average absolute oral bioavailability of ≈ 50%. Pharmacokinetics are linear over a dose range of 25 to 100 mg every 12 hours. A high fat meal decreases absorption, reducing AUC ≈ 20% and peak blood levels by ≈ 45%. The mean elimination half-life of riluzole is 12 hours after repeated doses. With multiple dose administration, riluzole accumulates in plasma by about 2–fold, and steady-state is reached in < 5 days. Riluzole is 96% bound to plasma proteins, mainly to albumin and lipoproteins.

Metabolism/Excretion – Riluzole is extensively metabolized to six major and a number of minor metabolites, not all of which have been identified. Some metabolites appear pharmacologically active in vitro. The metabolism is mostly hepatic and consists of cytochrome P450 dependent hydroxylation and glucuronidation.

There is marked inter-individual variability in the clearance of riluzole, probably attributable to variability of CYP 1A2 activity, the principal isozyme involved in N-hydroxylation.

In vitro studies using liver microsomes show that hydroxylation of the primary amine group producing N-hydroxyriluzole is the main metabolic pathway. Cytochrome P450 1A2 is the principal isozyme involved in N-hydroxylation. Whereas direct glucuroconjugation of riluzole (involving the glucurotransferase isoform UGT-HP4) is very slow in human liver microsomes, N-hydroxyriluzoe is readily conjugated at the hydroxylamine group resulting in the formation of O- (> 90%) and N-glucuronides.

Following a single 150 mg dose to six healthy males, 90% and 5% was recovered in the urine and feces, respectively, over 7 days. Glucuronides accounted for > 85% of the metabolites in urine. Only 2% was recovered in the urine as unchanged drug.

Special populations:

Hepatic/Renal disease – Because riluzole is extensively metabolized and subsequently excreted in the urine, it is likely that functional hepatic and renal impairment will reduce the clearance of riluzole and its metabolites and lead to higher plasma levels (see Warning).

Elderly – Age related decreased reanl function would be expected to give higher plasma levels of riluzole and metabolites. However, in controlled clinical trials, in which ≈ 30% of patients were > 65 years of age., there were no differences in adverse events between younger and older patients (see Warnings).

Gender – CYP 1A2 activity has been reported to be lower in women than in men. Therefore, a gender effect may result in higher blood concentrations of riluzole and its metabolites in women (see Precautions). No gender effect on favorable or adverse events of riluzole was seen in controlled trials, however.

Smoking – Cigarette smoking is known to induce CYP 1A2. Patients who smoke cigarettes would be expected to eliminate riluzole faster. However, there is no information on the effect of, or need for, dosage adjustment in these patients.

Race – Clearance of riluzole in Japanese subjects native to Japan was found to be 50% lower compared with Caucasians after normalizing for body weight. Although it is not clear if this differenc is due to genetic or environmental factors (eg, smoking, alcohol, coffee, dietary preferences), it is possible that Japanese subjects may possess a lower capacity (oxidative or conjugative) for metabolizing riluzole (see Precautions).

RILUZOLE

Clinical trials: The efficacy of riluzole as a treatment of ALS was established in two trials in which the time to tracheostomy or death was longer for patients randomized to riluzole than for those randomized to placebo. These studies admitted patients with either familial or sporadic ALS, a disease duration of < 5 years and a baseline forced vital capacity ≥ 60%. Although riluzole improved early survival in both studies, measures of muscle strength and neurological function did not show a benefit. Among the patients in whom treatment failed during the study (tracheostomy or death) there was a difference between the treatment groups in median survival of ≈ 60 to 90 days. There was no statistically significant difference in mortality at the end of the studies.

Indications:

Amyotrophic lateral sclerosis (ALS): Treatment of patients with ALS. Riluzole extends survival or time to tracheostomy.

Contraindications:

Severe hypersensitivity reacts to riluzole or any of the tablet components.

Warnings:

Neutropenia: Among ≈ 4000 patients given riluzole for ALS, there were three cases of marked neutropenia (absolute neutrophil < 500/mm^3), all seen within the first 2 months of treatment. In one case, neutrophil counts rose on continued treatment. In a second case, counts rose after therapy was stopped. A third case was more complex, with marked anemia as well as neutropenia and the etiology of both is uncertain. Warn patients to report any febrile illness to the physicians. The report of febrile illness should promt the checking of white blood cell coutns.

Renal function impairment: Use with caution in patients with concomitant renal insufficiency.

Hepatic function impairment: Use with care in patients with current evidence or history of abnormal liver function indicated by significant abnormalities in serum transaminase (SGPT, SGOT), bilirubin or gamma-glutamate transferase (GGT) levels. Baseline elevations of several LFTs (especially elevated bilirubin) should preclude the use of riluzole.

Riluzole, even in patients without a prior history of liver disease. causes serum aminotransferase elevations. Experience in almost 800 ALS patients indicates that ≈ 50% of riluzole-treated patients will experience at least one SGPT level above the upper limit of normaul (ULN), ≈ 8% will hve elevations > 3 × ULN and ≈ 2% will have elevations > 5 × ULN. A single non-ALS patient with epilepsy treated with concomitant carbamazepine and phenobarbital experienced marked, rapid elevations of liver enzymes with jaundice for four months after starting riluzole; these returned to normal 7 weeks after treatment discontinuation.

Maximum increases in serum SGPT usually occurred within 3 months after the start of therapy and were usually transient when < 5 × ULN. In trials, if SGPT levels were < 5 × ULN, treatment continued and SGPT levels usually returned to below 2 × ULN within 2 to 6 monhts. However, treatment in studies was discontinued if SGPT levels exceeded 5 × ULN, so that there is no experience with continued treatmetn of ALS patiens once GSPT values exceed 5 × ULN. There were rare instances of jaundice.

Monitor liver chemistries (see Precautions).

Fertility impairment: Riluzole imipaired fertility when administered to male and female rats prior to and during mating at an oral dose of 15 mg/kg or 1.5 times the maximum daily dose (see Pregnancy).

Elderly: Age-related compromised renal and hepatic function may cause a decrease in clearance of riluzole. In controlled clinical trials, ≈ 30% of patients were > 65 years old. There were no differences in adverse effects between younger and older patients.

Pregnancy: Category C. Administration of riluzole to pregnant animals during the period of organogenesis caused embryotoxicity in rats and rabbits at doses of 27 and 60 mg/kg, respectively, or 2.6 and 11.5 times, respectively, the respectively, the recommended maximum human daily dose. Evidence of maternal toxicity was also observed at these doses. When administered to rats prior to and during mating (males and females) and throughout gestation and lactation (females), riluzole produced adverse effects on pregnancy (decreased implantations, increased intrauterine death) and offspring viability and growth at an oral dose of 15 mg/kg.

There are no adequate and well controlled studies in pregnant women. Use during pregnancy only if the potential benefit justifies the potential risk to the fetus.

Lactation: In rat studies, riluzole was detected in maternal milk. It is not known whether riluzole is excreted in breast milk. Because the potential for serious adverse reactions in nursing infants from riluzole is unknown, advise women not to breastfeed during treatment with riluzole.

Children: The safety and efficacy in children have not been established.

Precautions:

Monitoring: Measure serum aminotransferases including SGPT levels before and during therapy. Evaluate serum SGPT levels every month during the first 3 months of treatment, every 3 months during the remainder of the first year and periodically thereafter. Evaluate serum SGPT levels more frequently in patients who develop elevations (see Warnings).

As noted in the Warnings section, there is no experience with continued treatment of patients once SGPT exceeds 5 × ULN. If a decision is made to continue to treat these patients, frequent monitoring (at least weekly) of complete liver function is recommended. Discontinue treatment if SGPT exceeds 10 × ULN or if clinical jaundice develops. Because there is no experience with rechallenge of patients who have had riluzole discontinued for SGPT > 5 × ULN, no recommendations about restarting riluzole can be made.

In the two controlled trials in patients with ALS, the frequency with which values for hemoglobin, hematocrit and erythrocyte counts fell below the lower limit of normal was greater in riluzole-treated patients than in placebo-treated patients; however, these changes were mild and transient. The proportions of patients observed with abnoramlly low values for these parameters showed a dose-response relationship. Only one patient was discontinued from treatment because of severe anemia. The significance of this finding is unknown.

Special populations: Females and Japanese patients may possess a lower metabolic capacity to eliminate riluzole compared with male and Caucasian subjects, respectively.

Drug Interactions:

Effect of other drugs on riluzole metabolism: In vitro studies using human liver microsomal preparations suggest that CYP 1A2 is the principal isozyme involved in the initial oxidative metabolism of riluzole and therefore potential interactions may occur when riluzole is given concurrently with agents that affect CYP 1A2 activity. Potential inhibitors of CYP 1A2 (eg, caffeine, theophylline, amitriptyline, quinolones) could decrease the rate of riluzole elimination, while inducers of CYP 1A2 (eg, cigarette smoke, charcoal-broiled food, rifampin, omeprazole) could increase the rate of riluzole elimination.

Drug/Food interactions: A high fat meal decreases absorption of riluzole, reducing AUC by ≈ 20% and peak blood levels by ≈ 45%.

Adverse Reactions:

The most commonly observed adverse reactions associated with the use of riluzole were: Asthenia, nausea, dizziness, diarrhea, anorexia, vertigo, somnolence, circumoral paresthesia (dose-related); decreased lung function; abdominal pain; pneumonia; vomiting.

Approximately 14% of patients with ALS who received riluzole in premarketing clinical trials discontinued treatment because of an adverse experience. Of those patients who discontinued due to adverse events, the most commonly reported were: Nausea, abdominal pain, constipation and SGPT elevations.

Riluzole Adverse Reactions (%)

Adverse Reaction	Riluzole 50 mg/day (n = 237)	Riluzole 100 mg/day (n = 313	Riluzole 200 mg/day (n = 244)	Placebo (n = 320)
Body as a whole				
Asthenia	14.8	19.2	20.1	12.2
Headache	8	7.3	7	6.6
Abdominal pain	6.8	5.1	7.8	3.8
Arthralgia	5.1	3.5	1.6	3.4
Back pain	1.7	3.2	4.1	2.5
Aggravation reaction	0.4	1.3	2	0.9
Malaise	0.4	0.6	1.2	0
Metabolic/Nutritional				
Weight loss	4.6	4.8	3.7	4.7
Peripheral edema	4.2	2.9	3.3	2.2
GI				
Nausea	12.2	16.3	20.5	10.6

RILUZOLE

Adverse Reaction	Riluzole 50 mg/day (n = 237)	100 mg/day (n = 313)	200 mg/day (n = 244)	Placebo (n = 320)
Vomiting	4.2	4.2	4.5	1.6
Dyspepsia	2.5	3.8	6.1	5
Anorexia	3.8	3.2	8.6	3.8
Diarrhea	5.5	2.9	9	3.1
Flatulence	2.5	2.6	2	1.9
Stomatitis	0.8	1	1.2	0
Tooth disorder	0	1	1.2	0.3
Oral moniliasis	0.4	0.6	1.2	0.3
CNS				
Hypertonia	5.9	6.1	5.3	5.9
Depression	4.2	4.5	6.1	5
Dizziness	5.1	3.8	12.7	2.5
Dry mouth	3	3.5	2	3.4
Insomnia	2.1	3.5	2.9	3.4
Somnolence	0.8	1.9	4.1	1.3
Vertigo	2.5	1.9	4.5	0.9
Circumoral paresthesia	1.3	1.6	3.3	0
Dermatologic				
Pruritus	3.8	3.8	2.5	3.1
Eczema	0.8	1.6	1.6	0.6
Alopecia	0	1	1.2	0.6
Exfoliative dermatitis	0	0.6	1.2	0
Respiratory				
Decreased lung function	13.1	10.2	16	9.4
Rhinitis	8.9	6.4	7.8	6.3
Increased cough	2.1	2.6	3.7	1.6
Sinusitis	0.4	1	1.6	0.9
Cardiovascular				
Hypertension	6.8	5.1	3.3	4.1
Tachycardia	1.3	2.6	2	13
Phlebitis	0.4	1	0.8	0.3
Palpitation	0.4	0.6	1.2	0.9
Postural hypotension	0.8	0	1.6	0.6
GU				
Urinary tract infection	2.5	2.6	4.5	2.2
Dysuria	0	1	1.2	0.3

Miscellaneous: Adverse events that occurred in > 2% of patients treated with 100 mg/day but equally or more frequently in the placebo group included: Accidental injury; apnea; bronchitis; constipation; death; dysphagia; dyspnea; flu syndrome; heart arrest; increased sputum; pneumonia; respiratory disorder. Dizziness did occur more commonly in females (11%) than in males (4%).

Body as a whole: Hostility (≥ 1); abscess, sespsis, photosensitivity reaction, cellulitis, face edema, hernia, peritonitis, attempted suicide, injection site reaction, chills, flu syndrome, intentional injury, enlarged abdomen, neoplasm (0.1% to 1%); acrodynia, hypothermia, moniliasis, rheumatoid arthritis (≤ 0.1%).

GI: Increased appetite, intestinal obstruction, fecal impaction, GI hemorrhage, GI ulceration, gastritis, fecal incontinence, jaundice, hepatitis, glossitis, gum hemorrhage, pancreatitis, tenesmus, esophageal stenosis (0.1% to 1%); cheilitis, cholecystitis, hematemesis, melena, biliary pain, proctitis, pseudomembranous enterocolitis, enlarged salivary gland, tongue discoloration, tooth caries (≤ 1%).

CNS: Agitation, tremor (≥ 1%); hallucinations, personality disorders, abnormal thinking, coma, paranoid reaction, manic reaction, ataxia, extrapyrimidal syndrome, hypokinesis, urinary retention, emotional ability, delusions, apathy, hypesthesia, incoordination, confusion, convulsion, leg cramps, amnesia, dysarthria, increased libido, stupor, subdural hematoma, abnormal gait, delirium, depersonalization, facial paralysis, hemiplegia, decreased libido, myoclonus (0.1% to 1%); abnormal dreams, acute brain syndrome, CNS depression, dementia, cerebral embolism, euphoria, hypotonia, ileus, peripheral neurities, psychosis, psychotic depression, schizophrenic reaction, trismus, wristdrop (≤ 0.1%).

Dermatologic: Skin ulceration, urticaria, psoriasis, seborrhea, skin disorder, fungal dermatitis (0.1% to 1%); engioedema, contact dermatitis, erythema multiforme, furunculosis, skin moniliasis, skin granuloma, skin nodule (≤ 0.1%).

Respiratory: Hiccough, pleural disorder, asthma, epistaxis, hemoptysis, yawn, hyperventilation, lung edema, hypoventilation, lung carcinoma, hypoxia, laryngitis, pleural effusion, pneumothorax, respiratory monoliasis, stridor (0.1% to 1%).

Cardiovascular: Syncope, hypotension, heart failure, migraine, peripheral vascular disease, angina pectoris, myocardial infarction, ventricular extrasystoles, cerebral hemorrhage, atrial fibrillation, bundle branch block, congestive heart failure, pericarditis, lower extremity embolus, myocardial ischemia, shock (0.1% to 1%); bradycardia, cerebral ischemia, hemorrhage, mesenteric artery occlusion, subarachnoid hemorrhage, supraventricular tachycardia, thrombosis, ventricular fibrillation, ventricular tachycardia (≤ 0.1%).

Metabolic/Nutritional: Gout, respiratory acidosis, edema, thirst, hypokalemia, hyponatremia, weight gain (0.1% to 1%); generalized edema, hypercalcemia, hypercholesteremia (≤ 0.1%).

Endocrine: Diabetes mellitus, thyroid neoplasia (0.1% to 1%); diabetes insipidus, parathyroid disorder (≤ 0.1%).

Hematologic/Lymphatic: Anemia, leukocytosis, leukopenia, ecchymosis (0.1% to 1%); neutropenia, aplastic anemia, cyanosis, hypochromic anemia, iron deficiency anemia, lymphadenopathy, petechiae, purpura (≤ 0.1%).

Musculoskeletal: Athrosis, myasthenia, bone neoplasm (0.1% to 1%); bone necrosis, osteoporosis, tetany (≤ 0.1%).

Special senses: Amblyopia, ophthalmitis (0.1% to 1%); blepharitis, cataract, deafness, diplopia, ear pain, glaucoma, hyperacusis, photophobia, taste loss, vestibular disorder (≤ 0.1%).

GU: Urinary urgency, urine abnormality, urinary incontinence, kidney calculus, hematuria, impotence, prostate carcinoma, kidney pain, metorrhagia, priapism (0.1% to 1%); amenorrhea, breast abscess, breast pain, nephritis, nocturia, pyelonephritis, enlarged uterine fibroids, uterine hemorrhage, vaginal moniliasis (≤ 0.1%).

Lab test abnormalities: Increased gamma glutamyl transferase, abnormal liver function/tests, increased alkaline phosphatase, positive direct Coombs test, increased gamma globulins (0.1% to 1%); increased lactic dehydrogenase (≤ 0.1%).

Overdosage:

No specific antidote or treatment information is available. In the event of overdose, discontinue therapy immediately. Treatment should be supportive and directed toward alleviating symptoms.

Patient Information:

Advise patients to report any febrile illness to their physicians.

Advise patients to take riluzole at the same time of day (eg, in the morning and evening) each day. If a dose is missed, take the next tablet as originally planned.

Warn patients about the potential for dizziness, vertigo or somnolence and advise them not to drive or operate machinery until they have gained sufficient experience on riluzole to gauge whether or not it affects their mental or motor performance adversely.

Whether alcohol increases risk of serious hepatotoxicity with riluzole is unknown; discourage riluzole-treated patients from drinking alcohol in excess.

Administration and Dosage:

Approved by the FDA on December 12, 1995.

The recommended dose is 50 mg every 12 hours. No increased benefit can be expected from higher daily doses, but adverse events are increased.

Take at least 1 hour before or 2 hours after a meal to avoid decreased bioavailability.

Storage/Stability: Protect from bright light.

Rx	**Rilutek** (Rhone-Poulenc Rorer)	**Tablets:** 50 mg	(RPR 202.) White. Capsule shape. Film coated. In 60s.

The following is a list of available diagnostic aids for professional office use or for use by patients at home (when noted). Those tests requiring special equipment and used primarily by commercial laboratories are not included. For complete information on specific uses, directions and characteristics of these products, consult the manufacturers' package literature.

ACETONE (Ketone) TESTS

To detect the presence of ketones.

For complete prescribing information, refer to the In Vitro Diagnostic Aids introduction.

Acetest (Bayer Corp)	**Reagent tablets** for urine, whole blood, serum or plasma tests	In 100s.
Chemstrip K (Boehringer Mannheim)	**Reagent strips** for urine tests	In 25s.
Ketostix (Bayer Corp)[1]	**Reagent strips** for urine tests	In 50s, 100s and UD 20s.

[1] For use by patient at home.

ALBUMIN TESTS

To detect the presence of protein.

For complete prescribing information, refer to the In Vitro Diagnostic Aids introduction.

Albustix (Bayer Corp)	**Reagent strips** for urine tests	In 100s.
Chemstrip Micral (Boehringer Mannheim)	**Reagent strips** for urine tests	In 30s.

BACTERIURIA TESTS

To detect nitrate, uropathogens, total bacterial or gram-negative bacterial counts.

For complete prescribing information, refer to the In Vitro Diagnostic Aids introduction.

Microstix-3 (Bayer Corp)	**Reagent strips** for urine tests	In test kits containing 25 reagent strips, 25 incubation pouches and 25 ID labels.
Uricult (Orion Diagnostica)	**Culture paddles** for urine tests	In 10s.
Isocult for Bacteriuria (Remel)	**Culture paddles** for urine tests	In 12s.

BILIRUBIN TESTS

To detect the presence of bilirubin.

For complete prescribing information, refer to the In Vitro Diagnostic Aids introduction.

Ictotest (Bayer Corp)	**Reagent tablets** for urine tests	In 100s.

BLOOD UREA NITROGEN TESTS

To estimate amounts of urea nitrogen.

For complete prescribing information, refer to the In Vitro Diagnostics introduction.

Azostix (Bayer Corp)	**Reagent strips** for whole blood tests	In 25s.

CANDIDA TESTS

To detect *Candida albicans.*

For complete prescribing information, refer to the In Vitro Diagnostics introduction.

Isocult for *Candida* (Remel)	**Culture paddles** for vaginal specimen tests	In 4s.
CandidaSure (Orion Diagnostica)	**Reagent slides** for vaginal specimen tests	In kits containing 20 slides.

CHLAMYDIA TRACHOMATIS TESTS

To detect and identify *Chlamydia trachomatis*.

For complete prescribing information, refer to the In Vitro Diagnostics introduction.

Chlamydiazyme (Abbott)	**Reagent kit** for enzyme immunoassay	In kits containing 100 and 500 tests.
MicroTrak *Chlamydia Trachomatis* (Syva)	**Slide tests** for urogenital, rectal, conjunctival or nasopharyngeal specimens	In kits containing 60 tests.
Amplicor (Roche Diagnostics Systems)	**Reagent kit** for endocervical, male urethral and male urine specimens	In kits containing 10, 96 and 100 tests.
Sure Cell Chlamydia (Kodak)	**Reagent kit** for endocervical, urethral, male urine or ocular specimens	In kits containing 10, 25 and 100 tests.
Clearview Chlamydia (Wampole)	**Color-label immunoassay** for endocervical specimens	In 20s.

CHOLESTEROL TESTS

To estimate cholesterol levels. For use by patient at home.

For complete prescribing information, refer to the In Vitro Diagnostics introduction.

Advanced Care Cholesterol Test (Johnson & Johnson)	**Cassette** for blood test	In kits containing test cassette, result chart, lancet, gauze pad, adhesive bandage, instruction booklet and question and answer booklet.

COLOR ALLERGY SCREENING TESTS

For determination of immunoglobulin E.

For complete prescribing information, refer to the In Vitro Diagnostics introduction.

CAST (Biomerica)	**Reagent sticks** for serum tests	In kits containing reagent sticks for 25 tests.

CRYPTOCOCCAL ANTIGEN TESTS

For the qualitative or quantitative determination of *Cryptococcus neoformans* antigen.

For complete prescribing information, refer to the In Vitro Diagnostics introduction.

Crypto-LA (Wampole)	**Slide tests** for CSF and serum	In 70s.

GASTROINTESTINAL TESTS

For determination of GI disorders.

For complete prescribing information, refer to the In Vitro Diagnostics introduction.

Entero-Test (HDC Corp)	**String capsules** for collection of duodenal fluid	In packages containing 25 capsules, pH sticks and color charts.
Entero-Test Pediatric Capsules (HDC Corp)	**String capsules** for collection of duodenal fluid	In packages containing 25 capsules, pH sticks and color charts.
Gastro-Test (HDC Corp)	**String capsules** for collection of stomach acid	In packages containing 25 capsules, pH sticks and color charts.
Pyloriset (Orion Diagnostica)	**Reagent kit** for serum test	In kits containing 20 latex reagents, positive and negative controls, dilution buffers, mixing sticks and test cards.

GLUCOSE, BLOOD TESTS

To determine blood glucose levels. For use by patient at home.

For complete prescribing information, refer to the In Vitro Diagnostics introduction.

Chemstrip bG (Boehringer Mannheim)	**Reagent strips** for blood tests	In 25s, 50s and 100s.
Dextrostix (Bayer Corp)		In 25s and 100s for use with bottle label color chart (provided) or *Glucometer Reflectance Photometer.*
Diascan (Home Diagnostics)		In 50s for use with *Diascan Color Chart* (provided) or *Diascan Blood Glucose Meter.*
Glucostix (Bayer Corp)		In 50s, 100s and UD 25s for use with bottle label color blocks, *Glucometer II, Glucometer II With Memory, Glucometer M* or *Glucometer QA Blood Glucose Meters.*
Glucofilm (Bayer Corp)		In 25s, 50s and 100s for use with *Glucometer 3, Glucometer QA* or *Glucometer M+ Blood Glucose Meters.*
Glucometer Encore (Bayer Corp)		In 50s for use with *Glucometer Encore Blood Glucose Meter*or *Glucometer M+ Blood Glucose Meters.*
Glucometer Elite (Bayer Corp)		In 25s and 50s with code strips for use with *Glucometer Elite Blood Glucose Meter.*
Accu-Chek Advantage (Boehringer Mannheim)		In 50s to be used with *Accu-Chek Advantage Blood Glucose Monitoring System.*
One Touch (LifeScan)		In 25s, 50s and 100s for use with *One Touch Basic Blood Glucose Monitoring System* or *One Touch II Blood Glucose Monitoring System.*
First Choice (Polymer Technology)		In 25s, 50s and 100s for use with *Glucometer II, Glucometer II With Memory, Glucometer 3, Diascan, One Touch, One Touch II* or *One Touch Basic Meters.*

GLUCOSE, URINE TESTS

To measure glucose in urine. For use by patient at home.

For complete prescribing information, refer to the In Vitro Diagnostic Aids introduction.

Clinitest (Bayer Corp)	**Reagent tablets** for urine tests	In 36s and 100s with color charts and sets containing 36 tablets, 1 test tube, 1 dropper and color chart.
Chemstrip bG (Boehringer Mannheim)	**Reagent strips** for urine tests	In 100s.
Chemstrip uG (Boehringer Mannheim)		In 100s.
Clinistix (Bayer Corp)		In 50s.
Diastix (Bayer Corp)		In 50s and 100s.
Tes-Tape (Lilly)		In packages containing tape, dispenser and color chart for 100 tests.

GONORRHEA TESTS

Used as a presumptive test for *Neisseria gonorrhoeae*.

For complete prescribing information, refer to the In Vitro Diagnostic Aids introduction.

Biocult-GC (Orion Diagnostica)	**Culture paddles** for endocervical, oropharyngeal, anterior urethra or anal cultures	In kits containing vials, CO_2-generating tablets, swabs, reagent and specimen ID labels.
Gonozyme Diagnostic (Abbott)	**Reagent kit** for urogenital swab specimens	In test kits containing reagent, reaction trays, assay tubes with identifying racks and cover seals for 100 tests.
LCx Neisseria gonorrhea Assay (Abbott)	**Reagent kit** in endocervical, male urethral and urine swab specimens.	Kit includes swabs, vials and reagent for 100 tests.
Isocult for *Neisseria gonorrhoeae* (Remel)	**Culture paddles** for endocervical, rectal and urethral cultures	In test kits containing culture tubes, CO_2-generating tablets, reagent and information sheet for 12 tests.
MicroTrak *Neisseria gonorrhoeae* Culture Confirmation Test (Syva)	**Reagent kit** for endocervical, urethral, rectal, conjunctival and pharyngeal cultures	In test kits containing reagent, reconstitution diluent and mounting fluid for 85 tests.

HEMATOCRIT/HEMOGLOBIN TESTS

To determine hematocrit/hemoglobin measurement.

For complete prescribing information, refer to the In Vitro Diagnostic Aids introduction.

Stat-Crit (Wampole)	**Electrode device** for blood samples	In 120s for use with *STAT-CRIT* instrument kit.

HUMAN IMMUNODEFICIENCY VIRUS (HIV) TESTS

For the detection of HIV.

For complete prescribing information, refer to the In Vitro Diagnostic Aids introduction.

	HIV-1 LA Recombigen HIV-1 Latex Agglutination Test (Cambridge Biotech)	**Reagent kit** for blood, serum, plasma or capillary sample tests.	In kits containing vial, diluent, card and transfer loop for 100 tests.
	HIVAB HIV-1 EIA (Abbott)	**Reagent kit** for serum or plasma tests	In kits containing reagents for 100 tests.
	HIVAG-1 (Abbott)	**Reagent kit** for serum or plasma tests	In kits containing reagents for 100 tests.
Rx	**Amplicor HIV-1 Monitor** (Roche)	**Reagent kits** for plasma HIV-1 tests.	In kits containing reagents for 24 tests.
otc	**Confide** (Direct Access Diagnostics)	**Reagent kit** for HIV blood tests.	In kit containing materials to draw blood sample, a test card and a protective mailer for 1 test.
	HIVAB HIV-1/HIV-2 (rDNA) E1A (Abbott)	**In vitro enzyme immunoassay** for qualitative detection of antibodies to human immunodeficiency viruses type 1 or type 2 in human serum or plasma.	In 100, 1000 and 5000 test kits.
	OraSure (Epitope)[1]	**Reagent kit** for oral fluid tests	In kit containing collection pad, vial and reagent for 1 test.
	OraSure HIV-1 (Epitope)	**Collection kit** for oral specimen collection	In kit containing cotton fiber on stick with collection vial.

[1] For use by patient at home.

MENINGITIS TESTS

For the qualitative detection of *Neisseria meningitidis* serogroups A/B/C/Y/W135 antigens for the diagnosis of meningitis.

For complete prescribing information, refer to the In Vitro Diagnostic Aids introduction.

Bactigen *N Meningitidis* (Wampole)	**Slide tests** for cerebrospinal fluid, serum, urine or blood cultures	In 54s.

MONONUCLEOSIS TESTS

For qualitative and quantitative identification of heterophilic antibodies for the diagnosis of infectious mononucleosis.

For complete prescribing information, refer to the In Vitro Diagnostics introduction.

Mono-Diff (Wampole)	**Reagent kit** for serum or plasma tests	In kits containing reagent, absorbent I and II, positive control serum, calibrated capillary tubes and bulbs, disposable stirrers and disposable card slides for 20 tests.
Mono-Latex (Wampole)	**Reagent kit** for serum or plasma tests	In kits containing reagent latex, positive control, negative control, capillary tubes and bulbs, black glass slide and disposable stirrers for 20 and 50 tests.
Mono-Plus (Wampole)	**Reagent kit** for serum or plasma tests	In kits containing *micro-plus* test devices and *mono-plus* developer solution for 30 tests.
Monospot (Meridian Diagnostics)	**Slide test** for serum or plasma	In kits containing reagents I and II, indicator cells, positive and negative control serum, glass slide, microcapillary pipettes, rubber bulbs, plastic pipettes and wooden applicators for 20 tests.
Monosticon Dri-Dot (Organon Teknika)	**Slide test** for serum, plasma or whole blood tests	In kits containing test slides, positive and negative I.M. serum controls, dropper bottle and *dispenstirs* for 25 and 100 tests.
Mono-Sure (Wampole)	**Slide test** for serum or plasma	In kits containing reagent, positive and negative control serums, absorbent I and II, calibrated capillary tubes and bulbs, glass slides, disposable stirrers and card slides for 40 and 100 tests.
Mono-Test (Wampole)	**Slide test** for serum or plasma	In kits containing reagent, positive and negative control serums, calibrated capillary tubes and bulbs, glass slides, disposable stirrers and card slides for 40 and 100 tests.
Quantaffirm (Organon Teknika)	**Reagent kit** for serum tests	In test kits containing vials and reagent for 4 tests.

OCCULT BLOOD SCREENING TESTS

To detect occult blood.

For complete prescribing information, refer to the In Vitro Diagnostic Aids introduction.

ColoCare (Helena Labs)[1]	**Kit** for fecal specimens	In kits containing 3 tests.
ColoScreen (Helena Labs)	**Slide tests** for fecal specimens	In kits containing slides, monitors, tape, developer, specimen applicators and mailing envelopes for 100 tests.
EZ Detect (Biomerica)[1]	**Kit** for fecal specimens	In kits containing 5 test tissues, control and control card for 48 tests.
Hemoccult II Dispensapak (SmithKline Diagnostics)[1]	**Slide tests** for fecal specimens	In kits containing slides, applicators and developer for 100 tests.
Hemoccult II Dispensapak Plus (SmithKline Diagnostics)[1]	**Slide tests** for fecal specimens	In kits containing slides, sample collection tissues, applicators and mailing pouch for 40 tests.
Hemoccult II (SmithKline Diagnostics)	**Slide tests** for fecal specimens	In kits containing developer and applicators for 102 and 1020 tests.
Hemoccult Slides (SmithKline Diagnostics)	**Slide tests** for fecal specimens	In kits containing developer and applicators for 100 and 1000 tests.

OCCULT BLOOD SCREENING TESTS

Hemoccult Tape (SmithKline Diagnostics)	**Tape** for fecal specimens	In kits containing tape dispenser and developer for 100 tests.
Hemoccult SENSA (SmithKline Diagnostics)	**Slide tests** for fecal specimens	In 100s and 1000s with developer and applicators.
Hemoccult II SENSA (SmithKline Diagnostics)	**Slide tests** for fecal specimens	In kits containing slides, tissues, applicators and mailing pouches for 40 tests.
HemeSelect Reagent (SmithKline Diagnostics)	**Reagent kit** for fecal specimens	In kits containing vials, diluent, Hb positive control, microtiter plate and droppers for 40 tests. *For use with HemeSelect Sample Collection Kit.*
HemeSelect Collection (Smith Kline Diagnostics)[1]	**Collection kit** for fecal specimens	In kits containing sample collection card, applicator, self-sealing sample bag and instructions. *For use with the HemeSelect Reagent Kit.*
Hema-Chek (Bayer Corp)[1]	**Slide tests** for fecal specimens	In kits containing slide pak, developer, control and applicator sticks for 100 and 300 tests.
Hematest (Bayer Corp)	**Reagent tablets** for fecal specimens	In packages containing reagent tablets and filter paper for 100 tests.
Hemastix (Bayer Corp)	**Reagent strips** for urine specimens	In 50s.
Gastroccult (SmithKline Diagnostics)	**Slide tests** for gastric specimens	In kits containing slides, developer and applicators for 40 tests.

[1] For use by patient at home.

OVULATION TESTS

To measure luteinizing hormone for prediction of ovulation.

For complete prescribing information, refer to the In Vitro Diagnostic Aids introduction.

Answer Ovulation (Carter Wallace)[1]	**Kit** for urine tests	In kits containing vial, droppers, clear tube, urine collection containers, test well, stand and clear tube holder for 5 tests.
Clearplan Easy (Whitehall)[1]	**Kit** for urine tests	In kits containing sticks for 5 tests.
OvuQUICK Self-Test (Quidel)[1]	**Kit** for urine tests	In kits containing urine cup, droppers, reconstitution buffer, enzyme conjugate, test pad labels, test pad, foil pouch, substrate and stop solution for 6 tests.
OvuKIT Self-Test (Quidel)[1]	**Kit** for urine tests	In kits containing test stick, vials, urine cups and test stick holder for 6 and 9 tests.
Color Ovulation Test (Biomerica)[1]	**Kit** for urine tests	In 9 day test kits.
First Response Ovulation Predictor (Carter Wallace)[1]	**Kit** for urine tests	In kits containing vial, droppers, clear tube, urine collection containers, test well, stand and clear tube holder for 5 tests.
Conceive Ovulation Predictor (Quidel)	**Cassettes** for urine tests	In kits containing cassettes, foil pouches, plastic cups and droppers for 5 tests.
QTest Ovulation (Quidel)	**Kit** for urine tests	In kits containing teststrips, teststrip holders, urine collection cups, glass vials, reagents, solutions and droppers for 5 tests.
OvuGen (BioGenex)	**Kit** for urine tests.	In kits of 6 and 10.

[1] For use by patient at home.

PREGNANCY TESTS

To detect the presence of human chorionic gonadotropin.

For complete prescribing information, refer to the In Vitro Diagnostic Aids introduction.

Advance (Ortho)[1]	**Stick** for urine test	In 1s.
Answer Plus (Carter Wallace)[1]	**Kit** for urine test	In kits containing urine collection cup, filter dropper, vial, test well, test tray and tube for 1 test.
Answer Quick & Simple (Carter Wallace)[1]	**Kit** for urine test	In kits containing dropper, tube and color key for 2 tests.
Conceive Pregnancy (Quidel)[1]	**Kit** for urine test	In kits containing tape cassette, dropper, plastic cup for 1 and 2 tests.
Clearblue Easy (Whitehall)[1]	**Stick** for urine test	In 1s.
e.p.t. Quick Stick (Parke-Davis)[1]	**Stick** for urine test	In 1s.
Fact Plus (Ortho)[1]	**Kit** for urine test	In kits containing test disk, urine collection cup and urine dropper.
First Response (Carter Wallace)[1]	**Stick** for urine test	In 1s.
Fortel Midstream (Bioamerica)	**Stick** for urine test	In 1s.
Fortel Plus (Bioamerica)[1]	**Kit** for urine test	In kits containing urine collection cup, test device, dropper and absorbent packet.
Midstream Pregnancy Test Kit (Goldline)	**Kit**: Stick for urine test. In 1s.	
One Step Midstream (Biocare International)[1]	**Stick** for urine test	In 1s.
Pregnosis (Roche)[1]	**Slide tests** for urine	In kits containing reagents, droppers, pipettes, applicator stick and slide for 50 and 200 tests.
Nimbus Quick Strip (Bioamerica)[1]	**Test strips** for urine	In 25s.
RapidVue (Quidel)[1]	**Kit** for urine test	In kits containing cup, dropper and test cassette.
QTest (Quidel)[1]	**Stick** for urine test	In kits containing vial, test stick, reagent, developer and solution for 1 test.
UCG Slide (Wampole)	**Slide tests** for urine	In kits containing latex reagent, antibody reagent, slide stirrers and plastic cup for 30, 100, 300 and 1000 tests.

PREGNANCY TESTS

Abbott TestPack hCG-Urine Plus (Abbott)	**Kit** for urine test	In kits containing reaction dish and transfer pipette. In 20s.
Nimbus (Biomerica)	**Kit** for urine test	In kits containing tube, conjugate and pipettes for 25, 50 and 100 tests.
Nimbus Plus (Bioamerica)	**Kit** for urine test	In kits containing test devices and droppers for 25 tests.
Unistep hCG (Orion Diagnostica)	**Kit** for urine test	In kits containing hCG reaction packs and droppers for 25 and 50 tests.
QuickVue (Quidel)	**Cassettes** for urine test	In kits containing test cassettes and pipettes 25 and 75 tests.
SureCell Pregnancy (Kodak)	**Kit** for urine test	In kits containing reagents for 10, 25 and 100 tests.
SureCell hCG-Urine Test (Kodak)	**Kit** for urine test.	In 10s, 25s and 100s.
UCG Beta-Slide Monoclonal II (Wampole)	**Slide tests** for urine	In kits containing slide test and reagent for 50, 100 and 300 tests.

[1] For use by patient at home.

RHEUMATOID FACTOR TEST

To detect rheumatoid factor in blood.

For complete prescribing information, refer to the In Vitro Diagnostic Aids introduction.

Rheumatex (Wampole)	**Slide tests** for blood	In kits containing reagents and slides for 100 and 200 tests.
Rheumaton (Wampole)	**Slide tests** for serum or synovial fluid	In kits containing reagent, positive and negative control, tubes, bulbs and slides for 20, 50 and 150 tests.

SICKLE CELL TEST

To detect hemoglobin S.

For complete prescribing information, refer to the In Vitro Diagnostic Aids introduction.

Sickledex (Ortho)	**Kit** for blood tests	In kits containing reagents and solution for 12 and 100 tests.

STAPHYLOCOCCUS TEST

To determine the presence of *Staphylococcus aureus*.

For complete prescribing information, refer to the In Vitro Diagnostic Aids introduction.

Isocult for *Staphylococcus aureus* (Remel)	**Culture paddles** for exudate	In kits containing reagents for 12 tests.

STREPTOCOCCI TESTS

To detect beta-hemolytic group A streptococci, group B streptococci, *streptococci pharyngitis*, antibodies to DNase-B, *Streptococcus pneumoniae* and streptococcal extracellular antigens.

For complete prescribing information, refer to the In Vitro Diagnostic Aids introduction.

Sure Cell Streptococci (Kodak)	**Kit** for the detection of Group A streptoccal antigen from throat swabs and blood	In kits containing test cells, extraction blocks, reagents, dye solutions, filter and swabs for 25 and 100 tests.
Culturette 10 Minute Group A Strep ID (Becton Dickinson)	**Slide test** for the detection of Group A streptoccal antigen from throat swabs	In kits containing reagents and test slides for 55 and 200 tests.
Isocult for *Streptococcal pharyngitis* (Remel)	**Culture paddles** for the detection of *streptococcal pharyngitis* from throat swabs	In kits culture paddles and reagents for 12 tests.
Respiracult-Strep (Orion Diagnostica)	**Culture paddles** for the detection of beta-hemolytic group A streptococci from throat and nasopharyngeal sources	In kits containing reagents and culture paddles for 25 and 50 tests.
Streptonase-B (Wampole)	**Kit** for the detection of antibodies to DNase-B in serum	In kits containing reagents and tubes for 10 tests.
Test Pack (Abbott)	**Kit** for the detection of Group A streptococci from throat specimens	In kits containing reagents, extraction tubes and swabs for 40 and 80 tests.
Bactigen Strep B (Wampole)	**Slide tests** for the detection of Group B streptococci from serum, urine, cerebrospinal fluid and blood	In kits containing slide, droppers, stirrers and reagents for 54 tests.
Bactigen B Streptococcus-CS (Wampole)	**Slide tests** for the detection of group B streptococcus antigen from vaginal and cervical swabs	In kits containing reagents, slides, droppers and stirrers for 48 tests.
Bactigen S Pneumonia (Wampole)	**Kit** for the detection of *Streptococcus pneumoniae* antigens in cerebrospinal fluid, blood and urine	In kits containing reagents, slides, droppers and stirrers for 54 tests.
Streptozyme (Wampole)	**Slide tests** for the detection of streptococcal extracellular antigens in blood, plasma and serum	In kits containing reagents, tubes, positive and negative control serum, bulbs and slides for 15, 50 and 150 tests.
Detect-A-Strep (Antibodies Inc.)	**Slide tests** for the detection of streptococcal antigen from throat swabs	In kits containing reagents and test plates for 6 tests.
Strep Detect (Navillus Inc.)	**Slide tests** for the detection of streptococcal antigen from throat swabs	In kits containing reagents and test plates for 6 tests.

TOXOPLASMOSIS TEST

To detect the presence of *Toxoplasma gondii* in blood.

For complete prescribing information, refer to the In Vitro Diagnostic Aids introduction.

TPM Test (Wampole)	**Kit** for blood test	In kits including reagents for 120 tests.

VIRUS TESTS, MISCELLANEOUS

To detect Human T-Lymphotropic Type 1, HSV–1, HSV–2, Herpes, Rotavirus, Rubella and C-Reactive Protein.

For complete prescribing information, refer to the In Vitro Diagnostic Aids introduction.

Human T-Lymphotropic Virus Type I EIA (Abbott)	**Reagent kit** for serum or plasma tests	In kits containing reagents, vials and reaction trays for 100 tests.	NA
MicroTrak HSV 1/HSV 2 Culture Identification/ Typing Test (Syva)	**Culture test** for tissue	1 test per kit.	NA
MicroTrak HSV1/ HSV2 Direct Specimen Identification/Typing Test (Syva)	**Slide test** for external lesions	In kits containing reagent for 60 tests.	NA
Sure Cell Herpes (Kodak)	**Reagent kit** for genital, rectal, oral or dermal swabs	In 10s and 25s.	7.5
Rubazyme for Rubella (Abbott)	**Reagent kit** for serum test	In kits containing reagents and diluent for 1 and 5 tests.	NA
Virogen Herpes (Wampole)	**Slide test** for the detection of herpes simplex virus antigens directly from lesions or cell culture	In kits containing reagents, stirrers, slides and slide covers for 100 tests.	5.7
Virogen Rotatest for Rotavirus (Wampole)	**Slide test** for fecal specimens	In kits containing reagents, extraction buffer and slides for 50 tests.	6.9
Immunex C-Reactive Protein (Wampole)	**Kit** for blood tests	In kits containing reagents and slides for 100 tests.	NA
Impact Rubella (Wampole)	**Slide test** for serum.	In kits containing reagents and slides for 100, 500 and 5000 tests.	2.4

COMBINATION TESTS

To detect a multiplicity of conditions, including *Haemophilus influenzae* type b, *Neissaria meningitidis* serogroups A/B/C/Y/W135, *Streptococcus pneumoniae, Salmonella, Schigella, N Gonorrhoeae, T vaginalis* and Candida.

For complete prescribing information, refer to the In Vitro Diagnostic Aids introduction.

Bactigen Meningitis Panel (Wampole)	**Slide test** for cerebrospinal fluid, serum, urine and blood	In 54s.
Bactigen *Salmonella-Shigella* (Wampole)	**Slide test** for cultures	In kits containing reagents, dispenser cannulae, droppers, slides and stirrers for 96 tests.
Isocult for *N gonorrhoeae* and Candida (Remel)	**Culture test** for endocervical rectal, urethral, pharyngeal and vaginal specimens	In 12s.
Isocult for *T vaginalis* and Candida (Remel)	**Culture test** for vaginal and urethral cultures	In kits containing culture tubes and reagents for 12 tests.

MISCELLANEOUS URINE TEST

Used for the quantitative detection of NA and pH in urine.

For complete prescribing information, refer to the In Vitro Diagnostic Aids introduction.

Nitrazine (Apothecon)	**Paper** for urine tests	In rolls.

MULTIPLE URINE TEST PRODUCTS

To make simultaneous determinations of two or more urine tests.

Product & Distributor	Glucose	Protein	pH	Blood	Ketones	Bilirubin	Urobilinogen	Nitrite	Leukocytes	How Supplied
Chemstrip 2 GP (Boehringer Mannheim)	X	X								In 100s.
Uristix (Bayer Corp)	X	X	X	X						In 100s.
Combistix (Bayer Corp)	X	X	X	X						In 100s.
Hema-Combistix (Bayer Corp)	X	X	X	X						In 100s.
Uristix 4 (Bayer Corp	X	X						X	X	In 100s.
Chemstrip 4 the OB (Boehringer Mannheim)	X	X		X					X	In 100s.
Chemstrip uGK (Boehringer Mannheim)	X				X					In 50s.
Keto-Diastix (Bayer Corp)	X				X					In 50s and 100s.
Chemstrip 6 (Boehringer Mannheim)	X	X	X	X	X				X	In 100s.
Labstix (Bayer Corp)	X	X	X	X	X					In 100s.
Bili-Labstix (Bayer Corp)	X	X	X	X	X	X				In 100s.
Chemstrip 7 (Boehringer Mannheim)	X	X	X	X	X	X			X	In 100s.
Multistix (Bayer Corp)	X	X	X	X	X	X	X			In 100s.
Multistix SG[1] (Bayer Corp)	X	X	X	X	X	X	X			In 100s.
Multistix 7 (Bayer Corp)	X	X	X	X	X			X	X	In 100s.
Multistix 8 SG[1] (Bayer Corp)	X	X	X	X	X			X	X	In 100s.
Chemstrip 8 (Boehringer Mannheim)	X	X	X	X	X	X	X		X	In 100s.
N-Multistix (Bayer Corp)	X	X	X	X	X	X	X	X		In 100s.
N-Multistix SG[1](Bayer Corp)	X	X	X	X	X	X	X	X		In 100s.
Multistix 9 SG[1](Bayer Corp)	X	X	X	X	X	X		X	X	In 100s.
Multistix 10 SG[1] (Bayer Corp)	X	X	X	X	X	X	X	X	X	In 100s.
Chemstrip 10 With SG[1] (Boehringer Mannheim)	X	X	X	X	X	X	X	X	X	In 100s.
Chemstrip 9 (Boehringer Mannheim)	X	X	X	X	X	X	X	X	X	In 100s.
Multistix 9 (Bayer Corp)	X	X	X	X	X	X	X	X	X	In 100s.
Chemstrip 2 LN (Boehringer Mannheim)								X	X	In 100s.
Multistix 2 (Bayer Corp)								X	X	In 100s.
Biotel Kidney (Biotel)		X		X						In 12s.

[1] Also tests specific gravity.

AMINOHIPPURATE SODIUM (PAH)

For the estimation of renal plasma flow and to measure the functional capacity of the renal tubular secretory mechanism.

For complete prescribing information, refer to the In Vivo Diagnostic Aids introduction.

Rx	**Aminohippurate Sodium** (Merck)	**Injection:** 20% aqueous solution	In 10 ml vials.

HYSTEROSCOPY FLUID

For use with the hysteroscope as an aid in distending the uterine cavity and in irrigating and visualizing its surfaces.

For complete prescribing information, refer to the In Vivo Diagnostic Aids introduction.

Rx	**Hyskon** (Pharmacia)	32% w/v dextran 70 in 10% w/v dextrose	In 100 and 250 ml.

INDIGOTINDISULFONATE SODIUM INJECTION

For localizing ureteral orifices during cystoscopy and ureteral catheterization.

For complete prescribing information, refer to the In Vivo Diagnostic Aids introduction.

Rx	**Indigo Carmine Solution Ampules** (American Regent)	0.8% aqueous solution	In 5 ml amps.

INDOCYANINE GREEN

For determining cardiac output, hepatic function and liver blood flow and for ophthalmic angiography.

For complete prescribing information, refer to the In Vivo Diagnostic Aids introduction.

Rx	**Cardio-Green** (Becton Dickinson)	**Powder**	In 25 and 50 mg vials w/solvent.

INULIN

For measurement of glomerular filtration rate (GFR).

For complete prescribing information, refer to the In Vivo Diagnostic Aids introduction.

Rx	**Inulin Injection** (Iso-Tex Diagnostics)	**Injection:** 100 mg per ml	In 50 ml vials.[1]

[1] With 0.9% Sodium Chloride in Water for Injection.

MANNITOL

For measurement of glomerular filtration rate (GFR). For therapeutic indications, refer to monographs in the Cardiovasculars and Anti-Infectives chapters.

For complete prescribing information, refer to the In Vivo Diagnostic Aids introduction.

Rx	**Mannitol IV** (Various, eg, Kendall McGaw)	**Injection:** 10%	In 1000 ml.
Rx	**Mannitol IV** (Various, eg, Abbott, Kendall McGaw)	**Injection:** 15%	In 150 and 500 ml.
Rx	**Mannitol IV** (Various, eg, Abbott, Kendall McGaw)	**Injection:** 20%	In 250 and 500 ml.
Rx	**Mannitol IV** (Various, eg, American Regent, Astra, IMS, Lyphomed, Pasadena, Schein, Steris)	**Injection:** 25%	In 50 ml vials and syringes.

D-XYLOSE

For evaluating intestinal absorption and diagnosing malabsorptive states.

For complete prescribing information, refer to the In Vivo Diagnostic Aids introduction.

otc	**Xylo-Pfan** (Adria)	**Powder**	In 25 g bottles.

Thyroid Function Tests

PROTIRELIN

Actions:

Pharmacology: Protirelin, a synthetic tripeptide, is probably structurally identical to the natural thyrotropin-releasing hormone produced by the hypothalamus. Protirelin increases release of thyroid stimulating hormone (TSH) from the anterior pituitary. Prolactin release is also increased. About 65% of acromegalic patients respond with a rise in circulating growth hormone levels; clinical significance is unclear.

Pharmacokinetics: Following IV administration, the mean plasma half-life is approximately 5 minutes. TSH levels rise rapidly and reach a peak in 20 to 30 minutes. The decline in TSH levels approaches baseline levels after approximately 3 hours.

Indications:

An adjunct in the diagnostic assessment of thyroid function, and an adjunct to other diagnostic procedures in patients with pituitary or hypothalamic dysfunction.

An adjunct to evaluate the effectiveness of thyrotropin suppression with a particular dose of T_4 in patients with nodular or diffuse goiter. A normal TSH baseline value and a minimal difference between the 30 minute and baseline response to protirelin injection indicates adequate suppression of the pituitary secretion of TSH.

May be used adjunctively for adjustment of thyroid hormone dosage in patients with primary hypothyroidism. A normal or slightly blunted TSH response, 30 minutes following injection, indicates adequate replacement therapy.

Warnings:

Blood pressure: Transient blood pressure changes are common. Measure blood pressure before and at frequent intervals during the first 15 minutes after administration. To minimize incidence or severity of hypotension, the patient should be supine before, during and after administration. If a clinically important change occurs, continue monitoring blood pressure until it returns to baseline. Increased systolic (usually < 30 mm Hg) or diastolic pressures (usually < 20 mm Hg) are observed more often than decreased pressure. These changes do not ordinarily persist > 15 min.

More severe degrees of hypertension or hypotension, with or without syncope, have occurred in a few patients. In patients in whom such changes would be hazardous, weigh the benefit/risk ratio carefully.

Pregnancy: Reproduction studies in rabbits at 1.5 and 6 times the human dose revealed an increased number of resorption sites. There are no studies in pregnant women; safety for use has not been established. Use only when clearly needed and when potential benefits outweigh potential hazards to the fetus.

Drug Interactions:

Adrenocortical drugs: Do not withdraw maintenance doses used in the therapy of documented hypopituitarism. Glucocorticoids at physiologic doses have no significant effect on the TSH response to thyrotropin-releasing hormone, but pharmacologic doses of steroids reduce the TSH response.

Aspirin: Therapeutic doses (2 to 3.6 g/day) inhibit the TSH response to protirelin. Aspirin ingestion caused the peak level of TSH to decrease approximately 30%, as compared to values obtained without aspirin administration. In both cases, the TSH peak occurred 30 minutes after protirelin administration.

Levodopa: Chronic administration of levodopa may inhibit TSH response to protirelin.

Thyroid hormones reduce TSH response to protirelin. Discontinue liothyronine (T_3) ≈ 7 days prior to testing and discontinue medications containing levothyroxine (T_4) (eg, desiccated thyroid, thyroglobulin or liotrix) at least 14 days before testing.

Do not discontinue hormone therapy when the test is used to evaluate the effectiveness of thyroid suppression with T_4 in patients with nodular or diffuse goiter, or for adjustment of thyroid dosage in patients with primary hypothyroidism.

Adverse Reactions:

Side effects, reported in about 50% of patients tested, are generally minor, occur promptly and persist for only a few minutes.

Cardiovascular: Blood pressure changes (see Warnings).

Endocrine: Breast enlargement and leakage in lactating women for up to 2 to 3 days.

Body as a whole:

Most frequent – Nausea; urge to urinate; flushed sensation; lightheadedness; bad taste in mouth; abdominal discomfort; headache; dry mouth.

Less frequent – Anxiety; sweating; tightness in the throat; pressure in the chest; tingling sensation; drowsiness; headaches (sometimes severe); transient amaurosis in patients with pituitary tumors. Rarely, convulsions may occur in patients with predisposing conditions (eg, epilepsy, brain damage).

Thyroid Function Tests

PROTIRELIN

Administration and Dosage:

Administer IV bolus over 15 to 30 seconds with the patient remaining supine for an additional 15 minutes; during this time, monitor blood pressure.

Draw one blood sample for TSH assay immediately prior to injection, and obtain a second sample 30 minutes after injection.

The TSH response to protirelin is reduced by repetitive administration. If the protirelin test is repeated, an interval of 7 days is recommended.

Elevated serum lipids may interfere with the TSH assay. Thus, fasting (except in patients with hypopituitarism) or a low-fat meal is recommended prior to the test.

Adults: 500 mcg IV (range 200 to 500 mcg); 500 mcg is the optimum dose to give the maximum response. Doses > 500 mcg are unlikely to elicit a greater TSH response.

Children (6 to 16 years old): 7 mcg/kg, up to 500 mcg.

Infants and children (up to 6 years): Experience is limited in this age group; doses of 7 mcg/kg have been administered.

Interpretation of test results: TSH test results vary with the laboratory; therefore, be familiar with the TSH assay method used and the normal range for the laboratory performing the assay.

Characterization of Thyroid Function with Protirelin

Thyroid function	Baseline serum TSH (microU/ml)	Change of serum TSH (microU/ml) at 30 minutes
Euthyroidism (normal thyroid function)	≤ 10 (usually ≤ 6; 20% have < 1.5)	≥2 (usually 6 to 30)
Hyperthyroidism	≤ 10 (usually ≤ 4)	< 2
Primary hypothyroidism (thyroidal)	> 10 (usually 15 to 200)	≥ 2 (usually ≥ 20)
Secondary hypothyroidism (pituitary)	≤ 10 (usually ≤ 6)	< 2 (59%) 2 to 50 (41%)
Tertiary hypothyroidism (hypothalamic)	≤ 10 (often < 2)	≥ 2

Primary (thyroidal) hypothyroidism – The diagnosis is frequently supported by the finding of clearly elevated baseline TSH levels; protirelin administration to these patients generally would not be expected to yield additional useful information. Since the same response in 30 minutes is also found in normal subjects, protirelin testing does not differentiate primary hypothyroidism from normal.

Secondary (pituitary) and tertiary (hypothalamic) hypothyroidism – In the presence of evidence of hypothyroidism, a baseline TSH level < 10 microU/ml should suggest secondary or tertiary hypothyroidism. A response > 2 microU/ml is not helpful in differentiating between secondary and tertiary hypothyroidism.

Establishing the diagnosis of secondary or tertiary hypothyroidism requires a careful history and physical examination along with appropriate tests of anterior pituitary or target gland function. Do not use the protirelin test as the only laboratory determinant for establishing these diagnoses.

Rx	**Thypinone** (Abbott)	**Injection:** 500 mcg per ml	In 1 ml amps.[1]
Rx	**Relefact TRH** (Ferring)		In 1 ml amps.

[1] With 0.9 mg sodium chloride.

Thyroid Function Tests

SODIUM IODIDE I^{123}

Actions:

Pharmacology: Sodium Iodide I^{123} ($Na^{123}I$) is readily absorbed from the upper GI tract. The iodide is distributed primarily within the extracellular fluid of the body. It is trapped and organically bound by the thyroid and concentrated by the stomach, choroid plexus and salivary glands. It is excreted by the kidneys.

The fraction of the administered dose that is accumulated in the thyroid gland may be a measure of thyroid function in the absence of unusually high or low iodine intake or use of certain drugs which influence iodine accumulation by the thyroid gland. Accordingly, question the patient carefully regarding previous medications or procedures involving radiographic media. Healthy subjects can accumulate ≈ 10% to 50% of the administered iodine dose in the thyroid gland; however, normal and abnormal ranges are established by individual physician's criteria.

Indications:

As a diagnostic procedure in evaluating thyroid function or morphology.

Warnings:

Pregnancy: Category C. It is not known whether Sodium Iodide I^{123} can cause fetal harm when administered to a pregnant woman or can affect reproductive capacity. Give to a pregnant woman only if clearly needed. Females of childbearing age should not be studied unless the benefits anticipated from the test outweigh the possible risk of exposure to the amount of ionizing radiation associated with the test. Ideally, perform examinations using radiopharmaceuticals, especially those elective in nature, during the first few (≈ 10) days following onset of menses.

Lactation: Since I^{123} is excreted in breast milk, substitute formula feeding for breastfeeding if the agent must be administered to the mother during lactation.

Children: Safety and efficacy aree not established. Children under age 18 should not be studied unless benefits anticipated from the test outweigh possible risk of exposure to the amount of ionizing radiation associated with the test.

Precautions:

Capsule contents are radioactive. Shield preparation adequately at all times.

Do not use after expiration time and date stated on the label. Administer prescribed Sodium Iodide I^{123} dose as soon as practical from time of receipt of product (ie, as close to calibration time as possible), in order to minimize the fraction of radiation exposure due to the relative increase of radionuclidic contaminants with time.

Handle with care. Use appropriate safety measures to minimize radiation exposure to clinical personnel. Take care to minimize radiation exposure to the patient consistent with proper patient management.

Radiopharmaceuticals should be used only by physicians who are qualified by training and experience in the safe use and handling of radionuclides, and whose experience and training have been approved by the appropriate government agency authorized to license the use of radionuclides.

Adverse Reactions:

Although rare, reactions include, in decreasing order of frequency: Nausea; vomiting; chest pain; tachycardia; itching skin; rash; hives.

Administration and Dosage:

The recommended oral dose for the average patient (70 kg) is 3.7 to 14.8 MBq (100 to 400 mcCi). The lower part of the dosage range is recommended for uptake studies alone, and the higher part for thyroid imaging. The determination of I^{123} concentration in the thyroid gland may be initiated at 6 hours after administering the dose; measure according to standardized procedures.

Measure the patient dose by a suitable radioactivity calibration system immediately prior to use. Can be given up to 30 hours after calibration time and date. Thereafter, discard according to standard safety procedures. User should wear waterproof gloves at all times when handling capsules or container.

Storage: The contents of the vial are radioactive and adequate shielding and handling precautions must be maintained. Dispense and preserve capsules in tightly closed containers that are adequately shielded. Control the storage and disposal of Sodium Iodide I^{123} capsules in a manner that is in compliance with the appropriate regulations of the government agency authorized to license the use of this radionuclide.

Rx	**Sodium Iodide I 123** (Mallinckrodt Diagnostic)	**Capsules:** 3.7 MBq	Sucrose. Red/white. In 1s, 3s, 5s.
		7.4 MBq	Sucrose. Green/white. In 1s, 3s, 5s.

Thyroid Function Tests

THYROTROPIN (Thyroid Stimulating Hormone; TSH)

Actions:

Pharmacology: Thyrotropin or thyroid stimulating hormone (TSH) is a highly purified and lyophilized thyrotropic isolated from bovine anterior pituitary. The potency is designated in International-Thyrotropin units and is free of significant amounts of adrenocorticotropic, gonadotropic, somatotropic, and posterior pituitary hormones. It is a glycoprotein with a molecular weight in the range of 28,000 to 30,000. Thyrotropin produces increased uptake of iodine by the thyroid, increased formation of thyroid hormone, increased release of thyroid hormone, and cellular hyperplasia of the thyroid on prolonged stimulation.

After injection, the effect on the thyroid in normal individuals is evident within 8 hours, reaching a maximum in 24 to 48 hours.

Indications:

As a diagnostic agent to differentiate thyroid failure and to establish a diagnosis of decreased thyroid reserve.

Thyrotropin can be used for PBI or I^{131} uptake determinations.

Contraindications:

Hypersensitivity to thyrotropin; coronary thrombosis; untreated Addison's disease.

Warnings:

Anaphylactic reactions have occurred with repeated administration.

Pregnancy: Category C. It is not known whether thyrotropin can cause fetal harm when administered to a pregnant woman or can affect reproduction capacity. Give to a pregnant woman only when clearly needed.

Lactation: It is not known whether this drug is excreted in breast milk. Exercise caution when administering thyrotropin to a nursing woman.

Children: Safety and efficacy for use in children have not been established.

Precautions:

Thyrotropin can stimulate thyroid secretion; use cautiously in patients with cardiac disease who are unable to tolerate additional stress.

Adverse Reactions:

Most common: Nausea; vomiting; headache; urticaria.

Cardiovascular: Transitory hypotension; tachycardia (probably related to sensitivity reaction).

Body as a whole: Anaphylactic reactions with patient collapse; thyroid gland swelling (particularly with doses > 10 IU).

Overdosage:

Symptoms: Headache; irritability; nervousness; sweating; tachycardia; increased bowel motility; menstrual irregularities. Angina pectoris or congestive heart failure may be induced or aggravated. Shock may develop. Excessive doses may result in symptoms resembling thyroid storm. Chronic excessive dosage will produce signs and symptoms of hyperthyroidism.

Treatment: Discontinue thyrotropin. In shock, consider supportive measures and treatment of unrecognized adrenal insufficiency.

Administration and Dosage:

Administer IM or SC.

Usual dose: 10 IU for 1 to 3 days. Follow by a radioiodine study 24 hours after the last injection. No response will occur in thyroid failure, but substantial response will occur in pituitary failure.

Storage: After reconstitution, store between 2° to 8°C (36° to 46°F), for not > 2 weeks.

Rx	**Thytropar** (Armour)	**Powder for Injection (lyophilized):** 10 IU of thyrotropic activity/vial	With vial of diluent.

GONADORELIN HCl

Actions:

Pharmacology: A synthetic luteinizing hormone releasing hormone (LH-RH), also referred to as gonadotropin releasing hormone (GnRH). It is structurally identical to natural LH-RH.

Gonadorelin has gonadotropin releasing effects on the anterior pituitary. Normal baseline luteinizing hormone (LH) levels are 5 to 25 mIU/ml in postpubertal males and postpubertal and premenopausal females, but levels vary with assay method.

In menopausal and postmenopausal females, the baseline LH levels are elevated; maximum LH increases are exaggerated when compared to premenopausal levels.

Patients with clinically diagnosed or suspected pituitary or hypothalamic dysfunction often had subnormal or no LH responses following administration.

Indications:

Evaluating functional capacity and response of the gonadotropes of the anterior pituitary; testing suspected gonadotropin deficiency; evaluating residual gonadotropic function of pituitary following removal of pituitary tumor by surgery or irradiation.

Unlabeled uses: Ovulation inhibition (contraceptive effect); treatment of precocious puberty. Gonadorelin acetate *(Lutrepulse)* is used for the induction of ovulation in women with primary hypothalamic amenorrhea. See individual monograph in Gonadotropin Releasing Hormones section.

Contraindications:

Hypersensitivity to gonadorelin or any of the components of the product.

Warnings:

Pregnancy: Category B. No adequate and well controlled studies have been conducted in pregnant women. Repetitive, high doses of gonadorelin may cause luteolysis and inhibition of spermatogenesis. Safety for use during pregnancy has not been established; use only when clearly needed.

Precautions:

Hypersensitivity and anaphylactic reactions have occurred following multiple-dose administration. Refer to Management of Acute Hypersensitivity Reactions.

Antibody formation has rarely occurred after chronic administration of large doses.

Drug Interactions:

Androgen, estrogen, glucocorticoid and progestin containing preparations directly affect pituitary secretion of the gonadotropins. Do not conduct tests during administration of these agents.

Digoxin and oral contraceptives may suppress gonadotropin levels.

Levodopa and spironolactone may transiently elevate gonadotropin levels.

Phenothiazines and dopamine antagonists which increase prolactin may blunt the response to gonadorelin.

Adverse Reactions:

Systemic (rare): Headache; nausea; lightheadedness; abdominal discomfort; flushing.

Local: Swelling, with occasional pain, and pruritus at the SC injection site may occur. Local and generalized skin rash have been noted after chronic SC administration. (See Warnings.)

Rare instances of hypersensitivity reaction (bronchospasm, tachycardia, flushing, urticaria, induration at injection site) and anaphylactic reactions have occurred following multiple-dose administration. (See Warnings.)

Overdosage:

Treat symptomatically. Refer to General Management of Acute Overdosage.

Administration and Dosage:

Adults: 100 mcg SC or IV. In females, perform the test in the early follicular phase (days 1 to 7) of the menstrual cycle.

For specific test methodology and interpretation of test results, refer to manufacturer's full prescribing product information.

Preparation of solution: Reconstitute 100 mcg vial with 1 ml and the 500 mcg vial with 2 ml of accompanying diluent. Prepare immediately before use. After reconstitution, store at room temperature (≈ 25°C; ≈ 77°F); use within 1 day. Discard unused solution and diluent.

Rx	**Factrel** (Wyeth-Ayerst)	**Powder for Injection:** 100 mcg (as HCl) per vial.[1]	With 2 ml sterile diluent.[2]
		500 mcg (as HCl) per vial.[1]	

[1] With 100 mg lactose.
[2] With 2% benzyl alcohol.

TOLBUTAMIDE SODIUM

Actions:

Pharmacokinetics: Patients with functioning insulinomas exhibit hypoglycemic responses to IV tolbutamide, which are distinctive from responses of normal individuals.

Administration of 1 g to healthy subjects results in a rapid fall in blood sugar levels for 30 to 45 minutes, followed by a secondary rise into the normal range in the ensuing 90 to 180 minutes. The initial hypoglycemia results from the rapid release of insulin from the pancreatic beta cells, while the secondary rise is due to activation of counter-regulatory factors. Serum insulin levels rise from a fasting mean value of 19 microU/ml to a peak mean value of ≈ 40 microU/ml (range, 27 to 89), 20 minutes after injection.

In contrast, patients with insulinomas exhibit tolbutamide-induced blood sugar decreases of greater magnitude associated with an excessive, prompt rise in serum insulin (118 to 1055 microU/ml). The magnitude of blood sugar fall in these patients is of greater significance than the persistence of hypoglycemia for 3 hours after administration. Persistent tolbutamide-induced hypoglycemia, rather than degree of blood sugar decrease, is important in the diagnosis of pancreatic islet cell adenomas.

Indications:

As an aid in the diagnosis of pancreatic islet cell adenoma. Accurate differential diagnosis of spontaneous hypoglycemia is essential to avoid subtotal pancreatic resection in patients in whom surgery is not indicated.

Contraindications:

Children (see Warnings); previous allergy to tolbutamide or related sulfonylureas.

Warnings:

False-positive responses occurred in a few patients with liver disease, alcohol hypoglycemia, idiopathic hypoglycemia of infancy, severe undernutrition, azotemia, sarcoma, and other extrapancreatic insulin-producing tumors.

Hypoglycemia may develop, particularly in patients with fasting hypoglycemic blood sugar levels. If it occurs, terminate the test immediately; inject 12.5 to 25 g glucose IV in a 25% to 50% solution.

Anaphylaxis: Epinephrine and other resuscitative drugs should be available. Refer to Management of Acute Hypersensitivity Reactions.

Renal/Hepatic function impairment: Use cautiously because severe and prolonged hypoglycemia following oral tolbutamide has occurred.

Pregnancy:

Category C. Teratogenic effects – Tolbutamide sodium was teratogenic in rats given doses 25 to 100 times the human dose (increased mortality in offspring and ocular and bony abnormalities). There are no adequate and well controlled studies in pregnant women. Tolbutamide is not recommended for the treatment of pregnant diabetic patients. Consider the possible hazards of the use in women of childbearing potential who might become pregnant while using the drug.

Nonteratogenic effects – Prolonged severe hypoglycemia (4 to 10 days) occurred in neonates born to mothers who were receiving a sulfonylurea drug at the time of delivery. This has occurred more frequently with the use of agents with prolonged half-lives. Use of the drug in pregnant patients is not recommended.

Lactation: Tolbutamide is excreted in small amounts in the breast milk of nursing mothers. Because of the potential for serious adverse reactions in nursing infants, discontinue nursing or discontinue the drug.

Children: Not recommended in children because of the lack of data to establish ideal dosage and the inability to interpret results.

Precautions:

Test dose-induced hypoglycemic symptoms are usually not severe; however, certain nondiabetics may develop moderate to severe symptoms. To avoid this occurrence, terminate the diagnostic test by administering carbohydrates immediately after obtaining the 30 minute blood sample, especially in the testing of persons with atherosclerosis.

Use only a true glucose procedure (Somogyi-Nelson, Modified Folin-Wu, AutoAnalyzer, or glucose oxidase) to eliminate highly variable amounts of nonglucose-reducing substances as a major source of error.

Drug Interactions:

Salicylates, sulfonamides, oxyphenbutazone, phenylbutazone, probenecid, and MAOIs may interfere with results of a tolbutamide tolerance test.

TOLBUTAMIDE SODIUM

Since the tolbutamide diagnostic test involves a single injection, drug interactions that may occur with chronic tolbutamide use may not occur in this situation. However, for further information refer to the Sulfonylureas monograph.

Drug/Lab test interactions: On rare occasions, urine containing the tolbutamide metabolite may give a false-positive reaction for albumin by the usual test (acidification after boiling). Circumvent this problem by using bromphenol reagent strips.

Adverse Reactions:

Rare: Mild shoulder pain or slight burning sensation along the course of the vein during the IV injection may occur. It lasts no more than 2 to 3 minutes, is attributed to venospasm and may be obviated by administering the solution over 2 to 3 min.

Thrombophlebitis with thrombosis of the injected vein occurs in 0.8% to 2.4% of patients. These are usually painless, detectable only by careful palpation and may not appear for 1 or 2 weeks after injection. No sequelae have been noted. The vein gradually shrinks or recanalizes.

Overdosage:

The dose which may cause hypoglycemia is variable; usual therapeutic doses have caused symptomatic hypoglycemia.

Symptoms: Overdose of sulfonylureas, including tolbutamide, will produce symptoms of hypoglycemia. Seizures may occur with marked hypoglycemia.

Mild – Sweating; trembling; weakness; fatigue; nervousness; hunger; nausea.

Severe – Lethargy; confusion; stupor; loss of consciousness; coma.

Treatment: Treat mild symptoms of hypoglycemia without loss of consciousness with oral glucose and adjustment in drug dosage and meal patterns. Continue monitoring until the patient is out of danger. Severe hypoglycemic reactions with coma, seizure or other neurological impairment are rare, but require immediate hospitalization; give a rapid IV injection of 50% dextrose solution. Repeat as needed. Follow by a continuous infusion of 10% dextrose solution to maintain the blood glucose level above 100 mg/dl. Closely monitor patients in hospital for a minimum of 24 to 48 hours, since hypoglycemia may recur after apparent clinical recovery.

Overdosage with sulfonylurea drugs has not responded to peritoneal dialysis or hemodialysis. Experience, however, is quite limited.

Administration and Dosage:

For IV use only.

Fajans test:

1.) Eat a high carbohydrate diet of 150 to 300 g/day for at least 3 days prior to test.
2.) On the morning of the test, after an overnight fast, obtain a fasting blood specimen.
3.) Inject 20 ml tolbutamide solution IV at a constant rate over 2 to 3 minutes.
4.) Withdraw blood specimens at the following intervals (in minutes) after the midpoint of the injection: 20, 30, 45, 60, 90, 120, 150, and 180. The determination of serum insulin levels before, and at 10, 20 and 30 minutes after the IV administration, provides a specific and safer test for insulinoma, and permits the performance of the test in the presence of moderate fasting hypoglycemia, since interpretation is not based on the decline of the blood glucose.
5.) Blood glucose determinations are made by the true glucose procedures.
6.) Terminate the procedure with readily assimilable carbohydrates or breakfast.

Interpretation of results:

Healthy subjects – A decrease in blood sugar (38% to 79% of the fasting level) may be expected. At 90 to 120 minutes, 78% to 100% of the initial level may be seen. Similar responses occur in patients with functional hyperinsulinism.

Insulinoma patients – Minimum blood sugar levels of 17% to 50% of fasting values are seen. In 90 to 180 minutes, levels range from 40% to 64%. Patients with liver disease may show the same type of blood glucose response as patients with insulinomas; use appropriate laboratory and clinical tests to distinguish between these conditions.

Inject 1 g IV at a constant rate over 2 to 3 minutes.

For specific test methodology (Fajans test) and interpretation of test results, refer to the manufacturer's full prescribing product information.

Storage: Use within 1 hour after reconstitution, but only if solution is complete and clear.

Rx	**Orinase Diagnostic** (Upjohn)	**Powder for Injection**: 1 g (as sodium) per vial with 20 ml amp of diluent.

METHACHOLINE CHLORIDE

Warning:

Methacholine is a bronchoconstrictor for diagnostic purposes only. Perform inhalation challenge under the supervision of a physician trained in and thoroughly familiar with all aspects of the technique, all contraindications, warnings and precautions of methacholine challenge and the management of respiratory distress. Have emergency equipment and medication immediately available to treat acute respiratory distress.

Administer only by inhalation; severe bronchoconstriction and reduction in respiratory function can result. Patients with severe hyperreactivity of the airways can experience bronchoconstriction at a dosage as low as 0.025 mg/ml (0.125 cumulative units). If severe bronchoconstriction occurs, reverse immediately by administration of a rapid-acting inhaled bronchodilator (β-agonist). Do not perform methacholine challenge in any patient with clinically apparent asthma, wheezing or very low baseline pulmonary function tests (ie, $FEV_1 < 1$ to 1.5 L or < 70% of the predicted values). Consult standard nomograms for predicted values.

Actions:

Pharmacology: Methacholine is a parasympathomimetic (cholinergic) bronchoconstrictor, the β-methyl homolog of acetylcholine, and differs from the latter primarily in its greater duration and selectivity of action. Bronchial smooth muscle contains significant parasympathetic innervation. Bronchoconstriction occurs when the vagus nerve is stimulated releasing acetylcholine from the nerve endings. Muscle constriction is essentially confined to the local site of release because acetylcholine is rapidly inactivated by acetylcholinesterase.Compared with acetylcholine, methacholine is more slowly hydrolyzed by acetylcholinesterase and is almost totally resistant to inactivation by nonspecific cholinesterase or pseudocholinesterase. Asthmatics are markedly more sensitive to inhaled methacholine-induced bronchoconstriction than are healthy subjects. This difference is the pharmacologic basis for the methacholine inhalation challenge.

Indications:

Bronchial airway hyperreactivity diagnosis: For the diagnosis of bronchial airway hyperreactivity in subjects who do not have clinically apparent asthma.

Contraindications:

Hypersensitivity to methacholine or other parasympathomimetics; repeated administration other than challenge with increasing doses; patients receiving any β-adrenergic blocking agent because, in such patients, responses to methacholine can be exaggerated or prolonged, and may not respond as readily to treatment.

Warnings:

Pregnancy: Category C. It is not known whether this drug can cause fetal harm when administered to a pregnant patient or can affect reproductive capacity. Give to a pregnant woman only if clearly needed. In females of childbearing potential, perform inhalation challenge either within 10 days following the onset of menses or within 2 weeks of a negative pregnancy test.

Lactation: It is not known whether inhaled methacholine is excreted in breast milk. Do not administer to nursing women.

Children: Safety and efficacy for use in children < 5 years of age have not been established.

Precautions:

Special risk patients: Do not administer to patients with epilepsy, cardiovascular disease accompanied by bradycardia, vagotonia, peptic ulcer disease, thyroid disease, urinary tract obstruction or other conditions that could be adversely affected by a cholinergic agent unless the benefit to the individual outweighs the potential risk.

Adverse Reactions:

Inhalation: Headache, throat irritation, lightheadedness, itching (one case each).

Oral/Injection: Nausea; vomiting; substernal pain or pressure; hypotension; fainting; transient complete heart block.

Overdosage:

Symptoms: When administered orally or by injection, overdosage with methacholine can result in a syncopal reaction with cardiac arrest and loss of consciousness.

Treatment: Treat serious toxic reactions with 0.5 to 1 mg atropine sulfate, IM or IV.

Patient Information:

Instruct patients about symptoms that may occur as a result of the test, and explain how to manage such symptoms.

METHACHOLINE CHLORIDE

Female patients should inform physician of pregnancy, the date of last onset of menses or the date and result of last pregnancy test.

Administration and Dosage:

Administer by inhalation only.

Before inhalation challenge is begun, perform baseline pulmonary function tests. The subject to be challenged must have an FEV_1 of at least 70% of the predicted value.

The target level for a positive challenge is a 20% reduction in the FEV_1 compared with the baseline value after inhalation of the control sodium chloride solution. Calculate and record the target value before challenge is started.

Procedure: Perform the challenge by giving a subject ascending serial concentrations of methacholine. At each concentration, five breaths are administered by a nebulizer that permits intermittent delivery time of 0.6 seconds by either a Y–tube or a breath-actuated timing device (dosimeter).

At each of five inhalations of a serial concentration, the subject begins at functional residual capacity (FRC) and slowly and completely inhales the dose delivered. Within 5 minutes, FEV_1 values are determined. The procedure ends either when there is a ≥ 20% reduction in the FEV_1 compared with the baseline sodium chloride solution value (ie, a positive response) or if 188.88 total cumulative units have been given (see table below) and FEV_1 has been reduced by ≤ 14% (ie, a negative response). If there is a reduction of 15% to 19% in FEV_1 vs baseline, either repeat the challenge at that concentration or give a higher concentration as long as dosage administered does not result in total cumulative units > 188.88.

The following is a suggested schedule for administration of methacholine challenge. Calculate cumulative units by multiplying number of breaths by concentration given. Total cumulative units is the sum of cumulative units for each concentration given.

Suggested Methacholine Administration Schedule

Vial	Serial concentration	Number of breaths	Cumulative units per concentration	Total cumulative units
E	0.025 mg/ml	5	0.125	0.125
D	0.25 mg/ml	5	1.25	1.375
C	2.5 mg/ml	5	12.5	13.88
B	10 mg/ml	5	50	63.88
A	25 mg/ml	5	125	188.88

An inhaled β-agonist may be administered after methacholine challenge to expedite the return of the FEV_1 to baseline and to relieve the discomfort of the subject. Most patients revert to normal pulmonary function within 5 minutes following bronchodilators or within 30 to 45 minutes without any bronchodilator.

Dilutions: (Do not inhale powder. Do not handle this material if you have asthma or hay fever.) Make all dilutions with 0.9% sodium chloride injection containing 0.4% phenol (pH 7). Use a bacterial-retentive filter (porosity 0.22 μ) when transferring solution from vial to nebulizer. After adding the sodium chloride solution, shake each vial to obtain a clear solution.

Vial A – Add 4 ml of 0.9% sodium chloride injection containing 0.4% phenol (pH 7) to the 5 ml vial containing 100 mg (25 mg/ml).

Vial B – Remove 3 ml from vial A, transfer to another vial and add 4.5 ml of the 0.9% sodium chloride solution (10 mg/ml). An alternative method of preparing vial B is to remove 1 ml from vial A and add 1.5 ml 0.9% sodium chloride solution.

Vial C – Remove 1 ml from vial A, transfer to another vial and add 9 ml of the 0.9% sodium chloride solution (2.5 mg/ml). This step depletes contents of vial A if the first dilution method under vial B directions is used.

Vial D – Remove 1 ml from vial C, transfer to another vial and add 9 ml of the 0.9% sodium chloride solution (0.25 mg/ml).

Vial E – Remove 1 ml from vial D, transfer to another vial and add 9 ml of the 0.9% sodium chloride solution (0.025 mg/ml).

Storage/Stability: Store dilutions A through D in refrigerator (36° to 46° F) for up to 2 weeks, then discard the vials. Freezing does not affect the stability of dilutions A through D. Vial E must be prepared on the day of the challenge. Store the unreconstituted powder at 59° to 86° F.

Rx	**Provocholine** (Roche)	**Powder for reconstitution of solution for inhalation:** 100 mg per 5 ml	In 5 ml vials.

TERIPARATIDE ACETATE

Actions:

Pharmacology: Teriparatide acetate (hPTH 1-34) is a synthetic polypeptide hormone consisting of the 1-34 fragment of human parathyroid hormone, the biologically active N-terminal region of the 84 amino acid native hormone.

Parathyroid hormone is secreted by the four parathyroid glands found on or embedded in the two lateral lobes of the thyroid gland. Human parathyroid hormone 1-34 acts on bone to mobilize calcium; it also acts on the kidney to reduce calcium clearance, increase phosphate excretion, stimulate the release of cyclic AMP in the urine, and stimulate the conversion of 25-hydroxyvitamin D_3 (25-OH-D_3) to the active form 1, 25-dihydroxyvitamin D_3 [1,25$(OH)_2D_3$].

The initial effect of teriparatide acetate on bone is to promote an increased rate of release of calcium from bone into blood.

The kidney effects, which may be due to a direct action of the hormone on its receptors, include a reduction of calcium clearance and an inhibition of tubular phosphate reabsorption as well as an increased excretion of sodium and potassium. Parathyroid hormone stimulates the conversion of 25-OH-D to 1,25$(OH)_2$D by the kidney.

Intestinal transport of calcium is increased by the PTH indirectly by increasing renal 1,25$(OH)_2$D production.

The primary mode of action is the stimulation of adenylate cyclase in the involved organ.

Indications:

Diagnostic agent to assist in establishing the diagnosis in patients presenting with clinical laboratory evidence of hypocalcemia due to either hypoparathyroidism or pseudohypoparathyroidism. The test will distinguish between hypoparathyroidism and pseudohypoparathyroidism, but not between these conditions and normal. The discriminant power of its effect on urinary cAMP is much greater than that of the effect on urinary phosphate.

Contraindications:

Hypersensitivity to teriparatide or any component of this preparation.

Warnings:

Hypercalcemia may develop with the administration of teriparatide. Teriparatide is not intended for recurrent or chronic use.

Allergic reactions: Because teriparatide acetate is a peptide, systemic allergic reactions are possible. This product may contain up to 35% extraneous peptides, the chemical structures of which have not been determined. Have epinephrine 1:1000 immediately available. Refer to Management of Acute Hypersensitivity Reactions.

Pregnancy: Category C. It is not known whether teriparatide can cause fetal harm when administered to a pregnant woman or can affect reproductive capacity. Give to a pregnant woman only if clearly needed.

Lactation: It is not known to what degree teriparatide is excreted in human milk, but the peptide would not be expected to be absorbed in an active form from the infant's GI tract. However, exercise caution when administering to a nursing woman.

Children: Use in children 3 years of age and older was uneventful and the response to the drug followed expected patterns. Limited data are available.

Adverse Reactions:

Hypertensive crisis occurred in one patient 8 hours after a study. This patient had experienced previous hypertensive episodes not related to teriparatide acetate injection.

Metabolic: Hypocalcemia was not reversed in one patient, and a hypocalcemic convulsion occurred 4½ hours following injection; this was corrected by calcium administration.

GI: Nausea, abdominal cramps, urge to defecate, diarrhea (< 2%).

Body as a whole: Tingling of the extremities, metallic taste and pain at the injection site during or shortly following the infusion (< 2%).

TERIPARATIDE ACETATE

Overdosage:

Repeated doses in excess of 500 units may produce hypercalcemia. In those who are borderline hypercalcemic (10.5 mg/dl), a dose of 200 units could produce mild hypercalcemia for a brief period. If hypercalcemia develops, discontinue the drug and ensure adequate hydration.

Administration and Dosage:

Diagnostic use in patients with hypocalcemia:

Adult dose – 200 units. Reconstitute by adding the 10 ml diluent to the 10 ml vial. The 10 ml of solution is infused IV over 10 minutes.

Children (≥ 3 years) – 3 units/kg (maximum of 200 units). Use reconstituted solution within 4 hours. Discard any unused portion.

Modified Ellsworth Howard test: Test subjects should be in a fasting state when starting the test period. Initiate and maintain an active urine output by the ingestion of 200 ml of water/hour for 2 hours prior to study and continuing through the study. Make a baseline urine collection in the 60 minute period preceding the infusion. Following the hPTH (1-34) infusion (time 0), collect urine as separate collections in the 0 to 30 minute, 30 to 60 minute and 60 to 120 minute postinfusion time periods. Confidence in the test will be influenced by adequate hydration and urine flow and complete collection of urine specimens.

Interpretation of test: The measurement of urinary cAMP and phosphate must be corrected for creatinine excretion.

Hypoparathyroidism patients – In the clinical trials, these patients showed a tenfold or greater increase over baseline of urinary cAMP at the 0 to 30 minute postinfusion period, and 92% of these patients showed a threefold or greater urinary phosphate excretion in the 0 to 60 minute collection.

Pseudohypoparathyroid patients with end-organ resistance pseudohypoparathyroidism showed a blunted response of less than sixfold increase of urinary cAMP excretion over baseline in the 0 to 30 minute period, and 88% showed a less than threefold increase in urinary phosphate excretion in the 0 to 60 minute collection period.

Although this test does not discriminate between normal and abnormal in most cases, it does discriminate between hypoparathyroidism and pseudohypoparathyroidism. The change in the urinary cAMP excretion in the 0 to 30 minute period is the most sensitive indicator for separation of hypoparathyroidisms.

Rx	**Parathar** (Rorer)	**Powder for Injection (lyophilized):** 200 units hPTH activity	In 10 ml vials[1] w/10 ml vial of diluent.

[1] With 20 mg gelatin.

Gastrointestinal Function Tests

PENTAGASTRIN

Actions:

Pharmacology: Pentagastrin contains the C-terminal tetrapeptide responsible for the actions of the natural gastrins and, therefore, acts as a physiologic gastric acid secretagogue. The recommended dose of 6 mcg/kg SC produces a peak acid output which is reproducible when used in the same individual. It stimulates gastric acid secretion approximately 10 minutes after SC injection, with peak responses occurring in most cases 20 to 30 minutes after administration. Duration of activity is usually between 60 and 80 minutes.

Indications:

A diagnostic agent to evaluate gastric acid secretory function in:

Anacidity: In suspected pernicious anemia, atrophic gastritis or gastric carcinoma.

Hypersecretion: In suspected duodenal ulcer or postoperative stomal ulcer; Zollinger-Ellison tumor.

It is also useful in determining the adequacy of acid-reducing operations for peptic ulcer.

Contraindications:

Hypersensitivity or idiosyncrasy to pentagastrin.

Warnings:

Effects on gastric acid secretion: In amounts in excess of the recommended dose, pentagastrin may cause inhibition of gastric acid secretion.

Pregnancy: Safety for use during pregnancy has not been established. Use only when clearly needed and when the potential benefits outweigh the unknown potential hazards to the fetus.

Children: Safety and efficacy for use in children have not been established.

Precautions:

Use with caution in patients with pancreatic, hepatic or biliary disease. Like gastrin, pentagastrin could, in some cases, have the physiologic effect of stimulating pancreatic enzyme and bicarbonate secretion, as well as biliary flow.

Adverse Reactions:

Causes fewer and less severe cardiovascular and other adverse reactions than histamine. The majority of reactions are related to the GI tract.

Allergic and hypersensitivity reactions may occur in some patients.

GI: Abdominal pain; urge to defecate; nausea; vomiting; borborygmi; blood-tinged mucus.

Cardiovascular: Flushing; tachycardia.

CNS: Dizziness; faintness; lightheadedness; drowsiness; sinking feeling; transient blurring of vision; tiredness; headache.

Body as a whole: Shortness of breath; heavy sensation in arms and legs; tingling fingers; chills; sweating; generalized burning sensation; warmth; pain at injection site; bile in collected specimens.

Overdosage:

In case of overdosage or idiosyncrasy, administer symptomatic treatment, as required.

Refer to General Management of Acute Overdosage.

Administration and Dosage:

Adults: 6 mcg/kg SC.

Rx	**Peptavlon** (Ayerst)	**Injection:** 0.25 mg (250 mcg) per ml	In 2 ml amps.

Gastrointestinal Function Tests

BENTIROMIDE

Actions:

Pharmacology: Bentiromide is a peptide which carries the marker para-aminobenzoic acid (PABA); 500 mg of bentiromide contains 170 mg PABA.

Pharmacokinetics: Following oral administration, bentiromide is selectively cleaved by pancreatic chymotrypsin with the liberation of PABA. PABA is readily absorbed through the intestinal mucosa under normal conditions, and is conjugated primarily by the liver and rapidly excreted in the urine. Under conditions of normal exocrine pancreatic function, gastric emptying, and gut and kidney function, over 50% of the PABA contained in bentiromide appears in the urine within 6 hours following administration. It is not known whether bentiromide or PABA crosses the placental barrier or the blood brain barrier.

PABA is detected in the urine using the Smith modification of the Bratton-Marshall test for arylamines, which detects both conjugated and unconjugated arylamines.

Indications:

Screening test for pancreatic exocrine insufficiency; to monitor the adequacy of supplemental pancreatic therapy.

Contraindications:

Hypersensitivity to bentiromide.

Warnings:

Hypersensitivity: A single case of bentiromide hypersensitivity has been reported (see Adverse Reactions). The frequency of sensitization is unknown. Following administration, patients should remain in a medical setting for observation.

Have epinephrine 1:1000 immediately available. Refer to Management of Acute Hypersensitivity Reactions.

Renal/Hepatic function impairment: May alter test interpretation due to altered handling of PABA.

Pregnancy: Category B. Reproduction studies in small animals revealed no evidence of impaired fertility or fetal harm due to bentiromide doses 50 and 100 times the human dose. Safety for use during pregnancy has not been established. Use only when clearly needed and when the potential benefits outweigh the unknown potential hazards to the fetus.

Lactation: It is not known whether this drug is excreted in breast milk. Safety for use in the nursing mother has not been established.

Children: Safety and efficacy for use in children < 6 years old are not established.

Precautions:

Proper use of bentiromide requires close attention to the technical details of drug administration and of urine collection, handling and assay for arylamine levels and awareness that "false-positive" and "false-negative" results can occur.

Schedule repeat dosings, if needed, at intervals of 7 days or more to assure complete metabolism and excretion of prior doses of the drug.

Diabetics: Insulin may need adjustment to accommodate the fasting patient.

GI absorption defects may falsely indicate decreased chymotrypsin secretion.

Laboratory tests: It has not been established whether concurrent GI diagnostic testing interferes with the results of this test; conduct GI testing at least 24 hours before or after dosing with bentiromide.

Drug Interactions:

Methotrexate may compete for binding sites with PABA.

Sulfa drugs: PABA interferes with antibacterial action.

Salicylates: Therapeutic and toxic effects may be increased with concurrent administration of PABA.

Assay Interactions: Drugs metabolized to primary arylamines may cause assay interference and falsely elevate test results. These drugs include: **Acetaminophen, benzocaine, chloramphenicol, lidocaine, procaine, procainamide**and **thiazide diuretics. PABA-containing drugs**such as sunscreens or certain multiple vitamins may also falsely elevate test results. Discontinue any of these drugs 3 days prior to bentiromide administration.

In adults, discontinue oral pancreatic enzyme supplements 5 days prior to bentiromide administration. In cystic fibrotic children, reduce the time interval to 1 day.

Gastrointestinal Function Tests

BENTIROMIDE

Adverse Reactions:

Most frequent: Diarrhea, headache (< 2%).

Rare: Flatulence, nausea, vomiting and weakness (0.6%) are transient and rarely require symptomatic therapy.

Acute respiratory distress and stridor requiring symptomatic therapy has been reported in one patient following a second dose of bentiromide; the patient developed coughing and choking after his first dose.

Causal relationship unknown: Abdominal pain; drowsiness; lightheadedness; heartburn; transient elevations of liver function tests.

Overdosage:

Treatment includes usual supportive measures. Refer to General Management of Acute Overdosage.

Patient Information:

Patient package insert available with product.

Fast after midnight before taking bentiromide.

Urinate before taking the drug.

Notify physician if you are taking any drugs that may interfere with the test (see Drug Interactions). Discontinue pancreatic supplements 5 days before the test.

Diarrhea, headache, nausea, vomiting, flatulence and weakness have been reported. If any discomfort or unusual change is experienced, notify physician.

Administration and Dosage:

Administer following an overnight fast. Urinate prior to drug administration. Administer a single 500 mg dose; follow immediately by 250 ml of water. In patients less than 12 years of age, calculate the dose on the basis of 14 mg/kg. Drinking water is encouraged to promote diuresis. Give the patient 250 ml of water at post-dosing hour 2 and up to an additional 500 ml during post-dosing hours 2 through 6. Obtain a total urine collection during 0 to 6 hours post-dosing. Measure the volume of the collection and retain a 10 ml sample for analysis. Break the fast following completion of urine collection. Should re-testing be necessary, separate subsequent administrations by at least 7 day intervals to avoid interference of test results by prior bentiromide dosings.

Analysis of urine: Use the Smith modification of the Bratton-Marshall test for arylamines.

A negative bentiromide test suggesting pancreatic exocrine insufficiency should not lead to termination of the search for a pancreatic etiology of maldigestion or other pancreatic disease. A good response to an oral pancreatic enzyme supplement would be confirmatory of a positive bentiromide test.

For test interpretations, see manufacturer's package insert.

Rx	**Chymex** (Adria)	**Solution:** 500 mg (170 mg PABA) in 40% propylene glycol	In 7.5 ml.

SECRETIN

Actions:

Pharmacology: The main action of secretin is to increase the volume and bicarbonate content of pancreatic juice. In one study of 6 healthy subjects, the elimination half-life was about 4 minutes and the clearance rate was 540 ml/min. Normal ranges and values for pancreatic secretory response to IV secretin in patients with specific pancreatic diseases can vary significantly from one investigator to another, presumably because of differences in technique. However, a constant and reliable response can be obtained. The results of a properly performed test when compared to results obtained in an adequate series of normal subjects will reliably identify pancreatic disease.

A set of typical values (± S.D.) for pancreatic secretory responses to secretin in normal subjects and patients with well documented pancreatitis is given in the table below:

Values for Pancreatic Secretory Responses to Secretin

Parameters	Normal Subjects	Pancreatitis
Volume (ml/hr)	235 ± 60	63 ± 42
Bicarbonate (mEq/L)	114 ± 20	71 ± 33
Bicarbonate output (mEq/kg/hr)	0.436 ± 0.141	0.105 ± 0.093

These values are derived from a single study. Use them as guidelines only. When performing secretin testing for diagnosis of pancreatic disease for the first time, begin by assessing normal subjects to develop proficiency in proper technique and to generate normal ranges for the three commonly assessed parameters of pancreatic exocrine response.

Secretin IV stimulates gastrin release in patients with gastrinoma (Zollinger-Ellison syndrome), and either does not affect, or produces small changes in, serum gastrin concentrations in normal subjects. It may produce a small decrease in gastrin in patients with duodenal ulcer disease. This action is the basis for its use as a provocative test in the evaluation of patients in whom gastrinoma is a diagnostic consideration.

Indications:

Diagnosis of pancreatic exocrine disease.

Diagnosis of gastrinoma (Zollinger-Ellison syndrome).

As an adjunct in obtaining desquamated pancreatic cells for cytopathologic examination.

Contraindications:

Do not give to patients with acute pancreatitis until the attack has subsided.

Warnings:

Pregnancy: It is not known whether secretin can cause fetal harm when administered to pregnant women or can affect reproductive capacity. Since fluoroscopic guidance is usually necessary to position the duodenal lumen of the double-lumen tube used for the pancreatic function test, postpone the test until after delivery in pregnant women.

Lactation: It is not known whether secretin is excreted in breast milk. Exercise caution when administering to the nursing mother. Normal values for pancreatic secretory and serum gastrin response to secretin have not been established for nursing mothers.

Precautions:

Test dose: Administer an IV test dose of 0.1 to 1 CU secretin, especially to patients with a history of atopic allergy or asthma. One minute later, if there has been no allergic reaction, administer the recommended dose by injection over approximately 1 minute.

Patients who have undergone vagotomy, who are receiving anticholinergics at the time of secretin testing, or who have inflammatory bowel disease may be hyporesponsive to secretin stimulation. This does not indicate pancreatic disease.

A greater than normal volume response to secretin stimulation, which can mask coexisting pancreatic disease, is occasionally encountered in patients with alcoholic or other liver disease.

Adverse Reactions:

None reported.

Gastrointestinal Function Tests

SECRETIN

Administration and Dosage:

Pancreatic function testing: Pass a Dreiling type, radiopaque, double-lumen tube through the mouth after a 12 to 15 hour fast. Under fluoroscopic guidance, place the proximal lumen of the tube in the gastric antrum and the distal lumen just beyond the papilla of Vater. Confirm the position of the tube and secure the tube in place prior to testing. Apply suction at a negative pressure of 25 to 40 mm Hg to both lumens and maintain throughout the test. Interruption of suction at intervals of about 1 minute improves the reliability of collection. When uncontaminated duodenal contents are obtained (ie, clear, although possibly bile stained, with a pH of 6 or higher), collect a baseline sample of duodenal fluid for 2 consecutive 10 minute periods. Subsequent to the baseline collections, slowly inject secretin in a dose of 1 CU/kg IV over approximately 1 minute. Then, collect duodenal fluid for 60 minutes after administration. The aspirate is fractioned into four collection periods, the first two at 10 minute intervals, and the last two at 20 minute intervals. Clear the duodenal lumen of the tube with an injection of air after collection of each fraction. Wide variations in volume of the aspirate suggest incomplete aspiration or contamination. Place each fraction of duodenal fluid on ice and subsequently analyze for volume and bicarbonate concentration. The duodenal aspirate may also be submitted for cytopathological examination.

Diagnosis of gastrinoma (Zollinger-Ellison syndrome): The patient should fast for 12 hours prior to the test. Prior to injection of secretin, draw 2 blood samples for determination of baseline serum gastrin levels. Subsequently, give 2 CU/kg IV over 1 minute and collect post-injection blood samples at 1, 2, 5, 10 and 30 minutes for determination of serum gastrin concentrations.

Gastrinoma is strongly suggested in patients with elevated fasting serum gastrin concentrations in the 120 to 500 pg/ml range (determined by RIA using an antibody to gastrin similar to that prepared by Rehfeld) and an increase in serum gastrin concentration of more than 110 pg/ml over basal level in response to IV secretin.

Preparation of solution: Prepare immediately prior to use. Dissolve contents of a vial in 7.5 ml Sodium Chloride Injection, to give a concentration of 10 CU/ml. Avoid vigorous shaking.

Storage: Store in freezer at -20°C. Can be stored at 25°C or below for up to 3 weeks.

Rx	**Secretin Ferring Powder** (Ferring)	**Powder for Injection:** 75 CU per vial (10 CU/ml when reconstituted w/7.5 ml)	In 10 ml vials.[1]

[1] With 1 mg l-cysteine HCl and 20 mg mannitol.

Gastrointestinal Function Tests

SINCALIDE

Actions:

Pharmacology: Sincalide IV substantially reduces gallbladder size by causing it to contract. The evacuation of bile that results is similar to the physiological response to endogenous cholecystokinin. Bolus IV administration causes a prompt contraction of the gallbladder that becomes maximal in 5 to 15 minutes. The stimulus of a fatty meal causes a progressive contraction that becomes maximal after approximately 40 minutes. A 40% reduction in radiographic area of the gallbladder is satisfactory.

Like cholecystokinin, sincalide given in conjunction with secretin stimulates pancreatic secretion; concurrent administration increases the volume of pancreatic secretion and the output of bicarbonate and protein (enzymes). This combined effect of secretin and sincalide permits the assessment of specific pancreatic function through measurement and analysis of the duodenal aspirate. The parameters determined are: Volume of the secretion; bicarbonate concentration; and amylase content (which parallels the content of trypsin and total protein).

Indications:

Used to provide a sample of gallbladder bile for analysis of its composition (eg, to determine the degree of cholesterol saturation).

Use in conjunction with secretin (see Administration and Dosage) to stimulate pancreatic secretion for analysis of its composition and examination of cytology (eg, in suspected cancer of the pancreas).

For postevacuation cholecystography, when this procedure is indicated but the physician wishes to avoid the fatty meal.

Contraindications:

Patients sensitive to sincalide.

Warnings:

Pregnancy: No teratogenic or antifertility effects were seen in animal studies. Data are inadequate to determine safety in human pregnancy. Use in pregnant women only when the benefits outweigh the possible risk to the fetus.

Children: The safety for use in children has not been established.

Precautions:

Stimulation of gallbladder contraction in patients with small gallbladder stones may lead to the evacuation of the stones, resulting in their lodging in the cystic duct or in the common bile duct. The risk is minimal because sincalide, when given as directed, does not ordinarily cause complete contraction of the gallbladder.

Adverse Reactions:

Gastrointestinal symptoms such as abdominal discomfort or pain and an urge to defecate frequently accompany the injection of sincalide. These phenomena are manifestations of the physiologic actions of the drug including delayed gastric emptying and increased intestinal motility. The reactions do not necessarily indicate a biliary tract abnormality unless there is other clinical or radiologic evidence of disease. Nausea, dizziness and flushing occur occasionally.

Administration and Dosage:

Contraction of the gallbladder: A dose of 0.02 mcg/kg (1.4 mcg/70 kg) is injected IV over 30 to 60 seconds; if satisfactory gallbladder contraction does not occur in 15 minutes, a second dose (0.04 mcg/kg) may be given. In cholecystography, roentgenograms are usually taken at 5 minute intervals after the injection. For visualization of the cystic duct, it may be necessary to take roentgenograms at 1 minute intervals during the first 5 minutes after the injection.

Secretin-Sincalide test of pancreatic function: A dose of 0.25 units/kg of secretin is infused IV over 60 minutes. Thirty minutes after initiating secretin, give a separate IV infusion of sincalide at a total dose of 0.02 mcg/kg over 30 minutes. For example, the total dose for a 70 kg patient is 1.4 mcg sincalide; therefore, dilute 1.4 ml reconstituted sincalide solution to 30 ml with Sodium Chloride Injection and administer at a rate of 1ml/minute.

Preparation of solution: To reconstitute, add 5 ml Sterile Water for Injection to the vial; the solution may be kept at room temperature. Use within 24 hours after reconstitution; discard any unused portion.

Storage: Store at room temperature prior to reconstitution.

Rx	**Kinevac** (Squibb)	**Powder for Injection**: 5 mcg per vial for reconstitution (1 mcg/ml when reconstituted).

BENZYLPENICILLOYL-POLYLYSINE

Actions:

Pharmacology: Benzylpenicilloyl-polylysine is a skin test antigen that reacts specifically with benzylpenicilloyl skin sensitizing antibodies (reagins: IgE class) to produce an immediate wheal and flare reaction at a skin test site. Individuals exhibiting a positive response possess reagins against the benzylpenicilloyl group.

Individuals who have previously received therapeutic penicillin may have positive skin test reactions to benzylpenicilloyl-polylysine and to other non-benzylpenicilloyl haptenes of minor determinants. The major metabolite of penicillin is the penicilloyl group; this "major determinant" is thought to be responsible for accelerated reactions, but not anaphylaxis. Other breakdown products or "minor determinants" are felt to be responsible for anaphylaxis and immediate systemic reactions. Virtually everyone who receives penicillin develops specific antibodies, but skin tests to penicillin and penicillin-derived reagents become positive in less than 10% of patients who have tolerated penicillin in the past; allergic responses are infrequent (< 1%).

Many individuals reacting positively will not develop a systemic allergic reaction on subsequent exposure to therapeutic penicillin; this skin test facilitates assessing the local allergic skin reactivity to benzylpenicilloyl.

Indications:

An adjunct in assessing the risk of administering penicillin (benzylpenicillin or penicillin G) in adults with a history of clinical penicillin hypersensitivity. A negative skin test is associated with an incidence of allergic reactions of < 5% after the administration of penicillin; the incidence may be > 20% in the presence of a positive skin test.

Contraindications:

Systemic or marked local reaction to previous administration. Do not test patients known to be extremely hypersensitive to penicillin.

Warnings:

Systemic allergic reactions rarely follow a skin test. Avoid by making the first application by scratch test. Use the intradermal route only if the scratch test is entirely negative. Do not perform skin testing with penicillin or other penicillin derived reagents simultaneously.

Pregnancy: Safety for use during pregnancy has not been established. Use only when clearly needed and when potential benefits outweigh unknown potential hazards.

Precautions:

Allergic reactions are predominantly dermatologic. Data are insufficient to document that a decreased incidence of anaphylactic reactions following penicillin administration will occur in patients with a negative skin test. Similarly, data are insufficient to determine the value of this skin test as a means of assessing the risk of administering therapeutic penicillin (when penicillin is the drug of choice) in adult patients with no history of clinical penicillin hypersensitivity or in pediatric patients.

No reagent, test or combination of tests will completely assure a reaction to penicillin therapy will not occur.

Data are insufficient to assess the potential danger of sensitization to penicillin from repeated skin testing.

There are no data to assess the clinical value of benzylpenicilloyl-polylysine skin test where exposure to penicillin is suspected as a cause of a drug reaction and in patients who are undergoing routine allergy evaluation.

There are no data relating the clinical value of skin tests to the risk of administering semisynthetic penicillins (phenoxymethyl penicillin, ampicillin, carbenicillin, dicloxacillin, methicillin, nafcillin, oxacillin) and cephalosporin-derived antibiotics.

Consider the following clinical outcomes when the decision to administer or not to administer penicillin is based in part on the skin test: (1) An allergic reaction to penicillin may occur in a patient with a negative skin test. (2) A patient may have an anaphylactic reaction to penicillin in the presence of a negative skin test and a negative history of clinical penicillin hypersensitivity. (3) If penicillin is the absolute drug of choice in a life-threatening situation, successful desensitization with therapeutic penicillin may be possible, despite a positive skin test or a positive history of clinical penicillin hypersensitivity.

BENZYLPENICILLOYL-POLYLYSINE

Adverse Reactions:

Local: Occasional intense inflammatory response at the skin test site.

Systemic: Generalized erythema, pruritis, urticaria, angioneurotic edema, dyspnea or hypotension. The usual methods of treating a skin test antigen-induced reaction (application of a venous occlusion tourniquet proximal to the skin test site and administration of epinephrine or antihistamine) are recommended and will usually control the reaction. Systemic allergic reactions following skin test procedures usually are of short duration and controllable, but observe the patient for several hours.

Hypersensitivity: Have epinephrine 1:1000 immediately available. Refer to Management of Acute Hypersensitivity Reactions.

Administration and Dosage:

Scratch testing: Perform skin testing on the inner volar aspect of the forearm. *Always* apply the skin test material first by the scratch technique. After preparing the skin surface, use a sterile 20 gauge needle to make a 3 to 5 mm scratch on the epidermis. Very little pressure is required to break the epidermal continuity. If bleeding occurs, prepare a second site and scratch more lightly with the needle, sufficient to produce a nonbleeding scratched surface. Apply a small drop of solution to the scratch and rub gently with an applicator, toothpick or the side of the needle.

Interpretation of test results – Observe for the appearance of a wheal, erythema and itching at the test site during the next 15 minutes, then wipe off the solution over the scratch. A positive reaction consists of development of a pale wheal, usually with pseudopods, surrounding the scratch site within 10 minutes. It varies in diameter from 5 to 15 mm (or more). This wheal may be surrounded by erythema and accompanied by itching. The most sensitive individuals develop itching instantly, and the wheal and erythema promptly appear. As soon as a positive response is clearly evident, wipe off the solution over the scratch. If the scratch test is either negative or equivocally positive (< 5 mm wheal, little or no erythema, no itching), perform an intradermal test.

Intradermal test: Using a tuberculin syringe with a ⅜" to ⅝", 26 to 30 gauge, short bevel needle, withdraw the contents of the ampule. Prepare a sterile skin test area on the upper, outer arm, sufficiently below the deltoid muscle to permit proximal application of a tourniquet, if necessary. Inject an amount of benzylpenicilloyl-polylysine sufficient to raise the smallest possible perceptible bleb. This volume will be 0.01 to 0.02 ml. Using a separate syringe and needle, inject a like amount of saline as a control at least 1½ inches from the test site.

Interpretation of test results – Most skin reactions develop within 5 to 15 minutes.

Negative (–): No increase in size of original bleb or no greater reaction than the control site.

Ambiguous (±): Wheal only slightly larger than initial injection bleb, with or without accompanying erythematous flare and larger than the control site.

Positive (+): Itching and marked increase in size of original bleb. Wheal may exceed 20 mm in diameter and exhibit pseudopods.

The control site should be completely reactionless. If it exhibits a wheal greater than 2 to 3 mm, repeat the test. If the same reaction is observed, consult a physician experienced with allergy skin testing.

Storage: Stable only when kept under refrigeration; discard test materials subjected to ambient temperatures for over a day.

Rx	**Pre-Pen** (Kremers-Urban)	**Solution:** 0.25 ml per amp.

DIPYRIDAMOLE

Dipyridamole oral is used as an antiplatelet agent. Refer to the individual monograph in the Blood Modifiers chapter.

Actions:

Pharmacology: Dipyridamole for IV injection is a coronary vasodilator used for the evaluation of coronary artery disease. The mechanism of vasodilation has not been fully elucidated, but may result from inhibition of adenosine uptake, an important mediator of coronary vasodilation. How dipyridamole-induced vasodilation leads to abnormalities in thallium distribution ventriculation function is also uncertain, but presumably represents a "steal" phenomenon in which relatively intact vessels dilate, and sustain enhanced flow, leaving reduced pressure and flow across areas of hemodynamically important coronary vascular constriction.

In a study of 10 patients with angiographically normal or minimally stenosed coronary vessels, IV dipyridamole 0.56 mg/kg infused over 4 minutes resulted in an average fivefold increase in coronary blood flow velocity compared to resting coronary flow velocity. The mean time to peak flow velocity was 6.5 minutes from the start of the 4 minute infusion. Cardiovascular responses, when given to patients in the supine position, include a mild but significant increase in heart rate of ≈ 20% and mild, but significant decreases in both systolic and diastolic blood pressure of ≈ 2% to 8%, with vital signs returning to baseline values in ≈ 30 minutes.

Pharmacokinetics: Plasma dipyridamole concentrations decline in a triexponential fashion following IV infusion with half-lives averaging 3 to 12 minutes, 33 to 62 minutes and 11.6 to 15 hours. The mean dipyridamole serum concentration is 4.6 ± 1.3 mcg/ml 2 minutes after a 4 minute 0.568 mg/kg infusion. The average plasma protein binding of dipyridamole is ≈ 99%, primarily to α_1-glycoprotein. Dipyridamole is metabolized in the liver to the glucuronic acid conjugate and excreted with the bile. Average total body clearance is 2.3 to 3.5 ml/min/kg, with apparent volume of distribution at steady state of 1 to 2.5 L/kg and a central apparent volume of 3 to 5 L.

Clinical trials: In a study of about 1100 patients who underwent coronary arteriography and IV dipyridamole-assisted thallium imaging, the sensitivity of the dipyridamole test (true positive dipyridamole divided by the total number of patients with positive angiography) was about 85%. The specificity (true negative divided by the number of patients with negative angiograms) was about 50%. In a subset of patients who had exercise thallium imaging as well as dipyridamole thallium imaging, sensitivity and specificity of the two tests were almost identical.

Indications:

As an alternative to exercise in thallium myocardial perfusion imaging for the evaluation of coronary artery disease in patients who cannot exercise adequately.

Contraindications:

Hypersensitivity to dipyridamole.

Warnings:

Cardiotoxicity and bronchospasm: Serious adverse reactions have included fatal and non-fatal myocardial infarction, ventricular fibrillation, symptomatic ventricular tachycardia, transient cerebral ischemia and bronchospasm.

In a study of 3911 patients given IV dipyridamole as an adjunct to thallium myocardial perfusion imaging, two types of serious adverse events occurred: Four cases of myocardial infarction (0.1%; two fatal, two non-fatal); and six cases of severe bronchospasm (0.2%). Although the incidence was small (0.3%; 10 of 3911), the potential clinical information to be gained through use of IV dipyridamole thallium imaging must be weighed against the patient risk. Patients with a history of unstable angina may be at a greater risk for severe myocardial ischemia, and patients with a history of asthma may be at a greater risk for bronchospasm.

When thallium myocardial perfusion imaging is performed with IV dipyridamole, parenteral aminophylline should be readily available for relieving adverse events such as bronchospasm or chest pain. Monitor vital signs during, and for 10 to 15 minutes following, the IV infusion of dipyridamole, and obtain an ECG tracing using at least one chest lead. Should severe chest pain or bronchospasm occur, administer parenteral aminophylline by slow IV injection (50 to 100 mg over 30 to 60 seconds) in doses ranging from 50 to 250 mg. In the case of severe hypotension, place the patient in a supine position with the head tilted down, if necessary, before administration of aminophylline. If 250 mg does not relieve chest pain symptoms within a few minutes, SL nitroglycerin may be administered. If chest pain continues despite use of aminophylline and nitroglycerin, consider the possibility of myocardial infarction. If the clinical condition of a patient with an adverse event permits a 1 minute delay in the use of aminophylline, thallium-201 may be injected and allowed to circulate for 1 minute before the injection of aminophylline. This will allow initial thallium perfusion imaging to be performed before reversal of the pharmacologic effects of dipyridamole on the coronary circulation.

DIPYRIDAMOLE

Fertility impairment: A significant reduction in number of corpora lutea with consequent reduced implantations and live fetuses occurred in rats after 1250 mg/day.

Pregnancy: Category B. There are no adequate and well controlled studies in pregnant women. Use during pregnancy only if clearly needed.

Lactation: Dipyridamole is excreted in breast milk.

Children: Safety and efficacy in children have not been established.

Drug Interactions:

Theophylline may abolish the coronary vasodilation induced by IV dipyridamole. This could lead to a false negative thallium imaging result.

Adverse Reactions:

Adverse reaction information is derived from a study of 3911 patients, from spontaneous reports and from the published literature.

IV Dipyridamole Adverse Reactions (>1%)	
Adverse Reaction	Incidence (%)
Chest pain/angina pectoris	19.7
Headache	12.2
Dizziness	11.8
ECG abnormalities/ST-T changes	7.5
ECG abnormalities/extrasystoles	5.2
Hypotension	4.6
Nausea	4.6
Flushing	3.4
ECG abnormalities/tachycardia	3.2
Dyspnea	2.6
Pain unspecified	2.6
Blood pressure lability	1.6
Hypertension	1.5
Paresthesia	1.3
Fatigue	1.2

Other adverse reactions (≤ 1%):

Cardiovascular – ECG abnormalities unspecified (0.8%); arrhythmia unspecified (0.6%); palpitation (0.3%); ventricular tachycardia (see Warnings), bradycardia (0.2%); myocardial infarction (see Warnings), AV block, syncope, orthostatic hypotension, atrial fibrillation, supraventricular tachycardia (0.1%); ventricular arrhythmia unspecified (see Warnings), heart block unspecified, cardiomyopathy, edema (0.03%).

CNS – Hypothesia (0.5%); hypertonia (0.3%); nervousness/anxiety (0.2%); tremor (0.1%); abnormal coordination, somnolence, dysphonia, migraine, vertigo (0.03%).

GI – Dyspepsia (1%); dry mouth (0.8%); abdominal pain (0.7%); flatulence (0.6%); vomiting (0.4%); eructation (0.1%); dysphagia, tenesmus, increased appetite (0.03%).

Respiratory – Pharyngitis (0.3%); bronchospasm (0.2%, see Warnings); hyperventilation, rhinitis (0.1%); coughing, pleural pain (0.03%).

Miscellaneous – Myalgia (0.9%); back pain (0.6%); injection site reaction unspecified, diaphoresis (0.4%); asthenia, malaise, arthralgia (0.3%); injection site pain, rigor, earache, tinnitus, vision abnormalities unspecified, dysgeusia (0.1%); thirst, depersonalization, eye pain, renal pain, perineal pain, breast pain, intermittent claudication, leg cramping (0.03%).

Overdosage:

It is unlikely that overdosage will occur because of the nature of use (ie, single IV administration in controlled settings).

Administration and Dosage:

Adjust dose according to weight of patient. Recommended dose is 0.142 mg/kg/min (0.57 mg/kg total) infused over 4 min. Although maximum tolerated dose is not determined, clinical experience suggests a total dose > 60 mg is not needed for any patient. Prior to IV use, dilute in at least a 1:2 ratio with 0.5N NaCl Injection, 1N NaCl Injection, or 5% Dextrose Injection for a total volume of ≈ 20 to 50 ml. Infusion of undiluted dipyridamole may cause local irritation. Inject thallium-201 within 5 minutes after the 4 minute dipyridamole infusion.

Storage: Avoid freezing. Protect from direct light.

Rx	**Persantine IV** (DuPont-Merck)	**Injection:** 10 mg[1]	In 2 ml amps.

[1] With 100 mg polyethylene glycol 600 and 4 mg tartaric acid.

SERMORELIN ACETATE

Actions:

Pharmacology: Sermorelin is for diagnostic use only. It increases plasma growth hormone (GH) concentrations by direct stimulation of the pituitary gland to release GH. Sermorelin is an acetate salt of a synthetic, 29-amino acid polypeptide that is the amino-terminal segment of the naturally occurring human growth hormone-releasing hormone (GHRH or GRH) consisting of 44 amino acid residues. Sermorelin appears to be equivalent to GRH (1-44) in its ability to stimulate growth hormone secretion in humans. It has also been called GRH (1-29) and GHRH (1-29).

Because baseline GH levels are generally very low (< 4 ng/ml), provocative tests may be useful in determining the functional GH-secreting capability of the pituitary somatotroph. Adults and children with normal responses to standard provocative tests of GH secretion were used to define the range of normal plasma GH-level responses to sermorelin. It was found that the absolute peak GH level following sermorelin infusion and the time elapsed from infusion to that peak are appropriate measures to evaluate the response to GH infusion. Doses used in children and adults in these studies ranged from 0.3 to 6.06 mcg/kg with a majority of patients receiving 1 mcg/kg. Based on these studies and published reports, 1 mcg/kg was chosen as the recommended dose for diagnostic purposes.

Clinical trials: A total of 71 sermorelin injection tests were performed on 47 boys and 24 girls who showed normal responses to standard, indirect provocative tests such as clonidine, L-dopa and arginine. The GH peak plasma response to sermorelin was 28 ± 15 ng/ml and the time to this peak was 30 ± 27 minutes.

Of all children who had GH responses of > 7 ng/ml to standard provocative tests, 96% also had responses to sermorelin of > 7 ng/ml. In 77 patients who failed to respond to standard provocative tests, mean GH peak responses to sermorelin were significantly lower compared to the mean GH peak response of normal control children. However, 53% of the children who failed to respond to standard tests had a GH response to sermorelin of > 7 ng/ml suggesting that clinical GH deficiency is frequently not due to somatotroph failure.

Preliminary studies have demonstrated an age-related decline in GH responsiveness to GRH in persons > 40 years old, but the normal range of GH response to sermorelin in older adults has not been established.

Indications:

As a single IV injection for evaluating the ability of the somatotroph of the pituitary gland to secrete growth hormone.

Contraindications:

Hypersensitivity to sermorelin or any of the excipients.

Warnings:

Antibody formation has occurred in humans after chronic SC administration of large doses of sermorelin. Approximately one in four patients given repeated doses of one or more of the three forms of GRH (1-29, 1-40 and 1-44) has developed antibodies to GRH. The clinical significance of these antibodies is unknown. One patient who developed antibodies to GRH (1-44) also experienced an allergic reaction described as severe redness, swelling and urticaria at the injection sites. No long-lasting effects from this reaction were reported. No symptomatic allergic reactions to GRH (1-29) have been reported.

GH deficiency: A normal plasma GH response to sermorelin demonstrates that the somatotroph is intact. However, a normal response does not exclude GH deficiency because this deficiency is frequently the result of hypothalamic dysfunction in the presence of an intact somatotroph. The sermorelin stimulation test is most easily interpreted when there is a subnormal response to conventional provocative testing and a normal response to sermorelin. Such findings suggest that hypothalamic dysfunction is the cause for the growth hormone deficiency. When both conventional and sermorelin testing result in subnormal GH responses, the site of dysfunction cannot be determined with certainty because some patients with GH deficiency due to hypothalamic dysfunction require repeated sermorelin administration before demonstrating a normal response.

Acromegaly: The sermorelin test has not been found useful in the diagnosis of acromegaly.

Hypersensitivity: Although hypersensitivity reactions have been observed with other polypeptide hormones, to date no such reactions have been reported following the administration of a single dose of sermorelin.

SERMORELIN ACETATE

Pregnancy: Category C. Sermorelin produces minor variations in fetuses of rats and rabbits when given in SC doses of 50, 150 and 500 mcg/kg. In the rat teratology study, external malformations (thin tail) were observed in the higher dose groups, and there was an increase in minor skeletal variants at the high dose. Some visceral malformations (hydroureter) were observed in all treatment groups, with the incidence greatest in the high-dose group. In rabbits, minor skeletal anomalies were significantly greater in the treated animals than in the controls. There are no adequate and well controlled studies in pregnant women. Use sermorelin during pregnancy only if the potential benefit justifies the potential risk to the fetus.

Lactation: It is not known whether this drug is excreted in breast milk. Exercise caution when administering to a nursing woman.

Precautions:

Subnormal GH response: Obesity, hyperglycemia and elevated plasma fatty acids generally are associated with subnormal GH responses to sermorelin.

Drug Interactions:

The sermorelin test should not be conducted in the presence of drugs that directly affect the pituitary secretion of somatotropin. These include preparations that contain or release somatostatin, insulin, glucocorticoids, or cyclooxygenase inhibitors such as aspirin or indomethacin. Somatotropin levels may be transiently elevated by clonidine, levodopa and insulin-induced hypoglycemia. Response to sermorelin may be blunted in patients who are receiving muscarinic antagonists (atropine) or who are hypothyroid or being treated with antithyroid medications such as propylthiouracil. Discontinue exogenous growth hormone therapy at least 1 week before administering the test.

Adverse Reactions:

The following adverse reactions, in decreasing order of frequency, have occurred following sermorelin administration: Transient warmth or flushing of the face; injection site pain; redness or swelling at injection site; nausea; headache; vomiting; strange taste in the mouth; paleness; tightness in the chest. Antibody formation has been reported (see Warnings).

Overdosage:

Changes of heart rate and blood pressure have occurred with the various GRH peptides in IV doses exceeding 10 mcg/kg. Cardiovascular collapse is a conceivable, but as of yet, unreported, complication of overdosage with GRH (1-29).

Administration and Dosage:

Approved by the FDA in 1991.

Individualize dosage for each patient according to weight. Administer in a single IV dose of 1 mcg/kg in the morning following an overnight fast.

Children (or subjects < 50 kg):

1.) Reconstitute the contents of one 50 mcg amp with a minimum of 0.5 ml of the accompanying sterile diluent.
2.) Draw venous blood samples for GH determinations 15 minutes before and immediately prior to administration.
3.) Administer a bolus of 1 mcg/kg IV followed by a 3 ml normal saline flush.
4.) Draw venous blood samples for GH determinations at 15, 30, 45 and 60 minutes after administration.

Adults (or subjects > 50 kg):

1.) Determine the number of amps needed, based on a dose of 1 mcg/kg.
2.) Reconstitute the contents of each amp with a minimum of 0.5 ml of the accompanying sterile diluent.
3.) Follow steps 2 through 4 in the Children's section.

Storage/Stability: The lyophilized product must be stored under refrigeration (2° to 8°C; 36° to 46°F). Use immediately after reconstitution. Discard unused material.

Rx	**Geref** (Serono Labs)	**Powder for Injection, lyophilized**: 50 mcg (as the acetate)[1]	In amps with 2 ml of 0.9% Sodium Chloride Injection, USP as a diluent in vials.

[1] With 5 mg mannitol, 0.66 mg monobasic sodium phosphate and 0.04 mg dibasic sodium phosphate; may contain up to 1% albumin (Human).

ADENOSINE

For information on the use of adenosine as an antiarrhythmic agent, refer to the monograph in the Cardiovasculars chapter.

Actions:

Pharmacology: Adenosine is an endogenous nucleoside occurring in all cells of the body. Adenosine is a potent vasodilator in most vascular beds, except in renal afferent arterioles and hepatic veins where it produces vasoconstriction. Adenosine is thought to exert its effects through activation of purine receptors (cell-surface A_1– and A_2–adenosine receptors). Although the exact mechanism by which adenosine receptor activation relaxes vascular smooth muscle is not known, there is evidence to support both inhibition of the slow inward calcium current reducing calcium uptake and activation of adenylate cyclase through A_2–receptors in smooth muscle cells. Adenosine may also lessen vascular tone by modulating sympathetic neurotransmission.

Myocardial uptake of thallium-201 is directly proportional to coronary blood flow. Since adenosine significantly increases blood flow in normal coronary arteries with little or no increase in stenotic arteries, adenosine causes relatively less thallium-201 uptake in vascular territories supplied by stenotic coronary arteries (ie, a greater difference is seen after adenosine between areas served by normal vessels and areas served by stenotic vessels than is seen prior to adenosine).

Hemodynamics – Adenosine produces a direct negative chronotropic, dromotropic and inotropic effect on the heart, presumably due to A_1-receptor agonism, and produces peripheral vasodilation, presumably due to A_2-receptor agonism. The net effect of adenosine in humans is typically a mild to moderate reduction in systolic, diastolic and mean arterial blood pressure associated with a reflex increase in heart rate. Rarely, significant hypotension and tachycardia have been observed.

Pharmacokinetics: Adenosine IV is rapidly cleared from the circulation via cellular uptake, primarily by erythrocytes and vascular endothelial cells. Intracellular adenosine is rapidly metabolized either via polyphorylation to adenosine monophosphate by adenosine kinase or via deamination to inosine by adenosine deaminase in the cytosol. These intracellular metabolites are not vasoactive. Inosine formed by deamination of adenosine can leave the cell intact or can be degraded to hypoxanthine, xanthine and ultimately uric acid. Adenosine monophosphate formed by phosphorylation of adenosine is incorporated into the high-energy phosphate pool. As adenosine requires no hepatic or renal function for its activation or inactivation, hepatic and renal failure would not be expected to alter its effectiveness or tolerability.

Indications:

Diagnostic aid: Adjunct to thallium-201 myocardial perfusion scintigraphy in patients unable to exercise adequately.

Contraindications:

Second- or third-degree AV block (except in patients with a functioning artificial pacemaker); sinus node disease, such as sick sinus syndrome or symptomatic bradycardia (except in patients with a functioning artificial pacemaker); suspected bronchoconstrictive or bronchospastic lung disease (eg, asthma); hypersensitivity to adenosine.

Warnings:

Cardiac effects: Fatal cardiac arrest, sustained ventricular tachycardia (requiring resuscitation) and nonfatal myocardial infarction have been reported coincident with adenosine infusion. Patients with unstable angina may be at greater risk.

Sinoatrial and atrioventricular nodal block – Adenosine exerts a direct depressant effect on the SA and AV nodes and has the potential to cause AV block, or sinus bradycardia. Approximately 6.3% of patients develop AV block with adenosine, including first-degree (2.9%), second-degree (2.6%) and third-degree (0.8%) heart block. All episodes of AV block have been asymptomatic and transient, and did not require intervention. Use with caution in patients with pre–existing first-degree AV block or bundle branch block and avoid in patients with high-grade AV block or sinus node dysfunction (except in patients with a functional artificial pacemaker). Discontinue in any patient who develops persistent or symptomatic high-grade AV block. Sinus pause has been rarely observed with adenosine infusions.

Hypotension – Adenosine is a potent peripheral vasodilator and can cause significant hypotension. Patients with an intact baroreceptor reflex mechanism are able to maintain blood pressure and tissue perfusion in response to adenosine by increasing heart rate and cardiac output. However, use with caution in patients with autonomic dysfunction, stenotic valvular heart disease, pericarditis or pericardial effusions, stenotic carotid artery disease with cerebrovascular insufficiency, or uncorrected hypovolemia, due to the risk of hypotensive complications in these patients. Discontinue in any patient who develops persistent or symptomatic hypotension.

ADENOSINE

Hypertension – Increases in systolic and diastolic pressure have been observed (as great as 140 mm Hg systolic in one case) concomitant with adenosine infusion; most increases resolved spontaneously within several minutes, but in some cases, hypertension lasted for several hours.

Bronchoconstriction: Adenosine is a respiratory stimulant and, with IV administration, increases minute ventilation (Ve) and reduces arterial PCO_2 causing respiratory alkalosis. Approximately 28% of patients experience breathlessness (dyspnea) or an urge to breathe deeply. These complaints are transient and rarely require intervention. Adenosine given by inhalation may cause bronchoconstriction in asthmatic patients, presumably due to mast cell degranulation and histamine release. These effects have not been observed in healthy subjects. Adenosine has been given to a limited number of patients with asthma and mild to moderate exacerbation of their symptoms has occurred. Respiratory compromise has occurred during adenosine infusion in patients with obstructive pulmonary disease. Use with caution in patients with obstructive lung disease not associated with bronchoconstriction (eg, emphysema, bronchitis) and avoid in patients with bronchoconstriction or bronchospasm (eg, asthma). Discontinue in any patient who develops severe respiratory difficulties.

Mutagenesis/Fertility impairment: Adenosine produces a variety of chromosomal alterations. In rats and mice, adenosine caused decreased spermatogenesis and increased numbers of abnormal sperm, a reflection of the ability of adenosine to produce chromosomal damage.

Pregnancy: Category C. It is not known whether adenosine can cause fetal harm when administered to pregnant women; use during pregnancy only if clearly needed.

Children: Safety and efficacy in patients < 18 years of age have not been established.

Drug Interactions:

Whenever possible, drugs that might inhibit or augment the effects of adenosine should be withheld for at least five half-lives, prior to the use of adenosine.

Adenosine Drug Interactions			
Precipitant drug	Object drug*		Description
Cardioactive agents	Adenosine	⬆	Because of the potential for additive or synergistic depressant effects on the SA and AV nodes, use with caution in the presence of these agents.
Methylxanthines (eg, caffeine and theophylline)	Adenosine	⬇	The vasoactive effect of adenosine is inhibited by adenosine receptor antagonists, such as methylxanthines.

* ⬆ = Object drug increased. ⬇ = Object drug decreased.

Adverse Reactions:

Despite the short half-life of adenosine, 10.6% of the side effects listed occurred several hours after the infusion terminated. Also, 8.4% of the side effects that began coincident with the infusion persisted for up to 24 hours after the infusion was complete. In many cases, it is not possible to know whether these late adverse events are the result of adenosine infusion.

Adenosine Adverse Reactions (≥ 1%) (n = 1421)	
Adverse reaction	%
Flushing	44
Chest discomfort	40
Dyspnea or urge to breathe deeply	28
Headache	18
Throat, neck or jaw discomfort	15
GI discomfort	13
Lightheadedness/dizziness	12
Upper extremity discomfort	4
ST segment depression	3
First-degree AV block	3
Second-degree AV block	3
Paresthesia	2
Hypotension	2
Nervousness	2
Arrhythmias	1

ADENOSINE

The following adverse events occurred in < 1% of patients:

Body as a whole: Back discomfort; lower extremity discomfort; weakness.

Cardiovascular: Nonfatal myocardial infarction; life-threatening ventricular arrhythmia; third-degree AV block; bradycardia; palpitation; sinus exit block; sinus pause; sweating; T-wave changes, hypertension (systolic blood pressure >200 mm Hg).

CNS: Drowsiness; emotional instablility; tremors.

GU: Vaginal pressure; urgency.

Pulmonary: Cough.

Special senses: Blurred vision; dry mouth; ear discomfort; metallic taste; nasal congestion; scotomas; tongue discomfort.

Overdosage:

The half-life of adenosine is < 10 seconds and side effects (when they occur) usually resolve quickly when the infusion is discontinued, although delayed or persistent effects have been observed. Methylxanthines, such as caffeine and theophylline, are competitive adenosine receptor antagonists and theophylline has been used to effectively terminate persistent side effects. In controlled clinical trials, theophylline (50 to 125 mg slow IV injection) was needed to abort adenosine side effects in < 2% of patients.

Administration and Dosage:

For IV infusion only. Safety and efficacy of the intracoronary route have not been established.

Adenosine should be given as a continuous peripheral intravenous infusion.

The recommended IV dose for adults is 140 mcg/kg/min infused for 6 minutes (total dose of 0.84 mg/kg).

Inject the required dose of thallium-201 at the midpoint of the adenosine infusion (ie, after the first 3 minutes of adenosine). Thallium-201 is physically compatible with adenosine and may be injected into the adenosine infusion set.

The injection should be as close to the venous access as possible to prevent an inadvertent increase in the dose of adenosine (the contents of the IV tubing) being administered.

The following adenosine infusion nomogram may be used to determine the appropriate infusion rate corrected for total body weight:

Adenosine Infusion Rate Based on Weight

Patient Weight		Infusion Rate
kg	lbs	ml/min
45	99	2.1
50	110	2.3
55	121	2.6
60	132	2.8
65	143	3
70	154	3.3
75	165	3.5
80	176	3.8
85	187	4
90	198	4.2

This nomogram was derived from the following general formula:

$$\frac{0.14 \text{ (mg/kg/min)} \times \text{total body weight (kg)}}{\text{Adenosine concentration (3 mg/ml)}} = \text{infusion rate (ml/min)}$$

Storage/Stability: Store at controlled room temperature 15° to 30°C (59° to 86°F). Do not refrigerate as crystallization may occur. If crystallization has occurred, dissolve crystals by warming to room temperature. The solution must be clear at the time of use.

Rx	**Adenoscan** (Fujisawa)	**Injection:** 3 mg/ml	Preservative-free. In 30 ml single-dose vials.

ARGININE HCl

Actions:

Pharmacology: Infusion IV often induces a pronounced rise in the plasma level of human growth hormone (HGH) in subjects with intact pituitary function. This rise is usually diminished or absent in patients with impairment of this function.

Indications:

Diagnostic aid: An IV stimulant to the pituitary for the release of HGH in patients where the measurement of pituitary reserve for HGH can be of diagnostic usefulness. It can be used as a diagnostic aid in such conditions as panhypopituitarism, pituitary dwarfism, chromophobe adenoma, postsurgical craniopharyngioma, hypophysectomy, pituitary trauma, acromegaly, gigantism and problems of growth and stature.

Contraindications:

Persons having highly allergic tendencies.

Warnings:

Arginine is a diagnostic aid and not intended for therapeutic use.

Route of administration: Always administer by IV injection due to the drug's hypertonicity.

Deficiency of pituitary reserve for HGH: If the insulin hypoglycemia test has indicated a deficiency of pituitary reserve for HGH, a test with arginine is advisable to confirm the negative response. This can be done after a waiting period of 1 day. As patients may not respond during the first test, the unresponsive patient should be tested again to confirm the negative result. A second test can be performed after a waiting period of 1 day. Some patients who respond to arginine do not respond to insulin and vice versa. The rate of false positive responses is approximately 32%, and the rate of false negatives is approximately 27%.

Hypersensitivity: Have a suitable antihistaminic drug available in case of an allergic reaction. Refer to Management of Acute Hypersensitivity Reactions.

Pregnancy: Category B. Do not use this drug during pregnancy.

Lactation: It is not known whether IV administration of arginine could result in significant quantities of arginine in breast milk. Systemically administered amino acids are secreted into breast milk in quantities not likely to have a deleterious effect on the infant. Nevertheless, exercise caution when arginine is administered to nursing women.

Precautions:

Arginine is a hypertonic (950 mOsmol/L) and acidic (average pH of 5.6) solution that can irritate tissues. Use care to ensure administration of arginine through a patent catheter within a patent vein.

Excessive infusion rates may result in local irritation and flushing, nausea or vomiting. Inadequate dosing or prolongation of the infusion period may diminish the stimulus to the pituitary and nullify the test.

Nitrogen: Arginine has a high content of metabolizable nitrogen; consider the temporary effect of a high load of nitrogen upon the kidneys when administered.

Chloride: The chloride ion content is 47.5 mEq/100 ml of solution; consider the effect of infusing this amount of chloride into patients with electrolyte imbalance before the test is undertaken.

Growth hormone levels: Basal and post-stimulation levels of growth hormone are elevated in patients who are pregnant or who are taking oral contraceptives.

Adverse Reactions:

Approximately 3% of patients reported nonspecific side effects consisting of nausea, vomiting, headache, flushing, numbness and local venous irritation.

One patient had an allergic reaction manifested as a confluent macular rash with reddening and swelling of the hands and face. The rash subsided rapidly after the infusion was terminated and 50 mg diphenhydramine was administered. One patient had an apparent decrease in platelet count from 150,000 to 60,000. One patient with a history of acrocyanosis had an exacerbation of this condition following infusion.

ARGININE HCl

Overdosage:

An overdosage may cause a transient metabolic acidosis with hyperventilation. The acidosis will be compensated and the base deficit will return to normal following completion of the infusion. If the condition persists, determine the deficit and correct by a calculated dose of an alkalizing agent.

Administration and Dosage:

Administer IV.

Dose:

Adults – 300 ml.
Children – 5 ml/kg.

Test procedure: For successful administration of the test for measurement of pituitary reserve of human growth hormone, clinical conditions and procedures should be as follows:

1. Schedule the test in the morning following a normal night's sleep and an overnight fast which should continue throughout the test period. Place patient at bed rest, and for at least 30 minutes before the infusion begins, take care to minimize apprehension and distress. This is particularly important in children.
2. Infuse through an indwelling needle or soft catheter placed in an antecubital vein or other suitable vein. Take blood samples by venipuncture from the contralateral arm. A desirable schedule for drawing blood samples is at –30, 0, 30, 60, 90, 120 and 150 minutes. Promptly centrifuge blood samples and store the plasma at –20°C (-4°F) until assayed by one of the published radioimmunoassay procedures.
3. Infuse arginine beginning at zero time at a uniform rate which will permit the recommended dose to be administered in 30 minutes.

Interpretation of results: Infusion IV often induces a pronounced rise in the plasma level of human growth hormone in subjects with intact pituitary function. This rise is usually diminished or absent in patients with impairment of this function.

Expected Plasma Levels of HGH with Arginine

Patient	Control range (ng/ml)	Range of peak response to arginine (ng/ml)
Normal	0-6	10-30
Pituitary deficient	0-4	0-10

The above ranges are based on the mean values of plasma HGH levels calculated from the data of several clinical investigators and reflect their experiences with various methods of radioimmunoassay. Upon gaining experience with this diagnostic test, each clinician will establish his own ranges for control and peak levels of HGH.

Diagnostic test results showing a deficiency of pituitary reserve for HGH should be confirmed by a second test with arginine, or confirmed with the insulin hypoglycemia test. A waiting period of 1 day is advised between tests.

Stability: Invert and inspect each bottle before use to be sure that its contents are clear. Discard any flask in which its contents are not clear or which lacks a vacuum.

Rx	**R-Gene 10** (Pharmacia)	**Injection:** 10% arginine HCl (950 mOsmol/L)	With 47.5 mEq chloride ion per 100 ml. In 300 ml.

RADIOPAQUE AGENTS

Radiopaque agents, except barium sulfate, include a number of iodinated compounds; these agents are used to visualize various organ systems upon x-ray examination. The radiopacity of these agents is a function of the percentage of iodine in the molecule and the concentration of compound present.

The most important characteristic of contrast media is the iodine content. The relatively high atomic weight of iodine contributes sufficient radiodensity for radiographic contrast with surrounding tissues. The enteral radiopaque agents are substituted, triiodinated, benzoic acid derivatives.

Parenteral radiopaque diagnostic agents are water soluble, triiodinated, benzoic acid salts. Due to organically bound iodine (5.1% to 48.25% by weight), the injectable radiopaque agents can opacify internal structures for x-ray visualization and fluoroscopy.

Nonionic vs ionic agents: Iohexol, iopamidol and metrizamide are nonionic iodine contrast media. The other iodinated contrast media currently available are ionic. The nonionic media have a lower osmolality than the ionic contrast media and are associated with a lower incidence of adverse effects. The nonionic media are also associated with a lower incidence of anaphylactoid reactions.

Anaphylactoid reactions occur in 1% to 2% of patients receiving radiopaque agents. Incidence increases to 17% to 35% if radiocontrast procedures are repeated in patients with a history of anaphylactoid reactions to radiopaque agents. Pretreating high risk patients with a regimen including diphenhydramine, prednisone and ephedrine has reduced the incidence of repeated and possibly more severe reactions to ≈ 3.1%. Use extreme caution. Refer to Management of Acute Hypersensitivity Reactions.

Tartrazine sensitivity: Some of these products contain tartrazine which may cause allergic-type reactions (including bronchial asthma) in certain susceptible individuals. Although the overall incidence of tartrazine sensitivity in the general population is low, it is frequently seen in patients who also have aspirin hypersensitivity. Specific products containing tartrazine are identified in the product listings.

Patient Information:

Oral and rectal iodinated agents: Take all medication with water after a fat-free dinner the evening before test. Thereafter, take only water until test is completed.

Inform physician of pregnancy or allergy to iodine, any foods or x-ray materials.

These agents may cause mild and transient abdominal cramping, nausea, vomiting, diarrhea, skin rashes, itching, heartburn, dizziness or headache.

Consult physician if thyroid tests are planned; iodine may interfere.

Parenteral iodinated agents: Prior to these procedures, notify physician if any of the following conditions exist: Pregnancy, diabetes, multiple myeloma, pheochromocytoma, homozygous sickle cell disease, thyroid disease, allergy to any drugs or food, reactions to previous injections of dyes used for x-ray procedures. Also notify physician if you are taking any other medications, including otc drugs.

These agents should be given only by personnel experienced in their use, and only in facilities with proper equipment to deal with possible untoward effects.

The table summarizes radiopaque agents and their uses. Due to specificity of use and multiplicity of administrations, this table and product listings in this section are not intended to provide comprehensive information necessary for their safe and effective use. Consult package literature for complete prescribing information.

Indications and Uses of the Radiopaque Agents

Radiopaque Agents	% Iodine (Approx.)	Cholecystography	Cholangiography	Gastrointestinal	Urography	Pyelography	Cystourethrography	Arthrography	Myelography	Angiography	Angiocardiography	Arteriography	Aortography	Ventriculography	Venography	Hysterosalpingography	Splenoportography	Computed Tomography	Lymphography
Oral Cholecystographics																			
Iocetamic acid	62	✓																	
Iopanoic acid	67	✓	✓																
Ipodate calcium	62	✓	✓																
Ipodate sodium	61	✓	✓																
Tyropanoate sodium	57	✓																	
GI Contrast																			
Barium	0			✓														✓	
Diatrizoate sodium 41.66%	25			✓															
Diatrizoate sodium powder	60			✓															
Diatrizoate meglumine 66%/ Diatrizoate sodium 10%	37			✓														✓	

RADIOPAQUE AGENTS

Indications and Uses of the Radiopaque Agents

Radiopaque Agents	% Iodine (Approx.)	Cholecystography	Cholangiography	Gastrointestinal	Urography	Pyelography	Cystourethrography	Arthrography	Myelography	Angiography	Angiocardiography	Arteriography	Aortography	Ventriculography	Venography	Hysterosalpingography	Splenoportography	Computed Tomography	Lymphography
Parenteral																			
Diatrizoate meglumine 30%	14				✓	✓									✓			✓	
Diatrizoate meglumine 60%[1]	28		✓		✓	✓		✓		✓		✓			✓		✓	✓	
Diatrizoate meglumine 76%	36				✓					✓		✓	✓						
Diatrizoate sodium 25%	15				✓													✓	
Diatrizoate sodium 50%	30		✓		✓					✓			✓		✓	✓	✓	✓	
Gadopentetate dimeglumine[2]	0																		
Iodamide meglumine 24%	11				✓	✓												✓	
Iodamide meglumine 65%	30				✓														
Iodipamide meglumine 10.3%	5	✓	✓																
Iodipamide meglumine 52%	26	✓	✓																
Iohexol	46				✓				✓	✓	✓	✓	✓	✓	✓			✓	
Iopamidol 26%	13									✓									
Iopamidol 41%	20				✓					✓	✓	✓	✓	✓	✓			✓	
Iopamidol 61%	30				✓					✓	✓	✓	✓	✓	✓			✓	
Iopamidol 76%	37				✓					✓	✓	✓	✓	✓	✓			✓	
Iothalamate meglumine 30%	14				✓					✓								✓	
Iothalamate meglumine 43%	20				✓	✓	✓			✓					✓			✓	
Iothalamate meglumine 60%[3]	28		–		✓			✓		✓		✓			✓			✓	
Iothalamate sodium 54.3%	33				✓														
Iothalamate sodium 66.8%	40				✓						✓		✓					✓	
Iothalamate sodium 80%	48										✓		✓						
Metrizamide[4]	48								✓		✓	✓		✓				✓	
Diatrizoate meglumine 28.5%/ Diatrizoate sodium 29.1%[5]	31				✓						✓	✓	✓		✓				
Diatrizoate meglumine 34.3%/ Diatrizoate sodium 35%[5]	37				✓						✓	✓	✓		✓				
Diatrizoate meglumine 50%/ Diatrizoate sodium 25%	39				✓					✓	✓		✓					✓	
Diatrizoate meglumine 52%/ Diatrizoate sodium 8%[1]	29		✓		✓			✓		✓		✓			✓		✓	✓	
Diatrizoate meglumine 60%/ Diatrizoate sodium 30%	46				✓					✓	✓		✓			✓		✓	
Diatrizoate meglumine 66%/ Diatrizoate sodium 10%	37				✓					✓	✓	✓	✓	✓	✓			✓	
Iothalamate meglumine 52%/ Iothalamate sodium 26%	40				✓					✓	✓	✓	✓					✓	
Ioxaglate meglumine 39.3%/ Ioxaglate sodium 19.6%	32				✓			✓		✓	✓	✓	✓	✓	✓	✓		✓	
Ioversol 34%	16									✓									
Ioversol 51%	24									✓					✓				
Ioversol 68%	32				✓					✓		✓	✓	✓				✓	
Miscellaneous																			
Diatrizoate meglumine 18%	9						✓												
Diatrizoate meglumine 30%	14					✓	✓												
Diatrizoate sodium 20%	12					✓													
Iothalamate meglumine 17.2%[6]	8						✓												
Iothalamate meglumine 43%[6]	20					✓	✓												
Diatrizoate meglumine 52.7%/ Iodipamide meglumine 26.8%	38															✓			
Ethiodized oil	37															✓			✓
Propyliodone oil[7]	34																		

[1] Also discography.
[2] With MRI for intracranial, spine and associated tissues.
[3] Also cholangiopancreatography.
[4] Also cisternography.
[5] Also venocavography.
[6] Also cystography.
[7] Also bronchography.

Oral Cholecystographic Agents

IOCETAMIC ACID (62% iodine)

For complete prescribing information, refer to the Radiopaque Agents group monograph.

Rx	**Cholebrine** (Mallinckrodt)	**Tablets:** 750 mg	White, scored. In 150s.

IOPANOIC ACID (66.68% iodine)

For complete prescribing information, refer to the Radiopaque Agents group monograph.

Rx	**Telepaque** (Winthrop Pharm.)	**Tablets:** 500 mg	Off-white, scored. In 150s.

IPODATE CALCIUM (61.7% iodine)

For complete prescribing information, refer to the Radiopaque Agents group monograph.

Rx	**Oragrafin Calcium** (Squibb Diagnostics)	**Granules for Oral Suspension:** 3 g/packet	Sucrose. In 25 g packets.

IPODATE SODIUM (61.4% iodine)

For complete prescribing information, refer to the Radiopaque Agents group monograph.

Rx	**Bilivist** (Berlex)	**Capsules:** 500 mg	D-sorbitol, lecithin. (162). In 120s.
Rx	**Oragrafin Sodium** (Squibb Diagnostics)		Tartrazine, lecithin. (455). Yellow. In 100s, 144s and UD 100s.

TYROPANOATE SODIUM (57.4% iodine)

For complete prescribing information, refer to the Radiopaque Agents group monograph.

Rx	**Bilopaque** (Winthrop Pharm.)	**Capsules:** 750 mg	Benzyl alcohol. In 100s.

GI Contrast Agents (Iodinated)

DIATRIZOATE SODIUM 41.66% (24.9% iodine)

For complete prescribing information, refer to the Radiopaque Agents group monograph.

Rx	**Hypaque Sodium** (Winthrop Pharm.)	**Solution**	In 120 ml.[1]

[1] Parabens, polysorbate 80, saccharin, sucrose.

DIATRIZOATE SODIUM (59.87% iodine)

For complete prescribing information, refer to the Radiopaque Agents group monograph.

Rx	**Hypaque Sodium** (Winthrop Pharm.)	**Powder**	In 10 and 250 g.[2]

[2] Polysorbate 80.

DIATRIZOATE MEGLUMINE 66% and DIATRIZOATE SODIUM 10% (37% iodine)

For complete prescribing information, refer to the Radiopaque Agents group monograph.

Rx	**Gastrografin** (Squibb Diagnostics)	**Solution**	Lemon flavor. In 120 ml.[3]
Rx	**MD-Gastroview** (Mallinckrodt)		Vanilla-lemon flavor. In 120 and 240 ml.[4]

[3] EDTA, polysorbate 80, saccharin.
[4] EDTA, saccharin.

GI Contrast Agents (Miscellaneous)

RADIOPAQUE POLYVINYL CHLORIDE

For complete prescribing information, refer to the Radiopaque Agents group monograph.

Rx	**Sitzmarks** (Konsyl Pharm)	**Capsules:** Contain 20 radiopaque rings (1 mm x 4.5 mm)	In 10s.

BARIUM SULFATE

For complete prescribing information, refer to the Radiopaque Agents group monograph.

Rx	**Baro-cat** (Lafayette Pharm.)	**Suspension:** 1.5%	Sorbitol. Pineapple-banana flavor. In 300, 900 and 1900 ml.
Rx	**Prepcat** (Lafayette Pharm.)		Sorbitol. Strawberry flavor. In 450 ml.
Rx	**Enecat** (Lafayette Pharm.)	**Concentrated Suspension:** 5%	Sorbitol. In 110 ml with 480 ml bottle for dilution.
Rx	**Tomocat** (Lafayette Pharm.)		Sorbitol. Strawberry flavor. In 145 ml with 480 ml bottle for dilution and 225 ml with two 1000 ml bottles for dilution.
Rx	**Entrobar** (Lafayette Pharm.)	**Suspension:** 50%	In 500 ml.
Rx	**Liquid Barosperse** (Lafayette Pharm.)	**Suspension:** 60%	Vanilla flavor. In 355 ml.
Rx	**HD 85** (Lafayette Pharm.)	**Suspension:** 85%	Raspberry flavor. In 150, 450 and 1900 ml.
Rx	**Barobag** (Lafayette Pharm.)	**Suspension:** 97%	In 340 and 454g kits.
Rx	**Liquipake** (Lafayette Pharm.)	**Suspension:** 100%	In 1850 ml.
Rx	**Flo-Coat** (Lafayette Pharm.)		In 1850 ml.
Rx	**Epi-C** (Lafayette Pharm.)	**Concentrated Suspension:** 150%	Spearmint flavor. In 450 ml.
Rx	**Barium Sulfate, USP** (Various, eg, Humco)	**Powder**	In 500 g, 1 lb and 5 lb.
Rx	**Baroflave** (Lannett)	**Powder**	Raspberry flavor. In 5 and 25 lb.
Rx	**Tonopaque** (Lafayette Pharm)	**Powder for Suspension:** 95%	Sorbitol. Strawberry flavor. In 180 and 1200 g.
Rx	**Baricon** (Lafayette Pharm.)	**Powder for Suspension:** 98%	Vanilla-lemon flavor. In UD 340 g.
Rx	**HD 200 Plus** (Lafayette Pharm.)		Strawberry flavor. In 312 g.
Rx	**Barosperse** (Lafayette Pharm.)	**Powder for Suspension:** 95% and suspending agent	Vanilla flavor. In UD 225 and 900 g.
Rx	**Anatrast** (Lafayette Pharm.)	**Paste:** 100%	In 500 g tubes.

Parenteral Agents

DIATRIZOATE MEGLUMINE 30% (14.1% iodine)

For complete prescribing information, refer to the Radiopaque Agents group monograph.

Rx	**Hypaque Meglumine 30%** (Winthrop Pharm.)	**Injection**	In 100 ml bottles[1] and 300 ml bottles[1] with or without infusion set.
Rx	**Reno-M-Dip** (Squibb Diagnostics)		In 300 ml bottles[1] with or without infusion set.
Rx	**Urovist Meglumine DIU/CT** (Berlex)		In 300 ml bottles[1] with or without infusion set.

DIATRIZOATE MEGLUMINE 60% (28% iodine)

For complete prescribing information, refer to the Radiopaque Agents group monograph.

Rx	**Angiovist 282** (Berlex)	**Injection**	In 50, 100, 150, 500, 1000 ml vials.[1]
Rx	**Hypaque Meglumine 60%** (Winthrop Pharm.)		In 20, 30, 50, 100 ml vials, 150, 200 ml bottles, 100 & 150 ml with infusion sets.[1]
Rx	**Reno-M-60** (Squibb Diagnostics)		In 10, 30, 50, 100 ml vials[1], 100, 150 ml bottles[1] with or without infusion sets.

DIATRIZOATE MEGLUMINE 76% (35.8% iodine)

For complete prescribing information, refer to the Radiopaque Agents group monograph.

Rx	**Diatrizoate Meglumine 76%** (Squibb Diagnostics)	**Injection**	In 50 ml vials.[1]

DIATRIZOATE SODIUM 25% (15% iodine)

For complete prescribing information, refer to the Radiopaque Agents group monograph.

Rx	**Hypaque Sodium 25%** (Winthrop Pharm.)	**Injection**	In 300 ml bottles with or without infusion set.[1]

DIATRIZOATE SODIUM 50% (30% iodine)

For complete prescribing information, refer to the Radiopaque Agents group monograph.

Rx	**Hypaque Sodium 50%** (Winthrop Pharm.)	**Injection**	In 20, 30, 50 ml vials[1], 150, 200 ml dilution bottles.[1]
Rx	**Urovist Sodium 300** (Berlex)		In 50 ml vials.[1]

GADOPENTETATE DIMEGLUMINE 46.9%

For complete prescribing information, refer to the Radiopaque Agents group monograph.

Rx	**Magnevist** (Berlex)	**Injection**	In 20 ml.

IODAMIDE MEGLUMINE 24% (11.1% iodine)

For complete prescribing information, refer to the Radiopaque Agents group monograph.

Rx	**Renovue-Dip** (Squibb Diagnostics)	**Injection**	In 300 ml bottles.[1]

IODAMIDE MEGLUMINE 65% (30% iodine)

For complete prescribing information, refer to the Radiopaque Agents group monograph.

Rx	**Renovue-65** (Squibb Diagnostics)	**Injection**	In 50 ml vials.[1]

IODIPAMIDE MEGLUMINE 10.3% (5.1% iodine)

For complete prescribing information, refer to the Radiopaque Agents group monograph.

Rx	**Cholografin Meglumine** (Squibb Diagnostics)	**Injection**	In 100 ml vials.[1]

Parenteral Agents

IODIPAMIDE MEGLUMINE 52% (25.7% iodine)

For complete prescribing information, refer to the Radiopaque Agents group monograph.

Rx	**Cholografin Meglumine** (Squibb Diagnostics)	**Injection**	In 20 ml vials.[1]

IOHEXOL (46.36% iodine)

For complete prescribing information, refer to the Radiopaque Agents group monograph.

Rx	**Omnipaque** (Winthrop Pharm.)	**Injection:** 140 mg/ml (intrathecal only)	In 50 ml vials and bottles.
		180 mg/ml	In 10, 20 ml vials.
		210 mg/ml	In 15 ml.
		240 mg/ml	In 10, 20, 50 ml vials & 50, 100, 150, 200 ml bottles.
		300 mg/ml	In 10, 30, 50 ml vials & 50, 100, 150 ml bottles.
		350 mg/ml	In 50 ml vials & 50, 75, 100, 125, 150, 175, 200 ml.

[1] With EDTA.

Parenteral Agents

IOPAMIDOL 26% (12.8% iodine)

For complete prescribing information, refer to the Radiopaque Agents group monograph.

Rx	**Isovue-128** (Squibb Diagnostics)	**Injection**	In 50 ml vials.[1]

IOPAMIDOL 41% (20% iodine)

For complete prescribing information, refer to the Radiopaque Agents group monograph.

Rx	**Isovue-200** (Squibb Diagnostics)	**Injection**	In 50 ml vials[1], 100 & 200 ml bottles.[1]
Rx	**Isovue-M 200** (Squibb Diagnostics)	**Injection**	In 20 ml vials.[1] *For intrathecal use.*

IOPAMIDOL 61% (30% iodine)

For complete prescribing information, refer to the Radiopaque Agents group monograph.

Rx	**Isovue-300** (Squibb Diagnostics)	**Injection**	In 30, 50, 75, 100, 150 ml.[2]
Rx	**Isovue-M 300** (Squibb Diagnostics)	**Injection**	In 15 ml vials.[2] *For intrathecal use.*

IOPAMIDOL 76% (37% iodine)

For complete prescribing information, refer to the Radiopaque Agents group monograph.

Rx	**Isovue-370** (Squibb Diagnostics)	**Injection**	In 20, 30, 50, 75, 100, 150, 175, 200 ml.[2]

IOTHALAMATE MEGLUMINE 30% (14.1% iodine)

For complete prescribing information, refer to the Radiopaque Agents group monograph.

Rx	**Conray 30** (Mallinckrodt)	**Injection**	In 50, 100, 150 and 300 ml[1].

IOTHALAMATE MEGLUMINE 43% (20.2% iodine)

For complete prescribing information, refer to the Radiopaque Agents group monograph.

Rx	**Conray 43** (Mallinckrodt)	**Injection**	In 50, 100, 150, 200 and 250 ml vials[1] and 50, 95, 125 ml prefilled syringes.[1]

IOTHALAMATE MEGLUMINE 60% (28.2% iodine)

For complete prescribing information, refer to the Radiopaque Agents group monograph.

Rx	**Conray** (Mallinckrodt)	**Injection**	In 20, 30, 50, 100, 150 and 200 ml vials[1]and 30, 50, 95 and 125 ml prefilled syringes.[1]

IOTHALAMATE SODIUM 54.3% (32.5% iodine)

For complete prescribing information, refer to the Radiopaque Agents group monograph.

Rx	**Conray 325** (Mallinckrodt)	**Injection**	In 30 and 50 ml vials[1] and 50 ml prefilled syringes.[1]

IOTHALAMATE SODIUM 66.8% (40% iodine)

For complete prescribing information, refer to the Radiopaque Agents group monograph.

Rx	**Conray 400** (Mallinckrodt)	**Injection**	In 25 and 50 ml vials[1] and 30 and 50 ml prefilled syringes.[1]

IOTHALAMATE SODIUM 80% (48% iodine)

For complete prescribing information, refer to the Radiopaque Agents group monograph.

Rx	**Angio Conray** (Mallinckrodt)	**Injection**	In 50 ml vials.[1]

Parenteral Agents

IOVERSOL 34% (16% iodine)

For complete prescribing information, refer to the Radiopaque Agents group monograph.

Rx	**Optiray 160** (Mallinckrodt)	**Injection**	In 50 and 100 ml vials.[2]

IOVERSOL 51% (24% iodine)

For complete prescribing information, refer to the Radiopaque Agents group monograph.

Rx	**Optiray 240** (Mallinckrodt)	**Injection**	In 50, 100 and 200 ml.[2]

IOVERSOL 68% (32% iodine)

For complete prescribing information, refer to the Radiopaque Agents group monograph.

Rx	**Optiray 320** (Mallinckrodt)	**Injection**	In 20, 30, 50, 100, 150 and 200 ml.[2]

METRIZAMIDE (48.25% iodine)

For complete prescribing information, refer to the Radiopaque Agents group monograph.

Rx	**Amipaque** (Winthrop Pharm.)	**Powder for Injection, lyophilized:**	
		13.5%	In 50 ml vial[2] w/diluent.
		18.75%	In 20 ml vial[2] w/diluent.

[1] With EDTA.

[2] With EDTA and tromethamine.

Parenteral Agents

DIATRIZOATE MEGLUMINE 28.5% and DIATRIZOATE SODIUM 29.1% (31% iodine)

For complete prescribing information, refer to the Radiopaque Agents group monograph.

Rx	**Renovist II** (Squibb Diagnostics)	**Injection**	In 30 and 60 ml vials.[1]

[1] With EDTA.

DIATRIZOATE MEGLUMINE 34.3% and DIATRIZOATE SODIUM 35% (37% iodine)

For complete prescribing information, refer to the Radiopaque Agents group monograph.

Rx	**Renovist** (Squibb Diagnostics)	**Injection**	In 50 ml vials.[1]

[1] With EDTA.

DIATRIZOATE MEGLUMINE 50% AND DIATRIZOATE SODIUM 25% (38.5% iodine)

For complete prescribing information, refer to the Radiopaque Agents group monograph.

Rx	**Hypaque-M, 75%** (Winthrop Pharm.)	**Injection**	In 20 and 50 ml vials.[1]

[1] With EDTA.

DIATRIZOATE MEGLUMINE 52% and DIATRIZOATE SODIUM 8% (29.3% iodine)

For complete prescribing information, refer to the Radiopaque agents group monograph.

Rx	**Angiovist 292** (Berlex)	**Injection**	In 30, 50 and 100 ml vials.[1]
Rx	**MD-60** (Mallinckrodt)		In 30 and 50 ml vials.[1]
Rx	**Renografin-60** (Squibb Diagnostics)		In 10, 30, 50 and 100 ml vials.[1]

[1] With EDTA.

DIATRIZOATE MEGLUMINE 60% and DIATRIZOATE SODIUM 30% (46.2% iodine)

For complete prescribing information, refer to the Radiopaque Agents group monograph.

Rx	**Hypaque-M, 90%** (Winthrop Pharm.)	**Injection**	In 50 ml vials.[1]

[1] With EDTA.

Parenteral Agents

DIATRIZOATE MEGLUMINE 66% and DIATRIZOATE SODIUM 10% (37% iodine)

For complete prescribing information, refer to the Radiopaque Agents group monograph.

Rx	**Angiovist 370** (Berlex)	**Injection**	In 50, 100, 150 and 200 ml vials & 500 ml w/infusion set.[1]
Rx	**Hypaque-76** (Winthrop Pharm.)		In 30, 50, 100, 150 and 200 ml.[1]
Rx	**MD-76** (Mallinckrodt)		In 50, 100, 150 and 200 ml vials and 95 and 125 ml syringes.[1]
Rx	**Renografin-76** (Squibb Diagnostics)		In 20, 50, 100 and 200 ml.[1]

[1] With EDTA.

IOTHALAMATE MEGLUMINE 52% and IOTHALAMATE SODIUM 26% (40% iodine)

For complete prescribing information, refer to the Radiopaque Agents group monograph.

Rx	**Vascoray** (Mallinckrodt)	**Injection**	In 50 ml vials and 100, 150 and 200 ml bottles.[1]

[1] With EDTA.

IOXAGLATE MEGLUMINE 39.3% and IOXAGLATE SODIUM 19.6% (32% iodine)

For complete prescribing information, refer to the Radiopaque Agents group monograph.

Rx	**Hexabrix** (Mallinckrodt)	**Injection**	In 20, 30 and 50 ml vials, 75 ml fill in 150 ml bottles, 100 ml fill in 150 ml, 200 ml fill in 250 ml, 150 ml bottles, 95 and 125 ml prefilled syringes.[1]

[1] With EDTA.

Miscellaneous Agents

DIATRIZOATE MEGLUMINE 18% (8.5% iodine)

For complete prescribing information, refer to the Radiopaque Agents group monograph.

NOT intended for intravascular administration.

Rx	**Cystografin Dilute** (Squibb Diagnostics)	**Injection**	In 300 and 500 ml[1] with or without administration sets.

[1] With EDTA.

DIATRIZOATE MEGLUMINE 30% (14.1% iodine)

For complete prescribing information, refer to the Radiopaque Agents group monograph.

NOT intended for intravascular administration.

Rx	**Cystografin** (Squibb Diagnostics)	**Injection**	In 100 and 300 ml.[1]
Rx	**Hypaque-Cysto** (Winthrop Pharm.)		In 100 ml in a pediatric 300 ml bottle[1] and 250 ml in a 500 ml bottle.[1]
Rx	**Reno-M-30** (Squibb Diagnostics)		In 50 and 100 ml.[2]
Rx	**Urovist Cysto** (Berlex)		In 100 ml in a pediatric 300 ml bottle[1] and 300 ml in a 500 ml bottle.[1]

[1] With EDTA.
[2] With EDTA and methyl and propyl parabens.

DIATRIZOATE SODIUM 20% (12% iodine)

For complete prescribing information, refer to the Radiopaque Agents group monograph.

NOT intended for intravascular administration.

Rx	**Hypaque Sodium 20%** (Winthrop Pharm.)	**Injection**	In 100 ml.[1]

[1] With EDTA.

IOTHALAMATE MEGLUMINE 17.2% (8.1% iodine)

For complete prescribing information, refer to the Radiopaque Agents group monograph.

NOT intended for intravascular administration.

Rx	**Cysto-Conray II** (Mallinckrodt)	**Injection**	In 250 and 500 ml.[1]

[1] With EDTA

IOTHALAMATE MEGLUMINE 43% (20.2% iodine)

For complete prescribing information, refer to the Radiopaque Agents group monograph.

NOT intended for intravascular administration.

Rx	**Cysto-Conray** (Mallinckrodt)	**Injection**	In 50 and 100 ml vials and 250 ml bottles and 50 ml prefilled syringes.[1]

[1] With EDTA.

DIATRIZOATE MEGLUMINE 52.7% & IODIPAMIDE MEGLUMINE 26.8% (38% iodine)

For complete prescribing information, refer to the Radiopaque Agents group monograph.

NOT intended for intravascular administration.

Rx	**Sinografin** (Squibb Diagnostics)	**Injection**	In 10 ml vials.[1]

[1] With EDTA.

ETHIODIZED OIL (37% iodine)

For complete prescribing information, refer to the Radiopaque Agents group monograph.

NOT intended for intravascular administration.

Rx	**Ethiodol** (Savage)	**Injection**	In 10 ml amps.

Miscellaneous Agents

PROPYLIODONE 60% in peanut oil (≈ 34% iodine)

For complete prescribing information, refer to the Radiopaque Agents group monograph.

NOT intended for intravascular administration.

Rx	**Dionosil Oily** (Allen & Hanburys)	**Suspension**	In 20 ml vials. *For intratracheal use.*

ISOSULFAN BLUE

For complete prescribing information, refer to the Radiopaque Agents group monograph.

NOT intended for intravascular administration.

Indications:

Delineates the lymphatic vessels. Adjunct to lymphography for visualization of the lymphatic system draining the region of injection.

Rx	**Lymphazurin 1%** (Hirsch Industries, Inc.)	**Injection:** 1% (10 mg/ml)	In 5 ml vials.

POTASSIUM PERCHLORATE

For complete prescribing information, refer to the Radiopaque Agents group monograph.

NOT intended for intravascular administration.

Indications:

To minimize the accumulation of pertechnetate Tc 99m in the choroid plexus and in the salivary and thyroid glands of patients receiving sodium pertechnetate Tc 99m for brain and blood pool imaging and placenta localization.

Unlabeled uses: Treatment of hyperthyroidism.

Rx	**Perchloracap** (Mallinckrodt)	**Capsules:** 200 mg	(19-N025) Opaque gray. In 100s.

ORPHAN DRUGS

The Orphan Drug Act defines an orphan drug as a drug or biological product for the diagnosis, treatment or prevention of a rare disease or condition. A rare disease is one which affects < 200,000 persons in the US or one which affects > 200,000 persons but for which there is no reasonable expectation that the cost of developing the drug and making it available will be recovered from sales of that drug in the US.

The FDA Office of Orphan Products Development (OPD) provides an information package that includes an overview of the FDA's orphan drug program, a brief description of the orphan products grant program and a current list of designated orphan products. OPD's information package also contains a directory sheet listing sources of information about the treatment of rare diseases, patient organizations and availability of orphan drugs. Requests for the Rare Disease Information Directory, or the entire orphan drugs information package, may be made by contacting OPD:

Office of Orphan Products Development (HF-35)
5600 Fishers Lane
Rockville, MD 20857
(301) 443–2043

Drug (*Trade name*)	Proposed use	Sponsor
Acetylcysteine (*Mucomyst*) (*Mucomyst 10 IV*)	IV for moderate to severe acetaminophen overdose	Apothecon
Aconiazide	Tuberculosis	Lincoln Diagnostics
Adeno-associated viral-based vector cystic fibrosis gene therapy	Cystic fibrosis	Targeted Genetics
Aerosol talc, sterile	Malignant pleural effusion	Bryan Corp
AI-RSA	Autoimmune uveitis	Autoimmune, Inc.
Albendazole (*Albenza*)	Hydatid disease (cystic echinococcosis due to E. granulosus larvae or alveolar echinococcosis due to E. multilocularis larvae; neurocysticercosis due to Taenia solium as: 1) chemotherapy of perenchymal, subarachnoidal and racemose (cysts in spinal fluid) neurocysticercosis in symptomatic cases and 2) prophylaxis of epilepsy and other sequelae in asymptomatic neurocysticercosis	S-K Beecham
Aldesleukin (*Proleukin*)	Metastatic renal cell carcinoma[1]/ melanoma; primary immunodeficiency disease associated with T-cell defects	Chiron
Alglucerase injection (*Ceredase*)	Replacement therapy in Gaucher's disease type I[1], II and III	Genzyme
Allopurinol sodium (*Zyloprim Injection*)	Management of leukemia, lymphoma and solid tumor malignancies in patients who cannot tolerate oral therapy and are receiving cancer therapy that causes elevations of serum and urinary uric acid levels[1]	Glaxo Wellcome
Alpha-1-antitrypsin (recombinant DNA origin)	Supplementation therapy for alpha-1-antitrypsin deficiency in the ZZ phenotype population	Chiron
Alpha-galactosidase A (*Fabrase*) (*CC-Galactosidase*)	Fabry's disease	Robert J. Desnick, MD David H. Calhoun, PhD
Alpha-1-proteinase inhibitor (*Prolastin*)	Replacement therapy in the alpha-1-proteinase inhibitor congenital deficiency state[1]	Miles

ORPHAN DRUGS

Drug (*Trade name*)	Proposed use	Sponsor
Alprostadil	Severe peripheral arterial occlusive disease (critical limb ischemia) in patients where other procedures, grafts or angioplasty, are not indicated	Schwarz Pharma
Altretamine (*Hexalen*)	Advanced ovarian adenocarcinoma[1]	U.S. Bioscience
Amifostine (*Ethyol*)	Chemoprotective agent for: Cisplatin in metastatic melanoma and advanced ovarian carcinoma[1]; cyclophosphamide in advanced ovarian carcinoma	U.S. Bioscience
Amiloride HCL solution for inhalation	Cystic fibrosis	Glaxo
Aminocaproic acid	Topical treatment of traumatic hyphema of the eye	Orphan Medical
Aminosalicylate sodium	Crohn's disease	Syncom
Aminosalicylic acid (*Pasar Granules*)	Tuberculosis infections[1]	Jacobus
4-Aminosalicylic acid (*Pamisyl*, Parke-Davis) (*Rezipas*, Squibb)	Mild to moderate ulcerative colitis in patients intolerant to sulfasalazine	Warren Beeken, MD
Aminosidine (*Gabbromicina*) (*Paromomycin*)	Tuberculosis; *Mycobacterium avium* complex; Visceral leishmaniasis (KALA-AZAR)	Thomas P. Kanyok, PharmD
Amiodarone (*Amio-Aqueous*) (*Cordarone*)	Incessant ventricular tachycardia; acute treatment[1] and prophylaxis of life-threatening ventricular tachycardia or ventricular fibrillation[1]	Academic Pharm Wyeth-Ayerst
Ammonium tetrathiomolybdate	Wilson's disease	George J. Brewer, MD
Amphotericin B lipid complex (*Abelcet*)	Invasive fungal infections[1]	Liposome Co.
Anagrelide (*Agrylin*)	Polycythemia vera; essential thrombocythemia[1]; thrombocytosis in chronic myelogenous leukemia	Roberts Pharm
Ananain, Comosain (*Vianain*)	For enzymatic debridement of severe burns	Genzyme
Anaritide acetate (*Auriculin*)	Improvement of early renal allograft function following renal transplantation; acute renal failure	Scios
Ancrod	Antithrombotic in patients with heparin-induced thrombocytopenia or thrombosis who require immediate and continued anticoagulation	Knoll Pharm
Antiepilepsirine	Drug-resistant generalized tonic-clonic epilepsy in children and adults	Children's Hospital, Columbus, OH
Antihemophilic factor, human (*Alphanate*) (*Humate P*)	Von Willebrand's disease	Alpha Ther Behringwerke Aktiengesellschaft
Antihemophilic factor (recombinant) (*Kogenate*)	Prophylaxis/treatment of bleeding in hemophilia A[1]; for prophylaxis when surgery is required in these patients[1]	Miles
Antithrombin III concentrate IV (*Kybernin*)	Prophylaxis/treatment of thromboembolic episodes in genetic AT-III deficiency	Centeon

ORPHAN DRUGS

Drug (*Trade name*)	Proposed use	Sponsor
Antithrombin III human (*Atnativ*) (*Thrombate* III) (*Antithrombin* III *human*)	Hereditary antithrombin III deficiency in connection with surgical or obstetrical procedures or thromboembolism[1]; replacement therapy in congenital deficiency of AT-III to prevent and treat thrombosis and pulmonary emboli[1]; to prevent/arrest episodes of thrombosis in patients with congenital AT-III deficiency or to prevent the occurrence of thrombosis in patients with AT-III deficiency who have undergone trauma or are about to undergo surgery or parturition	Kabivitrum Miles Red Cross
Anti-thymocyte serum (*Nashville Rabbit Anti-thymocyte serum*)	Allograft rejection, including solid organ (kidney, liver, heart, lung, pancreas) and bone marrow transplantation	Applied Medical Research
Antivenin, polyvalent crotalid (ovine) Fab (*CroTab*)	Treatment of the envenomations inflicted by North American crotalid snakes	Therapeutic Antibodies
Antivenom (crotalidae) purified (avian)	Treatment of envenomation by poisonous snakes belonging to the crotalidae family	Ophidian
APL 400-020	Cutaneous t-cell lymphoma	Apollon
Apomorphine HCl	Treatment of the on-off fluctuations associated with late-stage Parkinson's disease	Forum Products Pentech Pharm
Aprotinin (*Trasylol*)	Prophylaxis to reduce perioperative blood loss and the homologous blood transfusion requirement in patients undergoing repeat coronary artery bypass graft (CABG) surgery, and in selected cases of primary CABG surgery when the risk of bleeding is especially high or where transfusion is unavailable or unacceptable[1]	Miles
Arcitumomab (*99m Tc-labeled CEA-Scan*)	Diagnosis and localization of primary, residual, recurrent and metastatic medullary thyroid carcinoma	Immunomedics
Arginine butyrate	Beta-hemoglobinopathies and beta-thalassemia; sickle cell disease and beta-thalassemia	Susan P. Perrine, MD Vertex Pharm
Atovaquone (*Mepron*)	AIDS-associated *Pneumocystis carinii* pneumonia (PCP)[1]; prevention of PCP in high-risk, HIV-infected patients (defined by one or more episodes of PCP or a peripheral CD4+ lymphocyte count ≤ 200/mm^3); treatment/suppression of *Toxoplasma gondii* encephalitis; primary prophylaxis of HIV-infected persons at high risk for developing *T gondii* encephalitis	Glaxo Wellcome
Autolymphocyte therapy	Renal cell carcinoma	Cellcor
Bacitracin (*Altracin*)	Antibiotic-associated pseudomembranous enterocolitis caused by toxins A and B elaborated by *Clostridium difficile*	A.L. Labs

ORPHAN DRUGS

Drug (*Trade name*)	Proposed use	Sponsor
Baclofen (*Lioresal intrathecal*)	Intractable spasticity caused by spinal cord injury/multiple sclerosis and other spinal diseases (eg, spinal ischemia, spinal tumor, cerebral palsy, transverse myelitis, cervical spondylosis and degenerative myelopathy)[1]	Medtronic
Benzoate and phenylacetate (*Ucephan*)	Adjunctive therapy to prevent/treat hyperammonemia in patients with urea cycle enzymopathy due to carbamylphosphate synthetase, ornithine, transcarbamylase or arginosuccinate synthetase deficiency[1]	Kendall McGaw
Benzylpenicillin, benzylpenicilloic, benzylpenilloic acid (*Pre-Pen/MDM*)	To assess risk of penicillin use when it is the preferred drug in adults who previously received penicillin and have a history of sensitivity	Schwarz Pharma
Beractant (*Survanta Intratracheal Suspension*)	To prevent/treat neonatal respiratory distress syndrome[1]; full-term newborns with respiratory failure caused by meconium aspiration syndrome, persistent pulmonary hypertension of the newborn, or pneumonia and sepsis	Ross
Beta alethine (*Betathine*)	Multiple myeloma; metastatic melanoma	Dovetail Tech
Betaine (*Cystadane*)	Homocystinuria[1]	Orphan Medical
Bispecific antibody 520C9x22	In vivo serotherapy of ovarian cancer	Medarex
Bleomycin sulfate (*Blenoxane*)	Malignant pleural effusion[1]	Bristol-Myers Squibb
Botulinum toxin type A (*Botox*) (*Dysport*)	Blepharospasm and strabismus associated with dystonia in adults (≥ 12 years old)[1]; cervical dystonia; dynamic muscle contracture in pediatric cerebral palsy; essential blepharospasm; synkinetic closure of the eyelid associated with VII cranial nerve aberrant regeneration	Associated Synapse Allergan Porton
Botulinum toxin type B	Cervical dystonia	Athena Neurosciences
Botulinum toxin type F	Spasmodic torticollis (cervical dystonia); essential blepharospasm	Porton
Botulism immune globulin	Infant botulism	CA Dept. Health Service
Bovine colostrum	AIDS-related diarrhea	Donald Hastings, DVM
Bovine immunoglobulin concentrate, Cryptosporidium parvum (*Sporidin-G*)	Treatment/symptomatic relief of *Cryptosporidium parvum* infection of GI tract in immunocompromised patients	GalaGen
Bovine whey protein concentrate (*Immuno-C*)	Cryptosporidiosis caused by *Cryptosporidium parvum* in the GI tract of patients who are immunodeficient/immunocompromised or immunocompetent	Biomune Systems
Branched chain amino acids	Amyotrophic lateral sclerosis	Mount Sinai Medical Center
Bromhexine	Mild/moderate keratoconjunctivitis sicca in Sjogren's syndrome	Boehringer Ingelheim

ORPHAN DRUGS

Drug (*Trade name*)	Proposed use	Sponsor
Bromodeoxyuridine	Radiation sensitizer in the treatment of primary brain tumors	Neopharm, Inc
Buffered intrathecal electrolye/dextrose injection (*Elliotts B Solution*)	Diluent in intrathecal administration of methotrexate and cytarabine for prevention/treatment of meningeal leukemia or lymphocytic lymphoma	Orphan Medical
Buprenorphine HCl	Alone or with naloxone for treatment of opiate addictions	Reckitt and Coleman
Busulfan (*Busulfanex*)	Preparative therapy for malignancies treated with bone marrow transplantation	Sparta Orphan Medical
Butyrylcholinesterase	Reduction and clearance of toxic blood levels of cocaine in overdose; post-surgical apnea	Pharmavene
C1-Esterase-inhibitor (human)	Prevention/treatment of angioedema caused by C1-esterase inhibitor deficiency	Alpha Ther
C1-Esterase-inhibitor, human, pasteurized (*Berinert P*)	Prevention/treatment of acute attacks of hereditary angioedema	Behringwerke Aktiengesellschaft
C1-inhibitor (*C1-Inhibitor [human] Vapor Heated, Immuno*)	Treatment of acute attacks of angioedema; prevention of acute attacks of angioedema, including short-term prophylaxis for patients requiring dental or other surgical procedures	Osterreichisches Immuno
Caffeine (*Neocaf*)	Apnea of prematurity	OPR Development, LP
Calcitonin-human for injection (*Cibacalcin*)	Symptomatic Paget's disease (osteitis deformans)[1]	Ciba-Geigy
Calcium acetate (*Phos-Lo*)	Hyperphosphatemia in end-stage renal failure/disease[1]	Pharmedic Braintree
Calcium carbonate (*R&D Calcium Carbonate/600*)	Hyperphosphatemia in end-stage renal disease	R & D
Calcium gluconate gel **Calcium gluconate gel 2.5%** (*H-F Gel*)	Emergency topical treatment of hydrogen fluoride (hydrofluoric acid) burns	LTR Pharm Paddock
Carbovir	AIDS; symptomatic HIV infection and CD4 count < 200/mm^3	Glaxo
Cascara sagrada fluid extract	For oral drug overdosage to speed lower bowel evacuation	Intramed
Ceramide trihexosidase/ alpha-galactosidase A	Fabry's disease	Genzyme
Chenodiol (*Chenix*)	For radiolucent stones in well opacifying gallbladders, where elective surgery would be undertaken except for presence of increased surgical risk due to systemic disease or age[1]	Solvay
Chimeric A2 (human-murine) IgG monoclonal anti-TNF antibody (cA2)	Crohn's disease	Centocor
Chimeric (murine variable, human constant) Mab (C2B8) to CD20	Non-Hodgkin's B-cell lymphoma	Idec Pharm
Chlorhexidine gluconate mouthrinse (*Peridex*)	Amelioration of oral mucositis associated with cytoreductive therapy for conditioning patients for bone marrow transplantation	Procter & Gamble

ORPHAN DRUGS

Drug (*Trade name*)	Proposed use	Sponsor
Choline chloride	Choline deficiency, specifically the choline deficiency, hepatic steatosis, and cholestasis, associated with long-term parenteral nutrition	Orphan Medical
Chondroitinase	Patients undergoing vitrectomy	Storz Ophthalmics
Ciliary neutrotrophic factor	Amyotrophic lateral sclerosis	Regeneron Pharm
9-Cis retinoic acid	Treatment of promyelocytic leukemia; prevention of retinal detachment due to proliferative vitreoretinopathy	Allergan Ligand
Citric acid, glucono-delta-lactone and magnesium carbonate (*Renacidin Irrigation*)	Renal and bladder calculi of the apatite or struvite variety[1]	United-Guardian
Cladribine (*Leustatin Injection*)	Acute myeloid, hairy-cell[1] and chronic lymphocytic leukemias; non-Hodgkin's lymphoma; chronic multiple sclerosis	R.W. Johnson Res
Clindamycin (*Cleocin*)	Treatment/prevention of *Pneumocystis carinii* pneumonia associated with AIDS	Pharmacia & Upjohn
Clofazimine (*Lamprene*)	Lepromatous leprosy, including dapsone-resistant lepromatous leprosy and lepromatous leprosy complicated by erythema nodosum leprosum[1]	Ciba-Geigy
Clonazepam (*Klonopin*)	Hyperekplexia (startle disease)	Hoffman-La Roche
Clonidine (*Duraclon*)	For continuous epidural administration as adjunctive therapy with intraspinal opiates for pain in cancer patients toerant or unresponsive to intraspinal opiates	Fujisawa
Clostridial collagenase	Advanced (involutional or residual stage) Dupuytren's disease	L. Hurst, MD M. Badalamente, PhD
Clotrimidazole	Sickle cell disease	Carlo Brugnara, MD
Coagulation factor IX (*Mononine*)	Replacement/prophylaxis of hemorrhagic complications of hemophilia B[1]	Armour Pharm
Coagulation factor IX (human) (*AlphaNine*)	Replacement therapy in hemophilia B for prevention and control of bleeding episodes; during surgery to correct defective hemostasis[1]	Alpha Therapeutic
Coagulation factor IX (recombinant) (*BeneFix*)	Hemophilia B[1]	Genetics Institute
Colfosceril palmitate, cetyl alcohol, tyloxapol (*Exosurf Neonatal for Intratracheal Suspension*)	To prevent hyaline membrane disease (respiratory distress syndrome) in infants born at ≤ 32 weeks gestation[1]; to treat established hyaline membrane disease at all gestational ages[1]; adult respiratory distress syndrome	Glaxo Wellcome
Collagenase (lyophilized) for injection (*Plaquase*)	Peyronie's disease	Advance Biofactures
Corticorelin Ovine Triflutate (*Acthrel*)	To differentiate between pituitary and ectopic production of ACTH in ACTH-dependent Cushing's syndrome[1]	Ferring
Coumarin (*Oncostate*)	Renal cell carcinoma	Praevomed GmBH

ORPHAN DRUGS

Drug (*Trade name*)	Proposed use	Sponsor
Cromolyn sodium (*Gastrocrom*)	Mastocytosis[1]	Fisons
Cromolyn sodium 4% ophthalmic solution (*Opticrom*)	Vernal keratoconjunctivitis[1]	Fisons
Cryptosporidium hyperimmune bovine colostrum IgG concentrate	Diarrhea in AIDS patients caused by infection with *Cryptosporidium parvum*	ImmuCell
CY-1503	Post-ischemic pulmonary reperfusion edema following surgical treatment for chronic thromboembolic pulmonary hypertension	Cytel
CY-1899	Chronic active hepatitis B infection in HLA-A2 positive patients	Cytel
8 Cyclopentyl 1,3-dipropylxanthine	Cystic fibrosis	SciClone Pharm
Cyclosporine ophthalmic (*Optimmune*)	Severe keratoconjunctivitis sicca with Sjogren's syndrome	U of Georgia College of Veterinary Medicine
Cyclosporine 2% ophthalmic ointment	Treatment of patients at high risk of graft rejection following penetrating keratoplasty; corneal melting syndromes of known or presumed immunologic etiopathogenesis, including Mooren's ulcer	Allergan
Cysteamine (*Cystagon*)	Nephropathic cystinosis[1]	Jess Thoene, MD Mylan
Cystic fibrosis gene therapy	Cystic fibrosis	Genzyme
Cystic fibrosis transmembrane conductance regulator	Cystic fibrosis transmembrane conductance regulator protein replacement therapy in cystic fibrosis patients	Genzyme
Cystic fibrosis transmembrane conductance regulator gene	Cystic fibrosis	Genetic Therapy
Cystic fibrosis TR gene therapy (recombinant adenovirus) (*AdGVCFTR. 10*)	Cystic fibrosis	GenVec
Cytomegalovirus immune globulin (human) (*CytoGam*)	Prevention or attenuation of primary cytomegalovirus disease in immunosuppressed recipients of organ transplants[1]	MA Public Health Bio Labs
Cytomegalovirus immune globulin IV (human)	With ganciclovir sodium for the treatment of CMV pneumonia in bone marrow transplant patients	Miles
DAB_{389}IL-2	Cutaneous T-cell lymphoma	Seragen
Dapsone	Prophylaxis of toxoplasmosis in severely immunocompromised patients with CD4 counts < 100	Jacobus Pharm
Dapsone, USP (*Dapsone*)	Prophylaxis of *Pneumocystis carinii* pneumonia; with trimethoprim for treatment of PCP	Jacobus Pharm
Daunorubicin citrate liposome injection (*DaunoXome*)	Treatment of patients with advanced HIV-associated Kaposi's sarcoma[1]	NeXstar
Defibrotide	Thrombotic thrombocytopenic purpura	Crinos International
Dehydrex	Recurrent corneal erosion unresponsive to conventional therapy	Holles Labs

ORPHAN DRUGS

Drug (*Trade name*)	Proposed use	Sponsor
Dehydroepiandrosterone	Systemic lupus erythematosus (SLE) and reduction of steroid use in steroid-dependent SLE patients	Genelabs
Dehydroepiandrosterone sulfate sodium	Treat serious burns requiring hospitalization; accelerate re-epithelialization of donor sites in autologous skin grafting	Pharmadigm
2′-Deoxycytidine	Host-protective agent in acute myelogenous leukemia	Steven Grant, MD
Deoxycytidine, 5-Aza-2′	Acute leukemia	Pharmachemie USA
Depofoam encapsulated cytarabine	Neoplastic meningitis	DepoTech
Deslorelin (*Somagard*)	Central precocious puberty	Roberts Pharm
Desmopressin acetate	Mild hemophilia A and von Willebrand's disease[1]	Rhone-Poulenc Rorer
Dexrazoxane (*Zinecard*)	Prevention of cardiomyopathy associated with doxorubicin administration[1]	Pharmacia & Upjohn
Dextran and deferoxamine (*Bio-Rescue*)	Acute iron poisoning	Biomedical Frontiers
Dextran sulfate, (inhaled, aerosolized) (*Uendex*)	As an adjunct to the treatment of cystic fibrosis	Kennedy & Hoidal, MDs
Dextran sulfate sodium	AIDS	Ueno Fine Chemicals
3,4-Diaminopyridine	Lambert-Eaton myasthenic syndrome	Jacobus Pharm
Dianeal peritoneal dialysis solution with 1.1% amino acids (*Nutrineal Peritoneal Dialysis Solution with 1.1% Amino Acid*)	Nutritional supplement for malnourishment in patients undergoing continuous ambulatory peritoneal dialysis	Baxter Healthcare
Diazepam viscous solution, rectal	Rectal administration for acute repetitive seizures	Athena
Dibromodulcitol	Recurrent invasive or metastatic squamous cervical carcinoma	Biopharmaceutics
Diethyldithiocarbomate (*Imuthiol*)	AIDS	Connaught
Digoxin immune fab (Ovine) (*Digibind*) (*Digidote*)	Treatment of potentially life-threatening digitalis intoxication in patients refractory to management by conventional therapy[1]; life-threatening acute cardiac glycoside intoxication manifested by conduction disorders, ectopic ventricular activity and sometimes hyperkalemia	Glaxo Wellcome Boehringer Mannheim
5,6-Dihydro-5-azacytidine	Malignant mesothelioma	Ilex Oncology
Dihydrotestosterone (*Androgel-DHT*)	Weight loss in AIDS with HIV-associated wasting	Unimed
24,25 Dihydroxycholecalciferol	Uremic osteodystrophy	Lemmon
Dimethyl sulfoxide	Increased intracranial pressure in patients with severe, closed-head injury (traumatic brain coma) for whom no other effective treatment is available	Pharma 21
Dipalmitoylphosphatidylcholine/Phosphatidylglycerol (*ALEC*)	Prevention/treatment of neonatal respiratory distress syndrome	Forum Products

ORPHAN DRUGS

Drug (*Trade name*)	Proposed use	Sponsor
Disaccharide tripeptide glycerol dipalmitoyl (*ImmTher*)	Pulmonary and hepatic metastases in colorectal adenocarcinoma	Immuno Therapeutics
Disodium clodronate	Hypercalcemia of malignancy	Discovery Experimental & Development
Disodium clodronate tetrahydrate (*Bonefos*)	Increased bone resorption due to malignancy	Leiras Pharm
DMP 777	Therapeutic management of lung disease attributable to cystic fibrosis	Du Pont Merck
Dornase alfa (*Pulmozyme*)	Reduces mucous viscosity and enables the clearance of airway secretions in cystic fibrosis[1]	Genentech
Dronabinol (*Marinol*)	For the stimulation of appetite and prevention of weight loss in patients with a confirmed diagnosis of AIDS[1]	Unimed
Dynamine	Lambert-Eaton myasthenic syndrome; hereditary motor and sensory neuropathy type I (Charcot-Marie-Tooth disease)	Mayo Foundation
Eflornithine HCl (*Ornidyl*)	*Trypanosoma brucei gambiense* infection (sleeping sickness)[1]	Marion Merrell Dow
Elcatonin	Intrathecal treatment of intractable pain	Innapharma, Inc
Enadoline hydrochloride	Severe head injury	Warner-Lambert
Encapsulated porcine islet preparation (*BetaRx*)	Type I diabetic patients already on immunosuppression	VivoRx
Epidermal growth factor (human)	Acceleration of corneal epithelial regeneration and healing of stromal tissue in non-healing corneal defects	Chiron
Epoetin alpha (*Epogen*) (*Procrit*)	Anemia associated with end-stage renal disease or HIV infection or treatment[1]; myelodysplastic syndrome; anemia of prematurity in preterm infants	Amgen R. W. Johnson Res
Epoetin beta (*Marogen*)	Anemia associated with end-stage renal disease	Chugai-USA
Epoprostenol (*Flolan*)	Primary pulmonary hypertension	Glaxo Wellcome
Erwinia L-asparaginase (*Erwinase*)	Acute lymphocytic leukemia	Porton
Erythropoietin (recombinant human)	Anemia associated with end-stage renal disease	McDonnell Douglas
Ethanolamine oleate (*Ethamolin*)	Esophageal varices that have recently bled, to prevent rebleeding[1]	Block
Ethinyl estradiol, USP	Turner's syndrome	Bio-Technology
Etidronate disodium (*Didronel*)	Hypercalcemia of malignancy inadequately managed by dietary modification or oral hydration[1]	MGI Pharma
Etiocholanedione	Aplastic anemia; Prader-Willi syndrome	SuperGen
Exemestane	Hormonal therapy of metastatic carcinoma of the breast	Pharmacia & Upjohn

ORPHAN DRUGS

Drug (*Trade name*)	Proposed use	Sponsor
Factor VIIa (recombinant, DNA origin)	Hemophilia A and B with and without antibodies against Factors VIII/IX; von Willebrand's disease	Novo Nordisk
Factor XIII (plasma-derived) (*Fibrogammin P*)	Congenital Factor XIII deficiency	Behringwerke Aktiengesellschaft (AG)
Fampridine (*Neurelan*)	Symptoms of multiple sclerosis	Elan
Felbamate (*Felbatol*)	Lennox-Gastaut syndrome	Wallace
FGN-1	For suppression and control of colonic adematous polyps in adenomatous polyposis coli	Cell Pathways
FIAU	Adjunctive treatment of chronic active hepatitis B	Oclassen
Fibrinogen (human)	Control of bleeding and prophylactic treatment of patients deficient in fibrinogen	Alpha Therapeutic
Fibronectin (human plasma derived)	Non-healing corneal ulcers or epithelial defects unresponsive to conventional therapy (underlying cause has been eliminated)	Melville Biologics
Filgrastim (*Neupogen*)	Severe chronic neutropenia (absolute neutrophil count < 500/mm^3); neutropenia associated with bone marrow transplants; AIDS patients with CMV retinitis being treated with ganciclovir; mobilization of peripheral blood progenitor cells for collection in patients who will receive myeloablative or myelosuppressive chemotherapy; reduce duration of neutropenia, fever, antibiotic use and hospitalization following induction and consolidation for acute myeloid leukemia	Amgen
Fludarabine phosphate (*Fludara*)	Treatment/management of non-Hodgkin's lymphoma; chronic lymphocytic leukemia (CLL) including refractory CLL[1]	Berlex
Flumecinol (*Zixoryn*)	Hyperbilirubinemia in newborns unresponsive to phototherapy	Farmacon
Flunarizine (*Sibelium*)	Alternating hemiplegia	Janssen
Fluorouracil (*Adrucil*)	With interferon alpha-2a for esophageal or advanced colorectal carcinoma; with leucovorin for metastatic adenocarcinoma of the colon and rectum	Hoffman-LaRoche Lederle
Fomepizole (*Antizol*)	Methanol or ethylene glycol poisoning	Orphan Medical
Fosphenytoin (*Cerebyx*)	Acute treatment of patients with status epilepticus of the grand mal type	Warner-Lambert
Gabapentin (*Neurontin*)	Amyotrophic lateral sclerosis	Warner-Lambert
Gallium nitrate injection (*Ganite*)	Hypercalcemia of malignancy[1]	Solopak
Gamma-hydroxybutyrate	Narcolepsy and symptoms of cataplexy, sleep paralysis, hypnagogic hallucinations and automatic behavior	Biocraft Orphan Medical

ORPHAN DRUGS

Drug (*Trade name*)	Proposed use	Sponsor
Gammalinolenic acid	Juvenile rheumatoid arthritis	Robert B Zurier, MD
Ganaxolone	Infantile spasms	CoCensys
Ganciclovir intravitreal implant (*Vitrasert Implant*)	Cytomegalovirus retinitis	Chiron Vision
Gentamicin impregnated PMMA beads on surgical wire (*Septopal*)	Chronic osteomyelitis of post-traumatic, postoperative or hematogenous origin	Lipha
Gentamicin liposome injection (*Maitec*)	Disseminated *Mycobacterium avium-intracellulare* infection	Liposome Company
Glatiramer acetate (*Copaxone*)	Multiple sclerosis	Teva
Glutamine	With human growth hormone in treatment of short bowel syndrome (nutrient malabsorption from the GI tract resulting from an inadequate absorptive surface)	Nutritional Restart
Glyceryl trioleate **Glyceryl trierucate**	Adrenoleukodystrophy	Hugo W. Moser, MD
Gonadorelin acetate (*Lutrepulse*)	Ovulation induction in women with hypothalamic amenorrhea due to a deficiency or absence in quantity or pulse pattern of endogenous GnRH secretion[1]	Ferring Labs
Gossypol	Cancer of the adrenal cortex	Marcus M. Reidenberg, MD
GP 100 adenoviral gene therapy	Metastatic melanoma	Genzyme
Group B streptococcus immune globulin	Disseminated group B streptococcal infection in neonates	North American Biologicals
Growth hormone releasing factor	Long-term treatment of children who have growth failure due to a lack of adequate endogenous growth hormone secretion	ICN Pharm
Guanethidine monosulfate (*Ismelin*)	Moderate/severe reflex sympathetic dystrophy and causalgia	Ciba-Geigy
Gusperimus (*Spanidin*)	Acute renal graft rejection episodes	Bristol-Myers Squibb
Halofantrine (*Halfan*)	Mild to moderate acute malaria caused by susceptible strains of *Plasmodium falciparum* and *P. vivax*[1]	SK-Beecham
Heme arginate (*Normosang*)	Symptomatic stage of acute porphyria; myelodysplastic syndromes	Leiras
Hemin (*Panhematin*)	Amelioration of recurrent attacks of acute intermittent porphyria (AIP) temporarily related to menstrual cycle and similar symptoms that occur in other patients with AIP, porphyria variegata and hereditary coproporphyria[1]	Abbott
Hemin and zinc mesoporphyrin (*Hemex*)	Acute porphyric syndromes	Herbert L. Bonkovsky, MD
Heparin, 2-0-desulfated (*Aeropin*)	Cystic fibrosis	Kennedy & Hoidal, MDs

ORPHAN DRUGS

Drug (*Trade name*)	Proposed use	Sponsor
Hepatitis B immune globulin IV (*H-BIGIV*)	Prophylaxis against hepatitis B virus reinfection in liver transplant patients	NABI
Herpes simplex virus gene	Primary and metastatic brain tumors	Genetic Therapy, Inc.
Histrelin	Treatment of acute intermittent porphyria, hereditary coproporphyria and variegate porphyria	Karl E. Anderson, MD
Histrelin acetate (*Supprelin Injection*)	Central precocious puberty[1]	Roberts
Human acid alpha-glucosidase	Glycogen storage disease type II	Pharmain BV
Human growth hormone	With glutamine in the treatment of short bowel syndrome (nutrient malabsorption from the GI tract resulting from an inadequate absorptive surface)	Nutritional Restart
Human immunodeficiency virus immune globulin (*Hivig*)	AIDS; HIV-infected pregnant women and infants of HIV-infected mothers; HIV-infected pediatric patients	NABI
Humanized anti-tac (*Zenapax*)	Prevent acute renal allograft rejection; prevent acute graft-vs-host disease following bone marrow transplantation	Hoffmann-La Roche
Human thyroid stimulating hormone (THS) (*Thyrogen*)	Adjunct in the diagnosis of thyroid cancer	Genzyme
Human T-lymphotropic virus type III Gp 160 antigens (*Vaxsyn HIV-1*)	AIDS	MicroGeneSys
Hydroxocobalamin/Sodium thiosulfate	Severe acute cyanide poisoning	Alan H. Hall, MD
Hydroxyurea (*Hydrea*)	Treatment of patients with sickle cell anemia as shown by the presence of hemoglobin S	Bristol-Myers Squibb
Ibuprofen IV solution (*Salprofen*)	Prevention/treatment of patent ductus arteriosus	Farmacon
Idarubicin (*Idamycin*)	Myelodysplastic syndromes; chronic myelogenous leukemia	Pharmacia & Upjohn
Idarubicin HCl for injection (*Idamycin*)	Acute myelogenous leukemia (acute nonlymphocytic leukemia)[1]; acute lymphoblastic leukemia in pediatric patients	Adria Pharmacia & Upjohn
Idoxuridine	Nonparenchymatous sarcomas	NeoPharm
Ifosfamide (*Ifex*)	With other antineoplastics for third-line chemotherapy in the treatment of germ-cell testicular cancer[1]; bone sarcomas; soft tissue sarcomas	Bristol-Myers Squibb
Imciromab pentetate (*Myoscint*)	Detecting early necrosis as an indication of rejection of orthotopic cardiac transplants	Centocor
Imexon	Multiple myeloma	Amplimed
Imiglucerase (*Cerezyme*)	Replacement therapy in patients with types I, II and III Gaucher's disease[1]	Genzyme

ORPHAN DRUGS

Drug (*Trade name*)	Proposed use	Sponsor
Immune globulin IV (human) (*Gamimune N*) (*Immuno*) (*Iveegam*) (*Immue Globulin Intravenous [human] Immuno*)	Juvenile rheumatoid arthritis; infection prophylaxis in pediatric patients with HIV; acute myocarditis	Immuno Miles
Imported fire ant venom, allergenic extract	Skin testing of fire ant stings to confirm fire ant sensitivity and if positive, as immunotherapy for prevention of IgE-mediated anaphylactic reactions	ALK Labs
In-111 murine Mab (2B8-MX-DTPA) and Y-90 murine Mab (2B8-MXDTPA) (*Melimmune*)	B-cell non-Hodgkin's lymphoma	IDEC Pharm
Indium in 111 murine monoclonal antibody FAB to myosin (*Myoscint*)	Aid in diagnosis of myocarditis	Centocor
Inosine pranobex (*Isoprinosine*)	Subacute sclerosing panencephalitis	Newport
Insulin-like growth factor-1 (*Myotrophin*)	Amyotrophic lateral sclerosis	Cephalon
Interferon alfa-2a (*Roferon A*)	Chronic myelogenous leukemia	Hoffmann-La Roche
Interferon alfa-2a (recombinant) (*Roferon A*)	AIDS-related Kaposi's sarcoma[1]; renal-cell carcinoma; with fluorouracil for esophageal carcinoma or advanced colorectal cancer; with teceleukin for metastatic renal cell carcinoma or metastatic malignant melanoma	Hoffmann-LaRoche
Interferon alfa-2b (recombinant) (*Intron A*)	AIDS-related Kaposi's sarcoma[1]	Schering
Interferon alfa-NL (*Wellferon*)	Human papillomavirus in severe resistant/recurrent respiratory (laryngeal) papillomatosis	Glaxo Wellcome
Interferon beta-1a (*Avonex*) (*Rebif*)	Multiple sclerosis; secondary progressive multiple sclerosis	Biogen Serono
Interferon beta-1b (*Betaseron*)	Multiple sclerosis	Berlex Chiron
Interferon beta (recombinant) (*Rebif*) (*R-IFN-beta*)	Systemic treatment of cutaneous malignant melanoma, cutaneous T-cell lymphoma and metastatic renal-cell carcinoma; intralesional/systemic treatment of AIDS-related Kaposi's sarcoma; symptomatic patients with AIDS (including CD4 T-cell counts < 200 cells/mm^3)	Biogen Serono
Interferon beta (recombinant human) (*Avonex*)	Acute non-A, non-B hepatitis; primary brain tumors	Biogen
Interferon gamma-1b (*Actimmune*)	Chronic granulomatous disease[1]; renal cell carcinoma; severe congenital osteopetrosis	Genentech

ORPHAN DRUGS

Drug (*Trade name*)	Proposed use	Sponsor
Interleukin-1 receptor antagonist (human recombinant) (*Antril*)	Juvenile rheumatoid arthritis; prevention/treatment of graft-vs-host disease in transplant recipients	Amgen
Interleukin-2 (*Teceleukin*)	Alone or with interferon alfa-2a for metastatic renal-cell carcinoma and metastatic malignant melanoma	Hoffmann-La Roche
Iobenguane sulfate I-131	Diagnostic adjunct in patients with pheochromocytoma	CIS-US
Iodine I^{123} murine monoclonal antibody to alpha-fetoprotein	Detects hepatocellular carcinoma and hepatoblastoma and alpha-fetoprotein-producing germ-cell tumors	Immunomedics
Iodine I^{123} murine monoclonal antibody to hCG	Detection of hCG-producing tumors (eg, germ-cell and trophoblastic-cell tumors)	Immunomedics
Iodine I^{131} 6B-iodomethyl-19-norcholesterol	Adrenal cortical imaging	William Beierwaltes, MD
Iodine I^{131} murine monoclonal antibody IgG2a to B cell (*Immurait; L1-2-I-131*)	B-cell leukemia and B-cell lymphoma	Immunomedics
Iodine I^{131} murine monoclonal antibody to alpha-fetoprotein	Hepatocellular carcinoma and hepatoblastoma; alpha-fetoprotein-producing germ-cell tumors	Immunomedics
Iodine I^{131} murine monoclonal antibody to hCG	hCG-producing tumors (eg, germ-cell and trophoblastic-cell tumors)	Immunomedics
I-131 radiolabeled B1 monoclonal antibody	Non-Hodgkin's B-cell lymphoma	Coulter Pharm
Isobutyramide (*Isobutyramide Oral Solution*)	Beta-hemoglobinopathies and beta-thalassemia syndromes; sickle cell disease and beta-thalassemia	Susan P. Perrine, MD Alpha Ther
KL4-surfactant	Acute respiratory distress syndrome in adults; respiratory distress syndrome in premature infants; meconium aspiration syndrome in newborn infants	Acute Therapeutics
L-2-oxothiazolidine-4-carboxylic acid (*Procysteine*)	Adult respiratory distress syndrome; amyotrophic lateral sclerosis	Transcend Therapeutics
L-5 hydroxytryptophan	Postanoxic intention myoclonus	Circa
Lactobin	AIDS-associated diarrhea unresponsive to initial antidiarrheal therapy	Roxane
Lamotrigine (*Lamictal*)	Lennox-Gestaut syndrome	Glaxo Wellcome
L-baclofen (*Neuralgon*)	Trigeminal neuralgia; intractable spasticity from spinal cord injury or multiple sclerosis; intractable spasticity in children with cerebral palsy	Gerhard Fromm, MD WTD, Inc
L-cycloserine	Gaucher's disease	Meier Lev, MD
L-cysteine	Prevention and lessening of photosensitivity in erythropoietic protoporphyria	Tyson
Leflunomide	Prevention of acute and chronic rejection in patients with solid organ transplants	James W. Williams, MD
Lepirudin (*Refludan*)	Heparin-associated thrombocytopenia Type II	Behringwerke AG

ORPHAN DRUGS

Drug (*Trade name*)	Proposed use	Sponsor
Leucovorin **Leucovorin calcium** (*Wellcovorin*)	With 5-fluorouracil for metastatic colorectal cancer[1]; rescue use after high-dose methotrexate therapy in the treatment of osteosarcoma[1]	Glaxo Wellcome Immunex
Leupeptin	As an adjunct to microsurgical peripheral nerve repair	Neuromuscular Adjuncts
Leuprolide acetate (*Lupron*)	Central precocious puberty[1]	Tap Pharm
Levocarnitine (*Carnitor*)	Genetic carnitine deficiency[1]; primary and secondary carnitine deficiency of genetic origin[1]; treatment of manifestations of carnitine deficiency in patients with end-stage renal disease who require dialysis; prevention/treatment of secondary carnitine deficiency in valproic acid toxicity; pediatric cardiomyopathy	Sigma-Tau
Levomethadyl acetate HCl (*ORLAAM*)	Treatment of heroin addicts suitable for maintenance on opiate agonists[1]	Biodevelopment Corp.
Lidocaine patch 5% (*Lidoderm Patch*)	Post-herpetic neuralgia resulting frm Herpes zoster infection	Hind Health Care
Liothyronine sodium injection (*Triostat*)	Myxedema coma/precoma[1]	SmithKline-Beecham
Lipid/DNA human cystic fibrosis gene	Cystic fibrosis	Genzyme
Liposomal amphotericin B (*AmBisome*)	Cryptococcal meningitis; visceral leishmaniasis; histoplasmosis	Fujisawa
Liposomal prostaglandin E-1 injection	Acute respiratory distress syndrome	Liposome Co.
Liposome encapsulated recombinant interleukin-2	Brain and CNS tumors; kidney and renal pelvis cancers	Biomira
L-leucovorin (*Isovorin*)	With high-dose methotrexate in the treatment of osteosarcoma; in combination chemotherapy with the approved agent 5-fluorouracil in the palliative treatment of metastatic adenocarcinoma of the colon and rectum	Lederle
Lodoxamide tromethamine (*Alomide Ophthalmic Solution*)	Vernal keratoconjunctivitis[1]	Alcon
L-threonine (*Threostat*)	Amyotrophic lateral sclerosis; spasticity associated with familial spastic paraparesis	Tyson Interneuron
Mafenide acetate solution (*Sulfamylon Solution*)	To control bacterial colonization and prevent infectious graft loss under moist dressings over meshed autografts on excised burn wounds	Mylan
MART-1 adenoviral gene therapy for malignant melanoma	Metastatic melanoma	Genzyme
Matrix metalloproteinase inhibitor (*Galardin*)	Corneal ulcers	Glycomed
Mazindol (*Sanorex*)	Duchenne muscular dystrophy	Platon J. Collipp, MD

ORPHAN DRUGS

Drug (*Trade name*)	Proposed use	Sponsor
Mecasermin	Growth hormone insufficency syndrome	Genentech
Mefloquine HCl (*Lariam*) (*Mephaquin*)	Prevent/treat chloroquine-resistant falciparum malaria; acute malaria due to *Plasmodium falciparum* and *P. vivax*[1]; prophylaxis of resistant *P. falciparum*[1]	Mepha AG Hoffman-LaRoche
Megestrol acetate (*Megace*)	Anorexia, cachexia or significant weight loss (≥ 10% of body weight) with confirmed diagnosis of AIDS[1]	Bristol-Myers Squibb
Melanoma cell vaccine	Invasive melanoma	Donald L. Morton, MD
Melanoma vaccine (*Melacine*)	Stage III-IV melanoma	Ribi ImmunoChem Research
Melatonin	Circadian rhythm sleep disorders in blind people with no light perception	Robert Sack, MD
Melphalan (*Alkeran for Injection*)	Multiple myeloma when oral therapy is inappropriate[1]; hyperthermic regional limb perfusion to treat metastatic melanoma of the extremity	Glaxo Wellcome
Mesna (*Mesnex*)	Prophylactic to reduce the incidence of ifosfamide-induced hemorrhagic cystitis[1]; inhibition of the urotoxic effects induced by oxazaphosphorine compounds (eg, cyclophosphamide)	Asta Degussa Corp
Methionine L-methionine	AIDS myelopathy	Alessandro Di Rocco, MD
Methotrexate (*Rheumatrex*)	Juvenile rheumatoid arthritis	Wyeth-Ayerst
Methotrexate sodium (*Methotrexate*)	Osteogenic sarcoma[1]	Lederle
Methotrexate with laurocapram (*Methotrexate/Azone*)	Topical treatment of *Mycosis fungoides*	Durham Pharm
8-Methoxsalen (*Uvadex*)	In conjunction with the UVAR photopheresis to treat diffuse systemic sclerosis; prevention of acute rejection of cardiac allografts	Therakos, Inc.
Methylnaltrexone	Unresponsive chronic opioid-induced constipation	Univ. of Chicago
Metronidazole (*Flagyl*) (*Metrogel*)	Perioral dermatitis; grade III and IV, anaerobically infected, decubitus ulcers; acne rosacea[1]	Galderma Searle
Microbubble contrast agent (*Filmix Neurosonographic Contrast Agent*)	Intraoperative aid in the identification and localization of intracranial tumors	Cav-Con
Midodrine HCl (*Amatine*)	Symptomatic orthostatic hypotension	Roberts
Mitoguazone (*Zyrkamine*)	Diffuse non-Hodgkin's lymphoma including AIDS-related diffuse non-Hodgkin's lymphoma	ILEX Oncology
Mitolactol	Adjuvant therapy in the treatment of primary brain tumors	Biopharmaceutics
Mitomycin-C	Refractory glaucoma as an adjunct to ab externo glaucoma surgery	IOP Inc
Mitoxantrone HCl (*Novantrone*)	Hormone refractory prostate cancer[1]; acute myelogenous leukemia (acute nonlymphocytic leukemia)[1]	Immunex Lederle

ORPHAN DRUGS

Drug (*Trade name*)	Proposed use	Sponsor
Modafinil (*Provigil*)	Excessive daytime sleepiness in narcolepsy	Cephalon
Monoclonal antibodies PM-81 and AML-2-23	Exogenous depletion of CD14 and CD15 positive acute myeloid leukemic bone marrow cells from patients undergoing bone marrow transplantation	Medarex
Monoclonal antibody-B43.13 (*Ovarex Mab-B43.13*)	Epithelial ovarian cancer	AltaRex
Monoclonal antibody for immunization against lupus nephritis	Lupus nephritis	Medclone
Monoclonal antibody PM-81	Adjunctive treatment of acute myelogenous leukemia	Medarex
5A8, Monoclonal antibody to CD4	Post-exposure prophylaxis for occupational exposure to HIV	Biogen
Monoclonal antibody to cytomegalovirus (human)	Prophylaxis of cytomegalovirus disease in solid organ transplants; cytomegalovirus retinitis in AIDS	Protein Design Labs
Monoclonal antibody to hepatitis B virus (human)	Prophylaxis of hepatitis B reinfection in liver transplantation secondary to end-stage chronic hepatitis B infection	Protein Design Labs
Monolaurin (*Glylorin*)	Congenital primary ichthyosis	Cellegy Pharm
Monooctanoin (*Moctanin*)	Dissolution of cholesterol gallstones retained in the common bile duct[1]	Ethitek
Morphine sulfate concentrate (preservative free) (*Infumorph*)	For use in microinfusion devices for intraspinal administration for intractable chronic pain[1]	Elkins-Sinn
Mucoid exopolysaccharide pseudomonas hyperimmune globulin (*MEPIG*)	Prevent/treat pulmonary infections due to *Pseudomonas aeruginosa* in cystic fibrosis	North American Biologicals
Multi-vitamin infusion (neonatal formula)	Establish/maintain total parenteral nutrition in very low birth weight infants	Astra
Mycobacterium avium sensitin RS-10	For use in diagnosis of invasive *Mycobacterium avium* disease in immunocompetent individuals	Statens Seruminstitut
Myelin	Multiple sclerosis	AutoImmune
N-acetyl-procainamide	Prevent life-threatening ventricular arrhythmias in documented procainamide-induced lupus	NAPA of the Bahamas
Nafarelin acetate (*Synarel Nasal Solution*)	Central precocious puberty	Syntex (USA)
Naltrexone HCl (*Trexan*)	Blockade effects of exogenous opioids as an adjunct to maintain opioid-free state in detoxified formerly opioid-dependent individuals	Du Pont Pharm
Nebacumab (*Centoxin*)	Gram-negative bacteremia that has progressed to endotoxin shock	Centocor
Neurotrophin-1	Motor neuron disease/amyotrophic lateral sclerosis	Arthur Dale Ericsson, MD
NG-29 (*Somatrel*)	Diagnostic measure of the capacity of the pituitary gland to release growth hormone	Ferring Labs

ORPHAN DRUGS

Drug (*Trade name*)	Proposed use	Sponsor
Nifedipine	Interstitial cystitis	Jonathan Fleischmann, MD
Nitazoxanide	Immunocompromised patients with cryptosporidiosis	Unimed Pharm
Nitric oxide	Persistent pulmonary hypertension in the newborn; acute respiratory distress syndrome in adults	Ohmeda
9-Nitro-20-(S)-camptothecin (9-NC)	Pancreatic cancer	Stehlin Foundation
NTBC	Tyrosinemia type 1	Swedish Orphan Ab
N-trifuoroacetyladriamycin-14-valerate	Carcinoma in situ of of the urinary bladder	Anthra Pharm
Ofloxacin (*Ocuflox Ophthalmic Solution*)	Bacterial corneal ulcers	Allergan, Inc
OM 401 (*Drepanol*)	Prophylactic treatment of sickle cell disease	Omex International
Omega-3 (n-3) polyunsaturated fatty acid with all double bonds in the cis configuration	Prevent organ graft rejection	Research Triangle
OncoRad Ov103	Ovarian cancer	Cytogen
Orgotein for Injection	Familial amyotropic lateral sclerosis associated with a mutation of the gene (chromosome 21q) for copper, zinc superoxide dismutase	Oxis
Oxaliplatin	Ovarian cancer	Debio Pharm SA
Oxandrolone (*Hepandrin*) (*Oxandrin*)	Short stature associated with Turner's syndrome; constitutional delay of growth and puberty; adjunctive therapy for AIDS patients with HIV-wasting syndrome; moderate/severe acute alcoholic hepatitis and moderate protein calorie malnutrition	Bio-Technology
Oxymorphone HCl (*Numorphan HP*)	Relief of severe intractable pain in narcotic-tolerant patients	Du Pont Merck
Paclitaxel (*Taxol*)	AIDS-related Kaposi's sarcoma	Bristol-Myers Squibb
Patul-end	Patulous eustachian tube	Ear Foundation
Pegademase bovine (*Adagen*)	Enzyme replacement in ADA deficiency in patients with severe combined immunodeficiency [1]	Enzon
Pegaspargase (*Oncaspar*)	Acute lymphocytic leukemia[1]	Enzon
PEG-glucocerebrosidase (*Lysodase*)	Chronic enzyme replacement therapy in Gaucher's disease patients who are deficient in glucocerebrosidase	Enzon
PEG-interleukin-2	Primary immunodeficiencies associated with T-cell defects	Chiron
Pentamidine isethionate (*NebuPent*) (*Pentam 300*)	Treatment of *Pneumocystis carinii* pneumonia (PCP)[1]; PCP prevention in high-risk patients[1]	Fujisawa Rhone-Poulenc Rorer
Pentamidine isethionate (inhalation) (*Pneumopent*)	PCP prevention in high-risk patients	Fisons

ORPHAN DRUGS

Drug (*Trade name*)	Proposed use	Sponsor
Pentastarch (*Pentaspan*)	Adjunct in leukapheresis to improve the harvesting and increase the yield of leukocytes by centrifugal means[1]	Du Pont
Pentosan polysulphate sodium (*Elmiron*)	Interstitial cystitis	Baker Norton
Pentostatin Pentostatin injection (*Nipent*)	Chronic lymphocytic leukemia; hairy-cell leukemia[1]	Warner-Lambert
Phenylalanine ammonia-lyase (*Phenylase*)	Hyperphenylalaninemia	Ibex
Phosphocysteamine	Cystinosis	Medea Research
Physostigmine salicylate (*Antilirium*)	Friedreich's and other inherited ataxias	Forest
Pilocarpine HCl (*Salagen*)	Xerostomia induced by radiation therapy for head and neck cancer[1]; xerostomia and keratoconjunctivitis sicca in Sjogren's syndrome	MGI Pharma
Piracetum (*Nootropil*)	Myoclonus	UCB Pharm
Polifeprosan 20 with carmustine (*Gliadel*)	Malignant glioma	Guilford
Poloxamer 188 (*RheothRx Copolymer*)	Sickle cell crisis; severe burns requiring hospitalization	CytRx Corp
Poloxamer 331 (*Protox*)	Initial therapy of toxoplasmosis in AIDS patients	CytRx Corp
Poly-ICLC	Primary brain tumors	Andres Salazar, MD and Hilton Levy, PhD
Poly I: Poly C12U (*Ampligen*)	AIDS; renal cell carcinoma; chronic fatigue syndrome; invasive metastatic melanoma (stage IIB, III, IV)	HemispheRx Biopharma
Polymeric oxygen	Sickle cell anemia	Capmed USA
Porcine fetal neural dopaminergic cells or precursors (*NeuroCell-PD*)	Hoehn and Yahr stage 4 and 5 Parkinson's disease (prepared and coated with anti-MHC-1 Ab for intracerebral implantation)	Diacrin
Porcine fetal neural dopaminergic cells or precursors (*NeuroCell-PD*)	Hoehn and Yahr stage 4 and 5 Parkinson's disease (prepared for intracerebral implantation)	Diacrin
Porcine fetal neural gabaergic cells or precursors (*NeuroCell-HD*)	Huntington's disease (prepared and coated with anti-MHC-1 Ab for intracerebral implantation)	Diacrin
Porcine fetal neural gabaergic cells or precursors (*NeuroCell-HD*)	Huntington's disease (prepared for intracerebral implantation)	Diacrin
Porfimer sodium (*Photofrin*)	Photodynamic therapy of patients with primary or recurrent obstructing (either partially or completely) esophageal carcinoma and patients with transitional cell carcinoma in situ of urinary bladder	QLT Phototherapeutics
Porfiromycin (*Promycin*)	Head, neck and cervical cancer	OncoRx Vion Pharm

ORPHAN DRUGS

Drug (*Trade name*)	Proposed use	Sponsor
Potassium citrate (*Urocit-K*)	Prevention of uric acid nephrolithiasis[1]; prevention of calcium renal stones in patients with hypocitraturia[1]; avoidance of the complication of calcium stone formation in uric lithiasis[1]	Univ. of Texas Health Sciences
Prednimustine (*Sterecyt*)	Malignant non-Hodgkin's lymphomas	Pharmacia & Upjohn
Primaquine phosphate	With clindamycin HCl in the treatment of *Pneumocystis carinii* pneumonia associated with AIDS	Sanofi Winthrop
Progesterone	Establishment and maintenance of pregnancy in women undergoing in vitro fertilization or embryo transfer procedures	Watson Labs
Propamidine isethionate 0.1% ophthalmic solution (*Brolene*)	Acanthamoeba keratitis	Bausch & Lomb
Prostaglandin E1 in lipid emulsion	Ischemic ulceration of the lower limbs due to peripheral arterial disease	Alpha Ther
Protein C concentrate (*Protein C Concentrate [human] Vapor Heated, Immuno*)	For replacement therapy in patients with congenital or acquired protein C deficiency for the prevention/treatment of: Warfarin-induced skin necrosis during oral anticoagulation, thrombosis, pulmonary emboli and purpura fulminans; prevention/treatment of purpura fulminans in meningococcemia	Immuno
Protirelin	Prevention of infant respiratory distress syndrome associated with prematurity	UCB Pharm
Pulmonary surfactant replacement, porcine (*Curosurf*)	Prevention/treatment of respiratory distress syndrome in premature infants	Dey Labs
Purified type II collagen (*Colloral*)	Juvenile rheumatoid arthritis	AutoImmune
9-[3-pyridylmethyl]-9-deazaguanine	Cutaneous T-cell lymphoma	BioCryst Pharm
R-II Retinamide	Myelodysplastic syndromes	Sparta
R-VIII SQ (*Refacto*)	Long-term or hospital treatment of hemophilia A; hemophilia A in connection with surgical procedures	Pharmacia & Upjohn
Recombinant human CD4 immunoglobulin G	AIDS resulting from infection with HIV-1	Genentech
Recombinant human gelsolin	Respiratory symptoms of cystic fibrosis; acute and chronic respiratory symptoms of bronchiectasis	Biogen
Recombinant human insulin-like growth factor-I	Post-poliomyelitis syndrome	Cephalon
Recombinant human interleukin-11 (*Neumega rhIL-11 Growth Factor*)	Prevent severe chemotherapy-induced thrombocytopenia	Genetics
Recombinant human luteinizing hormone	With recombinant human follicle stimulating hormone for women with chronic anovulation due to hypogonadotropic hypogonadism	Serono

ORPHAN DRUGS

Drug (*Trade name*)	Proposed use	Sponsor
Recombinant human relaxin	Progressive systemic sclerosis	Connective Therapeutics
Recombinant human superoxide dismutase	Prevent bronchopulmonary dysplasia in premature neonates weighing < 1500 grams	Bio-Technology General
Recombinant methionyl brain-derived neurotrophic factor	Amyotrophic lateral sclerosis	Amgen
Recombinant methionyl human stem cell factor	With filgrastim to decrease the number of phereses required to collect peripheral blood progenitor cells capable of providing rapid multilineage hematopoietic reconstitution following myelosuppressive or myeloablative therapy; primary bone marrow failure	Amgen
Recombinant retroviral vector-glucocerebrosidase	Enzyme replacement therapy for types I, II or III Gaucher disease	Genetic
Recombinant secretory leucocyte protease inhibitor	Congenital alpha-1 antitrypsin deficiency; cystic fibrosis	Amgen
Recombinant soluble human CD4 (rCD4)	AIDS	Genentech
Recombinant vaccinia (human papillomavirus) (*TA-HPV*)	Cervical cancer	Cantab Pharm
Reduced L-glutathione (*Cachexon*)	AIDS-associated cachexia	Telluride
Respiratory syncytial virus immune globulin (human) (*Hypermune RSV*) (*Respigam*)	Treatment of respiratory syncytial virus lower respiratory tract infections in hospitalized infants and young children; prophylaxis of RSV lower respiratory tract infections in infants and young children at high risk of RSV disease	MedImmune
RGG0853, E1A lipid complex	Advanced ovarian cancer that overexpresses the HER/neu oncogene	Targeted Genetics
Rho (D) immune globulin intravenous (human) (*WinRho SD*)	Immune thrombocytopenic purpura[1]	Rh Pharmaceuticals
Ribavirin (*Virazole*)	Hemorrhagic fever with renal syndrome	ICN
Ricin (blocked) conjugated murine MCA (anti-B4)	B-cell leukemia and B-cell lymphoma; ex vivo purging of leukemic cells from bone marrow of non-T-cell ALL patients in complete remission	ImmunoGen
Ricin (blocked) conjugated murine MCA (anti-MY9)	Myeloid leukemia, including AML, and blast crisis of CML; ex vivo treatment of autologous bone marrow and subsequent reinfusion in acute myelogenous leukemia	ImmunoGen
Ricin (blocked) conjugated murine MCA (N901)	Small-cell lung cancer	ImmunoGen
Ricin (blocked) conjugated murine monoclonal antibody (CD6)	Cutaneous T-cell lymphomas, acute T-cell leukemia-lymphoma and related mature T-cell malignancies	ImmunoGen

ORPHAN DRUGS

Drug (*Trade name*)	Proposed use	Sponsor
Rifabutin (*Mycobutin*)	Treatment of disseminated *Mycobacterium avium* complex disease; prevention of disseminated MAC disease in advanced HIV infection[1]	Adria Pharmacia & Upjohn
Rifampin (*Rifadin IV*)	Antituberculosis treatment when oral doseform is not feasible[1]	Marion Merrell Dow
Rifampin, isoniazid, pyrazinamide (*Rifater*)	Short course treatment of tuberculosis[1]	Marion Merrell Dow
Rifapentin	Pulmonary tuberculosis; treatment of *mycobacterium avium* complex in patients with AIDS; prophylaxis of MAC in patients with AIDS and a CD4+ count ≤ 75/mm^3	Marion Merrell Dow
Riluzole (*Rilutek*)	Amyotrophic lateral sclerosis; Huntington's disease	Rhone-Poulenc Rorer
Roquinimex (*Linomide*)	Prolongs time to relapse in leukemia patients who have undergone autologous bone marrow transplantation	Pharmacia & Upjohn
Sacrosidase (*Sucraid*)	Congenital sucrase-isomaltase deficiency	Orphan Medical
Sargramostim (*Leukine*)	Neutropenia associated with bone marrow transplant, graft failure and delay of engraftment, and for promotion of early engraftment[1]; reduce neutropenia and leukopenia and decrease the incidence of death due to infection in patients with acute myelogenous leukemia[1]	Immunex
Satumomab pendetide (*Oncosinct CR/OV*)	Detection of ovarian carcinoma[1]	Cytogen
Secalciferol (*Osteo-D*)	Familial hypophosphatemic rickets	Lemmon
Secretory leukocyte protease inhibitor	Bronchopulmonary dysplasia	Synergen
Selegiline HCl (*Eldepryl*)	Adjuvant to levodopa/carbidopa in idiopathic Parkinson's disease (paralysis agitans), postencephalitic parkinsonism and symptomatic parkinsonism[1]	Somerset
Sermorelin acetate (*Geref*)	Idiopathic or organic growth hormone deficiency in children with growth failure; adjunct to gonadotropin in ovulation induction in anovulatory or oligo-ovulatory infertility after failure of clomiphene citrate or gonadotropin alone; AIDS-associated catabolism/weight loss	Serono
Serratia marcescens extract (polyribosomes) (*Imuvert*)	Primary brain malignancies	Cell Technology
Short chain fatty acid solution	Active phase of ulcerative colitis with involvement restricted to the left side of the colon	Orphan Medical

ORPHAN DRUGS

Drug (*Trade name*)	Proposed use	Sponsor
Sodium benzoate/sodium phenylacetate	Treatment of urea cycle disorders: Carbamylphosphate synthetase deficiency, ornithine transcarbamylase deficiency and argininosuccinic acid synthetase deficiency	Saul W. Brusilow, MD
Sodium dichloroacetate	Congenital lactic acidosis; lactic acidosis in severe malaria; homozygous familial hypercholesterolemia	Peter Stacpoole, PhD, MD
Sodium monomercaptoundecahydro-closo-dodecaborate (*Borocell*)	For use in boron neutron capture therapy (BNCT) in glioblastoma multiforme	Neutron Technology
Sodium phenylbutyrate (*Buphenyl*)	Sickling disorders including S-S, S-C and S-thalassemia hemiglobinopathy; urea cycle disorders: Carbamylphosphate synthetase deficiency, ornithine transcarbamylase deficiency and arginiosuccinic acid synthetase deficiency	Saul W. Brusilow, MD Ucyclyd Pharma
Sodium tetradecyl sulfate (*Sotradecol*)	Bleeding esophageal varices	Elkins-Sinn
Soluble recombinant human complement receptor type 1	Prevention/reduction of adult respiratory distress syndrome	T Cell Sciences
Somatostatin (*Zecnil*)	Adjunct to non-operative management of secreting cutaneous fistulas of the stomach, duodenum, small intestine (jejunum and ileum) or pancreas; bleeding esophogeal varices	Ferring UCB Pharm
Somatrem for injection (*Protropin*)	Long-term treatment of children with growth failure due to lack of adequate endogenous growth hormone secretion; short stature associated with Turner's syndrome	Genentech
Somatropin (*Genotropin/Genotonorm*) (*Humatrope*) (*Norditropin*) (*Nutropin*) (*Saizen*)	Long term treatment of children with growth failure due to lack of adequate endogenous growth hormone secretion[1]; growth failure in children with inadequate growth hormone secretion; idiopathic or organic growth hormone deficiency in children with growth failure; enhancement of nitrogen retention in hospitalized patients with severe burns; short stature in Turner's syndrome; adults with growth hormone deficiency	Eli Lilly Genentech Novo Nordisk Pharmacia & Upjohn Serono
Somatropin for injection (*Humatrope*) (*Nutropin*) (*Serostim*)	Long term treatment of children with growth failure due to inadequate secretion of normal endogenous growth hormone; short stature in Turner's syndrome[1]; growth retardation in chronic renal failure; catabolism/weight loss in AIDS; children with AIDS-associated failure to thrive including AIDS-associated wasting; replacement therapy for growth hormone deficiency in adults after epiphyseal closure	Eli Lilly Genentech Serono
Sotalol HCl (*Betapace*)	Treatment[1]/prevention of life-threatening ventricular tachyarrhythmias	Berlex

ORPHAN DRUGS

Drug (*Trade name*)	Proposed use	Sponsor
ST1-RTA immunotoxin (SR 44163)	Prevention of acute graft-vs-host disease in allogenic bone marrow transplantation; treatment of B-chronic lymphocytic leukemia	Sanofi Winthrop
SU-101	Malignant glioma; ovarian cancer	Sugen, Inc
Succimer (*Chemet*)	Lead poisoning in children[1]; prevention of cystine kidney stones in patients with homozygous cystinuria who are prone to stone development; mercury intoxication	Bock Pharmacal Sanofi Winthrop
Sucralfate	Oral mucositis and stomatitis following radiation for head and neck cancer	Fuisz Technologies
Sucralfate suspension	Oral complications of chemotherapy in bone marrow transplants; oral ulcerations and dysphagia in epidermolysis bullosa	Darby Pharm
Sulfadiazine	With pyrimethamine for *Toxoplasma gondii* encephalitis in patients with and without AIDS[1]	Eon Labs
Sulfapyridine	Dermatitis herpetiformis	Jacobus
Superoxide dismutase (human)	Protection of donor organ tissue from damage or injury mediated by oxygen-derived free radicals that are generated during the necessary periods of ischemia (hypoxia, anoxia) and especially reperfusion associated with the operative procedure	Pharmacia-Chiron Partnership
Superoxide dismutase (recombinant human)	Prevention of reperfusion injury to donor organ tissue	Bio-Technology
Surface active extract of saline lavage of bovine lungs (*Infasurf*)	Prevent/treat respiratory failure due to pulmonary surfactant deficiency in preterm infants	ONY
Synsorb PK	Verocytotoxogenic *E. coli* infections	Synsorb Biotech
T4 endonuclease V, liposome encapsulated	Prevent cutaneous neoplasms and other skin abnormalities in xeroderma pigmentosum	Applied Genetics
Technetium TC-99M anti-melanoma murine monoclonal antibody (*Oncotrac Melanoma Imaging Kit*)	Detecting, by imaging, metastases of malignant melanoma	NeoRx
Technetium TC-99M murine monoclonal antibody (IgG2a) to B cell (*LymphoScan*)	Diagnostic imaging in evaluating the extent of disease in patients with histologically confirmed diagnosis of non-Hodgkin's B-cell lymphoma, acute B-cell lymphoblastic leukemia (in children and adults) and chronic B-cell lymphocytic leukemia	Immunomedics
Technetium Tc-99M murine monoclonal antibody to hCG (*Immuraid, hCG-Tc-99m*)	Detection of hCG-producing tumors such as germ-cell and trophoblastic cell tumors	Immunomedics
Technetium Tc-99M murine monoclonal antibody to human AFP (*Immuraid, AFP-Tc-99m*)	Detection of hepatocellular carcinoma and hepatoblastoma; detection of alpha-fetoprotein producing germ-cell tumors	Immunomedics
Teniposide (*Vumon Injection*)	Refractory childhood acute lymphocytic leukemia[1]	Bristol-Myers Squibb

ORPHAN DRUGS

Drug (*Trade name*)	Proposed use	Sponsor
Teriparatide (*Parathar*)	Diagnostic agent for patients with clinical and laboratory evidence of hypocalcemia due to hypoparathyroidism or pseudohypoparathyroidism[1]	Rhone-Poulenc Rorer
Terlipressin (*Glypressin*)	Bleeding esophageal varices	Ferring
Testosterone (*Androgel*)	Weight loss in AIDS patients with HIV-associated wasting	Unimed
Testosterone propionate ointment 2%	Vulvar dystrophies	Star
Testosterone sublingual	Constitutional delay of growth and puberty in boys	Bio-Technology
Thalidomide (*Synovir*)	Prevent/treat graft-vs-host disease in bone marrow transplantation; treatment/maintenance of reactional lepromatous leprosy; prevent/treat graft-vs-host disease; clinical manifestations of mycobacterial infection caused by *Mycobacterium tuberculosis* and non-tuberculous mycobacteria; severe recurrent aphthous stomatitis and treatment and prevention of recurrent aphthous ulcers in severely, terminally immunocompromised patients; erythema nodosum leprosum; HIV-associated wasting syndrome	Andrulis Celgene Corp Pediatric Pharm
Thymosin alpha-1	Chronic active hepatitis B	SciClone
Tiopronin (*Thiola*)	Prevention of cystine nephrolithiasis in patients with homozygous cystinuria[1]	Charles Y.C. Pak, MD
Tiratricol (*Triacana*)	With levothyroxine to suppress thyroid stimulating hormone in patients with well differentiated thyroid cancer intolerant of adequate doses of levothyroxine alone	Marcofina Labs
Tizanidine HCl (*Zanaflex*)	Spasticity associated with multiple sclerosis and spinal cord injury	Athena
Tobramycin for inhalation	Bronchopulmonary infections of *Pseudomonas aeruginosa* in cystic fibrosis patients	Pathogenesis Corp.
Topiramate (*Topamax*)	Lennox-Gastaut syndrome	R. W. Johnson
Toremifene	Hormonal therapy of metastatic breast carcinoma; desmoid tumors	Orion
Transforming growth factor-beta 2	Full thickness macular holes	Celtrix
Treosulfan (*Ovastat*)	Ovarian cancer	Medac GmbH
Tretinoin (*Atragen*) (*Vesanoid*)	Squamous metaplasia of the ocular surface epithelia (conjunctiva or cornea) with mucous deficiency and keratinization; acute promyelocytic leukemia[1]; acute and chronic leukemia	Aronex Hannan Ophthalmic Hoffman-La Roche
Trientine HCl (*Cuprid*)	Wilson's disease intolerant or inadequately responsive to penicillamine[1]	Merck

ORPHAN DRUGS

Drug (*Trade name*)	Proposed use	Sponsor
Trimetrexate glucuronate (*Neutrexin*)	Metastatic carcinoma of head and neck (buccal cavity, pharynx, larynx); metastatic colorectal adenocarcinoma; pancreatic adenocarcinoma; *Pneumocytosis carinii* pneumonia (PCP) in AIDS[1]; advanced non-small cell carcinoma of the lung	US Bioscience
Trisaccharides A and B (*Biosynject*)	Moderate to severe hemolytic disease in newborns arising from placental transfer of antibodies against blood groups A and B; ABO-incompatible solid organ transplantation including kidney, heart, liver and pancreas; prevent ABO hemolytic reactions arising from ABO-incompatible bone marrow transplantation	Chembiomed
Trisodium citrate concentration (*Hemocitrate*)	For use in leukapheresis procedures	Hemotec Medical
Troleandomycin	Severe steroid-requiring asthma	Stanley M Szefler, MD
Tumor necrosis factor-binding protein I and II	Symptomatic patients with AIDS including CD4 counts < 200 cells/mm^3	Serono
Tyloxapol	Cystic fibrosis	Kennedy & Hoidal, MDs
Uridine 5′-triphosphate	Cystic fibrosis; facilitate removal of lung secretions in patients with primary ciliary dyskinesia	Inspire Pharm
Urofollitropin (*Metrodin*)	Ovulation induction in patients with polycystic ovarian disease who have an elevated LH/FSH ratio and who have failed to respond to adequate clomiphene citrate therapy[1]	Serono
Urogastrone	Acceleration of corneal epithelial regeneration and healing of stromal incisions from corneal transplant surgery	Chiron Vision
Ursodiol (*Actigall*) (*URSO*)	Treatment of primary biliary cirrhosis; management of clinical signs and symptoms associated with primary biliary cirrhosis	Axcan Pharma Ciba-Geigy
Valine, isoleucine and leucine (*VIL*)	Hyperphenylalaninemia	Leas Research
Vasoactive intestinal polypeptide	Acute esophageal food impaction	Research Triangle
Zalcitabine (*Hivid*)	AIDS[1]	National Cancer Inst Hoffman-La Roche
Zidovudine (*Retrovir*)	AIDS and AIDS-related complex[1]	Glaxo Wellcome
Zinc acetate (*Galzin*)	Wilson's disease	Lemmon

[1] Approved for marketing.

PHENFORMIN – Available under IND exemption.

The biguanide hypoglycemic agent, phenformin, was removed from the US market on October 23, 1977, as a result of concern over the unacceptably high risk of lactic acidosis associated with its use. Phenformin is now available only through an Investigational New Drug (IND) Application which must be filed with the US Food and Drug Administration. Use of phenformin is restricted to specific clearly defined situations and requires registration and reporting to the FDA. Complete information on use of phenformin, physician sponsor applications, patient consent forms and request forms for ordering phenformin tablets or capsules are available from:

Center for Drug Evaluation and Research
Division of Metabolism and Endocrine
Drug Products (HFD-510)
Room 14B03
5600 Fishers Lane
Rockville, Maryland 20857
301-443-3510

Indications: May be used only in adult-onset, nonketotic diabetics who meet all of the following criteria: In addition to elevated blood glucose, have symptoms such as polydipsia; symptoms are not controlled with diet and sulfonylureas or cannot take sulfonylureas because of nontolerance or allergy; symptoms are controlled by phenformin; no underlying risk factors which contraindicate the use; (a) occupation is such that the risk of hypoglycemia from insulin would threaten their jobs or be a hazard to them or others, or (b) cannot take insulin because of disability and have no practical way to receive assistance.

Phenformin is also available under a separate IND for a dermatological condition called atrophie blanche or livedo vasculitis.

Contraindications: Although there is no absolute way to predict the population at risk for lactic acidosis, the following are recognized contraindications: Insulin-dependent diabetes; hypersensitivity to phenformin; renal disease with even mild degrees of impaired renal function; liver disease; history of lactic acidosis; alcohol abuse; any acute medical situation such as cardiovascular collapse (shock), congestive heart failure, myocardial infarction, surgery or septicemia; disease states that may be associated with hypoxemia; complications of diabetes such as metabolic acidosis, coma, infection or gangrene; acute gastrointestinal disturbances (vomiting or diarrhea) which are likely to result in dehydration and prerenal azotemia.

Lactic acidosis in patients taking phenformin has been estimated to occur in 0.25 to 4 cases per 1000 phenformin treatment years. Lactic acidosis is characterized by elevated lactate levels, increased lactate-to-pyruvate ratio and decreased blood pH. In many of the reported cases, azotemia ranging from mild to severe was present.

Nausea, vomiting, hyperventilation, malaise or abdominal pain may herald the onset of lactic acidosis. Instruct the patient to discontinue phenformin and notify the physician immediately if any of these symptoms occur.

Warn patients against using alcohol while receiving phenformin, since ethanol and phenformin potentiate the tendency of each to cause elevated blood lactate levels.

Conclusions: Although phenformin has been removed from the market because of the potential for adverse effects, a select group of patients may require use of this agent. Careful patient selection is necessary to assure a reasonable risk-benefit ratio. Supplies of phenformin are available to practicing physicians from the FDA under an IND exemption.

Bibliography Available on Request

KETOTIFEN (*Zaditen* by Sandoz) – An antiasthmatic agent.

Pharmacology: Asthma is a chronic respiratory disease characterized by episodes of reversible airway obstruction due to bronchospasms. Although a variety of effective agents are available for the prophylaxis and treatment of asthmatic conditions, both the incidence of side effects and inconvenience of administration by inhalation encourage the search for new modes of therapy. Ketotifen is an orally active agent with significant antihistamine and antianaphylactic properties which may prove useful in asthma prophylaxis.

The factors responsible for intrinsic asthma are poorly understood. Extrinsic allergic asthma results from a series of events triggered by an allergen (antigen) which activates the release of chemical mediators of bronchoconstriction (histamine and the slow-reacting substance of anaphylaxis) from sensitized mast cells. Bronchodilators (beta-adrenergic agonists or theophylline) counteract these bronchoconstrictor effects. Antihistamines are somewhat useful in blocking the effects of histamine. The introduction of cromolyn sodium was the advent of a true prophylactic measure for allergic asthma. Although not effective during an acute asthma episode, chronic therapy with cromolyn stabilizes the mast cell membrane and inhibits the release of histamine and slow-reacting substance of anaphylaxis.

Ketotifen appears to act by the same pharmacological mechanism as cromolyn; however, it has the advantage of being active on oral administration. Ketotifen is a benzocycloheptathiophene derivative with antihistaminic and antianaphylactic activity. It is well absorbed orally; effects are sustained for up to 12 hours. As with cromolyn, the onset of its prophylactic activity is slow; 4 to 6 weeks are required to achieve full prophylactic value. Therapeutic serum levels range between 1 and 4 mcg/ml.

Clinical studies: Ketotifen, 1 mg orally, twice daily was found to be equivalent to 20 mg sodium cromolyn 4 times daily (via spinhaler). No statistically significant differences were demonstrated between the two drugs for daily peak respiratory flow rates and spirometry during the 3 months that each drug was administered to 35 skin test positive (allergic) asthmatic adults. Ketotifen prevented histamine-induced bronchoconstriction in 24 patients with mild to moderate extrinsic (allergic) asthma. Histamine challenge was used to evaluate bronchial reactivity following 1 week of treatment with theophylline and salbutamol spray. Ketotifen, 1 mg twice daily, was then added to the regimen. Patients were rechallenged with histamine after 4, 8 and 12 weeks of ketotifen therapy. Decrease in bronchial reactivity to histamine was noted at 4 weeks and maintained for 12 weeks.

In a double-blind study of 50 patients with allergic asthma, ketotifen, 1 or 2 mg twice daily, was added to existing inhalation therapy of salbutamol or corticosteroid. Ketotifen, 2 mg twice daily, slightly decreased the number of puffs per week of salbutamol and improved breathing. No improvement was noted in patients using inhaled corticosteroids. Ketotifen, 1 mg twice daily, failed to provide prophylaxis in adults with intrinsic (nonallergic) asthma; however, there was no deterioration of the condition.

In a double-blind study in 23 children with asthma, 0.5 to 0.94 mg/kg ketotifen failed to provide protection against bronchoconstriction. Ketotifen 1 mg twice daily for 3 days was compared to cromolyn 20 mg administered 15 minutes prior to exercise. Ketotifen was ineffective in preventing exercise-induced bronchospasm, while cromolyn was effective.

Side effects: The most frequently reported side effects, sedation and drowsiness, may require dosage reduction or discontinuation if the severity does not decrease with continued therapy. Alcohol may potentiate these adverse reactions. Weight gain, dry mouth, headache, dizziness and giddiness have also been reported. In addition, symptoms of overdosage have included: Mild abdominal pain, confusion, hyperexcitability, bradycardia, tachycardia, dyspnea, tachypnea, cyanosis, convulsions and unconsciousness.

Summary: Ketotifen appears to be a potential alternative in the prophylaxis of asthma; however, it is unlikely to replace established drugs. Several weeks of administration are required to produce maximum prophylactic effects; additionally, it frequently produces marked drowsiness. Ketotifen is long-acting and offers the convenience of oral administration which may be useful in individuals who develop bronchospasms following inhalation of other products. Ketotifen is available in Britain and Europe; Sandoz filed a New Drug Application (NDA) in November 1982 which is pending, and plans to market the drug under the name *Zaditen*.

Bibliography Available on Request

DOMPERIDONE (*Motilium* by Janssen Pharmaceutica) – An antiemetic.

Pharmacology: Acute nausea and vomiting induced by cytotoxic chemotherapy are frequent and serious toxicities distressful to cancer patients. Symptoms can be so pronounced and refractory that they interfere with therapeutic measures and patient nutrition. Available antiemetics block the chemoreceptor trigger zone (CTZ) (neuroleptics), sedate the vomiting centers (antihistamines), block afferent impulses at the vomiting center (anticholinergics), act peripherally and in the CNS (metoclopramide), or by less defined central mechanisms (cannabinoids). These agents are effective in most patients; however, side effects (eg, drowsiness, dry mouth, hypotension, extrapyramidal effects) are limitations. Domperidone, an investigational antiemetic, appears to act with minimum adverse effects.

Domperidone is chemically unrelated to the butyrophenones, phenothiazines or metoclopramide; however, it shares pharmacological properties with these agents. In the medulla it produces a direct blocking effect of dopamine receptors in the CTZ. Like metoclopramide and haloperidol, domperidone is a peripheral dopamine antagonist; however, it contrasts in that it does not cross the blood-brain barrier and produce CNS effects. It selectively blocks peripheral dopamine receptors in the gastrointestinal wall, thus enhancing normal synchronized GI peristalsis and motility in the proximal portion of the GI tract; it may also counteract anticholinergic-induced relaxation of the lower esophageal sphincter (LES).

Pharmacokinetics: Peak plasma levels are achieved within 30 minutes following IM or oral administration and between 1 to 4 hours after rectal administration. Approximately 40% of a dose is rapidly distributed into peripheral compartments. It is metabolized in the liver and eliminated in the urine, primarily as conjugates. Less than 1% appears in the urine as unchanged drug. Excretion is almost complete within 4 days. The duration of activity is between 2 and 4 hours following IV administration.

Clinical trials: The effectiveness of domperidone in the treatment of nausea and vomiting associated with cytotoxic chemotherapy has been evaluated. Several double-blind studies were conducted in patients with Hodgkin's disease. Domperidone 16 mg IV was preferred and superior to placebo; it was effective and well tolerated, and decreased the duration of nausea and vomiting by greater than ⅓ when injected 1 hour before the start of cytostatic treatment. Domperidone, 1 to 40 mg IV daily, was administered with chemotherapy infusion in 172 patients. Vomiting induced by agents considered to be moderate emetics (eg, cyclophosphamide, 5–fluorouracil, vinblastine) was reduced; however, patients with emesis induced by doxorubicin or mechlorethamine did not respond as well. The higher dosages of domperidone did not achieve a proportionally augmented response rate. In another study, domperidone 4 mg IV produced excellent or good response in 72% of patients receiving varied chemotherapy; poor responses occurred in patients receiving dacarbazine. When domperidone 12 mg IV was compared to metoclopramide 10 mg IV, both drugs produced a good or excellent response in 70% of patients; however, metoclopramide had a higher incidence of side effects. Domperidone 1 mg/kg IV or metoclopramide 0.5 mg/kg IV was used to prevent chemotherapy-induced nausea and vomiting in children. In the random crossover trial, domperidone decreased nausea and vomiting to a significantly greater extent than metoclopramide.

Domperidone has been compared favorably to cimetidine in 20 gastric ulcer patients; it may also have value in treating symptoms of gastroesophageal reflux and postoperative- or bromocriptine-induced nausea and vomiting.

Side effects: Domperidone does not appear to produce significant side effects or toxicities. Doses of 40 mg IV or 100 mg orally have not been reported to produce CNS or cardiovascular side effects, only facial flushing, headache, slight somnolence and dry mouth. Unlike metoclopramide, domperidone does not cross the blood-brain barrier; therefore, the incidence of extrapyramidal or psychotropic effects should be low. Yet there have been isolated reports of idiosyncratic extrapyramidal reactions. Domperidone does not stimulate aldosterone secretion.

Summary: Domperidone selectively blocks peripheral dopamine receptors both in the GI wall and in the CTZ. Its major advantage appears to be the lack of significant side effects; it may be an effective alternative to available antiemetics, including metoclopramide. Domperidone, like other antiemetics, produces variable effects on cytotoxic chemotherapy-induced nausea and vomiting, depending on the agent administered. There is limited or no data available comparing domperidone to more standard antiemetic agents other than metoclopramide. Domperidone was developed in Belgium by Janssen Pharmaceutica; it is available in Europe. Clinical trials are still in progress in the US; a New Drug Application (NDA) was filed in 1985.

Bibliography Available on Request

CLOBAZAM (*Frisium* by Hoechst-Roussel) and NITRAZEPAM (*Mogadon* by Roche) — Two (more) investigational benzodiazepines.

Clobazam and nitrazepam are investigational benzodiazepine derivatives. The profile of these agents parallels those of approved benzodiazepines; subtle differences account for individual product distinction.

Clobazam is structurally and pharmacologically related to approved benzodiazepines. Antianxiety and anticonvulsant properties are similar to diazepam; the usual adult dose is 20 to 30 mg daily. Initially, clobazam is effective against all varieties of epilepsy; however, efficacy decreases within a few days to a few weekc in approximately one-third of patients. Success has also been demonstrated in cyclic exacerbations of epilepsy associated with menstruation. Clobazam is a weak hypnotic agent.

The pharmacokinetics are independent of dose and concentration. Oral clobazam is 87% absorbed. Concomitant administration with alcohol increases clobazam's bioavailability by 50%. Food may slow the rate, but does not alter total absorption. Absorption is not influenced by age or sex. Clobazam is 85% bound to human serum protein; peak serum concentrations occur 1 to 4 hours after ingestion. It is metabolized via dealkylation and hydroxylation to a pharmacologically active metabolite, N–desmethylclobazam, and several inactive metabolites. The mean half-life of the unchanged drug is 18 hours, and up to 77 hours for metabolites. Clobazam is 81% to 97% excreted in the urine; accumulation is expected in impaired renal function.

The most frequent (10% to 44%) side effects include: Drowsiness, hangover effects, dizziness, weakness and lightheadedness. Less frequent (5% to 10%) adverse reactions include: Weight gain, orthostatic hypotension, syncope, headache, dry mouth and incoordination.

Nitrazepam has been widely used for many years in Europe and Canada as a sedative/hypnotic in doses of 2.5 to 10 mg, and in the management of myoclonic seizures of childhood epilepsy. Its structure and clinical effects are also analogous to other benzodiazepines.

Nitrazepam is 80% bioavailable following oral administration. Absorption is rapid: 0.5 to 5 hours to peak concentration; concomitant administration with food decreases peak levels by 30%. Nitrazepam is lipophilic and is widely distributed in the body; 10% to 15% is found in the cerebrospinal fluid; 85% to 90% is plasma protein bound. It crosses the placenta and is found in breast milk (50% and about 50% to 100% of maternal plasma concentration, respectively). Metabolism is extensive and excretion is urinary, primarily as inactive metabolites; only 1% is excreted as the unchanged drug. The elimination half-life is approximately 30 hours.

The frequency of adverse reactions increases with age and dosage, and parallels those of other benzodiazepines. The most common include: Fatigue, dizziness, lightheadedness, drowsiness, lethargy, mental confusion, staggering, ataxia and falling. Nightmares, insomnia, agitation, rash, pruritus, headache and GI disturbances have also been reported. The hangover effect is also common and may be a function of nitrazepam's long half-life.

Summary: Nitrazepam and clobazam appear to be safe and effective agents with antianxiety, anticonvulsant and hypnotic properties. These agents have long elimination half-lives; this enhances the potential for drug accumulation and increases the potential for residual side effects. These agents are unlikely to replace established benzodiazepine derivatives; however, they may provide viable therapeutic alternatives.

Bibliography Available on Request

ISOXICAM (*Maxicam* by Warner-Lambert) – A nonsteroidal anti-inflammatory drug.

Pharmacology: Isoxicam, like piroxicam *(Feldene),* is a member of the oxicam class of drugs. It is about one–tenth as potent (on a weight basis) as piroxicam and has a long duration of action which permits once-daily dosing. Clinical studies show it to be as effective as or superior to other NSAIDs. Isoxicam is well tolerated; GI disturbance is the most common side effect.

Rheumatoid arthritis (RA) and degenerative joint disease (DJD) are common chronic rheumatic disorders which cause considerable human suffering and disability. The NSAIDs are first-line agents for pain relief in both disorders and for the reduction of inflammation in RA. Salicylates have long been established as analgesic anti-inflammatory drugs and are usually drugs of first choice. However, since therapeutic failure and side effects are frequent, newer agents are steadily being introduced as alternatives.

Isoxicam has potent and prolonged antipyretic, analgesic and anti-inflammatory activity. It inhibits the synthesis of prostaglandins which may contribute to the development of the cardinal signs/symptoms of inflammation. It is also a potent inhibitor of platelet aggregation. This effect likely underlies its potentiation of sodium warfarin's anticoagulant action (see below).

Pharmacokinetics: Isoxicam is well absorbed orally and generally reaches peak plasma concentration 4 to 8 hours after administration. Both its rate and extent of absorption increase when given with meals.

Isoxicam is 95% to 98% protein bound. It is extensively metabolized with only 1% to 2% of the dose appearing in the urine as unchanged drug. This suggests that the drug's dose need not be changed in patients with renal dysfunction. Isoxicam has a half-life of approximately 31 hours (range, 21 to 70 hours) which permits once-daily dosing. Because of its long half-life, steady-state levels occur after 1 to 2 weeks of daily administration. As a result, a continual increase in response is expected until steady state is achieved.

Clinical trials: In a placebo controlled multicenter study, isoxicam was superior to placebo for the treatment of patients with RA or DJD. Morning stiffness was reduced by more than 60% in the isoxicam group, compared to 19% for patients in the placebo group; 52% of patients in the placebo group withdrew from the study because of lack of treatment efficacy, compared to 18% withdrawal in the isoxicam group.

An aspirin (3.6 g/day) and placebo controlled study of isoxicam (200 mg/day) in the treatment of RA found isoxicam superior to aspirin and placebo. Patient withdrawal rates for insufficient efficacy were 17.1%, 31.1% and 58.5% for isoxicam, aspirin and placebo, respectively.

In comparative studies of isoxicam (200 mg/day) vs naproxen (750 mg/day) and ibuprofen (1200 mg/day) in patients with RA, no significant efficacy differences were observed. In similar studies involving patients with DJD, isoxicam (200 mg/day) was as effective as naproxen (750 mg/day) and indomethacin (150 mg/day) in relieving pain and improving articular function. Patients on isoxicam experienced significantly fewer adverse effects than those on indomethacin.

Side effects: Isoxicam has so far been well tolerated and has caused few problems other than gastrointestinal effects. Other less commonly reported adverse effects include headache, dizziness and tinnitus. A higher than anticipated rate of skin reactions has occurred in foreign countries where isoxicam is available.

Drug interactions: The use of aspirin with NSAIDs is not generally recommended because of aspirin-induced reductions of NSAID blood levels and a lack of therapeutic advantage with concomitant use. However, the use of aspirin with isoxicam does not appear to lower plasma isoxicam levels, but the combination increases GI blood loss. It remains to be determined whether an isoxicam-aspirin combination offers any therapeutic advantage. When used with sodium warfarin, isoxicam potentiates warfarin's anticoagulant effect. Monitor the prothrombin time in patients on both agents more frequently and adjust the sodium warfarin dosage if needed. No interaction occurs between cimetidine and isoxicam.

Summary: Isoxicam is a novel NSAID of the oxicam class. It appears to be as effective as or superior to aspirin and nonaspirin agents for the treatment of common rheumatic disorders. The ability to administer isoxicam once a day is an important advantage. Parke-Davis (Warner-Lambert) submitted an NDA for isoxicam in August 1983, to be marketed under the name *Maxicam.* The drug was withdrawn from the European market in October 1985 following reports of adverse skin reactions during which time the NDA was pending in the US. In 1987, Warner-Lambert asked the FDA to reactivate the NDA since the skin reactions were apparently due to a manufacturing byproduct.

Bibliography Available on Request

L-5-HYDROXYTRYPTOPHAN (L-5HTP)

Pharmacology: L-5HTP is available as an "orphan" drug for the treatment of post-anoxic intention myoclonus. Myoclonus is an uncommon neuromuscular movement disorder characterized by involuntary, irregular muscle contraction; it is associated with a variety of brain lesions. There is evidence that at least some of these disorders are related to brain neurotransmitter levels or function, specifically serotonin. L-5HTP is an aromatic amino acid, the immediate precursor of serotonin.

L-5HTP is administered with carbidopa (see individual monograph), a peripheral dopa-decarboxylase inhibitor that decreases the conversion of L-5HTP to serotonin in the extracerebral tissues. This permits the administration of lower doses of L-5HTP and reduces the peripheral GI side effects such as diarrhea and nausea.

Pharmacokinetics: When administered orally with carbidopa (which produces a 5 to 15 fold increase in plasma L-5HTP), the systemic availability of L-5HTP is 47% to 84%; peak plasma concentrations of L-5HTP are reached at 1 to 3 hours. The biological half-life of L-5HTP, after pretreatment with carbidopa, is 2 to 7 hours. The major metabolic pathway of L-5HTP is decarboxylation to serotonin by L-aromatic amino acid decarboxylase; the highest activity is in the kidney, liver and small intestine. However, carbidopa-decarboxylase inhibition is incomplete; this may account for the GI side effects.

Indications: L-5HTP in combination with carbidopa is effective in the therapy of post-anoxic intention myoclonus. In 41 patients, 65% experienced a 50% or more improvement. However, patients with intention myoclonus associated with head trauma and methyl bromide toxicity, progressive myoclonus epilepsy, essential myoclonus and palatal myoclonus also show improvement. In addition, L-5HTP has shown some success in treating depression and in migraine prophylaxis.

Contraindications: L-5HTP/carbidopa is contraindicated in patients with renal disease, peptic ulcer, platelet disorders, scleroderma and Parkinson's disease.

Drug interactions: Do not give **monoamine oxidase inhibitors** or **reserpine** concurrently with L-5HTP/carbidopa. Discontinue these drugs at least 2 weeks prior to initiating treatment with L-5HTP/carbidopa.

Discontinue **tricyclic antidepressants** with a major serotonin reuptake inhibition mechanism (ie, imipramine) prior to L-5HTP/carbidopa therapy. Also, avoid serotonin receptor antagonists like **methysergide** or **cyproheptadine**, which may reduce the therapeutic effects of L-5HTP/carbidopa.

Fenfluramine releases brain serotonin from serotonergic nerve terminals and may potentiate L-5HTP/carbidopa.

Precautions: L-5HTP/carbidopa with caution in patients with severe emotional or psychiatric disorders because of occasional mental side effects. Mental depression has improved in some patients.

Adverse reactions:

Most common (GI) – Anorexia, nausea, diarrhea and vomiting. These can usually be avoided or minimized by gradual increases of L-5HTP dosage; they rapidly disappear when the dose is reduced or discontinued. The diarrhea will respond to therapy with diphenoxylate; the other GI symptoms respond to treatment with prochlorperazine or trimethobenzamide. These side effects eventually disappear or diminish.

Other adverse effects include mental changes (ie, euphoria) which may progress to hypomania, restlessness, rapid speech, anxiety, insomnia, aggressiveness and agitation; mydriasis, lightheadedness, sleepiness, blurring of vision and bradycardia. Dyspnea, sometimes accompanied by hyperventilation and lightheadedness, is rare. L-5HTP/carbidopa might unmask subclinical scleroderma in patients with an abnormality in kynurenine metabolism.

Overdosage of L-5HTP/carbidopa can produce respiratory difficulties and hypotension.

Administration and dosage: Begin with 25 mg L-5HTP 4 times daily; increase by 100 mg/day every 3 to 5 days if there are no significant side effects. If significant GI side effects develop, reduce the rate of increase to every 1 to 2 weeks. A reduction in myoclonus is usually first observed at 600 to 1000 mg/day (with carbidopa); the usual optimal dose of L-5HTP is between 1000 and 2000 mg/day in 4 divided doses.

Summary: L-5HTP is available through a treatment IND under the FDA's orphan drug program from Bolar Pharmaceuticals, Inc., 130 Lincoln Street, Copiague, NY 11726; (516) 842-8383. The drug will be beneficial to a small number of patients; further research may elucidate additional uses as we increase our understanding of the brain's complex chemistry. Carbidopa may be obtained for use with L-5HTP by contacting Audrey A. Geist, MD, Professional Information, MSD, West Point, PA 19486; (215) 661-7300.

Bibliography Available on Request

VINDESINE SULFATE (*Eldisine* by Lilly) – An antineoplastic.

Pharmacology: Vindesine sulfate (Lilly 99094, NSC-245467, DAVA, desacetyl vinblastine amide sulfate) is a synthetic vinca alkaloid derived from vinblastine sulfate, but more closely resembling the activity of vincristine.

A large number of studies support its utility in a diverse group of cancer types. Major and dose-limiting toxicities include myelosuppression and neurotoxicity.

The mechanism of vindesine's anticancer action is probably like that of the other vinca alkaloids; it is cell-cycle specific and blocks mitosis with metaphase arrest. Vinca alkaloids bind specifically to cellular microtubules of the mitotic apparatus and disrupt their function. This leads to inability of the dividing cell to correctly segregate chromosomes and ultimately, to cell death.

Pharmacokinetics: Vindesine sulfate appears to have similar pharmacokinetics to vincristine and vinblastine. The triphasic clearance profile of IV vindesine is summarized below:

IV Vindesine Clearance		
Phase	Half-life (minutes)	Volume of distribution (liters)
Alpha (α)	3 ± 1	5 ± 2
Beta (β)	99 ± 45	58 ± 51
Gamma (γ)	1213 ± 493	598 ± 294

Elimination in the urine in the first 24 hours accounts for 13.2% of the total dose administered. The remainder is sequestered in the body or eliminated in the bile.

Clinical trials: Overall, vindesine demonstrates good activity in difficult-to-treat and refractory cancer types. Responses to vindesine in patients who have received vincristine or vinblastine therapy suggest a lack of cross-resistance between these agents. Doses have ranged from 3 to 4.5 mg/m² as an IV bolus every 1 to 2 weeks *or* 1 to 2 mg/m²/day for 2 to 10 days every 2 to 3 weeks. The results of clinical studies are summarized below:

Vindesine Clinical Studies				
	Number of patients treated	Response rate		
Cancer type		Range (%)	Average (%)	Complete No. of patients
Lung	234	17-43	30	10
Esophageal	76	17-55	43	0
Colorectal	33	6	6	1
Metastatic breast	120	0-28	18	0
Lymphoma	61	34-50	41	4
Leukemias	26	15-61	38	4
TOTAL	550	0-61	29	19

Side effects: Major dose-limiting toxicities include myelosuppression and neuropathy. The primary *hematologic* toxicity is leukopenia, which is reversible with dosage reduction or discontinuation. Anemia and thrombocytopenia occur, but are rarely severe. *Neurotoxicity* appears to be a function of cumulative dose. Patients with hepatic dysfunction and those over 60 years old may be at greater risk. Neurotoxic manifestations include peripheral paresthesia, decreased tendon reflexes, muscle weakness and myalgia, headache, parotid and jaw pain, constipation and paralytic ileus.

Other side effects – Nausea; vomiting; stomatitis; hoarseness; transient hepatic dysfunction; inappropriate antidiuretic hormone secretion; fever; skin rash; alopecia; local cellulitis. Vindesine sulfate is a potent vesicant; avoid extravasation into the SC tissues.

Summary: Vindesine sulfate is a vinca alkaloid which demonstrates promise for a wide variety of cancer types; however, its full extent of activity remains to be determined. Its major toxicities are similar to those of its family, myelotoxicity and neurotoxicity. It was recommended for approval by FDA's Oncologic Drugs Advisory Committee in September 1982. A New Drug Application (NDA) is pending.

Bibliography Available on Request

PIRENZEPINE HCl (*Gastrozepine* by Boehringer Ingelheim) – An antiulcer agent.

Pharmacology: Pirenzepine is a tricyclic benzodiazepine antiulcer agent comparable to standard antiulcer agents such as cimetidine and ranitidine. However, its uniqueness and mechanism of action hinge on *selective* antimuscarinic activity for gastric acid secretory cells.

Pirenzepine selectively suppresses both basal and stimulated acid and pepsin secretion with lesser effects on other muscarinic sites (eg, salivary secretion) compared to atropine and other classic anticholinergic agents. Controlled trials show that 50 mg, 2 to 3 times daily, inhibits acid secretion at least up to 4.5 hours after dosing. Higher doses inhibit esophageal and colonic motility and decrease lower esophageal sphincter pressure. Pirenzepine may also have cytoprotective effects; however, this is of questionable significance since it has little or no effect on gastric mucus and endogenous gastric prostaglandin production.

Pharmacokinetics: Pirenzepine is a hydrophilic molecule which has systemic bioavailability after oral dosing of 20% to 30%. Approximately 10% of the drug is protein bound. Little drug is found in the brain; brain to serum concentration is 1 to 10.

At least 80% is renally excreted unchanged. Most metabolites are of a desmethyl variety. The parent molecule has a half-life of about 10 hours.

These data indicate the potential for few CNS effects and the need to adjust dosage in patients with impaired renal function.

Clinical studies: Numerous short-term (1 to 6 weeks) studies have been conducted comparing pirenzepine to placebo and other antiulcer drugs in ulcer patients. In small doses (50 to 75 mg/day) duodenal ulcer healing percentages with pirenzepine are not superior to placebo. Doses of 100 to 150 mg/day produce healing in 70% to 90% of patients. Statistically significant symptomatic improvement (decreased antacid use and pain) occurs with both dosage levels.

Short-term double-blind studies comparing duodenal ulcer healing rates of pirenzepine (100 to 150 mg/day) and cimetidine (1 g/day) produced similar results (60% to 79% for pirenzepine and 53% to 85% for cimetidine). A single study comparing pirenzepine (100 mg/day) to cimetidine (1 g/day) and ranitidine (300 mg/day) found similar rates of ulcer healing. However, pirenzepine showed a slower effect on symptom disappearance.

Fewer studies have been conducted in patients with gastric ulcer. Double-blind studies comparing pirenzepine to placebo show a need to use adequate doses (100 to 150 mg/day). Pirenzepine and cimetidine have produced similar healing rates (50% vs 48%) in patients with gastric ulcer, but more studies are indicated.

Trials were performed comparing maintenance doses of pirenzepine (30 to 50 mg/day) to placebo and cimetidine (400 mg/day) in duodenal ulcer patients for 12 months. Results indicate statistically significant reductions in ulcer recurrences for active treatment groups vs placebo (24% recurrence in active treatment group vs 80% in placebo-treated patients). No difference was demonstrated in recurrence rates between pirenzepine and cimetidine patients.

Combined use of pirenzepine with ranitidine or cimetidine shows more effective inhibition of gastric acid secretion than with use of a single agent. Such combinations may be useful in peptic ulcer conditions resistant to single drug therapy and in the Zollinger-Ellison syndrome.

Side effects: Pirenzepine is well tolerated with few reported adverse effects. Dry mouth is the most common effect, but nausea, vomiting, diarrhea, constipation, increased appetite, anorexia, tiredness and difficulty of accommodation have all occurred. Daily doses of less than 150 mg seem to significantly reduce the incidence of at least some of these problems.

Summary: In clinical studies, pirenzepine is equally effective as cimetidine in the treatment of peptic ulcer disease. Its low incidence of side effects and selective inhibition of muscarinic gastric acid secretion will make it a valuable addition to existing agents used to treat ulcers. Pirenzepine is currently available in some European countries; expected date of availability in the United States is unknown. A New Drug Application (NDA) is pending.

Bibliography Available on Request

INOSIPLEX (*Isoprinosine* by Newport) – An immunomodulating agent.

Pharmacology: Inosiplex (inosine pranobex, BAN) is a synthetic complex formed from the p–acetamidobenzoic acid salt of N–N dimethylamino-2-propanol and inosine in a 3:1 molar ratio. Early studies examined inosiplex as an antiviral agent. However, recent research has focused on its immunomodulating properties and suggests that its antiviral activity involves enhancement of host defenses rather than direct inhibition of viral replication. Inosiplex may be more appropriately classed with those agents that regulate immunity, eg, levamisole.

Inosiplex augments immunological events triggered by such agents as mitogens, antigens, phagocyte stimulants or lymphokines. Inosiplex alone does not appear to affect lymphocytes or macrophages. In the presence of triggering agents, it results in an increase in mitogen responses, T–lymphocyte differentiation, total rosette-forming T–cells, lymphotoxin production, virus-induced lymphoproliferative responses, lymphocyte cytotoxicity to viral-infected target cells and skin test responses. This augmentation of responses occurs at inosiplex levels of 0.1 to > 100 mcg/ml with a biphasic profile. Such a profile suggests action on more than one cell population or, more likely, a dual action on a single cell population which is concentration-dependent. Exactly how the drug acts on the lymphocyte to alter the magnitude of triggered responses is unclear. It may involve one or several cell surfaces and nuclear metabolic events linked to RNA metabolism, cyclic nucleotide levels or calcium ion flux. Inosiplex also potentiates interferon activity through mechanisms which remain unclear.

Pharmacokinetics: Inosiplex is rapidly metabolized after both oral and IV administration. The half-life of the inosine portion of the parent complex is 3 minutes after IV administration and 50 minutes after oral administration. In animal models, 90% of the inosine moiety is excreted in the urine as allantoin and uric acid, along with small amounts of hypoxanthine, xanthine and adenine. The p–acetamidobenzoic acid moiety and the N–N-dimethylamino-2-propanol moiety are excreted in the urine after glucuronidation and oxidation, respectively.

Clinical trials examining the use of inosiplex in a variety of viral disorders (eg, herpes zoster, herpes simplex, rhinovirus, influenza A and subacute sclerosing panencephalitis), rheumatoid arthritis and solid tumors have not been able to establish definite efficacy of the drug in any of these disorders. A preliminary study involving four patients with a pre-Acquired Immune Deficiency Syndrome (AIDS) complex (a prodrome of AIDS) and five patients with AIDS given 4 g inosiplex per day for 4 weeks showed enhancement of mitogen-induced lymphocyte proliferative responses in two patients with the pre-AIDS complex. These results agreed with data from an in vitro study of inosiplex's effect on lymphocytes from pre-AIDS patients, patients with AIDS and healthy heterosexual controls which demonstrated that inosiplex could partially restore some of the depressed lymphocyte functions associated with AIDS. The data also suggested, however, that this effect was likely to have clinical significance only in those patients with the milder, pre-AIDS condition. After examination of the combined preliminary results of three studies (unpublished data), Newport Pharmaceuticals reported to FDA officials that there appeared to be a trend toward a delay in the development of fully developed AIDS in pre-AIDS patients treated with inosiplex for 28 days. A multicenter study is in progress to evaluate the use of inosiplex in pre-AIDS patients.

Side effects: In tolerance studies involving healthy volunteers and in clinical trials involving various patient groups, no serious side effects were reported after continuous inosiplex administration for 1 week to 7 years at doses of 1 to 8 g/day. Occasional transient nausea was associated with the ingestion of large numbers of tablets; a transient rise in serum and urinary uric acid, related to the metabolism of the drug, occurred in a small number of patients. Initiate concomitant administration of drugs that increase uric acid levels with caution, since potential for additive effects has not been studied.

Summary: Inosiplex is a new immunomodulating agent. Preliminary data indicate that the compound may improve the immunologic status of some pre-AIDS patients and may delay progression of pre-AIDS to AIDS. Inosiplex could presumably be used long-term in these patients, since it is administered orally and has not been associated with serious side effects. However, more extensive clinical trials are needed to establish the safety and efficacy of the agent. Newport Pharmaceuticals submitted a New Drug Application (NDA) September 3, 1985, requesting approval of inosiplex *(Isoprinosine)* for immunorestoration in pre-AIDS patients, but it was rejected by the FDA in February 1986.

Bibliography Available on Request

FENOTEROL HBr (*Berotec* by Boehringer Ingelheim) - A β_2 agonist.

Pharmacology: Fenoterol HBr is a β_2-adrenergic agonist undergoing investigation in the US as a bronchodilating agent. It has been available outside the US since the early 1970s as a metered dose inhaler (MDI), a solution for nebulization, a powder for inhalation and an oral dosage form.

Stimulation of β_2-adrenoreceptors activates adenyl cyclase which converts adenosine triphosphate into cAMP. Increased levels of cAMP inhibit mediator release and produce bronchodilation. Although controversial, an increase in mucociliary transport may also occur. In addition, β_2 stimulation causes vasodilatation of peripheral blood vessels. This effect can result in a baroreceptor-mediated reflex-positive chronotropic response (increase in heart rate) and stimulation of skeletal muscle, leading to tremor. Fenoterol has greater β_2 selectivity than metaproterenol, but it is approximately equal in selectivity to albuterol and terbutaline. Bronchoselectivity is enhanced by administering fenoterol by inhalation; this allows for use of a lower dose to achieve a therapeutic effect and reduce dose-related side effects.

Usual therapeutic doses (200 to 400 mcg) of inhaled fenoterol do not significantly affect the cardiovascular system; however, marked cardiovascular effects have been observed after oral, SC, IM or IV administration. Fenoterol prevents immediate antigen-induced bronchospasm but does not prevent delayed allergic reactions. A transient reduction in serum potassium levels (representing the uptake of potassium into the intracellular space), and an increase in serum glucose levels have been observed, but the clinical significance remains unclear.

Pharmacokinetics: Approximately 60% of an oral dose is absorbed, with peak plasma levels reached in 2 hours. After inhalation, fenoterol appears to undergo a two-stage absorption process; the first stage is independent of dose, while the second is similar to that seen after oral administration. This is consistent with the observation that, when a drug is administered by inhalation, as much as 90% of the dose is swallowed. Fenoterol undergoes extensive first-pass metabolism. The half-life of total radioactive-labelled drug is 7 hours; however, this does not represent a true half-life for the parent compound. Although maximum effect of inhaled fenoterol is not achieved for 1 to 2 hours, 60% of the maximal response is seen within the first few minutes. The duration of action is $\approx$ 4 to 6 hours. However, since the lower therapeutic dose produces near maximal bronchodilatation, increasing the dose to near maximal effective concentrations will increase the duration of action without affecting the intensity of the peak response. After oral administration, < 2% of the dose is eliminated unchanged in the urine; the balance is excreted as acid conjugates in the urine and feces (40%).

Clinical trials: Clinical trials have established the efficacy of fenoterol for maintenance therapy in patients with moderate to severe asthma, therapy of chronic obstructive pulmonary disease (COPD), protection against exercise-induced asthma and treatment of acute asthma attacks. It is difficult to evaluate many of the studies because they are single-dose studies, or because they do not compare equipotent doses when evaluated against albuterol and terbutaline. However, at equipotent doses (1 puff fenoterol [200 mcg/puff] = 2 puffs albuterol [100 mcg/puff] = 2 puffs terbutaline [250 mcg/puff]), there appears to be no clinically significant difference in duration of action, bronchoselectivity or therapeutic efficacy among the three agents. The dose of fenoterol used to treat an acute asthma attack is 200 mcg (1 puff) repeated once in 5 minutes for children, and 1 to 3 puffs for adults. Maintenance therapy is 1 to 2 puffs 2 to 4 times daily for adults; give 1 puff twice daily to children. Increasing an inhaled dose of fenoterol to > 600 mcg (3 puffs) does not appear to increase the therapeutic response but may increase the incidence of side effects. In one study, an 800 mcg dose increased the heart rate 10% with a slow return to baseline over 2 hours. Although inhaled bronchodilators have many advantages, as many as 10% of the patients may not receive maximal therapeutic benefit due to improper MDI use.

Side effects: After inhalation of therapeutic doses of fenoterol, side effects are rare. After oral therapy, skeletal muscle tremor, tachycardia, palpitations and nervousness occur occasionally. Fenoterol is not recommended for use in patients with hyperthyroidism. Use with caution in patients with cardiovascular disease, diabetes mellitus and hepatic or renal dysfunction.

Summary: Fenoterol by inhalation appears to be a safe and effective treatment for prophylaxis of exercise-induced bronchospasm, acute attacks of mild to moderate asthma and maintenance therapy for chronic asthma or COPD. However, no apparent advantage of fenoterol over equipotent doses of the currently available β_2-selective agonists, albuterol or terbutaline, has yet been demonstrated. A New Drug Application (NDA) is pending. Fenoterol will be marketed as *Berotec* from Boehringer Ingelheim. Further information on this product can be received from Boehringer Ingelheim Canada.

Bibliography Available on Request

NITRENDIPINE (*Baypress* by Bayer): A Type II calcium channel blocking agent.

Pharmacology: Nitrendipine is a 1,4-dihydropyridine derivative calcium entry blocker, structurally similar to nifedipine. It is further classified as a Type II calcium antagonist because, at usual doses and concentrations, it is devoid of electrophysiologic effects, but is a potent peripheral vasodilator. Relaxation of peripheral vascular smooth muscle occurs as a result of inhibition of calcium influx across cellular membranes.

Nitrendipine causes a decrease in both systolic and diastolic blood pressure, primarily due to arteriolar dilatation. Significant peripheral venodilation is unlikely, since postural hypotension is usually not seen. Reflex increases in heart rate, AV nodal conduction and myocardial contractility occur frequently at therapeutic doses and may precipitate myocardial ischemia in patients with coronary artery disease. Plasma renin activity and catecholamine concentrations increase during therapy with nitrendipine; however, the fact that it reduces the pressor response to norepinephrine but affects no change in responses to angiotensin II may explain its greater effectiveness in the treatment of low-renin hypertension. Nitrendipine does not alter glomerular filtration rate (GFR), renal blood flow or plasma aldosterone levels. A short-term, modest diuretic and natriuretic effect has been observed on initiation of therapy.

The dose/response relationship for this effect appears to be flat; a 10 mg dose produces maximum diuresis. It is unlikely that this has any therapeutic implications during long-term therapy. Preliminary data suggest that nitrendipine has no effect on blood glucose, total cholesterol, triglyceride or uric acid levels.

Pharmacokinetics: Available pharmacokinetic data are based on experience with small numbers of patients using assays of varying sensitivity; data vary.

Nitrendipine appears to be well absorbed after oral administration. Peak serum concentrations are seen at 1 to 2 hours; peak effect is seen at approximately 4 hours. The distribution half-life ($t\frac{1}{2}$-α) is approximately 1 hour. Beta elimination half-life ($t\frac{1}{2}$-β) averages 8 to 11 hours. Nitrendipine is metabolized by the liver to an inactive pyridine analog and to several more polar metabolites that are excreted in the urine. Dosage adjustments appear to be necessary in patients with hepatic dysfunction, but specific guidelines are not established. A single-dose study in 16 patients with various degrees of renal dysfunction found no alterations in any kinetic parameters; dosage adjustments appear unnecessary in renal patients.

Clinical trials: Nitrendipine is effective in the treatment of mild to moderate hypertension (diastolic blood pressure 90 to 114 mm Hg). Initial data suggest that the drug is particularly useful in low-renin hypertension, which accounts for 20% to 30% of the hypertensive population. Doses of 10 to 80 mg/day have been used, administered as a single dose or in 2 to 3 divided doses per day. Although a single daily dose will decrease blood pressure for 24 hours, most patients require twice-daily dosing for optimal blood pressure control. Due to reflex increases in heart rate and contractility, concomitant β-blocker therapy may be required in some patients. It has not been determined whether nitrendipine, like verapamil and nifedipine, tends to be more effective in older patients.

Side effects: Nitrendipine has a side effect profile similar to nifedipine. The side effect reported most frequently is headache. Fatigue, peripheral edema, flushing, palpitations, dizziness, polyuria and mild elevations in liver function (in two patients) have also occurred.

Summary: Nitrendipine is a potent vasodilator which effectively reduces blood pressure when given 1 to 3 times daily. The drug appears most useful in low-renin hypertensives. Biochemical abnormalities common to other currently used antihypertensives (eg, hypokalemia, hyperglycemia, increased uric acid and lipids) are not seen with this class of drugs and may represent an advantage over β-blockers and diuretics. Although most patients will require twice-daily dosing, the only other available dihydropyridine (nifedipine) usually requires dosing 3 to 4 times a day.

A New Drug Application (NDA) is pending with the FDA for an antihypertensive indication. Nitrendipine will be co-marketed by Miles and Roche; however there are no plans to market nitrendipine at this time.

Bibliography Available on Request

PINACIDIL (*Pindac* by Lilly) – An antihypertensive agent.

Pharmacology: Pinacidil is a vasodilator under investigation for use as an antihypertensive agent. Pinacidil acts at the level of the precapillary, arteriolar (resistance) vessels, causing direct relaxation of vascular smooth muscle. Its vasodilator effect is not altered by blockade of β-adrenergic, cholinergic or histaminic receptors, or by the presence of prostaglandin inhibitors such as indomethacin.

When compared to other vasodilators with similar sites of action (eg, minoxidil [*Loniten*], guancydine, diazoxide [*Hyperstat*]), pinacidil, at comparable levels of blood pressure reduction, produces quantitatively identical increases in heart rate, reflex sympathetic mediated cardiac contractility and cardiac output. However, when compared to hydralazine (another precapillary arteriolar vasodilator), pinacidil, at doses which produce equivalent reductions in total peripheral resistance, is a more potent blood pressure lowering agent. Since blood pressure is a function of the cardiac output multiplied by the total peripheral resistance, this difference may be explained by the fact that hydralazine appears to have a direct (as well as the indirect) cardiostimulatory effect which offsets some of the blood pressure reduction caused by vasodilation. As would be expected from their differing effects on cardiac output, pinacidil produces less of an increase in myocardial oxygen consumption than hydralazine.

Although an active metabolite has been identified, it does not appear to contribute significantly to the overall antihypertensive activity.

There is a linear correlation between pinacidil drug levels and the fall in mean blood pressure and total peripheral resistance; minimal therapeutic levels are 50 ng/ml.

Pharmacokinetics:

Absorption/Distribution – Available data are complicated by the fact that at least two different oral formulations have been used in clinical trials. However, in general, bioavailability approaches 100% after oral administration, with both peak serum levels and effect occurring at 1 hour. Coadministration of food does not alter bioavailability but slightly delays absorption. Approximately 60% of a dose is protein bound.

Metabolism/Excretion – Pinacidil is metabolized by the liver to a number of metabolites, the most significant being the active metabolite, pinacidil N–oxide. Within the first 24 hours, 55% to 60% of an administered dose appears in the urine as pinacidil or the N–oxide, 20% to 30% is excreted in the urine as other metabolites and 3% is recovered in the feces. The elimination half-life ($t\frac{1}{2}$) varies between 1.5 to 3 hours. Average clearance values are 42 $\pm$ 5 L/hr.

Although exact dosage guidelines have not been established, patients with liver disease should have therapy initiated slowly, at low doses, and with careful blood pressure monitoring. Eight patients with chronic, stable cirrhosis showed a 50% reduction in clearance, prolongation of the half-life and a decrease in the percentage of parent compound converted to the N–oxide metabolite.

Clinical trials: Only a limited number of clinical studies, each involving only a few patients, have been published. This may reflect that pinacidil is not considered to be a first- or second-line drug in the stepped-care approach.

Pinacidil use has generally been confined to patients with moderate to severe hypertension. It is safe and effective, especially when added to a regimen of a diuretic and β-blocker in patients who failed the initial combination regimen. Pinacidil has been particularly effective in selected patients with renal impairment (both dialysis and non-dialysis patients) with drug-resistant, non-volume dependent hypertension.

Although most studies have used doses of 10 to 100 mg twice daily, some clinicians feel that the drug may require 3 times daily dosing. The most effective dose range appears to be 12.5 or 25 mg twice daily.

Side effects: Pinacidil appears to be well tolerated. Only a few reports of mild side effects (eg, dizziness, headache and facial flushing) have been noted.

Edema has occurred in 23.5% to 45.2% of patients on doses of pinacidil alone of 25 to 50 mg. Concomitant diuretics may be required in most patients.

Two patients developed positive anti-nuclear antibody (ANA) titers while receiving pinacidil. Neither had clinical manifestations of a lupus-like syndrome, and a direct cause and effect relationship could not be linked to pinacidil; further studies are necessary to investigate the potential for pinacidil to cause a drug-induced lupus syndrome.

Summary: Pinacidil appears to be a promising alternative agent for the treatment of moderate to severe hypertension. However, further studies are needed to clarify the drug's optimal dosing schedule, long-term side effects and optimal drug combinations.

The FDA's Cardio-Renal Drugs Advisory Committee recommended approval of pinacidil on May 28, 1987, with the stipulation that it be used concomitantly with diuretics. The drug was approved by the FDA in December 1989; however, Lilly has no plans to market pinacidil at this time.

Bibliography Available on Request

CARPROFEN (*Rimadyl* by Roche) – A nonsteroidal anti-inflammatory agent.

Pharmacology: Carprofen [(D,L)-6-chloro-alpha-methylcarbazole-2-acetic acid] is a member of the arylpropionic acid class of nonsteroidal anti-inflammatory drugs (NSAIDs) which includes ibuprofen (eg, *Motrin*), naproxen (eg, *Naprosyn*) and others. The drug also possesses analgesic and antipyretic activity.

Although the site and exact mechanism of action of the NSAIDs has not been fully elucidated, most investigators agree that these drugs owe their analgesic and anti-inflammatory activity, as well as their gastric irritant properties, to their ability to inhibit prostaglandin synthetase. Carprofen is considered to be a less potent inhibitor of prostaglandin biosynthesis than naproxen or ibuprofen, and is only 1% to 4% as potent as indomethacin (eg, *Indocin*).

Considerable evidence suggests that the anti-inflammatory activity of carprofen is due primarily to the D-isomer; the L-isomer is only about one-seventh as potent.

Pharmacokinetics:

Absorption/Distribution – Carprofen is rapidly and extensively absorbed after oral administration. Peak concentrations of approximately 6 to 12 mcg/ml are achieved in 1 to 3 hours; absolute bioavailability is approximately 90%. Ingestion of food results in a slight reduction in the rate of absorption as well as the peak plasma concentration. However, the total amount of the drug absorbed is not reduced. Peak plasma concentrations may be higher in the elderly. Carprofen is highly protein bound (> 98%). In patients with osteoarthritis (OA) or rheumatoid arthritis (RA), the drug enters the synovial fluid rapidly, where it may achieve concentrations in excess of plasma concentrations.

Metabolism – Approximately 65% to 70% of an administered dose is metabolized by direct conjugation to an ester glucuronide. The elimination half-life (t½) is between 13 to 25 hours. Despite the extensive hepatic metabolism, no difference has been observed in pharmacokinetics between cirrhotics and normal volunteers. Thus, dosage adjustments are unnecessary in patients with renal or hepatic insufficiency.

Excretion – Most of an orally administered dose of carprofen (65% to 70%) is eliminated in the urine as the glucuronide metabolite; only 3% to 12% of a dose is excreted unchanged. The remainder of the drug is excreted in the feces after undergoing extensive enterohepatic recycling.

Clinical trials: Carprofen is effective in a variety of clinical settings including treatment of rheumatoid arthritis, osteoarthritis, ankylosing spondylitis, extra-articular inflammatory processes (eg, tendonitis, bursitis), acute pain syndromes (eg, dental and post-traumatic pain) and acute gouty arthritis. Dosages have ranged from 150 to 600 mg/day in two or three divided doses. The few available comparative studies have usually shown carprofen to be equal to, or superior to, aspirin up to 3600 mg/day. Comparisons with indomethacin 75 to 150 mg/day have usually shown the lower doses (up to 300 mg/day) of carprofen to be slightly less effective but better tolerated than indomethacin. Larger doses of carprofen (400 to 600 mg/day) have been used in the treatment of OA; however, the use of larger doses may not produce any additional response over lower doses.

Side effects: Gastrointestinal effects have occurred in approximately 15% of patients. Pain, nausea, heartburn and dyspepsia are most common, while diarrhea is uncommon (approximately 1%). More serious GI side effects such as peptic ulceration are rare. Carprofen has been used along with antacids in patients with active peptic ulcer disease and has been well tolerated.

Renal or urinary adverse reactions including urinary frequency, dysuria, burning, hematuria, nephritis, proteinuria and acute renal failure occurred in 3.4% of 1521 patients in premarketing clinical trials.

Cutaneous reactions such as eczema, skin rash, urticaria and photosensitivity have occurred in 6% to 10% of patients.

Hepatic enzyme elevation occurred in 1.4% of patients in European trials and in as many as 14% of patients in large American trials. These enzyme elevations are usually asymptomatic.

Summary: Carprofen appears to be an effective NSAID which offers convenient twice daily dosing. Despite a low incidence of serious GI side effects, the drug does not appear superior to currently available agents.

Carprofen was approved by the FDA December 31, 1987. However, Roche has made a decision not to market carprofen at this time.

Bibliography Available on Request

ACECAINIDE HCl (*Napa* by Medco Research/Parke-Davis) – An antiarrhythmic agent.

Pharmacology: Acecainide (also known as N–acetylprocainamide, NAPA and acetylprocainamide) is an antiarrhythmic agent which was first identified as the major active metabolite produced by N–acetylation of procainamide (eg, *Pronestyl, Procan SR*). The drug has distinct electrophysiologic and pharmacologic effects which differ from the parent compound.

Acecainide is classified as a Type III (Vaughn-Williams classification) antiarrhythmic agent, along with amiodarone *(Cordarone)* and bretylium (eg, *Bretylol*), because of its ability to prolong atrial and ventricular action potential durations and refractory periods. This occurs without significant depression of conduction velocity. Sinus cycle length, sinus node recovery time, atrioventricular (AV) node refractory period and conduction intervals (eg, atrio-His, His-ventricular) are also not affected by therapeutic concentrations of the drug. Electrocardiographically, the PR interval and QRS duration show no significant changes during acecainide therapy. However, the rate corrected QT interval (QTc) is significantly increased at concentrations of the drug which produce arrhythmia suppression (12 to 35 mcg/ml).

Blood pressure and heart rate may be reduced, but this effect is not consistently seen. There is no significant effect on cardiac output or pulmonary artery wedge pressure. Several studies have shown that acecainide increases myocardial contractility.

Pharmacokinetics: Acecainide is well absorbed after oral administration, with bioavailability values ranging from 82% to 100% using capsule and tablet dosage formulations. Peak levels occur within 1 to 3 hours after oral administration. Protein binding averages 10% and is independent of plasma concentration.

Metabolism of acecainide is limited. A small amount (2% to 5%) is deacetylated back to the parent compound, procainamide, or converted to desethyl N–acetylprocainamide (< 1%). The majority of the drug (59% to 87%) is excreted unchanged in the urine, and there appears to be a strong correlation between renal clearance and creatinine clearance. Additional metabolic or excretion pathways are presumed to exist since approximately 10% to 15% of an administered dose cannot be accounted for in present studies.

The half-life ranges from 4 to 13 hours in patients with normal renal function to as long as 42 hours in functionally anephric patients. Elderly patients show a reduction in acecainide clearance which may reflect both age-related decrease in renal function and reduced renal tubular secretion of the drug.

Hemodialysis and continuous arteriovenous hemofiltration enhance clearance.

Clinical trials: The fact that acecainide produces electrophysiologic effects which are distinctly different from procainamide requires that the drug be evaluated separately. A positive response to procainamide is not necessarily predictive of a positive response to acecainide.

Acecainide has been used to suppress premature ventricular complexes (PVCs) and refractory ventricular arrhythmias. About 50% of patients with at least one PVC/minute achieved 50% suppression of arrhythmia; 40% achieved 75% suppression at plasma levels which averaged 22 mcg/ml. In the only published long-term trial of acecainide in drug refractory ventricular arrhythmias, 63% of patients were effectively controlled at 12 months.

Animal studies suggest acecainide may be useful in converting atrial flutter to sinus rhythm.

Side effects: Side effects are common, ≈ 45%. Discontinuation of therapy due to side effects, however, is only required in ≈ 10% of patients. Gastrointestinal disturbances are the most common (nausea, vomiting), followed by neurologic symptoms such as dizziness, lightheadedness, blurred vision, numbness and tingling.

Acecainide has little tendency to cause a drug-induced lupus-like syndrome which frequently limits the usefulness of procainamide. This reaction appears to be caused by the parent compound; however, a small amount of administered acecainide is converted back to procainamide. Like all antiarrhythmics, acecainide may have a proarrhythmic effect. Although not systematically studied in humans, reports of acecainide-induced torsade de pointes have been recorded.

Summary: Acecainide appears to be a potentially useful antiarrhythmic. The fact that it has little tendency to induce the lupus-like syndrome frequently associated with procainamide is of interest, but other alternatives to procainamide also exist. Additional studies are necessary to compare the efficacy of this drug to currently available agents and further define its place in therapy.

On December 10, 1993, Medco announced that development of acecainide has been discontinued since it appears to offer no increased benefit over currently available antiarrhythmic agents.

Bibliography Available on Request

CIFENLINE SUCCINATE (*Cipralan* by Hoffman-LaRoche) – An antiarrhythmic agent.

Pharmacology: Cifenline succinate (formerly cibenzoline) is a new antiarrhythmic agent. It is an imidazoline derivative, structurally unrelated to any other currently available antiarrhythmic.

Cifenline's primary electrophysiologic effects are similar to those produced by quinidine (eg, *Duraquin, Quinidex*). The drug acts predominantly on the fast sodium current, reducing the rate of rise of phase 0 of the action potential and prolonging the effective refractory period. These effects are characteristic of Class IA (Vaughn-Williams classification) agents such as quinidine, procainamide (eg, *Pronestyl, Procan SR*) and disopyramide (eg, *Norpace*).

The drug has also been shown to increase the action potential duration, a property of Class III agents, and may produce blockade of the slow inward calcium channel similar to the Class IV agents. The contribution of these secondary effects to the drug's clinical usefulness has not been clearly delineated.

The drug produces a plasma concentration-dependent prolongation of the QRS duration. Prolongation of the PR interval and the rate-corrected QT interval have not been consistently observed, but these effects are compatible with the drug's known electrophysiologic effects and may be seen at higher doses or in patients with underlying conduction disturbances.

Pharmacokinetics: Cifenline is well absorbed after oral administration. Absolute bioavailability is approximately 85%, with peak plasma concentrations occurring approximately 1.5 hours after administration. Coadministration with food slightly decreases the rate, but not the extent, of absorption. Approximately 55% of the drug is bound to plasma proteins, primarily albumin.

Following multiple doses, the elimination half-life of the drug is approximately 12 hours (range, 8 to 12 hours). As much as 60% of a dose is excreted unchanged in the urine, and total body clearance correlates closely with creatinine clearance. Therefore, in patients with chronic renal failure, dosage should be reduced. Older patients also clear the drug more slowly, probably as a result of age-related reductions in renal function. The plasma concentrations of unchanged drug are apparently responsible for its antiarrhythmic effect. Studies have shown that the antiarrhythmic response following twice-daily administration of cifenline is equivalent to a 4 times a day regimen.

Clinical trials: Cifenline is effective in suppressing a variety of ventricular arrhythmias, including complex PVCs and nonsustained ventricular tachycardia. In these applications, the drug has produced response rates similar to or higher than those for quinidine, procainamide, disopyramide and tocainide *(Tonocard)*. Data for patients with sustained ventricular tachycardia resistant to conventional therapy is limited; however, response rates of 25% have occurred. Long-term follow-up studies (12 to 24 months) have reported sustained therapeutic efficacy in 36% to 80% of initial responders.

Side effects: Cifenline appears to be well tolerated, especially when compared to the other Class IA antiarrhythmics. Gastrointestinal intolerance is the most common reason cited for discontinuation of therapy due to side effects. Other adverse effects reported include: Lightheadedness, dizziness, nervousness, tremulousness, blurred vision and dry mouth.

Worsening of preexisting left ventricular dysfunction has occurred. The drug should be used with caution in patients with CHF, especially if baseline ejection fraction is less than 30%. The proarrhythmic effect that may occur (as with all antiarrhythmic agents) has occurred in 10% to 15% of patients receiving cifenline.

No serious hematologic or laboratory abnormalities have been reported.

Summary: Cifenline is a unique antiarrhythmic agent which may offer similar efficacy with a more favorable side effect profile than currently available Class IA agents. The long half-life which permits twice-daily dosing may also be considered an advantage. Cifenline will be co-marketed as *Cipralan* by Roche and Glaxo. The NDA has been pending since December 1985. The official generic name was recently changed from cibenzoline to cifenline.

Bibliography Available on Request

TOLRESTAT (*Alredase* by Wyeth-Ayerst) – An aldose reductase inhibitor.

Pharmacology: Tolrestat, a carboxylic acid, is an aldose reductase inhibitor currently undergoing clinical trials to assess its value in controlling the biochemical abnormalities responsible for the late complications of diabetes (eg, diabetic neuropathy and retinopathy).

Diabetic neuropathy, characterized by postural hypotension, diarrhea, pain and tingling in muscle groups, impotence, etc, occurs in about 10% of diabetic patients with good glycemic control and in up to 70% of patients with poorly controlled diabetes. Diabetic retinopathy occurs in approximately 75% of long-standing (up to 20 years) diabetics. These late complications of insulin-dependent diabetes appear to be related to the accumulation of intracellular sorbitol and galactitol which results in cellular damage. A deficit of myo-inositol may also be involved, especially in the diabetic neuropathies.

Aldose reductase is the first enzyme in the sorbitol (polyol) pathway. This pathway is responsible for conversion of glucose to sorbitol, and of galactose to galactitol. Under conditions of hyperglycemia, sorbitol accumulation occurs. By inhibiting aldose reductase, tolrestat prevents the accumulation of intracellular sorbitol.

Pharmacokinetics: Tolrestat is almost completely absorbed after oral administration in healthy subjects. Bioavailability is reduced in diabetic patients, but the difference is not statistically significant. Peak plasma concentrations are achieved in 1 to 2 hours. Maximum decreases in red blood cell (RBC) sorbitol levels occur after 3 days of treatment with 100 mg twice daily. The distribution half-life averages 2 to 3 hours, whereas the elimination half-life averages 10 to 13 hours. Protein binding is extensive (99.5%).

Metabolism of tolrestat is minimal. The drug is excreted primarily by the kidneys as unchanged drug. The need for dosage reductions in patients with compromised renal function has not been established.

Clinical trials: The majority of published data on tolrestat involves animal or in vitro studies. However, a study of 23 diabetic patients receiving tolrestat 25 or 100 mg twice daily showed a dose-dependent reduction of RBC sorbitol levels of 21% and 57%, respectively.

In two unpublished clinical efficacy trials, tolrestat was administered to patients with diabetic neuropathy in a randomized, double-blind placebo controlled fashion. The short-term (8 week) trial in 260 patients compared placebo to 200 mg twice daily or 400 mg once daily; the long-term (1 year) trial in 548 patients compared placebo to 50, 100 or 200 mg once daily or 100 mg twice daily. Compared with placebo, 28% of patients in the long-term study receiving tolrestat 200 mg once daily showed improvement of nerve conduction velocity and paresthesias but not pain. Improvement was seen in both trials with a once-daily dose of 200 or 400 mg, but not when the same dose was given twice daily.

Side effects: The most common side effect reported by the manufacturer in unpublished clinical trials was dizziness, which occurred in 11% of patients receiving 200 mg tolrestat daily. Other adverse effects that have occurred include skin rash and liver enzyme elevations. A clear cause-and-effect relationship between tolrestat therapy and these adverse effects has not been established.

Drug interactions: Studies with warfarin (eg, *Coumadin*) indicated that no drug interaction occurred due to protein binding displacement at therapeutic doses. Salicylates at concentrations of 100 to 200 mcg/ml displace tolrestat (21% and 35%, respectively). Tolbutamide (eg, *Orinase*) also displaces tolrestat (22% displacement at tolbutamide concentrations of 160 mcg/ml).

Summary: Published data, although scant, suggest that tolrestat is safe and well tolerated. The ability of aldose reductase inhibition to decrease RBC sorbitol accumulation has been demonstrated in humans. Despite evidence for a favorable biochemical effect, supporting evidence for a beneficial clinical effect (ie, prevention of late complications of diabetes) has yet to be conclusively established. Furthermore, the groups most likely to benefit from this form of therapy, those with poor glycemic control or long-standing diabetes, present methodologic problems for assessing cause and effect relationships with any form of therapy.

The NDA for tolrestat was filed on April 4, 1986 for diabetic neuropathy. It is in Phase III trials for diabetic retinopathy. Tolrestat will be marketed as *Alredase* by Wyeth-Ayerst.

Bibliography Available on Request

DILEVALOL (*Unicard* by Key) – A β-adrenergic blocking agent.

Pharmacology: Dilevalol, a noncardioselective β-adrenergic blocking agent, is the R,R-isomer of labetalol *(Normodyne, Trandate),* one of four optical isomers of the drug. Although dilevalol is virtually devoid of α_1-blocking activity, having only one-fourth to one-third the activity of labetalol, it has ≈ 7 times the vasodilatory effect. However, this effect appears to be mediated via a β_2-agonist effect as opposed to an α_1-blocking effect. Dilevalol also has ≈ 4 times the β-blocking (β_1 and β_2) effect of labetalol. The degree of β_1 receptor blockade appears to be similar to propranolol (eg, *Inderal*).

The β-agonist activity of dilevalol appears to be selective for β_2 receptors. The vasodilatory response is blocked by propranolol, but not metoprolol *(Lopressor)* pretreatment, indicating the vasodilatory actions are mediated by β_2 receptor stimulation. Pindolol *(Visken),* which has significant intrinsic sympathomimetic activity (ISA), differs from dilevalol in that its agonist activity is not β_2 selective.

Dilevalol appears to decrease peripheral vascular resistance with no effect on cardiac output. The reflex increase in heart rate that might be expected with vasodilation is counteracted by the drug's β-blocking activity. In one study of 29 patients, heart rate actually decreased by 8 beats per minute compared to placebo. Dilevalol slightly decreased plasma renin activity in one study. In a study comparing dilevalol and metoprolol on the lipid profile of 309 patients, dilevalol increased HDL cholesterol and slightly decreased LDL cholesterol, a finding that is opposite that seen with other agents in this class besides pindolol and acebutolol (*Sectral*).

Pharmacokinetics:

Absorption/Distribution – Dilevalol is rapidly absorbed following oral administration, reaching peak levels within 1 hour. Following absorption, it is rapidly distributed in the extravascular system. In 12 volunteers, the mean maximum concentration was 62 ng/ml. Plasma levels appear to increase in a dose-related manner.

Metabolism/Excretion – Dilevalol undergoes extensive first-pass metabolism (85% to 95%), resulting in an absolute bioavailability of 11% to 14%. The half-life is ≈ 8 hours following oral administration, and 12 hours following IV, indicating dilevalol need only be given once daily. The metabolites are conjugated with glucuronides and are excreted in urine. Approximately 3% of the drug was excreted unchanged after an IV dose in 12 volunteers.

Plasma concentrations do not appear altered in severe renal impairment. In a study of six volunteers, only 0.007% (mean, 27 mcg) of a dose was excreted in breast milk over 48 hours.

Clinical trials: Dilevalol, in once-daily doses of 100 to 800 mg, is effective in the treatment of mild to moderate hypertension. Because of its vasodilatory effects, it may be more useful than other agents of this class in hypertensive patients with compromised myocardial function or peripheral vascular insufficiency. Since it does not affect glomerular filtration rate, renal plasma flow, renal blood flow or renal vascular resistance, it may be useful in patients with renal insufficiency. Some studies also indicate a possible benefit in black patients. It is effective when administered orally and IV. In several studies, dilevalol was equal to or greater than labetalol, metoprolol and atenolol (*Tenormin*) in antihypertensive efficacy, with less side effects. In one study comparing dilevalol with atenolol, patients receiving dilevalol showed a greater and longer-lasting decrease in mean arterial pressure.

Although only reported in two patients, dilevalol may be useful for the treatment of pheochromocytoma. It may also be useful, administered IV, in the management of severe hypertension. Further studies are needed.

Side effects: Dilevalol appears to be well tolerated. It has a relatively low incidence of CNS side effects, despite its lipid solubility. When compared to placebo, the most common side effects associated with dilevalol were dizziness, somnolence and nausea.

Drug interactions: In one study involving nine healthy subjects, cimetidine *(Tagamet)* slightly increased dilevalol's bioavailability. The clinical significance was not determined.

Summary: Dilevalol, an isomer of labetalol, is a noncardioselective β-adrenergic blocking agent with significant vasodilatory (β_2 agonist) activity; therefore, it may have advantages over other agents in this class in certain hypertensive patients with altered cardiac conduction. Black patients and patients with renal insufficiency may also benefit. It also appears to be well tolerated, with minimal side effects reported. It is usually administered once daily, and can be given orally or IV.

An NDA for the oral form was filed in 1986. In January 1990, the FDA's Cardio-Renal Advisory Committee recommended approval for dilevalol. However, due to an increasing incidence of hepatotoxicity, the manufacturer decided to withdraw the NDA and discontinue the worldwide marketing of the drug.

Bibliography Available on Request

INDECAINIDE HCl (*Decabid* by Eli Lilly) – An antiarrhythmic agent.

Pharmacology: Indecainide is a class IC antiarrhythmic agent that is structurally similar to the investigational agent aprindine. Other available class IC antiarrhythmics are encainide (*Enkaid*) and flecainide (*Tambocor*). This class of drugs markedly suppresses premature ventricular complexes (PVCs) and depresses intramyocardial conduction. Indecainide prolongs the PR and QRS intervals, significantly increasing intraventricular conduction time without significantly affecting atrial or ventricular refractoriness. There appear to be no significant hemodynamic effects.

Pharmacokinetics: Indecainide is completely absorbed following oral administration. In animals, the half-life is 3 to 5 hours; however, the half-life in patients is considerably longer (9 to 10 hours), suggesting that twice-daily dosing may be effective in some patients. Indecainide is metabolized in the liver to desisopropyl indecainide. This metabolite appears to have a longer half-life than the parent drug, although the plasma levels of the metabolite are only approximately 10% those of indecainide. It is not known if desisopropyl indecainide possesses any antiarrhythmic effects.
Approximately 63% of indecainide is recovered in the urine, with < 10% recovered as the metabolite. In one study, there was no correlation between percent suppression of ventricular ectopic depolarizations and plasma levels or half-life of either indecainide or the metabolite.

Clinical trials: Clinical information regarding the efficacy of indecainide is available only through several studies using small patient populations. Antiarrhythmic efficacy appears similar to encainide and flecainide. Efficacy was maintained in some patients for up to 2 years. Indecainide orally or IV markedly suppresses the frequency of PVCs, particularly repetitive forms. In one study, 63% to 82% of patients had suppression of PVCs, 60% to 82% had more than a 95% elimination of couplets, and 56% to 74% had complete elimination of ventricular tachycardia. The average suppression of PVCs with most available antiarrhythmics ranges from 50% to 75%. The degree of suppression was comparable to encainide and flecainide. Other studies have reported a 90% reduction in PVCs in approximately 85% of patients, and elimination of ventricular tachycardia in approximately 86% of patients. In a study involving 231 patients, indecainide reduced PVCs by 93%, while disopyramide reduced PVCs by 80%; suppression of runs of ventricular tachycardia were equivalent for both drugs. In a study of 11 patients, indecainide suppressed ventricular premature beats in 90% of patients, but suppression of ventricular tachycardia was achieved in only 45% of patients.

In data from five clinical trials through the manufacturer involving 792 patients, 70% receiving indecainide responded to ≤ 200 mg/day, and 90% responded to 300 mg/day.

Side effects: In clinical trials, the following side effects were noted: Dizziness (18% with the 200 mg dose, 12% with 150 mg and 9% with 100 mg); proarrhythmias (14.8%); congestive heart failure (3.9%). Each effect appeared to be dose-related. Other adverse reactions reported in the smaller patient population studies included headache, blurry vision, impotence, lightheadedness, confusion, thought disorders, nausea and constipation. Most reactions appear mild and may respond to dosage adjustment.

Drug interactions: In five patients receiving concurrent indecainide and digoxin, the digoxin concentration increased (range, 47% to 300%) in three of the five patients. The digoxin concentration decreased significantly when indecainide was discontinued. The clinical significance of this pharmacokinetic interaction was not determined.

Summary: Indecainide is an effective class IC antiarrhythmic agent that may offer an alternative for the patients who cannot tolerate the GI side effects of quinidine or the CNS effects of the other class IC agents. Lilly is recommending a dosage of 100 to 200 mg/day, and they plan to market only the twice-daily formulation (an immediate release form for 4 times daily administration was also tested in clinical trials).

Because of the recent findings of the Cardiac Arrhythmia Suppression Trial (CAST), which reduced the indications for encainide and flecainide to treatment of life-threatening arrhythmias only, Lilly is reviewing the CAST study data to determine if there is any potential relevance to indecainide.

In November, 1988, the FDA's Cardio-Renal Drugs Advisory Committee unanimously recommended approval for indecainide for sustained ventricular tachycardia, ventricular fibrillation, nonsustained ventricular and chronic benign PVCs. Indecainide was approved by the FDA in December, 1989. However, Lilly has made a decision not to market the drug at this time.

Bibliography Available on Request

DOTHIEPIN HCl (*Prothiaden* by Boots) – A tricyclic antidepressant.

Pharmacology: Dothiepin, a thio analog of amitriptyline (eg, *Elavil*), is a tricyclic antidepressant (TCA) used for the treatment of depression. It is also structurally related to doxepin (eg, *Sinequan*). The efficacy of dothiepin does not appear to differ significantly from other available TCAs, and it appears comparable in efficacy to other antidepressants including fluoxetine *(Prozac)* and trazodone (eg, *Desyrel*). The anticholinergic effects may be less than with amitriptyline, although the sedative and anxiolytic activity appears to be similar.

Dothiepin and its metabolites inhibit the neuronal uptake of norepinephrine in vitro, thereby facilitating noradrenergic neurotransmission. The drug may also enhance serotonergic neurotransmission by inhibiting serotonin uptake. In vitro, dothiepin is a potent antagonist of histamine H_1-receptors, an effect common with other antidepressants. As with other TCAs, the therapeutic effects may not occur for 2 to 4 weeks following initiation of therapy.

Pharmacokinetics: Following oral administration, dothiepin is rapidly and completely absorbed. Peak plasma concentrations are achieved in 2 to 4 hours, and reach steady-state concentrations within 12 days (1 or 3 times daily administration).

Dothiepin undergoes extensive hepatic metabolism resulting from N-demethylation and S-oxidation. Following the first-pass effect, oral bioavailability is ≈ 30%. In one study in healthy volunteers, peak plasma concentrations and AUC of dothiepin-S-oxide were higher than the parent drug; the peak plasma concentrations of the other two metabolites were lower. It is not known if the metabolites contribute to the therapeutic efficacy of the drug. The terminal elimination half-lives of dothiepin and its metabolites are: Dothiepin 14.4 to 23.9 hrs; dothiepin-S-oxide 22.7 to 25.5 hrs; northiaden 34.7 to 45.7 hrs; northiaden-S-oxide 24.2 to 33.5 hrs. In two subjects, within 96 hours of administration, ≈ 56% of a dothiepin dose was recovered in the urine, and 15% in the feces. Unchanged dothiepin accounted for only 0.5% of the dose.

In elderly subjects, the time to peak plasma concentration, elimination half-life and AUC of dothiepin are increased, and the absorption rate constant, volume of distribution and plasma clearance are decreased. Dothiepin also appears in the breast milk in a concentration of ≥ 1 mcg/dl (dose: 75 mg/day).

Clinical trials: In several noncomparative studies using dothiepin (75 to 300 mg/day for 4 to 24 weeks), a marked improvement in symptoms of depression occurred in a large percentage of patients. However, results are difficult to assess due to lack of controls and short duration of therapy in some cases. Although one study showed the efficacy of dothiepin (75 to 225 mg/day) to be greater with a single dose at night vs a 3 times daily regimen, others reported no significant difference in efficacy.

In randomized double-blind studies of amitriptyline and dothiepin (50 to 300 mg/day) for 4 to 12 weeks, no significant difference in efficacy was noted, although dothiepin may have a faster onset of action. Dothiepin is also comparable in efficacy to doxepin, imipramine (eg, *Tofranil*), maprotiline *(Ludiomil)*, fluoxetine and trazodone. In patients with mixed depression and anxiety symptoms, dothiepin is equally effective as alprazolam *(Xanax)*, and equal or superior to chlordiazepoxide (eg, *Librium*).

Dothiepin also appears to have significant analgesic activity and may be useful in patients with idiopathic fibromyalgia syndrome (eg, generalized musculoskeletal aching, multiple tender points, fatigue, stiffness, sleep disturbances), rheumatoid arthritis or psychogenic facial pain.

Side effects: The adverse effects are similar to those seen with other TCAs. The following occurred in data pooled from 12 studies (n = 5755): Dry mouth (24%); drowsiness (16.8%); GI disorders (10.8%); dizziness (10.3%); tremor (8.5%); sweating, insomnia (5.7%); blurred vision (4.5%); weight gain (3.5%); palpitations (2.8%); hypotension, headache (1.9); cardiac dysrhythmias (0.1%). Approximately 5% of patients withdrew from treatment due to side effects. Dothiepin appears to produce a lower incidence of anticholinergic, cardiac and sedative effects than amitriptyline; tolerability is similar to doxepin and imipramine.

Summary: Dothiepin is a TCA that is effective in the treatment of depression but appears to offer no significant advantage over existing agents. The lower incidence of anticholinergic effects compared to amitriptyline may make it more useful in elderly patients. The initial dosage appears to be 75 mg/day either divided 3 times daily or as a single nighttime dose. Dosage range appears to be 75 to 300 mg/day.

The NDA for dothiepin was originally submitted in 1979 by Boots licensee Marion. In 1982 the drug was recommended for approval by an FDA advisory committee; however, in 1987 the FDA requested additional safety information for the higher dosage ranges (200 to 300 mg) ≈ 6 months after Boots reacquired rights to the drug. Dothiepin will be marketed as *Prothiaden*. Dothiepin HCl is available in Europe.

Bibliography Available on Request

MIFEPRISTONE (RU 486) – An antiprogesterone.

Pharmacology: Mifepristone is a synthetic progesterone and glucocorticosteroid receptor antagonist.

Mifepristone's antagonist activity at the glucocorticosteroid receptor disrupts the negative pituitary feedback resulting from the normal morning rise in cortisol level.

When used as an abortifacient, mifepristone acts as an antagonist at progesterone receptors in the endometrium and the trophoblast, allowing prostaglandins to stimulate uterine contractions and causing the conceptus to detach from the uterine wall. Various vascular changes are produced which may decrease placental viability as well as decrease glandular secretory activity, accelerate degenerative changes, and increase stromal but not glandular mitotic activity in the endometrium causing sloughing of the endometrium.

Pharmacokinetics: Mifepristone is rapidly absorbed after oral administration. After a single dose of 25 mg and up to 25 mg/kg, peak plasma levels of 3.5 to 7.5 mcmol/L have been reported at 1 to 3 hours after administration. The drug is 94% bound to protein, with the majority (91%) bound to albumin. The volume of distribution is ≈ 1.5 L/kg. Cerebrospinal fluid levels equal to 4% of the plasma concentration have occurred. The half-life is 20 or 54 hours, depending on the method of pharmacokinetic analysis used in the study. Three active metabolites have been identified. Less than 0.5% of the drug is excreted in the urine.

Mifepristone also crosses the placental barrier, achieving levels equal to one-third of the maternal plasma levels in the fetal circulation.

Clinical trials: Clinical trials have demonstrated that mifepristone is an effective abortifacient in early pregnancy (< 56 days of amenorrhea). A variety of dosing regimens have been successful. Dosages from 25 mg twice daily for 4 days to 50 mg 3 times daily for 4 days have resulted in success rates of 61% to 85%. Once-daily administration of 50 to 100 mg for 7 days was successful in 50% to 73% of cases. A single 600 mg dose has a success rate of 72% to 100%. Menses typically begins within 5 days of initiation of therapy and continues for 1 to 2 weeks. Preliminary evidence suggests that the combination of a single dose of mifepristone followed within 48 hours by the administration of gemeprost, an investigational synthetic prostaglandin in vaginal suppository form, may improve the success rate by stimulating myometrial contraction, cervical softening and dilation. Patients are treated as outpatients unless complications occur.

Preliminary data suggest that the antiglucocorticosteroid action of mifepristone 20 mg/kg/day is useful in the treatment of Cushing's syndrome in some patients.

Mifepristone has also been used in patients with tamoxifen *(Nolvadex)* resistant breast cancer who have evidence of progesterone receptors. A dose of 200 mg/day resulted in a response rate of 18% at 3 months in one study.

Other uses under investigation are treatment of open-angle glaucoma, postcoital contraception (600 mg single dose within 72 hours of unprotected intercourse) and induction of labor. Due to the transplacental passage of mifepristone, the latter application requires further clarification of the drug's effect on a viable fetus.

Side effects: The most common side effect of mifepristone used as an abortifacient is heavy bleeding. Dilation and curettage or transfusion may be required to manage this side effect in some cases. The severity of bleeding is directly related to the use of higher doses (> 800 mg) and a longer duration of gestation before therapy.

Other common side effects include abdominal pain (80%), mild to moderate nausea and vomiting (43%), mild to moderate uterine pain (26%), headache (15%) and diarrhea (7.5%). These can usually be controlled with mild analgesics and antiemetic agents.

Summary: Mifepristone appears to be a safe and effective alternative to presently available forms of abortion. Efficacy is increased when used concurrently with a prostaglandin. It also shows promise in several disease states, such as Cushing's syndrome and breast cancer, which may respond to its specific receptor antagonist effects.

Mifepristone is currently marketed in France as *Mifegyne* by Roussel-Uclaf, and it also is approved in Sweden and the UK. On April 20, 1993, Roussel-Uclaf licensed the drug to the Population Council; this US research group will conduct large-scale clinical trials of the drug starting in October 1994 and establish selection criteria for a US firm to manufacture the product following FDA approval. Companies potentially interested in marketing mifepristone include Gynex, Cabot Medical and Adeza Biomedical. Roussel-Uclaf's parent company, Hoechst AG, will not allow them to manufacture the drug for the US market. The FDA is willing to accept foreign clinical trial data as evidence of safety and efficacy to speed the approval process. Mifepristone was recommended for approval by the FDA in July 1996.

Bibliography Available on Request

FLUPIRTINE MALEATE (by Carter-Wallace) – A nonnarcotic analgesic.

Pharmacology: Flupirtine maleate, a triaminopyridine derivative, is a nonnarcotic analgesic structurally unrelated to other analgesic agents. Although its exact mechanism of action is not known, flupirtine lacks affinity for any type of opiate receptor and therefore, has a mechanism that differs from the opiates. Flupirtine also appears to lack some of the side effects of the opiates including constipation, respiratory depression, withdrawal phenomena, development of tolerance and abuse potential. It is suggested that flupirtine is a medium to strong analgesic; its duration of action is comparable to codeine, and it is up to three times as potent as codeine and propoxyphene (eg, *Darvon*), up to twice as potent as meperidine (eg, *Demerol*) and approximately ten times as potent as acetaminophen (eg, *Tylenol*).

Pharmacokinetics: The pharmacokinetics of flupirtine have not been well defined. The drug appears to have linear kinetics. A dosage of 100 mg 3 times daily achieves average steady-state blood levels equivalent to the peak for a single 200 mg dose. In one study of 55 patients, the analgesic effect occurred within 45 minutes to 2 hours; the duration of action was 4 to 6 hours. The half-life of flupirtine appears to be 7 to 10 hours.

In 13 elderly patients receiving flupirtine 100 mg 3 times daily for 12 days, the mean elimination half-life was higher than in healthy young subjects (mean, 18.6 hours on day 12 vs 6.5 hours). This was associated with an increased maximum serum concentration and reduced clearance in the elderly subjects.

In 12 patients with renal impairment, the half-life of flupirtine was higher compared to healthy subjects (mean, 9.8 hours vs 6.5 hours) following a single oral 100 mg dose.

Flupirtine peak levels and area under the curve may be higher in patients with primary biliary cirrhosis. In a study of ten patients, flupirtine did not induce hepatic microsomal enzymes.

Clinical trials: Flupirtine is effective in the treatment of pain resulting from various procedures or conditions including episiotomy, cancer, and postoperative and dental pain. Dosages used have ranged from 100 to 600 mg/day; the most common dosages were 100 mg once daily or 100 mg 3 times daily. Capsules were used in most studies although the suppository form was also used. Analgesic efficacy of flupirtine was judged to be as effective as other analgesics used in the studies including acetaminophen, codeine, pentazocine *(Talwin NX)*, oxycodone plus acetaminophen (eg, *Percocet*), naproxen (eg, *Naprosyn*) and diclofenac *(Voltaren)*. Flupirtine appears to have no tolerance or addiction potential. In one study, the average number of capsules taken per month remained constant for 12 months, as did the analgesic effect.

Flupirtine significantly reduced seizure frequency in eight of nine patients with minimal side effects; however, since other derivatives of the drug may have greater activity, no further studies in the treatment of epilepsy are planned at this time.

Side effects: Flupirtine does not appear to share the common side effects of the opiates such as respiratory depression and constipation. The drug is generally well tolerated. In a study of 55 patients, the most common adverse effects were dizziness (11%), drowsiness (9% to 10%), pruritis (9%) and dry mouth (5%). Other side effects that occurred included: Pain in forehead; sensation of excessive fullness in stomach; muscular tremor; nausea; other GI disturbances (eg, vomiting, abdominal discomfort).

Summary: Flupirtine is a nonnarcotic analgesic that compares favorably in efficacy with other available analgesics. At this time, however, it offers no clear advantage over the nonsteroidal anti-inflammatory agents except perhaps in the GI and CNS side effect profile. It does offer an advantage over the opiates in side effect profile, abuse potential, withdrawal phenomena and development of tolerance. The average dose appears to be 100 mg 1 to 3 times daily. It has been used in both a capsule and suppository formulation.

An NDA was filed for flupirtine by Carter-Wallace in April 1986. At one time, a 1989 approval was anticipated; however, there has been no recent projected approval date and Carter-Wallace is no longer interested in pursuing this product. The company is also working with a combination product of flupirtine with codeine.

Bibliography Available on Request

CILAZAPRIL (*Inhibace* by Roche/Glaxo) – A non-sulfhydryl-containing ACE inhibitor.

Pharmacology: Cilazapril is a potent, structurally new, non-sulfhydryl-containing orally active angiotensin-converting enzyme (ACE) inhibitor prodrug under investigation for use in patients with hypertension and CHF. Following oral administration, cilazapril is de-esterified in the liver and other tissues to the active diacid form, cilazaprilat. Cilazaprilat is ≈ 10 times more potent than captopril *(Capoten)* and 5 times more potent than enalaprilat, the active form of enalapril *(Vasotec)*.

ACE inhibitors block the enzymatic conversion of angiotensin I to the potent vasoconstrictor angiotensin II. While this inhibition also results in reduced metabolism of bradykinin, alterations in the prostaglandin system and reductions in plasma aldosterone and antidiuretic hormone, these responses do not appear to be responsible for the primary therapeutic effects of these agents. Blockade of angiotensin II production reduces supine and standing blood pressure in hypertensive patients. In patients with CHF, the vasodilatory response reduces afterload, leading to an increase in cardiac output. These beneficial responses may be facilitated by the responses mentioned above.

After administration of cilazapril, ACE activity, angiotensin II and plasma aldosterone concentrations, total peripheral resistance, blood pressure (systolic, diastolic and mean), and the response to exogenous angiotension I are all reduced, while heart rate, baroreceptor reflex sensitivity, cardiovascular reflexes and glomerular filtration rate are usually unchanged.

Pharmacokinetics: Cilazapril is rapidly absorbed after oral administration, with peak levels of the parent compound achieved at ≈ 1 hour. Conversion to cilazaprilat, the active form, is rapid and extensive, with peak levels attained at ≈ 1.8 hours with 57% absolute bioavailability of the active compound. In contrast to some other ACEIs, the bioavailability is not significantly reduced by food. After single doses of 0.5, 1, 2.5 and 5 mg, peak plasma levels of cilazaprilat were 5.4, 12.4, 37.7 and 94.2 ng/ml, respectively, indicating that greater than proportional increases in the active compound are achieved over this dose range. The elimination of cilazaprilat is biphasic, with an initial half-life of 1 to 2 hours controlled by the rate of conversion to this active form, followed by a prolonged terminal elimination half-life of 30 to 50 hours. The volume of distribution is ≈ 20 L.

Clearance of cilazaprilat is almost exclusively renal. Patients with severe renal or hepatic impairment may require smaller or less frequent doses. One study suggests that hypertensive patients undergoing hemodialysis can be controlled on 0.5 mg cilazapril post-dialysis. Presence of CHF or advanced age has not been shown to significantly alter pharmacokinetic parameters.

Clinical trials: Clinical trials in > 4500 hypertensive patients have evaluated the efficacy of cilazapril. Single daily doses of 2.5 to 5 mg are as effective as single daily doses of: Hydrochlorothiazide (HCTZ; eg, *Esidrix*) 25 to 50 mg; atenolol *(Tenormin)* 50 to 100 mg; sustained release propranolol (eg, *Inderal LA*) 80 to 160 mg; and enalapril 10 to 20 mg. In patients with mild to moderate hypertension, a 5 mg cilazapril dose produces a maximal effect, which can be enhanced by the addition of 12.5 to 25 mg HCTZ. In patients with severe hypertension, including patients with left ventricular hypertrophy, the mean effective dose was 10 mg in combination with 12.5 to 25 mg of HCTZ daily.

Side effects: Cilazapril appears to be well tolerated. In controlled trials of cilazapril monotherapy in > 3500 patients, the most frequently reported side effects were: Headache (4.5%); dizziness (3.3%); fatigue (1.7%); cough (1.6%); chest pain (0.8%); rash, somnolence (0.6%). In patients ≥ 65 years of age, cough, dizziness, palpitations and somnolence occurred slightly more frequently than in younger patients. The addition of HCTZ in an additional 1000 patients resulted in a slightly higher incidence of dizziness, cough and somnolence, while the incidence of other side effects was comparable to cilazapril monotherapy.

Drug interactions: Indomethacin (eg, *Indocin*) considerably attenuates the antihypertensive activity of cilazapril. This attenuation was most pronounced when cilazapril was added to indomethacin, while the addition of indomethacin to a stable cilazapril regimen resulted in a degree of attenuation of effect which was considered to be clinically insignificant. Thus, the significance of this interaction appears to be dependent on the order of drug administration.

Summary: Cilazapril is a long-acting, potent ACE inhibitor. It appears to be well tolerated, while offering the advantage of once-daily dosing; this property may make it a useful addition to a class of drugs whose safety and efficacy continue to be confirmed in a variety of disease states. An NDA for cilazapril was filed in September 1989 for hypertension. Roche and Glaxo will comarket cilazapril as *Inhibace*. On August 13, 1992, the FDA classified cilazapril as "approvable".

Bibliography Available on Request

TERODILINE HCl (*Micturin* by Forest Labs) – An agent for urinary incontinence.

Pharmacology: Terodiline is a secondary amine which has non-selective anticholinergic and calcium blocking effects. Although originally investigated as an anti-anginal agent, terodiline is presently undergoing evaluation in the treatment of patients with bladder incontinence. Terodiline provides the advantage of both anticholinergic and calcium blocking effects within the same plasma concentration range, with anticholinergic effects predominating at lower plasma concentrations and calcium entry blocking action predominating at higher plasma concentrations.

The motor nerve supply to the bladder and urethra is from the parasympathetic system; the neurotransmitter active in this system is acetycholine. Therefore, anticholinergic agents have been used to treat incontinence, but side effects often limit their usefulness. In addition to parasympathetic activity, it appears that calcium entry from the extracellular space is important in the contractile activity of urinary tract smooth muscle. Calcium blockers reduce frequency and amplitude of detrusor contractions and improve bladder capacity; however, side effects associated with their use have prevented their use in treating incontinence.

Pharmacokinetics: Terodiline is well absorbed after oral administration with a bioavailability of ≈ 90%. Peak serum levels occur 2 to 8 hours (average, 4 hours) after administration. Although therapeutic levels have not been clearly established, a steady-state concentration of 0.6 mg/L is generally well tolerated. Higher concentrations of 0.8 to 1.1 mg/L can be maintained in some patients without serious adverse effects.

The volume of distribution is 500 L, ≈ 80% to 85% is bound to serum proteins, and the half-life is ≈ 60 hours. Due to the long half-life, maximum clinical effects will not be seen until ≈ 10 days after initiation of therapy.

Terodiline is extensively metabolized in liver. The major metabolite, parahydroxyterodiline, is minimally active compared to the parent. Approximately 15% of the drug can be recovered unchanged in urine.

Major pharmacokinetic changes occurred in patients with an average age of 85 years (eg, prolongation of half-life, decreased unbound drug fraction and body clearance, increased time to reach steady-state plasma concentrations). A 25 mg/day dose achieved similar plasma concentrations as a 37.5 to 50 mg/day dose in younger, healthier patients. This suggests that elderly patients should have therapy initiated at a dose not to exceed 12.5 mg twice daily, and increased doses should not occur prior to 4 weeks post-initiation.

Clinical trials: Terodiline 12.5 to 25 mg twice daily was effective in the treatment of some patients with urge urinary incontinence. Patients treated with terodiline have a decrease in both pre-micturition symptoms such as urgency and in urinary frequency. One study reported a decrease in voluntary micturitions from a mean of 10.8 to 7.9/day after 6 months of treatment. Another group reported a decrease in involuntary micturitions from 2.5 to 1.5/day with greater effects in those patients with higher baseline micturition frequency.

An increase in bladder capacity has been observed in several studies with one group reporting an average increase from 252 to 335 ml after 6 months of therapy.

A preliminary study suggests that terodiline may be effective in children 6 to 14 years of age involved in a bladder training program to correct urgency or urge incontinence.

Side effects: Up to 50% of patients in some studies reported side effects during the first 3 months of therapy vs 35% with placebo. Most side effects were mild, anticholinergic-related and decreased in frequency (34%) between 3 and 6 months of continuous therapy. The most commonly reported effect was dry mouth (27% during first 3 months, 19% between 3 and 6 months). Other side effects reported during the first 3 months include: Blurred vision (15%); tremor (14%); weight gain (11%); tachycardia (4%); ankle edema (2%). The incidence of these effects decreased between 3 and 6 months. One study reported a small increase (2 mm Hg) in resting diastolic blood pressure after 6 months. Other side effects include: Vertigo; headache; nausea; polymorphic ventricular tachycardia (PVT; reported in other countries).

Summary: Studies to date suggest that terodiline is a safe and effective agent for the treatment of urinary incontinence. Its unique combination of both anticholinergic and calcium blocking activity may provide an advantage over presently available treatments. However, further studies are required to clarify long-term safety and to identify those patients most likely to benefit from terodiline therapy. Forest Labs acquired US licensing rights for the oral tablets from KabiPharmacia in December 1987. Kabi temporarily discontinued the sale of terodiline world wide following reports of an association with PVT. Clinical trials in the US have been put on hold at the request of the FDA. Forest submitted an NDA on August 30, 1989. An anticipated approval date for the drug, which will be marketed as *Micturin*, is now unknown.

Bibliography Available on Request

CELIPROLOL HCl (*Selecor* by Upjohn/Rhone-Poulenc Rorer) – A cardioselective beta-adrenergic blocking agent.

Pharmacology: Celiprolol is a third-generation, cardioselective, hydrophilic beta-adrenoreceptor blocking agent. It possesses weak vasodilating and bronchodilating effects attributed to partial, selective β_2-adrenoreceptor agonist activity and, possibly, direct papaverine-like smooth muscle relaxation. There is evidence for intrinsic sympathomimetic activity (ISA) at the β_2-receptor. The drug is devoid of membrane stabilizing activity (MSA, or quinidine-like effect). Weak alpha$_2$-antagonist properties are also present but are not considered clinically significant at therapeutic doses.

At therapeutic doses, celiprolol reduces heart rate and blood pressure. While the drug dose not generally produce any ECG changes, it can increase the AV nodal functional refractory period. Celiprolol does not appear to alter pulmonary function, nor inhibit bronchodilation induced by agents such as aminophylline (eg, *Phyllocontin*), albuterol (eg, *Proventil*) and ipratropium *(Atrovent)*. Triglycerides, LDL cholesterol and total cholesterol are decreased in some patients while HDL is increased; it appears that total lipid levels are not increased. A reduction in fibrinogen levels has occurred, which may be of some benefit in hypertensive patients with hypercoagulability.

Pharmacokinetics: Following oral administration, absorption is non-linear and dose-dependent. Bioavailability ranges from 30% to 70% following a single 100 mg dose and averages 74% after a 400 mg dose. Single-dose bioavailability is reduced by chlorthalidone (eg, *Hygroton*), hydrochlorothiazide (eg, *Esidrix*) and theophylline (eg, *Theo-Dur*). Food has also reduced bioavailability in some studies, but data are conflicting. Peak plasma concentrations and pharmacodynamic activity are seen 2 to 4 hours after oral administration; pharmacodynamic activity persists for 24 hours. Protein binding is ≈ 25% and the drug follows a hydrophilic pattern of distribution.

Celiprolol is largely unmetabolized and is excreted unchanged in urine and feces. It does not undergo first-pass hepatic metabolism and there are no significant active metabolites. Approximately 15% (range, 3% to 22%) of an oral dose and 50% of an IV dose is recovered in the urine within 3 days, the rest being excreted in the feces. Steady-state concentrations are achieved after 2 to 3 days. The predominant mode of excretion of active drug is renal; renal dysfunction may cause a reduction in systemic clearance and the need for dose reduction. Bioavailability is decreased and the extent of renal elimination increased in patients with cirrhosis. The pharmacokinetics are not significantly different in the elderly. The elimination half-life averages 4 to 5 hours. Placental transfer averages 3% at steady state compared to 18% for propranolol (eg, *Inderal*) and 6% for atenolol *(Tenormin)*.

Clinical trials: Celiprolol is a safe and effective drug for treatment of hypertension and angina. In doses of 200 to 500 mg once daily in the morning, celiprolol reduces blood pressure to comparable levels seen with other β-blockers, calcium blockers and ACE inhibitors. In comparative trials in patients with mild to moderate hypertension, a 200 to 600 mg dose was similar in efficacy to 80 to 160 mg/day propranolol or 100 mg/day atenolol. In patients with angina, celiprolol 300 to 600 mg daily was as effective as propranolol 80 to 160 mg/day or atenolol 50 to 100 mg/day in improving exercise performance, reducing the number of angina attacks and nitroglycerin requirements, and increasing the time to, or reducing the degree of, ST segment depression. The addition of a diuretic to doses of 200 to 400 mg/day may be more effective at controlling blood pressure than the use of celiprolol monotherapy in doses of 300 to 600 mg/day.

Side effects: In a study of > 2300 patients, side effects were mild. GI symptoms (eg, nausea, abdominal discomfort, diarrhea), the most frequently reported complaints, were responsible for drug discontinuation in 13 patients. Cardiovascular symptoms included development of a modest degree of CHF, AV nodal block and bradycardia. Other side effects included: Headache (6%); fatigue (4%); dizziness (3%); insomnia (1%); Raynaud's phenomenon; orthostatic hypotension; bronchial obstruction; tremor; rash; muscle cramps; impotence.

Summary: Celiprolol appears to be well tolerated and effective for the treatment of hypertension and angina. Its combination of cardioselectivity, β_2-agonist activity, hydrophilicity and long duration of action make it unique among currently available drugs in this class. Whether these properties will be useful in the myriad of other applications for which β-blockers have been used (eg, post-MI prophylaxis, migraine, selected arrhythmias) will require additional experience. The NDA for celiprolol was filed by Rhone-Poulenc Rorer in June 1987 for long-term use in controlling hypertension and angina. The drug will be co-marketed by Upjohn under the name *Selecor*.

Bibliography Available on Request

TEICOPLANIN (*Targocid* by Marion-Merrell Dow) – A glycopeptide antibiotic.

Pharmacology: Teicoplanin (teichomycin A2) is a glycopeptide antibiotic complex structurally related to vancomycin (eg, *Vancocin*). It has a similar spectrum of activity but a longer half-life which allows less frequent dosing. It may be administered by IM and IV injection and brief (30 minute) infusion. Teicoplanin is a mixture of six closely related glycopeptide components designated as teicoplanin-A2 (1 through 5) and teicoplanin-A3. The components of the A2 complex account for 90% to 95% of teicoplanin. The drug interferes with cell wall synthesis in susceptible organisms by inhibiting peptidoglycan polymerization.

Like vancomycin, teicoplanin is active only against gram-positive organisms. It is bactericidal against most susceptible strains, with the possible exception of some coagulase-negative staphylococci (which may show reduced susceptibility), where it may be bacteriostatic. It has equivalent or superior activity (based on MIC data) to vancomycin against staphylococci, including both methicillin-sensitive and -resistant *S aureus, S epidermidis,* streptococci (including viridans group, and groups B, C, F and G), enterococci, and many anaerobic gram-positive bacteria, including *Clostridium difficile, C perfringens, Listeria monocytogenes* and *Corynebacterium jeikeium.* Vancomycin-resistant enterococci may be resistant to teicoplanin.

Teicoplanin is usually synergistic with aminoglycosides and imipenem, and additive with rifampin (eg, *Rifadin*). A post-antibiotic effect of 2.4 to 4.1 hours has been reported with both methicillin-sensitive and -resistant strains of *S aureus.*

Pharmacokinetics: Like vancomycin, teicoplanin is minimally absorbed after oral administration; this route is acceptable only for the treatment of pseudomembranous colitis. Following IM administration of 3 mg/kg, peak levels of 5 to 7 mcg/ml are achieved at 2 to 4 hours; bioavailability is 90%. Peak serum levels after IV administration are dependent on the dose and the method of administration. Following administration of 3 mg/kg, peak levels after a 30 second injection or a 30 minute infusion average 53 and 20 mcg/ml, respectively. Trough (24 hour) levels are not influenced. The drug is widely distributed in most tissues and fluids (with the exception of the CSF), although the rate and extent varies. Volume of distribution (Vd) at steady state averages 0.6 to 0.8 L/kg. Protein binding is 90%.

The drug does not appear to undergo metabolism and is excreted in the urine almost entirely by glomerular filtration. The terminal elimination half-life averages 45 to 70 hours. In patients with renal dysfunction and the elderly, the elimination half-life is increased but the Vd is unchanged. Current dosing recommendations for renal impairment state that usual doses be given for the first 3 days. Thereafter, either the dose is reduced or the interval prolonged, based on the degree of renal insufficiency according to the following scheme: Creatinine clearance (Ccr) 40 to 60 ml/min, half the dose or twice the interval; Ccr < 40 ml/min, one-third the dose or triple the interval.

Clinical trials: Reported response rates by type of infection are: Skin and soft tissue (90%); septicemia, bone and joint (89%); endocarditis (83%); respiratory tract (77%). Other applications in which the drug has demonstrated efficacy include: Endocarditis prophylaxis in dental surgery; Hickman catheter and other indwelling device-related infections; neurosurgical shunt ventriculitis; CAPD-related peritonitis (added to dialysate); surgical prophylaxis; presumed gram-positive infections in immunocompromised patients. The usual loading and maintenance doses of 6 mg/kg followed by 3 mg/kg/24 hours may need to be increased in children and in the treatment of *S aureus* endocarditis and septicemia. A reduction in efficacy has been noted in diabetics, immunocompromised patients and when foreign bodies are present.

Side effects: The overall incidence of side effects is 10.3%. Most commonly reported effects include: Non-specific complaints (fatigue, headache, diarrhea) (5.1%); injection site intolerance (pain, redness, phlebitis) (3%); hypersensitivity skin reactions (pruritus, urticaria, maculopapular rash) (2.4%); hematologic abnormalities (eosinophilia, reversible neutropenia, increased platelet count) (2.2%); transient elevation of LFTs (1.7%); nephrotoxicity (0.35% to 0.6%); high-frequency hearing loss which may be irreversible (0.28%); bronchospasm (0.2%); anaphylactoid reactions (0.07%). Teicoplanin does not appear to cause the dose or infusion rate-related histamine release associated with the "red man syndrome", as does vancomycin. Concomitant use of an aminoglycoside appears to increase the incidence of nephrotoxicity.

Summary: Teicoplanin appears to be a safe and effective alternative to vancomycin. Potential advantages appear to be the availability of IM administration, reduced infusion times and volume requirements, the lack of infusion-related reactions and once daily dosing. The NDA for teicoplanin was filed in March 1991. The FDA has given the drug a "1A" priority review rating. Teicoplanin is currently available in 13 countries. It will be available as *Targocid* by Marion Merrell Dow.

Bibliography Available on Request

REMOXIPRIDE (*Roxiam* by Astra/Merck) – An antipsychotic agent.

Pharmacology: Remoxipride, a substituted benzamide, is an atypical antipsychotic agent. It is a weak, but selective, dopamine-2 (D_2) receptor antagonist. D_2 receptors are thought to act in an inhibitory manner on adenylate cyclase, while dopamine-1 (D_1) receptors are associated with adenylate cyclase stimulation. The presynaptic dopamine "autoreceptors", which regulate the synthesis and release of dopamine, appear to be of the D_2 subtype. Many investigators have suggested that it is blockade of the D_2 receptor that mediates the clinical effects of most antipsychotic agents.

Remoxipride has a marked affinity for sigma receptors, which mediate opioid effects; clinical significance is unknown. There is a wide range between the dose that blocks apomorphine-induced hyperactivity and the dose that produces catalepsy, suggesting a favorable separation between the dose associated with antipsychotic effects and that producing extrapyramidal symptoms. The administration of remoxipride causes a significant, transient increase in prolactin release; however, prolonged administration (> 15 days) results in a reduction in this response.

Pharmacokinetics: Remoxipride is almost completely absorbed after oral administration with a bioavailability of 96% for both standard and controlled release (CR) formulations. There is no first-pass metabolism. Plasma levels peak within 1 to 2 hours after administration of standard formulations and within 2 to 6 hours after CR formulations and are linearly related to dose. Volume of distribution averages 0.5 to 0.7 L/kg. Protein binding averages 80%. CSF levels average 6% to 17% of total plasma levels. Breast milk concentrations are ≈ 30% of those in plasma.

Approximately 70% of an administered dose is metabolized in the liver to six inactive oxidized metabolites. Plasma concentrations of unchanged remoxipride are higher in slow debrisoquine metabolizers. Between 10% and 40% of an oral dose is excreted unchanged in the urine. Plasma elimination half-life averages 4 to 7 hours.

Remoxipride is a weak base (pKa 8.9). Urinary elimination is reduced and plasma half-life is prolonged in alkaline urine (pH 7.2). Conversely, acidification of urine (pH 5.2) results in increased urinary elimination and a reduction in half-life. Mean plasma concentrations are increased and the half-life is prolonged in the elderly, in patients with creatinine clearances < 25 ml/min, and in severe liver disease. Most investigators recommend initiating therapy with one-half the usual dose in the elderly.

Clinical trials: Remoxipride is an effective treatment for chronic schizophrenia and acute exacerbations of chronic schizophrenia. Improvement was documented in both positive (eg, thought disturbances, hostility/suspiciousness, hallucinations, delusions) and negative (eg, emotional withdrawal, motor retardation) symptoms. In doses of 150 to 600 mg/day, remoxipride had similar antipsychotic efficacy to haloperidol (eg, *Haldol*) 5 to 45 mg/day and thioridazine (eg, *Mellaril*) 150 to 750 mg/day.

In most clinical trials, therapy was initiated with 300 mg/day. Patients responded to total daily doses of 300 to 450 mg/day (maximum dose, 600 mg/day) during initiation of therapy, and were tapered to usual maintenance doses of 150 to 300 mg/day. Dosage adjustments were made no more frequently than every 3 days and were based on patient response.

Remoxipride may also be effective in the treatment of acute mania.

Side effects: Remoxipride, like other atypical antipsychotic agents (eg, clozapine [*Clozaril*]), causes less frequent extrapyramidal symptoms (EPS) than the classic antipsychotic agents (eg, haloperidol). Long-term, comparative trials reported an EPS incidence of 2% to 15% and 7% to 27% in the remoxipride- and haloperidol-treated groups, respectively. Pooled data from nine comparative trials with haloperidol also showed a lower incidence of insomnia, tiredness/drowsiness, difficulty in concentration and dry mouth in the remoxipride-treated group. Although isolated reports of cardiovascular effects such as postural hypotension are documented, they are not considered to be clinically significant.

Summary: Available data suggests that remoxipride is a safe and effective treatment for schizophrenia. Its favorable side effect profile makes it an important therapeutic option for patients unable to tolerate traditional antipsychotic agents. Additional comparative and long-term studies are necessary to clarify its overall role in the treatment of schizophrenia and evaluate its potential to cause tardive dyskinesia.

An NDA for remoxipride was filed in December 1988. It is currently in phase III clinical trials for the treatment of acute and chronic schizophrenia. However, because of recent reports of aplastic anemia, including one death, in European patients, Astra/Merck notified investigators to discontinue use of the drug. The company has recommended restricting the use of the drug to patients who have failed other antipsychotics. The drug, which will be marketed as *Roxiam* by Astra/Merck, is currently available in the UK, Denmark and Luxembourg. The NDA was withdrawn in December 1993.

Bibliography Available on Request

GEPIRONE HCl (by Bristol-Myers Squibb) – An anxiolytic and antidepressant.

Pharmacology: Gepirone, an azapirone, is chemically related to buspirone *(Buspar)* but unrelated to the benzodiazepines in structure or pharmacology. Gepirone does not directly or indirectly interact with the benzodiazepine-GABA receptor-chloride ion channel complex. Differing from buspirone, gepirone does not interact with dopamine receptors. Its principle effect relates to its action on brain serotonin activity.

The biochemical basis of psychiatric disorders of anxiety and depression may be viewed as a dynamic serotonergic continuum with anxiety representing a relative serotonin (5-HT) excess disease and depression a relative 5-HT deficit disease. Gepirone acts as a *total* agonist on presynaptic 5-HT_1A autoreceptors (inhibit neuronal firing and decrease 5-HT synthesis) and as a *partial* agonist at postsynaptic 5-HT_1A receptors (linked to cyclic-AMP and probably modulate signal transfer).

Partial agonists recognize and bind to receptors, but exert less activity than the *full* agonist. In the absence of the endogenous full agonist (serotonin), gepirone would exert its agonist effects. However, when full agonists are also present, partial agonists compete for receptors. When partial agonists (which have less intrinsic activity) displace full agonists from receptor sites, they decrease synaptic neurotransmission relative to what would have been achieved by the full agonist alone, and thus essentially act as functional antagonists. Therefore, the effects that 5-HT partial agonists (eg, buspirone, gepirone) ultimately exert on 5-HT neurotransmission depend on the serotonergic tone of the synapse in which the drug is working.

In the 5-HT excess state of anxiety, gepirone would act as an agonist on presynaptic 5-HT_1A receptors to decrease 5-HT synthesis and neuronal firing and on the postsynaptic 5-HT_1A receptor as a functional antagonist, resulting in a reduction of hyperserotonergic tone in the brain and an amelioration of anxiety symptomatology. However, effects of gepirone in the relative serotonin deficit disease of depression would be quite different. Gepirone would bind to presynaptic 5-HT_1A receptors and exert its agonist effects to decrease neuron activity. In the 5-HT-deficit state of depression, this action would allow 5-HT depleted neurons to replenish their serotonin stores and thus serve 5-HT homeostasis. Gepirone would also bind to postsynaptic 5-HT_1A receptors, but in the 5-HT-deficient state it would express its agonist effects thus causing normosensitization of postsynaptic 5-HT_1A receptors and restoration of postsynaptic serotonergic activity. This normalization of hyposerotonergic tone in depression would produce antidepressant effects and improvement of depressive symptoms.

Pharmacokinetics: Gepirone is rapidly absorbed after oral administration, reaching peak levels in about 1 hour. It undergoes extensive first-pass metabolism by the liver and has an oral bioavailability of only 15%. Both it and buspirone are hepatically metabolized to the major active metabolite 1-(2-pyrimidinyl) piperazine (1-PP). The plasma half-life of gepirone is 2 to 3 hours. No change in dosing would be anticipated in patients with renal insufficiency or failure.

Clinical trials: Gepirone 30 to 60 mg/day and placebo were compared in a 6 week double-blind trial in 30 outpatients with generalized anxiety disorder. According to various scales, gepirone was significantly superior to placebo and produced improvement in both somatic and psychic anxiety. Significant improvement was delayed and occurred after 2 to 3 weeks of treatment. Predictors of clinical improvement included high levels of baseline anxiety and length of time off anxiolytic therapy (ie, the longer the time off benzodiazepines, etc, the more likely a positive response).

Both a single blind study using doses of 25 to 75 mg/day and a double-blind, placebo controlled study using doses ranging from 5 to 90 mg/day found gepirone exerted significant antidepressant effects in patients with major depression.

Side effects: Gepirone is well tolerated with most side effects reported as mild to moderate. The most frequently reported adverse effects were dizziness, nausea, headache, drowsiness and weakness. Gepirone does not impair memory, verbal fluency or psychomotor performance. Like buspirone, gepirone does not appear to have a potential for causing physical dependence or addiction in humans, and it is expected that gepirone will not interact with alcohol or sedative/hypnotic drugs.

Summary: Gepirone is a nonbenzodiazepine drug similar in structure to buspirone. It lacks the sedative and adverse psychomotor and memory impairment effects of the benzodiazepines and does not appear to have the potential for causing physical dependence or addiction. Gepirone selectively affects the serotonergic system, targeting specifically the serotonin 5-HT_1A receptor subtype. Clinical studies indicate that it possesses both antianxiety and antidepressant properties and is well tolerated.

Gepirone is currently in Phase II/III clinical trials and will be available from Bristol-Myers Squibb. An anticipated approval date is unknown.

Bibliography Available on Request

VELNACRINE (*Mentane* by Hoechst-Roussel) – A cholinesterase inhibitor for Alzheimer's disease.

Pharmacology: Alzheimer's disease is associated with alterations in a number of central neurotransmitters, including norepinephrine, serotonin, somatostatin, corticotropin-releasing factor and acetylcholine. Of these, a disturbance in cholinergic function mediated by a specific deficit of neuronal choline acetyltransferase (an enzyme responsible for the formation of acetylcholine) plays a central role in the etiology of cognitive symptoms in Alzheimer's disease patients. As a result of this association, cholinomimetic compounds such as physostigmine *(Antilirium)* and the investigational agent tacrine (tetrahydroaminoacridine; THA; *Cognex*) have been evaluated with encouraging preliminary results.

Velnacrine (HP 029) is the maleate salt of an alcohol derivative of tacrine. It produces cholinergic-mediated physiological effects and inhibits true- and pseudocholinesterase. The cholinomimetic effects are not due to release of acetylcholine or to a direct muscarinic agonist effect.

Pharmacokinetics: Velnacrine is rapidly and extensively absorbed after oral administration. Peak plasma concentrations are achieved in approximately 1 hour, are linearly proportional to dose and tend to be slightly higher in the elderly (0.9 to 1.7 hours). There appears to be no correlation between plasma levels and therapeutic or adverse effects in individual patients. The drug undergoes conjugation in the liver; the fate and activity of these metabolites are not known. Approximately 11% to 30% of an administered dose is excreted unchanged in the urine. Renal clearance is markedly reduced in the elderly; however, accumulation has not been detected. The half-life is about 2 hours in younger volunteers and is slightly longer (2.5 to 3 hours) in elderly volunteers. Food appears to delay the rate but not extent of absorption.

Clinical trials: Cholinomimetic agents are most effective at improving memory (a core feature of Alzheimer's disease) and reversing scopolamine-induced dementia in animal models. Limited published data suggest that velnacrine, 150 to 225 mg/day in divided doses, produces modest benefit in cognitive function in up to two-thirds of patients, as judged by performance-based measures. Improvement tends to be greatest during dose titration, suggesting the potential for tolerance or the use of inadequate performance measures.

Current evidence suggests that the predominant neurotransmitter defect may vary from one patient to another. Attempts to identify subsets of patients most likely to benefit from cholinesterase inhibitors have yielded conflicting results. In addition, some patients may require combination therapy with different classes of drugs. Until markers are identified that will help predict response, single-drug efficacy trials in all Alzheimer's disease patients are likely to show only modest results.

Side effects: The side effect profile of velnacrine is similar to other cholinomimetic drugs. Nausea, diarrhea, flushing, headache, dizziness and abdominal cramping are reported most frequently and occur more commonly at the higher dose ranges (150 to 300 mg).

In the largest protocol group reported to date, 78% of the patients discontinuing the drug due to an adverse event did so because of elevated liver enzymes. The hepatotoxicity of velnacrine appears to be dose-related, mild and reversible, usually within 4 weeks of discontinuation. Clinical features of the enzyme elevation were consistent with a biochemical insult (70%), hypersensitivity (10%), or a mixture of both.

Summary: Velnacrine appears to be a promising agent for the treatment of Alzheimer's disease. Additional trials are needed to identify subsets of patients most likely to respond, demonstrate sustained efficacy, and assess its place in combination therapy.

An NDA was filed by Hoechst-Roussel in early 1992 for velnacrine *(Mentane)*. The FDA was considering a treatment IND for velnacrine; however, due to concerns over safety and efficacy, the FDA's Peripheral and Central Nervous System Drugs Advisory Committee unanimously decided not to recommend approval of the drug, even under treatment IND status.

Bibliography Available on Request

VILOXAZINE (*Catatrol* by Zeneca) – A bicyclic antidepressant.

Pharmacology: Viloxazine is a bicyclic antidepressant agent. It has noradrenergic reuptake blocking properties and acts, in part, as an amphetamine-like central stimulant. Overall sympathomimetic, sedative and anticholinergic activity is less than that seen with the tricyclic antidepressants (eg, imipramine [eg, Tofranil]). Conflicting data has been reported on the effects of viloxazine on the seizure threshold, with some reports indicating that seizure risk is greater, while others claiming it is less than that seen with traditional tricyclics. Rapid eye movement (REM) sleep and overall sleep time is markedly reduced with viloxazine. It does not appear to potentiate the effects of alcohol.

Pharmacokinetics: Viloxazine is rapidly and almost completely (85%) absorbed after oral administration in the small intestine. Peak blood levels occur 1 to 4 hours after ingestion; however, no correlation has been established between blood levels and clinical response. Volume of distribution averages 0.78 L/kg. The eliminiation half-life ranges from 2 to 5 hours. The drug is extensively metabolized by hydroxylation and oxidation to inactive metabolites in the liver. Only 12% to 15% of the parent compound is eliminated unchanged by the kidneys. In patients > 60 years of age, there appears to be a reduction in viloxazine clearance, possibly due to decreased hepatic metabolism. Specific dosage guidelines in the elderly and patients with hepatic dysfunction have not been established.

Clinical trials: Viloxazine was an effective antidepressant in controlled clinical trials of both hospitalized and outpatient populations with depression. Its efficacy appears to be equivalent to imipramine, with a 60% response rate. Published trials have not examined whether efficacy rates vary with specific types of depression. Viloxazine has also been studied in small groups of patients with narcolepsy and cataplexy (a form of narcolepsy characterized by periods of momentary paralysis); this appears to be a potential target population. Fewer sleep attacks were reported during treatment.

Side effects: Nausea is the most commonly reported side effect, with an average incidence of 19%, but some studies have reported an incidence as high as 50%. Nausea progressing to vomiting was reported in 4.7% of patients. These effects may be minimized by initiating therapy with low doses accompanied by slow, upward dose titration. Headache is also commonly reported. Less frequently reported side effects include: Insomnia; taste disturbances; hypomania; mania; dizziness; tachycardia; ataxia; tremor; confusion; restlessness; dry mouth; constipation; drowsiness; difficult micturition; seizures. The anticholinergic-related side effects appear to occur less frequently than with the tricyclic agents.

Drug interactions: Viloxazine decreases the elimination rate of theophylline (eg, *Theo-Dur*), carbamazepine (eg, *Tegretol*) and phenytoin (eg, *Dilantin*), possibly by competing for the same microsomal enzymes. When viloxazine was added to a stable regimen of these drugs, theophylline toxicity was reported (no levels available), carbamazepine levels increased by 55% and those of its active metabolite by 16%, and phenytoin levels increased by an average of 36%.

Summary: Viloxazine is a safe and effective antidepressant with a somewhat different side effect profile than the tricyclic antidepressants, although it is most likely to be used in patients with narcolepsy or cataplexy. Available data has not established whether viloxazine has any advantages over currently available agents. Additional studies in specific populations of patients are needed to establish its place in therapy. Viloxazine currently has orphan drug status for the treatment of cataplexy and narcolepsy. An NDA was filed in July 1987 for viloxazine, which will be available as *Catatrol* by Zeneca.

Bibliography Available on Request

HALOFANTRINE HCl (*Halfan* by SK Beecham) – A new antimalarial.

Pharmacology: Halofantrine, an antimalarial agent developed by the US Army Antimalarial Program, is active against multi-drug resistant *Plasmodium falciparum* malaria. It is a phenanthrenemethanol, structurally related to mefloquine *(Lariam)*. Halofantrine and its active metabolite, N-desbutylhalofantrine (DHF), are blood schizontocides active against the erythrocyte stages of *Plasmodium* sp. The mechanism of action has not been fully elucidated, but may be similar to other blood schizontocides or involve inhibition of a proton pump at the host-parasite interface. In vitro and clinical data suggest that cross-resistance occurs with mefloquine-resistant strains.

Pharmacokinetics: Following oral administration, absorption is erratic and variable, with a high degree of intra- and intersubject variability. Influencing factors appear to include dietary fat content and the presence or absence of active disease. Racial and genetic factors may also play a role. Since the cure rate appears to be influenced by plasma concentration, irregular absorption and variable peak drug concentrations may be responsible for some treatment failures.

The lack of an IV formulation due to poor solubility precludes accurate bioavailability data. However, the maximum plasma concentration (C_{max}) and area under the plasma concentration-time curve (AUC) of both the parent and active metabolite are significantly increased (up to 6 fold) following administration with a high fat meal. AUC and C_{max} are proportionally related to dose in the range of 250 to 500 mg, but do not increase proportionally when the dose is increased from 500 to 1000 mg. This may explain why single doses of 1.5 g are associated with a high relapse rate. In healthy subjects, half-lives of halofantrine and DHF are approximately 2 and 10 days (range, 4 to 13), respectively. In patients with active disease, the half-life for both compounds is approximately 4 days.

The drug is widely distributed in most tissues and is excreted mainly in the feces as unchanged drug.

Clinical trials: The risk of mortality associated with inadequately treated malaria and the documented efficacy of agents such as chloroquine (eg, *Aralen*) precludes the use of placebo controlled trials and limits comparative trials with halofantrine. Non-comparative trials, using oral doses of 500 mg every 6 hours for 3 doses in adults and children > 40 kg (8 mg/kg in smaller children), have shown the drug to be both safe and effective in the treatment of *P falciparum* infections. A second course of therapy, administered 7 days after initial treatment, is recommended for patients such as non-immune travelers or young children with no previous (or minimal) exposure to malaria.

Cure rates of 83% to 100% have been recorded in areas with high rates of *P falciparum* malaria resistant to chloroquine and sulfonamide/pyrimethamine (eg, *Fansidar*). Following treatment, many symptoms improve within the first day. Fever usually decreases within 18 to 100 hours while parasitemia clears within 34 to 78 hours in most cases. Resolution of splenomegaly and hepatomegaly occurs in approximately 75% of treated patients. A relapse rate of 5.8% has been reported, but it was noted that some of these cases may have represented reinfection. Experience in treatment of *P ovale* and *P malariae* is too limited to be conclusive. Present trials do not support halofantrine's use for prophylaxis.

Side effects: Abdominal pain, vomiting and diarrhea have occurred in 15% to 25% of treated patients. Whether these represent drug- or disease-related events is difficult to distinguish. Pruritus occurs in 2.3% of patients and represents an advantage for African populations, in which chloroquine-induced pruritus is intolerable in 8% to 20% of patients. The pruritus has been characterized as a generalized burning sensation, most pronounced on the soles of the feet, scalp and perineal areas. Onset is usually within the first 14 hours with resolution after 20 hours. Headache and rash have occurred. Anecdotal reports of neuromuscular spasm, mouth ulcers, seizures, ventricular ectopy (PVCs) and intravascular hemolysis have been attributed to halofantrine; cause and effect have not been established.

Summary: Halofantrine appears to be a safe and effective alternative to current therapy for *Plasmodium falciparum* malaria. Additional studies are needed to delineate the role of true drug resistance versus bioavailability factors as causes for treatment failures. Its role in the treatment of *P ovale, P vivax* and *P malariae* has not been determined. Halofantrine was approved by the FDA on July 24, 1992; however, it is not yet commercially available. A release date is unknown at this time.

Bibliography Available on Request

HEXOPRENALINE SULFATE (*Delaprem* by Altana) – A tocolytic agent.

Pharmacology: Hexoprenaline sulfate is a β_2-selective adrenergic agonist. Structurally, it is two norepinephrine molecules joined through their amino groups by a hexamethylene bridge. This compound, while retaining the catechol moiety, has a longer duration of action than classic catecholamines (eg, isoproterenol [eg, *Isuprel*]), and is orally active. Stimulation of uterine β_2-receptors results in a decrease in the frequency and intensity of uterine smooth muscle contractions, believed to be due to a decrease in myometrial cellular calcium. These local effects, as well as the systemic effects, are mediated by adenyl cyclase and cyclic adenosine 3'-5'-monophosoate (cAMP) and are antagonized by β-blocking compounds. Uterine activity and the frequency and intensity of uterine contractions following an IV bolus of 7.5 mcg are reduced by 70%, 40% and 50%, respectively; further reductions can be achieved with repeat boluses or administration of a continuous infusion. IV administration is associated with a dose-dependent increase in heart rate (> 20 to 30 beats/minute) and systolic blood pressure (mean,+13 mm Hg), and a reduction in diastolic blood pressure (mean, -21 mm Hg), producing a widening of the pulse pressure. At equivalent tocolytic doses, the increase in heart rate and systolic blood pressure is reported to be less than that seen with ritodrine *(Yutopar)*. Maternal glucose, insulin, glucagon and free fatty acid levels increase while serum potassium levels and pH may decrease.

Pharmacokinetics: A lack of published data in humans precludes an accurate description of the pharmacokinetic profile of hexoprenaline. However, certain characteristics may be inferred from available clinical trials. Following administration of an IV bolus of 7.5 mcg, the mean time to onset of stable uterine activity was 12.9 ± 6.9 minutes, with return to baseline activity at 33.7 ± 17.8 minutes. Similar values (34.9 ± 12.7 minutes) were reported for the time required for the heart rate to return to baseline. Return to uterine activity and heart rate baselines was similar following discontinuation of a continuous infusion of 0.38 mcg/min for 20 minutes (37.3 ± 13 minutes and 35.3 ± 13 minutes, respectively). In rats, two methylated metabolites have been identified, one of which is active.

Clinical trials: In available, published clinical trials, hexoprenaline is an effective tocolytic. When compared to ritodrine, equivalent tocolytic doses produced less maternal tachycardia and elevation of systolic blood pressure. It has also been used, as an IV bolus or bolus plus infusion, to control contraction-related fetal heart rate abnormalities, a marker of fetal distress. In this latter setting, the desired increase in fetal heart rate was attributed to control of uterine contractions and, possibly, an increase in placental blood flow, since <1% of hexoprenaline was shown to cross the placenta in rabbits and in an in vitro model.

Side effects: Hexoprenaline shares the side effect profile of the β_2-agonists such as tremor, tachycardia (maternal and fetal), arrhythmias (supraventricular and ventricular), myocardial ischemia, hypotension, hyperglycemia and hypokalemia. However, available data suggest that the frequency and severity of these adverse effects is less than that seen with β_2-agonist tocolytics currently in clinical use (eg, ritodrine, terbutaline [*Brethine, Bricanyl*]) and are usually only seen in the higher dose ranges. A recent report also describes non-cardiac pulmonary edema, a recognized complication of this form of therapy but not previously reported with hexoprenaline. As with the other β_2-agonist tocolytics, preexisting myocardial dysfunction, iatrogenic fluid overload and the concomitant administration of glucocorticoids appear to increase the risk of this complication.

Summary: Hexoprenaline appears to be a safe and effective agent for the treatment of premature uterine contractions. Limited available data suggest that, at doses that produce effective tocolysis, side effects, particularly maternal tachycardia, are less frequent or severe than those seen with currently used β_2-agonist tocolytics. Additional data are required to determine its relative place in therapy. An NDA has been filed by Altana and is currently pending. On February 2, 1990, the FDA's Fertility and Maternal Health Drugs Advisory Committee recommended approval for hexoprenaline for suppression of uterine contractions during premature labor. Hexoprenaline, which will be available as *Delaprem,* is currently available in several other countries.

Bibliography Available on Request

VIGABATRIN (*Sabril* by Marion Merrell Dow) - An anticonvulsant agent.

Pharmacology: Vigabatrin is a second generation antiepileptic which appears to exert its mechanism of action via increasing brain GABA levels by inhibition of GABA metabolism. These effects on GABA appear to be dose-related. Vigabatrin has an S(+)-enantiomer that inhibits GABA-T, whereas the R(-)-enantiomer has almost no effect. Vigabatrin's mechanism of action may also be attributed to its ability to decrease excitation-related amino acids, aspartate, glutamate and glutamine concentrations in the brain but these same changes do not occur in the CSF.

Pharmacokinetics: Although the exact bioavailability of vigabatrin is not known, following oral administration about 80% of the dose is recovered in the urine. In healthy volunteers, its absorption was rapid and peak plasma concentrations occurred within the first 2 hours. When vigabatrin was administered with food, its approximate bioavailability was 92% ± 11%. Vigabatrin has a volume of distribution of about 0.8 L/kg, is not bound to plasma proteins and distributes into the CSF. The drug does not appear to be metabolized by the liver, or influence hepatic metabolism. The elimination half-life observed in 24 volunteers was approximately 7 hours and does not appear to be significantly affected by single or multiple dosing, and appears to be similar in both adults and children. Dosing adjustments may be necessary in patients with renal impairment (Ccr less than 60 ml/min) and in the elderly.

Clinical trials: When traditional antiepileptic therapies including add on treatments are used, up to 25% of patients still experience seizures. The studies examining the efficacy of vigabatrin as an antiepileptic medication were primarily add-on trials in patients with resistant epilepsy. Reductions in seizure frequency have been observed in patients with partial and complex partial seizures, but reductions have been observed less frequently with primary generalized seizures, and no reductions (and even worsening) of absence and myoclonic seizures. In a meta-analysis of nine European trials, of the patients with complex partial seizures, 72% showed a > 25% decrease in seizure frequency over a 7 to 12 week period. When combining all clinical trials (including European studies) examining the efficacy of vigabatrin in treatment of resistant partial complex epilepsy, between 33% and 61% of patients experienced a > 50% reduction in seizure frequency at doses between 1 and 4 g/day.

The use of vigabatrin in doses ranging from 50 to 150 mg/kg/day has also been studied as add-on therapy in children with partial, generalized, Lennox-Gaustaut Syndrome and West Syndrome. Results appear similar to those in adults; children with partial seizures appeared to respond better with rates between 38% and 49% of patients experiencing between a 50 to 100 reduction in seizure frequency. Vigabatrin has also been examined in the use of intractable infantile spasms and was found to be effective in reducing spasms > 50% in 30 patients (71%), with complete relief of spasms in 16 patients (38%). Caution should be used in the interpretation of these results since great variability can occur with the incidence of infantile seizures over time.

Side effects: Vigabatrin appears to be well tolerated with minimal side effects and when they do occur, they are mild. In a trial of 254 patients who received vigabatrin from 12 months to > 2 years, up to 75% of patients reported no side effects. Data from pooled studies indicate that the most common side effects are: Somnolence; fatigue; irritability; dizziness; headache; depression; confusion; poor concentration; abdominal pain; anorexia (some trials have reported weight gain). In the studies involving children, the main side effects observed were agitation and insomnia, with a similar number of patients reporting a lack of side effects (79%).

Drug interactions: One of the major advantages of vigabatrin is the fact that it does not appear to be metabolized by the liver, nor influence hepatic metabolism. Therefore, the typical drug interactions observed with traditional anticonvulsants are not seen with vigabatrin. However, vigabatrin was shown to decrease phenytoin (eg, *Dilantin*) levels by 20% to 30% in clinical trials. No mechanism of action could account for the decreased levels; therefore, phenytoin levels should be monitored if vigabatrin is added. Vigabatrin does not appear to interact with phenobarbital, primidone, carbamazepine (eg, *Tegretol*) or valproate (eg, *Depakene*) to any clinically significant degree.

Summary: Vigabatrin appears to be effective in the treatment of complex partial seizures, less effective for primary generalized seizures and not effective (and may even worsen) absence and myoclonic seizures. The dosing range is from 1 to 4 g/day in adults, with 2 to 3 g appearing to be the most optimal and a dose of 50 to 150 mg/kg/day in children. Side effects are minimal and mild and there seems to be a lack of clinically significant drug interactions, except that observed with phenytoin.

Vigabatrin is already available in Europe. An anticipated approval date is unknown.

Bibliography Available on Request

VESNARINONE (*Arkin-Z* by Otsuka) - An inotropic agent for CHF.

Pharmacology: Vesnarinone, a quinolinone derivative, is an oral inotropic agent with little to no effect on heart rate or myocardial oxygen consumption. The mechanism of action is largely unknown. It may be related to a slight inhibition of PDE III which causes an increase in cyclic AMP and finally an increase in the inward calcium current. There is also a reduction in the potassium current.

In addition, vesnarinone inhibits the production and release of cytokines such as TNF-alpha, IL-1, IL-2 and IFN-gamma. This inhibition may relate directly to its efficacy as an inotropic agent. Increased concentrations of TNF-alpha are seen in patients with chronic heart failure. These increased concentrations depress myocardial contractility, alter muscle membrane potential, decrease blood pressure and precipitate pulmonary edema. Therefore, reducing the concentration of TNF-alpha is beneficial in patients with heart failure.

Interestingly, vesnarinone also inhibits the replication of HIV-1 in peripheral blood lymphocytes and in chronically infected macrophages, suggesting that it may be useful in treating patients with HIV-1 disease.

Pharmacokinetics: The pharmacokinetic parameters of vesnarinone were evaluated in 21 healthy male volunteers in a two-phase, nonblinded trial. In phase I, subjects received vesnarinone in a sequentially ascending single dose ranging from 7.5 to 240 mg. In phase II, three subjects received vesnarinone 30 mg daily for 15 days. The elimination half-life was 44.7 ± 1.2 hour and the clearance 0.284 ± 0.018 L/hr. The drug was fairly extensively metabolized, with only 11% to 27% (mean, 17.7%) being excreted unchanged in the urine. The authors concluded that elimination of vesnarinone is dose-dependent and that plasma concentrations are proportional to the dose administered.

Clinical trials: In two small, uncontrolled trials, vesnarinone was administered to a total of 20 patients with CHF; significant hemodynamic and functional improvement was seen. In a small, placebo controlled study, eight patients with chronic, stable, moderate CHF received vesnarinone 60 mg/day or placebo for 4 to 8 weeks. Patients were then crossed over to the alternate treatment group. Symptomatic improvement was noted in four patients while receiving vesnarinone. In addition, vesnarinone caused an increase in contractility of the left ventricle. Mild to moderate dyspnea and fatigue on exertion was seen in all patients while receiving placebo. In two placebo controlled double-blind trials, a total of 159 patients with CHF were randomized to receive vesnarinone 60 mg/day or placebo for 12 weeks. In both trials there was an improvement in the quality of life and a reduction in the severity or progression of heart failure in patients receiving vesnarinone.

The long-term use of vesnarinone was evaluated in a double-blind trial involving 477 patients with CHF. Patients were randomized to receive vesnarinone 60 mg/day or placebo for 6 months. Patients receiving vesnarinone experienced an improvement in their quality of life and a reduction in morbidity and mortality when compared to patients receiving placebo. In the initial design of this trial, patients could also be randomized to receive vesnarinone 120 mg/day. However, this treatment group was stopped after the first 253 patients had been enrolled because of a significant increase in mortality. These results suggest that vesnarinone may have a narrow therapeutic window.

Side effects: The primary side effect noted with vesnarinone use is reversible neutropenia seen in 2.5% of patients. Other reported side effects include: Reversible agranulocytosis; palpitations; dyspnea; gastric discomfort; nausea; headache; skin rash.

Summary: Vesnarinone is a new positive inotropic agent that appears to be effective in the management of CHF. Because of its unique mechanism of action involving inhibition of cytokines, vesnarinone may prove to be a useful alternative in the long-term management of this patient population. It appears to be well tolerated with the exception of the relatively high incidence of reversible neutropenia. Because of this potentially serious toxicity, the clinical utility of vesnarinone remains to be determined.

Although vesnarinone is currently available in Japan, all research ended in the US on July 31, 1996.

Bibliography Available on Request

TIRILAZAD (*Freedox* by Upjohn) - A 21-aminosteroid antioxidant.

Pharmacology: Tirilazad mesylate is a 21-aminosteroid (also referred to as lazaroids) with distinct antioxidant properties. It does not manifest glucocorticoid activity. Tirilazad acts as a cytoprotective agent that oxidizes peroxyl radicals and stabilizes cell membranes. It also helps to preserve the membrane content of vitamin E (alphatocopherol), another important antioxidant. As a result of its ability to prevent lipid peroxidation in cell membranes, tirilazad promotes tissue survival in the vicinity of a CNS injury.

Due to the high content of polyunsaturated lipids in neuronal membranes, the CNS is particularly susceptible to the destructive effects of oxygen radicals. Tissue injury occurring during CNS trauma or a stroke increases oxygen radical production, which in turn leads to damaging lipid peroxidation reactions. Such oxygen radical-mediated processes appear to be involved in posttraumatic brain edema, spinal axonal degeneration and microvascular damage. The progressive secondary tissue destruction which follows the precipitating event may be amenable to therapy with antioxidants.

Pharmacokinetics: Tirilazad is administered in a citrate solution as an IV infusion over not more than 30 minutes. It is a lipophilic substance that distributes extensively to tissue, with a volume of distribution of about 1.7 L/kg. The drug appears to follow a multi-compartment elimination pattern. Following a single dose, the half-life is approximately 3.75 hours. However, upon multiple dosing, a terminal elimination half-life of 35 hours has been observed. Elimination occurs via hepatic metabolism. The clearance of tirilazad is roughly equal to hepatic plasma flow.

Clinical trials: In numerous neurological studies of animal models, tirilazad has shown distinct promise as a useful therapeutic agent for brain and spinal injury, aneurysmal subarachnoid hemorrhage (SAH) and stroke. Phase III clinical trials are currently being conducted in each of these areas.

The second National Acute Spinal Cord Injury Study (NASCIS 2) demonstrated that patients treated with high-dose methylprednisolone (eg, *Solu-Medrol*; 8 to 9 g/day) within 8 hours of injury, experienced significantly greater neurological improvement than those treated with placebo. The efficacy of methylprednisolone in slowing the progression of CNS damage is believed to be due to its antioxidant properties rather than its glucocorticoid activity. For this reason, in NASCIS 3 (an ongoing follow-up study), one of the three treatment arms involves 2 g methylprednisolone bolus, followed by 2.5 mg/kg tirilazad infusion every 6 hours for a total of 48 hours.

To date, most of the clinical efficacy trials conducted with tirilazad have studied its use in SAH. Upjohn has submitted three double-blind, randomized, placebo controlled study results to the FDA in support of an NDA for tirilazad in the treatment of SAH. However, an FDA committee determined that these studies did not confirm efficacy; one study showed an improvement in males, but this was not replicated in another study, and there were no differences in females.

Tirilazad and newer, more potent antioxidants may also be studied in other neurologic conditions in which peroxidative mechanisms have been implicated. These include Alzheimer's disease, Parkinson's disease and multiple sclerosis.

Side effects: Tirilazad has been shown to be safe in elderly patients (average age, 66 years) with acute ischemic stroke at doses up to 6 mg/kg/day for 3 days. In healthy volunteers, tirilazad had no effect on cerebral blood flow or cerebral oxygen metabolism. Studies have failed to show any significant glucocorticoid effect to be caused by the drug. Up to 50% of subjects in one study exhibited a moderate, transient increase in serum alanine transaminase. Thus far, the most noted side effect has been mild to moderate pain at the injection site, occurring in 60% to 80% of patients.

Studies involving tirilazad and both nimodipine (*Nimotop*) and cimetidine (eg, *Tagamet*) have failed to identify a clinically significant drug interaction with either of those drugs.

Summary: Tirilazad is a potent antioxidant, similar in structure to other steroids, but without glucocorticoid activity. Due to its ability to prevent oxygen radical-mediated lipid peroxidation, it may prove to be useful in preventing progressive neuronal degeneration and associated complications following brain and spinal injury, SAH and stroke.

Upjohn submitted a new drug application in June 1994 for tirilazad with the indication of SAH. Due to the lack of serious side effects that have been documented thus far, and the considerable potential benefit that this drug possesses as a therapeutic agent in areas greatly in need of new treatment modalities, approval is anticipated. However, on September 26, 1994, the FDA's Peripheral and Central Nervous System Drugs Advisory Committee decided that the studies for tirilazad did not confirm efficacy and that further studies would be necessary. A Treatment IND program was discussed as a possibility.

Bibliography Available on Request

TIAGABINE (by Abbott/Novo Nordisk) - An antiepileptic.

Pharmacology: Evidence has shown that decreased GABAergic inhibition may be a cause or partial cause of epilepsy. There are several ways of increasing GABAergic inhibition; augmenting the synthesis of GABA (eg, valproic acid [eg, *Depakene*]); by giving drugs that act as GABA agonists; inhibition of GABA metabolism (eg, vigabatrin [*Sabril*; investigational]); stimulating the release of GABA; and inhibiting the uptake of GABA (eg, tiagabine). Tiagabine is a second generation antiepileptic which appears to prolong the action of GABA by increasing brain GABA levels via inhibition of the high-affinity uptake systems into presynaptic neurons and glia.

Pharmacokinetics: The exact bioavailability of tiagabine is not known. Following oral administration approximately 25% of the dose is recovered in the urine and 63% in the feces. Very little drug is recovered unchanged in the urine suggesting that tiagabine is extensively metabolized. The absorption of tiagabine is complete and rapid with peak plasma concentrations occurring within 0.5 to 1 hour after administration. Food reduces the rate, but not the extent of absorption of tiagabine. The elimination half-life of tiagabine is variable with a range from 4.5 to 13.4 hours (mean, 6.7) but does not appear to be dose-related or significantly affected by single or multiple dosing. Tiagabine does not influence hepatic metabolism of other antiepileptic agents but it may be metabolized by the cytochrome P450 system, and therefore its metabolism may be influenced by other antiepileptic agents. A study involving elderly subjects concluded that the pharmacokinetics of tiagabine are similar to younger subjects.

Clinical trials: Single or add-on therapy with traditional antiepileptic agents fails to control seizure frequency in up to 30% of epileptic patients. Studies examining the efficacy of tiagabine were primarily add-on trials in patients with resistant epilepsy. A few of the studies utilized a technique referred to as enrichment (Amery design). This design initially enrolls all subjects under open, dose escalation conditions for 4 to 8 weeks. Only those patients who respond at a preset percent reduction in seizure frequency and do not experience unacceptable adverse effects continue to the double-blind, crossover or parallel phase of the study where tiagabine is compared to placebo for up to 23 weeks. There are both advantages and disadvantages to this design. The main disadvantage is the difficulty in comparing results from this type of study to traditional clinical trials.

Reductions in seizure frequency have been observed in patients with complex partial, simple partial and secondarily generalized tonic-clonic seizures receiving other antiepileptic agents. Tiagabine doses ranged from 8 to 64 mg/day. When combining all clinical trials, 24% to 26% of subjects with complex partial seizures, 37% with simple seizures and 44% to 63% with tonic-clonic seizures involved in the double-blind phase of the studies showed a > 50% decrease in seizure frequency. In all cases, tiagabine was found to reduce seizure frequency significantly more than placebo. One study determined that the minimum effective dose for tiagabine is 32 mg/day.

Side effects: Tiagabine appears to be well tolerated with minimal, mild side effects. It does not cause any significant changes in vital signs or laboratory values. The incidence and severity of adverse effects appear to be dose related. Side effects are mild/moderate when patients are administered 12 mg/day; 24 mg/day leads to a higher incidence. Tiagabine has only been administered as add-on therapy, therefore it is difficult to determine the exact side effect profile. The incidence of side effects with tiagabine add-on therapy are similar to placebo. Data from pooled studies indicate that the most common side effects are: Dizziness; asthenia; headache; somnolence; ataxia; tiredness; poor concentration; abnormal thinking; depression; nervousness; tremor.

Drug interactions: Tiagabine does not influence hepatic metabolism, therefore it should not affect the metabolism of other antiepileptic agents. Several combinations of antiepileptic agents have been shown to affect the metabolism of tiagabine and therefore, adjustments in the dose of tiagabine are probably warranted. Combination administration of carbamazepine (eg, *Tegretol*) and phenytoin (eg, *Dilantin*), primidone (eg, *Mysoline*) or vigabatrin has been shown to induce the metabolism of tiagabine, although valproate has not been shown to cause this effect.

Summary: Tiagabine appears to be effective in the treatment of complex partial, simple partial and secondarily generalized tonic-clonic seizures. The dosing range used in studies was from 8 to 64 mg/day in adults, with a dose of 32 mg/day appearing to be the minimum effective dose.

Tiagabine is currently in late clinical trials. An anticipated approval date is unknown.

Bibliography Available on Request

TENIDAP (*Enable* by Pfizer) - An anti-inflammatory cytokine inhibitor.

Pharmacology: Tenidap sodium is an anti-inflammatory agent being developed for use in the treatment of rheumatoid arthritis and osteoarthritis. Whereas NSAIDs decrease prostaglandin synthesis by inhibiting cyclooxygenase, tenidap appears to inhibit both cyclooxygenase and 5-lipoxygenase, thus impairing production of both prostaglandins and leukotrienes.

Although the exact mechanism of action has not been determined, in vitro studies suggest that tenidap lowers concentrations of interleukin-1, interleukin-6, leukotriene B4, tumor necrosis factor and C-reactive proteins. It also inhibits the release of neutrophil collagenase.The arachidonic acid metabolites inhibited by tenidap are potent inflammatory mediators that profoundly augment leukocyte chemotaxis. The failure of NSAIDs to inhibit the lipoxygenase pathway partially explains their inability to significantly alter the progressive tissue destruction often associated with rheumatoid arthritis. Thus, the unique pharmacology of tenidap provides the drug with a distinct pharmacologic advantage over NSAIDs.

Pharmacokinetics: To date, pharmacokinetic data on tenidap have not been published. It is known that the drug is roughly 99% reversibly bound to albumin, and multiple dosing of 120 mg/day yields a serum concentration of approximately 5 to 15 mg/L.

Clinical trials: A recent report describes four separate studies comparing tenidap to naproxen (eg, *Naprosyn*) or placebo in treating rheumatoid arthritis (RA). Doses of tenidap ranged from 40 to 120 mg/day; naproxen dosage was 500 mg twice daily. Patients were allowed to remain on other medications, such as auranofin (*Ridaura*), penicillamine (*Cuprimine*; *Depen*), hydroxychloroquine (*Plaquenil Sulfate*) and prednisone (eg, *Deltasone*). Durations ranged from 2 weeks to 1 year. All four studies demonstrated a significantly greater reduction in C-reactive protein with tenidap than with naproxen or placebo.

In another study, 374 patients with RA treated previously with only NSAIDs were randomized to receive either tenidap 120 mg/day or auranofin 3 mg twice daily with diclofenac (*Cataflam*; *Voltaren*) 50 mg 3 times daily. Evaluation included patient and physician assessments of disease activity, number of painful joints, swollen joints and pain. After 9 months, there was no significant difference between the two therapies, though a higher rate of discontinuation was reported for auranofin due to diarrhea.

A similar trial involving 367 RA patients compared 120 mg/day of tenidap to piroxicam (eg, *Feldene*) 20 mg/day, alone and in combination with hydroxychloroquine 400 mg/day, for 2 years. Based on clinical evaluation, results indicated that tenidap therapy was more effective than piroxicam and equally as effective as the combination of piroxicam and hydroxychloroquine.

A 1-year multi-center study of 488 RA patients compared clinical efficacy of treatment with 40, 80 or 120 mg/day tenidap to treatment with 500, 750 or 1000 mg/day naproxen, beginning with the lowest dose and titrating to clinical response. Efficacy of the two treatments was not significantly different during the first 4 weeks, but tenidap became significantly more efficacious by 24 weeks. Reductions in all acute phase reactants were significantly greater in the tenidap-treated group.

Side effects: The most significant side effect reported in tenidap clinical trials has been reversible proteinuria of proximal tubular origin, occurring in ≤ 20% of patients. This has not been associated with renal function impairment. One study reported 24% GI side effects in patients receiving tenidap.

Summary: Studies conducted to date, both in vitro and in vivo, clearly suggest that tenidap is a unique anti-rheumatoid agent with disease modifying potential. Based on clinical and laboratory parameters, tenidap is more efficacious than NSAIDs and comparable to current mainstays of RA therapy. Tenidap appears to hold promise as a major new drug in the management of rheumatoid arthritis and osteoarthritis.

Pfizer filed an NDA with the FDA for tenidap on December 22, 1993. It will be available as *Enable*.

Bibliography Available on Request

SERTINDOLE (by Abbott Laboratories) - An antipsychotic agent.

Pharmacology: Sertindole is a new "atypical" antipsychotic agent with unique pharmacologic properties compared to traditional agents. The mechanism of action of sertindole is via its strong antagonism of dopamine D_2, serotonin 5-HT_2 and norepinephrine alpha$_1$ receptors. Sertindole appears to have low extrapyramidal symptoms (EPS) potential, does not cause anticholinergic side effects, does not inhibit cognitive functioning and has potent anxiolytic activity.

Pharmacokinetics:

Immunocompromised patients – Sertindole is slowly absorbed from the GI tract with a peak plasma concentration achieved after 8 to 10 hours. Following a single oral dose, the elimination half-life is approximately 60 hours, but there is great patient variability with 10% of subjects demonstrating half-lives > 100 hours after administration of a single dose. Due to sertindole's long half-life, steady-state concentrations are not reached until after 3 to 4 weeks. The long half-life of sertindole should allow for once-daily dosing. Sertindole is characterized by non-linear kinetics. Increasing the dose by 20% can increase plasma concentrations by approximately 40%. Sertindole is significantly bound to plasma proteins (> 99%), with only a small amount of the drug being renally excreted; therefore, sertindole will presumably not be eliminated by dialysis. In vitro studies have shown that sertindole is predominately metabolized by the hepatic cytochrome P450 3A4 isoform system and eliminated via the GI tract. Sertindole has two metabolites, norsertindole and Lu 28-092, but the activity of these metabolites has not been established.

Clinical trials: In seven phase I trials, over 100 healthy patients received sertindole 0.5 to 32 mg as a single dose or in escalating dosing for up to 14 days. These studies demonstrated that, overall, sertindole was safe and well tolerated.

Three phase II studies examined the efficacy of sertindole in doses of 4 to 24 mg/day. The first was a pilot, double-blind, randomized, placebo controlled, multi-center study designed to compare the efficacy of sertindole (n = 27) and placebo (n = 11) in patients diagnosed with schizophrenia or schizoaffective disorder. The study concluded that sertindole was effective in most patients at a dose of 16 or 20 mg/day and this therapy was associated with minimal adverse effects.

The second and third phase II studies were randomized, double-blind, multi-centered and placebo controlled with identical study designs except that each study had four different treatment groups: 8, 12 or 20 mg/day of sertindole or placebo in the second trial, and the third study had 4 or 12 mg/day sertindole, placebo or haloperidol (eg, *Haldol*) 8 mg twice daily. All patients taking sertindole were titrated upwards starting with 4 mg/day and increasing by 4 mg every third day until the desired dose was reached. The titration phase lasted 12 days and the maintenance phase period was 28 days. Patients enrolled in both studies had to have a previous response to antipsychotic drugs. There were 205 patients enrolled in the second trial and 109 in the third; 153 patients completed at least 13 of the total 40 days of the second trial and were included in the final analysis (107 completed the entire study). Only the 20 mg sertindole group significantly improved in all efficacy parameters compared to placebo. Sertindole 20 mg was equally efficacious to haloperidol but caused fewer side effects.

In a long term, open-label study, sertindole 4 to 24 mg/day was administered to 170 patients for up to 2 years to determine its safety and efficacy. The mean exposure to sertindole was 121 days (range, 2 to 532 days) and the most common dose administered was 20 mg/day (33%).

Side effects: Adverse effects observed during phase I trials included lethargy, drowsiness, nasal congestion, sexual dysfunction, GI complaints, dizziness, lightheadedness, mild tremor, orthostatic hypotension, syncope, dystonia, postural hypotension and cogwheel rigidity. No patients experienced EPS. The most common adverse effects experienced during phase II trials that occurred more often with sertindole 20 mg/day than with placebo included: Headache (26%); nasal congestion (26%); dry ejaculation (17%); constipation, dizziness, somnolence (11%). Dry ejaculation was the only side effect that was found to be significantly greater than placebo ($p < 0.05$). Adverse effects experienced during the long term study were similar, but incidence rates were higher.

Summary: Sertindole should provide an effective and safe alternative treatment when therapy with traditional antipsychotics have failed due to lack of efficacy or intolerable side effects. Additional trials are necessary to establish the long term safety, especially the incidence of tardive dyskinesia, and efficacy of sertindole. The drug, which will be available from Abbott may be " approvable" in 1997.

Bibliography Available on Request

PENCICLOVIR (SmithKline Beecham) - An antiherpes virus agent.

Pharmacology: Penciclovir is a potent, selective antiherpes virus agent that has activity in vitro against herpes simplex virus (HSV) type 1 and 2 and varicella-zoster virus (VZV). Its spectrum of antiviral activity is similar to that of acyclovir (*Zovirax*), but it has the advantage of a longer duration of effect.

Both acyclovir and penciclovir are efficient inhibitors of viral DNA replication. They are initially phosphorylated to the monophosphate salt, a reaction that is catalyzed by virus-induced thymidine kinase. There is then subsequent phosphorylation to the triphosphate ester (TPE) by cellular enzymes. In in vitro studies, both penciclovir and acyclovir were phosphorylated to the TPE in HSV-1, HSV-2 and VZV infected cells; only very low concentrations of the ester were noted in uninfected cells. The concentration of the TPE was much greater and was maintained for a longer period of time in all three viral strains treated with penciclovir vs acyclovir. The half-lives of the penciclovir-TPE were 10, 20 and 7 hours in HSV-1, HSV-2 and VZV infected cells, respectively, compared to approximately 1 hour for acyclovir. It is thought that the TPE of acyclovir is rapidly metabolized to the acylonucleoside which then diffuses out of the cell. In contrast, penciclovir maintains its activity even when blood levels decrease since this diffusion is not observed with its ester. It is the TPE of both agents that is an efficient inhibitor of viral replication. Unlike acyclovir, penciclovir is not an obligate DNA chain terminator. Inhibition of viral DNA polymerase is effective due to the high concentration of penciclovir in infected cells.

Pharmacokinetics: The pharmacokinetic parameters of penciclovir were studied in 15 healthy male subjects. A single dose was administered as a 60 minute infusion at doses of 10, 15 or 20 mg/kg. There were 5 subjects for each dosing level and escalation to the next dose only occurred if subjects tolerated the previous dose level. Penciclovir exhibited a linear pharmacokinetic profile in the dose range studied. The C_{max} was 12.1, 19.6 and 22.7 mcg/ml for doses of 10, 15 and 20 mg/kg, respectively. It is believed that penciclovir distributes into tissues because the volume of distribution for all three dose levels exceeded 100 L. Elimination was primarily renal with > 70% of the drug being recovered in the urine after 72 hours. Penciclovir has shown limited oral absorption in animal trials, so there have been a variety of prodrugs developed to facilitate oral administration. One such drug that is already commercially available is famciclovir (*Famvir*); > 50% of an oral dose of famciclovir is absorbed and is then rapidly converted to penciclovir. Famciclovir (125, 250, 500 and 750 mg) was administered to 20 healthy male subjects; at all four dose levels penciclovir was the major metabolite detected 15 to 30 minutes after oral administration. The C_{max} occurred at 0.5 to 0.75 hours after the dose was administered. Approximately 60% of the oral famciclovir dose was excreted as penciclovir in the urine within 24 hours.

Clinical trials: In vitro, penciclovir decreased HSV yield with a shorter period of exposure compared to acyclovir. In addition, HSV replication remained inhibited for several days after removal of penciclovir from the medium. This same effect has not been seen with acyclovir. In one trial, 20 isolates each of HSV-1 and HSV-2 were treated with acyclovir and penciclovir; the drugs had similar activity against both strains of HSV. One isolate of HSV-1 was intermediate to acyclovir but sensitive to penciclovir. Seven isolates of each HSV-1 and HSV-2 were then studied for the effect of in vitro pulse therapy; penciclovir was better than acyclovir at inhibiting viral replication. The activity of penciclovir has also been studied against 23 isolates of HSV that were either acyclovir-sensitive or -resistant. The activity of penciclovir paralleled that of acyclovir; isolates highly resistant to acyclovir were also highly resistant to penciclovir. Therefore, penciclovir does not show promise for the treatment of acyclovir-resistant strains of HSV. In vivo trials with penciclovir have not been published to date.

Side effects: In the dose-escalation, pharmacokinetic trial described above there were no significant adverse drug effects observed with penciclovir administration. One subject developed a mild headache 1 hour after dosing that lasted for 9 hours. There was a slight decrease in supine diastolic blood pressure 1 hour after the infusion and standing diastolic blood pressure 2 hours after the 20 mg/kg dose and a slight increase in creatinine clearance was also noted; however, the effects were not clinically significant.

Summary: Penciclovir is a new antiviral agent with similar activity to acyclovir. However, because it is able to achieve higher levels of the TPE within the viral cell and to sustain the levels for a longer period of time, it may offer the advantages of treatment with lower doses at less frequent intervals compared to acyclovir. Because of poor oral absorption, oral administration will require the use of prodrugs. In vivo clinical trials evaluating its efficacy are currently in progress. An anticipated approval date is unknown.

Bibliography Available on Request

LACIDIPINE (*Lacipil* by Glaxo) - A dihydropyridine calcium antagonist.

Pharmacology: Lacidipine, a 1,4 dihydropyridine calcium channel blocker, is a selective vasodilator which exerts little effect on myocardial contractility. The dose required to impair cardiac function is approximately 50 times greater than that needed for significant blood pressure reduction. Electrocardiographic studies indicate that it has no effect on SA node function or AV node conduction. Lacidipine effectively reduces blood pressure and decreases systemic vascular resistance by dilating peripheral and coronary arteries. This may lead to reflex tachycardia during the early stages of therapy. In addition to its cardiovascular effects, lacidipine has been shown in animal studies to have mild diuretic and natriuretic effects. In vitro studies have also demonstrated antioxidant activity and a possible tissue protective effect. As with other calcium channel blockers, there is some evidence to suggest activity toward inhibiting atherosclerosis. Lacidipine has been shown via a rat model to decrease infarct size following cerebral artery occlusion. The drug does not appear to affect carbohydrate or lipid metabolism.

Pharmacokinetics: Lacidipine is rapidly absorbed after oral administration and undergoes extensive first-pass metabolism. Virtually no parent drug is excreted in the urine or feces. Of the two primary metabolites, neither possesses pharmacologic activity. Due to the first-pass effect, the absolute bioavailability of lacidipine is < 20%. Its high lipophilicity results in a prolonged pharmacologic effect, thus facilitating a single daily dose regimen. The elimination half-life ranges from 2 to 10 hours after a single dose, but increases to 12 to 15 hours at steady state. Plasma protein binding exceeds 90%. Volume of distribution after a single dose is ≈ 1 to 2 L/kg.

Metabolism of lacidipine is decreased in elderly patients and in those with liver impairment. The elimination of the drug appears to be unaffected by renal function.

Clinical trials: Dose titration studies involving over 400 patients with mild to moderate hypertension demonstrate a minimum response rate of 77%, as defined by the achievement of a diastolic blood pressure (DBP) ≤ 90 mm Hg or a reduction in DBP of ≥ 15 mm Hg. Doses of lacidipine ranged from 2 to 8 mg, administered once daily. One study treated 96 hypertensive patients with lacidipine, starting at a dose of 4 mg for 1 month. If DBP was not controlled after 1 month, the dose was increased to 8 mg. If DBP was not controlled after the second month, a beta blocker was added to the regimen. At 2 months, mean values for DBP and systolic blood pressure (SBP) dropped significantly. After 5 months, 87% of the patients were controlled: 63% on 4 mg, 21% on 8 mg and 3% with combination therapy.

Studies have compared lacidipine 2 to 6 mg/day to hydrochlorothiazide (eg, *Esidrix*) 25 to 50 mg/day, atenolol (eg, *Tenormin*) 50 to 100 mg/day, sustained release nifedipine (eg, *Procardia XL*) 20 to 40 mg twice daily and enalapril (*Vasotec*) 10 to 20 mg/day. In all cases, the differences in mean decrease for both SBP and DBP were not significantly different. In studies comparing lacidipine 4 mg/day to other long-acting dihydropyridine calcium antagonists, lacidipine showed greater antihypertensive effect than amlodipine (*Norvasc*) 10 mg/day and similar efficacy to that of isradipine 5 mg/day; further study is needed to clarify this issue.

Side effects: Adverse effects for lacidipine correspond to those expected for the dihydropyridine calcium antagonists, due mostly to the vasodilatory properties of these drugs: Headache (15%); flushing (10%); edema (8%); dizziness (6%); palpitations (5%); fatigue (4%); gastric irritation (3%). Generally, the side effects are mild and diminish over time. In most cases, they appear to be dose-related. Less common effects include paresthesia, sexual impotence and changes in liver function tests. The tolerability of lacidipine compares favorably to nifedipine; further study is needed to compare lacidipine to newer long-acting drugs in the class (eg, amlodipine).

Summary: Lacidipine appears to be a safe, effective agent for first-line treatment of mild to moderate hypertension. The recommended starting dose is 2 to 4 mg, titrated as needed up to 8 mg/day. Elderly patients and those with liver impairment should be started at 2 mg daily. Future clinical trials may elucidate additional beneficial effects of lacidipine and perhaps define new therapeutic roles for the drug.

Lacidipine is marketed as an antihypertensive drug in Italy and Portugal by Glaxo. It is also available under license to Boehringer Ingelheim in both England and France. It can be found under a variety of trade names, including *Lacipil*, *Viapres*, *Lacirex*, and *Motens*. Future marketing plans in the US are uncertain, largely because lacidipine would compete with Sandoz's isradipine (*DynaCirc*), for which Glaxo also holds the marketing rights. Despite considerable use and investigation of lacidipine in other countries, it may be quite some time before it appears in the US.

Bibliography Available on Request

PROPIRAM (*Dirame* by Roberts Pharmaceuticals) — An opioid analgesic.

Pharmacology: Propiram, also known as Bay 4503, is an opioid analgesic with μ receptor partial agonist activities. It acts centrally at the receptor and has both agonist and weak antagonistic activities at the receptor.

Pharmacokinetics: Propiram has been studied in oral, rectal and injectable forms. The majority of literature available, however, evaluated the oral tablet formulation, propiram fumarate. Bioavailability of the oral formulation is > 97% with a T_{max} of 1.4 hours. Elimination half-life is 5.17 hours and 24% of an orally administered dose is excreted as the parent drug in the urine within 48 hours of administration, indicating extensive metabolism. Total body clearance is 444 ml/min and the V_d is 2.3 L/kg. Duration of action is 3 to 4 hours.

Clinical trials: Relative potencies between injectable propiram and morphine in a ratio of 10:1, and oral to injectable propiram of 150 mg to ≈ 100 mg were identified. Peak analgesic activity was seen at doses of 100 mg propiram (equivalent to 10 mg injectable morphine).

A limited number of clinical trials have been published, and most have been single-dose studies evaluating the efficacy of propiram in post-operative pain. One non-comparative trial, however, evaluated the efficacy of oral propiram 50 to 100 mg repeated as needed every 4 hours for postoperative ocular pain. Of patients enrolled, 64% received 1 or 2 tablets each day and duration of therapy was 1 to 2 days in 80% of those studied. While 93% of the patients rated their pain relief as excellent or good, the authors do not report the degree of relief the current "standard" analgesic provides.

Several single-dose studies have been performed in patients tolerating oral analgesics. Both 50 and 100 mg of oral propiram were shown to be more effective than codeine 60 mg and placebo for the treatment of episiotomy pain. Aspirin 650 mg orally, however, was more effective than 50 mg oral propiram in the treatment of dental pain post-impaction. Both aspirin and propiram proved to be more effective than 60 mg oral codeine or placebo.

One study found 50 mg oral propiram to be equivalent in analgesic efficacy to 50 mg oral pentazocine (*Talwin*) and 60 mg oral codeine; all therapies provided significantly better analgesia than placebo. A second study reported similar results using the same doses of codeine, propiram and placebo. However, a subset of patients in the second study were evaluable for 6 hours after the analgesic was administered; within this subset 50 mg propiram had a significantly better Pain Intensity Difference score at 5 hours than did 60 mg oral codeine sulfate. The patient populations in both of these trials included post-operative cholecystectomy, hemorrhoidectomy, gynecologic and orthopedic surgery patients.

Much of this literature was published during the 1970s and early 1980s and study design either is not well described or is of questionable scientific design in many of the trials. Questions include whether "randomization" included random order of administration in cross-over design studies; whether solid conclusions can be drawn about analgesia when baseline pain and the number of post-operative days when the patient is enrolled are not standardized; whether the study drugs were actually the first analgesic administered post-operatively; and when a drop-out rate/rate of incomplete data collection is considered high.

Side effects: The side effects of propiram are similar to other opioids and appear to be dose-related. The most common side effect, sedation, is reported to occur between 25% and 31%. Other side effects include nausea (5% to 6%) and dizziness (2.2% to 20%). With long-term administration both constipation and dry mouth are frequent side effects.

Despite statements throughout the literature regarding propiram's lower "abuse potential" than morphine or other μ agonists, use of propiram has resulted in display of drug-seeking behavior in non-tolerant addicts. Also, upon abrupt discontinuation of propiram, a mild withdrawal can be experienced by patients, supporting some degree of the development of physical dependence in patients.

Summary: Propiram, an oral partial agonist, appears to be a safe and effective analgesic and provides pain relief for a longer time period than 60 mg codeine. At this time, research on propiram is on hold.

Bibliography Available on Request

TROSPECTOMYCIN (*Spexil* by Upjohn) - An aminocyclitol antibiotic.

Pharmacology: Trospectomycin is a water soluble analog of spectinomycin (*Trobicin*) that is 8 to 10 times more potent and has a broader spectrum of activity. It has good gram-positive and gram-negative aerobic and anaerobic activity, including in vitro activity against *Staphylococci, Streptococci, Peptostreptococci, Peptococci, Haemophilus, Gardnerella, Neisseria, Bacteroides, Chlamydia, Mycoplasma* and *Ureaplasma.* It has moderate activity against Enterobacteriaceae and no activity against *Pseudomonas.*

Trospectomycin acts by binding to the 30S component of the ribosome unit thereby inhibiting protein synthesis. It has a greater affinity for the 30S ribosome unit than spectinomycin and therefore has higher activity. Cross-resistance to spectinomycin has been observed in vitro.

Pharmacokinetics: Patients (n = 128) were randomized to receive trospectomycin (75 to 1000 mg) by IM injection or by 20 minute IV infusion. The IM product was 100% bioavailable. The mean peak plasma concentration and AUC were linear relative to dose, and the half-life was 2.1 hours. Serum concentrations were < 2 mcg/ml 12 hours post-dose, suggesting 2 to 3 times daily dosing as the MIC for most organisms is between 2 to 4 mcg/ml. In another trial, trospectomycin was administered by IV infusion. While almost no drug was found in the feces, 48% to 62% was recovered in the urine during the first 48 hours, suggesting that the drug is slowly released from tissues. The half-life of 2.18 hours did not change with increasing dose.

Clinical trials: The in vitro activity of trospectomycin was compared to that of amikacin (eg, *Amikin*), cephalothin (eg, *Keflin*) and vancomycin (eg, *Vancocin*) against 342 gram-positive organisms. Vancomycin was the most active agent overall, and trospectomycin was better than amikacin, especially for *Staphylococci* and *Streptococci.*

The activity of trospectomycin, clindamycin (eg, *Cleocin*), metronidazole (eg, *Flagyl*), imipenem (*Primaxin*), cefoxitin (*Mefoxin*) and piperacillin (*Pipracil*) was evaluated against 72 strains of *Bacteroides.* Trospectomycin had very good activity and was comparable to imipenem and metronidazole. Its activity was greater than that of piperacillin and cefoxitin. In another trial, trospectomycin was comparable to clindamycin and cefoxitin against *Bacteroides fragilis,* and there was no cross-resistance between the three drugs. Of the organisms tested, 90% to 100% were resistant to ampicillin (eg, *Polycillin*) and cefaclor (eg, *Ceclor*), and > 50% were resistant to doxycycline (eg, *Vibramycin*). None of the organisms tested were resistant to trospectomycin.

The effect of trospectomycin and several other antibiotics was evaluated against *Mycoplasma pneumoniae, M hominis* and *Ureaplasma urealyticum.* Trospectomycin and spectinomycin were equivalent to tetracycline (eg, *Achromycin*) against *M pneumoniae* but less active against *M hominis.* It was concluded that trospectomycin is active against *Mycoplasma*-induced respiratory or genital infections.

To date, published in vivo trials with trospectomycin are limited. The efficacy of a single 1 g IM dose was evaluated in 10 men with uncomplicated *C trachomatis* urethritis. All were culture-positive at follow-up on days 4 to 8. On follow-up on days 21 to 28, six of the eight men were still culture-positive. It was concluded that a single IM dose for the treatment of uncomplicated *C trachomatis* urethritis is not effective.

Side effects: In one study, mild, transient and local reactions were seen in 20% of subjects receiving trospectomycin vs 22% with placebo; none of the reactions were thought to be drug-related. Overall, mild and transient side effects were seen in 32 of 64 subjects receiving trospectomycin; 12 had dizziness or lightheadedness and 17 who received > 600 mg had perioral/facial numbness. Results from a similar trial using IM injection were comparable.

In a multiple-dose trial involving 10 healthy males, trospectomycin caused significantly more pain at the injection site. There was also a significant increase in perioral paresthesias with increasing doses (especially at the 500 and 750 mg doses). Perioral paresthesias were mild and transient, were seen shortly after dosing and lasted about 1 to 2 hours. Tolerance did not develop over the 7 days of the study. Clinically significant orthostatic hypotension occurred after the first dose in patients receiving 500 or 750 mg but was not seen with subsequent dosing.

Summary: Trospectomycin is an injectable aminocyclitol aminoglycoside that is structurally related to spectinomycin. It has good gram-positive and gram-negative aerobic and anaerobic activity and may prove to be useful for the treatment of upper respiratory tract infections, bacterial vaginitis, pelvic inflammatory disease and gonorrhea. Overall, it appears to be well tolerated and the major side effects are pain at the injection site and perioral paresthesias.

Trospectomycin is currently in phase III clinical trials.

Bibliography Available on Request

RITANSERIN (Janssen) - A specific central serotonin S_2-antagonist.

Pharmacology: Ritanserin is a specific, long-acting central serotonin S_2-antagonist which does not affect norepinephrine, acetylcholine or central dopamine antagonism, but does antagonize peripheral histamine. Ritanserin improves sleep quality, decreases fatigue, increases energy levels, improves depressed mood and anxiety and appears to lack abuse potential. Ritanserin 10 mg twice daily also improves neuroleptic-induced akathisia in patients resistant to traditional therapy (eg, anticholinergics, benzodiazepines, beta-blockers). These actions of ritanserin have caused researchers to investigate its effects in the treatment of anxiety, schizophrenia, alcoholism, drug abuse, depressive disorders and Parkinsonism.

Pharmacokinetics: The oral bioavailability is about 75 . Following oral administration, very little drug is recovered unchanged in the urine after a 5 mg IV dose suggesting that it is extensively metabolized by the liver. In a study involving nine healthy volunteers, peak plasma concentrations occurred within 2.39 hours after oral administration. Steady-state plasma concentrations are achieved within 1 week after initiating dosing and the half-life is ≈ 40 hours. Ritanserin is usually administered with or after a meal to decrease the incidence of transient side effects (eg, dizziness, tiredness, lightheadedness) that have been reported in 10% of patients.

Clinical trials: A trial involving 33 patients was conducted to determine the effectiveness of ritanserin in decreasing the negative symptoms in type II schizophrenia over a 6 week period. Patients initially received 10 mg ritanserin. Doses were increased by 10 mg increments to 30 mg as tolerated. The average total dose at the end of the study was 26 mg. Ritanserin significantly improved several negative symptoms such as facial expressions, global affective flattening and relationships with friends and peers and also caused significant reductions in scores for emotional withdrawal and depressive mood compared to placebo. Three patients in the ritanserin group dropped out of the study because of lack of efficacy and one due to side effects (eg, unrest).

In another study, nine patients with acute schizophrenia received ritanserin 10 mg twice daily for 4 weeks. Five of the nine patients experienced a 50%decrease in comprehensive psychological rating scale scores, and scores for negative symptoms also decreased significantly from baseline. No extrapyramidal side effects or akathisia that could be attributed to ritanserin were reported.

Several studies have examined the ability of ritanserin to affect the motor symptoms of Parkinson's disease. Initial studies demonstrated that ritanserin significantly reduced tremor. In contrast, two recent studies determined that ritanserin (range, 5 to 30 mg/day) had a positive effect on dyskinesias but not tremor.

Ritanserin's effect on dysthymia has been studied compared to placebo, amitriptyline (eg, Elavil) and imipramine (eg, Tohranil). Ritanserin was superior to placebo and equal to amitriptyline and imipramine for up to 8 weeks ($n > 300$).

Several studies have determined that ritanserin is effective in relieving anxiety, decreasing fatigue and increasing energy in patients with generalized anxiety disorders compared to placebo, and ritanserin 10 mg appears to have equal efficacy to lorazepam (eg, Ativan). The antianxiety effects occurred after 2 to 4 weeks of treatment.

Ritanserin decreases craving for alcohol and cocaine. One study involving 39 patients concluded that ritanserin 5 mg decreased desire and craving for alcohol but did not change the amount of alcohol intake during 14 days of the study. Another small study (n = 5) suggested that patients receiving ritanserin 10 mg for 28 days not only had no desire to drink but also demonstrated improvement in mood. Several large scale double-blind studies that will include > 900 patients with various types of alcohol dependence are currently underway.

Slow wave sleep (SWS) patterns were significantly improved in several studies when ritanserin was given to patients with alcoholism and depressive disorders; one study found that ritanserin did not affect SWS in 12 depressed patients.

Side effects: Ritanserin appears to be well tolerated. Observed side effects in clinical trials were minimal, with 10% of patients reporting transient dizziness, tiredness and lightheadedness.

Summary: Although ritanserin shows promise in the treatment of a variety of psychiatric illnesses including anxiety, schizophrenia, alcoholism, drug abuse, depressive disorders and Parkinsonism, it is still undergoing clinical trials and has not been approved by the FDA. The dosing range used in the studies was from 5 to 30 mg per day in adults. Side effects are minimal and mild and there seems to be a lack of clinically significant changes in vital signs, laboratory values, ECGs or mood evaluations. An anticipated approval date for the drug, which will be available from Janssen, is unknown.

Bibliography Available on Request

AMIFLOXACIN (Sterling Winthrop)- A fluoroquinolone antibiotic.

Pharmacology: Amitlaxacin is a fluorinated quinolone-carboxylic acid that is structurally related to nalidixic acid *(NegGram)* and cinoxacin (eg, *Cinobac).* It has a broad spectrum of activity against many gram-positive and gram-negative organisms including *Escherichia coli, Klebsiella pneumoniae, Proteus vulgaris, Citrobacter freundii, Pseudomonas aeruginosa* and *Serratia marcescens.* Because of its high degree of renal excretion, it may be effective for the treatment Of urinary tract infections.

Pharmacokinetics: The pharmacokinetic parameters of multiple oral dosing of amifloxacin were evaluated in 48 men randomized to receive amiloxacin every 12 hours (200, 400 or 600 mg) or every 8 hours (400, 600 or 800 mg), orally for 10 days. Amifloxacin was rapidly absorbed with a T_{max} of 0.98 hours. Steady-state concentrations in the urine were > 100 mcg/ml for all doses exc,ept forge 200 mg every 12 hour regimen (where the concentration was > 40 mcg/ml). The half-life ranged from 4.25 to 5.78 hours, and the renal clearance ranged from 128 to 73 ml/hr/kg with the 200 mg ever 12 hour and 800 mg every 8 hour regimins respectively. The major route of elimination was renal with ≈ 54% of the administered dose excreted in the urine. Amifloxacin exhibited concentration-dependent, pharmacokinetics. Pharmacokinetic parameters were comparable to those of other quinolones.

A single oral dose of amifloxacin 200 mg was evaluated in 10 elderly subjects (aged 65 to 79 years). The time to maximum concentration was 1.6 hours, the half-life was 5.37 hours for men and 4.47 hours for women and 42% was excreted renally. Dose adjustment of amifloxacin in the elderly is probably not necessary.

Clinical trials: The in vitro activity of amiflaxacin was compared with that of ciprofloxacin *(Cipro)* and ofloxacin *(Floxin)* against 500 isolates of gram-positive and gram-negative bacteria. Overall, amifloxacin had high in vitro activity against a wide range of organisms, especially *Enterobacteriaceae.*

In another trial, the in vitro activity of amifloxacin against *Staphylococcus saprophyticus* and *E coli* was compared with that of other standard antibiotics used for the treatment of acute urinary tract infections. The drugs evaluated included amifloxacin, gentamicin (eg, *Garamycin*), amoxicillin (eg, *Amoxil*), cephalexin (eg, *Keflex*), trimethoprim (TMP; eg, *Trimpex*), trimethoprim-sulfamethoxazole (TMP-SMZ; eg, *Septra*) and cinoxacin (eg, *Cinobac*). Overall, the isolates were more susceptible to TMP-SMZ, TMP and amifloxacin than to the other drugs tested.

The in vitro activity of seven different quinolone antibiotics (ciprofloxacin, ofloxacin, amifloxacin, enoxacin, norfloxacin and two investigational agents) against 115 strains of MRSA was evaluated; all of the agents were effectively bactericidal.

n vivo trials with amifloxacin that have been published to date are limited. In one trial, the safety and efficacy of oral amifloxacin was compared with that of SMZ/TMP for the treatment of uncomplicated urinary tract infections in women (n = 153) with signs and symptoms of a UTI and bacteria in the urine. Patients received amifloxacin 200 mg every 12 hours (n = 52) or 400 mg every 12 hours (n = 54) orTMP 160 mg/SMZ 800 mg every 12 hours (n = 47) for 10 days. The outcomes were defined as bacteriologic cure, failure or superinfection, and clinical cure or improvement. There was no significant difference in bacteriologic cure rates at 5 to 9 days post-therapy between the two drugs. All evaluable patients showed clinical improvement or cure at the 5 to 9 day visit. Persistent cure was seen in almost all cases at the 4 to 6 week follow-up visit.

Side effects: In clinical trials the adverse effects seen with amifloxacin were mild and self-limited. In the multiple dose study, four patients required discontinuation of therapy due to amifloxacin; one developed pruritus and three experienced a 5- to 8-fold increase in serum ALT (above upper normal limits) that was asymptomatic and resolved spontaneously once the drug was discontinued. The primary adverse effects noted were nausea (15%), abdominal pain (8.3%), dyspepsia (6.7%), headache (8.3%), insomnia (3.3%), tinnitus (3.3%) and pruritus (5%). The renal (asymptomatic crystalluria) and hepatic adverse effects were seen in subjects receiving > 1200 mg daily. Doses < 1200 mg daily were well tolerated.

Summary: Amifloxacin is a fluoroquinolone antibiotic with activity and pharmacokinetics similar to other commercially available quinolones. Because it is primarily renally eliminated, it may be effective for the treatment of urinary tract infections. Overall, it appears to be well tolerated with the major side effects being GI in nature.

At this time, amifloxacin research has ended.

Bibliography Available on Request

TOPIRAMATE (*Topamax* by Ortho-McNeil) - An antiepileptic drug.

Pharmacology: Topiramate is a sulfamate-substituted monosaccharide which is structurally unique in comparison to other antiepileptic drugs. It is a weak carbonic anhydrase inhibitor, originally developed in a search for new antidiabeticagents. The presence of the sulfamate moiety, similar to that of acetazolamide (eg, Diamax), does not explain its antiepileptic effects. Topiramate appears to act by blocking the spread of seizure activity rather than raising seizure threshold, yet the exact mechanism of action remains to be defined. It does not significantly affect receptor binding or neuronal uptake of any of the major neurotransmitters, but does appear to block voltage-dependent sodium and calcium channels. Electrophysiologic studies suggest that topiramate reduces the frequency of repetitive neuronal firing.

The anticonvulsant profile of topiramate is similar to that of phenytoin (eg, *Dilantin*) and carbamazepine (eg, *Tegretol*). It has demonstrated effectiveness against simple and complex partial and generalized tonic clonic seizures. It has also proven to be efficacious in treating Lennox-Gastaut syndrome.

Pharmacokinetics: Topiramate is well absorbed after oral administration, with an absolute bioavailability > 75%. When administered with food, the rate of absorption is moderately slowed but extent of absorption is unaffected. Time to peak after an oral dose varies from about 2 to 4 hours. Topiramate is mainly excreted as unchanged drug in the urine; the fraction excreted unchanged ranges from 70% to 97%. The drug demonstrates linear pharmacokinetics over a wide range of doses, with an average elimination half-life of approximately 20 hours. Volume of distribution is 0.6 to 0.8 L/kg, and the extent of binding to serum proteins is only about 15%.

Topiramate does not appear to affect the metabolism of phenytoin, carbamazepine or valproic acid (eg, *Depakene*), although concomitant administration with any of these drugs tends to lower the AUC of topiramate by 15% to 50%. Topiramate increases the clearance of ethinyl estradiol (*Estinyl*) by 15% to 33%. As with carbamazepine, topiramate therapy must be initiated at low doses (about 50 mg/day) and gradually titrated upward, in order to minimize side effects.

Clinical trials: Clinical trials of topiramate have evaluated daily doses ranging from 200 to 1000 mg. Although most literature to date has been published in abstract form, the results of the studies have been impressive. Many such studies have been add-on trials in which patients who were refractory to prior therapy had topiramate added to the drug regimen. A placebo controlled, add-on trial of 356 patients showed at least a 50% reduction in seizure frequency for 58% of patients who received 600 mg. Another study conducted an add-on, double-blind, placebo controlled, parallel, multicenter study with 56 intractable partial seizure patients. At doses of 200 to 800 mg/day, 50% of the patients showed at least a 50% improvement in seizure frequency.

Two recent US dose-response studies compared doses of 400,600,800 and 1000 mg/day. Using a 50% seizure reduction as the definition of a positive response, 400 mg/day appeared to be the optimal dose, with 46.7% of the patients responding. Larger doses did not produce an enhanced therapeutic effect. Placebo response rates of the two studies were 17.8% and 8.5%, respectively. A long-term study was conducted of add-on topiramate therapy in 18 patients with refractory partial epilepsy. At a mean daily dose of 500 mg, 13 of the patients responded. Efficacy was maintained over a 2-year period. Another study reported results of topiramate monotherapy in 12 patients. Four showed 75% reduction in seizure frequency, and another four patients became seizure-free.

Side effects: Adverse effects caused by topiramate have been dose-related and reversible. The most common adverse reactions reported during clinical trials include sedation, dizziness/ataxia, paresthesia, visual disturbances, diarrhea, decreased appetite with weight loss and cognitive dysfunction. Most side effects attributed to topiramate have been relatively mild. Cognitive dysfunction, reported to be as high as 83% in one study, appears to be the most limiting adverse effect of the drug. Animal studies suggest that topiramate may be teratogenic.

Summary: Topiramate is a promising anticonvulsant drug which is currently undergoing phase III trials. It appears to have a unique mechanism of action which is as yet unknown, and seems to be most effective in treating partial seizures. The drug has been shown to have a relatively narrow therapeutic range, with the optimal dose being in the vicinity of 400 mg/day. Generally the drug is given in two divided doses. Over a dozen studies are currently in progress.

An NDA for topiramate was filed in December 1994. It will be available as *Topamax* by Ortho-McNeil. An anticipated approval date is unknown.

Bibliography Available on Request

TIZANIDINE (*Zanaflex* by Athena Neuroscience) - A centrally acting α2 agonist.

Pharmacology: Tizanidine is a centrally acting α2 agonist structurally similar to clonidine (eg, *Catapres*) used for treatment of spasticity in various conditions (eg, multiple sclerosis [MS], spinal cord injury). The antispasmodic activity of tizanidine is thought to be a result of indirect depression of polysynaptic reflexes by antagonizing the excitatory actions of spinal interneurons.

Pharmacokinetics: The pharmacokinetics of tizanidine were evaluated in two separate studies involving MS patients (n = 17) and spinal cord injury patients (n = 10). The researchers identified a linear relationship between dose and antispastic action with oral doses of 2 to 8 mg. Peak serum concentrations occurred between 1 and 2 hours. A difference from baseline spasticity was evident in both populations for 3 to 4 hours post-dose. A weak relationship was identified between subjects and plasma concentrations, indicating high interpatient variability. Elimination half-life is between 2.7 and 4.2 hours. Tizanidine undergoes first-pass effect (80%) and is nearly completely metabolized hepatically to metabolites which are primarily renally eliminated.

Clinical trials: Spasticity caused by multiple sclerosis - In one study, a greater improvement in muscle tone using the Ashworth Score was seen in the placebo arm of the trial than in the treatment arm (tizanidine) at the end of the titration phase and again at the study endpoint (13 weeks). After the study was completed, it was discovered that no consideration was given to timing of measurement of tonicity in relationship to the treatment. When comparing mean changes from baseline to 3 hours post-dose, a greater improvement was seen in the tizanidine patients. When blindly evaluating global efficacy and tolerability of the two treatments, tizanidine was significantly better than placebo.

In a 12-week study, muscle tone was reduced to a significantly greater extent in the tizanidine group vs placebo. Muscle strength was not affected by either therapy. Spasms and pain decreased in both treatment arms during the study.

One study compared the efficacy and side effects of tizanidine and baclofen (*Lioresal*) in patients with spasticity. Similar efficacy and tolerability of both agents were reported.

Spasticity caused by spinal cord injury - A study compared placebo and escalating doses of tizanidine. The Ashworth Scale and other outcome measures were assessed 1 to 2 hours after the study medication was administered so measurements would coincide with peak blood levels of tizanidine. A significantly greater decrease in muscle tone from baseline was seen in the tizanidine group than in the placebo group. A greater decrease in the frequency of spasms was also seen in the tizanidine-treated patients.

Meta-analysis data - A study reported summary data from 20 short-term studies dating back to 1977. Patients suffered from spasticity due to MS, cerebrovascular disorders and ALS. Analysis of patient-data revealed equal efficacy of tizanidine, baclofen and diazepam (eg, *Valium*) in decreasing muscle tone with significantly better muscle strength in the tizanidine-treated group.

Other - A trial comparing tizanidine with baclofen over a 12 month period found similar effectiveness for the treatment of spasticity in patients with cerebrovascular lesions. In one study, tizanidine was as effective as diazepam in the treatment of cerebral spasticity in patients following a cerebrovascular accident or cranial trauma.

Side effects: Side effects reported in clinical trials are similar to other α2 agonists. More common or potentially severe side effects include dry mouth (45% to 49%), drowsiness (48% to 54%), asthenia (41%), dizziness (16%), liver function abnormalities (< 1%) and hallucinations (1%). Hypotension and orthostatic hypotension may occur. Side effects have been found to be dose related and often resolve with a decrease in dose. Slow titration of doses appears to decrease the frequency of side effects.

Summary Tizanidine offers a novel mechanism of action for the treatment of spasticity in multiple sclerosis, spinal cord injury patients and other settings. Efficacy is comparable to baclofen. Although most studies use every 8 hour dosing, as needed dosing would be appropriate in the MS population. Side effects frequently occur and efficacy approaches good to excellent in only 24% and poor to fair in 76% of the population based on self-evaluation by the patient.

Tizanidine has been commercially available in the foreign market since 1984. Athena Neurosciences, Inc. has marketing rights in Canada, the UK and the US. Athena was denied an NDA in March 1995 and is proceeding with the reapplication process. The product will be marketed as an oral agent, *Zanaflex,* available in 4 mg tablets.

Bibliography Available on Request

ZILEUTON (*Leutrol* by Abbott) - A potent, selective 5-lipoxygenase inhibitor.

Pharmacology: Zileuton is a selective 5-lipoxygenase inhibitor that is being investigated to treat asthma, allergic rhinitis, arthritis, ulcerative colitis (UC) and systemic lupus erythematosus (SLE). 5-lipoxygenase causes the metabolism of arachidonic acid to form products (eg, leukotriene B_4) that have been speculated to cause narrowing of airways observed in asthma. It also exhibits anti-inflammatory activity and inhibits antigen induced contraction of the trachea and bronchospasm in guinea pigs. Although zileuton inhibits 5-lipoxygenase, it has no influence on myeloperoxidase activity, neutrophil degranulation, mast cell histamine release, cyclo-oxygenase products or phospholipase A_2 activity.

Pharmacokineics: Zileuton is rapidly absorbed with a t^{max} of about 1.5 to 4.5 hours and a half-life of 1.5 hours. Zileuton is eliminated primarily by hepatic glucuronidation, therefore, dosing adjustments may be warranted in patients with hepatic dysfunction. When zileuton was administered with sulfasalazine in patients with UC, the pharmacokinetic profile of sulfasalazine and its metabolites was not affected.

Clinical trials: A trial involving 139 patients was conducted to assess the efficacy of zileuton 600 mg 4 times daily or 800 mg twice daily in the treatment of mild-to-moderate asthma over a 4 week period. Zileuton 600 mg significantly increased FEV^1, compared with placebo beginning 1 hour after administration and continued to cause improvement throughout the study period. The group receiving 800 mg twice daily also showed improvement in FEV, compared with placebo, but this difference failed to reach statistical significance. Patients who received zileuton 2.4 g/day also had significant improvement in FVC, airway function and reported asthma symptoms compared with placebo. Zileuton 2.4 g/day caused a significant decrease (24%) in Q-agonist use compared with placebo (7%). In another study involving 8 aspirin-sensitive asthmatics, zileuton 600 mg 4 times daily not only prevented the development of nasal, GI and dermal symptoms associated with aspirin ingestion, but it also curtailed the maximum rise in urinary LTE_4 and averted the fall in FEV_1.

A study involving 8 patients with allergic rhinitis was conducted to assess the effects of zileuton 800 mg after two different nasal challenges. Nasal congestion induced by allergens was significantly decreased in the zileuton patients but prostaglandin D_2, histamine release and sneezing were not.

Zileuton has been studied in the treatment of UC since it has been acknowledged that leukotriene B4 is a prominent intermediary of mucosal inflammation. A study was conducted to examine the effects of zileuton 800 mg/day in decreasing the symptoms of UC in 11 Hispanic patients with mild to moderately active UC over a 28 day period. Ten patients were allowed to continue sulfasalazine therapy (1.5 to 4.5 g/day) since they were taking a constant dose prior to the start of the study. Eight of the 11 patients (73%) had improvement in the gross appearance in the sigmoidoscopy and 100% of the patients encountered a reduction in discomfort of symptoms of their UC. None of the patients experienced any histologic improvement.

A study was conducted to determine the effects of zileuton 600 mg 4 times daily in 40 patients with mild SLE over an 8 week period. Zileuton significantly improved the symptoms associated with SLE compared with placebo.

A study involving rheumatoid arthritis patients was conducted to determine the effect of zileuton on leukotriene generation and clinical response. At the end of 1 week of study, patients receiving zileuton had a 70% decrease in leukotriene synthesis and an improvement in clinical response.

Side effects: Zileuton appears to be well tolerated. In one clinical trial involving 139 asthma patients, observed side effects included headache (10% receiving 2.4 g/day, 16% receiving 1.6 g/day, 14% receiving placebo). Although one patient experienced hives and abnormal liver function tests 24 hours after initiating zileuton 800 mg twice daily therapy, these symptoms resolved after zileuton was suspended.

Summary Potential therapeutic uses of zileuton include asthma, allergic rhinitis, arthritis, ulcerative colitis and systemic lupus erythematosus. It shows promise in all of these diseases, but only asthma is currently being sought as an FDA indication.

On April 10, 1995, the Pulmonary-Allergy Drugs Product Advisory Committee voted to recommend the approval of zileuton for the treatment of asthma, provided that liver function tests be routinely monitored. However, on October 19, 1995, Abbott received a "not approvable" letter from the FDA concerning zileuton. The FDA stated that the NDA contained inadequate information pertaining to preclinical toxicity, especially liver test irregularities. Abbott will try to address the FDA's concerns and supply the necessary information in order to receive an "approvable" letter in the near future.

Bibliography Available on Request

CABERGOLINE (by Adria) - An antiparkinson agent.

Pharmacology: Cabergoline, a synthetic ergoline, is a dopamine agonist that has high specificity and affinity for the D_2 receptor. The continuous stimulation of dopamine receptors may make cabergoline useful for the treatment of motor fluctuations associated with Parkinson's disease (PD). It has also been used for the treatment of hyperprolactinemia, inhibitions of lactation, prolactinomas and acromegaly.

Pharmacokinetics: Cabergoline is well absorbed after oral administration. Administration with food does not affect the absorption or disposition of cabergoline. Peak plasma levels are seen between 0.5 and 4 hours. Once absorbed, cabergoline is widely distributed to well perfused organs and is approximately 41% plasma protein bound. Cabergoline Is extensively metabolized after oral administration to a number of inactive metabolites. Fecal excretion is the major route of elimination. There is no fecal excretion within 24 hours suggesting biliary excretion and enterohepatic recycling. Urinary excretion of unchanged drug accounts for < 14% of the administered dose. The estimated half-life in healthy volunteers is 63 to 68 hours.

Clinical trials: Initial treatment of PD with levodopa produces a dramatic response, but disease progression results in a shortening of response duration with clinical fluctuations. To date, bromocriptine *(Parlodel)* and pergolide *(Permax)*, direct-acting dopamine agonists, have helped alleviate this change in clinical response. However, they have a short duration of action requiring multiple daily doses. Cabergoline has the advantages of increased potency and a very long half-life allowing for once daily dosing.

The efficacy of cabergoline was studied in a randomized, double-blind study of 61 patients (44 males, 17 females) with PD who were stabilized on levodopa/carbidopa *(Sinemet)* but had response fluctuations. Cabergoline was initiated at 0.5 mg daily and Increased by 0.5 mg per week for 5 weeks until there were 12 patients in each dose group (0.5, 1, 1.5, 2, 2.5 mg/day). If patients improved by at least 25% on activities of daily living (ADL) and motor score on the Unified Rating Scale for PD (URSPD), then they continued on the assigned dose for an additional 8 weeks. If not, the dose was Increased by 0.5 mg per week until a 25% improvement occurred or a dose of 5 mg was reached. At the end of 5 weeks, the mean ADL on the URSPD decreased by 22%. Twenty-three patients (38%) had at least 25% improvement; 37 required a further dose adjustment. At week 13, the mean ADL decreased by 35%, and the percent "off" time decreased by 31%. Four patients withdrew early due to adverse effects (confusion, angina, heart failure, increased dyskinesias); not all of these were cabergoline-related.

In an open-label trial, 36 patients (27 males, 9 females) with PD stabilized on levodopa/carbidopa received cabergoline 0.5 to 1 mg initially with dose increases every 7 to 14 days until there was the best control of "off" periods. After 3 months of cabergoline (mean dose 9.2 mg), "off" time significantly decreased. A reduction in "off" hours continued after a mean period of 14.2 months of treatment. There was also a significant decrease in daily levodopa dose. Response was dramatic in 10 patients, moderate in 23 patients and 3 patients were considered treatment failures.

In a recent trial with a similar study design to those previously described (5 week double-blind dose escalation followed by 8 week evaluation), 41 patients with PD (mean duration, 9 years) were evaluated. Three patients dropped out of the trial, 2 due to cardiac conditions not related to cabergoline and 1 due to medication-related confusion. The mean cabergoline dose was 2.8 mg. There was an 18% reduction in mean total levodopa dose. Mean Parkinson motor score, timed finger tapping score and timed walking test scores all significantly improved. There was a 42% reduction in "off" time (6.2 VS 3.6 hr/day). When patients self-rated their response to therapy, 14 showed marked improvement, 7 moderate improvement and 6 mild improvement. Physician ratings showed 9 marked, 21 moderate and 6 mild improvements. No patients deteriorated during the trial.

Side effects: Cabergoline appears to be well tolerated with side effects similar to those seen with other dopamine agonists. In clinical trials involving patients with PD, the major adverse effects noted were mild and transient and included dizziness/vertigo, somnolence, headache, nausea, symptomatic orthostatic hypotension, vivid dreams, visual hallucinations, confusion, increased dyskinesias and nasal stuffiness. One case of pleuropulmonary disease has been reported in a PD patient receiving cabergoline.

Summary: Cabergoline is a dopamine agonist that is more potent and has a longer half-life than either bromocriptine or pergolide. These two features make it an attractive alternative for the treatment of response fluctuations in patients with PD. Clinical trials to date have shown promising results, and the drug has been well tolerated. Its major limiting adverse effect is hypotension. An anticipated approval date for cabergoline which will be available from Adria, is unknown.

Bibliography Available on Request

MEROPENEM (*Merrem* by Zeneca) - A broad-spectrum antibiotic.

Pharmacology: Meropenem is a parenteral carbapenem antibiotic similar in structure to imipenem. Because it is more stable than imipenem against inactivation by renal dehydropeptidase-1 (DHP-1), meropenem does not require concomitant administration with a DHP-1 inhibitor like cilastatin, as in the case of imipenem/cilastatin *(Primaxin)*. The bactericidal activity of meropenem results from a high affinity for binding to penicillin binding proteins and stability against beta-lactamase enzymes.

In vitro studies demonstrate an extremely broad range of antibacterial activity. Meropenem is more active than imipenem against gram-negative *Enterobacteriaceae, Hae mophilus* influenzae and *Neisseria gonorrhoeae,* with MIC_{90} values well below 1 mg/L. *Pseudomonas aeruginosa,* though usually susceptible, is not as sensitive, with an MIC_{90} in the range of 2 to 8 mg/L. Meropenem is active against gram-positive aerobes, including penicillin-resistant strains of *Streptococcus pneumonias,* but it is not active against methicillin-resistant strains of *Staphylococcus aureus.* Most strains of *Enterococcus faecalis* are susceptible, but strains of *E faecium* are generally resistant. MIC_{90} values for meropenem against gram-positive organisms are quite low, only slightly higher than for imipenem. Meropenem is highly active against anaerobes including *Bacteroides fragilis,* with MIC_{90} s below 1 mg/L, except for *Clostridium difficile,* which demonstrates sensitivity with an MIC_{90} of about 2 mg/L.

Pharmacokinetics: Meropenem can be administered by IV infusion over 30 minutes, IV push over 5 minutes or by IM injection. After IV infusion, meropenem achieves peak plasma concentrations > 50 mg/L with a 1 9 dose and 100 mg/L with a 2 9 dose. The volume of distribution is about 0.25 L/kg and protein binding is < 20%. More than 70% of meropenem elimination results from renal excretion of unchanged drug, mostly via glomerular filtration. Up to 30% of a dose is metabolized to a microbiologically inactive metabolite, then eliminated renally. Only 2% is excreted in the feces. The elimination half-life is 1 hour, assuming normal renal function, but dosing adjustments are needed when creatinine clearance (Ccr) falls below 50 ml/min The standard dose is usually 500 mg or 1 g every 8 hours. If the Ccr is 26 to 50 ml/min, the interval is 12 hours; if Ccr is 10 to 25 ml/min, half the standard dose is given every 12 hours; if the Ccr is < 10 ml/min, half the standard dose is given every 24 hours. Meropenem distributes into virtually all body tissues and fluids, including the CSF. Though tissue concentrations are characteristically low, as with other lactam antibiotics, concentrations are usually well above the MIC^{90} for common pathogens.

Clinical trials: Meropenem has been studied in > 3000 patients, covering a full range of infection sites and pathogens. The majority of controlled studies compared meropenem as monotherapy against a cephalosporin, such as ceftazidime (eg, *Fortez*), cefotaxime *(Claforan)* or ceftriaxone *(Rocephin)*, or a cephalosporin in combination with either an aminoglycoside, clindamycin *(Cleocin)* or metronidazole (eg, *Flapyl*). Some studies also included imipenem/cilastatin. Meropenem has demonstrated bacteriological and clinical efficacy comparable to standard antibiotic treatment regimens for intra-abdominal infections, febrile episodes in neutropenic patients, meningitis in both children and adults, lower respiratory tract infections including cystic fibrosis patients, urinary tract infections, skin and soft tissue infections, obstetric/gynecological infections and septicemia.

Pediatric clinical trials have been conducted with both neonates and children, at dosages ranging from 10 to 20 mg/kg 3 times daily (40 mg/kg for meningitis), with documented efficacy. Results suggest that meropenem provides effective monotherapy for moderate to severe infections, including meningitis, especially against resistant strains of *S pneumoniae, H influenzae* and other beta-lactamase producing gram-negative organisms.

Side effects: Trials indicate that meropenem is safer and better tolerated than imipenem/cilastatin. It does not seem to have the same propensity for causing seizures in patients with underlying neurological conditions or renal insufficiency. Commonly reported adverse effects include: Diarrhea, nausea (4%); rash, inflammation at injection site, headache (2%); pruritus (1%). Mild alterations in lab values have also been reported: Thrombocytosis (2%); eosinophilia (1%); liver enzyme elevations (ALT [7%] and AST [6%]). These laboratory changes were found to be reversible and not clinically significant. Adverse effects caused the withdrawal of therapy in 1.4% of patients.

Summary: Meropenem is a carbapenem antibiotic that seems to have empiric monotherapy use for a wide range of infections, including meningitis. Zeneca filed an NDA for *Merrem* in 1993, was approved by the FDA in July 1996. Please look for complete information in the next edition.

Bibliography Available on Request

SIBUTRAMINE (*Meridia* by Knoll) - Weight loss agent.

Pharmacology: Sibutramine is a novel monoamine reuptake inhibitor antidepressant that is being investigated as a weight loss agent. Its mechanism of action as a weight loss agent has not been explored. However, the mechanism of sibutramine and its desmethylated metabolites for depression is via inhibition of monoamine reuptake (not inhibition of monoamine oxidase), noradrenaline and 5-hydroxytryptamine (5-HT) and possibly inhibition of dopamine uptake. However, sibutramine lacks anticholinergic activity, central depressant effects and is nonsedating. These characteristics may cause sibutramine to have a more favorable side effect profile than other weight control products. In several models, sibutramine was shown to have a more rapid onset of antidepressant action after administration (several hours to 3 days) compared with other antidepressants, which can take several weeks to show an antidepressant effect.

Pharmacokineics: No published pharmacokinetic information is available.

Clinical trials: Unpublished phase I and II trials from Boots Phammaceuticals have shown that 15 nonobese volunteers receiving either 2.5 or 5 mg sibutramine per day for 15 weeks lost 3.3% of their initial weight without dieting. Another 15 volunteers in the study who received 5 to 10 mg/day lost 3.7% compared with nine volunteers who received placebo who lost 0.2% of their initial body weight. In another unpublished 6 week trial, 15 healthy nonobese volunteers who received sibutramine 30 mg lost 6% of their initial body weight compared to five patients receiving placebo who gained 0.5%. One last unpublished study involving depressed patients showed that 11 patients who received 2.5 to 5 mg/day lost 1.2% of their initial body weight, 14 patients receiving 5 to 10 mg lost 1.7% and 28 subjects who received 10 to 20 mg lost 2.1% compared to 25 subjects receiving placebo who gained 0.4%.

The only published study was a randomized, double-blind, placebo controlled trial to determine the safety and efficacy of sibutramine 5 and 20 mg administered as adjunctive therapy to caloric restriction (eg, 22 to 25 cal/kg IBW/day), behavior modification and exercise. Following an initial 3 week individualized diet, behavior modification and exercise period, 55 morbidly obese (between 130% to 180% overweight), otherwise healthy subjects received either sibutramine 5 mg (n = 18), sibutramine 20 mg (n = 18) or placebo (n = 19) for 8 weeks and then were followed up 1 week after discontinuing therapy. Sibutramine 5 and 20 mg caused an average weight loss of 2.9 kg (3%) and 5 kg (5.1%), respectively, vs placebo 1.4 kg (1.3%). Sibutramine 20 mg caused a significantly greater weight loss than sibutramine 5 mg and placebo. The authors stated that successful weight loss would include losing between 0.5 to 0.7 kg/week. Patients meeting or exceeding this criteria were as follows in each group: Placebo (n = 2), sibutramine 5 mg (n = 4), sibutramine 20 mg (n = 11). None of the participants receiving sibutramine 20 mg gained weight during the study, and only one subject receiving sibutramine 5 mg gained weight.

Side effects: Adverse effects noted in phase I and II clinical trials included: Insomnia, rapid heartbeat, and periodically, diastolic hypertension. One case of serious, reversible thrombocytopenia has occurred. In the one published trial including only obese, otherwise healthy subjects, sibutramine caused an increase in blood pressure, pulse and heart rate, which appeared similar to placebo, although the statistical significance was not determined. Other side effects noted in this trial included headache, sleep difficulty, irritability, dry mouth, rash or dry skin. Sibutramine users, especially those in the 20 mg group also reported CNS stimulation noted as clearheadedness, increased interest and alertness.

When single-dose sibutramine 30, 45 and 60 mg was compared with amitriptyline (eg, *Elavil*) 50 mg and placebo in six healthy male volunteers, sibutramine 60 mg caused statistically significant increases in heart rate and systolic blood pressure at 1, 2 and 6 hours after administration compared to both amitriptyline and placebo. With sibutramine 30 mg, this difference was only significant at 2 hours. More patients taking amitr.ptyline reported a decrease in salivation and an increase in drowsiness, whereas patients in the sibutramine group did not. Further studies will be required to determine sibutramine's cardiovascular effects.

Summary Although only one clinical trial has been published to date, sibutramine shows promise as an adjunctive weight loss therapy to diet and exercise. The weight loss effects of sibutramine may be dose-related. Additional clinical trials are necessary to establish the long-term safety and efficacy of sibutramine as a weight loss agent. Sibutramine, which will be available as *Meridia* from Knoll, is in late clinical trials for treatment of depression and obesity. Approval is anticipated in late 1997.

Bibliography Available on Request

ACETORPHAN (by Laboratoire Bioproject, Paris, France) - An enkephalinase inhibitor.

Pharmacology: Acetorphan is a lipophilic inhibitor of enkephalinase, a peptidase present in the gastrointestinal tract and the central nervous system. By inhibiting enkephalinase, endogenous enkephalin concentrations increase, giving acetorphan varied therapeutic indications.

Acetorphan is used for symptomatic treatment of acute diarrhea in adults Treatment should not last more than 7 days. Acetorphan administration does not obviate the need for hydration when relevant.

Pharmacokinetics: Available pharmacokinetic data in humans is limited to the dosing Information included below.

Clinical trials: A double-blind cross-over design evaluated the ability of acetorphan to prevent diarrhea in patients receiving castor oil. Acetorphan was administered 45 minutes after the castor oil. Castor oil was selected to induce an experimental "secretory diarrhea. Six subjects were studied. Prophylactic acetorphan significantly reduced the mean number of stools during the following 24 hours by 50% and the stool weight by 37%. No side effects other than nausea and discomfort, which were noted in all subjects, were reported.

One hundred ninty-nine patients randomly received acetorphan or placebo after being diagnosed wrth infectious diarrhea. Patients took two capsules (100 mg each) on enrollment into the study and one capsule aher each unformed stool for a maximum of 10 days. No other therapies were initiated during the trial, with the exception of acetaminophen as needed. Patients receiving acetorphan experienced a significantly shorter duration of diarrhea. Of the patients still experiencing diarrhea on day 10, 7% received acetorphan and 24% received placebo. Side effects were similar between the two groups.

One study compared the efficacy of acetorphan (100 mg three times daily) and loperamide (eg, *Imodium A-D;* 1.33 mg three times daily) in the treatment of infectious diarrhea. Therapy continued until resolution of diarrhea or for a maximum of 7 days. Thirty-seven patients received acetorphan, and 32 patients received loperamide. The mean duration of diarrhea did not differ between the two groups. Abdominal distension and constipation, however, were significantly more common in the loperamide group.

Another study compared the efficacy of acetorphan and clonidine (eg, *Catapres*) in suppressing opiate withdrawal symptoms. Nineteen heroin or synthetic opiate addicts were treated with 50 mg IV acetorphan twice daily or clonidine 0.075 mg five times dally if they displayed opioid withdrawal syndrome within 24 hours after a hospital admission. Changes In the overall Opiate Withdrawal Scale did not differ between the two groups; however, diarrhea and lacrimation were more improved in the acetorphan group. No side effects were noted in the acetorphan group; one clonidine patient experienced severe hypotension.

Published studies evaluating analgesic activity are only in the animal model. The potential for a new analgesic mechanism of action makes acetorphan a promising agent. Acetorphan has been shown to have minimal abuse potential and withdrawal is not precipitated upon abrupt discontinuation of the drug in animals.

Finally, a possible role in the treatment of gastroesophageal reflux disease (GERD) has been suggested based on the results of a study evaluating the drug's effects on the lower esophageal sphincter.

Side effects: No side effects significantly different from placebo have been identified in the clinical trials.

Summary Acetorphan is not commercially available in the US, but it is available in France as 100 mg capsules. Recent research, however, suggests it will provide a novel antidiarrheal agent with minimal side effects. Several potential additional indications are currently being investigated, such as the treatment of opioid withdrawal, GERD and analgesia.

Bibliography Available on Request

ROXATIDINE ACETATE (*Roxin* by Hoechst-Roussel) - An agent for peptic ulcers.

Pharmacology: Roxatidine acetate is a potent, selective, histamine H_2RA (H_2 receptor antagonist) that is structurally unrelated to cimetidine (eg, *Tagamet*) or ranitidine (eg, *Zantac*). Its potency is 3 to 6 times that of cimetidine and twice that of ranitidine. Basal gastric acid secretion is inhibited by > 90% 3 hours after a single 50 mg dose and by 86% 4 to 6 hours after a 75 mg dose. Unlike cimetidine, ranitidine or famotidine (eg, *Pepcid*), roxatidine has a mucosal protective effect in animal models. It has no direct effect on serum gastrin levels (unlike cimetidine or ranitidine) and no antiandrogenic effect.

Pharmacokinetics: Roxatidine acetate is well absorbed with a bioavailability of > 95%. After administration, it is rapidly converted to roxatidine, its active metabolite, by esterases in the small intestine, plasma and liver. The peak concentration occurs 3 hours after oral administration, with food and antacids having little or no clinical effect on its pharmacokinetics. Its volume of distribution is 3.2 L/kg after a single dose and 1.7 L/kg at steady state. Plasma protein binding is 6% to 7%. Elimination is primarily renal with 96% eliminated as roxatidine. The clearance is 21 to 29 L/hr and the half-life is 4 to 8 hours. Other than roxatidine, nine other inactive metabolites have been identified. Because it is renally eliminated, the dose of roxatidine must be adjusted in patients with severe renal dysfunction.

The pharmacokinetic parameters of a single dose of roxatidine 150 mg were evaluated in 31 patients with varying degrees of renal dysfunction (control group, mild chronic renal failure [CRF], moderate CRF, severe CRF or uremia). The half-life increased 12 hours in patients with uremia (Ccr < 7 ml/min), with the t_{max} doubling (2.08 hours vs 4.05 hours, respectively). In patients with renal failure, there can be an increase in half-life by 140% to 200% with peak plasma concentrations increasing by 50% to 70%. Data on the effects of hemodialysis are conflicting, ranging from no effect to a marked reduction in plasma concentration.

Clinical trials:

Duodenal ulcers (DU) - Roxatidine 75 mg twice daily is effective for the treatment of DU. Six-week healing rates were between 73% to 90%, with 8-week rates being between 87% to 95%.The efficacy of roxatidine was evaluated in 356 patients with active DU in a multicenter, double-blind trial. Patients were randomized to receive roxatidine (150 mg at bedtime, n = 170) or placebo (n = 170) for 4 weeks; antacids were administered as needed for pain relief. Four-week ulcer healing rates were 68% for patients receiving roxatidine compared with 30% for placebo; roxatidine was also better at decreasing abdominal pain.

Roxatidine is also effective as maintenance therapy for the prevention of DU. In one trial, 105 patients with healed duodenal ulcers received roxatidine 75 mg at bedtime for 6 months as preventive therapy. Ulcer relapse rates were 18% after 3 months and 35% after 6 months. Relapse rates were higher in smokers. In another trial evaluating 372 patients with healed duodenal ulcers, cumulative ulcer relapse rates at 12 months were 35% for patients receiving roxatidine (75 mg at bedtime) vs 66% for placebo. Most patients who relapsed did so within 6 months. When patients relapsed, they were asymptomatic in 26% of patients receiving roxatidine vs 16% of patients receiving placebo. The study showed that roxatidine 75 mg at bedtime is effective as preventive therapy for DU.

Gastric ulcers (GU) - In small, noncomparative trials in patients with gastric ulcers, roxatidine 75 mg twice daily had ulcer healing rates ranging from 77% to 96% at 8 weeks. In a double-blind, multicenter trial, patients with GU were randomized to receive roxatidine 75 mg twice daily (n = 172) or 150 mg at bedtime (n = 171). Both dosing regimens were found to produce symptomatic pain relief and to have comparable ulcer healing rates (84% and 86% at 8 weeks, respectively).

Side effects: The most common adverse effects are hypersensitivity reactions (rash), GI (diarrhea, constipation, nausea) or involve the CNS (headache, dizziness, fatigue).

Summary: Roxatidine acetate is a potent, selective H_2 receptor antagonist that is effective for both treatment of and maintenance therapy for duodenal and gastric ulcers. It is generally well tolerated with the primary side effects involving the GI, cutaneous or central nervous systems.

For the treatment of peptic ulcer disease, roxatidine should be dosed 75 mg twice daily or 150 mg at bedtime for 8 weeks. For prevention of DU or GU recurrence, the dose is 75 mg at bedtime. Decrease dose in patients with renal dysfunction; treatment doses of 75 mg once daily for a Ccr between 20 and 40 ml/min and 75 mg every other day for a CCr of < 20 ml/min have been suggested.

Hoechst-Roussel has filed an NDA for *Roxin,* and FDA approval is expected in 1997.

Bibliography Available on Request

PRAMIPEXOLE (by Pharmacia & Upjohn) - A dopamine agonist.

Pharmacology: Pramipexole is a potent dopamine agonist that binds preferentially to the D3 dopamine receptor. Though originally thought to be a selective D2 agonist, selectivity of pramipexole for D3 receptors is 5 times greater than for other dopamine receptor subtypes. Currently available dopamine agonists (bromocriptine, *Parlodel,* and pergolide, *Permax*) are more selective for the D2 dopamine receptor. These agents are indicated for adjunctive treatment of Parkinson's Disease (PD) with levodopa, and are used predominantly in the later stages of the disease. Pharmacia & Upjohn submitted a New Drug Application to the FDA for pramipexole on December 28, 1995. The NDA submission is based on clinical trials in which pramipexole was used to treat both early and late PD.

Because pramipexole stimulates presynaptic dopamine autoreceptors, it has been hypothesized to decrease postsynaptic dopamine activity in the mesolimbic system. For this reason, pramipexole is being investigated as a possible treatment for schizophrenia. By functioning as a postsynaptic dopamine receptor agonist in the nucleus accumbens, the drug has also demonstrated antidepressant properties.

Pharmacokinetics: Little has been published to date about the pharmacokinetic profile of pramipexole. One report suggests an elimination half-life of 11.7 hours and a time to peak plasma concentration of 1.8 hours.

Clinical trials: Pramipexole was evaluated against placebo for the treatment of early PD in a randomized, parallel-group, double-blind study. The 55 subjects (age range, 37 to 86) were diagnosed with early idiopathic PD (stages I to III by the Modified Hoehn and Yahr scale). Mean duration of illness was 2.3 years. All subjects received selegiline 5 mg twice a day throughout the trial and anticholinergics as needed. The pramipexole dose was administered on an ascending schedule for the first 6 weeks, starting at 0.1 mg three times a day and increasing up to 1.5 mg three times a day. Patients who experienced dose-limiting side effects were maintained at the highest tolerated dose. The maintenance dose phase lasted 3 weeks, followed by a 1-week dose reduction chase. Efficacy was measured by the Unified Parkinson's Disease Rating Scale (UPDRS) Parts II (Activities of Daily Living) and III (Motor Examination). Based on UPDRS Part II, the pramipexole group showed significantly greater ($p = 0.002$) improvements in daily activities especially hand writing, cutting food, dressing, hygiene and tremor. Though the pramipexole group showed a 44% greater improvement in UPDRS Part III, the difference was not significant ($p = 0.1$). Orthostatic hypotension occurred in all subjects, though none required treatment of symptoms. Nine patients experienced dose-limiting side effects.

Pramipexole was also compared with placebo for the treatment of advanced PD (stage II through IV) in an 11-week, single-blind, parallel-group study. The 24 patients (age range, 49 to 81) had a mean duration of illness of 11.9 years. All patients were experiencing motor fluctuations on levodopa (LD) therapy. The study consisted of a 3-week screening phase to optimize the dose of LD, followed by an 11-week treatment phase. The pramipexole dose was titrated from 0.1 mg three times a day to 1.5 mg three times a day during the first 7 weeks of treatment, followed by a 3-week maintenance phase and 1 week of dose reduction. Subjects were evaluated using the UPDRS. Results showed a significantly greater improvement ($p < 0.05$) in the "off" score of the treatment group for activities of daily living. UPDRS motor examination scores showed a greater reduction in "off" time for the treatment group, but results were not statistically significant ($p = 0.06$). The pramipexole-treated group experienced a significantly greater ($p = 0.004$) reduction in LD dose of 30%. No serious side effects were observed.

Side effects: Orthostatic hypotension is very common, though it is usually not symptomatic. Other dose-related adverse effects include confusion, dizziness, insomnia, hallucinations, visual disturbances, nausea, dry mouth and headache. In a study conducted on healthy male volunteers, pramipexole caused decreased levels of serum prolactin and thyrotropin, and increased levels of growth hormone and cortisol. These endocrine effects are similar to those observed with other dopamine agonists.

Summary: Pramipexole is a promising agent as adjunctive treatment of both early and advanced PD. It demonstrates a unique selectivity for the dopamine D3 receptor. It may also have potential benefit in treating psychiatric disorders. The side effect profile is similar to that of other dopamine agonists. An NDA for treating early and advanced PD was submitted on December 28, 1995.

Bibliography Available on Request

ORLISTAT, TETRAHYDROLIPSTATIN (*Xenical* by Roche)- A weight loss agent.

Pharmacology: Orlistat is a chemically produced derivative of the natural product, lipstatin, a potent irreversible lipase inhibitor that decreases the amount of ingested dietary fat that is absorbed and increases fecal fat excretion. Pancreatic lipase is the primary enzyme that allows for the digestion of dietary triglycerides by dividing free fatty acids from the glycerol backbone, thereby reducing triglyceride absorption. This, in turn, also affects cholesterol absorption. The unabsorbed triglycerides and cholesterol are then eliminated in the feces. Besides potentially causing weight loss, orlistat, in doses of 10 to 360 mg, has been shown to decrease total cholesterol levels by 4% to 11% and LDL by 5% to 10%.

Pharmacokineics: Because orlistat works in the GI tract, traditional bioavailability studies cannot be used. Instead, the amount of excreted fecal fat is measured. Both normal and obese subjects have received the drug in doses of 12.5 to 400 mg three times a day with diets ranging in fat content from 45 to 130 g/day. The amount of fecal fat excretion In excess of placebo ranged from 5% to 35.8% of ingested fat. The amount of fecal fat excreted does not depend on the amount of dietary fat or fiber ingested. The optimal dosage range appears to be from 100 to 400 mg three times a day. Doses higher than 400 mg three times a day have not shown improved efficacy. Orlistat can be administered before, during or after meals without affecting the amount of fat excreted. Orlistat does not significantly alter the kinetics of single oral doses of digoxin 0.4 mg and glyburide 5 mg.

Clinical trials: A double-blind, randomized, 12 week study investigated the weight loss potential of orlistat compared with placebo. Obese patients 20% to 50% above ideal body weight (IBW) received, in addition to a diet with 30% of calories from fat, orlistat 50 mg three times a day (n = 20) or placebo (n = 19). Patients were asked to record their dietary intake, physical activity and bowel movement activity. Patients receiving orlistat lost significantly more weight than patients on placebo, 43 kg and 2.1 kg, respectively (orlistat patients lost 0.3 lbs/week > placebo patients). In this group of normolipidemic patients, neither triglyceride nor cholesterol levels were affected. Vitamin E, but not vitamin A, levels were significantly lower in the orlistat group, but this did not necessitate treatment. Another study with a similar design and duration examined orlistat 10, 60 and 120 mg three times a day compared with placebo in 188 obese patients who engaged in "consistent regular physical activity." At the conclusion of the study, additional weight loss above that of placebo with orlistat 30 mg was 0.63 kg, 180 mg was 0.71 kg and 360 mg was 1.75 kg. Only the 360 mg group lost significantly more weight compared with placebo (0.32 lbs/week > placebo). This study demonstrated that the weight loss abilities of orlistat are also dose-dependent. In this group of normolipidemic patients, small but statistically significant decreases in total cholesterol levels, LDL levels and the LDL to HDL cholesterol ratio were noted, but not triglyceride or HDL levels. Vitamins E and D, but not vitamin A, levels were significantly lower in the orlistat 180 and 360 mg groups but did not necessitate treatment.

Side effects: The most common adverse effects are GI complaints, such as loose bowel movements, oily appearing stools, abdominal cramps, fecal incontinence and nausea. A few patients in the trials had to drop out due to intolerable GI complaints such as fecal incontinence. These side effects do not appear to be dose-related, but may be partially associated with the amount of dietary fat ingested. Vitamin A, D and E levels have been noted to decrease while patients are taking orlistat but supplementation does not appear to be warranted during short-term treatment.

Summary: Orlistat appears to have similar efficacy to other weight loss agents. Doses in the studies ranged from 12.5 to 400 mg three times a day. Doses between 100 and 400 mg three times a day appear to be optimal in most patients. Studies have shown no relationship between time of administration and fecal fat excretion.

Bibliography Available on Request

ENPROSTIL (*Gardrin* by Syntex) — An investigational agent for acute peptic ulcers. Enprostil, a synthetic analog of prostaglandin E_2, is a potent, long-lasting inhibitor of gastric acid secretion. It also has a mucosal protective effect. Enprostil has been studied for the treatment of duodenal ulcer, gastric ulcer and NSAID/aspirin-induced injury.

Pharmacology: Enprostil suppresses gastric acid secretion by ≤ 80% for 12 hours following a single dose of 35 or 70 mcg. Nocturnal acid secretion remains suppressed for 4 to 11 hours after single or multiple doses. Enprostil also decreases the secretion of pepsin. In patients with duodenal ulcer, pepsin secretion decreased by 63% after enprostil 70 mcg at bedtime and by 85% with 35 mcg twice daily. Unlike the H_2 receptor antagonists, enprostil inhibits basal and postprandial gastrin release. It also prevents the increase in serum gastrin that occurs secondary to food.

In a retrospective analysis of clinical trials in patients with ulcers, it was noted that enprostil produced at least a 10% decrease in total cholesterol in ≈ 65% of hypercholesterolemic subjects compared with 16% of subjects receiving placebo. The median percent change was 17% for patients who received enprostil 70 mcg and 13% for those receiving 35 mcg. In a double-blind, placebo controlled, crossover trial, enprostil 70 mcg was administered daily for 9 days to eight normal subjects. Total cholesterol and apolipoprotein B both decreased by 16%, and LDL cholesterol decreased by 22%. There was little to no change in HDL cholesterol. These results suggest the potential for enprostil use in the treatment of hyperlipidemia.

When enprostil was studied in 207 pregnant females (1st trimester), it was found that there were no drug-induced abortions; 4% of patients had vaginal bleeding. However, enprostil may induce uterine contractions and, therefore, its use in pregnancy should be avoided.

Pharmacokinetics: Data on the pharmacokinetic parameters of enprostil are limited. After a 1 mcg/kg dose, the mean plasma concentration occurred after 30 to 60 minutes and the half-life was 34 hours. The drug was primarily eliminated renally (53% in the urine after 48 hours); 34% was excreted in the feces after 144 hours.

Efficacy:

Duodenal ulcer – Enprostil 35 mcg twice daily for 4 weeks had healing rates between 65% and 85%, rates that are greater than those seen with placebo, equivalent to those seen with cimetidine 400 mg twice daily and less than those seen with ranitidine 150 mg twice daily. In a multicenter, double-blind trial, 127 patients with endoscopically diagnosed active duodenal, pyloric or prepyloric ulcers were randomized to receive enprostil 35 mcg twice daily or placebo for 4 weeks. The cumulative healing rates at 2 weeks were 25% for enprostil and 12% for placebo; at 4 weeks the rates were 59% and 33%, respectively.

Enprostil 35 mcg twice daily also was compared with misoprostol 200 mcg 4 times daily for 4 to 6 weeks in 214 patients with acute duodenal ulcers in a randomized, single-blind trial. There was no significant difference in ulcer healing rates between the two agents (≈ 80% at week 4 and 90% at week 6). Daytime and nighttime pain relief occurred in < 50% of subjects in both groups.

Gastric ulcer – Enprostil 35 or 70 mcg twice daily was compared with placebo for the treatment of gastric ulcers in 128 patients for 6 weeks. At week 6, ulcer healing rates were 82% for the 35 mcg dose, 70% for the 70 mcg dose and 50% for placebo. Enprostil 35 mcg twice daily has been shown to have ulcer healing rates comparable with cimetidine 200 mg 3 times daily plus 400 mg at bedtime in 57 patients. Healing rates at 8 weeks were 86% for enprostil vs 96% for cimetidine. Both agents produced similar pain relief.

NSAID/ASA-induced ulcer – Enprostil was equivalent in efficacy to cimetidine and sucralfate in reducing the total number of lesions secondary to aspirin administration, suggesting that enprostil may offer some protection to the GI mucosa.

Safety: In clinical trials, enprostil was generally well tolerated. The primary adverse effect was diarrhea, which occurred in ≈ 10% to 15% of subjects who received 35 mcg twice daily. The incidence of diarrhea increased with increasing doses. Other reported adverse effects include abdominal pain, flatulence, nausea, vomiting, dyspepsia and headache. Enprostil has been shown to have no drug interactions with theophylline or propranolol.

Summary: Enprostil is an investigational, synthetic analog of prostaglandin E_2 that has been shown to be effective for the treatment of gastric, duodenal and NSAID-induced ulcers. It has also been shown to reduce total cholesterol in hypercholesterolemic subjects. Its major adverse effect is diarrhea, which occurs in 10% to 15% of subjects. Other adverse effects are primarily gastrointestinal in nature.

Bibliography Available on Request

ATORVASTATIN (by Parke-Davis) - A new HMG-CoA reductase inhibitor.

Pharmacology: Atorvastatin is a potent inhibitor of 3-hydroxy-3-methylglutaryl-coenzyme A (HMG-CoA) reductase, the rate-limiting enzyme in cholesterol synthesis. It produces significant reductions in total cholesterol, low-density lipoprotein (LDL) cholesterol and apolipoprotein B. The drug also appears to increase high-density lipoprotein (HDL) cholesterol and decrease both triglycerides and very low-density lipoprotein (VLDL) cholesterol. The mechanism of action is similar to that of other reductase inhibitors: The direct inhibition of HMG-CoA and an up-regulation of LDL receptors. Whereas lovastatin (*Mevacor*) and simvastatin (*Zocor*) are inactive lactone prodrugs, atorvastatin, pravastatin (*Pravachol*) and fluvastatin (*Lescol*) are hydroxy acids that exist in active form. These lipid-lowering drugs are used predominantly to treat patients with hypercholesterolemia who are at risk of developing coronary artery disease.

Pharmacokinetics: Atorvastatin demonstrates significant first-pass metabolism in the liver. As with other reductase inhibitors, the drug undergoes extensive hepatic extraction following oral administration (range, 46% to 79%). The elimination half-life is ≈ 13 to 16 hours, considerably longer than other drugs in the class. Atorvastatin is 80% bound to plasma proteins.

Atorvastatin pharmacokinetics are affected by age, food and time of administration. When elderly subjects were compared with younger subjects, peak serum concentration (C_{max}) and half-life were 42.5% and 36.2% higher, respectively. In the presence of food (a medium-fat meal), C_{max} was lowered by 48% and area under the curve (AUC) was lowered by 13%. Food caused the time-to-peak to more than double but only slightly decreased the extent of absorption. Bioavailability of atorvastatin is 30% lower following evening administration compared with morning administration. Despite having a pharmacokinetic influence, the effects of age, food and time of administration have little or no impact on the clinical efficacy of the drug. This is probably because of the extensive first-pass effect, which results in high concentrations at the site of action (the liver) that do not correlate well with serum concentrations. Studies suggest that atorvastatin dose, rather than serum concentration, correlates to the lipid-lowering effects of the drug.

Clinical trials: In a randomized, double-blind, placebo controlled, parallel group, multicenter study, 56 patients with primary hypertriglyceridemia received either placebo or 5, 20 or 80 mg of atorvastatin for 4 weeks. Dietary counseling was maintained throughout the study. Results demonstrated a dose-dependent reduction in total triglycerides of 26.5%, 32.4% and 45.8% for the 5, 20 and 80 mg doses of atorvastatin, respectively. The placebo group showed a reduction of 8.9%. The groups treated with 20 and 80 mg of atorvastatin showed a statistically significant drop in total triglycerides, total cholesterol, LDL and VLDL compared with placebo. HDL increased by 12.7% in the 20 mg group, significantly more than placebo. The maximum lipid-lowering effect was generally observed by the second week. No patients withdrew due to adverse effects.

In a crossover study involving 16 normolipidemic subjects, a 40 mg dose of atorvastatin was administered at 6 p.m. for 15 days. After a 28–day washout phase, the same dose was administered at 7 a.m. for 15 days. Mean reductions were 34% in total cholesterol, 48% in LDL, 37% in VLDL and 25% in triglycerides. Differences between the morning and evening dose were not significant.

Side effects: Atorvastatin is generally well tolerated. The most commonly reported adverse effects in clinical trials included headache (5%), pain (myopathy, 5%), diarrhea (5%) and flatulence (5%), along with sporadic reports of nausea and insomnia. Modest elevations in alkaline phosphatase, ALT and AST have been reported. One subject experienced giddiness and mild confusion following a 120 mg dose. The symptoms resolved after 5 hours.

Drug interactions: Atorvastatin does not affect antipyrine clearance and, therefore, does not interfere with cytochrome P450 enzymes. No drug interactions have been reported thus far.

Summary: Atorvastatin shows promise as a single agent for treating patients with high LDL and VLDL. It appears to be more potent and efficacious than currently available HMG-CoA reductase inhibitors, has a similar safety profile and is unique in its ability to significantly lower total serum triglycerides. The manufacturer filed an NDA on June 17, 1996. A 1997 approval by the FDA is anticipated.

Bibliography Available on Request

TOREMIFENE (*Fareston* by Orion Corp) — for advanced breast cancer

Pharmacology: Toremifene is a triphenylethylene derivative differing from tamoxifen only by the addition of a chlorine atom. Under development since 1979, toremifene was designed in an effort to produce a more effective agent than tamoxifen that specifically bound to estrogen receptors and inhibited growth of estrogen receptor positive breast cancer cell lines. Overall, toremifene has anti-estrogen activity, weak estrogenic activity and an oncolytic effect. In both estrogen receptor-positive and estrogen receptor-negative cell lines, high levels of toremifene have been inhibitory while low levels have been stimulatory.

Pharmacokinetics: Toremifene is well absorbed orally, reaching peak serum concentration in 1 to 6 hours (mean, 3 hours). Steady state is reached within 1 to 5 weeks. Toremifene is highly plasma protein bound (99.7%). The mean distribution half-life of toremifene is 4 hours and the mean elimination half-life is 5 to 6 days. Toremifene undergoes extensive metabolism via the cytochrome P450 3A4 isozyme to N-demethyl, 4–hydroxyl and deaminohydroxy metabolites and other minor metabolites, many of which are active, possessing anti-estrogen activity comparable to toremifene. Toremifene undergoes enterohepatic circulation and is excreted primarily in the feces as metabolites.

Clinical trials: Toremifene was demonstarted to be as effective as tamoxifen in 648 postmenopausal patients with estrogen or progesterone receptor-positive or unknown metastatic breast cancer. Patients received toremifene 60 mg/day, tormifene 200 mg/day or tamoxifen 20 mg/day with 50%, 48% and 44% achieving complete or partial response or stability of disease, respectively. Patients in this study may have had prior adjuvant chemotherapy but had not had prior hormone or cytotoxic chemotherapy for recurrent/metastatic disease. Response rates, time to progression, survival times and response durations were comparable in the three treatment groups. Clinical tumor flare also occurred with a similar frequency in the three treatment groups.

Toremifene does not appear to be effective in estrogen receptor-negative breast cancer. Because several preclinical and early clinical studies suggested toremifene may have activity in estrogen receptor—negative or unknown breast cancer, a phase II study was undertaken to evaluate toremifene 400 mg daily in patients with estrogen receptor-negative metastatic breast cancer. In this study enrolling 21 patients, no objective responses were observed. Progressive disease was observed in 14 evaluable patients, and five of six patients with stable disease at 8 weeks had progressive disease at 11 to 33 weeks.

Side effects: Dose-related side effects of toremifene include nausea, vomiting and dizziness. Other adverse effects reported include sweating, peripheral edema, vaginal discharge, vaginal bleeding, hot flushes and hypercalcemia. At high doses, some patients have experienced moderate-to-severe vomiting, disorientation, hallucinations and vertigo. Elevated liver function tests have also been reported.

Dosing: The optimal dose of toremifene has not been clearly established, however, daily administration of 60 mg appears safe and effective. No advantage to administration of higher doses has been demonstrated.

Summary: Toremifene appears to offer an alternative to tamoxifen in the treatment of advanced breast cancer in postmenopausal patients. No advantage over tamoxifen has been established. Additional studies comparing toremifene with tamoxifen as adjuvant therapy and prophylactic therapy are necessary before this agent can be regarded as an alternative to tamoxifen for these indications.

Bibliography Available on Request

TROGLITAZONE (*Rezulin* by Warner-Lambert) — An oral antidiabetic agent.

Pharmacology: Troglitazone, a thiazolidinedione, is a novel oral antidiabetic agent that reduces hyperglycemia without increasing insulin secretion in patients with noninsulin-dependent diabetes mellitus (NIDDM). It improves insulin sensitivity by reducing peripheral and hepatic insulin resistance, thus, reducing hepatic glucose output, and improves glucose tolerance. Animal and in vitro studies have shown that troglitazone intensifies insulin activity at both the receptor and postreceptor sites in the peripheral as well as hepatic tissues. In vitro studies have shown that troglitazone not only increases insulin receptors but also increases insulin-stimulated glucose uptake. It can mimic the effects of insulin and increase insulin's actions. Thus, troglitazone may work by stimulating muscle and liver cells to increase glucose consumption and reduce glucose production. In addition to decreasing hyperglycemia, troglitazone may also have potential benefit in patients with NIDDM and hypertension, hyperlipidemia and hypertriglyceridemia. In vitro, it had a high antioxidative potency in restricting the lipid peroxidation of human plasma LDL and, thus, may reduce atherogenesis.

Pharmacokinetics: Available pharmacokinetic data have been extrapolated to humans from animal data. Troglitazone is metabolized in the liver to sulfate and glucuronide conjugates and is also partially oxidized to a quinone form. It is highly protein bound (> 99.8%) and distributes to a number of tissues.

Clinical trials: One study examined 11 patients with NIDDM to determine the metabolic effects of troglitazone 400 mg/day administered for 6 to 12 weeks. Eight of the 11 subjects were determined to be responders (ie, subjects had a decrease in fasting blood glucose [FBG]), whereas, three were labeled nonresponders (ie, no decrease in FBG). At the end of 6 to 12 weeks, FBG decreased from an average of 12.5 to 10.7 mM in all subjects and 12.7 to 8.3 mM in the responder group, although an improvement in insulin resistance was noted in the nonresponder group. A beneficial response in mean FBG was generally noted within 2 to 3 weeks and reached a peak effect within 4 to 6 weeks, although some patients had an initial delay until 5 to 6 weeks and achieved maximum benefit at 10 to 11 weeks. No change in total or LDL cholesterol levels was noted, but there was a modest increase in HDL cholesterol levels and a significant decrease in total triglyceride levels. The authors determined that troglitazone decreases both insulinemia and hepatic glucose production as well as improves insulin resistance and fasting and postprandial glycemia in patients with NIDDM. It also had a positive effect on HDL cholesterol and triglyceride levels.

A 12-week open-label study involving 146 patients with NIDDM who had failed to maintain adequate glycemic control (FBG > 140 mg/dl) by diet or oral hypoglycemic agents was conducted to determine the efficacy of adding troglitazone 200 or 400 mg/day. A beneficial response of mean FBG was noted within 2 weeks and HbA_{1c} within 8 weeks. At the end of the 12-week trial, FBG had decreased from an average of 192 to 155 mg/dl and HbA_{1c} decreased from 8.9% to 8.1%. In 39% of patients, FBG decreased by > 20% of the baseline value, with the 400 mg dose (46%) proving more effective than the 200 mg dose (25%). Troglitazone was also more effective in decreasing FBG (by > 20%) in obese patients (body mass index [BMI] > 25) (56%) than in normal weight individuals (BMI < 25) (30%). The efficacy of troglitazone was not different between those individuals who received other hypoglycemic agents and those who received troglitazone alone.

Side effects: Troglitazone does not affect insulin secretion but improves insulin sensitivity, thereby causing insulin to more effectively produce a decrease in glucose levels; therefore, it should not cause hypoglycemia. In clinical studies, side effects of troglitazone are absent or mild in nature. In one large clinical study, the most common side effects occurring with troglitazone more often than with placebo were dizziness (2.8%) and edema (2.1%). Edema resolved in all patients without discontinuing treatment. Hypoglycemia was observed in 1.4% of the troglitazone group and 0.7% of the placebo group, which was relieved by ingesting sugar or food. No significant difference was noted in the incidence of laboratory abnormalities between the troglitazone (9.2%) and the placebo group (5.1%). Five patients in the troglitazone group and four patients in the placebo group discontinued treatment due to side effects. Other side effects noted in clinical trials were nausea, vomiting, abdominal fullness, epigastralgia and diarrhea.

Summary: Troglitazone improves insulin resistance and HbA_{1c} in patients with NIDDM and obese patients with and without insulin resistance; therefore, it may play a role in the prevention of NIDDM. It may also have a positive effect on cholesterol and triglyceride levels as well as blood pressure. It was recommended for approval in December 1996.

Bibliography Available on Request

AMSACRINE (*Amsidyl* by Parke-Davis) - A dye derivative for the treatment of acute leukemia and lymphoma.

Pharmacology: Amsacrine is an acridine dye derivative for the treatment of acute leukemia and lymphoma. It inhibits DNA synthesis by a mechanism similar to the anthracyclines, via intercalation with base pairs in the DNA molecule. The precise mechanism of action is not well understood; however, it is thought that amsacrine may also interact with cellular membranes and interfere with the enzyme topoisomerase II.

Pharmacokinetics: Amsacrine has demonstrated biphasic elimination characteristics. Its distribution half-life is 0.15 to 1.4 hours. The terminal half-life is 4.7 to 9 hours. Elimination is via hepatic metabolism and biliary excretion. More than 80% of an administered dose is excreted via the biliary route into the feces. Approximately 2% to 10% of the dose is excreted in the urine unchanged. Changes in hepatic function significantly reduce clearance and increase the elimination half-life. In patients with severe hepatic dysfunction, the elimination half-life is 17.2 hours. The major metabolite, which appears inactive, is an amsacrine-glutathione 5′ conjugate.

The volume of distribution is 1.7 to 2.6 L/kg. Amsacrine is highly plasma protein bound (96.4% to 97.7%), however, 2 hours after administration 50% plasma protein binding has also been reported. High levels of amsacrine have been found distributed in the gallbladder, kidney and lower levels in the lung, testes, muscle, fat, spleen, bladder, pancreas, colon, prostate, brain and cerebrospinal fluid.

Clinical trials:

Acute myelogenous leukemia (AML) – Amsacrine and cytarabine were compared in 48 patients with AML in relapse. Patients were treated with either amsacrine 75 mg/m^2 daily for 7 days or high-dose cytarabine 3 g/m^2 every 12 hours for 6 days. Response rates in both groups were similar, with 3 of 23 amsacrine-treated patients and 3 of 25 cytarabine-treated patients achieving complete remission. All patients achieved remissions after only 1 course of therapy. Failures appeared to be primarily due to the inability to reduce the leukemic population (absolute drug resistance) or regrowth of leukemia (relative drug resistance), with over half the patients demonstrating drug resistance. Overall response rates with both agents were low. In another study, therapy with amsacrine administered as a continuous infusion at a dose of 90 mg/m^2/day for 5 days produced no complete responses in 21 patients with refractory or relapsed AML. Other studies have reported response rates of 15% to 29% for reinduction of complete remission.

Acute promyelocytic leukemia (APL) – An amsacrine, cytarabine and thioguanine regimen was compared with a daunorubicin, cytarabine, thioguanine regimen in a small number of patients with APL. Complete remission was achieved in 7 of 7 patients receiving the amsacrine regimen and 5 of 9 patients receiving the daunorubicin regimen, suggesting amsacrine may effectively replace daunorubicin in some APL chemotherapy regimens.

Acute lymphoblastic leukemia (ALL) – In patients with refractory or relapsed ALL, amsacrine alone was demonstrated to be as effective as a combination regimen with cytarabine and thioguanine. Complete remissions were achieved in 3 of 11 amsacrine-treated patients and 3 of 13 cytarabine-treated patients. Amsacrine plus high-dose cytarabine was also evaluated in ALL. As in other types of leukemia, this combination produced good remission rates but does not appear to impact long-term survival.

Side effects: Common adverse effects include myelosuppression, stomatitis/mucositis, nausea and vomiting, alopecia, phlebitis, diarrhea, hypersensitivity reactions, hepatoxicity, hyperbilirubinemia, hypoalbuminemia, mild hepatic dysfunction, elevations in alkaline phosphatase and transaminase levels, serious cardiac arrhythmias (ventricular tachycardia, supraventricular tachyarrhythmias), QT interval prolongation, hypokalemia, transient hypomagnesemia, acute myocardial necrosis, presented as an acute myocardial infarction, congestive heart failure, sudden death and seizures.

The most common adverse effects of the combination cytarabine and amsacrine regimens have included nausea and vomiting, ocular discomfort, mucositis, hepatic dysfunction, cutaneous erythremia and cerebellar dysfunction.

Summary: Amsacrine appears to be an active agent in the treatment of refractory/relapsed acute leukemia when administered alone or in combination with other chemotherapeutic agents, especially cytarabine. Amsacrine therapy has been demonstrated to improve the rate of complete remissions, but duration of survival has not been shown to improve. The role of amsacrine may be most effective in combination with other agents to induce remissions prior to bone marrow transplantation. A NDA has been filed with the FDA.

Bibliography Available on Request

BROMFENAC (*Duract* by Wyeth-Ayerst) — An anti-inflammatory analgesic.

Pharmacology: Bromfenac is a nonsteroidal anti-inflammatory agent (NSAID) under evaluation for use as an analgesic. Bromfenac is structurally related to diclofenac (eg, *Voltaren*) and ketoprofen (eg, *Orudis*). It is classified as a peripherally acting analgesic with anti-inflammatory, antipyretic and prostaglandinase-inhibiting properties.

Animal and in vitro studies indicate bromfenac to be 7.5 to 20 times more potent than indomethacin (eg, *Indocin*) in suppressing acute inflammation and 3.8 times more potent at suppressing chronic inflammation. Gastric and intestinal toxicity potency is comparable with and 1.8 times greater than indomethacin, respectively.

Pharmacokinetics: Peak levels of bromfenac are reached within 1 hour of oral administration. Bromfenac is extensively plasma protein bound (99%). The elimination half-life is 30 to 54 minutes. Overall, the pharmacokinetics of bromfenac are similar to other NSAIDs with short half-lives, particularly tolmetin (eg, *Tolectin*).

Clinical trials: Two studies compared bromfenac with aspirin 650 mg, ibuprofen 400 mg and placebo in the treatment of postoperative pain after surgical removal of impacted third molars. The first study used bromfenac 5, 10 and 25 mg in 241 patients, while the second study used bromfenac 10, 25, 50 and 100 mg in 280 patients. All active treatments were more effective than placebo. Bromfenac 5 mg was as effective as aspirin; bromfenac ≥ 10 mg and ibuprofen were more effective than aspirin; and bromfenac 25 mg was as effective as ibuprofen. The effects of bromfenac 5 mg and aspirin peristed until hour 3, and the effects of bromfenac 10 mg persisted until hour five. From hours 5 through 8 after dose administration, bromfenac 50 and 100 mg were more effective than bromfenac 25 mg, and bromfenac 100 mg was more effective than ibuprofen. Bromfenac demonstrated a linear dose response at doses ≤ 100 mg. Re-evaluation by another investigator suggested that linear dose response with bromfenac is not detectable at doses > 50 mg.

In another study, bromfenac 5, 10 and 25 mg were compared with acetaminophen 1 g and placebo in the treatment of postoperative orthopedic pain in 150 patients. Bromfenac 10 and 25 mg and acetaminophen 1 g were more effective than placebo. Bromfenac 25 mg produced a longer time to remedication than acetaminophen. All three bromfenac doses, but not the acetaminophen dose, produced a longer time to remedication than placebo. Completion of the 6–hour treatment period without requiring remedication occurred in 13% of the placebo-treated patients, 37% of the acetaminophen-treated patients and 37%, 50% and 63% of the bromfenac 5, 10 and 25 mg treated patients, respectively. Overall, bromfenac 10 mg appeared as effective as acetaminophen 1 g at producing pain relief.

Oral bromfenac 10 and 25 mg have been compared with sublingual buprenorphine (*Buprenex*) 0.2 and 0.4 mg in 91 patients for the treatment of moderate to severe pain following general surgical or orthopedic operations. Both bromfenac doses were more effective than the buprenorphine, and bromfenac was better tolerated. Buprenorphine 0.4 mg was more effective than buprenorphine 0.2 mg, while bromfenac 10 and 25 mg doses appeared equally effective.

Side effects: Side effects reported with bromfenac have been consistent with those reported for other NSAIDs and have included dizziness, lightheadedness, headache, sleepiness, nausea, vomiting and abdominal pain.

Drug interactions: Drug interactions with bromfenac have not been reported at this time but are expected to be comparable with those reported with other NSAIDs.

Summary: Bromfenac at doses of 10 to 100 mg appears to be an effective analgesic that is an alternative NSAID for the treatment of nonarthritic pain, providing it is priced competitively. The optimal dosage has not been reported at this time. Limited information is available on its renal and GI tolerance.

Bromfenac has been recommended for approval by an FDA Advisory Committee. At this time, it remains an investigational agent in the US.

Bibliography Available on Request

QUINUPRISTIN/DALFOPRISTIN (*Synercid* by Rhone-Poulenc Rorer) — A streptogramin antibiotic.

Pharmacology: Quinupristin/dalfopristin is the first of a new class of antimicrobial agents known as streptogramins. It was developed from pristinamycin, which was isolated from *Streptomyces pristinaespirales*. Both agents are bacteriostatic. When used in combination (30:70), they are synergistic and become bactericidal. It works by irreversibly binding to the 70S ribosome that results in the inhibition of protein synthesis. In vitro testing demonstrates a post-antibiotic effect of 2.2 to > 18 hours depending on the organism. The modifications that were made to form the semisynthetic streptogramins made them more water soluble while retaining the antibiotic activity. The provisional breakpoint is 4 mcg/ml. Additional tests indicate that quinupristin/dalfopristin is also effective against various organisms found in the mouth and could be useful in the treatment of dental sepsis or endocarditis prophylaxis. In addition, it has demonstrated in vitro effectiveness against several respiratory tract pathogens (*Moraxella catarrhalis, Streptococcus pneumoniae* and *S. pyogenes*), except *Haemophilus influenzae.*

The drug penetrates cardiac vegetation and reaches a concentration in the vegetation higher than that reached in cardiac tissue. Using an in vitro-infected fibrin clot model, quinupristin/dalfopristin was as effective as vancomycin in killing the *Staphylococcus aureus*. The combination of quinupristin/dalfopristin and vancomycin was even more effective. In animal studies, quinupristin/dalfopristin has shown the ability to penetrate infected fibrin clots and cardiac vegetations. The peak fibrin clot levels were achieved ≤ 1 hour. The peak level was 3.3 mcg/g. The clot levels had dropped to 1.2 mcg/g after 6 hours. Cross-resistance to quinupristin/dalfopristin and other antibiotic agents has not been documented.

Pharmacokinetics: The peak serum concentration of quinupristin/dalfopristin is 8.65 mg/L after a 12 mg/kg intravenous dose. The elimination half-life of quinupristin/dalfopristin is 1.27 to 1.53 hours. The maximum concentration in blister fluid is found at 1.7 hours and is 2.41 mg/L. This represents a penetration of 82.5% into noninflammatory interstitial fluid over 6 hours.

Clinical trials: The majority of the effectiveness data currently exists in the form of in vitro sensitivity and animal studies. Very limited information is published on the use of quinupristin/dalfopristin in humans. More than 500 adults and children have been treated via the emergency use program. A favorable result has been obtained in 70% of the 95 evaluable patients treated in the emergency use program. Phase III studies are underway at > 310 centers in the US and Europe.

Three patients with chronic ambulatory peritoneal dialysis-associated peritonitis caused by glycopeptide-resistant enterococci were treated with quinupristin/dalfopristin. The intravenous dose used was 10 to 20 mg/kg/day in two divided doses. The infection in two of the patients was rapidly and completely resolved. In the third, the condition improved and then relapsed. The condition responded after a second course of therapy and removal of the cannula. The infecting organism was *Enterococcus faecium* in all three cases. The MIC for vancomycin for these organisms was > 32 mg/L, and all three were resistant to teicoplanin. The MIC reported for quinupristin/dalfopristin was 0.3 mg/L.

Summary: Quinupristin/dalfopristin is a promising agent that can be used in the treatment of gram-positive infections unresponsive to other available antibiotic therapy, including vancomycin. Given the emergence of resistant micro-organisms to various antibiotics, quinupristin/dalfopristin should be reserved for those cases where vancomycin cannot be used.

Quinupristin/dalfopristin is in Phase III trials for the treatment of community-acquired pneumonia, complicated skin and skin-structure infections and nosocomial pneumonia. The product can be acquired for compassionate use by calling 610–454–3872.

Bibliography Available on Request

STERILE AEROSOL TALC (*Sclerosol* by Bryan Corp.)

Pharmacology: Although talc has been used in pleurodesis since 1935, a commercially available sterile product has yet to be FDA approved. In practice, a number of different formulations have been tried, including aerosolized talc and talc slurry. *Sclerosol* is a sterile, asbestos-free talc powder aerosol formulated with a chlorofluorocarbon propellant (dichlorodifluromethane) as a disposable, single-use spray canister. The canisters are sterilized by gamma radiation and packaged in a sterile pack with 15 and 25 cm hollow plastic delivery catheters. Talc is delivered at a maximun rate of 0.4 g/second as a fine mist. It is not a metered-dose delivery system, rather the dose depends on the extent and duration of manual compression of the nozzle.

Some facilities have chosen to manufacture their own sterile talc and package it in sterile plastic test tubes containing 1.2 or 2.5 g of sterile talc powder or double-package talc in 2.2 g packets in heat-sealed sterilization pouches. Unsterile USP grade talc obtained from chemical supply companies may contain bacteria or fungi. Sterilization with gamma irradiation, ethylene oxide gas or prolonged dry heat exposure is recommended. In some institutions, a combination of ethylene oxide and dry heat treatment have been used. Gamma irradiation is the most expensive sterilization method and the dry heat method is the least expensive; the product is administered by aerosolization, atomizer or bulb syringe at the time of thoracotomy or thoracostomy, or by using a slurry (sterile talc powder is diluted in 10 to 250 ml of normal saline solution and instilled via pleural trocar or chest tube).

Clinical trials: A comparison of talc and mustine found talc more effective in the treatment of pleural effusion. The talc was instilled using a Stanford Cade insufflator through an intercostal cannula. The talc was instilled until it discharged freely from the second cannula. Control of the effusion was obtained in 56% of those treated with mustine and 90% with talc.

An open-label study was conducted to compare the effectiveness of talc (n = 39), bleomycin (n = 44) and tetracycline (n = 41) in the treatment of malignant pleural effusions. In the patients treated with talc, a thoracentesis was performed the day before treatment. The talc used was pharmaceutical-grade, asbestos-free and heat-sterilized; 3 g of talc was insufflated into the pleural space through a rigid suction catheter with a pneumatic atomizer. A chest tube was left in place to facilitate fluid drainage. The other patients were treated with 60 units bleomycin (*Blenoxane*) or 1000 mg tetracycline (eg, *Achromycin*) diluted in 100 ml of normal saline solution. The solution was instilled into a tube thoracostomy after the fluid drainage had decreased to < 100 ml/day. After 30 days, there were 55 evaluable patients; no evidence of recurrent pleural effusion was found in 97% of those treated with talc, 64% of those treated with bleomycin and 33% in those treated with tetracycline. After 90 days these values were 95%, 70% and 47%, respectively.

Side effects: Problems previously reported with talc pleurodesis have included fever, pain, pulmonary talcoma, pachypleuritis (pleural inflammation and thickening), pulmonary insufficiency, acute pneumonitis and acute respiratory distress syndrome. Side effects that could be related to the surgical procedure but also could be caused by the talc include arrhythmias, cardiac arrest, chest pain, myocardial infarction, hypotension and death. The risk of granuloma, malignant mesothelioma and bronchogenic carcinoma has been a concern but may be related to historical contaminates, such as asbestos. The fever that has occurred with talc administration generally occurs within 4 to 12 hours after instillation and lasts for ≤ 72 hours. Whether these adverse effects occur with talc pleurodesis using *Sclerosol* remains to be determined.

Summary: Parenteral tetracycline is no longer available. Bleomycin tends to be more expensive and less effective than talc. Doxycycline (eg, *Vibramycin*), minocycline (*Minocin*) and *Corynebacterium parvum* are not as well studied and may be less effective. A facility looking at this product will need to consider if in-house production and sterilization will be less expensive and as convenient as the commercial product or other products for the treatment of pleural effusion (eg, bleomycin, doxycycline).

Sterile aerosol talc is awaiting FDA approval for administration intrapleurally by thoracoscopy in the treatment of malignant pleural effusions. The Bryan Corp. received an approvable letter August 9, 1996.

Bibliography Available on Request

LYME BORRELIOSIS VACCINE — Inactivated subunit vaccines against *Borrelia burgdorferi* (cause of Lyme Disease).

Pharmacology:

Epidemiology – Lyme disease results when infection with the spirochete *Borrelia burgdorferi* causes an inflammatory, multi-organ disorder. Infection classically begins with a bull's-eye shaped rash, called erythema migrans, and a "flu-like" illness. Later, chronic arthritis and other rheumatologic manifestations may develop. Other problems may include neurologic (eg, meningitis, neuritis, Bell's palsy), cardiac (eg, heart block, myocarditis) or hepatic dysfunction. Transmission to humans occurs via a tick vector (genus *Ixodes*), which in turn is a parasite of mice and deer. Lyme disease has been found in most US states, Europe, Australia and elsewhere. Between 11,000 and 13,000 cases were reported in the US in both 1994 and 1995, especially in the mid-Atlantic and northeastern regions, with the number of reports climbing since the beginning of this decade. Lyme borreliosis is the most commonly reported arthropod-borne disease of humans in the US.

Animal models – Candidate vaccines have already protected several species of animals against challenge with *Borrelia burgdorferi*. An inactivated *Borrelia* vaccine for dogs is commercially marketed by Fort Dodge Laboratories (Fort Dodge, Iowa), consisting of two doses 3 weeks apart, followed by annual revaccination.

Immunopharmacology – Osp subunits (see Clinical Trials) elicit neutralizing antibodies. The clinical trials will establish whether they are sufficient to protect people against infection. Such vaccines might control disease in a novel way: Antibodies and perhaps other serum factors ingested by the tick during a blood meal may reduce the bacterial inoculum before transmission to the host. Diversity of OspA proteins varies among *Borrelia burgdorferi* strains in Europe and may necessitate a vaccine consisting of several antigens.

Pharmacokinetics: In early testing, a single IM vaccine dose induced antibodies that persisted for only a few months. The minimum protective antibody level is not yet known. Several doses will probably be needed for protection, with the possibility of periodic booster doses needed to sustain immunity.

Clinical trials: Two subunit vaccines consisting of the outer suface protein A (OspA) of *Borrelia burgdorferi* are currently in human phase III clinical trials with tens of thousands of volunteers. These vaccines are sponsored by Pasteur-Merieux-Connought and SmithKline-Beecham. Each vaccine is prepared through recombinant DNA technology. Other vaccine candidates sponsored by other firms and using other immunologic technologies are in earlier stages of development.

Side effects: Most vaccine reactions reported to date involve local discomfort at the injection site, typical of most vaccines. Whether the human immune system responds to the vaccine antigens with autoimmune effects, similar to Lyme borreliosis, that target cross-reacting human antigens is being studied closely. Such events are considered less likely with a subunit vaccine than a whole-cell vaccine.

Summary: Licensing of a Lyme borreliosis vaccine is unlikely before the end of this decade. Safety concerns will require time and large test populations to resolve.

If one or more of these vaccines is found to be safe and effective in preventing Lyme borreliosis, rational discussion will be needed to determine who needs to be vaccinated: All or some children and adolescents, all or some adults. Who should pay for this vaccine: The public sector, private insurers or the people who choose vaccine for themselves. These policies will vary from place to place, depending on local incidence of the disease and public perceptions of risk.

Until Lyme borreliosis vaccines are licensed, effective protection consists of wearing socks, applying tick repellents containing N,N-diethyl-m-toluamide (DEET) to clothing or exposed skin according to manufacturers' instructions, checking thoroughly and regularly for ticks and removing attached ticks promptly. Acaracides containing permethrin that kill ticks on contact can safely be applied to clothing, but not skin.

Bibliography Available on Request

FENRETINIDE (by McNeil Pharmaceuticals) — A synthetic retinoid.

Pharmacology: Fenretinide (N-4–hydroxyphenylretinamide) is a synthetic retinoid currently under evaluation for use in prevention of breast, bladder, oral and skin cancer. It does not act like other retinoids, because its activity does not correlate with cellular retinoic acid-binding proteins. It is believed, however, that fenretinide is metabolized to an agent which competes for cellular retinoic acid-binding protein binding sites.

Pharmacokinetics: Peak levels are achieved in 3 to 9 hours following oral administration. Bioavailability is significantly increased by administration after a meal (189%), particularly after a high-fat meal (200% to 300%). The elimination half-life is 17.4 to 27 hours. Fenretinide was present in very low amounts (at the limits of detectability) 50 days after discontinuation of treatment for 1 year with 200 mg/day. Levels were undetectable 6 days after the last dose following 1 month of treatment at that dose. After 5 years of continuous treatment, fenretinide concentrations were at the limits of detectability at 6 and 12 months after discontinuation, while levels of the metabolite were 5 times higher. Retinol concentrations returned to baseline after 1 month.

Clinical trials: The effects of fenretinide were evaluated in 149 women who received fenretinide for at least 4 years in a breast cancer chemoprevention trial. Evaluation was done by mammographies performed at baseline and then once a year. The results of mammographies after 4 years of fenretinide therapy reported no substantial changes in breast parenchymal patterns, except in 1 patient who demonstrated improvement (P2 to P1 Wolfe's classification). Preliminary studies are evaluating the effects of combination tamoxifen (eg, *Nolvadex*) and fenretinide in patients with previously untreated metastatic breast cancer.

One trial involved patients with previously untreated homogenous or nonhomogenous oral leukoplakias that had a benign postoperative histology following laser resection. Patients were randomized to receive fenretinide 200 mg daily for a maximum of 52 weeks (with a 3–day drug holiday at the end of each month) or no treatment. Of 153 patients in this study (74 treated with fenretinide and 79 in the control group), 19 patients had recurrences (9 in the control group and 10 in the fenretinide group), and 15 had new localizations (12 in the control group and 3 in the fenretinide group). The overall risk of recurrence and new localization was 6% in the fenretinide group and 30% in the control group.

Another report described the treatment of oral lichen planus (2 patients) and leukoplakias (6 patients) with topical fenretinide. Eight patients applied fenretinide twice daily by opening a 100 mg capsule and applying its contents to the affected sites after brushing teethe. Responses were apparent in all patients within 15 days. After 1 month of therapy, 2 patients had complete response and the other 6 had a > 75% response. No side effects were observed.

Results of a small study evaluating fenretinide effects on the outcomes of previously-resected superficial bladder cancer have been reported. Twelve patients were treated with fenretinide 200 mg daily and were compared with 17 non-randomized, untreated controls. The proportion of patients with DNA aneuploid stemlines in bladder washed cells decreased from 7 of 12 (58%) to 5 of 11 (45%) in the fenretinide group, but increased from 7 of 17 (41%) to 10 of 17 (59%) in the control group. Positive or suspicious cytologic examinations were present in 3 of 12 fenretinide-treated patients prior to therapy, but all reverted to normal. Positive or suspicious cytologic examinations increased from 4 of 17 to 6 of 17 during the study in the control group. These data suggest fenretinide may affect DNA content and abnormal cytology in patients with previously-resected superficial bladder cancer. Additional studies are necessary to further evaluate the effects of fenretinide in bladder cancer, including patients with previous bladder papillomas or transitional cell carcinoma.

It has also been suggested that fenretinide be evaluated as chemoprevention in patients with cervical dysplasia or previous basal cell or squamous cell actinic keratoses.

Summary: Insufficient information on the effects of fenretinide in cancer chemoprevention are available at this time. Fenretinide does appear to be better tolerated than currently-available retinoids under evaluation for cancer chemoprevention. Fenretinide is currently in phase III trials by McNeil.

Bibliography Available on Request

Acquired Immune Deficiency Syndrome (AIDS) is an immunodeficiency state caused by an infection with the human immunodeficiency virus, HIV. This retrovirus has also been referred to as human T–cell lymphotropic virus, type III (HTLV-III), lymphadenopathy-associated virus (LAV) and the AIDS-related virus. There are several drugs being studied for HIV and AIDS. Listed below are some antiviral, cytokine and immunomodulating drugs currently undergoing clinical trials. To date, three types of HIV antivirals have been approved by the FDA: Reverse transcriptase inhibitors, non-nucleoside reverse trascriptase inhibitors and protease inhibitors (refer to the Antivirals section in the Anti-Infectives chapter).

AIDS Drugs in Development

Drug	Drug type	FDA status	Treatment sponsor
Acemannan (*Carrisyn*)	antiviral, immunomodulator	Phase I AIDS	Carrington Laboratories
Acetylcysteine (*Fluimucil*)	immunomodulator	Phase I HIV, AIDS	Zambon
Adefovir dipivoxil	antiretroviral	Phase II/III; HIV	Gilead Science
AIDS vaccine (eg, gp 120, rgp 160, rgp 160 MN, rp 24, *VaxSyn HIV-1*)	antiviral	Phase I to III AIDS, HIV prophylaxis and treatment	MicroGeneSys/ Genentech/Immuno/ Connaught/Virogenetics
AL-721	antiviral	Phase I/II AIDS, HIV	Matrix Laboratories
Aldesleukin[1] (interleukin-2; IL-2; *Proleukin*)	cytokine	Phase II with zidovudine for HIV	Cetus Oncology
Alvircept sudotox (sCD4-PE40)	antiviral	Phase II AIDS	Upjohn
Ampligen	immunomodulator	Phase II/III HIV	HEM Pharmaceutical
AR-121 (*Nystatin-LF I.V.*)	antiviral	Phase I/II HIV	Argus
AR177	integrase inhibitor	Phase I; HIV	Aronex
AS-101	immunomodulator	Phase I/II AIDS	Wyeth-Ayerst
Atevirdine mesylate	antiviral	Phase I HIV, AIDS	Upjohn
Azidouridine (AzdU)	antiviral	Phase I HIV-positive symptomatic, AIDS	Berlex
AZT-P-ddI (*Scriptene*)	antiviral	Phase I AIDS	Baker Norton
CD4, soluble human, recombinant	antiviral	Phase II AIDS	Biogen
CD4-IgG	antiviral	Phase I Maternal/fetal HIV transfer	Genentech
Cidofovir[1] (*Visitide*)	antiviral	Phase I/II, AIDS	Gilead
CI-1020	antiviral	IND, HIV	Warner Lambert
Curdlan sulfate (CRDS)	antiviral	Phase I/II HIV	Lenti-Chemico Pharmaceuticals
DAB_{389}IL-2 fusion toxin	cytokine	Phase I/II HIV	Seragen
Delavirdine mesylate	antiviral	Phase III HIV, AIDS	Upjohn
Deoxynojirimycin, n-butyl (DNJ)	antiviral	Phase II ARC, AIDS	Searle
Dextran sulfate (*Uendex*)	antiviral	Phase II AIDS, HIV-positive asymptomatic	Ueno Fine Chemicals Industry Ltd.
DHEA (EL10)	immunomodulator	IND approved; Phase I/II HIV	Elan

AIDS Drugs in Development

Drug	Drug type	FDA status	Treatment sponsor
Diethyldithio-carbamate (*Imuthiol*)	immunomodulator	Phase II/III AIDS, HIV, pediatric HIV	Connaught
Fiacitabine (FIAC)	antiviral	Phase I/II HIV, AIDS	Oclassen
Fialuridine (FIAU)	antiviral	Phase II HIV	Oclassen
Filgrastim[1] (granulocyte colony-stimulating factor; G-CSF; *Neupogen*)	cytokine	Phase III AIDS	Amgen
FK-565	immunomodulator	Phase I HIV	Fujisawa
Fluorothymidine (FLT)	antiviral	Phase II HIV, AIDS	Lederle
Ganciclovir[1] (*Cytovene*)	antiviral	Phase I/II, HIV prophylaxis	Roche
gp 120 vaccine (*Remune*)	vaccine	Phase I/II, HIV prophylaxis	Genevax
gp 160 vaccine	vaccine	Investigational; HIV prophylaxis	Micro Genesys
HIV immune globulin (*HIVIG*)	immunomodulator	Phase III Prevention of maternal/fetal HIV transfer	North American Biologicals
HIV immuno-therapeutic	antiviral	Phase I HIV (symptomatic)	Viagene
HIV immuno-therapeutic vaccine	antiviral	Phase II/III HIV asymptomatic	Immunization Products Ltd. (joint venture of RPR and Immune Response Corp.)
HIV vaccine (gp 120)	antiviral	Phase I AIDS	Chiron/Ciba-Geigy
HIV Vaccine (*Apollon*)	vaccine	HIV	Genevax
HIV Vaccine (*Genevax*)	vaccine	Phase I/II, HIV prophylaxis	Apollon
Hypericin (*VIMRxyn*)	antiviral	Phase I AIDS, HIV	VIMRx Pharm
Immune globulin IV[1] (IGIV; eg, *Gamimune-N*)	immunomodulator	Phase II/III Pediatric HIV; with zidovudine for AIDS	Miles
Imreg-1	immunomodulator	Phase III HIV	Imreg
Interferon alfa (*Wellferon*)	cytokine	Phase III with zalcitabine and zidovudine for HIV disease, non-AIDS	Glaxo Wellcome
Interferon, alfa-2b[1] (*Intron A*)	cytokine	Phase I/II with zidovudine for AIDS	Schering-Plough
Interferon, alfa-n3[1] (*Alferon N*; *Alferon LDO* [low-dose oral])	cytokine	Phase I/II ARC, AIDS, asymptomatic AIDS	Interferon Sciences
Interferon, beta (*Betaseron*)	cytokine	Phase II/III AIDS	Berlex
Interleukin-1 receptor, soluble	antiviral	Phase I HIV	Immunex
Interleukin-2 PEG	cytokine	Phase II with zidovudine for AIDS	Chiron
Interleukin-3, recombinant human	cytokine	Phase I HIV with cytopenia	Sandoz
Iscador	antiviral	Phase I HIV, AIDS	Hiscia

AIDS Drugs in Development			
Drug	Drug type	FDA status	Treatment sponsor
Lentinan (*Lentinan-Ajinomoto*)	immunomodulator	Phase II/ III with didanosine for AIDS HIV-positive (symptomatic/ asymptomatic), AIDS, pediatric AIDS	Lenti-Chemico Pharmaceuticals
Molgramostim (GM-CSF; *Leucomax*)	cytokine	Phase II/III With zidovudine for AIDS	Sandoz/Genetics Institute/Schering-Plough
Monoclonal antibody (MSL-109; MAb)	antiviral	Phase I AIDS	Sandoz
Nelfinavir (Viracept)	antiviral	Phase III	Agouron
Novapren	antiviral	Phase I HIV inhibitor	Novaferon Labs
PMEA (*GS 393*)	antiviral	Phase I/II HIV	Gilead Sciences
Ribavirin[1] (*Virazole*)	antiviral	Phase II/III Asymptomatic HIV positive; IND denied	Viratek/ICN
Roquinimex (*Linomide*)	immunomodulator	Phase II HIV	Kabi Pharmacia
Sargramostim[1] (granulocyte macrophage colony stimulating factor; GM-CSF; *Leukine*)	cytokine	Phase II HIV	Immunex
T4, soluble human, recombinant	antiviral	Phase I/II HIV	Biogen
TAT antagonist	antiviral	Phase I/II HIV	Hoffman LaRoche
Thymic humoral factor	immunomodulator	Phase I HIV	Adria
Thymopentin (*Timunox*)	immunomodulator	Phase III Asymptomatic HIV	Immunobiology Research Institute
Thymostimuline (*TP-1*)	immunomodulator	Phase III AIDS	Serono Laboratories
Trichosanthin (*GLQ223*; Compound Q)	antiviral	Phase II ARC, AIDS	Genelabs Technologies
Tumor necrosis factor (TNF)	antiviral	Phase I HIV	Immunex
Veldona	cytokine	Phase I AIDS	Veldona USA
VX478	antiviral	Investigational, AIDS	Glaxo Wellcome

[1] Approved for other indications; refer to individual monographs.

APPENDIX

APPENDIX

FDA New Drug Classification

The FDA developed an alpha-numeric drug classification to aid in the prioritization of a new drug review. The use of numbers identify the drug's chemical classification; letters identify the assessment of therapeutic potential or review priority. This system was revised in 1992. When the classification for a new drug is known, it is listed in parentheses following the approval date for the drug at the beginning of the Administration and Dosage section of the monograph.

FDA Classification System for Newly Approved Drugs	
Chemical Ranking	
1 =	New chemical entity not previously marketed in US
2 =	New salt form of a drug currently on US market
3 =	New dosage formulation of a drug currently on US market
4 =	New combination of drugs already available in US
5 =	New manufacturer (ie, generic drug)
6 =	New indication for drug already approved
7 =	Marketed drug without an approved NDA (drugs marketed prior to 1938)
Therapeutic Potential/Review Priority	
A =	Represents significant therapeutic gain over drugs currently available *(replaced by "P" ranking in 1992)*
AA =	Important therapeutic gain for drugs indicated for AIDS
B =	Represents modest therapeutic advances in drug therapy *(replaced by "P" ranking in 1992)*
C =	Represents little or no therapeutic gain in drug class *(replaced by "S" ranking in 1992)*
E =	Drug used to treat life-threatening or severely debilitated patients
P =	Priority; represents a therapeutic gain or provides improved treatment over marketed drugs OR has modest advantages compared to marketed agents (this category was initiated in first quarter of 1992)
S =	Standard; has similar therapeutic properties when compared to marketed drugs (this category was initiated in first quarter of 1992)

Canadian Trade Names

Canadian trade names are included in this publication. They are designated with a 🍁 in the product tables. For complete Canadian prescribing information and drug schedules, contact the listed Canadian Drug Manufacturer. **Only** United States prescribing information is contained in this publication.

Controlled Substances

The Controlled Substances Act of 1970 regulates the manufacturing, distribution and dispensing of drugs that have abuse potential. The Drug Enforcement Administration (DEA) within the US Department of Justice is the chief federal agency responsible for enforcement.

DEA Schedules: Drugs under jurisdiction of the Controlled Substances Act are divided into five schedules based on their potential for abuse and physical and psychological dependence. All controlled substances listed in *Drug Facts and Comparisons* are identified by schedule as follows:

Schedule I *(c-I):* High abuse potential and no accepted medical use (eg, heroin, marijuana, LSD).

Schedule II *(c-II):* High abuse potential with severe dependence liability (eg, narcotics, amphetamines, dronabinol, some barbiturates).

Schedule III *(c-III):* Less abuse potential than schedule II drugs and moderate dependence liability (eg, nonbarbiturate sedatives, nonamphetamine stimulants, limited amounts of certain narcotics).

Schedule IV *(c-IV):* Less abuse potential than schedule III drugs and limited dependence liability (eg, some sedatives, antianxiety agents, nonnarcotic analgesics).

Schedule V *(c-V):* Limited abuse potential. Primarily small amounts of narcotics (codeine) used as antitussives or antidiarrheals. Under federal law, limited quantities of certain *c-V* drugs may be purchased without a prescription directly from a pharmacist if allowed under state statutes. The purchaser must be at least 18 years of age and must furnish suitable identification. All such transactions must be recorded by the dispensing pharmacist.

Registration: Prescribing physicians and dispensing pharmacies must be registered with the DEA, PO Box 28083, Central Station, Washington, DC 20005.

Inventory: Separate records must be kept of purchases and dispensing of controlled substances. An inventory of controlled substances must be made every 2 years.

Prescriptions: Prescriptions for controlled substances must be written in ink and include: Date; name and address of the patient; name, address and DEA number of the physician. Oral prescriptions must be promptly committed to writing. Controlled substance prescriptions may not be dispensed or refilled more than 6 months after the date issued or be refilled more than five times. A written prescription signed by the physician is required for schedule II drugs. In case of emergency, oral prescriptions for schedule II substances may be filled; however, the physician must provide a signed prescription within 72 hours. Schedule II prescriptions cannot be refilled. A triplicate order form is necessary for the transfer of controlled substances in schedule II. Forms are available for the individual prescriber at no charge from the DEA.

State Laws: In many cases state laws are more restrictive than federal laws and therefore impose additional requirements (eg, triplicate prescription forms).

FDA Pregnancy Categories

The rational use of any medication requires a risk versus benefit assessment. Among the myriad of risk factors which complicate this assessment, pregnancy is one of the most perplexing.

The FDA has established five categories to indicate the potential of a systemically absorbed drug for causing birth defects. The key differentiation among the categories rests upon the degree (reliability) of documentation and the risk vs benefit ratio. Pregnancy Category X is particularly notable in that if any data exist that may implicate a drug as a teratogen and the risk vs benefit ratio does not support use of the drug, the drug is contraindicated during pregnancy. These categories are summarized below:

FDA Pregnancy Categories

Pregnancy Category	Definition
A	Adequate studies in pregnant women have not demonstrated a risk to the fetus in the first trimester of pregnancy and there is no evidence of risk in later trimesters.
B	Animal studies have not demonstrated a risk to the fetus but there are no adequate studies in pregnant women ... or ... Animal studies have shown an adverse effect, but adequate studies in pregnant women have not demonstrated a risk to the fetus during the first trimester of pregnancy and there is no evidence of risk in later trimesters.
C	Animal studies have shown an adverse effect on the fetus but there are no adequate studies in humans; the benefits from the use of the drug in pregnant women may be acceptable despite its potential risks ... or ... There are no animal reproduction studies and no adequate studies in humans.
D	There is evidence of human fetal risk, but the potential benefits from the use of the drug in pregnant women may be acceptable despite its potential risks.
X	Studies in animals or humans demonstrate fetal abnormalities or adverse reaction reports indicate evidence of fetal risk. The risk of use in a pregnant woman clearly outweighs any possible benefit.

Regardless of the designated Pregnancy Category or presumed safety, no drug should be administered during pregnancy unless it is clearly needed and potential benefits outweigh potential hazards to the fetus.

General Management of Acute Overdosage

Rapid intervention is essential to minimize morbidity and mortality in an acute toxic ingestion. Institute measures to prevent absorption and hasten elimination as soon as possible; however, symptomatic and supportive care takes precedence over other therapy. It is assumed that basic life support measures, ie, cardiopulmonary resuscitation (CPR), have been instituted. Specific antidotes are discussed in the overdosage section of individual drug monographs. The discussion below outlines procedures used in the management of acute overdosage of orally ingested systemic drugs.

Advanced Life Support Measures:

Adequate Airway must be established and maintained, generally via oropharyngeal or endotracheal airways, cricothyrotomy or tracheostomy.

Ventilation may then be performed via mouth-to-mouth insufflation, hand-operated bag (ambu bag) or a mechanical ventilator.

Circulation must be maintained.

- *Hypotension:* If hypotension/hypoperfusion occurs, place the patient in shock position (head lowered, feet elevated); specific therapy may include:

  Establish IV access and initiate IV fluids (eg, Normal [0.9%] Saline, 0.45% Saline, Lactated Ringer's Dextrose Solutions). A maintenance flow rate is generally 100 to 200 ml/hour; individualize as necessary.

  Plasma, plasma protein fractions, whole blood or plasma expanders may be required.

  Severe hypotension may require judicious use of cardiovascular active agents. The most commonly recommended agents are dopamine, dobutamine and norepinephrine.
- *Arrhythmia* treatment is dictated by the offending drug.
- *Hypertension,* sometimes severe, may occur. (See Agents for Hypertensive Emergencies.)

For specific information on individual drugs or drug classes, see individual or group monographs.

Seizures: Simple isolated seizures may require only observation and supportive care. Repetitive seizures or status epilepticus require therapy. Intravenous diazepam or fosphenytoin are generally the agents of choice; phenobarbital may also be considered.

Reduction of Drug Absorption:

Gastric emptying is generally recommended as soon as possible; however, this is generally not very effective unless employed within the first 1 to 2 hours after ingestion. Syrup of ipecac and gastric lavage are the two most commonly employed methods.

- *Syrup of ipecac* is the method of choice outside the hospital, but administer only on the advice of a qualified health-care professional.

- *Gastric lavage* is indicated in the comatose patient and for those in whom syrup of ipecac fails to produce emesis. Airway protection via endotracheal intubation is appropriate for the patient without a gag reflex. Position the patient on his left side and use a large bore tube. Instill warm water or saline 37° C (98.6° F), 100 to 300 ml per wash for adults; 10 ml/kg to a maximum of 250 ml for children, until lavage solution returns clear. Instill the fluid over 1 to 2 minutes, leave in place about 1 minute and drain over 3 to 4 minutes.

Adsorption, using activated charcoal after completion of emesis or lavage, is indicated for virtually all significant toxic ingestions. It adsorbs a wide variety of toxins and there are no contraindications. However, it adsorbs many orally administered antidotes as well, so space dosage properly.

Catharsis is sometimes recommended, generally using a saline or osmotic cathartic (eg, magnesium sulfate or citrate or sorbitol) to promote passage of the toxin through the GI tract.

Whole bowel irrigation (WBI) utilizes rapid administration of large volumes of lavage solutions, such as PEG. It may be most useful for removal of iron tablets and cocaine-containing condoms or balloons.

Elimination of Absorbed Drug:

Interruption of enterohepatic circulation by "gastric dialysis" uses scheduled doses of activated charcoal for 1 to 2 days. Gastric dialysis not only interrupts the enterohepatic cycle of some drugs, but also creates an osmotic gradient, drawing drug from the plasma back into the gastrointestinal lumen where it is bound by the charcoal and excreted in the feces.

Diuresis may be effective as identified in the individual drug monographs.

- *Forced diuresis* is occasionally useful. The most common agents employed are furosemide and osmotic diuretics.
- *Alkaline diuresis* is appropriate for certain compounds (eg, phenobarbital, salicylates) and is usually accomplished by the administration of IV sodium bicarbonate.
- *Acid diuresis* may be indicated (eg, in overdose with amphetamines, fenfluramine, quinine) but use with caution in patients with renal or liver disease. It is usually accomplished with oral or IV ascorbic acid or ammonium chloride.

Dialysis is indicated in a minority of severe overdose cases. Drug factors that alter dialysis effectiveness include volume of distribution, drug compartmentalization, protein binding and lipid/water solubility.

- *Peritoneal dialysis* and *hemodialysis* have been the most common methods used. *Charcoal or resin hemoperfusion* is a relatively new procedure with promising clinical potential (eg, with theophylline).

Poison Control Center:

Consultation with a regional poison control center is highly recommended.

Type I hypersensitivity reactions (immediate hypersensitivity or anaphylaxis) are immunologic responses to a foreign antigen to which a patient has been previously sensitized. Anaphylactoid reactions are not immunologically mediated; however, symptoms and treatment are similar.

Signs and Symptoms

Acute hypersensitivity reactions typically begin within 1 to 30 minutes of exposure to the offending antigen. Tingling sensations and a generalized flush may proceed to a fullness in the throat, chest tightness or a "feeling of impending doom". Generalized urticaria and sweating are common. *Severe* reactions include life-threatening involvement of the airway and cardiovascular system.

Treatment:

Appropriate and immediate treatment is imperative. The following general measures are commonly employed:

Epinephrine 1:1000, 0.2 to 0.5 mg (0.2 to 0.5 ml) SC is the primary treatment. In children, administer 0.01 mg/kg or 0.1 mg. Doses may be repeated every 5 to 15 minutes if needed. A succession of small doses is more effective and less dangerous than a single large dose. Additionally, 0.1 mg may be introduced into an injection site where the offending drug was administered. If appropriate, the use of a tourniquet above the site of injection of the causative agent may slow its absorption and distribution. However, remove or loosen the tourniquet every 10 to 15 minutes to maintain circulation.

Epinephrine IV (generally indicated in the presence of hypotension) is often recommended in a 1:10,000 dilution, 0.3 to 0.5 mg over 5 minutes; repeat every 15 minutes, if necessary. In children, inject 0.1 to 0.2 mg or 0.01 mg/kg/dose over 5 minutes; repeat every 30 minutes.

A conservative IV epinephrine protocol includes 0.1 mg of a 1:100,000 dilution (0.1 mg of a 1:1000 dilution mixed in 10 ml normal saline) given over 5 to 10 minutes. If an IV infusion is necessary, administer at a rate of 1 to 4 mcg/min. In children, infuse 0.1 to 1.5 (maximum) mcg/kg/min.

Dilute epinephrine 1:10,000 may be administered through an endotracheal tube, if no other parenteral access is available, directly into the bronchial tree. It is rapidly absorbed there from the capillary bed of the lung.

Airway: Ensure a patent airway via endotracheal intubation or cricothyrotomy (ie, inferior laryngotomy, used prior to tracheotomy) and administer oxygen. Severe respiratory difficulty may respond to IV aminophylline or to other bronchodilators.

Hypotension: The patient should be recumbent with feet elevated. Depending upon the severity, consider the following measures:

- Establish a patent IV catheter in a suitable vein.
- Administer IV fluids (eg, Normal Saline, Lactated Ringer's).
- Administer plasma expanders.

- Administer cardioactive agents (see group and individual monographs). Commonly recommended agents include dopamine, dobutamine, norepinephrine and phenylephrine.

Adjunctive therapy does not alter acute reactions, but may modify an ongoing or slow-onset process and shorten the course of the reaction.

- *Antihistamines: Diphenhydramine* – 50 to 100 mg IM or IV, continued orally at 5 mg/kg/day or 50 mg every 6 hours for 1 to 2 days. For children, give 5 mg/kg/day, maximum 300 mg/day.

  Chlorpheniramine – (adults, 10 to 20 mg; children, 5 to 10 mg) IM or slowly IV.

  Hydroxyzine – 10 to 25 mg orally or 25 to 50 mg IM 3 to 4 times daily.
- *Corticosteroids,* eg, hydrocortisone IV 100 to 1000 mg or equivalent, followed by 7 mg/kg/day IV or oral for 1 to 2 days. The role of corticosteroids is controversial.
- *H_2 antagonists: Cimetidine – Children,* 25 to 30 mg/kg/day IV in six divided doses; *adults,* 300 mg every 6 hours. *Ranitidine* – 50 mg IV over 3 to 5 minutes. May be of value in addition to H_1 antihistamines, although this opinion is not universally shared.

Calculations

To calculate milliequivalent weight: $mEq = \frac{\text{gram molecular weight/valence}}{1000}$

$mEq = \frac{mg}{\text{eq wt}}$ equivalent weight or eq wt = $\frac{\text{gram molecular weight}}{\text{valence}}$

Commonly used mEq weights			
Chloride	35.5 mg = 1 mEq	Magnesium	12 mg = 1 mEq
Sodium	23 mg = 1 mEq	Potassium	39 mg = 1 mEq
Calcium	20 mg = 1 mEq		

To convert temperature °C ↔ °F: $\frac{°C}{°F - 32} = \frac{5}{9}$ or $°C = \frac{5}{9}(°F - 32)$

$°F = 32 + \frac{9}{5}\,°C$

To calculate creatinine clearance (Ccr) from serum creatinine:

Male: $Ccr = \frac{\text{weight (kg)} \times (140 - \text{age})}{72 \times \text{serum creatinine (mg/dl)}}$ Female: $Ccr = 0.85 \times$ calculation for males

To calculate ideal body weight (kg):

Male = 50 kg + 2.3 kg (each inch > 5 ft)   Female = 45.5 kg + 2.3 kg (each inch > 5 ft)

To calculate body surface area (BSA) in adults and children:

1) *Dubois method:*

$SA\ (cm^2) = wt\ (kg)^{0.425} \times ht\ (cm)^{0.725} \times 71.84$

$SA\ (m^2) = K \times \sqrt[3]{wt^2}\ (kg)$ (common K value 0.1 for toddlers, 0.103 for neonates)

2) *Simplified method:*

$BSA\ (m^2) = \sqrt{\frac{ht\ (cm) \times wt\ (kg)}{3600}}$

To approximate surface area (m^2) of children from weight (kg):

Weight range (kg)	≈ Surface area (m^2)
1 to 5	(0.05 x kg) + 0.05
6 to 10	(0.04 x kg) + 0.10
11 to 20	(0.03 x kg) + 0.20
21 to 40	(0.02 x kg) + 0.40

Suggested Weights for Adults

Height*	Weight in pounds†
4′10″	91-119
4′11″	94-124
5′0″	97-128
5′1″	101-132
5′2″	104-137
5′3″	107-141
5′4″	111-146
5′5″	114-150
5′6″	118-155
5′7″	121-160
5′8″	125-164
5′9″	129-169
5′10″	132-174
5′11″	136-179
6′0″	140-184
6′1″	144-189
6′2″	148-195
6′3″	152-200
6′4″	156-205
6′5″	160-211
6′6″	164-216

* Without shoes.   † Without clothes.

The higher weights in the ranges generally apply to people with more muscle and bone. Source: Nutrition and Your Health: Dietary Guidelines for Americans, 4th ed, 1995. US Department of Agriculture, US Department of Health and Human Services. At press time, these new guidelines had not been officially released. It is possible some changes to this chart will occur.

The *Systeme international d 'unités* (International System of Units) or *SI* is a modernized version of the metric system. The primary goal of the conversion to SI units is to revise the present confused measurement system and to improve test-result communications.

The SI has 7 basic units from which other units are derived:

Base Units of SI		
Physical quantity	Base unit	SI symbol
length	meter	m
mass	kilogram	kg
time	second	s
amount of substance	mole	mol
thermodynamic temperature	kelvin	K
electric current	ampere	A
luminous intensity	candela	cd

Combinations of these base units can express any property although, for simplicity, special names are given to some of these derived units.

Representative Derived Units		
Derived unit	Name and symbol	Derivation from base units
area	square meter	m^2
volume	cubic meter	m^3
force	newton (N)	$kg \cdot m \cdot s^{-2}$
pressure	pascal (Pa)	$kg \cdot m^{-1} \cdot s^{-2}$ (N/m^2)
work, energy	joule (J)	$kg \cdot m^2 \cdot s^{-2}$(N•m)
mass density	kilogram per cubic meter	kg/m^3
frequency	hertz (Hz)	s^{-1}
temperature degree	Celsius (°C)	°C = °K − 273.15
concentration		
mass	kilogram/liter	kg/L
substance	mole/liter	mol/L
molality	mole/kilogram	mol/kg
density	kilogram/liter	kg/L

Prefixes to the base unit are used in this system to form decimal multiples and submultiples. The preferred multiples and submultiples listed below change the quantity by increments of 10^3 or 10^{-3}. The exceptions to these recommended factors are within the middle rectangle.

Prefixes and Symbols for Decimal Multiples and Submultiples		
Factor	Prefix	Symbol
10^{18}	exa	E
10^{15}	peta	P
10^{12}	tera	T
10^9	giga	G
10^6	mega	M
10^3	kilo	k
10^2	hecto	h
10^1	deka	da
10^{-1}	deci	d
10^{-2}	centi	c
10^{-3}	milli	m
10^{-6}	micro	μ
10^{-9}	nano	n
10^{-12}	pico	p
10^{-15}	femto	f
10^{-18}	atto	a

To convert drug concentrations to or from SI units:

Conversion factor (CF) $= \frac{1000}{\text{mol wt}}$

Conversion *to* SI units: μg/ml x CF = μmol/L

Conversion *from* SI units: μmol/L ÷ CF = μg/ml

Normal Laboratory Values

In the following tables, normal reference values for commonly requested laboratory tests are listed in traditional units and in SI units. The tables are a guideline only. Values are method dependent and "normal values" may vary between laboratories.

Blood, Plasma or Serum

Determination	Reference Value	
	Conventional Units	SI Units
Ammonia (NH_3)	10-80 mcg/dl	5-50 mcmol/L
Amylase	≤ 130 U/L	≤ 130 U/L
Antinuclear antibodies	negative at 1:10 dilution of serum	negative at 1:10 dilution of serum
Antithrombin III (AT III)	18-30 mg/dl	18-30 g/L
Bilirubin: conjugated	≤ 0.2 mg/dl	≤ 4 mcmol/L
total	0.1-1 mg/dl	2-18 mcmol/L
Calcitonin	< 100 pg/ml	< 100 ng/L
Calcium: female < 50 years old	8.8-10 mg/dl	2.2-2.5 mmol/L
female > 50 years old	8.8-10.2 mg/dl	2.2-2.56 mmol/L
male	8.8-10.3 mg/dl	2.2-2.58 mmol/L
all populations	4.4-5.1 mEq/L	2.2-2.56 mmol/L
Carbon dioxide content	22-28 mEq/L	22-28 mmol/L
Carcinoembryonic antigen	< 3 ng/ml	< 3 mcg/L
Chloride	95-105 mEq/L	95-105 mmol/L
Coagulation screen:		
Bleeding time	2-9 min	60-540 sec
Prothrombin time	10-12 sec	10-12 sec
Partial thromboplastin time (activated)	35-45 sec	35-45 sec
Protein C	0.4 mg/dl	0.4 g/L
Protein S	2.3 mg/dl	2.3 g/L
Copper, total	70-140 mcg/dl	11-22 mcmol/L
Corticotropin (ACTH adrenocorticotropic hormone)	20-100 pg/ml	4-22 pmol/L
Cortisol: 0800 hr	4-19 mcg/dl	110-520 nmol/L
1800 hr	2-15 mcg/dl	50-410 nmol/L
2400 hr	< 5 mcg/dl	< 140 nmol/L
Creatine phosphokinase, total (CK, CPK)	≤ 150 U/L	≤ 150 U/L
Creatine kinase isoenzymes, MB fraction	> 5% in MI	> 0.05 fraction of 1
Creatinine	0.6-1.2 mg/dl	50-110 mcmol/L
Fibrinogen (coagulation factor I)	150-350 mg/dl	1.5-3.5 g/L
Follicle stimulating hormone (FSH):		
female	2-15 mIU/ml	2-15 IU/L
peak production	20-50 mIU/ml	20-50 IU/L
male	1-10 mIU/ml	1-10 IU/L
Glucose, fasting	70-110 mg/dl	3.9-6.1 mmol/L
Haptoglobin	50-220 mg/dl	0.5-2.2 g/L
Hematologic tests:		
Hematocrit (Hct), female	33%-43%	0.33-0.43 fraction of 1
male	39%-49%	0.39-0.49 fraction of 1
Hemoglobin (Hb), female	14-18 g/dl	140-180 g/L
male	11.5-15.5 g/dl	115-155 g/L
Leukocyte count (WBC)	3200-9800/mm^3	3.2-9.8 x 10^9/L
Erythrocyte count (RBC), female	3.5-5 × $10^6/mm^3$	3.5-5 x 10^{12}/L
male	4.3-5.9 × $10^6/mm^3$	4.3-5.9 x 10^{12}/L

Blood, Plasma or Serum		
	Reference Value	
Determination	Conventional Units	SI Units
Erythrocyte sedimentation rate		
(sedrate, ESR), female	≤ 30 mm/hr	≤ 30 mm/hr
male	≤ 20 mm/hr	≤ 20 mm/hr
Ferritin	18-300 ng/ml	18-300 mcg/L
Folic acid: normal	> 3.8 ng/ml	> 8.4 nmol/L
Mean corpuscular volume (MCV)	76-100 mcm^3	76-100 fL
Mean corpuscular hemoglobin (MCH)	27-33 pg	27-33 pg
Mean corpuscular hemoglobin concentration (MCHC)	33-37 g/dl	330-370 g/L
Platelet count	130-400 × $10^3/mm^3$	130-400 × 10^9/L
Vitamin B_{12}	200-1000 pg/ml	150-750 pmol/L
Iron		
female	60-160 mcg/dl	11-29 mcmol/L
male	80-180 mcg/dl	14-32 mcmol/L
Iron binding capacity	250-460 mcg/dl	45-82 mcmol/L
Lactic acid (lactate)	0.5-2 mEq/L	0.5-2 mmol/L
Lactic dehydrogenase	50-150 U/L	50-150 U/L
Lead (toxic levels)	> 60 mcg/dl	> 2.9 mcmol/L
Lipids:		
Triglycerides		
Desirable	< 250 mg/dL	< 2.82 mmol/L
Borderline	250-500 mg/dL	2.82-5.65 mmol/L
High	> 500 mg/dL	> 5.65 mmol/L
LDL Cholesterol		
Desirable	< 130 mg/dL	< 3.36 mmol/L
Borderline	130-159 mg/dL	3.36-4.11 mmol/L
High	> 159 mg/dL	> 4.11 mmol/L
HDL Cholesterol		
High	< 35 mg/dL	< 0.91 mmol/L
Total Cholesterol		
Desirable	< 200 mg/dL	5.17 mmol/L
Borderline	200-239 mg/dL	5.17-6.18 mmol/L
High	> 239 mg/dL	> 6.18 mmol/L
Triglycerides	< 460 mg/dl	< 5.3 mmol/L
Magnesium	1.6-2.4 mEq/L	0.8-1.2 mmol/L
Osmolality	280-300 mOsm/kg	280-300 mmol/kg
Oxygen saturation (arterial)	96%-100%	0.96-1 fraction of 1
PCO_2, arterial	35-45 mmHg	4.7-6 kPa
pH, arterial	7.35-7.45	7.35-7.45
PO_2, arterial: Breathing room air	75-100 mmHg	10-13.3 kPa
Phosphatase (acid)	2-11 IU/L	3-183 mcKat/L ≤ 16.1 U/L
Phosphatase alkaline (ALP)	25-100 IU/L	4-1.7mcKat/L
Phosphorus, inorganic, (phosphate)	2.5-5 mg/dl	0.8-1.6 mmol/L
Potassium	3.5-5 mEq/L	3.5-5 mmol/L
Progesterone		
Follicular phase	< 2 ng/ml	< 6 nmol/L
Luteal phase	2-20 ng/ml	6-64 nmol/L
Prolactin	< 20 ng/ml	< 20 mcg/L
Protein: Total	5.5-9 g/dl	55-90 g/L
Albumin	3.5-5 g/dl	35-50 g/L
Globulin	2-3 g/L	20-30 g/L

Blood, Plasma or Serum		
	Reference Value	
Determination	Conventional Units	SI Units
Rheumatoid factor	< 80 IU/ml	< 80 kIU/L
Sodium	135-147 mEq/L	135-147 mmol/L
Testosterone: female	< 0.6 ng/ml	< 2 nmol/L
male	4-8 ng/ml	14-28 nmol/L
Thyroid Hormone Function Tests:		
Thyroid-stimulating hormone (TSH)	2-11 mcU/ml	2-11 mU/L
Thyroxine-binding globulin capacity	12-28 mcg/dl	150-360 nmol/L
Total triiodothyronine (T_3)	75-220 ng/dl	1.2-3.4 nmol/L
Total thyroxine (T_4)	4-11 mcg/dl	51-142 nmol/L
T_3 uptake	25%-35%	0.25-0.35 fraction of 1
Transaminase, AST (aspartate aminotransferase, SGOT)	≤ 35 U/L	≤ 35 U/L
Transaminase, ALT (alanine aminotransferase, SGPT)	≤ 35 U/L	≤ 35 U/L
Urea nitrogen (BUN)	8-18 mg/dl	3-6.5 mmol/L
Uric acid	2-7 mg/dl	120-420 mcmol/L
Vitamin A (retinol)	10-50 mcg/dl	0.35-1.75 mcmol/L
Zinc	75-120 mcg/dl	11.5-18.5 mcmol/L

Urine						
		Reference Value				
Determination		Conventional Units		SI Units		
Catecholamines: Epinephrine		< 10 mcg/day		< 55 nmol/day		
Norepinephrine		< 100 mcg/day		< 590 nmol/day		
Creatinine: female		14-22 mg/kg/24 h		0.12-0.19 mmol/kg/day		
male		20-26 mg/kg/24 h		0.18-0.23 mmol/kg/day		
Potassium (diet-dependent)		25-100 mEq/day		25-100 mmol/day		
Protein, quantitative		< 150 mg/day		< 0.15 g/day		
Steroids:		(mg/day)		(mcmol/day)		
	Age (yrs)	male	female	male	female	
17-Ketosteroids	10	1-4	1-4	3-14	3-14	
	20	6-21	4-16	21-73	14-56	
	30	8-26	4-14	28-90	14-49	
	50	5-18	3-9	17-62	10-31	
	70	2-10	1-7	7-35	3-24	
17-Hydroxycorticosteroids (as cortisol):						
female		2-8 mg/day		5-25 mcmol/day		
male		3-10 mg/day		10-30 mcmol/day		

Drug Levels†

	Drug Determination	Reference Value: Conventional Units	Reference Value: SI Units
Aminoglycosides (peak levels)	Amikacin	16-32 mcg/ml	nd
	Gentamicin	4-8 mcg/ml	nd
	Kanamycin	15-40 mcg/ml	nd
	Netilmicin	6-10 mcg/ml	nd
	Streptomycin	20-30 mcg/ml	nd
	Tobramycin	4-8 mcg/ml	nd
Antiarrhythmics	Amiodarone	0.5-2.5 mcg/ml	nd
	Bretylium	0.5-1.5 mcg/ml	nd
	Digitoxin	9-25 mcg/L	11.8-32.8 nmol/L
	Digoxin	0.5-2.2 ng/ml	0.6-2.8 nmol/L
	Disopyramide	2-8 mcg/ml	6-18 mcmol/L
	Flecainide	0.2-1 mcg/ml	nd
	Lidocaine	1.5-6 mcg/ml	4.5-21.5 mcmol/L
	Mexiletine	0.5-2 mcg/ml	nd
	Procainamide	4-8 mcg/ml	17-34 mcmol/ml
	Propranolol	50-200 ng/ml	190-770 nmol/L
	Quinidine	2-6 mcg/ml	4.6-9.2 mcmol/L
	Tocainide	4-10 mcg/ml	nd
	Verapamil	0.08-0.3 mcg/ml	nd
Anti-convulsants	Carbamazepine	4-12 mcg/ml	17-51 mcmol/L
	Phenobarbital	15-40 mcg/ml	65-172 mcmol/L
	Phenytoin	10-20 mcg/ml	40-80 mcmol/L
	Primidone	5-12 mcg/ml	25-46 mcmol/L
	Valproic acid	50-100 mcg/ml	350-700 mcmol/L
Antidepressants	Amitriptyline	110-250 ng/ml	nd
	Amoxapine	200-500 ng/ml	nd
	Bupropion	25-100 ng/ml	nd
	Clomipramine	80-100 ng/ml	nd
	Desipramine	125-300 ng/ml	nd
	Doxepin	100-200 ng/ml	nd
	Imipramine	200-350 ng/ml	nd
	Maprotiline	200-300 ng/ml	nd
	Nortriptyline	50-150 ng/ml	nd
	Protriptyline	100-200 ng/ml	nd
	Trazodone	800-1600 ng/ml	nd
Antipsychotics	Chlorpromazine	30-500 ng/ml	nd
	Fluphenazine	0.13-2.8 ng/ml	nd
	Haloperidol	5-20 ng/ml	nd
	Perphenazine	0.8-1.2 ng/ml	nd
	Thiothixene	2-57 ng/ml	nd
Miscellaneous	Amantadine	300 ng/ml	nd
	Amrinone	3.7 mcg/ml	nd
	Chloramphenicol	10-20 mcg/ml	31-62 mcmol/L
	Cyclosporine[1]	250-800 ng/ml (whole blood, RIA)	nd
		50-300 ng/ml (plasma, RIA)	nd
	Ethanol[2]	0 mg/dl	0 mmol/L
	Hydralazine	100 ng/ml	nd
	Lithium	0.5-1.5 mEq/L	0.5-1.5 mmol/L
	Salicylate	100-200 mg/L	724-1448 mcmol/L
	Sulfonamide	5-15 mg/dl	nd
	Terbutaline	0.5-4.1 ng/ml	nd
	Theophylline	10-20 mcg/ml	55-110 mcmol/L
	Vancomycin (peak)	30-40 ng/ml	nd

† The values given are generally accepted as desirable for achieving therapeutic effect without toxicity for most patients. However, exceptions are not uncommon.

[1] 24 hour trough values.

[2] Toxic: 50-100 mg/dl (10.9-21.7 mmol/L).

nd – No data available.

Standard Abbreviations

ac	before meals
bid	twice daily
°C	degrees Celsius
bpm	beats per minute
Ca	calcium
Cal	Calorie (kilocalorie)
Ccr	creatinine clearance
CDC	Centers for Disease Control
CHF	congestive heart failure
Cl	chloride
CNS	central nervous system
CPK	creatine phosphokinase
CSF	cerebrospinal fluid
cu	cubic
Cu	copper
dl	deciliter (100 ml)
DNA	Deoxyribonucleic acid
ECG or EKG	electrocardiogram
EEG	electroencephalogram
F	fluoride
°F	degrees Fahrenheit
FA	folic acid
FDA	Food and Drug Administration
Fe	iron
g	gram
G-6-PD	glucose-6-phosphate dehydrogenase
gal	gallon
GI	gastrointestinal
GU	genitourinary
h or hr	hour
hs	at bedtime
I	iodine
IM	intramuscular
IU	international units
IV	intravenous
K	potassium
kg	kilogram
L	liter
lb	pound
m	meter
m^2	square meter
mcg	microgram
mCi	millicurie
mEq	milliequivalent
mg	milligram
Mg	magnesium
MIC	minimum inhibitory concentration
min	minute
ml	milliliter
mm	millimeter
mm^3	cubic millimeter
Mn	manganese
Mo	molybdenum
mOsm	milliosmole
MRI	Magnetic resonance imaging
Na	sodium
NF	National Formulary
ng	nanogram
otc	over the counter (nonprescription)
oz	ounce
P	phosphorus
pc	after meals
po	by mouth
ppm	parts per million
prn	as needed
pt	pint
qid	four times daily
qt	quart
RDA	Recommended Dietary Allowance
RNA	ribonucleic acid
Rx	prescription only
SC	subcutaneous
Se	selenium
$t_{1/2}$	half-life
tid	three times daily
tbsp	tablespoon
tsp	teaspoon
U	unit
UD	unit dose package
USP	United States Pharmacopeia
V_d	Volume of distribution
WHO	World Health Organization
Zn	zinc

Manufacturer/Distributor Abbreviations

This listing includes only those manufacturers whose names are abbreviated in *Drug Facts and Comparisons.* It is not a complete list of all manufacturers whose products are listed in this book.

B-D	Becton, Dickinson & Co.
B-I	Boehringer Ingelheim
B-Mannheim	Boehringer Mannheim
B-M Squibb	Bristol-Myers Squibb
Hickam	Dow B. Hickam
Inter. Ethical	International Ethical Labs
IMS	International Medication Systems
J & J	Johnson & Johnson
McNeil-CPC	McNeil Consumer Products Company
Mead-J	Mead Johnson Nutritional
Merck	Merck & Co.
P-D	Parke-Davis
PBH	Pilkington Barnes Hind
PBI	Pharmaceutical Basics, Inc.
P & G	Procter & Gamble
RPR	Rhone-Poulenc Rorer
Schwarz Pharma K-U	Schwarz Pharma Kremers Urban
SK-Beecham, SKB	SmithKline Beecham
URL	United Research Labs
Warner-C	Warner Chilcott
Warner-L	Warner-Lambert
W-A	Wyeth-Ayerst

Trademark Glossary

Many companies use trademarks to identify specific dosage forms or unique packaging materials. The following list is provided as a guide to the interpretation of these descriptions.

Abbo-Pac (Abbott)
Unit dose package

Accu-Pak (Ciba-Geigy)
Unit dose blister pack

Act-O-Vial (Upjohn)
Vial system

ADD-Vantage (Abbott)
Sterile dissolution system for admixture

ADT (Upjohn)
Alternate day therapy

Arm-A-Med (Armour)
Single-dose plastic vial

Arm-A-Vial (Armour)
Single-dose plastic vial

Aspirol (Lilly)
Crushable ampule for inhalation

bidCAP (B-M Squibb)
Double strength capsule

Bristoject (B-M Squibb)
Unit dose syringe

Caplet (Various)
Capsule shaped tablet

Carpuject (Sanofi Winthrop)
Cartridge needle unit

Chronotab (Schering)
Sustained action tablet

Clinipak (Wyeth-Ayerst)
Unit dose package

ControlPak (Sandoz)
Unit dose rolls, tamper resistant

Detecto-Seal (Sanofi Winthrop)
Tamper resistant parenteral package

Dialpak (Ortho)
Compliance package

Dis-Co Pack (Robins)
Unit dose package

Disket (Lilly)
Dispersible tablet

Dispenserpak (Glaxo Wellcome)
Unit-of-use package

Dispertab (Abbott)
Particles in tablet

Dispette (Lederle)
Disposable pipette

Divide-Tab (Abbott)
Scored tablet

Dividose (Mead Johnson)
Tablet, bisected/trisected

Dosa-Trol Pack (B-M Squibb)
Unit-dose box packaging

Dosepak (Upjohn)
Unit-of-use package

Dosette (Elkins-Sinn)
Single dose ampule or vial

Drop Dose (Glaxo Wellcome)
Ophthalmic dropper dispenser

Drop-Tainer (Alcon)
Ophthalmic dropper dispenser

Dulcet (Abbott)
Chewable tablet

Dura-Tab (Berlex)
Sustained release tablet

Enseal (Lilly)
Enteric coated tablet

EN-tabs (Pharmacia)
Enteric coated tablet

Expidet (Wyeth-Ayerst)
Fast-dissolving doseform

Extentab (Robins)
Continuous release tablet

Fast-Trak (Wyeth-Ayerst)
Quick-loading hypodermic syringe

Filmlok (B-M Squibb)
Veneer coated tablet

Filmtab (Abbott)
Film coated tablet

Flo-Pack (Glaxo Wellcome)
Vial for preparation of IV drips

Gelseal (Lilly)
Soft gelatin capsule

Gradumet (Abbott)
Controlled release tablet

Gy-Pak (Ciba-Geigy)
Unit-of-issue package

Gyrocap (Rhone-Poulenc Rorer)
Timed release capsule

Hyporet (Lilly)
Unit dose syringe

Identi-Dose (Lilly)
Unit dose package

Infatab (Parke-Davis)
Chewable pediatric tablet

Inject-all (B-M Squibb)
Prefilled disposable dilution syringe

Inlay-Tabs (Sandoz)
Inlaid tablets

Isoject (Pfizer)
Unit dose syringe

Kapseal (Parke-Davis)
Banded (sealed) capsule

Kronocap (Ferndale)
Sustained release capsule

Lederject (Lederle)
Disposable syringe

Liquitab (Mission)
Chewable tablet

Memorette (Syntex)
Compliance package

Mix-O-Vial (Upjohn)
Two compartment vial

Mono-Drop (Sanofi Winthrop)
Ophthalmic plastic dropper

Ocumeter (Merck & Co.)
Ophthalmic dropper dispenser

Perle (Forest)
Soft gelatin capsule

Pilpak (Wyeth-Ayerst)
Compliance pack

Plateau CAP (Marion Merrell Dow)
Controlled release capsule

Pulvule (Lilly)
Bullet-shaped capsule

Redipak (Wyeth-Ayerst)
Unit dose or unit-of-issue package

Redi Vial (Lilly)
Dual compartment vial

Repetabs (Schering)
Extended release tablet

Rescue Pak (Glaxo Wellcome)
Unit dose packaging

Respihaler (Merck & Co.)
Aerosol for inhalation

SandoPak (Sandoz)
Unit dose blister package

Secule (Wyeth-Ayerst)
Single dose vial

Sequels (Lederle)
Sustained release capsule or tablet

SigPak (Sandoz)
Unit-of-use package

Snap Tabs (Sandoz)
Tablet with facilitated bisect

Solvet (Lilly)
Soluble tablet

Spansule (SmithKline Beecham)
Sustained release capsule

Stat-Pak (Adria)
Unit dose package

Steri-Dose (Parke-Davis)
Unit dose syringe

Steri-Vial (Parke-Davis)
Ampule

Supprette (PolyMedica)
Suppository

Tabloid (Glaxo Wellcome)
Branded tablet (with raised lettering)

Tamp-R-Tel (Wyeth-Ayerst)
Tubex, tamper resistant

Tel-E-Amp (Roche)
Single dose amp

Tel-E-Dose (Roche)
Unit dose strip package

Tel-E-Ject (Roche)
Unit dose syringe

Tel-E-Pack (Roche)
Packaging system

Tel-E-Vial (Roche)
Single dose vial

Tembids (Wyeth-Ayerst)
Sustained action capsule

Tempule (Armour)
Timed release capsule or tablet

Thera-Ject (SmithKline Beecham)
Unit dose syringe

Tiltab (SmithKline Beecham)
Tablet shape

Timecap (Schwarz Pharma Kremers Urban)
Sustained release capsule

Timecelle (Roberts Hauck)
Timed release capsule

Timespan (Roche)
Timed release tablet

Titradose (Wyeth-Ayerst)
Scored tablet

Traypak (Lilly)
Multivial carton

Tubex (Wyeth-Ayerst)
Cartridge-needle unit

Turbinaire (Adams)
Aerosol for nasal inhalation

UDIP (Marion Merrell Dow)
Unit dose indentification pack

U-Ject (Upjohn)
Disposable syringe

Uni-Amp (Sanofi Winthrop)
Single dose ampule

Unimatic (B-M Squibb)
Unit dose syringe

Uni-Nest (Sanofi Winthrop)
Ampule

UNI-Rx (Marion Merrell Dow)
Unit dose packages and containers

Unisert (Upsher-Smith)
Suppository

Vaporole (Glaxo Wellcome)
Crushable ampule for inhalation

Visipak (Upjohn)
Reverse numbered pack

Wyseals (Wyeth-Ayerst)
Film coated tablet

00089, 55298, 55326
3M Personal Healthcare Products
3M Center
Building 275-5W-05
St. Paul, MN 55133
612-733-1110

00089
3M Pharmaceutical
3M Center
Building 275-3E-09
St. Paul, MN 55133
612-736-4930

12463
Abana Pharmaceuticals, Inc.
See Jones Medical

00074
Abbott Diagnostics
Customer Support Center
Dept. 94P
Abbott Park, IL 60064
800-323-9100

00074
Abbott Hospital Products
1 Abbott Park Road
Abbott Park, IL 60064-3500
847-937-6100

00074
Abbott Laboratories
1 Abbott Park Road
Abbott Park, IL 60064-3500
847-937-6100

Able Laboratories, Inc.
6 Hollywood Ct.
South Plainfield, NJ 07080
908-754-2253

Academic Pharmaceuticals, Inc.
25720 Saunders Road North
Lake Forest, IL 60045

Acme United Corp.
75 Kings Highway Cutoff
Fairfield, CT 06430
203-332-7330

53014
Adams Laboratories
14801 Sovereign Road
Ft. Worth, TX 76155-2645
817-545-7791

Adolphs
75 Merritt Blvd.
Trumbull, CT 06611
203-381-3500

Adria Laboratories
See Pharmacia & Upjohn

00062
Advanced Care Products
Route 202
P.O. Box 610
Raritan, NJ 08869
908-218-8625

10888
Advanced Nutritional Technology
P.O. Box 3225
Elizabeth, NJ 07207
201-354-2740

Advanced Polymer Systems
3697 Haven Avenue
Redwood City, CA 94063
415-366-2626

Advanced Vision Research
7 Alfred Street,
Suite 330
Woburn, MA 01801
617-932-8327

Agouron Pharmaceuticals
10350 North Torrey Pines
La Jolla, CA 92037-1020
619-622-3000

A.H. Robins Consumer Products
See Wyeth-Ayerst

00031
A.H. Robins, Inc.
See Wyeth-Ayerst

17478
Akorn, Inc.
100 Akorn Drive
Abita Springs, LA 70420
504-893-9300

41383
AKPharma, Inc.
P.O. Box 111
Pleasantville, NJ 08232
609-645-5100

00065, 00998
Alcon Laboratories, Inc.
6201 South Freeway
Ft. Worth, TX 76134
817-293-0450

ALK Laboratories, Inc.
27 Village Lane
Wallingford, CT 06492
203-949-2727

38697
ALK Laboratories
2840 Eighth Street
Berkeley, CA 94710-2707
510-843-6846

A.L. Labs
One Executive Drive
P.O. Box 1399
Ft. Lee, NJ 07024
201-947-7774

00173
Allen & Hanburys
See Glaxo Wellcome

Allercreme
See Carme, Inc.

11980
Allergan America
2525 DuPont Drive
Irvine, CA 92715-9534
800-433-8871

00023
Allergan, Inc.
2525 DuPont Drive
Irvine, CA 92715-9534
800-433-8871

Allermed
7203 Convoy Ct.
San Diego, CA 92111
619-292-1060

Alliance Pharmaceuticals
3040 Science Park Road
San Diego, CA 92121
619-558-4300

54569
Allscrips
1033 Butterfield Road
Vernon Hills, IL 60061
708-680-3515

Alpha 1 Biomedicals, Inc.
6903 Rockledge Drive
Bethesda, MD 20817
301-564-4400

00472
Alpharma
333 Cassell Drive
Suite 3500
Baltimore, MD 21224
410-558-7250

Alpharma USPd
7205 Windsor Blvd.
Baltimore, MD 21244-2654
800-638-9096

49669
Alpha Therapeutic Corp.
5555 Valley Blvd.
Los Angeles, CA 90032
213-225-2221

51641
Alra Laboratories, Inc.
3850 Clearview Court
Gurnee, IL 60031
708-244-9440

Altana Incorporated
60 Baylis Road
Melville, NY 11747
516-454-7677

00731
Alto Pharmaceuticals, Inc.
P.O. Box 1910
Land O'Lakes, FL 34639-1910
813-949-7464

72959
Alva Laboratories
6625 Avondale Ave.
Chicago, IL 60631
312-792-0200

17314
Alza Corp.
950 Page Mill Road
Palo Alto, CA 94303-0802
415-494-5000

10038
Ambix Laboratories, Inc.
210 Orchard Street
East Rutherford, NJ 07073
201-939-2200

89709, 90605
Amcon Laboratories
40 N. Rock Hill Road
St. Louis, MO 63119
314-961-5758

Americal Pharmaceutical, Inc.
See Akorn, Inc.

51201
American Dermal Corp.
51 Apple Tree Lane
P.O. Box 900
Plumsteadville, PA 18949-0900
610-454-8000

57506
American Drug Industries, Inc.
5810 S. Perry Ave.
Chicago, IL 60621
312-667-7070

American Lecithin Company
115 Hurley Road, Unit 2B
Oxford, CT 06478
800-364-4416

00517
American Regent
1 Luitpold Drive
Shirley, NY 11967
516-924-4000

00539
American Urologicals, Inc.
7881 Hollywood Blvd.
Suite 4
Pembroke Pines, FL 33024
305-438-5070

55513
Amgen, Inc.
1840 Dehavilland Drive
Thousand Oaks, CA 91320-1789
805-499-5725

52152
Amide Pharmaceuticals, Inc.
101 E. Main Street
Little Falls, NJ 07424
201-890-1440

53926
Amsco Scientific
1002 Lufkin Road
P.O. Box 747
Apex, NC 27502
800-388-5155

Amswiss Scientific, Inc.
2170 Broadway
Suite 1200
New York, NY 10024

Anaquest
See Ohmeda Pharmaceuticals

Andrew Jergens
2535 Spring Grove
Cincinnati, OH 45214
513-421-1400

Andrulis Research Corp.
11800 Baltimore Ave.
Beltsville, MD 20705
301-419-2400

Anthra Pharmaceuticals, Inc.
19 Carson Road
Princeton, NJ 08540

Antibodies, Inc.
P.O. Box 1560
Davis, CA 95617
916-758-4400

48028
Aplicare Inc.
P.O. Box 237
Prichard, WV 25555
304-486-5656

Apotex Critical Care, Inc.
1776 Broadway
Suite 1900
New York, NY 10019
800-700-3092

Apothecary Products, Inc.
11531 Rupp Drive
Burnsville, MN 55337
612-890-1940

00003, 00015
Apothecon
P.O. Box 4500
Princeton, NJ 08543-4500
800-321-1335

48723
Apothecus, Inc.
20 Audrye Avenue
Oyster Bay, NY 11771
516-624-8200

Applied Biotech
10237 Flanders Ct.
San Diego, CA 92121
619-587-6771

Applied Genetics
205 Buffalo Ave.
Freeport, NY 11520
516-868-9026

Applied Medical Research
1600 Hayes Street
Nashville, TN 37203
615-327-0676

Approved Drug
See Health for Life Brands, Inc.

00070
Arcola Laboratories
500 Arcola Road
Collegeville, PA 19426
610-454-8000

00275
Arco Pharmaceuticals, Inc.
90 Orville Drive
Bohemia, NY 11716
516-567-9500

Argus Pharmaceuticals, Inc.
3400 Research Forest Drive
The Woodlands, TX 77381

Armour Pharmaceutical
See Centeon

48558
Arther, Inc.
P.O. Box 1455
W. Caldwell, NJ 07007
201-226-5288

61113
Astra Merck
725 Chesterbrook Blvd.
Wayne, PA 19087-5677
800-236-9933

00186
Astra USA, Inc.
50 Otis Street
Westborough, MA 01581
508-366-1100

59075
Athena Neurosciences, Inc.
800 Gateway Blvd.
South San Francisco, CA 94080
415-877-0900

59702
Atley Pharmaceuticals, Inc.
340 S. Richardson Road
Suite 1
Ashland, VA 23005
804-550-1979

Autoimmune, Inc.
128 Spring Street
Lexington, MA 02173
617-860-0710

Axion Pharmaceuticals
395 Oyster Point Blvd.
Suite 405
South San Francisco, CA 94080

44184
Bajamar Chemical, Inc.
9609 Dielman Rock Island
St. Louis, MO 63132
314-997-3414

58174
Baker Cummins Dermatologicals
50 Northwest 176 Street
Miami, FL 33169
800-842-6704

00575, 11414
Baker Norton Pharmaceuticals
8800 N.W. 36th Street
Miami, FL 33178-2404
305-590-2200

00304
J.J. Balan, Inc.
5725 Foster Ave.
Brooklyn, NY 11234
718-251-8663

00555
Barr Laboratories, Inc.
2 Quaker Road
Pomona, NY 01970
914-362-1100

10116
Bartor Pharmacal Co.
70 High Street
Rye, NY 10580
914-967-4219

58887
Basel Pharmaceuticals
See Novartis

10119
Bausch & Lomb Personal Products Division
1400 N. Goodman Street
P.O. Box 450
Rochester, NY 14692-0450
716-338-6000

24208, 57782
Bausch & Lomb Pharmaceuticals
8500 Hidden River Pkwy.
Tampa, FL 33637
813-975-7700

Baxter Healthcare
550 North Brand Blvd.
Glendale, CA 91203
818-956-3200

00944
Baxter Hyland
550 North Brand Blvd.
Glendale, CA 91203
818-956-3200

00118
Bayer Corp. (Allergy Div.)
P.O. Box 3145
Spokane, WA 99220
509-489-5656

00026, 00161, 00192
Bayer Corp. (Biological and Pharmaceutical Div.)
400 Morgan Lane
West Haven, CT 06516
203-937-2000

12843, 16500
Bayer Corp. (Consumer Div.)
P.O. Box 5967
Parsippany, NJ 07054
800-331-4536

00193
Bayer Corp. (Diagnostic Div.)
P.O. Box 3100
Elkhart, IN 46515-3100
800-248-2637

BDI Pharmaceuticals, Inc.
P.O. Box 78610
Indianapolis, IN 46278-0610
317-228-5008

00486
Beach Pharmaceuticals
P.O. Box 128
Conestee, SC 29636
803-277-7282

31280
Becton Dickinson & Co.
One Becton Drive
Franklin Lakes, NJ 07417-1881
201-847-6800

00011
Becton Dickinson Microbiology Systems
250 Schilling Circle
Cockeysville, MD 21031
410-771-0100

55390
Bedford Laboratories
300 Northfield Road
Bedford, OH 44146
216-232-3320

Behringwerke Aktiengesellschaft
500 Arcola Road
P.O. Box 1200
Collegeville, PA 19426-0107

10356
Beiersdorf, Inc.
P.O. Box 5529
S. Norwalk, CT 06856-5529
203-853-8008 956

50419
Berlex Laboratories, Inc.
300 Fairfield Road
Wayne, NJ 07470-2095
201-694-4100

58337
Berna Products Corp.
4216 Ponce De Leon Blvd.
Coral Gables, FL 33146
305-443-2900

Best Generics
See Goldline Laboratories, Inc.

00283
Beutlich, Inc.
1541 Shields Dr.
Waukegan, IL 60085
708-473-1100

00225
B. F. Ascher and Co.
15501 W. 109th St.
Lenexa, KS 66219
913-888-1880

Biocare International, Inc.
2643 Grand Avenue
Bellmore, NY 11710
516-781-5800

00332
Biocraft Laboratories, Inc.
See Teva Pharmaceuticals

Biocryst Pharmaceuticals, Inc.
2190 Parkway Lake Drive
Birmingham, AL 35244

59527
BioDevelopment Corp.
8180 Greensboro Drive
Suite 1000
McLean, VA 22102
703-506-0290

Biofilm, Inc.
3121 Scott Street
Vista, CA 92083-8323
619-727-9030

Biogen
14 Cambridge Center
Cambridge, MA 02142
617-679-2000

BioGenex Laboratories
4600 Norris Canyon Road
Suite 400
San Ramon, CA 94583
510-275-0550

Bioline Labs, Inc.
See Zenith Goldline Laboratories, Inc.

Biomedical Frontiers, Inc.
1095 10th Ave. S.E.
Minneapolis, MN 55414
612-378-0228

Biomerica, Inc.
1533 Monrovia Ave.
Newport Beach, CA 92663
714-645-2111

Biomune Systems, Inc.
40 East South Temple
Suite 310
Salt Lake City, UT 84111

Biopure Corp.
68 Harrison Ave.
Boston, MA 02111

52311
Biosearch Medical Products
P.O. Box 1700
Somerville, NJ 08876
908-722-5000

53191
Bio-Tech
P.O. Box 1992
Fayetteville, AR 72702
501-443-9148

Bio-Technology General Corp.
70 Wood Ave. South
Iselin, NJ 08830
908-632-8800

BIRA Corp.
2525 Quicksilver
McDonald, PA 15057
412-796-1820

50289
Birchwood Laboratories, Inc.
7900 Fuller Road
Eden Prairie, MN 53344
800-328-6156

12136
Bird Corp.
1100 Bird Center Drive
Palm Springs, CA 92262
619-778-7200

00165
Blaine, Inc.
1465 Jamike Lane
Erlanger, KY 41018-1878
606-283-9437

00154
Blair Laboratories
100 Connecticut Ave.
Norwalk, CT 06850-3590
203-853-0123

50486
Blairex Labs, Inc.
P.O. Box 2127
Columbus, IN 47202-2127
812-378-1864

10157
Blistex, Inc.
1800 Swift Drive
Oak Brook, IL 60521
708-571-2870

10158
Block Drug, Inc.
257 Cornelison Ave.
Jersey City, NJ 07302
201-434-3000

10160
Bluco Inc./Med. Discnt. Outlet
14849 W. McNichols
Detroit, MI 48235
313-273-0322

00563
Bock Pharmacal Co.
P.O. Box 419056
St. Louis, MO 63141-9056
314-579-0770

00597
Boehringer Ingelheim, Inc.
900 Ridgebury Road
Ridgefield, CT 06877
203-798-9988

50924

53169
Boehringer Mannheim Corp.
101 Orchard Ridge Drive
Gaithersburg, MD 20878
800-621-3784

Boehringer Mannheim Diags.
9115 Hague Road
P.O. Box 50100
Indianapolis, IN 46250-0100
800-428-5074

44437
Bolan Pharmaceutical, Inc.
P.O. Box 230
Hurst, TX 76053
817-268-6110

Boots Pharmaceuticals, Inc.
See Knoll Laboratories

00222
Boyle and Co. Pharm.
1613 Chelsea Rd.
San Marino, CA 91108
818-441-0284

00003
Bracco Diagnostics
P.O. Box 5225
Princeton, NJ 08543
609-897-4200

Bradley Pharmaceutical
See Kenwood Laboratories

52268
Braintree Laboratories, Inc.
60 Columbian
P.O. Box 361
Braintree, MA 02184
617-843-2202

51991
Breckenridge Pharmaceutical, Inc.
P.O. Box 206
Boca Raton, FL 33429
407-367-8512

72363
Brimms, Inc.
425 Fillmore Ave.
Tonawanda, NY 14150
716-694-7100

Bristol Laboratories
See Bristol-Myers Squibb

Bristol-Myers Oncology
P.O. Box 4500
Princeton, NJ 08543
609-897-2000

19810
Bristol-Myers Products
345 Park Ave. 4th Floor
New York, NY 10154
800-468-7746

00003, 00087
Bristol-Myers Squibb
P.O. Box 4000
Princeton, NJ 08543-4000
609-252-4000

Britannia Pharmaceuticals
Forum Hs Brighton Road Redhill
Surrey, UK RH 1 6YS

Burroughs Wellcome Co.
See GlaxoWellcome

00398
C & M Pharmacal, Inc.
1721 Maple Lane
Hazel Park, MI 48030-1215
313-548-7846

00132
C. B. Fleet, Inc.
4615 Murray Place
Lynchburg, VA 24506
804-528-4000

00463
C. O. Truxton, Inc.
P.O. Box 1594
Camden, NJ 08101
609-365-4118

10486
C. S. Dent & Co. Division
317 E. Eighth Street
Cincinnati, OH 45202
513-241-1677

55559
Calgon Vestal Laboratories
P.O. Box 147
St. Louis, MO 63166-0147
314-535-1810

California Department Health Service
2151 Berkeley Way
Berkeley, CA 94704

00147
Camall, Inc.
P.O. Box 307
Romeo, MI 48065-0307
313-752-9683

Cambridge Neuroscience, Inc.
1 Kendall Square
Building 700
Cambridge, MA 02139
617-225-0600

38083
Campbell Laboratories
P.O. Box 639
Deerfield Beach, FL 33443
305-570-9834

Can-Am Care Corp.
Cimetra Industrial Park
Chazy, NY 12921
800-461-7448

Cangene Corp.
104 Chancellor Matheson Road
Winnipeg, R3T 2N2
204-989-6850

Capmed USA
P.O. Box 14
Bryn Mawr, PA 19010

59046
Caprice-Greystoke
1259 Activity Drive
Vista, CA 92083
619-598-9300

57664
Caraco Pharmaceutical Labs
1150 Elijah McCoy Drive
Detroit, MI 48202
313-871-8400

Care Technologies, Inc.
55 Holly Hill Lane
Greenwich, CT 06830

Carme, Inc.
84 Galli
Novato, CA 94949
415-382-4000

Carnation
800 North Brand Blvd.
Glendale, CA 91203
800-628-2229

00086
Carnrick Laboratories, Inc.
65 Horse Hill Road
Cedar Knolls, NJ 07927
201-267-2670

46287
Carolina Medical Products
P.O. Box 147
Farmville, NC 27828
919-753-7111

Carrington Labs
1300 E. Rochelle Blvd.
Irving, TX 75062
214-518-1300

00164
Carter Products
Half Acre Road
P.O. Box 1001
Cranbury, NJ 08512-0181
609-655-6000

Cavitation-Control Technology
55 Knollwood Road
Farmington, CT 06032
203-673-0507

Celgene Corp.
7 Powder Horn Drive
Warren, NJ 07059
908-271-1001

Cellegy Pharmaceuticals, Inc.
371 Bel Marin Keys
Suite 210
Novato, CA 94949

Cell Pathways, Inc.
1700 Broadway
Suite 2000
Denver, CO 80290

Cell Technology
1668 Valtec Lane
Boulder, CO 80301
303-790-0587

Celtrix Pharmaceuticals, Inc.
3055 Patrick Henry Drive
Santa Clara, CA 95054

00053
Centeon
1020 First Avenue
King of Prussia, PA 19406-1310
800-683-1288

00268
Center Laboratories
35 Channel Drive
Port Washington, NY 11050
516-767-1800

Centers for Disease Control
1600 Clifton Road
Mail Stop D-09
Atlanta, GA 30333
404-639-3670

Centocor, Inc.
200 Great Valley Pkwy.
Malvern, PA 19355
610-651-6000

00131
Central Pharmaceuticals, Inc.
See Schwarz Pharma

00436
Century Pharmaceuticals, Inc.
10377 Hague Road
Indianapolis, IN 46256-3399
317-849-4210

Cephalon, Inc.
145 Brandywine Pkwy.
West Chester, PA 19380
215-344-0200

00173
Cerenex Pharmaceuticals
See Glaxo Wellcome

10223
Cetylite Industries, Inc.
9051 River Road
P.O. Box 90006
Pennsauken, NJ 08110
609-665-6111

54429
Chase Laboratories
280 Chestnut Street
Newark, NJ 07105-1598
201-589-8181

49447
Chattem Consumer Products
1715 W. 38th Street
Chattanooga, TN 37409
615-821-4571

Chembiomed, Ltd.
P.O. Box 8050
Edmonton, AB T6H4NP

52489
Chemi-Tech Laboratories
74-80 Marine Street
Farmingdale, NY 11735

00521
Chesebrough-Pond's, USA
33 Benedict Place
Greenwich, CT 06830
203-661-2000

Chiesi Pharmaceuticals, Inc.
150 Danbury Road
Ridgefield, CT 06877

53905
Chiron Therapeutics
4560 Horton Street
Emeryville, CA 94608
800-244-7668

Chiron Vision
500 Iolab Drive
Claremont, CA 91711
909-624-2020

Chugai-Upjohn, Inc.
6133 North River Road
Suite 800
Rosemont, IL 60018

00067, 00083

00083
Ciba-Geigy Pharmaceuticals
See Novartis

Ciba Self-Medication, Inc.
See Novartis

00346
Ciba Vision Ophthalmics
11460 Johns Creek Pkwy.
Duluth, GA 30136
404-418-4101

00677, 00725, 71114
Circa Pharmaceuticals, Inc.
33 Ralph Ave.
Copiague, NY 11726-0030
516-842-8383

00659
Circle Pharmaceuticals, Inc.
6320 B Rucker Road
Indianapolis, IN 46220
317-475-1921

City Chemical Corp.
132 W. 22nd Street
New York, NY 10011
201-653-6900

45802
Clay-Park Labs, Inc.
1700 Bathgate Ave.
Bronyx, NY 10457
212-901-2800

Clintec Nutrition
Three Pkwy. North
Suite 500
Deerfield, IL 60015
708-317-2800

Cocensys, Inc.
213 Technology Drive
Irvine, CA 92718
714-453-0131

Colgate Oral Pharmaceuticals
1 Colgate Way
Canton, MA 02021
617-821-2880

Collagen Corp.
2500 Faber Place
Palo Alto, CA 94303
415-856-0200

00837, 21406
Columbia Laboratories, Inc.
2665 South Bayshore Drive
Miami, FL 33133
305-860-1670

11509
Combe, Inc.
1101 Westchester Ave.
White Plains, NY 10604
914-694-5454

11793, 49281, 50361
Connaught Labs
See Pasteur-Mérieux-Connaught

00223
Consolidated Midland Corp.
20 Main St.
Brewster, NY 10509
914-279-6108

34044
Continental Consumer Products
770 Forest
Suite B
Birmingham, MI 48009
800-542-5903

33130
Continental Quest Research
220 W. Carmel Drive
Carmel, IN 46032
800-451-5773

00003
ConvaTec
P.O. Box 5254
Princeton, NJ 08543-5254
908-359-9200

00961
Cook-Waite Laboratories, Inc.
90 Park Ave.
New York, NY 10016
212-907-2000

Cooper Biomedical, Inc.
One Technology Court
Malvern, PA 19355
215-219-6300

Cooper Development Co.
455 East Middlefield Road
Mountain View, CA 94043
415-969-9030

59426
CooperVision
10 Faraday
Irvine, CA 92618
714-597-8130

38245
Copley Pharmaceutical, Inc.
25 John Road
Canton, MA 02021
617-821-6111

Cord Labs
See Geneva Pharmaceuticals

Coulter Corp.
11800 S.W. 147 Ave.
P.O. Box 169015
Miami, FL 33116
305-380-3800

50752
Creighton Products Corp.
59 Route 10
East Hanover, NJ 07936-1080
201-503-6099

CTRC Research Foundation
11812 Becket Street
Potomac, MD 20854

01020
Cumberland Packing Corp.
35 Old Ridgefield Road
P.O. Box 7688
Willton, CT 06897
203-762-7227

55326
Curatek Pharmaceuticals
See 3M Pharmaceuticals

Cutter Biologicals
See Bayer Corp. (Biological and Pharmaceutical Div.)

Cyclin Pharmaceuticals Inc.
429 Gammon Place
Madison, Wi 53715
608-833-8462

54799
Cynacon/OCuSOFT
P.O. Box 429
Richmond, TX 77406-0429
800-233-5469

Cytel Corp.
3525 John Hopkins Court
San Diego, CA 92121
619-552-3000

Cytogen
600 College Road East
Princeton, NJ 08540
609-987-8200

23731
Cytosol Laboratories
55 Messina Drive
Braintree, MA 02184

CytRx
150 Technology Pkwy.
Norcross, GA 30092
404-368-9500

55994
Dakryon Pharmaceuticals
2579 S. Loop
Suite 8
Lubbock, TX 79423-1400
806-745-2872

55425
Dal-Med Pharmaceuticals
5701 N. Pine Island Road
Tamarac, Fl 33321
800-543-9151

Danbury Pharmacal
See Schein Pharmaceutical, Inc.

00689
Daniels Pharmaceuticals, Inc.
See Jones Medical

Dapat Pharmaceuticals, Inc.
5040 Linbar Drive,
Suite 102
Nashville, TN 37211
615-833-2616

Darby Pharmaceuticals, Inc.
100 Banks Ave.
Rockville Centre, NY 11570

58869
Dartmouth Pharmaceuticals
19 Whaler's Way
North Dartmouth, MA 02747
508-636-5553

00938
Davis and Geck
One Cyanamid Plaza
Wayne, NJ 07470
201-831-2000

52041
Dayton Laboratories, Inc.
3307 NW 74th Ave.
Miami, FL 33122
305-594-0988

00744
Daywell Laboratories Corp.
78 Unquowa Place
Fairfield, CT 06430
203-255-3154

Degussa Corp.
65 Challenger Road
Ridgefield Park, NJ 07660
201-641-6100

48532
Delmont Laboratories, Inc.
P.O. Box 269
Swarthmore, PA 19081
215-543-3365

10310
Del Pharmaceuticals, Inc.
163 East Bethpage
Plainview, NY 11803
516-293-7070

00316
Del-Ray Laboratory, Inc.
22 20th Ave. N.W.
Birmingham, AL 35215
205-853-8247

00295
Denison Laboratories, Inc.
60 Dunnell Lane
P.O. Box 1305
Pawtucket, RI 02862
401-723-5500

00066
Dermik Laboratories, Inc.
500 Arcola Road
P.O. Box 1200
Collegeville, PA 19426
610-454-8000

50744
Dermol Pharmaceuticals, Inc.
3807 Roswell Road
Marietta, GA 30062
404-977-7779

49502
Dey Laboratories, Inc.
2751 Napa Valley Corporate Dr.
Napa, CA 94558
707-224-3200

Discovery Experimental & Development, Inc.
29949 SR 54 West
Wesley Chapel, FL 33543
813-973-7200

00777
Dista Products Co.
Lilly Corp. Center
Indianapolis, IN 46285
317-276-4000

10337
Doak Dermatologics
383 Route 46 West
Fairfield, NJ 07004-2402
201-882-1505

25358
Donell DerMedex
342 Madison Ave.
Suite 1422
New York, NY 10173
212-697-3800

00514
Dow B. Hickam, Inc.
P.O. Box 2006
Sugarland, TX 77487
713-240-1000

13723
Dr. Nordyke Footcare Products
1650 Palma Drive
Suite 102
Ventura, CA 93003
805-650-8333

00094
Du Pont Merck Pharmaceutical
4301 Lancaster Pike
Wilmington, DE 19805
302-892-7050

00056, 00590
Du Pont Pharma
P.O. Box 800723
Wilmington, DE 19880
800-474-2762

00217
Dunhall Pharmaceuticals, Inc.
P.O. Box 100
Gravette, AR 72736
501-787-5232

51285
Duramed Pharmaceuticals
5040 Lester Road
Cincinnati, OH 45213
513-731-9900

51479
Dura Pharmaceuticals
5880 Pacific Center Blvd.
San Diego, CA 92121-4202
619-457-2553

55516
Dyna Pharm, Inc.
P.O. Box 2141
Del Mar, CA 92014-2141
619-792-9523

10331
E. E. Dickinson Co.
2 Enterprise Drive
Shelton, CT 06484
203-929-1197

00168
E. Fougera and Co.
60 Baylis Road
Melville, NY 11747
516-454-6996

Eagle Vision, Inc.
6263 Poplar Ave.
Suite 650
Memphis, TN 38119
901-767-3937

Eastman Kodak Co.
10 Indigo Creek Drive
Rochester, NY 14650-0862
800-526-8811

Eaton Medical Corp.
2288 Dunn Ave.
Memphis, TN 38114
901-744-8024

19458
Eckerd Drug Co.
P.O. Box 4689
Clearwater, FL 34618
813-397-7461

38130
Econo Med Pharmaceuticals
4305 Sartin Road
Burlington, NC 27217-7522
919-226-1091

00095, 59010
ECR Pharmaceuticals
3981 Deep Rock Road
Richmond, VA 23233
804-527-1950

00485
Edwards Pharmaceuticals, Inc.
111 Mulberry Street
Ripley, MS 38663
601-837-8182

55806
Effcon Labs, Inc.
1800 Sandy Plains Pkwy.
Marietta, GA 30066
404-428-7011

Elan Corp.
1300 Gould Drive
Gainesville, GA 30504
404-534-8239

Elder
See Zeneca Pharmaceuticals

00002, 59075
Eli Lilly and Co.
Lilly Corp. Center
Indianapolis, IN 46285
317-276-2000

00641
Elkins-Sinn, Inc.
See Wyeth Ayerst

EM Industries, Inc.
5 Skyline Drive
Hawthorne, NY 10532
914-592-4660

60951
Endo Laboratories
P.O. Box 80390
Wilmington, DE 19880
800-462-4467

57665
Enzon, Inc.
40 Kingsbridge Road
Piscataway, NJ 08854-3998
908-980-4500

00185, 00536
Eon Labs Manufacturing, Inc.
227-15 North Conduit Ave.
Laurelton, NY 11413
718-276-8600

Epitope Inc.
8505 SW Creekside Place
Beaverton, OR 97008
503-641-6115

E.R. Squibb & Sons, Inc.
See Bristol-Myers Squibb

Escalon Ophthalmics, Inc.
182 Tamarack Circle
Skillman, NJ 08558
609-497-9141

00005, 59911
ESI Lederle Generics
P.O. Box 8299
Philadelphia, PA 19101
610-688-4400

58177
Ethex Corp.
10888 Metro Court
St. Louis, MO 63043-2413
314-567-3307

Ethicon, Inc.
Route 22 West
P.O. Box 151
Somerville, NJ 08876-0151
908-218-0707

54686
Ethitek Pharmaceuticals
7701 North Austin
Skokie, IL 60077
708-675-6611

00642
Everett Laboratories, Inc.
71 Glenwood Place
East Orange, NJ 07017
201-674-8455

Evreka
600 Montgomery Street
San Francisco, CA 94111
415-627-2040

Falcon Ophthalmics, Inc.
6201 S. Freeway
Fort Worth, TX 76134
800-343-2133

Farmacon, Inc.
90 Grove Street
Suite 109
Ridgefield, CT 06877-4118
203-431-9989

99766
Faulding USA
200 Elmora Ave.
Elizabeth, NJ 07207
800-526-6978

00496
Ferndale Laboratories, Inc.
780 W. Eight Mile Road
Ferndale, MI 48220-1218
313-548-0900

55566
Ferring Laboratories, Inc.
400 Rella Blvd.
Suite 201
Suffern, NY 10901
914-368-7900

31795
Fibertone Co.
14851 N. Scottsdale Road
Scottsdale, AZ 85254
800-462-7596

00729
Fidelity Halsom
1330 Farr Drive at Stanley
Dayton, OH 45404
800-356-3065

Fidia Pharmaceutical
1401 I Street N.W.
Washington, DC 20005
202-371-9898

00421
Fielding Co.
94 Weldon Pkwy.
Maryland Heights, MO 63043
314-567-5462

51687
Fischer Pharmaceuticals, Inc.
165 Gibraltar Court
Sunnyvale, CA 94089
408-747-1760

Fiske Industries
339 N. Main Street
New City, NY 10956
914-634-5099

Fisons Consumer Health
See Ciba Self-Medication, Inc.

00585
Fisons Corp.
See Medeva Pharmaceuticals

54323
Flanders, Inc.
P.O. Box 39143
Charleston, SC 29407-9143
803-571-3363

00256
Fleming & Co.
1600 Fenpark Drive
Fenton, MO 63026-2918
314-343-8200

00288
Fluoritab Corp.
P.O. Box 507
Temperance, MI 48182-0507
313-847-3985

00258, 00456, 00535
Forest Pharmaceutical, Inc.
13622 Lakefront Drive
St. Louis, MO 63045
314-344-8870

00494
Foy Laboratories
906 Penn Ave.
Wyomissing, PA 19610
215-678-9460

Free Radical Sciences, Inc.
245 First Street
Cambridge, MA 02142
617-374-1200

10432
Freeda Vitamins, Inc.
36 E. 41st Street
New York, NY 10017-6203
212-685-4980

Fuisz Technologies, Ltd.
3810 Concorde Pkwy.
Suite 100
Chantilly, VA 22021
703-803-3260

00469, 57317
Fujisawa USA, Inc.
3 Parkway North Center
Deerfield, IL 60015-2548
708-317-0600

00713
G & W Laboratories
111 Coolidge Street
South Plainfield, NJ 07080
908-753-2000

Galagen, Inc.
4001 Lexington Ave. North
Arden Hills, MN 55126-2998
612-481-2105

00299
Galderma Laboratories, Inc.
P.O. Box 331329
Ft. Worth, TX 76163
817-263-2600

00254
Gambro, Inc.
1185 Oak Street
Lakewood, CO 80215
800-525-2623

57844
Gate Pharmaceuticals
650 Cathill Road
Sellersville, PA 18960
800-292-4283

00386
Gebauer Co.
9410 St. Catherine Ave.
Cleveland, OH 44104
216-271-5252

00028
Geigy Pharmaceuticals
See Novartis

Gencon
6116 N. Central Expy. 200
Dallas, TX 75206
214-373-4665

52761
GenDerm Corp.
600 Knightsbridge Pkwy.
Lincolnshire, IL 60069-3657
708-634-7373

50242
Genentech, Inc.
460 Point San Bruno Blvd.
South San Francisco, CA 94080
415-225-1000

50272
General Generics, Inc.
P.O. Box 510
Oxford, MS 38655
601-234-0130

52584
General Injectables & Vaccines
U.S. Hwy. 52
Bastian, VA 24314
703-688-4121

00918
General Medical Corp.
8741 Landmark Road
Richmond, VA 23261
804-264-7500

Genetic Therapy, Inc.
938 Copper Road
Gaithersburg, MD 20878
301-590-2626

00781
Geneva Pharmaceuticals
2599 W. Midway Blvd.
P.O. Box 469
Broomfield, CO 80038-0469
800-525-8747

Gen-King
See Kinray

00703
Gensia Laboratories, LTD.
19 Hughes
Irvine, CA 92718-1902
800-331-0124

58468
Genzyme Corp.
One Kendall Square
Cambridge, MA 02139
617-252-7500

Geriatric Pharmaceutical Corp.
See Roberts Pharmaceuticals

Gilead Sciences, Inc.
333 Lakeside Drive
Foster City, CA 94404
800-445-3235

59366
Glades Pharmaceuticals
255 Alhambra Center
Suite 1000
Coral Gables, FL 33134
800-452-3371

00081, 00173
GlaxoWellcome
Five Moore Drive
Research Triangle Pk., NC 27709
919-248-2100

00516
Glenwood, Inc.
83 N. Summit Street
Tenafly, NJ 07670
201-569-0050

Global Source
3001 N. 29th Ave.
Hollywood, FL 33020
305-921-0006

Glycomed, Inc.
860 Atlantic Ave.
Alameda, CA 94501
510-523-5555

00182
Goldline Laboratories, Inc.
See Zenith Goldline

74684
Goody's Manufacturing Corp.
436 Salt Street
Winston Salem, NC 27108
910-723-1831

10481
Gordon Laboratories
6801 Ludlow Street
Upper Darby, PA 19082-1694
215-734-2011

12165
Graham Field
400 Rabro Drive East
Hauppauge, NY 11788
516-582-5900

00152
Gray Pharmaceutical Co.
100 Connecticut Ave.
Norwalk, CT 06856
203-853-0123

51301
Great Southern Laboratories
10863 Rockley Road
Houston, TX 77099
713-530-3077

Green Turtle Bay Vitamin Co.
P.O. Box 642
Summit, NJ 07902
908-277-2240

8225
Greenstone
Moors Bridge Road
Portage, MI 49002
800-447-3360

22840
Greer Laboratories, Inc.
P.O. Box 800
Lenoir, NC 28645-0800
704-754-5327

00327
Guardian Laboratories
230 Marcus Blvd.
Hauppauge, NY 11788
516-273-0900

54396
Gynex Pharmaceuticals, Inc.
1175 Corporate Woods Pkwy.
Vernon Hills, IL 60061
708-913-1144

54765
GynoPharma Laboratories
50 Division Street
Somerville, NJ 08876
908-725-3100

00879
Halsey Drug Co.
1827 Pacific Street
Brooklyn, NY 11233
718-467-7500

Hannan Ophthalmic Marketing Services, Inc.
163 Meetinghouse Road
Duxbury, MA 02332

51432
Harber Pharmaceutical Co.
350 Meadowlands Pkwy.
Secaucus, NJ 07094
201-348-3700

HDC Corporation
2109 O'Toole Ave.
San Jose, CA 95131
408-954-1909

Health & Medical Techniques
See Graham Field

50383
Health Care Products
369 Bayview Ave.
Amityville, NY 11701
516-789-8455

00598
Health for Life Brands, Inc.
1643 E. Genesee Street
Syracuse, NY 13210
315-478-6303

51662
Healthfirst Corp.
22316 70th Ave. W.
Mountlake Terrace, WA 98043
206-771-5733

59512
Healthline Laboratories, Inc.
835 Potts Ave.
Green Bay, WI 54304
414-497-3322

00586
Heather Drug, Inc.
1 Fellowship Road
Cherry Hill, NJ 08003
609-424-3663

Helena Laboratories
P.O. Box 752
Beaumont, TX 77704-0752
409-842-3714

HEM Research
1617 John F. Kennedy Blvd.
Philadelphia, PA 19103
215-988-0080

Hemacare Corp.
4954 Van Nuys Blvd.
Sherman Oaks, CA 91403
818-986-3883

Herald Pharmacal Inc.
6503 Warwick Rd.
Richmond, VA 23225
804-524-3112

Herbert Laboratories
See Allergan, Inc.

48017
Hermal Pharmaceutical Labs
163 Delaware Ave.
Delmar, NY 12054
518-475-0175

28105
Hill Dermaceuticals, Inc.
P.O. Box 149283
Orlando, FL 32814-9283
407-896-8280

17808
Himmel Pharmaceuticals, Inc.
P.O. Box 5479
Lake Worth, FL 33466-5479
407-585-0070

50673
Hirsch Industries, Inc.
4912 West Broad Street
Richmond, VA 23230-0964
804-355-4500

Hiscia
CH-4144, Arlesheim Kirshweg
Switzerland
4106172-2323

00839
H.L. Moore Drug Exchange, Inc.
389 John Downey Drive
New Britain, CT 06050
203-826-3600

00039, 00068, 00088
Hoechst-Marion Roussel
P.O. Box 9627
Kansas City, MO 64134
908-231-2000

58573
Hogil Pharmaceutical Corp.
1 Byram Brook Place
Armonk, NY 10504
914-273-9666

47992
Holles Laboratories, Inc.
30 Forest Notch
Cohasset, MA 02025-1198
617-383-0741

Hollister-Stier
See Bayer Corp. (Allergy Div.)

Home Diagnostics, Inc. (HDI)
51 James Way
Eatontown, NJ 07724
908-542-7788

Hope Pharmaceuticals
2961 W. MacArthur Blvd.
Santa Ana, CA 92704
714-556-4673

59630
Horizon Pharmaceutical Corp.
1125 Northmeadow Pkwy.
Roswell, GA 30076
404-442-9707

59229
Horus Therapeutics, Inc.
2320 Brighton-Henrietta Town
Rochester, NY 14623
716-292-4820

00196
Houba, Inc.
P.O. Box 190
Culver, IN 46511
219-842-3305

00556
H.R. Cenci Labs, Inc.
1420 E. Street
P.O. Box 12524
Fresno, CA 93778-2524
209-237-3346

58407
Huckaby Pharmacal, Inc.
104 E. Main Street
LaGrange, KY 40031
502-222-4700

25077
Hudson Corp.
90 Orville Drive
Bohemia, NY 11716
516-567-9500

00395
Humco Holding Group, Inc.
P.O. Box 2550
Texarkana, TX 75504
903-793-3174

Hybritech
P.O. Box 269006
San Diego, CA 92196-9006
619-455-6700

Hyland Therapeutics
See Baxter Hyland

Hynson, Westcott & Dunning
See Becton Dickinson
Microbiology Systems

00314
Hyrex Pharmaceuticals
P.O. Box 18385
Memphis, TN 38181-0385
901-794-9050

Iatric Corp.
2330 S. Industrial Park Drive
Tempe, AZ 85282-1893
602-966-7248

ICI Pharmaceuticals
See Zeneca Pharmaceuticals

00163, 00187
ICN Pharmaceuticals, Inc.
See Zeneca Pharmaceuticals

51244
I.C.P. Pharmaceuticals
P.O. Box 294
Cudahy, WI 53110
414-521-4647

IDEC Pharmaceuticals
11099 N. Torrey Pines Road #160
La Jolla, CA 92037
619-458-0600

Immucell Corp.
56 Evergreen Drive
Portland, ME 04103
207-878-2770

00205, 58406
Immunex Corp.
51 University Street
Seattle, WA 98101
206-587-0430

Immuno Clinical Research Corp.
155 East 56th Street
New York, NY 10022
212-759-3521

54129
Immuno U.S., Inc.
1200 Parkdale Road
Rochester, MI 48307-1744
313-652-7872

Immunobiology Research Inst.
Route 22 East
P.O. Box 999
Annandale, NJ 08801-0999
908-730-1700

ImmunoGen
148 Sidney Street
Cambridge, MA 02139
617-661-9312

Immunomedics
300 American Road
Morris Plains, NJ 07950
201-605-8200

Immunotherapeutics
3505 Riverview Circle
Morehead, MN 56560
701-232-9575

Imreg
144 Elk Place
Suite 1400
New Orleans, LA 70112
504-523-2875

00548
I.M.S., Ltd.
1886 Santa Anita Ave.
South El Monte, CA 91733
818-913-4660

Infusaid, Inc.
1400 Providence Highway
Norwood, MA 02062
617-769-8330

18686
InnoVisions, Inc.
6065 Frantz Road
Suite 202
Dublin, OH 43017
614-766-5477

Interchem Corp.
120 Route 17 North
Suite 115
Paramus, NJ 07652

Interfalk U.S., Inc.
25 Margaret
Plattsburgh, NY 12901

Interferon Sciences
783 Jersey Ave.
New Brunswick, NJ 08901
908-249-3250

11584
International Ethical Labs
Reparto Metropolitano
Rio Piedras, PR 00921
809-765-3510

00665
International Laboratories
901 Sawyer Road
Marietta, GA 30062
404-578-5583

Interneuron Pharmaceuticals
1 Ledgemont Center
99 Hayden Ave.
Lexington, MA 02173
617-861-8444

Interpro
P.O. Box 1823
Haverhill, MA 01831
508-373-2438

00814
Interstate Drug Exchange
1500 New Horizons Blvd.
Amityville, NY 11701-1130
516-957-8300

Intramed
102 Tremont Way
Augusta, GA 30907

52189
Invamed, Inc.
2400 Route 130N
Dayton, NJ 08810
908-274-1040

Inveresk Research
4470 Redwood Hwy.
San Rafael, CA 94903
415-491-6460

00258
Inwood Laboratories
300 Prospect Street
Inwood, NY 11696
516-371-1155

Iolab Pharmaceuticals
See Ciba Vision Ophthalmics

61646
Iomed
7425 Pebble Drive
Fort Worth, TX 76118
817-589-7257

11808
ION Laboratories, Inc.
7431 Pebble Drive
Ft. Worth, TX 76118
817-589-7257

IOP, Inc.
3100 Airway Ave.
Suite 106
Costa Mesa, CA 92626
714-549-1185

54921
IPR Pharmaceuticals, Inc.
P.O. Box 6000
Carolina, PR 00984
800-477-6385

50914
Iso Tex Diagnostics, Inc.
P.O. Box 909
Friendswood, TX 77546
713-482-1231

16837
J & J Merck Consumer Pharm.
Camp Hill Road
Ft. Washington, PA 19034
215-233-7000

88395
J. R. Carlson Laboratories
15 College Drive
Arlington Heights, IL 60004-1985
708-255-1600

49938
Jacobus Pharmaceutical Co.
37 Cleveland Lane
Princeton, NJ 08540
609-921-7447

50458
Janssen Pharmaceutical, Inc.
P.O. Box 200
Titusville, NJ 08560-0200
609-730-2000

JMI-Canton Pharmaceuticals
See Jones Medical Industries

56091
Johnson & Johnson Medical
P.O. Box 130
Arlington, TX 76004-0130
800-433-5009

00137
Johnson & Johnson
Grandview Road
Skillman, NJ 08558-9418
908-524-0400

00252, 52604, 00689
Jones Medical Industries
P.O. Box 46903
St. Louis, MO 63146-6903
314-576-6100

10106
J.T. Baker, Inc.
See Mallinckrodt-Baker

KabiVitrum, Inc.
See Pharmacia & Upjohn

Kanetta
90 Park Ave.
New York, NY 10016
212-907-2690

00588
Keene Pharmaceuticals, Inc.
P.O. Box 7
Keene, TX 76059-0007
817-645-8083

28851
Kendall Health Care Products
15 Hampshire Street
Mansfield, MA 02048
508-261-8000

Kendall-McGaw Labs, Inc.
See McGaw, Inc.

00482
Kenwood Laboratories
383 Rt. 46 W.
Fairfield, NJ 07006-2402
201-882-1505

00085
Key Pharmaceuticals
2000 Galloping Hill Road
Kenilworth, NJ 07033
908-298-4000

60793
King Pharmaceuticals Inc.
501 Fifth Street
Bristol, TN 37620
615-989-6232

55299
Kingswood Laboratories, Inc.
10375 Hague Road
Indianapolis, IN 46256
317-849-9513

Kinray
152-35 10th Ave.
Whitestone, NY 11357
718-767-1234

58223
Kirkman Sales, Inc.
P.O. Box 1009
Wilsonville, OR 97070-1009
503-694-1600

31600
Kiwi Brands, Inc.
447 Old Swede Road
Douglassville, PA 19518-1239
215-385-9322

KLI Corp.
1119 Third Ave. S.W.
Carmel, IN 46032
317-846-7452

00044, 00048, 00524
Knoll Laboratories
3000 Continental Drive North
Mt. Olive, NJ 07828-1234
201-426-2600

00044, 00048, 00524
Knoll Pharmaceuticals
3000 Continental Drive North
Mt. Olive, NJ 07828-1234
201-331-7633

Kodak Dental
343 State Street
Rochester, NY 14650

00224
Konsyl Pharmaceuticals
4200 South Hulen
Suite 513
Ft. Worth, TX 76109
817-763-8011

55505
Kramer Laboratories, Inc.
8778 S.W. 8th Street
Miami, FL 33174-9990
305-223-1287

La Haye Laboratories, Inc.
2205 152nd Ave. N.E.
Redmond, WA 98052
206-644-2020

Lacrimedics, Inc.
9008 Newby St.
Rosemead, CA 91770

41383
Lactaid, Inc.
7050 Camp Hill Road
Ft. Washington, PA 19034
215-233-7000

59081
Lafayette Pharmaceuticals, Inc.
P.O. Box 4499
Lafayette, IN 47903-4499
317-447-3129

Lake Pharmaceutical, Inc.
625 Forest Edge Dr.
Vernon Hills, IL 60061
708-793-0230

00527
Lannett, Inc.
9000 State Road
Philadelphia, PA 19136
215-333-9000

00277
Laser, Inc.
2200 W. 97th Place
P.O. Box 905
Crown Point, IN 46307
219-663-1165

10651
Lavoptik, Inc.
661 Western Ave.
St. Paul, MN 55103
612-489-1351

00005
Lederle Laboratories
North Middletown Road
Pearl River, NY 10965-1299
914-732-5000

53124
Lederle-Praxis Biologicals
North Middletown Road
Pearl River, NY 10965
914-272-7000

23558
Lee Pharmaceuticals
1444 Santa Anita Blvd.
South Elmonte, CA 91733
800-950-5337

Leeming
See Pfizer US Pharmaceutical Group

25332
Legere Pharmaceuticals, Inc.
7326 E. Evans Road
Scottsdale, AZ 85260
602-991-4033

19200
Lehn & Fink
See Reckitt & Coleman

Leiner Health Products
1845 W. 205th Street
Torrance, CA 90501
310-835-8400

Leiras Pharmaceuticals, Inc.
2345 Waukegan Road
Suite N-135
Bonnockburn, IL 60015

00093, 00332
Lemmon Co.
See Teva Pharmaceuticals

Lenti-Chemico Pharmaceuticals
500 Frank W. Burr Blvd.
Teaneck, NJ 07666
201-836-1196

00454
Lexis Laboratories
P.O. Box 202887
Austin, TX 78720
512-328-8484

Lifescan
1000 Gibraltar
Milpitas, CA 95035-6312
408-263-9789

Ligand Pharmaceuticals, Inc.
9393 Towne Centre Drive
San Diego, CA 92121
619-535-3900

00002, 59075
Eli Lilly and Co.
Lilly Corp. Center
Indianapolis, IN 46285
317-276-2000

Lincoln Diagnostics
P.O. Box 1128
Decatur, IL 62525
217-877-2531

60799
Liposome Co.
One Research Way
Princeton, NJ 08540
609-452-7060

54198
Liquipharm
10716 McCune Avenue
Los Angeles, Ca 90034
310-558-3344

Loch Pharmaceuticals
See Bedford Laboratories

00273
Lorvic Corp.
See Young Dental

59417
Lotus Biochemical
7335 Lee Highway
P.O. Box 3586
Radford, VA 24143-3586
703-633-3500

LTR Pharmaceuticals, Inc.
145 Sakonnet Blvd.
Narragansett, RI 02882

LuChem Pharmaceuticals, Inc.
See H.N. Norton Co.

00374
Lyne Laboratories
260 Tosca Drive
Stoughton, MA 02072
508-583-8700

00466
Macsil, Inc.
P.O. Box 29276
Philadelphia, PA 19125-0976
215-739-7300

00904
Major Pharmaceuticals
1640 W. Fulton
Chicago, IL 60612
312-666-9600

10106
Mallinckrodt-Baker
222 Red School Lane
Phillipsburg, NJ 08865
908-859-2151

00406
Mallinckrodt Chemical
16305 Swingley Ridge Drive
Chesterfield, Mo 63017
314-530-2058

00019
Mallinckrodt Medical, Inc.
675 McDonnell Blvd.
P.O. Box 5840
St. Louis, MO 63134
314-895-2000

10706
Manne
P.O. Box 825
Johns Island, SC 29457
800-517-0228

Marlin Industries
P.O. Box 560
Grover City, CA 93483-0560
805-473-2743

12939
Marlop Pharmaceuticals, Inc.
5704 Mosholu Ave.
P.O. Box 536
Bronx, NY 10471
800-345-7192

10712
Marlyn, Inc.
14851 N. Scottsdale Road
Scottsdale, AZ 85254
800-462-7596

00682
Marnel Pharmaceuticals, Inc.
206 Luke Drive
Lafayette, LA 70506
318-232-1396

00209
Marsam Pharmaceuticals, Inc.
P.O. Box 1022
Cherry Hill, NJ 08034
609-424-5600

52555
Martec Pharmaceutical, Inc.
P.O. Box 33510
Kansas City, MO 64120-3510
816-241-4144

11845
Mason Distributors, Inc.
5105 N.W. 159th Street
Hialeah, FL 33014-6370
305-624-5557

12758
Mason Pharmaceuticals, Inc.
4425 Jamboree
Suite 250
Newport Beach, CA 92660
714-851-6860

14362
Mass. Public Health Bio. Lab.
305 South Street
Jamaica Plains, MA 02130
617-522-3700

Matrix Laboratories
1430 O'Brian Drive
Suite G
Menlo Park, CA 94025
415-326-6100

00259
Mayrand, Inc.
915 Bridge Street
Winston Salem, NC 27101
910-765-4252

00264
McGaw, Inc.
P.O. Box 19791
Irvine, CA 92713-9791
714-660-2000

11089
McGregor Pharmaceuticals, Inc.
8420 Ulmenton Road
Suite 305
Largo, FL 34641
813-530-4361

49072
McGuff, Inc.
3617 W. MacArthur Blvd.
Suite 507
Santa Ana, CA 92704
800-854-7220

50185
McHenry Laboratories, Inc.
118 N. Wells, Lee Building
Edna, TX 77957
512-782-5438

00045
McNeil Consumer Products Co.
Camp Hill Road
Mail Stop 278
Ft. Washington, PA 19034-2292
215-233-7000

MCR American Pharmaceuticals
120 Summit Parkway,
Suite 101
Birmingham, AL 35209
205-942-6415

58607
ME Pharmaceuticals, Inc.
2800 Southeast Pkwy.
Richmond, IN 47375
800-637-4276

Mead Johnson Laboratories
See Bristol-Myers Squibb

00087
Mead Johnson Nutritionals
2404 Pennsylvania Street
Evansville, IN 47721
812-426-6000

Mead Johnson Oncology
See Bristol-Myers Oncology

Mead Johnson Pharmaceuticals
See Bristol-Myers Squibb

Medac GmbH c/o Princeton Regulatory Assoc.
65 South Main Street
Pennington, NJ 08534
609-951-9596

Medarex
1545 Rte. 22E
P.O. Box 953
Annandale, NJ 08801
908-713-6001

MedChem
232 W. Cummings Park
Woburn, MA 01801
800-451-4716

Medclone, Inc.
2435 Military Avenue
Los Angeles, CA 90064

11940
Medco Lab, Inc.
P.O. Box 864
Sioux City, IA 51102-0864
712-255-8770

Medco Research, Inc.
P.O. Box 13886
Research Triangle Park, NC
27709
919-549-8117

45565
Med-Derm Pharmaceuticals
P.O. Box 5193
Kingsport, TN 37663
615-477-3991

Medea Research Laboratories
200 Wilson Street
Port Jefferson, NY 11776
516-331-7718

00585
Medeva Pharmaceuticals
755 Jefferson Road
Rochester, NY 14623-0000
888-963-3382

Medi Aid Corp.
8250 S. Akron Street
Suite 205
Englewood, CO 80155
303-790-1655

00576
Medical Products Panamericana
647 West Flagler Street
Miami, FL 33130
305-545-6524

99207
Medicis Dermatologicals, Inc.
100 East 42nd Street, 15th Floor
New York, NY 10017-5613
212-599-2000

60574
Medimmune, Inc.
35 West Watkins Mill Road
Gaithersburg, MD 20878
301-417-0770

Medimorphics
245 East 6th Street
St. Paul, MN 55101
612-224-2800

17156
MediPhysics, Inc., Amersham Healthcare
2636 S. Clearbrook Drive
Arlington Heights, Il 60005
800-322-6334

Medi-Plex Pharm., Inc.
See ECR Pharmaceuticals

57480
Medirex, Inc.
20 Chapin Road
Pine Brook, NJ 07058
201-227-4774

61563
Medisan
400 Lanidex Plaza
Parsippany, NJ 07054
201-515-5300

MediSense, Inc.
266 Second Street
Waltham, MA 02154

53978
Med-Pro, Inc.
210 E. 4th Street
Lexington, NB 68850
308-324-4571

00348, 75137
Medtech Laboratories, Inc.
3510 N. Lake Creek
P.O. Box 1108
Jackson, WY 83011-1108
307-733-1680

58281
Medtronic
800 53rd Ave. N.E.
Minneapolis, Mn 55421
612-572-5000

87900
Menley & James Labs, Inc.
100 Tournament Drive
Horsham, PA 19044
215-441-6500

22200
Mennen Co.
Hanover Ave.
Morristown, NJ 07962-1928
201-631-9000

10742
Mentholatum, Inc.
1360 Niagara Street
Buffalo, NY 14213
716-882-7660

00006
Merck & Co.
P.O. Box 4
West Point, PA 19486
215-652-5000

00394
Mericon Industries, Inc.
8819 N. Pioneer Road
Peoria, IL 61615
309-693-2150

Merieux Institute, Inc.
See Pasteur-Mérieux-Connaught

30727
Merit Pharmaceuticals
2611 San Fernando Road
Los Angeles, CA 90065
213-227-4831

Michigan Department of Health
P.O. Box 30035
Lansing, MI 48909
517-335-8000

00682, 46672
Mikart, Inc.
2090 Marietta Blvd. N.W.
Atlanta, GA 30318
404-351-1125

52836
Milance Laboratories, Inc.
P.O. Box 368
Millington, NJ 07946
908-580-1591

Miles, Inc.
See Bayer Corp. (Consumer Div.)

Miles, Inc.
See Bayer Corp. (Diagnostic Div.)

00396, 34567
Milex Products, Inc.
5915 Northwest Hwy.
Chicago, IL 60631-1032
312-631-6484

17204
Miller Pharmacal Group, Inc.
350 Randy Road, Unit #2
Carol Stream, IL 60188
630-871-9557

53118
Millgood Laboratories, Inc.
250 D Arizona Ave.
P.O. Box 170159
Atlanta, GA 30317
404-377-6538

00276
Misemer Pharmaceuticals, Inc.
4553 S. Campbell
Springfield, MO 65810-5918
417-881-0660

00178
Mission Pharmacal Co.
P.O. Box 1676
San Antonio, TX 78296-1676
210-650-3273

53169
Monarch Pharmaceuticals
355 Beecham Street
Bristol, TN 37620
800-776-3637

Montgomery Medical Ventures
600 Montgomery Street
San Francisco, CA 94111

00426, 00832, 60432
Morton Grove Pharmaceuticals
6451 West Main Street
Morton Grove, IL 60053
708-967-5600

Morton Salt
100 N. Riverside Plaza
Chicago, IL 60606-1597
312-807-2000

MSD
See Merck & Co.

Mt. Vernon Foods, Inc.
13246 Wooster Road
Mt. Vernon, OH 43050
800-932-5525

54964
Murdock, Madaus, Schwabe
1400 Mountain Springs Pkwy.
Springvale, UT 84663
801-489-1500

00451
Muro Pharmaceutical, Inc.
890 East Street
Tewksbury, MA 01876-9987
508-851-5981

00150
Murray Drug Corp.
415 S. 4th Street
Murray, KY 42071
502-753-6654

53489
Mutual Pharmaceutical, Inc.
1100 Orthodox Street
Philadelphia, PA 19124
215-288-6500

00378
Mylan Pharmaceuticals
P.O. Box 4310
Morgantown, WV 26505
304-599-2595

05973
Nabi
5800 Park of Commerce Blvd.
Northwest
Boca Raton, FL 33487
305-625-5303

05745
Nastech Pharmaceutical, Inc.
129 Oser Ave.
Hauppauge, NY 11788
516-273-0101

National Patent Medical
P.O. Box 419
Dayville, CT 06241
800-243-1172

53983
Natren, Inc.
3105 Willow Lane
Westlake Village, CA 91361

Natures Bounty, Inc.
See NBTY, Inc.

74312
NBTY, Inc.
105 Orville Drive
Bohemia, NY 11716
516-567-9500

72559
NCI Medical Foods
5801 Ayala Ave.
Irwindale, CA 91706
818-812-3393

Neorx Corp.
410 West Harrison
Seattle, WA 98119
206-281-7001

00487
Nephron Pharmaceuticals Corp.
4121 S.W. 34th Street
Orlando, FL 32811-6458
407-246-1389

Nephro-Tech, Inc.
P.O. Box 14703
Lenexa, KS 66285
913-894-6646

NeuroGenesis/Matrix Tech., Inc.
100 Louisiana
Suite 600
Houston, TX 77002
800-345-8912

10812, 70501
Neutrogena Corp.
5760 W. 96th Street
Los Angeles, CA 90045-5595
310-642-1150

Neutron Technology Corp.
877 Main Street
Boise, ID 83702
208-345-3460

New World Trading Corp.
P.O. Box 952
DeBary, FL 32713
407-668-7520

Newport Pharmaceuticals
140 Columbia
Laguna Hills, CA 92656-1459
714-362-1330

56146
Nexstar
2860 Wilderness Place
Boulder, CO 80301
303-444-5893

59016
Niche Pharmaceuticals, Inc.
200 N. Oak Street
P.O. Box 449
Roanoke, TX 76262
807-491-2770

12934
Nion Corp.
15501 First Street
Irwindale, CA 91706
818-969-1932

23317
NMC Laboratories
70-36 83rd Street
Glendale, NY 11385
718-326-1500

51801
Nomax, Inc.
40 North Rock Hill Road
St. Louis, MO 63119
314-961-2500

Norcliff Thayer
See SmithKline Beecham
Consumer Healthcare

10118
Norstar Consumer Products
206 Pegasus Ave.
Northvale, NJ 07647
201-784-8155

North American Biologicals, Inc.
16500 N.W. 15th Ave.
Miami, FL 33169
305-625-5303

Novaferon Labs
2658 Patton Road
Roseville, MN 55713

00028, 00067, 00083, 58887
Novartis
556 Morris Ave.
Summit, NJ 07901
908-277-5000

Noven
11960 S.W. 144th Street
Miami, FL 33186
305-253-5099

00362
Novocol Chemical Mfr. Co.
P.O. Box 11926
Wilmington, DE 19850
302-328-1102

00169
Novo/Nordisk Pharm., Inc.
100 Overlook Center
Suite 200
Princeton, NJ 08540
800-727-6500

55953
Novopharm USA, Inc.
165 E. Commerce
Suite 100
Schaumberg, IL 60173-5326
708-882-4200

NPDC-AS101, Inc.
783 Jersey Avenue
New Brunswick, NJ 08901
716-636-9096

55499
Numark Laboratories, Inc.
P.O. Box 6321
Edison, NJ 08818
800-338-8079

34999
Nutraloric
350 N. Lantana, Unit G1
Camarillo, CA 93010
805-388-2811

NutraMax
9 Blackburn Drive
Gloucester, MA 01930
508-283-1800

Nutricia, Inc.
See Mt. Vernon Foods, Inc.

51081
Nutripharm Laboratories, Inc.
Salem Industrial Park
Building 5
Lebanon, NJ 08833
908-534-6267

00407
Nycomed Inc.
101 Carnegie Center
Princeton, NJ 08540-6231
609-514-6438

10797
Oakhurst Co.
3000 Hempstead Turnpike
Levittown, NY 11756
516-731-5380

55515
Oclassen Pharmaceuticals, Inc.
100 Pelican Way
San Rafael, CA 94901
415-258-4500

O'Connor, Inc.
See Columbia Laboratories, Inc.

51944
Ocumed, Inc.
119 Harrison Ave.
Roseland, NJ 07068
201-226-2330

Ohm Laboratories, Inc.
P.O. Box 7397
N. Brunswick, NJ 08902
908-297-3030

10019
Ohmeda Pharmaceuticals
110 Allen Road
Liberty Corner, NJ 07938
908-647-9200

12622
Olin Corp.
120 Long Ridge Road
Stamford, CT 06904-1355
203-356-2000

Omex International, Inc.
6001 Savoy
Suite 110
Houston, TX 77036
713-975-8325

Oncotherapeutics, Inc.
1002 East Park Blvd.
Cranbury, NJ 08512
609-655-5300

ONY, Inc.
1576 Sweet Home Road
Amherst, NY 14228
716-636-9096

Ophidian Pharmaceuticals, Inc.
2800 S. Fish Hatchery Road
Madison, WI 53711
608-271-0878

O.P.R. Development, LP
1501 Wakarusa Drive
Lawrence, KS 66047
913-749-0034

Optikem International, Inc.
2172 S. Jason Street
Denver, CO 80223
303-936-1137

50520
Optimox Corp.
2720 Monterey
Suite 406
Torrance, CA 90503
310-618-9370

52238
Optopics Laboratories, Corp.
32 Main Street
P.O. Box 210
Fairton, NJ 08320-0210
508-283-1800

00041
Oral-B Laboratories, Inc.
1 Lagoon Drive
Redwood City, CA 94065
415-961-8130

00052
Organon, Inc.
375 Mt. Pleasant Ave.
West Orange, NJ 07052
201-325-4500

Organon Teknika Corp.
100 Akzo Ave.
Durham, NC 27704
919-620-2000

Orion Diagnostica
71 Veronica Ave.
P.O. Box 218
Somerset, NJ 08875-0218
908-246-3366

Orphan Medical
13911 Ridgedale Drive
Minnetonka, MN 55305
612-513-6900

59676
Ortho Biotech, Inc.
700 US Hwy. 202
P.O. Box 670
Raritan, NJ 08869-0670
800-325-7504

00062
Ortho McNeil Pharmaceutical
Route 202
P.O. Box 600
Raritan, NJ 08869
908-218-6000

59148
Otsuka America Pharmaceutical
2440 Research Blvd.
Rockville, MD 98101
206-682-5300

Owen/Galderma
See Galderma Laboratories, Inc.

Oxis International
6040 N. Cutter Circle
Suite 317
Portland, OR 97212
503-283-3911

00574
Paddock Laboratories
3940 Quebec Avenue
North Minneapolis, MN 55427
612-546-4676

53159
Palisades Pharmaceuticals, Inc.
64 N. Summit Street
Tenafly, NJ 07670
201-569-8502

Pan America Labs
P.O. Box 8950
Mandeville, LA 70470-8950
504-893-4097

49884
Par Pharmaceuticals
One Ram Ridge Road
Spring Valley, NY 10977
914-425-7100

00071
Parke-Davis
201 Tabor Road
Morris Plains, NJ 07950
800-223-0432

00349
Parmed Pharmaceuticals, Inc.
4220 Hyde Park Blvd.
Niagara Falls, NY 14305
716-284-5666

50930
Parnell Pharmaceuticals, Inc.
Larkspur Landing Circle
Larkspur, CA 94939
415-461-4900

10865
Parthenon, Inc.
3311 W. 2400 South
Salt Lake City, UT 84119
801-972-5184

00418
Pasadena Research Labs
See Taylor Pharmaceuticals

11793, 49281, 50361
Pasteur-Mérieux-Connaught Labs
Route 611
P.O. Box 187
Swiftwater, PA 18370-0187
717-839-7187

00077
PBH Wesley Jessen
7976 Engineer Road
San Diego, CA 92111
619-614-7600

Pediatric Pharmaceuticals
718 Bradford Ave.
Westfield, NJ 07090
908-225-0989

00884
Pedinol Pharmacal, Inc.
30 Banfi Plaza North
Farmingdale, NY 11735
516-293-9500

10974
Pegasus Medical, Inc.
1 Technology Drive
Building 1C
Suite 525
Irvine, CA 92718-2325
714-753-9055

Pennex Pharmaceutical, Inc.
See Morton Grove Pharmaceuticals

Permeable Technologies, Inc.
712 Ginesi Drive
Morganville, NJ 07751
908-972-8585

00096
Person and Covey, Inc.
616 Allen Ave.
P.O. Box 25018
Glendale, CA 91221-5018
818-240-1030

00927
Pfeiffer Co.
43-45 N. Washington
P.O. Box 100
Wilkes-Barre, PA 18701
717-826-9000

Pfipharmecs
See Pfizer US Pharmaceutical Group

00069, 00663, 74300
Pfizer US Pharmaceutical Group
235 E. 42nd Street
New York, NY 10017-5755
800-438-1985

39822
Pharma Tek, Inc.
P.O. Box 1920
Huntington, NY 11743-0568
516-757-5522

58197
Pharmacel Laboratory, Inc.
203 South Coolidge Ave.
Tampa, FL 33609
813-289-2750

00121
Pharmaceutical Associates, Inc.
P.O. Box 128
Conestee, SC 29636
803-277-7282

Pharmaceutical Basics, Inc.
See Rosemont Pharmaceutical

51655
Pharmaceutical Corp.
12348 Hancock Street
Carmel, IN 46032
317-573-8000

21659
Pharmaceutical Labs, Inc.
1229 W. Corporate Drive
Arlington, TX 76006
817-633-1461

45334
Pharmaceutical Specialties, Inc.
P.O. Box 6298
Rochester, MN 55903
507-288-8500

Pharmachemie USA, Inc.
P.O. Box 145
Oradell, NJ 07049
201-265-1942

00013, 00016
Pharmacia & Upjohn
P.O. Box 16529
Columbus, OH 43216-6529
614-764-8100

PharmaControl
661 Palisade Ave.
P.O. Box 931
Englewood Cliffs, NJ 07632
201-567-9004

Pharmafair
See Bausch & Lomb Pharmaceuticals

55422
Pharmakon Laboratories, Inc.
6050 Jet Port Industrial Blvd.
Tampa, FL 33634
813-886-3216

Pharmaquest Corp.
See Inveresk Research

Pharmatec
County Road 2054
P.O. Box 730
Alachua, FL 32615
904-462-1210

Pharmavene, Inc.
35 West Watkins Mill Road
Gaithersburg, MD 20878
301-417-0033

Pharmedic Co.
28101 Ballard Road
Suite F
Lake Forest, IL 60045
708-549-8600

00813
Pharmics, Inc.
P.O. Box 27554
Salt Lake City, UT 84127
801-972-4138

Plexus Pharmaceuticals, Inc.
8122 Datapoint Drive
Suite 600
San Antonio, TX 78229

Plough, Inc.
See Schering-Plough Healthcare Products

00998
PolyMedica Pharmaceuticals
2 Constitution Way
Woburn, MA 01801
617-933-2020

47144
Polymer Technology Corp.
100 Research Drive
Wilmington, MA 01887
800-343-1445

Polymer Technology International
1595 N.W. Gilman Blvd.
Suite 17
Issaquah, WA 98027
206-391-2650

Porton Product Limited
See Speywood Pharmaceuticals, Inc.

Poythress
See ECR Pharmaceuticals

59012
Pratt Pharmaceuticals
235 E. 42nd Street
New York, NY 10017-5755
800-438-1985

Precision-Cosmet
500 Iolab Drive
Claremont, CA 91711
800-423-1871

Premier, Inc.
See Advanced Polymer Systems

00684
Primedics Laboratories
15524 S. Broadway
Gardenia, CA 90248
213-770-3005

Princeton Pharm. Products
See Bristol-Myers Squibb

37000
Procter & Gamble Co.
1 Procter & Gamble Plaza
Cincinnati, OH 45202
513-983-1100

00149
Procter & Gamble Pharm.
P.O. Box 191
Norwich, NY 13815-0191
607-335-2111

00034
Purdue Frederick Co.
100 Connecticut Ave.
Norwalk, CT 06850-3590
203-853-0123

00228
Purepac Pharmaceutical Co.
200 Elmora Ave.
Elizabeth, NJ 07207
908-527-9100

QLT Phototherapeutics, Inc.
401 North Middletown Road
Pearl River, NY 10965

00603
Qualitest Products, Inc.
1236 Jordan Road
Huntsville, AL 35811
205-859-4011

12225
Quality Formulations, Inc.
P.O. Box 827
Zachary, LA 70791-0827
504-654-6880

Quidel Corp.
10165 McKellar Court
San Diego, CA 92121
619-552-1100

54391
R & D Laboratories, Inc.
4640 Admiralty Way,
Suite 710
Marina Del Rey, CA 90292
310-305-8053

R & R Registrations
P.O. Box 262079
San Diego, CA 92196-2069
619-586-0751

00196
Rachelle Laboratories, Inc.
See Houba, Inc.

30103
Randob Laboratories, Ltd.
P.O. Box 440
Cornwall, NY 12518
914-699-3131

00686
Raway Pharmacal, Inc.
15 Granit Road
Accord, NY 12404-0047
914-626-8133

12496
Reckitt & Colman
1901 Huguenot Road
Suite 110
Richmond, VA 23235
804-379-1090

10952
Recsei Laboratories
330 S. Kellogg
Building M
Goleta, CA 93117-3875
805-964-2912

48028
Redi-Products Labs, Inc.
See Aplicare, Inc.

00021
Reed & Carnrick
See Schwarz Pharma

10956
Reese Chemical Co.
10617 Frank Ave.
Cleveland, OH 44106
216-231-6441

Regeneron Pharmaceuticals
777 Old Saw Mill River Road
Tarrytown, NY 10591-6707
914-347-7000

Reid Rowell
See Solvay

Remel, Inc.
12076 Santa Fe Drive
Lenexa, KS 66215

10961
Requa, Inc.
1 Seneca Place
P.O. Box 4008
Greenwich, CT 06830
203-869-2445

00433
Research Industries Corp.
6864 S. 300 West
Midvale, UT 84047
801-562-0200

Research Triangle Pharmaceuticals
4364 S. Alston Ave.
Durham, NC 27713
919-544-4029

60575
Respa Pharmaceuticals, Inc.
P.O. Box 88222
Carol Stream, IL 60188
708-462-9986

00122
Rexall Group
4031 N.E. 12th Terrace
Ft. Lauderdale, FL 33334
800-255-7399

Rexar Pharmaceuticals
See Richwood Pharmaceutical

RH Pharmaceuticals, Inc.
See Cangene Corp.

Rhone-Poulenc Rorer Consumer, Inc.
See Novartis

00075
Rhone-Poulenc Rorer Pharmaceuticals, Inc.
500 Arcola Road
P.O. Box 1200
Collegeville, PA 19426
610-454-8000

Ribi Immunochem Research
553 Old Corvallis Road
Hamilton, MT 59840-3131
406-363-6214

Richardson-Vicks, Inc.
See Procter & Gamble Co.

12071
Richie Pharmacal, Inc.
197 State Ave.
P.O. Box 460
Glasgow, KY 42141
800-626-0250

58521
Richwood Pharmaceutical, Inc.
P.O. Box 6497
Florence, KY 41022
800-974-4700

54807
R.I.D., Inc.
609 North Mednik Avenue
Los Angeles, CA 90022-1320
213-268-0635

54092
Roberts Pharmaceuticals
4 Industrial Way West
Eatontown, NJ 07724
908-389-1182

A.H. Robins Consumer Products
See Wyeth-Ayerst

00031
A.H. Robins, Inc.
See Wyeth-Ayerst

Roche Diagnostic Systems, Inc.
1080 U.S. Highway 202
Somerville, NJ 08876-3771
908-253-7200

00004, 00033, 00140, 18393, 42987
Roche Laboratories
340 Kingsland Street
Nutley, NJ 07110-1199
800-526-6367

00049
Roerig
See Pfizer

00832
Rosemont Pharmaceutical Corp.
301 South Cherokee Street
Denver, CO 80223
303-733-7207

00074
Ross Laboratories
6480 Busch Blvd.
Columbus, OH 43229
614-624-3333

00054
Roxane Laboratories, Inc.
P.O. Box 16532
Columbus, OH 43216-6532
614-276-4000

51875
Royce Laboratories, Inc.
16600 N.W. 54 Ave.
Miami, FL 33014
305-624-1500

00536
Rugby Labs, Inc.
898 Orlando Ave.
West Hempstead, NY 11552
516-536-8565

Russ Pharmaceuticals
See UCB Pharmaceuticals

46500
Rydelle Laboratories
1525 Howe Street
Racine, WI 53403-5011
414-631-2000

00263
Rystan, Inc.
P.O. Box 214
Little Falls, NJ 07424-0214
201-256-3737

00043
Sandoz Consumer
59 Route 10
East Hanover, NJ 07936
201-503-7500

00212
Sandoz Nutrition Corp.
5320 W. 23rd Street
Minneapolis, MN 55440
800-999-9978

00078
Sandoz Pharmaceuticals
59 Route 10
East Hanover, NJ 07936
201-503-7500

51353
Sanitube Co.
19 Concord Street
S. Norwalk, CT 06854
203-853-7856

00024
Sanofi Winthrop Pharmaceuticals
90 Park Ave.
New York, NY 10016
800-446-6267

00281
Savage Laboratories
60 Baylis Road
Melville, NY 11747-2006
800-231-0206

Scandinavian Natural Health & Beauty Products
13 N. 7th St.
Perkasie, PA 18944
215-453-2505

58914
Scandipharm, Inc.
22 Inverness Center Pkwy.
Suite 310
Birmingham, AL 35242
800-950-8085

11012
Schaffer Laboratories
1058 North Allen Ave.
Pasadena, CA 91104
818-798-8644

00364
Schein Pharmaceutical, Inc.
100 Campus Drive
Florham Park, NJ 07932
914-278-3724

00274
Scherer Laboratories, Inc.
16200 N. Dallas Pkwy.
Suite 165
Dallas, TX 75248
800-858-9888

00085
Schering-Plough Corp.
2000 Galloping Hill Road
Kenilworth, NJ 07033-0530
908-298-4000

00085
Schering-Plough Healthcare Products
110 Allen Road
Liberty Corner, NJ 07938
908-298-4000

Schiapparelli Searle
See SCS Pharmaceuticals

Schiff Products
P.O. Box 26708
Salt Lake City, UT 84126
801-975-1166

00234
Schmid Products Co.
P.O. Box 4703
Sarasota, FL 34230-4703
800-827-0987

Scholl, Inc.
See Schering-Plough Healthcare Products

00021, 00091
Schwarz Pharma
5600 W. County Line
Mequon, WI 53092
800-558-5114

Scios Nova, Inc.
2450 Bayshore Pkwy.
Mountain View, CA 94043
415-966-1550

00372
Scot-Tussin Pharmacal, Inc.
50 Clemence Street
P.O. Box 8217
Cranston, RI 02920-0217
800-638-7268

00905
SCS Pharmaceuticals
P.O. Box 5110
Chicago, IL 60680
800-323-1603

00014, 00025
Searle
Box 5110
Chicago, IL 60680-5110
847-982-7000

00551
Seatrace Pharmaceuticals
P.O. Box 363
Gadsden, AL 35902-0363
205-442-5023

Sequus Pharmaceuticals, Inc.
960 Hamilton Court
Menlo Park, CA 94025
415-833-7207

50694
Seres Laboratories
3331 Industrial Drive
P.O. Box 470
Santa Rosa, CA 95401
707-526-4526

44087
Serono Laboratories, Inc.
100 Longwater Circle
Norwell, MA 02061
617-982-9000

97692
S.G. Labs, Inc.
500 North Broadway
Jericho, NY 11753
516-822-2900

49731
Sherman Pharmaceuticals, Inc.
P.O. Box 1377
Mandeville, LA 70470-1377
504-893-0007

08884
Sherwood Medical
1915 Olive Street
St. Louis, MO 63103
314-621-7788

45809
Shionogi USA
3848 Carson Street
Suite 206
Torrance, CA 90503
310-540-1161

50111
Sidmak Laboratories, Inc.
P.O. Box 371
East Hanover, NJ 07936
201-386-5566

54482
Sigma-Tau Pharmaceuticals, Inc.
800 S. Frederick Avenue
Gaithersburg, MD 20877-4150
301-948-1041

54838
Silarx Pharmaceuticals, Inc.
19 West Street
Spring Valley, NY 10977
914-352-4020

08026
Smith & Nephew United
11775 Starkey Road
Largo, FL 34643
800-876-1261

00766
SmithKline Beecham Consumer Healthcare
1500 Littleton
Parsippany, NJ 07054-3884
201-631-8700

00007, 00029, 00108, 00128
SmithKline Beecham Pharmaceuticals
One Franklin Plaza,
P.O. Box 7929
Philadelphia, PA 19103
215-751-4000

00978
SmithKline Diagnostics
225 Baypoint Pkwy.
San Jose, CA 95134-1622
800-877-6242

Sola/Barnes-Hind
See Pilkington Barnes Hind

33984
Solgar, Inc.
410 Ocean Ave.
Lynbrook, NY 11563
516-599-2442

39769
SoloPak Pharmaceuticals, Inc.
1845 Tonne Road
Elk Grove Village, IL 60007-5125
847-806-0080

00032
Solvay Pharmaceuticals
901 Sawyer Road
Marietta, GA 30062-2224
770-578-9000

39506
Somerset Pharmaceuticals
5215 West Laurel Street
Tampa, FL 33607
813-223-7677

Sparta Pharmaceuticals
P.O. Box 13288
Research Triangle Park, NC 27709
919-361-3461

Spectra Pharmaceuticals
See Cooper Pharmaceuticals

38137
Spectrum Chemical Mfg. Corp.
14422 S. San Pedro Street
Gardena, CA 90248-9985
800-772-8786

00537
Spencer Mead, Inc.
100 Banks Ave.
Rockville Center, NY 11570
800-645-3737

55688
Speywood Pharmaceuticals, Inc.
27 Maple Street
Milford, MA 01757-2658
508-478-8900

Sphinx Pharmaceutical Corp.
P.O. Box 52330
Durham, NC 27717
919-489-0909

Squibb Diagnostic Division
See Bracco Diagnostics

00078
Stanback Co.
P.O. Box 1669
Salisbury, NC 28145-1669
704-633-9231

53385
Standard Drug Co.
P.O. Box 710
Riverton, IL 62561
217-629-9884

00076
Star Pharmaceuticals, Inc.
1990 N.W. 44th Street
Pompano Beach, FL 33064-1278
305-971-9704

51318
Stellar Pharmacal Corp.
1990 N.W. 44th Street
Pompano Beach, FL 33064
800-845-7827

00402
Steris Laboratories, Inc.
620 N. 51st Ave.
Phoenix, AZ 85043
602-278-1400

Sterling Health
See Bayer Corp. (Consumer Div.)

Sterling Winthrop
See Sanofi Winthrop Pharmaceuticals

00145
Stiefel Laboratories, Inc.
255 Alhambra Circle
Coral Gables, FL 33134
800-327-3858

89223
Stockhausen, Inc.
2408 Doyle Street
Greensboro, NC 27406
800-334-0242

41701
Stolle
6954 Cornell Road
Cincinnati, OH 45242
513-489-4235

57706
Storz Ophthalmics
3365 Tree Court Industrial
St. Louis, MO 63122-6694
314-225- 5051

58980
Stratus Pharmaceuticals, Inc.
P.O. Box 4632
Miami, FL 33265
800-442-7882

Stuart Pharmaceuticals
See Zeneca Pharmaceuticals

Sublingual Products International
See Pharmaceutical Labs, Inc.

11086
Summers Laboratories, Inc.
103 G.P. Clement Drive
Collegeville, PA 19426
610-454-1471

57267
Summit Pharmaceuticals
556 Morris Ave.
Summit, NJ 07901
908-277-5000

11704
Survival Technology, Inc.
2275 Research Blvd.
Rockville, MD 20850
301-926-1800

Syncom Pharmaceuticals, Inc.
155 Passaic Ave.
Fairfield, NJ 07004

Synergen, Inc.
1885 33rd Street
Boulder, CO 80301
303-938-6200

00033, 18393, 42987
Syntex Laboratories
3401 Hillview Ave.
Palo Alto, CA 94304
415-855-5050

Syntex-Synergen Neuroscience
1885 33rd Street
Boulder, CO 80301
303-442-1926

Syva Co.
929 Queensbridge
St. Louis, MO 63021
314-391-5374

Tag Pharmaceuticals
P.O. Box 904
Sellersville, PA 18960
215-723-5544

Tambrands, Inc.
777 Westchester Ave.
White Plains, NY 10604
914-696-6060

Tanning Research Labs, Inc.
1190 U.S. 1 North
Ormond Beach, FL 32174
904-677-9559

00300
Tap Pharmaceuticals
2355 Waukegan Road
Deerfield, IL 60015
800-621-1020

51672
Taro Pharmaceuticals USA, Inc.
Six Skyline Drive
Hawthorne, NY 10532-9998
914-345-9001

00418
Taylor Pharmaceuticals
P.O. Box 5136
San Clemente, CA 92674-5136
714-492-4030

83926
Tec Laboratories, Inc.
615 Water Ave. S.E.
P.O. Box 1958
Albany, OR 97321-0512
503-926-4577

Telluride Pharm. Corp.
146 Flanders Drive
Hillsborough, NJ 08876-4656
908-359-1375

00093, 00332
Teva Pharmaceuticals USA
650 Cathill Road
Sellersville, PA 18960

49158
Thames Pharmacal, Inc.
2100 Fifth Ave.
Ronkonkoma, NY 11779-6906
516-737-1155

Therakos, Inc.
201 Brandywine Pkwy.
West Chester, PA 19380
610-430-7900

Therapeutic Antibodies, Inc.
1500 21st Ave.
Suite 310
Nashville, TN 37212
615-327-1027

11290
Thompson Medical Co.
222 Lakeview Ave.
West Palm Beach, FL 33401
407-820-9900

T/I Pharmaceuticals, Inc.
See Fischer Pharmaceuticals

49483
Time-Cap Labs, Inc.
7 Michael Avenue
Farmingdale, NY 11735
516-753-9090

TNI Pharmaceuticals
5105 N. Pearl Street
Schiller Park, IL 60176
708-678-3067

93312
Trask Industries, Inc.
163 Farrell Street
Somerset, NJ 08873
908-214-9267

Triage Pharmaceuticals
See Health for Life Brands, Inc.

Triangle Labs, Inc.
1000 Robins Road
Lynchburg, VA 24504-3558
804-845-7073

53020
Trinity Technologies, Inc.
28510 Hayes
Roseville, MI 48066
313-778-5630

79511
Triton Consumer Products, Inc.
561 West Golf
Arlington Heights, IL 60005
708-228-7650

Tsumura Medical
1000 Valley Park Drive
Shakopee, MN 55379
612-496-4700

Tweezerman
55 Sea Cliff Ave.
Glen Cove, NY 11542-3695
516-676-7772

53335
Tyson & Associates, Inc.
12832 Chadron Ave.
Hawthorne, CA 90250-5525
310-675-1080

UAD Laboratories, Inc.
See Forest Pharmaceutical, Inc.

59640
UBI Corp.
2920 N.W. Boca Raton Blvd.
Boca Raton, FL 33431
407-367-1252

UCB Pharmaceuticals, Inc.
P.O. Box 4410
Hampton, VA 23664-0410
804-851-4618

62592
Ucyclyd Pharma, Inc.
10819 Gilroy Road,
Suite 100
Hunt Valley, MD 21031
410-584-0001

51079
UDL Laboratories, Inc.
P.O. Box 10319
Rockford, IL 61131-3019
815-282-1201

Ueno Fine Chemicals Industry
31 Koraibashi
Osaka 541, Japan
06-203-0761

00127
Ulmer Pharmacal Co.
2440 Fernbrook Lane
Plymouth, MN 55447-9987
612-559-0601

41785
Unimed
2150 E. Lake Cook Road
Buffalo Grove, IL 60089
800-541-3492

00677
United Research Laboratories
3600 Marshall Lane
P.O. Box 8546
Bensalem, PA 19020-8546
215-638-2626

48663
Unitek Corp.
2724 South Peck Road
Monrovia, CA 91016
818-445-7960

Univax Biologics
12280 Wilkins Ave.
Rockville, MD 20852
301-770-3099

00009
Upjohn Co.
See Pharmacia & Upjohn

00245
Upsher-Smith Labs, Inc.
14905 23rd Ave. N.
Minneapolis, MN 55447
612-473-4412

58178
US Bioscience
100 Front Street
Suite 400
West Conshohocken, PA 19428
800-447-3969

US Packaging Corp. Medical
506 Clay Street
LaPorte, IN 46350
219-362-9782

52747
US Pharmaceutical Corp.
2401-C Mellon Court
Decatur, GA 30035
(770) 987-4745

54627
ValMed, Inc.
203 Southwest Cutoff
Northboro, MA 01532
800-477-0487

00615
Vangard Labs, Inc.
P.O. Box 1268
Glasgow, KY 42142-1268
502-651-6188

17022
Veratex Corp.
1304 E. Maple Road
P.O. Box 4031
Troy, MI 48007
810-619-0800

Vertex Pharmaceuticals, Inc.
40 Allston Street
Cambridge, MA 02139-4211
617-576-3111

53258
VHA Supply Co.
300 Decker Drive
P.O. Box 160909
Irving, TX 75016
214-650-4444

23900
Vicks Health Care Products
See Procter & Gamble Co.

25866
Vicks Pharmacy Products
One Far Mill Crossing
Shelton, CT 06484
203-929-2500

Vintage Pharmaceuticals, Inc.
3241 Woodpark Blvd.
Charlotte, NC 28256
704-596-0516

Viratek
3300 Hyland Ave.
Costa Mesa, CA 92627
714-540-1866

54891
Vision Pharmaceuticals, Inc.
P.O. Box 400
Mitchell, SD 57301-0400
605-996-3356

54022
Vitaline Corp.
385 Williamson Way
Ashland, OR 97520
503-482-9231

Vita-Rx Corp.
P.O. Box 8229
Columbus, GA 31908
706-568-1881

00298
Vortech Pharmaceuticals
6851 Chase Road
Dearborn, MI 48126
313-584-4088

11444
W. F. Young, Inc.
111 Lyman Street
Springfield, MA 01102
413-737-0201

59310
Wakefield Pharmaceuticals, Inc.
1050 Cambridge Square
Suite C
Alpharetta, GA 30201
404-664-1661

00741
Walker, Corp. and, Inc.
P.O. Box 1320
Syracuse, NY 13201
315-463-4511

00619
Walker Pharmacal Co.
4200 Laclede Ave.
St. Louis, MO 63108
314-533-9600

00037
Wallace Laboratories
Halfacre Road
Cranbury, NJ 08512
609-655-6000

00017
Wampole Laboratories
Half Acre Road
P.O. Box 1001
Cranbury, NJ 08515-0181
609-655-6000

00047
Warner Chilcott Laboratories
182 Tabor Road
Morris Plains, NJ 07950
800-521-8813

11370
Warner Lambert Co.
201 Tabor Road
Morris Plains, NJ 07950
201-540-2000

59930
Warrick Pharmaceuticals, Corp.
1095 Morris Ave.
Union, NJ 07083
908-629-3600

00047, 52544
Watson Laboratories
311 Bonnie Circle Drive
Corona, CA 91720
909-270-1400

59196
WE Pharmaceuticals, Inc.
P.O. Box 1142
Ramona, CA 92065
619-788-9155

Wendt Laboratories
P.O. Box 128
Belle Plaine, MN 56011
800-328-5890

00917
Wesley Pharmacal, Inc.
114 Railroad Drive
Ivyland, PA 18974
215-953-1680

59591
West Point Pharma
P.O. Box 4
West Point, PA 19486-0004
212-652-2121

50893
Westport Pharmaceuticals, Inc.
1 Turkey Hill Road S.
Westport, CT 06880
203-226-0622

00143
West-Ward, Inc.
465 Industrial Way W.
Eatontown, NJ 07724
908-542-1191

00003, 00072
Westwood Squibb Pharmaceuticals
100 Forest Ave.
Buffalo, NY 14213
716-887-3400

50474
Whitby Pharmaceuticals, Inc.
See UCB Pharmaceuticals, Inc.

00031, 00573
Whitehall Robins Laboratories
Five Giralda Farms
Madison, NJ 07940-0871
201-660-5500

00317
Whorton Pharmaceuticals, Inc.
4202 Gary Ave.
Fairfield, AL 35064
205-786-2584

Willen Pharmaceuticals
See Baker Norton Pharmaceuticals

Winthrop Consumer
See Bayer Corp. (Consumer Div.)

Winthrop Pharmaceuticals
See Sanofi Winthrop Pharmaceuticals

12120
Wisconsin Pharmacal Co.
1 Repel Road
Jackson, WI 53037
414-677-4121

11428
Wonderful Dream Salve Corp.
18546 Old Homestead
Harper Woods, MI 48225
313-521-4233

Woodward Laboratories, Inc.
10357 Los Alamitos Blvd.
Los Alamitos, CA 90720
310-598-0800

WTD, Inc.
8819 N. Pioneer Road
Peoria, IL 61615
309-693-2150

00008
Wyeth-Ayerst Laboratories
P.O. Box 8299
Philadelphia, PA 19101
610-688-4400

50962
Xactdose, Inc.
722 Progressive Lane
South Beloit, IL 61080
815-624-8523

Xoma
2910 Seventh Street
Berkeley, CA 94710
510-644-1170

00116
Xttrium Laboratories, Inc.
415 West Pershing Road
Chicago, IL 60609
312-268-5800

64855
Young Again Products
43 Randolph Road
Suite 125
Silver Spring, MD 20904
301-622-1073

60077
Young Dental
13705 Shoreline Court E.
Earth City, MO 63045
314-344-0010

Young Pharmaceutical
1840 Berlin Turnpike
Wethersfield, CT 06109
203-529-7919

00310
Zeneca Pharmaceuticals
1800 Concord Pike
Wilmington, DE 19897
302-886-3000

00172
Zenith Goldline Pharmaceuticals
1900 W. Commercial Blvd.
Ft. Lauderdale, FL 33309
305-491-4002

05128
Zila Pharmaceuticals, Inc.
5227 N. 7th Street
Phoenix, AZ 85014-2817
602-266-6700

Zymogenetics, Inc.
1201 Eastlake Ave. E.
Seattle, WA 98102
206-547-8080

INDEX

C

D

T

U

NOTES

NOTES

NOTES

NOTES

NOTES

NOTES

NOTES

NOTES

NOTES

NOTES

NOTES

NOTES

NOTES

ISBN 1-57439-034-1

90000

9 781574 390346